$\mathscr{S}$ABISTON
TEXTBOOK OF
SURGERY

SABISTON
TEXTBOOK OF
SURGERY
The Biological Basis of Modern Surgical Practice

18th EDITION

COURTNEY M. TOWNSEND, JR., MD
Professor and John Woods Harris Distinguished Chairman
Department of Surgery
The University of Texas Medical Branch
Galveston, Texas

R. DANIEL BEAUCHAMP, MD
J. C. Foshee Distinguished Professor of Surgery
Chairman, Section of Surgical Sciences
Vanderbilt University Medical Center
Surgeon-in-Chief, Vanderbilt University Hospital
Nashville, Tennessee

B. MARK EVERS, MD
Professor, Departments of Surgery and of Biochemistry and Molecular Biology
Robertson-Poth Distinguished Chair in General Surgery
Director, Sealy Center for Cancer Cell Biology
Director, UTMB Comprehensive Cancer Center
The University of Texas Medical Branch
Galveston, Texas

KENNETH L. MATTOX, MD
Professor and Vice Chairman
Michael E. DeBakey Department of Surgery
Baylor College of Medicine
Chief of Staff and Chief of Surgery
Ben Taub General Hospital
Houston, Texas

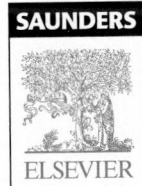

SAUNDERS

ELSEVIER

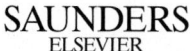

SAUNDERS
ELSEVIER

1600 John F. Kennedy Boulevard
Suite 1800
Philadelphia, PA 19103-2899

SABISTON TEXTBOOK OF SURGERY

Basic Edition ISBN: 978-1-4160-3675-3
Premium Edition ISBN: 978-1-4160-5233-3
International Edition ISBN: 978-0-8089-2401-2

Notice

Knowledge and best practice in this field are constantly changing. As new research and experience broaden our knowledge, changes in practice, treatment, and drug therapy may become necessary or appropriate. Readers are advised to check the most current information provided (i) on procedures featured or (ii) by the manufacturer of each product to be administered, to verify the recommended dose or formula, the method and duration of administration, and contraindications. It is the responsibility of the practitioner, relying on his or her own experience and knowledge of the patient, to make diagnoses, to determine dosages and the best treatment for each individual patient, and to take all appropriate safety precautions. To the fullest extent of the law, neither the Publisher nor the Editors assume any liability for any injury and/or damage to persons or property arising out of or related to any use of the material contained in this book.

The Publisher

Copyright © 2008, 2004, 2001, 1997, 1991, 1986, 1981, 1977, 1972, 1968, 1964, 1960, 1956 by Saunders, an imprint of Elsevier Inc.

Copyright 1949, 1945, 1942, 1939, 1936 by Elsevier Inc.

Copyright renewed 1992 by Richard A. Davis, Nancy Davis Reagan, Susan Okum, Joanne R. Artz, and Mrs. Mary E. Artz.

Copyright renewed 1988 by Richard A. Davis and Nancy Davis Reagan.

Copyright renewed 1977 by Mrs. Frederick Christopher.

Copyright renewed 1973, 1970, 1967, 1964 by W.B. Saunders Company.

Library of Congress Cataloging-in-Publication Data
Sabiston textbook of surgery: the biological basis of modern surgical practice.—18th ed. / editors, Courtney M. Townsend Jr. . . . [et al.].
   p. ; cm.
  Includes bibliographical references and index.
  ISBN 978-1-4160-3675-3
  1. Surgery. I. Sabiston, David C. II. Townsend, Courtney M. III. Title: Textbook of surgery.
  [DNLM: 1. Surgical Procedures, Operative. 2. Perioperative Care. 3. Surgery. WO 100 T3552 2008]
RD31.T473 2008
617–dc22
                      2007022754

Publishing Director: Judy Fletcher
Senior Developmental Editor: Scott Scheidt
Publishing Services Manager: Tina Rebane
Senior Project Manager: Amy L. Cannon

Printed in Canada

Last digit is the print number: 9 8 7 6 5 4 3 2 1

To our patients, who grant us the privilege of practicing our craft;

to our students, residents, and colleagues, from whom we learn;

and to our wives—Mary, Shannon, Karen, and June—

without whose support this would not have been possible.

Jose Acosta, MD
Associate Professor of Surgery, U.S. Naval Hospital, San Diego;
Associate Professor, Department of Surgery, University of
California–Irvine, Orange, California
Management of Acute Trauma

Charles A. Adams, Jr., MD
Medical Director, Surgical Intensive and Intermediate Surgical
Care Units, Rhode Island Hospital; Assistant Professor of
Surgery, Brown Medical School, Providence, Rhode Island
Surgical Critical Care

Louis H. Alarcon, MD
Assistant Professor, Departments of Critical Care Medicine and
Surgery and Associate Director, Trauma Surgery, University of
Pittsburgh School of Medicine, Pittsburgh, Pennsylvania
Mediators of the Inflammatory Response

Daniel A. Anaya, MD
Fellow, Surgical Oncology, The University of Texas, M. D.
Anderson Cancer Center, Houston, Texas
Surgical Infections and Choice of Antibiotics

Stanley W. Ashley, MD
Frank Sawyer Professor and Vice-Chairman, Department of
Surgery, Brigham and Women's Hospital, Boston,
Massachusetts
Acute Gastrointestinal Hemorrhage

Paul S. Auerbach, MD, MS
Clinical Professor of Surgery, Department of Surgery, Division
of Emergency Medicine, Stanford University School of
Medicine, Stanford, California
Bites and Stings

Ali Azizzadeh, MD
Assistant Professor, Department of Cardiothoracic and Vascular
Surgery, The University of Texas at Houston Medical School,
Houston, Texas
*Thoracic Vasculature With Emphasis on the Thoracic
Aorta*

Clyde F. Barker, MD
Donald Guthrie Professor of Surgery, Department of Surgery,
Hospital of the University of Pennsylvania, Philadelphia,
Pennsylvania
Transplantation of Abdominal Organs

B. Timothy Baxter, MD
Professor, Department of Surgery, University of Nebraska
Medical Center, Omaha, Nebraska
The Lymphatics

R. Daniel Beauchamp, MD
J. C. Foshee Distinguished Professor of Surgery and Chairman,
Section of Surgical Sciences, Vanderbilt University Medical
Center; Surgeon-in-Chief, Vanderbilt University Hospital,
Nashville, Tennessee
The Spleen

Paul R. Beery, MD
Clinical Assistant Professor, Department of Surgery, Ohio State
University Grant Medical Center, Columbus, Ohio
Surgery in the Pregnant Patient

Michael Belkin, MD
Division Chief, Vascular Surgery, Brigham and Women's
Hospital, Boston, Massachusetts
Peripheral Arterial Occlusive Disease

David H. Berger, MD
Professor of Surgery and Vice-Chair, Michael E. DeBakey
Department of Surgery, Baylor College of Medicine; Operative
Care Line Executive, Michael E. DeBakey Veterans Affairs
Medical Center, Houston, Texas
Surgery in the Elderly

Walter L. Biffl, MD
Associate Professor and Chief, Surgical Critical Care,
Department of Surgery, University of Colorado Health
Science Center, Denver, Colorado
Surgical Critical Care

John D. Birkmeyer, MD
George D. Zuidema Professor and Chair, Surgical Outcomes
Research, University of Michigan, Ann Arbor, Michigan
Critical Assessment of Surgical Outcomes

Steven J. Blackwell MD
Stephen R. Lewis Professor of Plastic Surgery, Division of
Plastic Surgery, Department of Surgery, The University of
Texas Medical Branch, Galveston, Texas
Plastic Surgery

Mark E. Brecher, MD
Professor and Vice-Chair, Department of Pathology
and Laboratory Medicine; Director of Transfusion Medicine,
University of North Carolina, Chapel Hill, North Carolina
Hematologic Principles in Surgery

Bruce D. Browner, MD
Gray-Gossling Professor and Chairman, Department of
Orthopedic Surgery, University of Connecticut School of
Medicine, Farmington, Connecticut
Emergency Care of Musculoskeletal Injuries

Brian B. Burkey, MD
Associate Professor, Department of Otolaryngology,
Vanderbilt–Bill Wilkerson Center for Otolaryngology and
Communication Sciences, Vanderbilt University Medical
Center, Nashville, Tennessee
Head and Neck

John L. Burns, MD
Clinical Instructor, Department of Plastic Surgery, University of
Texas Southwestern Medical Center, Dallas, Texas
Plastic Surgery

Kathleen E. Carberry, RN
Research Coordinator, Center for Clinical Outcomes Research,
Congenital Heart Surgery Service, Texas Children's Hospital,
Houston, Texas
Congenital Heart Disease

Ronald A. Carson, PhD
Harris L. Kempner Distinguished Professor, Institute for the
Medical Humanities, The University of Texas Medical Branch,
Galveston, Texas
Ethics in Surgery

Ravi S. Chari, MD
Professor of Surgery and Cancer Biology and Chief, Division of
Hepatobiliary Surgery and Liver Transplantation, Vanderbilt
University Medical Center, Nashville, Tennessee
Biliary System

Robert R. Cima, MD
Assistant Professor of Surgery, Division of Colon and Rectal
Surgery, Mayo Clinic College of Medicine, Rochester,
Minnesota
Anus

William G. Cioffi, MD
Surgeon-in-Chief, Department of Surgery, Rhode Island
Hospital; Professor and Chairman of Surgery, Brown Medical
School, Providence, Rhode Island
Surgical Critical Care

Raul Coimbra, MD
Professor of Surgery and Chief, Division of Trauma, Burns, and
Surgical Critical Care, University of California–San Diego, San
Diego, California
Management of Acute Trauma

Michael S. Conte, MD
Associate Professor of Surgery, Brigham and Women's
Hospital, Division of Vascular and Endovascular Surgery,
Harvard Medical School, Boston, Massachusetts
Peripheral Arterial Occlusive Disease

Michael D'Angelica, MD
Assistant Attending, Department of Surgery, Division of
Hepatobiliary Surgery, Memorial Sloan-Kettering Cancer
Center, New York, New York
The Liver

Alan Dardik, MD
Assistant Professor of Surgery, Yale University School of
Medicine; Chief, Surgical Research, Veterans Affairs
Connecticut Healthcare System, West Haven, Connecticut
Surgery in the Elderly

Merril T. Dayton, MD
Professor and Chairman, Department of Surgery, State
University of New York–Buffalo; Chief of Surgery, Kaleida
Health System, Buffalo General Hospital, Buffalo, New York
Surgical Complications

Joseph P. DeAngelis, MD
Resident, Department of Orthopedic Surgery, University of
Connecticut School of Medicine, Farmington, Connecticut
Emergency Care of Musculoskeletal Injuries

E. Patchen Dellinger, MD
Professor and Vice-Chairman, Department of Surgery and
Chief, Division of General Surgery, University of Washington
Medical Center, Seattle, Washington
Surgical Infections and Choice of Antibiotics

Christopher J. Dente, MD
Associate Chief of Trauma, Department of Surgery, Emory
University School of Medicine, Atlanta, Georgia
Ultrasound for Surgeons

Jose J. Diaz, MD
Associate Professor of Surgery and Medicine, Division of
Trauma and Surgical Care, Vanderbilt University Medical
Center, Nashville, Tennessee
Bedside Surgical Procedures

Magruder C. Donaldson, MD
Chairman of Surgery, MetroWest Medical Center, Framingham;
Associate Professor of Surgery, Division of Vascular and
Endovascular Surgery, Brigham and Women's Hospital, Harvard
Medical School, Boston, Massachusetts
Peripheral Arterial Occlusive Disease

Quan-Yang Duh, MD
Professor of Surgery, Surgical Service, San Francisco Veterans
Affairs Medical Center, San Francisco, California
The Adrenal Glands

Timothy J. Eberlein, MD
Bixby Professor and Chairman, Department of Surgery,
Washington University School of Medicine, St. Louis, Missouri
Tumor Biology and Tumor Markers

E. Christopher Ellison, MD
Associate Vice President for Health Sciences, Vice Dean of
Clinical Affairs, Robert M. Zollinger Professor, and Chair,
Department of Surgery, Ohio Sate University Medical Center,
Columbus, Ohio
Surgery in the Pregnant Patient

Stephen S. Entman, MD
Professor Emeritus, Obstetrics and Gynecology, Vanderbilt
University School of Medicine, Nashville, Tennessee
Gynecologic Surgery

Anthony L. Estrera, MD
Associate Professor, Department of Cardiothoracic and
Vascular Surgery, The University of Texas at Houston Medical
School, Houston, Texas
*Thoracic Vasculature With Emphasis on the Thoracic
Aorta*

Richard T. Ethridge, MD, PhD
Resident Surgeon, Division of Plastic Surgery, Department of Surgery, The University of Texas Medical Branch, Galveston, Texas
Wound Healing

Thomas R. Eubanks, DO
President, Portland Surgical Specialists, Portland, Oregon
Hiatal Hernia and Gastroesophageal Reflux Disease

B. Mark Evers, MD
Professor, Departments of Surgery and of Biochemistry and Molecular Biology; Robertson-Poth Distinguished Chair in General Surgery; Director, Sealy Center for Cancer Cell Biology; and Director, UTMB Comprehensive Cancer Center, The University of Texas Medical Branch, Galveston, Texas
Molecular and Cell Biology; Small Intestine

Timothy C. Fabian, MD
Harwell Wilson Alumni Professor and Chairman, Department of Surgery, University of Tennessee Health Science Center, Memphis, Tennessee
The Spleen

Samir M. Fakhry, MD
Chief, Trauma and Surgical Critical Care; Associate Chair for Research and Education, Department of Surgery, Inova Fairfax Hospital; Professor of Surgery, Virginia Commonwealth University–Inova Campus, Falls Church, Virginia
Hematologic Principles in Surgery

Victor A. Ferraris, MD, PhD
Tyler Gill Professor of Surgery, Division of Cardiovascular and Thoracic Surgery, University of Kentucky College of Medicine, Lexington, Kentucky
Acquired Heart Disease: Coronary Insufficiency

Mitchell P. Fink, MD
Professor and Chair, Department of Critical Care Medicine; Watson Professor of Surgery; and Associate Vice-Chancellor for Translational Research and Commercialization, Department of Critical Care, University of Pittsburgh, Pittsburgh, Pennsylvania
Mediators of the Inflammatory Response

Samuel R. G. Finlayson, MD, MPH
Associate Professor of Surgery, Dartmouth Medical School, Dartmouth-Hitchcock Medical Center, Lebanon, New Hampshire
Critical Assessment of Surgical Outcomes

Nicholas Fiore, MD
Assistant Professor of Surgery, Division of Plastic Surgery, Baylor College of Medicine, Houston, Texas
Hand Surgery

Josef E. Fischer, MD
William V. McDermott Professor of Surgery, Harvard Medical School; Surgeon-in-Chief, Beth Israel Deaconess Medical Center, Boston, Massachusetts
Metabolism in Surgical Patients

Yuman Fong, MD
Murray F. Brennan Chair in Surgery, Department of Surgery, Gastric and Mixed Tumor Service, Memorial Sloan-Kettering Cancer Center, New York, New York
The Liver

Robbi L. Franklin, MD
Resident, Department of Surgery, Division of Neurosurgery, The University of Texas Medical Branch, Galveston, Texas
Neurosurgery

Charles D. Fraser, Jr., MD
Chief and The Donovan Chair in Congenital Health Surgery, Texas Children's Hospital; Chief, Division of Congenital Heart Surgery, Michael E. DeBakey Department of Surgery, Baylor College of Medicine, Houston, Texas
Congenital Heart Disease

Julie A. Freischlag, MD
William Steward Halsted Professor and Chair, Department of Surgery, Johns Hopkins University, Baltimore, Maryland
Venous Disease

Robert D. Fry, MD
Professor of Surgery and Chair, Department of Surgery, Pennsylvania Hospital, Philadelphia, Pennsylvania
Colon and Rectum

Eric R. Frykberg, MD
Professor of Surgery, University of Florida College of Medicine; Chief, Division of General Surgery, Shands Jacksonville Medical Center, Jacksonville, Florida
The Surgeon's Role in Unconventional Civilian Disasters

David A. Fullerton, MD
Professor and Division Head, Cardiothoracic Surgery, University of Colorado at Denver and Health Sciences Center, Denver, Colorado
Acquired Heart Disease: Valvular

James J. Gallagher, MD
Assistant Professor of Surgery, The University of Texas Medical Branch, Shriners Hospital for Children, Galveston, Texas
Burns

Peter Gloviczki, MD
Director, Gonda Vascular Center, Mayo Clinic, Rochester, Minnesota
Aneurysmal Vascular Disease

Peter S. Goedegebuure, PhD
Research Assistant Professor, Department of Surgery, Washington University School of Medicine, St. Louis, Missouri
Tumor Biology and Tumor Markers

Joel E. Goldberg, MD
Associate Surgeon, Brigham and Women's Hospital; Instructor in Surgery, Harvard Medical School, Boston, Massachusetts
Acute Gastrointestinal Hemorrhage

Guillermo Gomez, MD
Associate Professor and Granville T. Hall Chair, Department of Surgery, The University of Texas Medical Branch, Galveston, Texas
Emerging Technology in Surgery: Informatics, Electronics, Robotics

Darla K. Granger, MD
Clinical Associate Professor of Surgery, St. John Hospital and Medical Center, Wayne State University, Detroit, Michigan
Transplantation Immunobiology and Immunosuppression

Edwin Gravereaux, MD
Instructor of Surgery, Division of Vascular and Endovascular Surgery, Brigham and Women's Hospital, Harvard Medical School, Boston, Massachusetts
Peripheral Arterial Occlusive Disease

Cornelia R. Graves, MD
Medical Director, Tennessee Maternal-Fetal Medicine and Consultant, Division of Maternal-Fetal Medicine, Obstetrics and Gynecology, Baptist Hospital, Nashville, Tennessee
Gynecologic Surgery

Carl E. Haisch, MD
Professor, Department of Surgery, Brody School of Medicine, East Carolina University, Greenville, North Carolina
Access and Ports

Fadi Hanbali, MD
Assistant Professor, Neurosurgery Division, Texas Tech University Health Science Center, School of Medicine, El Paso, Texas
Neurosurgery

John B. Hanks, MD
C. Bruce Morton Professor and Chief, Department of Surgery, University of Virginia, Charlottesville, Virginia
Thyroid

Alden H. Harken, MD
Chairman, Department of Surgery, University of California-San Francisco (East Bay), San Francisco, California
Acquired Heart Disease: Valvular

Jennifer A. Heller, MD
Assistant Professor and Surgery Director, Johns Hopkins Vein Center, Johns Hopkins Bayview Medical Center, Baltimore, Maryland
Venous Disease

David N. Herndon, MD
Chief of Staff, Shriners Burns Hospital for Children; Professor of Surgery and Jesse H. Jones Distinguished Chair in Burn Surgery, The University of Texas Medical Branch, Galveston, Texas
Burns

Asher Hirshberg, MD
Professor of Surgery, State University of New York Downstate College of Medicine; Director of Emergency Vascular Surgery, Kings County Hospital Center, Brooklyn, New York
Vascular Trauma

Ginger E. Holt, MD
Assistant Professor, Vanderbilt University Medical Center, Nashville, Tennessee
Bone Tumors

Michael D. Holzman, MD, MPH
Associate Professor of Surgery and Lester and Sara Jayne Williams Chair in Academic Surgery, General Surgery Division, Vanderbilt University Medical Center, Nashville, Tennessee
The Spleen

David B. Hoyt, MD
John E. Connolly Professor and Chairman of Surgery, Department of Surgery, University of California-Irvine, Orange, California
Management of Acute Trauma

J. Dirk Iglehart, MD
Chief, Division of Surgical Oncology, Anne E. Dyson Professor of Women's Cancer, Harvard Medical School; and Director of Women's Cancers Program, Dana-Farber Cancer Institute, Boston, Massachusetts
Diseases of the Breast

Suzanne T. Ildstad, MD
Director, Institute for Cellular Therapeutics; Jewish Hospital Distinguished Professor of Transplantation; and Professor of Surgery, University of Louisville, Louisville, Kentucky
Transplantation Immunobiology and Immunosuppression

Barry K. Jarnagin, MD
Associate Professor, Urogynecology, Obstetrics and Gynecology, Vanderbilt University School of Medicine, Nashville, Tennessee
Gynecologic Surgery

R. Scott Jones, MD
Director, Division of Research and Optimal Patient Care, American College of Surgeons, Chicago, Illinois; and Professor Emeritus, Department of Surgery, University of Virginia Health System, Charlottesville, Virginia
Surgical Patient Safety

Kimberly S. Kirkwood, MD
Associate Professor of Surgery, Department of Surgery, University of California-San Francisco, San Francisco, California
The Appendix

Tien C. Ko, MD
Professor of Surgery, The University of Texas Health Science Center and Chief of Surgery, Lyndon B. Johnson General Hospital, Houston, Texas
Molecular and Cell Biology

Mahmoud N. Kulaylat, MD
Associate Professor of Surgery, Department of Surgery, State University of New York-Buffalo, Buffalo General Hospital, Buffalo, New York
Surgical Complications

Matthew D. Kwan, MD
Post-Doctoral Fellow, Department of Surgery, Stanford
University School of Medicine, Stanford, California; General
Surgery Resident, Department of Surgery, Temple University
Hospital, Philadelphia, Pennsylvania
Regenerative Medicine

Terry C. Lairmore, MD
Professor of Surgery and Director, Division of Surgical
Oncology, Scott and White Memorial Hospital and Clinic,
Texas A&M University System Health Science Center College
of Medicine, Temple, Texas
The Multiple Endocrine Neoplasia Syndromes

Christine L. Lau, MD
Assistant Professor, Section of Thoracic Surgery, University of
Michigan, Ann Arbor, Michigan
The Mediastinum

Mimi Leong, MD
Assistant Professor, Plastic Surgery Division, Michael E.
DeBakey Department of Surgery, Baylor College of Medicine,
Houston, Texas
Wound Healing

Benjamin D. Li, MD
Professor and Chief, Division of Surgical Oncology,
Department of Surgery, Louisiana State University Health
Sciences Center, Shreveport, Louisiana
*Abdominal Wall, Umbilicus, Peritoneum, Mesenteries,
Omentum, and Retroperitoneum*

Michael T. Longaker, MD, MBA
Deane P. and Louise Mitchell Professor, Department of
Surgery, Stanford University School of Medicine,
Stanford and Deputy Director, The Stanford Institute for
Stem Cell Biology and Regenerative Medicine, Palo Alto,
California
Regenerative Medicine

Robert R. Lorenz, MD
Head, Section of Head and Neck Surgery, Laryngotracheal
Reconstruction/Oncology, Head and Neck Institute, Cleveland
Clinic, Cleveland, Ohio
Head and Neck

Jeanne M. Lukanich, MD
Staff, Division of Thoracic Surgery, Brigham and Women's
Hospital; Instructor of Surgery, Harvard Medical School,
Boston, Massachusetts
Chest Wall and Pleura

John Maa, MD
Assistant Professor, Department of Surgery, University of
California–San Francisco, San Francisco, California
The Appendix

Najjia Mahmoud, MD
Assistant Professor of Surgery, Division of Colon and Rectal
Surgery, Hospital of the University of Pennsylvania,
Philadelphia, Pennsylvania
Colon and Rectum

Mary Maish, MD
Surgical Director of the Esophageal Center, Department of
Surgery, Division of Thoracic Surgery, David Geffen School of
Medicine, University of California at Los Angeles, Los Angeles,
California
Esophagus

Mark A. Malangoni, MD
Professor of Surgery, Case Western Reserve University;
Chairperson, Department of Surgery; and Surgeon-in-Chief,
MetroHealth Medical Center, Cleveland, Ohio
Hernias

James F. Markmann, MD, PhD
Associate Professor of Surgery, Department of Surgery, Hospital
of the University of Pennsylvania, Philadelphia, Pennsylvania
Transplantation of Abdominal Organs

David J. Maron, MD
Assistant Professor of Surgery, Division of Colon and Rectal
Surgery, Hospital of the University of Pennsylvania,
Philadelphia, Pennsylvania
Colon and Rectum

Kenneth L. Mattox, MD
Professor and Vice Chairman, Michael E. DeBakey Department
of Surgery, Baylor College of Medicine; Chief of Staff and Chief
of Surgery, Ben Taub General Hospital, Houston, Texas
Vascular Trauma

Addison K. May, MD
Associate Professor of Surgery and Anesthesiology, Division of
Trauma and Surgical Critical Care, Vanderbilt University
Medical Center, Nashville, Tennessee
Bedside Surgical Procedures

John C. McDonald, MD
Chancellor and Dean, Professor of Surgery, Department of
Surgery, Louisiana State University Health Sciences Center,
Shreveport, Louisiana
*Abdominal Wall, Umbilicus, Peritoneum, Mesenteries,
Omentum, and Retroperitoneum*

Robert M. Mentzer, Jr., MD
Dean, Wayne State University School of Medicine, Detroit,
Michigan
Acquired Heart Disease: Coronary Insufficiency

David W. Mercer, MD
Professor and Vice Chairman, Department of Surgery, The
University of Texas Health Science Center at Houston,
Houston, Texas
Stomach

Dean J. Mikami, MD
Assistant Professor of Surgery, Department of Surgery, Ohio
State University Medical Center, Columbus, Ohio
Surgery in the Pregnant Patient

Charles C. Miller, III, PhD
Professor, Department of Cardiothoracic and Vascular Surgery,
The University of Texas at Houston Medical School, Houston,
Texas
*Thoracic Vasculature With Emphasis on the Thoracic
Aorta*

Jeffrey F. Moley, MD
Professor of Surgery and Chief, Section of Endocrine and
Oncologic Surgery, Washington University School of Medicine,
St. Louis, Missouri
The Multiple Endocrine Neoplasia Syndromes

Richard J. Mullins, MD
Professor of Surgery and Chief, Trauma/Critical Care, Oregon
Health and Science University, Portland, Oregon
Shock, Electrolytes, and Fluid

Ali Naji, MD, PhD
J. William White Professor of Surgery, Department of Surgery,
Hospital of the University of Pennsylvania, Philadelphia,
Pennsylvania
Transplantation of Abdominal Organs

Haring J. W. Nauta, MD, PhD
Professor, Chief, and Samuel R. Snodgrass Professor of
Neurosurgery, Division of Neurosurgery, Department of
Surgery, The University of Texas Medical Branch,
Galveston, Texas
Neurosurgery

Elaine E. Nelson, MD
Chairman, Department of Emergency Medicine, Regional
Medical Center of San Jose, San Jose, California
Bites and Stings

Heidi Nelson, MD
Professor of Surgery, Division of Colon and Rectal Surgery,
Mayo Clinic, Rochester, Minnesota
Anus

David Netscher, MD
Clinical Professor, Division of Plastic Surgery; Professor,
Department of Orthopedic Surgery, Baylor College of
Medicine; Chief of Hand Surgery, Texas Children's Hospital;
and Chief of Plastic Surgery, Veterans Affairs Medical Center,
Houston, Texas
Hand Surgery

James L. Netterville, MD
Director, Head and Neck Oncologic Surgery and Mark C. Smith
Professor, Department of Otolaryngology, Vanderbilt Medical
Center, Nashville, Tennessee
Head and Neck

Leigh Neumayer, MD
Professor of Surgery, Department of General Surgery,
University of Utah Health Sciences Center, Salt Lake City, Utah
Principles of Preoperative and Operative Surgery

Robert L. Norris, MD
Associate Professor, Department of Surgery and Chief, Division
of Emergency Medicine, Stanford University School of
Medicine, Palo Alto, California
Bites and Stings

Brant K. Oelschlager, MD
Associate Professor; Director, Center for Videoendoscopic
Surgery; and Director, Swallowing Center, Department of
Surgery, University of Washington, Seattle, Washington
Hiatal Hernia and Gastroesophageal Reflux Disease

Kim M. Olthoff, MD
Director of Liver Transplant Program, Children's Hospital of
Philadelphia, Hospital of the University of Pennsylvania,
Philadelphia, Pennsylvania
Transplantation of Abdominal Organs

Aria F. Olumi, MD
Assistant Professor of Surgery/Urology, Massachusetts General
Hospital, Harvard Medical School, Boston, Massachusetts
Urologic Surgery

Christopher D. Owens, MD
Instructor of Surgery, Division of Vascular and Endovascular
Surgery, Brigham and Women's Hospital, Harvard Medical
School, Boston, Massachusetts
Peripheral Arterial Occlusive Disease

Frank M. Parker, DO
Assistant Professor, Department of Vascular Surgery, Brody
School of Medicine, East Carolina University, Greenville, North
Carolina
Access and Ports

Joel T. Patterson, MD
Assistant Professor, Department of Surgery, Division of
Neurosurgery, The University of Texas Medical Branch,
Galveston, Texas
Neurosurgery

Carlos A. Pellegrini, MD
The Henry N. Harkins Professor and Chairman, Department of
Surgery, University of Washington Medical Center, Seattle,
Washington
Hiatal Hernia and Gastroesophageal Reflux Disease

Linda G. Phillips, MD
Truman G. Blocker, Jr., MD, Distinguished Professor and Chief,
Division of Plastic Surgery, Department of Surgery, The
University of Texas Medical Branch, Galveston, Texas
Wound Healing; Breast Reconstruction

Iraklis I. Pipinos, MD
Associate Professor, Vascular Surgery, Department of Surgery,
University of Nebraska Medical Center, Omaha, Nebraska
The Lymphatics

Eyal E. Porat, MD
Chairman, Department of Cardiothoracic Surgery, Rabin
Medical Center, Petah Tikva, Israel
*Thoracic Vasculature With Emphasis on the Thoracic
Aorta*

Russell G. Postier, MD
John A. Schilling Professor and Chairman, Department of
Surgery, University of Oklahoma Health Sciences Center,
Oklahoma City, Oklahoma
Acute Abdomen

Donald S. Prough, MD
Professor and Chair, Department of Anesthesiology, The
University of Texas Medical Branch, Galveston, Texas
*Anesthesiology Principles, Pain Management, and
Conscious Sedation*

Joe B. Putnam, Jr., MD
Ingram Professor of Surgery; Chairman, Department of
Thoracic Surgery; Program Director, Resident Education
in Thoracic Surgery; and Professor, Department of
Biomedical Informatics, The Vanderbilt Clinic, Nashville,
Tennessee
  *Lung (Including Pulmonary Embolism and Thoracic
  Outlet Syndrome)*

Gautam G. Rao, MD
Assistant Professor, Gynecologic Oncology, Obstetrics and
Gynecology, Vanderbilt University School of Medicine,
Nashville, Tennessee
  Gynecologic Surgery

Scott I. Reznik, MD
Assistant Professor of Surgery, Division of Cardiothoracic
Surgery, Section of General Thoracic Surgery, Scott and White
Memorial Hospital and Clinic, Texas A&M University Health
Science Center, College of Medicine, Temple, Texas
  *Lung (Including Pulmonary Embolism and Thoracic
  Outlet Syndrome)*

William O. Richards, MD
Ingram Professor of Surgery; Director, Laparoscopic General
Surgery; and Medical Director, Center for Surgical Weight
Loss, Vanderbilt University Medical Center, Nashville,
Tennessee
  Morbid Obesity

Kathryn A. Richardson, MD
Assistant Professor, Department of Surgery, Louisiana State
University Health Sciences Center, Shreveport, Louisiana
  *Abdominal Wall, Umbilicus, Peritoneum, Mesenteries,
  Omentum, and Retroperitoneum*

Jerome P. Richie, MD
Chief, Division of Urology, Elliott Carr Cutler Professor of
Surgery, Brigham and Women's Hospital, Boston,
Massachusetts
  Urologic Surgery

Joseph J. Ricotta, II, MD
Fellow in Vascular Surgery, Mayo Clinic, Rochester,
Minnesota
  Aneurysmal Vascular Disease

Layton F. Rikkers, MD
A. R. Curreri Professor and Chairman, Department of Surgery,
University of Wisconsin, Madison, Wisconsin
  *Surgical Complications of Cirrhosis and Portal
  Hypertension*

Thomas Stuart Riles, MD
Frank C. Spencer Professor of Surgery and Associate Dean for
Medical Education and Technology, New York University
School of Medicine, New York, New York
  Cerebrovascular Disease

Emily K. Robinson, MD
Associate Professor, Department of Surgery, University of
Texas Health Science Center at Houston, Houston, Texas
  Stomach

Caron B. Rockman, MD
Associate Professor, Department of Surgery, New York
University School of Medicine, New York, New York
  Cerebrovascular Disease

John Rombeau, MD
Professor, Department of Surgery, Temple University Hospital,
Philadelphia, Pennsylvania
  Colon and Rectum

Michael J. Rosen, MD
Assistant Professor of Surgery, Case Western Reserve
University, Cleveland, Ohio
  Hernias

Ronnie A. Rosenthal, MD
Associate Professor of Surgery, Yale University School
of Medicine, New Haven and Chief, Surgical Service,
Veterans Affairs Connecticut Healthcare System, West Haven,
Connecticut
  Surgery in the Elderly

Howard M. Ross, MD
Assistant Professor of Surgery, Division of Colon and Rectal
Surgery, Hospital of the University of Pennsylvania,
Philadelphia, Pennsylvania
  Colon and Rectum

Grace S. Rozycki, MD, RDMS
Chief of Trauma and Surgical Critical Care, Department of
Surgery, Emory University School of Medicine, Atlanta,
Georgia
  Ultrasound for Surgeons

Edmund J. Rutherford, MD
Associate Professor, Trauma and General Surgery, WakeMed
Faculty Physicians, Raleigh, North Carolina
  Hematologic Principles in Surgery

Ira M. Rutkow, MD, MPH, DrPH
Clinical Professor of Surgery, University of Medicine and
Dentistry of New Jersey, Newark, New Jersey
  History of Surgery

Hazim J. Safi, MD
Professor and Chairman, Department of Cardiothoracic and
Vascular Surgery, The University of Texas at Houston Medical
School, Houston, Texas
  *Thoracic Vasculature With Emphasis on the Thoracic
  Aorta*

Leslie J. Salomone, MD
Clinical Fellow, Division of Endocrinology and Metabolism,
University of Virginia Health System, Charlottesville, Virginia
  Thyroid

Bruce D. Schirmer, MD
Stephen H. Watts Professor of Surgery and Director, Residency
Program, Department of Surgery, University of Virginia Health
Sciences Center, Charlottesville, Virginia
  Morbid Obesity

Herbert S. Schwartz, MD
Professor, Vanderbilt University Medical Center, Nashville, Tennessee
Bone Tumors

Shimul A. Shah, MD
Assistant Professor of Surgery, Division of Organ Transplantation, University of Massachusetts Memorial Medical Center, Worcester, Massachusetts
Biliary System

Abraham Shaked, MD, PhD
Professor of Surgery, Hospital of the University of Pennsylvania, Philadelphia, Pennsylvania
Transplantation of Abdominal Organs

George F. Sheldon, MD
Zack D. Owens Distinguished Professor of Surgery and Social Medicine and Chair Emeritus, Department of Surgery, The University of North Carolina at Chapel Hill, Chapel Hill, North Carolina
Hematologic Principles in Surgery

Edward R. Sherwood, MD, PhD
Professor, Department of Anesthesiology, The University of Texas Medical Branch, Galveston, Texas
Anesthesiology Principles, Pain Management, and Conscious Sedation

Samuel Singer, MD
Chief, Sarcoma Disease Management Team, Department of Surgery, Memorial Sloan-Kettering Cancer Center, New York, New York
Soft Tissue Sarcomas

Barbara L. Smith, MD, PhD
Director, Breast Program, Division of Surgical Oncology, Massachusetts General Hospital Cancer Center, Boston, Massachusetts
Diseases of the Breast

W. Roy Smythe, MD
Chairman, Department of Surgery; Professor of Surgery, Medical Biochemistry and Genetics, Scott & White Hospital, Texas A & M University Health Sciences Center College of Medicine, Temple, Texas
Lung (Including Pulmonary Embolism and Thoracic Outlet Syndrome)

Seng-jaw Soong, PhD
Professor of Medicine, Comprehensive Cancer Center, Wallace Tumor Institute, Birmingham, Alabama
Melanoma and Cutaneous Malignancies

Julie Ann Sosa, MA, MD
Assistant Professor of Surgery and Clinical Epidemiology, Yale University School of Medicine, New Haven, Connecticut
The Parathyroid Glands

Ronald A. Squires, MD
Professor, Department of Surgery, University of Oklahoma Health Sciences Center, Oklahoma City, Oklahoma
Acute Abdomen

Michael L. Steer, MD
Chief, General Surgery and Vice Chairman, Department of Surgery, Tufts–New England Medical Center, Boston, Massachusetts
Exocrine Pancreas

Michael C. Stoner, MD
Assistant Professor, Department of Vascular Surgery, Brody School of Medicine, East Carolina University, Greenville, North Carolina
Access and Ports

David J. Sugarbaker, MD
Chief of Thoracic Surgery, Brigham and Women's Hospital, Boston, Massachusetts
Chest Wall and Pleura

Marcus C. B. Tan, MBBS (Hons)
Clinical Research Fellow, Department of Surgery, Washington University School of Medicine, St. Louis, Missouri
Tumor Biology and Tumor Markers

Ali Tavakkolizadeh, MD
Associate Surgeon, Brigham and Women's Hospital and Instructor in Surgery, Harvard Medical School, Boston, Massachusetts
Acute Gastrointestinal Hemorrhage

Nicholas E. Tawa, Jr., MD, PhD
Assistant Professor of Surgery (Cell Biology), Harvard Medical School and Associate in Surgery, Beth Israel Deaconess Medical Center, Boston, Massachusetts
Metabolism in Surgical Patients

James C. Thompson, MD
Department of Surgery, Shriners Hospital for Children, Galveston, Texas
Endocrine Pancreas

Courtney M. Townsend, Jr., MD
Professor and John Woods Harris Distinguished Chairman, Department of Surgery, The University of Texas Medical Branch, Galveston, Texas
Endocrine Pancreas

Richard H. Turnage, MD
Professor and Chairman, Department of Surgery, Louisiana State University Health Sciences Center, Shreveport, Louisiana
Abdominal Wall, Umbilicus, Peritoneum, Mesenteries, Omentum, and Retroperitoneum

Robert Udelsman, MD, MBA
William H. Carmalt Professor of Surgery and Oncology and Chairman, Department of Surgery, Yale University School of Medicine, New Haven, Connecticut
The Parathyroid Glands

Marshall M. Urist, MD
Professor and Vice-Chairman, Department of Surgery, University of Alabama at Birmingham, Birmingham, Alabama
Melanoma and Cutaneous Malignancies

Thomas K. Varghese, Jr., MD
Cardiothoracic Surgery Fellow, University of Michigan, Ann Arbor, Michigan
The Mediastinum

Daniel Vargo, MD
Assistant Professor of Surgery, Department of General Surgery, University of Utah Health Sciences Center, Salt Lake City, Utah
Principles of Preoperative and Operative Surgery

Derrick C. Wan, MD
Post-Doctoral Fellow, Department of Surgery, Stanford University School of Medicine, Stanford and General Surgery Resident, Department of Surgery, University of California–San Francisco, San Francisco, California
Regenerative Medicine

Brad W. Warner, MD
Apolline Blair Professor of Surgery, Washington University School of Medicine and Surgeon-in-Chief, St. Louis Children's Hospital, St. Louis, Missouri
Pediatric Surgery

Lawrence W. Way, MD
Professor, Department of Surgery, School of Medicine, University of California–San Francisco, San Francisco, California
Surgical Patient Safety

Jordan A. Weinberg, MD
Assistant Professor, Department of Surgery, University of Alabama at Birmingham, Birmingham, Alabama
The Spleen

Anthony D. Whittemore, MD
Professor of Surgery, Division of Vascular and Endovascular Surgery, Brigham and Women's Hospital, Harvard Medical School, Boston, Massachusetts
Peripheral Arterial Occlusive Disease

Bradon J. Wilhelmi, MD
Leonard Weiner Endowed Professor, Chief of Plastic Surgery, and Residency Program Director, Division of Plastic and Reconstructive Surgery, University of Louisville, Louisville, Kentucky
Breast Reconstruction

Courtney G. Williams, MD
Professor, Department of Anesthesiology, The University of Texas Medical Branch, Galveston, Texas
Anesthesiology Principles, Pain Management, and Conscious Sedation

Steven E. Wolf, MD
Professor of Surgery, University of Texas Health Science Center at San Antonio, San Antonio and Director of Burns, U.S. Army Institute for Surgical Research, Brooke Army Medical Center, Fort Sam Houston, Texas
Burns

Heidi Yeh, MD
Assistant Professor of Surgery, Department of Surgery, Hospital of the University of Pennsylvania, Philadelphia, Pennsylvania
Transplantation of Abdominal Organs

Michael W. Yeh, MD
Assistant Professor of Surgery, Endocrine Surgical Unit, Division of General Surgery, David Geffen School of Medicine, University of California at Los Angeles, Los Angeles, California
The Adrenal Glands

| FOREWORD

"To study the phenomena of disease without books is to sail an uncharted sea . . ."

SIR WILLIAM OSLER (1849–1919)

During the past 3 score and 7 years, this surgical text, edited successively by Christopher (5 editions), Davis (4 editions), Sabiston (6 editions), and now Townsend (3 editions), has charted the surgical seas for generations of surgeons throughout their careers as they progressed from students to practitioners and teachers. Dr. Townsend and his three associate editors have added to the innovations that they initiated in the 15th edition in recognition of the ever-increasing velocity of acquisition of knowledge, expansion of surgical practice, and application of new technology. This edition is organized into 13 sections—focused on basic principles of surgery, organ-specific general surgical care, and the surgical super-specialties—to recapitulate the content of the American Board of Surgery certifying examination. The editorial team has added more than 50 new members to the all-star cast of authors for the 77 chapters that provide global coverage of surgery.

Of all the surgical texts, this one most successfully integrates information from the laboratory to illuminate the rationale for surgical care. Each chapter begins with a chapter outline and contains other tables presenting checklists of key principles and practices. Abundant use is made of color in illustrative photographs and drawings and to emphasize important aspects of graphs and tables. A unique feature is the citation and brief summary of seminal articles, which are beyond the reach of short–time span search programs, designed to inform the reader how we arrived at the current state-of-the-art.

The new chapters about patient safety considerations, bedside procedures, and regenerative medicine provide the reader with charts of previously unexplored surgical seas. Dr. Townsend and his colleagues have further enhanced the value of this classic work by bringing it into the world of electronic education. Expert Consult will facilitate lifetime learning by giving access to the fully searchable complete book content online, along with updates, references linked to Medline, downloadable illustrations, and "bonus" articles from surgical periodicals, as well as review questions that can be used in preparing for examinations.

In sum total, this volume sets a new standard for surgical textbooks. The information contained in this, Dr. Townsend's 3rd and overall the 18th, edition of this venerable text ensures smooth sailing in the currently turbulent surgical seas.

BASIL A. PRUITT, JR., MD

PREFACE

Surgery continues to evolve as new technology, techniques, and knowledge are incorporated into the care of surgical patients. Safety is paramount in care of our surgical patients. We have included a new chapter in this edition of *Sabiston Textbook of Surgery* about our roles and responsibilities to ensure safety. Surgeons, traditional leaders in mass casualty situations, face new problems and challenges in the era of bioterrorism. Distant surgery, employing robotic and telementoring technology, has become a reality. Minimally invasive techniques are being employed in almost all invasive procedures. Increased understanding of molecular genetic abnormalities has expanded the application of preemptive surgical operations to prevent cancer.

The 18th edition of the *Sabiston Textbook of Surgery* reflects these exciting changes and new knowledge. We have incorporated 3 new chapters and more than 50 new authors to ensure that the most current information is presented. The goal of this new edition is to remain the most thorough, useful, readable, and understandable textbook presenting the principles and techniques of surgery. It is designed to be equally useful to students, trainees, and experts in the field. We are committed to maintaining this tradition of excellence begun in 1936. Surgery, after all, remains a discipline in which the knowledge and skill of a surgeon combine for the welfare of our patients.

COURTNEY M. TOWNSEND, JR., MD

| ACKNOWLEDGMENTS

We would like to recognize the invaluable contributions of editor Paul Waschka, publication coordinators Karen Martin, Steve Schuenke, and Eileen Figueroa, and administrator Barbara Petit. Their dedicated professionalism, tenacious efforts, and cheerful cooperation are without parallel. They accomplished whatever was necessary, often on short or instantaneous deadlines, and were vital for the successful completion of the endeavor.

Our authors, respected authorities in their fields and busy physicians and surgeons all, did an outstanding job in sharing their wealth of knowledge.

We would also like to acknowledge the professionalism of our colleagues at Elsevier: senior developmental editor Scott Scheidt, publication services manager Tina Rebane, senior project manager Amy Cannon, and publishing director Judith Fletcher.

CONTENTS

SURGICAL BASIC PRINCIPLES

CHAPTER 1

History of Surgery

Ira M. Rutkow, MD, MPH, DrPH

IMPORTANCE OF UNDERSTANDING SURGICAL HISTORY

It remains a rhetorical question whether an understanding of surgical history is important to the maturation and continued education and training of a surgeon. Conversely, it is hardly necessary to dwell on the heuristic value that an appreciation of history provides in developing adjunctive humanistic, literary, and philosophic tastes. Clearly, the study of medicine is a lifelong learning process that should be an enjoyable and rewarding experience. For a surgeon, the study of surgical history can contribute toward making this educational effort more pleasurable and can provide constant invigoration. Tracing the evolution of what one does on a daily basis and understanding it from a historical perspective become enviable goals. In reality, there is no way to separate present-day surgery and one's own clinical practice from the experience of all surgeons and all the years that have gone before. For budding surgeons, it is a magnificent adventure to appreciate what they are currently learning within the context of past and present cultural, economic, political, and social institutions. Active practitioners will find that study of the profession—dealing, as it rightly must, with all aspects of the human condition—affords an excellent opportunity to approach current clinical concepts in ways not previously appreciated.

In studying our profession's past, it is certainly easier to relate to the history of so-called modern surgery over the past 100 or so years than to the seemingly primitive practices of previous periods because the closer to the present, the more likely it is that surgical practices will resemble those of nowadays. Nonetheless, writing the history of modern surgery is in many respects more difficult than describing the development of surgery before the late 19th century. One significant reason for this difficulty is the ever-increasing pace of scientific development in conjunction with unrelenting fragmentation (i.e., specialization and subspecialization) within the profession. The craft of surgery is in constant flux, and the more rapid the change, the more difficult it is to obtain a satisfactory historical perspective. Only the lengthy passage of time permits a truly valid historical analysis.

HISTORICAL RELATIONSHIP BETWEEN SURGERY AND MEDICINE

Despite outward appearances, it was actually not until the latter decades of the 19th century that the surgeon truly emerged as a specialist within the whole of medicine to become a recognized and respected clinical practitioner. Similarly, it was not until the first decades of the 20th century that surgery could be considered to have achieved the status of a bona fide profession. Before this time, the scope of surgery remained quite limited. Surgeons, or at least those medical men who used the sobriquet *surgeon,* whether university educated or trained in private apprenticeships, at best treated only simple fractures, dislocations, and abscesses and occasionally performed amputations with dexterity but also with high mortality rates. They managed to ligate major arteries for common and accessible aneurysms and made heroic attempts to excise external tumors. Some individuals focused on the treatment of anal fistulas, hernias, cataracts, and bladder stones. Inept attempts at reduction of incarcerated and strangulated hernias were made, and hesitatingly, rather rudimentary colostomies or ileostomies were created by simply incising the skin over an expanding intra-abdominal mass, which represented the end stage of a long-standing intestinal obstruction. Compound fractures of the limbs with attendant sepsis remained mostly unmanageable, with staggering morbidity being a likely surgical outcome. Although a few bold surgeons endeavored to incise the abdomen in the hope of dividing obstructing bands and adhesions, abdominal and other intrabody surgery was virtually unknown.

Despite it all, including an ignorance of anesthesia and antisepsis tempered with the not uncommon result of the patient suffering from or succumbing to the effects of a surgical operation (or both), surgery was long considered an important and medically valid therapy. This seeming paradox, in view of the terrifying nature of surgical intervention, its limited technical scope, and its damning consequences before the development of modern conditions, is explained by the simple fact that surgical procedures were usually performed only for external difficulties that required an objective anatomic diagnosis. Surgeons or followers of the surgical cause saw what needed to be fixed (e.g., abscesses, broken bones, bulging tumors, cataracts, hernias) and would treat the problem in as rational a manner as the times permitted. Conversely, the physician was forced to render subjective care for disease processes that were neither visible nor understood. After all, it is a difficult task to treat the symptoms of illnesses such as arthritis, asthma, heart failure, and diabetes, to name but a few, if there is no scientific understanding or internal knowledge of what constitutes their basic pathologic and physiologic underpinnings.

With the breathtaking advances made in pathologic anatomy and experimental physiology during the 18th and the first part of the 19th centuries, physicians would soon adopt a therapeutic viewpoint that had long been prevalent among surgeons. It was no longer a question of just treating symptoms; the actual pathologic problem could ultimately be understood. Internal disease processes that manifested themselves through difficult-to-treat external signs and symptoms were finally described via physiology-based experimentation or viewed pathologically through the lens of a microscope. Because this reorientation of internal medicine occurred within a relatively short time and brought about such dramatic results

in the classification, diagnosis, and treatment of disease, the rapid ascent of mid-19th century internal medicine might seem more impressive than the agonizingly slow, but steady advance of surgery. In a seeming contradiction of mid-19th century scientific and social reality, medicine appeared as the more progressive branch, with surgery lagging behind. The art and craft of surgery, for all its practical possibilities, would be severely restricted until the discovery of anesthesia in 1846 and an understanding and acceptance of the need for surgical antisepsis and asepsis during the 1870s and 1880s. Still, surgeons never needed a diagnostic and pathologic revolution in the manner of the physician. Despite the imperfection of their scientific knowledge, the pre–modern era surgeon did cure with some technical confidence.

That the gradual evolution of surgery was superseded in the 1880s and 1890s by the rapid introduction of startling new technical advances was based on a simple culminating axiom—the four fundamental clinical prerequisites that were required before a surgical operation could ever be considered a truly viable therapeutic procedure had finally been identified and understood:

1. Knowledge of human anatomy
2. Method of controlling hemorrhage and maintaining intraoperative hemostasis
3. Anesthesia to permit the performance of pain-free procedures
4. Explanation of the nature of infection along with the elaboration of methods necessary to achieve an antiseptic and aseptic operating room environment

The first two prerequisites were essentially solved in the 16th century, but the latter two would not be fully resolved until the ending decades of the 19th century. In turn, the ascent of 20th century scientific surgery would unify the profession and allow what had always been an art and craft to become a learned vocation. Standardized postgraduate surgical education and training programs could be established to help produce a cadre of scientifically knowledgeable practitioners. Moreover, in a final snub to an unscientific past, newly established basic surgical research laboratories offered the means of proving or disproving the latest theories while providing a testing ground for bold and exciting clinical breakthroughs.

KNOWLEDGE OF HUMAN ANATOMY

Few individuals have had an influence on the history of surgery as overwhelmingly as that of the Brussels-born Andreas Vesalius (1514-1564) (Fig. 1-1). As professor of anatomy and surgery in Padua, Italy, Vesalius taught that human anatomy could be learned only through the study of structures revealed by human dissection. In particular, his great anatomic treatise *De Humani Corporis Fabrica Libri Septem* (1543) provided fuller and more detailed descriptions of human anatomy than any of his illustrious predecessors did. Most importantly, Vesalius corrected errors in traditional anatomic teachings propagated 13 centuries earlier by Greek and Roman authorities, whose

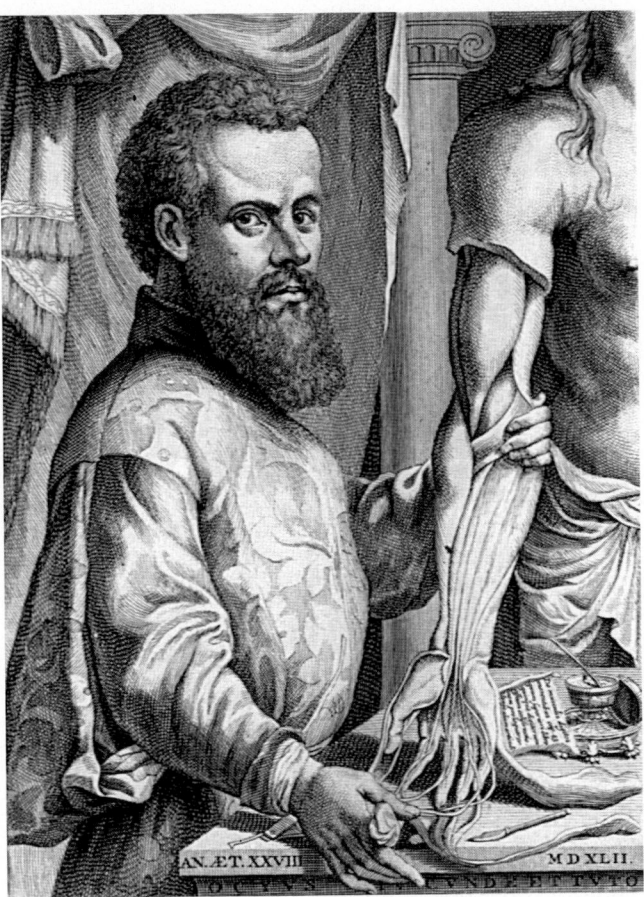

Figure 1-1 Andreas Vesalius (1514-1564).

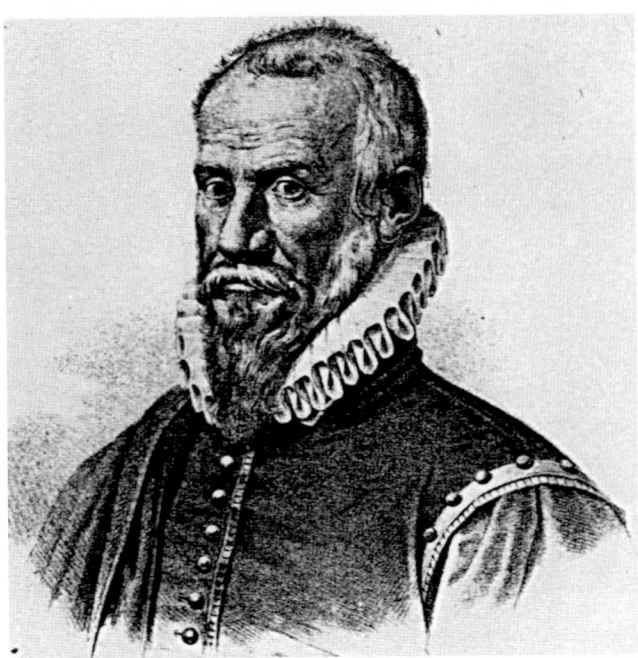

Figure 1-2 Ambroise Paré (1510-1590).

findings were based on animal rather than human dissection. Even more radical was Vesalius' blunt assertion that anatomic dissection must be completed by physician/surgeons themselves—a direct renunciation of the long-standing doctrine that dissection was a grisly and loathsome task to be performed by a diener-like individual while from on high the perched physician/surgeon lectured by reading from an orthodox anatomic text. This principle of hands-on education would remain Vesalius' most important and long-lasting contribution to the teaching of anatomy. Vesalius' Latin *literae scriptae* ensured its accessibility to the most well-known physicians and scientists of the day. Latin was the language of the intelligentsia and the *Fabrica* became instantly popular, so it was only natural that over the next 2 centuries the work would go through numerous adaptations, editions, and revisions, though always remaining an authoritative anatomic text.

METHOD OF CONTROLLING HEMORRHAGE

The position of Ambroise Paré (1510-1590) (Fig. 1-2) in the evolution of surgery remains of supreme importance. He played the major role in reinvigorating and updating Renaissance surgery and represents severing of the final link between surgical thought and techniques of the ancients and the push toward more modern eras. From 1536 until just before his death, Paré was either engaged as an army surgeon, during which he accompanied different French armies on their military expeditions, or performing surgery in civilian practice in Paris. Although other surgeons made similar observations about the difficulties and nonsensical aspects of using boiling oil as a means of cauterizing fresh gunshot wounds, Paré's use of a less irritating emollient of egg yolk, rose oil, and turpentine brought him lasting fame and glory. His ability to articulate such a finding in multiple textbooks, all written in the vernacular, allowed his writings to reach more than just the educated elite. Among Paré's important corollary observations was that when performing an amputation, it was more efficacious to ligate individual blood vessels than to attempt to control hemorrhage by means of mass ligation of tissue or with hot oleum. Described in his *Dix Livres de la Chirurgie avec le Magasin des Instruments Necessaires à Icelle* (1564), the free or cut end of a blood vessel was doubly ligated and the ligature was allowed to remain undisturbed in situ until, as a result of local suppuration, it was cast off. Paré humbly attributed his success with patients to God, as noted in his famous motto, "*Je le pansay. Dieu le guérit,*" that is, "I treated him. God cured him."

PATHOPHYSIOLOGIC BASIS OF SURGICAL DISEASES

Although it would be another 3 centuries before the third desideratum, that of anesthesia, was discovered, much of the scientific understanding concerning efforts to relieve discomfort secondary to surgical operations was based

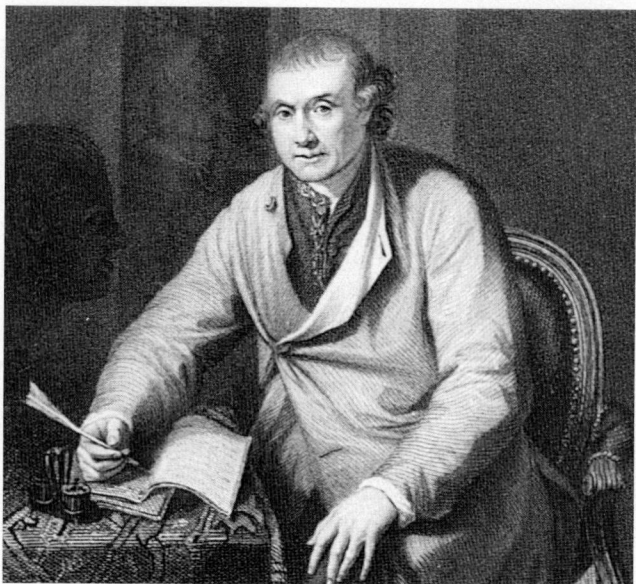

Figure 1-3 John Hunter (1728-1793).

on the 18th century work of England's premier surgical scientist, John Hunter (1728-1793) (Fig. 1-3). Considered one of the most influential surgeons of all time, his endeavors stand out because of the prolificacy of his written word and the quality of his research, especially in using experimental animal surgery as a way to understand the pathophysiologic basis of surgical diseases. Most impressively, Hunter relied little on the theories of past authorities but rather on personal observations, with his fundamental pathologic studies first described in the renowned textbook *A Treatise on the Blood, Inflammation, and Gun-Shot Wounds* (1794). Ultimately, his voluminous research and clinical work resulted in a collection of more than 13,000 specimens, which became one of his most important legacies to the world of surgery. It represented a unique warehousing of separate organ systems, with comparisons of these systems, from the simplest animal or plant to humans, demonstrating the interaction of structure and function. For decades, Hunter's collection, housed in England's Royal College of Surgeons, remained the outstanding museum of comparative anatomy and pathology in the world. That was until a World War II Nazi bombing attack of London created a conflagration that destroyed most of Hunter's assemblage.

ANESTHESIA

Since time immemorial, the inability of surgeons to complete pain-free operations had been among the most terrifying of medical problems. In the preanesthetic era, surgeons were forced to be more concerned about the speed with which an operation was completed than with the clinical efficacy of their dissection. In a similar vein, patients refused or delayed surgical procedures for as long as possible to avoid the personal horror of experiencing the surgeon's knife. Analgesic, narcotic, and soporific agents such as hashish, mandrake, and opium had been put to use for thousands of years. However, the systematic operative invasion of body cavities and the inevitable progression of surgical history could not occur until an effective means of rendering a patient insensitive to pain was developed.

As anatomic knowledge and surgical techniques improved, the search for safe methods to prevent pain became more pressing. By the early 1830s, chloroform, ether, and nitrous oxide had been discovered and so-called laughing gas parties and ether frolics were in vogue, especially in America. Young people were amusing themselves with the pleasant side effects of these compounds as itinerant so-called professors of chemistry traveled to hamlets, towns, and cities to lecture on and demonstrate the exhilarating effects of these new gases. It soon became evident to various physicians and dentists that the pain-relieving qualities of ether and nitrous oxide could be applicable to surgical operations and tooth extraction. On October 16, 1846, William T. G. Morton (1819-1868), a Boston dentist, persuaded John Collins Warren (1778-1856), professor of surgery at the Massachusetts General Hospital, to let him administer sulfuric ether to a surgical patient from whom Warren went on to painlessly remove a small, congenital vascular tumor of the neck. After the operation, Warren, greatly impressed with the new discovery, uttered his famous words: "Gentlemen, this is no humbug."

Few medical discoveries have been so readily accepted as inhalational anesthesia. News of the momentous event spread rapidly throughout the United States and Europe, and a new era in the history of surgery had begun. Within a few months after the first public demonstration in Boston, ether was used in hospitals throughout the world. Yet no matter how much it contributed to the relief of pain during surgical operations and decreased the surgeon's angst, the discovery did not immediately further the scope of elective surgery. Such technical triumphs awaited the recognition and acceptance of antisepsis and asepsis. Anesthesia helped make the illusion of surgical cures more seductive, but it could not bring forth the final prerequisite: all-important hygienic reforms.

Still, by the mid-19th century, both doctors and patients were coming to hold surgery in relatively high regard for its pragmatic appeal, technologic virtuosity, and unambiguously measurable results. After all, surgery appeared to some a mystical craft. To be allowed to consensually cut into another human's body, to gaze at the depth of that person's suffering, and to excise the demon of disease seemed an awesome responsibility. Yet it was this very mysticism, long associated with religious overtones, that so fascinated the public and their own feared but inevitable date with a surgeon's knife. Surgeons had finally begun to view themselves as combining art and nature, essentially assisting nature in its continual process of destruction and rebuilding. This regard for the natural would spring from the eventual, though preternaturally slow, understanding and use of Joseph Lister's (1827-1912) techniques (Fig. 1-4).

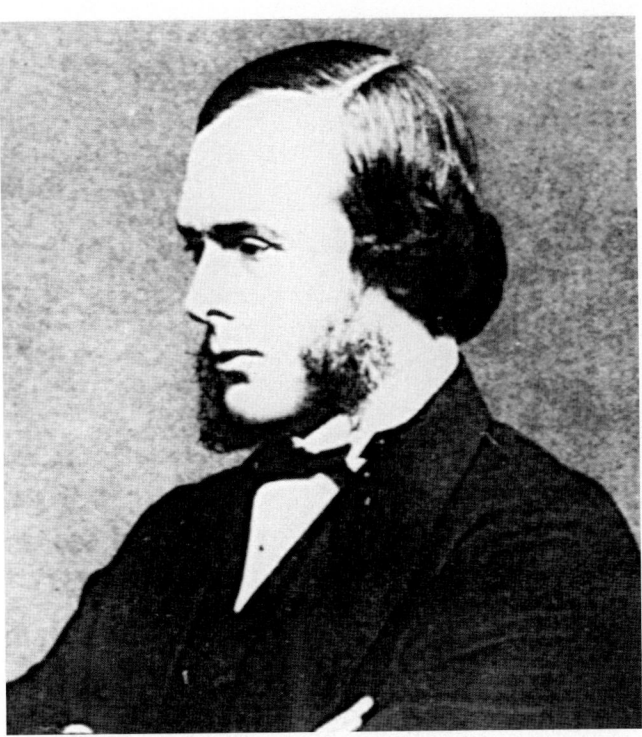

Figure 1-4 Joseph Lister (1827-1912).

ANTISEPSIS, ASEPSIS, AND UNDERSTANDING THE NATURE OF INFECTION

In many respects, the recognition of antisepsis and asepsis was a more important event in the evolution of surgical history than the advent of inhalational anesthesia was. There was no arguing that deadening of pain permitted a surgical operation to be conducted in a more efficacious manner. Haste was no longer of prime concern. However, if anesthesia had never been conceived, a surgical procedure could still be performed, albeit with much difficulty. Such was not the case with listerism. Without antisepsis and asepsis, major surgical operations more than likely ended in death rather than just pain. Clearly, surgery needed both anesthesia and antisepsis, but in terms of overall importance, antisepsis proved to be of greater singular impact.

In the long evolution of world surgery, the contributions of several individuals stand out as being preeminent. Lister, an English surgeon, can be placed on such a select list because of his monumental efforts to introduce systematic, scientifically based antisepsis in the treatment of wounds and the performance of surgical operations. He pragmatically applied others' research into fermentation and microorganisms to the world of surgery by devising a means of preventing surgical infection and securing its adoption by a skeptical profession.

It was evident to Lister that a method of destroying bacteria by excessive heat could not be applied to a surgical patient. He turned, instead, to chemical antisep-sis and, after experimenting with zinc chloride and the sulfites, decided on carbolic acid. By 1865, Lister was instilling pure carbolic acid into wounds and onto dressings. He would eventually make numerous modifications in the technique of dressings, the manner of applying and retaining them, and the choice of antiseptic solutions of varying concentrations. Although the carbolic acid spray remains the best remembered of his many contributions, it was eventually abandoned in favor of other germicidal substances. Lister not only used carbolic acid in the wound and on dressings but also went so far as to spray it in the atmosphere around the operative field and table. He did not emphasize hand scrubbing but merely dipped his fingers into a solution of phenol and corrosive sublimate. Lister was incorrectly convinced that scrubbing created crevices in the palms of the hands where bacteria would proliferate. A second important advance by Lister was the development of sterile absorbable sutures. He believed that much of the deep suppuration found in wounds was created by previously contaminated silk ligatures. Lister evolved a carbolized catgut suture that was better than any previously produced. He was able to cut the ends of the ligature short, thereby closing the wound tightly, and eliminate the necessity of bringing the ends of the suture out through the incision, a surgical practice that had persisted since the days of Paré.

The acceptance of listerism was an uneven and distinctly slow process, for many reasons. First, the various procedural changes that Lister made during the evolution of his methodology created confusion. Second, listerism, as a technical exercise, was complicated with the use of carbolic acid, an unpleasant and time-consuming nuisance. Third, various early attempts to use antisepsis in surgery had proved abject failures, with many leading surgeons unable to replicate Lister's generally good results. Finally and most important, acceptance of listerism depended entirely on an understanding and ultimate recognition of the veracity of the germ theory, a hypothesis that many practical-minded surgeons were loath to accept.

As a professional group, German-speaking surgeons would be the first to grasp the importance of bacteriology and the germ theory. Consequently, they were among the earliest to expand on Lister's message of antisepsis, with his spray being discarded in favor of boiling and use of the autoclave. The availability of heat sterilization engendered sterile aprons, drapes, instruments, and sutures. Similarly, the use of facemasks, gloves, hats, and operating gowns also naturally evolved. By the mid-1890s, less clumsy aseptic techniques had found their way into most European surgical amphitheaters and were approaching total acceptance by American surgeons. Any lingering doubts about the validity and significance of the momentous concepts that Lister had put forth were eliminated on the battlefields of World War I. There, the importance of just plain antisepsis became an invaluable lesson for scalpel bearers, whereas the exigencies of the battlefield helped bring about the final maturation and equitable standing of surgery and surgeons within the worldwide medical community.

X-RAYS

Especially prominent among other late 19th century discoveries that had an enormous impact on the evolution of surgery was research conducted by Wilhelm Roentgen (1845-1923), which led to his 1895 elucidation of x-rays. Having grown interested in the phosphorescence from metallic salts that were exposed to light, Roentgen made a chance observation when passing a current through a vacuum tube and noticed a greenish glow coming from a screen on a shelf 9 feet away. This strange effect continued after the current was turned off. He found that the screen had been painted with a phosphorescent substance. Proceeding with full experimental vigor, Roentgen soon realized that there were invisible rays capable of passing through solid objects made of wood, metal, and other materials. Most significant, these rays also penetrated the soft parts of the body in such a manner that the more dense bones of his hand were able to be revealed on a specially treated photographic plate. In a short time, numerous applications were developed as surgeons rapidly applied the new discovery to the diagnosis and location of fractures and dislocations and the removal of foreign bodies.

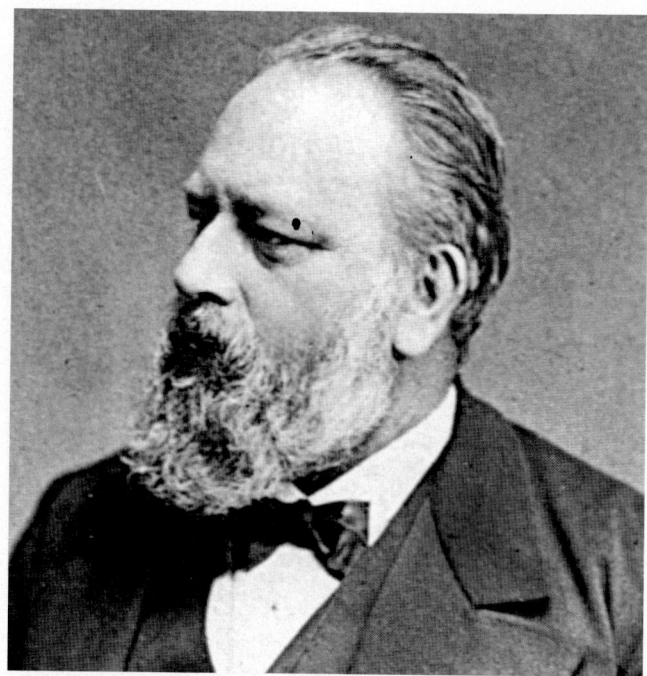

Figure 1-5 Theodor Billroth (1829-1894).

TURN OF THE 20TH CENTURY

By the late 1890s, the interactions of political, scientific, socioeconomic, and technical factors set the stage for what would become a spectacular showcasing of surgery's newfound prestige and accomplishments. Surgeons were finally wearing antiseptic-looking white coats. Patients and tables were draped in white, and basins for bathing instruments in bichloride solution abounded. Suddenly all was clean and tidy, with conduct of the surgical operation no longer a haphazard affair. This reformation would be successful not because surgeons had fundamentally changed but because medicine and its relationship to scientific inquiry had been irrevocably altered. Sectarianism and quackery, the consequences of earlier medical dogmatism, would no longer be tenable within the confines of scientific truth.

With all four fundamental clinical prerequisites in place by the turn of the century and highlighted with the emerging clinical triumphs of various English surgeons, including Robert Tait (1845-1899), William Macewen (1848-1924), and Frederick Treves (1853-1923); German-speaking surgeons, among whom were Theodor Billroth (1829-1894) (Fig. 1-5), Theodor Kocher (1841-1917) (Fig. 1-6), Friedrich Trendelenburg (1844-1924), and Johann von Mikulicz-Radecki (1850-1905); French surgeons, including Jules Peán (1830-1898), Just Lucas-Championière (1843-1913), and Marin-Theodore Tuffiér (1857-1929); the Italians, most notably Eduardo Bassini (1844-1924) and Antonio Ceci (1852-1920); and several American surgeons, exemplified by William Williams Keen (1837-1932), Nicholas Senn (1844-1908), and John Benjamin Murphy (1857-1916), scalpel wielders had essentially explored all cavities of the human body.

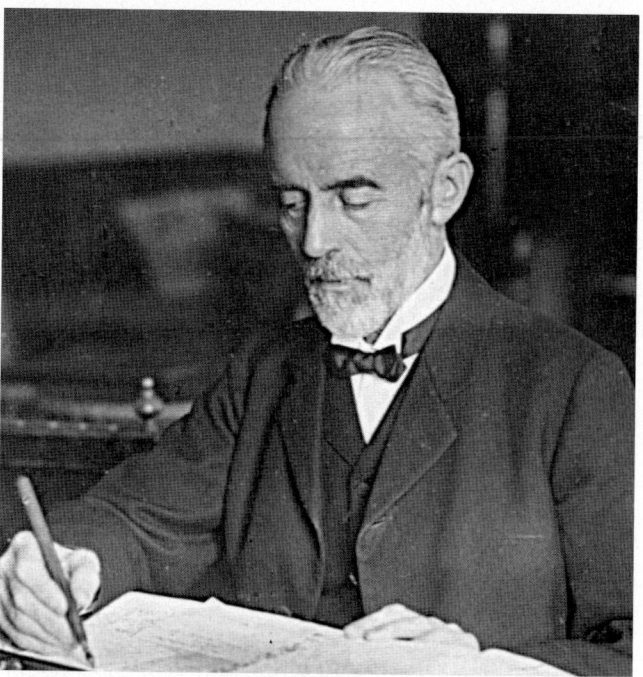

Figure 1-6 Theodor Kocher (1841-1917).

Nonetheless, surgeons retained a lingering sense of professional and social discomfort and continued to be pejoratively described by nouveau scientific physicians as *nonthinkers* who worked in little more than an inferior and crude manual craft.

It was becoming increasingly evident that research models, theoretical concepts, and valid clinical applications would be necessary to demonstrate the scientific basis of surgery to a wary public. The effort to devise new operative methods called for an even greater reliance on experimental surgery and absolute encouragement of it by all concerned parties. Most importantly, a scientific basis for therapeutic surgical recommendations—consisting of empirical data, collected and analyzed according to nationally and internationally accepted rules and set apart from individual authoritative assumptions—would have to be developed. In contrast to previously unexplainable doctrines, scientific research would triumph as the final arbiter between valid and invalid surgical therapies.

In turn, surgeons had no choice but to allay society's fear of the surgical unknown by presenting surgery as an accepted part of a newly established medical armamentarium. This would not be an easy task. The immediate consequences of surgical operations, such as discomfort and associated complications, were often of more concern to patients than was the positive knowledge that an operation could eliminate potentially devastating disease processes. Accordingly, the most consequential achievement by surgeons during the early 20th century was ensuring the social acceptability of surgery as a legitimate scientific endeavor and the surgical operation as a therapeutic necessity.

ASCENT OF SCIENTIFIC SURGERY

William Stewart Halsted (1852-1922) (Fig. 1-7), more than any other surgeon, set the scientific tone for this most important period in surgical history. He moved surgery

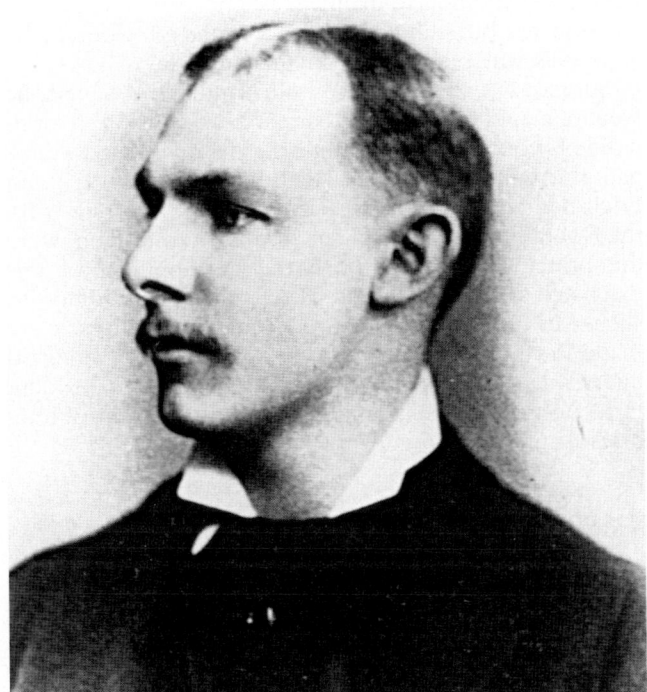

Figure 1-7 William Halsted (1852-1922).

from the melodramatics of the 19th century operating *theater* to the starkness and sterility of the modern operating *room,* commingled with the privacy and soberness of the research laboratory. As professor of surgery at the newly opened Johns Hopkins Hospital and School of Medicine, Halsted proved to be a complex personality, but the impact of this aloof and reticent man would become widespread. He introduced a new surgery and showed that research based on anatomic, pathologic, and physiologic principles and the use of animal experimentation made it possible to develop sophisticated operative procedures and perform them clinically with outstanding results. Halsted proved, to an often leery profession and public, that an unambiguous sequence could be constructed from the laboratory of basic surgical research to the clinical operating room. Most importantly, for surgery's own self-respect, he demonstrated during this turn-of-the-century renaissance in medical education that departments of surgery could command a faculty whose stature was equal in importance and prestige to that of other more academic or research-oriented fields such as anatomy, bacteriology, biochemistry, internal medicine, pathology, and physiology.

As a single individual, Halsted developed and disseminated a different system of surgery so characteristic that it was referred to as a *school of surgery.* More to the point, Halsted's methods revolutionized the world of surgery and earned his work the epithet *halstedian principles,* which remains a widely acknowledged and accepted scientific imprimatur. Halsted subordinated technical brilliance and speed of dissection to a meticulous and safe, albeit sometimes slow performance. As a direct result, Halsted's effort did much to bring about surgery's self-sustaining transformation from therapeutic subservience to clinical necessity.

Despite his demeanor as a professional recluse, Halsted's clinical and research achievements were overwhelming in number and scope. His residency system of training surgeons was not merely the first such program of its kind; it was unique in its primary purpose. Above all other concerns, Halsted desired to establish a school of surgery that would eventually disseminate throughout the surgical world the principles and attributes that he considered sound and proper. His aim was to train able surgical teachers, not merely competent operating surgeons. There is little doubt that Halsted achieved his stated goal of producing "not only surgeons but surgeons of the highest type, men who will stimulate the first youth of our country to study surgery and to devote their energies and their lives to raising the standards of surgical science." So fundamental were his contributions that without them, surgery might never have fully developed and could have remained mired in a quasi-professional state.

The heroic and dangerous nature of surgery seemed appealing in less scientifically sophisticated times, but now, surgeons were courted for personal attributes beyond their unmitigated technical boldness. A trend toward hospital-based surgery was increasingly evident, owing in equal parts to new, technically demanding operations and to modern hospital physical structures within which surgeons could work more effectively. The increasing complexity and effectiveness of aseptic surgery, the diagnostic necessity of the x-ray and clinical laboratory, the convenience of 24-hour nursing, and the availability of capable surgical residents living within a hospital were making the hospital operating room the most plausible and convenient place for a surgical operation to be performed.

It was obvious to both hospital superintendents and the whole of medicine that acute care institutions were becoming a necessity more for the surgeon than for the physician. As a consequence, increasing numbers of hospitals went to great lengths to supply their surgical staffs with the finest facilities in which to complete operations. For centuries, surgical operations had been performed under the illumination of sunlight or candles, or both. Now, however, electric lights installed in operating rooms offered a far more reliable and unwavering source of illumination. Surgery became a more proficient craft because surgical operations could be completed on stormy summer mornings, as well as on wet winter afternoons.

INTERNATIONALIZATION, SURGICAL SOCIETIES, AND JOURNALS

As the sophistication of surgery grew, internationalization became one of its underlying themes, with surgeons crossing the great oceans to visit and learn from one another. Halsted and Hermann Küttner (1870-1932), director of the surgical clinic in Breslau, Germany (now known as Wroclaw and located in southwestern Poland), instituted the first known official exchange of surgical residents in 1914. This experiment in surgical education was meant to underscore the true international spirit that had engulfed surgery. Halsted firmly believed that young surgeons achieved greater clinical maturity by observing the practice of surgery in other countries, as well as in their own.

An inevitable formation of national and international surgical societies and the emergence and development of periodicals devoted to surgical subjects proved to be important adjuncts to the professionalization process of surgery. For the most part, professional societies began as a method of providing mutual improvement via personal interaction with surgical peers and the publication of presented papers. Unlike surgeons of earlier centuries, who were known to closely guard so-called trade secrets, members of these new organizations were emphatic about publishing transactions of their meetings. In this way, not only would their surgical peers read of their clinical accomplishments, but a written record was also established for circulation throughout the world of medicine.

The first of these surgical societies was the Académie Royale de Chirurgie in Paris, with its *Mémoires* appearing sporadically from 1743 through 1838. Of 19th century associations, the most prominent published proceedings were the *Mémoires* and *Bulletins* of the Société de Chirurgie of Paris (1847), the *Verhandlungen* of the Deutsche

Gesellschaft für Chirurgie (1872), and the *Transactions* of the American Surgical Association (1883). No surgical association that published professional reports existed in 19th century Great Britain, and the Royal Colleges of Surgeons of England, Ireland, and Scotland never undertook such projects. Although textbooks, monographs, and treatises had always been the mainstay of medical writing, the introduction of monthly journals, including August Richter's (1742-1812) *Chirurgische Bibliothek* (1771), Joseph Malgaigne's (1806-1865) *Journal de Chirurgie* (1843), Bernard Langenbeck's (1810-1887) *Archiv für Klinische Chirurgie* (1860), and Lewis Pilcher's (1844-1917) *Annals of Surgery* (1885), had a tremendous impact on updating and continuing the education of surgeons.

WORLD WAR I

Austria-Hungary and Germany continued as the dominating forces in world surgery until World War I. However, results of the conflict proved disastrous to the central powers (Austria-Hungary, Bulgaria, Germany, and the Ottoman Empire), especially to German-speaking surgeons. Europe took on a new social and political look, with the demise of Germany's status as the world leader in surgery a sad but foregone conclusion. As with most armed conflicts, because of the massive human toll, especially battlefield injuries, tremendous strides were made in multiple areas of surgery. Undoubtedly, the greatest surgical achievement was in the treatment of wound infection. Trench warfare in soil contaminated by decades of cultivation and animal manure made every wounded soldier a potential carrier of any number of pathogenic bacilli. On the battlefront, sepsis was inevitable. Most attempts to maintain aseptic technique proved inadequate, but the treatment of infected wounds by antisepsis was becoming a pragmatic reality.

Surgeons experimented with numerous antiseptic solutions and various types of surgical dressing. A principle of wound treatment entailing débridement and irrigation eventually evolved. Henry Dakin (1880-1952), an English chemist, and Alexis Carrel (1873-1944) (Fig. 1-8), the Nobel prize–winning French American surgeon, were the principal protagonists in the development of this extensive system of wound management. In addition to successes in wound sterility, surgical advances were made in the use of x-rays in the diagnosis of battlefield injuries, and remarkable operative ingenuity was evident in reconstructive facial surgery and the treatment of fractures resulting from gunshot wounds.

AMERICAN COLLEGE OF SURGEONS

For American surgeons, the years just before World War I were a time of active coalescence into various social and educational organizations. The most important and influential of these societies was the American College of Surgeons, founded by Franklin Martin (1857-1935), a Chicago-based gynecologist, in 1913. Patterned after the

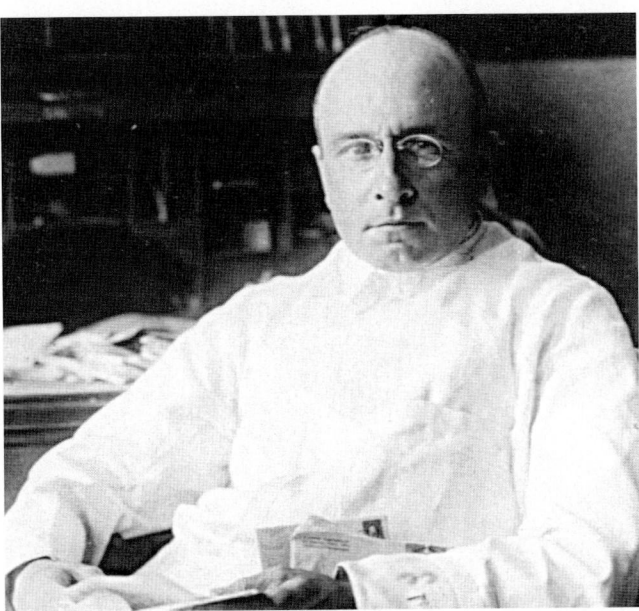

Figure 1-8 Alexis Carrel (1873-1944).

Royal Colleges of Surgeons of England, Ireland, and Scotland, the American College of Surgeons established professional, ethical, and moral standards for every graduate in medicine who practiced in surgery and conferred the designation *Fellow of the American College of Surgeons* (FACS) on its members. From the outset, its primary aim was the continuing education of surgical practitioners. Accordingly, the requirements for fellowship were always related to the educational opportunities of the period. In 1914, an applicant had to be a licensed graduate of medicine, receive the backing of three fellows, and be endorsed by the local credentials committee.

In view of the stipulated peer recommendations, many practitioners, realistically or not, viewed the American College of Surgeons as an elitist organization. With an obvious so-called blackball system built into the membership requirements, there was a difficult-to-deny belief that many surgeons who were immigrants, females, or members of particular religious and racial minorities were granted fellowships sparingly. Such inherent bias, in addition to questionable accusations of fee splitting along with unbridled contempt of certain surgeons' business practices, resulted in some very prominent American surgeons never being permitted the privilege of membership.

The 1920s and beyond proved to be a prosperous time for American society and its surgeons. After all, the history of world surgery in the 20th century is more a tale of American triumphs than it ever was in the 18th or 19th centuries. Physicians' incomes dramatically increased and surgeons' prestige, aided by the ever-mounting successes of medical science, became securely established in American culture. Still, a noticeable lack of standards and regulations in surgical specialty practice became a serious concern to leaders in the profession. The difficulties of World War I had greatly accentuated

this realistic need for specialty standards when many of the physicians who were self-proclaimed surgical specialists were found to be unqualified by military examining boards. In ophthalmology, for example, more than 50% of tested individuals were deemed unfit to treat diseases of the eye.

It was an unmistakable reality that there were no established criteria with which to distinguish a well-qualified ophthalmologist from an upstart optometrist or to clarify the differences in clinical expertise between a well-trained, full-time ophthalmologic specialist and an inadequately trained, part-time general practitioner/ophthalmologist. In recognition of the gravity of the situation, the self-patrolling concept of a professional examining board, sponsored by leading voluntary ophthalmologic organizations, was proposed as a mechanism for certifying competency. In 1916, uniform standards and regulations were set forth in the form of minimal educational requirements and written and oral examinations, and the American Board for Ophthalmic Examinations, the country's first, was formally incorporated. By 1940, six additional surgical specialty boards were established, including orthopedic (1934), colon and rectal (1934), urologic (1935), plastic (1937), surgical (1937), and neurologic (1940).

As order was introduced into surgical specialty training and the process of certification matured, it was apparent that the continued growth of residency programs carried important implications for the future structure of medical practice and the social relationship of medicine to overall society. Professional power had been consolidated, and specialization, which had been evolving since the time of the Civil War, was now recognized as an essential, if not integral part of modern medicine. Although the creation of surgical specialty boards was justified under the broad imprimatur of raising the educational status and evaluating the clinical competency of specialists, board certification undeniably began to restrict entry into the specialties.

As the specialties evolved, the political influence and cultural authority enjoyed by the profession of surgery were growing. This socioeconomic strength was most prominently expressed in reform efforts directed toward the modernization and standardization of America's hospital system. Any vestiges of so-called kitchen surgery had essentially disappeared, and other than numerous small private hospitals predominantly constructed by surgeons for their personal use, the only facilities where major surgery could be adequately conducted and postoperative patients appropriately cared for were the well-equipped and physically impressive modern hospitals. For this reason, the American College of Surgeons and its expanding list of fellows had a strong motive to ensure that America's hospital system was as up to date and efficient as possible.

On an international level, surgeons were confronted with the lack of any formal organizational body. Not until the International College of Surgeons was founded in 1935 in Geneva would such a society exist. At its inception, this organization was intended to serve as a liaison to the existing colleges and surgical societies in the various countries of the world. However, its goals of elevating the art and science of surgery, creating greater understanding among the surgeons of the world, and affording a means of international postgraduate study never came to full fruition, in part because the American College of Surgeons adamantly opposed the establishment—and continues to do so—of a viable American chapter of the International College of Surgeons.

WOMEN SURGEONS

One of the many overlooked areas of surgical history concerns the involvement of women. Until recent times, women's options for obtaining advanced surgical training were severely restricted. The major reason was that through the mid-20th century, only a handful of women had performed enough surgery to become skilled mentors. Without role models and with limited access to hospital positions, the ability of the few practicing female physicians to specialize in surgery seemed an impossibility. Consequently, women surgeons were forced to use different career strategies than men and to have more divergent goals of personal success to achieve professional satisfaction. Despite these difficulties and through the determination and aid of several enlightened male surgeons, most notably William Byford (1817-1890) of Chicago and William Keen of Philadelphia, a small cadre of female surgeons did exist in late 19th century America. Mary Dixon Jones (1828-1908), Emmeline Horton Cleveland (1829-1878), Mary Harris Thompson (1829-1895), Anna Elizabeth Broomall (1847-1931), and Marie Mergler (1851-1901) would act as a nidus toward greater equality of the genders in 20th century surgery.

AFRICAN AMERICAN SURGEONS

There is little disputing the fact that both gender and racial bias have influenced the evolution of surgery. Every aspect of society is affected by such discrimination, and African Americans, like women, were innocent victims of injustices that forced them into never-ending struggles to attain competency in surgery. As early as 1868, a department of surgery was established at Howard University. However, the first three chairmen were all white Anglo-Saxon Protestants. Not until Austin Curtis was appointed professor of surgery in 1928 did the department have its first African American head. Like all black physicians of his era, he was forced to train at so-called Negro hospitals, in Curtis' case Provident Hospital in Chicago, where he came under the tutelage of Daniel Hale Williams (1858-1931), the most influential and highly regarded of early African American surgeons. In 1897, Williams received considerable notoriety when he reported successful suturing of the pericardium for a stab wound of the heart.

With little likelihood of obtaining membership in the American Medical Association or its related societies, in 1895 African American physicians joined together to form the National Medical Association. Black surgeons identi-

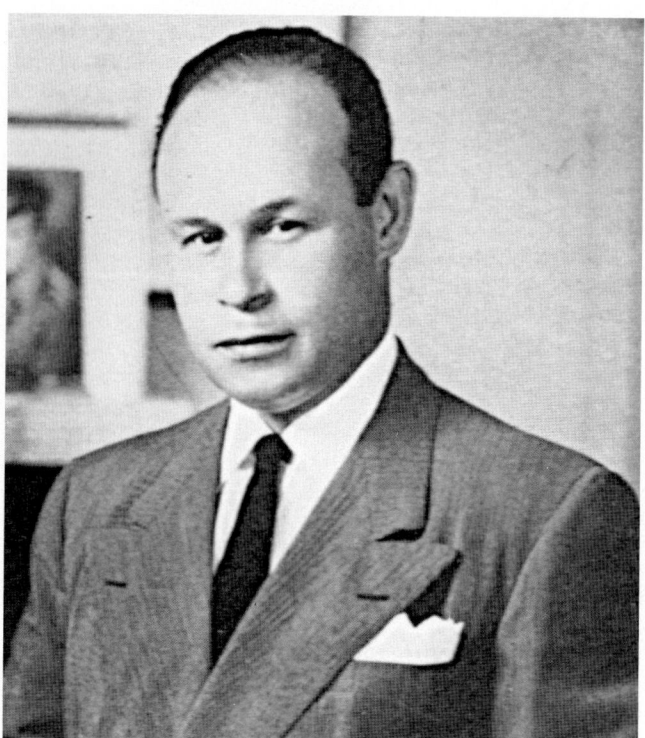

Figure 1-9 Charles Drew (1904-1950).

fied an even more specific need when the Surgical Section of the National Medical Association was opened in 1906. These National Medical Association surgical clinics, which preceded the Clinical Congress of Surgeons of North America, the forerunner to the annual congress of the American College of Surgeons, by almost half a decade, represented the earliest instances of organized so-called show-me surgical education in the United States.

Admittance to surgical societies and attainment of specialty certification were important social and psychological accomplishments for early African American surgeons. When Daniel Williams was named a Fellow of the American College of Surgeons in 1913, the news spread rapidly throughout the African American surgical community. Still, African American surgeons' fellowship applications were often acted on rather slowly, which suggested that denials based on race were clandestinely conducted throughout much of the country. As late as the mid-1940s, Charles Drew (1904-1950) (Fig. 1-9), chairman of the department of surgery at Howard University School of Medicine, acknowledged that he refused to accept membership in the American College of Surgeons because this so-called nationally representative surgical society had, in his opinion, not yet begun to freely accept capable and well-qualified African American surgeons. Claude H. Organ, Jr. (1926-2005) (Fig. 1-10), was a distinguished editor, educator, and historian. Among his books, the two-volume *A Century of Black Surgeons: The U.S.A. Experience* and the authoritative *Noteworthy Publications by African-American Surgeons* underscored the numerous contributions made by African American surgeons to the nation's health care system. In addition,

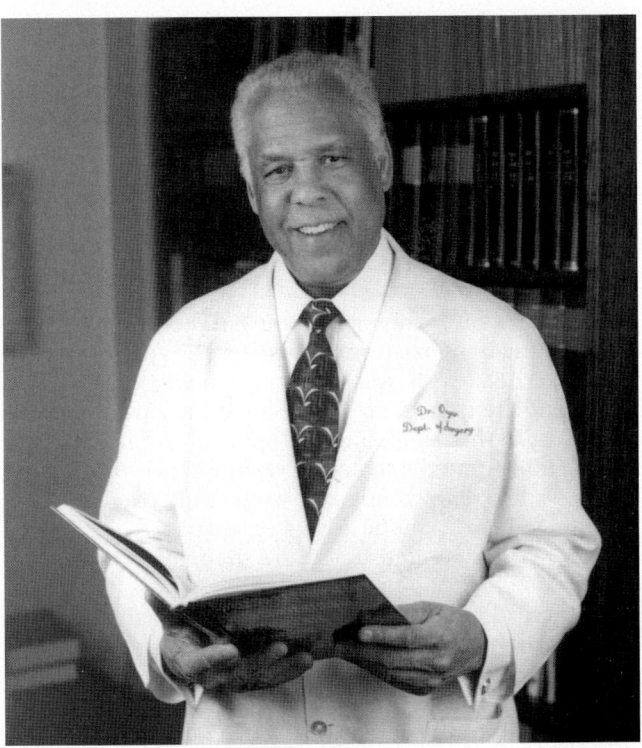

Figure 1-10 Claude H. Organ, Jr. (1926-2005). (Courtesy of the American College of Surgeons and Dr. James C. Thompson.)

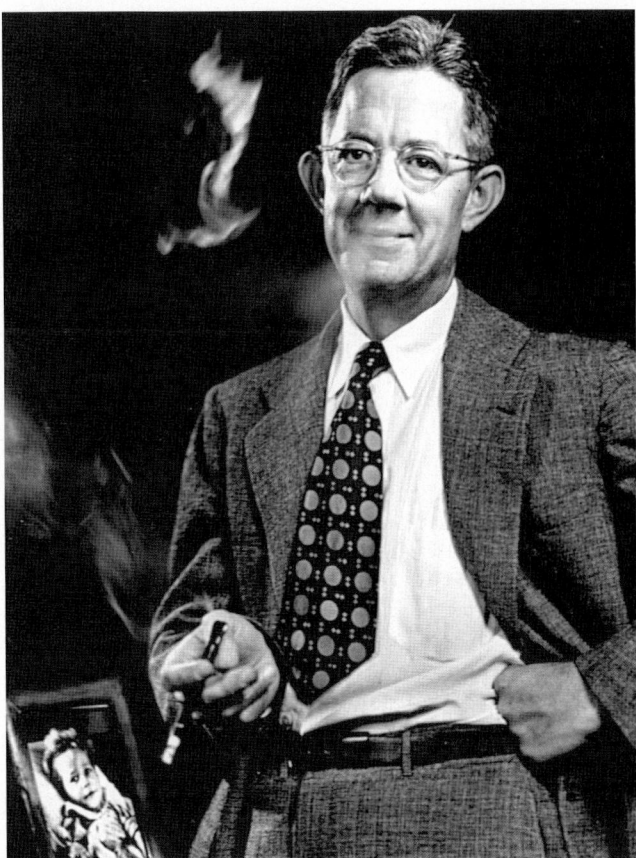

Figure 1-11 Alfred Blalock (1899-1964).

as the long-standing editor-in-chief of *Archives of Surgery*, as well as serving as president of the American College of Surgeons and chairman of the American Board of Surgery, Organ wielded enormous influence over the direction of American surgery.

MODERN ERA

Despite the global economic depression in the aftermath of World War I, the 1920s and 1930s signaled the ascent of American surgery to its current position of international leadership. Highlighted by educational reforms in its medical schools, Halsted's redefinition of surgical residency programs, and the growth of surgical specialties, the stage was set for the blossoming of scientific surgery. Basic surgical research became an established reality as George Crile (1864-1943), Alfred Blalock (1899-1964) (Fig. 1-11), Dallas Phemister (1882-1951), and Charles Huggins (1901-1997) became world-renowned surgeon-scientists.

Much as the ascendancy of the surgeon-scientist brought about changes in the way in which the public and the profession viewed surgical research, the introduction of increasingly sophisticated technologies had an enormous impact on the practice of surgery. Throughout the evolution of surgery, the practice of surgery—the art, the craft, and finally, the science of working with one's hands—had largely been defined by its tools. From the crude flint instruments of ancient peoples, through the simple tonsillotomes and lithotrites of the 19th century,

up to the increasingly complex surgical instruments developed in the 20th century, new and improved instruments usually led to a better surgical result. Progress in surgical instrumentation and surgical techniques went hand in hand.

Surgical techniques would, of course, become more sophisticated with the passage of time, but by the conclusion of World War II, essentially all organs and areas of the body had been fully explored. In fact, within a short half-century the domain of surgery had become so well established that the profession's foundation of basic operative procedures was already completed. As a consequence, there were few technical surgical mysteries left. What surgery now needed to sustain its continued growth was the ability to diagnose surgical diseases at earlier stages, to locate malignant growths while they remained small, and to have more effective postoperative treatment so that patients could survive ever more technically complex operations. Such thinking was exemplified by the introduction in 1924 of cholecystography by Evarts Graham (1883-1957) and Warren Cole (1898-1990). In this case, an emerging scientific technology introduced new possibilities into surgical practice that were not necessarily related solely to improvements in technique. To the surgeon, the discovery and application of cholecystography proved most important, not only because it brought about more accurate diagnoses of cholecystitis but also because it created an influx of surgical patients where few had previously existed. If surgery was to grow, large numbers of individuals with surgical diseases were needed.

It was an exciting era for surgeons, with important clinical advances being made both in the operating room and in the basic science laboratory. Among the most notable highlights were the introduction in 1935 of pancreaticoduodenectomy for cancer of the pancreas by Allen Oldfather Whipple (1881-1963) and a report in 1943 on vagotomy for operative treatment of peptic ulcer disease by Lester Dragstedt (1893-1976). Frank Lahey (1880-1953) stressed the importance of identifying the recurrent laryngeal nerve during the course of thyroid surgery; Owen Wangensteen (1898-1981) successfully decompressed mechanical bowel obstructions by using a newly devised suction apparatus in 1932; George Vaughan (1859-1948) successfully ligated the abdominal aorta for aneurysmal disease in 1921; Max Peet (1885-1949) presented his splanchnic resection for hypertension in 1935; Walter Dandy (1886-1946) performed intracranial section of various cranial nerves in the 1920s; Walter Freeman (1895-1972) described prefrontal lobotomy as a means of treating various mental illnesses in 1936; Harvey Cushing (1869-1939) introduced electrocoagulation in neurosurgery in 1928; Marius Smith-Petersen (1886-1953) described a flanged nail for pinning a fracture of the neck of the femur in 1931 and introduced Vitallium cup arthroplasty in 1939; Vilray Blair (1871-1955) and James Brown (1899-1971) popularized the use of split-skin grafts to cover large areas of granulating wounds; Earl Padgett (1893-1946) devised an operative dermatome that allowed calibration of the thickness of skin grafts in 1939; Elliott Cutler (1888-1947) performed a successful section of the mitral valve for relief of mitral stenosis in 1923; Evarts Graham completed the first successful removal of an entire lung for cancer in 1933; Claude Beck (1894-1971) implanted pectoral muscle into the pericardium and attached a pedicled omental graft to the surface of the heart, thus providing collateral circulation to that organ, in 1935; Robert Gross (1905-1988) reported the first successful ligation of a patent arterial duct in 1939 and resection for coarctation of the aorta with direct anastomosis of the remaining ends in 1945; and John Alexander (1891-1954) resected a saccular aneurysm of the thoracic aorta in 1944.

With such a wide variety of technically complex surgical operations now possible, it had clearly become impossible for any single surgeon to master all the manual skills as well as the pathophysiologic knowledge necessary to perform such cases. Therefore, by the middle of the century, a consolidation of professional power inherent in the movement toward specialization, with numerous individuals restricting their surgical practice to one highly structured field, had become among the most significant and dominating events in 20th century surgery. Ironically, the United States, which had been much slower than European countries to recognize surgeons as a distinct group of clinicians separate from physicians, would now spearhead this move toward surgical specialization with great alacrity. Clearly, the course of surgical fragmentation into specialties and subspecialties was

gathering tremendous speed as the dark clouds of World War II settled over the globe. The socioeconomic and political ramifications of this war would bring about a fundamental change in the way that surgeons viewed themselves and their interactions with the society in which they lived and worked.

LAST HALF OF THE 20TH CENTURY

The decades of economic expansion after World War II had a dramatic impact on surgery's scale, particularly in the United States. It was as though being victorious in battle permitted medicine to become big business overnight, with the single-minded pursuit of health care rapidly transformed into society's largest growth industry. Spacious hospital complexes were built that not only represented the scientific advancement of the healing arts but also vividly demonstrated the strength of American's postwar socioeconomic boom. Society was willing to give surgical science unprecedented recognition as a prized national asset.

The overwhelming impact of World War II on surgery was the sudden expansion of the profession and the beginnings of an extensive distribution of surgeons throughout the country. Many of these individuals, newly baptized to the rigors of technically complex trauma operations, became leaders in the construction and improvement of hospitals, multispecialty clinics, and surgical facilities in their hometowns. Large urban and community hospitals established surgical education and training programs and found it a relatively easy matter to attract interns and residents. For the first time, residency programs in general surgery were rivaled in growth and educational sophistication by those in all the special fields of surgery. These changes served as fodder for further increases in the number of students entering surgery. Not only would surgeons command the highest salaries, but society was also enamored of the drama of the operating room. Television series, movies, novels, and the more-than-occasional live performance of a heart operation on network broadcast beckoned the lay individual.

Despite lay approval, success and acceptability in the biomedical sciences are sometimes difficult to determine, but one measure of both in recent times has been awarding of the Nobel Prize in medicine and physiology. Society's continued approbation of surgery's accomplishments is seen in the naming of nine surgeons as Nobel laureates (Table 1-1).

CARDIAC SURGERY AND ORGAN TRANSPLANTATION

Two clinical developments truly epitomized the magnificence of post–World War II surgery and concurrently fascinated the public: the maturation of cardiac surgery as a new surgical specialty and the emergence of organ transplantation. Together, they would stand as signposts along the new surgical highway. Fascination with the

Table 1-1 Surgeons Named Nobel Laureates in Medicine and Physiology

SURGEON	COUNTRY	FIELD (YEAR OF AWARD)
Theodor Kocher (1841-1917)	Switzerland	Thyroid disease (1909)
Allvar Gullstrand (1862-1930)	Sweden	Ocular dioptrics (1911)
Alexis Carrel (1873-1944)	France and United States	Vascular surgery (1912)
Robert Bárány (1876-1936)	Austria	Vestibular disease (1914)
Frederick Banting (1891-1941)	Canada	Insulin (1922)
Walter Hess (1881-1973)	Switzerland	Midbrain physiology (1949)
Werner Forssmann (1904-1979)	Germany	Cardiac catheterization (1956)
Charles Huggins (1901-1997)	United States	Oncology (1966)
Joseph Murray (1919-)	United States	Organ transplantation (1990)

heart goes far beyond that of clinical medicine. From the historical perspective of art, customs, literature, philosophy, religion, and science, the heart has represented the seat of the soul and the wellspring of life itself. Such reverence also meant that this noble organ was long considered a surgical untouchable. Whereas the late 19th and 20th centuries witnessed a steady march of surgical triumphs in opening successive cavities of the body, the final achievement awaited the perfection of methods for surgical operations in the thoracic space.

Such a scientific and technologic accomplishment can be traced back to the repair of cardiac stab wounds by direct suture and the earliest attempts at fixing faulty heart valves. As triumphant as Luther Hill's (1862-1946) first known successful suture of a wound that penetrated a cardiac chamber was in 1902, it would not be until the 1940s that the development of safe intrapleural surgery could be counted on as something other than an occasional event. During World War II, Dwight Harken (1910-1993) gained extensive battlefield experience in removing bullets and shrapnel in or in relation to the heart and great vessels without a single fatality. Building on his wartime experience, Harken and other pioneering surgeons, including Charles Bailey (1910-1993) of Philadelphia and Russell Brock (1903-1980) of London, proceeded to expand intracardiac surgery by developing operations for the relief of mitral valve stenosis. The procedure was progressively refined and evolved into the open commissurotomy repair used today.

Despite mounting clinical successes, surgeons who operated on the heart had to contend not only with the quagmire of blood flowing through an area where difficult dissection was taking place but also with the unrelenting to-and-fro movement of a beating heart. Technically complex cardiac repair procedures could not be developed further until these problems were solved. John Gibbon (1903-1973) (Fig. 1-12) addressed this enigma by devising a machine that would take on the work of the heart and lungs while the patient was under anesthesia, in essence pumping oxygen-rich blood through the circulatory system while bypassing the heart so that the organ could be operated on at leisure. The first successful open heart operation in 1953, conducted with the use of a heart-lung machine, was a momentous surgical contri-

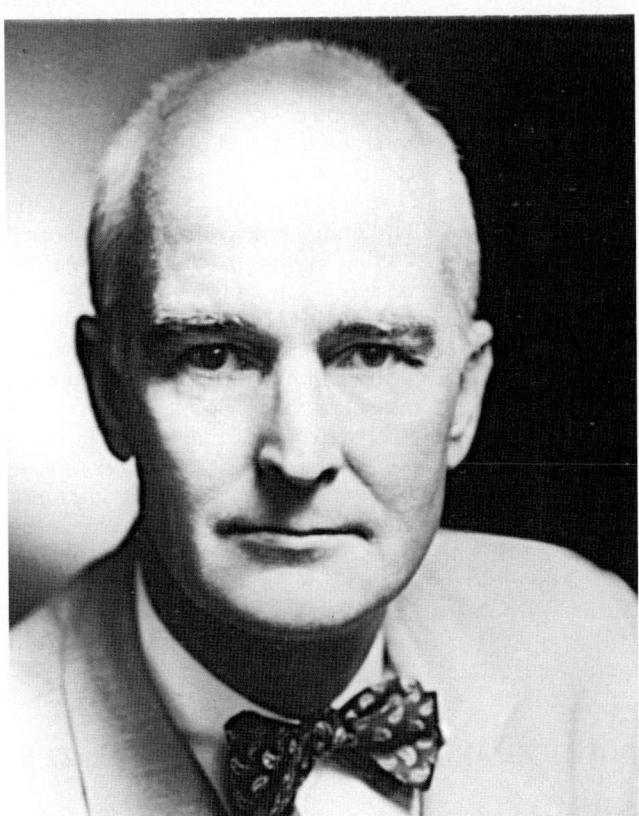

Figure 1-12 John Gibbon (1903-1973).

bution. Through single-mindedness of purpose, Gibbon's research paved the way for all future cardiac surgery, including procedures for correction of congenital heart defects, repair of heart valves, and transplantation of the heart.

Since time immemorial, the focus of surgery was mostly on excision and repair. However, beginning in the 20th century, the opposite end of the surgical spectrum—reconstruction and transplantation—became realities. Nineteenth century experience had shown that skin and bone tissues could be autotransplanted from one site to another in the same patient. It would take the horrendous and mutilating injuries of World War I to decisively advance skin transplants and legitimize the concept of surgery as a method of reconstruction. With Harold Gillies (1882-1960) of England and America's Vilray Blair establishing military-based plastic surgery units to deal with complex maxillofacial injuries, a turning point in the way in which society viewed surgery's raison d'être occurred. Now, not only would surgeons enhance nature's healing powers, but they could also dramatically alter what had previously been little more than one's physical foregone conclusion. For example, Hippolyte Morestin (1869-1919) described a method of mammaplasty in 1902. John Staige Davis (1872-1946) of Baltimore popularized a manner of splinting skin grafts and later wrote the first comprehensive textbook on this new specialty, *Plastic Surgery: Its Principles and Practice* (1919). Immediately after the war, Blair would go on to establish the first separate plastic surgery service in a civilian institution at Barnes Hospital in St. Louis. Vladimir Filatov (1875-1956) of Odessa, Russia, used a tubed pedicle flap in 1916, and in the following year, Gillies introduced a similar technique.

What about the replacement of damaged or diseased organs? After all, even at the midpoint of the century, the very thought of successfully transplanting worn-out or unhealthy body parts verged on scientific fantasy. At the beginning of the 20th century, Alexis Carrel developed revolutionary new suturing techniques to anastomose the smallest of blood vessels. Using his surgical élan on experimental animals, Carrel began to transplant kidneys, hearts, and spleens. Technically, his research was a success, but some unknown biologic process always led to rejection of the transplanted organ and death of the animal. By the middle of the century, medical researchers had begun to clarify the presence of underlying defensive immune reactions and the necessity of creating immunosuppression as a method to allow the host to accept the foreign transplant. Using high-powered immunosuppressant drugs and other modern modalities, kidney transplantation soon blazed the way, and it was not long before a slew of organs and even whole hands were being replaced.

POLITICAL AND SOCIOECONOMIC INFLUENCES

Despite the 1950s and 1960s witnessing some of the most magnificent advances in the history of surgery, by the 1970s, political and socioeconomic influences were starting to overshadow many of the clinical triumphs. It was the beginning of a schizophrenic existence for surgeons in that complex and dramatic lifesaving operations were completed to innumerable accolades, while concurrently, public criticism of the economics of medicine, in particular, high-priced surgical practice, portrayed the scalpel holder as an acquisitive, financially driven, selfish individual. This was in stark contrast to the relatively selfless and sanctified image of the surgeon before the growth of specialty work and the introduction of government involvement in health care delivery.

Although they are philosophically inconsistent, the dramatic and theatrical features of surgery that make surgeons heroes from one perspective and symbols of corruption, mendacity, and greed from the opposite point of view are the very reasons why society demands so much of its surgeons. There is the precise and definitive nature of surgical intervention, the expectation of success that surrounds an operation, the short time frame in which outcomes are realized, the high income levels of most surgeons, and the almost insatiable inquisitiveness of lay individuals concerning all aspects of the act of consensually cutting into another human's flesh. These phenomena, ever more sensitized in an age of mass media and instantaneous telecommunication, make surgeons seem more accountable than their medical colleagues and, simultaneously, symbolic of the best and the worst in medicine. In ways previously unimaginable, this vast social transformation of surgery controls the fate of the individual practitioner in the present era to a much greater extent than surgeons as a collective force are able to control it by their attempts to direct their own profession.

20TH CENTURY SURGICAL HIGHLIGHTS

Among the difficulties in studying 20th century surgery is the abundance of famous names and important written contributions—so much so that it becomes a difficult and invidious task to attempt any rational selection of representative personalities along with their significant journal or book-length writings. Although many justly famous names might be missing, the following description of surgical advances is intended to chronologically highlight some of the stunning clinical achievements of the past century.

In 1900, the German surgeon Hermann Pfannenstiel (1862-1909) described his technique for a suprapubic surgical incision. That same year, William Mayo (1861-1939) presented his results on partial gastrectomy before the American Surgical Association. The treatment of breast cancer was radically altered when George Beatson (1848-1933), professor of surgery in Glasgow, Scotland, proposed oophorectomy and the administration of thyroid extract as a possible cure (1901). John Finney (1863-1942) of The Johns Hopkins Hospital authored a paper on a new method of gastroduodenostomy, or widened pyloroplasty (1903). In Germany, Fedor Krause (1856-1937) was writing about total cystectomy and bilateral ureterosigmoidostomy. In 1905, Hugh Hampton Young (1870-1945) of Baltimore was presenting early studies of his radical prostatectomy for carcinoma. William Handley (1872-1962) was surgeon of the Middlesex Hospital in London when he authored *Cancer of the Breast and Its Treatment* (1906). In that work he advanced the theory that in breast cancer, metastasis is due to extension along lymphatic vessels and not to dissemination via the bloodstream. That same year, José Goyanes (1876-1964) of Madrid used vein grafts to restore arterial flow. William Miles (1869-1947) of England first wrote about his technique of abdominoperineal resection in 1908, the same year that Friedrich Trendelenburg (1844-1924) attempted pulmonary embolectomy. Three years later, Martin Kirschner (1879-1942) of Germany described a wire for skeletal traction and for stabilization of bone fragments or joint immobilization. Donald Balfour (1882-1963) of the Mayo Clinic provided the initial account of his important operation for resection of the sigmoid colon, as did William Mayo for his radical operation for carcinoma of the rectum in 1910.

In 1911, Fred Albee (1876-1945) of New York City began to use living bone grafts as internal splints. Wilhelm Ramstedt (1867-1963), a German surgeon, described a pyloromyotomy (1912) at the same time that Pierre Fredet (1870-1946) was reporting a similar operation. In 1913, Henry Janeway (1873-1921) of New York City developed a technique for gastrostomy in which he wrapped the anterior wall of the stomach around a catheter and sutured it in place, thereby establishing a permanent fistula. Hans Finsterer (1877-1955), professor of surgery in Vienna, improved on Franz von Hofmeister's (1867-1926) description of a partial gastrectomy with closure of a portion of the lesser curvature and retrocolic anastomosis of the remainder of the stomach to the jejunum (1918). Thomas Dunhill (1876-1957) of London was a pioneer in thyroid surgery, especially in his operation for exophthalmic goiter (1919). William Gallie (1882-1959) of Canada used sutures fashioned from the fascia lata in herniorrhaphy (1923). Barney Brooks (1884-1952), professor of surgery at Vanderbilt University in Nashville, Tennessee, initially introduced clinical angiography and femoral arteriography in 1924. Five years later, Reynaldo dos Santos (1880-1970), a Portuguese urologist, reported the first translumbar aortogram. Cecil Joll (1885-1945), professor of surgery in London, fully described the treatment of thyrotoxicosis by means of subtotal thyroidectomy in the 1930s.

In 1931, George Cheatle (1865-1951), professor of surgery in London, and Max Cutler (1899-1984), a surgeon from New York City, published their important treatise *Tumours of the Breast*. In that same year, Cutler detailed his systemic use of ovarian hormone in the treatment of chronic mastitis. Around the same time, Ernst Sauerbruch (1875-1951) of Germany completed the first successful surgical intervention for cardiac aneurysm, and his countryman Rudolph Nissen (1896-1981) removed an entire bronchiectatic lung. Geoffrey Keynes (1887-1982) of St. Bartholomew's Hospital in England articulated the basis for the opposition to radical mastectomy and his favoring of radium treatment in breast cancer (1932). The Irish surgeon Arnold Henry (1886-1962) devised an operative approach for femoral hernia in 1936. Earl Shouldice (1891-1965) of Toronto first began to experiment with a groin hernia repair based on overlapping layers brought together by a continuous wire suture during the 1930s. René Leriche (1879-1955) proposed an arteriectomy for arterial thrombosis in 1937 and, later, periarterial sympathectomy to improve arterial flow. Leriche also enunciated a syndrome of aortoiliac occlusive disease in 1940. In 1939, Edward Churchill (1895-1972) of the Massachusetts General Hospital performed a segmental pneumonectomy for bronchiectasis. Charles Huggins (1901-1997) (Fig. 1-13), a pioneer in endocrine therapy for cancer, found that antiandrogenic treatment consisting of orchiectomy or the administration of estrogens could produce long-term regression in patients with advanced prostatic

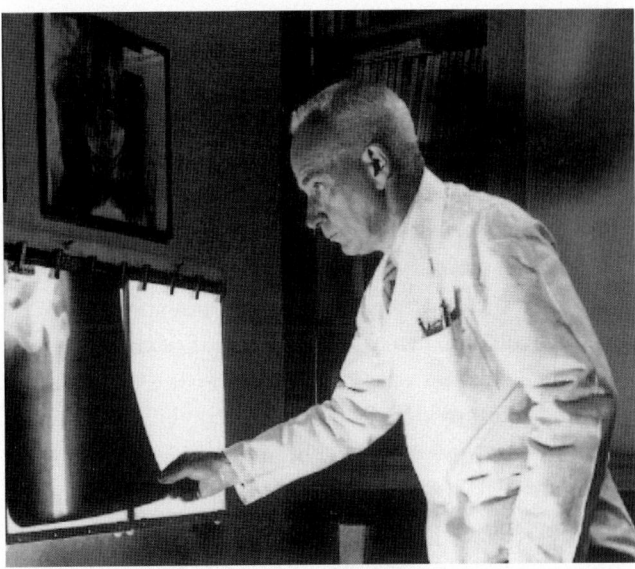

Figure 1-13 Charles Huggins (1901-1997). (Used with permission from the University of Chicago Hospitals.)

cancer. These observations formed the basis for the current treatment of prostate and breast cancer by hormonal manipulation; Dr. Huggins was awarded the Nobel Prize in 1966 for these monumental discoveries. Clarence Crafoord (1899-1984) pioneered his surgical treatment of coarctation of the aorta in 1945. The following year, Willis Potts (1895-1968) completed an anastomosis of the aorta to a pulmonary vein for certain types of congenital heart disease. Chester McVay (1911-1987) popularized a repair of groin hernias based on the pectineal ligament in 1948. Working at Georgetown University Medical Center in Washington, DC, Charles Hufnagel (1916-1989) designed and inserted the first workable prosthetic heart valve in a man (1951). That same year, Charles Dubost (1914-1991) of Paris performed the first successful resection of an abdominal aortic aneurysm and insertion of a homologous graft. Robert Zollinger (1903-1994) and Edwin Ellison (1918-1970) first described their eponymic polyendocrine adenomatosis in 1955. The following year, Donald Murray (1894-1976) completed the first successful aortic valve homograft. At the same time, John Merrill (1917-1986) was performing the world's first successful homotransplantation of the human kidney between identical twin brothers. Francis D. Moore (1913-2001) (Fig. 1-14) defined objectives of metabolism in surgical patients and in 1959 published his widely quoted book *Metabolic Care of the Surgical Patient*. Moore was also a driving force in the field of transplantation and pioneered the technique of using radioactive isotopes to locate abscesses and tumors. In the 1960s, Jonathan E. Rhoads (1907-2002) (Fig. 1-15), in collaboration with colleagues Harry Vars and Stan Dudrick, described the technique of total parenteral nutrition, which has become an important and lifesaving treatment in the management of a critically ill patient who cannot tolerate standard enteral feedings. James D. Hardy (1918-2003), at the University of Mississippi, performed the first lung (1963) and heart (1964) transplants in a human.

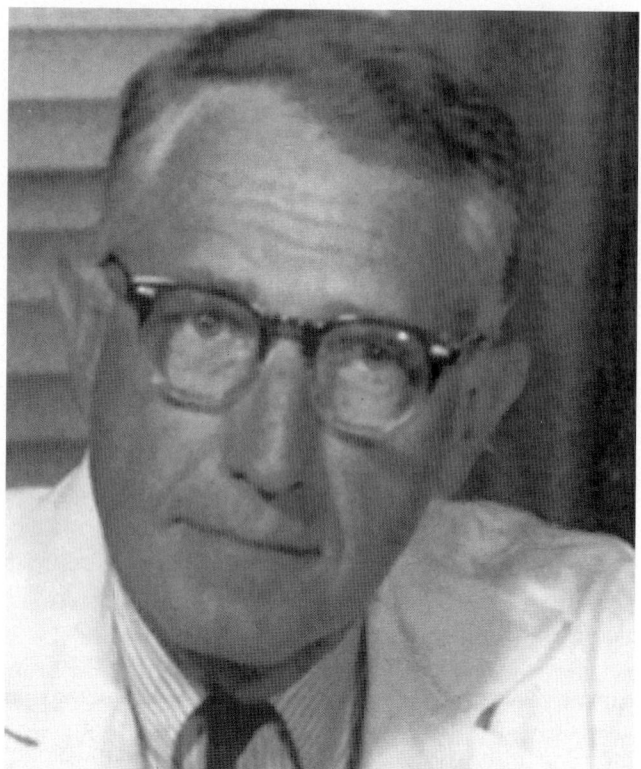

Figure 1-14 Francis D. Moore (1913-2001).

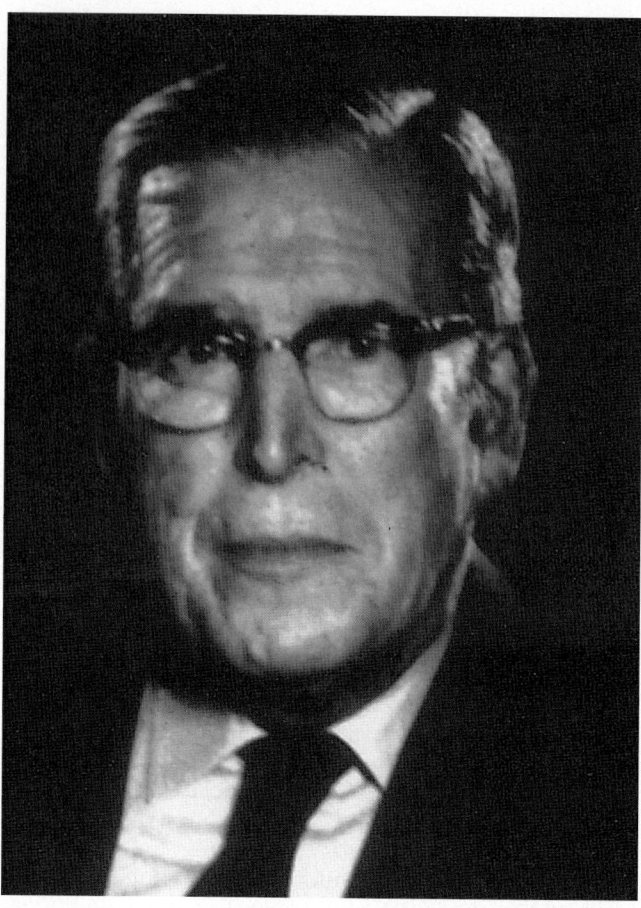

Figure 1-15 Jonathan Rhoads (1907-2002). (Courtesy of James C. Thompson, MD.)

FUTURE TRENDS

Throughout most of its evolution, the practice of surgery has been largely defined by its tools and the manual aspects of the craft. The last decades of the 20th century saw unprecedented progress in the development of new instrumentation and imaging techniques. These refinements have not come without noticeable social and economic cost. Advancement will assuredly continue, for if the study of surgical history offers any lesson, it is that progress can always be expected, at least relative to technology. There will be more sophisticated surgical operations with better results. Eventually, automation may even robotize the surgeon's hand for certain procedures. Still, the surgical sciences will always retain their historical roots as fundamentally a manually based art and craft.

In many respects, the surgeon's most difficult future challenges are not in the clinical realm but instead in better understanding the socioeconomic forces that affect the practice of surgery and in learning how to effectively manage them. Many splendid schools of surgery now exist in virtually every major industrialized city, but none can lay claim to dominance in all the disciplines that make up surgery. Likewise, the presence of authoritative individual personalities who help guide surgery is more unusual today than in previous times. National aims and socioeconomic status have become overwhelming factors in securing and shepherding the future growth of surgery

worldwide. In light of an understanding of the intricacies of surgical history, it seems an unenviable and obviously impossible task to predict what will happen in the future. In 1874, John Erichsen (1818-1896) of London wrote that "the abdomen, chest, and brain will forever be closed to operations by a wise and humane surgeon." A few years later Theodor Billroth remarked, "A surgeon who tries to suture a heart wound deserves to lose the esteem of his colleagues." Obviously, the surgical crystal ball is a cloudy one at best.

To study the fascinating history of our profession, with its many magnificent personalities and outstanding scientific and social achievements, may not necessarily help us predict the future of surgery. However, it does shed much light on the clinical practices of our own time. To a certain extent, if surgeons in the future wish to be regarded as more than mere technicians, the profession needs to better appreciate the value of its past experiences. Surgery has a distinguished heritage that is in danger of being forgotten. Although the future of the art, craft, and science of surgery remains unknown, it assuredly rests on a glorious past.

Selected References

Allbutt TC: The Historical Relations of Medicine and Surgery to the End of the Sixteenth Century. London, Macmillan, 1905.

An incisive and provocative address by the Regius Professor of Physic in the University of Cambridge concerning the sometimes strained relationships between early medical and surgical practitioners.

Billings JS: The history and literature of surgery. In Dennis FS (ed): System of Surgery, vol 1. Philadelphia, Lea Brothers, 1895, pp 17-144.

Surgeon, hospital architect, originator of *Index Medicus,* and director of the New York Public Library, Billings has written a comprehensive review of surgery, albeit based on a hagiographic theme.

Bishop WJ: The Early History of Surgery. London, Robert Hale, 1960.

This book by Bishop, a distinguished medical bibliophile, is best for its description of surgery in the Middle Ages, Renaissance, and 17th and 18th centuries.

Bliss M: Harvey Cushing, A Life in Surgery. New York, Oxford, 2005.

Prized as a fascinating biography of one of America's most influential surgeons. Bliss is a wonderful writer who provides an incisive and colorful description of surgery during the late 19th and early 20th centuries.

Cartwright FF: The Development of Modern Surgery from 1830. London, Arthur Barker, 1967.

An anesthetist at King's College Hospital in London, Cartwright has produced a work rich in detail and interpretation.

Cope Z: Pioneers in Acute Abdominal Surgery. London, Oxford University Press, 1939.
Cope Z: A History of the Acute Abdomen. London, Oxford University Press, 1965.

These two works by the highly regarded English surgeon provide overall reviews of the evolution of surgical intervention for intra-abdominal pathology.

Earle AS: Surgery in America: From the Colonial Era to the Twentieth Century. New York, Praeger, 1983.

A fascinating compilation of journal articles by well-known surgeons that trace the development of the art and science of surgery in America.

Edmondson JM: American Surgical Instruments. San Francisco, Norman Publishing, 1997.

Although a wealth of information is available about the practice of surgery and the men who performed it in colonial and 19th-century America, this book details the lost story of the instrument makers and dealers who supplied the all-important tools for these practitioners.

Gurlt EJ: Geschichte der Chirurgie und ihrer Ausübung (3 vols). Berlin, A Hirschwald, 1898.

A monumentally detailed history of surgery from the beginnings of recorded history to the end of the 16th century. Gurlt, a German surgeon, includes innumerable translations from ancient manuscripts. Unfortunately, this work has not been translated into English.

Hurwitz A, Degenshein GA: Milestones in Modern Surgery. New York, Hoeber-Harper, 1958.

The numerous chapters by these surgical attending physicians at Maimonides Hospital in Brooklyn contain prefatory information, including a short biography of various surgeons (with portrait) and a reprinted or translated excerpt of each one's most important surgical contribution.

Kirkup J: The Evolution of Surgical Instruments: An Illustrated History from Ancient Times to the Twentieth Century. Novato, CA, historyofscience.com, 2006.

Surgeons are often defined by their surgical armamentarium, and this treatise provides detailed discussions on the evolution of all manner of surgical instruments and the materials from which they are constructed.

Leonardo RA: History of Surgery. New York, Froben, 1943.
Leonardo RA: Lives of Master Surgeons. New York, Froben, 1948 [plus Lives of Master Surgeons, Supplement 1, Froben, 1949].

These texts by the eminent Rochester, New York, surgeon and historian together provide an in-depth description of the whole of surgery from ancient times to the mid-20th century. Especially valuable are the countless biographies of both famous and near-famous scalpel bearers.

Malgaigne JF: Histoire de la Chirurgie en Occident depuis de VIe Jusqu'au XVIe Siècle, et Histoire de la Vie et des Travaux d'Ambroise Paré. In Malgaigne JF (ed): Ambroise Paré, Oeuvres Complètes, vol 1, Introduction. Paris, JB Baillière, 1840-1841.

This history by Malgaigne, considered among the most brilliant French surgeons of the 19th century, is particularly noteworthy for its study of 15th and 16th century European surgery. This entire work was admirably translated into English by Wallace Hamby, an American neurosurgeon, in *Surgery and Ambrose Paré* by J. F. Malgaigne (Norman, University of Oklahoma Press, 1965).

Meade RH: An Introduction to the History of General Surgery. Philadelphia, WB Saunders, 1968.
Meade RH: A History of Thoracic Surgery. Springfield, IL, Charles C Thomas, 1961.

Meade, an indefatigable researcher of historical topics, practiced surgery in Grand Rapids, Michigan. With extensive bibliographies, his two books are among the most ambitious of such systematic works.

Porter R: The Greatest Benefit to Mankind, a Medical History of Humanity. New York, WW Norton, 1997.

A wonderful literary tour de force by one of the most erudite and entertaining of modern medical historians. Though more a history of the whole of medicine than of surgery specifically, this text has become an instantaneous classic and should be required reading for all physicians and surgeons.

Ravitch MM: A Century of Surgery: 1880-1980, The History of the American Surgical Association, 2 vols. Philadelphia, JB Lippincott, 1981.

Ravitch, among the first American surgeons to introduce mechanical stapling devices for use in the United States, was highly regarded as a medical historian. This text provides a year-by-year account of the meetings of the American Surgical Association, the most influential of America's numerous surgical organizations.

Rutkow IM: The History of Surgery in the United States, 1775-1900, 2 vols. San Francisco, Norman Publishing, 1988 and 1992.
Rutkow IM: Surgery, An Illustrated History. St Louis, Mosby–Year Book, 1993.
Rutkow IM: American Surgery, An Illustrated History. Philadelphia, Lippincott-Raven, 1998.

Rutkow IM: Bleeding Blue and Gray: Civil War Surgery and the Evolution of American Medicine, New York, Random House, 2005.

Using detailed descriptions, biographic compilations, and colored illustrations, these books explore the evolution of surgery, internationally and in the United States.

Thorwald J: The Century of the Surgeon. New York, Pantheon, 1956.
Thorwald J: The Triumph of Surgery. New York, Pantheon, 1960.

In a most dramatic literary fashion, Thorwald uses a fictional eyewitness narrator to create continuity in the story of the development of surgery during its most important decades of growth, the late 19th and early 20th centuries. Imbued with a myriad of true historical facts, these books are among the most enjoyable to be found within the genre of surgical history.

Wangensteen OH, Wangensteen SD: The Rise of Surgery, from Empiric Craft to Scientific Discipline. Minneapolis, University of Minnesota Press, 1978.

Not a systematic history but an assessment of various operative techniques (e.g., gastric surgery, tracheostomy, ovariotomy, vascular surgery) and technical factors (e.g., débridement, phlebotomy, surgical amphitheater, preparations for surgery) that contributed to or retarded the evolution of surgery. Wangensteen was a noted teacher of experimental and clinical surgery at the University of Minnesota and his wife, an accomplished medical historian.

Zimmerman LM, Veith I: Great Ideas in the History of Surgery. Baltimore, Williams & Wilkins, 1961.

Zimmerman, late professor of surgery at the Chicago Medical School, and Veith, a masterful medical historian, provide well-written biographic narratives to accompany numerous readings and translations from the works of almost 50 renowned surgeons of varying eras.

CHAPTER 2

Ethics in Surgery

Ronald A. Carson, PhD

Renewed public attention is being paid to ethics today. There are governmental ethics commissions, research ethics boards, and corporate ethics committees. Some of these institutional entities are little more than window dressing, whereas others are investigative bodies called into being, for example, on suspicion that financial records have been altered or data have been presented in a deceptive manner. However, many of these groups do important work, and the fact that they have been established at all suggests that we are not as certain as we once were, or thought we were, about where the moral boundaries are and how we would know if we overstepped them. In search of insight and guidance, we turn to ethics. In the professions, which are largely self-regulating, and especially in the medical profession, whose primary purpose is to be responsive to people in need, ethics is at the heart of the enterprise.

It is important to be clear at the outset about what ethics is and is not. Although physicians are expected to uphold such standards of professionalism as reporting impaired colleagues, medical ethics is not primarily about keeping transgressors in line. That is the domain of laws, courts, and boards of medical examiners. Ethics has to do with discerning where the lines should be drawn in the first place and to what we should aspire. It is about thinking through what we believe is good or bad or right or wrong and why we think that way. The emphasis is on reflecting and deliberating. Ethical reflection is especially useful in a social and cultural environment such as ours in which values often conflict.

The ethical precepts of the medical profession have traditionally been summarized in various oaths and codes. For example, it is still customary for students to repeat the Hippocratic Oath, or some contemporary adaptation of it, on graduation from medical school. The American College of Surgeons' Statements on Principles contains a fellowship pledge that includes a promise to maintain the College's historical commitment to "the ethical practice of medicine."[1] The American College of Obstetricians and Gynecologists (ACOG) subscribes to a code of ethics that governs the patient-physician relationship, physician conduct and practice, conflicts of interest, professional relationships, and societal responsibilities.[2] Moreover, ACOG's publication *Ethics in Obstetrics and Gynecology* is exemplary in its comprehensiveness and specificity in discussing ethical issues ranging from reproductive choice to end-of-life care.[3] Several other surgical subspecialties, as well as anesthesiology, have also given careful thought to ethical issues that arise in practice, research, education, and the introduction of innovative surgical technologies and techniques.[4-13]

Since 1847, the American Medical Association has promulgated a statement of ethical principles. Although this code has evolved over time to accommodate changes in society and medicine, it has always enunciated the ethical principles on which the profession perceives itself to be grounded. The most recent version of this statement of principles is more patient centered than ever before. It asserts that "a physician must recognize responsibility to patients first and foremost" and spells out this responsibility as the provision of "competent medical care, with compassion and respect for human dignity and rights." Principle VIII states, "A physician shall, while caring for a patient, regard responsibility to the patient as paramount."[14]

Responsibility to the patient in contemporary clinical ethics entails maximal patient participation, as permitted by the patient's condition, in decisions regarding the course of care. For the surgeon, this means arriving at an accurate diagnosis of the patient's complaint, making a treatment recommendation based on the best knowledge available, and then talking with the patient about the merits and drawbacks of the recommended course in light of the patient's life values. For the patient, maximal participation in decision making means having a conversation with the surgeon about the recommendation, why it seems reasonable and desirable, what the alternatives are, if any, and what the probable risks are of accepting the recommendation or pursuing an alternative course.

This view of ethically sound clinical care has evolved over the latter half of the 20th century from a doctor-knows-best ethic that worked reasonably well for both patients and physicians at a time when medical knowledge was limited and most of what medicine could do for patients could be carried in the doctor's black bag or handled in a small, uncluttered office or operating room.

The subsequent explosion of biomedical knowledge and the resulting proliferation of treatment options, many of them involving new technologic apparatus and interventions, were accompanied by a growing dissatisfaction with medical paternalism. As medicine grew more complex and doctors became more reliant on specialty knowledge and instrumentation, physicians and patients became less familiar with each other. Patients could no longer assume that they and their physicians shared a common set of personal values sufficient to guide physicians in judging what was best for their patients. For example, faced with a variety of treatment options, women in whom breast cancer is diagnosed and men in whom prostate cancer is diagnosed want to personally participate in decisions that will affect not only their bodies but also their lives.

In response to these new complexities and following on the various rights movements of the 1960s, some bioethicists began to advocate giving pride of place to patient autonomy (respecting patients' right to decide by seeking their consent to treatment) over physician beneficence (doing what, in the physician's judgment, is in the patient's best interest) in the hierarchy of principles governing ethical medicine (autonomy, nonmaleficence, beneficence, and justice).[15]

Consent is permission, granted by the patient to the surgeon, to make a diagnostic or therapeutic intervention on the patient's behalf. For consent to be valid, it must be informed. The patient must be provided all relevant information. To be valid, it must also be voluntary, that is, as free from coercion as possible while recognizing that in extremis the patient's condition itself may be inherently coercive. The surgeon's ethical objective is to judiciously provide the patient sufficient information with which to decide what course to follow. This entails selectively presenting all information pertinent to the patient's condition regarding benefits, risks, and alternatives while avoiding overwhelming the patient with extraneous data. To walk the line between what is pertinent and what is extraneous requires prudent judgment.

Informed consent has become a baseline best-practice ethical standard in modern medical care. It is a necessary but insufficient condition for ethically sound patient care. More moral work remains to be done if the physician-patient relationship is to be more than a contractual arrangement for rendering services. The ultimate goal is to achieve the best outcome, not only in terms of adherence to ethical principles of practice but also in keeping with patients' moral values, with what matters most to patients in their relationships and their lives. Achieving this goal certainly entails the provision of information and the granting of consent, but this exchange must take place in the context of a conversation about how the proposed intervention will affect a particular patient's life.

In 1984, Jay Katz foresaw the moral work that would be required to construct a contemporary medical ethic capable of overcoming what he termed a prevailing *silence* between doctors and patients. Katz was referring to the practice of physicians deciding what was best for patients and patients abiding by the decision. He proposed that this silence be supplanted by "meaningful conversation" based on "the humaneness of consenual understanding."[16(pxvii)]

Meaningful conversation requires conversation partners jointly committed to treating the patient's ailment in a context of mutual respect and understanding. In addition to enhancing mutuality and promoting understanding, meaningful conversation contributes to better health outcomes and to patients' satisfaction with their care. It stands to reason that patients whose doctors are responsive to their questions are likely to feel better. Is such attentiveness a luxury in today's time-conscious, monitored, and managed environment? On the contrary, studies show that when doctors miss clues to emotional and social matters that their patients cannot broach explicitly, visits tend to be prolonged as the patient continues to try to elicit an acknowledgment from the physician of concerns that may not seem immediately relevant to the patient's chief complaint.[17]

Anticipating the need for physicians to cultivate the ability to engage patients in meaningful conversation, the Accreditation Council for Graduate Medical Education (ACGME) has included ethical and professional skills and behavior among the general clinical competencies on which residency training programs are evaluated. Accreditation criteria for programs include adherence to accepted ethical principles of patient care, as well as respectful personal interactions with diverse patients, families, and other professionals.[18]

In the growing literature on diversity in clinical medicine it has become commonplace to use the shorthand concept of cultural competence. This may be a misnomer in that competence denotes mastery of a body of knowledge whereas what is wanted is improved cross-cultural interactions between patients and physicians. Culture is not a data set to be mastered and applied but a concept that is dynamic and personal and interpersonal. Culture plays a significant role in influencing the way we think about illness and health.

At its most basic, culture is a pattern of shared beliefs, values, and behavior. Culture includes, but is not limited to, the language we use, shared customs and practices, and the way we think about relationships. A culture may be religious, social, or professional (we speak, for example, of the culture of medicine), and it unquestionably affects interactions between patients and clinicians—often beneath the awareness of either party to the relationship. At its best, studied attention to cultural sensitivity in clinical medicine is aimed at raising physicians' awareness of the significance of cultural factors in their practice. Some efforts to increase cultural awareness generalize about the so-called Hispanic, African American, or Asian American patient. Knowledge of community values may be useful in caring for patients from different communities, but the risk of stereotyping is great if insufficient attention is paid to the individual patient from a particular community, whatever it is. Culturally competent care is no substitute for patient-centered care. Practically speaking, when cultural differences between patients and their physicians are not taken into account, patient dissatisfaction and poorer health outcomes may result.

In many cultures, patients traditionally are not told that they have cancer or other life-threatening conditions. In some cultures, disclosure of a grave prognosis is believed to cause patients to suffer unnecessarily, whereas withholding such information is believed to encourage hope. Being direct and explicit may be considered insensitive. Families may try to protect their loved one by taking on decision-making responsibility. It would be unfair to impose the standards of disclosure common in one culture on patients from another culture who may not want to know. This is all useful information that can contribute to culturally appropriate care—as long as one keeps in mind the caveat mentioned before, that patients are not solely the products of their culture and should therefore be related to as individuals who may share some of their culture's attitudes and beliefs but not others. Joseph Betancourt describes the case of an elderly Italian woman whose son asked her surgeon not to inform her that she had metastatic colon cancer for fear that it would sap her will to live.[19] Decision-making and truth-telling processes vary not only from culture to culture but also from family to family. Exploring the reasons for and the consequences of a preference for secrecy can lead to culturally sensitive and ethically appropriate care.

What practical steps can be taken by clinicians to evaluate patient attitudes and behavior relative to the patient's cultural context so that the physician and patient together can reach mutually desired goals of care? Marjorie Kagawa-Singer and her colleagues at the University of California, Los Angeles,[20] developed a useful tool for ascertaining patients' levels of cultural influence. It goes by the acronym RISK:

Resources: On what tangible resources can the patient draw, and how readily available are they?
Individual identity and acculturation: What is the context of the patient's personal circumstances and her degree of integration within her community?
Skills: What skills are available to the patient that allow him to adapt to the demands of the condition?
Knowledge: What can be discerned from a conversation with the patient about the beliefs and customs prevalent in her community and relevant to illness and health, including attitudes about decision making and other issues that may affect the physician-patient relationship?

RISK, therefore, encompasses resources, identity, skills, and knowledge.

Nowhere are respectful personal interactions more in demand than in the care of patients near the end of life.

In 1998 the American College of Surgeons adopted a *Statement on Principles Guiding Care at the End of Life,*[21(p46)] which includes the following principles:

- Respect the dignity of both patient and caregivers.
- Be sensitive to and respectful of the patient's and family's wishes.
- Use the most appropriate measures that are consistent with the choices of the patient or the patient's legal surrogate.
- Ensure alleviation of pain and management of other physical symptoms.
- Recognize, assess, and address psychological, social, and spiritual problems.
- Ensure appropriate continuity of care by the patient's primary and/or specialist physician.
- Provide access to therapies that may realistically be expected to improve the patient's quality of life.
- Provide access to appropriate palliative care and hospice care.
- Respect the patient's right to refuse treatment.
- Recognize the physician's responsibility to forgo treatments that are futile.

A Surgeons Palliative Care Workgroup was convened in 2001 to put these principles into operation and to introduce the precepts and techniques of palliative care into surgical practice and education by means of symposia, a palliative care website, and focused contributions to the surgical literature.

In a paper introducing a monthly series from members of the work group written for and by surgeons, Geoffrey P. Dunn and Robert A. Milch observe that caring for patients near the end of life offers surgeons an "opportunity to rebalance decisiveness with introspection, detachment with empathy," and thereby "restore the integrity of our relationships with our patients."[22(p328)] Other contributions to this series provide expert discussions of such ethically difficult issues as decision making in palliative surgery[23]; chronic pain management and opioid tolerance[24,25]; withdrawing life support, including tube feeding, hydration, and total parenteral nutrition[26,27]; management of dyspnea,[28] depression, and anxiety[29]; and attending to dying patients' spiritual needs.[30] Two themes thread their way through these discussions. Patients in a surgeon's care near the end of life stand not only to gain from the surgeon's cognitive and technical expertise as long as rescue is an option but also to benefit from the surgeon's attentiveness and guidance when what ails the patient cannot be remedied or reversed.[31] Moreover, surgeons themselves can derive satisfaction from staying the course with dying patients and their families, responding to their trust, seeing them through difficult times, and caring for them even when curative options are no longer indicated or available.[32]

Among other responsibilities articulated in the American Medical Association's Principles of Medical Ethics, two suggest a growing sense within the profession of medicine's role as a public-spirited profession:

1. Contributing to betterment of the health of the community
2. Supporting access to medical care for everyone

Additional evidence of public-spiritedness is to be found in the association's Declaration of Professional Responsibility, which was forged in response to the terrorist attacks on New York and Washington in September 2001. Subtitled *Medicine's Social Contract with Humanity,* this unprecedented oath contains the following declaration[33]:

We, the members of the world community of physicians, solemnly commit ourselves to

I. Respect human life and the dignity of every individual.
II. Refrain from supporting or committing crimes against humanity and condemn all such acts.
III. Treat the sick and injured with competence and compassion and without prejudice.
IV. Apply our knowledge and skill when needed, although doing so may put us at risk.
V. Protect the privacy and confidentiality of those for whom we care and breach that confidence only when keeping it would seriously threaten their health and safety and that of others.
VI. Work freely with colleagues to discover, develop, and promote advances in medicine and public health that ameliorate suffering and contribute to human well-being.
VII. Educate the public and polity about present and future threats to the health of humanity.
VIII. Advocate for social, economic, educational, and political changes that ameliorate suffering and contribute to human well-being.
IX. Teach and mentor those who follow us for they are the future of our caring profession.

We make these promises solemnly, freely, and on our personal and professional honor.

Recognizing the social value of volunteerism, the Governors' Committee on Socioeconomic Issues of the American College of Surgeons created the Giving Back project in the year 2000. Based on survey data from 500 fellows, the committee recommended that the college "Promote surgeon volunteerism as 'The right thing to do' and 'Part of being a physician.'"[34]

Taken together, these three documents, along with the emphasis on professional values in the medical ethics literature and the ACGME *General Competencies,* indicate a renewed commitment on the part of clinicians to competent, respectful, compassionate patient care and a growing awareness within the profession of the ethical obligations of physicians in their various roles as clinicians, researchers, educators, and citizens that arise from and extend beyond the traditional patient-physician relationship.[35-37]

Contemporary clinical ethics is evolving toward a relational understanding of interactions between doctors and patients. In the parlance of ethics, this means that ethical principles are being supplemented by moral virtues. Adherence to principles leads one to ask: What should I do? Attention to virtues prompts the question: What kind of person or doctor should I be? How to conduct oneself with patients in an economic and social environment that rewards haste, encourages narrow self-interest and inattention to the patient as a person, and is increasingly inhospitable to underserved populations is motivating a re-evaluation of medical professionalism not only at the bedside but in society as well.

Selected References

Barnard D, Boston P, Towers A, Lambrinidou Y: Crossing Over: Narratives of Palliative Care. New York, Oxford University Press, 2000.

Accounts of patients, families, and health care professionals working together to maintain hope in the face of incurable illness.

Cassell EJ: The Nature of Suffering and the Goals of Medicine. New York, Oxford University Press, 1991.

Experienced internist's reflections on suffering and the relationship between patient and doctor.

Gawande A: Complications: A Surgeon's Notes on an Imperfect Science. New York, Metropolitan Books, 2002.

A young surgeon's thoughts on fallibility, mystery, and uncertainty in surgical practice.

Jonsen AR, Siegler M, Winslade WJ: Clinical Ethics. New York, McGraw-Hill, 2002.

The standard physician's pocket guide to clinical-ethical decision making.

Juarez PM, Weinberg, AD: Cultural Competence in Cancer Care. Rockville, MD, Office of Minority Health, Department of Health and Human Services, 2004.

A useful pocket guide for clinicians with references to relevant websites and additional readings. Available from Baylor College of Medicine, Intercultural Cancer Council, 6655 Travis Street, Suite 322, Houston, TX 77030-1312.

Lynn J, Lynch Schuster J, Kabcenell A: Improving Care for the End of Life. New York, Oxford University Press, 2000.

A source book for improving health care practices and systems, with appendices containing helpful instruments for assessing pain, survival time, comfort, and grief.

May WF: The Physician's Covenant: Images of the Healer in Medical Ethics. Philadelphia, Westminster Press, 1983.

Reflections on the physician as parent, fighter, technician, and teacher.

McCullough LB, Jones JW, Brody BA: Surgical Ethics. New York, Oxford University Press, 1998.

Nineteen chapters on surgical ethics, varying from principles and practice through research and innovation to finances and institutional relationships.

Nuland SB: How We Die: Reflections on Life's Final Chapter. New York, Alfred A Knopf, 1994.

A national bestseller by a senior surgeon, writer, and historian of medicine.

Selzer R: Letters to a Young Doctor. New York, Simon & Schuster, 1982.

Sage advice for young surgeons from a seasoned surgeon-writer.

References

1. American College of Surgeons Statements on Principles. These statements were collated, approved by the Board of Regents, and initially published in 1974. They were last revised in October 1997. Retrieved April 30, 2003, from http://www.facs.org.
2. Code of Professional Ethics of the American College of Obstetricians and Gynecologists. Approved by the Executive Board of the American College of Obstetricians and Gynecologists. Retrieved April 28, 2003, from http://www.acog.org/.
3. American College of Obstetricians and Gynecologists: Ethics in Obstetrics and Gynecology. (2002). Retrieved April 30, 2003, from http://www.acog.org/.
4. Gates E: Ethical considerations in the incorporation of new technologies into gynecologic practice. Clin Obstet Gynecol 43:540-550, 2000.
5. Shaw A: Historical review of pediatric surgical ethics. Semin Pediatr Surg 10:171-178, 2001.
6. Boudreaux AM, Tilden SJ: Ethical dilemmas for pediatric surgical patients. Anesthesiol Clin North Am 20:227-240, 2002.
7. Frader JE, Flanagan-Klygis E: Innovation and research in pediatric surgery. Semin Pediatr Surg 10:198-203, 2001.
8. Levin AV: IOLs, innovation, and ethics in pediatric ophthalmology: Let's be honest. J AAPOS 6:133-135, 2002.
9. Day SH: Teaching ethics: A structured curriculum on ethics for ophthalmology residents is valuable. Arch Ophthalmol 120:963-964, 2002.
10. Wenger NS, Liu H, Lieberman JR: Teaching medical ethics to orthopaedic surgery residents. J Bone Joint Surg Am 80:1125-1131, 1998.
11. Capozzi JD, Rhodes R, Springfield DS: Ethical considerations in orthopaedic surgery. Instruct Course Lect 49:633-637, 2000.
12. Committee on Ethics of the American Society of Anesthesiologists: Syllabus on Ethics: Informed Consent (1997). Retrieved October 10, 2002, from http://www.asahq.org/wlm/Ethics.html.
13. ABIM Foundation, American Board of Internal Medicine, ACP-ASIM Foundation, American College of Physicians–American Society of Internal Medicine, European Federation of Internal Medicine: Medical professionalism in the new millennium: A physician charter. Ann Intern Med 136:243-246, 2002.
14. American Medical Association: E-Principles of Medical Ethics. Current Opinions of the Council on Ethical and Judicial Affairs (2001). Retrieved April 30, 2007, from http://www.ama-assn.org/ama/pub/category/8292.html.
15. Beauchamp TL, Childress JF: Principles of Biomedical Ethics, 5th ed. New York, Oxford University Press, 2001.
16. Katz J: The Silent World of Doctor and Patient. New York, Free Press, 1984.
17. Levinson W, Gorawara-Phat R, Lamb J: A study of patient clues and physician responses in primary care and surgical settings. JAMA 284:1021-1027, 2000.
18. Accreditation Council for Graduate Medical Education: General Competencies. Available at http://www.acgme.org/Outcome/.
19. Betancourt JR: Cultural competence—marginal or mainstream movement? N Engl J Med 351:953-955, 2004.
20. Kagawa-Singer M, Kassim-Lakha S: A strategy to reduce cross-cultural miscommunication and increase the likelihood of improving health outcomes. Acad Med 78:577-587, 2003.
21. Statement on principles guiding care at the end of life. American College of Surgeons' Committee on Ethics. Bull Am Coll Surg 83:46, 1998.
22. Dunn GP, Milch RA: Introduction and historical background of palliative care: Where does the surgeon fit in? J Am Coll Surg 193:325-328, 2001.
23. McCahill LE, Krouse RS, Chu DZJ, et al: Decision making in palliative surgery. J Am Coll Surg 195:411-422, 2002.
24. Lee KF, James B, Ray JB, Dunn GP: Chronic pain management and the surgeon: Barriers and opportunities. J Am Coll Surg 193:689-701, 2001.
25. Thompson AR, Ray JB: The importance of opioid tolerance: A therapeutic paradox. J Am Coll Surg 196:321-324, 2003.
26. Easson AM, Hinshaw DB, Johnson DL: The role of tube feeding and total parenteral nutrition in advanced illness. J Am Coll Surg 194:225-228, 2002.
27. Huffman JL, Dunn GP: The paradox of hydration in advanced terminal illness. J Am Coll Surg 194:835-839, 2002.
28. Mosenthal AC, Lees KF: Management of dyspnea at the end of life: Relief for patients and surgeons. J Am Coll Surg 194:377-386, 2002.
29. Hinshaw DB, Carnahan JM, Johnson DL: Depression, anxiety, and asthenia in advanced illness. J Am Coll Surg 195:271-277, 2002.
30. Hinshaw DB: The spiritual needs of the dying patient. J Am Coll Surg 195:565-568, 2002.
31. Little M: Invited commentary: Is there a distinctively surgical ethics? Surgery 129:668-671, 2001.
32. The Kaiser Family Foundation: 2001 National Survey of Physicians. Retrieved from http://www.kff.org/content/2003/3223/National_Survey_Physicians_Toplines_Revised.pdf.
33. American Medical Association: Declaration of Professional Responsibility. Retrieved April 30, 2007, from http://www.ama-assn.org/ama/pub/category/7491.html.
34. The American College of Surgeons: Volunteerism and Giving Back to Society Among Surgeons Project: Phase Three-Survey of ACS Fellows. Retrieved April 30, 2007, from http://www.facs.org/about/governors/phase3givingback.pdf.
35. Mechanic D: Managed care and the imperative for a new professional ethic. Health Affairs 19:100-111, 2000.
36. Bloche MG: Clinical loyalties and the social purpose of medicine. JAMA 281:268-274, 1999.
37. Little M: Ethonomics: The ethics of the unaffordable. Arch Surg 135:17-21, 2000.

3 CHAPTER |

Molecular and Cell Biology

Tien C. Ko, MD   and   B. Mark Evers, MD

Human Genome
Recombinant DNA Technology
Cell Signaling
Cell Division Cycle
Apoptosis
Human Genome Project
Novel Treatment Strategies
Ethical, Psychological, and Legal Implications

Since the 1980s there has been an explosion in knowledge regarding molecular and cellular biology. These advances will transform the practice of surgery to one that is based on molecular techniques for prevention, diagnosis, and treatment of many surgical diseases. This has been made possible by achievements of the Human Genome Project, which is intended to reveal the complete genetic instruction of humans. The core knowledge of molecular and cellular biology has been presented in detail in several textbooks.[1,2] An overview of the field is presented here, with emphasis on basic concepts and techniques.

HUMAN GENOME

Mendel first defined *genes* as information-containing elements that are distributed from parents to offspring. Genes contain the design that is essential for the development of each human. The field of molecular biology began in 1944 when Avery demonstrated that DNA was the hereditary material that made up genes. Translation of this genetic information into RNA and then protein leads to the expression of specific biologic characteristics or phenotypes. Major advances made in the field of molecular biology are listed in Table 3-1. In this section the structure of genes and DNA are reviewed, as are the

processes by which genetic information is translated into biologic characteristics.

Structure of Genes and DNA

DNA is composed of two antiparallel strands of unbranched polymer wrapped around each other to form a right-handed double helix (Fig. 3-1).[3] Each strand is composed of four types of deoxyribonucleotides containing the bases adenine (A), cytosine (C), guanine (G), and thymine (T). The nucleotides are joined together by phosphodiester bonds that join the 5′ carbon of one deoxyribose group to the 3′ carbon of the next. Whereas the sugar-phosphate backbone remains constant, the attached bases can vary to encode different genetic information. The nucleotide sequences of the opposing strands of DNA are complementary to each other, thus allowing the formation of hydrogen bonds that stabilize the double-helix structure. Complementary base pairs require that A always pair with T and C always pair with G. For example, if the sense strand (5′-3′ direction) of DNA has the nucleotide sequence GAATTC, the complementary antisense strand (3′-5′ direction) has the sequence CTTAAG.

The entire human genetic information, or human genome, contains 3×10^9 nucleotide pairs. However, less than 10% of the DNA sequences are copied into either messenger RNA (mRNA) molecules, which encode proteins, or structural RNA, such as transfer RNA (tRNA) or ribosomal RNA (rRNA) molecules. Each nucleotide sequence in a DNA molecule that directs the synthesis of a functional RNA molecule is called a *gene* (Fig. 3-2). DNA sequences that do not encode genetic information may have structural or other unknown functions. Human genes commonly contain more than 100,000 nucleotide pairs, yet most mRNA molecule–encoding proteins consist of only 1000 nucleotide pairs. Most of the extra nucleotides consist of long stretches of noncoding sequences called *introns* that interrupt the relatively short segments of coding sequences called *exons*. For example, the thyroglobulin gene has 300,000 nucleotide bases and 36

26

introns, whereas its mRNA has only 8700 nucleotide bases. The processes by which genetic information encoded in DNA is transferred to RNA and protein molecules are discussed later.

The human genome contains 24 different DNA molecules; each DNA has 10^8 bases and is packaged in a separate chromosome. Thus, the human genome is organized into 22 different autosomes and 2 different sex chromosomes. Because humans are diploid organisms, each somatic cell contains 2 copies of each different autosome and 2 sex chromosomes for a total of 46 chromosomes. One copy of chromosomes is inherited from the mother and one is inherited from the father. Germ cells contain only 22 autosomes and 1 sex chromosome. Each chromosome contains three types of specialized DNA sequences that are important in the replication or segregation of chromosomes during cell division (Fig. 3-3). To replicate, each chromosome contains many short, specific DNA sequences that act as *replication origins*. A second sequence element, called a *centromere,* attaches DNA to the mitotic spindle during cell division. The third sequence element is a *telomere,* which contains G-rich repeats located at each end of the chromosome. During DNA replication, one strand of DNA becomes a few bases shorter at its 3′ end because of limitation in the replication machinery. If this is not remedied, DNA molecules will become progressively shorter in their telomere segments with each cell division. This problem is solved by an enzyme called *telomerase,* which periodically extends the telomerase sequence by several bases.

Each chromosome, when stretched out, would span the cell nucleus thousands of times. To facilitate DNA

Table 3-1   Major Events in Molecular Biology

YEAR	EVENT
1941	Genes are found to encode proteins
1944	DNA is determined to carry the genetic information
1953	DNA structure is determined
1962	Restriction endonucleases are discovered
1966	Genetic code is deciphered
1973	DNA cloning technique is established
1976	First oncogene is discovered
1977	Human growth hormone is produced in bacteria
1978	Human insulin gene is cloned
1981	First transgenic animal is produced
1985	Polymerase chain reaction is invented
	First tumor suppressor gene is discovered
1990	Human Genome Project is created
1998	First mammal is cloned

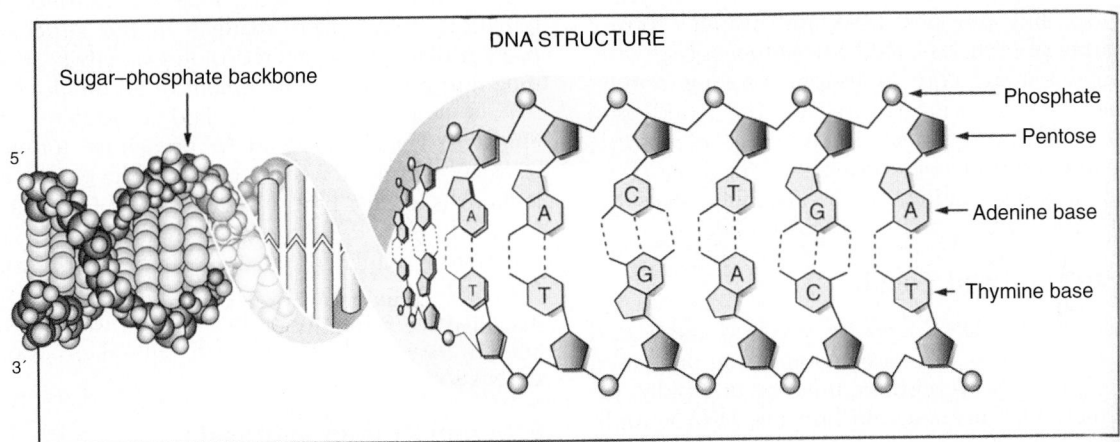

Figure 3-1 DNA double-helix structure. The sequence of four bases (guanine, adenine, thymine, and cytosine) determines the specificity of genetic information. The bases face inward from the sugar-phosphate backbone and form pairs (*dashed lines*) with complementary bases on the opposing strand. (Adapted from Rosenthal N: DNA and the genetic code. N Engl J Med 331:39, 1994. Copyright © 1994 Massachusetts Medical Society. All rights reserved.)

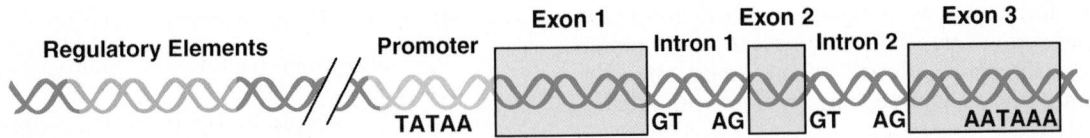

Figure 3-2 Gene structure. The DNA sequences that are transcribed as RNA are collectively called *the gene* and include exons (expressed sequences) and introns (intervening sequences). Introns invariably begin with the nucleotide sequence GT and end with AG. An AT-rich sequence in the last exon forms a signal for processing the end of the RNA transcript. Regulatory sequences that make up the promoter and include the TATA box occur close to the site where transcription starts. Additional regulatory elements are located at variable distances from the gene. (Adapted from Rosenthal N: Regulation of gene expression. N Engl J Med 331:932, 1994. Copyright © 1994 Massachusetts Medical Society. All rights reserved.)

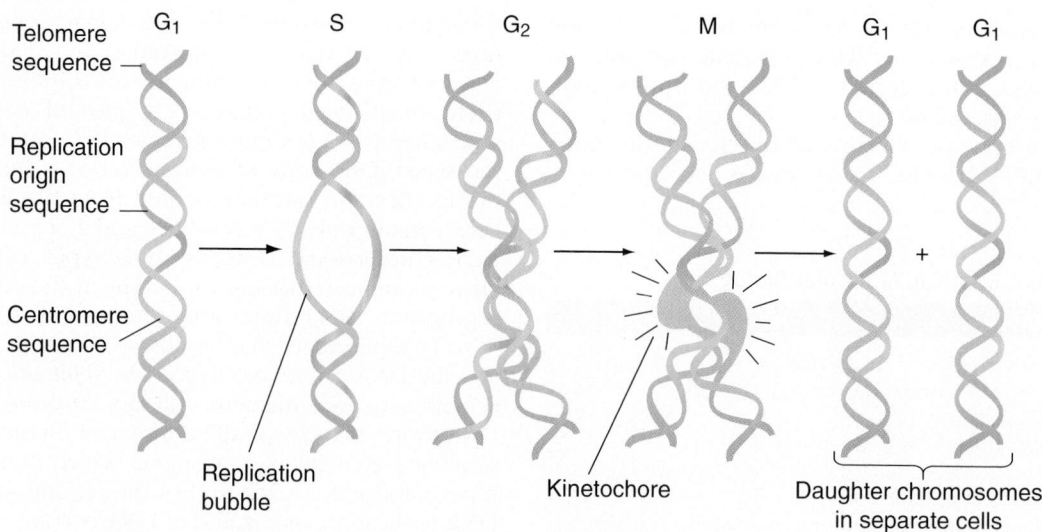

Figure 3-3 Chromosome structure. Each chromosome has three types of specific sequences that facilitate its replication during the cell cycle. Origins of replication are located throughout each chromosome to facilitate DNA synthesis. The centromere holds the duplicated chromosome together and is attached to the mitotic spindle through a protein complex called a *kinetochore*. Telomere sequences are located at each end of the chromosome and are replicated in a special way to preserve chromosome integrity.

replication and segregation, each chromosome is packaged into a compact structure with the aid of special proteins, including histones. DNA and histones form a repeated array of particles called *nucleosomes;* each consists of an octomeric core of histone proteins around which the DNA is wrapped twice. The condensed complex of DNA and proteins is known as *chromatin.* Not only does chromosome packaging facilitate DNA replication and segregation, but it also influences the activity of genes, which will be discussed later.

DNA Replication and Repair

Before cell division, DNA must be precisely duplicated such that a complete set of chromosomes can be passed to each progeny. DNA replication must occur rapidly, yet with extremely high accuracy. In humans, DNA is replicated at the rate of approximately 50 nucleotides per second with an error rate of one in every 10^9 base pair replications. This efficient replication of genetic material requires an elaborate replication machinery consisting of several enzymes. Because each strand of DNA double helix encodes nucleotide sequences complementary to its partner strand, both strands contain identical genetic information and serve as templates for the formation of an entirely new strand. DNA replication occurs in the 5'-to-3' direction along each strand by the sequential addition of complementary deoxyribonucleoside triphosphates.

Eventually, two complete DNA double helices are formed that contain identical genetic information. The fidelity of DNA replication is of critical importance because any mistake, called a *mutation,* will result in wrong DNA sequences being copied to daughter cells. Change in a single base pair is called a *point mutation,* which can result in one of two types of mutation (Fig.

3-4). A single amino acid change as the consequence of a point mutation is called a *missense mutation*. Missense mutations may cause changes in the structure of the protein that lead to altered biologic activity. If the point mutation results in replacement of an amino acid codon with a stop codon, it is called a *nonsense mutation*. Nonsense mutations lead to premature termination of translation and often result in loss of the encoded protein. If there is an addition or deletion of a few base pairs, it is called a *frameshift mutation,* which leads to the introduction of unrelated amino acids or a stop codon (see Fig. 3-4). Some mutations are silent and will not affect the function of the organism. Several proofreading mechanisms are used to eliminate mistakes during DNA replication.

RNA and Protein Synthesis

In the early 1940s, geneticists demonstrated that genes specify the structure of individual proteins. The transfer of information from DNA to protein proceeds through the synthesis of an intermediate molecule known as *RNA.* RNA, like DNA, is made up of a linear sequence of nucleotides composed of four complementary bases. RNA differs from DNA in two respects:

1. Its sugar-phosphate backbone contains ribose instead of deoxyribose sugar
2. Thymine (T) is replaced by uracil (U), a closely related base that pairs with adenine (A)

RNA molecules are synthesized from DNA by a process known as *DNA transcription,* which uses one strand of DNA as a template. DNA transcription differs from DNA replication in that RNA is synthesized as a single-stranded molecule and is relatively short in comparison to DNA. Several classes of RNA transcripts are made, including

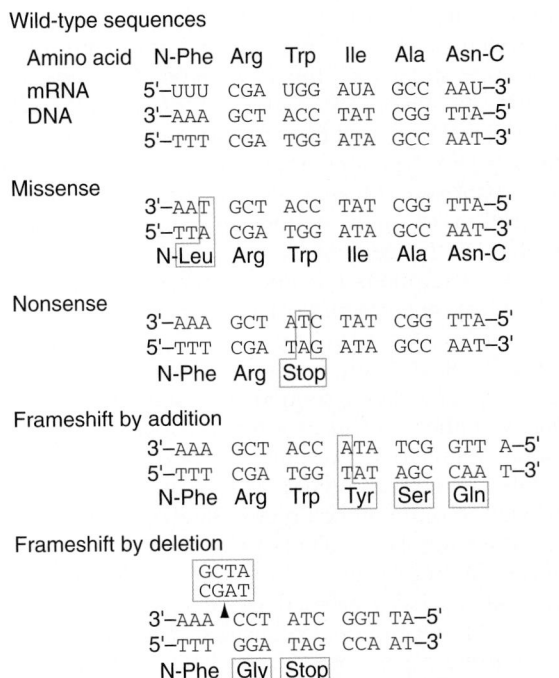

Wild-type sequences

Amino acid	N-Phe	Arg	Trp	Ile	Ala	Asn-C
mRNA	5'-UUU	CGA	UGG	AUA	GCC	AAU-3'
DNA	3'-AAA	GCT	ACC	TAT	CGG	TTA-5'
	5'-TTT	CGA	TGG	ATA	GCC	AAT-3'

Missense

3'-AA[T] GCT ACC TAT CGG TTA-5'
5'-TT[A] CGA TGG ATA GCC AAT-3'
N-[Leu] Arg Trp Ile Ala Asn-C

Nonsense

3'-AAA GCT A[T]C TAT CGG TTA-5'
5'-TTT CGA T[A]G ATA GCC AAT-3'
N-Phe Arg [Stop]

Frameshift by addition

3'-AAA GCT ACC [A]TA TCG GTT A-5'
5'-TTT CGA TGG [T]AT AGC CAA T-3'
N-Phe Arg Trp [Tyr] [Ser] [Gln]

Frameshift by deletion

[GCTA]
[CGAT]
3'-AAA ▲CCT ATC GGT TA-5'
5'-TTT GGA TAG CCA AT-3'
N-Phe [Gly] [Stop]

Figure 3-4 Different types of mutations. Point mutations involve alteration in a single base pair. Small additions or deletions of several base pairs directly affect the sequence of only one gene. A wild-type peptide sequence and the mRNA and DNA encoding it are shown at the *top*. Altered nucleotides and amino acid residues are enclosed in a *box*. Missense mutations lead to a change in a single amino acid in the encoding protein. In a nonsense mutation, a nucleotide base change leads to the formation of a stop codon that results in premature termination of translation, thereby generating a truncated protein. Frameshift mutations involve the addition or deletion of any number of nucleotides that is not a multiple of three, thus causing a change in the reading frame. (From Lodish HF, Baltimore D, Berk A, et al (eds): Molecular Cell Biology, 3rd ed. New York, Scientific American, 1998, p 267, with permission.)

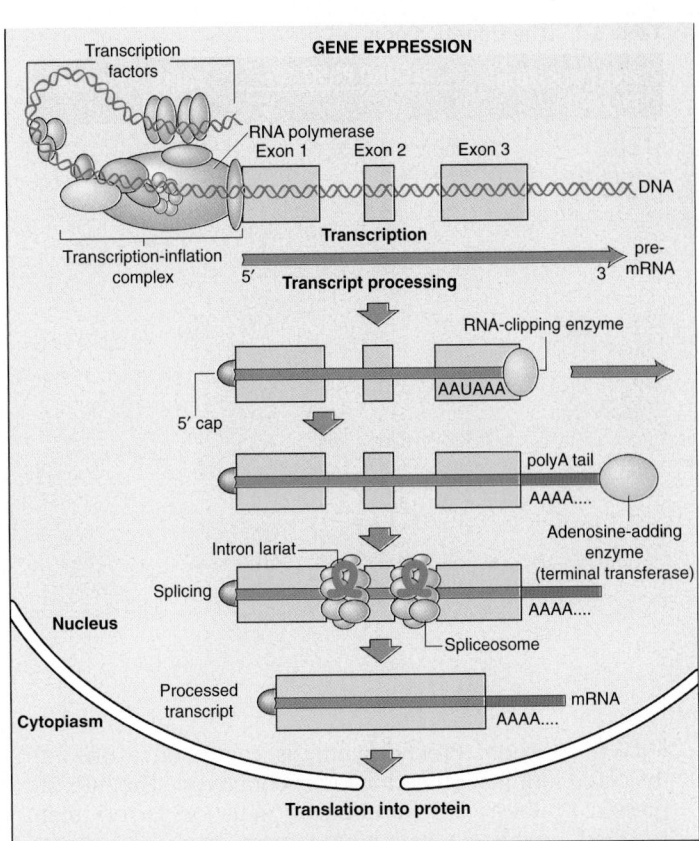

Figure 3-5 Process of gene transcription. Gene expression begins with binding of multiple protein factors to enhancer sequences and promoter sequences. These factors help form the transcription-initiation complex, which includes the enzyme RNA polymerase and multiple polymerase-associated proteins. The primary transcript (pre-mRNA) includes both exon and intron sequences. Post-transcriptional processing begins with changes at both ends of the RNA transcript. At the 5′ end, enzymes add a special nucleotide cap; at the 3′ end, an enzyme clips the pre-mRNA approximately 30 base pairs after the AAUAAA sequence in the last exon. Another enzyme adds a polyadenylate (polyA) tail, which consists of as many as 200 adenine nucleotides. Next, spliceosomes remove the introns by cutting the RNA at the boundaries between exons and introns. The process of excision forms lariats of the intron sequences. The spliced mRNA is then mature and can leave the nucleus for protein translation in the cytoplasm. (Adapted with permission from Rosenthal N: Regulation of gene expression. N Engl J Med 331:932, 1994. Copyright © 1994 Massachusetts Medical Society. All rights reserved.)

mRNA, tRNA, and rRNA. Even though all these RNA molecules are involved in the translation of information from RNA to protein, only mRNA serves as the template. RNA synthesis is a highly selective process, with only about 1% of the entire human DNA nucleotide sequence transcribed into functional RNA sequences. DNA nucleotide sequences that code for proteins are called *exons* and are separated by noncoding sequences called *introns* (see Fig. 3-2). After RNA transcription, intron sequences are removed by RNA-processing enzymes (Fig. 3-5). This RNA-processing step, called *RNA splicing,* occurs in the nucleus. Although each cell contains the same genetic material, only specific genes are transcribed. RNA transcription is controlled by regulatory proteins that bind to specific sites on DNA close to the coding sequence of a gene. The complex regulation of gene transcription occurs during development and tissue differentiation and allows differential patterns of gene expression.

Once in the cytoplasm, RNA directs the synthesis of a particular protein through a process called *RNA translation.* The sequence of nucleotides in mRNA is translated into the amino acid sequence of a protein. Each triplet of nucleotides forms a codon that specifies one amino acid. Because RNA is composed of four types of nucleotides, there are 64 possible codon triplets (4×4×4). However, only 20 amino acids are commonly found in proteins, so most amino acids are specified by several codons. The rule by which different codons are translated into amino acids is called the *genetic code* (Table 3-2).

Protein translation requires a ribosome, which is composed of more than 50 different proteins and several rRNA molecules. Ribosomes bind an mRNA molecule at the initiation codon (AUG) and begin translation in the

Table 3-2 The Genetic Code

FIRST POSITION (5′ END)	SECOND POSITION				THIRD POSITION (3′ END)
	U	C	A	G	
U (uracil)	Phe	Ser	Tyr	Cys	U
	Phe	Ser	Tyr	Cys	C
	Leu	Ser	Stop	Stop	A
	Leu	Ser	Stop	Trp	G
C (cytosine)	Leu	Pro	His	Arg	U
	Leu	Pro	His	Arg	C
	Leu	Pro	Gln	Arg	A
	Leu	Pro	Gln	Arg	G
A (adenine)	Ile	Thr	Asn	Ser	U
	Ile	Thr	Asn	Ser	C
	Ile	Thr	Lys	Arg	A
	Met	Thr	Lys	Arg	G
G (guanine)	Val	Ala	Asp	Gly	U
	Val	Ala	Asp	Gly	C
	Val	Ala	Glu	Gly	A
	Val	Ala	Glu	Gly	G

5′-to-3′ direction. Protein synthesis ceases once one of the three termination codons is encountered. The rate of protein synthesis is controlled by initiation factors that respond to the external environment, such as growth factor and nutrients. These regulatory factors help coordinate cell growth and proliferation.

Control of Gene Expression

The human body is made up of millions of specialized cells, each performing predetermined functions. This is characteristic of all multicellular organisms. In general, different human cell types contain the same genetic material (i.e., DNA), yet they synthesize and accumulate different sets of RNA and protein molecules. This difference in gene expression determines whether a cell is a hepatocyte or a cholangiocyte. Gene expression can be controlled at six major steps in the synthetic pathway from DNA to RNA to protein.[4,5] The first control is at the level of gene transcription, which determines when and how often a given gene is transcribed into RNA molecules. The next step is RNA processing control, which regulates how many mature mRNA molecules are produced in the nucleus. The third step is RNA transport control, which determines which mature mRNA molecules are exported into the cytoplasm where protein synthesis occurs. The fourth step involves mRNA stability control, which determines the rate of mRNA degradation. The fifth step involves translational control, which determines how often mRNA is translated by ribosomes into proteins. The final step is post-translational control, which regulates the function and fate of protein molecules.

Control of gene transcription is the best studied step of regulation for most genes. RNA synthesis begins with assembly and binding of the *general transcription machinery* to the *promoter* region of a gene (see Fig. 3-5). The promoter is located upstream of the transcription initiation site at the 5′ end of the gene and consists of a stretch of DNA sequence primarily composed of T and A nucleotides (i.e., the *TATA box*). The general transcription machinery is composed of several proteins, including RNA polymerase II and general transcription proteins. These general transcription factors are abundantly expressed in all cells and are required for the transcription of most mammalian genes. The rate of assembly of the general transcription machinery to the promoter determines the rate of transcription, which is regulated by *gene regulatory proteins*. In contrast to the small number of general transcription proteins, there are thousands of different gene regulatory proteins. Most bind to specific DNA sequences, called *regulatory elements*, to either activate or repress transcription.

Gene regulatory proteins are expressed in small amounts in a cell, and different selections of proteins are expressed in different cell types. Similarly, different combinations of regulatory elements are present in each gene to allow differential control of gene transcription. Many human genes have more than 20 regulatory elements; some bind transcriptional activators, whereas others bind transcriptional repressors. Ultimately, the balance between transcriptional activators and repressors determines the rate of transcription, which can vary by a factor of more than 10^6 between genes that are expressed and those that are repressed. Most regulatory elements are located at a distance (i.e., thousands of nucleotide bases) away from the promoter. These distant regulatory elements are brought into the proximity of the promoter through DNA bending, thus enabling control of promoter activity. In summary, the combination of regulatory elements and the types of gene regulatory proteins expressed determines where and when a gene is transcribed.

Post-translational control is another important step in the regulation of gene expression because most proteins are modified in one form or another.[6] Modifications such as proteolytic cleavage, disulfide formation, glycosylation, lipidation, and biotinylation allow the protein to achieve the proper structural conformation essential for its biologic activity. The complexity of regulation is greatly increased by additional amino acid modifications that can occur at multiple sites of a protein. Examples of amino acid modification include phosphorylation, acetylation, methylation, ubiquitination, and sumoylation.

RECOMBINANT DNA TECHNOLOGY

Advances in recombinant DNA technology, beginning in the 1970s, have greatly facilitated study of the human genome. It is now routine practice in molecular laboratories to excise a specific region of DNA, produce unlimited copies of it, and determine its nucleotide sequences. Furthermore, isolated genes can be altered (engineered) and transferred back into cells in culture or into the germline of an animal or plant so that the altered gene is inherited as part of the organism's genome. The most important recombinant DNA technology includes the ability to cut DNA at specific sites by restriction nucleases, rapidly amplify DNA sequences, quickly determine the nucleotide sequences, clone a DNA fragment, and create a DNA sequence.[7]

Restriction Nucleases

Restriction nucleases are bacterial enzymes that cut the DNA double helix at specific sequences of four to eight nucleotides. More than 400 restriction nucleases have been isolated from different species of bacteria and they recognize over 100 different specific sequences. Restriction enzyme protects the bacterial cell from foreign DNA, whereas native DNA is protected from cleavage by methylation at vulnerable nucleotides. Commonly used restriction enzymes often recognize a six–base pair palindromic sequence, such as GAATTC. Each restriction nuclease will cut a DNA molecule into a series of specific fragments. These fragments have either cohesive or blunt ends, depending on the restriction nuclease, and can be rejoined to other DNA fragments with the same cohesive ends (Fig. 3-6, top panel). By using a combination of different restriction enzymes, a restriction map of each DNA can be created, thus facilitating the isolation of individual genes. Restriction nucleases have also been used for the manipulation of individual genes.

Polymerase Chain Reaction

An ingenious technique to rapidly amplify a segment of a DNA sequence in vitro was developed in 1985 by Saiki and coworkers.[8] This method, called *polymerase chain reaction (PCR),* can enzymatically amplify a segment of DNA a billion-fold.[9] The PCR technique is made possible by the availability of purified heat-stable DNA polymerase from bacteria and the ability to synthesize small segments of DNA (oligonucleotides). The principle of the PCR technique is illustrated in the bottom panel of Figure 3-6.

To amplify a segment of DNA, two single-stranded oligonucleotides, or primers, must be synthesized, each designed to complement one strand of the DNA double helix and lying on opposite sides of the region to be amplified. The PCR reaction mixture consists of the double-stranded DNA sequence (the template), two DNA oligonucleotide primers (heat stable), DNA polymerase, and four types of deoxynucleotide triphosphate. Each round of amplification involves three thermally controlled steps. First, the reaction mixture is briefly heated to 94°C to separate the double-helix structure of the DNA template into two single strands. Next, the reaction mixture is cooled to below 55°C, which results in hybridization of the two DNA primers to complementary sequences on each strand of the DNA template. Finally, the reaction is heated to 72°C to allow DNA synthesis downstream of each primer. Each round of PCR requires only about 5 minutes and results in a doubling of the double-stranded DNA molecules, which serve as templates for subsequent reactions. After only 32 cycles, more than a billion copies of the desired DNA segment is produced. Not only is the PCR technique extremely powerful, but it is also the most sensitive technique to detect a single copy of a DNA or RNA molecule in a sample. To detect RNA molecules, they must first be transcribed into complementary DNA

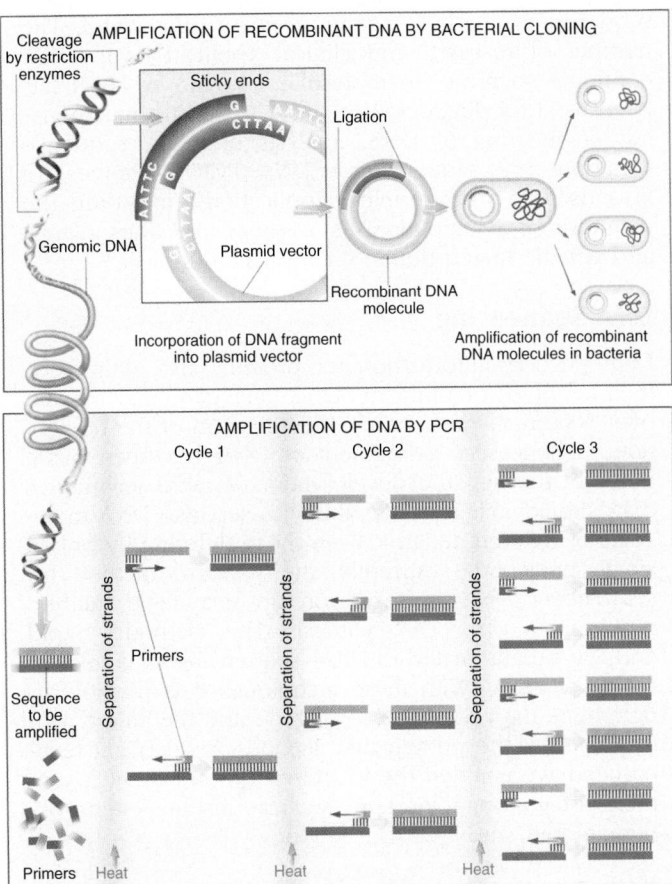

Figure 3-6 Amplification of recombinant DNA and amplification by polymerase chain reaction (PCR). At the *top*, the DNA segment to be amplified is separated from surrounding genomic DNA by cleavage with a restriction enzyme. The enzymatic cuts often produce staggered or "sticky" ends. In the example shown, the restriction enzyme *Eco*RI recognizes the sequence GAATTC and cuts each strand between G (guanine) and A (adenine); the two strands of genomic DNA are shown as *black* (C denotes cytosine and T denotes thymine). The same restriction enzyme cuts the circular plasmid DNA (*gray*) at a single site, thereby generating sticky ends that are complementary to the sticky ends of the genomic DNA fragment. The cut genomic DNA and the remainder of the plasmid, when mixed together in the presence of a ligase enzyme, form smooth joints on each side of the plasmid-genomic DNA junction. This new molecule—recombinant DNA—is carried into bacteria, which replicate the plasmid as they grow in culture. At the *bottom*, the DNA sequence to be amplified is selected by primers, which are short, synthetic oligonucleotides that correspond to sequences flanking the DNA to be amplified. After an excess of primers is added to the DNA, together with a heat-stable DNA polymerase, the strands of both the genomic DNA and the primers are separated by heating and allowed to cool. A heat-stable polymerase elongates the primers on either strand, thus generating two new identical double-stranded DNA molecules and doubling the number of DNA fragments. Each cycle takes just a few minutes and doubles the number of copies of the original DNA fragment. (From Rosenthal N: Tools of the trade—recombinant DNA. N Engl J Med 331:316, 1994. Copyright © 1994 Massachusetts Medical Society. All rights reserved.)

sequences with the enzyme *reverse transcriptase*. The number of research and clinical applications for PCR continues to grow. In molecular laboratories, PCR has been used for direct cloning of DNA, in vitro mutagenesis, engineering of DNA, analysis of allelic sequence variations, and sequencing of DNA. PCR techniques are also used in many clinical applications, including the diagnosis of genetic diseases, assay of infectious agents, and genetic fingerprinting for forensic samples.

DNA Sequencing

DNA encodes information for proteins and, ultimately, the phenotype of a human being. Each gene may contain over 3000 nucleotide bases. Identification of the nucleotide sequences of a fragment of DNA has been made possible through the development of rapid techniques that take advantage of the ability to separate DNA molecules of different lengths, even those differing by only a single nucleotide. Currently, the standard method for sequencing DNA is based on an enzymatic method requiring in vitro DNA synthesis. This method is rapid and can be automated to allow sequencing of large segments of DNA. With these techniques it is possible to determine the boundaries of a gene and the amino acid sequence of the protein that it codes. Sequencing techniques have enabled the identification and in vitro synthesis of important proteins such as insulin, interferon, hemoglobin, and growth hormones.

DNA Cloning

DNA cloning techniques allow identification of a gene of interest from the human genome. First, DNA fragments are generated by digesting the entire DNA content of a cell with a restriction nuclease. The DNA fragments are joined to a self-replicating genetic element (a virus or a plasmid) that is also digested with the same restriction nuclease. Viruses or plasmids are small circular DNA molecules that occur naturally and can replicate rapidly when introduced into bacterial cells. They are extremely useful vectors for propagating a segment of DNA. Once the DNA fragments are inserted into viruses or plasmids, they are introduced into bacterial cells that have been made transiently permeable to DNA. These transfected cells are able to produce large copies of viruses or plasmids containing the DNA fragment. With this method a collection of bacteria plasmids containing the entire human genome can be created. This human DNA library can then be used to identify genes of interest.

DNA Engineering

One of the most important outcomes of recombinant DNA technologies is the ability to generate new DNA molecules of any sequence through DNA engineering. New DNA molecules can be synthesized either by the PCR method or by using automated oligonucleotide synthesizers. PCR can be used to amplify any known segment of the human genome and to redesign its two ends. Automated oligonucleotide synthesizers enable the rapid production of DNA molecules up to about 100 nucleotides in length. The sequence of such synthetic DNA molecules is entirely determined by the experimenter. Larger DNA molecules are formed by combining two or more DNA molecules that have complementary cohesive ends created by restriction enzyme digestion. One powerful application of DNA engineering is the synthesis of large quantities of cellular proteins for medical application. Most cellular proteins are produced in small amounts in human cells, which makes it difficult to purify and study these proteins. However, with DNA engineering, it is possible to place a human gene into an expression vector that is engineered to contain a highly active promoter. When the vector is transfected into bacterial, yeast, insect, or mammalian cells, it will initiate the production of a large amount of mRNA of the human gene, thereby leading to the production of a large quantity of protein. With these expression vectors it is possible to make a single protein that accounts for 1% to 10% of the total cellular protein. The protein can easily be purified and used for scientific studies or clinical applications. Medically useful proteins, such as human insulin, growth hormone, interferon, and viral antigens for vaccines, have been made by engineering expression vectors containing these genes of interest.

DNA engineering techniques are also important for solving problems in cell biology. One of the fundamental challenges of cell biology is to identify the biologic functions of the protein product of a gene. With the use of DNA engineering techniques, it is now possible to alter the coding sequence of a gene in order to alter the functional properties of its protein product or the regulatory region of a gene and thus produce an altered pattern of its expression in the cell. The coding sequence of a gene can be changed in such subtle ways that the protein encoded by the gene has only one or a few alterations in its amino acid sequence. The modified gene is then inserted into an expression vector and transfected into the appropriate cell type to examine the function of the redesigned protein. With this strategy one can analyze which parts of the protein are important for fundamental processes such as protein folding, enzyme activity, and protein-ligand interactions.

Transgenic Animals

The ultimate test of the function of a gene is to either overexpress the gene in an organism and see what effect it has or delete it from the genome and evaluate the consequences. It is much easier to overexpress a gene of interest than to delete it from the genome of an organism.[10] To overexpress a gene, the DNA fragment encoding the gene of interest, or the *transgene*, must be constructed with recombinant DNA techniques.[9,11] The DNA fragment must contain all the components necessary for efficient expression of the gene, including a promoter and a regulatory region that drives transcription.

The type of promoter used can determine whether the transgene is expressed in many tissues of the transgenic animal or in a specific tissue. For example, selective expression in the acinar pancreas can be achieved by placing the amylase promoter 5′ upstream of the coding sequence of the transgene. The transgene DNA fragments are then introduced into the male pronucleus of a fertilized egg via microinjection techniques. Typically, 2% to 6% of injected embryos will have the transgene integrated into their germline DNA. Animals are then screened for the presence of the transgene. Analysis of these animals has provided important insight into the functions of many human genes, as well as animal models of human diseases. For example, transgenic animals engineered to overexpress a mutant form of the gene for β-amyloid protein precursor (the *APP* gene) have neuropathologic changes similar to those in patients with Alzheimer's disease. This transgenic model not only supports the role of the *APP* gene in the development of Alzheimer's disease but is also a model for testing methods of prevention or treatment of Alzheimer's disease.

A major disadvantage of using transgenic animals is that they will reveal only dominant effects of the transgene because these animals still retain two normal copies of the gene in their genome. Therefore, it is extremely useful to produce animals that do not express both copies of the gene of interest.[12] These *knockout* animals are much more difficult to develop than transgenic animals and require gene-targeting techniques. To knock out a gene, it is important to modify the gene of interest by DNA engineering to create a nonfunctioning gene. This altered gene is inserted into a vector and then inserted into germ cell lines. Although most mutated genes are inserted randomly into one of the chromosomes, rarely a mutated gene will replace one of the two copies of the normal gene by *homologous recombination.* Germ cells with one copy of the normal gene and one copy of the mutated gene will give rise to heterozygous animals. Heterozygous males and females are generated and can then be bred to produce animals that are homozygous for the mutated gene. These knockout animals can be studied to determine which cellular functions are altered in comparison to normal animals, thereby identifying the biologic function of the gene of interest. The ability to produce knockout animals that lack a known normal gene has greatly facilitated studies of the functions of specific mammalian genes.

RNA Interference

Because the majority of the approximately 30,000 to 40,000 human genes encoding potential proteins have unknown function, uncovering their biologic activities has been an area of intense investigation. The most effective way to assess the function of a gene is by using reverse genetics (i.e., target deletion of the expression of a specific gene) and examining the biologic consequences. Until recently, only a few reverse genetic approaches have been available, such as homologous recombination and antisense oligonucleotide strategies. Each of these technologies has significant limitations that make reverse genetic studies both slow and costly. However, a new powerful tool was developed in 1998 by Andrew Fire and Craig Mello that is based on silencing of specific genes by double-stranded RNA (dsRNA).[13] This

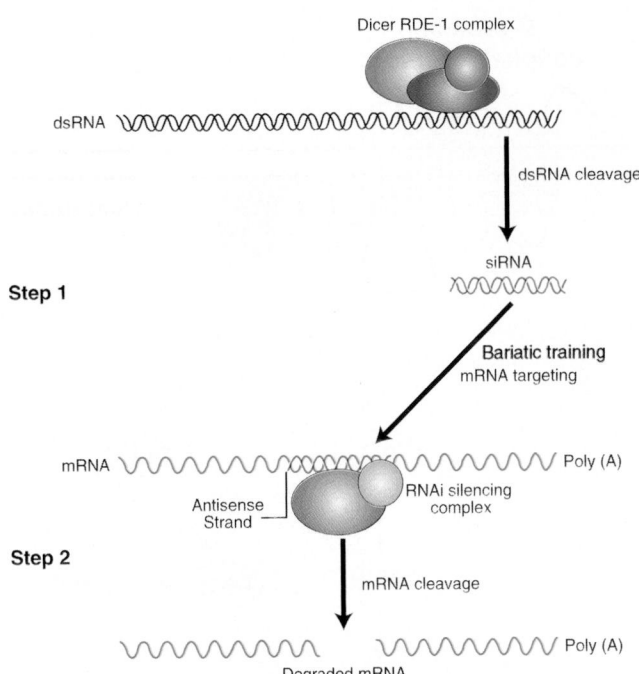

Figure 3-7 RNA interference. Long double-stranded RNA (dsRNA) is processed by the Dicer-RDE-1 complex to form short interfering RNA (siRNA). The antisense strand of siRNA is used by an RNA interference (RNAi) silencing complex to guide specific mRNA cleavage, thus promoting mRNA degradation. RDE-1, RNAi deficient-1.

technology, termed *RNA interference* (RNAi), requires the synthesis of a dsRNA that is homologous to the target gene.[14] Once taken up by the cells, the dsRNA is cleaved into 21- to 23-nucleotide-long RNA molecules called *short interfering RNAs* (siRNAs) by an enzyme complex (Dicer-RDE-1) (Fig. 3-7).[15] The antisense strand of the siRNA binds to the target mRNA, which leads to its degradation by an RNAi silencing complex. Recent advancement has allowed the direct design and synthesis of siRNAs, as well as placement of these siRNAs into viral vectors. Not only will this technology transform future studies in the analysis of gene function, but potentially, siRNAs may also be used as gene therapy to silence the function of specific genes.

CELL SIGNALING

The human body is composed of billions of cells that must be coordinated to form specific tissues. Both neighboring and distant cells influence the behavior of cells through intercellular signaling mechanisms. Whereas normal cell signaling ensures the health of the human, abnormal cell signaling can lead to diseases such as cancer. Through powerful molecular techniques, the sophisticated signaling mechanisms used by mammalian cells are becoming better understood. This section reviews the general principles of intercellular signaling and examines the signaling mechanisms of two main families of cell surface receptor proteins.[16]

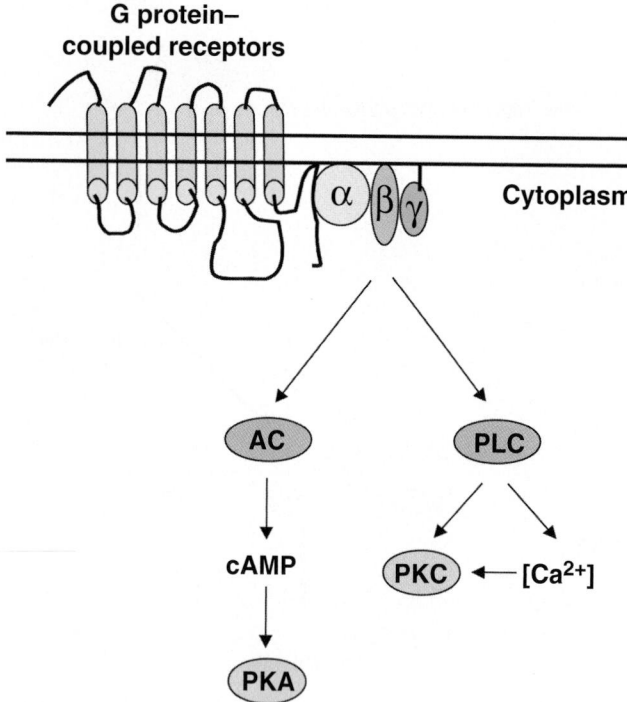

Figure 3-8 G protein-coupled receptor signaling pathway. G protein-coupled receptors are seven-transmembrane domain proteins that are activated by the binding of ligands. Activated receptors initiate a cascade of events leading to amplification of the original signal. First, the receptor activates a trimer G protein consisting of α, β, and γ subunits. G proteins can activate adenylyl cyclase (AC) to generate cyclic adenosine monophosphate (cAMP) or phospholipase C (PLC) to release intracellular calcium. cAMP can activate protein kinase A (PKA), whereas PLC or intracellular calcium can activate protein kinase C (PKC).

Ligands and Receptors

Cells communicate with one another by means of multiple signaling molecules, including proteins, small peptides, amino acids, nucleotides, steroids, fatty acid derivatives, and even dissolved gases such as nitric oxide and carbon monoxide. Once these signaling molecules are synthesized and released by a cell, they may act on the signaling cell (autocrine signaling), affect adjacent cells (paracrine signaling), or enter the systemic circulation to act on distant target cells (endocrine signaling). These signaling molecules, also called *ligands,* bind to specific proteins, called *receptors,* expressed in either the plasma membrane or the cytoplasm of the target cells. On ligand binding, the receptor becomes activated and generates a cascade of intracellular signals that alter the behavior of the cell. Each human cell is exposed to hundreds of different signals from its environment, but it is genetically programmed to respond to only specific sets of signals. Cells may respond to one set of signals by proliferating, to another set by differentiating, and to another by achieving cell death. Furthermore, different cells may respond to the same set of signals with different biologic activities.

Most extracellular signals are mediated by hydrophilic molecules that bind to receptors on the cell surface of the target cells. These cell surface receptors are divided into three classes based on the transduction mechanism used to propagate signals intracellularly. *Ion channel–coupled receptors* are involved in rapid synaptic signaling between electrically excitable cells. These receptors form gated ion channels that open or close rapidly in response to neurotransmitters. *G protein–coupled receptors* regulate the activity of other membrane proteins through a guanosine triphosphate–binding regulatory protein called *G protein.*[17] *Enzyme-coupled receptors* either act directly as enzymes or are associated with enzymes.[18,19] Most of these receptors are protein kinases or are associated with protein kinases that phosphorylate specific proteins in the cell.

Some extracellular signals are small hydrophobic molecules, such as steroid hormones, thyroid hormones, retinoids, and vitamin D. They communicate with target cells by diffusing across the plasma membrane and binding to intracellular receptor proteins. These cytoplasmic receptors are structurally related and constitute the intracellular receptor superfamily. On ligand activation, the intracellular receptors enter the nucleus, bind specific DNA sequences, and regulate transcription of the adjacent gene.

Some dissolved gases, such as nitric oxide and carbon monoxide, act as local signals by diffusing across the plasma membrane and activating intracellular enzymes in the target cells. In the case of nitric oxide, it binds and activates the enzyme guanylyl cyclase, which leads to production of the intracellular mediator cyclic guanosine monophosphate (cGMP).

G Protein–Coupled Receptors

G protein–coupled receptors are the largest family of cell surface receptors and mediate cellular responses to a broad range of signaling molecules, including hormones, neurotransmitters, and local mediators.[20] These receptors include β-adrenergic receptors, α$_2$-adrenergic receptors, and glucagon receptors. They share a similar structure with an extracellular domain that binds ligand and an intracellular domain that binds to a specific trimeric G protein. There are at least six distinct trimeric G proteins based on their intracellular signaling mechanisms; each is composed of three different polypeptide chains, called α, β, and γ.[17] Upon ligand binding, the G protein–coupled receptor activates its trimeric G protein (Fig. 3-8). Activated trimeric G protein alters the concentration of one or more small intracellular signaling molecules, referred to as *second messengers.*

Two major second messengers regulated by G protein–coupled receptors are cyclic adenosine monophosphate (cAMP) and calcium. cAMP is synthesized by the enzyme adenylyl cyclase and can be rapidly degraded by cAMP phosphodiesterase.[21] Intracellular calcium is stored in the endoplasmic reticulum and released into the cytoplasm upon proper signaling. Some trimeric G proteins can activate adenylyl cyclase, whereas others inhibit its activity. Trimeric G protein can also activate the enzyme phospholipase C, which produces the necessary signal molecules to activate release of calcium from the endoplasmic reticulum. Activation of phospholipase C can also lead to activation of protein kinase C (PKC), which initiates a cascade of kinases. Changes in cAMP or calcium concentrations in the cell directly affect the activities of specific kinases that phosphorylate target proteins. The end result is altered biologic activity of these target proteins, which leads to a specific biologic response to the initial signal molecule. Despite the differences in signaling details, all G protein–coupled receptors use a complex cascade of intracellular mediators to greatly amplify the biologic response to the initial extracellular signals.

Enzyme-Coupled Receptors

Enzyme-coupled receptors are a diverse family of transmembrane proteins with similar structure. Each receptor has an extracellular ligand-binding domain and a cytosolic domain that either has intrinsic enzyme activity or is associated directly with an enzyme. Enzyme-coupled receptors are classified according to the type of enzymatic activity used for their intracellular signal transduction. Some receptors have guanylyl cyclase activity and generate cGMP as an intracellular mediator. Others have tyrosine kinase activity or are associated with tyrosine kinase proteins that phosphorylate specific tyrosine residues on intracellular proteins to propagate intracellular signals. Finally, some enzyme-coupled receptors have serine/threonine kinase activity and can phosphorylate specific serine or threonine residues to transduce intracellular signals.

The receptors for most known growth factors belong to the tyrosine kinase receptor family.[18,19] These include receptors for epidermal growth factor (EGF), platelet-derived growth factor (PDGF), fibroblast growth factor (FGF), hepatocyte growth factor (HGF), insulin, insulin-like growth factor-I (IGF-I), vascular endothelial growth factor (VEGF), and macrophage colony-stimulating factor (M-CSF). These growth factor receptors play crucial roles during normal development and tissue homeostasis. Furthermore, many of the genes that encode proteins in the intracellular signaling cascades that are activated by receptor tyrosine kinases were first identified as oncogenes in cancer cells. Inappropriate activation of these proteins causes a cell to proliferative excessively.

Similar to G protein–coupled receptors, tyrosine kinase receptors use a complex cascade of intracellular mediators to propagate and amplify the initial signals (Fig. 3-9). Upon ligand binding, the tyrosine kinase receptor dimerizes, which activates the kinase. Activated receptor kinase initiates an intracellular relay system, first by cross-phosphorylation of tyrosine residues of the cytoplasmic domain of the receptor. Next, small intracellular signaling proteins bind to phosphotyrosine residues on the receptor and form a multiprotein signaling complex from which the signal propagates to the nucleus. The Ras proteins serve as crucial links in the signaling cascade.[22] Upon activation, Ras proteins initiate a cascade of serine/threonine phosphorylation that converges on mitogen-activated protein (MAP) kinases. Activated MAP kinases relay signals downstream by phosphorylating transcrip-

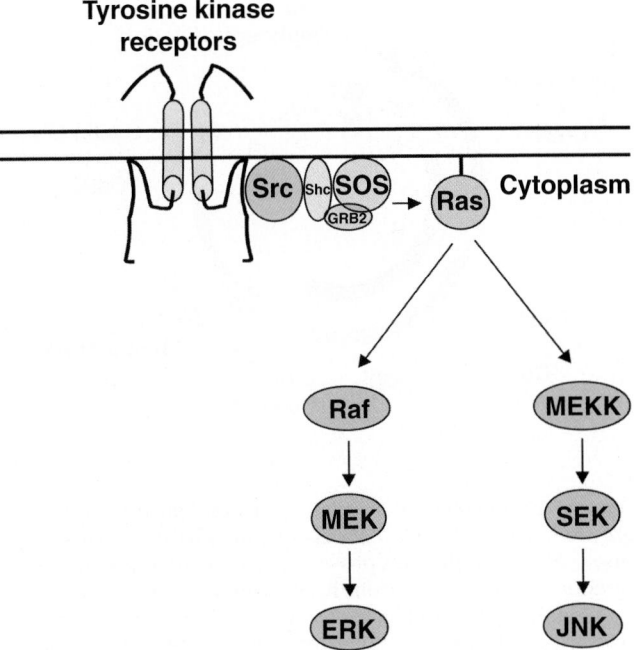

Figure 3-9 Tyrosine kinase receptor signaling pathway. Tyrosine kinase receptors are single transmembrane proteins that form a dimer on ligand binding. The activated receptors bind to several proteins (Src, Shc, SOS, GRB2) to form a multiprotein signal complex. This protein complex can activate Ras, which can initiate several kinase cascades. One kinase cascade includes the Raf, MEK, and ERK members, whereas another includes the MEKK, SEK, and JNK proteins.

tion factors, thereby leading to regulation of gene expression.

As mentioned previously, human cells integrate many different extracellular signals and respond with biologic behaviors such as proliferation, differentiation, and programmed cell death. In the following sections we review the mechanisms governing these important biologic processes.

CELL DIVISION CYCLE

The cell division cycle is the fundamental means by which organisms propagate and by which normal tissue homeostasis is maintained. The cell division cycle is an organized sequence of complex biologic processes that is traditionally divided into four distinct phases (Fig. 3-10). Replication of DNA occurs in the S phase (S=synthesis), whereas nuclear division and cell fission occur in the mitotic phase, or M phase. The intervals between these two phases are called the G_1 and G_2 phase (G=gap). After division, cells enter the G_1 phase, where they are able to receive extracellular signals and a determination is made whether to proceed with DNA replication or to exit the cell cycle. In this section we review the proteins that regulate progression through each phase of the cell cycle and how they control key checkpoints of the cell cycle. Then we discuss how many cell cycle proteins are mutated or deleted in human cancers.

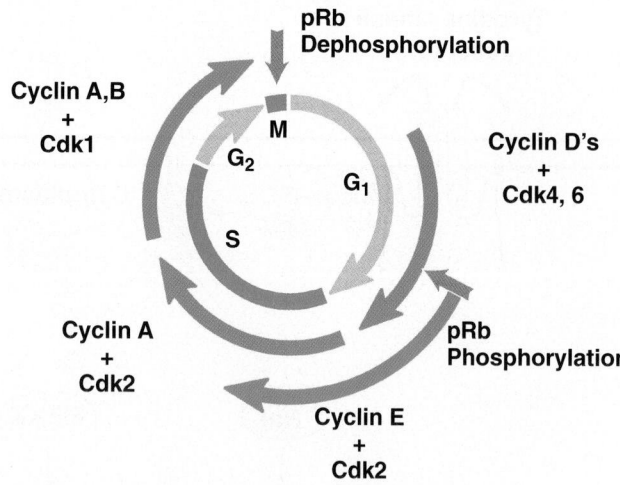

Figure 3-10 Mechanisms regulating mammalian cell cycle progression. The cell cycle consists of four phases: G_1 (first gap) phase, S (DNA synthetic) phase, G_2 (second gap) phase, and M (mitotic) phase. Progression through the cell cycle is regulated by a highly conserved family of serine/threonine protein kinases that are composed of a regulatory subunit (the cyclins) and a catalytic subunit (the cyclin-dependent kinases [Cdks]). Cell cycle progression can be inhibited by a class of regulators called the *cyclin kinase inhibitors* and by phosphorylation of the retinoblastoma (pRb) protein.

Regulation of the Cell Division Cycle by Cyclin, Cyclin-Dependent Kinase, and Cdk Inhibitory Proteins

Progression of the mammalian cell cycle through these specific phases is governed by the sequential activation and inactivation of a highly conserved family of regulatory proteins, cyclin-dependent kinases (Cdks).[23] Cdk activation requires the binding of a regulatory protein (cyclin) and is controlled by both positive and negative phosphorylation. Cdk activities are inhibited by Cdk inhibitory proteins (CKIs). The active cyclin/Cdk complex is involved in the phosphorylation of other cell cycle regulatory proteins. Cyclin proteins are classified according to their structural similarities. Each cyclin exhibits a cell cycle/phase–specific pattern of expression. In contrast, Cdk proteins are expressed throughout the cell cycle. The cyclins, Cdks, and CKIs form the fundamental regulatory units of the cell cycle machinery.

Cell Cycle Checkpoints

In proliferating cells, cell cycle progression is regulated at two key checkpoints, the G_1/S and the G_2/M transitions. Progression through early to mid G_1 is dependent on Cdk4 and Cdk6, which are activated by association with one of the D-type cyclins, D1, D2 or D3.[23] Progression through late G_1 and into the S phase requires the activation of Cdk2, which is sequentially regulated by cyclins E and A, respectively. The subsequent activation of Cdk1 (cdc2) by cyclin B is essential for the transition from G_2 into the M phase. There are two families of CKIs: the CIP/KIP family and the INK family. The four known

INK proteins (p15[INK4B], p16[INK4A], p18[INK4C], and p19[INK4D]) selectively bind and inhibit Cdk4 and Cdk6 and are expressed in a tissue-specific pattern. The three members of the CIP/KIP family (p21[CIP1], p27[KIP1], and p57[KIP2]) share a conserved amino-terminal domain that is sufficient for both binding to cyclin/Cdk complexes and inhibition of Cdk-associated kinase activity. Each CIP/KIP protein can inhibit all known Cdks. One of the key targets of the G_1 Cdks is the retinoblastoma tumor suppressor protein (pRb), which belongs to the Rb family of pocket proteins (pRb, p107, p130).[24] In their hypophosphorylated form, pocket proteins can sequester cell cycle regulatory transcription factors, including heterodimers of the E2F and DP families of proteins.[25] Phosphorylation of pRb, first by cyclin D–dependent kinases and then by cyclin E/Cdk2 during late G_1, leads to release of E2F/DP and subsequent activation of genes that participate in the entry into S phase.

Oncogenes and Tumor Suppressor Genes

The genes encoding cell cycle regulatory proteins are often targets of mutation during neoplastic transformation. If the mutated gene is cancer causing, it is referred to as an *oncogene* and its normal counterpart is called a *proto-oncogene*. Many proto-oncogenes have been identified and they are typically involved in relay of stimulatory signals from growth factor receptors to the nucleus. They include the intracellular signaling protein Ras, as well as the cell cycle regulatory protein cyclin D1. Mutation of a single copy of a proto-oncogene is sufficient to bring about increased cellular proliferation, one of the hallmarks of cancer. Several antiproliferative gene–encoding proteins such as pRb, p15, and p16 also negatively control the cell division cycle. These genes are often referred to as *tumor suppressor genes* because they prevent excess and uncontrolled cellular proliferation. These genes are inactivated in some forms of cancer to bring about loss of control of proliferation. However, unlike proto-oncogenes, both copies of a tumor suppressor gene must be deleted or inactivated during malignant transformation.

APOPTOSIS

Cell proliferation must be balanced by an appropriate process of cell elimination to maintain tissue homeostasis. Physiologic cell death is a genetic program pathway and is called *apoptosis*. Apoptosis has been implicated in various physiologic functions, including the remodeling of tissues during development, removal of senescent cells and cells with genetic damage beyond repair, and maintenance of tissue homeostasis. In this section we review the biologic and morphologic features of apoptosis and the molecular machinery that controls apoptosis.

Biochemical and Morphologic Features of Apoptosis

Apoptosis is a physiologic process of cell elimination, in contrast to another form of cell death called *necrosis*.

Necrosis is a passive, adenosine triphosphate–independent form of cell death that requires an acute nonphysiologic injury (i.e., ischemia, mechanical injury, or toxins) and results in destruction of the cytoplasmic and organelle membranes with subsequent cellular swelling and lysis.[15] Lysis of necrotic cells releases cytoplasmic and organelle contents into the extracellular milieu, thereby resulting in inflammation with surrounding tissue necrosis and destruction. In contrast, apoptosis is a highly regulated energy-requiring form of cell death that is genetically programmed. Apoptotic cells undergo the following sequence of morphologic and biochemical events:

1. In the early phase of apoptosis, cells exhibit a shrunken cytoplasm and detach from neighboring cells. One of the earliest biochemical features of apoptotic cells is the externalization of phosphatidyl serine residues on the plasma membrane. It has been proposed that these signaling intermediates may be involved in alerting surrounding cells to the occurrence of apoptosis.
2. Middle events include chromatin condensation with resultant crescent-shaped nuclei and subsequent nuclear fragmentation. During this phase, activation of endonuclease results in the fragmentation of DNA into 180– to 200–base pair internucleosomal sized fragments.
3. Late in apoptosis, the cells begin to fragment into discrete plasma membrane–bound vesicles termed *apoptotic bodies,* which are then phagocytized by neighboring cells and macrophages without inducing an inflammatory response.

The molecular machinery that governs apoptosis can be divided into three parts (Fig. 3-11):

1. Signaling of apoptosis by a stimulus
2. Regulation by proapoptotic and antiapoptotic factors
3. The execution machinery

These molecular events result in the morphologic and biochemical characteristics of the apoptotic cell.

Apoptotic Stimuli

Many stimuli activate the process of apoptosis (see Fig. 3-11), including DNA damage through ionizing radiation, growth factor and nutritional deprivation, activation of certain death receptors (e.g., Fas receptor [FasR] and tumor necrosis factor receptor [TNF-R1]), metabolic or cell cycle perturbations, oxidative stress, and many chemotherapeutic agents. Signal sensors proximal in the apoptotic pathway recognize these stimuli and include cell surface receptors requiring ligand binding and intracellular sensors detecting the loss of an advantageous environment for survival or irreparable damage. The nerve growth factor (NGF)/TNF receptor family is the typical example of membrane receptor signal sensors and includes the FasR and TNF-R1 receptors.[26] FasR is a 45-kd protein expressed at the surface of activated T cells, hepatocytes and enterocytes and can be found expressed in tissues, including the liver, heart, lung, kidney, and small intestine.

Extensive studies with the T-cell model have revealed the downstream events of receptor activation. Binding of a death-promoting ligand to the receptor triggers the death signal, which results in a conformational change in the intracellular region of the receptor. This change in protein structure allows binding of cytoplasmic adapter proteins. These receptor-adapter protein complexes, such as the Fas-activated death domain (FADD), catalyze the activation of downstream proteases involved in the execution phase of apoptosis. Intracellular signal sensors include the p53 tumor suppressor gene. The identification of DNA damage activates p53 functional activity and results in G_1 phase cell cycle arrest to allow DNA repair; however, irreparable damage commits the cell to death by apoptosis.[27] This differential function may be a result of the intracellular expression levels of p53. Finally, the lack of certain survival factors results in decreased cytoplasmic signals from cell surface receptors, such as interleukin-2 (IL-2) receptors, on activated T cells. This loss of exogenous survival signals culminates in activation of the endogenous death program. Similar results have been seen with serum withdrawal or growth factor receptor blockade, both of which induce apoptosis. Regardless of the many different signals and signal sensors involved in the activation of apoptosis, each of these pathways converge to activate a common central execution process, the caspase cascade.

Caspases

Caspases, or *c*ysteine *asp*artate prote*ases*, are highly conserved proteins first recognized as the *ced-3* gene product from the nematode *Caenorhabditis elegans*.[28] The sequence of Ced-3 exhibits homology to the mammalian IL-1β converting enzyme (ICE), which is now known as *caspase 1.* To date there are 14 known mammalian caspases, each of which is intimately involved in the conserved biochemical pathway that mediates apoptotic cell death. These proteolytic enzymes are synthesized as inactive proenzymes that require cleavage for activation. Each activated caspase has specific functions that may overlap with those of other caspases. This overlap in function shows the evolutionary significance of apoptosis. The protein substrates cleaved by activated caspases play a functional role in the morphologic and biochemical features seen in apoptotic cells.

As indicated in Figure 3-11, activated caspases result in the destruction of cytoskeletal and structural proteins (α-fodrin and actin), nuclear structural components (NuMA and lamins), and cell adhesion factors (FAK). They induce cell cycle arrest through Rb cleavage, cytoplasmic release of p53 by cleavage of the regulatory double minute 2 (MDM2) protein, and subsequent nuclear translocation and activation of PKC-δ. DNA repair enzymes, such as poly (adenosine diphosphate [ADP]-ribose) polymerase and the 140-kd component of DNA replication complex C, are inactivated by caspase proteolysis. Finally, DNA fragmentation is induced by the activation and nuclear translocation of a 45-kd cytoplasmic protein called *DNA fragmentation factor (DFF).* Although there is no known caspase involved in the

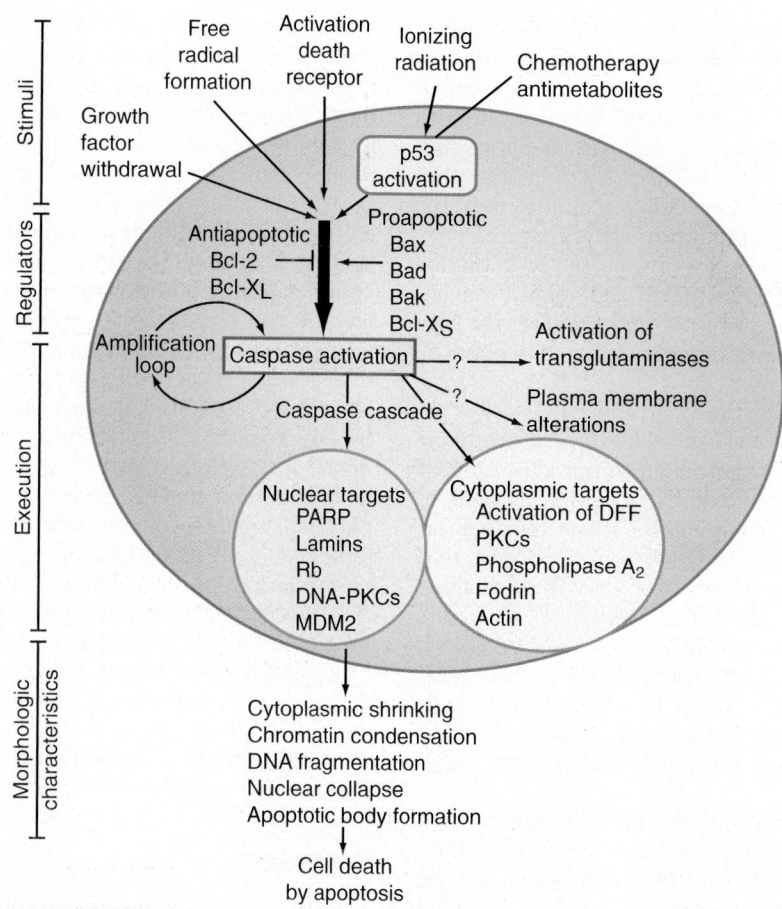

Figure 3-11 The apoptotic pathway of cell death. The molecular mechanisms involved in apoptosis are divided into three parts. First, stimuli of the apoptotic pathway include DNA damage by ionizing radiation or chemotherapeutic agents (p53 activation), activation of death receptors such as Fas and tumor necrosis factor-α, free radical formation, and loss of growth factor signaling. Second, progression of these stimuli to the central execution pathway is either positively or negatively regulated by expression of the Bcl-2 family of proteins. Third, the execution phase of apoptosis involves the activation of a family of evolutionarily conserved proteases called *caspases.* Caspase activation targets various nuclear and cytoplasmic proteins for activation or destruction, thereby leading to the morphologic and biochemical characteristics of apoptosis. (From Papaconstantinou HT, Ko TC: Cell cycle and apoptosis regulation in GI cancers. In Evers BM [ed]: Molecular Mechanisms in Gastrointestinal Cancer. Austin, TX, RG Landes, 1999, p 59, with permission.)

redistribution of phosphatidyl serine residues on the plasma membrane, caspase inhibitors have been shown to block this event. Overall, the net effect of caspase activation is to halt cell cycle progression, disable homeostatic and repair mechanisms, initiate detachment of the cell from its surrounding tissue structures, disassemble structural components, and mark the dying cell for engulfment by surrounding cells and macrophages.

Bcl-2 Family

The process of apoptosis is regulated by the expression of certain intracellular proteins belonging to the *Bcl-2* family of genes (see Fig. 3-11).[29] Bcl-2 is a potent inhibitor of apoptosis and is predominantly expressed in cholangiocytes, colonic epithelial cells, and pancreatic duct cells. The precise mechanism of apoptotic inhibition by

Bcl-2 is not known, but this protein is found on organelle membranes and may function as an antioxidant, protease inhibitor, or gatekeeper to prevent the apoptotic machinery from entering a target organelle. Other proteins in this family include Bcl-x_L, Bcl-x_s, Bax, Bak, and Bad. Bcl-x_L is another inhibitor of apoptosis. Bcl-x_s, Bax, Bak, and Bad function as proapoptotic regulators by dimerizing with Bcl-2 and Bcl-x_L and inhibiting their function. Furthermore, it has been shown that the proapoptotic protein Bax exhibits channel-forming activity in lipid membranes, which is blocked by Bcl-2. Increasing evidence suggests that the balance or ratio of these proapoptotic and antiapoptotic proteins is important for signaling the cell to commit to or inhibit apoptosis.

The complex molecular machinery of apoptosis, involving signaling, regulation of activation, promotion, or inhibition, and then execution, is a carefully choreographed process. Perturbations in this process at any of these three phases can result in loss of the apoptotic cell elimination pathway. Because apoptosis is a key regulator of cell number and therefore tissue homeostasis, it is easy to see how dysregulation of apoptosis can result in diseases.

HUMAN GENOME PROJECT

One of the most significant scientific undertakings of all times involves identification and sequencing of the entire human genome. The Human Genome Project was initiated in 1990, and the first versions of the DNA sequences of the human genome were published in 2001.[30,31] The Human Genome Project has had a significant impact on the field of medicine by providing clinicians with an unprecedented arsenal of genetic information that will, it is hoped, lead to a better understanding and treatment of a variety of genetic diseases. As an example, the Human Genome Project is providing new information on the genetic variations in the human population by identifying DNA variants such as single nucleotide polymorphisms (SNPs), which occur about once every 300 to 500 bases along the 3 billion-base human genome.[32] SNPs are thought to serve as genetic markers for identifying disease genes by linkage studies in families or by the discovery of genes involved in human diseases. These findings may lead to better screening and help implement preventive medical therapy in the hope of reducing the development of certain diseases in patients found to have predisposing conditions. It is anticipated that knowing the sequence of human DNA will allow scientists to better understand a host of diseases. With new information and techniques to unravel the mysteries of human biology, this knowledge will dramatically accelerate the development of new strategies for the diagnosis, prevention, and treatment of disease, not just for single-gene disorders, but for more common complex diseases, such as diabetes, heart disease, and cancer, for which genetic differences may contribute to the risk of contracting the disease and the response to particular therapies.

The transition from genetics to genomics marks the evolution from an understanding of single genes and their individual functions to a more global understanding of the actions of multiple genes and their control of biologic systems. Technology emanating from the Human Genome Project is currently available to assess an array of genes that may change (either increase or decrease) over time or with treatment. Such technology using so-called DNA chips provides one of the most promising approaches to large-scale studies of genetic variations, detection of heterogeneous gene mutations and gene expression. DNA chips, which are also called *microarrays,* generally consist of a thin slice of glass or silicone about the size of a postage stamp on which threads of synthetic nucleic acids are arrayed.[33,34] Literally thousands of genes can be assessed on a single DNA chip. A clinical example of the use of microarrays includes the detection of human immunodeficiency virus (HIV) sequence variations, p53 gene mutations in breast tissue, and expression of cytochrome P-450 genes. In addition, microarray technology has been applied to genomic comparisons across species, genetic recombination, and large-scale analysis of gene copy number and expression, as well as protein expression in cancers.

As genome technology moves from the laboratory to the clinical setting, new methods will make it possible to read the instructions contained in an individual person's DNA. Such knowledge may predict future disease and alert patients and their health care providers to initiate preventive strategies. Individual DNA profiles, as well as the DNA profiles of tumors, may provide better stratification of patients for cancer therapies. The Human Genome Project is certain to have an important impact on all areas of clinical medicine. All surgical disciplines will be directly affected by this information. We focus on some specific examples where we foresee major developments that will greatly influence our clinical management.

Transplantation

Despite the remarkable advances made in transplantation, organ procurement, and immunosuppression, a significant impediment remains the availability of suitable organs. The level of organ and tissue demand cannot be met by organ donation alone. Xenotransplantation has been proposed as a possible solution to the problem of organ availability and suitability for transplantation. A number of investigators have examined the possibility of using xenotransplanted organs. However, although short-term successes have been reported, there have been no long-term survivors with the use of these techniques. Data obtained from the Human Genome Project may enable transplant investigators to genetically engineer animals to potentially have more specific combinations of human antigens. It is anticipated that in the future, animals can be developed whose immune systems have been engineered to more closely resemble that of humans, thus eliminating dependence on organ donors.

Another possibility to address the organ donation problem is the potential for organ cloning. With the recent cloning of sheep and cattle, this topic has received a considerable amount of attention. Although the issue of whole-animal cloning is fascinating, the area that offers the greatest hope for transplant patients is the growing field of stem cell biology. By identifying stem cells of interest, the information gathered from the Human Genome Project could enable scientists to develop organ-cloning techniques that will revolutionize the field of transplantation. These pluripotent stem cells have the ability to divide without limit and to give rise to many types of differentiated and specialized tissues with a specific purpose. It is anticipated that the identification of stem cells and the potential modification of these cells by gene therapy may allow investigators to genetically engineer tissues of interest.

Oncology

The results of the Human Genome Project will have far-reaching effects on diagnostic studies, treatment, and counseling of cancer patients and family members.[34]

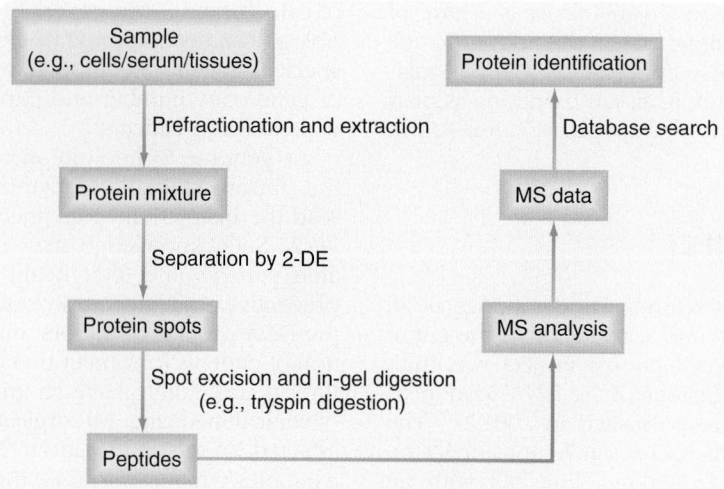

Figure 3-12 Basic approach of proteomics-based research. 2-DE, two-dimensional gel electrophoresis; MS, mass spectrometry. (From Lam L, Lind J, Semsarian C: Application of proteomics in cardiovascular medicine. Int J Cardiol 108:12-19, 2006.

Genetic testing is currently available for many disorders, including Tay-Sachs disease and cystic fibrosis. New tests have been developed to detect predispositions to Alzheimer's disease, colon cancer, breast cancer, and other conditions. Identification of the entire human genome will provide an unprecedented and powerful modality to increase our ability to screen high-risk groups and the general population.

With identification of certain high-risk groups for the development of cancer, surgeons will play an ever-increasing role in both genetic assessment and ultimate therapy. Prophylactic surgery may soon become more prevalent as a first-line treatment in the fight against cancer. For example, discovery of the association between mutations of the *ret* proto-oncogene and hereditary medullary thyroid carcinoma has allowed surgeons to identify patients in whom medullary thyroid cancer will eventually develop. Genetic screening for mutations of the *ret* proto-oncogene in patients with the multiple endocrine neoplasia type II allows prophylactic thyroidectomy to be performed at an earlier stage of the disease process than traditional biochemical screening does. Other areas of active interest include testing of patients with familial adenomatous polyposis, in which the timing and extent of therapy may be based on the exact location of adenomatous polyposis coli (APC) mutations. Furthermore, additional testing will allow investigators to better determine other genes that may contribute to this syndrome. Another area of controversy concerns the treatment of patients with mutations of the breast cancer susceptibility genes *BRCA1* and *BRCA2*. As more information becomes known regarding mutations of these genes and the clinical implications of these mutations, cancer treatment protocols will be altered accordingly.

Pediatric and Fetal Surgery

Identification of the human genome will further aid in prenatal diagnostic testing and screening. With the iden-

tification of fetuses at risk for a number of identifiable genetic diseases, the Human Genome Project will increase research and activity in the field of fetal surgery by expanding the current knowledge of genetic diseases and the rate of fetal surgical interventions involving not only current techniques but also the combination or use of somatic gene therapy. In utero manipulation of identifiable genetic defects may, in the future, become a common intervention.

Proteomics

An important offshoot of the Human Genome Project is the realization for the need to examine the expression and function of the end product of the gene (i.e., the protein). This has led to development of the field of proteomics, which is the study of the proteome. The term *proteome* was first coined by Marc Wilkins in 1995 to describe the entire collection of proteins of an organism.[35] The importance of proteomics is underscored by the fact that virtually all cellular phenotypes and activities are directed by proteins.

Protein expression and modifications are regulated under normal physiologic conditions (e.g., differentiation, apoptosis, and aging); they are altered during pathophysiologic stresses and lead to the development and progression of disease. However, the human proteome is both complex and dynamic, and examination of it requires the development of new tools and technologies. The basic steps in proteomic studies consist of sample preparation, protein separation, protein imaging, and protein identification. Protein separation usually involves two-dimensional gel electrophoresis and protein identification by mass spectrometry (Fig. 3-12).[36] With the use of proteomic technologies, investigators have begun to elucidate patterns of protein changes between health and disease states by profiling complex biologic samples such as serum, urine, and tissues.[37,38] The field of proteomics is advancing rapidly with the development of new and more powerful technologies to examine complex protein interactions and protein modifications. These advancements will lead to better detection and risk assessment, therapeutic targeting, and patient-tailored therapy for human diseases.

NOVEL TREATMENT STRATEGIES

Gene Therapy

The ability to alter specific genes of interest represents an exciting and powerful tool in the potential treatment of a wide array of diseases.[39-41] Instead of giving a patient a drug to treat or control the symptoms of a genetic disorder, physicians may be capable of treating the basic problem by altering the genetic makeup of the patient's cells. Several methods are currently available to introduce new genetic material into mammalian cells. Typically, two strategies have been considered: germline and somatic cell gene therapy. In the germline strategy, foreign DNA is introduced into the zygote or early embryo with the expectation that the newly introduced material will contribute to the germline of the recipient and will therefore be passed to the next generation. In contrast, somatic cell gene therapy models represent the introduction of genetic material into somatic cells, which is then not transmitted to the germ cells.

A wide array of somatic cell gene therapy protocols designed to treat single-gene diseases, a variety of cancers, or HIV are currently under development, with some gene therapy protocols in clinical trials. The goals of human somatic gene therapy are generally one of the following: repair or compensate for a defective gene, enhance the immune response directed at a tumor or pathogen, protect vulnerable cell populations against treatments such as chemotherapy, or kill tumor cells directly.[42,43]

Several single-gene disorders are candidates for gene therapy, and a number of protocols have been developed. In addition, current thinking has expanded from the treatment of single-gene disorders to include the treatment of acquired immunodeficiency syndrome and atherosclerosis with gene therapy techniques. Moreover, many protocols for the treatment of cancer are under evaluation, particularly for otherwise untreatable conditions. Strategies include alteration of cancer cells or other host cells to produce cytokines or other molecules to alter the host response to the malignancy, expression of antigens on cancer cells to induce a host immune response, insertion of tumor suppressor genes or their sequences to slow cell growth, and introduction of drug-resistant genes into normal cells to facilitate more aggressive chemotherapy.

Although a number of in vitro experiments have shown great promise, current in vivo trials have failed to match the in vitro results, partly as a result of the vehicles used for transfecting the DNA into cells. A repertoire of viral-based vectors have been analyzed, with each generation showing more promise than the previous modification.[44] Initially, retroviruses were used as vectors and are still used in certain instances. However, other potential vectors include adenovirus, herpesvirus, vaccinia, and other viruses. Nonviral systems, such as liposomes, DNA-protein conjugates, and DNA–protein–defective virus conjugates, also appear promising.[45] Safety issues, improvement of in vivo gene delivery, efficiency, and gene regulation after cellular transduction are the difficult issues that must be resolved in vector design. However exciting and appealing the prospects of gene therapy may appear, this technique is still in the experimental stages.

Short Interfering RNA

The recent discovery of siRNA as a method of gene silencing has provided another novel treatment strategy by targeting disease-causing genes. This powerful tool has already been tested in experimental conditions of viral infectious diseases and cancers. In infectious diseases, siRNAs against hepatitis B virus, HIV-1, and respiratory syncytial virus have been shown to inhibit viral replication.[46] Silencing of oncogenes such as K-*ras* and HER-2/*neu* has been shown to inhibit cancer cell growth. Although siRNA-based therapy holds great promise because of its potential for high selectivity and less toxicity, its clinical applications require overcoming the problem of the short half-life of siRNA and effective delivery to target tissues. Scientists are developing modifications of siRNA that will extend its half-life and improve cellular uptake.

Drug Design

Based on information from the fields of genomics and structural biology, rational drug design can be devised to treat a host of diseases.[47] This technique has been used to generate potent drugs, many of which are currently in use or under study. For example, a rational design based on crystallographic data has led to the development of new classes of anti-HIV agents targeted against HIV protease. Once the critical proteins accounting for a disease are identified and their abnormal function understood, drugs can be designed to stimulate, inhibit, or substitute function.

Identification of human genetic variations will eventually allow clinicians to subclassify diseases and adapt therapies that are appropriate to the individual patient.[48] There may be differences in the effectiveness of medicines from one patient to the next. Furthermore, toxic reactions can occur that may be a consequence of genetically encoded host factors. These observations have spawned the field of pharmacogenomics, which attempts to use information on genetic variations in patients to predict responses to drug therapies. In addition to genetic tests that will predict responsiveness to therapies currently available, these genetic approaches to disease prevention and treatment should provide an expanding array of gene products that will be used in developing future drug therapies.

Genetic Engineering of Antibodies

Monoclonal antibodies directed against specific antigens have been generated by using hybridoma techniques and are widely used in a number of fields of medicine, including oncology and transplantation. However, a major drawback is the fact that repeated treatment with murine antibodies results in an immune response directed against the antibody. Genetic engineering techniques have allowed the modification of mouse monoclonal antibodies to reduce the immune response directed against them by human recipients and to provide nonhuman resources for human antibodies.[49] This modification involves cloning either the variable or the hypervariable regions of the antibody from the mRNA of a hybridoma and fusing them with a human constant region, thus resulting in clones that can be expressed in human cell lines to produce large amounts of modified antibody. It is anticipated that such techniques will become more commonplace in the future and provide a ready source of antibodies directed against a wide array of antigens.

ETHICAL, PSYCHOLOGICAL, AND LEGAL IMPLICATIONS

The possibilities of genetic-based medicine are endless, and one can predict that in the next decade our lives will be greatly altered because of these rapid advances.[30,50] A number of ethical, psychological, and legal implications can be envisioned and will need to be addressed.[51,52] Such issues include ownership of the genetic information and who should have access to this information.[53] Another issue is how to correctly counsel both the patient and other family members based on information obtained from genetic testing.

The surgeon of the future will need to actively participate and be knowledgeable in these emerging technologies because our management of specific problems will be greatly altered by the new knowledge gained from analysis of the human genome.[50,54,55] Most assuredly, these rapid advances will continue to alter current treatment strategies and challenge existing dogmas. Surgeons have the opportunity to be active participants and leaders in the research and complex decision-making process that will affect our treatment of patients with surgical diseases. Surgeons, as well as all physicians, must rise to the occasion or otherwise be relegated to bystander status, with these complex clinical and ethical decisions being made by nonclinicians.

Selected References

Alberts B, Johnson A, Lewis J, et al (eds): Molecular Biology of the Cell, 4th ed. New York, Garland, 2002.

This textbook provides an excellent primer for the reader to better understand the fundamental concepts of molecular biology.

Calvo KR, Liotta LA, Petricoin EF: Clinical proteomics: From biomarker discovery and cell signaling profiles to individualized personal therapy. Biosci Rep 25:107-125, 2005.

Extensive review of proteomics and its potential applications in clinical practice.

Collins FS: Shattuck Lecture—Medical and societal consequences of the Human Genome Project. N Engl J Med 341:28-37, 1999.

This paper by the leader of the Human Genome Project provides an assessment of the progress toward completing this project, as well as future implications regarding human disease prevention and treatment.

Fadeel B, Orrenius S: Apoptosis: A basic biological phenomenon with wide-ranging implications in human disease. J Intern Med 258:479-517, 2005.

Review of the mechanism of apoptosis and its implication in medicine.

Malumbres M, Barbacid M: Mammalian cyclin-dependent kinases. Trends Biochem Sci 30:630-641, 2005.

Excellent review of the proteins that regulate cell cycle progression.

Papaconstantinou HT, Ko TC: Cell cycle and apoptosis regulation in GI cancers. In Evers BM (ed): Molecular Mechanisms of Gastrointestinal Cancers. Austin, TX, Landes Bioscience, 1999, pp 49-78.

This chapter provides an excellent review for the reader to better understand regulation of the cell cycle and apoptosis.

Rychahou PG, Jackson LN, Farrow BJ, et al: RNA interference: Mechanisms of action and therapeutic consideration. Surgery 140:719-725, 2006.

Review of recent progress in RNA interference technology and its potential clinical applications.

Sambrook J, Russell D (eds): Molecular Cloning: A Laboratory Manual, 3rd ed. Plainview, NY, Cold Spring Harbor Laboratory Press, 2001.

This manual is a collection of laboratory protocols, including detailed discussion of DNA recombinant technology.

The Chipping Forecast. Nat Genet 21(Suppl), 1999.

This entire supplement provides an excellent primer for the reader to better understand and appreciate the vast scientific potential and utility of microarray (i.e., gene chip) technology. A basic description of these techniques and possible limitations are discussed.

References

1. Alberts B, Johnson A, Lewis J, et al: Molecular Biology of the Cell. New York, Garland Publishing, 2002.
2. Lodish HF, Berk A, Matsudaira P, et al: Molecular Cell Biology. New York, WH Freeman, 2003.
3. Rosenthal N: DNA and the genetic code. N Engl J Med 331:39-41, 1994.
4. Rosenthal N: Regulation of gene expression. N Engl J Med 331:931-933, 1994.
5. Mata J, Marguerat S, Bahler JA: Post-transcriptional control of gene expression: A genome-wide perspective. Trends Biochem Sci 30:506-514, 2005.
6. Yang XJ: Multisite protein modification and intramolecular signaling. Oncogene 24:1653-1662, 2005.
7. Rosenthal N: Tools of the trade—recombinant DNA. N Engl J Med 331:315-317, 1994.
8. Saiki RK, Scharf S, Faloona F, et al: Enzymatic amplification of beta-globin genomic sequences and restriction site analysis for diagnosis of sickle cell anemia. Science 230:1350-1354, 1985.

9. Templeton NS: The polymerase chain reaction. History, methods, and applications. Diagn Mol Pathol 1:58-72, 1992.

10. Yamamura K: Overview of transgenic and gene knockout mice. Prog Exp Tumor Res 35:13-24, 1999.

11. Hofker MH, Breuer M: Generation of transgenic mice. Methods Mol Biol 110:63-78, 1998.

12. Majzoub JA, Muglia LJ: Knockout mice. N Engl J Med 334:904-907, 1996.

13. Fire A, Xu S, Montgomery MK, et al: Potent and specific genetic interference by double-stranded RNA in *Caenorhabditis elegans.* Nature 391:806-811, 1998.

14. McManus MT, Sharp PA: Gene silencing in mammals by small interfering RNAs. Nat Rev Genet 3:737-747, 2002.

15. Perl M, Chung CS, Ayala A: Apoptosis. Crit Care Med 33: S526-S529, 2005.

16. Nishizuka Y: Signal transduction: Crosstalk. Trends Biochem Sci 17:367-443, 1992.

17. Wettschureck N, Offermanns S: Mammalian G proteins and their cell type specific functions. Physiol Rev 85:1159-1204, 2005.

18. Perona R: Cell signaling: Growth factors and tyrosine kinase receptors. Clin Transl Oncol 8:77-82, 2006.

19. Roskoski R Jr: Src protein tyrosine kinase structure and regulation. Biochem Biophys Res Commun 324:1155-1164, 2004.

20. Marinissen MJ, Gutkind JS: G-protein–coupled receptors and signaling networks: Emerging paradigms. Trends Pharmacol Sci 22:368-376, 2001.

21. Hurley JH: Structure, mechanism, and regulation of mammalian adenylyl cyclase. J Biol Chem 274:7599-7602, 1999.

22. Campbell SL, Khosravi-Far R, Rossman KL, et al: Increasing complexity of Ras signaling. Oncogene 17:1395-1413, 1998.

23. Malumbres M, Barbacid M: Mammalian cyclin-dependent kinases. Trends Biochem Sci 30:630-641, 2005.

24. Tonini T, Hillson C, Claudio PP: Interview with the retinoblastoma family members: Do they help each other? J Cell Physiol 192:138-150, 2002.

25. DeGregori J: The genetics of the E2F family of transcription factors: Shared functions and unique roles. Biochim Biophys Acta 1602:131-150, 2002.

26. Lavrik I, Golks A, Krammer PH: Death receptor signaling. J Cell Sci 118:265-267, 2005.

27. Vousden KH, Lu X: Live or let die: The cell's response to p53. Nat Rev Cancer 2:594-604, 2002.

28. Lavrik IN, Golks A, Krammer PH: Caspases: Pharmacological manipulation of cell death. J Clin Invest 115:2665-2672, 2005.

29. Adams JM, Cory S: The Bcl-2 protein family: Arbiters of cell survival. Science 281:1322-1326, 1998.

30. Lander ES, Linton LM, Birren B, et al: Initial sequencing and analysis of the human genome. Nature 409:860-921, 2001.

31. Venter JC, Adams MD, Myers EW, et al: The sequence of the human genome. Science 291:1304-1351, 2001.

32. Wang DG, Fan JB, Siao CJ, et al: Large-scale identification, mapping, and genotyping of single-nucleotide polymorphisms in the human genome. Science 280:1077-1082, 1998.

33. The Chipping Forecast. Nature Genet 21(Suppl), 1999.

34. Khan J, Bittner ML, Chen Y, et al: DNA microarray technology: The anticipated impact on the study of human disease. Biochim Biophys Acta 1423:M17-M28, 1999.

35. Wilkins MR, Sanchez JC, Gooley AA, et al: Progress with proteome projects: Why all proteins expressed by a genome should be identified and how to do it. Biotechnol Genet Eng Rev 13:19-50, 1996.

36. Lam L, Lind J, Semsarian C: Application of proteomics in cardiovascular medicine. Int J Cardiol 108:12-19, 2006.

37. Colantonio DA, Chan DW: The clinical application of proteomics. Clin Chim Acta 357:151-158, 2005.

38. Plebani M: Proteomics: The next revolution in laboratory medicine? Clin Chim Acta 357:113-122, 2005.

39. Prieto J, Herraiz M, Sangro B, et al: The promise of gene therapy in gastrointestinal and liver diseases. Gut 52(Suppl 2):ii49-ii54, 2003.

40. Meyerson SL, Schwartz LB: Gene therapy as a therapeutic intervention for vascular disease. J Cardiovasc Nurs 13:91-109, 1999.

41. Petrie NC, Yao F, Eriksson E: Gene therapy in wound healing. Surg Clin North Am 83:597-616, vii, 2003.

42. Lee JH, Klein HG: Cellular gene therapy. Hematol Oncol Clin North Am 9:91-113, 1995.

43. Crystal RG: In vivo and ex vivo gene therapy strategies to treat tumors using adenovirus gene transfer vectors. Cancer Chemother Pharmacol 43(Suppl):S90-S99, 1999.

44. Mah C, Byrne BJ, Flotte TR: Virus-based gene delivery systems. Clin Pharmacokinet 41:901-911, 2002.

45. Niidome T, Huang L: Gene therapy progress and prospects: Nonviral vectors. Gene Ther 9:1647-1652, 2002.

46. Rychahou PG, Jackson LN, Farrow BJ, et al: RNA interference: Mechanisms of action and therapeutic consideration. Surgery 140:719-725, 2006.

47. Bailey DS, Bondar A, Furness LM: Pharmacogenomics—it's not just pharmacogenetics. Curr Opin Biotechnol 9:595-601, 1998.

48. Evans WE, McLeod HL: Pharmacogenomics—drug disposition, drug targets, and side effects. N Engl J Med 348:538-549, 2003.

49. Brekke OH, Sandlie I: Therapeutic antibodies for human diseases at the dawn of the twenty-first century. Nat Rev Drug Discov 2:52-62, 2003.

50. Hernandez A, Evers BM: Functional genomics: Clinical effect and the evolving role of the surgeon. Arch Surg 134:1209-1215, 1999.

51. Vineis P: Ethical issues in genetic screening for cancer. Ann Oncol 8:945-949, 1997.

52. Grady C: Ethics and genetic testing. Adv Intern Med 44:389-411, 1999.

53. Nowlan W: Human genetics. A rational view of insurance and genetic discrimination. Science 297:195-196, 2002.

54. Vogelstein B: Genetic testings for cancer: The surgeon's critical role. Familial colon cancer. J Am Coll Surg 188:74-79, 1999.

55. Moulton G: Surgeons have critical role in genetic testing decisions, medical, legal experts say. J Natl Cancer Inst 90:804-805, 1998.

4 CHAPTER |

Mediators of the Inflammatory Response

Louis H. Alarcon, MD   and   Mitchell P. Fink, MD

Basic Definitions and Classification Systems

Interferon-γ

Interleukin-1 and Tumor Necrosis Factor

Interleukin-6 and Interleukin-11

Interleukin-8 and Other Chemokines

Interleukin-12

Interleukin-18

Interleukin-4, Interleukin-10, and Interleukin-13

Transforming Growth Factor-β

Macrophage Migration Inhibitory Factor

Complement

Endogenous Danger Signals

Eicosanoids (Thromboxane, Prostaglandins, and
  Leukotrienes)

Nitric Oxide

Carbon Monoxide

Reactive Oxygen Species

Celsus is credited with describing the cardinal signs of inflammation: *calor* (warmth), *dolor* (pain), *tumor* (swelling), and *rubor* (redness). Classically, the term *inflammation* was used to denote the pathologic reaction whereby fluid and circulating leukocytes accumulate in extravascular tissue in response to injury or infection. Today, inflammation connotes not only localized effects, such as edema, hyperemia, and leukocytic infiltration, but also systemic phenomena, for example, fever and increased synthesis of certain acute phase proteins and mediators of inflammation. The inflammatory response is closely interrelated with the processes of healing and repair. In fact, wound healing is impossible in the absence of inflammation. Accordingly, inflammation is involved in virtually every aspect of surgery because proper healing of traumatic wounds, surgical incisions, and various kinds

of anastomoses is entirely dependent on the expression of a tightly orchestrated and well-controlled inflammatory process.

Inflammation is fundamentally a protective response that has evolved to permit higher forms of life to rid themselves of injurious agents, remove necrotic cells and cellular debris, and repair damage to tissues and organs. However, the mechanisms used to kill invading microorganisms or to ingest and destroy devitalized cells as part of the inflammatory response can also be injurious to normal tissue. Thus, inflammation is a major pathogenic mechanism underlying numerous diseases and syndromes. Many of these pathologic conditions, such as inflammatory bowel disease (IBD), sepsis, and adult respiratory distress syndrome (ARDS), are of importance in the practice of surgery.

Initiation, maintenance, and termination of the inflammatory response are extremely complex processes involving numerous different cell types, as well as hundreds of different humoral mediators. A thorough account of the cellular and humoral mediators of inflammation is beyond the scope of a single chapter in a text covering many other topics. Accordingly, the objective of this chapter is to provide an overview of the properties and functions of the mediators of humoral inflammatory, namely, the diverse group of proteins called *cytokines*, as well as other small molecules involved in inflammatory signaling.

For the purpose of describing the inflammatory process, this overview will use a single, albeit complicated clinical entity—septic shock—as a paradigm of the inflammatory response. *Septic shock* is the clinical manifestation of a systemic inflammatory response run amok. Sepsis is the most common cause of mortality in patients requiring care in an intensive care unit. Severe sepsis, which occurs in about 750,000 people in the United States every year, carries a mortality rate close to 30%. It is generally believed that the incidence of sepsis and septic shock is increasing, probably as a result of advances in many fields of medicine that have extended the use of complex invasive procedures and potent immunosuppressive agents. Given the importance of sepsis as a public health problem, effort has been made to translate improvements in our understanding of inflammation and inflammatory mediators into the development of useful therapeutic agents. Some of these therapeutic agents are mentioned in the context of the overall discussion of inflammation.

BASIC DEFINITIONS AND CLASSIFICATION SYSTEMS

Cytokines are small proteins or glycoproteins secreted for the purpose of altering the function of target cells in an endocrine (uncommon), paracrine, or autocrine fashion. In contrast to classic hormones such as insulin or thyroxine, cytokines are not secreted by specialized glands but, instead, are produced by cells individually (e.g., lymphocytes or macrophages) or as components of a tissue (e.g., the intestinal epithelium). Many cytokines are pleiotropic; these cytokines are capable of inducing many different biologic effects, depending on the target cell types involved and the presence or absence of other modulating factors. Redundancy is another characteristic feature of cytokines; that is, several different cytokines can exert very similar biologic effects.

Cytokines can be classified according to several different schemes, all of which are somewhat arbitrary and not completely satisfactory. In an older nomenclature, cytokines were classified according to the type of cell responsible for their synthesis; cytokines produced by lymphocytes were called *lymphokines*, whereas cytokines secreted by macrophages or monocytes were called *monokines*. However, cytokines can be produced by more than one type of cell. Thus, the terms lymphokine and monokine are rarely used today.

Another way that cytokines can be categorized is on the basis of structure. Thus, *type I* cytokines are a large group of proteins that share a characteristic tertiary structure consisting of a bundle of four α helices. The receptors for type I cytokines also share structural similarities and are referred to as *type I cytokine receptors*. Type I cytokines include the following proteins: interleukin-2 (IL-2), IL-3, IL-4, IL-5, IL-6, IL-7, IL-9, IL-11, IL-13, IL-15, and granulocyte colony-stimulating factor (G-CSF). *Type II* cytokines, including interferon-α (IFN-α), IFN-β, IFN-γ, and IL-10, are a second structurally related group of proteins. *Type II cytokine receptors* are also structurally related.

Yet another way of grouping cytokines is based on the recognition that naive CD4$^+$ T cells (T$_H$0 cells) can differentiate into either of two T helper (T$_H$) subsets called T$_H$1 and T$_H$2. T$_H$1 cells, responsible for directing the cell-mediated immune responses necessary for the eradication of intracellular pathogens, favor macrophage activation. T$_H$2 cells have been implicated in the pathogenesis of atopy and allergic inflammation and favor B-cell growth and differentiation. T$_H$1 cells produce IL-2, as well as the potent proinflammatory cytokines IFN-γ and lymphotoxin-α (LT-α). T$_H$2 cells produce IL-4, IL-5, IL-6, IL-9, IL-10, and IL-13. The actions of IL-4, IL-10, IL-13, and to some extent, IL-6 are largely anti-inflammatory in nature. Thus, T$_H$1 cytokines are often viewed as being proinflammatory, whereas T$_H$2 cytokines are thought of as being anti-inflammatory. The cytokine IL-12 drives T$_H$1 differentiation, whereas IL-4 induces T$_H$2 differentiation.[1]

Chemokines are a special family of cytokines that consist of small proteins with molecular weights in the range of 8 to 11 kd. The chemokines have as their primary biologic activity the ability to act as chemoattractants for leukocytes or fibroblasts. Another cytokine subclass is a group of proteins that act primarily to stimulate the growth or differentiation (or both) of hematopoietic progenitor cells; these mediators are collectively referred to as *colony-stimulating factors*. Other growth and differentiation factors, including the various platelet-derived growth factors, epidermal growth factor, and keratinocyte growth factor, also fit into the broad category of cytokines.

Overall, hundreds of soluble proteins involved in cell-to-cell signaling, variously called *cytokines, chemokines, interleukins, colony-stimulating factors,* and *growth factors,* have been identified and characterized. An exhaustive account of each and every one of these mediators is beyond the scope of this chapter and would be a futile exercise in any event given the rapid pace of discovery in this broad field of research. Some pertinent facts about some of the most important cytokines are provided in Table 4-1. Some of these mediators are discussed in greater detail in the sections that follow.

INTERFERON-γ

The immune response to infection has two broad components. *Innate* responses, which occur early and are not antigen specific, depend largely on proper functioning of natural killer (NK) cells and phagocytic cells, such as monocytes, macrophages, and neutrophils. *Acquired* responses, which develop later after antigen processing and the clonal expansion of T- and B-cell subsets, are antigen specific. A number of cytokines, including transforming growth factor-β (TGF-β), tumor necrosis factor (TNF), IL-1, IL-6, IL-10, IL-12, and IL-18, are synthesized by cells of the innate immune system and contribute to the ability of the host to mount an early, innate immune response to an infectious challenge. Another group of cytokines, the interferons, are also key components of the innate immune system.

The *interferons,* named for their ability to interfere with viral infection, were initially discovered in the 1950s as soluble factors secreted by leukocytes. The type 1 interferons, IFN-α and IFN-β, are primarily involved as mediators of innate (and acquired) immune responses to viral infection. IFN-γ, though also important in the immune response to viral infection, has much broader activity as a proinflammatory mediator.

For the most part, IFN-γ is produced by three types of cells: CD4$^+$ T$_H$1 cells, CD8$^+$ T$_H$1 cells, and NK cells. IFN-γ, along with two other cytokines, IL-12 and IL-18, plays a

Table 4-1 Cellular Sources and Important Biologic Effects of Selected Cytokines

CYTOKINE	ABBREVIATION	MAIN SOURCES	IMPORTANT BIOLOGIC EFFECTS
Tumor necrosis factor	TNF	Mφ, others	See Table 4-3
Lymphotoxin-α	LT-α	T_H1, NK	Same as TNF
Interferon-α	IFN-α	Leukocytes	Increases expression of cell surface class I MHC molecules; inhibits viral replication
Interferon-β	IFN-β	Fibroblasts	Same as IFN-α
Interferon-γ	IFN-γ	T_H1	Activates Mφ; promotes differentiation of CD4+ T cells into T_H1 cells; inhibits differentiation of CD4+ T cells into T_H2 cells
Interleukin-1α	IL-1α	Keratinocytes, others	See Table 4-3
Interleukin-1β	IL-1β	Mφ, NK, PMN, others	See Table 4-3
Interleukin-2	IL-2	T_H1	In combination with other stimuli, promotes proliferation of T cells; promotes proliferation of activated B cells; stimulates secretion of cytokines by T cells; increases cytotoxicity of NK cells
Interleukin-3	IL-3	T cells	Stimulates pluripotent bone marrow stem cells, thereby increasing production of leukocytes, erythrocytes, and platelets
Interleukin-4	IL-4	T_H2	Promotes growth and differentiation of B cells; promotes differentiation of CD4+ T cells into T_H2 cells; inhibits secretion of proinflammatory cytokines by Mφ
Interleukin-5	IL-5	T cells, mast cells	Induces production of eosinophils from myeloid precursor cells
Interleukin-6	IL-6	Mφ, T_H2, enterocytes, others	Induces fever; promotes B-cell maturation and differentiation; stimulates hypothalamic-pituitary-adrenal axis; induces hepatic synthesis of acute phase proteins
Interleukin-8	IL-8	Mφ, endothelial cells, others	Stimulates chemotaxis by PMN; stimulates oxidative burst by PMN
Interleukin-9	IL-9	T_H2	Promotes proliferation of activated T cells; promotes immunoglobulin secretion by B cells
Interleukin-10	IL-10	T_H2, Mφ	Inhibits secretion of proinflammatory cytokines by Mφ
Interleukin-11	IL-11	Neurons, fibroblasts, others	Increases production of platelets; inhibits proliferation of enterocytes
Interleukin-12	IL-12	Mφ	Promotes differentiation of CD4+ T cells into T_H1 cells; enhances IFN-γ secretion by T_H1 cells and NK cells
Interleukin-13	IL-13	T_H2, others	Inhibits secretion of proinflammatory cytokines by Mφ
Interleukin-18	IL-18	Mφ, others	Co-stimulation with IL-12 of IFN-γ secretion by T_H1 cells and NK cells
Monocyte chemotactic protein-1	MCP-1	Mφ, endothelial cells, others	Stimulates chemotaxis by monocytes; stimulates oxidative burst by macrophages
Granulocyte-macrophage colony-stimulating factor	GM-CSF	T cells, Mφ, endothelial cells, others	Enhances production of granulocytes and monocytes by bone marrow; primes Mφ to produce proinflammatory mediators after activation by another stimulus
Granulocyte colony-stimulating factor	G-CSF	Mφ, fibroblasts	Enhances production of granulocytes by bone marrow
Erythropoietin	EPO	Kidney cells	Enhances production of erythrocytes by bone marrow
Transforming growth factor-β	TGF-β	T cells, Mφ, platelets, others	Stimulates chemotaxis by monocytes and fibroblasts; induces synthesis of extracellular matrix proteins by fibroblasts; inhibits secretion of cytokines by T cells; inhibits immunoglobulin secretion by B cells; down-regulates activation of NK cells

Mφ, cells of the monocyte-macrophage lineage; MHC, major histocompatibility complex; NK, natural killer cells; PMN, polymorphonuclear neutrophils; T_H1, T_H2, subsets of differentiated CD4+ T helper cells.

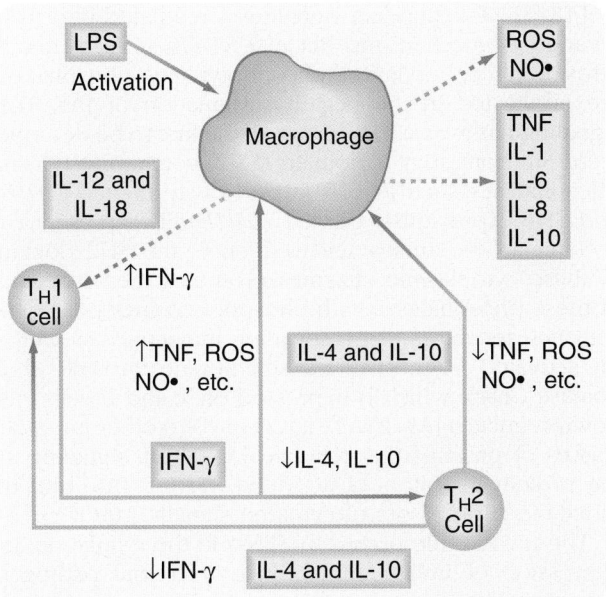

Figure 4-1 Simplified representation of the responses of three important cell types (macrophages, T helper cells with a T$_H$1 phenotype, and T helper cells with a T$_H$2 phenotype) involved in the inflammatory response to an archetypic proinflammatory stimulus, namely, exposure to lipopolysaccharide (LPS), a component of the outer cell wall of gram-negative bacteria. In response to stimulation by LPS, macrophages secrete the cytokines interleukin-12 (IL-12) and IL-18. IL-12 promotes the differentiation of naive CD4$^+$ T cells (T$_H$0 cells) into T$_H$1 cells capable of producing interferon-γ (IFN-γ) after activation, and IL-12 and IL-18 together stimulate secretion of IFN-γ by T$_H$1 cells. IFN-γ, in turn, further up-regulates the production of proinflammatory cytokines, such as tumor necrosis factor (TNF), IL-1, IL-6, and IL-8, and other proinflammatory mediators, such as reactive oxygen species (ROS) and nitric oxide (NO·), by LPS-stimulated macrophages. IFN-γ also down-regulates the production of anti-inflammatory cytokines (IL-4 and IL-10) by T$_H$2 cells. IL-4 and IL-10 act to down-regulate the production of IFN-γ by T$_H$1 cells and the production of proinflammatory cytokines and other proinflammatory mediators by macrophages. IL-10 is not only produced by T$_H$2 cells but is also secreted by stimulated macrophages as well, thus creating an autocrine negative feedback loop.

critical role in promoting the differentiation of CD4$^+$ T cells to the T$_H$1 phenotype. Because T$_H$1 cells also produce IFN-γ, the potential exists for a positive feedback loop. IL-12 and IL-18, produced by monocytes and macrophages, stimulate the production of IFN-γ by T$_H$1 and NK cells (Fig. 4-1). In turn, IFN-γ further activates monocytes and macrophages, thereby creating another positive feedback loop.

In addition to promoting the differentiation of uncommitted CD4$^+$ T cells into T$_H$1 cells, IFN-γ inhibits the differentiation of lymphocytes into cells with the T$_H$2 phenotype. Because T$_H$2 cells secrete the counter-regulatory cytokines IL-4 and IL-10, the effect of IFN-γ to down-regulate the production of these cytokines by T$_H$2 cells further promotes the development of an inflammatory response to an invading pathogen. In target cells, such as macrophages or enterocytes, IFN-γ induces the expres-

sion or activation of a number of key proteins involved in the innate immune response to microbes. Among these proteins are other cytokines, such as TNF and IL-1, and enzymes, such as inducible nitric oxide synthase (iNOS) and the reduced form of the nicotinamide adenine dinucleotide phosphate (NADPH) oxidase complex. Thus, IFN-γ stimulates the release of a number of other proinflammatory mediators, including cytokines such as TNF and small molecules such as superoxide radical anion (O$_2^-$·), an oxidant produced by NADPH oxidase, and nitric oxide (NO·), produced by iNOS. Secretion of these inflammatory mediators by activated macrophages and other cell types is inhibited by IL-4 and IL-10. Accordingly, IFN-γ–mediated down-regulation of the T$_H$2 phenotype—and thereby production of IL-4 and IL-10—further promotes the development of an inflammatory response.

The crucial role of IFN-γ in the host's innate immune response to microbial invasion, particularly by intracellular pathogens, has been emphasized by experiments using transgenic mice with targeted disruption of the genes coding for IFN-γ or the ligand-binding subunit of the IFN-γ receptor (IFN-γR). These knockout mice manifest increased susceptibility to infections caused by *Listeria monocytogenes, Mycobacterium tuberculosis,* or bacille Calmette-Guérin.

When responsive target cells are exposed to IFN-γ, a number of genes are activated within minutes and without the synthesis of new copies of intermediate signaling proteins. IFN-γ–induced signal transduction occurs through the activation of a protein tyrosine phosphorylation cascade known as the *JAK-STAT pathway.* JAK initially stood for *j*ust *a*nother *k*inase because the biologic role of these proteins was not established when they were initially discovered. Because these receptor-associated kinases look both outside and inside the cell, JAK has now come to stand for *Janus kinases,* after the two-faced Roman god. The moniker STAT, an acronym for *s*ignal *t*ransducers and *a*ctivators of *t*ranscription, was appropriately chosen because in medical parlance, an action to be carried out immediately is a *stat* order and signaling involving these proteins similarly occurs without delay. In addition to IFN-γ, a large number of other cytokines, including IL-6 and IL-11 (see later), also use versions of the JAK-STAT signaling mechanism. In mammals there are seven STAT proteins (STAT1, STAT2, STAT3, STAT4, STAT5A, STAT5B, and STAT6) and four JAK proteins (JAK1, JAK2, JAK3, and TYK2).

IFN-γR is a heterodimer that consists of a 90-kd glycoprotein, the α chain, which is required for binding of the ligand, and a transmembrane protein, the β chain, which is required for signaling. Associated with the receptor are two members of the JAK family of kinases, JAK1 and JAK2. Interaction of IFN-γ with its receptor results in dimerization of IFN-γR, which brings JAK1 and JAK2 into close association and leads to mutual phosphorylation and activation (Fig. 4-2). The activated JAK kinases then catalyze the phosphorylation of tyrosine residues on the α chains of IFN-γR, which results in docking to the receptor complex by the transcription factor STAT1. After tyrosine phosphorylation, two copies

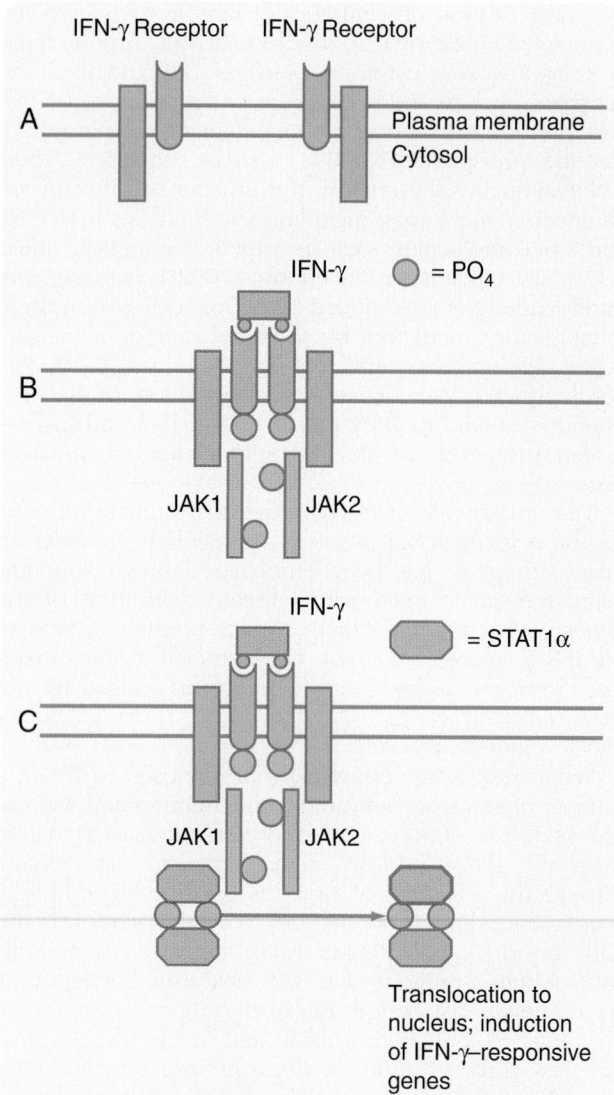

Figure 4-2 Simplified representation of intracellular signaling mediated by binding of interferon-γ (IFN-γ) to its receptor (IFN-γR). IFN-γR is a dimer that consists of a ligand-binding α chain and a transmembrane signaling β chain (*A*). Binding of IFN-γ leads to dimerization of IFN-γR and brings two signaling proteins, JAK1 and JAK2, into association with the receptor complex (*B*). The association of JAK1 and JAK2 with the receptor leads to mutual tyrosine phosphorylation of these proteins, as well as phosphorylation of tyrosine residues on the ligand-binding chains of IFN-γR, and docking of two copies of the preformed transcription factor STAT1α to the receptor complex (*C*). After tyrosine phosphorylation, STAT1α forms a homodimer. The homodimer dissociates from the receptor complex and translocates to the nucleus, where binding to the promoter regions of various IFN-γ–responsive genes leads to transcriptional activation.

of STAT1 form a homodimer (IFN-γ activation factor [GAF]) that subsequently dissociates from the receptor complex and translocates to the nucleus, where binding to the regulatory regions of target genes containing the IFN-γ activation site (GAS) nucleotide sequence leads to transcriptional activation.

JAK/STAT-dependent signaling is regulated in cells by a variety of mechanisms. Because STATs are activated by tyrosine phosphorylation, phosphotyrosine phosphatases are implicated in the negative regulation of JAK/STAT signaling pathways. In this regard, the first to be described were Src homology 2 domain (SH2)-containing tyrosine phosphatases such as SHP1 (previously named *PTP1C*) and SHP2 (previously named *PTP1D*). The presence of a characteristic amino acid sequence, the SH2 domain, in these cytoplasmic enzymes promotes the association of these phosphatases with phosphotyrosines present on activated receptors or on signaling molecules, as well as on activated JAKs.[2] The transmembrane tyrosine phosphatase CD45, which is expressed on T and B cells, also down-regulates JAK/STAT signaling. Two other important classes of proteins that regulate JAK/STAT signaling are the protein inhibitors of activated STAT (PIAS) and the inducible suppressors of cytokine signaling (SOCS).

The pivotal role played by IFN-γ in the regulation and expression of innate immunity to microbial pathogens led investigators to use this cytokine as a therapeutic agent to increase host resistance to infection, particularly for patients with congenital or acquired immunosuppression. For example, prophylactic treatment with recombinant IFN-γ has been shown to markedly reduce the frequency of infections in patients with chronic granulomatous disease, a life-threatening condition caused by an inherited defect in NADPH oxidase, the enzyme complex responsible for generating reactive oxygen species (ROS) in phagocytes. IFN-γ has been approved for this indication by the U.S. Food and Drug Administration (FDA). Severe trauma and burns are associated with defects in host antibacterial and antifungal defense, and in animal models of these conditions, treatment with IFN-γ has been found to increase resistance to infection. Three major clinical trials of prophylactic IFN-γ treatment were conducted in patients with multiple trauma or major thermal injury. Unfortunately, in all three studies, the incidence of infection and mortality was similar in cytokine- and placebo-treated patients.

It is unclear why treatment with IFN-γ failed to improve outcome in these trials. However, treatment with IFN-γ was not individualized according to immunologic phenotype, and thus some of the deleterious effects of inflammation might have been fostered in certain subjects by administration of this potent proinflammatory cytokine. This notion is supported by results from an uncontrolled trial wherein patients with sepsis and laboratory findings indicative of excessive immunosuppression (down-regulation of HLA-DR expression on circulating monocytes) were treated with IFN-γ.[3] In this small study, administration of IFN-γ resulted in resolution of sepsis in eight of nine patients. A small pilot study evaluated the use of prophylactic perioperative IFN-γ therapy to decrease the risk for infection in anergic high-risk patients undergoing major operations.[4] Another approach may be to substitute granulocyte-macrophage colony-stimulating factor (GM-CSF) for IFN-γ. GM-CSF, a hematopoietic growth factor that promotes an increase in the number of circulating polymorphonuclear neutrophils (PMNs), has a number if IFN-γ–like features, including the use of

Table 4-2 Partial List of the Physiologic Effects Induced by Infusing Interleukin-1 or Tumor Necrosis Factor Into Human Subjects

EFFECT	IL-1	TNF
Fever	+	+
Headache	+	+
Anorexia	+	+
Increased plasma adrenocorticotropic hormone level	+	+
Hypercortisolemia	+	+
Increased plasma nitrite/nitrate levels	+	+
Systemic arterial hypotension	+	+
Neutrophilia	+	+
Transient neutropenia	+	+
Increased plasma acute phase protein levels	+	+
Hypoferremia	+	+
Hypozincemia		+
Increased plasma level of IL-1RA	+	+
Increased plasma level of TNF-R1 and TNF-R2	+	+
Increased plasma level of IL-6	+	+
Increased plasma level of IL-8	+	+
Activation of coagulation cascades	−	+
Increased platelet count	+	−
Pulmonary edema	−	+
Hepatocellular injury	−	+

Table 4-3 Partial List of the Effects of Interleukin-1 and Tumor Necrosis Factor on Various Target Cells

CELL TYPE	IMPORTANT EFFECTS	IL-1	TNF
T cell	IL-2 synthesis	↑	↑
	IL-2R expression	↑	↑
Monocyte/ macrophage	IL-1 synthesis	↑	
	TNF synthesis	↑	
	IL-6 synthesis	↑	↑
	IL-10 synthesis	↑	
	GM-CSF synthesis	↑	→
	G-CSF synthesis	↑	↑
	Prostaglandin synthesis	↑	→
	Tissue factor expression	↑	↑
Neutrophils	Complement receptor 3 expression	→	↑
	IL-8 synthesis	↑	↑
	Priming for increased oxidant production	↑	↑
Endothelial cells	GM-CSF synthesis	↑	↑
	G-CSF synthesis	↑	↑
	Prostacyclin synthesis	↑	↑
	E-selectin expression	↑	↑
	VCAM-1 expression	↑	↑
	ICAM-1 expression	↑	↑
	Tissue factor expression	↑	↑
Hepatocytes	Albumin synthesis	↓	↓
	C-reactive protein synthesis	↑	↓
	Insulin-like growth factor-I synthesis	↓	↓
	Complement component 3	↑	↑
	Inducible nitric oxide synthase expression	↑	→
Fibroblasts	Hepatocyte growth factor synthesis	↑	↑
	Vascular endothelial growth factor synthesis	↑	→

G-CSF, granulocyte colony-stimulating factor; GM-CSF, granulocyte-macrophage colony-stimulating factor; ICAM-1, intercellular adhesion molecule-1; VCAM-1, vascular cell adhesion molecule-1.

JAK-STAT signaling pathways. A randomized trial of adjuvant treatment with GM-CSF in neonates with sepsis and neutropenia showed that survival was significantly improved in the group treated with the cytokine/growth factor.[5] Similarly, in a single-center randomized controlled trial, adjuvant treatment with recombinant GM-CSF significantly shortened hospital stay and decreased the number of infectious complications in patients with intra-abdominal sepsis.[6]

INTERLEUKIN-1 AND TUMOR NECROSIS FACTOR

IL-1 and TNF are structurally dissimilar pluripotent cytokines. Although these compounds bind to different cellular receptors, their multiple biologic activities overlap considerably, as can be appreciated by inspecting Tables 4-2 and 4-3. Table 4-2 summarizes some of the biologic effects observed when human subjects are injected with recombinant IL-1 or TNF. Table 4-3 summarizes some important effects observed when certain representative cell types are incubated in the presence of IL-1 or TNF in vitro. Through their ability to potentiate the activation of helper T cells, IL-1 and TNF can promote nearly all types of humoral and cellular immune responses. Furthermore, both these cytokines are capable of activating neutrophils and macrophages and inducing the expression of many other cytokines and inflammatory mediators. Many of the biologic effects of either IL-1 or TNF are greatly potentiated by the presence of the other cytokine. The molecular basis for these synergistic actions remains poorly understood because many of the signal transduction pathways that are activated by the two cytokines are the same.

Interleukin-1 and the Interleukin-1 Receptor/Toll-like Receptor Superfamily of Receptors

IL-1 was first described as a *lymphocyte-activating factor* produced by stimulated macrophages. IL-1 is not a single compound, but rather a family of three distinct proteins, IL-1α, IL-1β, and IL-1 receptor antagonist (IL-1RA), which are products of different genes located close to one another on the long arm of human chromosome 2. The genes for the two receptors for IL-1, IL-1RI and IL-1RII, are also located on chromosome 2. IL-1α and IL-1β are peptides composed of 159 and 153 amino acids, respectively. Although IL-1α and IL-1β are structurally distinct—only 26% of their amino acid sequences are homologous—the two compounds are virtually identical from a functional standpoint. IL-1RA, the third member of the IL-1 family of proteins, is biologically inactive but competes with IL-1α and IL-1β for binding to IL-1 receptors on cells and thereby functions as a competitive inhibitor to limit IL-1–mediated effects.

IL-1 is synthesized by a wide variety of cell types, including monocytes, macrophages, B lymphocytes, T lymphocytes, NK cells, keratinocytes, dendritic cells, fibroblasts, neutrophils, endothelial cells, and enterocytes. Compounds that can trigger the production of IL-1 by monocytes, macrophages, or other cell types include microbial cell wall products, such as lipopolysaccharide (LPS; from gram-negative bacteria), lipoteichoic acid (from gram-positive bacteria), or zymosan (from yeast). Production of IL-1 can also be stimulated by other cytokines, including TNF, GM-CSF, and IL-1 itself.

Although many cell types express genes for both IL-1α and IL-1β, most cells produce predominantly one form of the cytokine. For example, human monocytes produce mostly IL-1β, whereas keratinocytes produce predominantly IL-1α. The two forms of IL-1 are both initially synthesized as 31-kd precursors (pro–IL-1α and pro–IL-1β), which are then post-translationally modified to create the carboxyl-terminal 17-kd peptide forms of the mature cytokines. IL-1α is stored in the cytoplasm as pro–IL-1α or, after being phosphorylated or myristoylated, in a membrane-bound form. Whereas both pro–IL-1α and membrane-bound IL-1α are biologically active, pro–IL-1β is devoid of biologic activity. Pro–IL-1α is converted to the mature peptide by calpain and other nonspecific extracellular proteases. Pro–IL-1β is cleaved to its mature active form by a specific intracellular cysteine protease called *IL-1β converting enzyme* (ICE), or *caspase-1*. Like IL-1β, ICE is stored in cells in an inactive form and must be proteolytically cleaved to become enzymatically active. Transgenic mice deficient in ICE are resistant to endotoxic shock and manifest an impaired ability to mount a local inflammatory response to intraperitoneal zymosan, a known inducer of sterile peritonitis.[7] Various ICE-like enzymes, the caspases, have been identified as being important mediators of the process of programmed cell death, or apoptosis.

The mature 17-kd form of IL-1β lacks a secretory signal peptide and is not secreted via the classic exocytic pathway used for the secretion of most proteins (including most other cytokines) from cells. ICE-dependent processing of pro–IL-1β and the secretory step appear to occur at the same time. Secretion of the leaderless mature peptide apparently occurs through the action of a specific transporter called *ABC1*, which can be inhibited by the oral hypoglycemic agent glyburide.

Similar to the other members of the IL-1 family, IL-1RA can be produced by a variety of cell types. However, unlike IL-1α and IL-1β, IL-1RA is synthesized with a leader peptide that allows normal secretion of the protein. A specialized form of IL-1RA, intracellular IL-1RA, is synthesized without a leader peptide sequence and therefore accumulates intracellularly in certain cell types. In some tissues, such as intestinal epithelium, the formation of intracellular IL-1RA may serve a counter-regulatory function to limit inflammation and thereby confer mucosal

protection. Moreover, an imbalance between the production of IL-1 and IL-1RA may promote the development of chronic inflammation in certain pathologic conditions such as Crohn's disease. Cellular production of IL-1 and IL-1RA is differentially regulated. Certain cytokines, notably IL-4, IL-10, and IL-13, which function in many ways as counter-regulatory cytokines, serve as anti-inflammatory mediators, in part by promoting the synthesis of IL-1RA. IL-6, though not usually thought of as an anti-inflammatory cytokine, is also capable of triggering the production of IL-1RA.

The importance of IL-1β as a proinflammatory cytokine and IL-1RA as an anti-inflammatory cytokine is emphasized by experiments using transgenic mouse strains deficient in IL-1RA, IL-1α, IL-1β, or both IL-1α and IL-1β (double *knockout* mice). In these studies, IL-1α knockout mice were able to mount a normal inflammatory response, whereas the IL-1β knockout animals manifested an impaired ability to mount a normal inflammatory response. In contrast, mice functionally deficient in IL-1RA manifested an exaggerated response to a systemic proinflammatory stimulus (intraperitoneal injection of turpentine).

There are two distinct IL-1 receptors, *IL-1RI* and *IL-1RII*. IL-1RI is an 80-kd transmembrane protein with a long cytoplasmic tail. In contrast, IL-1RII, a 60-kd protein, has only a very short cytoplasmic tail and is incapable of signaling. As a consequence, IL-1RII is actually a *decoy receptor* that serves a counter-regulatory role by competing with IL-1RI, the fully functional IL-1 receptor, for IL-1 in the extracellular space. IL-1RI is present on a wide variety of cell types, including T cells, endothelial cells, hepatocytes, and fibroblasts. IL-1RII is the predominant IL-1 receptor found on B cells, monocytes, and neutrophils. The extracellular domains of IL-1RI and IL-1RII are shed by activated neutrophils and monocytes. The shed receptors can act as a sink for secreted IL-1 and, thus, along with IL-1RA, represent an important counter-regulatory component of the inflammatory response.

In 1991, Gay and Keith noted that the cytosolic region of IL-1RI is homologous to a protein, Toll, found in the fruit fly *Drosophila melanogaster*.[8] In the fruit fly, Toll plays a role in both development and host defense against infection. In mammalian cells, a large family of Toll homologues—the IL-1R/Toll-like receptor (TLR) superfamily—are involved in the recognition of microbial components, as well as endogenous ligands induced during the inflammatory response.[1,9] Whereas the cytoplasmic portions of all the members of this superfamily of transmembrane proteins are homologous, the extracellular domains fall into two main subdivisions. In one subdivision, the extracellular portion of the molecule contains three immunoglobulin-like domains and is homologous to the structure of IL-1RI. In the other subdivision, which includes 10 (human) or 11 (mouse) different TLRs (i.e., TLR1 to TLR10), the extracellular domain contains leucine-rich repeats.

One of the members of the TLR family, TLR4, has been shown to be important for the activation of inflammatory cells by LPS (endotoxin), a proinflammatory component of the cell wall of gram-negative bacteria. LPS is a complex glycolipid composed of a polysaccharide tail attached to a lipophilic domain called *lipid A*. The polysaccharide portion of the molecule tends to be structurally different in different species and strains of gram-negative bacteria, whereas the structure of lipid A (as well as a few neighboring sugar residues) is highly conserved across different species and strains of gram-negative microorganisms. A complex of LPS and a serum protein, LPS-binding protein (LBP), initiates the activation of monocytes and macrophages by binding to a surface protein, CD14. Being a glycophosphatidylinositol-anchored membrane protein, CD14 lacks a cytosolic domain and is unable to directly initiate intracellular signaling. Accordingly, investigators sought to identify another protein that presumably participates with CD14 to initiate the cellular response to LPS. The putative LPS coreceptor was ultimately identified as TLR4 by studying an inbred strain of mice, C3H/HeJ, that is congenitally hyporesponsive to endotoxin. Subsequently, TLR4 knockout mice were generated and shown to be as hyporesponsive to LPS as C3H/HeJ mice are, thus confirming the concept that expression of functional TLR4 is necessary for the activation of macrophages and monocytes by endotoxin.[10] TLR4 mutations are also associated with endotoxin hyporesponsiveness in humans.[11] MD-2, another protein that is associated with the extracellular domain of TLR4, is required for LPS responsiveness.

In addition to LPS, other microbial products are recognized by various TLRs. For example, TLR2 recognizes various bacterial lipoproteins, as well as peptidoglycan derived from gram-positive bacteria.[1] TLR5 recognizes flagellin, a 55-kd protein found in the flagella of certain bacteria. TLR9 recognizes certain oligonucleotides containing unmethylated CpG motifs that are more common in bacterial DNA than in mammalian DNA.[1]

Because the cytoplasmic domains of all these TLRs are homologous to the cytoplasmic region of IL-1RI, it is not surprising that shared mechanisms are responsible for downstream signaling (Fig. 4-3). In all cases, an adapter protein, MyD88, links the receptor to another protein called *IL-1 receptor–associated kinase* (IRAK). On binding of the ligand to the TLR (or IL-1RI), IRAK is phosphorylated and dissociates from the receptor complex, thereby allowing it to interact with another signaling protein, *TNF receptor–activated factor 6* (TRAF6). This process results in activation of nuclear factor κB (NF-κB), the key proinflammatory transcription factor, as well as the phosphorylation signaling cascades involving *mitogen-activated protein kinases* (MAPKs).[1]

In the case of activation of this signaling pathway by the binding of IL-1β to IL-1RI, the ligand-receptor interaction does not initiate signal transduction without the association of another transcytoplasmic protein called *IL-1 receptor accessory protein* (IL-1RAcP). Interestingly, the interaction of IL-18 (structurally related to IL-1) with IL-18R (another member of the IL-1R/TLR superfamily) does not trigger downstream signal transduction without the cooperation of a similar accessory protein called *IL-18RAcP* (or AcPL).

TLR4 may also be involved in activation of the innate immune response secondary to tissue injury, even in the

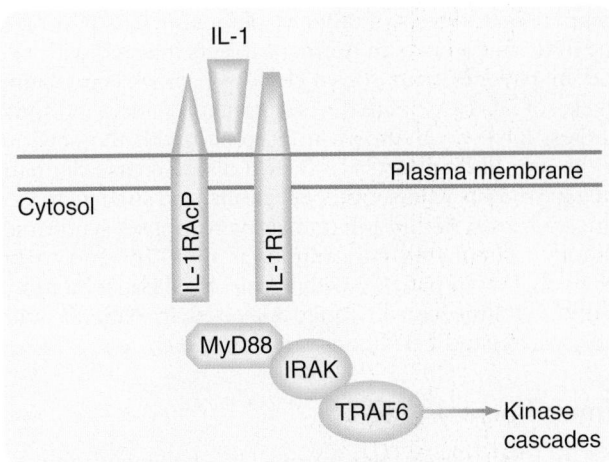

Figure 4-3 Simplified representation of the intracellular signal transduction initiated by the binding of interleukin-1 (IL-1) to its receptor. There are two IL-1 receptors called *IL-1RI* and *IL-1RII*. Only IL-1RI participates in signal transduction, and signaling via this receptor requires the participation of another transcytoplasmic protein called *IL-1 receptor accessory protein* (IL-1RAcP). The interaction of IL-1 with IL-1RI and IL-1RAcP leads to the formation of a trimolecular complex, which in turn results in the docking of yet another protein, called *IL-1 receptor–associated kinase* (IRAK). As a result of its interaction with MyD88, IRAK is phosphorylated and activates another signaling protein, TRAF6. The IRAK/TRAF6 complex activates various downstream kinase cascades, ultimately leading to activation of key transcription factors, such as nuclear factor κB, and transcriptional activation of various IL-1–responsive genes.

absence of infection. Three likely candidates for triggering this pathway for immune cell activation are the proteins heat shock protein 60 (HSP60), HSP70, and high mobility group box 1 (HMGB1). Signaling through TLR4 by these so-called endogenous danger signals is discussed in more detail later in the chapter.

IL-1 is an extremely potent mediator. Injecting healthy humans with as little as 1 ng/kg of recombinant IL-1β induces symptoms. Many IL-1–induced physiologic effects occur as a result of enhanced biosynthesis of other inflammatory mediators, including prostaglandin E$_2$ (PGE$_2$) and NO·. Thus, IL-1 increases expression of the enzyme cyclooxygenase-2 (COX-2) in many cell types, thereby leading to increased production of PGE$_2$. IL-1–induced hyperthermia is mediated by enhanced biosynthesis of PGE$_2$ within the central nervous system and can be blocked by the administration of cyclooxygenase inhibitors. IL-1 induces the enzyme iNOS in vascular smooth muscle cells, as well as other cell types. Induction of iNOS, which leads to increased production of the potent vasodilator NO· in the vascular wall, probably plays a key role in mediating hypotension triggered by the production of IL-1 and other cytokines released in response to LPS or other bacterial products.

Elevated circulating concentrations of IL-1β have been detected in normal human volunteers injected with tiny doses of LPS and in patients with septic shock. However, in subjects with acute endotoxemia or septic shock, circulating concentrations of IL-1β are relatively low in comparison to levels of other cytokines such as IL-6, IL-8, and TNF. In contrast, in normal subjects injected with LPS and in patients with sepsis or septic shock, circulating levels of IL-1RA increase substantially and, in some studies, have been shown to correlate with the severity of disease. Plasma levels of IL-1RII also increase dramatically in patients with serious infections, and such increases can lead to systemic inflammatory response syndrome. Although circulating concentrations of IL-1β tend to be relatively low in patients with sepsis, local concentrations of the cytokine can be quite elevated in patients with sepsis or related conditions such as ARDS.

Tumor Necrosis Factor

TNF was initially obtained from LPS-challenged animals and identified as a serum factor that was capable of killing tumor cells in vitro and causing necrosis of transplantable tumors in mice. The gene coding for the protein was sequenced and cloned shortly thereafter. At about the same time, another protein, named *cachectin,* was identified in supernatants from LPS-stimulated macrophages on the basis of its ability to suppress the expression of lipoprotein lipase and other anabolic hormones in adipocytes. TNF and cachectin were later demonstrated to be the same protein. Administration of a large dose of TNF/cachectin to mice was shown to induce a lethal shocklike state remarkably similar to that induced by the injection of LPS, and passive immunization with antibodies to cachectin/TNF was shown to protect mice from endotoxin-induced mortality. Thus, a modern version of Koch's postulates was satisfied, and TNF/cachectin was identified as a pivotal mediator of endotoxic shock in animals. Gradually, the term cachectin was abandoned; the name TNF has survived. TNF is sometimes called *TNF-α* because it is structurally related to another cytokine that was originally called *TNF-β* but is now generally referred to as LT-α. TNF and LT-α are both members of a large family of ligands that activate a corresponding family of structurally similar receptors. Other members of the TNF family include Fas ligand (FasL), receptor activator of NF-κB ligand (RANKL), CD40 ligand (CD40L) and TNF-related apoptosis-inducing ligand (TRAIL).[12] Although cells of the monocyte/macrophage lineage are the major sources of TNF, other cell types, including mast cells, keratinocytes, T cells, and B cells, are also capable of releasing the cytokine. A wide variety of endogenous and exogenous stimuli can trigger induction of TNF expression (Box 4-1). LT-α is produced by lymphocytes and NK cells.

TNF is initially synthesized as a 26-kd cell surface–associated molecule that is anchored by an N-terminal hydrophobic domain. This membrane-bound form of TNF possesses biologic activity. The membrane-bound form of TNF is cleaved to form a soluble 17-kd form by a specific TNF converting enzyme that is a member of the matrix metalloproteinase family of proteins. Like most of the other members of the TNF family of ligands, the soluble form of TNF exists as a homotrimer, a feature that is important for the cross-linking and activation of TNF receptors.

Box 4-1   Partial List of Stimuli Known to Initiate Release of Tumor Necrosis Factor

Endogenous Factors

Cytokines (TNF-α, IL-1, IFN-γ, GM-CSF, IL-2)
Platelet-activating factor
Myelin P2 protein
HMGB1
HSP70
HSP60

Microbe-Derived Factors

Lipopolysaccharide
Zymosan
Peptidoglycan
Streptococcal pyrogenic exotoxin A
Streptolysin O
Lipoteichoic acid
Staphylococcal enterotoxin B
Staphylococcal toxic shock syndrome toxin-1
Lipoarabinomannan
Bacterial (CpG) DNA
Flagellin

GM-CSF, granulocyte-macrophage colony-stimulating factor; HMGB1, high mobility group box 1; HSP70, heat shock protein 70; IFN-γ, interferon-γ; IL-1, interleukin-1; TNF, tumor necrosis factor.

TNF and LT-α are both capable of binding to two different receptors, TNFR1 (p55) and TNFR2 (p75). Both these receptors, like other receptors in the TNF receptor family, are transmembrane proteins that consist of two identical subunits. The extracellular domains of TNFR1 and TNFR2 are relatively homologous and manifest similar affinity for TNF, but the cytoplasmic regions of the two receptors are distinct. Accordingly, TNFR1 and TNFR2 signal through different pathways. Both receptors are present on most cell types except erythrocytes, but TNFR1 tends to be quantitatively dominant on cells of nonhematopoietic lineage.

The precise functions of the two TNF receptors remain to be elucidated. Nevertheless, considerable information about the roles of TNFR1 and TNFR2 has already been gleaned from experiments using genetically engineered strains of mice lacking one or the other or both of the TNF receptors. TNFR1 knockout mice are relatively resistant to LPS-induced lethality but manifest increased susceptibility to mortality caused by infection with the intracellular pathogens *L. monocytogenes* and *Salmonella typhimurium.* TNFR2 knockout mice are relatively resistant to lethality induced by large doses of recombinant TNF but have an exaggerated circulating TNF response and manifest exacerbated pulmonary inflammation after intravenous (IV) challenge with LPS. Double knockout mice deficient in both TNFR1 and TNFR2 are phenotypically similar to mice lacking only TNFR1.

Most of the members of the TNF family of ligands are involved primarily in the regulation of cellular proliferation or the converse process, programmed cell death (apoptosis). For example, interaction of FasL with the Fas

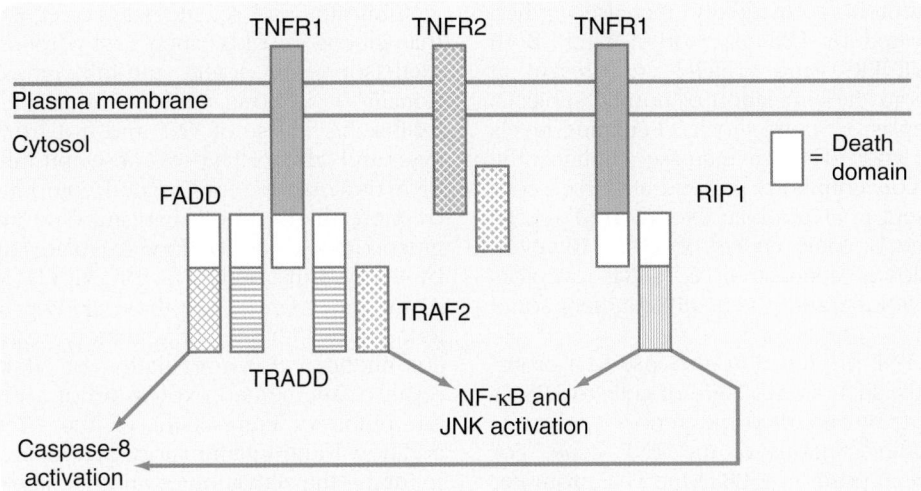

Figure 4-4 Simplified view of intracellular signal transduction events initiated by binding of tumor necrosis factor (TNF) to its cellular receptors. There are two TNF receptors, called *TNFR1* and *TNFR2*. Both receptors are homodimeric transmembrane proteins. Although both TNFR1 and TNFR2 are capable of initiating signal transduction, different pathways are involved. After TNF binds to TNFR1, a number of proteins, including receptor interacting protein (RIP), Fas-associated death domain (FADD), and TNF receptor–associated death domain (TRADD), associate with the receptor. The intracytoplasmic tail of TNFR1 and portions of these other signaling molecules share a highly conserved sequence of about 80 amino acids, which is called the *death domain*. Homotypic interactions among the death domains of these various proteins are essential for formation of the functional signaling complex. After docking to the receptor complex, TRADD recruits other proteins (e.g., TRAF2 and MADD), which in turn initiate protein kinase pathways leading to activation of the nuclear transcription factor NF-κB and the protein kinase c-Jun N-terminal kinase (JNK). TRAF2 can also interact with TNFR2. Association of FADD with the TNFR1 receptor complex leads to activation of the proteolytic enzyme caspase-8, which is the proximal element in a signaling cascade leading to apoptosis (so-called programmed cell death).

receptor is essential for the normal process of apoptosis in T lymphocytes. TNF itself is somewhat different from other members of the TNF family of ligands in that it is both an initiator of apoptosis and a potent proinflammatory mediator. Activation of inflammation by TNF depends, at least in part, on activation of the transcription factor NF-κB. Because activation of NF-κB tends to suppress apoptosis, it is generally necessary to suppress the synthesis of new proteins to observe TNF-mediated induction of apoptosis.

TNF-mediated signaling is initiated by trimerization of receptor subunits. The subsequent downstream events involved in TNF-mediated signaling are different for the two TNF receptors because the cytoplasmic domains for TNFR1 and TNFR2 are distinct. After ligand-induced trimerization of TNFR1, the first protein recruited to the receptor complex is *TNFR1-associated death domain protein* (TRADD). Subsequently, three more proteins are recruited to the receptor complex: *receptor-interacting protein 1* (RIP1), *Fas-associated death domain protein* (FADD), and *TNF receptor–associated factor 2* (TRAF2). When TNFR2 is trimerized after association of the ligand with the receptor, TRAF2 is recruited directly. TRAF1 then associates with TRAF2. The cytoplasmic domains of Fas, TNFRI, FADD, and TRADD all share a highly conserved sequence of about 80 amino acids called the *death domain,* which seems to serve as a mediator of critical protein-protein interactions involved in Fas- and TNFR1-mediated signaling.

The downstream events leading to activation of caspase (i.e., apoptosis) or gene transcription (i.e., inflammation) after recruitment of TRADD or TRAF2, or both, are exceedingly complex. A deliberately oversimplified model is depicted in Figure 4-4. In the proapoptotic pathway, TRADD interacts with FADD, which in turn interacts with a protein called *caspase-8* (also known as *Fas-associated death domain–like IL-1β converting enzyme* [FLICE]), the proximal element in the caspase cascade leading to programmed cell death. In the proinflammatory pathway induced by activation of TNFR1 or TNFR2, TRAF2 plays a central role in the early events that lead to activation of NF-κB and two important MAPK pathways, namely, those involving the proteins p38 MAPK and *c-Jun N-terminal kinase* (JNK). Overexpression of TRAF2 in engineered cells is sufficient to activate signaling pathways leading to activation of NF-κB, as well as another proinflammatory transcription factor, *activator protein-1* (AP-1).[12] By triggering the association of FADD with the receptor complex, the interaction of FasL with Fas directly leads to the induction of apoptosis, whereas recruitment of FADD to the TNF/TNFR1 receptor complex requires an adaptor protein, TRADD, and thus initiates apoptotic processes less directly. Furthermore, the FasL/Fas interaction does not lead to activation of NF-κB, whereas signaling through NF-κB can apparently be initiated by TNF through more than one pathway (TRAF2 and RIP1).[12]

The extracellular domains of TNFR1 and TNFR2 are constitutively released by monocytes, and release of these soluble receptors is markedly increased when the cells are activated by LPS or phorbol ester. Both soluble TNFR1 (sTNFR1) and sTNFR2 are present at low concentrations in the circulation of normal subjects. In patients with sepsis or septic shock, circulating levels of both sTNF-R1 and sTNF-R2 increase significantly. Moreover, higher concentrations portend a worse prognosis.[13] When present in great molar excess, sTNF receptors can inhibit the biologic effects of TNF. However, when present at lower concentrations, sTNF receptors can stabilize the cytokine and potentially augment some of its actions.

The amount of TNF produced in response to a proinflammatory stimulus, such as exposure of cells to LPS, is determined, in part, by inherited differences (polymorphisms) in noncoding regions of the TNF gene. For example, if the base at position −308 in the TNF promoter is adenine (A), in vitro spontaneous and stimulated TNF production by monocytes is greater than if the base at this position is guanine (G). The more common allelic form of the TNF gene (*TNF1*) has guanine at position −308, whereas the less common allele (*TNF2*) has adenine at this position. Some studies suggest that presence of the *TNF2* allele markedly increases the risk for mortality in patients with septic shock,[14] although other data dispute this notion. Interestingly, a G-to-A substitution at position +250 in the LT-α gene is likewise associated with increased production of TNF by stimulated mononuclear cells, and patients carrying this allele are also at higher risk for mortality from septic shock. In patients with community-acquired pneumonia (a relatively homogeneous population of patients with infection), the risk for development of septic shock is greatest for those who are homozygous for the so-called high TNF secretor genotype (i.e., AA) at position +250 in the LT-α gene.[15] Data such as these suggest that genotyping of patients may prove to be valuable in the coming years for tailoring anticytokine and other forms of adjuvant therapy for critically ill patients.

Interleukin-1 and Tumor Necrosis Factor as Targets for Anti-inflammatory Therapeutic Agents

In view of the central importance of IL-1 and TNF as mediators of the inflammatory response, investigators have regarded blocking the production or the actions of these cytokines as a reasonable strategy for treating a variety of conditions associated with excessive or poorly controlled inflammation. Though clearly different in many respects from sepsis in humans, the shocklike syndrome induced in rodents by injecting LPS IV or intraperitoneally has served as a useful paradigm for evaluating various anti-inflammatory strategies. In this model system, survival is improved when animals are treated with any one of a variety of different pharmacologic, immunologic, or genetic strategies that either block the release of TNF or prevent this cytokine from interacting with its receptors after it is released. To a lesser extent, the same statement also applies to IL-1.

Clinicians and scientists have recognized for decades that glucocorticoids, such as hydrocortisone and dexamethasone, are potent anti-inflammatory agents. Additionally, it is now well established that corticosteroids inhibit the release of TNF and IL-1 from activated monocytes and other cell types. These anti-inflammatory actions of hydrocortisone and related compounds are mediated by more than one mechanism. One important action of glucocorticoids is to down-regulate signaling mediated by a key transcription factor, NF-κB, known to activate many genes (including those coding for TNF and IL-1) associated with the inflammatory response. Glucocorticoid-induced down-regulation of NF-κB activation is a result of augmented expression of a protein, IκB, that is an inhibitory component of the NF-κB complex. An additional anti-inflammatory action of glucocorticoids is to inhibit the activation of another signaling pathway, the JNK/SAPK cascade, which leads to decreased translation of TNF mRNA and thus decreased production of TNF. Still another mechanism whereby glucocorticoids inhibit inflammation is through decreased expression of the enzyme ICE, required for post-translational processing of pro–IL-1β, and thus decreased secretion of mature IL-1β.

In experimental models of sepsis, early treatment with high doses of a potent synthetic glucocorticoid, such as methylprednisolone or dexamethasone, improves survival. Unfortunately, several large clinical trials failed to confirm the benefit of high-dose glucocorticoid therapy for the adjuvant treatment of patients with septic shock or the related condition ARDS.[16-18] As a result, the notion of using glucocorticoids for these indications seemed to be a dead issue. However, the concept of using glucocorticoids as anti-inflammatory agents in the management of ARDS or septic shock has been resurrected. Several small studies have shown that prolonged therapy with relatively low doses of hydrocortisone or methylprednisolone can improve systemic hemodynamics or pulmonary function, or both, in patients with ARDS or septic shock.[19,20] These findings were confirmed by the results obtained in a 300-patient multicentric randomized clinical trial carried out in a single country (France).[21] Though somewhat controversial, the results of this study support the view that administration of a relatively low dose of hydrocortisone (50 mg IV every 6 hours for 7 days) improves survival in patients with volume-unresponsive pressor-dependent septic shock and an inadequate cortisol response to an injection of adrenocorticotropic hormone (ACTH). It is not clear whether hydrocortisone is effective in this setting because many patients with septic shock are functionally adrenally insufficient (i.e., hydrocortisone is functioning as replacement therapy) or because administration of the glucocorticoid modulates the inflammatory response. Of course, these two potential mechanisms are not mutually exclusive. Although some earlier studies suggested that administration of corticosteroids might be beneficial in the late (so-called fibroproliferative) phase of ARDS, results from a multicentric randomized trial refute this notion.[22]

Glucocorticoids are a broad-spectrum and nonselective way to block IL-1– or TNF-mediated proinflammatory effects. As our understanding of the role of cytokines as mediators of inflammation has progressed, newer and more specific pharmacologic anti-inflammatory strategies have been developed and evaluated as adjunctive therapy for the treatment of sepsis in placebo-controlled prospective clinical trials. Unfortunately, results in these trials were disappointing. Positive results were obtained in only a single study, an open-label trial of recombinant IL-1RA that enrolled a relatively small number of patients. With the exception of this study, none of the agents tested significantly improved survival. Indeed, in one trial, treatment of septic patients with a so-called fusion protein incorporating the extracellular domain of TNFR2 resulted in increased mortality, particularly in patients with gram-positive infection.[23]

Despite the negative results obtained in sepsis trials, several agents designed to neutralize the effects of secreted TNF[24] or IL-1β[25] revealed significant clinical efficacy in other important inflammatory conditions such as Crohn's disease and rheumatoid arthritis. Infliximab, a monoclonal anti-TNF antibody, has been approved by the FDA for administration to patients to provide long-term remission-level control of the debilitating symptoms of Crohn's disease. Infliximab was approved for use, in combination with methotrexate, to reduce the signs and symptoms, inhibit the progression of structural damage, and improve physical function in patients with moderately to severely active rheumatoid arthritis who have had an inadequate response to methotrexate. Adalimumab, another monoclonal anti-TNF antibody, was approved by the FDA for administration with or without methotrexate to patients with rheumatoid arthritis to ameliorate symptoms and disability. Etanercept, the TNFR2 fusion protein evaluated unsuccessfully for the treatment of sepsis, has been approved by the FDA for the management of psoriatic arthritis; it can reduce the signs and symptoms and inhibit the progression of structural damage in patients with moderately to severely active rheumatoid arthritis, as well as reduce the signs and symptoms in patients 4 years and older with moderately to severely active polyarticular-course juvenile rheumatoid arthritis. Anakinra (recombinant human IL-1RA) was approved by the FDA for administration alone or with other drugs (except TNF-modifying agents) to reduce the symptoms and modify the progression of structural damage in patients with moderate or severe rheumatoid arthritis who have failed one or more other disease-modifying antirheumatic drugs. TNF expression is up-regulated in patients with severe asthma, and etanercept has been shown to decrease bronchial hyperreactivity in this condition.[26] Thus, cytokine-specific approaches to managing inflammatory conditions moved from the research bench to the clinic and occupy an important role in the clinical management of common clinical conditions, even though this approach has not yet panned out for the treatment of sepsis and septic shock.

The network of cytokines associated with the inflammatory response interacts at multiple points with another component of the host's defense against injury and infection, namely, the coagulation system. Thrombosis and coagulation help contain the invading organisms to a limited area. TNF, IL-1, and IL-6 (as well as some other proinflammatory cytokines) can activate the extrinsic pathway of coagulation, in part by promoting expression of tissue factor (TF), a transmembrane 45-kd protein, on endothelial cells and monocytes. In addition, these cytokines also down-regulate the expression of an important endogenous inhibitor of coagulation, thrombomodulin, on the surface of endothelial cells. Thus, TNF, IL-1, and IL-6 promote activation of the coagulation cascade. Numerous studies have documented that the extrinsic coagulation pathway is activated in patients with sepsis, even in the absence of frank, clinically evident disseminated intravascular coagulation (DIC).

Key components of the coagulation cascade are a group of proteins that function as endogenous anticoagulants and thus help provide counter-regulatory balance to the system. It is therefore noteworthy that the inflammatory response leads to not only TF-mediated activation of coagulation but also down-regulation of these natural anticoagulant pathways. The result is a hypercoagulable state that in its most severe form is characterized by DIC.

Three major anticoagulant pathways exist and all can be inhibited by the inflammatory cascade: antithrombin, the protein C system, and TF pathway inhibitor. Antithrombin is a serine protease inhibitor that antagonizes thrombin and factor Xa. During severe inflammatory responses, antithrombin levels are markedly decreased as the result of consumption, impaired synthesis (negative acute phase response), and degradation by elastase from activated neutrophils.

Protein C is activated by thrombin bound to thrombomodulin. During systemic inflammation, protein C levels are reduced because of impaired synthesis and degradation by neutrophil elastase. Furthermore, the protein C system is inhibited by decreased expression of thrombomodulin induced by TNF and IL-1β. In addition to its role in regulating coagulation, the protein C system also modulates the inflammatory response. Activated protein C binds to the endothelial protein C receptor. Activation of this signaling pathway inhibits LPS-induced NF-κB nuclear translocation and thereby inhibits secretion of TNF, IL-1β, IL-6, and IL-8 by monocytes.

Circulating levels of protein C decrease in patients with severe sepsis or septic shock, and a marked deficiency of protein C in these patients is a prognostic indicator for an unfavorable outcome. Various strategies to inhibit excessive activation of the coagulation system were extensively evaluated both in animal models of endotoxemia and sepsis and in clinical trials. One of these approaches, the administration of recombinant human activated protein C, also called *drotrecogin alfa (activated)*, was shown in a large multicentric randomized clinical trial to significantly improve survival in patients with severe sepsis.[27] Drotrecogin alfa (activated) has been approved for this indication by the FDA. Understandably, bleeding complications can occur with the use of drotrecogin alfa (activated). Furthermore, this agent was not beneficial for septic patients with an Acute Physiology and Chronic Health Evaluation II (APACHE II) score lower than 25, postoperative patients with single–

organ system dysfunction,[28] or pediatric patients with severe sepsis.[29]

INTERLEUKIN-6 AND INTERLEUKIN-11

IL-6 and IL-11 warrant consideration together because along with several other proteins (e.g., oncostatin M), both these cytokines use a specific transmembrane protein, gp130, for receptor function. IL-6 consists of 184 amino acids plus a 28–amino acid hydrophobic signal sequence. The protein is variably phosphorylated and glycosylated before secretion. IL-11 is translated as a precursor protein containing 199 amino acids, including a 21–amino acid leader sequence.

Like IL-1 and TNF, IL-6 is a pluripotent cytokine intimately associated with the inflammatory response to injury or infection. IL-6 can be produced not only by immunocytes (e.g., monocytes, macrophages, and lymphocytes) but also by many other cell types, including endothelial cells and intestinal epithelial cells. Factors known to induce expression of IL-6 include IL-1, TNF, platelet-activating factor, LPS, and reactive oxygen metabolites. The promoter region of the IL-6 gene contains functional elements capable of binding NF-κB, as well as another important transcription factor, CCAAT/enhancer binding protein (C/EBP), previously called *NF–IL-6*. The cellular and physiologic effects of IL-6 are diverse and include induction of fever, promotion of B-cell maturation and differentiation, stimulation of T-cell proliferation and differentiation, promotion of differentiation of nerve cells, stimulation of the hypothalamic-pituitary-adrenal axis, and induction of the synthesis of acute phase proteins (e.g., C-reactive protein) by hepatocytes. Plasmacytosis and hypergammaglobulinemia develop in transgenic mice that overexpress IL-6. Conversely, IL-6 knockout mice have an impaired acute phase response to inflammatory stimuli, abnormal B-cell maturation, deficient mucosal IgA production, and impaired host resistance to the intracellular pathogen *L. monocytogenes*. In other murine models of inflammation, the effects of genetic IL-6 deficiency proved highly variable. For example, in a murine model of acute pancreatitis induced by repetitive injections of cerulein, inflammation was exacerbated in IL-6 knockout mice as compared with wild-type controls, a finding that emphasizes the anti-inflammatory effects of IL-6.[30] In contrast, in a murine model of hemorrhagic shock and resuscitation, IL-6 knockout mice exhibited less pulmonary inflammation and lung and gut mucosal injury than wild-type controls did, findings that emphasize the proinflammatory effects of IL-6.[31] Although IL-6 knockout mice were not protected from the lethal effects of sepsis, treatment of septic wild-type mice with a carefully calibrated dose of an anti–IL-6 antibody improved survival.

IL-11 is expressed in a variety of cell types, including neurons, fibroblasts, and epithelial cells. Although constitutive expression of IL-11 can be detected in a range of normal adult tissues, expression of IL-11 can also be up-regulated by IL-1, TGF-β, and other cytokines or growth factors. Regulation of IL-11 expression is under both transcriptional and translational control. From a functional standpoint, IL-11 is a hematopoietic growth factor with particular activity as a stimulator of megakaryocytopoiesis and thrombopoiesis. IL-11 can also interact with epithelial cells in the gastrointestinal tract and inhibit the proliferation of enterocytic cell lines in vitro.

The mechanisms whereby IL-6– or IL-11–induced signals are transduced in target cells have been studied extensively. Activation of target cells via the IL-6 or IL-11 receptor complexes requires the cooperation of two distinct proteins. In the case of IL-6, the ligand-binding subunit is called *IL-6R*, whereas in the case of IL-11, the ligand-binding subunit is called *IL-11R*. For both receptors, a distinct protein, called *gp130*, is required for signal transduction. Intracellular signal transduction involves association of the IL-6/IL-6R complex or the IL-11/IL-11R complex with gp130. Dimerization of gp130 leads to downstream signaling via members of the JAK family of protein tyrosine kinases. JAK kinase activation in turn leads to phosphorylation and activation of STAT3, a member of the STAT family of signaling proteins. Phosphorylation of STAT proteins leads to dimerization, translocation to the nucleus, binding to DNA, and transcriptional activation.

Circulating concentrations of IL-6 increase dramatically after tissue injury, for example, as a consequence of elective surgical procedures, accidental trauma, or burns. Elevated plasma levels of IL-6 are consistently observed in patients with sepsis or septic shock. The degree to which circulating IL-6 levels are elevated after tissue trauma or during sepsis has been shown to correlate with the risk for postinjury complications or death. Although it remains to be established whether high circulating IL-6 levels are directly or indirectly injurious to patients with sepsis or are simply a marker of the severity of illness, the observation that immunoneutralization of IL-6 improves outcome in experimental bacterial peritonitis suggests that elevated concentrations of this cytokine are deleterious.

Circulating levels of IL-11 increase in patients with DIC and sepsis. IV or oral administration of recombinant IL-11 improves survival in neutropenic rodents with sepsis, possibly by preserving the integrity of the intestinal mucosal barrier.[32]

INTERLEUKIN-8 AND OTHER CHEMOKINES

Chemotaxis is the term used to denote the directed migration of cells toward increasing concentrations of an activating substance (chemotaxin). The ability to recruit leukocytes to an inflammatory focus by promoting chemotaxis is the primary biologic activity of a special group of cytokines called *chemokines*. More than 40 of these small proteins have been identified. Each contains about 70 to 80 amino acids, including three or four conserved cysteine residues. Four chemokine subgroups have been described. The subgroups are defined by the degree of separation of the first two NH2-terminal cysteine residues. In the CXC or α-chemokines, the first two cysteine moieties are separated by a single nonconserved amino acid residue, whereas in the CC or β-chemokines, the NH$_2$-terminal cysteines are directly adjacent to each other. The C chemokine subgroup is characterized by the presence of only a single NH$_2$-terminal cysteine moiety. The CX$_3$C subgroup has only one member (fractalkine); in this chemokine, the NH$_2$-terminal cysteine residues are separated by three intervening amino acids. A subclass of the CXC chemokines, exemplified by IL-8, contains a characteristic amino acid sequence (glutamate-leucine-arginine) near the NH$_2$-terminal end of the protein; these chemokines act primarily on PMNs. Other chemokines, including the CC chemokines and members of CXC subgroup not containing the glutamate-leucine-arginine sequence, act, for the most part, on monocytes, macrophages, lymphocytes, or eosinophils. Many different cell types are capable of secreting chemokines; cells of the monocyte-macrophage lineage and endothelial cells are particularly important in this regard. Numerous proinflammatory stimuli, including cytokines such as TNF and IL-1 and bacterial products such as LPS, can stimulate the production of chemokines.

IL-8, the prototypical CXC chemokine, was first identified as a chemotactic protein by Yoshimura and associates in 1987.[33] IL-8 is translated as a 99–amino acid precursor and is secreted after cleavage of a 20–amino acid leader sequence. In addition to attracting neutrophils along a chemotactic gradient, IL-8 also activates these cells by triggering degranulation, increased expression of surface adhesion molecules, and the production of reactive oxygen metabolites. There are at least two distinct IL-8 receptors: CXCR1 (IL-8R1) and CXCR2 (IL-8R2). CXCR1 is predominantly expressed on neutrophils. Like other chemokine receptors, CXCR1 and CXCR2 are coupled to G proteins, and binding of ligand to these receptors leads to intracellular signal transduction via the generation of inositol triphosphate, activation of protein kinase C, and perturbations in intracellular ionized calcium concentrations.

Increased circulating concentrations of IL-8 were detected in experimental animal models of infection or endotoxemia and in patients with sepsis.[34] Treatment of experimental animals with antibodies against IL-8 improves survival or prevents pulmonary injury in models of sepsis or ischemia/reperfusion injury.[35] These observations support the view that IL-8–mediated activation of neutrophils plays an important role in the pathogenesis of organ system damage in these syndromes.

Monocyte chemotactic protein-1 (MCP-1), the prototypical CC chemokine, was identified in the same year by two groups of investigators. MCP-1 is a chemotaxin for monocytes (but not neutrophils) and also activates monocytes by triggering the production of reactive oxygen metabolites and the expression of β$_2$ integrins (cell surface adhesion molecules). Elevated circulating concentrations of MCP-1 have been detected in endotoxemic mice and patients with sepsis. Pretreatment of mice with a polyclonal anti–MCP-1 antiserum ameliorates LPS-induced lung injury, thus suggesting an important role for this chemokine in the pathogenesis of sepsis-induced ARDS.

INTERLEUKIN-12

IL-12, a cytokine produced primarily by antigen-presenting cells, is a heterodimeric protein composed of two disulfide-linked peptides (p35 and p40) that are encoded by distinct genes. Both subunits are required for biologic activity. The IL-12 receptor is expressed on T cells and NK cells. The most important biologic activity associated with IL-12 is to promote T$_H$1 responses by helper T cells. In this regard, IL-12 promotes the differentiation of naive T cells into T$_H$1 cells capable of producing IFN-γ after activation and serves to augment IFN-γ secretion by T$_H$1 cells responding to an antigenic stimulus. Stimulation of IFN-γ production by IL-12 can be synergistically enhanced by the presence of other proinflammatory cytokines, notably TNF, IL-1, or IL-2. Conversely, counter-regulatory cytokines, such as IL-4 and IL-10, are capable of inhibiting IL-12–induced IFN-γ secretion.

The immunologic responses governed by T$_H$1 cells are central to the development of cell-mediated immunity necessary for appropriate host resistance to intracellular pathogens. It is not surprising, therefore, that transgenic mice deficient in IL-12 manifest increased susceptibility to infections caused by a number of intracellular pathogens, including *Mycobacterium avium* and *Cryptococcus neoformans*.

IL-12 may be a key factor in some of the deleterious inflammatory responses to LPS and gram-negative bacteria. Elevated circulating levels of IL-12 were measured in endotoxemic mice and baboons infused with viable *Escherichia coli*. Elevated plasma levels of IL-12 were also detected in children with meningococcal septic shock and were correlated with outcome. However, in patients with postoperative sepsis, circulating IL-12 levels were lower than those in control subjects without sepsis and did not correlate with outcome.[36] Defective production of IL-12 by peripheral blood mononuclear cells after stimulation with IFN-γ and LPS is associated with an increased risk for the development of postoperative sepsis in preoperative patients.[37]

IL-12 has also been implicated in the pathogenesis of IBD. T cells eluted from the lamina propria of intestinal resection specimens from patients with Crohn's disease secrete cytokines consistent with a T$_H$1-like profile. In addition, IL-12–secreting macrophages are present in large numbers in tissue specimens from patients with Crohn's disease but are rare in histologic sections from appropriate control subjects. Treatment with anti–IL-12 antibodies ameliorates the severity of disease in certain murine models of IBD. Treatment of patients with refractory IBD with thalidomide, a potent anti-inflammatory agent, decreases the production of both TNF and IL-12 by mononuclear cells isolated from the lamina propria of gut mucosal biopsy samples and decreases disease activity.[38]

Although excessive production of IL-12 has been implicated in the pathogenesis of acute inflammatory conditions such as septic shock and chronic inflammatory states such as Crohn's disease, adequate production of IL-12 appears to be essential for orchestration of the normal host response to infection. When antibodies to

IL-12 are administered to mice with fecal peritonitis induced by cecal ligation and perforation, mortality is increased and clearance of the bacterial load is impaired. Conversely, pretreatment or even post-treatment with recombinant IL-12 has been shown to improve survival in a murine model of bacterial peritonitis.[39]

INTERLEUKIN-18

IL-18 is structurally related to IL-1β and is functionally a member of the T_H1-inducing family of cytokines. Like IL-1β, IL-18 is translated in the form of a precursor protein (pro–IL-18). This precursor molecule requires cleavage by the same converting enzyme that activates IL-1β (i.e., ICE) to form biologically active IL-18. The two cytokines, IL-1β and IL-18, are also similar with respect to the way that intracellular signaling occurs after association of the cytokine with its receptor on target cells. Binding of IL-18 to its receptor initiates a cascade of events that involves participation by a number of the same accessory proteins required for IL-1β–induced signaling, including IRAK, TRAF6, and MyD88.

IL-18 is constitutively expressed by human peripheral blood mononuclear cells and murine intestinal epithelial cells, but IL-18 production can also be stimulated by a variety of proinflammatory microbial products. The main biologic activity of IL-18 is to induce production of IFN-γ by T cells and NK cells. In this regard, IL-18 acts most potently as a co-stimulant in combination with IL-12. Indeed, IL-12–induced IFN-γ expression appears to depend on the presence of IL-18 inasmuch as transgenic mice (or cells from mice) deficient in IL-18 or ICE produce little IFN-γ in response to appropriate stimulation, even in the presence of ample IL-12.[40] In addition to stimulating IFN-γ production, IL-18 induces the production of CC and CXC chemokines from human mononuclear cells and activates neutrophils, an effect that may contribute to organ injury and dysfunction in conditions such as sepsis and ARDS. Circulating concentrations of IL-18 are higher in patients with sepsis than in those with just injuries, and high levels of this cytokine are associated with a fatal outcome in patients with postoperative sepsis.[41]

INTERLEUKIN-4, INTERLEUKIN-10, AND INTERLEUKIN-13

IL-4, IL-10, and IL-13 can be regarded as *inhibitory, anti-inflammatory,* or *counter-regulatory* cytokines. All three of these cytokines are produced by T_H2 cells and, among other roles, serve to modulate the production and effects of proinflammatory cytokines such as TNF and IL-1.

IL-4, originally described as a B-cell growth factor, is a 15- to 20-kd glycoprotein that is synthesized by T_H2 cells, mast cells, basophils, and eosinophils. IL-4 has many biologic actions that promote expression of the T_H2 phenotype, characterized by down-regulation of proinflammatory and cell-mediated immune responses and up-regulation of humoral (B-cell–mediated) immune responses. IL-4 induces differentiation of CD4$^+$ T cells into T_H2 cells and, conversely, down-regulates differentiation of CD4$^+$ T cells into T_H1 cells. IL-4 inhibits the production of TNF, IL-1, IL-8, and PGE$_2$ by stimulated monocytes or macrophages and down-regulates endothelial cell activation induced by TNF. IL-4 acts as a comitogen for B cells and promotes expression of the class II major histocompatibility complex (MHC) on B cells.

IL-10, originally called *cytokine synthesis inhibitory factor,* was first isolated from supernatants of cultures of activated T cells. This cytokine is an 18-kd protein that is produced primarily by T_H2 cells, but it is also released by activated monocytes and other cell types. IL-10 acts to down-regulate the inflammatory response through numerous mechanisms. For example, IL-10 inhibits the production of numerous proinflammatory cytokines, including IL-1, TNF, IL-6, IL-8, IL-12, and GM-CSF, by monocytes and macrophages; on the other hand, it increases synthesis of the counter-regulatory cytokine IL-1RA by activated monocytes. In addition, IL-10 down-regulates the proliferation and secretion of IFN-γ and IL-2 by activated T_H1 cells, primarily by inhibiting the production of IL-12 by macrophages or other accessory cells. Conversely, IFN-γ down-regulates IL-10 production by monocytes. At least some of the inhibitory effects of IL-10 are mediated by blocking IFN-γ–induced tyrosine phosphorylation of STAT1α, a key protein in the signal transduction pathway for IFN-γ.

The importance of IL-10 as a regulatory cytokine was illustrated in experiments using transgenic mice deficient in IL-10. Such animals manifest increased resistance to the intracellular bacterial pathogen *L. monocytogenes,* thus suggesting that IL-10–mediated suppression of the T_H1-type phenotype can impair the host's ability to eradicate certain types of infection. In contrast to these results, IL-10 knockout mice succumbed to the lethal effects of excessive inflammation when infected with another intracellular pathogen, the protozoan parasite *Toxoplasma gondii.* Results have been variable in mice with severe sepsis, but a genetic deficiency of IL-10 production most likely alters the kinetics of the inflammatory process without affecting long-term survival.[42] In IL-10–deficient mice, a form of enterocolitis spontaneously develops that is reminiscent of IBD in humans. Because the IBD-like syndrome in these animals can be suppressed by treating the animals with either exogenous IL-10 or a neutralizing anti–IFN-γ antibody, the enterocolitis associated with IL-10 deficiency is thought to be caused by excessive expression of the T_H1-type phenotype.

Production of IL-10 by peripheral blood mononuclear cells and CD4$^+$ T cells is increased in trauma patients, and elevated circulating concentrations of this cytokine have been measured in patients with trauma or sepsis. Moreover, in trauma and burn patients, increased production of IL-10 has been associated with a greater risk for serious infection and, in patients with sepsis, a greater risk for mortality or shock. These findings support the view that although excessive production of proinflammatory mediators may be deleterious in trauma and sepsis, development of the T_H2 phenotype, characterized by increased production of IL-10 and IL-4 and decreased expression of the MHC type II antigen HLA-DR on monocytes, may lead to excessive immunosuppression and deleteriously affect the outcome on this basis. Evidence has been presented supporting the view that HLA-DR expression on monocytes is post-translationally down-regulated by IL-10 in patients with sepsis.[43]

Administering exogenous IL-10 in an effort to blunt excessive inflammation has led to mixed results in experimental models of sepsis or septic shock. In models in which experimental animals are challenged with IV LPS, treatment with recombinant IL-10 ameliorates fever and improves survival. In models such as cecal ligation and perforation wherein the sepsis syndrome is induced by infection with viable bacteria, administration of exogenous IL-10 is either beneficial[44] or without effect.[45] However, in mice with pneumonia caused by *Pseudomonas aeruginosa*, survival is improved when the animals are treated with an anti–IL-10 antibody to neutralize endogenous IL-10.[46] Thus, although the use of recombinant IL-10 as an adjuvant treatment of sepsis is appealing, caution will need to be exercised in the design and conduct of clinical trials because excessive immunosuppression could adversely affect antibacterial defense mechanisms.

IL-13 is 12-kd protein closely related to IL-4. The two proteins have about 25% homology and share many structural characteristics. IL-13 is produced by T_H2 cells and also undifferentiated CD4[+] T cells and CD8[+] T cells. The IL-13 receptor consists of two chains, one of which binds IL-4 but not IL-13, and another that binds IL-13 with high affinity. Binding of either IL-4 or IL-13 to their respective receptors induces signaling by activating the same JAK kinases, JAK1 and Tyk2. IL-4, but not IL-13, also activates JAK3. The biologic activities of IL-13 are very similar to those of IL-4 with respect to B-cell function, although unlike IL-4, IL-13 does not have any direct affects on T cells. IL-13 down-regulates the production of proinflammatory cytokines (e.g., IL-1, TNF, IL-6, IL-8, IL-12, G-CSF, GM-CSF, and MIP-1α) and PGE_2 by activated monocytes and macrophages and, by the same token, increases the production of anti-inflammatory proteins, including IL-1RA and IL-1RII, from these cells. Additional anti-inflammatory properties of IL-13 include inhibition of induction of the enzyme COX-2, required for the production of prostaglandins, and induction of an enzyme, 15-lipoxygenase, that catalyzes the formation of a lipid mediator (lipoxin A4) with anti-inflammatory properties. Treatment of mice with recombinant IL-13 has been shown to prevent LPS-induced lethality and to decrease circulating levels of TNF and other proinflammatory cytokines.[47] Conversely, treatment of septic mice with an anti–IL-13 antibody has been shown to increase mortality.[48]

TRANSFORMING GROWTH FACTOR-β

The TGF-β family of mediators exerts a number of effects on most cell types, including modulation of cell growth, inflammation, matrix synthesis, and apoptosis. Although more than 45 peptides in the TGF-β family have been isolated, TGF-β1 was the first identified and is the isoform most associated with modulation of immune function. The bioactive forms of the TGF-β proteins are produced from 50-kd monomers that dimerize to form the 100-kd TGF-β precursor. The TGF-β precursor undergoes intracellular cleavage by furin proteases to yield the active 25-kd TGF-β homodimer. This active TGF-β remains associated with the remaining portion of its pro-form, latency-associated peptide (LAP). This complex has been called *latent TGF-β* and is secreted in this inactive form into the extracellular matrix. This unusual mode of secretion allows the latent TGF-β complex to be considered an extracellular sensor. Latent TGF-β can be activated by the disassociation and degradation of LAP via proteolysis (catalyzed by plasmin or matrix metallopeptidases) or the nonenzymatic activity of integrins, thrombospondin-1, oxygen and nitrogen free radicals, or low pH. These activating factors are often perturbations of the extracellular matrix that are associated with phenomena such as angiogenesis, wound repair, inflammation, or cell growth. Thus, post-translational extracellular activation of TGF-β is the most important regulatory mechanism for this cytokine, a mode of activation that is unique among the cytokines.

Once activated, TGF-β–mediated signaling involves a cell surface heteromeric complex of transmembrane serine/threonine kinase receptors. Each receptor complex contains a pair of both TGF-β type I (TβRI) and type II (TβRII) receptors, which are activated by TGF-β binding and are regulated by a number of intracellular proteins that directly interact with the receptor complex in either a constitutive or ligand-induced manner. The intracellular signal transduction pathway responsible for gene induction or repression involves a family of structurally related proteins termed Smads. TGF-β receptor–activated Smads are phosphorylated by TβRI, form a heterotrimeric complex with the common partner Smad4, and translocate to the nucleus where they can either repress or activate transcription. From multiple studies using transgenic and knockout mice, TGF-β1 was found to play an important role in leukocyte development and function, wound healing, inflammation, suppression of tumorigenesis, and organogenesis and homeostasis in liver, kidney, pancreas, and lung tissues, among others. Furthermore, TGF-β1 administration reduces LPS-induced hypotension and mortality in a murine model of sepsis, and in trauma patients, lower circulating TGF-β1 levels are associated with the development of liver and kidney dysfunction, whereas higher TGF-β1 circulating levels 6 hours after admission to the intensive care unit are associated with an increased risk for sepsis.[49]

MACROPHAGE MIGRATION INHIBITORY FACTOR

Macrophage migration inhibitory factor (MIF) was the first functional cytokine described. MIF is produced by monocytes and macrophages and acts in an autocrine and paracrine fashion to activate various cell types during inflammation. Immunostimulated macrophages secrete MIF. MIF appears to function proximally in the inflammatory cascade because MIF knockout mice exhibit a global reduction in the production of other inflammatory mediators such as TNF, IL-1β, and PGE₂.[50]

MIF is encoded by a unique gene that displays very high sequence conservation across species. MIF is constitutively expressed, and after translation, preformed MIF remains in cytoplasmic pools and is readily released from macrophages after inflammatory stimulation. The rapid release of preformed MIF is unlike most other cytokines, which are typically released after transcriptional activation and translation of new protein. The receptor for MIF, CD74, is also distinct from the other cytokine receptor superfamilies.

Apoptosis is an important mechanism for resolution of the inflammatory response via the removal of activated monocytes and macrophages, and the proinflammatory action of MIF is due, in part, to suppression of apoptosis. MIF also up-regulates the expression of TLR4 on macrophages, thereby amplifying the response of the innate immune system to LPS (and possibly other proinflammatory substances such as HMGB1). Circulating MIF levels are increased in patients with sepsis and septic shock, but not in noninfected trauma patients.[51] In mice with peritonitis, treatment with a neutralizing anti-MIF antibody improves survival.[52]

COMPLEMENT

Complement was first identified as a heat-labile component in serum that complemented the function of humoral immunity in the killing of microorganisms. Rather than a single factor, complement is a complex system of more than 30 plasma and membrane-bound proteins. The nomenclature used to describe the multiple elements in the complement cascade follows their order of discovery rather than their sequential activation. Complement functions in consort with proteins of the coagulation, fibrinolysis, and kinin systems to augment the response to pathogenic stimuli via a series of catalytic reactions. The complement system is evolutionarily well preserved, thus suggesting that it represents a common ancestral host defense system. Although the complement system plays a key role in the host's defense against pathogenic microbes, dysregulated activation of the complement cascade can be deleterious and excessive complement activation has been implicated in the pathogenesis of a wide variety of immune and inflammatory conditions ranging from ARDS and sepsis to asthma.[53]

Activation of complement occurs via three distinct pathways: the classical pathway is activated by antigen-antibody (IgG or IgM) complexes, the alternative pathway is initiated by recognition of certain bacterial cell surface markers such as LPS, and the lectin-binding pathway is activated by detection of bacterial surface sugars such as mannose (Fig. 4-5). Most of the complement proteins circulate in inactive form until they are cleaved by an

upstream protease, which in turn activates their proteolytic activity. Thus, sequential activation of catalytically active proteins produces an escalating cascade of activity (similar to the coagulation system). Regardless of the activation pathway, the most important active products are the anaphylatoxins C3a and C5a and the membrane attack complex C5b-C9, which causes lysis of gram-negative bacteria. C3a induces the release of histamine from mast cells and causes smooth muscle cell contraction. C5a binds to its receptor (C5aR) on neutrophils and macrophages and triggers intracellular signaling, chemotaxis, enzyme release, and the generation of ROS, which participate in the killing of microorganisms.

Activation of the classical pathway is triggered by the interaction of antigen-antibody complexes with C1, which is a 790-kd complex composed of a recognition protein C1q and a Ca2q-dependent tetramer consisting of two copies each of two proteases: C1r and C1s. Binding of C1 to a cellular or molecular target is mediated by C1q and results in the self-activation of C1r, which subsequently activates C1s. C1s then cleaves C4 and C2, thereby resulting in their activation. At this point, all pathways converge at C3 and lead to activation of C3a and C5a and the terminal membrane attack complex C5b-C9, which creates pores in prokaryotic cell membranes that lead to bacterial cell lysis. Genetic defects in the classical pathway result in increased susceptibility to bacterial infections caused by organisms such as *Neisseria meningitidis, Haemophilus influenzae,* and *Streptococcus pneumoniae.*

The alternative pathway, triggered by bacterial products such as LPS, results in the sequential activation of C3a, C5a, and the membrane attack complex. The lectin-binding pathway, triggered by binding of bacterial sugars such as mannose to mannose-binding lectin protein, activates C4a and C5a and then joins the common pathway for activation of the membrane attack complex.

Activated complement products exert a number of biologic functions. C3b opsonizes pathogenic bacteria, which results in their enhanced phagocytosis by macrophages and neutrophils. Immune complexes bind to C3a and are then removed by binding with complement receptor 1 (CR1, discussed later). Clearance of necrotic and apoptotic cells may be facilitated by interaction with C1q. Complement factor deficiencies, which result in inadequate clearance of immune complexes and dead cells, may give rise to the development of autoimmunity.

Many of the effects of complement activation are mediated by the binding of activated complement products to specific receptors. Some receptors bind several different complement factors with varying affinity, thereby resulting in a variety of effects on different cells. Binding of C3b, C4b, and C1q by CR1, also known as CD35, results in the cleavage of C3 and C5 convertases, clearance of C3b-bound immune complexes, and activation of T lymphocytes. CR2, also known as CD21, is present on B and T lymphocytes and some endothelial cells. CR2 binds iC3b and C3d (C3b cleavage products) and causes stimulation of B lymphocytes and antibody production. Epstein-Barr virus also binds to CR2. CR3 and CR4 are

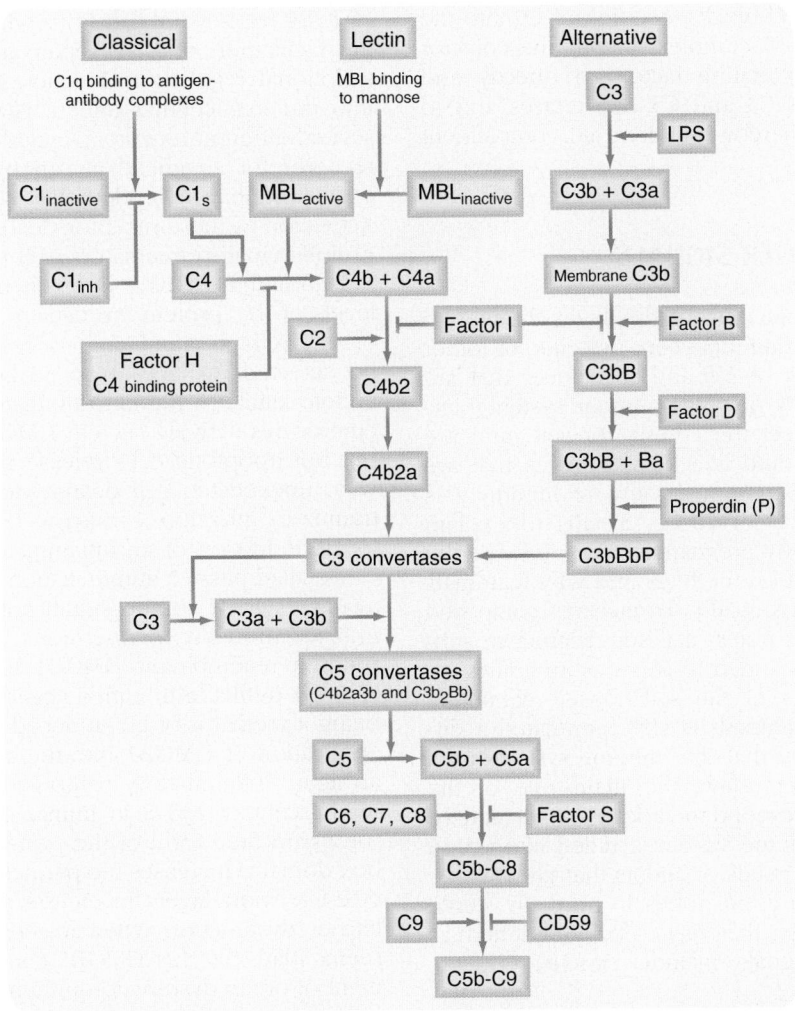

Figure 4-5 Activation of the complement cascade via the classical, lectin, or alternative pathways leads to formation of the membrane attack complex (C5b-C9). Various complement inhibitors antagonize several steps in the cascade: C1 inhibitor (C1$_{inh}$), factor I, factor H, C4-binding protein, factor S, and CD59, among others not shown here. LPS, lipopolysaccharide; MBL, mannose-binding lectin.

members of the integrin family and are expressed on myeloid cells. CR3 and CR4 bind iC3b, C3b, fibrinogen, intercellular adhesion molecule-1 (ICAM-1), and other ligands. Binding of ligands to these receptors enhances antibody-mediated phagocytosis by neutrophils and macrophages. Although a number of different ligands bind to complement receptors 1 through 4, C3a and C5a bind to specific receptors (C3aR and C5aR, respectively). Both these receptors are present on a wide variety of cell types. Binding of C3a or C5a to their respective receptors activates intracellular signaling cascades involving MAPK pathways.

Detrimental actions of the complement system on the host are mediated by the overproduction of C3a and C5a during complement activation and the excessive formation of membrane attack complexes. In rodent models of sepsis, treatment with a neutralizing anti-C5a antibody improves survival and also decreases circulating levels of TNF and IL-6, thus suggesting that activation of C5 receptors is associated with the release of these other mediators.[54]

Several inhibitors are present in plasma or are membrane bound to prevent uncontrolled activation of the complement system. C1 inhibitor is present in plasma and prevents the activation of C1s and C1r, thereby antagonizing the classical pathway. In addition, C1 inhibitor also inhibits the lectin pathway. Heterozygous deficiency of C1 inhibitor results in life-threatening angioedema. Factor H and C4-binding protein are plasma proteins that inhibit C3 and C4 activation, thereby inhibiting all complement activation pathways. Factor I is a serine protease that inactivates C3b and C4b and therefore C3 and C5 convertases. C3a and C5a are also antagonized by carboxypeptidase N. S protein, fibronectin, and clusterin are plasma proteins that prevent insertion of C5b-C9 into cellular membranes. The membrane-bound complement inhibitors act at several points in the complement pathways. CD59 is a glycoprotein that prevents polymerization of C9 and blocks insertion of C9 into the membrane-bound C5b-C9 complex. Membrane cofactor protein and decay-accelerating factor act directly and with factor I to inhibit C3 and C5 convertases and to cleave C3b and C4b, thereby inhibiting all complement pathways.

ENDOGENOUS DANGER SIGNALS

Traditionally, the immune system has been thought to function by discriminating between proteins or other substances that are part of *self* and substances that are *nonself*. According to this view, the immune system tolerates substances that meet the criteria for self (and are identified early in life) and attacks substances that are nonself. Although this traditional view of immunity is consistent with many observations, it fails to explain many others, such as why pregnant mothers tolerate the *nonself* antigens present on the fetus and why mammals fail to respond immunologically to vaccines composed of inert foreign proteins unless a tissue-destructive substance, such as alum, is added to serve as an adjuvant.

Prompted by failures of the self/nonself paradigm, Polly Matzinger[55] and Kenneth Rock[56] formulated a different notion of the way that the immune system functions. According to their view, the main role of the immune response is to respond to various danger signals; in other words, the immune system is called into action when it senses injured tissues or agents that are capable of injuring tissues, such as microbes in normally sterile places. Some substances that have been identified as endogenous danger signals include HMGB1, HSP60, HSP70, and uric acid.

High Mobility Group B1

When mice are injected with a lethal bolus dose of LPS, circulating levels of TNF peak about 60 to 90 minutes later and are virtually undetectable within 4 hours. Although the mice show clinical signs of endotoxemia (e.g., decreased activity and ruffled fur) within a few hours after the injection of LPS, mortality typically does not occur until more than 24 hours later, long after circulating levels of the so-called alarm phase cytokines (TNF and IL-1β) have retuned to normal. These observations suggested the possibility to Tracey and colleagues that LPS-induced lethality might be mediated by a previously unidentified factor that is released much later than TNF or IL-1β.[57] Prompted by this idea, these investigators carried out a prolonged search for the putative late-acting mediator. This research program ultimately resulted in the identification of HMGB1 (formerly called *HMG-1*) as a novel mediator of LPS-induced lethality.

HMGB1 was originally identified in 1973 as a nonhistone nuclear protein with high electrophoretic mobility. A characteristic feature of the protein is the presence of two folded DNA-binding motifs termed the *A domain* and the *B domain*. Both these domains contain a characteristic grouping of aromatic and basic amino acids within a block of 75 residues termed the HMG box.

HMGB1 has several functions within the nucleus, including facilitation of DNA repair and support of the transcriptional regulation of genes. When released by cells into the extracellular milieu, HMGB1 can interact with several different receptors, including TLR2, TLR4, and the receptor for advanced glycation end products (RAGE), on macrophages, endothelial cells, and enterocytes.[58] Activation of these receptors leads to the release of other proinflammatory mediators such as TNF and NO.

Although HMGB1 is normally not secreted by cells and levels of this protein are usually undetectable in plasma or serum, high circulating concentrations of HMGB1 can be detected in mice 16 to 32 hours after the onset of endotoxemia.[59] Immunostimulated macrophages and enterocytes actively secrete HMGB1. Moreover, necrotic but not apoptotic cells release nuclear HMGB1. In this way, unexpected cell death, such as that secondary to trauma or infection, can act as a danger signal and lead to the induction of an inflammatory response.

Delayed passive immunization of mice with antibodies against HMGB1 confers significant protection against LPS-induced mortality. Furthermore, administration of highly purified recombinant HMGB1 to mice is lethal. Thus, HMGB1 fulfills (a modified version) of Koch's criteria for being a mediator of LPS-induced lethality in mice. Direct application of HMGB1 into the airways of mice initiates an acute inflammatory response and lung injury that is reminiscent of ARDS in humans.[60] In addition, HMGB1 (or a truncated form of the protein including only the B box domain) increases the permeability of human enterocyte-like monolayers in culture and promotes intestinal barrier dysfunction when injected into mice.[61] Thus, it seems plausible that HMGB1 contributes to the development of organ dysfunction in human sepsis, a notion that is supported by the observation that circulating HMGB1 concentrations are significantly higher in patients with ultimately fatal sepsis than in patients with a less severe form of the syndrome. Ethyl pyruvate, a compound that blocks the release of HMGB1 from LPS-stimulated murine macrophage-like cells and inhibits release of the mediator in vivo, improves survival in mice with bacterial peritonitis, even when treatment with the compound is delayed for 24 hours after the onset of infection.[62]

Heat Shock Proteins

The heat shock proteins were first identified as a family of proteins that are induced when cells or experimental animals are subjected to sublethal thermal stress. These proteins are also induced by many other stimuli, such as inflammation, oxidative stress, and infection. The primary role of heat shock proteins is to serve as molecular chaperones to facilitate the proper folding of nascent proteins.

Like HMGB1, heat shock proteins are normally found inside cells, but under certain conditions these proteins can be detected in the extracellular milieu. For example, elevated circulating levels of HSP70 have been found in trauma patients and patients in the immediate period after coronary artery bypass graft surgery. In addition, immunostimulated monocytes appear to be capable of actively secreting HSP70. Extracellular HSP60 and HSP70 can activate innate immune cells via mechanisms that may depend on signaling through TLR4 and TLR2. Thus, like HMGB1, these proteins may serve as endogenous danger signals and trigger activation of the inflammatory response after damage to tissues.

EICOSANOIDS (THROMBOXANE, PROSTAGLANDINS, AND LEUKOTRIENES)

The prostaglandins, including PGE_2 and PGI_2 (prostacyclin), and thromboxane A_2 (TxA_2) are lipid mediators derived from the unstable intermediate compound PGG_2. Formation of PGG_2 depends on the activity of two families of enzymes. First, isoforms of the enzyme phospholipase A_2 liberate the polyunsaturated fatty acid arachidonate from membrane phospholipids. Second, the two cyclooxygenase isoforms COX-1 and COX-2 catalyze the stereospecific oxidation of arachidonate to form the cyclic endoperoxide PGG_2. Both these reactions are major regulatory steps in the formation of prostaglandins and TxA_2.

COX-1 is expressed constitutively in a variety of tissues, and mediators produced by this isoform are thought to be important in various homeostatic processes, such as regulating renal perfusion and salt and water handling, maintaining hemostasis by modulating platelet aggregation, and preserving gastrointestinal mucosal integrity. COX-2, however, is an inducible enzyme. Expression of COX-2 is induced by a number of stimuli, including various growth factors and proinflammatory cytokines. In cells subjected to inflammatory stimuli, activation of COX-2 is thought to be mediated by the powerful oxidant $ONOO^-$, thereby providing a tight functional linkage between the NO· and prostaglandin mediator systems.

Once expressed and activated, COX-2 promotes the formation of PGG_2 and PGH_2 and, ultimately, various prostaglandins and TxA_2. These mediators, in turn, interact with cell surface receptors belonging to the G protein–coupled receptor superfamily. Interaction of these receptors with cytosolic signaling pathways leads to rapid alterations in cell physiology manifested as physiologic or pathophysiologic phenomena such as vasodilation and increased microvascular permeability. Pharmacologic inhibition of cyclooxygenase activity is the basis for the anti-inflammatory actions of the class of compounds called *nonsteroidal anti-inflammatory drugs* (NSAIDs). Whereas the anti-inflammatory effects of NSAIDs are thought to be mediated by blocking the enzymatic activity of COX-2, some of adverse side effects of these agents (e.g., gastric mucosal ulceration) are thought to be mediated by inhibition of COX-1. Accordingly, identification of COX-2 as the so-called inflammatory isoform of cyclooxygenase led to intense efforts to develop drugs selective for the inducible enzyme. Selective COX-2 inhibitors were initially widely prescribed by clinicians. However, data from large multicentric trials of rofecoxib, one of the compounds in this class, showed that treatment with this agent was associated with an increased risk for death from cardiovascular complications.[63,64] As a result of these findings, rofecoxib was withdrawn from the market. The increased risk for cardiovascular complications associated with rofecoxib, however, does not seem to be peculiar to only this specific agent but rather is thought to be a class effect associated with therapy with all isoform-selective COX-2 inhibitors, possibly as a result of greater inhibition of the synthesis of PGI_2 (a vasodilator and inhibitor of platelet aggregation) relative to inhibition of the synthesis of TxA_2 (a potent vasoconstrictor and promoter of platelet aggregation).[65]

NITRIC OXIDE

Many of the downstream actions of the proinflammatory cytokines occur as a result of increased expression of two key enzymes, iNOS (NOS-2) and COX-2. These enzymes share some common features and are both centrally involved in many aspects of the inflammatory response. iNOS is one of three isoforms of an enzyme, nitric oxide synthase (NOS), that catalyzes conversion of the amino acid L-arginine to the free radical gas NO·. One of the simplest stable molecules in nature, NO· is produced by many different types of cells and serves as both a signaling and an effector molecule in mammalian biology. Whereas NOS-1 (also called *neuronal NOS* or *nNOS*) and NOS-3 (also called *endothelial* or *eNOS*) tend to be expressed constitutively in various cell types, iNOS is expressed for the most part only after stimulation of cells by proinflammatory cytokines (particularly IFN-γ, TNF, and IL-1) or LPS. NOS-1 and NOS-2 produce small puffs of NO· in response to transient changes in the intracellular ionized calcium concentration. In contrast, iNOS, once induced, produces large quantities of NO· for a prolonged period.

All three NOS isoforms require L-arginine as a substrate and, in a complex five-electron redox reaction, convert one of the guanidino nitrogens of the amino acid into NO·. In addition to L-arginine, the redox reaction catalyzed by the various NOS isoforms requires the presence of molecular oxygen and a number of cofactors, including flavin mononucleotide, flavin adenine dinucleotide, iron-protoporphyrin IX, and tetrahydrobiopterin (BH_4). The rate-limiting step in the biosynthesis of BH_4 is the reaction catalyzed by guanosine triphosphate (GTP) cyclohydrolase I, an enzyme that like iNOS, is induced in certain cell types by cytokines or LPS, or both.

Many of the biologic actions of NO·, including vasodilation, induction of vascular hyperpermeability, and inhibition of platelet aggregation, are mediated through activation of the enzyme soluble guanylyl cyclase (sGC). Binding of NO· to the heme moiety of sGC activates the enzyme, thereby enabling it to catalyze the conversion of GTP to cyclic guanosine monophosphate (cGMP). NO· is not the only ligand that is capable of activating sGC; carbon monoxide (CO), another small gaseous molecule produced by mammalian cells, has also been shown to activate this enzyme. Signal transduction via the NO·-sGC (or the CO-sGC) pathway entails the activation of various cGMP-dependent protein kinase (PKG) isoforms. In vascular smooth muscle cells, NO·-induced vasodilation occurs as a result of PKG-mediated opening of high-con-ductance calcium and voltage-activated potassium chan-nels. Excessive production of NO· as a result of iNOS induction in vascular smooth muscle cells is thought to be a major factor contributing to the loss of vasomotor tone and the loss of responsiveness to vasopressor agents (*vasoplegia*) in patients with septic shock. Treatment with a drug that blocks production of NO·, such as N^G-mono-methyl-L-arginine (L-NMMA), ameliorates hypotension in patients with septic shock.[66] Unfortunately, treatment of septic patients with L-NMMA actually worsens survival, possibly because the drug does not selectively inhibit iNOS but also inhibits NOS-3 as well and therefore inter-feres with the normal regulation of microcirculatory per-fusion. Some,[67,68] but not all,[69,70] studies suggest that iNOS knockout mice are partially resistant to the lethal effects of acute endotoxemia. In contrast, one study showed that iNOS knockout mice are more susceptible than wild-type controls to lethality induced by bacterial peritonitis,[71] possibly because enhanced NO· production is important for the host's defense against infection. In contrast, iNOS knockout mice are protected from sepsis-induced acute lung injury.[72]

Signaling via the sGC-PKG pathway is not the only way that NO· functions as an inflammatory mediator. In addition, NO· reacts rapidly with another free radical, superoxide anion (O_2^-·), to form peroxynitrite anion ($ONOO^-$), the conjugate base of the weak acid peroxyni-trous acid (ONOOH). Being a potent oxidizing and nitro-sating agent, $ONOO^-$/ONOOH is thought to be responsible for many of the toxic effects of NO·. For example, $ONOO^-$/ONOOH is capable of oxidizing sulfhydryl groups on various proteins at a rapid rate, peroxidizing membrane lipids, and inactivating mitochondrial aconitase. $ONOO^-$/ONOOH is also capable of damaging nuclear DNA, thus setting up a chain of events that ultimately leads to acti-vation of the enzyme poly(adenosine ribose diphosphate) polymerase-1 (PARP-1). On activation, PARP-1 catalyzes the poly(adenosine diphosphate) ribosylation of proteins, a reaction that consumes oxidized nicotine adenine dinu-cleotide (NAD^+) and leads to energetic failure in cells.[73] Treatment with pharmacologic agents that do the follow-ing has been shown to improve organ system function or survival (or both) in certain experimental models of inflammation, such as acute endotoxemia, mesenteric ischemia and reperfusion, hemorrhagic shock and resus-citation, and stroke:

1. Scavenge $ONOO^-$/ONOOH
2. Selectively block iNOS (without blocking NOS-1 or NOS-3)
3. Block the activity of PARP-1

CARBON MONOXIDE

CO has been identified as a poisonous substance since the mid-19th century. The importance of CO as an endog-enous signaling molecule has been recognized only in the past few years. The toxicity of CO relates to its ability to impair the oxygen-carrying capacity of hemoglobin.

Two mechanisms are involved. First, CO binds to hemo-globin with 250-fold greater affinity than O_2 does, thereby inhibiting O_2 binding and transport. Second, CO causes a conformational change in the hemoglobin molecule that impairs its ability to release bound O_2, thus shifting the oxyhemoglobin dissociation curve to the left. In addi-tion, CO binds to and inactivates cytochrome a_3, thereby impairing mitochondrial respiration.

The concentrations of endogenously generated CO are far below the toxic level. Endogenously generated CO is a product of heme catabolism. The CO-generating reac-tion is catalyzed by a family of enzymes called *heme oxygenases.* There are three isoforms of heme oxygenase called *HO-1, HO-2,* and *HO-3,* although only HO-1 and HO-2 have been widely studied. HO-2 is constitutively expressed, whereas HO-1 is an inducible enzyme. HO-1 expression is induced by a wide variety of agents, includ-ing heme itself, heat shock stress, ROS, LPS, heavy metals, and ultraviolet radiation. HO-1 plays an important role in the defense of cells against oxidative stress, and both products of the degradation of heme by HO-1, namely, bilirubin and CO, are important in this regard.

CO exerts a variety of physiologic effects. It causes relaxation of smooth muscle cells, which results in vaso-dilation and bronchodilation. CO inhibits the activation and aggregation of platelets. Like NO·, CO functions as a neurotransmitter. Finally, CO exerts a number of cyto-protective effects. Pretreatment of rodents with 250 ppm of inhaled CO ameliorates the development of acute lung injury after subsequent exposure to LPS or hyperoxia.[74] CO also has antiproliferative effects on tumor cells and vascular endothelial and smooth muscle cells. Finally, CO has an anti-inflammatory role mediated via the MAPK pathway that results in suppression of TNF release and up-regulation of IL-10 secretion.

Similar to NO·, CO mediates its effects by binding to the ferrous heme moieties of hemoproteins. Although the affinity of heme for NO· is higher than that for CO, the off rate for dissociation of CO from heme is much slower, so CO displaces NO· from heme over time. Thus, CO can modulate the effects of NO· in this manner. Binding of CO to the heme moiety of sGC results in the activation of sGC and is the primary mechanism responsible for many of the biologic effects of CO.

REACTIVE OXYGEN SPECIES

ROS are reactive, partially reduced derivatives of molecu-lar oxygen (O_2). Important ROS in biologic systems include superoxide radical anion (O_2^-·), hydrogen perox-ide (H_2O_2), and hydroxyl radical (OH·). Closely related species include the hypohalous acids, particularly hypo-chlorous acid (HOCl); chloramine (NH_2Cl) and substi-tuted chloramines (RNHCl or R'R"NCl); and singlet oxygen ($^1O_2$). Free radicals are atomic or molecular species with unpaired electrons. As a consequence of these unpaired electrons, free radicals are usually highly reactive and capable of modifying a wide range of cellular constitu-ents, including lipids, proteins, and nucleic acids. ROS that are also free radicals include $O_2^-\cdot$, OH·, peroxyl radical (RO_2), and hydroxyperoxyl radical (HO_2).

A variety of enzymatic and nonenzymatic processes can generate ROS in mammalian cells. Nevertheless, a few key reactions or processes constitute the main sources of these reactive species:

- NADPH oxidase catalyzes a one-electron reduction of O_2 to form $O_2^-\cdot$ according to the following equation: $2O_2 + NADPH \rightarrow 2O_2^-\cdot + NADP + 2H^+$. NADPH oxidase is an enzyme complex that is assembled and activated after the activation of phagocytes by microbes or microbial products (e.g., LPS) or various proinflammatory mediators such as leukotriene B_4, platelet activating factor, TNF, or IL-8. In resting cells, the components of NADPH oxidase are present in the cytosol and the membranes of various intracellular organelles. When the cell is activated, the components are assembled on a membrane-bound vesicle, which then fuses with the plasma membrane, and $O_2^-\cdot$ is released outward into the extracellular milieu and inward into the phagocytic vesicle. The reaction catalyzed by NADPH oxidase is critical for the formation of ROS in phagocytic cells, such as macrophages and PMNs. NADPH oxidase, however, is present in other cell types as well, including vascular smooth muscle cells and endothelial cells.
- Superoxide dismutase (SOD) catalyzes the conversion (dismutation) of two moles of O_2^- to form one mole each of O_2 and H_2O_2. Two forms of SOD are present in cells. Copper-zinc SOD (CuZn-SOD) is a constitutive enzyme localized to the cytoplasm, whereas manganese SOD (Mn-SOD) is an inducible enzyme present in mitochondria. Increased expression of Mn-SOD is induced by oxidant stress or various proinflammatory cytokines.
- In the presence of free ionized iron or copper in a low oxidation state (i.e., Fe^{2+} or Cu^+, respectively), H_2O_2 reacts nonenzymatically to form OH· and hydroxyl anion: $H_2O_2 + Fe^{2+} \rightarrow OH\cdot + OH^- + Fe^{3+}$. The lower oxidation state of the transition metal cation can then be regenerated by the action of any number of reducing agents within the cellular milieu (e.g., ascorbic acid) and the cycle then repeated. This cycle constitutes the so-called Fenton reaction.
- Myeloperoxidase (MPO) is an enzyme present in phagocytes that catalyzes oxidation of the halide ions chloride (Cl^-), bromide (Br^-), and iodide (I^-) by H_2O_2 to form the corresponding hypohalous acids (HOCl, HOBr, and HOI, respectively). MPO, a colored heme-containing enzyme, is responsible for the greenish tint that is sometimes noticeable in purulent exudates.
- Xanthine oxidase (XO) catalyzes the oxidation of xanthine (or hypoxanthine) by molecular oxygen to form uric acid and $O_2^-\cdot$: $xanthine + H_2O + 2O_2 \rightarrow uric\ acid + 2O_2^- + 2H^+$. An enzyme related to XO, xanthine dehydrogenase (XDH), uses reduced nicotinamide adenine dinucleotide (NADH) as a cofactor and converts xanthine (or hypoxanthine) to uric acid without forming partially reduced forms of molecular oxygen.

During episodes of tissue ischemia, XDH is proteolytically converted to XO, and adenosine triphosphate is degraded to xanthine and hypoxanthine. During reperfusion, O_2 is available and XO acts on the accumulated substrates (xanthine and hypoxanthine), which leads to a burst in the production of ROS.

- Although the various NOS isoforms ordinarily catalyze the formation of NO· and L-citrulline from L-arginine, these enzymes can generate $O_2^-\cdot$ if L-arginine availability is limiting.
- ROS are also produced as a by-product of the normal metabolism of oxygen in mitochondria and have important roles in cell signaling.

To counter the activity of ROS, cells are equipped with a number of antioxidant systems, including SOD, catalase, glutathione, glutathione peroxidase, ascorbic acid (vitamin C), α-tocopherol (vitamin E), and thioredoxin. Under normal circumstances, the reducing milieu in cells prevents ROS-induced cellular damage. However, during times of stress, ROS production can increase dramatically and overwhelm normal antioxidant defenses, thereby leading to so-called oxidative stress and damage to cells and tissues on this basis.

Sepsis is associated with oxidative stress. Low plasma ascorbate levels are predictive of the development of multiorgan dysfunction in septic patients, and some data show a reduction in the incidence of organ failure when antioxidants are administered to critically ill surgical patients.[75]

Selected References

Angus DC, Linde-Zwirble WT, Lidicker J, et al: Epidemiology of severe sepsis in the United States: Analysis of incidence, outcome, and associated costs of care. Crit Care Med 29:1303-1310, 2001.

A large observational cohort study that estimates that the incidence of severe sepsis is over 750,000 cases per year in the United States, with an expected growth rate of 1.5% per annum. It is also estimated that 215,000 patients with severe sepsis die annually, a number roughly equal to that associated with acute myocardial infarction.

Annane D, Sebille V, Charpentier C, et al: Effect of treatment with low doses of hydrocortisone and fludrocortisone on mortality in patients with septic shock. JAMA 288:862-871, 2002.

Important contribution to the evidence-based critical care literature demonstrating that treatment with low doses of mineralocorticoids and glucocorticosteroids significantly reduces mortality in patients with septic shock and relative adrenal insufficiency.

Bernard GR, Vincent J-L, Laterre PF, et al: Efficacy and safety of recombinant human activated protein C for severe sepsis. N Engl J Med 344:699-709, 2001.

Large, multicentric randomized trial demonstrating that treatment with recombinant human activated protein C (rhAPC) reduces mortality in patients with severe sepsis. The incidence of serious bleeding events was higher in the group that received rhAPC, but this did not reach statistical significance.

Carswell EA, Old LJ, Kassel RL, et al: An endotoxin-induced serum factor that causes necrosis of tumors. Proc Natl Acad Sci U S A 72:3666-3670, 1975.

Landmark paper that identified tumor necrosis factor as the agent responsible for the tumor-necrosing activity of endotoxin.

Matzinger P: The danger model: A renewed sense of self. Science 296:301-305, 2002.

The classic view of the immune system proposed that an immunologic distinction is made between self and nonself. This article proposes a paradigm shift in this concept. In fact, the immune system may be more concerned with entities that do damage than with those that are foreign, and the release of so-called danger signals from dead or dying cells may alert the immune system to such substances.

References

1. Akira S, Takeda K, Kaisho T: Toll-like receptors: Critical proteins linking innate and acquired immunity. Nat Immunol 2:675-680, 2001.
2. Valentino L, Pierre J: JAK/STAT signal transduction: Regulators and implication in hematological malignancies. Biochem Pharmacol 71:713-721, 2006.
3. Docke WD, Randow F, Syrbe U, et al: Monocyte deactivation in septic patients: Restoration by IFN-gamma treatment. Nat Med 3:678-681, 1997.
4. Schinkel C, Licht K, Zedler S, et al: Perioperative treatment with human recombinant interferon-gamma: A randomized double-blind clinical trial. Shock 16:329-333, 2001.
5. Bilgin K, Yaramis A, Haspolat K, et al: A randomized trial of granulocyte-macrophage colony-stimulating factor in neonates with sepsis and neutropenia. Pediatrics 107:36-41, 2003.
6. Orozco H, Arch J, Medina-Franco H, et al: Molgramostim (GM-CSF) associated with antibiotic treatment in nontraumatic abdominal sepsis: A randomized, double-blind, placebo-controlled clinical trial. Arch Surg 141:150-153, 2006.
7. Fantuzzi G, Ku G, Harding MW, et al: Response to local inflammation of IL-1 beta–converting enzyme–deficient mice. J Immunol 158:1818-1824, 1997.
8. Gay N, Keith F: *Drosophila* Toll and IL-1 receptor. Nature 351:355-356, 1991.
9. Bowie A, O'Neill LA: The interleukin-1 receptor/Toll-like receptor superfamily: Signal generators for pro-inflammatory interleukins and microbial products. J Leukoc Biol 67:508-514, 2000.
10. Hoshino K, Takeuchi O, Kawai T, et al: Cutting edge: Toll-like receptor 4 (TLR4)-deficient mice are hyporesponsive to lipopolysaccharide: Evidence for TLR4 as the Lps gene product. J Immunol 162:3749-3752, 1999.
11. Arbour NC, Lorenz E, Schutte BC, et al: TLR4 mutations are associated with endotoxin hyporesponsiveness in humans. Nat Genet 25:187-191, 2000.
12. Baud V, Karin M: Signal transduction by tumor necrosis factor and its relatives. Trends Cell Biol 11:372-377, 2001.
13. Gogos CA, Drosou E, Bassaris HP, et al: Pro- versus anti-inflammatory cytokine profile in patients with severe sepsis: A marker for prognosis and future therapeutic options. J Infect Dis 181:176-180, 2000.
14. Tang GJ, Huang SL, Yien HW, et al: Tumor necrosis factor gene polymorphism and septic shock in surgical infection. Crit Care Med 28:2733-2736, 2000.
15. Waterer GW, Quasney MW, Cantor RM, et al: Septic shock and respiratory failure in community-acquired pneumonia have different TNF polymorphism associations. Am J Respir Crit Care Med 163:1599-1604, 2001.
16. Veterans Administration Systemic Sepsis Cooperative Study Group: Effect of high-dose glucocorticoid therapy on mortality in patients with clinical signs of systemic sepsis. N Engl J Med 317:659-665, 1987.
17. Bone RC, Fisher CJ Jr, Clemmer TP, et al: A controlled clinical trial of high-dose methylprednisolone in the treatment of severe sepsis and septic shock. N Engl J Med 317:653-658, 1987.
18. Bernard GR, Luce JM, Sprung CL, et al: High-dose corticosteroids in patients with the adult respiratory distress syndrome. N Engl J Med 317:1565-1570, 1987.
19. Briegel J, Forst H, Haller M, et al: Stress doses of hydrocortisone reverse hyperdynamic septic shock: A prospective, randomized, double-blind, single-center study. Crit Care Med 27:723-732, 1999.
20. Bollaert P-E, Charpentier C, Debouverie M, et al: Reversal of late septic shock with supraphysiologic doses of hydrocortisone. Crit Care Med 26:645-650, 1998.
21. Annane D, Sebille V, Charpentier C, et al: Effect of treatment with low doses of hydrocortisone and fludrocortisone on mortality in patients with septic shock. JAMA 288:862-871, 2002.
22. Steinberg KP, Hudson LD, Goodman RB, et al: Efficacy and safety of corticosteroids for persistent acute respiratory distress syndrome. N Engl J Med 354:1671-1684, 2006.
23. Fisher CJ Jr, Agosti JM, Opal SM, et al: Treatment of septic shock with the tumor necrosis factor receptor:Fc fusion protein. N Engl J Med 334:1697-1702, 1996.
24. Present DH, Rutgeerts P, Targan S, et al: Infliximab for the treatment of fistulas in patients with Crohn's disease. N Engl J Med 340:1398-1405, 1999.
25. Cohen SB, Moreland LW, Cush JJ, et al: A multicentre, double blind, randomised, placebo controlled trial of anakinra (Kineret), a recombinant interleukin 1 receptor antagonist, in patients with rheumatoid arthritis treated with background methotrexate. Ann Rheum Dis 63:1062-1068, 2004.
26. Berry MA, Hargadon B, Shelley M, et al: Evidence of a role of tumor necrosis factor alpha in refractory asthma. N Engl J Med 354:697-708, 2006.
27. Bernard GR, Vincent J-L, Laterre PF, et al: Efficacy and safety of recombinant human activated protein C for severe sepsis. N Engl J Med 344:699-709, 2001.
28. Abraham E, Laterre PF, Garg R, et al: Drotrecogin alfa (activated) for adults with severe sepsis and a low risk of death. N Engl J Med 353:1332-1341, 2005.
29. Goldstein B, Nadel S, Peters M, et al: ENHANCE: Results of a global open-label trial of drotrecogin alfa (activated) in children with severe sepsis. Pediatr Crit Care Med 7:200-211. 2006.
30. Cuzzocrea S, Mazzon E, Dugo L, et al: Absence of endogenous interleukin-6 enhances the inflammatory response during acute pancreatitis induced by cerulein in mice. Cytokine 18:274-275, 2002.
31. Yang R, Han X, Uchiyama T, et al: IL-6 is essential for development of gut barrier dysfunction after hemorrhagic shock and resuscitation in mice. Am J Physiol Gastrointest Liver Physiol 285:G621-G629, 2003.
32. Opal SM, Keith JC, Jhung J, et al: Orally administered recombinant human interleukin-11 is protective in experimental neutropenic sepsis. J Infect Dis 187:70-76, 2003.
33. Yoshimura T, Matsushima K, Tanaka S, et al: Purification of a human monocyte-derived neutrophil chemotactic factor that has peptide sequence similarity to other host defense cytokines. Proc Natl Acad Sci U S A 84:9233-9237, 1987.

34. Marty C, Misset B, Tamion F, et al: Circulating interleukin-8 concentrations in patients with multiple organ failure of septic and nonseptic origin. Crit Care Med 22:673-679, 1994.

35. Carvalho GL, Wakabayashi G, Shimazu M, et al: Anti–interleukin-8 monoclonal antibody reduces free radical production and improves hemodynamics and survival rate in endotoxic shock in rabbits. Surgery 122:60-68, 1997.

36. Emmanuilidis K, Weighardt H, Matevossian E, et al: Differential regulation of systemic IL-18 and IL-12 release during postoperative sepsis: High serum IL-18 as an early predictive indicator of lethal outcome. Shock 18:301-305, 2002.

37. Weighardt H, Heidecke CD, Westerholt A, et al: Impaired monocyte IL-12 production before surgery as a predictive factor for the lethal outcome of postoperative sepsis. Ann Surg 235:560-567, 2002.

38. Bauditz J, Wedel S, Lochs H: Thalidomide reduces tumour necrosis factor alpha and interleukin 12 production in patients with chronic active Crohn's disease. Gut 50:196-200, 2002.

39. Ono S, Ueno C, Aosasa S, et al: Severe sepsis induces deficient interferon-gamma and interleukin-12 production, but interleukin-12 therapy improves survival in peritonitis. Am J Surg 182:491-497, 2001.

40. Fantuzzi G, Puren AJ, Harding MW, et al: Interleukin-18 regulation of interferon gamma production and cell proliferation as shown in interleukin-1β–converting enzyme (caspase-1)-deficient mice. Blood 91:2118-2125, 1998.

41. Oberholzer A, Steckholzer U, Kurimoto M, et al: Interleukin-18 plasma levels are increased in patients with sepsis compared to severely injured patients. Shock 16:411-414, 2001.

42. Latifi SQ, O'Riordan MA, Levine AD: Interleukin-10 controls the onset of irreversible septic shock. Infect Immun 70:4441-4446, 2002.

43. Fumeaux T, Pugin J: Role of interleukin-10 in the intracellular sequestration of human leukocyte antigen-DR in monocytes during septic shock. Am J Respir Crit Care Med 166:1475-1482, 2002.

44. Matsumoto T, Tateda K, Miyazaki S, et al: Effect of interleukin-10 on gut-derived sepsis caused by *Pseudomonas aeruginosa* in mice. Antimicrob Agents Chemother 42:2853-2857, 1999.

45. Remick DG, Garg SJ, Newcomb DE, et al: Exogenous interleukin-10 fails to decrease the mortality or morbidity of sepsis. Crit Care Med 26:895-904, 1998.

46. Steinhauser ML, Hogaboam CM, Kunkel SL, et al: IL-10 is a major mediator of sepsis-induced impairment in lung antibacterial host defense. J Immunol 162:392-399, 1999.

47. Muchamuel T, Menon S, Pisacane P, et al: IL-13 protects mice from lipopolysaccharide-induced lethal endotoxemia: Correlation with down-modulation of TNF-alpha, IFN-gamma, and IL-12 production. J Immunol 158:2898-2903, 1997.

48. Matsukawa A, Hogaboam CM, Lukacs NW, et al: Expression and contribution of endogenous IL-13 in an experimental model of sepsis. J Immunol 164:2738-2744, 2000.

49. Laun RA, Schroder O, Schoppnies M, et al: Transforming growth factor-beta1 and major trauma: Time-dependent association with hepatic and renal insufficiency. Shock 19:16-23, 2003.

50. Bozza M, Satoskar AR, Lin G, et al: Targeted disruption of migration inhibitory factor gene reveals its critical role in sepsis. J Exp Med 189:341-346, 1999.

51. Beishuizen A, Thijs LG, Haanen C, et al: Macrophage migration inhibitory factor and hypothalamo-pituitary-adrenal function during critical illness. J Clin Endocrinol Metab 86:2811-2816, 2001.

52. Calandra T, Echtenacher B, Roy DL, et al: Protection from septic shock by neutralization of macrophage migration inhibitory factor. Nat Med 6:164-170, 2000.

53. Guo RF, Ward PA: Role of C5a in inflammatory responses. Annu Rev Immunol 23:821-852, 2005.

54. Riedemann NC, Guo RF, Neff TA, et al: Increased C5a receptor expression in sepsis. J Clin Invest 110:101-108, 2002.

55. Matzinger P: The danger model: A renewed sense of self. Science 296:301-305, 2002.

56. Shi Y, Zheng W, Rock KL: Cell injury releases endogenous adjuvants that stimulate cytotoxic T cell responses. Proc Natl Acad Sci U S A 97:14590-14595, 2000.

57. Yang H, Wang H, Tracey KJ: HMG-1 rediscovered as a cytokine. Shock 15:247-253, 2001.

58. Lotze MT, Tracey KJ: High-mobility group box 1 protein (HMGB1): Nuclear weapon in the immune arsenal. Nat Rev Immunol 5:331-342, 2005.

59. Wang H, Bloom O, Zhang M, et al: HMG-1 as a late mediator of endotoxin lethality in mice. Science 285:248-251, 1999.

60. Abraham E, Arcaroli J, Carmody A, et al: HMG-1 as a mediator of acute lung inflammation. J Immunol 165:2950-2954, 2000.

61. Sappington PL, Yang R, Yang H, et al: HMGB1 B box increases the permeability of Caco-2 enterocytic monolayers and impairs intestinal barrier function in mice. Gastroenterology 123:790-802, 2002.

62. Ulloa L, Ochani M, Yang H, et al: Ethyl pyruvate prevents lethality in mice with established lethal sepsis and systemic inflammation. Proc Natl Acad Sci U S A 99:12351-12356, 2002.

63. Bresalier RS, Sandler RS, Quan H, et al: Cardiovascular events associated with rofecoxib in a colorectal adenoma chemoprevention trial. N Engl J Med 352:1092-1102, 2005.

64. Curfman GD, Morrissey S, Drazen JM: Expression of concern: Bombardier et al., "Comparison of upper gastrointestinal toxicity of rofecoxib and naproxen in patients with rheumatoid arthritis," N Engl J Med 343:1520-1528, 2000. N Engl J Med 353:2813-2814, 2005.

65. Grosser T, Fries S, FitzGerald GA: Biological basis for the cardiovascular consequences of COX-2 inhibition: Therapeutic challenges and opportunities. J Clin Invest 116:4-15, 2006.

66. Grover R, Zaccardelli D, Colice G, et al: An open-label dose escalation study of the nitric oxide synthase inhibitor, N(G)-methyl-L-arginine hydrochloride (546C88), in patients with septic shock. Glaxo Wellcome International Septic Shock Study Group. Crit Care Med 27:913-922, 1999.

67. MacMicking JD, Nathan C, Horn G, et al: Altered responses to bacterial infection and endotoxic shock in mice lacking inducible nitric oxide synthase. Cell 81:641-650, 1995.

68. Wei X-Q, Charles IG, Smith A, et al: Altered immune responses in mice lacking inducible nitric oxide synthase. Nature 375:408-411, 1995.

69. Nicholson SC, Grobmeyer SR, Shiloh MU, et al: Lethality of endotoxin in mice genetically deficient in the respiratory burst oxidase, inducible nitric oxide synthase, or both. Shock 11:253-258, 1999.

70. Laubach VE, Shesely EG, Smithies O, et al: Mice lacking inducible nitric oxide synthase are not resistant to lipopolysaccharide-induced death. Proc Natl Acad Sci U S A 92:10688-10692, 1995.

71. Cobb JP, Hotchkiss RS, Swanson PE, et al: Inducible nitric oxide synthase (iNOS) gene deficiency increases the mortality of sepsis in mice. Surgery 126:438-442, 1999.

72. Wang LF, Patel M, Razavi HM, et al: Role of inducible nitric oxide synthase in pulmonary microvascular protein leak in murine sepsis. Am J Respir Crit Care Med 165:1634-1639, 2002.

73. Fink MP: Cytopathic hypoxia: Mitochondrial dysfunction as a mechanism contributing to organ dysfunction in sepsis. Crit Care Clin North Am 17:219-237, 2001.

74. Otterbein LE, Mantell LL, Choi AM: Carbon monoxide provides protection against hyperoxic lung injury. Am J Physiol 276:L688-L694, 1999.

75. Nathens AB, Neff MJ, Jurkovich GJ, et al: Randomized, prospective trial of antioxidant supplementation in critically ill surgical patients. Ann Surg 236:814-822, 2002.

CHAPTER 5

Shock, Electrolytes, and Fluid

Richard J. Mullins, MD

Body Water and Solute Composition
Acid-Base Balance
Extracellular Fluid Distribution Between Plasma Volume
   and Interstitial Lymphatic Volume
Cellular Aerobic Function and Dysfunction
Physiologic Control of Perfusion Pressure
The Surgeon's Response to Shock
Hypovolemic Shock
Septic Shock
Cardiogenic Shock
Shock Associated With Adrenal Insufficiency

The body is composed of multiple water compartments separated by membranes, with substantial differences in solute composition within the compartments. In health, balance is maintained across the membranes that separate the compartments, and this balance, or homeostasis, is sustained by the consumption of energy. Inside cells, aerobic metabolism, or the consumption of oxygen and production of carbon dioxide, continually generates the energy required to maintain equipoise. In health, an individual depends on a group of physiologic systems functioning as a coordinated network. Specifically, carefully modulated flow of blood, lymph, water, and solutes delivers substrates and oxygen in aqueous solution to cells while at the same time, flow of water clears waste products to the kidney and lungs for excretion.

Homeostasis is at risk when fluctuations in the external environment alter the availability of essential substrates, particularly oxygen. Multiple physiologic mechanisms are available to enable the body to adjust to changes. Physiologic systems can accelerate or decelerate, depending on the imposed work needs. Homeostasis is intricately regulated as a result of modulated interactions among multiple physiologic systems. Claude Bernard was a 19th

century French physician whose studies of function led him to propose the concept of milieu intérieur: physiologic function is adjusted for the purpose of maintaining the optimal internal environment within cells. Survival of the individual is dependent on cells having access to energy. Shock is a circumstance in which homeostasis is disrupted because of failure of the normal physiologic systems to deliver oxygen. A universal physiologic threat to a patient in shock is deficient oxygen delivery to the mitochondria of cells. As a consequence, aerobic metabolism cannot be sustained at the rate needed to maintain cell function. The cell cannot recover from sustained interruption of aerobic metabolism. As cells die, organ failure ensues. Shock occurs because blood volume is lost, cardiac activity is impaired, or unmitigated vasodilation develops. Although each mechanism may differ, the end result that threatens a patient is deficient cellular energy to sustain the balance that characterizes homeostasis. Multiple treatments tailored to treat the range of clinical syndromes that share the basic problem of disruption in homeostasis are available to surgeons. Although surgical procedures treat problems at the level of organs, a favorable outcome is determined by whether the surgeon can effectively intervene with treatments that restore homeostasis and sustain cellular function. This chapter first describes the composition and function of the cellular and physiologic events that contribute to homeostasis and are altered in patients treated by surgeons. Common syndromes of dysfunction and failure of these systems are discussed. Priority in this chapter is given to information with a clinical basis. Information on normal human structure and function is reviewed, as well as pathologic conditions encountered in clinical practice. The mechanisms by which homeostasis is maintained are described, and the role that shock plays in disruption of these normal balances is defined. Therapy is described in the context of restoring the capacity of the body's physiologic systems to maintain the normal milieu intérieur. Focus is on the challenge of diagnosis and treatment of shock. In other chapters in this textbook, details are presented regarding blood transfusion, nutritional support, and management of specific disease.

BODY WATER AND SOLUTE COMPOSITION

Body Water Composition

Total Body Water

Water is a major component of body mass and has multiple compartments. Total body water (TBW) constitutes between 40% and 60% of the total body weight in most adults. Body fat content influences the proportion of body weight that is water. As body fat increases (a growing problem in modern society), water declines as a proportion of body weight. As muscle mass increases (as occurs in an athlete taking anabolic steroids), water increases as a proportion of body weight. Women have a lower proportion of body weight that is water than men do when matched for age, height, and weight. The proportion of body weight that is fat generally increases with age (Table 5-1).[1] In older patients, TBW is a lower proportion of body weight. For example, a 20-year-old man weighing 70 kg is estimated to have 42 L of TBW. That same man reaching the age of 70 years would be expected to have 31 L of TBW. This 11-L difference corresponds to primarily a reduction in muscle mass. TBW is measured by indicator dilution methods. The indicators used in clinical research are deuterium oxide (D_2O, an isotope of water), tritium, and nonradioactive water enriched with ^{18}O, the heavy isotope of oxygen. TBW was determined by serial D_2O measurements in a cohort of adults who had long-term follow-up. Subjects ingested a known mass of D_2O, and at 3 hours the concentration of the isotope in plasma was used to estimate its volume of distribution. Predicting body composition in an individual patient is done with models that include, as independent predictor variables, age, gender, and race, as well as

standard measures of stature such as height and weight.[1]

Two Major Body Water Compartments

Body water can be divided into two major compartments. Intracellular fluid (ICF) is the largest compartment and is estimated to be 55% of TBW (Fig. 5-1). Extracellular fluid (ECF) is 45% of TBW. The solutes in the ICF and ECF compartments are different. Energy is consumed during active transport of electrolytes across cell membranes. In ICF the principal cation is potassium and the anions are phosphates and bicarbonate, but the anions are primarily the negatively charged sites on organic molecules. In ECF the principal cation is sodium, and chloride and bicarbonate are the anions. ECF can be further divided into subcompartments defined by membranes and tissue composition. Water and solutes in the plasma fluid compartment are filtered across the microvascular membrane and become interstitial fluid, which subsequently flows through the lymphatics and returns to plasma. Water in bone and in dense connective tissue such as cartilage and tendons is fixed and does not readily flow with ECF in the interstitium and lymphatics. Transcellular water (TCW) is secreted from cells, with most TCW being located in the lumen of the gastrointestinal tract and a small proportion found in the synovial, cerebrospinal, and intraocular spaces. The volume of water in the gas-

Table 5-1 Body Composition* Estimated in Younger and Older Women of Similar Height and Weight, Separated by Race, as a Percentage of Body Weight

COMPARTMENT	AGE 20 YEARS		AGE 70 YEARS	
	Black	White	Black	White
ICW	30.3	30.7	26.3	25.1
ECW	19.9	19.0	13.4	12.8
TBW	50.2	49.7	39.7	37.9
Protein	15.1	14.8	13.4	12.8
Fat	29.6	30.7	36.2	37.5
Mineral	5.0	4.7	3.9	3.6

*Total body water (TBW) was measured as the dilution volume of an ingested dose of tritiated water. Extracellular water (ECW) was measured as the delayed gamma neuron activation for total body chloride. Intracellular water (ICW) was the difference TBW−ECW. Total body protein was calculated from total body nitrogen by gamma neutron activation. Total body fat was calculated from total body carbon measured in vivo by neutron inelastic scattering and total body nitrogen.

Adapted from Aloia JF, Vaswani A, Flaster E, Ma R: Relationship of body water compartments to age, race, and fat-free mass. J Lab Clin Med 132:483-490, 1998.

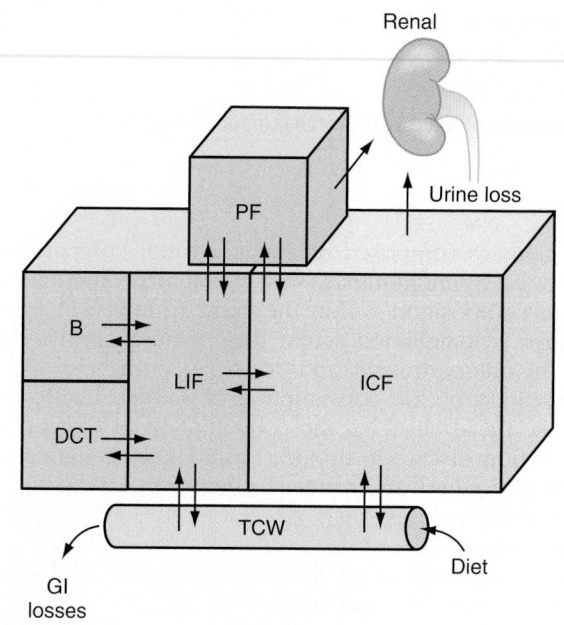

Figure 5-1 Total body water is divided into intracellular fluid (ICF), 55% of body water, with potassium being the predominant cation solute, and extracellular fluid (ECF), 45% of body water, with sodium being the predominant cation solute. ECF is divided into lymphatic and interstitial fluid (LIF, 20% of body water), water in bone (B, 7.5% of body water), water in dense connective tissues (DCT) such as cartilage and tendons (DCT, 7.5% of body water), and water in plasma fluid (PF, 7.5% of body water). Transcellular water (TCW, 2.5% of body water) is located in the lumen of the gastrointestinal (GI) tract.

trointestinal tract is increased by drinking and eating. Water and nutrients consumed in a diet are distributed in the water of the ECF and ICF compartments. These nutrients support metabolism. Waste products released from cells diffuse or are transported from the ICF to the ECF and through the lymphatics to the plasma compartment, where they are excreted primarily through renal function, except for carbon dioxide, which is exhaled in respiratory gases. Variable amounts of water and solutes can also be eliminated in evacuated stool, water in respiratory gases, and water and electrolytes in sweat. These latter three types of excretion are not tightly regulated. Renal function is modulated by a complex interaction of local regulatory factors and systemic hormones and is critical to the homeostasis of ECF and ICF. The size and composition of these compartments are determined by the volume of water and solutes excreted in urine.

Indicator dilution methods can be used to measure the volumes of extracellular and plasma fluid. Indicators are injected into ECF and given time to reach equilibrium by being distributed in the available volume. With knowledge of the mass of the indicator injected and the final concentration, the distribution volume can be calculated. The charge and molecular size of the indicator influence the measurement. ECF measured as the distribution volume of NaBr is 20% larger than ECF measured with $^{35}SO_4$, perhaps because of the difference in these two molecules' ability to gain access to bone and dense connective tissue water spaces. Investigators use simultaneous measurement with two separate indicators for TBW and ECF to calculate ICF volume as TBW minus ECF. Indicator dilution measurements are expensive and require meticulous technique, and in current clinical practice they are limited to research applications. Accurate indicator dilution measurements of body water compartments are best achieved in patients in a steady state and without rapidly changing pathologic conditions such as ascites, pleural effusions, or subcutaneous edema.

Bioimpedance Methods for Measuring Total Body Water

Bioimpedance spectroscopy, also called *bioelectrical impedance analysis,* is a clinically applicable method for estimating the volume of water in a body. Sensors are applied to a wrist and an ankle, and total body impedance is measured over a range of alternating sinusoidal current impulses that are imperceptible to the patient. Conduction of electric current through soft tissues is a function of the electrolyte concentrations in water, with bone and fat being poor conductors. Biophysical models applied to data collected during bioimpedence spectroscopy enable the clinician to estimate an individual's TBW, and with a measure of the individual's total body weight, the clinician calculates an estimate of body fat. The prevalence of obesity in modern society is increasing, and surgeons have a growing need to evaluate the bariatric surgical procedures. Cox-Reijven and colleagues reported that bioimpedence spectroscopy could precisely define changes in body composition during weight loss.[2] Bioimpedence spectroscopy has been validated by indicator dilution measurements in normal men and women.

Bioimpedence has been used to measure body composition in critically ill patients, but reliability of the estimates is reduced in overhydrated patients, a condition common in the intensive care unit (ICU). The expanded use of bioimpedence technology to assist surgeons in their care of critically ill patients will depend on the derivation and validation of new equations.

Measurement of Intracellular Fluid With Potassium

Investigators measure the volume of ICF by determining the total body's content of potassium at a relatively fixed concentration of 140 mEq/L. More than 90% of potassium in the human body is a solute inside cells. Potassium 40 (^{40}K) is a naturally occurring isotope, and the total body mass of ^{40}K can be measured with a scintillation counter composed of an array of ^{32}NaI detectors in a heavily shielded room. To calculate ICF volume, the investigator determines the volume of ECF by using indicator dilution methods and multiplies this measured volume by the concentration of ^{40}K in a serum sample to determine the mass of ^{40}K in ECF. ^{40}K in ECF is subtracted from the total body ^{40}K value (as measured with a scintillation counter), and the investigator measures the mass of ^{40}K in cells. This assessment method is particularly useful in serial measurements of body composition. Investigators assumed that the concentration of ^{40}K in cells is essentially unchanged over a wide range of conditions, and thus an increase or decrease in calculated ICF ^{40}K mass correspondingly reflects an increase or decrease in ICF volume. Finn and associates used ^{40}K to study body composition in patients and found that over a period of 3 weeks, severe stress from injury or sepsis led to cell shrinkage in patients in an ICU.[3] In this study, TBW was measured by tritium dilution and ECW was measured with both bromide tracers and bioimpedence spectroscopy. The authors observed that even though the patients had an expanded ECF volume, they still suffered from cellular dehydration (Figs. 5-2 and 5-3).

Control of Body Water Distribution Between Intracellular and Extracellular Fluid by Osmolality

Osmolality is a measure of the total number of solutes per mass of water and is clinically measured in units of millimoles per kilogram of water (mmol/kg H_2O). The principal osmoles in ICF are the electrolytes potassium, bicarbonate, the organic molecules (DNA, RNA, creatine phosphate, adenosine triphosphate [ATP], adenosine diphosphate [ADP], and phospholipids), and the uncharged metabolite molecules glucose and urea. The principal osmoles in ECF are the electrolytes sodium, chloride, and bicarbonate. Inorganic species (sulfate, phosphate) and uncharged metabolite molecules of glucose and urea are also present in ECF, but at substantially lower concentration, and thus have minimal impact on osmolality (Fig. 5-4). A fundamental principle of body fluid homeostasis is that TBW moves across cell membranes and distributes between ICF and ECF until the osmolality in these two compartments is the same. Cell membranes are readily permeable to water, and water shifts rapidly between ECF and ICF to achieve balance in osmolality. In contrast to water, the majority of solutes,

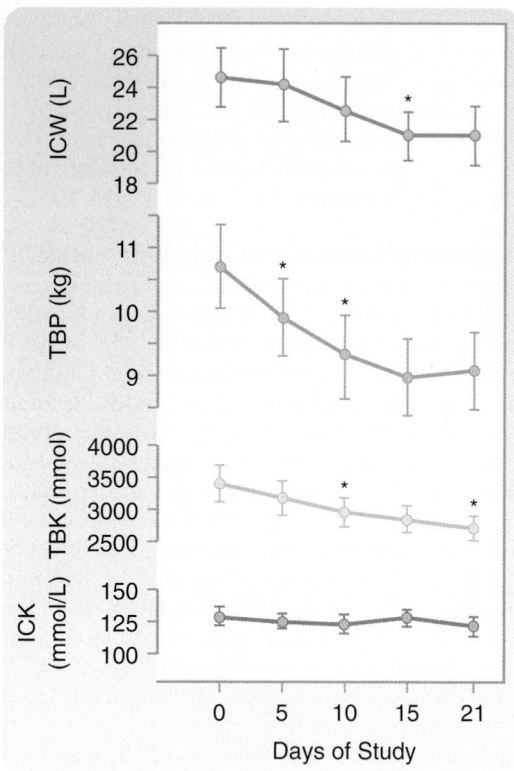

Figure 5-2 Sequential measurements of intracellular water (ICW), total body protein (TBP), total body potassium (TBK), and intracellular potassium (ICK) concentration in nine multiply injured patients. *Asterisks* (*) indicate significant change from the preceding measurement. (From Finn PJ, Plank LD, Clark MA, et al: Progressive cellular dehydration and proteolysis in critically ill patients. Lancet 347:654-656, 1996.)

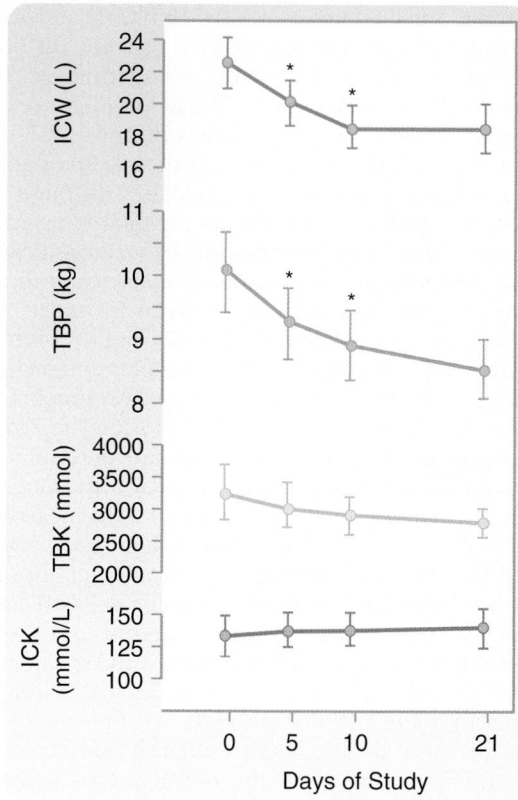

Figure 5-3 Sequential measurements of intracellular water (ICW), total body protein (TBP), total body potassium (TBK), and intracellular potassium (ICK) concentration in 11 patients with severe sepsis. *Asterisks* (*) indicate significant change from the preceding measurement. (From Finn PJ, Plank LD, Clark MA, et al: Progressive cellular dehydration and proteolysis in critically ill patients. Lancet 347:654-656, 1996.)

which determine osmolality in the two fluid compartments, cross the cell membrane only through regulated transport mechanisms. Active transport mechanisms, which depend on consumption of biochemical energy, move electrolytes across the cell membrane.

Renal function regulates the size of the ICF and ECF compartments by control of the excretion of solutes in urine and control of the osmolality of urine (Fig. 5-5). Renal control of sodium excretion (and with it the anion chloride) determines the size of the ECF compartment. Renal function in which sodium is retained and total body sodium mass is increased expands the size of the ECF compartment. Renal function controls the volume of TBW by producing urine with a range of osmolality from 100 to 1200 mmol/kg H_2O.

The concentration of urine produced is determined by the concentration of antidiuretic hormone (ADH) released from the pituitary. ADH is also called *arginine vasopressin* (AVP). ADH is a peptide synthesized in the hypothalamic region of the brain, stored in the pituitary, and released in response to several stimuli, including an increase in the osmolality of ICF and ECF greater than 285 mmol/kg H_2O. As the concentration of ADH in plasma increases, the osmolality of urine increases. If no ADH is circulating in plasma, the osmolality of urine

produced by the kidney can be less than 100 mmol/kg H_2O. This osmolality is a third of the osmolality of ECF, and the consequence for TBW balance is a net loss of water. If a maximum level of ADH is circulating in plasma, the osmolality of urine produced by the kidney can exceed 1200 mmol/kg H_2O. Production of urine with maximum osmolality means that TBW balance is positive and dilution of the osmolality of ECF and ICF is occurring. The sensation of thirst is another powerful factor that controls the osmolality of ECF and ICF by compelling an individual whose TBW is contracted with an elevation in osmolality to drink. As osmolality increases, a strong conscious desire to drink fluids is generated, thereby increasing the hydration of ECF. At the bedside, urine specific gravity is used to measure urine osmolality. A urine specific gravity of 1.010 units or less is a dilute urine and suggests that ADH levels are low. A urine specific gravity greater than 1.030 units suggests that the urine being produced is close to maximum osmolality.

Disorders of Body Water Balance

Disorders of water balance can be defined by pathologic changes in the production or release of ADH from the hypothalamus and pituitary, exogenous overproduction

DISTRIBUTION OF SOLUTES

Extracellular		Intracellular	
Na⁺	142	Na⁺	10
K⁺	4	K⁺	140
CL⁻	110	CL⁻	3
HCO₃⁻	24	HCO₃⁻	10
Inorganic⁻	12	*Organic⁻	137
Glucose	3	Glucose	2.5
OSM	300 ⟷ 300		
UREA ⟷ UREA			
(ETOH) ⟷ (ETOH)			

Units: mmol/kg of water, except organic⁻
*Units: mEq/kg of water

Figure 5-4 The cell membrane forms a selective barrier to electrolyte solutes. The osmolality (mmol/kg of water) of intracellular and extracellular water is equivalent because water can freely cross the cell membrane. Organic anions in intracellular water are macromolecules with multiple sites of phosphate ester charge per molecule. These organic anions include DNA, RNA, creatine phosphate, adenosine triphosphate, and phospholipids. Urea and ethanol can, like water, equilibrate rapidly by diffusion across the cell membrane. (From Halperin ML, Goldstein M: Fluid, Electrolyte, and Acid-Base Physiology: A Problem-Based Approach, 3rd ed. Philadelphia, WB Saunders, 1999.)

THE NEPHRON

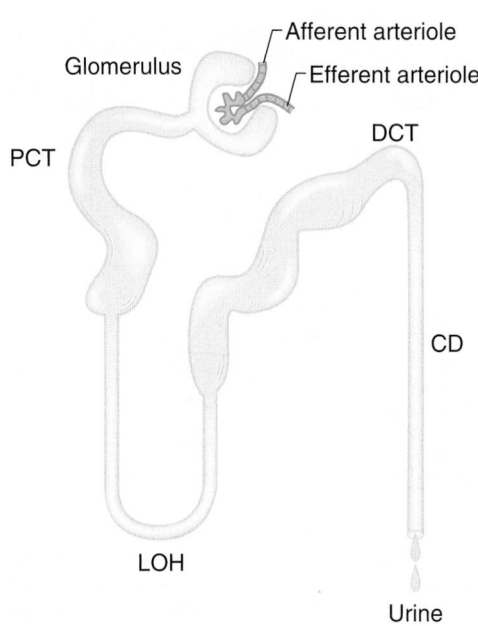

Figure 5-5 The major components of the nephron are the glomerulus, where plasma delivered in afferent arterioles is filtered; the proximal convoluted tubule (PCT); the loop of Henle (LOH); the distal convoluted tubule (DCT); and the collecting duct (CD). Different components of renal function occur along the nephron. A normal glomerular filtration rate of 125 mL/min would generate 180 L/day of filtrate containing 27,000 mmol of sodium. Approximately two thirds of the filtered sodium is absorbed in the PCT, 20% in the LOH, 7% in the DCT, and 3% in the CD; the net excretion of urinary sodium per day, as a fraction of the total sodium filtered load, is less than 1%.

of ADH, or failure of the renal tubular cells to respond to the hormone ADH. Brain-injured patients are one group who can suddenly stop synthesizing ADH because the hypothalamus or pituitary is destroyed. Typically, within a few hours of the cessation of release of ADH into plasma, these injured patients are producing dilute urine at flow rates in excess of 1 L/hr. This clinical syndrome is designated diabetes insipidus. Without ADH, the urine has a fixed osmolality of less than 100 mmol/kg H₂O. These patients will urinate at high flow rates, hyperosmolality will develop rapidly, and their serum sodium concentration will exceed 150 mEq/L. A patient with diabetes insipidus will continue to have high urine flow rates until the ECF is depleted and blood volume is reduced sufficiently to cause a drop in mean arterial blood pressure. The diuresis of diabetes insipidus stops when the patient is in shock and there is insufficient perfusion pressure to maintain renal function. Excessive production of ADH produces a syndrome of overhydration. These patients have a measured osmolality in ECF of less than 285 mmol/kg H₂O, yet they continue to produce urine that has an osmolality in excess of 300 mmol/kg H₂O. This syndrome is discussed in detail in the section of this chapter on hyponatremia, which is the essential finding in patients who have hypo-osmolality.

Body Solute Composition and Electrolyte Composition of Extracellular and Intracellular Fluid

Distribution of Solutes Between Intracellular and Extracellular Fluid

Sodium is the predominant cation in ECF and associates with the anions chloride and bicarbonate. These three electrolytes account for more than 90% of the active osmoles in ECF. The predominant cation in ICF is potassium, which is electrochemically balanced primarily by organic phosphates. In addition, DNA, RNA, ATP, ADP, and creatine phosphate are anionic and provide a negative charge to balance the positive charge of potassium in intracellular water (ICW). The difference in electrolyte composition between ICF and ECF is sustained by the activity of transport enzymes embedded in the cell membrane. These enzymes can actively transport sodium from ICW to extracellular water (ECW) in exchange for potassium. The enzyme Na⁺,K⁺-ATPase plays a key role in sustaining the difference in electrolyte composition between ECF and ICF (Fig. 5-6). Na⁺,K⁺-ATPase binds three sodium ions in ICW and uses the energy provided by hydrolysis of ATP to ADP to change its conformation and move three sodium molecules out of the cell while

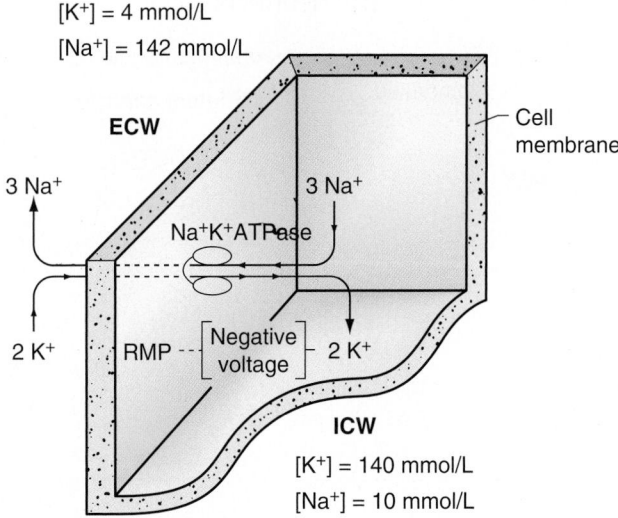

[K⁺] = 4 mmol/L
[Na⁺] = 142 mmol/L

ECW

Cell membrane

3 Na⁺   3 Na⁺

Na⁺K⁺ATPase

2 K⁺   RMP   Negative voltage   2 K⁺

ICW

[K⁺] = 140 mmol/L
[Na⁺] = 10 mmol/L

Figure 5-6 The resting membrane potential (RMP) within cells of a negative charge is established by the cell membrane enzyme Na⁺/K⁺-ATPase, which uses energy to pump three sodium molecules out of the cell for every two potassium molecules transported into the cell. ECW, extracellular water; ICW, intracellular water.

concurrently two potassium ions in ECF enter the cell. With three cations transported out and two cations transported into the cell, the electrochemical consequence of Na⁺,K⁺-ATPase activity is a net negative intracellular charge. The net negative charge within ICF is designated the resting membrane potential. In ICF the majority of anionic molecules are large and cannot diffuse across the cell membrane. Restricted to ICF, these negatively charged macromolecules contribute to the resting membrane potential. The voltage of the resting membrane potential is essential for cell function and is the basis for nerve cell conduction and muscle cell contraction.

Control of Na⁺,K⁺-ATPase involves multiple factors. An increase in ICF sodium concentration occurs during an action potential, when a pore opens in the cell membrane to allow sodium to transiently shift along its concentration gradient into the cell. The response to an increase in intracellular sodium concentration is accelerated Na⁺,K⁺-ATPase activity. Regulation of the electrolyte concentration is a critical function for survival and is accomplished within cells by local feedback mechanisms along with circulating hormones, including aldosterone and adrenergic agents. The substantial difference between potassium concentrations in ICF and ECF favors diffusion of potassium along a concentration gradient to the ECF. Transport of potassium along this gradient is passive, with no energy being required. However, the negative charge of the resting membrane potential powerfully favors potassium to remain intracellular. In normal cells, the ICF sodium concentration is 10 mmol/L and the potassium concentration is 150 mmol/L. Conversely, in ECW, the sodium concentration is 140 mmol/L and the potassium concentration averages 4 mmol/L. The Na⁺,K⁺-ATPase pump is constantly active and continuously con-

sumes the energy in ATP to sustain the resting membrane potential. In circumstances in which insufficient oxygen is available to sustain aerobic metabolism and, consequently, cellular ATP levels fall, the sodium pump function is impaired. One reason that cell dysfunction and death occur in patients in shock is that the intracellular sodium concentration increases and the resting membrane potential declines.

Sodium

The normal serum sodium ion concentration [Na⁺] ranges between 138 and 145 mEq/L. Hyponatremia can be classified as mild, moderate, or severe. Mild hyponatremia is present when [Na⁺] lies between 130 and 138 mEq/L, and moderate hyponatremia is present when [Na⁺] declines to the range of 120 to 130 mEq/L. Patients with mild to moderate hyponatremia rarely have signs or symptoms of their hyponatremia, and these patients are identified on serial laboratory testing. A falling [Na⁺] prompts the surgeon to evaluate the patient for reversible causes of the decline in [Na⁺]. *Severe hyponatremia* is defined as an [Na⁺] less than 120 mEq/L. A falling [Na⁺] indicates that the osmolality in ECF and ICF is also falling, which means that cells are swelling because osmoles inside cells cannot be readily transported out to the ECF. Intracranial cell swelling in patients with acute severe hyponatremia causes headaches and lethargy, and these patients may rapidly progress to coma or have seizures. Patients with coexisting brain injury, infection, or tumor in whom moderate hyponatremia develops are at risk for deteriorated neurologic function.

Acute dilution of osmolality can occur if patients with an ECF deficit are given sodium-free water. Acute hyponatremia develops in patients who rapidly incur a deficit in ECF that is replaced with either an enterally or intravenously (IV) infused hypo-osmotic fluid. IV infusion of 5% dextrose in water rapidly produces hyponatremia in patients who have hemorrhaged or suffered an acute bout of diarrhea or in patients with pancreatitis or a burn wound in whom inflammatory edema has developed. The hyponatremia problem is exacerbated in patients with a contracted blood volume because the hypothalamus of these patients is stimulated by the shock to release ADH. The normal hypothalamic-pituitary response to hyponatremia is suppression of ADH release, and as the dilute urine is excreted, there is a corrective increase in serum [Na⁺]. A moderate or severely hyponatremic patient should have undetectable blood levels of ADH. However, release of ADH can be stimulated by both elevated ECF osmolality and a reduction in ECF volume. Patients with a contracted blood volume have activation of their baroreceptors, which provide feedback to the hypothalamus. ADH is released from the pituitary if the patient is hypovolemic, even if ECF osmolality is diluted. Preservation of normal ECF has higher precedence than maintenance of normal osmolality.

A syndrome has been described in which patients experience a rapid onset of severe hyponatremia after a surgical procedure. Patients with small body stature, particularly menstruating females, have been described by

Arieff as individuals at high risk for this syndrome of hyponatremia.[4] Arieff described 15 women in whom [Na$^+$] declined from a mean of 138 to 108 mEq/L by the second postoperative day. Decreased responsiveness, seizures, and catastrophic respiratory arrest were the first clinical indications of hyponatremia in many of the patients. Arieff measured an average urine sodium concentration of 68 mEq/L and an average urine osmolality of 501 mOsm/L at the time when [Na$^+$] was at its nadir, which indicates that these patients had elevated levels of serum ADH despite having an ECF osmolality substantially less than 300 mmol/kg H$_2$O.

Acute hyponatremia can complicate a diuretic-induced, forced diuresis. Loop diuretics and IV infusion of mannitol, which increase urine flow and reduce plasma volume, can lead not only to an increase in ADH but also to excessive loss of sodium in urine. Sustained hyperglycemia can induce an osmotic diuresis that depletes ECF water. Hyponatremia can be a very challenging problem to correct in patients with a substantial increase in ECF, especially ascites and pleural effusions, but who have a contracted blood volume. In these patients the surgeon may need to accept as routine an [Na$^+$] in the range of mild to moderate hyponatremia.

Renal loss of sodium can lead to hyponatremia in patients who have excessive release of natriuretic peptides related to brain injury or disease. Cerebral salt wasting occurs in patients with a variety of brain lesions. Berendes and associates studied a group of patients with subarachnoid hemorrhage whom they aggressively infused with sodium to maintain a normal [Na$^+$].[5] They noted high urine output of 4 to 6 L/day and renal sodium excretion rates that were twice normal. They correlated days of elevated brain natriuretic peptide levels in plasma with elevated sodium levels in urine in hyponatremic patients and hypothesized that excessive renal loss of sodium accounted for the development of moderate hyponatremia in these patients. Treatment of patients with cerebral salt wasting requires the administration of sufficient daily sodium to sustain normal total body sodium balance. An additional cause of hyponatremia in patients with impaired consciousness is that many are given enteral nutrition with tube feeding formulations low in sodium. Hyponatremic patients with salt loss can receive sodium replacement therapy guided by 24-hour urinary sodium excretion. In brain-injured patients at risk that even mild hyponatremia can cause minimal, but pathologically significant cerebral swelling, IV infusion of isotonic or even 3% hypertonic saline solutions is required to prevent hyponatremia.

Acute water intoxication as a complication of a surgical procedure is a rare cause of hyponatremia. Water intoxication has developed during endoscopic procedures performed with hypo-osmotic irrigation fluids, including transcervical endometrial resection and transurethral resection of the prostrate. These patients can suffer an abrupt onset of severe hyponatremia with potentially lethal neurologic complications.

Successful treatment of acute hyponatremia usually requires the surgeon to IV infuse isotonic saline to expand a contracted ECF volume. The urgency for correction of [Na$^+$] is greatest in patients with severe hyponatremia who are at risk for seizures. The recommended rate of infusion of sodium-containing solutions in patients with acute hyponatremia and [Na$^+$] less than 120 mEq/L is one that increases serum [Na$^+$] not more rapidly than 0.25 mEq/L/hr.

Chronic Hyponatremia

The syndrome of inappropriate release of antidiuretic hormone (SIADH) has been a carefully studied cause of chronic hyponatremia. The diagnosis of SIADH can be made only in euvolemic patients. Patients with SIADH have a serum osmolality of less than 270 mmol/kg H$_2$O along with inappropriately concentrated urine. A hyponatremic patient with a urine osmolality greater 350 mmol/kg H$_2$O is producing ADH. If the patient is hypovolemic, the elevated ADH is an appropriate response. If the patients is euvolemic or even has an expanded blood volume, the cause of the patient's hyponatremia is probably SIADH. Inappropriate production of ADH by the hypothalamus at an ECF osmolality of less than 285 mmol/kg H$_2$O may indicate a resetting of the osmolality threshold of cells. Patients with indisputable SIADH are those with an ADH-secreting tumor, usually a carcinoid or small cell carcinoma of the lung. ADH can also be inappropriately released from the hypothalamus as a result of cerebral injury, infection, or tumor. Up to 35% of patients with acquired immunodeficiency syndrome (AIDS) admitted to the hospital with an active infection have hyponatremia and meet the criteria for SIADH. Renal dysfunction can be the primary cause of hyponatremia. Patients with chronic renal disease may have an impaired capacity to retain sodium, and hyponatremia associated with a contraction in the ECF volume subsequently develops. Renal diagnoses associated with obligatory sodium loss include medullary cystic disease, polycystic kidney disease, analgesic nephropathy, chronic pyelonephritis, and obstructive uropathy postdecompression syndromes. These patients require supplemental sodium as well as fluid to maintain normal ECF volume and compensate for daily fixed loss of sodium and water.

Rapid correction of [Na$^+$] in patients with chronic hyponatremia can lead to central pontine myelinolysis, a severe, permanent neurologic disorder characterized by spastic quadriparesis, pseudobulbar palsy, and depressed levels of consciousness. Although patients with acute, severe hyponatremia often have evidence of neurologic dysfunction, individuals with chronic, severely depressed levels of [Na$^+$] are often neurologically normal. To avoid the complications of central pontine myelinolysis, the maximal rate of sodium correction should not exceed 0.25 mEq/L/hr. Thus, the rate of increase in serum [Na$^+$] should not exceed 8 mEq/kg/day. Serum sodium correction rates should remain slow when serum [Na$^+$] exceeds 120 mEq/L. Additional factors should be kept in mind during correction of chronic hyponatremia. The compensatory depletion of intracellular potassium during prolonged hyponatremia requires that as ECF sodium is repleted, large amounts of supplemental potassium also

Table 5-2   Given a Patient With Hypernatremia (Serum [Na⁺]=160 mEq/L), the Estimated Change in [Na⁺] After Infusion of 1 L

$$\frac{\text{Change In [Na}^+]}{\text{L}} = \frac{(\text{Infusate [Na}^+] - \text{Serum [Na}^+])}{\text{TBW} + 1}$$

INFUSATE	WOMAN, AGE 70 YEARS 50 kg×0.45=22.5 L TBW	MAN, AGE 20 YEARS 80 kg×0.60=48.0 L TBW
D₅W	$\frac{(0-160)}{22.5+1} = -6.8$	$\frac{(0-160)}{48+1} = -3.3$
D₅ 0.2% NaCl	$\frac{(34-160)}{22.5+1} = -5.3$	$\frac{(34-160)}{48+1} = -2.6$
D₅ 0.45% NaCl	$\frac{(77-160)}{22.5+1} = -3.5$	$\frac{(77-160)}{48+1} = -1.7$

D₅W, 5% dextrose in water.

be administered to restore the ICF deficit. Patients with mild and moderate hyponatremia can be treated by restricting intake of water.

Hypernatremia and Syndromes of Hypertonicity

An acute onset of hypernatremia increases ECF osmolality and contracts the size of the ICF compartment. Patients have moderate hypernatremia if their serum [Na⁺] is 146 to 159 mEq/L. Patients with [Na⁺] greater than 160 mEq/L have severe, life-threatening hypernatremia.[6] Water loss is the most common explanation for acute hypernatremia. For example, hypernatremia can develop in patients who do not replace the water lost after excessive sweating in a hot environment or unregulated loss of hypo-osmotic gastrointestinal fluids. Neurologic damage as a result of contraction of brain cell volume is the primary risk associated with hypernatremia. As [Na⁺] exceeds 160 mEq/L, patients have an altered level of consciousness and seizures, and coma and intracerebral hemorrhage can develop. Although severe hypernatremia may not be associated with hypotension in a supine patient, postural hypotension, dry mucous membranes, and decreased skin turgor are clinical findings indicating that a hypernatremic patient has a significant contraction in ECF volume. The normal renal response to increased [Na⁺] is for the nephron to generate hyperosmolar urine and retain water. However, renal correction of hypernatremia depends on the patient having access to water. Severe hypernatremia rarely occurs in conscious patients because relentless thirst compels them to drink water. In contrast, severe hypernatremia can develop in pharmacologically sedated patients, disoriented patients with severe agitation from drug intoxication, or patients in delirium tremens.

Endocrine syndromes caused by failure to synthesize and release ADH or failure of the renal tubular cells to respond to ADH can result in hypernatremia. Hypernatremia can develop in patients with diabetes insipidus who have sustained a large water loss. In one clinical series, 50% of patients with diabetes insipidus had a pathologic condition identified that could explain the failure to produce ADH, including brain injury, intracerebral hemorrhage, skull base or pituitary surgery, or cerebral infection. Idiopathic diabetes insipidus can be due to an autoimmune mechanism. Patients with hypernatremia have been studied who appear to have adjusted the osmolality threshold in their hypothalamus from a normal level of 285 mmol/kg H₂O to a higher value. *Nephrogenic diabetes insipidus* is defined as an impaired capacity of the renal tubules to respond to ADH and concentrate urine. Moderate hypernatremia develops in patients with nephrogenic diabetes insipidus when they lose water in dilute urine despite having elevated plasma levels of ADH. The diagnosis of nephrogenic diabetes insipidus can be established if an infusion of exogenous ADH does not increase urine osmolality. Several pathologic conditions have been identified as causing nephrogenic diabetes insipidus. Renal tubular cells may be poorly responsive to AVP after decompression of chronically obstructed ureters. Nephrogenic diabetes insipidus can also develop in patients with sickle cell nephropathy and medullary cystic disease. Lithium, glyburide, demeclocycline, and amphotericin B can all induce nephrogenic diabetes insipidus. Hypercalcemia and severe hypokalemia impair the capacity of renal tubular cells to reabsorb Na⁺ from tubule fluid. Patients with end-stage renal dysfunction and low glomerular filtration rates may produce a fixed volume of 2 to 4 L/day of iso-osmolar urine. These patients, in hot and arid environments, are particularly susceptible to dehydration and the development of hypernatremia. Hypernatremia can also emerge rapidly in patients as a result of excessive and uncontrollable loss of hypotonic fluids. Geriatric patients with serious infections are at higher risk for hypernatremia on admission to the hospital. Hypernatremia is rarely caused by the IV infusion of a large sodium load, as might occur in patients resuscitated from shock with hypertonic saline or who received IV injections with multiple doses of sodium bicarbonate.

Treatment of Hypernatremia

Treatment of patients with hypernatremia secondary to dehydration involves IV or oral administration of water. Hypernatremic patients typically have significantly reduced blood volumes, and these patients are treated by the IV infusion of isotonic saline solutions until the contracted ECF has been restored. Then the patients should receive sufficient electrolyte-free water to enable their renal function to produce concentrated urine and correct the hypernatremia. A rapid decline in ECF osmolality in a severely hypernatremic patient can lead to cerebral injury as a result of cellular swelling. [Na⁺] should be lowered at a rate not to exceed 8 mEq/day. The optimal replacement fluid in patients with hypernatremia can be estimated by body size and electrolyte composition (Table 5-2). Patients with hypernatremia may also have deficits in total body potassium related to shrinkage of ICW. Serial serum chemistry studies are needed during correction of severe hypernatremia to monitor the response to therapy. Correction of hypernatremia caused by unregulated water loss should be achieved with a fluid replacement protocol that offsets the ongoing water loss. Patients with central diabetes insipidus who are producing urine at hundreds of milliliters per hour are treated with desmopressin. Desmopressin (1-desamino-8-D-arginine vasopressin [DDAVP]) is a synthetic analogue of ADH that has a half-life of several hours after IV injection. It is the agent of choice for treating patients with central diabetes insipidus because the drug increases water movement out of the collecting duct but does not have the vasoconstrictive effects of ADH. Patients with partial ADH deficiency typically have mild diabetes insipidus and are successfully managed with intranasal desmopressin and copious water intake. Patients with central diabetes insipidus treated with drugs on an outpatient basis risk the rapid development of hypernatremia in the event of a surgical emergency and discontinuation of desmopressin.

Potassium

The normal potassium concentration ([K^+]) in ECF is 4.5 mmol/L. [K^+] can neither increase nor decrease more than 3 mmol/L from the normal value without endangering the patient's life. Tight control of [K^+] is essential. More than 98% of the body's potassium is located in the ICF compartment. A substantial proportion of the daily consumption of oxygen by the body is used to maintain N^+,K^+-ATPase activity. In the daily intake of a diet, an individual consumes 50 to 100 mmol of potassium. Renal function controls the day-to-day [K^+] in ECF by ensuring that the excess potassium consumed in the diet is cleared in urine. Normal renal function can excrete a range of potassium in a day's urine, from less than 20 to greater than 400 mmol. The renin-angiotensin-aldosterone hormone axis plays a key role in renal control of potassium clearance. As the concentration of the hormone aldosterone increases in plasma, the concentration of potassium in urine increases.

Hyperkalemia

Hyperkalemia is defined as [K^+] that exceeds 5.0 mmol/L. As [K^+] exceeds 6 mmol/L, alterations occur in the resting cell membrane potential that impair normal depolarization and repolarization. Cardiac arrhythmias caused by the rapid onset of hyperkalemia often prove lethal. Electrocardiographic changes may provide the first clinical indication of hyperkalemia. Hyperkalemia in the range of 6 to 7 mmol/L may be associated with tall T waves. Symmetrically peaked T waves indicate dangerous hyperkalemia, particularly if the T waves are higher than the R wave in more than one lead (Fig. 5-7). As [K^+] exceeds 7 mmol/L, P-wave amplitudes on the electrocardiogram decrease, PR segments increase, and the QRS complex widens. As [K^+] exceeds 8 mmol/L, suddenly lethal arrhythmias ensue, such as asystole, ventricular fibrillation, or a wide pulseless idioventricular rhythm.

An acute onset of renal dysfunction or renal failure is the most common clinical cause of a rapid onset of hyperkalemia.[7] Patients with renal dysfunction may be protected from the development of hyperkalemia because they have an adequate fixed volume of urine output that enables clearance of their daily ingested potassium load.

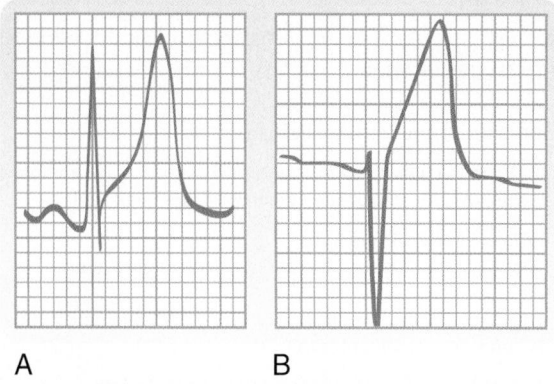

Figure 5-7 A, Electrocardiographic (ECG) changes indicating hyperkalemia. The T wave is tall, narrow, and symmetrical. **B,** ECG changes indicating acute myocardial infarction. The T wave is tall but broad-based and asymmetric. (From Somers MP, Brady WJ, Perron AD, Mattu A: The prominent T wave: Electrocardiographic differential diagnosis. Am J Emerg Med 20:243-251, 2002.)

However, patients with oliguric renal dysfunction or renal failure are at risk for a rapid increase in [K^+]. Patients in acute renal failure may experience a sudden release of potassium from ICF related to injury or sepsis. Patients with loss of more than 80% of normal renal function cannot respond to even markedly elevated levels of aldosterone in plasma to achieve urinary potassium excretion. Impaired release of aldosterone in a patient with normal renal function can lead to hyperkalemia. Injury or damage to the adrenals, including hemorrhagic infarction of both adrenal glands, can result in hyperkalemia, although typically these patients have only a modest elevation in serum [K^+] because other renal mechanisms are activated and stimulate the excretion of excess potassium in urine. Drugs with a direct effect on renal tubular cells that increase [K^+] include the diuretics spironolactone and triamterene, β-blockers, and cyclosporine and tacrolimus, immunosuppression drugs used in organ transplantation. Drugs are usually a contributing factor to hyperkalemia and not a primary cause.

Sudden release of potassium from ICF can cause hyperkalemia by overloading the capacity of renal function to clear potassium. Reperfusion of ischemic skeletal muscle is a clinical syndrome that has been recognized to incite a reperfusion injury that can lead to rhabdomyolysis and release of K^+. Reperfusion injury occurs at the completion of arterial injury repair and when the delay in achieving reperfusion exceeds 4 to 6 hours and the mass of skeletal muscle is large (i.e., an entire leg). In these circumstances, sufficient potassium can be washed out to produce immediate life-threatening hyperkalemia. To prevent cardiac arrest in this circumstance, bolus IV infusion of sodium bicarbonate is given immediately before reperfusion of the ischemic tissues by release of the arterial clamp. The bicarbonate shifts potassium from the ECF across the cell membrane into ICF. Precipitous hyperkalemia can follow the IV injection of succinylcholine, a depolarizing paralytic agent, when used in patients

---

Box 5-1 Guidelines for Treatment of Adult Patients With Hyperkalemia

FIRST: Stop all infusion of potassium

ECG EVIDENCE OF PENDING ARREST: Loss of P wave and broad slurring of QRS; immediate effective therapy indicated

1. IV infusion of calcium salts
   10 mL of 10% calcium chloride over a 10-minute period
   or
   10 mL of 10% calcium gluconate over a 3- to 5-minute period
2. IV infusion of sodium bicarbonate

   50-100 mEq over a 10- to 20-minute period; benefit proportional to extent of pretherapy acidemia

ECG EVIDENCE OF POTASSIUM EFFECT: Peaked T waves; prompt therapy needed

1. Glucose and insulin infusion
   IV infusion of 50 mL of $D_{50}W$ and 10 units of regular insulin; monitor glucose
2. Immediate hemodialysis

BIOCHEMICAL EVIDENCE OF HYPERKALEMIA AND NO ECG CHANGES: Effective therapy needed within hours

1. Potassium-binding resins into the gastrointestinal tract, with 20% sorbitol
2. Promotion of renal kaliuresis by loop diuretic

$D_{50}W$, 50% dextrose in water; ECG, electrocardiographic; IV, intravenous.

---

with muscle atrophy from disuse, neurologic denervation syndromes, severe burns, direct muscle trauma, or rhabdomyolysis syndromes or in patients after prolonged bed rest. Succinylcholine induces a sustained reduction of resting membrane potential in myocytes, and without a negative charge in the cell there is accelerated movement of K^+ from skeletal muscle cells into ECW. It is best to use a paralytic agent other than succinylcholine in high-risk patients.[8]

Treatment of Acute Hyperkalemia

Several interventions are useful in patients at risk for cardiac arrhythmias from hyperkalemia. IV calcium can immediately reduce the risk for arrhythmia in hyperkalemic patients with characteristic electrocardiographic changes. Calcium antagonizes the depolarization effect of elevated $[K^+]$. Sodium bicarbonate infusion buffers ECW protons and allows net transfer of cytosolic protons across the cell membrane via carbonic acid. The shift of protons out of the cell is associated with a shift of potassium into ICF. Bicarbonate therapy is most effective in hyperkalemic patients with metabolic acidemia. Insulin and glucose infusions prompt an increase in Na^+/K^+-ATPase activity and a decline in ECW potassium concentration as the ECW potassium is pumped into the ICW. Patients who suffer aldosterone deficiency as well as hyperkalemia will increase renal excretion of potassium if treated with a mineralocorticoid drug such as 9α-fludrocortisone. Hemodialysis is the most reliable method for controlling hyperkalemia in patients with acute renal

failure. Continuous filtration methods clear K^+ from ECF at a slower rate than hemodialysis does. Chronic hyperkalemia associated with renal dysfunction can be managed by oral or rectal administration of sodium polystyrene sulfonate, a cation exchange resin that binds potassium in the gut lumen. Rectally administered binding resins are particularly effective because the colonic mucosa can excrete mucus with large amounts of potassium. Surgeons should have a process for managing hyperkalemia clearly established because patients can have a rapidly escalating potassium level that is an immediate threat and requires rapidly delivered effective therapy (Box 5-1).

Hypokalemia

Patients with hypokalemia have a $[K^+]$ lower than 3.5 mmol/L. Generalized symptoms commonly associated with depressed serum levels include fatigue, weakness, and ileus. Rarely, rhabdomyolysis may occur in patients whose $[K^+]$ drops below 2.5 mmol/L. Flaccid paralysis with respiratory compromise can occur as $[K^+]$ decreases to less than 2 mmol/L. Hypokalemia is a common problem in hospitalized patients. Patients with persistent vomiting or who drain large volumes via gastric tubes, diarrhea, or high-output enteric or pancreatic fistulas can lose large amounts of potassium. Hypokalemia is a common problem in patients with congestive heart failure managed with multiple drugs. Hypokalemia develops in patients treated with diuretics that force renal function to excrete urine with an elevated potassium concentration. Long-term diuretic therapy can produce a sustained negative potassium balance and reduce ICW potassium levels. One consequence of impaired conduction in patients with chronic potassium deficiency is cardiac rhythm disturbance.[9] The electrocardiogram of patients with hypokalemia will show depressed T waves and U waves. Hypokalemia leads to cardiac arrhythmias, particularly atrial tachycardia with or without block, atrioventricular dissociation, ventricular tachycardia, and ventricular fibrillation. The risk for hypokalemia-associated arrhythmia is higher in patients treated with digoxin, even when potassium concentrations are in the low normal range.

Treatment of Acute Hypokalemia

Hypokalemic patients require potassium replacement. Potassium therapy is given as the chloride salt because hypokalemia is commonly associated with a contraction in ECW, where chloride is the predominant anion. Potassium in foods is linked to phosphate. Potassium phosphate salts may need to be given via IV, particularly when expansion of ICW is anticipated. To reduce the risk for serious cardiac arrhythmias in patients with cardiac disease or after cardiac surgery who have a serum value less than 3.5 mmol/L, serum $[K^+]$ should be promptly corrected to a level greater than 4.0 mmol/L.[8] Potassium infusion should not exceed a rate of 0.3 mmol/kg/hr to avoid overcorrection. High concentrations of potassium in IV fluids can be irritating to peripheral small veins, and infusions may therefore require a central venous catheter. Patients rarely require more than 200 mmol of potassium in 1 day. Patients with substantial and continuing gastrointestinal loss of potassium require extraordinary potassium replacement to achieve correction of hypokalemia.

Hypokalemic patients with concurrent acidemia are treated with potassium replacement before correction of pH by the administration of bicarbonate. Diabetics in ketoacidosis may initially have normal [K+], but hypokalemia rapidly develops as insulin is administered and glucose shifts into cells. Potassium supplements should be added to the resuscitation fluid of diabetic patients in ketoacidosis once the physician is confident that renal function is adequate. Patients in whom hypokalemia develops while undergoing diuretic therapy can be treated with additional drugs that reduce renal loss of potassium. Triamterene or spironolactone are two drugs that block the effect of aldosterone and cause a reduction in potassium loss in urine. Hypokalemic patients may also need magnesium, which is an important cofactor for potassium uptake and maintenance of intracellular potassium levels. In addition, supplemental magnesium reduces the risk for arrhythmia. Hypokalemia not caused by diuretics may be caused by a rare endocrine disorder, including primary hyperaldosteronism and renin-secreting tumors.

Calcium and Magnesium

Calcium, a divalent cation, is a critical component of many extracellular and intracellular reactions. It is an essential cofactor in the coagulation cascade, and intracellular ionized calcium participates in the regulation of neuronal, myocardial, and renal cellular function. The calcium concentration in ECF is assayed as the total serum calcium concentration (normally, 8.5-10.5 mg/dL). Calcium in ECF is present in three molecular forms: protein-bound calcium, diffusible calcium complexed to anions (bicarbonate, phosphate, and acetate), and freely diffusible calcium as ionized calcium (iCa^{2+}). The biochemically active species is iCa^{2+}, and it constitutes approximately 45% of total serum calcium. More than 80% of protein-bound calcium is attached to albumin, and thus the total calcium concentration in serum will decrease in hypoalbuminemia. Acidemia decreases iCa^{2+} binding to albumin. Electrodes are used to measure [iCa^{2+}] in anaerobic samples of blood or plasma, with normal [iCa^{2+}] ranging between 1.1 and 1.4 mmol/L. [iCa^{2+}] is substantially lower in ICF than in ECF, although intracellular concentrations fluctuate as a function of calcium shifts across the cell membrane, including in muscle cells during the process of contraction. Calcium functions in the cytosol as a second messenger. The increase in [iCa^{2+}] is controlled by cell membrane enzymes that transport calcium out of the cell. In muscle cells, ionized calcium is stored in the sarcoplasmic reticulum, from which it can be quickly released into ICF, where it has a key role in the molecular events that cause muscle contraction.

Tight control of [iCa^{2+}] in ECF is essential. The serum calcium concentration is controlled by the interaction of parathyroid hormone (PTH), calcitonin, and vitamin D. PTH and calcitonin are hormones subject to regulatory release by endocrine cells, whereas vitamin D is either consumed in diet or formed in the skin as cholecalciferol in response to ultraviolet irradiation. Bone contains an enormous reservoir of calcium in the form of a matrix of calcium and other molecules. Turnover of calcium salts in bone is constant and integral to maintaining a stable [iCa^{2+}] in ECF. Receptors in the membranes of parathyroid cells release PTH when [iCa^{2+}] in ECF declines. PTH activates osteoclasts in bones, which release calcium from the structural matrix of bone. PTH stimulates tubule cells in the proximal nephron to both absorb calcium from the filtrate and excrete phosphates. PTH with vitamin D enhances calcium absorption from the lumen of the gut. Calcitonin has effects on calcium metabolism opposite those of PTH. As calcitonin levels in ECF increase because of excretion of the hormone from type C cells of the thyroid, [iCa^{2+}] declines as more calcium is bound to bone matrix. Vitamin D circulating in blood is converted in the liver to 25-hydroxycholecalciferol (25D). Circulating in blood, 25D encounters kidney cells that further hydroxylate the sterol to 1,25-dihydroxycholecalciferol (1,25D), which is the most potent calcium-modulating hormone. 1,25D increases the transport of calcium and phosphate from the lumen of the bowel into the ECF of the intestine. Furthermore, with PTH, 1,25D increases bone resorption and thus increases the calcium concentration in ECF. In summary, multiple hormonal mechanisms produce a balance of influences on the concentration of calcium in ECF.

Magnesium is an essential cation in ICF. The normal concentration of magnesium [Mg^{2+}] in plasma ranges between 1.4 and 2.0 mEq/L, and approximately 20% is bound to proteins. Less than 1% of the total body magnesium content is found in ECF. The magnesium concentration in ICF can be measured first by osmotic rupture of erythrocytes to release the magnesium and then measurement of [Mg^{2+}] in the supernatant. Patients with ICF [Mg^{2+}] of less than 4.4 mEq/L will typically have a substantial total body magnesium deficiency, perhaps the result of a prolonged deficiency in the diet. Several diseases that deplete magnesium have parallel effects on calcium. Furthermore, these two divalent cations have similar effects on biochemical reactions. Patients with low ECF [Mg^{2+}] exhibit spasticity and hyperreflexia and have symptoms similar to those of patients with a depressed ECF calcium concentration.

Hypercalcemia

Mild hypercalcemia is suspected when total serum calcium levels are in the range of 10.5 to 12 mg/dL. Patients with a serum calcium concentration of 12 to 14.5 mg/dL have moderate hypercalcemia. Patients with transient modest elevations in serum calcium levels are generally asymptomatic. Those with sustained elevations in renal calcium excretion are susceptible to the development of renal lithiasis. Patients have severe hypercalcemia when serum calcium levels exceed 15 mg/dL. These patients have symptoms of weakness, stupor, and central nervous system dysfunction. A renal concentrating defect also occurs in hypercalcemic patients and leads to polyuria and loss of sodium and water. Indeed, many hypercalcemic patients suffer from dehydration. Hypercalcemic crisis is a syndrome in which total serum calcium levels exceed 17 mg/dL. These patients are subject to life-threatening cardiac tachyarrhythmia, coma, acute renal failure, and ileus with abdominal distention.

Several clinical syndromes or circumstances account for the majority of hypercalcemic cases. Hyperparathyroidism, or unregulated PTH secretion, is a common cause of significant hypercalcemia. Bone demineralization is found in patients with severe and prolonged hyperparathyroidism. Eighty-five percent of patients with this syndrome are found to have a solitary hyperfunctioning adenoma in one parathyroid gland, and the remainder have excessive PTH release as a result of hyperplasia of all four glands. PTH induces phosphaturia and depresses serum phosphate concentrations, a laboratory finding that corroborates the diagnosis of primary hyperparathyroidism. Secondary hyperparathyroidism, an endocrine disease characterized by hyperplasia of the parathyroid glands, develops in patients with chronic renal failure. Decreased renal function results in impaired synthesis of 1,25D. Although patients have low serum calcium, their osteomalacia indicates excessive PTH secretion. Surgical removal of most of the parathyroid tissue may be required to control elevated PTH levels in patients with secondary hyperparathyroidism.

In patients with malignancies, hypercalcemia can develop independent of the hormone PTH. Selected tumors have been demonstrated to produce a PTH-related peptide that shares 8 of its first 13 amino acids with PTH; this peptide induces release of calcium from bone and reduces calcium loss in urine. Multiple myeloma and lymphoma and solid tumors metastatic to bone (particularly breast, lung, and prostate cancer) cause hypercalcemia by excessive osteoclastic activity. Tumors that directly invade bone increase the release of calcium and cause hypercalcemia by nonhormonal mechanisms involving cytokines (interleukin-1, tumor necrosis factor, interleukin-6) that activate osteoclasts. Drugs can also cause hypercalcemia, including thiazide diuretics and extraordinarily high doses of vitamins A and D. Young, normally active patients with high bone turnover rates are subject to the development of hypercalcemia when suddenly forced into immobility, as may occur during forced bed rest after injury or major illness. This hypercalcemia of immobilization resolves with return to normal activity.

Definitive management of hypercalcemia depends on correction of the primary problem. Thus, patients with hyperparathyroidism secondary to a parathyroid adenoma or hyperplasia are cured of hypercalcemia by excision of the diseased parathyroid tissue. Hypercalcemic patients taking thiazide drugs should be converted to alternative therapies. Patients with a malignancy and hypercalcemia may respond to surgical excision, radiation therapy, or chemotherapy. Symptomatic patients with malignancy-related severe hypercalcemia can be quickly and effectively treated by saline infusion to expand ECW, followed by the administration of a loop diuretic (i.e., furosemide) to induce a saline diuresis with associated urinary calcium clearance. In fact, patients with severe hypercalcemia frequently suffer a contracted ECW volume and thus isotonic saline infusion is essential. Hypercalcemic patients in renal failure who cannot benefit from drug-induced diuresis can be managed by hemodialysis.

Severe hypercalcemia related to release of calcium from bone by tumor can be managed by administration of bisphosphonates. These drugs have a potent capacity to reduce osteoclast-mediated release of calcium from bone. Several formulations of bisphosphonates are available (in order of preference, zolendronic acid, pamidronate disodium, etidronate disodium), all of which produce a slow decline in [iCa^{2+}] over a period of several days. Bisphosphonates given as long-term prophylactic agents to patients with metastatic breast cancer and administered at a regular dosage have been proved to effectively prevent hypercalcemia. Calcitonin is the calcium-lowering hormone produced by parafollicular cells of the thyroid gland. Administration of exogenous calcitonin effectively induces renal excretion of calcium and suppresses reabsorption of bone by osteoclasts. Although calcitonin therapy for hypercalcemia is often initially effective, long-term therapy frequently leads to tachyphylaxis, possibly related to the development of antibodies to the exogenous calcitonin. Chelating agents (ethylenediaminetetraacetic acid or phosphate salts) that bind and neutralize ionized calcium are rarely indicated because of their association with the complications of metastatic calcification and acute renal failure and the risk that [iCa^{2+}] may be depressed to hypocalcemic levels.

Hypocalcemia

Acute hypocalcemia can be a life-threatening event. This condition impairs transmembrane depolarization, and [iCa^{2+}] below 0.8 mEq/L can lead to central nervous system dysfunction. Hypocalcemic patients complain of paresthesias and muscle spasms (including tetany), and seizures can develop. As [iCa^{2+}] declines, patients complain of numbness, paresthesias of the distal extremities, and painful muscle spasms. Patients may exacerbate the condition if they hyperventilate and induce a respiratory alkalosis, which further reduces [iCa^{2+}]. Cardiac dysfunction occurs in patients with hypocalcemia. Patients with low [iCa^{2+}] may require IV infusion of calcium to restore cardiac function. Hypocalcemic patients have a prolonged QT interval on electrocardiograms that may progress to complete heart block or ventricular fibrillation.

Tumor lysis syndrome is a constellation of electrolyte abnormalities that include hypocalcemia, hyperphosphatemia, hyperuricemia, and hyperkalemia. These electrolyte aberrations occur when antineoplastic therapy causes a sudden surge in tumor cell death and release of cytosolic contents. Solid tumors and lymphomas have been associated with this problem. Acute renal failure occurs in patients suffering from tumor lysis syndrome and prevents spontaneous correction of the electrolyte abnormalities; emergency dialysis may be the only therapy that provides comprehensive correction of the problems. Acute hypocalcemia is noted frequently after resuscitation from shock. In a study of patients in burn shock, Wray and associates hypothesized that a major factor contributing to the development of hypocalcemia was depressed levels of 1,25D, perhaps caused by a sudden lack of vitamin D in the diet.[10] In patients with severe pancreatitis, the fall in calcium is speculated to be the consequence of ionized extracellular calcium becoming linked to fats in the peripancreatic inflammatory phlegmon. Rapid infusion of a citrate load during the transfusion of blood products (particularly platelet concentrates and fresh frozen plasma) may also lead to acute severe hypocalcemia ([iCa^{2+}] < 0.62 mmol/L) and hypotension. Rapid increases in serum phosphate can occur after improper administration or excessive dosing of phosphate-containing cathartics, and as the phosphate concentration increases, severe hypocalcemia ensues.

In the ICU, where multiple blood tests are continuously monitored, mild hypocalcemia is common. Although replacement therapy is appropriate in a symptomatic hypocalcemic patient, it is controversial whether correcting to an [iCa^{2+}] value of 0.8 to 1.1 mmol/L is beneficial. Patients with severe hypocalcemia ([iCa^{2+}] <0.62 mmol/L) who are at risk for impending cardiac failure or fatal arrhythmia are treated with IV calcium salt infusions. Infusion of 10 mL of a 10% CaCl$_2$ solution provides 272 mg of calcium (equivalent to 13.6 mmol of ionized calcium), whereas the same volume of 10% calcium gluconate contains only 90 mg of calcium (equivalent to 4.5 mmol of ionized calcium). IV calcium infusion should be performed with caution because rapid shifts in ECF [iCa^{2+}] can cause cardiac arrhythmias, particularly in patients treated with digoxin. Also, in patients with low [iCa^{2+}] but elevated serum phosphate, rapid calcium infusion can result in the widespread precipitation of calcium. Furthermore, IV calcium preparations are caustic, and infiltration through a peripheral vein leads to necrosis of skin, so they are best administered rapidly through central venous catheters.

Hypermagnesemia and Hypomagnesemia

Hypermagnesemia is an electrolyte abnormality most often seen in patients with renal failure. It can be exacerbated by the ingestion of magnesium-containing drugs, particularly antacids, and such agents should be avoided. Magnesium blocks the shift of calcium into myocardial cells, and patients with severe hypermagnesemia show evidence of heart failure. Intracellular hypomagnesemia can develop in patients with chronic diarrhea syndrome or those who undergo prolonged aggressive diuretic therapy. Magnesium deficiency is also common in patients with heavy ethanol intake. Diabetic patients with persistent osmotic diuresis from glycosuria commonly have hypomagnesemia. These categories of patients often benefit from the addition of magnesium salts to resuscitation fluids. Correction of hypomagnesemia is accomplished by the IV infusion of magnesium sulfate (MgSO$_4$). Severe hypomagnesemia (<1.0 mEq/L) requires sustained therapy because of the slow equilibration of extracellular magnesium with intracellular stores. Correction of hypomagnesemia can also reduce the risk for cardiac arrhythmias. Frequently, the magnitude of magnesium deficiency parallels the magnitude of hypocalcemia. Hypocalcemia in patients with magnesium deficiency is resistant to calcium replacement alone, and these patients should therefore receive magnesium concurrently.

ACID-BASE BALANCE

Definition of Proton

A proton has a single positive charge, the lowest elemental molecular weight, and protons are distributed throughout body water.[9] The molar concentration of protons (H$^+$) in ECF is 40 nmol/L. In ICF the molar concentration of protons is 80 nmol/L. The concentration of protons measured in units of nanomoles per liter is less by a factor of 1 million than the concentration in units of millimoles per liter of the principal electrolytes in ECF (Na$^+$ and Cl$^-$) and ICF (K$^+$ and phosphate). Protons have a very low concentration in ICF and ECF, yet the proton concentration has a major influence on multiple biochemical reactions. The tolerable range of proton concentrations in ICF is severely restricted. As the proton concentration in ICF exceeds 80 nmol/L, protons bind in greater numbers to anionic sites on proteins. Enzyme function declines as proton binding increases. The concentration of protons in ICF changes little during normal biochemical activity despite the fact that every hour large numbers of protons are released and bound in biochemical reactions. An adult who ingests a normal Western diet daily adds 50 to 100 mmol of protons to their body fluids. Changes in proton concentration in ECF and ICF do not occur despite this large daily intake of protons because renal function excretes sufficient protons in urine in a modulated manner to maintain the proton concentration in ECF in the normal range.

Buffer systems in ICF and ECF play a vital role in reducing fluctuations in proton concentration. Cells are destroyed and ultimately the individual dies if there are even modest deviations in proton concentration outside the tolerable range in ICF of 60 to 100 nmol/L. Buffer systems protect body fluids from sudden increases or decreases in the number of protons by binding or releasing protons and thereby blunting fluctuations in the concentration of protons. The principal buffer in ECF is bicarbonate. Furthermore, bicarbonate is a major buffer in ICF, although imidazole sites on proteins in ICF and phosphates also buffer protons in ICF. Buffers have a capacity to bind or release excess protons, and though highly effective at fluid concentrations normally sustained in ECF or ICF, as the number of excess protons increases or as the deficit in protons expands, the capacity of buffers to preserve normal proton concentrations is impaired. The critical role played by buffers is that vital biochemical reactions are sustained during an acute change in proton concentration. Buffers provide the time needed for renal or pulmonary function to provide a sustained correction.

The Principal Buffer That Controls the Proton Concentration Is Bicarbonate

Bicarbonate is a dominant buffer system in biologic systems. The bicarbonate buffer system is important in both ICF and ECF and is key to enabling proton transport across cell membranes (Table 5-3). Two chemical reactions link five molecules of the bicarbonate buffer system.

Table 5-3 **Buffers as a Total Percentage of Buffer Capacity Active in Intracellular and Extracellular Water***

	HCO_3^-	$H_2PO_4^{2-}$	IMIDAZOLE ON PROTEINS
ECW	95%	4%	1%
ICW	42%	6%	52%

*It is estimated that a 70-kg person has 400 mmol of buffer in extracellular water (ECW) and 800 mmol of buffer in intracellular water (ICW).

Adapted from Halperin ML, Goldstein M: Fluid, Electrolyte, and Acid-Base Physiology: A Problem-Based Approach, 3rd ed. Philadelphia, WB Saunders, 1999.

A cationic proton binds to an anionic bicarbonate and forms carbonic acid, which has no charge. Carbonic acid is converted to the dissolved gas carbon dioxide and water. The enzyme carbonic anhydrase is capable of accelerating the transformation of carbonic acid to carbon dioxide and water.

Renal function　　　　　　　　Lung function
⇕　　⇕　　　　　　　　　　　⇕
Proton + bicarbonate ⇔ carbonic acid ⇔ $PaCO_2$ and water

Three components of the bicarbonate buffer system are critical in control of the proton concentration. First, bicarbonate binds or releases protons within the range of proton concentrations normally present in ECF and ICF. Thus, if the proton concentration increases from a baseline value between 40 and 80 nmol/L, the excess protons bind to available bicarbonate and produce carbonic acid. If there is a decline in proton concentration, carbonic acid dissociates back toward the left side of the equation, and a proton and bicarbonate are released. The second component of the buffer system that is vitally important is that charged molecules, protons and bicarbonate, are converted to uncharged molecular species, specifically CO_2, that readily cross cell membranes. Charged molecules cross cell membranes by energy-consuming reactions, but the chargeless CO_2 diffuses readily. This movement of CO_2 is the key to ICF and ECF having compensatory changes in proton concentration in circumstances in which one or the other fluid proton concentration suddenly changes. The third component of the bicarbonate buffer system that is vital to life is that bicarbonate and protons in ECF can be cleared from the body by the function of the pulmonary and renal systems. These two organ systems control the proton concentration, but the mechanisms used by the pulmonary and renal systems are substantially different. The renal tubule cells consume biochemical energy and pump protons into urine, thereby enabling net excretion of protons (principally as NH_4^+), or the renal tubule cells cannot recover the bicarbonate filtered at the glomerulus, thereby allowing loss of bicarbonate in an alkaline urine. By increasing or decreasing alveolar ventilation the pulmonary system can increase or decrease the loss of CO_2 in respiratory gases and consequently reduce the partial pressure of carbon dioxide ($PaCO_2$) in ECF. Timeliness is a critical distinction between these two physiologic systems. The renal system can correct the proton concentration in ECF in hours, whereas the pulmonary system can correct the proton concentration in ECF in minutes.

In 1909 Henderson observed that there was a fixed relationship between the proton concentration in ECF and the ratio of carbonic acid to bicarbonate. Substituting $PaCO_2$, a molecular species that is readily measured in arterial blood, for carbonic acid, the Henderson equation becomes

$$H^+ = 23.9 \times PaCO_2 / HCO_3^-$$

This equation can be used to comprehend four paradigms of acute change in acid-base balance. Many clinicians prefer to analyze the acid-base status of arterial blood with the Henderson-Hasselbalch equation, which involves the relationship of proton concentration, bicarbonate buffer, and $PaCO_2$. Acidemia, an increase in protons, occurs if there is an acute increase in $PaCO_2$ or a decline in bicarbonate concentration. Alkalemia occurs if there is an acute decrease in $PaCO_2$ or an increase in bicarbonate concentration. These paradigms of acidemia and alkalemia are a simplification because in physiologic systems, an immediate compensatory adjustment often takes place in response to an acute acid-base change to correct the proton concentration to normal. For example, the acute increase in ECF protons that occurs in shock produces an instantaneous decline in bicarbonate as the anion is consumed while buffering the proton, and this decline in buffer is followed within minutes by hyperventilation in response to acidemia and by a reduction in $PaCO_2$, which helps by reducing the proton concentration. Nonetheless, it is useful to consider these paradigms as representing examples of the first step produced by a change in one component of the Henderson equation. In clinical practice, the second step is a compensatory physiologic change that shifts the proton concentration toward 40 nmol/L in ECF. A common observation in clinical practice is for the initial pathologic changes in proton concentration to be followed by a compensatory change that soon converts the patient's acid-base status to a mixed effect of pathology and compensatory physiology.

In addition to the bicarbonate system, two other buffer systems are vital to control of the ICF proton concentration (see Table 5-3). Protons can be bound by the imidazole site in the amino acid histidine, which is a component amino acid in proteins. Proteins are an effective buffer system, but excessive proton loads can overload histidine sites and alter protein function. Inorganic phosphates are the third system for intracellular buffering of protons. Dibasic phosphate is converted to a monobasic phosphate with the addition of a proton. Two thirds of ICF inorganic phosphate is normally present as monovalent HPO_4^- and can readily assist in blunting an increase in protons. The inorganic phosphate buffer system accounts for less than 10% of the intracellular buffer capacity and makes only a minimal contribution to control of protons in ECW.

The difference in proton concentration between ICF and ECF is based on movement of carbon dioxide across the cell membrane. The carbon dioxide produced during aerobic metabolism in mitochondria shifts first to ICF and then across the cell membrane to ECF, where the carbon dioxide is eventually exhaled as a gas. Movement of carbon dioxide is linked to the bicarbonate buffer system. In addition to flux of carbon dioxide out of the cell, the bicarbonate buffer system is critical in the movement of protons from ICF out of the cell to ECF, where excess protons are excreted in urine. Carbon dioxide can readily cross the cell membrane. This ability is a key step in achieving clearance of protons from ICF. The charged molecules bicarbonate and protons do not readily cross the cell membrane. In cells in which these ionic species do cross (i.e., renal tubule cells, parietal cells in the stomach), active transport is accomplished by membrane mechanisms that depend on the energy of ATP. For movement of protons out of the cell when they accumulate, the bicarbonate buffer system shifts toward increased production of dissolved carbon dioxide, which then moves across the membrane. In ECF, as carbon dioxide accumulates, the bicarbonate buffer system shifts toward conversion of the carbon dioxide to a proton and a bicarbonate species.

Renal Function and Clearance of Protons

Renal function is the principal physiologic mechanism for control of excess protons in ECF. At the glomerulus, a filtrate of ECF enters the nephron tubules (see Fig. 5-5). Tubule cells pump protons into the renal tubule fluid while simultaneously pumping bicarbonate into ECF. In the ICF of tubule cells the bicarbonate buffer system is a key component in enabling the luminal side of the cell to transport protons outward, whereas on the abluminal side of the cell, there is net transport of bicarbonate to the ECF through diffusion of carbon dioxide across the cell membrane. One type of drug that can alter renal excretion of protons is carbonic anhydrase inhibitors, which impede the rapid conversion of carbonic acid to carbon dioxide and water. Patients given carbonic anhydrase inhibitors slow the rate of transport of bicarbonate out of the tubule cell, thereby impairing the tubule cell's capacity to transport protons into urine. The amount of bicarbonate flowing into the glomerular filtrate exceeds the amount of protons pumped into the tubule fluid, and the net result with the administration of carbonic anhydrase inhibitor is production of an alkaline fluid. Renal tubule cells have cell membrane transport enzymes that via an energy-consuming process, pump protons against a concentration gradient into tubule fluid. The molecule ammonium is a critical buffer in urine that enables the renal tubule cells to excrete 50 to 100 mmol of protons daily. Protons transported into the tubule fluid bind to ammonium and produce NH_4^+, which buffers the increase in proton concentration and enables additional protons to be excreted into urine. Phosphates are also a major buffer of protons in tubule fluid. The proximal tubule is where all the filtered bicarbonate entering the tubule fluid at the glomerulus is reabsorbed. The distal convoluted tubule (DCT) is where the sodium in tubule fluid is transported to the ECF while protons or potassium is pumped into urine. This exchange is regulated by the hormone aldosterone. Aldosterone is released from the adrenal medulla and is designated a mineralocorticoid.

An increase in aldosterone causes accelerated loss of potassium and protons into urine.

Renal function is quantitatively measured as the glomerular filtration rate. Normal glomerular filtration rates are 100 to 150 mL/min. Patients with rates of 30 to 100 mL/min are considered to have renal dysfunction. Although an increase in blood urea levels may occur in patients with renal dysfunction, most patients with renal dysfunction can sustain excretion of potassium and protons. Patients with a glomerular filtration rate less than 30 mL/min have renal failure, and unless renal replacement therapy is instituted, they will die of hyperkalemia or uremia. Acidemia develops in patients with renal failure secondary to accumulation of protons consumed in the diet.

Acid-Base Clinical Disorders

Acid-base disorders are a frequent and potentially lethal problem for patients. Patients are acidotic if they have an excess number of protons in their body fluids. Patients are alkalotic if they have a significant deficit in protons in their body fluids. Acidemia means that the proton concentration in ECF exceeds 40 nmol/L, whereas alkalemia means the proton concentration in ECF is less than 40 nmol/L. Surgeons need to intervene as patients become acidotic or alkalotic to avoid catastrophic irreversible dysfunction of multiple biochemical reactions. The goal of the next section, Clinical Syndromes of Acid-Base Disorders, is to describe common acid-base disorders encountered by surgeons. The pathophysiologic mechanisms will be described, as well as interventions that are usually successful in treating a given acid-base disorder.

pH and Measurement of Proton Concentration

Clinicians use blood tests to assess total body acid-base balance. The most informative blood test is arterial blood gas analysis, whereas less sensitive indicators of acid-base status are venous blood gas analysis and measurement of the total carbon dioxide in a venous blood sample. Blood gas tests report three components of a patient's acid-base status: pH, $Paco_2$, and the bicarbonate concentration (HCO_3^- in units of mEq/L). pH is a measure of the proton concentration and is calculated as the log to the base 10 of 1 divided by the proton concentration. $Paco_2$ is a measure of the partial pressure of carbon dioxide in ECF and is influenced by the rate of carbon dioxide production in aerobic energy metabolism and the rate of clearance of carbon dioxide during pulmonary alveolar ventilation.

Electrodes in blood gas machines enable direct measurement of pH and $Paco_2$, whereas bicarbonate is measured with a reagent assay. Hasselbalch added to the Henderson equation by proposing that the log to the base 10 of an inverted form of Henderson's formula be used in acid-base analyses. The Henderson-Hasselbalch formula (pH = pK_a + log [bicarbonate ÷ carbon dioxide]) has the analytic advantage that pH has a linear relationship to bicarbonate (Box 5-2). pK_a reflects a constant that is fixed by the units of measurement and the chemical relationship of pH and the other components measured in arterial blood gas samples. The variable used in the formula to measure carbon dioxide ($0.03 \times PaCO_2$) reflects the relationship between the carbonic acid concentration and the partial pressure of carbon dioxide. The Henderson-Hasselbalch equation implies that two factors, bicarbonate and $PaCO_2$, determine a patient's acid-base status.

Clinical Interpretation of Arterial Blood Gas

Surgeons rely on an arterial blood sample to determine a patients' acid-base status. For the blood gas measurement to be reliable, an arterial blood sample is collected with minimal exposure to ambient air and immediately processed. Surgeons can analyze an arterial blood gas sample by using a six-step process (Table 5-4). The surgeon first determines from the pH of the arterial blood gas sample whether the patient has acidemia, alkalemia, or normal status. A patient has acidemia if arterial blood pH is less than 7.35. A patient has alkalemia if the pH is greater than 7.45. The surgeon's second step is to determine from the $PaCO_2$ whether the patient's respiratory function is contributing or compensating for the acidemia or alkalemia. This second step may lead a surgeon treating a patient who is mechanically ventilated to increase or decrease minute ventilation to correct the pH toward

---

Box 5-2 Four Paradigms of Acid-Base Disorder Interpreted With the Henderson-Hasselbalch Equation

Normal Components of the Henderson-Hasselbalch Equation

$pH = 6.1 + \log[(HCO_3^-)/(0.03 \times PaCO_2)]$
pH is the log to base 10 of the proton concentration in nmol/L
HCO_3^- is the bicarbonate concentration in mEq/L
$PaCO_2$ is the partial pressure of carbon dioxide in an arterial blood sample in mm Hg. Partial pressure multiplied by 0.03 predicts the carbonic acid concentration

Normal Arterial Blood Gas

$$pH = 7.40 = 6.1 + \log(24/1.33)$$

Acidemia

Metabolic acidemia: Abrupt addition of sufficient protons to reduce the bicarbonate buffer 50%

$$pH = 7.10 = 6.1 + \log(12/1.33)$$

Respiratory acidemia: Sudden reduction in alveolar ventilation causing an increase in $PaCO_2$ to 50 mm Hg

$$pH = 7.30 = 6.1 + \log(24/1.5)$$

Alkalemia

Metabolic alkalemia: Abrupt addition of sufficient bicarbonate to increase the buffer concentration to 30 mEq/L

$$pH = 7.45 = 6.1 + \log(30/1.33)$$

Respiratory alkalemia: Sudden increase in alveolar ventilation causing a decrease in $PaCO_2$ to 20 mm Hg

$$pH = 7.70 = 6.1 + \log(24/0.6)$$

---

normal. The surgeon's third step in arterial blood gas analysis is to determine whether the patient has a bicarbonate deficit or excess. This calculation is made by the arterial blood gas machine and is an estimated value. Blood gas machines use the measured pH, $PaCO_2$, and bicarbonate level to estimate what the patient's bicarbonate level would be if the arterial blood sample had a $PaCO_2$ of 40 mm Hg. Surgeons use the difference between the calculated bicarbonate in ideal circumstance and the expected concentration of 24 mEq/L to categorize a patient's acid-base status. Specifically, the difference between observed and expected bicarbonate buffer indicates that the patient has either an excess or a deficit of bicarbonate buffer. Patients who have a shortage of bicarbonate have an excess number of protons, whereas patients who have an excess of bicarbonate have a reduction in protons. Surgeons must choose what mathematical sign they prefer when using arterial blood gas data to categorize a patient's bicarbonate buffer status. If the surgeon chooses to consider a patient as having an excess of bicarbonate, commonly termed *base excess* in the medical literature, the base excess is calculated as estimated bicarbonate at normal $PaCO_2$ minus 24. Thus, a patient with acute acidosis and an increase in ECF proton concentration would have a fall in ECF bicarbonate as these molecules buffer protons. This patient's arterial blood gas analysis would report a base excess that has a negative value. As the patient's acidosis worsens, the base excess would become a more negative number. An advantage to determining whether the patient has a calculated bicarbonate excess or deficit if their blood were equilibrated to a $PaCO_2$ of 40 is that independent of the actual arterial pH, this calculation of available buffer indicates to the surgeon whether interventions are needed to increase or decrease bicarbonate available as buffer. For example, a patient with less than normal bicarbonate (metabolic acidosis) may be agitated and hyperventilate, thereby producing a superimposed respiratory alkalemia. The concept of base excess is useful to clinicians who are planning therapy for patients with acid-base disorders. Patients with severe acidemia (pH < 7.20) and a large bicarbonate excess (< −10 mEq/L) are treated by the IV infusion of sodium bicarbonate. In patients with severe alkalemia (pH > 7.60) and an excess of estimated bicarbonate defined as a positive bicarbonate excess (> 10 mEq/L), the therapy would be IV infusion of HCl.

Anion Gap

The anion gap is useful in evaluating patients with acidemia. The anion gap is calculated from the ECF concentration of the cation sodium minus the concentration of the anions chloride and bicarbonate ($Na^+ - [Cl^- + HCO_3^-]$). Generally, the anions chloride and bicarbonate provide more than 90% of the anions needed to achieve electroneutrality with Na^+. Patients normally have an anion gap of 12 mEq/L. The anions that constitute the gap are phosphate, sulfates, and anionic sites on proteins. The anion gap is useful in determining the cause of acidemia. For example, a postoperative patient in whom acidemia with an elevated anion gap develops will have either lactic

Table 5-4 Six-Step Sequential Approach to the Interpretation of Arterial Blood Gas With Supplemental Information From Serum Sodium, Potassium, and Chloride Concentrations*

OBSERVATION	INTERPRETATION	INTERVENTION
Is the pH other than 7.40?	Acidosis if <7.35 Alkalosis if >7.45	Clinical evaluation for the causal disease
Is the pH<7.20 or >7.55?	Severe disorder	Prompt correction required
Is the PaCO$_2$ other than 40 mm Hg?	Ventilation compensates or contributes to the disorder	Change the ventilation so that PaCO$_2$ compensates
Is the base deficit other than zero?	Bicarbonate loss/gain compensates or contributes to the disorder	Infuse NaCO$_3$ or HCl to correct the proton concentration
Does the urine pH reflect acidosis/alkalosis?	Acid/alkaline urine indicates that renal function compensates or contributes	Renal-active drugs or electrolyte replacement so that the nephron contributes
Is the anion gap[†] <12 mmol/L?	Values above 12 mmol/L suggest lactic or ketoacidosis	Correct the primary metabolic problem

*The goal is to achieve a normal pH of 7.40.
[†]Anion gap = [Na$^+$]+[K$^+$]−[Cl$^−$].

acidemia secondary to impaired aerobic metabolism or ketoacidemia associated with uncontrolled diabetes mellitus. In the presence of acidemia and a normal anion gap, patients have a bicarbonate deficit, which can occur in patients with an enteric fistula draining bicarbonate-containing gastrointestinal fluid.

The Stewart Approach to Acid-Base Balance

Stewart derived an alternative approach to the Henderson-Hasselbalch method for understanding acid-base status.[11] In the Henderson-Hasselbalch approach, bicarbonate is the sole buffer, whereas Stewart's method of analysis is based on the quantity of all buffers. In practical terms this means that a clinician using the Stewart approach to interpret acid-base status must combine information from both the arterial blood gas and a peripheral venous sample. Three groups of variables are combined to enable the clinician to classify a patient's pH status. Stewart's method calls for the clinician to look at the strong ion difference, defined as the sum of cationic charges (sodium, potassium, calcium, magnesium) minus the sum of anion salts (lactate and chloride). The strong ion difference should be between 10 and 12 mEq. Stewart's method also incorporates the concentration of weak buffers (proteins and phosphates) in the interpretation of a patient's pH. Weak buffers differ from bicarbonate by the fact that bicarbonate buffer can be discharged from ECF by increasing ventilation and clearance of carbon dioxide as a gas. The Stewart approach to acid-base analysis depends on PaCO$_2$.

Several authors champion Stewart's approach because even though it is more complicated in the steps needed to analyze an arterial blood gas sample than those needed with the Henderson-Hasselbalch approach, the Stewart approach provides greater precision. The traditional Henderson-Hasselbalch method, which links all acid-base disorders to alterations in the bicarbonate buffer system, has difficulty precisely defining the cause of certain clinically important acid-base disorders. For example, the acidemia that is observed in a patient after resuscitation from hemorrhage by infusion of normal saline can be differentiated into excess protons caused by the hypoxia and replacement of the lost bicarbonate anion by chloride anion. Surgeons analyzing an arterial blood gas sample should recognize that the blood sample is a reflection of the acid-base status of arterial blood in ECF. A change in the pH of ECF, where the bicarbonate buffer system dominates, may not be equivalent in magnitude to changes in the pH of ICF. The Henderson-Hasselbalch equation does not reliably inform the clinician of the acid-base status of the intracellular environment, where pH is lower and buffer systems other than bicarbonate influence pH. Alterations in extracellular pH that occur over a period of hours usually directly reflect similar pH trends within the cytosol. However, in circumstances of a rapid change in proton concentration in ICF, the pH of ECF may not concurrently change in parallel. For example, hypoxia can cause a rapid and possibly fatal accumulation of protons in ICF with only a modest decline in the pH of an arterial blood gas sample.

Clinical Syndromes of Acid-Base Disorders

Frequently, acid-base disorders develop in patterns that correspond to specific clinical circumstances. Understanding these patterns enables the surgeon to select the treatment that not only corrects the acid-base disorder but also treats the primary cause of the metabolic disorder. An individual patient's acid-base status is defined by analysis of arterial blood gas, a measure of the acid-base status in ECF. However, the initial event that increases or decreases the proton concentration in ECF is usually a biochemical disorder in ICF. In these discussions patients with acidemia (arterial blood gas=ECF pH<7.35) will be categorized as having primarily a metabolic (also meaning a deficiency in bicarbonate) or respiratory (an elevation in PaCO$_2$) acid-base disorder based on the initial event that led to the disorder. In the same way, patients who have alkalemia (arterial blood gas=ECF pH>7.45) will be categorized as having primarily a metabolic (meaning excess bicarbonate) or respiratory (a decrease in $PaCO_2$) acid-base disorder.

Metabolic Acidemia Caused by Insufficient Delivery of Oxygen

Surgeons encounter acidemia when treating seriously ill and injured patients who are in shock. These patients have insufficient transport of oxygen from the pulmonary alveolus to the mitochondria of the body's cells. Biochemical reactions that generate ATP cannot be sustained at the needed rate if the partial pressure of oxygen is not maintained in mitochondria. Oxidative phosphorylation converts oxygen to carbon dioxide, and the biochemical energy released is used to convert ADP, protons, and phosphate to ATP. In a normal adult, mitochondria consume 12 mmol of oxygen per minute to support the oxidative phosphorylation needed to sustain life. Protons accumulate in ICF when there is impaired oxidative phosphorylation, and as the intracellular proton concentration increases, cell enzymes are impaired, a factor that contributes to the rapid deterioration in cellular function when oxygen delivery is insufficient. In addition to oxygen, oxidative phosphorylation depends on delivery of fuel in the form of carbon-carbon bonds in carbohydrates and fats. Glycolysis is a series of chemical reactions in ICF that convert the six-carbon glucose molecule to a pair of three-carbon pyruvate molecules. In circumstances of adequate oxygen delivery, pyruvate enters the citric acid cycle and produces molecules that are needed to support oxidative phosphorylation in mitochondria. When inadequate oxygen delivery occurs, the pyruvate cannot proceed forward into the citric acid cycle. As pyruvate levels increase in ICF, enzymes shunt pyruvate into lactate plus protons. Lactate and protons exit the ICF in proportion to the severity of the oxygen deficit in mitochondria. Thus, the degree of elevation of proton and lactate concentrations in ECF in patients in shock is usually an indication of the severity of the anaerobic insult inside cells.

Lactate that leaves ICF and enters ECF is taken up by the liver, where it participates in gluconeogenesis and is converted to glucose. The elevation in lactate levels in patients in shock with acidemia is a function of both the rate of production of lactate in cells with inadequate oxygen and clearance by liver cells. In patients with a mild to moderate decrease in oxygen delivery, modest acidemia (pH 7.20-7.35), a bicarbonate deficit, and no increase in the anion gap occur. With a sustained or severe metabolic acidemia pattern in patients in shock (pH<7.20), lactate levels increase. Multiple studies have established that the risk for death is proportional to the increase in lactate concentration and the severity of the acidemia.

Surgeons treat patients with lacticacidemia secondary to impaired delivery of oxygen by performing interventions that increase oxygen delivery. The acid-base status of patients in shock with lacticacidemia improves after interventions that restore delivery of oxygen to cells. Some specific causes of shock are a substantial depletion of blood volume, cardiac dysfunction causing impaired cardiac output, and a profound vasodilation that shunts blood away from vital organs that have high oxygen consumption (i.e., cardiac muscle, kidney, and brain). Success in correction of the acidemia is achieved by resuscitation that corrects the primary cause of the shock. Treatment of patients in shock depends on targeted therapy such as restoring blood volume in a patient in hypovolemic shock, infusion of inotropic drugs that improve cardiac function, and infusion of vasoconstrictive agents in a vasodilated patient that shift blood flow from nonvital organs to the heart and brain. In addition to impaired oxygen delivery secondary to cardiovascular failure, acidemia develops in patients whose blood oxygen content is low. In injured patients with an obstructed airway who are unable to ventilate, profound hypoxemia develops within 8 minutes, and irreversible damage to cells occurs because oxidative phosphorylation suddenly cannot be sustained. Patients who drown are sometimes resuscitated after longer periods of hypoxia because they are immersed in nearly freezing water and profound hypothermia rapidly develops, which is protective in the event of anaerobic stress. Lacticacidemia can develop when only one of the organ systems has impaired oxygen delivery. For example, patients with mesenteric arterial occlusion in whom a segment of bowel becomes ischemic will have evidence on arterial blood gas analysis of progressive worsening metabolic acidemia combined with an elevation in serum lactate. In these patients, correction of the acidemia requires excision of the dead organ.

The most effective treatment in patients with lacticacidemia is to restore aerobic metabolism. Patients whose pH is less than 7.20 are given IV sodium bicarbonate to correct their acidemia. Treatment of acid-base abnormalities in ECF may not have the desired effect on ICF. Rapid IV infusion of sodium bicarbonate solutions to improve the pH of a patient with profound acidemia should generate a large amount of carbonic acid in ECF as the bicarbonate buffer binds to the protons. In circumstances in which the rate of increase in the ECF carbonic acid concentration exceeds the capacity of alveolar ventilation to exhale carbon dioxide, the excess carbon dioxide shifts into the cell and there is the paradoxical effect of an increase in ICF proton concentration after bicarbonate therapy. To avoid this paradoxical ICF acidosis after injection of bicarbonate into the ECF, a surgeon administering IV bicarbonate therapy should infuse it slowly.

Dilutional Acidemia After Infusion of Isotonic Normal Saline to Replace Blood Loss

Not all patients resuscitated from shock have acidemia secondary to lactic acid. Dilutional metabolic acidemia occurs in situations in which large volumes of isotonic sodium chloride solutions have been rapidly infused. The rapid repletion by isotonic sodium chloride restores ECW but dilutes the bicarbonate concentration. Patients with this type of acidemia have a depressed bicarbonate concentration, an elevated chloride level, and a normal or decreased anion gap. Patients with this form of postresuscitation hyperchloremic acidemia correct their pH to normal by renal tubular excretion of bicarbonate and $NH_4^+Cl^-$, which results in a loss of protons and chloride from ECF to urine. Clinicians have recommended avoiding this form of hyperchloremic acidemia by using a balanced electrolyte solution (e.g., lactated Ringer's) for resuscitation fluid.[12]

Acidemia Related to Sepsis

In patients with severe sepsis and septic shock who require treatment with catecholamine infusions to sustain perfusion pressure, profound lacticacidemia has been noted to develop despite high cardiac output and increased delivery of oxygen to tissues. Lactic acidosis in septic patients is a multifactor process consistent with reduced mitochondrial oxygen availability and dysfunction of normal biochemical processes in the cytosol. More than 12 hours of septic shock and lacticacidemia leads to global and irreversible failure of cell functions with subsequent organ failure and death. Luchette and associates[13] carefully examined the acidemia in patients in shock and concluded that lactic acidosis during shock is in part a catecholamine-mediated accelerated anaerobic glycolysis. They have provided experimental evidence that elevations in circulating epinephrine associated with shock induce increased cell membrane enzyme activity, which in turn drives glycolysis and excess pyruvate production. As the pyruvate concentration increases in the cytosol, it is diverted into lactic acid. Successful treatment of lacticacidemia in patients in septic shock depends not only on resuscitation of the patient but also on effective treatment of the infection, including appropriate antibiotics and control of the source of sepsis.

Diabetic Ketoacidemia

Patients with diabetes mellitus have a deficiency of insulin that leads to dysfunction of two major ICF biochemical pathways, with the result that ketones accumulate in ECF. Patients with depressed insulin levels have accelerated lipolysis. Triglycerides in fat cells are broken down into glycerol and free fatty acids and are released into the circulation. Free fatty acids are converted in the liver into two ketoacids: α-hydroxybutyric acid and acetoacetic acid. These ketoacids can function as fuels by entering the citric acid cycle and supporting oxidative phosphorylation in selected cells. However, oxidative phosphorylation of ketoacids in mitochondria is slowed in patients without sufficient insulin to maintain glucose transport across cell membranes. In the cytosol, depressed glycolysis leads to an inability to metabolize ketones in the citric acid cycle. Failure of delivery of sufficient fuel to the mitochondria leading to impaired oxidative phosphorylation contributes to the acidemia of diabetic ketoacidemia. Serum and urine ketone levels become markedly elevated as acidemia develops. A patient with diabetic ketoacidemia on arterial blood gas analysis has a low pH and bicarbonate deficit. These patients have an increased anion gap acidemia because the excess ketoacids add to the anions in ECF. Patients with diabetic ketoacidemia hyperventilate with a Kussmaul respiration pattern, in which the patient ventilates with rapid, large tidal volumes. During hyperventilation, $PaCO_2$ may fall below 20 mm Hg as the patient attempts to increase the low pH caused by the diabetic ketoacidemia.

Treatment of diabetic ketoacidosis requires an IV infusion of insulin to accelerate transport of glucose from the ECF to the ICF. Increased glucose levels in ICF enable the excess ketones to enter the citric acid cycle and be used in support of oxidative phosphorylation. In the first hours of IV insulin infusion clinicians can monitor the success of insulin therapy in patients with ketoacidosis by measuring a decrease in serum or urine ketones. In contrast to the precipitous onset of lactic acidosis from shock, diabetics experience a slow onset of ketoacidosis over a period of hours. Patients with diabetic ketoacidemia have sustained hyperglycemia in ECF, and elevated levels of glucose lead to an osmotic diuresis that depletes the ECF. Therefore, in addition to ordering sufficient insulin to lower blood glucose levels, the clinician must anticipate a need to infuse several liters of a balanced electrolyte solution to restore ECF when treating adult patients with diabetic ketoacidemia. In patients with diabetes mellitus who take insufficient insulin, hyperglycemia develops first and then ketoacidemia over a span of several days. However, in a patient with diabetes mellitus who experiences a sudden severe stress related to an injury or illness, ketoacidosis can develop rapidly. These patients have elevated epinephrine and glucocorticoids related to their stress, and these hormones block the action of insulin. Successful correction of diabetic ketoacidemia in a patient with stress requires a combination of insulin therapy, restoration of ECF volume to normal, and delivery of adequate fuel and oxygen to cells.

Alcoholic Patients With Acidemia

Patients who consume large amounts of ethanol are at higher risk for acidemia. A specific pathophysiologic mechanism for lactic acidosis in alcoholic patients is thiamine deficiency. This vitamin deficiency is a clinical problem in alcoholics who consume a diet deficient in vegetables. Thiamine deficiency leads to lactic acidosis because pyruvate dehydrogenase requires thiamine as a critical cofactor. Without thiamine, pyruvate levels build up and are shifted to lactate and protons. Patients with thiamine deficiency are subject to the development of cardiac dysfunction, but it is easily treated by thiamine replacement therapy. A ketoacidosis syndrome can develop in alcoholics who continuously drink large amounts of ethanol over a several-day period. Alcohol consumption without food intake leads to a sustained fall in insulin, lipolysis, and hepatic conversion of free fatty acids to ketones. At the same time, intoxicated individuals have diuresis and their ECF is contracted. The increase in sympathetic tone that occurs, associated with elevated levels of circulating epinephrine, contributes to the acidemia. This constellation of biochemical events in an alcoholic sets the stage for the onset of ketoacidosis. Surgeons encounter ketoacidosis in alcoholic patients when injury or an acute surgical emergency such as pancreatitis or an invasive infection suddenly interrupts a period of sustained heavy ethanol ingestion. Ketoacidosis should be suspected in alcoholic patients with acidemia if they exhibit an increased anion gap. These patients will correct their acid-base disorder if they are treated with glucose, given thiamine, and infused with a balanced electrolyte solution to restore ECF volumes to normal.

Metabolic Acidemia Caused by Loss of Bicarbonate From the Gastrointestinal Tract

Patients with drainage from a proximal gastrointestinal fistula or diarrhea exceeding 4 L/day can loose large amounts of bicarbonate, and acidemia can develop from a deficit in ECF bicarbonate. Pancreatic fluid contains bicarbonate secreted by the exocrine glands of the pancreas. Consequently, large volumes of duodenal, proximal small bowel, and pancreatic fistula drainage can lead to ECF deficits of bicarbonate, sodium, and other electrolytes. Arterial blood gas analysis reveals these patients with gastrointestinal fluid loss to have acidemia and a bicarbonate deficit associated with a normal anion gap. Patients with cholera can die within hours because their voluminous stools lead to the rapid onset of a substantial contraction in ECF volume associated with severe acidemia related to the loss of bicarbonate. Patients with acidemia caused by gastrointestinal loss of bicarbonate often have deficits of sodium and potassium and are treated by the rapid IV infusion of isotonic saline solutions that contain supplemental bicarbonate, the amount of which is based on the severity of the bicarbonate deficit determined by arterial blood gas analysis. These infusions restore ECF volume and increase perfusion of the kidneys, and renal function can contribute to restoration of the bicarbonate deficit. Occult acidemia can develop when several liters of pancreatic fluid flow into the lumen of the bowel but the patient is neither vomiting nor has diarrhea. For example, patients with the rapid onset of a proximal small bowel obstruction have fluid-filled loops of jejunum containing fluid with a high bicarbonate concentration and thus have an acidemia secondary to occult loss of gastrointestinal fluid.

Acidemia Caused by Acute Renal Failure

Acidemia is a hallmark of renal failure. Patients with low glomerular filtration rates are susceptible to acidemia because they cannot clear into urine protons ingested in the daily diet and those formed as a consequence of normal metabolic activity. Patients with acute renal failure and uremia have an acidemia associated with an increased anion gap because there is an increase in the anions phosphate and sulfate in ECF. Treatment of the acidemia associated with acute renal failure is IV bicarbonate therapy. The acidemia can be corrected during renal replacement therapy. Generally, adult patients in renal failure need at least 50 mmol/day of bicarbonate. Renal tubular acidosis syndromes are rare causes of mild to moderate acidemia. The acidosis is caused by impaired capacity of the tubular cells to excrete protons and synthesize bicarbonate. Specifically, these cells are unable to generate and secrete sufficient ammonium into tubules to buffer the excreted protons. Another mechanism of renal tubular acidosis involves an inability to generate a high proton gradient across the abluminal membrane of tubular cells; most of these patients suffer a mild acidemia.

Metabolic Alkalosis

Metabolic alkalosis with an arterial blood gas pH higher than 7.50 can develop when surgeons resuscitating a patient from shock infuse excessive amounts of sodium bicarbonate. In these patients the infused bicarbonate corrects the acidemia, but when perfusion to cells is reinstated, restoration of normal aerobic metabolism consumes the excess protons. Consequently, after recovery from shock, a patient infused with excessive amounts of bicarbonate exhibits alkalemia. Sudden correction of a chronic hypoventilation syndrome can lead to alkalemia. Patients who have chronic respiratory failure and sustained elevation of $PaCO_2$ (as occurs in restrictive lung disease or morbid obesity) will correct the respiratory acidemia through renal function, which increases the bicarbonate concentration in ECF until the pH is normal. If these patients undergo endotracheal intubation and are suddenly mechanically ventilated and their $PaCO_2$ is quickly restored to a normal 40 mm Hg, they will have an alkalemia associated with an excess of bicarbonate. This complication can be avoided if mechanical ventilation is modulated to achieve a slow return to normal $PaCO_2$.

Vomiting-Induced Hypochloremic, Hypokalemic Metabolic Alkalosis

Patients with gastric outlet obstruction represent the classic clinical scenario for metabolic alkalosis in which a deficiency of chloride and potassium in ECF is also present. Parietal cells in the stomach mucosa produce gastric fluid that has a high hydrochloric acid concentration. For each proton pumped into gastric fluid, bicarbonate is added to ECF by the parietal cell. Patients who lose large amounts of gastric fluid deplete their ECF of protons and chloride, as well as potassium. Renal function plays a key role in hypochloremic, hypokalemic metabolic alkalosis. In these alkalemic patients urine pH can be lower than 7. Such patients paradoxically produce an acid urine despite having alkalemia because of three phenomena. These patients have lost large amounts of ECF, and consequently the renin-angiotensin-aldosterone hormonal axis is activated. As aldosterone levels increase, patients have an accelerated exchange of tubule sodium for potassium and protons in the DCT of the nephron. A second phenomenon contributing to the paradoxical production of an acidic urine in a patient with alkalemia is depletion of chloride, which has the renal consequence that with less chloride available in the proximal segments of the nephron, there is less capacity to reabsorb sodium with chloride and consequently delivery of sodium ions to the DCT is increased. Finally, loss of potassium in gastric fluid contributes to the paradoxical production of acidic urine in these patients because with less potassium available in the tubule cells of the DCT, the capacity to exchange potassium for a sodium molecule in the tubule fluid is impaired. In the circumstance of hypokalemia, the tubule cells are driven by aldosterone to make greater use of protons as the exchange cation for the sodium transported out of the tubule fluid. Surgeons correct the alkalemia of hypochloremic, hypokalemic metabolic alkalosis by IV infusions of electrolyte-containing solutions. Isotonic saline fluids are given to expand the ECF to normal. Supplemental KCl is administered to restore the potassium concentration to normal. One indication that a patient has been fully resuscitated is that the urine pH becomes appropriately alkaline. Rarely, patients with severe alkalemia need to be given a carbonic anhydrase inhibitor drug to reduce the renal tubule cell's capacity to generate protons for transport to urine. Surgeons cure patients with hyperchloremic, hypokalemic metabolic alkalemia by performing a surgical procedure that eliminates the foregut obstruction. For example, surgeons cure patients with gastric outlet obstruction caused by duodenal ulcer disease and alkalemia related to vomiting by performing a pyloroplasty.

Diuretic-Induced Alkalemia
Diuretic therapy can also produce metabolic alkalemia. Loop diuretics that alter tubule cell function in the loop of Henle increase urinary excretion of sodium chloride and can reduce plasma volume in patients with heart failure or hepatic cirrhosis, even in the presence of increased ECW caused by edema or ascites. Hypokalemia develops because elevated aldosterone promotes high loss of potassium in the distal nephron. Administration of a potassium-sparing diuretic (e.g., spironolactone) inhibits sodium absorption in the distal nephron and dampens the loss of protons and potassium in urine. A rare clinical form of metabolic alkalosis occurs in patients who ingest huge amounts of calcium carbonate to control peptic acid–related symptoms. Patients with severe alkalemia (pH>7.60) may require infusion of hydrochloric acid to correct the elevated bicarbonate concentration by converting it to carbonic acid and exhaling carbon dioxide. Alternatively, patients can be given a carbonic anhydrase inhibitor, which quickly establishes an elevated bicarbonate concentration in urine.

Respiratory Alkalosis
A sudden significant increase in alveolar ventilation reduces the $PaCO_2$ in an arterial blood sample and produces an acute increase in pH.[14] Respiratory alkalemia, also termed *acute hypocapnia,* can cause arterial vasoconstriction. Acute respiratory alkalosis is used as an emergency intervention to reduce the sudden onset of increased intracranial pressure. In alkalemia, cerebral blood vessels constrict, cerebral blood flow and blood volume decline, and intracranial pressure can be temporarily relieved. Guidelines developed for the prophylactic treatment of patients with brain injury recommend against the routine use of hyperventilation. Acute hypocapnia has been demonstrated to be associated with evidence of coronary vasoconstriction.[15] Most of the vasoconstrictive effects of hypocapnia are thought to be related to a reduction in the proton concentration in ECF and less to the fall in $PaCO_2$. The oxyhemoglobin dissociation curve is shifted to the left by hypocapnia and alkalosis, which reduces the capacity of oxygen to be released from hemoglobin in the microcirculation of tissues. Medical conditions that cause hyperventilation and acute respiratory alkalosis include pain, fever, anxiety, and hypoxia (hypocapnia is an early indication of the onset of acute respiratory distress syndrome). A common cause of iatrogenic respiratory alkalosis is excessive mechanical ventilation after endotracheal intubation. The respiratory rate and tidal volume ventilator settings needed to achieve a normal arterial $PaCO_2$ depend on multiple factors and are difficult to predict in an individual. The influence of mechanical ventilation on $PaCO_2$ is best determined by analysis of a patient's arterial blood gas obtained after 30 minutes of mechanical ventilation at a selected rate. An alternative method for monitoring whether hypocapnia is developing in a mechanically ventilated patient is continuous monitor in exhaled gases the partial pressure of CO_2. In the individual patient, calibration of the relationship between end-tidal CO_2 and $PaCO_2$ needs to be defined because it is influenced by the extent of an individual's pulmonary dysfunction. Patients with normal renal function who have sustained hyperventilation associated with alkalemia related to acute hypocapnia reduced their elevated pH toward 7.40 by renal excretion of alkaline urine. Hypocapnia induced by acute hyperventilation during mechanical ventilation should be considered an adverse event to be avoided in most patients.

Respiratory Acidemia
An abrupt decline in alveolar ventilation leads to an acute increase in $PaCO_2$. Acute hypercapnia leads to a decline in ECF pH and respiratory acidemia. Because carbon dioxide readily crosses the cell membrane, patients with acute hypercapnia have an associated decline in ICF pH. Two physiologic mechanisms provide reflex feedback stimulation to ventilation centers located in the brainstem that control the reflex mechanism for increasing minute ventilation. Central chemoreceptor cells in the brainstem respond to higher proton concentrations in ICF and stimulate an efferent signal that increases the respiratory rate. However, chronic hypercapnia blunts chemoreceptor responsiveness, and these patients depend instead on arterial hypoxemia-stimulating cells in the carotid bodies to increase the drive to ventilate. Patients with neurologic dysfunction may not have the usual reflex increase in pulmonary ventilation when an increase in their $PaCO_2$ occurs. Patients at risk for central hypoventilation syndromes are individuals with brain injury, infection, and a suppressed level of consciousness caused by the administration of sedatives, narcotics, and tranquilizers. Patients given large doses of narcotics after major surgery have died from respiratory arrest as a result of coma caused by markedly increased $PaCO_2$ (>70 mm Hg). Patients at higher risk for being overnarcotized are individuals with preexisting hypoventilation syndromes. Patients with chronic hypoventilation achieve correction of their acidemia by renal retention of excess bicarbonate, and thus they may have compensated mild to moderate hypercapnia ($PaCO_2$ 50-70 mm Hg) with a pH of 7.40 in arterial blood. Chronically hypoventilating patients have impaired central nervous system reflexes to a rise in $PaCO_2$ and rely on hypoxia as the drive for increased ventilation. Patients with chronic hypercapnia who are

given narcotics and high concentrations of inhaled oxygen can sustain a marked elevation in $PaCO_2$ without the development of hypoxia. Deep coma can develop as a result of hypercapnia, and when hypoxia finally occurs near death, they do not respond with spontaneous ventilation. Acute hypercapnia, acidemia, and respiratory depression can also occur in patients treated with an epidural anesthetic administered as patient-controlled anesthesia.

Surgeons can cause hypercapnia by their ventilator settings during mechanical ventilation. The respiratory acidemia in these patients is usually corrected by increasing tidal volume or the respiratory rate or rarely by reducing dead space. Occasionally, hypoventilated patients improve if a hemopneumothorax is evacuated by a chest tube. Intentional underventilation of patients with adult respiratory distress syndrome has been selected as the preferred method of ventilation to avoid distention of airways in patients with poorly compliant lungs. Kregenow and colleagues[16] observed that in patients with respiratory failure who are being mechanically ventilated, hypercapnic acidosis was an independent factor associated with reduced mortality. Nonetheless, permissive hypercapnia is a strategy that is beneficial because it temporarily reduces, in selected patients, baro-trauma in lungs that are poorly compliant due to injury or disease.

As the proportion of the population who are morbidly obese increases, surgeons are increasingly encountering chronically hypercapnic patients who require a surgical procedure. These patients are at high risk for a further increase in their $PaCO_2$ with acidemia if they are subjected to a surgical procedure. Chronic respiratory failure with hypercapnia has been successfully managed in obese patients with mask-based respiratory assist devices used with a bilevel mode of pressure support ventilation.[17]

EXTRACELLULAR FLUID DISTRIBUTION BETWEEN PLASMA VOLUME AND INTERSTITIAL LYMPHATIC VOLUME

Control of Fluid Movement Across the Capillary

Regulated flow of fluids through the ECF is essential for maintaining homeostasis. Blood flow delivers oxygen to arterioles, capillaries, and venules and clears waste products of metabolism. A second flow of fluid important to organ function is filtration of plasma across the microcirculation into the interstitial lymphatic compartment of the ECF. Multiple mechanisms regulate this flow and the distribution of ECF between the plasma volume and interstitial lymphatic fluid compartments (see Fig. 5-1). More than 100 years ago Ernest Starling described the hypothesis that there exists a balance of driving forces across the capillary membrane. Starling's hypothesis proposed that elevated hydrostatic pressure in the lumen of the capillary favors the flow of plasma into the interstitium whereas the oncotic pressure generated from protein solutes in plasma favors the flow of fluid from the interstitium to the plasma compartment. Starling's concept was that normally, the balance of forces across the capil-

lary membrane produces a net flow of fluid from the plasma compartment to the interstitial lymphatic compartments. Furthermore, because the endothelial membrane is semipermeable, water crosses the capillary wall more readily than the protein solutes in plasma do. The large size of the proteins and the small diameter of pores and pathways in the endothelial membrane mean that the concentration of small solutes such as sodium, chloride, and glucose is the same in plasma and interstitial lymphatic fluid but that the concentration of proteins, predominantly albumin, in plasma is substantially higher than the concentration of these proteins in interstitial lymphatic fluid. As a consequence of the difference in protein concentration, the oncotic pressure of plasma is higher than that of interstitial fluid. Starling's hypothesis was that the hydrostatic pressure forcing plasma to filter across the capillary membrane normally exceeds the difference in oncotic pressure between interstitial and plasma fluid such that a net flow of fluid into the interstitium occurs in most tissues. Lymph flows through a system of conduits that include lymph nodes, and eventually the lymph returns to the venous compartment, principally through the thoracic duct into the superior vena cava.

Flow of fluid into the interstitium is matched in steady-state conditions by the flow of lymph out of tissues, with the net result that the volume of fluid in the plasma volume and the interstitial lymphatic compartment does not change. Maintaining plasma volume and thus blood volume is a priority in regulation of the distribution of ECF. Multiple factors participate in physiologic processes to ensure that blood volume is kept close to normal. Starling forces play a dominant role in control of the shift of fluid between the plasma compartment and the interstitial lymphatic compartments. Starling forces that reduce the size of the plasma volume are an increase in hydrostatic pressure in capillaries and a decrease in plasma oncotic pressure. Correspondingly, Starling forces that favor an increase in plasma volume are a reduction in hydrostatic pressure in the capillary and an increase in plasma oncotic pressure. Another factor that can influence the size of the plasma compartment is the permeability characteristics of the capillary membrane. An increase in permeability of the capillary membranes to water or plasma proteins can reduce plasma volume as more fluid shifts into the interstitial lymphatic compartments. Hormones, endogenous proteins, and inflammatory agents can increase the permeability of the capillary membrane.[18] Factors that influence lymphatic flow are less clearly understood but also influence the proportion of ECF in the plasma compartment versus the interstitial lymphatic compartment.

An important function of the second circulation is unidirectional flux of soluble proteins from plasma to the interstitium and through the lymphatics back to the venous circulation. Eugene Renkin estimated that the total circulating protein mass (primarily albumin, immunoglobulins, and fibrinogen) could be 450 g in a 65-kg man (Fig. 5-8).[19] Located in the 3 L of plasma volume is 210 g of protein. Residing in the 12 L of interstitial lymphatic fluid is 240 g of protein. Thus, the majority of albumin in

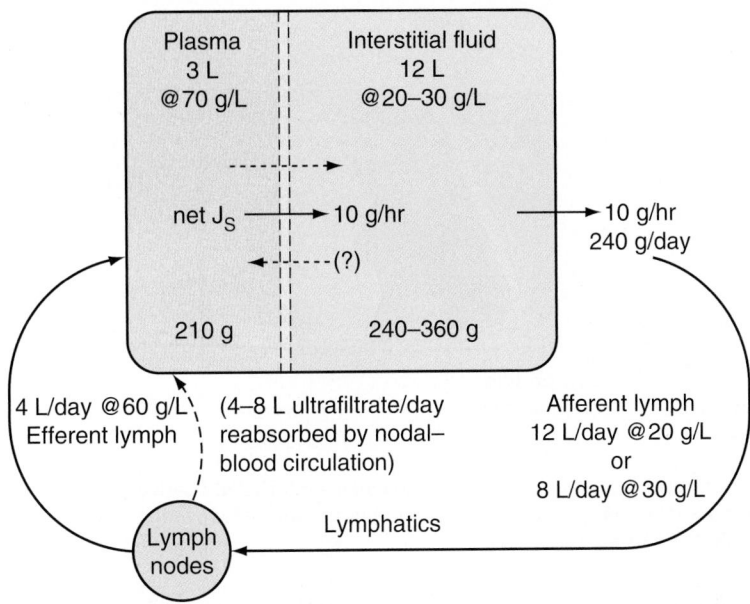

Figure 5-8 Magnitudes of lymphatic turnover of fluid and plasma protein. (From Renkin EM: Some consequences of capillary permeability to macromolecules: Starling's hypothesis reconsidered. Am J Physiol 250:H706, 1986.)

the body is located in the interstitium. In the daily filtration of fluid from plasma to the interstitium, Renkin concludes that approximately every 24 hours approximately half the plasma protein mass flows out of the capillary, through the interstitial lymphatic compartment, and returns to the plasma compartment as thoracic duct lymph at a flow rate of 4 to 6 L/day. This summation of fluid flow and protein flux should not obscure the fact that each organ has unique capillary permeability characteristics. There is negligible interstitial fluid and no lymph flow from the brain. Skin and skeletal muscle, which contain the largest proportion of interstitial volume, have relatively impermeable microvascular membranes, a rich network of lymphatics, and a compliant interstitial volume. Hepatic microvascular membranes are highly permeable, and lymph flow from the liver is high. In addition to variability in the characteristics of the endothelial barrier related to organs, factors can also modulate the characteristics of the endothelial membrane to change flow rates.

Endothelial cells attached to a basement membrane constitute the capillary wall. Endothelial cells are fused in a continuous monolayer, with gaps at junctions between adjacent cells. The basement membrane is a layer of macromolecules that form a barrier, particularly to highly charged proteins. The endothelial cell layer combines with the basement membrane to constitute the semipermeable barrier that separates the plasma compartment from the interstitial lymphatic compartment.[20] Permeability at the arteriole end of the capillary membrane is less than the permeability characteristics at the venule end of the capillary. Plasma water and solutes flow across endothelial cells through several types of passages, and the variable characteristics of these passages contribute to the semipermeable characteristics of the endothelial membrane (Fig. 5-9).

An equation that summarizes a contemporary model of Starling's hypothesis indicates that the flow of fluid across the capillary membrane is influenced by the balance of driving forces, the permeability characteristics of the capillary membrane, and the available capillary membrane surface area:

$$Jv = Lp \ S \ [(Pc - Pi) - \sigma(COPc - COPi)]$$

In steady-state conditions, a defined mass of tissue has a net flow (Jv) of plasma filtrate into the interstitial lymphatic space that is equivalent to the lymph flow draining fluid from the tissue. The driving forces responsible for water flow are presented in the equation as P and COP, which correspond to hydrostatic and colloid oncotic pressure, respectively. The model indicates that four types of pressure influence Jv. Pc, or hydrostatic pressure in the capillary, minus Pi, or hydrostatic pressure in the interstitium, generates the flow of fluid out of the capillary lumen. The equation factor ($COPc - COPi$) represents the force attributed to the osmotic pressure of proteins in a solution in millimeters of mercury, which favors water retention on the plasma side of the membrane. The normal colloid osmotic pressure of plasma is 25 to 30 mm Hg, and more than 50% of that is attributed to albumin, whereas the colloid osmotic pressure of interstitial fluid varies with tissues. Sigma, σ, has a value between 0 and 1 and corresponds to the effectiveness of the microvascular membrane as a barrier to plasma proteins. The more permeable the microvascular membrane to plasma proteins (i.e., the closer σ is to 0), the less effective the difference in colloid osmotic pressure between plasma and interstitial fluid. The σ of capillaries in skin and skeletal muscle exceeds 0.9, and the colloid osmotic pressure of plasma proteins effectively retains plasma water within these capillaries. In contrast, the σ in liver capillaries approaches 0, and colloid pressure has limited influence. High lymph flow and a tightly restrictive liver capsule prevent liver edema.

The term *Lp S* has two components. Lp represents the permeability of the capillary membrane to water, also

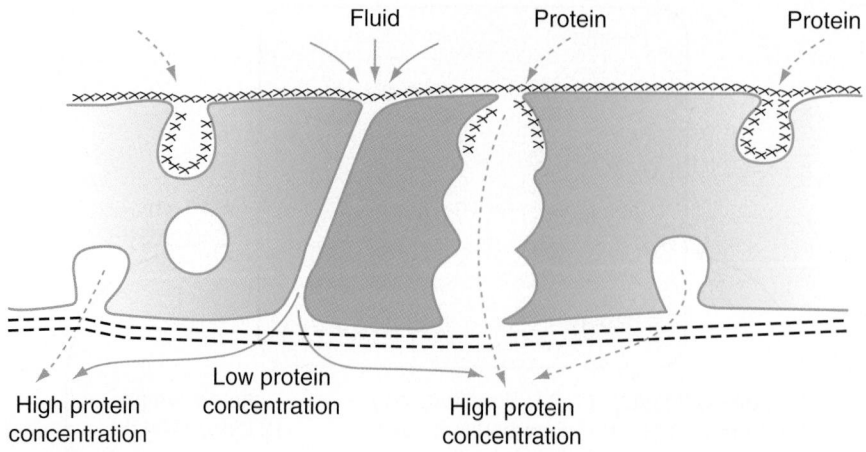

Figure 5-9 Diagrammatic representation of the microvascular endothelial barrier showing separate pathways for fluid and protein to cross from the plasma space to the interstitium. (From Michel CC, Curry FE: Microvascular permeability. Physiol Rev 79:703-761, 1999.)

designated as hydraulic conductivity. S refers to the capillary membrane surface area available for water to move across. Thus, tissues with many capillaries have large surface areas. Arteriolar vasomotor tone is a physiologic mechanism that not only adjusts Pc but also controls the surface area within the microcirculation of a specific tissue. Vasoconstriction reduces blood flow to a capillary bed, decreases Pc, and diminishes the surface area available for filtration, all of which lead to a decline in Jv. Ninety percent of hydraulic conductivity in the microcirculation can be attributed to small pores large enough to allow a water molecule to pass but too small to accommodate albumin and other plasma proteins. Circulating hormones can modulate the hydraulic conductivity of the capillary membrane.[21]

Pathologic Changes in Interstitial Volume: Dehydration and Edema

The size of the plasma volume is regulated by multiple physiologic factors that favor maintenance of normal blood volume. The distribution of fluid and proteins between plasma and the interstitium favors the plasma volume in dehydrated patients (i.e., patients with a contracted ECF volume). In contrast, in overhydrated patients with an expanded ECF volume, plasma volume is maintained close to normal while the majority of the excess ECF is edema in the interstitium or fluid in the pleural and peritoneal cavities.

Plasma volume is restored after acute hemorrhage by a shift of interstitial fluid with albumin and other proteins into the plasma compartment. Decreased capillary hydrostatic pressure leads to reduced plasma fluid transport across the microvascular membrane. Thoracic duct flow is sustained, and for a transient period, return of interstitial fluid and proteins exceeds filtration of plasma, with the consequence that plasma volume is restored. Small volumes of hypertonic saline have been successfully used to resuscitate patients in hemorrhagic shock. Hypertonic saline works in part because after IV infusions, the osmolality of ECF increases, water shifts from the ICF,

and the net result is a greater increase in plasma volume than is accomplished by the equivalent infusion of isotonic saline. In patients with heart failure, there is an increase in venous pressure that is transmitted retrogradely to the capillaries and causes greater filtration of plasma into the interstitium. As long as the flow of lymph compensates for the rate of filtration across the microvascular membrane, edema does not develop. However, in patients with end-stage congestive heart failure and markedly elevated left atrial pressure, filtration of fluid into the pulmonary interstitium can exceed the rate of lymphatic clearance, with the result that fluid accumulates in the parenchyma of the lung and produces pulmonary edema with hypoxia. Pulmonary edema in patients with congestive heart failure can be corrected with diuretics to reduce plasma volume, decrease left atrial pressure, and return the rate of plasma filtration in the pulmonary microcirculation to a rate that can be equaled by lymph drainage.

There is considerable interest in the edema produced in response to an inflammatory insult because this edema is typically caused by an increase in microvascular membrane permeability to proteins. For example, in skin capillaries more than 85% of colloid proteins in plasma do not cross the microvascular membrane at the time that water and smaller electrolyte solutes cross. In patients with a burn wound, capillary permeability is increased, and more than 50% of colloids have ready access to the interstitium. Not only does edema develop, but the interstitial fluid also has a substantial increase in proteins such as albumin. The consequence for total body homeostasis is that high-permeability edema is associated with a substantial reduction in plasma colloid oncotic pressure, which further increases the development of edema. Two endogenously produced molecules, histamine and the polypeptide bradykinin, can cause gaps to develop between venule endothelial cells that lead to increased permeability of the microvascular membrane. These drugs have a reversible effect on permeability, thus highlighting that the increases in permeability are more a phenomenon of physiologic fluctuation than an irreversible change in microvascular membrane permeability characteristics.

The interstitial space contains a gel matrix of collagen and glycosaminoglycans. Collagen fibers that attach to fibroblasts resist hydration because as interstitial volume increases, the collagen fibers come under tension. Water molecules and small solutes can hydrate the interstices of the tightly interwoven glycosaminoglycans, but large protein solutes, such as albumin, cannot gain access. This exclusion of albumin is a factor that increases the effective oncotic pressure of colloids in interstitial fluid. Also influencing hydration of the interstitial space is the magnitude of lymphatic pumping. Terminal lymphatics are open endothelial-lined tubes, and interstitial hydrostatic fluid pressure drives fluid into the lymphatics. Prenodal lymphatics drain into the cortical surface of a lymph node. The fluid percolates through lymphoid tissue, where its composition may be altered, and then drains into a lymphatic vessel that exits from the node's hilum. Larger lymphatics are lined with smooth muscle that can contract and propel lymph toward the thoracic duct.

CELLULAR AEROBIC FUNCTION AND DYSFUNCTION

Shock in patients is fundamentally a problem of dysfunction of intracellular energy metabolism. Patients in shock do not deliver sufficient oxygen to their mitochondria to sustain aerobic metabolism, and cell functions are impaired by energy deficits. Sustained failure to enable normal aerobic metabolism to occur kills cells, and consequently there is lethal organ failure. Therapies for patients in shock have focused on restoring organ function, for example, return of perfusion pressure, cardiac output, renal function, and neurologic function to normal. These organ-targeted therapies have led to improved survival of patients in shock. Nonetheless, in the future the development of new therapies for shock may depend on the discovery of interventions that directly reverse the cellular energy deficit and restore normal metabolism to cells.

Cellular Energy Metabolism

Cellular metabolism depends primarily on hydrolysis of the high-energy bond in ATP. The phosphoanhydride bond between the terminal phosphate and ADP is the source of chemical energy for most cellular work. Cellular work performed with ATP includes contraction of actin and myosin, transport of electrolytes across cell membranes, synthesis of constitutive molecules, and generation of heat. ATP is hydrolyzed to ADP, and with cleavage of the terminal phosphate bond, energy is released.

$$ATP \rightleftharpoons ADP + H^+ + PO_4^- + H_2O + Energy$$

Each mole of ATP converted to ADP, phosphate, a proton, and water releases 12,000 calories. ATP is constantly replenished by respiration, a sequence of biochemical reactions in cells that extract energy from fuels (primarily the carbon-to-carbon bond of glucose and fats) and

oxygen. Glycolysis is a process that occurs in the cytosol in which the six-carbon glucose is converted to a pair of three-carbon pyruvate molecules. Without consuming oxygen, glycolysis can produce 2 mol of ATP for each mole of glucose. This reaction is critical to temporarily sustain minimal amounts of ATP in a cell suddenly deprived of oxygen. In normal conditions with available oxygen, pyruvate enters the citric acid cycle, where biochemical reactions release electrons to coenzymes, which move to the mitochondria. In mitochondria the electrons and oxygen support oxidative phosphorylation in which ATP is formed and oxygen is reduced and converted to carbon dioxide and water. Complete oxidation of 1 mol of glucose generates 38 mol of ATP. When insufficient oxygen is available to support oxidative phosphorylation, the pyruvate is diverted away from the citric acid cycle to a reaction that generates lactate and protons. These molecules leave the ICF, and patients with impaired oxidative phosphorylation have elevated lactate and proton concentrations in their ECF.

Clinical Signs of Cellular Energy Failure

Direct measurement of cellular function during shock is complex and in clinical practice unreliable. Surgeons treating patients in shock measure levels of lactate in blood samples, as well as indications of acidemia in arterial blood gases, to determine the magnitude of impairment in intracellular aerobic metabolism. Several clinical investigators have reported that the risk for death in patents in shock is proportional to the severity of acidemia as measured by the calculated bicarbonate deficit on an arterial blood gas sample. Among trauma patients who sustained severe injury, Kaplan and Kellum reported that in comparison to survivors, nonsurvivors had more severe acidemia (pH 7.06 versus 7.34), more depressed base excess (−18 versus −3 mEq/L), and higher lactate levels (11 versus 4 mmol/L).[22] Patients treated with catecholamines to resuscitate them from septic shock commonly have elevated lactate levels that are attributed to underperfusion. Moribund patients had a substantially higher lactate level (12 versus 5 mmol/L) than did patients who were in shock but survived. There is a strong, consistently reported association between the lethality of shock and the extent of elevation in lactate and the severity of acidemia. These laboratory findings indicate that shock leads to an impaired cytoplasmic and mitochondrial redox state. However, as Pal and coauthors recently reported, the association with acidemia does not have a strong enough predictive value to assist the surgeon at the bedside in prospectively identifying a high-risk patient.[23] Pal and coauthors examined the association of elevated lactate levels in seriously injured patients admitted to a tertiary care trauma center. They observed that although lactate levels were higher in patients who died, by using receiver operating curves they determined that lactate levels had an area under the curve of only 0.73. Furthermore, the positive predictive value for an elevated lactate concentration (>2.0 mmol/L) and death was only 5.2%. Pal and coauthors confirmed that there was greater predictive value in the trend in lactate levels after resuscitation. The value of trends in the clearance of lactate was emphasized by Claridge and coworkers, who identified among multiply injured patients those who were at higher risk for orthopedic surgery. Patients who had sustained elevations in lactate indicating a persistent occult hypoperfusion state were at higher risk for death and complications.[24] Surgeons should evaluate patients in shock for untreated injuries if their elevated lactic acid levels do not resolve.

In patients who experience an anaerobic insult, an oxygen debt is hypothesized to develop. Clinical scientists have proposed that patients who have significant shock need a period of supernormal oxygen delivery at the start of their resuscitation to facilitate correction of their oxygen debt. Several randomized controlled trials intended to test this hypothesis have been conducted. The specific protocols varied, but in general, patients randomized to supernormal resuscitation were transfused with blood until the hemoglobin level exceeded 10 g/dL, were IV infused with fluid until their intravascular volume was high, and were treated with vasoactive drugs until their cardiac output, and thus oxygen delivery to tissues, was supernormal. The results of these randomized controlled trials either have failed to show benefit from increasing oxygen delivery to supernormal levels or, in one study, worsened the outcome. In a 2000 report, by Velmahos and colleagues, injured patients in shock were resuscitated to the end point of an oxygen delivery index greater than $600 \, mL/min/m^2$.[25] The investigators observed no difference in any of the outcomes, including hospital death, complications, or hospital length of stay. The trials of supernormal oxygen delivery have consistently observed that moribund patients cannot respond to attempts to increase oxygen delivery. New therapies are needed to improve the resuscitation of patients in shock. Moore and coworkers have proposed that novel interventions need to be developed that rapidly reverse shock and are effective in modulating the exaggerated systemic inflammatory response to shock and transfusion.[26]

PHYSIOLOGIC CONTROL OF PERFUSION PRESSURE

The autonomic nervous system is pivotal in modulating the hemodynamic response to shock. The response to hypotension is vasoconstriction. Baroreceptors located in the aortic arch and carotid arteries are stimulated by changes in perfusion pressure, identified as a decline in the stretch of vessel walls during systole. Both increases and decreases in systolic pressure prompt the transmission of afferent reflex signals to vascular control centers located in the brainstem. These centers control release of the catecholamines norepinephrine from terminal sites of sympathetic nerves adjacent to vascular smooth muscle and epinephrine from the adrenal medulla. Sympathetic postganglionic neurons release norepinephrine into synaptic junctions, and binding to α-adrenergic receptors increases perivascular smooth muscle constriction. In

response to increased sympathetic tone, receptors in the heart cause an increase in the heart rate and contractility. Furthermore, epinephrine released from the adrenal medulla circulates in blood and can bind α- and β-adrenergic receptors throughout the body. Baroreceptors stimulated in response to hypotension release ADH from the supraoptic and paraventricular nuclei of the hypothalamus, which circulates and contributes to constrict arterioles. Vasopressin has an additional longer acting compensatory response to hypotension because as a hormone it increases renal water absorption and expands ECF volume. Baroreceptors respond to hypertension by stimulating a reflex reduction in catecholamine release.

The kidney is both an endocrine organ and the body's location for filtration and clearance of ECF. The renal response to hypotension includes release of renin from the juxtaglomerular apparatus. The renin-angiotensin-aldosterone axis participates in modulating the response to hypotension through vasoconstriction by angiotensin II and through retention of sodium and water by the nephron. A fall in renal perfusion pressure activates mechanisms that adjust intrarenal blood flow. During shock, a greater proportion of blood flowing through the renal arteries is diverted to juxtamedullary nephrons to increase the kidneys' capacity to produce concentrated urine. The initial renal response to shock is to produce a small amount of very concentrated urine. During shock, renal tubule cells consume large amounts of oxygen to generate the ATP needed to produce concentrated urine through the transport of sodium and other solutes. A sustained period of hypotension and renal underperfusion can lead to acute renal failure because the renal tubule cells sustain an anaerobic insult.

Patients in shock can be categorized according to their hemodynamic response patterns. The three major categories are shock associated with a reduction in blood volume (and typically also associated with vasoconstriction), shock associated with impaired cardiac function, and shock attributable to excessive vasodilation. To categorize a patient in shock, invasive hemodynamic monitoring is needed. Surgeons monitor patients in shock by continuous measurement of arterial pressure with arterial catheters and continuous measurement of ventricular filling pressure with pulmonary artery catheters that have the capacity to use a thermodilution procedure for measurement of cardiac output. An alternative method of measuring cardiac output that is noninvasive is measurement of cardiac output by thoracic bioimpedance.[25] The pattern of shock guides the treatment. However, surgeons should recognize that it is common for patients with severe illness or injury to evolve through several patterns of hemodynamic instability over the first few days of treatment. For example, a patient in hemorrhagic shock who is treated with blood transfusions after surgery to control hemorrhage may have a vasodilatory pattern of shock related to an exaggerated inflammatory response to reperfusion. The basic information provided by a pulmonary artery catheter to a surgeon selecting treatment for a patient in shock is filling pressure, cardiac index, and calculation of systemic vascular resistance (SVR).

Table 5-5 Vasoactive Drugs Reported as Therapeutic in Adults in Shock*

DRUG	DOSE RANGE	PRINCIPAL MECHANISM[†]
Inotropic (May Be Chronotropic)		
Dobutamine	2-20 μg/kg/min	β₁-adrenergic
Dopamine (low dose)	5-10 μg/kg/min	β₁-adrenergic; dopaminergic
Epinephrine (low dose)	0.06-0.20 μg/kg/min	β₁- and β₂-adrenergic; less α
Vasoconstrictor and Inotropic		
Dopamine (high dose)	>10 μg/kg/min	α-adrenergic; less dopaminergic
Epinephrine (high dose)	0.21-0.42 μg/kg/min	α-adrenergic; less β₁ and β₂
Norepinephrine	0.02-0.45 μg/kg/min	α-adrenergic; less β₁ and β₂
Vasoconstrictor		
Phenylephrine	0.2-2.5 μg/kg/min	α-adrenergic
Vasopressin	0.01-0.04 U/min	V1 receptor
Vasodilator		
Milrinone	0.4-0.6 μg/kg/min	Phosphodiesterase inhibitor[‡]
Dopamine (very low dose)	1-4 μg/kg/min	Dopaminergic

*An individual patient's response to a given drug is variable.
[†]α and β refer to adrenergic agonists. β₁-adrenergic effects are inotropic and increase contractility. β₂-adrenergic effects are chronotropic.
[‡]After a loading dose of 50 μg/kg over a 10-minute period.

Pharmacologic Treatment of Shock

Drugs can play a vital role in supporting patients in shock (Table 5-5). However, because the pathophysiology of shock states varies, selection of the appropriate drug for specific circumstances should be guided by what intervention would restore delivery of oxygen to critical cells and not just the simplistic goal of increasing systolic pressure. The first step in resuscitation of most patients in shock involves IV infusion of isotonic fluid to expand plasma volume and therefore blood volume, with the beneficial consequence that increased return of blood to the right-sided cardiac chambers will increase cardiac output. Surgeons can evaluate the response to volume infusion by monitoring changes in right and left ventricular filling pressure. As a general guideline, full expansion of blood volume is achieved when central venous pressure exceeds 15 mm Hg or pulmonary artery catheter occlusion pressure stabilizes between 15 and 20 mm Hg. Balanced electrolyte solutions are the preferred resuscitation fluids for patients with shock, unless they are anemic with a hemoglobin content of 7 g/dL or less, in which case red cell transfusion is appropriate. Surgeons can use the information provided by pulmonary artery catheters to derive a more complex metric of end-diastolic filling: an increase in left ventricular stroke work index (LVSWI) in response to volume loading. The surgeon could conclude that intravascular volume has been fully restored if the patient does not have a further increase in LVSWI as a consequence of infusing additional resuscitation fluid.

Surgeons select vasoactive drugs for infusion into patients whose perfusion to vital organs is not restored by the IV infusion of fluids. Selection of a drug for a specific patient should be based on the intended effect.

There are four categories of hemodynamically active drugs: inotropic (and possibly chronotropic) agents, which increase cardiac contractility; inotropic and vasoconstrictive drugs; vasoconstrictive agents, which increase vascular resistance; and vasodilatory agents, which relax arteriole constriction in patients with severe vasoconstriction (see Table 5-5). Vasoactive drugs can have multiple effects, and the response of an individual patient to a specific drug varies. Nonetheless, surgeons can use these four categories of drug action as a general guideline for what drug should be initially used to treat shock in an individual patient. Surgeons infuse inotropic agents into patients in shock if their pulmonary artery wedge pressure is elevated and the cardiac response to the increased pressure is suboptimal. Dopamine, dobutamine, and epinephrine are the three most commonly used inotropic agents. The pharmacologic mode of action of these three drugs varies. Epinephrine and dobutamine increase cardiac contractility through β-adrenergic mechanisms, and these agents will commonly produce some degree of increased heart rate. Whereas dobutamine is solely a β-adrenergic agent, epinephrine has both β- and α-adrenergic receptor agonist effects and may increase vasoconstriction of vascular smooth muscle. Evidence indicates that dobutamine is the agent of choice to increase cardiac output in patients with cardiac dysfunction associated with septic shock, but it may dangerously increase cardiac oxygen consumption in a patient with coronary artery disease. Dopamine functions as an inotropic agent, depending on the dose at which it is infused. Dopamine binds dopaminergic receptors at low doses (0-5 μg/kg/min) and may increase blood flow to renal and mesenteric vascular beds. At midrange doses (5-10 μg/kg/min), β-adrenergic receptors are activated, which leads to positive inotropic and chronotropic effects on the myocardium. Dopamine was hypothesized to preserve renal function in patients with shock because of its renal vascular dilation effect. In several randomized controlled trials, dopamine infusions have been determined to not improve renal function and should not be infused for that purpose.

Dopamine and epinephrine at lower doses are expected to have predominantly an inotropic effect and at higher doses to have a combined inotropic and arteriole vasoconstrictive effect because these drugs bind to α-adrenergic agents (see Table 5-5).[27] Norepinephrine is a drug with potent α-adrenergic effects that also has an inotropic effect through β-adrenergic receptor effects. Infusion of norepinephrine has been reported to be particularly beneficial in patients with septic shock when surgeons attempt to increase mean aortic pressure by selective vasoconstriction of noncritical vascular beds (e.g., skin and skeletal muscle). In these patients the increase in mean aortic pressure improves perfusion of the renal, cerebral, and cardiac circulations.

Two drugs used to achieve only vasoconstriction are phenylephrine, a potent, pure α-adrenergic agonist, and vasopressin. In several studies reporting multiple-drug therapy for treatment of the hemodynamic consequences of septic shock, phenylephrine was successfully added to inotropic agents to improve perfusion. Infusion of vasopressin has been reported to be an effective treatment of vasodilatory shock refractory to the infusion of α-adrenergic agents. V1 receptors on the surface of smooth muscle cells surrounding blood vessels bind circulating vasopressin and induce contraction of smooth muscle cells surrounding arterioles. Skin, skeletal muscle, and fat are three tissues that contain arterioles responsive to vasopressin. Evidence indicates that patients with sustained septic shock (over a period of hours) deplete their endogenous vasopressin stores. These observations explain why infusion of vasopressin into patients with catecholamine-resistant septic shock can reverse vasodilation.

Vasodilators are the fourth category of vasoactive drugs used to improve the delivery of oxygen to cells in patients in shock. One group of patients with severe vasoconstriction encountered by surgeons are those with end-stage severe congestive heart failure in whom a surgical emergency develops. In patients with sustained periods of low cardiac output, increased SVR can develop as a result of intense baroreceptor-mediated constriction. In patients with intense vasoconstriction, the infusion of low-dose (0-5 μg/kg/min) dopamine, milrinone, or nitroprusside will improve blood flow to tissues. Optimal use of vasodilator therapy requires intensive hemodynamic monitoring combined with adjustments in infusion rates of the drugs so that the desired effect of an afterload reduction is combined with avoidance of hypotension and worsening renal function. Milrinone is a phosphodiesterase inhibitor that improves cardiac output by enhancing cardiac contractility through the β-adrenergic signaling pathway, as well as being a potent vasodilator. Nitroprusside is a smooth muscle–relaxing agent that vasodilates arterioles and improves symptoms through a reduction in cardiac preload. A new category of vasodilatory drugs

that may be effective are recombinant engineered B-type atrial natriuretic peptides.

THE SURGEON'S RESPONSE TO SHOCK

Venous Access and Hemodynamic Monitoring

Surgeons treating patients in shock rely on accurate measurements of a patient's pulse rate, rhythm, and mean arterial perfusion pressure. Noninvasive methods for monitoring vital signs have the lowest complication rates, but they are not reliable in hypotensive patients. Transcutaneous pulse oximetry enables continuous monitoring of oxygen saturation in capillary blood and provides a measure of the pulse rate. The pulse oximeter determines oxygen saturation by transmitting light through skin and a capillary and measuring the absorption of light at two wavelengths. Pulse oximetry calculates the percentage of saturated hemoglobin. It is reliable in circumstances of brisk pulsatile blood flow through the capillary bed. Pulse oximetry is less reliable in hypotensive patients, particularly those with extensive vasoconstriction. Transcutaneous oxygen saturation is falsely depressed by anemia, a preponderance of fetal hemoglobin, or IV injected dyes such as indigo carmine. Patients with carboxyhemoglobinemia can have falsely elevated oxygen saturation on pulse oximetry.

Arterial Catheters

Surgeons insert arterial catheters via the Seldinger technique in which a needle is passed through an artery and slowly withdrawn until pulsatile blood flows from the needle. A guidewire is inserted through the needle into the vessel, and the catheter is advanced over the wire into the artery over the guidewire. Arterial catheters enable continuous measurement of systolic, diastolic, and mean arterial pressure. Patterns in the arterial pressure waveform can be informative. For example, substantial fluctuations in mean arterial pressure corresponding to positive pressure ventilation cycles suggest that the patient is hypovolemic or that the tidal volume in a mechanically ventilated patient is high. Arterial catheters enable painless and reliable sampling of arterial blood for determination of pH and the partial pressure of respiratory gases. The radial artery is the most commonly used access site for an arterial line in adults. The risk of hand ischemia is less than 0.1%, but thrombosis of the radial artery can lead to amputation in patients whose ulnar artery is not patent. Thus, patency of the ulnar artery is confirmed before insertion of a catheter into the radial artery. The dorsalis pedis artery is an alternative site for arterial catheterization, although this vessel should not be used in patients with peripheral vascular disease or diabetes. Peripheral arterial cannulation can be difficult to perform in patients in shock. Furthermore, the pressure tracing from the radial artery is often damped because of excessive vasoconstriction occurring in patients who are in shock. Femoral artery catheters are useful in patients with profound vasoconstriction, unless the patient has occlusive vascular disease of the aorta or iliac vessels. Although femoral artery catheters are safe for 1 to 2 days, these catheters have a higher prevalence of serious catheter-related infections, probably because of the heavy bacterial contamination of groin skin.

Central Venous Catheters

Reliable venous access to enable rapid infusion of fluid, blood products, and drugs is essential in the treatment of patients in shock. Large-bore catheters can be inserted percutaneously into upper extremity veins. In desperate situations, saphenous vein cannulation can be performed through a venotomy created under direct vision after surgical exposure of the saphenous vein at the ankle or groin. Saphenous vein cut-down may be the most rapid method for securing a large IV line in a patient in profound shock. However, many surgeons prefer to resuscitate patients with catheters inserted in central veins. Three sites commonly used to achieve central venous catheter insertion are the femoral vein, the subclavian vein, and the internal jugular vein. Each site has advantages and disadvantages, depending on the cause of the patient's shock. Experienced surgeons can secure central venous access rapidly in the majority of patients who are in shock. Surgeons insert either multiple-lumen catheters (usually three channels) that permit simultaneous infusion of fluid and medications or large-diameter catheters (8.5 French) with a single lumen, which is ideally suited for the infusion of large volumes of resuscitation fluid and blood. An alternative venous access technique limited to application in infants and children is use of an interosseus catheter, usually inserted into the proximal end of the tibia of a child in profound shock.

Central venous catheters are inserted with sterile technique. Complications associated with insertion of central venous catheters include damage to an adjacent artery and failure to insert the catheter into the vein such that fluids and drugs given through the line extravasate into tissues. In the case of subclavian and internal jugular catheters, two serious complications requiring additional treatment are pneumothorax and hemopneumothorax. Proper insertion technique can reduce complication rates. The subclavian vein is punctured beneath the clavicle, where the vein courses anterior to the subclavian artery. The internal jugular vein is punctured in the lower third of the neck, where the vein is located beneath the sternocleidomastoid muscle and lateral to pulsation of the common carotid artery. Injury to the carotid artery is reduced if the surgeon identifies the location and depth of the internal jugular vein with an ultrasound device and inserts the needle under visual guidance (Fig. 5-10). A catheter successfully inserted into the right internal jugular vein of an adult has an exceptionally high likelihood of being correctly positioned above the right atrium in the superior vena cava. Femoral vein access is an attractive option for initial central venous access in patients in shock. The rationale for selecting a femoral vein catheterization site includes avoidance of pulmonary injury and less chance of major arterial injury leading to hemorrhage. Contraindications to femoral vein access sites are bleeding from pelvic or inferior vena cava wounds and

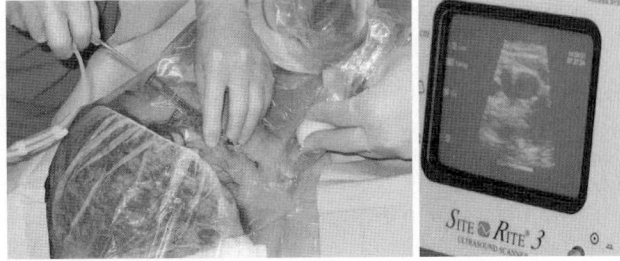

Figure 5-10 Cannulation of a right internal jugular vein guided by an ultrasound image of the position of the distended internal jugular vein in relation to the common carotid artery.

vein thrombosis. Surgeons treating a complex patient with multiple risk factors follow a strategy of first rapidly cannulating the femoral vein for the initial 24 hours and then, when the patient has become stable, inserting a new catheter under optimal sterile technique. Catheter-associated infection with bacteremia can be a life-threatening complication of central venous catheters. To reduce the risk for catheter-related infections, surgeons should insert catheters by following maximal sterile barrier precautions (i.e., wear a mask and cap, sterile gown, and gloves and have a large sterile drape).

Monitoring Central Venous and Pulmonary Artery Catheter Pressure

Central venous pressure monitoring can be useful during the resuscitation of selected patients in shock. The transducer used to measure central venous pressure is zeroed to a point 5 cm posterior to the sternum. Patients in shock with a central venous pressure lower than 5 mm Hg are hypovolemic. Patients in shock with a central venous pressure higher than 20 mm Hg could have a number of problems, including cardiac tamponade, acute pulmonary embolism, or tension pneumothorax. Generally, changes in central venous pressure in response to therapeutic interventions (e.g., infusion of 250 or 500 mL of a crystalloid fluid or a unit of red cells) are more useful to the surgeon treating a patient in shock than a single value is.

Detailed hemodynamic information can be obtained in patients with pulmonary artery catheters. Pulmonary artery catheters are passed from the superior vena cava while the surgeon observes pressures recorded from the port located at the end of the catheter. With the catheter in the superior vena cava, the balloon at the end of the catheter is inflated and the catheter floats through the right atrium (low-pressure atrial contractions), through the right ventricle (higher pressure with ventricular contractions), and across the pulmonic valve into the pulmonary artery (indicated by conversion of end-diastolic pressure from nearly zero to a higher level). Further advancement of the catheter with the balloon inflated results in the catheter being wedged in a pulmonary artery. The recorded pressure tracing flattens as pressure in the occluded vessel equilibrates across the pulmonary microcirculation with mean left atrial pressure.

Pulmonary artery catheters are manufactured with a temperature probe near the tip that enables thermodilution methods to be used for measurement of cardiac output. In addition, pulmonary artery catheters are manufactured to include a fiberoptic bundle to enable continuous assessment of the oxygen saturation of pulmonary artery blood. The range of information provided by pulmonary artery catheters enables surgeons to categorize the hemodynamic pattern in patients with shock and select targeted therapies. Serious complications related to inserting pulmonary artery catheters can occur, including bleeding and pneumothorax associated with insertion of the introducer used for inserting the pulmonary artery catheter in the vena cava, development of arrhythmia when the catheter irritates the myocardium, and perforation of the ventricle wall.

Perhaps the most worrisome complication of pulmonary artery catheters is the selection of needless or even harmful treatments intended to correct an abnormal hemodynamic value measured with the pulmonary artery catheter. The value of information provided to physicians and surgeons from pulmonary artery catheters has been debated. Martin and colleagues reported that pulmonary artery catheters were informative and provided details that influenced treatment decisions.[28] Richard and coworkers concluded that the information provided from the routine use of pulmonary artery catheters is not helpful when physicians select therapy.[29] Transthoracic or transesophageal ultrasound is an alternative diagnostic test that enables surgeons to reliably evaluate cardiac function in detail; in addition, it has the advantage of not requiring the insertion of venous catheters.

Risks associated with central venous catheters are infection and thrombosis. Central venous and pulmonary artery catheters have a 2% to 8% risk of infection. The most common pathogen is *Staphylococcus aureus*. Patients with infected catheters can have bloodstream infections with bacteria or fungi, and septic shock can develop. Interventions and best practices can reduce the risk for catheter-related infections. The Healthcare Infection Control Practices Advisory Committee of the Centers for Disease Control and Prevention has published recommendations for reducing infections, including instructions for optimal insertion techniques, use of chlorhexidine skin cleanser, and insertion of catheters impregnated with antimicrobial agents.[30] Insertion of catheters into central veins can lead to venous thrombosis. Catheters that remain in the femoral vein for several days are more likely to be associated with thrombosis of the vein at the access site than are catheters inserted through the subclavian vein.

HYPOVOLEMIC SHOCK

Hypovolemic shock is a syndrome of reduced cardiac output caused by a reduction in blood volume. As blood volume contracts, less blood returns to the heart, end-diastolic volume in the right and left ventricle declines, and hypotension ensues as cardiac output declines below a critical value. Surgeons routinely encounter hypovole-

mic shock, with hemorrhage being the most frequent specific cause. Hemorrhagic shock commonly has a rapid onset. The severity of hemorrhagic shock can be defined in terms of the proportional deficit of blood volume. Patients whose blood loss exceeds 40% of their blood volume are at imminent risk of death. Hypovolemic shock occurs if there are large shifts of plasma fluid and protein into inflammatory tissues. For example, liters of plasma fluid can shift into the skin and subcutaneous tissues of patients with second-degree burns on greater than 20% of their body surface area. A reduction in intravascular volume is often a contributing factor to hypotension in patients with septic shock. Patients with peritonitis after perforation of a duodenal ulcer accumulate several liters of inflammatory fluid in their peritoneal cavity, much of which has shifted out of the plasma compartment. After inflammatory edema, hypovolemic patients may have a high hematocrit indicative of loss of plasma volume. Substantial loss of gastrointestinal fluid can cause hypovolemic shock. In patients with small bowel obstruction, hypovolemic shock can develop as a result of shift of fluid into the bowel lumen.

A surgeon treating a patient in hypovolemic shock faces two concurrent challenges. First, the surgeon must restore intravascular volume to normal. Second, the surgeon must identify the cause of the patient's hypovolemic shock and decide whether immediate surgical therapy is needed. Hypotension is the hallmark of severe hypovolemic shock; however, hypotension elicits compensatory responses, including stimulation of neuroendocrine reflexes. The compensatory response of an individual in hypovolemic shock parallels the magnitude of the deficit in blood volume. Vasoconstriction is caused by greater sympathetic tone and release of ADH from the pituitary. Consequently, patients may be in hypovolemic shock despite having mean arterial pressure in the normal range. Riddez and associates studied normal adults with controlled hemorrhage of 900 mL of blood.[31] These investigators made serial measurements of blood volume as these subjects restored their blood volume through autotransfusion of fluid and protein from the interstitium to the plasma volume. Based on hematocrit dilution, they estimated that fluid shifts into the plasma compartment compensated for up to 50% of shed blood. Although many studies of animal models in hemorrhagic shock have been performed, the results of these studies have the limitation that in clinical practice, patients in hypovolemic shock are promptly resuscitated. Thus, in these patients the syndrome of hypovolemic shock is often transformed into a complex physiologic condition that reflects the mixed effects of both shock and treatment.

Hemorrhagic Shock

Hemorrhagic shock can be categorized into three grades of severity based on the magnitude of blood loss: compensated shock, uncompensated shock, and lethal exsanguination. Compensated shock syndrome occurs if the blood loss is less than 20% of the blood volume. Patients in compensated shock maintain adequate perfusion of the brain and heart and normal mean arterial pressure because vasoconstriction mediated by neuroendocrine reflexes decreases blood flow to the skin and skeletal muscle. With mild to moderate compensated shock patients can readily survive if they drink liquids. Those in compensated shock who cannot drink water can shift fluid within their ECF compartment. Patients with less than a 20% deficit in blood volume over a period of a few hours can adjust the flow of fluid through the interstitial-lymphatic compartment and achieve net transfer of fluid from the interstitium to the plasma compartment. Patients with uncompensated shock syndrome are hypotensive after acute hemorrhage in which losses are equivalent to 20% to 40% of their blood volume. This magnitude of blood loss in a 70-kg man corresponds to the loss of 1 to 2 L from an estimated blood volume of 5 to 6 L. Patients in uncompensated shock cannot sustain mean aortic pressure by vasoconstriction, have low cardiac output, are subject to anaerobic stress, and have acidemia that is proportional to the severity of their shock insult. Patients in uncompensated shock for hours are at risk for death. Those threatened by exsanguinating hemorrhage rapidly lose more than 40% of their blood volume and profound hypotension develops. With severely reduced blood flow to their brain, these patients become comatose within minutes and die of cardiac arrest.

The concept that hemorrhagic shock has three levels of severity suggests that surgeons treating patients in hemorrhagic shock should escalate the intensity of treatment, depending on the severity of an individual patient's insult. Patient in compensated shock can readily be resuscitated by the IV infusion of balanced electrolyte solutions. After complete resuscitation from compensated hemorrhage, patients dilute their red cells, and the fall in their hematocrit is inversely proportional to the volume of resuscitation fluid required to restore blood volume. Patients in uncompensated shock would be susceptible to lethal anemia after full resuscitation, so these patients need to be transfused with blood to be fully resuscitated. Those with exsanguinating hemorrhage not only need immediate massive transfusion but also frequently require prompt performance of a surgical procedure to control the hemorrhage. Ultimately, a patient's survival after any category of hemorrhagic shock requires that the site or sites of hemorrhage be identified and the bleeding controlled.

Clinical Diagnosis of Hemorrhagic Shock

Surgeons are most effective and successful at treating patients in hemorrhagic shock if the diagnosis is established promptly. Preventable deaths from hemorrhagic shock have occurred because surgeons have failed to recognize that a bleeding patient was in compensated shock. Changes in vital signs are the principal clinical indication that a patient is in hemorrhagic shock. Those in hypovolemic shock are described in textbooks as being hypotensive with an increased heart rate. These physiologic events reflect baroreceptor-mediated increased sympathetic tone and stimulated release of epinephrine. Diaphoresis and skin pallor caused by vasoconstriction of cutaneous arteries are additional indications on physical examination that a patient is in hemorrhagic shock. In severe shock, as blood flow to the brain declines, an ominous indication that the patient is nearing death is the presence of symptoms of cerebral ischemia, including confusion, agitation, and depressed levels of consciousness.

Burri and coworkers reported a correlation between the magnitude of blood loss and systolic blood pressure. Most patients who lost less than 25% of blood volume had systolic pressure greater than 110 mm Hg. Subjects with estimated blood loss of 25% to 33% had systolic pressure approximating 100 mm Hg. When losses exceeded 33% of blood volume, most patients had systolic pressure lower than 100 mm Hg; however, there was considerable variance in this population.[32] Clinical studies of patients in hemorrhagic shock after trauma have determined that the pulse rate is not a sensitive predictor of shock. Tachycardia may develop in hypovolemic patients with increased circulating levels of epinephrine. *Bradycardia,* defined as a heart rate lower than 100 beats per minute, occurs in patients with hypovolemia because they have markedly increased parasympathetic tone and, consequently, a vagally mediated decrease in heart rate. Tachycardia occurs in injured patients without hypovolemia because they are in pain or fear. These opposing neuroendocrine influences on heart rate explain why the pulse rate is neither a sensitive nor a specific indication of the severity of hemorrhagic shock. The vital signs of well-conditioned young adults can be deceptive. These patients may lose more than 30% of their blood with little alteration in their vital signs. They have a precipitous decline in blood pressure with a relatively small further reduction in blood volume when their compensatory mechanisms are exhausted. In contrast, in patients with marginal cardiac function who are treated with vasodilator and β-blocker medications, hypotension may develop after modest hemorrhage.[33] In summary, surgeons establish the diagnosis of hemorrhagic shock in an individual patient by review of a sequence of vital signs, not just a single value, combined with a systematic and through physical examination to look for sites of blood loss.

Acidemia is used as a measure of the severity of hemorrhagic shock. Acidemia develops in patients in hemorrhagic shock primarily because insufficient oxygen is delivered to support aerobic metabolism. A calculated bicarbonate excess from an arterial blood gas sample that is −10 mEq/L or less in a hypovolemic patient is an indication that the patient has uncompensated shock and is at risk for death if resuscitation and corrective therapies are not implemented. Clinical investigators have repeatedly demonstrated that the severity of hemorrhagic shock in injured patients is related to the patient's extent of acidemia, although it is debated whether pH, calculated base excess, or serum lactate is the most informative measure. Patients whose initial base excess was less than −6 mmol/L and, in some respects more important than the initial acid-base status, those whose acidemia did not correct by 24 hours had death rates that exceeded 50%. Surgeons can use either arterial blood gas data or consecutive lactate measures to monitor a patient's recovery from the anaerobic insult of an episode of hemorrhagic shock.

Treatment of Hemorrhagic Shock

Surgeons save the lives of patients in hemorrhagic shock by completion of a series of interventions. After securing reliable IV access, the first attempts at resuscitation of the patient are made with balanced electrolyte solutions. Adult patients who do not respond to 2 to 4 L of balanced electrolyte solution (children are given 20 mL/kg) and remain hypotensive usually require blood transfusions. The surgeon must identify the potential sites of active hemorrhage in an irreversibly hypotensive patient and decide whether a surgical intervention is needed. Promptly performed hemostatic interventions are paramount in the successful treatment of patients in uncompensated hypovolemic shock. For most patients in hemorrhagic shock, resuscitation involves only restoration of blood volume deficits. However, hemorrhagic shock can occur in patients with preexisting cardiac dysfunction. In these patients continuous monitoring of their hemodynamic response enables the surgeon to decide whether resuscitation should be guided by measurement of central venous pressure or, in complex patients, by the spectrum of hemodynamic data available from pulmonary artery catheters. Patients with complex comorbid conditions and hemorrhagic shock may require pharmacologic interventions. Furthermore, continuous monitoring of detailed information in the hours after recovery from hemorrhagic shock is useful in identifying changes in baroreceptor-mediated reflexes in response to hypotension. The vascular tone of patients in hemorrhagic shock increases, and in one study it was noted to transition back to normal in the 4 to 12 hours after an episode of shock reversed by resuscitation.[34] After shock, patients are at risk for additional life-threatening problems. Organ system (cardiac, renal, pulmonary, neurologic) dysfunction and failure can develop after shock. Reasons for this organ failure include delayed or incomplete resuscitation from shock, a reperfusion injury that incites an exaggerated endogenous inflammatory response, or the development of invasive infection. Thus, patient survival after an episode of hemorrhagic shock requires the surgeon to make a series of decisions that include, but are not limited to, rapid resuscitation, timely hemostasis, and postresuscitation support of organ function.

Controversy surrounds the timing of resuscitation in actively hemorrhaging patients. Bickell and associates studied the merits of delayed resuscitation in patients with penetrating torso trauma and shock by comparing a group of patients in whom IV fluid infusions for resuscitation from hemorrhagic shock were started in the emergency department with patients who did not receive fluid infusions until the operation to control hemorrhage had begun.[35] Patients who had delayed resuscitation had superior outcomes. The inferior outcome in patients whose IV fluid infusions were begun on arrival at the emergency department was associated with a higher net positive fluid balance, and the investigators hypothesized that this edema may have contributed to the inferior

survival rates and more complications in this group of early resuscitation patients. Hypotensive resuscitation has been advocated by other clinical investigators, although most caution that any hypotension is best avoided in patients with blunt trauma or brain injury. These studies all demonstrated that attempts to restore blood volume during active hemorrhage from large vessels are futile and possibly detrimental. The surgeon's most effective intervention for a hypotensive patient in hemorrhagic shock is to achieve hemostasis.

Debate continues regarding the composition of the ideal resuscitation fluid to treat patients in hemorrhagic shock. Substantial clinical experience over the past 50 years has established that rapid infusion of isotonic electrolyte solutions can effectively resuscitate a large proportion of patients in hemorrhagic shock. If large volumes of normal saline are used for resuscitation, hyperchloremic acidemia develops as a result of replacement of the bicarbonate in shed blood with chloride. Several clinical trials have demonstrated that infusion of balanced electrolyte solutions (e.g., lactated Ringer's) results in less of a bicarbonate deficit. Massive blood transfusions are often required in patients with severe hemorrhage. Coagulopathy may develop as a complication of massive transfusion, and selected blood components (i.e., coagulation factors, fresh frozen plasma, cryoprecipitate, and platelet concentrates) may be necessary to replenish coagulation factors, as well as restore blood volume. Colloid-containing solutions are advocated as being superior to isotonic saline solutions because more of the infusion is retained in the blood compartment. Schierhout and Roberts reported a systematic review of 26 randomized controlled trials that compared the use of crystalloid with colloid fluid in critically ill patients, including those with hemorrhagic shock.[36] The authors calculated that colloid infusion was associated with a 4% increased risk for death, and they concluded that colloid fluids are not indicted for resuscitation of patients in shock.

A substantial proportion of the patients treated by surgeons for hemorrhagic shock are injured patients. Shock in injured patients is commonly a complex phenomenon that involves more than a reduction in blood volume because of hemorrhage. Substantial hemorrhage can occur acutely in one of five locations: into the chest (identified by chest radiograph), into the peritoneal cavity (identified by abdominal ultrasound, diagnostic peritoneal lavage, or abdominal computed tomography [CT]), associated with a pelvic fracture (suggested by a pelvic radiograph but identified by abdominal-pelvic CT), into long bone fractures (indicated by radiography), and out of the patient's body from wounds. Surgeons evaluating an injured patient in shock need to quickly complete a systematic review of the patient to identify where a hypotensive patient may be experiencing hemorrhage. Other causes of shock in trauma patients include tension hemopneumothorax leading to impaired return of venous blood to the chest, cardiac tamponade, and neurologic shock caused by damage to the spinal cord and loss of sympathetic tone. Although the majority of trauma patients with hypotension need to have their blood volume restored to normal, surgeons treating these patients must remain vigilant and look for other correctable causes of hypotension.

Exsanguinating Shock and Damage Control Surgery

Success in the treatment of patients with exsanguinating hemorrhagic shock hinges on the surgeon's capacity to stop the bleeding. Many of these patients require massive transfusion and are susceptible to the development of coagulopathy and hypothermia. There is convincing evidence from multiple clinical series that a damage control strategy can be lifesaving in patients with severe injury. With such a strategy the surgeon limits interventions during the first operation to those that stop the bleeding and enable the patient to be resuscitated from hemorrhagic shock. In damage control, the surgeon selects a point in the first operation when the basic life-threatening problems have been managed and then decides to stop operating and return the patient to the ICU for resuscitation and correction of body temperature, acidemia, and coagulation disorders. Coagulopathy is common in patients with exsanguinating hemorrhagic shock, and selection of the proper blood product to rapidly correct bleeding disorders is guided by specific tests of coagulation function. The usual blood products used to correct coagulopathy include fresh frozen plasma to reduce the international normalized ratio, cryoprecipitate to restore fibrinogen, and platelet concentrates. Recently, anecdotal reports of synthetic procoagulant factors suggest that there will be a growing role for these drugs derived from recombinant technology.

Events After Resuscitation From Shock

After resuscitation of patients from hemorrhagic shock, restoration of the patient's blood volume to normal may not reestablish the patient's homeostasis. Recovery from an episode of hemorrhagic shock requires time. Typically, as the acidemia and increased sympathetic tone dissipate, there is a period of several hours when patients mount an inflammatory response. Moore and colleagues have provided evidence that after a period of hemorrhagic shock, a patient's immune system is activated, and if the patient is subjected to a second inflammatory insult, such as open reduction and internal fixation of a fracture in a trauma patient or blood transfusion, the activated immune system has an exaggerated response.[26] Transfusion of red cells and other blood products is a common treatment required to resuscitate patients in hemorrhagic shock. There is debate regarding the hematocrit threshold that surgeons should use as a guideline for transfusion. Authors have advocated in manuscripts published over the past 40 years that patients be transfused after hemorrhagic shock with the goal of keeping the blood hemoglobin level above 10 g/dL. This concept has been superseded in recent years, and several authorities advocate that the optimal transfusion trigger is a hemoglobin level between 6 and 7 g/dL. The rationale for lower transfusion thresholds has been supported by recent studies suggesting that transfusion of blood has adverse immunologic consequences.

In a sequence of manuscripts on a large population of patients treated for hemorrhagic shock, Lucas and Ledgerwood proposed that the optimal events after resuscitation from shock should correspond to three phases.[37] Phase I starts at the time of the patient's arrival in the emergency department. It ends when the operation or procedure needed to control the bleeding is complete. During phase I, patients are typically receiving fluid and blood to replace losses from hemorrhage, and there may be a contraction in the interstitial volume as fluids shift to compensate for shock. Phase II starts at the end of surgery and is characterized as a period in which more fluid needs to be infused than is lost. During phase II patients were infused with primarily balanced electrolyte solutions to maintain perfusion pressure. Typically, during phase II urine output is low, and patients gain weight. Patients may retain fluid during phase II equivalent to as much as 10% of their ideal body weight. Using tracer distribution methods, Lucas and Ledgerwood have determined that during phase II the majority of this excess fluid is located in the interstitial lymphatic compartment of ECF. The final phase corresponds to recovery. During phase III of the Lucas and Ledgerwood model of postresuscitation events, the investigators observed that patients who were recovering from their injuries usually had diuresis in which the excess fluid gained during phase II was excreted as urine. The diuresis is usually spontaneous. However, in patients with preexisting heart failure, the diuresis of phase III may need to be stimulated with a diuretic such as furosemide. In their detailed study of a large group of patients who recovered from hemorrhagic shock, Lucas and Ledgerwood demonstrated that those who remain in shock after the initial isotonic saline infusion are likely to have ongoing hemorrhage. These patients will require a therapeutic procedure that stops the bleeding, as well as transfusion of blood; management of blood transfusion and coagulopathy is discussed in detail in another chapter of this text.

Abdominal Compartment Syndrome

In patients who receive large volumes of fluid during resuscitation from hemorrhagic shock, abdominal compartment syndrome (ACS) may develop.[38] Patients with ACS have an excessive volume of water within their abdomen, typically interstitial fluid in the bowel wall, mesentery, and omentum, but also ascites or distended loops of bowel. The problem with ACS is that tight pressure within the abdominal cavity leads to organ dysfunction. As abdominal compartment pressure increases, blood flow to viscera within the peritoneal cavity declines. Reasons why ACS develops include a sudden accumulation of ascites, excessive bowel edema, bleeding into the peritoneal cavity or retroperitoneum, and gaseous distention of bowel. Secondary ACS can develop in patients with injury or infection outside the abdomen after massive infusions of fluid for resuscitation. Indications that ACS has developed are low urine output, a tense and hard abdomen, or the development of respiratory distress in a spontaneously ventilating patient or an increase in peak airway pressure in a mechanically ventilated patient. ACS is confirmed by measuring pressure within the bladder as a proxy for abdominal pressure. Abdominal pressure can be conveniently determined at the bedside by

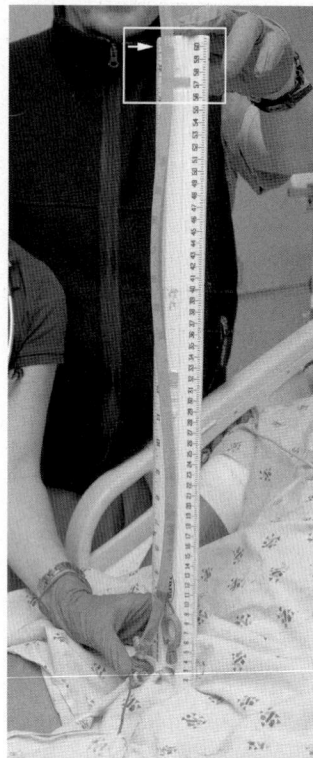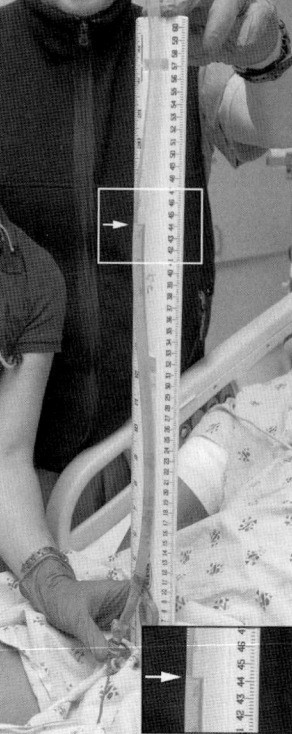

Initial   At equilibrium

Figure 5-11 Measuring the height of a column of urine above the pubic symphysis is a direct and reliable method of determining whether a patient has elevated bladder pressure consistent with abdominal compartment syndrome. In the image on the *left*, the urinary catheter tube filled with urine is initially held up next to the ruler resting on the patient's pubic symphysis. In the image on the *right*, the meniscus of urine has stabilized at the height at which the meniscus fluctuates with ventilation. Patients with a urine column height of less than 20 cm do not have abdominal compartment syndrome. Patients with a urine column height between 20 and 30 cm are at risk. Those with a urine column height higher than 30 cm are at high risk, and most patients with a urine column height higher than 40 cm need an intervention to reduce their abdominal compartment pressure.

---

measuring the height of a urine column above the pubic symphysis (Fig. 5-11). Patients with ACS require decompression. A patient's risk for the development of ACS after laparotomy can often be anticipated by the extent of visceral edema and increase in end-inspiratory pressure when an attempt is made to close the abdomen. In these high-risk patients the surgeon should avoid ACS by selecting a tension-free method of closing the abdomen.

SEPTIC SHOCK

Shock associated with the sepsis syndrome is a common cause of death in surgical ICUs. In 2001 an estimated 700,000 patients with sepsis were hospitalized, 210,000 of whom died. Sepsis is a particularly challenging problem in older patients, and as the proportion of the older

---

> ### Box 5-3 Criteria for Four Categories of the Systemic Inflammatory Response Syndrome
>
> #### Systemic Inflammatory Response Syndrome (SIRS)
>
> Two or more of the following:
>
> - Temperature (core) >38°C or <36°C
> - Heart rate >90 beats/min
> - Respiratory rate of >20 breaths/min for patients spontaneously ventilating or a $PaCO_2$ <32 mm Hg
> - White blood cell count >12,000 cells/mm^3 or <4000 cells/mm^3 or >10% immature (band) cells in the peripheral blood smear
>
> #### Sepsis
>
> Same criteria as for SIRS but with a clearly established focus of infection
>
> #### Severe Sepsis
>
> Sepsis associated with organ dysfunction and hypoperfusion
>
> Indicators of hypoperfusion:
>
> - Systolic blood pressure <90 mm Hg
> - >40 mm Hg fall from normal systolic blood pressure
> - Lacticacidemia
> - Oliguria
> - Acute mental status changes
>
> #### Septic Shock
>
> Patients with severe sepsis who
>
> - Are not responsive to intravenous fluid infusion for resuscitation
> - Require inotropic or vasopressor agents to maintain systolic blood pressure

population in the United States gets larger, it is reasonable for surgeons to expect that they will be treating more patients with shock caused by sepsis. A surgeon treating a patient with shock and infection must manage several issues. First, the surgeon orders the infusion of fluids and, if necessary, infusion of the appropriate vasoactive drugs to resuscitate the patient from shock. Second, the surgeon selects an antimicrobial agent that kills the bacteria causing the infection. Third, the surgeon considers whether the patient needs a surgical intervention to control the focus of sepsis. Finally, the surgeon orders additional medications consistent with evidence-based guidelines for the treatment of patients with life-threatening sepsis.

Humans respond to invasive infection with an immune response that involves multiple mediators. These mediators enable the patient's inflammatory processes to destroy the organisms at the site of infection. These same mediators can damage the individual's organs if they produce an exaggerated systemic inflammatory response syndrome (SIRS). In 1992, Bone and colleagues convened a consensus conference on the problem of organ damage caused by exaggerated activation of the endogenous inflammatory response (Box 5-3).[39] They defined four sepsis-related clinical syndromes. These four syndromes were defined in pathophysiologic terms as a hierarchy corresponding to four steps of increasingly exaggerated inflammatory responses. The first category of SIRS is caused by mediators released from lymphocytes, macrophages, granulocytes, and vascular endothelial cells. These activated immune cells release cytokines, enzymes, and oxygen radicals that are beneficial because they can destroy invading microorganisms. These immune mediators also initiate coagulation cascades, amplify the release of additional cytokines and vasoactive agents, and increase capillary membrane permeability. Patients with SIRS have fever, tachycardia, and tachypnea. SIRS occurs in patients with and without confirmed culture-positive infection. For example, SIRS can develop in response to the sterile insults of pancreatitis, aspiration pneumonia, and burn injury. To meet the criteria for SIRS, patients must have two or more of the clinical conditions identified in the consensus conference and subsequently validated in clinical studies. Patients are categorized as having the second level of the systemic inflammatory response, sepsis, if they meet the criteria for SIRS and have a confirmed focus of infection. Although in most cases of sepsis the invading organisms are bacteria, sepsis can also occur in patients with infections caused by fungal, viral, and parasitic pathogens. Patients meet the criteria for severe sepsis, the third level of systemic response, if they have established infection and hypotension develops. Patients with severe sepsis may have evidence of organ dysfunction, including lacticacidemia, oliguria, and a depressed level of consciousness. Surgeons treat the hypotension of patients with severe sepsis by the IV infusion of a balanced electrolyte solution. Patients with severe sepsis who respond to resuscitation fluids have an increase in blood pressure that is associated with a corresponding improvement in organ function. Septic shock is the fourth level and the most severe category of SIRS. Patients meet the criteria for septic shock if they have severe sepsis and remain hypotensive despite IV infusion of fluids. Patients in septic shock need an IV infusion of vasoactive drugs to restore perfusion pressure. The organ dysfunction in patients in septic shock may progress to organ failure.[40] Patients with SIRS have a life-threatening problem. The risk for death in patients with sepsis is 16%. The risk for death in patients with severe sepsis or septic shock is 20% and greater than 46%, respectively (Table 5-6). Among patients who met the criteria for SIRS, within 1 month 55% had progressed and met the criteria for sepsis, severe sepsis developed in 35% of patients with SIRS, and septic shock developed in 15% with severe sepsis. Surgeons treating patients with serious infection must typically base selection of antibiotic therapy on clinical patterns and before culture and sensitivity results are available. Identifying the pattern of infection in a patient can assist in the empirical selection of antibiotics. The four most prevalent sites of infection in ICU patients with serious infection are, in order of prevalence, pulmonary, bloodstream, genitourinary tract, and intra-abdominal wounds, and these sites should be routinely cultured before the administration of antibiotics. In patients with sepsis or severe sepsis, blood cultures were positive in 17% of patients with sepsis, in 25% of patients with severe sepsis, and in

Table 5-6 Categories of Systemic Inflammatory Response Syndrome Among 857 Patients Treated in Surgical Intensive Care Settings

	CULTURE POSITIVE*	CULTURE NEGATIVE*	DEATH RATE (%)†
Sepsis	305	165	16-10
Severe sepsis	260	130	20-16
Septic shock	40	22	46

*Indicates incidence density as episodes per 1000 patient-days.
†Death rates for culture-positive and culture-negative subgroups.
Adapted from Rangel-Frausto MS, Pitter D, Costigan M, et al: The natural history of the systemic inflammatory response syndrome. JAMA 273:117, 1995.

69% of patients with septic shock. In a cohort of patients with severe sepsis and septic shock who also had positive blood cultures, 44% of the cohort had gram-positive species, 44% had gram-negative species, 3% had fungemia (only *Candida* species), and the remaining 9% of patients had a mixed species of infecting organisms on culture. The top three gram-positive organisms included *S. aureus, Enterococcus* species, and coagulase-negative *Staphylococcus* species. The three most prevalent gram-negative species were *Escherichia coli, Klebsiella* species, and *Pseudomonas aeruginosa*. Organisms likely to be cultured from infected patients in a specific ICU are largely determined by the bacterial and fungal species endemic in that unit. Surgeons treating a patient with severe sepsis and septic shock should initially order broad-spectrum antibiotics that have a high likelihood of being effective. Empirical antifungal therapy should be included in immunosuppressed patients who have received previous courses of antibiotics. The antibiotic therapy should be adjusted once the results of culture reveal the specific characteristics of the infecting organism.

Treatment of Hypotension in Severe Sepsis and Septic Shock

The pathophysiology of shock in sepsis is multidimensional and complex because of the interaction of multiple physiologic and inflammatory events (Fig. 5-12). The majority of patients with severe sepsis or septic shock have hypotension associated with arterial vasodilation.[40] A minority of patients in septic shock are hypovolemic as a result of inflammatory edema or fluid loss and have a hemodynamic pattern of marked vasoconstriction and low-flow shock (Table 5-7). Typically, patients in vasodilatory septic shock have cardiac output twofold or greater than normal associated with a mean arterial pressure less than 65 mm Hg. The reduction in SVR in these patients is attributed to vasodilation in organs with high capillary density, such as skin and skeletal muscle. Experimental evidence indicates that excessive production of nitric oxide, a potent vasodilator, is a primary mechanism for the pattern of low SVR in patients with septic shock. Because of the induction of a potent enzyme system, patients with severe sepsis and septic shock produce large amounts of nitric oxide, and elevated

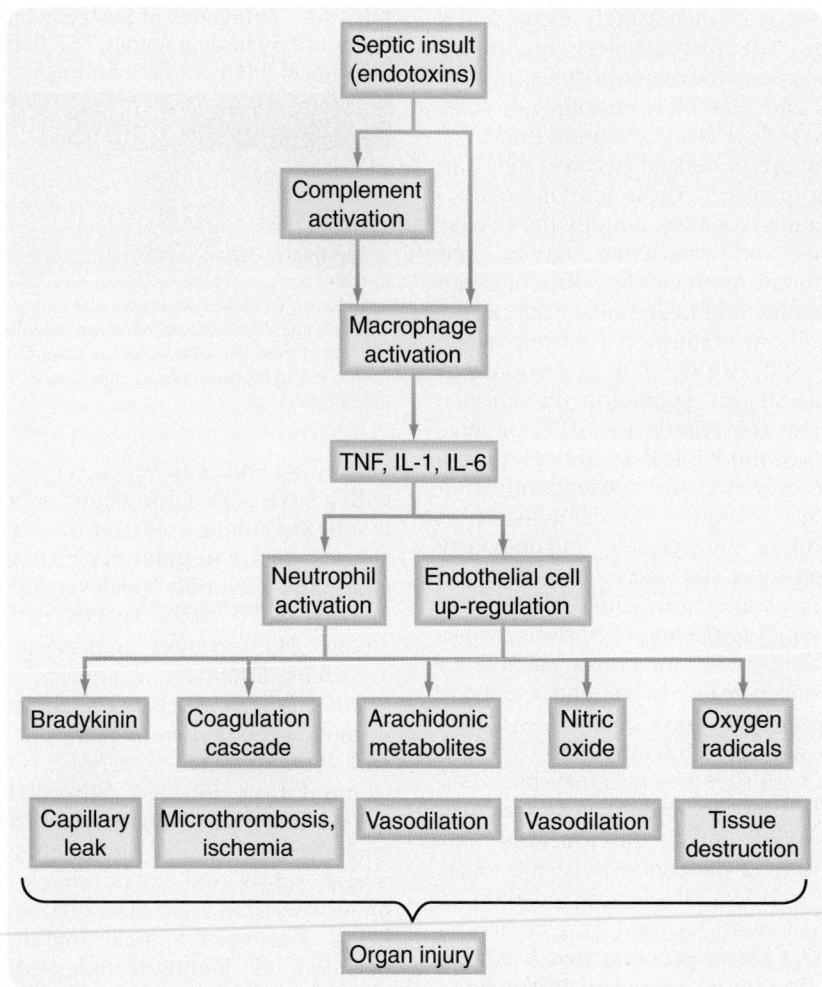

Figure 5-12 Septic shock–mediated inflammatory cascade. IL-1, interleukin-1; TNF, tumor necrosis factor.

Table 5-7 Hemodynamic Characteristics of Patients in Septic Shock*

CHARACTERISTIC	MEAN	MINIMUM	MAXIMUM
Heart rate (beats/min)	121	47	142
MAP (mm Hg)	60	48	66
PCWP (mm Hg)	14	8	20
CI (L/min/m²)	4.2	3.0	5.6
SVRI (dynes/cm⁵/sec/m²)	868	675	1110
O₂ delivery (mL/min/m²)	498	344	573
O₂ consumption (mL/min/m²)	141	101	183

*Average of mean values reported in 11 manuscripts describing findings in patients with severe sepsis or septic shock.

CI, cardiac index; MAP, mean arterial pressure; O₂ consumption, cardiac index multiplied by arterial oxygen content minus venous oxygen content; O₂ delivery, cardiac index multiplied by arterial oxygen content; PCWP, pulmonary capillary wedge pressure; SVRI, systemic vascular resistance index calculated as mean systemic arterial pressure minus right atrial pressure divided by cardiac index.

concentrations of nitric oxide generated near vascular smooth muscle overwhelm the vasoconstrictive effects of the endogenous vasoconstricting hormones (α-adrenergic catecholamine, angiotensin II, and vasopressin). Nitric oxide is a potent, but evanescent vasodilator. In clinical trials, treatment of patients in vasodilatory shock with inhibitors of nitric oxide synthesis did not improve their outcome.[40] Further research is needed to identify treatments that effectively modify the adverse influence of nitric oxide in septic shock.

Persistently and profoundly hypotensive septic patients who meet the criteria for severe sepsis or septic shock are first resuscitated by the IV infusion of isotonic crystalloid fluids to expand their intravascular volume. Surgeon's choices for the volume of infused fluid and vasoactive drugs are guided by invasive hemodynamic monitoring, including pulmonary artery catheters. IV fluid infusions are given until pulmonary artery wedge pressure stabilizes between 15 and 20 mm Hg. Patients in septic shock should be transfused with red cells if their hemoglobin drops below 7 g/dL. Septic shock patients infused with

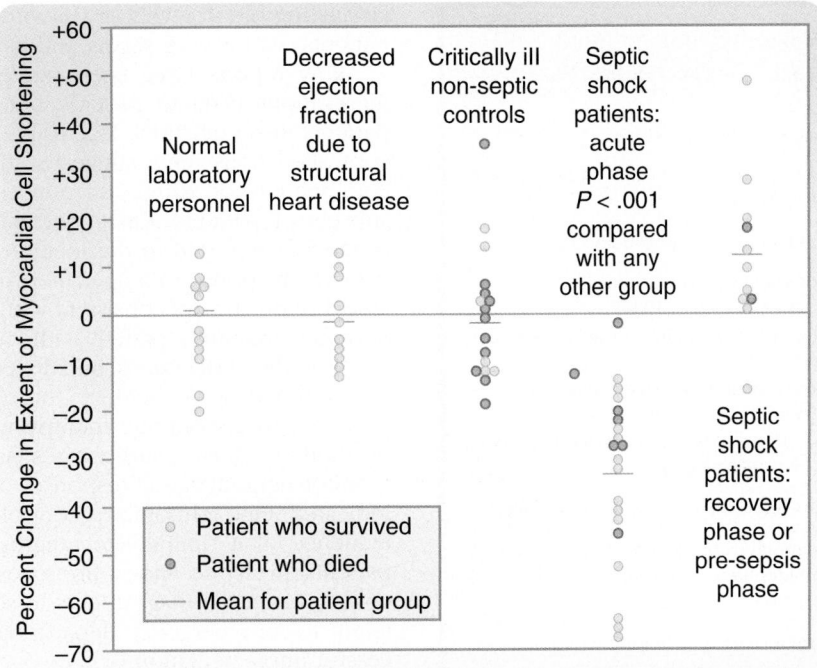

Figure 5-13 Suppression of myocardial cell function specifically by the serum of patients in septic shock. (From Parrillo JE, Burch C, Shelhamer JH, et al: A circulating myocardial depressant substance in humans with septic shock: Septic shock patients with a reduced ejection fraction have a circulating factor that depresses in vitro myocardial cell performance. J Clin Invest 76:1539-1553, 1985. Copyright 1985, Journal of Clinical Investigation. Reproduced with permission in the format Textbook via Copyright Clearance Center.)

balanced electrolyte solutions may require large volumes. Patients in septic shock are thought to have increased microvascular membrane permeability and need crystalloid fluid infusions equal in volume to 10% of their body weight to restore central venous pressure. Choi and coauthors reported that in a detailed review of the literature on the topic of colloid versus crystalloid resuscitation, there was no difference in outcome.[41] Patients with severe sepsis and septic shock have impaired cardiac function. Parrillo and colleagues identified dilated dysfunctional right and left ventricles in patients with septic shock (Fig. 5-13). Patients in septic shock who have received adequate intravascular volume expansion and who remain hypotensive are treated by the infusion of two categories of vasoactive agents: inotropic drugs and vasoconstrictors. Dopamine, norepinephrine, and epinephrine are three drugs given to patients in septic shock as inotropic agents. Increases in mean arterial pressure, cardiac stroke work index, or cardiac index are indicators that these drugs have had a favorable influence on cardiac contractility. Tachycardia is a common complication of the infusion of inotropic agents in patients with septic shock. Infusion of vasoconstrictor drugs in patients with septic shock has been reported to be an effective method for improving mean arterial pressure. Surgeons infusing vasoconstrictor drugs to treat septic shock can monitor the calculated SVR as a measure of the patient's response. Vasoconstrictors are infused to achieve an SVR index that exceeds 500 dynes/cm⁵/sec/m². To induce α-adrenergic–mediated vasoconstriction, norepinephrine and phenyl-

ephrine are infused. In patients who remain vasodilated despite the infusion of α-adrenergic agents, clinical observations have been published that vasopressin can increase SVR and restore perfusion pressure in those with refractory vasodilatory septic shock. Although vasoconstrictor agents can increase mean arterial pressure, surgeons treating patients with these drugs continuously monitor the patients because as a source of infection comes under control and the level of inflammatory mediators in blood decreases, the need for vasoconstriction declines. Patients in septic shock can sustain serious damage to organs (kidney, liver, skin, and skeletal muscle) while being treated with vasoconstrictive agents. Surgeons should look for evidence of improved perfusion in a patient being treated for septic shock, such as resolution of acidemia and improved urine flow, because evidence that shock is resolving provides an opportunity to wean the patient off the vasoconstrictor drugs.

Multiple clinical studies published in the medical literature have reported that a specific vasoactive drug, or combination of vasoactive drugs, provides a superior outcome in patients with septic shock.[40] Norepinephrine has repeatedly been reported as being effective in increasing the blood pressure of patients in septic shock. Infusion of norepinephrine has been noted in clinical trials to cause primarily an α-adrenergic–mediated vasoconstrictor effect that increases SVR. Norepinephrine infusion induces vasoconstriction in skin and skeletal muscle, which increases mean aortic pressure and consequently improves perfusion of the renal, cerebral, and cardiac

---

Box 5-4 Protocol for Resuscitation of Adult Hypotensive Patients With Suspected Sepsis

Culture relevant body fluids, including blood.

Infuse a balanced electrolyte solution of 500 mL/15 min. Monitor the systolic blood pressure response.

Insert a central venous or pulmonary artery catheter.

- If after a 500-mL bolus of saline the patient remains hypotensive and CVP is <8-12 mm Hg or PAWP is <8-12 mm Hg, infuse another 500-mL bolus of fluid; repeat as needed.
- If CVP is >15 or PAWP is 15-20 and the patient remains hypotensive (<65 mm Hg), start an infusion of the inotrope dobutamine or dopamine. The goal is a mean systemic pressure >65 mm Hg and a pulse rate <120 beats/min.

Determine the cardiac index and systemic vascular resistance.

- If after infusion of fluid and inotropes SVR is <600, infuse a vasopressor—either norepinephrine or vasopressin—to increase SVR.

Monitor mixed venous oxygen saturation and urine output as an indication that therapeutic interventions have improved perfusion.

CVP, central venous pressure; PAWP, pulmonary artery wedge pressure; SVR, systemic vascular resistance.

---

circulations. Some studies have suggested superior outcomes when norepinephrine is combined with an inotrope such as dopamine or dobutamine. An alternative to norepinephrine reported to be successful in increasing SVR in patients with septic shock has been phenylephrine, which has only an α-adrenergic effect. Epinephrine, usually infused in doses of 1 to 20 μg/min, acts as a powerful α- and β-adrenergic agonist. Patients in septic shock who were infused with epinephrine experienced improvements in hemodynamic status as a result of both increased inotropic activity and vasoconstriction (see Table 5-5). Dopamine is an effective inotropic agent in selected patients, and Levy and colleagues suggested that failure to respond to dopamine is a valuable means of identifying the subset of septic shock patients at very high risk for death.[42] One established guideline regarding the use of vasoactive drugs in patients with septic shock has been based on the results of several clinical trials designed to determine whether infusion of low doses of dopamine reduces the risk for renal failure. These studies have been negative, and current evidence-based guidelines state that low-dose dopamine infusion should not be used as a renal-sparing drug.[40] A minority of patients with septic shock have minimal or no vasoconstrictor response to α-adrenergic agents. Vasopressin has been demonstrated to be an alternative vasoconstrictor agent in these patients with refractory shock. Vasopressin causes vascular smooth muscle to contract by attaching to V1 receptors on the surface of smooth muscle cells. This mechanism is separate from the α-adrenergic–mediated effect and is one reason that vasopressin can achieve an increase in SVR. Several clinical trials have suggested that

circulating blood levels of vasopressin are suppressed in patients with severe sepsis and septic shock.

Many reports have been published on the range of medications used to provide hemodynamic support to patients in septic shock (see Table 5-5), and randomized controlled trials have suggested that a specific drug or combination of drugs is more effective in particular subsets of patients. One conclusion from the multiple drug trials reported in the literature is that an individual patient's response to a specific drug is generally predictable, but not always consistent with the average response. Surgeons treating a patient with vasoactive drugs should monitor the individual's initial hemodynamic response, adjust the dose to achieve the desired effect, and be prepared to discontinue therapy with one drug in favor of another. Thus, a surgeon resuscitating a patient must monitor hemodynamic responses and adjust therapies as indicated. One randomized controlled trial has published evidence that immediate aggressive resuscitation of patients in septic shock improves survival. Rivers and colleagues noted that patients in septic shock who were taken to an emergency department benefited from successful implementation of a protocol intended to rapidly achieve a balance of oxygen delivery and demand.[43] Patients in the protocol were resuscitated within 6 hours of arrival in the emergency department and compared with those whose resuscitation began when admitted to the ICU. The death rate for protocol patients was 30%, less than 45% in the control group. Patients in shock from sepsis who were resuscitated according to an efficient protocol were protected from a prolonged insult and avoided irreversible cellular damage. Guiding principles in the resuscitation of any patient in septic shock must include adjustment of fluid infusions, selection of vasoactive drugs, and modulation of drug doses based on the individual patient's response (Box 5-4). Thus, invasive hemodynamic monitoring is essential in complex patients to determine the effectiveness of interventions intended to restore delivery of oxygen to tissues. As a final consideration in the treatment of any patient in septic shock, resuscitation is often futile without effective treatment of the source of the sepsis. A patient's survival from an episode of sepsis often hinges on prompt and effective performance of a surgical procedure.

Immunomodulating and Anti-inflammatory Treatment of Severe Sepsis and Septic Shock

Considerable clinical research effort has been expended to determine whether the high risk for death in patients with severe sepsis and septic shock can be reduced by the administration of anti-inflammatory agents. The hypothesis of these studies was that because SIRS started as part of an exaggerated immune response to infection, patients who were at risk for organ injury could be spared by treatment with an anti-inflammatory agent. The majority of studies found no clear benefit in terms of survival. Deans and colleagues reported a review of 27 randomized controlled trials in which mediator-specific anti-inflammatory therapies were evaluated.[44] Among individual studies or even groups of studies examining similar drugs, these therapies did not show efficacy. However, in a meta-analysis applied to a composite of all 27 studies, a small significant improvement in survival was detected. In more detailed analyses of subsets of patients, Deans and colleagues observed that benefits from targeted anti-inflammatory agents appear to occur only in septic shock patients with a high risk for death. Patients enrolled in these anti-inflammatory mediator studies who had a low risk for death either did not benefit or perhaps were harmed by treatment with these drugs. Investigators have always expressed concern that a risk associated with anti-inflammatory drugs might be suppression of the capacity to eliminate the infection. Although no evidence from any of the multiple trials of anti-inflammatory agents has shown that treating patients with a specific anti-inflammatory agent is effective in reducing the risk for death and complication, it is reasonable to anticipate that further research will identify specific subsets of septic shock patients who will benefit from targeted therapy.

One anticoagulant therapy has been demonstrated to be effective in patients with septic shock.[44] The association between activation of the coagulation cascades in patients with severe sepsis and septic shock and autopsy evidence of diffuse microthrombi led investigators to hypothesize that anticoagulant agents might improve the outcome of these high-risk patients. Although several anticoagulant drugs have been evaluated in large randomized controlled trials, it was the administration of drotrecogin alfa (activated) (activated protein C) that improved patients' hospital survival rates. The patients with the greatest dysfunction at the time of treatment with activated protein C were the group most likely to benefit from this new and expensive form of therapy. Subsets of septic patients who benefited were those with a high risk for death. Two additional observations have been made regarding activated protein C. First, patients being treated with heparin at initiation of therapy did not have a reduction in the risk for death. Second, in long-term follow-up survival analyses, at 1 year the risk for death was increased in patients treated with activated protein C if their risk for death when they entered the study was less than 25% based on an Acute Physiology, Age, and Chronic Health Evaluation (APACHE) score. As clinical experience with activated protein C has increased, the risk for serious bleeding as a complication has been noted, as well as a suggestion that early (within 24 hours) treatment is beneficial. In a repetition of the conclusion regarding anti-inflammatory therapy, more research is needed to identify the subset of patients who will benefit from therapies intended to neutralize the procoagulant events induced by sepsis.[44]

Randomized controlled trials have demonstrated that patients in septic shock have improved survival if they are given glucocorticoids in physiologic doses. Evidence indicates that a subset of patients in septic shock have an impaired adrenal response to increased adrenocorticotropic hormone (ACTH) and thus have sepsis-associated adrenal insufficiency. In several trials, IV cortisol at a dose of 100 mg every 8 to 12 hours tapered over 5 to 11 days benefited these patients because this dose compensates for the low plasma cortisol levels caused by sepsis-induced suppression of adrenal cortical function. Patients had the dose of cortisol tapered over the course of treatment. There is debate whether cortisol replacement therapy in patients with vasopressor-dependent septic shock should be guided by patients' response to a corticotropin stimulation test. Advocates of the 250-μg corticotropin stimulation test report that patients who are nonresponders, defined as an increase in serum cortisol of less than 9 μg/dL, should receive the full course of glucocorticoids whereas responders who do achieve a greater than 9 μg/dL increase in cortisol do not need to be supplemented. Current guidelines regarding treatment of patients with vasopressor-dependent septic shock indicate that patients should be given supplemental glucocorticoids independent of their response to the corticotropin stimulation test.[44] Additional benefit is achieved in many patients by adding a mineralocorticoid, enteral fludrocortisone at a dose of 50 μg/day for 7 days, to the IV supplemental hydrocortisone. Patients with severe sepsis, and not septic shock, should not receive hydrocortisone based on current published data.

In a group of critically ill patients, Van den Berghe and associates demonstrated that a protocol of infusing insulin via IV to keep blood glucose levels tightly controlled between 80 and 110 mg/dL had several benefits.[45] The tightly control group of patients were compared with those who received insulin only when blood glucose exceeded 215 mg/dL. Benefits in the tightly controlled group included less organ dysfunction, a reduced prevalence of the onset of serious infection, and improved survival. One benefit from the infusion of insulin may be that more glucose gains access to the cytosol and supports cell function.

CARDIOGENIC SHOCK

Cardiogenic shock is failure of the cardiac ventricles to pump blood at a flow rate sufficient to maintain body perfusion pressure. The most common cause of cardiogenic shock is occlusion of a coronary artery in which a plaque in the coronary artery ruptures, combined with the formation of an intraluminal thrombus. Impaired cardiac muscle contractility secondary to ischemia is followed within hours by infarction of myocardial muscle. Cardiogenic shock develops in 7% to 10% of patients with acute myocardial infarction caused by coronary artery occlusion. Cardiogenic shock is lethal. Published series of patients with cardiogenic shock report death rates of between 40% and 70%. Six hours is the average interval between onset of the signs and symptoms of myocardial infarction and the development of cardiogenic shock. Hemodynamic patterns in patients with cardiogenic shock are a lowest mean systolic pressure of 88 mm Hg, mean pulse rate of 102 beats/min, mean pulmonary capillary wedge pressure of 24 mm Hg, a mean cardiac index of 1.75 L/min/m^2, and a mean ejection fraction of 31% (Table 5-8). The key to improving survival of patients in cardiogenic shock is to promptly reestablish blood flow at the site of the coronary artery occlusion.[46]

Table 5-8 Hemodynamic Characteristics of Patients in Cardiogenic Shock

Anterior myocardial infarction	60.5%
Median time from myocardial infarction to shock	5.6 hr
Lowest systolic blood pressure	88 mm Hg
Lowest diastolic blood pressure	54 mm Hg
Heart rate	102 beats/min
Pulmonary capillary wedge pressure	24 mm Hg
Cardiac index	1.75 L/min/m²
Left ventricular ejection fraction	31%
Number of diseased coronary vessels	
1	13%
2	23%
3	64%
Left main coronary artery disease	20%

Adapted from Hochman JS, Webb JG, et al: Early revascularization in acute myocardial infarction complicated by cardiogenic shock. SHOCK Investigators. Should we emergently revascularize occluded coronaries for cardiogenic shock? N Engl J Med 341:625-634, 1999.

Surgeons can suspect an acute coronary artery syndrome in patients who complain of a chest pain syndrome consistent with angina pectoris. On electrocardiography, ST segment elevation, a new onset of left bundle branch block, or the development of Q waves indicates that a myocardial infarction is imminent and interventions are required immediately. Suspecting an acute coronary thrombosis can be difficult in surgical patients who are intubated and anesthetized in the operating room or heavily sedated in an ICU. The first indication of myocardial ischemia may be the onset of hypotension or an arrhythmia. Protocols have been established for the treatment of patients with acute myocardial infarction. Patients should be given aspirin and a β-blocker and immediately receive an IV dose of a plasminogen activator. Alternatively, within 1 hour patients with acute myocardial infarction should undergo diagnostic catheterization of their coronary arteries, which could be extended to include balloon angioplasty with deployment of stents across areas of coronary stenosis. Depending on the number and location of coronary artery occlusions, selected patients are best managed by emergency coronary artery bypass surgery. These three definitive treatments of acute myocardial infarction—fibrinolysis, deployment of coronary artery stents, and surgery—are all effective therapy for preserving myocardium and preventing cardiogenic shock, but all have the associated risk of bleeding. Fibrinolytic therapy is contraindicated for at least 4 weeks after most surgical procedures. The risk associated with heparin or antiplatelet therapy in patients with acute injury or a surgical wound has not been determined in a manner that stratifies for the type and age of the wound. Clearly, the risk of anticoagulant therapy in patients with recent wounds is influenced by the location and the consequences of bleeding in the wound. When managing patients with an uncomplicated acute myocardial infarction, surgeons and cardiologists need to balance the risks and benefits of interventions to restore coronary perfusion.

On clinical examination, patients with acute myocardial infarction in whom cardiogenic shock develops have dyspnea and signs and symptoms of pulmonary edema. These patients have distended neck veins, a weakly palpable pulse, and a clamped down appearance in the cutaneous circulation of the fingers and toes. Patients in profound cardiogenic shock have a cyanotic face, are diaphoretic, have a decreased level of consciousness, and look desperately ill. Cardiologists depend on echocardiography to determine the extent of cardiac dysfunction in patients with an acute myocardial infarction. In patients with cardiogenic shock, echocardiography can not only identify poorly contracting ventricular wall motion but also determine the cardiac segments involved, which implies the coronary vessel that has occluded. An additional advantage of echocardiography is that other processes contributing to shock can be identified, including mitral regurgitation caused by tears in the chordae tendineae and rupture of the myocardial septum or ventricular wall producing cardiac tamponade. An elevation in the serum concentration of troponin, a protein released from damaged myocardial cells, is diagnostic of acute myocardial infarction. However, troponin levels have the disadvantage that there can be a delay of hours between myocardial ischemia and an increase in troponin levels. Cardiogenic shock can develop in patients with a cardiac arrhythmia, and prompt conversion of the patient to normal sinus rhythm can correct the shock.

Patients in cardiogenic shock need a prompt diagnostic workup to determine an effective therapy. IV fluid is infused to expand blood volume and optimize end-diastolic filling pressure in the impaired ventricle. Infusion of inotropic agents and other vasoactive drugs may be necessary but is done under guidance of the detailed hemodynamic information provided by the pulmonary artery catheter. The problem with inotropic drugs is that an increase in cardiac performance is associated with increased oxygen consumption by a heart already made ischemic. An intra-aortic balloon pump can sustain perfusion to vital organs in patients with cardiogenic shock and saves lives. It can support the patient while therapeutic interventions to restore coronary blood flow are being performed.[46]

In the large randomized controlled SHOCK trial, investigators determined that patients with cardiogenic shock after acute myocardial infarction benefited if within 6 hours of the onset of shock they underwent an intervention that restored coronary blood flow, as opposed to medical stabilization and delayed intervention.[47] Two interventions used to restore coronary blood flow were immediate coronary artery bypass surgery and immediate percutaneous coronary interventions that included transluminal angioplasty and deployment of endoluminal stents to prevent reocclusion of the coronary artery. Optimal management of a patient in cardiogenic shock requires coordinated decision making between the surgeon, whose goal is to avoid the development of a bleeding complication, and cardiology and cardiac surgery providers, whose goal is to achieve immediate reperfusion of hibernating myocardium to successfully restore ventricular contractile function.

Shock Caused by Cardiac Contusion

Injury to the heart caused by a blow to the anterior aspect of the chest that transmits substantial energy to the myocardium can cause myocardial hemorrhage and tissue edema. Cardiac contusion may be a common cause of immediate death in patients who sustain chest trauma in such high-energy circumstances as a motor vehicle crash. However, cardiac contusion is rarely the cause of shock in a blunt trauma patient who is hypotensive on arrival at an emergency department. Although several blood tests have been advocated for making the diagnosis of acute cardiac contusion, cardiac echocardiography is the most specific. Hypotensive patients who sustained chest trauma and have, by echocardiography, a dilated ventricular chamber associated with poor contractility of the wall have either a ventricular contusion or proximal main coronary artery occlusion and acute myocardial infarction in association with their injury. Infusion of dobutamine, epinephrine, or dopamine may improve myocardial contraction in a patient with cardiac contusion and profound pump dysfunction. An intra-aortic balloon pump may provide temporary support while the contused cardiac muscle recovers.

Shock Caused by Cardiac Tamponade

Cardiac tamponade occurs when fluid or blood accumulates between the pericardium and heart and the fluid compresses the ventricles during the diastolic filling phase of the cardiac cycle and causes impaired ejection of blood and inadequate aortic perfusion pressure. Cardiac tamponade can be divided into the clinical syndromes of acute cardiac tamponade and chronic cardiac tamponade. Acute cardiac tamponade occurs after a penetrating wound to the heart, with rupture of the myocardium after trauma, or as a result of rupture of an infarcted segment of the ventricular wall.[48] Acute cardiac tamponade is always suspected after gunshot or stab wounds to the chest in the vicinity of the sternum. Patients with acute cardiac tamponade have hypotension, distended neck veins, and distant heart wounds, but chest radiography may be nondiagnostic because as blood accumulates over the minutes after the cardiac wound, the poorly distensible pericardium does not stretch to enable the pericardium to distend. This means that less than 200 mL of blood in the pericardium can lead to lethal pericardial tamponade.

An additional physical finding in patients with cardiac tamponade is *pulsus paradoxus,* defined as a greater than 10 mm Hg decline in systolic pressure at the end of the inspiratory phase of respiration, a phenomenon that is best observed on pressure tracings from an arterial line. Echocardiography and helical CT are two imaging methods that can establish the diagnosis of not just excess fluid in the pericardium but also compression of the atria, which indicates that pressure in the pericardium is about to reach the critical stage. Patients with acute cardiac tamponade need immediate surgery to decom-

press the pericardium and prevent precipitous cardiac arrest. Additionally, patients with penetrating trauma require surgical control of their heart wound. The preferred incision for exploring the heart of patients with cardiac tamponade is a sternotomy. However, for patients who arrive at the emergency department with a precipitous loss of vital signs, thoracotomy through a left submammary incision between ribs is indicated because it can be accomplished quickly and enables the pericardial tamponade to be evacuated and the heart wound covered.

Chronic cardiac tamponade occurs in patients when an exudative or transudative fluid collection develops in the pericardium. Chronic tamponade can develop in a wide spectrum of clinical conditions, including pericarditis, uremia, tuberculosis, and in some patients, penetrating cardiac wounds with a sterile or infected pericardial collection in which treatment is delayed. Because the fluid accumulates over a period of days, the pericardium is able to stretch, and these patients can have more than a liter of fluid in their pericardium without the catastrophic hemodynamic consequences of considerably smaller volumes of fluid in acute cardiac tamponade syndromes. Chest radiographs do have a diagnostic appearance. Patients with chronic cardiac tamponade have a syndrome consisting of dyspnea, fatigue, chronic cough, and on physical examination, distended neck veins. Passage of a pulmonary artery catheter from the superior vena cava to the pulmonary artery through the right atrium and ventricle shows equalization of pressures, which is an indication that a patient with pericardial fluid has hemodynamically significant cardiac tamponade. Aspiration of fluid or blood from the pericardial space can temporarily relieve the cardiac compression and improve systolic pressure.

Shock From Massive Pulmonary Embolism

Massive pulmonary embolism can cause an acute onset of shock. A large clot that becomes impacted at the bifurcation, or a central saddle pulmonary embolus, obstructs the flow of blood into the pulmonary artery. With an embolus there is insufficient delivery of blood to the left side of the heart, and systemic hypotension occurs. Clinical examination reveals distended neck veins and a tricuspid regurgitation murmur. Electrocardiographic findings indicate right ventricular strain with an $S_1Q_3T_3$ pattern, which means a prominent S wave in lead I and Q-wave and T-wave inversion in lead III. Echocardiography reveals acute right heart distention and strain. Patients who are hypotensive with acute heart failure after acute pulmonary embolism may benefit from the infusion of inotropic agents to sustain cardiac output pending dissolution or removal of the emboli. The effectiveness of thrombolytic therapy for massive pulmonary embolism has been established.[49] Studies have shown that IV injected recombinant tissue plasminogen activator can be an effective thrombolysis agent. In patients with recent wounds or incisions, bleeding complications are a substantial risk associated with thrombolytic therapy, and embolectomy is a preferable alternative therapy for massive pulmonary embolism. Retrieval of the obstructing saddle embolus can be performed through a sternotomy with the patient on cardiopulmonary bypass or by using percutaneous intraluminal techniques. Embolectomy may be lifesaving only if performed within minutes of the onset of symptoms, thus indicating the value of prompt diagnosis of this condition in an acutely ill patient by echocardiography.

SHOCK ASSOCIATED WITH ADRENAL INSUFFICIENCY

The adrenal glands synthesize hormones essential for life. Cortisol is released from cells in the zona fasciculata of the adrenal cortex in response to stimulation by ACTH released from the pituitary. Cortisol plays a key role in sustaining biochemical reactions (e.g., amino acid mobilization, gluconeogenesis, lipolysis with release of fatty acids). Aldosterone is released from cells located in the zona glomerulosa of the adrenal cortex in response to stimulation by angiotensin II. Aldosterone is a powerful mineralocorticoid that modulates renal function by increasing recovery of sodium and excretion of potassium. The adrenal medulla secretes epinephrine, a powerful α- and β-adrenergic agonist that accelerates cardiac function and sustains vasomotor tone. During stress (e.g., pain, hypotension, hypoglycemia, altered body temperature), patients depend on accelerated release of adrenal hormones. For patients in shock to achieve optimal survival, the three adrenal hormones must be secreted in large amounts for a sustained period.

The brain and kidney control the release of adrenal hormones. The hypothalamic-pituitary interface leads to ACTH being released from the anterior pituitary. ACTH circulates in blood to the adrenals and stimulates the release of cortisol. In the presence of low perfusion pressure, the renin-angiotensin-aldosterone axis stimulates cells of the juxtaglomerular apparatus of the kidney to produce renin. Renin is an enzyme that generates angiotensin I, which is modified by angiotensin-converting enzyme located on endothelial cells of the pulmonary arteries to produce angiotensin II. As the concentration of angiotensin II in plasma increases, more aldosterone is released from the adrenal cortex. Cardiovascular control centers in the brainstem are activated by baroreceptors generating afferent neuronal signals that perfusion pressure has declined. The cardiovascular control centers respond to evidence of hypotension by transmitting an efferent neuronal signal through the sympathetic nerves to stimulate release of epinephrine by the adrenal. Epinephrine circulating in plasma alters body perfusion by increasing cardiac function and raising sympathetic vasoconstrictive tone.

Primary and Secondary Acute Adrenal Failure

The adrenal glands fail to function in patients with primary adrenal insufficiency, whereas in patients with secondary adrenal insufficiency, defective release of agonist hormone mediators such as ACTH and angiotensin II occurs. The critical nature of adrenal function is dramatically demonstrated by the rapid clinical deterioration of patients who have a sudden loss of adrenal function. Destruction or removal of both adrenal glands leads to the abrupt onset of primary adrenal insufficiency. Patients with meningococcal bacteremia have bilateral adrenal hemorrhage. Hemorrhagic infarction of both adrenal glands after thrombosis of the adrenal veins occurs in postoperative patients who have antiphospholipid antibody syndrome or heparin-associated thrombocytopenia. Invasive infections associated with AIDS can destroy the adrenal glands and lead to primary adrenal insufficiency. Tuberculosis is a commonly encountered cause of primary adrenal insufficiency in the developing world. Replacement therapy is essential for patients with primary adrenal insufficiency and stress. These patients have a combined deficit of both glucocorticoids and mineralocorticoids, and treatment should replace both hormones. Secondary adrenal insufficiency occurs in patients in whom the pituitary or hypothalamus is injured or diseased. Brain injury involving the skull base or pituitary surgery can suddenly terminate release of ACTH from the pituitary. A confounding event in these patients may be the onset of diabetes insipidus because AVP is neither synthesized in the hypothalamus nor released from the pituitary. Postpartum pituitary necrosis is a rare cause of acute secondary adrenal insufficiency.

The clinical finding in patients in whom sudden acute adrenal insufficiency develops can be nonspecific. If plasma cortisol levels precipitously decline to nil, an abdominal pain syndrome, vomiting, and a tender abdomen will occur and progress to prostration, coma, and hypotension unresponsive to catecholamine infusion. Signs and symptoms of a gradual reduction in cortisol function include malaise, fatigue, and hyponatremia with hyperkalemia. Patients with complete loss of circulating glucocorticoid die within hours of irreversible hypotension. It is difficult to quickly establish the diagnosis of adrenal insufficiency in critically ill patients. Laboratory tests confirm that plasma levels of the hormones are depressed, but the results of these tests take hours to return. Surgeons treat patients suspected of having adrenal insufficiency with hormone replacement pending return of the laboratory tests. Treatment of glucocorticoid deficiency in adults is an IV infusion of 100 mg of hydrocortisone, which has an onset of action within 1 to 2 hours and duration of action of 8 hours. Thus, the commonly recommended replacement dose in an adult is 100 mg hydrocortisone IV infused every 8 hours with a rapid taper over the subsequent days as the patient's condition stabilizes and the results of laboratory tests become available. Other glucocorticoids used for IV replacement therapy include methylprednisolone and dexamethasone, which have been determined to have an anti-inflammatory milligram-per-milligram potency of 5 and 25, respectively, relative to 1.0 for hydrocortisone. Patients with destruction of the adrenal glands may also require replacement of mineralocorticoids. Patients with primary adrenal failure should be treated with 50 to 200 μg/day of fludrocortisone.

Adrenal Insufficiency Syndromes

Adrenal glucocorticoid insufficiency, but not complete failure, occurs in patients with impaired function of their hypothalamic-pituitary-adrenal axis. These patients produce limited amounts of corticosteroids, and clinical problems develop when they are stressed by hypovolemia from hemorrhage, onset of an infection, fear, or hypothermia. Thus, chronic adrenal insufficiency may be initially diagnosed when a patient is found to have intractable hypotension during evaluation for a surgical emergency. Pathologic causes of chronic adrenal insufficiency include autoimmune destruction of the adrenal gland and adrenalitis, in which cytotoxic lymphocytes gradually destroy cortisol-synthesizing cells in the adrenal cortex. Fatigue, inanition, weight loss, and postural dizziness symptoms gradually develop in patients with adrenalitis. These patients may have as a chief complaint vague cramping abdominal pain, nausea, and a change in bowel habits. Laboratory findings suggesting adrenal insufficiency are hyperkalemia, acidemia, hyponatremia, and an elevation in the serum creatinine level. The diagnosis of adrenal insufficiency secondary to end-organ failure is established by demonstration of a disproportionate elevation in ACTH in comparison to cortisol levels.

Adrenal insufficiency occurs in patients who have received long-term glucocorticoid therapy.[50] Patients are given these drugs as immunosuppression after transplantation or to treat inflammatory conditions, including autoimmune diseases, inflammatory bowel disease, reactive airway disease, and arthritis. Regulatory cells in the hypothalamus of patients taking glucocorticoids experience sustained elevations of circulating corticosteroids with suppressed synthesis of corticotropin-releasing hormone, which leads to a reduction in release of ACTH by the pituitary. Without ACTH, cells that synthesize cortisol in the adrenal cortex atrophy. Consequently, when stress occurs, the patient's adrenal cortex cannot respond to ACTH stimulation by increased release of glucocorticoid. Surgeons treat patients experiencing stress with IV infused cortisol if they have a history of recent sustained exposure to glucocorticoid therapy.

Selected References

Lucas CE, Ledgerwood AM: Physiology of colloid-supplemented resuscitation from shock. J Trauma 54:S75-S81, 2003.

These clinical investigators, who have conducted a series of landmark clinical studies on the optimal fluid for resuscitation of patients in shock, provide an informative summary of their observations of the course of events during the resuscitation, fluid uptake, and diuresis phases of patients who survive resuscitation from shock.

Moore FA, McKinley BA, Moore EE: The next generation in shock resuscitation. Lancet 363:1988-1996, 2004.

These experienced investigators in the pathophysiology of hemorrhagic shock propose that future improvements in the outcome of patients with shock will depend on standardized protocols for resuscitation and new therapies that modulate the exaggerated systemic inflammatory response elicited by inflammation and transfusion of blood products.

Pal JD, Victorino GP, Twomey P, et al: Admission serum lactate levels do not predict mortality in the acutely injured patient. J Trauma 60:583-589, 2006.

This manuscript presents an analysis of the predictive value of lactate levels in a very large population of seriously injured patients. Although the authors confirmed that there were statistical differences in lactate levels between survivors and nonsurvivors, they present the cogent argument that lactate levels are not useful in guiding surgeons during their initial decisions when evaluating trauma patients.

Sanborn TA, Feldman T: Management strategies for cardiogenic shock. Curr Opin Cardiol 19:608-612, 2004.

This review provides surgeons evidence-based guidelines that should be applied to patients in cardiogenic shock. The key goal is revascularization by endovascular interventions or, if that fails, by coronary bypass surgery.

Schrier RW, Wang W: Acute renal failure and sepsis. N Engl J Med 351:159-169, 2004.

In this detailed review the pathophysiology of acute renal failure is discussed, along with a summary of current evidence on effective interventions to reduce the risk for acute renal failure.

References

1. Aloia JF, Vaswani A, Flaster E, Ma R: Relationship of body water compartments to age, race, and fat-free mass. J Lab Clin Med 132:483-490, 1998.
2. Cox-Reijven PL, van Kreel B, Soeters PB: Accuracy of bioelectrical impedance spectroscopy in measuring changes in body composition during severe weight loss. JPEN J Parenter Enteral Nutr 26:120-127, 2002.
3. Finn PJ, Plank LD, Clark MA, et al: Progressive cellular dehydration and proteolysis in critically ill patients. Lancet 347:654-656, 1996.
4. Arieff AI: Hyponatremia, convulsions, respiratory arrest, and permanent brain damage after elective surgery in healthy women. N Engl J Med 314:1529-1535, 1986.
5. Berendes E, Van Aken H, Raufhake C, et al: Differential secretion of atrial and brain natriuretic peptide in critically ill patients. Anesth Analg 93:676-682, 2001.
6. Adrogue HJ, Madias NE: Hypernatremia. N Engl J Med 342:1493-1499, 2000.
7. Halperin ML, Goldstein M: Fluid, Electrolyte, and Acid-Base Physiology: A Problem-Based Approach, 3rd ed. Philadelphia, WB Saunders, 1999.
8. Gronert GA: Cardiac arrest after succinylcholine: Mortality greater with rhabdomyolysis than receptor upregulation. Anesthesiology 94:523-529, 2001.
9. Wahr JA, Parks R, Boisvert D, et al: Preoperative serum potassium levels and perioperative outcomes in cardiac surgery patients. Multicenter Study of Perioperative Ischemia Research Group. JAMA 281:2203-2210, 1999.
10. Wray CJ, Mayes T, Khoury J, et al: The 2002 Moyer Award. Metabolic effects of vitamin D on serum calcium, magnesium, and phosphorus in pediatric burn patients. J Burn Care Rehabil 23:416-423, 2002.
11. Sirker AA, Rhodes A, Grounds RM, Bennett ED: Acid-base physiology: The "traditional" and the "modern" approaches. Anaesthesia 57:348-356, 2002.
12. Prough DS, White RT: Acidosis associated with perioperative saline administration: Dilution or delusion? Anesthesiology 93:1167-1169, 2000.
13. Luchette FA, Jenkins WA, Friend LA, et al: Hypoxia is not the sole cause of lactate production during shock. J Trauma 52:415-419, 2002.

14. Laffey JG, Kavanagh BP: Hypocapnia. N Engl J Med 347:43-53, 2002.

15. Rutherford JJ, Clutton-Brock TH, Parkes MJ: Hypocapnia reduces the T wave of the electrocardiogram in normal human subjects. Am J Physiol 289:R148-R155, 2005.

16. Kregenow DA, Rubenfeld GD, Hudson LD, Swenson ER: Hypercapnic acidosis and mortality in acute lung injury. Crit Care Med 34:1-7, 2006.

17. Berger KI, Ayappa I, Chatr-Amontri B, et al: Obesity hypoventilation syndrome as a spectrum of respiratory disturbances during sleep. Chest 120:1231-1238, 2001.

18. Curry FR: Atrial natriuretic peptide: An essential physiological regulator of transvascular fluid, protein transport, and plasma volume. J Clin Invest 115:1458-1461, 2005.

19. Renkin EM: Some consequences of capillary permeability to macromolecules: Starling's hypothesis reconsidered. Am J Physiol 250:H706-H710, 1986.

20. Michel CC, Curry FE: Microvascular permeability. Physiol Rev 79:703-761, 1999.

21. Victorino GP, Newton CR, Curran B: Dose-dependent actions and temporal effects of angiotensin II on microvascular permeability. J Trauma 55:527-530, 2003.

22. Kaplan LJ, Kellum JA: Initial pH, base deficit, lactate, anion gap, strong ion difference, and strong ion gap predict outcome from major vascular injury. Crit Care Med 32:1120-1124, 2004.

23. Pal JD, Victorino GP, Twomey P, et al: Admission serum lactate levels do not predict mortality in the acutely injured patient. J Tauma 60:583-589, 2006.

24. Claridge JA, Crabtree TD, Pelletier SJ, et al: Persistent occult hypoperfusion is associated with a significant increase in infection rate and mortality in major trauma patients. J Trauma 48:8-14, 2000.

25. Velmahos GC, Demetriades D, Shoemaker WC, et al: Endpoints of resuscitation of critically injured patients: Normal or supranormal? A prospective randomized trial. Ann Surg 232:409-418, 2000.

26. Moore FA, McKinley BA, Moore EE: The next generation in shock resuscitation. Lancet 363:1988-1996, 2004.

27. Beale RJ, Hollenberg SM, Vincent JL, Parrillo JE: Vasopressor and inotropic support in septic shock: An evidence-based review. Crit Care Med 32:S455-S465, 2004.

28. Martin RS, Kincaid EH, Russell HM, et al: Selective management of cardiovascular dysfunction in posttraumatic SIRS and sepsis. Shock 23:202-208, 2005.

29. Richard C, Warszawski J, Anguel N, et al: French Pulmonary Artery Catheter Study Group. Early use of the pulmonary artery catheter and outcomes in patients with shock and acute respiratory distress syndrome: A randomized controlled trial. JAMA 290:2713-2720, 2003.

30. O'Grady NP, Alexander M, Dellinger EP, et al: Guidelines for the prevention of intravascular catheter–related infections. Centers for Disease Control and Prevention. MMWR Recomm Rep 51(RR-10):1-29, 2002.

31. Riddez L, Hahn RG, Brismar B, et al: Central and regional hemodynamics during acute hypovolemia and volume substitution in volunteers. Crit Care Med 25:635-640, 1997.

32. Burri C, Henkemeyer H, Passler HH, Allgower M: Evaluation of acute blood loss by means of simple hemodynamic parameters. Prog Surg 11:108-131, 1973.

33. Auerbach AD, Goldman L: Beta-blockers and reduction of cardiac events in noncardiac surgery: Scientific review. JAMA 287:1435-1444, 2002.

34. Miyagatani Y, Yukioka T, Ohta S, et al: Vascular tone in patients with hemorrhagic shock. J Trauma 47:282-287, 1999.

35. Bickell WH, Wall MJ Jr, Pepe PE, et al: Immediate versus delayed fluid resuscitation for hypotensive patients with penetrating torso injuries. N Engl J Med 331:1105-1109, 1994.

36. Schierhout G, Roberts I: Fluid resuscitation with colloid or crystalloid solutions in critically ill patients: A systematic review of randomized trials. BMJ 316:961-964, 1998.

37. Lucas CE, Ledgerwood AM: Physiology of colloid-supplemented resuscitation from shock. J Trauma 54:S75-S81, 2003.

38. Mayberry JC, Mullins RJ, Crass RA, Trunkey DD: Prevention of abdominal compartment syndrome by absorbable mesh prosthesis closure. Arch Surg 132:957-961; discussion 961-962, 1997.

39. Bone R, Balk R, Cerra F, et al: Definitions for sepsis and organ failure and guidelines for the use of innovative therapies in sepsis. The ACCP/SCCM Consensus Conference Committee. American College of Chest Physicians/Society of Critical Care Medicine. Chest 101:1644-1655, 1992.

40. Schrier RW, Wang W: Acute renal failure and sepsis. N Engl J Med 351:159-169, 2004.

41. Choi PT, Yip G, Quinonez LG, Cook DJ: Crystalloids vs. colloids in fluid resuscitation: A systematic review. Crit Care Med 27:200-210, 2001.

42. Levy B, Dusang B, Annane D, et al: College Interregional des Reanimateurs du Nord-Est. Cardiovascular response to dopamine and early prediction of outcome in septic shock: A prospective multiple-center study. Crit Care Med 33:2172-2177, 2005.

43. Rivers E, Nguyen B, Havstad S, et al: Early goal-directed therapy in the treatment of severe sepsis and septic shock. N Engl J Med 345:1368-1377, 2001.

44. Deans KJ, Haley M, Natanson C, et al: Novel therapies for sepsis: A review. J Trauma 58:867-874, 2005.

45. Van den Berghe G, Wouters P, Weekers F, et al: Intensive insulin therapy in critically ill patients. N Engl J Med 345:1359-1367, 2001.

46. Sanborn TA, Feldman T: Management strategies for cardiogenic shock. Curr Opin Cardiol 19:608-612, 2004.

47. Hochman JS, Sleeper LA, Webb JG, et al: Early revascularization in acute myocardial infarction complicated by cardiogenic shock. SHOCK Investigators. Should we emergently revascularize occluded coronaries for cardiogenic shock? N Engl J Med 341:625-634, 1999.

48. Spodick DH: Acute cardiac tamponade. N Engl J Med 349:684-690, 2003.

49. Konstantinides S, Geibel A, Kasper W: Submassive and massive pulmonary embolism: A target for thrombolytic therapy? Thromb Haemost 82(Suppl 1):104-108, 1999.

50. Coursin DB, Wood KE: Corticosteroid supplementation for adrenal insufficiency. JAMA 287:236-240, 2002.

CHAPTER 6

Hematologic Principles in Surgery

Edmund J. Rutherford, MD   Mark E. Brecher, MD   Samir M. Fakhry, MD
and   George F. Sheldon, MD

Background
Hemostasis and Coagulation
Disorders of Hemostasis and Coagulation
Congenital Hemorrhagic Disorders
Acquired Hemorrhagic Disorders
Disseminated Intravascular Coagulation
Thrombotic Disorders
Preparation of Blood Components
Clinical Indications and Use of Blood Components
Risks Associated With Blood Transfusion
Massive Transfusion
Blood Substitutes and Alternatives to Transfusion

Management of bleeding disorders and administration of blood products are important therapeutic modalities used by surgeons caring for patients with acute and chronic problems. When used with a thorough understanding of appropriate indications, risks, and benefits, blood transfusion is safe and effective. Surgeons encounter congenital and acquired bleeding disorders in many clinical settings. Congenital conditions such as hemophilia present challenges for both elective and emergency operations. Acquired bleeding disorders are associated with conditions such as inflammatory states, massive transfusion, hypothermia, malnutrition, liver dysfunction, and drugs. Knowledge of the fundamentals of normal and deranged hemostasis is critical to successful operative procedures and complete care of surgical patients.

In this chapter, normal hemostatic mechanisms are discussed and appropriate diagnostic and therapeutic measures for disorders of surgical bleeding are reviewed. The indications for and use of blood components, potential risks associated with blood products, and alternatives to blood transfusion are reviewed. Because blood products are a limited resource with potential serious adverse effects, knowledge of appropriate indications, potential risks, and available alternatives allow clinicians to exercise judgment in using this important resource.

BACKGROUND

Though now routine, the ability to transfuse blood successfully is relatively recent. Accounts of bloodletting and phlebotomy appear in many early historical references and were recommended for many ailments. Jean-Baptiste Denis in France and Richard Lower in England recorded the first known successful transfusion to humans in 1667. Denis gave 3 pints of sheep blood to a patient with no apparent ill effects. Subsequent attempts to give blood to this young man "to mollify his fiery nature" failed, and the patient died shortly after the transfusion. A lawsuit resulted, and Denis went to trial but was ultimately exonerated. The Paris medical faculty subsequently forbade blood transfusions, which led to bans on transfusion throughout France and Italy that lasted until modern times. In 1795, Dr. Philip Syng Physick of Philadelphia performed the first successful transfusion of human blood.

Discovery of the A, B, and O blood types by Karl Landsteiner in 1900 and the AB blood type by Alfred Decastello and Adriano Sturli in 1902 began the era of modern blood transfusion. The first blood bank was established in the United States in 1937, and the introduction of plastic storage containers and centrifugation instruments made component therapy possible. By the 1940s, techniques of crossmatching, anticoagulation, and storage of blood and the establishment of blood banks made routine blood transfusion feasible.

Replacing blood intraoperatively is an important prerequisite in modern surgical practice, with a majority of blood products being transfused during or near surgery. Blood component therapy has made successful surgery possible in patients with symptomatic anemia, thrombocytopenia, or coagulopathy. Approximately 14 million units of red blood cells (packed RBCs and whole blood) were transfused in the United States in 2001,[1] an 11.8%

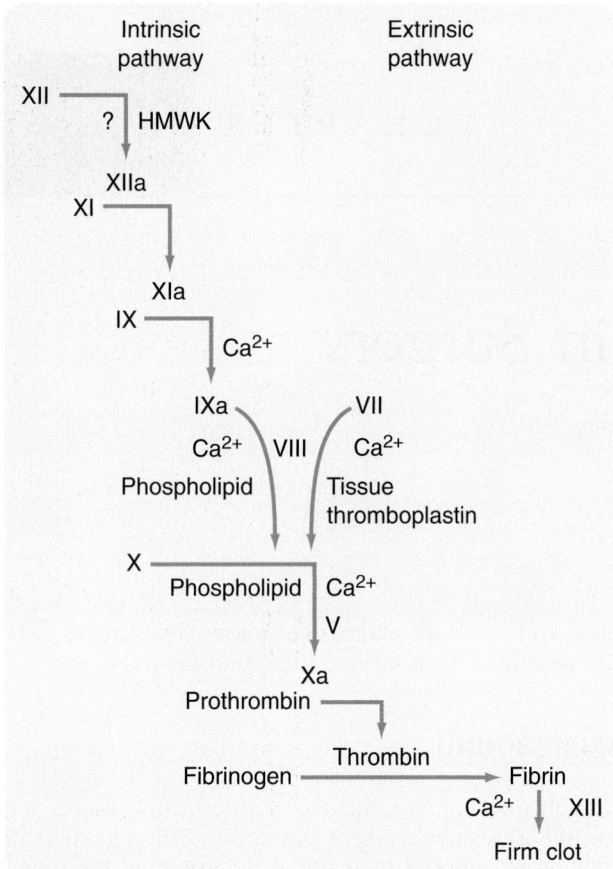

Figure 6-1 Traditional schematic version of the coagulation system. HMWK, high-molecular-weight kininogen.

increase since 1999 and an astonishing 56% increase since 1980.[2] The use of other components, especially platelets, has also increased. Because only 5% to 6% of eligible donors ever donate blood, future increases may exacerbate shortages.[2]

HEMOSTASIS AND COAGULATION

Traditional concepts of coagulation held that two pathways exist by which coagulation could occur: the intrinsic pathway and the extrinsic pathway (Fig. 6-1). In this cascade model, the two pathways converge to a common pathway. The clinical relevance of the intrinsic pathway is not associated with clinically significant bleeding in vivo, although it does produce aberrations in tests of coagulation. In particular, deficiencies of factor XII or prekallikrein are not associated with a bleeding tendency in humans, whereas patients with deficiencies of factor VIII or factor IX exhibit pronounced bleeding disorders (hemophilia A and B, respectively).

Deficiencies in the cascade model and recent discoveries have prompted a model of cell-based coagulation,[3] with tissue factor (TF)-bearing cells and platelets being at the center (Fig. 6-2). When the integrity of the blood vessel wall is disrupted, exposure of cells expressing TF

to plasma activates the coagulation system. The distribution of TF is highly cell specific and includes adventitial cells, outer layers of the epidermis, other squamous epithelial cells, and myoepithelial cells. This corresponds to a hemostatic envelope surrounding blood vessels and organs.[4] Endothelial cells also express TF. Monroe and associates describe three phases of cell-based coagulation: initiation, priming, and propagation.[3] In the first phase, factor VII binds to TF and is rapidly activated (VIIa). The TF/VIIa complex catalyzes the activation of factor IX (IXa). In addition, the TF/VIIa complex can directly activate factor X (Xa). The TF/VIIa/Xa complex binds activated factor V (Va) and converts prothrombin to thrombin. The relatively small amount of thrombin formed serves to further enhance platelet activation and accelerate the coagulation response. Platelets, already primed by exposure to collagen, are synergistically primed by the addition of thrombin. In the second or priming phase, platelets release granules containing factor V, which is cleaved to factor Va. Thrombin cleaves factor VIII from von Willebrand's factor (vWF), thereby converting it to factor VIII'. In the propagation phase, the activated primed platelets are now able to rapidly bind activated factors V, VIII, and IX. On the platelet membrane, a factor VIII'/IXa complex is formed. This complex is the major activator of factor X and is estimated to be 50 times more efficient than the TF/VIIa complex. Factor Xa binds with factor Va to form the major converter of prothrombin to thrombin. It is believed that complexes formed on the platelet surface are more efficient because they are protected from blood-borne inhibitors.[3] The significant amount of thrombin produced serves to form a stable fibrin clot. This revised scheme of blood coagulation explains the observed clinical syndromes of deficiency of various factors and clarifies the relatively limited role that factor XII plays in coagulation in vivo.

Coagulation is strictly regulated at different steps through the process. Tissue factor pathway inhibitor (TFPI) blocks the TF/VIIa/Va/Xa complex by binding to factor Xa.[5] TFPI is present in small amounts usually, but more is released in the presence of heparin.[5] Antithrombin III (AT-III) is a member of the serine protease inhibitor superfamily and a weak inhibitor of the TF/VIIa complex. AT-III more effectively neutralizes coagulation system enzymes such as activated factors IX, X, and XI, thus affecting thrombin production. Heparin accelerates these inhibitory reactions by causing a conformational change in AT-III. Thrombin is inactivated by AT-III in the presence of heparin. Heparin cofactor 2 is similar to AT-III as a naturally occurring anticoagulant; however, it inhibits only thrombin. The activity of heparin cofactor 2 is enhanced by both heparin and dermatan sulfate. Deficiency of AT-III is also associated with a tendency to venous thrombosis. Thrombin binds thrombomodulin on the cell surface of endothelial cells. The thrombin-thrombomodulin complex activates protein C in the presence of its cofactor protein S. Activated protein C competitively binds activated factors V and VIII, thereby limiting the production of factor Xa and thrombin. As a clinically important anticoagulant pathway in humans, either protein C or protein S deficiency is known to cause a significant tendency toward thrombosis. Activated protein C has also been used to treat patients with significant systemic inflammatory response syndrome; such patients appear to have a procoagulant state with decreased expression of thrombomodulin and decreased levels of protein C.[6]

Blood Vessels and Endothelial Cells

Hemostasis is the physiologic cessation of bleeding. Under normal circumstances, blood maintains its fluidity because of the balance of procoagulant and anticoagulant influences, including interactions at the blood-endothelium interface and many circulating factors.[3] When a vessel is injured, TF and collagen are exposed. Platelets adhere to the site of injury and undergo a release phenomenon with further platelet aggregation, and a platelet plug forms.

Vasoconstriction occurs in response to the release of vasoactive substances from platelets (e.g., thromboxane A_2 and serotonin) and endothelin from endothelial cells. Thromboxane A_2 is produced locally at the site of injury and is a very potent constrictor of smooth muscle, especially in smaller and medium-sized vessels. Larger vessels constrict in response to innervation and circulating constrictive factors, such as norepinephrine.

Endothelial cells are highly active cells with many important products and effects, including both procoagulant and antithrombotic effects.[4] Under normal conditions, endothelial cells are crucial in the maintenance of a nonthrombogenic interface between vessels and circulating blood. Among the contributory mechanisms identified thus far are elaboration of prostacyclin (a potent inhibitor of platelet aggregation), nitric oxide, thrombomodulin, and tissue plasminogen activator (tPA) and binding of the anticoagulant AT-III to heparin sulfate on the endothelial cell surface. Endothelial cell injury exposes subendothelial TF and collagen, reduces the availability of thrombomodulin, increases phospholipid sites for coagulation protein binding, and leads to expression of TF on the cell surface. These changes promote the procoagulant effect of injury. During inflammatory states, agents such as endotoxin, interleukin-1, and tumor necrosis factor promote the expression of TF on the endothelial cell surface and down-regulation of thrombomodulin, which leads to procoagulant effects.[4]

Platelets

Platelets participate in hemostasis through a sequence of adherence to the site of injury, release of the contents of their alpha and dense granules, aggregation to form a platelet plug, and promotion of coagulation by providing a procoagulant surface on their phospholipid membranes.[3] Platelets rapidly adhere to exposed subendothelial collagen and other basement membrane proteins. The presence of fibrinogen and vWF is important for the successful adherence of platelets. vWF is a large protein that produces several important effects in hemostasis and coagulation. In addition to its role in the adhesion of platelets to injured vessel walls, it is a carrier for factor VIII in plasma, thus protecting it from degradation.

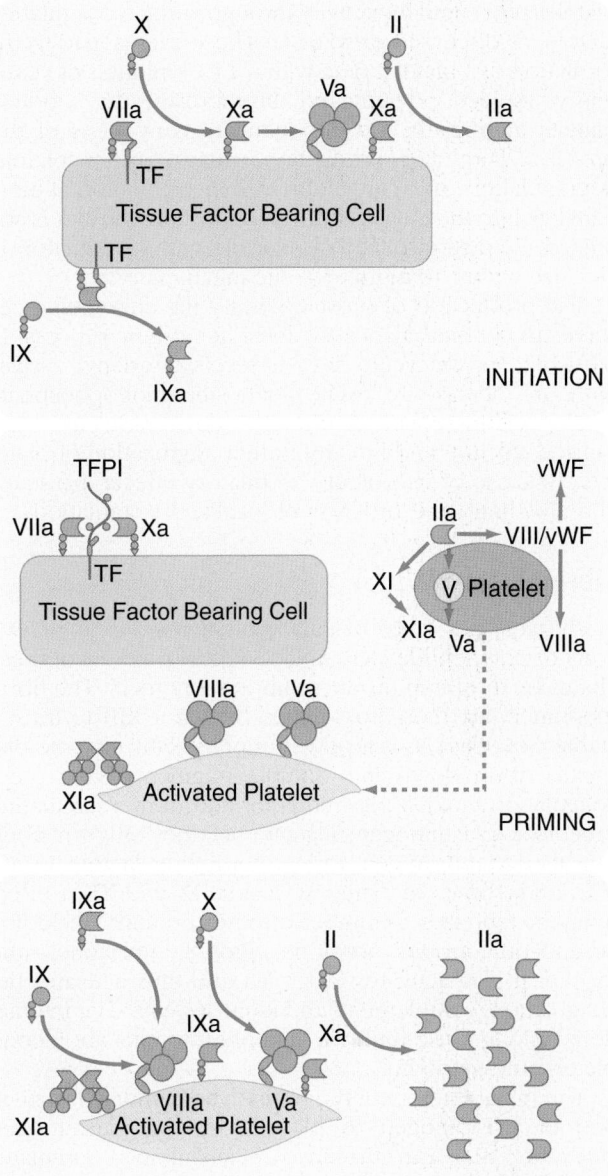

Figure 6-2 Cell-based model of coagulation. TF, tissue factor; TFPI, tissue factor pathway inhibitor; vWF, von Willebrand's factor. (From Monroe DM, Hoffman M, Roberts HR: Platelets and thrombin generation. Arterioscler Thromb Vasc Biol 22:1381-1389, 2002.)

vWF binds to collagen, undergoes a conformational change, and binds the platelet surface receptor glycoprotein Ib/IX. After adhering to the subendothelium, platelets form pseudopods. Platelets are activated with release of the contents of their alpha granules (platelet factor 4, β-thromboglobulin, thrombospondin, platelet-derived growth factor, fibrinogen, vWF) and dense granules (adenosine diphosphate, serotonin). With the release of platelet granule contents, particularly adenosine diphosphate, further platelet aggregation at the site of injury takes place. The glycoprotein IIb/IIIa receptors on adjacent platelets are joined by fibrinogen. Platelet activation also produces platelet procoagulant activity through surface coagulation factors, as discussed previously. These events lead to the formation of a platelet plug within 1 to 3 minutes of vessel injury. Ionized calcium and thromboxane A$_2$, a potent platelet aggregator, are important in many steps of this process. Thrombin production causes further platelet degranulation and aggregation with incorporation of more platelets into the clot. As fibrin is deposited, the clot is stabilized. Retraction of the clot occurs with a reduction in clot size within 10 minutes of the initial injury.

The production of prostacyclin by the endothelial cell serves to counterbalance the local hemostatic process. In particular, prostacyclin elevates levels of adenyl cyclase with an increase in cyclic adenosine monophosphate levels within platelets, thereby decreasing available ionized calcium and limiting further aggregation of platelets. Because of its potent vasodilatory effects, prostacyclin also limits the progress of localized coagulation.

Fibrinolysis

Fibrinogen is a large plasma protein composed of two pairs of polypeptide chains. Cleavage of portions of these chains by thrombin produces fibrin monomers. The fibrin monomers are then cross-linked by factor XIII to form a stable clot. Plasmin is a powerful proteolytic enzyme that breaks fibrin down into soluble fragments. Like other coagulation factors, plasmin is formed from a circulating precursor, plasminogen. Plasmin acts not only on fibrin but also on fibrinogen and prothrombin, factors V and VIII, and, some data suggest, factors IX and XI. It effectively metabolizes a number of other proteins, including adrenocorticotropic hormone, growth hormone, and insulin. It also activates factor XII and thus activates the coagulation, complement, and kinin systems. The interactions among these multiple, complex systems are incompletely understood.

The main reaction of the fibrinolytic pathway is activation of plasminogen to plasmin by the plasminogen activators tPA and urokinase. Plasminogen circulates in plasma at relatively high concentrations, whereas the activators are found in concentrations a hundred thousand–fold lower.[7] Plasma tPA concentrations are markedly increased by release from endothelial cells in response to stress and injury. Activation of plasminogen by tPA is inefficient in the absence of fibrin. In the presence of fibrin, activation proceeds rapidly, thus providing an important regulatory role for fibrin in the process of its degradation. Urokinase efficiently activates plasminogen in the absence of fibrin, but plasma levels of urokinase are low and its role in hemostasis is poorly defined. Epithelial cells lining excretory ducts of the body (e.g., renal tubules, mammary ducts) secrete urokinase, which is the physiologic activator initiating lysis of any fibrin that may be formed in these areas. Streptokinase, a bacterial product, is a potent activator of plasminogen and has been used to induce fibrinolysis therapeutically.

The reactions of the fibrinolytic cascade are catalyzed by serine proteases in a manner analogous to the coagulation cascade. These reactions are believed to occur on the surface of endothelial cells. The serine proteases are regulated by inhibitors from the serine protease inhibitor superfamily, which act as pseudosubstrates for the proteases. Fibrin helps regulate fibrinolysis, in addition to serving as its major substrate. Physiologic fibrinolysis is a reparative process that occurs in response to hemostatic plug or thrombus formation. The final enzymatic step, fibrin proteolysis, results from a coordinated interaction of enzymes and inhibitors, which produces effective action at the site of the process and spares the proteins of the blood or uninvolved parts of the vascular system.

The major inhibitor of plasminogen activation is plasminogen activator inhibitor (PAI-1), a substance found in low concentration in plasma but at higher concentration within platelets. Plasma PAI-1 is probably synthesized in endothelial cells or hepatocytes, or both. Levels of this inhibitor of the fibrinolytic system increase after trauma and surgery. Synthesis of PAI-1 is affected by many compounds, including endotoxin, thrombin, transforming growth factor-β, interleukin-1, and tumor necrosis factor-α. The major inhibitor of plasmin, α$_2$-antiplasmin or plasmin inhibitor, circulates in plasma at relatively high concentrations and can neutralize large amounts of plasmin. Plasmin inhibitor binds fibrin during the process of fibrin cross-linking by activated factor XIII and protects the thrombus from fibrinolysis.[8] Plasmin inhibitor also interferes with plasminogen and inhibits the effect of plasminogen activators.[8] The proenzyme thrombin activatable fibrinolysis inhibitor (TAFI) is activated by thrombin, thus providing a link between coagulation and fibrinolysis. The main mechanism of action of TAFI involves interference of plasminogen binding to degrading fibrin, but interference of plasmin binding and direct plasmin inhibition have also been demonstrated.[7]

Degradation of cross-linked fibrin creates distinctive products characterized by cross-linked (factor XIIIa induced) derivatives such as D-dimer. Disease states occurring after abnormalities in the fibrinolytic system include both hemorrhagic disorders, resulting from excessive fibrinolysis, and thrombotic disorders, resulting from deficient fibrinolysis. Hyperfibrinolysis can be induced by pharmacologic administration of activators such as streptokinase, urokinase, and tPA or by defective inhibition produced by α$_2$-antiplasmin deficiency. Thrombosis can result from hereditary defects of plasminogen or from pharmacologic inhibition of fibrinolysis, such as with ε-aminocaproic acid. Laboratory evaluation of fibrinolysis can aid in the assessment of thrombotic disorders, including specific measurements of plasminogen activators, plasminogen, plasmin inhibitors, and circulating fibrinogen and products of cross-linked fibrin degradation.

DISORDERS OF HEMOSTASIS AND COAGULATION

The surgeon may encounter disorders of hemostasis and coagulation either in the preoperative evaluation of patients for elective surgery or in the perioperative care of patients with acute bleeding disorders. Diagnosis of the specific disorder involved requires a detailed evaluation of the patient's history, review of medical records related to risk factors for bleeding or previously obtained laboratory data, physical examination, and appropriate laboratory tests.[9]

An accurate history and physical examination of a patient scheduled to undergo elective surgery offer the most valuable source of information regarding the risk for bleeding. A patient with a history of bleeding, easy bruising (either spontaneous or traumatic), frequent or unusual mucosal bleeding, metromenorrhagia (irregular, prolonged, and excessive menstrual flow), hematuria, epistaxis, previous history of significant or life-threatening hemorrhage associated with invasive procedures, or a family history may be at risk. Any intake of medications must always be elicited. Especially important are drugs such as aspirin and nonsteroidal anti-inflammatory drugs (NSAIDs); patients may not consider their intake important to mention when interviewed unless specifically asked. In addition, a history of liver dysfunction, renal dysfunction, or a major metabolic or endocrine disorder is useful in directing preoperative screening. Excessive bruising, joint deformities, petechiae or ecchymosis, adenopathy, hepatosplenomegaly, hypermobility of joints, and increased elasticity of the skin are symptoms of disorders associated with excessive perioperative bleeding. Evidence of amyloidosis (e.g., thickening of the skin or tongue), multiple myeloma, or other hematologic malignancies can also affect hemostasis and coagulation.

Screening Tests for Bleeding Disorders

The extent of laboratory testing needed for patients with a normal history and physical examination findings has been debated. For most patients undergoing either minor operations or procedures that do not involve extensive dissection, laboratory testing is unlikely to provide additional information over that obtained with a properly performed history and physical examination. Preoperative laboratory screening may be useful for patients undergoing major procedures, especially those involving body cavities or operations requiring significant dissection and the creation of raw surfaces, or for patients with an abnormal history or physical examination findings. Patients with infection, systemic inflammatory response syndrome, sepsis syndrome, malnutrition, organ failure, and other major systemic disorders also warrant preoperative screening. Commonly obtained tests include the prothrombin time (PT), the activated partial thromboplastin time (aPTT), a complete blood cell count with platelet count, and occasionally, a bleeding time. The PT measures the function of factor VII, as well as factor X, prothrombin/thrombin, fibrinogen, and fibrin. Prolongation of the PT occurs when levels of factors V, VII, or X fall below 50% of normal. A prothrombin level less than 30% of normal also prolongs the PT. Warfarin therapy and vitamin K deficiency deplete the vitamin K–dependent proteins (prothrombin; factors VII, IX, and X; protein C and S) and prolong the PT.

The aPTT detects decreased levels of high-molecular-weight kininogen, prekallikrein, and factors XII, XI, IX, and VIII, as well as fibrinogen, prothrombin, and factors

V and X. Factor levels of 30% or less are usually required to affect the aPTT. The anticoagulant heparin is a commonly used drug that causes prolongation of the aPTT without significantly prolonging the PT by depleting the intrinsic pathway factors.

The PT and aPTT can be used together in an attempt to localize coagulation defects. A normal PT with an abnormal aPTT suggests deficiency of the proximal intrinsic pathway factors. A prolonged PT with a normal aPTT suggests abnormalities of the vitamin K–dependent factors such as factor VII. An abnormal PT or aPTT may indicate the presence of an inhibitor (e.g., lupus anticoagulant, heparin, or an inhibitor of a specific factor). To differentiate an inhibitor from deficiency of a factor, the patient's plasma is mixed in a 1:1 ratio with normal plasma and the PT or aPTT is repeated. If the abnormal value corrects to the normal range, the presence of a coagulation factor deficiency in the patient's plasma is indicated. If the abnormality does not correct, an inhibitor is presumed to exist.

The platelet count identifies numbers of platelets, whereas the bleeding time estimates qualitative platelet function. None of the commonly recommended screening tests measures fibrinolytic function. Additional screening tests that may be used include a fibrinogen level and the thrombin time (TT). The TT detects abnormalities in globulin and fibrinogen, excess fibrinolysis, and heparin-like substances. In patients suspected of having platelet dysfunction, additional assessments include platelet function tests (aggregation with epinephrine, adenosine diphosphate, collagen, and ristocetin). If a deficiency or specific factor is suspected, as in patients with a family history of hemophilia, specific factor assays must be performed.

The bleeding time is a crude screening test for platelet function that also reflects endothelial cell function. This test is performed by placing a standardized cut in the skin of either the forearm (Ivy's method) or the earlobe (Duke's method). Because the bleeding time is affected by many variables, including the manner in which the cut is placed, the location of the cut, endothelial cell function, platelet counts, and overall platelet function, it is a difficult test to standardize. Data suggest that although the bleeding time may be useful in evaluating patients with bleeding disorders, it has no role in the preoperative evaluation of a normal patient.[9]

Patients with familial thrombocytopenia (May-Hegglin anomaly) have an autosomal dominant disorder associated with petechiae and hyperpigmentation of the distal aspect of the lower extremities. These patients may have abnormal bleeding as a result of decreased platelet numbers. Patients with Marfan's syndrome, Ehlers-Danlos syndrome, or osteogenesis imperfecta may have abnormal bleeding and poor wound healing despite normal screening test results. Other bleeding disorders often missed by routine coagulation testing include mild von Willebrand's disease, platelet function defect, factor XIII deficiency, hyperglobulinemic states, α_2-antiplasmin deficiency, and amyloidosis.

If a patient scheduled for an elective procedure has a history of a significant risk for bleeding, abnormal findings on physical examination, or deranged screening laboratory test results, the procedure is postponed pending a more complete evaluation and treatment. Patients about to undergo emergency operative procedures may require urgent correction of their hemostatic abnormalities before and during surgery (see guidelines in Clinical Indications and Use of Blood Components).

CONGENITAL HEMORRHAGIC DISORDERS

Congenital disorders of coagulation usually involve a single coagulation protein. The diagnosis depends on the history, physical examination, PT and aPTT determinations, and assay of factor levels. If available, a history of bleeding problems before the current manifestation usually suggests the presence of the disease. Careful management includes specific factor replacement, meticulous intraoperative hemostasis, and careful monitoring of blood coagulation in the perioperative period. Early consultation with a coagulation specialist is important.

Hemophilia

Hemophilia A (classic hemophilia) is a congenital coagulation disorder that results from a deficiency or abnormality of factor VIII. It is transmitted as an X-linked recessive disorder, with males being affected almost exclusively. A female patient with laboratory abnormalities consistent with hemophilia A is uncommon but may represent a carrier state, an unusual chromosomal aberration, or another rare disorder. A large number of different mutations accounting for the genetic abnormality have been identified, with up to 30% of cases representing spontaneous mutations. The severity of the disease can be categorized according to the functional levels of factor VIII (factor VIII:C), in contradistinction to factor VIII:Ag, which refers to the antigenic level. Patients generally have severe bleeding with factor levels less than 2%, moderate bleeding with levels between 2% and 5%, and mild disease with levels in the range of 5% to 30%. A patient with hemophilia A generally has large hematomas and hemarthroses, as opposed to the mucosal bleeding commonly noted with platelet disorders. Bleeding is often delayed by hours or days after injury because the platelet plug is the first line of defense against bleeding, followed later by thrombus formation.

Laboratory evaluation of patients with hemophilia A reveals a prolonged aPTT with decreased factor VIII:C and normal PT, bleeding time, and vWF antigen levels, which excludes the diagnosis of von Willebrand's disease. Inhibitors or IgG antibodies to factor VIII:C develop in a small proportion of patients with hemophilia A (10%-20%). Inhibitors can be detected with a mixing study.

Hemophilia B, also known as Christmas disease, is an inherited X-linked bleeding disorder that reflects a deficiency or defect in factor IX. Patients manifest deep bleeding and hemarthroses. The severity of symptoms correlates directly with the level of circulating factor IX. Laboratory diagnosis of hemophilia B consists of detection of an abnormal aPTT with decreased factor IX levels in a male patient with a normal PT, bleeding time, platelet count, and factor VIII and VIIIR antigen levels. Because factor IX

is a vitamin K–dependent factor, vitamin K deficiency may produce depressed levels; however, the PT is prolonged and levels correct with the administration of exogenous vitamin K. As with hemophilia A, inhibitors can develop to factor IX and are diagnosed in similar fashion.

Desmopressin (DDAVP) may temporarily raise factor VIII levels in a patient with mild hemophilia A (basal factor VIII levels of 5%-10%). Administration of desmopressin to such patients after minor trauma or before elective dental surgery may obviate or reduce the need for replacement therapy. An intravenous (IV) dose of 0.3 μg/kg raises factor VIII levels 2- to 10-fold. Intranasal desmopressin is also effective and raises factor VIII levels twofold to threefold. Desmopressin is ineffective in treating severe hemophilia A. Antifibrinolytic therapy with ε-aminocaproic acid or tranexamic acid has also been effective in combination with desmopressin in decreasing bleeding, particularly after dental procedures and in pediatric patients. Both ε-aminocaproic acid and tranexamic acid can be administered IV or orally and can be given in combination with factor replacement. They are contraindicated when prothrombin complex concentrates are used because of the increased risk for thrombosis.[10] Although plasma contains factors VIII and IX, sufficient whole plasma cannot be given to patients with severe hemophilia, unless plasma exchange is performed, to raise factor VIII or IX concentrations to levels that effectively prevent or control bleeding episodes. Cryoprecipitate is a good source of factor VIII but is rarely used now that specific factor VIII concentrates are available. Two types of concentrates are available for the treatment of hemophilia A: plasma-based factor VIII preparations and recombinant preparations. Plasma-based preparations are available in intermediate- and high-purity strength and are significantly less costly than recombinant preparations. One unit of factor VIII activity is the amount in 1 mL of normal plasma. In general, 1 U/kg of factor VIII raises levels by 2%. Although the concentration of factor VIII in individual bags of cryoprecipitate varies, a bag may be assumed to contain 80 units of factor VIII. In general, levels can be achieved by administering 50 U/kg and then about 30 U/kg every 8 hours for the first 2 days after surgery or injury. Subsequent infusions given every 12 hours are adjusted on the basis of serum factor VIII assays.

For the treatment of hemophilia B, the traditional therapy is prothrombin complex concentrate, which contains not only factor IX but also all of the vitamin K–dependent factors. High-purity factor IX concentrate is now available. For unknown reasons, only about half of factor IX units listed on a bottle of prothrombin complex concentrate can be recovered after infusion. Therefore, when prothrombin complex concentrate is given for factor IX replacement therapy, an amount double that calculated as being necessary is given. Because prothrombin complex concentrate may contain variable amounts of activated factors, patients receiving repeated doses of factor IX concentrate are at increased risk for disseminated intravascular coagulation (DIC) and, paradoxically, thrombosis. For this reason, heparin (5-10 units) is often added to each milliliter of reconstituted prothrombin complex concentrate.

Levels of factors VIII or IX are raised transiently to about 30% to protect against bleeding after dental extraction or to abort incipient joint hemorrhage, to 50% if major joint or intramuscular bleeding is already evident, and to 100% in patients with life-threatening bleeding or before major surgery. Transmission of human immunodeficiency virus (HIV) to the hemophilic population through replacement blood products was a major complication of transfusion therapy, with 55% of hemophiliacs being infected with HIV-1 by the mid 1980s; this complication has been mitigated by viral inactivation procedures, mandatory blood donor screening for HIV, and the use of recombinant products.

In hemophiliacs with a factor VIII inhibitor who are bleeding, treatment with factor VIII will stimulate further production of antibodies; therefore, consultation with a coagulation specialist is necessary. Special preparations of prothrombin complex concentrates that bypass the role of factor VIII in coagulation are available but expensive. Recombinant factor VIII preparations are also often effective in patients with inhibitors.

Recombinant activated factor VII (rFVIIa) has been used successfully to stop active bleeding in hemophilia patients and nonhemophilia patients with antibodies to factor VIII. Although the exact mechanism of action has not been elucidated, TF-independent activation of platelets appears to be taking place. Normally, 1% of total-body factor VII is circulating in activated form, and after injury this activated factor VII forms a complex with exposed subendothelial TF. With the administration of high doses of factor VIIa, platelet activation occurs with the formation of stable thrombin, independent of other clotting factors. Several randomized trials have demonstrated the effectiveness of rFVIIa in producing hemostasis in hemophilia patients with life- or limb-threatening hemorrhage and inhibitors to factors VIII, IX, and XI.[11] Administration of a single dose of rFVIIa given at 90 to 120 µg/kg IV over a period of 3 to 5 minutes has been shown to induce immediate hemostasis. Repeated doses can be given every 2 to 3 hours without laboratory monitoring.

von Willebrand's Disease

von Willebrand's disease is the most common congenital bleeding disorder; its frequency is estimated to be as high as 1%. Most patients have a mild bleeding disorder. The symptoms of von Willebrand's disease are related to the role of vWF as an important stimulus to platelet aggregation at the site of tissue injury and as the major carrier protein for circulating factor VIII. A large number of subtypes of the disease have been described, most of which are rare. The three major groups are type I, inherited as an autosomal dominant trait and characterized by a quantitative decrease in an otherwise normally functioning vWF; type II, which is variably inherited and characterized by qualitative defects in vWF; and type III, an autosomal recessive severe bleeding disorder with essentially absent levels of vWF. The bleeding encountered in patients with von Willebrand's disease is similar to that of patients with bleeding as a result of platelet dysfunction and consists of mucosal bleeding, petechiae, epistaxis, and menorrhagia.

The laboratory diagnosis of von Willebrand's disease varies by subtype. Type I von Willebrand's disease is characterized by a normal PT, a mildly prolonged aPTT, an abnormal bleeding time, a normal platelet count, and a mild reduction in factors VIII : C and VIII : Ag. The reduction in factor VIII : C occurs because vWF is the serum carrier for factor VIII. Patients with blood type O have lower normal levels of factors VIII : C and VIII : Ag and may be erroneously thought to have mild type I von Willebrand's disease. The diagnosis of type II von Willebrand's disease is complicated by many subgroups. In general, decreased functional activity of vWF produces a depressed ristocetin cofactor assay (vWF : Cof), which measures the effectiveness of vWF in agglutinating platelets when stimulated with the antibiotic ristocetin. A further subtype of type II von Willebrand's disease, called *pseudo–von Willebrand's disease,* is a platelet disorder characterized by the presence of very large platelets that aggregate in the presence of cryoprecipitate. Nearly complete absence of factors VIII : C, VIII : Ag, and VIIIR : C characterizes type III von Willebrand's disease. These patients have a prolonged aPTT, abnormal bleeding times, and low platelet counts. The help of a coagulation specialist is important in determining the subtype and treatment.

Administration of desmopressin, 0.3 µg/kg, induces an increase in plasma levels of vWF and factor VIII and potentiation of hemostasis. The cellular mechanism of action remains incompletely understood.[12] This effect lasts 8 to 10 hours, and two to four repeated doses can be administered every 12 to 24 hours, if necessary. Factor VIII levels are monitored. In patients who are not candidates for desmopressin treatment, replacement of vWF by infusion of cryoprecipitate is effective in the control or prevention of bleeding in von Willebrand's disease. Virus-inactivated plasma concentrates that contain both factor VIII and vWF are considered to be safer and preferable.[13]

Other Congenital Deficiencies

Other congenital deficiencies may rarely be encountered, including deficiencies of factors XI and XII, prekallikrein, and high-molecular-weight kininogen, also called the *contact factors.* Deficiencies of factors VII and V and prothrombin have been described but are extremely rare. Disorders of fibrinogen, including afibrinogenemia, hypofibrinogenemia, and dysfibrinogenemia, may occur. The bleeding disorder in these patients ranges from mild to severe, depending on the level and function of the factor in circulation. Factor XIII deficiency creates abnormalities in the cross-linking of fibrin monomers. This rare autosomal recessive disorder is characterized by poor wound healing and delayed bleeding. Because standard laboratory testing is not diagnostic, determination of factor XIII levels is necessary for diagnosis.

ACQUIRED HEMORRHAGIC DISORDERS

Many coagulation abnormalities may be present in a surgical patient. Acquired defects are more common than congenital ones.

Vitamin K Deficiency

Vitamin K is necessary for the reaction that attaches a carboxyl group to glutamic acid, and the proteins containing carboxyglutamic acid residues are therefore called *vitamin K–dependent clotting factors* (including prothrombin; factors VII, IX, and X; and proteins C and S). When synthesized in the absence of vitamin K, these proteins, lacking carboxyglutamic acid residues, cannot bind calcium normally. This is also the site of action of warfarin. Causes of vitamin K deficiency may be inadequate dietary intake, malabsorption, lack of bile salts, obstructive jaundice, biliary fistula, oral administration of antibiotics, or parenteral alimentation. A number of broad-spectrum antibiotics can cause a vita-min K–dependent coagulopathy, including cephalosporins, quinolones, doxycycline, and trimethoprim-sulfamethoxazole.

Vitamin K may be administered parenterally and corrects clotting times within 6 to 12 hours. Up to 5 mg IV is given slowly as an initial dose. Older preparations of vitamin K were less purified than those used at present, and anaphylaxis and death were reported with the IV administration of these older agents. The more purified forms are less likely to cause complications, but IV vitamin K must be given cautiously. Intramuscular or subcutaneous vitamin K may be administered in doses of 10 to 25 mg/day. Repeated doses of intramuscular or subcutaneous vitamin K allow total-body repletion (10-25 mg/day for 3 days). Administration of plasma rapidly corrects the coagulation deficit, and thus plasma is given with vitamin K to patients with ongoing bleeding.

Anticoagulant Drugs

Warfarin acts by blocking the synthesis of vitamin K–dependent factors, prolongs the PT, and causes a slight elevation in the aPTT by reducing levels of prothrombin and factors VII, IX, and X. A loading dose of 5 mg is generally recommended; the international normalized ratio (INR) is checked on day 3, with further adjustments based on the INR.[14] Warfarin has a half-life of 40 hours, and treatment of major bleeding caused by warfarin consists of administration of vitamin K, infusion of plasma for life-threatening bleeding, and possibly administration of rFVIIa.

Unfractionated heparin (UFH) blocks the activation of factor X by binding with AT-III and thrombin. All coagulation tests can be affected by UFH, including the PT, but the aPTT is most sensitive. A dose of UFH is cleared from the blood in approximately 6 hours, but clearance varies, depending on other factors such as hepatic function, body temperature, and shock. A weight-based nomogram (e.g., 80 U/kg followed by 18 U/kg/hr) is generally superior to non–weight-based nomograms in time to achieve the desired aPTT. Subsequent dose adjustments are based on the aPTT. UFH can be neutralized with IV protamine sulfate (100 units of UFH is equal to 1 mg of protamine).

Heparin-induced thrombocytopenia (HIT) can be caused by UFH in up to 5% of patients as a result of the formation of IgG antibodies to heparin–platelet factor 4 complexes. The platelet count decreases by at least 50% of the preheparin level in most patients with HIT. This usually occurs after 4 to 5 days of heparin therapy but can occur within 24 hours if heparin had been given in the previous 100 days. HIT can be induced by heparin flushes and even minute amounts eluted from heparin-bonded catheters.[15] Secondary arterial and venous thrombosis can develop for the first time up to 4 to 6 weeks after heparin therapy has been discontinued.[15] In any patient who has a decrease in platelet count by 30% to 50%, all heparin is withdrawn immediately and another anticoagulant such as lepirudin or argatroban initiated if necessary.

Low-molecular-weight heparins (LMWHs) derived from UFH have more selective anti-Xa activity than UFH does. LMWH has been associated with less bleeding complications and has become the first-line therapy for prophylaxis and treatment of deep venous thrombosis (DVT) and acute coronary syndromes. The risk for DVT ranges from 0.4% in low-risk to 80% in the highest-risk surgical patients. The risk for pulmonary embolism (PE) ranges from 0.2% to 10%, with up to 5% of episodes being fatal (Table 6-1).[16] The PT is not usually affected by LMWH, and anti-Xa activity is measured if dose efficacy is questioned. LMWH can also cause HIT (<1%). Fondaparinux does not appear to react with platelet factor 4 and may be a possible first-line treatment of HIT.[15]

Hepatic Failure

Liver diseases, including major hepatic trauma, cirrhosis, and biliary obstruction, can impair coagulation. The liver is the major site of synthesis of all the coagulation factors except factor VIII. Hemostasis may be further impaired by an associated thrombocytopenia or platelet dysfunction, which also occurs frequently with liver disease. Thrombocytopenia has been attributed to decreased platelet production, splenic sequestration of platelets, circulating antiplatelet antibodies, and viral hepatitis (particularly hepatitis C [HCV]). The prolonged bleeding times frequently seen in cirrhotic patients can be improved by the administration of desmopressin.[12] Desmopressin is often ineffective in patients with thrombocytopenia or congenital platelet dysfunction. The hyperfibrinolysis in cirrhosis also contributes to coagulopathy. The liver is important in clearing blood of the activated metabolites of both fibrinolysis and coagulation, and the coagulation system may be pushed toward either coagulation or bleeding in patients with liver dysfunction.

Liver disease is commonly associated with a low level of serum fibrinogen, a prolonged PT,[17] and a normal to slightly increased aPTT. An elevated TT usually indicates abnormal or decreased fibrinogen. In patients with severe liver dysfunction, large volumes of plasma may be required to maintain normal factor levels. Up to 2 units of plasma may be needed every 2 hours in patients with complete liver failure to maintain adequate coagulation factor levels.

Renal Failure

Renal disease and uremia cause a reversible bleeding disorder related to platelet dysfunction. There is a decrease in aggregation and adhesiveness of platelets and levels

Table 6-1 Levels of Risk for Thromboembolism and Prevention Strategies

LEVEL OF RISK		DVT		PE		PREVENTION STRATEGIES
		Calf	Proximal	Clinical	Fatal	
Low risk	Minor surgery in patients <40 years with no additional risk factors	2%	0.4%	0.2%	<0.01%	No specific prophylaxis, early and "aggressive" mobilization
Moderate risk	Minor surgery in patients with additional risk factors	10%-20%	2%-4%	1%-2%	0.1%-0.4%	LDUH (q12h)
	Surgery in patients 40-60 years of age with no additional risk factors					LMWH (<3400 units daily) GCS IPC
High risk	Surgery in patients >60 years old or 40-60 years old with additional risk factors (previous VTE, cancer, hypercoagulopathy)	20%-40%	4%-8%	2%-4%	0.4%-1.0%	LDUH (q8h) LMWH (>3400 units daily) IPC
Highest risk	Surgery in patients with multiple risk factors (age >40, cancer, previous VTE) Hip or knee arthroplasty, hip fracture operation Major trauma, spinal cord injury	40%-80%	10%-20%	4%-10%	0.2%-5%	LMWH (>3400 units daily) Fondaparinux Oral vitamin K antagonist (INR=2-3) IPC/GCS+LDUH/LMWH

DVT, deep venous thrombosis; GCS, graded compression stockings; INR, international normalized ratio; IPC, intermittent pneumatic compression; LDUH, low-dose unfractionated heparin; LMWH, low-molecular-weight heparin; PE, pulmonary embolism; VTE, venous thromboembolism.

Adapted from Geerts WH, Pineo GF, Heit JA, et al: Prevention of venous thromboembolism: The seventh ACCP conference on antithrombotic and thrombolytic therapy. Chest 126:338S-400S, 2004.

of platelet factor II, which results in a prolonged bleeding time. The nature of the lesion caused by renal insufficiency is not known. Administration of desmopressin helps decrease bleeding problems after procedures in these patients.[12] IV desmopressin, 0.3 µg/kg, decreases the bleeding time, increases platelet retention on glass beads, and enhances the activity of factor VIII. Cryoprecipitate and conjugated estrogens can also shorten the bleeding time.

Thrombocytopenia

Normal platelet counts range from 150,000 to 400,000/mm^3. A platelet count less than 100,000/mm^3 generally constitutes thrombocytopenia. With platelet counts between 40,000 and 100,000/mm^3, bleeding may occur after injury or surgery, but spontaneous bleeding is uncommon. Spontaneous bleeding may occur with platelet counts between 10,000 and 20,000/mm^3; with counts below 10,000/mm^3, spontaneous bleeding is frequent and often severe. Thrombocytopenia may be secondary to failure of production of platelets, splenic sequestration, increased destruction of platelets, increased use of platelets, or dilution. Defects in platelets often cause spontaneous bleeding into the skin, as manifested by petechiae, purpura, or confluent ecchymoses. Thrombocytopenia also causes mucosal bleeding and excessive bleeding after surgery. Heavy gastrointestinal bleeding and bleeding into the central nervous system may be life-threatening manifestations of thrombocytopenia. Thrombocytopenia does not generally cause massive bleeding into tissues or hemarthrosis.

Drugs (e.g., quinidine, sulfa preparations, H$_2$ blockers, oral antidiabetic agents, gold salts, rifampin, and heparin) can cause thrombocytopenia. Contributing factors include a recent blood transfusion (post-transfusion purpura), heavy consumption of alcohol (alcohol-induced thrombocytopenia), and underlying immunologic disease (e.g., arthralgia, Raynaud's phenomenon, unexplained fever). The presence or absence of fever is an important point of the differential diagnosis. Fever is usually present in thrombocytopenia secondary to infection or active systemic lupus erythematosus and in thrombotic thrombocytopenic purpura but absent in idiopathic thrombocytopenic purpura and drug-related thrombocytopenia. Size of the spleen on physical examination is a second important diagnostic point. The spleen is not palpably enlarged in most thrombocytopenia caused by increased destruction of platelets (e.g., idiopathic thrombocytopenic purpura, drug-related immune thrombocytopenia), whereas it is usually palpably enlarged in thrombocytopenia secondary to splenic sequestration of platelets and often in patients with thrombocytopenia secondary to lymphoma or a myeloproliferative disorder.

The peripheral blood smear and cell count provides clues to the diagnosis and severity of thrombocytopenia. An increased proportion of large platelets suggests compensatory increased production of platelets and is frequently found in thrombocytopenia secondary to increased destruction or use of platelets. The bleeding time is prolonged in severe thrombocytopenia of any cause. Bone marrow aspiration is useful.

Management of thrombocytopenia secondary to decreased production is directed toward correcting its cause. Platelet concentrates can raise the platelet count temporarily; however, repeated use reduces their effectiveness because of the development of platelet alloantibodies. If rapid correction of bone marrow failure is not expected, transfusions of platelets are often reserved to treat an active bleeding episode. Corticosteroids have not proved beneficial in the management of patients with thrombocytopenia secondary to bone marrow failure.

Thrombocytopathy

Platelet dysfunction can be secondary to drugs, congenital disorders, and metabolic derangement. Drugs to consider with important effects on platelets include chemotherapeutic agents, thiazide diuretics, alcohol, estrogen, antibiotics such as the sulfa agents, quinidine and quinine, methyldopa, and gold salts. The most common drugs that block platelet function are prostaglandin inhibitors, particularly aspirin, indomethacin, and other NSAIDs. Aspirin and other NSAIDs act by blocking prostaglandin metabolism in platelets. Aspirin permanently acetylates cyclooxygenase, and affected platelets remain dysfunctional throughout their 7-day life span after exposure to aspirin. NSAIDs cause a reversible defect that lasts 3 to 4 days. Desmopressin may be effective in normalizing the prolonged bleeding time caused by aspirin.[18] A normal platelet count with dysfunctional platelets can occur in congenital disorders such as Glanzmann's thrombasthenia (glycoprotein IIb/IIIa dysfunction) and Bernard-Soulier syndrome (platelet glycoprotein Ib/IX/V receptor deficiency) and with metabolic derangement.

Hypothermia

Hypothermia is one of the most common and least well recognized causes of altered coagulation in surgical patients, especially those receiving massive transfusion. It is exacerbated in patients who have an open thoracic or abdominal cavity, which accelerates heat loss. The coagulation system consists of a series of proteolytic enzymes, the activity of which decreases with decreasing temperature. Hypothermia is characterized by a marked increase in fibrinolytic activity, thrombocytopenia, impaired platelet function, a decrease in collagen-induced platelet aggregation, and increased affinity of hemoglobin for oxygen. Hypothermia has been associated with hepatic dysfunction and increased levels of blood citrate and hypocalcemia with transfusion, an effect exacerbated by shock. If blood is being rapidly infused through a central line with its tip near the sinoatrial node, fatal dysrhythmias can result.

Hypothermia and bleeding usually occur in a patient who undergoes large-volume resuscitation during an extensive surgical procedure or in the perioperative period. Body temperatures as low as 30°C to 34°C can be associated with coagulopathy, even if levels of factors and platelets are normal. Nonmechanical bleeding can occur and be uncontrollable and lethal. The best course is to terminate the surgical procedure as expeditiously as possible, pack the bleeding areas as needed, close the surgical incision, and attempt to rewarm the patient as rapidly as possible in the intensive care unit. Damage control celiotomy for trauma, which includes an abbreviated celiotomy with control of gross bleeding, overt enteric contamination, packing and staged delayed definitive repair of injuries, and abdominal closure, has become key in preventing the triangle of death: hypothermia, acidosis, and coagulopathy. Continued administration of plasma, platelets, and other blood products can worsen the hypothermia with continued bleeding. Warming IV fluids before they are given can ameliorate hypothermia. Care must be taken to not heat RBCs above 40°C because shortened survival or acute hemolysis can result. Hemorrhage accounts for 90% of deaths after abdominal injury, and half of these deaths are secondary to recalcitrant coagulopathy.[19]

DISSEMINATED INTRAVASCULAR COAGULATION

DIC is a syndrome rather than a specific disease. Much confusion and controversy surround its diagnosis and treatment. Although DIC is generally considered a hemorrhagic disorder because of the obvious bleeding problems encountered, it is important to recognize the sequelae resulting from the microvascular (and sometimes large-vessel) thrombosis that accompanies DIC and leads to end-organ failure and death. DIC is a systemic thrombohemorrhagic disorder with evidence of coagulant activation, deposition of fibrin, fibrinolytic activation, consumption of coagulation factor and platelets, and end-organ dysfunction that is seen in many clinical situations.[20] The disorder may have a spectrum of manifestations, from *low-grade DIC,* with minimal symptoms and minor laboratory abnormalities, to *fulminant DIC,* with life-threatening bleeding and coagulation abnormalities producing end-organ dysfunction and death. Conditions associated with DIC include hemolysis, massive transfusion, amniotic fluid embolism, placental abruption, retained fetus, gram-negative and gram-positive sepsis, viremia, burns, crush injury and tissue destruction, leukemia, malignancy (especially metastatic), liver disease, and miscellaneous inflammatory and autoimmune conditions, including vasculitis. Although the diagnosis of DIC is often attached to patients who are undergoing massive transfusion, platelet dysfunction as a result of hypothermia or a specific factor deficiency is excluded before making a diagnosis of DIC. In most cases, such patients will respond to rewarming and replenishment of coagulation factors and platelets (see Massive Transfusion).

With activation of the coagulation and fibrinolytic systems, both thrombin and plasmin are in circulation. Thrombin converts fibrinogen to fibrin monomers by cleaving fibrinopeptide A and B from fibrinogen. These fibrin monomers form soluble fibrin clots, which cause microvascular thrombosis with entrapment and depletion of platelets. Simultaneous degradation of these factors by plasmin takes place. Depressed levels of fibrinogen and elevated levels of fibrinogen degradation products (fibrin split products) result. These degradation products inhibit the normal coagulation of blood by delaying polymerization of fibrin. Fibrin degradation products may also interpose themselves between fibrin and polymers and form a weak fibrin clot. Fibrin degradation products include X, Y, D, and E fragments; platelet dysfunction is attributable to the latter two fragments. Plasmin also degrades factors V, VIII, IX, and XI and activates the complement system. These changes produce the clinically observed alterations characteristic of DIC.

Laboratory abnormalities in DIC are variable and related to the many diseases associated with this condition. Common abnormalities include an abnormal PT and aPTT with depressed fibrinogen levels and abnormal platelet counts. Levels of fibrin degradation products and D-dimer are elevated. The peripheral smear reveals fragmented RBCs, but this finding is not specific. Because of the continued activation of coagulation, thrombin/antithrombin complexes will be formed. Levels of thrombin/antithrombin and AT-III are depressed. Fragments of coagulation factor degradation are elevated, including F1.2 and FpA. Because of activation of the fibrinolytic system, plasminogen and α_2-antiplasmin inhibitor levels are decreased.

Low-grade DIC generally responds to management of the underlying disorder. The appropriate therapy for fulminant DIC remains controversial, compounded by the lack of objective studies and many underlying causes. The assistance of a physician experienced in managing DIC is valuable. Treatment of the underlying condition is critical to successful management of DIC. Also important is treatment of the thrombotic intravascular process that causes end-organ failure. Treatment with heparin has never demonstrated beneficial effects in controlled trials. The most logical anticoagulant would be directed against TF activity, such as recombinant TFPI, inactivated factor VIIa, and recombinant NAPc2.[20] Antithrombin concentrates administered to attain a serum level of 125% of normal have been useful in some patients. Continued bleeding may be related to depletion of components, but random administration of blood products, especially those containing fibrinogen, may exacerbate the syndrome. Washed RBCs, platelets, AT-III concentrate, and crystalloid and colloid volume expanders may be used. If other therapeutic measures are unsuccessful, inhibition of fibrinolysis may be attempted. ε-Aminocaproic acid may be given along with heparin. Despite improved diagnostic and therapeutic modalities, mortality from DIC remains high and closely related to the underlying disorder.

THROMBOTIC DISORDERS

Hypercoagulable disorders, or thrombophilias, are most frequently encountered in surgical practice as DVT or, less often, PE. Although a ready explanation based on Virchow's triad may be available for the majority of surgical patients, other potential causes must be considered. Thrombophilia may be caused by a decrease in antithrombotic proteins or an increase in prothrombotic proteins. The former include antithrombin deficiency, protein C deficiency, and protein S deficiency. The latter include factor V Leiden, prothrombin gene mutation (G20210A), and increased levels of factors VII, VIII, IX, and XI or vWF.

Antithrombin deficiency is an autosomal dominant genetic disorder that affects an estimated 1.1% of unselected patients with venous thromboembolism. Antithrombin levels range from 40% to 70% of normal, with as many as 85% of affected patients suffering a thrombotic event by 50 years of age. These patients are generally believed to be at greater risk than patients with other types of thrombophilia.[21]

Protein C is a vitamin K–dependent glycoprotein synthesized by the liver that inactivates factors Va and VIIIa. Protein C deficiency is also an autosomal dominant genetic disorder that affects 3.2% of unselected patients with venous thromboembolism. Up to 50% of affected patients will experience a thromboembolic event by the age of 50.[21]

Protein S is also a vitamin K–dependent glycoprotein that acts as a cofactor to inactivate factors Va and VIIIa. Protein S deficiency affects 2.2% of unselected patients with thromboembolism, with up to 50% experiencing their first event by 25 years of age.[21]

Factor V Leiden is a single–base pair mutation (Arg506→Gln) of the factor V gene that results in activated protein C resistance. Factor V Leiden is found in 4% to 6% of the general population and in 6% to 33% of unselected patients with venous thromboembolism. There is a threefold to sevenfold increase risk for thromboembolism, with 30% suffering an event by the age of 60.[21]

The prothrombin gene mutation G20210A is a glycine-to-arginine mutation in the factor II (prothrombin) gene. This mutation is identified in 6.2% of unselected patients with thrombotic events. A substantial number of these patients also carry the factor V Leiden mutation.[21]

Increased levels of factors VII, VIII, IX, and XI or vWF (>150 IU/dL) are associated with a 2.2- to 4-fold increase risk for thrombotic events and a 1.08 relative risk for each 10-IU/dL increase. The causes of these elevations remain unclear but may have a genetic basis.[21]

In addition to these inherited disorders, acquired disease processes associated with thrombotic events include pregnancy; cancer; sepsis; trauma; major operations, particularly those involving the pelvis; nephrotic syndrome; myeloproliferative disorders; drugs such as oral contraceptives, hormonal therapy, and chemotherapy; and malnutrition, including folic acid and vitamin B_{12} and B_6 deficiency. Arterial thromboembolic events are difficult to separate from underlying atherosclerotic disease. Disorders include hypercysteinemia; paradoxical embolism through a patent foramen ovale or an atrial or ventricular septal defect; and inherited thrombophilia. Treatment of thrombotic events includes correction of the underlying process and anticoagulation. The duration of anticoagulation remains controversial and depends on the magnitude of the event, ongoing risk for thrombosis and treatment-associated risks, and anticipated future circumstances. Prophylaxis for patients at risk is based on the underlying disorder, magnitude of the risk, and anticipated requirements.

PREPARATION OF BLOOD COMPONENTS

Component therapy is the accepted standard for optimal management of the blood supply. Blood is separated into its individual components (packed RBCs, plasma, platelets) to optimize therapeutic potency (Table 6-2). This strategy maximizes the benefit derived from each individual unit while minimizing the risk to each recipient. Blood is withdrawn from the donor and mixed with a citrate solution to prevent coagulation by binding calcium.

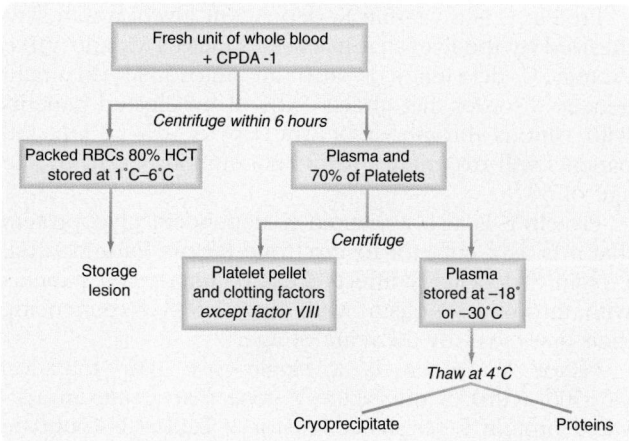

Figure 6-3 Preparation of blood components. CPDA-1, citrate phosphate dextrose adenine; HCT, hematocrit; RBC, red blood cell.

The solutions used commonly are citrate phosphate dextrose (CPD), citrate phosphate double dextrose (CP2D), and citrate phosphate dextrose adenine (CPDA-1). Solutions containing some combination of dextrose, adenine, sodium chloride, and either phosphate (AS-3) or mannitol (AS-1 and AS-5) extend the storage life of red cells. The unit is gently centrifuged (Fig. 6-3) to pack the RBCs and leave about 70% of the platelets suspended in plasma. The platelet-rich plasma is removed and centrifuged again at a faster speed to sediment the platelets. All but 35 mL of supernatant plasma is removed and rapidly frozen at a temperature lower than −30°C. The platelets are resuspended to yield platelet concentrate. Frozen plasma that is stored at a temperature lower than −18°C is termed *fresh frozen plasma*. If the frozen plasma is allowed to thaw at 4°C, the precipitate that remains can be collected to yield cryoprecipitate. Proteins such as albumin can be isolated from the remaining supernatant plasma by ethanol fractionation.

Automated cell separators (apheresis) can be used to collect leukocytes, platelets, or plasma. In apheresis procedures, blood is withdrawn in either a continuous or discontinuous flow from the donor. The blood is separated by centrifuge, and the desired component is removed. The remaining blood is then returned to the donor. Large numbers of units of leukocytes or platelets can be removed in a relatively short period.

The storage and refrigeration of packed RBCs create progressive changes, known as *storage lesions,* which include altered affinity of hemoglobin for oxygen; decrease in pH; changes in RBC deformability; hemolysis; an increase in the concentration of potassium, phosphate, and ammonia; development of microaggregates; release of vasoactive substances; and denaturation of proteins. The survival of RBCs is shorter the longer cells are stored. This shortened survival is associated with a decrease in both intracellular 2,3-diphosphoglycerate (2,3-DPG) and adenosine triphosphate (ATP). Transfusion of cold blood may also contribute to the development of hypothermia, especially in patients receiving large volumes of banked blood rapidly. Many of the changes described may be reversed within a short time after transfusion and may cause metabolic patterns different from those predicted.

CLINICAL INDICATIONS AND USE OF BLOOD COMPONENTS

Transfusion based on sound physiologic principles and an understanding of the relative risks and benefits provides maximal benefit to the patient, along with efficient use of a valuable and finite resource. A consensus conference reviewed the existing literature and developed 11 policies for surgical blood management and proposed interventions.[22] The standards, guidelines, and options are summarized in Table 6-3. The specific needs of some patients may require consultation with specialists in transfusion medicine.

Whole Blood

Storage of whole blood precludes the production of components and is highly inefficient. Whole blood is thus unavailable in most blood banks in the United States because oxygen-carrying capacity and replacement of volume can be achieved with packed RBCs and crystalloid solutions. There are currently few indications for whole blood, and many U.S. blood banks do not routinely store this product.

Red Blood Cells

Packed RBCs can be stored in additive solution (AS) with a shelf life of 42 days. With longer storage, less than 75% of the RBCs remain viable in circulation 24 hours after transfusion, which is the current U.S. Food and Drug Administration (FDA) definition of an outdated unit. Platelets degenerate at refrigerator temperatures, so banked packed RBCs contain essentially no functioning platelets. Levels of factors V and VIII decrease significantly at 1°C to 6°C ($T_{1/2} = 10$-14 days and 7 days, respectively), although levels of other factors remain essentially unchanged ($T_{1/2} > 21$ days). Only approximately 35 mL of plasma is present in a unit of AS red cells.

Packed RBCs provide oxygen-carrying capacity and maintain oxygen delivery provided that intravascular volume and cardiac function are adequate. The decision to transfuse and the amount to transfuse depend on the clinical situation. Use of a hematocrit of 30% (or a hemoglobin level of 10 g/dL) as a *transfusion trigger* is no longer acceptable. Oxygen delivery is maintained by a series of complex interactions and compensatory mechanisms when red cell mass (measured by hemoglobin or hematocrit) falls. Such mechanisms include increased cardiac output, increased extraction ratio, rightward shift of the oxyhemoglobin curve, and expansion of volume. Many chronically anemic patients tolerate hemoglobin levels of 7 to 8 g/dL or less, as has been demonstrated in chronic renal failure and Jehovah's Witnesses. Cardiac output does not increase until hemoglobin falls below approximately 7 g/dL. Young healthy patients tolerate acute anemia to hemoglobin levels of 7 g/dL or less, provided that they have normal intravascular volume and

Text continued on p 127

Table 6-2 Requirements for Storage, Transportation, and Expiration

ITEM NO.	COMPONENT	STORAGE	TRANSPORT	EXPIRATION[1]	ADDITIONAL CRITERIA
Whole Blood Components					
1	Whole blood	1°C-6°C. If intended for room temperature components, then store at 1°C-6°C within 8 hours.	Cooling toward 1°C-10°C. If intended for room temperature components, cooling toward 20°C-24°C.	ACD/CPD/CP2D: 21 days CPDA-1: 35 days	
2	Whole blood irradiated	1°C-6°C	1°C-10°C	Original expiration or 28 days from date of irradiation, whichever is sooner	
Red Blood Cell Components					
3	Red blood cells	1°C-6°C	1°C-10°C	ACD/CPD/CP2D: 21 days CPDA-1: 35 days Additive solution: 42 days Open system: 24 hours	
4	Deglycerolized RBCs	1°C-6°C	1°C-10°C	Open system: 24 hours or as FDA approved Closed system: 14 days or as FDA approved	
5	Frozen RBCs 40% glycerol	≤–65°C if 40% glycerol or as FDA approved	Maintain frozen state	10 years (A policy shall be developed if rare frozen units are to be retained beyond this time)	Open system: Frozen within 6 days of collection without an additive Frozen prior to red blood cell expiration if with an additive approved for this purpose Closed system: Frozen within 6 days
6	RBCs irradiated	1°C-6°C	1°C-10°C	Original expiration or 28 days from date of irradiation, whichever is sooner	
7	RBCs leukocytes reduced	1°C-6°C	1°C-10°C	ACD/CPD/CP2D: 21 days CPDA-1: 35 days Additive solution: 42 days Open system: 24 hours	
8	Rejuvenated RBCs	1°C-6°C	1°C-10°C	CPD, CPDA-1: 24 hours AS-1: freeze after rejuvenation	Follow manufacturer's written instructions
9	Deglycerolized rejuvenated RBCs	1°C-6°C	1°C-10°C	24 hours or as approved by FDA	Follow manufacturer's written instructions
10	Frozen rejuvenated RBCs	≤–65°C	Maintain frozen state	10 years AS-1: 3 years (A policy shall be developed if rare frozen units are to be retained beyond this time)	Follow manufacturer's written instructions
11	Washed RBCs	1°C-6°C	1°C-10°C	24 hours	
12	Apheresis RBCs	1°C-6°C	1°C-10°C	CPDA-1: 35 days Additive solution: 42 days Open system: 24 hours	
13	Apheresis RBCs leukocytes reduced	1°C-6°C	1°C-10°C	CPDA-1: 35 days Additive solution: 42 days Open system: 24 hours	
Platelet Components					
14	Platelets	20°C-24°C with continuous gentle agitation	20°C-24°C (as close as possible to)	24 hours to 5 days, depending on collection system	Maximum time without agitation 24 hours
15	Platelets irradiated	20°C-24°C with continuous gentle agitation	20°C-24°C (as close as possible to)	No change from original expiration date	Maximum time without agitation 24 hours
16	Platelets leukocytes reduced	20°C-24°C with continuous gentle agitation	20°C-24°C (as close as possible to)	Open system: 4 hours Closed system: No change in expiration	Maximum time without agitation 24 hours
17	Pooled platelets leukocytes reduced	20°C-24°C with continuous gentle agitation	20°C-24°C (as close as possible to)	Open system: within 4 hours of opening the system Closed system: 4 hours after pooling or 5 days following collection[2]	Maximum time without agitation 24 hours
18	Pooled platelets (or open system)	20°C-24°C with continuous gentle agitation	20°C-24°C (as close as possible to)	Open system: 4 hours	

Continued

Table 6-2   Requirements for Storage, Transportation, and Expiration—cont'd

ITEM NO.	COMPONENT	STORAGE	TRANSPORT	EXPIRATION[1]	ADDITIONAL CRITERIA
19	Apheresis platelets	20°C-24°C with continuous gentle agitation	20°C-24°C (as close as possible to)	24 hours to 5 days, depending on collection system	Maximum time without agitation 24 hours
20	Apheresis platelets irradiated	20°C-24°C with continuous gentle agitation	20°C-24°C (as close as possible to)	No change from original expiration date	Maximum time without agitation 24 hours
21	Apheresis platelets leukocytes reduced	20°C-24°C with continuous gentle agitation	20°C-24°C (as close as possible to)	Open system: within 4 hours of opening the system Closed system: 5 or 7 days[3]	Maximum time without agitation 24 hours
Granulocyte Components					
22	Apheresis granulocytes	20°C-24°C	20°C-24°C (as close as possible to)	24 hours	Transfuse as soon as possible
23	Apheresis granulocytes irradiated	20°C-24°C	20°C-24°C (as close as possible to)	No change from original expiration date	Transfuse as soon as possible
Plasma Components					
24	Cryoprecipitated AHF	≤−18°C	Maintain frozen state	12 months from original collection	Thaw the FFP at 1°C-6°C Place cryoprecipitate in the freezer within 1 hour
25	Thawed cryoprecipitated AHF	20°C-24°C	20°C-24°C (as close as possible to)	Open system or pooled: 4 hours Single unit: 6 hours	Thaw at 30°C-37°C
26	Fresh froze plasma (FFP)	≤−18°C or ≤−65°C	Maintain frozen state	≤−18°C: 12 months ≤−65°C: 7 years	Placed in freezer within 8 hours of collection in CPD, CP2D, CPDA-1, or within 6 hours of collection in ACD or as FDA-cleared Storage at ≤−65°C requires FDA approval
27	Thawed FFP	1°C-6°C	1°C-10°C	24 hours	Thaw at 30°C-37°C or using an FDA-cleared device
28	Plasma frozen within 24 hours after phlebotomy	≤−18°C	Maintain frozen state	12 months from original collection	Placed in freezer within 24 hours of collection
29	Thawed plasma frozen within 24 hours after phlebotomy	1°C-6°C	1°C-10°C	24 hours	Thaw at 30°C-37°C or using an FDA-cleared device
30	Thawed plasma	1°C-6°C	1°C-10°C	5 days from beginning of thawing of original product	
31	Plasma cryoprecipitate reduced	≤−18°C	Maintain frozen state	12 months from original collection	
32	Thawed plasma cryoprecipitate reduced	1°C-6°C	1°C-10°C	5 days	Thaw at 30°C-37°C
33	Liquid plasma	1°C-6°C	1°C-10°C	5 days after expiration of RBCs	21 CFR 640.34(c) applies
34	Recovered plasma (plasma for manufacture), liquid or frozen	Refer to short supply agreement	Refer to short supply agreement	Refer to short supply agreement	Requires a short supply agreement[4]
Tissue and Derivatives					
35	Tissue	Conform to source facility's written instructions	Conform to source facility's written instructions	Conform to source facility's written instructions	
36	Derivatives	Conform to manufacturer's written instructions	Conform to manufacturer's written instructions	Conform to manufacturer's written instructions	

[1]If the seal is broken during processing, components stored at 1°C to 6°C shall have an expiration time of 24 hours and components stored at 20°C to 24°C shall have an expiration time of 4 hours, unless otherwise indicated.
[2]Storage beyond 4 hours requires an FDA-cleared system.
[3]Storage beyond 5 days requires participation in a monitoring program defined by the FDA.
[4]21 CFR 601.22.
From Silva MA: Standards for Blood Banks and Transfusion Services, 24th ed. Bethesda, MD, AABB, 2006, pp 53-60.

Table 6-3 Blood Management Policies* and Interventions

POLICIES/INTERVENTIONS	SETTINGS		
	Preop	Intraop	Postop
Transfusion need should be assessed on a case-by-case basis	X	X	X
Blood should be transfused 1 U at a time, followed by an assessment of benefit and further need	X	X	X
Exposure to allogeneic blood should be limited to appropriate need	X	X	X
Modify the "transfusion trigger" according to the hemoglobin/hematocrit level (option)	X	X	X
Consider the use of directed-donor blood (option)	X	X	X
Perioperative blood loss should be prevented or controlled	X	X	X
Consider stopping treatment with aspirin, nonsteroidal anti-inflammatory drugs, warfarin, heparin, similar anticoagulant drugs, and thrombolytic agents before surgery (standard)	X		
Identify and address any existing coagulopathy (standard)	X	X	X
Restrict perioperative phlebotomy to necessary tests (standard)	X	X	X
Consider the use of regional anesthesia (option)		X	
Consider the use of hypotensive anesthesia (option)		X	
Maintain careful surgical hemostasis (standard)		X	
Modify the surgical approach (option)		X	
Use locally acting agents that encourage clotting, such as fibrin glue, collagen, and topical thrombin (option)		X	
Use fibrinolytic drugs such as aprotinin, aminocaproic acid, desmopressin acetate, and tranexamic acid (option)	X	X	X
Use drugs designed specifically to reduce or stop bleeding in gynecologic conditions (option)	X	X	X
Before resorting to surgery, consider tumor embolization via angiographic techniques (option)	X		
Autologous blood should be considered for use as an alternative to allogeneic transfusion	X	X	X
Consider preoperative autologous blood procurement (option/guideline)	X		
Consider intraoperative acute normovolemic hemodilution (option/guideline)		X	
Consider intraoperative autologous blood salvage and autotransfusion (option/guideline)		X	
Consider postoperative autologous blood salvage and autotransfusion (option)			X
Effort should be made to maximize oxygen delivery in a surgical patient	X	X	X
Treat any underlying cardiopulmonary disease (standard)	X	X	X
Red blood cell mass should be increased or restored by means other than red blood cell transfusion	X		X
Replace iron stores in patients with documented iron deficiency (standard)	X		X
Consider the use of epoetin alfa to increase or restore red blood cell mass (guideline)	X		X
The patient should be involved in the transfusion decision	X		X
The reasons for and results of the transfusion decision should be documented contemporaneously in the patient's record	X	X	X
Hospital transfusion policies and procedures should be developed as a cooperative effort that includes input from all those involved in the transfusion decision	X		X
Transfusion practices, both individual and institutional, should be reassessed yearly or more often	X		X

*Boldface rows are practice policies.
Intraop, intraoperative; Preop, preoperative; Postop, postoperative.
Reprinted from American Journal of Surgery, Vol. 170, No. 6A, supplement, Spence RK, Surgical red blood cell transfusion practice policies. pp. 3S-15S. Copyright 1995, with permission from Excerpta Medica Inc.

high arterial oxygen saturation. The primary compensation in this setting is increased cardiac output (heart rate and stroke volume). Response to the lowered RBC mass and the need for RBC transfusion can be assessed by clinical criteria, such as ongoing blood loss, increased heart rate, dizziness, decreased urinary output, base deficit, lactic acidosis, mixed venous oxygen saturation, and oxygen delivery, and then weighed against potential untoward effects.

In a multicenter, randomized, controlled study of transfusion in 838 patients in the critical care setting, a liberal transfusion strategy (transfusion for hemoglobin <10 g/dL) was compared with a restrictive strategy (transfusion for hemoglobin <7 g/dL). The restrictive strategy was found to be at least as effective as the liberal strategy, with the possible exception of patients with acute myocardial infarction and unstable angina.[23]

In patients with significant cardiopulmonary disease, transfusion may be considered because increases in cardiac output may cause myocardial ischemia. Stable, asymptomatic patients should not receive packed RBCs solely for a hematocrit below 30% (Box 6-1). Each unit

---

Box 6-1 Suggested Transfusion Guidelines for Red Blood Cells

Hemoglobin <8 g/dL or acute blood loss in an otherwise healthy patient with signs and symptoms of decreased oxygen delivery and two or more of the following:

- Estimated or anticipated acute blood loss of >15% of total blood volume (750 mL in a 70-kg male)
- Diastolic blood pressure <60 mm Hg
- Systolic blood pressure drop >30 mm Hg from baseline
- Tachycardia (>100 beats/min)
- Oliguria/anuria
- Mental status changes

Hemoglobin <10 g/dL in patients with a known increased risk for coronary artery disease or pulmonary insufficiency who have sustained or are expected to sustain significant blood loss

Symptomatic anemia with any of the following:

- Tachycardia (>100 beats/min)
- Mental status changes
- Evidence of myocardial ischemia, including angina
- Shortness of breath or dizziness with mild exertion
- Orthostatic hypotension

Unfounded/questionable indications:

- To increase wound healing
- To improve the patient's sense of well-being
- Hemoglobin between 7 and 10 g/dL (or hematocrit from 21%-30%) in an otherwise stable, asymptomatic patient
- Mere availability of predonated autologous blood without medical indication

---

Box 6-2 Suggested Transfusion Guidelines for Platelets

- Recent (within 24 hours) platelet count <10,000/mm^3 (for prophylaxis)
- Recent (within 24 hours) platelet count <50,000/mm^3 with demonstrated microvascular bleeding ("oozing") or a planned surgical/invasive procedure
- Demonstrated microvascular bleeding and a precipitous fall in the platelet count
- Adult patients in the operating room who have had complicated procedures or have required more than 10 units of blood *and* have microvascular bleeding. Giving platelets assumes that adequate surgical hemostasis has been achieved
- Documented platelet dysfunction (e.g., prolonged bleeding time >15 minutes; abnormal platelet function tests) with petechiae, purpura, microvascular bleeding ("oozing"), or a surgical/invasive procedure

Unwarranted indications:

- Empirical use with massive transfusion when the patient is not exhibiting clinically evident microvascular bleeding ("oozing")
- Prophylaxis in patients with thrombotic thrombocytopenic purpura/hemolytic-uremic syndrome or idiopathic thrombocytopenic purpura
- Extrinsic platelet dysfunction (e.g., renal failure, von Willebrand's disease)

---

of packed RBCs usually raises the hematocrit 2% to 3% in a 70-kg adult, although this varies with the donor, the recipient's fluid status, the method of storage, and its duration of storage.

Leukocyte-Reduced Red Blood Cells

An association between immunosuppression and allogeneic transfusion has been noted and subsequently challenged. This effect, termed *transfusion-related immunomodulation*, is thought to be principally related to exposure to leukocytes and may be decreased or prevented with leukocyte-reduced components. Despite significant cost and the lack of a definitive conclusion, the Blood Products Advisory Committee of the U.S. FDA has recommended that "the benefit-to-risk ratio associated with leukoreduction is sufficiently great to justify requiring the universal leukoreduction of all non-leukocyte cellular transfusion blood components."[24(p16)] A University HealthSystem Consortium Expert Panel reviewed the literature and identified four indications for leukocyte-reduced blood components[25]:

1. To decrease the incidence of subsequent refractoriness to platelet transfusion caused by HLA alloimmunization in patients requiring long-term platelet support
2. To provide blood components with reduced risk for transmission of cytomegalovirus (CMV)
3. To prevent subsequent febrile nonhemolytic transfusion reactions in patients who have had one documented episode

4. To decrease the incidence of HLA alloimmunization in nonhepatic solid-organ transplant candidates

Other indications lack evidence for benefit and may adversely affect the risk:benefit ratio secondary to increased financial burden. The majority of RBC and platelet transfusions in the United States are currently leukocyte reduced. Pre-storage leukocyte reduction is preferred to post-storage leukocyte reduction to minimize the accumulation of cytokines and leukocyte degradation products (e.g., histamine) in the stored units.

Platelets

Platelet transfusions (Box 6-2) are indicated for patients suffering from or at significant risk for bleeding as a result of thrombocytopenia or platelet dysfunction, or both. Two types of platelet concentrate are available. A single, random-donor unit of platelets is prepared from a single donation of whole blood from one donor (see Fig. 6-3). Apheresis platelets are harvested from one donor, and the platelet yield is equivalent to that of 6 to 10 single random-donor units. Multiple-unit, single-donor platelets can be obtained by apheresis from donors who are selected by HLA type to yield HLA-matched platelets. Besides monitoring the patient for evidence of improved hemostasis, follow-up platelet counts at 1 hour and 12 or 24 hours can provide an estimate of platelet survival. After platelet transfusion, the platelet count obtained at 1 hour should increase at least 5000 platelets/mm^3 for each unit of platelets transfused. Patients may experience a lesser response, especially after repeated transfusion and the development of alloimmunization or as a result of fever, sepsis, splenomegaly, or drug effects. When alloimmunization causes the poor response, platelets from a donor of an HLA type chosen to match the recipient or avoid the HLA antibodies present in the patient may also be needed.

Platelets are not transfused prophylactically in the absence of microvascular bleeding, a low platelet count in a patient undergoing a surgical procedure, or a platelet count that has fallen below 10,000/mm^3 (see Box 6-2). The following specific triggers for platelet transfusion in surgical patients have been proposed: DIC: 20,000 to 50,000/mm^3; major surgery in leukemia: 50,000/mm^3; thrombocytopenia secondary to massive transfusion: 50,000/mm^3; invasive procedures in cirrhotic patients: 50,000/mm^3; cardiopulmonary bypass: 50,000 to 60,000/mm^3; liver biopsy: 50,000 to 100,000/mm^3; and neurosurgery: 100,000/mm^3.[26] Hypothermia depresses platelet function, and platelet transfusion is generally ineffective. Restoration of a normal temperature returns platelet function to normal and ameliorates microvascular bleeding.

Granulocyte Concentrate

Granulocyte transfusions have been used for profound granulocytopenia (<500/mm^3) with evidence of infection (e.g., positive blood culture, persistent temperature higher than 38.5°C) unresponsive to antibiotic therapy. Daily transfusions are given until the infection is under control or the granulocyte count is greater than 1000/mm^3. Because leukocyte concentrate is usually prepared by apheresis from donors typically premedicated with granulocyte colony-stimulating factor (to stimulate granulocyte production) and corticosteroids (to increase the number of circulating granulocytes via demargination of cells), along with the use of hydroxyethyl starch to enhance the separation of cells, there is more risk to the donor than with a routine blood donation. Such products have a shelf life of 24 hours and are not routinely available. Consultation with specialists in infectious disease is recommended.

Plasma

Plasma products come in several varieties, and in many hospitals fresh frozen plasma is no longer available. Plasma is used to replace labile factors in patients with coagulopathy and documented factor deficiency (Box 6-3). This condition may derive from liver dysfunction, congenital absence of factors, or transfusion of factor-deficient blood products. A unit of plasma contains nearly normal levels of all factors, including about 400 mg of fibrinogen, and increases factor levels by about 3%. Adequate clotting is usually achieved with factor levels above 30%, although higher levels are advisable in patients undergoing operative or invasive procedures. The PT and the aPTT can be used to assess patients for plasma transfusion and to monitor the efficacy of administered plasma.

Documentation of factor deficiency or an abnormal PT or aPTT in a patient with clinical bleeding minimizes the unnecessary use of plasma. Plasma is not administered routinely by a preset formula after RBC transfusion (e.g., 2 units of plasma for every 5 units of packed RBCs) or *prophylactically* after cardiac bypass or other procedures. With equally effective but safer and less expensive crystalloids, plasma is not used as a volume expander. The following criteria are generally accepted indications for plasma transfusion: an INR greater than 1.5 with an anticipated invasive procedure or surgery, massive hemorrhage (>1 blood volume) with an INR higher than 1.5, treatment of thrombotic thrombocytopenic purpura, inherited coagulopathies in which a specific factor concentrate is not available, and emergency reversal of anticoagulant therapy.[27]

Solvent detergent (SD)-treated plasma was approved by the U.S. FDA to inactivate enveloped viruses, particularly HIV, hepatitis B virus (HBV), and HCV. Because of reports of deaths from thromboembolic complications or severe bleeding, SD plasma is not used in patients with severe liver disease and a known coagulopathy or in patients undergoing liver transplantation. The American Red Cross has discontinued supplying the product, and SD plasma is no longer available in the United States.

Cryoprecipitate

Cryoprecipitate is useful in treating factor deficiency (hemophilia A), von Willebrand's disease, and hypofibrinogenemia and may help treat uremic bleeding. Each 5- to 15-mL unit contains more than 80 units of factor VIII and about 200 mg of fibrinogen. Because the proteins mentioned previously are in relatively high concentration, a smaller volume may be given than would be required if plasma were used. Cryoprecipitate is usually administered as a transfusion of 10 single units.

Perioperative Transfusion

The decision to transfuse a patient before surgery addresses several factors. No specific hematocrit is an indication for preoperative transfusion in a stable patient. A symptomatic patient with anemia who is about to undergo a procedure that involves significant blood loss may benefit from perioperative transfusion. If the patient is anemic with a low (or normal) reticulocyte count, transfusion may be the only way to raise the hemoglobin level before surgery. Patients with chronic anemia whose condition is otherwise stable are not transfused on the basis of a hematocrit of 30%. The goal of transfusion in a symptomatic patient is relief of symptoms. Previously, single-unit transfusion was condemned; however, if 1 unit is sufficient to alleviate symptoms, no additional transfusion is given because each unit adds to the risk.

The maximal surgical blood order schedule was designed to minimize the use of perioperative RBC-containing products and is usually based on the institution's or physician's record of transfusion for certain operative procedures. When a surgeon requests blood preoperatively, a *type-and-screen* procedure is performed to determine the patient's ABO and D types and to detect preformed antibodies to RBC antigens. If the antibody screen is negative and the probability that the patient will require blood in the operating room is less than 10%, RBCs are not crossmatched unless the patient needs blood during the procedure. An abbreviated crossmatch is then performed within a few minutes. If the probability of transfusion is greater than 10%, blood is crossmatched preoperatively. The number of units prepared is a function of the number of units transfused during the procedure in the past. Typically, the number of units crossmatched is the number that would cover 90% of such procedures. In operations in which blood is frequently used, such as open heart or vascular procedures, the minimal number of units is crossmatched and additional units are made available if they are needed. When a procedure is completed, blood is held for 24 to 48 hours and then automatically released for other patients. This process allows the most efficient use of blood products and avoids the full, three-phase crossmatch.

Transfusion of Patients in Shock

During World War I, it was believed that toxins caused vascular collapse in injured patients. Experiments in the 1930s by Dallas B. Phemister and Alfred Blalock showed that fluid was lost from the circulation into damaged tissues—the concept of a *third space*. In World War II, plasma was the resuscitation solution of choice. Although solutions containing electrolytes were used for children with diarrhea and advances had increased understanding of the metabolic and endocrine changes seen with injury, the use of plasma solutions prevailed until the Korean conflict. Subsequent experimental work indicated that extracellular fluids shifted into the intracellular space after significant hemorrhage with shock. Providing volume resuscitation in excess of shed blood became standard practice to maintain adequate circulation.

During World War II, acute tubular necrosis was a common consequence of hypovolemic shock. As fluid resuscitation became more prevalent during the Korean and Vietnam conflicts, the incidence of acute tubular necrosis decreased. Although acute tubular necrosis after hypovolemic shock became less common with better fluid resuscitation, adult respiratory distress syndrome became increasingly common. The lung injury in adult respiratory

distress syndrome, however, is a function of the shock state rather than the resuscitation solution used.

The goal of resuscitation from shock is prompt restoration of adequate perfusion and transport of oxygen. The American College of Surgeons Committee on Trauma developed a classification of shock that permits useful guidelines for resuscitation. Crystalloid is infused at a 3:1 ratio for every unit of RBCs administered, and therapy is monitored by hemodynamic response. Because crystalloid solutions are universally available and some delay is required to prepare blood products, crystalloid is the proper initial resuscitation fluid. Resuscitation proceeds with the use of blood products, depending on the patient's response. The choice of a colloid solution (e.g., albumin, plasma) or a crystalloid solution (e.g., lactated Ringer's solution) has been controversial. Both can expand the extracellular space and provide effective resuscitation. Crystalloid solutions are favored because they are less expensive, need not be crossmatched, do not transmit disease, and probably create less fluid accumulation in the lung. No experimental data indicate that using colloid rather than crystalloid solutions can prevent pulmonary edema. An updated review of randomized controlled trials of albumin found no evidence of reduced mortality in hypovolemic patients or in critically ill patients with burns and hypoalbuminemia.[28]

Several crystalloid solutions are available for resuscitation, but isotonic solutions are used to avoid overload of free water. Lactated Ringer's solution is recommended as initial therapy. Metabolic alkalosis is common after successful resuscitation with lactated Ringer's solution and blood products because the lactate in Ringer's solution and the citrate in banked blood are both converted to bicarbonate in the liver. Lactated Ringer's solution contains calcium, and if it is mixed with a blood product, the blood may clot in the bag. Normal saline solution is an acceptable alternative to lactated Ringer's solution, but large volumes can produce hyperchloremic metabolic acidosis, which may complicate the use of base deficit in resuscitation.

RISKS ASSOCIATED WITH BLOOD TRANSFUSION

Physicians need to exercise judgment when prescribing a blood transfusion; a transfusion that is not clearly indicated is contraindicated. A transfusion of incompatible RBCs is potentially fatal, but other significant concerns exist when a patient receives blood products, including infectious hazards and immunologic effects. With the introduction of predonation screening for risk factors for hepatitis and HIV infection, as well as donor blood testing, the risk of viral transmission has fallen dramatically since the early 1980s. Administrative error leading to ABO incompatibility, bacterial contamination, and transfusion-related lung injury are the three leading causes of fatality after blood transfusion.[29] To the public, HIV infection and viral hepatitis remain the major risks associated with transfusion. Other transfusion risks include nonhemolytic reactions, graft-versus-host disease, volume overload, and immunomodulation. Physicians prescribing transfusions need to recognize these transfusion-related complications and be prepared to discuss these risks with patients and their families.

Transfusion Reactions

Transfusion reactions can be categorized broadly into acute (<24 hours) and delayed (>24 hours) reactions (Table 6-4). Hemolytic reactions are caused by complement-mediated destruction of transfused RBCs secondary to preexisting antibodies, and the severity of the reaction is determined by the degree of complement activation and cytokine release.[30] Severe acute hemolytic reactions generally involve the transfusion of ABO-incompatible blood, with fatalities occurring in 1 in 600,000 units.[31] As the RBCs are rapidly destroyed, peptides derived from complement are released and produce hypotension, compromise renal blood flow, activate coagulation, and lead to DIC. Signs and symptoms include pain and redness along the infused vein, chest tightness and pain, a feeling of doom, hypotension, oozing from IV sites, oliguria, chills, fever, hemoglobinemia, and hemoglobinuria. In an unconscious patient, hypotension, hemoglobinuria, and diffuse oozing may be the only clues.

When a transfusion reaction is suspected, the infusion must be stopped immediately and the label on the unit checked against the recipient's wristband. The unit, with all attached IV solutions and tubing, is sent to the blood bank along with blood samples drawn from a remote site. The blood needs to be tested for hemoglobinemia, and the urine need to be tested for free hemoglobin. The blood bank checks all samples and records and performs a direct antiglobulin test. The patient must receive aggressive fluid resuscitation to correct hypotension and maintain renal blood flow. A brisk diuresis may be initiated with furosemide, and agents that increase renal blood flow need to be considered. Patients in whom hypotension and DIC develop early are at greatest risk for death.

Delayed hemolytic reactions tend to occur 5 to 10 days after transfusion,[30] with a significant hemolytic reaction developing in approximately 1 in 260,000 patients.[2] The degree of hemolysis may be significant in a patient whose total RBC mass has been replaced by massive transfusion. A transfused patient in whom an unexplained fall in hematocrit, fever, or jaundice develops needs to be evaluated for the possibility of a hemolytic reaction. The workup is similar to that for acute hemolytic reactions, and the need for clinical intervention is less likely.

Allergic nonhemolytic reactions are generally believed to be caused by recipient antibodies to infused donor plasma proteins. The manifestations vary from a slight rash or urticaria to hemodynamic instability with bronchospasm and anaphylaxis. Allergic reactions may be prevented by premedication with antihistamines (e.g., diphenhydramine). Recipient antibodies against antigens on donor leukocytes or platelets cause febrile nonhemolytic reactions. Fevers and chills characterize these reactions shortly after the transfusion has started. An acute hemolytic reaction and bacterial contamination of the unit must be excluded. Treatment consists of antipyretics

and transfusion of leukocyte-depleted blood components when pharmacotherapy fails.

Transmission of Infection

Infections transmitted by blood transfusion include bacteria, Epstein-Barr virus, CMV, hepatitis viruses, HIV and human T-cell leukemia virus (HTLV) types I and II, parvovirus B19, human herpesvirus 8, TT (transfusion transmitted) virus, mad cow disease (bovine spongiform encephalopathy), and West Nile virus (Table 6-5). Since March 1999, pooled nucleic acid amplification testing (NAT) has been used to test for HIV and HCV; NAT involves pooling of 16 to 24 individual blood samples and polymerase chain reaction or other amplification techniques to test for HIV and HCV nucleic sequences. Bacterial and protozoal diseases include syphilis, malaria, and infection with *Babesia microti, Trypanosoma cruzi, Yersinia enterocolitica, Serratia marcescens, Staphylococcus aureus, Staphylococcus epidermidis,* and *Klebsiella pneumoniae.*[2] *T. cruzi* causes Chagas' disease, but transmission of this infection is very rare in the United States.

Bacterial Contamination

Bacterial contamination of blood is the most frequent cause of transfusion-transmitted infectious disease.[32] After hemolytic reactions and transfusion-related acute lung injury (TRALI), it is the most frequently reported cause of transfusion-related fatalities to the U.S. FDA.[33] The agents most often implicated in packed RBC bacteremia were *Serratia* and *Yersinia.* For platelets, *S. aureus, Escherichia coli, Enterobacter,* and *Serratia* species were more frequently identified. Fever, chills, hypotension, tachycardia, and shock after transfusion should raise suspicion of bacterial contamination, and blood cultures of the patient and unit must be obtained. Platelets stored at 20°C to 24°C are a good growth medium for bacteria. Platelets are now screened for bacterial contamination in the United States.

Transfusion-Related Acute Lung Injury

Fatal pulmonary edema associated with transfusion was first described in 1951 by Barnard, and the term *TRALI* was coined in 1983 by Popovsky. Its incidence is estimated to be one case per 5000 units transfused,[2] but the syndrome is often underdiagnosed. It is now known to be the most common cause of fatal transfusion reactions.[34] TRALI is a clinical syndrome associated with the transfusion of all blood components, especially platelets and plasma. TRALI is characterized by the onset of dyspnea, hypotension, hypoxemia, fever, and bilateral noncardiogenic pulmonary edema within 6 hours of transfusion. The diagnosis is one of exclusion after volume overload, cardiogenic pulmonary edema, or acute respiratory distress syndrome has been ruled out. The pathophysiology is thought to be due to the transfusion of donor leukocyte antibodies or biologically active lipids from donor blood cell membranes into recipients.[2] Some recipients are more susceptible to development of the syndrome, such as those with infection, cytokine admin-

Text continued on p 135

Table 6-4 Categories and Management of Adverse Transfusion Reactions

TYPE	INCIDENCE	ETIOLOGY	MANIFESTATION	DIAGNOSTIC TESTING	THERAPEUTIC/PROPHYLACTIC APPROACH
Acute (<24 Hours) Transfusion Reactions—Immunologic					
Hemolytic	1:38,000-1:70,000	Red cell incompatibility	Chills, fever, hemoglobinuria, hypotension, renal failure with oliguria, DIC (oozing from IV sites), back pain, pain along the infusion vein, anxiety	Clerical check DAT Visual inspection (free hemoglobin) Repeat patient ABO, pre- and post-transfusion sample Further tests as indicated to define possible incompatibility Further tests to detect hemolysis (LDH, bilirubin, etc.)	Keep urine output >100 mL/hr Analgesics (may need morphine) Pressors for hypotension Hemostatic components (platelets, cryoprecipitate, plasma) for bleeding
Fever/chill, nonhemolytic	RBCs: 1:200-1:17 (0.5%-6%) Platelets: 1:100-1:3 (1%-38%)	Antibody to donor WBCs Accumulated cytokines in platelet unit	Fever, chills/rigors, headache, vomiting	Rule out hemolysis (DAT, inspect for hemoglobinemia, repeat patient ABO) Rule out bacterial contamination WBC antibody screen	Antipyretic premedication (acetaminophen, no aspirin) Leukocyte-reduced blood
Urticarial	1:100-1:33 (1%-3%)	Antibody to donor plasma proteins	Urticaria, pruritus, flushing	No testing needed	Antihistamine, treatment or premedication (PO or IV) May start unit slowly after antihistamine if symptoms resolve
Anaphylactic	1:20,000-1:50,000	Antibody to donor plasma proteins (includes IgA, haptoglobin, C4)	Hypotension, urticaria, bronchospasm (respiratory distress, wheezing), local edema, anxiety	Rule out hemolysis (DAT, inspect for hemoglobinemia, repeat patient ABO) Anti-IgA IgA, quantitative	Trendelenburg position Fluids Epinephrine (adult dose: 0.3-0.5 mL of 1:1000 solution SC or IM; in severe cases, 1:10,000 IV) Antihistamines, corticosteroids, β_2-agonists IgA-deficient blood components
Transfusion-related acute lung injury	1:5000-1:190,000	WBC antibodies in donor (occasionally in recipient), other WBC-activating agents in components	Hypoxemia, respiratory failure, hypotension, fever, bilateral pulmonary edema	Rule out hemolysis (DAT, inspect for hemoglobinemia, repeat patient ABO) WBC antibody screen in donor and recipient. If positive, antigen typing may be indicated WBC crossmatch Chest x-ray	Supportive care until recovery Defer implicated donors

Table 6-4   Categories and Management of Adverse Transfusion Reactions—cont'd

TYPE	INCIDENCE	ETIOLOGY	MANIFESTATION	DIAGNOSTIC TESTING	THERAPEUTIC/PROPHYLACTIC APPROACH
Acute (<24 Hours) Transfusion Reaction—Nonimmunologic					
Transfusion-associated sepsis	Varies by component	Bacterial contamination	Fever, chills, hypotension	Gram stain Culture of component Patient culture Rule out hemolysis (DAT, inspect for hemoglobinemia, repeat patient ABO)	Broad-spectrum antibiotics (until sensitivity testing completed) Treat complications (e.g., shock)
Hypotension associated with ACE inhibition	Dependent on clinical setting	Inhibited metabolism of bradykinin with infusion of bradykinin (negatively charged filters) or activators of prekallikrein	Flushing, hypotension	Rule out hemolysis (DAT, inspect for hemoglobinemia, repeat patient ABO)	Withdraw ACE inhibition Avoid albumin volume replacement for plasmapheresis Avoid bedside leukocyte filtration
Circulatory overload	<1%	Volume overload	Dyspnea, orthopnea, cough, tachycardia, hypertension, headache	Chest x-ray	Upright posture Oxygen IV diuretic (furosemide) Phlebotomy (250-mL increments)
Nonimmune hemolysis	Rare	Physical or chemical destruction of blood (heating, freezing, hemolytic drug or solution added to blood)	Hemoglobinuria, hemoglobinemia	Rule out patient hemolysis (DAT, inspect for hemoglobinemia, repeat patient ABO) Test unit for hemolysis	Identify and eliminate cause
Air embolus	Rare	Air in infusion line	Sudden shortness of breath, acute cyanosis, pain, cough, hypotension, cardiac dysrhythmia	X-ray for intravascular air	Place patient on left side with legs elevated above chest and head
Hypocalcemia (ionized calcium)	Dependent on clinical setting	Rapid citrate infusion (massive transfusion of citrated blood, delayed metabolism of citrate, apheresis procedures)	Paresthesia, tetany, dysrhythmia	Ionized calcium Prolonged QT interval on electrocardiogram	Slow calcium infusion while monitoring ionized calcium levels in severe cases PO calcium supplement for mild symptoms during apheresis procedures
Hypothermia	Dependent on clinical setting	Rapid infusion of cold blood	Cardiac dysrhythmia	Central body temperature	Use blood warmer

Continued

Table 6-4   Categories and Management of Adverse Transfusion Reactions—cont'd

TYPE	INCIDENCE	ETIOLOGY	MANIFESTATION	DIAGNOSTIC TESTING	THERAPEUTIC/PROPHYLACTIC APPROACH
Delayed (>24 Hours) Transfusion Reactions—Immunologic					
Alloimmunization, RBC antigens	1:100 (1%)	Immune response to foreign antigens on RBCs, WBCs, or platelets (HLA)	Positive blood group antibody screening test	Antibody screen DAT	Avoid unnecessary transfusions Leukocyte-reduced blood
Alloimmunization, HLA antigens	1:10 (10%)	Immune response to foreign antigens on RBCs, WBCs, or platelets (HLA)	Platelet refractoriness, delayed hemolytic reaction, hemolytic disease of the newborn	Platelet antibody screen Lymphocytotoxicity test	Avoid unnecessary transfusions Leukocyte-reduced blood
Hemolytic	1:5000-1:11,000	Anamnestic immune response to red cell antigens	Fever, decreasing hemoglobin, new positive antibody screening test, mild jaundice	Antibody screen DAT Tests for hemolysis (visual inspection for hemoglobinemia, LDH, bilirubin, urinary hemosiderin as clinically indicated)	Identify antibody Transfuse compatible red cells as needed
Graft-versus-host disease	Rare	Donor lymphocytes engraft in recipient and mount attack on host tissues	Erythroderma, maculopapular rash, anorexia, nausea, vomiting, diarrhea, hepatitis, pancytopenia, fever	Skin biopsy HLA typing	Corticosteroids, cytotoxic agents Irradiation of blood components for patients at risk (including related donors and HLA-selected components)
Post-transfusion purpura	Rare	Recipient platelet antibodies (apparent alloantibody, usually anti–HPA-1) destroy autologous platelets	Thrombocytopenic purpura, bleeding 8-10 days after transfusion	Platelet antibody screen and identification	IGIV HPA-1–negative platelets Plasmapheresis
Immunomodulation	Unknown	Incompletely understood interaction of donor WBC or plasma factors with recipient immune system	Increased renal graft survival, infection rate, postresection tumor recurrence rate (controversial)	None specific	Avoid unnecessary transfusions Autologous transfusion Leukocyte-reduced red cells and platelets
Delayed (>24 Hours) Transfusion Reactions—Nonimmunologic					
Iron overload	Typically after >100 RBC units	Multiple transfusions with obligate iron load in transfusion-dependent patient	Diabetes, cirrhosis, cardiomyopathy	Serum ferritin Liver enzymes Endocrine function tests	Deferoxamine (iron chelator)

ACE, angiotensin-converting enzyme; DAT, direct antiglobulin test; DIC, disseminated intravascular coagulation; HPA-1, human platelet antigen-1; IGIV, intravenous immunoglobulin; IM, intramuscular; IV, intravenous; LDH, lactate dehydrogenase; PO, per os; RBC, red blood cell; SC, subcutaneous; WBC, white blood cell.

Adapted from Brecker ME (ed): Technical Manual, 15th ed. Bethesda, MD, AABB, 2005, p 634-638.

Table 6-5   Risk of Infection Associated With Blood Transfusion in the United States

INFECTIOUS AGENT OR OUTCOME	ESTIMATED RISK PER UNIT TRANSFUSED	ESTIMATED PERCENTAGE OF INFECTED UNITS THAT TRANSMIT OR CAUSE CLINICAL SEQUELAE
Viruses		
HIV-1 and -2	1:1,400,000-1:2,400,000	90
HTLV-I and -II	1:256,000-1:2,000,000	30
HAV	1:1,000,000	90
HBV	1:58,000-1:147,000	70
HCV	1:872,000-1:1,700,000	90
B19 parvovirus	1:3300-1:40,000	Low
Bacteria		
RBCs	1:1000	1:10,000,000 fatal
Platelets (screened by Gram stain, pH, or glucose concentration)	1:2000-1:4000	>40% result in clinical sequelae
Platelets (screened by early aerobic culture)	<1:10,000	Unknown
Parasites		
Babesiosis and malaria	<1:1,000,000	Unknown
Trypanosoma cruzi	Unknown	<20

HAV, hepatitis A virus; HBC, hepatitis B virus; HCV, hepatitis C virus; HIV, human immunodeficiency virus; HTLV, human T-cell leukemia virus; RBC, red blood cell.

Adapted from Brecker ME (ed): Technical Manual, 15th ed. Bethesda, MD, AABB, 2005, p 700. See reference for other data sources.

istration, recent surgery, and massive transfusion. The donor antibodies attack recipient leukocytes that localize to the pulmonary microvasculature and release cytokines that lead to an increase in vascular permeability and fluid exudation. Biologically active lipids serve to prime the recipient's neutrophils and lead to similar effects on the pulmonary microcirculation. Treatment of TRALI is mainly supportive and consists of hemodynamic and respiratory support. Overall mortality is 5% to 10%.[35] The blood bank must be notified so that the donated blood can be tested for anti-HLA or antigranulocyte antibodies, or both. Blood donations from multiparous women have been implicated as a contributor to the disease.[35]

Hepatitis

Transmission of the infectious agents for hepatitis is among the most serious risks associated with blood transfusion. Past estimates of post-transfusion hepatitis were approximately 10%. Current data suggest that the risk of becoming infected with hepatitis is less than 0.01% per unit transfused.[2] All blood is screened for HBV with tests for hepatitis B surface antigen (HBsAg) and antibody to hepatitis B core antigen (anti-HBc). In addition, blood is screened for HCV with anti-HCV testing. Transfusion-associated HBV infection occurs in approximately 1 in 30,000 to 250,000 units transfused.[30] With the development of pooled NAT for HCV, the window period has decreased, and the risk of transmitting HCV is now as low as 1 in 1 million.[29] Not a single new case of transfusion-associated HCV infection has been detected by the Centers for Disease Control and Prevention (CDC) Senti-

nel Counties Viral Hepatitis Surveillance System since 1994.

Symptoms develop in approximately half the blood recipients who contract HBV infection. A much smaller percentage require hospitalization. In approximately half the patients who contract post-transfusion HCV infection, a chronic form of the disease develops. Significant liver dysfunction, including cirrhosis, eventually develops in many of these patients.

Human Immunodeficiency Virus

The risk of HIV transmission from blood transfusion has decreased dramatically since the early 1980s despite an increasing incidence of HIV infection in the general population. The window period from initial infection to development of antibody to the virus poses a problem in the ability to detect all seropositive donors. With pooled NAT, the window period for detection of HIV has been reduced by 30% to 50%, and the risk of HIV transmission is estimated to be as low as 1 in 2 million units.[29]

Human T-Cell Leukemia Virus

In addition to transmission of CMV, hepatitis infection, and HIV, blood transfusion carries the risk of transmission of HTLV-I and HTLV-II infection. Transmission of the virus, especially to immunocompromised patients, may cause illnesses such as T-cell leukemia, spastic paraparesis, and myelopathy and has prompted routine screening of donors in the United States since 1989. The risk of HTLV-I and HTLV-II transmission is estimated to be 1 in 641,000 units.

Herpesviruses

CMV infection is endemic, so routine screening is not performed in the United States. About 20% of blood donors are infected with CMV by 20 years of age, and approximately 70% are infected by the age of 70. The infection is carried in white blood cells. Most patients who encounter problems with CMV are immunocompromised, especially transplant recipients taking immunosuppressive drugs. Such patients require transfusion with blood products that have reduced risk for CMV infection (leukocyte reduced or seronegative) to avoid transmission of this viral infection. Human herpesvirus 8 causes Kaposi's sarcoma and lymphoma in patients with acquired immunodeficiency syndrome and other immunosuppressed states such as transplantation.

Graft-Versus-Host Reaction

Blood transfusion exposes the recipient to many cells and proteins from the donor. When immunologically competent lymphocytes are introduced into an immunocompromised patient, a graft-versus-host reaction can occur.[30] The functional donor lymphocytes attack recipient tissues, notably the bone marrow, and cause aplasia. Patients have fever, rash, nausea, vomiting, diarrhea, liver function test abnormalities, and depressed cell counts. This complication is fatal in as many as 90% of cases. The prevalence of this complication in the United States is not known but it is thought to be rare. Rare cases have also been reported with familial-directed donations and with HLA-matched platelets. Gamma-irradiation of blood products eliminates this risk.

Immunomodulation

Allogeneic blood transfusion may alter the immune response in individuals and susceptibility to infection, tumor recurrence, and reactivation of latent viruses. It has been known since 1974 that transfusion of packed RBCs depresses the immune response in patients undergoing renal transplantation; however, it is unclear to what extent these immunosuppressive effects are present in other recipients. Contradictory evidence exists about an increased incidence of infections in patients given allogeneic blood transfusions. Similar controversy also exists regarding the exact relationship of blood transfusions to increased recurrence of tumor and poor prognosis. Early studies on colorectal cancer showed decreased survival and increased tumor recurrence in patients who were heavily transfused. Since then, studies on many tumors have been performed and have not yielded a decisive answer. The possibility exists that blood transfusion may represent a covariable because very ill patients and those undergoing more difficult procedures for more extensive disease are more likely to receive blood transfusion. In light of the immunomodulating effects of allogeneic blood transfusion, leukocyte-depleted transfusions have been suggested as an alternative. In view of the data on immunosuppression from blood transfusion, it would seem reasonable to adopt a policy of blood conservation in the perioperative period in the absence of clear indications and acute symptoms. Leukocyte reduction of blood products is thought to decrease the risk for immunomodulation.[36]

MASSIVE TRANSFUSION

Massive transfusion is defined as replacement of the patient's blood volume with packed RBCs in 24 hours or transfusion of more than 10 units of blood over a period of a few hours. Massive transfusion can create significant changes in the patient's metabolic status because of the infusion of large volumes of cold citrate-containing blood that has undergone changes during storage. When blood is stored at 1°C to 6°C, changes occur over time, including leakage of intracellular potassium, decrease in pH, reduced levels of intracellular ATP and 2,3-DPG in RBCs with increased affinity of hemoglobin for oxygen, degeneration of functional granulocytes and platelets, and deterioration of factors V and VIII. If a large volume of stored blood is infused rapidly, significant effects may be seen in the recipient. Many of the expected changes can be reversed after transfusion or may produce metabolic patterns different from those predicted. Consequently, the use of standard formulas for the infusion of plasma, platelets, calcium, bicarbonate, and other substances for a specific number of units of packed RBCs transfused is unwarranted and may subject the patient to increased risk.

Acid-Base Changes

Even though stored RBCs and whole blood have an acid pH (~6.3), alkalosis is the usual result of massive transfusion. Sodium citrate, the anticoagulant in blood products, is converted to sodium bicarbonate in the liver. The alkalosis increases the oxygen affinity of hemoglobin. Because alkalosis stimulates enzymes in the Embden-Meyerhof pathway of glycolysis, the net effect is to increase intracellular 2,3-DPG and restore RBC transport of oxygen. Post-transfusion pH may range from 7.48 to 7.50 and is associated with increased excretion of potassium. Routine administration of bicarbonate with large transfusion volumes is contraindicated because it causes more severe alkalosis with undesirable effects on myocardial contractility and greater affinity of hemoglobin for oxygen.

Changes in 2,3-Diphosphoglycerate

Because 2,3-DPG is greatly reduced in RBCs after about 3 weeks of storage, massive transfusion of a patient with blood near the end of its storage life may decrease oxygen off-loading. Rapid correction occurs in most cases after the RBCs are transfused and rewarmed (50% by 12 hours and 100% by 24 hours).

Changes in Potassium

Hyperkalemia is theoretically possible with massive blood transfusion because stored blood has elevated potassium concentrations, as high as 30 to 40 mEq/L by 3 weeks of storage. Unless the transfusion rate exceeds 100 to 150 mL/min, clinical problems associated with potassium are rare. Most patients requiring rapid transfusion are in shock and have an increase in aldosterone, antidiuretic hormone, and permissive steroid hormones that causes hypokalemia unless renal function ceases. Hyperkalemia may cause peaked T waves on the electrocardiogram. Hyperkalemia, especially if associated with hypocalcemia, may significantly alter cardiac function. Immediate treatment of hyperkalemia is aimed at depressing the membrane threshold potential with calcium, 5 mmol given IV over a 5-minute period. Somewhat paradoxically, hypokalemia is often seen after massive transfusion as the red cells rewarm and begin to absorb potassium.

Hypocalcemia

Massive transfusion of citrated blood products can lead to transiently decreased levels of ionized calcium. The effects of hypocalcemia include hypotension, narrowed pulse pressure, and elevated left ventricular end-diastolic pulmonary artery and central venous pressure. Electrocardiographic abnormalities (e.g., prolonged QT intervals) also occur. Most normothermic adults who are not in shock can withstand the infusion of 1 unit of RBCs every 5 minutes without requiring calcium supplementation. Indiscriminate administration of calcium can produce transient hypercalcemia and needs to be avoided.

Hemostasis

Dilutional thrombocytopenia may occur in a patient who is massively transfused because the number of viable platelets is almost nonexistent in blood stored for 24 hours at 1°C to 6°C. The decrease is often less than expected on the basis of simple dilution. This effect is not completely understood. Release of platelets from the spleen and bone marrow may account for part of the difference.

Despite the fact that platelet counts may fall with massive transfusion, dilutional thrombocytopenia alone does not usually account for microvascular bleeding. Prophylactic use of platelet concentrate in a massively transfused patient is not justified without evidence of microvascular bleeding. Platelet concentrate contains significant amounts of all factors except V and VIII (24%-35% and 39%-70%, respectively, after 5 days of storage). Patients receiving large-volume blood transfusion who experience microvascular bleeding unrelated to hypothermia are best treated with platelet concentrate, which provides factors in addition to platelets. The PT and aPTT provide a reliable indicator for the need for plasma and factor replacement. The prophylactic use of plasma along with transfusion of RBCs is no longer acceptable in light of convincing data and the added risk of transfusion. In patients in whom DIC develops, large doses of platelet concentrate, plasma, and cryoprecipitate may be required. Infusion of plasma is often not indicated unless the PT or PTT is greater than 1.5 times the normal value. It is also important to note that it is virtually impossible to completely normalize the PT and PTT with plasma infusions alone.

Some major changes in massively transfused patients are opposite what might be expected based on the changes that occur during the storage of RBCs. In patients requiring massive transfusion, packed RBCs are transfused to provide oxygen-carrying capacity, platelets are given for microvascular bleeding in a normothermic patient, and crystalloid solution is infused to restore intravascular volume. In most instances, the addition of bicarbonate or calcium and prophylactic transfusion of plasma are not warranted.

BLOOD SUBSTITUTES AND ALTERNATIVES TO TRANSFUSION

Autologous Blood

Patients scheduled for elective procedures in which significant blood loss requiring transfusion is expected may be considered for autologous blood donation. Autologous blood transfusion has many advantages, including compatibility and the lack of viral transmission risk. If the patient is free of infection and severe cardiac disease and has a hematocrit of at least 30%, predonation should be possible. Usually, 2 to 3 units can be obtained. Disadvantages of autologous blood donation are higher cost than for allogeneic blood transfusion, postoperative anemia, increased risk for allogeneic blood transfusion,[2] and a discard rate of 20% to 73% of the units (Table 6-6).[37] Because acute normovolemic hemodilution (ANH) is effective and less costly than preoperative donation, ANH is more likely to be used in future blood-conserving strategies.[38]

Acute Normovolemic Hemodilution

ANH involves the removal of 1 to 3 units of the patient's blood and replacement with crystalloid or colloid (or both) to restore intravascular volume. Performed after induction of anesthesia but before commencement of the operative procedure, ANH is tolerated well in most patient populations. The withdrawn blood is anticoagulated and maintained at room temperature for up to 4 hours. It is reinfused into the patient as needed during the surgical procedure. If ANH is combined with autologous predonation, 6 or more units of blood can be available for a procedure in which significant blood loss is expected. Studies comparing ANH with preoperative autologous blood donation show equal rates of the necessity for allogeneic blood transfusion, but ANH costs are lower.[37,38] There is no role for this technique in acute hemorrhage.

Autologous Cell Salvage

Salvage of intraoperative blood loss can minimize the need for blood transfusion. This technique has had successful applications in many operative procedures, including cardiac surgery, spine surgery, liver transplantation, trauma, and vascular surgery. Blood is suctioned from the field, washed or filtered (or both), and returned to

Table 6-6   **Alternatives to Allogeneic Transfusion**

TECHNIQUE	PRODUCT	DISADVANTAGES/STATUS
Autologous blood		Requires donation days to weeks before planned blood loss Potential for clerical error Cost
Acute normovolemic hemodilution		No role in acute hemorrhage Increased logistic requirements
Autologous cell salvage	Cell saver Chest tube Drains	Potential for contamination Cost
Iron supplementation	Ferrous gluconate Ferrous sulfate	Constipation/diarrhea False-positive fecal occult blood test Requires days to weeks for effect
Epoetin alfa (recombinant human erythropoietin)	Epogen (Amgen) Procrit (Ortho Biotech)	Hypertension, seizures, thrombotic events Cost
Antifibrinolytic agents	Aprotinin (Trasylol, Bayer) Tranexamic acid (Cyklokapron, Pharmacia and Upjohn) Aminocaproic acid (Amicar, Wyeth-Ayerst)	Thromboembolic events such as myocardial infarction and stroke (mostly reported with aprotinin) and renal dysfunction
Recombinant activated factor VII	NovoSeven (Novo Nordisk)	Cost
Oxygen Carriers		
Perflubron (perfluorocarbon)	Oxygent HT (Alliance Pharmaceutical)	Increased rate of strokes, trials halted
Hemoglobin-based substitutes (bovine)	Hemopure (Biopure)	Hypertension, increased amylase and lipase Phase III trials
	PEG-hemoglobin (Enzon)	Early-phase trials as radiosensitizer
Hemoglobin-based substitutes (human)	Diaspirin cross-linked hemoglobin/HemAssist (Baxter)	Increased mortality in phase III trials Trials closed
	PolyHeme (Northfield)	Elevated bilirubin and amylase Phase III trials
	Hemolink (Hemosol)	Increased rate of myocardial infarcts, trials halted
	PHP (Apex Bioscience)	Trials terminated
	Hemospan (Sangart)	Phase II trials
Hemoglobin-based substitute (recombinant)	Optro (Somatogen/Baxter)	All phase I trials terminated

PEG, polyethylene glycol.

the patient. Relative contraindications include fields with gross bacterial contamination, ascitic or amniotic fluid, and free tumor tissue.[2] Filtration plus irradiation has been proposed to further eliminate tumor cells.[37] Risks associated with intraoperative cell salvage include air embolism, dilutional coagulopathy, and hemolysis. The procedure is cost-effective when at least 2 shed units can be salvaged.[2]

Iron Supplementation

Oral iron supplementation with either ferrous gluconate or ferrous sulfate is indicated for iron deficiency anemia. It is inexpensive and generally well tolerated, but it can cause constipation or diarrhea and may also be associated with a false-positive reaction on occult fecal blood testing.

Erythropoietin

Erythropoietin is a glycoprotein that acts on bone marrow to selectively increase erythropoiesis. It is produced predominantly in the kidney in response to hypoxia, but extrarenal production sites such as the liver have been identified. Recombinant human erythropoietin (rHuEPO) is commercially available and commonly used to treat anemia associated with renal insufficiency, cancer-related anemia, and anemia in the critically ill.[31] Preoperative rHuEPO administration has been shown to decrease the need for allogeneic blood transfusion in orthopedic, urologic, and cardiothoracic procedures.[31,39]

Adverse effects, including hypertension, seizures, and thrombotic events, are few. The major disadvantages of erythropoietin are cost and the interval required for effect, which limits its usefulness in acute hemorrhagic conditions.

Antifibrinolytic Agents

Antifibrinolytic therapy has been used to reduce blood loss after surgery, particularly cardiac surgery, and after trauma. Agents used include aprotinin (Trasylol), tranexamic acid (Cyklokapron), and ε-aminocaproic acid (Amicar). Adverse effects include thromboembolic events, such as myocardial infarction and stroke, and renal dysfunction. An analysis of randomized controlled trials suggested that tranexamic acid and ε-aminocaproic acid were as effective as aprotinin in decreasing red cell transfusion and the need for reoperation and were significantly cheaper.[40] Mangano and colleagues found a doubling of the risk for renal failure and an increased incidence of myocardial infarction or heart failure and stroke or encephalopathy in patients treated with aprotinin.[41] Similarly, Karkouti and associates found an association between aprotinin and renal dysfunction.[42] After these two publications, the FDA issued a Public Health Advisory for aprotinin. Insufficient data are available from randomized controlled trials of antifibrinolytic agents in trauma.[43]

Recombinant Activated Factor VII

rFVIIa is FDA indicated for the treatment of bleeding episodes in hemophilia A or B patients with inhibitors to factor VIII or factor IX, for prevention of bleeding in surgical interventions or invasive procedures in hemophilia A or B patients with inhibitors to factor VIII or factor IX, for the treatment of bleeding episodes in patients with congenital factor VII deficiency, and for prevention of bleeding in surgical interventions or invasive procedures in patients with congenital factor VII deficiency. The use of rFVIIa in hemophilia has been discussed previously (see Hemophilia). Though not an FDA-approved indication, rFVIIa has shown potential as therapy for life-threatening hemorrhage secondary to acquired coagulopathy after major surgery or trauma.[44] rFVIIa is effective in improving clotting ability in patients with impaired liver function, thrombocytopenia, and functional platelet defects.[45,46] For nonemergency anticoagulant reversal, a dose of 20 to 40 µg/kg is recommended. For all other indications, 41 to 90 µg/kg is recommended. Uses of rFVIIa are summarized in Table 6-7.[47]

Red Blood Cell Substitutes

Concern over the short supply of donated blood and the risk of transmitting infection has driven the development of RBC substitutes. At this time, RBC transfusion is the only available clinical method for increasing oxygen-carrying capacity. Several substances that have been considered as RBC substitutes can be divided into two general groups:

1. Synthetic molecules, such as the porphyrins and the perfluorocarbon compounds
2. Molecules that incorporate hemoglobin in their structure, such as conjugated and polymerized stroma-free hemoglobin solutions

Acceptable RBC substitutes must be able to carry at least as much oxygen as hemoglobin normally carries (1.34 mL of oxygen/g of hemoglobin). In addition, these molecules should be stable and have an acceptable half-life. The RBC substitute should have properties that allow it to be completely saturated with oxygen at a normal fraction of inspired oxygen while unloading substantial portions of its transported oxygen at tissue oxygen partial pressure levels. Solutions prepared must be highly purified and free of contaminants and endotoxins.

Perfluorocarbons efficiently transport significant quantities of oxygen and carbon dioxide and have the potential to be an effective RBC substitute. Perfluorocarbons can transport 40 to 50 mL of oxygen/100 mL of solution, which is greater than twice the quantity of oxygen that completely saturated hemoglobin carries in a normal adult. Unfortunately, the loading and unloading of oxygen is linear and not sigmoid as with native hemoglobin. Several perfluorocarbon molecules have been tested in humans, but they are not currently approved in the context of acute hemorrhage. At present, perfluorocarbons are no longer in clinical trials.

Early attempts to prepare hemoglobin solutions consisted of pooling outdated blood, breaking the RBCs open, and extracting the hemoglobin molecules. This solution is termed *stroma-free hemoglobin.* Limitations to the use of stroma-free hemoglobin included its very short half-life in the circulation, relatively low oxygen-carrying capacity, and clearance through the kidneys, with vasoconstriction and direct toxic effects on the kidney. To circumvent these problems, the hemoglobin tetramer was stabilized, polymerized, or pyridoxylated. The resultant hemoglobin-based oxygen carriers (HBOCs) have the same oxygen-carrying capacity as normal blood and stay in circulation 4 to 5 days without being cleared through the kidneys. Subsequent trials in healthy volunteers demonstrated the safety of these solutions in humans. Clinical trials are being conducted to determine the efficacy of HBOCs for acute blood loss and perioperative applications.[48]

Most HBOCs have been found in trials to have a clinical hypertensive or pressor effect, the mechanisms of which are not entirely understood. HBOCs bind available nitric oxide, which may lead to a surplus of vasoconstrictive agents. Alternatively, the lower viscosity of HBOCs decreases flow velocity and shear stress on the endothelial lining, thereby resulting in a decrease in endothelial relaxation factors.[49] Another theory postulates that the decreased oxygen affinity of HBOCs leads to lower oxygen concentration at the tissue level. Autoregulatory mechanisms result in subsequent vasoconstriction,[49] which causes a decrease in cardiac output. A major advantage of most HBOCs is their lack of ability to prime neutrophils as seen with allogeneic blood, thereby resulting in fewer immunomodulatory effects.[48]

HBOCs have been produced from bovine hemoglobin, human hemoglobin, and recombinant hemoglobin (see Table 6-6).[50] They have been tested in animals and humans, but so far only one product (Hemopure) has been licensed for human use in South Africa. Hemopure, produced by Biopure, is a bovine HBOC that has been

Table 6-7 **Recommendations for the Use of Recombinant Factor VIIa (NovoSeven) Therapy**

FDA Indications

Treatment of bleeding episodes in patients with hemophilia A or B and inhibitors to factor VIII or factor IX

Prevention of bleeding in surgical interventions or invasive procedures in patients with hemophilia A or B and inhibitors to factor VIII or factor IX

Treatment of bleeding episodes in patients with congenital factor VII deficiency

Prevention of bleeding in surgical interventions or invasive procedures in patients with congenital factor VII deficiency

Off-Label Use

Closed-space bleeding	Nontraumatic intracranial bleeding	<4 hours since symptom onset	Not taking warfarin or LMWH	Appropriate
			Taking warfarin or LMWH	Appropriate
		≥4 hours since symptom onset	Not taking warfarin or LMWH	Inappropriate
			Taking warfarin or LMWH	Uncertain
	Isolated traumatic head injury	No evidence of expanding bleeding	Not taking warfarin or LMWH	Inappropriate
			Taking warfarin or LMWH	Uncertain
		Evidence of expanding bleeding	Not taking warfarin or LMWH	Uncertain
			Taking warfarin or LMWH	Appropriate
	Retroperitoneal bleeding	Not taking warfarin or LMWH	No significant clotting factor replacement	Inappropriate
			Attempted significant clotting factor replacement*	Uncertain
		Taking warfarin or LMWH	No significant clotting factor replacement	Inappropriate
			Attempted significant clotting factor replacement*	Appropriate
Rescue therapy for surgical patients	Cardiac surgery		No significant clotting factor replacement	Inappropriate
			Attempted significant clotting factor replacement*	Appropriate
	Aortic surgery	Thoracic	No significant clotting factor replacement	Inappropriate
			Attempted significant clotting factor replacement*	Appropriate
		Abdominal	No significant clotting factor replacement	Inappropriate
			Attempted significant clotting factor replacement*	Uncertain
	Hepatic resection or liver transplantation		No significant clotting factor replacement	Uncertain
			Attempted significant clotting factor replacement*	Appropriate
	Nontraumatic high blood loss in orthopedic surgery	Spine	No significant clotting factor replacement	Inappropriate
			Attempted significant clotting factor replacement*	Appropriate
		Large-joint replacement	No significant clotting factor replacement	Inappropriate
			Attempted significant clotting factor replacement*	Inappropriate
Other uses	Postpartum period and after hysterectomy		No significant clotting factor replacement	Inappropriate
			Attempted significant clotting factor replacement*	Appropriate
	Severe multiple trauma		Ongoing bleeding and coagulopathy despite surgical intervention and ≥10 units of blood in 6 hours	Appropriate
	Active GI bleeding			Inappropriate
	Hepatic failure with GI bleeding or pending invasive procedure		No significant clotting factor replacement	Inappropriate
			Attempted significant clotting factor replacement*	Appropriate
	Thrombocytopenia with severe bleeding refractory to conventional treatment			Uncertain
	Prophylactic use before major surgery			Inappropriate

For nonemergency anticoagulant reversal, a dose of 20 to 40 μg/kg is recommended. For all other indications, 41 to 90 μg/kg is recommended.

*Give 20 mL/kg or 6 units of plasma or 6 units of platelets×2 if the platelet count is less than 50,000/mm^3 or 10 bags of cryoprecipitate×2 if fibrinogen was low or clotting factor replacement was not a feasible alternative because of time or volume constraints.

FDA, Food and Drug Administration; GI, gastrointestinal; LMWH, low-molecular-weight-heparin.

Adapted from Shander A, Goodnougaph LT, Ratko T, et al: Consensus recommendations for the off-label use of recombinant human factor VIIa (NovoSeven) Therapy. Pharmacy Therapeutics 30:644-658, 2005. Available at http://www.ptcommunity.com/ptJournal/journalView.cfm.

tested in animals and humans and found to enhance oxygen utilization and erythropoiesis. At present this product is in phase III trial in the United States. Polyethylene glycol (PEG)-modified hemoglobin (Enzon) is also a bovine HBOC that is being studied as a sensitizer in radiation therapy.

Human HBOCs have been produced and tested by Baxter and Northfield. The Baxter product, HemAssist or diaspirin cross-linked hemoglobin, has been studied in multiple animal models and limited human studies. In both animals and humans, diaspirin cross-linked hemoglobin demonstrates a potent vasopressor effect. A phase I study demonstrated the product to be well tolerated, but a phase III trial with diaspirin cross-linked hemoglobin in trauma patients was closed because of increased mortality in the study group. The Northfield product, PolyHeme, has not been associated with vasoactive or toxic side effects. In trauma patients, PolyHeme demonstrated effective oxygen transport and safety and a decreased requirement for allogeneic blood transfusions.[51] PolyHeme is currently in phase III trials in the United States.

Selected References

Geerts WH, Pineo GF, Heit JA, et al: Prevention of venous thromboembolism: The seventh ACCP conference on antithrombotic and thrombolytic therapy. Chest 126:338S-400S, 2004.

Literature review and evidence-based guidelines on the prevention and treatment of venous thromboembolism.

Goodnough LT, Brecher ME, Kanter MH, AuBuchon JP: Transfusion medicine. Parts 1 and 2. N Engl J Med 340:438-447, 525-533, 1999.

Review article in two parts covering blood transfusion and blood conservation. Risks of transfusion, indications for transfusion, alternatives to transfusion, and emerging developments in transfusion medicine are discussed.

Goodnough LT, Shander A, Brecher ME: Transfusion medicine: Looking to the future. Lancet 361:161-169, 2003.

Review of the evolution of transfusion medicine, including blood safety, alternatives, and emerging technologies.

Monroe DM, Hoffman M, Roberts HR: Platelets and thrombin generation. Arterioscler Thromb Vasc Biol 22:1381-1389, 2002.

This article reviews the major role of platelets in thrombin generation and presents a cell-based model of coagulation.

Moore EE: Blood substitutes: The future is now. J Am Coll Surg 196:1-17, 2003.

The Scudder Oration on Trauma presented at the American College of Surgeons' 88th Annual Clinical Congress, San Francisco, October 8, 2002. This is an excellent review of the background leading up to and the latest clinical experience with blood substitutes.

Shander A, Goodnough LT, Ratko T, et al: Consensus recommendations for the off-label use of recombinant human factor VIIa (NovoSeven) therapy. Pharmacy Therapeutics 30:644-658, 2005. Available at http://www.ptcommunity.com/ptJournal/journalView.cfm.

Literature review and consensus recommendations for the use of recombinant activated factor VII.

References

1. Report on blood collection and transfusion in the United States in 2001, National Blood Data Resource Center, 2003.
2. Goodnough LT, Brecher ME, Kanter MH, AuBuchon JP: Transfusion medicine. Parts 1 and 2. N Engl J Med 340:438-447, 525-533, 1999.
3. Monroe DM, Hoffman M, Roberts HR: Platelets and thrombin generation. Arterioscler Thromb Vasc Biol 22:1381-1389, 2002.
4. Levi M, ten Cate H, van der Poll T: Endothelium: Interface between coagulation and inflammation. Crit Care Med 30:S220-S224, 2002.
5. Mann KG, Butenas S, Brummel K: The dynamics of thrombin formation. Arterioscler Thromb Vasc Biol 23:17-25, 2003.
6. Bernard GR, Vincent JL, Laterre PF, et al: Recombinant human protein C: Efficacy and safety of recombinant human activated protein C for severe sepsis. Worldwide Evaluation in Severe Sepsis (PROWESS) study group. N Engl J Med 344:699-709, 2001.
7. Rijken DC, Sakharov DV: Basic principles of thrombolysis: Regulatory role of plasminogen. Thromb Res 103:S41-S49, 2001.
8. Sidelmann JJ, Gram J, Jespersen J, Kluft C: Fibrin clot formation and lysis: Basic mechanisms. Semin Thromb Hemost 26:605-618, 2000.
9. Cobas M: Preoperative assessment of coagulation disorders. Int Anesthesiol Clin 39:1-15, 2001.
10. Triplett DA: Coagulation and bleeding disorders: Review and update. Clin Chem 46:1260-1269, 2000.
11. Bern MM, Sahud M, Zhukov O, Mitchell W Jr: Treatment of factor XI inhibitor using recombinant activated factor VIIa. Haemophilia 11:20-25, 2005.
12. Levi MM, Vink R, de Jonge E: Management of bleeding disorders by prohemostatic therapy. Int J Hematol 76:139-144, 2002.
13. Mannucci PM: Treatment of von Willebrand's disease. N Engl J Med 351:683-694, 2004.
14. Regal RE, Tsui V: Optimal understanding of warfarin: Beyond the nomogram. Pharmacy Therapeutics 29:652-656, 2004. Available at http://www.ptcommunity.com/ptJournal/journalView.cfm.
15. Davoren A, Aster RH: Heparin-induced thrombocytopenia and thrombosis. Am J Hematol 81:36-44, 2006.
16. Geerts WH, Pineo GF, Heit JA, et al: Prevention of venous thromboembolism: The seventh ACCP conference on antithrombotic and thrombolytic therapy. Chest 126:338S-400S, 2004.
17. Amitrano L, Guardascione MA, Brancaccio V, et al: Coagulation disorders in liver disease. Semin Liver Dis 22:83-96, 2002.
18. Kottke-Marchant K, Corcoran G: The laboratory diagnosis of platelet disorders. Arch Pathol Lab Med 126:133-146, 2002.
19. Eddy VA, Morris JA: Early issues in the intensive care unit: The second golden hour. Surg Clin North Am 80:845-854, 2000.
20. Levi M: Disseminated intravascular coagulation: What's new? Crit Care Clin 21:449-467, 2005.
21. Tran M, Spencer FA: Thromboepidemiology: Identifying patients with heritable risk for thrombin-mediated thromboembolic events. Am Heart J 149(Suppl):S9-S18, 2005.
22. Spence RK: Surgical red blood cell transfusion practice policies. Am J Surg 170:3S-15S, 1995.
23. Hebert PC, Wells G, Blajchman MA, et al: A multicenter, randomized, controlled clinical trial of transfusion requirements in critical care. N Engl J Med 340:409-417, 1999.

24. American Association of Blood Banks: Blood Products Advisory Committee recommends universal leukoreduction. AABB News Briefs 20:16, 1998.

25. Ratko TA, Cummings JP, Oberman HA, et al: Evidence-based recommendations for the use of WBC-reduced cellular blood components. Transfusion 41:1310-1319, 2001.

26. Rebulla P: Platelet transfusion trigger in difficult patients. Transfus Clin Biol 9:249-254, 2002.

27. Clark P, Mintz PD: Transfusion triggers for blood components. Curr Opin Hematol 8:387-391, 2001.

28. Alderson P, Bunn F, Lefebvre C, et al: Human albumin solution for resuscitation and volume expansion in critically ill patients. Cochrane Database Syst Rev 4:CD001208, 2004.

29. Strong DM: Infectious risks of blood transfusions. America's Blood Centers Blood Bulletin 4(2), 2001.

30. Snyder E: Transfusion reactions. In Hoffman R, Benz EJ, Shattil SJ, et al (eds): Hematology: Basic Principles and Practice, 3rd ed. New York, Churchill Livingstone, 2000.

31. Goodnough LT: Erythropoietin therapy versus red cell transfusion. Curr Opin Hematol 8:405-410, 2001.

32. Reading FC, Brecher ME: Transfusion-related bacterial sepsis. Curr Opin Hematol 8:380-386, 2001.

33. Kuehnert MJ, Roth VR, Haley NR, et al: Transfusion-transmitted bacterial infection in the United States, 1998 through 2000. Transfusion 41:1493-1499, 2001.

34. http://www.ashi-hla.org/publicationfiles/ASHI_Quarterly/28_3_2004/TRALI.pdf.

35. Shander A, Popovsky MA: Understanding the consequences of transfusion-related acute lung injury. Chest 128:598S-604S, 2005.

36. Blajchman MA: Immunomodulation and blood transfusion. Am J Ther 9:389-395, 2002.

37. Spahn DR, Casutt M: Eliminating blood transfusions: New aspects and perspectives. Anesthesiology 93:242-255, 2000.

38. Brecher ME, Goodnough LT: The rise and fall of preoperative autologous blood donation. Transfusion 41:1459-1462, 2001.

39. Ng T, Marx G, Littlewood T, Macdougall I: Recombinant erythropoietin in clinical practice. Postgrad Med J 79:367-376, 2003.

40. Henry DA, Moxey AJ, Carless PA, et al: Anti-fibrinolytic use for minimising perioperative allogeneic blood transfusion. Cochrane Database Syst Rev 1:CD001886, 2001.

41. Mangano DT, Tudor JC, Dietzel C, et al: The risk associated with aprotinin in cardiac surgery. N Engl J Med 354:353-365, 2006.

42. Karkouti K, Beattie WS, Dattilo KM, et al: A propensity score case-control comparison of aprotinin and tranexamic acid in high-transfusion-risk cardiac surgery. Transfusion 46:327-338, 2006.

43. Coats T, Roberts I, Shakur H: Antifibrinolytic drugs for acute traumatic injury. Cochrane Database Syst Rev 4:CD004896, 2004.

44. Barletta JF, Ahrens CL, Tyburski JG, Wilson RF: A review of recombinant factor VII for refractory bleeding in nonhemophilic trauma patients. J Trauma 58:646-651, 2005.

45. Hedner U, Erhardtsen E: Potential role for rFVIIa in transfusion medicine. Transfusion 42:114-124, 2002.

46. Goodnough LT, Lublin DM, Zhang L, et al: Transfusion medicine service policies for recombinant factor VIIa administration. Transfusion 44:1325-1331, 2004.

47. Shander A, Goodnough LT, Ratko T, et al: Consensus recommendations for the off-label use of recombinant human factor VIIa (NovoSeven) therapy. Pharmacy Therapeutics 30:644-658, 2005. Available at http://www.ptcommunity.com/ptJournal/journalView.cfm.

48. Stowell CP: Hemoglobin based oxygen carriers. Curr Opin Hematol 9:537-543, 2002.

49. Winslow RM: Blood substitutes: Curr Opin Hematol 9:146-151, 2002.

50. Spahn DR, Kocian R: Artificial O_2 carriers: Status in 2005. Curr Pharm Des 11:4099-4114, 2005.

51. Moore EE: Blood substitutes: The future is now. J Am Coll Surg 196:1-17, 2003.

CHAPTER 7

Metabolism in Surgical Patients

Nicholas E. Tawa, Jr., MD, PhD   and   Josef E. Fischer, MD

OVERVIEW

Artificial Nutrition—Importance and History

Among advances in surgery achieved in the 20th century, nutritional support, along with antibiotics, blood transfusion, critical care monitoring, advances in anesthesia, organ transplantation, and cardiopulmonary bypass, ranks high. During this time, parenteral nutrition has evolved from initial enthusiastic acceptance to more critical review, with demands for efficacy. Dudrick and associates in 1968 first demonstrated that intravenous (IV) nutrition would support normal growth rates in puppies, and parenteral alimentation began to be widely applied in the United States. In the 1960s and 1970s, it was standard practice to feed patients 3000 to 5000 kcal/day (*hyperalimentation*) in an effort to attain an anabolic state. It was not appreciated at that time that such overfeeding practices were potentially dangerous and that with excessive carbohydrate and lipid infusion, the body's ability to metabolize these nutrients was exceeded, thus predisposing patients to iatrogenic immune and hepatic dysfunction.

Today, nutrition is provided in more moderate amounts, and nutritional needs in specific disease states have been explored. Some investigators have also proposed the use of specific nutrient components as drugs (termed *nutritional pharmacology*), an approach that will be validated only when its pathophysiologic mechanisms are better defined. Although modern practice is to make aggressive use of the gut for nutritional support, IV nutrition remains a critical therapy in instances in which enteral support cannot be achieved, either because the gut cannot be used or because caloric requirements cannot be met by the gut alone and must be supplemented parenterally. Studies of body composition in critical illness show, however, that even current approaches to IV nutrition remain unsatisfactory. Thus, in a normal individual, body tissue is compartmentalized as approximately 30% adipose, 30% lean body mass (protein), and 30% extracellular fluid (water). In catabolic illness, extracellular fluid increases to 50% to 60% of total body mass secondary to sodium retention, whereas fat and lean body tissue decrease to approximately 20% each. Although IV nutrition can clearly retard the loss of lean body mass under such conditions, it has proved difficult to induce net accumulation of body protein in a nongrowing adult host without strenuous exercise. Increasing the amount of IV nutrition beyond basal requirements, without exercise, insulin, or other hormonal alterations, in an effort to enhance lean body mass only increases total body water and fat content further, with no beneficial effect on body protein.[1] This is particularly true in patients with sepsis. Furthermore, in patients with malignancy, efforts to nourish the host may increase growth of the tumor.

Clinical Sequelae of Impaired Nutrition

Numerous studies have clearly shown an increased incidence of nosocomial infection, longer hospital stay, and increased mortality in patients with significant unintentional weight loss (>10%) before their acute illness. Even in an individual with initially normal nutritional status, after 7 to 10 days of inanition, the body's ability to heal wounds and to support normal immune function begins to be impaired. Such deficits include diminished complement and immunoglobulin production, poor cellular immunity, and impairment of various aspects of leukocyte action, including chemotaxis, phagocytosis, and oxidative burst. Other consequences of inadequate nutrition in the postoperative period include poor tissue repair and wound healing and loss of muscle function and strength as a result of progressive muscle wasting, which may contribute to reduced ventilatory performance and prolonged ventilator dependence. Overall, malnutrition will be limiting to all aggressive surgical and medical therapies.

Incidence of Malnutrition in Hospitalized Patients

In the early 1970s, the widespread prevalence of malnutrition in hospitalized medical and surgical patients was recognized and suggested to have a major influence on clinical outcome.[2] Today, it is estimated that as many as 50% of hospitalized patients may be malnourished. In the usual U.S. hospital setting, starvation is generally the result of either anorexia, such as occurs in cancer, sepsis, or liver disease, or poor intake caused by esophageal or gastrointestinal (GI) obstruction. Other conditions, such as scleroderma, motility disorders or pseudo-obstruction, major gastric resection, inflammatory bowel disease, and short-bowel syndrome, may result in inadequate absorption of nutrients. Inadequate nutrition may also be due to excessive loss, as in patients with GI fistulas or protein-losing enteropathies. However, the most common cause of in-hospital malnutrition is poor food served without assistance to frail individuals and timed for the benefit of personnel rather than patients. Patients are also given

nothing by mouth for the most trivial reasons (e.g., radiologic studies), and diets are often not advanced rapidly even after minor operations.

METABOLIC ADAPTATIONS IN CATABOLIC STATES AND REGULATION OF NITROGEN BALANCE

Amino Acid Metabolism and Transport

Roles of Specific Amino Acids

Amino acids have a core configuration of an amino and a carboxyl group adjacent to a carbon atom, from which a side chain extends, and are thus zwitterions. Amino acids are grouped according to electrical charge and the side chain. The neutral amino acid group includes the following 12 amino acids: glycine and alanine; the hydroxyamino acids serine and threonine; the branched-chain amino acids (BCAAs) valine, leucine, and isoleucine; the aromatic amino acids phenylalanine, tyrosine, and tryptophan; and the sulfur-containing amino acids methionine and cysteine. Aspartate and glutamate are diacidic amino acids, whereas arginine, lysine, and histidine are dibasic. These features largely determine transport across membranes. The essential or indispensable amino acids are those whose carbon skeleton cannot be synthesized by the body; such amino acids include valine, leucine, isoleucine, lysine, methionine, phenylalanine, threonine, and tryptophan. Cysteine and tyrosine may be essential in that they are synthesized from the essential amino acids methionine and phenylalanine, respectively. The remaining 10 amino acids, alanine, arginine, aspartate, asparagine, glutamate, glutamine, glycine, histidine, proline, and serine, are not essential. Though not classically essential, histidine, proline, glutamine, and arginine may become conditionally essential under catabolic conditions, when needs are increased and synthetic rates fall short of increased requirements. This concept of conditionally essential amino acids remains controversial and is discussed later in this chapter. Three major fates of amino acids follow:

1. Protein synthesis
2. Oxidation by the tricarboxylic acid (TCA) cycle, either for production of energy or ultimately leading to

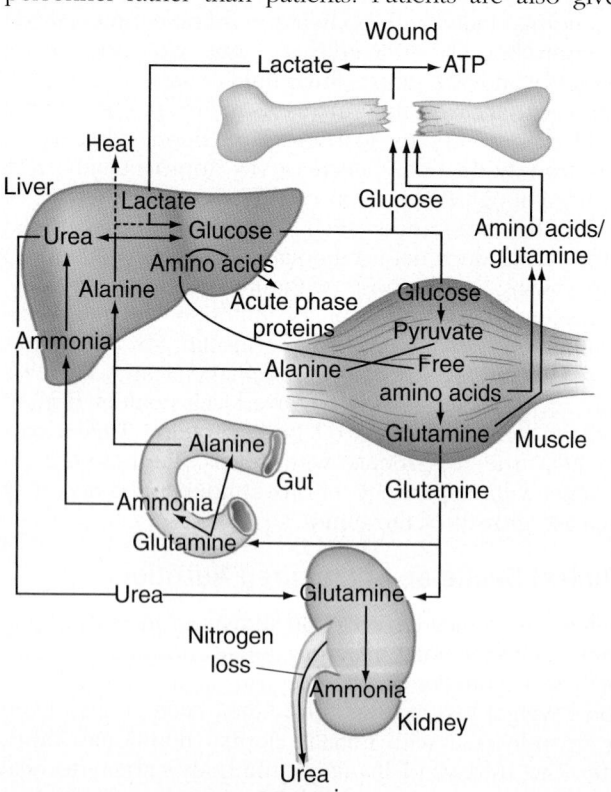

Figure 7-1 Overall scheme of the metabolic response to illness. This scheme includes the metabolic relationship among organs. This relationship has heretofore not been prominently addressed but is now receiving increased attention. One of the articles of faith is that such responses occur as a reaction to injury and are teleologically correct and beneficial. Thus, the wound requires glucose, probably glutamine, and certainly arginine with respect to certain cellular elements. Movement of amino acids from the periphery (muscle) to the liver presumably results in the secretion of acute phase protein, the purpose of which, in turn, is to fight infection. The muscle-gut-liver-alanine-glutamine-glucose cycle is prominently displayed. ATP, adenosine triphosphate. (Adapted from Bessey PQ: Metabolic response to critical illness. In Wilmore DW, Cheung LY, Harken AH, et al [eds]: Scientific American Surgery, Section II, Subsection 11. Healtheon/WebMD, New York, 2000. All rights reserved.)

storage as carbohydrate or fat, with the production of urea and carbon dioxide
3. Synthesis of nonessential amino acids and other small molecules such as purines and pyrimidines

The plasma amino acid pool is regulated by exchange of amino acids among skeletal muscle, the liver, and other viscera (kidney and lung). Of the essential amino acids, 7 of the 10 are degraded by the liver, the exceptions being the BCAAs, for which skeletal muscle plays a major role in catabolism. Two amino acids, alanine and glutamine, are carriers for organ exchange of nitrogen, in a complex process discussed later (Fig. 7-1).

Amino Acid Transport

Transport of free amino acids across cell membranes has been studied in only a few types of cells; it is probably universal. Christensen[3] proposed several transport systems:

1. The A-system is an energy- and sodium-dependent system with high affinity for alanine and other neutral amino acids, including the synthetic amino acid α-aminoisobutyric acid. It is concentrative against a gradient and is stimulated by insulin. Insulin stimulates amino acid transport into muscle via the A-system by recruiting specific sodium-dependent amino acid transporters to the plasma membrane (also see later).[4]
2. The L-system is sodium independent and transports the BCAAs (leucine, isoleucine, and valine) and the aromatic amino acids (phenylalanine, tyrosine, and tryptophan), as well as probably methionine and histidine. It operates by exchange for intracellular amino acids and is competitive.
3. Two transport systems are available for the basic amino acids. The carriers for transport of dibasic amino acids and the L-system may be linked in some as yet unknown way.
4. Dicarboxylic amino acids have their own transport system.

Current knowledge about amino acid transport in muscle is summarized in Table 7-1.

Amino Acid Metabolism in the Liver and Viscera

The liver is the major site in the body for the degradation and synthesis of amino acids and is the most important organ for regulation of plasma amino acid levels. The liver processes and stores ingested nutrients delivered by the portal venous system and releases them in response to neural and hormonal signals. The liver may extract

between 75% and 100% of all portal vein nutrients in one pass, with only 25% of ingested protein reaching the general (nonportal) circulation as free amino acids. Most (almost 60%) is converted to urea, a small amount (6%) is used for the synthesis of plasma protein, and 14% becomes liver protein. Although K_m values for hepatic amino acid degradation are high and those for synthesis are low, thus favoring net synthesis, excessive postprandial accumulation of plasma amino acids is prevented, which helps, for example, in avoiding rapid and possibly disruptive increases in amino acid brain neurotransmitter precursors. It is not clear whether the large postprandial urea production from absorbed amino acids is wasteful or is somehow required for hepatic functional integrity. During starvation, the liver metabolizes amino acids released by proteolysis in muscle to form glucose in the process of gluconeogenesis (see later). In parenteral nutrition, nutrients are first supplied to the systemic rather than the portal circulation and thus override the liver. Furthermore, as the normal postprandial production of gut hormones (which may have a role in anabolic signaling) is bypassed by parenteral feeding, overall nutrient disposal is probably less efficient and this phenomenon may contribute to the difficulty in achieving positive nitrogen balance discussed earlier.

The role of the kidney in amino acid homeostasis has not been as well studied as that of muscle or the liver but is probably more important than heretofore supposed. Amino acids in the kidney can have several fates, including the following:

1. Production of urea (with the liver) from ammonia by means of the argininosuccinate cycle
2. Production of ammonia (from glutamine) for urinary acid-base balance
3. Metabolism of other amino acids, such as the BCAAs
4. Participation with the liver in gluconeogenesis from muscle-derived glutamine (see later)

The lung may also have a greater role in the regulation of amino acid levels than has been appreciated, especially when the liver is bypassed or diseased and is thus incapable of modifying portal flow. For example, in sepsis, the lung, in addition to skeletal muscle, can become a major source for glutamine production.

Amino Acid Metabolism in Muscle

Skeletal muscle and cardiac muscle are the major sites in the body for the catabolism of several amino acids, most

Table 7-1 Amino Acid Transporters in Muscle

TRANSPORTER	Na COUPLING	TYPICAL SUBSTRATES	COMMENTS
X-A,G	Yes	Glutamate, aspartate	Insulin insensitive
y+	No	Lysine, cystine, arginine, ornithine	Insulin insensitive
L	No	Neutral amino acids	Insulin insensitive
A	Yes	Short-chain neutral amino acids	Insulin sensitive, reduced by starvation
ASC	Yes	Alanine, cysteine, serine, threonine	Insulin insensitive
N^m	Yes	Glutamine, histidine, asparagine	Insulin sensitive

notably leucine, isoleucine, and valine, and for the synthesis of others, specifically alanine and glutamine.[5] By contrast, muscle does not degrade the carbon skeletons of other amino acids found in plasma to any significant extent.

Branched-Chain Amino Acid Oxidation

The rate of degradation of BCAAs in muscle is greater than in the liver, and given that muscle accounts for up to 40% of body mass, it is probably the major site for degradation of BCAAs. Unlike most ingested amino acids, the BCAAs are not efficiently extracted from the portal circulation by the liver and pass directly into the systemic circulation to be taken up by peripheral tissues. Although leucine is readily oxidized by muscle, it is also degraded by the kidney, adipose tissue, and brain. The physiologic significance of BCAA metabolism in these tissues is probably distinct from that in skeletal muscle. For example, in adipose tissue, leucine degradation serves an anabolic function by providing precursors for triglyceride synthesis, whereas in muscle, leucine is degraded to acetyl coenzyme A moieties, which are then oxidized in the TCA cycle to provide energy.

In certain catabolic states, including fasting, diabetes, and after traumatic injury, rates of degradation of the BCAAs increase markedly in skeletal and cardiac muscle and in the kidney, whereas the liver and brain show no such effects. This increased oxidation in muscle is regulated by glucocorticoids and other stimuli.[6] Because leucine can serve as an alternative energy source for muscle during fasting, it can also reduce glucose utilization in this tissue. Therefore, during fasting, when leucine levels rise in blood and muscle, its degradation in muscle increases, and gluconeogenic precursor molecules such as pyruvate are preserved.[7]

Production and Release of Alanine

The breakdown of BCAAs in muscle generates amino groups whose accumulation could be toxic. Unlike the liver, muscle lacks the enzymes necessary to dispose of ammonia as urea. Instead, alanine and glutamine are released in much greater amounts than would be expected simply by the net breakdown of muscle proteins. Amino groups generated by the degradation of BCAAs and aspartate contribute to the de novo synthesis of alanine and glutamine in muscle.[5] Alanine production by this tissue seems to play an important role in the maintenance of blood glucose in the fasted state. The liver is very active in extracting alanine from the blood, and in the liver alanine is the most important amino acid used for gluconeogenesis.

Felig in the mid-1970s proposed the existence of a so-called glucose-alanine cycle, in which alanine derived from amino acid metabolism in muscle is carried in the circulation to the liver for conversion to urea and glucose. The glucose synthesized by the liver can then be taken up again by muscle and be converted back to alanine. This flux of alanine between muscle and liver is similar to that of lactate in the Cori (glucose-lactate) cycle, but in addition, alanine helps ferry potentially toxic amino groups to the liver for disposal as urea. Because alanine is derived from preexistent glucose, this cycle does not allow the generation of new carbohydrate from muscle proteins, and overall, as an amino group is ultimately lost, the glucose-alanine cycle is not a true metabolic cycle. However, in fasting, glucose is spared by the oxidation of leucine and prevention of pyruvate degradation in muscle.

Glutamine Production by Muscle and Interorgan Relationships

Skeletal muscle and cardiac muscle synthesize and release glutamine in similar or even greater amounts than they do alanine. Studies in isolated muscles[5] and more recent experiments in humans have shown that the carbon atoms in glutamine originate primarily from protein-derived amino acids that can enter the TCA cycle and are mainly converted to glutamine, which is then released from muscle. This process is an important initial step in gluconeogenesis from muscle protein. It has been estimated that about 87% of the glutamine released from muscle is derived from de novo synthesis rather than being liberated as a result of proteolysis. The glutamine released by muscle is an important energy source for many cells. For example, glutamine is extensively oxidized by leukocytes and fibroblasts. It is taken up from blood primarily by the kidney, where it serves as a precursor for urinary ammonia, and its carbon skeleton may be used for either gluconeogenesis or energy production, or some of the carbons are released into blood as alanine. In addition, as originally described by Windmueller and Spaeth,[8] the small intestine takes up and metabolizes large amounts of glutamine; in turn, it releases appreciable amounts of alanine. The liver then uses the released alanine for glucose production. This complex multiorgan process appears to play an important role in net gluconeogenesis from the five amino acids originating in proteins and converted to glutamine in muscle.

The level of glutamine within different tissues is determined by the relative activities of glutamine synthase and glutaminase. Transcription of glutamine synthase is strongly activated by corticosteroids in lung and muscle tissue. This leads to enhanced glutamine production and underlies the increased production and release of glutamine from muscle in starvation and disease states such as sepsis or other critical illnesses in which glucocorticoid levels are high.[9] As indicated earlier, the lung also has high capacity for synthesizing glutamine, and this process rises in sepsis. For example, after induction of a sepsis-like state with lipopolysaccharide in experimental animals and in studies measuring lung flux via pulmonary artery catheters in human patients with sepsis, release of glutamine by the lung at least doubles, presumably as a result of increased levels of glutamine synthase. Under these conditions, uptake of glutamine by the small intestine decreases and uptake by the liver increases dramatically. The benefit of these changes is not clear (see Controversies in Artificial Nutrition later).

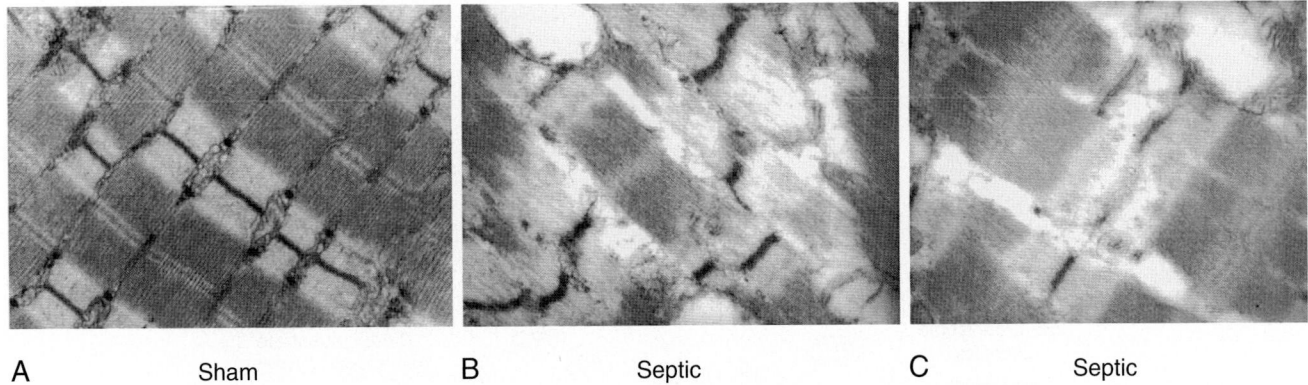

A   Sham   B   Septic   C   Septic

Figure 7-2 Electron micrographs of extensor digitorum longus (EDL) muscles from sham-operated (**A**) and septic (**B** and **C**) rats. Note the loss of registry between adjacent sarcomeres in septic muscles. Z disks were thickened, fragmented, or completely lost in septic muscles (×33,200). (**A** and **B**, From Williams AB, deCourten-Myers GM, Fischer JE, et al: Sepsis stimulates release of myofilaments in skeletal muscle by a calcium-dependent mechanism. FASEB J 13:1435, 1999.)

Regulation of Intracellular Protein Synthesis and Degradation

Physiologic Significance of Protein Turnover

Classic experiments by Schoenheimer in the 1940s with ^{15}N-labeled amino acids demonstrated that cellular proteins are synthesized and degraded continuously. Net mobilization of muscle protein can provide amino acids for metabolism by other tissues, for example, during fasting, whereas net uptake of amino acids by muscle plus incorporation of them into protein is a form of energy storage. However, there is no generic protein store; muscle may serve that purpose, but not perfectly.

A major technical factor limiting the study of protein metabolism in muscle and other tissues has been problems involving measurement of degradative rates. A variety of in vivo methods are available, but all are subject to a number of potential artifacts. Urinary urea or total nitrogen excretion is often regarded as an index of muscle protein breakdown, but these measurements actually represent processes of amino acid catabolism and will be influenced by amino acids released from nonmuscle tissues and from the diet. One useful method for estimating rates of degradation of certain muscle proteins in vivo is measurement of urinary *N*-methylhistidine excretion. This amino acid is formed by a post-translational modification of histidine residues in actin and myosin. When generated by proteolysis, it cannot be reincorporated into protein or significantly metabolized, and therefore its release in urine must reflect breakdown of these contractile proteins. However, actin and myosin also exist in other tissues, and the skin, GI tract, and possibly other organs, besides muscle, may contribute significantly to urinary excretion of *N*-methylhistidine. To analyze rates of protein degradation under controlled conditions, in vitro techniques involving the use of thin rodent muscles offer many advantages. Similar techniques have been applied for measuring rates of protein synthe-

sis and degradation in human muscle biopsy samples. Rates of protein synthesis are determined by measuring rates of incorporation of [^{14}C]-tyrosine or phenylalanine into muscle protein, whereas rates of protein degradation are estimated by measuring the release of tyrosine from muscle.

Biochemical Pathways for Intracellular Protein Breakdown

Several pathways for intracellular proteolysis have been identified, and each pathway uses a unique complement of proteases, including the acid-dependent proteases (cathepsins) in lysosomes and proteases active at neutral pH and found in the cytosol. This latter group includes the calcium-dependent calpains, the caspases, and the adenosine triphosphate (ATP)-dependent ubiquitin-proteasome pathway. It is now well established that the proteasome is responsible for the majority of protein degradation in mammalian cells, including skeletal muscle.[10] Seminal work by Alfred L. Goldberg and coworkers has yielded considerable evidence that the ubiquitin-proteasome pathway is responsible for the majority of accelerated proteolysis in many different catabolic conditions characterized by muscle wasting.[11,12] However, calpains may have a complementary role, as explored by Williams and colleagues in rats wasting as a result of sepsis. Calcium-dependent release of myofibrils plus disintegration of the Z band, along with increased mRNA levels for calpains 1, 2 and 3, was noted. This finding suggests that in sepsis, calpains might be important in releasing myofibrils from the contractile apparatus, and these then presumably serve as substrate for ubiquitination and degradation by the proteasome (Fig. 7-2).[13]

The importance of the ATP-dependent ubiquitin-proteasome pathway in muscle atrophy is now well established.[11] The majority of the acceleration in proteolysis induced by a variety of catabolic conditions, including

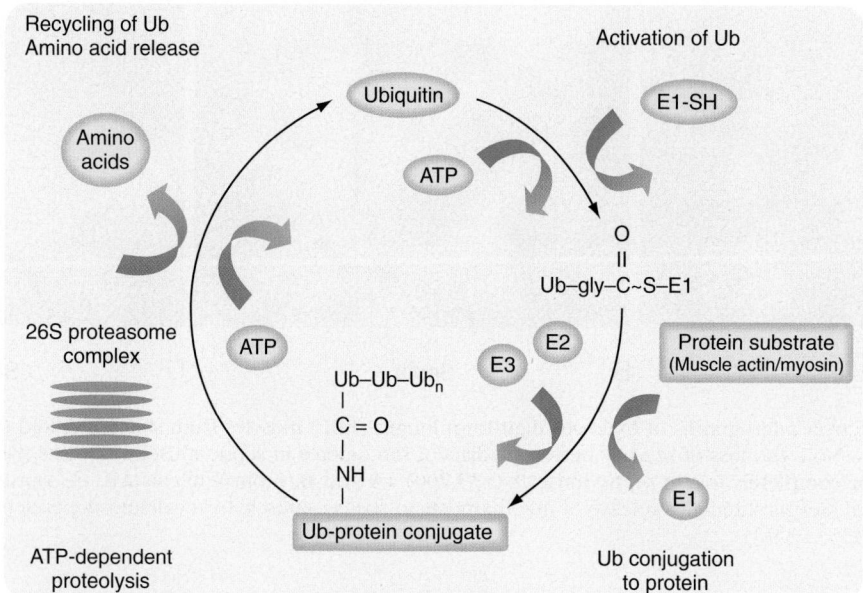

Figure 7-3 The adenosine triphosphate (ATP)-dependent ubiquitin (Ub)-proteasome pathway for protein degradation. In this energy-requiring process, ATP is hydrolyzed (1) during Ub conjugation to protein substrates (2) to allow formation of the proteasome complex and (3) to support the degradative function of the proteasome. *Activation of ubiquitin:* A high energy thiol-ester bond is formed between the C-terminal glycine of the polypeptide Ub and the Ub-activating enzyme E1. *Ub conjugation to protein:* With the participation of E2 and E3 proteins, Ub is transferred to the protein substrate targeted for degradation. Multiple Ub molecules may be attached to each other and to one or more lysine residues on the target protein via isopeptide bonds formed between the carboxyl-terminus of Ub and the ε-amino group of lysine. *ATP-dependent proteolysis:* The proteasome is assembled from proteolytic and regulatory elements and the protein substrate is degraded with the release of short peptides. *Recycling of Ub and amino acid release:* Ub is regenerated by the isopeptidase activity associated with the proteasome and is reused for the degradation of other proteins. Peptides generated by the proteasome are further degraded to amino acids, which in muscle can be released into the circulation for gluconeogenesis or to support protein synthesis in other tissues.

diabetes, acidosis, sepsis, thyroid hormone treatment, and denervation atrophy, can be blocked by proteasome inhibitors.[14] These muscles also show dramatic increases in ubiquitin-protein conjugates, which are intermediates in proteolysis via this pathway, as well as increases in mRNA encoding components of the ubiquitin-proteasome pathway.[11,12] Degradation of proteins via the ubiquitin-proteasome pathway is a multistep process that requires the hydrolysis of ATP, in addition to the 8-kd protein cofactor ubiquitin and the 26S proteasome (Fig. 7-3).[10] The 26S proteasome is a very large (2 Md) complex made up of at least 50 subunits.

Unlike typical proteases, the proteasome requires ATP for the degradation of proteins; in particular, ATP hydrolysis is thought to be needed to drive the unfolding and translocation of globular proteins into the proteolytic compartment. The majority of protein substrates are marked for degradation by covalent linkage of a chain of ubiquitin molecules to an internal lysine of the protein substrate. Discovery of the role of ubiquitination in protein breakdown led to awarding of the Nobel Prize in Chemistry to Hershko, Ciechanover, and Rose in 2004. Ubiquitination is now also recognized to underlie many other cell signaling processes not directly related to proteolysis. ATP-dependent proteolysis mediated by ubiqui-

tination requires at least three enzymes, the so-called E1, E2, and E3 enzymes. The E3 ubiquitin-protein ligase can bind only specific protein substrates and ubiquitinates these proteins with the aid of a specific E2 enzyme. However, which E2 and E3 enzymes are involved in the accelerated proteolysis during muscle wasting is still incompletely understood.[12] Very recently, genomic approaches have been used to identify genes regulated during muscle atrophy. These exciting studies have revealed E3 enzymes that appear to be directly involved in accelerated proteolysis in a number of different conditions. For example, mRNA levels for one new E3 enzyme increase severalfold in fasting, diabetes, cancer, and uremia[15] and during immobilization or denervation.[16] The importance of this E3 enzyme in muscle wasting was highlighted by studies showing that when muscles from transgenic knockout mice lacking the functional E3 gene were denervated, they lost half as much mass as muscles from wild-type mice did.[16]

Nutrients and Hormones Regulating Nitrogen Balance

The hormonal milieu of the body provides for either a storage state or a breakdown state. Insulin, the dominant anabolic signal, inhibits lipolysis and increases accrual of nitrogen in muscle, liver, and other tissues. In addition

---

Table 7-2 Hormones Influencing Energy Use and Nitrogen Balance

HORMONE	MUSCLE PROTEIN DEGRADATION	MUSCLE PROTEIN SYNTHESIS	GLUCOSE UTILIZATION	EFFECT ON GROWTH
Insulin	Decrease	Increase	Increase	Anabolic
Glucocorticoids	Increase	Decrease	Decrease	Catabolic
Cytokines	Increase	Decrease	Decrease	Catabolic
IGF-I	Decrease	Increase	Increase	Anabolic
Growth hormone	No change	Increase	Decrease	Anabolic
Thyroid hormone	Increase	Increase	Increase	Anabolic
Leucine	Decrease	Increase	Decrease	Anabolic
Fasting	Increase	Decrease	Decrease	Catabolic
Long-term fasting	Decrease	Decrease	Decrease	Catabolic
Protein deficiency	Decrease	Decrease	Unknown	Catabolic

IGF, insulin-like growth factor.

to hormonal and nutrient factors, lack of tension or disuse is a major signal activating muscle proteolysis, a phenomenon of considerable relevance clinically. Great advances have been made in understanding the signaling mechanisms mediating the effects of various nutrients and anabolic hormones (Table 7-2). In particular, two protein kinases, Akt and mTOR (the latter inhibited by the immunosuppressive drug rapamycin), appear to be particularly important in regulating mRNA translation and thus protein synthesis in response to various growth factors and nutrients.

It has been known for some time that leucine has regulatory effects on muscle protein balance. Studies from several laboratories have shown that BCAAs stimulate protein synthesis and reduce protein breakdown in isolated skeletal and cardiac muscle. Leucine appears to stimulate protein synthesis and mRNA translation principally via the pathway that involves mTOR, although the inhibitory effects of leucine on protein degradation have been less extensively investigated. However, this action of leucine is not related to its role as a metabolic fuel inasmuch as other carbon sources such as alanine and pyruvate fail to have the same anabolic effects despite being consumed by cells.

Insulin stimulates amino acid transport into muscle (see earlier),[4] increases rates of protein synthesis, and inhibits muscle protein breakdown. Thus, the rise in insulin after meals promotes net protein accumulation in muscle, whereas in the postabsorptive state, when insulin is low, there is net loss of protein and release of amino acids from muscle. Binding of insulin to its receptor on the plasma membrane leads to activation of phosphatidylinositol-3 kinase (PI3K), followed by Akt and S6 kinase, and ultimately initiation of enhanced translation. Insulin can have a limited role in promoting protein synthesis in some catabolic conditions such as after burns. In addition to its effects on protein synthesis, insulin inhibits protein degradation in many tissues.[17] Insulin's direct inhibition of protein breakdown in liver and muscle results largely from inhibition of lysosomal proteolysis. However, the systemic effects of low-insulin

states such as fasting or diabetes include muscle wasting as a result of accelerated proteolysis via the ATP-dependent ubiquitin-proteasome pathway, a process that appears to be insensitive to insulin. Under these conditions, glucocorticoids clearly contribute to activation of the ubiquitin-proteasome pathway and are required for muscle wasting. Possibly insulin somehow inhibits this catabolic response to glucocorticoids.

Glucose by itself can inhibit protein degradation in isolated muscle and the liver without affecting overall protein synthesis. This effect of glucose in muscle is not simply due to supplying energy to the tissue because fatty acids or ketone bodies do not reduce proteolysis despite their rapid oxidation. Therefore, elevated plasma levels of insulin and glucose after food intake together promote the accumulation of amino acids in muscle.

Hypophysectomy of young animals prevents growth, including skeletal muscle growth. When hypophysectomized animals are treated with growth hormone, overall body growth is reinitiated and rates of protein synthesis in muscle increase. Growth hormone does not appear to suppress proteolysis directly. Rather, the polypeptide insulin-like growth factors IGF-I and IGF-II, synthesized in part via stimulation by growth hormone, mediate the reduction in proteolysis. IGF-I has well-documented insulin-like effects and enhances protein synthesis by activating the PI3K/Akt/mTOR pathway, which accelerates the initiation of translation. In addition to enhancing protein synthesis, IGF-I and IGF-II inhibit protein breakdown in muscle. For example, the increase in protein degradation in isolated muscle after burn injury can be reversed by IGF-I, but this effect was not seen in muscle from septic animals, where IGF-I increased protein synthesis but had no effect on protein degradation rates.[18] The inhibition of protein breakdown by IGF-I is thought to involve suppression of the lysosomal process, as shown previously for insulin. However, recent evidence suggests that IGF-I, but not growth hormone, can reduce mRNA levels for components of the ubiquitin-proteasome pathway, and this might be an additional mechanism to reduce proteolysis.

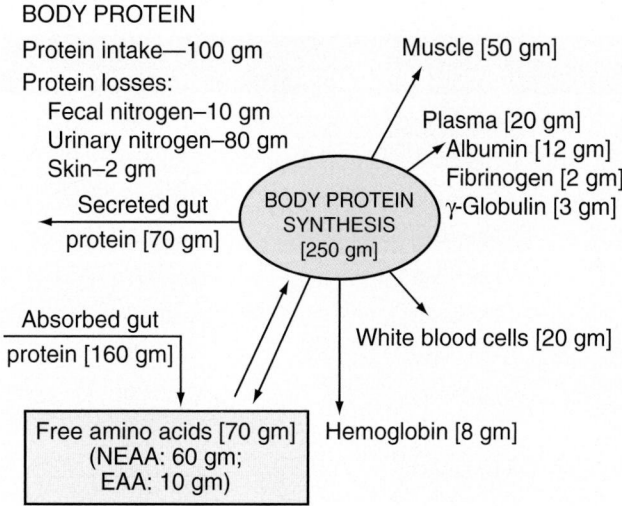

BODY PROTEIN

Protein intake—100 gm
Protein losses:
 Fecal nitrogen–10 gm
 Urinary nitrogen–80 gm
 Skin–2 gm
Secreted gut
protein [70 gm]

BODY PROTEIN
SYNTHESIS
[250 gm]

Absorbed gut
protein [160 gm]

Free amino acids [70 gm]
(NEAA: 60 gm;
 EAA: 10 gm)

Muscle [50 gm]

Plasma [20 gm]
Albumin [12 gm]
Fibrinogen [2 gm]
γ-Globulin [3 gm]

White blood cells [20 gm]

Hemoglobin [8 gm]

Figure 7-4 Daily flux of amino acids in the body of a 70-kg man. Total body protein synthesis is 250 g per 24 hours, 50 g of which is muscle; proteolysis contributes approximately the same. Thus, with adequate amounts of energy, nitrogen equilibrium is the result. EAA, essential amino acids; NEAA, nonessential amino acids. (Data from Munro HN: Parenteral nutrition: Metabolic consequences of bypassing the gut and liver. In Clinical Nutrition Update: Amino Acids. Chicago, American Medical Association, 1977, p 141.)

Glucocorticoids are another class of hormones that influence muscle size. For instance, the overproduction of adrenal steroids in Cushing's syndrome or the high levels used clinically lead to marked muscle weakness and wasting. Glucocorticoids act in several complex ways to retard growth and promote the release of amino acids from muscle, including decreasing DNA and protein synthesis and reducing amino acid uptake by muscle. In the fasted state, glucocorticoids play an important physiologic role in promoting the net breakdown of muscle protein, and this response appears to be important in the regulation of blood glucose. This action of glucocorticoids thus complements the other so-called permissive actions of cortisol in enhancing gluconeogenesis in the liver and kidney.

It is now clear that the accelerated proteolysis caused by glucocorticoids in experimental animals is largely due to activation of the ubiquitin-proteasome pathway in muscle, and in general, pale (glycolytic) muscle fibers appear to be more sensitive to these catabolic effects than dark (oxidative) fibers do. In addition to fasting, glucocorticoids are also important for the increase in proteolysis seen in other physiologic or pathologic states. Thus, the increased ATP-dependent protein breakdown occurring in the muscles of rats with metabolic acidosis, diabetes, or sepsis[19] is dependent on this class of hormone. However, it should be noted that in human studies, no increase in transcripts for components of the proteolytic pathway have been demonstrated, either after short exposure to high-dose prednisolone, which induces proteolysis,[20] or in those with untreated Cushing's disease. Recent experiments to define the effects of glucocorticoids on protein synthesis have shown that these hormones appear to antagonize the stimulatory effects of

insulin and leucine on the PI3K/Akt/mTOR pathway described earlier.

Physiologic Adaptations to Food Deprivation

Short-Term Fasting

Complete food deprivation leads to mobilization of body protein to support energy needs. Although the normal turnover of protein is 2.5% to 3% of lean body mass per day (Fig. 7-4), in starvation as much as 300 g of protein per day may be lost initially in humans. Early in fasting, release of amino acids from skeletal muscle increases as a result of a decrease in protein synthesis and a marked rise in protein degradation. These adaptive changes in muscle protein metabolism seem to result from the low level of circulating insulin, although glucocorticoids also play an essential permissive role (see earlier). Early in fasting, under the influence of decreased insulin and elevated glucagon, hepatic glycogenolysis provides a limited store (≤100 g) for maintenance of systemic glucose. However, fat constitutes the bulk of calories available (Table 7-3), and lipolysis and release of free fatty acids occur in response to the low insulin levels. For example, the average adult fat reserve is approximately 10 kg, or 100,000 kcal, 60 times hepatic glycogen stores.

In peripheral tissues during fasting, utilization of free fatty acids and ketone bodies for production of ATP increases, whereas glucose oxidation is inhibited. As discussed earlier, BCAA oxidation in muscle rises, thus sparing glucose. Most importantly, gluconeogenesis in the liver and kidney is activated via muscle-derived glutamine and alanine, lactate, and glycerol released from lipid oxidation, with increased production of urea. This process, in addition to metabolic cycles such as the glucose-alanine or glucose-lactate cycle (see earlier), maintains blood glucose levels for tissues that are highly dependent on glucose for energy, such as the brain, erythrocytes, and the kidney.

In the liver, the accelerated proteolysis induced by fasting occurs largely in lysosomes. However, in muscle tissue, activation of the ATP-ubiquitin–dependent proteolytic pathway is primarily responsible for the increased protein degradation in fasting. In rodents deprived of food for 48 hours, levels of total ubiquitin mRNA in muscle and the mRNA for several proteasome subunits increase coordinately threefold to sixfold.[11,12] Muscles from fasted animals also contain higher amounts of proteins conjugated to ubiquitin than do muscles of fed controls. This finding suggests an increased rate of ubiquitin conjugation in muscle during fasting, and it correlates with activation of the ATP-ubiquitin–dependent pathway in isolated muscles. Further detailed analysis of the transcriptional adaptations occurring in muscles of mice fasted for 48 hours has recently been performed with cDNA microarrays by Jagoe and coworkers.[21] This technique allows simultaneous measurement of changes in mRNA levels for several thousand genes (the so-called transcriptosome) and has revealed a number of important new alterations in gene expression that had not been noted before. One markedly induced gene, subsequently proven to be the new ubiquitin ligase, or E3, is atrogin-

Table 7-3 Normal Stores of Available Energy and Rates of Use in a Man Weighing 65 kg

| | TOTAL BODY CONTENT (g) | AVAILABLE STORE | | | DAILY UTILIZATION* (g) | EXHAUSTION TIME (DAYS) |
		g	mJ	kcal		
Carbohydrate	500	150	2.5	600	All used in first 24 hr	<1
Protein	11,000	2400	40	9,600	60	About 40[†]
Fat	9,000	6500	235	58,500	150	About 40[†]

*Assuming energy expenditure of about 6.7 mJ (1600 kcal)/day.

[†]Experience in voluntary starvation suggests that the limit of resting starvation in young men in excellent physical condition may be as much as 60 to 70 days (Maize Prison, Northern Ireland).

From Passmore R, Robson JS: A Companion to Medical Studies, vol 3. Oxford, Blackwell Scientific, 1974.

1[15,16] and was discussed earlier. Other features in fasting include reduced transcripts for many of the enzymes involved in later stages of glycolysis and coordinated changes in mRNA encoding translation initiation factors that might favor the translation of a subset of stress-related proteins.

Long-Term Fasting and Dietary Protein Deficiency

In prolonged fasting, gluconeogenesis from body proteins and loss of muscle mass are gradually reduced. The most important factor reducing glucose needs during fasting is a decrease in the brain's requirement for glucose, with ketone bodies being used instead for a large part of ATP production by the brain. As the use of alternative fuels to glucose increases, muscle proteolysis falls below levels seen early in starvation, and eventually proteolysis is lower than in the fed state. In humans, 1 week of fasting is necessary for this adaptation, as indicated by a diminished forearm arteriovenous difference in amino acids and by decreased urinary *N*-methylhistidine excretion. Both the lysosomal and nonlysosomal ATP-dependent pathways are suppressed in muscle of rats fasted for prolonged periods, and very similar reductions in muscle proteolysis occur in animals fed a protein-deficient diet.[22] It remains likely that these nutritional states share common signals and mechanisms for reducing proteolysis, for example, through reduced thyroid status, although additional mechanisms may also be important for these adaptations.

Physiology of Inflammation and Sepsis

Changes in Energy Metabolism and Protein Turnover

Sepsis is the major cause of surgical mortality. The metabolic tragedy of sepsis is that the suppression of proteolysis seen in prolonged starvation does not occur and breakdown of protein continues. In fact, lean tissue loss can approximate 900 g/day in patients with severe sepsis, traumatic injuries, closed head injury, or major burns, and generalized muscle wasting ensues. In humans and animals with sepsis, there is clear evidence of increased proteolysis and net release of amino acids from muscle, and furthermore, most of the increased proteolysis results from activation of the ubiquitin-proteasome pathway. Pale glycolytic muscles (*fast twitch*) appear to be far more sensitive to sepsis than dark oxidative ones are. For example, ubiquitin mRNA increases severalfold in pale extensor digitorum longus muscle from septic rats, where

ATP-dependent proteolysis also rises, but it does not change in dark soleus muscles (gravitational or *slow twitch*), in which ATP-dependent proteolytic activity is unchanged.[23] The mRNA for many other components of the ubiquitin-proteasome pathway increases in muscle in experimental models of sepsis[19,24] and in septic patients. Sepsis increases rates of ubiquitination of muscle proteins,[12] and inhibitors of the proteasome dramatically reduce total and myofibrillar proteolysis in muscle from septic animals.[14] Although they contribute little to overall proteolysis, other pathways, in addition to the ubiquitin-proteasome pathway, may also have a role in the muscle wasting in sepsis. For example, increased mRNA levels for cathepsin B and calpain have been found in muscle during sepsis, and the calpains also appear to play a role (see earlier).

Sepsis leads to reduced protein synthesis, especially in fast-twitch muscles, as a result of reduced rates of initiation of translation. Furthermore, the response to stimuli that normally promote increased protein synthesis, such as BCAAs or insulin, is diminished. In contrast, hepatic protein synthesis, largely of acute phase reactant proteins found in plasma, is increased in the septic state, but hepatic synthesis of structural components is not.

As discussed earlier, insulin normally inhibits gluconeogenesis. However, in sepsis and other inflammatory states, gluconeogenesis continues despite the administration of either fat or carbohydrate, and peripheral insulin resistance with impaired skeletal muscle uptake of glucose occurs. For these reasons, hyperglycemia in response to IV feeding during sepsis is common, particularly in patients predisposed to diabetes. This insulin resistance or stress-induced hyperglycemia is caused by multiple factors, including elevated counter-regulatory hormones (catecholamines, glucagon, and glucocorticoids) and cytokines (primarily tumor necrosis factor [TNF]; also see later) (Fig. 7-5). Numerous strategies have been proposed to counter hyperglycemia while providing IV nutrition to patients with sepsis or severe inflammation, such as that resulting from burn injury. One approach is lipid supplementation. However, whether lipid metabolism continues normally in sepsis is controversial. Perhaps in moderate sepsis fat continues to be used, whereas in severe sepsis fat is used inefficiently. To truly understand why these metabolic profiles are altered will require a better understanding of the effect of the various mediators released during severe inflammation and sepsis on the pancreatic beta cell and peripheral tissues.

INTEGRATED CONCEPT OF SEPSIS

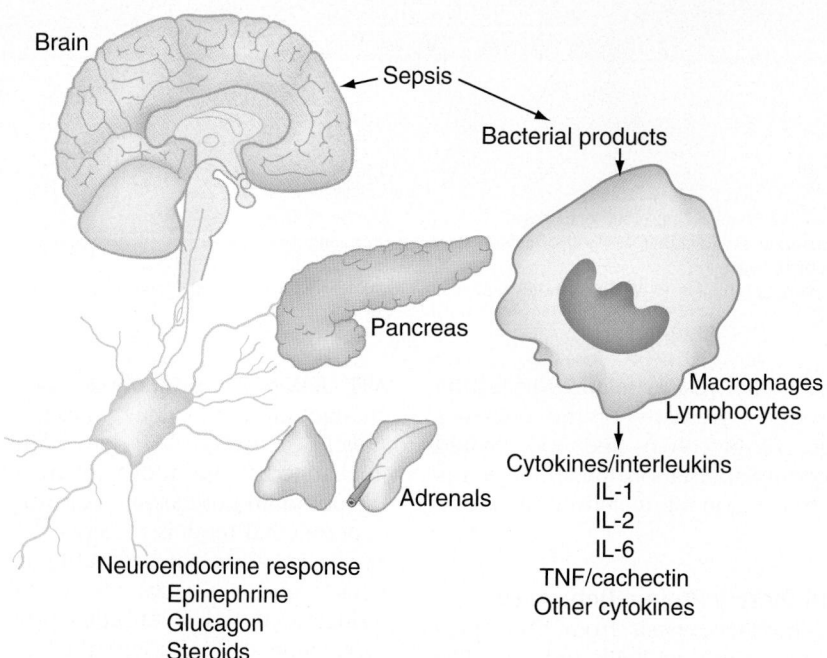

Figure 7-5 An emerging concept of the response to stress and sepsis. In previous years the neurosympathetic response to sepsis was emphasized, with the secretion of epinephrine, glucagon, and corticosteroids—the so-called counter-regulatory hormones. It is now clear that this is but half of the efferent limb and that cytokines are extremely important. IL, interleukin; TNF, tumor necrosis factor.

Role of Cytokines and Other Mediators in the Response to Sepsis

Many of the systemic manifestations of sepsis are mediated by cytokines, levels of which rise in the blood in infection and other inflammatory states such as burn injury (see Fig. 7-5) (for a complete discussion of the biology of cytokines and inflammation, the reader is directed to Chapter 4). Clowes, a general surgeon, in 1983 proposed for the first time that a so-called proteolysis inducing factor (most likely an interleukin split product) was responsible for increased muscle proteolysis and hepatic protein synthesis in sepsis, and this proposal stimulated broad interest in the cytokines as mediators of these processes. Although probably more than 100 products of macrophages exist, attention has focused largely on only a few, primarily interleukin-1 (IL-1), IL-6, TNF, and interferon-γ (IFN-γ). Enterocytes, in addition to inflammatory cells, may also serve as a source of these cytokines. In muscle, activation of proteolysis by TNF and other cytokines appears to depend, at least in part, on activation of a nuclear transcription factor termed NF-κB that serves as a common signaling pathway for inflammation. An increasingly commonly held view is that cytokine release is an appropriate response to a modest-sized insult but that sustained enormous cytokine release is deleterious and may contribute to the so-called multiple organ failure syndrome, the end-stage physiologic state accompanying sepsis.

Elucidation of the roles of particular cytokines in the activation of muscle proteolysis during sepsis has proved

difficult. Although many of the cytokines mentioned have, when administered in recombinant form to intact animals, been shown singly or in combination to activate the ATP-dependent ubiquitin-proteasome pathway of muscle proteolysis,[25] in isolated muscle preparations their actions are less clear. Interestingly, unlike IL-1, TNF, or IFN-γ, IL-6 does not induce changes in muscle mRNA for ubiquitin,[25] and this is consistent with the observation in Dr. Fischer's laboratory that in IL-6–deficient mice the sepsis-related acceleration in proteolysis still occurs. One important factor present in intact animals but perhaps lacking during in vitro experiments is the corticosteroids. Studies from Dr. Fischer and Dr. Hasselgren's laboratory strongly suggest that in septic animals, glucocorticoids are required for full activation of the ubiquitin-proteasome pathway in muscle and thus appear to be a permissive factor for the response to cytokines[19] and in particular TNF, whose actions are blocked by RU-486, a glucocorticoid antagonist. Inhibition of TNF production in sepsis and other conditions may be of benefit in inhibiting muscle wasting. For example, recent experiments with a xanthine derivative, torbafylline, demonstrated inhibition of proteolysis via the ubiquitin-proteasome pathway and prevented muscle wasting in animal models of cancer cachexia and sepsis.[26]

Both IL-1 and TNF elicit the release of prostaglandin E_2 from muscle. Although prostaglandin E_2 had been proposed to be critical for increased muscle proteolysis in septic models, no decrease in ATP-dependent proteolysis or ubiquitin mRNA levels occurred in muscles from endotoxin-treated rats that received naproxen, a potent inhibitor of prostaglandin E_2 production. To summarize both in vivo and in vitro studies, prostaglandins do not appear to be necessary for the rise in muscle proteolysis during infection.[11]

Another signal for increased proteolysis in muscle during systemic infection is fever. Studies of the influence of temperature on protein degradation and synthesis in isolated muscles by V. Baracos and A. Goldberg in 1984 demonstrated a linear increase in the rate of proteolysis but relatively unchanged protein synthesis. Therefore, in febrile animals, the rise in body temperature induced by cytokines and their direct catabolic effects on skeletal muscle appear to act synergistically to induce amino acid release and promote muscle wasting.

The effects of cytokines on the liver are complex. IL-1 is associated with increased hepatic protein synthesis of some of the complement intermediates, whereas synthesis of transferrin is steroid dependent. IL-6 appears to increase the synthesis of certain α-glycoproteins, but undoubtedly other cytokines are involved as well.

Role of Oxidizing Agents

Oxidizing agents such as nitric oxide (NO) and hydroxyl radicals are generated in a variety of tissues and play important roles in metabolic regulation. NO, a mediator of diverse physiologic processes, is a short-lived free radical gas and oxidant derived from arginine by nitric oxide synthase (NOS).[27] Three NOS isoforms have been identified in cells. Endothelial and neuronal NOS (ecNOS and ncNOS) are constitutively expressed and are Ca^{2+}-calmodulin dependent, whereas the largely inducible Ca^{2+}-independent NOS isoform (iNOS) is expressed in immunologically activated cells. A classic action of ecNOS is the cyclic guanosine monophosphate–dependent vasodilation mediated by the endothelium, whereas ncNOS-derived NO functions as a neurotransmitter in numerous pathways. NO reacts avidly with oxygen-derived free radicals, thiols, and the active metal centers of proteins, and a complex chemistry governs its functions in cell signaling and in altering metabolic activity. Of the three isoforms, iNOS is most important because once it is induced by lipopolysaccharide, cytokines, or other factors, large and sustained amounts of NO may be produced. The increase in NO production in sepsis has been proposed to mediate increased hepatic protein synthesis, killing of pathogens, and programmed cell death (apoptosis).[28] Various studies have also shown that skeletal muscle produces NO and that NOS activity in this tissue is influenced by contraction[29] and cytokines. In fact, our recent studies in incubated muscles have shown that NO donors or hydroxyl radicals activate proteolysis by up to 80%.[30] These mediators may therefore be important for the accelerated muscle proteolysis during strenuous exercise or ischemia, after muscle injury, and in inflammatory states.

Cachexia of Cancer

Patients with neoplastic disease may suffer profound weight loss and generalized cachexia. Many factors probably contribute to this response, including reduced food intake, altered metabolic rate, endocrine abnormalities, and the effects of anticancer treatments, but various cytokines and other circulating factors have been identified that undoubtedly play a role, such as TNF, IL-1, IL-6, and IFN-γ.[31] Anorexia is common, even when the tumor is small, a finding suggesting deranged central nervous system satiety mechanisms (see later). Marked muscle wasting is a debilitating feature of advanced cancer. In rats bearing tumors, severe muscle wasting occurs, apparently mediated by TNF and resulting primarily from an increased rate of ATP-dependent proteolysis with increased levels of mRNA for ubiquitin and subunits of the proteasome, especially in the pale muscle fibers, which atrophy most profoundly. However, additional proteolytic pathways may also be activated and different cytokines or other circulating factors are frequently implicated in the genesis of cachexia.[31] One other factor implicated in some types of cancer cachexia is proteolysis-inducing factor (PIF). This substance was identified first in tumor-bearing mice and, when injected into healthy mice, produced profound weight loss. Purified PIF induces catabolism in muscle cells and activates the ubiquitin-proteasome pathway in muscle.[32] PIF has also been found in the urine of a large proportion of patients with weight loss secondary to pancreatic cancer, and treatment with eicosapentaenoic acid (EPA), which blocks the formation of 15-hydroxyeicosatetraenoic acid by PIF in muscle cells, inhibits weight loss even in those with advanced disease.[33] However, whether these mechanisms have broad applicability in cancer remains unclear.

New Concepts in the Regulation of Body Energy Expenditure

In the past decade, exciting insights have been achieved in interrelated areas of mechanisms regulating body size and resting energy expenditure, satiety, and the metabolic phenomena thought to be relevant to aging.[34] These findings have relevance to diverse disease entities, including the etiology of insulin resistance (e.g., in sepsis), type II diabetes mellitus, and morbid obesity. One surprising realization has been that adipose tissue is not just a storage depot for calories, but via a complex network of hormonal and neuronal signals, this tissue also plays an important role in endocrine regulation. Beginning with the discovery by J. Friedman in 1994 of the adipocyte-derived circulating hormone leptin, adipose tissue is now known to be an important source of endocrine mediators, including TNF, angiotensinogen, resistin, and adiponectin. In conjunction with gut hormones such as ghrelin, cholecystokinin, PYY, and insulin, the adipocyte-derived hormones interact in the brain, in particular at the arcuate nucleus, to control food intake and energy expenditure. In the arcuate nucleus, two sets of neurons appear to interact with opposing effects. Activation of agouti-related peptide (AgRP)/neuropeptide Y (NPY) neurons increases appetite and metabolism, whereas activation of POMC/CART neurons has the opposing effect of inhibiting eating, in part by causing the release of α-melanocyte–stimulating hormone (α-MSH), a satiety signal. Such mechanisms are clearly relevant to understanding the inanition accompanying advanced cancer, and some evidence suggests that appetite-promoting agents such as ghrelin may find clinical use in this regard. How these newly described regulatory pathways influence the metabolism of particular nutrients or nitrogen balance remains poorly understood.

Recent discoveries in aging research appear to be connected, if indirectly, to the metabolic signaling pathways described earlier. It is now well accepted that in experimental animals and lower organisms, dietary caloric restriction enhances longevity and may have other desirable effects such as a reduction in primary tumors. Similar genetic mechanisms may underlie such responses, beginning with the discovery by L. Guarente and coworkers of the *Sir2* gene in yeast and the discovery by G. Ruvkun and colleagues of the daf-2 genetic pathway in *Caenorhabditis elegans*. These mechanisms appear to involve changes in nicotinamide adenine dinucleotide (NAD)-dependent functions such as histone acetylation, in insulin signaling, and in cellular responses to reactive oxygen species generated in the mitochondria. These exciting studies will undoubtedly contribute to our future understanding of overall metabolism, carcinogenesis, and free radical–induced injury.

FUNDAMENTALS OF ARTIFICIAL NUTRITION

General Indications for Nutrition Support and Choice of the Route of Administration

Indications for nutritional support should consider the following:

1. The patient's premorbid state (healthy or otherwise)
2. Poor nutritional status (current oral intake meeting <50% of total energy needs)
3. Significant weight loss (initial body weight less than usual body weight by 10% or more or a decrease in inpatient weight by more than 10% of the admission weight
4. The duration of starvation (>7 days' inanition)

5. An anticipated duration of artificial nutrition (particularly total parenteral nutrition [TPN]) of longer than 7 days
6. The degree of the anticipated insult, surgical or otherwise
7. A serum albumin value less than 3.0 g/dL measured in the absence of an inflammatory state
8. A transferrin level of less than 200 mg/dL
9. Anergy to injected antigens

Each practitioner must choose the criteria in a given patient. Obviously, in critically ill patients, nutritional supplementation should be undertaken more readily than in patients who are less severely stressed. Finally, when patients are either malnourished or in the postinjury stressed state, there is no obvious harm and there may be a clinical benefit to the initiation of immediate enteral feeding, particularly in more critically ill patients (see later).

Two routes of administration are possible: the enteral route, via the stomach or preferably the small intestine, and the parenteral route. The enteral route is considered to be more physiologic in that the liver is not bypassed, thereby allowing this organ to efficiently process and store various portally supplied nutrients, and the release of gut hormones and insulin is facilitated, presumably leading to more efficient nutrient disposal in the periphery. However, despite these and other putative advantages, the relative benefits of enteral versus parenteral nutrition in humans remain unclear (see Controversies in Artificial Nutrition later).

Nutritional Assessment

Nutritional assessment is a process by which changes in body nutritional composition are estimated, in part to predict risk for surgery or other stressful therapeutic activity. Ideally, valid methods of assessment should facilitate patient selection for instituting artificial nutrition and for determining the efficacy of nutritional interventions. Although functional measures of lean body mass, such as skeletal muscle strength, respiratory and cardiac performance, hepatic synthetic function, renal status, and immunologic reactivity, seem most desirable, in practice, such approaches have proved difficult (see later). Acceptable studies of nutritional assessment techniques should be randomized, prospective, and blinded. However, most published studies are retrospective for selected patients, usually those judged to be severely at risk. Studies that emphasize hepatic synthesis of short-lived or immunologically active proteins and those that measure neutrophil function may be more successful in identifying patients at risk for infection. In several studies, a careful history plus physical examination by a seasoned clinician yields the same accuracy as extensive testing for the estimation of nutritional risk, particularly when functionality is assessed (Box 7-1).

Clinical History

Weight loss, anorexia, weakness, inability to carry out normal functions, or a disease process that interferes with

---

Box 7-1   Methods of Nutritional Assessment

■ Clinical history
  Weighing, subjective assessment
■ Body composition analysis
  Bioelectrical impedance, exchange of labeled ions, neutron activation analysis
  Cross-sectional imaging (magnetic resonance imaging, computed tomography)
■ Indirect calorimetry
  Oxygen consumption, determination of respiratory quotient
■ Anthropomorphic measurements
  Ideal body weight, skinfold thickness
■ Biochemical measurements
  Albumin, transferrin, prealbumin
■ Measurement of nitrogen balance
■ Measurements of immunologic function

intake, such as esophageal carcinoma, should alert the examiner to the possibility of malnutrition. Certain disorders such as burns, sepsis, head injury, and pancreatitis are particularly catabolic and must be anticipated to raise caloric requirements significantly. The clinical criteria described earlier for the degree of acceptable body weight loss and duration of inanition must be calculated. Finally, on physical examination, muscle wasting, loose or otherwise abnormal skin, the edema of hypoproteinemia, weakness, loss of body fat, and pallor should suggest the diagnosis of malnutrition.

Body Composition Analysis

Accumulation of lean body mass is the principal objective of nutritional support; thus, determination of lean body mass is the most appropriate means of nutritional assessment. Such determinations are usually available only on a research basis.

Bioelectrical Impedance

This method estimates total body water and lean muscle mass by measuring electrical resistance at various surface locations. Though simple to perform, the values derived are often inaccurate and poorly reproducible. In addition, although bioelectrical impedance may be accurate in a normal individual, its accuracy in patients with abnormal body composition has not been verified.

Displacement

Probably the most sensitive determination of lean body mass is displacement. Various body components are estimated by displacement of water volume.

Exchange of Labeled Ions

Total body water may be determined by the administration of tritiated water. Lean body mass is estimated by exchangeable potassium (^{42}K) and extracellular water by total exchangeable sodium (^{22}Na). Shizgal suggested that a ratio of exchangeable sodium to exchangeable potassium greater than 1.2 is an indication of the increased extracellular water and decreased body mass accompanying malnutrition. Shizgal also proposed derivative ratios to estimate total body fat, but because of compounded error, these ratios are probably inaccurate.

Neutron Activation Analysis

This technique is accurate but requires sophisticated apparatus in which the body is bombarded with activated neutrons. Nitrogen, indicative of lean body mass, is then measured. Other ions may also be determined.

Total Body Counters

These large devices measure spontaneous decay of naturally occurring isotopes such as ^{40}K, which reflects lean body mass. However, these measurements are not suitable for patients who are ill because subjects must remain stationary within the counter for prolonged periods.

Magnetic Resonance Imaging

Magnetic resonance imaging may accurately measure lean body mass, although most current work has focused on energy metabolism and the relationship between high-energy phosphate stores in starvation and refeeding. For example, in rats, phosphocreatine is decreased after 6 to 8 days of starvation. Other studies suggest a possible decrease in ATP synthetic efficiency in the starved muscle, presumably secondary to insufficient stores of phosphocreatine to maintain ATP.

Computed Tomography

Computed tomography (CT) with three-dimensional reconstruction can yield accurate values for organ size and volume. Radiographic tissue density can also be used to monitor the response to therapy. For example, studies by Buchman and associates have shown that the hepatic steatosis that commonly occurs during long-term TPN administration can be at least partially reversed by supplementation of the TPN solution with carnitine or choline, as shown by a reduction in hepatic fat content (with increased radiographic density) on serial CT scanning.[35] Other workers have related hepatic steatosis to an abnormal portal vein insulin-to-glucagon ratio, and in experimental animals hepatic steatosis can be cleared by administration of glucagon (see later).

Indirect Calorimetry

Indirect calorimetry, performed with a bedside metabolic cart, is being used increasingly to measure energy balance and to estimate caloric requirements. The measurement is carried out with the patient in the resting state, and in general, 15% should be added for activity. Oxygen consumption can be determined directly and caloric expenditure calculated. In addition, if carbon dioxide production is measured simultaneously, the respiratory quotient (RQ) can be estimated for assessment of overfeeding. An alternative method for determination of oxygen consumption involves placement of a pulmonary artery catheter. If cardiac output is measured by thermodilution and the oxygen content in arterial and mixed venous blood is measured, the Fick equation can then be used to calculate $\dot{V}o_2$. In certain patient populations, particularly after severe burn injury, direct measurement of $\dot{V}o_2$ has proved very useful in estimating caloric needs because in these patients, standard formulas such as the Harris-Benedict equation (see Practical Approach to Artificial Nutrition later) often prove particularly inaccurate.

Metabolic carts can also determine which fuel is being consumed in a clinical setting. An RQ of 1 indicates pure carbohydrate utilization, 0.8 indicates pure protein oxidation, and 0.7 is consistent with pure fat utilization. Theoretically, the RQ with lipogenesis can be as high as 9. Although an RQ greater than 1 is rarely seen, such data are indicative of overfeeding of glucose or fat, or both, whereas an RQ less than 0.7 indicates ketogenesis. Without such measurements, when fat is administered, indirect measures of utilization, such as the absence of plasma lipemia and the presence of ketone bodies, are necessary to confirm efficient metabolism. Although indirect calorimetry is an attractive approach, a recent multicenter study of RQs derived by this method suggests that in practice, low sensitivity and specificity may limit its efficacy as an indicator of overfeeding or underfeeding.[36]

Anthropomorphic Measurements

These parameters are controversial with regard to normative values and their relevance to nitrogen depletion. Characteristic measurements include the creatinine-height index, triceps skinfold thickness, and arm muscle circumference. Although these values may be proportional to muscle or fat stores, they do not reflect function. A more practical anthropomorphic approach is the calculation of ideal body weight (IBW), particularly when usual body weight, or weight of the patient before the onset of illness, is unknown. IBW can be found in standardized tables developed by the insurance industry that relate height to expected weight, or IBW can be estimated by the following equations:

- For males: 106 lb for the first 5 ft and 6 lb for each inch thereafter.
- For females: 100 lb for the first 5 ft and 5 lb for each inch thereafter.

Because these tables were derived from population norms in the 1950s, before the current trend toward obesity in Americans, they tend to underestimate weight. However, in keeping with the general principle of avoiding excessive provision of calories during artificial feeding, use of the IBW for calculating caloric needs is not harmful and is commonly done (see Practical Approach to Artificial Nutrition).

Functional Studies of Muscle Function

Because many of the tests described earlier are not readily available, muscle strength has been evaluated either by handgrip dynamometry, force-frequency characteristics, or the rate of recovery from fatigue after electrical stimulation of the ulnar nerve. When properly conducted, such studies provide a functional counterpart of severe protein-calorie malnutrition, and they may be used to assess for a beneficial response to nutritional or other anabolic interventions. For example, an ongoing study at Beth Israel Deaconess Medical Center suggests that handgrip strength may improve in elderly patients administered growth hormone. In most studies, however, patients with deficits in hand dynamometry are easily identifiable by other means such as a simple functional history, physical examination, or global nutritional assessment. The importance of functional studies was recently emphasized by the work of Herridge and colleagues (see the accompanying editorial also), who demonstrated residual muscle wasting and weakness for up to 1 year after discharge from the intensive care unit (ICU) and treatment of acute respiratory distress syndrome (ARDS).[37]

Biochemical Measurements

A variety of biochemical approaches have been described for determining malnutrition. Though useful, such methods are often inaccurate and do not usually give added value when compared with a clinical approach to nutritional assessment.

Serum Proteins

Measurement of serum proteins, in particular albumin, is often used as an index of malnutrition, with an albumin concentration of less than 3.0 g/dL being the usual indicator. The half-life of albumin is as long as 14 to 18 days, and for this reason other more short-lived proteins, such as prealbumin (half-life 3-5 days) or transferrin (<200 mg/dL, half-life 7 days), have been proposed as more sensitive indicators of rapid changes in nutritional status. However, the meaning of the lowered serum albumin concentration in patients who are malnourished and at risk has always been controversial. Some investigators have attributed the low serum albumin to decreased synthesis, possibly as a result of low-grade sepsis or stress, and others have attributed it to increased degradation. In a model of long-term sepsis, von Allmen and associates[38] found that whereas albumin synthesis was decreased for the first 24 hours, after 4 days' synthesis this protein actually rose to normal levels. These results suggest that decreased albumin synthesis because of down-regulation may not be tenable in long-term malnutrition. In malnutrition one generally expects an increase in extravascular volume. With greater extravascular volume, a greater amount of albumin is likely to be present in the extravascular space, where it appears to be degraded more rapidly. Thus, increased albumin in the extravascular space with an increased rate of degradation may well explain the lowered serum albumin in patients who are at risk.

Nitrogen Balance

Measurement of nitrogen balance is a tedious technique that requires determination of all integumentary, wound, and excretory losses. Overall, such measurements tend to be inaccurate and will often favor the erroneous conclusion that positive nitrogen balance has been achieved. In the clinical setting, nitrogen balance is determined by measuring 24-hour urinary and GI losses. Because most patients receiving parenteral nutrition do not eat, stool nitrogen can be assumed to be 1 g/day, or it can be disregarded altogether. The 24-hour urine collection must be accurate, as monitored by measuring urinary creatinine. The value for the rate of nitrogen loss is compared with nitrogen intake, and nitrogen balance is thus obtained. Therefore,

$$\text{Nitrogen balance} = \text{Intake} - \text{Loss (urine 90\%, stool 5\%, integument 5\%)}$$

or

$$= (\text{Protein intake [g]}/6.25) - \text{Urinary urea (g)} - 2 \text{ (for stool and skin)} - 2 \text{ (for nonurea nitrogen)}$$

Measurement of Protein Breakdown

Nitrogen turnover, particularly that of lean body mass, can be estimated by urinary excretion of 3-methylhistidine, as described earlier. However, 3-methylhistidine measures not only the breakdown of muscle but also the breakdown of a more rapidly turning over protein pool derived from the gut and skin, thus invalidating it as a measurement of turnover of skeletal muscle protein alone. Short of actual in vitro measurement in isolated muscle tissue (see earlier), common in vivo approaches to the measurement of protein breakdown include pulse-chase and other isotopic methods that involve the infusion of ^{15}N-labeled amino acids and other metabolites. All these methods, unfortunately, are highly derivative and subject to a variety of artifacts.

Measurements of Immunologic Function

Delayed cutaneous hypersensitivity or anergy, most commonly tested by delayed reaction to skin recall antigens, was widely used in early studies of nutritional assessment and is a manifestation of cell-mediated immunity. Although most studies showed a statistical relationship between anergy and mortality, investigators have concluded that delayed cutaneous hypersensitivity is without value for measuring specific nutritional or operative risk. In contrast, more recent data suggest that when skin testing is carefully performed by trained personnel and done at defined times (e.g., on admission rather than at random throughout the hospital course), skin reactivity may have some value. For example, in patients admitted after trauma or with infection, anergy to injected cutaneous recall antigens is associated with high mortality and morbidity. These patients are probably those with severe malnutrition. However, not all malnourished patients are at risk and the defect is immunologic, not nutritional. Furthermore, delayed cutaneous hypersensitivity is complicated by extraneous factors such as surgery, which is followed by immediate anergy in many patients. Patients with cancer are also anergic, and this condition may be reversed after resection. Thus, the significance of delayed cutaneous hypersensitivity must be assessed in concert with other tests. Another method for determining immunologic function in the clinical setting is neutrophil function, but this approach appears to be even less relevant to nutritional status than assays of cell-mediated immunity are.

Specific Fuels

The sources of calories in a normal diet and during artificial feeding are carbohydrate, lipid, and protein. We will discuss each of these fuels, with particular emphasis on their relative roles during IV feeding and adjustments needed for concurrent illness such as diabetes and liver or renal failure.

Carbohydrate

Glucose is the preferred carbohydrate source in traditional TPN. Glucose administration during fasting or stress appears to decrease urinary urea production, the so-called protein-sparing effect, with a minimum of 100 g of glucose per 24 hours being required for this response based on Gamble's classic lifeboat ration studies of the 1940s. It was not until the late 1970s that the metabolism of exogenously supplied carbohydrate was evaluated in detail. The nitrogen-sparing effect of infused glucose was found to occur through two mechanisms. First, hepatic gluconeogenesis is suppressed, so protein need not be broken down to generate gluconeogenic precursors. Second, glucose itself is used as an energy substrate, so fewer amino acids need be oxidized for energy. Wolfe and coworkers showed that maximum suppression of gluconeogenesis is achieved at infusion rates of 4 mg/kg/min (~400 g/day for a 70-kg man) and that glucose infusion beyond this level has minimal effects in further suppressing glucose production during TPN administration in postoperative surgical patients.[39] In this work, although any additional nitrogen-sparing effects of glucose would be expected to be derived from its direct oxidation, at infusions rates higher than 9 mg/kg/min all glucose was degraded by nonoxidative pathways, specifically, those leading to net synthesis of lipid.

Toxicity of Hyperglycemia and Excessive Calorie Administration

When provided in excess, carbohydrate is converted to fat in the liver, a consequence that is referred to as de novo lipogenesis and probably contributes to TPN-related liver dysfunction (see later). In addition, the accompanying increase in Vco_2, as reflected by an elevated RQ (see earlier), may lead to impaired ventilatory function in patients with already compromised pulmonary status. Finally, the resultant hyperglycemic state, most pronounced with a blood glucose concentration greater than 300 mg/dL, leads to immunosuppression and an increased frequency of nosocomial infections. Hyperglycemia is a prevalent metabolic disorder that can be particularly pronounced in the ICU setting and postinjury state and is clearly exacerbated by excessive administration of dextrose.

The immunosuppressive effects of hyperglycemia have been well studied. In vitro data suggest that hyperglycemia leads to immune cell dysfunction as a result of impaired chemotaxis, adherence, phagocytosis, and bactericidal function. In prospective studies, tight postoperative glycemic control has been shown to significantly decrease nosocomial infections in diabetic patients. In the ICU setting, fastidious glycemic control achieved through intensive insulin therapy has been shown to dramatically improve patient outcomes.

In the prospective, randomized study of Van den Berghe and colleagues,[40] 1548 cardiac surgery ICU patients were randomized to either standard glycemic control (to maintain blood glucose at 180-200 mg/dL) or tight glycemic control (insulin infusion to maintain glucose at 80-110 mg/dL). All patents were fed 25 kcal/kg by either enteral or parenteral routes. By maintaining blood glucose in the 80 to 110 mg/dL range, these investigators demonstrated significant improvement in various clinical outcomes and a 42% decrease in overall mortality. This landmark study highlights the importance of maintaining normoglycemia during feeding because otherwise, the benefits of nutritional intervention may be negated by the detrimental consequences associated with the hyperglycemic state. In contrast, in a more recent publication in which a nonsurgical ICU population was studied,[41] Van den Berghe and coworkers failed to demonstrate improved mortality with vigorous glycemic control, and the incidence of clinically significant hypoglycemia attributable to aggressive insulin use was appreciable. In our own cardiac surgical unit, where maintenance of normoglycemia is prioritized, the incidence of mediastinitis is very low, although other initiatives were undertaken simultaneously.

In an effort to avoid the potential complications of overfeeding, one reasonable short-term option is the practice of hypocaloric feeding. The clinician must often balance the optimal administration of nutrition with a patient's overall clinical status. One could easily envision the desire to limit the volume of TPN received by a diabetic patient with difficult-to-control blood sugar, by a massively volume overloaded patient in renal failure who is not being dialyzed, or by a patient with poor oxygenation who is being maintained on high ventilatory support. In this setting it appears reasonable to provide goal protein (1.5 g/kg/day, see later) while limiting total calories to approximately 1000 kcal/day. This practice will decrease net protein catabolism while still allowing mobilization of endogenous fat stores to close the expected caloric gap and will limit excessive volume administration. This approach is particularly acceptable when applied over a limited time course such as 1 to 2 weeks and in the obese patient population, who have an abundance of lipid available for mobilization, but it is not a viable option for standard nutrition support. It is also unclear whether hypocaloric feeding in patients with renal failure has a similar outcome as nutritional supplementation with essential amino acids and hypertonic dextrose (see later).

Additional Sources of Dextrose

One must be careful to recognize all sources of exogenous dextrose administration, in addition to the patient's feeding solution, because significant amounts of dextrose can be found in the following:

- IV fluids containing 5% dextrose (50 g/L)
- Medications mixed in 5% dextrose instead of normal saline
- Patients undergoing continuous venovenous dialysis, who often have 5% solutions as return fluid
- Patients undergoing peritoneal dialysis with dextrose in the dialysate.

Alternative Carbohydrate Sources

Carbohydrate sources other than glucose have not achieved popularity in the United States. Fructose, which some investigators have proposed for use in glucose resistance, may cause fatal lactic acidosis. The polyalcohols xylitol and sorbitol also undergo transformation to glucose, but xylitol may be hepatotoxic and has probably contributed to several deaths in the literature. Glycerol, another potential source of glucose, is potentially advantageous in that it may be sterilized in solution with amino acids, without caramelization, and its osmolality is low. The safety as well as efficacy of glycerol was studied in patients recovering from major trauma or surgery.[42] In one group, nitrogen equilibrium was achieved with combined lipid and glycerol administration. However, glycerol in large doses may cause renal failure in experimental animals, and thus caution is appropriate.

Lipid

In starvation, fat provides the bulk of calories in the form of free fatty acids and as ketone bodies manufactured by the liver from long-chain fatty acids. Net lipolysis during fasting or stress is promoted by steroids, catechols, glucagon, and some cytokines and is extremely sensitive to inhibition by insulin. Under normal circumstances or in moderate stress, fat and carbohydrate are indistinguishable with respect to their positive effects on nitrogen balance, with 25% of nonprotein calories as fat seemingly being optimal for hepatic protein synthesis. What is not clear is at which point in stress or during sepsis that fat utilization becomes impaired. Most investigators agree that whereas hepatic manufacture of ketone bodies is reduced early in sepsis, fat clearance remains relatively normal until comparatively late, even though fat oxidation is clearly impaired at a previous stage. Many sources of lipid are available for IV use.

Nomenclature and Structure of Fatty Acids

Fatty acids consist of a carboxyl group with a hydrophobic carbon side chain of variable length. The convention for describing fatty acid structure is X (the total number of carbons, including the carboxyl carbon): Y (the total number of unsaturated bonds). So-called desaturases remove two hydrogens to yield a methylene group (double bond between carbons), whereas so-called elongases insert two sequential carbons into an existing fatty acid chain. The most abundant fatty acids contain 14 to 22 carbons, and 16 and 18 predominate. The most common saturated fatty acids are palmitic (C16:0) and stearic (C18:0) acids, with oleic acid (C18:1) being the most common monounsaturated fatty acid. Further complicating fatty acid nomenclature is the "n" or "ω" (omega) numbering system used to describe unsaturated fatty acids. Both "n" and "ω" are interchangeable and refer to the number of carbons between the terminal noncarboxyl carbon and the closest double bond. For the example of oleic acid, because the solitary double bond occurs adjacent to the 10th carbon thus leaving nine carbons at the end of the side chain, the complete nomenclature is C18:1 n-9 or C18:1 ω-9. For the polyunsaturated essential fatty acid linoleic acid, there are two double bonds with six terminal saturated carbons, which gives rise to C18:2 n-6. Lengthening of an unsaturated fatty acid side chain to produce longer derivatives of the essential fatty acid precursors linoleic and α-linolenic acid requires sequential cycles of two-carbon elongation followed by desaturation. These synthetic enzymes prefer substrates with terminal carbon chains of the n-3 > n-6 > n-9 configuration, in that order, which gives rise to the n-3, n-6, and n-9 series of polyunsaturated fatty acids (PUFAs). The most complete nomenclature for naming unsaturated fatty acids also includes the location of the double bonds. For the preceding example of linoleic acid, the double bonds are after the 9th carbon and the 12th carbon. The most complete description for linoleic acid is therefore C18:2 Δ9, 12, or in the "n" system, C18:2 n-6.

Long-Chain Triglycerides

Safe administration of IV lipid became a reality in the late 1970s when an emulsion (Intralipid) consisting of soybean oil and egg lecithin and containing predominantly long-chain triglycerides (LCTs) became commercially available in the United States. Though initially administered as a source of essential fatty acids (linoleic acid and α-linolenic acid), these n-3 and n-6 LCT emulsions now serve as a valuable caloric source in parenteral alimentation. Lipid emulsions are particularly versatile because they are calorically dense (9 kcal/g) and can be safely infused via a peripheral vein. Their role as a supplemental caloric source is particularly valuable when blood sugar is difficult to control or when carbohydrate administration reaches safe limits.

Medium-Chain Triglycerides

Because of the potential adverse effect of LCT emulsions (see later), alternative lipid fuels have been considered. In comparison to LCTs, medium-chain triglycerides (MCTs), which contain only 8 to 10 carbons, are cleared more rapidly from plasma, are oxidized more rapidly, do not require a carnitine-dependent transport system to enter liver mitochondria, and are more soluble in TPN solutions. MCTs may also have a favorable effect on protein metabolism leading to improved nitrogen balance. However, MCTs can be neurotoxic in patients with cirrhosis who cannot adequately clear them, and overall, mixed MCT-LCT emulsions are thought to be most desirable. Mixed emulsions may be of particular benefit in patients with inflammatory disorders because they contain approximately 50% fewer n-6 LCTs than the traditional Intralipid does. Such LCTs may serve as precursors of potentially deleterious prostaglandins (see later).

Structured Lipids

Structured lipids are a synthetic triglyceride molecule in which medium-chain and long-chain fatty acids are esterified to the same glycerol backbone. The composition of the three fatty acid side chains can vary randomly or can be chemically defined by a specific enzymatic re-esterification process. Studies have proved structured lipids to be safe and to carry the metabolic advantages seen with MCT-LCT physical mixtures. Future studies will determine their role in the routine clinical setting.

Essential or Unsaturated Fatty Acids

Unsaturated fatty acids can be classified as monounsaturated or polyunsaturated, depending on the location of their double bond. The three families of PUFAs (n-3, n-6, and n-9) start as the essential 18-carbon unsaturated fatty acids α-linolenic acid (C18:3 n-3) and linoleic acid (C18:2 n-6) and as the nonessential oleic acid (C18:2 n-9). Both linolenic and linoleic acids are abundant in plants but do not occur naturally in animal tissue. Via sequential steps of elongation and desaturation, the n-6 precursor linoleic acid is converted to arachidonic acid, whereas the n-3 precursor α-linolenic acid is converted to EPA and docosahexaenoic acid (DHA) (Fig. 7-6). As indicated earlier, these desaturase and elongase enzymes are found predominantly in the liver and have as their order of pre-

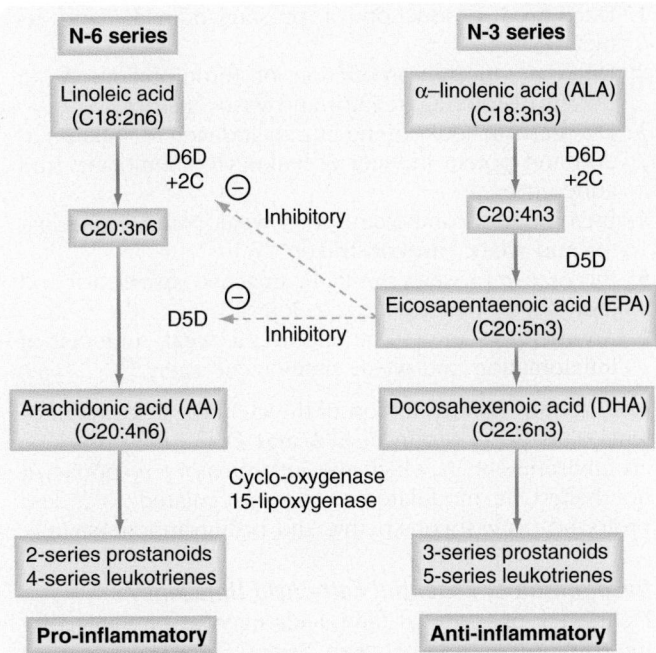

Figure 7-6 Pathways for the synthesis of essential polyunsaturated fatty acids. The important intermediate species leading to formation of the prostanoids and leukotrienes are shown. 2C, two-carbon elongation; D6D, δ-6-desaturase; D5D, δ-5-desaturase. The essential fatty acid precursors linoleic (n-6 series) and linolenic (n-3 series) acid are found only in plants, whereas the n-3 series intermediates eicosapentaenoic acid and docosahexaenoic acid are present at high levels in fish.

ferred substrate n-3>n-6>n-9. This process is under tight control and the enzymes δ-5-desaturase and δ-6-desaturase appear to be key regulatory points. Interestingly, EPA, the intermediate in the n-3 pathway, appears to be inhibitory for the action of these desaturases on substrates of the n-6 pathway, and therefore elevated levels of EPA can negatively regulate the synthesis of arachidonate. EPA and DHA can be derived only from the direct ingestion of nutrients such as fish oil, where they are abundant, or by synthesis from dietary α-linolenic acid.

Arachidonic acid and EPA are precursors of the eicosanoids, namely, the prostaglandins, thromboxanes, and leukotrienes. More specifically, arachidonic acid is the precursor of the 2-series of prostaglandins and thromboxanes and the 4-series of the leukotrienes. EPA and DHA are the precursors of the 3-series of prostaglandins and thromboxanes and the 5-series of leukotrienes. Therefore, at the level of the cyclooxygenase and lipoxygenase enzymes, which are critical for eicosanoid synthesis, there exists competition between arachidonic acid and EPA. With the ingestion of fish or fish oil, the primary dietary source of ω-3 fatty acids (or alternatively, the n-3 fatty acids), EPA and DHA levels rise and these lipids can displace arachidonic acid in the membranes of cells active in eicosanoid synthesis, namely, platelets, erythrocytes, neutrophils, monocytes, and liver cells. As a result, with ω-3 fatty acid administration there are the following:

1. Decreased production of prostaglandin E_2 and its metabolites
2. Decrease in the production of thromboxane A_2, a potent platelet aggregator and vasoconstrictor
3. Decrease in leukotriene B_4, an inducer of inflammation and potent inducer of leukocyte chemotaxis and adherence
4. Increase in thromboxane A_3, a weak platelet aggregator and weak vasoconstrictor
5. Increase in prostacyclin PGI_3, an active vasodilator and inhibitor of platelet aggregation
6. An increase in leukotriene B_5, a weak inducer of inflammation and weak chemotactic agent.[43]

Accordingly, administration of the ω-3 fatty acids (α-linolenic acid or its products EPA and DHA) may produce an environment in which the inflammatory response, if not halted, is modulated or down-regulated to a less profound provasoconstrictive and prothrombotic state.

Recognition of Essential Fatty Acid Deficiency

Deficiency of essential fatty acids may be prevented by the administration of between 2% and 5% of daily calories as either soybean or safflower oil fat emulsion or a minimum of 30 to 50 g of lipid emulsion weekly. Plasma alterations, which occur within 1 week of administration of fat-free parenteral nutrition, include decreases in the n-6 fatty acids linoleic and arachidonic acid and increased levels of the n-9 fatty acid 5,8,11-eicosatrienoic acid, also known as *Mead acid* (C20:3 n-9). These changes result from the relative deficiency of n-3 and n-6 precursors such that the desaturase/elongation enzymes begin to produce products derived from n-9 fatty acids by default. The so-called triene-to-tetraene ratio, or the Holman index, refers to the ratio of Mead acid (20:3 n-9) to arachidonic acid (20:4 n-6) and is normally less than 0.2. If the ratio is greater than this value and other data are suggestive, essential fatty acid deficiency may be suspected. A common clinical sign is dry, flaky skin with small reddish papules and alopecia. Patients with essential fatty acid deficiency absorb essential fatty acids through the skin, but this approach is not practical except in infants. Patients who have excess adipose tissue can live for months without exogenous essential fatty acid administration because they maintain a mobilizable depot of linolenic acid in their adipose tissue.

Omega-3 Fatty Acids in the Clinical Settin

Omega-3 and ω-6 PUFAs are important components of human cell membranes. Their composition within the cell membrane is primarily determined by dietary intake because the ω-3–to–ω-6 ratio changes with changes in dietary consumption. As indicated earlier, the ω-3 fatty acids EPA and DHA play important roles in prostaglandin metabolism, thrombosis and atherosclerosis, immunology and inflammation, and membrane function. Once epidemiologists recognized that the paucity of heart disease in Greenland Inuits was due to a diet high in long-chain n-3 fatty acids, subsequent human studies examining n-3 supplementation have documented their important role in the prevention and treatment of coronary artery disease,

hypertension, arthritis, inflammatory and autoimmune disorders, and cancer.

In the clinical setting, the benefits of ω-3 fatty acid administration to surgical patients have been realized when given as a key component of immune-modulating enteral feeding formulas. This topic is discussed in more detail elsewhere in this chapter. The use of IV n-3 lipid emulsions to modulate the immune system is only now being studied in clinical trials in the United States. Because lipid emulsions containing n-3 fatty acids inhibit triglyceride hydrolysis by lipoprotein lipase, fish oil cannot be infused alone or in combination only with LCTs. Instead, n-3 fatty acids must be combined with MCTs and LCTs in a solution composed of 50% MCT, 40% soybean (LCT), and 10% fish oil. Clinical studies in which this combined lipid solution has been administered have confirmed an increase in the ratio of 5-series to 4-series leukotrienes in peripheral leukocytes, an improvement in inflammatory disorders such as atopic dermatitis, and an attenuated inflammatory response in experimental models of both pancreatic injury and acute colitis.[43]

Supplementation of ω-3 may be particularly advantageous in cirrhosis and liver dysfunction. For example, it is well accepted that patients with end-stage liver disease have very low serum and possibly tissue levels of PUFAs. Several investigators have demonstrated low levels of long-chain PUFAs, namely, arachidonic acid, EPA, and DHA, in patients with advanced cirrhosis, and these deficiencies appear to serve as independent predictors of mortality. Patients with end-stage liver disease cannot mount an appropriate inflammatory response when faced with a severe insult or injury, and cirrhotic patients have a well-documented defect in T-cell–mediated immune function. These phenomena may in part be due to a deficiency in second messengers important in the inflammatory cascade, specifically, low levels of long-chain PUFAs and derived eicosanoids. In fact, one of the principal consequences of essential fatty acid deficiency in animals and humans is reduced resistance to infection. As described later (see Metabolic Complications of Long-Term Administration of Total Parenteral Nutrition), ω-3 fatty acids may also be effective in reversing hepatic steatosis in infants with TPN-associated liver disease.[44]

Potential Toxicities of Lipid Administration

Recent reviews of the literature reveal that no adverse effects related to LCT administration have been observed when IV lipids are administered in modest amounts, as long as infusion rates are lower than 0.1 g/kg/hr or 1 kcal/kg/hr. Before this critical level was determined, many adverse effects ensued when LCT solutions were infused at excessive rates and quantities. Lipid accumulating in the liver may inhibit the reticuloendothelial system, the major site of this system, by overloading and impairing Kupffer cell phagocytosis with lipid micelles. The phospholipid-emulsifying agent used in lipid solutions can also interfere with the action of lipoprotein lipase and potentially lead to a clinically relevant hypertriglyceridemic state. Therefore, lipid emulsions are not administered when serum triglyceride levels are greater than 400 mg/dL. The possibility of hypertriglyceride-related pancreatitis also arises when serum triglyceride levels reach the 800- to 1000-mg/dL range. Excessive lipid may also have deleterious effects in patients with severe pulmonary disease such as ARDS. The downstream prostaglandin products of lipid emulsion precursors, such as thromboxane A_2 or PGE_2, can suppress lymphocyte proliferation and natural killer cell activity while reversing hypoxic vasoconstriction in patients with ARDS, thus further worsening pulmonary gas diffusion, oxygenation, and resistance to infection. Impaired plasma clearance of lipids can result in fat overload syndrome, a particularly significant problem in children manifested as fever, back pain, chills, pulmonary insufficiency, and blocking of the reticuloendothelial system. Fat overload syndrome can result from the administration of a stable fat emulsion over a brief interval or from more modest doses of lipid, which might be physicochemically unstable, and is avoided when fat is administered at a limit of 2 g/kg/day. In infants, up to 4 g/kg/day of fat is tolerated.

Protein

A 70-kg man has between 10 and 11 kg of protein, otherwise referred to as lean body mass. In the fed state, daily protein turnover amounts to between 250 and 300 g, or 3%. The gut is the largest component of this turnover, the source of nitrogen loss being shed enterocytes and secreted digestive enzymes. After digestion of food, all amino acids are absorbed, save 1 g of nitrogen excreted in stool. Although intracellular proteolysis accounts for 50 to 70 g of amino acids being added to the amino acid pool daily, if adequate energy is present, most of these amino acids are reincorporated into protein. The nonessential amino acids can be synthesized from carbon skeletons, and sources of nitrogen such as glutamine can be synthesized through transamination. Twenty grams of plasma protein, 8 g of hemoglobin, 20 g of white blood cells, and a few grams of skin constitute the remainder of total body protein synthesis (see Fig. 7-4). Protein turnover decreases markedly with age. Thus, protein turnover in a neonate approximates 25 g/kg/24 hr and decreases to 7 g/kg/24 hr at 1 year, and in adults, turnover falls to 3 g/kg/24 hr.

Determining Protein Requirements

The minimal intake of protein required for neutral nitrogen balance can be determined empirically by two approaches. The first method involves measuring all nitrogen losses while the human or animal subject is fed a calorically adequate, but protein-free diet. In general, this approach will underestimate the true protein requirement, particularly when a superimposed stressor is present. For example, after several days of a protein-free diet in humans, 37 mg/kg of nitrogen is excreted into urine and 12 mg/kg is lost in feces. Integumentary losses account for another 5 mg/kg, with an additional 2 to 3 mg/kg of nitrogen lost by evaporation, for a total of 56 to 57 mg of nitrogen per kilogram, or in terms of whole protein, 0.34 g of protein per kilogram is lost per day. This latter value is well below commonly accepted norms for the daily protein requirement in humans. A second approach that appears to be more relevant to clinical practice is to determine the minimal quantity of ingested protein necessary to maintain nitrogen equilibrium. When derived in this manner, with various corrections, the average normal requirement is 0.8 g of protein per kilogram, or between 56 and 60 g of protein per day. Trauma, infection, and other catabolic conditions will increase this requirement. In addition, in the postinjury state, the increased rate of whole body protein catabolism appears to be unusually resistant to exogenous supplementation with amino acids. However, this obligate protein loss, driven by the overexpression of catecholamines and cytokines during the systemic inflammatory response, can be offset to some degree by protein administration, with the rate of net protein catabolism decreased to about a fourth of the rate seen in the absence of TPN. The extensive studies of whole body protein turnover by Graham Hill and Robert Wolfe during the 1980s documented that exogenous protein administration of 1.5 g/kg/day achieves maximal protein sparing and that when amounts exceeding this value are administered, no further incorporation of nitrogen into protein is possible, with the excess protein being converted to urea and excreted, at least in relatively normal patients. Accordingly, it is most common to administer protein during artificial nutrition, whether enteral or parenteral, at a value of 1.5 g/kg/day. It is not clear in patients with severe protein loss, such as after major burns, whether limiting protein intake to this level is efficacious, and many centers have attempted to administer even greater amounts of protein (e.g., 2 g/day) to correct measured deficits.

Alterations for Liver and Renal Failure

Patients who are intolerant of nitrogen in the surgical setting usually manifest renal or hepatic impairment, and patients with advanced hepatic failure may have both hepatic and renal insufficiency, the so-called hepatorenal syndrome. Both groups of patients tend to be hypercatabolic, and sepsis is a common accompaniment. In some patients, for example, after an episode of hypotension, a crush injury involving muscle, or dye toxicity in radiologic procedures, the renal failure will, one hopes, be self-limited. In this latter instance the goal is to decrease the rise in blood urea nitrogen (BUN), thus avoiding dialysis, which in turn may add to the mortality associated with an accompanying surgical condition. There are good data in the literature suggesting that essential amino acids are a useful treatment in acute renal failure. In the case of hepatic failure, a BCAA-enriched, aromatic amino acid–deficient solution, given in an effort to avoid encephalopathy but containing sufficient protein in these particularly hypercatabolic patients, is the approach that is also supported by much experimental and clinical data.

Renal Failure

The practice of administering essential amino acids and hypertonic dextrose in a restricted volume, usually in the surgical setting with superimposed acute tubular necrosis, is based on studies published independently in the early 1950s by Giordano and Giovannetti. This work attempted to decrease the frequency of dialysis in chronic renal failure patients. Substantial protein equivalents are lost during dialysis, but in the surgical setting, dialysis is usually thought to be necessary when BUN approaches 90 or 100 (at which point coagulopathy and other azotemic complications may occur). In addition, encephalopathy may be seen, which may or may not be correlated with the rise in BUN in a given patient. Giordano and Giovannetti found that patients with chronic renal failure who were given protein high in biologic value, such as egg albumin, along with adequate calories required less frequent dialysis. Whether this approach might also decrease damage to the few remaining functioning nephrons by decreasing their filtered load, a concept promoted by Brenner, currently lacks scientific support. According to the Giordano-Giovannetti hypothesis, urea was not an end product, as had been commonly supposed, but diffused into the GI tract and was converted to ammonia by urease-producing bacteria. If one supplied essential amino acids with protein high in biologic value and adequate calories, the hypothesis continued, the ammonia could be reincorporated into nonessential amino acids. Accordingly, a full complement of amino acids would result, thus supporting protein synthesis and adequate nutrition. This hypothesis, however, ultimately proved incorrect. In retrospect, most of the effect of essential amino acids on BUN appears to be the consequence of decreased urea generation resulting from their administration.

Although essential amino acids seemed helpful in the chronic setting, the question was whether they would work in a surgical patient with acute renal failure. A series of studies by Wilmore, Dudrick, Abel, Abbot, Fischer, and coworkers in the late 1960s and early 1970s demonstrated conclusively that when such patients were treated with essential amino acids and hypotonic dextrose, a number of beneficial effects could be demonstrated:

1. Hyperkalemia was improved.
2. Dialysis was averted in patients treated with essential amino acids and hypertonic dextrose, as opposed to hypertonic dextrose alone.
3. Survival was improved, especially in patients with some urine production.
4. There was a lower incidence of pneumonia, GI bleeding, and other complications, thus contributing to the improvement in survival.
5. The incidence of encephalopathy was decreased.

In patients after major procedures, such as repair of a ruptured abdominal aortic aneurysm in which the peritoneum has not sealed, essential amino acids and hypertonic dextrose may also be sufficient to tide the patient over until hemodialysis can be tolerated hemodynamically or, if desired, peritoneal dialysis initiated.

Other investigators, without satisfactory studies, have advocated increasing the complexity of amino acids from the essential eight (namely, the BCAAs isoleucine, leucine, and valine; the aromatic amino acids phenylalanine, tyrosine, and tryptophan; and the sulfur-containing amino acids methionine and cysteine) to include histidine and arginine, semiessential amino acids for which rates of synthesis may be insufficient to support the patient during acute stress. However, by adding these additional amino acids, the ability of the solution to hold the rise in BUN down is diminished. Other practices, such as giving BCAAs in large amounts with standard solutions, have little support in the literature. Using much reduced amounts of standard amino acid solutions, as advocated by some, resulted in one study in considerably worsened survival than in patients treated with essential amino acids. Other studies failed to show any difference in patients given dilute standard solutions or essential amino acids, but numbers of subjects were small.

One should be alert to the possibility of hyperammonemia (e.g., as heralded by mental status changes) in patients receiving only essential amino acids for a prolonged period. In infants, arginine deficiency may develop or the enzymes for conversion of arginine to ornithine may be insufficiently mature. The amino acids histidine, isoleucine, and leucine, if abundant, may suppress arginosuccinate synthetase, which is necessary for the conversion of arginine to ornithine. Whatever the mechanism, when ornithine stores are depleted, it can no longer serve its role as a carrier amino acid in the urea cycle, and as a result, ammonia is no longer detoxified in the liver and hyperammonemia may ensue. Therefore, when essential amino acid solutions are administered, particularly over prolonged periods, it is important that sufficient quantities of ornithine be included and serum ammonia levels monitored. Because this ordinarily does not happen, there is little reason to fear.

When used, the average duration of therapy with essential amino acids in hypertonic (35%) dextrose is generally 10 to 14 days. Once the patient is maintained on dialysis, a more complete amino acid solution is appropriate. In the outpatient setting, protein intake of 0.5 to 0.6 g/kg has been shown to slow the progression of chronic renal insufficiency. However, in renal failure patients with an acute superimposed illness or in those maintained on hemodialysis, protein intake of up to 1.2 g/kg is recommended, with most recent studies supporting improved patient outcome when adequate nutrition is administered, even if more frequent or even daily hemodialysis is required to clear the accumulated urea.

Hepatic Insufficiency

Patients with hepatic insufficiency are protein intolerant as well, but here the result of excessive protein administration is potentially severe encephalopathy. In the surgical setting, most such patients manifest sudden hepatic insufficiency, for example, as a result of cirrhosis with acute decompensation secondary to GI bleeding, sepsis, hepatic resection or transplantation, or portal venous diversion with resulting encephalopathy. The situation is doubly difficult because these patients are hypercatabolic, with a protein requirement of 1.1 g/kg/day, approximately double the minimal 0.55 g/kg/day adequate for a patient with well-compensated cirrhosis. Although it is generally acknowledged that patients with hepatic failure who are receiving IV amino acid solutions tolerate these solutions better than oral protein, most patients with significant liver disease do not tolerate 1.5 or even 1.1 g/

kg/day of amino acids when effort is made to achieve nitrogen equilibrium. Many practitioners confronted with these patients believe that an aromatic amino acid–deficient, BCAA-enriched solution is efficacious, and it is not unusual with such an approach to achieve levels of up to 120 g of amino acids per day, for example, and be rewarded not only by adequate nutrition but also by the absence of hepatic encephalopathy.

The basis for using enriched branched-chain and deficient aromatic amino acid solutions is the so-called false neurotransmitter hypothesis, in which hepatic encephalopathy is not a nonspecific toxic phenomenon, as heretofore had been thought, but instead results from abnormalities in brain synaptic function. The basis for this phenomenon is an abnormal plasma amino acid profile, as demonstrated by James, Fischer, and coworkers in the 1970s. In patients with hepatic failure, decreased circulating levels of BCAAs and increased aromatic amino acids, including phenylalanine, tyrosine, methionine, and tryptophan, appear to result in abnormal amine neurotransmitter products in which norepinephrine and dopamine are replaced by compounds such as octopamine and phenylethanolamine. These so-called false neurotransmitters are postulated to be responsible for the disturbances in consciousness known as hepatic encephalopathy. Accordingly, if the deranged plasma amino acid pattern can be normalized by increasing BCAAs and decreasing aromatic amino acids, the L-system transport pathway of the blood-brain barrier will be presented with an improved amino acid pattern, and a more functional brain amino acid profile will result. Glutamine may also play some role inasmuch as levels of glutamine in the brain reflect the availability of ammonia ion and glutamine is used for exchange of ammonia across the blood-brain barrier. The unified hypothesis of hepatic encephalopathy proposes that the deranged levels of plasma amino acids resulting from decreased hepatic function or anatomic shunting of blood flow, coupled with increased ammonia (glutamine) within the central nervous system, are synergistic in altering transport of amino acids across the blood-brain barrier.

Other workers have suggested the use of increased BCAAs alone in standard amino acid solutions instead of the modified amino acid solution described earlier. However, there is no evidence to support efficacy. The addition of BCAAs to standard solutions also creates a solution containing excessive concentrations of many aromatic amino acids, which with the decreased albumin present in most of these patients, results in increased free plasma and brain tryptophan. Thus, the only formula for which data are adequate is a HepatAmine type of solution consisting of 35% BCAAs and decreased aromatic amino acids. Numerous randomized prospective trials have clearly shown that encephalopathy is well treated by such formulas. Although some trials, particularly one in which glucose was used as the primary calorie source, resulted in increased survival in the group receiving these special solutions when compared with neomycin alone, other trials have not. Furthermore, a large meta-analysis did not support increased overall survival as a beneficial effect of such practices, even though encephalopathy

was improved. This topic is further discussed later (see Controversies in Artificial Nutrition).

Plasma Electrolytes

Abnormalities in plasma electrolytes are minimized by careful monitoring. At least 50 mEq of sodium and 20 to 40 mEq of potassium should be administered daily to most patients receiving parenteral nutrition. The daily maintenance requirement is 0.2 to 0.3 mEq/kg/day for calcium, 0.35 to 0.45 mEq/kg/day for magnesium, and 30 to 40 mmol/day for phosphate. Patients who are rapidly anabolic, such as extremely cachectic patients during the initiation of TPN, may require additional potassium, magnesium, and phosphorus (the so-called phosphate steal or refeeding syndrome). One must also be careful to limit sodium and volume administration because these patients are sodium avid and volume overload and congestive heart failure can easily develop. Acid-base imbalance is prevented by adding acetate to TPN solutions when acidosis or hyperchloremia is present, or conversely, solutions are supplemented with potassium chloride when gastric or other GI losses are significant. If potassium chloride is insufficient to prevent metabolic alkalosis, as in patients with gastric outlet obstruction, administration of dilute hydrochloric acid or arginine hydrochloride may also be necessary. In general, in the face of changing fluid and electrolyte requirements, it is generally possible to use the TPN solution to address such needs, unless instability is volatile. However, frequent changes in volume or electrolyte requirements are best dealt with by an alternative route of IV administration to minimize wastage of TPN solutions.

Vitamins and Micronutrients

In the modern era, micronutrient deficiencies in parenteral nutrition are rarely seen but result from inadequate provision of essential fatty acids (see earlier), trace elements, or vitamins (Table 7-4). Such mineral deficiencies are avoided with modern additives, and the available assays for deficiency are often unreliable and not very useful. Therefore, routine testing is not indicated. Some agents require portal passage for metabolic conversion or activation, which is potentially bypassed during parenteral infusion. Furthermore, in short-bowel syndrome or after extensive ileal resection, substances that normally require the enterohepatic circulation for maximal absorption and utilization, such as zinc, copper, manganese, selenium, and many vitamins (cobalamin, folate, and the fat-soluble vitamins A, D, E, and K), are particularly vulnerable. Fat malabsorption, as induced by pancreatic insufficiency, for example, can also lead to inadequate uptake of fat-soluble micronutrients.

Thiamine

Severe thiamine deficiency leads to the classic nutritional disease beriberi, characterized by refractory lactic acidosis as a result of a deficit of the thiamine needed to facilitate entry of glucose into the TCA cycle. The clinical syndrome consists of disturbed mentation, diabetes

Table 7-4 Suggested Dosage of Vitamins and Trace Metals During Severe Illness

VITAMINS AND TRACE METALS	SUGGESTED DAILY DOSAGE
Vitamin	
Water soluble	
Thiamine	25 mg
Riboflavin	25 mg
Niacin	200 mg
Pantothenic acid	50 mg
Pyridoxine	50 mg
Folic acid*	2.5 mg
Vitamin B$_{12}$[†]	5 mg
Fat soluble	
A[†]	5000 µg
D[†]	400 µg
E[†]	100 µg
K*	10 mg
Trace Metal	
Zinc	10-20 mg
Copper	0.5-2.0 mg
Chromium	20 µg
Selenium	70-150 µg
Manganese	2-2.5 mg
Iron	25 mg

*Inactivated (oxidized) by addition to hypertonic glucose amino acid solutions.

[†]Sufficient stores of these vitamins exist, so deficiency states are unlikely during short-term (2- to 4-week) parenteral nutrition. In practice, however, it is wise to provide them.

insipidus, hyperbilirubinemia, thrombocytopenia, and lactic acidosis mimicking sepsis. The plasma amino acid pattern is distorted, with high levels of proline and hydroxyproline. Thiamine deficiency in patients receiving normal amounts of thiamine has occasionally been seen, usually in a depleted patient given a sudden carbohydrate load. Once this condition is recognized, thiamine deficiency is easily treated with 100 mg of thiamine per day. One of the authors (J.E.F.) observed such a case when the Food and Drug Administration withheld the source of multivitamins for several months.

Biotin

Because biotin is ubiquitous, deficiency hardly ever occurs in patients taking anything by mouth, although biotin deficiency has been reported in patients entirely dependent on TPN.

Vitamin D

Deficiency of vitamin D is primarily an issue during long-term TPN administration or in the face of concurrent metabolic bone disease, such as severe osteoporosis (see Metabolic Complications of Long-Term Administration of Total Parenteral Nutrition later). Most standard multivitamin solutions used routinely in TPN contain 200 units of vitamin D. When assayed, aberrations in vitamin D levels (25-hydroxyvitamin D in normal subjects or 1,25-hydroxyvitamin D in chronic renal failure) should be

evaluated and levels of parathyroid hormone (PTH) measured concurrently. If vitamin D is to be repleted, oral administration is best (50,000 U/wk for 6 to 8 weeks) because IV replacement can be dangerous, with vitamin D overload and osteomalacia likely.

Vitamin K

In patients who maintain some oral intake in addition to TPN, vitamin K deficiency is unlikely. However, for patients who are entirely dependent on TPN, supplementation weekly with 10 mg vitamin K IV is necessary. In addition, if chronic warfarin (Coumadin) therapy is required, such as for a history of catheter-related superior vena cava syndrome, having a baseline amount of vitamin K in the TPN solution is probably helpful in buffering the inhibitory effect of warfarin on post-translation carboxylation of the coagulation proteins. In this way, large variations in the warfarin requirement can be avoided. Conversely, other practitioners avoid vitamin K entirely under such circumstances.

Zinc

Zinc deficiency may develop in patients who are extremely catabolic or who have excessive diarrhea. Massive diarrhea and malabsorption may increase losses to as great as 10 mEq Zn per liter of stool. Neither plasma zinc nor hair zinc is an accurate reflection of total body stores, which may be markedly depleted even when blood levels appear normal. Three milligrams to 6 mg of elemental zinc per day is required in patients with normal stool losses, and between 12 and 20 mg is required in patients with short-bowel syndrome or excessive diarrhea. Zinc deficiency has numerous manifestations, including alopecia, poor wound healing, immunosuppression, night blindness or photophobia, impaired taste or smell (anosmia), neuritis, and a variety of skin disorders (generalized eruptions, perioral pustular rash, darkening of the skin creases), and is similar to the syndrome of zinc deficiency seen in sheep (acrodermatitis enteropathica).

Copper

Copper deficiency has been observed in a few patients receiving long-term parenteral nutrition and is manifested as microcytic anemia, pancytopenia, depigmentation, and osteopenia. The microcytic anemia may be mistaken for pyridoxine deficiency. In standard mineral solutions used for TPN, up to 2 mg of copper per day is given as the sulfate.

Chromium

Deficiency of chromium is also likely to occur only in patients receiving long-term TPN with minimal or no oral intake. Chromium is necessary for adequate utilization of glucose, and deficiency is often manifested as a sudden diabetic state in which blood sugar is difficult to control, along with peripheral neuropathy and encephalopathy. A total of 15 to 20 µg/day of chromium is adequate to meet daily requirements. To treat chromium deficiency, 150 µg of chromium per day is given for several days.

Molybdenum

This metal is a cofactor for the enzymes superoxide dismutase and xanthine oxidase. The rare deficiency state is characterized by the toxic accumulation of sulfur-containing amino acids and encephalopathy.

Selenium

Selenium deficiency has not been clearly established and is clearly rare. Selenium deficiency may result in diffuse skeletal myopathy and cardiomyopathy (with abnormalities in basement and plasma membranes on muscle biopsy), loss of pigmentation, and erythrocyte macrocytosis.

Iron

Calcium, iron, and other metals are absorbed in the duodenum. Consequently, duodenal bypass (as after a Billroth II gastrectomy) or resection (as after a Whipple procedure) often results in long-term deficiencies of these ions. Iron deficiency can be classified as early (no anemia, serum Fe and ferritin decreased, transferrin increased), intermediate (no anemia, transferrin saturation <15%, ferritin <12 μg/L), or late (hypochromic microcytic anemia). The daily requirement for oral iron is 15 mg/day, 5% to 10% of which is absorbed. Therefore, the parenteral requirement is 1 to 2 mg/day. Despite obligate iron losses from desquamation of skin and gut mucosa, overall there is limited ability to excrete parenteral iron when administered in excess, and iron overload will develop in a significant number of patients given iron routinely. Patients most likely to manifest iron deficiency are premenopausal women (menstruation may increase Fe loss by an additional 1 mg/day), patients receiving more than 50% of their total caloric needs from TPN, patients with chronic GI bleeding (e.g., Crohn's disease in females), and patients maintained on hemodialysis (especially with concurrent erythropoietin therapy). Iron replacement should be avoided in the face of a concurrent inflammatory state or active infection because in these conditions iron utilization is poor and such supplementation may have immunosuppressant activity or may promote bacterial growth. In addition, in shortgut syndrome, some patients appear to carry out iron absorption in the intact duodenum and proximal jejunum too avidly and may be at risk for iron overload. Finally, concurrent inherited hemochromatosis must be recognized inasmuch as 0.2% to 0.7% of the population are homozygotic and 8% to 14% are heterozygotes. Even heterozygotic subjects appear to be predisposed to atherosclerosis, the possible mechanism being iron excess and increased free radical generation. A full discussion of iron deficiency and strategies for iron repletion in TPN is found elsewhere.[45]

PRACTICAL APPROACH TO ARTIFICIAL NUTRITION

A major change in nutritional support over the past decade is the realization that enteral nutrition may be more efficacious, particularly in patients with burns or

---

other trauma, than parenteral nutrition. This topic is explored more thoroughly later in this chapter (see Controversies in Artificial Nutrition) and is discussed briefly earlier as well (see Fundamentals of Artificial Nutrition). Historically, enteral nutrition has not been emphasized as much as parenteral nutrition because it has been assumed that in many disease states the gut will not function to allow adequate nutrient absorption.

In contrast, it is now clear that enteral feeding is often well tolerated, even in severe illness, although it may not provide total nutritional support in all cases. Nonetheless, use of the gut for partial nutritional support probably has significant benefit in areas of immunologic and hepatic function and should be encouraged. As little as 20% of overall nutrient calories administered to the gut was sufficient to show benefit versus TPN alone in certain studies. Therefore, one should approach nutritional support with two goals in mind:

1. To use the gut if possible
2. If total nutritional supplementation cannot be provided by the GI tract, to administer at least 20% of the caloric and protein requirements enterally while reaching goal support with TPN until the GI tract returns to full functionality (Box 7-2)

Principles of Enteral Feeding

The stomach is the principal defense against an enteral osmotic load. After bolus administration of hyperosmotic fluid, gastric motility is inhibited and gastric secretion proceeds until the gastric contents are isosmotic, at which point transfer across the pylorus begins. The small bowel is less able to dilute and tolerate large osmotic loads when they are administered directly. The small intestine is the principal area for nutrient absorption, with the products of protein digestion (i.e., dipeptides, oligopeptides, and single amino acids) being completely absorbed in the first 120 cm of jejunum. With short or diseased bowel, dipeptides may have an absorptive advantage. Carbohydrate is also absorbed high in the jejunum, with simple sugars being preferred. Complex sugars, such as disaccharides, require additional enzymatic cleavage.

A common difficulty in patients who are ill is acquired lactase deficiency, which often corrects itself in time, although in the early recovery phase lactose-containing foods may cause diarrhea. Fat is most difficult to absorb because it depends on proper release and mixing of bile and pancreatic enzymes. After gastrectomy, pancreatic resection, or complex upper abdominal operations, such relationships are disturbed, and proper mixing of bile and pancreatic enzymes does not occur. Thus, fat absorption is diminished after a Billroth II gastrectomy and less so after Billroth I procedures. Aside from mechanical issues related to the feeding tube (see later), the most common complications of enteral feedings result from solute overload. Inappropriately rapid administration of hyperosmolar solutions may result in diarrhea, dehydration, electrolyte imbalance, and hyperglycemia, as well as loss of potassium, magnesium, and other ions through diarrhea. If aggressive administration of hyperosmolar solute continues, pneumatosis intestinalis with bowel necrosis and perforation and potentially death will result. Hyperosmolar, nonketotic coma can also occur with enteral feedings as with parenteral nutrition.

Routes for Administration of Enteral Feeding

Patients with a functioning GI tract who cannot achieve adequate nutritional intake orally and are malnourished or at risk for the development of malnutrition are candidates for feeding tube placement. The choice of access route and device must be tailored to the individual by considering the disease process and how long the patient will probably require nutritional support.

Nasoenteric and Postpyloric Feeding

Nasoenteric feeding (gastric, duodenal, or jejunal) is the least expensive and most widely used modality of enteral nutrition. Most commonly, postsurgical patients have nasogastric tubes in place. These tubes are reasonable for the short term because they are typically large bored, do not clog easily, and allow gastric residuals to be checked in assessing GI tolerance. However, the traditional 16- or 18-French nasogastric tube (intended for gastric drainage) is uncomfortable and may promote relatively greater gastroesophageal reflux by holding the lower esophageal sphincter open more than occurs with a narrower tube. Such smaller-caliber feeding tubes (e.g., the Dobhoff tube, 8-10 French) are more comfortable and less erosive to the nasopharynx and esophagus, but they can clog when not carefully maintained and also collapse easily, thus making it difficult to monitor gastric residuals. Though generally considered to be relatively innocuous, nasoenteric feeding tubes are associated with multiple adverse consequences, including tube migration, esophageal and gastric mucosal erosions, pulmonary aspiration, sinusitis, pneumothorax, esophageal stricture, esophageal perforation, and fatal arrhythmias. In particular, feeding tubes with an indwelling removable metal stylet to aid their passage, although used often, appear to be particularly dangerous. In ventilated patients with indwelling endotracheal tubes, malposition in the bronchus with perforation into the pleural cavity seems to be associated most commonly with such stylet-type tubes. A more promising design, though not widely available, is the use of a rigid plastic overtube from which a narrower, soft feeding tube may be deployed after satisfactory gastric positioning. Many of these complications are avoidable with care. For example, aspiration may be minimized by positioning the patient head-up and by monitoring gastric residuals, which should generally be less than 150 mL, although some authors have advocated a more aggressive approach, such as tolerance of residuals as great as 300 to 400 mL.

Many enteral feeding studies are handicapped by the high prevalence of GI intolerance leading to inadequate protein and calorie administration. Such intolerance, in particular that attributable to elevated gastric residual volumes, can affect up to 60% of patients. A variety of approaches have been tried in an attempt to address poor gastric emptying in critically ill patients, including the use of promotility agents such as metoclopramide or erythromycin. Another strategy proposed as a means of bypassing the region of gastroduodenal ileus is postpyloric feeding. Nasoenteric feeding tubes can be placed with their tip positioned in the duodenum or jejunum, either under fluoroscopic guidance or by endoscopic manipulation and visualization. The hypothesis is that the jejunum may be more tolerant of continuous feeding and that by administering nutrients beyond the ligament of Treitz, the risk for aspiration is lessened. However, when these putative advantages have been studied in prospective randomized trials, there did not appear to be any difference when compared with intragastric feeding practices. In fact, in studies involving the use of radiolabeled feeding,[46] regurgitation of postpylorically delivered nutrients and the incidence of actual aspiration or clinically definable pneumonia were no different than in patients fed gastrically. It seems reasonable to assume that in most instances, whether the tube tip terminates prepylorically or postpylorically, because all tubes are introduced nasally, the lower esophageal sphincter is held open regardless, and this is probably the most important mechanism to allow aspiration.

As for feeding tolerance, there also does not appear to be any clear benefit attributable to postpyloric feeding. When aggressive advancement protocols are followed, nasogastrically fed patients, despite having higher gastric residual volumes, receive amounts of enteral nutrition equivalent to those fed nasojejunally. This finding has been confirmed in two separate prospective randomized trials that included 180 patients.[47,48] On the other hand, in postoperative trauma patients, Montecalvo and associates[49] showed that patients who received jejunal feeding attained a significantly higher percentage of their daily caloric goal than did patients fed intragastrically. In conclusion, although the concept of postpyloric feeding remains controversial, it appears reasonable to obtain postpyloric access in patients with specific indications, such as those suffering from significant gastroparesis or with severe pancreatitis (see later). Such access can easily be obtained at the time of surgery directed toward the primary disease process, when a well–carried out feeding jejunostomy obviates most of the risk for aspiration, and will anticipate gastric ileus if sepsis ensues.

Gastrostomy

If long-term access to the stomach will be needed, a permanent gastrostomy can be placed. This goal can be achieved either by the open approach or by percutaneous techniques, the latter using endoscopic, radiologic, or laparoscopic methods. The Stamm gastrostomy, which requires a small laparotomy incision, is the most widely used open technique for insertion of a gastric tube. Either inhalational or, in many cases, awake IV sedation with local anesthesia is an acceptable anesthetic approach for this procedure.

In more recent years, the percutaneous endoscopic gastrostomy (PEG) technique has become the procedure of choice for many patients because it is generally considered less expensive and less morbid, although some studies indicate that open gastrostomy and PEG carry equivalent perioperative risk. Necrosis of the gastric wall, attributable to excessive tension, is a recognized but avoidable complication of percutaneous gastrostomy. Percutaneous gastric tubes can also be placed by the interventional radiologist, which although seemingly less invasive than other procedures for gastrostomy insertion and being used with increasing frequency, actually appears to have a slightly higher incidence of complications and need for open revision than do surgical or endoscopic approaches. On the other hand, for moribund patients or those requiring gastric drainage with no attractive operative approach (e.g., in the face of intestinal obstruction as a result of terminal carcinomatosis), the radiologic technique can be an ideal solution. An important factor limiting any percutaneous gastrostomy insertion is a history of previous upper abdominal surgery, which is associated with the potential for adhesions and superimposition of structures such as the colon between the stomach and the abdominal wall. Perforation of the colon, which may go unrecognized for many days, is a well-described complication of all percutaneous techniques. In such circumstances a Stamm gastrostomy performed via a left upper quadrant incision can usually be carried out. Another drawback of gastrostomy tubes of all types is that they generally do not lie in a dependent position, so it is difficult to aspirate and check gastric residual volumes.

Jejunostomy

Jejunal or small bowel feeding tube access can be achieved by open jejunostomy (either at the time of laparotomy or as a separate procedure), percutaneously by extension through an existing gastrostomy tube (often termed a *G-J tube*), by a laparoscopic approach, or very rarely as a percutaneous jejunostomy placed under fluoroscopic or CT guidance by the interventional radiologist. This latter procedure has an undefined but presumably high frequency of complications and is of dubious value. True percutaneous jejunostomies (as opposed to G-J tubes), though often lifesaving, are complicated more frequently than desired by dislodgement, occlusion, bowel obstruction, and small bowel ischemia. Furthermore, because the small bowel does not accommodate bolus feeding, nutrients delivered to the jejunum must

be delivered in continuous fashion while carefully watching for signs of intolerance such as abdominal distention, abdominal pain or tenderness, diarrhea, or constipation. In a critically ill patient, hypo-osmolar or at most iso-osmolar solutions should generally be used. Hyper-osmolar solutions are often not tolerated in critical illness because the bowel is stressed to begin with and such solutions are much more likely to result in pneumatosis, necrosis, perforation, and death.

Management of Tube Tract Infections

A complication common to any percutaneous feeding tube is chronic infection or erosion of the tube tract as it traverses the abdominal wall. As indicated earlier, excessive traction, particularly in the case of PEG, may induce frank gastric wall necrosis and free perforation of the stomach. More commonly, patients may experience chronic drainage, erythema, or excessive buildup of granulation tissue with intermittent bleeding. Factors contributing to such phenomena appear to involve excessive tube motion, the choice of catheter material (latex being less desirable than silicone), and chronic bacterial colonization. Simple hygiene and antibacterial ointment daily usually suffice.

Enteral Formulas and Approach to Feeding Advancement

Mortality from enteral feeding is largely the result of aspiration or, as indicated earlier, occasionally results from hyper-osmolar feeding. Patients should be infused constantly, with the bolus technique reserved for special situations. To prevent reflux and aspiration, patients should be kept at a 30-degree angle because reflux may occur even with postpyloric feeding. In general, there is no commonly agreed on protocol for advancing enteral feeding. For gastric feeding, first osmolality and then volume are increased, usually beginning with solutions that are slightly hypo-osmolar. Most commonly, feeding is started at 10 to 20 mL/hr and gastric residual volumes checked every 4 to 6 hours.

As long as gastric residual volumes remain less than 100 to 150 mL, feeding is advanced in 10- to 20-mL increments until the goal rate is attained. Unfortunately, this conservative protocol often results in unnecessary cessation of feeding and thus leads to slow or inadequate provision of nutrition. Several investigators have had better success when feeding is advanced more aggressively and when standardized protocols that outline rules for feeding advancement and cessation are followed. Such practices, which tolerate gastric residual volumes as high as 250 to 300 mL and increase infusion rates in increments of 20 mL every 2 to 4 hours, have allegedly not resulted in increased complication rates or adverse outcomes. If administration is into the small bowel, volume is increased first, then osmolality. Most patients do not tolerate small bowel administration of tube feeding containing greater than 300 to 400 mOsm, especially when critically ill. Dehydration is prevented by carefully increasing osmolality and using kaolin-pectin (Kaopectate) and opioids to slow the diarrhea, as well as by the addition of free water. Pneumatosis, bowel necrosis, perforation, and mortality usually occur when hyperosmolar feeding persists in the face of voluminous diarrhea or when blood supply to the intestine is inadequate (the so-called challenged bowel), whether caused by reduced cardiac output or atherosclerotic vascular disease.

Enteral Formulas

Many different enteral products are available, and almost all are hyperosmolar (Table 7-5). Most formulas provide 1 kcal/mL, although some higher-calorie formulas (1.5-2 cal/mL) are also available and allow smaller volumes of administration. These high-density formulas tend to have greater proportions of fat and relatively less protein (e.g., Nepro, a formula optimized for renal failure). For patients with normal gut function, an inexpensive tube feeding analogous to a blenderized meal (e.g., a hydrolysate) is well tolerated. Some products have various degrees of complexity ranging from oligopeptides to individual amino acids. The carbohydrate source varies from dextrose to complex starches, the latter solving a major problem in gut feeding—hyperosmolality. Modular diets are those in which the protein, fat, and carbohydrate components can be individually supplied. In patients with reasonably normal gut function, elemental diets (e.g., Vivonex) appear to have no

advantage over hydrolysates. Elemental formulations (e.g., dipeptides and oligopeptides) may be more efficiently absorbed in patients suffering from short-gut syndrome or in those with chronic diarrhea, although this idea is unproven. Finally, a recent development is the formulation of tube feeding solutions with potential immune-enhancing properties (e.g., Impact), which is discussed subsequently (see Controversies in Artificial Feeding).

Parenteral Feeding

When enteral feeding is poorly tolerated or impossible to deliver, parenteral nutrition administered safely is the only alternative (Box 7-3). If the parenteral route is chosen, concentrated TPN (>900 mOsm/L) delivered to a large central vein (termed *central TPN*), with the line tip in the superior vena cava, is the preferred method. The potential sources of calories (e.g., carbohydrate, lipid, and protein) have been discussed in detail earlier. In the absence of central access, a less concentrated formula (dextrose not to exceed 5%) may be delivered via a peripheral vein (termed *peripheral TPN*). This latter method is usually for a short term only (4-7 days) and provides less than optimal calories, although nitrogen loss may be retarded. If lipid is included (250-500 mL of a 20% fat emulsion daily) and up to 3 L of dilute solution can be tolerated, peripheral TPN can satisfy the daily caloric requirement. However, the needs of sick patients are rarely satisfied by this approach, and to date, no clinical trials have attributed any benefit to the routine use of peripheral IV alimentation. As discussed earlier, there is some experimental evidence to support the provision of (hypocaloric) amino acids and 5% dextrose or glycerol in an attempt to minimize nitrogen breakdown for limited periods. However, in a European trial by Culebras and coworkers, a limited 14-hour infusion of amino acids and 5% dextrose after operations of modest severity did not show improved nitrogen balance.

Practical Approach to Calculation of the Ideal Parenteral Formula

Physicochemical Considerations

Today, most TPN solutions are administered as a total nutrient admixture (TNA or 3-in-1 solution) with lipid emulsions incorporated into the final solution, as opposed to the older method of a separate piggyback infusion of lipid. The TNA protocol is clinically advantageous because it does the following:

1. Limits the number of central venous catheter violations and chance for contamination
2. Produces a hyperosmolar environment in the TNA solution that protects against bacterial growth
3. Allows continuous infusion, thereby ensuring lipid administration at a safe rate (<0.11 g/kg/hr)

It is important to recognize that TPN is generally compounded in the pharmacy from concentrated stock solutions, which in turn can limit the range of individual solute concentrations achievable. These factors often lead

Table 7-5   **Enteral Nutrition Products**

DESCRIPTOR	PRODUCT							
	Criticare HN	Vivonex TEN	Peptamen VHP	Impact With Fiber	Impact	Respalor	Nepro	Promod (100 g)
Calories (kcal/mL)	1.06	1.00	1.0	1.00	1.00	1.52	2.00	424
Protein (g/L)	38 (14.4%)	38.2 (15%)	62.5 (25%)	56 (22%)	56 (22%)	75 (20%)	70 (14%)	76 (72%)
Carbohydrate (g/L)	220 (81%)	206 (82%)	104.5 (42%)	133 (53%)	130 (53%)	146 (40%)	215 (43%)	10 (10%)
Fat (g/L)	5.3 (4.5%)	2.8 (3%)	39 (33%)	28 (25%)	28 (25%)	68 (40%)	96 (43%)	9 (19%)
Fat as MCT (%)	0	0	70%	27%	27%	30%	0%	0
Osmolality (mOsm/L)	650	630	300 unflavored/ 430 flavored	375	375	400	665	—
Free water (mL/L)	850	853	840	868	853	770	699	—
Sodium (mEq/L)	27	20	24	48	48	55	37	10
Potassium (mEq/L)	34	20	38	33	36	38	27	25
Calcium (mg/L)	530	500	800	800	800	1000	1370	607
Phosphorus (mg/L)	530	500	700	800	800	1000	695	500
Magnesium (mg/L)	210	200	300	270	270	400	215	—
Vitamin K (mg/L)	131	22	50	67	67	84	85	—
Dietary fiber (g/L)	0	0	0	10	0	0	0	—
Volume for 100% DRI (mL)	1890	2000	1500	1500	1500	1000	947	NA
Comments	Elemental amino acids and peptides, ready to feed, gluten- and lactose-free	Elemental amino acids and peptides, oral or tube feeding, 4.9 g/L glutamine, requires mixing, gluten- and lactose-free	Semielemental high-protein oral or tube feeding, 4.6 g/L glutamine, gluten- and lactose-free	Immune-enhancing tube feeding for critical care; with fiber, high protein, fish oil, RNA, arginine; gluten- and lactose-free	See Impact (no fiber)	For respiratory failure (low carbohydrate, volume restricted), oral or tube feeding, gluten- and lactose-free	For renal failure (low electrolyte, Mg, Pi; volume restricted), oral or tube feeding, gluten- and lactose-free	Protein supplement, gluten-free, low residue; 4.5 g/100 g lactose
Flavors	Unflavored	+ Flavor packets	+ Flavor packets	Unflavored	Unflavored	Vanilla	Vanilla, pecan	NA
Cost per 1500 kcal	$13.50	$13.80	$23.50	$27.00	$25.50	$3.16	$4.90	—

Continued

Table 7-5 **Enteral Nutrition Products—cont'd**

	PRODUCT							
DESCRIPTOR	Boost	Boost Plus	Boost High Protein	Ultracal	Promote	Promote With Fiber	Probalance	Deliver 2.0
Calories (kcal/mL)	1.01	1.52	1.01	1.06	1.0	1.0	1.20	2.00
Protein (g/L)	43 (17%)	61 (16%)	61 (24%)	44 (17%)	62.5 (25%)	62.5 (25%)	54 (18%)	75 (15%)
Carbohydrate (g/L)	170 (67%)	190 (50%)	139 (55%)	123 (46%)	130 (52%)	138 (50%)	156 (52%)	200 (40%)
Fat (g/L)	18 (16%)	57 (34%)	23 (21%)	45 (37%)	26 (23%)	28 (25%)	40.8 (30%)	102 (45%)
Fat as MCT (%)	0	0	0	40	19	19	20	30
Osmolality (mOsm/L)	590	630-670	650	310	340	380	450	640
Free water (mL/L)	840	780	850	850	830	830	810	710
Sodium (mEq/L)	24	37	40	40	43	57	33	35
Potassium (mEq/L)	43	38	54	41	51	51	40	43
Calcium (mg/L)	1270	850	1010	850	1200	1200	1250	1010
Phosphorus (mg/L)	1060	850	930	850	1200	1200	1000	1010
Magnesium (mg/L)	420	340	380	340	400	400	400	400
Vitamin K (mg/L)	127	68	240	68	80	80	80	250
Dietary fiber (g/L)	0	<4	0	14	0	14	10	0
Volume for 100% DRI (mL)	1590	1180	1060	1250	1000	1000	1000	1000
Comments	Oral supplement only, gluten- and lactose-free	Oral, nutrient dense, may be used as tube feeding, gluten- and lactose-free	Standard high-protein oral or tube feeding, gluten- and lactose-free	Standard tube feeding with fiber, gluten- and lactose-free	Standard high-protein oral or tube feeding, lactose- and gluten-free, low residue	See Promote With Fiber	Higher-calorie (1.2 cal/mL) oral or tube feeding with fiber, gluten- and lactose-free	Volume-restricted oral or tube feeding, gluten- and lactose-free
Flavors	Vanilla, chocolate, strawberry	Vanilla, chocolate, strawberry	Vanilla, chocolate	Unflavored	Vanilla	Vanilla	Many	Vanilla
Cost per 1500 kcal	$1.20	$0.80	$1.20	$3.50	$3.40	$3.40	$2.60	$2.10

MCT, medium-chain triglyceride; DRI, daily recommended intake.

Table 7-6   Allowable Additive Supplementation (at the University of Cincinnati Hospital, Cincinnati, Ohio)*

ADDITIVES	AVAILABLE PRODUCTS (INJECTION)	MAXIMAL ALLOWABLE TOTAL PER LITER
Calcium	Calcium gluconate Calcium chloride	9 mEq
Magnesium	Magnesium sulfate	12 mEq
Phosphate	Sodium phosphate Potassium phosphate	15 mmol
Potassium	Potassium chloride Potassium acetate	80 mEq
Sodium	Sodium chloride Sodium acetate	Patient tolerance and/or need
Chloride	Sodium chloride Calcium chloride Potassium chloride	Limited by amount of cation
Acetate	Sodium acetate Potassium acetate	Limited by amount of cation
Insulin	Regular insulin	100 units (in conjunction with fingerstick blood sugar determination)

*Some points to remember: (1) Bicarbonate salts must not be added to parenteral nutrition formulations because they create certain incompatibilities and are ineffective given in this manner. (2) Medicinal agents not mentioned must not be admixed or administered with parenteral nutrition formulations unless compatibility data are available. (3) Phosphate supplementation must be ordered in terms of millimoles of phosphate. Phosphate is available only as the sodium or potassium salt, and when the potassium salt is used for "added" phosphate, it must not exceed the maximum allowable concentration of potassium (i.e., 80 mEq).

to a requirement for greater volumes of solution to be delivered than initially might seem apparent. For example, common stock solutions are 70% dextrose, 10% to 20% amino acids, and 20% lipid. Therefore, for 1 L of solution in the absence of fat, the maximal achievable concentrations are 7% amino acids (70 g/L) and 21% dextrose (210 g/L). These amounts become even lower when fat is added to a 3-in-1 mixture. In addition, the pharmacist must take into account the physical-chemical stability of the 3-in-1 solution with respect to the effect of mineral additives and the relative proportions of caloric sources on the stability of the lipid emulsion and on overall solubility (Table 7-6).

Estimation of Energy Needs

In an earlier section (Nutritional Assessment), a variety of approaches were described to estimate energy needs, including indirect calorimetry, use of the IBW, and calculation by standard methods such as the Harris-Benedict equation. Determination of the resting energy expenditure or basal metabolic rate (BMR) by the Harris-Benedict equation relies on the following formulas:

Male BMR $= 66 + (13.7 \times$ wt in kg$) + (5 \times$ ht in cm$)$
$$-(6.8 \times \text{age in yr})$$

Female BMR $= 65.5 + (9.6 \times$ wt in kg$) + (1.7 \times$ ht in cm$)$
$$-(4.7 \times \text{age in yr})$$

The weight used for this calculation should be the subject's actual body weight. The value obtained for BMR must then be corrected for normal activity, for example, ambulation and the work of breathing (+15%), and for stress. The added caloric expenditure, or relevant stress factor, is 10% for an uncomplicated postoperative patient; 10% to 30% for peritonitis; and 30% to 50% for sepsis, respiratory failure, or trauma. In burns, caloric requirements may be 50% to 100% greater than normal. Additional stress factors include fever (hyperthermia), for which each 1°C increment in body temperature causes a 5% to 8% increase in BMR, and conditions of uncontrolled heat loss, pain, sleep deprivation, and anxiety (Fig. 7-7).

Caloric requirements for TPN administration can also be estimated by using normative values consisting of body weight and the accepted parameter of 25 to 35 kcal/kg/day for the rate of caloric infusion. This latter approach is safe, easy, and the most commonly used in clinical practice. However, because patients can be at, below, or above IBW (as defined in Nutritional Assessment earlier), one must have a method of choosing an appropriate weight that will be used to calculate nutritional goals. This weight is called the *feeding weight* and is calculated by first determining IBW, as found in standardized tables or estimated by using the equations given earlier. Second, IBW is compared with actual body weight (ABW). In comparing IBW and ABW,

- If the patient is underweight, use ABW as the feeding weight.
- If the patient is obese (ABW is >120% of IBW), add 25% of the difference between ABW and IBW to the IBW as the feeding weight.
- If no reliable weight is available, use IBW alone.

Formulation of the TPN Solution

For the calculation of caloric content in TPN, glucose contains 3.4 kcal/g, protein contains 4 kcal/g, and fat contains 9 kcal/g. In general, minimal fluid requirements in the absence of GI or other losses are 25 to 35 mL/kg/day. Using the example of a 70-kg person as the feeding weight, one first calculates the overall caloric goal and the proportion contributed by protein, usually:

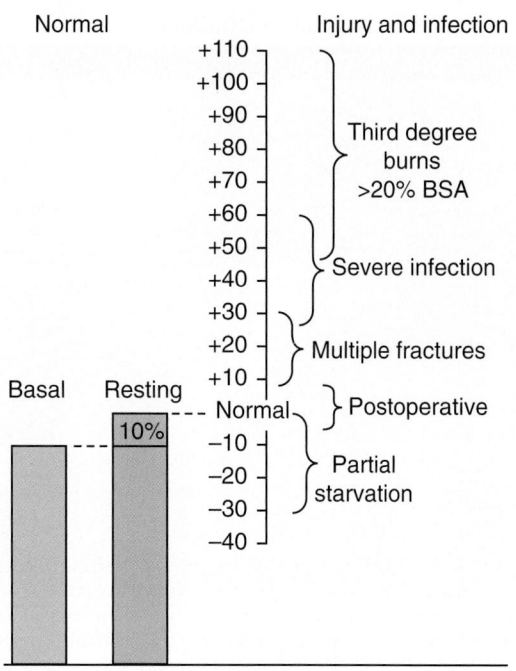

Figure 7-7 Increases in resting energy expenditure that have been shown to occur during the acute catabolic phase of injury or infection in comparison to the decreases that develop during partial starvation. BSA, body surface area. (From Kinney JM: The application of indirect calorimetry to clinical studies. In Kinney JM [ed]: Assessment of Energy Metabolism in Health and Disease. Columbus, OH, Ross Laboratories, 1980.)

Total kilocalories (25-35 kcal/kg/day): $30 \times 70 = 2100$ kcal

Protein (1.5 g/kg/day): $1.5 \times 70 = 105$ g amino acids

1. For TPN formulated without lipid (2-in-1 solution):

   Total kilocalories = 2100 kcal

   Calories from amino acids = 105 g $\times 4$ kcal/g = 420 kcal

   Remaining calories = $2100 - 420 = 1680$ kcal

   Then make up the difference with dextrose:

   1680 kcal $\div 3.4$ kcal/g = 494 g dextrose

   However, remember that as demonstrated by Wolfe (see earlier), 400 g dextrose/24 hr is probably the maximum that can be safely used.

2. For TPN formulated with lipid (3-in-1 solution):

   Total kilocalories = 2100 kcal

   Provide 20% of the total calories as

   $$\text{Lipid} = 2100 \times 0.2 = 420 \text{ kcal}$$

   Then

   $$420 \text{ kcal} \div 9 \text{ kcal/g} = 47 \text{ g lipid}$$

   Calories from amino acids:

   $$105 \text{ g} \times 4 \text{ kcal/g} = 420 \text{ kcal}$$

   Remaining calories:

   $$2100 - 420 - 420 = 1260 \text{ kcal}$$

   Then make up the difference with dextrose:

   $$1260 \text{ kcal} \div 3.4 \text{ kcal/g} = 370 \text{ g dextrose}$$

Final volume (for 3-in-1, maximally concentrated):

Amino acids (10% stock solution): 105 g = 1050 mL

Dextrose (70% stock solution): 370 g = 528 mL

Lipids (20% stock solution): 47 g = 235 mL

Total volume = 1813 mL/day

The final concentrations (wt/vol) is 5.8% amino acids, 20.4% dextrose, and 2.6% lipid.

For critically ill patients who may have unusually high caloric requirements or who require fine adjustment of the glucose or amino acid content in the TPN solution, it is important to facilitate the clinician's writing of the custom TPN order as just described, if necessary. On the other hand, in the hospital setting most providers have minimal experience managing TPN. For this reason and to avoid the inefficiencies and waste caused by inappropriately formulated TPN, our institution has implemented a weight-based standard TPN ordering process (Fig. 7-8). Values of 25 kcal/kg/day for total kilocalories and 1.5 g/kg/day for amino acids are assumed, and either a non-lipid 2-in-1 formula or a lipid-containing 3-in-1 formula (2% lipid, or 18% of the total calories from lipid) is provided in 10-kg ranges for weight. The order form also provides a suggested schedule for caloric advancement (see later), and the entire process has now been computerized in a Web/HTML-based format. For individuals who desire higher calories, the orders can and should be adjusted upward. In many institutions a very similar, but somewhat different approach to standardized TPN ordering is taken. A uniform, maximally concentrated solution is provided, for example, 7% amino acids/21% dextrose for 2-in-1 formulas, with caloric intake individualized by continuously varying the rate of infusion (versus the step-wise increments described earlier). This latter approach may best minimize wastage of solutions (Fig. 7-9).

Schedule for Advancement

The most important aspect of TPN administration is to ensure that it is delivered in a safe manner, one that prevents the development of hyperglycemia and metabolic derangements (Table 7-7). At our institution, on the first day TPN is initiated as a starter solution containing 70 g amino acids and 150 g dextrose in 1000 mL. Tolerance of the infusion is carefully monitored by assessing blood glucose every 6 hours and electrolytes daily and monitoring for signs of volume overload. If well tolerated, the solution is advanced to the day 2 formula, which consists of 70 g amino acids and 210 g dextrose. On the third day, protein is advanced to goal levels, lipids are added if desired, and dextrose is advanced gradually toward goal amounts by increments of 50 to 100 g/day. If blood sugar rises to levels greater than 150 mg/dL, the dextrose content of the TPN is not increased until glycemic control is secured. In institutions that use a single standard solution, the initial infusion may start at 40 mL/hr and advance in 20-mL/hr daily increments until the desired level of caloric intake is reached.

1954-0711-0279

Beth Israel Deaconess Medical Center
Adult Central Parenteral Nutrition (TPN) Order

Orders must be faxed to Pharmacy daily by 1300   Fax #: 2-8950
PN order has a 24 hr automatic stop time

☐ **DAY 1–2 / STARTER TPN**
A standard parenteral nutrition formulation that can be used
initially while assessing glucose and volume tolerance

Amino acid	70 g
Dextrose	150 g
Total volume	1000 ml (providing 800 Kcal)

☐ **DAY 2 AND/OR THEREAFTER: INTERMEDIATE TPN**
An advanced TPN formulation for patients who have demonstrated glucose
tolerance to Day 1 TPN. If the patient demonstrates tolerance to this TPN, the
patient can be advanced to goal with a Central Standard formula or continued
with this formulation for up to 10 days without adverse clinical consequence.

Amino acid	70 g
Dextrose	210 g
Total volume	1000 ml (providing 1000 Kcal)

DAY 3 AND/OR THEREAFTER: CENTRAL STANDARD FORMULAS:
The Central Standard TPNs are weight-based parenteral nutrition formulas providing protein 1.5g/kg/day and 25 kcal/kg/d. Select either the **2-in-1** formula (amino acid/ dextrose) or the **3-in-1** "mixed fuel" formula (amino acid/ dextrose/ lipid) based on the calculated feeding weight. *(See reverse side for calculation. Round to nearest 10 kg.)* For patients with a calculated feeding weight greater than 80 kg or for obese patients (greater than 130% IBW) consult the Nutrition Support Team for patient-specific recommendations.

CENTRAL STANDARD 2-in-1 TPN

	Feeding Weight	TPN Volume	Amino Acid (g/d)	Dextrose (g/d)	Kcal/day
☐	40 kg	1000	60	223	1000
☐	50 kg	1250	75	279	1250
☐	60 kg	1500	90	335	1500
☐	70 kg	1750	105	390	1750
☐	80 kg (or greater)	2000	120	446	2000

CENTRAL STANDARD 3-in-1 TPN

	Feeding Weight	TPN Volume	Amino Acid (g/d)	Dextrose (g/d)	Fat (g/d)	Kcal/day
☐	40 kg	1000	60	170	20	1000
☐	50 kg	1250	75	213	25	1250
☐	60 kg	1500	90	255	30	1500
☐	70 kg	1750	105	298	35	1750
☐	80 kg (or greater)	2000	120	340	40	2000

NON-STANDARD TPN: **Nutrition Support consult recommended.** *See reverse side for general recommendations.*
For patients with liver and/or kidney failure, protein and volume restriction may be required.

☐ Volume_____ ml/d   Amino Acid_____g/d   50% Branched-chain AA_____g/d   Dextrose_____g/d   Fat_____g/d

ADDITIVE OPTIONS

Vitamin / Trace Element Additives:	☐ Standard electrolytes Total amount below will be added per day.	☐ Non-standard electrolytes Designate amount to be added **per day.**	☐ Other Additives *See reverse side for general recommendations.*
Parenteral Multivitamins will be added daily Trace Elements will be added daily unless specified: ☐ No Vitamin K 10 mg will be added each Monday unless specified: ☐ No	Na 70 mEq K 40 mEq Ca 9 mEq Mg 10 mEq Cl 40 mEq Ac 30 mEq PO$_4$ 30 mM	NaCl_____mEq (60–150 mEq/day) NaAc_____mEq (as required) NaPO$_4$_____mEq (30–60 mEq/day) KCl_____mEq (60–100 mEq/day) KAc_____mEq (as required) KPO$_4$_____mEq (as required) MgSO$_4$_____mEq (10–20 mEq/day) CaGluc_____mEq (10–20 mEq/day)	Heparin_____units (usual range: 3000-6000 units/day) Rantidine_____mg Insulin_____units (Regular Human) Zinc_____mg Other_____

RATE OPTION:
☐ Total volume of solution per 24 hours. Rate of continuous infusion determined by pharmacy-SEE TPN label.
☐ Cycle over_____hrs. Start at:_ _ _ _
Decrease rate to _____ ml/h at:_ _ _ _ Stop at: _ _ _ _ Plug and flush line with_____units heparin.

Date:_____ Physician Signature_____ MD   Beeper:_____
Time Posted:_____ by_____ RN

White - MEDICAL RECORDS   Yellow - PHARMACY

Figure 7-8 Order form for the parenteral formulation used at the Beth Israel Deaconess Medical Center, Boston, MA.

Management of Insulin

All patients started on TPN must be provided a subcutaneous sliding-scale regimen for regular insulin administration or, in some cases, an IV regular insulin infusion. The choice depends on the patient's baseline insulin requirement (e.g., concurrent diabetes mellitus) and the presence of factors leading to insulin resistance (steroids, stress), along with the available level of nursing care. In general, it is safe to add an initial 10 units of regular insulin to every bag of TPN because this dose is below the basal rate of insulin production by the pancreatic beta cells and some insulin will be lost as a result of unavoidable binding to plastic components of the infusion equipment. The key to maintaining blood

UNIVERSITY OF CINCINNATI HOSPITAL
**PARENTERAL NUTRITION
ORDER FORM**
Deadline for orders at 9:30 A.M.

Date: _____ Time: _____

UMC-375, 8/92

STEP 1: SELECT BASE FORMULA:
Total Nutrient Admixture (TNA) contains: Fat emulsion, Dextrose, and Amino acids.
Non-TNA contains: Dextrose and Amino acids.

Standard Formula: **High Dextrose Formula:**

☐TNA ☐ NON-TNA   ☐TNA ☐ NON-TNA

Each liter contains: Each liter contains:
Non-protein Calorie: N   119   67   Non-protein Calorie: N   141   89
Total kcal/ml   1.1   0.71   Total kcal/ml   1.3   0.88

Dextrose   (15%)   150 gm   Dextrose   (20%)   200 gm
Amino Acids (5%)   50 gm   Amino Acids (5%)   50 gm
Fat Emulsion (4%)   40 gm (as TNA)   Fat Emulsion (4%)   40 gm (as TNA)

MVI-12 (10 ml) and Trace elements-5 (3 ml) daily   MVI-12 (10 ml) and Trace elements-5 (3 ml) daily
Vit K   5 mg weekly   Vit K   5 mg weekly

Standard Electrolytes (mEq/L)   Standard Electrolytes (mEq/L)

Na	K	Ca	Mg	P(mM)	Cl	Acetate
30	18	4.5	5	10	37	55

Na	K	Ca	Mg	P(mM)	Cl	Acetate
30	18	4.5	5	10	37	55

STEP 2: ORDER TOTAL ADDITIVES IF DIFFERENT FROM ABOVE:

Total Na _____ mEq/L   Other per Liter:
Total K _____ mEq/L   _____
Total Ca _____ mEq/L   _____
Total Mg _____ mEq/L   _____
Total Phos_____ mM/L   _____
Reg. Insulin_____ units/L _____

MAXIMUM TOTAL CONC/LITER		DAILY TRACE ELEMENTS	
K+	80 mEq	Zn	3.0 mg
Ca	9.4 mEq	Cu	1.2 mg
Mg	12 mEq	Cr	12 mcg
Phos	15 mM	Mn	0.3 mg
Ac	80 mEq	Se	60 mcg

STEP 3: SELECT INFUSION RATE:
INFUSE AT _____ ml/hr or Cycle:_____ ml Total Volume

PHYSICIAN SIGNATURE _____   PAGER #: _____

White–CHART   Yellow–PHARMACY

Figure 7-9 Order form for the parenteral formulation used at the University of Cincinnati Medical Center, Cincinnati, OH. The variety of solutions minimizes the chance of error and enables one to handle almost any metabolic situation. The various possible contents of each solution are given.

sugar in the normal range lies in the following maneuvers:

1. Never increase the amount of dextrose in the TPN solution until blood sugar is well controlled (i.e., <150 mg/dL).
2. Determine the amount of sliding-scale insulin administered over the previous 24 hours and add half to two thirds of that amount to the new TPN solution for the ensuing 24 hours.
3. When advancing the dextrose content of the TPN solution, advance the insulin concentration proportionally. For example, if a TPN solution contains 200 g dextrose and 10 units of insulin and the dextrose will be

advanced to 300 g, add 15 units of insulin to the solution. Be quick to convert to a constant insulin infusion if it is difficult to gain control with subcutaneous insulin, especially in the setting of critical illness.

It is important to remember that the insulin added to the TPN solution should cover only the dextrose in the TPN. This insulin should not be used to treat elevated blood sugar resulting from additional sources of dextrose, such as that contributed by an enteral feeding formula administered concurrently. For instance, if the enteral feeding was stopped for any reason, the patient would be at risk for the development of hypoglycemia from the excessive insulin in the TPN solution.

Table 7-7   Suggested Sequence for the Initiation of Parenteral Nutrition Therapy

PARAMETER	DAY 1	DAY 2	DAY 3
Volume (mL/24 hr)	1000	1000-1500	1500-2000
Calories (% of goal)	50%	75%, may add fat	100%
Dextrose (g/24 hr)	100-150	150-200	200-350
Amino acids (% of total)	50%-100%	100%	100%, check BUN
Fat	No	Perhaps	Often (3%-5%, 30-50 g/24 hr)
Insulin	Give separately	Add 50% to TPN	Add 50% to TPN

Note: Electrolytes should begin at a low range (total mEq/24 hr for Na^+=40 to 75, K^+=10 to 40). Insulin is initially given subcutaneously or otherwise separately from the TPN. Half of the preceding 24-hour requirement for insulin can then be added to the TPN solution each day until a stable dosage of insulin in the TPN is reached.

BUN, blood urea, nitrogen; TPN, total parenteral nutrition.

Mandatory Monitoring During Intravenous Nutrition

It is important to monitor a variety of parameters in a patient receiving IV feeding, both to ensure tolerance and to potentially witness a beneficial response (e.g., appropriate weight gain). These parameters are monitored by clinical observations and blood analysis:

Clinical: Daily fluid balance, body weight, evidence of infection

Laboratory:
Baseline: Electrolytes, BUN, creatinine, glucose, calcium, magnesium, inorganic phosphate, liver function (bilirubin, alanine transaminase, aspartate transaminase, alkaline phosphatase), triglyceride, albumin, prothrombin time
Every 6 to 12 hours: Glucose, usually for the initial 3 to 5 days or until stable
Daily until stable: Electrolytes, BUN, creatinine, glucose, calcium, magnesium, PO_4
Weekly: Liver function, triglyceride, albumin, prothrombin time

Catheter Issues in Parenteral Nutrition

Many different types of venous catheters are available for central infusion, and which is most appropriate for a given patient depends on many factors. We focus here on aspects particularly relevant to TPN patients. The most important issue is patient safety. Therefore, avoidance of surgical complications related to catheter placement, avoidance of infection, and prevention of late complications (e.g., thrombosis) are paramount. Current recommendations to aid in the prevention of nosocomial infections attributable to central venous catheters are summarized in a recent publication from the Centers for Disease Control and Prevention.[50]

Catheter Choice and Rationale

In choosing a catheter for TPN administration, the first consideration should be the anticipated duration of therapy. In the inpatient setting, the traditional percutaneous central line, introduced via the subclavian or internal jugular vein and often containing multiple lumens (e.g., the so-called triple-lumen catheter), is most common. As the number of lumens increases, infection rates will rise proportionally, thus arguing in favor of single-lumen catheters when the device is intended solely for TPN administration. A more recent trend is to use peripherally inserted central catheters (PICCs) introduced via the basilic vein, both in the inpatient setting and also for longer-term outpatient therapy. When evaluated in controlled trials, PICC lines show similar rates of line sepsis as traditional central catheters but have an increased incidence of local complications such as leakage, thrombophlebitis, and malpositioning. At best, a PICC line in the outpatient setting has a lifetime of 4 to 6 weeks before malfunctioning or becoming infected. Therefore, for long-term TPN administration, a more permanent solution is needed. The devices available consist of either subcutaneously tunneled central catheters (Hickman, Broviac, Groshong) or self-contained implantable chambers that connect to the central venous system (portacath). The catheter of these devices can be inserted into the vein percutaneously (e.g., the subclavian, internal jugular, or femoral) and then tunneled to the final skin exit site (or to connect to the portacath chamber). Alternatively, access may be obtained by venous cut-down, for example, the cephalic vein within the deltopectoral groove, the external or internal jugular vein, the saphenous vein, or a branch of the subclavian vein within the axilla.

The principle underlying tunneled catheters is that the subcutaneous tract forms a barrier to bacterial encroachment and colonization, thus discouraging a so-called tunnel or tract infection, although a competing mode of infection for these or any other catheters, with resultant bacteremia, is by an intraluminal route. Tunneled catheters are desirable when frequent access is required, or perhaps if a high incidence of infection is anticipated, because they are easily removed. However, these devices are disfiguring and proper care of the exit site usually implies an inability to fully bathe or swim. The portacath is completely subcutaneous and thus obviates some of the limitations of the Hickman design (improved appearance, ability to immerse the body totally). However, when accessed, these devices require percutaneous insertion of a special low-profile needle (Huber needle), which then passes through the self-sealing diaphragm of the device into the chamber. Particularly if accessed frequently, the portacath may have a higher rate of infection and overall rate of failure than tunneled catheters in the setting of TPN, as opposed to other common scenarios such as when used for chemotherapy.

Catheter Sepsis

Catheter sepsis is potentially the most lethal complication in patients receiving TPN.[50] This problem is directly related to catheter care and the incidence of hyperglycemia attributable to TPN and can be reduced to an acceptable minimum of less than 1% per year by attention to detail, avoidance of multiuse catheters, and careful metabolic management. Organisms causing line infections are generally 80% *Staphylococcus* (50:50 *aureus* versus *epidermidis*), 15% yeast, and 5% gram-negative bacteria. Staphylococcal infections are generally related to catheter care, whereas yeast probably reaches the catheter through the gut. Additional factors influencing the incidence of line sepsis include the presence of a percutaneous stoma (e.g., a colostomy or tracheostomy), preexistent malnutrition with an increased susceptibility to infection, corticosteroid administration, recent broad-spectrum antibiotic therapy, concurrent chemotherapy, or severe neutropenia (e.g., in acute leukemia). The absence of a protocol for inpatient line care is also very important because in the ideal circumstance of a hyperalimentation team and a rigid protocol, sepsis rates may be as low as 0.6%.

If fever or signs suggestive of bacteremia develop in a patient receiving TPN, the TPN bottle should be taken down. Blood cultures, both from the central catheter and peripherally, should be performed, and a thorough search should be made for other possible sources of fever, such as pneumonia, an intra-abdominal abscess, the urinary tract, or a wound infection. If the fever persists or blood cultures suggest an infected catheter, the catheter should be removed and the tip cultured quantitatively by rolling it on an agar plate. Such tip cultures are considered positive if more than 15 colonies of organisms appear. Whether a percutaneous central line is simply removed under these circumstances or exchanged over a wire depends on many factors, as does the decision to treat such an incident with antibiotics and for what duration. Fungemia is the most serious type of line infection, with the entry site of *Candida,* the most common fungal pathogen, most probably being the GI tract. It is important to treat colonization with yeast (defined as two positive site cultures, e.g., urine and skin) in a critically ill patient aggressively with either fluconazole or amphotericin to avoid further complications such as line sepsis.

In the instance of a permanent catheter (Hickman, portacath), these devices may sometimes be salvaged in the setting of confirmed bacteremia (usually with gram-negative organisms) by prolonged antibiotic therapy, usually of 2 weeks' duration. For patients receiving long-term TPN who may have limited access options remaining because of multiple previous lines, line salvage becomes even more attractive. For *S. epidermidis* or gram-negatives, antibiotic therapy is effective in 60% to 70% of patients. At times a fibrin sheath at the catheter tip may be a nidus, and dissolution with tissue plasminogen activator or urokinase may be useful. Line tract infections can be more difficult to eradicate. In general, if *Staphylococcus aureus* or yeast is documented on blood culture, the line should simply be removed and IV anti-microbial therapy subsequently administered because these organisms are too virulent and dangerous to treat in lesser fashion. Though beyond the scope of this chapter, additional approaches to the avoidance of line infection are the use of impregnated catheters (e.g., with silver or bonded antibiotics) or the so-called antibiotic lock. The latter consists of antibiotics in high concentration, such as rifampicin, instilled into the catheter at the time that it is disconnected from the infusion, either as prophylaxis or, in some centers, as definitive therapy for line colonization.

Catheter Thrombosis and Other Complications

Catheter failure as a result of clogging and lack of function because of an intraluminal thrombus or a fibrin tip sheath is quite common. This problem can often be corrected by instillation of tissue plasminogen activator or urokinase and can be avoided by administering long-term prophylactic low-dose heparin (usually 6000 U/bag) or by the use of low-dose warfarin (1-2 mg/day), as shown effective in randomized trials.[51] Thrombosis of the great veins (subclavian, superior vena cava) occurs much less frequently, although some series report an incidence as high as 5% to 10%. Signs include upper arm, neck, or facial swelling or pain, or both. When thrombosis of the great veins is suspected, the catheter should be removed, and after confirmation of the diagnosis, thrombolytic therapy should be initiated. Heparin should then be continued, followed by warfarin therapy for 6 months or indefinitely.

Other catheter complications include pneumothorax, vascular injuries (arterial or venous lacerations, delayed arteriovenous fistulas), brachial plexus injury, chronic pain, thoracic duct injury after left-sided cannulation, air embolism, and catheter embolism. Erosion of the catheter into the bronchus, right atrium, or other structures may occur. Septic venous thrombosis is a life-threatening complication, and if antibiotics and anticoagulation are not successful, excision of the involved vein or Fogarty catheter embolectomy may occasionally be successful. Hydrothorax results from catheter malposition and administration of fluid into the thoracic cavity. This problem is particularly common with the more rigid percutaneous triple-lumen temporary central venous catheters, especially when introduced via the left subclavian vein. Such catheters should be 20 cm long, as opposed to the 16-cm catheter manufactured for placement in the right side of the chest or neck. If too short and thus allowing the line tip to terminate or rub against the wall of the superior vena cava, erosion of the catheter tip into the left pleural cavity can result.

Home Parenteral Nutrition

A major contribution of parenteral nutrition has been the ability to maintain patients in a functional state for decades with minimal oral intake. Unlike the continuous-infusion approach appropriate for a hospitalized patient, home parenteral alimentation is generally cycled and performed overnight over an 8- to 14-hour period.

Common Indications for Long-Term Parenteral Nutrition

The most appropriate patients receiving home parenteral nutrition suffer from short-gut syndrome after having lost a large portion of the GI tract either by repeated resections for Crohn's disease or by massive small bowel resection after midgut volvulus or mesenteric thrombosis, or both. Additional indications may include GI motility disorders (chronic pseudo-obstruction, sprue, scleroderma), management of a high-output enterocutaneous fistula, intractable chylous ascites, active Crohn's disease, cystic fibrosis, and chronic pancreatitis. Although home TPN for patients with cancer seems to rarely be indicated (see Controversies in Artificial Nutrition later), Medicare data indicate that an increasing proportion of patients receiving home TPN carry this diagnosis (18% in 1984, 39% in 1988).

The best candidates appear to be those with either (1) a curable malignancy requiring aggressive treatment resulting in anorexia, ileus, or intolerance to GI feeding or (2) a cured patient with residual bowel dysfunction secondary to radiation enteritis or short-gut syndrome. For these patients, survival rates and TPN-related complications appear to be similar to those in TPN patients without cancer. On the other hand, if an incurable cancer is present or the overall prognosis is poor, only 15% of patients placed on TPN will survive 1 year. Human immunodeficiency virus (HIV) infection is a rare indication for TPN, usually in the presence of intractable diarrhea or treatment-related pancreatitis. However, although a prospective, randomized trial showed improvements in global nutritional assessment, subjective health feelings, and Karnofsky performance index in HIV-infected patients receiving TPN for 2 months, there was no difference in survival.[52]

Economic Aspects and Outcome Measures in Home Total Parenteral Nutrition

A variety of statistical sources, including the OASIS (Oley-ASPEN Information System) database, Medicare, and the Mayo Clinic, suggest that the primary disease process of patients receiving home TPN, rather than complications of TPN administration alone, have the strongest influence on survival and rehabilitation. Most deaths are related to the primary disease, with only 8% being related to TPN (e.g., superior vena cava thrombosis, sepsis, or liver failure). For the most favorable candidates, the average rehospitalization rate is one per patient per year, 50% of which are for sepsis, and at least one in six patients will eventually discontinue TPN. Advanced age alone does not appear to be a reason to deny TPN. Overall, the predicted quality of survival at home for several months, rather than a specific diagnosis, seems to be the best justification for prolonged TPN. In view of the profound impact of such therapies on lifestyle, quality-of-life measures are reduced in patients receiving chronic TPN and are comparable to those reported for patients with chronic renal failure treated by dialysis.[53] Home hyperalimentation is a costly proposition. Depending on the area of the United States and the technique used, such costs may

run from $30,000 to $60,000 per year for home therapy, with an annual cost of up to $140,000 for hospitalization. Clearly, patient function, rehabilitation, quality of life, and other considerations enter the cost-to-benefit ratio. Patients managed by home TPN who do not have a concurrent or chronic illness are usually extremely well motivated, and many work or have returned to their premorbid situation, or both.

Metabolic Complications of Long-Term Administration of Total Parenteral Nutrition

A variety of problems can arise when TPN is administered over prolonged periods, particularly in patients who have little if any oral intake and are therefore completely dependent on the solution for the provision of essential vitamins, minerals, and fatty acids. The rare deficiency states involving these nutrients and mechanical and infectious disease considerations relevant to the TPN catheter and common in the outpatient population have been discussed earlier.

Liver Disease

Hepatic dysfunction is commonly observed in patients receiving TPN, and these disorders occupy a spectrum ranging from simple elevations in liver function test results to cirrhosis. Most often, if hyperbilirubinemia occurs acutely in a patient receiving TPN, the cause is generally sepsis. Factors responsible for liver disease attributable primarily to TPN administration, as opposed to other causes, remain unclear and are a source of controversy. Hepatic steatosis, cholestasis (presumably from lack of enteral stimulation and reduced release of cholecystokinin), and the presence of chronic inflammation have all been implicated as relevant mechanisms. Predisposing factors include short-gut syndrome (ileal disease or resection), a history of bacterial overgrowth, and recurrent sepsis or a chronic inflammatory state. For example, in a study of patients with severe short-gut syndrome requiring duodenocolostomy, the risk for TPN-induced liver disease appeared to be higher than if some jejunum or ileum remained.[54] However, short-bowel syndrome alone seemed an insufficient risk factor unless combined with a chronic inflammatory state such as Crohn's disease. TPN-specific factors include excessive glucose or insulin administration (with increased hepatic lipogenesis), excessive lipid administration (sequestration in hepatocytes), and alterations in fatty acid metabolism leading to the release of arachidonate-derived inflammatory leukotrienes.[55] For example, a recent study at our institution has suggested that levels of inflammatory mediators such as TNF and C-reactive protein are chronically elevated in patients receiving long-term TPN when compared with normal subjects.[56] One possible mechanism for these alterations is increased generation of inflammatory prostanoids derived from the n-6 fatty acids (e.g., arachidonate), which are prevalent in standard lipid emulsions. However, whether TNF, prostanoids, or other second messengers play a role in the hepatocyte damage occurring in patients receiving TPN is unknown. Nussbaum and coworkers proposed an altered portal vein insulin-to-glucagon ratio in chronic TPN patients and were able to ameliorate hepatic steatosis in rats maintained on TPN by administering glucagon. Deficiencies in particular nutrients, such as carnitine, choline, taurine, cysteine, and *S*-adenosyl methionine, have also been implicated in TPN-related liver disease. However, although the studies of Buchman and colleagues (see Fundamentals of Artificial Nutrition earlier) have shown that hepatic steatosis and enzymatic abnormalities can be improved by supplementation of TPN solutions with carnitine or choline,[35] these workers have not shown histologic or other evidence for reversal of TPN-induced liver damage. Based on this work, the addition of 1 to 2 g of carnitine to standard TPN, especially during long-term administration, is well tolerated and should be recommended. The use of oral ursodeoxycholic acid (e.g., 500 mg at bedtime or twice daily) is also usually without significant sequelae (although mild diarrhea may occur), and this agent may be useful to help resolve cholestasis when liver function test abnormalities are observed during chronic TPN administration.

In infants dependent on TPN, hepatic dysfunction is a more serious and potentially lethal disease, and it may have a pathophysiology different from that seen in adults. It is frequently associated with cholestasis. Even when enteral feeding is begun and TPN is discontinued, hepatic dysfunction may persist and progress to cirrhosis and death. Whether translocation of gut bacteria or their products across the immature gut, immaturity of other enzyme systems, or other factors may play a role is not clear. The ultimate solution to TPN-induced liver failure in children, if other maneuvers are unsuccessful (e.g., reduced caloric intake, avoidance of inflammation, carnitine supplementation), is combined liver and small bowel transplantation, an extreme intervention with disappointing outcomes at present. Recent exciting work by Puder and associates[44] demonstrated reversal of cholestasis in two infants with intestinal failure and parenteral nutrition–associated liver disease by substitution of a conventional IV fat emulsion with one containing primarily ω-3 fatty acids, thus suggesting that fat emulsions made from fish oils may be an effective means of treating and preventing this often fatal condition. These observations may lend credence to the inflammatory hypothesis discussed earlier. Accordingly, our group is currently testing whether dietary supplementation with ω-3 fatty acids in adult patients receiving long-term TPN may be effective in improving their deleterious pattern of inflammatory mediators and potential liver dysfunction (also see Fundamentals of Artificial Nutrition earlier).

Metabolic Bone Disease

In various studies, 40% to nearly 100% of patients administered TPN over prolonged periods have decreased bone mineral density (BMD) or histologic evidence of bone disease. Some individuals can be shown to have increased urinary calcium or phosphate excretion, decreased PTH levels, or vitamin D deficiency as possible mechanisms, but even in these patients there is poor correlation with BMD.[57] Patients at greatest risk are postmenopausal women, patients with long-standing malnutrition or malabsorption (e.g., Crohn's disease), those with preexisting liver disease, or patients receiving steroids. Some TPN-specific mechanisms postulated to contribute to bone loss are TPN-induced hypercalciuria, in which fixed acids generated by metabolism are buffered by bone calcium carbonate, and calcium diuresis induced by hyperglycemia or excessive sodium. TPN-associated deficiency states, such as calcium or magnesium (magnesium deficiency may decrease PTH release and vitamin D formation), copper (a cofactor for lysyl oxidase and collagen synthesis), boron, or silicon, have also been suggested to play a role. Given that reduced BMD is so common in long-term TPN patients, routine evaluation is probably unnecessary. However, in the patient population at greatest risk, annual assessment of BMD by neutron activation, possibly with measurement of urinary *N*-telopeptides (a marker of bone resorption), is a valid approach. If BMD is markedly decreased (e.g., >2 SD from average), a search for easily corrected problems (vitamin D deficiency, PTH excess or deficiency) is carried out. A relatively new, but unproven intervention in such patients is the use of bisphosphonates, synthetic nonbiodegradable analogues of pyrophosphate that decrease osteoclast-mediated bone resorption. Pamidronate, a second-generation agent shown to be effective in randomized trials in inhibiting postmenopausal osteoporosis, can be administered IV to TPN patients in the outpatient setting (30 mg/200 mL 5% dextrose in water over a 2-hour period) every 3 months, with minimal toxicity.

Artificial Nutrition in Specific Disease States

Pediatrics

Requirements for pediatric patients differ from those for adults. Growth is more rapid, and the distribution of visceral versus lean body mass is considerably different in an infant, who has very little muscle in comparison to an adult. Enzyme systems are incompletely developed, and excessive administration of certain amino acids may result in abnormally high concentrations of potentially toxic amino acids in the brain and perhaps in other viscera. The requirement for protein is far in excess of that for adults and decreases progressively with age. Energy requirements are also greater than for adults but may be decreased by providing a thermoneutral environment. The amount of lipid that can safely be administered is approximately 4 g/kg in an infant, whereas the upper limit of normal in an adult is thought to be 2 g/kg. Whether this difference results from proportionally larger amounts of viscera in neonates, the caloric requirements of whom are largely met by fat, is unclear. Vitamins and trace metals must be carefully administered because the ability to store these substances is limited and the opportunity for toxicity is greater. Venous access is a problem; use of the umbilical artery or vein is mentioned only to be condemned because catheter sepsis at this site is a disaster. In certain catastrophes, such as meconium ileus, gastroschisis, and neonatal enterocolitis, the increased survival now seen is almost certainly the result of aggressive nutritional support, as well as improved perioperative care. However, the contribution of nutritional support to the survival of low-birth-weight babies, though suggestive, remains unproven. Requirements for nutritional support in infants are presented in Table 7-8.

Pancreatitis

Severe pancreatitis has traditionally been treated with bowel rest and IV feeding on the assumption that gut-derived hormones released with enteral feeding (secretin, cholecystokinin) would have the deleterious effect of stimulating pancreatic secretion, thus worsening pancreatic inflammation. In addition, there is an unfounded belief that lipid-containing TPN may aggravate pancreatitis in some way whereas a 2-in-1 solution will not. Where this has seemingly occurred has been with the use of Intralipid, which raises the possibility that inflammatory mediators derived from n-6 essential fatty acids are the cause (see earlier). However, aside from avoiding severe hypertriglyceridemia, a known precipitant of pancreatitis, there is no evidence to support a negative effect of IV lipid on the course of this disease. Furthermore, pancreatitis is often accompanied by glucose intolerance, particularly when sepsis is concurrent, and in this regard, substitution of fat for dextrose in the TPN solution can be very useful. McClave and coworkers[58] have championed the use of early postpyloric enteral feeding in acute pancreatitis. These workers have provided evidence that decreasing degrees of stimulation of the pancreas occur as the site of feeding descends in the GI tract, and results of randomized trials in acute pancreatitis suggest that jejunal feeding is at least as safe and well tolerated as TPN. Whether early gut feeding in this setting is beneficial in any other way, such as by decreasing the incidence of nosocomial infections (see later), is unproven. However, one of the authors (J.E.F.), in two separate studies in two different institutions, both with rigorous catheter care protocols, found an increased incidence of catheter infection in patients with pancreatitis.

CONTROVERSIES IN ARTIFICIAL NUTRITION

Advantages of Enteral Versus Parenteral Feeding

It is increasingly being accepted that enteral feeding is associated with improved clinical outcomes when compared with parenteral feeding alone and, furthermore, that early enteral feeding (i.e., after surgery or traumatic injury) is more efficacious than when such feeding is delayed. In addition, enteral feeding solutions for critically ill patients are now commonly formulated with conditional nutrients thought to have special properties for enhancing immune function, reducing inflammation, and improving nitrogen balance. However, this area of inquiry is confused by a lack of clarity in proposed mechanisms and by potentially overlapping or unrelated explanations for the effectiveness of a given intervention. For example, in studies proposing a benefit with arginine supplementation (see later), does this agent improve immune function directly, or does it promote anabolism by enhancing growth hormone or insulin release, with a

Table 7-8 **Nutritional Requirements in Infants**

Protein (g/kg/day)	
Newborn to 6 mo	2.5-3
6-12 mo	2.0-2.5
School age	1.75
Adolescent	1.2
kcal/nitrogen	150:1
Calories (kcal/kg/day)	
Newborn or premature infant	120
Infant ≤10 kg	100
Infant 10-20 kg	100+50
Infant >20 kg	100+50+20
Fat	? 35% of calories (≤3.5g/kg/day)
Electrolytes (mEq/kg/day)	
Na$^+$	24
K$^+$	1-2
Urine Na$^+$:K$^+$	>1.0 adequate
Trace elements (per day)	
Term infants	
Ca^{2+}	500-600 mg/L
Mg^{2+}	50-70 mg/L
P	400-450 mg/L
Zn	800 µg/L
Cu	100 µg/L
Children >1 year	
Ca^{2+}	200-400 mg/L
Mg^{2+}	20-40 mg/L
P	150-300 mg/L
Vitamins (per day)	
A	2000 IU
C	80 mg
D	400 IU
B$_1$	1.2 mg
B$_2$	1.4 mg
B$_6$	1.0 mg
E	7 IU
Niacin	17 mg
Dexpanthenol	5 mg
Folic acid	40 µg
B$_{12}$	50 µg
K	200 µg

nonspecific secondary improvement in immune and other physiologic functions? Moreover, when immune function appears to be improved by a nutritional intervention (the most common claim), does this mean that a specific biologic effect was documented, or as in most studies, was simply the overall incidence of infection or another clinical parameter such as length of stay in the ICU studied? Finally, if the frequency of infection is lessened by enteral feeding, is it because of some laudatory effect on the permeability of the intestine to bacteria, or are the relevant mechanisms more poorly defined?

Translocation Hypothesis and the Role of Gut Mucosa

Translocation is a process by which live bacteria or their by-products (e.g., lipopolysaccharide) gain access to the lymphatic system or portal circulation by passing across the intestinal mucosa. This phenomenon is now fairly well accepted to occur in animal studies after burns and perhaps in hemorrhagic shock, but not in other catabolic states such as starvation alone. Whereas translocated bacteria are normally cleared by the lymph nodes, bacterial products persisting in the portal or systemic circulation under pathologic conditions are postulated to contribute to hepatic dysfunction, nosocomial infection, and multiple organ system failure.[59]

One problem with the translocation hypothesis as a whole is that any beneficial result of enteral feeding or dietary supplementation with particular nutrients (e.g., glutamine; see later) is automatically attributed to an improvement in gut mucosal integrity, often with little or no evidence. Conversely, increased substrate supply to the liver and improved hepatic acute phase protein synthesis may be another mechanism by which outcome is improved by enteral feeding. Alexander and coworkers[60] provided the initial evidence that gut feeding early in burn injury in guinea pigs and subsequently in human patients could ameliorate the usual catabolic response. The working hypothesis was that gut feeding prevented bacterial translocation, with a resultant decrease in the release of catecholamines and other negative stimuli, and thus prevented catabolism. In trauma patients, several prospective randomized studies suggest that early gut feeding lowers mortality and septic complications (see later).[61] Kudsk and colleagues,[62] in a series of studies in traumatized patients, concluded that early jejunal feeding results in a lower rate of sepsis than in patients receiving parenteral nutrition, but their results remain controversial because of differences in nutrient administration and glycemic control (see later). These authors promoted the concept of total mucosal immunity, that is, improved barrier function of gut, respiratory, and nasal mucosa, and provided some evidence that this immunity is mediated through IgA.

Although it is probably true that a breakdown in gut mucosal integrity leading to bacteremia can occur in patients close to death or in those with defined ischemic colitis, clinically significant loss of gut mucosal integrity has been demonstrated only in patients with burns, trauma, and perhaps hemorrhagic shock. In addition, although bacterial translocation probably does occur in humans, there is little evidence that it is either reduced by the use of enteral nutrition or increased in patients given parenteral nutrition (as suggested by some). It is also interesting to note that in humans supported with parenteral nutrition, remaining without enteral feeding has no substantial effect on mucosal architecture or permeability,[63] whereas chronic starvation and malnutrition do. Furthermore, when illness results in increased intestinal permeability, there remains no clear association between changes in permeability and actual bacterial translocation.[64]

Benefit of Early Enteral Feeding Versus Parenteral Nutrition

It is often said that enteral nutrition is safer and more efficacious than the parenteral route. However, a preliminary note of caution is raised from observations in experimental animals, which concluded that outcomes of enteral and parenteral nutrition were equivalent when animals

with catheter sepsis were eliminated. Numerous studies have shown that it is safe to feed the gut in the immediate postoperative period and that this practice does not place the integrity of intestinal anastomoses at risk. Early feeding has been studied primarily in two patient populations: those who have undergone GI surgery and traumatically injured or critically ill persons.

A recent meta-analysis reviewed 11 prospective randomized controlled trials that compared the practice of early enteral feeding with no oral intake (NPO) after elective GI surgery.[65] This analysis of 837 patients concluded that there is no clear advantage to keeping patients NPO postoperatively and that early feeding may be of benefit in decreasing infections and shortening postoperative length of stay. However, closer evaluation of these data reveals that the length of stay was reduced by only 0.84 days, and although there was an increase in any type of infection in the NPO group, when considered individually, no difference was found in the incidence of anastomotic dehiscence, wound infections, pneumonia, intra-abdominal abscess, or mortality. In 2001 Marik and Zaloga performed a meta-analysis of 15 randomized controlled trials involving 753 subjects in which early was compared with delayed enteral nutrition in critically ill surgical patients.[66] Early enteral nutrition was associated with a significantly lower incidence of infection (relative risk reduction of 0.45) and reduced length of hospital stay (2.2 days less). There were no differences in noninfectious complications or mortality. The authors concluded that early initiation of enteral feeding was beneficial, but this result must be interpreted with caution because of substantial heterogeneity between studies.

The studies that compared enteral and parenteral nutrition in the trauma population,[61,62] as discussed earlier, concluded that enteral nutrition was superior because of an attenuated inflammatory response and a decrease in septic morbidity. When these studies are examined more closely, it is clear that patients who were fed enterally usually received significantly less calories than those fed parenterally. This discrepancy of relative overfeeding in the TPN groups led in many instances to hyperglycemia, presumably predisposing patients to immune dysfunction and nosocomial infection. Thus, poor glucose control alone may account for the observed differences in outcome. In more contemporary studies in which feeding is carefully advanced in a manner that avoids hyperglycemia and groups are fed equivalent protein and calories, there appears to be little difference in clinical outcome between the enteral and parenteral routes of feeding.[67] Enteral nutrition can also endanger patient safety in unique ways. Deaths in persons receiving enteral nutrition are often due to aspiration, for example, when gastric motility is suddenly impaired with the onset of sepsis. One death from aspiration is equivalent to the mortality over 2 to 3 years of a well-operated parenteral nutrition program despite the danger of catheter sepsis, which in well-operated units is now less than 1% to 3%.

In conclusion, when possible the gut should be used preferentially for the following reasons:

1. Enteral feeding is much less expensive, with cost as low as $25 to $50 per day as compared with up to $200 per day for parenteral nutrition
2. It probably improves hepatic function and mimics the normal ingress of nutrients to the liver
3. Gut mucosal integrity is probably maintained, particularly in patients with burns and hemorrhagic shock
4. Enteral nutrition may have beneficial effects on non-intestinal mucosa, possibly mediated by IgA secretion by the liver

It seems fair to say that when delivered appropriately, both forms of nutritional support can be expected to improve organ function, immune competence, and wound healing equally in appropriately selected patients. The two forms of nutrition should be considered complementary; patients should be fed both enterally and parenterally to ensure adequate delivery of protein and calories, with the goal of progressively converting to full enteral feeding when safely tolerated by the patient.

Modulation of the Immune Response by Diet, or Immunonutrition

Major injury, whether traumatic or induced by surgery, results in significant suppression of immune function, which may influence patient recovery. Specific nutrients, such as arginine, nucleotides (discussed later), and ω-3 fatty acids (see Fundamentals of Artificial Nutrition earlier), have been shown to modulate the host response in experimental animals, with potential improvements in immune function. The working hypothesis is that clinical use of a solution containing increased amounts of arginine stimulates T lymphocytes and provides a substrate for the generation of NO, whereas the inclusion of ω-3 fatty acids promotes the synthesis of more favorable prostaglandins and inclusion of RNA nonspecifically enhances immune competence. A variety of clinical trials have evaluated the efficacy of enteral formulas supplemented with such immune-modulating substances.

In 1992 Daly and coworkers[68] (also see Daly et al., 1988[69]) were the first to study the clinical effects of immune-enhancing diets by prospectively randomizing 85 patients undergoing surgery for upper GI malignancies to either a standard (Osmolite) or experimental (Impact) enteral formula. Postoperative nutrition was delivered via a jejunostomy tube starting on day 1 and continuing until the seventh postoperative day. Patients administered the immune-modulating diet experienced a significant improvement in both postoperative wound healing and infectious complications, along with a shorter length of hospital stay. A potential flaw in this study is that although patients were fed isocalorically, the diets were not isonitrogenous (15.6 versus 9.0 g of nitrogen per day), thus leaving it possible that the findings may be partially explained by greater protein administration in the subjects given Impact. A prospective, randomized, double-blinded, multicenter study of 296 critically ill ICU patients was conducted by Bower and associates[70] in 1995. Subjects stratified as having either sepsis or systemic inflammatory response syndrome were administered enteral feeding within 48 hours of the precipitating study entry

event (trauma, surgery, new onset of infection) that consisted of Impact or a control diet (Osmolite HN). Feeding formulas were not equivalent because the patients given Impact received more nitrogen and fewer calories. There were no statistically significant differences noted overall. However, patients stratified as septic and receiving the immune-modulating formula experienced a significant reduction in hospital length of stay (by 10 days) and a reduction in acquired infections. On subgroup analysis, the patients who received a minimum of 821 mL/day for at least 7 days experienced the greatest decrease in hospital stay.

Braga and coworkers[71] in 1999 showed fairly convincingly that administration of an immune-enhancing diet perioperatively yields significant clinical benefit. These workers randomized 206 candidates undergoing elective surgery for malignancies of the colon, rectum, stomach, or pancreas to receive either an immune-enhancing formula (Impact) or a control formula that was isonitrogenous and isocaloric. Patients were administered 1 L/day for 7 days preoperatively, followed by jejunal infusions of the same formula postoperatively starting 6 hours after surgery and continuing until postoperative day 7. The immunonutrition group experienced significantly fewer postoperative infections (14% versus 30%) and a shorter hospital length of stay (11.1 versus 12.9 days). These findings did not appear to be influenced by the baseline nutritional status of the patient. The authors concluded that attaining adequate intake before the surgical insult gives perioperative immunonutrition metabolic and immunologic advantages over less aggressive approaches to feeding. Despite this positive finding, subsequent studies were less consistent, and therefore several meta-analyses were performed between 1999 and 2001 to further delineate the efficacy of immune-enhancing diets in clinical practice.[72] Common to these meta-analyses was the universal finding of shorter hospital length of stay and an overall reduction in numbers of infectious complications. Although positive conclusions overall were reached in each of these more recent meta-analyses, the heterogeneity of the data makes broad recommendations about the use of immune-enhancing diets tentative.[73,74] What does appear clear is that if it is possible to give immune-modifying nutritional support early in the course of illness and to give it in rather large amounts, its benefits are more easily detected.[75]

Nutritional Pharmacology: Conditionally Essential and Other Special Metabolites in Critical Illness

Nutritional pharmacology is a poorly defined, but often used term that emphasizes the role of particular nutrients to change the pathophysiology of a disease process, presumably by distinct molecular mechanisms. Early examples include the administration of essential amino acids to patients in acute renal failure and using modified amino acid mixtures for the treatment of patients with hepatic failure.

As just discussed, one major area of potential advance in nutritional pharmacology has been the use of immunity-enhancing enteral formulas. However, many other proposed approaches in this area remain unproven. In some instances, nutritional pharmacology appears to refer to agents that although not metabolically limiting, may be useful if given in supranormal amounts, for example, the beneficial changes in lipid metabolism induced by ω-3 fatty acids. Another interpretation is the use of substances that may be metabolized with improved efficiency under conditions of stress, such as BCAAs. Yet another definition of nutritional pharmacology involves the concept of *conditionally essential* amino acids, nucleosides, or other substances that presumably become rate-limiting for protein or nucleic acid synthesis during stress but are sufficiently abundant under normal conditions. The classic example of the latter is glutamine, an amino acid easily synthesized in many cells and normally present in high levels in the circulation. However, despite some literature supporting a relative deficiency of glutamine during stress (see the next section), even under such conditions, circulating and intracellular levels of glutamine remain well above the K_m for glutamyl transfer RNA and other relevant enzymes.

Glutamine

Within 24 hours of surgery or trauma, levels of free intracellular glutamine fall in many tissues and do not return to normal until as long as 8 weeks later. The significance of this glutamine export is not clear. Glutamine has received much attention as a fuel for enterocytes. It has been proposed that in pathologic conditions, such as after traumatic injury or during infection, energy production from the glutamine released from muscle is critical for maintaining function of GI and immune cells.[1] Furthermore, it has also been suggested that under these conditions a state of glutamine deficiency may exist and that administration of supplemental glutamine in such circumstances is beneficial.[1] Glutamine's effects in either preventing or healing chemotherapeutic or radiation toxicity and in promoting mucosal regrowth after massive small bowel resection are most impressive when it is given enterally. In severe stress, such as after bone marrow transplantation, beneficial effects of glutamine in decreasing hospital stay, improving nitrogen balance, and decreasing infection have been demonstrated.[76] These effects have been attributed to improved gut barrier function, but improved gut protein and hepatic protein synthesis are equally possible.

Although most studies of gut histology with supplemental glutamine have involved enteral delivery, some investigators have proposed that the addition of glutamine to parenteral solutions may prevent the gut atrophy that often accompanies IV feeding. In certain animal studies, the addition of glutamine to parenteral nutrition solutions resulted in maintenance of small intestinal mucosal thickness, protein content, and DNA when compared with glutamine-free solutions, but other investigators failed to show any difference in gut protein, RNA, or wall thickness.[77] These inconclusive experimental results may explain the lack of enthusiasm for glutamine-supplemented parenteral nutrition in clinical practice. Glutamine is also very unstable when added to TPN solutions, thus limiting its practical use. An additional potential concern in neoplastic disease is the observation that glutamine is preferentially metabolized by many tumors, with the potential for augmented tumor growth.

Another putative beneficial effect of glutamine is improved nitrogen balance, particularly in muscle. Attempts to prevent depletion of free glutamine pools in muscle by glutamine supplementation in parenteral nutrition solutions have shown some glutamine sparing. Glutamine supplementation can also raise levels of TCA cycle intermediates, and although this response does not appear to increase energy production or endurance in healthy skeletal muscle, there is some evidence to suggest improved functioning of ischemic heart muscle.[78] Administration of high amounts of glutamine with parenteral nutrition has been reported to promote protein accretion in skeletal muscle.[1] However, although the marginal improvements in nitrogen balance are statistically significant, they seem unlikely to improve clinical outcome.

Arginine

A deficiency of arginine and dibasic amino acids in the plasma of patients with overwhelming sepsis was observed as early as 1978. Although arginine was thought to be a nonessential amino acid, investigators now recognize that the ability to synthesize arginine in the presence of increased requirements may be exceeded and thus it is probably semiessential. Aside from its metabolic functions, arginine supplementation in critical illness may be beneficial by at least two potential mechanisms: (1) by improving immune function and (2) by stimulating growth hormone and insulin secretion, a recognized action of this amino acid. Arginine is also known to enhance the responsiveness of T lymphocytes to mitogenic stimulation in vitro. In the study of immune-enhancing enteral diets by Daly and associates discussed earlier,[69] T-cell proliferation in response to concanavalin A or phytohemagglutinin was improved in arginine-supplemented patients, although nitrogen balance was no different between the two groups. Such clinical studies are difficult to interpret with respect to effects attributable to arginine alone because additional substances (e.g., fish oil) are usually present in the experimental formulas.

Ketone Bodies

The ketone bodies acetoacetate, propionate, and butyrate have been considerably investigated in experimental studies with respect to their beneficial effect on the gut and especially the effect of butyrate on the ileum and colon. No clinical studies involving exogenous administration of ketone bodies or other short-chain fatty acids are available, however. Acetoacetate, propionate, and butyrate are produced by the fermentation of soluble pectin by colonic bacteria. Because short-chain fatty acids are not synthesized endogenously, the colonic mucosa can obtain these metabolites only from bacterial fermentation. When compared with other fuels, butyrate appears to be the principal energy source for the colonic mucosa, with acetoacetate, glutamine, and glucose following in order of importance. Diminished short-chain fatty acid oxidation may therefore disrupt the colonic mucosal barrier and presumably, though certainly not proven in human patients, its immune function.

In experimental studies, IV butyrate results in wall thickening and increased protein content of both the colon and the ileum, and short-chain fatty acids derived from soluble pectin prevent and heal chemotherapy-related gut mucosal damage in animals, as well as improve diversion colitis. Some investigators have proposed a deficiency of short-chain fatty acids in colonocytes as a precursor to ulcerative colitis, but evidence to support this concept is lacking.[79]

Branched-Chain Amino Acids

For many years the experimental observations that BCAAs promote positive nitrogen balance in muscle and are preferentially oxidized by this tissue (see Metabolic Adaptations in Catabolic States and Regulation of Nitrogen Balance earlier) have stimulated broad interest in using BCAAs as nutritional supplements in critical illness, particularly for the management of hepatic encephalopathy and uremia. However, despite many attempts, little proof of clinical efficacy for BCAAs is available. As discussed elsewhere in this chapter, BCAAs do appear to be helpful in improving severe hepatic encephalopathy, but only in patients to whom a solution deficient in aromatic amino acids is given. However, in incubated muscles from septic animals or humans, BCAAs do not decrease protein breakdown even when present in pharmacologic quantities (5 mM). IV feeding with solutions enriched in BCAAs appears to reduce proteolysis in experimental animals with sepsis, but in septic patients, prospective randomized trials using solutions high in BCAAs (up to 50% of total amino acids) or containing leucine show marginal efficacy in preventing breakdown of lean body mass, perhaps increasing hepatic protein synthesis slightly, but only in severely ill patients. No difference in outcome was seen. Similar results have been obtained in patients undergoing bone marrow transplantation.

Essential Amino Acids

Most amino acids can be recycled, provided that energy is adequate. Thus, small amounts of essential amino acids with adequate energy are sufficient for nitrogen equilibrium. In infants, 40% to 50% of protein intake should be essential amino acids, whereas in adults in nitrogen equilibrium without stress, sepsis, or trauma, 19% to 20% is sufficient. The percentage of essential amino acids should increase with injury or depletion. The use of essential amino acids in the management of renal failure is discussed elsewhere in this chapter.

Purines and Pyrimidines

These nucleic acid precursors have been proposed to be conditionally essential under conditions of stress, potentially limiting cell division and the generation of new immune or other cells. For example, immune-enhancing enteral formulas such as *Impact* contain mRNA for this reason. However, as in the case of glutamine, it seems extremely unlikely that these nucleotides would ever be rate limiting given the numerous salvage pathways available in the cell to regenerate them.

Who Benefits From Parenteral Nutrition?

Indications for parenteral nutrition may be organized into three categories, depending on the desired outcome:

1. Primary therapy, in which parenteral nutrition is thought to influence the disease process beneficially
2. Supportive therapy, in which nutritional support is important but does not alter the primary disease process
3. Controversial indications or those under ongoing study

In most cases, the efficacy of IV feeding remains controversial because of the limited availability of prospective, randomized trials capable of answering such questions.

Primary Therapy: Efficacy Shown
Gastrointestinal-Cutaneous Fistulas

Patients with GI-cutaneous fistulas represent the classic indication for TPN because in general, increased oral intake increases fistula output. Two longitudinal reviews of fistulas concluded the following:

1. TPN increases spontaneous closure of fistulas.
2. TPN has not resulted in decreased mortality in centers experienced in the treatment of fistulas. The major decrease in mortality in the series at Massachusetts General Hospital and the University of California at San Francisco occurred in the 1960s, probably the result of improved intensive care, including monitoring, respiratory care, and better fluid and electrolyte balance.
3. TPN has probably contributed to decreased mortality in patients with fistulas in most other institutions.
4. Treatment of patients with fistulas has been altered by nutritional support. If spontaneous closure does not occur, patients are in better condition for surgery after being supported by TPN.

Respectable rates of fistula closure are also achieved with enteral nutrition, although these rates are slightly lower than with TPN. Initially, fistula drainage increases and then decreases toward closure. A useful compromise, if total caloric replacement is not possible enterally, is to give 20% to 30% of calories enterally, a method that is likely to give all the benefits of enteral feeding, and to give the remainder parenterally.

Renal Failure

TPN results in decreased mortality in patients with acute renal failure, but controversy persists concerning the amino acid solution to use. In 1973, Abel and coworkers, using a mixture of essential amino acids with hypertonic dextrose, largely in patients with surgically related renal failure, reported a decreased appearance of urea, earlier diuresis, and a statistically significant improvement in survival in treated patients versus those receiving dextrose alone. Other investigators have argued for a more complete amino acid formula and for dealing with the rise in BUN by dialysis. Whereas a few studies have attempted to compare the two formulas, no study with adequate patients concurrently studied is available. A useful compromise is to use essential amino acids early in an effort to avoid dialysis, but once dialysis is required, a complete formulation is used (see earlier discussion in Fundamentals of Artificial Nutrition).

Short-Bowel Syndrome

Repeated small bowel resections for Crohn's disease and major enterectomy after mesenteric thrombosis or volvulus are the major causes of short-bowel syndrome. No randomized prospective trials have been undertaken, but patients with short-bowel syndrome have no alternative to long-term home TPN. Patients receiving home TPN who would otherwise almost certainly have died commonly survive for 10 to 20 years or even longer. Some patients undergo sufficient hypertrophy of the remaining small bowel that the need for home TPN is ultimately decreased or obviated. If a patient is left with 1.5 ft of small bowel anastomosed to the left colon, hypertrophy in 1 or 2 years will, in most cases, enable survival without daily parenteral nutritional support, although twice-weekly supplementation may be necessary. Efforts to promote more rapid hypertrophy of the small bowel by using gut-specific hormones, fuels, and isotonic solutions have been reported.

Burns

The sharp decrease in mortality from 1965 to 1970 in patients with burns was probably the result of aggressive nutritional support. Early aggressive nutritional support in patients with major burns is associated with improved survival,[60] and aggressive enteral feeding within 3 hours of burn injury is increasingly being practiced. Parenteral nutritional support is reserved for those few patients in whom enteral nutrition cannot meet their caloric needs. Moreover, as discussed earlier, nutritional pharmacology is increasingly being used in enteral diets specifically designed for burned patients and most likely has contributed to lower rates of sepsis, fewer days of bacteremia, lower mortality, and shorter hospital stay.[70]

Hepatic Failure

Improved survival is also seen in patients with hepatic failure who are given aggressive nutritional support. Patients with liver disease are often malnourished secondary to excessive alcohol ingestion and decreased food intake and have decreased tolerance to stress. Protein is the important nutritional component that they require, but these patients are specifically protein intolerant if hepatic encephalopathy is present (see earlier discussion in Fundamentals of Artificial Nutrition). Of the seven randomized prospective trials thus far reported, in the five in which hypertonic dextrose was used as the caloric source, branched chain–enriched amino acid solutions were at least as effective as lactulose or neomycin in the treatment of hepatic encephalopathy. In two studies, improved survival was seen. For reasons that are unclear, in studies in which the major caloric source was fat, efficacy for BCAAs was not seen.[80]

Fan and associates[59] randomized 124 patients undergoing hepatic resection for hepatocellular carcinoma. Half the patients received only oral nutrition, whereas the other half received perioperative IV nutritional support with a branched chain–enriched solution. Dextrose and lipid were the caloric sources, with MCTs accounting for 50% of the lipids. A statistically significant reduction in the overall postoperative morbidity rate occurred in the perioperative nutrition group as compared with the control group (34% versus 55%), predominantly because of fewer septic complications (17% versus 37%). In addition, there was a reduced need for diuretic agents to control ascites (25% versus 50%), less weight loss (0 versus 1.4 kg), and less deterioration in liver function as measured by indocyanine green clearance (−2.8% versus 4.8%). However, the difference in mortality (5 of 64 in the perioperative nutrition group and 9 of 60 in the control group) did not reach statistical significance. Thus, during hepatectomy, outcome can be considerably improved by perioperative parenteral nutrition.

Primary Therapy: Efficacy Not Shown
Inflammatory Bowel Disease

In patients with inflammatory bowel disease, oral intake often provokes diarrhea, protein-losing enteropathy, bleeding, and abdominal pain. Although TPN and bowel rest are useful in the treatment of Crohn's disease (particularly disease limited to the small bowel, in which a remission rate of 75% can be expected), such therapy has not been subjected to a randomized prospective trial. The mean duration of remission is approximately 11 months. Patients with colonic involvement do less well; their rates of initial remission and duration are considerably lower than those of patients with small bowel disease alone. Patients with extensive, severe, and chronically recurrent Crohn's disease are suitable for home hyperalimentation, particularly when surgical therapy would leave the patient almost anenteric. Patients with ulcerative colitis should not receive long-term TPN to induce remission because definitive resection with a sphincter-saving operation (e.g., an ileoanal pouch or Soave procedure) produces a long-term cure. On the other hand, TPN for usually less than 2 weeks, in conjunction with IV antibiotics, may allow the rectal mucosa to heal and thus facilitates rectal mucosal stripping.

Anorexia Nervosa

Patients with anorexia nervosa starve to a moribund state, with enormous loss of lean body mass, tissue, and protein. Anorectic patients are difficult to treat and can be self-destructive, for example, by disconnecting their IV lines and thus inviting air embolism. A prospective trial has not been carried out in patients with anorexia nervosa.

Supportive Therapy: Efficacy Shown
Acute Radiation Enteritis or Chemotherapy Toxicity

Acute radiation enteritis or GI complications of chemotherapy, or both, may prevent oral intake. TPN must be administered until the gut mucosa heals and clearly enables the patient to survive. Chronic radiation enteritis with multiple strictures may render the patient a candidate for home parenteral nutrition or, rarely, enteral feeding with minimal-residue diets, provided that the original neoplasm has been cured. Some data suggest that enteral glutamine may alleviate acute radiation enteritis, chemotherapy-induced mucositis, or intestinal graft-versus-host disease in bone marrow transplant recipients, but because glutamine is a metabolic source for malignant cells, one should be certain that no malignancy persists.

Prolonged Ileus

Prolonged ileus after an abdominal procedure may necessitate a course of TPN until the ileus subsides. Obviously, this therapy is only supportive.

Supportive Therapy: Efficacy Probably Present
Weight Loss Preliminary to Major Surgery (Perioperative Parenteral Nutrition)

Four important questions concern the use of parenteral nutrition in patients experiencing weight loss before major surgical procedures: (1) Are operative complications of surgery increased in patients who have lost weight? (2) If so, can these patients be identified? (3) If these patients are identified, does short-term parenteral nutrition change the outcome? (4) If all these conditions are met, what mode of nutritional repletion should be used and for how long?

1. Are surgical complications of major operative procedures increased in patients who have lost weight? In an older review analyzing 18 randomized and nonrandomized studies, Detsky and colleagues[81] concluded that the case had not yet been made for the use of TPN before major surgery. In contrast, a critical Veterans Affairs study, one of the best randomized, controlled, prospective studies available in the entire field of parenteral nutrition, appears to identify a group at risk, namely, patients who lost more than 15% of their body weight before surgery.[82] In this group the incidence of surgical complications was greater and was ameliorated by TPN.

2. Can this group be identified? Observations as early as those of Studley in 1936 suggested that patients with profound (20%) weight loss and a low serum albumin level experienced increased complications and mortality after gastrectomy. Thus, identification of the group at risk requires a careful history and global assessment. A history of greater than 10% or certainly 15% weight loss and an albumin value of less than 3 g/100 mL would place these patients in a high-risk group. Delayed cutaneous hypersensitivity testing by injecting antigens, hand dynamometry, and serum transferrin are confirmatory and optional.

3. Does short-term nutritional intervention change the outcome? It does, provided that nutritional intervention is limited to the group with severe malnutrition and immunologic dysfunction. In the Veterans Affairs multicenter trial,[82] preoperative nutritional intervention for 7 to 10 days decreased operative septic complications in patients who were judged to be severely malnourished and who had lost more than 15% of

their body weight. However, in the group stratified as having mild to moderate malnutrition, the decrease in surgical complications was more than offset by the increase in catheter-related infectious complications. The total energy intake of the TPN group was 46 kcal/kg (2944 kcal/day), whereas the ad libitum group consumed 20 kcal/kg (1280 kcal/day). With this degree of TPN-induced hyperglycemia, the immunosuppressive effects would be great enough to negate any potential benefit of preoperative feeding, with the exception of the subgroup that was severely malnourished. Thus, improperly administered TPN increased the risk of catheter- and non–catheter-related infection. Whether fewer calories or a shorter period of preoperative repletion would have resulted in greater benefit to the minimally or moderately malnourished group is not clear.

4. How long should preoperative repletion last? In previous studies, with 3 days of parenteral nutritional support before surgery, the trend was toward decreased sepsis, but statistical significance was not achieved because of the small number of patients. With preoperative repletion, patients begin to feel better at approximately 5 days, a point that generally coincides with an increase in the shortest-turnover proteins, that is, retinol-binding protein and thyroxin-binding prealbumin. In the Veterans Affairs cooperative study,[82] the duration of preoperative parenteral nutrition was between 7 and 10 days, and efficacy was seen. Thus, a period of 5 to 7 days should be used for preoperative nutritional repletion.

Cancer

In the 1980s, the initial enthusiasm for nutritional support in patients with cancer waned as evidence suggested that tumor growth is stimulated by such intervention and that nutritional supplementation of patients undergoing chemotherapy or radiation therapy (or both) might decrease survival or the remission-free interval. This important area is plagued by a lack of uniformity in studies, by the inclusion of both malnourished and normally nourished patients in studies, and by the finding that responses to nutritional support may differ depending on whether the treatment modality is to be radiation therapy, chemotherapy, or resection. The sources of calories supplied in standard feeding regimes may also be inappropriate in a patient with cancer because glucose rather than fat may be used preferentially by many tumors. Randomized prospective trials in patients with cancer have shown efficacy for preoperative IV nutritional support only in severely malnourished patients with upper GI tumors. For example, in the Veterans Affairs study discussed earlier, patients with carcinoma of the esophagus or the gastric cardia benefited from perioperative nutritional support and had decreased mortality and morbidity without apparent stimulation of the tumor.[82] In addition, several studies in patients with cancer have suggested that postoperative nutritional support via so-called immunologically active tube feeding may improve postoperative outcomes in general (see Immunonutrition earlier).

Cardiac Surgery

Patients with cardiac cachexia are at increased risk for complications and mortality after cardiac surgery. The conventional wisdom is based on Starling's pronouncement in 1912 that the heart is spared the ravages of starvation. This is not true. Protein depletion in experimental animals results in decreased myocardial contractility, with distortion of cardiac histology manifested as edema and necrosis of myofibrils, conditions that are not totally reversed even after prolonged nutritional repletion. In the single prospective randomized trial in which nutritional supplementation was begun on the day of surgery (and thus unlikely to show efficacy), no improvement in outcome was seen. A study in which patients with cardiac cachexia about to undergo surgical treatment are subjected to prolonged nutritional repletion has yet to be done. Anecdotal clinical evidence suggests that patients with cardiac cachexia require nutritional supplementation for at least 2 to 3 weeks and perhaps as long as 6 weeks before surgery, a finding supported by experimental evidence. Fluid limitations in such patients require more concentrated solutions.

Respiratory Failure and Requirements for Prolonged Respiratory Support

No evidence indicates that pulmonary function itself, rather than the muscles of respiration, is improved by nutritional support. Although some information is available concerning the metabolic needs of the alveolar cells responsible for surfactant production and gas exchange, a tailored IV solution has not appeared. Whereas weaning from ventilators may improve with nutritional support, a potential deleterious effect of hypertonic dextrose is overproduction of carbon dioxide. Although this phenomenon is extensively discussed in the ICU setting, it is not common; occasionally, in patients with marginal pulmonary function, carbon dioxide overproduction may require replacing glucose with fat to promote weaning from the ventilator. Carbon dioxide production and RQ can be measured in most intensive care settings, as described earlier.

Large Wounds and Other Sources of Nitrogen Loss

Many patients with large wounds such as decubitus ulcers are unable to eat. Provision of nutritional support to improve wound healing is logical, but no randomized studies exist.

HIV Infection

The place of TPN in the treatment of patients with acquired immunodeficiency syndrome is controversial[52] and was discussed in an earlier section in the context of home TPN.

FUTURE DIRECTIONS IN ARTIFICIAL NUTRITION: NOVEL APPROACHES FOR REDUCING CACHEXIA

Besides the primarily nutritional approaches described earlier and designed to promote positive nitrogen balance and improved overall outcome in critically ill patients, additional strategies are available and are a focus of present and future research. Certain initially promising approaches, such as administration of growth hormone, have not been clearly shown to be of clinical benefit, whereas others, such as pharmacologic inhibition of protein breakdown, are in their infancy.

Inhibition of the Stress Response

A variety of approaches have been used to inhibit the actions of the inflammatory mediators and catabolic hormones that are released under conditions of stress and are presumably responsible for protein loss and cachexia. Included in this category are the ω-3 fatty acids, which have been amply discussed in earlier sections and which continue to show promise as therapeutic agents. Unfortunately, alternative strategies, such as the use of neutralizing antibodies to TNF or to endotoxin during sepsis, have either been shown to be ineffective or, in some cases, actually seem to cause increased mortality in clinical trials. An attractive drug is the glucocorticoid receptor antagonist RU-486, but no data are available for this agent in cachectic patients, perhaps in part because of societal unease with the identity of RU-486 as an abortifacient. An important issue for all such approaches is whether the signals commonly thought to be harmful in conditions of stress (e.g., the cytokines) should be interpreted in such a simple manner or, alternatively, whether these mediators serve critical and useful functions during the stress response as well.

Administration of Anabolic Factors

Gut-Derived Hormones

Studies have suggested that glucagon-like peptide-2 (GLP-2) has a robust effect on stimulating gut hypertrophy, DNA, and wall thickness in animals receiving parenteral nutrition. In one of the authors' (J.E.F.) preliminary studies, the effects of GLP-2 have been impressive in the sense that continued administration of GLP-2 in rats receiving TPN results in gut hypertrophy exceeding that seen in orally fed animals. It is hoped that clinical trials will take place within several years.

Growth Hormone and Insulin-like Growth Factors

In experimental studies discussed earlier, growth hormone and IGFs promoted positive nitrogen balance in muscle. Furthermore, the IGFs inhibit muscle proteolysis and stimulate protein synthesis directly (unlike growth hormone), and during systemic administration the IGFs may be less diabetogenic than growth hormone. These agents may also have beneficial effects on lipolysis. These anabolic effects have led to the clinical use of cloned human growth hormone. Pharmacologic levels of this hormone given with hypocaloric TPN to humans can promote positive nitrogen balance in sepsis and after major injury.[1] The increase in protein degradation in isolated muscles after burn injury can also be reversed by IGF-I in a dose-dependent manner,[83] but this effect was not seen in muscles from septic animals, where IGF-I increased protein synthesis but had no effect on protein degradation rates.[18,83] Although the role of growth hormone in clinical practice remains poorly defined, a cautionary note is raised by a recent clinical trial of growth hormone administration to ventilated ICU patients,[84] in which mortality, the duration of ventilator dependence, and length of stay were seemingly worsened, not improved, by the hormone.

Anabolic Steroids

The increased secretion of testosterone in males at puberty is thought to determine the increased skeletal muscle mass that occurs at this stage in development and is maintained into adult life. Accordingly, suppressing testosterone in healthy young men reduces fat-free mass and fractional muscle protein synthesis, and androgen supplementation to normal physiologic levels in androgen-deficient men leads to increased muscle mass and strength.[85] The potential therapeutic use of testosterone has also been explored in a number of studies. There is some evidence for the use of testosterone to reverse the loss of muscle mass and strength that occurs in normal aging in males.[85] In HIV-infected men with weight loss and low testosterone levels, testosterone supplements led to improved strength, and injections of testosterone after severe burn injury reduced muscle loss by improving protein synthetic efficiency and reducing muscle protein degradation rates.

Catecholamines

Catecholamines appear to exert an anabolic effect on muscle principally by reducing calcium-dependent proteolysis and by increasing protein synthesis. The anabolic effect of catecholamines can also be mimicked by the β$_2$-adrenergic agonist clenbuterol. Numerous studies in animals have shown that clenbuterol treatment increases carcass and muscle weight, and furthermore, clenbuterol can inhibit wasting caused by hind limb suspension or denervation in rats and can also attenuate cachexia after scald injury. In addition, clenbuterol improved lean body mass and muscle size in animals with experimental tumors while increasing the utilization of lipid.[86] The exact mechanism by which drugs such as clenbuterol promote positive nitrogen balance in vivo remains unclear. For example, a pure β-antagonist, propranolol, was shown by Herndon and colleagues to improve protein balance and reduce energy expenditure in children with severe burns randomized to 2 weeks of oral therapy.[87]

Inhibition of Proteolysis

Pharmacologic Inhibition

An extremely attractive approach to the treatment of muscle wasting is direct inhibition of intracellular proteolysis. As knowledge of the biochemical pathways for protein breakdown in muscle and other tissues grows, the potential for such intervention increases. Low-molecular-weight active-site inhibitors of the proteasome are now available,[12,14] and newer-generation inhibitors have been shown to be fairly safe in humans during initial trials of their use as antineoplastic agents, for example,

in treating multiple myeloma. More recently, specific E3s induced in muscle under catabolic conditions have been identified,[15,16] and these enzymes may offer tissue-specific targets for inhibition of ubiquitination and proteolysis during future drug development. Such specificity will probably prove important in avoiding toxicity inasmuch as intracellular protein breakdown has fundamental and pleotropic functions, including regulation of the cell cycle, antigen presentation, and prevention of the accumulation of abnormal proteins in cells.

Lessons From Nature

Muscle proteolysis is suppressed in certain physiologic conditions, including dietary protein deficiency and prolonged fasting.[22] Muscles from such animals are also resistant to many catabolic signals, such as the proteolysis induced by denervation. An improved understanding of the intracellular mechanisms and endocrine signals responsible for these adaptations should suggest new strategies relevant to clinical practice and useful for reducing muscle wasting in ill patients.

SUMMARY

One of the most important therapeutic modalities of the 20th century has been nutritional support, in particular, IV feeding. As investigators are trained who are equally familiar with the operating room and with modern cell biology, the basic mechanisms underlying disease states relevant to surgical patients are increasingly being elucidated at the molecular level. The ability to intervene in and correct nutritional deprivation states that cause significant mortality in patients will continue to improve as our knowledge of nutrition and metabolism becomes increasingly sophisticated.

Selected References

Abel RM, Beck CH Jr, Abbott WM, et al: Improved survival from acute renal failure after treatment with intravenous essential L-amino acids and glucose: Results of a prospective, double-blind study. N Engl J Med 288:695-699, 1973.

> An early, randomized, double-blinded trial showed improved survival after the application of techniques of parenteral nutrition and administration of a specialized solution to patients with renal failure. The eight essential L-amino acids were administered in hypertonic dextrose to patients with renal failure, and these patients were compared with a group receiving isocaloric hypertonic dextrose alone. Improved survival and perhaps early healing of the renal lesion were seen.

Clowes GH Jr, George BC, Villee CA Jr, Saravis CA: Muscle proteolysis induced by a circulating peptide in patients with sepsis or trauma. N Engl J Med 308:545-552, 1983.

> Few articles have inspired as much interest and excitement as this description of a 4200-d protein isolated in the plasma of patients with sepsis. This hypothetic cytokine, PIF, increased hepatic protein synthesis and muscle breakdown. Subsequent experiments revealed that the particular conditions used in these experiments may have contributed to these findings. Nonetheless, this article probably contributed more to research on the effect of cytokines during surgical procedures than any other and inspired a great deal of work over the subsequent years.

Cuthbertson DP: Observations on the disturbance of metabolism produced by injury to the limbs. Q J Med 1:233-246, 1932.

> This study may well have begun contemporary nutritional support. This classic description of loss of nitrogen and breakdown of lean body mass after injury is a careful study in a classic tradition.

Dominioni L, Trocki O, Mochizuki H, et al: Prevention of severe postburn hypermetabolism and catabolism by immediate intragastric feeding. J Burn Care Rehabil 5:106-112, 1984.

> The first demonstration that changes in gut flora and translocation of bacteria or absorption of bacterial products after thinning of the mucosa in burns contribute to hypermetabolism is presented. With the confirmation of similar results in patients with burns, it is clear that this hypothesis with respect to gut products is operant in other patients as well.

Dudrick SJ, Wilmore DW, Vars HM, Rhoads JE: Long-term total parenteral nutrition with growth, development, and positive nitrogen balance. Surgery 64:134-142, 1968.

> This is one of the classic articles originally describing high-glucose central TPN from which stems the current popularity of parenteral nutrition in the United States. In this ambitious project, the biochemical requirements for growth in puppies were investigated with astounding results: normal growth comparable to that seen in puppies who were eating freely could be achieved without any oral intake, provided that one infused the necessary nutrients by vein.

Fischer JE (ed): Total Parenteral Nutrition, 2nd ed. Boston, Little, Brown, 1991.

> This book represents an attempt to standardize the practical approach to TPN.

Fischer JE (ed): Nutrition and Metabolism in Surgical Patients. Boston, Little, Brown, 1996.

> The basic science and practical knowledge relevant to surgical nutrition are presented in one volume. The various chapters also address the efficacy of parenteral nutrition.

Fischer JE, Rosen HM, Ebeid AM, et al: The effect of normalization of plasma amino acids on hepatic encephalopathy in man. Surgery 80:77-91, 1976.

> An approach to liver disease and intolerance to protein in patients with hepatic encephalopathy is described. This study represents the culmination of a hypothesis of hepatic encephalopathy depending on altered plasma amino acid patterns, changes subsequently discovered to be amplified by alterations in the blood-brain barrier secondary to the disturbed metabolism in liver disease. It represents an early anecdotal attempt to enable patients with severe hepatic deficiency to receive adequate nutrition at the same time as awakening from hepatic encephalopathy; these patients received increased protein equivalent in the form of a branched-chain–enriched (to 36%) amino acid solution now commercially available as HepatAmine.

Rombeau JL, Rolandelli RH (eds): Clinical Nutrition, 3rd ed. Philadelphia, WB Saunders, 2001.

> This is the most recent large textbook on enteral and parenteral nutrition. It is well done and has been updated, with many specialized chapters.

Ryan JA Jr, Abel RM, Abbott WM, et al: Catheter complications in total parenteral nutrition: A prospective study of 200 consecutive patients. N Engl J Med 290:757-761, 1974.

> A study of the complications of parenteral nutrition was conducted in a large hospital with one of the first centralized nutritional support teams. This study confirmed that rigid asepsis in the care of catheters and minimizing catheter manipulation were the most important factors in preventing catheter line sepsis.

Wilmore DW, Dudrick SJ: Treatment of acute renal failure with intravenous essential L-amino acids. Arch Surg 99:669-673, 1969.

> This study represents the earliest approach to disease-specific parenteral nutrition. The principle of attempting to define the metabolic abnormalities in a given patient and infusing an appropriate nutritional substrate was first proposed in this study. The intravenous equivalent of a Giordano-Giovanetti diet containing only the eight essential L-amino acids (an oral diet of high biologic value) was used.

Van den Berghe G, Wouters P, Weekers F, et al: Intensive insulin therapy in the surgical intensive care unit. N Engl J Med 345:1359-1367, 2001.

> This carefully conducted study emphasizes the importance of stringent control of blood glucose for the prevention of sepsis and other complications in critically ill patients.

References

1. Wilmore DW: Catabolic illness. Strategies for enhancing recovery. N Engl J Med 325:695-702, 1991.
2. Bistrian BR, Blackburn GL, Vitale J, et al: Incidence of malnutrition in general medical patients. JAMA 235:1567-1570, 1976.
3. Christensen HN: Role of amino acid transport and counter transport in nutrition and metabolism. Physiol Rev 70:43-77, 1990.
4. Hyde R, Peyrollier K, Hundal HS: Insulin promotes the cell surface recruitment of the SAT2/ATA2 system A amino acid transporter from an endosomal compartment in skeletal muscle cells. J Biol Chem 277:13628-13634, 2002.
5. Goldberg AL, Chang TW: Regulation and significance of amino acid metabolism in skeletal muscle. Fed Proc 37:2301-2307, 1978.
6. Price SR, Wang X, Bailey JL: Tissue-specific responses of branched-chain alpha-ketoacid dehydrogenase activity in metabolic acidosis. J Am Soc Nephrol 9:1892-1898, 1998.
7. Goldberg AL, Tischler ME: Regulatory effects of leucine on carbohydrate and protein metabolism. In Walser M, Williamson JR (eds): Metabolism and Clinical Implications of Branched Chain Amino and Ketoacids. New York, Elsevier, 1981, pp 205-216.
8. Windmueller HG, Spaeth AE: Respiratory fuels and nitrogen metabolism in vivo in small intestine of fed rats. Quantitative importance of glutamine, glutamate, and aspartate. J Biol Chem 255:107-112, 1980.
9. Karinch AM, Pan M, Lin CM, et al: Glutamine metabolism in sepsis and infection. J Nutr 131:2535S-2538S, 2001.
10. Schwartz AL, Ciechanover A: The ubiquitin-proteasome pathway and pathogenesis of human diseases. Annu Rev Med 50:57-74, 1999.
11. Mitch WE, Goldberg AL: Mechanisms of muscle wasting. The role of the ubiquitin-proteasome pathway. N Engl J Med 335:1897-1905, 1996.
12. Jagoe RT, Goldberg AL: What do we really know about the ubiquitin-proteasome pathway in muscle atrophy? Curr Opin Clin Nutr Metab Care 4:183-190, 2001.
13. Williams AB, DeCourten-Myers GM, Fischer JE, et al: Sepsis stimulates release of myofilaments in skeletal muscle by a calcium-dependent mechanism. FASEB J 13:1435-1443, 1999.
14. Tawa NE Jr, Odessey R, Goldberg AL: Inhibitors of the proteasome reduce the accelerated proteolysis in atrophying rat skeletal muscles. J Clin Invest 100:197-203, 1997.

15. Gomes MD, Lecker SH, Jagoe RT, et al: Atrogin-1, a muscle-specific F-box protein highly expressed during muscle atrophy. Proc Natl Acad Sci U S A 98:14440-14445, 2001.

16. Bodine SC, Latres E, Baumhueter S, et al: Identification of ubiquitin ligases required for skeletal muscle atrophy. Science 294:1704-1708, 2001.

17. Larbaud D, Balage M, Taillandier D, et al: Differential regulation of the lysosomal, Ca^{2+}-dependent and ubiquitin/proteasome-dependent proteolytic pathways in fast-twitch and slow-twitch rat muscle following hyperinsulinaemia. Clin Sci (Lond) 101:551-558, 2001.

18. Hobler SC, Williams AB, Fischer JE, et al: IGF-I stimulates protein synthesis but does not inhibit protein breakdown in muscle from septic rats. Am J Physiol 274:R571-576, 1998.

19. Tiao G, Fagan J, Roegner V, et al: Energy-ubiquitin-dependent muscle proteolysis during sepsis in rats is regulated by glucocorticoids. J Clin Invest 97:339-348, 1996.

20. Lofberg E, Gutierrez A, Wernerman J, et al: Effects of high doses of glucocorticoids on free amino acids, ribosomes and protein turnover in human muscle. Eur J Clin Invest 32:345-353, 2002.

21. Jagoe RT, Lecker SH, Gomes MD, et al: Patterns of gene expression in atrophying skeletal muscles: Response to food deprivation. FASEB J 16:1697-1712, 2002.

22. Tawa NE Jr, Kettelhut IC, Goldberg AL: Dietary protein deficiency reduces lysosomal and nonlysosomal ATP-dependent proteolysis in muscle. Am J Physiol 263:E326-E334, 1992.

23. Attaix D, Taillandier D, Temparis S, et al: Regulation of ATP-ubiquitin-dependent proteolysis in muscle wasting. Reprod Nutr Dev 34:583-597, 1994.

24. Hobler SC, Williams AB, Fischer D, et al: Activity and expression of the 20S proteasome are increased in skeletal muscle during sepsis. Am J Physiol 277:R434-440, 1999.

25. Llovera M, Carbo N, Lopez-Soriano J, et al: Different cytokines modulate ubiquitin gene expression in rat skeletal muscle. Cancer Lett 133:83-87, 1998.

26. Combaret L, Tilignac T, Claustre A, et al: Torbafylline (HWA 448) inhibits enhanced skeletal muscle ubiquitin-proteasome-dependent proteolysis in cancer and septic rats. Biochem J 361:185-192, 2002.

27. Nathan C, Xie QW: Nitric oxide synthases: Roles, tolls, and controls. Cell 78:915-918, 1994.

28. Billiar TR, Simmons RL: Arginine and nitric oxide. In Fischer JE (ed): Surgical Nutrition, 2nd ed. Boston, Little Brown, 1996.

29. Kobzik L, Reid MB, Bredt DS, et al: Nitric oxide in skeletal muscle. Nature 372:546-548, 1994.

30. Tawa NE Jr, Warren MS: Activation of intracellular protein breakdown in skeletal muscle by nitric oxide and oxygen free radicals. Surg Forum 48:30-32, 1997.

31. Baracos VE: Regulation of skeletal-muscle-protein turnover in cancer-associated cachexia. Nutrition 16:1015-1018, 2000.

32. Lorite MJ, Smith HJ, Arnold JA, et al: Activation of ATP-ubiquitin-dependent proteolysis in skeletal muscle in vivo and murine myoblasts in vitro by a proteolysis-inducing factor (PIF). Br J Cancer 85:297-302, 2001.

33. Wigmore SJ, Barber MD, Ross JA, et al: Effect of oral eicosapentaenoic acid on weight loss in patients with pancreatic cancer. Nutr Cancer 36:177-184, 2000.

34. Flier JS: Neuroscience. Regulating energy balance: The substrate strikes back. Science 312:861-864, 2006.

35. Buchman AL, Ament ME, Sohel M, et al: Choline deficiency causes reversible hepatic abnormalities in patients receiving parenteral nutrition: Proof of a human choline requirement: A placebo controlled trial. JPEN J Parenter Enteral Nutr 25:260-268, 2001.

36. McClave SA, Lowen CC, Kleber MJ, et al: Clinical use of the respiratory quotient obtained from indirect calorimetry. JPEN J Parenter Enteral Nutr 27:21-26, 2003.

37. Herridge MS, Cheung AM, Tansey CM, et al: One-year outcomes in survivors of the adult respiratory distress syndrome. N Engl J Med 348:683-693, 2003.

38. von Allmen D, Hasselgren PO, Fischer JE: Hepatic protein synthesis in a modified septic rat model. J Surg Res 48:476-480, 1990.

39. Wolfe RR, O'Donnell TF, Stone MD, et al: Investigation of factors determining the optimal glucose infusion rate in total parenteral nutrition. Metabolism 29:892-900, 1980.

40. Van den Berghe G, Wouters P, Weekers F, et al: Intensive insulin therapy in critically ill patients. N Engl J Med 345:1359-1367, 2001.

41. Van den Berghe G, Wilmer A, Hermans G, et al: Intensive insulin therapy in the medical ICU. N Engl J Med 354:449-461, 2006.

42. Waxman K, Day AT, Stellin GP, et al: Safety and efficacy of glycerol and amino acids in combination with lipid emulsion for peripheral parenteral nutrition support. JPEN J Parenter Enteral Nutr 16:374-378, 1992.

43. Lee S, Gura KM, Kim S, et al: Current clinical applications of ω-6 and ω-3 fatty acids. Nutr Clin Pract 21:323-341, 2006.

44. Gura KM, Duggan CP, Collier SB, et al: Reversal of parenteral nutrition–associated liver disease in two infants with short bowel syndrome using parenteral fish oil: Implications for future management. Pediatrics 118:e197-e201, 2006.

45. Khaodhiar L, Keane-Ellison M, Tawa NE, et al: Iron deficiency anemia in patients receiving home total parenteral nutrition. JPEN J Parenter Enteral Nutr 26:114-119, 2002.

46. Esparza J, Boivin MA, Hartshorne MF, et al: Equal aspiration rates in gastrically and transpylorically fed critically ill patients. Intensive Care Med 27:660-664, 2001.

47. Davies AR, Froomes PR, French CJ, et al: A randomized comparison of nasojejunal and nasogastric feeding in critically ill patients. Crit Care Med 30:586-590, 2001.

48. Montejo JC, Grau T, Acosta J, et al: Multicenter, prospective, randomized, single-blind study comparing the efficacy and gastrointestinal complications of early jejunal feeding with early gastric feeding in critically ill patients. Crit Care Med 30:796-800, 2002.

49. Montecalvo MA, Steger KA, Farber HW, et al: Nutritional outcome and pneumonia in critical care patients randomized to gastric versus jejunal tube feedings. Crit Care Med 20:1377-1387, 1992.

50. O'Grady NP, Alexander M, Dellinger EP, et al: Guidelines for the prevention of intravascular catheter–related infections. Centers for Disease Control and Prevention (CDC). MMWR Recomm Rep 51(RR-10):1-29, 2002.

51. Bern MM, Lokich JJ, Wallach SR, et al: Very low doses of warfarin can prevent thrombosis in central venous catheters. A randomized prospective trial. Ann Intern Med 112:423-428, 1990.

52. Melchior JC, Chastang C, Gelas P, et al: Efficacy of 2-month total parenteral nutrition in AIDS patients: A controlled randomized prospective trial. The French Multicenter Total Parenteral Nutrition Cooperative Group Study. AIDS 10:379-384, 1996.

53. Jeppesen PB, Langholz E, Mortensen PB: Quality of life in patients receiving home parenteral nutrition. Gut 44:844-852, 1999.

54. Chan S, McCowen KC, Bistrian BR, et al: Incidence, prognosis, and etiology of end-stage liver disease in patients receiving home total parenteral nutrition. Surgery 126:28-34, 1999.

55. Ling PR, Ollero M, Khaodhiar L, et al: Disturbances in essential fatty acid metabolism in patients receiving long-term home parenteral nutrition. Dig Dis Sci 47:1679-1685, 2002.

56. Ling PR, Khaodhiar L, Bistrian BR, et al: Inflammatory mediators in patients receiving long-term home parenteral nutrition. Dig Dis Sci 46:2484-2489, 2001.

57. Saitta JC, Ott SM, Sherrard DJ, et al: Metabolic bone disease in adults receiving long-term parenteral nutrition: Longitudinal study with regional densitometry and bone biopsy. JPEN J Parenter Enteral Nutr 17:214-219, 1993.

58. McClave SA, Spain DA, Snider HL: Nutritional management in acute and chronic pancreatitis. Gastroenterol Clin North Am 27:421-434, 1998.

59. Fan ST, Lo CM, Lai ECS, et al: Perioperative nutritional support in patients undergoing hepatectomy for hepatocellular carcinoma. N Engl J Med 331:1547-1552, 1994.

60. Jenkins M, Gottschlich M, Alexander JW, et al: Effect of immediate enteral feeding on the hypermetabolic response following severe burn injury. JPEN J Parenter Enteral Nutr 13:12S, 1989.

61. Moore FA, Feliciano DV, Andrassy RJ, et al: Early enteral feeding, compared with parenteral, reduces postoperative septic complications: The results of a meta-analysis. Ann Surg 216:172-183, 1992.

62. Kudsk KA, Croce MA, Fabian TC, et al: Enteral versus parenteral feeding: Effects on septic morbidity after blunt and penetrating abdominal trauma. Ann Surg 215:503-511; discussion 511-513, 1992.

63. Reynolds JV, Kanwar S, Welsh FK, et al: Does the route of feeding modify gut barrier function and clinical outcome in patients after major upper gastrointestinal surgery? JPEN J Parenter Enteral Nutr 21:196-201, 1997.

64. Gennari R, Alexander JW, Gianotti L, et al: Granulocyte macrophage colony-stimulating factor improves survival in two models of gut-derived sepsis by improving gut barrier function and modulating bacterial clearance. Ann Surg 220:68-78, 1994.

65. Lewis SJ, Egger M, Sylvester PA, et al: Early enteral feeding versus "nil by mouth" after gastrointestinal surgery: Systematic review and meta-analysis of controlled trials. BMJ 323:1-5, 2001.

66. Marik PE, Zaloga GP: Early enteral nutrition in acutely ill patients: A systematic review. Crit Care Med 29:2264-2270, 2001.

67. Pacelli F, Bossola M, Papa V, et al: Enteral vs. parenteral nutrition after major abdominal surgery: An even match. Arch Surg 136:933-936, 2001.

68. Daly JM, Lieberman MD, Goldfine J, et al: Enteral nutrition with supplemental arginine, RNA, and omega-3 fatty acids in patients after operation: Immunologic, metabolic, and clinical outcome. Surgery 112:56-67, 1992.

69. Daly JM, Reynolds J, Thom A, et al: Immune and metabolic effects of arginine in the surgical patient. Ann Surg 208:512-523, 1988.

70. Bower RH, Cerra FB, Bershadsky B, et al: Early enteral administration of a formula (Impact) supplemented with arginine, nucleotides and fish oil in intensive care unit patients: Results of a randomized prospective clinical trial. Crit Care Med 23:436-449, 1995.

71. Braga M, Gianotti L, Radaelli G, et al: Perioperative immunonutrition in patients undergoing cancer surgery: Results of a randomized double-blind phase 3 trial. Arch Surg 134:428-433, 1999.

72. Heyland DK, Novak F, Drover JW, et al: Should immunonutrition become routine in critically ill patients? A systematic review of the evidence. JAMA 286:944-953, 2001.

73. Montejo JC, Zarazaga A, Lopez-Martinez J, et al: Immunonutrition in the intensive care unit. A systematic review and consensus statement. Clin Nutr 22:221-233, 2003.

74. Kreymann KG, Berger MM, Deutz NE, et al: ESPEN guidelines on enteral nutrition: Intensive care. Clin Nutr 25:210-223, 2006.

75. Kudsk KA: Immunonutrition in surgery and critical care. Annu Rev Nutr 26:463-479, 2006.

76. Ziegler TR, Young LS, Benfell K, et al: Clinical and metabolic efficacy of glutamine-supplemented parenteral nutrition after bone marrow transplantation: A randomized, double-blind, controlled study. Ann Intern Med 116:821-828, 1992.

77. Li S, Nussbaum MS, McFadden DW, et al: Addition of L-glutamine to total parenteral nutrition (TPN) and its effects on portal insulin and glucagon and the development of hepatic steatosis in rats. J Surg Res 48:421-426, 1990.

78. Rennie MJ, Bowtell JL, Bruce M, et al: Interaction between glutamine availability and metabolism of glycogen, tricarboxylic acid cycle intermediates and glutathione. J Nutr 131:2488S-2490S, 2001.

79. Roediger WEW: The place of SCFAs in colonocyte metabolism in health and ulcerative colitis: The impaired colonocyte barrier. In Cummings JH, Sakata T, Rombeau JL (eds): Physiologic and Clinical Aspects of Short-Chain Fatty Acids, Cambridge, England, Cambridge University Press, 1993.

80. Naylor CD, O'Rourke K, Detsky AS, Baker JP: Parenteral nutrition with branched-chain amino acids in hepatic encephalopathy: A meta-analysis. Gastroenterology 97:1033-1042, 1989.

81. Detsky AS, Baker JP, O'Rourke K, Joel V: Perioperative parenteral nutrition: A meta-analysis. Ann Intern Med 107:195-203, 1987.

82. Buzby GP: Perioperative total parenteral nutrition in surgical patients. The Veterans Affairs Total Parenteral Nutrition Cooperative Study Group. N Engl J Med 325:525-532, 1991.

83. Fang CH, Li BG, Wang JJ, et al: Insulin-like growth factor 1 stimulates protein synthesis and inhibits protein breakdown in muscle from burned rats. JPEN J Parenter Enteral Nutr 21:245-251, 1997.

84. Takala J, Ruokonen E, Webster NR, et al: Increased mortality associated with growth hormone treatment in critically ill adults. N Engl J Med 341:785-792, 1999.

85. Bhasin S, Woodhouse L, Storer TW: Proof of the effect of testosterone on skeletal muscle. J Endocrinol 170:27-38, 2001.

86. Chance WT, Cao L, Zhang FS, et al: Clenbuterol treatment increases muscle mass and protein content of tumor-bearing rats maintained on total parenteral nutrition. J Parenter Enteral Nutr 15:530-535, 1991.

87. Herndon DN, Hart DW, Wolf SE, et al: Reversal of catabolism by beta blockade after severe burns. N Engl J Med 345:1223-1229, 2001.

CHAPTER 8

Wound Healing

Richard T. Ethridge, MD, PhD   Mimi Leong, MD   and   Linda G. Phillips, MD

The treatment and healing of wounds are some of the oldest subjects discussed in the medical literature. The same events, in the same order, occur in every healing process regardless of the tissue type or the inciting injury. Knowledge of the steps involved allows physicians to manipulate wounds to achieve optimal results in a short period. The surgical and anesthetic advances of the 18th and 19th centuries resulted in improved surgical outcomes. With the recent basic science discoveries of the 1980s and 1990s, physicians can now manipulate the wound with cellular and molecular biology techniques and thus improve outcomes. Even with recent advances, the exact mechanisms underlying wound healing are not completely understood.

TISSUE INJURY AND RESPONSE

Wound repair is the effort of injured tissues to restore their normal function and structural integrity after injury. During the effort to restore barriers to fluid loss and infection, reestablish normal blood and lymphatic flow patterns, and restore the mechanical integrity of the injured system, oftentimes flawless repair is sacrificed because of the urgency to return to function. *Regeneration,* in contrast, is perfect restoration of the preexisting tissue architecture in the absence of scar formation. Although regeneration is the goal of wound healing, it is found only in embryonic development, in lower organisms such as the stone crab and salamander, or in certain tissue compartments such as bone and liver. In wound healing in adult humans, however, the accuracy of regeneration is sacrificed for the speed of repair. A key concept in wound healing is that all tissues proceed through the same series of events, and for ease of understanding, these events are divided into specific stages. However, these phases overlap in both time and activity; that is, a single wound may have regions that are in several different phases at once.

All wounds undergo the same basic steps of repair. Acute wounds proceed in an orderly and timely reparative process to achieve sustained restoration of structure and function. A chronic wound, in contrast, does not proceed to restoration of functional integrity. It is stalled in the inflammatory phase as a result of a variety of causes and does not proceed to closure.

Wound closure types are divided into *primary, secondary,* and *tertiary* repair (Fig. 8-1). In *primary,* or first-intention, closure, the wounds are sealed immediately with simple suturing, skin graft placement, or flap closure, such as closure of the wound at the end of a surgical procedure. Closure by *secondary,* or spontaneous, intention involves no active intent to seal the wound. Generally, this type of repair is associated with a highly contaminated wound and will close by re-epithelialization, which results in contraction of the wound. Wound closure by *tertiary* intention is also referred to as *delayed primary closure.* A contaminated wound is initially treated by repeated débridement, systemic or topical antibiotics, or negative pressure wound therapy for several days to control infection. Once the wound is assessed as being ready for closure, surgical intervention, such as suturing, skin graft placement, or flap design, is performed.

WOUND-HEALING PHASES

The three phases of wound healing are inflammation, proliferation, and maturation. The immediate response to injury is the *inflammatory* (also called *reactive*) *phase.*

Primary Healing

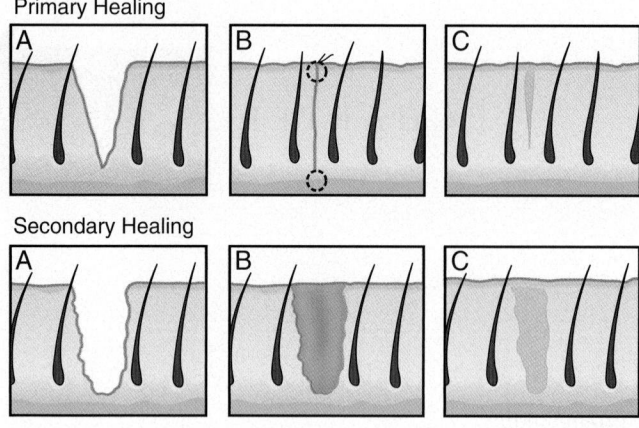

Secondary Healing

Figure 8-1 Wound closure types. **Top,** Primary or first-intention closure. A clean incision is made in the tissue (A) and the wound edges are reapproximated (B) with sutures, staples, or adhesive strips. C, Minimal scarring is the end result. **Bottom,** Healing by secondary intention. The wound is left open to heal (A and B) by a combination of contraction, granulation, and epithelialization. C, A large scar results.

The body's defenses are aimed at limiting the amount of damage and preventing further injury. The *proliferative* (also called *regenerative* or *reparative*) *phase* is the reparative process and consists of re-epithelialization, matrix synthesis, and neovascularization to relieve the ischemia of the trauma itself. The final *maturational (or remodeling) phase* is the period of scar contraction with collagen cross-linking, shrinking, and loss of edema. In a large wound such as a pressure sore, the eschar or fibrinous

exudate reflects the inflammatory phase, the granulation tissue is part of the proliferative phase, and the contracting or advancing edge is part of the maturational phase. All three phases may occur simultaneously, and the phases with their individual processes may overlap (Fig. 8-2).

Inflammatory Phase

During the immediate reaction of the tissue to injury, hemostasis and inflammation occur. This phase represents an attempt to limit damage by stopping the bleeding, sealing the surface of the wound, and removing any necrotic tissue, foreign debris, or bacteria present. The inflammatory phase is characterized by increased vascular permeability, migration of cells into the wound by chemotaxis, secretion of cytokines and growth factors into the wound, and activation of the migrating cells (Fig. 8-3).

Hemostasis and Inflammation

During an acute tissue injury, blood vessel damage results in exposure of subendothelial collagen to platelets, which leads to platelet aggregation and activation of the coagulation pathway. Initial intense local vasoconstriction of arterioles and capillaries is followed by vasodilation and increased vascular permeability (Fig. 8-4). Cessation of hemorrhage is aided by plugging of capillaries with erythrocytes and platelets, which adhere to the damaged capillary endothelium. Activation of these platelets by binding to the exposed type IV and V collagen from the damaged endothelium results in platelet aggregation. The initial contact between platelets and collagen requires von Willebrand's factor (vWF) VIII, a heterodimeric

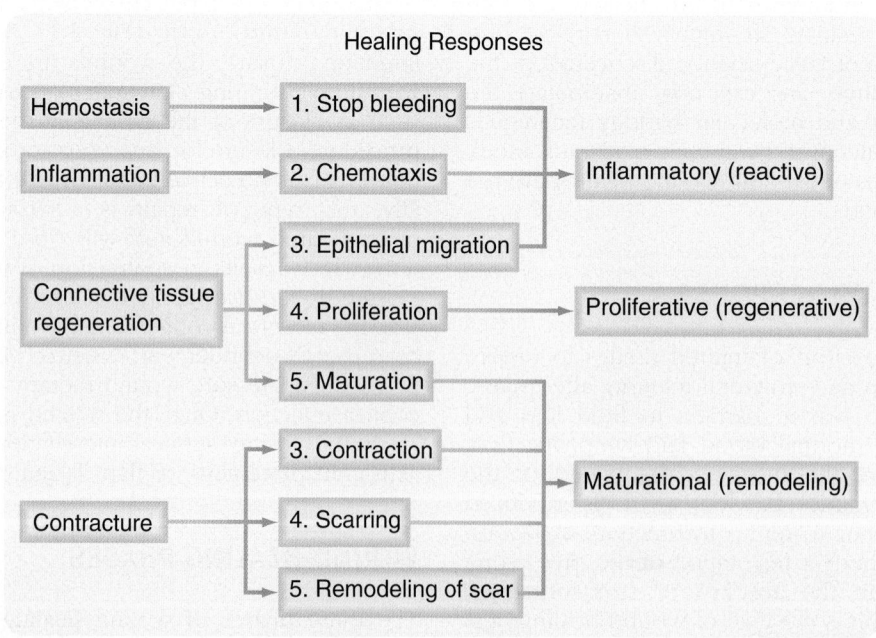

Figure 8-2 Schematic diagram of the wound-healing continuum.

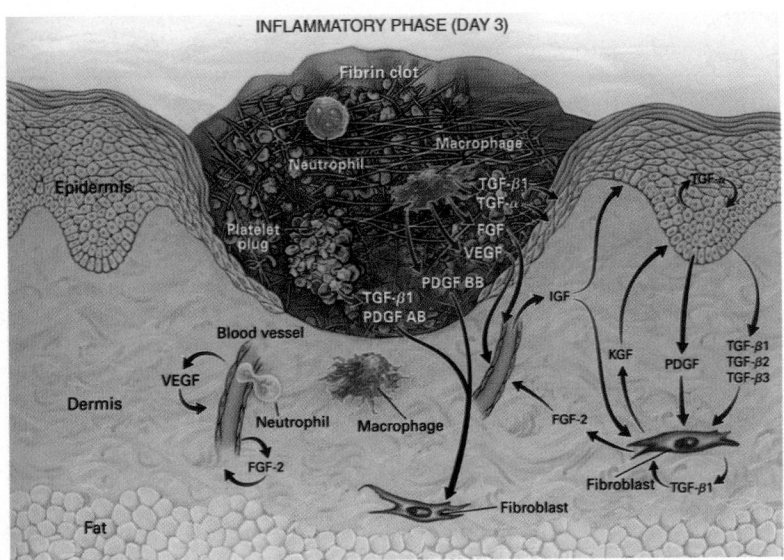

Figure 8-3 A cutaneous wound 3 days after injury. The cells and growth factors necessary to facilitate cell migration into the wound are shown. FGF, fibroblast growth factor; IGF, insulin-like growth factor; KGF, keratinocyte growth factor; PDGF, platelet-derived growth factor; TGF, transforming growth factor; VEGF, vascular endothelial growth factor. (From Singer AJ, Clark RAF: Mechanisms of disease: Cutaneous wound healing. N Engl J Med 341:738, 1999.)

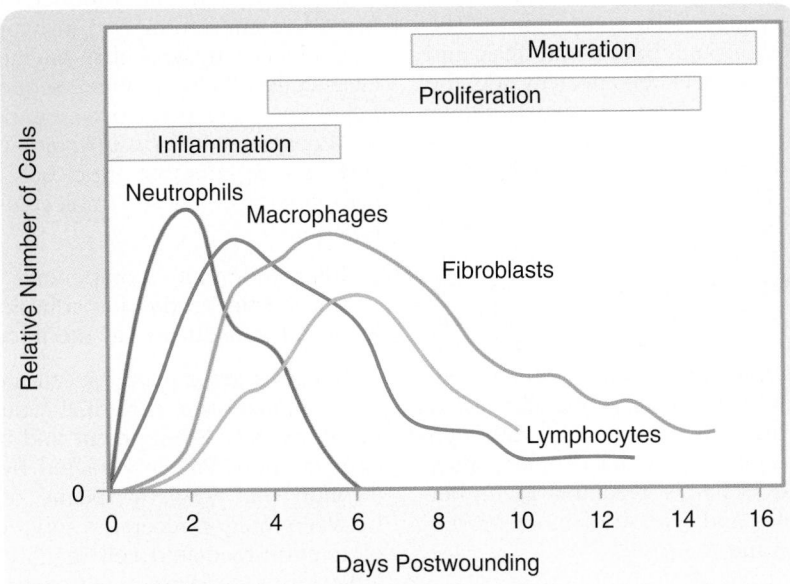

Figure 8-4 Time course of the appearance of different cells in the wound during healing. Macrophages and neutrophils are predominant during the inflammatory phase (peak at days 3 and 2, respectively). Lymphocytes appear later and peak at day 7. Fibroblasts are the predominant cells during the proliferative phase. (Modified from Witte MB, Barbul A: General principles of wound healing. Surg Clin North Am 77:512, 1997.)

protein synthesized by megakaryocytes and endothelial cells. Platelet adhesion to the endothelium is primarily mediated through the interaction between high-affinity glycoprotein receptors and the integrin receptor GPIIb-IIIa (αIIbβ_3). In addition, platelets express other integrin receptors that mediate direct binding to collagen ($\alpha_2\beta_1$) and laminin ($\alpha_6\beta_1$) or indirect binding by attaching to subendothelial matrix-bound fibronectin ($\alpha_5\beta_1$), vitronectin ($\alpha_v\beta_3$), and other ligands.

Increased Vascular Permeability
Platelet binding results in conformational changes in platelets that trigger intracellular signal transduction pathways that lead to platelet activation and the release of

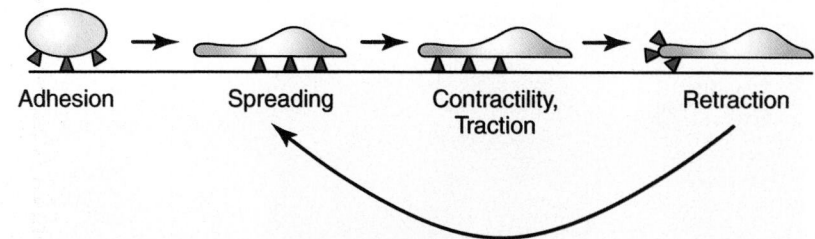

Adhesion   Spreading   Contractility,   Retraction
                                 Traction

Figure 8-5 Schematic of a cycle of integrin-mediated cell migration. Migration is a cyclic process involving integrins at each step. Entry into the migration cycle can take place at either of the first two steps. For example, nonadherent cell types such as lymphomas and circulating carcinomas begin the migration cycle at the first step of attachment, whereas adherent cells such as fibroblasts and solid tumors may begin the cycle at the spreading step. Regardless of the cell type, however, cells must maintain attachment to the extracellular matrix once the cycle has begun. (Modified from Holly SP, Larson MK, Parise LV: Multiple roles of integrins in cell motility. Exp Cell Res 261:72, 2000.)

biologically active proteins. Platelet alpha granules are storage organelles that contain platelet-derived growth factor (PDGF), transforming growth factor-β (TGF-β), insulin-like growth factor type I (IGF-I), fibronectin, fibrinogen, thrombospondin, and vWF. The dense bodies contain vasoactive amines, such as serotonin, that cause vasodilation and increased vascular permeability. Mast cells adherent to the endothelial surface release histamine and serotonin, thereby affecting the permeability of endothelial cells and causing leakage of plasma from the intravascular space to the extracellular compartment. The clotting cascade is initiated through both the intrinsic and extrinsic pathways. As the platelets become activated, the membrane phospholipids bind factor V, which allows interaction with factor X. Membrane-bound prothrombinase activity is generated and potentiates thrombin production exponentially. The thrombin itself activates platelets and catalyzes the conversion of fibrinogen to fibrin. The fibrin strands trap red blood cells to form the clot and seal the wound. The lattice framework that results will be the scaffold for endothelial cells, inflammatory cells, and fibroblasts. Thromboxane A_2 and prostaglandin $F_{2\alpha}$, formed from the degradation of cell membranes in the arachidonic acid cascade, also assist in platelet aggregation and vasoconstriction. Although these activities serve to limit the amount of injury, they can also cause localized ischemia resulting in further damage to cell membranes and release of more prostaglandin $F_{2\alpha}$ and thromboxane A_2.

Polymorphonuclear Cells

The release of histamine and serotonin leads to vascular permeability of the capillary bed. Complement factors such as C5a and leukotriene B_4 promote neutrophil adherence and chemoattraction. In the presence of thrombin, endothelial cells exposed to leukotriene C_4 and D_4 release platelet-aggregating factor, which further enhances neutrophil adhesion. Monocytes and endothelial cells produce the inflammatory mediators interleukin-1 (IL-1) and tumor necrosis factor-α (TNF-α), and these mediators also further promote endothelial-neutrophil adherence. The increased capillary permeability and the various chemotactic factors facilitate diapedesis of neu-

trophils into the inflammatory site. As the neutrophils begin their migration, they release the contents of their lysosomes and enzymes such as elastase and other proteases into the extracellular matrix (ECM), which facilitates migration of the neutrophils. The combination of intense vasodilation and increased vascular permeability leads to clinical findings of inflammation, *rubor* (redness), *tumor* (swelling), *calor* (heat), and *dolor* (pain). Local tissue swelling is further promoted by the deposition of fibrin, a protein end product of coagulation, and the fibrin becomes entrapped in lymphatic vessels.

Evidence suggests that migration of polymorphonuclear cells (PMNs) requires sequential adhesive and deadhesive interactions between β_1 and β_2 integrins and ECM components.[1] *Integrin* molecules are a family of cell surface receptors that are closely coupled with the cell's cytoskeleton. These molecules serve two major functions:

1. Interaction with components of the ECM, such as fibronectin, to provide adhesion
2. Signal transduction to the interior of the cell

Integrins are crucial for cell motility and are required in inflammation and normal wound healing, as well as in embryonic development and tumor metastases. After extravasation, PMNs, attracted by chemotaxins, migrate through the ECM by means of transient interactions between integrin receptors and their ligands. Four phases of integrin-mediated cell motility have been described: adhesion, spreading, contractility or traction, and retraction. Activation of specific integrins though ligand binding has been shown to increase cell adhesion and activate reorganization of the cell's actin cytoskeleton.[1] Spreading is characterized by the development of lamellipodia and filopodia. Traction at the leading edge of the cell develops through binding of integrin, followed by translocation of the cell over the adherent segment of the plasma membrane. The integrin is shifted to the rear of the cell and releases its substrate, thereby permitting cell advancement (Fig. 8-5).[1] Regulation of integrin function by adhesive substrates offers a mechanism for local control of migrant cells. Within the assembled framework of the ECM, binding sites for integrins have been identified on collagen, laminin, and fibronectin.[1]

The chemotactic agent mediates the PMN response through signal transduction as the chemotaxin binds to receptors on the cell surface. Bacterial products such as *N*-formyl-methionyl-leucyl-phenylalanine bind to induce cyclic adenosine monophosphate (cAMP), but if there is maximal receptor occupancy, superoxide is produced at peak rates. Neutrophils also possess receptors for IgG and the complement proteins C3b and C3bi. As the complement cascade is released and bacteria are opsonized, binding of these proteins to cell receptors on neutrophils allows recognition by the neutrophils and phagocytosis of the bacteria. When neutrophils are stimulated, they express more CR1 and CR3 receptors, thereby permitting more efficient binding and phagocytosis of these bacteria.

Functional activation occurs after migration of PMNs into the wound site, which may induce new cell surface antigen expression, increased cytotoxicity, or enhanced production and release of cytokines. These activated neutrophils scavenge for necrotic debris, foreign material, and bacteria and generate free oxygen radicals with electrons donated by the reduced form of nicotinamide adenine dinucleotide phosphate (NADPH). The electrons are transported across the membrane into lysosomes, where superoxide anion (O_2^-) is formed. Superoxide dismutase catalyzes the formation of hydrogen peroxide (H_2O_2), which is then degraded by myeloperoxidase in the azurophilic granules of neutrophils. This interaction oxidizes halides with the formation of by-products such as hypochlorous acid. The iron-catalyzed reaction between H_2O_2 and O_2^- forms hydroxyl radicals ($OH\cdot$). This very potent free radical is bactericidal, but it is also toxic to neutrophils and surrounding viable tissues.

Migration of PMNs stops when wound contamination has been controlled, usually within the first few days after injury. PMNs do not survive longer than 24 hours. After 24 to 48 hours, the predominance of cells in the wound cleft shifts to mononuclear cells. If wound contamination persists or secondary infection occurs, continuous activation of the complement system and other pathways provides a steady supply of chemotactic factors that results in sustained influx of PMNs into the wound. Besides the delay in healing, this prolonged inflammation can be deleterious in terms of destruction of normal tissue, with progression to tissue necrosis, abscess formation, and possibly systemic infection. PMNs are not essential for wound healing because their role in phagocytosis and antimicrobial defense may be taken over by macrophages. Sterile incisions will heal normally without the presence of PMNs.

Macrophages

The macrophage is the one cell that is truly crucial to wound healing in that it serves to orchestrate the release of cytokines and stimulate many of the subsequent processes of wound healing (Fig. 8-6). Macrophages in the wound appear at the same time that neutrophils disappear. Macrophages induce apoptosis of PMNs. Chemotaxis of migrating blood monocytes occurs within 24 to 48 hours. Chemotactic factors specific for monocytes include bacterial products, complement degradation products (C5a), thrombin, fibronectin, collagen, TGF-β, and PDGF-BB. Monocyte chemotaxis is also facilitated by the interaction of integrin receptors on the monocyte surface with ECM proteins such as fibrin and fibronectin. The β integrin receptor also transduces the signal for macrophage phagocytic activity. Activated integrin expression promotes adhesion-mediated gene induction in monocytes that transforms them into wound macrophages; such transformation results in increased phagocytic activity and selective expression of cytokines and signal transduction elements by messenger RNA (mRNA), including the early growth response genes *EGR2* and *c-fos*.[2] Macrophages have specific receptors for IgG (Fc receptor), C3b (CR1 and CR3), and fibronectin (integrin receptors) that permit surface recognition of opsonized pathogens and facilitate phagocytosis.[2]

Bacterial debris such as lipopolysaccharide can activate monocytes to release free radicals and cytokines that mediate angiogenesis and fibroplasia.[3] The presence of IL-2 increases the release of free radicals and thus enhances bactericidal activity, and the activity of the free radicals is potentiated by IL-2. In addition, the free radicals generate bacterial debris, which further potentiates the activation of monocytes. Activated wound macrophages also produce nitric oxide (NO), a substance that has been demonstrated to have many functions other than antimicrobial properties.

As the monocyte or macrophage is activated, phospholipase is induced, cell membrane phospholipids are enzymatically degraded, and thromboxane A_2 and prostaglandin $F_{2\alpha}$ are released. The macrophage also releases leukotrienes B_4 and C_4 and 15- and 5-hydroxyeicosatetraenoic acid. Leukotriene B_4 is a potent chemotaxin for neutrophils and increases their adherence to endothelial cells.

Wound macrophages release proteinases, including matrix metalloproteinases (MMP-1, MMP-2, MMP-3, and MMP-9) (Fig. 8-7),[2] that degrade the ECM and are crucial for removing foreign material, promoting cell movement through tissue spaces, and regulating ECM turnover. For example, macrophages secrete collagenase when activated by bacterial degradation by-products such as lipopolysaccharide or activated lymphocytes. This activity is dependent on the cAMP pathway and thus can be blocked by nonsteroidal anti-inflammatory or glucocorticoid drugs. Colchicine and retinoic acid appear to decrease collagenase production as well.

Macrophages secrete numerous cytokines and growth factors (Tables 8-1 and 8-2). IL-1, a proinflammatory cytokine, is an acute phase response cytokine. In experimental wound models, IL-1 levels become detectable within the first 24 hours, peak at 72 hours, and then rapidly decline throughout the first week. This endogenous pyrogen causes lymphocyte activation and stimulation of the hypothalamus, thereby inducing the febrile response. It also directly affects hemostasis by inducing the release of vasodilators and stimulating coagulation. IL-1's effect is further amplified as endothelial cells produce it in the presence of TNF-α and endotoxin. IL-1 has numerous effects: enhancement of collagenase production, stimulation of cartilage degradation and bone

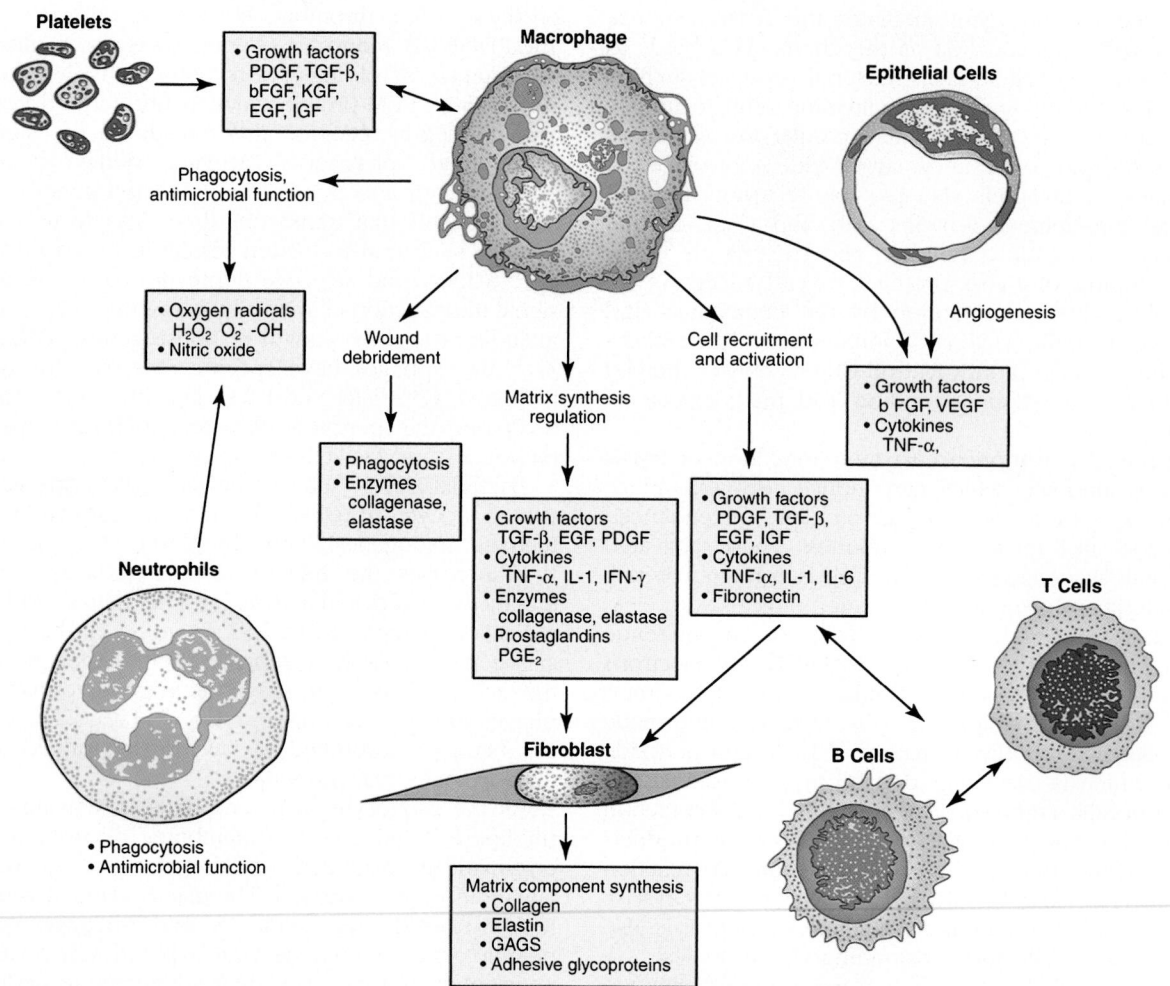

Figure 8-6 Interaction of cellular and humoral factors in wound healing. Note the key role of the macrophage. bFGF, basic fibroblast growth factor; EGF, epidermal growth factor; GAGs, glycosaminoglycans; H_2O_2, hydrogen peroxide; IFN-γ, interferon-γ; IGF, insulin-like growth factor; IL, interleukin; KGF, keratinocyte growth factor; O_2^-, superoxide; PDGF, platelet-derived growth factor; PGE_2, prostaglandin E_2; TGF-β, transforming growth factor-beta; TNF-α, tumor necrosis factor-α; VEGF, vascular endothelial growth factor. (Modified from Witte MB, Barbul A: General principles of wound healing. Surg Clin North Am 77:513, 1997.)

reabsorption, activation of neutrophils, regulation of adhesion molecules, and promotion of chemotaxis. It stimulates other cells to secrete proinflammatory cytokines. IL-1's effects also extend into the proliferative phase, during which it increases fibroblast and keratinocyte growth and collagen synthesis. Studies have demonstrated increased levels of IL-1 in chronic nonhealing wounds, thus suggesting its role in the pathogenesis of poor wound healing.[4] The early beneficial responses of IL-1 in wound healing appear to be maladaptive if elevated levels last beyond the first week after injury.

Microbial by-products induce macrophages to release TNF (previously called *cachectin*). TNF-α is crucial in initiating the response to injury or bacteria. TNF is chemotactic for the cellular components of inflammation. It up-regulates cell surface adhesion molecules that promote the interaction of immune cells and endothelium. TNF-α is detected in the wound within 12 hours and peaks after

72 hours. Its effects include hemostasis, increased vascular permeability, and enhanced endothelial proliferation. Like IL-1, TNF-α induces fever, increased collagenase production, reabsorption of cartilage and bone, and release of PDGF, as well as the production of more IL-1. Excessive production of TNF-α, however, has been associated with multisystem organ failure and increased morbidity and mortality in inflammatory disease states, partly through its effects on activating macrophages and neutrophils. Recent studies have observed elevated levels of TNF-α in nonhealing versus healing chronic venous ulcers.[4] Thus, as in the case of IL-1, TNF-α appears to be essential in the early inflammatory response required for wound healing, but local and systemic persistence of this cytokine may lead to impaired wound maturation.

IL-6, which is produced by monocytes and macrophages, is involved in stem cell growth, activation of B and T cells, and regulation of the synthesis of hepatic

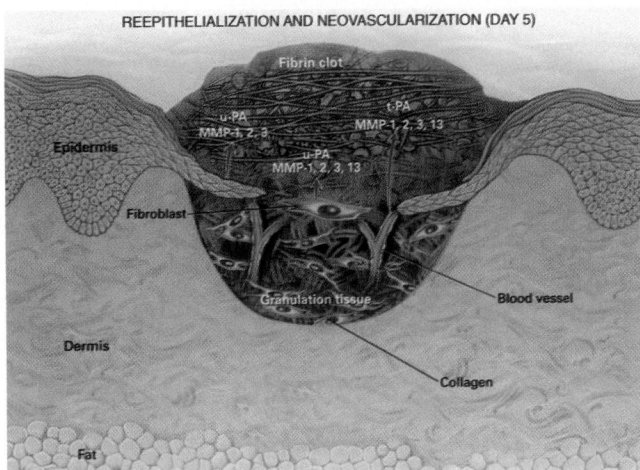

Figure 8-7 A cutaneous wound 5 days after injury. Blood vessels are seen sprouting into the fibrin clot as epidermal cells resurface the wound. Some of the proteinases involved in cell movement at this time point are shown. MMP-1, 2, 3, and 13, matrix metalloproteinases 1, 2, 3, and 13 (collagenase 1, gelatinase A, stromelysin 1, and collagenase 3, respectively); t-PA tissue plasminogen activator; u-PA, urokinase-type plasminogen activator. (Adapted from Singer AJ, Clark RAF: Mechanisms of disease: Cutaneous wound healing. N Engl J Med 341:738, 1999.)

Table 8-1 Cytokine Activity in Wound Healing

CYTOKINE	CELL SOURCE	BIOLOGIC ACTIVITY
Proinflammatory Cytokines		
TNF-α	Macrophages	PMN margination and cytotoxicity, with or without collagen synthesis; provides metabolic substrate
IL-1	Macrophages Keratinocytes	Fibroblast and keratinocyte chemotaxis, collagen synthesis
IL-2	T lymphocytes	Increases fibroblast infiltration and metabolism
IL-6	Macrophages PMNs Fibroblasts	Fibroblast proliferation, hepatic acute phase protein synthesis
IL-8	Macrophages Fibroblasts	Macrophage and PMN chemotaxis, keratinocyte maturation
IFN-γ	T lymphocytes Macrophages	Activates macrophages and PMNs, retards collagen synthesis and cross-linking, stimulates collagenase activity
Anti-inflammatory Cytokines		
IL-4	T lymphocytes Basophils Mast cells	Inhibition of TNF, IL-1, IL-6 production; fibroblast proliferation, collagen synthesis
IL-10	T lymphocytes Macrophages Keratinocytes	Inhibition of TNF, IL-1, IL-6 production; inhibition of macrophage and PMN activation

IFN-γ, interferon-γ; IL, interleukin; PMNs, polymorphonuclear leukocytes; TNF, tumor necrosis factor.

From Rumalla VK, Borah GL: Cytokines, growth factors, and plastic surgery. Plast Reconstr Surg 108:719-733, 2001.

acute phase proteins. Within acute wounds, IL-6 is also secreted by PMNs and fibroblasts, and its rise parallels the increase in PMN count locally. IL-6 is detectable within 12 hours of experimental wounding and may persist at high concentrations for longer than a week. It also works synergistically with IL-1, TNF-α, and endotoxins. It is a potent stimulator of fibroblast proliferation and is decreased in aging fibroblasts and fetal wounds.[5]

IL-8, another important proinflammatory cytokine after injury, is secreted primarily by macrophages and fibroblasts in the acute wound with peak expression within the first 24 hours. Its major effects include increased PMN and monocyte chemotaxis, PMN degranulation, and expression of endothelial cell adhesion molecules. In vitro experiments on the effect of recombinant human IL-8 revealed enhanced keratinocyte proliferation with an increased number of cells in S phase and overexpression of the integrin subunit α6.[6] In vivo, topical application of IL-8 to human skin grafts in a chimeric mouse model enhanced re-epithelialization over controls as a result of elevated numbers of mitotic keratinocytes.[6] In contrast, other investigators found that IL-8 levels were elevated in delayed human burn wound healing and appeared to inhibit keratinocyte replication. These findings suggest that IL-8 may have a role in keratinocyte maturation but that excessive levels may be detrimental.

Interferon-γ (IFN-γ), another proinflammatory cytokine, is secreted by T lymphocytes and macrophages. Its major effects are macrophage and PMN activation and increased cytotoxicity. It has also been shown to reduce local wound contraction and aid in tissue remodeling. IFN-γ has been used in the treatment of hypertrophic and keloid scars, possibly by its effect in slowing collagen

production and cross-linking while collagenase (MMP-1) production increases.[7] Experimentally, however, it has been shown to impair re-epithelialization and wound strength in a dose-dependent manner when applied either locally or systemically. These findings suggest that administration of IFN-γ may improve scar hypertrophy by decreasing the strength of the wound.

Macrophages also release growth factors that stimulate fibroblast, endothelial cell, and keratinocyte proliferation and are important in the proliferative phase (see Table 8-2). Macrophage-secreted PDGF stimulates collagen and proteoglycan synthesis. PDGF exists as three isomers—PDGF-AA, PDGF-AB, and PDGF-BB; however, the PDGF-BB isomer is the only growth factor preparation approved by the U.S. Food and Drug Administration and is the most widely studied clinically. Topical application of recombinant PDGF improved wound-breaking strength and healing time in both human and murine models of acute wounding.[8] Administration of PDGF-BB improved wound closure in chronic and diabetic nonhealing ulcers in both humans and rodents but did not have the same effect in steroid-treated animals.

Table 8-2   Cytokines That Affect Wound Healing

CYTOKINE	ABBREVIATION	SOURCE	FUNCTIONS
Platelet-derived growth factor	PDGF	Platelets, macrophages, endothelial cells, keratinocytes	Chemotactic for PMNs, macrophages, fibroblasts, and smooth muscle cells; activates PMNs, macrophages, and fibroblasts; mitogenic for fibroblasts, endothelial cells; stimulates production of MMPs, fibronectin, and HA; stimulates angiogenesis and wound contraction; remodeling
Transforming growth factor-β (including isoforms β1, β2, and β3)	TGF-β	Platelets, T lymphocytes, macrophages, endothelial cells, keratinocytes, fibroblasts	Chemotactic for PMNs, macrophages, lymphocytes, and fibroblasts; stimulates TIMP synthesis, keratinocyte migration, angiogenesis, and fibroplasia; inhibits production of MMPs and keratinocyte proliferation; induces TGF-β production
Epidermal growth factor	EGF	Platelets, macrophages	Mitogenic for keratinocytes and fibroblasts; stimulates keratinocyte migration
Transforming growth factor-α	TGF-α	Macrophages, T lymphocytes, keratinocytes	Similar to EGF
Fibroblast growth factor-1 and -2 family	FGF	Macrophages, mast cells, T lymphocytes, endothelial cells, fibroblasts	Chemotactic for fibroblasts; mitogenic for fibroblasts and keratinocytes; stimulates keratinocyte migration, angiogenesis, wound contraction, and matrix deposition
Keratinocyte growth factor (also called FGF-7)	KGF	Fibroblasts	Stimulates keratinocyte migration, proliferation, and differentiation
Insulin-like growth factor	IGF-I	Macrophages, fibroblasts	Stimulates synthesis of sulfated proteoglycans, collagen, keratinocyte migration, and fibroblast proliferation; endocrine effects similar to those of growth hormone
Vascular endothelial cell growth factor	VEGF	Keratinocytes	Increases vasopermeability; mitogenic for endothelial cells

HA, hyaluronic acid; MMPs, matrix metalloproteinases; PMNs, polymorphonuclear leukocytes; TIMP, tissue inhibitor of matrix metalloproteinase.
Modified from Schwartz SI (ed): Principles of Surgery, 7th ed. New York, McGraw-Hill, 1999, p 269.

TGF-α and TGF-β are both released by activated monocytes. TGF-α stimulates epidermal growth and angiogenesis. TGF-β itself stimulates monocytes to express other peptides such as TGF-α, IL-1, and PDGF. TGF-β, which is also released by platelets and fibroblasts within wounds, exists as at least three isomers—β1, β2, and β3—and its effects include fibroblast migration and maturation and ECM synthesis. TGF-β1 has been shown to play an important role in collagen metabolism and healing of gastrointestinal injuries and anastomoses. In experimental models, TGF-β1 accelerated wound healing in normal, steroid-impaired, and irradiated animals. TGF-β is the most potent stimulant of fibroplasia, and its strong mitogenic effects have been implicated in the fibrogenesis seen in disease states such as scleroderma and interstitial pulmonary fibrosis. Enhanced expression of TGF-β1 mRNA is found in both keloid and hypertrophic scars.[7] In contrast, fetal wounds have been demonstrated to have a paucity of TGF-β, thus suggesting that the scarless repair seen in utero occurs because of low or absent amounts of TGF-β. Studies of the three isomers suggest that although TGF-β1 and TGF-β2 play an important role in tissue fibrosis and postinjury scarring, TGF-β3 may limit scarring. As the concentration of TGF-β rises in the inflammatory site, fibroblasts are directly stimulated to produce collagen and fibronectin, thus leading to the proliferative phase.

Lymphocytes

T lymphocytes appear in significant number in the wound at around the fifth day, with a peak occurring at approximately the seventh day. B lymphocytes do not appear to play a significant role in wound healing but seem to be involved in down-regulating healing as the wound closes.[9] Lymphocytes exert most of their effects on fibroblasts by producing stimulatory cytokines, such as IL-2 and fibroblast-activating factor, and inhibitory cytokines, such as TGF-β, TNF-α, and IFN-γ. Initially, lymphocytes were thought to play a minimal role in acute wound healing, particularly in the absence of excessive inflammation. The macrophage processes foreign debris such as bacteria or enzymatically degraded host proteins and serves as an antigen-presenting cell to lymphocytes. This interaction stimulates lymphocyte proliferation and release of cytokines. T cells produce IFN-γ, which stimulates the macrophage to release a cascade of cytokines, including TNF-α and IL-1. IFN-γ also causes decreased synthesis of prostaglandins, which enhances the effect of inflammatory mediators. In addition, IFN-γ suppresses collagen synthesis and inhibits macrophages from leaving the site of injury. Thus, IFN-γ appears to be an important mediator of chronic nonhealing wounds, and its presence suggests that T lymphocytes are primarily involved in chronic wound healing.

Recent studies, however, question the belief that lymphocytes are not essential for acute wound healing. Drugs that suppress T-lymphocyte function and proliferation, such as steroids and immunosuppressive agents (cyclosporine and tacrolimus), have been found to result in impaired wound healing in experimental wound models, possibly through decreased NO synthesis. In vivo lymphocyte depletion suggests the existence of an incompletely characterized T-cell lymphocyte population that is neither CD4+ nor CD8+, and it is this subset that seems to be responsible for the promotion of wound healing.[10]

Proliferative Phase

As the acute responses of hemostasis and inflammation begin to resolve, the scaffolding is laid for repair of the wound through angiogenesis, fibroplasia, and epithelialization. This stage is characterized by the formation of granulation tissue, which consists of a capillary bed, fibroblasts, macrophages, and a loose arrangement of collagen, fibronectin, and hyaluronic acid.

Multiple studies have used growth factors to modify granulation tissue, particularly fibroplasia. Adenoviral transfer, topical application, and subcutaneous injection of PDGF, TGF-β, keratinocyte growth factor (KGF), vascular endothelial growth factor (VEGF), and epidermal growth factor (EGF) have been tested to increase the proliferation of granulation tissue.[11]

Angiogenesis

Angiogenesis is the process of new blood vessel formation and is necessary to support a healing wound environment. After injury, activated endothelial cells degrade the basement membrane of postcapillary venules, thereby allowing the migration of cells through this gap. Division of these migrating endothelial cells results in tubule or lumen formation. Eventually, deposition of the basement membrane occurs and results in capillary maturation.

After injury, the endothelium is exposed to numerous soluble factors and comes in contact with adhering blood cells. These interactions result in up-regulation of the expression of cell surface adhesion molecules, such as vascular cell surface adhesion molecule-1 (VCAM-1). Matrix-degrading enzymes, such as plasmin and the metalloproteinases, are released, activated, and degrade the endothelial basement membrane. Fragmentation of the basement membrane allows migration of endothelial cells into the wound, promoted by fibroblast growth factor (FGF), PDGF, and TGF-β. Injured endothelial cells express adhesion molecules, such as the integrin $\alpha_v\beta_3$, which facilitates attachment to fibrin, fibronectin, and fibrinogen and thus facilitates endothelial cell migration along the provisional matrix scaffold. Platelet endothelial cell adhesion molecule-1 (PECAM-1), also found on endothelial cells, modulates their interaction with each other as they migrate into the wound.[2]

Capillary tube formation is a complex process that involves cell-cell and cell-matrix interactions, modulated by adhesion molecules on endothelial cell surfaces. PECAM-1 has been observed to mediate cell-cell contact, whereas β_1 integrin receptors may aid in stabilizing these contacts and forming tight junctions between endothelial cells. Some of the new capillaries differentiate into arterioles and venules, whereas others undergo involution and apoptosis, with subsequent ingestion by macrophages.[2] Regulation of endothelial apoptosis is not well understood.

Angiogenesis appears to be stimulated and manipulated by a variety of cytokines predominantly produced by macrophages and platelets. As the macrophage produces TNF-α, it orchestrates angiogenesis during the inflammatory phase. Heparin, which can stimulate the migration of capillary endothelial cells, binds with high affinity to a group of angiogenic factors. VEGF, a member of the PDGF family of growth factors, has potent angiogenic activity. It is produced in large amounts by keratinocytes, macrophages, and fibroblasts during wound healing. Cell disruption and hypoxia, hallmarks of tissue injury, appear to be strong initial inducers of potent angiogenic factors at the wound site, such as VEGF and its receptor.

Both acidic and basic FGFs, or FGF-1 and FGF-2, are released from disrupted parenchymal cells and are early stimulants of angiogenesis. FGF-2 provides the initial angiogenic stimulus within the first 3 days of wound repair, followed by a subsequent prolonged stimulus mediated by VEGF from days 4 through 7.[12] There is a dose-dependent effect of VEGF and FGF-2 on angiogenesis.[12] Recent investigations to develop collateral circulation by the introduction of VEGF and FGF-2 or their genes have shown promise in preclinical models and even in clinical trials. Both TGF-α and EGF stimulate endothelial cell proliferation. TNF-α is chemotactic for endothelial cells; it promotes formation of the capillary tube and may mediate angiogenesis through its induction of hypoxia-inducible factor-1 (HIF-1).[13] It regulates the expression of other hypoxia-responsive genes, including inducible NO synthase and VEGF. HIF-1α mRNA is prominently present in wound inflammatory cells during the initial 24 hours, and HIF-1α protein is present in cells isolated from the wound 1 and 5 days after injury in vitro.[13] Data also suggest that there is a positive interaction between endogenous NO and VEGF, with endogenous NO enhancing VEGF synthesis.[14] Similarly, VEGF has been shown to promote NO synthesis in angiogenesis, thus suggesting that NO mediates aspects of VEGF signaling required for endothelial cell proliferation and organization. An in vivo study of NO on wound healing that examined the effect of the NO synthase inhibitor aminoguanidine in murine burn wounds demonstrated greater epithelial proliferation, collagen formation, and granulation tissue with rich capillaries in the control group than in the group that received aminoguanidine intraperitoneally.[15]

TGF-β is a chemoattractant for fibroblasts and probably assists angiogenesis by signaling the fibroblast to produce FGFs. Other factors that have been shown to induce angiogenesis include angiogenin, IL-8, and lactic acid.[16] Several of the matrix materials, such as fibronectin and hyaluronic acid from the wound site, are angiogenic. Fibronectin and fibrin are produced by macrophages and damaged endothelial cells. Collagen appears to interact by causing tubular formation of endothelial cells in vitro. Angiogenesis thus results from the complex interaction of ECM material and cytokines.

Fibroplasia

Fibroblasts are specialized cells that differentiate from resting mesenchymal cells in connective tissue; they do not arrive in the wound cleft by diapedesis from circulating cells. After injury, the normally quiescent and sparse fibroblasts are chemoattracted to the inflammatory site, where they divide and produce the components of the ECM. After stimulation by macrophage- and platelet-derived cytokines and growth factors, the fibroblast, which is normally arrested in the G_0 phase, undergoes replication and proliferation. Platelet-derived TGF-β stimulates fibroblast proliferation indirectly by releasing PDGF. The fibroblast can also stimulate replication in an autocrine manner by releasing FGF-2. To continue proliferating, fibroblasts require further stimulation by factors such as EGF or IGF-I.[17] Although fibroblasts require growth factors for proliferation, they do not need growth factors to survive. Fibroblasts can live quiescently in growth factor–free media in either monolayers or three-dimensional cultures.

The primary function of fibroblasts is to synthesize collagen, which they begin to produce during the cellular phase of inflammation. The time required for undifferentiated mesenchymal cells to differentiate into highly specialized fibroblasts accounts for the delay between injury and the appearance of collagen in a healing wound. This period, generally 3 to 5 days, depending on the type of tissue injured, is called the *lag phase* of wound healing. Fibroblasts begin to migrate in response to chemotactic substances such as growth factors (PDGF, TGF-β), C5 fragments, thrombin, TNF-α, eicosanoids, elastin fragments, leukotriene B$_4$, and fragments of collagen and fibronectin.[2]

The rate of collagen synthesis declines after 4 weeks and eventually balances the rate of collagen destruction by collagenase (MMP-1). At this point the wound enters a phase of collagen maturation. The maturation phase continues for months or even years. Glycoprotein and mucopolysaccharide levels decrease during the maturation phase, and new capillaries regress and disappear. These changes alter the appearance of the wound and increase its strength.

Epithelialization

The epidermis serves as a physical barrier to prevent fluid loss and bacterial invasion. Tight cell junctions within the epithelium contribute to its impermeability, and the basement membrane zone gives structural support and provides attachment between the epidermis and the dermis. The basement membrane zone consists of several layers:

1. The lamina lucida (electron clear), consisting of laminin and heparan sulfate
2. The lamina densa (electron dense), containing type IV collagen
3. Anchoring fibrils, consisting of type IV collagen, which secure the epidermodermal interface and connect the lamina densa to the dermis

The basal layer of the epidermis attaches to the basement membrane zone by hemidesmosomes. Re-epithelialization of wounds begins within hours after injury. Initially, the wound is rapidly sealed by clot formation and then by epithelial (epidermal) cell migration across the defect. Keratinocytes located at the basal layer of the residual epidermis or in the depths of epithelium-lined dermal appendages migrate to resurface the wound. Epithelialization involves a sequence of changes in wound keratinocytes: detachment, migration, proliferation, differentiation, and stratification. If the basement membrane zone is intact, epithelialization proceeds more rapidly. The cells are stimulated to migrate. Attachments to neighboring and adjoining cells and to the dermis are loosened, as demonstrated by intracellular tonofilament retraction, dissolution of intercellular desmosomes and hemidesmosomes linking the epidermis to the basement membrane, and the formation of cytoplasmic actin filaments.[2]

Epidermal cells express integrin receptors that allow them to interact with ECM proteins such as fibronectin. The migrating cells dissect the wound by separating the desiccated eschar from viable tissue. This path of dissection is determined by the integrins that the epidermal cells express on their cell membranes. Degradation of the ECM, required if epidermal cells are to migrate between the collagenous dermis and fibrin eschar, is driven by epidermal cell production of collagenase (MMP-1) and plasminogen activator, which activates collagenase and plasmin. The migrating cells are also phagocytic and remove debris in their path. Cells behind the leading edge of migrating cells begin to proliferate. The epithelial cells move in a leapfrog and tumbling fashion[2] until the edges establish contact. If the basement membrane zone is not intact, it will be repaired first. The absence of neighboring cells at the wound margin may be a signal for the migration and proliferation of epidermal cells. Local release of EGF, TGF-α, and KGF and increased expression of their receptors may also stimulate these processes.[17] Topical application of KGF-2 in both young and aged animals accelerated re-epithelialization. Basement membrane proteins, such as laminin, reappear in a highly ordered sequence from the margin of the wound inward. After the wound is completely re-epithelialized, the cells become columnar and stratified again while firmly attaching to the reestablished basement membrane and underlying dermis.

Extracellular Matrix

The ECM exists as a scaffold to stabilize the physical structure of tissues, but it also plays an active and complex role by regulating the behavior of cells that contact it.

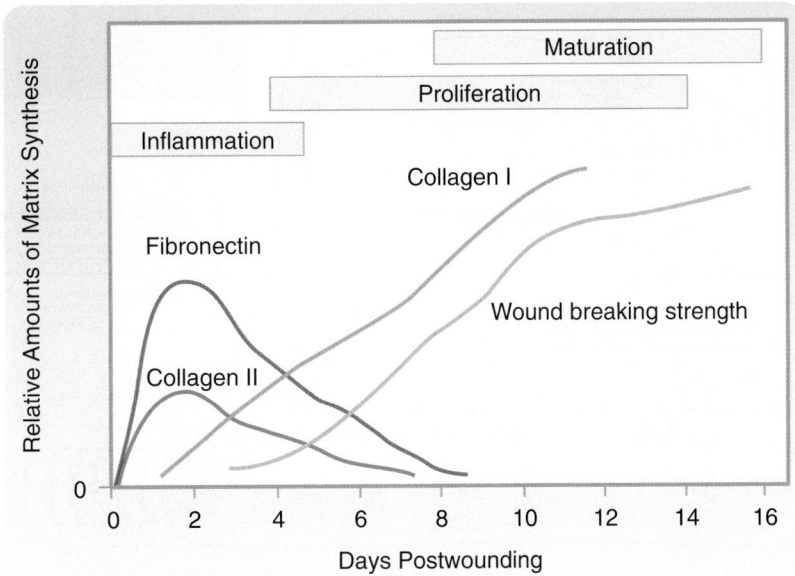

Figure 8-8 Wound matrix deposition over time. Fibronectin and type III collagen constitute the early matrix. Type I collagen accumulates later and corresponds to the increase in wound-breaking strength. (Adapted from Witte MB, Barbul A: General principles of wound healing. Surg Clin North Am 77:515, 1997.)

Cells within it produce the macromolecular constituents, including the following:

1. Glycosaminoglycans (GAGs), or polysaccharide chains, usually found covalently linked to protein in the form of proteoglycans
2. Fibrous proteins such as collagen, elastin, fibronectin, and laminin[18]

In connective tissue, proteoglycan molecules form a gel-like ground substance. This highly hydrated gel allows the matrix to withstand compressive force while permitting rapid diffusion of nutrients, metabolites, and hormones between blood and tissue cells. Collagen fibers within the matrix serve to organize and strengthen it, whereas elastin fibers give it resilience and matrix proteins have adhesive functions.[18]

The wound matrix accumulates and changes in composition as healing progresses, balanced between new deposition and degradation (Fig. 8-8). The provisional matrix is a scaffold for cellular migration and is composed of fibrin, fibrinogen, fibronectin, and vitronectin. GAGs and proteoglycans are synthesized next and support further matrix deposition and remodeling. Collagens, which are the predominant scar proteins, are the end result.[3] Attachment proteins, such as fibrin and fibronectin, provide linkage to the ECM through binding to cell surface integrin receptors.

Stimulation of fibroblasts by growth factors induces up-regulated expression of integrin receptors, thereby facilitating cell-matrix interactions. Ligand binding induces clustering of integrin into focal adhesion sites.[19] Regulation of integrin-mediated cell signaling by the extracellular divalent cations Mg^{2+}, Mn^{2+}, and Ca^{2+} is perhaps due to induction of conformational changes in the integrins.

A dynamic and reciprocal relationship exists between fibroblasts and the ECM. Cytokine regulation of fibroblast responses is altered by variations in the composition of the ECM. For example, expression of matrix-degrading enzymes, such as the MMPs, is up-regulated after cytokine stimulation of fibroblasts. Collagenolytic MMP-1 is induced by IL-1 and down-regulated by TGF-β.[2] Activation of plasminogen to plasmin by plasminogen activator and procollagenase to collagenase by plasmin results in matrix degradation and facilitates cell migration. Modulation of these processes provides additional mechanisms by which the cell-matrix interaction can be regulated during wound healing. Matrix modulation is also seen in tumor metastasis. Neoplastic cells lose their dependence on anchorage, mediated mainly by integrins; this is probably due to decreased production of fibronectin and subsequent decreased adhesion, and as a result these cells can break away from the primary tumor and metastasize.

An example of the necessary dynamic interactions occurring in the provisional matrix during wound healing is the effect of TGF-β on incisional wounds sealed with fibrin sealant. Fibrin sealant is a derivative of plasma components that mimics the last step in the coagulation cascade. Commercially available fibrin sealant has an approximately 10-fold greater concentration of fibrin than plasma does and consequently provides a more airtight, waterproof seal. Fibrin sealant may serve as a mechanical barrier to the early cell-mediated events occurring in wound healing. Supplementation of fibrin sealant with TGF-β has been demonstrated to reverse the inhibitory effects of fibrin sealant on wound healing and increase tensile strength as compared with sutured wounds.[20] The increased tensile strength may be a result of improved

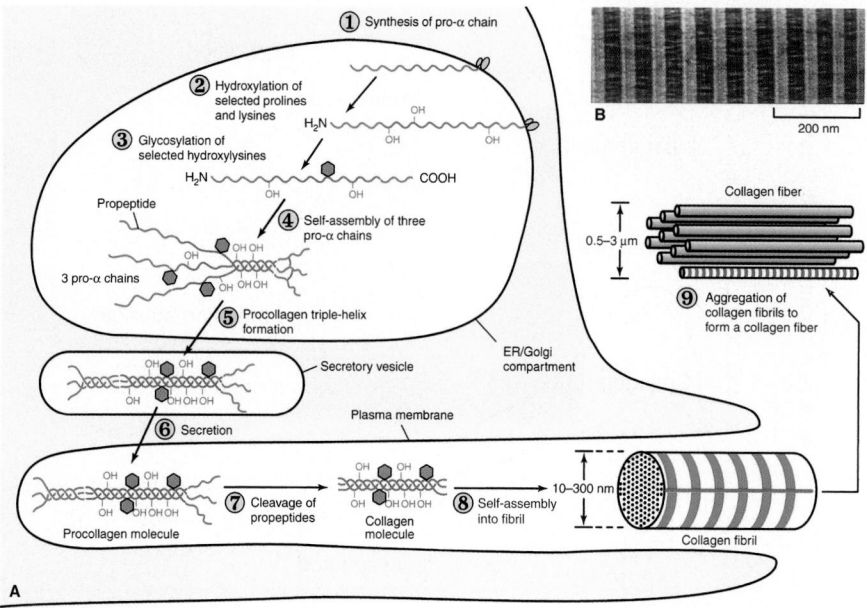

Figure 8-9 Intracellular and extracellular events in the formation of a collagen fibril. **A,** Collagen fibrils are shown assembling in the extracellular space contained within a large infolding in the plasma membrane. As one example of how collagen fibrils can form ordered arrays in the extracellular space, they are shown further assembling into large collagen fibers, which are visible with a light microscope. The covalent cross-links that stabilize the extracellular assemblies are not shown. **B,** Electron micrograph of a negatively stained collagen fibril revealing its typical striated appearance. ER, endoplasmic reticulum. (**A,** From Alberts B, Johnson A, Lewis J, et al [eds]: Molecular Biology of the Cell, 4th ed. New York, Garland, 2002, p 1100; **B,** Courtesy of Robert Horne.)

cell migration into the wound site, more rapid clearance of fibrin sealant, suppression of gelatinase (MMP-9), and enhancement of ECM synthesis in TGF-β–supplemented wounds.

Collagen Structure

Collagens are found in all multicellular animals and are secreted by a variety of cell types. They are a major component of skin and bone and constitute 25% of the total protein mass in mammals. The proline- and glycine-rich collagen molecule is a long, stiff, triple-stranded helical structure that consists of three collagen polypeptide α chains wound around one another in a ropelike superhelix. With its ringlike structure, proline provides stability to the helical conformation in each α chain, whereas glycine, because of its small size, allows tight packing of the three α chains to form the final superhelix. There are at least 20 types of collagen, the main constituents of connective tissue being types I, II, III, V, and XI. Type I is the principal collagen of skin and bone and is the most common.[18] In adults, the skin is approximately 80% type I and 20% type III. In newborns, the content of type III collagen is greater than that found in adults. In early wound healing there is also increased expression of type III collagen. Type I collagens are the fibrillar, or fibril-forming, collagens. They are secreted into the extracellular space, where they assemble into collagen fibrils (10-300 nm in diameter), which then aggregate into larger, cable-like bundles called *collagen fibers* (several micrometers in diameter).

Other types of collagens include types IX and XII (fibril-associated collagens) and types IV and VII (network-forming collagens). Types IX and XII are found on the surface of collagen fibrils and serve to link the fibrils to one another and to other components in the ECM. Type IV molecules assemble into a meshlike pattern and are a major part of the mature basal lamina. Dimers of type VII form anchoring fibrils that help attach the basal lamina to the underlying connective tissue and are especially abundant in the skin.

Type XVII and XVIII collagens are two of a number of collagen-like proteins. Type XVII has a transmembrane domain and is found in hemidesmosomes. Type XVIII is located in the basal laminae of blood vessels. The peptide endostatin, which inhibits angiogenesis and shows promise as an anticancer drug, is formed by cleavage of the C-terminal domain of type XVIII collagen.[21]

Collagen Synthesis

Collagen polypeptide chains are synthesized on membrane-bound ribosomes and enter the endoplasmic reticulum (ER) lumen as pro-α chains (Figs. 8-9 and 8-10). These precursors have amino-terminal signal peptides to direct them to the ER, as well as propeptides at both the N- and C-terminal ends. Within the lumen of the ER, some of the prolines and lysines undergo hydroxylation to form hydroxyproline and hydroxylysine. Hydroxylation results in the stable triple-stranded helix through the formation of interchain hydrogen bonds. The pro-α chain then combines with two others to form procollagen, a hydrogen-bonded, triple-stranded helical molecule. In conditions such as vitamin C (ascorbic acid) deficiency (scurvy), proline hydroxylation is prevented, thereby resulting in the formation of unstable triple helices secondary to the synthesis of defective pro-α chains. Vitamin C deficiency is characterized by the gradual loss of preexisting normal collagen, which leads to fragile blood vessels and loose teeth.

After secretion into the ECM, specific proteases cleave the propeptides of the procollagen molecules to form collagen monomers. These monomers assemble to form collagen fibrils in the ECM, driven by collagen's tendency to self-assemble. Covalent cross-linking of the lysine residues provides tensile strength. The extent and type of cross-linking vary from tissue to tissue. In tissues such as tendons, where tensile strength is crucial, collagen cross-linking is extremely high. In mammalian skin, the fibrils are organized in a basket-weave pattern to resist multidirectional tensile stress. In tendons, on the other hand, fibrils are in parallel bundles aligned along the major axis of tension.[3,18]

Multiple factors can affect collagen synthesis. Vitamin C (ascorbic acid), TGF-β, IGF-I, and IGF-II increase collagen synthesis.[17] IFN-γ decreases type I procollagen mRNA synthesis, and glucocorticoids inhibit procollagen gene transcription, thereby leading to decreased collagen synthesis.[22]

Several genetic disorders are caused by abnormalities in collagen fibril formation. In *osteogenesis imperfecta,* deletion of one procollagen α_1 allele results in weak and easily fractured bones. Ehlers-Danlos syndrome is a result of mutations affecting type III collagen and is characterized by fragile skin and blood vessels and hypermobile joints.

Elastic Fibers

Tissues such as skin, blood vessels, and lungs require strength and elasticity to function. Elastic fibers in the ECM of these tissues provide the resilience to allow recoil after transient stretching.

Elastic fibers are predominantly composed of elastin, a highly hydrophobic protein (~750 amino acids long). Soluble tropoelastin is secreted into the extracellular space, where it forms lysine cross-links to other tropoelastin molecules to generate a large network of elastin fibers and sheets. Elastin is composed of hydrophobic and alanine- and lysine-rich α-helical segments that alternate along the polypeptide chain. The hydrophobic segments are responsible for the molecule's elastic properties. The alanine- and lysine-rich α-helical segments form cross-links between adjacent molecules. Although the proposed conformation of elastin molecules is controversial, the predominant theory is that the elastin polypeptide chain adopts a random coil conformation that allows the network to stretch and recoil like a rubber band. Elastic fibers consist of an elastin core covered by a sheath of microfibrils, which are composed of several distinct glycoproteins such as fibrillin. Elastin-binding fibrillin is essential for integrity of the elastic fibers.

Microfibrils appear before elastin in developing tissues and seem to form a scaffold on which the secreted elastin

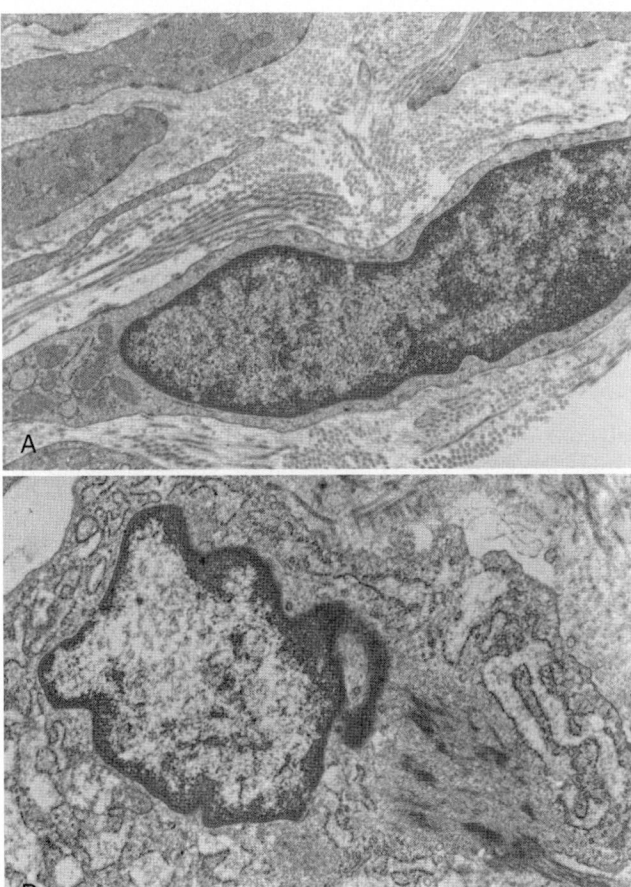

Figure 8-10 A, Normal resting fibroblast from human connective tissue. Note the large, smooth, oval nucleus; normal mitochondria; and small amount of rough endoplasmic reticulum. The cell is surrounded by collagen fibrils cut in longitudinal and cross section. The cell fragments seen in the upper left are typical smooth muscle cells (electron micrograph, ×22,000). **B,** Myofibroblast from a patient with plantar fasciitis. In contrast to the fibroblast, note the highly irregular nucleus, the large amount of rough endoplasmic reticulum, and the dense collection of myofilaments. There are numerous dense bodies adjacent to and intermingled with the myofilaments. No basal lamina is seen, and the cell is surrounded by numerous collagen fibrils. This cell has ultrastructural features typical of both a fibroblast and a smooth muscle cell (electron micrograph, ×25,000). (Courtesy of Edward C. Carlson, PhD.)

molecules are deposited. Elastin is produced early in life, stabilizes, and does not undergo much further synthesis or degradation, with a turnover that approaches the life span.[23] Age-related modification is a result of progressive degradation as the elastic fibers gradually become tortuous, frayed, and porous. Scanning electron microscopy shows that in humans, the elastic meshwork grows largely undistorted during postnatal growth, where fibers seem to enlarge in synchrony with growth of the tissue. In nonwounded circumstances, there is very little elastin degradation, probably because of elastin's hydrophobic nature, which makes the interior of this highly folded protein inaccessible. As a result of this high degree of three-dimensionality and extensive cross-linking, cleavage must be considerable before there is much loss of elasticity. Both IGF-1 and TGF-β stimulate the production of elastin. Glucocorticoids and basic FGF reduce adult skin cell production of elastin.

Mutations causing a deficiency of elastin protein result in arterial narrowing as a consequence of excessive smooth muscle cell proliferation in the arterial wall (intimal hyperplasia). These findings suggest that the normal elasticity of an artery is needed to prevent proliferation of these cells. Gene mutations in fibrillin result in Marfan's syndrome; severely affected individuals are prone to aortic rupture.[24]

Glycosaminoglycans and Proteoglycans

GAGs are unbranched polysaccharide chains composed of repeating disaccharide units: a sulfated amino sugar (*N*-acetylglucosamine or *N*-acetylgalactosamine) and uronic acid (glucuronic or iduronic). GAGs are highly negatively charged because of the sulfate or carboxyl groups on most of their sugars. Four types of GAGS exist[18]:

1. Hyaluronan
2. Chondroitin sulfate and dermatan sulfate
3. Heparan sulfate
4. Keratan sulfate

The GAGs in connective tissue usually constitute less than 10% of the weight of the fibrous proteins. Their highly negative charge attracts osmotically active cations, such as Na^+, which causes large amounts of water to be incorporated into the matrix. This results in porous hydrated gels and is responsible for the turgor that enables the matrix to withstand compressive force.[18]

Hyaluronan is the simplest of the GAGs. It is composed of repeating nonsulfated disaccharide units and is found in adult tissues, but it is especially prevalent in fetal tissues. Its abundance in fetal wounds is believed to be a factor in the scarless wound healing seen in fetal tissues.[25] Unlike the other GAGs, hyaluronan is not covalently attached to any protein and is synthesized directly from the cell surface by an enzyme complex embedded in the plasma membrane.

Hyaluronan serves several different roles because of its large hydration shell. It is produced in large quantities during wound healing, where it facilitates cell migration by physically expanding the ECM and allowing cells additional space for migration; it also reduces the strength of adhesion of migrating cells to matrix fibers. Hyaluronan synthesized from the basal side of epithelium creates a cell-free space for cell migration, as during embryogenesis and formation of the heart and other organs. When cell migration finishes, the excess hyaluronan is degraded by hyaluronidase.

Proteoglycans are a diverse group of glycoproteins with functions mediated by both their core proteins and GAG chains. The number and types of GAGs attached to the core protein can vary greatly, and the GAGs themselves can be modified by sulfonation. Because of their GAGs, proteoglycans provide hydrated space around and between cells. They also form gels of different pore size and charge density to regulate the movement of cells and molecules. Perlecan, a heparan sulfate proteoglycan, serves this role in the basal lamina of the kidney glomerulus. Decreased levels of perlecan are believed to play a role in diabetic albuminuria.

Proteoglycans function in chemical signaling by binding various secreted signal molecules, such as growth factors, and modulating their signaling activity. Proteoglycans can also bind other secreted proteins, such as proteases and protease inhibitors. Such binding allows proteoglycans to regulate proteins by the following[26]:

1. Immobilizing the protein and restricting its range of action
2. Providing a reservoir of the protein for delayed release
3. Altering the protein to allow more effective presentation to cell surface receptors
4. Prolonging the protein's action by protecting it from degradation
5. Blocking the activity of the protein

Proteoglycans can be components of plasma membranes and have a transmembrane core protein or are attached to the lipid bilayer by a glycosylphosphatidylinositol anchor. These proteoglycans act as coreceptors that work with other cell surface receptor proteins in binding cells to the ECM and initiating the response of cells to extracellular signaling proteins. For example, the syndecans are transmembrane proteoglycans that are located on the surface of many cells, including fibroblasts and epithelial cells. In fibroblasts, syndecans are found in focal adhesions, where they interact with fibronectin on the cell surface and with cytoskeletal and signaling proteins inside the cell. Mutations leading to inactivation of these coreceptor proteoglycans result in severe developmental defects.[18]

The ECM has other noncollagen proteins, such as the fibronectins, that have multiple domains and can bind to other matrix macromolecules and cell surface receptors. These interactions help organize the matrix and facilitate cell attachment. Fibronectin is important in animal embryogenesis.

Fibronectin exists as soluble and fibrillar isoforms. Soluble plasma fibronectin circulates in various body fluids and enhances blood clotting, wound healing, and phagocytosis. The highly insoluble fibrillar forms assemble on cell surfaces and are deposited in the ECM. The fibronectin fibrils that form on the surface of fibroblasts are usually coupled with neighboring intracellular actin stress fibers. The actin filaments promote assembly of the fibronectin fibril and influence fibril orientation. Integrin transmembrane adhesion proteins mediate these interactions. The contractile actin and myosin cytoskeleton pulls on the fibronectin matrix and generates tension.[18]

Basal Lamina

Basal laminae are flexible, thin (40-120 nm–thick) mats of specialized ECM that separate cells and epithelia from the underlying or surrounding connective tissue. In skin, the basal lamina is tethered to the underlying connective tissue by specialized anchoring fibrils. This composite of basal lamina and collagen is the basement membrane.

The basal lamina acts in numerous ways:

1. As a molecular filter to prevent the passage of macromolecules (i.e., in the kidney glomerulus)
2. As a selective barrier to certain cells (i.e., the lamina beneath the epithelium prevents fibroblasts from contacting epithelial cells, but does not stop macrophages or lymphocytes)
3. As a scaffold for regenerating cells to migrate
4. As an important element in tissue regeneration in locations where the basal lamina survives

Although its composition may vary from tissue to tissue, most mature basal laminae contain type IV collagen, perlecan, and the glycoproteins laminin and nidogen. Type IV collagen has a more flexible structure than the fibrillar collagens do; its triple-stranded helix is interrupted, thereby allowing multiple bends.

Laminins, in general, consist of three long polypeptide chains (α, β, and γ). Mice lacking the laminin γ_1 chain die during embryogenesis because they cannot make a basal lamina. The laminin in basement membranes consists of several domains that bind to perlecan, nidogen, and laminin receptor proteins found on cell surfaces. The type IV collagen and laminin networks are connected by nidogen and perlecan, which act as stabilizing bridges. Many of the cell surface receptors for type IV collagen and laminin are members of the integrin family. Another important type of laminin receptor is dystroglycan, a transmembrane protein that together with integrins may organize assembly of the basal lamina.[27]

Degradation of the Extracellular Matrix

Regulated turnover of the ECM is crucial to many biologic processes. ECM degradation occurs during metastasis when neoplastic cells migrate from their site of origin to distant organs via the bloodstream or lymphatics. In injury or infection, localized degradation of the ECM occurs so that cells can migrate across the basal lamina to reach the site of injury or infection. Locally secreted cellular proteases, such as MMPs or serine proteases, degrade the ECM components. Matrix proteolysis helps the cell migrate in the following ways:

1. Clearing a path through the matrix
2. Exposing binding sites, thereby promoting cell binding or migration
3. Facilitating cell detachment so that a cell can move forward
4. Releasing signal proteins that promote cell migration

Proteolysis is tightly regulated. Many proteases are secreted as inactive precursors that are activated when required. In addition, cell surface receptors bind these proteases to ensure that they act only on sites where they are needed. Finally, protease inhibitors, such as the tissue inhibitors of metalloproteinase (TIMP), can bind these enzymes and block their activity.

Maturational Phase

Wound *contraction* occurs by centripetal movement of the whole thickness of the surrounding skin and reduces the amount of disorganized scar. Wound *contracture,* in contrast, is a physical constriction or limitation of function and is a result of the process of wound contraction. Contractures occur when excessive scar exceeds normal wound contraction, and it results in a functional disability. Scars that traverse joints and prevent extension or scars that involve the eyelid or mouth and cause an ectropion are examples of contractures.

Wound contraction appears to take place as a result of a complex interaction of the extracellular materials and fibroblasts, which is not completely understood. Using a fibroblast-populated collagen lattice, Ehrlich demonstrated that aborted cell locomotion appears to cause bunching and contraction of the collagen fibers.[28] In this in vitro model, trypsinized collagen is populated by fibroblasts that adhere to it in culture. If normal dermal fibroblasts are cultured, they attempt to move but are trapped by the collagen fibers. The tractional forces cause the lattice to bunch and contract.

Numerous studies have shown that fibroblasts in a contracting wound undergo change to stimulated cells, referred to as *myofibroblasts.* These cells have both function and structure in common with fibroblasts and smooth muscle cells and express alpha smooth muscle actin in bundles called *stress fibers.* The actin appears at day 6 after wounding, persists at high levels for 15 days, and is gone by 4 weeks when the cell undergoes apoptosis.[3] It appears that a stimulated fibroblast develops contractile ability related to the formation of cytoplasmic actin-myosin complexes. When this stimulated cell is placed in the fibroblast-populated collagen lattice, contraction occurs even faster. The tension that is exerted by the fibroblasts' attempt at contraction appears to stimulate the actin-myosin structures in their cytoplasm. If colchicine, which inhibits microtubules, or cytochalasin D, which inhibits microfilaments, is added to the tissue culture, the result is minimal contraction of the collagen gels. Fibroblasts develop a linear arrangement in the line of tension that when removed, causes the cells to round up.

Stimulated fibroblasts, or myofibroblasts, are found to be a constant feature present in abundance in diseases involving excessive fibrosis. Such diseases include hepatic cirrhosis, renal and pulmonary fibrosis, Dupuytren's contracture, and desmoplastic reactions induced by neoplasia. The actin microfilaments are arranged linearly along the long axis of the fibroblast. They are associated with dense bodies that allow attachment to the surrounding ECM. Fibronexus is the attachment entity that connects the cytoskeleton to the ECM and spans the cell membrane in doing so.

MMPs also appear to be important for wound contraction. It has been demonstrated that stromelysin-1 (MMP-3) strongly affects wound contraction. MMPs may be necessary to allow cleavage of the attachment between the fibroblast and the collagen so that the lattice can be made to contract. Different populations of fibroblasts, from different organs, respond to the contraction stimulus in a heterogeneous fashion. It is likely that the stromelysin-1, with the participation of β_1 integrins, allows modification of attachment sites between fibroblasts and the collagen fibrils. Similarly, cytokines such as TGF-β1 affect contraction by increasing the expression of β_1 integrin.

Remodeling

The fibroblast population decreases and the dense capillary network regresses. Wound strength increases rapidly within 1 to 6 weeks and then appears to plateau up to 1 year after the injury (see Fig. 8-8). When compared with unwounded skin, tensile strength is only 30% in the scar. An increase in breaking strength occurs after approximately 21 days, mostly as a result of cross-linking. Although collagen cross-linking causes further wound contraction and an increase in strength, it also results in a scar that is more brittle and less elastic than normal skin. Unlike normal skin, the epidermodermal interface in a healed wound is devoid of rete pegs, the undulating projections of epidermis that penetrate into the papillary dermis. Loss of this anchorage results in increased fragility and predisposes the neoepidermis to avulsion after minor trauma.

ABNORMAL WOUND HEALING

In such a complex series of interweaving events as wound healing, multiple factors can impede the outcome (Box 8-1). The amount of tissue lost or damaged, the amount of foreign material or bacterial inoculation, and the length of exposure to toxic factors affect the time to recovery. The greater the insult, the longer the reparative process and the greater the amount of residual scar. Intrinsic factors such as chemotherapeutic agents, atherosclerosis, cardiac or renal failure, and location on the body all affect wound healing. The blood supply in the lower extremity is the worst in the body; that on the face and hands is the best. The older the patient, the slower the healing.

Ultimately, the type of scar—whether it be adequate, inadequate, or proliferative—is dictated by the amount

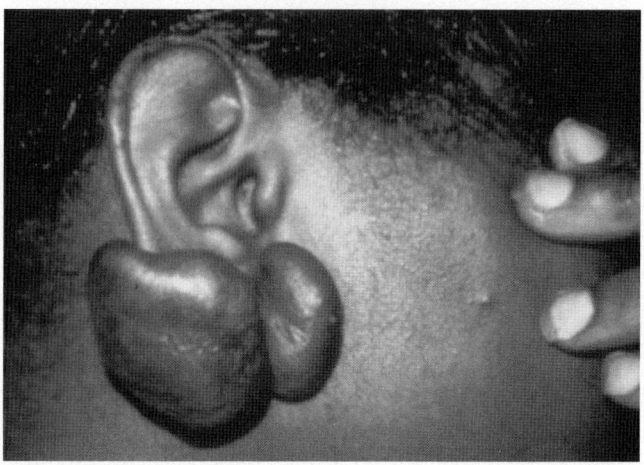

Figure 8-11 Keloids caused by ear piercing.

of collagen deposition and balanced by the amount of collagen degradation. If the balance is tipped in either direction, the result is poor.

Hypertrophic Scars and Keloids

An example of a proliferative scar is a hypertrophic scar or keloid (Fig. 8-11). Pathologic scarring in other areas of the body can cause hepatic cirrhosis, pulmonary fibrosis, scleroderma, retrolental fibroplasia, diabetic retinopathy, or osteoarthritis, among other conditions. Both keloids and hypertrophic scars are characterized by excessive collagen deposition versus collagen degradation. *Keloids* are defined as scars that grow beyond the borders of the original wounds, and these scars rarely regress with time. Keloids are more prevalent in patients with more darkly pigmented skin; they develop in 15% to 20% of African Americans, Asians, and Hispanics. Keloids appear to have a genetic predisposition. Keloid scars tend to occur above the clavicles, on the trunk, on the upper extremities, and on the face. They cannot be prevented at this time and are often refractory to medical and surgical intervention. Hypertrophic scars, in contrast, are raised scars that remain within the confines of the original wound and frequently regress spontaneously. A hypertrophic scar can occur anywhere on the body. These scars also differ histologically from normal scars. Keloids and hypertrophic scars have stretched collagen bundles aligned in the same plane as the epidermis, as opposed to normal scar tissue, where the collagen bundles are randomly arrayed and relaxed. In addition, keloid scars have thicker, more abundant collagen bundles that form acellular nodelike structures in the deep dermal portion of the keloid lesion. The center of keloid lesions also contains a paucity of cells in comparison to hypertrophic scars, which have islands composed of aggregates of fibroblasts, small vessels, and collagen fibers throughout the dermis.

Hypertrophic scars are in many cases preventable. Prolonged inflammation and insufficient resurfacing, such as can occur with a burn wound, lead to hypertrophic scars. It appears that the tension that signals the forma-

---

Box 8-1   Factors That Inhibit Wound Healing

Infection
Ischemia
   Circulation
   Respiration
   Local tension
Diabetes mellitus
Ionizing radiation
Advanced age
Malnutrition
Vitamin deficiencies
   Vitamin C
   Vitamin A
Mineral deficiencies
   Zinc
   Iron
Exogenous drugs
   Doxorubicin (Adriamycin)
   Glucocorticosteroids

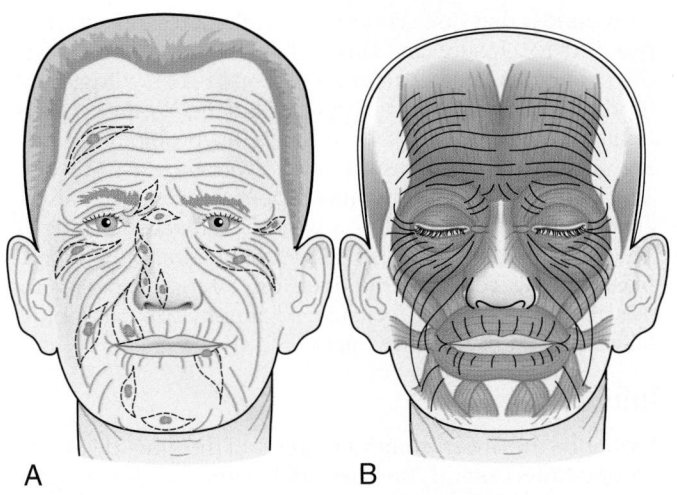

Figure 8-12 The preferred orientation for elective skin incisions (**A**) is parallel to lines of facial expression (**B**). (From Kraissl CJ: The selection of appropriate lines for elective surgical incisions. Plast Reconstr Surg 8:1-28, 1951.)

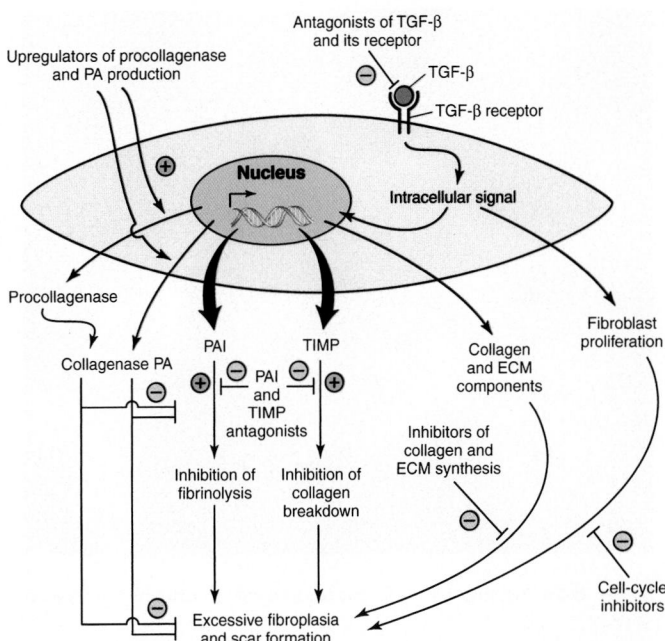

Figure 8-13 Pathways in causing excessive fibroplasia by transforming growth factor-β (TGF-β) and means for therapeutic intervention. TGF-β increases the cellular production of extracellular matrix (ECM) proteins, such as fibronectin and collagen, and also increases the cellular expression of integrins (not shown). Furthermore, the synthesis of inhibitors of degrading enzymes of plasminogen activator inhibitor (PAI) and tissue inhibitor of matrix metalloproteinases (TIMP) is also increased by TGF-β, whereas expression of collagenase and plasminogen activator (PA) is decreased. This up-regulation of inhibitor synthesis plus down-regulation of protease synthesis further augments the accumulation of ECM proteins induced by TGF-β and is the basis for fibrotic tissue formation secondary to excessive action of TGF-β. Possible means of therapeutic intervention are highlighted. Antagonists of TGF-β and its receptor would shift the ECM equilibrium toward degradation, as would up-regulators of PA production and PAI antagonists. Inhibitors of collagen and ECM synthesis would prevent excessive ECM deposition. Cell cycle inhibitors would prevent the proliferation of fibroblasts. (From Tuan TL, Nichter LS: The molecular basis of keloid and hypertrophic scar formation. Mol Med Today 41:21, 1998.)

tion of activated fibroblasts also causes excessive collagen to be deposited. Scars that are perpendicular to the underlying muscle fibers tend to be flatter and narrower, with less collagen formation than when they are parallel to the underlying muscle fibers. The position of an elective scar can be chosen in such a way to make a narrower and less obvious scar in the distant future (Fig. 8-12). As muscle fibers contract, the wound edges become reapproximated if they are perpendicular to the underlying muscle. If, however, the scar is parallel to the underlying muscle, contraction of that muscle tends to cause gaping of the wound edges and leads to more tension and scar formation.

At this time there is some indication of biochemical differences between proliferative scars and normal wound scars. Hypertrophic scars represent a hyperproliferative phenotype that develops after multiple stimulatory effects. This phenotype can be reversed once the stimulation, such as excessive skin tension or growth factors, is removed. Keloids, however, represent a unique phenotype that appears to be genetically predisposed to changes in ECM production and is switched on irreversibly by factors such as TGF-β. Expression of the isoforms TGF-β1 and TGF-β2 is increased in human keloid cells in comparison to normal human dermal fibroblasts. Hypertrophic scar fibroblasts produce more TGF-β1.[29] The addition of exogenous TGF-β2 activates proliferative scar fibroblasts from both keloids and burn hypertrophic scars. In contrast to the elevated collagen synthesis seen in these scars, collagen degradation is low. Both MMP-1 (collagenase) and MMP-9 (gelatinase involved in early tissue repair) are decreased in hypertrophic scars and keloids. MMP-2 (gelatinase in late tissue remodeling) is significantly elevated in hypertrophic scars and keloids. Studies involving antibodies to TGF-β show that its activity can be blocked and fibrosis decreased.[30] Recently, studies examining the genetic susceptibility of certain individuals

to keloid and hypertrophic scar formation have been reported, yet the findings failed to demonstrate an association between plasma levels of TGF-β1 and the common polymorphisms with increased keloid and hypertrophic scars.[31] Growth factors have also been implicated in fibrosis and are being studied as targets for the blockade of fibrosis. IFN-γ, which suppresses collagen synthesis, has been tested clinically in keloid scars and has produced an average 30% reduction in scar thickness (Fig. 8-13).

Chronic Nonhealing Wounds

Chronic wounds, like other abnormal wounds, appear to have derangements in various stages of wound healing and unusually elevated or depressed levels of cytokines, growth factors, or proteinases. Chronic wound fluid,

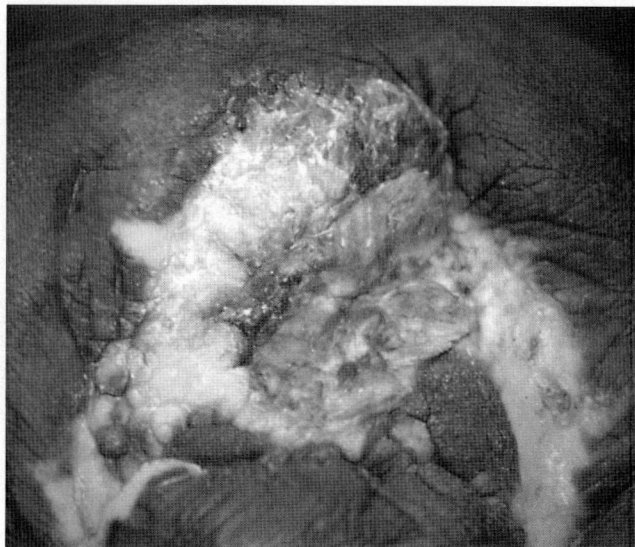

Figure 8-14 Squamous cell carcinoma in a chronic pressure sore.

unlike acute wound fluid, has been demonstrated to have greater levels of IL-1, IL-6, and TNF-α; levels of these proinflammatory cytokines decreased as the wound healed.[4] In addition, an inverse relationship between TNF-α and essential growth factors such as EGF and PDGF has been demonstrated.[4]

The amount of normal wound ECM is determined by a dynamic balance between overall matrix synthesis, deposition, and degradation. Proteolytic degradation of ECM is an essential feature of repair and remodeling during cutaneous repair. Current evidence suggests that proteolytic degradation in the wound environment is a major cause of failure to heal. MMPs are a family of structurally related enzymes that have the ability to degrade ECM components and are differentiated by their substrate specificity and inhibited by TIMPs. TNF-α has been shown to increase the production of MMPs while inhibiting the production of TIMPs. Conversely, inhibition of MMPs results in decreased levels of TNF-α in wound fluid and decreased inflammatory cell numbers while increasing wound tensile strength and levels of TGF-β.

Studies in chronic wounds, such as pressure ulcers in both human and animal models, have demonstrated elevated levels of MMPs, particularly MMP-1, MMP-2, MMP-8, and MMP-9, and decreased levels of TIMPs.[32] This finding has led many investigators to conclude that a chronic wound is a result of persistently elevated levels of MMPs and depressed levels of their inhibitors. These MMPs have been shown to degrade the adhesive substrates for cell migration and signaling molecules, such as growth factors and cytokines. In addition, excessive proteolysis may cause the release of high levels of breakdown products of connective tissue that will inappropriately activate inflammatory cell processes. With increased inflammation of the wound, there is less likelihood that the wound will progress to healing. The balance is slanted in favor of collagen degradation rather than collagen synthesis.

Wounds that are chronically inflamed and do not proceed to closure are susceptible to the development of squamous cell carcinoma (Fig. 8-14). Originally reported in chronic burn scars by Marjolin,[33] other conditions have also been associated with this problem, including osteomyelitis, pressure sores, venous stasis ulcers, and hidradenitis. The wound appears irregular, raised above the surface, and has a white, pearly discoloration. The premalignant state is pseudoepitheliomatous hyperplasia. If this report is obtained on a biopsy specimen, the biopsy is repeated because squamous cell carcinoma may be present in other areas.

Infection

Probably the most common cause of healing delays is wound infection. If the bacterial count in the wound exceeds 10^5 organisms per gram of tissue or if any β-hemolytic streptococci are present, the wound will not heal by any means, including flap closure, skin graft placement, or primary suture.[34] Bacteria prolong the inflammatory phase and interfere with epithelialization, contraction, and collagen deposition. The endotoxins themselves stimulate phagocytosis and release of collagenase, which contributes to collagen degradation and destruction of surrounding, previously normal tissue. Treatment to decrease the bacterial count, either mechanically or with the use of systemic antibiotics, therefore limits the amount of inflammation and allows closure of the wound.

Bacteria may accelerate the expression or increase concentrations of MMPs, growth factors, and cytokines in chronic-type wounds; their role, as yet, has not been clearly defined. Neutrophils release pro–MMP-8, and fibroblasts and macrophages express pro–MMP-1 and pro–MMP-9. These inactive precursors are activated by bacterial proteinases of the thermolysin family (*Pseudomonas, Vibrio,* and *Serratia*), thus supporting the role of bacteria in remodeling the ECM. Bacterial phospholipase C can disrupt normal re-epithelialization by decreasing cell-cell contact and increasing cell migration, possibly by altering integrin expression and by up-regulating MMP-9. However, some studies refute the importance of bacterial induction of MMPs in chronic wounds. Murphy and associates[4] performed quantitative bacteriology on tissue biopsy samples from 10 nonhealing and healing leg ulcers and did not find any significant difference in the number of bacteria present in the two groups of wounds.

Hypoxia

Molecular oxygen is essential for collagen formation. Ischemia can be caused by atherosclerosis, cardiac failure, or simple wound tension preventing localized perfusion. Under hypoxic conditions, energy derived from glycolysis may be sufficient to initiate collagen synthesis, but the presence of molecular oxygen is critical for post-translational hydroxylation of the prolyl and lysyl residues required for triple-helix formation and cross-linking of collagen fibrils. Although hypoxia will stimulate angiogenesis, this essential step in collagen fibril assembly proceeds poorly when PO_2 falls below 40 mm Hg. Optimal PO_2 for collagen synthesis is present at the periphery of the wound while the center remains hypoxic.

The role of anemia in wound healing has long been attributed to be predominantly secondary to hypoperfusion. However, recent work evaluating colonic anastomoses in a crystalloid-resuscitated hemorrhagic shock model demonstrated altered histologic parameters (decreased white blood cell infiltration, angiogenesis, fibroblast production, and collagen production).[35] Use of tobacco products has a similar impact on wound healing because of both the vasoconstriction that occurs with smoking and elevated carbon monoxide serum levels, which can limit the oxygen-carrying capacity of blood.

Diabetes

Diabetes mellitus impairs wound healing at all stages of the process. A diabetic patient with associated neuropathy and atherosclerosis is prone to tissue ischemia, repetitive trauma, and infection. Tissue hypoxia, as indicated by reduced dorsal foot transcutaneous oxygen tension, is a consequence of vascular disease and has been well demonstrated in diabetic patients. In addition to large-vessel disease, many diabetic patients have abnormalities at the microvascular level. The thickened basement membrane of the capillaries causes decreased perfusion in the microenvironment, and there is increased perivascular localization of albumin, which suggests that these capillaries are leaky. Diabetic patients are prone to repeated trauma as a result of the diabetic neuropathy that affects both sensory and motor function in both the somatic and autonomic pathways. Furthermore, diabetics are susceptible to infection because of an attenuated inflammatory response, impaired chemotaxis, and inefficient bacterial killing. Infection also increases local tissue metabolism, thus further imposing a burden on an already tenuous blood supply and thereby amplifying the risk for tissue necrosis. Lymphocyte and leukocyte function is impaired, and there is increased collagen degradation and decreased collagen deposition. The collagen that is formed is more brittle than normal collagen, probably because of glycosylation from the increased levels of glucose present in the ECM.

Ionizing Radiation

Ionizing radiation causes endothelial cell injury with endarteritis and results in atrophy, fibrosis, and delayed tissue repair. Unlike most hypoxic wound beds, angiogenesis is not initiated. Because its greatest effect is on cells in the G_2 through M phase, rapidly dividing cell populations are most sensitive to radiation. Such cells include keratinocytes and fibroblasts during wound healing, injury to which impairs epithelialization and the formation of granulation tissue.

Aging

Elderly patients are more likely to sustain surgical wound rupture and delayed healing than younger patients are. With aging, collagen undergoes qualitative and quantitative changes. Dermal collagen content decreases with aging, and aging collagen fibers show distorted architecture and organization. Up-regulation of MMP-2 and MMP-9 was enhanced in elderly healthy subjects after experimental wounding as compared with young controls.[36] Studies in aged animals have also demonstrated decreased re-epithelialization, depressed collagen synthesis, and impaired angiogenesis with decreased levels of multiple growth factors, including the proangiogenic factors FGF-2 and VEGF. Other studies have suggested that the early inflammatory period of wound healing is altered in the elderly, including impaired macrophage activity with reduced phagocytosis and delayed infiltration of macrophages and B lymphocytes into wounds.[36] In addition, with aging there is a decrease in response to hypoxia, as demonstrated by decreased MMP activation and TGF-β1 receptor expression by keratinocytes isolated from aged donors.[37]

Malnutrition

Malnutrition has an impact on wound healing. Protein catabolism can result in a delay in wound healing. A hypoalbuminemic patient can experience wound-healing delay or even dehiscence, although the albumin level must be lower than 2.0 g/dL to have an effect on wound healing. Protein supplements can reverse this deficiency.

Vitamin deficiencies affect wound healing primarily as a result of their effect as cofactors. Delayed healing can occur in as few as 3 months of vitamin C deprivation. This deficiency can be reversed by the administration of 100 to 1000 g/day. Deficiency of vitamin A impedes monocyte activation and deposition of fibronectin, thus further affecting cellular adhesion, and impairs TGF-β receptors. Vitamin A contributes to lysosomal membrane destabilization and directly counteracts the effect of glucocorticoids. The main effect of vitamin K deficiency is to limit the synthesis of prothrombin and factors VII, IX, and X. Vitamin K metabolism is impeded by antibiotics. Patients who have chronic or recurrent infections need to have their clotting parameters checked before surgical procedures.

A few minerals, if deficient in the diet, adversely affect wound healing. Zinc deficiency is rare, except in patients with conditions such as large burns, severe multiple trauma, and hepatic cirrhosis. Zinc is a necessary cofactor for RNA polymerase and DNA polymerase. Deficiency of zinc results in early wound healing delays. Iron deficiency anemia is a debatable cause of wound healing delay. Although the ferrous ion is a cofactor needed to convert proline to hydroxyproline, reports are conflicting regarding the effects that acute and chronic anemia have on wound healing. In general, patients benefit most by a well-rounded diet consisting of adequate protein intake and caloric value plus vitamin and mineral supplementation.

Drugs

Some exogenous drugs directly inhibit wound healing. Doxorubicin (Adriamycin) is a potent inhibitor,

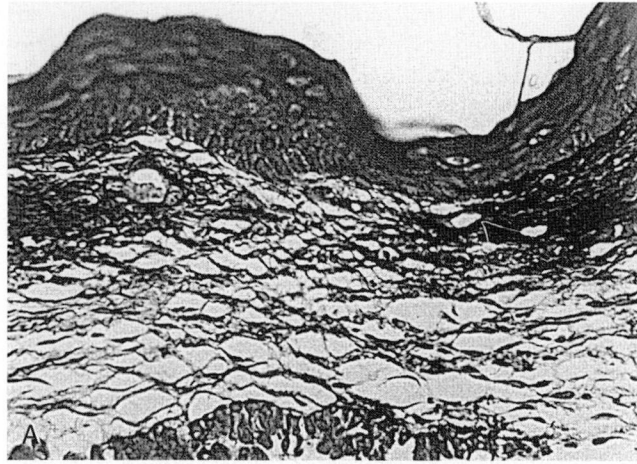

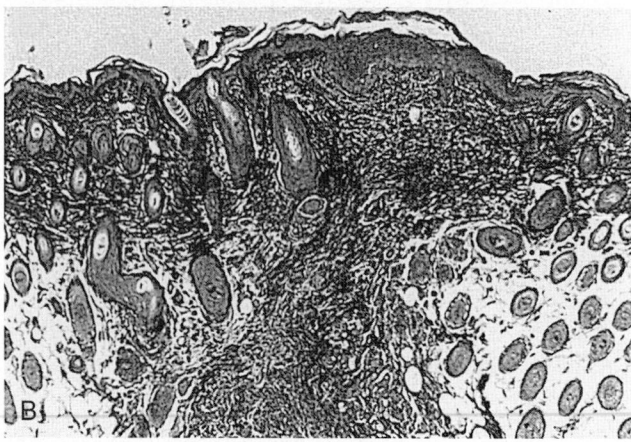

Figure 8-15 Comparison of scar-free repair and healing with scarring by Mallory trichrome staining. **A,** A healed skin wound in a 2-day-old opossum in the pouch, 2 days after wounding, illustrates the absence of scar formation in the dermis and the very rapid repair process. Epithelial thickening is apparent at the wound site, as well as a fine reticular collagen pattern in the healed dermis. **B,** A wound in a 28-day-old opossum in the pouch, 7 days postoperatively, demonstrates extensive scarring in the dermis, as well as abnormal orientation of the collagen fibers perpendicular to the dermis.

particularly if administered preoperatively. Although clinical studies have shown little impairment, experimental models have indicated that nitrogen mustard, cyclophosphamide, methotrexate, bis-chloroethyl-nitrosourea (BCNU), and doxorubicin are the most potent wound inhibitors. These chemotherapeutic agents reduce mesenchymal cell proliferation and reduce the number of platelets, inflammatory cells, and growth factors available, especially if given preoperatively. Tamoxifen, an antiestrogen, is known to decrease cellular proliferation. In addition, there appears to be a dose-dependent decrease in wound-breaking strength associated with tamoxifen. This effect may be due to decreased TGF-β production. Glucocorticosteroids impair fibroblast proliferation and collagen synthesis. The amount of granulation tissue formed is also decreased. Steroids stabilize the lysosomal membranes. This particular effect can be reversed by the administration of vitamin A. The decrease in breaking strength caused by the administration of exogenous steroids appears to be both time and dose related. High doses of nonsteroidal anti-inflammatory drugs have been reported to delay healing, but doses in the therapeutic range are unlikely to have an effect.[38]

FETAL WOUND HEALING

Fetal skin wounds heal rapidly and without the scarring and inflammation that are characteristic of adult skin wounds (Fig. 8-15). As a result, a great deal of wound-healing research has focused on fetal wounds. It was thought that fetal wound healing represented ideal tissue repair and that understanding fetal wound healing would provide surgeons the tools to regulate and control the different steps in adult wound healing. In adult cutaneous healing as opposed to fetal healing, dermal appendages such as hair follicles, sweat glands, and sebaceous glands fail to regenerate. Furthermore, there are changes in collagen in adult wounds, with the healed wound demonstrating densely packed collagen bundles oriented perpendicular to the wound surface, unlike that of normal uninjured skin and fetal skin, both of which have a reticular pattern.

Fetal wounds re-epithelialize faster with less neovascularization and a faster increase in strength. Fetal wound research has demonstrated that fetal wounds differ from adult wounds in inflammatory responses, ECM components, and growth factor expression and responses.

Fetal repair is dependent on both gestational age and wound size. There may be a wound size threshold (the diameter of excised skin at which 50% of wounds heal scarlessly at a given gestational age). The wound size threshold for 60- and 70-day-gestation animals is 6 to 10 mm and 4 to 6 mm for 80- and 90-day-gestation animals. It has been suggested that larger wounds may extend the time of the healing response and expose wound tissue to a different ECM and growth factor profile. Larger excisional wounds may also stimulate the formation of myofibroblasts in the wound and thereby result in scar formation. The transition from scarless to scarring repair occurs near the end of the second trimester and the beginning of the third. Wounds heal faster in a fetus than in a neonate, and they heal slowest in adults. Normal development of skin appendages occurs when fibroblasts of the dermis induce the epithelium to form hair follicles or glands. Wounds created early in gestation heal scarlessly and with dermal appendages, thus suggesting tissue regeneration versus repair. Late-gestation wounds, in contrast, heal with scarring and without dermal appendages. The transition from scarless healing to healing without dermal appendages suggests that the fetal fibroblast loses its ability to induce the epithelium to form dermal appendages with advancing gestational age.

Investigators have cited intrinsic (i.e., oxygen tension of the human fetus) and extrinsic (amniotic fluid environment) differences between fetal and adult wound healing, with most stating that the intrinsic differences are the key determinants in whether wounds will heal with scars.[39]

Intrinsic differences include fetal oxygen tension, which is markedly decreased (fetal sheep, mean PaO_2 of 20 mm Hg) when compared with adult animals (adult sheep, mean PaO_2 of 116 mm Hg).[40] This decrease in fetal oxygenation is partially compensated by the relative affinity of fetal hemoglobin for oxygen.

The fetal environment, an extrinsic difference between fetal and adult wounds, is characterized by a hyaluronic acid–rich amniotic fluid. Studies suggest that the increased number of hyaluronic acid receptors and increased amount of hyaluronic acid may create a permissive environment in which fibroblast movement is facilitated and thereby results in the increased rate and efficiency of fetal healing.[39]

Much of fetal wound-healing research has focused on the role of fibroblasts. Fetal fibroblasts appear to have characteristics quite different from those of adult fibroblasts. Proline hydroxylation is a rate-limiting step in collagen synthesis by dermal cells; early-gestation fetal human fibroblasts have increased prolyl hydroxylase activity, which gradually falls off to adult levels after 20 weeks of gestation. Collagens I, III, V, and VI appear earlier and the ratio of type III to type I is greater in fetal wounds, which is consistent with the higher prevalence of type III collagen in normal fetal tissue. Fetal fibroblasts in vitro have higher collagen production than their adult counterparts do. This may be secondary to the unique regulatory mechanism for prolyl hydroxylase and may explain why there is higher fibroblast activity in fetuses younger than 20 weeks' gestation.

Collagen synthesis falls to adult levels after 20 weeks' gestation. There appears to be an increase in collagen degradation as a function of gestational age. Recent work has found marked increases in the gene expression of MMP-1, MMP-3, and MMP-9 that correlated with the onset of scar formation in nonwounded fetal skin.[41] These findings suggest that late-gestational fetal rat skin undergoes an adult type of tissue remodeling after wounding that leads to the scarring seen in adult skin.

There are also differences in the components of the ECM of fetal and adult wounds. After injury, fibronectin levels are similar in adults and fetuses, but tenascin, an inhibitor of fibronectin, increases earlier and returns to normal more rapidly in the fetus. Larger amounts of fibronectin in fetal wounds stimulate immediate cell attachment, whereas the more rapid deposition of tenascin in the fetus allows cells to migrate and fully epithelialize the wound more rapidly and thus decreases wound-healing time.

Levels of hyaluronic acid are persistently elevated in fetal wounds. During gestation, decreasing levels of hyaluronic acid correlate with increasing scarring potential. The unique ECM composition of fetal tissues may influence collagen fibril deposition by facilitating cell mobility and migration, thereby leading to the loose collagen pattern seen in healed fetal wounds as opposed to the dense collagenous pattern seen in adult scars. However, few studies have examined the effect of modifying the ECM components.

Differences in fetal wound healing also occur in the inflammatory phase. The fetus exhibits a reduced inflammatory response with a lack of neutrophil infiltration and decreased infiltration of endogenous immunoglobulins. The paucity of macrophages and a difference in the temporal appearance of macrophages in a fetal wound may explain why there are differences in growth factor profiles between adult and fetal wounds and why there is a reduced inflammatory response. These studies cite a direct correlation between increased macrophage recruitment in older fetuses and the development of increased scarring.

Fetal wounds have been demonstrated to have minimal levels of TGF-β and FGF-2 by immunohistochemistry. Furthermore, PDGF in fetal wounds disappears more rapidly than in adult wounds. This lack of growth factors may be explained by the decreased inflammatory cell recruitment. Normal inflammatory (adult-type) wound healing may have evolved to reduce the risk of infection at the expense of healing quality.

TGF-β is the growth factor that has been most extensively studied in fetal wound repair. TGF-β1 has been shown to induce rapid healing and scar formation when added to adult rat wounds and induce inflammation and fibrosis when added to fetal rabbit wounds. TGF-β production may be blunted in hypoxemic conditions, and this has led to the theory that the decreased oxygen tension in the fetal environment inhibits TGF-β production and results in decreased scar formation. More recent work has suggested that differential expression of the different TGF-β isoforms, rather than the mere presence of TGF-β, may be important in explaining the differences in repair.

Growth factor manipulation to make wounds more fetal-like with less angiogenesis, less fibrosis, and improved ECM migratory ability has not resulted in completely scarless healing, and there is still failure of regeneration of dermal appendages. These findings suggest that the mechanisms of scarless fetal wound healing have yet to be completely elucidated. Some inconsistencies in fetal wound healing are not clearly understood. It has been shown that there are differences in species with regard to scarless fetal wound healing and that not all fetal tissues are capable of scarless healing. For example, fetal lamb diaphragm and gastric wounds scar, whereas concurrent skin wounds heal scarlessly.

Studies have demonstrated a correlation between the presence of myofibroblasts and scar formation; this suggests that a transition in fibroblast phenotype may contribute to the onset of scarring. Excisional wounds in 75-day-gestation fetal lambs show an absence of scar formation and alpha smooth muscle actin expression. Alpha smooth muscle actin appears after 100 days of gestation along with scar formation. Although attempts to make wounds more fetal-like has failed to reproduce scarless healing, the differences in fetal and adult wounds have not yet been completely elucidated.

WOUND DRESSINGS

Wound dressings have been used since the time of antiquity. Treatment of wounds originally consisted of homemade remedies and evolved very little for many years, but in 1867, Lister introduced antiseptic dressings by soaking lint and gauze in carbolic acid. Currently, there are many more sophisticated dressings to help speed the healing process and decrease the bacterial load present in some wounds.

In treating a wound in a nonsurgical, conservative manner, certain characteristics are important in the wound dressing. First, the dressing needs to protect the wound from trauma and contamination by bacteria. The dressing helps with absorption of the wound exudate. In addition, the dressing helps obliterate dead space and provides compression to assist in decreasing edema. Other dressings provide immobilization to allow stable scar formation (i.e., bolster over a skin graft). Nonadherence to the wound is also important to prevent decreased disruption of healing tissues. It is important to note that not all dressings can provide all the aforementioned characteristics and not all wounds require all these functions. It is essential that the choice of dressing match the specific wound conditions.

Two concepts that are critical in selecting appropriate dressings for wounds are occlusion and absorption. The concept of occlusion is a relatively new idea that came about after Winter and colleagues[42] published a study demonstrating that the rate of epithelialization under an occlusive dressing was twice that of a wound that was left uncovered and allowed to dry. Placement of an occlusive dressing over the wound provides a mildly acidic pH and low oxygen tension on the wound surface. The steep oxygen gradient is a good environment for proliferation of fibroblasts and formation of granulation tissue. A relatively occlusive dressing is a good choice for many wounds; however, other options would be beneficial in wounds that have a significant amount of exudate or wounds with high bacterial counts. First, if the wound has a heavy amount of exudate, it is crucial to have a dressing that has a degree of absorption. The skin surrounding the wound can become macerated with large amounts of uncontrolled exudate. These wounds require a dressing that reduces the bacterial load within the wound while removing the exudate produced. Placement of a pure occlusive dressing without bactericidal properties will allow bacterial overgrowth and worsen the infection.

An in-depth discussion on the types of wound dressings exceeds the scope of this text, but it is important to mention the various classes of dressings. Wound dressings can be categorized into four classes: nonadherent fabrics; absorptive dressings; occlusive dressings; and creams, ointments, and solutions. A brief discussion of the categories of dressings follows.

Nonadherent fabrics are generally fine-mesh gauze supplemented with a substance to augment its occlusive properties or antibacterial abilities. An example of this type of dressing is Scarlet Red, a relatively nonocclusive dressing that is impregnated with *O*-tolylazo-*O*-tolylazo-B-naphthol, which has some antimicrobial abilities. Another example of this class is Xeroform, a relatively occlusive, hydrophobic dressing containing 3% bismuth tribromophenate in a petrolatum base.

The absorptive class is used mainly for wounds that produce a significant amount of exudate. As previously described, exudate collects and can contribute to wound maceration, thus slowing wound healing, if not removed from the wound bed. Wide-mesh gauze is the oldest of this type of dressing and is very absorbent, but it loses its effectiveness when saturated. Newer materials such as foam dressings provide the absorbent qualities to remove large quantities of exudate and have a nonadherant quality to prevent disruption of newly formed granulation tissue on removal. Examples of these foams are Lyofoam (Convatec, Princeton, NJ), Allevyn (Smith and Nephew, Largo, FL), Curafoam (The Kendall Company, Mansfield, MA), Flexzan (Dow Hickam, Sugar Land, TX), and Vigi-FOAM (Bard, Murray Hill, NJ). Wound healing beneath absorptive dressings appears to be slower than under occlusive dressings, possibly because of wicking of cytokines from the wound bed or decreased keratinocyte migration.[43]

The occlusive dressing class provides moisture retention, mechanical protection, and a barrier to bacteria. The occlusive class can be divided into biologic and nonbiologic dressings. Examples of biologic dressings are allograft, xenograft, amnion, and skin substitutes. Homograft is a graft transplanted between genetically unique humans, whereas a xenograft is a graft transplanted between species. Pigskin is the most commonly used xenograft. Homografts and xenografts are temporary dressings in that both are rejected if left on a wound for an extended period. Amnion is derived from human placentas and is another effective biologic wound dressing. These dressings are often used in the treatment of burn wounds; however, they can be used as a temporary measure in other types of wounds as well.

The newest type of wound dressings are skin substitutes that can be used for structural support and scaffolding for regeneration. Examples include Integra (Integra LifeSciences Corp, Plainsboro, NJ), Apligraf (Novartis, Basel), and AlloDerm (Lifecell, Branchburg, NJ). We will briefly discuss these three examples of skin substitutes. Integra is a bilayer membrane system for skin replacement. The first layer is made of a porous matrix of cross-linked bovine tendon collagen and a GAG (chondroitin 6-sulfate). The second layer is made of synthetic polysiloxane polymer (silicone) and functions to control moisture loss from the wound. The first layer serves as a template for the infiltration of fibroblasts, macrophages, lymphocytes, and capillaries from the wound bed. During the healing process, a new collagen matrix is deposited by fibroblasts and the dermal layer of the template is degraded. Once vascularization of the dermal layer is complete, a thin autograft can be applied after removal of the silicone layer. AlloDerm is an acellular dermal matrix derived from donated human skin tissue. It provides the matrix for revascularization and incorporation into host tissue. Apligraf is a living, bilayered biologic dressing that has been designed to simulate normal skin. Initially, neonatal-derived dermal fibroblasts are cultured in a collagen matrix for 6 days. Human keratinocytes are then cultured on top of this neodermis. The dressing contains matrix proteins and expresses cytokines;

however, it does not contain melanocytes, Langerhans cells, macrophages, lymphocytes, or the adnexal structures normally present in human skin. These are only three examples of the types of skin substitutes that are currently available. Many other substitutes are in development and will continue to provide options for the surgeon.

The final class of wound dressings consists of creams, ointments, and solutions. This is a broad category that extends from traditional materials, such as zinc oxide paste, to cutting-edge preparations containing growth factors. The various categories include those with antibacterial properties such as acetic acid, Dakin's solution, silver nitrate, mafenide (Sulfamylon), silver sulfadiazine (Silvadene), iodine-containing ointments (Iodosorb), and bacitracin. Application of these products is indicated when clinical signs of infection, such as an increase in exudate or cellulitis, are present or if quantitative culture demonstrates greater than 10^5 organisms per gram of tissue.

Many types of wound dressings are available to the surgeon and the number is increasing constantly. The characteristics of the wound dictate the types of wound dressings that are necessary, and the requirements often change. The surgeon must have a baseline knowledge of the types of options that exist to allow effective wound management.

NEW HORIZONS

Negative Pressure–Assisted Wound Closure

In the past 10 years there have been significant advances in complex acute and chronic wound management. One of the largest discoveries was the improvement in wounds with negative pressure–assisted wound closure (Fig. 8-16). With this technology, the surgeon now has additional options besides immediate closure of wounds (i.e., adjunctive therapy before or after surgery or an alternative to surgery in the extremely ill).

The original description of negative pressure–assisted wound closure was presented by Argenta and associates in 1997.[44] This study described a method of applying subatmospheric pressure to a wide variety of wounds. By applying this negative pressure, they demonstrated removal of chronic edema, an increase in local blood flow, and stimulation of granulation tissue. This technique may be used on acute, subacute, and chronic wounds. The authors treated 300 wounds with negative-pressure therapy; 296 wounds responded favorably with an increased rate of granulation tissue.

Additional studies have demonstrated significant improvement in wound depth in chronic wounds treated with negative-pressure therapy as compared with wounds treated with saline wet to moist dressings.[45] In addition, treatment with negative pressure results in faster healing times with fewer associated complications.

The exact mechanism of the improvement in healing with negative-pressure therapy has yet to be determined. Many authors initially believed that the reason for increased wound healing is the removal of wound exudates while keeping the wound moist. As originally hypothesized by Argenta and colleagues,[44] with negative-pressure therapy, there is a fivefold increase in blood flow to cutaneous tissues.[46] Further studies have shown an increase in capillary caliber and stimulated endothelial proliferation and angiogenesis.[47] Interestingly, it is well know that increased bacterial loads result in slowed wound healing; however, despite increased wound healing with negative-pressure therapy, it has been shown to result in increased bacterial counts.[48]

Even though the mechanisms behind the improvement achieved with negative-pressure therapy have yet to be elucidated, such treatment represents a significant improvement in cost-effectiveness and has decreased length of stay after acute and chronic wounds. In fact, there have been reports of a 78% decrease in hospital stay and a 76% decrease in cost with negative-pressure therapy. The cost decrease and effectiveness of wound treatment with negative-pressure therapy have translated to home health care treatment of Medicare patients.

Since publication of the original description, numerous studies have reported many uses for subatmospheric pressure. Although the most natural use for negative-pressure wound therapy was in treating the complex wounds that are commonplace in plastic surgery practice, the technique has bridged into all surgical subspecialties. For instance, treatment of the post–coronary artery bypass complication post-sternotomy mediastinitis has resulted in significant improvements and avoidance of additional procedures.[49] Moreover, wounds in which it is notoriously difficult to achieve closure, such as orthopedic wounds with exposed hardware, have benefited from this therapy.[50]

Currently, this technique has helped in the management of complex wounds. However, the mechanisms behind negative pressure–assisted wound closure are relatively unknown. Further knowledge of these mechanisms will allow manipulation of wound conditions and

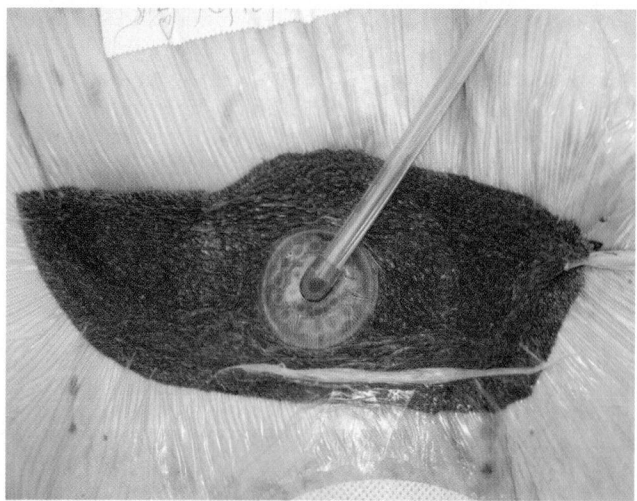

Figure 8-16 Negative pressure–assisted wound closure sponge in place on a patient's abdomen.

lead to further improvements in healing times, thus providing additional options as adjunct therapy for surgeons.

Scaffolds

When dressings alone fail to achieve healing, the clinician now has a variety of advanced therapeutics to turn to. Topical application of growth factors to chronic wounds has not been as beneficial as anticipated, presumably because they are degraded by proteases in the wound fluid. Researchers are now investigating whether localized gene therapy may be a better delivery system for providing growth factors to the wound bed. In addition, dressings that actively alter the wound matrix are currently being developed. One such device, oxidized regenerated cellulose/collagen, has been found to promote human dermal fibroblast proliferation and cell migration, accelerate wound closure in diabetic mice, and possibly sequester or inactivate proteases.[51,52] Biodegradable scaffolds, either natural or synthesized, may also alter the wound milieu to be more favorable. Porcine small intestinal submucosa has been demonstrated in a number of applications to provide a scaffold for tissue repair and reconstruction. Though xenogeneic, this acellular scaffold is minimally immunogenic and has been shown to be completely degraded and replaced by host tissue.[53] Hyaluronic acid conjugated with glycidyl methacrylate, chondroitin sulfate, or gelatin has been shown to have vulnerary effects on wound-healing parameters.[54,55]

The addition of live cells to scaffolds is a promising therapy for chronic wounds that are very difficult to heal. Whether using actual cultured skin with both fibroblasts and keratinocytes or fibroblasts integrated into a dermal matrix, the neonatal cells provide growth factors and matrix elements consistent with rapid healing. They are currently cost prohibitive for large wounds and are primarily applicable only to shallow ulcerations.

In summary, the choice of dressings needs to be based on the basics of wound bed preparation and modified according to the characteristics of the wound. Despite the availability of many dressings on the market, there have been no substantial studies showing a difference in healing between dressings of the same category. Thus, a systematic approach that addresses débridement, exudate management, and bacterial burden should be the standard of clinical practice and can be accomplished even in situations with limited resources.

Selected References

Alberts B, Johnson A, Lewis J, et al (eds): Cell junctions, cell adhesion, and the extracellular matrix. In The Molecular Biology of the Cell, 4th ed. New York, Garland, 2002, pp 1091-1114.

This chapter gives a comprehensive review of matrix and integrin biology and their critical role in biologic processes, including tissue repair.

Banwell PE, Musgrave M: Topical negative pressure therapy: Mechanisms and indications. Int Wound J 1:95-106, 2004.

Up-to-date review of negative-pressure wound closure topics and uses.

Dang C, Ting K, Soo C, et al: Fetal wound healing: Current perspectives. Clin Plast Surg 30:13-23, 2003.

This review article discusses the morphologic, cellular, and molecular aspects of scarless fetal wound healing.

Lionelli, G, Lawrence W: Wound dressings. Surg Clin North Am 83:617-638; 2003.

Thorough discussion of classes and uses of wound dressings.

Rohrich R (ed): Current concepts in wound healing. Plast Reconstr Surg 117(Suppl 7S):1S, 2006.

Recent comprehensive supplement with many clinical correlates.

Rumalla VK, Borah GL: Cytokines, growth factors, and plastic surgery. Plast Reconstr Surg 108:719-733, 2001.

The authors review the critical role of cytokines and growth factors in wound healing.

Schultz GS, Sibbald RG, Falanga V, et al: Wound bed preparation: A systematic approach to wound management. Wound Repair Regen 11(2 Suppl):S1-S28, 2003.

This monograph reviews the current status, role, and key elements in wound bed preparation. It gives an analysis of acute and chronic wound environments and how healing can take place in these settings.

Singer AJ, Clark, RAF: Mechanisms of disease: Cutaneous wound healing. N Engl J Med 341:738-746, 1999.

Comprehensive review of the cellular and molecular aspects of wound healing.

References

1. Giagulli C, Ottoboni L, Caveggion E, et al: The Src family kinases Hck and Fgr are dispensable for inside-out, chemoattractant-induced signaling regulating beta 2 integrin affinity and valency in neutrophils, but are required for beta 2 integrin–mediated outside-in signaling involved in sustained adhesion. J Immunol 177:604-611, 2006.
2. Nwometh BC, Olutoye OO, Diegelmann RF, et al: The basic biology of wound healing. J Surg Pathol 2:143-162, 1997.
3. Witte MB, Barbul A: General principles of wound healing. Surg Clin North Am 77:509-528, 1997.
4. Murphy MA, Joyce WP, Condron C, Bouchier-Hayes D: A reduction in serum cytokine levels parallels healing of venous ulcers in patients undergoing compression therapy. Eur J Vasc Endovasc Surg 23:349-352, 2002.
5. Liechty KW, Adzick NS, Crombleholme TM: Diminished interleukin 6 (IL-6) production during scarless human fetal wound repair. Cytokine 12:671-676, 2000.
6. Rennekampff HO, Hansbrough JF, Kiessig V, et al: Bioactive interleukin-8 is expressed in wounds and enhances wound healing. J Surg Res 93:41-54, 2000.
7. Tredget EE, Wang R, Shen Q, et al: Transforming growth factor-beta mRNA and protein in hypertrophic scar tissues and fibroblasts: Antagonism by IFN-alpha and IFN-gamma in vitro and in vivo. J Interferon Cytokine Res 20:143-151, 2000.
8. Smith PD, Kuhn MA, Franz MG, et al: Initiating the inflammatory phase of incisional healing prior to tissue injury. J Surg Res 92:11-17, 2000.

9. Boyce DE, Jones WD, Ruge F, et al: The role of lymphocytes in human dermal wound healing. Br J Dermatol 143:59-65, 2000.

10. Barbul A, Regan MC: Immune involvement in wound healing. Otolaryngol Clin North Am 28:955-968, 1995.

11. Deodato B, Arsic N, Zentilin L, et al: Recombinant AAV vector encoding human VEGF165 enhances wound healing. Gene Ther 9:777-785, 2002.

12. Nissen NN, Polverini PJ, Koch AE, et al: Vascular endothelial growth factor mediates angiogenic activity during the proliferative phase of wound healing. Am J Pathol 152:1445-1452, 1998.

13. Hellwig-Burgel T, Stiehl DP, Wagner AE, et al: Review: Hypoxia-inducible factor-1 (HIF-1): A novel transcription factor in immune reactions. J Interferon Cytokine Res 25:297-310, 2005.

14. Dulak J, Jozkowicz A, Dembinska-Kiec A, et al: Nitric oxide induces the synthesis of vascular endothelial growth factor by rat vascular smooth muscle cells. Arterioscler Thromb Vasc Biol 20:659-666, 2000.

15. Akcay MN, Ozcan O, Gundogdu C, et al: Effect of nitric oxide synthase inhibitor on experimentally induced burn wounds. J Trauma 49:327-330, 2000.

16. Liu S, Yu D, Xu ZP, et al: Angiogenin activates Erk1/2 in human umbilical vein endothelial cells. Biochem Biophys Res Commun 287:305-310, 2001.

17. Rumalla VK, Borah GL: Cytokines, growth factors, and plastic surgery. Plast Reconstr Surg 108:719-733, 2001.

18. Alberts B, Johnson A, Lewis J, et al (eds): Cell junctions, cell adhesion, and the extracellular matrix. In The Molecular Biology of the Cell, 4th ed. New York, Garland, 2002, pp 1091-1114.

19. Romer LH, Birukov KG, Garcia JG: Focal adhesions: Paradigm for a signaling nexus. Circ Res 98:606-616, 2006.

20. Petratos PB, Felsen D, Trierweiler G, et al: Transforming growth factor-beta2 (TGF-beta2) reverses the inhibitory effects of fibrin sealant on cutaneous wound repair in the pig. Wound Repair Regen 10:252-258, 2002.

21. Cattaneo MG, Pola S, Francescato P, et al: Human endostatin-derived synthetic peptides possess potent antiangiogenic properties in vitro and in vivo. Exp Cell Res 283:230-236, 2003.

22. Laato M, Heino J, Gerdin B, et al: Interferon-gamma–induced inhibition of wound healing in vivo and in vitro. Ann Chir Gynaecol Suppl (215):19-23, 2001.

23. Bailey AJ: Molecular mechanisms of ageing in connective tissues. Mech Ageing Dev 122:735-755, 2001.

24. Nollen GJ, Groenink M, van der Wall EE, et al: Current insights in diagnosis and management of the cardiovascular complications of Marfan's syndrome. Cardiol Young 12:320-327, 2002.

25. Kennedy CI, Diegelmann RF, Haynes JH, et al: Proinflammatory cytokines differentially regulate hyaluronan synthase isoforms in fetal and adult fibroblasts. J Pediatr Surg 35:874-879, 2000.

26. Iozzo RV: Matrix proteoglycans: From molecular design to cellular function. Annu Rev Biochem 67:609-652, 1998.

27. Ghohestani RF, Li K, Rousselle P, et al: Molecular organization of the cutaneous basement membrane zone. Clin Dermatol 19:551-562, 2001.

28. Ehrlich HP: Wound closure: Evidence of cooperation between fibroblasts and collagen matrix. Eye 2:149-157, 1988.

29. Colwell AS, Phan TT, Kong W, et al: Hypertrophic scar fibroblasts have increased connective tissue growth factor expression after transforming growth factor-beta stimulation. Plast Reconstr Surg 116:1387-1390, 2005.

30. Lu L, Saulis AS, Liu WR, et al: The temporal effects of anti–TGF-beta1, 2, and 3 monoclonal antibody on wound healing and hypertrophic scar formation. J Am Coll Surg 201:391-397, 2005.

31. Bayat A, Bock O, Mrowietz U, et al: Genetic susceptibility to keloid disease and hypertrophic scarring: Transforming growth factor beta1 common polymorphisms and plasma levels. Plast Reconstr Surg 111:535-546, 2003.

32. Ladwig GP, Robson MC, Liu R, et al: Ratios of activated matrix metalloproteinase-9 to tissue inhibitor of matrix metalloproteinase-1 in wound fluids are inversely correlated with healing of pressure ulcers. Wound Repair Regen 10:26-37, 2002.

33. Marjolin J-N: Ulce̊re. Dictionnaire de Medecine, vol 21, Pratique, 1828.

34. Robson MC, Heggers JP: Surgical infection. II. The beta-hemolytic streptococcus. J Surg Res 9:289-292, 1969.

35. Buchmiller-Crair TL, Kim CS, Won NH, et al: Effect of acute anemia on the healing of intestinal anastomoses in the rabbit. J Trauma 51:363-368, 2001.

36. Ashcroft GS, Horan MA, Herrick SE, et al: Age-related differences in the temporal and spatial regulation of matrix metalloproteinases (MMPs) in normal skin and acute cutaneous wounds of healthy humans. Cell Tissue Res 290:581-591, 1997.

37. Xia YP, Zhao Y, Tyrone JW, et al: Differential activation of migration by hypoxia in keratinocytes isolated from donors of increasing age: Implication for chronic wounds in the elderly. J Invest Dermatol 116:50-56, 2001.

38. Radi ZA, Khan NK: Effects of cyclooxygenase inhibition on bone, tendon, and ligament healing. Inflamm Res 54:358-366, 2005.

39. Dang C, Ting K, Soo C, et al: Fetal wound healing current perspectives. Clin Plast Surg 30:13-23, 2003.

40. Scheid A, Wenger RH, Christina H, et al: Hypoxia-regulated gene expression in fetal wound regeneration and adult wound repair. Pediatr Surg Int 16:232-236, 2000.

41. Peled ZM, Phelps ED, Updike DL, et al: Matrix metalloproteinases and the ontogeny of scarless repair: The other side of the wound healing balance. Plast Reconstr Surg 110:801-811, 2002.

42. Winter GD: Formation of the scab and the rate of epithelization of superficial wounds in the skin of the young domestic pig. Nature 193:293-294, 1962.

43. Salisbury RE, Bevin AG, Dingeldein GP, et al: A clinical and laboratory evaluation of a polyurethane foam: A new donor site dressing. Arch Surg 114:1188-1192, 1979.

44. Argenta LC, Morykwas MJ: Vacuum-assisted closure: A new method for wound control and treatment: Clinical experience. Ann Plast Surg 38:563-576; discussion 577, 1997.

45. Joseph E, Hamori CA, Bergman S, et al: A prospective randomized trial of vacuum-assisted closure versus standard therapy of chronic nonhealing wounds. Wounds 12:60-67, 2000.

46. Timmers MS, Le Cessie S, Banwell P, et al: The effects of varying degrees of pressure delivered by negative-pressure wound therapy on skin perfusion. Ann Plast Surg 55:665-671, 2005.

47. Chen SZ, Li J, Li XY, et al: Effects of vacuum-assisted closure on wound microcirculation: An experimental study. Asian J Surg 28:211-217, 2005.

48. Weed T, Ratliff C, Drake DB: Quantifying bacterial bioburden during negative pressure wound therapy: Does the wound VAC enhance bacterial clearance? Ann Plast Surg 52:276-279; discussion 279-280, 2004.

49. Obdeijn MC, de Lange MY, Lichtendahl DH, et al: Vacuum-assisted closure in the treatment of poststernotomy mediastinitis. Ann Thorac Surg 68:2358-2360, 1999.

50. Defranzo AJ, Argenta LC, Marks MW, et al: The use of vacuum-assisted closure therapy for the treatment of lower-extremity wounds with exposed bone. Plast Reconstr Surg 108:1184-1191, 2001.

51. Hart J, Silcock D, Gunnigle S, et al: The role of oxidised regenerated cellulose/collagen in wound repair: Effects in vitro on fibroblast biology and in vivo in a model of compromised healing. Int J Biochem Cell Biol 34:1557-1570, 2002.

52. Veves A, Sheehan P, Pham HT: A randomized, controlled trial of Promogran (a collagen/oxidized regenerated cellulose dressing) vs standard treatment in the management of diabetic foot ulcers. Arch Surg 137:822-827, 2002.

53. Badylak SF: Small intestinal submucosa (SIS): A biomaterial conducive to smart tissue remodeling. In Bell E (ed): Tissue Engineering: Current Perspectives. Cambridge, MA, Burkhauser, 1993, pp 179-189.

54. Park SN, Lee HJ, Lee KH, et al: Biological characterization of EDC-crosslinked collagen–hyaluronic acid matrix in dermal tissue restoration. Biomaterials 24:1631-1641, 2003.

55. Baier Leach J, Bivens KA, Patrick CW Jr, et al: Photocrosslinked hyaluronic acid hydrogels: Natural, biodegradable tissue engineering scaffolds. Biotechnol Bioeng 82:578-589, 2003.

CHAPTER 9

Regenerative Medicine

Derrick C. Wan, MD   Matthew D. Kwan, MD   and   Michael T. Longaker, MD, MBA

Stem Cell Sources
Stem Cell Applications in Regenerative Medicine
Conclusions and Future Outlook

For centuries, the debilitating effects of soft and hard tissue defects have plagued patients and surgeons alike, with removal of diseased tissue, including amputation, often being the only solution available. The advent of antibiotics, improved hygiene and diet, and a better understanding of several disease processes have all led to increased life expectancy, but the attendant need for tissue repair has become ever more prominent. Treatment of tissue loss and organ failure in an increasingly aging population already represents a significant biomedical burden, and as human longevity increases, these socioeconomic costs can only be expected to escalate.

Although current strategies have undoubtedly improved the quality of life for millions of patients, solutions such as artificial heart valves, joint prostheses, and arterial stents are not ideal given their limited durability. Even though the design and construction of new implants can incorporate the use of more lasting and biologically inert compounds, this often comes at the price of poor integration and biocompatibility. The principal challenge facing both clinicians and scientists, therefore, is the need to repair organ and tissue loss in a functional and lasting manner. Such a challenge can best be addressed through a shift in paradigm from one of tissue replacement to one of tissue regeneration.

The fundamental ineffectiveness of current synthetic implants to fully mimic the ability of living tissues to adapt and remodel in response to environmental cues is perhaps the single most important factor contributing to overall unsatisfactory results. Consequently, novel strategies must use more biologically active materials to better guide a regenerative response at the site of injury. Com-

bining these materials with competent cellular elements will allow the creation of tissue able to dynamically respond to the external environment while simultaneously meeting a functional demand. Such is the core premise of regenerative medicine, with restoration of defects achieved through the coalescence of tissue-specific building blocks, molecular and environmental cues, and biomimetic scaffolding. This regenerative strategy is in direct contradistinction to replacement by nonfunctioning fibrous scar tissue or poorly functional alloplastic materials prone to infection and mechanical failure.

With an increasingly aging population shifting patient demographics, the potential applications for regenerative medicine are rapidly burgeoning. Orthopedic joint replacement has proved to be one of the greatest triumphs in tissue replacement, with more than 500,000 hospital discharges for total hip or knee replacement in 2003 alone.[1] Despite dramatic improvements in quality of life, however, implant survival has been hampered by frictional damage and loosening of the prosthesis.[2] The development of a biologic bone and cartilaginous tissue regeneration scheme would thus undoubtedly assist in prolonging the durability of contemporary implants and perhaps eventually supplant current approaches for musculoskeletal repair/replacement. Craniofacial bone deficit, whether from trauma, tumor resection, or congenital malformations, may similarly benefit from regenerative strategies, with endogenous tissue engineering through distraction osteogenesis already being widely used clinically for the treatment of maxillary and mandibular hypoplasia. Finally, wide-ranging conditions such as coronary heart disease, diabetes, gastrointestinal disorders, and neurodegenerative disorders, whether from trauma or disease, may also be improved through the incorporation of modalities designed to promote regeneration. Importantly, the cornerstone in each of these strategies remains the careful selection of an optimal cell source from which to engineer living tissue. Establishment of an ideal cellular unit devoid of biologic and ethical concerns has thus been an active area of investigation over the past decade.

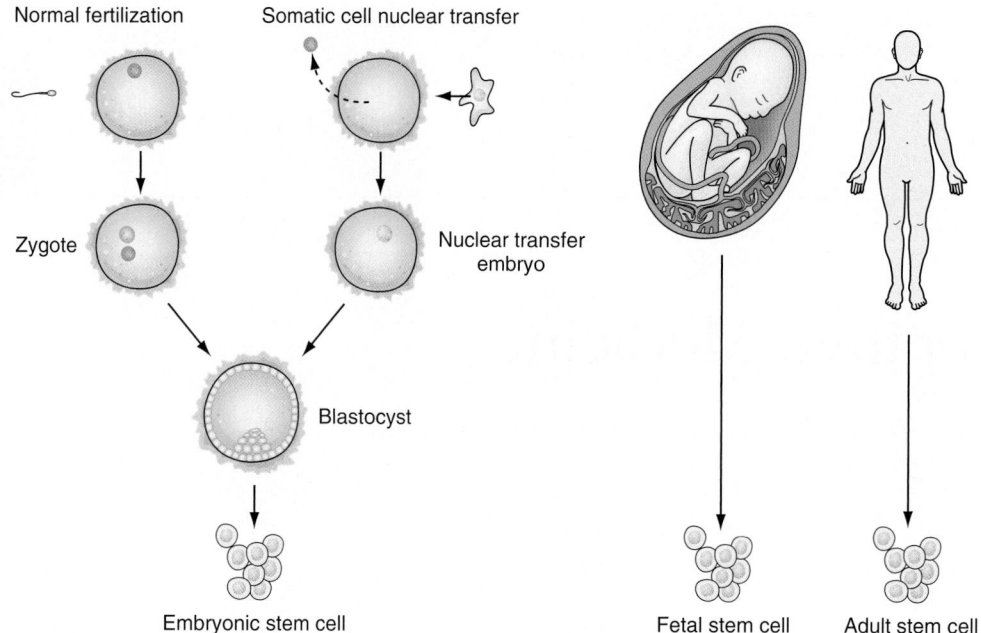

Figure 9-1 Derivation of stem cells through normal fertilization or nuclear transfer, as well as from fetal or adult sources.

Advancements in this field have and will continue to make an impact on management and options for surgical patients.

STEM CELL SOURCES

Contentious debate has surrounded the identification of a consummate cellular building block with which to base therapy for tissue repair. Irrespective of this controversy, however, the promise of regeneration through cell-based modalities has made this approach ever more appealing for the reconstruction of tissue defects. Current investigations involve the use of embryonic stem (ES) cells, genetically matched stem cell lines created through somatic cell nuclear transfer, fetal stem cells, and multipotent adult stem cells (Fig. 9-1).

Embryonic Stem Cells

ES cells are derived from totipotent cells of the early mammalian blastocyst that have the capacity to differentiate into a wide range of adult tissues from all three embryonic germ layers.[3] Isolation of a primate ES cell line was first described by Thomson and colleagues,[4,5] with subsequent work demonstrating the ability to identify similar cells in human embryos. After derivation, human ES cells can be maintained indefinitely on feeder layers composed of mitotically inactive murine embryonic fibroblasts. When cultured in suspension, these cells readily differentiate into multicellular aggregates resembling early postimplantation embryos.[6] Several studies investigating both mouse and human ES cells have demonstrated an in vitro capacity to form cardiomyocytes, hematopoietic progenitors, neurons, skeletal myocytes and smooth muscle cells, adipocytes, osteocytes, chondrocytes, endothelial cells, and pancreatic islet cells when cultured in specific growth factor conditions.[7-10] With the ability to generate a variety of postmitotic, terminally differentiated cell types, ES cells thus represent a potentially advantageous cell source for tissue regeneration.

Multiple limitations currently exist, however, with regard to the use of human ES cells in regenerative strategies. Aside from the significant political and ethical hurdles that have encumbered further investigations, concern has recently been raised over the acquisition of immunogenic, nonhuman sialic acid residues secondary to culture on mouse feeder cells.[11] Furthermore, although ES cells can differentiate in vitro into a multitude of adult cell types, their capacity for in vivo organogenesis has yet to be fully investigated. At this time, the limited number of lines available and the restrictions placed on scientific inquiry into human ES cells have generally precluded significant progress, thus raising the demand for alternative solutions.

Somatic Cell Nuclear Transfer

Although controversy surrounds the derivation of stem cells through somatic cell nuclear transfer, this modality still represents a promising means by which to generate genetically matched stem cell lines. Somatic cell nuclear transfer, also referred to as therapeutic cloning, involves the transfer of nuclei from postnatal cells into an enucleated ovum. Activation of the subsequent construct then generates a blastocyst from which ES cells can be derived.

Like other ES cells described earlier, products of somatic cell nuclear transfer are totipotent, with the capacity to give rise to products from all three germ layers. In addition, therapeutic cloning theoretically obviates the issues of nonself recognition and host immune responses to implanted tissues. However, in many ways similar to human ES cells, somatic cell nuclear transfer is currently embroiled in an ethically complex debate. The technical limitations of this procedure have also dampened early enthusiasm, with several studies reporting less than 10% efficiency in the derivation of nuclear transfer ES cells.[12]

Fetal Stem Cells

Though less prominently discussed, fetal stem cells represent another source for a regenerative building block with dramatic clinical potential. The identification of circulating mesenchymal stem/progenitor cells within first-trimester human fetuses has made possible the notion of in utero treatment with autologous cells.

Fetal stem cells comprise a population of adherent fibroblast-like cells, which can be found at a frequency of 8.2 per 1 million nucleated blood cells.[13] Although these cells have also been identified in fetal liver and bone marrow, in all cases, their frequency substantially declines with advancing gestational age.[13,14] Fetal stem cells have been found to expand in culture for at least 20 passages, and their capacity for adipogenic, osteogenic, and chondrogenic differentiation has been demonstrated under appropriate culture conditions. In addition, transplantation into a xenogeneic sheep model has shown the ability of these cells to engraft and undergo site-specific tissue differentiation.[14]

Despite these promising findings, however, significant debate has been raised over the issue of using cells from fetuses and the attendant risks associated with intrauterine procedures. Nonetheless, fetal stem cells may still provide a novel means by which future autogenous in utero cellular and genetic therapies can be devised.

Adult Stem Cells

The ability of many adult tissues to repair or regenerate has long hinted at the potential existence of stem or progenitor cell involvement. No more apparent has this been exemplified than in the liver. Although the hepatocyte represents the main functional element of the liver, in states of injury, studies have shown the ability of these cells to undergo clonal expansion.[15] Moreover, when agents have been used to impair the regenerative ability of hepatocytes, an alternative stem cell source of biliary origin has been identified. These oval cells possess bipotential capacity, with the ability to generate both new hepatocytes and biliary epithelia.[16] Similar to the liver, several studies have shown apparent stem cell involvement in pancreatic regeneration—including new islet formation—after partial pancreatectomy. In vitro manipulation of human pancreatic ductal cells has revealed the capacity to yield three-dimensional ductal cysts from which insulin-secreting endocrine cells have also been observed to arise.[17] This transduction may be regulated by the homeodomain transcription factor PDX-1, thus providing further support for a progenitor-like role of ductal cells in the pancreas.[18]

Recent doubt has been cast, however, on the true contribution of these cells to in vivo islet formation, with some reports suggesting that terminally differentiated beta cells retain the ability to regenerate.[19] Given the need for transplantable human islets, though, ductal tissue may still represent a potential source for glucose-responsive endocrine elements. Finally, in one of the most rigidly constructed systems of the body with minimal capacity for repair, stem cells have also been identified within specific areas of the brain. Cells isolated from the subventricular zone and hippocampus have been shown to clonally expand and differentiate in vitro into neurons, oligodendrocytes, and astrocytes.[20] Although these cells are generally incapable of mending most neurologic damage, future strategies may be developed for the use of these progenitors to enhance regenerative efforts.

In contrast to these adult stem cells, which have been found to primarily propagate cells found only within the tissue of origin, significant work has defined greater multipotency for other elements. These studies have focused on mesenchymal stem cells (MSCs) found within the stromal fraction of adult bone marrow. Using aspirates from more than 350 human donors, Pittenger and colleagues were able to demonstrate lineage-specific in vitro differentiation of these bone marrow–derived MSCs into fat, cartilage, and bone under appropriate culture conditions.[21] Furthermore, these cells exhibited the ability to clonally proliferate while maintaining a stable undifferentiated phenotype, thus making them a provocative cell source for potential tissue-engineering applications.[21] However, although great promise surrounds the use of bone marrow–derived MSCs in regenerative medicine, much of the excitement has been curbed by several limiting factors. With a frequency estimated to be as low as 1 in 27,000 nucleated cells harvested, large volumes of bone marrow aspirate are commonly necessary to obtain enough usable MSCs.[22] Given the painful nature of this procedure, general or spinal anesthesia may be necessary. In addition, concern over donor age–associated changes in cellular biology has left bone marrow–derived MSCs a potentially suboptimal solution for a large segment of the population.[23]

As an alternative to stem cells harvested from bone marrow, MSCs have also been identified within the stromal fraction of postnatal adipose tissue.[24] Unlike their bone marrow counterpart, adipose-derived mesenchymal cells (AMCs) represent a more readily accessible, expandable building block for tissue engineering. Procurement of adipose tissue through lipoaspiration is subject to less whole blood contamination than seen with bone marrow, thereby significantly raising the yield of harvested AMCs.[25] This ability for large-volume procurement has made AMCs particularly well suited for regenerative strategies. From a biologic perspective, mesenchymal cells obtained from fat demonstrate similar growth kinetics and gene transduction capacity as those derived from marrow stroma.[22] Characterization of these cells by Zuk and associates[24] has suggested AMCs to be true multipotent stem cells capable of lineage-specific differentiation. In the presence of various induction factors, tissues, including fat, cartilage, muscle, and bone, have all been shown to

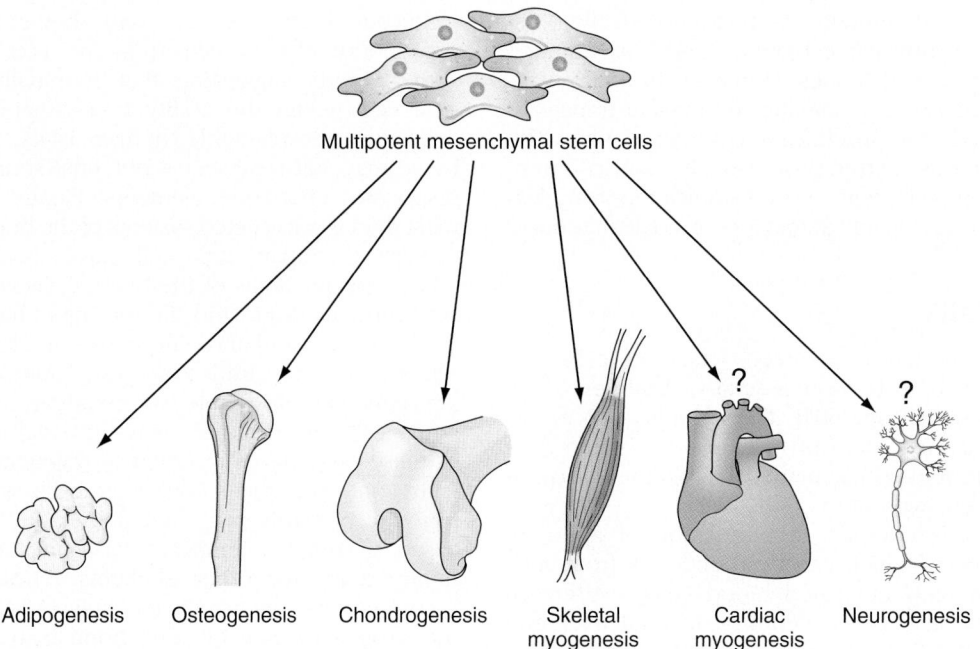

Figure 9-2 Adult multipotent mesenchymal stem cells have the capacity to undergo adipogenesis, osteogenesis, chondrogenesis, and skeletal myogenesis. In addition, they may potentially contribute to cardiac myogenesis and neurogenesis.

form. In view of the relative abundance and ease by which AMCs can be obtained, the design of future therapeutic approaches incorporating fat-derived MSCs may be particularly desirable.

STEM CELL APPLICATIONS IN REGENERATIVE MEDICINE

Over the past century, dramatic advancements have been made in almost every aspect of medicine, including the treatment of extensive soft and hard tissue defects. Several regenerative modalities, including distraction osteogenesis, bone morphogenetic protein therapy, and microsurgical nerve repair, have already been used, with proven success, to enhance both cosmetic and functional outcomes. By combining recent developments in molecular biology, organogenesis, and material sciences with the strong tissue engineering potential of stem cells, however, new strategies have begun to evolve that offer even better results. In particular, the use of adult multipotent MSCs has increasingly proved valuable in a variety of clinical settings, given their ready availability and unfettered ethical status (Fig. 9-2). Such current and future regenerative treatment options will undoubtedly expand the surgeon's armamentarium to more effectively address problematic conditions associated with complex tissue defects.

Adipogenesis

The need for soft tissue augmentation has long been a challenging problem in both reconstructive and cosmetic surgery. Correction of traumatic and postablative defects,

hemifacial microsomia, and Romberg's hemifacial atrophy all collectively represent only a small segment of the many clinical situations requiring both skeletal reconstruction and significant soft tissue repair. Although current techniques of fat grafting—including harvest, processing, and transplantation—continue to evolve, the ability to use autogenous cells precisely contoured for soft tissue reconstruction has increasingly become a reality. Both bone marrow–derived MSCs and AMCs have been shown to undergo in vitro adipogenic differentiation in the presence of insulin and other specific induction factors.[21,24]

Recent studies have exploited this capacity to promote in vivo adipogenesis as well. A variety of vehicles, including natural collagen and synthetic poly(lactic-co-glycolic acid) scaffolds, have been used to deliver predifferentiated human or mouse AMCs for the purpose of inducing ectopic formation of fat.[26] Importantly, however, most studies to date have generally agreed on the need for a period of in vitro priming before implantation for the induction of significant adipogenesis. Nonetheless, the ability to engineer constructs to precise shape and volume specifications makes this approach particularly valuable for the reestablishment of contour in both reconstructive and aesthetic cases. Ongoing studies will begin to identify more optimal scaffolds capable of promoting both cell proliferation and subsequent adipogenic differentiation, thereby obviating the need for a period of ex vivo culture.

Osteogenesis

For decades, autologous bone grafting and vascularized free flaps represented the most effective means by which surgeons could reconstruct large skeletal defects. Studies in regenerative medicine, however, have introduced a variety of novel modalities, many of which may ultimately prove superior to contemporary approaches. First described by Codivilla in 1905 and later consolidated by Ilizarov,[27] distraction osteogenesis has revolutionized the treatment of bony hypoplasia or deficiencies in both the craniofacial and appendicular skeleton. By the gradual separation of osteogenic fronts, distraction osteogenesis represents a powerful form of endogenous tissue engineering to promote the deposition of mineralized bone in the intervening gap. Clinical application of this technique has led to the evolution of new methods for limb salvage and more favorable results in the treatment of several midface and mandibular deficiencies.

In similar fashion, the discovery of bone morphogenetic proteins by Marshall Urist[28] has also led to the development of new strategies for bone tissue engineering, with particular benefits seen in promoting fracture healing and spinal fusion. Despite the enormous potential of these modalities for the generation of de novo bone, however, the need for skeletal repair after trauma or resection often cannot be met by current strategies alone. With the demonstration that adult multipotent MSCs have osteogenic capacity, recent studies have begun to explore the delivery of these cells to sites in need of bone regeneration.

The ability of bone marrow– and adipose tissue–derived MSCs to give rise to osteoblasts has been demonstrated by several groups. Under certain culture conditions, these cells have been shown to express markers associated with an osteoblast phenotype, including runx2/cbfa1, alkaline phosphatase, collagen I, osteopontin, and osteocalcin.[21,24] Furthermore, a variety of in vitro assays have shown both bone marrow–derived MSCs and AMCs to readily form mineralized matrix.[21,24] Multiple investigators have also explored the capacity of MSCs to promote bone formation in vivo. AMCs have been shown to regenerate critical-sized calvarial defects by 8 to 12 weeks in mice when delivered on an apatite-coated poly(lactic-co-glycolic acid) scaffold.[29] In addition, when human-derived AMCs are seeded on various osteoinductive or osteoconductive vehicles, significant osteogenesis has been noted after subcutaneous implantation into immunodeficient mice.[30] Importantly, these findings have already proved to be particularly germane from a clinical standpoint, given the multitude of case reports already demonstrating their translational utility.

In the setting of long bone distraction, injection of MSCs into the callus was found to potentially shorten the overall treatment period in three patients through acceleration of bone regeneration.[31] Likewise, AMCs, in combination with bone chips harvested from the iliac crest, have been used to repair a large post-traumatic calvarial defect in a 7-year-old child.[32] Collectively, these studies engender significant enthusiasm for the use of MSCs in the repair of skeletal defects. In settings in which guided distraction and cytokine therapy are incapable of generating the necessary bone, novel methods using stem cell–based modalities may very well become the gold standard.

Chondrogenesis

Few options currently exist that offer durable treatment results for the repair of articular cartilage defects. Limited success has been noted with periosteal, perichondral, or osteochondral autografts, with potential complications ranging from surface incongruity to donor site morbidity and insufficient stability when mechanically loaded.[33] Furthermore, in sites of diffuse disease secondary to osteoarthritis, inflammatory arthropathy, or avascular necrosis, many of these modalities are generally contraindicated.[33] As an alternative, autogenous chondrocyte implantation has become increasingly popular for the treatment of cartilaginous defects since its clinical introduction in 1994.[34] This technique involves the harvest of normal hyaline cartilage and ex vivo expansion of chondrocytes before reimplantation in suspension or on a scaffold. Animal models using this method have demonstrated over 88% of cartilaginous defects to be filled by reparative tissue.[35] Less than 50% of this tissue, however, was observed to be true hyaline cartilage, and on mechanical testing, compressive stiffness was far below that of native articular cartilage.[35] In addition, with a density of 30 million cells/mL generally used clinically for implantation, the amount of harvested cartilage necessary to generate these numbers can be far from trivial.[33] Given the attendant donor site morbidity and suboptimal results currently reported with autologous chondrocyte implantation, further refinement of this technique is therefore necessary.

Investigations with adult multipotent MSCs have furnished a potential cellular surrogate, thereby obviating the need for the acquisition of normal cartilage. Culturing either bone marrow–derived MSCs or AMCs in high-density micromass environments, several studies have demonstrated large amounts of in vitro cartilage-related extracellular matrix protein production, including aggregan, proteoglycans, and collagen II and IV.[21,24,36] Furthermore, by juxtaposing chondrogenically and osteogenically differentiated murine MSCs in culture, osteochondral constructs have been fabricated within a hydrogel scaffold.[37] Subcutaneous implantation resulted in two stratified, yet integrated layers of cartilaginous and osseous tissue, histologically resembling an articular condyle.[37] Though still biomechanically inferior to healthy, intact tissue, engineered cartilage from MSCs nevertheless harbors several advantages over autologous chondrocyte implantation. Most significantly, the use of a far more abundant cell source such as AMCs may allow the potential for a single-stage procedure, thereby eliminating the need for multiple arthrotomies and disruption of otherwise normal cartilage.[33] These findings therefore highlight the dramatic potential for the use of MSCs in cartilage tissue engineering. Future studies will continue to elucidate the molecular mechanisms behind stem cell chondrogenesis in an effort to more efficiently regenerate both articular and nonarticular cartilage with optimal site-specific biomechanical profiles.

Skeletal Myogenesis

Functional impairment has generally ensued from muscular injuries and defects after resection or trauma. A more comprehensive understanding of mechanics, however, has led to the development of several strategies to restore mobility, including muscular transposition and microvascular muscle grafts. Although these techniques have immeasurably enhanced the quality of life for many, such procedures inevitably come at the cost of some loss of function at the site of muscle harvest.

Recent advances in regenerative medicine have enabled a more elegant approach to the need for muscle repair, with multiple studies demonstrating a myogenic potential for adult multipotent MSCs. In vitro culture of these cells with dexamethasone and hydrocortisone has been shown to induce the expression of key regulatory factors for muscle differentiation, including MyoD1 and myogenin, as well as late markers of differentiation such as myosin heavy chain.[21,24] Animal studies have also shown both bone marrow–derived MSCs and AMCs to actively participate in muscle repair under various conditions.[38,39] In one of the most compelling studies, Bacou and colleagues[38] reported that autotransplantation of rabbit AMCs into damaged tibialis anterior muscles could promote significant muscle regeneration. Functional studies revealed heavier muscles with larger cross-sectional area and greater contractile force generation.[38] Collectively, these studies all point to the emerging utility of stem cells in muscle repair. Although investigations demonstrating true clinical translation are still lacking, such findings continue to drive prudent optimism in this field.

Cardiac Myogenesis

Cardiovascular disease remains one of the leading causes of morbidity and mortality and accounts for almost 30% of deaths annually in the United States.[40] Current treatment paradigms have focused on the preservation of injured myocardium, with pharmacologic therapy and revascularization representing the most effective instruments to accomplish this aim. In recent years, reports of mesenchymal cell transdifferentiation along a cardiomyogenic lineage have incited a considerable amount of investigation regarding their potential application in postinfarct myocardial regeneration. Adult MSCs harvested from both bone marrow and fat have been shown to be capable of in vitro formation of cardiac myocytes when cultured in the presence of 5-azacytidine.[41] Subsequent studies by Orlic and associates[42] in which they evaluated direct injection of bone marrow–derived MSCs into the myocardial ischemic border zone after ligation of the left anterior descending artery in mice revealed potential myocardial repair, with 68% of the infarct region composed of new donor cell–derived myocardium 9 days after implantation. A number of subsequent reports have cast doubt on these findings, however, with Balsam and colleagues[43] demonstrating only transient engraftment at best.

Interestingly, although few donor bone marrow cells were identified at the site of infarct 30 days after initial transplantation, functional studies revealed preservation of left ventricular contractility and protection against myocardial remodeling.[43] Similar findings have been noted in clinical trials using either intracoronary or intramyocardial delivery of autologous bone marrow–derived MSCs in patients after acute myocardial infarction.[44] Although no demonstration of true engraftment was shown in any of these studies, left ventricular ejection fraction and myocardial tissue perfusion were observed to increase.[44] Speculation about how MSCs may enhance recovery has recently centered on alternative mechanisms, including augmentation of blood flow to ischemic tissue, regulation of inflammation, reduction of cardiac myocyte apoptosis, and recruitment of local endogenous stem cells already residing within the myocardium.[45] Therefore, even though MSCs may not directly contribute to myocardial regeneration after infarction, their delivery to sites of injury may still be of functional benefit to patients.

Neurogenesis

Attempts at nerve regeneration have been described for more than 400 years, with a variety of materials such as fat sheaths, bone, and gauze all being unsuccessfully used.[46] Advances in microsurgery and interfascicular nerve grafting represented a quantum leap in the repair of peripheral nerve lesions, and these techniques still remain the treatment of choice in multiple clinical settings.[47] Although favorable results can be achieved with various contemporary conduits, nerve transfers, nerve grafts, or any combination of these techniques, the ingress of stem cell research into this field has provided prospects for even better outcomes.

Similar to cardiac myogenesis, the ability of MSCs to undergo differentiation along a nonmesenchymal neuronal lineage has been demonstrated by several groups.[24,48] In vitro culture of bone marrow–derived MSCs or AMCs with β-mercaptoethanol has been shown to result in rapid assumption of neuronal morphology with the expression of nestin, neuron-specific enolase, and neuron-specific protein, all markers of early neural differentiation.[48] Importantly, however, studies have yet to describe the expression of more definitive neuronal markers by these cells. Nonetheless, several groups have already evaluated the ability of these cells to promote neural regeneration in animal models of cerebral ischemia.

Recent reports have demonstrated improved sensorimotor function after the implantation of human MSCs (either bone marrow or fat derived) into sites of cortical ischemia in rats.[49] Histologic analysis revealed these gains to be associated with some evidence of astrocytic, oligodendrocytic, and neuronal differentiation by transplanted stem cells, but in all cases, evidence supporting incorporation of these cells into the native cerebral architecture was notably absent. Akin to the functional improvements engendered by injection of MSCs into injured myocardium, indirect mechanisms have thus been proffered to account for the observed neurologic recovery. Implanted cells may elaborate angiogenic or antiapoptotic factors that help promote the survival of compromised tissue or stimulate resident neural stem cells to undergo differentiation and participation in repair.[50] In such a capacity, MSCs may emerge as an invaluable tool in the development of future treatment strategies for both central and peripheral neurologic disease.

CONCLUSIONS AND FUTURE OUTLOOK

Regenerative approaches to the treatment of disease could revolutionize nearly every aspect of surgery by allowing the development of tissue repair strategies with considerable promise. Research into the myriad of imaginable applications for multipotent stem cells has supplanted more antiquated paradigms focused on replacement of damaged tissue alone. Many obstacles still exist, however, between current studies and their translation into clinical practice. The political and ethical debate surrounding ES cells and somatic nuclear transfer will undoubtedly continue to fetter the use of these cells in regenerative strategies. As a consequence, therapeutic modalities using cellular elements will probably embrace adult multipotent mesenchymal cells for the reconstruction of tissue defects.

Further work must also be performed to define modes of delivery and optimal conditions for site-specific growth and differentiation. Finally, the mechanisms involved in the development of stem cells into solid-organ tissue remain poorly understood. Despite these concerns, clinical studies into the benefits of stem cell therapy continue, and it is this translational research that will ultimately bridge extraordinary potential with the development of practicable treatment strategies. Undoubtedly, surgeon-investigators will play critical roles in the development, implementation, and translation of these discoveries to new applications for the treatment of surgical patients.

Selected References

Balsam LB, Wagers AJ, Christensen JL, et al: Haematopoietic stem cells adopt mature haematopoietic fates in ischaemic myocardium. Nature 428:668-673, 2004.

Balsam and colleagues provide evidence that adult bone marrow cells, whether delivered exogenously or circulating endogenously, do not contribute significantly to myocardial regeneration in mice.

Beltrami AP, Barlucchi L, Torella D, et al: Adult cardiac stem cells are multipotent and support myocardial regeneration. Cell 114:763-776, 2003.

Beltrami and colleagues present data describing a stem cell population among cardiac cells and challenge the idea that the heart is a terminally differentiated organ. In a rat model of myocardial infarction, they were able to demonstrate myocardial regeneration and improved cardiac function after local injection of these cells.

Campagnoli C, Roberts IA, Kumar S, et al: Identification of mesenchymal stem/progenitor cells in human first-trimester fetal blood, liver, and bone marrow. Blood 98:2396-2402, 2001.

Campagnoli and colleagues document the presence of multipotent cell populations within human fetal blood, liver, and bone marrow. These multipotent cells could be induced to differentiate along adipogenic, osteogenic, and chondrogenic lineages.

Cowan CM, Shi YY, Aalami OO, et al: Adipose-derived adult stromal cells heal critical-size mouse calvarial defects. Nat Biotechnol 22:560-567, 2004.

Cowan and coworkers report on the in vivo capability of stromal cells from mouse adipose tissue, seeded on apatite-coated, poly(lactic-co-glycolic acid) scaffolds, to differentiate into bone and heal calvarial defects. Mesenchymal cells derived from adipose tissue reossified calvarial defects with the same efficacy as bone marrow mesenchymal cells did. By chromosomal detection, the implanted cells were found to make up 84% to 99% of the new bone.

Dezawa M, Kanno H, Hoshino M, et al: Specific induction of neuronal cells from bone marrow stromal cells and application for autologous transplantation. J Clin Invest 113:1701-1710, 2004.

This paper demonstrates that human and rat bone marrow mesenchymal stem cells have the capability of differentiating into cells with the electrophysiologic and biochemical properties of neurons. Dezawa and colleagues report increased induction efficiency after transfecting mesenchymal stem cells with the intracellular domain of Notch. Transplantation of these cells into the striatum of rats with a model of Parkinson's disease led to improved motor control on functional testing.

Erickson GR, Gimble JM, Franklin DM, et al: Chondrogenic potential of adipose tissue–derived stromal cells in vitro and in vivo. Biochem Biophys Res Commun 290:763-769, 2002.

Erickson and colleagues document the ability of adipose-derived stromal cells to differentiate along a chondrogenic lineage in vitro and to form cartilage matrix molecules when implanted subcutaneously in nude mice.

Pittenger MF, Mackay AM, Beck SC, et al: Multilineage potential of adult human mesenchymal stem cells. Science 284:143-147, 1999.

Pittenger and associates report on the capability of clonal lines of mesenchymal cells isolated from adult human bone marrow to differentiate along adipogenic, chondrogenic, and osteogenic lineages with the proper cues.

Thomson JA, Itskovitz-Eldor J, Shapiro SS, et al: Embryonic stem cell lines derived from human blastocysts. Science 282:1145-1147, 1998.

This paper was the first to describe an embryonic cell line derived from human blastocysts. Thomson and colleagues described the ability of these cell lines to remain undifferentiated while proliferating, yet retain the ability to differentiate into tissues of endodermal, mesodermal, and ectodermal origin.

Zuk PA, Zhu M, Ashjian P, et al: Human adipose tissue is a source of multipotent stem cells. Mol Biol Cell 13:4279-4295, 2002.

This paper describes a multipotent population isolated from the stromal component of adipose tissue. Zuk and associates demonstrated the capability of clonal isolates from this population to be induced along osteogenic, adipogenic, myogenic, and chondrogenic lineages. They also showed that this population of cells from adipose tissue expressed CD marker antigens similar to those of mesenchymal stem cells.

References

1. Steiner C, Elixhauser A, Schnaier J: The healthcare cost and utilization project: An overview. Eff Clin Pract 5:143-151, 2002.
2. Bajs ID, Saric V, Opalic M: Investigation of hip joint prosthesis damage. Coll Antropol 25:263-268, 2001.

3. Odorico JS, Kaufman DS, Thomson JA: Multilineage differentiation from human embryonic stem cell lines. Stem Cells 19:193-204, 2001.

4. Thomson JA, Kalishman J, Golos TG, et al: Isolation of a primate embryonic stem cell line. Proc Natl Acad Sci U S A 92:7844-7848, 1995.

5. Thomson JA, Itskovitz-Eldor J, Shapiro SS, et al: Embryonic stem cell lines derived from human blastocysts. Science 282:1145-1147, 1998.

6. Itskovitz-Eldor J, Schuldiner M, Karsenti D, et al: Differentiation of human embryonic stem cells into embryoid bodies compromising the three embryonic germ layers. Mol Med 6:88-95, 2000.

7. Rohwedel J, Maltsev V, Bober E, et al: Muscle cell differentiation of embryonic stem cells reflects myogenesis in vivo: Developmentally regulated expression of myogenic determination genes and functional expression of ionic currents. Dev Biol 164:87-101, 1994.

8. Poliard A, Nifuji A, Lamblin D, et al: Controlled conversion of an immortalized mesodermal progenitor cell towards osteogenic, chondrogenic, or adipogenic pathways. J Cell Biol 130:1461-1472, 1995.

9. Bain G, Kitchens D, Yao M, et al: Embryonic stem cells express neuronal properties in vitro. Dev Biol 168:342-357, 1995.

10. Wang Y, Yates F, Naveiras O, et al: Embryonic stem cell–derived hematopoietic stem cells. Proc Natl Acad Sci U S A 102:19081-19086, 2005.

11. Martin MJ, Muotri A, Gage F, Varki A: Human embryonic stem cells express an immunogenic nonhuman sialic acid. Nat Med 11:228-232, 2005.

12. Perry AC: Progress in human somatic-cell nuclear transfer. N Engl J Med 353:87-88, 2005.

13. Campagnoli C, Roberts IA, Kumar S, et al: Identification of mesenchymal stem/progenitor cells in human first-trimester fetal blood, liver, and bone marrow. Blood 98:2396-2402, 2001.

14. Gotherstrom C, Ringden O, Tammik C, et al: Immunologic properties of human fetal mesenchymal stem cells. Am J Obstet Gynecol 190:239-245, 2004.

15. Overturf K, al-Dhalimy M, Ou CN, et al: Serial transplantation reveals the stem-cell–like regenerative potential of adult mouse hepatocytes. Am J Pathol 151:1273-1280, 1997.

16. Alison M: Liver stem cells: A two compartment system. Curr Opin Cell Biol 10:710-715, 1998.

17. Bonner-Weir S, Taneja M, Weir GC, et al: In vitro cultivation of human islets from expanded ductal tissue. Proc Natl Acad Sci U S A 97:7999-8004, 2000.

18. Noguchi H, Kaneto H, Weir GC, Bonner-Weir S: PDX-1 protein containing its own antennapedia-like protein transduction domain can transduce pancreatic duct and islet cells. Diabetes 52:1732-1737, 2003.

19. Dor Y, Brown J, Martinez OI, Melton DA: Adult pancreatic beta-cells are formed by self-duplication rather than stem-cell differentiation. Nature 429:41-46, 2004.

20. Reynolds BA, Weiss S: Generation of neurons and astrocytes from isolated cells of the adult mammalian central nervous system. Science 255:1707-1710, 1992.

21. Pittenger MF, Mackay AM, Beck SC, et al: Multilineage potential of adult human mesenchymal stem cells. Science 284:143-147, 1999.

22. De Ugarte DA, Morizono K, Elbarbary A, et al: Comparison of multi-lineage cells from human adipose tissue and bone marrow. Cells Tissues Organs 174:101-109, 2003.

23. Stenderup K, Justesen J, Clausen C, Kassem M: Aging is associated with decreased maximal life span and accelerated senescence of bone marrow stromal cells. Bone 33:919-926, 2003.

24. Zuk PA, Zhu M, Ashjian P, et al: Human adipose tissue is a source of multipotent stem cells. Mol Biol Cell 13:4279-4295, 2002.

25. Batinic D, Marusic M, Pavletic Z, et al: Relationship between differing volumes of bone marrow aspirates and their cellular composition. Bone Marrow Transplant 6:103-107, 1990.

26. Patrick CW Jr, Chauvin PB, Hobley J, Reece GP: Preadipocyte seeded PLGA scaffolds for adipose tissue engineering. Tissue Eng 5:139-151, 1999.

27. Ilizarov GA: The tension-stress effect on the genesis and growth of tissues. Part I. The influence of stability of fixation and soft-tissue preservation. Clin Orthop Relat Res 238:249-281, 1989.

28. Urist MR: Bone: Formation by autoinduction. Science 150:893-899, 1965.

29. Cowan CM, Shi YY, Aalami OO, et al: Adipose-derived adult stromal cells heal critical-size mouse calvarial defects. Nat Biotechnol 22:560-567, 2004.

30. Hicok KC, Du Laney TV, Zhou YS, et al: Human adipose-derived adult stem cells produce osteoid in vivo. Tissue Eng 10:371-380, 2004.

31. Kitoh H, Kitakoji T, Tsuchiya H, et al: Transplantation of marrow-derived mesenchymal stem cells and platelet-rich plasma during distraction osteogenesis—a preliminary result of three cases. Bone 35:892-898, 2004.

32. Lendeckel S, Jodicke A, Christophis P, et al: Autologous stem cells (adipose) and fibrin glue used to treat widespread traumatic calvarial defects: Case report. J Craniomaxillofac Surg 32:370-373, 2004.

33. Alford JW, Cole BJ: Cartilage restoration, part 1: Basic science, historical perspective, patient evaluation, and treatment options. Am J Sports Med 33:295-306, 2005.

34. Brittberg M, Lindahl A, Nilsson A, et al: Treatment of deep cartilage defects in the knee with autologous chondrocyte transplantation. N Engl J Med 331:889-895, 1994.

35. Lee CR, Grodzinsky AJ, Hsu HP, Spector M: Effects of a cultured autologous chondrocyte-seeded type II collagen scaffold on the healing of a chondral defect in a canine model. J Orthop Res 21:272-281, 2003.

36. Erickson GR, Gimble JM, Franklin DM, et al: Chondrogenic potential of adipose tissue–derived stromal cells in vitro and in vivo. Biochem Biophys Res Commun 290:763-769, 2002.

37. Alhadlaq A, Mao JJ: Tissue-engineered osteochondral constructs in the shape of an articular condyle. J Bone Joint Surg Am 87:936-944, 2005.

38. Bacou F, el Andalousi RB, Daussin PA, et al: Transplantation of adipose tissue–derived stromal cells increases mass and functional capacity of damaged skeletal muscle. Cell Transplant 13:103-111, 2004.

39. Ferrari G, Cusella-De Angelis G, Coletta M, et al: Muscle regeneration by bone marrow–derived myogenic progenitors. Science 279:1528-1530, 1998.

40. Kochanek KD, Murphy SL, Anderson RN, Scott C: Deaths: Final data for 2002. Natl Vital Stat Rep 53(5):1-115, 2004.

41. Makino S, Fukuda K, Miyoshi S, et al: Cardiomyocytes can be generated from marrow stromal cells in vitro. J Clin Invest 103:697-705, 1999.

42. Orlic D, Kajstura J, Chimenti S, et al: Bone marrow cells regenerate infarcted myocardium. Nature 410:701-705, 2001.

43. Balsam LB, Wagers AJ, Christensen JL, et al: Haematopoietic stem cells adopt mature haematopoietic fates in ischaemic myocardium. Nature 428:668-673, 2004.

44. Wollert KC, Meyer GP, Lotz J, et al: Intracoronary autologous bone-marrow cell transfer after myocardial infarction: The BOOST randomised controlled clinical trial. Lancet 364:141-148, 2004.

45. Beltrami AP, Barlucchi L, Torella D, et al: Adult cardiac stem cells are multipotent and support myocardial regeneration. Cell 114:763-776, 2003.

46. Evans GR: Approaches to tissue engineered peripheral nerve. Clin Plast Surg 30:559-563, viii, 2003.

47. Klug CN, Millesi-Schobel GA, Millesi W, et al: Preprosthetic vertical distraction osteogenesis of the mandible using an L-shaped osteotomy and titanium membranes for guided bone regeneration. J Oral Maxillofac Surg 59:1302-1308; discussion 1309-1310, 2001.

48. Dezawa M, Kanno H, Hoshino M, et al: Specific induction of neuronal cells from bone marrow stromal cells and application for autologous transplantation. J Clin Invest 113:1701-1710, 2004.

49. Kang SK, Lee DH, Bae YC, et al: Improvement of neurological deficits by intracerebral transplantation of human adipose tissue–derived stromal cells after cerebral ischemia in rats. Exp Neurol 183:355-366, 2003.

50. Li Y, Chen J, Chen XG, et al: Human marrow stromal cell therapy for stroke in rat: Neurotrophins and functional recovery. Neurology 59:514-523, 2002.

Critical Assessment of Surgical Outcomes

Samuel R. G. Finlayson, MD, MPH   and   John D. Birkmeyer, MD

Two Main Applications of Outcomes Research
Data Sources
Is the Study Valid?
Is the Study Focusing on the Right Outcome Measure?
Is the Intervention Cost-Effective?
Critical Assessment of Studies of Surgical Quality

Studies assessing outcomes and quality of surgical care have become ubiquitous in the medical literature, and a wide range of research tools and methodologies collectively known as *outcomes research* have been used.[1] Outcome studies take many forms. In addition to more traditional prospective clinical studies, surgical journals now publish an increasing number of population-based studies derived from administrative data and clinical registries that are designed to assess and improve quality of care. Methodologically, outcomes research also applies an ever-broadening range of quality-of-life measures and economic end points. Some focus on evaluating the effectiveness of a clinical intervention, whereas others focus on quality of care or broader policy issues.

Despite the increasing popularity of outcome studies, the quality of this research is highly variable. Many studies have limited validity because they fail to adequately account for the role of chance, bias, or confounding or because their findings cannot be generalized to other settings. Other surgical outcome studies fail to use the most appropriate outcome measures or fail to consider clinical benefits in the context of cost-effectiveness. To judge the usefulness of published studies, surgeons must consider these basic issues.

In this chapter we provide a framework for critical assessment of surgical outcome studies. In the process

we describe many of the common methodologies and data sources used by outcomes researchers and illustrate, when appropriate, their strengths and weaknesses.

TWO MAIN APPLICATIONS OF OUTCOMES RESEARCH

No perfect taxonomy has been devised for categorizing the very heterogeneous field of outcomes research. Instead, we consider the field according to its two main applications: study of the effectiveness of a clinical intervention and assessment of quality of care.

Studies Assessing the Effectiveness of a Clinical Intervention

The most prevalent surgical outcome studies are aimed at making inferences about the effectiveness of a clinical intervention. In this context, evaluation of a clinical intervention may imply assessment of an existing procedure (e.g., surgery versus medical therapy in patients with carotid stenosis), modification of an existing procedure (e.g., open versus laparoscopic appendectomy), or adjunctive surgical care (e.g., prophylactic perioperative antibiotics versus no antibiotics). Each case, however, involves an explicit (or sometimes implicit) comparison between two or more interventions.

A variety of different study designs are used in making such comparisons (Table 10-1). Many consider the gold standard to be the randomized controlled trial (RCT), in which patients are assigned in prospective, random fashion to treatment and control groups. By ensuring that patients are as similar as possible between comparisons groups, RCTs minimize the risk that observed differences in outcomes are attributable to other factors (confounding). Cohort studies, which are observational

Table 10-1   **Common Types of Studies Used to Assess the Effectiveness of Interventions**

STUDY TYPE	DESCRIPTION	STRENGTHS	WEAKNESSES	EXAMPLE: DOES FUNDOPLICATION SURGERY PREVENT BARRETT'S ESOPHAGUS IN PATIENTS WITH GERD?
Case series	Measure outcomes of an intervention in a single case or in a series of cases	Simple, inexpensive	No comparison group	Perform surgery on patients with GERD and measure the proportion progressing to Barrett's esophagus
Case-control study	Identify subjects with and without the outcome of interest and then look back in time to find factors that might predict the difference in outcome	Useful for studying rare outcomes; relatively inexpensive; retrospective, therefore no prolonged follow-up	Potential sampling bias, as well as bias measuring predictors; limited to one outcome variable	Identify a group of patients with GERD and Barrett's esophagus and a group with GERD but without Barrett's esophagus to compare the proportion in each group who have previously undergone surgery
Cohort study Retrospective	Select a population to study and then measure predictor variables and outcomes by *looking back in time*	Inexpensive, events already happened and just need to be analyzed	Less control over selection of subjects and measurement of variables, limited to using existing data	Select population of patients with GERD and look back over time to discover whether those who underwent surgery are less likely to have Barrett's esophagus
Prospective	Select a population to study and then measure predictor variables and outcomes by *monitoring the subjects over time*	More control over selection of subjects and measurement of variables	Expensive, requires prolonged follow-up	Select a population of patients with GERD but not Barrett's esophagus and monitor them through time to discover whether those who undergo surgery are less likely to progress to Barrett's esophagus
Randomized controlled trial	Randomly assign patients to different interventions and then compare outcomes	Avoids confounding; strongest evidence for cause and effect	Patients may not be willing to randomize, relatively expensive, difficult to study rare outcomes	Randomize patients with GERD to surgical or nonsurgical treatment and compare proportions in each group who progress to Barrett's esophagus

GERD, gastroesophageal reflux disease.

in nature, are much more common, however. They may be either prospective (study and research questions established before data are collected and analyzed) or retrospective. With cohort studies, investigators use a variety of control groups for their comparisons. These groups may include patients with the same clinical condition who are not undergoing the treatment of interest during the study period (concurrent controls) or similar patients from an earlier period (historical controls). Many studies (i.e., case series) lack explicit control groups and instead make inferences based on contrasts between their findings and the results of previously published studies.

Studies Assessing Quality of Care

An increasing number of surgical outcome studies focus on assessing the quality of surgical care. Such studies are inherently observational in nature. They often involve direct comparisons across individual hospitals or surgeons, for example, variation in mortality rates after coronary artery bypass graft surgery across New York State hospitals.[2] Others involve comparisons in which providers are aggregated according to specific characteristics. Common examples include studies examining the effects of procedure volume or surgeon specialty on patient outcomes.[3,4]

More recently, clinical registries and studies designed to assess and improve the quality of surgical care have garnered increased attention. Among the best known of the clinical registries is the National Surgical Quality Improvement Program (NSQIP), which was initially administered solely in the Veterans Administration but has now been implemented in many private sector hospitals through an alliance with the American College of Surgeons.[5] Although efforts such as the NSQIP are designed to provide a comprehensive view of surgical quality, other data collection efforts focus on quality as reflected in specific dimensions of care, such as compliance with recommended practices known to be associated with better outcomes.[6]

DATA SOURCES

A variety of data sources are used in outcome studies assessing the effectiveness of a clinical intervention. Many studies rely exclusively on clinical data from a single institution or a small number of selected institutions. For studies assessing quality of care, however, large data sets involving large numbers of patients and providers are required. These are typically either large clinical registries or administrative data sets. Understanding the advantages and disadvantages of these data sources is crucial for critically assessing a surgical outcome study.

Clinical Registries

Large clinical registries contain medical information collected for purposes of research or quality improvement, or both. Clinical registries are occasionally population based (capture all patients in a defined geographic region), such as cardiac surgery registries maintained by state departments of health in New York or California. In other instances, clinical registries capture all patients within a defined health care system or consortium, such as the NSQIP. Some clinical registries are voluntary in nature, with data captured from participating members of professional societies or other groups. For example, in the outcomes initiative managed by the Society of American Gastrointestinal and Endoscopic Surgeons (SAGES), participating surgeons submit data on outcomes of their laparoscopic cases. The level of clinical detail captured in various clinical registries varies widely.

Administrative Data

A large number of studies focusing on the quality of surgical care rely on administrative data—clinical and nonclinical information collected for purposes other than research (most often billing). Large, administrative databases are produced and maintained by the federal and state government, as well as many private health payers and providers (Box 10-1).

Most studies using administrative data to examine surgical outcomes rely on hospital discharge abstract files, although more recently some limited ambulatory surgical administrative databases have become available.[7] By far the most frequently used administrative data sets are from

---

Box 10-1   Administrative Databases Commonly Used for Surgical Outcomes Research

National Level

Medicare population (Center for Medicare and Medicaid Services files)
  MEDPAR and Inpatient files (hospital discharge abstracts for acute care hospitalizations)
  Part B file (contains claims for all physicians services based on CPT codes)
  Provider files (information about characteristics of physicians participating in the Medicare program)
Health Care Utilization Project (Agency for Healthcare Quality and Research)
  Nationwide Inpatient Sample (all-payer database containing hospital discharge abstracts from a large number of states)
  Analogous files pertaining to ambulatory surgery, emergency care, and pediatrics
Department of Veterans Affairs
  Patient Treatment File (use and outcomes of inpatient services)
  Outpatient File
Vital and Health Statistics Databases
  National Death Index (collates death certificate information from all 50 states)

State Level

Medicaid management system
State hospital discharge or ambulatory surgery databases (all-payer databases maintained by most but not all states)
Birth and death certificate data

Private/Proprietary Databases

Large insurer databases, e.g., Blue Cross/Blue Shield
Provider network, managed care organization databases (content and availability vary widely)

CPT, Current Procedural Terminology; MEDPAR, medical provider analysis and review.

---

national Medicare files or samples of state-level files (e.g., Nationwide Inpatient Sample). Within each of the databases based on discharge abstracts, a uniform set of information is collected for every patient experiencing an acute care hospitalization. Because hospitalization is required for inclusion in discharge data sets, these files are generally useful only for studying surgical procedures with (at least) overnight hospital stays. Data collected for each hospital discharge abstract includes demographic information—age, sex, race/ethnicity, and patient residence. Administrative data include admission and discharge dates, total charges and amount reimbursed, expected payment source, admission type (elective, urgent, emergency), and discharge disposition (including vital status).

Based on their Unique Physician Identification Numbers (UPINs), attending physicians and operating physicians are also identified. Hospital discharge abstracts contain codes and dates for at least nine diagnoses reflecting the reason for admission or surgery (principal diagnosis), preexisting conditions (secondary diagnoses), and complications occurring during hospitalization. They

Table 10-2   Critical Assessment of Surgical Outcome Studies

QUESTIONS TO ASK	THINGS TO WATCH FOR
Are the conclusions valid? Chance—could the findings be simply "luck of the draw?"	Use of appropriate statistical tests for studies reporting "significant" effects (i.e., to avoid type I errors) Adequate sample sizes for studies reporting no effect (i.e., to rule out type II errors)
Bias—were there systematic errors in how study subjects were selected or assessed?	Process of selecting study subjects that does not distort treatment outcomes across comparison groups (i.e., selection bias) Process of collecting outcomes information or other data that does not favor one of the comparison groups (i.e., information bias)
Confounding—could findings be explained by other differences in patient groups?	Comparison groups similar in their baseline risks and likelihood of experiencing outcomes (independent of intervention) Risk factors adequately measured and accounted for with appropriate risk adjustment techniques Observed differences in outcomes large enough to rule out important confounding by unmeasured risk factors
Generalizability (external validity)—can the findings be extrapolated to general clinical practice?	Study population or providers representative enough to reflect outcomes in the "real world"
Is the study focusing on the right outcome measure?	Use of primary outcome measure that reflects the most important outcome from a clinical and/or patient perspective Appropriate instruments used to capture general health status, disease-specific quality of life, or patient preferences
Is the intervention cost-effective?	Benefits of the intervention sufficiently large to justify its cost (relative to other commonly accepted clinical practices)

also contain fields for the principal and other procedures (at least five). Both diagnoses and procedures are classified by codes from the *International Classification of Diseases, Ninth Revision, Clinical Modification* (ICD-9-CM).

There are distinct trade-offs associated with using administrative data for clinical research.[8-12] Among the advantages, administrative databases contain large amounts of longitudinal data already collected for other purposes, which makes these data relatively inexpensive to obtain. They tend to be very accurate for identifying patients undergoing surgical interventions and for assessing so-called hard end points (e.g., mortality). Many administrative databases are very large (which ensures that studies have adequate power) and contain information about a wide range of surgical conditions and interventions. Patient-level files can be linked to databases containing information about characteristics of hospitals and surgeons, which is ideal for studying issues related to health care delivery and quality. Because they are generally population based and often national in scope, administrative databases are often the only way to study surgical outcomes in the real world (i.e., effectiveness rather than efficacy).

However, several pitfalls are associated with using administrative data for clinical research. Most are related to the relative lack of specificity of the clinical information contained in these files. ICD-9-CM codes can be very imprecise, with heterogeneous clinical conditions (or procedures) often aggregated under a single code. They do not adequately account for severity (e.g., mild stable angina or end-stage ischemic heart disease). There is

wide variability in coding practices across hospitals and a generally tendency to undercode clinical diagnoses, particularly preexisting conditions. Such problems in coding and coding accuracy create obvious limitations in the ability to perform risk adjustment, which is particularly relevant in studies focusing on quality of care. For example, in a study of quality of surgical care among hospitals in the Veterans Administration, mortality prediction models constructed from administrative data were understandably weaker than models based on prospectively collected clinical data from the NSQIP.[13]

Finally, administrative data lack specificity about the timing of clinical events and are thus limited in their ability to distinguish between preexisting conditions and surgical complications. Thus, administrative data are not well suited to assessing nonfatal outcomes of surgical interventions.

IS THE STUDY VALID?

Despite the heterogeneity of published studies, critical readers must consider several basic questions as they make inferences from studies assessing the effectiveness of a clinical intervention or quality of care (Table 10-2). The first question is most fundamental to clinical research: Is the study valid? Validity reflects the degree to which an observed association (e.g., between a given intervention and outcome) cannot be attributed to alternative explanations. Factors that can lead to erroneous inferences include *chance* (luck of the draw), *bias* (there is a systematic error in how study subjects were selected or assessed), and

Table 10-3 Simple Overview of Statistical Tests for Evaluating the Role of Chance in Studies Comparing Outcome Data of Different Types

TYPE OF OUTCOME DATA BEING COMPARED	COMMON STATISTICAL APPROACH/TEST	EXAMPLE
Proportions		
Unadjusted	Chi-square test (Fisher exact test if small number of observations)	Compare proportions of smokers and nonsmokers who contract lung cancer
Risk adjusted	Logistic regression	Compare proportions of smokers and nonsmokers who contract lung cancer after adjusting for age, race, and gender
Means		
Within individuals	Paired t-test	Compare mean hemoglobin A_{1c} levels in diabetic patients before and after pancreas transplantation
Between groups	Unpaired t-test	Compare mean hemoglobin A_{1c} levels between diabetic patients with a transplanted pancreas and diabetic patients without a transplanted pancreas
Risk adjusted	Linear regression	Compare hemoglobin A_{1c} levels as above after adjusting for age, race, and gender
Survival Time		
Unadjusted	Life table analysis or Kaplan-Meier plots	Compare 3-year survival with cryosurgery versus radiofrequency ablation for hepatoma
Risk adjusted	Cox proportional hazards	Compare 3-year survival as above after adjusting for age, race, and gender

confounding (the findings are due to other differences in patient groups). These three potential sources of error are generally considered criteria for internal validity. External validity refers to *generalizability*—the extent to which findings from a given study can be generalized to other patient populations and settings.

Chance

In clinical research, inference involves making a generalization about a larger group (or universe) of patients based on observations from a smaller subset or sample. Whenever inferences are based on samples, there is always the possibility that the results could be inaccurate because of chance alone. For studies comparing outcomes across groups, there are two types of chance-related error: type I and type II. Each is best defined relative to the *null hypothesis*—the assumption that there is no difference in outcomes between comparison groups. With type I errors, the null hypothesis is erroneously rejected; that is, outcomes are asserted to differ by group when in reality they are equivalent. With type II errors, the null hypothesis is erroneously accepted; that is, the outcomes are asserted to be equivalent when they are really different.

Type I Errors

Although type I errors (also called α errors) can occur with any study, they are particularly prevalent in those involving multiple comparisons, for example, studies comparing operative mortality rates across a very large number of hospitals or surgeons. In such cases it is virtually certain that some providers will be outliers (good or bad) by chance alone.

The likelihood of a type I error is quantified by statistical testing. A P value reflects the probability that the dif-

ferences seen between groups would be observed by chance alone, under the assumption that the comparison groups are truly equivalent (the null hypothesis). Thus, a P value of .05, the conventional threshold for statistical significance, signifies that the likelihood of observing differences of at least that magnitude by chance alone is 5 out of 100. Confidence intervals (e.g., 95% CIs), an alternative to P values, reflect the degree of statistical imprecision by bracketing the observed difference between groups in a range of values that might be expected if the same study were repeated an infinite number of times.

A variety of statistical tests can be used to calculate both P values and confidence intervals. Tests are generally selected according to the following criteria (Table 10-3):

1. How many groups are being compared?
2. Is one group being compared with different groups, or is a single group being compared with itself after an intervention or event?
3. Is risk adjustment required?
4. What kind of numerical data are being analyzed (e.g., continuous versus categorical)?

Although a detailed discussion about choosing the appropriate test is beyond the scope of this chapter, Glantz's *Primer on Biostatistics* is a useful text.[14]

Type II Errors

Type II errors occur when studies erroneously conclude no difference in outcomes between comparison groups when such a difference really does exist. A large proportion of surgical studies lack sufficient sample size to detect small but clinically important benefits of a clinical intervention.[15] When the sample size in a study is too small to detect a meaningful difference in outcomes, the study can be said to lack sufficient statistical power. Type II errors are also prevalent in studies assessing quality of care. Detecting small but clinically meaningful differences in outcomes (e.g., a 1% versus 2% stroke rate with carotid endarterectomy) requires thousands of patients, sample sizes often available only with administrative data. Type II errors are best avoided by assessing statistical power before conducting the study to ensure that a sufficient number of patients are enrolled in the study. Type II errors cannot be addressed in any way by statistical testing after the study is complete.

Bias

Bias refers to any systematic error in a clinical study that results in an incorrect estimate of differences in outcomes between comparison groups. Bias reflects problems with the design and conduct of the study, not with how the analysis is performed once the data are collected. There are two general categories of bias:

1. *Selection bias* (errors arising from the process of choosing study populations)
2. *Information bias* (errors related to the process of ascertaining outcomes and other pertinent data)

Selection bias can occur whenever the manner in which study subjects are identified influences the likelihood of the outcome of interest (independent of the treatment being studied). For example, consider a hypothetic cohort study at a single academic center in which the effectiveness of antireflux surgery is assessed by comparing long-term quality of life in medical and surgical patients with gastroesophageal reflux disease. If the medical arm consisted of patients identified from a gastroenterology clinic, the study might be preferentially including patients most bothered by their reflux (enough to seek care by a specialist).

Selection bias, usually at the provider level, can also occur in studies focusing on quality of care. This is a particular problem for databases that do not include outcomes for all patients and providers from a defined population (i.e., are not population based). For example, in clinical registries based on voluntary participation, surgeons with better than average outcomes may be more predisposed to share their data than other surgeons.

Information bias refers to a broad category of problems that arise from the process by which information about outcomes is collected. For example, bias can be introduced by the technique used to ascertain outcomes. Consider the same study (described earlier) of outcomes after medical and surgical therapy for gastroesophageal reflux. Patients might respond one way to their surgeon about their satisfaction with surgery but another way to an anonymous survey. For studies assessing the effectiveness of a clinical intervention, information bias is best avoided by prospective studies with standardized outcome definitions and, when possible, by blinded assessment of treatment outcomes.

Information bias can occur even with hard end points. For example, consider a study comparing hospital mortality rates after a given procedure, with in-hospital death used to reflect operative mortality. In this case, in-hospital mortality rates would be biased with regard to length of stay (LOS), which varies widely by hospital. Hospitals with relatively short LOS would be predisposed to fewer in-hospital deaths; those with longer LOS would be biased toward higher observed mortality. This type of information bias would be avoided by the use of a uniform outcome measure (e.g., 30-day mortality).

Confounding

Confounding occurs when outcomes differ because of differences in the baseline risks of the comparison groups (often as a result of selection bias). Consider a hypothetic study comparing mortality rates between open and laparoscopic cholecystectomy. Although laparoscopy may have an independent (protective) effect on mortality, it is also true that patients undergoing open cholecystectomy are more likely to have acute cholecystitis and, independent of the surgical approach, are more likely to die after surgery than patients without this condition. Thus, disease severity (acute cholecystitis) confounds the observed relationship between treatment choice and outcome. Of course, confounding can also occur in studies assessing quality of care: some hospitals may have higher mortality rates because their patients are sicker at the outset.

Confounding is optimally addressed by randomized controlled clinical trials—randomization ensures that potentially confounding patient characteristics are equally distributed between the study groups. Restricting patient eligibility criteria is another study design option, for example, restricting the study sample, as in the earlier example, to patients with acute cholecystitis. Although randomization or restriction may be feasible for prospective studies assessing the effectiveness of an intervention, these approaches are rarely feasible for studies focusing on quality of care, which are inherently observational in nature.

For these reasons, outcome studies most commonly deal with potential confounding by using analytic techniques collectively known as risk adjustment. Risk adjustment refers to a variety of statistical approaches used to control for patient mix. Typically, potentially confounding patient characteristics are entered as independent variables into multivariable regression equations that best predict the outcome of interest. For studies focusing on quality of care (e.g., mortality), these equations adjust observed mortality rates according to the average baseline risk of patients treated by each provider—downward for providers caring for sicker than average patients, upward for providers with healthier patients. There is a large body of literature addressing various issues related to risk adjustment in studies investigating quality of care.[16-18] In general, the statistical approach is less important than the completeness and quality of data used for risk adjustment.

Critical readers must be able to assess the adequacy of risk adjustment and, equally important, whether risk adjustment is important in the first place. To address these issues, surgeons should ask the follow questions:

How Reliably Are the Important Risk Factors Measured?

In studies based on clinical data, information collected about patient characteristics (potential confounders) is generally accurate. Thus, the main question about clinical registries is their completeness. Administrative databases reliably capture some important predictors of surgical outcomes, such as patient age and procedure type. However, such data are particularly limited in their ability to reflect surgical indication and procedure acuity (elective versus emergency). In addition, preexisting comorbid conditions (e.g., diabetes, coronary artery disease) tend to be underreported, frequently misclassified, and often difficult to distinguish from postoperative complications.[19-21]

Do Important Risk Factors Vary Between Comparison Groups

Regardless of the strength of its relationship with the outcome measure or how well it is measured, a variable can be an important confounder only if it varies across comparison groups. For measured risk factors, this question can be addressed directly by comparing the distribution of patient characteristics (or predicted mortality rates) across providers. For unmeasured variables, surgeons must consider the a priori likelihood that the case mix varies between comparison groups.

How Large Are the Observed Outcome Differences?

Finally, in judging the likelihood of confounding, surgeons should consider the magnitude of reported differences in outcomes across comparison groups. In practice, differences in patient mix can readily explain small differences in outcomes (e.g., 4% versus 5% mortality rates with lower extremity bypass in high- and low-volume hospitals).[22] However, confounding would be a very implausible explanation for large differences (e.g., 4% versus 16% mortality rates with pancreatic resection in high- and low-volume hospitals).

Generalizability

In any surgical outcome study, observations from a specific study population are used to make broader inferences about effectiveness or quality in the broader population of patients or providers. Thus, it is important to judge the extent to which a study's findings can be safely generalized to other settings.

In assessing generalizability, critical readers should first focus on the patients. In many studies, the study subjects do not adequately represent patients from the general population. Patients who volunteer for clinical trials are often more motivated and thus tend to have better outcomes than other patients do. Study populations may also do better for more obvious reasons. In the Asymptomatic Carotid Artery Stenosis (ACAS) trial,[23] for example, study patients were substantially younger and healthier than most patients undergoing carotid end-

arterectomy. As a result, their risk for perioperative mortality (0.1%) was considerably lower than that observed in other patients at the same centers and in the general population.[24] Because the net benefit of carotid endarterectomy was ultimately relatively small in this trial, even small differences in procedure-related risks could dramatically alter conclusions about the effectiveness of this procedure.

In considering generalizability, it is also important to focus on the providers and the care that patients are receiving, particularly in studies focusing on quality of care. Clinical trials generally imply careful, standardized protocols for patient selection, operative and perioperative care, and follow-up, often very different from the variable care that patients receive in real-world clinical practice. For obvious reasons, many surgical outcome studies are conducted at large academic centers. Outcomes at these centers tend to be systematically better than those achieved in the real world. For example, hospitals participating in the ACAS trial had markedly lower mortality rates than other U.S. hospitals did.[24] Although some of this difference was attributable to hospital procedure volume, ACAS hospitals also had lower mortality rates than other high-volume hospitals did. Thus, the special attributes of study populations or providers can sometimes make it unsafe to extrapolate the findings of a study to the general population.

IS THE STUDY FOCUSING ON THE RIGHT OUTCOME MEASURE?

Clinical research in surgery has traditionally focused on intermediate outcomes (biologic or physiologic measures) and clinical end points (mortality or specific complications). Physiologic measures are useful for exploring the mechanisms underlying an intervention's effectiveness and for improving the precision and statistical power of a study. For example, in assessing the effectiveness of peripheral arterial stenting, a study focusing on ankle-brachial indices, a continuous measure obtained in all patients, would have much more power than one centered on limb amputations, which occur much less commonly. Clinical end points also have the advantage of being discrete and generally simple to measure.

Despite these strengths, however, intermediate outcomes and clinical end points may not always correlate with what matters to patients. Thus, these measures may not reflect the relative success of interventions aimed at improving quality of life. For example, 24-hour pH probe results or mortality rates will provide a very incomplete picture of the effectiveness of laparoscopic fundoplication in patients with gastroesophageal reflux.

For this reason, surgical outcome studies rely on a heterogeneous collection of instruments and techniques for assessing outcomes important to patients, so-called patient-centered outcomes. These surgical outcomes measures can be grouped according to five different aspects of health-related quality of life: general health status, disease-specific symptom scores, pain, utilities, and satisfaction (Table 10-4).

Table 10-4 Common Measures of Health Status and Health-Related Quality of Life

MEASURE	DEFINITION	MOST COMMON ASSESSMENT TOOLS
General health status	Overall health status, assessed as a composite of broad domains of physical and mental health	Previously developed and validated survey instruments (e.g., MOS SF-36, Activities of Daily Living scale)
Disease-specific symptoms	Effect of specific condition on health and quality of life	Symptom scores using either off-the-shelf or project-specific survey instruments
Pain	Component of health status particularly relevant in assessing outcomes of surgery	Visual analog scale
Utilities	Quantitative expressions of patient preferences for a particular state of health, important for decision analysis and cost-effectiveness analysis	Visual analog scale, time trade-off, standard gamble
Satisfaction	What patients think about the health care or intervention itself	Survey with Likert-style questions

MOS SF-36, 36-question Medical Outcomes Study Short-Form survey

General Health Status

General health status, which is most commonly assessed with survey instruments, is the broadest measure of health-related quality of life. Several well-tested and well-known health status surveys are used widely in clinical research. Though beyond the scope of this chapter, detailed summaries and critiques of these instruments are available elsewhere.[25]

Among the best known general health surveys is the Medical Outcomes Study Short-Form survey, which consists of 36 questions (SF-36) or, in its abridged version, 12 questions.[26,27] We describe it here in more detail because it has become a standard tool for assessing baseline health status or outcomes (or both) in clinical trials involving surgical interventions. The 36 questions are distributed across eight health domains—physical functioning (10 questions), role limitations (4), bodily pain (2), general health (5), emotional functioning (4), social functioning (2), role limitations because of emotional problems (3), and mental health (5)—and a single item on perceptions of health changes over the past 12 months. Typical questions take the following form: "In general, would you say your health is excellent, very good, good, fair, or poor?" In scoring the SF-36, "subscale" scores are calculated for each of the eight domains and rolled up to create separate summary scores for physical and mental function. Scores are transformed to a linear, 100-point scale by using population-based weights (mean score, 50).

Many surgical outcome studies focus on patient disability, a component of general health status. The most widely used scale to measure activities of daily living is the Activities of Daily Living scale developed by Katz.[28] Designed primarily for elderly or institutionalized patients, it summarizes the degree of independence in bathing, dressing, using the toilet, moving around the house, continence, and eating. Each function is rated on a three-point scale ranging from complete dependence to independence. The survey is scored according to the number of functions associated with dependence.

Disease-Specific Symptom Scores

Although general health status surveys have the advantage of generalizability and broadly capture the implications of a given disease on overall health, they often lack the sensitivity and precision necessary to assess clinically meaningful changes in how patients experience a single clinical condition. For example, in a trial of therapy for gastroesophageal reflux disease, heartburn symptoms that are very bothersome to patients may not be sufficient to produce large effects on overall health-related quality of life as measured by the SF-36.

For this reason, many surgical outcome studies apply instruments that measure symptoms and quality of life specific to the clinical condition under study. A large number of symptom classification scores have been developed and widely tested for various clinical conditions.[25]

Pain

Pain, whether disease or procedure related, is an essential outcome measure in many surgical studies. Most studies rely on instruments that assess pain in a summary (or global) sense. Among the most commonly used methods for measuring pain is the visual analog scale, in which patients mark a continuous 10-cm line with "no pain" on one end and "worst pain" on the other. Some survey instruments assess pain in multiple dimensions.[29]

Utilities

Utilities, or quantitative expressions of patient preferences for a particular state of health, are most commonly used in the context of decision analysis and cost-effectiveness analysis (described later in this chapter). Although both reflect quality of life, utilities should be distinguished from measures of health status described earlier in this chapter, which generally describe how patients are affected by a given clinical condition, what they can and cannot do, and so forth. Instead, utilities reflect how patients feel about or value living in a specific state of health.[30] Techniques for assessing utilities, which are usually measured on a scale from 0 (death or worst health imaginable) to 1 (best health), include the visual analog scale, the time trade-off, and standard gamble methods.

Satisfaction

Patient satisfaction surveys assess what patients think about the health care or intervention itself, not its effects on an underlying disease process. In general terms, patient satisfaction surveys ask patients to judge their actual care against their underlying expectations. Most surgical outcome studies rely on relatively simple instruments, often based on Likert-style questions (e.g., How satisfied were you with your surgical procedure: not at all, somewhat satisfied, satisfied, or very satisfied?). Studies focusing on patient satisfaction as a primary outcome often use surveys that assess satisfaction in multiple dimensions.[31,32]

IS THE INTERVENTION COST-EFFECTIVE?

As resources available for health care become increasingly constrained, accepting a new intervention as standard practice requires more than scientific evidence of its effectiveness. Unless the intervention is cost-effective, limited health care dollars may be better spent elsewhere.

Cost-effectiveness analysis is a systematic approach to assessing whether an intervention provides sufficient bang for the buck. It is appropriate only for assessing interventions that produce benefit at some additional cost. It is not useful for interventions that are (1) not effective (which should not be adopted regardless of cost) or (2) both effective and cost saving (which should always be adopted).

The cost-effectiveness of a medical intervention is determined as the ratio of its net costs to its net benefits. Net costs are determined by comparing the direct and indirect costs associated with the intervention versus those associated with treating the same condition without it (i.e., current practice). Net benefits, which are assessed in similar fashion, are usually expressed in terms of quality-adjusted life years (QALYs) A QALY is a composite measure reflecting both quality and quantity of life and is obtained by multiplying the length of time spent in a given health state by its associated utility. For example, 15 years of life with a stroke (average utility, hypothetically 0.5) would be equivalent to 7.5 QALYs. Although cost-effectiveness analyses are becoming increasingly common components of prospective clinical

Table 10-5 League Table of Selected Cost-Effectiveness Analyses of Interest to Surgeons

INTERVENTION	COST-EFFECTIVENESS (DOLLARS PER QALY)*
Primary closure of contaminated appendectomy wound versus delayed primary or secondary closure with a perforated or gangrenous appendicitis	Cost saving
Endoscopic surveillance with esophagectomy for high-grade dysplasia versus endoscopic surveillance with esophagectomy for cancer in Barrett's esophagus	Cost saving
Total hip arthroplasty versus no surgery for osteoarthritis	Cost saving
Carotid endarterectomy versus medical management for asymptomatic patients with >60% internal carotid stenosis	$8300
Coronary artery bypass grafting versus medical therapy for a male with 3-vessel disease and normal ventricular function	$13,000
Breast-conserving surgery versus modified radical mastectomy in women with stage I and II breast cancer	$21,000
Elective surgical repair of asymptomatic, unruptured intracranial aneurysms versus expectant management	$26,000
Heart transplantation versus optimal conventional treatment	$46,000
Biennial breast cancer screening from age 40 versus biennial screening from age 50	$70,000
Ursodiol versus elective cholecystectomy for symptomatic gallstones	$77,000
Lithotripsy versus cholecystectomy for symptomatic gallstones	$84,000
Simultaneous pancreas-kidney transplantation versus kidney transplantation alone in type 1 diabetics with end-stage renal disease	$280,000
Prostate biopsy versus no biopsy in men with abnormally high prostate-specific antigen levels but low cancer probabilities	Dominated
Shunt surgery versus propranolol in cirrhotic patients with nonbleeding esophageal varices	Dominated

*"Cost saving" indicates that the intervention costs less and is more effective than the alternative. "Dominated" indicates that the intervention costs more and is less effective.

QALY, quality-adjusted life year.

From Chapman RH, Stone PW, Sandberg EA, et al: A comprehensive league table of cost-utility ratios and a sub-table of 'panel-worthy' studies. Med Decis Making 20:451-467, 2000.

trials, cost-effectiveness analysis is most frequently conducted with decision analysis models that simulate costs and benefits in hypothetic cohorts of patients.[33]

Cost-effectiveness ratios are only interpretable in relative terms. Although there is considerable disagreement about where to set the bar, interventions that cost less than $50,000 to $100,000 per QALY saved are generally considered cost-effective. For comparative purposes, Table 10-5 lists estimates of cost-effectiveness for several common surgical procedures.

CRITICAL ASSESSMENT OF STUDIES OF SURGICAL QUALITY

In recent years, studies of surgical quality have increased both in number and in level of attention. This is explained not only by the proliferation of registries and quality improvement consortiums but also by heightened interest in quality seen among health care payers, the federal government, and consumers.[34,35] Unlike much of outcomes research that is limited to the realm of assessing specific clinical interventions, studies of surgical quality often focus on specific providers of care and carry implications that might potentially influence surgical market share, referral patterns, and institutional accreditation. Because of the many competing interests in play and the far-reaching policy implications that studies of surgical quality can bring to bear, objective critical assessment of these studies can be as challenging as it is important.

Research and reporting in the area of surgical quality typically rely on methods and data sources similar to those of other types of outcome studies and are therefore subject to similar potential weaknesses, including chance, bias, and confounding. However, among studies that attempt to compare overall surgical quality across providers, statistical power is of particular concern.

As noted previously, statistical power depends on adequate sample size. Because the unit of analysis in studies of surgical quality is usually the provider, sample sizes are generally limited by providers' surgical volume. Studies assessing quality of care across providers are therefore particularly susceptible to type II errors. This limitation is greatest when the outcomes being measured are relatively rare events (e.g., surgical mortality).[36]

Because risk adjustment has the effect of further dampening statistical power, its use in studies of surgical quality can hamper efforts to show differences across providers of surgical care, even when sample sizes are relatively large. When the surgical care being studied is broad based (i.e., heterogeneous populations and procedures), risk adjustment is particularly limiting because of the extent to which it must be used. When providers not only care for different patient populations but also provide different types of surgical services, comparisons of outcomes require adjustment for both patient mix and procedure mix. Under these circumstances, there is greater risk of failing to identify providers of surgical care who perform better or worse than their peers.

Efforts to study quality of surgical care continue to evolve in the face of ongoing challenges. For example, the NSQIP, which was once limited to assessment of the surgical care of veterans, has been adapted and validated for use in broader populations in the private sector.[37] Other developments, such as the cooperative involvement of payers, are likely to move this important field forward by bringing greater resources to bear.[38] In view of the growth and the broad implications of these efforts, the surgeon's ability to knowledgeably and critically assess studies of surgical quality is becoming increasingly important.

Selected References

Birkmeyer JD: Using administrative data for clinical research. In Souba WW, Wilmore DW (eds): Surgical Research. San Diego, CA, Academic Press, 2002, pp 127-136.

This chapter provides a broad overview of administrative databases used for clinical research, as well as a description of the potential pitfalls associated with their use.

Dimick JB, Welch HG, Birkmeyer JD: Surgical mortality as an indicator of hospital mortality: The problem with small sample size. JAMA 292:847-851, 2004.

This journal article clearly and convincingly illustrates the statistical pitfalls of trying to use mortality rates to identify hospitals of better or worse quality.

Glantz SA: Primer of Biostatistics. New York, McGraw-Hill, 2002.

This popular primer introduces the fundamentals of biostatistics, uses many examples from the medical literature, and is written in a manner that is both enjoyable and accessible to the uninitiated.

Gold M, Siegel JE, Russell LB, Weinstein MC: Cost-effectiveness in Health and Medicine. New York, Oxford University Press, 1996.

This concise and highly readable book was written by a panel of experts charged by the U.S. Public Health Service with the task of creating guidelines for the appropriate conduct of cost-effectiveness analysis.

Iezzoni LI: The risks of risk adjustment. JAMA 278:1600-1607, 1997.

This paper examines the history and current practices of risk adjustment with particular reference to the implications for quality assessment across hospitals.

McDowell I, Newell C: Measuring Health: A Guide to Rating Scales and Questionnaires. New York, Oxford University Press, 1996.

This book describes in detail a wide variety of patient-based surveys and other health measurement instruments that are commonly used in clinical outcomes research.

Torrance GW: Utility approach to measuring health-related quality of life. J Chronic Dis 40:593-603, 1987.

This landmark article describes the rationale and use of utility assessment, a technique that measures the so-called bottom line of health from the patients' perspective: how patients feel about or value living in a specific health state.

Ware JE Jr, Snow KK, Kosinski M, et al: SF-36 Health Survey: Manual and Interpretation Guide. Boston, The Health Institute, New England Medical Center, 1993.

This publication describes in detail the most ubiquitous and widely accepted general health assessment tool—the Medical Outcome Study SF-36—along with an overview of health dimension scores and their interpretation.

References

1. Birkmeyer JD: Outcomes research and surgeons. Surgery 124:477-483, 1998.
2. Hannan EL, Kilburn H Jr, O'Donnell JF, et al: Adult open heart surgery in New York State. An analysis of risk factors and hospital mortality rates. JAMA 264:2768-2774, 1990.
3. Begg CB, Cramer LD, Hoskins WJ, Brennan MF: Impact of hospital volume on operative mortality for major cancer surgery. JAMA 280:1747-1751, 1998.
4. Porter GA, Soskolne CL, Yakimets WW, Newman SC: Surgeon-related factors and outcome in rectal cancer. Ann Surg 227:157-167, 1998.
5. Khuri SF: The NSQIP: A new frontier in surgery. Surgery 138:837-842, 2005.
6. Flum DR, Fisher N, Thompson J, et al: Washington State's approach to variability in surgical processes/outcomes: Surgical Clinical Outcomes Assessment Program (SCOAP). Surgery 138:821-828, 2005.
7. Centers for Disease Control National Center for Health Statistics (February 2, 2005). National Survey of Ambulatory Surgery Description. Available from http://www.cdc.gov/nchs/about/major/hdasd/nsasdes.htm. Retrieved April 15, 2006.
8. Birkmeyer JD: Using administrative data for clinical research. In Souba WW, Wilmore DW (eds): Surgical Research. San Diego, CA, Academic Press, 2002, pp 127-136.
9. Iezzoni LI: Assessing quality using administrative data. Ann Intern Med 127:666-674, 1997.
10. Paul JE, Weis K, Epstein RA: Data bases for variations research. Med Care 31:S96-S102, 1993.
11. Mitchell JB, Bubolz T, Paul JE, et al: Using Medicare claims for outcomes research. Med Care 32:S38-S51, 1994.
12. Epstein MH: Guest alliance: Uses of state-level hospital discharge databases. J Am Health Inform Manage Assoc 63:32-39, 1992.
13. Gordon HS, Johnson ML, Wray NP, et al: Mortality after noncardiac surgery: Prediction from administrative versus clinical data. Med Care 43:159-167, 2005.
14. Glantz SA: Primer of Biostatistics. New York, McGraw-Hill, 2002.
15. Dimick JB, Diener-West M, Lipsett PA: Negative results of randomized clinical trials published in the surgical literature: Equivalency or error? Arch Surg 136:796-800, 2001.
16. Iezzoni LI, Ash AS, Shwartz M, et al: Predicting who dies depends on how severity measured: Implications for evaluating patient outcomes. Ann Intern Med 123:763-770, 1995.
17. Iezzoni LI: An introduction to risk adjustment. Am J Med Qual 11:S8-S11, 1996.
18. Iezzoni LI: The risks of risk adjustment. JAMA 278:1600-1607, 1997.
19. Concato J, Horwitz RI, Feinstein AR, et al: Problems of comorbidity in mortality after prostatectomy. JAMA 267:1077-1082, 1992.
20. Fisher ES, Whaley FS, Krushat WM, et al: The accuracy of Medicare's hospital claims data: Progress has been made, but problems remain. Am J Public Health 82:243-248, 1992.
21. Roos LL, Stranc L, James RC, Li J: Complications, comorbidities, and mortality: Improving classification and prediction. Health Serv Res 32:229-242, 1997.
22. Birkmeyer JD, Siewers AE, Finlayson EVA, et al: Hospital volume and surgical mortality in the United States. N Engl J Med 346:1128-1137, 2002.
23. Executive Committee for the Asymptomatic Carotid Atherosclerosis Study: Endarterectomy for asymptomatic carotid artery stenosis. JAMA 273:1421-1428, 1995.
24. Wennberg DE, Lucas FL, Birkmeyer JD, et al: Variation in carotid endarterectomy mortality in the Medicare population: Trial hospitals, volume, and patient characteristics. JAMA 279:1278-1281, 1998.
25. McDowell I, Newell C. Measuring Health: A Guide to Rating Scales and Questionnaires, 2nd ed. New York, Oxford University Press, 1996.
26. Ware JE Jr, Snow KK, Kosinski M, et al: SF-36 Health Survey: Manual and Interpretation Guide. Boston, The Health Institute, New England Medical Center, 1993.
27. Ware JE Jr, Kosinski M, Keller SD: A 12-Item Short-Form Health Survey: Construction of scales and preliminary tests of reliability and validity. Med Care 34:220-233, 1996.
28. Katz S, Ford AB, Moskowitz RW, et al: Studies of illness in the aged: The index of ADL—a standardized measure of biological and psychosocial function. JAMA 185:914-919, 1963.
29. Melzack R, Casey K: Sensory, motivational, and central control determinants of pain: A new conceptual model. In Kenshalo D (ed): The Skin Senses. Springfield, IL, Charles C Thomas, 1968, pp 423-443.
30. Torrance GW: Utility approach to measuring health-related quality of life. J Chronic Dis 40:593-603, 1987.
31. Pascoe G: Patient satisfaction in primary health care: A literature review and analysis. Eval Progam Plan 6:185-210, 1983.
32. Ware JE Jr, Snyder MK, Wright WR, et al: Defining and measuring patient satisfaction with medical care. Eval Program Plan 6:247-263, 1983.
33. Gold M, Siegel JE, Russell LB, Weinstein MC: Cost-effectiveness in Health and Medicine. New York, Oxford University Press, 1996.
34. Rosenthal MB, Fernandopulle R, Song HR, Landon B: Paying for quality: Providers' incentives for quality improvement. Health Aff 23:127-141, 2004.
35. Kahn J: HealthGrades: Playing doctor on the Web. Fortune 140(11):318, 1999.
36. Dimick JB, Welch HG, Birkmeyer JD: Surgical mortality as an indicator of hospital mortality: The problem with small sample size. JAMA 292:847-851, 2004.
37. Fink AS, Campbell DAJ, Mentzer RMJ, et al: The National Surgical Quality Improvement Program in non–Veterans Administration hospitals: Initial demonstration of feasibility. Ann Surg 236:344-353, 2002.
38. Birkmeyer NJ, Share D, Campbell DAJ, et al: Partnering with payers to improve surgical quality: The Michigan plan. Surgery 138:815-820, 2005.

CHAPTER 11

Surgical Patient Safety

R. Scott Jones, MD   and   Lawrence W. Way, MD

History
The Patient Safety Problem
The Science of Safety and Joint Cognitive Systems
Safer Surgical Systems

HISTORY

Adverse events and errors have accompanied surgical care since antiquity. The ancient Mesopotamian Code of Hammurabi (1795-1750 BC) recognized adverse surgical outcomes and surgical errors.[1] Over centuries, the public and medical profession have accepted the risks associated with disease and its surgical treatment. During the 20th century, health care became increasingly effective but increasingly more complex, more dangerous, and error prone. Because of contemporary knowledge and technology, modern society expects error-free health care. Although no human endeavor will ever become error free, today's health care, including surgical care, has abundant opportunities for improving its safety.

Brennan and colleagues focused attention on adverse events and medical negligence in hospitalized patients and defined an adverse event as an injury caused by medical management that prolonged hospitalization, produced a disability at the time of discharge, or both.[2] Negligence is care falling below the standard expected of physicians in their community.

Their study of 30,121 randomly selected patient records in 51 acute care hospitals in the state of New York revealed adverse events in 3.7% of cases, with negligence causing 27.6% of these adverse outcomes. Of all adverse events, 70% caused disability for up to 6 months, 2.6% caused permanent disability, and 13% resulted in death.[2] A companion publication by Leape and associates revealed that 19% of the adverse events involved drug

complications, 14% involved wound complications, and technical complications caused 13%. Forty-eight percent of adverse events in that study accompanied surgical operations. Most negligence was related to diagnostic mishaps, noninvasive therapeutic mishaps, and events in the emergency department.[3]

Another study by Gawande and colleagues focused on surgical adverse events in a 1992 review of 15,000 non–psychiatric hospital discharges in Colorado and Utah. Surgical care produced 66% of all adverse events in this cohort. Adverse events accompanied 3% of operations and deliveries. The investigators judged 54% of surgical adverse events to be preventable. Eight types of operations had high risk for preventable adverse events. Surgical adverse events were associated with 5.6% mortality and accounted for 12.2% of hospital deaths. Technique-related complications, wound infections, and postoperative bleeding produced nearly half of all surgical adverse events.[4]

Reducing surgical errors requires awareness of their various types of venues. Regarding venues, the operating room is the highest risk site for surgical errors, followed by the surgical intensive care unit (ICU), the ward, ambulatory care sites, and finally, consulting sites. The emergency department provides a very high-risk environment for errors. Because a large portion of surgical errors, particularly serious errors, arise from care in the operating room, safety improvement efforts should concentrate on operating room care. High-risk areas have the following characteristics: multiple individuals involved in the care of individual patients, high acuity, multiple distractions and interruptions, need for rapid decisions, narrow margins for safety, high volume and unpredictable patient flow, communication obstacles, and an instructional setting.[5]

Common operations have different levels of adverse events ranging from 4.4% for hysterectomy to 18.9% for repair of an abdominal aortic aneurysm. Eight operations have a high risk for preventable adverse events: lower extremity bypass graft (11.0%), abdominal aortic aneurysm repair (8.1%), colon resection (5.9%), coronary artery bypass graft/valve surgery (4.7%), transurethral resection (3.9%), cholecystectomy (3.0%), hysterectomy (2.8%), and appendectomy (1.5%). Serious errors tend to occur in operating rooms, ICUs, and emergency departments.[4] Box 11-1 presents the types of errors described by Leape and colleagues.[6] Surgeons sometimes summarize these as errors in diagnosis, errors in technique, and errors in judgment.

THE PATIENT SAFETY PROBLEM

The Institute of Medicine (IOM) conducted a comprehensive study of medical errors and safety in health care. In its report To Err Is Human, Building a Safer Health System,[7] the IOM defined safety as freedom from accidental injury. It defines error as failure of a planned action to be completed as intended or the use of a wrong plan to achieve an objective. Reason states that errors depend on two kinds of failure: either the correct action does not proceed as intended (an error of execution), or the original intended action is not correct (an error of planning). Not all errors produce harm. Large systems fail because recognized or unrecognized multiple faults occur together to cause an accident. An accident damages the system and disrupts the system's output.[8]

All human endeavors have a constant risk for error. Complex systems may experience active errors or latent errors. Active errors occur at the point of care, and the involved personnel recognize active errors almost immediately. Reason calls this the sharp end. At the blunt end,

latent errors occur remote from the point of care and include poor design, incorrect installation, faulty maintenance, bad management decisions, and poorly structured organizations.[8] Practitioners at the sharp end—surgeons, anesthesiologists, nurses, and technicians—directly engage the hazardous process close to the patient. The blunt end affects system safety, with its constraints and resources allocated to practitioners at the sharp end. The blunt end includes government regulators, hospital administrators, nursing managers, and insurance companies.[9]

Extrapolation from the New York and Utah/Colorado studies suggest that 44,000 to 98,000 hospital patients die each year as a result of medical errors, which makes medical errors the eighth leading cause of death in the United States, with a total national cost of $17 to $29 billion. We have the opportunity not only to prevent deaths and suffering but also to reduce substantially the national cost burden of health care.[4,7,10] These studies addressed inpatient surgical care, whereas ambulatory surgery centers and office surgery went unexamined.

According to the latest data from the National Center for Health Statistics, 40.3 million inpatient surgical procedures were performed in the United States in 1996, followed closely by 31.5 million outpatient procedures.[11,12] A large proportion of operations are performed in ambulatory surgery centers or in surgeons' offices. This deserves special attention because procedures performed in unregulated doctors' offices have a 10-fold increased risk for adverse events and mortality than do procedures performed in accredited facilities.[13]

These studies document adverse events and negligence in hospital care and, in particular, surgical care in both inpatient and outpatient settings. More importantly, we have good reason to believe that behavior modifications throughout the health care industry can prevent more than half of surgical adverse events. To Err Is Human received wide recognition among politicians, business, the public, and the medical profession. It prompted substantial government funding for health care safety improvement, organization of committees, educational programs, and publications—an extraordinary effort. Yet in the 15 years since Brennan's landmark publication and in the 7 years since publication of To Err Is Human, no credible evidence has appeared to suggest that health care in general and surgical care in particular has become safer.

What explains this observation? Perhaps our profession has not assumed its responsibility to protect the interests of the sick. This happens in part because our profession fails to understand errors and how and why they occur. To correct this matter will require incorporating an understanding of safety into the mind of every surgeon. These questions and assertions reveal a remarkable paradox. Because of the high risks associated with surgical care, surgeons devote a majority of their professional energy to avoiding errors, adverse events, and complications. This effort begins on the first day of surgical residency.

The sociologist Charles Bosk provided a detailed and scholarly analysis of this topic in his carefully researched book *Forgive and Remember: Managing Medical Failure.* This study, published in 1979, exerted no impact on surgical errors. Why not? It clearly documented the admirable professional, technical, moral, ethical, and personal attributes and dedication of surgeons and surgical trainees of an elite academic department of surgery. It also documented a rigid hierarchy of autonomous superordinates who promoted disdain for outcome data, clinical trials, and scientific thought.[14]

> In general, surgeons believed that the only protection for patients, the only guarantee of high-quality care, was the individual surgeon's personal standards of attention to detail, honesty, and adequate training. They took every opportunity to instill residents with the proper professional values and to model proper professional conduct. At the same time they did virtually nothing to inculcate a sense of corporate or collective responsibility for outcomes. The patterns of assessment and surveillance suggested a hypertrophy of individual responsibility for outcomes and an atrophy of collective responsibility. This pattern reinforced and reflected the values of personal autonomy and the superiority of clinical over scientific judgment.[15(p168)]

Certainly, safe surgery requires well-informed, skilled, dedicated, conscientious, honest, trustworthy surgeons and much more (Box 11-2). Safe surgery requires teamwork among all health care professionals interacting effectively with other stakeholders in the health care industry and with available physical resources to form accountable, high-reliability organizations. High-reliability organizations develop a so-called systems approach to understand errors or accidents and to support decisions in complex health care. Such organizations create an open flow of information, learn to eliminate the culture of blame, and in addition, build partnerships among health care stakeholders to resolve differences and agree on common goals. According to Woods,

> High reliability organizations created safety by anticipating and planning for unexpected events and future surprises. These organizations did not take past successes as a reason for confidence. Instead, they continued to invest in anticipating the changing potential for failure because of the deeply held understanding that their knowledge base was fragile in the face of the hazards inherent in their work and the changes omnipresent in their environment. Safety for these organizations was not a commodity but a value that required continuing reinforcement and investment. The learning activities at the heart of this process depend on the open flow of information about the changing potential for failure.[16(p490)]

Health care in the United States does not possess the characteristics of a high-performance organization. The medical profession remains a cottage industry operating under the direction of powerful corporations and a powerful government. A safe health care system will require realignment of all health care professionals into a high-performance organization with a defined infrastructure.

Box 11-2 Characteristics of Safety

- Systems, not individuals, make safety.
- Designs for safety require a detailed understanding of the technical work.
- Safety is dynamic, not static; it is constantly renegotiated.
- Trade-offs compromise the core of safety.
- Adding complexity (e.g., technology) can compromise safety.
- People constantly create safety.

Adapted from Cook RI, O'Connor M, Reader M, et al: Operating at the sharp end: The human factors of complex technical work and its implications for patient safety. In Manuel BM, Nora P (eds): Surgical Patient Safety. Chicago, American College of Surgeons, 2004, pp 19-30.

W. Edwards Deming, a respected scholar in the field of quality control, stated, "We have learned to live in a world of mistakes and defective products as if they were necessary to life. It is time to develop a new philosophy in America."[17]

Deming established 14 points for management in industry or business. Those points and the Deming program contributed to improvement of goods and services in industry worldwide.[18] Although Deming's points addressed quality, we believe that they can apply to improving safety in surgical care. Six of the points modified to apply to surgical care can serve as a foundation or guiding principle for the discussions to follow in this chapter:

1. Appoint leaders who make as their top priorities helping people whom they supervise and improving the services that those individuals provide.
2. Break down the barriers between departments and specialties so that each professional who cares for a patient is part of a team and is able to foresee problems that may be encountered during the course of treatment.
3. Drive out fear so that everyone may work effectively in partnership.
4. Institute on-the-job safety training by using a practice-based approach to lifelong learning.
5. Institute a vigorous program of education and self-improvement.
6. Put everybody in the institution or office to work to accomplish the transformation. The transformation is everybody's job.[19]

THE SCIENCE OF SAFETY AND JOINT COGNITIVE SYSTEMS

During the past 3 decades, cognitive psychologists and systems engineers working in industry have examined the problem of errors in detail and revealed that most errors occur as a result of flaws in systems. We can apply their knowledge and the principles they defined to improving surgical safety. A system is an arrangement of components, people, and functions organized and managed to accomplish tasks or goals (Box 11-3). Hollnagel and Woods define a cognitive system as a system that can modify its behavior on the basis of experience

---

Box 11-3 Systems

A system has two or more parts and the following features:

- It has a function or purpose.
- Each part can affect the other parts.
- Subsets of the system's parts can function alone but cannot perform total system tasks.
- The function of any part depends on at least one other part.
- In large complex systems, certain events cannot be attributed to any single part.

Adapted from Hollnagel E, Woods DD: Joint Cognitive Systems: Foundations of Cognitive Systems Engineering. Boca Raton, FL, Taylor & Francis, 2005.

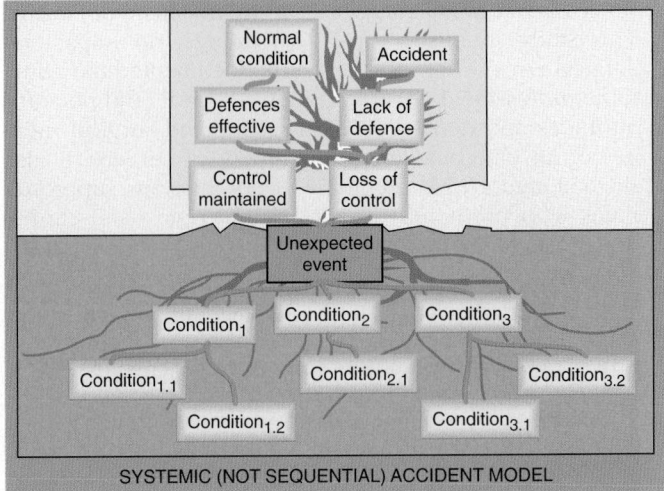

SYSTEMIC (NOT SEQUENTIAL) ACCIDENT MODEL

Figure 11-1 This Hollnagel accident model, which focuses on examination of the system, provides a higher probability of improving safety than sequential accident models do. (From Hollnagel E: Barriers and Accident Prevention. Aldershot, UK, Ashgate, 2004.)

to achieve specific antientropic ends. Entropy is the amount of energy in a system unavailable for work or, viewed in another way, the amount of disorder in a system. Some systems, called *cognitive systems,* can maintain order in the presence of disruptions. Accordingly, a joint cognitive system (JCS) can control what it does and is defined by what it does. A cognitive system has two or more parts, each part can affect the other parts, and the way that any part behaves depends largely on at least one other part.[20]

Some system disruptions permit errors. Scholars challenge the notion of *human error.* Human error may be a post hoc rationalization starting from the assumption that all effects must have causes.[20,21] Although there are no medical errors, many errors occur in medical settings. We can predict the probability of errors, but we cannot predict when errors occur. Undetected or uninterrupted errors lead to accidents and perhaps injury. Cognitive systems engineering (CSE) states that one cannot understand why something fails without first understanding why it usually goes right. Efforts to make work safe should start from an understanding of the normal variability of human and system performance rather than from putative error mechanisms.

According to conventional thought, complex systems fail when multiple small failures, called *latent errors,* align to allow an accident. This so-called Swiss cheese accident model is being increasingly criticized because it is too linear, defects are more often transient, and the whole process is more dynamic than the model suggests. Sequential accident models inevitably lead to a root cause, which is the basis of the root cause analysis. The search for a root cause, often a human, tends to perpetuate the blame-the-person outcome. It may also suggest, incorrectly, that eliminating a root cause will solve the problem. Postaccident reviews frequently identify human error as the so-called cause of failure because of hindsight bias. That is, outcome knowledge made the failure seem foreseeable when it was not foreseen and not foreseeable. The work of Hollnagel reveals that comprehensive detailed inquiries often find multiple parallel factors leading to the event first considered a root cause (Fig. 11-1). This model focuses on examination of the system and provides a higher probability of improving safety than the other models do. Blaming a person has a poor

track record of safety improvement because it leaves the faulty system uncorrected.[22]

CSE addresses the following themes:

1. How people cope with the complexity produced by technologic and sociotechnical developments
2. How people use artifacts in their work
3. How humans and artifacts form a JCS to focus on how humans and technology work together effectively

Hence, a JCS consists of purposeful human and technologic interactions. A JCS can recognize issues and understand events within the context of their occurrence. Proper system performance requires control of processes and events, and loss of control or loss of the ability to solve performance aberrations produces system instability. A JCS can deal with unexpected events best when they occur infrequently. The ability of a JCS to deal with and control complexity depends on a degree of orderliness or predictability, the time available, knowledge, competence, and resources.

A JCS can modify its behavior on the basis of experience to achieve its goals effectively. It can control what it does. CSE concerns a JCS with the following features:

1. Functioning is complex
2. The artifact (i.e., machinery, equipment, patient) functions unpredictably
3. The artifact has a dynamic process (i.e., it changes with time)

CSE recognizes other important features of a JCS:

1. Cognition is distributed among all system participants so that cooperation and coordination can become ubiquitous
2. Rapidly growing technologic development leads to more data, options, modes, displays, and the like, as well as ultimately to more complexity

THE SAFETY SPACE

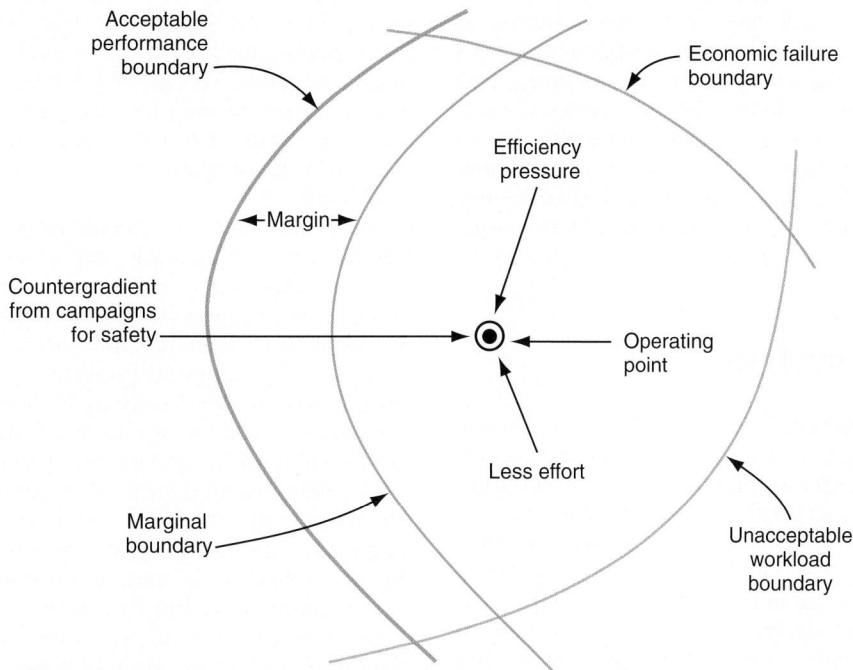

Figure 11-2 Rasmussen's dynamic safety model as depicted by Cook and Rasmussen describes a relationship among workload, economic boundaries, and accident risk boundaries. The model suggests that increasing workload or economic pressure increases the potential for accidents. In addition, pressure to avoid accidents pushes back on the workload and economic boundaries. From Cook R, Rasmussen J: "Going solid": A model of system dynamics and consequences for patient safety. Qual Saf Health Care 14:130-134, 2005.)

3. Growth of system complexity produces failures, currently called *human error*

Only cooperation and congruence of the participants allow control and smooth functioning of a JCS. The effectiveness of the system affects throughput capacity, efficiency, quality, safety, and organization culture.[20]

Surgical teams in busy hospitals must often manage around impediments in the smooth flow of patients into and through their system. Any single system component, such as the ICU, filled to capacity will require additional unit management. Frequently, another hospital unit can allow work flow to continue, for example, holding a patient in the recovery room until an ICU bed becomes available. When additional units reach capacity, management of the system becomes increasingly difficult. Cognitive systems engineers coined the phrase *tight coupling* to describe a deficiency of redundancy among the components of a system.

Tight coupling connects parts of the system so rigidly that actions at one place are immediately transmitted throughout. Prediction and control become harder, and accidents increase. Tight coupling promotes errors. Everyday examples of tight coupling include no hospital beds, no ICU beds, inadequate nurse staffing, overbooked operating room schedule, shortage of surgical instruments, delay in procedures, inadequate resources to staff operating room procedures, lengthy queues for operations, elective surgery in off-hours, and long queues for routine outpatient appointments. Tight coupling results from failure to recognize production limits that match production capacity. With all units filled to capacity, or maximal tight coupling, events in one hospital unit have an impact on the operation of all other units in the system. Cook and Rasmussen called this situation *going solid*. Going solid produces situations both hazardous and difficult to control. Though not directly producing accidents, it makes accidents more likely and more difficult to deflect and makes recovery more complicated. Conversely, although going solid may be difficult to manage, it can improve the hospital's financial performance considerably. The fact that more accidents do not occur when health systems become tightly coupled or go solid is a tribute to the health care professionals providing knowledge, technical skill, judgment, dedication, and commitment at the sharp end.[23]

A surgical system's operating space resides within three boundaries: the risk-of-economic-failure boundary, the risk-of-unacceptable-workload boundary, and the acceptable-performance (accident-free) boundary. Consequently, increasing economic pressure and increasing workload pressure can perturb the acceptable-performance boundary in ways to increase the risk for accidents (Fig. 11-2). High-reliability organizations develop accurate, precise, and shared understanding of the balance among economic, workload, and performance boundaries. Low-reliability organizations have inaccurate, imprecise, and divergent understanding of these boundaries. High-reliability organizations frequently anticipate accidents, whereas low-reliability organizations are often surprised by accidents. The increased complexity of tightly coupled systems makes system behavior unpredictable and increases the risk for accidents. However, tight coupling gains efficiency and economy. Tightly coupled system failures have produced large-scale power outages, for example.[23]

SAFER SURGICAL SYSTEMS

Surgical services represent JCSs amenable to improved effectiveness, improved efficiency, and improved safety with focused management practices and professional leadership. Improving surgical safety, particularly operating room safety, will require surgeons to assume their responsibility to lead the surgical JCS. Many surgeons currently lead efforts to improve surgical safety. The following paragraphs describe some of these efforts and delineate additional opportunities to prevent adverse events, errors, and accidents.

Team Development

Systems include people working with artifacts to accomplish goals: teams. Consequently, addressing systems of care begins with an examination of the people in the system forming the team. In surgical care the team includes surgeons, anesthesiologists, anesthetists, nurses, allied health personnel, and administrators. To work effectively in surgical teams the people require competency, proficiency, continued learning, and skill development. Competency refers to the cognitive skills and knowledge required to practice a profession. Proficiency is the ability to execute a task at a consistently optimum level and outcome. Learning is the acquisition of new knowledge. Maintaining surgical competency and proficiency requires a long-term, perhaps endless process that begins with the selection of trainees. Because some individuals learn and acquire skill faster than others do, the training process should possess continual, objective, standardized assessments of cognition and technical skills. These processes should then continue beyond the training period into continuing professional practice to provide continuing assessment of established surgeons for revalidation and recertification. Practicing surgical professionals of all disciplines require opportunities for continuing acquisition of new knowledge and new technical skills. Because of the rapidly increasing volume of new knowledge and new technology, learning and development of new skills assume increasing importance for maintaining patient safety.[24]

Surgical professionals need reliable performance assessment in the form of regularly provided outcome data such as morbidity rates, mortality rates, cure rates,

and patient postoperative quality-of-life assessments. In addition, some system for analyzing and evaluating anonymous incident, error, and accident reports could promote safety in surgical practice. The U.S. Congress enacted laws permitting collection of such data without risk of legal discovery. The Agency for Healthcare Research and Quality is developing federal regulations to permit health care organizations to form patient safety organizations for the purpose of examining data on medical errors and accidents.

Surgeons have a special responsibility to promote safety by providing leadership to surgical teams. Surgeon leaders must have sufficient experience and surgical volume to sustain a high level of proficiency. A surgeon leader who understands the system will implement good team management and promote optimal performance of all involved professionals by focusing on the interests of the patient. Leadership requires the physical presence of the surgeon in the operating room.

A safety-oriented surgical system would include measures to identify impaired members of the team, including surgeons, anesthesiologists, anesthetists, nurses, allied health professionals, and administrators. These problems occur infrequently but can pose threats to patient safety when they occur. Our profession has not addressed this matter as well in the past as it must in the future. Team leaders should develop processes for recognizing impaired members. Impairments include substance abuse, mental illness, and physical illness. In addition, recognition and correction of declining competency and proficiency should promote safety. Teams should also recognize and correct behavioral problems causing disruption in the workplace. Professionals who cannot work effectively with others or who are abusive to others, including personnel and patients, must undergo rehabilitation. Institutional or team leaders should identify problem staff members early and take corrective action in a timely manner. A system of professional accountability must be objective, based on data; it must be fair and apply to everyone in the system; and it must respond with prompt and effective treatment with the goal of enabling all to continue professional practice.[25]

Surgeons, anesthesiologists, nurses, and allied health professionals recognize the importance of teamwork in the operating room. For many operations, pathologists play a crucial role in safe, effective surgery and smooth conduct of surgical procedures. A high-performance operating room requires good communication among all surgical team members because breakdowns in communication can lead to errors, adverse events, and accidents compromising patient safety. Medical team training can improve communication in the operating room. Operating room teams can use crew resource management (CRM) principles to enhance communication and patient safety. CRM principles include didactic instruction, interactive participation, role-playing, training films, and clinical vignettes. Awad and coworkers investigated CRM quantitatively and concluded, "Medical team training using CRM principles can improve communication in the operating room, ensuring a safer environment that leads to decreased adverse events."[26(p773)]

Preoperative Checklist–General Surgery
(To be Filled in by Chief Resident the Day Before the Operation)

Patient: _____   Date of Operation: _____

Operation: _____   Attending: _____

1. Outpatient H&P available ☐

2. Office records available ☐

3. Signed consent form here ☐

4. Signed blood consent form here ☐

5. Pertinent x-rays here ☐

6. Pre-op chest x-ray, EKG and lab tests reviewed ☐

7. Outside path slides read at UCSF; no discrepancy ☐

8. Results of preop consults checked; recommendations implemented ☐

9. SFP Admit Form checked for other details ☐

10. Beta-blocker protocol implemented ☐

11. Regimen for venous thrombosis prophylaxis implemented ☐

12. Prophylactic antibiotics decided & ordered ☐

13. Resident assignments made ☐

Special protocols:

13. Glucose control in insulin-dependent diabetics ☐

14. Patients on chronic anticoagulation ☐

15. Splenectomy immunization ☐

Initial the box or write n/a if a step is not applicable.

Signed and checked by   Date

Figure 11-3 Checklists such as this one can maximize effective communication at gaps and during handoffs along the continuum of surgical care. (Courtesy of the Department of Surgery, University of California, San Francisco.)

Gap Protection

Cook and colleagues introduced the useful concept of gaps and recognized that gaps provide opportunities for errors and accidents.[27] Gaps, or discontinuities, may produce loss of information, loss of momentum, or interruptions in delivery of care. Fortunately, gaps rarely lead to failure or produce errors because nurses, technicians, clerks, or physicians anticipate, identify, and bridge most gaps.

Organizational boundaries, changes in authority or responsibility, different roles of professionals, and divisions of labor produce gaps. For example, shift changes, patient transfer to different units within a hospital, patient transfer between hospitals, discharge to a rehabilitation facility, and discharge home produce gaps in care. Gaps can occur within the activities of a single practitioner, for example, when a nurse divides attention between two or more patients. Organizational change or the introduction of new technology can cause new gaps or disrupt bridges spanning established gaps. System complexity creates gaps in care, and information can be lost. Every transition

in care constitutes a gap. The increasing fragmentation of medical care produces more gaps. Structured handoff routines and checklists can decrease information loss at gaps. A dozen or more gaps or handoffs can occur between evaluation in the clinic, surgical admission unit, operating room, recovery room, ICU, and surgical ward and discharge from the hospital. Each gap requires a handoff.

Handoff routines can include reading back orders and instructions, face-to-face review of clinical information, or handoff information technology resources. Checklists and standardized orders can also minimize loss of information at handoffs. Checklists can simplify preoperative planning, operating room scheduling, admission scheduling, night-before instructions, preoperative details (briefing), and postoperative care (Fig. 11-3). A system can apply standardization to admission and preoperative orders, postoperative orders, transition orders, discharge orders, and discharge instructions. Guidelines, clinical pathways, protocols, and algorithms can also facilitate bridging of gaps. All these gap transition artifacts prompt routine, necessary action at system gaps, can be

Box 11-4 JCAHO *Time-Out* Immediately Before Starting a Procedure

Must be conducted in the location where the procedure will be performed, just before starting the procedure. It must involve the entire operative team, use active communication, be briefly documented, such as in a checklist (the organization should determine the type and amount of documentation), and must, at the least, include the following:

- Correct patient identity
- Correct site and side
- Agreement on the procedure to be performed
- Correct patient position
- Availability of correct implants and any special equipment or special requirements

  The organization should have processes and systems in place for reconciling differences in staff responses during the time-out

Adapted from the Joint Commission on Accreditation of Healthcare Organizations. Universal Protocol, 2006. Available at http://jointcommission.org?PatientSafety/UniversalProtocol. Retrieved October 27, 2006.

Box 11-5 Goals of the National Health Information Infrastructure

- National platform for standards
- Confidentiality
- Electronic medical records
- Computerized physician order entry
- Electronic prescriptions
- Quality improvement databases
- Repositories of best evidence
- Computer-assisted decision support
- Prompts and reminder systems

From U.S. Department of Health and Human Services. National Health Information Infrastructure (NIIH 2002-2004), 2006. Available at http://aspe.hhs.gov/sp/NHII/index.html. Retrieved October 27, 2006.

customized for individual patients, and are effective, inexpensive, low-tech, and efficient.[27]

The Joint Commission for Accreditation of Healthcare Organizations (JCAHO), the American College of Surgeons (ACS), and the Veterans Administration Health System (VAHS) recommend processes for preoperative review to promote safety and eliminate errors in patient and surgical site identification, as well as other important considerations.[28-30] The ACS, JCAHO, and VAHS endorse a preoperative briefing or *time-out* before every surgical procedure. Box 11-4 shows the JCAHO recommendations for its time-out procedure. This guide stipulates essential topics for preoperative discussion by all members of the surgical team and a checklist to verify that all personnel, all necessary equipment, and all necessary processes have been accomplished or are in place before making the incision or beginning the procedure. Development of a preoperative briefing guide and the related checklists can begin with the patient's first encounter with the surgical team. This first encounter can initiate an iterative process that produces a checklist for review by members of the surgical team on the preoperative evening in elective cases. The preoperative time-out in the operating room will then verify all items on the list. After the operation, members of the surgical team will bridge the gap between the operating room and the recovery room or the ICU.

Improvements in Information Technology

Federal and state governments and all health industry stakeholders assign high priority to the application of information technology for increasing the safety and quality of health care. With the leadership of the Department of Health and Human Services, 13 government agencies, professional organizations, private foundations, providers, and vendors formed an organization, the National Health Information Infrastructure (NHII), to promote the development and implementation of information technology systems and programs to support the development of a national health care system. Box 11-5 lists the goals and objectives of a national health information technology system. This task will require unprecedented leadership from government, industry, and the health professions. In addition, the project faces substantial financial challenges. As it develops over time, a national health information infrastructure will undoubtedly improve the quality and safety of health care.[31] However, the health care industry should introduce new information technology with care and deliberation because such new technology could create tighter coupling in the system and produce unforeseen challenges in system control and unanticipated opportunities for error.[23]

Nonetheless, computerized physician order entry and computerized prescription writing already show promise for reducing medical errors. Information technology provides multiple opportunities for improving patient safety; for example, computerized rounding and sign-out systems have the potential to improve the continuity of care and facilitate the bridging of gaps. Van Eaton and associates, working in an academic medical center, developed a centralized, Web-based computerized rounding and sign-out system that securely stores information, automatically downloads patient data, and prints the data to rounding, sign-out, and progress note templates. Authorized users could access the system from any hospital workstation or from their own computers. The centralized computer allowed residents to organize patient lists, enter detailed sign-out information, and compile "to do" lists. Residents could add patient data to other team's lists when cross-covering or consulting. The system produced sign-out reports and rounding lists that included clinical data and laboratory values downloaded from the hospital clinical information systems. This team evaluated the system in a prospective randomized trial involving six general surgery services and eight internal medicine services. Helping residents cope with the limitations of the 80-hour work week motivated this project, which succeeded in this objective by decreasing rounding time. However, the system also enhanced patient care by decreasing the number of patients missed on resident rounds and improved the continuity of care. Although a teaching hospital developed this system, the method and the principles developed should work in any hospital.[32]

Observational Studies of Perioperative Systems

Most efforts to improve surgical safety have relied on retrospective reviews of health records, administrative data, or malpractice claims. Recent prospective observational studies conducted in the perioperative period with particular focus on intraoperative events have provided new insight into safety in the operating room and have revealed opportunities for improving surgical safety. Because accidents, adverse events, and errors of consequence occur during or after operations, observations in the operating room can provide abundant opportunities for improving patient safety.[33] Christian and colleagues organized a multidisciplinary research team of surgeons and human factors experts experienced in investigating high-risk work environments. They developed a hierarchic coding scheme for system factors and human factors for each observation. They annotated, classified, and entered their field notes into a relational database with a custom software application. The investigators met the patient and the surgical team in the preoperative holding area and recorded detailed observations during the care from that time until completion of the operation. Of 10 cases, 9 were completed with preoperative, intraoperative, and postoperative observations. The surgeon cancelled one case in the preoperative phase.

Sixty-three hours of observation provided 4500 observations for analysis. Table 11-1 shows the quantitative analysis of communications/information flow and its influence on performance and safety. The 10 study cases had an average of nine instances of information loss or information degradation per case. These lapses caused delays in case progression, increased team workload, uncertainty in patient management, waste of resources, increased exposure of patients to injury, and cancellation of a case. Handoffs occurred during each case an average of 4.8 times, or once every hour during each case. The surgical team spent an average of 43 minutes, or 17.3% of the operating time, waiting for communication from pathology.

Table 11-2 presents a quantitative analysis of workload and auxiliary tasks and their influence on performance and safety in cases that progressed to the intraoperative phase. Note that the circulating nurse left the operating room an average of 33 times per case, or 7.5 times per hour of incision time. Instruments or other materials were added to the operative field 14.6 times per case. The routine of counting sponges and instruments attracted the attention of the investigators. During each procedure the team spent 35 minutes on counting activities, or 14.5% of the incision time. If the results of these counting activities were inconsistent or incorrect, it increased workload for non-nursing personnel, required radiographic confirmation in two cases, and exposed patients to injury. This study revealed that communication breakdown and infor-

Table 11-1 Quantitative Analysis of Communication/Information Flow and Its Influence on Performance and Safety (*N*=10)

Instances of Information Loss or Degradation	
Aggregate number of instances across all cases	88
Per-case mean	9
Influence of Information Loss on Performance or Safety (Total Instances Across All Cases)	
Delay in case progression	19
Increased workload	15
Increased uncertainty in patient management for others	29
Overuse of material resources	6
Increased exposure to injury (patient)	6
Cancellation of case	1
No influence detected	12
Handoff of Patient Care Across Provider Groups	
Mean number per case	
All provider groups	4.8
Nursing staff	2.8
Anesthesia staff	1.8
Surgeons	0.4
Frequency of handoffs	1 per 60 minutes of operation
Communication With Pathology	
Mean time waiting for a pathologist's response	43 minutes
Mean percentage of incision time waiting for a response	17.3%

Adapted from Christian CR, Gustafson M, Roth EM, et al: A prospective study of patient safety in the operating room. Surgery 139:159-172, 2006.

mation loss, as well as high workload and multiple competing tasks, can compromise patient safety. Direct field observations such as this have the potential to provide better understanding of the processes and systems of operative care and thereby improve patient safety and reduce errors.[34]

The airline industry implemented a program called *Line Operations Safety Audits* (LOSA) that used methods similar to those described earlier to evaluate aviation safety. On April 4, 2006, the Federal Aviation Agency issued an Advisory Circular on LOSA. The program has a trained pilot observer on board the aircraft to complete a targeted observation form. LOSA is totally voluntary and the observations remain unidentified and confidential. LOSA is designed to permit crews to recognize opportunities for improving safety and decreasing the risk for error. It is possible that a similar, voluntary nonthreatening program could promote patient safety, improve processes of operative care, and reduce errors in operating rooms.[35]

Systems Engineers

Previous work has revealed that collaboration between surgeons and systems engineers can provide useful

Table 11-2 Quantitative Analysis of Workload and Auxiliary Tasks and Their Influence on Performance and Safety in Cases That Progressed to the Intraoperative Phase (*N*=9)

Circulating Nurse Exits for Procurement of Resources	
Aggregate number of exits across all cases	299
Per-case average number of exits	33
Mean frequency of exits	7.5 per hour of incision time
Addition of Instruments or Materials to the Operative Field After Start of the Procedure	
Aggregate number of objects added across all cases	131
Per-case average number of objects added	14.6
Mean frequency of addition to the field	1 per 27 minutes of incision time
Counting Activities	
Mean time spent on counting	35 minutes
Mean percentage of incision time spent on counting	14.5%
Influence of Counting Activities on Performance or Safety	
Aggregate number of performance issues during counting	28
Errors or inconsistencies in the count	17
Increased workload for non-nursing providers	11
Interruption of the procedure to take a radiograph after failure to resolve inconsistencies	2
Increased exposure to injury (patient)	2

Adapted from Christian CR, Gustafson M, Roth EM, et al: A prospective study of patient safety in the operating room. Surgery 139:159-172, 2006.

insight into understanding surgical system improvement. Systems engineers have the competency and proficiency that surgeons, anesthesiologists, and nurses lack in analyzing and quantifying system performance, human factors, communication, equipment design, and situation awareness. These skills will help health care professionals analyze, monitor, and manage their care systems to promote safety, minimize errors, improve the quality of care, and maintain a healthy satisfying workplace.

Operating Room Safety Committee

Most hospitals maintain an operating room committee to advise operating managers on asset allocation, equipment, scheduling, purchasing, and budgeting. Is there evidence that operating room committees effectively address surgical safety, perioperative systems, tight coupling, going solid, queuing, and elective cases after hours? Because traditional work flow consumes the operating room committee and because patient safety in the operating room deserves high priority, hospitals should consider forming operating room safety committees. Perhaps complex organizations bog down with too many com-

mittees and other forms of bureaucracy. However, *To Err Is Human* tells us that we can reduce errors by 50% by applying attention to our health system and to our operating rooms in particular. Focusing on operating room systems and safety remains a fruitful opportunity to save lives.

Fellowships in Surgical Safety

Careful examination reveals critical underfunding of research in surgical disciplines. Surgeons compete ineffectively with nonsurgeons and basic scientists in seeking research funding from the National Institutes of Health and other funding agencies. Improving surgical safety without high-quality research and scientific rigor will remain as ineffective in the future as it has in the past.[36] Improving surgical safety will require funding for surgeons, anesthesiologists, and nurses to develop research skills and will require funding for their research. Young surgeons, anesthesiologists, and nurses will require opportunities to work and study with systems engineers, human factors experts, and other scholars relevant to system safety. Health professional investigators should receive encouragement and academic recognition for revealing new knowledge and new insights about human factors, communication, equipment design, and the principles of CSE and management of JSCs. Editors of surgical journals can promote surgical safety by publishing the work of surgical safety researchers. Changing the culture of safety in surgery will require a cadre of devoted researchers and scholar experts in the field.

Selected References

Brennan TA, Leape L, Laird NM, et al: Incidence of adverse events and negligence in hospitalized patients: Results of the Harvard Medical Practice Study I. N Engl J Med 324:370-376, 1991.

This publication and its companion called attention to the frequency of medical errors and the magnitude of the problem.

Christian CK, Gustafson ML, Roth EM, et al: A prospective study of patient safety in the operating room Surgery 139:158-73, 2006.

The authors of this work demonstrated the effectiveness of a multidisciplinary team and that a well-structured prospective study protocol can reveal threats to patient safety in the operating room.

Cook R, Rasmussen J: "Going solid": A model of system dynamics and consequences for patient safety. Qual Saf Health Care 14:130-134, 2005.

This interesting publication examines the tensions among workload, financial pressures, and the risks of errors.

Cook R, Render M, Woods DD: Gaps in the continuity of care and progress on patient safety. BMJ 320:791-794, 2000.

The authors reveal that gaps or discontinuity in care processes create vulnerabilities and opportunities for error. Checklists and other standardizations of handoffs can minimize the risk for error in those circumstances.

Hollnagel E, Woods D: Joint Cognitive Systems: Foundations of Cognitive Systems Engineering. Boca Raton, FL, Taylor & Francis, 2005.

> This book provides detailed discussions of errors and how understanding systems can improve patient safety.

Leape L, Brennan TA, Laird NM, et al: The nature of adverse events in hospitalized patients: Results of the Harvard Medical Practice Study II. N Engl J Med 324:377-384, 1991.

> This publication, like its companion, provided new knowledge about medical errors and adverse events.

Reason J: Human Error. Cambridge, England, Cambridge University Press, 1990.

> This book provides a scholarly and detailed analysis of errors.

References

1. Code of Hammurabi. Available at http://www.wsu.edu/~dee/MESO/CODE.HTM.
2. Brennan TA, Leape L, Laird NM, et al: Incidence of adverse events and negligence in hospitalized patients. N Engl J Med 324:370-376, 1991.
3. Leape LL, Brennan T, Laird NM, et al: The nature of adverse events in hospitalized patients. N Engl J Med 324:377-384, 1991.
4. Gawande AA, Thomas EJ, Zinner MJ, et al: The incidence and nature of surgical adverse events in Utah and Colorado. Surgery 126:66-75, 1999.
5. Aspden P, Corrigan J, Wolcott J, et al: Patient Safety: Achieving a New Standard for Care. Washington, DC, National Academies Press, 2004.
6. Leape L, Lawthers A, Brennan TA, et al: Preventing medical injury. Qual Rev Bull 19(5):144-149, 1993.
7. Kohn LT, Corrigan J, Donaldson MS: To Err Is Human: Building a Safer Health System. Washington, DC, National Academy Press, 1999.
8. Reason J: Human Error. Cambridge, England, Cambridge University Press, 1990.
9. Cook R, Woods D: Operating at the sharp end: The complexity of human error. In Bogner S (ed): Human Error in Medicine. Hillsdale, NJ, Lawrence Erlbaum, 1994, pp 255-310.
10. Thomas EJ, Studdert DM, Newhouse JP, et al: Costs of medical injuries in Utah and Colorado. Inquiry 36:255-264, 1999.
11. Centers for Disease Control and Prevention. Available at http://www.cdc.gov/nchs/fastats/insurg.htm.
12. Centers for Disease Control and Prevention. Available at http://www.cdc.gov/nchs/data/series/sr_13/sr_13_139.pdf.
13. Vila H, Soto R, Cantor AB, et al: Comparative outcomes analysis of procedures performed in physician offices and ambulatory surgery centers. Arch Surg 138:991-995, 2003.
14. Bosk C: Forgive and Remember: Managing Medical Failure. Chicago, University of Chicago Press, 1979.
15. Bosk CL, Frader JE: It's not easy wearing green: The art of surgical innovation and the science of clinical trials. In Reitsma AM, Moreno JD (eds): Ethical Guidelines for Innovative Surgery. Hagerstown, MD, University Publishing Group, 2006, p 168.
16. Leadership Institute, Inc. Available at: http://www.lii.net/deming.html.
17. Woods DD: Conflicts between learning and accountability in patient safety. DePaul Law Review 54:485-502, 2005.
18. Deming WE: Out of the Crisis. Cambridge, MA, MIT Press, 1982.
19. Manuel BM, Nora P: Surgical Patient Safety: Essential Information for Surgeons in Today's Environment. Chicago, American College of Surgeons, 2004.
20. Hollnagel E, Woods D: Joint cognitive Systems: Foundations of Cognitive Systems Engineering. Boca Raton, FL, Taylor & Francis, 2005.
21. Dekker S: Ten Questions about Human Error: A New View of Human Factors and System Safety. Mahwah, NJ, Lawrence Erlbaum, 2005.
22. Hollnagel E: Barriers and Accident Prevention. Aldershot, UK, Ashgate, 2004.
23. Cook R, Rasmussen J: "Going solid": A model of system dynamics and consequences for patient safety. Qual Saf Health Care 14:130-134, 2005.
24. Cuschieri A: Medical errors, incidents, accidents, and violations. Minim Invasive Ther Allied Technol 12:111-120, 2006.
25. Leape LL, Fromson J: Problem doctors: Is there a system-level solution? Ann Intern Med 144:107-115, 2006.
26. Awad SS, Fagan S, Bellows C, et al: Bridging the communication gap in the operating room with medical team training. Am J Surg 190:770-774, 2005.
27. Cook R, Render M, Woods DD: Gaps in the continuity of care and progress on patient safety. BMJ 320:791-794, 2000.
28. Joint Commission for Accreditation of Healthcare Organizations. Available at http://www.jointcommission.org/PatientSafety/UniversalProtocol/.
29. American College of Surgeons. Available at http://www.facs.org/fellows_info/statements/st-41.html.
30. Veterans Administration. Available at http://www1.va.gov/vhapublications/ViewPublications.asp?pub_ID=1106.
31. National Healthcare Information Infrastructure. Available at http://aspe.hhs.gov/sp/NHII/index.html.
32. Van Eaton EG, Horvarth K, Lober WB, et al: A randomized controlled trial evaluating the impact of a computerized rounding and sign-out system on continuity of care and resident work hours. J Am Coll Surg 200:538-545, 2005.
33. Guerlain S, Adams R, Turrentine FB, et al: Assessing team performance in the operating room: Development and use of a "black box" recorder and other tools for the intraoperative environment. J Am Coll Surg 200:29-37, 2005.
34. Christian CK, Gustafson M, Roth EM, et al: A prospective study of patient safety in the operating room. Surgery 139:159-172, 2006.
35. Federal Aviation Administration. Available at http://homepage.psy.utexas.edu/Homepage/Group/HelmreichLAB/Aviation/LOSA/LOSA.html.
36. Jones RS, Debas H: Research: A vital component of optimal patient care in the United States. Ann Surg 240:573-577, 2004.

PERIOPERATIVE MANAGEMENT

CHAPTER 12

Principles of Preoperative and Operative Surgery

Leigh Neumayer, MD   and   Daniel Vargo, MD

PREOPERATIVE PREPARATION OF THE PATIENT

The modern preparation of a patient for surgery is epitomized by the convergence of the art and science of the surgical discipline. The context in which preoperative preparation is conducted ranges from an outpatient office visit to hospital inpatient consultation to emergency department evaluation of a patient. Approaches to preoperative evaluation differ significantly, depending on the nature of the complaint and the proposed surgical intervention, patient health and assessment of risk factors, and the results of directed investigation and interventions to optimize the patient's overall status and readiness for surgery. This chapter reviews the components of risk assessment applicable to the evaluation of any patient for surgery and attempts to provide some basic algorithms to aid in the preparation of patients for surgery.

Determining the Need for Surgery

Patients are often referred to surgeons with a suspected surgical diagnosis and the results of supporting investigations in hand. In this context, the surgeon's initial encounter with the patient may be largely directed toward confirmation of relevant physical findings and review of the clinical history and laboratory and investigative tests

that support the diagnosis. A recommendation regarding the need for operative intervention can then be made by the surgeon and discussed with the patient's family members. A decision to perform additional investigative tests or consideration of alternative therapeutic options may postpone the decision for surgical intervention from this initial encounter to a later time. It is important for the surgeon to explain the context of the illness and the benefit of different surgical interventions, further investigation, and possible nonsurgical alternatives, when appropriate.

The surgeon's approach to the patient and family during the initial encounter should be one that fosters a bond of trust and opens a line of communication among all participants. A professional and unhurried approach is mandatory, with time taken to listen to concerns and answer questions posed by the patient and family members. The surgeon's initial encounter with a patient should result in the patient being able to express a basic understanding of the disease process and the need for further investigation and possible surgical management. A well-articulated follow-up plan is essential.

Perioperative Decision Making

Once the decision has been made to proceed with operative management, a number of considerations must be addressed regarding the timing and site of surgery, the type of anesthesia, and the preoperative preparation necessary to understand the patient's risk and optimize the outcome. These components of risk assessment take into account both the perioperative (intraoperative period through 48 hours postoperatively) and the later postoperative (up to 30 days) periods and seek to identify factors that may contribute to patient morbidity during these periods.

Preoperative Evaluation

The aim of preoperative evaluation is not to screen broadly for undiagnosed disease but rather to identify and quantify any comorbidity that may have an impact on the operative outcome. This evaluation is driven by findings on the history and physical examination suggestive of organ system dysfunction or by epidemiologic data suggesting the benefit of evaluation based on age, gender, or patterns of disease progression. The goal is to uncover problem areas that may require further investigation or be amenable to preoperative optimization (Table 12-1).[1] Routine preoperative testing is not cost-effective and, even in the elderly, is less predictive of perioperative morbidity than the American Society of Anesthesiologists (ASA) status or American Heart Association (AHA)/American College of Cardiology (ACC) guidelines for surgical risk.

The preoperative evaluation is determined in light of the planned procedure (low, medium, or high risk), the planned anesthetic technique, and the postoperative disposition of the patient (outpatient or inpatient, ward bed, or intensive care). In addition, the preoperative evaluation is used to identify patient risk factors for postoperative morbidity and mortality. The National Surgical Quality Improvement Program (NSQIP) has been used to develop predictive models for postoperative morbidity and mortality, and several factors have consistently been found to be independent predictors of postoperative events (Table 12-2).[2]

If preoperative evaluation uncovers significant comorbidity or evidence of poor control of an underlying disease process, consultation with an internist or medical subspecialist may be required to facilitate the workup and direct management. In this process, communication between the surgeon and consultants is essential to define realistic goals for this optimization process and to expedite surgical management.

SYSTEMS APPROACH TO PREOPERATIVE EVALUATION

Cardiovascular

Cardiovascular disease is the leading cause of death in the industrialized world, and its contribution to perioperative mortality during noncardiac surgery is significant. Of the 27 million patients undergoing surgery in the United States every year, 8 million, or nearly 30%, have significant coronary artery disease or other cardiac comorbid conditions. One million of these patients will experience perioperative cardiac complications, with substantial morbidity, mortality, and cost.[3] Consequently, much of the preoperative risk assessment and patient preparation centers on the cardiovascular system.

One of the first anesthesia risk categorization systems was the ASA classification. It has five stratifications:

I—Normal healthy patient
II—Patient with mild systemic disease
III—Patient with severe systemic disease that limits activity but is not incapacitating
IV—Patient who has incapacitating disease that is a constant threat to life

V—Moribund patient not expected to survive 24 hours with or without an operation

Even though the system seems subjective, it continues to be a significant independent predictor of mortality.[2]

Later assessment tools for stratification of anesthetic risk involved more easily defined and measured parameters and were enhanced by multivariate statistical methodology. The premiere example is Goldman's criteria (Table 12-3).[4] This strategy, designed by multivariate analysis, assigns points to easily reproducible characteristics. The points are then added to yield a total, which has been correlated with perioperative cardiac risk. One of the more important contributions of this work was the inclusion of functional capacity, clinical signs and symptoms, and operative risk assessment to estimate the patient's overall risk and plan preoperative interventions. This concept has been further refined in the Revised Cardiac Risk Index, which uses six predictors of complications to estimate cardiac risk in noncardiac surgical patients (see Table 12-3). In addition, several other investigators have proposed cardiac risk indices, many of which were expensive and time consuming.

In an attempt to best assess and optimize the cardiac status of patients undergoing noncardiac surgery, a joint committee of the ACC and the AHA has developed an easily used tool (Fig. 12-1).[5] This methodology takes into account previous coronary revascularization and evaluation and clinical risk assessment, which are divided into major, intermediate, and minor clinical predictors. The next factor taken into account is the patient's functional capacity, which is estimated by obtaining a history of the patient's daily activities. The earlier-mentioned variables and the type of surgery are then used to determine whether the pretest probability can be altered by noninvasive testing. The standard exercise stress test with or without thallium for perfusion imaging can be limited by the functional capacity of the patient. Patients not able to exercise to an acceptable stress level may require pharmacologic stress testing with dipyridamole; thereafter, perfusion defects can be assessed via thallium or a dobutamine-induced stress, followed by functional evaluation with echocardiography. Angiography can then be used to exactly define the anatomic abnormalities contributing to the ischemia. Although no prospective, randomized trial has been conducted to determine whether following these guidelines has improved outcomes for patients, several studies suggest that there is utility in doing so.[4]

Once these data have been obtained, the surgeon and consultants need to weigh the benefits of surgery against the risk and determine whether any perioperative intervention will reduce the probability of a cardiac event. This intervention usually centers on coronary revascularization via coronary artery bypass or percutaneous transluminal coronary angioplasty but may include modification of the choice of anesthetic or the use of invasive intraoperative monitoring. Patients who have undergone a percutaneous coronary intervention with stenting need to have elective noncardiac procedures delayed for 4 to 6 weeks, although the delay may be shortened

Table 12-1   Suggestions for Adult Preoperative Testing

The table groups conditions into three categories:

- **BASIC: MINOR SURGERY IN HEALTHY PATIENT (WITHIN 90 DAYS)**
- **Surgical Procedures (Within 90 Days)**
- **ADDITIVE SURGICAL AND MEDICAL FACTORS** — Clinically Significant and Changing Disorders and/or Medications (Shaded = Within 90 Days; Light = Test for Disorder Probably Should Be Performed Within 30 Days)

Condition	ECG	CBC+platelets	Electrolytes	BUN/creatinine	Glucose	LFTs	Calcium	PT/PTT	U/A, culture	CXR	Hormone levels	Bleeding time	Pregnancy	Drug levels	Tumor markers	Clot
BASIC: MINOR SURGERY IN HEALTHY PATIENT																
Healthy Adult <45 y/o																
H45-54 y/o	M															
55-69 y/o	Y	Y														
>70 y/o	Y	Y	Y	Y	Y											
Surgical Procedures																
Cardiac/Thoracic	Y	Y	Y	Y	Y			Y		Y						
Vascular	Y	Y	Y	Y	Y											
Major Intraperitoneal/abdominal	Y	Y	Y	Y	Y	±										
Anticipated >2 U EBL	Y	Y	Y	Y	Y			Y								
Intracranial	Y	Y	Y	Y	Y			Y					S			
Orthopedic Prosthesis		Y	Y	Y	Y				S							
TURP, Hysterostomy		Y	Y	Y	Y											
Hypertension	Y		Y	Y												
Smoking	Y	Y														
Morbid Obesity	Y	Y	Y	Y	Y											
h/o Stroke	Y	Y	Y	Y	Y											
Cancer (?Metastatic)	Y	Y	Y	Y	Y					S					S	
Seizure Medications			Y			Y								S		
ADDITIVE SURGICAL AND MEDICAL FACTORS																
Cardiovascular	Y	Y	Y	Y	Y											
Respiratory	Y	Y	Y	Y	Y					Y						
Diabetes		Y	Y	Y	Y											
Hepatic		Y	Y	Y	Y			Y								
Renal		Y	Y	Y	Y			Y								
Fluid or Electrolyte Loss	±	Y	Y	Y												
Autoimmune/Lupus	Y	Y	Y	Y				Y	Y							
EtOH/Drug Abuse	Y	Y	Y	Y	Y	Y		Y						±		
Steroids/Cushing's Syndrome	Y	Y	Y	Y	Y	Y										
HIV	Y	Y	Y	Y	Y	Y				S						
Parathyroid	Y	Y	Y	Y	Y		Y									
Unstable Thyroid	Y	Y	Y	Y	Y		Y				Y					
Anticoagulant/Bleeding								Y		Y		±				
Suspected Pregnancy													Y*			
Clot	Depends primarily on extensiveness of proposed surgery, as per Blood Bank MSBOS guidelines															

Note: (1) Times and test listings are suggestions; they are not absolute and should not preclude other testing in given settings, nor should they prevent a case from proceeding if the anesthesiologist and surgeon deem it to be appropriate. (2) Testing for a given disorder depends on the severity of the disorder in the context of the planned surgery; that is, are the tests likely to generate potentially clinically significant information and provide information that would be an important component of the history and physical examination.

*At a minimum, a urine pregnancy test should be performed on the morning of surgery in any woman of childbearing age, unless the uterus or ovaries are surgically absent.

Shaded area, timing of test is not typically critical; results from 90 days (and possibly 180 days) may be acceptable. *Light area*, typically best to obtain within 30 days of surgery.

BUN, blood urea nitrogen; CBC, complete blood count; CXR, chest x-ray; EBL, estimated blood loss; ECG, electrocardiogram; EtOH, ethanol; HIV, human immunodeficiency virus; h/o, history of; LFTs, liver function tests; M, usually indicated for male; MSBOS, maximum surgical blood order schedule; PT/PTT, prothrombin time/partial thromboplastin time; S, may be requested (and reviewed) by the surgeon as part of surgical workup; TURP, transurethral resection of the prostate; U/A, urinalysis; Y, usually indicated; ±, if situation acute/severe.

Adapted from Halaszynski TM, Juda R, Silverman DG: Optimizing postoperative outcomes with efficient preoperative assessment and management. Crit Care Med 32(Suppl):S76-S86, 2004.

Table 12-2 Patient Risk Factors Most Predictive of Postoperative Mortality and Morbidity, National Surgical Quality Improvement Program

	MORTALITY		MORBIDITY	
PATIENT RISK FACTOR	No. of Times in Model	Average Order of Entry	No. of Times in Model	Average Order of Entry
Serum albumin	9/9	1.9	9/9	1.2
ASA class	9/9	3.6	9/9	2.9
Functional status			9/9	4.6
Emergency surgery	8/9	5.0	7/9	6.6
Disseminated cancer	8/9	6.5		
Age	8/9	6.6	7/9	9.7
DNR status	8/9	7.4		
Platelets ≤150,000	6/9	7.5	6/9	13.8
Weight loss >10%	6/9	8.2		
Operative complexity score	6/9	8.8	9/9	3.4
BUN >40 mg/dL	4/9	5.0		
Hematocrit ≤38%			7/9	12.4
WBC >11,000			7/9	12.4
Ventilator dependence			6/9	8.0

ASA, American Society of Anesthesiologists; BUN, blood urea nitrogen; DNR, do not resuscitate; WBC, white blood cell count.

Table 12-3 Cardiac Risk Indices

CARDIAC RISK INDEX WITH VARIABLES	POINTS	COMMENTS
Goldman Cardiac Risk Index, 1977		**Cardiac Complication Rate**
1. Third heart sound or jugular venous distention	11	0-5 points = 1%
2. Recent myocardial infarction	10	6-12 points = 7%
3. Nonsinus rhythm or premature atrial contraction on ECG	7	13-25 points = 14%
4. >5 premature ventricular contractions	7	>26 points = 78%
5. Age >70 years	5	
6. Emergency operations	4	
7. Poor general medical condition	3	
8. Intrathoracic, intraperitoneal, or aortic surgery	3	
9. Important valvular aortic stenosis	3	
Detsky Modified Multifactorial Index, 1986		**Cardiac Complication Rate**
1. Class 4 angina	20	>15 = high risk
2. Suspected critical aortic stenosis	20	
3. Myocardial infarction within 6 mo	10	
4. Alveolar pulmonary edema within 1 wk	10	
5. Unstable angina within 3 mo	10	
6. Class 3 angina	10	
7. Emergency surgery	10	
8. Myocardial infarction >6 mo ago	5	
9. Alveolar pulmonary edema resolved >1 wk ago	5	
10. Rhythm other than sinus or PACs on ECG	5	
11. >5 PVCs any time before surgery	5	
12. Poor general medical status	5	
13. Age >70 yr	5	
Eagle's Criteria for Cardiac Risk Assessment, 1989		
1. Age >70 yr	1	<1, no testing
2. Diabetes	1	1-2, send for noninvasive test
3. Angina	1	≥3, send for angiography
4. Q waves on ECG	1	
5. Ventricular arrhythmias	1	
Revised Cardiac Risk Index		
1. Ischemic heart disease	1	Each increment in points increases the risk for
2. Congestive heart failure	1	postoperative myocardial morbidity
3. Cerebral vascular disease	1	
4. High-risk surgery	1	
5. Preoperative insulin treatment of diabetes	1	
6. Preoperative creatinine >2 mg/dL	1	

ECG, electrocardiogram; PAC, premature atrial contraction; PVC, premature ventricular contraction.
Adapted from Akhtar S, Silverman DG: Assessment and management of patients with ischemic heart disease. Crit Care Med 32(Suppl):S126-S136, 2004.

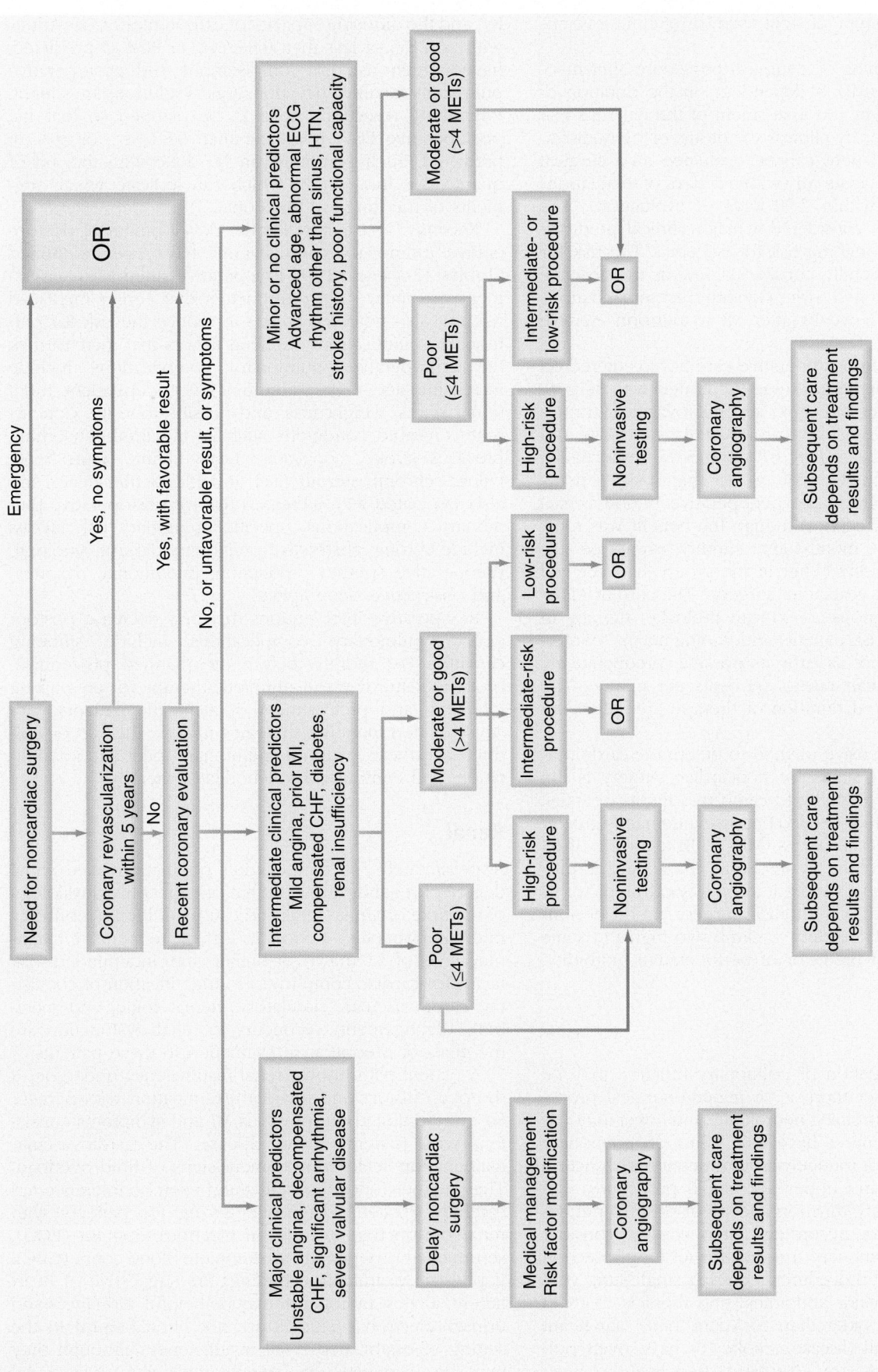

Figure 12-1 Stepwise approach to preoperative cardiac assessment. An abbreviated list of metabolic equivalents (METs) includes the following: 1—take care of yourself, eat, dress, and so forth; 4—light housework; 5—climb a flight of stairs or walk up a hill; 10—strenuous sports. *Procedure risks* are defined as the following: *high*—emergency major operations, aortic surgery, other vascular surgery, large blood loss; *intermediate*—carotid, head and neck, intraperitoneal, intrathoracic, orthopedic, or prostate surgery; *low*—all others. CHF, congestive heart failure; ECG, electrocardiogram; MI, myocardial infarction; OR, operating room. (Adapted from Eagle KA, Berger PB, Calkins H, et al: ACC/AHA guideline update for perioperative cardiovascular evaluation for noncardiac surgery—executive summary: A report of the American College of Cardiology/American Heart Association Task Force on Practice Guidelines [Committee to Update 1996 Guidelines on Perioperative Cardiovascular Evaluation for Noncardiac Surgery]. J Am Coll Cardiol 39:542-553, 2002.)

depending on the type of stent used (drug eluting versus non–drug eluting).[4]

The optimal timing of a surgical procedure after myocardial infarction (MI) is dependent on the duration of time since the event and assessment of the patient's risk for ischemia, either by clinical symptoms or by noninvasive study. Any patient can be evaluated as a surgical candidate after an acute MI (within 7 days of evaluation) or a recent MI (within 7-30 days of evaluation). The infarction event is considered a major clinical predictor in the context of ongoing risk for ischemia. The risk for reinfarction is generally considered low in the absence of such demonstrated risk. General recommendations are to wait 4 to 6 weeks after MI to perform elective surgery.[5]

Improvements in postoperative care have centered on decreasing the adrenergic surge associated with surgery and halting platelet activation and microvascular thrombosis. Perioperative risk for cardiovascular morbidity and mortality was decreased by 67% and 55%, respectively, in ACC/AHA-defined medium- to high-risk patients receiving β-blockers in the perioperative period versus those receiving placebo. Although the benefit was most noticeable in the 6 months after surgery, event-free survival was significantly better in the group that received β-blockers up to 2 years after surgery.[6] The current AHA/ACC recommendations are to start β-blocker therapy in medium- to high-risk patients undergoing major- to intermediate-risk surgery as early as possible preoperatively and titrate to a heart rate of 60 beats per minute. The choice of agent and duration of therapy are still being debated.

An easy, inexpensive method to determine cardiopulmonary functional status for noncardiac surgery is the patient's ability or inability to climb two flights of stairs. Two flights of stairs is needed because it demands greater than 4 metabolic equivalents (METs). In a review of all studies of stair climbing as preoperative assessment, prospective studies have shown it to be a good predictor of mortality associated with thoracic surgery.[7] In major noncardiac surgery, an inability to climb two flights of stairs is an independent predictor of perioperative morbidity, but not mortality.

Pulmonary

Preoperative evaluation of pulmonary function may be necessary for either thoracic or general surgical procedures. Whereas extremity, neurologic, and lower abdominal surgical procedures have little effect on pulmonary function and do not routinely require pulmonary function studies, thoracic and upper abdominal procedures can decrease pulmonary function and predispose to pulmonary complications. Accordingly, it is wise to consider assessment of pulmonary function for all lung resection cases, for thoracic procedures requiring single-lung ventilation, and for major abdominal and thoracic cases in patients who are older than 60 years, have significant underlying medical disease, smoke, or have overt pulmonary symptomatology.[8] Necessary tests include forced expiratory volume in 1 second (FEV_1), forced vital capac-

ity, and the diffusing capacity of carbon monoxide. Adults with an FEV_1 of less than 0.8 L/sec, or 30% of predicted, have a high risk for complications and postoperative pulmonary insufficiency; nonsurgical solutions are sought. Pulmonary resections need to be planned so that the postoperative FEV_1 is greater than 0.8 L/sec, or 30% of predicted. Such planning can be done with the aid of quantitative lung scans, which can indicate which segments of the lung are functional.

Recently, risk factors for the development of postoperative pulmonary complications have been identified (Tables 12-4 and 12-5).[8] Preoperative pulmonary assessment determines not only factors that confer increased risk but also potential targets to reduce the risk for pulmonary complications. General factors that increase risk for postoperative pulmonary complications include increasing age, lower albumin level, dependent functional status, weight loss, and possibly obesity. Concurrent comorbid conditions such as impaired sensorium, previous stroke, congestive heart failure, acute renal failure, chronic steroid use, and blood transfusion are also associated with increased risk for postoperative pulmonary complications. Specific pulmonary risk factors include chronic obstructive pulmonary disease, smoking, preoperative sputum production, pneumonia, dyspnea, and obstructive sleep apnea.

Preoperative interventions that may decrease postoperative pulmonary complications include smoking cessation (>2 months before the planned procedure), bronchodilator therapy, antibiotic therapy for preexisting infection, and pretreatment of asthmatic patients with steroids. Perioperative strategies include the use of epidural anesthesia, vigorous pulmonary toilet and rehabilitation, and continued bronchodilator therapy.[8]

Renal

Approximately 5% of the adult population have some degree of renal dysfunction that can affect the physiology of multiple organ systems and cause additional morbidity in the perioperative period. In fact, a preoperative creatinine level of 2.0 mg/dL or higher is an independent risk factor for cardiac complications. Identification of coexisting cardiovascular, circulatory, hematologic, and metabolic derangements secondary to renal dysfunction are the goals of preoperative evaluation in these patients.

A patient with known renal insufficiency undergoes a thorough history and physical examination with particular questioning about previous MI and symptoms consistent with ischemic heart disease. The cardiovascular examination seeks to document signs of fluid overload. The patient's functional status and exercise tolerance are carefully elicited. Diagnostic testing for patients with renal dysfunction include an electrocardiogram (ECG), serum chemistry panel, and complete blood count (CBC). If physical examination findings are suggestive of heart failure, a chest radiograph may be helpful. Urinalysis and urinary electrolyte studies are not often helpful in the setting of established renal insufficiency, although they may be diagnostic in patients with new-onset renal dysfunction.

Table 12-4 Risk Factors for the Development of Postoperative Pneumonia and Respiratory Failure

RISK FACTORS	POSTOPERATIVE PNEUMONIA RISK INDEX (OR [95% CI])	POINT VALUE	RESPIRATORY FAILURE RISK INDEX (OR [95% CI])	POINT VALUE
Type of surgery				
AAA repair	4.29 (3.34-5.50)	15	14.3 (12.0-16.9)	27
Thoracic	3.92 (3.36-4.57)	14	8.14 (7.17-9.25)	21
Upper abdominal	2.68 (2.38-3.03)	10	4.21 (3.80-4.67)	14
Neck	2.30 (1.73-3.05)	8	3.10 (2.40-4.01)	11
Neurosurgical	2.14 (1.66-2.75)	8	4.21 (3.80-4.67)	14
Vascular	1.29 (1.10-1.52)	3	4.21 (3.80-4.67)	14
Emergency surgery	1.33 (1.16-1.54)	3	3.12 (2.83-3.43)	11
General anesthesia	1.56 (1.36-1.80)	4	1.91 (1.64-2.21)	—
Age				
>80 yr	5.63 (4.62-6.84)	17	—	—
70-79 yr	3.58 (2.97-4.33)	13	—	—
60-69 yr	2.38 (1.98-2.87)	9	—	—
50-59 yr	1.49 (1.23-1.81)	4	—	—
<50 yr	1.00 (referent)	—	—	—
≥70 yr	—	—	1.91 (1.71-2.13)	6
60-69 yr	—	—	1.51 (1.36-1.69)	4
<60 yr	—	—	1.00 (referent)	—
Functional status				
Totally dependent	3.83 (2.33-3.43)	10	1.92 (1.74-2.11)	7
Partially dependent	1.83 (1.63-2.06)	6	1.92 (1.74-2.11)	7
Independent	1.00 (referent)	—	1.00 (referent)	—
Albumin				
<3.0 g/dL	—	—	2.53 (2.28-2.80)	9
>3.0 g/dL	—	—	1.00 (referent)	—
Weight loss >10% (within 6 mo)	1.92 (1.68-2.18)	7	1.37 (1.19-1.57)*	—
Chronic steroid use	1.33 (1.12-1.58)	3	—	—
Alcohol—>2 drinks/day (within 2 wk)	1.24 (1.08-1.42)	2	1.19 (1.07-1.33)*	—
Diabetes—insulin treated	—	—	1.15 (1.00-1.33)*	—
History of COPD	1.72 (1.55-1.91)	5	1.81 (1.66-1.98)	6
Current smoker				
Within 1 yr	1.28 (1.17-1.42)	3	—	—
Within 2 wk	—	—	1.24 (1.14-1.36)*	—
Preoperative pneumonia	—	—	1.70 (1.24-2.13)*	—
Dyspnea				
At rest	—	—	1.69 (1.36-2.09)*	—
With minimal exertion	—	—	1.21 (1.09-1.34)*	—
No dyspnea	—	—	1.00 (referent)	—
Impaired sensorium	1.51 (1.26-1.82)	4	1.22 (1.04-1.43)*	—
History of CVA	1.47 (1.28-1.68)	4	1.20 (1.05-1.38)*	—
History of CHF	—	—	1.25 (1.07-1.47)*	—
Blood urea nitrogen				
<8 mg/dL	1.47 (1.26-1.72)	4	1.00 (referent)	—
8-21 mg/dL	1.00 (referent)	—	1.00 (referent)	—
22-30 mg/dL	1.24 (1.11-1.39)	2	1.00 (referent)	—
>30 mg/dL	1.41 (1.22-1.64)	3	2.29 (2.04-2.56)	8
Preoperative renal failure	—	—	1.67 (1.23-2.27)*	—
Preoperative transfusion (>4 units)	1.35 (1.07-1.72)	3	1.56 (1.28-1.91)*	—

*Risk factor was statistically significant in multivariable analysis but was not included in the Respiratory Failure Risk Index.

AAA, abdominal aortic aneurysm; CHF, congestive heart failure; CI, confidence interval; COPD, chronic obstructive pulmonary disease; CVA, cerebrovascular accident; OR, odds ratio.

Adapted from Arozullah AM, Khuri SF, Henderson WG, et al: Development and validation of a multifactorial risk index for predicting postoperative pneumonia after major noncardiac surgery. Ann Intern Med 135:847-857, 2001; and Arozullah AM, Daley J, Henderson WG, Khuri SF: Multifactorial risk index for predicting postoperative respiratory failure in men after major noncardiac surgery. Ann Surg 232:242-253, 2000, with permission.

Table 12-5   Pulmonary Risk Class Assignment

RISK CLASS	POSTOPERATIVE PNEUMONIA RISK INDEX (POINT TOTAL)	PREDICTED PROBABILITY OF PNEUMONIA (%)	RESPIRATORY FAILURE RISK INDEX (POINT TOTAL)	PREDICTED PROBABILITY OF RESPIRATORY FAILURE (%)
1	0-15	0.2	0-10	0.5
2	16-25	1.2	11-19	2.2
3	26-40	4.0	20-27	5.0
4	41-55	9.4	28-40	11.6
5	>55	15.3	>40	30.5

Adapted from Arozullah AM, Khuri SF, Henderson WG, et al: Development and validation of a multifactorial risk index for predicting postoperative pneumonia after major noncardiac surgery. Ann Intern Med 135:847-857, 2001; and Arozullah AM, Daley J, Henderson WG, Khuri SF: Multifactorial risk index for predicting postoperative respiratory failure in men after major noncardiac surgery. Ann Surg 232:242-253, 2000, with permission.

Laboratory abnormalities are often seen in a patient with advanced renal insufficiency. Some metabolic derangements in a patient with advanced renal failure may be mild and asymptomatic and are revealed by electrolyte or blood gas analysis. Anemia, when present in these patients, may range from mild and asymptomatic to that associated with fatigue, low exercise tolerance, and exertional angina. Such anemia can be treated with erythropoietin or darbepoietin preoperatively or perioperatively. Because the platelet dysfunction associated with uremia is often a qualitative one, platelet counts are usually normal. A safe course is to communicate with the anesthesiologist the potential need for agents to be available in the operating room to assist in improving platelet function. A patient with end-stage renal disease frequently requires additional attention in the perioperative period. Pharmacologic manipulation of hyperkalemia, replacement of calcium for symptomatic hypocalcemia, and the use of phosphate-binding antacids for hyperphosphatemia are often required. Sodium bicarbonate is used in the setting of metabolic acidosis not caused by hypoperfusion when serum bicarbonate levels are below 15 mEq/L. It can be administered in intravenous (IV) fluid as 1 to 2 ampules in a 5% dextrose solution. Hyponatremia is treated by volume restriction, although dialysis is commonly required within the perioperative period for control of volume and electrolyte abnormalities.

Patients with chronic end-stage renal disease undergo dialysis before surgery to optimize their volume status and control the potassium level. Intraoperative hyperkalemia can result from surgical manipulation of tissue or transfusion of blood. Such patients are often dialyzed on the day after surgery as well. In the acute setting, patients who have stable volume status can undergo surgery without preoperative dialysis, provided that no other indication exists for emergency dialysis.[9] Prevention of secondary renal insults in the perioperative period include the avoidance of nephrotoxic agents and maintenance of adequate intravascular volume throughout this period. In the postoperative period, the pharmacokinetics of many drugs may be unpredictable, and adjustments in dosage need to be made according to pharmacy recommendation. Notably, narcotics used for postoperative pain control may have prolonged effects despite hepatic clearance, and nonsteroidal agents are avoided in patients with renal insufficiency.

Hepatobiliary

Hepatic dysfunction may reflect the common pathway of a number of insults to the liver, including viral-, drug-, and toxin-mediated disease. A patient with liver dysfunction requires careful assessment of the degree of functional impairment, as well as a coordinated effort to avoid additional insult in the perioperative period (Fig. 12-2).[10]

A history of any exposure to blood and blood products or exposure to hepatotoxic agents is obtained. Patients frequently know whether hepatitis has been diagnosed and need to be questioned about when the diagnosis was made and what activity led to the infection. Although such a history may not affect further patient evaluation, it is important to obtain in case an operative team member is injured during the planned surgical procedure. A review of systems specifically inquires about symptoms such as pruritus, fatigability, excessive bleeding, abdominal distention, and weight gain. Evidence of hepatic dysfunction may be seen on physical examination. Jaundice and scleral icterus may be evident with serum bilirubin levels higher than 3 mg/dL. Skin changes include spider angiomas, caput medusae, palmar erythema, and clubbing of the fingertips. Abdominal examination may reveal distention, evidence of fluid shift, and hepatomegaly. Encephalopathy or asterixis may be evident. Muscle wasting or cachexia can be prominent.

A patient with liver dysfunction undergoes standard liver function tests. Elevations in hepatocellular enzymes may suggest a diagnosis of acute or chronic hepatitis, which can be investigated by serologic testing for hepatitis A, B, and C. Alcoholic hepatitis is suggested by lower transaminase levels and an aspartate/alanine transaminase ratio (AST/ALT) greater than 2. Laboratory evidence of chronic hepatitis or clinical findings consistent with cirrhosis is investigated with tests of hepatic synthetic function, notably serum albumin, prothrombin, and fibrinogen. Patients with evidence of impaired hepatic synthetic function also have a CBC and serum electrolyte analysis. Type and screen is indicated for any procedure in which blood loss could be more than minimal.

In the event of an emergency situation requiring surgery, such an investigation may not be possible. A patient with acute hepatitis and elevated transaminases is managed nonoperatively, when feasible, until several

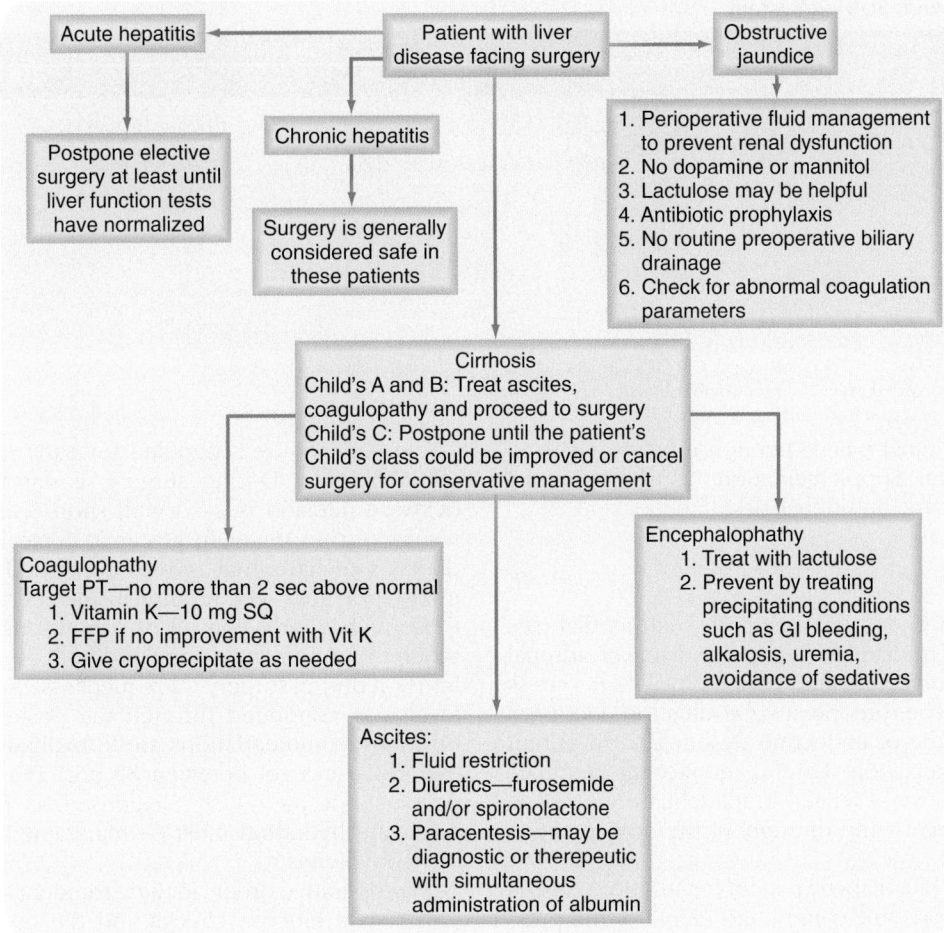

Figure 12-2 Approach to a patient with liver disease. GI, gastrointestinal; FFP, fresh frozen plasma; PT, prothrombin time; SQ, subcutaneous. (Adapted from Rizvon MK, Chou CL: Surgery in the patient with liver disease. Med Clin North Am 87:211-227, 2003.)

weeks beyond normalization of laboratory values. Urgent or emergency procedures in these patients are associated with increased morbidity and mortality. A patient with evidence of chronic hepatitis may often safely undergo surgery. A patient with cirrhosis may be assessed with the Child-Pugh classification, which stratifies operative risk according to a score based on abnormal albumin and bilirubin levels, prolongation of the prothrombin time (PT), and the degree of ascites and encephalopathy (Table 12-6). This scoring system was initially applied to predict mortality in cirrhotic patients undergoing porta-caval shunt procedures, although it has been shown to correlate with mortality in cirrhotic patients undergoing a wider spectrum of procedures as well. Data generated 20 years ago showed that patients with Child's class A, B, and C cirrhosis had mortality rates of 10%, 31%, and 76%, respectively, during abdominal operations; these figures have been validated more recently.[10] Although the figures may not represent current risk for all types of abdominal operations, little doubt exists that the presence of cirrhosis confers additional risk for abdominal surgery and that this risk is proportional to the severity of disease. Other factors that affect outcomes in these patients are the emergency nature of a procedure, pro-

longation of the PT greater than 3 seconds above normal and refractory to correction with vitamin K, and the presence of infection.

Two common problems requiring surgical evaluation in a cirrhotic patient are hernia (umbilical and groin) and cholecystitis. An umbilical hernia in the presence of ascites is a difficult management problem because spontaneous rupture is associated with increased mortality rates. Elective repair is best after the ascites has been reduced to a minimum preoperatively, although the procedure is still associated with mortality rates as high as 14%.[11] Repair of groin hernias in the presence of ascites is less risky in terms of both recurrence and mortality.[12]

Several recent reports have shown decreased rates of complication with laparoscopic procedures performed in cirrhotic patients. Among the best-described procedures is laparoscopic cholecystectomy performed in patients with Child's class A through C. When compared with open cholecystectomy, less morbidity in terms of blood loss and wound infection has been observed.[13]

Malnutrition is common in cirrhotic patients and is associated with a reduction in hepatic glycogen stores and reduced hepatic protein synthesis. Patients with advanced liver disease often have a poor appetite, tense

Table 12-6 Child-Pugh Scoring System

	POINTS		
	1	**2**	**3**
Encephalopathy	None	Stage I or II	Stage III or IV
Ascites	Absent	Slight (controlled with diuretics)	Moderate despite diuretic treatment
Bilirubin (mg/dL)	<2	2-3	>3
Albumin (g/L)	>3.5	2.8-3.5	<2.8
PT (prolonged seconds)	<4	4-6	>6
INR	<1.7	1.7-2.3	>2.3

Class A = 5-6 points; Class B = 7-9 points; Class C = 10-15 points.
INR, international normalized ratio; PT, prothrombin time.

ascites, and abdominal pain. Attention must be given to appropriate enteral supplementation, as done for all patients at significant nutritional risk.

Endocrine

A patient with an endocrine condition such as diabetes mellitus, hyperthyroidism or hypothyroidism, or adrenal insufficiency is subject to additional physiologic stress during surgery. The preoperative evaluation identifies the type and degree of endocrine dysfunction to permit preoperative optimization. Careful monitoring identifies signs of metabolic stress related to inadequate endocrine control during surgery and throughout the postoperative course.

The evaluation of a diabetic patient for surgery assesses the adequacy of glycemic control and identifies the presence of diabetic complications, which may have an impact on the patient's perioperative course. The patient's history and physical examination document evidence of diabetic complications, including cardiac disease, circulatory abnormalities, and the presence of retinopathy, neuropathy, or nephropathy. Preoperative testing may include fasting and postprandial glucose and hemoglobin A_{1c} levels. Serum electrolyte, blood urea nitrogen, and creatinine levels are obtained to identify metabolic disturbances and renal involvement. Urinalysis may reveal proteinuria as evidence of diabetic nephropathy. An ECG is considered in patients with long-standing disease. The existence of neuropathy in diabetics may be accompanied by cardiac autonomic neuropathy, which increases the risk for cardiorespiratory instability in the perioperative period.

A diabetic patient requires special attention to optimize glycemic control perioperatively. Non–insulin-dependent diabetics need to discontinue long-acting sulfonylureas such as chlorpropamide and glyburide because of the risk for intraoperative hypoglycemia; a shorter-acting agent or sliding-scale insulin coverage may be substituted in this period. The use of metformin is stopped preoperatively because of its association with lactic acidosis in the setting of renal insufficiency. An insulin-dependent diabetic is told to withhold long-acting insulin preparations (Ultralente preparations) on the day of surgery; lower dosages of intermediate-acting insulin (NPH or Lente) are substituted on the morning of surgery.

These patients are scheduled for early morning surgery, when feasible. During surgery, a standard 5% or 10% dextrose infusion is used with short-acting insulin or an insulin drip to maintain glycemic control. A patient with diabetes mellitus that is well controlled by diet or oral medication may not require insulin perioperatively, but those with poorer control or patients taking insulin may require preoperative dosing and both glucose and insulin infusion during surgery.[14] Frequent assessments of glucose levels are continued through the postoperative period. Current recommendations are to maintain the perioperative glucose level between 80 and 150 mg/dL, even in patients not previously diagnosed as being diabetic.[15] Adequate hydration must be maintained with avoidance of hypovolemia.

Postoperative orders include frequent (every 2-4 hours) finger stick glucose checks and the use of short-acting insulin in the form of sliding-scale coverage. Twice-daily doses of intermediate-acting insulin can be supplemented with sliding-scale coverage until the patient is eating and can resume the usual regimen. Postoperative cardiac events can occur with unusual manifestations in these patients. Although chest pain needs to be evaluated with ECG and serum troponin levels, this same evaluation may need to be done for new-onset dyspnea, blood pressure alterations, or a decrease in urine output. Adequate prophylaxis for deep venous thrombosis (DVT) is essential because of the increased risk for thrombosis. The adequacy of perioperative glycemic control has an impact on wound healing and the risk for surgical site infection.

Perioperative Diabetic Management

Management of diabetic patients has evolved over the past several years. The introduction of new drugs for non–insulin-dependent diabetics, in addition to new types of insulin and new insulin delivery systems in insulin-dependent diabetics, has changed the way that these patients are approached in the perioperative period.

Insulin is available in several types and is typically classified by its length of action (Table 12-7). Rapid-acting (Lispro) and short-acting (Regular) insulin preparations are usually withheld when the patient stops oral intake (NPO) and are used for acute management of hyperglycemia during the NPO period. Intermediate-acting (NPH Lente) and long-acting (Ultralente, Glargine) insulin preparations are administered at two thirds the normal PM

Table 12-7   Insulin Types

TYPE OF INSULIN	ONSET OF ACTION	PEAK EFFECT	DURATION OF ACTION
Rapid acting (Lispro)	15-30 minutes	30-90 minutes	3-4 hours
Short acting (Regular)	30-60 minutes	2-4 hours	6-10 hours
Intermediate acting (NPH Lente)	1-4 hours	4-12 hours	12-24 hours
Long acting			
Ultralente	1-2 hours	8-20 hours	24-30 hours
Glargine	1 hour	3-20 hours	24 hours

From Ahmed Z, Lockhart CH, Weiner M, et al: Advances in diabetic management: Implications for anesthesia. Anesth Analg 100:666-669, 2005.

dose the night before surgery and half the normal AM dose the morning of surgery, with frequent bedside glucose determinations and treatment with short-acting insulin as needed. An infusion of 5% dextrose is initiated the morning of surgery. If the planned procedure is expected to take a long time, an insulin infusion can be administered, again with frequent monitoring of blood glucose.

Insulin pumps are used by some patients as their method of glucose management. These pumps use short-acting insulin and have a variable delivery rate that can be programmed to more closely simulate endogenous insulin production. On the day of surgery, the patient continues with the basal insulin infusion. The pump is then used to correct the glucose level as it is measured. Patients generally have a correction or sensitivity factor that will decrease their glucose by 50 mg/dL. It is important to know this factor before the planned surgical procedure so that glucose can be managed in the operating room.[16]

Patients who take oral hypoglycemic agents typically withhold their normal dose the day of surgery. Patients can resume their oral agent once diet is resumed. Coverage for hyperglycemia is with a short-acting insulin preparation based on blood glucose monitoring. An exception is metformin. If the patient has altered renal function, this agent needs to be discontinued until renal function either normalizes or stabilizes.[15]

A patient with known or suspected thyroid disease is evaluated with a thyroid function panel. Evidence of hyperthyroidism is addressed preoperatively and surgery deferred until a euthyroid state is achieved, when feasible. These patients need to have their electrolyte levels determined and an ECG performed as part of their preoperative evaluation. In addition, if the physical examination suggests signs of airway compromise, further imaging may be warranted. A patient with hyperthyroidism who takes antithyroid medication such as propylthiouracil or methimazole is instructed to continue this regimen on the day of surgery. The patient's usual doses of β-blockers or digoxin are also continued. In the event of urgent surgery in a thyrotoxic patient at risk for thyroid storm, a combination of adrenergic blockers and glucocorticoids may be required and are administered in consultation with an endocrinologist. Patients with newly diagnosed hypothyroidism generally do not require preoperative treatment, although they may be subject to

increased sensitivity to medications, including anesthetic agents and narcotics. Severe hypothyroidism can be associated with myocardial dysfunction, coagulation abnormality, and electrolyte imbalance, notably hypoglycemia. Severe hypothyroidism needs to be corrected before elective operations.

A patient with a history of steroid use may require supplementation for a presumed abnormal adrenal response to perioperative stress (Box 12-1). Patients who have taken more than 5 mg of prednisone (or equivalent) per day for more than 3 weeks within the past year are considered at risk when undergoing major surgery. Lower doses of steroid or minor procedures are not generally associated with adrenal suppression.

The adequacy of the hypothalamic-pituitary response to adrenocorticotropic hormone (ACTH) can be tested in any patient who may have some degree of suppression secondary to chronic or intermittent steroid use. A low-dose (1 μm) ACTH stimulation test may demonstrate abnormal response to adrenal stimulation and suggest the need for perioperative steroid supplementation. Recent guidelines suggest titrating the dosage of glucocorticoid replacement to the degree of surgical stress (see Box 12-1). Minor operations such as hernia repair under local anesthesia may not require any additional steroid. Moderate operations such as open cholecystectomy or lower extremity revascularization require 50 to 75 mg/day of hydrocortisone equivalent for 1 or 2 days. Major operations such as colectomy or cardiac surgery are covered with 100 to 150 mg/day of hydrocortisone equivalent for 2 to 3 days. Inadequacy of the hypothalamic-pituitary-adrenal axis in the perioperative period can lead to unexplained hypotension.

Patients with pheochromocytoma require preoperative pharmacologic management to prevent intraoperative hypertensive crises or hypotension leading to cardiovascular collapse. The state of catecholamine excess associated with pheochromocytoma is controlled by a combination of α-adrenergic and β-adrenergic blockade before surgery. One to 2 weeks is generally required to achieve adequate therapeutic effect by α-blockade; this can be accomplished with either a nonselective agent such as phenoxybenzamine or a selective α_1-adrenergic agent such as prazosin. α-Blockade usually uncovers a vascular volume deficit that is not apparent clinically. In addition, patients have generally been placed on a sodium-restricted diet as part of their hypertension man-

Box 12-1 Perioperative Supplemental Glucocorticoid Regimens

No HPA Axis Suppression

Less than 5 mg of prednisone or equivalent per day for any
duration

Alternate-day single morning dose of short-acting glucocorticoid
of any dose or duration

Any dose of glucocorticoid for less than 3 weeks
   Rx: Give the usual daily glucocorticoid dose during the
      perioperative period

HPA Axis Suppression Documented or Presumed

More than 20 mg of prednisone or equivalent per day for 3
weeks or longer

Cushingoid appearance

Biochemical adrenal insufficiency on a low-dose ACTH
stimulation test

Minor procedures or local anesthesia
   Rx: Give the usual glucocorticoid dose before surgery
   No supplementation

Moderate surgical stress
   Rx: 50 mg hydrocortisone IV before induction of anesthesia,
      25 mg hydrocortisone every 8 hours thereafter for 24-48
      hours, then resume usual dose

Major surgical stress
   Rx: 100 mg hydrocortisone IV before induction of anesthesia,
      50 mg hydrocortisone every 8 hours thereafter for 48-72
      hours, then resume usual dose

HPA Axis Suppression Uncertain

5-20 mg of prednisone or its equivalent for 3 weeks or longer

5 mg or greater of prednisone or its equivalent for 3 weeks or
more in the year before surgery

Minor procedures or local anesthesia
   Rx: Give the usual glucocorticoid dose before surgery
   No supplementation

Moderate or major surgical stress

Check the low-dose ACTH stimulation test to determine HPA axis
suppression or

Give supplemental glucocorticoids as though suppressed

ACTH, adrenocorticotropic hormone; HPA, hypothalamic-pituitary-
adrenal axis.

Adapted from Schiff RL, Welsh GA: Perioperative evaluation and
management of the patient with endocrine dysfunction. Med Clin North
Am 87:175-192, 2003.

agement. Liberalization of sodium in the diet may aid in replenishing plasma volume. β-Blockade is initiated several days after the α-adrenergic agent is begun and serves to inhibit the tachycardia that accompanies nonselective α-blockade, as well as to control arrhythmia. Patients with pheochromocytoma may undergo surgery when pharmacologic blood pressure control is achieved.

Immunologic

The approach to a patient with suspected immunosuppression is the same, regardless of whether this state results from antineoplastic drugs in a cancer patient or immunosuppressive therapy in a transplant patient or is the result of advanced disease in patients with acquired immunodeficiency syndrome. The goal is to optimize immunologic function before surgery and to minimize the risk for infection and wound breakdown.

Preoperative assessment includes a thorough history of the patient's underlying disease and current functional status; a history of immunosuppressive treatment, including names of medications and duration of treatment; and a history of recent changes in weight. The physical examination seeks to document any signs of organ dysfunction that may underlie progression of the disease or be related to its treatment. Laboratory assessment includes a CBC with differential, electrolyte determination, and liver function tests, and an ECG and chest radiograph are obtained when age or physical findings suggest risk. Possible sites of infection must be investigated, including examination of any indwelling catheters, and a complete workup of any suspected infectious focus may be warranted. Additional studies of T-cell, B-cell, polymorphonuclear, or complement function may be helpful to delineate the degree of immune system compromise. Neutropenia, anemia, or thrombocytopenia may accompany the underlying disease process or result from treatment of the condition with immunosuppressive medication. Decisions regarding red blood cell transfusion or the use of synthetic erythropoietin or colony-stimulating factors are often based on the degree of dysfunction and other patient risk factors. Careful attention is paid to nutritional deficiency in this patient population, with supplementation indicated in the perioperative period. Appropriate antibiotic prophylaxis is critical.

Patients who are immunocompromised may be at risk for wound complications, especially if receiving exogenous steroid therapy. When taken within 3 days of surgery, steroids reduce the degree of wound inflammation, epithelialization, and collagen synthesis, which can lead to wound breakdown and infection.

Human Immunodeficiency Virus–Infected Patients and Surgery

As morbidity and mortality continue to decrease with improved medical management of human immunodeficiency virus (HIV), more HIV-infected patients are requiring surgery. It is important to understand how the agents that are used to treat HIV will affect the patient during surgery.

HIV treatment involves antiretroviral drugs from one of four classes: protease inhibitors, fusion inhibitors, nucleoside/nucleotide reverse transcriptase inhibitors (NRTIs), and non-nucleoside reverse transcriptase inhibitors (NNRTIs). It is important to note that these drugs are not immunosuppressive agents but work directly on the pathway of HIV cell integration and reproduction. For this reason, they do not have a significant effect on wound-healing or infection rates. The patient's white blood cell count or, more specifically, the absolute neutrophil count, in addition to the direct HIV titer, is more predictive of postoperative complications. One specific finding with NRTIs is that of lacticacidosis as a result of mitochondrial toxicity.[17] This condition needs to be added to the differential diagnosis of a critically ill patient with known HIV infection who has a persistently elevated lactate concentration. Hypoperfusion is ruled out initially, but drug complication needs to be investigated. Treatment is discontinuation of the agent.

Hematologic

Hematologic assessment may lead to the identification of disorders such as anemia, inherited or acquired coagulopathy, or a hypercoagulable state. Substantial morbidity may derive from failure to identify these abnormalities preoperatively. The need for perioperative prophylaxis for venous thromboembolism must be carefully reviewed in every surgical patient.

Anemia is the most common laboratory abnormality encountered in preoperative patients. It is often asymptomatic and can require further investigation to understand its cause. The history and physical examination may uncover subjective complaints of energy loss, dyspnea, or palpitations, and pallor or cyanosis may be evident. Patients are evaluated for lymphadenopathy, hepatomegaly, or splenomegaly, and pelvic and rectal examinations are performed. A CBC, reticulocyte count, and serum iron, total iron-binding capacity, ferritin, vitamin B_{12}, and folate levels are obtained to investigate the cause of anemia. Preoperative treatment and optimization are appropriate for an anemic patient. The decision to transfuse a patient perioperatively is made with consideration of the patient's underlying risk factors for ischemic heart disease and the estimated magnitude of blood loss during surgery. Generally, patients with normovolemic anemia without significant cardiac risk or anticipated blood loss can be managed safely without transfusion, with most healthy patients tolerating hemoglobin levels of 6 or 7 g/dL (Box 12-2).[18]

All patients undergoing surgery are questioned to assess their bleeding risk. Coagulopathy may result from inherited or acquired platelet or factor disorders or may be associated with organ dysfunction or medications. The inquiry begins with direct questioning about a personal or family history of abnormal bleeding. Supporting information includes a history of easy bruising or abnormal bleeding associated with minor procedures or injury. A history of liver or kidney dysfunction or recent common bile duct obstruction needs to be elicited, as well as an assessment of nutritional status. Medications are carefully reviewed, and the use of anticoagulants, salicylates, nonsteroidal anti-inflammatory drugs (NSAIDs), and antiplatelet drugs are noted. Physical examination may reveal bruising, petechiae, or signs of liver dysfunction. Patients with thrombocytopenia may have qualitative or quantitative defects as a result of immune-related disease, infection, drugs, or liver or kidney dysfunction. Qualitative defects may respond to medical management of the underlying disease process, whereas quantitative defects may require platelet transfusion when counts are less than 50,000 in a patient at risk for bleeding. Although coagulation studies are not routinely ordered, patients with a history suggestive of coagulopathy undergo coagulation studies before surgery. Coagulation studies are also obtained before the procedure if considerable bleeding is anticipated or any significant bleeding would be catastrophic. Patients with documented disorders of coagulation may require perioperative management of factor deficiencies, often in consultation with a hematologist.

Patients receiving anticoagulation therapy usually require preoperative reversal of the anticoagulant effect. In patients taking warfarin, the drug is withheld for four scheduled doses preoperatively to allow the international normalized ratio (INR) to fall to the range of 1.5 or less (assuming that the patient is maintained at an INR of 2.0-3.0). Additional recommendations for specific diagnoses requiring chronic anticoagulation are based on risk-benefit analysis. Patients with a recent history of venous thromboembolism or acute arterial embolism frequently require perioperative IV heparinization because of an increased risk for recurrent events in the perioperative period. Systemic heparinization can often be stopped within 6 hours of surgery and restarted within 12 hours postoperatively. When possible, surgery is postponed in the first month after an episode of venous or arterial thromboembolism. Patients taking anticoagulants for less than 2 weeks for pulmonary embolism (PE) or proximal DVT are considered for inferior vena cava filter placement before surgery (Table 12-8).[19]

All surgical patients are assessed for their risk for venous thromboembolism and receive adequate prophylaxis according to current guidelines (Table 12-9).[20] Patients are questioned to elicit any personal or family history suggestive of a hypercoagulable state. Levels of protein C, protein S, antithrombin III, and antiphospholipid antibody can be obtained. Risk factor stratification is achieved by considering multiple factors, including age, type of surgical procedure, previous thromboembolism, cancer, obesity, varicose veins, cardiac dysfunction, indwelling central venous catheters, inflammatory bowel disease, nephrotic syndrome, pregnancy, and estrogen or tamoxifen use. A number of regimens may be appropriate for prophylaxis of venous thromboembolism, depending on assessed risk (see Table 12-9). Such regimens include the use of unfractionated heparin, low-

---

Box 12-2   Guidelines for Red Blood Cell Transfusion for Acute Blood Loss

- Evaluate the risk for ischemia
- Estimate/anticipate the degree of blood loss. Less than 30% rapid volume loss probably does not require transfusion in a previously healthy individual
- Measure the hemoglobin concentration: <6 g/dL, transfusion usually required; 6-10 g/dL, transfusion dictated by clinical circumstance; >10 g/dL, transfusion rarely required
- Measure vital signs/tissue oxygenation when hemoglobin is 6-10 g/dL and the extent of blood loss is unknown. Tachycardia and hypotension refractory to volume suggest the need for transfusion; O_2 extraction ratio >50%, decreased Vo_2, suggest that transfusion is usually needed

Adapted from Simon TL, Alverson DC, AuBuchon J, et al: Practice parameters for the use of red blood cell transfusions: Developed by the Red Blood Cell Administration Practice Guideline Development Task Force of the College of American Pathologists. Arch Pathol Lab Med 122:130-138, 1998.

Table 12-8 Recommendations for Perioperative Anticoagulation in Patients Taking Oral Anticoagulants

INDICATION	PREOPERATIVE	POSTOPERATIVE
Acute venous thromboembolism		
Month 1	IV heparin	IV heparin
Months 2 and 3	No change	IV heparin
Recurrent venous thromboembolism	No change	SC heparin
Acute arterial embolism		
Month 1	IV heparin	IV heparin
Mechanical heart valve	No change	SC heparin
Nonvalvular atrial fibrillation	No change	SC heparin

IV, intravenous; SC, subcutaneous.
Adapted from Kearon C, Hirsh J: Management of anticoagulation before and after elective surgery. N Engl J Med 336:1506, 1997.

molecular-weight heparin, intermittent compression devices, and early ambulation. Initial prophylactic doses of heparin can be given preoperatively, within 2 hours of surgery, and compression devices are in place before induction of anesthesia.

ADDITIONAL PREOPERATIVE CONSIDERATIONS

Age

Older adults account for a disproportionate percentage of surgical patients. Risk assessment must carefully consider the effect of comorbid illness in this population. Although age has been reported as an independent risk factor for postoperative mortality, this observation may represent the unmeasured aspects of comorbid disease and the severity of illness.[2]

In an older adult patient, the preoperative evaluation seeks to identify and quantify the magnitude of comorbid disease and optimize the patient's condition before surgery when possible. Preoperative testing is based on findings suggested in the history and physical examination. Generally, elderly patients have an ECG, chest radiograph, CBC, and determination of glucose, creatinine, blood urea nitrogen, and albumin levels. Additional preoperative studies are based on the criteria discussed earlier for evaluation of patient and procedural risk.

Predicting and preventing postoperative delirium are important aspects of the perioperative care of the elderly. Patients with three or more of the following have a 50% risk for postoperative delirium: 70 years or older; self-reported alcohol abuse; poor cognitive status; poor functional status; markedly abnormal preoperative serum sodium, potassium, or glucose level; noncardiac thoracic surgery; and aortic aneurysm surgery.[21] This risk is explained to the patient and the family along with the symptoms of postoperative delirium. If delirium does occur, metabolic and infectious causes need to be investigated before labeling the event as *sundowning*.

Nutritional Status

Evaluation of the patient's nutritional status is part of the preoperative evaluation. A history of weight loss greater than 10% of body weight over a 6-month period or 5% over a month is significant. Albumin or prealbumin levels and immune competence (as assessed by delayed hypersensitivity reaction) may help identify patients with some degree of malnutrition, and physical findings of temporal wasting, cachexia, poor dentition, ascites, or peripheral edema may be corroborative. The degree of malnutrition is estimated on the basis of weight loss, physical findings, and plasma protein assessment. The adequacy of a nutritional regimen can be confirmed with a number of serum markers. Albumin (half-life, 14-18 days), transferrin (half-life, 7 days), and prealbumin (half-life, 3-5 days) levels can be determined on a regular basis in hospitalized patients. These proteins are responsive to stress conditions, however, and their synthesis may be inhibited in the immediate perioperative period. Once a patient is on a stable regimen and in the anabolic phase of recovery, these markers reflect the adequacy of nutritional efforts.

The effect of perioperative nutritional support on outcomes has been studied in a number of trials. Patients with *severe malnutrition* (as defined by a combination of weight loss, visceral protein indicators, and prognostic indices) appear to benefit most from preoperative parenteral nutrition, as demonstrated in study groups treated with total parenteral nutrition for 7 to 10 days before surgery for gastrointestinal malignancy. The majority of studies show a reduction in the rate of postoperative complications from approximately 40% to 30%. The use of total parenteral nutrition postoperatively in similar groups of patients is associated with an approximately 10% increase in complication rates.[22] Well-nourished patients undergoing surgery do not appear to benefit from aggressive perioperative nutritional support; parenteral nutrition is additionally associated with increased septic complications. Generally, nutritional support begins within 5 to 10 days after surgery in all patients unable to resume their normal diet. Such support may take the form of nasoenteric feeding, parenteral nutrition, or a combination of the two.

Obesity

The perioperative mortality rate is significantly increased in patients with clinically severe obesity (body mass index [BMI] >40 kg/m^2 or BMI >35 kg/m^2 with significant

Table 12-9 Levels of Risk for Thromboembolism in Surgical Patients Without Prophylaxis and Successful Prevention Strategies

LEVEL OF RISK	DEFINITION OF RISK LEVEL	CALF DVT (%)	PROXIMAL DVT (%)	CLINICAL PE (%)	FATAL PE (%)	PREVENTION STRATEGY
Low	Minor surgery in patients <40 yr with no additional risk factors	2	0.4	0.2	0.002	No specific measures Aggressive mobilization
Moderate	Minor surgery in patients with additional risk factors; nonmajor surgery in patients 40-60 yr with no additional risk factors; major surgery in patients <40 yr with no additional risk factors	10-20	2-4	1-2	0.1-0.4	LDUH q12h, LMWH, ES, or IPC
High	Nonmajor surgery in patients >60 yr or with additional risk factors; major surgery in patients >40 yr or with additional risk factors	20-40	4-8	2-4	0.4-1.0	LDUH q8h, LMWH, or IPC
Highest	Major surgery in patients >40 yr plus previous VTE, cancer, or molecular hypercoagulable state; hip or knee arthroplasty, hip fracture surgery; major trauma; spinal cord injury	40-80	10-20	4-10	0.2-5	LMWH, oral anticoagulants, IPC/ES+LDUH/ LMWH or ADH

ADH, adjusted-dose heparin; DVT, deep venous thrombosis; ES, elastic stockings; IPC, intermittent pneumatic compression; LDUH, low-dose unfractionated heparin; LMWH, low-molecular-weight heparin; PE, pulmonary embolus; VTE, venous thromboembolism.
Adapted from Geerts WH, Heit JA, Clagett GP, et al: Prevention of venous thromboembolism. Chest 119:132S-175S, 2001.

comorbid conditions). The goal of preoperative evaluation of an obese patient is to identify risk factors that might modify perioperative care of the patient. Clinically severe obesity is associated with a higher frequency of essential hypertension, pulmonary hypertension, left ventricular hypertrophy, congestive heart failure, and ischemic heart disease. Patients with no or one of these risk factors receive a β-blocker preoperatively for cardioprotection. Patients with two or more risk factors undergo noninvasive cardiac testing preoperatively.[23]

Obesity is also a risk factor for postoperative wound infection. The rate of wound infections is much lower with laparoscopic surgery in this group, which could have a bearing on selection of the operative approach. Obesity is an independent risk factor for DVT and PE; therefore, appropriate prophylaxis is instituted in these patients.

PREOPERATIVE CHECKLIST

The preoperative evaluation concludes with a review of all pertinent studies and information obtained from investigative tests. Documentation of this review is made in the chart, which represents an opportunity to ensure that all necessary and pertinent data have been obtained and appropriately interpreted. Informed consent after discussion with the patient and family members regarding the indication for the anticipated surgical procedure, as well as its risks and proposed benefits, are documented in the chart. The preoperative checklist also gives the surgeon an opportunity to review the need for β-blockade, DVT prophylaxis, and prophylactic antibiotics.

Preoperative orders are written and reviewed. The patient receives written instructions regarding the time of

surgery and management of special perioperative issues such as fasting, bowel preparation, and medication use.

Antibiotic Prophylaxis

Appropriate antibiotic prophylaxis in surgery depends on the most likely pathogens encountered during the surgical procedure. The type of operative procedure (Table 12-10) is helpful in deciding the appropriate antibiotic spectrum and is considered before ordering or administering any preoperative medication. Prophylactic antibiotics are not generally required for clean (class I) cases, except in the setting of indwelling prosthesis placement or when bone is incised. Patients who undergo class II procedures benefit from a single dose of an appropriate antibiotic administered before the skin incision. For abdominal (hepatobiliary, pancreatic, gastroduodenal) cases, cefazolin is generally used. Contaminated (class III) cases require mechanical preparation or parenteral antibiotics with both aerobic and anaerobic activity. Such an approach is taken in the setting of emergency abdominal surgery, as for suspected appendicitis, and in trauma cases. Dirty or infected cases often require the same antibiotic spectrum, which can be continued into the postoperative period in the setting of ongoing infection or delayed treatment.

The appropriate antibiotic is chosen before surgery and administered before the skin incision is made (Table 12-11).[24] Repeat dosing occurs at an appropriate interval, usually 3 hours for abdominal cases or twice the half-life of the antibiotic, although the patient's renal function may alter the timing (Table 12-12).[25] Perioperative antibiotic prophylaxis generally is not continued beyond the day of surgery. With the advent of minimal-access surgery, the use of antibiotics seems less justified because the risk for wound infection is extremely low. For example, routine antibiotic prophylaxis in patients undergoing

Table 12-10 National Research Council Classification of Operative Wounds and Rates of Wound Infection

Clean (class I)	Nontraumatic No inflammation No break in technique Respiratory, alimentary, or genitourinary tract not entered	2.1%
Clean-contaminated (class II)	Gastrointestinal or respiratory tract entered without significant spillage	3.3%
Contaminated (class III)	Major break in technique Gross spillage from the gastrointestinal tract Traumatic wound, fresh Entrance into the genitourinary or biliary tracts in the presence of infected urine or bile	6.4%
Dirty and infected (class IV)	Acute bacterial inflammation encountered, without pus Transection of "clean" tissue for the purpose of surgical access to a collection of pus Traumatic wound with retained devitalized tissue, foreign bodies, fecal contamination, or delayed treatment, or all of these, or from a dirty source	7.1%

Adapted from Cruse PJE: Wound infections: Epidemiology and clinical characteristics. In Howard RJ, Simmons RL (eds): Surgical Infectious Disease, 2nd ed. Norwalk, CT, Appleton & Lange, 1988.

laparoscopic cholecystectomy for symptomatic cholelithiasis is of questionable value. It may have a role, however, in cases that result in prosthetic graft (i.e., mesh) placement, such as laparoscopic hernia repair.

The Surgical Care Improvement Project (SCIP) is a national quality partnership of organizations committed to improving the safety of surgical care through a reduction in postoperative complications. The ultimate goal of the partnership is to save lives by reducing the incidence of surgical complications by 25% by the year 2010. The guidelines developed as part of SCIP will be monitored in every hospital (Table 12-13).[26]

Preoperative Mechanical Bowel Cleansing

Mechanical bowel preparation with the addition of oral antibiotics was the standard of care for several decades for any intestinal surgery. More recent studies have evaluated the need for both oral antibiotics and mechanical cleansing. Oral antibiotics confer no benefit to the patient and may increase the risk for postoperative infection with *Clostridium difficile*. In addition, although it seems intuitive that removal of bulk fecal material would decrease the risk for anastomotic and infectious complications, the opposite is true. A recent meta-analysis showed that both of these events are not decreased and may be increased with mechanical cleansing.[27]

Review of Medications

Careful review of the patient's home medications is a part of the preoperative evaluation before any operation; the goal is to appropriately use medications that control the patient's medical illnesses while minimizing the risk associated with anesthetic-drug interactions or the hematologic or metabolic effects of some commonly used medications and therapies. The patient is asked to name all medications, including psychiatric drugs, hormones, and alternative/herbal medications, and to provide dosages and frequency.

In general, patients taking cardiac drugs, including β-blockers and antiarrhythmics, pulmonary drugs such as

inhaled or nebulized medications, or anticonvulsants, antihypertensives, or psychiatric drugs are advised to take their medications with a sip of water on the morning of surgery. Parenteral forms or substitutes are available for many drugs and may be used if the patient remains NPO for any significant period postoperatively. It is important to return patients to their normal medication regimen as soon as possible. Two notable examples are the additional cardiovascular morbidity associated with the perioperative discontinuation of β-blockers and rebound hypertension with abrupt cessation of the antihypertensive clonidine. Medications such as lipid-lowering agents or vitamins can be omitted on the day of surgery.

Some drugs are associated with an increased risk for perioperative bleeding and are withheld before surgery. Drugs that affect platelet function are withheld for variable periods: aspirin and clopidogrel (Plavix) are withheld for 7 to 10 days, whereas NSAIDs are withheld between 1 day (ibuprofen and indomethacin) and 3 days (naproxen and sulindac), depending on the drug's half-life. Because the use of estrogen and tamoxifen has been associated with an increased risk for thromboembolism, they probably need to be withheld for a period of 4 weeks preoperatively.[28]

The widespread use of herbal medications has prompted review of the effects of some commonly used preparations and their potential adverse outcomes in the perioperative period. These substances may fail to be recorded in the preoperative evaluation, although important metabolic and hematologic effects can result from their regular use (Table 12-14).[29] Generally, the use of herbal medications is stopped preoperatively, but this needs to be done with caution in patients who report the use of valerian, which may be associated with a benzodiazepine-like withdrawal syndrome.

Preoperative Fasting

The standard order of "NPO past midnight" for preoperative patients is based on the theory of reduction of volume and acidity of the stomach contents during surgery.

Table 12-11 Antimicrobial Prophylaxis for Surgery

NATURE OF OPERATION	COMMON PATHOGENS	RECOMMENDED ANTIMICROBIALS	ADULT DOSAGE BEFORE SURGERY[1]
Cardiac	*Staphylococcus aureus,* *S. epidermidis*	cefazolin or cefuroxime OR vancomycin[3]	1-2 g IV[2] 1.5 g IV[2] 1 g IV
Gastrointestinal			
Esophageal, gastroduodenal	Enteric gram-negative bacilli, gram-positive cocci	*High risk[4] only:* cefazolin[7]	1-2 g IV
Biliary tract	Enteric gram-negative bacilli, enterococci, clostridia	*High risk[5] only:* cefazolin[7]	1-2 g IV
Colorectal	Enteric gram-negative bacilli, anaerobes, enterococci	*Oral:* neomycin + erythromycin base[6] OR metronidazole[6] *Parenteral:* cefoxitin[7] OR cefazolin + metronidazole[7] OR ampicillin/sulbactam	 1-2 g IV 1-2 g IV 0.5 g IV 3 g IV
Appendectomy, non-perforated[8]	Enteric gram-negative bacilli, anaerobes, enterococci	cefoxitin[7] OR cefazolin + metronidazole[7] OR ampicillin/sulbactam	1-2 g IV 1-2 g IV 0.5 g IV 3 g IV
Genitourinary	Enteric gram-negative bacilli, enterococci	*High risk[9] only:* ciprofloxacin	500 mg PO or 400 mg IV
Gynecologic and Obstetric			
Vaginal, abdominal, or laparoscopic hysterectomy	Enteric gram-negative bacilli, anaerobes, Gp B strep, enterococci	cefoxitin[7] or cefazolin[7] OR ampicillin/sulbactam[7]	1-2 g IV 3 g IV
Cesarean section	same as for hysterectomy	cefazolin[7]	1-2 g IV after cord clamping
Abortion	same as for hysterectomy	*First trimester, high risk[10]:* aqueous penicillin G OR doxycycline *Second trimester:* cefazolin[7]	2 mill units IV 300 mg PO[11] 1-2 g IV
Head and Neck Surgery			
Incisions through oral or pharyngeal mucosa	Anaerobes, enteric gram-negative bacilli, *S. aureus*	clindamycin + gentamicin OR cefazolin	600-900 mg IV 1.5 mg/kg IV 1-2 g IV
Neurosurgery	*S. aureus, S. epidermidis*	cefazolin OR vancomycin[3]	1-2 g IV 1 g IV
Ophthalmic	*S. epidermidis, S. aureus,* streptococci, enteric gram-negative bacilli, *Pseudomonas spp.*	gentamicin, tobramycin, ciprofloxacin, gatifloxacin, levofloxacin, moxifloxacin, ofloxacin, or neomycin-gramicidin-polymyxin B cefazolin	multiple drops topically over 2 to 24 hours 100 mg subconjunctivally
Orthopedic	*S. aureus, S. epidermidis*	cefazolin[12] or cefuroxime[12] OR vancomycin[3,12]	1-2 g IV 1.5 g IV 1 g IV
Thoracic (Non-Cardiac)	*S. aureus, S. epidermidis,* streptococci, enteric gram-negative bacilli	cefazolin or cefuroxime OR vancomycin[3]	1-2 g IV 1.5 g IV 1 g IV
Vascular			
Arterial surgery involving a prosthesis, the abdominal aorta, or a groin incision	*S. aureus, S. epidermidis,* enteric gram-negative bacilli	cefazolin OR vancomycin[3]	1-2 g IV 1 g IV
Lower extremity amputation for ischemia	*S. aureus, S. epidermidis,* enteric gram-negative bacilli, clostridia	cefazolin OR vancomycin[3]	1-2 g IV 1 g IV

[1]Parenteral prophylactic antimicrobials can be given as a single IV dose begun 60 minutes or less before the operation. For prolonged operations (>4 hours) or those with major blood loss, additional intraoperative doses should be given at intervals 1-2 times the half-life of the drug for the duration of the procedure in patients with normal renal function. If vancomycin or a fluoroquinolone is used, the infusion should be started 60-120 minutes before the initial incision in order to minimize the possibility of an infusion reaction close to the time of induction of anesthesia and to have adequate tissue levels at the time of incision.

[2]Some consultants recommend an additional dose when patients are removed from bypass during open heart surgery.

[3]Vancomycin is used in hospitals in which methicillin-resistant *S. aureus* and *S. epidermidis* are frequent causes of postoperative wound infection, for patients previously colonized with MRSA, or for those who are allergic to penicillins or cephalosporins. Rapid IV administration may cause hypotension, which could be especially dangerous during induction of anesthesia. Even when the drug is given over 50 minutes, hypotension may occur; treatment with diphenhydramine (Benadryl and others) and further slowing of the infusion rate may be helpful. Some experts would give 15 mg/kg of vancomycin to patients weighing more than 75 kg, up to a maximum of 1.5 g, with a slower infusion rate (90 minutes for 1.5 g). To provide coverage against gram-negative bacteria, most *Medical Letter* consultants would also include cefazolin or cefuroxime in the prophylaxis regimen for patients not allergic to cephalosporins; ciprofloxacin, levofloxacin, gentamicin, or aztreonam, each one in combination with vancomycin, can be used in patients who cannot tolerate a cephalosporin.

[4]Morbid obesity, esophageal obstruction, decreased gastric acidity, or gastrointestinal motility.

[5]Age >70 years, acute cholecystitis, non-functioning gall bladder, obstructive jaundice, or common duct stones.

[6]After appropriate diet and catharsis, 1 g of neomycin plus 1 g of erythromycin at 1 PM, 2 PM, and 11 PM or 2 g of neomycin plus 2 g of metronidazole at 7 PM and 11 PM the day before an 8 AM operation.

[7]For patients allergic to penicillins and cephalosporins, clindamycin with gentamicin, ciprofloxacin, levofloxacin, or aztreonam is a reasonable alternative.

[8]For a ruptured viscus, therapy is often continued for about 5 days. Ruptured viscus in postoperative setting (dehiscence) requires antibacterials to include coverage of nosocomial pathogens.

[9]Urine culture positive or unavailable, preoperative catheter, transrectal prostatic biopsy, placement of prosthetic material.

[10]Patients with previous pelvic inflammatory disease, previous gonorrhea, or multiple sex partners.

[11]Divided into 100 mg 1 hour before the abortion and 200 mg $^1/_2$ hour after.

[12]If a tourniquet is to be used in the procedure, the entire dose of antibiotic must be infused prior to its inflation.

From Antimicrobial prophylaxis for surgery. Med Lett 4(52):84-85, 2006.

Table 12-12 Suggested Initial Dose and Time Until Redosing of Antimicrobial Drugs Commonly Used for Surgical Prophylaxis

ANTIMICROBIAL	RENAL HALF-LIFE (hr)		RECOMMENDED INFUSION DURATION	STANDARD DOSE	WEIGHT-BASED DOSE RECOMMENDATION*	RECOMMENDED REDOSING INTERVAL† (hr)
	Patients With Normal Renal Function	Patients With End-Stage Renal Disease				
Aztreonam	1.5-2	6	3-5 min,‡ 20-60 min§	1-2 g IV	2 g maximum (adults)	3-5
Ciprofloxacin	3.5-5	5-9	60 min	400 mg IV	400 mg	4-10
Cefazolin	1.2-2.5	40-70	3-5 min,‡ 15-60 min§	1-2 g IV	20-30 mg/kg (if <80 kg, use 1 g; if >80 kg, use 2 g)	2-5
Cefuroxime	1-2	15-22	3-5 min,‡ 15-60 min§	1.5 g IV	50 mg/kg	3-4
Cefamandole	0.5-2.1	12.3-18‖	3-5 min,‡ 15-60 min§	1 g IV		3-4
Cefoxitin	0.5-1.1	6.5-23	3-5 min,‡ 15-60 min§	1-2 g IV	20-40 mg/kg	2-3
Cefotetan	2.8-4.6	13-25	3-5 min,‡ 20-60 min§	1-2 g IV	20-40 mg/kg	3-6
Clindamycin	2-5.1	3.5-5.0¶	10-60 min (do not exceed 30 mg/min)	600-900 mg IV	If <10 kg, use at least 37.5 mg; if >10 kg, use 3-6 mg/kg	3-6
Erythromycin base**	0.8-3	5-6	NA	1 g PO 19, 18, and 9 hr before surgery	9-13 mg/kg	NA
Gentamicin	2-3	50-70	30-60 min	1.5 mg/kg IV#	—#	3-6
Neomycin**	2-3 (3% absorbed under normal gastrointestinal conditions)	12-24 or longer	NA	1 g PO 19, 18, and 9 hr before surgery	20 mg/kg	NA
Metronidazole	6-14	7-21; no change	30-60 min	0.5-1 g IV	15-mg/kg initial dose (adult); 7.5 mg/kg on subsequent doses	6-8
Vancomycin	4-6	44.1-406.4 (CCR<10 mL/min)	1 g over 60-min period (use longer infusion time if dose >1 g)	1 g IV	10-15 mg/kg (adult)	6-12

*Data are primarily from published pediatric recommendations.

†For procedures of long duration, antimicrobials should be readministered at intervals of one to two times the half-life of the drug. The intervals in the table were calculated for patients with normal renal function.

‡Dose injected directly into a vein or via running intravenous fluids.

§Intermittent intravenous infusion.

‖In patients with a serum creatinine level of 5 to 9 mg/dL.

¶The half-life of clindamycin is the same or slightly increased in patients with end-stage renal disease as those with normal renal function.

#If a patient's body weight is more than 30% higher than ideal body weight (IBW), the dosing weight (DW) can be determined as follows: DW=IBW=0.4×(total body weight−IBW).

**Routine oral antibiotic preparation can be omitted in most operations on the colon if intravenous antibiotics are used.

CCR, creatinine clearance rate.

Adapted from Bratzler DW, Honck PM: Antimicrobial prophylaxis for surgery: An advisory statement from the National Surgical Infection Prevention Project. Clin Inf Dis 38:1706-1715, 2004.

Recently, guidelines have recommended a shift to allow a period of restricted fluid intake up to a few hours before surgery. The ASA recommends that adults stop intake of solids for at least 6 hours and clear fluids for 2 hours. When the literature was recently reviewed by the Cochrane group, they found 22 trials in healthy adults that provided 38 controlled comparisons.[30] There was no evidence that the volume or pH of gastric contents differed with the length and type of fasting. Though not reported in all the trials, there did not appear to be an increased risk for aspiration/regurgitation with a shortened period of fasting. Very few trials investigated the fasting routine in patients at higher risk for regurgitation/aspiration (pregnant, elderly, obese, or those with stomach disorders). There is also increasing evidence that preoperative carbohydrate supplementation is safe and may improve a patient's response to perioperative stress.[31,32] Surgeons and anesthesiologists should evaluate the evidence and consider adjusting their standard fasting policies.

POTENTIAL CAUSES OF INTRAOPERATIVE INSTABILITY

Anaphylaxis/Latex Allergy

Intraoperative anaphylactic reactions may occur as frequently as 1 in every 4500 surgical procedures and carry a 3% to 6% risk for mortality.[33] Causative agents are most often muscle relaxants, latex, anesthetic induction agents such as etomidate and propofol, and narcotic drugs. Additional agents administered while patients are under anesthesia that may be associated with anaphylaxis include dyes (e.g., isosulfan blue dye for sentinel node procedures), colloid solutions, antibiotics, blood products, protamine, and mannitol.

The manifestations of anaphylactic reactions occurring under anesthesia may range from mild cutaneous eruptions to hypotension, cardiovascular collapse, bronchospasm, and death. When suspected, use of the offending agent is discontinued and the patient is given epinephrine, 0.3 to 0.5 mL of a 1:1000 solution subcutaneously; with severe anaphylaxis it is given IV and repeated at 5- to 10-minute intervals as needed. Histamine-1 (H_1) blockade with diphenhydramine, 50 mg IV or intramuscularly, plus H_2 blockade with ranitidine, 50 mg IV, as well as hydrocortisone, 100 to 250 mg IV every 6 hours, is usually required. Additional supportive measures in the setting of hemodynamic or respiratory collapse may include fluid boluses, pressors, orotracheal intubation, and nebulized β_2-agonists or racemic epinephrine. Postoperative monitoring in the intensive care unit is generally required for a patient who has had a severe intraoperative anaphylactic reaction.

Latex sensitivity is the second most common cause of anaphylactic reactions (after muscle relaxants) and must be screened for in the medical history. Although the incidence of such sensitivity may be less than 5% in the general population, higher-risk groups, including those with a genetic predisposition (atopic conditions) or chronic exposure to latex, and individuals with spina

Table 12-13 Surgical Care Improvement Project (SCIP) Guidelines

	GUIDELINE
SCIP INF 1	Prophylactic antibiotic received within 1 hour before surgical incision
SCIP INF 2	Prophylactic antibiotic selection for surgical patients
SCIP INF 3	Prophylactic antibiotics discontinued within 24 hours after surgery completion time (48 hours for cardiac patients)
SCIP INF 4	Cardiac surgery patients with controlled 6 AM postoperative serum glucose
SCIP INF 5	Postoperative wound infection diagnosed during index hospitalization (outcome)
SCIP INF 6	Surgery patients with appropriate hair removal
SCIP INF 7	Colorectal surgery patients with immediate postoperative normothermia

INF, infection guideline.

bifida may have rates as high as 72%.[34] Those who give a history consistent with possible latex sensitivity undergo skin testing before anticipated operative procedures. Appropriate intraoperative measures to ensure a latex-free environment obviates most perioperative risk in a patient with latex allergy.

Malignant Hyperthermia

The incidence of malignant hyperthermia (MH) is higher in children and young adults than in adults; a rate of 1 in 15,000 has been estimated in the group at highest risk, boys younger than 15 years.[35] MH represents an acute episode of hypermetabolism and muscle injury related to the administration of halogenated anesthetic agents or succinylcholine. Susceptibility to MH is inherited according to an autosomal dominant pattern, with apparent incomplete penetrance. The patient may therefore fail to reveal familial knowledge of the trait, and a personal history of muscle disorder may not be evident.

An acute episode of MH may be recognized by increased sympathetic nervous system activity, muscle rigidity, and high fever. Associated derangements include hypercapnia, arrhythmia, acidosis, hypoxemia, and rhabdomyolysis. When suspected, MH is treated by discontinuing inhalational anesthetic agents and succinylcholine, completely changing the anesthesia circuit, and administering dantrolene sodium at doses of 2 to 3 mg/kg IV. This drug may be titrated to the abatement of symptoms. Additional supportive measures include active or passive cooling and pharmacologic treatment of arrhythmia, hyperkalemia, and acidosis.

PRINCIPLES OF OPERATIVE SURGERY

Proper operative technique is of paramount importance for optimizing outcome and enhancing the wound-

Table 12-14 Perioperative Concerns and Recommendations for Eight Herbal Medicines

COMMON NAME OF HERB	PERIOPERATIVE CONCERNS	PREOPERATIVE RECOMMENDATIONS
Echinacea	Allergic reactions; decreased effectiveness of immunosuppressants; potential for immunosuppression with long-term use	No data
Ephedra	Risk for myocardial ischemia and stroke from tachycardia and hypertension; ventricular arrhythmias with halothane; long-term use depletes endogenous catecholamines and may cause intraoperative hemodynamic instability; life-threatening interaction with monoamine oxidase inhibitors	Discontinue at least 24 hr before surgery
Garlic	Potential to increase risk for bleeding, especially when combined with other medications that inhibit platelet aggregation	Discontinue at least 7 days before surgery
Ginkgo	Potential to increase risk for bleeding, especially when combined with other medications that inhibit platelet aggregation	Discontinue at least 36 hr before surgery
Ginseng	Hypoglycemia; potential to increase risk for bleeding; potential to decrease anticoagulative effect of warfarin	Discontinue at least 7 days before surgery
Kava	Potential to increase sedative effect of anesthetics; potential for addiction, tolerance, and withdrawal after abstinence unstudied	Discontinue at least 24 hr before surgery
St. John's wort	Induction of cytochrome P-450 enzymes, with effect on cyclosporine, warfarin, steroids, protease inhibitors, and possibly benzodiazepines, calcium channel blockers, and many other drugs; decreased serum digoxin levels	Discontinue at least 5 days before surgery
Valerian	Potential to increase sedative effect of anesthetics; benzodiazepine-like acute withdrawal; potential to increase anesthetic requirements with long-term use	No data

Adapted from Ang-Lee MK, Moss J, Yuan C-S: Herbal medicines and perioperative care. JAMA 286:208-216, 2001.

healing process. There is no substitute for a well-planned and conducted operation to provide the best possible surgical outcome. One of the most reliable means of ensuring that surgeons provide quality care in the operating room is through participation in high-quality surgical training programs, which provide opportunities for repetitive observation and performance of surgical procedures in a well-structured environment. With their participation, young surgeons-in-training can progressively develop the technical skills necessary to perform the most demanding and complex operative procedures.

THE OPERATING ROOM

Preparation for surgery does not end with evaluation of the patient and selection of the operative procedure. It is the responsibility of the surgeon to ensure that all things needed for the procedure are available on the day of surgery, including any special equipment required to carry out the operation and the availability of any implants, blood, blood products, or special medications.

To run an operating room efficiently requires well-trained surgeons, anesthesiologists, and operating room staff, as well as an operating room equipped with an easily maneuverable operating table, good lighting, and ample space for personnel and equipment. The room is cleaned and the table checked for malfunction before and after each case. It is extremely costly and stressful to replace the operating table or other equipment with the patient already in the operating room. Preoperative communication among surgeons, anesthesiologists, and operating room staff is vitally important. Such communication helps save time, prevents confusion and undue frustration in the management of equipment use, accounts

for patient needs and personnel requirements, and makes planned procedures progress in a safe and efficient manner. The modern operating room for a trauma service has a temperature control panel that allows room temperature to be modified rapidly to avoid hypothermia. Patients are positioned and secured on the table. Position-related neuromuscular or orthopedic injury are prevented with careful positioning and padding. Barriers consisting of sterile drapes and gowns are established between the surgeon, patient, and other operating room staff. The barriers need to be impermeable to water and other body fluids. Finally, a hands-free communication system (e.g., intercom, voice-activated speaker phone) must be functioning in the room to facilitate communication between surgeons and pathologists, radiologists, blood bank, pharmacy, and the patient's family members. Most important, should an unexpected situation arise, help can be summoned immediately.

Maintenance of Normothermia

Hypothermia averaging only 1.5°C below normal is associated with adverse outcomes that add hospitalization costs of $2500 to $7000 per surgical patient. Many factors increase the risk for perioperative hypothermia: extremes of age, female sex, ambient room temperature, length and type of surgical procedure, cachexia, preexisting conditions, significant fluid shifts, use of cold irrigants, and use of general or regional anesthesia. *Normothermia* is defined as a core temperature between 36°C and 38°C. Preventive warming measures are used to avoid hypothermia. Passive insulation includes warmed cotton blankets, socks, head covering, limited skin exposure, circulating water mattresses, and an increase in ambient room temperature (68°F-75°F). Some patients may require active

Table 12-15 Comparison of Absorbable Sutures

SUTURE	TYPES	RAW MATERIAL	TENSILE STRENGTH RETENTION IN VIVO	TISSUE REACTION
Surgical Gut Suture	Chromic	Collagen derived from healthy beef and sheep	Individual patient characteristics can affect rate of tensile strength loss.	Moderate reaction
Monocryl Suture (poliglecaprone 25)	Monofilament	Copolymer of glycolide and epsilon-caprolactone	~50%-60% (violet: 60%-70%) remains at 1 week. ~20%-30% (violet 30%-40%) remains at 2 weeks. Lost within 3 weeks (violet: 4 weeks).	Minimal acute inflammatory reaction
Coated Vicryl Suture (polyglactin 910)	Braided Monofilament	Copolymer of lactide and glycolide coated with 370 and calcium stearate	~75% remains at 2 weeks. ~50% remains at 3 weeks. 25% at 4 weeks.	Minimal acute inflammatory reaction
PDS II Suture (polydioxanone)	Monofilament	Polyester polymer	~70% remains at 2 weeks ~50% remains at 4 weeks ~25% remains at 6 weeks	Slight reaction

Adapted from Ethicon Wound Closure Manual, Somerville, NJ, Ethicon, 2007.

warming, which includes use of a forced air convection warming system, humidified warmed anesthetic gases, and warmed IV fluids. The greatest temperature decline occurs during the first hour of surgery. Therefore, even in short cases, temperature monitoring is indicated.[36]

Preoperative Skin Preparation

Preoperative skin preparation of both the patient and surgeon is important in preventing surgical site infection. The effectiveness of the preparation is dependent on both the type of antiseptic used and the method of application. The Centers for Disease Control and Prevention recommends that the size of the area prepared be sufficient, the solution be applied in concentric circles, the applicator be discarded once the periphery has been reached, and time be allowed for the solution to dry, especially when alcoholic solutions are used because they are flammable. The Association of Operating Room Nurses adds that the applicator needs to be sterile and the solution needs to be applied with the use of friction and extend from the incision site to the periphery. A recent Cochrane review of this subject revealed six evaluable studies; however, all described a unique comparison and thus could not be combined for meta-analysis.[37] They concluded that there is insufficient evidence to recommend one skin preparation antiseptic over another. In fact, only one small study has shown superiority of chlorhexidine over povidone-iodine. Hair removal, if needed, is accomplished by clipping with electric clippers rather than shaving with a razor.

Hemostasis

Minimizing blood loss is an important technical aspect of surgery. Increased blood loss exacerbates the stress of surgery and resuscitation; less blood loss allows the performance of a technically superior operation. In the presence of adequate hemostasis, one can conduct a more precise dissection and shorten both operating time and recovery time of the patient. Avoidance of blood transfusion obviates the risk for transfusion-related complications and transmission of blood-borne diseases.[38]

Essential operative technique dictates that larger vessels (>1 mm) be tied, clipped, or sealed with monopolar or bipolar electrocautery or high-frequency ultrasonic devices. Major named vessels, in particular, not only are tied but also undergo suture ligation. Hemoclip application is acceptable, especially in an operating field with an extremely confined space or when dealing with delicate vessels such as portal vein branches. With limited-access procedures such as those performed with minimal-access techniques, clip application seems to be a better choice than knot tying. At times it is necessary to use hemoclips, such as when performing an oncologic procedure in which outlining of margins provides a radio-opaque marker for postoperative irradiation.

In the event of catastrophic bleeding, such as when confronted with an unexpected intraoperative major vessel injury, intraperitoneal rupture of an aortic aneurysm, or bleeding from major intra-abdominal trauma, temporary occlusion of the aorta at the esophageal hiatus with a compression device such as a sponge on a stick or vascular clamp or manual compression is considered. Such a maneuver may be lifesaving by allowing anesthesia staff to catch up with blood loss by aggressive resuscitation. It also allows the surgeon to remove intraperitoneal blood and clots with lap sponges or suction devices until the exact bleeding site can be identified, controlled, and repaired primarily or with an interposition graft. Occasionally, a partial vascular injury may need to be extended or converted to a complete transection to allow a better repair. This approach is particularly applicable to injury of the aorta and vena cava.

Bleeding that occurs from multiple sites in a trauma patient, such as liver laceration or pelvic fracture, or both, especially in a hypothermic patient, may best be treated with packing alone or in conjunction with angiographic embolization to achieve temporary control followed by a second-look operation. This maneuver of damage control is of paramount importance. It may be the only way that a patient's life can be saved. In fact, this principle of damage control can and should be applied beyond the trauma patient to all surgical procedures when unexpected bleeding is encountered or a second-look laparotomy will be necessary. Other adjuncts that may be helpful in dealing with wide areas of surface tissue oozing include microwave coagulation, laser coagulation, and the application of topical hemostatic agents (i.e., Surgicel, thrombin, Gelfoam, and fibrin glue).

Table 12-16   Comparison of Nonabsorbable Sutures

SUTURE	TYPES	RAW MATERIAL	TENSILE STRENGTH RETENTION IN VIVO	TISSUE REACTION
Perma-Hand Silk Suture	Braided	Organic protein called *fibroin*	Progressive degradation of fiber may result in gradual loss of tensile strength over time.	Acute inflammatory reaction
Ethilon Nylon Suture	Monofilament	Long-chain aliphatic polymers Nylon 6 or Nylon 6,6	Progressive hydrolysis may result in gradual loss of tensile strength over time.	Minimal acute inflammatory reaction
Nurolon Nylon Suture	Braided	Long-chain aliphatic polymers Nylon 6 or Nylon 6,6	Progressive hydrolysis may result in gradual loss of tensile strength over time.	Minimal acute inflammatory reaction
Mersilene Polyester Fiber Suture	Braided Monofilament	Poly (ethylene terephthalate)	No significant change known to occur in vivo.	Minimal acute inflammatory reaction
Ethibond *Excel* Polyester Fiber Suture	Braided	Poly (ethylene terephthalate) coated with polybutilate	No significant change known to occur in vivo.	Minimal acute inflammatory reaction
Prolene Polypropylene Suture	Monofilament	Isotactic crystalline stereoisomer of polypropylene	Not subject to degradation or weakening by action of tissue enzymes.	Minimal acute inflammatory reaction
Pronova Poly (hexafluoropropylene-VDF Suture)	Monofilament	Polymer blend of poly (vinylidene fluoride) and poly (vinylidene fluoride-cohexafluoropropylene)	Not subject to degradation or weakening by action of tissue enzymes.	Minimal acute inflammatory reaction

Adapted from Ethicon Wound Closure Manual, Somerville, NJ, Ethicon, 2007.

Wound Closure

Wound closure can be temporary or permanent; the latter can be primary or secondary. Critical factors in making this decision are the patient's condition, the clinical setting, the area of the body involved, the condition of the wound itself, and the disease process or injury that led to surgical intervention.

Various methods can be chosen to close wounds in different parts of the body, depending on the clinical circumstance. In general, clean, noncontaminated wounds with healthy local tissue conditions are best closed by primary permanent closure. In a patient with a condition requiring re-exploration or one suffering from abdominal compartment syndrome, temporary closure is preferable. Heavily contaminated extremity or trunk wounds are left open with packing. Heavily contaminated abdominal wounds are best served by fascial closure alone, with skin left open and packed. The principle of eliminating dead space to reduce the risk for seroma and hematoma formation is important and can be achieved internally with sutures or a suction device or externally with a compression appliance.

Permanent closure can be achieved with either running or interrupted sutures. Suture can be monofilament or multifilament, braided or nonbraided, and dissolvable or nondissolvable (Tables 12-15 and 12-16). In general, when proven infection or contamination is a concern, monofilament, nonbraided suture is preferred. For abdominal wall closure in a debilitated, malnourished cancer patient, permanent closure with nondissolvable suture seems prudent. In a cirrhotic patient with established ascites or a patient with potential for the development of postoperative ascites, the abdomen is closed with running suture, and a multilayer, watertight closure must be achieved.

Temporary closure of the abdominal wall may be appropriate in the setting of a multiply injured patient or one with intra-abdominal hypertension. This can be achieved with a vacuum suction device or a prosthesis bridging technique using either a sterile IV bag or polypropylene mesh (Table 12-17). The vacuum suction technique (so-called Vac Pac) uses a two-sided temporary closing material made of a biodrape over a blue towel. The biodrape faces the intestine and prevents adhesion to the blue towel. The membrane is tucked beneath the abdominal wall with the blue towel side facing up to

Table 12-17   Types of Synthetic Mesh and Their Uses

TYPE OF MESH	TRADE NAME	TYPE	COMMENTS
Nonabsorbable			
Polypropylene	Marlex, Prolene, Atrium	Monofilament	Highly elastic, withstands infection well; widely used for abdominal wall reconstruction, hernia repair
Polytetrafluoroethylene (PTFE)	Teflon	Multifilament	"Nonexpanded" mesh; associated with a large number of complications; limited utility
Expanded PTFE	Gore-Tex	Multifilament	Greatest elongation in comparison to other nonabsorbable meshes; minimal tissue incorporation; multiple uses in abdominal, vascular reconstruction
Polyethylene terephthalate	Mersilene, Dacron	Multifilament	Polyester fiber mesh with broad utility in abdominal wall, hernia repair; less extensively used than polypropylene
Absorbable			
Polyglycolic acid	Dexon	Multifilament	Useful for temporary abdominal closure; resists infection
Polyglactin 910	Vicryl	Multifilament	Useful for temporary abdominal closure; resists infection

Adapted from Fenner DE: New surgical mesh. Clin Obstet Gynecol 43:650-658, 2000.

provide retention and prevent potential loss of domain. The central portion of the drape is fenestrated before placement. Suction catheters and gauze dressings are placed beneath a second biodrape that covers the entire abdominal wall and seals the closure (Fig. 12-3). This technique has a number of advantages: it is quick and easy to use, the temporary closure can be constructed from materials that are readily available in the operating room, no suturing is required and therefore the integrity of the abdominal fascia is maintained for later permanent closure, and the applied suction prohibits fluid from accumulating in the abdominal cavity. Disadvantages include an inability to inspect the intestine (as with an IV bag) at the bedside and increased complexity of fluid and electrolyte balance because of potentially large fluid losses. It has been our practice to return these patients to the operating room every 3 to 4 days for replacement of the temporary closure. If possible, interrupted permanent fascial closure sutures are placed at the superior and inferior ends of the fascia to gradually (over the course of up to four trips to the operating room) close the fascia.

Two other new ideas in abdominal surgery include the use of adhesion reduction barriers and synthetic biomembranes for abdominal wall closure. Two types of adhesion reduction barriers are available: hyaluronic acid/carboxymethylcellulose and oxidized regenerated cellulose. Both these materials are applied to the raw surface of the bowel before abdominal closure, and within an hour they turn to a gelatinous substance.[39] Although the use of these membranes does not totally obviate adhesions, they have been demonstrated in clinical trials to decrease their severity.[40]

The second innovation is that of engineered tissue matrices that can be used for abdominal wall closure. These materials are constructed from donor integumentary tissue and processed to remove the epidermal and dermal cellular portions and thus the antigenic component of the allograft. The resulting product is a collagen-based matrix with its native tensile strength intact but its capacity to generate an immune response abrogated. The interstices of the allograft are then colonized by cellular populations from the recipient.[41] This material promises to yield an adjunct to closure of a complex abdominal wall defect that has good strength and is more resistant to infection than is the case with synthetic materials such as polypropylene mesh.

Staplers

Surgical staplers have changed the practice of surgery in a profound way, most notably within the field of minimally invasive technology. Several different devices are available for stapling:

1. Skin staplers
2. Ligating and dividing staplers (LDSs)
3. Gastrointestinal anastomosis (GIA) staplers
4. Thoracoabdominal (TA) staplers
5. End-to-end anastomosis (EEA) staplers
6. Laparoscopic hernia mesh tackers
7. Open hernia mesh staplers
8. Endo-GIA

A modification of the GIA stapler for laparoscopic use, the endo-GIA, has particularly broad utility. It can facili-

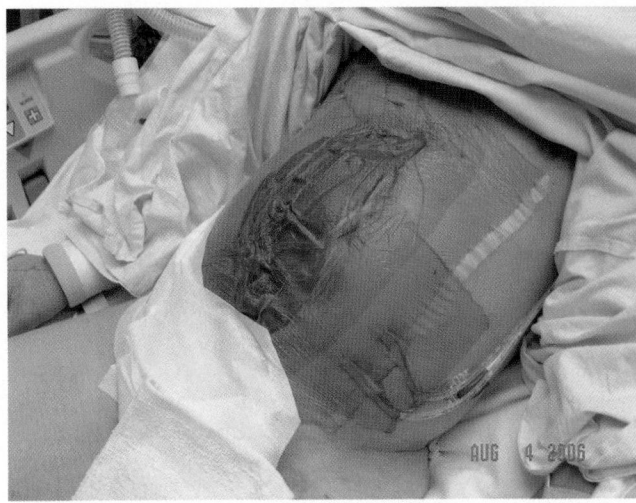

Figure 12-3 Vac Pac temporary abdominal wound closure. This closure method allows easy reentry into the abdomen and does not compromise the fascia. To fashion, place a surgical towel between two medium sticky drapes. Then place it in the abdomen and tuck the edges underneath the fascia with a several-centimeter overlap. Closed suction drains are next placed along the edges and brought out through the skin. Another surgical towel is then placed over the open portion of the wound and a large sticky drape is used to cover the entire abdomen. The drains are immediately connected to wall suction to provide adequate compression of the dressing.

tate the ligation and transection of major vascular pedicles in laparoscopy, as in the performance of splenectomy, nephrectomy, or hepatectomy, or facilitate gastrointestinal anastomosis or transection of solid organs such as the pancreas. In a video-assisted thoracoscopic surgical procedure, it can aid in wedge resection of injured or diseased lung. The GIA (endo-GIA or standard version) may aid in the transection of thick or indurated mesentery during intestinal resection in patients with inflammatory bowel disease.

Surgical Adhesives

Surgical adhesives have been widely used in modern surgery. They can be used for a simple task such as skin closure or for more complex wound problems. Many agents are clinically available and are used for a variety of purposes. Fibrin seal adhesive has been used to close fistulas, prevent lymphatic leakage after complete lymphadenectomy in the axilla or groin, and prevent leakage from tissue surfaces that have been newly transected, such as staple lines of the lung or pancreatic resection. It also has been adapted to seal the terminal bronchus via bronchoscopy as a noninvasive means of treating a small subset of patients with pneumothorax. Fibrin seal adhesive has become the preferred way to treat pseudoaneurysms in the groin or axilla that result from arterial puncture. Ultrasound-guided direct injection into such lesions has been reported to be successful with low complication rates.[42] Adhesives can also be used as an adjunct to reinforce and provide a watertight seal to a delicate gastrointestinal anastomosis, such as one involving the biliary tract or pancreas.

Surgical adhesives work by admixing a two-component agent derived from whole blood; each is secured in separate containers for shipping and storage. When mixed, the components form a viscous semiliquid tissue glue that can be applied onto a suture line, fistula tract or cavity, or other raw tissue surface or potential small dead space. When set, it becomes a solid adhesive biomembrane, sealant, or plug that will be self-retained. Major obstacles to its widespread use are cost and the potential for complications related to disease transmission with the use of blood products.

Two other commonly used agents are 2-octylcyanoacrylate (Dermabond) and butyl-2-cyanoacrylate (Histoacryl). Cyanoacrylate has been used for repair of organs and as an adhesive in many orthopedic procedures. Dermabond has been demonstrated to be an adequate replacement for the traditional suture closure of simple skin lacerations. Dermabond also allows the patient to resume showering within a few hours of closure of the wound.

SURGICAL DEVICES AND ENERGY SOURCES

Electrosurgery and Electrocautery

In 1928, Cushing first published a series of 500 neurosurgical procedures performed with an electrocautery device that was developed by Bovie. Since that time, electrocautery and electrosurgery have become the most important and basic surgical tools in the operating room.

High-frequency alternating current can be delivered in either unipolar or bipolar fashion. The unipolar (or monopolar) device is composed of a generator, an electrode for application, and an electrode for the returning current to complete the circuit. The patient's body becomes part of the circuit when the system is activated. Because the effectiveness of energy conversion into heat is inversely related to the area of contact, the application electrode is designed to be small to generate heat efficiently, and the returning electrode is designed to be large to disperse energy and prevent burn injury. The heat generated is dependent on three other factors in addition to the size of the contact area: the power setting/frequency of the current, the length of activation time, and whether the waveform released from the generator is continuous or intermittent. Unipolar devices can be used to incise tissue when activated with a constant waveform and to coagulate when activated with an intermittent waveform. In the cutting mode, much heat is generated relatively quickly over the target with minimal lateral thermal spread. As a result, the device cuts through tissue without coagulating any underlying vessels. In contrast, in the coagulation mode, electrocautery generates less heat on a slower frequency, with the potential for large lateral thermal spread. Such spread results in tissue dehydration and vessel thrombosis. A blended waveform can be chosen that will be able to take advantage of both the cutting and coagulation modes. A large grounding pad must be placed securely on the patient for the unipolar electrosurgical/electrocautery device to function properly and to prevent thermal burn injury at the current reentry electrode site.

Bipolar electrocautery establishes a short circuit between the tips of the instrument, whether a tissue grasper or forceps, without the requirement for a grounding pad. The tissue grasped between the tips of the instrument completes the circuit. In generating heat that affects only the tissue within the short circuit, it provides precise thermal coagulation. Bipolar electrocautery is more effective than the monopolar instrument in coagulating vessels because it adds the mechanical advantage of compression of tissue between the tips of the instrument to the thermal coagulation. Bipolar electrocautery is particularly useful when conducting a procedure in which lateral thermal injury or an arcing phenomenon needs to be avoided.

Lasers

Lasers use photons to excite the chromophore molecules within target tissue and generate kinetic energy that is released as heat, which causes protein denaturation and coagulation necrosis. This effect occurs without much collateral damage to surrounding tissue. It can be applied to the surface of target tissue or interstitially with a fiber-optic probe placed under precision image guidance. The energy generated and the depth of tissue penetration can be varied with the power setting selected and the photon chosen for the particular task. The laser effect can be enhanced by photosensitizing agents. The most common types of laser in use today are the argon, carbon dioxide, and neodymium:yttrium-aluminum-garnet (Nd-YAG) lasers. The depth of energy penetration within the target organ is least with the argon laser, moderate with the carbon dioxide laser, and deepest with the Nd-YAG laser.

Interstitial laser photocoagulation is a recently adopted laser treatment technology. With a precisely placed optic fiber (or fibers) inside target tissue, laser light is delivered and absorbed by the surrounding structure and tissue. The degree of absorption within and around the target tissue depends on the wavelength of the laser chosen and the specific optical properties of the tissue. The optical properties of different tumors or tissues are markedly different and depend on their tissue composition and density, degree of parenchymal fibrosis, vascularity, and the presence or absence of necrosis.

Argon Beam Coagulator

The argon beam coagulator creates a monopolar electric circuit between a hand-held probe and the target tissue by establishing a steady flow of electrons through a channel of electrically activated and ionized argon gas. This high-flow argon gas conducts electrical current to the target tissue and generates thermal coagulation of this tissue. The depth of the thermal penetration of tissue varies from fractions of a millimeter to a maximum of 6 mm, depending on three factors:

1. Power setting
2. Distance between the probe and the target
3. Length of its application

The hand-held control is usually combined with the regular Bovie, which can provide much more focused tissue coagulation for any such vessels. Because the argon gas blows blood away from the surface or paren-chyma of the target organ, coagulation is more effective in this setting. Visibility is also improved by the same mechanism. It is most commonly used to treat parenchy-mal hemorrhage of an organ, particularly the liver, but it can be used on the spleen, kidney, or any other solid organs with surface oozing.

Photodynamic Therapy

Photodynamic therapy is a new treatment that allows destruction of cancer cells and has recently been expanded to the eradication of metaplastic cells. It begins with the administration of a target-specific photosensi-tizer that is eventually concentrated in the target tissue. The photosensitizing agent is then activated with a wave-length-specific light energy source, which leads to the generation of free radicals cytotoxic to the target tissue. Photodynamic therapy has been used to treat different types of late-stage cancer, mainly in a palliative setting, but it has also been used in the treatment of some che-moresistant tumors. Applications reported in the literature include treating early radiographically detected non–small cell lung cancer, pancreatic cancer, squamous cell and basal cell carcinoma of the skin, recurrent superficial bladder cancer, chest wall involvement from breast cancer, and even chest wall recurrence of breast cancer.[43,44] Its utility has recently expanded to include the treatment of noncancer conditions such as Barrett's esophagus and psoriasis.[44,45]

High-Frequency Sound Wave Techniques

Ultrasound has had a strong impact on the practice of modern medicine. It has different functions, depending on the frequency of ultrasound generated by the machine. At a low power level, it causes no tissue damage and is mainly used for diagnostic purposes. With a high-fre-quency setting, ultrasound can be used to dissect, cut, and coagulate. Several high-frequency ultrasonic devices are available for surgical practice.

Another beneficial manipulation of acoustic wave technology is that of extracorporeal shock wave litho-tripsy. It has been used in treating cholelithiasis and nephrolithiasis. In this modality, the patient is placed in a water bath and a high-energy acoustic shock wave is generated by piezoelectric or electromagnetic technology and focused. The water-tissue interface allows the wave to pass through normal tissue without injuring it. The energy of the shock wave is focused on the offending stone by ultrasound and causes disruption and fragmen-tation of the calculus, which is then passed via the ureter.

Harmonic Scalpel

The harmonic scalpel is an instrument that uses ultra-sound technology to dissect tissue in bipolar fashion with only minimal collateral tissue damage. The device vibrates at a high frequency, usually around 55,000 times per second, to cut tissue. The high-frequency vibration of tissue molecules generates stress and friction in the tissue, which in turn generate heat and denaturation of protein.

Because of this unique capability to dissect tissue and coagulate small blood vessels all at once with minimal energy transfer to surrounding tissue, the device has gained recognition among surgeons. It has been used in many different types of minimally invasive surgery, and its application has recently been extended to many open procedures as well.

Ultrasonic Cavitation Devices

The Cavitron ultrasonic surgical aspirator is an ultrasonic instrument that uses lower-frequency ultrasound energy to fragment and dissect tissue of low fiber content. It is basically an ultrasound probe combined with an aspira-tor, so it functions as an acoustic vibrator and suction device at the same time. The Cavitron ultrasonic surgical aspirator has a variety of applications. Because the instru-ment fragments and aspirates tissue of low collagen and high water content, it can be an effective surgical instru-ment for liver and pancreas procedures without causing damage to surrounding tissue. When compared with the dissection technique of other instruments such as the scalpel or cautery, the advantages of using this device are less blood loss, improved visibility, and reduced col-lateral tissue injury. The device has been used for resect-ing lesions in a noncirrhotic liver and pancreatic tumors, especially small endocrine tumors within a soft normal pancreas without fibrosis. It has also been used for partial nephrectomy, salvage splenectomy, head and neck pro-cedures, and treatment of many gynecologic tumors as well.

Radiofrequency Ablation

Radiofrequency energy can be used for tissue ablation either in a curative or in a palliative attempt to treat dif-ferent cancers. It is also effective in treating benign condi-tions such as neuralgia, bone pain, and cardiac arrhythmias (e.g., atrial fibrillation). The basic method of radiofre-quency application is to place an electrode or electrodes into or over the target tissue to transmit a high-frequency alternating current to the tissue in the range of 350 to 500 kHz. Rapid alternating directional movement of ions results in the release of kinetic energy. It can raise the temperature of the target tissue to higher than 100°C and cause protein denaturation, desiccation, and coagulation necrosis; it has a built-in sensor for automatically termi-nating transmission of the current at a particular set point to prevent overheating and unwanted collateral damage. The main use of this modality is for tumors in the liver parenchyma. Its applications have been expanded to tumors in the lung, kidney, adrenal gland, breast, thyroid, pancreas, and bone. The indications for radiofrequency ablation will continue to grow in the future because it is inexpensive and can be reliably used to destroy a larger tumor mass.[47-53]

Cryoablation

Cryotherapy can be applied topically to treat skin condi-tions or tumors or interstitially for the ablation of liver lesions. It destroys cells by the process of freezing and thawing. With liquid nitrogen or argon circulating through a probe placed over or within the target lesion, the tissue can be frozen to a temperature of −35°C or lower. Cell damage occurs as a result of disruption of subcellular structures with ice crystal formation in the freezing phase and degradation during the thawing process. Ischemia of the tissue from focal disruption of the circulation, shifting of water and electrolyte content in situ, and protein denaturation also contribute to the tissue damage induced by cryotherapy. Lesions that contact major vessels can be difficult to treat with this modality because of the heat-sink effect introduced by circulating blood. Nonetheless, it has been reported to be effective in treating both primary and secondary lesions of the liver that are unresectable. The major disadvantage of interstitial cryotherapy is its cost. Patients usually need general anesthesia for the procedure, the equipment is more expensive than a radiofrequency system, and the process itself is time consuming. Complications such as hemorrhage from tissue fracture are a concern. With the availability of multiple alternative image-guided tissue ablation techniques, cryotherapy will have limited application in the future.[53]

Microwave Ablation and Radiosurgery

Microwave coagulation is achieved by using a generator to transmit microwave energy at a frequency of 2450 MHz via a probe placed under image guidance within target organs or tissue. A rapidly alternating electrical field is created within the target tissue to induce motion of polar molecules in the tissue, such as water. Kinetic energy is dissipated as heat, which causes coagulation necrosis. Its use was initially for lesions in the liver; however, its application has been expanded to the treatment of cardiac rhythm disturbances, prostatic hyperplasia, endometrial bleeding, sterilization of bony margins, and partial nephrectomy. The major limiting factor is that the area that can be ablated with the current equipment is very small, thus necessitating multiple insertions of the microwave probe to treat a single lesion.[47]

The premiere tool in radiosurgery is the gamma knife, and its principal area of use is in neurosurgery. This tool allows more than 200 separate sources of high-energy gamma radiation, arranged in a circular fashion, to be stereotactically focused onto a minute area within the brain. Essential to avoiding injury to normal brain tissue is that the head be held motionless by an external fixation device. This ability to destroy finite areas within the brain has been applied to the treatment of benign and malignant brain neoplasms, arteriovenous malformations, and epilepsy.[54-56]

OUTPATIENT SURGERY

Over the past 20 years, outpatient surgery has become more commonplace. It is estimated that up to 75% of elective surgical procedures are now performed in an outpatient setting, which means that patients do not experience an overnight stay around the time of the procedure. Even patients who will need a postoperative inpatient stay after the procedure are usually admitted to the hospital *after* the surgery. Outpatient surgery can take place in operating rooms associated with a large hospital, in a freestanding outpatient surgery center, or even in a physician's office. Preoperative evaluation of the patient usually takes place on an ambulatory basis, and more coordination is required by the surgeon to ensure that the evaluation is completed and acted on in timely fashion. Patients with significant comorbid conditions are evaluated by anesthesia staff at least 1 day before the planned procedure (Box 12-3).[57] The standards for perioperative monitoring are similar regardless of the setting and are tailored to the complexity of the procedure and the comorbid conditions of the patient. In addition, the patient's postoperative disposition takes into account the distance from the place of surgery, as well as who will be around to monitor the patient.

In general, procedures performed under local anesthesia without sedation are of a magnitude that patients can be discharged home under their own recognizance. The need for postoperative pain control with narcotic-based agents may alter patients' suitability for transporting themselves and thus is considered when making decisions about disposition.

Any patient who receives sedation or a general anesthetic, or both, at a minimum needs to have a ride home. Ideally, the patient will have a responsible individual staying overnight in the same residence. Again, the patient's ability to perform tasks at home will be influenced by the need for narcotics, as well as any restrictions or limitations dictated by the procedure. Patients who will be unable to maintain oral intake after surgery (because of either the operation itself or the need for postoperative ventilatory support) or who will need IV or other nonoral pain medication will require postoperative hospitalization. The need for postoperative care will have a bearing on the type of facility in which the surgeon chooses to carry out the procedure.

Selected References

Cohn SL (ed): Preoperative medical consultation. Med Clin North Am, vol 87, January 2003.

An overview of the components of risk assessment and an organized approach to medical consultation for preoperative evaluation.

Eagle KA, Berger PB, Calkins H, et al: ACC/AHA guideline update on perioperative cardiovascular evaluation for noncardiac surgery: A report of the American College of Cardiology/American Heart Association Task Force on Practice Guidelines (Committee to Update the 1996 Guidelines on Perioperative Cardiovascular Evaluation for Noncardiac Surgery). Circulation 105:1257-1267, 2002.

Evidence-based guidelines for perioperative cardiovascular evaluation for noncardiac surgery, updated in 2002 by the American College of Cardiology/American Heart Association Task Force on Practice Guidelines.

Geerts WH, Heit JA, Clagett GP, et al: Prevention of venous thromboembolism. Chest 119:132S-175S, 2001.

Evidence-based guidelines for the prevention of venous thromboembolism in patients of various risk groups published by the American College of Chest Physicians.

Gulec SA, Wang YZ, Reinbold RB, et al: Selected technologies in general surgery. In O'Leary P (ed): The Physiologic Basis of Surgery, 3rd ed. Philadelphia, Lippincott Williams & Wilkins, 2002.

An overview of the basic principles behind the technology commonly used in the operating room and for diagnostic purposes.

Klein S, Kinney J, Jeejeebhoy K, et al: Nutrition support in clinical practice: Review of published data and recommendations for future research directions. JPEN J Parenter Enteral Nutr 21:133-156, 1997.

Summary of nutritional support data relevant to the treatment of patients requiring all levels of nutritional support.

Litaker D: Preoperative screening. Med Clin North Am 83:1565-1581, 1999.

A discussion of how to understand risk in preoperative patients and a review of effective screening tools to highlight sources of risk from the IMPACT (Internal Medicine Preoperative Assessment, Consultation, and Treatment) Center and Department of General Internal Medicine, The Cleveland Clinic.

Mack MJ: Minimally invasive and robotic surgery. JAMA 285:568-572, 2001.

Overview of emerging technologies relevant to practitioners-in-training in the surgical fields.

Napolitano LM (ed): Perioperative issues for surgeons: Improving patient safety and outcomes. Surg Clin North Am, vol 85, December 2005.

Overview of the perioperative concerns of patients, surgeons, and anesthesiologists, including topics addressing risk adjustment, hospital systems, and patient safety.

References

1. Halaszynski TM, Juda R, Silverman DG: Optimizing postoperative outcomes with efficient preoperative assessment and management. Crit Care Med 32:S76-S86, 2004.
2. Khuri SF, Daley J, Henderson W, et al: The Department of Veterans Affairs' NSQIP: The first national, validated, outcome-based, risk-adjusted, and peer-controlled program for the measurement and enhancement of the quality of surgical care. National VA Surgical Quality Improvement Program. Ann Surg 228:491-507, 1998.
3. Mangano DT, Goldman L: Preoperative assessment of patients with known or suspected coronary disease. N Engl J Med 333:1750-1756, 1995.
4. Akhtar S, Silverman DG: Assessment and management of patients with ischemic heart disease. Crit Care Med 32:S126-S136, 2004.
5. Eagle KA, Berger PB, Calkins H, et al: ACC/AHA guideline update for perioperative cardiovascular evaluation for noncardiac surgery—executive summary: A report of the American College of Cardiology/American Heart Association Task Force on Practice Guidelines (Committee to Update the 1996 Guidelines on Perioperative Cardiovascular Evaluation for Noncardiac Surgery). J Am Coll Cardiol 39:542-553, 2002.
6. Mangano DT, Layug EL, Wallace A, et al: Effect of atenolol on mortality and cardiovascular morbidity after noncardiac surgery. Multicenter Study of Perioperative Ischemia Research Group. N Engl J Med 335:1713-1720, 1996.
7. Biccard BM: Relationship between the inability to climb two flights of stairs and outcome after major non-cardiac surgery: Implications for the pre-operative assessment of functional capacity. Anaesthesia 60:588-593, 2005.
8. Arozullah AM, Conde MV, Lawrence VA: Preoperative evaluation for postoperative pulmonary complications. Med Clin North Am 87:153-173, 2003.
9. Joseph AJ, Cohn SL: Perioperative care of the patient with renal failure. Med Clin North Am 87:193-210, 2003.

10. Rizvon MK, Chou CL: Surgery in the patient with liver disease. Med Clin North Am 87:211-227, 2003.

11. Maniatis AG, Hunt CM: Therapy for spontaneous umbilical hernia rupture. Am J Gastroenterol 90:310-312, 1995.

12. Hurst RD, Butler BN, Soybel DI, et al: Management of groin hernias in patients with ascites. Ann Surg 216:696-700, 1992.

13. Yerdel MA, Koksoy C, Aras N, et al: Laparoscopic versus open cholecystectomy in cirrhotic patients: A prospective study. Surg Laparosc Endosc 7:483-486, 1997.

14. Schiff RL, Welsh GA: Perioperative evaluation and management of the patient with endocrine dysfunction. Med Clin North Am 87:175-192, 2003.

15. Turina M, Christ-Crain M, Polk HC Jr: Impact of diabetes mellitus and metabolic disorders. Surg Clin North Am 85:1153-1161, ix, 2005.

16. Ahmed Z, Lockhart CH, Weiner M, et al: Advances in diabetic management: Implications for anesthesia. Anesth Analg 100:666-669, 2005.

17. Carr A, Cooper DA: Adverse effects of antiretroviral therapy. Lancet 356:1423-1430, 2000.

18. Simon TL, Alverson DC, AuBuchon J, et al: Practice parameters for the use of red blood cell transfusions: Developed by the Red Blood Cell Administration Practice Guideline Development Task Force of the College of American Pathologists. Arch Pathol Lab Med 122:130-138, 1998.

19. Kearon C, Hirsh J: Management of anticoagulation before and after elective surgery. N Engl J Med 336:1506-1511, 1997.

20. Geerts WH, Heit JA, Clagett GP, et al: Prevention of venous thromboembolism. Chest 119:132S-175S, 2001.

21. Marcantonio ER, Goldman L, Mangione CM, et al: A clinical prediction rule for delirium after elective noncardiac surgery. JAMA 271:134-139, 1994.

22. Klein S, Kinney J, Jeejeebhoy K, et al: Nutrition support in clinical practice: Review of published data and recommendations for future research directions. National Institutes of Health, American Society for Parenteral and Enteral Nutrition, and American Society for Clinical Nutrition. JPEN J Parenter Enteral Nutr 21:133-156, 1997.

23. Abir F, Bell R: Assessment and management of the obese patient. Crit Care Med 32:S87-S91, 2004.

24. Bratzler DW, Houck PM, Richards C, et al: Use of antimicrobial prophylaxis for major surgery: Baseline results from the National Surgical Infection Prevention Project. Arch Surg 140:174-182, 2005.

25. Weed HG: Antimicrobial prophylaxis in the surgical patient. Med Clin North Am 87:59-75, 2003.

26. SCIPWebsite:http://www.medqic.org/dcs/ContentServer?cid=1089815967030&pagename=Medqic%2FMeasure%2FMeasuresHome&parentName=Topic&level3=Measures&c=MQParents. Accessed June 24, 2006.

27. Wille-Jorgensen P, Guenaga KF, Castro AA, et al: Clinical value of preoperative mechanical bowel cleansing in elective colorectal surgery: A systematic review. Dis Colon Rectum 46:1013-1020, 2003.

28. Mercado DL, Petty BG: Perioperative medication management. Med Clin North Am 87:41-57, 2003.

29. Ang-Lee MK, Moss J, Yuan CS: Herbal medicines and perioperative care. JAMA 286:208-216, 2001.

30. Brady M, Kinn S, Stuart P: Preoperative fasting for adults to prevent perioperative complications. Cochrane Database Syst Rev 4:CD004423, 2003.

31. Diks J, van Hoorn DE, Nijveldt RJ, et al: Preoperative fasting: An outdated concept? JPEN J Parenter Enteral Nutr 29:298-304, 2005.

32. Melis GC, van Leeuwen PA, von Blomberg-van der Flier BM, et al: A carbohydrate-rich beverage prior to surgery prevents surgery-induced immunodepression: A randomized, controlled, clinical trial. JPEN J Parenter Enteral Nutr 30:21-26, 2006.

33. Lieberman P: Anaphylactic reactions during surgical and medical procedures. J Allergy Clin Immunol 110:S64-S69, 2002.

34. Ricci G, Gentili A, Di Lorenzo F, et al: Latex allergy in subjects who had undergone multiple surgical procedures for bladder exstrophy: Relationship with clinical intervention and atopic diseases. BJU Int 84:1058-1062, 1999.

35. Rosenbaum HK, Miller JD: Malignant hyperthermia and myotonic disorders. Anesthesiol Clin North Am 20:623-664, 2002.

36. Jeran L: Patient temperature: An introduction to the clinical guideline for the prevention of unplanned perioperative hypothermia. J Perianesth Nurs 16:303-304, 2001.

37. Edwards PS, Lipp A, Holmes A: Preoperative skin antiseptics for preventing surgical wound infections after clean surgery. Cochrane Database Syst Rev 3:CD003949, 2004.

38. Hebert PC, Wells G, Tweeddale M, et al: Does transfusion practice affect mortality in critically ill patients? Transfusion Requirements in Critical Care (TRICC) Investigators and the Canadian Critical Care Trials Group. Am J Respir Crit Care Med 155:1618-1623, 1997.

39. DeCherney AH, diZerega GS: Clinical problem of intraperitoneal postsurgical adhesion formation following general surgery and the use of adhesion prevention barriers. Surg Clin North Am 77:671-688, 1997.

40. Vrijland WW, Tseng LN, Eijkman HJ, et al: Fewer intraperitoneal adhesions with use of hyaluronic acid–carboxymethylcellulose membrane: A randomized clinical trial. Ann Surg 235:193-199, 2002.

41. Mizuno H, Takeda A, Uchinuma E: Creation of an acellular dermal matrix from frozen skin. Aesthetic Plast Surg 23:316-322, 1999.

42. Friedman SG, Pellerito JS, Scher L, et al: Ultrasound-guided thrombin injection is the treatment of choice for femoral pseudoaneurysms. Arch Surg 137:462-464, 2002.

43. Tanaka H, Hashimoto K, Yamada I, et al: Interstitial photodynamic therapy with rotating and reciprocating optical fibers. Cancer 91:1791-1796, 2001.

44. Allison R, Mang T, Hewson G, et al: Photodynamic therapy for chest wall progression from breast carcinoma is an underutilized treatment modality. Cancer 91:1-8, 2001.

45. Lim KN, Waring PJ, Saidi R: Therapeutic options in patients with Barrett's esophagus. Dig Dis 17:145-152, 1999.

46. Salo JA, Salminen JT, Kiviluoto TA, et al: Treatment of Barrett's esophagus by endoscopic laser ablation and antireflux surgery. Ann Surg 227:40-44, 1998.

47. Izumi N, Asahina Y, Noguchi O, et al: Risk factors for distant recurrence of hepatocellular carcinoma in the liver after complete coagulation by microwave or radiofrequency ablation. Cancer 91:949-956, 2001.

48. Pearson AS, Izzo F, Fleming RY, et al: Intraoperative radiofrequency ablation or cryoablation for hepatic malignancies. Am J Surg 178:592-599, 1999.

49. Wood BJ, Abraham J, Hvizda JL, et al: Radiofrequency ablation of adrenal tumors and adrenocortical carcinoma metastases. Cancer 97:554-560, 2003.

50. Dupuy DE, Monchik JM, Decrea C, et al: Radiofrequency ablation of regional recurrence from well-differentiated thyroid malignancy. Surgery 130:971-977, 2001.

51. Izzo F, Thomas R, Delrio P, et al: Radiofrequency ablation in patients with primary breast carcinoma: A pilot study in 26 patients. Cancer 92:2036-2044, 2001.

52. Maessen JG, Nijs JF, Smeets JL, et al: Beating-heart surgical treatment of atrial fibrillation with microwave ablation. Ann Thorac Surg 74:S1307-S1311, 2002.
53. Bilchik AJ, Wood TF, Allegra D, et al: Cryosurgical ablation and radiofrequency ablation for unresectable hepatic malignant neoplasms: A proposed algorithm. Arch Surg 135:657-662; discussion 662-654, 2000.
54. Weil MD: Stereotactic radiosurgery for brain tumors. Hematol Oncol Clin North Am 15:1017-1026, 2001.
55. Hartford AC, Loeffler JS: Radiosurgery for benign tumors and arteriovenous malformations of the central nervous system. Front Radiat Ther Oncol 35:30-47, 2001.
56. McKhann GM 2nd, Bourgeois BF, Goodman RR: Epilepsy surgery: Indications, approaches, and results. Semin Neurol 22:269-278, 2002.
57. Pasternak LR: Preoperative screening for ambulatory patients. Anesthesiol Clin North America 21:229-242, vii, 2003.

Ultrasound for Surgeons

Christopher J. Dente, MD and Grace S. Rozycki, MD, RDMS

Although the scientific principles underlying ultrasonography (US) were first elucidated in the 19th century, it was not until the second half of the 20th century that this technology could be effectively applied to medicine. Surgeons, first in Europe and more recently in the United States, have now embraced US as a key diagnostic tool in many areas of clinical practice. Because US is noninvasive, portable, rapid, and easily repeatable, it is especially well suited to surgical practice. In many hospitals and offices across the country, US machines are owned by surgeons and are often part of standard equipment in the trauma resuscitation area and intensive care unit (ICU). Use of this diagnostic tool as an extension of the physical examination allows the surgeon to receive immediate information about the patient's disease process and thus permits expedited patient management. In addition, computer-enhanced high-resolution imaging and multifrequency specialized transducers have made US increasingly user-friendly, which has extended its applicability to a variety of surgical settings.

The objectives of this chapter include an introduction to some of the basic principles of US technology with both a discussion of the physics of US and definitions of the common terminology used, followed by brief descriptions of the current use of US in various clinical settings, including the office, operating room, trauma resuscitation room, and ICU. Also included is a discussion of the opportunities for training in US available to surgical residents and surgeons in practice.

PHYSICS AND INSTRUMENTATION

Nowhere in diagnostic imaging is an understanding of wave physics more important than in US because US is highly operator dependent. To perform an US examination correctly, a surgeon must be able to interpret echo patterns, determine artifacts, and adjust the machine appropriately to obtain the best images.

In diagnostic US, the transducer or probe interconverts electrical and acoustic energy (Fig. 13-1). To accomplish this interconversion, the transducer contains the following essential components:

1. An *active element*. Electrical energy is applied to the piezoelectric crystals within the transducer, and a US pulse is thereby generated via the piezoelectric effect. The pulse distorts the crystals, and an electrical signal is produced. This signal causes a US image to form on the screen via the reverse piezoelectric effect.
2. *Damping* or *backing material*. An epoxy resin absorbs the vibrations and reduces the number of cycles in a pulse, thereby improving resolution of the US image.
3. A *matching layer*. This substance (generally a US gel) reduces the reflection that occurs at the transducer-tissue interface. The great difference in density (i.e., the impedance mismatch) between soft tissue and the transducer results in reflection of the US waves. The matching material decreases this reflection and facilitates transit of the US waves through the body and into the target organ.

Table 13-1 Commonly Used Ultrasound Frequencies

FREQUENCY (MHz)	CLINICAL APPLICATION
2.5-3.5	Abdominal, aorta, renal
5.0	Transvaginal, pediatric abdominal, testicular
7.5	Vascular, superficial soft tissue, thyroid
10-12	Intravascular ultrasound, endoscopic ultrasound

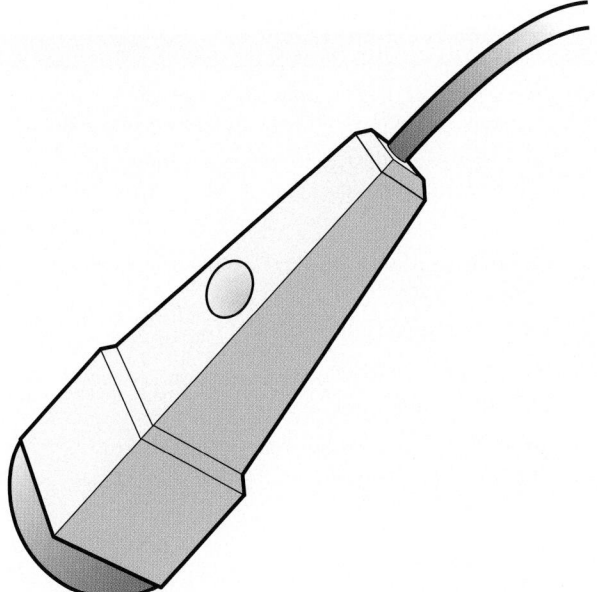

Figure 13-1 Standard curved-array ultrasound probe. The *circle* on the probe is an example of an indicator that allows probe orientation.

Transducers are classified according to (1) the arrangement of the active elements (array) contained within the transducer and (2) the frequency of the US wave produced. Transducer arrays contain closely packed piezoelectric elements, each with its own electrical connection to the US instrument. These elements can be excited individually or in groups to produce the US beam. There are four main transducer arrays:

1. *Rectangular linear array:* yields a rectangular image
2. *Curved array:* yields a trapezoidal image
3. *Phased array:* a small transducer in which the sound pulses are generated by activating all the elements in the array
4. *Annular array:* the elements are arranged in circular fashion

Transducer arrays allow the US beam to be focused and electronically steered without any moving mechanical parts (except for the annular array). In the clinical setting, this arrangement allows the operator to adjust the focal zone so that a large organ (e.g., the liver) can be accurately imaged while still being able to obtain fine details of a lesion.

The frequency of the transducer is determined by the thickness of the piezoelectric elements within the transducer: the thinner the piezoelectric elements, the higher the frequency. Although diagnostic US makes use of transducer frequencies ranging from 1 to 20 Megahertz (MHz), the most commonly used frequencies for medical diagnostic imaging are those between 2.5 and 10 MHz (Table 13-1). US beams of different frequencies have different characteristics: higher frequencies penetrate tissue poorly but yield excellent resolution, whereas lower frequencies penetrate well but at the cost of compromised resolution. Accordingly, transducers are generally chosen on the basis of the depth of the structure to be imaged. For example, a 7.5-MHz transducer is a suitable choice for imaging a superficial organ such as the thyroid, but a 3.5-MHz transducer would be preferable for imaging a deep structure such as the abdominal aorta.

US machines vary in complexity, but each has the following essential components:

1. A *transmitter* to control electrical signals sent to the transducer.
2. A *receiver* or *image processor* that admits the electrical signal returning from the transducer.
3. A *transducer* to interconvert electrical and acoustic energy. Each transducer has an indicator to allow orientation of the probe.
4. A *monitor* to display the US image.
5. An *image recorder* to produce copies of the US images.

Finally, there are three scanning modes, A, B, and M; these modes evolved over a period of several years. A mode (amplitude modulation), the most basic form of diagnostic US, yields a one-dimensional image that displays the amplitude or strength of the wave along the vertical axis and the time along the horizontal axis. Therefore, the greater the signal returning to the transducer, the higher the spike. B mode (brightness modulation), the mode most commonly used today, relates the brightness of the image to the amplitude of the US wave. Thus, denser structures appear brighter (i.e., whiter, more echogenic) on the image because they reflect the US waves better. M mode relates the amplitude of the US wave to the imaging of moving structures, such as cardiac muscle. Before real-time imaging became available, M-mode scanning formed the basis for echocardiography.

A summary of technical terms used commonly in US physics and their definitions are found in Table 13-2. Essential US principles are listed in Table 13-3 and clinical terminology is found in Table 13-4. Finally, a summary of scanning planes is listed in Table 13-5.

CLINICAL USES OF ULTRASOUND

As an extension of the physical examination, US is a valuable adjunct to surgical practice in the office, emergency department, operating room, and surgical ICU. Once surgeons have learned the essential principles of US, they can readily build on this experience and extend the use of this technology to various specific aspects of

Table 13-2 Ultrasound Physics Terminology

TERM	DEFINITION	CLINICAL APPLICATION
Frequency	Number of cycles/sec*	Increasing frequency improves resolution. Diagnostic ultrasound uses frequencies of 1-20 MHz
Wavelength	Distance traveled by the wave per cycle	Shorter wavelengths yield better resolution but poorer penetration[†]
Amplitude	Strength or height of the wave	
Attenuation	Decrease in amplitude and intensity of the wave as it travels through a medium	The time-gain compensation circuit compensates for attenuation
Absorption	Conversion of sound energy to heat	Method of attenuation
Scatter	Redirection of the wave as it strikes a rough boundary	Method of attenuation
Reflection	Return of the wave toward the transducer	Method of attenuation
Propagation speed	Speed at which the wave passes through soft tissue (1540 m/sec)	Speed is greater in solids than in liquids and greater in liquids than in gases

*10^6 cycles/sec = 1 MHz.
[†]As frequency increases, wavelength decreases.

surgery. What follows is a list and description of several clinical areas in which surgeon-performed US has proved to be an effective diagnostic and interventional tool.

Outpatient Setting

Breast

US-directed biopsy of breast lesions is now a common office procedure for general surgeons. The increase in the number of screening mammograms performed since the late 1970s has led to the detection of more nonpalpable breast lesions. The traditional choice for further evaluation of such masses has been open surgical excision, but the yield of malignancies with this approach has been only about 20%. Advances in US technology, including automated biopsy needles, high-resolution transducers, and computer-aided diagnosis programs,[1]

have prompted a surge of interest in fine-needle and core biopsy tissue sampling as an alternative to open biopsy. Such procedures are appealing because they are minimally invasive, are about as accurate as open biopsy, and can be performed by the surgeon in the office setting.[2] Essentially, surgeons can use US as an extension of their physical examination to evaluate the breast for a solid or cystic lesion and also to identify characteristics of the lesion that suggest whether it is benign or malignant. Characteristics suggestive of malignancy in a breast mass include an indistinct, jagged margin; posterior shadowing (as opposed to posterior enhancement); internal echoes (nonhomogenicity); and noncompressibility.

Current indications for breast US include the following[3]:

1. Evaluation of a nonpalpable, new growing mass or microcalcifications detected on mammography

Table 13-3 Principles of Ultrasound

PRINCIPLE	EXPLANATION
Piezoelectric effect	Piezoelectric crystals expand and contract to interconvert electrical and mechanical energy
Pulse-echo principle	When ultrasound waves contact tissue, some of the signal is reflected and some is transmitted. The waves that are reflected back to the crystals generate an electrical impulse comparable to the strength of the returning wave
Acoustic impedance	Defined as the density of tissue × the speed of sound in tissue. The strength of the returning echo depends on the difference in density between structures imaged. Structures with significant differences in acoustic impendence are easy to distinguish from one another (e.g., bile and gallstone)

Table 13-4 Ultrasound Clinical Terminology

TERM	DEFINITION
Echogenicity	Degree to which a tissue reflects ultrasound waves (reflected in images as the degree of brightness)
Anechoic	No internal echoes, appearing dark or black
Isoechoic	Having similar appearance to surrounding tissue
Hypoechoic	Less echoic (darker) than surrounding tissue
Hyperechoic	More echoic (whiter) than surrounding tissue
Resolution	The ability to distinguish between two adjacent structures; may be lateral (width of structure) or axial (depth of structure)

2. Evaluation of duct size in the presence of nipple discharge
3. Assessment of a dense breast or a vaguely palpable mass, especially in younger women
4. Differentiation between a solid palpable mass and a cystic one
5. Guidance of percutaneous drainage of a cyst or an abscess

US is especially useful in younger women with suspected breast pathology. Indeed, a recent study of 296 women younger than 30 years who underwent surgeon-performed breast sonography revealed 254 masses in 224 patients. These masses were an average of 2.2 cm in size, and all patients were able to undergo immediate biopsy during the same office visit. The most common finding was fibroadenoma (72%), followed by fibrocystic change (8%), phylloides tumor (6%), cyst (4%), and abscess (3%). In 2% of cases, malignancy was detected (four invasive carcinomas and one malignant phylloides tumor).[4] Thus, US may be extremely helpful, especially in younger women, in whom most masses are benign, physical examination is difficult, and mammography is unreliable.

It is important to note, however, that US-guided biopsy is not infallible. One recent report of 715 patients revealed a sensitivity of 96% for US-guided core needle biopsy for the diagnosis of cancer. Of the 12 patients who had false-negative (benign) findings on needle biopsy, 9 underwent open surgical biopsy because of indeterminate findings (*n* = 2) or discordant radiologic/pathologic results (*n* = 7) and thus had no appreciable delay in the time to diagnosis of cancer. However, three patients (two lobular cancers, one tubular cancer) had the diagnosis of cancer delayed between 16 and 27 months because of false-negative US-guided biopsies, although all still had early-stage cancer at final diagnosis.[5] Thus, like any other modality, US must be used in context with other physical findings, radiologic results, and patient preferences if the number of missed diagnoses is to be minimized.

Other well-described uses of US for evaluation of the breasts include not only postoperative follow-up for hematomas, seromas, and prostheses but also US-guided interventions such as cyst aspiration, biopsy of solid lesions, preoperative needle localization, axillary lymph node fine-needle aspiration (FNA), and peritumoral injection for sentinel lymph node biopsy. Indeed, as experience with US diagnosis of malignant lymph nodes has increased, certain characteristics suggestive of malignancy have been described. Suspicious lymph nodes are generally round or ovoid, have a hypoechoic core, are larger than 5 mm, and have an irregular cortex that is generally greater than 2 mm in thickness.[6] Based on these criteria, US-guided FNA is now being used by certain groups with some success to avoid sentinel node biopsy.[7]

Rizzatto reported that high-resolution US can demonstrate intraductal spread of tumors and their multiple foci. Because of new technologies and contrast agents, perfusion studies show enhanced contrast resolution that increases the sensitivity of US for small nodal metastases.[2] It is clear that the use of breast US in office practice has

Table 13-5 Ultrasound Scanning Planes

PLANE	EXPLANATION
Sagittal	Divides the body into right and left sections parallel to the long axis (the transducer indicator points to the patient's head)
Transverse	Divides the body into superior and inferior sections perpendicular to the long axis (the transducer indicator points to the patient's right side)
Coronal	Divides the body into anterior and posterior sections perpendicular to the sagittal plane and parallel to the long axis (the transducer indicator points toward the patient's head)

become more sophisticated and has allowed more patients to have their diagnosis and management expedited.

Gastrointestinal Tract

Endoscopic US (EUS) and endorectal US have added a new dimension to the preoperative assessment and treatment of many gastrointestinal lesions. EUS involves visualization of the gastrointestinal tract via a high-frequency (12-20 MHz) US transducer placed through an endoscope. With the transducer near the target organ, images of the gut wall and the surrounding parenchymal organs can be obtained that are detailed enough to define the depth of tumor penetration with precision and detect the presence of involved lymph nodes as small as 2 mm.

Indications for EUS include the following[8]:

1. Preoperative staging of esophageal, gastric, and rectal malignancies
2. Preoperative localization of pancreatic endocrine tumors, particularly insulinomas
3. Evaluation of submucosal lesions of the gastrointestinal tract
4. Guidance of imaging during interventional procedures (e.g., tissue sampling and drainage of a pancreatic pseudocyst)

Recently, EUS has been used to facilitate FNA for biopsy of submucosal lesions of the gastrointestinal tract, as well as lesions of the pancreas. EUS-guided FNA accurately detects neoplastic pancreatic cysts and may therefore assist in decision making for either a medical or surgical approach in these patients.[9]

EUS for staging of tumors of the esophagus and stomach has become more and more commonplace. Two recent reports[10,11] of EUS for gastric cancer have quoted accuracy rates for T stage to be between 65% and 92% and accuracy rates for N stage to be between 50% and 90%. Accuracy is best for stage T3 and worst for T2 lesions, which seem to be more commonly overstaged than understaged. US findings suggestive of lymph node metastases include size greater than 10 mm, round shape, sharp demarcation, and a hypoechoic center.[11] It is theorized, but not well documented, that the addition of FNA to EUS will improve diagnostic accuracy.

Endorectal US is used in the evaluation of patients with benign and malignant anal and rectal conditions. It

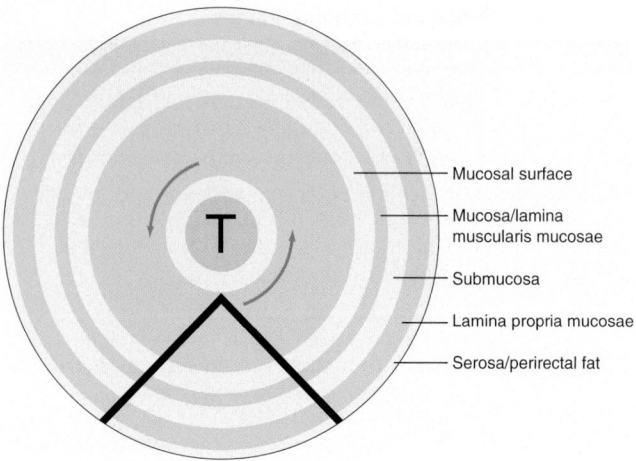

Mucosal surface

Mucosa/lamina
muscularis mucosae

Submucosa

Lamina propria mucosae

Serosa/perirectal fat

Figure 13-2 Five-layer rectal wall anatomy as delineated by endorectal ultrasonography. (From Wong WK: Endorectal ultrasonography for benign disease. In Staren ED, Arregui ME [eds]: Ultrasound for the Surgeon. Philadelphia, Lippincott-Raven, 1997, p 66.)

is commonly performed with an axial 7.0- or 10.0-MHz rotating transducer that produces a 360-degree horizontal cross-sectional view of the rectal wall. This special transducer is 24 cm long and is covered with a water-filled latex balloon. After the transducer is advanced above the rectal lesion, the balloon that surrounds the transducer is filled with water to create an acoustic window for US imaging. The transducer is gradually withdrawn while the examiner views the layers of the rectal wall by means of real-time imaging (Fig. 13-2).[12] These layers are important landmarks in US staging, just as they are in postoperative pathologic staging. For example, if the middle white line (i.e., the submucosa) is intact, a lesion may be adequately removed via submucosal resection.

The sensitivity of US in determining the depth of tumor invasion is about 85% to 90%; however, it can sometimes overestimate the extent of invasion in the presence of tissue inflammation and edema.[12] Errors in staging are likely to occur with tumors that invade the muscularis mucosae or are associated with inflammation of the lamina propria. The accuracy of EUS after neoadjuvant chemoradiation therapy is somewhat less, with a recent report suggesting an accuracy of 72% and 80% for T stage and N stage, respectively, in this setting.[13]

Finally, endoanal US may play an important role in the evaluation of benign anal disease such as anal incontinence and fistula in ano; US is capable of detecting defects in the internal and external sphincters. The study is performed in much the same way as endorectal US, except that the 10-MHz transducer is covered with a sonolucent hard plastic cone instead of a water-filled balloon. Although endoanal US does not measure sphincter function, US-detected sphincter disruption correlates well with pressure measurements and operative findings.[14]

Endoanal US may also be used to assess a fistulous track to determine its course relative to the sphincters and assist in locating its internal opening. In one study,

US was able to detect 100% of tracks; however, only 86% of these studies led to accurate preoperative assessment of the fistula's relationship to the sphincters. Moreover, only 60% had the internal opening identified accurately.[15] A second study reported an overall accuracy of around 70% for determining the level and internal opening of the fistula.[16] Thus, although US may be helpful for complex or recurrent disease, its use is probably still not warranted for routine management of fistula in ano.

Vascular System

Color flow duplex imaging and endoluminal US have significantly expanded the diagnostic and therapeutic aspects of vascular imaging. Vascular diagnostic imaging is commonly used for diagnosing arterial disease or deep vein thrombosis (DVT); however, it is also helpful for the diagnosis of other disorders such as Raynaud's disease and thoracic outlet syndrome. In the office, surgeons use US to screen for abdominal aortic aneurysm or to monitor patients with a known aneurysm because it is capable of detecting changes in aortic diameter as small as a few millimeters. In patients who have undergone repair of an abdominal aortic aneurysm, color flow duplex imaging is highly specific for the diagnosis of anastomotic false aneurysms. Duplex US was compared with B-mode US, computed tomography (CT), digital subtraction arteriography, and magnetic resonance imaging and emerged as the diagnostic test of choice when accuracy, cost, safety, and availability of each method were assessed.[17]

Color flow duplex scanning is also used to examine the patency and size of the portal vein and the hepatic artery in patients who have undergone liver transplantation, assess the resectability of pancreatic tumors, diagnose superior mesenteric artery occlusion, and diagnose a pseudoaneurysm or an arteriovenous fistula after percutaneous arterial catheterization.

Duplex imaging of the lower extremity is used to assess the patency of the deep venous system and is capable of detecting DVT reliably. The addition of color flow imaging facilitates the examination by making the artery and its associated vein easier to identify. By performing serial duplex venous US imaging to detect DVT, one group of investigators was able to identify a subgroup of injured patients who were at highest risk for pulmonary embolism; they suggested that these patients be given DVT prophylaxis and undergo close surveillance with duplex imaging.[18]

Endocrine System

The thyroid and parathyroid, being superficial structures, are easily visualized by high-frequency US. Indeed, the modality was used more than 30 years ago to distinguish cystic from solid lesions of the thyroid.[19] US is commonly being used to identify nodules for FNA, to plan excision of thyroid cancers, and to evaluate cervical lymph nodes.[20] The group at the Cleveland Clinic reported their experience with 5703 US examinations of the neck. All were performed at the initial office visit by the surgeon for a variety of indications, including identifying suspected and unexpected pathology, distinguishing solid from cystic as well as benign from malignant lesions, distinguishing thyroid lesions from other neck pathology, localizing parathyroid adenomas, guiding interventions (FNA, ethanol ablation), and resident education.[21] Most studies were performed for thyroid (42%) or parathyroid (57%) disease. Accuracy in determining site- and side-specific parathyroid adenomas was 72% and 74%, respectively, as compared with 50% and 68% for sestamibi scanning. Another study reported an overall 91% accuracy of US in the detection of abnormal parathyroid glands.[22]

Intraoperative Use of Ultrasound

Breast
There are an increasing number of reports of the use of intraoperative US for nonpalpable breast lesions. Advantages include ease of scheduling the surgical procedure (without having to involve mammography), potential cost savings, lessening of pain and anxiety for the patient, and equivalent accuracy.[23]

One study reported on 100 patients who had nonpalpable lesions visualized by US in the outpatient clinic.[24] This subpopulation was derived from 207 patients who had nonpalpable disease. At surgery, US was able to correctly localize all lesions in the patients who had lesions visualized on US in the clinic. Negative margins at the initial operation were obtained in 90% of cases. The authors identified four requirements for intraoperative US to be effective: the mass must be visualized preoperatively, US films must be available in the operating room, the breast surgeon must be able to document experience with US, and the surgeon needs to be able to repeat the original US pictures immediately preoperatively.[24]

Gastrointestinal Tract
Examination with intraoperative or laparoscopic US is an integral part of many hepatic, biliary, and pancreatic surgical procedures. With this tool, surgeons can detect previously undiscovered lesions or bile duct stones, avoid unnecessary dissection of vessels or ducts, clarify tumor margins, and perform biopsy and cryoablation procedures. When compared with other preoperative imaging modalities, intraoperative US is much more sensitive in detecting malignant or benign lesions. The precision with which intraoperative US can delineate small lesions (5 mm) and define their relationship to other structures facilitates resection, reduces operative time, and frequently alters the surgeon's operative strategy.

Intraoperative US makes use of both contact scanning and so-called standoff scanning for imaging. In contact scanning, the transducer is directly applied to the organ so that the deepest part of the organ is accurately depicted. This technique is most often used for imaging large organs (e.g., the liver). In standoff scanning, the transducer is placed about 1 to 2 cm away from the structure in a pool of sterile saline solution to permit transmission of the US waves. This technique is often used to image blood vessels, bile ducts, or the spinal cord; it allows good visualization of the structure without compression by the transducer. The size, shape, and type of US transducer used for intraoperative scanning depend on the anatomic structure to be examined. For example, a pencil-like 7.5-MHz transducer is used for scanning the common bile duct, whereas a side-viewing T-shaped 5-MHz transducer is preferable for imaging a cirrhotic liver. Intraoperative US examinations must be conducted systematically to ensure that no subtle pathology is missed and that the examination is reproducible. For example, the liver may be imaged sequentially according to a system based on Couinaud's anatomic segments.

Similar principles apply to laparoscopic US, except that the transducers are made to adapt to the laparoscopic equipment. Indications for this modality include detection of common bile duct stones, staging of pancreatic cancer to prevent unnecessary celiotomy, and resection or cryoablation of hepatic metastases.

Vascular and Endocrine Systems
Intraoperative duplex imaging can be used to detect technical errors in vascular anastomoses, as well as abnormalities in flow. Although arteriography also assesses the patency of an anastomosis and measures distal arterial runoff, it is significantly more invasive. Intraoperative duplex imaging, in contrast, permits rapid visualization of the anatomic and hemodynamic aspects of a vascular reconstruction, and it is noninvasive, easily repeatable, and less time consuming than arteriography. Intravascular US is being used for a variety of indications, including the evaluation of coronary plaques, assistance in endovascular stent placement, and facilitation of the placement of vena cava filters.

Intraoperative US is also a useful modality for the endocrine surgeon. For example, US is an extremely valuable tool to assist in the intraoperative localization of endocrine tumors of the pancreas. Furthermore, parathyroid pathology and cervical lymph node abnormalities may also be identified and localized intraoperatively. In one study, 70 of 87 patients were able to undergo a directed parathyroidectomy based on a combination of preoperative US and sestamibi imaging, as well as intraoperative US. Seventeen patients required conversion to bilateral neck exploration based on the intraoperative findings.[25] All in all, intraoperative US is potentially a very useful tool in a surgeon's armamentarium.

Trauma Resuscitation

FAST Examination
*F*ocused *a*ssessment of the *s*onographic examination of the *t*rauma patient (FAST) is a rapid diagnostic examination to assess patients with potential thoracoabdominal injuries. The test sequentially surveys for the presence or absence of blood in the pericardial sac and dependent abdominal regions, including the right upper quadrant (RUQ), left upper quadrant (LUQ), and pelvis. Surgeons perform FAST during the American College of Surgeons' advanced trauma life support (ATLS) secondary survey. Although minimal patient preparation is needed, a full urinary bladder is ideal to provide an acoustic window for visualization of blood in the pelvis.

FAST is designed to assess fluid accumulation (presumed to be blood) in dependent areas of the pericardial sac and abdomen while the patient is in the supine position. It is important to note that FAST needs to be performed in a specific sequence. The pericardial area is visualized first so that blood within the heart can be used as a standard to set the gain. Most modern US machines have presets so that gain does not need to be reset each time that the machine is turned on. Periodically, however, especially if multiple types of examinations are performed with different transducers, gain needs to be checked to make sure that intracardiac blood appears

anechoic. This maneuver ensures that hemoperitoneum will also appear anechoic and will therefore be readily detected on the US image. The abdominal part of FAST begins with a survey of the RUQ, which is the location within the peritoneal cavity where blood most often accumulates and is therefore readily detected with FAST. Investigators from four level I trauma centers examined true-positive US images of 275 patients who sustained either blunt (220 patients) or penetrating (55 patients) injuries. They found that regardless of the injured organ (with the exception of patients who had an isolated perforated viscus), blood was most often identified on the RUQ image of FAST.[26] This can be a time-saving measure because when hemoperitoneum is identified on a FAST examination in a hemodynamically unstable patient, that image alone, in combination with the patient's clinical picture, is sufficient to justify an immediate abdominal operation.[26]

The technique of performing FAST is well documented. US transmission gel is applied to four areas of the thoracoabdomen, and the examination is conducted in the following sequence: pericardial area, RUQ, LUQ, and pelvis (Fig. 13-3). A 3.5-MHz convex transducer is oriented for sagittal views and positioned in the subxiphoid region to identify the heart and examine for blood in the pericardial sac. Normal and abnormal views of the pericardial area are shown in Figure 13-4. The subcostal image is not usually difficult to obtain, but a severe chest wall injury, a very narrow subcostal area, subcutaneous emphysema, or morbid obesity can prevent a satisfactory examination. Both of the latter conditions are associated with poor imaging because air and fat reflect the wave too strongly and prevent penetration into the target organ. If the subcostal pericardial image cannot be obtained or is suboptimal, a parasternal US view of the heart is performed (Fig. 13-5).

Next, the transducer is placed in the right midaxillary line between the 11th and 12th ribs to identify the liver, kidney, and diaphragm in the sagittal section (Fig. 13-6). The presence or absence of blood is sought in Morison's

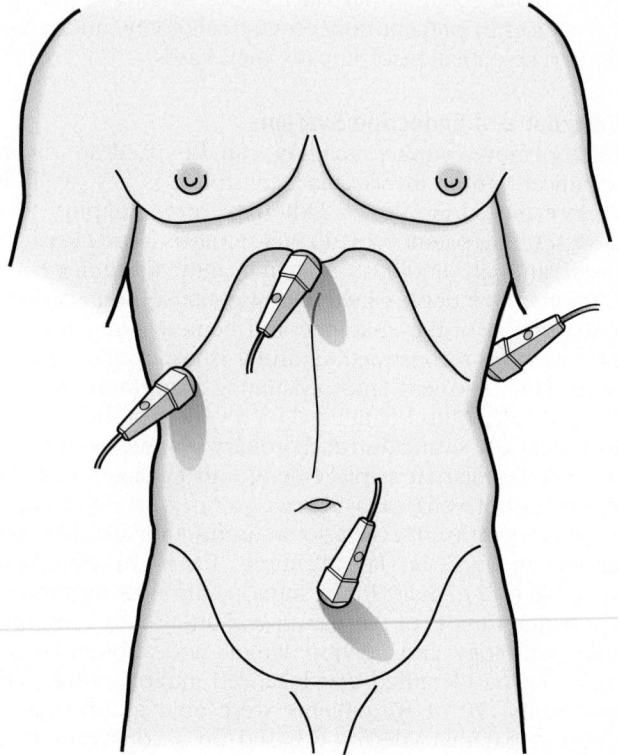

Figure 13-3 Transducer positions for FAST: pericardial, right upper quadrant, left upper quadrant, and pelvis.

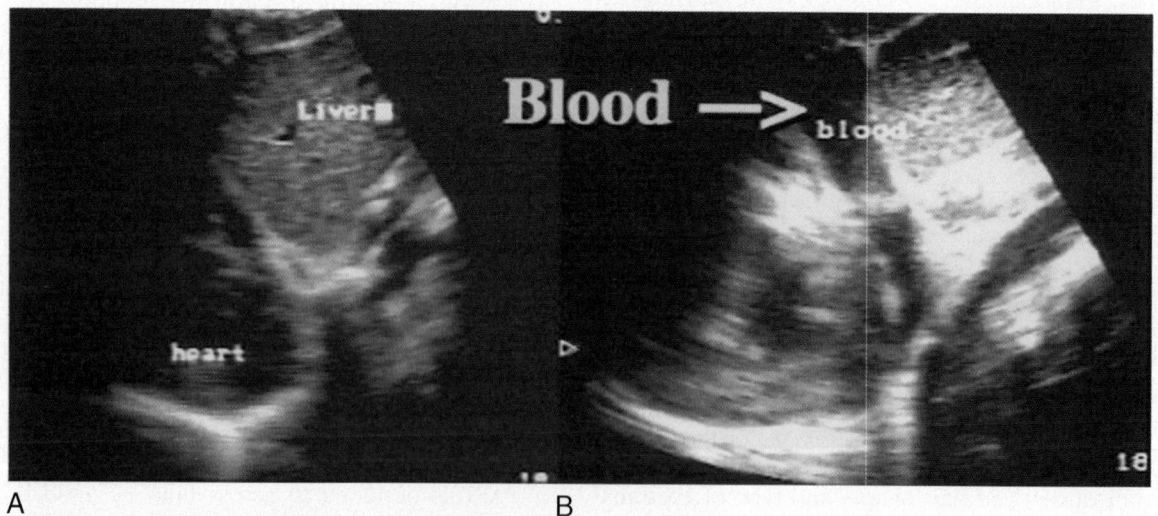

Figure 13-4 Normal (**A**) and abnormal (**B**) pericardial windows in FAST.

pouch and in the subphrenic space. With the transducer positioned in the left posterior axillary line between the 10th and 11th ribs, the spleen and kidney are visualized and blood is sought between the two organs and in the subphrenic space (Fig. 13-7). Finally, the transducer is directed for a transverse view and placed about 4 cm cephalad to the symphysis pubis. It is swept inferiorly to obtain a coronal view of the full bladder and the pelvis to examine for the presence or absence of blood (Fig. 13-8).

FAST is probably the surgeon-performed US examination that has the most literature support. However, factors such as improper technique, inexperience of the examiner, and inappropriate use of US are known to have an adverse impact on US imaging. In addition, the cause of injury, the presence of hypotension on admission, and

select associated injuries have been shown to influence the accuracy of this modality.[27] Failure to consider these factors has led to inaccurate assessment of the accuracy of FAST by inappropriately comparing it with a CT scan and not recognizing its role in the evaluation of patients with penetrating torso trauma. Indeed, both false-positive and false-negative pericardial US examinations have been reported to occur in the presence of massive hemothorax or mediastinal blood.[27] Repeating FAST after insertion of a tube thoracostomy improves visualization of the pericardial area, thereby decreasing the number of false-positive and false-negative studies. Notwithstanding these circumstances, a rapid focused US survey of the subcostal pericardial area is a very accurate method to detect hemopericardium in most patients with penetrating wounds in the so-called cardiac box. In another large study involving patients who sustained either blunt or penetrating injuries, FAST was 100% sensitive and 99.3% specific for detecting hemopericardium in patients with precordial or transthoracic wounds.[28] Furthermore, the use of pericardial US has been shown to be especially helpful in the evaluation of patients who have no overt signs of pericardial tamponade. This was highlighted in a study in which 10 of 22 patients with precordial wounds and hemopericardium on US examinations had admission systolic blood pressure higher than 110 mm Hg and were relatively asymptomatic.[26] Based on these signs and the lack of symptoms, it is unlikely that the presence of cardiac wounds would have been strongly suspected in these patients, and therefore this rapid US examination provided an early diagnosis of hemopericardium before the patients underwent physiologic deterioration.

FAST is also very accurate when it is used to evaluate hypotensive patients with blunt abdominal trauma. In this scenario, US is so accurate that when FAST is positive, immediate surgery is justified.[27] However, because FAST is a focused examination for the detection of blood in dependent areas of the abdomen, its results must not be compared with those of a CT scan because FAST does not readily identify intraparenchymal or retroperitoneal

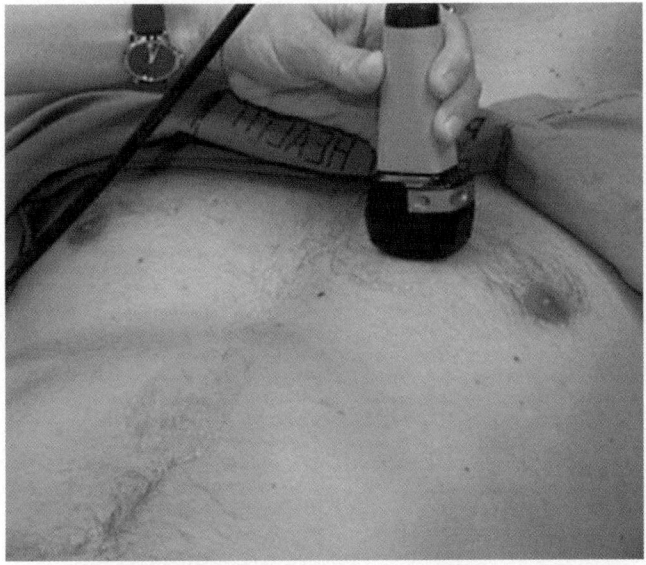

Figure 13-5 Transducer position for a sagittal view of the pericardial area.

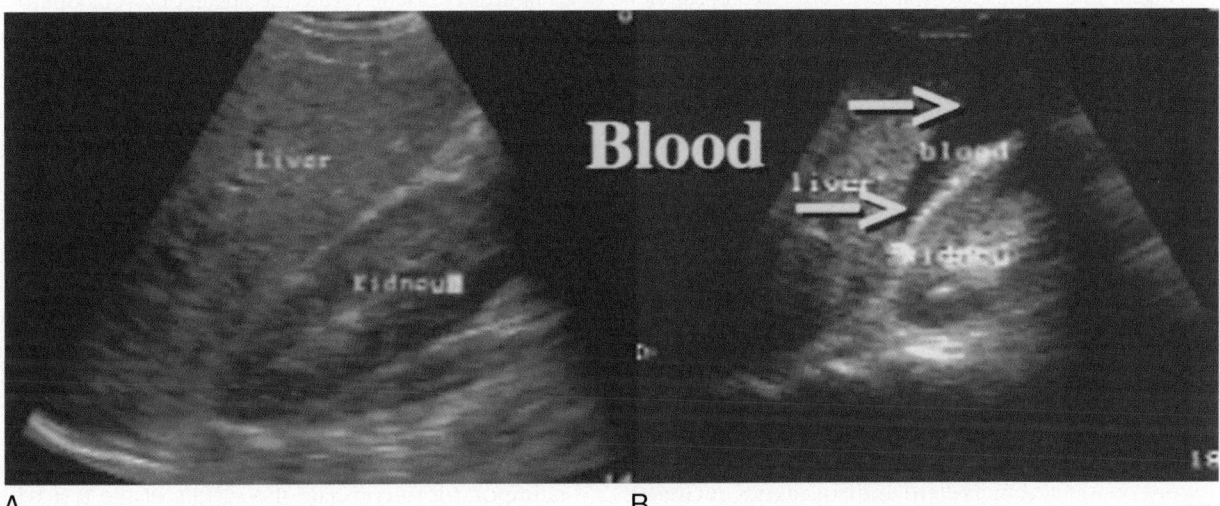

Figure 13-6 Normal (**A**) and abnormal (**B**) sagittal views of the liver, kidney, and diaphragm.

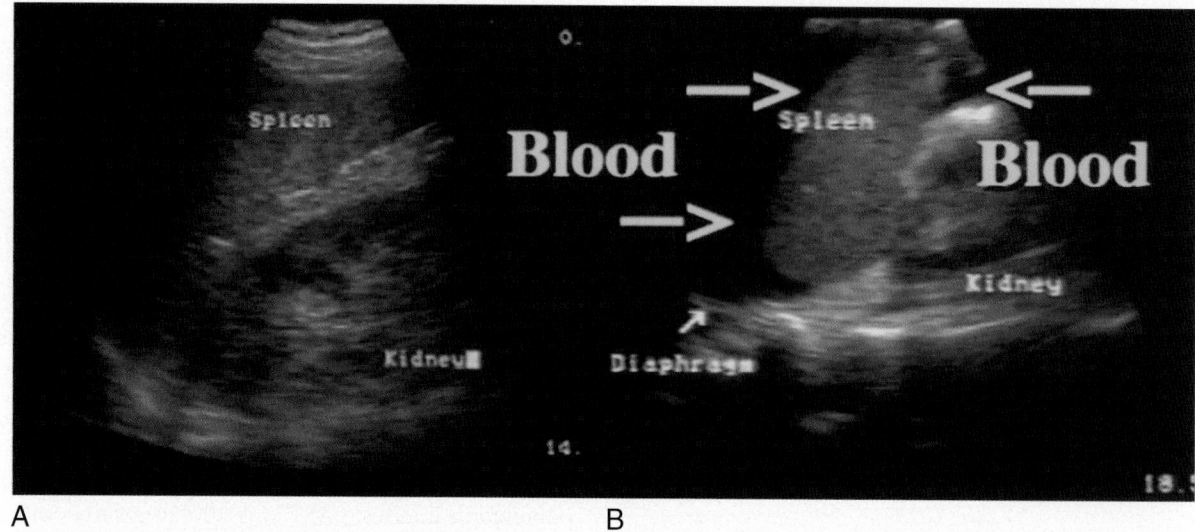

Figure 13-7 Normal (**A**) and abnormal (**B**) sagittal views of the spleen, kidney, and diaphragm. Note the blood above the spleen and between the spleen and kidney.

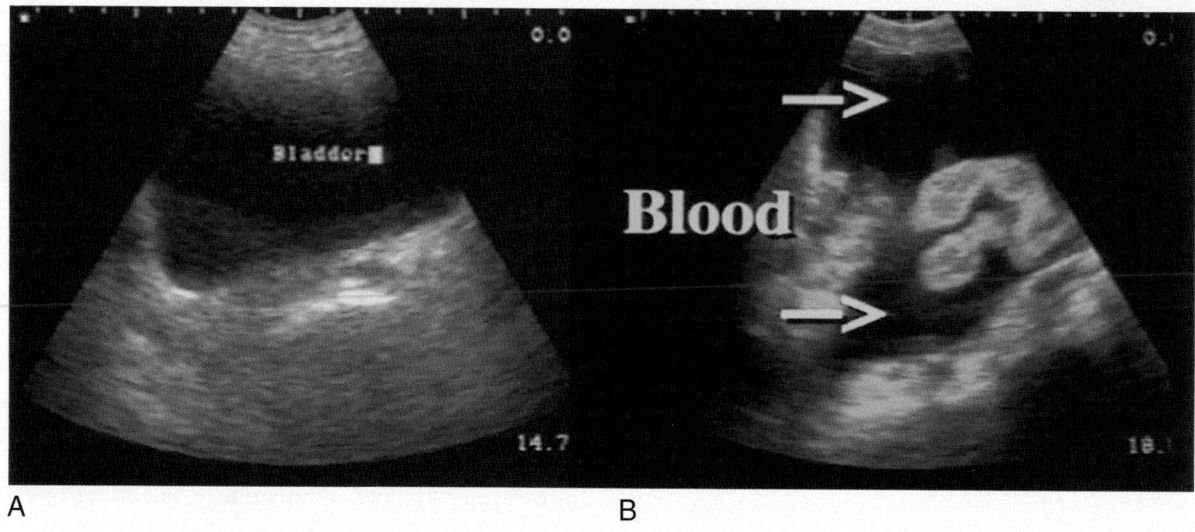

Figure 13-8 Normal (**A**) and abnormal (**B**) coronal views of a full urinary bladder. Note the floating bowel loops in **B**.

injuries. Therefore, select patients considered to be at high risk for occult intra-abdominal injury undergo a CT scan of the abdomen when the results of FAST are negative. Such patients include those with fractures of the pelvis or thoracolumbar spine, major thoracic trauma (pulmonary contusion, lower rib fractures), or hematuria. These recommendations are based on the results of two studies from Chiu in 1997 and Ballard in 1999.[29,30] Chiu and colleagues reviewed their data on 772 patients who underwent FAST after sustaining blunt torso injury. Of the 772 patients, 52 had intra-abdominal injury, but 15 (29%) of them had no hemoperitoneum on the admitting FAST examination or on CT scan of the abdomen.[29] In other work conducted by Ballard and colleagues at Grady Memorial Hospital,[30] an algorithm was developed and tested over a 3.5-year period to identify patients who

were at high risk for occult intra-abdominal injuries after sustaining blunt thoracoabdominal trauma. Of the 1490 patients admitted with severe blunt trauma, 102 (70 with pelvic fractures, 32 with spine injuries) were considered to be at high risk for occult intra-abdominal injuries. Although there was only one false-negative FAST examination in the 32 patients who had spine injuries, there were 13 false-negatives in those with pelvic fractures. Based on these data, the authors concluded that patients with pelvic fractures have a CT scan of the abdomen regardless of the result of FAST. Both studies provide guidelines to decrease the number of false-negative FAST studies, but as with the use of any diagnostic modality, it is important to correlate the results of the test with the patient's clinical picture. Suggested algorithms for the use of FAST are depicted in Figure 13-9A and B.

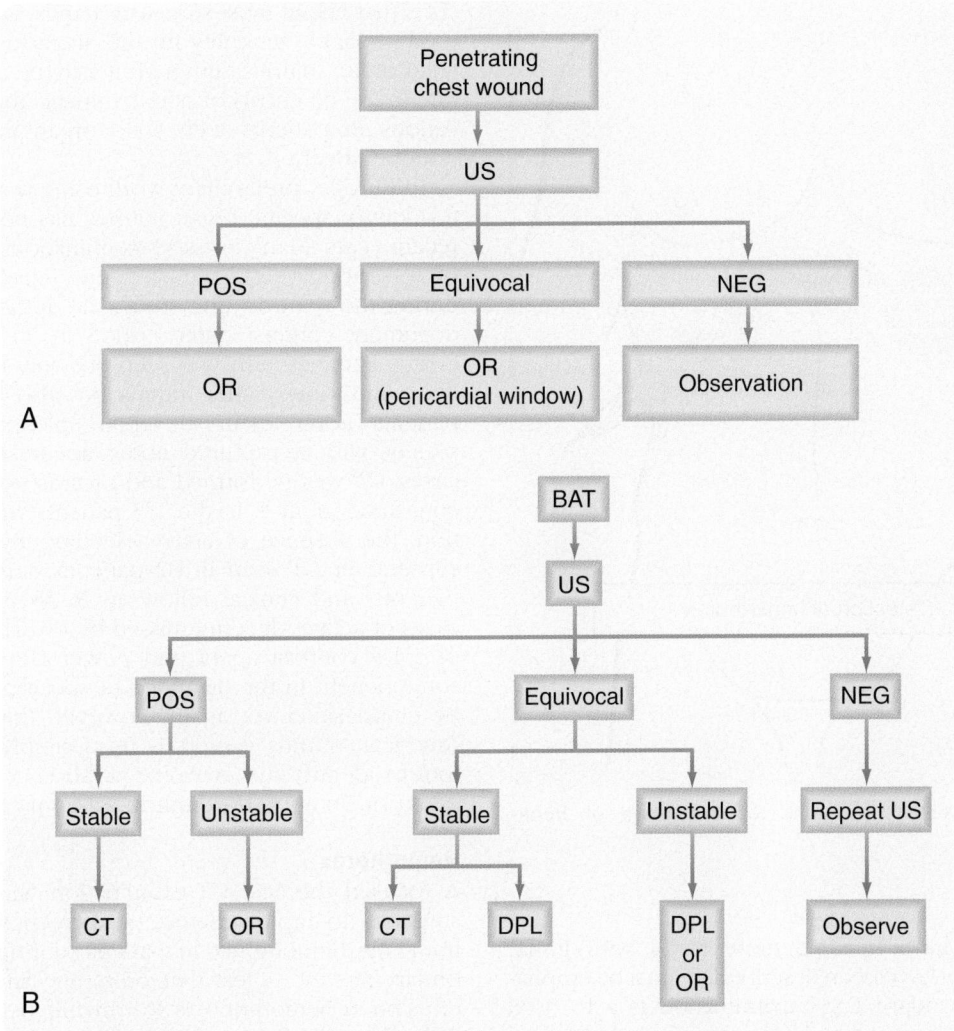

Figure 13-9 A, Algorithm for the use of ultrasound in penetrating chest wounds. **B,** Algorithm for the use of ultrasound in blunt abdominal trauma (BAT). CT, computed tomography; DPL, diagnostic peritoneal lavage; NEG, negative; OR, operating room; POS, positive; US, ultrasound.

The amount of blood detected on an abdominal CT scan or in a diagnostic peritoneal lavage aspirate (or effluent) has been shown to predict the need for operative intervention. Similarly, the quantity of blood that is detected with US may be predictive of a therapeutic operation.[31,32] Huang and associates[31] developed a scoring system based on the identification of hemoperitoneum in specific areas such as Morison's pouch or the perisplenic space, with each abdominal area being assigned a score from 1 to 3. The authors found that a total score of 3 or higher corresponded to more than 1 L of hemoperitoneum and had a sensitivity of 84% for determining the need for an immediate abdominal operation. Another scoring system developed and prospectively validated by McKenney and colleagues[32] examined patients' admission blood pressure, base deficit, and the amount of hemoperitoneum present on the US examination of 100 patients. The hemoperitoneum was categorized by its measurement and distribution in the peritoneal cavity, with a score of 1 being considered a minimal amount of hemoperitoneum but a score greater than 3 being a large hemoperitoneum. Forty-six of the 100 patients had a score higher than 3 and 40 (87%) of them underwent a therapeutic abdominal operation. Their scoring system had a sensitivity, specificity, and accuracy of 83%, 87%, and 85%, respectively. The authors concluded that an US score greater than 3 is statistically more accurate than a combination of the initial systolic blood pressure and base deficit for determining which patients will undergo therapeutic abdominal surgery. Although the quantification of hemoperitoneum is not exact, it can provide valuable information about the need for an abdominal operation and its potential to be therapeutic.

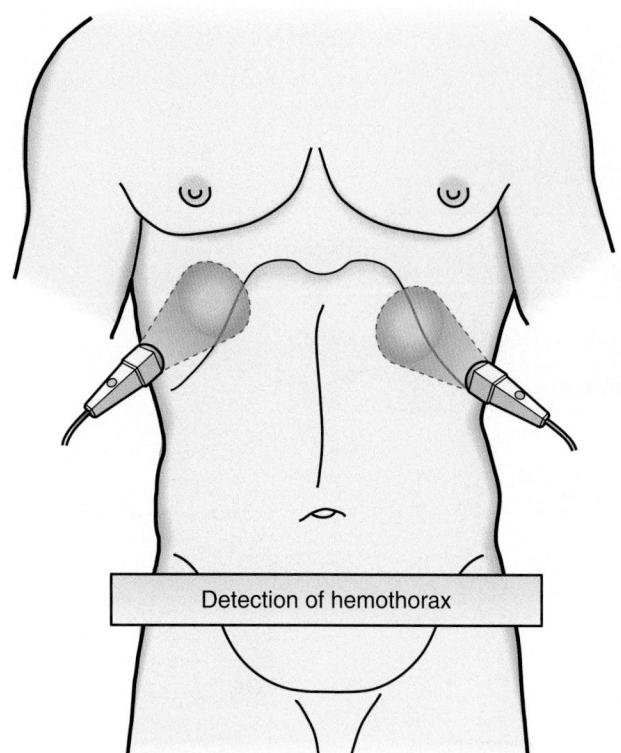

Detection of hemothorax

Figure 13-10 Transducer positions for evaluation of hemothorax.

As surgeons have become more facile with FAST, certain extensions have been described. It must be emphasized that the standard FAST examination is a focused attempt to answer two simple questions: is there fluid within the peritoneal cavity and is there fluid in the pericardial sac? The examinations described in the following text represent extensions that are beyond the purview of standard FAST and, as such, are less well studied.

A recent prospective, multicenter trial conducted by the Western Trauma Association[33] reported on the use of US to serially evaluate patients with documented solid organ injuries after trauma. The so-called BOAST examination, or bedside organ assessment with sonography after trauma, was performed by a limited number of experienced surgeon-sonographers in 126 patients with 135 solid organ injuries in four American trauma centers. This study, performed over a period of nearly 2 years, was designed to be a more thorough abdominal US examination with multiple views obtained of each solid organ (kidneys, liver, and spleen). Overall, only 34% of injuries to solid organs were seen with BOAST, for an error rate of 66%. None of the 34 grade I injuries and only 13 (31%) of the grade II injuries were identified. Sensitivities for grade III and IV injuries ranged from 25% to 75%, and only one grade V injury (to the liver) was examined and positively identified. It was noted, however, that 16 intra-abdominal complications (8 pseudoaneurysms, 4 bilomas, 3 abscesses, and 1 necrotic organ) developed in 11 patients and 13 (81%) were identified by the sonographers. This study empha-

sizes that US, in most surgeons' hands, cannot be considered a reliable modality for the diagnosis and grading of solid organ injuries, although it may be acceptably accurate in the diagnosis of post-traumatic abdominal complications in patients with solid organ injuries managed nonoperatively.

In Europe, preliminary work using power Doppler US to identify specific organ injuries has been published in recent years. Many of these examinations include the use of a sonographic contrast agent injected peripherally during the scan. In one study, the authors were able to document contrast extravasation in 20 of 153 patients (13%). Extravasation was seen not only from the spleen, liver, and kidney after trauma but also in postoperative patients (aortic aneurysm repair, splenectomy) and in a patient with a ruptured aortic aneurysm.[34] In 9 of 20 cases, CT was performed and contrast extravasation was confirmed in all 9. In the 133 patients without extravasation, the absence of active bleeding was inferred by a subsequent CT scan in 82 patients, surgical data in 13 patients, and clinical follow-up in 38 patients, with no cases of active bleeding missed by US. Thus, the addition of a US contrast agent and power Doppler may be of some benefit in the diagnosis of specific injuries. It must be emphasized yet again, however, that FAST in most American trauma centers is used simply as a screening tool to identify the presence or absence of hemoperitoneum or hemopericardium in a trauma patient.

Hemothorax

A focused thoracic US examination was developed by surgeons to rapidly detect the presence or absence of traumatic hemothorax in patients during the ATLS secondary survey. A test that promptly detects a traumatic effusion or hemothorax is worthwhile because it dramatically shortens the interval from the diagnosis of hemothorax to tube thoracostomy insertion and thus facilitates patient management.

Not only is the technique for this examination similar to that used to evaluate the upper quadrants of the abdomen in FAST, but it also uses the same type and frequency of transducer and is performed with the patient in the supine position. US transmission gel is applied to the right and left lower thoracic areas in the mid to posterior axillary lines between the 9th and 10th intercostal spaces (Fig. 13-10). The transducer is slowly advanced cephalad to identify the hyperechoic diaphragm and to interrogate the supradiaphragmatic space for the presence or absence of fluid (Fig. 13-11A and B), which appears anechoic. In a positive thoracic US examination, the hypoechoic lung can be seen floating amidst the fluid. The same technique can be used to evaluate a critically ill patient for a pleural effusion, as discussed later in this chapter.

Surgeons have examined the accuracy of this examination in 360 patients with blunt and penetrating torso injuries.[35] They compared the time and accuracy of US with that of supine portable chest radiography and found both to be very similar, 97.4% sensitivity and 99.7% specificity observed for thoracic US versus 92.5% sensitivity and 99.7% specificity for portable chest radiography.

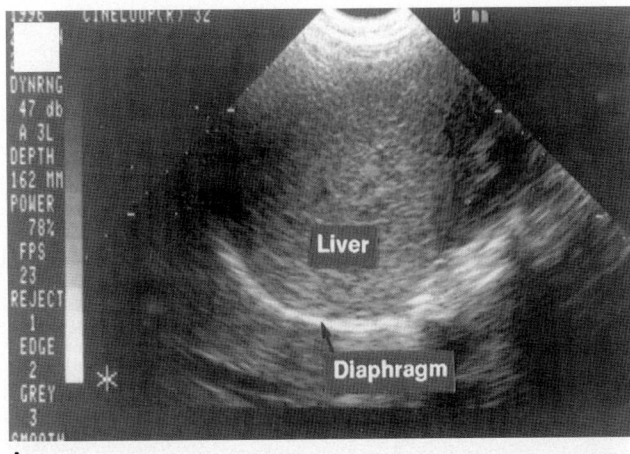

A

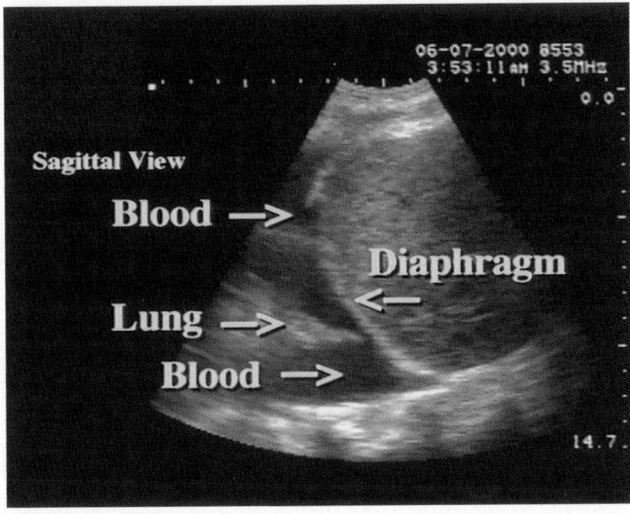

B

Figure 13-11 A, Sagittal view of the liver, kidney, and diaphragm plus the supradiaphragmatic area without evidence of effusion. **B,** Sagittal view of the liver and diaphragm with a large hemothorax. Note the lung floating in anechoic fluid.

Performance times, however, for the thoracic US examinations were statistically much faster ($P < .0001$) than those for the portable chest radiograph. Although it is not recommended that the thoracic US examination replace the chest radiograph, its use can expedite treatment in many patients and decrease the number of chest radiographs obtained.

Pneumothorax

The use of US for detection of pneumothorax is not a new concept; it has been reported by several authors, including Knudtson and coworkers.[36] This examination is useful to the surgeon for evaluation of a patient for a potential pneumothorax if any of the following are true:

1. Bulky radiology equipment is not readily available
2. Inordinate delays in obtaining a chest radiograph are anticipated

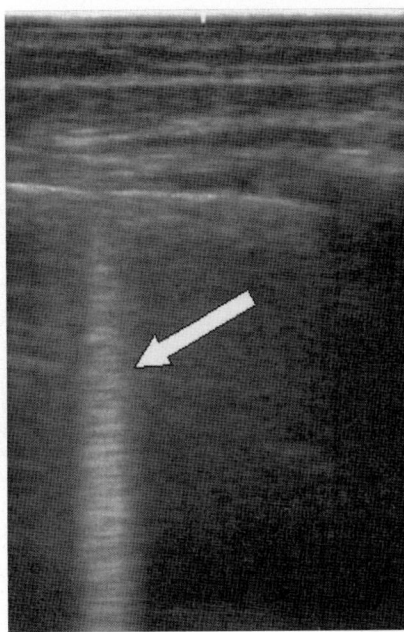

Figure 13-12 Comet tail artifact during pleural examination for pneumothorax with a linear-array probe (*arrow*).

3. Numerous injured patients (mass casualty situation) must be rapidly assessed and triaged

Although useful in the trauma resuscitation area, surgeons may also find this examination helpful to detect pneumothorax in a critically ill patient maintained on a ventilator, after a thoracentesis procedure, or after discontinuing the suction on a Pleurovac.

A 5.0- to 7.5-MHz linear-array transducer is used to evaluate a patient for the presence of pneumothorax. The examination may be performed while the patient is in the erect or the supine position. US transmission gel is applied to the right and left upper thoracic areas at about the third to fourth intercostal space in the midclavicular line, and the presumed unaffected thoracic cavity is examined first. The transducer is oriented for longitudinal imaging, is placed perpendicular to the ribs, and is slowly advanced medially toward the sternum and then laterally toward the anterior axillary line. A normal examination of the thoracic cavity identifies the rib (seen as black on the US image because of a refraction artifact), pleural sliding, and a comet tail artifact. Pleural sliding is identification of the visceral and parietal layers of the lung seen as hyperechoic superimposed pleural lines. When pneumothorax is present, air becomes trapped between the visceral and parietal pleura and does not allow transmission of the US waves. Therefore, the visceral pleura is not imaged and pleural sliding is not observed. The comet tail artifact is generated because of the interaction of two highly reflective opposing interfaces: air and pleura (Fig. 13-12). When air separates the visceral and parietal pleura, the comet tail artifact is not visualized. If desired, the examination may be repeated with the transducer oriented for transverse views, with images obtained with the probe parallel to the ribs.

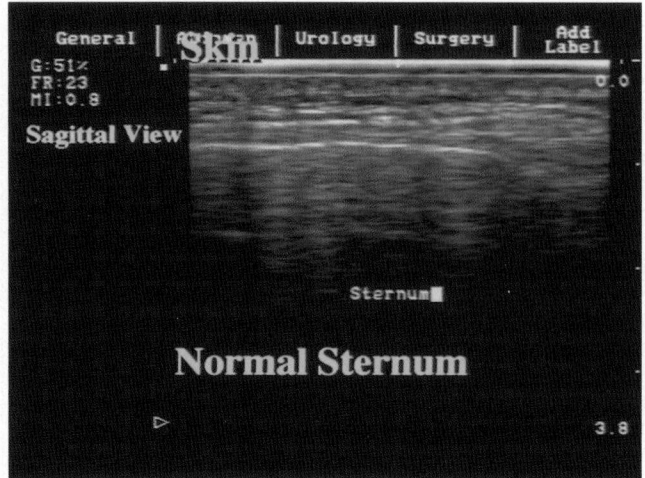

Figure 13-13 Sagittal view of a normal sternum (high-frequency linear-array probe).

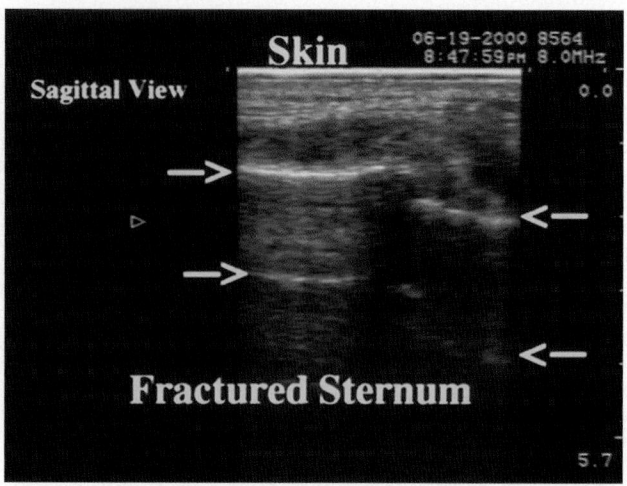

Figure 13-14 Sagittal view of a fractured sternum. Note the disrupted anterior and posterior cortex (*arrows*).

Several studies have documented the sensitivity and specificity of US for the detection of pneumothorax. Dulchavsky and colleagues showed that US can be used successfully by surgeons to detect pneumothorax in injured patients.[37] Of the 382 patients (364 trauma, 18 spontaneous) evaluated with US, 39 had pneumothorax and US successfully detected 37 of them, for a sensitivity of 95%. Pneumothorax could not be detected in two patients as a result of the presence of subcutaneous emphysema because air reflects the sound wave and does not allow through transmission. The authors recommended that when a portable chest radiograph cannot be readily obtained, use of this bedside US examination for the identification of pneumothorax can expedite patient management.

Sternal Fracture

Fractures of the sternum are visualized on a lateral x-ray view of the chest, but this film may be difficult to obtain in a multisystem-injured patient. For this reason, US examination of the sternum can rapidly detect a fracture while the patient is still in the supine position and therefore avoid the need to obtain a radiograph.

US examination of the sternum is performed by using a 5.0- or 8.0-MHz linear-array transducer that is oriented for sagittal or longitudinal views. US transmission gel is applied over the sternal area while the patient is in the supine position. Beginning at the suprasternal notch, the transducer is slowly advanced caudad to interrogate the bone for a fracture, and then the examination is repeated with the transducer oriented for transverse views. Examination of an intact sternum is shown in Figure 13-13. The sternal fracture is identified on US examination as a disruption of the cortical reflex (Fig. 13-14).

Austere Settings

Ultrasound on Deployment

The portability of US makes it ideal for use in forward settings. In fact, routine training courses are in place to teach military surgeons the use of FAST, and hand-held US is now routinely deployed within the British Defence Medical Services. Although up to 90% of war wounds are penetrating, US may allow quicker, more accurate triage decisions so that patients with penetrating abdominal trauma and no or minimal hemoperitoneum may be transferred to the next echelon of care, where the study may be repeated or additional diagnostic maneuvers undertaken. In a recent small series,[38] FAST was used with excellent results in a British military hospital in Iraq. Fifteen casualties were evaluated by serial FAST and 14 had negative examinations at admission and again at 6 hours. One patient underwent laparotomy based on trajectory and had no intraperitoneal fluid, but two small holes were detected in the cecum that required repair. The other 13 patients recovered without sequelae. One examination was positive and led to immediate laparotomy in a patient with a grade V liver injury after a motor vehicle collision.

Because US is portable enough to use in active combat situations, research is ongoing to evaluate the best method to teletransmit images obtained in the field. Several different satellite transmission systems have been evaluated, and high-quality images were able to be obtained in the majority of cases, although balance between the weight of the system and minimum image quality has still not been completely achieved. It is noted, however, that images can be transmitted from up to 1500 ft from the antennas without significant degradation.[39] As technology advances, one would expect imaging systems to continue to become smaller and lighter with improved image quality, thus making US even more appealing as a modality for use in the forward setting.

Ultrasound in Space

Many of the same qualities that make US appealing for use in combat make it equally appealing as a diagnostic modality in space, where an injury might require abortion of a multimillion dollar mission. Indeed, US is one of the only feasible diagnostic modalities on space missions, given their size and weight restrictions. US examinations are easily taught and images can be relayed with minimal delay to physicians on the ground. Furthermore, ATLS procedures are also feasible in space, and thus lifesaving procedures could be performed on the basis of US findings.

US has been used in space for several decades. Indeed, it has been US technology that has taught us much about the physiologic effects of microgravity, especially the fluid shifts associated with space travel. As early as 1982, cardiac US was used to evaluate left ventricular systolic function and cardiac chamber size in cosmonauts. The first American US system in space was the American flight echograph from Advanced Technology Laboratories (Bothel, WA), which first flew in 1984 and was eventually capable of three-dimensional images with the use of a tilt frame device. Currently, the Human Research Facility aboard the International Space Station (ISS) is equipped with a state-of-the-art Philips HDI 5000 (Philips Medical, Bothel WA).[40]

Because surface tension and capillary action are the principal physical forces in space, scientists questioned whether images obtained on the standard FAST examination would be useful in microgravity. There are now several published studies of US performed on parabolic flights onboard the NASA Microgravity Research Facility, a KC-135 aircraft. This aircraft can generate 25- to 30-second intervals of weightlessness with the use of serial parabolic trajectories. In the first of a series of experiments, a porcine model of intra-abdominal hemorrhage was created on the ground and studied during parabolic flights.[40] More than 2000 US segments were recorded, with 80% of them considered feasible for diagnosis of the presence or absence of abdominal fluid. The sonographers believed that the examination was no more difficult than one done on the ground, as long as the sonographer and patient were adequately restrained. For the intraperitoneal portion of the examination, a fourth view (the midline abdominal sweep) was added, and with this addition FAST was able to reliably detect even relatively small amounts of intraperitoneal fluid. The Morison pouch view remained the most sensitive window for detection of fluid. Studies evaluating the diagnosis of hemothorax and pneumothorax have also been published, with similar encouraging results.[41]

Recently, astronauts aboard the ISS performed FAST examinations that were transmitted with a 2-second satellite delay to directors on the ground, who were able to provide them with real-time instructions for probe position and system adjustments. Examinations were able to be completed in roughly 5 minutes, with adequate images obtained in all views.[42]

In summary, US fulfills all the necessary criteria for a diagnostic modality in austere settings. It is sufficiently portable, teletransmittable, teachable, and accurate. It will probably continue to be the only feasible technology to assist in medical diagnoses on space missions in the near future.

Intensive Care Unit

A surgeon's use of US is particularly applicable to the evaluation of critically ill patients for the following reasons[27]:

1. Many patients have depressed mental status, thus making it difficult to elicit pertinent signs of infection
2. Physical examination is hampered by tubes, drains, and monitoring devices
3. The clinical picture often changes, thus necessitating frequent reassessment
4. Transportation to other areas of the hospital is not without inherent risks
5. Complications frequently develop in these patients, which if diagnosed and treated early, may lessen morbidity and length of stay in the ICU

Both diagnostic and therapeutic US examinations can be performed by the surgeon while on rounds in the ICU. However, these focused examinations must be done with a specific purpose and as an extension of the physical examination, not as its replacement.

Surgeons most commonly use bedside US examination in the ICU to detect pleural effusions, intra-abdominal and soft tissue fluid collections, hemoperitoneum, and femoral vein thrombosis, as well as being a guide for the cannulation of central veins in patients with difficult access. Advantages of interventional US include the following:

1. Visualization in real-time imaging allows direct placement of a catheter and confirmation of complete drainage of a fluid collection
2. Performance at the patient's bedside avoids transport
3. US is safe, minimally invasive, and repeatable, if necessary

Contraindications to the performance of a US-guided interventional procedure include the lack of a safe pathway, the presence of coagulopathy, and an uncooperative patient.

Larger needles and those that are Teflon coated produce more echogenicity and are easier to visualize with US. Although minor procedures may be done with minimal preparation, basic principles of sterility must be followed for major interventional procedures.

Soft Tissue Infections

Soft tissue infections may be difficult to assess by physical examination because the signs of infection may be only superficial and not reflect the status of the entire wound. With the US transducer in hand, the surgeon can assess the presence, depth, and extent of an abscess at the patient's bedside and determine the appropriate treatment. Furthermore, the collection can be localized to ensure complete drainage of it, especially if it is loculated. In the postoperative period, wounds can be imaged to examine for hematomas or seromas. Because the fascia can be precisely delineated with US, fascial dehiscence (Fig. 13-15) can also be diagnosed at an early stage.

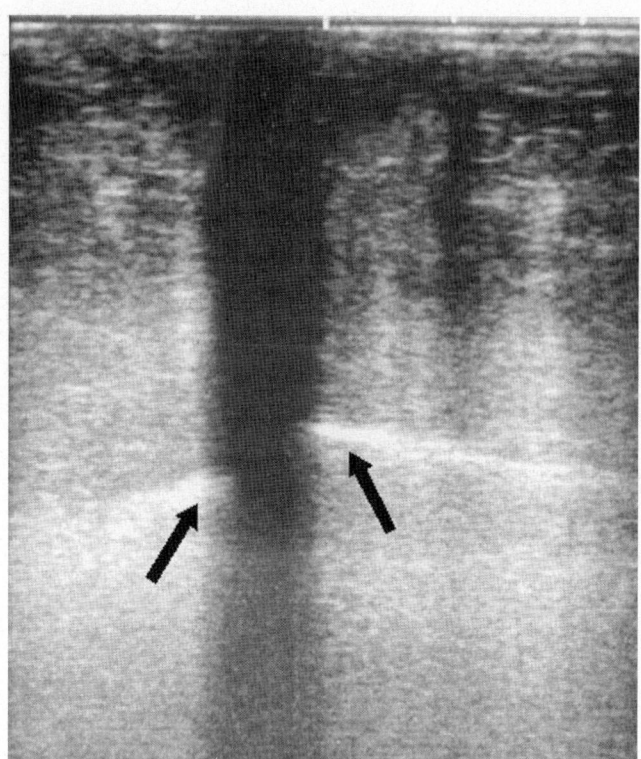

Figure 13-15 Fascial dehiscence as seen with a high-frequency linear-array probe (*arrows*).

US examination of soft tissue is performed with a 5.0- to 8.0-MHz linear-array transducer. The area of inflammation is scanned in both the transverse and longitudinal views to accurately assess the depth and extent of the fluid collection. The depth is measured so that a needle of appropriate length is chosen. Once the fluid collection is assessed, US-guided needle aspiration may be performed. Aspiration of the collection is undertaken after the planned point of needle insertion is marked with a felt-tipped pen. The field is prepared and draped, and an 18- or 20-gauge needle attached to a 10- or 12-mL syringe is inserted into the tissue at the marked site. An alternative method involves using real-time US imaging with sterile transmission gel and a sterile plastic cover for the transducer. The US transducer is held in the nondominant hand and the area is imaged as the needle is directed into the fluid collection. The advantage of this method is that the surgeon visualizes active drainage of the entire fluid collection and collapse of the cavity.

Pleural Effusions

The use of US for detection of a pleural effusion is similar to that described earlier in this chapter for detection of traumatic hemothorax. Although the technique for focused thoracic US examination has already been described, the following is the technique used for US-guided thoracentesis.

The head of the bed is elevated to a 45- to 60-degree angle (if the patient's spine is not injured), or the patient may be supine if spine precautions are needed. A 3.5- or 5.0-MHz convex-array transducer is oriented for sagittal views and placed in the midaxillary line at the sixth or seventh intercostal region. The liver (or spleen) and diaphragm are identified, and then the thoracic cavity is interrogated for the presence of pleural fluid. After the fluid is localized, the area adjacent to the transducer is marked with a felt-tipped pen and the chest is prepared and draped. A local anesthetic is injected into the skin near the mark and infiltrated into the underlying subcutaneous tissue and parietal pleura. The pleural space is entered with an 18-gauge needle obtained from a central line kit, and fluid from the pleural space is aspirated in its entirety. For large effusions, a guidewire is passed through the needle into the pleural cavity via the Seldinger technique. A small skin incision is made around the guidewire and, if necessary, the stiff dilator is passed just through the dermis to allow easy passage of the catheter but minimize the risk for pneumothorax. A standard central line catheter is placed in the pleural space and a three-way stopcock is connected to the port so that the pleural fluid can be aspirated entirely and collected into a separate container. The central line catheter is removed from the pleural space while applying constant suction with a syringe, and an occlusive dressing is placed over the small incision. Real-time US imaging can also be used for the detection and aspiration of small or loculated fluid collections because the needle is observed as it enters the collection and collapse of the space confirms that the fluid has been removed entirely.

Intraperitoneal Fluid/Blood

A sudden decrease in a patient's blood pressure or persistent metabolic acidosis despite continued resuscitation is a common indication to reassess the peritoneal cavity as the source of hemorrhage. FAST can be performed as needed at the patient's bedside to exclude hemoperitoneum as a potential source of hypotension. It may be applied to a critically ill patient who has multisystem injuries or one receiving anticoagulation therapy. US is also used to evaluate a patient with cirrhosis who has abdominal pain. In addition, US-guided aspiration of ascites can be performed, thus minimizing the risk of injury to the bowel.

Central Venous Catheter Insertion

Placement of a central venous catheter is a commonly performed procedure in critically ill patients. Although surgical residents are generally adept at the insertion of central lines, US-guided procedures may be helpful when the resident is initially learning the technique or when the patency of a vessel is uncertain. US-guided central line insertion is especially useful in patients with anasarca or morbid obesity and for an immobilized patient with a potential cervical spine injury. In the past decade, several studies have evaluated the use of US as an aid for central line placement in order to reduce the risk of complications. These studies suggest that the use of US results in a decreased number of cannulation attempts and complications for subclavian and internal jugular venous catheter procedures. A recent study reported similar excellent results with US-guided percutaneous access of the cephalic vein in the deltopectoral groove.[43]

The central veins in the cervical and upper thoracic region may be imaged with a 7.5-MHz linear-array transducer so that the skin insertion site can be marked before creating a sterile field or the procedure may be performed with real-time imaging. Cannulation of the subclavian vein is slightly more difficult because of its location beneath the clavicle, and therefore color flow duplex and Doppler may be helpful to identify the vein before cannulation. Patency of the vein is determined by its ability to be easily compressed with the US transducer. The vein is then imaged about 2 to 3 cm medial to the point of the planned insertion site. The transducer is held in the nondominant hand, and the cannulating needle is followed during real-time imaging as it traverses the soft tissue toward the vein. Once the vein is cannulated, the remainder of the procedure is completed with the standard Seldinger technique.

Common Femoral Vein Thrombosis

Despite the administration of prophylactic agents and routine screening by duplex imaging, DVT still occurs in high-risk patients. The characteristics of venous thrombosis as seen on duplex imaging include the following: dilation, incompressibility, echogenic material within the lumen, absence or decreased spontaneous flow, and loss of phasic flow with respiration. Although each US characteristic of a thrombosed vein is important in making the diagnosis of DVT, loss of compressibility of a thrombus-filled vein is the most useful, with the other criteria considered supportive of the diagnosis.

Focused US examination of the femoral veins is based on the following principles:

1. Most lethal pulmonary emboli originate from the iliofemoral veins.
2. The common femoral artery is identified as a pulsatile vessel lateral to the common femoral vein on B-mode (brightness mode) US and provides a consistent anatomic landmark.
3. B-mode US can be used to evaluate for incompressibility of the vein, echogenic material (thrombus) within the lumen of the vein, and dilation of the vein.
4. Surgeons are familiar with B-mode US because it is frequently used to detect hemopericardium, hemoperitoneum, and pleural effusion/traumatic hemothorax in critically ill patients, hence enhancing its practical applicability in this setting.

A focused US examination of the common femoral veins is performed with the patient in the supine position as an extension of the physical examination. A 7.5-MHz linear-array transducer is used to examine the common femoral veins according to the following protocol as described by Lensing and colleagues[44]:

1. The transducer is oriented for transverse imaging, and the right common femoral vein and artery are visualized.

2. The vein is examined for the presence or absence of intraluminal echogenicity (consistent with thrombus) and for ease of compressibility.
3. The transducer is positioned for sagittal images, and a view of the common femoral vein is identified. The vein is inspected for intraluminal thrombus and adequate compressibility. The diameter of the vein is measured just distal to the saphenofemoral junction.
4. The same examination (1 through 3) is then conducted on the left lower extremity.

A positive study is defined as dilation of the common femoral vein (>10% increase) when compared with the same vein in the opposite extremity, incompressibility of the vein, or the presence of echogenic foci consistent with an intraluminal thrombus (or any combination of the three). A negative study is the presence of a normal-caliber vein with good compressibility and absence of an echogenic intraluminal thrombus.

Insertion of Inferior Vena Cava Filters

Because critically ill surgical patients are at significant risk for DVT and many have contraindications to anticoagulation, therapeutic and prophylactic inferior vena cava filters (IVCFs) are being used ever more frequently. Although the topic is quite controversial, some authors recommend prophylactic insertion of an IVCF within 48 hours in critically ill patients who are at high risk for DVT and have a contraindication to anticoagulation. Although many other authors are less apt to be this aggressive, enough critically ill surgical patients require this procedure that a bedside technique for insertion would be ideal. In fact, with improvements in technology and the advent of intravascular US (IVUS), bedside insertion of an IVCF is now possible.

Both transabdominal duplex US and IVUS have been used to insert vena cava filters successfully and safely at the bedside. Ashley and coauthors[45] reported their experience with bedside insertion of 29 IVCFs via IVUS in the trauma ICU. All patients were able to have their vena cava diameter measured and renal veins located. All filters were successfully deployed in good position without complication. Follow-up CT scans in 27 of the 29 patients were available and indicated proper placement (in reference to the renal veins) in all 27 patients. A much larger experience with bedside IVCF insertion was recently published, with similarly excellent results.[46]

SURGEON EDUCATION IN ULTRASOUND

Although many approaches have been shown to be effective in teaching these focused US examinations, surgeons need to have a solid understanding of the physics principles of US imaging as an integral part of their education process. Furthermore, these principles must be emphasized each time that the examinations are taught.

The first educational model for how surgeons can learn US was published by Han and colleagues from Emory University.[47] Incoming interns took a pretest and then attended a lecture and videotape about the FAST examination. After completion of the ATLS laboratory session, three swine had diagnostic peritoneal lavage catheters reinserted to infuse fluid and produce so-called positive US examinations. Two fresh swine were so-called negatives; however, all five swine were draped similarly to disguise interventions. Incoming interns were tested individually by surgeon sonographers to determine whether the US image was positive or negative. The interns completed a post-test that showed a statistically significant improvement from the pretest ($P < .001$). The authors concluded that incoming interns could learn the essential US principles of FAST and that swine are feasible models for learning it.

Other paradigms that have been used as educational models include cadavers whose peritoneal cavities were instilled with saline and simulators that had data stored in three-dimensional images. Knudson and Sisley[48] conducted a prospective cohort study involving residents from two university trauma centers. They compared the post-test results of residents trained on a real-time US simulator and those trained in a traditional hands-on format. The main outcome measured was the residents' performance on a standardized post-test, which included interpretation of US cases recorded on videotape. They did not find any significant difference between residents trained on the simulator and those trained on models or patients. From their study, the authors concluded that the use of a simulator is a convenient and objective method of introducing US to surgery residents.[48]

Another issue is that of the learning curve. One of the best studies to address this issue for FAST was conducted by Shackford and colleagues.[49] The authors questioned the recommendations that various numbers of US examinations are completed under supervision before a surgeon is considered qualified to perform them. They calculated the primary and adjusted error rates and then determined the potential clinical utility of FAST and found that although the clinician's (nonradiologists) initial error rate was 17%, it fell to 5% after 10 examinations were performed. Additionally, in that study the authors proposed recommendations for credentialing[49]:

1. The process for credentialing of surgeons in the use of US occurs within the department of surgery, either by surgeons or by a committee composed of surgeons and nonsurgeons that reports to the chairperson of the department of surgery.
2. A formal course with 4 hours of didactic and 4 hours of hands-on training is adequate. The curriculum for performance of US in trauma, recently developed by the American College of Surgeons, is strongly recommended.
3. Competency in performance of FAST is determined on the basis of the error rate with respect to the prevalence of the target disease in the series.
4. *Control* or repeat scans are allowed during the proctored experience.
5. After completion of proctoring, an ongoing process for monitoring error rates and causes of indeterminate studies via the department of surgery's quality improvement program is essential.

Teaching of surgeon-performed US is now an integral part of the American College of Surgeons' educational program. Modular courses begin with an US basics course, which is now available on compact disk. Advanced courses in many topics, including an acute/trauma module, are taught at American College of Surgeons' meetings and across the country each year. A very recent survey of surgeons participating in these courses show that they have been a tremendous success.[50]

Experience with US is now a mandated part of residency training. In a recent published survey, 95% of all residency programs are teaching US, either in a didactic or in a clinical form. FAST and general abdominal and breast US were being taught in both academic and community-based programs. Academic centers additionally reported significant resident experience with IVUS and laparoscopic and endocrine US. These data suggest that US is being incorporated to a larger and larger extent into surgical training programs.[51]

SUMMARY

As the role of the surgeon continues to evolve, the surgeon's use of US will surely influence practice patterns. With the use of real-time imaging, the surgeon receives instantaneous information to augment the physical examination, narrow the differential diagnosis, or initiate an intervention. This is of benefit in elective, outpatient settings, as well as acute, inpatient settings. As surgeons become more facile with US, it is anticipated that other uses will develop to further enhance its value for the assessment of patients in various clinical settings.

Selected References

Dulchavsky SA, Schwarz KL, Kirkpatrick A, et al: Prospective evaluation of thoracic ultrasound in the detection of pneumothorax. J Trauma 50:201-205, 2001.

This series establishes US's use beyond the FAST examination in trauma patients and serves as a springboard for the use of US in remote locations for the diagnosis of injuries outside the abdomen.

Han DC, Rozycki GS, Schmidt JA, et al: Ultrasound training during ATLS: An early start for surgical interns. J Trauma 41:208-213, 1996.

One of the earlier descriptions of training surgical residents in the use of FAST, it establishes a steep learning curve even for trainees early in their career.

Hedrick WR, Hykes L, Starchman DE: Ultrasound Physics and Instrumentation. St Louis, CV Mosby, 1995.

This text is a comprehensive resource for readers interested in further information on the technical and theoretical background of US principles.

Kirkpatrick AW, Hamilton DR, Nicolaou S, et al: Focused assessment with sonography for trauma in weightlessness: A feasibility study. J Am Coll Surg 196:833-844, 2003.

This paper describes the first in a series of experimental models that establishes the feasibility and accuracy of US in space exploration.

Milas M, Stephen A, Berber E, et al: Ultrasonography for the endocrine surgeon: A valuable clinical tool that enhances diagnostic and therapeutic outcomes. Surgery 138:1193-1201, 2005.

> This large series in a tertiary referral center for endocrine surgery details their experience with high-frequency US for the diagnosis and management of various endocrine disorders.

Passman MA, Dattilo JB, Guzman RJ, et al: Bedside placement of inferior vena cava filters by using transabdominal duplex ultrasonography and intravascular ultrasound imaging. J Vasc Surg 42:1027-1032, 2005.

> This paper is one of the largest published series on bedside insertion of inferior vena cava filters under intravascular US guidance.

Rozycki GS, Ballard RB, Feliciano DV, et al: Surgeon-performed ultrasound for the assessment of truncal injuries: Lessons learned from 1,540 patients. Ann Surg 228:557-567, 1998.

> One of the largest series of FAST examinations published, this report highlights the technical aspects of performance of FAST, as well as its potential shortcomings.

Schaffzin DM, Wong WD: Surgeon-performed ultrasound: Endorectal ultrasound. Surg Clin North Am 84:1127-1149, 2004.

> This review article contains clear descriptions of US's use in benign and malignant rectal pathology, with emphasis on technical issues and a comprehensive list of references.

Staren ED, Knudson MM, Rozycki GS, et al: An evaluation of the American College of Surgeons' ultrasound education program. Am J Surg 191:489-496, 2006.

> This report contains a description of and results from the modular US courses currently offered by the American College of Surgeons.

Staren ED, Skjoldbye B: General interventional ultrasound. In Staren ED (ed): Ultrasound for the Surgeon. Philadelphia, Lippincott-Raven, 1997.

> General reference for readers interested in learning more about techniques of interventional US applicable to the intensive care unit.

References

1. Chang R, Kuo W, Chen D, et al: Computer-aided diagnosis for surgical office–based breast ultrasound. Arch Surg 135:696-699, 2000.
2. Rizzatto G: Towards a more sophisticated use of breast ultrasound. Eur Radiol 11:2423-2435, 2001.
3. Gufler H, Buitrago-Tellez C, Madjar H, et al: Ultrasound demonstration of mammographically detected microcalcifications. Acta Radiol 41:217-221, 2000.
4. Vargas HI, Vargas MP, Eldrageely K, et al: Outcomes of surgical and sonographic assessment of breast masses in women younger than 30. Am Surg 71:716-719, 2005.
5. Crystal P, Koretz M, Shcharynsky S, et al: Accuracy of sonographically guided 14-gauge core-needle biopsy: Results of 715 consecutive breast biopsies with at least two-year follow-up of benign lesions. J Clin Ultrasound 33:47-52, 2005.
6. Deurloo EE, Tanis PJ, Gilhuijs KG, et al: Reduction in the number of sentinel lymph node procedures by preoperative ultrasonography of the axilla in breast cancer. Eur J Cancer 39:1068-1073, 2003.
7. van Rijk MC, Deurloo EE, Nieweg OE, et al: Ultrasonography and fine-needle aspiration cytology can spare breast cancer patients unnecessary sentinel lymph node biopsy. Ann Surg Oncol 13:31-35, 2005.
8. Chen C, Yang C, Yeh Y: Preoperative staging of gastric cancer by endoscopic ultrasound: The prognostic usefulness of ascites detected by endoscopic ultrasound. J Clin Gastroenterol 35:321-327, 2002.
9. Hernandez L, Mishra G, Forsmarck C, et al: Role of endoscopic ultrasound (EUS) and EUS-guided fine needle aspiration in the diagnosis and treatment of cystic lesions of the pancreas. Pancreas 25:222-228, 2002.
10. Ganpathi S, So BY, Ho KY: Endoscopic ultrasonography for gastric cancer. Does it influence treatment? Surg Endosc 20:559-562, 2006.
11. Tsendsuren T, Jun SM, Mian XH: Usefulness of endoscopic ultrasonography in preoperative TNM staging of gastric cancer. World J Gastroenterol 12:43-47, 2006.
12. Schaffzin DM, Wong WD: Surgeon-performed ultrasound: Endorectal ultrasound. Surg Clin North Am 84:1127-1149, 2004.
13. Maor Y, Nadler M, Barshack I, et al: Endoscopic ultrasound staging of rectal cancer: Diagnostic value before and following chemoradiation. J Gastroenterol Hepatol 21:454-458, 2006.
14. Falk PM, Blatchford GJ, Cali RL: Transanal ultrasound and manometry in the evaluation of fecal incontinence. Dis Colon Rectum 37:468-472, 1994.
15. Ortiz H, Marzo J, Jimenez G, et al: Accuracy of hydrogen peroxide–enhanced ultrasound in the identification of internal openings of anal fistulas. Colorect Dis 4:280-283, 2002.
16. Lindsey I, Humphreys MM, George BD, et al: The role of anal ultrasound in the management of anal fistulas. Colorect Dis 4:118-122, 2002.
17. Bastounis E, Georgopoulos S, Maltezos C, et al: The validity of current vascular imaging methods in the evaluation of aortic anastomotic aneurysms developing after abdominal aortic aneurysm repair. Ann Vasc Surg 10:537-545, 1996.
18. Knudson MM, Collins JA, Goodman SB, et al: Thromboembolism following multiple trauma. J Trauma 32:2-11, 1992.
19. Levine RA: Something old and something new: A brief history of thyroid ultrasound technology. Endocr Pract 10:227-233, 2004.
20. Senchenkov A, Staren ED: Ultrasound in head and neck surgery: Thyroid, parathyroid and cervical lymph nodes. Surg Clin North Am 84:973-1000, 2004.
21. Milas M, Stephen A, Berber E, et al: Ultrasonography for the endocrine surgeon: A valuable clinical tool that enhances diagnostic and therapeutic outcomes. Surgery 138:1193-1201, 2005.
22. Solorzano CC, Carneiro-Pla DM, Irvin GL III: Surgeon-performed ultrasonography as the initial and only localizing study in sporadic primary hyperparathyroidism. J Am Coll Surg 202:18-24, 2005.
23. Kaufman CS, Jacobson L, Bachman B, et al: Intraoperative ultrasound facilitates surgery for early breast cancer. Ann Surg Oncol 9:988-993, 2002.
24. Kaufman CS, Jacobson L, Bachman B, et al: Intraoperative ultrasonography guidance is accurate and efficient according to results in 100 breast cancer patients. Am J Surg 186:378-382, 2003.
25. Burkey SH, Snyder WH III, Nwariaku F, et al: Directed parathyroidectomy: Feasibility and performance in 100 consecutive patients with primary hyperparathyroidism. Arch Surg 138:604-609, 2003.
26. Rozycki GS, Ochsner MG, Feliciano DV, et al: Early detection of hemoperitoneum by ultrasound examination of the

right upper quadrant: A multicenter study. J Trauma 45:878-880, 1998.

27. Rozycki GS, Ballard RB, Feliciano DV, et al: Surgeon-performed ultrasound for the assessment of truncal injuries: Lessons learned from 1,540 patients. Ann Surg 228:557-567, 1998.

28. Rozycki GS, Feliciano DV, Ochsner MG, et al: The role of ultrasound in patients with possible penetrating cardiac wounds: A prospective multicenter study. J Trauma 46:543-552, 1999.

29. Chiu WC, Cushing BM, Rodriguez A, et al: Abdominal injuries without hemoperitoneum: A potential limitation of focused abdominal sonography for trauma (FAST). J Trauma 42:617-625, 1997.

30. Ballard RB, Rozycki GS, Newman PG, et al: An algorithm to reduce the incidence of false-negative FAST examinations in patients at high risk for occult injury. J Am Coll Surg 189:145-151, 1999.

31. Huang M, Liu M, Wu J, et al: Ultrasonography for the evaluation of hemoperitoneum during resuscitation: A simple scoring system. J Trauma 36:173-177, 1994.

32. McKenney KL, McKenney MG, Cohn SM, et al: Hemoperitoneum score helps determine the need for therapeutic laparotomy. J Trauma 50:650-656, 2001.

33. Rozycki GS, Knudson MM, Shackford SR, Dicker R: Surgeon-performed Bedside organ assessment with sonography after trauma (BOAST): A pilot study from the WTA Multicenter Group. J Trauma 59:1356-1364, 2005.

34. Catalano O, Sandomenico F, Raso MM, et al: Real-time, contrast-enhanced sonography: A new tool for detecting active bleeding. J Trauma 59:933-939, 2005.

35. Sisley AC, Rozycki GS, Ballard RB, et al: Rapid detection of traumatic effusion using surgeon-performed ultrasound. J Trauma 44:291-297, 1998.

36. Knudtson JL, Dort JM, Helmer SD, et al: Surgeon-performed ultrasound for pneumothorax in the trauma suite. J Trauma 56:527-530, 2004.

37. Dulchavsky SA, Schwarz KL, Kirkpatrick A, et al: Prospective evaluation of thoracic ultrasound in the detection of pneumothorax. J Trauma 50:201-205, 2001.

38. Brooks AJ, Price V, Simms M: FAST on operational military deployment. Emerg Med J 22:263-265, 2005.

39. Strode CA, Rubal BJ, Gerhardt RT, et al: Wireless and satellite transmission of prehospital focused abdominal sonography for trauma. Prehosp Emerg Care 7:375-359, 2003.

40. Kirkpatrick AW, Hamilton DR, Nicolaou S, et al: Focused Assessment with Sonography for Trauma in weightlessness: A feasibility study. J Am Coll Surg 196:833-844, 2003.

41. Hamilton DR, Sargsyan AE, Kirkpatrick AW, et al: Sonographic detection of pneumothorax and hemothorax in microgravity. Aviat Space Environ Med 75:272-277, 2004.

42. Sargsyan AE, Hamilton DR, Jones JA, et al: FAST at MACH 20: Clinical ultrasound aboard the International Space Station. J Trauma 58:35-39, 2005.

43. LeDonne J: Percutaneous cephalic vein cannulation (in the deltopectoral groove), with ultrasound guidance. J Am Coll Surg 200:810-811, 2005.

44. Lensing AW, Prandoni P, Brandjes D, et al: Detection of deep-vein thrombosis by real-time B-mode ultrasonography. N Eng J Med 320:342-345, 1989.

45. Ashley DW, Gamblin TC, McCampbell BL, et al: Bedside insertion of vena cava filters in the intensive care unit using intravascular ultrasound to locate renal veins. J Trauma 57:26-31, 2004.

46. Passman MA, Dattilo JB, Guzman RJ, et al: Bedside placement of inferior vena cava filters by using transabdominal duplex ultrasonography and intravascular ultrasound imaging. J Vasc Surg 42:1027-1032, 2005.

47. Han DC, Rozycki GS, Schmidt JA, et al: Ultrasound training during ATLS: An early start for surgical interns. J Trauma 41:208-213, 1996.

48. Knudson MM, Sisley AC: Training residents using simulation technology: Experience with ultrasound for trauma. J Trauma 48:659-665, 2000.

49. Shackford SR, Rogers FB, Osler TM, et al: Focused abdominal sonogram for trauma: The learning curve of nonradiologist clinicians in detecting hemoperitoneum. J Trauma 46:553-564, 1999.

50. Staren ED, Knudson MM, Rozycki GS, et al: An evaluation of the American College of Surgeons' ultrasound education program. Am J Surg 191:489-496, 2006.

51. Freitas ML, Frangos SG, Frankel HL: The status of ultrasonography training and use in general surgery residency programs. J Am Coll Surg 202:453-458, 2006.

Surgical Infections and Choice of Antibiotics

Daniel A. Anaya, MD   and   E. Patchen Dellinger, MD

Surgical Site Infections
Specific Surgical Infections
Pathogens in Surgical Infections
Antimicrobials

During the second half of the 19th century many operations were developed after anesthesia was introduced by Morton in 1846, but advances were few for many years because of the high rate of infection and the high mortality that followed infections. By the beginning of the 20th century, following the work of Ignaz Philipp Semmelweis and later with the introduction of antisepsis into the practice of medicine by Joseph Lister, reduced infection rates and mortality in surgical patients were seen. The work of Holmes, Pasteur, and Kocher in infectious diseases, as well as the operating room (OR) environment and discipline established by Halsted, continued to prove the aseptic and antiseptic theory to be the first effective measure for preventing infections in surgical patients.

These initial principles helped change surgical therapy from a dreaded event, with infection and death commonplace, to one that alleviates suffering and prolongs life with predictable success when carefully performed. With the introduction of antibiotic therapy in the middle of the 20th century, a new adjunctive method to treat and prevent surgical infections was discovered, and hope for final elimination of infections was fostered. However, not only have postoperative wound and hospital-acquired infections continued, but widespread antibiotic therapy has also often made prevention and control of surgical infections more difficult. The present generation of surgeons has seen increasing numbers of serious infections related to a complex combination of factors, including the performance of more complicated and longer operations, an increase in the number of geriatric patients with accompanying chronic or debilitating diseases, many new surgical procedures with implants made of foreign materials, a rapidly expanding number of organ transplants requiring the use of immunosuppressive agents, and increased use of diagnostic and treatment modalities that cause greater bacterial exposure or suppression of normal host resistance.

The modern surgeon cannot escape the responsibility of dealing with infections and, when dealing with them, of having knowledge of the appropriate use of aseptic and antiseptic technique, proper use of prophylactic and therapeutic antibiotics, and adequate monitoring and support with novel surgical and pharmacologic modalities, as well as nonpharmacologic aids. Basic understanding of how the body defends itself against infection is essential to the rational application of surgical and other therapeutic principles to the control of infection.

SURGICAL SITE INFECTIONS

Surgical site infections (SSIs) are infections present in any location along the surgical tract after a surgical procedure. In 1992 the Surgical Wound Infection Task Force published a new set of definitions for wound infections that included changing the term to SSI. Unlike surgical wound infections, SSIs involve postoperative infections occurring at any level (incisional or deep) of a specific procedure. SSIs are divided into incisional superficial (skin, subcutaneous tissue), incisional deep (fascial plane and muscles), and organ/space related (anatomic location of the procedure itself). Examples of organ/space SSIs include intra-abdominal abscesses, empyema, and mediastinitis.[1]

SSIs are the most common nosocomial infection in our population and constitute 38% of all infections in surgical patients. By definition, they can occur anytime from 0 to 30 days after the operation or up to 1 year after a procedure that has involved the implantation of a foreign material (mesh, vascular graft, prosthetic joint, and so on). Incisional infections are the most common; they account for 60% to 80% of all SSIs and have a better

Table 14-1   Risk Factors for Surgical Site Infection According to the Three Main Determinants of Such Infection

MICROORGANISM	LOCAL WOUND	PATIENT
Remote site infection	Surgical technique:	Age
Long-term care facility	Hematoma/seroma	Immunosuppression
Recent hospitalization	Necrosis	Steroids
Duration of the procedure	Sutures	Malignancy
Wound class	Drains	Obesity
Intensive care unit patient	Foreign bodies	Diabetes
Previous antibiotic therapy		Malnutrition
Preoperative shaving		Multiple comorbid conditions
Bacterial number, virulence, and antimicrobial resistance		Transfusions
		Cigarette smoking
		Oxygen
		Temperature
		Glucose control

prognosis than organ/space-related SSIs do, with the latter accounting for 93% of SSI-related mortalities.[1-3]

The microbiology of SSI is related to the bacterial flora present in the exposed anatomic area after a particular procedure and has been relatively fixed during the past 30 years, as shown by the National Nosocomial Infection Surveillance System (NNIS) established by the Centers for Disease Control and Prevention (CDC). The CDC is in the process of revising and renaming this program as the National Healthcare Safety Network (NHSN). This study has shown that *Staphylococcus aureus* remains the most common pathogen in SSIs, followed by coagulase-negative staphylococci, enterococci, and *Escherichia coli*. However, for clean-contaminated and contaminated procedures, *E. coli* and other Enterobacteriaceae are the most common cause of SSI. In addition, some emerging organisms have become more common in recent years. Vancomycin-resistant enterococci (VRE) and gram-negative bacilli with unusual patterns of resistance have been isolated more frequently. Of particular interest is the growing frequency of *Candida* species as a cause of SSI and surgical infections in general.[2]

Understanding the microbiology of SSIs is important to guide initial empirical therapy for infections in a specific patient, as well as for identification of outbreaks and selection of strategies for the management of prophylactic antibiotics, as discussed later in this chapter.

Causes and Risk Factors

Multiple risk factors for SSI have been identified over time and can all be compiled within one or more of the three major determinants of SSI: bacterial factors, local wound factors, and patient factors (Table 14-1). The interaction between these three is what determines the risk for SSI as a complication of surgery. Most of these factors have been shown to be associated with SSI; however, it is difficult to prove an independent association between every specific risk factor and SSI, particularly when looking at different groups of surgical patients (i.e., different patient population, different procedures).

Bacterial factors include virulence and bacterial load in the surgical site. The development of infection is affected by the toxins produced by the microorganism and the microorganism's ability to resist phagocytes and intracellular destruction. Several bacterial species have surface components that contribute to their pathogenicity by inhibiting phagocytosis (e.g., the capsules of *Klebsiella* and *Streptococcus pneumoniae*, the slime of coagulase-negative staphylococci). Gram-negative bacteria have surface components (endotoxin or lipopolysaccharide) that are toxic, and others, such as certain strains of clostridia and streptococci, produce powerful exotoxins that enable them to establish invasive infection after smaller inocula than needed for other pathogens and to evolve much more rapidly. Thus, although most wound infections do not become clinically evident for 5 days or longer after the operation, streptococcal or clostridial infections may become severe within 24 hours.

Studies of traumatic wounds in healthy subjects have shown that bacterial contamination with more than 10^5 organisms frequently causes infection whereas contamination with less than 10^5 organisms usually does not, although β-hemolytic streptococci can cause infection with many fewer organisms. The normal defense mechanisms are therefore of great importance in preventing infection at its inception, but wound infection is inevitable if the bacterial inoculum is sufficiently large. This observation led, in the 1990s, to a wound classification system in which wounds are classified and presumed to have different number and type of bacteria according to the anatomic areas entered and the aseptic and antiseptic techniques used (Table 14-2). Length of preoperative stay, remote site infection at the time of surgery, and duration of the procedure have also been associated with an increased bacterial load and SSI rate.[4] Preoperative shaving has been shown to increase the incidence of SSI after clean procedures as well. This practice increases the infection rate about 100% as compared with removing the hair by clippers at the time of the procedure or not removing it at all, probably secondary to bacterial growth in microscopic cuts. Therefore, the patient is not shaved

Table 14-2 Surgical Wound Classification According to Degree of Contamination

WOUND CLASS	DEFINITION
Clean	An uninfected operative wound in which no inflammation is encountered and the respiratory, alimentary, genital, or infected urinary tract is not entered. Wounds are closed primarily and, if necessary, drained with closed drainage. Surgical wounds after blunt trauma should be included in this category if they meet the criteria
Clean-contaminated	An operative wound in which the respiratory, alimentary, genital, or urinary tract is entered under controlled conditions and without unusual contamination
Contaminated	Open, fresh, accidental wounds. In addition, operations with major breaks in sterile technique or gross spillage from the gastrointestinal tract and incisions in which acute, nonpurulent inflammation is encountered are included in this category
Dirty	Old traumatic wounds with retained devitalized tissue and those that involve existing clinical infection or perforated viscera. This definition suggests that the organisms causing postoperative infection were present in the operative field before the operation

Table 14-3 NNIS Score and Risk for SSI

Risk Factors
Procedure time >75th percentile
Contaminated or dirty wound
ASA III, IV, V

NUMBER OF POSITIVE RISK FACTORS	RISK FOR SSI
0	1.5%
1	2.9%
2	6.8%
3	13.0%

ASA, American Society of Anesthesiologists class; NNIS, National Nosocomial Infection Surveillance; SSI, surgical site infection.

Table 14-4 Comparison of NNIS Score and Wound Classification for Predicting Risk for SSI

WOUND CLASS	NNIS RISK SCORE				
	0	1	2	3	All
Clean	1.0	2.3	5.4	—	2.1
Clean-contaminated	2.1	4.0	9.5	—	3.3
Contaminated	—	3.4	6.8	13.2	6.4
Dirty	—	3.1	8.1	12.8	7.1
All	1.5	2.9	6.8	13.0	—

NNIS, National Nosocomial Infection Surveillance; SSI, surgical site infection.
Adapted from: Dellinger EP, Ehrenkranz NJ: Surgical Infections. In Bennett JV, Brachman PS (eds): Hospital Infections, 4th ed. Philadelphia, Lippincott-Raven, 1998.

before an operation. Extensive removal of hair is not needed, and any hair removal that is done is performed by electric clippers with disposable heads at the time of the procedure and in a manner that does not traumatize the skin.[5]

Local wound factors are related to the invasiveness of an operation and to specific surgeon's practices and surgical technique. The fact that an operation breaks basic barrier defense mechanisms such as skin and gastrointestinal mucosa is a factor clearly associated with SSI. Good surgical technique while managing tissues (local wound) in the most appropriate manner and using sutures, drains, and foreign bodies only with adequate indication is the best way to avoid SSIs.

Patient-related factors include age, immunosuppression, steroids, malignancy, obesity, perioperative transfusions, cigarette smoking, diabetes, other preexisting illness, and malnutrition, among others. It is hard to perform a study in which independent association with SSI can be proved while controlling for all other factors; however, patient-related factors seem to play a very important role in SSI, and preventive measures are starting to focus on manipulating these factors, as discussed later in this section. Recent data suggest that maintaining normothermia in the perioperative period and delivering an FIO_2 of 80% or higher in the OR and postanesthesia

care unit will reduce the rate of SSI by improving O_2 tension and white blood cell function in the surgical incision. In addition, data suggest that control of glucose levels in the perioperative period and up to 48 hours later in both diabetic and nondiabetic patients can reduce rates of SSI and decrease overall postoperative mortality.[6-13]

Risk Scores for Surgical Site Infection

SSI risk has traditionally been correlated to wound class. The accepted range of infection rates has been 1% to 5% for clean, 3% to 11% for clean-contaminated, 10% to 17% for contaminated, and greater than 27% for dirty wounds. Wound class, as discussed earlier, is a significant risk factor for SSI; however, it assesses only the bacterial factors related to wound infection and is thus an imprecise method of including different types of procedures and different kinds of patients in one category.

More recently, the NNIS score, published by Culver and associates in 1991[2,14] and recently validated,[15] includes additional factors that have an independent relationship with SSI (Table 14-3). The NNIS score includes the wound class, the American Society of Anesthesiologists (ASA) class, and the duration of the procedure in comparison to national averages for the same operation. This combination of factors differentiates the risk for SSI more accurately than the previous wound classification system does when used alone (Table 14-4).

Table 14-5   Preventive Measures for Surgical Site Infection

| TIMING OF ACTION | DETERMINANT IN WHICH THE PREVENTIVE MEASURE ACTS | | |
	Microorganism	Local	Patient
Preoperative	Shorten preoperative stay Antiseptic shower preoperatively Appropriate preoperative hair removal or no hair removal Avoid or treat remote site infections Antimicrobial prophylaxis	Appropriate preoperative hair removal or no hair removal	Optimize nutrition Preoperative warming Tight glucose control (insulin drip) Stop smoking
Intraoperative	Asepsis and antisepsis Avoid spillage in gastrointestinal cases	Surgical technique: Hematoma/seroma Good perfusion Complete débridement Dead spaces Monofilament sutures Justified drain use (closed) Limit use of sutures/foreign bodies Delayed primary closure when indicated	Supplemental oxygen Intraoperative warming Adequate fluid resuscitation Tight glucose control (insulin drip)
Postoperative	Protect incision for 48-72 hours Remove drains as soon as possible Avoid postoperative bacteremia	Postoperative dressing for 48-72 hours	Early enteral nutrition Supplemental oxygen Tight glucose control (insulin drip) Surveillance programs

Prevention

Understanding risk factors and preventive measures promotes better control with lower infection rates. Two *milestones* in preventing SSI have been defined by specific preventive measures: first, the aseptic and antiseptic technique introduced by Lister and, second, the proper use of prophylactic antibiotics. A third *milestone* is currently being defined by practices that optimize and maximize the patient's own ability to prevent infection. Microorganisms are a necessary part of the human microenvironment, and even clean wounds have small numbers of bacteria present at the end of the operation. Most of the early preventive measures implemented were focused on controlling the bacterial factors for wound infection. In recent years research has focused on manipulating host (patient) factors to assist the body in dealing with fixed bacterial factors (assuming that all preventive measures have been applied appropriately). The future in the control of infection will focus on patient factors and the body's ability to counteract the obligatory presence of microorganisms. Finally, as we practice in the era of *health care management and quality assurance,* an additional and recently emphasized key component in preventing SSI has become the ability to implement and translate known preventive measures into everyday practice.[16,17]

Preventive measures can be also classified according to the three determinants of wound infection and the timing at which the measures are implemented (preoperatively, intraoperatively, and postoperatively) (Table 14-5).

Microorganism Related

Microorganisms causing SSI can be either exogenous or endogenous. Exogenous microorganisms come from the operating team or from the environment around the surgical site (OR, equipment, air, water, and so on). Endogenous microorganisms come either from the bacteria present in the patient at the surgical site or from bacteria present at a different location (e.g., remote site infection, nasal colonization). Two primary measures exist to control the bacterial load in the surgical site: aseptic and antiseptic methods and antimicrobial prophylaxis.[16]

Aseptic and Antiseptic Methods

Specific environmental and architectural characteristics of the OR help reduce the bacterial load in the OR itself, although it has not been proved to decrease the incidence of SSI, except in refined clean procedures such as joint replacement. Basic principles include size of the OR, air management (filtered flow, positive pressure toward the outside, and air cycles per hour), equipment handling (disinfection and cleansing), and traffic rules. All OR personnel wear clean scrubs, caps, and masks, and traffic in and out of the OR is minimized. Exogenous sources of bacteria causing SSI are rare when standard measures are followed and are important only in cases of outbreaks, such as those that follow failure of sterilization procedures or are traced to OR personnel who shed bacteria. Specific air-filtering mechanisms and other high-tech measures for environmental control in the OR play a significant role in wound infection control only in clean cases in which prostheses are implanted. However, a minimum of basic traffic, environment, and OR behavior rules is followed by staff in the surgical pool as part of a discipline that keeps the team aware of potential causes of infection in surgical patients.

Surgical site preparation, on the other hand, is an important measure in preventing SSI. Preoperative showers the night before surgery with chlorhexidine have not been shown to affect the frequency of SSI, although they do reduce the bacterial colony count on skin. The CDC recommends the use of chlorhexidine showers, and it is reasonable to implement such a policy, particularly in patients who have been in the hospital for a few days and in those in whom an SSI will cause significant morbidity (cardiac, vascular, and prosthetic procedures). Skin preparation of the surgical site is done with a germicidal antiseptic such as tincture of iodine, povidone-iodine, or chlorhexidine. An alternative preparation is the use of antimicrobial incise drapes applied to the entire operative area. Traditionally, the surgical team has scrubbed their hands and forearms for at least 5 minutes the first time in the day and for 3 minutes every consecutive time. Popular antiseptics used are povidone-iodine and chlorhexidine. Recent data have shown that the use of alcohol hand rub solutions is as effective as the aforementioned antiseptics while being faster and kinder to the skin of the surgical team. The use of sterile drapes and gowns is a way of maintaining every surface in contact with the surgical site as sterile as possible.

As many as 90% of an operative team puncture their gloves during a prolonged operation. The risk increases with time, as does the risk for contamination of the surgical site if the glove is not changed at the moment of puncture. The use of double gloving is becoming a popular practice to avoid contamination of the wound, as well as exposure to blood by the surgical team. Double gloving is recommended for all surgical procedures.[18] Instruments that will be in contact with the surgical site are sterilized in standard fashion, and protocols for flash sterilization or emergency sterilization, or both, must be well established to ensure the sterility of instruments and implants.

Antimicrobial Prophylaxis

Systemic antimicrobial prophylaxis is a potentially powerful preventive measure for SSI that is frequently delivered in an ineffective manner, more because of lack of a reliable process in the hospital and operating room than because of lack of understanding. Experience has shown that the effectiveness of antibiotic prophylaxis depends on an organized system to ensure its delivery in an effective manner. If a system is not in place, the results are haphazard failures. Recent national surveys have documented suboptimal prophylactic antibiotic use in 40% to 50% of operative procedures. It is clear that the administration of therapeutic doses of antimicrobial agents can prevent infection in wounds contaminated by bacteria sensitive to the agents. The decision to use prophylactic antibiotic therapy, however, must be based on balancing possible benefit against possible adverse effects. Indiscriminate use of antibiotics is discouraged because it may lead to the emergence of antibiotic-resistant strains of

organisms or serious hypersensitivity reactions. In particular, prolonged use of *prophylactic* antibiotics may also mask the signs of established infections, thus making diagnosis more difficult and causing an increase in the number of resistant pathogens recovered from surgical patients.[19]

Prophylactic systemic antibiotics are not indicated for patients undergoing low-risk, straightforward clean surgical operations in which no obvious bacterial contamination or insertion of a foreign body has occurred. When the incidence of wound infections is less than 1% and the consequences of SSI are not severe, the potential for reducing this low infection rate does not justify the expense and side effects of antibiotic administration. Prophylactic antibiotic therapy is no substitute for careful surgical technique using established surgical principles, and indiscriminate or general use of prophylactic therapy is not in the best interest of the patient. Antibiotic agents can be used effectively only as adjuncts to adequate surgery.

In several clinical situations the administration of prophylactic systemic antibiotic therapy is usually beneficial. Such situations almost always involve a brief period of contamination by organisms that can be predicted with reasonable accuracy. As examples, prophylactic systemic antibiotics reduce infection and are clinically beneficial in the following circumstances:

1. High-risk gastroduodenal procedures, including operations for gastric cancer, ulcer, obstruction, or bleeding; operations when gastric acid production has been suppressed effectively; and gastric operations for morbid obesity
2. High-risk biliary procedures, including operations in patients older than 60 years and those for acute inflammation, common duct stones, or jaundice and in patients with previous biliary tract operations or endoscopic biliary manipulation
3. Resection and anastomosis of the colon or small intestine (see later)
4. Cardiac procedures through a median sternotomy
5. Vascular surgery of the lower extremities or abdominal aorta
6. Amputation of an extremity with impaired blood supply, particularly in the presence of a current or recent ischemic ulcer
7. Vaginal or abdominal hysterectomy
8. Primary cesarean section
9. Operations entering the oral pharyngeal cavity
10. Craniotomy
11. Implantation of any permanent prosthetic material
12. Any wound with known gross bacterial contamination
13. Accidental wounds with heavy contamination and tissue damage. In such instances the antibiotic is given intravenously as soon as possible after injury. The two best-studied situations are penetrating abdominal injuries and open fractures
14. Injuries prone to clostridial infection because of extensive devitalization of muscle, heavy contamination, or impairment of the blood supply

Whether prophylactic antibiotics are given for so-called clean operations not involving the implantation of prosthetic materials has been controversial. A well-designed trial demonstrated a reduction in infection risk when patients undergoing breast procedures or groin hernia repairs received prophylactic antibiotics versus placebo.[20] However, these procedures are not universally considered valid indications for prophylaxis. Some have proposed that such clean operations with one or more NNIS risk points be considered for prophylactic antibiotic administration.

Administration of oral nonabsorbable antibiotics to suppress both aerobic and anaerobic intestinal bacteria before scheduled operations on the colon has also been successful in controlled trials. Neomycin plus erythromycin given only on the day before surgery, 19, 18, and 9 hours before the scheduled start of the procedure, is the most well-established combination at the present time. Neomycin plus metronidazole is also an effective combination. Thorough mechanical cleansing of the intestinal tract is an important component of the oral regimen.[21] Controversies regarding the benefit of mechanical and oral antimicrobial bowel preparation have recently resurfaced. Multiple meta-analyses have shown no effect of mechanical bowel preparation on the incidence of SSI in the absence of oral antibiotics, and some have shown an increased incidence of anastomotic leaks, thus questioning its true benefit even more.[22-24] However, several reports demonstrated a reduced infection rate with the combination of oral nonabsorbable and intravenous antibiotics, and this is the most common practice among colorectal surgeons in the United States. Future recommendations regarding this practice may well change over the next few years.

Prophylactic antibiotic therapy is clearly more effective when begun preoperatively and continued through the intraoperative period, with the aim of achieving therapeutic blood levels throughout the operative period. This produces therapeutic levels of antibiotic agents at the operative site in any seromas and hematomas that may develop. Antibiotics started as late as 1 to 2 hours after bacterial contamination are markedly less effective, and it is completely without value to start prophylactic antibiotics after the wound is closed. Failure of prophylactic antibiotic agents occurs in part through neglect of the importance of the timing and dosage of these agents, which are critical determinants.

For most patients undergoing elective surgery, the first dose of prophylactic antibiotics are given intravenously at the time that anesthesia is induced. It is unnecessary and may be detrimental to start them more than 1 hour preoperatively, and it is unnecessary to give them after the patient leaves the operating room. A single dose, depending on the drug used and length of the operation, is often sufficient. For operations that are prolonged, the prophylactic agent chosen is given in repeated doses at intervals of one to two half-lives for the drug being used. Prophylactic antibiotic coverage for more than 12 hours for a planned operation is never indicated. In addition, for obese patients there are studies showing benefit of higher initial doses and more frequently repeated doses

(including continuous antibiotic drips) to achieve appropriate tissue levels throughout the operation.[25-27] No evidence supports the practice of continuing prophylactic antibiotics until central lines, drains, and chest tubes are removed. There is evidence, however, that this practice increases the recovery of resistant bacteria.

Many patients fail to receive needed prophylactic antibiotics because the system for their administration is complex at the time of multiple events just before a major operation. This problem has been made worse by the trend of admitting patients directly to the operating room for planned operations, which intensifies the pressure to accomplish a large number of procedures during a short interval before the operation. The possibility that prophylactic antibiotics will unintentionally be omitted can be minimized by establishing a system with a checklist. One member of the operative team (usually the preoperative nurse or a member of the anesthesia team) is responsible for initialing a portion of the operative record that states either that the patient received indicated prophylactic antibiotics or that the surgeon has determined that antibiotics are not indicated for the procedure.

Many antibiotics effectively reduce the rate of postoperative SSI when used appropriately for indicated procedures. No antibiotic has been reliably superior to another when each possessed a similar and appropriate antibacterial spectrum. The most important determinant is whether the planned procedure is expected to enter parts of the body known to harbor obligate colonic anaerobic bacteria (*Bacteroides* species). If anaerobic flora are anticipated, such as during operations on the colon or distal ileum or during appendectomy, an agent effective against *Bacteroides* species, such as cefotetan, must be used. Cefoxitin is an alternative with a dramatically shorter half-life. Cefazolin combined with metronidazole is another alternative choice. If anaerobic flora are not expected, cefazolin is the prophylactic drug of choice.

For patients who are allergic to cephalosporins, clindamycin or, in settings in which methicillin-resistant *S. aureus* (MRSA) is common, vancomycin can be used. Prophylactic use of vancomycin is minimized as much as possible to reduce environmental pressure favoring the emergence of vancomycin-resistant enterococci and staphylococci. If an intestinal procedure is planned in such an allergic patient, a regimen with activity against gram-negative rods and anaerobes must be used, such as an aminoglycoside or a fluoroquinolone combined with clindamycin or metronidazole or aztreonam combined with clindamycin.

The use of topical antibiotics often effectively diminishes the incidence of infection in contaminated wounds. However, the combination of topical agents and parenteral agents is not more effective than either one alone, and topical agents alone are inferior to parenteral agents in complex gastric procedures. As a general rule, topical agents do not cause any harm if one adheres to the following rules:

1. Do not use any agent in wounds or in the abdomen that would not be suitable for parenteral administration.

2. Do not use more of the agent than would be acceptable for parenteral administration.

In considering the amount used, any drug being given parenterally must be added to the amount being placed in the wound. Topical agents used for burn wounds (discussed elsewhere) may be used in large open wounds in selected patients.

Prophylactic antibiotic therapy is generally ineffective in clinical situations in which continuing contamination is likely to occur. Examples follow:

1. In patients with tracheostomies or tracheal intubation to prevent pulmonary infections
2. In patients with indwelling urinary catheters
3. In patients with indwelling central venous lines
4. In patients with wound or chest drains
5. In most open wounds, including burn wounds

Local Wound Related

Most of the preventive measures related to the local wound are determined by the good judgment and surgical technique of the surgeon. Intraoperative measures include appropriate handling of tissue and assurance of satisfactory final vascular supply, but with adequate control of bleeding to prevent hematomas/seromas. Complete débridement of necrotic tissue plus removal of unnecessary foreign bodies is recommended, as well as avoiding the placement of foreign bodies in clean-contaminated, contaminated, or dirty cases. Monofilament sutures have proved in experimental studies to be associated with a lower rate of SSI. Sutures are foreign bodies that are used only when required. Suture closure of dead space has not been shown to prevent SSI. Large potential dead spaces can be treated with the use of closed-suction systems for short periods, but these systems provide a route for bacteria to reach the wounds and may cause SSI. Open drainage systems (e.g., Penrose) increase rather than decrease infections in surgical wounds and are avoided unless used to drain wounds that are already infected.

In heavily contaminated wounds or wounds in which all the foreign bodies or devitalized tissue cannot be satisfactorily removed, delayed primary closure minimizes the development of serious infection in most instances. With this technique, the subcutaneous tissue and skin are left open and dressed loosely with gauze after fascial closure. The number of phagocytic cells at the wound edges progressively increases to a peak about 5 days after the injury. Capillary budding is intense at this time, and closure can usually be accomplished successfully even with heavy bacterial contamination because phagocytic cells can be delivered to the site in large numbers. Experiments have shown that the number of organisms required to initiate an infection in a surgical incision progressively increases as the interval of healing increases, up to the fifth postoperative day.

Finally, adequate dressing of the closed wound isolates it from the outside environment. Providing an appropriate dressing for 48 to 72 hours can decrease wound contamination. However, dressings after this period increase the subsequent bacterial count on adjacent skin by altering the microenvironment underneath the dressing.

Patient Related

Host resistance is abnormal in a variety of systemic conditions and diseases, including leukemia, diabetes mellitus, uremia, prematurity, burn or traumatic injury, advanced malignancy, old age, obesity, malnutrition, and several diseases of inherited immunodeficiency. In surgical patients who have these or similar problems, extra precautions are taken to prevent the development of wound infections, including correction or control of the underlying defect whenever possible.

Malnutrition and low albumin levels are associated with an increased rate of SSI. Optimizing nutritional status before surgery and early in the postoperative periods with specific immunonutrition (arginine, nucleotides, ω-3 fatty acids) formulas may decrease the incidence of SSI in patients with upper gastrointestinal tract cancer.[28-30] Recent studies have also demonstrated that maintaining a higher partial pressure of oxygen by delivering a higher inspired fraction of oxygen with adequate fluid resuscitation is associated with a decreased rate of SSI. The presumed mechanism is more oxygen available for white blood cells to kill bacteria present in the wound at the time of the operation. Preoperative warming was also demonstrated in two recent prospective randomized controlled trials to reduce SSI rates. Other studies have shown that increasing tissue temperature by 4°C results in increased perfusion and oxygen delivery to the incision. Finally, in critically ill patients, aggressive perioperative insulin therapy with the use of insulin drips to maintain glucose levels between 80 and 110 mg/dL was associated with decreased mortality in this set of patients. Other studies of patients undergoing cardiac and gastrointestinal surgery have demonstrated an increased rate of SSI when perioperative blood glucose levels exceeded 200 mg/dL, regardless of whether the patients were diabetic.[6-13]

System-Based Prevention

The need for efficient resource utilization and cost containment, as well as the new era of managed health care and quality assurance, has raised new interest in the prevention of SSI. Recently, delivery processes for preventive strategies have been studied and shown to be well under ideal standards. The most illustrative example has been the use of prophylactic antibiotics. The Surgical Infection Prevention Project (SIPP)—a national effort led by the Center for Medicare and Medicaid Services (CMS) to achieve lower rates of SSI—showed that in more than 32,000 surgical procedures performed in different centers around the United States, only 55.7% of patients were given prophylactic antibiotics within 1 hour of the incision time. A collaborative (the SIPP Collaborative) was created to maximize delivery of this preventive strategy through educational and system-related changes, among others. The project was carried out over a 12-month period in more than 50 U.S. hospitals, and the timing of antibiotic prophylaxis, as well as other measures, improved significantly, with a relative 27% reduction in

SSIs being achieved. This constitutes a good example of the current system-related obstacles in controlling SSI and a method to overcome the problem and is one of many other models to follow as part of the strategy to decrease the incidence of SSI.[17,31,32] The CMS has recently begun to alter and make payment rates dependent on hospitals reporting their success in this and other preventive measures.

It is the modern surgeon's responsibility, as the leader of the surgical delivery system, to implement all known and proven measures that reduce the incidence of SSI. Wound infection surveillance systems have proved to be an important measure in controlling SSI rates, and perhaps this is achieved by permanent and continuous awareness by surgeons and surgical teams of the risk and the measures that can be used to avoid this common complication.[33-35] Surveillance of SSI includes a determination for each SSI of whether all accepted preventive measures were provided for that patient and procedure. If they were not, the SSI can be classified as *potentially preventable*. If all appropriate preventive measures were provided, the SSI is *apparently unpreventable*. The goal of surgical practice and surveillance is to have no potentially preventable SSI. As our knowledge regarding SSI prevention increases, the definition of potentially preventable could expand.[36]

Treatment

Treatment of SSI follows standard principles of management for all surgical infections, as explained later. In general, the mainstay of treatment is source control or draining of the infected area. For a superficial SSI this involves opening the wound at the skin and subcutaneous levels and cleansing the wound, along with dressing changes twice or three times a day. Occasionally, sharp débridement to allow healing of the open wound is necessary. Once the wound infection has been controlled, wound-suctioning devices can also be used to minimize the discomfort from more frequent dressing changes and possibly to accelerate wound healing. For organ/procedure-related SSI, source control can generally be achieved with percutaneous drainage. It is imperative to ensure that the infection is well controlled with percutaneous drainage; if it involves a more diffuse area of a human cavity (i.e., diffuse peritonitis, mediastinitis), surgical drainage is encouraged and would include repair of any anatomic cause of infection (e.g., anastomotic leak) if present. The use of antibiotics is not the standard for treatment of incisional SSI. They are recommended only as adjunctive therapy when surrounding cellulitis occurs or when treating a deep SSI (organ/procedure related).

SPECIFIC SURGICAL INFECTIONS

Surgical infections are those that occur as a result of a surgical procedure or those that require surgical intervention as part of their treatment. They are characterized by a breech of mechanical/anatomic defense mechanisms (barriers) and are associated with greater morbidity, significant mortality, and increased cost of care.[37]

Some generalizations can be made concerning typical differences between surgical and medical infections. In common community-acquired medical infections, such as primary pneumonia, general host defenses are usually intact. Some exceptions to intact host defenses occur in patients undergoing systemic therapy for malignancy or for transplant rejection and patients infected with human immunodeficiency virus (HIV). Most surgical infections, in contrast, are the result of damaged host defenses, especially injury to the epithelial barrier that normally protects the sterile internal environment from endogenous and exogenous bacteria. Immunologic defects may be acquired, through either trauma (accidental or surgical) or tumor. Nonmechanical host defense defects are global and caused by nutritional deficiency or the systemic effects of trauma, or both.

The pathogens found in medical infections are usually single and aerobic. They either derive from exogenous sources or are present only in a minority of asymptomatic normal hosts. Typically, they possess virulence properties that allow them to invade and infect despite an intact epithelial barrier. Examples include β-hemolytic streptococci, *S. pneumoniae, Shigella, Salmonella,* and *Vibrio cholerae.* The pathogens causing surgical infections, in contrast, are frequently mixed, involving both aerobes and anaerobes, and generally originate from the patient's own endogenous flora. These pathogens are opportunistic and often depend on an acquired epithelial defect to cause infection.

The primary principle when treating surgical infections is *source control,* which refers to drainage of the infection or correction of the predisposing cause (or both). Typical types of source control include draining an abscess, resecting or débriding dead tissue, diverting bowel, relieving obstruction, and closing a perforation. Antibiotic treatment of a surgical infection without this mechanical solution will not resolve the infection. The most important aspect of the initial approach to a surgical infection is the recognition that operative intervention is required. Antibiotic treatment and systemic support are only adjunctive therapies that will help the patient overcome the infectious insult once appropriate source control has been achieved.

Non-Necrotizing Soft Tissue Infections

The distinction between surgical and medical infections in superficial tissues depends on the recognition of dead tissue or pus, or both, in surgical infections. The most obvious example of a surgical infection is a subcutaneous abscess, an infectious process characterized by a necrotic center without a blood supply and composed of debris from local tissues, dead and dying white blood cells, components of blood and plasma, and bacteria. This semiliquid central portion (pus) is surrounded by a vascularized zone of inflammatory tissue. An abscess will not resolve unless the pus is drained and evacuated. It is recognized clinically as a localized swelling with signs of inflammation and tenderness. An abscess must be distinguished from cellulitis, which is a soft tissue infection with an intact blood supply and viable tissue that is marked by an acute inflammatory response with small vessel engorgement and stasis, endothelial leakage with interstitial edema, and polymorphonuclear leukocyte infiltration; it is typically located in a more superficial plane. Cellulitis resolves with appropriate antibiotic therapy alone if treatment is initiated before tissue death occurs.

An abscess may be mistaken for cellulitis when the central necrotic portion is located deep beneath overlying tissue layers and it cannot be readily detected by physical examination. It may also be disguised in anatomic locations where fibrous septa join skin and fascia and divide subcutaneous tissue into compartments that limit the local expression of fluctuance while leading to high pressure that causes ischemia and promotes early tissue death. Examples of such infections include perirectal abscesses, breast abscesses, carbuncles on the posterior of the neck and upper part of the back, and infections in the distal phalanx of the finger (felon).

Knowledge of the local anatomy and pathophysiology of these special abscesses helps provide optimal treatment. A perirectal abscess is often associated with a fistula communicating with the anus at a crypt. The perirectal abscess must be drained, and if a fistula is not found acutely, the surgeon needs to be alert for its occurrence in the postoperative period. A felon is drained through a lateral incision to avoid a painful scar on the pressure-bearing distal pulp. At the time of incision and drainage of a felon, all fibrous septa in the infected pulp must be broken to resolve the infection.

Superficial abscesses on the trunk and on the head and neck are most commonly caused by *S. aureus,* often combined with streptococci. Abscesses in the axillae frequently have a prominent gram-negative component. Abscesses below the waist, especially on the perineum, are often found to harbor mixed aerobic and anaerobic gram-negative flora.

Traumatic wounds, when closed and infected, become a surgical complication that needs to be opened, drained, and treated with antibiotics if associated with cellulitis or systemic compromise. Wounds older than 6 hours, those with significant contamination (dirty, including human and animal bites), wounds associated with necrotic or ischemic tissue, puncture wounds, those classified as stab wounds or gunshot wounds, and wounds caused by a significant crush mechanism or avulsion are not closed. These wounds, as well as those deeper than 1 cm and wounds caused by burns or a frostbite mechanism, receive tetanus prophylaxis if the most recent tetanus booster occurred 5 or more years earlier. The use of antibiotics for simple extremity lacerations has not been proved to reduce the risk for infection after closure.

Necrotizing Soft Tissue Infections

Necrotizing soft tissue infections (NSTIs) are less common than subcutaneous abscesses and cellulitis but are much more serious conditions whose severity may initially be unrecognized. They typically involve deep subcutaneous tissue, superficial or deep fascia, or muscle, or any combination of the three.

NSTIs are characterized by the absence of clear local boundaries or palpable limits. This lack of clear boundaries accounts for both the severity of the infection and the frequent delay in recognizing its surgical nature. Anatomically, these infections are marked by a layer of necrotic tissue that is not walled off by a surrounding inflammatory reaction and thus is not typically manifested as an abscess unless it is the initiating factor. In addition, the overlying skin has a relatively normal appearance in the early stages of infection, and the visible degree of involvement is substantially less than that of the underlying tissues.

NSTIs have been described by a variety of different labels, including *gas gangrene* and *necrotizing fasciitis.* A substantial number of classifications based on anatomic location, microbiology, and depth of infection, among others, have also been described. The wide range of classifications makes understanding of this entity rather confusing, when the only important factor to be determined is the presence or absence of a necrotic component requiring surgical intervention. If suspected, the approach to diagnosis and management of all patients is the same, thus making detailed classification schemes even less useful. We encourage applying the term NSTI to all infections that fit this category.[38-40]

In advanced stages of the disease, patients usually have overt signs of systemic compromise and septic physiology. Local findings include tense and tender soft tissues associated with ecchymoses or blistering of the skin, or both. The presence of gas detected either by physical examination (crepitus) or by radiographs has been recognized as a grave finding and can be associated with virtually any bacteria, as opposed to the common perception of its unique association with clostridial infections. Most bacteria, especially facultative gram-negative rods such as *E. coli,* make insoluble gases whenever they are forced to use anaerobic metabolism. Thus, the presence of gas in a soft tissue infection implies anaerobic metabolism. Because human tissue cannot survive in an anaerobic environment, gas associated with infection implies dead tissue and therefore a surgical infection. At this stage the disease advances rapidly and must be diagnosed and treated as soon as possible; however, progression from cellulitis or abscess to NSTI may take several days, which can confuse the clinical picture and delay diagnosis. In patients with chronic infections (e.g., diabetic foot), obese patients, and those at the early stage of the disease, making the diagnosis of NSTI is not straightforward. Different strategies to allow earlier diagnosis and surgical débridement have been proposed. Frozen biopsy and imaging with either computed tomography (CT) or magnetic resonance imaging may be helpful in these scenarios.[38-41] However, imaging studies, though sensitive, are nonspecific, and if one has sufficient suspicion to perform a biopsy, the evidence is usually clear to the eye when the incision for biopsy is made.

Wall and colleagues[42] described the association of NSTI with leukocytosis greater than 15,400/mL^3 together with a serum sodium level less than 135 mEq/L, and more

Table 14-6 **Comparison of Clostridial and Nonclostridial Infections**

	CLOSTRIDIAL MYONECROSIS	NONCLOSTRIDIAL NECROTIZING INFECTIONS
Erythema	Usually absent	Present, often mild
Swelling/edema	Mild to moderate	Moderate to severe
Exudate	Thin	"Dishwater" to purulent
White cells	Usually absent	Present
Bacteria	GPR ± others	Mixed ± GPR
		May be GPC alone
Advanced signs	Hypesthesia	Hypoesthesia
	Bronze discoloration	Ecchymoses
	Hemorrhagic bullae	Bullae
	Dermal gangrene	Dermal gangrene
	Crepitus	±Crepitus
Deep involvement	Muscle > skin	Subcutaneous tissue ± fascia ± muscle (uncommon) > skin
Histology	Minimal inflammation	Acute inflammation
	Muscle necrosis	Microabscesses
		Viable muscle
Physiology	Rapid onset of tachycardia, hypotension, volume deficit, ± intravascular hemolysis	Variable to minimal tachycardia, hypotension, and volume deficit
Treatment		
General	Aggressive cardiopulmonary resuscitation	Aggressive cardiopulmonary resuscitation
Antibiotics	Penicillin G plus broad-spectrum antibiotic	Third-generation cephalosporin or fluoroquinolone plus antianaerobic agent
	Clindamycin may be useful for inhibiting toxin production	Clindamycin may be useful for inhibiting toxin production
Hyperbaric O₂	If it does not delay other treatment	No
Surgery	Aggressive removal of infected tissue; amputation of extremity often required	Débridement and exposure; not much removal required; usually no amputation
Antitoxin	No	No

GPC, gram-positive cocci; GPR, gram-positive rods.
Adapted from Dellinger EP: Crepitus and gangrene. In Platt R, Kass EH (eds): Current Therapy in Infectious Diseases, 3rd ed. Philadelphia, BC Decker, 1990. Reprinted with permission of B.C. Decker, Inc.

recently, Wong and associates[43] created a score (laboratory risk indicator for necrotizing fasciitis [LRINEC]) to distinguish NSTI from non-necrotizing soft tissue infections by using the following variables: C-reactive protein, leukocytosis, hemoglobin, sodium, creatinine, and glucose levels. Use of these scores can certainly help guide the management of patients with suspected NSTI. However, whenever in doubt, an incision over the compromised area for exploration of the site in the OR is mandatory. Typical intraoperative findings consistent with NSTI include a dishwater-like exudate, dusky tissues, thrombosed vessels, and lack of clear boundaries allowing finger dissection to spread through the compromised plane abnormally easily.

NSTIs are typically polymicrobial in nature. Staphylococcal and streptococcal species are relatively common causative organisms in combination with anaerobes. *Vibrio* and fungal (mucormycosis) pathogens have also been described as causing NSTI. Clostridial infections are worth special mention. They are typically monomicrobial, although they can be seen in combination with other bacteria. They are often characterized by infection and necrosis of muscles (myonecrosis) and are associated with a significantly worse prognosis.[44] Clostridial infections are more common in patients with intravenous drug use and are accompanied by a very high white blood cell count. These infections require very expeditious and

repeated débridement together with supportive care in the intensive care unit (ICU). Table 14-6 lists a series of differences between clostridial and nonclostridial NSTIs. The most common organisms associated with clostridial infections are *Clostridium perfringens, Clostridium novyi,* and *Clostridium septicum.* The only other bacteria commonly reported as the sole cause of nonclostridial NSTI is β-hemolytic *Streptococcus pyogenes.* Although it has been popularized by the media as so-called flesh-eating bacteria and it does cause a rapidly spreading NSTI, its prognosis over the last few years has improved when compared with other more common causes of NSTI.

Treatment of NSTI always includes débridement, and additional support is provided by broad-spectrum antibiotics, monitoring, and systemic support. Débridement of all necrotic tissue must be done promptly, with *scheduled* repeat débridement every 24 hours or sooner if indicated by clinical deterioration. Major amputations may be required to achieve appropriate source control or when the infection spreads to involve the entirety of a limb. Antibiotic choices include agents with broad activity against facultative gram-negative rods, gram-positive cocci, and anaerobes. Combination regimens include an aerobic and anaerobic agent, as demonstrated in Table 14-7, as well as coverage of gram-positive and gram-negative organisms. In addition, if MRSA is thought to probably be a pathogen in the patient being treated, an

Table 14-7 Antibiotics With Predominantly Aerobic or Anaerobic Broad-Spectrum Activity

AEROBIC COVERAGE	ANAEROBIC COVERAGE
Gentamicin	A penicillin with a β-lactamase
Tobramycin	inhibitor
Amikacin	Clindamycin
Netilmicin	Metronidazole*
Cefotaxime	Chloramphenicol
Ceftizoxime	
Ceftriaxone	
Ceftazidime	
Cefepime	
Aztreonam*	
Ciprofloxacin	
Ofloxacin	
Levofloxacin	

*Do not use aztreonam alone with metronidazole.

Table 14-8 Prognostic Score to Predict Mortality in Patients With Necrotizing Soft Tissue Infection at the Time of First Assessment

VARIABLE (ON ADMISSION)	NO. OF POINTS
Heart rate >110 beats/min	1
Temperature <36°C	1
Creatinine >1.5 mg/dL	1
Age >50 yr	3
White blood cell count >40,000	3
Hematocrit >50	3

GROUP CATEGORIES	NO. OF POINTS	MORTALITY RISK
1	0-2	6%
2	3-5	24%
3	≥6	88%

From Anaya DA, Bulger EM, Kwon YS, et al: Predicting mortality in necrotizing soft tissue infections: A clinical score. Paper presented at the 25th Annual Meeting of the Surgical Infection Society and the 2nd Joint Meeting with the Surgical Infection Society—Europe, May 5-7, 2005, Miami.

antibiotic that covers this organism needs to be added. Typical empirical treatments include triple (penicillin, clindamycin, and aminoglycoside/quinolone) or quadruple (plus vancomycin) antibiotic regimens. When starting empirical antibiotic treatment, combinations that include the use of high-dose clindamycin is strongly considered. Clindamycin has been shown to block exotoxin production from bacteria, one of the key bacterial factors that perpetuates and leads to spreading of the infection through tissues. Narrower antibiotic regimens can be given once a definitive culture with specific sensitivity results is available. Appropriate single agents include imipenem/cilastatin, meropenem, ertapenem, tigecycline, and piperacillin/tazobactam.

The mortality associated with NSTI has been in the range of 16% to 45%. Multiple prognostic factors have been identified, including the presence of clostridial infection. More recently, Anaya and coworkers created a score to predict mortality in patients with NSTI at the time of initial assessment. In this study we reported our experience in 350 patients with NSTI from two referral centers (unpublished data). Mortality in our series was 16.6%. Table 14-8 lists the variables and points assigned for determining the predictive score. This tool helps establish which patients may benefit from more aggressive surgical intervention (early amputation), evaluating novel therapeutic approaches, and selecting patients for future trials.

Intra-abdominal and Retroperitoneal Infections

Most serious intra-abdominal infections require surgical intervention for resolution. In this context, surgical intervention includes percutaneous drainage of intra-abdominal abscesses. Specific exceptions to the requirement for surgical intervention include pyelonephritis, salpingitis, amebic liver abscess, enteritis (e.g., *Shigella, Yersinia*), spontaneous bacterial peritonitis, some cases of diverticulitis, and some cases of cholangitis. However, all these *exceptions* can be diagnosed pre-

sumptively with a rapid initial evaluation. If the diagnosis of one of these exceptions cannot be made, a patient with fever and abdominal pain is not given antibiotics without a plan leading to surgery or other drainage procedure. Administration of antibiotics in this setting before diagnosis may obscure subsequent findings and delay diagnosis and will certainly delay definitive operative management. If too sick to go without antibiotic therapy, the patient is also too sick to avoid operative intervention and definitive diagnosis and treatment.

Despite modern antibiotics and intensive care, mortality from serious intra-abdominal or retroperitoneal infection remains high (5%-50%) and morbidity is substantial. The systemic response to intra-abdominal or retroperitoneal infection is accompanied by fluid shifts similar to that seen in patients with major burns. Fever, tachycardia, and hypotension are common, and a severe hypermetabolic, catabolic response is universal. If a corrective operation and effective antibiotics are not delivered promptly, the sequence of events termed *multiple-organ dysfunction syndrome* may ensue and cause the patient to die even after the primary focus of infection has been controlled. Regardless of the initial antibiotic choice and operative procedure, there is a significant chance that a change in antibiotics may be required and that a reoperation may be necessary. A physician caring for a patient with an intra-abdominal infection must be alert to these possibilities and be diligent in monitoring and re-examining the patient and examining the antimicrobial susceptibility of the recovered pathogens so that this decision can be made at the earliest possible time.

Outcome is improved by early diagnosis and treatment. The risk for death and complications increases with increased age, preexisting serious underlying diseases, and malnutrition.[45] The risk of death or failure to control the abdominal source of infection is also related to the normal homeostatic balance of the patient at the time of diagnosis and initiation of definitive therapy. This balance can be measured by scales designed to quantitate the number of physical findings and laboratory test results that are abnormal. One of the most widely used scales is the Acute Physiology and Chronic Health Evaluation (APACHE) scoring system. The higher the score, the more abnormal test results and findings are present and the greater the risk for death.[46]

When an intra-abdominal infection is diagnosed, initial treatment consists of cardiorespiratory support, antibiotic therapy, and operative intervention. In most cases the responsible bacteria are not known for at least 24 hours, and sensitivity information is not available for 48 to 72 hours after samples are obtained for culture during the operative procedure. Because most intra-abdominal infections yield three to five different aerobic and anaerobic pathogens, specific, targeted antibiotic therapy is not possible at first, and the initial choice must be empirical and designed to cover a range of possible organisms. In recent years, numerous new antibiotics have widened the available choices. For infections acquired in the community with a small likelihood of resistant gram-negative rods and for a patient not severely ill, empirical therapy can be initiated with cefoxitin, cefotetan, ticarcillin/clavulanate, ertapenem, or ampicillin/sulbactam. For the more severely ill or a patient who has been in the hospital or has recently been treated with antibiotics, a more comprehensive antimicrobial spectrum is needed. Imipenem, meropenem, piperacillin/tazobactam, or a combination chosen from Table 14-7 is useful; one antibiotic is taken from the aerobic column and one from the anaerobic column (see later for discussion of specific antibiotics).[47,48]

Operative Intervention

The goal of operative intervention in patients with intra-abdominal infection is source control, that is, to correct the underlying anatomic problem that either caused the infection or perpetuates it. The cause of the peritonitis must be corrected. Foreign material in the peritoneal cavity that inhibits white blood cell function and promotes bacterial growth (feces, food, bile, mucin, blood) must be removed. Large deposits of fibrin that entrap bacteria and thereby allow bacterial growth and prevent phagocytosis are removed.[49,50]

An intra-abdominal or retroperitoneal abscess requires drainage. CT scans provide precise localization of intra-abdominal abscesses, thus permitting selected abscesses to be drained percutaneously under radiologic or ultrasound guidance. If the abscess is single and has a straight path to the abdominal wall that does not transgress the bowel, it can be drained percutaneously. Such drainage is accomplished by needle puncture, and a small sample of pus is aspirated to confirm the location and diagnosis. Subsequently, a guidewire is passed through the needle, which is then removed. The guidewire allows dilation of the tract, followed by placement of a drainage catheter. The progress of abscess closure can be monitored by plain radiographs after the instillation of contrast material or by repeat CT scans. If percutaneous drainage is not successful, an open operation may be required.[51]

If a patient has multiple abscesses or abscesses combined with underlying disease that requires operative correction or if a safe percutaneous route to the abscess is not present, open, operative drainage may be required. A single abscess in the subphrenic or subhepatic position may be drained by an extraperitoneal subcostal or posterior 12th rib approach, which provides open drainage without exposing the entire peritoneal cavity to the abscess contents. Likewise, most retroperitoneal abscesses are drained from a retroperitoneal approach. However, most pancreatic abscesses, which in reality more often consist of diffusely infected, necrotic, peripancreatic retroperitoneal tissue, require transabdominal surgery and débridement. Recent reports demonstrate that many cases of necrotizing pancreatitis can be débrided and drained with minimally invasive techniques aided by laparoscopy. A pelvic abscess may be amenable to transrectal or transvaginal drainage.

Prosthetic Device–Related Infections

As the ability to replace parts of the body has increased, so has the potential for infectious complications associated with these replacement parts. Some of the most significant complications associated with vascular grafts, cardiac valves, pacemakers, and artificial joints are caused by infections at the site of implantation. The presence of the foreign material (the prosthetic device) impairs local host defenses, especially polymorphonuclear leukocyte function, and allows certain bacteria with specific virulence factors (*S. epidermidis*—slime) to stick to foreign surfaces and colonize and cause infections. Accordingly, most such infections resist treatment short of removing the offending device. The morbidity and mortality associated with these infections is high. Some success can be obtained by intensive antibiotic therapy, removal of the infected device under antibiotic coverage, and replacement with a new uninfected device, followed by prolonged antibiotic treatment. This approach is warranted when the device is life sustaining, as in the case of a cardiac valve, or prevents severe disability, as in the case of a prosthetic joint.

Nonsurgical Infections in Surgical Patients

Postoperative patients are at increased risk for a variety of nonsurgical postoperative nosocomial infections, the most common of which is urinary tract infection (UTI). Any patient who has had an indwelling urinary catheter is at increased risk for a UTI. Despite the benign course of most UTIs, the occurrence of one in a surgical patient is associated with a threefold increase in death during hospitalization. The best prevention is to use urinary catheters sparingly and for specific indications and short durations and to adhere to strict closed drainage techniques for those that are used.

Lower respiratory tract infections are the third most common cause of nosocomial infection in surgical patients (after SSIs and UTIs) and are the leading cause of death from nosocomial infection. The diagnosis is usually relatively straightforward in a patient who is breathing spontaneously. However, a patient who is intubated and being ventilated because of adult respiratory distress syndrome presents an extremely difficult diagnostic problem.

Patients with this syndrome commonly have abnormal chest x-ray findings, abnormal blood gas values, and elevated temperatures and white blood cell counts, even in the absence of infection. Both false-positive and false-negative diagnoses of pneumonia are common. New chest x-ray infiltrates with signs of infection constitute a good indication for bronchoalveolar lavage, a method that is being used to diagnose and identify bacteria causing ventilator-associated pneumonia; it has been proved to minimize the indiscriminant use of antibiotics and possesses higher specificity than seen with previous methods. Preventive methods to reduce the risk for postoperative pneumonia in intubated patients include elevation of the head of the bed and specific protocols for weaning from the ventilator.

As part of the workup for fever in a surgical patient, central lines used for monitoring or treatment are always considered. Catheter-related sepsis is diagnosed when an organism is isolated from blood culture and from a segment of the catheter in question, without any other source of septicemia and with clinical findings consistent with sepsis. Infection of the catheter site is defined as the presence of erythema, warmth, tenderness, or pus (or any combination) at the catheter insertion site. Both require removal of the catheter, and if a new central line is needed, a new puncture is warranted. Further treatment usually depends on the organism isolated. Placement of lines is done in accordance with standard aseptic and antiseptic technique, including wide drapes and full gown and glove for the inserting physician. Still, the best way to minimize these infections is to avoid placement of unnecessary lines and remove them as soon as possible, once the indication is not present anymore. Routine change of central lines has not proved to reduce infection rates.

Other types of nosocomial infection that can develop in surgical patients include sinusitis and meningitis. These infections do not occur as frequently but must always be considered, particularly in high-risk patients.

Postoperative Fever

Approximately 2% of all primary laparotomies are followed by an unscheduled operation for intra-abdominal infection, and roughly 50% of all serious intra-abdominal infections are postoperative. Wound infections are more common but less serious. Postoperative fever occurs more frequently and may be a source of concern to the physician and patient. Fever is associated with infection, and empirical prescription of antibiotics is a common response to fever. However, most febrile postoperative patients are not infected, and indeed a significant proportion of infected patients may not be febrile, depending on the definition of *fever*. Because fever is common in the absence of infection, it is important to consider causes of postoperative fever other than infection and to make a presumptive diagnosis before instituting antibiotic treatment.[52]

The most common nonsurgical causes of postoperative infection and fever—UTI, respiratory tract infection, and intravenous catheter–associated infection—are all readily diagnosed. The other important causes of postoperative infection and fever—wound infection and intra-abdominal infection—require operative treatment and are not properly managed with antibiotics in the absence of operative treatment. The most sensitive test for detecting these infections and determining their location continues to be history taking and physical examination conducted by a conscientious physician. The physician with the most detailed understanding of the relevant history in a postoperative patient is the operating surgeon. Supportive laboratory and x-ray evaluation, including a white blood cell count, blood cultures, and CT, can supplement the physical examination. Fever in the first 3 days after surgery most likely has a noninfectious cause. However, when the fever starts or continues 5 or more days postoperatively, the incidence of SSI exceeds the incidence of undiagnosed fever. Neither prolongation of perioperative prophylactic antibiotics nor initiation of empirical therapeutic antibiotics is indicated without a presumptive clinical diagnosis and a plan for operative intervention when needed.

Only two important infectious causes of fever are likely in the first 36 hours after laparotomy. Both can be diagnosed readily if they are suspected and appropriate examinations are conducted. The first is an injury to bowel with intraperitoneal leakage, which is characterized by marked hemodynamic changes—first tachycardia and then hypotension and falling urine output. Fluid requirements are substantial, and physical examination reveals diffuse abdominal tenderness. The other early cause of fever and infection is an invasive soft tissue infection beginning in the wound and caused either by β-hemolytic streptococci or by clostridial species (most commonly *C. perfringens*). This event is diagnosed by inspection of the wound and Gram stain of wound fluid, which shows either gram-positive cocci or gram-positive rods. White blood cells are often present with streptococcal infections but are usually absent with clostridial infection. A rare cause of infection in the first 48 hours after surgery is wound toxic shock syndrome. This occurs when certain toxin-producing *S. aureus* species grow in a wound. Less than 1% of all toxic shock cases reported to the CDC were from wounds, and half of them occurred within 48 hours of surgery. Initial symptoms include fever, diarrhea, vomiting, erythroderma, and hypotension. Desquamation follows later. Physical findings of wound infection were often unimpressive or absent. Wound drainage and antibiotics are recommended, but the best treatment is not known. Administration of clindamycin may be helpful for its inhibition of exotoxin production.

PATHOGENS IN SURGICAL INFECTIONS

This discussion of pathogens commonly responsible for surgical infections is not intended to be a complete review. Rather, it focuses on some broad distinctions and classifications that help organize the vast body of data concerning the usual bacterial flora of different surgical infections and the antibiotic susceptibility patterns of

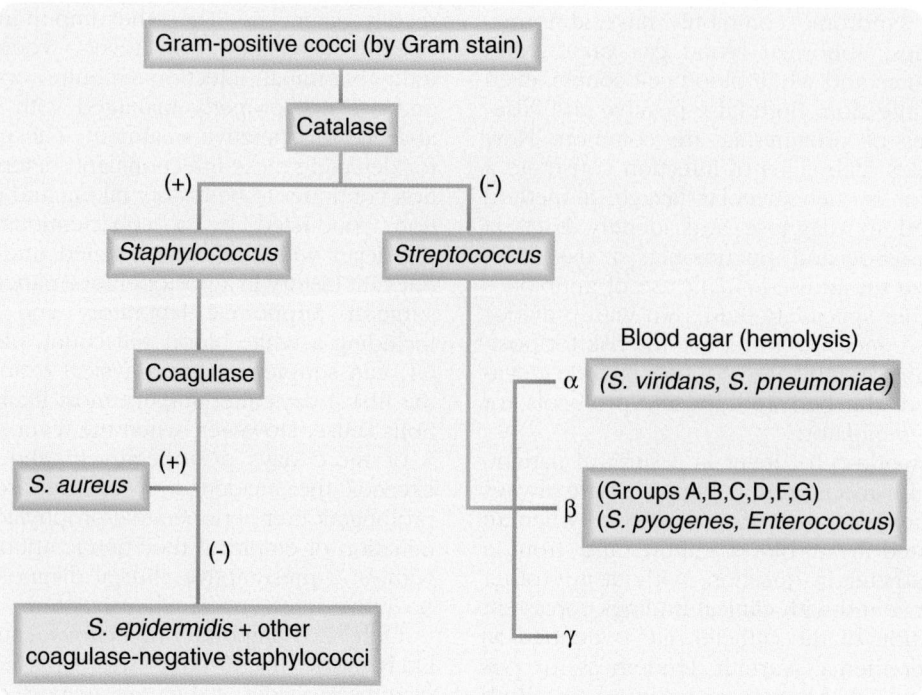

Figure 14-1 Biochemical tests used to identify specific pathogens within gram-positive cocci.

these pathogens. Bacteria important in surgical infections are broadly divided into aerobic and facultative bacteria in one group and anaerobic bacteria in the other, into gram-positive and gram-negative bacteria, and into bacilli (rods) and cocci.

It is important to recognize that the vast majority of infections occurring in surgical patients are caused by endogenous bacteria. Specific bacteria are found in specific parts of the body, and the exposed anatomic areas during a surgical procedure are usually the source of microorganisms that cause infection. It is helpful to know the normal microbial flora of the body because such knowledge helps direct prophylactic antibiotics, start intelligent empirical therapy, and suspect the origin of an unknown source of infection in patients with positive blood cultures.

It is also helpful to be familiar with the different classifications of bacteria because it can take up to 72 hours for a final culture to give the result as to specific bacteria; however, Gram stain and biochemical tests can help in providing earlier guidance regarding which group of bacteria may be responsible for an infection (Figs. 14-1 and 14-2).

Gram-Positive Cocci

Gram-positive cocci of importance to surgeons include staphylococci and streptococci. Staphylococci are divided into coagulase-positive and coagulase-negative strains. *S. aureus,* a coagulase-positive staphylococcus, is the most common pathogen associated with infections in wounds and incisions not subject to endogenous contamination. Coagulase-positive staphylococci are assumed to be

resistant to penicillin and require treatment with a penicillinase-resistant antibiotic. Extensive use of penicillinase-resistant β-lactam antibiotics in the past has encouraged the emergence of MRSA. These organisms do not seem to have intrinsic pathogenicity greater than that of other staphylococci, but they are more difficult to treat because of antibiotic resistance. The prevalence of MRSA varies considerably by geographic region but has been increasing during the past 2 decades. MRSA was initially seen primarily in hospitalized patients but is now found in an increasing number of community-acquired infections. The incidence of MRSA recovery is increased in patients coming from long-term care facilities, patients previously hospitalized or treated with antibiotics, and those with diabetes or on dialysis. These organisms are especially common in endocarditis associated with intravenous drug use. MRSA must be treated with vancomycin, quinupristin/dalfopristin, daptomycin, or linezolid. Recent years have seen the introduction of *S. aureus* strains with decreased susceptibility to vancomycin, and more recently *S. aureus* strains have been found with high-level resistance to vancomycin. If the history of other pathogens and antimicrobial agents repeats itself, the number of such strains will increase in the future.

For many years, coagulase-negative staphylococci were considered contaminants and skin flora incapable of causing serious disease. However, in the correct clinical setting, coagulase-negative staphylococci can cause serious disease, most commonly in patients who have been compromised by trauma, extensive surgery, or metabolic disease or who have invasive vascular devices in place. Coagulase-negative staphylococci are the most common organisms recovered in nosocomial bacteremia

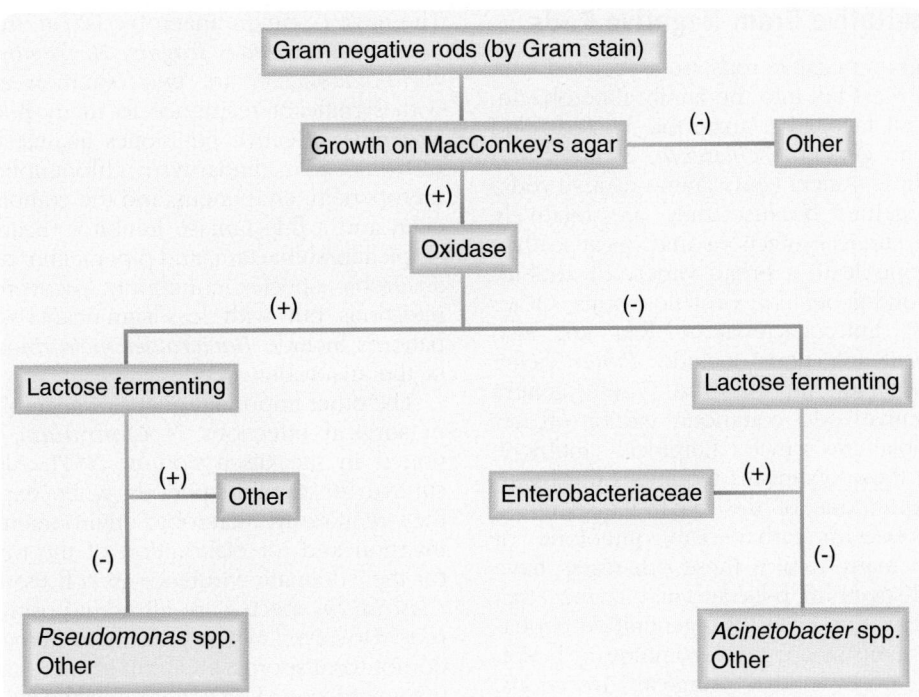

Figure 14-2 Biochemical tests used to identify specific pathogens within gram-negative rods.

and are frequently associated with clinically significant infections of intravascular devices. Coagulase-negative staphylococci are also found in endocarditis, prosthetic joint infections, vascular graft infections, and postsurgical mediastinitis. Most coagulase-negative staphylococci are methicillin resistant. Although the majority of infections associated with intravascular devices are cured simply by removing the device, if empirical antibiotic therapy is indicated, vancomycin, quinupristin/dalfopristin, daptomycin, or linezolid is chosen.

The streptococcal species include β-hemolytic streptococci (especially group A or *S. pyogenes*), *S. pneumoniae,* and other α-hemolytic streptococci. These species were initially uniformly sensitive to penicillin G and almost all other β-lactam antibiotics. Penicillin-resistant *S. pneumoniae* is now found in most urban communities. The β-hemolytic streptococci alone, though not commonly recovered from soft tissue wounds, can cause life-threatening infections. *S. pneumoniae* is a common cause of community-acquired pneumonia but is a less common pathogen in hospitalized surgical patients. The other α-hemolytic streptococci or viridans streptococci are rarely significant pathogens in a surgical setting. They are commonly found on mucous membranes and skin and may be recovered from the peritoneal cavity after upper gastrointestinal perforations, but they are almost never found as the sole cause of significant surgical infections.

The precise significance of enterococci in surgical infections is controversial. Enterococci are commonly recovered as part of a mixed flora in intra-abdominal infections. It is rare to recover enterococci alone from a surgical infection. In animal models of infection, entero-

cocci clearly can increase the virulence of other bacteria. Enterococcal bacteremia in association with a surgical infection carries a grave prognosis. The occurrence of the bacteremia itself probably signals a profound compromise of host defenses. Enterococci clearly do cause significant disease in the urinary and biliary tract and are a cause of subacute bacterial endocarditis, and they probably contribute to morbidity and mortality from intra-abdominal infections in high-risk patients with serious underlying diseases or protracted illnesses with impairment of host defenses. One recent report of patients with intra-abdominal infection found a significantly higher treatment failure rate in patients in whom enterococci were initially isolated. The stimulus for discussing the pathogenic significance of enterococci derives from the relative resistance of these species to antibiotic therapy. No single antibiotic is reliably effective in eradicating deep-seated infections or bacteremia. The most effective antibiotic combination for treating enterococcal infections is gentamicin combined with either ampicillin (or another advanced-generation penicillin) or vancomycin. However, enterococci resistant to all known antibiotics, including gentamicin and vancomycin (VRE), have been isolated in increasing numbers in most major medical centers in the United States. Isolation of VRE is especially common and carries a grave prognosis in liver transplant patients. Between 1989 and 1993 the incidence of VRE reported to the CDC increased 26-fold, whereas the incidence in ICUs increased 34-fold. The incidence of VRE infection and colonization in hospitalized patients is increased after therapy with third-generation cephalosporins and vancomycin.

Aerobic and Facultative Gram-Negative Rods

A great variety of gram-negative rods are associated with surgical infections. Most fall into the family Enterobacteriaceae. They are all facultative anaerobic bacteria and include the familiar genera *Escherichia, Proteus,* and *Klebsiella.* These three genera (*easy* gram-negative rods) are considered together because they are relatively common in mixed surgical infections and because they are generally susceptible to a broad variety of antibiotics, especially second-generation cephalosporins. Other genera within the Enterobacteriaceae that are also common in surgical infections include *Enterobacter, Morganella, Providencia,* and *Serratia.* These genera (*difficult* gram-negative rods) commonly exhibit greater intrinsic antimicrobial resistance. Empirical antibiotic therapy directed at these organisms requires a third-generation cephalosporin, one of the expanded-spectrum penicillins, a monobactam, carbapenem, quinolone, or aminoglycoside. In many locales these organisms have acquired extended-spectrum β-lactamase enzymes that are capable of inactivating even third-generation cephalosporins. These organisms are more common in hospital-acquired and postoperative surgical infections. Gram-negative rods recovered from infections originating in the community, such as uncomplicated appendicitis or diverticulitis, are less likely to involve antibiotic-resistant strains.

Obligate aerobic gram-negative rods that can be found in surgical infections include *Pseudomonas* and *Acinetobacter* species. These organisms are most commonly seen in hospital-associated pneumonia in surgical patients but may also be recovered from the peritoneal cavity or severe soft tissue infections. These species are often antibiotic resistant and require treatment with specific antipseudomonal antibiotics such as ceftazidime, cefepime, aztreonam, imipenem/cilastatin, meropenem, ciprofloxacin, an acylureidopenicillin, or an aminoglycoside. *Acinetobacter* species are resistant to aztreonam. A significant proportion of these species exhibit strains resistant to even the most effective antibiotics, and patients with such pathogens are probably best treated empirically with two antibiotics until in vitro susceptibility testing becomes available. Even after susceptibility data are known, critically ill patients may benefit from treatment with two effective agents. Bacteria from both these genera have a tendency to develop resistance to antibiotics during therapy. Although using two agents may not reduce this process, it does leave the patient with at least one effective drug when it occurs. *Stenotrophomonas maltophilia* (previously *Pseudomonas* or *Xanthomonas*) is uniformly resistant to carbapenems (imipenem, meropenem, and ertapenem) and is most commonly encountered as an emerging organism when one of these agents is used for empirical treatment of a serious infection.

Anaerobes

Anaerobic bacteria are the most numerous inhabitants of the normal gastrointestinal tract, including the mouth.

The most common anaerobic isolate from surgical infections is *Bacteroides fragilis. B. fragilis* and *Bacteroides thetaiotaomicron* are two common anaerobic species with significant resistance to many β-lactam antibiotics. The most effective antibiotics against these species are metronidazole, clindamycin, chloramphenicol, imipenem, meropenem, ertapenem, and the combinations of a penicillin and a β-lactamase inhibitor (ticarcillin/clavulanate, ampicillin/sulbactam, and piperacillin/tazobactam). Other anaerobic species commonly recovered from surgical infections but with less significant bacterial resistance patterns include *Bacteroides melaninogenicus* and most of the anaerobic cocci.

The other important genus of anaerobic bacteria found in surgical infections is *Clostridium,* previously mentioned in the discussion of NSTI. Although they can survive for variable periods while exposed to oxygen, they require an anaerobic environment for growth and invasion and for elaboration of the toxins that account for their dramatic virulence in soft tissue infections. The *Clostridium* species are all gram-positive, spore-forming rods. However, when present in human infections they do not form spores, so Gram-stained material from a soft tissue infection shows gram-positive rods without spores. *Clostridium difficile* belongs to this family, and *Clostridium tetani* is responsible for tetanus. Prevention of tetanus is accomplished solely through active and passive immunization, not through antibiotic administration.

Anaerobic bacteria have a special importance in relation to surgical infections. These strains grow only in settings with low oxidation-reduction potential, which is incompatible with the survival of mammalian tissue. Thus, recovery of anaerobes from a soft tissue infection or even from blood implies their growth and multiplication in a focus of dead tissue. The predominant source of anaerobic bacteria is the gastrointestinal tract; thus, an anaerobic infection implies a defect in the anatomic integrity of the gastrointestinal tract. Both these conditions (dead tissue and a defect in the gastrointestinal tract) require surgical correction, so the great majority of anaerobic infections (other than lung abscess) call for surgical intervention. Certainly, anaerobic bacteremia always prompts a search for an abscess or for an enteric lesion that requires surgical intervention.

Fungi

Fungi are infrequently the primary pathogens in deep-seated surgical infections. *Candida,* however, has become a relatively frequent pathogen in surgical infections over the past years. NNIS data show that it is now the fourth leading cause of bloodstream infection in hospitalized patients in the United States, and other studies show that it can be present as a source of intra-abdominal infection in 8% of cases.

Pathogens from the *Candida* genus may be seen frequently as an opportunistic invader in patients with serious surgical infections who have received broad-spectrum antibiotic treatment that suppresses normal endogenous flora. These infections are best avoided through the judicious use of systemic broad-spectrum antibiotics and by prophylaxis with oral nystatin or keto-conazole when broad-spectrum antibacterial therapy is required. *Candida* species recovered from open wounds usually represent contamination, not true invasion. Recovery of *Candida* from peptic ulcer perforations also does not usually require treatment. However, recovery of *Candida* from an established intra-abdominal abscess or from urine and sputum in an otherwise compromised patient may warrant therapy. Intra-abdominal *Candida* infections are more common in association with infections after severe pancreatitis.

Therapy for *Candida* infections in patients with multiple sites colonized or in patients with well-drained abscesses formerly required the use of amphotericin at a total dose of 3 to 5 mg/kg over a 10- to 14-day period, with all the intrinsic complications derived from the use of this nephrotoxic antimycotic. Fluconazole and the newly developed triazole voriconazole have allowed better control of *Candida* infections with more liberal indications for treatment and fewer side effects or complications. A newer drug is caspofungin. Fluconazole is usually adequate treatment of *Candida albicans*. However *Candida krusei, Candida glabrata,* and occasionally *Candida lusitaniae,* which are becoming more frequent in surgical infections, are species resistant to fluconazole, in which case the use of voriconazole, caspofungin, or amphotericin is indicated.

Virus

Viruses do not cause any infections that require surgery for resolution and thus are not discussed in any detail here. As a result of immunosuppression to prevent rejection, transplant patients are at significant risk for viral infection, especially with cytomegalovirus. Viral infections of most relevance to other surgical patients are blood-borne viruses that may be transmitted via blood transfusion: hepatitis B virus (HBV), hepatitis C virus (HCV), and HIV. Transmission of HBV and HIV by transfusion is unusual because of the use of accurate tests for screening infected units of blood. Previously, HCV was one of the most common viruses transmitted by transfusion in the medical setting, but a new serologic test for HCV has greatly reduced that risk. Cytomegalovirus is also commonly transmitted by transfusions. However, other, currently unknown blood-borne viruses are likely to be described in the future. Therefore, it is good medical practice to limit blood transfusion to circumstances clearly requiring it.

ANTIMICROBIALS

This discussion of antibiotics is not intended to be exhaustive. Rather, it focuses on the antibiotics that are most commonly indicated for the treatment of patients with surgical infections. Table 14-9 lists these antibiotics with their relative half-lives, mechanism of action, important toxicities, and general antibacterial spectra. Several handy references are updated yearly and provide more detailed information regarding all commercially available antibiotics, including doses and dose ranges, pharmacokinetic data, sensitivity patterns, incompatibilities, and excretion data.

General Principles

Whichever antibiotics are administered, the goal of therapy is to achieve antibiotic levels at the site of infection that exceed the minimum inhibitory concentration for the pathogens present. For mild infections, including most that can be handled on an outpatient basis, this concentration may be achievable with oral antibiotics when appropriate choices are available. For severe surgical infections, however, the systemic response to infection may make gastrointestinal absorption of antibiotics unpredictable and thus antibiotic levels unreliable. In addition, for intra-abdominal infections, gastrointestinal function is often directly impaired. For this reason, most initial antibiotic therapy for surgical infections is begun intravenously.

Each patient with a serious infection is evaluated daily or more frequently to assess response to treatment. If obvious improvement is not seen within 2 to 3 days, one often hears the question, "Which antibiotic should we add/switch to?" That question is appropriate, however, only after the following question has been addressed: Why is the patient failing to improve? Probable answers include the following:

1. The initial operative procedure was not adequate.
2. The initial procedure was adequate but a complication has occurred.
3. A superinfection has developed at a new site.
4. The drug choice is correct, but not enough is being given.
5. Another or a different drug is needed.

The choice of antibiotics is not the most common cause of failure unless the original choice was clearly inappropriate, such as failing to provide coverage for anaerobes with an intra-abdominal infection.

As the patient improves, one must decide when to stop antibiotic therapy. For most surgical infections there is no specific duration of antibiotics that is known to be ideal. Antibiotics generally support local host defenses until the local responses are sufficient to limit further infection. When an abscess is drained, the antibiotics prevent invasive bacterial infection in the fresh tissue planes opened in the course of drainage. After 3 to 5 days, the local responses of new capillary formation and inflammatory infiltrate provide a competent local defense. For deep-seated or poorly localized infections, longer treatment may be needed. A reliable guideline is to continue antibiotics until the patient has shown obvious clinical improvement based on clinical examination and has had a normal temperature for 48 hours or longer. Signs of improvement include improved mental status, return of bowel function, resolution of tachycardia, and spontaneous diuresis. A shorter course of antibiotics may be sufficient, but data supporting a specific duration are not available.

Text continued on p 322

Table 14-9   Antibiotics Commonly Used in Surgical Infections

DRUG CLASS AND NAME	MECHANISM OF ACTION	COMMENT	HALF-LIFE	TOXICITY	ANTIBACTERIAL SPECTRUM
Penicillins					
Penicillin G	β-Lactam mechanism: inhibits bacterial cell wall by binding to penicillin-binding proteins (PBPs). It inhibits the final transpeptidation step of peptidoglycan synthesis in the bacterial cell wall	Prototype. Hydrolyzed by all β-lactamases	Short	Low, but rarely an allergic reaction may be life threatening	Streptococcal species except enterococci and penicillin-resistant pneumococci, *Neisseria* species except lactamase-producing gonococci
Antistaphylococcal					
Methicillin	β-Lactam mechanism. Also penicillinase resistant and acid stable	First antistaphylococcal drug	Short	Interstitial nephritis	Staphylococcal species (methicillin sensitive) and streptococcal species except enterococcus
Oxacillin			Short	Interstitial nephritis	Narrow spectrum; generally used for staphylococcal infections only
Nafcillin			Short	Interstitial nephritis	
"Easy" gram-negative					
Ampicillin	β-Lactam mechanism	Hydrolyzed by all β-lactamases	Short	Low; diarrhea and rash	Streptococcal species, including many enterococci, *Neisseria* species (non–lactamase producing), *Haemophilus influenzae* (non–lactamase producing), some *Escherichia coli* and *Proteus mirabilis*
Amoxicillin			Medium		
Expanded spectrum					
Carbenicillin	β-Lactam mechanism	Hydrolyzed by all β-lactamases	Short	High sodium load. Inhibition of platelet aggregation	Greatly expanded gram-negative spectrum while still active against streptococcal species, including enterococci. Moderate antianaerobe activity. May not be reliable as the sole agent for established gram-negative rod infections
Ticarcillin	β-Lactam mechanism	Same	Short		Same, but less activity against enterococci
Very advanced spectrum					
Mezlocillin	β-Lactam mechanism	Hydrolyzed by all β-lactamases	Short	Low	Same as expanded-spectrum penicillins but with more activity against *Pseudomonas, Acinetobacter,* and *Serratia* species
Piperacillin		Same	Short	Low	

Table 14-9 Antibiotics Commonly Used in Surgical Infections—cont'd

DRUG CLASS AND NAME	MECHANISM OF ACTION	COMMENT	HALF-LIFE	TOXICITY	ANTIBACTERIAL SPECTRUM
β-Lactamase inhibitor combination	β-Lactam mechanism, plus			Low; same as constituent β-lactam	
Clavulanic acid plus	Clavulanic acid mechanism: β-lactamase inhibitor that increases the antibacterial activity of β-lactam antibiotics				
Ticarcillin			Short		Same as ticarcillin or amoxicillin plus staphylococci (methicillin sensitive), lactamase-positive *H. influenzae* and some lactamase-producing gram-negative rods, and anaerobes
Amoxicillin		Oral only	Medium		
Sulbactam plus	β-Lactam mechanism, plus	IV only	Short		
Ampicillin	Sulbactam mechanism: forms enzyme-sulbactam complex that inhibits β-lactamases				Similar to cefoxitin with activity against enterococci
Tazobactam plus	β-Lactam mechanism, plus		Short		
Piperacillin	Tazobactam mechanism: inhibits β-lactamases. More potent than sulbactam or clavulanic acid				Similar to piperacillin plus staphylococci (methicillin sensitive), some lactamase-producing gram-negative rods, and anaerobes
Cephalosporins					
"First" generation	β-Lactam mechanism				Streptococcal species except enterococci, staphylococcal species (methicillin sensitive), and "easy" gram-negative rods
Short half-life					
Cephalothin		Prototype of class	Short	Low	
Cephapirin			Short	Low	
Longer half-life					
Cefazolin			Medium	Low	
"Second" generation	β-Lactam mechanism				Same as first-generation cephalosporins with expanded gram-negative activity not including *Pseudomonas, Acinetobacter,* or *Serratia*
Poor anaerobic activity					
Shorter half-life					
Cefamandole			Short	Low	
Cefuroxime			Medium	Low	
Longer half-life					
Ceforanide			Long		
Cefonicid		Reduced antistaphylococcal activity	Long		

Continued

Table 14-9   Antibiotics Commonly Used in Surgical Infections—cont'd

DRUG CLASS AND NAME	MECHANISM OF ACTION	COMMENT	HALF-LIFE	TOXICITY	ANTIBACTERIAL SPECTRUM
Good anaerobic activity					Same as above, plus many anaerobes
Short half-life					
Cefoxitin			Short	Low	
Longer half-life					
Cefmetazole			Medium	Low	
Cefotetan			Long	Prolonged prothrombin times	
"Third" generation	β-Lactam mechanism				Very active against most gram-negative rods except *Pseudomonas, Acinetobacter,* and *Serratia.* Poor against anaerobes. Less activity against streptococcal and staphylococcal species than first- and second-generation cephalosporins.
Poor *Pseudomonas* activity					
Short half-life					
Cefotaxime			Short	Low	
Ceftizoxime			Medium	Low	
Long half-life					
Ceftriaxone			Long	Low	
Good *Pseudomonas* activity					
Cefoperazone			Medium	Low	Same as above plus activity against many *Pseudomonas, Acinetobacter,* and *Serratia* species
Ceftazidime			Medium	Low	
Cefepime			Medium	Low	Same as above with increased activity against gram-positive cocci
Monobactams					
Aztreonam	β-Lactam mechanism: preference to PBP-3 of gram-negative bacteria. Very stable against β-lactamases	Safe for most patients with penicillin allergy	Short	Low	Excellent activity against most gram-negatives, including *Pseudomonas* and *Serratia.* Inactive against gram-positive cocci, anaerobes, and most *Acinetobacter* strains
Carbapenems	β-Lactam mechanism, plus				
Imipenem/cilastatin	Cilastatin mechanism: inactivates dehydropeptidases, which would normally break the β-lactam ring of imipenem in the proximal tubule	Provided in combination with cilastatin to prevent renal breakdown and renal toxicity	Short	Low. Seizures in certain high-risk patients	Extremely broad gram-positive and gram-negative aerobic and anaerobic. Modest activity against enterococci. Inactive against *Stenotrophomonas* (formerly *Xanthomonas*) *maltophilia*
Meropenem		Provided alone without cilastatin	Short	Reduced potential for seizures	Same activity as imipenem

Table 14-9   Antibiotics Commonly Used in Surgical Infections—cont'd

DRUG CLASS AND NAME	MECHANISM OF ACTION	COMMENT	HALF-LIFE	TOXICITY	ANTIBACTERIAL SPECTRUM
Ertapenem		Provided alone without cilastatin	Long	Low	Better activity against Enterobacteriaceae, less activity against gram-positive cocci, *Pseudomonas, Acinetobacter,* and anaerobes
Quinolones					
Poor anaerobic activity	Inhibit bacterial enzyme DNA-gyrase, thus inhibiting DNA replication				
Norfloxacin		Oral only; urine levels only	Long	Low Interaction leads to accumulation of theophylline	Very broad Gram-negative activity. Gram-positive and very broad gram-negative activity, including *Pseudomonas, Acinetobacter,* and *Serratia.* Poor activity against anaerobes
Ciprofloxacin		Oral and intravenous (applies to all below)	Long		
Ofloxacin		Racemic mixture of levofloxacin (active) and dextrofloxacin (inactive)	Long		
Levofloxacin			Long		
Better anaerobic activity Gatifloxacin			Very long		As above plus better gram-positive and anaerobe coverage
Moxifloxacin			Very long		Broad spectrum against gram-positive, gram-negative, and anaerobes
Aminoglycosides	Bind to a specific protein in the 30S subunit of the bacterial ribosome, which leads to faulty alignment or recognition by RNA during initiation of microbial peptide chain formation	All have a low ratio of therapeutic-to-toxic levels. All are frequently underdosed. All exhibit a significant postantibiotic effect*	Medium	Nephrotoxicity and nerve VIII toxicity, both auditory and vestibular	Extremely broad coverage of gram-negative rods. Poor activity against streptococci. Some synergism with penicillin or vancomycin against enterococci. No activity against anaerobes
Gentamicin		See above	Medium	See above	Most active against enterococci and *Serratia* spp.
Tobramycin		See above	Medium	Statistically but questionably clinically significant decrease in nephrotoxicity	More active against *Pseudomonas* spp.
Amikacin		See above	Medium	See above (aminoglycosides)	Active against a significant number of gentamicin- and tobramycin-resistant organisms

Continued

Table 14-9 Antibiotics Commonly Used in Surgical Infections—cont'd

DRUG CLASS AND NAME	MECHANISM OF ACTION	COMMENT	HALF-LIFE	TOXICITY	ANTIBACTERIAL SPECTRUM
Netilmicin		See above	Medium	See above (aminoglycosides)	See above (aminoglycosides)
Other Antianaerobes					
Chloramphenicol	Inhibits bacterial protein synthesis by reversibly attaching to the 50S subunit of the 70S bacterial ribosome	Oral or IV	Long[†]	Dose-dependent, reversible bone marrow suppression Rare (1/25000-40000) irreversible bone marrow aplasia	Many gram-positive and easy gram-negative rods, *H. influenzae,* most anaerobes
Clindamycin	Inhibits bacterial protein synthesis by attaching to the 50S subunit of the bacterial ribosome	Oral or IV	Long[†]	Linked to *Clostridium difficile* diarrhea	Streptococcal species except enterococci, staphylococci, most anaerobes. Inactive against gram-negative rods
Metronidazole	Not fully elucidated Seems to produce cytotoxic effects on anaerobes by a reduction reaction (nitro group of metronidazole)	Oral or IV	Very long[†]	Disulfiram-type (Antabuse) reaction. Peripheral neuropathy with prolonged use	Very active against most anaerobes. Inactive against facultative and aerobic bacteria. Active against protozoa (amoebae and *Giardia*)
Glycopeptides					
Vancomycin	Inhibits cell wall synthesis by binding to carboxyl subunits on peptide subunits containing free D-alanyl-D-alanine (different site from β-lactams—no cross resistance), plus may affect permeability of membrane, plus may inhibit RNA synthesis	Only IV. No oral absorption	Very long	Hypotension and histamine release phenomena (redman syndrome) during infusion. Nephrotoxicity and ototoxicity	Streptococcal species, including many enterococci, staphylococci (including methicillin-resistant strains), *Clostridium* species. No activity against gram-negative rods
Streptogramins					
Quinupristin/dalfopristin	Binds to different sites on the 50S subunit of bacterial ribosomes A 5- to 10-fold decrease in the dissociation constant of quinupristin is seen in the presence of dalfopristin	Significant postantibiotic effect*	Medium	Reversible transaminase elevations	Most gram-positive pathogens, including vancomycin-resistant *Enterococcus faecium,* methicillin-resistant *Staphylococcus aureus* and *Staphylococcus epidermidis,* and penicillin-resistant *Streptococcus pneumoniae* but not *Enterococcus faecalis*
Oxazolidinones					
Linezolid	Attaches to the 50S subunit of the bacterial ribosome and inhibits protein synthesis	Oral or IV	Long	Reversible monoamine oxidase inhibition with the potential to interact with adrenergic or	Most gram-positive bacteria, including methicillin-resistant *S. aureus* and vancomycin-resistant enterococci

Table 14-9 Antibiotics Commonly Used in Surgical Infections—cont'd

DRUG CLASS AND NAME	MECHANISM OF ACTION	COMMENT	HALF-LIFE	TOXICITY	ANTIBACTERIAL SPECTRUM
				serotoninergic drugs and cause hypertension Reversible myelosuppression with thrombocytopenia, anemia, and leukopenia	
Macrolides Erythromycin	Attaches to the 50S subunit of the bacterial ribosome and may interfere with translocation reactions of the peptide chains	Oral or IV	Medium	Cholestasis with estolate (IV) form	Most gram-positive, *Neisseria*, *Campylobacter*, *Mycoplasma*, *Chlamydia*, *Rickettsia*, *Legionella*
Tetracyclines Tetracycline	Inhibit protein synthesis by attaching to the 30S subunit of the bacterial ribosome	Oral or IV	Long	Stain teeth of children	Many gram-positive, easy gram-negative rods, some anaerobes, *Rickettsia*, *Chlamydia*, *Mycoplasma*
Doxycycline		Oral or IV	Very long	Same	
Glycylcyclines Tigecycline	Inhibit protein synthesis by attaching to the 30S subunit of the bacterial ribosome	IV	Long	No major toxicities described yet	Good against multidrug-resistant staphylococci and streptococci (including enterococci). No *Pseudomonas* coverage
Antifungal Triazoles Fluconazole	Inhibition of cytochrome P-450–dependent ergosterol synthesis	Oral or IV	Very long	Elevation of liver function test result	Most fungi except *Candida krusei*, *Candida glabrata*
Voriconazole			Long	Visual disturbances, fever	Most fungi
Polyenes Amphotericin B	Binds to sterols of cell wall and interferes with permeability	IV	Very long	Nephrotoxicity, fevers and chills	Most fungi
Echinocandins Caspofungin	Inhibits β-glucan synthase, disrupts integrity of the cell wall, and causes cell lysis	IV	Very long	Fever. Infusion-related complications	Most fungi

Drugs have been grouped into those with short, medium, long, and very long half-lives. Drugs with a short half-life usually have a half-life of 1 hour or less and are commonly administered every 3 to 6 hours, depending on the severity of the infection and the sensitivity of the pathogen. Drugs with a medium half-life usually have half-lives of 1 to 2 hours and are administered every 6 to 12 hours, most commonly every 8 hours. Drugs with a long half-life have half-lives longer than 2 hours and are usually administered every 12 to 24 hours. Drugs with a very long half-life usually have half-lives longer than 6 to 8 hours and can safely be administered every 24 hours in most cases. Amphotericin with a half-life of approximately 24 hours can be administered every other day.

*Postantibiotic effect is an effect of certain antibiotics that results in inhibition of bacterial growth for several hours *after* the antibiotic levels have fallen below the minimum inhibitory concentration.

‡Chloramphenicol, clindamycin, and metronidazole all have half-lives longer than 2 hours but have traditionally been administered at 6- to 8-hour intervals because of historical factors rather than pharmacokinetics.

The recent availability of potent systemic antibiotics that can be given orally has led to some studies demonstrating that patients with intra-abdominal and other serious infections can be treated initially with parenteral antibiotics and then switched to oral antibiotics to complete their antibiotic course. This practice has the potential to reduce overall costs of antibiotic treatment, but it also carries the risk of unnecessarily increasing the duration of antibiotic treatment. Some physicians have succumbed to the temptation to send patients home with oral antibiotics because it is easy, when previously, the same patient would have been sent home without any antibiotics at all. This temptation needs to be resisted.

The white blood cell count may not have returned to normal when antibiotic therapy is stopped. If the white blood cell count is normal, the likelihood of further infectious problems is small. If the white blood cell count is elevated, further infections may be detected, but in most cases they will not be prevented by continuing antibiotics. Rather, a new infection requires drainage or different antibiotics for a new, resistant pathogen in a different location. In this case, the best approach is to stop the existing drugs and observe the patient closely for subsequent developments.

When choosing an antibiotic for empirical treatment, follow these guidelines:

1. Ensure coverage of the presumed microorganisms involved. This usually means starting broad-spectrum antibiotics, which can then be tailored and narrowed to the specific microorganism isolated. Avoid anaerobic-spectrum antibiotics when possible because this group of bacteria plays an important role in maintaining the gastrointestinal tract microenvironment.
2. Choose an antibiotic that is able to reach the site of the infection. Specifically, for UTI and cholangitis, choose antibiotics with high renal and biliary concentrations, respectively. Consider skin, lung, and central nervous system tissue concentrations for infections at these sites.
3. Consider toxicity, particularly in critically ill patients, in whom bioavailability and the range of therapeutic and toxic levels are harder to predict. Once an antimicrobial with significant toxic side effects is started, closely monitor blood levels and organ function.
4. Whenever an infection that will need antibiotics is identified, aggressively dose the antibiotics. The volume of redistribution of these patients is unpredictable because they have usually undergone aggressive fluid replacements as part of their support or resuscitation.
5. Whenever starting an antibiotic regimen, set a time limit for the period the antibiotic will be given.

Superinfection

A superinfection is a new infection that develops during antibiotic treatment of the original infection. Whenever antibiotics are used, they exert selective pressure on the endogenous flora of the patient and on exogenous bacteria that colonize sites at risk. Bacteria that remain are resistant to the antibiotics being used and become the pathogens in superinfection. Respiratory tract infections are common superinfections that occur during the treatment of intra-abdominal infection. The greater the severity of the abdominal infection and the greater the risk of a poor outcome, the greater the risk for pneumonia as well.

Careful surveillance of hospitalized patients reveals superinfections in 2% to 10% of antibiotic-treated patients, depending on their underlying risk factors. The best preventive action is to limit the dose and duration of antibiotic treatment to what is obviously required and to be alert to the possibility of superinfection. The use of increasingly powerful and broad-spectrum antibiotics during the past 2 decades has also led to an increasing incidence of fungal superinfections.

Antibiotic-associated colitis is another significant superinfection that can occur in hospitalized patients with mild to serious illness. This entity is caused by the enteric pathogen *C. difficile* and has been reported after treatment with every antibiotic except vancomycin. *C. difficile* colitis can vary from a mild, self-limited disease to a rapidly progressive septic process culminating in death. The most important step in treating this disease is to suspect it. The diagnosis is best accomplished by detecting *C. difficile* toxin in stool. In severe cases, endoscopy to reveal the typical mucosal changes of inflammation, ulceration, and plaque formation can lead to more rapid diagnosis of the severe form of the disease, pseudomembranous colitis. Treatment is supportive and consists of fluid and electrolytes, withdrawal of the offending antibiotic if possible, and oral metronidazole to treat the superinfection. Reserve vancomycin for metronidazole failures. In rare instances when overwhelming colitis does not respond to medical management, emergency colectomy may be required.

Antibiotic Resistance

Antibiotic resistance is an escalating problem, particularly in patients in ICUs. Its implications include longer length of stay, higher cost of care, and more importantly, increased morbidity and mortality derived from infections treated unsuccessfully.

Resistance has been broadly divided into two forms, intrinsic resistance, in which a specific species is inherently resistant to a specific antibiotic (e.g., gram-negative bacteria resistant to vancomycin), and acquired resistance, in which a change in the genetic composition of the bacteria occurs. This acquired resistance can be the result of intrinsic changes within the native genetic material of the pathogen or can be transferred from another species.

The molecular mechanisms by which bacteria acquire resistance to antibiotics can be broadly classified into four categories[53]:

1. Decreased intracellular concentration of antibiotic, either by decreased influx or increased efflux. Most antibiotics are susceptible to this mechanism (*Pseudomonas*/Enterobacteriaceae to β-lactams).

2. Neutralization by inactivating enzymes. This is the most common mechanism of antibiotic resistance and affects all β-lactam antibiotics (e.g. β-lactamases from gram-positive and gram-negative bacteria).
3. Alteration of the target at which the antibiotic will act. This category affects all antibiotics and is the main resistance mechanism for some specific bacteria (*Pneumococcus* to penicillin or MRSA to all β-lactam antibiotics).
4. Complete elimination of the target at which the antibiotic will act. Some specific bacteria develop the ability to create new metabolic pathways and completely eliminate a specific target (e.g., VRE).

Antibiotic resistance is usually achieved by a combination of these different mechanisms. However, the presence of one of them may confer resistance to one or more different group of antibiotics.

The bacterial genome is divided into chromosomal DNA, which gives specific characteristics and metabolic pathways to the bacteria, and smaller, circular and independent DNA elements (plasmids) that encode information for supplemental bacterial activities such as virulence factors and resistance mechanisms. Most resistance mechanisms are plasmid mediated, although they can interchange with chromosomal information (with the aid of transposons, or mobile DNA elements) conferring more fixed mechanisms, which will be transmitted vertically. However, plasmids can also be transmitted horizontally through conjugation, transduction, and transformation processes in which different bacteria are exposed to a specific plasmid.

Risk factors for antibiotic resistance in a specific patient include the use of antibiotics, prolonged hospital stay, administration of broad-spectrum antibiotics, use of invasive devices (endotracheal tubes, central lines, Foley catheters, etc.), and the presence of outbreaks, which may reflect ineffective infection control policies. The population at highest risk are ICU patients, in whom the potential absence of effective antibiotic treatment correlates with higher mortality rates.

Prevention strategies have been studied, and although it is difficult to establish a clear relationship between their practice and decreased resistance, such strategies need to be part of a discipline that not only reduces the incidence of antibiotic resistance but also follows a logical practice for infection control and use of antibiotics. Some of these strategies include guidelines for the use of antibiotics (hospital formulary restriction, use of narrow-spectrum antibiotics, antibiotic cycling, use of new antibiotics), assessment of infection risk and quantitative cultures, consultation with infectious disease specialists, and area-specific use of antibiotics (outpatients versus nosocomial, hospital-to-hospital difference, etc.). Nonantibiotic strategies include prevention of nosocomial infections (general and specific measures) and prevention of hospital transmission (hand washing, contact precautions). The battle against antibiotic resistance is definitely multidisciplinary and involves the development of new antibiotics, as well as strategies in the everyday care of patients from all health care personnel.[53,54]

Specific Antimicrobials

Penicillins

The penicillins are broadly divided into those that are stable against staphylococcal penicillinase and all others. The antistaphylococcal penicillins are active against methicillin-susceptible staphylococcal species but have reduced activity against streptococcal species and essentially no activity against gram-negative rods or anaerobic bacteria. All the remaining penicillins are readily hydrolyzed by staphylococcal penicillinase and are therefore unreliable for treating staphylococcal infections. They all have excellent activity against other gram-positive cocci except for enterococci, which are variably resistant. The major difference among these penicillins is in their spectrum of aerobic and facultative gram-negative rod activity. The more advanced acylureidopenicillins are very active against this group, including the *difficult* gram-negative rods.

Recently, various penicillins have been combined with one of the β-lactamase inhibitors clavulanic acid, sulbactam, or tazobactam. These combinations provide antibiotic compounds that retain their broad gram-negative activity while also acting against methicillin-sensitive staphylococci and anaerobes, facultative species, and aerobic bacteria that are resistant to the penicillins by virtue of β-lactamase production. The β-lactamases produced by some *E. coli* and by *Pseudomonas, Enterobacter, Citrobacter,* and *Serratia* species, however, are not susceptible to these inhibitors, so these organisms are not susceptible to antibiotic combinations that rely on β-lactamase inhibition unless they are susceptible to the antibiotic alone.

Cephalosporins

The cephalosporin class is the largest and most frequently used group of antibiotics. It is commonly divided into three *generations,* but there are also important differences between members within each generation. The first-generation cephalosporins have excellent activity against methicillin-susceptible staphylococci and all streptococcal species, but not against enterococci. No cephalosporin in any generation has reliable activity against enterococci, and indeed many cephalosporins seem to encourage enterococcal overgrowth. The first-generation cephalosporins also have modest activity against the *easy* Enterobacteriaceae, such as *E. coli, Proteus mirabilis,* and many *Klebsiella* species. The only important difference between members of the first generation is in half-life. Cefazolin, with its longer half-life, can be given every 8 hours rather than every 4 to 6 hours and maintains more reliable serum and tissue levels when used for prophylaxis than the other members of this class do.

The second-generation cephalosporins have expanded gram-negative activity when compared with the first generation but still lack activity against many gram-negative rods. They can be used when susceptibility patterns are known or when community-acquired infections with a low probability of antibiotic-resistant bacteria are being treated. This class of antibiotics is not reliable for empirical treatment of hospital-acquired gram-negative rod infections. The most important distinction within the second generation is between antibiotics with good activity against anaerobes (cefoxitin and cefotetan) and those without important anaerobic activity (cefamandole, cefuroxime, ceforanide, and cefonicid). Within each of these groups are antibiotics with relatively short half-lives (cefamandole and cefoxitin) and with relatively longer half-lives (cefuroxime, cefotetan, ceforanide, and cefonicid).

The third-generation cephalosporins have greatly expanded activity against gram-negative rods, including many resistant strains, and rival the aminoglycosides in their coverage while having a much more favorable safety profile. In exchange for this gram-negative coverage, most members of this group have significantly less activity against staphylococcal and streptococcal species than first- and second-generation cephalosporins do. Anaerobic coverage is generally rather poor as well. The important distinction in the third-generation cephalosporins is between those with significant activity against *Pseudomonas* species (cefoperazone, ceftazidime, and cefepime) and those without (cefotaxime, ceftizoxime, and ceftriaxone). The use of third-generation cephalosporins has been associated with an increased incidence of VRE in critically ill patients. Their use against specific gram-negative rods has also been shown to promote the release of endotoxin and increase the concentration of tumor necrosis factor, which is related to a so-called septic response after the antibiotic has been given. These disadvantages are becoming more important and could potentially be avoided with the use of a different type of antibiotic that has a similar or even broader spectrum—something worth considering once an antibiotic is going to be chosen.

Monobactams

Aztreonam is the only currently available member of the class of monobactams. It has gram-negative coverage, including many *Pseudomonas* species, similar to the aminoglycosides, and like the aminoglycosides lacks significant activity against gram-positive cocci and anaerobes. It also lacks activity against most *Acinetobacter* species. Aztreonam has the safety profile of other β-lactam antibiotics but does not cross-react in patients who are allergic to penicillins or cephalosporins.

Carbapenems

Imipenem and meropenem are the first representatives of the class of carbapenems. They have a very broad spectrum of antibacterial activity with excellent activity against all gram-positive cocci except for methicillin-resistant staphylococci and only modest activity against enterococci. They are very active against all anaerobic bacteria, with broad activity against gram-negative rods, including most *Pseudomonas* species, but they are inactive against *Pseudomonas cepacia* and *S. maltophilia* (formerly *Pseudomonas* or *Xanthomonas*), and strains of indole-positive *Proteus* are often resistant. As with all other antibiotics, *Pseudomonas* species have an unfortunate propensity to develop resistance during treatment. Imipenem is provided only in combination with the enzyme inhibitor cilastatin, which prevents its hydrolysis

in the kidneys and resultant nephrotoxicity. Meropenem is given without a renal enzyme inhibitor. More recently, ertapenem, a newer carbapenem, has become available. It differs from its predecessors in that it has to be given only once a day because it has a longer half-life. It does not require cilastatin because it is resistant to hydrolysis in the kidneys and its spectrum seems to be better against most enterobacteria but less active than imipenem against some gram-positive cocci, *Pseudomonas* species, and *Acinetobacter* species.

Quinolones

In recent years a large number of new fluoroquinolone antibiotics have been developed, with six currently available. The currently available members of this class are norfloxacin, which has useful levels only in urine, and ciprofloxacin, ofloxacin, levofloxacin, gatifloxacin, and moxifloxacin, which are effective against sensitive pathogens throughout the body. As a class, the fluoroquinolones are marked by extremely broad activity against gram-negative rods, including many *Pseudomonas* species. This activity has, however, decreased in recent years with increasing numbers of resistant gram-negative rods. Most also have relatively broad activity against gram-positive cocci, including some methicillin-resistant staphylococci, although there is insufficient clinical information to recommend their routine use against methicillin-resistant staphylococci. Activity against anaerobes is poor for all fluoroquinolones except moxifloxacin, which has good activity in this area, as well as against gram-positive cocci (better than other quinolones), although its spectrum against some Enterobacteriaceae and *Pseudomonas* species may be reduced in comparison to ciprofloxacin. The fluoroquinolones other than norfloxacin are distinguished by excellent tissue penetration and comparable serum and tissue levels with either intravenous or oral administration.

Aminoglycosides

For many years the aminoglycoside class of antibiotics was the only reliable class of drugs for the empirical treatment of serious gram-negative infections. The availability of third-generation cephalosporins, advanced-generation penicillins, monobactams, carbapenems, and now fluoroquinolones has greatly reduced the instances in which aminoglycosides must be used. As a class, aminoglycosides have very broad activity against aerobic and facultative gram-negative rods. They have relatively indifferent activity against gram-positive cocci but are an important component of synergistic therapy against some enterococci when combined with a penicillin or vancomycin. Aminoglycosides have no activity against anaerobes or against facultative bacteria in an anaerobic environment.

Clinically, aminoglycosides are difficult to use because the ratio of therapeutic levels to toxic levels is low, approximately 2:3. The primary toxicities are nephrotoxicity and eighth nerve damage, both auditory and vestibular. Aminoglycosides distribute in interstitial fluid, a body compartment that varies significantly with disease and is greatly enlarged in patients with life-threatening infections. Therefore, aminoglycoside doses and intervals of administration need to be tailored to the individual patient, and the results must be confirmed by determination of serum levels. No nomogram or dosing scheme has been sufficiently reliable to recommend without such testing. In routine clinical practice it has been far more common to find inadequate levels of aminoglycosides than toxic levels. Because of these difficulties, many clinicians now reserve aminoglycosides for specific treatment of known resistant organisms or as part of a synergistic combination to treat serious enterococcal infections or certain gram-negative rod infections. More recent data suggest that once-daily administration of aminoglycosides is as effective as the more traditional dosing of two or three times per day and is less toxic.

Antianaerobes

The antibiotics with important antianaerobic activity are not logically grouped except by this characteristic. The oldest effective antianaerobic drug is chloramphenicol. It is still very active against most anaerobic pathogens by in vitro testing but is uncommonly used because of its potential for bone marrow toxicity. Clindamycin possesses activity against most anaerobic bacteria, as well as most gram-positive bacteria. Its complete lack of activity against gram-negative aerobic and facultative rods means that it must be used in combination with another antibiotic to cover the pathogens that commonly accompany anaerobes in clinical infections. Its spectrum against *Bacteroides* species is not as good as that of metronidazole. In animal models, clindamycin improves the outcome of infections caused by toxin-producing clostridia, streptococci, or staphylococci, presumably by inhibiting the production and release of exotoxins.

Metronidazole currently possesses the most complete activity against all anaerobic pathogens. However, it has no activity against any aerobic or facultative pathogens, either gram-negative or gram-positive, so it must always be combined with another antibiotic for complete coverage. Because it has no activity against gram-positive cocci, as clindamycin does, its combination with aztreonam in the treatment of mixed aerobic and anaerobic infections leaves this potentially important group of pathogens uncovered. For this reason, metronidazole is theoretically better combined with a third-generation cephalosporin or a fluoroquinolone. Metronidazole is active against *C. difficile*. Other antibiotics with important antianaerobic activity, including cefoxitin, cefotetan, the penicillin–β-lactamase inhibitor combinations, the carbapenems, tigecycline, and moxifloxacin, are discussed elsewhere.

Macrolides

Erythromycin is a macrolide antibiotic with only modest antianaerobic activity in the concentrations that can be achieved systemically. It has found widespread use, however, as an oral agent (erythromycin base) in combination with an aminoglycoside to reduce numbers of bacteria in the lumen of the bowel before operations on the colon. In the concentrations achieved within the lumen of the colon, it markedly suppresses anaerobic growth. Erythromycin is also active against many gram-positive cocci and *Neisseria* species. For this reason it is sometimes used as an alternative agent for patients allergic to penicillins. In addition, it has significant activity against *Mycoplasma, Chlamydia, Legionella* species, and *Rickettsia.* It is also an effective antibiotic against *Campylobacter jejuni.* Clarithromycin and azithromycin are two more recent macrolides with expanded antimicrobial spectra that are available only in oral formulations.

Tetracyclines

Tetracyclines were previously an important class of antibiotics with significant antianaerobic activity. In addition to activity against anaerobes, tetracyclines possess modest activity against easy gram-negative rods and many gram-positive cocci. Currently, other agents are preferable as first and second choices for the overwhelming majority of surgical infections

Glycylcyclines

The first glycylcycline, a class related to tetracyclines, is tigecycline. It is a new class of antibiotics with good gram-positive and gram-negative coverage. One of its advantages is that its activity extends to multidrug-resistant *S. aureus, S. pneumoniae,* and vancomycin-resistant enterococci and staphylococci with reduced susceptibility to glycopeptides. It allows single-agent therapy for soft tissue and some intra-abdominal infections. Its main limitation is its poor activity against *Pseudomonas* species.

Glycopeptides

Vancomycin is the only glycopeptide antibiotic available in the United States, whereas teicoplanin is also available in Europe. It is active against essentially all gram-positive cocci, especially methicillin-resistant staphylococci, for which it is one of only four reliable antibiotics. It also has moderate activity against enterococci. Vancomycin is active against most *Clostridium* species, especially *C. difficile,* the primary pathogen responsible for antibiotic-associated diarrhea. However, it is not used as a first-line agent against *C. difficile* diarrhea because of the risk that the incidence of VRE will be increased. Several new glycopeptide antibiotics are in development, and some of them may be effective against vancomycin-resistant staphylococci and enterococci.

Streptogramins

The first water-soluble streptogramin antibiotic is actually a combination, quinupristin/dalfopristin. It is active against nearly all gram-positive pathogens, including vancomycin-resistant *E. faecium* (but not *E. faecalis*), multidrug-resistant *S. aureus,* and penicillin-resistant *S. pneumoniae.*

Oxazolidinones

The first representative of the class oxazolidinone is linezolid. This drug is active against nearly all gram-positive bacteria, including VRE and vancomycin-intermediate *S. aureus.* In addition, linezolid is quite active against many anaerobic bacterial species. It is available in both parenteral and oral forms.

Antifungals

Triazoles are a type of antifungal that acts on cell wall function through inhibition of cytochrome P-450–dependant ergosterol synthesis. Fluconazole is the triazole most commonly used in surgical patients. It has a good spectrum against *Cryptococcus* and most *Candida* species, although *C. krusei* and other subtypes have been reported to be resistant to this drug. Its use in surgical patients includes treatment of systemic *Candida* infection, as well as prophylaxis in high-risk patients. Voriconazole is a newly developed triazole with a broader spectrum than fluconazole. It has excellent activity against all *Candida* species, including *C. krusei, C. glabrata, C. tropicalis,* and *C. parapsilosis,* which often exhibit significant resistance against fluconazole. This new antifungal has enabled appropriate treatment of some lethal fungal infections without the toxicity of amphotericin B. It also has very good activity against *Aspergillus* infections. Both of these triazoles are available in oral and parenteral preparations.

Amphotericin B is a polyene antifungal with broad activity but significant toxicity. It acts by binding to the sterols of the cell wall and interfering with membrane permeability. It has been used traditionally for the treatment of lethal infections only (given its toxicity), usually secondary to *Candida, Aspergillus,* and *Histoplasma.*

Caspofungin, an echinocandin derivative, is a systemic antifungal agent. It acts by inhibiting β-glucan synthase and thus disrupts the integrity of the cell wall and causes cell lysis. It is indicated in the treatment of refractory systemic fungal infections caused by *Aspergillus* and *Candida.*

Annotated References

Fry DE (ed): Surgical Infections. Boston, Little, Brown, 1995.

This is a complete textbook devoted to the prevention, diagnosis, and treatment of surgical infections. It is comprehensive, well written, and an invaluable resource for more detailed information regarding surgical infections.

Gilbert DN, Moellering RC, Sande MA, The Sanford Guide to Antimicrobial Therapy. Hyde Park, VT, Antimicrobial Therapy Inc, 2006.

This handy guide to indications and doses of all available antimicrobial agents is updated every year. It comes in pocket-sized text or can be downloaded to personal digital assistants. It tends to be more up to date on doses and new indications than a regular textbook.

Gorbach SL, Bartlett JG, Blacklow NR, et al (eds): Infectious Diseases. Philadelphia, WB Saunders, 1998.

This is a comprehensive textbook of infectious diseases with specific chapters devoted to surgical site infections and to the evaluation of postoperative fever. It also has more extensive information regarding specific pathogens and specific antimicrobial drugs.

Wilmore DE, Cheung LY, Harken AH, et al (eds): American College of Surgeons Surgery. New York, WebMD, 2002.

This comprehensive, on-line, frequently updated surgical textbook emphasizes perioperative care of the surgical patient. It has an entire section with multiple chapters devoted to all aspects of surgical infection.

References

1. Horan TC, Gaynes RP, Martone WJ, et al: CDC definitions of nosocomial surgical site infections, 1992: A modification of CDC definitions of surgical wound infections. Infect Control Hosp Epidemiol 13:606-608, 1992.
2. Culver DH, Horan TC, Gaynes RP, et al: Surgical wound infection rates by wound class, operative procedure, and patient risk index. National Nosocomial Infections Surveillance System. Am J Med 91(Suppl 3B):152S-1527S, 1991.
3. Cruse PJE, Foord R: The epidemiology of wound infection: A 10-year prospective study of 62,939 wounds. Surg Clin North Am 60:27-40, 1980.
4. Haley RW, Culver DH, Morgan WM, et al: Identifying patients at high risk of surgical wound infection. A simple multivariate index of patient susceptibility and wound contamination. Am J Epidemiol 121:206-215, 1985.
5. Alexander JW, Fischer JE, Boyajian M, et al: The influence of hair-removal methods on wound infections. Arch Surg 118:347-352, 1983.
6. Melling AC, Ali B, Scott EM, et al: Effects of preoperative warming on the incidence of wound infection after clean surgery: A randomized controlled trial. Lancet 358:876-880, 2001.
7. Kurz A, Sessler DI, Lenhardt R, et al: Perioperative normothermia to reduce the incidence of surgical-wound infection. N Engl J Med 334:1209-1215, 1996.
8. Greif R, Akca O, Horn EP, et al: Supplemental perioperative oxygen to reduce the incidence of surgical-wound infection. N Engl J Med 342:161-167, 2000.
9. Belda FJ, Aguilera L, Garcia de la Asuncion J, et al: Supplemental perioperative oxygen and the risk of surgical wound infection: A randomized controlled trial. JAMA 294:2035-2042, 2005.
10. Dellinger EP: Increasing inspired oxygen to decrease surgical site infection: Time to shift the quality improvement research paradigm. JAMA 294:2091-2092, 2005.
11. Van Den Berghe G, Wouters P, Weekers F, et al: Intensive insulin therapy in critically ill patients. N Engl J Med 345:1359-1367, 2001.
12. Furnary AP, Zerr KJ, Grunkemeier GL, et al: Continuous intravenous insulin infusion reduces the incidence of deep sternal wound infection in diabetic patients after cardiac surgical procedures. Ann Thorac Surg 67:352-360; discussion 360-362, 1999.
13. Latham R, Lancaster AD, Covington JF, et al: The association of diabetes and glucose control with surgical-site infections among cardiothoracic surgery patients. Infect Control Hosp Epidemiol 22:607-612, 2001.
14. Emori TG, Culver DH, Horan TC, et al: National Nosocomial Infections Surveillance System (NNIS): Description of surveillance methodology. Am J Infect Control 19:19-35, 1991.
15. Gaynes RP, Culver DH, Horan TC, et al: Surgical site infection (SSI) rates in the United States, 1992-1998: The National Nosocomial Infections Surveillance System basic SSI risk index. Clin Infect Dis 33(Suppl 2):S69-S77, 2001.
16. Mangram AJ, Horan TC, Pearson ML, et al: Guidelines for prevention of surgical site infection. Centers for Disease Control and Prevention Hospital Infection Control Practices Advisory Committee. Am J Infect Control 26:97-134, 1999.
17. Anaya DA, Dellinger EP: Challenges in the prevention of surgical site infections. Infect Med 23:120-126, 2006.
18. Quebbeman EJ, Telford GL, Wadsworth K, et al: Double gloving. Protecting surgeons from blood contamination in the operating room. Arch Surg 127:213-216, 1992.

19. Dellinger EP, Gross PA, Barrett TL, et al: Quality standard for antimicrobial prophylaxis in surgical procedures. Clin Infect Dis 18:422-427, 1994.

20. Platt R, Zucker JR, Zaleznik DF, et al: Perioperative antibiotic prophylaxis and wound infection following breast surgery. J Antimicrob Chemother 31(Suppl B):43-48, 1993.

21. Clarke JS, Condon RE, Bartlett JG, et al: Preoperative oral antibiotics reduce septic complications of colon operations: Results of prospective, randomized, double-blind clinical study. Ann Surg 186:251-259, 1977.

22. Slim K, Vicaut E, Panis Y, et al: Meta-analysis of randomized clinical trials of colorectal surgery with or without mechanical bowel preparation. Br J Surg 91:1125-1130, 2004.

23. Bucher P, Mermillod B, Gervaz P, et al: Mechanical bowel preparation for elective colorectal surgery: A meta-analysis. Arch Surg 139:1359-1364; discussion 1365, 2004.

24. Guenaga KF, Matos D, Castro AA, et al: Mechanical bowel preparation for elective colorectal surgery. Cochrane Database Syst Rev 1:CD001544, 2005.

25. Forse RA, Karam B, MacLean LD, et al: Antibiotic prophylaxis for surgery in morbidly obese patients. Surgery 106:750-756; discussion 756-757, 1989.

26. Edmiston CE, Krepel C, Kelly H, et al: Perioperative antibiotic prophylaxis in the gastric bypass patient: Do we achieve therapeutic levels? Surgery 136:738-747, 2004.

27. Anaya DA, Dellinger EP: The obese surgical patient: A susceptible host for infection. Surg Infect (Larchmt) 7:473-480, 2006.

28. Braga M, Gianotti L, Radaelli G, et al: Perioperative immunonutrition in patients undergoing cancer surgery: Results of a randomized double-blind phase 3 trial. Arch Surg 134:428-433, 1999.

29. Braga M, Gianotti L, Vignali A, et al: Preoperative oral arginine and n-3 fatty acid supplementation improves the immunometabolic host response and outcome after colorectal resection for cancer. Surgery 132:805-814, 2002.

30. Bozzetti F, Braga M, Gianotti L, et al: Postoperative enteral versus parenteral nutrition in malnourished patients with gastrointestinal cancer: A randomized multicentre trial. Lancet 358:1487-1492, 2001.

31. Bratzler DW, Houck PM, Richards C, et al: Use of antimicrobial prophylaxis for major surgery: Baseline results from the National Surgical Infection Prevention Project. Arch Surg 140:174-182, 2005.

32. Dellinger EP, Hausmann SM, Bratzler DW, et al: Hospitals collaborate to decrease surgical site infections. Am J Surg 190:9-15, 2005.

33. Haley RV, Culver DH, White WJ, et al: The efficacy of infection surveillance and control programs in preventing nosocomial infections in the US hospitals. Am J Epidemiol 121:182-205, 1985.

34. Olson M, O'Connor MO, Schwartz ML: A 5-year prospective study of 20,193 wounds at the Minneapolis VA Medical Center. Ann Surg 199:253-259, 1984.

35. Consensus paper on the surveillance of surgical wound infections. The Society for Hospital Epidemiology of America; the Association for Practitioners in Infection Control; the Centers for Disease Control; the Surgical Infection Society. Infect Control Hosp Epidemiol 13:599-605, 1992.

36. Lee JT: Wound infection surveillance. Infect Dis Clin North Am 6:643-656, 1992.

37. Dellinger EP, Ehrenkranz NJ: Surgical infections. In Bennett JV, Brachman PS (eds): Hospital Infections, 4th ed. Philadelphia, Lippincott-Raven, 1998, pp 571-585.

38. Green RJ, Dafoe DC, Raffin TA: Necrotizing fasciitis. Chest 110:219-229, 1996.

39. Majeski JA, John JF: Necrotizing soft tissue infections: A guide to early diagnosis and initial therapy. South Med J 96:900-905, 2003.

40. Kuncir EJ, Tillou A, Petrone P, et al: Necrotizing soft-tissue infections. Emerg Med Clin North Am 21:1075-1087, 2003.

41. Ma LD, Frassica FJ, Bluemke DA, et al: CT and MRI evaluation of musculoskeletal infection. Crit Rev Diagn Imaging 38:535-568, 1997.

42. Wall DB, Klein SR, Black S, et al: A simple model to help distinguish necrotizing fasciitis from non-necrotizing soft tissue infection. J Am Coll Surg 191:227-231, 2000.

43. Wong CH, Khin LW, Heng KS, et al: The LRINEC (Laboratory Risk Indicator for Necrotizing Fasciitis) score: A tool for distinguishing necrotizing fasciitis from other soft tissue infections. Crit Care Med 32:1535-1541, 2004.

44. Anaya DA, McMahon K, Nathens AB, et al: Predictors of mortality and limb loss in necrotizing soft tissue infections. Arch Surg 140:151-157, 2005.

45. Anaya DA, Nathens AB: Risk factors for severe sepsis in secondary peritonitis. Surg Infect (Larchmt) 4:355-362, 2003.

46. Christou NV, Barie PS, Dellinger EP, et al: Surgical Infection Society intra-abdominal infection study: Prospective evaluation of management techniques and outcome. Arch Surg 128:193-199, 1993.

47. Mazuski JE, Sawyer RG, Nathens AB, et al: The Surgical Infection Society guidelines on antimicrobial therapy for intra-abdominal infections: Evidence for the recommendations. Surg Infect (Larchmt) 3:175-233, 2002.

48. Mazuski JE, Sawyer RG, Nathens AB, et al: The Surgical Infection Society guidelines on antimicrobial therapy for intra-abdominal infections: An executive summary. Surg Infect (Larchmt) 3:161-173, 2002.

49. Koperna T, Schulz F: Relaparotomy in peritonitis: Prognosis and treatment of patients with persisting intraabdominal infection. World J Surg 24:32-37, 2000.

50. Seiler CA, Brugger L, Forssmann U, et al: Conservative surgical treatment of diffuse peritonitis. Surgery 127:178-184, 2000.

51. Levison MA: Percutaneous versus open operative drainage of intra-abdominal abscesses. Infect Dis Clin North Am 6:525-544, 1992.

52. Dellinger E: Approach to the patient with postoperative fever. In Gorbach S, Bartlett J, Blacklow N (eds): Infectious Diseases in Medicine and Surgery. Philadelphia, WB Saunders, 1998, pp 903-909.

53. Kaye KS, Fraimow HS, Abrutyn E: Pathogens resistant to antimicrobial agents; epidemiology, molecular mechanisms and clinical management. Infect Dis Clin North Am 14:293-319, 2000.

54. Kollef MH, Fraser VJ: Antibiotic resistance in the intensive care unit. Ann Intern Med 134:298-314, 2001.

15 CHAPTER

Surgical Complications

Mahmoud N. Kulaylat, MD   and   Merril T. Dayton, MD

Surgical complications remain a frustrating and difficult aspect of the operative treatment of patients. Regardless of how technically gifted and capable surgeons are, all will have to deal with complications that occur after operative procedures. The cost of surgical complications in the United States runs into millions of dollars; in addition, such complications are associated with lost work productivity, disruption of family life, and stress to employers and society in general. Frequently, the functional results of the operation are compromised by complications; in some cases the patient never recovers to the preoperative level of function. The most significant and difficult part of complications is the suffering borne by a patient who enters the hospital anticipating an uneventful operation but is left suffering and compromised by the complication.

Complications can occur for a variety of reasons. A surgeon can perform a technically sound operation in a patient who is severely compromised by the disease process and still have a complication. Similarly, a surgeon who is sloppy or careless or hurries through an operation can make technical errors that account for the operative complications. Finally, the patient can be healthy nutritionally, have an operation performed meticulously, and yet suffer a complication because of the nature of the disease. The possibility of postoperative complications remains part of every surgeon's mental preparation for a difficult operation.

Surgeons can do much to avoid complications by careful preoperative screening. When the surgeon sees the surgical candidate for the first time, a host of questions come to mind, such as the nutritional status of the patient and the health of the heart and lungs. The surgeon will make a decision regarding performing the appropriate operation for the known disease. Similarly, the timing of the operation is often an important issue. Some operations can be performed in a purely elective fashion, whereas others must be done in an urgent fashion. Occasionally, the surgeon will require that the patient lose weight before the operation to enhance the likelihood of a successful outcome. At times a wise surgeon will request preoperative consultation from a cardiologist or pulmonary specialist to make certain that the patient will be able to tolerate the stress of a particular procedure.

Once the operation has begun, the surgeon can do much to influence the postoperative outcome. Surgeons must handle tissues gently, dissect meticulously, and honor tissue planes. Performing the technical portions of the operation carefully will lower the risk for a significant complication. At all costs, surgeons must avoid the temptation to rush, cut corners, or accept marginal technical results. Similarly, the judicious use of antibiotics and other preoperative medications can influence the outcome. For a seriously ill patient, adequate resuscitation may be necessary to optimize the patient before giving a general anesthetic.

Once the operation is completed, compulsive postoperative surveillance is mandatory. Thorough and careful rounding on patients on a regular basis postoperatively gives the operating surgeon an opportunity to be vigilant and seek postoperative complications at an early stage when they can be most effectively addressed. During this process the surgeon will carefully check all wounds, evaluate intake and output, check temperature profiles, ascertain what the patient's activity levels have been, evaluate nutritional status, and check pain levels. Over years of experience, the clinician can begin to assess the aforementioned parameters and detect deviations from the normal postoperative course. Expeditious response to a complication makes the difference between a brief, inconvenient complication and a devastating, disabling one. In summary, a wise surgeon will deal with complications quickly, thoroughly, and appropriately.

SURGICAL WOUND COMPLICATIONS

Seroma

Etiology

A seroma is a collection of liquefied fat, serum, and lymphatic fluid under the incision. The fluid is usually clear, yellow, and somewhat viscous and is found in the subcutaneous (SC) layer of the skin. Seromas represent the most benign complication after an operative procedure and are particularly likely to occur when large skin flaps are developed in the course of the operation, as is often seen with mastectomy, axillary dissection, groin dissection, and large ventral hernias.

Presentation and Management

A seroma is usually manifested as a localized and well-circumscribed swelling, pressure or discomfort, and occasional drainage of clear liquid from the immature surgical wound.

Prevention of seroma formation may be achieved by placing suction drains under the skin flaps or in potential dead space created by lymphadenectomy. Premature removal of drains frequently results in large seromas that require aspiration under sterile conditions, followed by placement of a pressure dressing. A seroma that reaccumulates after at least two aspirations is evacuated by opening the incision and packing the wound with saline-moistened gauze to allow healing by secondary intention. In the presence of synthetic mesh, the best option is open drainage in the operating room with the incision closed to avoid exposure and infection of the mesh; closed suction drains are generally placed. An infected seroma is also treated by open drainage. The presence of synthetic mesh in these cases will prevent the wound from healing. Management of the mesh depends on the severity and extent of infection. In the absence of severe sepsis and spreading cellulitis and the presence of localized infection, the mesh can be left in situ and removed at a later date when the acute infectious process has resolved. Otherwise, the mesh must be removed and the wound managed with open wound care.

Hematoma

Etiology

A hematoma is an abnormal collection of blood, usually in the SC layer of a recent incision or in a potential space in the abdominal cavity after extirpation of an organ, for example, splenic fossa hematoma after splenectomy or pelvic hematoma after proctectomy. Hematomas are more worrisome than seromas because of the potential for secondary infection. Hematoma formation is related to inadequate hemostasis, depletion of clotting factors, and the presence of coagulopathy. A host of disease processes can contribute to coagulopathy, including myeloproliferative disorders, liver disease, renal failure, sepsis, clotting factor deficiencies, and medications. Medications most commonly associated with coagulopathy are antiplatelet drugs, such as aspirin, clopidogrel bisulfate (Plavix), ticlopidine hydrochloride (Ticlid), eptifibatide (Integrilin), and abciximab (ReoPro), and anticoagulants, such as ultrafractionated heparin, low-molecular-weight heparin (LMWH: enoxaparin [Lovenox], dalteparin sodium [Fragmin], tinzaparin [Innohep]), and warfarin sodium.

Presentation and Management

The clinical manifestations of a hematoma vary with its size and location. A hematoma may appear as an expanding, unsightly swelling or pain in the area of a surgical incision, or both. In the neck a large hematoma may cause compromise of the airway; in the retroperitoneum it may cause paralytic ileus, anemia, and ongoing bleeding because of local consumptive coagulopathy; and in the extremity and abdominal cavity it may result in compartment syndrome. On physical examination, a hematoma appears as a localized soft swelling with purplish/blue discoloration of the overlying skin. The swelling varies from small to large and may be tender to palpation or associated with drainage of dark red fluid out of the fresh wound.

Hematoma formation is prevented preoperatively by correcting any clotting abnormalities and discontinuing medications that alter coagulation. Antiplatelet medications and anticoagulants are given to patients undergoing surgery for a variety of reasons: after implantation of a coronary stent, for the treatment of coronary artery disease (CAD) and stroke, after implantation of a mechanical mitral valve, and in the presence of atrial fibrillation, venous thromboembolism, and hypercoagulable states. These medications must be discontinued before surgery. One must balance the risk of significant bleeding due to uncorrected medication-induced coagulopathy and the risk of thrombosis after discontinuation of therapy. In patients at high risk for thrombosis who are scheduled to undergo an elective major surgical procedure, warfarin must be discontinued 3 days before surgery to allow the international normalized ratio (INR) to be less than 1.5. Then they are given heparin intravenously (IV) or an equivalent dose SC. Those receiving standard heparin can have the medication discontinued 2 to 3 hours before surgery and those receiving LMWH (variable half-life), 12 to 15 hours before surgery. Anticoagulants are then

Box 15-1   Factors Associated With Wound Dehiscence

Technical error in fascial closure
Emergency surgery
Intra-abdominal infection
Advanced age
Wound infection, hematoma, and seroma
Elevated intra-abdominal pressure
Obesity
Chronic corticosteroid use
Previous wound dehiscence
Malnutrition
Radiation therapy and chemotherapy
Systemic disease (uremia, diabetes mellitus)

resumed 24 to 48 hours after surgery. Patients taking clopidogrel must have the medication withheld 5 to 6 days before surgery; otherwise, the surgery must be delayed. During surgery, adequate hemostasis must be achieved with ligature, electrocautery, fibrin glue, or topical bovine thrombin before closure. Closed suction drainage systems are placed in large potential spaces and removed postoperatively when output is not bloody and scant.

Evaluation of a patient with a hematoma, especially one that is large and expanding, includes assessment of preexisting risk factors and coagulation parameters (prothrombin time, partial thromboplastin time, INR, platelet count). A small hematoma does not require any intervention and will eventually resorb. Most retroperitoneal hematomas can be managed by expectant waiting after correction of the associated coagulopathy. A large or expanding hematoma in the neck is managed in similar fashion and best evacuated in the operating room urgently after securing the airway if there is any respiratory compromise. Similarly, hematomas detected soon after surgery, especially those developing under skin flaps, are best evacuated in the operating room.

Acute Wound Failure (Dehiscence)

Etiology

Acute wound failure (wound dehiscence or a burst abdomen) refers to postoperative separation of the abdominal musculoaponeurotic layers. It is among the most dreaded complications faced by surgeons and of greatest concern because of the risk of evisceration, the need for immediate intervention, and the possibility of repeat dehiscence, surgical wound infection, and incisional hernia formation.

Acute wound failure occurs in approximately 1% to 3% of patients who undergo an abdominal operation. Dehiscence most often develops 7 to 10 days postoperatively but may occur anytime after surgery from 1 to more than 20 days. A multitude of factors may contribute to wound dehiscence (Box 15-1). Acute wound failure is often related to technical errors in placing sutures too close to the edge, too far apart, or under too much tension. A deep wound infection is one of the most

common causes of localized wound separation. Increased intra-abdominal pressure and factors that adversely affect wound healing are often cited as contributing to the complication. In healthy patients, the rate of wound failure is similar whether closure is accomplished with a continuous or interrupted technique. In high-risk patients, however, continuous closure is worrisome because suture breakage in one place weakens the entire closure.

Presentation and Management

Acute wound failure may occur without warning and evisceration makes the diagnosis obvious. Sudden, dramatic drainage of a relatively large volume of a clear, salmon-colored fluid precedes dehiscence in a fourth of patients. Probing the wound with a sterile, cotton-tipped applicator or gloved finger may detect the dehiscence.

Prevention of acute wound failure is largely a function of careful attention to technical detail during fascial closure. For very high-risk patients, interrupted closure is often the wisest choice. Alternative methods of closure must be selected when primary closure is not possible without undue tension. Although retention sutures were used extensively in the past, their use is less common today, with some surgeons opting to use a synthetic prosthesis or tissue graft.

Once dehiscence is diagnosed, treatment depends on the extent of fascial separation and the presence of evisceration or significant intra-abdominal contamination (intestinal leak, peritonitis). A small dehiscence in the proximal aspect of an upper midline incision 10 to 12 days postoperatively can be managed conservatively by packing the wound with saline-moistened gauze and using an abdominal binder. In the event of evisceration, the eviscerated intestines must be covered with a sterile, saline-moistened towel and preparations made to return to the operating room after a very short period of fluid resuscitation. Once in the operating room, thorough exploration of the abdominal cavity is performed to rule out the presence of a septic focus or an anastomotic leak that may have predisposed to the dehiscence. Treatment of the infection is of critical importance before attempting closure. Management of the incision is a function of the condition of the fascia. When technical mistakes are made and the fascia is strong and intact, primary closure is warranted. If the fascia is infected or necrotic, débridement is performed. If after débridement the edges of the fascia cannot be approximated without undue tension, consideration needs to be given to closing the wound with absorbable mesh or the recently developed biologic prostheses (decellularized porcine submucosa and dermis and human cadaveric dermis). Attempts to close the fascia under tension guarantee a repeat dehiscence and possible intra-abdominal hypertension. Definitive surgical repair to restore the integrity of the abdominal wall will eventually be required if absorbable mesh is used but not if a biologic prosthesis is used.

Absorbable mesh and biologic prostheses protect from evisceration, maintain the abdominal domain, and provide a barrier to prevent bowel desiccation, bacterial invasion, and nonadherent, potentially permanent closure. Autologous skin grafts are used to reconstitute the epithelial barrier, and flaps (local/regional or free) are used to reconstruct the abdominal wall.

For short-term management of a dehisced wound, a wound vacuum system can be used that consists of open-cell foam placed on the tissue, semiocclusive drape to cover the foam and skin of the patient, and suction apparatus. The wound vacuum system provides immediate coverage of the abdominal wound and acts as a dressing that minimizes heat loss and does not require suturing to the fascia. By using negative pressure, the device removes interstitial fluid and thus lessens bowel edema, decreases wound size, reduces bacterial colonization, increases local blood perfusion, and induces the healing response.[1-3] Successful closure of the fascia can be achieved in 85% of cases of abdominal wound dehiscence. The technique, however, may be associated with evisceration, intestinal fistulization, and hernia formation.

Surgical Site Infection (Wound Infection)

Etiology

Surgical site infections continue to be a significant problem for surgeons in the modern era. Despite significant improvements in antibiotics, better anesthesia, superior instruments, earlier diagnosis of surgical problems, and improved techniques for postoperative vigilance, wound infections continue to occur. Although some may view the problem as a merely cosmetic one, that view represents a very shallow understanding of this problem, which causes significant patient suffering, morbidity and even mortality, and a financial burden to the health care system. Currently, in the United States wound infections account for almost 40% of hospital-acquired infections among surgical patients.

The surgical wound encompasses the area of the body, both internally and externally, that involves the entire operative site. Wounds are thus categorized into three general groups:

1. Superficial, including the skin and SC tissue
2. Deep, including the fascia and muscle
3. Organ space, including the internal organs of the body if the operation includes that area

The Centers for Disease Control and Prevention has proposed specific criteria for the diagnosis of surgical site infection (Box 15-2).[4]

A host of factors may contribute to the development of a surgical site infection (Table 15-1).[5] Surgical site infection is caused by bacterial contamination of the surgical site, which can occur in a variety of ways: violation of integrity of the wall of a hollow viscus, skin flora, and a break in the surgical sterile technique that allows exogenous contamination from the surgical team, the equipment, or the surrounding environment. The pathogens associated with a surgical site infection reflect the area that provided the inoculum for the infection to develop. *Staphylococcus aureus* and coagulase-negative *Staphylococcus* remain the most common bacteria colonized from wounds (Table 15-2). However, at locations where high volumes of gastrointestinal (GI) operations

---

> ### Box 15-2 Centers for Disease Control and Prevention Criteria for Defining a Surgical Site Infection
>
> #### Superficial Incisional
>
> Infection less than 30 days after surgery
> Involves skin and subcutaneous tissue only, *plus* one of the following:
> - Purulent drainage
> - Diagnosis of superficial surgical site infection by a surgeon
> - Symptoms of erythema, pain, local edema
>
> #### Deep Incisional
>
> Less than 30 days after surgery with no implant and soft tissue involvement
> Infection less than 1 year after surgery with an implant; involves deep soft tissues (fascia and muscle), *plus* one of the following:
> - Purulent drainage from the deep space but no extension into the organ space
> - Abscess found in the deep space on direct or radiologic examination or on reoperation
> - Diagnosis of a deep space surgical site infection by the surgeon
> - Symptoms of fever, pain, and tenderness leading to dehiscence of the wound or opening by a surgeon
>
> #### Organ Space
>
> Infection less than 30 days after surgery with no implant
> Infection less than 1 year after surgery with an implant and infection; involves any part of the operation opened or manipulated, *plus* one of the following:
> - Purulent drainage from a drain placed in the organ space
> - Cultured organisms from material aspirated from the organ space
> - Abscess found on direct or radiologic examination or during reoperation
> - Diagnosis of organ space infection by a surgeon
>
> Modified from Mangram AJ, Horan TC, Pearson ML, et al: Guidelines for prevention of surgical site infection. Infect Control Hosp Epidemiol 20:252, 1999.

---

are performed, the predominant bacteria will include *Enterobacter* species and *Escherichia coli*. In most studies, group D *Enterococcus* continues to be a common pathogen isolated from surgical site infections. Surgical wounds are classified into clean, clean-contaminated, contaminated, and dirty according to the relative risk for development of a surgical site infection (Table 15-3).

Presentation and Management

Surgical site infections most commonly occur 5 to 6 days postoperatively but may develop sooner or later than that. About 80% to 90% of all postoperative infections occur within 30 days after the operative procedure. With the increased utilization of outpatient surgery and decreased length of stay in hospitals, 30% to 40% of all wound infections have been shown to occur after hospital discharge. Nevertheless, although less than 10% of surgical patients are hospitalized for 6 days or less, 70% of postdischarge infections occur in that group.

Table 15-1   Risk Factors for Postoperative Wound Infection

PATIENT FACTORS	ENVIRONMENTAL FACTORS	TREATMENT FACTORS
Ascites	Contaminated medications	Drains
Chronic inflammation	Inadequate	Emergency procedure
Undernutrition	disinfection/sterilization	Inadequate antibiotic coverage
Obesity	Inadequate skin antisepsis	Preoperative hospitalization
Diabetes	Inadequate ventilation	Prolonged operation
Extremes of age	Presence of a foreign body	
Hypercholesterolemia		
Hypoxemia		
Peripheral vascular disease		
Postoperative anemia		
Previous site of irradiation		
Recent operation		
Remote infection		
Skin carriage of staphylococci		
Skin disease in the area of infection		
Immunosuppression		

Data from National Nosocomial Infections Surveillance Systems (NNIS) System Report: Data summary from January 1992–June 2001, issued August 2001. Am J Infect Control 29:404-421, 2001.

Table 15-2   Pathogens Isolated From Postoperative Surgical Site Infections at a University Hospital

PATHOGEN	PERCENTAGE OF ISOLATES
Staphylococcus (coagulase negative)	25.6
Enterococcus (group D)	11.5
Staphylococcus aureus	8.7
Candida albicans	6.5
Escherichia coli	6.3
Pseudomonas aeruginosa	6.0
Corynebacterium	4.0
Candida (non-*albicans*)	3.4
α-Hemolytic *Streptococcus*	3.0
Klebsiella pneumoniae	2.8
Vancomycin-resistant *Enterococcus*	2.4
Enterobacter cloacae	2.2
Citrobacter species	2.0

From Weiss CA, Statz CI, Dahms RA, et al: Six years of surgical wound surveillance at a tertiary care center. Arch Surg 134:1041, 1999.

Superficial and deep surgical site infections are accompanied by erythema, tenderness, edema, and occasionally drainage. The wound is often soft or fluctuant at the site of infection, which is a departure from the firmness of the healing ridge present elsewhere in the wound. The patient may have leukocytosis and a low-grade fever. According to the Joint Commission on Accreditation of Healthcare Organizations, a surgical wound is considered infected if it meets the following criteria:

1. Grossly purulent material drains from the wound
2. The wound spontaneously opens and drains purulent fluid

3. The wound drains fluid that is culture positive or Gram stain positive for bacteria
4. The surgeon notes erythema or drainage and opens the wound after deeming it to be infected

Treatment of surgical site infection starts with the implementation of preventive measures before and during surgery. Patients who are heavy smokers are encouraged to stop smoking around the time of the operation. Obese patients must be encouraged to lose weight if the procedure is elective and there is time to achieve significant weight loss. Tight control of glucose levels, especially in diabetics, will lower the risk for wound infection.[6] Similarly, patients who are taking high doses of corticosteroids will have lower infection rates if they are weaned off corticosteroids or are at least taking a lower dose. The night before surgery, patients are encouraged to take a shower or bath in which an antibiotic soap may be used. Patients undergoing major intra-abdominal surgery are administered bowel preparation in the form of lavage solutions or strong cathartics, followed by oral, nonabsorbable antibiotics, particularly for surgery on the colon and small bowel. Such preparation lowers the patient's risk for infection from that of a contaminated case (25%) to a clean-contaminated case (5%).

Preoperative antibiotics for prophylaxis are given selectively. For dirty or contaminated wounds, the use of antibiotics is for therapeutic intentions rather than for prophylaxis. For clean cases, prophylaxis is controversial. However, a small but significant benefit may be achieved with the prophylactic administration of a first-generation cephalosporin for certain types of clean surgery (e.g., mastectomy and herniorrhaphy). For clean-contaminated procedures, administration of preoperative antibiotics is indicated. The appropriate preoperative antibiotic is a function of the most likely inoculum based on the area being operated on. For example, when a prosthesis may be placed in a clean wound, preoperative antibiotics would include something to protect against *S. aureus* and *Streptococcus* species.

Table 15-3 Classification of Surgical Wounds

CATEGORY	CRITERIA	INFECTION RATE
Clean	No hollow viscus entered Primary wound closure No inflammation No breaks in aseptic technique Elective procedure	1%-3%
Clean-contaminated	Hollow viscus entered but controlled No inflammation Primary wound closure Minor break in aseptic technique Mechanical drain used Bowel preparation preoperatively	5%-8%
Contaminated	Uncontrolled spillage from viscus Inflammation apparent Open, traumatic wound Major break in aseptic technique	20%-25%
Dirty	Untreated, uncontrolled spillage from viscus Pus in operative wound Open suppurative wound Severe inflammation	30%-40%

A first-generation cephalosporin, such as cefazolin, would be appropriate in this setting. For patients undergoing upper GI tract surgery, complex biliary tract operations, or elective colonic resection, administration of a second-generation cephalosporin such as cefoxitin or a penicillin derivative with a β-lactamase inhibitor is more suitable. The surgeon will give a preoperative dose, appropriate intraoperative doses approximately 4 hours apart, and two postoperative doses appropriately spaced. Timing of administration of prophylactic antibiotics is critical. To be most effective, the antibiotic is administered IV within 30 minutes before the incision so that therapeutic tissue levels are present when the wound is created and exposed to bacterial contamination. Most often, a period of anesthesia induction, preparation, and draping takes place that is adequate to allow tissue levels to build up to therapeutic levels before the incision is made. Of equal importance is making certain that the prophylactic antibiotic is not administered for extended periods postoperatively. To do so in the prophylactic setting is to invite the development of drug-resistant organisms, as well as serious complications such as *Clostridium difficile* colitis.

At the time of surgery the operating surgeon plays a major role in reducing or minimizing the presence of postoperative wound infections. The surgeon must be attentive to personal hygiene (hand scrubbing) and that of the entire team.[7] In addition, the surgeon must make certain that the patient undergoes a thorough skin preparation with appropriate antiseptic solutions and is draped in a sterile careful fashion. During the operation, steps that have a positive impact on outcome are followed:

1. Careful handling of tissues
2. Meticulous dissection, hemostasis, and débridement of devitalized tissue
3. Compulsive control of all intraluminal contents
4. Preservation of blood supply of the operated organs
5. Elimination of any foreign body from the wound
6. Maintenance of strict asepsis by the operating team (no holes in gloves, avoidance of the use of contaminated instruments, avoidance of environmental contamination such as debris falling from overhead)
7. Thorough drainage and irrigation of any pockets of purulence in the wound with warm saline
8. Ensuring that the patient is kept in a euthermic state, well monitored, and fluid resuscitated
9. At the end of the case, a judgment with regard to closing the skin or packing the wound

The use of drains remains somewhat controversial in preventing postoperative wound infections. In general, there is virtually no indication for drains in this setting. However, placing closed suction drains in very deep, large wounds and wounds with large wound flaps to prevent the development of a seroma or hematoma is a worthwhile practice.

Once a surgical site infection is suspected or diagnosed, management depends on the depth of the infection. For both superficial and deep surgical site infections, skin staples are removed over the area of the infection, and a cotton-tipped applicator may be easily passed into the wound with efflux of purulent material and pus. The wound is gently explored with the cotton-tipped applicator or a finger to determine whether the fascia or muscle tissue is involved. If the fascia is intact, débridement of any nonviable tissue is performed, and the wound is irrigated with normal saline solution and packed to its base with saline-moistened gauze to allow healing of the wound from the base anteriorly and prevent premature skin closure. If widespread cellulitis is noted, administration of IV antibiotics must be considered. However, if the fascia has separated or purulent material appears to be coming from deep to the fascia, there is obvious concern about dehiscence or an intra-abdominal abscess that may require drainage or possibly a reoperation.

Wound cultures are controversial. If the wound is small, superficial, and not associated with cellulitis or tissue necrosis, culture may not be necessary. However, if fascial dehiscence and a more complex infection are present, material is sent for culture. A deep surgical site infection associated with grayish, dishwater-colored fluid, as well as frank necrosis of the fascial layer, raises suspicion for the presence of a necrotizing type of infection. The presence of crepitus in any surgical wound or gram-positive rods (or both) suggests the possibility of infection with *Clostridia perfringens*. Rapid and expeditious surgical débridement is indicated in these settings.

Most postoperative infections are treated with healing by secondary intention (allowing the wound to heal from the base anteriorly, with epithelialization being the final event). In some cases when there is a question about the amount of contamination, delayed primary closure may be considered. In this setting, close observation of the wound for 5 days may be followed by closure of the skin if the wound looks clean and the patient is otherwise doing well.

Recently, wound vacuum systems have been used in large, deep, or moist wounds with generally successful outcomes. Their advantage is a decrease in the nursing time previously required for dressing changes, as well as less pain for the patient.

Chronic Wounds

Etiology

A chronic wound is a wound that has not healed completely within 30 to 90 days of the operative procedure. These wounds are commonly found in patients taking high doses of corticosteroids, cancer patients treated with immunosuppressants, patients who are undergoing chemotherapy, patients who have had radiation therapy, malnourished patients, morbidly obese patients with huge wounds, or those in whom wound dehiscence occurred and there is a large granulating base. Nonhealing perineal wounds can occur in patients with previous radiation therapy, Crohn's disease, acquired immunodeficiency syndrome (AIDS), or cancer.

Presentation and Management

Chronic wounds may be large and are usually covered with shaggy granulation tissue, exuberant granulation tissue, or areas of purulent fibrinous exudation. Meticulous wound care, débridement, and the use of a fenestrated skin graft, rotation flaps, or a wound vacuum device may accelerate healing of these chronic wounds. Quantitative wound cultures may be helpful in selecting more targeted antibiotic therapy. Reducing corticosteroid doses, improving nutritional status, and the use of epidermal growth factor preparations may help heal some types of chronic wounds.

Preventing large chronic wounds is often difficult, but in situations in which one can, avoiding an operation in an irradiated field, encouraging obese patients to lose weight or improve their nutritional status before surgery,

and having patients cease smoking may all contribute to prevention of a chronic wound infection.

COMPLICATIONS OF THERMAL REGULATION

Hypothermia

Etiology

Optimal function of physiologic systems in the body occurs within a narrow range of core temperatures. A 2°C drop in body temperature or a 3°C increase signifies a health emergency that is life threatening and requires immediate intervention. Hypothermia can result from a number of mechanisms preoperatively, intraoperatively, or postoperatively. A trauma patient with injuries in a cold environment can suffer significant hypothermia, and paralysis leads to hypothermia because of loss of the shiver mechanism.

Hypothermia develops in patients undergoing rapid resuscitation with cool IV fluids or transfusions or intracavitary irrigation with cold irrigant and in patients undergoing a prolonged surgical procedure with low ambient room temperature and a large, exposed operative area subjected to significant evaporative cooling. Virtually all anesthetics impair thermoregulation and render the patient susceptible to hypothermia in the typically cool operating room environment.[8,9] Advanced age and opioid analgesia also reduce perioperative shivering.[8,9] Propofol causes vasodilation and significant redistribution hypothermia. Postoperatively, hypothermia can result from cool ambient room temperature, rapid administration of IV fluids or blood, and failure to keep patients covered when they are only partially responsive. More than 80% of elective operative procedures are associated with a drop in body temperature, and 50% of trauma patients are hypothermic on arrival in the operating suite.

Presentation

Hypothermia is uncomfortable because of the intense cold sensation and shivering. It may also be associated with profound effects on the cardiovascular system, coagulation, wound healing, and infection.[7,8] A core temperature lower than 35°C after surgery triggers a significant peripheral sympathetic nervous system response consisting of increased norepinephrine, vasoconstriction, and elevated arterial blood pressure. Patients in shock or with severe illnesses often have associated vasoconstriction that results in poor perfusion of peripheral organs and tissues, an effect accentuated by hypothermia. In a high-risk patient a core temperature lower than 35°C is associated with a twofold to threefold increase in the incidence of early postoperative ischemia and a similar increase in the incidence of ventricular tachyarrhythmia. Hypothermia also impairs platelet function and reduces the activity of coagulation factors, thereby resulting in an increased risk for bleeding.[8] Hypothermia results in impaired macrophage function, reduced tissue oxygen tension, and impaired collagen deposition, which predisposes wounds to poor healing and infection.[8] Other complications of hypothermia include a relative diuresis, compromised hepatic function, and some neurologic manifestations.

Similarly, the patient's ability to manage acid-base abnormalities is impaired. In severe cases the patient can have significant cardiac slowing and may be comatose with low blood pressure, bradycardia, and a very low respiratory rate.

Treatment

Prevention of hypothermia entails monitoring core temperature, especially in patients undergoing body cavity surgery or surgery lasting longer than 1 hour, children and the elderly, and patients in whom general-epidural anesthesia is being conducted.[9] Sites of monitoring include pulmonary artery blood, the tympanic membrane, the esophagus and pharynx, the rectum, and the urinary bladder.[8] While the patient is being anesthetized and during skin preparation, significant evaporative cooling can take place; the patient is kept warm by increasing the ambient temperature and using heated humidifiers and warmed IV fluid. After the patient is draped, room temperature can be lowered to a more comfortable setting. A forced-air warming device that provides active cutaneous warming is placed on the patient.[8,9] Passive surface warming is not effective in conserving heat. There is some evidence that a considerable amount of heat is lost through the head of the patient, so simply covering the patient's head during surgery may prevent significant heat loss.

In the perioperative period, mild hypothermia is commonplace and patients usually shiver because the anesthesia impairs thermoregulation. Many patients who shiver after anesthesia, however, are hypothermic. Treatment of the hypothermia with forced-air warming systems and radiant heaters will also reduce the shivering.[8,9] In a severely hypothermic patient who does not require immediate operative intervention, attention must be directed toward rewarming by the following methods:

1. Immediate placement of warm blankets, as well as currently available forced-air warming devices
2. Infusion of blood and IV fluids through a warming device
3. Heating and humidifying inhalational gases
4. Peritoneal lavage with warmed fluids
5. Rewarming infusion devices with an arteriovenous system
6. In rare cases, cardiopulmonary bypass

Special attention must be paid to cardiac monitoring during the rewarming process because cardiac irritability may be a significant problem. Similarly, acid-base disturbances must be aggressively corrected while the patient is being rewarmed. Once in the operating room, measures previously mentioned to keep the patient warm are applied.

Malignant Hyperthermia

Etiology

Malignant hyperthermia (MH) is a life-threatening hypermetabolic crisis that is manifested during or after exposure to a triggering general anesthetic in susceptible individuals. It is estimated that MH occurs in 1 in 30,000 to 50,000 adults. Mortality from MH has decreased to less than 10% in the past decade as a result of improved monitoring standards that allow early detection of MH, the availability of dantrolene, and increased use of susceptibility tests.

Susceptibility to MH is inherited as an autosomal dominant disease with variable penetrance. To date, two MH susceptibility genes have been identified in humans and four mapped to specific chromosomes but not definitely identified.[10] The mutation results in altered calcium regulation in skeletal muscle in the form of enhanced efflux of calcium from the sarcoplasmic reticulum into the myoplasm. Halogenated inhalational anesthetic agents (halothane, enflurane, isoflurane, desflurane, and sevoflurane) and depolarizing muscle relaxants (succinylcholine and suxamethionine) cause a rise in the myoplasmic Ca^{2+} concentration. When an MH-susceptible individual is exposed to a triggering anesthetic, there is abnormal release of Ca^{2+}, which leads to prolonged activation of muscle filaments culminating in rigidity and hypermetabolism. Uncontrolled glycolysis and aerobic metabolism give rise to cellular hypoxia, progressive lactic acidosis, and hypercapnia. The continuous muscle activation with adenosine triphosphate breakdown results in excessive generation of heat. If untreated, myocyte death and rhabdomyolysis result in hyperkalemia and myoglobulinuria. Eventually, disseminated coagulopathy, congestive heart failure (CHF), bowel ischemia, and compartment syndrome develop.

Presentation and Management

Prevention of MH can be accomplished by identifying at-risk individuals before surgery. MH susceptibility is suspected preoperatively in a patient with a family history of MH or a personal history of myalgia after exercise, a tendency for the development of fever, muscular disease, and intolerance to caffeine. In these cases, creatine kinase is checked, and a caffeine and halothane contraction test (or an in vitro contracture test developed in Europe) may be performed on a muscle biopsy specimen from the thigh.[11] MH-susceptible individuals confirmed by abnormal skeletal muscle biopsy findings or individuals with suspected MH susceptibility who decline a contracture test are given a trigger-free anesthesia (barbiturates, benzodiazepines, opioids, propofol, etomidate, ketamine, nitrous oxide, and nondepolarizing neuromuscular blockers).

Unsuspected MH-susceptible individuals may manifest MH for the first time during or immediately after the administration of a triggering general anesthetic. The clinical manifestations of MH are not uniform and vary in onset and severity. Some patients manifest the abortive form of MH (tachycardia, arrhythmia, raised temperature, and acidosis). Others, after intubation with succinylcholine, demonstrate loss of twitches on neuromuscular stimulation, and muscle rigidity develops. An inability to open the mouth as a result of masseter muscle spasm is a pathognomonic early sign and indicates susceptibility to MH. Other manifestations include tachypnea, hypercapnia, skin flushing, hypoxemia, hypotension, electrolyte abnormalities, rhabdomyolysis, and hyperthermia.

Once MH is suspected or diagnosed, steps outlined in Box 15-3 are followed. Dantrolene is a muscle relaxant.

Box 15-3   Management of Malignant Hyperthermia

Discontinue the triggering anesthetic
Hyperventilate the patient with 100% oxygen
Administer alternative anesthesia
Terminate surgery
Give dantrolene, 2.5 mg/kg as a bolus and repeat every 5 minutes, then 1 to 2 mg/kg/hr until normalization or disappearance of symptoms
Check and monitor arterial blood gas, creatine kinase, electrolytes, lactate, and myoglobin
Monitor the electrocardiogram, vital signs, and urine output
Adjunctive and supportive measures are carried out:
    Volatile vaporizers are removed from the anesthesia machine
    Carbon dioxide canisters, bellows, and gas hoses are changed
    Surface cooling is achieved with ice packs and core cooling with cool parenteral fluids
    Acidosis is monitored and treated with sodium bicarbonate
    Arrhythmias are controlled with β-blockers or lidocaine
    Urine output greater than 2 mL/kg/hr is promoted: furosemide (Lasix) or mannitol and a glucose-insulin infusion (0.2 U/kg in a 50% glucose solution) are given for hyperkalemia, hypercalcemia, and myoglobulinuria
The patient is transferred to the intensive care unit to monitor for recurrence

Table 15-4   Causes of Postoperative Fever

INFECTIOUS	NONINFECTIOUS
Abscess	Acute hepatic necrosis
Acalculous cholecystitis	Adrenal insufficiency
Bacteremia	Allergic reaction
Decubitus ulcers	Atelectasis
Device-related infections	Dehydration
Empyema	Drug reaction
Endocarditis	Head injury
Fungal sepsis	Hepatoma
Hepatitis	Hyperthyroidism
Meningitis	Lymphoma
Osteomyelitis	Myocardial infarction
Pseudomembranous colitis	Pancreatitis
Parotitis	Pheochromocytoma
Perineal infections	Pulmonary embolus
Peritonitis	Retroperitoneal hematoma
Pharyngitis	Solid organ hematoma
Pneumonia	Subarachnoid hemorrhage
Retained foreign body	Systemic inflammatory
Sinusitis	response syndrome
Soft tissue infection	Thrombophlebitis
Tracheobronchitis	Transfusion reaction
Urinary tract infection	Withdrawal syndromes
	Wound infection

When given via IV, it blocks up to 75% of skeletal muscle contraction. Side effects reported with dantrolene therapy include muscle weakness, phlebitis, respiratory failure, GI discomfort, hepatotoxicity, dizziness, confusion, and drowsiness.

Postoperative Fever

Etiology

One of the most concerning clinical findings in a patient postoperatively is the development of fever. Fever refers to a rise in core temperature, modulation of which is managed by the anterior hypothalamus. Fever may result from bacterial invasion or their toxins, which stimulate the production of cytokines.[12] Trauma (including surgery) and critical illness also invoke a cytokine response. Fever after surgery is reported to occur in up to two thirds of patients, and infection is the cause of fever in about a third of cases. Numerous disease states can cause fever in the postoperative period (Table 15-4).

The most common infections, however, are health care–associated infections: surgical site infection, urinary tract infection, intravascular catheter–related infection, and pneumonia. Pneumonia may be acquired early (within 4-5 days of admission to the hospital). Aspiration of oropharyngeal and gastric contents is the most common cause of health care–associated pneumonia. Early pneumonia is commonly caused by *E. coli, Klebsiella* species, *Streptococcus pneumoniae, Haemophilus influenzae,* and *S. aureus,* and late onset pneumonia is typically caused by methicillin-resistant *S. aureus* and *Pseudomonas aeruginosa.*[13] Urinary tract infections are mostly catheter-associated infections and are commonly caused by *E. coli.* Coagulase-negative *S. aureus,* gram-negative bacilli, and

Candida species are the most frequent cause of catheter-related infection.

Presentation and Management

In evaluating a patient with fever, one has to take into consideration the type of surgery performed, the patient's immune status and the underlying primary disease process, the duration of hospital stay, and the epidemiology of hospital infections.

High fever that fluctuates or is sustained and that occurs 5 to 8 days after surgery is more worrisome than fever that occurs early postoperatively. In the first 48 to 72 hours after abdominal surgery, atelectasis is often believed to be the cause of the fever. Occasionally, clostridial or streptococcal surgical site infections can be manifested as fever within the first 72 hours of surgery. Temperatures that are elevated 5 to 8 days postoperatively demand immediate attention and, at times, intervention. Evaluation involves studying the six W's: wind (lungs), wound, water (urinary tract), waste (lower GI tract), wonder drug (e.g., antibiotics), and walker (e.g., thrombosis). The patient's symptoms usually point to the organ system involved with infection: cough and productive sputum suggest pneumonia, dysuria and frequency point to a urinary tract infection, watery foul-smelling diarrhea develops as a result of infection with *C. difficile,* pain in the calf may be due to deep venous thrombosis (DVT), and flank pain may be due to pyelonephritis. Physical examination may show a surgical site infection; phlebitis; tenderness on palpation of the abdomen, flank, or calf; or cellulitis at the site of a central venous catheter.

A complete blood count, urinalysis and culture, radiograph of the chest, and blood culture are essential initial tests. A chest radiograph may show a progressive infiltrate suggestive of the presence of pneumonia. Urinalysis showing greater than 10^5 colony-forming units per milliliter (CFU/mL) in a noncatheterized patient and greater than 10^3 CFU/mL in a catheterized patient indicates a urinary tract infection.[14] Peripheral blood cultures showing bacteremia and isolation of 15 CFUs or 10^2 CFUs from an IV catheter indicate the presence of a catheter-related infection.[15] In patients with valvular heart disease and *S. aureus* bacteremia, catheter-related infection requires evaluation by transesophageal echocardiography to check for vegetations. Patients who continue to have fever, slow clinical progress, and no discernible external source may require computed tomography (CT) of the abdomen to look for an intra-abdominal source of infection.

Management of postoperative fever is dictated by the results of a careful workup. Attempts to bring the temperature down with antipyretics are recommended. If pneumonia is suspected, empirical broad-spectrum antibiotic therapy is started and then altered according to culture results. Urinary tract infection is treated by removal of the catheter and administration of broad-spectrum antibiotics because most offending organisms exhibit resistance to several antibiotics. Patients with catheter-related infection are treated with vancomycin or linezolid. Empirical coverage of gram-negative bacilli and *Candida* species and removal of the catheter are essential in patients with severe sepsis or immunosuppression. Treatment is continued for 10 to 14 days. For patients with septic thrombosis or endocarditis, treatment is continued for 4 to 6 weeks.

PULMONARY COMPLICATIONS

A host of factors contribute to abnormal pulmonary physiology after an operative procedure. First, loss of functional residual capacity is present in virtually all patients. This loss may be due to a multitude of problems, including abdominal distention, a painful upper abdominal incision, obesity, a strong smoking history with associated chronic obstructive pulmonary disease, prolonged supine positioning, and fluid overload leading to pulmonary edema. Virtually all patients who undergo an abdominal incision or a thoracic incision have a significant alteration in their breathing pattern. Vital capacity may be reduced up to 50% of normal for the first 2 days after surgery for reasons that are not completely clear. The use of narcotics substantially inhibits the respiratory drive, and anesthetics may take some time to wear off. The majority of patients who have respiratory problems postoperatively have mild to moderate problems that can be managed with aggressive pulmonary toilet. However, in a portion of patients, severe postoperative respiratory failure develops and may require intubation and ultimately be life threatening.

Two types of respiratory failure are commonly described. Type I, or hypoxic, failure results from abnormal gas exchange at the alveolar level. This type is characterized by a low PaO_2 with a normal $PaCO_2$. Such hypoxemia is associated with ventilation-perfusion ($\dot{V}/\dot{Q}$) mismatching and shunting. Clinical conditions associated with type I failure include pulmonary edema and sepsis. Type II respiratory failure is associated with hypercapnia and is characterized by a low PaO_2 and high $PaCO_2$. These patients are unable to adequately eliminate CO_2. This condition is often associated with excessive narcotic use, increased CO_2 production, altered respiratory dynamics, and adult respiratory distress syndrome (ARDS). The overall incidence of pulmonary complications exceeds 25% in surgical patients. Twenty-five percent of all postoperative deaths are due to pulmonary complications, and pulmonary complications are associated with a fourth of the other lethal complications. Thus, it is of critical importance that the surgeon anticipate and prevent serious respiratory complications from occurring.

One of the most important elements of prophylaxis is careful preoperative screening of patients. The majority of patients have no pulmonary history and need no formal preoperative evaluation. However, patients with a history of heavy smoking, patients maintained on home oxygen, patients who are unable to walk one flight of stairs without severe respiratory compromise, patients with a previous history of major lung resection, and elderly patients who are malnourished all must be carefully screened with pulmonary function tests. Similarly, patients managed by chronic bronchodilator therapy for asthma or other pulmonary conditions need to be assessed carefully as well. Although there is some controversy about the value of perioperative assessment, most careful clinicians will study a high-risk pulmonary patient before making an operative decision. The assessment may start with posteroanterior and lateral chest radiographs to evaluate the appearance of the lungs. It serves as a baseline if the patient should have problems postoperatively.

Similarly, a patient with polycythemia or chronic respiratory acidosis warrants careful assessment. A room-temperature arterial blood gas analysis is obtained in high-risk patients. Any patient with a PaO_2 less than 60 mm Hg is at increased risk. If the $PaCO_2$ is greater than 45 to 50 mm Hg, perioperative morbidity might be anticipated. Spirometry is a simple test that high-risk patients undergo before surgery. Probably the most important parameter in spirometry is forced expiratory volume in 1 second (FEV_1). Studies demonstrate that any patient with an FEV_1 greater than 2 L will probably not have serious pulmonary problems. Conversely, patients with an FEV_1 less than 50% of the predicted value will probably have exertional dyspnea. If bronchodilator therapy demonstrates an improvement in breathing patterns by 15% or more, bronchodilation is considered. Consultation with the patient includes a discussion about cessation of cigarette smoking 48 hours before the operative procedure, as well as a careful discussion about the importance of pulmonary toilet after the operative procedure.

Atelectasis and Pneumonia

The most common postoperative respiratory complication is atelectasis. As a result of the anesthetic, abdominal incision, and postoperative narcotics, the alveoli in the periphery collapse and a pulmonary shunt may occur. If appropriate attention is not directed to aggressive pulmonary toilet with the initial symptoms, the alveoli remain collapsed and a buildup of secretions occurs and becomes secondarily infected with bacteria. The risk appears to be particularly high in patients who are heavy smokers, are obese, and have copious pulmonary secretions.

Pneumonia may develop early (i.e., 2-5 days after admission to the hospital) or late (i.e., >5 days) and is referred to as health care–related pneumonia.[13] Aspiration of oropharyngeal and gastric contents is the leading cause of health care–related pneumonia.

Presentation and Management

The most common cause of a postoperative fever in the first 48 hours after the procedure is atelectasis. The patients has a low-grade fever, malaise, and diminished breath sounds in the lower lung fields. Very often the patient is uncomfortable from the fever but has no other overt pulmonary symptoms. Atelectasis is so common postoperatively that a formal workup is not usually required. However, if not aggressively managed, frank development of pneumonia is likely. A patient with pneumonia, on the other hand, will have a high fever, occasionally mental confusion, and the production of a thick secretion with coughing, leukocytosis, and a chest radiograph that reveals infiltrates. If the condition is not expeditiously diagnosed and treated, the patient may rapidly progress to respiratory failure and require intubation.

Prevention of atelectasis and pneumonia is associated with pain control, which allows the patient to take deep breaths and cough. A patient-controlled analgesia device seems to be associated with better pulmonary toilet, as does the use of an epidural infusion catheter, particularly in patients with epigastric incisions. Respiratory care, otherwise, begins preoperatively. The patient must be instructed in use of the incentive spirometer and be held accountable by nurses and physicians during rounds. Encouraging the patient to cough while applying counterpressure with a pillow on the abdominal incision site is most helpful. Rarely, other modalities such as intermittent positive pressure breathing and chest physiotherapy may be required. Encouraging the patient to breathe deeply and cough is the single most valuable management approach in preventing and resolving atelectasis and pneumonia.

Patients in whom pneumonia develops in the postoperative period are managed with aggressive pulmonary toilet, induced sputum for culture and sensitivity testing, and empirical broad-spectrum IV antibiotic therapy while awaiting culture results. Once the organisms are cultured from sputum, a specific antibiotic must be used as indicated.

Aspiration Pneumonitis and Aspiration Pneumonia

Etiology

Aspiration of oropharyngeal or gastric contents into the respiratory tract is a serious complication of surgery. Aspiration pneumonitis (Mendelson's syndrome) describes acute lung injury that results from the inhalation of regurgitated gastric contents, whereas aspiration pneumonia results from the inhalation of oropharyngeal secretions that are colonized by pathogenic bacteria. Although there is some overlap between the two disease entities with regard to predisposing factors, their clinicopathologic features are distinct.

Factors that predispose patients to regurgitation and aspiration include impairment of the esophageal sphincters (upper and lower) and laryngeal reflexes, altered GI motility, and absence of preoperative fasting. A host of iatrogenic maneuvers place the patient at increased risk for aspiration in a hospital setting.[13] In the perioperative period, aspiration is more likely with urgent surgery, in patients with altered levels of consciousness, and in patients with GI and airway problems. Trauma patients and patients with peritonitis and bowel obstruction may have a depressed level of consciousness and airway reflexes, a full stomach as a result of a recent meal or gastric stasis, or GI pathology that predisposes to retrograde emptying of intestinal contents into the stomach. Patients with depressed levels of consciousness as a result of high doses of narcotics and patients with cerebrovascular accidents are obtunded and have neurologic dysphagia and dysfunction of the gastroesophageal junction. Anesthetic drugs lower esophageal sphincter tone and depress the level of consciousness of the patient. Diabetics have gastroparesis and gastric stasis. Patients with an increased bacterial load in the oropharynx and depressed defense mechanisms as a result of an altered level of consciousness are at risk for aspiration pneumonia.

The elderly are particularly susceptible to oropharyngeal aspiration because of an increased incidence of dysphagia and poor oral hygiene. Patients with a nasogastric (NG) tube or debility are also at risk for aspiration because they have difficulty swallowing and clearing their airway. The risk for aspiration pneumonia is similar in patients receiving feeding via an NG, nasoenteric, or gastrostomy tube (patients receiving nutrition via a gastrostomy tube frequently have scintigraphic evidence of aspiration of gastric contents). The critically ill are at an increased risk for aspiration and aspiration pneumonia because they are in a supine position, have an NG tube in place, exhibit gastroesophageal reflux even with the absence of an NG tube, and have altered GI motility. Prophylactic H_2 antagonists or proton pump inhibitors that increase gastric pH and allow the gastric contents to become colonized by pathogenic organisms, tracheostomy, reintubation, and previous antibiotic exposure are other factors associated with an increased risk for health care–related pneumonia.[13] The risk of aspiration is high after extubation because of the residual effect of sedation, the NG tube, and oropharyngeal dysfunction.

The pathophysiology of aspiration pneumonitis is related to pulmonary intake of gastric contents at a low pH associated with particulate matter. The severity of lung injury increases as the volume of aspirate increases and its pH decreases. The process often progresses very rapidly, may require intubation soon after the injury occurs, and later sets the stage for bacterial infection. The infection is refractory to management because of the combination of infection occurring in an injured field. The pathophysiology of aspiration pneumonia is related to bacteria gaining access to the lungs.

Presentation and Diagnosis

A patient with aspiration pneumonitis often has associated vomiting, may have received general anesthesia, or had an NG tube placed. The patient may be obtunded or have altered levels of consciousness. Initially, the patient may have associated wheezing and labored respiration. Many patients who aspirate gastric contents have a cough or a wheeze. Some patients, however, have silent aspiration suggested by an infiltrate on a radiograph of the chest or decreased PaO_2. Others have cough, shortness of breath, and wheezing that progressively progress to pulmonary edema and ARDS. In the great majority of patients with aspiration pneumonia, on the other hand, the condition is diagnosed after a chest radiograph shows an infiltrate in the posterior segments of the upper lobes and the apical segments of the lower lobes in a susceptible patient.

Treatment

Prevention of aspiration in patients undergoing surgery is achieved by instituting measures that reduce gastric contents, minimize regurgitation, and protect the airway. For adults, a period of no oral intake, usually 6 hours after a night meal, 4 hours after clear liquids, and a longer period for diabetics, is necessary to reduce gastric contents before elective surgery.[16] Routine use of H_2 antagonists or proton pump inhibitors to reduce gastric acidity and volume has not been shown to be effective in reducing the mortality and morbidity associated with aspiration and hence is not recommended.[14] When a difficult airway is encountered, awake fiberoptic intubation is performed. In emergency situations in patients with a potentially full stomach, preoxygenation is accomplished without lung inflation, and intubation is performed after applying cricoid pressure during rapid-sequence induction. In the postoperative period, identification of an elderly or overly sedated patient or a patient whose condition is deteriorating mandates maneuvers to protect the patient's airway. Postoperatively, it is important to avoid the overuse of narcotics, encourage the patient to ambulate, and cautiously feed a patient who is obtunded, elderly, or debilitated.

A patient who sustains aspiration of gastric contents needs to be immediately placed on oxygen and have a chest radiograph to confirm the clinical suspicions. A diffuse interstitial pattern is usually seen bilaterally and is often described as bilateral, fluffy infiltrates. Close surveillance of the patient is absolutely essential. If the patient is maintaining oxygen saturation via facemask without an excessively high work of breathing, intubation may not be required. However, if the patient's oxygenation deteriorates or the patient is obtunded, the work of breathing increases as manifested by an increased respiratory rate, and prompt intubation must be accomplished. After intubation for suspected aspiration, suc-

tioning of the bronchopulmonary tree will confirm the diagnosis and remove any particulate matter. Administration of antibiotics shortly after aspiration is controversial except in patients with bowel obstruction or other conditions associated with colonization of gastric contents. Administration of empirical antibiotics is also indicated in a patient with aspiration pneumonitis that does not resolve or improve within 48 hours of aspiration. Corticosteroid administration does not provide any beneficial effects to patients with aspiration pneumonitis.

Antibiotic therapy with activity against gram-negative organisms is indicated in patients with aspiration pneumonia.

Pulmonary Edema, Acute Lung Injury, and Adult Respiratory Distress Syndrome

Etiology

A wide variety of injuries to the lungs or cardiovascular system, or both, may result in acute respiratory failure. Three of the most common manifestations of such injury are pulmonary edema, acute lung injury, and ARDS. The clinician's ability to recognize and distinguish between these conditions is of critical importance because clinical management of these three entities varies considerably.

Pulmonary edema is a condition associated with accumulation of fluid in the alveoli. As a result of the fluid in the lumen of the alveoli, oxygenation cannot take place and hypoxemia occurs. As a consequence, the patient must increase the work of breathing, including an increased respiratory rate and exaggerated use of the muscles of breathing. Pulmonary edema is usually due to increased vascular hydrostatic pressure associated with CHF and acute myocardial infarction (MI). It is also commonly associated with fluid overload as a result of overly aggressive resuscitation (Box 15-4).

A recent consensus conference identified acute lung injury and ARDS as two separate grades of respiratory failure secondary to injury. In contrast to pulmonary edema, which is associated with increased wedge and right-sided heart pressure, acute lung injury and ARDS are associated with hypo-oxygenation because of a pathophysiologic inflammatory response that leads to the accumulation of fluid in the alveoli, as well as thickening in the space between the capillaries and the alveoli. Acute lung injury is associated with a PaO_2/FIO_2 ratio of less than 300, bilateral infiltrates on chest radiography, and a wedge pressure less than 18 mm Hg. It tends to be shorter in duration and not as severe. On the other hand, ARDS is associated with a PaO_2/FIO_2 ratio of less than 200 and also has bilateral infiltrates and a wedge pressure less than 18 mm Hg.

Presentation and Management

Patients with pulmonary edema often have a corresponding cardiac history or a recent history of massive fluid administration (or both). In the presence of a frankly abnormal chest radiograph, invasive monitoring in the form of a Swan-Ganz catheter for evaluation of pulmonary capillary wedge pressure is indicated. Patients with an elevated wedge pressure are managed by fluid

Box 15-4 Conditions Leading to Pulmonary Edema, Acute Lung Injury, and Adult Respiratory Distress Syndrome

Increased Hydrostatic Pressure

Acute left ventricular failure
Chronic congestive heart failure
Obstruction of the left ventricular outflow tract
Thoracic lymphatic insufficiency
Volume overload

Altered Permeability State

Acute radiation pneumonitis
Aspiration of gastric contents
Drug overdose
Near-drowning
Pancreatitis
Pneumonia
Pulmonary embolus
Shock states
Systemic inflammatory response syndrome and multiple organ failure
Sepsis
Transfusion
Trauma and burns

Mixed or Incompletely Understood Pathogenesis

Hanging injuries
High-altitude pulmonary edema
Narcotic overdose
Neurogenic pulmonary edema
Postextubation obstructive pulmonary edema
Re-expansion pulmonary edema
Tocolytic therapy
Uremia

Table 15-5 Criteria for Weaning From the Ventilator

PARAMETER	WEANING CRITERIA
Respiratory rate	<25 breaths/min
PaO_2	>70 mm Hg (FIO_2 of 40%)
$PaCO_2$	<45 mm Hg
Minute ventilation	8-9 L/min
Tidal volume	5-6 mL/kg
Negative inspiratory force	−25 cm H_2O

ARDS is initially placed on an FIO_2 of 100% and then weaned to 60% as healing takes place. Positive end-expiratory pressure is a valuable addition to ventilator management of patients with this injury. Similarly, tidal volume needs to be 6 to 8 mL/kg with peak pressure kept at 35 cm H_2O. Tidal volume is set at 10 to 12 mL/kg of body weight and the respiratory rate chosen to produce a $PaCO_2$ near 40 mm Hg. In addition, the inspiratory-to-expiratory ratio is set at 1:2. Most patients will require heavy sedation and pharmacologic paralysis during the early phases of recuperation.

Careful monitoring of oxygenation, improvement of the respiratory rate with intermittent mandatory ventilation, and general alertness will suggest when the patient is ready to be extubated. Criteria for extubation are listed in Table 15-5.

Pulmonary Embolism and Venous Thromboembolism

Etiology

Venous thromboembolism describes DVT and pulmonary embolism (PE). PE is a serious postoperative complication that represents a source of preventable morbidity and mortality in the United States and is responsible for 5% to 10% of all in-hospital deaths. Undiagnosed PE has a hospital mortality rate as high as 30%, which falls to 8% if diagnosed and treated appropriately.

Venous thromboembolism is caused by a perturbation of the homeostatic coagulation system induced by intimal injury, stasis of blood flow, and a hypercoagulable state. Risk factors for the development of venous thromboembolism are listed in Table 15-6.[17,18]

Thrombophilia describes hereditary and acquired biochemical states that predispose to venous thromboembolism. One in four fatal PE cases occurs in surgical patients. Survivors of venous thromboembolism are at increased risk for recurrence. The highest risk for venous thromboembolism occurs in patients hospitalized for surgery. The prevalence of PE in patients with malignancy is 11%; that of DVT and PE in patients with inflammatory bowel disease is about 5% and 3%, respectively; and in major trauma victims the incidence of DVT is 50%, with fatal emboli occurring in 0.4% to 2% of cases. The critically ill have multiple risk factors and are at higher risk for venous thromboembolism. Central venous catheter–related thrombosis is more common with femoral placement. The frequency of thrombosis ranges from 4% to 28% after subclavian vein cannulation and 4% to 33%

restriction and aggressive diuresis. Administration of oxygen via facemask in mild cases and intubation in more severe cases is also clinically indicated. In most cases, the pulmonary edema resolves quickly after diuresis and fluid restriction.

Patients with acute lung injury and ARDS generally have tachypnea, dyspnea, and increased work of breathing, as manifested by exaggerated use of the muscles of breathing. Cyanosis is associated with advanced hypoxia and is an emergency. Auscultation of the lung fields reveals very poor breath sounds associated with crackles and, occasionally, with rales. Arterial blood gas analysis will reveal the presence of a low PaO_2 and a high $PaCO_2$. Administration of oxygen alone does not usually result in improvement in the hypoxia.

In patients with impending respiratory failure, including tachypnea, dyspnea, and air hunger, management of acute lung injury and ARDS is initiated by immediate intubation plus careful administration of fluids and invasive monitoring with a Swan-Ganz catheter to assess wedge pressure and right-sided heart pressure. The strategy is one of maintaining the patient on the ventilator with assisted breathing while healing of the injured lung takes place. A patient with severe acute lung injury or

Table 15-6 Risk Factors for Venous Thromboembolism

CATEGORY	FACTORS
General factors	Advancing age Hospitalization or nursing home (with or without surgery) Indwelling venous catheters Neurologic disease (plegia and paresis) Cardiomyopathy, myocardial infarction, or heart failure secondary to valve disease Acute pulmonary disease (adult respiratory distress syndrome and pneumonia) Chronic obstructive lung disease Varicose veins
Inherited thrombophilia	Protein C deficiency Protein S deficiency Antithrombin III deficiency Dysfibrinogenemia Factor V Leiden mutation Prothrombin gene mutation Hyperhomocystinemia Anticardiolipin antibody Paroxysmal nocturnal hemoglobinemia
Acquired thrombophilia	Malignancy Inflammatory bowel disease Heparin-induced thrombocytopenia Trauma Major surgery Pregnancy/postpartum Nephrotic syndrome Behçet's syndrome Systemic lupus erythematosus History of venous thromboembolism

Box 15-5 Symptoms and Signs of Pulmonary Embolism

Pleuritic chest pain*
Sudden dyspnea*
Tachypnea
Hemoptysis*
Tachycardia*
Leg swelling*
Pain on palpation of the leg*
Acute right ventricular dysfunction
Hypoxia
Fourth heart sound*
Loud second pulmonary sound*
Inspiratory crackles*

*More common with pulmonary embolism.

after internal jugular catheterization. In patients with subclavian or axillary vein thrombosis, PE is reported in 9.4%.

The majority of PE originates from an existing DVT in the legs, and the iliofemoral venous system is the site from which most clinically significant pulmonary emboli arise. PE develops in about 50% of patients with proximal DVT. Rare causes of PE include a fat embolus associated with fractures of long bones and air embolism, often associated with operative procedures and central lines.

Presentation and Diagnosis

The physiologic response to PE depends on the size of the thrombus, coexisting cardiopulmonary disease, and various neurohormonal effects. More than 50% of DVTs are silent, and PE may be the first manifestation of the disease. Most symptoms and signs associated with symptomatic PE are nonspecific and may be encountered with other disease states such as MI, pneumothorax, and pneumonia (Box 15-5). Chest radiography has limited value in the diagnosis of PE and is mainly used to rule out other causes of a patient's symptoms.[19] Massive PE that results in hemodynamic instability (hypotension with or without shock) and death develops in about 5% to

10% of patients. The probability of an individual having PE (pretest probability) is assessed by the sum of points given to risk factors for venous thromboembolism (see Table 15-6) and the patient's symptoms, signs, and laboratory results (electrocardiogram [ECG], chest radiograph, and arterial blood gas) most likely to be associated with PE. In general, patients with the aforementioned symptom complex (see Box 15-5) are thought to require workup for PE if their P_{CO_2} is less than 36 mm Hg, their P_{O_2} is less than 60 mm Hg, and the ECG shows characteristic changes of PE (right bundle branch block, right-axis deviation, P-wave pulmonale). With the use of various scoring systems, patients are categorized into low, moderate, and high probability.[20]

Establishing the diagnosis of PE requires confirmatory tests ($\dot{V}/\dot{Q}$ lung scan, helical CT angiogram scan) or a pulmonary angiogram and ancillary tests (venous duplex ultrasound and a D-dimer assay). A $\dot{V}/\dot{Q}$ scan was commonly used as the initial test of choice in patients with suspected PE in the recent past. However, CT angiography has rendered $\dot{V}/\dot{Q}$ scans obsolete in most institutions.[19] Helical CT, which is also known as spiral CT or CT pulmonary angiography, is more accurate than $\dot{V}/\dot{Q}$ scans, has high specificity (92%) and sensitivity (86%), and is especially accurate for central PE (main pulmonary artery or subsegmental branches).[19] Spiral CT also allows diagnosis of other pulmonary causes of a patient's symptoms.[19] However, the test is invasive; requires IV contrast; may not be available after normal working hours; requires a cooperative patient to avoid artifacts; may miss emboli in subsegmental arteries, which account for 20% of all pulmonary emboli; and may be inconclusive in about 10% of cases. Pulmonary angiography is the gold standard test because it directly visualizes the arterial tree and detects intravascular filling defects. It is used less commonly, however, because it is invasive, requires expertise, and after-hours availability is limited. Echocardiography is a rapid, noninvasive, available bedside test that provides quick results in a critically ill or hemodynamically unstable patient. Transthoracic imaging shows the hemodynamic consequences of acute ventricular pressure overload, namely, right ventricular dysfunction (hypokinesia and dilation), interventricular septal flattening and paradoxical motion, elevated tricuspid gradient, pulmonary hypertension, and a patent foramen ovale.[21] Echocardiography also rules out other causes of shock such as pericardial tamponade. Transesophageal echocardiography is not always available and requires specialty training.

Venous ultrasound of the extremities is used as an indirect test for diagnosing PE. About a third of patients with PE will demonstrate lower extremity findings consistent with DVT, and 80% of patients with PE have a DVT on venography. D-dimer is a degradation product of a cross-linked fibrin blood clot. Levels are typically elevated in patients with acute thromboembolism. Of the many D-dimer tests, enzyme-linked immunosorbent assay (ELISA) is the most sensitive with quick results. A negative test excludes the diagnosis, but a positive test does not rule in the diagnosis.

Based on the pretest clinical probability, a patient suspected of having PE requires a chest radiograph, ECG, arterial blood gas analysis, and D-dimer assay. If leg symptoms are present, venous ultrasound is performed, and if positive, the patient is considered to have PE and receives anticoagulant medication (because treatment is similar to that for PE). If leg symptoms are not present, the spiral CT scan approach may be used. If the findings on spiral CT are suboptimal or negative and there is a high clinical probability of PE, an angiogram is obtained. This approach is not appropriate for patients with iodinated-dye allergy.

In the critically ill with high suspicion for PE and patients with suspected massive PE, the workup depends on hemodynamic stability. In stable patients, anticoagulation is started if there are no contraindications, venous ultrasound is performed, and a spiral CT scan approach is followed. In unstable patients, anticoagulation is started and venous ultrasound and echocardiography are performed. If the echocardiographic results are positive, thrombolytic therapy is started, and if negative, a pulmonary angiogram is obtained.

Treatment

The most commonly used medications in the management of venous thromboembolism are the heparins and vitamin K antagonists. Heparin prevents the formation of new thrombi and stops propagation of the thrombi, ultrafractionated heparin enhances the antithrombotic activity of antithrombin III and factor Xa, and LMWH primarily inactivates factor Xa. Vitamin K antagonists (warfarin) have a delayed onset of action and the potential to interact with other medications. Synthetic pentasaccharide anticoagulant (fondaparinux) is a newly introduced medication that selectively inhibits factor Xa. Thrombolytic agents (streptokinase, urokinase, and recombinant tissue plasminogen activator) are used in the treatment of massive PE.

Treatment of PE starts with prevention. Because the great majority of emboli originate from existing clots in the deep venous system of the legs in at-risk patients, identifying patients at risk for DVT plus applying preventive measures is the only way to decrease the morbidity and mortality associated with venous thromboembolism.[22] In the critically ill, heparin is the first line of prophylaxis, with low-dose ultrafractionated heparin being administered SC every 8 hours or LMWH given as a daily dose. Overt bleeding and thrombocytopenia are contraindications to chemical prophylaxis. In patients undergoing surgery, low-dose ultrafractionated heparin is administered (5000 U 1-2 hours preoperatively and then every 8 hours). Fondaparinux is emerging as an alternative prophylaxis after major orthopedic surgery. Nonpharmacologic prophylaxis can be achieved with elastic stockings, graduated compression stockings, intermittent pneumatic compression devices, or venous foot pumps. They produce a satisfactory reduction in risk for DVT in high-risk surgical patients. The presence of leg ulcers and peripheral vascular disease precludes the use of mechanical devices. In patients with a contraindication to anticoagulation, placement of an inferior vena cava filter protects against PE. Ultrafractionated heparin is given IV (a bolus of 70 U/kg followed by 1000 U/hr) to achieve a partial thromboplastin time 1.5 to 2 times the control value.[21] Ultrafractionated heparin is easily reversible and hence the agent of choice. LMWH is given SC once or twice daily (enoxaparin, 1.5 mg/kg/day, or dalteparin, 10,000-18,000 U/day, depending on weight). Monitoring of LMWH is not necessary. Warfarin is given orally and therapy allowed to overlap with heparin therapy until the INR is therapeutic for 2 consecutive days before heparin is discontinued. Therapy is continued for more than 3 months with the goal of reaching an INR of 2.5.

In massive PE the goal of therapy is to maintain hemodynamic stability, enhance coronary flow, and minimize right ventricular ischemia. Once suspected, resuscitation is initiated, oxygen administered, and IV ultrafractionated heparin therapy started. In the hemodynamically unstable, IV vasoactive medications are required. Thrombolytic therapy, if not contraindicated, has the advantage of dissolving the clot rapidly with rapid improvement in pulmonary perfusion, hemodynamic alterations, gas exchange, and right ventricular function. The role of surgical embolectomy is controversial. A transcatheter technique (with or without low-dose thrombolytic therapy) is another therapeutic approach. Placement of an inferior vena cava filter reduces the risk for recurrence of PE.

CARDIAC COMPLICATIONS

Postoperative Hypertension

Etiology

Hypertension is a serious problem that can cause devastating complications in the preoperative, intraoperative, and postoperative periods. Perioperative hypertension (or hypotension) occurs in a quarter of patients undergoing surgery. The risk for hypertension is related to the type of surgery performed; cardiovascular, thoracic, and intra-abdominal procedures are most commonly associated with hypertensive events. Preoperatively, most hypertension is essential hypertension; much less common are cases associated with renovascular causes and even rarer, vasoactive tumors. Intraoperatively, fluid overload and pharmacologic agents may cause hypertension. Postoperatively, a host of factors are associated with hypertension, including pain, hypothermia, hypoxia, fluid overload in the postanesthesia period caused by mobilization of fluid from the extravascular compartment, and discontinuation of chronic antihypertensive therapy before surgery. Other causes of postoperative hypertension include intra-abdominal bleeding, head trauma, clonidine withdrawal syndrome, and pheochromocytoma crisis.

Presentation and Management

Most cases of hypertension are detected during the routine preoperative workup. An observant surgeon will consider hypertension in the preoperative screening of patients because failure to detect significant problems with hypertension can lead to needless hypertension-related complications. By definition, any patient who has a diastolic blood pressure greater than 110 mm Hg must be assessed and treated preoperatively if elective surgery is being contemplated. Patients taking chronic antihypertensive medications who are undergoing elective surgery are instructed to continue taking the medication up to the day of surgery. Patients receiving oral clonidine can be switched to a clonidine patch for at least 3 days before surgery. In emergency cases, the medications administered during induction and maintenance of anesthesia will assist in bringing the blood pressure down. Intraoperatively, the anesthesiologist must carefully monitor blood pressure, make certain that it stays within acceptable limits, and avoid fluid overload, hypoxia, and hypothermia. In the postoperative period, the patient is given adequate analgesia and long-term antihypertensive medications are resumed. In patients who are not able to take oral medications, β-blockers, angiotensin-converting enzyme (ACE) inhibitors, calcium channel antagonists, or diuretics are given parenterally or clonidine as a transdermal patch.

Although hypertension in the postoperative period is common, a hypertensive crisis is uncommon, especially after noncardiac surgery. A hypertensive crisis is characterized by severe elevation of blood pressure associated with organ dysfunction: cerebral and subarachnoid hemorrhage and stroke, acute cardiac events, renal dysfunction, and bleeding from the operative wound. This appears to be particularly the case in carotid endarterectomy, aortic aneurysm surgery, and many head and neck procedures. Diastolic hypertension (>110 mm Hg) is significantly associated with cardiac complications, and systolic hypertension (>160 mm Hg) is associated with an increased risk for stroke and death. In patients with new-onset or severe perioperative hypertension and patients with a hypertensive emergency, treatment with agents that have a rapid onset of action, short half-life, and few autonomic side effects to lower blood pressure is essential. Medications most commonly used in this setting include nitroprusside and nitroglycerin (vasodilators), labetalol and esmolol (β-blockers),) enalaprilat (useful in patients receiving long-term ACE inhibitors), and nicardipine (calcium channel blocker). It is crucial in the acute setting to not decrease blood pressure more than 25% to avoid ischemic strokes and hypoperfusion injury to other organs.

Perioperative Ischemia and Infarction

Etiology

Approximately 30% of all patients taken to the operating room have some degree of CAD. Patients at risk for an acute cardiac event in the perioperative period are the elderly, those with peripheral artery disease, and patients undergoing vascular, thoracic, major orthopedic, and upper abdominal procedures. Although management of nonoperative MI has improved, the mortality associated with perioperative MI remains around 30%. Perioperative myocardial complications result in at least 10% of all perioperative deaths. In the 1970s, the risk for recurrence of MI within 3 months of an MI was reported to be 30%, and if a patient underwent surgery within 3 to 6 months of infarction, the reinfarction rate was 15%. Six months postoperatively the reinfarction rate was only 5%. However, improved preoperative assessment, advances in anesthesia and intraoperative monitoring, and the availability of more sophisticated intensive care unit (ICU) monitoring have resulted in improvement in the outcome of patients at risk for an acute cardiac event. Individuals undergoing an operation within 3 months of an infarction have an 8% to 15% reinfarction rate; between 3 and 6 months postoperatively the reinfarction rate is only 3.5%. The general mortality associated with MI in patients without a surgical procedure is 12%.

Presentation

The risk for myocardial ischemia and MI is greatest in the first 48 hours after surgery, and it may be difficult to make the diagnosis. The classic manifestation, chest pain radiating into the jaw and left arm region, is often not present. Patients may have shortness of breath, an increased heart rate, hypotension, or respiratory failure. Perioperative myocardial ischemia and MI are often silent, and when they occur, they are marked by shortness of breath (heart failure, respiratory failure), an increased heart rate (arrhythmias), a change in mental status, or excessive hyperglycemia in diabetics. Many perioperative MIs are non–Q wave, non–ST segment elevation MIs.

Treatment

Preventing coronary ischemia is a function of prospectively identifying patients at risk for a perioperative cardiac complication. This will allow improvement of the condition of patients and possibly lower their risk, selection of patients for invasive or noninvasive cardiac testing, and identification of patients who will benefit from more intensive perioperative monitoring. Preoperative cardiac risk assessment includes adequate history taking, physical examination, and basic diagnostic tests. The history is important for identifying patients with cardiac disease or those at risk for cardiac disease, including previous cardiac revascularization, MI, or stroke and the presence of valvular heart disease, heart failure, arrhythmia, hypertension, diabetes, and lung and renal disease. Unstable

Table 15-7 Clinical Predictors of Increased Perioperative Cardiovascular Risk Leading to Myocardial Infarction, Heart Failure, or Death

Major Risk Factors
Unstable coronary syndromes
  Acute or recent myocardial infarction with evidence of considerable ischemic risk as noted by clinical symptoms or noninvasive studies
  Unstable or severe angina (Canadian class III or IV)
Decompensated heart failure
Significant arrhythmias
  High-grade atrioventricular block
  Symptomatic ventricular arrhythmias in the presence of underlying heart disease
  Supraventricular arrhythmias with an uncontrolled ventricular rate
Severe valve disease

Intermediate Risk Factors
Mild angina pectoris (Canadian class I or II)
Previous myocardial infarction identified by history or pathologic evidence
Q waves
Compensated or previous heart failure
Diabetes mellitus (particularly insulin dependent)
Renal insufficiency

Minor Risk Factors
Advanced age
Abnormal electrocardiogram (e.g., left ventricular hypertrophy, left bundle branch block, ST-T abnormalities)
Rhythm other than sinus (e.g., atrial fibrillation)
Low functional capacity (e.g., inability to climb one flight of stairs with a bag of groceries)
History of stroke
Uncontrolled systemic hypertension

Table 15-8 Cardiac Risk Stratification for Noncardiac Surgical Procedures

RISK	FACTOR
High (cardiac risk often >5%)	Emergency major operations, particularly in the elderly; Aortic and other major vascular surgery; Peripheral vascular surgery; Anticipated prolonged surgical procedures associated with large fluid shifts and blood loss
Intermediate (cardiac risk generally <5%)	Carotid endarterectomy; Intraperitoneal and intrathoracic surgery; Orthopedic surgery; Prostate surgery
Low (cardiac risk generally <1%)	Endoscopic procedures; Superficial procedures; Cataract surgery; Breast surgery

Reprinted with permission. *ACC/AHA 2002 Guideline Update on Perioperative Cardiovascular Evaluation for Noncardiac Surgery—Executive Summary.* ©2002, American Heart Association, Inc.

chest pain, especially crescendo angina, warrants careful evaluation and postponement of an elective operation. Physical examination may reveal uncontrolled hypertension, evidence of peripheral artery disease, arrhythmia, or clinical stigmata of heart failure. Chest radiographs may show pulmonary edema, the ECG may show an arrhythmia, blood gas analysis may reveal hypercapnia or a low PaO_2, and blood tests may show abnormal kidney function. "Guidelines for Perioperative Cardiovascular Evaluation for Noncardiac Surgery," recently published by the American College of Cardiology (ACA) and the American Heart Association (AHA), stratifies clinical predictors of increased perioperative cardiovascular risk leading to MI, CHF, or death into major, intermediate, and minor (Table 15-7) and stratifies cardiac risk into high, intermediate, and low (Table 15-8).[23]

The ACC/AHA guidelines permit more appropriate use of preoperative testing (echocardiography, dipyridamole myocardial stress perfusion imaging, traditional exercise stress test, or angiography) and β-blocker therapy with probable canceling of the elective operative procedure.[24]

An algorithm for perioperative cardiovascular evaluation is presented in Figure 15-1.

Patients identified as being at high risk for myocardial events in the perioperative period are managed with β-blockers, careful monitoring intraoperatively, maintenance of perioperative normothermia and vital signs, and continued pharmacologic management postoperatively, including the administration of adequate pain medication. Given several days before surgery and continued for several days afterward, β-blockers (atenolol) have been shown to reduce perioperative myocardial ischemia by 50% in patients with CAD or risk factors for CAD.[25] Patients with chronic stable angina continue with their antianginal medications, and β-blockers are continued to the time of surgery and thereafter. An ECG is obtained before, immediately after, and for 2 days after surgery. Patients are monitored for 48 hours after surgery—5 days for very high-risk patients—and cardiac enzyme levels are also checked. Invasive hemodynamic monitoring is appropriate in patients with left ventricular dysfunction, fixed cardiac output, and unstable angina or recent MI.

Shortness of breath and chest pain remain the two postoperative symptoms that must always be carefully evaluated and never written off as postoperative discomfort. Subtle changes in the ST segment and T wave hint of possible ischemia or MI. Evaluation of a patient suspected of having an intraoperative or postoperative MI includes immediate assessment by ECG, as well as serum troponin levels. Constant monitoring of the ECG is required so that the development of any potentially lethal arrhythmia can be immediately treated. Cardiac-specific troponin levels begin to rise by 3 hours after myocardial

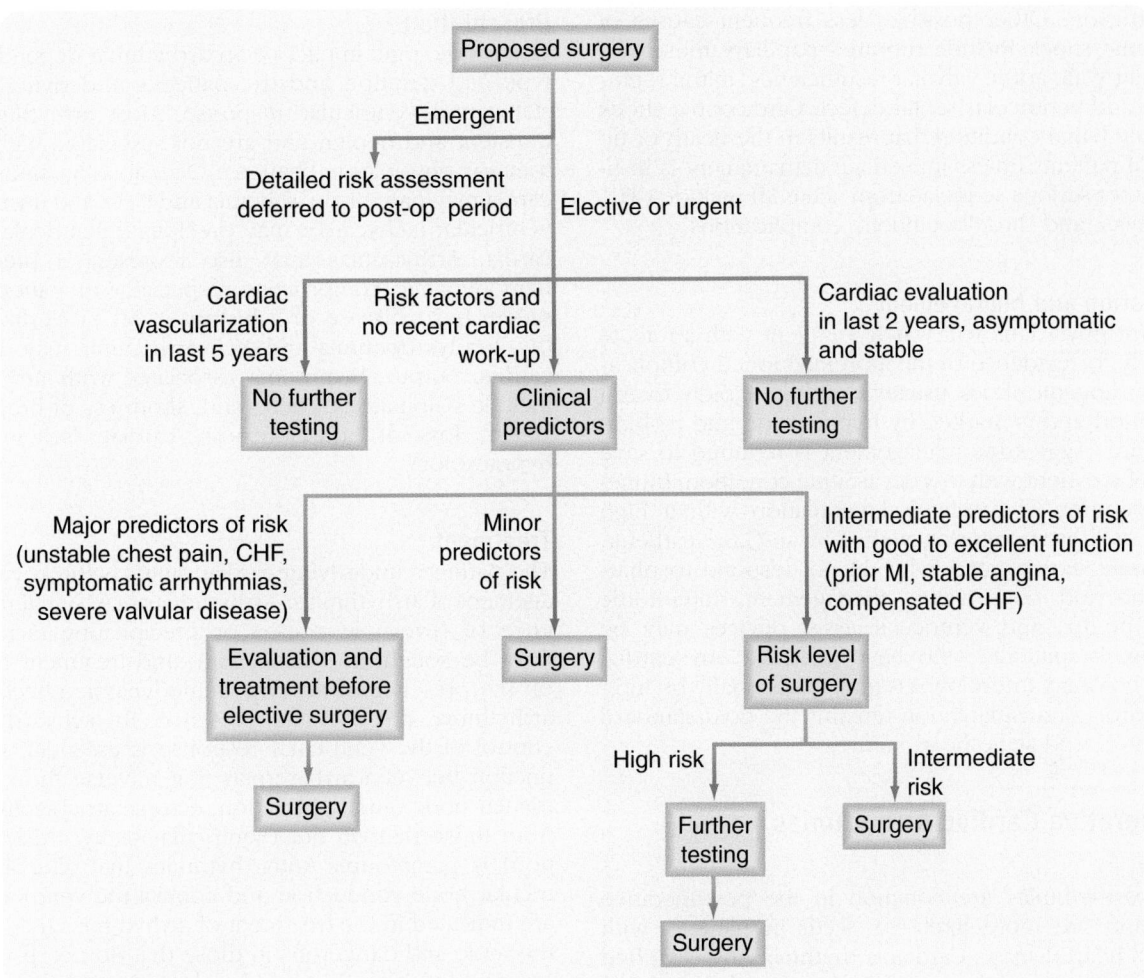

Figure 15-1 Algorithm for perioperative cardiovascular evaluation for noncardiac surgery. Patients with major predictors of risk and patients with intermediate predictors of risk and a planned high-risk procedure undergo additional testing and resultant indicated treatment before elective surgery. CHF, congestive heart failure; MI, myocardial infarction. (Modified from Eagle KA, Brundage BH, Chaitman BR, et al: Guidelines for perioperative cardiovascular evaluation for noncardiac surgery. Report of the American College of Cardiology/American Heart Association Task Force on Practice Guidelines. J Am Coll Cardiol 27: 910-945, 1996.)

injury. A troponin I level greater than 1 ng/mL is specific, and elevations persist for 7 to 10 days. Troponin T elevations persist for 10 to 14 days after MI. If the level of cardiac function is a concern, echocardiography is considered. Medical management of myocardial ischemia and MI includes immediate administration of high-flow oxygen, transfer to the ICU, and early involvement of a cardiologist. The goal of management of myocardial ischemia is to preserve the maximal amount of myocardial muscle possible, as well as improve coronary blood flow and decrease myocardial work. Immediate administration of β-blockers and aspirin (160-325 mg) is essential. β-Blockers are not indicated in patients with bradycardia, hypotension, severe left ventricular dysfunction, heart block, or severe bronchospastic disease. Nitroglycerin (given as a continuous IV infusion after a loading dose) alleviates pain and is beneficial in patients with MI complicated by heart failure or pulmonary edema. Systemic heparinization (or SC LMWH), if not contraindicated, is administered. In most cases, thrombolytic therapy is contraindicated in the postoperative period and can be used only in situations in which minor surgery is performed. ACE inhibitors may be given early after MI (especially anterior MI or with low-ejection left ventricular function) and probably continued as a long-term therapy. Angiography must be strongly considered if the patient has ongoing myocardial ischemia that does not respond to pharmacologic therapy.

Cardiogenic Shock

Etiology

Cardiogenic shock is one of the most serious sequelae of acute MI. Presumably, 50% or more of left ventricular muscle mass is irreversibly damaged, thereby leading to a substantial reduction in cardiac output and resultant hypoperfusion. Other possible, less frequent causes of cardiogenic shock include ruptured papillary muscle or ventricular wall, aortic valvular insufficiency, mitral regurgitation, and ventricular septal defect. Cardiogenic shock is a highly lethal condition that results in the death of up to 75% of patients unless immediate management is instituted. Other serious sequelae from acute MI include CHF, arrhythmias, and thromboembolic complications.

Presentation and Management

Observant physicians will watch a patient with an acute MI closely for evidence of the aforementioned complications. Cardiogenic shock usually develops rapidly over a short period and is marked by hypotension and respiratory failure. Aggressive management is required to save the life of a patient with this devastating condition. Immediate institution of mechanical ventilation with a high FIO_2, as well as monitoring with a Swan-Ganz catheter, is important. For patients who do not respond to pharmacologic and conservative management, intra-aortic balloon pumps and ventricular assist devices may be lifesaving. In patients who have adequate myocardial reserve, coronary artery bypass may occasionally be indicated. Cardiac transplantation remains the gold standard treatment of end-stage heart failure.

Postoperative Cardiac Arrhythmias

Etiology

Cardiac arrhythmias are common in the postoperative period and are more likely to occur in patients with structural heart disease. Cardiac arrhythmias are classified into tachyarrhythmia, bradyarrhythmia, and heart block. Tachyarrhythmia is further subdivided into supraventricular (sinus, atrial, nodal) and ventricular (premature ventricular contraction [PVC], ventricular tachycardia, ventricular fibrillation). Sustained supraventricular arrhythmia in patients undergoing major noncardiac surgery may be associated with increased risk for a cardiac event (heart failure, MI, unstable angina) and cerebrovascular event.[26] Risk factors associated with increased risk for supraventricular arrhythmias are increasing age, a history of heart failure, and the type of surgery performed. Sinus tachycardia and atrial flutter/fibrillation are the most common types of tachyarrhythmia. Sinus tachycardia is caused by pain, fever, hypovolemia, anemia, anxiety, and less commonly, heart failure, MI, thyrotoxicosis, and pheochromocytoma. Atrial flutter/fibrillation occurs commonly in patients with electrolyte imbalance, a history of atrial fibrillation, and chronic obstructive lung disease.

Ventricular ectopy occurs in a third of patients after major noncardiac surgery, and risk factors associated with an increased risk for PVCs include the presence of preoperative PVC, a history of CHF, and cigarette smoking.[27] Postoperative risk factors include hypoxia, acute hypokalemia, and hypercapnia. Ventricular arrhythmias consist of largely benign and sustained ventricular tachycardia and fibrillation. Nonsustained ventricular tachycardia occurs commonly during or after major vascular procedures.

Presentation

The physiologic impact of an arrhythmia depends on its type and duration and the patient's underlying cardiac status and ventricular response. Most arrhythmias are transient and benign and are not associated with symptoms or physiologic changes. Occasionally, sinus tachycardia may precipitate ischemia and PVC, and unsustained ventricular tachycardia may precipitate ventricular tachycardia. Arrhythmias may also represent a prelude to hemodynamic compromise, especially in patients with severe heart disease or a history of MI or cardiomyopathy. Bradyarrhythmia and tachyarrhythmia may decrease cardiac output. Symptoms associated with arrhythmias include palpitations, chest pain, shortness of breath, dizziness, loss of consciousness, cardiac ischemia, and hypotension.

Treatment

The patient's underlying cardiac status is the key to management of arrhythmias. Arrhythmias may signal the presence of reversible causes or precipitating factors that must be sought and dealt with, and treatment is based on the presence of adverse hemodynamic effects of the arrhythmia, not its mere presence. In tachyarrhythmia, control of the ventricular response is essential, and distinction between arrhythmias that traverse the atrioventricular node (atrial fibrillation, ectopic atrial tachycardia) from those that do not (ventricular tachycardia, fibrillation) is paramount. Antiarrhythmics that alter atrioventricular node conduction and control the ventricular rate are indicated in the treatment of arrhythmias that traverse the node and dangerous in those that do not. β-Blockers are avoided in patients with a low ejection fraction and bronchospastic lung disease. The ultimate goal of therapy is to achieve sinus rhythm, and if not possible, prevention of complications associated with arrhythmias must be addressed (e.g., anticoagulants given to patients with atrial fibrillation for more than 48 hours). Management of postoperative arrhythmias is outlined in Box 15-6.

Postoperative Heart Failure

Etiology

Heart failure is a clinical syndrome characterized by any structural or functional cardiac disorder that impairs the ability of the ventricle to fill with or eject blood.[28] Several risk factors predispose to the development of heart failure, the most significant of which are CAD, hypertension, and increasing age. Poorly controlled heart failure represents one of the most serious cardiac risk factors for a preoperative patient, whereas patients with well-managed heart failure generally do well during an operation. A multitude of factors can lead to new-onset heart failure or decompensation of preexisting heart failure in the perioperative period, including perioperative myocardial ischemia or MI, volume overload, hypertension, sepsis, occult cardiac valvular disease, PE, and new-onset atrial fibrillation. The risk for heart failure is greatest immediately after surgery and in the first 24 to 48 hours after surgery.

Box 15-6   Management of Postoperative Cardiac Arrhythmias

Cardiology consultation

Monitoring of the patient on a telemetry floor or in the intensive care unit

A 12-lead electrocardiogram and a long strip to differentiate between atrial and ventricular arrhythmia

Clinical assessment
  Vital signs
  Peripheral perfusion
  Cardiac ischemia and congestive heart failure
  Level of consciousness

Treatment of arrhythmia
  Tachyarrhythmia
    Unstable: Cardioversion
    Stable
      Supraventricular tachyarrhythmia: β-blockers (esmolol), ibutilide, or alternatives (digoxin, calcium channel blockers, amiodarone)
      Paroxysmal supraventricular tachyarrhythmia: vagal stimulation or adenosine. Digoxin, amiodarone, or calcium channel blocker if adenosine fails
      Multifocal atrial tachycardia: β-blocker, calcium channel blocker, or amiodarone
      Ventricular tachycardia: lidocaine, procainamide, or amiodarone
  Bradyarrhythmia
    Sustained: atropine or β-agonist
    Transient: no therapy
  Heart block: persistent high-grade second- or third-degree block: insertion of a permanent pacemaker

---

Presentation

Patients with poorly controlled heart failure or new-onset heart failure suffer from shortness of breath and wheezing. Physical examination often reveals tachycardia, a narrow pulse pressure, low pressure or orthostatic hypotension, jugular venous distention, peripheral edema, rales, and general evidence of poor peripheral perfusion. An ECG may reveal an MI, ventricular hypertrophy, atrial enlargement, or arrhythmias. A chest radiograph may show cardiomegaly, pulmonary edema, and pleural effusion. An echocardiogram assesses ventricular function and provides information about regional wall motion and valve function.

Treatment

Management of patients with heart failure is directed at optimizing preload, afterload, and myocardial contractility. Afterload reduction is accomplished by lowering the vascular resistance against which the heart must contract, and ACE inhibitors are one of the cornerstones of therapy for heart failure.[29] Nitrates (venodilator) and hydralazine (vasodilator) reduce excessive preload and are used as an alternative in patients who cannot tolerate ACE inhibitors. β-Adrenergic blockade (selective or nonselective) for heart failure has proved effective in reducing mortality in patients with ischemic and nonischemic heart failure.[30] Digoxin (sympatholytic agent) has been used tradition-

ally for patients with heart failure in sinus rhythm. Its use has decreased given the superior and definitive beneficial effects of ACE inhibitors and β-blockers. Diuretics are necessary in all patients with heart failure for the management of volume overload and relief of symptoms of congestion. Calcium channel blockers are used only for the treatment of hypertension or angina not adequately controlled with other agents such as ACE inhibitors or β-blockers. Inotropes increase cardiac contractility and are used in the critically ill and patients with end-stage heart failure.

RENAL AND URINARY TRACT COMPLICATIONS

Urinary Retention

Etiology

Inability to evacuate a urine-filled bladder is referred to as urinary retention. Urinary retention is a common postoperative complication seen with particularly high frequency in patients undergoing perianal operations and hernia repair. Urinary retention may also occur after operations for low rectal cancer when an injury to the nervous system affects bladder function. Most commonly, however, the complication is a reversible abnormality resulting from discoordination of the trigone and detrusor muscles as a result of increased pain and postoperative discomfort. Urinary retention is also occasionally seen after spinal procedures and may occur after overly vigorous IV administration of fluid. Benign prostatic hypertrophy and, rarely, a urethral stricture may also be the cause of urinary retention.

Presentation and Management

Patients with postoperative urinary retention will complain of a dull, constant discomfort in the hypogastrium. Urgency and actual pain in this area occur as the retention worsens. Percussion just above the pubis reveals fullness and tenderness.

To prevent urinary retention, the population at greatest concern, the elderly and patients who have undergone low anterior resection, must be watched carefully. Adequate management of pain, including postoperative injection of local anesthetics, may also diminish the incidence of urinary retention. Judicious administration of IV fluids during the procedure and in the immediate postoperative period, especially in patients who have undergone anorectal surgery for benign disease, may similarly diminish the likelihood of postoperative urinary retention. Furthermore, awareness of the time from the last voiding to the present time is crucial in preventing acute retention. Most patients should not go more than 6 to 7 hours without passing some urine, and an observant clinician will make certain that no patient goes longer than that before undergoing straight catheterization.

General management principles for acute urinary retention include initial straight catheterization or placement of a Foley catheter, especially in the elderly and patients who have undergone anterior resection because they may be unable to sense the fullness associated with

Table 15-9 Causes of Postoperative Acute Renal Failure

INFLOW OR PRERENAL	PARENCHYMAL OR RENAL	OUTFLOW OR POSTRENAL
Sepsis	Renal ischemia	Cellular debris (acute tubular necrosis)
Medications	Drugs (aminoglycosides, amphotericin)	Crystals
Nonsteroidal anti-inflammatory drugs	Iodinated contrast media	Uric acid
Angiotensin-converting enzyme	Interstitial nephritis	Oxylate
inhibitors		Pigment
Intravascular volume contraction		Myoglobin
Hypovolemia		Hemoglobin
Hemorrhage		
Dehydration		
Atherosclerotic emboli		
Third spacing		
Cardiac failure		

retention. In high-risk patients, cystoscopy and cystometry may be required.

Acute Renal Failure

Etiology

Acute renal failure (ARF) is characterized by a sudden reduction in renal output that results in the systemic accumulation of nitrogenous wastes. This hospital-acquired renal insufficiency is more prevalent after major vascular procedures (ruptured aneurysm), renal transplantation, cardiopulmonary bypass procedures, major abdominal cases associated with septic shock, and major urologic operations. It may also occur in cases in which there is major blood loss, with transfusion reactions, in serious diabetics undergoing operations, in life-threatening trauma, with major burn injuries, and in multiple organ system failure. Hospital-acquired renal insufficiency adversely affects surgical outcomes and is associated with significant mortality, especially when dialysis is required. Two types of ARF have been identified: oliguric and nonoliguric. Oliguric renal failure refers to urine in which volumes of less than 480 mL are seen in a day. Nonoliguric renal failure involves output exceeding 2 L/day and is associated with large amounts of isosthenuric urine that clears no toxins from the bloodstream. Factors leading to ARF can be inflow, parenchymal, or outflow, historically referred to as prerenal, renal, or postrenal, respectively (Table 15-9).

In normal kidneys, effective perfusion of the glomeruli is maintained by an autoregulatory mechanism involving the afferent and efferent arterioles. Any factor that interferes with or disrupts this mechanism results in ARF. Afferent constriction or efferent dilation decreases the glomerular filtration rate. Inflow, or prerenal, failure is secondary to hypotension, which causes afferent arteriolar constriction and efferent dilation; nonsteroidal anti-inflammatory drugs (NSAIDs), which inhibit afferent vasodilation; and gram-negative sepsis, which causes decreased peripheral vascular resistance while increasing renal vasoconstriction. Renal vascular stenosis and thrombosis can also be causes, though much less commonly. Outflow, or postrenal, ARF is caused by tubular obstruction from debris, crystals, or pigments; ureteric obstruc-

tion; or urinary bladder outflow obstruction. Ischemia, toxins, or nephritis cause parenchymal ARF.

The incidence of contrast-induced nephropathy is on the rise. Tubular damage can occur within 48 hours of dye administration.[31] Diabetic patients with vascular disease are at risk for major renal injury when contrast agents are administered. Administration of contrast to hypovolemic patients and those with preexisting renal dysfunction guarantees some degree of renal injury. The tubular injury is generally self-limited and reversible. Diabetic patients with creatinine clearance less than 50 mL/min who receive 100 mL of contrast dye, however, can sustain severe tubular damage and may require dialysis. Blunt trauma with associated crush injuries places the patient at risk for ARF because of high serum levels of hematin and myoglobin, both of which are injurious to the renal tubules. ARF is a prominent feature in patients with acute compartment syndrome.[32,33] Growing awareness of this problem has led surgeons to intervene surgically, often resulting in dramatic improvement in renal function and preservation of renal filtering capacity.

Presentation and Management

Prevention of hospital-acquired renal insufficiency requires identification of patients with preexisting renal dysfunction; avoidance of hypovolemia, hypotension, and medications that depress renal function; and judicious use of nephrotoxic drugs. In the presence of renal impairment, the dose of antibiotics given for serious infections must be adjusted. The risk for contrast-induced nephropathy is reduced by adequate hydration and premedication with a free radical scavenger (N-acetylcysteine) or the use of alternative contrast (gadolinium). Renal hypoperfusion is avoided by optimizing cardiac output and volume expansion. Administration of fluid must be particularly judicious in patients with a history of heart failure. Monitoring renal function, at times including creatinine clearance, in all surgical patients is a sound clinical practice. Early intervention in cases of postrenal obstruction and abdominal compartment syndrome can obviate the development of renal injury.

Anuria that suddenly develops postoperatively in an otherwise healthy individual with no preexisting renal

Table 15-10   Diagnostic Evaluation of Acute Renal Failure

PARAMETER	PRERENAL	RENAL	POSTRENAL
Urine osmolality	>500 mOsm/L	=Plasma	Variable
Urinary sodium	<20 mOsm/L	>50 mOsm/L	>50 mOsm/L
Fractional excretion of sodium	<1%	>3%	Variable
Urine/plasma creatinine	>40	<20	<20
Urine/plasma urea	>8	<3	Variable
Urine/plasma osmolality	<1.5	>1.5	Variable

disease is postrenal in nature until proved otherwise. A kink in the Foley catheter or obstruction must be cleared. In patients who have undergone major pelvic surgery, ligation of the ureters is suspect. If renal ultrasound or a CT scan shows hydronephrosis, immediate surgical treatment is indicated. Postrenal causes of ARF are the most dramatic and straightforward to diagnose and treat, with significant immediate improvement after treatment.

ARF is otherwise diagnosed when there is a rise in serum creatinine, decrease in creatinine clearance, and urine output less than 400 mL/day (<20 mL/hr). Distinguishing between prerenal and renal azotemia, however, is complicated. Careful history taking may identify patients with preexisting renal dysfunction. Patients with large fluid losses from the GI tract (e.g., diarrhea, vomiting, fistula, high ileostomy output) often have associated profound dehydration. In such cases, the rise in blood urea nitrogen (BUN) is usually greater than the rise in creatinine, and the ratio of BUN to creatinine is greater than 20. Examination of the patient may reveal distended neck veins, rales in the lungs, and a cardiac gallop—all signs that a failing heart may be underperfusing the kidneys as the cause of the oliguria. Brown urine in the Foley bag in a trauma patient raises suspicion of myoglobinuria and requires rapid hydration, diuresis, and alkalinization of the urine. Evaluation of spun urine is helpful. The presence of hyaline casts indicates hypoperfusion, and the presence of course granular casts indicates acute tubular necrosis. Lipoid casts are found with NSAID- and contrast-induced nephropathy and white and red cell casts with pyelonephritis. In patients with prerenal azotemia, the concentrating ability of the nephrons is normal, thereby resulting in normal urine osmolality and fractional excretion of sodium (>500 mOsm and FE_{Na}<1%, respectively). Conversely, with acute tubular necrosis, the concentrating ability of the kidney is lost and the patient produces urine with an osmolality equal to that of serum and high urine sodium levels (350 mOsm and >50 mg/L, respectively) (Table 15-10). The best laboratory test for discriminating prerenal from renal azotemia is probably FE_{Na}. In prerenal patients FE_{Na} is 1% or less, whereas in renal azotemia patients, it often exceeds 3%.

Once ARF is diagnosed, one has to ascertain whether the hypoperfusion of the kidney is due to hypovolemia or cardiac failure. Distinguishing the two is critical because giving heart failure patients more fluid exacerbates an already failing system. Similarly, giving diuretics to a hypovolemic patient can worsen the renal failure. If the prerenal patient has no history of cardiac disease, administration of isosmotic fluid (normal saline or lactated Ringer's solution or blood in patients who have hemorrhaged) is indicated. The IV fluid can be given rapidly (1 L over a 20- to 30-minute period) in young patients with healthy hearts and a Foley catheter in place to measure hourly urine output and must be administered until the patient is producing a minimum of 30 to 40 mL of urine per hour. If fluid administration does not result in improvement of the oliguria, placement of a central venous pressure or Swan-Ganz catheter is indicated to measure left- or right-sided heart filling pressure. In the presence of CHF, diuretics, fluid restriction, and appropriate cardiac medications are indicated. Ultrasound may show renal atrophy reflecting the presence of chronic metabolic disease.

Treatment of ARF includes management of fluid and electrolyte imbalance, careful monitoring of fluid administration, avoidance of nephrotoxic agents, provision of adequate nutrition, and adjustment of doses of renally excreted medications until recovery of renal function. Most urgent in management of ARF is treating hyperkalemia and fluid overload. Hyperkalemia can be managed with a sodium/potassium exchange resin, insulin plus glucose, an aerosolized β_2-adrenergic agonist, and calcium gluconate. Insulin and β_2-agonists shift potassium intracellularly. Hyperkalemia-associated cardiac irritability (prolonged PR interval or peaked T waves) is urgently treated with the administration of a 10% calcium gluconate solution over a 15-minute period, as well as simultaneous IV administration of glucose and insulin (10-unit IV bolus with 50 mL of a 50% dextrose solution, followed by continuation of glucose to prevent hypoglycemia). A β_2-adrenergic agonist is given as a nebulizer containing 10 to 20 mg in 4 mL of saline over a period of 10 minutes or as IV infusion containing 0.5 mg. Calcium gluconate is given as 10 mL of a 10% solution over a 5-minute period to reduce arrhythmia. Refractory hyperkalemia associated with metabolic acidosis and rhabdomyolysis requires hemodialysis. In less severe hyperkalemia, ion exchange resin (Kayexalate) in enema form will help lower potassium levels. Phosphate levels also require careful monitoring. Hypophosphatemia can induce rhabdomyolysis and respiratory failure and is treated with the oral administration of Fleet Phospho-Soda. Hyperphosphatemia with hypercalcemia increases the risk for calciphylaxis and is treated with the administration of phosphorus binders (calcium carbonate) or dialysis. IV fluids are monitored with an emphasis on fluid restriction and occasional use of catheters to measure

---

Box 15-7   Indications for Hemodialysis

Serum potassium >5.5 mEq/L
Blood urea nitrogen >80-90 mg/dL
Persistent metabolic acidosis
Acute fluid overload
Uremic symptoms (pericarditis, encephalopathy, anorexia)
Removal of toxins
Platelet dysfunction causing bleeding
Hyperphosphatemia with hypercalcemia

Box 15-8   Rapid Adrenocorticotropic Hormone Stimulation Test in Patients With Adrenal Insufficiency

Determine baseline serum cortisol

Give 250 µg cosyntropin intravenously (or intramuscularly)
Measure serum cortisol levels 30 to 60 minutes after cosyntropin is given

Results

Normal adrenal function: basal or postcorticotropin plasma cortisol concentration at least 18 µg/dL (500 nmol/L) or preferably 20 µg/dL (550 nmol/L)
Primary adrenal insufficiency: cortisol secretion is not increased
Severe secondary adrenal insufficiency: cortisol levels increase a little or not at all because of adrenocortical atrophy

---

right- and left-sided heart filling pressure to avoid fluid overload.

When supportive measures fail, consideration must be given to hemodialysis.[34,35] Indications for hemodialysis are listed in Box 15-7. Although some hemodynamic instability may occur during dialysis, it is usually transient and may be treated with fluids. Dialysis may be continued on an intermittent basis until renal function has returned, which occurs in the vast majority of cases.

ENDOCRINE GLAND DYSFUNCTION

Adrenal Insufficiency

Etiology

Adrenal insufficiency is an uncommon but potentially lethal condition associated with failure of the adrenal glands to produce adequate glucocorticoids. Cortisol, the predominant corticosteroid secreted from the adrenal cortex, is under the influence of adrenocorticotropic hormone released from the pituitary gland, which in turn is under the influence of hypothalamic corticotropin-releasing hormone, and both hormones are subject to negative feedback by cortisol itself. Cortisol is a stress hormone.

Chronic adrenal insufficiency may result from primary destruction of the adrenal gland or be secondary to a disease state or disorder involving the hypothalamus or anterior pituitary gland. Primary adrenal insufficiency is most frequently due to autoimmune adrenalitis (Addison's disease), in which the adrenal cortex is destroyed by cytotoxic lymphocytes. Secondary adrenal insufficiency is most commonly caused by long-term administration of pharmacologic doses of glucocorticoids. Chronic use of glucocorticoids causes suppression of the hypothalamic-pituitary-adrenal axis (HPA), induces adrenal atrophy, and results in isolated adrenal insufficiency.

Acute adrenal insufficiency may occur as a result of abrupt cessation of pharmacologic doses of chronic glucocorticoid therapy, surgical excision or destruction of the adrenal gland (adrenal hemorrhage, necrosis, or thrombosis in patients with sepsis or antiphospholipid syndrome), or surgical excision or destruction (postpartum necrosis) of the pituitary gland. In addition, so-called functional or relative acute adrenal insufficiency may develop in critically ill and septic patients.[36]

Presentation and Diagnosis

The clinical manifestations of adrenal insufficiency depend on the cause of the disease and associated endocrinopathies.[36] Symptoms and signs of chronic primary and secondary adrenal insufficiency are similar and nonspecific (fatigue, weakness, anorexia, weight loss, orthostatic dizziness, abdominal pain, diarrhea, depression, hyponatremia, hypoglycemia, eosinophilia, decreased libido and potency). Patients with primary hypoadrenalism also show manifestations of elevated plasma levels of corticotropin (hyperpigmentation of the skin and mucous membrane). Patients with secondary disease, in contrast, initially have neurologic or ophthalmologic symptoms (headaches, visual disturbances) before showing signs of HPA axis disease (hypopituitarism). Manifestations of HPA axis suppression include hypoadrenalism, decreased levels of corticotropin, and manifestations of other hormone deficiencies (pallor, loss of hair in androgen-dependent areas, oligomenorrhea, diabetes insipidus, hypothyroidism).

Laboratory test abnormalities, including hyponatremia, hyperkalemia, acidosis, hypoglycemia or hyperglycemia, normocytic anemia, eosinophilia, and lymphocytosis, are present to a variable extent. The diagnosis is, however, established by measuring the morning plasma cortisol concentration. A concentration greater than 19 µg/dL (525 nmol/L) rules out adrenal insufficiency and less than 3 µg/dL (83 nmol/L) indicates its presence. A basal plasma corticotropin level exceeding 100 pg/mL (22 nmol/L), a low or low normal basal aldosterone level, and an increased renin concentration are indicative of primary hypoadrenalism. The rapid corticotropin stimulation test to determine adrenal responsiveness is the diagnostic procedure of choice in testing for primary adrenal insufficiency. The test is conducted as shown in Box 15-8.

To confirm the diagnosis of secondary adrenal insufficiency the metyrapone test is performed. An insufficient increase in plasma 11-deoxycortisol and a low plasma cortisol concentration (<8 µg/dL) after the oral administration of metyrapone indicate the presence of secondary adrenal insufficiency. Magnetic resonance imaging (MRI) allows evaluation of the pituitary-hypothalamic region in patients with neurologic and ophthalmologic symptoms, and a CT scan is used to evaluate the adrenal glands in patients with primary hypoadrenalism.

The diagnosis of acute adrenal insufficiency can be especially difficult to make in the critically ill. The condition is suspected in patients exhibiting manifestations of preexisting or undiagnosed chronic adrenal insufficiency in whom unexplained hypotension or hemodynamic instability develops despite fluid resuscitation, as well as ongoing evidence of inflammation without an obvious source of infection. Hyponatremia is usually present and does not respond to saline infusion. A sodium level of less than 120 mmol/L is dangerous and may lead to delirium, coma, and seizures. Hypoglycemia and azotemia may also be present. An ECG will occasionally reveal low voltage and peaked T waves. To diagnose the condition, cortisol and corticotropin concentrations are checked and the short corticotropin stimulation test performed.

Treatment

Prevention and avoidance of adrenal insufficiency are achieved by a thorough preoperative history, detailed instruction of patients receiving chronic corticosteroid therapy regarding the dangers of abrupt termination of the medication, and adequate perioperative corticosteroid administration. Specific patients with rheumatoid arthritis, inflammatory bowel disease, or autoimmune disease and recipients of organ transplants are targeted. In the critically ill, a high index of suspicion can prevent a fatal outcome. A stress dose of hydrocortisone (100 mg) may be given with induction of anesthesia. For minor surgical procedures, usual maintenance dose is continued postoperatively. For major surgical procedures, a stress dose (100 mg) is continued every 8 hours until stable or free of complications and then tapered to the usual maintenance dose.

Symptomatic patients are treated with hydrocortisone or cortisone. Fludrocortisone (substitute for aldosterone) is also administered to patients with primary disease. Patients who have received more than 20 mg of prednisone daily (or equivalent dose of another corticosteroid) (Table 15-11) for more than 3 weeks within the previous

Table 15-11 Relative Corticosteroid Potency Compared With Hydrocortisone

	GLUCOCORTICOID ACTIVITY	MINERALOCORTICOID ACTIVITY
Short Acting		
Hydrocortisone	1	1
Cortisone	0.8	0.8
Intermediate Acting		
Prednisone	4	0.25
Prednisolone	4	0.25
Methylprednisolone	5	Trace
Triamcinolone	5	Trace
Long Acting		
Dexamethasone	20	Trace

Modified from Druck P, Andersen DK: Diabetes mellitus and other endocrine problems. In Stillman RM (ed): Surgery: Diagnosis and Therapy. New York, Lange, 1989, p 205.

year and patients with Cushing's syndrome who are undergoing surgery are presumed to have HPA suppression and must be treated in a similar fashion.

Treatment of functional acute adrenal insufficiency involves immediate, rapid administration of high-dose hydrocortisone or methylprednisolone with appropriate monitoring until clinical improvement is seen. Hypovolemia and hyponatremia are corrected with saline infusion.

Hyperthyroid Crisis
Etiology

Hyperthyroidism refers to a sustained increase in the synthesis of thyroid hormones, and thyrotoxicosis is a clinical syndrome that results from abnormal elevation of circulating levels of thyroid hormone, regardless of cause. Thyroid hormones are under the influence of pituitary gland thyroid-releasing hormone, which in turn is under the influence of hypothalamic thyrotropin-releasing hormone, and both hormones are subject to negative feedback by the thyroid hormones. Thyroid hormones have physiologic effects on many organ systems, but the greatest effect is on the cardiovascular system.

Thyroid crisis is a medical emergency that occurs in thyrotoxic patients with toxic adenoma or toxic multinodular goiter, but most often in patients with Grave's disease. The crisis is frequently precipitated by a stressful event and characterized by exacerbation of hyperthyroidism and decompensation of one or more organ systems. Mortality is high, ranging from 20% to 50% if the crisis is unrecognized and left untreated.

Presentation and Diagnosis

Clinical manifestations of hyperthyroidism include nervousness, fatigue, palpitations, heat intolerance, weight loss, atrial fibrillation (in the elderly), and ophthalmopathy characterized by eyelid retraction or lag, periorbital edema, and proptosis. The onset of thyroid crisis is sudden and characterized by accentuation of the symptoms and signs of thyrotoxicosis and organ system dysfunction, including hyperpyrexia, tachycardia out of proportion to fever, dehydration and collapse, central nervous system dysfunction (delirium, psychosis, seizure, coma), cardiac manifestations, GI symptoms, and liver dysfunction.

The diagnosis of thyrotoxicosis requires demonstration of elevated levels of circulating thyroid hormone and suppressed thyroid-stimulating hormone (TSH) levels and identification of the cause of the thyrotoxicosis. Free thyroxin (T_4) and triiodothyronine (T_3) represent the small unbound fraction of total thyroxin that is biologically active and correlate directly with the presence and severity of thyroid dysfunction. Thyroid scintigraphy with technetium pertechnetate ($^{99m}TcO_4^-$) or iodine 123 (^{123}I) provides information about the functional anatomy of the gland. In Grave's disease there is diffuse uptake; in Plummer's gland (toxic multinodular goiter) there is an inhomogeneous pattern with hot, cold, and warm areas; and with Goetsch's disease (toxic solitary nodule) there is intense activity in the area of the nodule with suppression of paranodular tissue.

Box 15-9   Management of Thyroid Crisis

Identification and treatment of the precipitating factor
Supportive care
  Oxygen
  Intravenous fluid therapy
  Sedation (chlorpromazine)
  Venous thromboembolism prophylaxis with heparin
  Dexamethasone
Fever: antipyretics and cooling
Heart failure: digoxin and diuretics
Atrial fibrillation: intravenous heparin
β-Blockers: Oral propranolol, 60-80 mg/4 hr (or diltiazem), to reduce the heart rate below 100 beats/min. In very sick patients esmolol is given intravenously, and reserpine is given to patients refractory to large doses of propranolol
Propylthiouracil or methimazole
Lugol's solution given 4 hours after propylthiouracil
Plasmapheresis and charcoal plasma perfusion or exchange transfusion reserved for recalcitrant cases if there is no response in 24-48 hours
Once euthyroidism is achieved, definitive therapy must be considered to prevent a second crisis

---

Treatment

In addition to identification and treatment of the precipitating factor or factors and supportive care, specific medications (iodine, propylthiouracil, β-adrenergic blockers, dexamethasone) that target hormonal synthesis and release and block peripheral effects of the hormone are administered (Box 15-9).[37] Steroids are required to block peripheral conversion of T_4 to T_3 and as a supplement because there is increased steroid demand and turnover and decreased physiologic effectiveness. Cardioversion for supraventricular tachyarrhythmia is ineffective during the thyrotoxic storm.

Definitive therapy for Graves' disease is accomplished with either radioactive iodine or surgery. Radioactive iodine has obvious advantages in elderly high-risk patients but needs to be avoided in children, pregnant women, and patients with large toxic adenomas. By using doses of ^{123}I in the range of 10 mCi (5-15 mCi) and subsequent levothyroxine, thyrotoxicosis can be successfully managed in 85% to 90% of patients. The main side effect of radioactive iodine is hypothyroidism. Surgery usually includes one of two operations, either total thyroidectomy or a lobectomy on one side with subtotal lobectomy on the other side. Total thyroidectomy is associated with a lower recurrence rate than subtotal thyroidectomy is (4%-15%) but does require lifelong thyroxine replacement postoperatively. Excision of the lesion is indicated for toxic adenoma, whereas total thyroidectomy is indicated for toxic multinodular goiter. Before surgery, patients must be made euthyroid with antithyroid drugs, and iodine is given for 7 days before surgery.

Hypothyroidism

Etiology

Hypothyroidism is characterized by low systemic levels of thyroid hormone and may be exacerbated in the post-operative period in patients with preexisting chronic hypothyroidism or as a result of severe stress. Severe illness, physiologic stress, and drugs may inhibit peripheral conversion of T_4 to T_3 and induce a hypothyroid-like state. Hypothyroidism may be primary (surgical removal, ablation, or disease of the thyroid gland), secondary (hypopituitarism), or tertiary (hypothalamic disease).

Presentation and Diagnosis

Patients with chronic hypothyroidism may be asymptomatic or rarely have the severe form (myxedema coma) characterized by coma, loss of deep tendon reflexes, cardiopulmonary collapse, and high (~40%-50%) mortality. The majority, however, demonstrate cold intolerance, constipation, brittle hair, dry skin, sluggishness, weight gain, and fatigue. The impact of hypothyroidism is greatest on the cardiovascular system, with effects such as bradycardia, hypotension, impaired cardiac function, conduction abnormalities, pericardial effusion, and increased risk for CAD. In the critically ill (trauma, sepsis), hypothyroidism is associated with worsening of pulmonary function, a predisposition to pleural effusion, and susceptibility to hypothermia.

The ECG usually shows bradycardia, low voltage, and prolonged PR, QRS, and QT intervals. In patients with primary hypothyroidism, serum total T_4, free T_4, and free T_3 levels are low, whereas TSH is elevated. In secondary disease, TSH, the free T_4 index, and free T_3 are low. Distinguishing the two is important because adrenal insufficiency is present in secondary disease and administration of levothyroxine must be accompanied by cortisol or the disease could be exacerbated.

Treatment

Patients with known hypothyroidism who are receiving replacement hormonal therapy and are in the euthyroid state do not require any special treatment before surgery but are instructed to continue taking their medications. In patients with symptomatic chronic hypothyroidism, surgery is postponed until a euthyroid state is achieved.

Patients with myxedema coma or those showing clinical signs of significant hypothyroidism (severe postoperative hypothermia, hypotension, hypoventilation, psychosis, and obtundation) are immediately treated with thyroid hormone, concomitant with the IV administration of hydrocortisone, to avoid an addisonian crisis. IV levothyroxine or triiodothyronine may be given until oral intake is possible.

Syndrome of Inappropriate Antidiuretic Hormone Secretion

Etiology

The syndrome of inappropriate antidiuretic hormone secretion (SIADH) is the most common cause of chronic normovolemic hyponatremia. Hyponatremia is defined as a serum sodium concentration of less than 135 mmol/L. SIADH is diagnosed in any patient who remains hyponatremic despite all attempts to correct the imbalance in the presence of persistent antidiuretic activity from elevated arginine vasopressin. Vasopressin is a naturally occurring antidiuretic hormone that regulates free water excretion. It is synthesized in the hypothalamus, transported to the posterior pituitary, and stored until specific stimuli cause it to be secreted into the bloodstream. Thirst, hypovolemia, nausea, hypoglycemia, and drugs are among the many stimuli for vasopressin. Disorders and conditions that predispose to this relatively rare condition include trauma, stroke, antidiuretic hormone–producing tumors, drugs (ACE inhibitors, dopamine, NSAIDs), and pulmonary conditions.

Presentation

Clinical characteristics of SIADH include anorexia, nausea, vomiting, obtundation, and lethargy. With more rapid onset, seizures, coma, and death can result. Clinical expression of the syndrome is caused by hyponatremia and is a function of the degree of hyponatremia, as well as the rapidity of its onset. The cardinal criteria of SIADH include hyponatremia with hypotonicity of plasma, urine osmolality in excess of plasma osmolality, increased renal sodium excretion, absence of edema or volume depletion, and normal renal function.

Treatment

Management of SIADH includes treatment of the underlying disease process and removal of excess water (i.e., treatment of the hyponatremia). Fluid restriction is the mainstay of management of chronic SIADH. IV administration of normal saline is used only in significantly symptomatic patients with chronic SIADH or those with symptomatic acute SIADH with a duration of less than 3 days. Correction must occur at a rate of 0.5 mmol/L/hr until the serum sodium concentration is 125 mg/dL or higher. Rapid correction leads to serious permanent neurologic damage. Diuretics such as furosemide occasionally help correct the imbalance. In some cases, IV administration of 3% saline solution may be required, but correction must be done in a constant, sustained fashion because overly rapid correction can result in seizure activity.

GASTROINTESTINAL COMPLICATIONS

Ileus and Early Postoperative Bowel Obstruction

Etiology

Early postoperative bowel obstruction denotes obstruction occurring within 30 days after surgery. The obstruction may be functional (i.e., ileus), due to inhibition of propulsive bowel activity, or mechanical as a result of a barrier. Ileus that occurs immediately after surgery in the absence of precipitating factors and resolves within 2 to 4 days is referred to as *primary* or *postoperative ileus*.[38] On the other hand, ileus that occurs as a result of a precipitating factor and is associated with a delay in return of bowel function is referred to as *secondary* or *adynamic* or *paralytic ileus*.[38] Mechanical bowel obstruction may be caused by a luminal, mural, or extraintestinal barrier.

> **Box 15-10   Causes of Intestinal Paralytic Ileus**
>
> Pancreatitis
> Intra-abdominal infection (peritonitis or abscess)
> Retroperitoneal hemorrhage and inflammation
> Electrolyte abnormalities
> Lengthy surgical procedure and prolonged exposure of abdominal contents
> Medications (narcotics, psychotropic agents)
> Pneumonia
> Inflamed viscera

The precise mechanism and etiology of postoperative ileus are not completely understood. Several events that occur during an abdominal surgical procedure and in the perioperative period may interfere with or alter the contractile activity of the small bowel, which is governed by a complex interaction between the enteric nervous system, central nervous system, hormones, and local molecular and cellular inflammatory factors.[39] Surgical stress and manipulation of the bowel result in sustained inhibitory sympathetic activity and release of hormones and neurotransmitters, as well as activation of a local molecular inflammatory response that results in suppression of the neuromuscular apparatus.[40] In the immediate postoperative period, restricted oral intake and postoperative narcotic analgesia also contribute to altered small bowel motility. Opiates and opioid peptides in the enteric nervous system suppress neuronal excitability. After transection and reanastomosis of the small bowel, the distal part of the bowel does not react to the pacemaker (found in the duodenum), and the frequency of contractions decreases. Other conditions listed in Box 15-10 are associated with or result in adynamic ileus.

Mechanical early postoperative small bowel obstruction is commonly caused by adhesions (92%), a phlegmon or abscess, internal hernia, intestinal ischemia, or intussusception. Intussusception occurring in the postoperative period is relatively uncommon and a rare occurrence after colorectal surgery. A phlegmon or abscess may be caused by leakage of intestinal contents from a disrupted anastomosis or by iatrogenic injury to the bowel during enterolysis or closure of laparotomy incision. With mechanical obstruction there is an increased incidence of discrete, clustered contractions proximal to the obstruction that propel the intestinal contents past the point of obstruction (in cases of partial obstruction) and result in cramps. In high-grade or complete obstruction, the contents do not move distally, they accumulate in the proximal part of the bowel, and they initiate retrograde contractions that empty the small bowel contents into the stomach in preparation for expulsion during vomiting.

Presentation

Postoperative ileus affects the stomach and colon primarily. After laparotomy, small bowel motility returns within several hours, gastric motility within 24 to 48 hours, and colonic motility in 48 to 72 hours. Secretions and swallowed air are not emptied from the stomach, and gastric dilation and vomiting may occur. Return of bowel activity is heralded by the presence of bowel sounds, flatus, and bowel movements.

Patients with early postoperative small bowel obstruction either do not show manifestations of bowel activity or have temporary return of bowel function. In adynamic ileus, the stomach, small bowel, and colon are affected. In mechanical obstruction, the obstruction may be partial or complete, may occur in the proximal part of the small bowel (high obstruction) or in the distal part of the small bowel (low obstruction), and may be a closed-loop or open-ended obstruction.[41] There is stasis and progressive accumulation of gastric and intestinal secretions and gas, and the bowel may lose its tone and dilate, thereby resulting in abdominal distention, pain, nausea and vomiting, and obstipation. The extent of the clinical manifestations varies with the cause, degree, and level of obstruction. Patients with high mechanical small bowel obstruction vomit early in the course and usually have no or minimal distention. The vomitus is generally bilious. Patients with distal obstruction, on the other hand, vomit later in the course and have more pronounced abdominal distention. The vomitus may initially be bilious then becomes more feculent. Differentiation between adynamic ileus and mechanical obstruction can be very difficult. With adynamic ileus patients have diffuse discomfort but no sharp colicky pain and a distended abdomen. They often have a quiet abdomen with few bowel sounds detected on auscultation with a stethoscope. With mechanical obstruction, high-pitched, tinkling sounds may be detected. Fever, tachycardia, manifestations of hypovolemia, and sepsis may also develop.

The diagnosis of bowel obstruction is usually based on clinical findings and plain radiographs of the abdomen.[41] However, in the postoperative period, differentiation between adynamic ileus and mechanical obstruction is imperative because the treatment is completely different. A CT scan, abdominal radiographs, and small bowel follow-through are variably used to establish the diagnosis and assist in treatment decision making.[4] In adynamic ileus, abdominal radiographs reveal diffusely dilated bowel throughout the intestinal tract with air in the colon and rectum. Air-fluid levels may be present, and the amount of dilated bowel varies greatly. With mechanical bowel obstruction there is small bowel dilation with air-fluid levels and thickened valvulae conniventes in the bowel proximal to the point of obstruction and little or no gas in the bowel distal to the obstruction. A CT scan is more accurate in differentiating functional from mechanical obstruction by identifying the so-called transition point or cutoff at the obstruction site in cases of mechanical obstruction. It also determines the level (high or low) and degree of obstruction (partial versus high grade or complete), differentiates between uncomplicated and complicated (compromised bowel, perforation) obstruction, and identifies specific types of obstruction (closed-loop obstruction, intussusception). In addition, CT may identify other associated disease states (bowel ischemia, phlegmon, abscess, pancreatitis). Small bowel follow-through is indicated if the clinical picture

of postoperative small bowel obstruction is confusing, radiographs of the abdomen are not diagnostic, or the response to expectant management is inadequate. A standard battery of laboratory tests is also obtained, including a complete blood cell count with differential; amylase, lipase, electrolyte, magnesium, and calcium levels; and urinalysis.

Treatment
Preventive measures must be started intraoperatively and continued in the immediate postoperative period. A concerted effort must be made during any abdominal operation to minimize injury to the bowel and other peritoneal surfaces—the recognized source of adhesion formation. During the operation, the surgeon must handle the tissues gently and limit peritoneal dissection to only what is essential. The bowel must not be allowed to desiccate by prolonged exposure to air without protection. Moist laparotomy pads must be used to cover the bowel and must be moistened frequently if contact with bowel is prolonged. Instrument injury to the bowel must be avoided. Given the importance of adhesion formation and the large magnitude of serious problems related to adhesions, adjunctive measures such as antiadhesion barriers may be considered. A number of antiadhesion barriers are available, including an oxidized cellulose product and a product that is a combination of sodium hyaluronate and carboxymethyl cellulose. These agents may inhibit adhesions wherever they are placed. However, a decrease in the number of adhesions at the site of application does not necessarily translate into a decrease in the rate of small bowel obstruction.

In the postoperative period, electrolytes are monitored and any imbalance corrected. Alternative analgesia to narcotics, such as NSAIDs and placement of a thoracic epidural with local anesthetic, may be used when possible. Intubation of the stomach with an NG tube needs to be applied selectively. Routine intubation does not confer any appreciable effect and is associated with discomfort, inhibits ambulation, and predisposes to aspiration, sinusitis, otitis, esophageal injury, and electrolyte imbalance. The use of prokinetic agents does not alter the outcome after colorectal surgery, and other pharmacologic manipulations such as parasympathetic agents, adrenergic blocking agents, and metoclopramide also do not have an impact on resolving postoperative ileus.[40] The role of early postoperative feeding remains unclear.[39]

Once early postoperative obstruction is suspected or diagnosed, a three-step approach is essential to guarantee a favorable outcome: resuscitation, investigation, and surgical intervention.[41] Emergency relaparotomy is performed if there is a closed-loop, high-grade, or complicated small bowel obstruction, intussusception, or peritonitis. Adynamic ileus is treated by resolving some of the abnormalities listed in Box 15-10 and expectantly waiting for resolution, with surgery not usually being required. Partial mechanical small bowel obstruction is also initially managed expectantly and for a longer period, 7 to 14 days, if the patient is stable and clinical and radiologic improvement continues.[41] During this time nutritional support is initiated and surgical intervention is performed if there are signs of deterioration or no improvement.

Acute Abdominal Compartment Syndrome

Etiology

Specific parameters have been proposed to describe the syndrome of abdominal compartment syndrome: consistently increased intra-abdominal pressure greater than 12 mm Hg associated with rising peak airway pressure, hypoxia, difficult ventilation, and oliguria or anuria that improve with decompression.

Abdominal compartment syndrome is most commonly encountered in the multiple trauma and ICU setting.[33] Factors that predispose a victim of multiple trauma to intra-abdominal hypertension and abdominal compartment syndrome include ileus as a result of bowel edema and contamination, coagulopathy, packing used to control bleeding, capillary leak, and massive fluid resuscitation and transfusion. In the nontrauma setting, intra-abdominal hypertension and abdominal compartment syndrome have been reported to occur in patients with ascites, retroperitoneal hemorrhage, pancreatitis after reduction of chronic hernias that have lost their domain, repair of ruptured abdominal aortic aneurysms, complex abdominal procedures, and liver transplantation. Closure of noncompliant abdominal wall under tension in these situations is associated with intra-abdominal hypertension in 100% of cases.

Normal intra-abdominal pressure is around 5 mm Hg (range, 0.2-16.2 mm Hg). With an increase in intra-abdominal pressure, deleterious effects are observed in the intra- and extra-abdominal organs and the abdominal wall.[32,33] Upward displacement of the diaphragm results in decreased thoracic volume and compliance, which leads to an increase in peak airway pressure, $\dot{V}/\dot{Q}$ mismatch, hypoxia, hypercapnia, and acidosis. When intra-abdominal pressure reaches 25 mm Hg, compression of the inferior vena cava and portal vein occurs and results in decreased venous return and increased peripheral vascular resistance. As a consequence, cardiac output, the cardiac index, and right atrial and pulmonary artery occlusion pressure decrease. Systemic delivery of oxygen decreases and whole body oxygen consumption is significantly reduced. Direct compression of the kidneys and obstruction of venous outflow result in a decrease in the glomerular filtration rate and urine output. Compression of the mesenteric vasculature leads to a decrease in splanchnic perfusion, mesenteric venous hypertension and severe intramucosal acidosis, intestinal edema, and visceral swelling. Elevated central venous pressure interferes with venous cerebral outflow and leads to an increase in intracerebral pressure. Finally, blood flow to the abdominal wall decreases with a progressive increase in intra-abdominal pressure. This reduced blood flow may result in impaired healing and an increased rate of abdominal wound complications.

Presentation

Patients with intra-abdominal hypertension and abdominal compartment syndrome have difficulty breathing and exhibit elevated peak airway pressure, hypoxia, worsening hypercapnia, and deteriorating compliance. Oliguria rarely occurs in the absence of respiratory dysfunction or failure. The abdomen becomes distended and tense, cardiac output is reduced, and vasopressor therapy is often required. Neurologic deterioration may occur. Central venous, pulmonary capillary wedge, and peak airway pressure become elevated and acidosis develops. Anuria, exacerbation of pulmonary failure, cardiac decompensation, and death ultimately occur.

Treatment

Prevention of abdominal compartment syndrome requires identifying patients at risk for intra-abdominal hypertension and assessing their organ function, measuring and monitoring their intra-abdominal hypertension, and intervening in timely fashion to relieve the intra-abdominal hypertension (Box 15-11).[32,33] A urinary bladder catheter is the gold standard indirect method used to measure intra-abdominal pressure; a regular Foley catheter, a three-way Foley catheter with saline injected into one port and pressure measured through the other, or a regular Foley catheter serially connected to a three-way stopcock and a transducer can be used. Recently, new measurement kits have become commercially available.

Box 15-11   Prevention of Abdominal Compartment Syndrome

Patients at risk for intra-abdominal hypertension and abdominal compartment syndrome are identified (major trauma, complex abdominal procedure)

Organ function is monitored and assessed:

Lungs: hypercapnia, hypoxia, difficult ventilation, elevated pulmonary artery pressure, drop in PaO_2/FIO_2 ratio, decreased compliance, intrapulmonary shunt, increased dead space

Heart: decreased cardiac output and cardiac index and need for vasopressors

Kidneys: oliguria unresponsive to fluid therapy

Central nervous system: Glasgow Coma Scale score less than 10 or neurologic deterioration in the absence of neurotrauma

Abdomen: distention. Computed tomography scan to check for fluid collections, narrowing of the inferior vena cava, compression of the kidneys, and rounding of the abdomen

Intra-abdominal pressure is measured and monitored with a urinary bladder or gastric catheter

Other tests to check organ dysfunction:

Gastric mucosal pH

Near-infrared spectroscopy to measure muscle and gastric tissue oxygenation

Abdominal perfusion pressure = mean arterial pressure − intra-abdominal pressure

Renal filtration gradient = mean arterial pressure − 2 × intra-abdominal pressure

Computed tomography scan

Measures to lower intra-abdominal hypertension:

Drainage of intra-abdominal fluid collections

Muscle relaxation

Avoid primary closure of the incision—laparostomy or mesh, Bogota bag, biomesh, or vacuum-assisted closure

Once measured, the pressure is graded into GI (IAP = 10-15 cm H$_2$O); GII (IAP = 16-25 cm H$_2$O), GIII (IAP = 26-35 cm H$_2$O), and GIV (IAP >36 cm H$_2$O).[33]

The decision to intervene surgically is not based on intra-abdominal hypertension alone but rather on the presence of organ dysfunction in association with intra-abdominal hypertension. Few patients with a pressure of 12 mm Hg have any organ dysfunction, whereas intra-abdominal pressure greater than 15 to 20 mm Hg is significant in every patient. With grade III intra-abdominal hypertension, decompression may be considered when the abdomen is tense and signs of extreme ventilatory dysfunction and oliguria develop.

Decompression is an emergency and is performed in the operating room. Decompression results in washout of the by-products of anaerobic metabolism from below the diaphragm, which in turn results in respiratory alkalosis, a drop in effective preload, and a bolus of acid, potassium, and other by-products delivered to the heart, where they cause arrhythmia or asystolic arrest. Hence, decompression is performed after adequate preload with volume is established. Once stable, the patient may be returned to the operating room for primary closure. If primary closure is not possible, closure may be achieved with a synthetic prosthesis, tissue graft, or wound vacuum system.

Postoperative Gastrointestinal Bleeding

Etiology

Postoperative GI bleeding is one of the most worrisome complications encountered by general surgeons. Possible sources in the stomach include peptic ulcer disease, stress erosion, a Mallory-Weiss tear, and gastric varices; in the small intestine, arteriovenous malformations and bleeding from an anastomosis; and in the large intestine, anastomotic hemorrhage, diverticulosis, arteriovenous malformations, and varices.

In the critically ill, GI bleeding secondary to stress ulceration is a serious complication. The incidence of bleeding from stress ulceration has decreased in the past decade, mainly because of improved supportive care and enhanced resuscitative measures. Clinically significant bleeding that leads to hemodynamic instability, a need for transfusion of blood products, and occasionally operative intervention occurs in less than 5% of cases and is associated with significant mortality. Risk factors for stress ulceration are listed in Box 15-12.

Box 15-12 Risk Factors for the Development of Stress Erosions

Multiple trauma
Head trauma
Major burns
Clotting abnormalities
Severe sepsis
Systemic inflammatory response syndrome
Cardiac bypass
Intracranial operations

Presentation and Diagnosis

When considering the source of the hemorrhage, a previous history is important in assessing the patient. A history of peptic ulcer disease and previous upper GI bleeding lead one to consider a duodenal ulcer. Severe trauma, major abdominal surgery, central nervous system injury, sepsis, or MI may be associated with stress ulceration. An antecedent history of violent emesis points to consideration of a Mallory-Weiss tear, and a history of portal hypertension or variceal bleeding is a hint to the presence of esophageal varices. A previous history of diverticulosis may indicate that the hemorrhage is diverticular in nature. With a recent surgical history of intestinal anastomosis, oozing from the suture or staple line may be the source of GI bleeding. In distal colorectal anastomoses, bleeding may be the first sign of anastomotic breakdown. A previous history of aortic aneurysm repair may indicate the presence of an aortoduodenal fistula. A history of intake of NSAIDs or anticoagulant or platelet inhibitor therapy will identify patients at high risk for postoperative bleeding.

In general, bright red blood is considered to come from a colonic or distal small bowel source. Melanotic stools suggest a gastric cause of the bleeding. However, rapid bleeding at any site may result in bright red blood. Bleeding from the anastomosis may be a slow ooze or a rapid hemorrhage that can lead to hypotension. Patients who appear to have lost a significant amount of blood have associated tachycardia or hypotension or have a significant drop in hematocrit.

Treatment

To prevent stress ulceration and decrease the risk for bleeding, patients at risk must receive aggressive fluid resuscitation to improve oxygen delivery and prophylaxis that neutralizes or reduces gastric acid. Patients with respiratory failure and coagulopathy benefit the most from prophylaxis. Maintaining gastric pH above 4 is essential to minimize gastric mucosal injury and propagation of injury by acid. This can be achieved with antacids, H$_2$ blockers, M$_1$ cholinoreceptor antagonists, sucralfate, or proton pump inhibitors.

The basic principles of management of postoperative GI bleeding include the following:

1. Fluid resuscitation and restoration of intravascular volume
2. Checking and monitoring clotting parameters and correcting abnormalities as needed
3. Identification and treatment of aggravating factors
4. Transfusion of blood products
5. Identification and treatment of the source of the bleeding

In general, management of GI bleeding is best conducted in the ICU setting. Fluid resuscitation with isosmotic crystalloids is begun after securing venous access. Blood samples are sent to assess the hematocrit, platelet count, prothrombin time, partial thromboplastin time, and INR. If the INR is elevated, vitamin K and fresh frozen plasma are administered. Platelet transfusion is administered to patients with a prolonged bleeding time or to those who have been taking antiplatelet drugs; desmopressin acetate may also be given to patients in renal failure. Hypothermia, if present, is corrected.

Blood transfusion is recommended when tachycardia and hypotension refractory to volume expansion are present with a hemoglobin concentration in the 6- to 10-g/dL range and the extent of blood loss is unknown, a hemoglobin concentration less than 6 g/dL, and rapid blood loss greater than 30%, as well as in patients at risk for ischemia or those with an oxygen extraction ratio greater than 50% with a decrease in Vo_2.[42] An NG tube is placed and the effluent checked for the presence of blood. Nonbloody bilious drainage virtually rules out a gastroduodenal source of the bleeding. If blood is present, lavage with saline at room temperature is performed.

Identification and treatment of the source of bleeding can be achieved with endoscopy, angiography, or occasionally, laparotomy. Endoscopic control of bleeding can be achieved with an injection of epinephrine, electrocoagulation, laser coagulation, heater probe, argon plasma coagulator, clip application, or banding (or any combination of these modalities), depending on the source of bleeding. Visceral angiography is indicated in patients who are actively bleeding or when endoscopy fails to control the bleeding. Once an actively bleeding vessel is identified, embolization (with Gelfoam, autologous blood clot, coils) often controls the bleeding. Infusion of vasopressin may be used in patients with severe stress ulceration, diverticulosis, and ongoing bleeding. Bleeding from an intestinal anastomosis and stress ulceration usually cease with expectant management. Rarely, a patient with an anastomosis may require a reoperation to resect the anastomosis and reconnect the bowel. Similarly, surgery for stress ulceration is reserved for patients who fail medical management. Usually, a generous gastrotomy is performed to evacuate the blood clots and oversew sites of active bleeding; uncommonly, total or subtotal gastrectomy, with or without vagotomy, is performed. Recurrence with both approaches is prevented in 50% to 80% of cases.

Stomal Complications

Etiology
Stomas are widely used in the treatment of colorectal, intestinal, and urologic diseases. An intestinal stoma can be an ileostomy, colostomy, or urostomy; end, loop, or end-loop; temporary or permanent; diverting or decompressing; or continent or incontinent. A tube cecostomy and a blowhole are considered temporary decompressing colostomies performed in emergencies. Stomal complications are the result of several factors. Technical factors are most important in minimizing the complication rate of stoma construction and are largely preventable. Stomal complications are numerous (Table 15-12) and range from a bothersome problem with fit of the stomal appliance to major skin erosion and bleeding. Early complications are considered those that occur within 30 days after surgery.

Table 15-12 Stomal Complications

CATEGORY	COMPLICATION	
	Early	Late
Stoma	Poor location	Prolapse
	Retraction*	Stenosis
	Ischemic necrosis	Parastomal hernia
	Detachment	Fistula formation
	Abscess formation*	Gas
	Opening wrong end	Odor
Peristomal skin	Excoriation	Parastomal varices
	Dermatitis*	Dermatoses
		Cancer
		Skin manifestations of inflammatory bowel disease
Systemic	High output*	Bowel obstruction Nonclosure

*May also develop as a late complication.

Presentation and Diagnosis
Ischemic necrosis results from impaired perfusion to the terminal portion of the bowel as a result of a tight aperture, overzealous trimming of mesentery, or mesenteric tension. Stomal retraction occurs early as a result of tension on the bowel or ischemic necrosis of the stoma. Late retraction is due to increased thickness of the abdominal wall with weight gain. Stenosis occurs as a result of a small aperture, so-called natural maturation, ischemia, recurrence of Crohn's disease, or the development of carcinoma. Mucocutaneous separation develops as a result of ischemia, inadequate approximation of mucosa to the dermal layer of skin, excessive bowel tension, or peristomal infection.

Stomal prolapse is mostly alarming to the patient and can result in incomplete diversion of stool, interfere with the stoma appliance, lead to leakage of stool, or become associated with obstructive symptoms and incarceration. Parastomal hernia formation occurs to some degree in most patients. A peristomal fistula is often a sign of Crohn's disease, may result from a deep suture used to mature the stoma, or may be due to trauma from appliances.

Chemical dermatitis is caused by contact of the stoma effluent with peristomal skin as a result of a large opening in the faceplate or leakage from an ill-fitted faceplate. Chemical dermatitis is initially manifested as erythema, ulceration (ileostomy effluent), encrustation (urostomy effluent), and pseudoepitheliomatous hyperplasia. Infectious dermatitis may be caused by fungus, bacteria, tinea corporis, or *Candida albicans*. Allergic dermatitis may be related to any of the stoma equipment (faceplate, tape, belt, etc.), with skin manifestations appearing at the site of contact. Traumatic dermatitis occurs during change of the stoma device, from stripping of adhesive, or as a result of friction or pressure from the stoma device or supportive belt. Traumatic dermatitis is manifested as erythema, erosion, and ulceration.

Stoma patients are at risk for diarrhea and dehydration. The risk for dehydration depends on the type of stoma, the underlying primary disease process, and any concomitant bowel resection and commonly occurs in the elderly, in hot weather, during strenuous exercise, and in association with short-bowel syndrome.

Cutaneous manifestations of the disease may develop in the damaged peristomal skin in patients afflicted with certain skin conditions such as psoriasis. Pyoderma gangrenosa may develop in patients with inflammatory bowel disease, and parastomal varices may develop in patients with liver disease.

Treatment

To prevent the majority of stomal complications, adherence to sound surgical technique is imperative. Application of the technical points shown in Box 15-13 ensures the construction of a healthy and well-positioned stoma in patients undergoing surgery. In emergencies and difficult cases such as the obese, distended bowel, and shortened mesentery, to ensure delivery of a viable stoma free of tension, the fascial aperture may be made larger, the bowel may have to be extensively mobilized, the ileocolic artery and inferior mesenteric artery may have to be divided at their origin, windows may need to be created in the mesentery, the stoma may be brought out

---

Box 15-13   Technical Aspects of Stoma Construction

Abdominal Wall Aperture

Excision of a circular piece of skin about 2 cm in size
Preservation of subcutaneous fat to provide support for the stoma
Transrectus muscle placement of the stoma
Fascial aperture to admit two fingers

Stoma

Selection of normal bowel for the stoma
Adequate mobilization of bowel to avoid tension on the stoma
Preservation of blood supply to the end of bowel (the marginal artery of the colon and the last vascular arcade of the small bowel mesentery must be preserved)
The small bowel serosa must not be denuded of more than 5 cm of mesentery

Maturation

Primary maturation of the end stoma or the afferent limb of the loop ileostomy
Avoidance of traversing the skin with sutures during maturation

Other Maneuvers*

Tunneling of bowel through the extraperitoneal space of the abdominal wall
Mesenteric-peritoneal closure
Fixation of mesentery/bowel to the fascial ring
Use of a supportive rod with loop stomas

*May be performed but have not been proved to be effective in preventing postoperative complications.

---

at a site with less SC fat (above the umbilicus), or alternative stomas may be selected.

After construction of a stoma, a dusky appearance indicates some degree of ischemia. The ischemia may be mucosal or full thickness, and the extent and depth of ischemia dictate the need for immediate revision of the stoma. Viability of the stoma is checked with a test tube and a flashlight or endoscopy. Necrosis extending to and beyond the fascia requires immediate reoperation. Ischemia limited to a few millimeters is observed and may not result in any long-term sequelae. Repair of stomal retraction often requires laparotomy.

Skin-level stenosis can be repaired locally and stenoses from other causes via laparotomy. Complete separation or detachment usually requires revision. Repair of end-stoma prolapse can be achieved locally by making a circumferential incision at the mucocutaneous junction, excision of redundant bowel, and rematuration. Repair of loop-stoma prolapse is achieved by local revision to an end-stoma. Laparotomy may be required for the treatment of recurrent prolapse and prolapse associated with a parastomal hernia. Large permanent or complicated parastomal hernias are treated by relocating the stoma or reinforcing the fascia ring with mesh (synthetic or biomaterial).[43] Treatment of peristomal fistula entails resection of the diseased/involved segment of bowel and relocation of the stoma. Treatment of mucosal islands ranges from ablation with electrocautery to relocation of the stoma.

Treatment of chemical dermatitis entails cleaning the damaged skin, the use of barriers, and a properly fitting stoma management system. *Candida* dermatitis is best treated with nystatin powder. Allergic dermatitis is treated by removal of the offending item and symptomatic relief with oral antihistamine or topical or oral steroid therapy. Traumatic dermatitis is treated by patient education and application of a skin barrier under the tape used to secure the faceplate in place. Occasionally, in cases of severe dermatitis, the patient will have to be admitted to the hospital and placed on total parenteral nutrition (TPN) while the skin around the stoma heals enough to allow subsequent placement of an appliance.

Clostridium difficile Colitis

Etiology

C. difficile colitis is an inflammatory bowel disease caused by toxins produced by unopposed proliferation of the bacterium *C. difficile*. Several factors are associated with increased risk for *C. difficile* colitis (Table 15-13). The incidence of *C. difficile* colitis has increased by more than 30% in the past decade. Overall mortality has also increased from 3.5% to 15.3%, in part because of the increased number of elderly and immunocompromised individuals infected with the bacterium and altered host immunity.

C. difficile colitis is closely associated with nosocomial transmission of toxigenic strains of *C. difficile*. The organism may be present endogenously or acquired from exogenous sources. Antibiotic use continues to precede nearly all cases of infection. Of the patients contracting *C. diffi cile* colitis, 90% have received antibiotic therapy and 70% were treated with multiple antibiotics.⁴⁴ Patients receiving prolonged courses of antibiotic therapy are particularly susceptible. Intensive care and long-term facility units house critically ill and vulnerable patients; impaired host immune defense as a result of advanced age, surgery, immunosuppressive medications, infection with human immunodeficiency virus, and chemotherapy is a major risk factor. Surgical patients account for 45% to 55% of *C. difficile* colitis, and the highest rates of infection are noted in patients undergoing general and vascular surgery.⁴⁴ *C. difficile* is a gram-positive anaerobic spore-forming bacillus that has the capability to produce toxins A and B. The spore is heat resistant, persists in the environment for months and years in a dormant phase, and survives on inanimate objects. About 3% to 5% of the general population has the organism in their stool.

Antibiotic use leads to a disturbance in the microflora of the colon and allows the nosocomial organism to grow, proliferate, and produce toxins. Toxin A, an enterotoxin, causes cell rounding, mucosal damage and inflammation, and release of inflammatory mediators. Toxin B is a potent cytotoxin that causes identical cell rounding and activates the release of cytokines from human monocytes.

Presentation and Diagnosis

Overgrowth of toxigenic strains of *C. difficile* results in a variety of disease states with varied clinical courses, ranging from asymptomatic carrier to self-limited colitis, pseudomembranous colitis, fulminant colitis to toxic megacolon. Watery diarrhea is the hallmark symptom and usually starts during or shortly after antibiotic use. One dose of antibiotic can result in the disease, but the incidence with prophylactic antibiotics increases with extended use of antibiotics beyond the recommended period. Stools are foul smelling and may be positive for the presence of occult blood. In mild to moderate cases, systemic signs of infection are absent or present to a mild degree. In severe colitis, the diarrhea becomes associated with abdominal cramps and anorexia, abdominal tenderness, dehydration, tachycardia, and a raised leukocyte (white blood cell) count. Pseudomembranous colitis is the more dramatic form of the disease and develops in 40% of patients who are significantly symptomatic.

ELISA for detection of toxin A or B in stool is a highly sensitive and specific diagnostic test. Unlike the stool cytotoxic test, which required 24 to 48 hours, results with ELISA are obtained within hours, and the test is less expensive and does not require specific training. Endoscopy reveals nonspecific colitis (mucosal edema and patchy erythema) in moderate disease or pseudomembranes in severe disease. Radiographs of the abdomen may be normal or show adynamic ileus, colonic dilation, thumb printing, or haustral thickening. CT may show thickened and edematous colon wall and free peritoneal fluid.

Fulminant colitis may develop in about 2% to 5% of patients despite timely medical therapy, and such patients may succumb to cytokine-mediated cardiovascular collapse and death.⁴⁵ At-risk patients are the immunocompromised or those taking multiple antibiotics, patients with a previous diagnosis of *C. difficile* infection, patients with severe vascular disease, the elderly, those with chronic obstructive pulmonary disease, and patients with renal failure. In fulminant colitis, abdominal cramps, distention, and tenderness become more prominent and associated with systemic signs of toxicity. Diarrhea may be absent in 5% to 12% of cases, and the white blood cell count may be depressed but is most commonly increased with a rapid elevation (>20,000 cells/mm³) and bandemia (>30%). Toxic megacolon may develop and is characterized by obstipation, a dilated colon, and systemic toxicity. Sigmoidoscopy shows pseudomembranes in 90% of cases (versus 23% in mild cases). CT scan is diagnostic and typically shows a boggy, edematous, thick-walled colon. Other findings include the presence of pancolitis, ascites, pericolic inflammation, and megacolon.

Treatment

Treatment of *C. difficile* colitis starts with prevention. Judicious use of antibiotics, use of disposable gloves and single-use disposable thermometers, and in outbreaks, ward closure and decontamination are measures important in decreasing the mortality and morbidity associated with *C. difficile* colitis.

Once a diagnosis of *C. difficile* colitis is made, medical therapy and timely surgical intervention improve recovery and lower the mortality rate. Infections with *C. difficile* usually follow a benign course. Whereas some patients respond to discontinuation of antibiotic therapy, others require treatment and respond within 3 to 4 days. Vancomycin is given orally or as an enema, or metronidazole is given orally or IV for 2 weeks. Antimotility agents and narcotics are avoided. In the absence of ileus, oral intake is allowed. Recurrent disease develops in about 25% to 30% of patients as a result of reinfection with a second strain or reactivation of toxigenic spores that persist in the colon. Treatment of relapse is similar to that of the primary infection. In patients with recurrent attacks, pulsed vancomycin therapy, combination vancomycin and rifampicin therapy, or the administration of

Table 15-13 Factors Associated With Increased Risk for *Clostridium difficile* Colitis

CATEGORY	RISK FACTORS
Patient-related factors	Increasing age Preexisting renal disease Preexisting chronic obstructive lung disease Impaired immune defense Underlying malignancy Underlying gastrointestinal disease
Treatment-related factors	Preoperative bowel cleansing Antibiotic use Immunosuppressive therapy Surgery Prolonged hospital stay
Facility-related factors	Intensive care units Caregivers Long-term facilities

Table 15-14 Risk Factors Associated With Anastomotic Leak

DEFINITIVE FACTORS	IMPLICATED FACTORS

Technical aspects:
  Blood supply
  Tension on the suture line
  Airtight and water-tight
    anastomosis
	Mechanical bowel
	  preparation
	Drains
	Advanced malignancy
	Shock and coagulopathy

Location in the
  gastrointestinal tract:
  Pancreaticoenteric
  Colorectal
    Above the peritoneal
      reflection
    Below the peritoneal
      reflection
	Emergency surgery
	
	Blood transfusion
	Malnutrition
	Obesity
	
	Sex

Local factors:
  Septic environment
  Fluid collection
	Smoking
	Steroid therapy
	Neoadjuvant therapy

Bowel-related factors:
  Radiotherapy
  Compromised distal lumen
  Crohn's disease
	Vitamin C, iron, zinc, and
	  cysteine deficiency
	Stapler-related factors:
	  Forceful extraction of
	    the stapler
	  Tears caused by anvil
	    or gun insertion
	  Failure of the stapler to
	    close

competitive organisms (*Lactobacillus acidophilus* and *Saccharomyces cerevisiae*) may be tried.

Obvious indications for surgical intervention are colonic perforation and toxic megacolon. Failure of medical therapy, the presence of systemic toxicity, adynamic ileus, worsening of colitis identified on CT, and an immunocompromised state of the patient are criteria that mandate surgical intervention. The procedure of choice is total abdominal colectomy and ileostomy.

Anastomotic Leak

Etiology

Numerous factors can cause or are associated with an increased risk for anastomotic leak (Table 15-14). Mechanical bowel preparation has long been considered a critical factor in preventing infectious complications after elective colorectal surgery.[46] With decreased morbidity rates as a result of effective antibiotic prophylaxis, modern surgical techniques, and advances in patient care, the need for mechanical bowel preparation has been questioned.[47] Although there may be a trend toward elimination of cleansing of the colon in elective and emergency colon resection, one must be cautioned against abandoning the practice completely, especially for anterior resections, where the presence of stool in the rectum poses a problem with the use of staplers.

The level of the anastomosis in the GI tract is important. Although small bowel, ileocolic, and ileorectal anastomoses are considered safe, esophageal, pancreaticoenteric, and colorectal anastomoses are considered high risk for leakage. In the esophagus, lack of serosa appears to be a significant contributing factor. In the pancreas, the texture of the gland and the size of the pancreatic duct are implicated. In the rectum, the highest leak rate is found in anastomoses in the distal part of the rectum.

Adequate microcirculation at the resection margins is crucial for the healing of any anastomosis. In colorectal anastomoses, relative ischemia in the rectal remnant is a factor because its blood supply is derived from the internal iliac artery via the inferior hemorrhoidal vessels and contribution from the middle hemorrhoidal artery is minimal. Total mesorectal excision, neoadjuvant therapy, and extended lymphadenectomy with high ligation of the inferior mesenteric artery are additional contributing factors.

Intraluminal distention is believed to be responsible for rupture of an anastomosis. The mechanical strength of the anastomosis is important and, in the early period, is dependent on sutures or staples. Construction of a water-tight and airtight anastomosis is therefore essential. Antiadhesive agents may predispose to leaks because they isolate the anastomosis from the peritoneum and omentum, decrease anastomotic bursting pressure and hydroxyproline levels.[48] In the pelvis, some studies have shown that drains are associated with higher leak rates than the use of no drains is. Local sepsis has a negative impact on the integrity of the anastomosis because it reduces collagen synthesis and increases collagenase activity, which results in increased lysis of collagen at the anastomosis. Defunctioning or protective stomas do not decrease the overall leak rate but rather minimize the severity and sequelae of perianastomotic contamination and decrease the reoperation rate.[49]

Emergency bowel surgery is associated with high morbidity and mortality, in part because of sepsis and anastomotic leakage. This is related to the poor nutritional status of the patient, an immunocompromised state, and the presence of intra-abdominal contamination/sepsis. Obesity increases the difficulty and complexity of the surgery, has been shown to be associated with increased postoperative complications, and is an independent factor for an increasing leakage rate, especially after a low colorectal anastomosis. Steroids affect healing by decreasing collagen synthesis and reducing production of transforming growth factor-β and insulin-like growth factor in wounds, which are essential for wound healing.

Presentation and Diagnosis

Anastomotic leak is a dreadful complication to encounter. It results in sepsis and enteric fistula formation, leads to reoperation and a possible permanent stoma, increases the local recurrence rate after curative resection of cancer, and possibly leads to death.[50]

The clinical manifestations are the result of a cascade of events that start with loss of integrity of the anastomosis and leakage of intestinal contents. The leakage may be diffuse throughout the peritoneal cavity (uncontrolled leak) or become walled off by omentum or loops of small bowel. If the fluid collection is drained surgically or percutaneously, there is an initial discharge of purulent material followed by feculent material heralding the formation of an enterocutaneous fistula (controlled fistula). If the effluent is allowed to drain through the surgical incision or abdominal wall, surgical wound infection and dehiscence with evisceration or an abdominal wall abscess may occur. If the fluid collection burrows into a contiguous structure such as the urinary bladder or vagina, spontaneous drainage occurs with the formation of an enterovesical or enterovaginal fistula.

The early warning signs of anastomotic leak are malaise, fever, abdominal pain, ileus, localized erythema around the surgical incision, and leukocytosis. Bowel obstruction and induration and erythema in the abdominal wall may also develop. In addition, patients may experience pneumaturia, fecaluria, and pyuria.

Sepsis is a prominent feature of anastomotic leakage and results from diffuse peritonitis or localized abscess, abdominal wall infection, or contamination of a sterile site with intestinal contents.

Treatment

Treatment of anastomotic leakage starts with prevention. In emergencies, especially in hemodynamically unstable, immunocompromised, and nutritionally depleted patients and in the presence of fecal peritonitis, significant bowel dilation, and edema, an anastomosis is best avoided because a leak may prove fatal. Mechanical and chemical bowel preparations are still recommended before elective colorectal resection.

Construction of an anastomosis that is at low risk for disruption requires the following:

1. Adequate exposure, gentle handling of tissues, aseptic precautions, and meticulous, careful dissection
2. Adequate mobilization so that the two attached organs have a tension-free anastomosis
3. Correct technical placement of sutures or staples with very little variance
4. Matching of the lumens of the two organs to be connected with hand-sewn anastomoses
5. Preservation of blood supply to the ends of structures to be anastomosed.

For intestinal and colorectal anastomoses, there is no difference in the rate of anastomotic leakage between hand-sewn and stapled anastomoses and between various stapling techniques, provided that sound surgical technique is followed. Since the advent of stapling devices, such anastomoses, especially deep in the pelvis, have usually been stapled. In low anterior resection, the omentum may be advanced to the pelvis and around the colorectal anastomosis; this maneuver may lower the rate of anastomotic leak/disruption. Drainage of colorectal anastomoses is advisable in difficult cases or when neoadjuvant therapy has been used. Defunctioning stomas are used for extraperitoneal anastomoses, when technical difficulties are encountered, and after neoadjuvant therapy.

When constructing a pancreaticoenteric anastomosis, end-to-side/duct-to-mucosa pancreaticojejunostomy is associated with a lower rate of leakage than end-to-end/invaginating pancreaticojejunostomy is.[51] Drains and octreotide can be used for anastomoses to a soft pancreas with a small duct.

Once an anastomotic leak is suspected or diagnosed, resuscitation is started immediately. Intravascular volume is restored with crystalloid fluids and blood transfusion if anemia is present. Oral intake is stopped and the bowel is put at rest to decrease luminal contents and GI stimulation and secretion. An NG tube is placed if obstructive symptoms are present. Infected surgical wounds are opened, and any abdominal wall abscesses are incised and drained. Reoperation is indicated if there is diffuse peritonitis, intra-abdominal hemorrhage, suspected intestinal ischemia, major wound disruption, or evisceration. Primary closure of the leaking point is avoided because failure is certain. Management of jejunal, ileal, and colorectal leaking anastomoses depends on the severity and duration of contamination, the condition of the bowel, and the hemodynamic stability of the patient. In a critically ill and unstable patient, especially one with fecal peritonitis, a damage control type of procedure is performed (i.e., the anastomosis is taken down, the ends of the bowel are stapled, peritoneal lavage is performed, and the incision is left open). A second-look laparotomy with stoma formation is performed in 24 to 48 hours or once the patient is more stable. Otherwise, in the small bowel, an anastomosis may be performed or the ends of the bowel are delivered as stomas; in the colon, the proximal end of the colon is brought out as a colostomy and the distal end closed or brought out as a mucus fistula; and in the rectum, the distal end is closed and the proximal end of the colon delivered as a stoma. A proximal diverting stoma with drainage of the pelvis is not adequate treatment of leaking colorectal anastomoses associated with diffuse peritonitis.

Multiple abscesses require open drainage, a single intra-abdominal abscess can be drained percutaneously, and a pelvic abscess can be drained transrectally/transvaginally. If percutaneous drainage fails to control sepsis, reoperation is indicated. At the time of open drainage of a pelvic abscess, if there is any doubt about the origin of the abscess, a defunctioning stoma is constructed unless there is complete disruption of the anastomosis, in which case the ends of the bowel are exteriorized as a stoma. A pancreaticojejunostomy leak, if small, can probably be drained and a drain placed next to the leak. However, for an anastomosis that has virtually fallen apart, the patient will probably require completion pancreatectomy. A patient who has a bile duct leak will require drainage of the infection and placement of a drain next to the leak or, in the case of a large leak, may require bile duct reconstruction.

Intestinal Fistula

Etiology

A fistula represents an abnormal communication between two epithelialized surfaces, one of which is a hollow organ. In the GI tract, a fistula may develop between any two digestive organs or between a hollow organ and the skin and may be developmental or acquired. Acquired fistulas account for the majority of GI fistulas and can be traumatic, spontaneous, or postoperative in nature.

GI fistulas are most commonly iatrogenic, develop after an operation, and may occur anywhere in the GI tract. They commonly occur as a result of anastomotic breakdown, dehiscence of a surgically closed segment of stomach or bowel, or unrecognized iatrogenic bowel injury after adhesiolysis or during closure of a laparotomy incision. Occasionally, they develop after instrumentation or drainage of a pancreatic, appendiceal, or diverticular fluid collection or abscess. The presence of intrinsic intestinal disease, such as Crohn's disease, radiation enteritis, distal obstruction, or a hostile abdominal environment, such as an abscess or peritonitis, is a predisposing factor for fistula formation.

Gastric fistulas are uncommon and frequently occur after resection for cancer and less commonly after resection for peptic ulcer disease. Pancreatic fistulas develop as a result of disruption of the main pancreatic duct or its branches secondary to trauma or postoperatively after pancreatic surgery. Intestinal fistulas develop after resection for cancer, diverticular disease, or inflammatory bowel disease.

Presentation and Diagnosis

Patients with an intestinal fistula have the clinical manifestations of leakage of intestinal contents as discussed in the previous section. The seriousness and severity of these manifestations depend on the surgical anatomy and physiology of the fistula. Anatomically, the fistula may originate from the stomach, duodenum, small bowel (proximal or distal), or large bowel. The tract of the fistula may erode into another portion of the intestines (enteroenteric fistula) or another hollow organ (enterovesical), thus forming an internal fistula, or into the body surface (enterocutaneous and pancreatic fistula) or vagina (enterovaginal fistula), thus forming an external fistula. Physiologically, the fistula is classified into high and low output on the basis of the volume of discharge in 24 hours. The exact definition of high and low output varies from 200 to 500 mL/24 hr. However, three different categories are recognized—low output (<200 mL/24 hr), moderate output (200-500 mL/24 hr), and high output (>500 mL/24 hr). The ileum is the site of the fistula in 50% of high-output fistulas.

Sepsis is a prominent feature of postoperative intestinal fistulas and is present in 25% to 75% of cases. Loss of intestinal contents through the fistula results in hypovolemia and dehydration, electrolyte and acid-base imbalance, loss of protein and trace elements, and malnutrition. In a high intestinal fistula it also results in loss of the normal inhibitory effect on gastric secretion, thus giving rise to a gastric hypersecretory state. In gastroduodenal and proximal small bowel fistulas the output is high and the fluid loss, electrolyte imbalance, and malabsorption are profound. In distal small bowel and colonic fistulas the output is low and dehydration, acid-base imbalance, and malnutrition are uncommon.

Skin and surgical wound complications develop as a result of contact of GI effluent with skin or the wound. Effluent dermatitis results from the corrosive effect of intestinal contents, which cause irritation, excoriation, ulceration, and infection of the skin. The pain and itching caused by contact of effluent with unprotected skin is intolerable and affects the morale of the patient.

Treatment

In the past the main themes of management were suctioning of the intestinal effluent and early surgical intervention. This approach has proved ineffective and is associated with significant patient morbidity and mortality and a high reoperation rate. At the present time, management requires the involvement of a surgeon, nutritionist, enterostomal therapist, interventional radiologist, and a gastroenterologist and entails initial medical management to allow spontaneous healing of the fistula and planned definitive surgery for patients whose fistulas have failed to heal. Although spontaneous closure occurs in 40% to 80% of cases, operative intervention may be required in 30% to 60% of cases.

Should a fistula form, management involves several phases that are applied systematically and simultaneously. Once a leak is diagnosed, resuscitation is of paramount importance because patients have been without nutrition, have a contracted intravascular volume secondary to loss of intestinal contents, and may have electrolyte imbalance. Intravascular volume is restored with crystalloids and the electrolyte imbalance is corrected. Oral intake is stopped and the bowel is put at rest, thus decreasing luminal contents and reducing GI stimulation and secretion. In the presence of infection, broad-spectrum IV antibiotic therapy is started.

Treatment with H_2 antagonists or proton pump inhibitors decreases fistula output. Accurate measurement of output from all orifices and the fistula is paramount in maintaining fluid balance. Effective control of all sources of sepsis is important because continued sepsis is a major source of mortality. Infected surgical wounds are opened and drained, and intra-abdominal fluid collections are drained percutaneously or surgically.

Nutrition is one of the most important factors contributing to a successful outcome in the management of intestinal fistulas. TPN must be started early after correction of electrolyte imbalance and repletion of volume. TPN allows bowel rest, which decreases output, eliminates negative nitrogen balance, increases the rate of recovery, and may slightly improve the closure rate once sepsis is controlled. TPN is the initial nutritional support in any patient with a fistula and is continued in patients with high-output fistulas or those who cannot tolerate oral intake. Somatostatin analogues help in management of the fistula by reducing GI secretions and inhibiting GI motility. Enteral nutrition is administered to patients with low-output small bowel and colonic external fistulas. Fistuloclysis (i.e., infusion of nutrition directly through the fistula into the bowel distal to the fistula) is another option to deliver enteral nutrition to patients whose fistula has not healed spontaneously.[52]

Skin protection achieved with barriers, sealants, adhesives, and pouches has proved effective in containing the effluent, protecting the integrity of the perifistula skin, and promoting healing of damaged skin. Early involvement of an enterostomal therapist and wound care team cannot be overemphasized.

Diagnostic studies are performed to define the pathology of the fistula and the condition of the bowel and to evaluate resolution of the intra-abdominal abscess. A fis-

Table 15-15 Factors Affecting Healing of External Intestinal Fistulas

FACTORS	FAVORABLE	UNFAVORABLE
Surgical anatomy of the fistula	Long tract, >2 cm Single tract No other fistulas Lateral fistula Nonepithelialized tract Origin (jejunum, colon, duodenal stump, and pancreaticobiliary) No adjacent large abscess	Short tract, <2 cm Multiple tracts Associated internal fistulas End fistula Epithelialized tract Origin (lateral duodenum, stomach, and ileum) Adjacent large abscess
Status of the bowel	No intestinal disease No distal bowel obstruction Small enteral defect, <1 cm	Intrinsic intestinal disease (Crohn's disease, radiation enteritis, recurrent or incompletely resected cancer) Distal bowel obstruction Large enteral defect, >1 cm
Condition of the abdominal wall	Intact Not diseased No foreign body	Disrupted (fistula opens into the base of the disrupted incision) Infiltrated with malignancy or intestinal disease Foreign body (mesh)
Physiology of the patient	No malnutrition No sepsis	Malnutrition Sepsis
Output of the fistula	No influence	Influence

tulogram delineates the anatomy of the fistula and identifies associated cavities, other fistulas, and distal obstruction. A contrast enema demonstrates the presence of a colocutaneous fistula in 90% of cases, a colovesical fistula in 34%, and a coloenteric fistula in the majority of cases. Enteroclysis allows evaluation for intrinsic intestinal disease. Cystoscopy identifies the fistula opening in 40% of enterovesical fistulas. GI endoscopy permits direct visualization of colonic, intestinal, and gastroduodenal mucosa. A CT scan allows evaluation of the resolution of intra-abdominal abscesses and the presence of intrinsic intestinal disease.

Factors associated with spontaneous healing are depicted in Table 15-15. After control of sepsis, about 60% to 90% of external intestinal fistulas with favorable factors will close spontaneously with medical management. Fistulas that do not close will require definitive surgical intervention. There are no well-established guidelines to help in determining the timing of surgery. However, the experience of the surgeon, the general condition of the patient, the softness of the abdominal wall, and the surgical anatomy of the fistula must be taken into consideration. A simple fistula can be closed 12 weeks after the index surgery. A complex fistula (i.e., one associated with other internal fistulas or a large abscess cavity or one that opens into the base of a disrupted wound) is closed 6 to 12 months after the index surgery.

The aim of a definitive surgical procedure is to resect the fistulizing segment, reestablish continuity of the GI tract, and close or reconstruct the abdominal wall. The laparotomy incision is closed primarily or with a synthetic prosthesis, tissue graft, or wound vacuum system.

New innovative approaches such as percutaneous management or management with a wound vacuum device, endoscopic tissue sealant application, and porcine small intestinal submucosa have been used in recalcitrant

cases or as an adjunctive therapy to hasten healing of the intestinal fistula, with some success. The indications and appropriateness of their use are awaiting further studies.

Pancreatic Fistulas

Overall, the physiologic classification, diagnosis, management, and outcome of postoperative external pancreatic fistulas are similar to that for external intestinal fistulas. Diagnosis of the fistula is heralded by increased surgical drain output of serous to cloudy fluid with a high amylase content.

Once a pancreatic fistula has formed, medical management results in spontaneous closure in almost all fistulas. Octreotide therapy is beneficial because it significantly reduces fistula output and decreases the time until fistula closure. Endoscopic retrograde cholangiopancreatography (ERCP) is valuable because it allows the placement of a stent to bypass the high resistance of the sphincter of Oddi. The stent may also block the ductal opening of the fistula. Operative treatment of a benign pancreaticocutaneous fistula depends on the location of the fistula (proximal versus distal portion of the pancreas) and the status of the pancreatic duct (dilated versus stenotic duct). High excision of the fistula with fistuloenterostomy is associated with the best results.

HEPATOBILIARY COMPLICATIONS

Bile Duct Injuries

Etiology

The most dreaded complication of gallbladder surgery is injury to the extrahepatic bile duct system. Cholecystectomy accounts for the great majority of postoperative biliary injuries and strictures. The rate of major bile duct injury after laparoscopic cholecystectomy ranges from 0.4% to 0.7%, as opposed to 0.2% after open cholecystectomy.[53] Bile leak may be due to a bile duct injury, cystic duct stump leak, divided accessory duct, or injury to the intestine. Acute cholecystitis, a foreshortened cystic duct, anomalies of the biliary tree, hemorrhage from injury to the cystic or hepatic artery, dissection with thermal instruments in the triangle of Calot, and failure to clearly define the anatomy in the triangle of Calot are among the most important factors associated with a higher frequency of duct injury after laparoscopic cholecystectomy.

The most common injury sustained during the laparoscopic procedure is complete transection at or below the hepatic duct bifurcation. Other less complex injuries include occlusion of the duct with a clip, thermal injury, avulsion of the cystic duct, and partial laceration.

Presentation and Diagnosis

Most bile duct injuries are not identified at the time of surgery. Early in the postoperative period patients may have manifestations related to a bile leak or later have signs of a bile duct stricture. Bile leaking from a lacerated, divided duct may accumulate in the subhepatic space and form a biloma or seep into the peritoneal cavity and result in bile ascites. Patients in this situation have right upper quadrant pain, fever, nausea, abdominal distention, and malaise. The bile, on the other hand, may drain through an intraoperatively placed drain and be manifested as a bile leak. In this setting patients may have leukocytosis and slightly elevated bilirubin. Patients with a clipped bile duct do not usually have symptoms but do have elevated liver enzymes. Bile duct strictures are usually accompanied by cholangitis, pain, fever, chills, and jaundice.

Diagnosis of bile duct injury requires the use of nuclear medicine imaging to demonstrate the presence of a leak or obstruction, a CT scan to identify bile collections or ascites, and ERCP to accurately define the type and level of injury. Percutaneous transhepatic cholangiography is indicated in cases of complete transection to define the proximal anatomy and site of injury. Magnetic resonance cholangiopancreatography is becoming the test of choice to diagnose late strictures and define the bile duct anatomy.

Treatment

Prevention of bile duct injury starts with proper surgical technique and adequate identification of the anatomy. The anatomic variability associated with severe inflammation creates a low threshold for converting a laparoscopic to an open cholecystectomy. During laparoscopic cholecystectomy, the infundibulum of the gallbladder must be retracted laterally and inferiorly to expose the triangle and widen the cystic–common bile duct angle. Dissection of the cystic duct and artery must commence close to the infundibulum of the gallbladder. The cystic duct and artery are divided once the anatomy is clearly delineated. Excessive traction on the gallbladder must be avoided because it will result in tenting of the common duct. If there is bleeding in the area of the cystic duct, blind clipping and cautery must be avoided, and adequate exposure must be achieved even if placement of another port is required. If there is an unexpected bile leak, unusual anatomy, or a second bile duct identified or when technical difficulties and excessive bleeding are encountered, intraoperative cholangiography helps identify the anatomy and any injuries. Early conversion to an open procedure must also be considered.

Once a leak is diagnosed intraoperatively, immediate repair must be performed. The procedure is converted to an open one and the extent of duct injury is assessed. An accessory duct can be ligated, partial transection of the common duct is repaired over a T-tube, a divided duct or nearly circumferential transection of the common duct is repaired with an end-to-end anastomosis over a T-tube, and a high injury is repaired with a Roux-en-Y biliary-enteric anastomosis. If repair of a high duct injury is difficult, drains are placed in the subhepatic space and the patient is referred to a tertiary center.

A leak or injury identified early in the postoperative period is treated as follows: the biloma is drained percutaneously, and a sphincterotomy is performed or a stent is placed (or both) if ERCP demonstrates a leak or partial narrowing. Surgical intervention is indicated in patients with major obstruction of the bile duct, a major injury, or suspicion of a bowel injury. After adequate resuscitation, administration of antibiotics, and adequate drainage, patients are watched for a few days to make certain that they are not septic at the time of the operation. If there is evidence of adequate control of the leak, the surgeon may wait up to 5 to 7 days for inflammation in the area to subside before undertaking operative repair. Meticulous and careful dissection is required in this area because there is usually loss of common bile duct substance. After identifying the source of the bile extravasation, dissection plus débridement of nonviable common bile duct is prudent. Once it is ascertained that there is tissue with good integrity, a Roux-en-Y limb can be anastomosed to the common bile duct. Multiple drains are left around the site of the repair.

NEUROLOGIC COMPLICATIONS

Delirium, Cognitive Disorder, and Psychosis

Etiology

Delirium refers to a state of acute confusion and is a common complication of surgery. Numerous factors are implicated in causing delirium (Box 15-14). The presence of a structural brain disorder (infarct) increases the individual's susceptibility to delirium. Anticholinergic medications and conditions that decrease the production of acetylcholine can precipitate delirium. In addition, a planned operation with loss of the patient's routine schedule, stress of the disease process, fear of the operation, loss of personal control, placement in an unfamiliar environment, the addition of mind-altering pain medications, and pain can all lead to dramatic alterations in behavior in postoperative patients. At particularly high risk for behavioral disorders in the postoperative period are the elderly, patients with a previous history of substance abuse or psychiatric disorders, and children.

Presentation and Diagnosis

Early in the postoperative period a patient may become acutely agitated, uncooperative, and confused. Patients with a previous psychiatric disorder may, however, become more withdrawn and depressed. Some patients may become noncommunicative and emotionally flat and may withdraw from any emotional exchange. Patients may also show an altered level of consciousness and changes in cognition. They have reduced ability to focus, decreased levels of awareness, and difficulty with attention. In addition, they may have hallucinations and altered psychomotor activity and sleep-wake cycle. These changes have a tendency to fluctuate during the course of the day and are worse at night (sundowning). The severity of these manifestations depends on the underlying cause.

The incidence of postoperative delirium and cognitive disorders in geriatric patients varies with the type of surgery performed and preexisting dementia. Postoperative anemia (secondary to acute blood loss), electrolyte imbalance, sepsis, malnutrition, bladder catheterization, physical restraints, extended duration of anesthesia, infection, and respiratory complications are significant precipitating factors.

The most immediately threatening disorder encountered by physicians is delirium tremens, which may occur 48 hours to 14 days after acute alcohol withdrawal. In addition, delirium tremens is associated with extreme autonomic hyperactivity. Early signs of delirium tremens include fever, tremor, and tachycardia, and late signs include confusion, psychosis, agitation, and seizures. Because of the serious underlying nutritional and medical deficiencies, these patients have moderately high mortality that approaches 20% in some series.

Treatment

Management of delirium and cognitive disorders in a postoperative patient is a frustrating and challenging clinical scenario. Prevention starts with identification of high-risk individuals before surgery and careful follow-up thereafter. Minimizing the dose or eliminating medications that cause interruption in mental function must be considered. Optimizing fluid status, providing nutrition and adequate pain control, and removing restraints early, including the Foley catheter, are essential. Early ambulation and transfer from the ICU are encouraged.

Treatment of patients with acute confusion or a sudden change in behavior after surgery requires the following:

1. Recognition of the disorder
2. Close observation and monitoring
3. Identification and elimination of the precipitating factor
4. Treatment of any associated laboratory abnormalities
5. Selective use of imaging or other studies to rule out an organic brain lesion
6. Application of measures to protect the patient and staff
7. Treatment

A history of drug or alcohol abuse and a history of cardiac, pulmonary, renal, or liver disease or psychiatric

---

Box 15-14 Causes of Acute Delirium

Advanced age
Alcohol intoxication and withdrawal
Drugs (overdose or withdrawal):
    Anticholinergic drugs (tricyclic antidepressants, antihistamine)
    Oral hypoglycemic agents
    Antibiotics (cephalosporins)
    Histamine receptor blocking agents
    Anti-inflammatory drugs (steroidal, nonsteroidal)
    Anticonvulsant medications
    Anxiolytics (diazepam)
    Narcotics
    Cardiac medications (β-blockers, digoxin)
Structural brain abnormalities (edema, transient ischemic attack, neoplasm)
Metabolic and hemodynamic disturbances
    Electrolyte imbalance
    Hypoglycemia
    Hypoxemia
    Hypovolemia
Endocrine dysfunction
    Thyrotoxicosis
    Hypothyroidism
    Adrenocortical insufficiency
Sepsis and infections
Respiratory dysfunction (respiratory failure, pulmonary embolism, chronic obstructive pulmonary disease)
Liver, renal, and cardiac disease (congestive heart failure, renal failure)
Trauma (surgical or otherwise)
Critical illness and intensive care unit stay

---

illness must be sought. A list of medications used in the perioperative period must be checked. Clinical evaluation is performed to look for evidence of sepsis or a recent neurologic event. A thorough neurologic examination is performed while focusing on the level of consciousness and the presence of focal neurologic deficits, ataxia, paresis, or paralysis. Cognitive tests are conducted. Blood samples are sent to check for evidence of infection and to identify metabolic, electrolyte, nutritional, and blood gas abnormalities. A radiograph of the chest and urinalysis are performed to look for a source of infection. An ECG is obtained to look for evidence of MI. CT or MRI and occasionally a spinal tap may be helpful in select cases.

Measures to protect the patient and staff may include the occasional use of physical restraints, reassurance by speaking to the patient, and allowing family members to be involved in patient care. Medical therapy includes haloperidol, a neuroleptic (0.5-2 mg given IV or intramuscularly to achieve a rapid effect then orally for maintenance therapy). Benzodiazepines are the drug of choice for acute alcohol withdrawal. Other medications, including haloperidol (to control psychosis), β-blockers (to control autonomic manifestations), and clonidine (to control hypertension) are given in addition to benzodiazepine to patients with acute alcohol withdrawal.

Seizure Disorders

Etiology

Seizures are caused by paroxysmal electrical discharges from the cerebral cortex and may be primary or secondary. Primary causes of seizure include intracranial tumor, hemorrhage, trauma, or idiopathic seizure activity. Secondary causes of seizure include metabolic derangement, sepsis, systemic disease processes, and pharmacologic agents. Patients at particularly high risk for postoperative seizure include those with a previous history of epilepsy and patients acutely withdrawing from alcohol or medications or receiving other pharmacologic agents, including antidepressants, hypoglycemic agents, and lidocaine.

Presentation and Management

Seizures characterized by convulsions, rhythmic myoclonic activity, loss of consciousness, and a change in mental status are often associated with fecal and urinary incontinence, lack of neurologic responsiveness, and postevent amnesia. On recognizing evidence of seizure activity, the patient must be carefully restrained so that injury is not sustained during convulsions and carefully observed. Administration of IV benzodiazepines is essential to stop the seizure activity and is the standard for immediate care. Phenytoin (Dilantin) is the most commonly used anticonvulsant for a new onset of generalized or focal seizures. It may be administered IV during acute convulsions or orally for maintenance. Phenytoin has several side effects, including rash and liver dysfunction. Occasionally, phenobarbital may be used but, because of sedation, is not an agent of choice. The two most commonly used agents for maintenance after seizures or for someone with status epilepticus are carbamazepine (Tegretol) and valproic acid. Neither of these agents can be given IV and thus are used for maintenance only. Gabapentin can be administered when the patient's condition is refractory to other agents. After adequate control of the seizure, a diagnostic workup for its cause is initiated. The workup includes a detailed history and physical examination, history of previous medication and drug use, white blood cell count to rule out occult infection, and electrolyte and metabolic assessment. CT or MRI is indicated for a patient with new onset of seizure activity because tumors are often the cause. Similarly, an electroencephalogram is obtained at some point to look for abnormal waveform activity.

Stroke and Transient Ischemic Attacks

Etiology

A stroke in the perioperative period is devastating and correlates with the type of operative procedure performed, the age of the patient, and the presence of risk factors for cardiovascular disease. Strokes are more commonly associated with cardiovascular procedures. Although the elderly with cardiovascular disease are at a higher risk for a stroke, the young are not exempt, especially those with an underlying inherited thrombophilia.

Postoperative strokes may be ischemic or hemorrhagic in nature. Ischemic strokes most commonly result from perioperative hypotension or overzealous control of hypertension or from cardioemboli in patients with atrial fibrillation. Other sources of cardioemboli include MI and bacterial endocarditis. An embolus arising from DVT and traversing a patent foramen ovale (i.e., paradoxical embolization) may be responsible for strokes of unknown cause. Hemorrhagic strokes are less common and are mostly related to therapy with anticoagulants. Factors related to coagulation disorders, such as chronic abuse of alcohol, AIDS, cocaine use, bleeding diathesis, and preexisting cerebrovascular anomalies, are associated with an increased risk for hemorrhagic stroke.

Presentation and Management

In all cases of stroke, the neurologic changes represent a dramatic departure from normal patient function. A focal alteration in motor function, an alteration in mental status, aphasia, or occasionally unresponsiveness may be noted. Hemorrhagic strokes are uncommon, and their effect can be more devastating than ischemic strokes that are either transient (occurring for seconds to minutes) or reversible (occurring for minutes to hours). In truly irreversible injury, the impact on the patient's overall health is immeasurable, and the patient's ability to function and to enjoy good quality of life is severely compromised.

Prevention of a perioperative stroke starts with the identification of at-risk patients. Patients with hypertension must receive adequate treatment, and overzealous correction must be avoided. Patients with atrial fibrillation benefit from prophylaxis with anticoagulants. Patients with a carotid bruit must be evaluated with noninvasive vascular studies and treated accordingly. Patients undergoing a high-risk surgical procedure (e.g., carotid endarterectomy) may be monitored intraoperatively with transcranial Doppler and electroencephalography. Adequate hydration and monitoring in the perioperative period to avoid hypotension and fluctuations in blood pressure are essential to avoid ischemic strokes.

On recognizing the clinical signs and symptoms of a stroke, the patient must have an IV line placed and be monitored for cardiac arrhythmias. Coagulation parameters are assessed for the presence of a coagulopathy, and blood is sent for culture and determination of the sedimentation rate to check for bacteremia and bacterial endocarditis. A diagnostic workup is started immediately to distinguish between hemorrhagic and ischemic stroke with a CT scan or MRI of the brain. Further tests depend on the clinical scenario: an echocardiogram to assess the heart for structural disease, a carotid duplex scan to assess patency of the carotid artery, and a cerebral angiogram to evaluate for vascular anomalies. Therapy is dictated by the underling mechanism of the stroke. A hypertensive hemorrhagic stroke is treated by aggressive control of the hypertension, an embolic stroke (cardiogenic or secondary to inherited thrombophilia) is treated by anticoagulation (in the absence of a contraindication to anticoagulation) to prevent recurrence, and a hemorrhagic stroke is treated by reversal of the coagulopathy with protamine (if secondary to heparin) or platelet transfusion (if secondary to antiplatelet therapy). Mannitol and dexamethasone are given to reduce cerebral swelling.

Treatment of any underlying cardiac arrhythmia is imperative to prevent recurrent embolization. Surgical intervention is indicated in patients with a localized hematoma or vascular anomaly, depending on the location and size of the hematoma, status of the patient, and accessibility of the aneurysm. Thrombolytic therapy (recombinant tissue plasminogen activator) is effective in restoring cerebral blood flow and minimizing brain injury if instituted early after the onset of an embolic event. Otherwise, low-dose aspirin therapy is the standard for acute ischemic infarction, and in patients who continue to have symptoms, antiplatelet agents (clopidogrel bisulfate [Plavix] and ticlopidine hydrochloride [Ticlid]) are added.

EAR, NOSE, AND THROAT COMPLICATIONS

Epistaxis

Epistaxis may be associated with primary blood dyscrasias such as leukemia and hemophilia, excessive anticoagulation, and hypertension. Epistaxis is divided into two general categories: anterior and posterior. Anterior trauma is often caused by contusion or laceration of the nasal septum or turbinates during insertion of an NG or endotracheal tube.

Firm pressure applied between the thumb and index finger to the nasal ala and held for 3 to 5 minutes is generally successful in stopping most cases of anterior epistaxis. Occasionally, packing with strip gauze for 10 to 15 minutes will aid in a particularly refractory case. If the bleeding fails to stop, packing for an extended period with petrolatum-covered strip gauze may be required. Removal of the packing in 1 to 3 days is usually associated with successful treatment of refractory epistaxis, along with treatment of the underlying condition or reversal of anticoagulation.

A more serious scenario is posterior nasal septal bleeding, which on occasion can be life threatening. If all attempts to stop anterior nasal septal bleeding are unsuccessful, one may infer the probability of a posterior nasal hemorrhage, which may necessitate placement of a posterior pack of strip gauze covered in petrolatum ointment. For particularly refractory cases, a Foley catheter with a 30-mL balloon can be passed through the nasal passages, and after the pack is placed, pressure can be applied to the pack by pulling on the Foley catheter. This type of epistaxis may require concomitant anterior nasal packing to be successful. The packs on a difficult hemorrhage such as this may need to be left in place for 2 to 3 days. For epistaxis that defies all attempts at conservative management, ligation of the sphenopalatine artery or the anterior ethmoidal artery may be required.

Acute Hearing Loss

Abrupt loss of hearing in the postoperative period is an uncommon event. An immediate physical examination is performed to ascertain the degree of hearing loss. Unilateral hearing loss is generally associated with obstruc-

tion or edema related to an NG or feeding tube. Bilateral hearing loss is more often neural in nature and is usually associated with pharmacologic agents such as aminoglycosides and diuretics. Examination with an otoscope will often reveal the presence of cerumen impaction or edema from a middle ear infection. If the otologic examination is completely normal, one needs to suspect neural injury related to the agents just mentioned. These agents need to be discontinued immediately and hearing monitored over the ensuing 2 to 3 days to see whether recovery occurs. For cerumen impaction, use of a delicate speculum under direct vision is indicated. If the hearing loss is associated with edema related to an NG tube, merely removing the NG tube will result in resolution of the edema.

Nosocomial Sinusitis

Nosocomial sinusitis is a recently recognized complication in the critically ill. Left untreated, sinusitis may be complicated by brain abscess formation, postorbital cellulitis, and nosocomial pneumonia. Patients at high risk for sinusitis are those receiving ventilatory support via a nasotracheal tube and those with nasal colonization with gram-negative bacteria. Also at risk are patients with facial trauma, those with an NG or feeding tube, and patients who have received antibiotic therapy.

The majority of nosocomial sinusitis occurs in the second week of hospitalization, and the maxillary sinuses are the most commonly affected. The classic signs encountered with community-acquired sinusitis (i.e., facial pain, malaise, fever, and purulent nasal discharge) may not be present because the patient is usually unconscious and intubated, has other sources of infection, and is receiving analgesics and antipyretics. The diagnosis is often made when a CT scan is performed to look for a source of fever and the sinuses are included in the cuts. The CT scan generally shows thickened mucosa and the presence of an air-fluid level or opacification of the sinus.

Once diagnosed or suspected, nasal tubes are removed, decongestant is administered, and antibiotic therapy targeting the two most common organisms, *S. aureus* and *Pseudomonas* species, is given. Other organisms that play a major role in nosocomial infections, such as methicillin-resistant *S. aureus,* vancomycin-resistant *Enterococcus,* and *Acinetobacter* species, are also included in the coverage. With such treatment, clinical response occurs in 48 hours and clinical and radiologic cure occurs in two thirds of patients. Failure of medical therapy leads to surgical drainage of the sinus involved. In rare cases, severe intractable sinusitis may require a drainage procedure via an operative technique.

Parotitis

Parotitis most commonly occurs in an elderly man with poor oral hygiene and poor oral intake with an associated decrease in saliva production. The pathophysiology involves obstruction of the salivary ducts or an infection in a diabetic or immunocompromised patient. The patient is noted to have significant edema and focal tenderness surrounding the parotid gland, which eventually progresses to involve edema of the floor of the mouth. If left undiagnosed and untreated, the parotitis can cause life-threatening sepsis. In the worst-case scenario, the infection can dissect into the mediastinum and cause stridor from partial airway obstruction. Patients with advanced parotitis will have dysphagia and some respiratory occlusion. If the diagnosis of parotitis is being entertained, the patient receives IV, high-dose, broad-spectrum antibiotics with good coverage of *Staphylococcus* (the most common agent cultivated from this disease). In the presence of a fluctuant area, incision plus drainage is indicated, with care taken to avoid the facial nerve. On rare occasion, advanced disease may even require emergency tracheostomy. Most patients with parotitis will have the condition arise 4 to 12 days after the initial operation. Because of the rapid progression of this disease, one must be aware of the diagnosis and, when present, institute immediate therapy, including emergency surgery on occasion for patients with an obvious fluctuant area.

Selected References

ACCP Consensus Committee on Pulmonary Embolism, American College of Chest Physicians: Opinions regarding the diagnosis and management of venous thromboembolic disease. Chest 113:499-504, 1998.

This paper is the result of a consensus conference held by the ACCP regarding pulmonary embolism. The paper discusses the appropriate way to manage pulmonary embolism and the current recommendations regarding diagnosis and prevention.

Almanaseer Y, Mukherjee D, Kline-Rogers EM, et al: Implementation of the ACC/AHA guidelines for preoperative risk assessment in a general medicine preoperative clinic: Improving efficiency and preserving outcomes. Cardiology 103:24-29, 2005.

This paper describes the clinical predictors of increased cardiovascular risk leading to acute cardiac events in surgical patients. Implementation of these predictors may also allow better selection of patients who require more specific preoperative cardiac evaluation and β-blocker therapy.

Dronge AS, Perkal MF, Kancir S, et al: Long-term glycemic control and postoperative infectious complications. Arch Surg 141:375-380, 2006.

This paper addresses the importance of "glycemic" control as it relates to postoperative infections.

Cooper MS, Stewart PM: Current concepts: Corticosteroid insufficiency in acutely ill patients. N Engl J Med 348:727-734, 2003.

The authors in this paper discuss the topic of "functional adrenal insufficiency" in critically ill patients and outline the workup and treatment strategies.

Eagle KA, Berger PB, Calkins H, et al: ACC/AHA Guideline Update for Perioperative Cardiovascular Evaluations for Noncardiac Surgery—Executive Summary. A report of the American College of Cardiology/American Heart Association Task Force on Practice Guidelines. (Committee to Update the 1996 Guidelines on Perioperative Cardiovascular Evaluation for Noncardiac Surgery). Anesth Analg 94:1052-1064, 2002.

This important report from the ACC and AHA carefully outlines the management of patients with cardiac risk factors who will undergo a noncardiac operation.

Heller L, Levin SL, Butler CE: Management of abdominal wound dehiscence using vacuum assisted closure in patients with compromised healing. Am J Surg 191:165-172, 2006.

This paper deals with the concept of integration of vacuum-assisted closure systems in the management of wound dehiscence.

Mangram AJ, Horan TC, Pearson ML, et al: Guideline for prevention of surgical site infection, 1999. Hospital Infection Control Practices Advisory Committee. Infect Control Hosp Epidemiol 20:250-278, 1999.

This fairly comprehensive review article delineates guidelines for wound infections postoperatively. It thoroughly treats the topic of preoperative antibiotics and current recommendations regarding their use in various operations.

Migneco A, Ojetti V, Testa A, et al: Management of thyrotoxic crisis. Eur Rev Med Pharmacol Sci 9:69-74, 2005.

This paper outlines the manifestations and treatment of an uncommon, but potentially devastating complication of thyrotoxicosis.

Moore AFK, Hargest R, Martin M, et al: Intra-abdominal hypertension and the abdominal compartment syndrome. Br J Surg 91:1102-1110, 2004.

This paper is important because it details the pathophysiology of intra-abdominal hypertension and abdominal compartment syndrome and attempts to provide guidelines for medical and surgical management of patients in whom these complications develop.

Perry SL, Ortel TL: Clinical and laboratory evaluation of thrombophilia. Clin Chest Med 24:153-170, 2003.

The authors in this review outline the etiology and workup of patients with a hypercoagulable state and provide recommendations for testing of this high-risk group of patients.

Simon TL, Alverson DC, AuBuchon J, et al: Practice guidelines for the use of red blood cell transfusions: Developed by the Red Blood Cell Administration Practice Guideline Development Task Force of the College of American Pathologists. Arch Pathol Lab Med 122:130-138, 1998.

This paper is the result of a consensus conference held by the College of American Pathologists regarding blood transfusion and its utility in the treatment of surgical patients.

Slim K, Vicaut E, Panis Y, et al: Meta-analysis of randomized clinical trials of colorectal surgery with or without mechanical bowel preparation. Br J Surg 91:1125-1130, 2004.

This paper sheds light on the usefulness of mechanical bowel preparation before colorectal surgery.

References

1. Suliburk JW, Ware DN, Balogh Z, et al: Vacuum-assisted wound closure achieves early fascia closure of open abdomens after severe trauma. J Trauma 55:1155-1160, 2003.
2. Heller L, Levin SL, Butler CE: Management of abdominal wound dehiscence using vacuum assisted closure in patients with compromised healing. Am J Surg 191:165-172, 2006.

3. Helton WS, Fisichella PM, Berger R, et al: Short-term outcomes with small intestinal submucosa for ventral abdominal hernia. Arch Surg 140:549-562, 2005.
4. Mangram AJ, Horan TC, Pearson ML, et al: Guidelines for prevention of surgical site infection, 1999. Hospital Infection Control Practices Advisory Committee. Infect Control Hosp Epidemiol 20:250-278, 1999.
5. National Nosocomial Infections Surveillance Systems (NNIS) System Report: Data summary from January 1992–June 2001, issued August 2001. Am J Infect Control 29:404-421, 2001.
6. Dronge AS, Perkal MF, Kancir S, et al: Long-term glycemic control and postoperative infectious complications. Arch Surg 141:375-380, 2006.
7. Parienti JJ, Thibon P, Heller R, et al: Hand-rubbing with an aqueous alcohol vs. traditional surgical hand scrubbing and 30-day surgical site infection rates: A randomized equivalence study. JAMA 288:722-727, 2002.
8. Frank SM, Tran KM, Fleisher LA, et al: Clinical importance of body temperature in the surgical patient. J Thermal Biol 25:141-155, 2000.
9. Buggy DJ, Crossley AWA: Thermoregulation, mild perioperative hypothermia and post-anesthesia shivering. Br J Anesth 84:615-628, 2000.
10. McCarthy TV, Quane KA, Lynch PJ: Ryanodine receptor mutations in malignant hyperthermia and central core disease. Hum Mutat 15:410-417, 2000.
11. Rosenberg H, Antognini JF, Muldoon S: Testing for malignant hyperthermia. Anesthesiology 96:232-237, 2002.
12. Jawa RS, Kulaylat MN, Bauman H, et al: What is new in cytokine research related to trauma/critical care? J Intensive Care Med 21:63-85, 2006.
13. Hospital-acquired pneumonia in adults: Diagnosis, assessment of severity, initial antimicrobial therapy, and preventive strategies. A consensus statement. American Thoracic Society, November 1995. Am J Respir Crit Care Med 153:1711-1725, 1996.
14. Maki DG, Tambyah PA: Engineering out the risk for infection with urinary catheters. Emerg Infect Dis 7:342-347, 2001.
15. Mermel LA, Farr BM, Sheretz RJ, et al: Guidelines for the management of intravascular catheter–related infections. Clin Infect Dis 32:1249-1272, 2001.
16. American Society of Anesthesiologists Task Force on Preoperative Fasting: Practice guidelines for preoperative fasting and the use of pharmacologic agents to reduce the risk of pulmonary aspiration: Application to healthy patients undergoing elective procedures. Anesthesiology 79:482-485, 1999.
17. Heit JA, Silverstein MD, Mohr DN, et al: Risk factors for deep vein thrombosis and pulmonary embolism: A population-based case-control study. Arch Intern Med 160:809-815, 2000.
18. Perry SL, Ortel TL: Clinical and laboratory evaluation of thrombophilia. Clin Chest Med 24:153-170, 2003.
19. Powell T, Muller NL: Imaging of acute pulmonary thromboembolism: Should spiral computed tomography replace the ventilation-perfusion scan? Clin Chest Med 24:29-38, 2003.
20. Wells PS, Anderson DR, Rodger MA, et al: Derivation of a simple clinical model to categorize patients' probability of pulmonary embolism: Increasing the models utility with the SimpliRED D-dimer. Thromb Haemost 83:416-420, 2000.
21. Goldhaber SZ: Echocardiography in the management of pulmonary embolism. Ann Intern Med 136:691-700, 2002.
22. ACCP Consensus Committee on Pulmonary Embolism. American College of Chest Physicians: Opinions regarding the diagnosis and management of venous thromboembolic disease. Chest 113:499-504, 1998.
23. Eagle KA, Berger PB, Calkins H, et al: ACC/AHA Guideline Update for Perioperative Cardiovascular Evaluations for Noncardiac Surgery—Executive Summary. A report of the American College of Cardiology/American Heart Association Task Force on Practice Guidelines (Committee to Update the 1996 Guidelines on Perioperative Cardiovascular Evaluation for Noncardiac Surgery). Anesth Analg 94:1052-1064, 2002.
24. Almanaseer Y, Mukherjee D, Kline-Rogers EM, et al: Implementation of the ACC/AHA guidelines for preoperative risk assessment in a general medicine preoperative clinic: Improving efficiency and preserving outcomes. Cardiology 103:24-29, 2005.
25. Mangano DT, Layug EL, Wallace A, et al: Effect of atenolol on mortality and cardiovascular morbidity after noncardiac surgery. Multicenter Study of Perioperative Ischemia Research Group. N Engl J Med 335:1713-1720, 1996.
26. Polanzky CA, Goldman L, Marcantonia ER, et al: Supraventricular arrhythmias in patients having noncardiac surgery: Clinical correlates and effect on length of stay. Ann Intern Med 129:279-285, 1998.
27. O'Kelly B, Browner WS, Massie B, et al: Ventricular arrhythmias in patients undergoing noncardiac surgery. The Study of Perioperative Ischemia Research Group. JAMA 268:217-221, 1992.
28. Hunt SA, Baker DW, Chin MH, et al: ACC/AHA guidelines for the evaluation and management of chronic heart failure in the adult: Executive summary. J Heart Lung Transplant 21:189-203, 2002.
29. Tamura T, Said S, Harris J, et al: Reverse remodeling of cardiac myocyte hypertrophy in hypertension and failure by targeting the renin-angiotensin system. Circulation 102:253-259, 2000.
30. Bonet S, Agusti A, Arnau JM, et al: Beta-adrenergic blocking agents in heart failure: Benefits of vasodilating and non-vasodilating agents according to patients' characteristics: A meta-analysis of clinical trials. Arch Intern Med 160:621-627, 2000.
31. Murphy SW, Barrett BJ, Parfrey PS: Contrast nephropathy. J Am Soc Nephrol 11:177-182, 2000.
32. Moore AFK, Hargest R, Martin M, et al: Intra-abdominal hypertension and the abdominal compartment syndrome. Br J Surg 91:1102-1110, 2004.
33. Malbrain MLNG, Deeren D, De Potter TJR: Intra-abdominal hypertension in the critically ill: It is time to pay attention. Curr Opin Crit Care 11:156-171, 2005.
34. Karsou SA, Jaber BL, Pereira BJ: Impact of intermittent hemodialysis variables on clinical outcomes in acute renal failure. Am J Kidney Dis 35:980-991, 2000.
35. Kumar VA, Craig M, Depner TA, et al: Extended daily dialysis: A new approach to renal replacement for acute renal failure in the intensive care unit. Am J Kidney Dis 36:294-300, 2000.
36. Cooper MS, Stewart PM: Current concepts: Corticosteroid insufficiency in acutely ill patients. N Eng J Med 348:727-734, 2003.
37. Migneco A, Ojetti V, Testa A, et al: Management of thyrotoxic crisis. Eur Rev Med Pharmacol Sci 9:69-74, 2005.
38. Postoperative Ileus Management Council: Proceedings of Consensus Panel to Define Postoperative Ileus. Colorectal Surgery Consensus Report. Atlanta, Thomson American Health Consultants, May 1, 2006.

39. Luckey A, Livingston E, Tache Y: Mechanisms and treatment of postoperative ileus. Arch Surg 138:206-214, 2003.

40. Schwartz NT, Kalff JC, Turler A, et al: Selective jejunal manipulation causes postoperative pan-enteric inflammation and dysmotility. Gastroenterology 126:159-169, 2004.

41. Kulaylat MN, Doerr RJ: Small bowel obstruction. In Holzheimer RG, Mannick JA (eds): Surgical Treatment—Evidence-Based and Problem-Oriented. New York, Zuckschwerdt, 2001, pp 102-113.

42. Simon TL, Alverson DC, AuBuchon J, et al: Practice guidelines for the use of red blood cell transfusions: Developed by the Red Blood Cell Administration Practice Guideline Development Task Force of the College of American Pathologists. Arch Pathol Lab Med 122:130-138, 1998.

43. Carne PW, Robertson GM, Frizelle FA: Parastomal hernia. Br J Surg 90:784-793, 2003.

44. Morris AM, Jobe BA, Stoney M, et al: *Clostridium difficile* colitis—an increasing aggressive iatrogenic disease. Arch Surg 137:1096-1100, 2002.

45. Dallal RM, Harbrecht BG, Boujoukas AJ, et al: Fulminant *Clostridium difficile:* An underappreciated and increasing cause of death and complications. Ann Surg 235:363-372, 2002.

46. Salem L, Flum DR: Primary anastomosis or Hartmann's procedure for patients with diverticular peritonitis: A systematic review. Dis Colon Rectum 47:1953-1964, 2004.

47. Slim K, Vicaut E, Panis Y, et al: Meta-analysis of randomized clinical trials of colorectal surgery with or without mechanical bowel preparation. Br J Surg 91:1125-1130, 2004.

48. Uzunkoy A, Akinci F, Coskun A, et al: Effects of antiadhesive agents on the healing of intestinal anastomosis. Dis Colon Rectum 43:370-375, 2000.

49. Wong NY, Eu KW: A defunctioning ileostomy does not prevent clinical anastomotic leak after a low anterior resection: A prospective, comparative study. Dis Colon Rectum 48:2076-2079, 2005.

50. Branagan G, Finnis D: Prognosis after anastomotic leakage in colorectal surgery. Dis Colon Rectum 48:1021-1026, 2005.

51. Stojadinovic A, Brooks A, Hoos A, et al: An evidence-based approach to the surgical management of resectable pancreatic adenocarcinoma. J Am Coll Surg 196:954-964, 2003.

52. Teubner A, Farrer K, Ravishankar H, et al: Fistuloclysis can successfully replace parenteral feeding in the nutritional support of patients with enterocutaneous fistulas. Br J Surg 31:625-631, 2004.

53. Krahenbuhl L, Sclabas G, Wente MN, et al: Incidence, risk factors, and prevention of biliary tract injuries during laparoscopic cholecystectomy in Switzerland. World J Surg 25:1325-1330, 2001.

CHAPTER 16

Surgery in the Elderly

David H. Berger, MD   Alan Dardik, MD   and   Ronnie A. Rosenthal, MD

Aging and Surgery
Physiologic Decline
Preoperative Assessment
Specific Considerations

The population of the United States has increased significantly over the past two generations, primarily as a result of the increase in life expectancy that accompanied the implementation of public health and medical interventions such as improved sanitation, vaccinations, nutrition and lifestyle modifications, and antibiotics. Until the 1980s it was thought that life expectancy would increase to a point where survival curves would become nearly rectangular, with the majority of the population dying within a few years of a fixed maximum life span. Recent evidence suggests, however, that the maximum life expectancy may also be increasing, with survival curves remaining nearly rectangular but shifting to the right (Fig. 16-1).[1]

These improvements in life expectancy—and perhaps life span—combined with aging of the baby boomer generation will result in a rapid increase in the population older than 65 years in the next few decades (Fig. 16-2). It is expected that by 2030 one in five people will be older than 65 years, with the most rapidly growing segment of this older population being persons older than 85. This number is expected to increase fivefold and reach 20 million by 2050.

Social security, Medicare, and Medicaid benefits to the elderly currently account for more than a third of U.S. spending and have the potential to consume the entire federal budget by the year 2012. As a result, the simple increase in the number of older persons is going to stress the health care industry even though the actual cost for care of older persons is relatively low when compared with their younger counterparts.[2]

AGING AND SURGERY

As the number of persons reaching old age continues to grow, there will be a concomitant need to provide surgical care to an increasing number of older patients. Over the past 2 decades alone, the percentage of operations in which the patient was older than 65 increased from 19% of all operations to 35%. When obstetric procedures are excluded, this portion rises to 43%. The proportion of the surgical workload across age groups in the specialties in non–federally funded hospitals is shown in Table 16-1.

This increase in the percentage of operations in which the patient is older than 65 years is not entirely due to the increase in the number of older patients. It is also a reflection of a greater willingness to offer surgical treatment to the elderly. Over the past several decades, advances in surgical and anesthetic techniques have allowed us to operate with much greater control and safety. Operative mortality in older patients has declined sharply. As a result, the risk associated with surgery has become somewhat less of a concern than the need to provide maximal disease management.

The pattern of surgical management of malignant disease in the elderly is an example of the changing views on surgery in this age group. Data from the National Cancer Institute's Surveillance, Epidemiology and End Results (SEER) Program indicate a decrease in the gap between the percentage of younger and older patients treated surgically for certain cancers. For early-stage breast, colon, and rectal cancer, in which the chance of surgical cure is high, the percentage of older patients receiving surgical treatment has approached that of younger patients. For localized gastric, pancreatic, lung, and liver cancer, operative percentages still decline sharply with age (Fig. 16-3). At present it is still unclear whether this decline is the result of appropriate decision making based on the overall health of the patient and patient treatment preference or whether it is a reflection

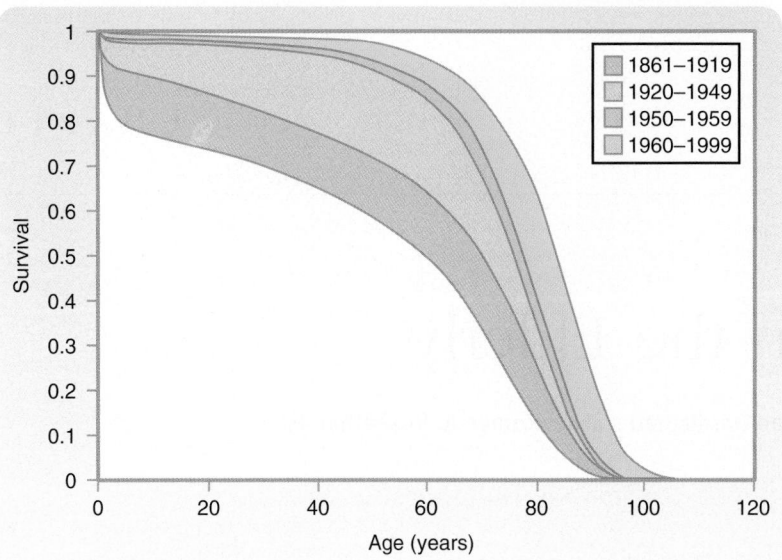

Figure 16-1 Survival curves in Sweden since 1861. Rectangularization of the survival curve occurred until 1950. From then onward, the curves remained parallel and shifted to the right, indicative of an increasing maximal life expectancy. (Adapted from Westendorp RGJ: What is healthy aging in the 21st century? J Clin Nutr 83(Suppl):404S-409S, 2006.)

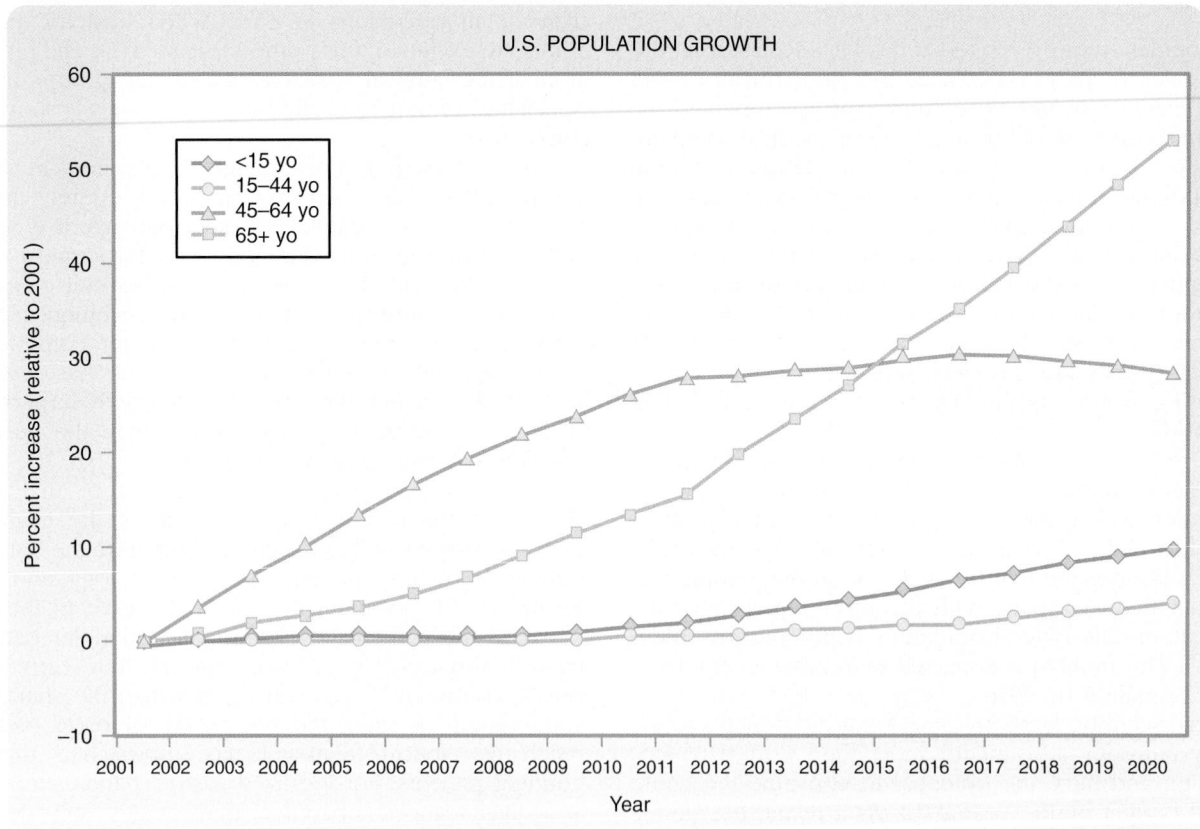

Figure 16-2 Growth in the U.S. population by age group. (Adapted from Etzioni DA, Liu JH, Maggard MA, Ko CY: The aging population and its impact on the surgery workforce. Ann Surg 238:170-177, 2003.)

of vestigial prejudice and age bias resulting in patients not being referred for cancer surgery.

However, additional data from the SEER database indicate that even in the oldest elderly, those 90 years and older, cancer treatment is worthwhile. After the first year from diagnosis, *relative survival* (defined as the ratio of observed survival over a specific period to expected survival) is identical for older and younger cancer patients for up to 10 years (Fig. 16-4).[3] Most of the difference seen in the first year occurs in the first few months, and the only factor that positively influences first year survival is whether the patient underwent surgical treatment of the cancer or other major surgery. This finding may be the result of selection bias inasmuch as only the healthiest 90-year-olds may have been offered surgery. However, this serves to emphasize the fact that age alone should not be the sole reason to deny surgical treatment of cancer.

It is also important to remember that the pattern of symptoms and the natural history of the surgical disease in older patients may not be identical to that seen in their younger counterparts. The absence of typical signs and symptoms often leads to errors in diagnosis and delays in treatment. As a result, it is not unusual for an acute complication to be the first indication of disease. This situation is unfortunate because emergency operative mortality is 3- to 10-fold higher than in comparable elective cases.

There is no doubt that increasing age appears to have a negative effect on the outcome of surgery. However,

Table 16-1 **Distribution of Procedure Types (by Age Group) Performed in Non–Federally Funded Hospitals**

TYPE OF PROCEDURE	AGE			
	<15 Years	15-44 Years	45-65 Years	>65 Years
Ophthalmologic	12%	26%	28%	34%
Otolaryngologic	24%	36%	19%	21%
Thoracic	6%	16%	30%	48%
Cardiovascular	3%	10%	36%	51%
Gastrointestinal	4%	24%	29%	43%
Urologic	5%	19%	31%	45%
Gynecologic	1%<	58%	30%	11%
Neurosurgical	18%	31%	25%	26%
Orthopedic	4%	23%	34%	39%
All	5%	36%	26%	35%

Data from DeFrances CJ, Podgornik MN: 2004 National Hospital Discharge Survey. Adv Data 4(371):1-19, 2006.

most studies have indicated that chronologic age alone has little effect on outcome. Rather, it is the age-related decline in physiologic reserves and increase in comorbidity that is responsible for this observation. Even a compromised older patient can tolerate a surgical experience well if the procedure is carefully conducted and the postoperative course is uncomplicated. However, if even

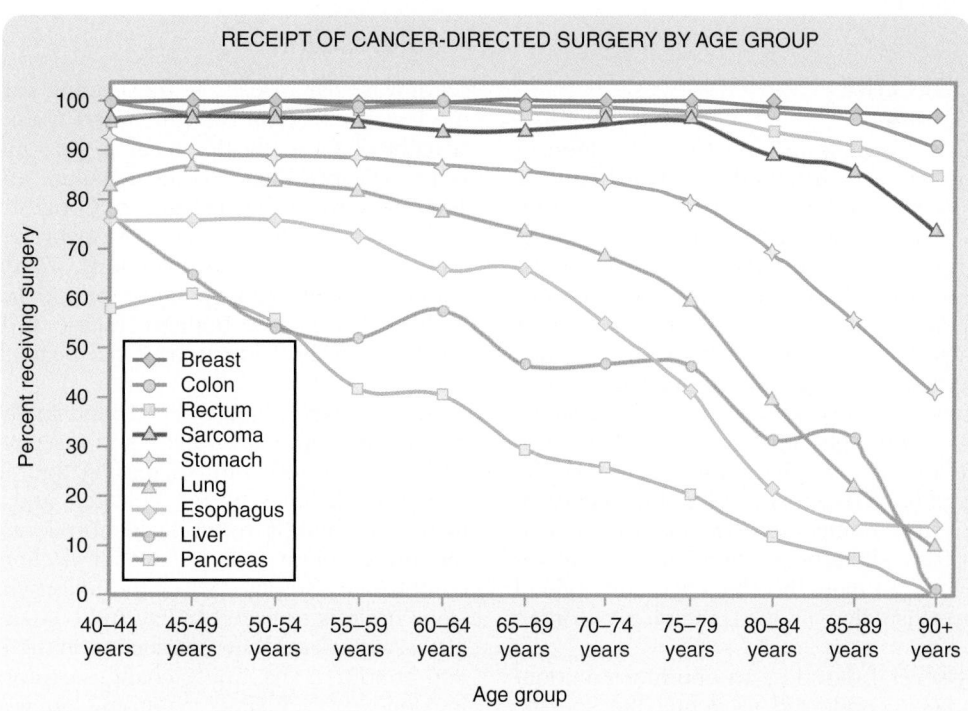

Figure 16-3 **Age distribution of patients receiving cancer-directed surgery for local stage disease.** (Adapted from O'Connell JB, Maggard MA, Ko CY: Cancer-directed surgery for localized disease: Decreased use in the elderly. Ann Surg Oncol 11:962-969, 2004.)

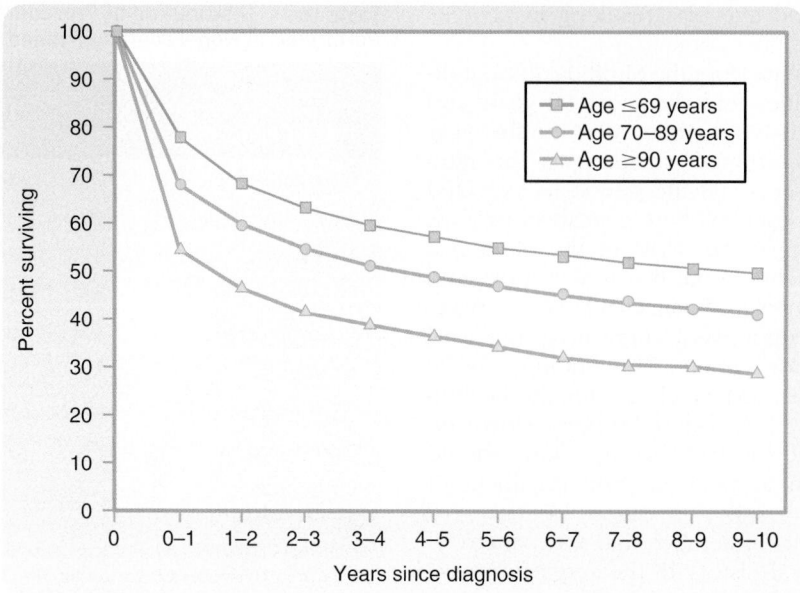

Figure 16-4 Cumulative relative survival of cancer patients by age group from the SEER database, 1973 to 1998. Note that after the first year, survival curves are parallel for even the oldest old. (Adapted from Saltzstein SL, Behling CA: 5- and 10-year survival in cancer patients aged 90 and older: A study of 37,318 patients from SEER. J Surg Oncol 81:113-116, 2002.)

one complication occurs, mortality increases significantly. In a study of more than 26,000 patients older than 80 years undergoing major noncardiac surgery in Veterans Affairs Hospitals, mortality rose from 3.7% in patients with no complications to 26.1% in patients in whom one complication occurred.[4]

PHYSIOLOGIC DECLINE

With aging there is a decline in physiologic function in all organ systems, but the magnitude of this decline is variable among organs and individuals. In the resting state, this decline usually has minimal functional consequence, although physiologic reserves may be used just to maintain homeostasis. However, when physiologic reserves are required to meet the additional challenges of surgery or acute illness, overall performance may deteriorate. This progressive age-related decline in organ system homeostatic reserves, known as *homeostenosis,* was first described by the physiologist Walter Cannon in the 1940s. Figure 16-5 is a graphic representation of the present concepts of homeostenosis.[5] With older age there is increased use of physiologic reserves just to maintain normal homeostasis. Therefore, when stressed, fewer reserves are available to meet the challenge, and overall function may be pushed over the precipice of organ failure or death.

Over the past several decades, an enormous amount of research has been conducted to define the specific changes in organ function that are directly attributable to aging. This task is inherently difficult because aging is also accompanied by increased vulnerability to disease. It is often difficult to determine whether an observed

decline in function is secondary to aging per se or to disease associated with aging. The overall effect, however, is still the same: a much smaller margin for error in the care of older patients. Understanding the changes in organ function can help minimize these errors.

Cardiovascular

Cardiovascular disease is the leading cause of death in the United States in both men and women. Eighty-three percent of these deaths occur in persons older than 65 years. The prevalence of heart failure approaches 10 in 1000 persons in this age group. Congestive heart failure is a risk factor for several postoperative complications, including surgical site infections. Cardiac events are common in the postoperative period in older patients and are attributable both to disease and to changes in the structure and function of the heart that accompany aging.

Morphologic changes are found in the myocardium, conducting pathways, valves, and vasculature of the heart and great vessels with increasing age. The number of myocytes declines as the collagen and elastin content increases, thereby resulting in fibrotic areas throughout the myocardium and an overall decline in ventricular compliance. Nearly 90% of the autonomic tissue in the sinus node is replaced by fat and connective tissue, and fibrosis interferes with conduction in the intranodal tracts and bundle of His. These changes contribute to the high incidence of sick sinus syndrome, atrial arrhythmia, and bundle branch block. Sclerosis and calcification of the aortic valve are common but usually of no functional significance. Progressive dilation of all four valvular annuli is probably responsible for the multivalvular regur-

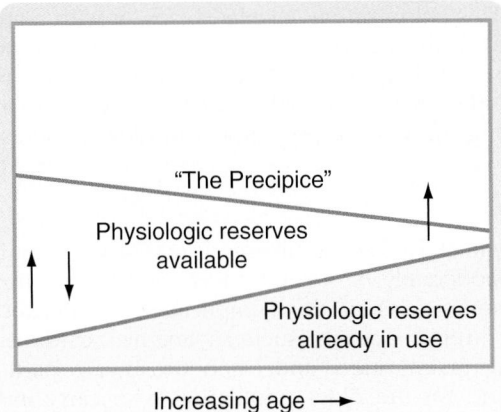

Figure 16-5 Graphic representation of homeostenosis. With advancing age, physiologic reserves are increasingly being used to maintain homeostasis. *Vertical arrows* represent challenges such as surgical stress or acute illness. Because reserves are already used, there are fewer available to meet these challenges. As a result, the precipice is crossed by a stress that would easily be tolerated in younger age. This precipice may be any relevant clinical marker such as organ dysfunction or failure or death. (Adapted from Taffert GE: Physiology of aging. In Cassel CK, Leipzig RM, Cohen HJ, et al [eds]: Geriatric Medicine: An Evidence-Based Approach, 4th ed. New York, Springer, 2003.)

Box 16-1   Indications for Perioperative β-Blockade

Any of the Following

- High-risk operation
- Ischemic heart disease
- Cerebrovascular disease
- Creatinine >2.0 mg/dL
- Diabetics taking insulin

Two of the Following

- Age >65 years
- Hypertension
- Current smoker
- Cholesterol >240 mg/dL
- Diabetics not taking insulin

Adapted from McGory ML, Maggard MA, Ko CY: A meta-analysis of perioperative beta blockade: What is the actual risk reduction? Surgery 138:171-179, 2005.

---

gitation demonstrated in healthy older persons. Finally, there is a progressive increase in rigidity and decrease in distensibility of both the coronary arteries and the great vessels. Changes in the peripheral vasculature contribute to increased systolic blood pressure, increased resistance to ventricular emptying, and compensatory loss of myocytes with ventricular hypertrophy.

The direct functional implications of these changes are difficult to accurately assess because age-related changes in body composition, metabolic rate, general state of fitness, and underlying disease all influence cardiac performance. It is now generally accepted that *systolic* function is well preserved with increasing age. Cardiac output and ejection fraction are maintained despite the increase in afterload imposed by stiffening of the outflow tract.[6] The mechanism by which cardiac output is maintained during exercise, however, is somewhat different. In younger persons, output is maintained by increasing the heart rate in response to β-adrenergic stimulation. With aging there is a relative hyposympathetic state in which the heart becomes less responsive to catecholamines, possible secondary to declining receptor function. The aging heart therefore maintains cardiac output not by increasing its rate but by increasing ventricular filling (preload). Because of the dependence on preload, even minor hypovolemia can result in significant compromise in cardiac function.

Diastolic function, however, which depends on relaxation rather than contraction, is affected by aging. Diastolic dysfunction is responsible for up to 50% of cases of heart failure in patients older than 80 years.[7] Myocardial relaxation is more energy dependent and therefore requires more oxygen than contraction does. With aging there is a progressive decrease in the partial pressure of oxygen. Consequently, even mild hypoxemia can result in prolonged relaxation, higher diastolic pressure, and pulmonary congestion. Because early diastolic filling is impaired, maintenance of preload becomes even more reliant on atrial kick. Loss of the atrial contribution to preload can result in further impairment of cardiac function.

It is also important to remember that the manifestation of cardiac disease in the elderly may be nonspecific and atypical. Although chest pain is still the most common symptom of myocardial infarction, nonclassic symptoms such as shortness of breath, syncope, acute confusion, or stroke will occur in as many as 40% of older patients.

The use of β-blockade in the perioperative period has been shown to be of value in decreasing the negative impact of cardiac comorbidity on surgical outcome in patients with risk factors for cardiac complications. These factors are shown in Box 16-1.

Respiratory

Chronic lower respiratory disease is the fourth leading cause of death after heart disease, cancer, and stroke. Respiratory problems are the most common postoperative complications in older patients. Both disease- and age-related changes in lung structure and function contribute to this vulnerability.

With aging there is a decline in respiratory function that is attributable to changes in both the chest wall and the lung. Chest wall compliance decreases secondary to changes in structure caused by kyphosis and exaggerated by vertebral collapse. Calcification of the costal cartilage and contractures of the intercostal muscles result in a decline in rib mobility. Maximum inspiratory and expiratory force decreases by as much as 50% as a result of a progressive decrease in the strength of the respiratory muscles.

In the lung there is loss of elasticity, which leads to increased alveolar compliance with collapse of the small airways and subsequent uneven alveolar ventilation with air trapping. Uneven alveolar ventilation leads to

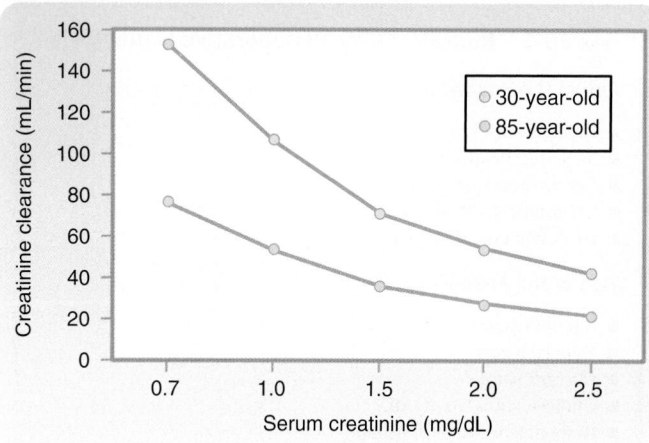

Figure 16-6 Correlation between creatinine clearance and serum creatinine in younger and older persons. (Adapted from Luckey AE, Parsa CJ: Fluid and electrolytes in the aged. Arch Surg 138:1055-1060, 2003.)

ventilation-perfusion mismatches, which in turn cause a decline in arterial oxygen tension of approximately 0.3 or 0.4 mm Hg per year. The partial pressure of CO_2 does not change despite an increase in dead space. This may be due, in part, to the decline in production of CO_2 that accompanies the falling basal metabolic rates. Air trapping is also responsible for an increase in residual volume, or the volume remaining after maximal expiration.

Loss of support of the small airways also leads to collapse during forced expiration, which limits dynamic lung volumes and flow rates. Forced vital capacity decreases by 14 to 30 mL/yr, and forced expiratory volume in 1 second (FEV_1) decreases by 23 to 32 mL/yr (in males). The overall effect of loss of elastic inward recoil of the lung is balanced somewhat by the decline in chest wall outward force. Total lung capacity therefore remains unchanged, and there is only a mild increase in resting lung volume, or functional residual capacity. Because total lung capacity remains unchanged, the increase in residual volume results in a decrease in vital capacity.

Control of ventilation is also affected by aging. Ventilatory responses to hypoxia and hypercapnia fall by 50% and 40%, respectively. The exact mechanism of this decline has not been well defined but it may be due to declining chemoreceptor function at either the peripheral or central nervous system level.[8]

In addition to these intrinsic changes, pulmonary function is affected by alterations in the ability of the respiratory system to protect against environmental injury and infection. There is a progressive decrease in T-cell function (see later), a decline in mucociliary clearance, and a decrease in several components of swallowing function. Loss of the cough reflex secondary to neurologic disorders, combined with swallowing dysfunction, may predispose to aspiration. The increased frequency and severity of pneumonia in older persons have been attributed to these factors and to an increased incidence of oropharyngeal colonization with gram-negative organ-

isms. This colonization correlates closely with comorbidity and with the ability of older patients to perform activities of daily living (ADLs). This fact lends support to the idea that functional capacity is a crucial factor in assessing the risk for pneumonia in older patients.

Renal

Approximately 25% of all Americans 70 years and older have moderately or severely decreased kidney function. The implications of the complications associated with chronic renal disease, such as anemia, cardiovascular disease, malnutrition, and osteoporosis, are particularly profound for the older population who carry independent risk factors for these comorbid conditions.

Between the ages of 25 and 85 there is a progressive decrease in the renal cortex. Over time, approximately 40% of the nephrons become sclerotic. The remaining functional units hypertrophy in a compensatory manner. Sclerosis of the glomeruli is accompanied by atrophy of the afferent and efferent arterioles and by a decrease in renal tubular cell number. Renal blood flow also falls by approximately 50%. Functionally, there is a decline in the glomerular filtration rate (GFR) of approximately 45% by 80 years of age. This decrease is reflected in a decline in creatinine clearance of 0.75 mL/min/yr in healthy older men. The serum creatinine value, however, may remain unchanged as a result of a concomitant decrease in lean body mass and, thus, a decrease in creatinine production (Fig. 16-6).[9]

To account for the effects of age, sex, and ethnic origin on the correlation between serum creatinine and GFR, the use of derived formulas is recommended. The most commonly used formulas are the Cockcroft-Gault equation and the Modification of Diet in Renal Disease (MDRD) equation (Fig. 16-7). Although neither equation has been validated in elderly people with a broad range of creatinine values, the MDRD equation appears to be more consistently reliable. Caution must be exercised when applying these formulas to critically ill patients or those taking medications that directly affect renal function. Additionally, both equations tend to underestimate GFR in older women and patients with normal renal function.

Renal tubular function also declines with advancing age. The ability to conserve sodium and excrete hydrogen ion falls, thereby resulting in a diminished capacity to regulate fluid and acid-base balance. Dehydration becomes a particular problem because losses of sodium and water from nonrenal causes are not compensated for by the usual mechanisms of increased renal sodium retention, increased urinary concentration, and increased thirst. The inability to retain sodium is believed to be due to a decline in activity of the renin-angiotensin system. The increasing inability to concentrate urine is related to a decrease in end-organ responsiveness to antidiuretic hormone. The marked decline in the subjective feeling of thirst is also well documented but not well understood. Alterations in osmoreceptor function in the hypothalamus may be responsible for the failure to recognize thirst despite significant elevations in serum osmolality.

<table>
<tr><td colspan="2" align="center">**Cockroft-Gault equation**</td></tr>
</table>

$$C_{cr} = [(140 - \text{Age in years}) \times \text{Weight in kilograms}]/(72 \times \text{Serum creatinine in mg/dL})$$

MDRD study equation

$$\text{GFR} = 175 \times (\text{Standardized serum creatinine in mg/dL})^{-1.154} \times (\text{Age in years})^{-0.203}$$

Figure 16-7 Equations for calculation of creatinine clearance.

Alterations in renal function have important implications for the type and dosage of drugs used in older patients. Although drugs are handled by the kidney in several different ways, most changes in renal drug processing parallel the decline in GFR. Therefore, creatinine clearance can be used to determine the appropriate clearance of most agents processed by the kidney.

The lower urinary tract also changes with increasing age. In the bladder, increased collagen content leads to limited distensibility and impaired emptying. Overactivity of the detrusor secondary to neurologic disorders or idiopathic causes has also been identified. In women, decreased circulating levels of estrogen and decreased tissue responsiveness to this hormone cause changes in the urethral sphincter that predispose to urinary incontinence. In males, prostatic hypertrophy impairs bladder emptying. Together, these factors lead to urinary incontinence in 10% to 15% of elderly persons living in the community and 50% of those in nursing homes. There is also an increased prevalence of asymptomatic bacteriuria with age that varies from 10% to 50%, depending on gender, level of activity, underlying disorders, and place of residence. Urinary tract infections alone are responsible for 30% to 50% of all cases of bacteremia in older patients. Alterations in the local environment and declining host defenses are thought to be responsible. Because of the lack of symptoms in elderly patients with bacteriuria, preoperative urinalysis is important.

The elderly are among the fastest-growing cohorts of individuals starting renal replacement therapy. In the year 2000 the mean age of the dialysis population was reported to be 61.5 years, an increase of more than 3 years from the mean age reported in 1990. The mean survival of patients undergoing renal replacement therapy is 31 months. The 3-year survival rate of patients older than 75 maintained on hemodialysis is 45%. Cardiovascular disease is the main cause of death in these patients. Vascular access may be an obstacle in caring for such patients. The elderly have an increased incidence of peripheral vascular disease and inadequate venous systems for placement of fistulas and synthetic grafts. Despite these limitations, there appears to be no increased risk for access thrombosis or decrease in 5-year fistula survival in older patients. Kidney transplantation in elderly patients with end-stage renal disease remains a subject of debate and investigation (see later).

Hepatobiliary

Hepatic function is well preserved overall with aging. However, there is as much as a fourfold increase in liver disease–related mortality in persons between the ages of 45 and 85 years.[10] Morphologic changes include a decrease in the number of hepatocytes and a reduction in overall weight, size, and volume. There is, however, a compensatory increase in cell size and proliferation of bile ducts. Functionally, hepatic blood flow falls by approximately 0.3% to 1.5% per year to 40% to 45% of earlier values after 65 years of age.

The synthetic capacity of the liver, as measured by standard tests of liver function, remains unchanged. However, the metabolism of and sensitivity to certain kinds of drugs is altered. Drugs requiring microsomal oxidation (phase I reactions) before conjugation (phase II reactions) may be metabolized more slowly, whereas those requiring only conjugation may be cleared at a normal rate. Drugs that act directly on hepatocytes, such as warfarin (Coumadin), may produce the desired therapeutic effects at lower doses in the elderly because of an increased sensitivity of cells to these agents. Some recent data also suggest that aging may be associated with a decline in the ability of the liver to protect against the effects of oxidative stress.

The most significant correlate of altered hepatobiliary function in the aged is the increased incidence of gallstones and gallstone-related complications. Gallstone prevalence rises steadily with age, although there is variability in the absolute percentages, depending on the population. Stones have been demonstrated in as many as 80% of nursing home residents older than 90 years. Biliary tract disease is the single most common indication for abdominal surgery in the elderly population (see later).

Immune Function

Immune competence, like other physiologic parameters, declines with advancing age. This immunosenescence is characterized by enhanced susceptibility to infections, an increase in autoantibodies and monoclonal immunoglobulins, and an increase in tumorigenesis. In addition, like other physiologic systems, this decline may not be apparent in the nonchallenged state. For example, there is no decline in neutrophil count with age, but the ability of the bone marrow to increase neutrophil production in

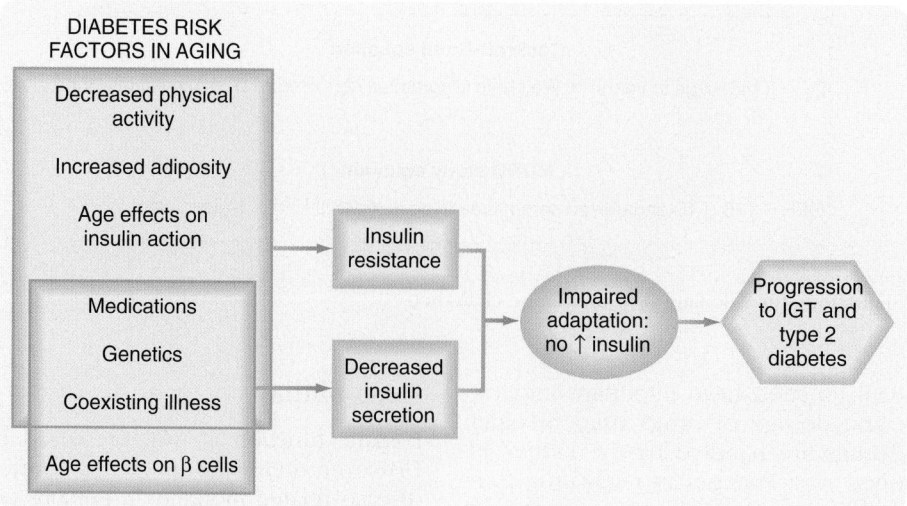

Figure 16-8 The normal response to hyperglycemia is for the beta cell to adapt and secrete sufficient insulin to restore euglycemia. In aging, there is a decrease in insulin secretion and a probable increase in insulin resistance, which when combined with comorbid illness, genetic factors, and medications, leads to failure of this glucoregulatory process. (IGT, impaired glucose tolerance.) (Adapted from Change AM, Halter JB: Aging and insulin secretion. Am J Physiol Endocrinol Metab 284:E7-12, 2003.)

response to infection may be impaired. Elderly patients with major infections frequently have normal white blood cell (WBC) counts, but the differential count will show a profound shift to the left with a large proportion of immature forms.

With aging, there is a decline in the hematopoietic stem cell pool in the bone marrow that leads to decreased production of naive T cells from the thymus and B cells from the bone marrow. Moreover, involution of the thymus gland with a decline in thymic hormones further impairs the production and differentiation of naive T cells and leads to an increased proportion of memory T cells. This change in the population of T cells leaves the elderly host less able to respond to new antigens. Furthermore, recent data suggest that chronic infection with viruses such as cytomegalovirus produces nonfunctional T-cell clonal expansions that may limit the space available for proliferating T cells.[11]

Some B-cell defects have recently been identified, although it is thought that the functional deficits in antibody production are related to altered T-cell regulation rather than intrinsic B-cell changes. In vitro, there is increased helper T-cell activity for nonspecific antibody production, as well as decreased ability of suppressor T cells from old mice to recognize and suppress specific antigens from self. This is reflected in an increase in the prevalence of autoantibodies to greater than 10% by 80 years of age. The mix of immunoglobulins also changes: IgM levels decrease, whereas IgG and IgA increase slightly.

Changes in the immune system with aging are similar those seen in chronic inflammation and cancer. In addition to the reduced mitogenic responses of T cells, there

is an increase in the levels of acute phase proteins. It is hypothesized that persistently elevated levels of inflammatory cytokines may be responsible for down-regulation of interleukin-2 production by chronically stimulated T cells. Markers of inflammation such as interleukin-6 have recently been shown to be increased in older patients. Chronic inflammation has been implicated in the syndrome of frailty, which is characterized by loss of muscle mass (sarcopenia), undernutrition, and impaired mobility.[12] Inflammatory cytokines are also implicated in the normocytic anemia that is common in frail elders.

The clinical implications of these changes are difficult to determine. When superimposed on the known immunosuppression caused by the physical and psychological stress of surgery, insufficient immunologic responses are to be expected in the elderly. The increased susceptibility to many infectious agents in the postoperative period, however, is more likely the result of a combination of stress and comorbid disease rather than physiologic decline alone.

Glucose Homeostasis

Data from the National Health and Nutrition Examination Survey show a clear rise in the prevalence of disorders of glucose homeostasis with age such that more than 20% of persons older than 60 have type 2 diabetes. An additional 20% have glucose intolerance characterized by normal fasting glucose and a postchallenge glucose level of greater than 140 mg/dL but less than 200 mg/dL. This glucose intolerance may be the result of a decrease in insulin secretion, an increase in insulin resistance, or both (Fig. 16-8).[13]

There is now general consensus that beta cell function declines with age. This change is manifested by failure of the beta cell to adapt to the hyperglycemic milieu with an appropriate increase in insulin response. The question of insulin resistance is more controversial. Although insulin action has been shown to decrease in the aged, this change is thought to be more a function of changing body composition, with increased adipose tissue and decreased lean body mass, rather than age per se. Others believe that there is an increase in insulin resistance directly attributable to aging, as manifested by a decrease in insulin-mediated glucose utilization in muscle that is normally regulated by the glucose transporter GLUT-4. There is also an increase in intracellular lipid accumulation, which interferes with normal insulin signaling. These changes may be associated with the decline in mitochondrial function that also accompanies aging.[13]

The aforementioned factors, combined with comorbid illness, medications, and genetic predisposition, come together to render older surgical patients at particularly high risk for uncontrolled hyperglycemia when subjected to the usual insulin resistance that accompanies the physiologic stress of surgery. Both the endogenous glucose response to traumatic stress and the glycemic response to an exogenous glucose load are exaggerated in injured older patients.

Recent evidence has confirmed that uncontrolled hyperglycemia in the perioperative period is associated with an increase in mortality and morbidity. Furthermore, tight control of blood sugar to the normal range with continuous infusion of insulin has been shown to improve a variety of outcomes, including mortality in critically ill patients in the surgical intensive care unit.[14] Attention to control of perioperative hyperglycemia is particularly important in the elderly because of the increased likelihood for hyperglycemia in the face of acute physiologic stress.

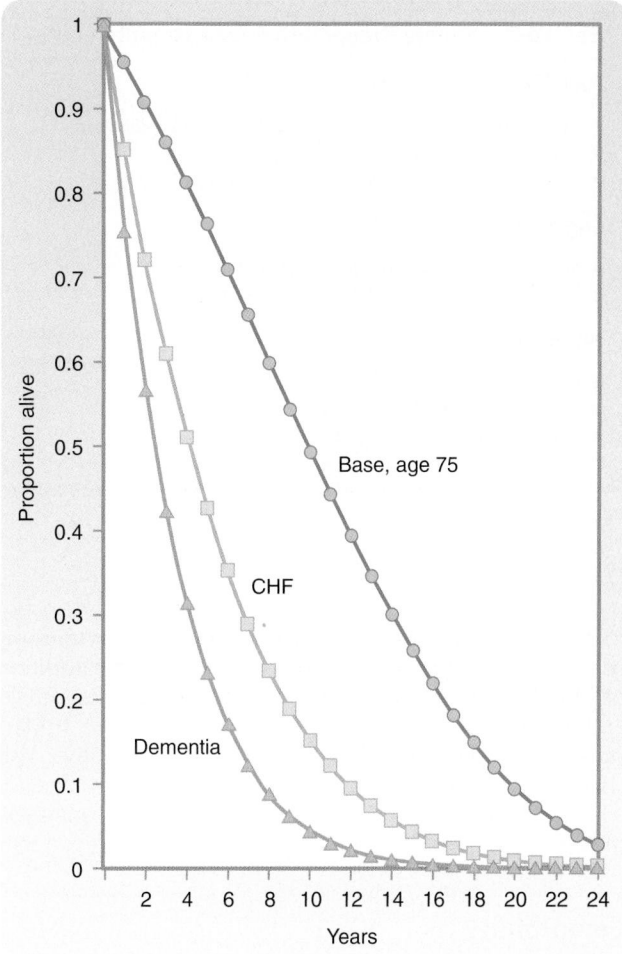

Figure 16-9 Survival at 75 years of age at baseline *(circles)*, with congestive heart failure (CHF) *(squares)*, and with dementia *(triangles)*. Median survival is 10, 4, and 2.5 years, respectively. (Adapted from Robinson B, Beghe C: Cancer screening the older patient. Clin Geriatr Med 13:97-118, 1997.

PREOPERATIVE ASSESSMENT

Although physiologic decline is common in older patients, the functional sequelae of this decline are rarely sufficient to cause a negative outcome in the elective, uncomplicated surgical setting. The presence of coexisting disease, however, strongly influences surgical outcome in any setting. Comorbidity also influences overall life expectancy and is therefore an important consideration in risk-benefit discussions. For example, the mean life expectancy for the total population of 75-year-olds is 10 years. In those with congestive heart failure or dementia, life expectancy falls to 4 and 2.5 years, respectively (Fig. 16-9).[15]

The prevalence of diseases in organ systems other than that for which the older patient is seeking surgical care clearly increases with age. Numerous studies have documented the impact of comorbidity on outcome.[4]

Like the surgical disease itself, the manifestations of comorbid illnesses in the elderly are frequently less typical than in younger patients. For example, more than 40% of the myocardial infarctions in patients older than 75 to 84 years are silent or unrecognized, as opposed to less than 20% in patients between the ages of 45 and 54. Cognitive and nutritional deficits occur frequently in the aged, but as many as two thirds and one half, respectively, are overlooked unless a specific assessment is undertaken. Swallowing disorders are also not uncommon but are often unrecognized.

The goal of preoperative assessment of an elderly patient is to define the extent of decline and identify and characterize coexisting diseases. Extensive testing for disease in every organ system is neither cost-effective, practical, nor necessary for most patients. A thorough history and physical examination will provide information to direct further workup if necessary. It is important, however, to adjust the history and physical examination

---

Box 16-2   Simple Preoperative Assessment Tools

Function

- American Society of Anesthesiologists (ASA) classification
- Activities of daily living (ADLs)
- Exercise capacity in metabolic equivalents (METs)

Cognition

- Mini-Cog (three-item recall + clock-drawing task)
- Folstein's Mini Mental Status examination

Nutrition

- Risk factor assessment
- Subjective Global Assessment
- Mini Nutritional Assessment
- Serum albumin/body mass index

to carefully look for the risk factors, signs, and symptoms of the more common comorbid conditions. The addition of simple tools for assessment of functional, cognitive, and nutritional status will significantly enhance understanding of the individual patient's true operative risk (Box 16-2). When initial evaluation identifies disease or risk factors for disease, further workup may be indicated.

Comorbidity

Of all comorbid conditions, cardiovascular disease is the most prevalent and cardiovascular events are a leading cause of severe perioperative complications and death. For this reason the main thrust of preoperative evaluation, in general, has focused on identifying patients at risk for cardiac complications. The American College of Cardiology and the American Heart Association Task Force on Practice Guidelines first published an in-depth set of guidelines for preoperative cardiac evaluation in 1996, with an update in 2002.[16] These guidelines provide a stepwise bayesian strategy for determining which patients will need further testing to clarify risk or further treatment to minimize risk. Stratification is based on factors related to the patient and the type of surgery. For elderly patients with known cardiac disease, rigorous workup may be necessary. For most patients, assessment of exercise tolerance and functional capacity is an accurate method of predicting the adequacy of cardiac and pulmonary reserves (see later).

Although the main focus of preoperative evaluation has been cardiac status, in older patients pulmonary complications are at least as common as cardiac complication, if not more so. Risk factors for pulmonary complications are not nearly as well studied as those for cardiac complications, although many of the same issues apply to both. Poor exercise capacity and poor general health predict pulmonary as well as cardiac complications. Poor nutrition, preexisting pulmonary disease,

smoking, obesity, and the type of incision have also been implicated.[17] Though less well studied, subtle cognitive and swallowing abnormalities are likewise common in the elderly and are associated with aspiration pneumonia and other negative outcomes.

In a recent review of strategies to reduce postoperative pulmonary complications, only lung expansion interventions, such as incentive spirometry, were shown by good evidence to have an effect. The selective use of nasogastric decompression (rather than routine use) and short-acting (as opposed to long-acting) intraoperative neuromuscular blockade was supported by fair evidence. Evidence supporting smoking cessation, epidural anesthesia and analgesia, laparoscopic versus open approaches, and nutritional supplementation was insufficient or conflicting.[18]

Functional Status

Assessment of functional status, by a variety of methods, is an extremely reliable means of predicting postoperative outcome. For decades, the physical status classification of the American Society of Anesthesiologists (ASA) has been used successfully to stratify operative risk. This simple classification ranks patients according to the functional limitations imposed by coexisting disease. When curves for mortality versus ASA class are examined with regard to age, there is little difference between younger and older patients. This indicates that mortality is a function of coexisting disease rather than chronologic age. ASA classification has been shown to accurately predict postoperative mortality, even in patients older than 80. In a large, multicenter Department of Veterans Affairs study (National Surgical Quality Improvement Program [NSQIP]), surgical patients were assessed prospectively for operative risk, and risk-adjusted models were then created to allow comparison of the quality of surgical care among different institutions. Of the 68 variables studied, the ASA functional classification was the factor most predictive of postoperative morbidity and the second most predictive of mortality.[19] There is also good evidence to support an ASA classification of II or greater and functional dependence, among other factors, as predictors of pulmonary complications.

Other standard measures of functional capacity, such as the ability to perform ADLs (e.g., feeding, continence, transferring, toileting, dressing, and bathing), have also been correlated with postoperative mortality and morbidity. Inactivity has been associated with a higher incidence of all major surgical complications. Postoperative mortality in severely limited patients has been reported to be nearly 10 times higher than mortality in active patients. Preoperative functional deficits also contribute to postoperative immobility, as well as associated complications such as atelectasis and pneumonia, venous stasis and pulmonary embolism, and multisystem deconditioning. Deconditioning is an important clinical entity that leads to further functional decline despite improvement in the acute illness. In a more recent study of functional recovery after major elective open abdominal operations,

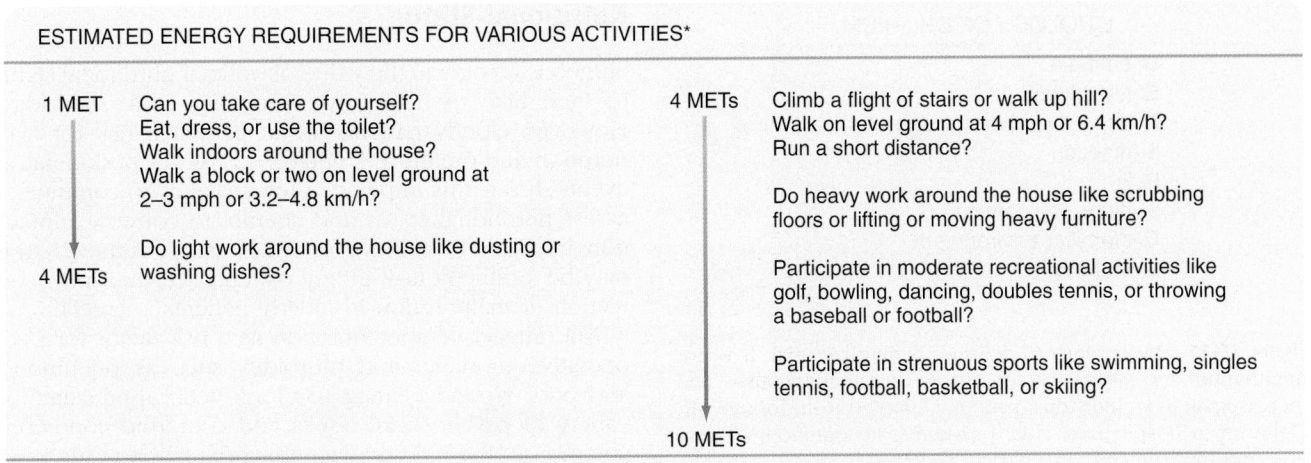

ESTIMATED ENERGY REQUIREMENTS FOR VARIOUS ACTIVITIES*

1 MET → 4 METs
- Can you take care of yourself?
- Eat, dress, or use the toilet?
- Walk indoors around the house?
- Walk a block or two on level ground at 2–3 mph or 3.2–4.8 km/h?
- Do light work around the house like dusting or washing dishes?

4 METs → 10 METs
- Climb a flight of stairs or walk up hill?
- Walk on level ground at 4 mph or 6.4 km/h?
- Run a short distance?
- Do heavy work around the house like scrubbing floors or lifting or moving heavy furniture?
- Participate in moderate recreational activities like golf, bowling, dancing, doubles tennis, or throwing a baseball or football?
- Participate in strenuous sports like swimming, singles tennis, football, basketball, or skiing?

*MET, metabolic equivalent (see text).

Figure 16-10 Estimated energy requirements for various activities. With increasing activity the number of metabolic equivalents (METs) increases. An inability to function above 4 METs has been associated with increased perioperative cardiac events and long-term risk. (**Reprinted with permission.** *ACC/AHA 2002 Guideline Update on Perioperative Cardiovascular Evaluation for Noncardiac Surgery—Executive Summary.* ©2002, American Heart Association, Inc.)

better recovery and short time to recovery of ADLs and instrumental activities of daily living (IADLs) were nearly always predicted by a better preoperative physical performance status, as measured by three simples tests of strength and mobility.[20]

Of all the methods of assessing overall functional capacity, exercise tolerance is the most sensitive predictor of postoperative cardiac and pulmonary complications in the elderly. In a frequently quoted study comparing exercise tolerance and a variety of other assessment techniques, Gerson and associates demonstrated that an inability to raise the heart rate to 99 beats/min while performing 2 minutes of supine bicycle exercise was the most sensitive predictor of postoperative cardiac and pulmonary complications and death.[21]

Formal exercise testing, however, is not necessary in every elderly patient. The metabolic requirements for many routine activities have already been determined and are quantitated as metabolic equivalents (METs). One *MET,* defined as 3.5 mL/kg/min, represents the basal oxygen consumption of a 70-kg, 40-year-old man at rest. Estimated energy requirements for various activities are shown in Figure 16-10. An inability to function above 4 METs has been associated with increased perioperative cardiac events and long-term risk. By asking appropriate questions about the level of activity, functional capacity can be accurately determined without the need for additional testing.

Cognitive Status

Although many people experience healthy aging without significant impairments, a number of sensory, cognitive, and functional declines can occur with age and threaten independence. In cases of extreme sensory or cognitive loss, as seen with both vascular and Alzheimer's dementia, the capacity to perform ADLs (e.g., toileting, eating, bathing, and very basic aspects of mobility) can be compromised. These age-associated changes in cognitive function may have profound effects on postsurgical recovery and outcome. In addition, poor biologic function is often associated with lower cognitive performance. The importance of preoperative cognitive status as a risk factor for negative postoperative outcomes in elderly patients is often overlooked. Cognitive assessment is rarely a part of the preoperative history and physical examination, and there are no widely accepted guidelines for such evaluation in surgical patients. Yet cognitive deficits can persist for as long as 6 months after surgery.

Most importantly, preoperative cognitive deficits are a major risk factor for delirium in the postoperative period (see later). Assessment of cognitive status is essential for recognition of elderly patients at risk. There are several methods for evaluating baseline cognitive function. The Folstein Mini Mental Status Evaluation (MMSE) has traditionally been used because of its ease of administration and reliability. Recent studies suggest that the Mini-Cog detects clinically significant cognitive impairment as well as if not better than the MMSE in multiethnic elderly individuals. It is easier to administer to non–English-speaking patients and is less biased by low education and literacy. The Mini-Cog combines a three-item word-learning and recall task (0 to 3 points; each correctly recalled word = 1 point), with a simple clock-drawing task (abnormal clock = 0 points; normal clock = 2 points) used as a distraction before word recall. Total possible Mini-Cog scores range from 0 to 5, with 0 to 2 suggesting high and 3 to 5 suggesting a low likelihood of cognitive impairment.[22]

ETIOLOGY OF DELIRIUM

D ementia
E lectrolytes
L ungs, liver, heart, kidney, brain
I nfection
R x
I njury, pain, stress
U nfamiliar environment
M etabolic

Figure 16-11 The etiology of delirium is multifactorial. It is not uncommon for several factors to exist simultaneously and increase risk in an individual patient. (Adapted from Inouye SK: Delirium in hospitalized elderly patients: Recognition, evaluation and management. Conn Med 57:309-312, 1993.)

Postoperative delirium, an acute disorder of cognition and attention, is among the most common and potentially devastating complications seen in elderly patients. Postoperative delirium is associated with high morbidity and mortality, longer length of hospital stay, and a high rate of institutionalization after discharge. The incidence of postoperative delirium in older patients varies with the type of procedure: up to 5.1% after major abdominal surgery, 33% after abdominal aortic aneurysm repair, and 37% after operations for repair of a hip fracture.

The etiology of delirium in hospitalized patients is multifactorial (Fig. 16-11). Postoperative delirium may be the manifestation of an unrecognized preexisting disease or the result of intraoperative or postoperative events. Risk factors associated with delirium include older age, cognitive impairment, sensory impairment, poor functional status, depression, preoperative psychotropic drug use, psychopathologic symptoms, institutional residence, and greater comorbidity.[23] Alcohol consumption, severity of illness, malnutrition, hypoxia, metabolic disturbances, use of bladder catheters, and use of physical restraints have also been identified as risk factors. A variety of medications, including certain antibiotics, analgesics, antihypertensives, β-blockers, and tranquilizers, have additionally been shown to precipitate delirium. Intraoperative and postoperative factors have likewise been studied. No association has been found with the route of anesthesia (epidural versus general) or the occurrence of intraoperative hemodynamic complications. However, intraoperative blood loss, the need for blood transfusion, and postoperative hematocrit less than 30% are associated with a significantly increased risk for postoperative delirium.[24] Alterations in the wake-sleep cycle after surgery have also been associated with delirium.

It is most important to recognize that mental status changes in elderly surgical patients are often the earliest signs of a postoperative complication. Therefore, tests for cognitive impairment are essential components of the routine postoperative evaluation. If an adequate preoperative mental status examination has been conducted, postoperative assessment only requires brief observations of behavior and a comparison to baseline.

Nutritional Status

Surgeons recognize the value of optimal nutritional status to minimize perioperative mortality and morbidity. However, elderly patients are at particular risk for malnutrition and therefore at increased risk for perioperative events. It remains imperative for surgeons to continue to assess nutritional status and attempt to correct malnutrition in order to achieve optimal results. Although this may be a difficult task in any patient, detection plus correction of malnutrition in elderly patients is crucial.

The impact of poor nutrition as a risk factor for perioperative mortality and morbidity such as pneumonia and poor wound healing has long been appreciated. A variety of psychosocial issues and comorbid conditions common to the elderly place this population at high risk for nutritional deficits. Malnutrition is estimated to occur in approximately 0% to 15% of community-dwelling elderly persons, 35% to 65% of older patients in acute care hospitals, and 25% to 60% of institutionalized elderly.[25] Factors that lead to inadequate intake and utilization of nutrients in this population include the ability to get food (e.g., financial constraints, availability of food, limited mobility), the desire to eat food (e.g., living situation, mental status, chronic illness), the ability to eat and absorb food (e.g., poor dentition, chronic gastrointestinal disorders such as gastroesophageal reflux disease [GERD] or diarrhea), and medications that interfere with appetite or nutrient metabolism (Box 16-3). In the frail elderly, multiple factors contribute to neuroendocrine dysregulation of the signals that control appetite and satiety and lead to what is termed *the anorexia of aging*. Although the anorexia of aging is a complex interaction of many interrelated events and systems, the result is chronic undernutrition and loss of muscle mass.

Measurement of nutritional status in the elderly, however, is difficult. Standard anthropomorphic measures do not take into account the changes in body composition and structure that accompany aging. Immune measures of nutrition are influenced by age-related changes in the immune system in general. Furthermore, criteria for the interpretation of biochemical markers in this age group have not been well established. Complicated markers and indices of malnutrition exist but are not necessary in the routine surgical setting. Subjective assessment by history and physical examination, in which risk factors and physical evidence of malnutrition are evaluated, has been shown to be as effective as objective measures of nutritional status (see Box 16-2). The Subjective Global Assessment (SGA) is a relatively simple, reproducible tool for assessing nutritional status from the history and physical examination. SGA ratings are most strongly influenced by loss of subcutaneous tissue, muscle wasting, and weight loss. The Mini Nutritional Assessment (MNA), which measures 18 factors, including BMI, weight history, cognition, mobility, dietary history, and self-assessment, among others, is also a reliable method for assessing nutritional status. Nutritional status, as determined by both the SGA and the MNA, has been shown to predict outcome in both outpatient and hospitalized geriatric medical patients.[26]

Serum albumin has been implicated as a strong predictor of outcome, both perioperative mortality and morbidity, in surgical patients. Recent evidence demonstrates that low serum albumin in elderly patients correlates with increased length of stay, increased rates of readmission, unfavorable disposition, and increased all-cause mortality. In the Veterans Affairs NSQIP study mentioned earlier,[19] low serum albumin was the most important predictive factor for mortality. This suggests that low serum albumin is a sensitive marker of outcome, regardless of whether it is directly related to poor nutritional status or to unidentified complex chronic illness. In a study of octogenarians undergoing surgical treatment of gastrointestinal malignancy, low serum albumin was a strong independent predictor of postoperative complications.[27]

Although good data from large randomized trials on preoperative nutritional restoration do not exist, amelioration of malnutrition with protein or immune-enhancing supplementation may improve outcome in some groups of elderly patients.

Box 16-3   Historical Findings Associated With an Increased Risk for Nutritional Deficiency

Recent weight loss
Restricted dietary intake
Limited variety, food avoidances
Psychosocial situation
Depression, cognitive impairment, isolation, economic difficulties
Problems with eating, chewing, swallowing
Previous surgery
Increased losses secondary to gastrointestinal disorders such as malabsorption and diarrhea
Systemic disease interfering with appetite or eating (chronic lung, liver, heart, and renal disease; abdominal angina; cancer)
Excessive alcohol use
Medications that interfere with appetite or nutrient metabolism, or both

Reprinted with permission from Rosenberg IH: Nutrition and aging. In Hazzard WR, Bierman EL, Blass JP, et al (eds): Principles of Geriatric Medicine and Gerontology, 3rd ed. New York, McGraw-Hill, 1994.

SPECIFIC CONSIDERATIONS

Endocrine Surgery

Breast Disease

Epidemiology

In Western countries the incidence of breast cancer increases with age. Breast cancer is the most common cancer in women and the second leading cause of cancer death in women. In the United States the risk for breast cancer in women younger than 40 years is 1 in 229; in women aged 40 to 59 years, 1 in 24; and in women 60 to 79 years of age, 1 in 13. Breast cancer mortality also rises with increasing age. In fact, most deaths from breast cancer occur in women older than 65 years. It is expected that as life expectancy continues to improve in Western countries, both the proportion and the absolute number of older women with breast cancer will rise dramatically.

Clinical Features and Screening

The clinical findings of breast cancer are similar in both the older and younger populations. A painless mass is the most common symptom. In older women, a new breast lump is likely to represent a malignancy. Breast pain, skin thickening, breast swelling, or nipple discharge or retraction needs to be vigorously pursued with biopsy. The breast become less dense with aging, thus making clinical examination easier in older women. This difference also translates to an improved positive predictive value of an abnormal mammogram in women older than 65 years. The American Cancer Society recommends monthly breast self-examination, annual clinical breast examination, and annual mammography beginning at age 40, with no upper age limit as long as a woman remains in good health. If a woman's life expectancy is

estimated to be less than 3 to 5 years, if severe functional limitations are present, or if a woman has multiple comorbid conditions that are likely to impair survival, discontinuation of screening is appropriate. The American Geriatrics Society position statement recommends annual or at least biennial mammography to age 75. Beyond the age of 75, mammography is performed biennially or at least every 3 years if life expectancy is greater than 4 years.[28]

Pathology and Treatment Overview

Overall, breast cancer in elderly patients tends to be associated with more favorable pathologic prognostic factors. Tumors in older women have more frequent expression of hormone receptors, lower rates of tumor cell proliferation, a greater frequency of diploidy, and lower expression of the epidermal growth factor receptor and HER-2 (c-erb-B2).[29] Despite the presence of these more favorable tumor markers, stage per stage, survival in elderly women with breast cancer is similar to that seen in younger women. In fact, women 70 years and older may have lower distant disease-free survival rates at 10 years than women aged 40 to 70 years.

Older women are often undertreated in comparison to younger women, in part because of the belief that their tumors are more indolent. Older women are less likely to receive definitive surgery, postlumpectomy radiotherapy, adjuvant hormonal therapy, and adjuvant chemotherapy.[30]

Breast cancer trials in the United States have a disproportionately low enrollment of elderly women. Women 65 years and older are less likely than stage- and physician-matched younger women to be offered participation in breast cancer trials. Therefore, most recommendations for treatment of elderly women with breast cancer are derived from studies conducted in women younger than 70 years. Unlike the treatment of younger women with breast cancer, a central concept in decision making in elderly patients is that of life expectancy. Accurate predictions and knowledge of life expectancy are inherently important in decisions regarding screening older populations with mammography, treatment of the primary lesion, and use of systemic adjuvant therapy. Currently available treatment options often carry short-term risks and toxicities in older women that are not mitigated by long-term survival gains.

Surgery

Surgical resection of the primary tumor is recommended for all elderly patients unless they are poor surgical candidates, and breast-conserving therapy is recommended when possible. Despite evidence that age is not a contraindication to breast-conserving surgery, older women have historically had lower rates of breast-conserving cancer surgery than younger women. Tamoxifen alone is a reasonable treatment option for women with early-stage breast cancer who are not surgical candidates. Although tamoxifen is less effective than surgery in achieving durable local control, there is no effect on overall survival for women whose life expectancy is limited. Recently, aromatase inhibitors have been used in this setting and may be superior to tamoxifen.

The role of axillary lymph node dissection (ALND) in the management of women with breast cancer has evolved over the last 10 to 15 years. Although ALND decreases axillary recurrence in younger women, it is not clear that it is as effective in older women. Elderly women have an increased incidence of significant side effects from ALND, including lymphedema, decreased extremity function, and impaired quality of life. Therefore, ALND is recommended for clinically node-negative older women only if the results would affect the choice of adjuvant chemotherapy. Sentinel lymph node biopsy is nearly as accurate as formal ALND and has been shown to decrease lymphedema and pain when compared with ALND. For older women with clinically or pathologically positive axillary lymph nodes who are candidates for surgery, ALND remains the procedure of choice.

Radiation Therapy

For women 70 years or older who have early, estrogen receptor–positive breast cancer, the addition of adjuvant radiation therapy to tamoxifen does not significantly decrease the rate of mastectomy for local recurrence, increase the survival rate, or increase the rate of freedom from distant metastases. Therefore, tamoxifen alone is a reasonable choice for adjuvant treatment in such women. For older women with small, node-negative tumors, the decision to include breast irradiation after lumpectomy is made on a case-by-case basis after careful discussion of the risk for locoregional recurrence and the side effects of radiation therapy. Alternatively, partial-breast irradiation with multicatheter interstitial brachytherapy, balloon catheter brachytherapy, three-dimensional conformal external beam radiotherapy, and intraoperative radiotherapy can be an option in selected older patients. Older women treated with mastectomy are offered chest wall irradiation if they have tumors larger than 5 cm or more than four involved axillary lymph nodes.

Chemotherapy

Tamoxifen and aromatase inhibitors, such as anastrozole, improve overall survival, reduce local recurrence, and decrease the risk for contralateral breast cancer in older women with hormone-sensitive tumors. Both tamoxifen and anastrozole have side effects that can reduce their tolerance. Tamoxifen is associated with deep venous thrombosis, pulmonary emboli, cerebrovascular events, endometrial carcinoma, vaginal discharge and bleeding, and hot flashes. There are considerably more musculoskeletal complaints, including arthralgias and fractures, with anastrozole. The added value of chemotherapy in older women who receive endocrine therapy is influenced greatly by comorbidity and life expectancy. Models for estimating the benefits of chemotherapy in hormone receptor–positive older women have been developed. These models demonstrate that a high risk of recurrence is needed to achieve a small survival benefit with adjuvant chemotherapy. For example, to reduce mortality risk at 10 years by 1% with chemotherapy, the risk for breast recurrence at 10 years has to be at least 25% for a 75-year-old in average health. These data suggest that chemotherapy for older women with hormone receptor–positive breast cancer is offered only to node-positive patients who are in reasonable health and have a high risk of recurrence and a life expectancy of more than 5 years. Older node-negative patients are unlikely to benefit from chemotherapy unless they have large hormone receptor–positive tumors with adverse pathologic characteristics or hormone receptor–negative tumors larger than 2 cm. An Internet-based tool that incorporates age, health status, and tumor characteristics is available to determine the potential benefit of adjuvant chemotherapy for breast cancer patients.[31]

Thyroid Disease

Hypothyroidism occurs in 10% of women and 2% of men older than 60 years, and hyperthyroidism occurs in 0.5% to 6% of persons older than 55. Hypothyroidism is caused by autoimmune disease, previous radioablation or surgery, and drugs that interfere with the synthesis of thyroid hormone, such as amiodarone.[32] Hyperthyroidism is usually caused by toxic multinodular goiter, with Grave's disease being less common than it is in younger persons.[33] Medical treatment of hypothyroidism in old age is similar to that in youth. Surgical treatment of hyperthyroidism may be necessary for large goiters compressing the trachea. It is most important to remember that as with disorders of many other organ systems, symptoms of both hypothyroidism and hyperthyroidism in this age group are easily overlooked or attributed to other causes. Failure to recognize the presence of either can result in serious problems in the perioperative period.

The incidence of thyroid nodules increases throughout life, whether detected by physical examination, ultrasound, or autopsy, although physical examination is less sensitive because of fibrosis of the soft tissues of the neck and the gland. The incidence of nodules in autopsy series is 50%. Thyroid nodules are four times more common in females, but the risk for cancer in a nodule is higher in males. Most thyroid nodules are single when detected. Thyroid nodules change slowly over the short term. Prospective studies have shown, however, that up to a quarter of colloid nodules can shrink over a period of 2 to 3 years and may disappear.

After exposure to ionizing radiation, the incidence of new nodules increases at 2% per year, with the peak incidence being reached at 15 to 25 years. The highest risk occurs in patients younger than 20 years, not the elderly. Because radiation treatment of benign diseases such as tonsillitis, hemangiomas, thymic enlargement, and lymphadenopathy has not been practiced for many years, the majority of patients with such a history are now in the elderly cohort. The effect of radiation-induced thyroid disease from atomic bombs or accidental discharge from nuclear power plants is currently being examined. Early data suggest a similar pattern.

Well-differentiated thyroid cancer is divided into papillary and follicular subtypes. Sporadic papillary thyroid cancer has an almost bell-shaped distribution of age at diagnosis, with a decreasing trend in patients older than 60. Age is a negative prognostic factor for survival and other variables. Patients older than 60 years have an increased risk for local recurrence, and patients younger than 20 and older than 60 have a higher risk for the development of distant metastasis. Similar results have been noted for follicular cancer. Increasing patient age correlates with increased risk for death by approximately twofold over a span of 20 years. Because age is a significant prognostic factor, most scoring system of differentiated thyroid cancer, including the AMES classification (age, distant metastases, extent, size), have age as a component.

Parathyroid Disease

The incidence of primary hyperparathyroidism increases with age, and it affects approximately 2% of elderly persons, with a 3:1 female preponderance (1 in 1000 postmenopausal women). The disease is characterized by elevated serum calcium, often within 1 mg of normal, in the presence of elevated parathyroid hormone (PTH) to levels 1.5 to 2.0 times normal. The majority of cases in the elderly are solitary adenomas.

Until the 1970s the disease was often symptomatic with nephrolithiasis (stones), overt skeletal disease (bones), and neuropsychiatric complaints (psychic groans). With the advent of routine calcium testing as part of automated chemistry analysis, this pattern has changed and now 80% of cases are asymptomatic. A careful history, however, will frequently reveal the presence of less obvious psychological and emotional symptoms. Other subtle symptoms in older persons include memory loss, personality changes, inability to concentrate, exercise fatigue, and back pain. Several studies have shown that only 5% to 8% of patients are truly asymptomatic.

In response to the controversy regarding treatment of asymptomatic hyperparathyroidism, the National Institutes of Health (NIH) consensus conference in 1990 offered parameters for care. Participants agreed that truly asymptomatic patients, with serum calcium levels only mildly elevated, no previous history of life-threatening hypercalcemia, and normal renal, bone, and mental status, can be safely observed without surgery. Patients with creatinine clearance decreased 30% over age-matched controls, 24-hour urinary calcium excretion of more than 400 mg, and decreased bone mass more than 2 standard deviations from age- and race-matched controls are offered surgical treatment.

Further indications for surgery include primary hyperparathyroidism in patients younger than 50 years and hyperparathyroidism in patients for whom close follow-up would be difficult or for whom significant concomitant illness complicates management. At a more recent NIH workshop in 2002, a panel reconsidered therapy for asymptomatic primary hyperparathyroidism. The threshold for parathyroidectomy was reduced to include patients with a serum calcium level greater than 1 mg/dL above the upper limits of normal. This definition still leaves uncertain whether weakness and depression indicate symptomatic disease, although roughly 40% of patients with hyperparathyroidism have one or both complaints. No medical treatment of hyperparathyroidism is available, so there is no means of predicting when or whether severe complications of the disease such as nephrocalcinosis or bone disease will develop. Because the risk for morbidity and mortality associated with surgery is low, even in older patients, parathyroidectomy remains the treatment of choice unless other comorbid conditions preclude surgery.

Minimally invasive parathyroid surgery has gained acceptance with the adoption of sestamibi-directed surgery, intraoperative PTH assay, and videoscopic surgery. Cure rates in patients older than 70 years at one center have risen from 84% in the pre–minimally invasive era (before 2001) to 98% after the introduction of radioguided minimally invasive surgery under regional anesthesia.[34]

Gastrointestinal Surgery

Esophagus

The esophagus undergoes characteristic changes with aging. There is a progressive decrease in amplitude of the primary peristaltic waves after deglutition, with octogenarians exhibiting only 50% of the amplitude of younger controls and nonagenarians, 20%. Although lower esophageal sphincter resting pressure is normal and relaxes appropriately after deglutition, the sphincter fails to rapidly contract back to baseline, thereby resulting in prolonged decreased tone.

There is also an increased incidence of hernias at the hiatus. Sliding hiatal hernias, probably caused by laxity at the gastroesophageal junction, in addition to delayed gastric emptying, predispose to GERD. Although it is uncertain whether the incidence and prevalence of GERD are higher in older persons, age appears to be a risk factor for more severe forms of the disease. In an Italian study of patients 18 to 101 years of age, classic symptoms of heartburn, pain, and indigestion decreased with age, whereas nonspecific symptoms of dysphagia, anorexia,

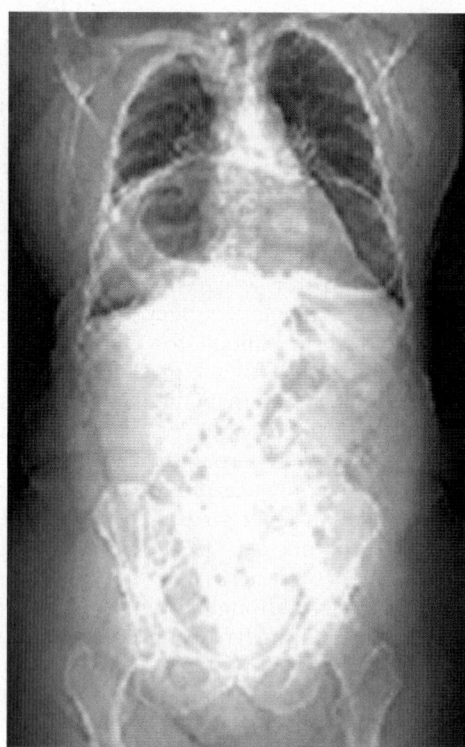

Figure 16-12 Scout film for a CT scan showing a giant paraesophageal hernia with the entire stomach in the chest, rotated in an organoaxial direction.

anemia, weight loss, and vomiting increased.[35] The degree of esophagitis also increased, with a larger percentage of older patients having grade III to IV disease. Age, male sex, and size of the hernia correlated with the severity of esophagitis, whereas nonsteroidal anti-inflammatory drug (NSAID) use, *Helicobacter pylori* infection, and the presence of hernia did not.

As a result of the atypical symptom pattern or reluctance on the part of primary care practitioners to refer older patients for surgery, or both, the duration of symptoms before referral of patients older than 60 years is more than 14 years as opposed to 4 years in younger patients. Consequently, older patients undergo surgery more frequently with a complication such as bleeding, stricture, aspiration, or Barrett's esophagus. The recent success of laparoscopic Nissen fundoplication for correction of GERD in older patients provides a viable alternative to lifelong medications, which may also be less effective in older patients. As many as 90% of older patients report relief of symptoms, particularly vomiting and aspiration, after a Nissen procedure.

Paraesophageal hernias also increase with advancing age and can reach enormous size without symptoms (Fig. 16-12). In the past, the fear of gastric volvulus with subsequent strangulation mandated immediate repair of paraesophageal hernias, even in the absence of symptoms. Recent evidence supports watchful waiting rather than immediate surgery for asymptomatic hernias, with a 1.1% annual probability of requiring an emergency operation.

Dysmotility of the cricopharyngeus (upper esophageal sphincter) with increasing age can give rise to Zenker's diverticulum. Failure of the cricopharyngeus to relax results in herniation of mucosa between it and the thyropharyngeus above. Cricopharyngeal myotomy to relieve the underlying motor dysfunction is the treatment of choice. For large pouches, many, but not all surgeons combine myotomy with stapled resection of the diverticulum. Endoscopic approaches have also been used with excellent results.

Resection for esophageal cancer is a complicated issue because of its low cure rate and high operative morbidity and mortality. Most studies show no difference in morbidity related to age, although some have shown increased complication and death rates. Overall 5-year survival rates for curative resection are 14% to 25%, similar to that observed in younger patients.

Stomach

Progressive cephalad migration of the antral-fundic junction occurs with age. Studies have shown that between 25% and 80% of elderly persons have fasting achlorhydria because of progressive loss of parietal cells and decreased antral and serum concentrations of gastrin. Achlorhydria results in derangements in folate, iron, and vitamin B_{12} absorption.

The incidence of peptic ulcer disease increases with age. Up to 80% of peptic ulcer–related deaths occur in patients older than 65. Other factors that increase the risk for peptic ulcer disease in the elderly population are the use of NSAIDs and infection with *H. pylori*. NSAIDs are well-established inducers of peptic ulcer disease, the mechanism being inhibition of the formation of prostaglandins, essential components of the gastric mucosal barrier. NSAID use has increased markedly over the past few years, especially in the elderly population. Use of NSAIDs increases the risk for development of complicated peptic ulcer disease in the elderly when compared with younger patients. Despite an overall decline in peptic ulcer disease, the incidence of duodenal and gastric ulcer bleeding has not changed between 1989/1990 and 1999/2000, probably because of increased NSAID use in elderly patients. Actual NSAID use is also a useful prognostic indicator; the mortality rate from peptic ulcer disease in elderly patients who take NSAIDs is twice that of those who do not. Similarly, 80% of all ulcer-related deaths occurred in patients taking NSAIDs. Despite this finding, NSAIDs are frequently prescribed to older patients, even those with previous gastrointestinal problems.

H. pylori infections are believed to occur at a rate of 1% per year, so a substantial percentage of the elderly population harbors such infection. Some have postulated that a cohort of patients who were infected during childhood earlier in the 20th century are now aged and experiencing complications of the infection. *H. pylori* screening and treatment have increased significantly in recent years, whereas counseling about the risks associated with NSAID therapy has not. Yet in one study, treatment of *H. pylori* did not reduce the risk for rehospitalization or death within 1 year of initial hospitalization, whereas counseling about NSAIDs did both.[37]

Elderly patients are typically referred for surgical correction of peptic ulcer disease in delayed fashion and thus have more advanced disease. This translates to statistically significant increases in operative mortality for elderly patients undergoing surgery for complicated peptic ulcer disease. Age alone has not been shown to be an independent predictor of surgical risk. Multivariate analysis reveals that there are three risk factors for operative mortality in patients with a perforated ulcer: concomitant disease, preoperative shock, and the presence of perforation for longer than 48 hours. Age, amount of peritoneal soilage, and duration of ulcer disease do not appear to be significant risks. However, in a study of patients with bleeding duodenal ulcer, multivariate logistic regression analysis revealed that age does plays a role in determining outcome.

The incidence of gastric cancer rises progressively with age, with most patients being between 50 and 70 years of age at diagnosis. Cases in patients younger than 30 years are very rare. Risks include diet (pickled vegetables, salted fish, nitrates, and nitrites), occupation (metal, asbestos, and rubber workers), and geography (Asia versus the Western Hemisphere). Chronic atrophic gastritis, previous gastric surgery, and chronic *H. pylori* infection, more frequently found in older patients, are associated with increased risk as well. Chronic atrophic gastritis and *H. pylori* infection are also risk factors for gastric lymphoma and its precursor, mucosa-associated lymphoid tissue (MALT). These patients are typically initially seen in the sixth decade of life. The manifestation of gastric cancer is changing in older persons, with a trend toward a need for more aggressive surgery. Elderly patients have a predominance of intestinal-type tumors rather than the more aggressive diffuse type. There is also a progression of the location of the tumor to more proximal areas of the stomach. As a result, total gastrectomy for cure in this population is now required in 13% to 34% of cases. No difference in resectability or the rate of positive lymph nodes found at surgery has been noted between young and older patients.

Liver

Tumors of the liver are 20 times more likely to arise from metastatic disease than from primary cancer. Metastatic tumors from gastrointestinal tract primaries are the most common type referred for resection. Patients with colon cancer have a 35% risk for recurrence in the liver, but only 10% to 20% of those identified have resectable disease. Patients resected have upward of a 30% 5-year survival rate, versus 0% if not resected.

Over the past 20 years the mortality associated with liver resection in patients older than 65 has decreased. Today, the rates in young and older patients are comparable.[38] Results are so similar that age alone is not necessarily a contraindication to simultaneous resection of colorectal malignancy and liver metastases.

In addition to surgical resection, treatments of hepatic cancer include radiologic embolization, cryotherapy, and radiofrequency ablation therapy, which can be performed operatively or transcutaneously.

Biliary Tract Disease

Biliary tract disease is the single most common cause of acute abdominal complaints and accounts for approximately a third of all abdominal operations in the elderly. In nearly all populations, the prevalence of gallstones increases with increasing age, although the magnitude of this increase varies with the population. By 65 years of age, 90% of female Pima Indians have gallstones as compared with 23% of female civil servants in Rome, Italy.

Although the majority of gallstones in the United States are cholesterol stones, the proportion of pigment stones increases with advancing age. A study of U.S. veterans (90% male) demonstrated that 63% of stones found in patients younger than 50 years were predominately cholesterol whereas 59% of stones in patients older than 70 years were predominantly pigment. Bacteria were present in 69% of pigment stones and only 9% of pure cholesterol stones. Biliary bacteria also increased with age, from 31% in patients younger than 50 years to 65% in those older than 70 years. The presence of biliary bacteria correlated with the severity of illness, with 46% of patients with bacteria having severe disease. Therefore, it is not surprising that a higher incidence of complicated disease (acute cholecystitis, choledocholithiasis/cholangitis, and biliary pancreatitis) is reported at the time of cholecystectomy in septuagenarians (40%) and octogenarians (55%).[39]

The increased frequency of gallstones in the elderly is thought to result from both changes in the composition of bile and impaired biliary motility. Alterations in the composition of bile with advancing age include an increase in the activity of 3-hydroxy-3-methylglutaryl coenzyme A (HMG-CoA; the rate-limiting enzyme in the synthesis of cholesterol) and a decrease in the activity of 7α-hydroxylase (the rate-limiting enzyme in the synthesis of bile salts from cholesterol). This results in supersaturation of bile with cholesterol and a decrease in the primary bile salt pool. The ratio of secondary to primary bile salts also increases. It is postulated that these secondary bile salts promote cholesterol gallstone formation by enhancing cholesterol synthesis, increasing the protein content of bile, decreasing nucleation time, and increasing the production of specific phospholipids that are thought to effect the production of mucin. It has also been suggested that the increase in secondary bile salts in the aged may promote recycling of bilirubin, which in turn leads to the unconjugated bilirubin supersaturation necessary for pigment stone formation.

Alterations in gallbladder motility and bile duct motility are thought to be central to the development of cholesterol and brown pigment stones, respectively. The role of motility in black pigment stone formation, however, is less clear. Biliary motility is a complex interaction of hormonal and neural factors, but the major stimulus for gallbladder emptying is cholecystokinin (CCK). The sensitivity of the gallbladder wall to CCK has been shown to decrease with increasing age in animal models. In humans, gallbladder sensitivity to CCK is also decreased. However, there is a compensatory increase in the production of CCK in response to a stimulus that results in normal gallbladder contraction. The significance of this observation with regard to gallstone formation, though, is undetermined.

The indications for treatment of gallstone disease in older persons are the same as in younger patients, although complications of the disease rather than biliary colic are more common in advanced age. The increased rate of complicated disease seen in older patients may be attributable to the increased severity of the disease or to an increased prevalence of comorbid illnesses (or both). However, it is more likely to be due to a combination of factors, including delays in diagnosis and treatment caused by the frequent *absence* of typical biliary tract symptoms. Biliary colic, or episodic right upper quadrant pain radiating to the back, precedes the development of a complication only half as often in older as in younger patients. Even in the presence of acute cholecystitis, as many as a quarter of older patients may have no abdominal tenderness, a third no elevation in temperature or WBC count, and as many as a half no peritoneal signs in the right upper quadrant. Unfortunately, mortality in the emergency setting is at least three times that in the elective setting. Until predictors of impending complications other than symptoms are identified, improving the outcome of biliary tract disease in the elderly will be difficult. Increased awareness of the atypical manifestations of gallstone-related illness in this age group is essential.

Treatment of acute cholecystitis in the elderly is somewhat controversial. Whereas some authors support early laparoscopic cholecystectomy, others favor percutaneous drainage, followed by delayed laparoscopic cholecystectomy. In patients older than 80 years, rates of conversion and complications of laparoscopic cholecystectomy are higher than in patients aged 65 to 79 years, even in the elective setting.

The presence of common bile duct (CBD) stones increases the likelihood of postoperative complications and death. In the prelaparoscopic era, bile duct stones were addressed at the time of cholecystectomy. Although open CBD exploration was extremely successful in clearing the bile duct of stones, it was associated with a significant increase in operative mortality and morbidity over simple cholecystectomy alone. Most clinicians now agree that if CBD stones are suspected, either from a dilated duct on ultrasound or from abnormal liver or pancreatic test results, a preoperative attempt at sphincterotomy and extraction via endoscopic retrograde cholangiopancreatography is made. Successful duct clearance by this approach is reported in more than 90% of cases. Recurrence of CBD stones after sphincterotomy, however, even with antecedent or subsequent cholecystectomy, is higher in older than in younger patients (20% versus 4%).[40] Risk factors for recurrence include a dilated CBD, duodenal diverticulum, angulation of the CBD, and previous cholecystectomy.

Management of the gallbladder after successful endoscopic treatment of CBD stones in patients without coincident acute cholecystitis is still controversial. Several studies indicate that a complication related to the gallbladder will eventually develop in 4% to 24% of patients managed by endoscopic sphincterotomy alone and that 5.8% to 18% will require subsequent cholecystectomy. Unfortunately, because patients managed in this fashion are frequently the oldest and most frail, the mortality related to subsequent acute cholecystitis in these patients can be as high as 25%.

Special consideration must be given to the treatment of gallstones found at the time of laparotomy for an unrelated condition. The addition of cholecystectomy to the primary procedure usually adds little increased morbidity or mortality. Although some controversy still exists, many surgeons would proceed with incidental cholecystectomy if the patient were stable, exposure was appropriate, and the cholecystectomy added little additional operative time. In the past, stronger arguments for incidental cholecystectomy were based on concerns that the symptoms of acute postoperative cholecystitis might be unrecognized in the setting of a recent laparotomy incision. With better postoperative monitoring, more accurate imaging techniques, and percutaneous methods for decompressing the gallbladder should postoperative cholecystitis occur, these concerns have diminished.

Small Bowel Obstruction

Small bowel obstruction (SBO) is by far the most common and surgically relevant disorder of small intestinal function encountered in the aged. Although the exact incidence of SBO in the elderly is difficult to ascertain, lysis of adhesions is the third most common gastrointestinal procedure after cholecystectomy and partial excision of the large bowel. Fifty percent of the deaths associated with SBO occur in patients older than 70 years.

In Western countries, adhesions are responsible for a substantial majority of SBOs, followed by incarcerated hernias, neoplasms, and inflammatory bowel disease. It has been noted that the age of patients with incarcerated hernias is slightly older than that of patients with adhesive obstruction. In addition, certain kinds of hernias, such as those that occur through the obturator foramen, are found almost exclusively in the elderly and are particularly difficult to diagnose. Luminal obstruction, other than from deliberately ingested objects, accounts for less than 5% of cases. However, the majority of this type of obstruction occurs in the elderly. The two most common objects obstructing the lumen in adults are phytobezoars and gallstones. Phytobezoars, or large concretions of poorly digested fruit and vegetable matter, form with increased frequency in the stomach of elderly patients with poor dentition, decreased gastric acid, impaired gastric motility, and previous gastrectomy. In the stomach these masses can become enormous without any symptoms. However, when a portion breaks free and migrates into the small bowel, obstruction ensues. Gallstones enter the small bowel usually through a fistula between the gallbladder and the duodenum. *Obturation of the small bowel lumen by an aberrantly located gallstone,* incorrectly termed *gallstone ileus,* accounts for 1% to 3% of all

SBOs but has been implicated in as many as 25% of obstructions in patients older than 65 with no abdominal wall hernia or history of previous surgery.

The pathophysiology, diagnosis, and treatment of SBO are discussed elsewhere in the text. It is important to note, however, that two important issues that determine management strategy—distinguishing functional (ileus) from mechanical obstruction and distinguishing simple from strangulated obstruction—are even more complex in elderly patients.

Many of the factors associated with ileus, such as systemic infections, intra-abdominal infections, metabolic abnormalities, and medications that affect motility, are more common in older persons. The relevance of these factors to the finding of abdominal distention is not always appreciated. Signs and symptoms of underlying infections such as pneumonia, urinary tract infection, or appendicitis may be subtle. Bowel distention may be erroneously considered the primary problem rather than a secondary event. Vomiting from a variety of nonobstructive causes can rapidly lead to dehydration and subsequent electrolyte abnormalities in the elderly. The constellation of vomiting and bowel distention can easily be mistaken for obstruction.

In patients of all ages suspected of having adhesive SBO, initial nonoperative management with nasogastric decompression and intravenous (IV) hydration is standard. Although rates vary, only about 30% of patients with adhesive SBO will require surgery, usually for failure to progress or fear of strangulation. However, accurate distinction between strangulated and simple mechanical SBO is difficult to make, particularly in the elderly, because there are no objective markers that consistently identify which patient will require small bowel resection for ischemia at the time of surgery for SBO. Clinical findings of fever, tachycardia, elevated WBC count, and focal tenderness are notoriously misleading, particularly in the elderly, in whom the risk for strangulation is the highest.

Several additional considerations are important in the elderly. Although the natural reflex is to avoid unnecessary operations in sick older patients, prolonged conservative management can present new problems. Prolonged bed rest is associated with an increased incidence of venous stasis, pulmonary complications, and deconditioning. Prolonged nasogastric intubation is associated with an increased incidence of aspiration and pneumonia. Even a short period of nutritional deprivation may present a significant risk to an elderly patient with a baseline nutritional deficit. These factors together may result in a poor outcome should surgery become necessary after a prolonged attempt to avoid it.

In a review of more than 32,000 patients treated for SBO in California, 24% required surgery on the index admission. Although length of stay was longer for those who had operations, mortality was lower, readmissions for SBO were fewer, and the time interval to readmission for SBO was longer. The authors specifically stated that further research is needed to determine the importance of time to surgery on outcomes for the oldest and sickest patients.[41]

In elderly patients who have undergone previous abdominal operations for malignant disease, the decision about when to operate is even more difficult. Metastatic obstruction presents several technical and ethical problems. Obstructing lesions are frequently found at multiple points in the bowel and resection may not be possible. Bypass of long, partially obstructed segments may be technically feasible but can leave the patient with a functionally short gut. Thirty-day operative mortality rates for this form of obstruction in elderly patients exceed 35%, and the majority of all patients die within 6 months. This discouraging outcome has led some to advocate prolonged periods of nonoperative decompression. Unfortunately, this approach produces only transient relief of obstructive symptoms. Furthermore, a previous history of malignancy is not an absolute indication that the obstruction is due to metastatic disease. In 10% to 38% of patients with suspected malignant obstruction, a benign cause is found at the time of surgery.

Over the past decade there has been increasing interest in using minimally invasive techniques to diagnose and treat SBO. At first glance the laparoscopic approach in the elderly has considerable appeal. Early intervention with minimal surgical stress would seem ideal. There are now numerous relatively small series by very experienced laparoscopic surgeons that show diagnostic success in more than 90% of cases and total therapeutic success rates of 50% to 90%. However, laparoscopy in this setting can be technically challenging and not without complications. It is unclear at present how widely this option will be adopted as more surgeons become skilled in these advanced laparoscopic techniques.

Appendicitis

Although appendicitis typically develops in the second and third decades of life, 5% to 10% of cases occur in old age. Appendicitis in the elderly has increased in recent decades while the incidence in younger patients is declining. Inflammation of the appendix now accounts for 2.5% to 5% of acute abdominal disease in patients older than 60 to 70 years. The overall mortality from appendicitis is only 0.8%, but the vast majority of deaths occur in the very young and the very old. In adults, the mortality rate after appendectomy is strongly related to age and ranges from 0.07 per 1000 appendectomies in patients 20 to 29 years old to 164 per 1000 in nonagenarians.

The classic manifestation of appendicitis—periumbilical pain that localizes over a period of several hours to the right lower quadrant, fever, anorexia, and leukocytosis—is present in less than 33% of elderly patients with appendicitis. Although nearly all elderly patients with acute appendicitis will have abdominal pain, only 50% to 75% will have pain localized to the right lower quadrant. Nearly a third of patients will have diffuse nonlocalizable abdominal pain. Because vague abdominal pain is a common complaint in older persons, its significance may be overlooked and thereby result in delays in treatment. The most frequent misdiagnosis in this patient group is bowel obstruction. Other signs of acute appendicitis are also unreliable in the elderly. The WBC count and temperature are normal in 20% to 50% of older patients. Nausea, vomiting, and anorexia are also found less frequently in older patients.

The indolent and nonspecific nature of the initial symptoms of appendicitis in the elderly usually leads to delays of 48 to 72 hours before medical attention is sought. These delays are compounded by a delay in diagnosis once the patient reaches the hospital. In only 30% to 70% of cases is the correct diagnosis made on admission. Delays of greater than 24 hours until surgery are three times more likely to occur in older than in younger patients. A potential result of this delay in diagnosis and treatment is an increased risk for appendiceal perforation. In fact, rates of perforation increase directly with age; by 70 years of age, perforation will be present in 50% to 60% of patients. Elderly patients undergoing appendectomy for perforated appendicitis have a higher risk for complications (24.9% versus 12.7%) and death (4.0% versus 0.7%) than those undergoing simple appendectomy for appendicitis without peritonitis.

Elderly patients may benefit from a laparoscopic approach for the treatment of acute appendicitis. In a retrospective study of 2722 elderly patients from North Carolina, significant reductions in length of stay were seen in the laparoscopic appendectomy (LA) group as compared with the open appendectomy (OA) group. Although LA did not result in statistically fewer complications than OA in elderly patients with perforated appendicitis, it did result in statistically fewer complications in the nonperforated appendicitis group. More impressive was the higher likelihood of discharge home versus discharge to a skilled or nonskilled nursing facility and reduced mortality rates in the LA patients.[42]

Because of the atypical manifestation of appendicitis in the elderly and the expanded differential diagnosis, a computed tomography (CT) scan is often helpful. If there is a suspicion of perforation and periappendiceal abscess, CT is performed before surgery. Percutaneous drainage and IV antibiotics are often preferable to exploration in the presence of a large abscess. In younger patients, this approach is followed by interval appendectomy approximately 6 weeks after the abscess has resolved. In the elderly, recurrent appendicitis after resolution of the abscess is uncommon, and therefore interval appendectomy is not necessary in all cases. However, the possibility of perforated cancer in this age group does mandate a thorough evaluation of the colon when the acute process is controlled. An elderly patient with signs and symptoms of acute appendicitis but with a longer duration of symptoms and a lower hematocrit than expected raises concern for colon or appendiceal cancer.

Carcinoma of the Colon and Rectum

Colorectal cancer is predominantly a disease of aging and is a major cause of morbidity and mortality in the elderly population. The overall incidence of colon cancer is 17 cases per 100,000 population, but this incidence rises sharply after 50 years of age. The annual incidence of colon cancer is nearly 40 times higher in those older than

85 than in individuals 40 to 44 years of age. Carcinoma of the colon and rectum accounts for two thirds of all gastrointestinal malignancies in patients older than 70.

With increasing age there is a progressive increase in the percentage of right-sided colon cancer, which is offset by a decrease in the percentage of rectal cancer (Fig. 16-13). Although there has been debate on the impact of age on stage at diagnosis, a large published review of the surgical literature demonstrated that older patients were more likely than younger patients to initially be seen with more advanced disease. In addition, the proportion of unstaged cancers increased with age from 3.9% in those younger than 65 years to 6.1% in the 65- to 74-year-old group, to 9.0% in the 74- to 84-year-old group, and to 17.3% in those 85 years and older.[43]

The initial signs and symptoms of colorectal cancer do not vary substantially with age, although some report more local symptoms in younger patients and more anorexia in older patients with rectal cancer. The response to these signs and symptoms, however, may be different. Right-sided lesions tend to cause microcytic anemia from occult bleeding, which may be manifested as lassitude, weakness, syncope, or a fall. Left-sided neoplasms tend to be manifested as changes in bowel habit or stool caliber. Because fatigue, falls, constipation, and bowel dysfunction are accepted as common sequelae of aging, these symptoms are frequently ignored by both the patient and physician. The diagnosis is therefore often not made until a complication occurs.

With advancing age, an increasing proportion of patients with colorectal cancer require emergency surgery. In fact, the proportion of patients undergoing emergency surgery for colorectal cancer is more than twice as high in those 85 years or older than in those 65 years or younger. A diminishing proportion of patients undergo curative surgery for colorectal cancer with advancing age. The proportion of patients who do not undergo surgery (presumably because they were thought unfit) rises with age from 4% in those younger than 65 years to 21% in those 85 years and older. These findings might be attributed to age-related differences in seeking medical advice, recognition of symptoms, or primary care referral patterns.

Operative mortality for colorectal cancer is determined by the same two factors that influence operative mortality in the elderly in general: the presence of coexisting disease and the need for emergency surgery. In patients with little or no comorbidity, operative mortality is similar regardless of age. When surgery is performed as an emergency, mortality increases threefold to fourfold over elective mortality for similar procedures. Even in patients older than 80 years, elective operative mortality rates are only approximately 2%. Length of hospital stay and hospital cost, however, are increased with advanced age and an emergency setting. In addition, survivors of elective operations are twice as likely to return to independent living as those surviving emergency surgery.[43] The increase in emergency surgery has an impact on 5-year survival in elderly patients. The 5-year survival rate after elective resection is 33.6% as compared with 14.7% after an emergency procedure.[44]

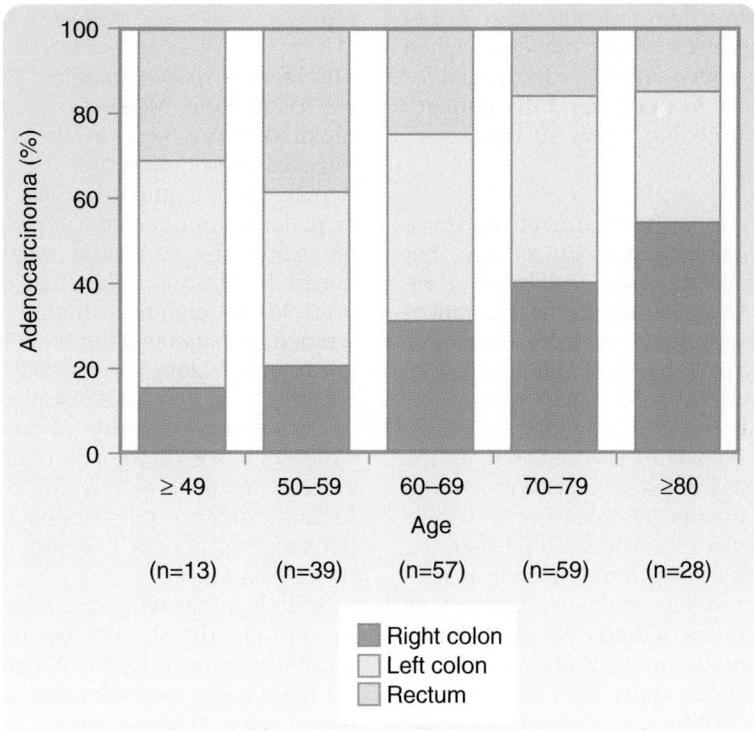

Figure 16-13 Location of colorectal carcinoma with increasing age. With age there is a progressive increase in right-sided colon cancer and a decrease in rectal cancer. (From Okamoto M, Shiratori Y, Yamaji Y, et al: Relationship between age and site of colorectal cancer based on colonoscopy findings. Gastrointest Endosc 55:548-551, 2002.)

Survival after a diagnosis of colorectal cancer in the elderly is disproportionately poor in comparison to that in younger patients. Methodology taking into account competing causes of death establishes that elderly patients die more frequently of colorectal cancer, over and above expected age-related rates of death. In elderly patients with both colon and rectal cancer, 5-year mortality after surgical resection is 1.5 to 2.5 times greater than that in younger patients.[44] The poorer survival seen in elderly patients with colorectal cancer may be a result of the reduced use of adjuvant therapy in this group. Despite demonstrated efficacy and tolerance, elderly patients with stage III colon cancer are less likely to receive adjuvant chemotherapy. Although 80% of patients aged 65 to 69 with stage III colorectal cancer receive adjuvant chemotherapy, only 28% of those aged 75 to 79 receive this recommended treatment. Similarly, there is decreased use of radiation therapy for elderly patients with stage II and III rectal cancer.

Screening

Screening for colorectal cancer in average-risk individuals begins at age 50; however, no upper age limit for colorectal cancer screening has been determined. Recommendations for screening include annual fecal occult blood testing and flexible sigmoidoscopy every 5 years (with full colonoscopy for positive occult blood or adenomatous polyps on flexible sigmoidoscopy) or colonoscopy every 5 to 10 years. Because elderly patients have an increased incidence of right-sided cancer and more than half of patients with right-sided cancer have no lesions within reach of the flexible sigmoidoscope, colonoscopy may be a more effective screening tool in older patients. The potential benefits of colorectal cancer screening may decrease with age and increasing comorbidity as competing risks for mortality become more prominent. In addition, the potential for harm related to screening, such as colonoscopy-related complications, may increase in older patients and those with significant comorbidity. Therefore, in some patient subgroups, the potential harm related to screening may outweigh any potential benefit in reducing cancer-specific mortality. Although colorectal cancer incidence rates increase with age, the cumulative lifetime risk for colorectal cancer death actually decreases in men and women with advancing age and increasing comorbidity. For example, the risk for colorectal cancer death is 1.8% in men aged 80 to 84 years with average health status versus 2.3% for similar men aged 50 to 54 years. It is assumed that colorectal cancer screening is unlikely to benefit individuals whose life expectancy is less than 5 years. Based on this assumption and published estimates of life expectancy, the following groups would not benefit from colorectal cancer screening: men aged 75 to 84 years with poor health, men 85 years and older with average or poor health, women aged 80 to 89 years with poor health, and women 90 years and older with average or poor health. Older individuals are not to be denied colorectal cancer screening; however, when pondering the decision to screen any older individual for colorectal cancer it is crucial to understand the patient's comorbid conditions and probable 5-year survival.

Surgery

In general, surgical resection is the treatment of choice for resectable colorectal cancer regardless of age. For tumors of the abdominal colon, only prohibitive anesthetic risk secondary to severe comorbidity influences this choice. There has been some concern, however, about the ability of elderly patients to tolerate resectional procedures for low rectal cancers. Such procedures include abdominoperineal resection, low anterior resection, and sphincter-saving coloanal anastomosis. Over the past 15 years, resection plus coloanal anastomosis with a J pouch for low rectal tumors has been more widely accepted. Though technically more demanding than the traditional abdominoperineal resection, coloanal anastomosis provides a sphincter-saving alternative that is well tolerated by the elderly in terms of both operative mortality and postoperative complications. Both are equally effective for cure provided that there is at least a 2-cm distal resection margin. Although abdominoperineal resection obligates patients to a permanent colostomy, coloanal reconstruction can achieve continence in nearly 80% of elderly individuals. Assessment of anal function is extremely important in patient selection for low rectal anastomosis. Fecal incontinence may be far worse for quality of life than a well-controlled end-sigmoid colostomy.

Several studies comparing laparoscopic (LC) with open colectomy (OC) have been completed; however, few studies have been performed in which outcomes in the elderly have been examined. Meta-analysis demonstrates that on average, LC takes more than 30% longer to perform but has an associated morbidity rate at least 30% lower than OC does. This is most significant for wound complications. In the elderly, there is no significant difference between the two groups in perioperative mortality rates, need for blood transfusion, or incidence of reoperation. Gastrointestinal and respiratory recovery is quicker after LC. After LC patients report less pain, require less narcotic analgesia, experience a shorter hospital stay, and are more likely to return to independent status. Adequacy of oncologic clearance is similar in both treatment groups.

Local excision of low-lying rectal cancers may be an option for patients with early-stage cancer with a favorable prognosis. Although the local recurrence rate is significantly higher with local excision, overall 5-year survival is similar. For a frail elderly or high-risk patient, lesser procedures, including transanal excision and fulguration, can provide local control of the tumor without disrupting continence. Local control of rectal tumors with chemoradiation therapy is also possible for management of pain and bleeding in poor-risk patients with metastatic disease and short life expectancy. Recently, the use of colon stents has been advocated to palliate poor surgical candidates with impending obstruction.

Hernia

The lifetime risk for inguinal hernia is 27% for men and 3% for women. More than 600,000 inguinal hernias are repaired every year in the United States. There is a bimodal distribution for the development of inguinal hernia. Most inguinal hernias develop for the first time in patients younger than 1 year and in those aged 55 to 85 years. The estimated incidence of abdominal wall hernia in persons older than 65 is 13 per 1000, with a fourfold to eightfold higher incidence in men than women. In patients older than 70 years, 65% of all hernias are inguinal, 20% are femoral, 10% are ventral, 3% are umbilical, and 1% are esophageal hiatal. Whereas the overwhelming majority of all groin hernias occur in males, 80% of femoral hernias occur in females.[41] The elderly are also at risk for the more occult types of hernias, such as paraesophageal hernias and obturator hernias, that do not become apparent until a complication has occurred.

It is clear that symptomatic groin and umbilical hernias in the elderly should be repaired electively. Open, tension-free mesh repair of inguinal, femoral, and umbilical hernias can be performed as an outpatient procedure under either epidural anesthesia or local anesthesia with IV sedation. Mortality rates are very low, even in patients with concomitant medical disease, and many reports demonstrate mortality rates of 0%. Laparoscopic repair requires a general anesthetic in most cases, takes more operative time to complete, and incurs greater hospital costs. In the elderly, the decreased economic benefit to society of an earlier return to normal activities and work seems to obviate the overall cost benefit of the laparoscopic operation. The trend in most centers is for laparoscopic repair to be restricted to bilateral and recurrent inguinal hernias, for which the results are excellent.[45]

The issue of watchful waiting of asymptomatic and mildly symptomatic hernia remains controversial. A recent randomized study[46] comparing watchful waiting and surgery for minimally symptomatic inguinal hernias, in which a third of the patients were older than 65, found the incarceration rate to be only 1.8 per 1000 cases per year over as long a period as 4.5 years. The authors concluded that watchful waiting was safe. In a similar recent study[47] in which all the patients were older than 55 years, there were several adverse outcomes in the observation group and more than 25% of these patients crossed over to the repair group by 15 months. These authors suggested that repair may improve health and decrease possible serious morbidity. Both studies agree that the incidence of incarceration is low over the several-year period of observation. However, should emergency surgery become necessary in the elderly, particularly the frail elderly, morbidity and mortality rates are high, largely because of the high incidence of bowel incarceration and strangulation found at surgery. Intestinal resection is required in up to 12% to 20% of incarcerated inguinal hernias and as many as 40% of incarcerated femoral hernias.[45] The decision to operate for asymptomatic or mildly symptomatic hernias is made on an individual basis by balancing the patient's concerns with the risks.

However, care should be taken to determine whether the patient has limited activities to avoid mild discomfort. Decreased activity presents much more of a risk to the overall health of most older persons than the operative risk associated with inguinal hernia repair does.

Vascular Surgery

The most frequent peripheral vascular diseases seen in elderly patients are abdominal aortic aneurysms, carotid artery disease, and peripheral arterial occlusive disease. Under elective conditions and in patients with well-managed concomitant disease, vascular surgery remains safe and effective; in some cases, endovascular technology is changing patterns of intervention.

In patients 65 years and older, mortality from elective aneurysm repair is less than 5% despite the high incidence of comorbidity in this age group.[48] Emergency repair for rupture remains associated with an operative mortality rate higher than 50% and an extremely high morbidity rate in those who do survive. Although elective surgery has been shown to be safe, older studies often lead to conservative care for elderly patients. Twenty-five years ago only about half of internists and family practitioners would refer a patient with an aneurysm to surgery, and only half of those would do so for an aneurysm smaller than 8 cm. It is unclear whether that attitude has changed, although there have been many reports in the past 25 years suggesting that aneurysm repair is safe, specifically in octogenarians. It is likely that the increased availability of minimally invasive techniques, such as aortic endograft placement, will encourage more referrals for early aneurysm repair and may even reduce the mortality associated with repair of ruptured aneurysms as experience grows.[49] An early report of endovascular aneurysm repair in octogenarians demonstrated no perioperative deaths or cardiac complications; although the long-term durability of endovascular aneurysm repair is still questionable, the medium-term results appear to be durable and may suit elderly patients with limited life expectancy.

The perception of excess risk in elderly patients by medical professionals is also present in cases of carotid artery disease. As many as 28% of internists do not refer an octogenarian for surgery despite the fact that multiple studies have shown that endarterectomy is safe, has minimal mortality, and can prevent strokes. In patients older than 65 to 80 years, the stroke rate from surgery is 2.8% and the mortality rate is 2.4%. Survival of patients older than 80 after endarterectomy is similar to that in the general population. Similarly, the incidence of neurologic symptoms after endarterectomy is lower than in an unoperated patient (13% versus 33%), and the incidence of late stroke is much lower as well (2% versus 17%), thus confirming the efficacy of endarterectomy in elderly patients. Proper indications in octogenarians are similar to those in younger patients and include high-grade carotid lesions, hemispheric symptoms, and well-controlled concomitant disease.[50] Recent application of endovascular stenting to the carotid artery may provide a less invasive method for treating carotid artery disease.

At present, this procedure is indicated only for high-risk patients or complex technical situations. There is no level I evidence to suggest that stenting should replace open surgery in the routine setting for any patients. In fact, octogenarians have been shown to experience a higher rate of stroke with carotid stenting than with standard carotid endarterectomy.

Peripheral vascular surgery for limb salvage is indicated for ischemic pain at rest, nonhealing ulcers, or frank gangrene. This too can be safely performed in elderly patients. In patients older than 80 years, the mortality rate associated with surgery is 4.6%, and limb salvage rates over a period of 3 to 5 years are 50% to 87%. Five-year graft patency rates have been reported to be better in older than in younger patients with both prosthetic (55% versus 36%) and autologous (82% versus 72%) graft material. Endovascular approaches can also be used in the periphery in elderly patients, with reasonable durability in those with limited life expectancy. Angioplasty of the superficial femoral artery has a 5-year cumulative primary patency rate higher than 50% and a secondary patency rate of 70% in elderly patients in some series. It is unclear whether these results will lead to increased treatment of elderly claudicants as it has in younger patients.

Quality of life and preservation or restoration of functional independence are most important considerations in older patients. Amputation can be performed safely in elderly patients, with rates of perioperative mortality less than 10%. However, long-term survival after amputation is poor, with 1-year survival rates of approximately 50%; independent risk factors for mortality include high-level amputation, congestive heart failure, and inability to ambulate in the community.[51] These functionally poor results of amputation lead many surgeons to continue to offer an aggressive approach to limb salvage in elderly patients.

Cardiothoracic Disease

Cardiovascular disease has been the leading cause of death in the United States for almost 100 years. In the new millennium, cardiovascular disease is still present in approximately 64 million Americans, or 23% of the population.[12] Most deaths attributable to cardiovascular disease occur in elderly patients.

Cardiac surgery is usually a dramatic event for patients and, accordingly, is one of the most frequently studied surgical procedures. Elderly patients have excellent results after cardiac surgery; as minimally invasive treatment of cardiac atherosclerosis changes patterns of referral to cardiac surgeons, patients are becoming older with more frequent and severe comorbid conditions. Nevertheless, the uniformly good results with both coronary artery bypass and valve replacement have encouraged continued performance of cardiac surgery, even in marginal candidates.

Coronary Artery Disease

The number of coronary artery bypass graft (CABG) procedures performed on patients older than 65 years rose from 2.6 operations per 1000 population in 1980 to 13.0 operations per 1000 population in 1993. Over the last decade, with the increasing use of coronary artery stents, the rate in persons older than 65 has fallen to 8.9 per 1000 population, whereas the rate in males older than 75 in 2001 was 11.4 per 1000. Patients who are now referred for bypass usually have more complex disease or have failed alternative procedures. More than 55% of CABG procedures are now performed on patients older than 65 years. As the mortality and morbidity associated with cardiac surgical procedures have decreased, there has been a growing willingness to offer surgical therapy to older patients with reconstructible coronary artery disease. Unfortunately, elderly patients referred for cardiac surgery have a higher incidence of advanced disease (triple-vessel disease, left main or main equivalent disease, and poor left ventricular function) and more symptomatic disease (90% of octogenarians are preoperatively classified as New York Heart Association [NYHA] functional class III or IV) and require emergency or urgent procedures more often.

Comorbid disease must be considered in elderly patients and may be extensive in some patients. Several preoperative risk factors for mortality after coronary bypass surgery have been identified, including an emergency procedure, severe left ventricular dysfunction, mitral insufficiency requiring a combined procedure, NYHA functional class IV, elevated preoperative creatinine, chronic pulmonary disease, anemia (hematocrit <34%), and previous vascular surgery. Further risk factors for morbidity include obesity, diabetes mellitus, aortic stenosis, and cerebrovascular disease. These risk factors must be taken in the context of global patient comorbidity and considered as part of informed decision making for an individual patient. Risks attributable to patient age of 70 to 79 are not significantly differently from those in patients younger than 60 years; however, patients older than 80 years have increased age-associated risk, equivalent to the presence of shock or acute (<6 hours) myocardial infarction.

Even in individuals older than 80 years, coronary artery bypass surgery is associated with an acceptable overall mortality of 7% to 12%, with mortality after elective procedures being lower than 3%. Early elective surgery is clearly preferable to emergency surgery, which is associated with 2 to 10 times higher mortality. Unfortunately, with persistent reluctance to offer elective operations to many elderly patients, some series continue to report a significant percentage, as many as 40%, of elderly patients requiring urgent or emergency operations.

Morbidity after coronary surgery in the elderly is quite high in many series. Pulmonary failure requiring prolonged intubation, neurologic events such as cardiovascular accidents and delirium, and sternal wound infections increase with age and are associated with postoperative mortality. Other complications, including reoperation for bleeding, need for pacemaker insertion, perioperative myocardial infarction, and superficial wound infections, occur with equal frequency in both age groups, although some studies have noted a slightly higher incidence of sternal wound infection in elderly patients.

The effectiveness of coronary artery bypass surgery versus medical management in octogenarians has been assessed in terms of cost per quality life year survival, and good late functional results have been demonstrated in elderly patients.[52] The cost per quality life year saved was only $10,424, less than the cost for many common procedures such as screening mammography. The survival rate in the surgery group was 80% and 69% at 3 and 4 years respectively, whereas in the medical group, comparable survival rates were 64% and 32%. Using a validated health status assessment tool, the EurQol Questionnaire, the authors assessed quality of life in five domains: pain, activity, mobility, self-care, and depression/anxiety. In all areas, quality of life was better in the surgically treated than in the medically treated groups. Quality of life in the group of octogenarians who selected CABG was found to be equal to that of an average 55-year-old in the general population.

Elderly patients with end-stage heart failure have traditionally been excluded from the option of cardiac transplantation because of both the scarcity of donor hearts and an inability to easily tolerate pharmacologic immunosuppression. Recent reports of partial left ventriculectomy are encouraging, with mortality and functional outcome in patients older than 65 years similar to that in younger patients.

Valve Replacement

Since 1975, much data have accumulated that support the safety and efficacy of aortic valve replacement in the elderly. Operative mortality is 3% to 10% (mean, 7.7%), and the long-term survival rate is approximately 75% to 80%. Although mortality in older patients in several series is slightly higher than that in younger patients, most differences were not statistically significant. In addition, the vast majority of elderly patients receiving new aortic valves have great improvement in their quality of life.[53] As many as 90% of elderly patients who were classified as NYHA functional class III or IV preoperatively and survive are reclassified postoperatively as class I or II. Because the average life expectancy for a healthy 70-year-old is approximately 13 years and that for an 80-year-old is approximately 8 years, safe aortic valve replacement surgery is preferable to the 80% 4-year mortality associated with untreated calcific aortic stenosis.

Mitral valve disease in the elderly has been less well investigated, partly because it is less common but also because the natural history is less well defined and the outcome of surgical therapy is less favorable; in one study, operative mortality after mitral valve replacement was 16.7% as opposed to 11.8% for aortic valve replacement in octogenarians.[54] Left ventricular reserve is often compromised in the elderly with mitral insufficiency because of the frequently associated ischemic disease. Low cardiac output is a particular problem after mitral valve replacement. Frequently, both aortic and mitral valve replacement is accompanied by additional procedures. There is some debate about whether valve replacement plus CABG or multiple valve replacement in the very elderly is too risky to justify the combined procedures. Many believe that with appropriate patient selection, even multiple procedures can be performed with relative safety, but the number of patients who meet the selection criteria is small. In centers that perform mitral valvuloplasty to repair the valve in patients with low ejection fractions, results in elderly patients are similar to those in younger patients.

The choice of valve material is also an important consideration in older patients. Mechanical valves are extremely durable but require lifelong anticoagulation. In patients older than 75, the mortality from long-term anticoagulation alone is nearly 10% per year. Bioprosthetic valves do not require anticoagulation and are somewhat less durable, but they may suffice for patients with life expectancy less than a decade.[55]

Lung Cancer

Lung cancer, most commonly either adenocarcinoma or squamous cell carcinoma, remains a leading cause of death in industrialized countries; more than 150,000 deaths are still due to lung cancer in the United States annually. Smoking remains the most important risk factor for lung cancer, and smoking cessation is an appropriate preventive measure for all patients. Appropriate therapy is critically dependent on accurate staging, and CT and ^{18}F-fluorodeoxyglucose positron emission tomography are playing increasing roles in modern diagnosis.

The incidence of non–small cell lung cancer (NSCLC) increases with age. There is still bias that elderly patients with early-stage (I to III) NSCLC do poorly with surgical resection, and thus these patients are often referred for limited resection or radiation therapy; aggressive chemotherapy, particularly platinum-based adjuvant therapy, is often poorly tolerated in elderly patients. Stage IV disease is initially diagnosed in the majority of patients with NSCLC, and they are treated with combined chemotherapy and radiation therapy; however, elderly patients are not generally considered candidates for this therapy. Some recent studies have shown that lower-dose chemotherapy might be safe in elderly patients, but well-performed controlled trials await publication.

Some recent reports suggest improved outcomes in elderly patients after surgical treatment of lung cancer. A retrospective review of 379 elderly patients undergoing surgical therapy for lung cancer between 1985 and 2004 was recently reported from the Mayo Clinic.[56] Operative mortality was 6.3% and was predicted by congestive heart failure and previous myocardial infarction but not by diabetes or renal insufficiency. However, morbidity occurred in 48% of patients and included atrial fibrillation, pneumonia, and retained secretions requiring bronchoscopy. Interestingly, asymptomatic patients were significantly less likely to have a perioperative complication.

Video-assisted thoracic surgery (VATS) is finding increased application in thoracic surgery, with some surgeons performing VATS for lung resection for cancer. The potential for less operating time and blood loss, as well as short hospital length of stay associated with improved recovery time, holds great promise for all patients, especially the elderly. One California group reported a series of 159 octogenarians treated with VATS, the majority (96%) undergoing lobectomy.[57] Mortality was 1.8%, and there were only two conversions to open thoracotomy. Morbidity was 18% and was most commonly due to arrhythmia (5%). The mean hospital length of stay was only 4 days. Results such as these suggest that VATS may increase the number of elderly patients who will be candidates for surgical therapy.

It is likely that future reports will define combinations of adjuvant and neoadjuvant therapy that will increase the number of elderly patients who will be surgical candidates and achieve disease-free survival. However, the outlook for elderly patients with preexisting pulmonary disease or other severe comorbid conditions remains poor.

Trauma

Trauma is currently the fifth leading cause of death in the elderly. Persons older than 65 years account for up to a third of trauma cases and 30% to 40% of trauma deaths, with more recent rates being the highest. Older patients have increased mortality, longer hospital stays, increased morbidity, and worse functional outcomes than younger patients do, even when severity-of-illness scores are lower.[58] Motor vehicle accidents are the most common form of fatal injury in patients younger than 80, and falls are the most frequent fatal injury after the age of 80. Interestingly, the incidence of death from motor vehicle accidents in the elderly is the same whether they are passengers or pedestrians.

Older persons are at increased risk for blunt trauma and its complications. Age-associated central nervous system changes decrease coordination and mobility and increase the risk for accidents. Cerebral atrophy and decreased viscoelastic properties within the cranial vault make the brain more susceptible to blunt injury. Increased bone fragility results in an increased tendency for fracture. Decreased cardiac reserve and inability to increase cardiac output prevent escape from accidents. Concomitant use of drugs such as anticoagulants and antiplatelet agents increases the morbidity associated with traumatic events in elderly patients.

Significant injury can result from even simple falls from a level surface to the ground. The incidence of fracture or serious injury from such a fall is as high as 40% in an older person. After a fall with injury there is significant morbidity. Of those hospitalized after a fall, up to 43% wind up being discharged from the hospital to a nursing facility, and only 50% are alive 1 year later.

Elderly patients have increased morbidity and mortality after head trauma, particularly when taking anticoagulant medications.[59] Older people have increased rates of traumatic brain injury after head trauma and have longer disability. They take much longer to recover from head trauma than younger people do and require more intensive rehabilitation. Blunt head trauma in an elderly person carries particularly high mortality. Mortality in older patients with a Glasgow Coma Scale score of 5 is more than twice that of patients aged 20 to 40 years.

Importantly, only 2% of elderly patients had a favorable recovery as compared with 38% of younger patients.

Injury from burns accounts for 8% of trauma in elderly patients. The elderly are at particular risk for burns because of impaired vision, decreased reaction time, depressed alertness, and decreased sensation of pain. In 81% of elderly burn victims, injuries occurred as a result of actions during ADLs: scalding, cooking accidents with flame, and electrical burns. Although survival from burns is directly related to the total body surface area affected, this is more pronounced in the elderly. In general, burns involving more than 40% of the total body surface area in older persons have a very poor prognosis. Reasons for the increased mortality are concomitant medical disease, burn wound sepsis, and multisystem failure. For survivors of serious burns aged 59 or older, fewer than half are discharged to independent living, a third to assisted living at home, and a fifth to nursing facilities.

Elderly patients, whether they live with relatives or are institutionalized, are at risk for trauma as a result of elder abuse. It is estimated that 5% of elders living in the community are subject to this kind of maltreatment.[60] It has also been shown that only 1 in 13 or 14 cases of elder abuse is reported. Maltreatment of elders can take one or more of six basic forms: physical abuse, sexual abuse, neglect, psychological abuse, financial exploitation, and violation of rights. As the elderly population increases, surgeons treating older trauma victims must learn to detect and report signs of physical and sexual elder abuse, in addition to providing physical care of the patient's injuries, much as they have been mandated to do with children.

Transplantation

In 1946, the first successful renal transplantation was performed. Early results with cadaveric renal transplants in patients older than 45 years were poor. The introduction of cyclosporine in the 1980s led to dramatic improvement, particularly in high-risk patients. As experience at transplant centers has grown and the population of persons older than 60 years has increased, the number of elderly patients who could potentially benefit from transplantation has also increased.[61] In fact, over the past 2 decades the rate of persons older than 65 requiring renal replacement therapy in the United States has doubled and the rate in those older than 75 years has tripled.

The results of renal transplantation in the elderly in terms of survival and quality of life justify extension of the age limit for this procedure. In one recent study[62] of renal transplantation, patients older than 60 years had more delayed graft function and longer initial hospital stay, but the incidence of acute rejection episodes was lower. Patient survival, graft survival, and death-censored graft survival did not differ between older and younger patients, although follow-up of older patients was shorter (4.1 versus 6.7 years). The main cause of organ loss in older patients was death with a functioning kidney. Other studies show that 10-year allograft survival is higher in

elderly patients than in patients younger than 60 years. However, the survival rate at 10 years in those older than 60 is 44% versus 81% for younger patients. Given the shortage of organ donors, the ethics of transplantation in elderly individuals with a higher likelihood of dying with a functioning allograft is questioned, although many believe that the evidence does not justify denying transplantation on the basis of age alone.

The number of older persons requiring liver transplantation has also increased. The percentage of liver recipients older than 65 has increased from 4.9% in 1991 to 6.8% in 2002. Although age has been identified as a risk factor for a poorer outcome after liver transplantation, when patients are in better health (i.e., living at home at the time of transplantation), age is not a factor. Many studies support liver transplantation in low-risk, properly evaluated seniors.[63]

As the number of elderly transplant patients has increased, one important factor has emerged. The rate of both acute and chronic rejection is clearly lower in older patients. This has been attributed to the overall decline in immunocompetence with age. However, this decline also renders elderly patients more susceptible to infection and malignancy. The high incidence of lymphoproliferative disorders in older transplant patients in general and the high rate of recurrent hepatitis C in older liver transplant patients in particular may be the result of excessive immunosuppression in this already compromised population. Decreasing immunosuppression in older patients may in fact improve both long- and short-term survival.

Selected References

Chang AM, Halter JB: Aging and insulin secretion. Am J Physiol Endocrinol Metab 284:E7-E12, 2003.

> Excellent review of the effects of aging on glucose regulation.

Dasgupta M, Drumbrell AC: Preoperative risk assessment for delirium after noncardiac surgery: A systematic review. J Am Geriatr Soc 54:1578-1589, 2006.

> Delirium is associated with a poor outcome after surgical procedures in the elderly. This is a thorough review of the factors associated with postoperative delirium.

Eagle KA, Berger PB, Calkins H, et al: ACC/AHA guideline update for perioperative cardiovascular evaluation for noncardiac surgery—executive summary: A report of the American College of Cardiology/American Heart Association Task Force on Practice Guidelines (Committee to Update the 1996 Guidelines on Perioperative Cardiovascular Evaluation for Noncardiac Surgery). J Am Coll Cardiol 39:542-553, 2002.

> This is the updated guideline for the preoperative cardiac evaluation of patients undergoing noncardiac surgery.

Gerson MC, Hurst JM, Hertzberg VS, et al: Prediction of cardiac and pulmonary complications related to elective abdominal and noncardiac thoracic surgery in geriatric patients. Am J Med 88:101-107, 1990.

> Classic reference demonstrating the predictive value of exercise tolerance in assessing preoperative cardiopulmonary risk in the elderly.

Giordano S, Hortobagyi G, Kau SW, et al: Breast cancer treatment guidelines in older women. J Clin Oncol 23:783-791, 2005.

> This study demonstrates how even in a single cancer center, age older than 75 years was associated with a decrease in concordance with treatment guidelines for breast cancer.

Smetana GW: Perioperative pulmonary assessment of the older adult. Clin Geriatr Med 19:35-55, 2003.

> Excellent review of the perioperative evaluation of elderly patients.

Sollano JA, Rose EA, Williams DL, et al: Cost-effectiveness of coronary artery bypass surgery in octogenarians. Ann Surg 228:297-306, 1998.

> Excellent study of the cost-effectiveness of coronary bypass grafting in terms of quality life years saved. This is a good example of how appropriate studies can clarify the value of major surgery in the elderly.

Van den Berghe G, Wouters P, Weekers F, et al: Intensive insulin therapy in critically ill patients. N Engl J Med 345:1350-1367, 2001.

> This is the landmark study that demonstrated the value of tight glucose control for surgical critical care patients.

Westendorp RGJ: What is healthy aging in the 21st century? Am J Clin Nutr 83(Suppl)404S-409S, 2006.

> Interesting overview of longevity and aging.

References

1. Westendorp RGJ: What is healthy aging in the 21st century? J Clin Nutr 83(Suppl):404S-409S, 2006.
2. Rowe JW: Health care myths at the end of life. Bull Am Coll Surg 81:11-18, 1996.
3. Saltzstein SL, Behling CA: 5- and 10-year survival in cancer patients aged 90 and older: A study of 37,318 patients from SEER. J Surg Oncol 81:113-116, 2002.
4. Hamel MB, Henderson WG, Khuri SF, Daley J: Surgical outcomes for patients aged 80 and older: Morbidity and mortality from major noncardiac surgery. J Am Geriatr Soc 53:424-429, 2005.
5. Taffett GE: Physiology of aging. In Cassel CK, Leipzig RM, Cohen HJ, et al (eds): Geriatric Medicine. An Evidence-Based Approach, 4th ed. New York, Springer-Verlag, 2003.
6. Lewis JF, Maron BJ: Cardiovascular consequences of the aging process. Cardiovasc Clin 22:25-34, 1992.
7. Tresch DD, McGough MF: Heart failure with normal systolic function: A common disorder in older people. J Am Geriatr Soc 43:1035-1042, 1995.
8. Campbell EJ: Physiologic changes in respiratory function. In Rosenthal RA, Zenilman ME, Katlic MR (eds): Principles and Practice of Geriatric Surgery. New York, Springer-Verlag, 2000.
9. Luckey AF, Parsa CJ: Fluids and electrolytes in the aged. Arch Surg 138:1055-1060, 2003.
10. Schmucker DL: Age-related changes in liver structure and function: Implications for disease? Exp Gerontol 40:650-659, 2005.
11. Pawelec G, Koch S, Franceschi C, Wikby A: Human immunosenescence. Does it have an infectious component? Ann N Y Acad Sci 1067:56-65, 2006.
12. Roubenoff R: Catabolism of aging. Is it an inflammatory process? Curr Opin Clin Nutr Metab Care 6:295-299, 2003.
13. Chang AM, Halter JB: Aging and insulin secretion. Am J Physiol Endocrinol Metab 284:E7-E12, 2003.
14. Van den Berghe G, Wouters P, Weekers F, et al: Intensive insulin therapy in critically ill patients. N Engl J Med 345:1350-1367, 2001.
15. Robinson B, Beghe C: Cancer screening in older patients. Clin Geriatr Med 13:97-118, 1997.
16. Eagle KA, Berger PB, Calkins H, et al: ACC/AHA guideline update for perioperative cardiovascular evaluation for noncardiac surgery—executive summary: A report of the American College of Cardiology/American Heart Association Task Force on Practice Guidelines (Committee to Update the 1996 Guidelines on Perioperative Cardiovascular Evaluation for Noncardiac Surgery). J Am Coll Cardiol 39:542-553, 2002.
17. Smetana GW: Perioperative pulmonary assessment of the older adult. Clin Geriatr Med 19:35-55, 2003.
18. Lawrence VA, Cornell JE, Smetana GW; American College of Physicians: Strategies to reduce postoperative pulmonary complications after noncardiothoracic surgery: Systematic review for the American College of Physicians. Ann Intern Med 144:596-608,2006.
19. Khuri SF, Daley J, Henderson W, et al: Risk adjustment of the postoperative mortality rate for the comparative assessment of the quality of surgical care: Results of the National Veterans Affairs Surgical Risk Study. J Am Coll Surg 185:315-327, 1997.
20. Lawrence VA, Hazuda HP, Cornell JE, et al: Functional independence after major abdominal surgery in the elderly. J Am Coll Surg 199:762-772, 2004.
21. Gerson MC, Hurst JM, Hertzberg VS, et al: Prediction of cardiac and pulmonary complications related to elective abdominal and noncardiac thoracic surgery in geriatric patients. Am J Med 88:101-107, 1990.
22. Borson S, Scanlan JM, Watanabe J, et al: Simplifying detection of cognitive impairment: Comparison of the Mini-Cog and Mini-Mental State Examination in a multiethnic sample. J Am Geriatr Soc 53:871-874, 2005.
23. Dasgupta M, Drumbrell AC: Preoperative risk assessment for delirium after noncardiac surgery: A systematic review. J Am Geriatr Soc 54:1578-1589, 2006.
24. Marcantonio ER, Goldman L, Orav JE, et al: The association of intraoperative factors with the development of postoperative delirium. Am J Med 105:380-384, 1998.
25. Kagansky N, Berner Y, Koren-Morag N, et al: Poor nutritional habits are predictors of poor outcome in very old hospitalized patients. Am J Clin Nutr 82:784-791, 2005.
26. Persson MD, Brismar KE, Katzarski KS, et al: Nutritional status using mini nutritional assessment and subjective global assessment predict mortality in geriatric patients. J Am Geriatr Soc 50:1996-2002, 2002.
27. Marrelli D, Roviello F, De Stefano A, et al: Surgical treatment of gastrointestinal carcinomas in octogenarians: Risk factors for complications and long-term outcome. Eur J Surg Oncol 26:371-376, 2000.
28. American Geriatirc Society Clinical Practice Committee: AGS position statement: Breast cancer screening in older women. J Am Geriatr Soc 48:842-844, 2000.
29. Diab SG, Elledge RM, Clark GM: Tumor characteristics and clinical outcome of elderly women with breast cancer. J Natl Cancer Inst 92:550-556, 2000.
30. Giordano S, Hortobagyi G, Kau SW, et al: Breast cancer treatment guidelines in older women. J Clin Oncol 23:783-791, 2005.
31. Holmes CE, Muss HB: Diagnosis and treatment of breast cancer in the elderly. CA Cancer J Clin 53:227-244, 2003.

32. Laurberg P, Andersen S, Pedersen IB, Carle A: Hypothyroidism in the elderly: Pathophysiology, diagnosis and treatment. Drugs Aging 22:23-38, 2005.

33. Diez JJ: Hyperthyroidism in patients older than 55 years: An analysis of etiology and management. Gerontology 49:316-323, 2003.

34. Pruhs AM, Starling JR, Chen H: Changing trends for surgery in elderly patients with hyperparathyroidism at a single institution. J Surg Res 127:59-62, 2005.

35. Pilotto A, Franceschi M, Leandro G, et al: Clinical features of reflux esophagitis in older people: A study of 840 consecutive patients. J Am Geriatr Soc 54:1537-1542, 2006.

36. Tedesco P, Lobo PM, Way L, Patti MG: Laparoscopic fundoplication in elderly patients with gastroesophageal reflux disease. Arch Surg 141:289-292, 2006.

37. Brock J, Sauaia A, Ahnen D, et al: Process of care and outcomes for elderly patients hospitalized with peptic ulcer disease. JAMA 286:1985-1993, 2001.

38. Petrowky H, Clavien PA: Should we deny surgery for malignant hepato-pancreatico-biliary tumors to elderly patients? World J Surg 29:1093-1100, 2005.

39. Bingener J, Richards ML, Schwesinger WH, et al: Laparoscopic cholecystectomy for elderly patients. Gold standard for the golden years? Arch Surg 138:526-531, 2003.

40. Keitzman D, Shalom MI, Konikoff FM: Recurrent symptomatic common duct stones after endoscopic stone extraction in elderly patients. Gastrointest Endosc 64:60-65, 2006.

41. Foster NM, McGory ML, Zingmond DS, Ko CY: Small bowel obstruction: A population-based appraisal. J Am Coll Surg 203:170-176, 2006.

42. Harrell AG, Lincourt AE, Novitsky YW, et al: Advantages of laparoscopic appendectomy in the elderly. Am Surg 72:474-480, 2006.

43. Colorectal Cancer Collaborative Group: Surgery for colorectal cancer in elderly patients: A systematic review. Lancet 356:968-974, 2000.

44. Clark AJ, Stockton D, Elder A, et al: Assessment of outcomes after colorectal cancer resection in the elderly as a rationale for screening and early detection. Br J Surg 91:1345-1351, 2004.

45. Arenal JJ, Rodriguez-Vielba P, Gallo E, Tinoco C: Hernias of the abdominal wall in patients over the age of 70 years. Eur J Surg 46:111-116, 2003.

46. Fitzgibbon RJ, Giobbie-Hurder A, Gibbs JO, et al: Watchful waiting vs repair of inguinal hernia in minimally symptomatic men: A randomized clinical trial. JAMA 295:285-292, 2006.

47. O'Dwyer PJ, Norrie J, Alani A, et al: Observation or operation for patients with an asymptomatic inguinal hernia: A randomized clinical trial. Ann Surg 244:167-173, 2006.

48. Dainese L, Barili F, Spirito R, et al: Abdominal aortic aneurysm repair in octogenarians: Outcomes and predictors. Eur J Vasc Endovasc Surg 31:464-469, 2006.

49. Lange C, Leurs LJ, Buth J, Myhre HO, EUROSTAR collaborators: Endovascular repair of abdominal aortic aneurysm in octogenarians: An analysis based on EUROSTAR data. J Vasc Surg 42:624-630, discussion 630, 2005.

50. Alamowitch S, Eliasziw M, Algra A, et al, for the North American Symptomatic Carotid Endarterectomy Trial (NASCET) Group: Risk, causes and prevention of ischaemic stroke in elderly patients with symptomatic internal-carotid artery stenosis. Lancet 357:1154-1160, 2001.

51. Wong MW: Predictors for mortality after lower-extremity amputations in geriatric patients. Am J Surg 191:443-447, 2006.

52. Sollano JA, Rose EA, Williams DL, et al: Cost-effectiveness of coronary artery bypass surgery in octogenarians. Ann Surg 228:297-306, 1998.

53. Langanay T, Verhoye JP, Ocampo G, et al: Current hospital mortality for aortic valve replacement in octogenarians. J Heart Valve Dis 15:630-637, 2006.

54. Avery GJ 2nd, Ley SJ, Hill JD, et al: Cardiac surgery in the octogenarian: Evaluation of risk, cost, and outcome. Ann Thorac Surg 71:591-596, 2001.

55. Suttie SA, Jamieson WR, Burr LH, Germann E: Elderly valve replacement with bioprostheses and mechanical prostheses. Comparison by composites of complications. J Cardiovasc Surg (Torino) 47:191-199, 2006.

56. Dominguez-Ventura A, Allen MS, Cassivi SD, et al: Lung cancer in octogenarians: Factors affecting morbidity and mortality after pulmonary resection. Ann Thorac Surg 82:1175-1179, 2006.

57. McVay CL, Pickens A, Fuller C, et al: VATS anatomic pulmonary resection in octogenarians. Am Surg 71:791-793, 2005.

58. Grossman MG, Scaff DW, Miller D, et al: Functional outcomes in octogenarian trauma. J Trauma 55:26-32, 2003.

59. Franko J, Kish KO, O'Connell BG, et al: Advanced age and preinjury warfarin anticoagulation increase the risk of mortality after head trauma. J Trauma 61:107-110, 2006.

60. Colins KA: Elder maltreatment: A review. Arch Pathol Lab Med 130:1290-1296, 2006.

61. Feng S, Tomlanovich SL, Fraser K, et al: Transplantation in elderly patients. In Rosenthal RA, Zenilman ME, Katlic MR (eds): Principles and Practice of Geriatric Surgery. New York, Springer-Verlag, 2000.

62. Pedroso S, Martins L, Fonseca I, et al: Renal transplantation in patients over 60 years of age: A single-center experience. Transpl Proc 38:1885-1889, 2006.

63. Keswani RN, Ahmed A, Keefe EB: Older age and liver transplantation: A review. Liver Transpl 10:957-967, 2004.

CHAPTER 17

Morbid Obesity

William O. Richards, MD and Bruce D. Schirmer, MD

The surgical treatment of morbid obesity is known as *bariatric surgery*. It has its origin in the 1950s, when malabsorptive operations were first performed for severe hyperlipidemia syndromes. Subsequently, jejunoileal bypass to produce weight loss began to be performed sporadically during the 1960s, then more frequently in the 1970s. This operation, however, produced unacceptable metabolic complications. Bariatric surgeons developed myriad operations, few of which proved effective in the long term for providing safe and durable weight loss.

This process has clearly pointed out two very unique aspects of the field of bariatric surgery. The first is that this surgery involves the alteration of metabolic processes, not just simply weight loss. The effects of any bariatric operation on metabolic processes need to be fully understood before the operation's effectiveness and safety can be determined. The second is that long-term follow-up is required to adequately assess the merits of

an operation. Durability of weight loss is as important, ultimately, as the amount of weight loss achieved. Similarly, some consequences of an operation may be fully appreciated only after a long period of follow-up.

OBESITY: THE MAGNITUDE OF THE PROBLEM

Morbid obesity is defined as being either 100 lb above ideal body weight, twice ideal body weight, or a body mass index (BMI, measured as weight in kilograms divided by height in meters squared) of $40 \, kg/m^2$. The latter definition is more accepted internationally and has essentially replaced the former ones for all practical and scientific purposes. A consensus conference by the National Institutes of Health (NIH) in 1991 suggested that the term *severe obesity* is more appropriate for defining people of such size.[1] This term shall be used interchangeably with *morbid obesity* in the remainder of this chapter.

It is estimated that approximately 5% of the U.S. adult population, or more than 23 million people, are morbidly obese or clinically severely obese,[2] the highest percentage of obesity in the population of any country. Patients undergoing bariatric surgery in the United States have average BMIs that are significantly higher than those reported in Europe. Australia, however, is not far behind, according to Australian bariatric surgeons. Even Europe, where severely obese individuals are not common in crowds, is now experiencing an overall enlargement of the population. Studies of adolescent obesity have estimated the incidence of obesity (40% above ideal body weight) as being in the 35% range for adolescents in the United States but more than 20% in most European countries. The problem is also growing at an alarmingly rapid rate in the United States. In 1985, when statistics of national obesity were first measured by the Centers for Disease Control and Prevention according to individual states, many states had no such data available. Of the roughly half that did, more than half reported a less than

10% incidence of people with a BMI greater than 30 kg/m². By 1990, when most states' data were known, 60% of the states reported BMI higher than 30 kg/m² in more than 10% of the population. By 1995, half the states had a greater than 15% incidence of BMI higher than 30 kg/m². By 2000, 21 states reported that incidence had risen to higher than 20%, with all but 1 of the remaining states having an incidence greater than 15%.[3] This alarming rate of increasing obesity outstrips any theory that the disease has a solely genetic component to it.

Obesity is estimated to cause 280,000 deaths annually in the United States, whereas the total number of deaths annually from both breast and colon cancer is only about 90,000 per year.[3] After tobacco use, obesity is the second leading cause of preventable death in the United States and is second to smoking on the list of preventable factors responsible for increased health care costs. It is a sobering thought to realize that a 25-year-old morbidly obese man has a 22% reduction in life expectancy, or 12 years of life lost, when compared with a normal-sized man.[3] There is speculation that within the next decade, obesity may overtake tobacco as the leading cause of preventable medical expense in the United States.

PATHOPHYSIOLOGY AND ASSOCIATED MEDICAL PROBLEMS

The pathophysiology of severe obesity is poorly understood. Debate is ongoing regarding the relative genetic versus environmental components of the disease. There is a clear familial predisposition; it is rare for a single family member to have severe obesity. The rapid increase in obesity from 1980 to 2006 emphasizes the considerable environmental component that contributes to the problem as well.

Although there is no definitive answer to the pathophysiology of severe obesity, it is clear that a severely obese individual has, in general, persistent hunger that is not satiated by amounts of food that satisfy the nonobese. This lack of satiety or maintenance of satiety may be the single most important factor in the process. The capacity to eat large amounts is greatly increased in the morbidly obese. Others eat or "nibble" for prolonged periods of the day, usually later in the day, with resultant increased caloric intake greatly in excess of metabolic needs.

Basic scientific understanding of the roles played by hormones, peptides, or other factors on satiety is incomplete. Cholecystokinin and ghrelin, produced largely in the proximal part of the stomach by the presence of food, are involved in satiety. Increased levels of ghrelin seem to produce increased food intake, and increased levels develop in individuals following low-calorie diets. Patients with gastric inflow restricted but allowing food to pass through the stomach have normal to elevated ghrelin levels postoperatively. In contrast, patients undergoing gastric bypass probably have suppressed postoperative levels of ghrelin,[4] although measurements have differed. The role of ghrelin in the lack of hunger after gastric bypass or recovery of appetite is not clear.

Morbid obesity is a metabolic disease associated with numerous medical problems, some of which are virtually unknown in the absence of obesity. Box 17-1 lists the most common. These problems must be carefully considered when one is contemplating offering a patient weight reduction surgery. The most frequent problem is the combination of arthritis and degenerative joint disease, present in at least 50% of patients seeking surgery for severe obesity. The incidence of sleep apnea is high. Asthma is present in more than 25%, hypertension in more than 30%, diabetes in more than 20%, and gastroesophageal reflux in 20% to 30% of patients. The incidence of these conditions increases with the duration of severe obesity and age.

The *metabolic syndrome* includes type 2 diabetes mellitus, impaired glucose tolerance, dyslipidemia, and hypertension. Patients with this constellation of problems are generally obese, with central body obesity being the primary body feature. The syndrome is thought to result in impaired hepatic uptake of insulin, systemic hyperinsulinemia, and subsequent tissue resistance to insulin.

Not listed in Box 17-1 are the associated societal discriminatory problems that severely obese individuals face. Public facilities in terms of seating, doorways, and restroom facilities often make access to events held in such settings unavailable to a severely obese person. Travel on public transportation is sometimes difficult if not impossible. Employment discrimination clearly exists for these individuals. Finally, the combination of low self-esteem, a frequent history of sexual or physical abuse, and these social difficulties coalesce to create a very high incidence of depression in the severely obese patient population.

MEDICAL VERSUS SURGICAL THERAPY

Medical therapy for severe obesity has limited short-term success and almost nonexistent long-term success. Once severely obese, the likelihood that a person will lose enough weight by dietary means alone and remain at a BMI below 35 kg/m² is estimated at 3% or less. The NIH consensus conference recognized that for this patient population, medical therapy has been uniformly unsuccessful in treating the problem.[1]

Despite this limited success, it is generally agreed that a severely obese patient needs to be given the chance to comply with a medically supervised diet program to see whether any success can be achieved. A 10% weight loss attained over a period of months at a rate of 0.5 to 2 lb/wk is the initial goal of medical therapy. Maintenance of the weight loss for 6 months defines the initial medical success with medical therapy (NIH), and further weight loss through a reduction in calories and increase in physical activity is encouraged. Insurance funding for surgery has traditionally been linked to such an attempt or, for some insurance companies, a well-documented history of several such attempts. However, data showing any efficacy of the need for a prolonged diet attempt as positively influencing outcomes after bariatric surgery are lacking.

Very low-calorie diets fall into two categories: those that primarily restrict fat intake and those that primarily restrict carbohydrate intake. Both diets produce weight loss that is insufficient to affect any major change in health status.

Pharmacologic therapy in 2007 focused on two medications. Sibutramine blocks presynaptic receptor uptake of both norepinephrine and serotonin, thereby potentiating their anorexic effect in the central nervous system. Orlistat inhibits pancreatic lipase and thereby reduces absorption of up to 30% of ingested dietary fat. A maximum weight loss of up to 10% of body weight has been noted in unselected individuals taking either or both drugs; however, weight is regained within 12 to 18 months.[5] For a severely obese individual, neither drug has proved to be effective therapy alone.

PREOPERATIVE EVALUATION AND SELECTION

Eligibility

Preoperative selection of patients for weight reduction surgery is based strictly on currently accepted NIH guidelines.[1] Patients must have a BMI greater than 40 kg/m^2 without associated comorbid medical conditions or a BMI greater than 35 kg/m^2 with an associated comorbid medical problem. They must have also failed dietary therapy. Beyond this, the NIH guidelines are not specific. However, it has been our experience that several practical criteria must also be used as guidelines for indications for surgery, including psychiatric stability, motivated attitude, and ability to comprehend the nature of the operation and its resultant changes in eating behavior and lifestyle. The criteria used at our institutions for eligibility for bariatric surgery are given in Box 17-2. An inability to fulfill these criteria is a contraindication to bariatric surgery.

One criterion not listed in Box 17-2 that unfortunately is often a significant issue for a severely obese patient is insurance coverage for the operation. The cost of hospitalization alone for bariatric surgery can easily approach $20,000 and may be significantly higher if any complications arise. This figure makes the cost prohibitive for most individuals without insurance coverage. The criteria of individual insurance companies are as varied as the number of companies in existence. The Centers for Medicare and Medicaid Services (CMS), the federal agency that sets Medicare guidelines, has recently established criteria for coverage of open and laparoscopic gastric bypass, laparoscopic adjustable gastric banding (AGB), and duodenal switch (DS) operations.[6] A controversial aspect of the ruling is the requirement that bariatric surgery be performed only by surgeons in hospitals that are designated as either Centers of Excellence by the American Society of Bariatric Surgeons or level I centers by the American College of Surgeons. These unique requirements for Medicare beneficiaries were at least partly due to concern by policymakers that the morbidity and mortality associated with bariatric surgery was high and that the explosive growth in the number of hospitals and

---

Box 17-1 Medical Conditions Associated With Severe Obesity

Cardiovascular

Hypertension
Sudden cardiac death
Cardiomyopathy
Venous stasis disease
Deep venous thrombosis
Pulmonary hypertension
Right-sided heart failure

Pulmonary

Obstructive sleep apnea
Hypoventilation syndrome of obesity
Asthma

Metabolic

Type 2 diabetes
Hyperlipidemia
Hypercholesterolemia
Nonalcoholic steatotic hepatitis

Gastrointestinal

Gastroesophageal reflux disease
Cholelithiasis

Musculoskeletal

Degenerative joint disease
Lumbar disk disease
Osteoarthritis
Ventral hernias

Genitourinary

Stress urinary incontinence
End-stage renal disease (secondary to diabetes and hypertension)

Gynecologic

Menstrual irregularities

Skin/Integumentary System

Fungal infections
Boils, abscesses

Oncologic

Cancer of the uterus, breast, colon, kidney, prostate

Neurologic/Psychiatric

Pseudotumor cerebri
Depression
Low self-esteem
Stroke

Social/Societal

History of physical abuse
History of sexual abuse
Discrimination for employment
Social discrimination

Box 17-2   Indications for Bariatric Surgery

Patients must meet the following criteria for consideration for bariatric surgery:

- BMI >40 kg/m² or BMI >35 kg/m² with an associated medical comorbidity worsened by obesity
- Failed dietary therapy
- Psychiatrically stable without alcohol dependence or illegal drug use
- Knowledgeable about the operation and its sequelae
- Motivated individual
- Medical problems not precluding probable survival from surgery

---

Box 17-3   The Bariatric Multidisciplinary Team

Surgeon
Assisting surgeon
Nutritionist
Anesthesiologist
Operating room nurse
Operating room scrub tech/nurse
Nurse care coordinator/educator
Secretary/administrator
Psychiatrist/psychologist
Primary care physician
Medical specialists for cardiac, pulmonary, gastrointestinal, endocrine, musculoskeletal, and neurologic conditions as indicated

---

surgeons performing the operations did not match the hospital oversight of these procedures and the resulting complications. Data substantiating these allegations have never been published. Regardless, this marks a watershed moment in surgery, where increasingly payers are demanding that surgeons and hospitals meet stringent requirements for infrastructure, training of personnel, and ultimately, results of the procedures.

Medical contraindications to bariatric surgery are not clear. All patients with comorbid conditions are at greater risk. The surgeon must ensure that these risks are well understood by all patients before bariatric surgery, especially those at high risk. Ideally, several family members are included in these discussions. There are certain individuals who have end-stage organ dysfunction of the heart, lungs, or both. These patients are unlikely to gain the benefit of longevity and improved health.

Patients who cannot walk have greater risk than those who can ambulate, even for short distances. Although nonambulatory status is not an absolute contraindication to surgery, it does place the patient at increased risk for deep venous thrombosis (DVT), pulmonary failure, and sacral decubitus ulcers, among other problems.

Patients who weigh more than 600 lb are at increased risk for mortality and have more complications. Many options for diagnostic testing, such as computed tomography (CT), are exceeded by this weight limit. At this weight, operating room tables, moving and lift equipment and teams, blood pressure cuffs, sequential compression device (SCD) boots, and any sort of invasive bedside procedures such as central venous catheters become extraordinarily difficult or problematic. It has been our practice to strongly encourage patients weighing more than 600 lb to lose weight down to that level by nonoperative methods, even if it means enforced hospitalization.

Prader-Willi syndrome is an absolute contraindication. No surgical therapy affects the constant need to eat in these patients.

Age is a controversial contraindication to bariatric surgery. For adolescents, most pediatric/bariatric surgeons recommend that the operation be performed after the major growth spurt (mid to late teens), thus allowing increased maturity on the part of the patient. Simple restrictive operations are thought to be most appropriate

for patients in this age group. In the United States, although the laparoscopic AGB procedure (LAP-BAND) has been approved by the Food and Drug Administration (FDA) only for patients 18 years or older, several groups have modest experiences using this device under FDA guidelines.[7] Increasing experience will be required to determine which operation is most effective in adolescents.

Although in our practice we have generally set the age of 60 as a rough cutoff for performing gastric bypass, patients between the ages of 60 and 65 have been individually evaluated. Such evaluations focus on the patient's relative physiologic age and potential for longevity rather than chronologic age. The duration and degree of obesity are the most important factors in evaluating an older patient. In general, the longer and more severe the degree of obesity, the more comorbid medical problems exist and the lower the potential for such individuals to benefit from bariatric surgery.

Preoperative Evaluation

Preoperative assessment of a bariatric surgical patient involves two distinct areas. One is a specific preoperative assessment of candidacy for bariatric surgery and evaluation for comorbid conditions. The second is a general assessment and preoperative preparation as for any major abdominal surgery, which is discussed in depth in Chapter 12 of this textbook.

General Bariatric Preoperative Evaluation and Preparation

A team approach is required for optimal care of a morbidly obese patient. Box 17-3 lists the key personnel for the bariatric multidisciplinary team.

Box 17-4 summarizes the steps and tests routinely performed for the preoperative evaluation of bariatric patients in the authors' clinics. After a complete history and physical examination at the initial assessment, arterial blood gas analysis is performed in selected patients, upper endoscopy in patients with symptomatic gastroesophageal reflux disease (GERD) or other upper digestive symptoms, and ultrasound of the gallbladder.

Proper preoperative patient education is essential, and attendance at educational sessions is mandatory. Family members are encouraged to attend. After preoperative testing is completed, a final counseling session with the surgeon and an education session with the nurse educator and nutritionist are held.

A first-generation cephalosporin, in a dose appropriate for weight, is given preoperatively, and antibiotics are continued for only 24 hours. Three major measures are used for prophylaxis against DVT and pulmonary embolism: ambulation within 4 to 6 hours of surgery, SCD stockings or shoe sleeves, and subcutaneous low-molecular-weight heparin on call in the operating room and then administered twice daily until discharge. High-risk patients (e.g., those with history of DVT, venous stasis ulcers, known or highly suspected pulmonary hypertension, hypoventilation syndrome of obesity, or a need for reoperation during the initial hospitalization) are given subcutaneous injections of heparin at home for a full 2-week course. Prophylactic vena cava filters are inserted, if possible on a temporary basis, in patients at extremely high risk for DVT and pulmonary embolism. Data support the use of preoperative antibiotics, but no data have established the optimal regimen for DVT prophylaxis. Despite aggressive prophylactic programs, pulmonary embolism remains one of the most common causes of death after bariatric surgery.

Evaluation of Specific Comorbid Conditions

Cardiovascular evaluation of a bariatric patient must include a history of recent chest pain and functional assessment of activity in relation to cardiac function. Patients with a history of recent chest pain or a change in exercise tolerance need to undergo a formal cardiology assessment, including stress testing as indicated. We almost never resort to invasive central monitoring with a Swan-Ganz catheter because central venous and pulmonary hypertension is the norm and must not be interpreted as volume overload. The use of transesophageal echocardiography intraoperatively is occasionally helpful in patients with cardiomyopathy.

Pulmonary assessment includes a search for obstructive sleep apnea. A 32% incidence of sleep apnea has been reported in morbidly obese individuals undergoing bariatric surgery.[8] A history of falling asleep while driving or while at work or a history of feeling tired after a night's sleep, coupled with a history of snoring or even witnessed apnea, is strongly suggestive of the condition. Patients with suggestive histories of clinically significant sleep apnea need to undergo preoperative sleep study testing. If found to have the condition, use of a continuous or bilevel positive airway pressure apparatus postoperatively while sleeping can eliminate the stressful periods of hypoxia that would otherwise result in these patients. Though tolerated under normal circumstances, these hypoxic episodes in the immediate postoperative period are more dangerous because other factors affecting hemodynamic stability are at work.

Reactive asthma is another common problem of the severely obese and one that is under-recognized. It requires less preoperative preparation in terms of testing than sleep apnea does and is less dangerous.

Box 17-4 Preoperative Evaluation

Before the Clinic Visit

- Documented, medically supervised diet
- Counseling and referral from the primary care physician
- Reading a comprehensive written brochure and/or attendance at a seminar regarding operative procedures, expected results, and potential complications

Initial Clinic Visit

- Group presentation on information in the booklet
- Group presentation on preoperative and postoperative nutritional issues by the nutritionist
- Individual assessment by the surgeon's team
- Individual counseling session with the surgeon
- Individual counseling session with the nutritionist
- Screening blood tests

Subsequent Events/Evaluations

- Full psychological assessment and evaluation as indicated
- Medical specialist evaluations as indicated
- Insurance approval for coverage of the procedure
- Screening flexible upper endoscopy as indicated
- Screening ultrasound of the gallbladder (if present)
- Arterial blood gas analysis as indicated

Subsequent Clinic Visits

- Counseling session with the surgeon (including selection of the date for surgery)
- Education session with the nurse educator
- Preoperative evaluation by the anesthesiologist
- Final paperwork by the preadmissions center

Hypoventilation syndrome of obesity (pickwickian syndrome) is a diagnosis that is often suspected by the patient's clinical appearance. The condition is usually limited to the super-obese patient population with a BMI higher than $60 \, kg/m^2$. Individuals with this diagnosis have plethoric faces, may appear clinically cyanotic, and clearly exhibit difficulty in normal respiratory efforts at baseline or with mild exertion. Arterial blood gas analysis reveals $PaCO_2$ higher than PaO_2 and an elevated hematocrit. Pulmonary artery pressure is greatly elevated. These patients have extremely high cardiopulmonary morbidity and mortality and are among the few subsets of patients who, in our experience, require planned intensive care admission postoperatively. Prolonged ventilator support is often required, and management of intravascular volume is based on the patient's baseline status.

Because there is a considerable incidence of hypertension or diabetes in patients with concomitant renal disease, the serum creatinine value is an excellent preoperative screening test for baseline renal function.

Musculoskeletal conditions, especially arthritis and degenerative joint disease, are the most common group of comorbid diseases found in severely obese patients. Over half the patients have some form of these conditions, often to an advanced degree. Limited ambulation, joint replacement, severe back pain, and other sequelae are not uncommon. Before surgery, it is important for patients to understand that any preexisting structural damage cannot be reversed by weight loss. Fortunately, significant weight loss often alleviates or even reverses the chronic pain or disability from such conditions.

Metabolic problems are common in severely obese patients, particularly hyperlipidemia, hypercholesterolemia, and type 2 diabetes mellitus. All are easily screened for by simple blood tests. Twenty percent to 30% of severely obese patients undergoing bariatric surgery have clinically significant type 2 diabetes. Diabetes needs to be controlled preoperatively to reduce the incidence of perioperative morbidity.

Skin must be examined for fungal infection and venous stasis changes. Sugerman and colleagues[9] report that venous stasis disease is associated with a greatly increased incidence of postoperative DVT.

Umbilical or ventral hernias may be present. Decisions on how to best deal with large hernias must be made preoperatively because the approach and incision may be affected by the presence of hernias.

Cholelithiasis is the most prevalent of the several gastrointestinal conditions and must be sought before bariatric surgery. Gallstone formation occurs during periods of rapid weight loss. The incidence of gallstone or sludge formation after gastric bypass is approximately 30%. If gallstones are present, most surgeons agree that cholecystectomy needs to be performed simultaneously with the bariatric surgery. For patients undergoing malabsorptive operations, gallstone formation is so frequent that prophylactic cholecystectomy is a standard part of these procedures. However, for restrictive operations, screening ultrasound is recommended, particularly in patients undergoing Roux-en-Y gastric bypass (RYGB), because endoscopic retrograde cholangiopancreatography is not possible. Ursodeoxycholic acid, 300 mg twice daily for 6 months postoperatively, reduces the incidence of gallstone formation to 3% in patients who follow this treatment plan.[10] Our current recommendations for patients undergoing laparoscopic bariatric surgery are simultaneous cholecystectomy if gallstones are present and ursodiol therapy for 6 months after surgery if the gallbladder is normal.

GERD is common in severely obese patients because of the increased abdominal pressure and shortened lower esophageal sphincter. Preoperative upper endoscopy is indicated in all patients who have GERD to detect Barrett's esophagus and the presence of hiatal hernias and to evaluate the lower part of the stomach in patients undergoing RYGB.[11]

A patient with nonalcoholic steatotic hepatitis (NASH) presents a potential problem. The size of the left lobe of the liver often determines the ability to complete an operation laparoscopically. Patients with known enlarged fatty livers may benefit from caloric restriction, especially carbohydrate restriction, for a period of several weeks preoperatively. Bariatric surgery is beneficial for NASH; weight loss improves the prognosis. NASH is not a contraindication to bariatric surgery if there is no cirrhosis and portal hypertension or hepatocellular decompensation. Liver biopsy is performed at the time of bariatric surgery in any patient whose liver appears abnormal.

SPECIAL EQUIPMENT

Clinic

The clinic for evaluating bariatric patients must be constructed with the needs of the patient in mind. The waiting area must contain comfortable benches with backs, not standard-size chairs. Doorways must be extra wide to accommodate wheelchairs. This is true for bathrooms as well, which must be equipped with toilets on the floor, not mounted on the wall. A scale that can weigh up to 1000 lb is necessary. Large-sized gowns, wide examining tables stable enough for large patients, and wide blood pressure cuffs are needed. A large room with appropriate seating is needed for the patient group education session.

Operating Room

The operating room needs to contain a hydraulically operated operating room table that can accommodate up to 800 lb. Side attachments to widen the table as needed are required. Foam cushioning, extra large SCD stockings, wide and secure padded straps for the abdomen and legs, and a footboard for the operating room table are all essential to safely secure the patient for placement in a steep reverse Trendelenburg position during surgery.

Video telescopic equipment as used for any laparoscopic abdominal procedure is necessary. Two monitors, one near each shoulder, and high-flow insufflators able to maintain pneumoperitoneum are essential.

We have found a 45-degree telescope, extra long staplers, atraumatic graspers, and other instruments to be most useful. Extra long trocars may be needed. An ultrasonic scalpel is most helpful in gastric dissection, particularly along the lesser curvature of the stomach.

A fixed retractor device secured to the operating room table for clamping and holding the liver retractor is also essential. This can pose one of the most difficult technical challenges in patients with a large thick liver. Sometimes, two retractors may be necessary for a large liver.

Box 17-5 Bariatric Operations: Mechanism of Action

Restrictive

Vertical banded gastroplasty (VBG) (historic purposes only)
Laparoscopic adjustable gastric banding (LAGB)

Largely Restrictive/Mildly Malabsorptive

Roux-en-Y gastric bypass (RYGB)

Largely Malabsorptive/Mildly Restrictive

Biliopancreatic diversion (BPD)
Duodenal switch (DS)

OPERATIVE PROCEDURES

Bariatric operations are performed via either an open or laparoscopic approach. Data confirm advantages of the laparoscopic approach, including a reduced rate of incisional hernias and decreased hospitalization.[12]

Bariatric operations produce weight loss as a result of two factors. One is restriction of oral intake. The other is malabsorption of ingested food. Some operations involve the use of only one mechanism for weight loss, whereas others combine the two. Box 17-5 lists the major procedures to be described.

Vertical Banded Gastroplasty

This procedure has now largely been abandoned in favor of other operations because of poor long-term weight loss, a high rate of late stenosis of the gastric outlet, and a tendency for patients to adopt a high-calorie liquid diet, thereby leading to regain of weight.

Adjustable Gastric Banding

The AGB procedure may be performed with any of three types of adjustable bands. The only band approved for use by the FDA in the United States is the LAP-BAND (INAMED Health, Santa Barbara, CA). The Swedish Adjustable Gastric Band (Obtech Medical, Baar, Switzerland), the MIDBAND (Medical Innovation Development, Villeurbanne, France), and the Heliogast Band (Helioscopie, Vienna, France) are other banding systems used in Europe and elsewhere. The techniques of placement of the bands are similar; only the locking mechanisms,

band shape and configuration, and adjustment schedules vary somewhat for the different types of bands. They all work on the principle of restriction of oral intake by limiting the volume of the proximal part of the stomach. Their advantage over the traditional vertical banded gastroplasty is adjustability.

Trocar placement for AGB is shown in Figure 17-1. The surgeon stands to the patient's right, the assistant is to the patient's left, and the camera operator is adjacent to the surgeon. Most surgeons place the patient in the supine position, but some prefer to have the patient's legs spread so that the surgeon can stand between the legs.

The technique for placement of the AGB system is described in detail by Fielding and Allen.[13] The peritoneum at the angle of His is divided to create an opening in the peritoneum between the angle of His and the top of the spleen (Fig. 17-2A). The telescope is placed through the left upper quadrant port for this part of the operation to maximally view the angle of His area.

The *pars flaccida* technique has become the approach of choice for placing the adjustable band and begins with dividing the gastrohepatic ligament in its thin area just over the caudate lobe of the liver. The anterior branch of the vagus nerve is spared, and any aberrant left hepatic artery is preserved. The base of the right crus of the diaphragm is identified. Care must be taken to clearly identify the crus because occasionally the vena cava can lie close to the caudate lobe. The surgeon gently follows the surface of the right crus posterior and inferior to the esophagus while aiming for the angle of His (see Fig. 17-2B). A gentle spreading and pushing technique is used

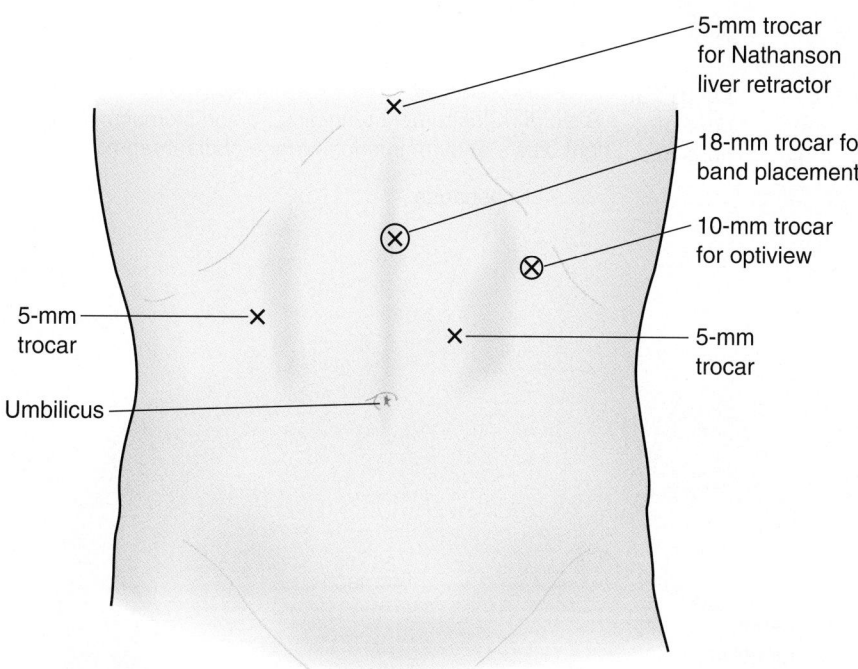

Figure 17-1 Trocar location for adjustable gastric banding.

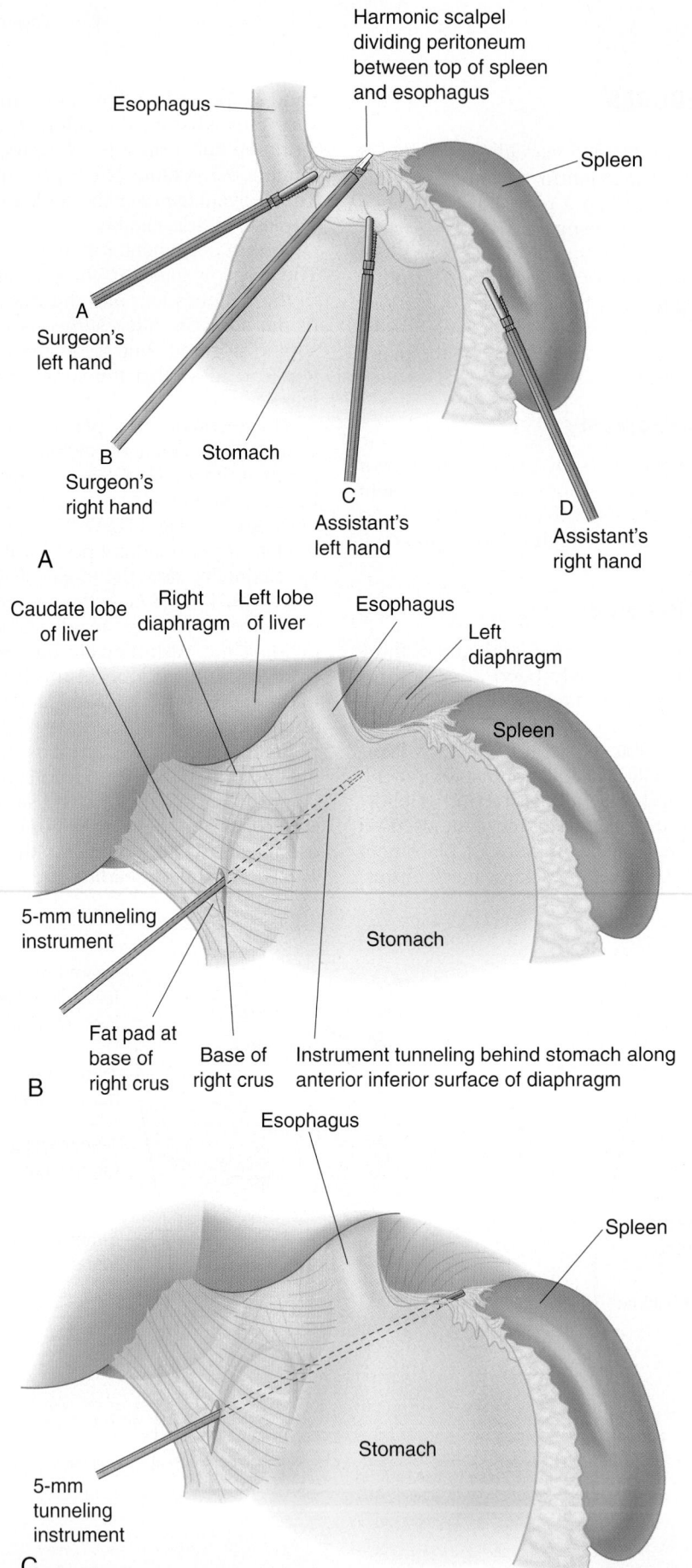

Figure 17-2 **A,** Dividing the peritoneum at the angle of His. **B,** Pars flaccida technique in which the fat pad is divided at the base of the right crus. **C,** Tunnel posterior to the stomach completed.

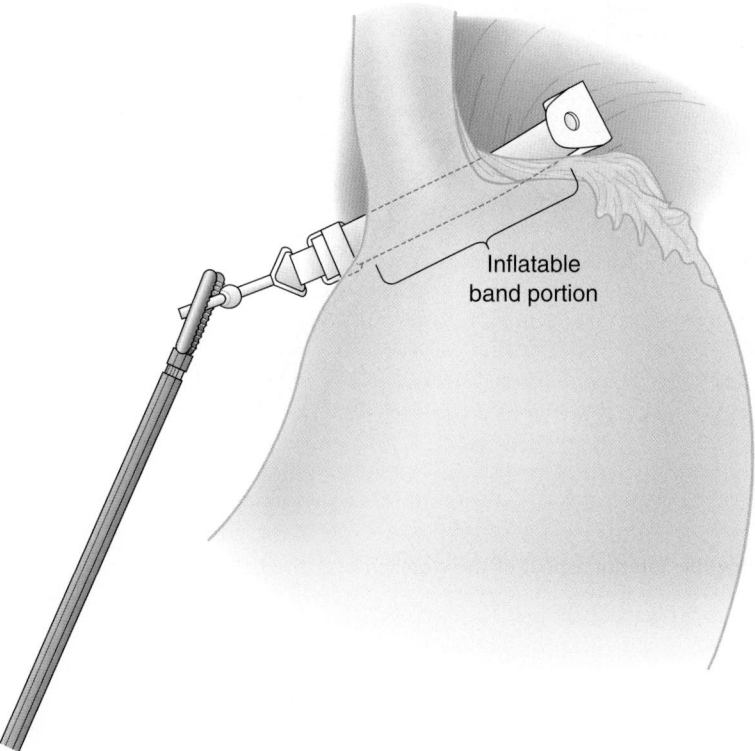

Figure 17-3 Pulling the LAP-BAND through the tunnel.

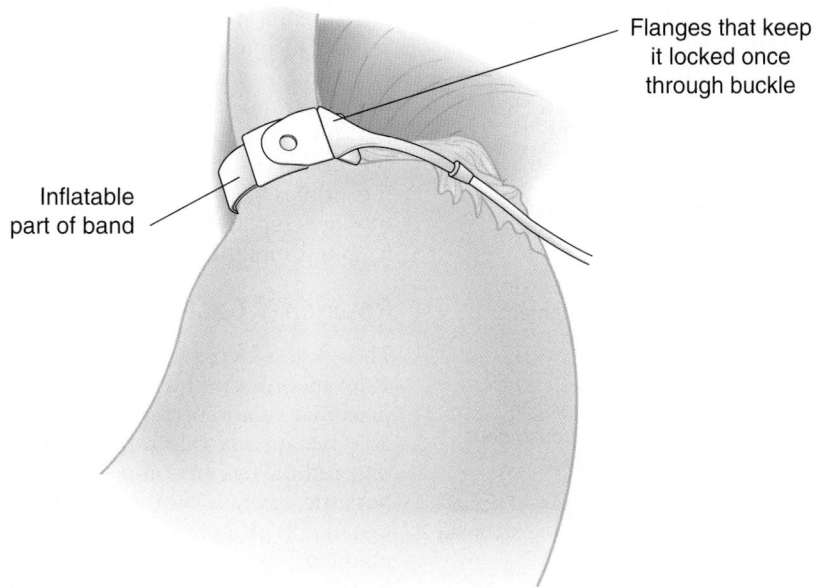

Figure 17-4 Locking the LAP-BAND.

to create an avascular tunnel along this plane. Once the tip of the tunneling instrument is seen near the top of the spleen, it is gently pushed through any remaining peritoneal layers to complete the tunnel (see Fig. 17-2C). The adjustable band has already been placed in the peritoneal cavity through the large 15-mm trocar located in the right upper quadrant before dissection of the pars flaccida. The narrow end of the band itself is grasped by the tunneling instrument and pulled through the tunnel from the greater to the lesser side of the stomach (Fig. 17-3). That end is then threaded through the locking mechanism of the band, after which the band is locked. Once the band has been locked in place, the buckle is adjusted to lie on the lesser curvature side of the stomach (Fig. 17-4). A 5-mm grasper inserted between the band and stomach ensures that the band is not too tight.

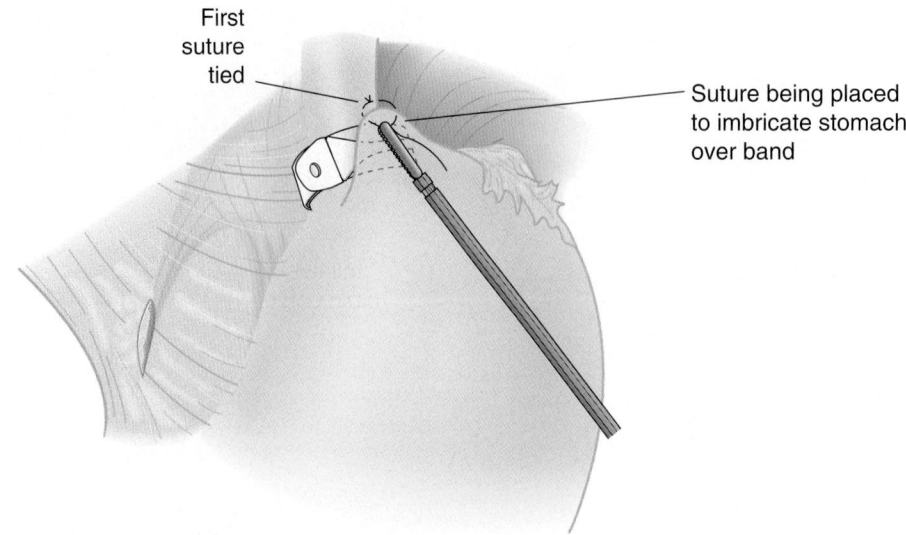

Figure 17-5 Imbricating the anterior aspect of the stomach over the LAP-BAND.

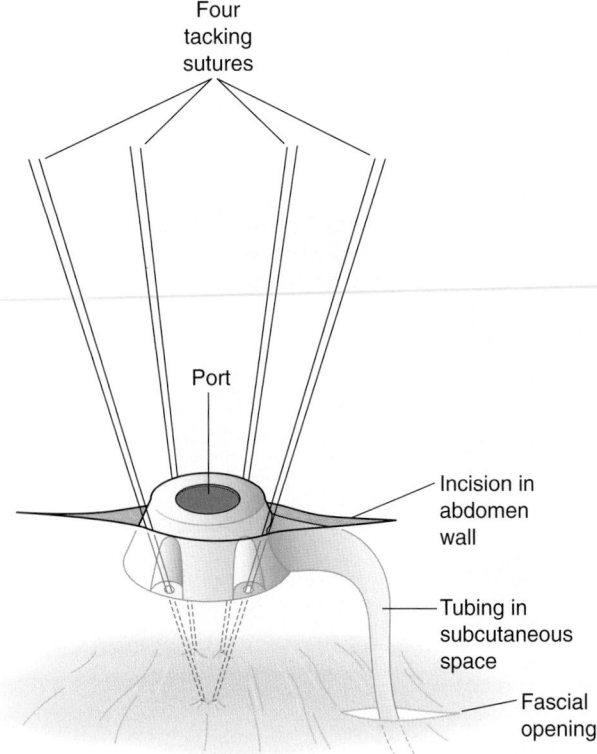

Figure 17-6 Passing the inflation tubing through the abdominal wall sufficiently far from the port site to prevent acute kinking of the tubing.

The anterior gastric wall is imbricated over the band with four interrupted, nonabsorbable sutures (Fig. 17-5). There needs to be just enough stomach above the level of the band for incorporating that tissue into the suture. Suturing is carried as far posterolaterally as possible because this region has been the most frequent area of fundus herniation through the band. The band is thus ideally secured about 1 cm below the gastroesophageal junction with this technique.

The Silastic tubing leading from the band is pulled through the 15-mm trocar site in the right upper quadrant paramedian area to complete the laparoscopic portion of the operation. The trocar site incision is enlarged to reveal the anterior rectus fascia, which is exposed approximately 2 to 4 cm lateral to the existing fascial defect for the trocar, and the access port is connected to the inflation tubing. Four sutures inserted through the four holes on the access port are placed in the fascia, after which the port is tied to the fascia (Fig. 17-6). The redundant tubing is replaced in the abdominal cavity with care taken to avoid kinking.

Roux-en-Y Gastric Bypass

The gastric bypass first described by Mason and Ito in 1969 incorporated a loop of jejunum anastomosed to a proximal gastric pouch. This operation proved unacceptable because of bile reflux, and RYGB, which eliminates bile reflux, has become the most commonly performed bariatric operation in the United States.

Described here is one technique that incorporates many of these modifications. There are certainly many variations of this technique, and many, if not most, will give excellent results.[14] Essential principles of the operation are listed in Box 17-6.

We have found the left subcostal region, near the midclavicular line, to be an ideal location for placement of the first trocar under direct vision; either a bladed trocar (United States Surgical Corporation, Norwalk, CT) or an optical trocar (Optiview, Ethicon Endosurgery, Cincinnati, OH) that dilates a tract under direct vision can be used. Subsequent trocars are placed under laparoscopic vision to achieve the configuration shown in Figure 17-7.

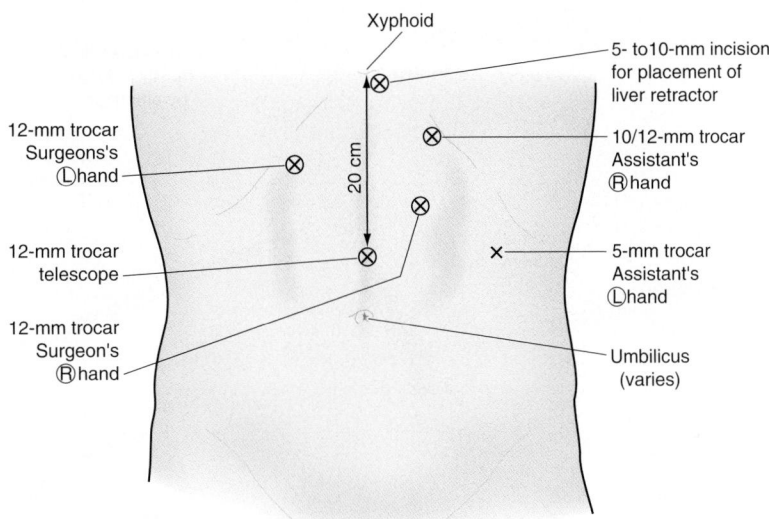

Figure 17-7 Trocar configuration for laparoscopic Roux-en-Y gastric bypass.

Once the omentum is mobilized, the ligament of Treitz is identified. A location approximately 30 to 40 cm distal to the ligament is chosen for division of the jejunum with an endoscopic stapler (Fig. 17-8). The mesentery is then further divided with staples or a harmonic scalpel. The proximal end of the Roux limb is now marked by suturing a small, ¼-inch Penrose drain to it.

The length of the Roux limb is influenced in our practices by patient weight. Patients with a BMI in the 40s will be well served with a Roux limb of 80 to 120 cm, whereas patients with a BMI significantly in excess of 50 are usually given a Roux limb of approximately 150 cm.[15] The proximal jejunum is left to lay to the patient's right side, and the Roux limb is lifted cephalad and coiled in the curve of the transverse colon mesentery (Fig. 17-9). This technique allows the proximal jejunum to be aligned directly alongside the designated point on the Roux limb for the distal anastomosis. The stapler is placed through the surgeon's left-hand port because the bowel segments are easily aligned to facilitate placement of the stapler into enterotomies created in each segment of bowel at the desired location of the anastomosis (Fig. 17-10). Once the anastomosis is created, the stapler defect is closed with a single layer of suture. We have found that stapling predisposes to obstruction or stenosis. The mesenteric defect between the loops of small bowel is now closed with running permanent suture (Fig. 17-11).

The Roux limb may be passed toward the proximal gastric pouch through a retrocolic or antecolic pathway. The retrocolic route may then take either a retrogastric or antegastric pathway, whereas the antecolic route always takes an antegastric pathway. All routes seem to work well. We use a retrocolic, retrogastric approach because this is the shortest distance between the small intestine and the proximal gastric pouch and the likelihood of tension on the anastomosis is decreased, which may reduce leaks at the gastrojejunostomy.[16] Passage of the Roux limb through the transverse colon mesentery to

---

Box 17-6   Essential Components of Roux-en-Y Gastric Bypass

Small proximal gastric pouch
Gastric pouch constructed from the cardia of the stomach to prevent dilation and minimize acid production
Gastric pouch divided from the distal part of the stomach
Roux limb at least 75 cm in length
Enteroenterostomy constructed to avoid stenosis or obstruction
Closure of all potential spaces for internal hernias

---

a retrogastric position can be challenging. Creating an opening in the transverse colon mesentery just to the left and slightly above the ligament of Treitz generally provides a view of the inferior aspect of the greater curvature of the stomach. The stomach is then grasped and held upward to allow passage of first the Penrose drain and then the attached proximal end of the Roux limb (Fig. 17-12). Care must be taken to ensure that the Roux limb is passed with the mesentery downward and not twisted.

The left lobe liver retractor is now placed and the patient placed in the reverse Trendelenburg position. Exposure of the angle of His allows division of the peritoneum between the top of the spleen and the gastroesophageal junction with the ultrasonic scalpel. The lesser sac is entered through the gastrohepatic ligament, 3 to 4 cm below the gastroesophageal junction. The blue load of the linear stapler is now fired multiple times to create a 10- to 15-mL proximal gastric pouch based on the upper lesser curvature of the stomach (Fig. 17-13). Once the gastric pouch is created, the drain is used to help pass the Roux limb to a position adjacent to the proximal gastric pouch. The blue load of the linear stapler is then used to create the proximal anastomosis (Fig. 17-14). The stapler defect is closed, the entire anas-

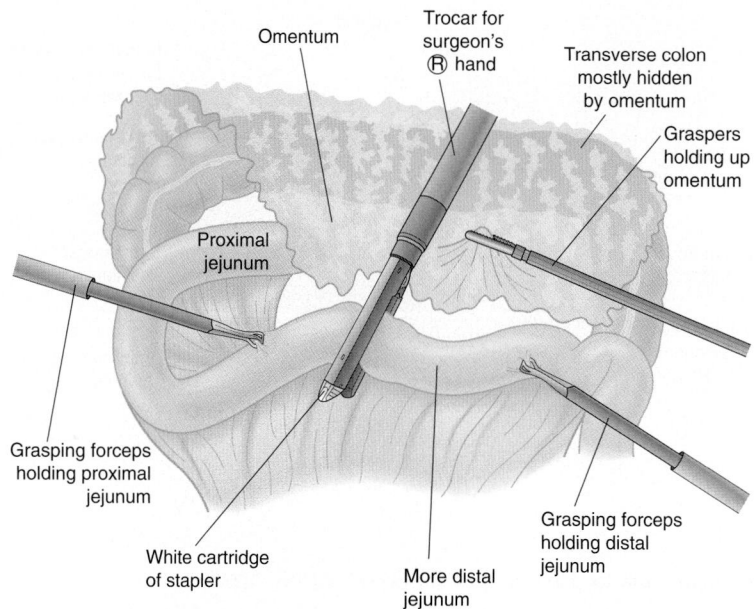

Figure 17-8 Placing a stapler to divide the jejunum for creation of the Roux limb.

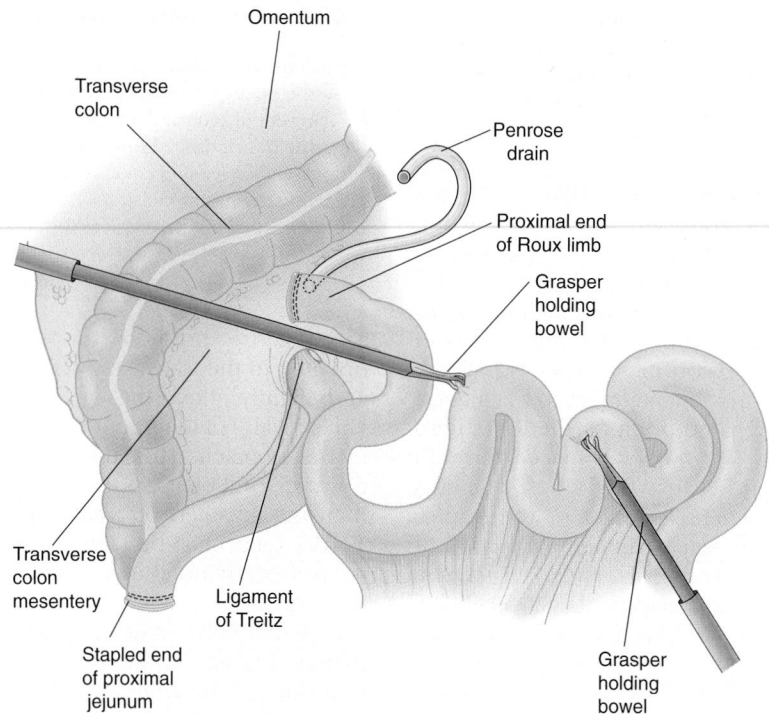

Figure 17-9 Measuring and laying out the jejunum to set up a distal anastomosis for the length of the Roux-en-Y gastric bypass.

tomosis is irrigated with saline, and a member of the operative team uses the endoscope to monitor occlusion of the Roux limb with an atraumatic 10-mm bowel clamp. Even the smallest leaks of air can be identified and closed with this technique. Studies have shown that use of this technique can dramatically reduce the incidence of post-operative leaks to very low levels.[16] Alternatively, the gastrojejunostomy may be performed with a circular stapler or a hand-sutured technique.[17]

The final step of the operation involves closing the mesenteric defects. Retrogastric herniation of the Roux limb was a problem because sutures often pulled through

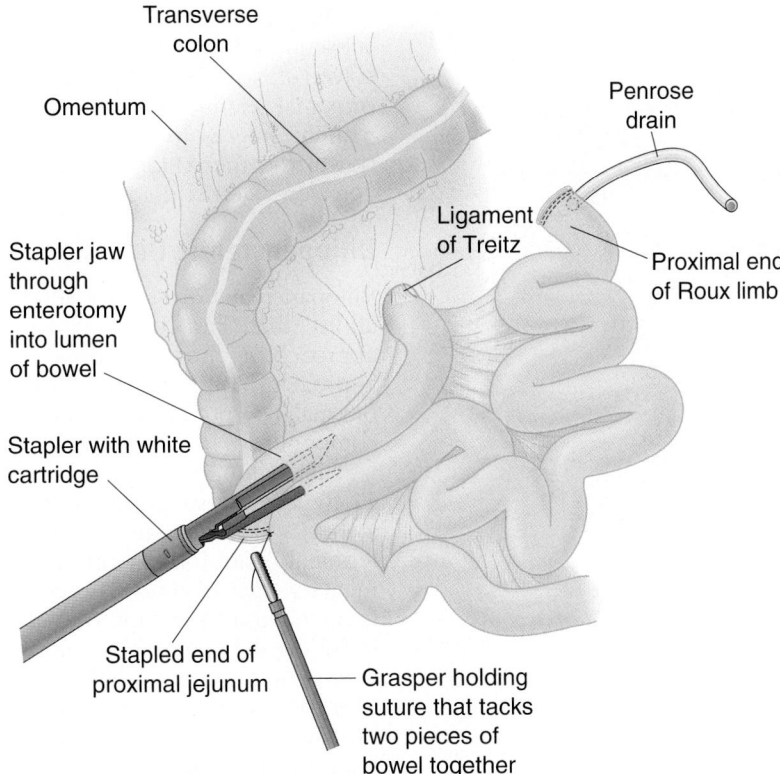

Figure 17-10 Placing the stapler to create an enteroenterostomy.

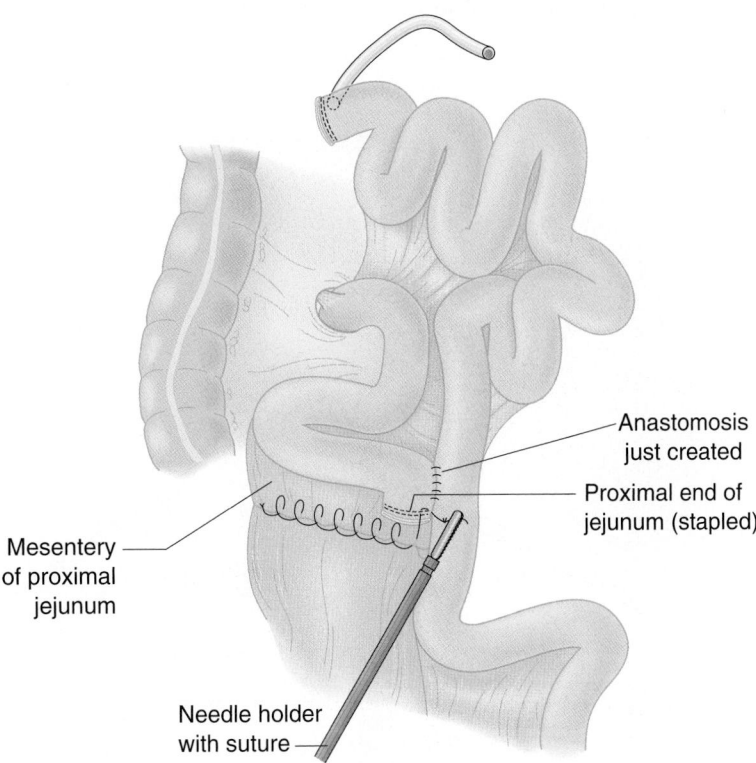

Figure 17-11 Sewing the mesenteric defect and placing an antiobstruction stitch.

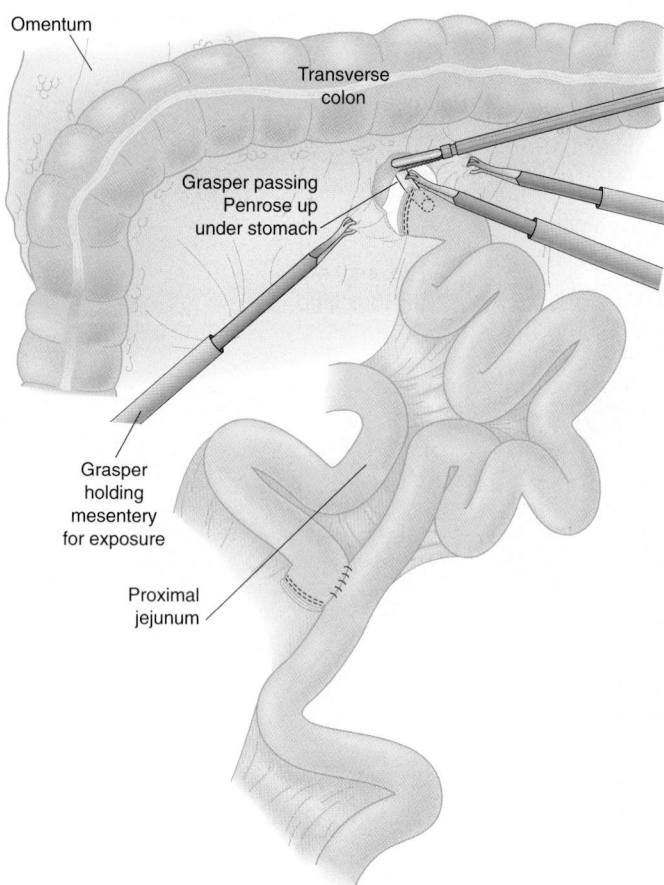

Omentum

Transverse colon

Grasper passing Penrose up under stomach

Grasper holding mesentery for exposure

Proximal jejunum

Figure 17-12 Passing the Roux limb into a retrocolic, retrogastric position.

the fatty mesentery of the transverse colon and allowed subsequent bowel herniation and obstruction.[18] We have solved this problem by attaching the Roux limb to the proximal jejunum near the ligament of Treitz with permanent sutures to fix a segment of the two pieces of bowel together (Fig. 17-15). This technique also closes Petersen's hernia defect.

Biliopancreatic Diversion

Biliopancreatic diversion (BPD), like most bariatric operations that had been performed through an open approach, is now performed through a laparoscopic approach.[19] BPD produces weight loss based primarily on malabsorption, but it does have a mild restrictive component.

The anatomic configuration of BPD is shown in Figure 17-16. The intestinal tract is reconstructed to allow only a short so-called common channel of the distal 50-cm of terminal ileum for absorption of fat and protein. The alimentary tract beyond the proximal part of the stomach is rearranged to include only the distal 200 cm of ileum, including the common channel. The proximal end of this ileum is anastomosed to the proximal end of the stomach after performing a distal hemigastrectomy. The ileum proximal to the end that is anastomosed to the stomach is in turn anastomosed to the terminal ileum within the 50- to 100-cm distance from the ileocecal valve, depending on the surgeon's preference and the patient's size.

The laparoscopic procedure is performed with a trocar alignment as shown in Figure 17-17. The initial portion of the operation involves exposing the terminal ileum and cecum. Appendectomy is optional. The terminal

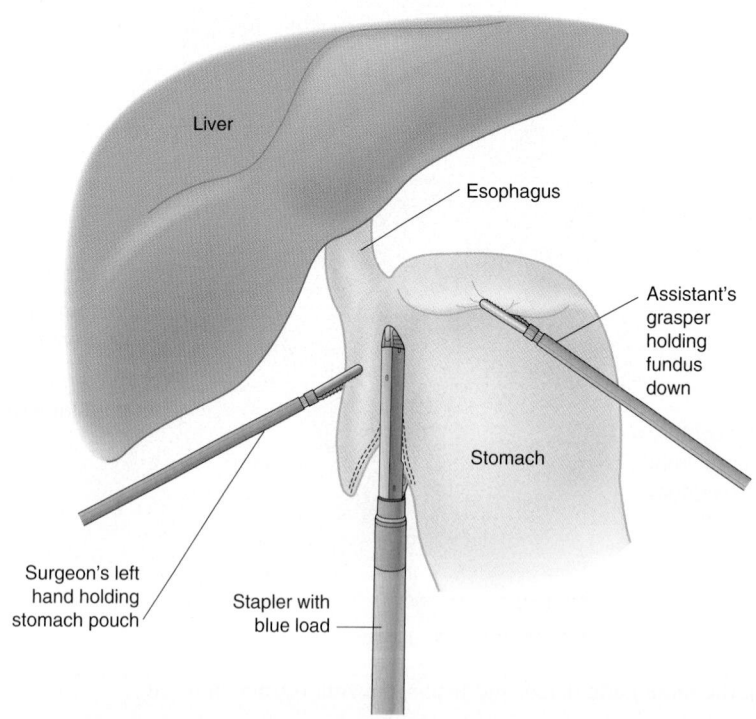

Liver

Esophagus

Assistant's grasper holding fundus down

Stomach

Surgeon's left hand holding stomach pouch

Stapler with blue load

Figure 17-13 Firing the stapler to create the proximal gastric pouch.

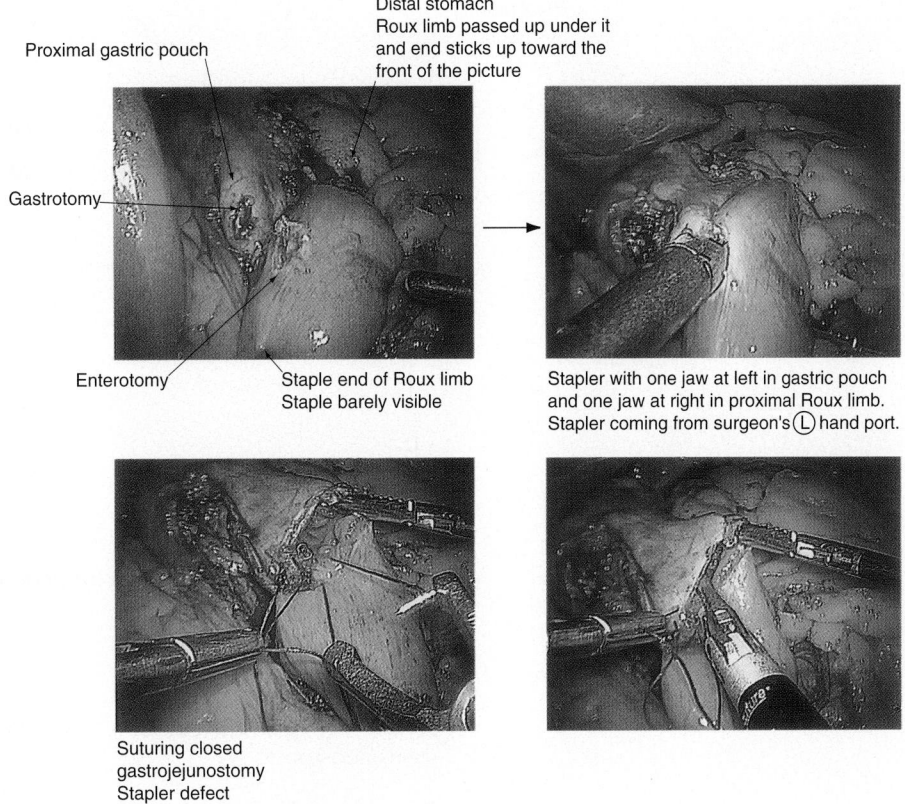

Figure 17-14 Creating the proximal anastomosis.

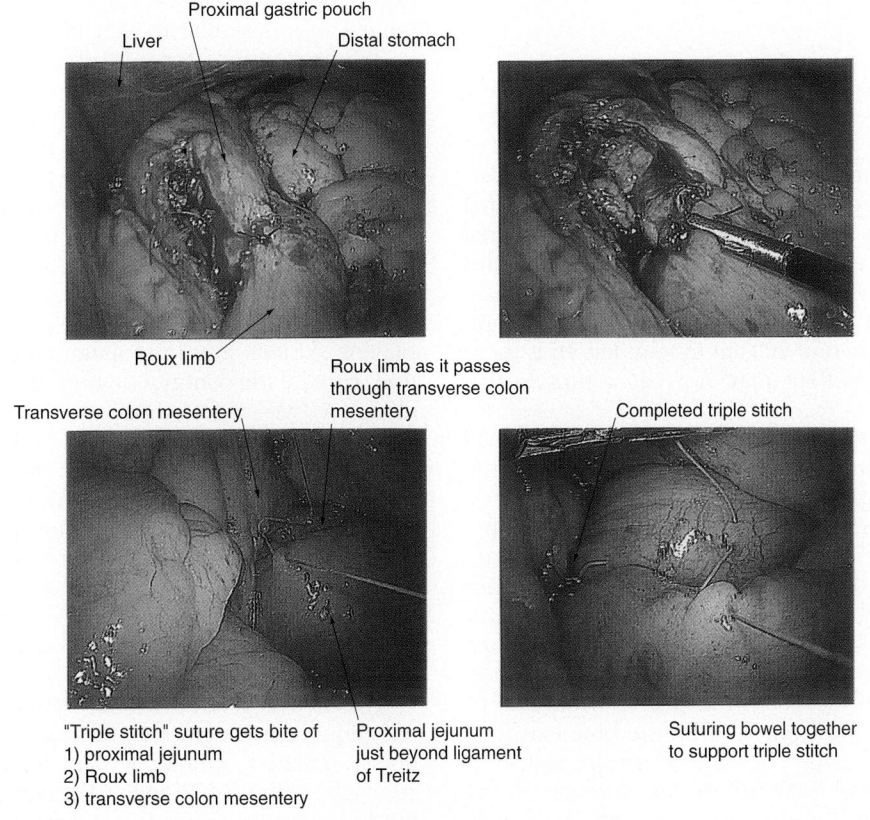

Figure 17-15 Placing the "triple stitch" to close the mesenteric defects.

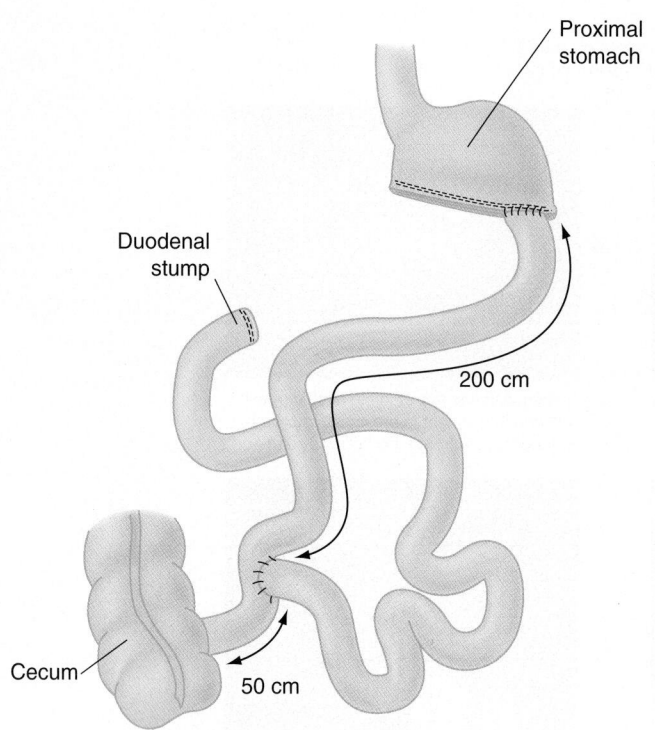

Alimentary channel = 250 (± 50) cm
Common channel = 50 cm

Figure 17-16 Anatomic configuration of biliopancreatic diversion.

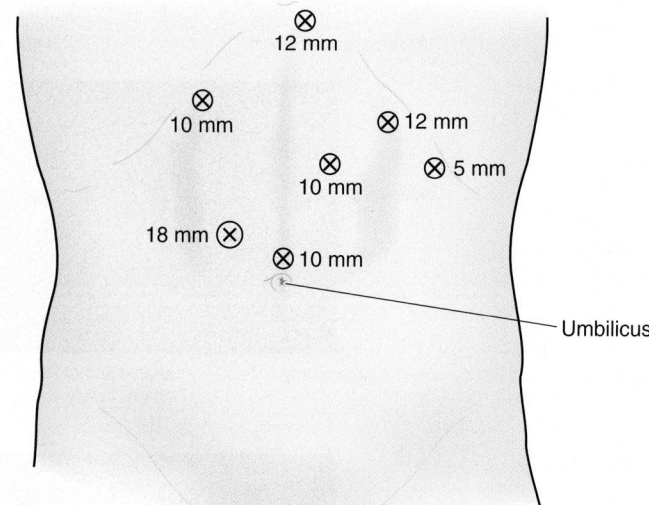

Figure 17-17 Location of trocars for performing a laparoscopic biliopancreatic diversion.

suture to prevent kinking of the bowel at the gastroileostomy.

Duodenal Switch

The DS configuration is shown in Figure 17-22. This modification was developed to help lessen the high incidence of marginal ulcers after BPD. The mechanism of weight loss is similar to that of BPD.

Trocar locations for performing the operation laparoscopically are shown in Figure 17-17. An appendectomy is followed by measurement of the terminal ileum. Notably in the DS procedure, the common channel is 100 cm and the entire alimentary tract is 250 cm. However, the major difference between DS and BPD is the gastrectomy and the proximal anatomy. Instead of a distal hemigastrectomy, a sleeve gastrectomy of the greater curvature of the stomach is performed. This procedure is done as the initial part of the operation because if the patient exhibits any intraoperative instability, the operation can be discontinued after the sleeve gastrectomy alone. A two-stage DS has been used in patients who have an extremely high BMI and are high operative risks.[20] The sleeve gastrectomy alone usually produces enough weight loss to make the second stage of the operation technically easier. This approach lowers the mortality rate despite the need to undergo two operative procedures. Others have found weight loss after the initial sleeve gastrectomy to be sufficient to preclude subsequent conversion to a DS, although the long-term results are not known.[21]

The sleeve gastrectomy is performed with a stapling technique that begins at the mid antrum, and a staple line is created parallel to the lesser curvature of the stomach, with a 60-French Maloney dilator placed along the lesser curve to prevent narrowing. The staple line is

ileum is measured to a length of 50 cm, with a marking suture placed for the location of the anastomosis. After placing the marking suture, a total length of 200 cm of ileum is measured, and at this point the ileum is divided with the vascular staple load (Fig. 17-18). The proximal end of the bowel is then anastomosed to the terminal ileum at the site of the marking suture with a standard linear stapling technique, and the mesenteric defects are closed with suture (Fig. 17-19). The alimentary tract limb can be lengthened beyond 200 cm in total length if there is concern that the patient may not eat a protein-rich diet.

Attention is now turned toward the stomach. A distal gastrectomy is performed with serial applications of the blue load of the stapler (Fig. 17-20). The duodenum is stapled and divided distal to the pylorus. Gastric volume may be tailored to the patient's degree of obesity, with larger volumes of 250 mL being created for patients with a BMI less than 50 kg/m² and smaller pouches to a lower limit of 150 mL for patients with a BMI greater than 50 kg/m². The proximal end of the 200-cm length of terminal ileum is anastomosed to the posterior surface of the proximal end of the stomach with the blue cartridge of the linear stapler (Fig. 17-21). The stapler defect is closed and the bowel secured to the surface of the stomach beyond the anastomosis with an anchoring

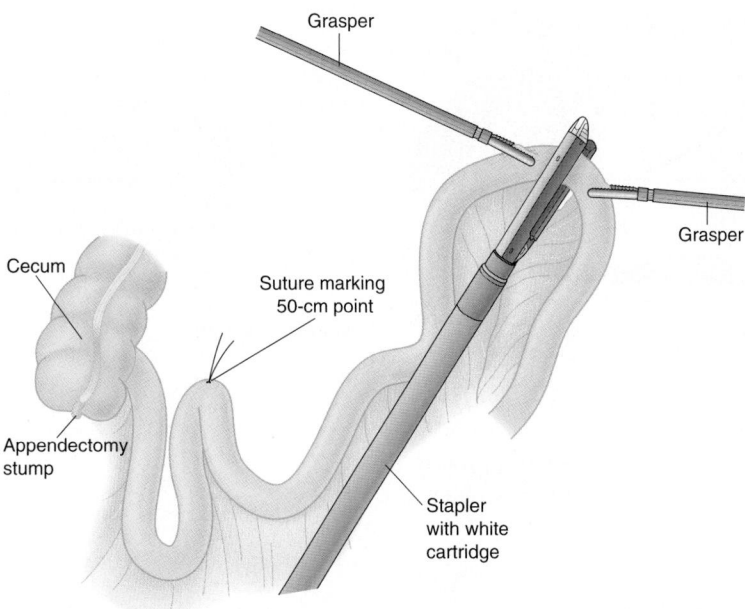

Figure 17-18 Dividing the ileum at the 200-cm location proximal to the ileocecal valve after having already marked the 50-cm location.

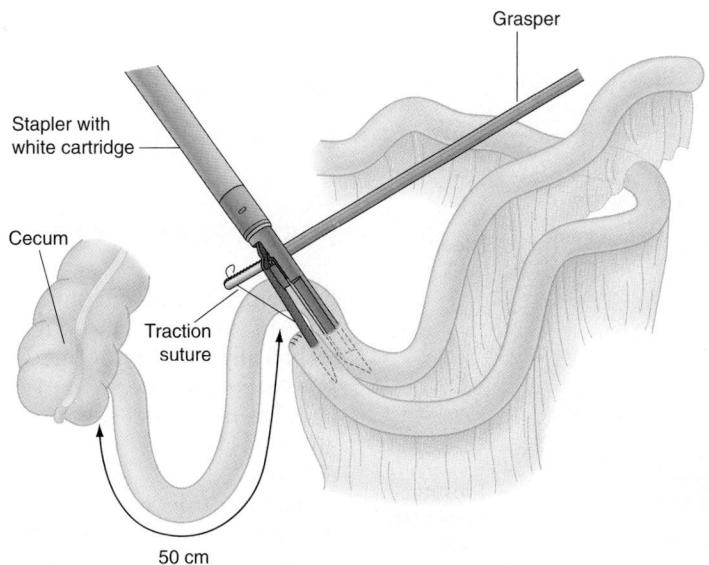

Figure 17-19 Creating the ileoileostomy for the biliopancreatic diversion.

created with multiple firings of the stapler until the angle of His is reached (Fig. 17-23). The goal is to produce a lesser curvature gastric sleeve with a volume of 150 to 200 mL.

After sleeve gastrectomy, or preceding it in smaller patients, the duodenum is divided with the stapler approximately 2 cm beyond the pylorus. The distal connections are performed as for BPD. The distal anastomosis is created at the 100-cm point proximal to the ileocecal valve. The proximal anastomosis is created between the proximal end of the 250 cm of terminal ileum and the first portion of the duodenum. The duodenoileostomy is an antecolic end-to-side duodenoenterostomy. This anastomosis is the most tenuous part of the operation and is performed with a circular stapler because of the nature of the relatively narrow first portion of duodenum (Fig. 17-24). The anvil is directly inserted through the staple line of the duodenal stump via a gastrotomy under suture guidance or through an oral approach with a nasogastric tube.

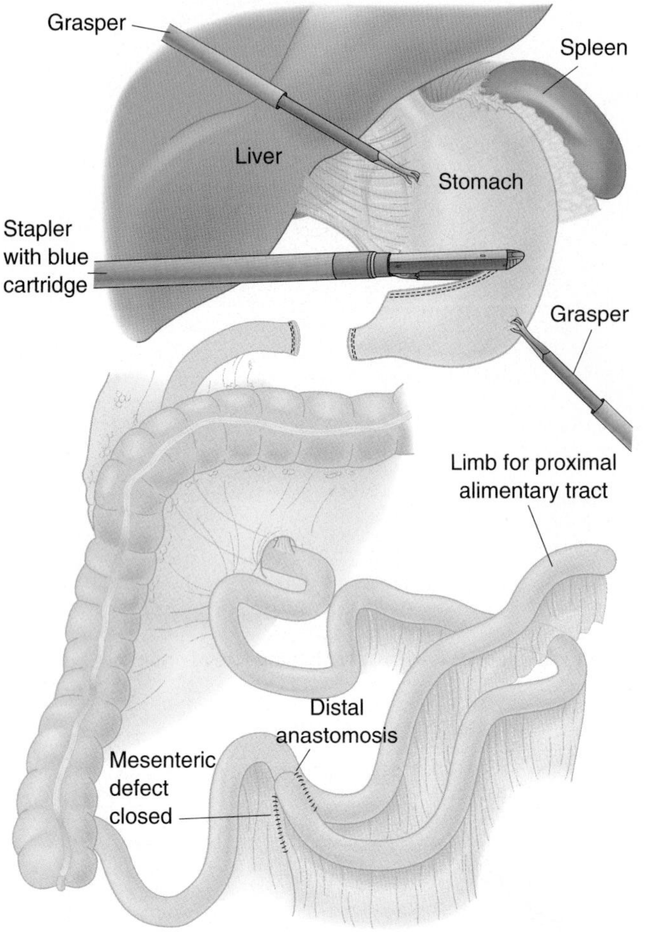

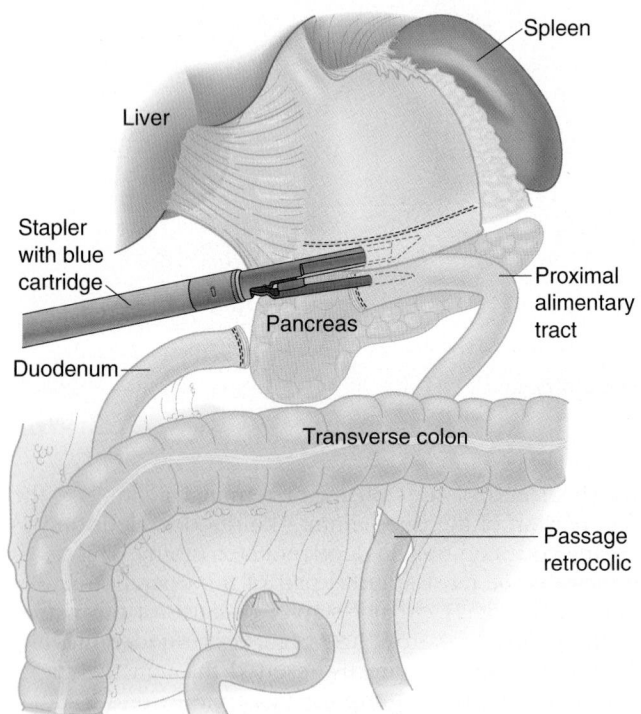

Figure 17-20 Performing the distal gastrectomy.

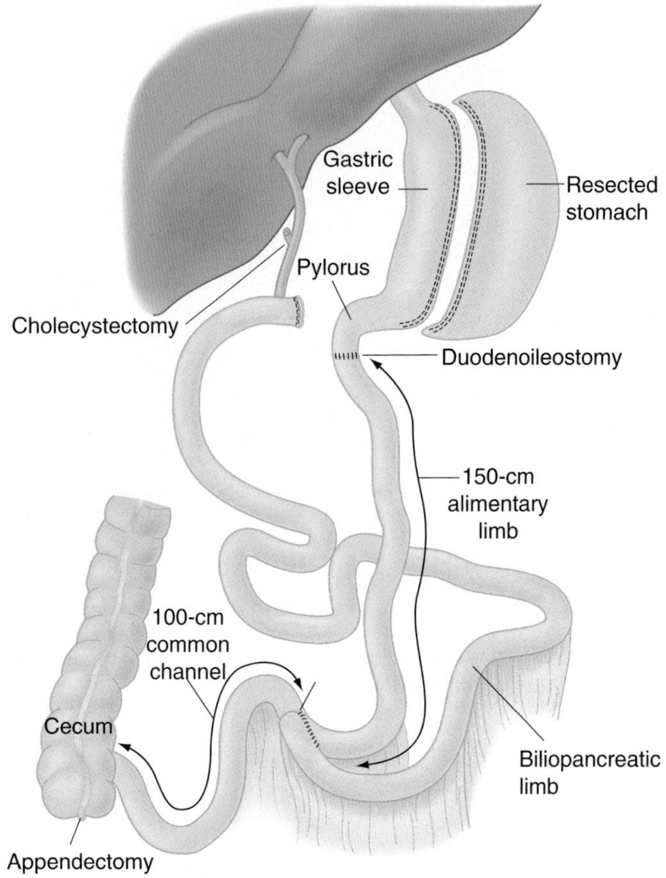

Figure 17-22 Configuration of the duodenal switch.

Figure 17-21 Creation of the gastrojejunostomy between the ileum and proximal part of the stomach.

POSTOPERATIVE CARE AND FOLLOW-UP

Excellent surgical outcomes require the appropriate selection of patients, thorough preoperative preparation, technically well-performed operations, and attentive postoperative care. A bariatric patient requires particularly attentive and special postoperative care in several areas above and beyond that of the average surgical patient.

The most dreaded complication after bariatric surgery is a leak from the gastrointestinal tract. Tachycardia, at times accompanied by tachypnea or agitation, is often the only manifestation of this severe intra-abdominal problem. A severely obese patient may not be subject to the development of fever or signs of peritonitis, as would a patient with a normal body habitus.

Appropriate fluid resuscitation is essential. A 200-kg patient who undergoes open gastric bypass can easily require 6 to 10 L of fluid for replacement of maintenance, third-space, and operative fluid or blood losses. Our postoperative protocol after open surgery calls for 400 mL/hr of a balanced salt solution (usually lactated Ringer's), with boluses given as needed for low urine output. A Foley catheter is used for the first 24 hours. Patients undergoing laparoscopic surgery usually have much less third-space and operative blood loss than do patients undergoing open surgery and can be managed

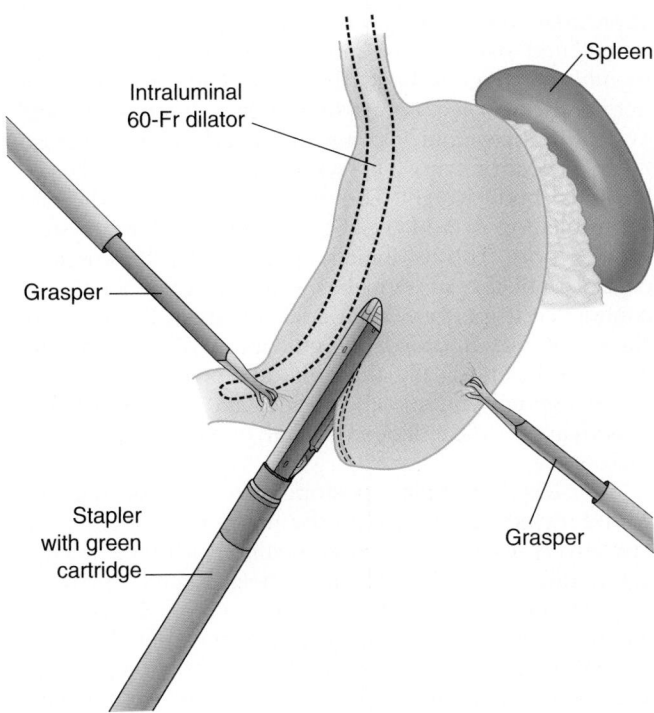

Figure 17-23 Creation of the sleeve gastrectomy during a laparoscopic duodenal switch procedure.

with 200 mL/hr of intravenous fluids. Urine output intraoperatively is normally low because of the pneumoperitoneum and usually improves in the recovery room area. Some patients who have been taking diuretics for many years will not have adequate urine output without diuretic use, but the surgeon must ensure that the patient is adequately volume resuscitated before giving diuretics. Higher than expected fluid requirements, oliguria, and tachycardia are a constellation of postoperative findings suggesting intra-abdominal problems.

Adequate pain control is essential. Narcotic requirements are decreased with a laparoscopic approach. A patient-controlled analgesia pump is appropriate and helpful. The value of an epidural catheter for pain relief is controversial. It has been our experience that such catheters in the severely obese population are often difficult to place and easy to dislodge. In addition, the use of low-molecular-weight heparin for DVT prophylaxis may preclude safe placement.

DVT prophylaxis is important. Pulmonary embolism is one of the leading causes of death after bariatric surgery. No data have substantiated one regimen of prophylaxis to be better than another. We use a combination of early ambulation (the same day as surgery, generally within 4 to 6 hours), the use of SCDs, and subcutaneous administration of low-molecular-weight heparin (enoxaparin).

Our standard practice procedure is to obtain a radiographic study of the gastrointestinal tract on the first postoperative day at one institution (University of Virginia) and, at the other (Vanderbilt), only if there are clinical signs of a leak, which include a temperature higher than 100°C or a heart rate greater than 100 beats/min. If neither are present, we start a water trial and

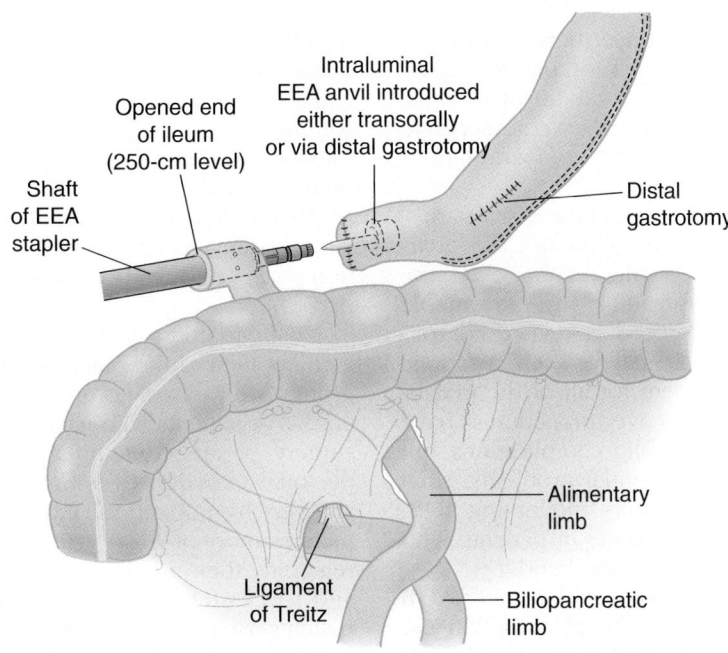

Figure 17-24 Creation of the duodenoenterostomy. EEA, end-to-end anastomosis.

Table 17-1 Results of the Three Major Bariatric Procedures

PARAMETER	BUCHWALD[25]	MAGGARD[26]
AGB weight loss (kg)	39.7 (42.2-37.2)	34.8 (29.5-40.1)
AGB EWL (%)	61.2 (64.4-58.1)	
AGB mortality	0.1% (2297 patients)	0.02% (9222) patients)
RYGB weight loss (kg)	43.5 (48.1-38.8)	41.5 (37.4-45.6)
RYGB EWL (%)	61.6 (66.5-56.7)	
RYGB mortality	0.5% (5644 patients)	0.3% (11,290 patients)
BPD/DS weight loss (kg)	46.4 (51.6-41.2)	53.1 (47.4-58.8)
BPD/DS EWL (%)	70.1 (73.9-66.3)	
BPD/DS mortality	1.1% (3030 patients)	0.9% (2808 patients)

AGB, adjustable gastric banding; BPD, biliopancreatic diversion; DS, duodenal switch; EWL, excess weight loss; RYGB, Roux-en-Y gastric bypass.

progress the diet to liquids. No data from randomized, prospective trials support either approach, however. The greatest value of a postoperative study is to document pouch size and identify patients with partial obstruction of the distal anastomosis, which is usually a result of edema but on occasion is due to technical reasons. The latter requires early reoperation.

Discharge, regardless of the bariatric operation, occurs when the patient is mobile, is tolerating an oral liquid diet, has adequate pain control with oral analgesics, and exhibits no signs of problems (e.g., fever or wound cellulitis). The timing of discharge, once these criteria are met, is often influenced by cultural issues, patient expectation, or distance between home and the hospital. Thus, the duration of hospitalization is not always an accurate reflection of optimal outcomes when comparing published studies in the literature.

Although the schedule of postoperative visits varies, all patients must undergo long-term follow-up. This guarantees that the surgeon will obtain feedback on the operative results and helps ensure that any preventable long-term metabolic or other procedure-related complications will be avoided. The potential for such metabolic complications is inherently present for all of the malabsorptive procedures. The restrictive procedures have minimal health risks from metabolic complications but instead have their own set of potential problems, such as band slippage or erosion in patients undergoing AGB. Moreover, improved weight loss occurs in patients who see their surgeon for adjustments to the band.[22]

A typical regimen for monitoring a patient after AGB would be to have the initial visit take place within the first month postoperatively to evaluate oral intake, food tolerance, and wound healing and to determine whether

appropriate restriction has resulted from placement of the noninflated band. Subsequent visits, usually scheduled monthly to bimonthly in the beginning and then less frequently, involve counseling with a nutritionist and evaluation of weight loss and the need for band adjustment. A goal of 1- to 2-kg/wk of weight loss is adjusted for initial body weight. Less weight loss is an indication for instillation of additional saline into the band system via the port. This is initially done under fluoroscopic control until the surgeon has sufficient experience and confidence to perform such adjustments in the office or clinic without fluoroscopic guidance. Blood tests are performed periodically throughout the patient's follow-up, depending on metabolic indications, the patient's underlying medical illnesses, and other indications for such tests.

After RYGB, a typical postoperative checkup regimen would include a visit within the first 2 to 3 weeks postoperatively to assess wound healing, advance from a liquid diet to solid food, and check overall recovery. Subsequent visits are scheduled at 6 weeks, 3 months, 6 months, and 1 year after surgery and then annually. Visits during the first year are for monitoring weight loss; those after the first year are for checking maintenance of weight loss and nutritional competence. The risk for iron, folate, vitamin A, vitamin D, or vitamin B_{12} deficiency exists for life.

Patients undergoing malabsorptive operations must understand the necessity of meticulous compliance with a strict follow-up plan. After BPD or DS, a patient is seen within the first 2 weeks to be certain that diarrhea is not too prolific and dehydration has not resulted. The patient must be taught the signs of dehydration and plans for its treatment. Replacement of fat-soluble vitamins is mandatory, and patient compliance must be documented. Initial visits after the first month take place monthly for the first several months until the risk of dehydration, poor protein intake, and significant metabolic consequences of rapid weight loss has lessened. The potential for protein-calorie malnutrition exists after these procedures, and it will usually be manifested during this time. Thereafter, as weight loss slows, periodic visits separated by 3-month intervals are indicated for the first year and then semiannually thereafter. Weight loss will taper after the first 12 to 18 months. Lifelong follow-up to assess fat-soluble vitamin deficiencies, as well as protein levels, liver function tests, and metabolic stability, is indicated after BPD or DS.

Most bariatric practices use patient support groups as a component of the postoperative support system. These groups are variously organized and managed but usually consist of patients who have undergone weight reduction surgery or are contemplating it; they meet to discuss personal experiences with respect to their surgery and recovery from it and the experience of losing weight and maintenance of lost weight. Although no data exist regarding their medical benefit, groups that are vigorous and successful seem to provide an excellent forum for patients to exchange information, as well as provide psychological and emotional support and encouragement to patients both before and after surgery.

Table 17-2 **Results of Laparoscopic Adjustable Gastric Banding Procedures**

CRITERIA	STUDY			
	O'Brien[28]	Buchwald[25]	Maggard[26]	Ponce[29]
Number of patients	709	1848	5562 (1 yr)	1014
Age (yr)	41	NR	NR	NR
Body mass index (kg/m²)	45	NR	NR	NR
Operating room time (min)	56	NR	NR	NR
Conversion (%)	1.0	NR	NR	NR
Follow-up (yr)	0.25-6	NR	1/>3	1/4
% Excess weight loss/yr	54/5	47.5/NR	NR	41/1, 64/4
Weight loss, kg (yr)	NR	28.6/NR	30 (1)/35 (>3)	NR

NR, not reported.

RESULTS

There is no consensus on the definition of success for any of these operations in terms of percentage of weight loss or extent of reversal of comorbid conditions, but there is now considerable data demonstrating that bariatric procedures are effective in achieving long-term weight loss and improvement in comorbid diseases. Several studies have shown improved survival or improvement in cardiovascular risk in patients undergoing bariatric surgery as compared with a matched set of individuals who did not undergo such surgery.[23,24] Resolution and improvement of comorbid conditions after all types of bariatric surgery have been confirmed in two meta-analyses, as shown in Table 17-1.[25,26]

The most striking evidence of efficacy comes from trials comparing morbidly obese diabetics who undergo bariatric surgery with those who do not and are treated medically. A Swedish study[24] showed an 80% decrease in the annual mortality of diabetic individuals in the surgical weight loss group versus a group of control patients not undergoing surgery (9% mortality at 9 years versus 28% mortality in a control group). The decrease in mortality is not limited to diabetic subjects undergoing bariatric surgery. In a study comparing matched control subjects with those who underwent bariatric surgery in Canada, Christou and colleagues[23] demonstrated that weight loss surgery reduced the relative risk of mortality by 89% (95% confidence interval, 73%-96%) 5 years later. It appears to be self-evident to these authors that the continued reports of improvement in cardiovascular risk factors, such as diabetes, hypertension, and dyslipidemia, seen after bariatric surgery will lead to a reduction in cardiovascular mortality.

Results of operations can be determined only after adequate long-term follow-up and with adequate numbers of operations performed by a variety of surgeons. The applicability of some operations may vary depending on patient factors, such as size or previous abdominal surgery; however, there is considerable variation in the regional use of bariatric surgery that does not appear to be related to the prevalence of morbid obesity in that region.[27]

Adjustable Gastric Banding

Patients undergoing AGB experience an operation that may last as little as 1 hour in experienced hands. Discharge from the hospital after an overnight stay is the norm, with a few reports of same-day discharge but more frequent reports of longer discharge based on cultural norms and acceptance. Table 17-2 gives the results of laparoscopic AGB in several large reported series in the literature with long-term follow-up.

The band is initially placed without adding any saline to distend it. Saline is added in 1.0- to 1.5-mL increments to produce a desired weight loss of 1 to 2 kg/wk. Excess weight loss may lead to actual removal of a small amount of saline, whereas inadequate weight loss is an indication for the addition of more saline to the system to increase restriction of the band. The incidence of metabolic problems is low after AGB because there is no disruption of the normal gastrointestinal tract. One potential problem is esophageal dilation from chronic obstruction secondary to band slippage.

Weight loss after AGB averaged 39.7 kg (61.2% excess weight loss [EWL]) and 34.8 kg in two meta-analyses of bariatric surgery (see Table 17-1).[25,26] The pattern of weight loss is such that weight loss continues after the first year, up to a maximal amount usually achieved by the third year. Series with 5-year follow-up confirm that the weight loss may even improve slightly further after 3 years. In series with longer than 5-year follow-up,[28,29] baseline BMI decreased from an average of 42 to 46 kg/m² to 30 to 36 kg/m² at 5 years.

The LAP-BAND has been shown to resolve type 2 diabetes in 47.9% and improve the condition in 80.8% of patients in the meta-analyses published.[25] Hypertension was resolved in 42% and improved in 70.8% of patients after this procedure.[25] Improvement in dyslipidemia was also noted in 58.9%. Other comorbid conditions such as obstructive sleep apnea, GERD, and venous stasis improved or resolved after weight loss with AGB.[29]

Table 17-3 Results of Roux-en-Y Gastric Bypass

CRITERIA	STUDY			
	Pories	Buchwald	Maggard	Sugerman
Number of patients	1160	4204	1281	1025
Age (yr)	NR	NR	NR	39
Body mass index (kg/m²)	50	NR	NR	51
Follow-up (yr)	4	NR	1/>3	10-12
Excess weight loss (%)	49	62	NR	52
Weight loss (kg)	NR	43	43/41	NR
Resolution/improvement (%)	NR	NR	NR	NR
Diabetes mellitus type 2	NR	93	NR	83
Hypertension	NR	87	NR	69
Obstructive sleep apnea	NR	95	NR	NR
Osteoarthritis	NR	NR	NR	18

NR, not reported.

Quality-of-life testing measures parameters that include the physical, mental, and psychological well-being of patients. A group of 459 patients undergoing a LAP-BAND procedure had scores 1 year after surgery that were in the normal values for the community on the Medical Outcomes Trust Short Form-36 test.[30]

Roux-en-Y Gastric Bypass

RYGB has an established track record longer than that of any other operation. Its performance has been modified over the years, and the results presented in Table 17-3 reflect data from series in the era of its performance as both an open and a laparoscopic procedure. Recovery after RYGB is improved after a laparoscopic approach, as has been demonstrated for several other abdominal operations. This improvement is largely related to the decrease in postoperative pain experienced by patients after laparoscopic RYGB versus open RYGB. One prospective randomized study compared open and laparoscopic RYGB.[12] In that study, patients were monitored for 1 year, at which time weight loss with both approaches was comparable (68% loss of excess weight for laparoscopic RYGB versus 62% loss of excess weight for open RYGB). Nguyen and colleagues[12] reported a shorter length of hospitalization and more rapid return to activities of daily living with laparoscopic RYGB. Although the early (3 months postoperatively) improvement in quality of life reported by Nguyen and colleagues[12] after laparoscopic RYGB was greater than with open RYGB, the data were comparable for the two groups at 6 months after surgery, thus suggesting that the major recovery benefit with a laparoscopic approach is limited to the first 3 months postoperatively.

Another important advantage of the laparoscopic approach for RYGB is a decrease in the incidence of wound complications and incisional hernia seen after RYGB. Long-term follow-up of a prospective randomized trial comparing laparoscopic and open gastric bypass found a much higher rate of incisional hernias in the open surgery group.[31] There was, however, no difference in the rate resolution of comorbid conditions or weight loss between the two procedures. Maggard and coworkers[26] also found laparoscopic RYGB to be superior to the open procedure for incisional hernias and respiratory and wound complications.

The duration of hospitalization has decreased in all patients undergoing RYGB. Patients undergoing laparoscopic RYGB are usually hospitalized for about 2 days. Since the advent of laparoscopic RYGB, we have seen patients who undergo open RYGB or who require conversion to open RYGB discharged within 1 day of patients after laparoscopic RYGB, probably because of protocols in place to encourage early ambulation and oral intake after RYGB that did not exist before the era of laparoscopic RYGB.

Two meta-analyses of long-term follow-up studies have shown that RYGB provides weight loss of 43.5 kg and 41.5 kg (see Table 17-1).[25,26] Long-term follow-up studies show 58% loss of excess weight at 5 years and 49% at 14 years after RYGB.

Resolution of comorbid conditions after open and laparoscopic RYGB has generally been excellent. Meta-analysis of the effects of RYGB on diabetes showed resolution in 83.7% and improvement in 93.2%.[25] Schauer and associates[32] showed that glycosylated hemoglobin levels returned to normal in 83% of their patients, and a reduction in the use of insulin was seen in 79%. Diabetes for more than 5 years, more severe forms of diabetes, or less weight loss postoperatively were all factors that contributed to lack of resolution of the problem. Torquati and colleaguess[33] showed a substantial reduction in hemoglobin A_{1c} and resolution of diabetes in 74% of diabetics undergoing laparoscopic RYGB. Preoperative factors that predicted failure of diabetes to resolve were need for insulin preoperatively or waist circumference greater than 50 inches in men and 40 inches in women. All series demonstrated that resolution of diabetes begins immediately after surgery and that it must be related to enteric factors regulating glucose metabolism rather than sheer

Table 17-4 Results of Malabsorptive Operations (Biliopancreatic Diversion and Duodenal Switch)

	STUDY		
	Scopinaro	Buchwald	Maggard
Number of patients (BPD)/(DS)	1356	2480	735
Age (yr)	37	NR	NR
Body mass index (kg/m^2)	47	NR	NR
Follow-up (yr)	12	NR	1/>3
Loss of excess weight (%)	78	70	NR
Number of bowel movements/day	2-4	NR	NR
Weight loss (kg)	NR	46	52/53
Resolution/improvement (%)	NR	NR	NR
Diabetes mellitus type 2	100	98.9	NR
Hypertension	87	83.4	NR
Cholesterol	100	87	NR

NR, not reported.

weight loss alone because a similar amount of weight loss after low-calorie diets produces no such high incidence of resolution of diabetes.

Metabolic syndrome is cured or ameliorated with gastric bypass.[34,35] Mattar and associates showed that gastric bypass was also very effective in improving NASH.[35]

The meta-analysis of the effect of RYGB on comorbid conditions shows remarkable improvement in every disease studied.[25] Hypertension resolved in 67.5% and improved in 87.2%. Obstructive sleep apnea resolved in 80.4% and improved in 94.8%. Hyperlipidemia, hypercholesterolemia, and hypertriglyceridemia improved in 96.9%, 94.9%, and 91.2%, respectively, of patients undergoing RYGB.

RYGB has also been shown to resolve the symptoms of pseudotumor cerebri, as well as cure the difficult problem of venous stasis ulcers.

Immediate resolution of symptoms of GERD occurs in more than 90% of cases. The extremely small gastric pouch has a limited reservoir for holding gastric juice, and the cardia is a low acid-producing area of the stomach.

One large comparison study of laparoscopic RYGB versus laparoscopic AGB showed that laparoscopic RYGB achieved greater weight loss at all times during the comparison until 18 months postoperatively. At 12 months, laparoscopic RYGB patients had lost 67% of their excess weight versus 33% for AGB. However, the AGB series was older, and long-term follow-up of the AGB group showed 58% loss of excess weight at 4 years.[36]

Biliopancreatic Diversion/Duodenal Switch

Most malabsorptive procedures performed in the United States are the DS modification of BPD, so this section will discuss the results of both operations. EWL after BPD/DS is the highest of the bariatric operations dis-

cussed in this chapter, with a mean weight loss of 46.4 and 53.1 kg found by meta-analysis (see Table 17-1). Percent EWL for BPD/DS was 70.1%, also the highest for any of the procedures discussed in this chapter.[25,26]

In a recent study comparing morbidly obese patients with a BMI greater than 50 kg/m^2, there was significantly more EWL at 12, 18, and 24 months postoperatively after DS than after RYGB. Twelve months postoperatively, EWL was 65% in the DS group and 57% in the RYGB group.[37] Thus, some surgeons argue that super-obese patients fare better and maintain weight loss better in the long term after undergoing DS than after other bariatric operations. Others point out that side effects, mortality, and morbidity are much higher with DS and therefore the incremental improvements in EWL are not justified.

BPD/DS has also been highly effective in treating comorbid conditions, including hypertension, diabetes, lipid disorders, and obstructive sleep apnea. Lipid disorders and type 2 diabetes are almost uniformly resolved after BPD/DS, as shown in Table 17-4. Hypertension is cured in 83.4% and obstructive sleep apnea resolves in 91.9% of patients.[25]

After BPD, patients typically have between two and four bowel movements per day. Excessive flatulence and foul-smelling stools are the rule. Relatively selective malabsorption of starch and fat provides the major mechanism of weight loss, although the partial gastric resection does contribute a restrictive component to the operation.

Surgeons caring for these patients must be alert to measure protein levels for confirmation of adequate absorption. When protein malnutrition does occur, the common channel may need to be lengthened with a reoperation. Patients must also be aware that their ability to absorb simple sugars, alcohol, and short-chain triglycerides is good and that overindulgence of sweets, milk products, soft drinks, alcohol, and fruit may produce excess weight gain.

Table 17-5   Comparison of Complications After Laparoscopic and Open Roux-en-Y Gastric Bypass

ADVERSE EVENT AND TYPE OF PROCEDURE	ADVERSE EVENT RATE (%)	ODDS RATIO (95% CI)	PATIENTS
Respiratory (including pneumonia, atelectasis, and respiratory insufficiency) Open vs. laparoscopic	3.0 vs. 1.9	1.54 (0.17-19.42)	101 vs. 104
Surgical, preventable and not preventable (including wound, hernia, splenic injury, repeated operation, anastomotic events, and others) Open vs. laparoscopic	31.1 vs. 26.1	1.32 (0.72-2.43)	122 vs. 134
Wound, all Open vs. laparoscopic	13.1 vs. 0.0	Not estimable	122 vs. 134
Wound infection, major Open vs. laparoscopic	3.0 vs. 0.0	Not estimable	101 vs. 104
Wound infection, minor Open vs. laparoscopic	14.3 vs. 0.0	Not estimable	21 vs. 30
Incisional hernia Open vs. laparoscopic	8.2 vs. 0.0	Not estimable	122 vs. 134
Internal hernia Open vs. laparoscopic	0.0 vs. 1.3	0.00 (0.00-40.40)	76 vs. 79
Reoperation Open vs. laparoscopic	0.0 vs. 4.0	0.00 (0.00-38.94)	25 vs. 25
Deep venous thrombosis, pulmonary embolism, or both Open vs. laparoscopic	1.0 vs. 0.9	1.22 (0.02-96.69)	97 vs. 109

From Maggard MA, Shugarman LR, Suttorp M, et al: Meta-analysis: Surgical treatment of obesity. Ann Intern Med 142:547-559, 2005.

Major considerations for achieving excellent results in patients offered BPD/DS include the ability to reliably monitor these patients, as well as confirm that they are being compliant with the recommendations to take appropriate vitamin supplements. Supplements include multivitamins, as well as at least 2 g of oral calcium per day. Supplemental fat-soluble vitamins, including D, K, and A, are indicated monthly as well.

The reported experience with laparoscopic DS has been limited. Prachand and coworkers[37] reported results in 185 DS procedures, the majority of which were performed laparoscopically. The patients in this series, having been selected because they had a BMI greater than 50 kg/m^2, were larger than patients in most selected series. A median loss of 73% of excess weight was noted at 18 months after surgery. There was a 0.5% mortality rate (one patient), which is the lowest ever reported for BPD/DS.

Because of a high incidence of morbidity and mortality (23% and 6.5%) in patients with a BMI greater than 60 kg/m^2 undergoing laparoscopic DS, surgeons developed the two-stage DS, with sleeve gastrectomy alone performed as the first stage to decrease morbidity in this super-obese patient population. Milone and colleagues reported their findings in a group of 18 patients in whom both stages of the operation were performed within 1 year, with a mean interval between operations of 196 days and a mean decrease in BMI from 65 to 51 kg/m^2 between stages. Mean loss of excess weight in the group at 6 months was 71%, with no mortality and two complications (5.6%).[20]

COMPLICATIONS

The various procedures are associated with complications that can occur with any intra-abdominal operation, such as pulmonary embolism. However, each operation has unique complications, as well as different incidences of some of the shared common complications seen after any abdominal operation.

Maggard and colleagues[26] have shown laparoscopic procedures to be associated with less respiratory, surgical wound, and thrombotic complications. The differences taken from the meta-analysis are detailed in Table 17-5. It is clear that respiratory, surgical wound, and thrombotic complications related to the upper abdominal incision and postoperative pain have been reduced with the minimally invasive laparoscopic approach. The benefits touted for laparoscopic surgery go beyond the cosmetic and really do influence postoperative complication rates, which makes the laparoscopic technique our preferred approach in virtually every patient, including remedial operations.

Adjustable Gastric Banding

The mortality associated with AGB (0.02%-0.1%) has been significantly lower than that for RYGB (0.3%-0.5%)

Table 17-6 **Complications After Laparoscopic Adjustable Gastric Banding**

CRITERIA	O'BRIEN	BUCHWALD	MAGGARD	PONCE
Number of patients	1120	2297	9222	1014
Mortality	0	0.1%	0.04	0
Postoperative complications	1.5		13.2	
Slippage	13.9			21 (PG)/1.4 (PF)
Erosions	3			0.2
Port complications	5.4			1.2
Reoperations	25.3		7.7	
Perforations	0			0
Pulmonary embolism	0			
Wound infection	0.9			

All numbers except number of patients represent percentages.
PF, pars flaccida; PG, perigastric.

or either of the malabsorptive operations (0.9%-1.1%).[25,26] Complications for the procedure are described in this section and summarized in Table 17-6. A major complication of either RYGB or BPD/DS is the risk of leakage from the anastomosis, which does not occur with AGB; however, from the meta-analysis it appears that the need for reoperation and complications related to surgery occur in all types of bariatric procedures.

Large series of AGB procedures report an overall complication rate of 11%.[38] The rate of perioperative complications for laparoscopic AGB was 1.5%. The rate of band slippage or prolapse was 13.9%, the rate of erosion was 3%, and port access problems occurred in 5.4%.

A common complication that plagued AGB in the mid to late 1990s was the high incidence of band slippage, which was reported in 15% of patients in one series,[39] a figure that was comparable to other reports for the initial perigastric band placement. Before the *pars flaccida* technique, the band was placed around the proximal part of the stomach, with the posterior portion of the band free within the lesser sac, a technique termed the perigastric approach. This allowed much more movement of the stomach, and despite the anterior imbricating sutures, the fundus of the stomach herniated up through the band in a significant percentage of cases. In a randomized trial of the two techniques, O'Brien and colleagues showed that use of the pars flaccida technique was associated with a much lower rate of slippage than use of the perigastric technique was (4% versus 15%).[39] The pars flaccida technique has subsequently become the preferred approach.

This so-called slippage is usually manifested as the sudden development of food intolerance or occasionally gastroesophageal reflux. The latter symptom is also indicative of any form of obstruction at the site of the band. Slippage is by far the most common cause of obstruction, but on occasion, erosion and fibrosis can also cause similar symptoms. A patient with obstructive symptoms or food intolerance has a plain radiograph of the abdomen taken. In its appropriate position, the band is oriented in a diagonal direction, along the 1- to 7-o'clock or the 2- to 8-o'clock axis in the epigastric region. A plain film showing the band in a horizontal or a 10- to 4-o'clock position is diagnostic of slippage and altered band position. Slippage or any other obstructive process at the band site will give rise to functional stenosis of the gastrointestinal tract at the proximal end of the stomach. As a result, esophageal dilation can occur if this situation is not fixed.

Erosion of the band into the lumen of the stomach is a far less frequent complication but requires reoperation. The incidence of erosion may increase with the passage of time. At this time, however, the incidence remains below 1% for many large series and up to 3% as noted earlier in the Australian collected experience.[38] Erosion may be manifested as abdominal pain or as a port access site infection. In cases in which the band does erode into the stomach, it is presumed that the band is either too tight or the stomach was imbricated too close to the buckle of the band, which will cause erosion over time. Surprisingly, this complication is rarely life threatening, and there are many reports in the literature describing removal of the eroded band, repair of the stomach, and replacement of a new band at the same operative setting.

Port access site problems are the most numerous of the complications that occur after AGB. These problems also require reoperative therapy in most cases, but the procedure can often be performed under local anesthesia and does not involve the peritoneal cavity. Leakage of the access tubing is a common problem that occurs in up to 11% of cases. In addition, kinking of the tubing as it passes through the fascia is another relatively common reason for port access difficulties. Port site infection is the least common port access problem (<1%) but needs to be evaluated with upper endoscopy to be certain that band erosion has not occurred.

Roux-en-Y Gastric Bypass

Mortality rates after RYGB have generally been in the 0.3% to 1.0% range for large reported series. Meta-

Table 17-7 Complications After Roux-en-Y Gastric Bypass

CRITERIA	SUGERMAN	MAGGARD	BUCHWALD
Number of patients	1025	11290	5644
Mortality (%)	0.9	0.3	0.5
Gastrointestinal bleeding (%)		2.0	
Leak/major wound complications (%)	3	2.2	

analysis showed a 30-day mortality rate of 0.3% to 0.5% for RYGB (see Table 17-1).[25,26]

Causes of mortality have varied but include pulmonary embolism, anastomotic leak, cardiac events, intra-abdominal abscess, and multiorgan failure. Mortality rates are obviously influenced heavily by patient selection. Male gender is also associated with an increased risk for morbidity and mortality in many published series in which this has been analyzed.[40] Overall complication rates from RYGB vary greatly depending on the reporting. Liu and coworkers[41] reviewed the incidence of complications after RYGB in California, during which time the incidence of serious complications decreased from 15.1% to 7.6%. The authors identified male gender, presence of comorbidity, and low hospital volume of the procedure as independent predictors of complications. Overall complication rates in the authors' series of open RYGB approached 40%, including a 15% to 24% incidence of incisional hernias, depending on the time of analysis of the series, and a wound seroma/hematoma rate approaching 8%. The wound infection rate of all severity was in the 7% range. As noted earlier, the use of a laparoscopic approach has greatly lessened the incisional hernia and wound complication rates.[12] Anastomotic leak/complication occurred in 2.2%, and the reoperation rate was 1.6% in the meta-analysis.[26] Table 17-7 summarizes data regarding complications after RYGB.

Pulmonary embolism is one of the most feared complications after any form of bariatric surgery, and its incidence in large reported series of open RYGB sometimes exceeds 1%. Thrombotic complications such as DVT and pulmonary embolism appear to be less frequently associated with laparoscopic surgery than with open gastric bypass.

Improvement in postoperative morbidity after laparoscopic procedures is not limited to incisional hernia, as detailed in Table 17-5. Specifically, postoperative atelectasis/pneumonia and respiratory insufficiency are 1.54 times more common after open bariatric than after laparoscopic procedures.[26]

Although nausea and vomiting are not unusual in isolated circumstances after RYGB, especially in relation to a patient's adaptation to food restriction, if persistent these symptoms can lead to the obvious problem of dehydration. This must be aggressively treated in the postoperative period or when associated with a viral or other gastrointestinal illness compounding the problem

and further limiting oral intake. Intravenous fluids are indicated when in doubt. This is the case for all bariatric operations, not just RYGB.

One specific problem that may arise with persistent vomiting after *any* of the bariatric operations and that is *imperative* for the surgeon to remember and treat is Wernicke's encephalopathy from prolonged vomiting. This neurologic deficit is preventable with appropriate administration of parenteral thiamine (vitamin B_1) when the patient has persistent and severe vomiting. If the neurologic symptoms become significant, they may often not be fully reversed despite thiamine therapy.

Because depression is so frequent in the patient population undergoing bariatric surgery, severe postoperative depression may develop after any of the bariatric operations as well. When it does occur, the patient may totally stop eating, thereby producing what at first seems like wonderful weight loss, but soon, when gone beyond its desired end point, it progresses to loss of critical visceral and musculoskeletal protein mass, which can be life threatening.

Complications specific to RYGB include anastomotic leaks from the proximal or distal anastomosis. Leaks from the gastrojejunostomy are more common and are generally the cause of a significant percentage of the life-threatening complications and deaths in any large series of patients. Data suggest that a surgeon's experience will influence the leak rate, especially early in the laparoscopic experience with RYGB. Most large series of open RYGB procedures reported a leak rate of 1% to 2%, whereas some laparoscopic surgeons early in their experience were observing a leak rate approaching 5%. Maggard and colleagues found a leak rate of 2.2% in open and laparoscopic RYGB.[26] Fortunately, this appears to be a transient phenomenon of learning for some surgeons; most large series of laparoscopic RYGB now report anastomotic leak rates of 1% to 2%, and some have treated large series without a leak.[16]

Another specific life-threatening complication that may result after RYGB is that of bowel obstruction. Patients who have a clinical or radiographic picture of small bowel obstruction after RYGB need a reoperation. The potential for internal hernias after this operation makes strangulation obstruction a frequent type of bowel obstruction. Patients with bowel obstruction and not ileus in the immediate postoperative period (we perform CT with contrast or an upper gastrointestinal series to confirm or rule out obstruction) *must* be promptly operated on. Retrograde distention of the biliopancreatic limb and distal part of the stomach can result in rupture of the distal gastric staple line with subsequent peritonitis.

Stenosis of the gastrojejunostomy may occur after RYGB and has been reported in 2% to 14% of patients in various series. The higher incidence seems to be associated with circular stapler versus suture-type anastomoses. Postoperative anastomotic stenosis is usually manifested at 4 to 6 weeks postoperatively as progressive intolerance to solids and then liquids in a setting in which they were previously tolerated. The problem is quite successfully treated with endoscopic or fluoroscopic balloon dilation. Unless a marginal ulcer is associated

Table 17-8   Complications After Malabsorptive Operations (Biliopancreatic Diversion and Duodenal Switch)

CRITERIA	SCOPINARO	BUCHWALD	MAGGARD	REN
Number of patients	1356	3030	2808	170
Mortality	0.7	1.1	0.9	
Leak	0.1		1.8	
DVT/PE	?/0.07			
Medical problems/malnutrition				
Iron deficiency anemia	40			
Vitamin A deficiency				69
Vitamin K deficiency				68
Vitamin D deficiency				63

All numbers except number of patients represent percentages.
DVT, deep venous thrombosis; PE, pulmonary embolism.

with the stenosis, the problem does not require a reoperation.

A marginal ulcer occurs after 2% to 10% of RYGB procedures. The incidence can be decreased by preoperative treatment of patients for *Helicobacter pylori* colonization of the stomach. Patients with a marginal ulcer typically have continuous boring epigastric pain. Treatment consists of medical therapy with proton pump inhibitors. Medical treatment resolves all marginal ulcers unless the ulcer has fistulized to the lower part of the stomach and created an ongoing source of acid to exacerbate the ulcer.

Short-term metabolic complications after RYGB can include dehydration. Another problem in both the short and long term may be severe dumping. This is initially addressed by diet modification to avoid sweets and highly concentrated foods, as well as separating eating and drinking. Should the dumping be uncontrollable with these measures, subcutaneous octreotide is generally highly successful in reversing the symptoms of severe postoperative dumping. The medication may need to be administered for several months, after which the drug can usually be tapered over a several-month interval.

Iron and vitamin B_{12} deficiencies are the two most common long-term metabolic complications of RYGB. The incidence of iron insufficiency varies among reported series. Iron is preferentially absorbed in the duodenum and proximal jejunum. Hence, RYGB bypasses the area of maximal iron absorption in the gut. The iron deficiency, based on serum values, is between 15% and 40%, whereas actual iron deficiency anemia occurs in as many as 20% of patients after RYGB. This problem is easily treated in most cases with oral iron supplements. The gluconate form of iron is best absorbed in a nonacid environment.

The incidence of vitamin B_{12} deficiency after RYGB is reported as being 15% to 20%, although it rarely causes anemia. Peripheral neural complications from low vitamin B_{12} after RYGB are virtually unknown. Vitamin B_{12} deficiency is due to inefficient absorption because of delayed mixing with intrinsic factor. Several preparations include intrinsic factor and will maximize absorption in the terminal ileum. Other routes of vitamin B_{12} administration include sublingual medication, nasal spray, and parenteral injections.

Laparoscopic RYGB has been associated with overall complications similar to those after open RYGB in many areas but has differed significantly in some. The incidence of associated splenectomy, wound infection, incisional hernia, respiratory complications, and DVT/pulmonary embolism was lower with laparoscopic RYGB than with open RYGB.[26] In contrast, the incidence of bowel obstruction, especially early bowel obstruction, appears to be higher in patients undergoing laparoscopic RYGB.

Biliopancreatic Diversion

Mortality rates after BPD/DS were reported to be 1.1% in the meta-analysis of Buchwald and colleagues and 0.9% in Maggard and associates' study.[25,26] Surgical wound complications occur in 5.9% of patients, leaks develop in 1.8%, and reoperations occur 4.2% of the time, as summarized in Table 17-8.[26]

The most significant and specific long-term complication seen after BPD is protein malnutrition, which occurs in 11.9% of patients. Treatment is hospitalization with 2 to 3 weeks of parenteral nutrition. This particular problem is usually manifested within the first few months after surgery, but it can occur sporadically, though less frequently, after surgery. In one series, 4% of patients eventually required a reoperation to either reverse the BPD completely or lengthen the common channel. The revision rate was approximately 0.1% annually for the first 6 years, and the rehospitalization rate for malabsorption or diarrhea was 0.93% annually during that time. The percentage of patients averaging more than three bowel movements per day was 7%, and 34% believed that the unpleasant odor of stools and flatus was a problem. Abdominal bloating was experienced in a third of patients more than once weekly. Bone pain was reported in 29% of patients. Metabolic complications and side effects included iron deficiency in 9%, low ferritin level in 25%, low calcium concentration in 8%, and low level of vitamin A in 5%. Elevated parathyroid hormone levels were present in 17%.

Malabsorption of fat-soluble vitamins is one of the major problems associated with BPD/DS. Ren and associates[42] showed that levels of vitamins D and A 2 years after BPD were significantly depressed, with vitamin D deficiency in 63%, vitamin A deficiency in 69%, evidence of bone resorption in 3%, and all patients having essential fatty acid deficiency. Lack of clinical correlation with these levels suggests that the problem may be more prevalent than originally reported or suspected from past series.

Although the complication of protein malnutrition and poor intake is theoretically most likely to occur soon after BPD/DS, the fact that late deaths occur from protein malnutrition and Wernicke's encephalopathy suggests that these patients may always be at risk for these problems.

Marginal ulcers are a distinct problem of BPD, but with revision of the anastomotic technique and the use of H₂ blockers, they can be substantially reduced.

Perhaps it is the overall difficulty of the operation, as well as the potential dangers of the operation, that has left BPD the least popular operation performed in the United States. Even the DS modification does not represent more than 10% of bariatric operations. Further studies are needed to evaluate the long-term consequences of BPD and DS to justify the performance of such operations as a primary procedure.

REOPERATIVE SURGERY

A controversial topic is the appropriateness of performing repeat bariatric operations for failed previous ones. There are no specific rules to govern the appropriateness of repeat bariatric surgery. The absolute definition of a failed operation is unclear, but most surgeons would accept return to the criteria listed in Box 17-2 as appropriate when considering reoperation. If a patient has undergone an operation that has proved by mass experience to be ineffective, a repeat operation for failure of that procedure is appropriate. Complications of procedures, such as stenosis causing gastric outlet obstruction after vertical banded gastroplasty or metabolic complications after jejunoileal bypass, are obvious indications for revisional surgery. One mistake frequently made by a nonbariatric surgeon in correcting a complication of a bariatric operation is to simply perform a procedure that corrects the complication but does not provide for continued weight restriction. In these circumstances, a typical long-term course is for patients to slowly regain weight to their degree of obesity before the initial bariatric procedure and then seek further surgical assistance.

In assessing a patient for the appropriateness of reoperative surgery, the surgeon must determine whether the original bariatric operation is intact and anatomically still appropriate for maintaining weight loss. If not, consideration for reoperation is appropriate. However, a patient who has failed an anatomically intact and well-constructed bariatric operation is, in our opinion, at high risk to fail a second or revisional bariatric operation. Although little has been reported, there are no reports contradicting this logic. It is known that the incidence of infection, organ ischemia, anastomotic leakage, blood transfusion, and other severe intra-abdominal complications is increased in revisional surgery.

All bariatric operations have some incidence of failure. A figure of approximately 10% is often used in discussions regarding the failure rate of various well-established operations considered effective, including all operations described in this chapter. The definition of *failure* is varied and may include inadequate weight loss, inadequate resolution of medical comorbid conditions, the development of side effects negatively influencing lifestyle and satisfaction, the development of complications requiring medical or surgical intervention, or complications requiring alteration or reversal of the operation.

Jejunoileal bypass, a relic of history, still exists in a small number of patients, who need to have it reversed to prevent progression to cirrhosis/liver failure and other severe metabolic consequences. Any reversal must include a replacement weight reduction operation.

Use of AGB as a revision procedure has been successful in several centers. Failed RYGB has been treated by adding a malabsorptive component to the original procedure by reconnecting the efferent end of the RYGB halfway down the length of the alimentary bowel and thereby decreasing the alimentary tract in half. Although patients experience a decrease in BMI, protein malnutrition can develop in a significant number. Conversion of patients after failed open or laparoscopic gastroplasty to RYGB has been shown to decrease BMI. The use of laparoscopic BPD to treat patients with failed weight loss after laparoscopic AGB was reported by Fielding.[43] Other sporadic reports of small case series in the literature suggest that even reoperations can, under appropriate circumstances, be performed laparoscopically and give relatively good results, although not with as low a complication rate as the initial surgery.

CONTROVERSIES IN BARIATRIC SURGERY

Controversy exists concerning morbidity and mortality after bariatric surgery in routine practice versus the published results usually reported by experienced surgeons. Flum and associates[44] accessed the Medicare database for all bariatric surgical procedures from 1997 to 2002 and found that the 30-day mortality was 2.0%—much higher than the rate reported in the two meta-analyses. Mortality also increased to 4.8% in patients older than 65 years versus a rate of 1.7% in those younger than 65. Patients 75 years or older had five times the risk of death than those aged 65 to 74. The risk of death 90 days postoperatively was greater for men than women (4.8% versus 2.1%) and for patients whose surgeon performed less than the median number of bariatric procedures (odds ratio of 1.6 at 90 days postoperatively). They found high mortality within the first 30 days, but also a surprisingly high death rate (4.6%) within the first year after surgery. Their conclusion was that mortality rates were much higher in real-life practice than those reported in retrospective case review or prospective studies.[44] The increased mortality rates in this patient population point out the inherent risks of operating on patients already declared disabled on the basis of comorbid conditions arising often directly from their obesity. Finally, the very high mortality rate during the year after surgery, especially in male groups older than 30 years, is related to the decreased life expectancy of the group in general once such a severely diseased state is present.

Nguyen and colleagues[45] showed that high-volume academic hospitals had a lower mortality rate, length of hospital stay, complication rate, and cost. In patients older than 55 years, mortality was 3.1% at low-volume hospitals and 0.9% at high-volume centers. These reports of high morbidity and mortality after bariatric surgery and the reduction in rates in high-volume centers led to a spate of editorials and policy changes aimed at reducing the risk associated with bariatric surgery. One of the most important developments has been the medical policy decision handed down by CMS for Medicare beneficiaries in February 2006, which is notable for the dramatic step of requiring that surgery be performed only in Centers of Excellence as certified by the American College of Surgeons[46] or the American Society of Bariatric Surgeons.[47] The requirement for surgeons and the hospitals in which the surgery is performed to go through a significant vetting process, demonstration of surgical results, and demonstration of the processes and readiness of the facilities to take care of the needs of morbidly obese patients is a seminal event in the practice of surgery in the United States. The future most certainly holds the surgeon and the hospital more accountable to be able to demonstrate the outcome of their surgical care of patients in both the short and long term. The current CMS decision, though perhaps made as a means of recognizing the validity of bariatric surgery performed at high-volume centers, has had the unfortunate effect of limiting the access of many federally insured patients to care.

INVESTIGATIONAL BARIATRIC PROCEDURES

A number of procedures have been investigated for weight loss surgery but have not been totally accepted by the surgical community. Several surgeons have proposed a two-stage procedure for a super-obese patient, who often has a large liver that precludes safe retraction for gastric bypass, because of the recognition that the DS procedure has been associated with much higher mortality and morbidity rates in the super-obese (BMI >60 kg/m^2).[20,21] They have proposed performance of a sleeve gastrectomy as the first stage, and then months afterward, in a second procedure, they convert the sleeve gastrectomy to either

a gastric bypass or a DS. When this technique was used, operative mortality was lowered dramatically during the first stage of surgery. Now, reports of vertical sleeve gastrectomy (VSG) alone suggest that weight loss is sufficient to preclude conversion to gastric bypass or DS. EWL was 58.5% at 12 months and 83.1% at 24 months after VSG.[48] The weight loss resulting from VSG was comparable to that in patients undergoing DS or RYGB and has led them to conclude that VSG produces adequate weight loss with morbidity comparable to that after AGB. Long-term weight loss data will be essential in confirming the efficacy of this procedure.

Gastric pacing has been performed in several trials but has not gained widespread acceptance. The concept is to stimulate gastric smooth muscle by implanting a pacemaker in the body of the stomach to induce early satiety, which reduces caloric intake and therefore results in weight loss. Animal studies have shown that pacing by gastric electrical stimulation with a gastric pacemaker can induce delayed gastric emptying, reduce caloric intake, and induce weight loss. The actual physiology of the reduction in food intake is still poorly understood and has not been particularly actively investigated. Human trials have been only partially successful and have aimed at pacing at a level just below what it takes to induce nausea. Clinical trials show EWL of 23% after 16 months, and selected patients (preoperative screening algorithm) have a better outcome with almost 40% EWL.[49]

Increasingly, surgeons are observing effects of bariatric operations not just on the physical reduction of caloric intake or malabsorption. Alteration in comorbid conditions caused by metabolic processes may prove equally as important. For example, bariatric operations may have important metabolic components that alter the hormonal/cytokine/metabolic rate of patients.[50]

THE BARIATRIC REVOLUTION AND COUNTERREVOLUTION

Bariatric surgery is literally in the midst of a revolution. In many U.S. hospitals, bariatric surgical procedures are the most commonly performed operation on the general surgical service.[51]

There are several reasons for this rapid revolution. The most important one, which temporally corresponds with the rapid rise in patient demand for bariatric surgery, is the use of a laparoscopic approach for operations. Although a laparoscopic approach was more commonplace in Europe and Australia in the mid-1990s with advent of the popularity of laparoscopic AGB on those continents, use of the laparoscopic approach for RYGB in the United States really began only in 1999. Before then, just a very few medical centers were offering that approach. Laparoscopic AGB was not performed in the United States until 2001, but it is rapidly becoming the most common bariatric procedure performed in some U.S. centers.

Mass media and the rapid dissemination of information are also a major factor in the bariatric revolution. Patients may now access many sites on the Internet where information about bariatric surgery is available. Television stations show videos of actual operations. Internet chat groups in which former and prospective patients discuss the topic of bariatric surgery are common, and many patients participate in these groups both before and after surgery. Media and television personalities have undergone bariatric surgery, with superb results that they have been quite willing to share with the public. The combination of all these factors has led to a patient population that is more informed and more aware of the potential of such surgery to treat their morbid obesity.

Finally, the surgical community itself has adjusted its perception of bariatric surgery. It is now a desirable area of specialization for graduating residents, who enjoy the technical challenge of advanced laparoscopic surgery combined with the rewards of performing a life-altering and usually highly successful operation for their patients.

CONCLUSION

Surgical treatment of morbid obesity is no longer considered out of the mainstream of general surgery and is now a component of most surgical residents' training programs. It currently represents the fastest growing area of general surgery. Patient demand for the procedure has vastly increased; at present, surgeons operate annually on only 1% of the eligible patients who would benefit from bariatric surgery. This chapter has discussed all aspects of the performance of bariatric surgery in current surgical practice, including the most commonly performed procedures at this time. The disease process of morbid obesity is unfortunately both poorly understood and rapidly increasing. Surgical therapy is currently the only effective treatment of morbid obesity.

Selected References

Buchwald H, Avidor Y, Braunwald E, et al: Bariatric surgery: A systematic review and meta-analysis. JAMA 292:1724-1737, 2004.

The authors reviewed the literature and selected 136 studies (22,094 patients) that they reviewed and subjected to meta-analysis. Bariatric surgery was found to be very effective in weight loss and resulted in improvement or cure of serious comorbid conditions (diabetes, dyslipidemia, hypertension, and sleep apnea) in the majority of patients. This comprehensive meta-analysis provides the most compelling data on the effectiveness and beneficial results of bariatric surgery in the literature.

Christou NV, Sampalis JS, Liberman M, et al: Surgery decreases long-term mortality, morbidity, and health care use in morbidly obese patients. Ann Surg 240:416-423; discussion 423-414, 2004.

In a study comparing matched control subjects with subjects who underwent bariatric surgery in Canada, Christou and coauthors demonstrated that weight loss surgery reduced the relative risk for mortality by 89% (95% confidence interval, 73% to 96%) 5 years after surgery. This is one of the substantial arguments for the effectiveness of bariatric surgery to not only reduce weight but to also ameliorate or cure the comorbid conditions, which increases survival.

Maggard MA, Shugarman LR, Suttorp M, et al: Meta-analysis: Surgical treatment of obesity. Ann Intern Med 142:547-559, 2005.

The authors assessed 147 studies on bariatric surgery to analyze weight loss, mortality, and complications. They found that laparoscopic gastric bypass resulted in fewer wound complications, incisional hernias, and respiratory complications than the open approach did. They concluded from the analysis of weight loss and resolution of comorbid conditions that bariatric surgery was more effective than medical treatment in patients with a BMI of 40 kg/m^2 or greater. This study amplifies the growing body of data supporting bariatric surgery as being safe and effective.

Nguyen NT, Goldman C, Rosenquist CJ, et al: Laparoscopic versus open gastric bypass: A randomized study of outcomes, quality of life, and costs. Ann Surg 234:279-289; discussion 289-291, 2001.

The first prospective randomized trial comparing laparoscopic with open gastric bypass. Patients were monitored for 1 year, at which time weight loss with both approaches was comparable (68% loss of excess weight for laparoscopic RYGB versus 62% loss of excess weight for open RYGB), but the laparoscopic approach had a shorter length of hospitalization and more rapid return to activities of daily living than the open procedure did.

Sjostrom L, Lindroos AK, Peltonen M, et al: Lifestyle, diabetes, and cardiovascular risk factors 10 years after bariatric surgery. N Engl J Med 351:2683-2693, 2004.

This study compared a group of patients undergoing bariatric surgery with a group of matched control subjects and monitored them for 10 years. They found an 80% decrease in the annual mortality of diabetic individuals in the surgical weight loss group as compared with control patients not undergoing surgery (9% mortality at 9 years versus 28% mortality in the control group). This is the best long-term study indicating that bariatric surgery results in sustained weight loss, resolution of comorbid conditions, and increased survival in comparison to standard medical treatment.

References

1. Gastrointestinal surgery for severe obesity: National Institutes of Health Consensus Development Conference Statement. Am J Clin Nutr 55(Suppl 2):S615-S619, 1992.
2. Flegal KM, Carroll MD, Ogden CL, et al: Prevalence and trends in obesity among US adults, 1999-2000. JAMA 288:1723-1727, 2002.
3. Fontaine KR, Redden DT, Wang C, et al: Years of life lost due to obesity. JAMA 289:187-193, 2003.
4. Cummings DE, Weigle DS, Frayo RS, et al: Plasma ghrelin levels after diet-induced weight loss or gastric bypass surgery. N Engl J Med 346:1623-1630, 2002.
5. Weigle DS: Pharmacological therapy of obesity: Past, present, and future. J Clin Endocrinol Metab 88:2462-2469, 2003.
6. Centers for Medicare and Medicaid Services: Decision Memo for Bariatric Surgery for the Treatment of Morbid Obesity (CAG-00250R) (website). Available at http://www.cms.hhs.gov/mcd/viewdecisionmemo.asp?id=160. Accessed October 19, 2006.
7. Dolan K, Creighton L, Hopkins G, et al: Laparoscopic gastric banding in morbidly obese adolescents. Obes Surg 13:101-104, 2003.
8. Simard B, Turcotte H, Marceau P, et al: Asthma and sleep apnea in patients with morbid obesity: Outcome after bariatric surgery. Obes Surg 14:1381-1388, 2004.
9. Sugerman HJ, Sugerman EL, Wolfe L, et al: Risks and benefits of gastric bypass in morbidly obese patients with severe venous stasis disease. Ann Surg 234:41-46, 2001.

10. Sugerman HJ, Brolin RE, Fobi MAL, et al: Prophylactic ursodeoxycholic acid prevents gallstone formation following gastric bypass–induced rapid weight loss: A multicenter, placebo controlled, randomized, double-blinded, prospective trial. Am J Surg 169:91-97, 1995.

11. Schirmer B, Erenoglu C, Miller A: Flexible endoscopy in the management of patients undergoing Roux-en-Y gastric bypass. Obes Surg 12:634-638, 2002.

12. Nguyen NT, Goldman C, Rosenquist CJ, et al: Laparoscopic versus open gastric bypass: A randomized study of outcomes, quality of life, and costs. Ann Surg 234:279-289; discussion 289-291, 2001.

13. Fielding GA, Allen JW: A step-by-step guide to placement of the LAP-BAND adjustable gastric banding system. Am J Surg 184:26S-30S, 2002.

14. Schauer P, Ikramuddin S, Hamad G, et al: The learning curve for laparoscopic Roux-en-Y gastric bypass is 100 cases. Surg Endosc 17:212-215, 2003.

15. Brolin RE, Kenler HA, Gorman JH, Cody RP: Long-limb gastric bypass in the superobese: A prospective randomized study. Ann Surg 215:387-395, 1992.

16. Sekhar N, Torquati A, Lutfi R, et al: Endoscopic evaluation of the gastrojejunostomy in laparoscopic gastric bypass. A series of 340 patients without postoperative leak. Surg Endosc 20:199-201, 2006.

17. Gonzalez R, Lin E, Venkatesh KR, et al: Gastrojejunostomy during laparoscopic gastric bypass: Analysis of 3 techniques. Arch Surg 138:181-184, 2003.

18. Scott JR, Miller A, Miller M, et al: Retrocolic herniation following laparoscopic Roux-en-Y gastric bypass: Potential prevention? Obes Surg 13:230, 2003.

19. Scopinaro N, Marinari GM, Camerini G: Laparoscopic standard biliopancreatic diversion: Technique and preliminary results. Obes Surg 12:362-365, 2002.

20. Milone L, Strong V, Gagner M: Laparoscopic sleeve gastrectomy is superior to endoscopic intragastric balloon as a first stage procedure for super-obese patients (BMI > or = 50). Obes Surg 15:612-617, 2005.

21. DeMaria EJ, Schauer P, Patterson E, et al: The optimal surgical management of the super-obese patient: The debate. Presented at the annual meeting of the Society of American Gastrointestinal and Endoscopic Surgeons, Hollywood, Florida, USA, April 13-16, 2005. Surg Innov 12:107-121, 2005.

22. Ren CJ: Controversies in bariatric surgery: Evidence-based discussions on laparoscopic adjustable gastric banding. J Gastrointest Surg 8:396-397; discussion 404-395, 2004.

23. Christou NV, Sampalis JS, Liberman M, et al: Surgery decreases long-term mortality, morbidity, and health care use in morbidly obese patients. Ann Surg 240:416-423; discussion 423-414, 2004.

24. Sjostrom L, Lindroos AK, Peltonen M, et al.: Lifestyle, diabetes, and cardiovascular risk factors 10 years after bariatric surgery. N Engl J Med 351:2683-2693, 2004.

25. Buchwald H, Avidor Y, Braunwald E, et al: Bariatric surgery: A systematic review and meta-analysis. JAMA 292:1724-1737, 2004.

26. Maggard MA, Shugarman LR, Suttorp M, et al: Meta-analysis: Surgical treatment of obesity. Ann Intern Med 142:547-559, 2005.

27. Poulose BK, Holzman MD, Zhu Y, et al: National variations in morbid obesity and bariatric surgery use. J Am Coll Surg 201:77-84, 2005.

28. O'Brien PE, Dixon JB, Brown W, et al: The laparoscopic adjustable gastric band (Lap-Band): A prospective study of medium-term effects on weight, health and quality of life. Obes Surg 12:652-660, 2002.

29. Ponce J, Paynter S, Fromm R: Laparoscopic adjustable gastric banding: 1,014 consecutive cases. J Am Coll Surg 201:529-535, 2005.

30. Dixon JB, O'Brien PE: Changes in comorbidities and improvements in quality of life after LAP-BAND placement. Am J Surg 184:51S-54S, 2002.

31. Puzziferri N, Austrheim-Smith IT, Wolfe BM, et al: Three-year follow-up of a prospective randomized trial comparing laparoscopic versus open gastric bypass. Ann Surg 243:181-188, 2006.

32. Schauer PR, Burguera B, Ikramuddin S, et al: Effect of laparoscopic Roux-en-Y gastric bypass on type 2 diabetes mellitus. Ann Surg 238:467-484; discussion 484-465, 2003.

33. Torquati A, Lutfi R, Abumrad N, et al: Is Roux-en-Y gastric bypass surgery the most effective treatment for type 2 diabetes mellitus in morbidly obese patients? J Gastrointest Surg 9:1112-1116; discussion 1117-1118, 2005.

34. Madan AK, Orth W, Ternovits CA, et al: Metabolic syndrome: Yet another co-morbidity gastric bypass helps cure. Surg Obes Relat Dis 2:48-51; discussion 51, 2006.

35. Mattar SG, Velcu LM, Rabinovitz M, et al: Surgically-induced weight loss significantly improves nonalcoholic fatty liver disease and the metabolic syndrome. Ann Surg 242:610-617; discussion 618-620, 2005.

36. Biertho L, Steffen R, Ricklin T, et al: Laparoscopic gastric bypass versus laparoscopic adjustable gastric banding: A comparative study of 1,200 cases. J Am Coll Surg 197:536-544; discussion 544-535, 2003.

37. Prachand VN, DaVee RT, Alverdy JC: Duodenal switch provides superior weight loss in the superobese (BMI >50) compared to gastric bypass. Paper presented at a meeting of the American Surgical Association, April 22, 2006, Boston.

38. O'Brien PE, Dixon JB: Weight loss and early and late complications—the international experience. Am J Surg 184:42S-45S, 2002.

39. O'Brien PE, Dixon JB, Laurie C, et al: A prospective randomized trial of placement of the laparoscopic adjustable gastric band: Comparison of the perigastric and pars flaccida pathways. Obes Surg 15:820-826, 2005.

40. Poulose BK, Griffin MR, Moore DE, et al: Risk factors for post-operative mortality in bariatric surgery. J Surg Res 127:1-7, 2005.

41. Liu JH, Zingmond D, Etzioni DA, et al: Characterizing the performance and outcomes of obesity surgery in California. Am Surg 69:823-828, 2003.

42. Ren CJ, Siegel N, Williams T, et al: Fat-soluble nutrient deficiency after malabsorptive operations for morbid obesity. J Gastrointest Surg 8:48-55; discussion 54-55, 2004.

43. Fielding GA: Laparoscopic biliopancreatic diversion with or without duodenal switch as revision for failed lap band. Surg Endosc 17:S187, 2003.

44. Flum DR, Salem L, Elrod JA, et al: Early mortality among Medicare beneficiaries undergoing bariatric surgical procedures. JAMA 294:1903-1908, 2005.

45. Nguyen NT, Paya M, Stevens CM, et al: The relationship between hospital volume and outcome in bariatric surgery at academic medical centers. Ann Surg 240:586-593; discussion 593-584, 2004.

46. http://www.facs.org/cqi/bscn/index.html.

47. http://www.surgicalreview.org/.

48. Lee CM, Feng JJ, Cirangle PT, et al: Laparoscopic vertical sleeve gastrectomy for morbid obesity in 216 patients: Report of two-year results. Paper presented at the annual

meeting of the Society of American Gastrointestinal and Endoscopic Surgeons, April 2006.

49. Shikora SA: "What are the yanks doing?" The U.S. experience with implantable gastric stimulation (IGS) for the treatment of obesity—update on the ongoing clinical trials. Obes Surg 14(Suppl 1):S40-S48, 2004.

50. le Roux CW, Aylwin SJ, Batterham RL, et al: Gut hormone profiles following bariatric surgery favor an anorectic state, facilitate weight loss, and improve metabolic parameters. Ann Surg 243:108-114, 2006.

51. Nguyen NT, Root J, Zainabadi K, et al: Accelerated growth of bariatric surgery with the introduction of minimally invasive surgery. Arch Surg 140:1198-1202; discussion 1203, 2005.

CHAPTER 18

Anesthesiology Principles, Pain Management, and Conscious Sedation

Edward R. Sherwood, MD, PhD   Courtney G. Williams, MD
and   Donald S. Prough, MD

Pharmacologic Principles
Anesthesia Equipment
Patient Monitoring During and After Anesthesia
Preoperative Evaluation
Selection of Anesthetic Techniques and Drugs
Airway Management
Regional Anesthesia
Conscious Sedation
Postanesthesia Care
Acute Pain Management
Conclusion

The relatively brief history of anesthesiology began only a little more than 150 years ago with administration of the first ether anesthetic. Throughout much of the subsequent history, the risk of anesthesia-related mortality and morbidity was unacceptably high as a consequence of primitive equipment, complication-prone drugs, and lack of adequate monitors. However, during the past 4 decades, rapid technologic and pharmacologic progress has resulted in the ability to provide anesthesia safely for complex surgical procedures, even in patients with severe underlying disease.

The most notable advances in anesthesia equipment have been the development of anesthetic machines that reduce the possibility of providing hypoxic gas mixtures, vaporizers that provide more accurate doses of potent inhalational agents, and intraoperative anesthesia ventilators that provide more precise physiologic support. Pharmacologic advances have generally consisted of shorter-acting drugs with fewer important side effects. However, the greatest advances have been in monitoring devices. Monitoring devices of particular value include in-circuit oxygen analyzers, capnometers, pulse oximeters, and anesthetic vapor–specific analyzers. Although these monitors do not guarantee a successful outcome, they markedly increase its probability. This chapter first sets the stage for discussing anesthetic management by reviewing the unique aspects of the anesthetic environment: the drugs, equipment, and monitors that are the basis for safe practice. Subsequent sections address preanesthetic assessment and preparation for anesthesia, selection of anesthetic techniques and drugs, airway management, conscious sedation, postanesthetic care, and management of acute postoperative pain.

PHARMACOLOGIC PRINCIPLES

The initial practice of anesthesiology used single drugs such as ether or chloroform to abolish consciousness, prevent movement during surgery, ensure amnesia, and provide analgesia. In contrast, current anesthesia practice combines multiple agents, often including regional techniques, to achieve specific end points. Although inhalational agents remain the core of modern anesthetic combinations, most anesthesiologists initiate anesthesia with intravenous (IV) induction agents and then maintain anesthesia with inhalational agents supplemented by IV opioids and muscle relaxants. Benzodiazepines are often added to induce anxiolysis and amnesia.

Inhalational Agents

The original inhalational anesthetics—ether, nitrous oxide, and chloroform—had important limitations. Ether was characterized by notoriously slow induction and equally delayed emergence but could produce unconsciousness, amnesia, analgesia, and lack of movement without the addition of other agents. In contrast, both induction and emergence were rapid with nitrous oxide,

Table 18-1 **Important Characteristics of Inhalational Agents**

ANESTHETIC	POTENCY	SPEED OF INDUCTION AND EMERGENCE	SUITABILITY FOR INHALATIONAL INDUCTION	SENSITIZATION TO CATECHOLAMINES	METABOLIZED (%)
Nitrous oxide	Weak	Fast	Insufficient alone	None	Minimal
Diethyl ether	Potent	Very slow	Suitable	None	10
Halothane	Potent	Medium	Suitable	High	20+
Enflurane	Potent	Medium	Not suitable	Medium	<10
Isoflurane	Potent	Medium	Not suitable	Minimal	<2
Sevoflurane	Potent	Rapid	Suitable	Minimal	<5
Desflurane	Potent	Rapid	Not suitable	Minimal	0.02

but the agent lacked sufficient potency to be used alone. Nitrous oxide is still used in combination with other agents. Chloroform was associated with hepatic toxicity and, occasionally, fatal cardiac arrhythmias.

Subsequent drug development has emphasized inhalational agents that facilitate rapid induction and emergence and are nontoxic. Such drugs include halothane, isoflurane, enflurane, sevoflurane, and desflurane. The important aspects of each drug can be summarized in terms of key clinical attributes (Table 18-1). Two of the most important characteristics of inhalational anesthetics are the blood/gas (B/G) solubility coefficient and the minimum alveolar concentration (MAC). The B/G solubility coefficient is a measure of the uptake of an agent by blood. In general, less soluble agents (lower B/G solubility coefficients), such as nitrous oxide and desflurane, are associated with more rapid induction and emergence. MAC is the concentration of agent required to prevent movement in response to a skin incision in 50% of patients and is a way of describing the potency of a volatile anesthetic. A higher MAC represents a less potent volatile anesthetic.

Nitrous Oxide

Nitrous oxide provides only partial anesthesia at atmospheric pressure because its MAC is 104% of inspired gas at sea level. Nitrous oxide minimally influences respiration and hemodynamics. In addition, it has low solubility in blood. Therefore, it is often combined with one of the potent volatile agents to permit a lower dose of the potent volatile agent, thus limiting side effects, reducing cost, and facilitating rapid induction and emergence. The most important clinical problem with nitrous oxide is that it is 30 times more soluble than nitrogen and diffuses into closed gas spaces faster than nitrogen diffuses out. Because nitrous oxide increases the volume or pressure of these spaces, it is contraindicated in the presence of closed gas spaces such as pneumothorax, small bowel obstruction, or middle ear surgery, as well as in retinal surgery in which an intraocular gas bubble is created. Because nitrous oxide gradually accumulates in the pneumoperitoneum, some clinicians prefer to avoid its use during laparoscopic procedures. However, periodic venting can prevent buildup, and some investigators have

suggested that nitrous oxide might be preferable to carbon dioxide as the insufflated gas.[1]

Halothane

Introduced in the mid-1950s, halothane has a pleasant odor that facilitates mask induction and has a variety of useful clinical characteristics (see Table 18-1). Halothane is the most potent volatile anesthetic in modern practice, with a MAC of 0.74 vol% in adults. A potent bronchodilator, halothane was previously the inhalational agent of choice in patients at risk for bronchospasm, although other agents have subsequently been shown to provide equivalent bronchodilation.

Halothane has numerous shortcomings that have contributed to its almost complete replacement by newer agents. First, the drug is a powerful cardiac depressant that could potentially precipitate acute decompensation in patients with severe left ventricular dysfunction (Table 18-2). Second, halothane sensitizes the myocardium to catecholamines, which is a particular problem when epinephrine is added to local anesthetics for infiltration into the surgical site. Third, halothane is associated with a rare form of fulminant hepatitis that is manifested as postoperative fever and jaundice and is microscopically indistinguishable from viral hepatitis. The incidence, about 1 in 35,000, is thought to be due to metabolites of halothane.

Halothane is not a direct hepatotoxin. However, in adults the incidence of hepatitis is increased sevenfold if halothane anesthesia is repeated within 3 months. Therefore, halothane is best avoided in adults who have received the agent within the preceding year. Because halothane hepatitis has not been reported in children younger than 8 years, halothane can be used repeatedly in children. Prudence suggests that halothane be avoided in cases in which there is a potential for postoperative liver injury (e.g., trauma, history of viral hepatitis, or liver surgery) or if the patient has taken enzyme-inducing drugs such as phenobarbital and isoniazid. Although the majority of halothane is eliminated through the lungs, as are other inhalational anesthetics, approximately 20% is metabolized, primarily to nontoxic compounds. Like all other potent inhalational agents, halothane can trigger malignant hyperthermia, a rare but serious metabolic disease.[2]

Table 18-2   Cardiopulmonary Effects of Inhalational Anesthetics

INHALATIONAL AGENT	BLOOD PRESSURE	HEART RATE	CARDIAC OUTPUT	SENSITIZATION TO CATECHOLAMINES	VENTILATORY DEPRESSION	BRONCHODILATION
Nitrous oxide	Little effect	Little effect	Little effect	No	Minimal	No
Halothane	Marked dose-dependent decrease	Moderate decrease	Marked dose-dependent decrease	Marked	Moderate dose-dependent effect	Moderate
Enflurane	Marked dose-dependent decrease	Moderate decrease	Moderate dose-dependent decrease	Moderate	Marked dose-dependent effect	Minimal
Isoflurane	Moderate dose-dependent decrease	Variable increase	Minimal decrease	Minimal	Marked dose-dependent effect	Moderate
Sevoflurane	Moderate dose-dependent decrease	Little effect	Moderate dose-dependent decrease	Minimal	Moderate dose-dependent effect	Moderate
Desflurane	Minimal decrease	Variable; marked increase with rapid increase in concentration	Minimal decrease	Minimal	Marked dose-dependent effect	Moderate

Enflurane

Introduced in the 1970s as an alternative to halothane, enflurane failed to achieve wide popularity. Although enflurane is less soluble than halothane and produces less cardiac sensitization to catecholamines, the drug is metabolized to fluoride (F^-) and, after prolonged administration, especially in obese patients, is associated with mild renal dysfunction. In addition, enflurane is relatively contraindicated in patients with seizure disorders because it induces epileptiform electroencephalographic changes that are most pronounced at high concentrations and with hypocapnia.

Isoflurane

Approved by the Food and Drug Administration (FDA) in 1979, isoflurane rapidly replaced halothane as the most commonly used potent inhalational agent. Despite the recent release of sevoflurane and desflurane, isoflurane is commonly used in modern operating rooms, at least in part because the cost of the now-generic compound is well below that of the newer agents. Isoflurane has several advantages over halothane, including less reduction in cardiac output, less sensitization to the arrhythmogenic effects of catecholamines, and minimal metabolism. However, isoflurane-induced tachycardia, a variable response, can increase myocardial oxygen consumption. Careful observation of the heart rate is necessary when it is used in patients with coronary artery disease (CAD). In concentrations of 1.0 MAC or less, isoflurane causes little increase in cerebral blood flow and

intracranial pressure (ICP) and depresses cerebral metabolic activity more than halothane or enflurane does. Its pungent odor virtually precludes use for inhalational induction.

Sevoflurane

Sevoflurane's relatively low solubility facilitates rapid induction and emergence. Sevoflurane is associated with faster emergence than isoflurane is, especially in longer cases, although its slightly faster emergence does not result in earlier discharge after outpatient surgery. Sevoflurane is associated with a lower incidence of postoperative somnolence and nausea in the postanesthesia care unit (PACU) and in the first 24 hours after discharge than isoflurane is. Unlike isoflurane, sevoflurane is pleasant to inhale, thus making it suitable for inhalational induction in children. However, the clinical differences between halothane and sevoflurane are subtle. In premedicated pediatric patients undergoing bilateral myringotomy and tube placement and randomized to receive sevoflurane or halothane, anesthesiologists correctly identified the agent (to which they were blinded) in only 56.6% of cases.

Sevoflurane is clinically suitable for outpatient surgery, mask induction of patients with potentially difficult airways, and maintenance of patients with bronchospastic disease. When sevoflurane, halothane, and isoflurane were compared with thiopental/nitrous oxide anesthesia, all three of the potent agents decreased respiratory resistance in endotracheally intubated nonasthmatics;

Table 18-3 Clinical Characteristics of Intravenous Induction Agents

IV INDUCTION AGENT	DOSE (mg/kg)	COMMENTS	SIDE EFFECTS	SITUATIONS REQUIRING CAUTION	RELATIVE INDICATIONS
Thiopental	2-5	Inexpensive Slow emergence after high doses	Hypotension	Hypovolemia Compromised cardiac function	Suitable for induction in many patients
Ketamine	1-2	Psychotropic side effects controllable with benzodiazepines Good bronchodilator Potent analgesic at subinduction doses	Hypertension Tachycardia	Coronary disease Severe hypovolemia	Rapid-sequence induction of asthmatics, patients in shock (reduced doses)
Propofol	1-2	Burns on injection Good bronchodilator Associated with low incidence of postoperative nausea and vomiting	Hypotension	Coronary artery disease Hypovolemia	Induction of outpatients Induction of asthmatics
Etomidate	0.1-0.3	Cardiovascularly stable Burns on injection Spontaneous movement during induction	Adrenal suppression (with continuous infusion)	Hypovolemia	Induction of patients with cardiac contractile dysfunction Induction of patients in shock (reduced doses)
Midazolam	0.15-0.3	Relatively stable hemodynamics Potent amnesia	Synergistic ventilatory depression with opioids	Hypovolemia	Induction of patients with cardiac contractile dysfunction (usually in combination with opioids)

sevoflurane reduced airway resistance more than halothane or isoflurane did.[3] Another advantage of sevoflurane is that its cardiovascular side effects are minimal.

However, considerable metabolic transformation of sevoflurane takes place and results in increases in the serum fluoride ion concentration and, in the presence of soda lime or Baralyme, production of *compound A,* a metabolite that is toxic in experimental animals. However, β-lyase, the enzyme responsible for the formation of compound A,[4] has 8 to 30 times greater activity in rat kidneys than in human kidney tissue. Therefore, the toxicity of compound A in humans appears to be theoretical and not clinically important.

Desflurane

Desflurane is rapidly taken up and eliminated. After anesthesia lasting more than 3 hours, desflurane was associated with more rapid recovery than isoflurane was.[5] The most volatile and least potent of the volatile anesthetics, desflurane must be administered through electrically heated vaporizers that release pure desflurane vapor, which then mixes with carrier gas to produce specific inspired concentrations. However, its pungent odor precludes inhalational induction. In addition, desflurane is associated with tachycardia and hypertension if the concentration is increased too rapidly.

When exposed to dry carbon dioxide absorbent, desflurane, isoflurane, and enflurane are partially converted to carbon monoxide. Desflurane, enflurane, and isoflurane produce more carbon monoxide than halothane or

sevoflurane does. Carbon monoxide production is greater with dry CO_2 absorbent, with Baralyme than with soda lime, at higher temperatures, and at higher anesthetic concentrations.[6] Because continued gas flow in an unused machine will desiccate the CO_2 absorbent, turning gas flow off in anesthesia machines when they are not in use can reduce carbon monoxide production.

Intravenous Agents

Since the introduction of thiopental, IV agents have become an indispensable component of modern anesthetic practice. IV agents are used primarily for induction of anesthesia and as part of a multidrug combination to produce anesthesia.

Induction Agents

Most adult patients and many older children prefer IV induction to inhalational induction. IV induction is rapid, pleasant, and safe for the vast majority of patients, although there are situations in which IV induction introduces hazards. The five IV agents most commonly used in the United States for induction of anesthesia are sodium thiopental, ketamine, propofol, etomidate, and midazolam.

Induction with thiopental, the oldest IV induction agent, is rapid and pleasant. Although the drug is remarkably well tolerated by a wide variety of patients, several clinical situations necessitate caution (Table 18-3). In hypovolemic patients and those with congestive heart failure, thiopental-induced vasodilation and cardiac depression can lead to severe hypotension unless doses are markedly reduced. In such patients, etomidate or ketamine is an alternative agent. Although thiopental does not directly precipitate bronchospasm, bronchospasm may develop in patients with reactive airway disease in response to the intense airway stimulation produced by endotracheal intubation. Consequently, propofol or ketamine is often chosen as an alternative for induction in patients with reactive airway disease.

In the usual doses used for induction of anesthesia, thiopental is associated with rapid emergence because of redistribution of the agent from the brain to peripheral tissues, particularly fat. In higher doses, circulating blood levels increase and the action of thiopental must be terminated by hepatic metabolism, which eliminates only about 10% per hour.

Ketamine, which produces a dissociative state of anesthesia, is the only IV induction agent that increases blood pressure and heart rate and decreases bronchomotor tone. Usually associated with increased sympathetic tone, ketamine causes direct cardiac depression that may become evident if given to patients with high preanesthetic sympathetic tone, as in patients in hemorrhagic shock. In markedly reduced doses (15%-20% of the usual induction dose), ketamine is an appropriate choice for IV induction of severely hypovolemic patients, in whom it causes the least fall in blood pressure of any of the induction agents. Ketamine is an appropriate agent for IV induction of asthmatic patients because it reduces the increase in bronchomotor tone associated with endotracheal intubation. Among the IV induction agents, ketamine also causes the least amount of ventilatory depression and loss of airway reflexes. However, because of the induction of copious oropharyngeal secretions, a drying agent such as glycopyrrolate is generally administered with ketamine.

Ketamine can be used as the sole anesthetic for brief, superficial procedures because it produces profound amnesia and somatic analgesia. It is less useful, however, for abdominal cases or delicate surgery because it produces no muscular relaxation, does not control visceral pain, and may not completely control patient movement. The potent pain-relieving effects of ketamine have been exploited for preemptive analgesia. In patients in whom ketamine was infused continuously before incision and continued through wound closure, postoperative morphine consumption was significantly lower on postoperative days 1 and 2 than in patients who did not receive ketamine.[7]

In patients with CAD, ketamine is usually avoided because tachycardia and increased blood pressure may cause myocardial ischemia. In patients with increased ICP (e.g., after traumatic brain injury), ketamine may further increase ICP because it is the only IV agent that increases cerebral blood flow. Another clinically important side effect of ketamine is emergence delirium. In adults and older children, supplemental benzodiazepines or volatile agents are generally effective in preventing emergence delirium.

Propofol, commonly used as an induction agent for ambulatory surgery, is a short-acting induction agent that is associated with smooth, nausea-free emergence. Small doses are also useful for short-term sedation during brief procedures such as retrobulbar or peribulbar eye blocks. The primary limitations of propofol are pain on injection and blood pressure reduction. The latter precludes use in patients who may be hypovolemic and prompts caution in patients who may tolerate hypotension poorly, such as those with severe CAD.

Propofol also produces excellent bronchodilation. In asthmatic patients, 0% of those who received propofol wheezed at 2 or 5 minutes after intubation versus 45% of those who received a thiobarbiturate and 26% of those who received an oxybarbiturate.[8] In nonasthmatic patients, three quarters of whom smoked, airway resistance was less after induction with propofol than after induction with thiopental or etomidate. Brown and Wagner[9] demonstrated that the bronchodilatory effects of propofol and ketamine are mediated through blockade of vagus nerve–mediated cholinergic bronchoconstriction.

Etomidate is an imidazole compound that produces minimal hemodynamic changes. Because it preserves blood pressure in most patients, etomidate is often chosen as an alternative for induction of patients with cardiovascular disease. Major drawbacks include burning pain on injection, abnormal muscular movements (myoclonus), and adrenal suppression when given as a prolonged infusion for sedation of critically ill patients.

Midazolam is sometimes used for induction because it usually causes minimal cardiovascular side effects and has a much shorter duration of action than diazepam does. Its onset of action is acceptably rapid and, even in smaller doses, induces profound amnesia for painful or anxiety-producing events. Midazolam is frequently selected for induction of patients for cardiovascular surgery. Because midazolam combines powerful anxiolytic and amnesic effects, smaller doses are also commonly used to premedicate anxious patients and as a component of a multidrug anesthetic.

Opioids

Opioids are used in the majority of patients undergoing general anesthesia and are given systemically to many patients receiving regional or local anesthesia. As a component of a multifaceted anesthetic, opioids produce profound analgesia and minimal cardiac depression. Their disadvantages include ventilatory depression and inconsistent hypnosis and amnesia, which must usually be provided by other agents.

Several reasons explain the universal popularity of opioids in anesthetic management. First, they reduce the MAC of potent inhalational agents. For example, fentanyl (3 ng/mL plasma concentration) decreased the MAC of sevoflurane by 59% and reduced MAC_{awake} (the alveolar concentration at which an emerging patient responds to commands) by 24%.[10] Second, they blunt the hypertension and tachycardia associated with manipulations such as endotracheal intubation and surgical incision. Third, they provide analgesia that extends through the early postemergence interval and facilitates smoother awakening from anesthesia. Fourth, in doses 10 to 20 times the analgesic dose, opioids act as complete anesthetics in a high proportion of patients by providing not only analgesia but also hypnosis and amnesia. This characteristic has prompted their use in cardiac surgery patients, sometimes as sole anesthetic agents and more often as a major component of the anesthetic. Finally, they are now often added to local anesthetic solutions in epidural and intrathecal blocks to improve the quality of analgesia.

Morphine, hydromorphone, and meperidine are inexpensive, intermediate-acting agents that are less commonly used for maintenance of anesthesia than for postoperative analgesia. Fentanyl, a synthetic opioid that is 100 to 150 times more potent than morphine, is commonly used for maintenance of anesthesia because of its shorter duration of action and rapid onset. Newer synthetic, short-acting opioids, including sufentanil and alfentanil, are also used during anesthesia because they are quickly metabolized and excreted. Remifentanil, an opioid metabolized by serum esterases, is particularly short acting. Remifentanil does not accumulate during prolonged infusions and is therefore often used as part of IV anesthetics.

Neuromuscular Blockers

Fifty years ago, anesthesia was typically conducted with single potent inhalational agents that produced all the components of general anesthesia, including whatever degree of muscle relaxation was necessary for the conduct of surgery. Among the drawbacks of this approach was the fact that the depth of anesthesia necessary to produce profound muscle relaxation was much deeper than that necessary to provide hypnosis and amnesia. The addition of muscle relaxants afforded the opportunity to deliver only enough of the inhalational and IV agents to achieve hypnosis, amnesia, and analgesia while still providing satisfactory operating conditions.

The two categories of neuromuscular blockers in clinical use are depolarizing (noncompetitive) and nondepolarizing (competitive) agents. The depolarizing agents exert agonistic effects at the cholinergic receptors of the neuromuscular junction, initially causing contractions evident as fasciculations, followed by an interval of profound relaxation. The nondepolarizing neuromuscular blockers compete for receptor sites with acetylcholine, with the magnitude of block dependent on the availability of acetylcholine and the affinity of the agent for the receptor.

Succinylcholine, the only depolarizing agent still in use, remains popular for endotracheal intubation because of its rapid onset and short duration of action. However, it is associated with serious hazards, including hyperkalemia and malignant hyperthermia, in a small proportion of patients. The drug can be administered in a relatively high dose for intubation because it is rapidly metabolized by plasma pseudocholinesterase, except in a small fraction of patients with atypical or absent pseudocholinesterase. Because its duration of action is only 5 minutes, a patient who cannot be successfully intubated can be ventilated by mask for a short time until spontaneous respiration resumes. However, a patient who cannot be ventilated by mask will not resume spontaneous breathing before the onset of life-threatening hypoxemia.[11]

Side effects of succinylcholine include bradycardia, especially in children, and severe, life-threatening hyperkalemia in patients with burns, paraplegia, quadriplegia, and massive trauma. Succinylcholine, when combined with a volatile agent, is also implicated in triggering malignant hyperthermia in susceptible individuals. Therefore, it is best avoided in patients at risk for malignant hyperthermia, including those with muscular dystrophy or a family history of malignant hyperthermia. Some anesthesiologists avoid succinylcholine in children because masseter spasm is a common occurrence that may presage malignant hyperthermia, but it is usually a benign effect. Because succinylcholine is a depolarizing agent that causes visible muscle fasciculations, it has been implicated in causing postoperative muscle pain, which can be reduced by pretreatment with a small, precurarizing dose of a nondepolarizing agent. As a result of the multiple sporadic problems associated with the use of succinylcholine, some anesthesiologists now reserve its use only for situations in which an airway must be rapidly secured (i.e., rapid-sequence induction). In other situations, nondepolarizing agents, chosen largely on the basis of their mode of excretion and duration of action, are preferable. For instance, cisatracurium is largely metabolized in serum by Hoffman degradation and is suitable for patients with reduced renal function, in whom pancuronium and vecuronium would be unsuitable because they are partially eliminated by the kidneys.

Nondepolarizing relaxants are used when succinylcholine is contraindicated, as an alternative to succinylcholine for patients in whom easy endotracheal intubation is anticipated, and when intraoperative relaxation is required to facilitate surgical exposure. Knowledge of the side effects of individual agents (often related to vagolysis or release of histamine) and routes of metabolism plays a major role in the selection of specific agents for individual cases. Doses required to provide satisfactory operating conditions are summarized in Table 18-4. Dosing of nondepolarizing agents requires knowledge of several important characteristics. First, the use of neuromuscular blockers prevents movement in response to noxious stimuli. Therefore, chemical paralysis can mask the signs of inadequate anesthesia (or sedation or analgesia in postoperative patients). Medicolegal claims of intraoperative awareness during general anesthesia were more than twice as frequent in patients receiving intraoperative muscle relaxants.[12] Second, higher doses are required to provide satisfactory conditions for intubation than for surgical relaxation. Therefore, if a nondepolarizer is used only after intubation, smaller doses are required. Third, other anesthetic drugs potentiate the actions of nondepolarizing agents. Succinylcholine used for intubation decreases subsequent requirements for nondepolarizers. Potent inhalational agents dose-dependently potentiate the effects of competitive neuromuscular blockers. The newer inhalational agent desflurane potentiates the effects of vecuronium approximately 20% more than isoflurane

Table 18-4 Dose-Response Relationships of Nondepolarizing Neuromuscular Blocking Drugs in Humans

DRUG	DURATION	ED$_{50}$ (mg/kg)	ED$_{95}$ (mg/kg)	INTUBATING DOSE (mg/kg)
d-Tubocurarine	Long	0.23 (0.16-0.26)	0.48 (0.34-0.56)	0.5-06
Pancuronium	Long	0.036 (0.022-0.042)	0.067 (0.059-0.080)	0.08-0.12
Vecuronium	Intermediate	0.027 (0.015-0.031)	0.043 (0.037-0.059)	0.1-0.2
Cisatracurium	Intermediate	0.026 (0.15-0.31)	0.04 (0.32-0.55)	0.15-0.2
Mivacurium	Short	0.039 (0.027-0.052)	0.067 (0.045-0.081)	0.15-0.2
Rocuronium	Intermediate	0.147 (0.069-0.220)	0.305 (0.257-0.521)	0.6-1.0

ED$_{50}$, dose effective for surgical relaxation in 50% of patients; ED$_{95}$, dose effective for surgical relaxation in 95% of patients; mean (95% confidence limits). Somewhat larger doses are required to facilitate endotracheal intubation.

Modified from Naguib M, Lien CA: Pharmacology of muscle relaxants and their antagonists. In Miller RD, Fleisher LA, Johns RA, et al (eds): Anesthesia, 6th ed. Philadelphia, Churchill Livingstone, 2005, pp 481-572.

does.[13] Fourth, individual responses to muscle relaxants vary widely, with patients demonstrating both markedly increased and markedly decreased neuromuscular blockade in comparison to expected levels.

Fifth and most important, subtle blockade can be difficult to detect and can be associated with postoperative problems. The importance of subtle residual paralysis has recently been quantified by using the train-of-four (TOF) fade ratio, a semiquantitative monitoring technique used to assess the adequacy of neuromuscular blockade and the adequacy of pharmacologic reversal. At the conclusion of anesthesia, a TOF ratio greater than 0.70 has been considered adequate return of neuromuscular function. This ratio means that the fourth of four muscle twitches in response to supramaximal stimuli delivered at 0.5-second intervals to the ulnar nerve is at least 70% of the magnitude of the first twitch. A 1997 report characterized the symptoms of volunteers receiving graded doses of muscle relaxants at various TOF ratios.[14] A sustained 5-second head lift (a commonly used clinical index of adequate reversal) was achieved if the TOF ratio was greater than 0.60. At TOF ratios greater than 0.70, all subjects maintained patent airways and oxygen saturation greater than 96%. However, in a 2003 study, at TOF ratios less than 0.90, subjects had diplopia and difficulty tracking objects in all directions. The ability to strongly oppose the incisors did not return until the TOF ratio was higher than 0.90. The authors concluded that satisfactory return of neuromuscular function requires return of the TOF ratio to greater than 0.90 and ideally to 1.0.[15] In patients who received the intermediate-acting neuromuscular blockers atracurium, vecuronium, or rocuronium only for endotracheal intubation, the TOF ratio was lower than 0.9 in 37% of patients 2 hours after receiving the muscle relaxant.[15]

The use of neuromuscular blocking agents in general and nondepolarizing agents in particular necessitates a strategy to ensure adequate muscular function at the conclusion of anesthesia. Many of the complications associated with neuromuscular blockers relate to inadequate reversal at the conclusion of cases or inadequate assessment of reversal. Nondepolarizing relaxants are generally pharmacologically reversed with an anticholinesterase (neostigmine or edrophonium), accompanied by atropine or glycopyrrolate to counteract the muscarinic

effects of the anticholinesterase. However, recovery depends both on the intensity of neuromuscular blockade at the time that reversal is attempted and on the effects of the reversal agent. At the end of anesthesia, profound neuromuscular blockade may preclude reliable antagonism by an anticholinesterase within 5 to 10 minutes.

With the longer-acting muscle relaxants, residual blockade can potentially complicate postoperative recovery. In a clinical trial of reversal of muscle relaxation, 691 patients undergoing abdominal, gynecologic, or orthopedic surgery under general anesthesia were randomized to receive pancuronium, vecuronium, or atracurium. After reversal with neostigmine, a higher proportion (26%) of patients who had received pancuronium had residual neuromuscular blockade (TOF <0.70) than did patients who had received vecuronium or atracurium (5.3% combined).[16] Patients who received pancuronium and had a TOF ratio less than 0.70 had a higher incidence of atelectasis or pneumonia on postoperative chest radiographs (16.9% of 59 patients in that category). There was no association between postoperative pulmonary complications and residual blockade with the other two muscle relaxants.

One key factor determining recovery from neuromuscular blockade is the ability to metabolize and excrete the drugs. In patients with renal disease, the half-lives of *d*-tubocurarine, rocuronium, vecuronium, and pancuronium are prolonged. In such patients, alternative drugs include atracurium or cisatracurium, which are metabolized by Hoffman degradation and thus do not have prolonged half-lives in patients with renal dysfunction.

ANESTHESIA EQUIPMENT

Anesthesia equipment has undergone rapid development over the past few decades. Despite many years of improving design, hazards of gas delivery systems must still be considered. The primary concern is inadvertent delivery of a hypoxic gas mixture. Adverse anesthetic outcomes were associated with gas delivery equipment in 72 of 3791 cases in the American Society of Anesthesiologists

Box 18-1 Routine and Specialized Electronic Monitors Used in Anesthetic Practice and Their Indications

Routine Monitors

Pulse oximetry
  Measure blood oxygen saturation
  Heart rate
Automated blood pressure cuff
  Blood pressure
Electrocardiography
  Heart rhythm
  Heart rate
  Monitor of myocardial ischemia
Capnography
  Adequacy of ventilation
  Intratracheal placement of endotracheal tube
Oxygen analyzer
  Monitoring of delivered oxygen concentration
Ventilator pressure monitor
  Ventilator disconnection during general anesthesia
  Monitoring of airway pressure
Temperature monitoring

Specialized Monitors

Monitoring of urine output (Foley catheter)
  Gross indicator of intravascular volume status and renal
    perfusion
Arterial catheter
  Continuous measurement of arterial blood pressure
  Sampling of arterial blood
Central venous catheter
  Continuous measurement of central venous pressure
  Delivery of centrally acting drugs
  Rapid administration of fluids and blood
Pulmonary artery catheter
  Measurement of pulmonary artery pressure
  Measurement of left ventricular pressure
  Measurement of cardiac output
  Measurement of mixed venous oxygenation
Precordial Doppler
  Detection of air embolism
Transesophageal echocardiography
  Evaluation of myocardial performance
  Assessment of heart valve function
  Assessment of intravascular volume
  Detection of air embolism
Esophageal Doppler
  Assessment of descending aortic blood flow
  Assessment of cardiac preload
Transpulmonary indicator dilution
  Measurement of cardiac output
  Measurement of preload
Esophageal and precordial stethoscope
  Auscultation of breathing and heart sounds

(ASA) closed claims database. Misuse of equipment occurred in 75% of incidents, and 78% could have been detected with monitoring of pulse oximetry or capnography.[17] The essential elements of an anesthesia machine are gas sources (oxygen, nitrous oxide, and air), flowmeters, and a flow-proportioning device. In most cases,

gases are delivered to the anesthesia machine through a bank of large H cylinders housed in a central area within the hospital. A backup system of E cylinders is attached directly to the anesthesia machine and provides a source of gases, particularly oxygen, if the central gas source becomes unavailable. The flowmeters allow independent administration of individual gases. So-called fail-safe valves that require pressurization of the oxygen line before nitrous oxide can be delivered and flow-proportioning devices that automatically reduce the flow of nitrous oxide if the flow of oxygen is reduced below a safe concentration are present to minimize the chance of delivering a hypoxic gas mixture.

The most commonly used anesthetic circuit is a circle system with one-way valves that properly direct inspired and expired gas flow. The typical circuit includes a carbon dioxide absorber containing either soda lime (sodium hydroxide, calcium hydroxide, and potassium hydroxide) or Baralyme (a combination of barium hydroxide and calcium hydroxide). Gas flow is adjusted to provide sufficient oxygen for metabolism and adequate delivery of anesthetic vapor. Gas-scavenging systems are attached to the exhaust valve of anesthetic circuits to permit the elimination of anesthetic gases and vapors that otherwise would contaminate the operating room environment. Although the health risks of operating room contamination are poorly quantified, the general consensus is that exhausting gases into the operating room risks potential harm to personnel and their offspring. The gas is exhausted into the air outside the hospital or ambulatory surgery center, where the dilution with ambient air is so great that no health risks are considered to be present.

PATIENT MONITORING DURING AND AFTER ANESTHESIA

Effective monitoring is a critical aspect of anesthesia care. The essential components of monitoring include observation and vigilance, instrumentation, data analysis, and institution of corrective measures, if indicated. The goal of patient monitoring is to provide optimal anesthetic management and detect abnormalities early in their course so that corrective measures can be instituted before serious or irreversible injury occurs. Although it is difficult to directly relate improved patient outcomes with specific monitors, the reduction in anesthesia-related morbidity and mortality has paralleled the institution of current monitoring practices.

The indications as well as risks and benefits associated with the use of noninvasive and invasive electronic monitors must be assessed for each individual patient (Box 18-1). These decisions are guided by the patient's medical condition, the type of surgery, and the potential complications associated with invasive monitoring. However, the proliferation of electronic monitoring devices does not circumvent the need for clinical skills such as observation, inspection, auscultation, and palpation. The ASA has established standards for basic anesthetic monitoring.[18] These standards are designed to integrate clinical skills and electronic monitoring with the goal of enhancing patient safety.

Standard I asserts that a qualified anesthesia care provider must be continuously present in the operating room during the administration of anesthesia. The practitioner must continuously monitor the status of the patient and alter anesthesia care based on the patient's response to the dynamic changes associated with anesthesia and surgery.

Standard II mandates continuous assessment of ventilation, oxygenation, circulation, and temperature during all anesthetics. Specific requirements include the following:

1. The use of an oxygen analyzer with a low–oxygen concentration alarm during general anesthesia.
2. Quantitative assessment of blood oxygenation such as by pulse oximetry.
3. The adequacy of ventilation must be continuously ensured by clinical evaluation. Quantitative monitoring of the CO_2 content in expired gas and the volume of expired gas is strongly recommended.
4. Clinical assessment and monitors to determine the presence of CO_2 in expired gases to ensure correct endotracheal tube placement after intubation. A device capable of detecting disconnection of breathing system components during mechanical ventilation must be in continuous use. This device must give an audible signal when its alarm threshold is exceeded.
5. The electrocardiogram must be continuously monitored during anesthesia, and blood pressure and the heart rate must be evaluated at least every 5 minutes. In patients undergoing general anesthesia, adequacy of circulatory function must be continuously monitored by electronic means, palpation, or auscultation.
6. A means of temperature evaluation must be readily available in the operating room and is used during periods of intended or expected changes in body temperature.

Blood Pressure Monitoring

Blood pressure monitoring is required during all anesthetics. Noninvasive blood pressure monitoring is appropriate for the majority of surgical cases, and most modern operating rooms are equipped with automated oscillometric blood pressure analyzers. Indications for invasive blood pressure monitoring include intraoperative use of deliberate hypotension, continuous blood pressure assessment in patients with significant end-organ damage or during high-risk surgical procedures, anticipation of wide perioperative blood pressure swings, need for multiple blood gas analyses, and inadequacy of noninvasive blood pressure measurements, such as in morbidly obese patients. Several sites for arterial cannulation are available, each with inherent advantages and potential for complications. The radial artery is most commonly cannulated because of its superficial location, relative ease of cannulation, and in most patients, adequate collateral flow from the ulnar artery. Other potential sites for percutaneous arterial cannulation include the femoral, brachial, axillary, ulnar, dorsalis pedis, and posterior tibial arteries. Possible complications of intra-arterial monitoring include hematoma, neurologic injury, arterial embolization, limb ischemia, infection, and inadvertent intra-arterial injection of drugs. Intra-arterial catheters are not placed in extremities with potential vascular insufficiency. However, with proper patient selection, the complication rate associated with intra-arterial cannulation is low and its benefits can be important.

Electrocardiography

Electrocardiographic (ECG) monitoring is a standard of care during the administration of anesthesia. Information regarding dysrhythmias and cardiac ischemia can be readily obtained from ECG data. Analysis of ECG tracings is the cornerstone of cardiopulmonary resuscitation protocols.

Ventilation Monitoring

Sedation and opioid administration and the induction of general or regional anesthesia can depress or abolish spontaneous ventilation and thus necessitate intraoperative ventilatory support. Several means are available to assess the adequacy of ventilation, among which are physical assessment of chest expansion, auscultation of breath sounds, and evaluation for evidence of upper airway obstruction and stridor. Precordial and esophageal stethoscopes provide continuous input regarding air movement and the development of wheezing. During mechanical ventilation, monitors of airway pressure and minute ventilation alert the anesthesiologist to conditions that can impair ventilation, such as disconnection of the ventilatory circuit, dislodgement of the endotracheal tube, obstruction of the gas delivery system, and changes in airway resistance or compliance, or both.

The advent of end-tidal carbon dioxide ($ETCO_2$) monitoring has greatly enhanced the monitoring of ventilation and detection of esophageal intubation. In normal individuals, the difference between $ETCO_2$ and $PaCO_2$ is 2 to 5 mm Hg. The gradient between end-tidal and arterial CO_2 reflects dead space ventilation, which is increased in cases of decreased pulmonary blood flow, such as pulmonary air embolism or thromboembolism and decreased cardiac output. Therefore, $ETCO_2$ monitoring can also provide important information regarding systemic perfusion.

Oxygenation Monitoring

Monitoring of FIO_2 and hemoglobin oxygen saturation is a standard of care during all general anesthetics. Modern anesthesia machines are equipped with oxygen analyzers that detect the delivered oxygen concentration (FIO_2). This monitor, in combination with fail-safe devices, low–oxygen delivery alarms, and oxygen ratio monitors, greatly decreases the chance of delivering a hypoxic gas mixture during anesthesia.

Temperature Monitoring

Temperature is monitored in all patients undergoing general anesthesia. The site of measurement is dependent on the surgical procedure and the physical characteristics of the patient. Esophageal temperature is most commonly measured during general anesthesia. Other sites of temperature monitoring include rectal, cutaneous, tympanic membrane, bladder, nasopharynx, and in patients with pulmonary artery catheters, the pulmonary artery. Because of the potential morbidity associated with hypothermia and hyperthermia, it is important to monitor body temperature and institute measures to maintain temperature as close to normal as possible.

Neuromuscular Blockade Monitoring

Because of variability in sensitivity to neuromuscular blockers among patients, it is essential to monitor neuromuscular function in patients receiving intermediate- and long-acting muscle relaxants. The most common sites of monitoring are at the ulnar or orbicularis oculi muscles. The basis of neuromuscular monitoring is assessment of muscle activity after proximal nerve stimulation (Box 18-2). This evaluation gives an indication of acetylcholine receptor blockade at the neuromuscular junction. The degree of neuromuscular blockade is indicated by a decreased evoked response to twitch stimulation.

Central Nervous System Monitoring

Awareness during anesthesia is an uncommon, but disturbing complication. Many years of experience with intraoperative electroencephalogram (EEG) signal processing has resulted in development of the bispectral array (BIS), which is believed to monitor awareness

during anesthesia. The monitor is essentially a modified EEG that assesses brain wave activity and reports numbers from 0 to 100, which correlate with the level of awareness. A value of 100 represents complete awareness and 0 represents complete suppression of brain wave activity. Data suggest that BIS is an accurate indicator of the depth of anesthesia.[19] Monitoring the depth of anesthesia may improve time to awakening and discharge in the outpatient setting. In addition, BIS monitors are gaining acceptance as a means of assessing awareness in locations such as emergency departments and intensive care units.

PREOPERATIVE EVALUATION

The ASA has developed basic standards for preanesthetic care in which an anesthesiologist is required to evaluate the medical status of the patient, derive a plan for anesthetic care, and discuss the plan with the patient.[20] The Joint Commission for Accreditation of Healthcare Organizations requires that all patients receiving anesthesia undergo a preanesthetic evaluation. Because a decreasing percentage of patients are admitted to the hospital on the day before surgery, preoperative testing clinics have been developed to facilitate preoperative evaluation. Optimally, preoperative clinics need to be efficient, predictable, and thorough.

The anesthesia evaluation serves multiple purposes. First, the patient has the opportunity to meet an anesthesiologist and discuss the expected impact of anesthesia, including the patient's fears and concerns regarding anesthesia and postoperative pain management. Second, the preanesthetic interview focuses on the type of surgery, the underlying conditions necessitating surgery, any history of previous anesthetics, and the presence of coexisting diseases. The preoperative interview allows evaluation of the patient's medical status to determine whether additional medical evaluation or treatment is needed before surgery. This process requires a focused history, physical examination, and laboratory evaluation. Current medications must be reviewed to anticipate potential drug interactions and manage medical problems during the perioperative period.

A well-focused history will allow the practitioner to perform targeted physical and laboratory examinations. Overall, the patient's age and gender and the type of surgery dictate the need for preoperative testing. Laboratory tests performed within 1 year of surgery probably do not need to be repeated unless a significant change in the patient's medical status has occurred. Healthy patients undergoing elective procedures may not need any preoperative laboratory testing (Table 18-5).

In the current climate of cost containment, preoperative testing must be minimized but effective. Therefore, a skilled preoperative evaluation minimizes unproductive testing yet uncovers and effectively evaluates conditions that have a high probability of resulting in perioperative morbidity or mortality. Ferschl and colleagues[21] reported that development of an anesthesia preoperative evaluation clinic in a teaching hospital reduced day-of-surgery cancellations and delays.

Table 18-5 Preoperative Testing Recommendations for Asymptomatic Patients Undergoing Elective Surgery

| AGE | GENERAL ANESTHESIA | | MAC OR REGIONAL TECHNIQUE (MEN AND WOMEN) | LOCAL (MEN AND WOMEN) |
	Men	Women		
<40 years	None	Hb or Hct Pregnancy test?	None	None
40-50 years	ECG	Hb or Hct Pregnancy test?	None	None
50-64 years	Hb or Hct ECG	Hb or Hct ECG Pregnancy test?	Hb or Hct*	None
65-74 years	Hb or Hct ECG Creatinine/BUN	Hb or Hct ECG Creatinine/BUN	Hb or Hct* ECG	Hb or Hct*
>74 years	Hb or Hct ECG Creatinine/BUN Glucose Chest x-ray?	Hb or Hct ECG Creatinine/BUN Glucose Chest x-ray?	Hb or Hct* ECG Creatinine/BUN Glucose	Hb or Hct* ECG Creatinine/BUN

*Within 6 months.
BUN, blood urea nitrogen; ECG, electrocardiogram; Hb, hemoglobin; Hct, hematocrit; MAC, monitored anesthesia care.
Modified from Roizen M, Cohn S: Preoperative evaluation for elective surgery: What laboratory tests are needed? In Stoelting R, Barash P, Gallagher J (eds): Advances in Anesthesia, vol 10. Chicago, Mosby–Year Book, 1993, pp 25-43.

Investigation of conditions associated with increased perioperative morbidity is important for reducing the risks related to anesthesia and surgery. Coexisting conditions that must be carefully evaluated include intravascular volume status, airway abnormalities, cardiovascular disease, pulmonary disease, neurologic disease, renal and hepatic disease, and disorders of nutrition, endocrinology, and metabolism. Preoperative pregnancy testing is controversial. The rationale for performing preoperative pregnancy testing is the potential for spontaneous abortion and birth anomalies associated with surgery and anesthesia. There is no clear evidence to demonstrate an association of anesthetic drugs with the development of fetal anomalies in humans, but animal studies have shown that some anesthetics, such as nitrous oxide, may cause developmental abnormalities. A clear sexual history and documentation of the last menstrual cycle is obtained in women of childbearing age. In ambiguous situations, a preoperative pregnancy test is indicated.

Airway Examination

Assessing the airway is a crucial step in developing an anesthetic plan. Even if regional anesthesia is planned, general anesthesia and the need to maintain a patent airway could be necessary. The goal of the airway examination is to identify characteristics that could hinder assisted mask ventilation or tracheal intubation. A history of diseases or conditions that are associated with airway closure or difficult laryngoscopy will alert the practitioner to potential airway difficulties. Review of previous anesthetic records can provide invaluable information regarding previous airway management. The airway examination is completed by systematic inspection of the mouth opening, thyromental distance, neck mobility, and the

---

Box 18-3 Important Factors in Performing an Airway Examination

Patient History

Previous anesthetic history
Medical history (e.g., history of oropharyngeal mass, pharyngeal disease)
Review of the chart to assess prior airway management with previous anesthesia

Physical Examination

Mouth opening (should be 6-8 cm [3-4 fingerbreadths])
Cervical spine mobility
Mallampati classification
Thyromental distance (should be 6-8 cm [3-4 fingerbreadths])
Frontal and profile view
Assessment for disease-associated airway abnormalities

---

size of the tongue in relation to the oral cavity (Box 18-3). The patient is observed in both frontal and profile views. Many airway abnormalities, such as a receding mandible, will not be evident from a frontal view. The size of the tongue in relation to the oral cavity can be graded by using the Mallampati classification (Fig. 18-1). The examination is performed with the patient sitting and the head in a neutral position, the mouth opened as wide as possible, and the tongue protruded maximally. The observer views the oral and pharyngeal structures that are evident. In general, a patient in whom the uvula, tonsillar pillars, and soft palate are visible (class I) will be easy to mask ventilate and intubate. Patients in whom only the hard palate is visible, a class IV airway, have a higher likelihood of being difficult to mask ventilate and

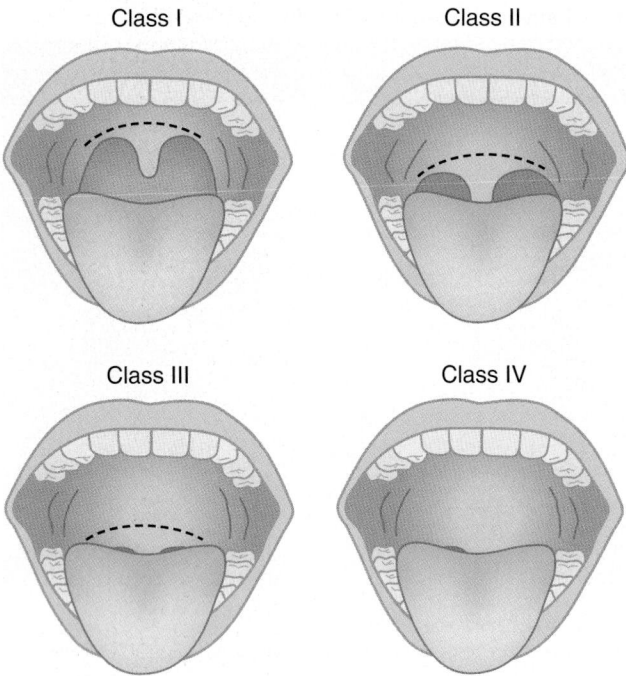

Class I Class II

Class III Class IV

Figure 18-1 The Mallampati classification relates tongue size to pharyngeal size. This test is performed with the patient in the sitting position, the head held in a neutral position, the mouth wide open, and the tongue protruding to the maximum. The subsequent classification is assigned according to the pharyngeal structures that are visible: class I, visualization of the soft palate, fauces, uvula, anterior and posterior pillars; class II, visualization of the soft palate, fauces, and uvula; class III, visualization of the soft palate and the base of the uvula; and class IV, soft palate not visible at all. (From Mallampati SR, Gatt SP, Gugino LD, et al: A clinical sign to predict difficult tracheal intubation: A prospective study. Can Anaesth Soc J 32:429-434, 1985.)

intubate. However, the Mallampati classification is only one component of the airway examination and needs to be used in conjunction with other aspects of airway examination and the patient's history to provide a complete airway assessment. Shiga and coauthors[22] recently reported that single end points aimed at predicting airway difficulties have poor predictive value. However, a combination of end points significantly improved sensitivity and specificity.

Cardiovascular Disease

The risk for perioperative myocardial ischemia and infarction and the risk for cardiac death have become important issues as progressively more complex surgery has been offered to patients with increasingly severe systemic disease. The apparent incidence of perioperative myocardial ischemia depends on the perspective of the study (prospective or retrospective), the sensitivity of the markers used, and the type of surgical procedure. Major clinical predictors of perioperative cardiac morbidity are listed:

1. Unstable coronary syndromes
2. Decompensated congestive heart failure

3. Significant arrhythmias
4. Severe valvular disease

The preanesthetic evaluation identifies potentially serious cardiovascular disorders, including CAD, congestive heart failure, and arrhythmias. The American College of Cardiology (ACC) and the American Heart Association (AHA) have published guidelines for the evaluation and treatment of CAD in noncardiac surgical patients.[23] These guidelines focus on the patient's history of CAD and exercise tolerance and the type of surgery (Fig. 18-2). Patients with known CAD are at increased risk for perioperative cardiac ischemia and myocardial infarction. The ACC/AHA task force suggests that patients who have suffered a myocardial infarction within 30 days of the proposed surgery are at highest risk. Other important factors to consider are a history of previous coronary revascularization, the presence of stable or unstable angina, evidence of congestive heart failure, patient age, the presence of diabetes mellitus or hypertension, and the current medical regimen for the treatment of CAD. Clinical indicators of increased cardiac risk are shown in Box 18-4.

Patients with CAD who have undergone previous myocardial revascularization are at lower risk than patients who have been medically managed. Among 24,959 patients in the Coronary Artery Surgery Study (CASS) database, 3368 required noncardiac surgery during more than 10 years of follow-up.[24] Of these, abdominal, vascular, thoracic, and head and neck surgery each had a combined rate of myocardial infarction or death exceeding 4% in patients who had not undergone myocardial revascularization; in patients who had undergone previous revascularization, both the myocardial infarction and death rates were significantly reduced to 0.8% and 1.7%, respectively, versus 2.7% and 3.3% in patients who were medically managed.

Exercise tolerance is an important indicator of myocardial performance and coronary reserve. Excellent exercise tolerance is a good indicator that the myocardium will not become dysfunctional during the stress of anesthesia and surgery. However, poor exercise tolerance indicates impaired cardiac reserve that may require evaluation and treatment before surgery. As proposed by the AHA, patients who can undertake activities requiring greater than four metabolic equivalents, equivalent to doing light housework or walking up one flight of stairs, are considered to have moderate to excellent exercise tolerance. High-risk procedures such as aortic aneurysm repair and pulmonary resection are associated with greater perioperative stress and require optimization of cardiac status. The ACC/AHA task force has proposed cardiac risk stratification for specific procedures (Box 18-5).

Investigators have extensively studied the implications of noninvasive cardiovascular testing as a guide to perioperative risk. Review of the literature indicates that the negative predictive value of dobutamine echocardiography and myocardial perfusion tests is nearly 100%.[25] However, the positive predictive value is only about 20%. Therefore, a negative noninvasive test predicts a low

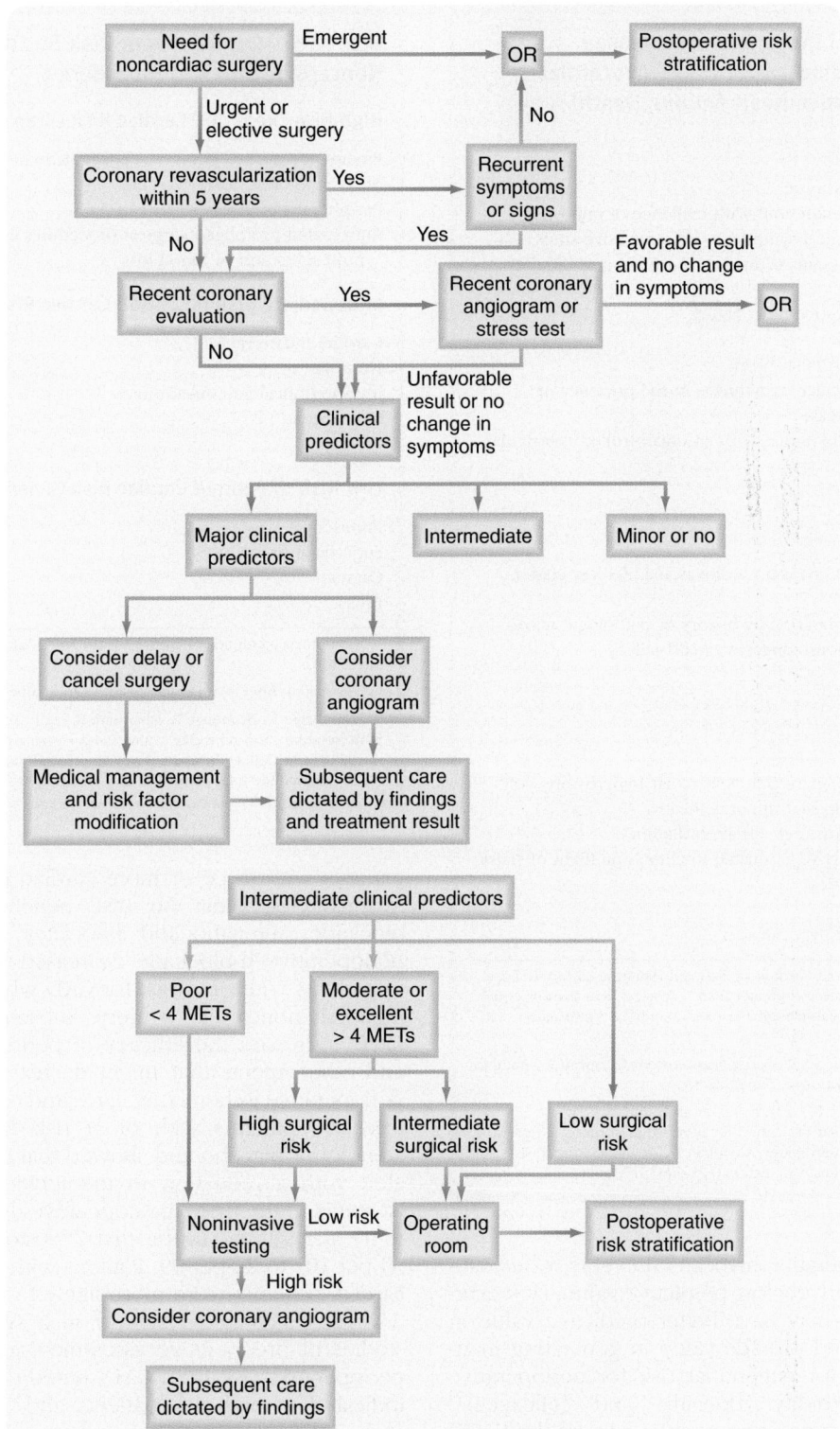

Figure 18-2 Algorithm for preoperative evaluation of patients with cardiac disease who are undergoing noncardiac surgery. METs, metabolic equivalents. (From Eagle K, Brundage B, Chaitman B, et al: Guidelines for perioperative cardiovascular evaluation for noncardiac surgery. A report of the American College of Cardiology/American Heart Association Task Force on practice guidelines. Circulation 93:1278-1317, 1996.)

incidence of perioperative myocardial events, whereas a positive test has relatively low predictive value. However, noninvasive testing may have better predictive value in high-risk patients and provide value in generating management strategies for patients at risk for perioperative cardiovascular morbidity. Boersma and colleagues[26] reported that dobutamine stress echocardiography (DSE) was not able to identify patients who would suffer perioperative cardiac events associated with major vascular surgery in those with two or fewer risk factors for perioperative cardiac morbidity. However, DSE had much higher positive predictive value in patients with three or more cardiac risk factors. Patients in this group with reversible ischemia on DSE had a significantly higher incidence of perioperative cardiac events than did patients without evidence of reversible ischemia. In addition,

patients with three or more cardiac risk factors without reversible ischemia on DSE benefited most from β-blockade. Mangano and associates[27] first reported that perioperative β-blockade decreased long-term mortality in patients with or at risk for CAD who were undergoing high-risk noncardiac surgery. Subsequent investigations have addressed the efficacy of perioperative β-blockers and other agents that might decrease the likelihood of perioperative ischemia. Wallace and coworkers[28] randomized 200 patients with or at risk for CAD to receive atenolol or placebo and showed that atenolol was associated with a reduction in the incidence of myocardial ischemia in the first 2 postoperative days from 34 per 101 to 17 per 99 and in the first 7 postoperative days from 39 per 101 to 24 per 99. Patients with perioperative myocardial ischemia were more likely to die within the next 2 years. Palda and Detsky,[29] in a systematic review of studies of preoperative assessment and management of perioperative risk from CAD, noted that β-blockers were indicated in high-risk patients and that cancellation of such patients was occasionally necessary, but that the role of catheterization and myocardial revascularization was unclear. Intermediate-risk patients undergoing vascular surgery are better stratified by pharmacologic stress testing or echocardiography, but such tests have not been shown to have a role in nonvascular surgery.

Hypertension is a common disorder that can be associated with end-organ damage, relative hypovolemia, and if inadequately treated, intraoperative blood pressure lability. In hypertensive patients, assessment of cardiovascular, neurologic, and renal function is necessary to quantify the extent of end-organ impairment. The preoperative antihypertensive regimen and compliance with that regimen is also reviewed. In general, antihypertensive medications are continued throughout the perioperative period.

Endocarditis Prophylaxis

Some patients with congenital or valvular heart disease are at increased risk for the development of bacterial endocarditis.[30] The guidelines for endocarditis prophylaxis have changed several times during the past 15 years. The prophylaxis guidelines provided here are the most current recommendations of the AHA. Dental procedures and surgery on the respiratory, gastrointestinal, and genitourinary tracts cause significant release of organisms into the circulation that have a high affinity for causing bacterial endocarditis (Box 18-6). Therefore, patients with high to moderate risk for the development of endocarditis need to receive antibiotics for prophylaxis during these procedures (Box 18-7).

Pulmonary Disease

Surgical patients often have obstructive or restrictive pulmonary disease. The preoperative history focuses on functional status, exercise tolerance, severity of the disease, and current medications. Recent worsening of symptoms needs to be closely evaluated. A thorough chest physical examination must be performed. Findings on the history and physical examination, as well as an understanding of the planned surgical procedure, suggest appropriate preoperative testing, which may include chest radiography, arterial blood gas analysis, and pulmonary function testing. The goal of preoperative evaluation is to detect and treat reversible pulmonary pathology, optimize medical management, and allow planning for postoperative ventilatory support, if indicated.

The perioperative risk associated with preexisting pulmonary disease has been extensively studied. Qaseem and coworkers,[31] reviewing the topic of preoperative pulmonary evaluation, identified patient-related risk factors, factors related to the surgical site, and other factors related to surgery, such as the duration of surgery, the choice of general anesthesia, and intraoperative use of pancuronium (Table 18-6). Major patient-associated risk factors are ASA class greater than II, age older than 60 years, functional dependence, and the presence of chronic obstructive pulmonary disease or congestive heart failure. A serum albumin concentration of less than 3.5 g/dL was also a strong predictor of pulmonary complications. Unadjusted rates of pulmonary complications were 27% and 7% in patients with low or normal serum albumin concentrations, respectively.[32] Current smoking was a minor predictor of pulmonary complications. The presence of obesity or mild to moderate asthma was not significantly associated with perioperative pulmonary complications.

In a cohort of patients in whom asthma was diagnosed and who subsequently required surgery at the Mayo Clinic (general or regional anesthesia), perioperative

---

Box 18-6   Guidelines for Endocarditis Prophylaxis

Patients at Risk for the Development of Bacterial Endocarditis

High Risk

Prosthetic cardiac valves, including bioprosthetic and homograft valves
Previous bacterial endocarditis
Complex congenital heart disease (e.g., single-ventricle states, transposition of the great arteries, tetralogy of Fallot)
Surgically constructed systemic pulmonary shunts or conduits

Moderate Risk

Most other congenital cardiac malformations (other than above)
Acquired valvular dysfunction (e.g., rheumatic heart disease)
Hypertrophic cardiomyopathy
Mitral valve prolapse with valvular regurgitation and/or thickened leaflets

Procedures Associated With Increased Risk of Causing Bacterial Endocarditis

Dental Procedures for Which Endocarditis Prophylaxis Is Recommended

Dental extractions
Periodontal procedures, including surgery, scaling and root planing, probing, and recall maintenance
Endodontic (root canal) instrumentation or surgery only beyond the apex
Subgingival placement of antibiotic fibers or strips
Initial placement of orthodontic bands but not brackets
Intraligamentary local anesthetic injections
Prophylactic cleaning of teeth or implants when bleeding is anticipated

Other Procedures for Which Endocarditis Prophylaxis Is Recommended

Respiratory tract
  Tonsillectomy and adenoidectomy
  Surgical procedures that involve the respiratory mucosa
  Bronchoscopy with a rigid bronchoscope
Gastrointestinal tract
  Sclerotherapy for esophageal varices
  Dilation of esophageal strictures
  Endoscopic retrograde cholangiography
  Biliary tract surgery
  Surgical operations that involve the intestinal mucosa
Genitourinary tract
  Prostatic surgery
  Cystoscopy
  Urethral dilation

---

bronchospasm was documented in 1.7% (confidence interval, 0.9%-3%).[33] All attacks were treated successfully, and there were no episodes of pneumothorax, pneumonia, or death. The risk was greatest in patients who were older, had recently used antiasthmatic medications, had recent asthma symptoms, and had recently required physician attention for bronchospasm or required hospitalization.[33]

The other major factors predicting perioperative pulmonary complications are related to surgical and

Table 18-6 Risk Factors Associated With Postoperative Pulmonary Complications

PATIENT-ASSOCIATED RISK FACTORS	RELATIVE RISK ASSOCIATED WITH FACTOR	PROCEDURE-ASSOCIATED RISK FACTORS	RELATIVE RISK ASSOCIATED WITH FACTOR
Age >60 yr	2.1-3.0	Surgery >3 hr	2.1
Functional dependence	2.5		
ASA class > II	4.9	General anesthesia	1.8
Congestive heart failure	2.9		
Smoking	1.3	Emergency surgery	2.2
Obesity	1.3		
COPD	1.8		

ASA, American Society of Anesthesiologists; COPD, chronic obstructive pulmonary disease.
Modified from Qaseem A, Snow V, Fitterman N, et al: Risk assessment for strategies to reduce perioperative pulmonary complications for patients undergoing non-cardiovascular surgery: A guideline from the American College of Physicians. Ann Intern Med 144:575-580, 2006.

Box 18-7 Recommended Antibiotic Regimens for Endocarditis Prophylaxis

Standard general prophylaxis for patients at risk:
  Amoxicillin—Adults, 2 g (children, 50 mg/kg) given orally 1 hour before the procedure
Unable to take oral medications:
  Ampicillin—Adults, 2 g (children, 50 mg/kg) given intramuscularly or intravenously 30 minutes before the procedure
Amoxicillin/ampicillin/penicillin-allergic patients:
  Clindamycin—Adults, 600 mg (children, 20 mg/kg) given orally 1 hour before the procedure
    or
  Cephalexin—Adults, 2 g (children, 50 mg/kg) orally 1 hour before the procedure*
    or
  Azithromycin or clarithromycin—Adults, 500 mg (children, 15 mg/kg) orally 1 hour before the procedure
Amoxicillin/ampicillin/penicillin-allergic patients who cannot take oral medications
  Clindamycin—Adults, 600 mg (children, 20 mg/kg) 30 minutes before the procedure
    or
  Cefazolin—Adults, 1 g (children, 25 mg/kg) 30 minutes before the procedure*

---
*Cephalosporins should not be used in an individual with a history of anaphylaxis, angioedema, or urticaria with penicillin or ampicillin.
A follow-up dose is no longer recommended.

---

anesthetic interventions and include surgery lasting longer than 3 hours, emergency surgery, and the use of general anesthesia. Procedures with an increased risk for pulmonary complications include abdominal surgery, thoracic surgery, neurosurgery, head and neck surgery, and vascular surgery.

Pulmonary function testing remains controversial, in part because of changing expectations regarding the ability of patients with chronic pulmonary disease to tolerate extensive surgery. Pulmonary function testing has variable predictive value, cannot define a threshold above which the risk associated with surgery is prohibitive, and identifies no group at high risk but without clinical evidence of pulmonary disease. Arterial blood gas analysis also does not identify a group for whom the risk of surgery is prohibitive. Spirometry may be helpful in a patient who has unexplained cough, dyspnea, or exercise intolerance or if there is a question regarding optimal improvement of airflow obstruction. Warner and associates[34] compared 135 patients who had undergone spirometry, were undergoing abdominal surgery, and met objective criteria for obstructive pulmonary disease (mean forced expiratory volume in 1 second, 0.9 ± 0.2 L) with 135 patients matched for gender, surgical site, smoking history, and age. Although there was a significantly greater incidence of bronchospasm, the incidence of prolonged endotracheal intubation, prolonged intensive care unit admission, or readmission was no different. These results are reiterated in the meta-analysis performed by Qaseem and colleagues.[31]

Renal and Hepatic Disease

Renal and hepatic dysfunction alter the metabolism and disposition of many anesthetic agents, as well as impair many systemic functions. Patients with acute renal or hepatic insufficiency do no undergo elective surgery until these conditions can be adequately stabilized. Chronic renal insufficiency (CRI) provides many perioperative management challenges, including acid-base abnormalities, electrolyte disturbances, and coagulation disorders. A thorough history must include the cause of CRI, the presence of systemic complications related to CRI, and other systemic diseases. Current daily urinary output, the type and frequency of dialysis, and dialysis-related complications must also be evaluated. The physical examination focuses on identifying systemic complications of CRI, including evidence of altered volume status, coagulopathy, anemia, pericardial effusion, and encephalopathy. Laboratory evaluation includes assessment of anemia, electrolyte abnormalities, coagulopathy, and cardiovascular disease. Dialysis is performed 18 to 24 hours before surgery to avoid the fluid and electrolyte shifts that occur immediately after dialysis.

A patient with chronic liver disease poses many perioperative challenges. The presence of liver disease alters anesthetic drug metabolism, and hypoalbuminemia increases the free fraction of many drugs, thus making these patients sensitive to both the acute and long-term effects of many anesthetics. The perioperative risks associated with anesthesia and surgery are dependent on the severity of hepatic dysfunction. The preoperative evaluation focuses on hepatic synthetic and metabolic function and the presence of coagulopathy, encephalopathy, and ascites, as well as the nutritional status of the patient.

Nutrition, Endocrinology, and Metabolism

Diabetes mellitus warrants discussion because of its high prevalence and potential for comorbidity. Preanesthetic evaluation focuses on the duration and type of diabetes, as well as the current medical regimen. Review of end-organ function with emphasis on autonomic dysfunction, cardiovascular disease, renal insufficiency, retinopathy, and neurologic complications is mandatory. Patients with diabetes are considered to have delayed gastric emptying and to be at risk for gastroesophageal reflux. Perioperative plasma glucose levels need to be well controlled, yet hypoglycemia must be prevented. Appropriate control of perioperative blood sugar in diabetics is difficult to define. Over the long term there is compelling evidence of a correlation between hyperglycemia and long-term diabetic complications. It is much less clear whether blood sugar must be tightly controlled during the acute stress of surgery. However, there is a strong correlation between mortality and tight control of glucose in critically ill patients, including surgical patients.[35]

In diabetic patients undergoing surgery, several principles of management are generally accepted.

1. Substitute shorter-acting for longer-acting insulin.
2. Provide a reduced dose of insulin on the morning of surgery.
3. Once a diabetic who is receiving nothing by mouth is given insulin, provide glucose in IV fluids.
4. In patients with type 2 diabetes, long-acting sulfonylurea drugs such as chlorpropamide are stopped and shorter-acting agents are substituted.
5. Metformin is always stopped because of a slight risk for perioperative drug-induced lacticacidosis. Perioperative insulin requirements vary depending on body weight, liver disease, steroid therapy, infection, and the use of cardiopulmonary bypass.

Patients who have received systemic glucocorticoids during the year before surgery may not be able to respond adequately to surgical stress. Because of the remote risk for adrenal insufficiency during anesthesia, patients who receive chronic glucocorticoids generally receive perioperative steroid coverage. Recommendations regarding identification of patients at risk and appropriate dosing are based on anecdote. Newer recommendations are based on the preoperative dosage of glucocorticoid, the duration of therapy, and the type of surgery. For minor surgical stress, the equivalent of 25 mg of hydrocortisone on the operative day is recommended; for moderate surgical stress, 50 to 75 mg equivalent for 1 to 2 days; and for major surgical stress, 100 to 150 mg/day for 2 to 3 days.

Fasting Before Surgery

Pulmonary aspiration of gastric contents during anesthesia is an uncommon, but serious complication. To prevent aspiration, *nil per os* (NPO) guidelines have been developed for patients scheduled for anesthesia and surgery. Traditionally, orders for "NPO after midnight" forbade any intake of liquids and solids. However, applying the same guidelines for clear liquids (gastric emptying time, 1-2 hours) and solids (gastric emptying time, 6 hours) has been questioned. The ASA adopted guidelines in 1998 that recommended a minimum fasting period of 2 hours after the ingestion of clear liquids and 6 hours for solids and nonclear liquids such as milk or orange juice. *Clear liquids* are defined as liquids that you can see through and do not contain solids or particulates. The routine use of gastrointestinal stimulants, gastric acid secretion blockers, antacids, and antiemetics is not recommended. However, many patients have medical conditions that cause decreased gastric emptying. In these patients the use of agents to improve gastric emptying and neutralize gastric acid may be warranted. In addition, precautions are instituted to decrease the risk for aspiration during anesthesia in patients undergoing emergency procedures.

The reported incidence of aspiration during anesthesia in various studies has varied from 1.4 to 11 per 10,000 anesthetics. A higher incidence has been noted during emergency surgery and in patients with underlying disease processes that cause decreased gastric emptying. Interestingly, some reports suggest that aspiration is at least as common during emergence from anesthesia as during the induction phase. Of patients in whom aspiration is suspected, less than half exhibit evidence of pulmonary injury. In one study, approximately a third of patients with suspected aspiration during anesthesia required postoperative intubation and ventilation. Most of these patients were extubated within 6 hours of surgery. About 10% of patients required intubation and ventilation for 24 hours or longer. Approximately half the patients requiring ventilation for longer than 24 hours after aspiration of gastric contents died of pulmonary complications.

Assessment of Physical Status

The ASA has developed a graded, descriptive scale as a means of categorizing preoperative comorbidity. The classification is independent of operative procedure and serves as a standardized method of communicating patient physical status to anesthesiologists and other health care providers. Patients are categorized as follows:

ASA I—No organic, physiologic, biochemical, or psychiatric disturbance.
ASA II—A patient with mild systemic disease that results in no functional limitation. Examples are well-controlled hypertension and uncomplicated diabetes mellitus.

ASA III—A patient with severe systemic disease that results in functional impairment. Examples are diabetes mellitus with vascular complications, previous myocardial infarction, and uncontrolled hypertension.

ASA IV—A patient with severe systemic disease that is a constant threat to life. Examples are congestive heart failure and unstable angina pectoris.

ASA V—A moribund patient who is not expected to survive with or without the surgery. Examples are ruptured aortic aneurysm and intracranial hemorrhage with elevated ICP.

ASA VI—A declared brain-dead patient whose organs are being harvested for transplantation.

E—Emergency surgery is required. For example, *ASA IE* represents an otherwise healthy patient undergoing emergency appendectomy.

SELECTION OF ANESTHETIC TECHNIQUES AND DRUGS

Selection of anesthetic techniques and drugs begins with the preoperative anesthetic evaluation. Recognition of important preexisting conditions and chronic medication use may suggest that certain approaches are preferable. Then the requirements of the surgical procedure and surgeon are considered. What is the operative site? How will the patient be positioned? What is the expected duration of surgery? Is the patient expected to return home after an ambulatory procedure or is hospital admission anticipated? Finally, in this era of cost constraints, are the costs of newer drugs justified by probable clinical benefit? Evidence of the increasing safety of anesthesia is the fact that multiple options can often be used safely and effectively for the same procedure and the same patient.

After completing the preanesthetic evaluation, the anesthesiologist discusses various options regarding anesthetic care with the patient. Together, sometimes with input from the patient's surgeon, the anesthesiologist and patient choose an anesthetic technique (Box 18-8). Continued progress in the pharmacology of anesthetic drugs, improvements in the accuracy and applicability of monitoring devices, and parallel improvements in the management of chronic disease processes have resulted in the ability to extensively customize the anesthetic management of individual patients.

Risk of Anesthesia

Patients often desire information regarding the risk of death or major complications associated with anesthesia. However, because perioperative death and major complications have become so uncommon, the risk associated with anesthesia is difficult to quantify. The risk for cardiac arrest attributable to anesthesia appears to be less than 1 in 10,000 cases.[36,37] Schwilk and colleagues[38] prospectively studied preoperative risk factors as predictors of perioperative adverse events in 26,907 patients undergoing noncardiac surgery. Fourteen variables proved to be independent risk factors, including gender, age, ASA status, general condition, nutritional state, coronary disease, airway and lung pathology, Mallampati classification, fluid and electrolyte balance, metabolic state, grade of urgency, operative site, duration of surgery, and anesthetic technique (lower risk with regional than with general anesthesia). With the use of a point system, patients could be reliably separated into low- and high-risk groups.

Because so many surgical procedures are now performed without admission to the hospital, the risk associated with ambulatory anesthesia is particularly important. To assess this risk, 38,598 patients who had undergone 45,090 consecutive ambulatory surgical procedures were contacted within 72 hours and 30 days of surgery (99.94% and 95.9% of patients, respectively). No patient died of a medical complication within 1 week of surgery.[39] The total death rate was 1 in 11273 (4 deaths), and the total complication rate was 1 in 1366.

Selection of a Specific Technique

The first step in selecting a specific anesthetic technique (see Box 18-8) for an individual patient is to consider whether the procedure can be appropriately performed with monitored anesthesia care (also sometimes abbreviated as MAC, to be distinguished from the identical abbreviation for minimum alveolar concentration), regional anesthesia (including regional upper and lower extremity blocks, subarachnoid blocks, and epidural anesthesia), or general anesthesia. Monitored anesthesia care supplements local anesthesia performed by surgeons. Anesthesiologists usually participate because an individual patient or procedure requires higher doses of potent sedatives or opioids or because an acutely or chronically ill patient requires close monitoring and hemodynamic or respiratory support. Regional anesthesia (discussed in detail in a later section) is useful for operations on the upper and lower extremities, pelvis, and lower part of the abdomen. Certain other procedures, such as carotid endarterectomy and so-called awake craniotomy, can also be successfully performed under a regional or field block. Patients receiving regional anesthesia can generally remain awake and, if needed, can receive IV sedation or analgesics. Although regional anesthesia avoids general anesthesia and intuitively appears to be safer, hazards specific to regional anesthesia must be considered. Such hazards include, among others, post–dural puncture headache, local anesthetic toxicity, and peripheral nerve injury. In addition, an inadequate regional anesthetic may require rapid transition to heavy sedation or general anesthesia.

General anesthesia is a reversible state of unconsciousness. Although the mechanism of general anesthetics remains speculative and controversial, the four components of general anesthesia (amnesia, analgesia, inhibition of noxious reflexes, and skeletal muscle relaxation) are usually achieved in modern anesthesia by a combination of IV anesthetics and analgesics, inhalational anesthetics, and frequently muscle relaxants. Because the drugs that produce these components cause both desirable and undesirable physiologic changes, the pharmacologic effects of the agents must be matched to the pathophysiology of the patient's medical problems. The major adverse changes associated with anesthetic drugs are respiratory depression, cardiovascular depression, and loss of airway maintenance and protection. Important complications of general anesthesia include hypoxemia (with possible central nervous system [CNS] damage), hypotension, cardiac arrest, and aspiration of acidic gastric contents (which can lead to severe pulmonary damage). Dental damage is more frequent but not life-threatening.

Regardless of the suitability of a particular technique for a specific surgical procedure, other factors, including the patient's preferences, must be considered. For instance, regional anesthesia might not be chosen if a patient were extremely anxious or could not communicate effectively because of a language barrier. Monitored anesthesia care might be inappropriate if a patient were unlikely to lie quietly during delicate or prolonged surgery. Any procedure planned under regional anesthesia or monitored anesthesia care can require conversion to general anesthesia if the original choice proves unsatisfactory.

AIRWAY MANAGEMENT

Airway management is perhaps the most critical skill in anesthesia. As discussed earlier, the preoperative evaluation focuses on recognition of patients who may be difficult to mask ventilate or intubate. Facility with various techniques for establishment of a patent airway constitutes the central group of skills that are critical for the safe practice of anesthesiology. Fortunately, the incidence of difficult intubations is low. Difficult direct laryngoscopy occurs in 1.5% to 8.5% of general anesthetics, and failed intubation occurs in 0.13% to 0.3% of general anes-

thetics. The laryngeal mask airway, the Combitube, the lighted stylet, and the Bullard laryngoscope are recent developments that make ventilation and intubation possible in many patients who have failed intubation with a conventional laryngoscope. The fiberoptic bronchoscope is an additional tool for the management of a difficult airway.

Because of the importance of a prompt, effective response to difficult intubation, the ASA has developed guidelines for managing difficult airways (Fig. 18-3). A key factor is the initial airway examination and recognition of patients with potentially difficult airways. If the practitioner suspects that mask ventilation and tracheal intubation will be difficult, it is recommended that spontaneous ventilation be preserved. Approaches to these patients include awake intubation or the use of anesthetic techniques that preserve spontaneous ventilation. In some cases, establishment of a surgical airway in an awake patient under local anesthesia may be indicated. However, some patients are found to have a difficult airway only after anesthesia and muscle relaxation have been induced. This is an emergency situation that must be rectified quickly to avoid hypoxemia, brain injury, or death. A variety of airway adjuncts are available to preserve ventilation and facilitate tracheal intubation. The practitioner always must call for assistance in these situations to optimize patient care and consider reestablishment of spontaneous ventilation.

REGIONAL ANESTHESIA

Regional anesthesia is an attractive anesthetic option for many types of operative procedures and can provide excellent postoperative pain management in selected patients. However, like any anesthetic technique, the risks and benefits associated with regional anesthesia must be assessed for each individual. Several regional techniques are in common use, including spinal, epidural, and peripheral nerve blocks. Each technique has specific benefits and risks, which depend in part on the choice of local anesthetic drugs.

Local Anesthetic Drugs

Local anesthetics have played a critical role in intraoperative anesthesia almost since they were first described. The two classes of local anesthetic drugs in common use are aminoesters and aminoamides (often described as *esters* and *amides*). The mechanism of action of local anesthetics is dose-dependent blockade of sodium currents in nerve fibers. Local anesthetic drugs differ in terms of their physicochemical characteristics. Of these characteristics, the most important are pK_a, protein binding, and the degree of hydrophobicity. pK_a refers to the pH at which half the drug exists in the basic uncharged form and half exists in the cationic form. In general, agents with a lower pK_a have a faster onset than do agents with a higher pK_a, although some agents, such as chloroprocaine, can be given at much higher concentrations, thereby offsetting the effects of a high pK_a. Because all commonly used

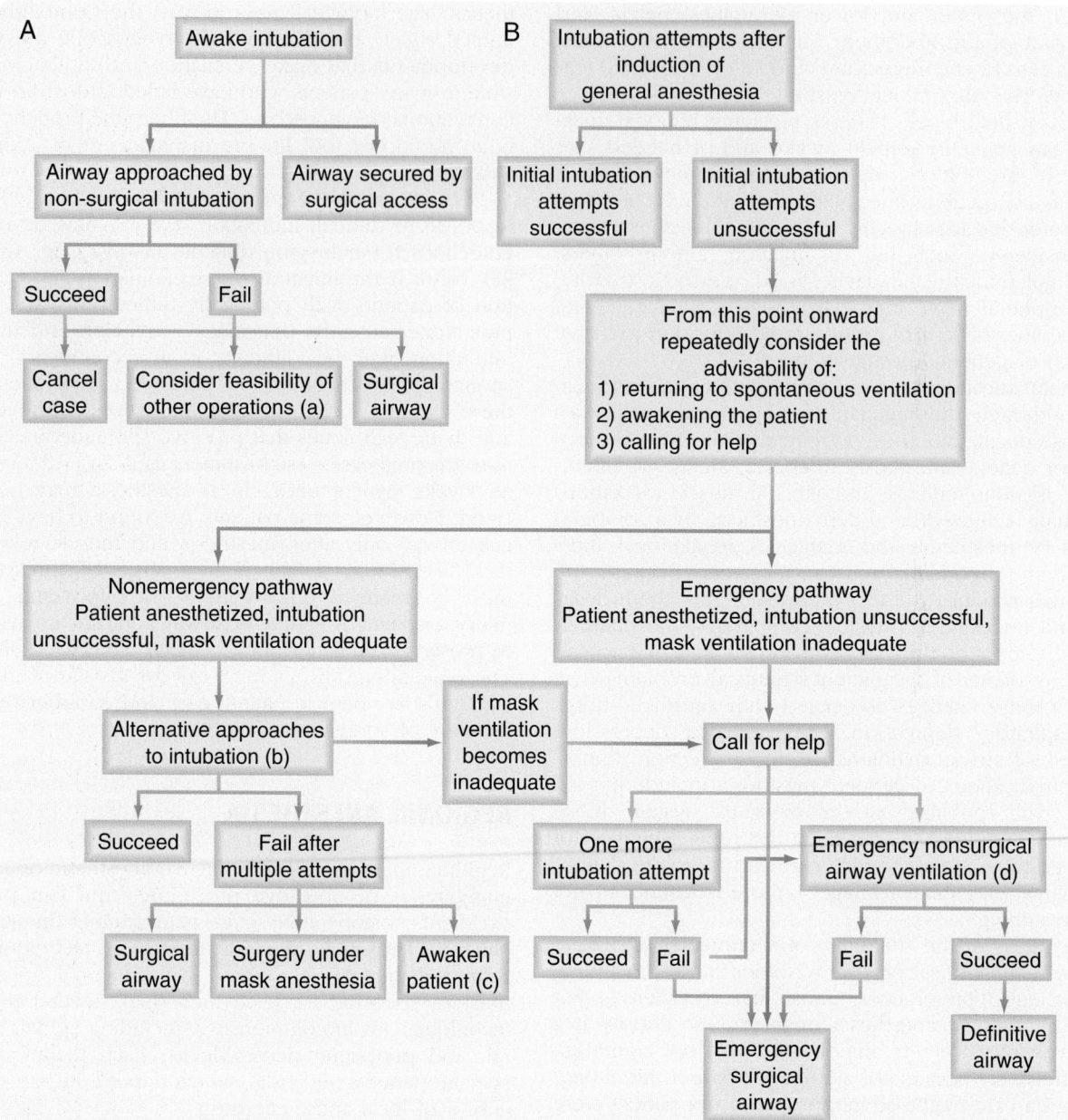

Figure 18-3 American Society of Anesthesiologists difficult airway algorithm. The likelihood and clinical impact of basic management problems such as difficult intubation, difficult mask ventilation, and difficulty with patient cooperation or consent should be assessed in all patients in whom airway management is being contemplated. The clinician should consider the relative merits and feasibility of basic management choices, including the use of awake intubation techniques, preservation of spontaneous ventilation, and the use of surgical approaches to establish a secure airway. Primary and alternative strategies should be considered: (a) other options include, but are not limited to surgery under mask anesthesia, surgery under local infiltration or nerve block, and intubation attempts after induction of general anesthesia; (b) alternative approaches include the use of different laryngoscope blades, awake intubation, blind oral or nasal intubation, fiberoptic intubation, an intubating stylet or tube changer, light wand, retrograde intubation, and surgical airway access; (c) see awake intubation; (d) options for an emergency nonsurgical airway include transtracheal jet ventilation, laryngeal mask airway, and Combitube. (From American Society of Anesthesiologists: Practice guidelines for management of the difficult airway: A report by the American Society of Anesthesiologists task force on management of the difficult airway. Anesthesiology 78:597-602, 1993.)

Table 18-7   Important Characteristics of Local Anesthetics for Major Nerve Blocks

LOCAL ANESTHETIC	AMINOAMIDE OR AMINOESTER	SPEED OF ONSET (min)	DURATION OF ACTION (min)	MAXIMAL DOSE* (AXILLARY BLOCK)
Lidocaine	Aminoamide	10-20	60-180	5 mg/kg
Mepivacaine	Aminoamide	10-20	60-180	5 mg/kg
Bupivacaine	Aminoamide	15-30	180-360	3 mg/kg
Chloroprocaine	Aminoester	10-20	30-50	Not generally used

*Maximal dose without epinephrine; doses of lidocaine and mepivacaine can be increased to 7 to 8 mg/kg if epinephrine is added. Lower doses may be toxic if infiltrated subcutaneously, as for intercostal nerve blocks; larger doses of lidocaine and mepivacaine may be tolerated if given by epidural injection.

local anesthetics have relatively high pK_a values, they are largely ineffective in acidotic (inflamed) environments, in which local anesthetics exist primarily in the ionized form, which does not penetrate nerves. In general, greater hydrophobicity is associated with greater potency, and increased protein binding correlates with a longer duration of action. The speed of onset, duration of action, and typical doses of agents commonly used for regional anesthesia or local anesthesia are summarized in Table 18-7.

In using local anesthetics clinically, the priority is to prevent local anesthetic toxicity. When used for regional anesthesia, the toxicity of local anesthetics is dependent on the site of injection and the speed of absorption. Inadvertent intravascular injection of local anesthetics will produce toxicity with much smaller doses. The main symptoms of local anesthetic toxicity involve the CNS and cardiovascular system. The earliest signs of an overdose or inadvertent intravascular injection are numbness or tingling of the tongue or lips, a metallic taste, light-headedness, tinnitus, or visual disturbances. Signs of toxicity can progress to slurred speech, disorientation, and seizures. With higher doses of local anesthetics, cardiovascular collapse will ensue.

The best defenses against local anesthetic toxicity are aspiration to detect unplanned vascular entry before injecting large doses of local anesthetics and knowledge of the maximal safe dose of the drug being injected. Adding epinephrine, which slows absorption, also decreases the likelihood of a toxic response secondary to rapid absorption. The primary treatments of local anesthetic toxicity are oxygen and airway support. If a seizure does not terminate spontaneously, a benzodiazepine (e.g., midazolam) or thiopental is given. Cardiovascular support may be needed.

Cardiovascular toxicity from bupivacaine may be particularly difficult to treat. One approach intended to reduce the cardiovascular toxicity of bupivacaine (a racemic mixture of the *levo* and *dextro* isomers) has been to produce a solution consisting of only the *levo* isomer. In healthy male volunteers, slow IV infusion of levobupivacaine reduced the mean stroke index, acceleration index, and ejection fraction less than racemic bupivacaine did. Ropivacaine, a newer potent amide local anesthetic, was compared with bupivacaine and lidocaine in volunteers receiving a slow IV infusion until CNS symptoms

first occurred. Echocardiography and electrocardiography were used to quantify systolic, diastolic, and electrophysiologic effects. Bupivacaine increased QRS width during sinus rhythm as compared with the other two treatments and reduced both systolic and diastolic function, whereas ropivacaine reduced only systolic function.

An area of intense research interest has been the use of α_2-adrenergic agents to potentiate or substitute for local anesthetics. Regional anesthesia was first produced with cocaine (also a local anesthetic) for subarachnoid block in the late 1800s, although the specific receptors involved were not established until much later. The α_2-adrenergic drug clonidine was first used epidurally in 1984 after extensive characterization in animals. Despite side effects such as hypotension, bradycardia, and sedation, experience in thousands of patients has demonstrated considerable safety when used alone or with local anesthetics or opioids for epidural anesthesia and analgesia, subarachnoid block, or peripheral nerve block. In general, clonidine prolongs or intensifies the effects of local anesthetics or opioids and produces pain relief when used alone.

Spinal Anesthesia

Spinal anesthesia or subarachnoid block has many applications for urologic, lower abdominal, perineal, and lower extremity surgery. Spinal anesthesia is induced by the injection of local anesthetic, with or without opiates, into the subarachnoid space. A well-performed subarachnoid block provides excellent sensory and motor blockade below the level of the block. The block generally has a relatively rapid and predictable onset. Several factors determine the level, speed of onset, and duration of spinal blockade.

1. Local anesthetic agent. Local anesthetics have varying potencies, durations of action, and speeds of onset after subarachnoid administration. Typical doses and durations of action are shown in Table 18-8. These properties are determined by the lipid solubility, protein binding, and pK_a of each agent.

2. Volume and dose of the local anesthetic. Increasing the dose will generally increase the extent of cephalad spread and duration of subarachnoid blockade. Eighteen volunteers received one of three doses (4, 8, or 12 mg) of bupivacaine and one of three doses of

Table 18-8 Local Anesthetics Used for Subarachnoid Block

DRUG	USUAL CONCENTRATION (%)	USUAL VOLUME (mL)	TOTAL DOSE (mg)	BARICITY	GLUCOSE CONCENTRATION (%)	USUAL DURATION (MIN)
Lidocaine	1.5, 5.0	1-2	30-100	Hyperbaric	7.5	30-60
Tetracaine	0.25-1.0	1-4	5-20	Hyperbaric	5.0	75-200
	0.25	2-6	5-20	Hypobaric	0	75-200
	1.0	1-2	5-20	Isobaric	0	75-200
Bupivacaine	0.5	2-4	10-20	Isobaric	0	75-200
	0.75	1-3	7.5-22.5	Hyperbaric	8.25	75-200

From Berde CB, Strichartz GR: Local anesthetics. In Miller RD (ed): Anesthesia, 5th ed. Philadelphia, Churchill Livingstone, 2000, pp 491-522.

ropivacaine for subarachnoid analgesia. Ropivacaine is half as potent and in equipotent doses has a similar profile with a higher incidence of side effects, such as a 28% incidence of pain on injection. Rapidly injecting local anesthetic solutions leads to turbulent flow and unpredictable spread.

3. Patient position and local anesthetic baricity. Local anesthetic solutions can be prepared as hypobaric, isobaric, and hyperbaric solutions. Cerebrospinal fluid (CSF) has low specific gravity (i.e., only slightly greater than that of water). Local anesthetic solutions prepared in water have slightly lower specific gravity than CSF does and will therefore ascend within CSF. Plain local anesthetic solutions are isobaric, and local anesthetics mixed in 5% dextrose are hyperbaric relative to CSF. The baricity of the local anesthetic solution and the position of the patient at the time of injection and until the local anesthetic firmly binds to nervous tissue will determine the level of block. For example, administration of hyperbaric bupivacaine at the low lumbar level to a patient in the sitting position will result in intense lumbosacral blockade. The longer the patient remains in the sitting position, the less the cephalad spread of the block.

4. Vasoconstrictors. The addition of epinephrine, particularly to short-acting local anesthetics, will increase the duration of action.

5. Addition of opioids. The addition of small doses of fentanyl (e.g., 20 μg) or morphine (e.g., 0.25 mg) will prolong the duration of analgesia and increase the duration of analgesia and tolerance for tourniquet pain.

6. Anatomic and physiologic factors. A higher than expected level of spinal anesthesia can result from anatomic factors that decrease the relative volume of the subarachnoid space, such as obesity, pregnancy, increased intra-abdominal pressure, previous spine surgery, and abnormal spinal curvature. Elderly patients tend to be more sensitive to intrathecally injected local anesthetics.

Spinal anesthesia provides the advantage of avoiding manipulation of the airway and the potential complication of tracheal intubation, as well as the potential side effects of general anesthetics such as nausea, vomiting, and prolonged emergence or drowsiness. Spinal anesthesia also provides advantages for several types of surgery, including endoscopic urologic procedures, particularly transurethral resection of the prostate, in which an awake patient provides a valuable monitor for assessment of hyponatremia or bladder perforation. Less confusion and postoperative delirium have been reported in elderly patients after repair of hip fractures under spinal anesthesia. Intrathecal opiate administration can provide high-quality postoperative analgesia for patients undergoing abdominal, lower extremity, urologic, and gynecologic procedures.

In most cases, spinal anesthesia is administered as a single bolus injection. Therefore, the block is of limited duration and is not suitable for prolonged procedures. The practice of continuous spinal anesthesia with the use of small-bore catheters has largely been abandoned because of neurologic complications associated with local anesthetic toxicity. However, continuous spinal anesthesia with relatively large-bore epidural catheters can provide the advantages of incremental titration and the ability to administer additional doses in selected elderly patients. Unfortunately, this technique has a high likelihood of inducing a post–dural puncture headache in young patients.

Complications of subarachnoid block include hypotension (sometimes refractory), bradycardia, post–dural puncture headache, transient radicular neuropathy, backache, urinary retention, infection, epidural hematoma, and excessive cephalad spread resulting in cardiorespiratory compromise. Frank neurologic injury, though recently described with continuous techniques using small-bore catheters, is quite rare. Hypotension, which occurs as a consequence of sympathectomy, usually responds readily to fluids and small doses of pressors such as ephedrine. The efficacy of fluid preloading in providing prophylaxis against hypotension is controversial.

Post–dural puncture headache occurs after a small proportion of subarachnoid blocks. Factors that increase its incidence include female gender, younger age, and larger needles. Epidural analgesia would appear to avoid the complication but, if the dura is inadvertently punctured, leaves a much larger dural rent. When compared with epidural anesthesia, spinal anesthesia has a quicker onset, is more predictably satisfactory for surgery, and is less frequently associated with backache. Transient radicular neuropathy, a painful but usually self-limited condition, recently became evident in association with an increase in enthusiasm for the use of lidocaine for subarachnoid block.

When cardiac arrest results from excessive cephalad spread of subarachnoid block or protracted hypotension, cardiopulmonary resuscitation is notoriously difficult. Patients who suffer cardiac arrest during subarachnoid block have poor survival, possibly because the profound sympathectomy causes difficulty in generating adequate coronary perfusion pressure. Relatively large doses of epinephrine may be necessary to achieve adequate perfusion pressure during cardiopulmonary resuscitation after spinal anesthesia. Absolute contraindications to spinal anesthesia include sepsis, bacteremia, infection at the site of injection, severe hypovolemia, coagulopathy, therapeutic anticoagulation, increased ICP, and patient refusal.

Epidural Anesthesia

Epidural block, another form of neuraxial regional block, has application in a wide variety of abdominal, thoracic, and lower extremity procedures. Induction of epidural anesthesia or analgesia results from injection of local anesthetics, with or without opiates, into the lumbar or thoracic epidural space. Generally, a catheter is inserted after the epidural space has been located with a needle. The presence of the catheter provides several advantages. First, local anesthetic can be added in a controlled fashion so that the time to onset of the block can be well controlled. Second, the catheter can be use for repeated dosing so that anesthesia can be provided for the duration of lengthy procedures. Third, local anesthetics or opiates can be administered for several days to provide postoperative analgesia.

Epidural anesthesia has specific advantages for thoracic surgery, peripheral vascular surgery, and gastrointestinal surgery. Epidural anesthesia has also been shown to decrease blood loss and deep venous thrombosis during total joint arthroplasty. Postoperative epidural analgesia for thoracic surgery provides superior pain control, less sedation, and better pulmonary function than parenteral opiates do.

Christopherson and coworkers[40] randomized 100 patients undergoing major elective vascular reconstruction to receive either epidural anesthesia followed by postoperative epidural analgesia or general anesthesia followed by patient-controlled analgesia (PCA). Epidural anesthesia was associated with a lower rate of reoperation for vascular insufficiency (2 versus 11 in the general anesthesia group). Other morbidity and mortality were similar. However, the choice of anesthesia does not apparently influence overall morbidity in patients undergoing peripheral vascular surgery.

The use of low concentrations of local anesthetics in conjunction with epidural opiates has been associated with earlier ambulation and less postoperative ileus after abdominal surgery. Thoracic epidural anesthesia, but not lumbar epidural anesthesia, appears to be associated with more rapid recovery of gastrointestinal function after major abdominal surgery. However, because intraoperative IV lidocaine also resulted in more rapid return of bowel function (flatus and bowel movement), circulating systemic lidocaine may account for at least some of the effects of epidural anesthesia on postoperative bowel function. A continuing controversy relates to whether epidural or subarachnoid analgesia reduces subsequent analgesic requirements after the block has resolved (so-called preemptive analgesia).

The complications and contraindications associated with epidural anesthesia are similar to those for spinal anesthesia. However, a special cautionary note is indicated regarding epidural anesthesia and anticoagulation. Because of the risk of spinal hematoma, placement and removal of epidural catheters in patients receiving oral or parenteral anticoagulation is performed in conjunction with an anesthesiologist. The recent advent of low-molecular-weight heparin (LMWH) for prophylaxis of deep venous thrombosis has resulted in an increase in the incidence of epidural hematomas associated with the removal or placement of epidural catheters. Although LMWH is effective as prophylaxis against venous thromboembolism, spinal hematomas have occurred in association with perioperative use of LMWH in patients given neuraxial anesthesia. The timing of catheter placement and removal in the setting of LMWH use is critical to avoiding this rare but catastrophic complication. A high index of suspicion of epidural hematoma must be maintained in patients undergoing neuraxial blockade who have received or will receive LMWH. All persons involved in the care of patients receiving continuous epidural analgesia need to be aware of the signs of epidural hematoma, including back pain, lower extremity sensory and motor dysfunction, and bladder and bowel abnormalities. To reduce the risk, needle placement is not done less than 10 to 12 hours after the last dose, and subsequent dosing is delayed at least 2 hours. Epidural catheters are withdrawn at least 10 to 12 hours after the last dose of LMWH.

A final rare complication, epidural abscess, is considered in patients in whom back pain develops after epidural injection; magnetic resonance imaging is an effective diagnostic tool in such patients.

Peripheral Nerve Blocks

Blockade of the brachial plexus, lumbar plexus, and specific peripheral nerves is an effective means of providing surgical anesthesia and postoperative analgesia for many surgical procedures involving the upper and lower extremities. The advantage of peripheral nerve blocks is reduced physiologic stress in comparison to spinal or epidural anesthesia, avoidance of airway manipulation and the potential complications associated with endotracheal intubation, and avoidance of the potential side effects associated with general anesthesia. However, successful nerve block anesthesia requires a cooperative patient, an anesthesiologist skilled in peripheral nerve blocks, and a surgeon who is accustomed to operating on awake patients. All patients undergoing peripheral nerve block receive full preoperative evaluation under the assumption that general anesthesia could be used if the block is inadequate.

Improvements in nerve block equipment and methodology, as well as the availability of a wide range of local anesthetics, have greatly improved the effectiveness and safety of peripheral nerve blocks. In addition to providing surgical anesthesia, peripheral nerve blocks and the placement of indwelling catheters for a prolonged nerve block provide excellent analgesia for many types of upper extremity surgery and trauma. An additional application of indwelling catheters is enhancement of blood flow after reattachment of amputated limbs and in patients with peripheral vascular disease. Each particular block has specific associated risks and benefits. However, general complications of peripheral nerve blocks include local anesthetic toxicity, neurologic injury, inadvertent neuraxial block, and intravascular injection of local anesthetics.

CONSCIOUS SEDATION

When anesthesiologists participate in the sedation of patients undergoing surgical procedures, the procedure is termed *monitored anesthesia care.* Monitored anesthesia care encompasses a wide range of depths of sedation ranging from minimal sedation to brief intervals of complete unconsciousness (for instance, during placement of a retrobulbar block by an ophthalmologist). When non-anesthesia personnel administer sedation for surgical procedures, the process is generally termed *conscious sedation,* although the term *moderate sedation* is preferable. Moderate sedation implies that the patient can respond purposefully to verbal or tactile stimulation, has a patent airway requiring no intervention, demonstrates adequate spontaneous ventilation, and has maintained cardiovascular function. There is a narrow margin between minimal sedation, which may be inadequate for surgery to continue, and deep sedation, which may result in airway compromise and cardiovascular and ventilatory depression. Because of the risks associated with moderate sedation, the Joint Commission for Accreditation of Healthcare Organizations requires that patients be managed with precautions similar to what they would receive if an anesthesiologist were managing the sedation. Important factors include the necessity for preprocedure evaluation, continuous presence of a trained monitoring assistant who has no other responsibilities throughout the procedure, immediate availability of airway and resuscitation equipment, monitoring after the procedure until the effects of sedation have resolved, and specific written postoperative instructions. Physicians who perform procedures under conscious sedation are granted privileges in line with their training and experience in the appropriate resuscitative procedures.

Drugs used for moderate sedation usually consist of opioids such as fentanyl or morphine, often combined with an anxiolytic such as midazolam. Titration of these agents requires careful assessment of a patient's level of pain or anxiety and the requirements for the surgical procedure. In general, IV induction agents such as propofol introduce an added element of risk and increase the need for caution because of the ease with which the administration of additional agent may result in progression to deep sedation or even general anesthesia. Most hospitals now have specific policies and procedures governing moderate sedation. Those who use moderate sedation outside hospitals (e.g., in office-based surgical practices) need to follow the same precautions as practiced in the hospital environment.

POSTANESTHESIA CARE

The PACU is the area designated for the care of patients recovering from the immediate physiologic and pharmacologic consequences associated with anesthesia and surgery. The PACU ideally is located close to the operating rooms. Monitors for the assessment of ventilation, oxygenation, and circulation need to be available for all recovering patients. The extent of monitoring depends on the condition of the patient. The ASA has established standards of postanesthesia care,[41] which mandate the following:

1. All patients undergoing general, regional, or monitored anesthesia care will receive appropriate postanesthesia care as dictated by the responsible anesthesiologist.
2. An anesthesia provider who is aware of the patient's condition will accompany the patient to the PACU.
3. On arrival in the PACU, the patient's condition will be reassessed and a report given to the care provider assuming responsibility for care.
4. The patient's condition will be evaluated continually in the PACU.
5. A physician is responsible for discharge of the patient from the PACU.

Recovery from anesthesia is usually uneventful and routine. Most patients stay in the PACU for 30 to 60 minutes until they are fully reactive and can move to a second-stage recovery area (for ambulatory patients who are returning home that day) or to a bed on a surgical floor. However, several criteria need to be met before the patient can be safely discharged from the PACU. All patients must be awake and oriented and have stable vital signs. Patients must be breathing without difficulty, able to protect their airways, and oxygenating appropriately. Pain, shivering, nausea, and vomiting must be adequately controlled. Patients receiving regional anesthesia must be observed for resolution of the block. There can be no evidence of surgical complications such as postoperative bleeding.

Several types of anesthesia-related complications can be encountered in the PACU and must be promptly recognized and treated to prevent serious injury.

Postoperative Agitation and Delirium

Pain and anxiety are often manifested as postoperative agitation. However, agitation may also signal serious physiologic disturbances such as hypoxemia, hypercapnia, acidosis, hypotension, hypoglycemia, surgical complications, and adverse drug reactions. Serious underlying conditions must be excluded as the cause of agitation before empirically treating patients with pain medications, sedatives, or physical restraints.

Respiratory Complications

Respiratory problems are the most frequently occurring major complications in the PACU. Airway obstruction is most commonly due to obstruction of the oropharynx by the tongue or oropharyngeal soft tissues as a result of the residual effects of general anesthetics, pain medications, or muscle relaxants. Other causes of airway obstruction include laryngospasm; blood, vomitus, or debris in the airway; glottic edema; vocal cord paralysis; and external compression of the airway by a hematoma, dressing, or cervical collar. Oxygen must be administered to a patient with airway obstruction as measures are taken to relieve the obstruction. The characteristic physical signs of airway obstruction are sonorous respiratory sounds and paradoxical chest movement.

Many obstructions can be relieved by applying a head-tilt and jaw-thrust maneuver with or without placement of an oral or nasopharyngeal airway. Suctioning the airway may also be beneficial, and the patient needs to be examined for evidence of external airway compression. In cases of laryngospasm, continuous positive airway pressure (CPAP) is applied, followed by the administration of 10 to 20 mg of succinylcholine if CPAP is ineffective. Patients may require mask ventilation and endotracheal intubation if the laryngospasm does not resolve promptly. In children, glottic edema or postextubation croup can result in airway obstruction. Mild cases are treated with humidified oxygen. Refractory obstruction may require the administration of systemic steroids and racemic epinephrine by nebulization. Reintubation may also be required.

Hypoxemia is a surprisingly common problem. The incidence of mild hypoxemia (SpO_2 of 86%-90%) and severe hypoxemia ($SpO_2 \leq 85\%$) was 7% and 0.7%, respectively, in the PACU for patients undergoing superficial elective plastic surgery; 38% and 3%, respectively, for patients undergoing upper abdominal surgery; and 52% and 20%, respectively, for patients undergoing thoracoabdominal surgery.[42] Hypoxemia can result from hypoventilation, ventilation-perfusion mismatching, or right-to-left intrapulmonary shunting. Reluctance to inspire deeply after abdominal or thoracic surgery may also result in hypoxemia. Clinically, hypoxemia must be suspected as an underlying problem in patients exhibiting restlessness, tachycardia, or cardiac irritability. Bradycardia, hypotension, and cardiac arrest are late signs. Hypoxemia in the PACU may be secondary to atelectasis, which may respond to incentive spirometry or vigorous encouragement to inspire deeply and cough. Treatment of hypoxemia requires the administration of oxygen, assurance of adequate ventilation, and treatment of the underlying causes.

Hypoventilation (synonymous with hypercapnia) can result from airway obstruction, central respiratory depression caused by the residual effects of anesthetic agents, hypothermia, CNS injury, or restriction of ventilation secondary to muscle relaxants, abdominal distention, and electrolyte abnormalities. Signs can include prolonged somnolence, a slow (or rapid) respiratory rate, airway obstruction, shallow breathing, tachycardia, and arrhythmias. Severe hypoventilation can result in hypoxemia, although augmented inspired oxygen will limit the severity of hypoventilation-induced hypoxemia. Treatment is aimed at identification and treatment of the underlying problem. In all cases, ventilation must be supported until corrective measures are instituted. Obtundation, circulatory depression, and severe respiratory acidosis are indications for endotracheal intubation and ventilatory support.

Postoperative Nausea and Vomiting

Perhaps one of the most annoying problems for both patients and personnel in the PACU is postoperative nausea and vomiting. Agents used to prevent or treat postoperative nausea and vomiting include propofol for induction of anesthesia; droperidol, an inexpensive agent that is often effective in subsedative doses; ondansetron and related drugs, which are expensive agents that are marginally more effective; and metoclopramide, which increases gastric motility. No technique has yet proved to be both uniformly therapeutic and cost-effective. One important complication related to the IV coadministration of ondansetron and metoclopramide has been the production of bradyarrhythmias, including a slow junctional escape rhythm and ventricular bigeminy. More recently, the U.S. FDA has placed a so-called black box warning on the use of droperidol in which additional ECG monitoring is required before and after administration of the drug because of an alleged increase in serious cardiac arrhythmias caused by QT prolongation. The FDA warning has been controversial because of the good safety profile of droperidol during the past 30 years and relative lack of scientific evidence to support the recommendation.[43] A recent study comparing droperidol and saline did not show a significant effect of either intervention on the QT interval during or after anesthesia.[44] Nevertheless, the FDA recommendation has caused a significant reduction in the use of droperidol for the treatment of postoperative nausea and vomiting.

The approach to the prophylaxis and treatment of postoperative nausea and vomiting are guided by an understanding of the mechanisms causing nausea and vomiting. Areas in the brainstem that control nausea and vomiting reflexes, such as the chemoreceptor trigger zone, contain receptors for dopamine, acetylcholine, histamine, and serotonin. Binding of all of these receptors

Table 18-9 Commonly Used Antiemetic Agents

DRUG CLASS	COMMON SIDE EFFECTS
Dopamine Receptor Antagonists (DA-2)	
Phenothiazines	
Fluphenazine	
Chlorpromazine	
Prochlorperazine	Sedation
Butyrophenones	Dissociation
Droperidol	Extrapyramidal effects
Haloperidol	
Substituted benzamide	
Metoclopramide	
Antihistamines (H$_1$)	
Diphenhydramine	Sedation
Promethazine	Dry mouth
Anticholinergics	
Scopolamine	Sedation
Atropine	Dry mouth
	Tachycardia
Serotonin Receptor Antagonists	
Ondansetron	Headache
Dolasetron	
Corticosteroids	
Dexamethasone	Glucose intolerance
Methylprednisolone	Altered wound healing
Hydrocortisone	Immunosuppression
	Renal effects

may precipitate nausea or vomiting, or both. Effective pharmacologic approaches to the treatment of postoperative nausea and vomiting include the use of anticholinergics, serotonin receptor antagonists, antidopaminergics, and antihistamines (Table 18-9). The use of any particular agent is based on efficacy, potential side effects, and cost.

Hypothermia

Hypothermia has been extensively studied as a perioperative complication. The most important issues related to perioperative hypothermia include the risk of increased oxygen consumption postoperatively and the possibility that hypothermia could increase the rate of surgical infections. Increased oxygen consumption could be a particular problem in patients with CAD, in whom shivering could trigger myocardial ischemia. However, the risk associated with mild hypothermia has not been well defined in otherwise healthy patients.

Circulatory Complications

Hypotension in the PACU is most commonly due to hypovolemia, left ventricular dysfunction, or arrhythmias. Other causes include anaphylaxis, transfusion reactions, cardiac tamponade, pulmonary emboli, adverse drug reactions, adrenal insufficiency, and hypoxemia. Treatment involves support of the circulation with fluids,

administration of inotropic agents, use of the Trendelenburg position, and delivery of oxygen until the underlying cause is diagnosed and treated.

Hypertension is a common finding in the PACU. Common causes include pain, anxiety, and inadequately managed essential hypertension. Hypoxemia and hypercapnia always need to be ruled out. Other less common causes include hypoglycemia; drug reactions; diseases such as hyperthyroidism, pheochromocytoma, or malignant hyperthermia; and bladder distention. The fundamental goal in control of postoperative hypertension is to identify and correct the underlying cause.

ACUTE PAIN MANAGEMENT

Pain, one of the most common symptoms experienced by surgical patients, has historically been poorly evaluated and frequently undertreated. There have been important changes in medical care with respect to pain management, with inclusion of pain management in medical school curricula, establishment of institutional protocols and procedures for pain management, development of the subspecialty of pain medicine, creation of organizations focused on pain, and increased interest on the part of governmental and third-party payers. These changes will continue into the future, and medical personnel must continue to increase their knowledge of pain control and their commitment to provide optimal analgesia as a key component of patient care. Surveys demonstrate that continued improvement is necessary to further reduce the high incidence of moderate to severe acute postoperative pain.

Acute pain occurs frequently in the setting of surgery and trauma. The pain experience may be part of the symptom complex that prompts the patient to seek medical care, or it may be caused by tissue injury sustained as a result of surgery or trauma. The term *acute* refers to pain that is expected to be of relatively short duration and that should resolve with tissue healing or withdrawal of the noxious stimulus. Acute pain generally resolves within minutes, hours, or days. *Chronic pain,* which can persist for years, is defined as pain that persists for at least 1 month beyond the usual course of an acute disease or beyond a reasonable time in which an injury would be expected to heal. The acute stress response associated with acute pain serves a useful function, although undertreatment may result in harmful pathophysiologic changes. Chronic pain serves no useful function and is now recognized not only as a part of certain disease processes such as cancer but also often as a disease itself.

Mechanisms of Acute Pain

The International Association for the Study of Pain defines *pain* as "an unpleasant sensory and emotional experience associated with actual or potential tissue damage or described in terms of such damage." This definition emphasizes not only the sensory experience but also the affective component of pain. The tissue injury that leads to the complaint of pain results in a process called *nociception*, which has four steps: transduction, transmission, modulation, and perception (Fig. 18-4). With transduction, the noxious stimulus is converted into an electrical signal at free nerve endings, which are also known as nociceptors. Nociceptors are widely distributed throughout the body in both somatic and visceral tissues.

With transmission, the electrical signal is sent via nerve pathways toward the CNS. Nerve pathways include primary sensory afferents (primarily Aδ and C fibers) that project to the spinal cord, ascending tracts (including the spinothalamic tract) to the brainstem and thalamus, and thalamocortical pathways to the cortex. Modulation, the process that either enhances or suppresses the pain signal, occurs primarily in the dorsal horn of the spinal cord, in particular, the substantia gelatinosa. Perception, the final step in the nociceptive process, occurs when the pain signal reaches the cerebral cortex. The first three steps in nociception are important for the sensory and discriminative aspects of pain. The fourth step, perception, is integral to the subjective and emotional experience.

Methods of Analgesia

Multiple agents, routes of administration, and modalities are available for effective management of acute pain. Analgesic agents include opioids, nonsteroidal anti-inflammatory drugs (NSAIDs), acetaminophen, and local anesthetics. Less traditional agents that may be used more frequently in the future include clonidine, dexmedetomidine, dextromethorphan, and gabapentin. Routes of administration include the oral, parenteral, epidural, and intrathecal routes. The oral route is the preferred route for analgesic delivery. Patients experiencing mild to moderate acute pain and who can receive agents orally can obtain effective analgesia. Parenteral administration is preferred for patients experiencing moderate to severe pain, patients who require rapid control of pain, and those who cannot receive agents through the gastrointestinal tract. The IV route is preferred over intramuscular and subcutaneous injections when the parenteral route is indicated. Intramuscular injections are painful, result in erratic absorption, and lead to variable blood levels of the administered agent.

Opioids

Opioids are potent analgesic agents that are effective but frequently underused. By binding to opioid receptors in the CNS and probably also in peripheral tissues, opioids modulate the nociceptive process. The best-characterized opioid receptors are μ1, μ2, δ, κ, ε, and σ receptors. The μ1 receptors are involved in supraspinal analgesia. The δ and κ receptors are involved in spinal analgesia. Opioids can be administered by multiple routes, including oral, parenteral, neuraxial, rectal, and transdermal.

Opioids have varying degrees of potency. Strong opioids are ideal for moderate to severe pain and for pain that is constant in frequency. Weak opioid agents are suitable for mild to moderate pain that is intermittent in frequency. Morphine, the prototype strong opioid, can

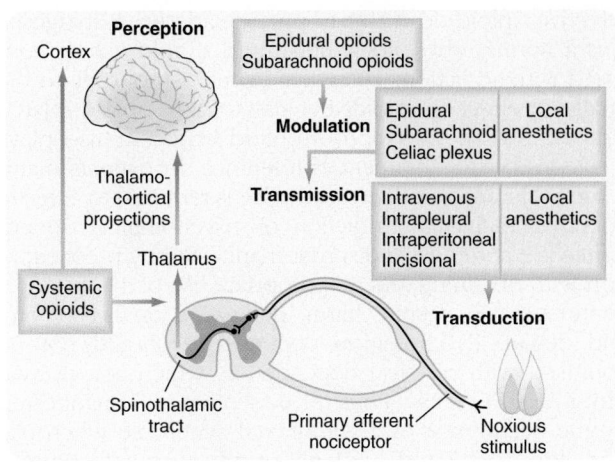

Figure 18-4 Schematic diagram outlining the nociceptive pathway for transmission of painful stimuli. Interventions that prevent nociceptive transmission are shown at the points in the pathway that are thought to be their sites of action. (From Ferrante FM, VadeBoncouer TR: Postoperative Pain Management. New York, Churchill Livingstone, 1993.)

be delivered by a variety of routes and techniques. Other strong opioids include hydromorphone, fentanyl, and meperidine. Morphine is metabolized to morphine-3-glucoronide and morphine-6-glucoronide, which can accumulate in patients who have renal impairment. For moderate to severe pain in patients with renal dysfunction, fentanyl and hydromorphone are more suitable agents. Historically, meperidine has frequently been the preferred strong opioid. This practice has declined because meperidine is metabolized to normeperidine, a unique toxic metabolite that can accumulate and cause seizure-like activity. Patients who are particularly vulnerable to this side effect include the elderly, patients who are dehydrated, and those with renal impairment. Fentanyl is available in a transdermal preparation, but this route is not recommended for acute pain management.

Weak opioid agents, such as hydrocodone and codeine, are commonly combined with aspirin or acetaminophen. Tramadol is an analgesic that is a nonopioid but has some opioid-like effects. It is a centrally acting agent that is administered orally and can be used for mild to moderate pain. Common opioid-related side effects include nausea, pruritus, sedation, mental clouding, decreased gastric motility, urinary retention, and respiratory depression. Appropriate selection of agents, monitoring, and treatment can prevent or ameliorate these side effects.

One major barrier to the effective use of opioid agents by patients, physicians, and other health care providers is the fear of addiction, which can be manifested as underdosing, use of excessively wide dosing intervals, administration of weak opioids for moderate to severe pain, and underreporting of pain. In the setting of acute postoperative pain, the use of opioids has not been shown to be a risk factor for the development of an addiction disorder. Key terms to understand include *tolerance, addiction* (psychological dependence), and *physical dependence*. Tolerance occurs when a previously effective opioid dose fails to provide adequate analgesia. It is a normal physiologic effect and should not be confused with addiction. Tolerance develops not only to the analgesic effect of opioids but also to most opioid-related side effects. The duration of opioid exposure also plays a role in the development of tolerance. In patients manifesting tolerance, an increased dose is required to achieve effective analgesia. Addiction or psychological dependence is a compulsive disorder manifested by preoccupation with obtaining and inappropriate use of a substance, continued use despite harm, decreased quality of life, and denial. Psychological dependence should not be confused with physical dependence, which is a normal physiologic process. Physical dependence is manifested by the occurrence of a withdrawal syndrome when use of a drug is stopped suddenly or when an antagonist is given. The duration of opioid treatment is a factor in the development of physical dependence. The short-term use of opioids in the perioperative period rarely results in physical dependence. Slow tapering of opioids generally prevents withdrawal symptoms.

Nonsteroidal Anti-Inflammatory Agents

NSAIDs are an important component of perioperative analgesia that, when used as a part of the analgesic regimen, reduce pain and can decrease opioid consumption. Their mechanism of action is achieved through inhibition of cyclooxygenase (COX) enzyme activity, which results in decreased production of prostaglandins. Prostaglandins are potent mediators of pain that act directly at nociceptors and also increase nociceptor sensitivity. Inhibition of prostaglandin production results in analgesia but can also lead to side effects such as gastric ulceration, bleeding, and renal injury. These side effects have limited the used of NSAIDs in the perioperative period. Contrary to previous evidence that NSAIDs act mainly in peripheral tissues, there is now evidence that NSAIDs also work in the CNS.

There is a wide range of compounds in this analgesic class with differing chemical structures. Most of these agents are intended for oral administration, which limits their use perioperatively. Ketorolac is available for parenteral administration and has been shown to be effective for analgesia and safe with appropriate patient selection. Ketorolac is avoided in patients with a history of gastropathy, platelet dysfunction, or thrombocytopenia; in those with a history of allergy to the agent; and in patients with renal impairment or hypovolemia. It is used with caution in elderly patients. A loading dose of 30 mg IV, followed by 15 mg IV every 6 hours for a short course, can provide effective analgesia for mild to moderate pain or can be a useful adjunct for moderate to severe pain when combined with opioids or other analgesic techniques.

The most recent advance in this analgesic category involves the introduction of agents that are selective in their inhibition of subtypes of the COX enzyme. There are at least two subtypes of this enzyme: COX-1 (constitutive) and COX-2 (inducible). Traditional NSAIDs are nonselective inhibitors of COX. The newer agents (celecoxib, rofecoxib, valdecoxib) are selective COX-2 inhibitors. COX-2 inhibitors appear to offer similar analgesia with a somewhat reduced risk of causing gastrointestinal bleeding, bleeding diathesis, and renal compromise.[45] They have mostly been studied and used clinically in the management of arthritis-related pain but are becoming more frequently used in the perioperative period. Currently available COX-2 inhibitors are for oral administration. Parecoxib is being studied for parenteral use. There are indications that COX-2 inhibitors are associated with a lower incidence of gastropathy. They are increasingly being used in the perioperative period and may have preemptive analgesic effects.[46] In patients undergoing total knee replacement, oral administration of rofecoxib from 24 hours before surgery through the fifth postoperative day increased knee flexion and decreased both pain and postoperative opioid consumption.[47] Concerns about the use of these selective NSAIDs include the risk for cardiovascular events and their effects on bone healing. Some of these agents (rofecoxib, valdecoxib) have been removed from the market because of the risk for cardiovascular complications. Valdecoxib was removed from commercial distribution because of the risk for severe skin reaction and cardiovascular complications.

Local Anesthetics for the Management of Acute Pain

Local anesthetics work by blocking conduction in nerve fibers, the second step in the process of nociception. These agents are used to provide regional anesthesia for surgery, but their effects last into the postoperative period and contribute to preemptive analgesia. Local anesthetics used in doses lower than that required for anesthesia can also provide analgesia by a variety of application techniques, including local infiltration, topical application, epidural infusion, and peripheral nerve infusion. Local infiltration of local anesthetic before the surgical incision may reduce the sensitization of nociceptors and thereby result in reduced conduction of pain signals to the CNS. This may be manifested as decreased postoperative pain and analgesic requirements. Local infiltration on wound closure may also be helpful. Topical application of local anesthetic includes the use of agents such as eutectic mixture of local anesthetics (EMLA cream), which contains prilocaine and lidocaine. This agent can be used for superficial procedures and can be placed before the surgical incision. Placement of peripheral nerve catheters for local anesthetic infusion is becoming a frequently used technique for postoperative pain management. The development of disposable and lightweight infusion pumps is leading to the increasing use of peripheral nerve infusion in the ambulatory setting. Peripheral nerve infusion analgesia has been shown to provide improved postoperative pain control when compared with opioid administration.[48]

Combination Analgesic Therapy

By combining agents from different analgesic classes, synergy may be obtained. Synergy results in potentiation of effect and reduced dosage of each individual agent with fewer and less severe side effects from each agent. Common combinations include opioids and NSAIDs in an analgesic regimen or epidural administration of a local anesthetic with an opioid. The choice of agent and technique depends on factors such as the patient's medical history, the patient's preference, the extent of surgery, the expected degree of postoperative pain, the experience of the staff providing care for the patient, and the postoperative setting in which the patient will recover. Gabapentin, an anticonvulsant used for the management of chronic neuropathic pain, has shown efficacy for analgesia in the acute postoperative period, including improved pain control and reduced opioid-related side effects.[49]

The concept of preemptive analgesia continues to be actively explored and used in the perioperative period. Induced by a variety of agents and techniques, the goal of preemptive analgesia is to influence the analgesic process before initiation of the noxious stimulus (e.g., surgical incision). This minimizes sensitization of the nervous system and moderates the process of nociception described previously. Effective preemptive analgesia results in decreased postoperative pain, reduced postoperative analgesic requirement, decreased side effects from analgesics, increased compliance with postoperative rehabilitation, and decreased incidence of chronic postsurgical pain syndromes.

Neuraxial Analgesia

Neuraxial routes of administration include the epidural and intrathecal (subarachnoid) routes. These modes of administration require consultation from acute pain specialists, usually anesthesiologists who receive specialized training in use of the neuraxial route for the administration of anesthesia and analgesia. Neuraxial agents are delivered by a single injection into the epidural or subarachnoid space, by intermittent injections through an indwelling epidural catheter, by continuous infusion through an indwelling epidural catheter, or by patient-controlled epidural analgesia through an indwelling catheter. Indwelling subarachnoid catheters are rarely used for acute pain. An important consideration in selecting patients for neuraxial analgesia is the presence of abnormal coagulation, including concurrent use of antiplatelet and anticoagulant agents. Knowledge of such coagulation issues is important to minimize the risk for intraspinal bleeding and spinal hematoma formation, which can lead to severe neurologic injury. The neuraxial route requires education of the medical and nursing staff and the use of protocols and guidelines. In general, patients can be managed on surgical floors with these analgesic techniques. However, monitoring procedures need to be in place to minimize the development of side effects and enhance patient safety.

Agents such as opioids and local anesthetics are given via the neuraxial route to achieve analgesia. Other agents that have been used neuraxially include clonidine, neostigmine, and acetaminophen. Opioids, when delivered by the neuraxial route, provide analgesia by their action at opioid receptors located in the dorsal horn of the spinal cord. An important determinant of opioid action when delivered by the neuraxial route is the drug's degree of lipid solubility. Morphine is hydrophilic, which accounts for its slow onset of analgesia, long duration of

action, ability to provide analgesia over a wide dermatomal distribution, and the risk for late respiratory depression. Fentanyl is lipophilic, which accounts for its fast onset and short duration of action, ability to provide segmental analgesia, and limited risk for late respiratory depression. A hydrophilic opioid such as morphine, when delivered into the epidural or subarachnoid space, remains in the CSF longer than a lipophilic opioid does. The drug can travel rostrally to the brain and influence the respiratory centers hours after initial delivery.

Local anesthetics, when used for neuraxial analgesia, provide analgesia by blocking nerve conduction. To achieve neuraxial analgesia, local anesthetics are delivered in smaller doses and weaker concentrations than those required to achieve surgical anesthesia. This resulting sensory blockade is sufficient to provide analgesia but not sufficiently profound to interfere with motor function and mask complications. Analgesic concentrations of local anesthetics also cause less impairment of sympathetic tone. Bupivacaine and ropivacaine are the most commonly used local anesthetics for epidural analgesia and peripheral nerve infusion analgesia. They affect sensory fibers more than motor fibers (differential blockade) and have a lower incidence of tachyphylaxis (tolerance to local anesthetic action). Neuraxial analgesia for acute pain commonly combines opioids and local anesthetics. Each agent has a different mechanism of action; combining these agents produces synergistic analgesia and thereby results in reduced doses of each agent and a decreased incidence and severity of side effects. A recent meta-analysis of the efficacy of postoperative epidural analgesia concluded that epidural analgesia, regardless of agent, location of catheter placement, and type of pain assessment, provided analgesia superior to that of parenteral opioids.[50]

Intravenous Patient-Controlled Analgesia

An increasingly popular and effective modality using the parenteral route of administration is IV PCA. This modality minimizes the steps involved in the delivery of analgesia and increases patient autonomy and control. Opioids are the agent of choice for IV PCA. In comparing IV PCA with conventional intermittent nurse-administered opioid delivery, patients obtain prompt analgesia, receive smaller doses of opioids at more frequent intervals, can maintain blood concentration of drug in the analgesic range, and have a lower incidence of drug-related side effects. Candidates for IV PCA are patients who can understand the basic steps involved in use of the device, who are willing to assume control of their analgesia, and who are physically capable of activating the device. Such patients include children as young as 4 years of age and most adults, including geriatric patients.

The preferred agents for IV PCA are opioids, with morphine sulfate most commonly chosen. Other opioids used for IV PCA include hydromorphone, fentanyl, and meperidine. Methadone IV PCA has been described. Physicians' orders for IV PCA must specify the drug, drug concentration, loading dose, bolus dose, continuous infusion rate (basal rate), lockout interval, and dose limits. Selection of these parameters is based on the patient's age, medical status, and level of pain. The routine use of a continuous basal infusion rate with IV PCA remains controversial. With a continuous infusion, drug is delivered to the patient regardless of demand, thus resulting in the potential for a higher incidence of drug-related side effects, including respiratory depression. It is safest to restrict the use of basal infusions to patients in special categories, including those with severe pain from extensive surgery or trauma and patients who are tolerant because of chronic opioid use.

The use of structured protocols and guidelines is encouraged for facilities using IV PCA. The medical and nursing staff need to receive training in the care of patients using this modality. There is an increased risk for complications if staff members are not trained to understand the concept of IV PCA; to perform appropriate patient selection, education, and assessment; to use appropriate drug and dose selection; and to establish appropriate monitoring requirements and protocols for management of side effects.

Selection of Methods of Postoperative Analgesia

The choice of postoperative pain management strategies is a function of patient factors, surgeon preferences, the anesthesiologist's skills, and the availability of resources for postoperative care and monitoring.

Chronic Pain

In a subset of patients, pain persists after the expected healing time despite the lack of sufficient pathology to account for the pain. Pain that persists for 1 month beyond the expected time for recovery or initial onset is considered evidence of a chronic pain syndrome. Such patients with persistent pain frequently use words such as *burning, shooting,* and *shock-like* to describe their pain, which is generally associated with a neuropathic pain syndrome. Neuropathic pain syndromes occur when there has been injury to the nervous system (central, peripheral, or both). Central sensitization is believed to underlie the development of neuropathic pain. Examples include patients with persistent pain after head and neck surgery, thoracotomy, mastectomy, hernia repair, and amputation. Certain factors that may increase the risk for chronic pain include infection at the surgical site, intraoperative trauma to nerves, diabetes mellitus, and nerve entrapment by cancer. There is some evidence that preemptive analgesia may help minimize the occurrence of these syndromes.

Because chronic pain syndromes can be difficult to diagnose in the early postoperative period, it is important for physicians to perform appropriate pain assessment during postoperative follow-up. For instance, after amputation, patients might consider it strange to continue to feel sensation and pain in the location of an amputated limb and might be reluctant to volunteer information that they believe could suggest psychological instability. In such circumstances, appropriate questioning may elicit the complaint and result in patient reassurance and appropriate treatment. Referral to a pain medicine consultant is appropriate when the diagnosis of a chronic

postoperative pain syndrome is made. Treatment modalities include the use of adjuvant medications such as antidepressants and anticonvulsants, nerve blocks, physical therapy, and psychological techniques.

Specific Types of Acute Pain Patients

Patients With a History of Chronic Pain

Patients who have a history of chronic pain may experience acute pain as a result of surgery or trauma differently from patients who have no history of chronic pain. Their experience of pain is affected by their experience with chronic pain. Some of these patients may be receiving chronic opioid therapy as a part of their chronic pain management. It is likely that these patients will manifest tolerance to opioid therapy and have a decreased pain threshold, which may result in the patient reporting higher levels of pain and the physician increasing the opioid dose. Obtaining a pain history preoperatively, choosing anesthetic and surgical techniques to minimize tissue trauma and the response to trauma, and appropriate planning for postoperative analgesia can assist in achieving effective analgesia.

Patients With a History of Substance Abuse

Patients with a history of substance abuse are frequently undertreated for acute pain complaints. The stigma associated with drug abuse, misunderstanding on the part of health care providers, and inappropriate pain behavior contribute to undertreatment in this patient population. Effective analgesia can be obtained with strict guidelines, patient education, and appropriate use of consultants and modalities such as regional analgesia.

Pediatric Patients

Pediatric patients experience similar severity of acute postoperative and post-traumatic pain as adults. A major historical myth that has been refuted is the belief that neonates, infants, and children do not perceive pain as adults do. Effective analgesia for a pediatric patient experiencing acute pain can be achieved with pain assessment tools that are tailored for this population and the use of modalities and agents similar to those used for adults. Dosage selection in a pediatric patient must be guided by calculations based on patient weight. With neonates, nurse-controlled analgesia is standard. Older children can effectively use PCA. Regional anesthesia is increasingly being used for pediatric surgery, with the benefits of analgesia extending into the postoperative period and reduced opioid requirements. Epidural analgesia, usually via a caudally placed catheter or a single injection into the caudal canal, can provide effective analgesia. Placement of a peripheral catheter for infusion of local anesthetics can also be used. Topical anesthesia with local anesthetics such as the application of EMLA cream can likewise minimize pain from IV catheter placement and superficial procedures.

Elderly Patients

As the proportion of elderly in the general population increases, a growing percentage of geriatric patients are undergoing surgery or being treated for trauma. These patients will require pain assessment and evaluation tailored to their mental status and cognitive abilities. The modalities and agents used to manage acute pain in this population must take into consideration underlying disease states and decreased organ function.

CONCLUSION

Modern anesthesia is safe and effective for the vast majority of patients, in large part because of important advances in anesthesia equipment, monitors, and drugs. With a wide variety of specific techniques to choose from, selection of anesthetic and postoperative pain regimens for each patient can be based on the requirements of the surgical procedure, the patient's preferences, and the experience and expertise of the anesthesiologist.

Selected References

Benumof JL, Dagg R, Benumof R: Critical hemoglobin desaturation will occur before return to an unparalyzed state following 1 mg/kg intravenous succinylcholine. Anesthesiology 87:979-982, 1997.

Using a combination of pharmacologic and physiologic information from the literature, the authors provide a detailed discussion of factors that influence the rate at which clinically important hypoxemia occurs in relation to the expected duration of succinylcholine. This contributes an important counter to the common misconception that succinylcholine will be metabolized before hypoxemia-induced harm occurs.

Debaene B, Plaud B, Dilly MP, et al: Residual paralysis in the PACU after a single intubating dose of nondepolarizing muscle relaxant with an intermediate duration of action. Anesthesiology 98:1042-1048, 2003.

In a study of 526 patients who received a single dose of vecuronium, rocuronium, or atracurium to facilitate tracheal intubation, received no more relaxant thereafter, and did not undergo reversal of neuromuscular blockade, residual paralysis was present in 45% overall and 37% after 2 hours. The authors emphasize the importance of quantitative measurement of neuromuscular transmission.

Eagle KA, Berger PB, Calkins H, et al: ACC/AHA Guideline Update for Perioperative Cardiovascular Evaluation for Noncardiac Surgery—Executive Summary. A report of the American College of Cardiology/American Heart Association Task Force on Practice Guidelines (Committee to Update the 1996 Guidelines on Perioperative Cardiovascular Evaluation for Noncardiac Surgery). Circulation 105:1257-1267, 2002.

In this extensive review, a joint task force of the American College of Cardiology and the American Heart Association reports guidelines for evaluation of patients scheduled for surgery. They thoroughly examine the importance of the history, physical findings, available tests, and the influence of various types of surgery. This is a valuable update of a consensus approach to this difficult topic.

Mangano DT, Layug EL, Wallace A, et al: Effect of atenolol on mortality and cardiovascular morbidity after noncardiac surgery. N Engl J Med 335:1713-1720, 1996.

This landmark study randomized 200 patients with coronary artery disease or at risk for coronary artery disease to receive placebo or atenolol intravenously preoperatively and postoperatively and orally

for the remainder of hospitalization. Atenolol increased survival over the first 2 years of the study, an effect that was particularly evident in the first 6 months (0% versus 8% in the first 6 months after hospital discharge).

Qaseem A, Snow V, Fitterman N, et al: Risk assessment for strategies to reduce perioperative pulmonary complications for patients undergoing non-cardiovascular surgery: A guideline from the American College of Physicians. Ann Intern Med 144:575-580, 2006.

Report of a consensus conference that reviewed the topic of preoperative pulmonary evaluation. This group identified patient-related risk factors, factors related to the surgical site, and other factors related to surgery, such as the duration of surgery, choice of general anesthesia, and intraoperative use of pancuronium. Major patient-associated risk factors were ASA class greater than 2, age older than 60 years, functional dependence, and the presence of chronic obstructive pulmonary disease or congestive heart failure. A serum albumin concentration of less than 3.5 g/dL was also a strong predictor of pulmonary complications.

Sprung J, Warner ME, Contreras MG, et al: Predictors of survival following cardiac arrest in patients undergoing noncardiac surgery—a study of 518,294 patients at a tertiary referral center. Anesthesiology 99:259-269, 2003.

Cardiac arrest occurred in 223 of 518,294 patients (4.3 per 10,000) undergoing noncardiac surgery between January 1, 1990, and December 31, 2000. The frequency of arrest in patients receiving general anesthesia decreased over time (7.8 per 10,000 during 1990-1992; 3.2 per 10,000 during 1998-2000). The immediate survival rate after arrest was 46.6%, and the hospital survival rate was 34.5%. Twenty-four patients (0.5 per 10,000) had cardiac arrest related primarily to anesthesia.

White PF, Song D, Abrao J, et al: Effect of low-dose droperidol on the QT interval during and after general anesthesia: A placebo-controlled study. Anesthesiology. 102:1101-1105, 2005.

The FDA has issued a "black box" warning concerning the use of droperidol for the treatment postoperative nausea and vomiting because of reported prolongation of the QT interval and the potential development of ventricular arrhythmias. This study showed that the use of droperidol (0.625-1.25 mg intravenously) for antiemetic prophylaxis during general anesthesia was not associated with a statistically significant increase in the QTc interval when compared with saline.

References

1. Diemunsch PA, Van Dorsselaer T, Torp KD, et al: Calibrated pneumoperitoneal venting to prevent N_2O accumulation in the CO_2 pneumoperitoneum during laparoscopy with inhaled anesthesia: An experimental study in pigs. Anesth Analg 94:1014-1018, 2002.
2. Rosenbaum HK, Miller JD: Malignant hyperthermia and myotonic disorders. Anesthesiol Clin North Am 20:623-664, 2002.
3. Rooke GA, Choi JH, Bishop MJ: The effect of isoflurane, halothane, sevoflurane, and thiopental/nitrous oxide on respiratory system resistance after tracheal intubation. Anesthesiology 86:1294-1299, 1997.
4. Spracklin DK, Kharash ED: Evidence for metabolism of fluoromethyl 2,2-difluoro-1-(trifluoromethly)vinyl ether (compound A), a sevoflurane degradation product, by cysteine conjugate β-lyase. Chem Res Toxicol 9:696-702, 1996.
5. Beaussier M, Deriaz H, Abdelahim Z, et al: Comparative effects of desflurane and isoflurane on recovery after long lasting anaesthesia. Can J Anaesth 45:429-434, 1998.

6. Fang ZX, Eger EI II, Laster MJ, et al: Carbon monoxide production from degradation of desflurane, enflurane, isoflurane, halothane, and sevoflurane by soda lime and Baralyme. Anesth Analg 80:1187-1193, 1995.

7. Fu ES, Miguel R, Scharf JE: Preemptive ketamine decreases postoperative narcotic requirements in patients undergoing abdominal surgery. Anesth Analg 84:1086-1090, 1997.

8. Eames WO, Rooke GA, Sai-Chuen R, et al: Comparison of the effects of etomidate, propofol, and thiopental on respiratory resistance after tracheal intubation. Anesthesiology 84:1307-1311, 1996.

9. Brown RH, Wagner EM: Mechanisms of bronchoprotection by anesthetic induction agents. Propofol versus ketamine. Anesthesiology 90:822-828, 1999.

10. Katoh T, Ikeda K: The effects of fentanyl on sevoflurane requirement for loss of consciousness and skin incision. Anesthesiology 88:18-24, 1998.

11. Benumof JL, Dagg R, Benumof R: Critical hemoglobin desaturation will occur before return to an unparalyzed state following 1 mg/kg intravenous succinylcholine. Anesthesiology 87:979-982, 1997.

12. Domino KB, Posner KL, Caplan RA, et al: Awareness during anesthesia. A closed claims analysis. Anesthesiology 90:1053-1061, 1999.

13. Wright PMC, Hart P, Lau M, et al: The magnitude and time course of vecuronium potentiation by desflurane versus isoflurane. Anesthesiology 82:404-411, 1995.

14. Kopman AF, Yee PS, Neuman GG: Relationship of the train-of-four fade ratio to clinical signs and symptoms of residual paralysis in awake volunteers. Anesthesiology 86:765-771, 1997.

15. Debaene B, Plaud B, Dilly MP, et al: Residual paralysis in the PACU after a single intubating dose of nondepolarizing muscle relaxant with an intermediate duration of action. Anesthesiology 98:1042-1048, 2003.

16. Berg H, Viby-Mogensen J, Roed J, et al: Residual neuromuscular block is a risk factor for postoperative pulmonary complications. Acta Anaesthesiol Scand 41:1095-1103, 1997.

17. Caplan RA, Vistica MF, Posner KL, et al: Adverse anesthetic outcomes arising from gas delivery equipment. Anesthesiology 87:741-748, 1997.

18. Standards for basic anesthetic monitoring. ASA standards, guidelines and statements web page, 1998. American Society of Anesthesiologists. Approved by House of Delegates on October 21, 1986; last amended October 23, 1996.

19. Kreuer S, Bruhn J, Larsen R, et al: A-line, bispectral index, and estimated effect-site concentrations: A prediction of clinical end-points of anesthesia. Anesth Analg 102:1141-1146, 2006.

20. Basic standards of pre-anesthesia care. ASA standards, guidelines and statements web page, 2005. Approved by the House of Delegates Oct 17, 2001; amended Oct. 15, 2003.

21. Ferschl MB, Tung A, Sweitzer B, et al: Preoperative clinical visits decrease room cancellation and delays. Anesthesiology 103:855-859, 2005.

22. Shiga T, Wajima Z, Inoue T, Sakamoto A: Predicting difficult intubation in apparently normal patients: A meta-analysis of bedside screening performance. Anesthesiology 103:429-437, 2005.

23. Eagle KA, Berger PB, Calkins H, et al: ACC/AHA Guideline Update for Perioperative Cardiovascular Evaluation for Noncardiac Surgery—Executive Summary. A report of the American College of Cardiology/American Heart Association Task Force on Practice Guidelines (Committee to Update the 1996 Guidelines on Perioperative Cardiovascular Evaluation for Noncardiac Surgery). Circulation 105:1257-1267, 2002.

24. Eagle KA, Rihal CS, Mickel MC, et al: Cardiac risk of noncardiac surgery. Influence of coronary disease and type of surgery in 3368 operations. Circulation 96:1882-1887, 1997.

25. Wesoriak DH, Eagle KA: The preoperative cardiovascular evaluation of the intermediate risk patient: New data, changing strategies. Am J Med 118:1413E1-1413E9, 2005.

26. Boersma E, Polderman D, Bax J, et al: Predicting cardiac death after major vascular surgery: Role of clinical characteristics, dobutamine echocardiography and β blocker therapy. JAMA 285:1665-1673, 2001.

27. Mangano DT, Layug EL, Wallace A, et al: Effect of atenolol on mortality and cardiovascular morbidity after noncardiac surgery. N Engl J Med 335:1713-1720, 1996.

28. Wallace A, Layug B, Tateo I, et al: Prophylactic atenolol reduces postoperative myocardial ischemia. Anesthesiology 88:7-17, 1998.

29. Palda VA, Detsky AS: Perioperative assessment and management of risk from coronary artery disease. Ann Intern Med 127:313-328, 1997.

30. Seto TB, Kwiat D, Taira DA, et al: Physicians' recommendations to patients for use of antibiotic prophylaxis to prevent endocarditis. JAMA 284:68-71, 2000.

31. Qaseem A, Snow V, Fitterman N, et al: Risk assessment for strategies to reduce perioperative pulmonary complications for patients undergoing non-cardiovascular surgery: A guideline from the American College of Physicians. Ann Intern Med 144:575-580, 2006.

32. Smetana GW: Preoperative pulmonary evaluation. N Engl J Med 340:937-944, 1999.

33. Warner DO, Warner MA, Barnes RD, et al: Perioperative respiratory complications in patients with asthma. Anesthesiology 85:460-467, 1996.

34. Warner DO, Warner MA, Offord KP, et al: Airway obstruction and perioperative complications in smokers undergoing abdominal surgery. Anesthesiology 90:372-379, 1999.

35. Van den Burghe G, Wouters P, Weekers F, et al: Intensive insulin therapy in the critically ill patients. N Engl J Med 345:1359-1367, 2001.

36. Newland MC, Ellis SJ, Lydiatt CA, et al: Anesthetic-related cardiac arrest and its mortality: A report covering 72,959 anesthetics over 10 years from a US teaching hospital. Anesthesiology 97:108-115, 2002.

37. Sprung J, Warner ME, Contreras MG, et al: Predictors of survival following cardiac arrest in patients undergoing noncardiac surgery—A study of 518,294 patients at a tertiary referral center. Anesthesiology 99:259-269, 2003.

38. Schwilk B, Muche R, Treiber H, et al: A cross-validated multifactorial index of perioperative risks in adults undergoing anesthesia for non-cardiac surgery. J Clin Monit Comput 14:283-294, 1998.

39. Warner MA, Shields SE, Chute CG: Major morbidity and mortality within 1 month of ambulatory surgery and anesthesia. JAMA 270:1437-1441, 1993.

40. Christopherson R, Beattie C, Frank SM, et al: Perioperative morbidity in patients randomized to epidural or general anesthesia for lower extremity vascular surgery. Anesthesiology 79:422-434, 1993.

41. Practice guidelines for postanesthesia care. ASA Task Force on Postanesthesia Care. Anesthesiology 96:742-752, 2002.

42. Xue FS, Li BW, Zhang GS, et al: The influence of surgical sites on early postoperative hypoxemia in adults undergoing elective surgery. Anesth Analg 88:213-219, 1999.

43. White PF, Abrao J: Drug-induced prolongation of the QT interval: What's the point? Anesthesiology 104:386-387, 2006.

44. White PF, Song D, Abrao J, et al: Effect of low-dose droperidol on the QT interval during and after general anesthesia: A placebo-controlled study. Anesthesiology 102:1101-1105, 2005.

45. Gilron I, Milne G, Hong M: Cyclooxygenase-2 inhibitors in postoperative pain management: Current evidence and future directions. Anesthesiology 99:1198-1208, 2003.

46. Reuben SS, Bhopatkar S, Maciolek H, et al: The preemptive analgesic effect of rofecoxib after ambulatory arthroscopic knee surgery. Anesth Analg 94:55-59, 2002.

47. Buvanendran A, Kroin JS, Tuman KJ, et al: Effects of perioperative administration of a selective cyclooxygenase-2 inhibitor on pain management and recovery of function after knee replacement. A randomized controlled trial. JAMA 290:2411-2418, 2003.

48. Richman JM, Liu SS, Courpas G, et al: Does continuous peripheral nerve block provide superior pain control to opioids? A meta-analysis. Anesth Analg 102:248-257, 2006.

49. Turan A, White PF, Karamanlioglu B, et al: Gabapentin: An alternative to the cyclooxygenase-2 inhibitors for perioperative pain management. Anesth Analg 102:175-181, 2006.

50. Block BM, Liu SS, Rowlingson AJ, et al: Efficacy of postoperative epidural analgesia: A meta-analysis. JAMA 290:2455-2463, 2003.

Emerging Technology in Surgery: Informatics, Electronics, Robotics

Guillermo Gomez, MD

Minimally Invasive Surgery and Robotics
Concept and Functions of Surgical Robots
Classification of Surgical Robots

Informatics, electronics, and robotics are intermingled fields that constantly change the way we experience our lives and practice medicine. For instance, we order and receive our journals through Internet connections, we enter orders on computerized sheets, we go on rounds with the pharmacopeia in a pocket PC, we obtain scrubs from a dispensing robot, our patients are imaged by robotic computed tomography (CT) and magnetic resonance imaging (MRI) scanners, and we read clinical results on high-resolution, interactive video displays (just to mention some examples of our reliance on technology). From the user's point of view, it is not practical to discuss these fields separately. Despite many decades of technologic developments, the performance of surgical operations (the cutting and suturing by the artisan) remained unchanged. The advent of minimally invasive surgery (MIS), however, brought about a major deviation from traditional surgery.[1,2] The traditional premise that large surgical problems require large incisions for adequate treatment is no longer sustainable. MIS is here to stay and will continue to embody a growing portion of surgery. At the forefront of MIS is robotics.[3] Robotic surgery is aimed at improving surgical outcomes through increased precision in a setting of minimal invasiveness. In addition, robotics is creating fertile ground for the gestation of telementoring and telepresence in the surgery of the 21st century.[3] The focus in this chapter is on concepts and technologic developments that have reached clinical application. The description of different robotic systems provides insight for the understanding of surgical robotics and its applications.

MINIMALLY INVASIVE SURGERY AND ROBOTICS

The principle *first do no harm* is central to the practice of medicine. In surgery, however, wounding is an inseparable component of the operation itself. Indeed, in many instances the trauma inflicted by surgical access alone is greater or adds significantly more injury than the tissue damage caused by dissection of the organ to be operated on. Typically, the surgical access (e.g., laparotomy, thoracotomy) on its own is responsible for significant pain and morbidity. The development of MIS (or minimal access surgery), therefore, has been a logical and ethically justified process. Advantages of MIS were clearly demonstrated by pioneer surgeons such as Kurt Semm, who performed the first laparoscopic appendectomy in a human in 1980, and Eric Mühe, who performed the first laparoscopic cholecystectomy in a human in 1985.[4] Technologic and dogmatic limitations of that time, however, placed constraints on the progress of MIS. In 1985, a major technologic leap took place with invention of the solid-state, charged-couple device (CCD), which allowed the manufacturing of miniature video cameras. Digital video has transformed the operating room such that the entire team can observe simultaneously, in the same direction, a magnified surgical field.

In 1987, laparoscopic cholecystectomy was reintroduced by Philippe Mouret and other pioneers,[4] but in a new environment—the digital era; from there on, the so-called laparoscopic revolution took place around the world. In a relatively short period, several operations were adapted to MIS technique (e.g., appendectomy, antireflux procedures, hernia repairs, adrenalectomy, splenectomy).[1,2] In many aspects these MIS operations yielded better outcomes than their open counterparts did: less pain, decreased blood loss, fewer wound complications, shorter hospital stay, faster recovery, and better cosmetics. In general, a better quality of life was obtained without compromising the primary outcome of the surgical procedure. In addition, reduced surgical stress, less impairment of physiologic functions, and improved immune responses with MIS expanded the indications for MIS to include the elderly and high-risk patients. Not unexpectedly, the educated public has become a major advocate of MIS. However, other more complex operations have not found an easy transition to MIS (e.g., colectomy, pancreatectomy, coronary bypass). In part, the problem has been due to the technical limitations inherent in the videoscopic platforms. In brief, videoscopic surgery is hindered by the following[3,5]:

1. Replacement of the normal open three-dimensional (3-D) view by a two-dimensional (2-D) vision of the field displayed on a monitor
2. Unstable video camera positioning
3. Operative ergonomics inferior to that of open surgery
4. Loss of the normal degrees of freedom for manipulation of surgical instruments

Robotic technology has been envisioned as the way to overcome the physical obstacles of MIS and improve on the surgeon's natural limitations.[5] In relation to these advances, research on surgical robots was begun before the advent of videoscopic MIS.[6]

CONCEPT AND FUNCTIONS OF SURGICAL ROBOTS

The term *robot* is derived from the Czechoslovakian word *robata,* which is translated as "forced labor" or "worker."[3] The term *surgical robot* is refuted by some because a robot is generally considered a machine that is programmed to perform tasks autonomously. The terms *computer enhanced* and *computer assisted* have been coined in reference to surgical systems that operate without autonomy. However, the idea of having a humanoid machine (as seen in science fiction books and movies) replace the surgeon is not the intent of a surgical robot. For instance, surgical robots are not capable of clinical judgment. Robots do not have the compassion to establish a humane patient-physician relationship or the requirement to earn continuous medical education credits. A *surgical robot* has been defined as a powered, computer-controlled device that can be programmed to aid in the positioning and manipulation of surgical instruments.[6] The central requirement for a surgical system to be classified as a robot is to be self-powered. In a broad sense, surgical robots represent sophisticated powered instruments that enable the surgeon to carry out more complex tasks.

Common tasks given to industrial robots include the execution of repetitive, tiresome, or hazardous motions

and handling of specialized tools with high precision. Similar applications have been given to surgical robots, but the development of these robots has been more complex because of constraints imposed by human safety and functionality (e.g., sterilization, interference with medical equipment, restricted room space). Examples of surgical tasks assigned to robotic systems include percutaneous biopsy of solid organs (e.g., brain, prostate, kidney), high-precision drilling or cutting (e.g., bone), automated resection of solid organs (e.g., prostate), image processing (e.g., magnification) and reproduction of 3-D vision, microsurgery (e.g., motion scaling), suturing in MIS, endoscope holding, and surgery under biohazardous conditions (e.g., radiosurgery, brachytherapy). Furthermore, surgical robots are becoming integral components of a more comprehensive network of clinical information.[7,8] Integrated robotic systems will be capable of assisting in the preoperative, intraoperative, and postoperative management of surgical patients. A surgical robot linked to another robotic system such as a CT or MRI scanner can have access to imaging studies for importation into the operative theater. Robots have the potential to assist not only with the preoperative planning but also with the rehearsal of individualized operations.[7,8] In fact, current robots such as Robodoc (see later) function by using the patient's actual anatomy obtained by preoperative imaging examinations.

Surgical training has changed little in more than a century despite several leaps of technologic progress. Surgical training remains lengthy because there are a minimal number of cases to complete to achieve competency. Surgical experience continues to a significant extent to be the product of a trial-error exercise in patients. Learning curves are said to be steep, and there is an inherent rate of morbidity and mortality with each operation. Most residency programs do not offer training in cutting-edge MIS. The relative magnitude of these problems is not acceptable for an indeterminate amount of time. Robotic technologies offer feasible solutions for updating our methods of surgical training and improving outcomes in patient care. New technologic disciplines such as virtual reality have emerged and are approaching a practical realm thanks to rapid growth in computational power and software capabilities. Similar to the aerospace industry (e.g., aircraft simulators), purpose-designed robots in surgical simulation may become invaluable tools for surgical training and licensing procedures.[8]

Progress in telecommunications has made telemedicine practical. Telementoring, a class of telemedicine, has been carried out successfully in surgery via standard means of transmission over various distances. Short-distance telementoring (e.g., between adjacent operating theaters) has been accomplished by linking video monitors with fixed coaxial cables. Short-distance telementoring has been shown to be a feasible and safe method for supervision and assessment of the competency of trainees during laparoscopic cholecystectomy.[9] Long-distance telementoring (e.g., over thousands of miles apart) has been accomplished successfully with standard telephone, cellular, and satellite systems. For example, laparoscopic inguinal hernia repairs were performed aboard the

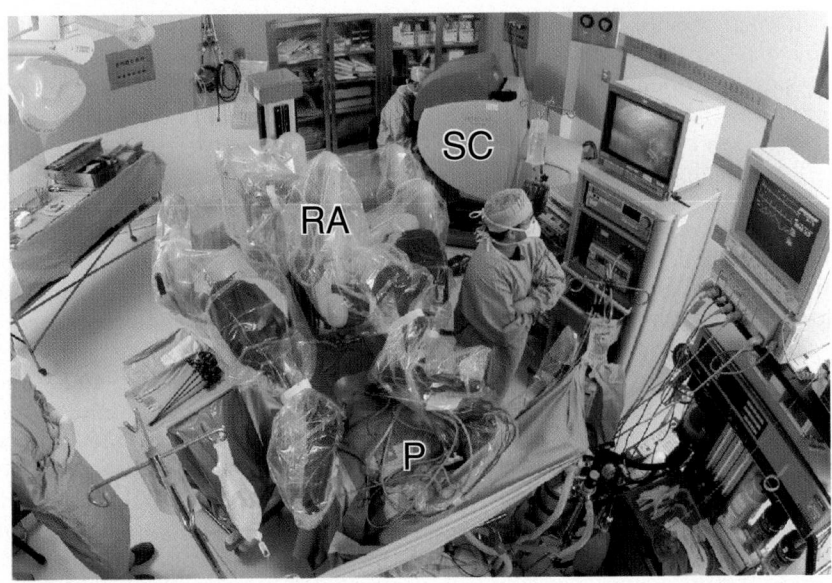

Figure 19-1 Telepresence surgery at the University of Texas Medical Branch. The surgeon operates at a distance from the patient, seated at the surgeon's console (SC). The robotic arms (RA) are positioned and docked to the patient (P). The assistants stand at the patient's side, sterile and ready to perform the changes of instruments.

aircraft carrier USS *Abraham Lincoln* under telementoring from land-based laparoscopic surgeons,[10] and laparoscopic cholecystectomy was performed in Ecuador under expert telementoring from New Haven, Connecticut.[11] A more active system of surgical telementoring has been attained by linking a robot to a telecommunications system. Via custom software and fast data transfer (integrated services digital network [ISDN] lines), a telementor had control over a robotic arm, video cameras, electrosurgical generator, and a drawing pen/pad assembly that were used by a mentored surgeon operating several thousand miles away.[12] With this setup, advanced laparoscopic operations (e.g., varicocelectomy, nephrectomy, and adrenalectomy) were telementored from Baltimore, Maryland, to Bangkok (Thailand), Innsbruck (Austria), Rome, and Singapore.[12] Telementoring represents a feasible method of conveying proctorship and expert consultation in MIS.

Telepresence surgery has traversed the portal of the MIS suite in the 21st century. In telepresence surgery, the surgeon does not operate in direct contact with but rather at a distance from the patient (Fig. 19-1). The distance can be a few meters or thousands of kilometers away. The surgeon is immersed in a virtual representation of the surgical field by observing a video display mounted in an ergonomic console. In return, the surgeon telecasts manual commands to the robotic instruments, which are positioned over the surgical field at the patient's side.[13] The robots used for telepresence surgery are called *telerobots*. Jacques Marescaux and coworkers provided an elegant demonstration of telepresence surgery.[14] They successfully performed a transatlantic telerobotic cholecystectomy in July 2001. In that operation the operating surgeon was in New York City and the patient was in Strasbourg, France (appropriately supervised by assistant surgeons).

The surgeon-side and the patient-side components of the telerobot were connected by a high-speed terrestrial optic fiber (asynchronous transfer mode [ATM] technology); the mean total delay time in the circuit was 155 ms. Remote telepresence surgery is not intended to interfere with the art of the patient-physician relationship or with local and international regulation of medical practice. Telepresence surgery, however, stands as a viable channel to outreach underserved areas in need of surgical expertise.[13] For this purpose, human telesurgery has already been practiced in Ontario, Canada, through a broad-bandwidth Internet protocol. Mehran Anvari and associates established a remote telesurgery service between a university hospital in Hamilton and a rural hospital located in North Bay, some 400 kilometers away. This Canadian group has reported successful completion of remote telerobotic operations such as fundoplication, sigmoidectomy, right hemicolectomy, and inguinal hernia repair, all without conversion or significant complications derived from the robotic technology itself. Despite this promising pioneering work, most telepresence surgery today is readily conducted within the same operative theater (i.e., single operating room).

Wide implementation of remote telerobotic surgery will require significant adjustments in current systems framing the practice of medicine: management of health information, medical liability, professional licensing and credentialing, and billing and reimbursement, among others. On a daily basis, telerobots can be used to overcome the shortcomings of traditional MIS. Telerobots enable the surgeon to do the following:

1. Take personal control of the optical system (e.g., camera positioning, zooming, and magnification)
2. Operate with 3-D vision

3. Increase precision (e.g., dumping of tremor and scaling of motion)
4. Improve dexterity (e.g., increased degrees of freedom)

The term *degrees of freedom* refers to the maximum possible motions at a joint. Furthermore, telerobots may be used to maximize the surgeon's safety when operating in hazardous environments (infectious, radioactive).[3]

CLASSIFICATION OF SURGICAL ROBOTS

Passive Robots

In passive robots, the energy to propel the system is provided by the surgeon; in turn, the system provides information about tracking and relative position of the device with regard to the target.[6] Passive robots function to hold a fixture at a desired location through which the surgeon introduces an instrument into an area in which access is difficult. The first passive robot appeared in 1985; it was a modified industrial robot, Puma 560 (Unimation Limited), and was used to guide drills and needles for intracranial biopsies. Another early surgical robot was a modified Scara robot (IBM) that was used to cut bone in the proximal end of the femur for total hip replacement; this robot found veterinary applications only.

In the beginning of laparoscopy, existing passive retractors were adapted to assist in holding the camera and other laparoscopic instruments. These devices, however, are considered prerobotic devices. In general, these prerobots attach to the side rail of the table and have joints and links that are deployed in the most unobtrusive manner; positioning, locking, and release functions are facilitated by mechanical, electromagnetic, or pneumatic brakes controlled by hand or foot pedals. Examples of prerobots include the Omni-Lapo Tract (Omnitract), the Iron Intern (Automated Medical Products), the Surgassistant (Solos Endoscopy), the Trocar Sleeve Stabilizer (Richard Wolfe), the Bookwalter retraction systems (Codman), the Robotrac system (Aesculap), the First Assistant (Leonard Medical, Inc.), and the Endex laparoscopic holder (Andronic Medical, Ltd.). Prerobots are useful because they can be used as adjuncts to current robotic devices.

Semiactive and Synergistic Robots

Semiactive robots are devices that combine the capability of some autonomous function with other actions carried out by the surgeon.

One example is LARS (Laparoscopic Assistant Robotic System, Johns Hopkins University and IBM).[15] LARS is a robotic arm that has 4 degrees of freedom for positioning a video camera or retracting instruments and is fitted with sensors that monitor force and torque. The arm is driven by the operator, but should the force exceed the programmed safety thresholds (e.g., tissue resistance), the robot halts the motion until the operator corrects the position. The arm is mounted in a cart that is rolled to the side of the operating table. LARS has been used for experimental surgery only.

Synergistic robots are devices simultaneously powered by both the robot's engine and the surgeon. This hybrid platform establishes a partnership between the skills and experience of the surgeon and the geometric accuracy of a tireless machine. ACROBOT (Active Constraint Robot, Imperial College, London) is an example of a synergistic robot. ACROBOT was designed to cut bone with maximum precision and safety in preparation for knee replacement. After the knee is immobilized and the robot is registered to the target, the area of resection is calculated and transferred to ACROBOT. The surgeon then manually drives a motorized cutter, thus having complete force feedback from the procedure but restricted to move within a preprogrammed spatial framework. Another example of a synergistic robot is the Steady Hand robot (Johns Hopkins). The Steady Hand robot is a device under development with the purpose of enhancing the ability of the human hand to perform micromanipulations.

Active Robots

Active surgical robots are powered devices that can function with significant independence from the surgeon. These robots carry the greatest safety concerns and have been developed for specific purposes.

Camera Holder Robots

Frequently, in traditional laparoscopy, the camera person is a less experienced member of the team who stands in an uncomfortable position. The result is an unstable, improperly centered, and rotated picture that misses important anatomic details and causes motion sickness (among other things). If the surgeon has to take over the camera, one of the hands needed for two-handed maneuvers is lost. Therefore, robots for camera holding were the first active robots to be developed for commercial use. Furthermore, these robots have fewer safety concerns because the telescope is not a cutting tool and they can also be operated in a passive mode. AESOP (Automated Endoscopic System for Optimal Positioning, Computer Motion, Inc.) and EndoAssist (Armstrong Healthcare, Ltd.)[16] are the better-known robotic camera holder systems around the world. They have successfully replaced the camera assistant and have allowed solo performance of surgery.

AESOP was the first laparoscopic robot to gain approval by the U.S. Food and Drug Administration. This system is composed of a control computer, a power system, and an articulated, electromechanical arm for holding and maneuvering the telescope. The arm attaches to the operating table, and its action can be controlled by foot pedals, hand controls, or a voice activation/recognition system. The voice activation platform has been the preferred technique. The arm provides 7 degrees of freedom and centers at the point where the telescope enters the patient (e.g., abdominal or chest cavity). AESOP has been used extensively to assist in urologic (e.g., nephrectomy, prostatectomy), gynecologic (e.g., hysterectomy), gastrointestinal (e.g., cholecystectomy, colectomy, Nissen fundoplication), and thoracic (e.g., internal mammary artery) videoscopic operations. Several authors have reported that the use of AESOP significantly reduces smudging, fogging, need for cleaning, and inadvertent movements of the telescope.[17-19] The use of a robot camera holder has not increased but has sometimes reduced operative time.[17]

EndoAssist is another robot for camera holding that differs from AESOP in the commanding mechanism. EndoAssist is a head-mounted navigation system that allows the laparoscopic camera to follow the surgeon's head movements by tracking a headband sensor. The robot is in active mode only when a foot switch is pressed by the surgeon. In active mode, any glance of the operator in one direction on the video monitor causes the camera to pan in the same direction (left/right, up/down, zoom in/out).

Orthopedic Robots

One of the first active robots was designed for orthopedic surgery. Orthopedic operations are especially suited for automated tasks because the target site can be effectively stabilized. Included among the goals for using robots in orthopedic surgery are decreased frequency of iatrogenic fractures, more precise bone drilling, better alignment of fragments and prostheses, improved contact areas, better bone ingrowth, and hopefully, improved long-term performance.

Robodoc (Integrated Surgical Systems) has been developed for primary total hip replacement, revision hip replacement, and total knee replacement. Manual bone milling produces a rough and uneven cavity for cementless implantation of prostheses. The average contact area created by manual drilling is about 23%. In contrast, the contact area achieved with Robodoc is 98% (or better). Robodoc is a computer-controlled mechanical arm capable of 5 degrees of freedom and force sensing in all axes. The tip of the arm holds a rotary bone cutter. Robodoc functions in coordination with a preoperative planning station, Orthodoc (Integrated Surgical Systems). Orthodoc is a computer workstation that converts actual CT images into a 3-D reconstruction of the joint to be replaced. Via computer modeling, the surgeon can choose the prosthesis (from a software library) with the best fit and can simulate the joint replacement (virtual surgery). At the time of surgery, the patient is clamped to a rigid framework and the joint is exposed by conventional means. Robodoc is then moved next to the patient and is registered (by using preoperative imaging and fiducial markers) to the intraoperative location of the target. The robot then cuts and shapes the bone for a precise fit of the prosthesis according to a plan determined preoperatively. The procedure is constantly monitored for the sequence of motions, applied force, and any displacement of the bone. The robot stops immediately if there is any deviation from the preoperative plan.

Other computer-assisted robotic systems are under development for different orthopedic applications that integrate image reconstruction and guidance; some examples include CASPAR,[20] CRIGOS,[21] and the Loughborough manipulator.[22]

Neurosurgery Robots

The rigid structure of the skull and the delicateness of access to specific regions in the cranial cavity stimulated the use of robots in neurosurgery since the early 1980s. Initially, passive robots were used as stereotactic frames only. Today, powered, computer-assisted, image-guided devices have been developed to assist in active, frameless neuronavigation.

Minerva is a powered neurosurgery robot that functions under the guidance of a dedicated CT imaging system.[23] Specifically designed instruments loaded onto a rotary carrousel can carry out the entire operation without assistance from the surgeon.[23] Minerva was developed at the University of Lausanne and has not been commercialized.

NeuroMate (Integrated Surgical Systems) is a computer-assisted, image-guided device for stereotactic procedures in neurosurgery.[24] It consists of a mechanical arm, an image-planning computer station, and a head stabilizer. Preoperatively, CT, MRI, or other images are correlated to the individual characteristics of the patient. With the use of a system of spatial coordinates, the robot is registered to the patient at the time of the operation. During the operation, the robot moves and positions the instruments as programmed preoperatively. The surgeon can manually drive instruments to preselected areas of the central nervous system by using the fixture provided by the robot (semantically, because the surgeon takes active part in portions of the operation, NeuroMate also classifies as a semiactive robot).

PathFinder (Armstrong-Healthcare, Ltd.) is a powered, image-guided robot used for accurate positioning of stereotactic instruments. PathFinder consists of a planning workstation and a gyratory mechanical arm mounted on a wheeled trolley. The workstation accepts standard output formats from CT and MRI scanners and enables the surgeon to view and mark images to plan the path to a designated target within the brain; the preoperative planning also includes a demarcation of "no-go" zones for safety purposes. To allow registration, preoperative images have to be acquired with titanium fiducial markers placed on the surface of the head. The robotic arm has 6 degrees of freedom and a camera. PathFinder uses the preoperative images and the camera picture for registration and intraoperative navigation. The algorithm also calculates the error of fit, and the surgeon can enter instructions for reregistration, if necessary. Other built-in safety features of PathFinder include an interlock mechanism (to prevent motion of the robot when an instrument is active) and contact sensors (to stop motion in case of collision). The robot moves and positions the arm and the effector under its own power according to the preoperative plan. The surgeon can then proceed in a semiactive mode by inserting an instrument manually, or motorized drivers can be mounted to let the robot complete the procedure autonomously. The maximum error between the specified position and the actual position of a tool is 1 mm.

CyberKnife (Accuray) is an advanced system for stereotactic radiosurgery.[25] It is composed of a computer-controlled robotic arm, a compact 6-MV linear accelerator, and an image guidance system. The linear accelerator is mounted on the robot arm, and the arm has 6 degrees of freedom. The maneuverability of the system enables nonisocentric delivery of radiotherapy, thus limiting radiation exposure of normal tissue. The imaging system (built into the treatment room) uses the body's skeletal structure and small implanted fiducial markers as a reference frame, thus avoiding the pinning associated with external rigid stereotactic frames. The image guidance system uses preoperative CT or MRI scans, along with intraoperative radiographs and video cameras, to register the target and monitor any movements of the patient; any displacement of the target is compensated by repositioning of the robot arm. CyberKnife can be used for any other parts of the body.

Urology Robots

The prostate and the kidney are relatively fixed solid organs that are amenable to minimally invasive access.

The prostate is readily accessible through the urethra. Transurethral resection of the prostate (TURP) is accomplished by passing a diathermy cutter under endoscopic guidance (resectoscope). TURP is a repetitive, manual debulking procedure. Preventable complications from TURP include incontinence, damage to the sphincter muscles and nerves, bleeding from the capsule, and rectal injury. Therefore, TURP is a good candidate procedure for automation to improve precision.

Probot (Mechatronics in Medicine, Imperial College)[26] is a powered, image-guided, computer-controlled robot for TURP. It moves in four axes to carry out TURP within the constraints of the size of the prostate exclusively. The surgeon docks Probot to the patient and measures the length of the prostate under direct endoscopic visual cues. The prostate is then imaged with transurethral, thin-cut ultrasound scanning. In a computer station, specific software uses the ultrasound images to create a 3-D reconstruction of the prostate, and the surgeon can specify the cavity to be cut. Probot carries out TURP by cutting tissue cones in a sequence of concentric rings, starting at the bladder neck and moving toward the verumontanum. The operation is completely performed by Probot under supervision of the surgeon. The surgeon follows the progression of the procedure at the workstation and can adjust the cutting parameters or stop the robot at any time. If there is a system failure, the surgeon can complete the operation. Further refinements may render Probot an invaluable tool for training in TURP.

Percutaneous access to the kidney is a common procedure. The RCM robot (Remote Center of Motion, Brady Urological Institute, Johns Hopkins University) was developed for radiologic percutaneous access for MIS interventions and delivery of therapy. Initially developed for percutaneous access to the kidney (PAKY), the device has also been referred to as the PAKY-RCM robot. The RCM robot is a three-module system consisting of the RCM unit, the PAKY unit, and a passive mechanical arm. The mechanical arm mounts on the operating table,

confers 7 degrees of freedom for positioning, and accommodates both the RCM and the PAKY units. The RCM unit has 2 degrees of freedom for motorized rotation in two planes (x and y directions) around the RCM point. The PAKY unit is a motorized needle driver that holds and inserts the trocar needle. PAKY is radiolucent, thus making it compatible with radiographic imaging. The low and flexible profile of the robot makes it compatible with CT scanners and C-arms in operating rooms. The RCM and PAKY units are activated in sequence. The RCM unit is used first to align the needle under radiologic guidance. After alignment is complete, the RCM unit is deactivated and the PAKY unit is activated to insert the needle. The RCM robot is able to insert a needle to a precise depth with minimal deflection and in a shorter time than possible with the traditional manual procedure. Therefore, radiation exposure of the patient and surgical team is reduced. The RCM robot can be used in manual or automatic mode.

Master-Slave Robots

Master-slave robots are powered, computer-controlled devices that do not perform autonomous tasks but are completely governed by the surgeon, thus the term *master-slave* system in which the surgeon is the "master" and the robot is the "slave." The master surgeon is seated at a control console, and the slave robotic arm is located at the surgical field over the patient (see Fig. 19-1). They are also called *telemanipulators,* which implies that the master and the slave are separated from each other by a distance but communicate through data cables. At the console, the surgeon observes the surgical field on a video display and actuates his hands not on traditional surgical instruments but on mechanical transducers (masters or joysticks) (Fig. 19-2). The surgeon's motions are telecast from the console to the robotic arms, which in turn manipulate instruments (needle drivers, forceps, scissors) and the telescope (Fig. 19-3). The surgeon's console also holds commands for special functions (e.g., focusing, motion scaling) and accessory equipment (e.g., electrosurgical and ultrasonic units).

The separation between master and slave components may vary from a few meters (e.g., inside the same operating room) to several kilometers apart (e.g., transatlantic or interhospital operation).[14] These systems provide unique advantages for MIS when compared with conventional laparoscopic or thoracoscopic surgery:

1. The surgeon holds control of a stable camera-telescope platform, thus eliminating dependence on a camera assistant.
2. The surgical field is presented to the surgeon in a 3-D display.
3. The robotic instruments have articulations near the tip that increase the degrees of freedom to function more like a human hand.
4. The computer eliminates hand tremor and the scale of motion is programmable.
5. The console provides a more ergonomic operating position for the surgeon.

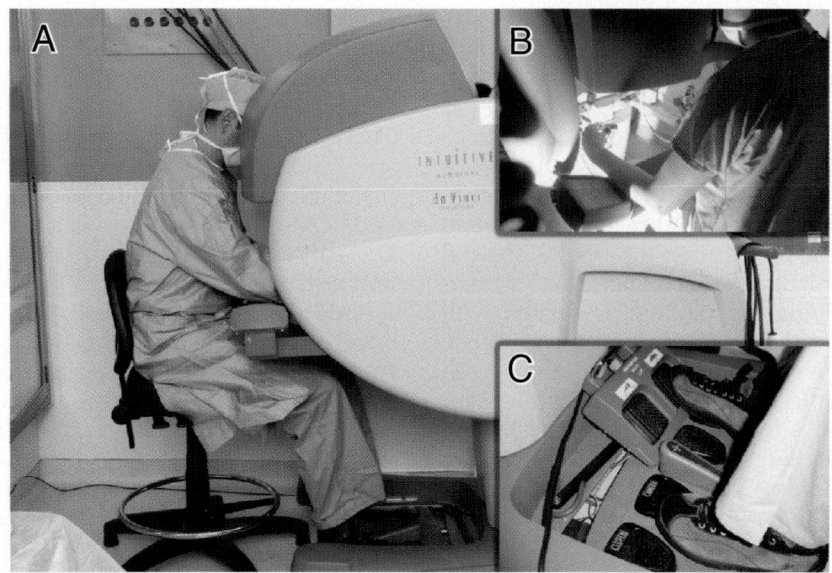

Figure 19-2 Surgical console of a master-slave robot (da Vinci system). **A,** The surgeon sits at the console in an ergonomic position and observes the surgical field in a three-dimensional video display; his eyes and hands are aligned with the field. **B,** The surgeon actuates his hands on mechanical transducers or "masters"; the surgeon's motions are telecasted to the robotic arms, which in turn manipulate the instruments and the telescope. **C,** Foot pedals function in concert to transfer the action of the "masters" to take control of the instruments or the telescope, to realign the masters, or to activate energy sources.

Taken together, these computer-enhanced functions add precision and dexterity to the MIS surgeon, particularly when performing microsurgical procedures.[27]

The master-slave robots of today, however, have significant limitations[27]:

1. The major drawback is the lack of tactile feedback, and therefore application of the force exerted during tissue dissection and suturing must rely on visual cues exclusively.
2. A scant number of instruments are available.
3. The hardware is extremely bulky and heavy and easily clutters the operating room

Special technical features of current systems, da Vinci and Zeus, are presented in the following paragraphs. A brief synopsis of these robotic technologies is of general interest, but a detailed comparison between them is not necessary because the Zeus system is not in production anymore (after merging of the companies Intuitive Surgical and Computer Motion).

The da Vinci robotic surgical system (Intuitive Surgical) gives a true 3-D view of the surgical field by using a dual-lens, three-chip digital camera system. The dual-lens system is bundled into one large telescope. Each camera transmits to separate cathode ray tube (CRT) screens located inside the console, and each screen projects separately to an individual eye (i.e., binocular system). A synchronizer keeps both cameras in phase. At the surgeon's console, the binocular viewer is anatomically aligned with the position of the masters (i.e., the hands). Such an arrangement creates the feeling of being immersed in the surgical field, much like the situation in open surgery. Both the instruments and the telescope are driven by the masters, and control is switched from one to the other with the press of a clutch. The robotic arms of the da Vinci system are floor mounted and therefore the patient cannot be moved after the robotic arms become attached to the cannulas. Any repositioning of the patient requires undocking of the system. Initially developed for cardiovascular surgery, both thoracic and abdominal operations have been performed with the da Vinci system.

The Zeus robotic surgical system (Computer Motion) produces 3-D views of the field by merging right and left video frames (from right and left cameras) over a single video monitor fitted with an active matrix and polarizing filters. The broadcast alternates between right and left frames that synchronize with clockwise or counterclockwise polarization filters, respectively. The surgeon wears glasses fitted with different polarizing filters, a clockwise filter for the right eye and a counterclockwise filter for the left eye. This arrangement causes the right eye to see right video frames only and the left eye to see left video frames only. The telescope is driven by a voice activation system. The robotic arms are mounted on the operating table, and therefore it is possible to change the patient's position without undocking the robot. Thoracic and abdominal operations have been performed with Zeus.

The ARTEMIS (Advanced Robotics and Telemanipulator System for Minimally Invasive Surgery, Karlsruhe Research Center) consists of two master-slave units for manipulation of surgical instruments and a guiding system for a 3-D endoscope. ARTEMIS is still a project under development for both abdominal and thoracic MIS.

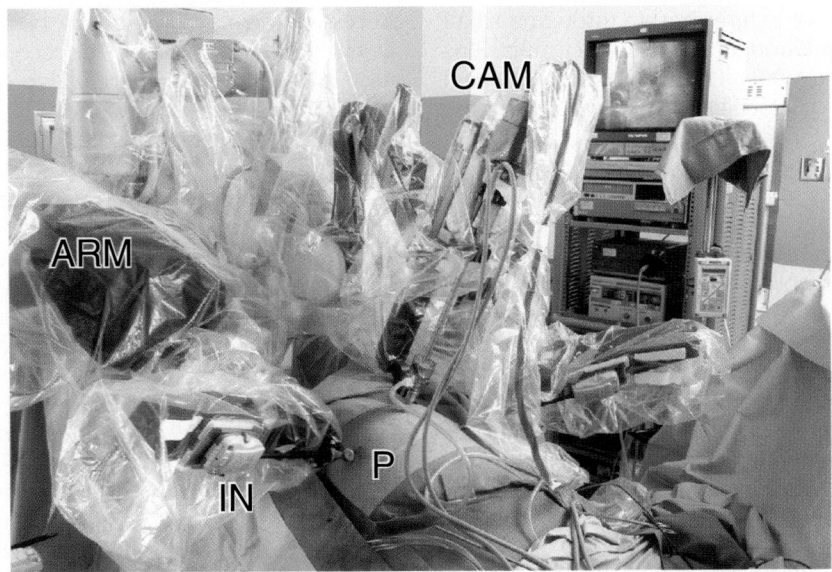

Figure 19-3 Arms of a master-slave robot (da Vinci system). The robotic arms covered with sterile drapes are positioned over the patient (P). The arms are connected to laparoscopic cannulas; the center arm holds the telescope and camera (CAM), and the lateral arms (ARM) hold exchangeable instruments (IN).

Robotic Abdominal Surgery

The technical pitfalls of laparoscopic surgery have been discussed already; robotic technology promises to solve these hindrances. In fact, the increased dexterity and fidelity conferred by master-slave telemanipulators is leading to increased acceptance of them for abdominal MIS. The first telerobotic operation was a cholecystectomy performed with an early version of the da Vinci system in 1997. Since then, both the da Vinci and the Zeus systems have been successfully used for a broad spectrum of interventions in general surgery, gynecology, and urology. Abdominal telerobotic operations that have been well described include cholecystectomy,[28-30] antireflux procedures,[30,31] Heller's cardiomyotomy,[32-34] distal pancreatectomy,[32] gastrojejunostomy,[34] esophagectomy,[32,34] gastric bypass,[34] gastric banding,[35] pyloroplasty,[33] colectomy,[36] adrenalectomy,[34] splenectomy,[32,37] salpingo-oophorectomy,[38] hysterectomy,[39] tubal reanastomosis,[40] nephrectomy,[34,41] radical prostatectomy,[42,43] and pelvic lymph node dissection.[44]

In general, these series are of the case report and feasibility type of studies and have been conducted to determine the safety of telerobotic technology. Telerobotic operations were found to confer the same advantages of laparoscopic operations over open surgery but have not been shown to be superior to their laparoscopic counterparts, at least by the arbitrary end points classically used for comparison (e.g., operative time, blood loss, postoperative pain, hospital stay, conversion rates). Two small prospective randomized studies have compared laparoscopic versus robotic-assisted Nissen fundoplication and transabdominal adrenalectomy; in both cases the classic laparoscopic technique was superior to the robotic approach. However, telerobotic surgery offers new possibilities for which the measure of success is not a comparison with standard laparoscopic outcomes. One

example is remote telerobotic surgery, such as the telesurgical service implemented in Ontario, Canada. Thanks to robotic technology, many patients at a remote location can enjoy the benefits of MIS.

Another area for progress in robotic surgery is training in MIS itself. The learning curve of complex laparoscopic operations may be significantly reduced by using a robotic platform, first for the acquisition of psychomotor skills and afterward for telementoring of an inexperienced surgeon in practice. For example, robotic assistance has been shown to allow novice trainees to perform complex laparoscopic operations such as radical prostatectomy and gastric bypass with outcomes equal to those of experienced surgeons. In the future, more surgeons might become adept at practicing complex MIS, and in turn, more patients may benefit from the advantages of MIS.

Robotic Cardiothoracic Surgery

Despite well-established benchmarks of safety and technical outcomes of current open chest surgery, there is still significant morbidity from the median sternotomy used for access (e.g., thoracic cage deformation and fractures, pain, prolonged rehabilitation time, large amount of blood loss, ventilatory problems, sternitis, mediastinitis) and from the cardiopulmonary bypass (CPB) needed to obtain a stable and dry operative field (e.g., hemolysis, complement activation, immunosuppression, and impairments of visual, memory, and intellectual functions, among others). Therefore, MIS techniques have been actively pursued in cardiovascular surgery to improve on both access and dependence on CPB.

A major obstacle to minimizing the size of access in cardiothoracic surgery is the inherent rigidity of the chest wall and mediastinum. Mediastinal structures cannot be displaced for exposure or exteriorization through a small thoracotomy. Working through small thoracic incisions greatly limits exposure and technical dexterity. Digital technology, however, has facilitated substantial progress in cardiothoracic MIS (CT-MIS). A high-resolution videoscope introduced into the chest can reach targets and replace or even improve the classic open exposures. For instance, the 10× to 20× optic magnification capability of the digital video camera is more powerful than the typical 2.5× to 3× magnification provided by conventional surgical glasses. Furthermore, 3-D video displays have been refined to eliminate the lack of depth perception inherent in conventional 2-D videoscopic systems. In addition, when the videoscope is mounted on a robotic arm, control of the visual field is at the personal command of the surgeon via voice- or hand-mediated mechanisms. Finally, robotic articulated instruments (e.g., the da Vinci and Zeus systems) have been developed that permit working at a distance with the natural 7 degrees of freedom of the human hand; indeed, scaling of motion and filtering of tremor can augment hand dexterity. Digital technology has made totally endoscopic and closed chest cardiothoracic operations a reality.

Loulmet and coworkers[45] from Paris and Mohr and coworkers from Leipzig, Germany, have reported the first human cases of robot-assisted CT-MIS since 1998; the procedures included repair of an atrial septal defect, repair or replacement of the mitral valve, and coronary artery bypass. Surgical robots have been used for heart valve surgery (e.g., valve replacement, leaflet resection and reconstruction, papillary muscle reconstruction, and cord insertion), dissection of the internal mammary artery, anastomosis in coronary bypass graft surgery, and correction of atrial septal defects; both the da Vinci and Zeus systems have been used in various phases of development of these procedures.[46,47] In fact, robotic telemanipulators were initially targeted for CT-MIS. At the cutting edge of CT-MIS is totally endoscopic coronary artery bypass (TECAB), in which both conduit preparation (e.g., for dissection of the internal mammary artery) and anastomosis for single- or two-vessel disease are completed through a three-port operation.[48] A sternotomy or limited thoracotomy has been included in preliminary trials for safety purposes.

Carpentier and Loulmet have proposed a classification of increasing complexity for the development and implementation of CT-MIS. In level I CT-MIS, or the direct vision/mini-incision approach, the procedure is performed under direct vision through small incisions by conventional means. A number of mini-access approaches have been developed and described under different acronyms, such as LAST (limited anterior small thoracotomy) and MIDCAB (minimally invasive direct coronary artery bypass); these techniques, however, suffer from the limited access itself and have obvious restricted applications.[49]

In level II CT-MIS, or the video-assisted/micro-incision approach, a videoscope is passed through the incision to function as a secondary visual aid for portions of the operation; an intracardiac minicamera has been used to add lighting and a magnified view of anatomic details.

Accessory operative ports can be added to pass surgical instruments. This type of videoscopic assistance has been used successfully for mitral valve surgery and harvesting of the internal mammary artery.

In level III CT-MIS, or the video-directed/port incision approach, most of the operation is conducted videoscopically and instruments are passed through operative ports. A helmet-mounted 3-D videoscopic system (Vista Medical Technologies, Becton, MA) driven by an assistant or docked to an AESOP mechanical arm has been used successfully to improve visualization and dexterity.[49] This video-directed/port incision technique has been used in mitral valve surgery and has achieved outcomes that challenge the conventional open approach, but with faster recovery times and significant cost savings.[46]

The level IV, or video-directed/robot-assisted, approach represents the current cutting edge of CT-MIS; at this level of technologic sophistication and skill, complex procedures are performed through port incisions only by using 3-D video displays and robotic articulated micro-instruments (e.g., DeBakey forceps, Potts scissors, microclips).

Important to mention here are the alternatives to conventional CPB that have been developed to permit closed chest cardiothoracic surgery. The Port-Access (Heartport, Redwood City, CA) is a device for femorofemoral CPB and endovascular balloon clamping of the aorta. The Heartport system allows antegrade and retrograde perfusion of the systemic and coronary circulation. Proper positioning of the Heartport is guided by contrast fluoroscopy or by transesophageal echocardiography. The Heartport technology has proved to be an invaluable adjunct in performing videoscopic valve surgery, as well as coronary bypass.[46,47] Another more striking alternative is the off-pump or beating-heart technique; at this moment, however, this technique has been applicable to coronary bypass only. For this purpose, a myocardial stabilizer (e.g., Genzyme, Intuitive Surgical) is deployed over the target coronary artery to be anastomosed. Kappert and coworkers from Dresden, Germany, have already achieved off-pump TECAB with bilateral harvest of the internal mammary artery for single-and double-vessel coronary disease.[48]

In summary, robotic technology holds great promise to expand the spectrum of MIS—not only the technical aspects of surgery itself but also in the areas of training and telesurgery. The rapidly growing computational power and dedicated instrument design are expected to address unresolved technical pitfalls such as lack of tactile feedback and shortage of specific tools. Surgical technique and diagnostic imaging technology can be integrated in the operative theater to facilitate image-guided surgery by using the patient's actual anatomic data. To this point, however, all the studies have documented and proved the feasibility and safety of these emerging technologies as used under ideal conditions. Although early results are encouraging, the cost-effectiveness of them has not been established, and they do not represent the standard of care. One major hurdle to overcome is the high cost of the technology itself. Future trials with outcome and cost analysis will help determine the place of surgical robots in MIS. However, it is said that one picture may be worth a thousand words. Today, the ability to perform laparoscopic surgery with 3-D vision and 7 degrees of freedom may be enough for more surgeons to embrace the development of robotic surgery.

Selected References

Ballantyne GH: The pitfalls of laparoscopic surgery: Challenges for robotics and telerobotic surgery. Surg Laparosc Endosc Percutan Tech 12:1-5, 2002.

A concise presentation of the triumph and pitfalls of laparoscopic surgery; how robotic technology offers solutions for the advancement of MIS.

Chitwood WR Jr: Endoscopic robotic coronary surgery: Is this reality or fantasy? J Thorac Cardiovasc Surg 118:1-3, 1999.

Objective review of the use of current robotic systems (da Vinci and Zeus) in coronary bypass surgery.

Davies B: A review of robotics in surgery. Proc Inst Mech Eng [H] 214:129-140, 2000.

A comprehensive introduction to the world of surgical robots, their history, and classification.

Kappert U, Cichon R, Schneider J, et al: Robotic coronary artery surgery—the evolution of a new minimally invasive approach in coronary artery surgery. Thorac Cardiovasc Surg 48:193-197, 2000.

Remarkable pioneering work toward totally endoscopic, robotic, and off-pump coronary bypass surgery.

Marescaux J, Leroy J, Gagner M, et al: Transatlantic robot-assisted telesurgery. Nature 413:379-380, 2001.

A landmark publication that illustrates the introduction of modern digital technology into the art and science of surgery.

Périssat J, Collet D, Monguillon N: Advances in laparoscopic surgery. Digestion 59:606-618, 1998.

Comprehensive and authoritative review of the origins of MIS and its projections for the modern practice of surgery.

Reynolds W Jr: The first laparoscopic cholecystectomy. JSLS 5:89-94, 2001.

The real story of the operation that revolutionized the practice of surgery; a tribute to our pioneers.

Vanermen H, Wellens F, De Geest R, et al: Video-assisted port-access mitral valve surgery: from debut to routine surgery. Will trocar-port-access cardiac surgery ultimately lead to robotic cardiac surgery? Semin Thorac Cardiovasc Surg 11:223-234, 1999.

Comprehensive review and analysis of the progress in minimally invasive mitral valve surgery, including techniques for minimizing the access and alternatives for cardiopulmonary bypass.

References

1. Périssat J, Collet D, Monguillon N: Advances in laparoscopic surgery. Digestion 59:606-618, 1998.
2. Himal HS: Minimally invasive (laparoscopic) surgery. Surg Endosc 16:1647-1652, 2002.
3. Kavic MS: Robotics, technology, and the future of surgery. JSLS 4:277-279, 2000.
4. Reynolds W Jr: The first laparoscopic cholecystectomy. JSLS 5:89-94, 2001.
5. Ballantyne GH: The pitfalls of laparoscopic surgery: Challenges for robotics and telerobotic surgery. Surg Laparosc Endosc Percutan Tech 12:1-5, 2002.
6. Davies B: A review of robotics in surgery. Proc Inst Mech Eng [H] 214:129-140, 2000.
7. Mack MJ: Minimally invasive and robotic surgery. JAMA 285:568-572, 2001.
8. Satava RM: Emerging technologies for surgery in the 21st century. Arch Surg 134:1197-1202, 1999.
9. Byrne JP, Mughal MM: Telementoring as an adjunct to training and competence-based assessment in laparoscopic cholecystectomy. Surg Endosc 14:1159-1161, 2000.
10. Cubano M, Poulose BK, Talamini MA, et al: Long distance telementoring: A novel tool for laparoscopy aboard the USS Abraham Lincoln. Surg Endosc 13:673-678, 1999.
11. Rosser JC Jr, Bell RL, Harnett B, et al: Use of mobile low-bandwidth telemedical techniques for extreme telemedicine applications. J Am Coll Surg 189:397-404, 1999.
12. Lee BR, Moore R: International telementoring: A feasible method of instruction. World J Urol 18:296-298, 2000.
13. Bowersox JC: Telepresence surgery. Br J Surg 83:433-434, 1996.
14. Marescaux J, Leroy J, Gagner M, et al: Transatlantic robot-assisted telesurgery. Nature 413:379-380, 2001.
15. Poulose BK, Kutka MF, Mendoza-Sagaon M, et al: Human vs robotic organ retraction during laparoscopic Nissen fundoplication. Surg Endosc 13:461-465, 1999.
16. Yavuz Y, Ystgaard B, Skogvoll E, et al: A comparative experimental study evaluating the performance of surgical robots AESOP and EndoAssist. Surg Laparosc Endosc Percutan Tech 10:163-167, 2000.
17. Mettler L, Ibrahim M, Jonat W: One year of experience working with the aid of a robotic assistant (the voice-controlled optic holder AESOP) in gynaecological endoscopic surgery. Hum Reprod 13:2748-2750, 1998.
18. Omote K, Feussner H, Ungeheuer A, et al: Self-guided robotic camera control for laparoscopic surgery compared with human camera control. Am J Surg 177:321-324, 1999.
19. Merola S, Weber P, Wasielewski A, et al: Comparison of laparoscopic colectomy with and without the aid of a robotic camera holder. Surg Laparosc Endosc Percutan Tech 12:46-51, 2002.
20. Siebert W, Mai S, Kober R, et al: Technique and first clinical results of robot-assisted total knee replacement. Knee 9:173-180, 2002.
21. Brandt G, Zimolong A, Carrat L, et al: CRIGOS: A compact robot for image-guided orthopedic surgery. IEEE Trans Inf Technol Biomed 3:252-260, 1999.
22. Bouazza-Marouf K, Browbank I, Hewit JR: Robotic-assisted internal fixation of femoral fractures. Proc Inst Mech Eng [H] 209:51-58, 1995.
23. Glauser D, Fankhauser H, Epitaux M, et al: Neurosurgical robot Minerva: First results and current developments. J Image Guid Surg 1:266-272, 1995.
24. Li QH, Zamorano L, Pandya A, et al: The application accuracy of the NeuroMate robot—a quantitative comparison with frameless and frame-based surgical localization systems. Comput Aided Surg 7:90-98, 2002.
25. Adler JR Jr, Chang SD, Murphy MJ, et al: The Cyberknife: A frameless robotic system for radiosurgery. Stereotact Funct Neurosurg 69:124-128, 1997.

26. Arambula Cosio F, Davies BL: Automated prostate recognition: A key process for clinically effective robotic prostatectomy. Med Biol Eng Comput 37:236-243, 1999.

27. Hashizume M, Konishi K, Tsutsumi N, et al: A new era of robotic surgery assisted by a computer-enhanced surgical system. Surgery 131:S330-S333, 2002.

28. Marescaux J, Smith MK, Folscher D, et al: Telerobotic laparoscopic cholecystectomy: Initial clinical experience with 25 patients. Ann Surg 234:1-7, 2001.

29. Ruurda JP, Broeders IA, Simmermacher RP, et al: Feasibility of robot-assisted laparoscopic surgery: An evaluation of 35 robot-assisted laparoscopic cholecystectomies. Surg Laparosc Endosc Percutan Tech 12:41-45, 2002.

30. Chitwood WR Jr, Nifong LW, Chapman WH, et al: Robotic surgical training in an academic institution. Ann Surg 234:475-484; discussion 484-476, 2001.

31. Cadiere GB, Himpens J, Vertruyen M, et al: Evaluation of telesurgical (robotic) NISSEN fundoplication. Surg Endosc 15:918-923, 2001.

32. Melvin WS, Needleman BJ, Krause KR, et al: Computer-enhanced robotic telesurgery: Initial experience in foregut surgery. Surg Endosc 16:1790-1792, 2002.

33. Shah J, Rockall T, Darzi A: Robot-assisted laparoscopic Heller's cardiomyotomy. Surg Laparosc Endosc Percutan Tech 12:30-32, 2002.

34. Horgan S, Vanuno D: Robots in laparoscopic surgery. J Laparoendosc Adv Surg Tech A 11:415-419, 2001.

35. Cadiere GB, Himpens J, Vertruyen M, et al: The world's first obesity surgery performed by a surgeon at a distance. Obes Surg 9:206-209, 1999.

36. Weber PA, Merola S, Wasielewski A, et al: Telerobotic-assisted laparoscopic right and sigmoid colectomies for benign disease. Dis Colon Rectum 45:1689-1694; discussion 1695-1686, 2002.

37. Chapman WH III, Albrecht RJ, Kim VB, et al: Computer-assisted laparoscopic splenectomy with the da Vinci surgical robot. J Laparoendosc Adv Surg Tech A 12:155-159, 2002.

38. Gutt CN, Markus B, Kim ZG, et al: Early experiences of robotic surgery in children. Surg Endosc 16:1083-1086, 2002.

39. Diaz-Arrastia C, Jurnalov C, Gomez G, et al: Laparoscopic hysterectomy using a computer-enhanced surgical robot. Surg Endosc 16:1271-1273, 2002.

40. Falcone T, Goldberg JM, Margossian H, et al: Robotic-assisted laparoscopic microsurgical tubal anastomosis: A human pilot study. Fertil Steril 73:1040-1042, 2000.

41. Guillonneau B, Jayet C, Tewari A, et al: Robot-assisted laparoscopic nephrectomy. J Urol 166:200-201, 2001.

42. Abbou CC, Hoznek A, Salomon L, et al: Laparoscopic radical prostatectomy with a remote controlled robot. J Urol 165:1964-1966, 2001.

43. Guillonneau B, Vallancien G: Laparoscopic radical prostatectomy: The Montsouris experience. J Urol 163:418-422, 2000.

44. Guillonneau B, Cappele O, Martinez JB, et al: Robotic assisted, laparoscopic pelvic lymph node dissection in humans. J Urol 165:1078-1081, 2001.

45. Loulmet D, Carpentier A, d'Attellis N, et al: Endoscopic coronary artery bypass grafting with the aid of robotic-assisted instruments. J Thorac Cardiovasc Surg 118:4-10, 1999.

46. Chitwood WR Jr: Video-assisted and robotic mitral valve surgery: Toward an endoscopic surgery. Semin Thorac Cardiovasc Surg 11:194-205, 1999.

47. Damiano RJ Jr, Reichenspurner H, Ducko CT: Robotically assisted endoscopic coronary artery bypass grafting: Current state of the art. Adv Card Surg 12:37-57, 2000.

48. Kappert U, Cichon R, Schneider J, et al: Robotic coronary artery surgery—the evolution of a new minimally invasive approach in coronary artery surgery. Thorac Cardiovasc Surg 48:193-197, 2000.

49. Reichenspurner H, Boehm D, Reichart B: Minimally invasive mitral valve surgery using three-dimensional video and robotic assistance. Semin Thorac Cardiovasc Surg 11:235-243, 1999.

TRAUMA AND CRITICAL CARE

CHAPTER 20

Management of Acute Trauma

David B. Hoyt, MD   Raul Coimbra, MD   and   Jose Acosta, MD

Trauma is a major worldwide public health problem. It is one of the leading causes of death and disability in both industrialized and developing countries. Globally, injury is the seventh leading cause of death, with 5.8 million deaths attributable to trauma in 2006. In the United States, trauma is the leading cause of death in children and adults up to 44 years of age, and it kills more Americans 1 to 34 years of age than all diseases combined. Injury fatalities, however, represent only a small fraction of the scope of injury. During 2003 there were 148,000 injury fatalities in the United States. Another 2.5 million patients were hospitalized for their injuries, and still another 40.4 million were treated at local emergency departments and released. An estimated 89.9 million patients were treated by primary care physicians or self-doctored at home. The total cost of injury in the United States is estimated to be more than $200 billion per year, and these costs only continue to rise.

MORTALITY AFTER TRAUMATIC INJURY

Trauma deaths occur at traditionally recognized time points after injury (Fig. 20-1). Approximately half of trauma deaths occur within seconds or minutes after injury and are caused by injury to the aorta, heart, brainstem, or spinal cord or by acute respiratory distress. Very few of these patients can be saved by trauma systems, and these deaths must be addressed by improved injury prevention and control strategies.[1]

The second mortality peak occurs within hours of injury and accounts for approximately 30% of deaths. Half of these deaths are caused by hemorrhage and the other half by central nervous system (CNS) injury. Most of these deaths can be averted by treatment during the so-called golden hour. Trauma system and acute patient care has the greatest impact on this group of injured patients. Recent analysis of trauma system efficacy suggests at least a 10% reduction in preventable deaths as a result of trauma systems. Reduction in mortality through a statewide trauma system has been demonstrated; nonetheless, only approximately 50% of the United States is served by trauma systems.[2,3]

The third peak in mortality represents deaths that occur 24 hours after injury and includes late mortality from infection and multiple organ failure. Traditionally, this peak has accounted for 10% to 20% of trauma-related deaths.[1] Recent analyses suggest that this incidence is closer to 10%. Pulmonary embolism has emerged as an important late cause of death as well.[1]

Further improvements in mortality reduction will require a different strategy for each peak. Early deaths can be reduced by injury prevention and control programs, active legislation, and behavior modification. Regional planning and trauma system development will make an impact on the second mortality peak most effectively. Late deaths will be affected only as we better

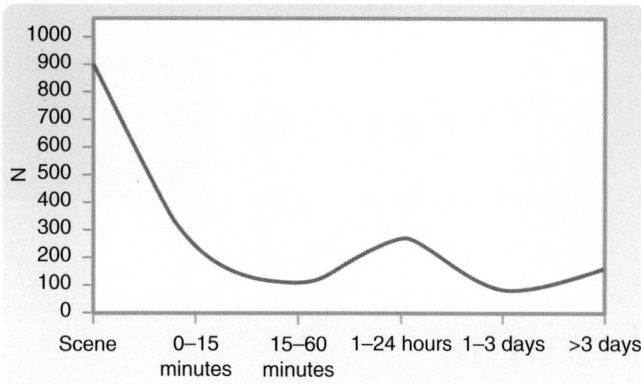

Figure 20-1 Trimodal distribution of death. The time to mortality for a population of trauma patients admitted to a single trauma center from a unified geographic area over a 10-year period is shown. All deaths at the scene and hospital deaths are included. (From Acosta JA, Yang JC, Winchell RJ, et al: Lethal injuries and time to death in a level I trauma center. J Am Coll Surg 186:528-533, 1998.)

understand the pathophysiology of multiple organ failure and delayed treatment of secondary brain injury.

DEVELOPMENT OF TRAUMA CARE

The development of modern trauma care has evolved from the close association of surgery and casualty management in times of war. Many important concepts, including prehospital transport, volume resuscitation, wound management, enteric injury management, and critical care, have been advanced as a result of observations during military conflict. These management principles have been refined in the civilian sector and have led to advances such as primary repair of colonic injuries rather than colostomy and early revascularization of ischemic limbs rather than amputation.[4]

Major progress in the development of trauma systems has occurred in civilian practice because of the efforts of federal agencies, professional organizations, and individual institutions, which have led the development of regional trauma centers. Advancements in acute care, critical care, and rehabilitation have been realized as a result of these specialized centers.

The American College of Surgeons, with establishment of the Committee on the Treatment of Fractures, recognized the importance of injury more than 80 years ago. Formal recognition of multidisciplinary trauma care and establishment of the American College of Surgeons Committee on Trauma occurred only during the past 50 years. The first organized trauma unit opened in 1961 at the University of Maryland. It was not until 1966 that the National Academy of Sciences and the National Research Council published "Accidental Death and Disability: The Direct Disease of Modern Society."[5] This landmark paper documented how little progress in applying what was known had been made in injury control. In 1985 the National Research Counsel again analyzed the status of

trauma care in the United States in the report "Injury in America: A Continuing Health Problem." *Injury* was once more identified as "the principal health problem in America," highlighted by the fact that more than 2.5 million Americans had died of injuries since the 1966 report. Most recently, the Institute of Medicine again documented the importance of injury in the report "Reducing the Burden of Injury: Advancing Prevention and Treatment." Each of these reports over the past 35 years emphasized the same essential elements to effectively reduce and treat injury. Despite these clear mandates, we still have much to accomplish, although much progress has been made.

These analyses have acknowledged the need for a coordinated national approach to trauma care. Regional trauma centers integrated with public education, injury prevention, prehospital care, quality assurance, and rehabilitation form the basis of a trauma system's approach to trauma care.

Historically, trauma centers were inner-city county hospitals that had de facto trauma center status. In the 1970s, an evolution in the initial development of trauma systems began. The elements necessary to establish a trauma system have been defined and include four primary patient needs: access to care, prehospital care, hospital care, and rehabilitation. Additional issues that require both social and political solutions to supplement the medical efforts include prevention, disaster medical planning, patient education, research, and rational financial planning. Through recent reappropriation of federal legislation and the National Highway Traffic Safety Administration's technical assistance program, an organized process for trauma system planning has occurred. The Trauma Office of the Human Resources and Services Administration now works to complete trauma system development throughout the United States. The American College of Surgeons has also developed a trauma system consultation process based on a multidisciplinary collaboration. The trauma system consultation document defines the elements of a trauma system, including its administrative, operational, and clinical components.

ACCESS AND EMERGENCY MEDICAL SERVICES RESPONSE

The vital components of prehospital care include committed medical control, established lines of communication, tested triage criteria, effective transportation, and a cadre of prehospital providers well trained in specific field interventions. Hospitals were first developed by the Romans for the care of military legions; however, prehospital care or field care of injured victims can be traced back to the *Edwin Smith Surgical Papyrus* (3000-1600 BC), in which procedures for treatment of injuries are specifically described.

Most of the history of medicine pertains to the field care of injured patients, which consists primarily of first aid. Modern emergency medical services (EMS) training can perhaps be traced to 1962, when the Chicago Committee on Trauma and the Chicago Fire Department collaborated to develop a prehospital trauma school. In 1966, the National Highway Safety Act authorized the U.S. Department of Transportation to fund ambulance services, communications systems, and training programs to address the needs of trauma victims before reaching the hospital. In 1969, the U.S. Department of Transportation published the first manual for emergency medical technician—ambulance (EMT-A) training based on the Chicago Trauma School program. Subsequent programs were developed in collaboration with the American Academy of Orthopedics for the training of paramedics (EMT-P).

An integral component of the EMS system is active physician involvement in establishing, directing, and monitoring emergency medical care. The 1973 Emergency Medical Services Systems Act authorized federal funding for EMS in which prehospital emergency care was regionalized through a series of interrelated components and physician involvement was identified as an essential element. Since that time, state and community governments have assumed responsibility for EMS development and its medical control. There still remains wide regional variability in policies, procedures, and authority of medical control of EMS. The basic premise of medical control is physician-directed assurance of quality emergency care. In caring for trauma patients, surgeons must be involved along with emergency physicians to ensure quality trauma care based on knowledge and active participation. The National Highway Traffic Safety Administration's EMS Agenda for the Future attempts to further define and set standards for each aspect of medical control. Progress toward the development of trauma systems has, however, remained slow.[6]

After the events of September 11, 2001, the need for an organized approach to mass casualty events has increased. This commitment to readiness will increase the focus to complete the process of EMS and trauma system implementation.

TRIAGE

The term *triage,* derived from the French word meaning "to sort," in its military application involves prioritizing victims into categories based on their severity of injury, likelihood of survival, and urgency of care. The goal of civilian prehospital triage is to identify high-risk injured patients who would benefit from the resources available in a trauma center. This is debated to be between 5% and 10% of all injured patients. As such, a second goal of triage is to limit the excessive transport of nonseverely injured patients so that the trauma center is not overwhelmed.

The ideal tool to accomplish these two divergent tasks does not exist. Assessment must be made quickly, often under difficult conditions with limited resources, and current schemes are of limited accuracy. Although it is easy to identify patients with severe injuries based on abnormal physiology, a more difficult problem is identification of high-risk patients whose initial physiologic status is normal. Perhaps the most useful currently available system is that advocated by the Committee on Trauma of the American College of Surgeons, which assesses four components simultaneously: physiologic response, injury anatomy, injury biomechanics, and comorbid factors (Fig. 20-2).

The goal of a trauma system is to prevent unnecessary death, and thus a certain degree of over-triage is acceptable and even desirable. Under-triage, however, is always to be avoided because the benefits of trauma center care are withheld from a patient who is thus misclassified. Many studies have tried to determine and adjust the optimal ratio of under- and over-triage. Conventional wisdom suggests that a 50% over-triage rate may be required to minimize under-triage. Although this figure seems high, the additional number of patients going to trauma centers represents only about 5% of all paramedic transports when analyzed over a large geographic area. The accepted norm for under-triage is less than 3%.

Triage can take on differing forms as the situation demands. As medical care resources become limited, alternative triage schemes may be used so that the greatest number of patients may be treated. Such schemes may be seen in situations of multiple or mass casualties. In these cases the "most good is applied to the greatest number of patients." This is different from our present triage scheme, whereby the most seriously injured patient receives the majority of the medical care while the less seriously injured wait for care.

The military uses a triage scheme in which patients are classified for transport as immediate, delayed, or expectant.

The method of triage widely used by municipalities is the START triage scheme, which stands for simple triage and rapid treatment. This is accomplished by color tagging of patients. The color red is first priority and signifies a critical patient, yellow (urgent) is second priority, green (minor) is a third-priority patient, whereas black represents expectant or dead patients. The initial triage assessment components include the ability of the patient to ambulate, respiratory function, systemic perfusion, and level of consciousness. Patients are classified into transport categories on the basis of these assessments.

PREHOSPITAL CARE

The principles of prehospital care of a trauma victim follow:

1. Securing the area
2. Determining the need for emergency treatment
3. Initiating treatment according to protocols for medical direction
4. Communicating with medical control
5. Rapid transfer of the patient to a trauma center

Treatment at the scene varies according to the severity of injury, local medical practice, and the training experience of prehospital providers. The complexity of prehospital care that is appropriate is debated but is generally agreed to be different from that of a medical arrest victim. The goal in prehospital care of a trauma patient is to deliver the patient to the hospital for definitive care as

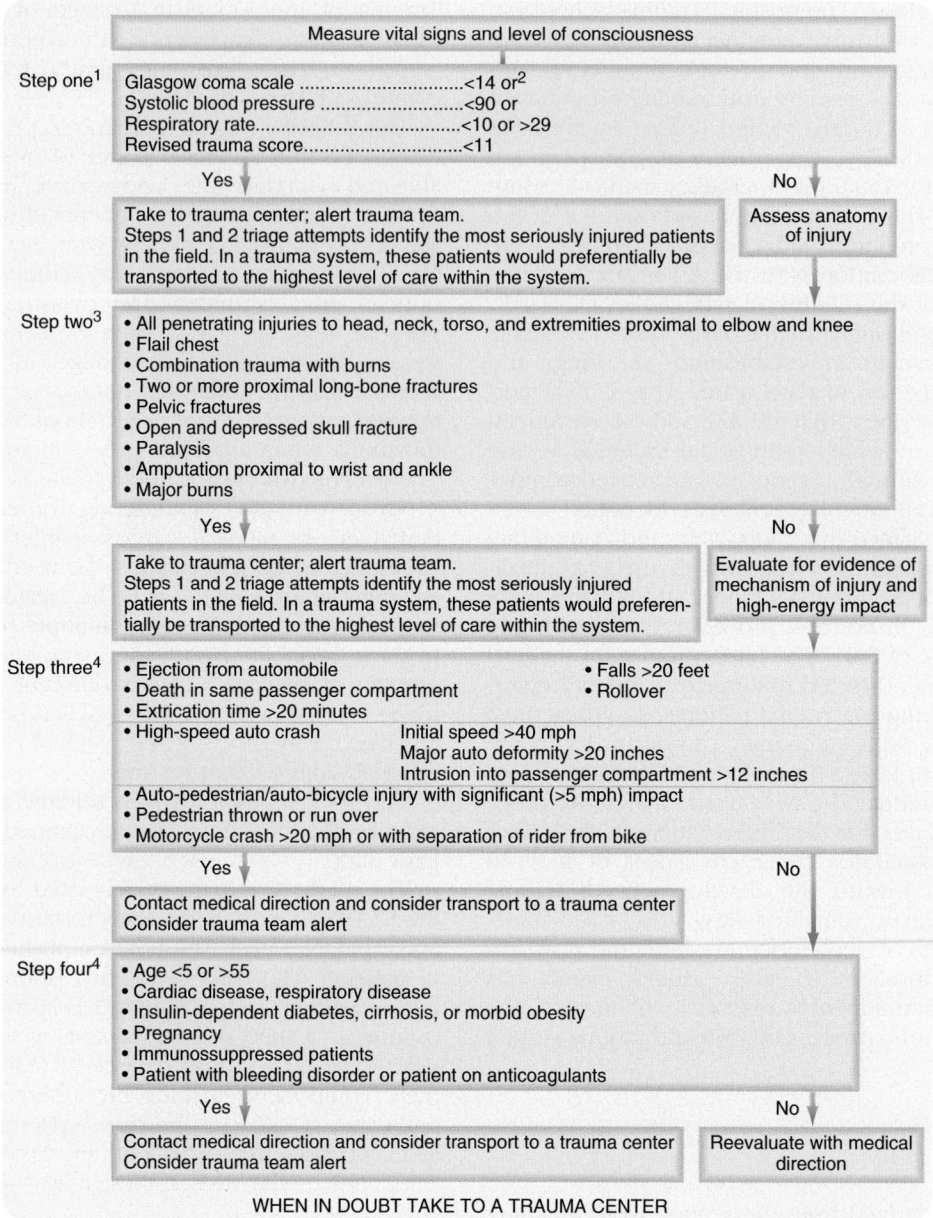

Figure 20-2 **American College of Surgeons field triage algorithm.** (From Resources for Optimal Care of the Injured Patient: 1999. Chicago, Committee on Trauma, American College of Surgeons, 1999).

rapidly as possible. In this context, the role of advanced life support (ALS) interventions is debated.

The efficacy of immediate evacuation (scoop and run) versus scene resuscitation (stay and play) has been argued repeatedly over the past 20 years. The use of prehospital airway control via endotracheal intubation continues to be debated. Several studies indicate that endotracheal intubation and excessive ventilation may increase mortality.[7] Nonetheless, when indicated, adequate control of the airway, to include suctioning, jaw thrust, placement of an oral pharyngeal airway, and bag mask ventilation, should be applied as needed to ensure adequate oxygenation of injured patients. The need for prehospital administration of intravenous (IV) fluid has

recently been challenged, and the use of military anti-shock trousers (MAST) has largely been abandoned.[8] New strategies to provide fluid resuscitation, including hyperosmolar solutions, modified crystalloids, and hemoglobin solutions, will require study before being put into practice.

TRANSPORTATION

Rapid transportation of patients to a trauma center probably originated with Napoleon's chief surgeon, Dominic Jean Larrey. He developed horse-drawn carts, or "flying ambulances," to transport the wounded to medical care behind the battle lines. By World War I, horse-drawn ambulances had been replaced by motorized vehicles, although the first use of motorized ambulances was during the 1906 San Francisco earthquake. The Korean conflict introduced the helicopter, and its use was expanded during the Vietnam War. Civilian aeromedical transport has been possible via military helicopters since 1970 in accordance with the Military Assistance to Safety and Traffic Program. The first hospital-based aeromedical transport program in the United States was established in Denver in 1972, and the rapid development of helicopter access has spread to virtually every region in the United States.

The best method for transportation depends on the patient's condition, distance to the regional trauma center, accessibility of the scene, and weather conditions. In general, ground ambulances serve the majority of needs in the urban setting, although at times, with traffic congestion and natural barriers, the use of a helicopter is more appropriate. In rural or remote areas, the time and distance to a regional trauma center may be prolonged and the prehospital care provider may be faced with a choice of either transporting the patient to a closer non-trauma hospital or calling for a remote aeromedical transport. The development of transportation guidelines is part of a regionalized trauma care system. Such guidelines must be flexible to accommodate regional variability in personnel, facilities, and geography. In general, if transport distances are greater than 20 to 30 miles or if 15 to 20 minutes of prehospital time can be saved, use of a helicopter seems justified.

HOSPITAL CARE

Trauma center care consists of care provided in the emergency department, the operating room, the intensive care unit, and the floor and may even extend to rehabilitation in some hospitals. In 1979, the American College of Surgeons Committee on Trauma published the *Optimal Hospital Resources for the Care of the Seriously Injured*. This has undergone several revisions and the current version, *Resources for Optimal Care of the Injured Patient: 2006*, stratifies hospitals into levels of resources depending on specific criteria, including specific hospital and equipment resources, personnel resources, volume of experience in treating trauma patients, and requirements for programs such as quality improvement, education, and research.

The importance of predesignated trauma team members with assigned duties cannot be overemphasized. Equally important is the team leader, who accepts the responsibility of leadership and is responsible for making overall assessment and management decisions. This team approach enables the resuscitative process to be continually coordinated and ensures that no details are neglected or overlooked so that the resuscitation is timely and focused. The overall coordinated team approach to critically ill trauma patients is one of the most significant and compelling examples of excellence in modern health care. The effects of a trauma care

program on a hospital are far reaching, and the decision to commit to becoming a trauma center is one of the most challenging and satisfying decisions that a hospital will ever make.

REHABILITATION

Rehabilitation, the long-term component of trauma care, is as important as prehospital and hospital care, although it is traditionally undeveloped. Too often, rehabilitation is ignored in regional plans despite the fact that it ultimately plays an integral role in returning patients to productive life. For each trauma-related death, two or three patients, or 350,000 patients annually, experience associated permanent or partial disability. The long-term functional recovery of patients after injury is poorly understood. Recent data suggest that post-traumatic depression is a significant problem, even for moderately injured patients.

Many patients have difficulty returning to their preinjury activities. Those who return to work after a serious injury may function at a lower level than before. Quality-of-life evaluations are lower in this group of patients.[9]

A challenge to those practicing trauma care is that despite the development of sophisticated prehospital and hospital care systems, too many patients obtain post-traumatic rehabilitation in inadequate facilities. One exception is the excellent spinal cord rehabilitation centers that have been developed. Rehabilitation of spinal cord injuries can significantly reduce the number of patients requiring institutionalization and decrease associated costs. This example should serve as a model for incorporating regionalized rehabilitation into global trauma center care.

PREVENTION AND INJURY CONTROL

Because 50% of trauma deaths occur within seconds or minutes of injury, with little chance of organized trauma system care reducing this mortality, programs in prevention and injury control must be a priority. The term *accident prevention* is no longer used because it leads one to conclude that injuries are a result of events that we cannot control or modify. This is not true because most injuries are preventable or the results of the injury are modifiable. The field of *injury prevention* focuses on reduction of the events that may result in injury. *Injury control* is an area concerned with modification of the event to minimize traumatic injury.

There are four main tenets of injury prevention and control: education, engineering, enactment, and enforcement. The target population must be educated about the problem of a specific type of injury and how to prevent it from occurring. Engineering improvements help reduce the likelihood of an injury, as well as its severity. For example, better street lighting may reduce motor vehicle crashes or accidents involving pedestrians. Padded dashes and front and side air bags have lessened the potential for injury during a motor vehicle crash. Enactment of

Table 20-1 Haddon Matrix

| PHASES | HOST | FACTORS | | |
		Agent	Physical Environment	Sociocultural Environment
Pre-event phase	Alcohol treatment programs	Antilock brakes	Safer roads	55 mph speed limit
Event	Seat belt use	Airbags	Guard rails	Automatic call systems
Postevent phase	General physical condition	Explosion-resistant gas tanks	Distance to trauma center	Trauma systems

A matrix made by arraying the factors and phases of an injury allows analysis of potential interventions.

laws to improve the safety of products aids in injury prevention. In-home smoke detectors and flame-retardant children's wear are examples of legislated prevention initiatives. Enforcement of existing safety standards and laws is central to injury prevention and control. For example, at least half of motor vehicle–related deaths in the United States involve intoxicated drivers, and as many as 80% of intentional penetrating trauma deaths occur in intoxicated individuals. The relationship of handgun availability and homicide rates is well established and should be addressed by legislation. The mandatory use of seat belts has resulted in a significant reduction in motor vehicle fatalities.

To alert researchers to factors contributing to the incidence and severity of injury and the timing involved in these factors, Haddon devised a matrix of broad categories of factors and phases of injury (Table 20-1). The Haddon matrix analyzes each injury by phase and factors and uses this methodology to identify potential opportunities for intervention.

Concurrent with broadening of the scope of injury control is a shift from active to passive approaches to prevention. Active strategies are those requiring active, continued cooperation on the part of the individual, whereas passive strategies are effective without requiring special response from an individual. Passive approaches, or a combination of passive and active approaches, have on the whole proved to be much more successful in reducing the toll from injuries than has sole reliance on active strategies. Whereas motor vehicle occupant injuries can be prevented by the use of seat belts or air bags, the latter is a much more effective option, particularly for teenagers or intoxicated drivers because it works automatically and does not require action by the individual. Similarly, tap water scalding in young children can be prevented by constant and close parental supervision for the first 5 years of life or, alternatively, by factory preset regulation of water heater temperature to lower than 125°F.

Legislation can be successful in injury control. Motorcycle and bicycle helmet laws have been successful in increasing helmet use. Increasingly, states have adopted mandatory child seat restraint legislation and mandatory seat belt use for drivers and other passengers. It is estimated that these laws have resulted in a 9% to 12% reduction in occupant fatalities. Recent studies have shown that postinjury intervention is effective in reducing alcohol consumption and recurrent injury over time.

SURGEON'S ROLE IN A TRAUMA SYSTEM

The key individual in the development of a system of trauma care is the general surgeon. A general surgeon is the best suited and most widely trained person capable of participating in and supervising all aspects of trauma care. The surgeon should be involved in the development of trauma systems, assessment of local needs, prehospital management protocols, and evaluation of prehospital services. During resuscitation the surgeon should maintain involvement in the initial management of injured patients and the application of advanced trauma life support (ATLS) protocols while working together with emergency physicians and other members of the trauma team in resuscitation areas. It is essential for the surgeon to maintain active involvement in the initial resuscitation and to prioritize and orchestrate the sequence of evaluation and management of complex injuries. Because the greatest source of preventable death and morbidity occurs during the initial phase of care related to rapid operative intervention, the essential role of the surgeon is obvious. Equally important, postinjury critical care, including ventilatory management, hemodynamic support, management of organ failure, and nutrition, are within the armamentarium of the general surgeon and further defines the surgeon's essential involvement.[10]

INITIAL MANAGEMENT

The initial management of a severely injured patient requires the surgeon to make rapid choices between various diagnostic and therapeutic interventions. In patients with a single severe injury, there is a single set of priorities. In sharp contrast, a patient with critical injuries to several different organ systems often presents conflicting priorities in management. Thoughtful and accurate ordering of diagnostic and therapeutic interventions is critical to provide the optimal outcome and is perhaps the most important task of a trauma surgeon.

Priorities in Initial Management

It is essential to begin with the assumption that the physiologic state of the patient is likely to deteriorate, perhaps abruptly, and that more than one serious injury is present. It is also essential to realize that the most obvious or most dramatic injury may not be the most critical one. A trauma surgeon must adopt a very focused approach in which problems are addressed in strict order of their threat to life and function. Even a small delay to treat a more minor injury cannot be tolerated.

Initial Evaluation of a Trauma Patient

The initial evaluation of a trauma patient consists of a rapid primary survey aimed at identifying and treating immediately life-threatening problems. The primary survey should be completed in no more than 5 to 10 minutes. After all critical issues in the primary survey have been addressed, a full head-to-toe secondary survey is undertaken, with the goal of carefully examining the entire patient and identifying all injuries. The primary survey is conducted according to the mnemonic ABCDE: airway, breathing, circulation, disability, exposure.

Airway

The crucial first step in managing an injured patient is securing an adequate airway. Mechanical removal of debris and the chin-lift or jaw-thrust maneuver, both of which pull the tongue and oral musculature forward from the pharynx, are often useful in clearing the airway of less severely injured patients. However, if there is any question about the adequacy of the airway, if there is evidence of severe head injury, or if the patient is in profound shock, more definitive airway control is necessary and appropriate. In the majority of patients this is accomplished by endotracheal intubation.

Endotracheal intubation must be done rapidly, under the assumption of cervical spine instability, and in a fashion that does not induce increased intracranial pressure (ICP) in patients with head injury. Intubation is best accomplished by a technique borrowed from surgical anesthesia, known as rapid-sequence induction. In rapid-sequence induction the patient is given a fast-acting anesthetic agent, followed by a neuromuscular blocking agent. This combination of deep sedation and muscular relaxation allows careful intubation without cervical hyperextension and with minimal physiologic impact. The technique can be used with a number of different pharmacologic agents, depending on the knowledge and preferences of the individual practitioner. It is incumbent on the individual responsible for the procedure to be fully aware of the dosage, risks, and indications associated with the agents chosen. Excessive ventilation must be avoided after intubation, particularly in a hypovolemic patient because excessive ventilation will increase mean intrathoracic pressure and compromise cardiac filling.[11]

Although nasotracheal intubation had been widely suggested as a central modality for emergency airway control in the past, it should now be used only rarely in the initial management of an injured patient. Nasotracheal intubation has a number of drawbacks, and the goal of safe endotracheal intubation with cervical spine precautions can better be accomplished by orotracheal intubation after rapid-sequence induction. Our approach to airway control is outlined in Figure 20-3.

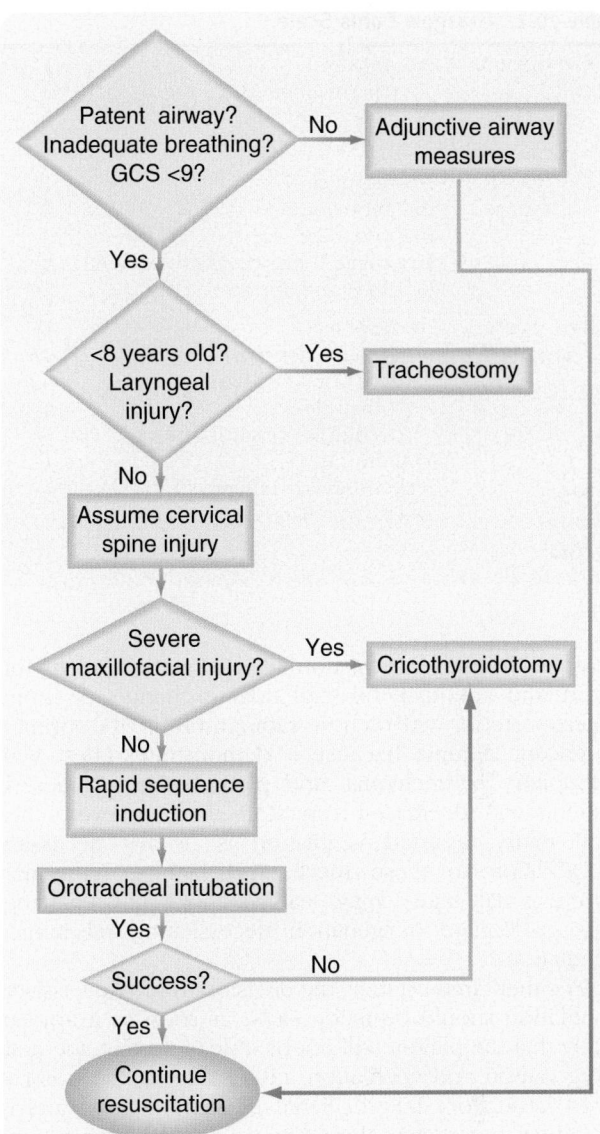

Figure 20-3 Algorithm for airway management in a trauma patient. GCS, Glasgow Coma Scale score.

In a few patients endotracheal intubation is either impractical or impossible, and a surgical airway is required. Indications for a surgical airway include massive maxillofacial trauma, anatomic distortion as a result of neck injury, and inability to visualize the vocal cords because of the presence of blood, secretions, or airway edema. Cricothyroidotomy is the preferred emergency procedure in the majority of circumstances. Actual tracheotomy may be indicated in select patients, such as those with laryngeal injuries. Either surgical procedure may be preceded by needle cricothyroidotomy with jet insufflation to improve oxygenation and allow the surgical procedure to be performed in more orderly fashion.

Breathing

After a secure airway has been established, the nature and adequacy of tidal ventilation are assessed. Inspection, palpation, and auscultation of the chest will dem-

Table 20-2 Glasgow Coma Scale

Eye opening	No response	1
	To painful stimulus	2
	To verbal stimulus	3
	Spontaneous	4
Best verbal response	No response	1
	Incomprehensible sounds	2
	Inappropriate words	3
	Disoriented, inappropriate content	4
	Oriented and appropriate	5
Best motor response	No response	1
	Abnormal extension (decerebrate posturing)	2
	Abnormal flexion (decorticate posturing)	3
	Withdrawal	4
	Purposeful movement	5
	Obeys commands	6
Total		**3-15**

onstrate the presence of normal, symmetrical ventilatory effort and adequate bilateral tidal exchange. A supine anteroposterior (AP) chest radiograph is the primary diagnostic adjunct because it demonstrates chest wall, pulmonary parenchymal, and pleural abnormalities. In patients with decreased respiratory drive or severe chest wall injury, assisted ventilation is usually necessary. In addition to these mechanical factors, pulmonary parenchymal injury may lead to poor gas exchange and inadequate oxygenation necessitating mechanical ventilation.

In either circumstance, the decision to provide assisted ventilation should be made early, as soon as it appears likely that the patient will not be able to sustain adequate oxygenation and ventilation, rather than at the point of overt ventilatory failure. Serial measurement of arterial blood gas parameters should be used to monitor patients who are at risk and to assist in appropriate adjustment of the ventilator. It is especially important to prevent episodes of hypoxemia and hypoventilation in patients with associated head injury. There is also a body of evidence suggesting that hyperventilation may be detrimental to cerebral perfusion, thus accentuating the need for accuracy in ventilator management and vigilance in monitoring pH and $PaCO_2$.

Circulation

Once the airway is secured and adequate breathing has been established, focus shifts to the circulatory system. The primary goal is identification and control of hemorrhage. External hemorrhage is controlled by direct pressure on the wound while the possibility of hemorrhage into the chest, abdomen, or pelvis is rapidly assessed. In patients with a known pelvic fracture, a pneumatic anti-shock garment may be applied or circumferential compression can be accomplished with a bed sheet wrapped around the pelvis.

While steps are being taken to control hemorrhage, at least two large-bore IV lines should be inserted to allow

fluid resuscitation. These lines are generally placed percutaneously in the vessels of the arm. If peripheral upper extremity access is inadequate, alternative routes include placement of a large-bore venous line in the femoral vein at the groin or cutdown on the greater saphenous vein at the ankle. The subclavian vein is a poor site for emergency access in a hypovolemic patient and should be used only when other sites are not available. In small children, intraosseous infusion is the preferred alternative route if peripheral access cannot be established. Fluid resuscitation begins with a 1000-mL bolus of lactated Ringer's solution for an adult and 20 mL/kg for a child. Response to therapy is monitored by clinical indicators, including blood pressure, skin perfusion, urinary output, and mental status. If there is no response or only a transient response to the initial bolus, a second bolus should be given. If ongoing resuscitation is required after two boluses, it is likely that transfusion will be required and should be initiated early. It is essential to remember that the primary goal is control of hemorrhage and that fluid resuscitation is of value only if active measures to control hemorrhage are in progress.

The clinician must be vigilant for possible causes of hypotension that require immediate intervention during the primary survey, such as pericardial tamponade or tension pneumothorax. If the pattern of injury and clinical findings raise suspicion for such injuries, immediate steps must be taken, often before the chest radiograph is available. For example, if a patient is profoundly hemodynamically unstable and tension pneumothorax is highly suspected, needle catheter decompression of the affected hemithorax should be performed immediately, without radiologic confirmation. Needle catheter decompression can be done with relative impunity, even bilaterally, in patients who are intubated and maintained on positive pressure ventilation. Much greater care must be taken in patients who are breathing spontaneously because the process of needle catheter decompression can induce pneumothorax and worsen ventilatory dysfunction, especially if done on both sides of the chest.

Disability

The next step is a rapid examination to determine the presence and severity of neurologic injury. Level of consciousness measured by the Glasgow Coma Scale (GCS) score (Table 20-2), pupillary response, and movement of extremities are evaluated and recorded. Assessment of neurologic function can be complicated by endotracheal intubation and administration of neuromuscular blocking agents. Pupillary response can still be assessed in a paralyzed patient, but a GCS score measured under these circumstances is of no value. Intubation interferes with assessment of the verbal component of the GCS, and there is no standard method for interpretation. If the GCS is used in intubated and paralyzed patients, notation should be made about the circumstances of the assessment to signify that the score may be inaccurate.

Exposure

The final step in the primary survey is to completely undress the patient and perform a rapid head-to-toe examination to identify any injuries to the back, perineum, or other areas that are not easily seen in the supine, clothed position. Evidence of blunt trauma, fracture, and unexpected penetrating injuries is likely to be discovered.

After completion of the primary survey and once all immediately life-threatening injuries have been addressed, a complete physical examination is performed. This secondary survey is often done in a head-to-toe manner and includes ordering and collecting data from appropriate laboratory and radiologic tests. This period also allows placement of additional lines, catheters (e.g., a nasogastric tube or Foley catheter), and monitoring devices. Data accumulated can then be used to reset priorities and plan definitive management of all injuries.

A number of minor injuries may not become apparent until the patient has been under medical care for 12 to 24 hours. By this time, competing pain from other major injuries has often subsided, and the patient has had an opportunity to take inventory of all body complaints. It is very important for the physician to return and perform a tertiary survey, which is another complete head-to-toe physical examination aimed at identifying injuries that may have escaped notice in the first several hours.

MANAGEMENT OF SPECIFIC INJURIES

Head Injury

Brain injury, either alone or in combination with other injuries, is the major determinant of survival and functional outcome in most cases of blunt trauma. Traumatic brain injury (TBI) affects 1.5 million patients a year in the United States. Approximately 50,000 patients will die of TBI, whereas another 80,000 to 90,000 will have long-term neurologic impairment.[12] TBI is the leading cause of death in trauma patients and is responsible for more than 50% of all traumatic deaths.[1] Falls and motor vehicle crashes account for 80% of TBI.

It is critical to optimize the early care of a patient with head injury. The overall trauma to the brain is believed to consist of a primary injury and subsequent secondary injuries. The primary injury is the anatomic and physiologic disruption that occurs as a direct result of the external trauma. Secondary injury consists of extension of the primary injury and may result from local swelling, increased ICP, hypoperfusion, hypoxemia, or other factors. The type and severity of the primary injury can be affected only through measures aimed at injury prevention and through the increased use of safety equipment. Acute care of a patient with head injury is focused on prompt recognition and treatment of TBI and prevention of secondary injury.

Resuscitative Priorities

Secondary TBI is primarily due to cerebral ischemia. Hypotension and hypoxemia have proved to be the most significant factors leading to a poor neurologic outcome or death. Hypotension appears to be more deleterious than hypoxemia and in one study resulted in a twofold increase in mortality from closed head injuries. A goal of

Table 20-3 Classification of Head Injury Severity

CLASSIFICATION	RANGE OF GLASGOW COMA SCALE SCORE
Mild	GCS ≥13
Moderate	9 ≤ GCS ≤12
Severe	GCS ≤8

a systolic blood pressure of 90 mm Hg or greater is of prime importance.[13] Adequate oxygenation and ventilation are essential to the management of these patients. A PaO_2 greater than 60 mm Hg and prevention of elevated $PaCO_2$ are also essential to management. Elevated $PaCO_2$ may lead to cerebral vasodilation and increased cerebral blood volume. In patients with elevated ICP, this small increase in blood volume may result in a sharp increase in ICP (Monro-Kellie doctrine). Both the initial treatment and later definitive care are primarily intended to prevent these secondary injuries.

Assessment of Injury Severity

The severity of brain injury can be rapidly estimated by determining the level of consciousness and the presence or absence of lateralizing signs of CNS dysfunction, including pupillary changes and motor findings.

Level of consciousness is most commonly assessed by the GCS score. Although this system was initially developed for the evaluation of chronic coma, it has almost universally been applied to patients with acute brain injury. The GCS consists of evaluation of eye opening, best motor response, and verbal response (see Table 20-2). The GCS score is determined by summation of the best response in each category (motor, verbal, and eye movement). The GCS score ranges from 3 to 15. Head injury is often classified as severe, moderate, or mild based on the GCS score, as illustrated in Table 20-3. The GCS score is an indicator of the overall prognosis and is also predictive of the likelihood of neurosurgical intervention. In a study done at an urban level I trauma center, patients with a GCS score less than 8 had a 19% rate of craniotomy, those with a score between 8 and 13 had a 9% rate, and those with a score higher than 13 required craniotomy in only 3% of cases.

The GCS score is useful because it is simple and objective and can be repeated serially. A decrease of even 1 or 2 points in the GCS score is indicative of a significant change in neurologic status and demands prompt re-evaluation and treatment. The GCS score should be assessed in the field or by the first responders and then reassessed frequently during resuscitation and treatment.

The GCS is heavily weighted toward higher cognitive function, and the presence of acute drug or alcohol intoxication can greatly lower scores in the eye-opening and verbal categories, even in the absence of brain injury. Changes in the motor component of the GCS are most predictive of serious anatomic injury to the brain and correlate most strongly with outcome. It is impossible to have a GCS score in the severe head injury range (GCS score <8) without changes in the motor component.

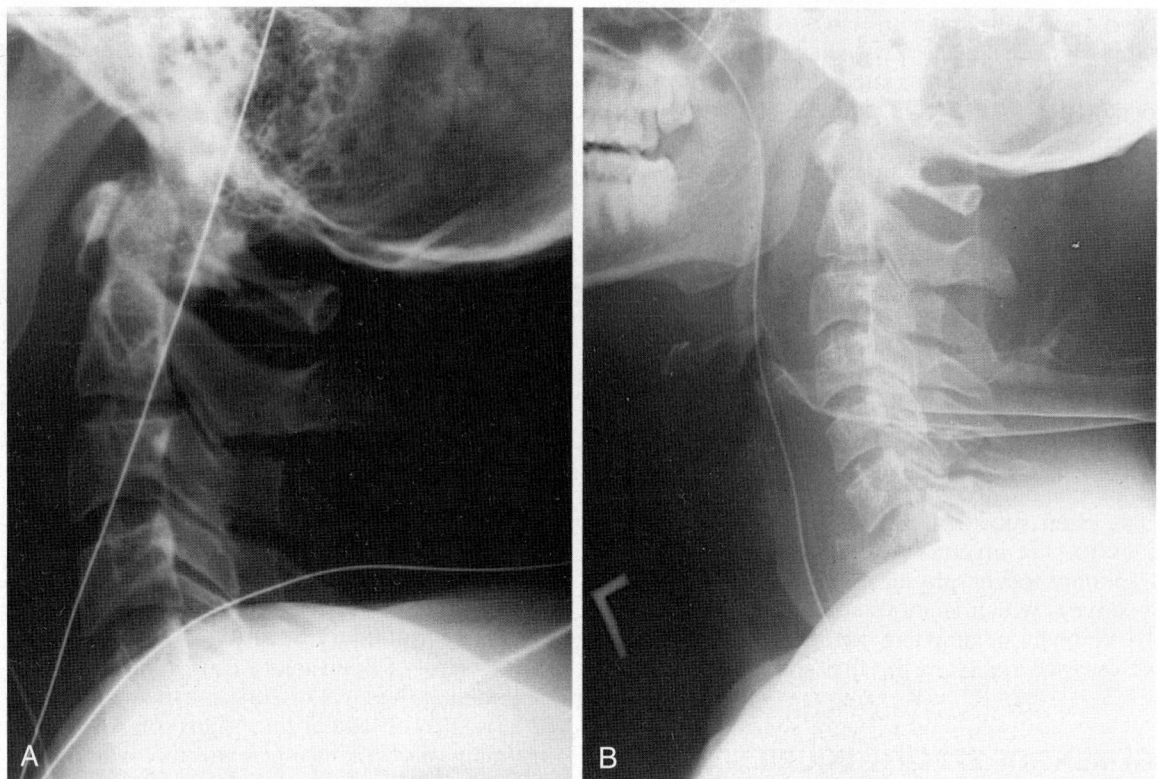

Figure 20-4 Importance of a complete lateral view of the cervical spine. The importance of completely visualizing all seven cervical vertebrae in a cross-table lateral cervical spine radiograph is illustrated in these two photoradiographs. **A,** Inadequate cross-table lateral cervical spine radiograph (C7 not visualized). **B,** A repeat lateral film on the right demonstrates a burst fracture of C7.

Signs of CNS dysfunction that are unilateral or asymmetric, so-called lateralizing signs, are highly suggestive of focal intracranial lesions that may require surgical intervention. Pupillary function is assessed by the size, equality, and response to bright light. Regardless of whether an ocular injury has occurred, any pupillary asymmetry greater than 1 mm must be attributed to intracranial injury unless proved otherwise. Often, the largest pupil is on the side of the mass lesion, but such localization is inadequate for accurate surgical planning. It is essential to obtain a computed tomography (CT) scan of the head as rapidly as possible to ensure accurate localization of the lesion. Lateralized extremity weakness is detected by testing motor power in patients able to cooperate or by observing symmetry of movement in response to a painful stimulus. In patients with a markedly decreased level of consciousness, lateralized weakness can be quite difficult to appreciate, and small differences in response to stimuli may be important. Lateralizing signs of either type, motor or pupillary, are relatively uncommon, but when seen they must lead to a very high priority for CT of the head and subsequent neurosurgical evaluation, even in patients with other severe injuries.

Definitive Management Strategy

The key to therapy for patients with severe head injury is maintenance of existing cerebral function and prevention of further secondary injury. Evidence-based guidelines for the management of severe head injury were published in 1995 and have been revised.[14] Institutions that adhere to these guidelines and are aggressive in their management principles may have better outcomes than institutions with a more empirical approach. Multiply injured patients with both TBI and extracranial trauma have been considered to be at increased risk for secondary brain insults. Recently, there are institutions reporting similar outcomes in both groups of patients. Close neurologic monitoring to guide goal-directed therapy for increased ICP and cerebral perfusion pressure and delayed operative management of extracranial lesions are cornerstones of this management strategy.[15]

Patients with focal intracranial pathology that is causing a significant mass effect require urgent surgical evacuation of the mass lesion. Because the outcome in these patients is improved by rapid decompression, time is of the essence. Craniotomy takes precedence over or must be performed simultaneously with any other necessary interventions. In general, any epidural or subdural hematoma that is causing a significant mass effect, especially in a patient with poor mental status, should be evacuated. The threshold for surgical evacuation of intraparenchymal contusions causing a mass effect is somewhat more controversial, but large lesions or smaller frontal, temporal contusions that are likely to increase in size should be approached aggressively. Failure of nonoperative management of CNS trauma is more common with frontal and temporal contusions and occipital bleeding. Serial neurologic assessment in the intensive care unit with liberal use of head CT is mandatory for nonoperative management of these lesions.[12] Management of diffuse axonal injury and postoperative management of patients undergoing surgical decompression involve measures aimed at maintaining cerebral perfusion and overall homeostasis. ICP monitoring is widely used in patients with severe injury, as are other invasive monitors, including arterial catheters and pulmonary artery catheters.

Vertebrae and Spinal Cord

Approximately 11,000 new cases of spinal cord injury are diagnosed each year. The permanent nature of some of these injuries has resulted in 200,000 patients living with spinal cord disability in the United States. A study published in 1990 reported that approximately 6% of injury hospitalizations result from vertebral injuries whereas only 1% are the result of spinal cord injury. Despite this low incidence, spinal cord injuries are often devastating in both their socioeconomic and psychological impact. Patients with high spinal cord injuries require intensive initial hospital care, long-term rehabilitation, and lifelong care. The prognosis for patients with incomplete neurologic injury can be fairly good, and many patients will regain significant function with appropriate rehabilitation.

Resuscitative Priorities

High cervical spinal injuries can result in acute ventilatory decompensation secondary to loss of phrenic nerve function (roots C3-5) and intercostal muscle function (primarily the thoracic roots). As always, patency of the airway must be ensured and the adequacy of ventilation assessed. Patients with injuries above C3 are often completely apneic, thus necessitating early intubation in the field as a lifesaving measure. Patients with injuries between C3 and C5 may initially have good ventilatory function but are likely to deteriorate as a result of fatigue and difficulty clearing secretions. An aggressive approach to early endotracheal intubation is warranted, especially if the patient has other injuries.

High spinal cord injuries can also result in systemic hypotension because of loss of sympathetic tone. The patient will usually have hypotension and relative bradycardia and will show evidence of good peripheral perfusion on physical examination. The term *neurogenic shock* is used but is somewhat of a misnomer because these patients are typically hyperdynamic, with high cardiac output secondary to loss of sympathetic vascular tone. After hemorrhagic causes of hypotension have been ruled out, the hypotension associated with high spinal injury can be treated by the administration of an α-agonist such as phenylephrine.

The essential priority in the initial care of patients with a potential spinal cord injury is to maintain strict immobilization of the entire spine. Such immobilization is most often initiated in the field. As soon as practical and often before extrication is complete, the neck is immobilized in a cervical collar and the patient is secured to a full-length backboard. In the cervical spine it is essential for

Table 20-4 **Motor Function of the Spinal Roots**

NERVE ROOT	MUSCLE	MOTOR EXAMINATION
Upper Extremity		
C5	Deltoid	Shoulder abduction
C6	Biceps	Elbow flexion
C7	Triceps	Elbow extension
C8	Flexor carpi ulnaris	Wrist flexion
T1	Lumbricales	Finger abduction
Lower Extremity		
L2	Iliopsoas	Hip flexion
L3	Quadriceps	Knee extension
L4	Tibialis anterior	Ankle dorsiflexion
L5-S1	Extensor hallucis longus	Great toe extension
S1	Gastrocnemius	Ankle plantar flexion

the radiographs to include all seven cervical vertebrae, down to and including the articulation between C7 and T1. The lower portion of the cervical spine is frequently difficult to visualize well on lateral views, especially in large patients. If the region of C7 to T1 is not visualized, there is potential for dramatic missed injury (Fig. 20-4). In these circumstances or in situations in which the findings on plain films are equivocal, CT is a useful adjunct. Likewise, if a cervical fracture is identified on any cervical spine radiograph, further evaluation of the neck should be accomplished with a CT scan. Subtle movement of the cervical spine has been demonstrated while obtaining further films, including the lateral swimmer's view. A small group of patients will have spinal cord injury without radiographic abnormality (SCIWORA). Originally described in pediatric patients, SCIWORA is now seen more frequently in adults. The use of magnetic resonance imaging (MRI) in these patients will reveal the cause of the injury in many patients.

Assessment of Injury Severity

Injury to the spinal cord may occur as a result of direct compression from a bony fragment, subluxation of a vertebra onto the cord, distraction, disk protrusion, cord contusion, hematoma, or ischemia. Whenever possible, injury assessment begins with determination of the history, including the mechanism of injury and any weakness, loss of sensation, tingling, or other neurologic symptoms noted in the field. A careful physical examination of the spine is performed, including palpation of the entire dorsal spine to look for areas of tenderness, deformity, or swelling.

All patients at risk for spinal injury should undergo a thorough neurologic examination with assessment of both motor and sensory function for all major nerve roots. Table 20-4 illustrates the basic physical examination steps for motor evaluation, and Table 20-5 illustrates the steps for sensory evaluation. Motor strength is measured on a scale of 0 to 5 as outlined in Table 20-6. Sensation is generally assessed with a combination of pinprick and light touch. In patients with neurologic deficits, the presence of low spinal cord reflexes is also assessed. This examination includes testing for anal

Table 20-5 Sensory Assessment of the Spinal Roots

NERVE ROOT	SITE OF ASSESSMENT
C2	Occipital region
C3	Supraclavicular region, near the head of the clavicle
C4	Top of the shoulder, near the acromion
C5	Lateral aspect of the arm, just above the elbow
C6	Dorsum of the thumb
C7	Dorsum of the middle finger
C8	Dorsum of the little finger
T1	Medial aspect of the arm, just above the elbow
T2	Axilla
T4	Thorax at the level of the nipples
T10	Abdomen at the level of the umbilicus
L1	Region of the femoral pulse
L2	Medial aspect of the thigh, mid-femur
L3	Medial aspect of the knee
L4	Medial aspect of the leg, above the medial malleolus
L5	Dorsum of the great toe
S1	Lateral aspect of the heel
S2	Popliteal fossa
S3	Medial gluteal region
S4-5	Perianal region

sphincter tone, anal wink, and the bulbocavernosus reflex. The motor and sensory findings should be fully documented in the medical record, including the time of the assessment because changes from this baseline examination are of critical importance in determining the course of therapy.

If the injury appears to be complete, the presence of spinal cord reflexes, especially the sacral reflexes, yields important prognostic information. After acute spinal cord injury, a transient phenomenon known as *spinal shock* is seen in which all cord function is absent below the level of injury. The affected muscle groups are flaccid and areflexic. As time progresses, the spinal reflex arcs return, and the muscle groups become hyperreflexic because of loss of inhibition. Therefore, lack of reflexes, particularly sacral reflexes such as the bulbocavernosus, indicate the presence of spinal shock and leave hope that the actual degree of anatomic injury may be less than initially perceived. Once the spinal reflexes have returned, the examination is more likely to represent the true extent of cord damage.

As a general rule, complete cord lesions are fixed and permanent, with little hope for major recovery of distal function. Restoration of spinal canal anatomy and decompression of the spinal cord do not improve the neurologic outcome because the lesion in the spinal cord is fixed.

These are devastating injuries, especially in the high cervical spine. A single–motor level change in the cervical spine has an enormous impact on functional outcome, and thus every effort must be made to ensure that the level of injury does not ascend as a result of therapeutic intervention. In the thoracic and lumbar spine the precise level is of less importance because ventilatory and upper extremity function is unaffected.

The second pattern of spinal cord injury is an incomplete injury. In these circumstances the patient will exhibit some sensory and motor function below the level of injury. Incomplete injuries have a much better prognosis for recovery of function, and most will improve with time. In addition, in certain circumstances, restoration of the anatomy of the spinal canal and decompression of the spinal cord may lead to an improved outcome. Therefore, in a patient with an incomplete injury it is essential that careful sequential neurologic examinations be performed to determine whether the deficit is worsening, stable, or improving. Patients with findings on examination that are stable or improving are monitored closely, whereas patients with findings that are deteriorating are candidates for emergency surgical intervention.

Incomplete cord injuries most often present a mixed picture of sensory and motor findings. In the minority of cases, the findings represent well-defined clinical syndromes that are related to the type of injury. Most common is central cord syndrome. A patient with central cord syndrome will have motor weakness and sensory loss primarily involving the distal muscles of the upper extremities. The proximal muscles of the upper extremities and function of the lower extremities are preserved. Frequently, there is no radiologically identifiable fracture of the spinal column. Central cord syndrome is thought to be an ischemic lesion in which hyperflexion or hyperextension of the neck leads to interference with blood flow in the spinal arteries. This results in hypoperfusion of the cord and loss of function in a watershed distribution, most often affecting tissue in the central portion of the cord. These anatomic data provide the rationale for the clinical findings. The neurologic elements controlling the distal portion of the upper extremity are in the most central portions of the cord and are most affected, whereas the structures controlling the lower extremity are more lateral and nearly always preserved. Function of the proximal aspect of the upper extremity is variable. Central cord syndromes can be functionally quite significant because the muscles most affected are the small muscles of the hand and the distal part of the arm. Usually, the neurologic changes are transient and will improve with time, but there may still be a degree of permanent impairment.

A second clinical syndrome is the Brown-Séquard syndrome, anatomically interesting but uncommon in clinical practice. Brown-Séquard syndrome results from partial transection of the cord and yields a split motor and sensory deficit. Motor function is lost on the ipsilateral side, and sensory function is lost on the contralateral side. This is due to an anatomic difference in the level of midline crossing between motor and sensory neural tracts. Motor tracts cross over at the level of the brainstem, whereas sensory tracts cross near the level of the spinal root.

Assessment of the severity of injury to the spinal column itself is independent of the nature and type of spinal cord injury. The primary question that must be answered is one of stability. The initial evaluation should be based on at least three views of the cervical spine (lateral, AP, and odontoid) and two views (lateral and AP) of the thoracolumbar spine. In alert patients with normal plain radiographs but persistent symptoms, flexion-extension views, especially of the cervical spine, can be obtained to look for ligamentous instability.

The spinal column is generally conceptualized as having three columns: the anterior spinal ligament and anterior walls of the vertebral bodies, the posterior spinal ligament and posterior walls of the vertebral bodies, and the posterior elements of the vertebral column. Injuries involving only one column are thought to be stable; those involving two or three columns are unstable. Many spine fractures are difficult to visualize with standard radiographs. CT of the spine and, more recently, MRI provide much better detail of bony and ligamentous structures, respectively. These more detailed studies should be performed whenever there is a suspicion of injury on plain radiographs. Careful examination of the plain radiographs, augmented by CT or MRI of the spine, provides the data, but final assessment of stability is based on the judgment of the physician.

Definitive Care

There is little that can be done to repair an anatomic injury to the spinal cord, and acute therapy for spinal cord injury is targeted at preservation of remaining function. General support of the patient's cardiovascular function is important to optimize spinal cord perfusion and prevent ischemic secondary injury. Some advocate the use of inotropic support or vasoactive infusions to maintain spinal cord perfusion pressure in a manner analogous to that used in brain injury, although data on the efficacy of this approach are lacking. The use of high-dose corticosteroids for the first 24 hours after spinal cord injury has become nearly universal in the United States as a result of a placebo-controlled clinical trial published in 1990. This trial showed a statistically significant improvement in function in the steroid-treated group, although the practical significance of the improvement is open to debate. To be efficacious, steroid therapy must be initiated within a few hours of injury and consists of a bolus of 30 mg/kg of methylprednisolone infused over a 1-hour period, followed by an infusion of 5.4 mg/kg/hr for the next 23 hours. If more than 3 hours but less than 8 hours has elapsed since the injury, steroids should be continued for a total of 48 hours.[16]

Surgical therapy for lesions of the spinal cord is limited to restoration of spinal canal anatomy, removal of foreign bodies, and removal of any bone, disk, or hematoma that may be compressing the cord. Therefore, decompressive surgery is unlikely to be of benefit in complete lesions and is rarely performed. In patients with incomplete injury, the decision to operate requires mature judgment.

Table 20-6 Assessment of Motor Strength

SCORE	FUNCTIONAL ABILITY
0	No contraction of muscle
1	Palpable muscle contraction, no limb movement
2	Able to move in a gravity-neutral plane
3	Able to move against gravity
4	Diminished strength
5	Normal strength

Injuries believed to be relatively stable or unstable in only one column can be managed by immobilization only. For significant fractures, immobilization involves the use of a halo brace for the cervical spine and an orthosis, usually a molded jacket, for the thoracic and lumbar spine. Unstable injuries usually require surgical stabilization. Stabilization can be achieved by the placement of hardware posteriorly, by the use of hardware and bone grafting anteriorly, or in some cases by the use of both techniques simultaneously. The anterior approach allows better access to the vertebral body and better decompression of the spinal canal. Three-column injuries will generally require both anterior and posterior stabilization.

The benefits of early spinal stabilization in patients with complete injury are primarily related to the prevention of complications of long-term immobilization. Data show fewer complications in patients whose spinal injuries are fixed early, although there are no compelling survival differences. Therefore, spinal column injuries should be fixed as early as practical once the patient is physiologically stable and no longer at risk to suffer deterioration of neurologic function, either from exacerbation of brain injury or as a result of manipulation of the spinal cord.

Neck Injuries

The neck contains multiple vital structures with little anatomic protection provided by overlying bone, muscle, and soft tissue. Most severe neck injuries are caused by penetrating wounds and may present an immediate threat to life as a result of airway compromise or hemorrhage. Neck injuries can also result from blunt trauma, and the diagnosis is often more difficult to make because of the more subtle manifestation of blunt injuries. As a consequence of the high likelihood of injury to the airway or major blood vessels, accurate and aggressive initial evaluation and treatment are required to optimize outcome.

In evaluating penetrating injuries of the neck, it is important to consider location in both an AP and craniocaudal direction. On an anatomic basis, the neck is divided into anterior and posterior triangles (Fig. 20-5). The major vascular and aerodigestive structures in the neck are located in the anterior triangle, and all are deep to the platysma. Therefore, the platysma and the sternocleidomastoid muscle are useful anatomic boundaries. Injuries that do not penetrate the platysma can be considered superficial, and no further investigation is needed. Wounds that penetrate the platysma must be further evaluated. Injuries that are anterior to the sternocleido-

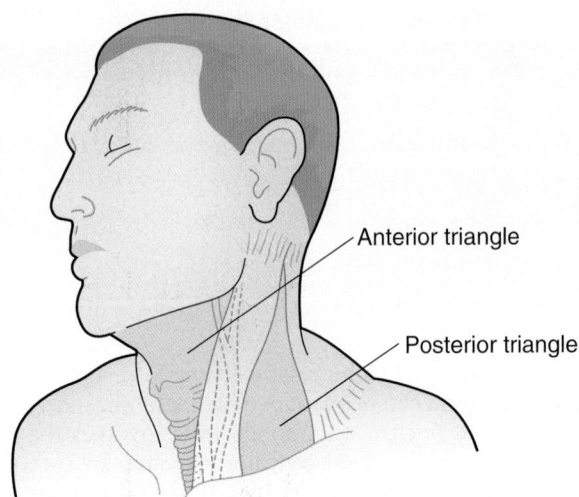

Figure 20-5 Anatomic triangles of the neck. The anterior and posterior anatomic triangles of the neck are defined by the sternocleidomastoid muscle. The major vascular and aerodigestive structures in the neck are contained in the anterior triangle. Wounds involving only the posterior triangle have a low probability of injury requiring urgent surgical intervention.

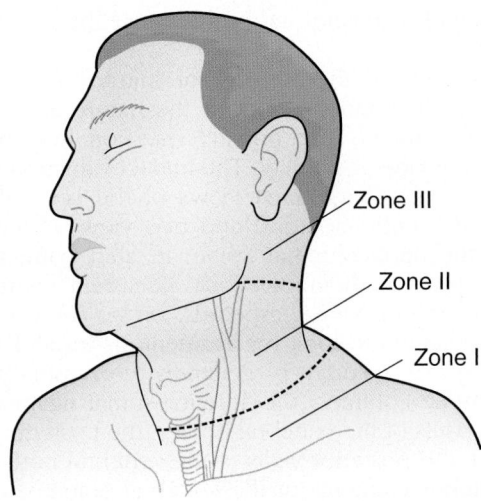

Figure 20-6 Zones of the neck. The border between zone I and zone II is at the level of the cricoid cartilage. The border between zone II and zone III is at the angle of the mandible. These zones are primarily useful in the management of injuries to the anterior triangle of the neck.

mastoid present a high likelihood of significant injury, whereas those that track posterior to the sternocleidomastoid are unlikely to involve major vascular or aerodigestive structures. Penetrating injuries to the posterior triangle should raise concern about trauma to the cervical spine and spinal cord.

In analyzing wounds based on craniocaudal location, the neck is commonly divided into three horizontal zones (Fig. 20-6). Zone I is the thoracic inlet and extends roughly from the sternal notch to the cricoid cartilage. Injuries in this zone carry the highest mortality because of the presence of the great vessels and the difficult surgical approach. Zone II is the midportion of the neck and it extends from the cricoid cartilage to the angle of the mandible. Injuries in this zone are usually clinically apparent, and vascular control is relatively straightforward. Zone III extends from the angle of the mandible to the base of the skull. Exposure in this zone, particularly of the distal carotid artery, can be quite difficult to manage. Penetrating wounds may traverse more than one zone and require evaluation of all possible structures in all affected zones.

Resuscitative Priorities

Significant injuries to the neck are often an immediate threat to life because of airway compromise. Airway obstruction can be caused by direct injury to the larynx or trachea, an expanding hematoma within the neck, or bleeding into the airway. Patients may initially have a patent airway, only to become compromised a short time later. It is essential to obtain early definitive control of the airway as the top priority in all patients with major neck injuries. Progressive bleeding or neck swelling may produce a circumstance in which orotracheal intubation is no longer possible. What might have been a routine intubation in the first 15 minutes of the resuscitation may

become a difficult emergency surgical airway procedure. If the airway is not in jeopardy, intubation may be deferred, but this course should be chosen only if the perceived likelihood of significant injury is very low.

Neck injuries also present the threat of hemorrhage from the carotid artery, jugular vein, and great vessels. After the airway has been controlled, the potential for major vascular injury must be assessed. Injuries in zone II are usually clinically apparent, with significant hematoma or frank external hemorrhage. These injuries are approached by immediate surgical exploration, with direct pressure used to maintain hemostasis until vascular control can be achieved. Based on the potential for great vessel injury and the difficulty of vascular exposure in both zone I and zone III, radiographic vascular imaging is mandatory before surgical exploration in all but the most unstable patients. If no vascular injury is found, radiographic vascular imaging may preclude the need for surgical exploration.

The potential for blunt injury to the larynx, trachea, or carotid arteries must be kept in mind in any patient with evidence of a blunt impact to the neck. Such injuries often have subtle findings, and the workup must be based on appropriate clinical suspicion consistent with the mechanism of injury.

Assessment of Injury Severity

Patients with overt clinical signs of vascular or aerodigestive tract injury require surgical exploration of the neck. Such clinical signs include significant external hemorrhage, a large or expanding hematoma, air movement through the wound with breathing, crepitance in the neck, voice changes, dysphagia, and odynophagia (Box 20-1). Preoperative workup in this subset of patients is minimal. Patients with penetrating injuries in zone II are generally taken directly to surgery, whereas patients with injuries in zone I and zone III should undergo preopera-

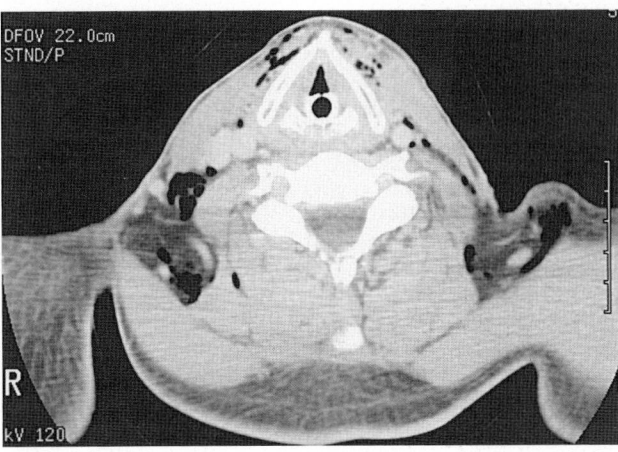

Figure 20-7 Use of computed tomography in blunt neck trauma. The study shows a fracture of the thyroid cartilage, with significant airway swelling and air in the soft tissues surrounding the larynx.

tive radiographic vascular imaging, if possible. Workup of the aerodigestive tract is undertaken at the time of surgical exploration. Neck injuries not requiring operative exploration may need to have the aerodigestive tract evaluated with CT, bronchoscopy, upper endoscopy, or esophagography to exclude injury.

Significant controversy exists regarding the optimal approach to patients with injuries that penetrate the platysma in zone II but who exhibit no suspicious clinical findings.[17] One school of thought favors mandatory surgical exploration for all penetrating injuries because of a low rate of complications and the potentially devastating effect of delay in the diagnosis of aerodigestive tract injuries. The second school of thought favors selective exploration based either on the results of extensive evaluation, including angiography, esophagoscopy, and esophagography, or on progression of clinical symptoms. Proponents of this course of action cite the high rate of negative exploration in asymptomatic patients and the low incidence of devastating complications associated with delay. Current data show similar outcomes for both approaches and do not favor one approach over the other. Some centers advocate thin-slice CT scanning of the neck with IV contrast to determine the track of a penetrating object, such as a knife or gunshot wound. Knowledge of the trajectory of penetration permits determination of anatomic structures at risk for injury. The presence of contrast extravasation or nonvisualization of vascular structures, or free air in the tissue planes, suggests tissue injury.[18] Thin-slice CT scanning may also provide information about injuries to the cervical spine and aerodigestive tract. We favor an aggressive CT imaging approach to asymptomatic zone II injuries. Patients with zone I and zone III injuries who are asymptomatic should also undergo CT imaging and be observed if this study is negative.

Nonsurgical evaluation of potential vascular injury is relatively straightforward. In penetrating injuries and blunt trauma with clinical evidence of carotid injury, full four-vessel evaluation of the neck must be done, as well as assessment of the arch and great vessels included in the wound trajectory if considered suspicious. Careful biplanar films are mandatory because the signs of vascular injury can be quite subtle. In asymptomatic patients with blunt injuries, duplex ultrasound or thin-slice CT scanning is used as a screening examination before angiography. Duplex ultrasound has been evaluated for application in penetrating trauma but is not in widespread use.

Nonsurgical evaluation of the aerodigestive tract must include the pharynx, larynx, trachea, and esophagus. Screening for potential injuries may initially be carried out by thin-slice CT. If this study is equivocal, further evaluation may require a combination of direct laryngoscopy, bronchoscopy, and esophagoscopy. Early endotracheal intubation may complicate evaluation of the larynx and proximal trachea. There has been some controversy regarding the use of rigid versus flexible esophagoscopy, but the utility of either approach appears to be operator dependent. Clinical data support the efficacy of both modalities. Contrast esophagography is a complementary examination, and its use probably improves diagnostic accuracy over esophagoscopy alone.

Blunt injury to the neck often involves the larynx, and these injuries are difficult to assess by direct laryngoscopy. Furthermore, the examination itself poses a risk of worsening the injury. Therefore, CT of the neck is commonly used to assess the larynx in blunt injury (Fig. 20-7). Blunt injury to the esophagus is exceedingly uncommon, and clinical observation is probably sufficient in asymptomatic patients with no clinical signs of esophageal injury. Patients with symptoms referable to the aerodigestive tract must be aggressively evaluated. Blunt vascular injuries to the carotid or vertebral arteries are more difficult to diagnose. These lesions may be asymptomatic on initial evaluation and tend to be arterial dissections, flaps, or thrombosis rather than frank bleeding. A suspicion of injury based on mechanism or the association of adjacent injuries may be the only clue to an occult vascular injury. Screening criteria should include the following[19]:

1. Le Fort facial fractures
2. Cervical spine injury
3. Basilar skull fracture
4. Abnormal neurologic examination unexplained by CT findings

Patients with evidence of either significant vascular injury or injury to the aerodigestive tract will probably require surgical repair. Patients with no clinical findings and negative evaluation of both the vascular and aerodigestive systems can safely be observed.

Definitive Therapy

Technique of Neck Exploration

Regardless of whether one adopts a policy of mandatory or selective exploration for penetrating injuries of the neck, once a decision to operate has been made, the approach is the same. From a strategic point of view it is important to remember that the goal is to explore the structures of the neck to identify injuries, not to explore the wound per se. In the case of unilateral injury, an oblique incision along the anterior border of the sterno-cleidomastoid muscle will provide access to all of the critical structures in the neck. The trajectory and depth of any suspicious wounds will become clear after the major vessels and midline structures have been visualized. Wounds that approach the carotid sheath or the midline must be followed to the end of the wound tract to rule out injury. Those that do not approach the carotid sheath or the midline do not need to be fully explored. If bilateral exploration is necessary, a modified collar-type incision carried up along the sternocleidomastoid muscle on both sides will allow complete bilateral exposure.

Intraoperative endoscopy is a very useful adjunct in cases in which there is high suspicion of aerodigestive injury but no injury is immediately identified during surgical exploration. The ability to simultaneously observe the esophagus or trachea from both the inside and outside allows the surgeon to most reliably identify an injury or exclude the possibility of injury. Esophageal instillation of methylene blue or other dyes may rule out injury.

Vascular Injuries

Vascular injuries are common in penetrating wounds of the neck and occur in approximately 20% of cases. Blunt injuries to the carotid are relatively uncommon; they account for only about 3% of all carotid injuries and occur in just a small percentage of all patients with blunt neck injury. The general approach to major vascular injuries in the neck is the same as that for vascular injuries elsewhere in the body.[20] In brief, hemostasis should be maintained by direct pressure or digital occlusion until proximal and distal control of the vessel can be achieved. If possible, proximal and distal control should be ensured before a large contained hematoma is entered. Arterial

injuries should be débrided and repaired primarily, if possible. In most circumstances, primary repair will not be practical because of loss of length, and a short inter-position graft should be used. The choice of graft material should be based primarily on size match. Although there is a small theoretical preference for autologous vein, it is often difficult to find an appropriate match for the common carotid or proximal internal carotid. In practice, a correctly sized synthetic graft, usually polytetrafluoroethylene, will commonly be used. Major injuries to the external carotid can be safely treated by ligation. Ligation of the common or internal carotid carries much more functional significance and should be done only for uncontrollable hemorrhage or if repair is technically impossible. The advisability of revascularization after a period of ischemia has been debated, but the concerns appear to be primarily theoretical. Existing clinical data show improved outcome with repair in all subsets of patients except those with frank coma, in whom both repair and ligation groups do poorly. Extracranial-intracranial bypass has been suggested in patients requiring ligation of the common or internal carotid, but experience is limited. Major venous injuries should be repaired primarily when practical and ligated under other circumstances. There is probably no role for interposition grafting to repair a unilateral internal jugular injury.

Several retrospective series have documented the use of endovascular stents in patients with blunt carotid dissection or defined penetrating carotid injuries. The role of stents remains to be demonstrated in prospective studies. It is now accepted by most that antithrombotic therapy/anticoagulation should be the initial treatment of significant blunt carotid injuries.[21]

Airway Injuries

Penetrating injuries to the airway are either clinically overt, with bubbling and air movement through the wound, or found at the time of neck exploration performed for other indications. In blunt laryngotracheal injuries the diagnosis is generally established through a combination of neck CT, direct laryngoscopy, and bronchoscopy. Almost all tracheal lacerations and disruptions should be repaired. The need for operative intervention for laryngeal trauma is determined by the degree of anatomic derangement and mucosal integrity in the larynx.

In general, tracheal injuries should be débrided and closed primarily. Simple lacerations of the trachea can frequently be repaired by direct suture. The use of non-absorbable suture is often suggested, but absorbable suture can be used in this setting as well. If there is significant tissue loss, the trachea can usually be mobilized sufficiently to allow for the loss of about two tracheal rings without undue difficulty. Loss of a larger portion of trachea may necessitate tracheostomy or complex reconstructive procedures. Laryngeal injuries are treated by closure of mucosal lacerations and reduction of cartilaginous fractures. The structure of the larynx is important to glottic function, and careful anatomic reconstruction, if possible, is critical. Injuries involving the larynx can be difficult to treat, and there is significant controversy regarding the timing of repair, the operative technique,

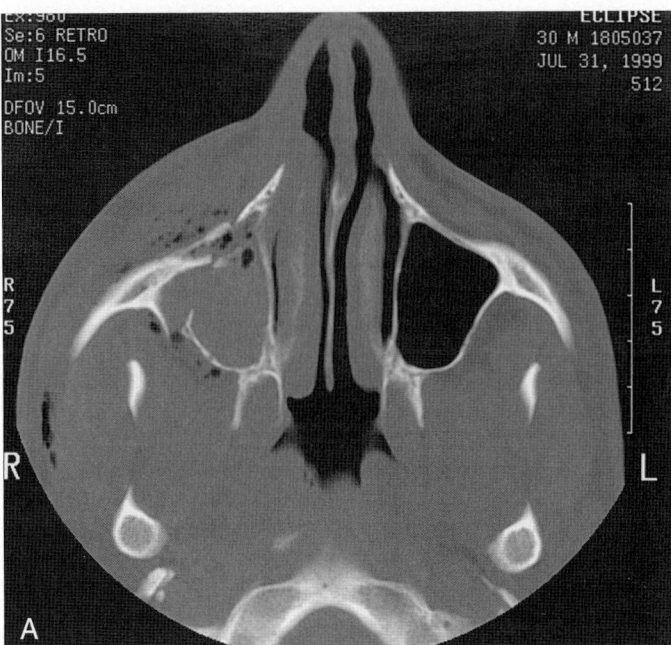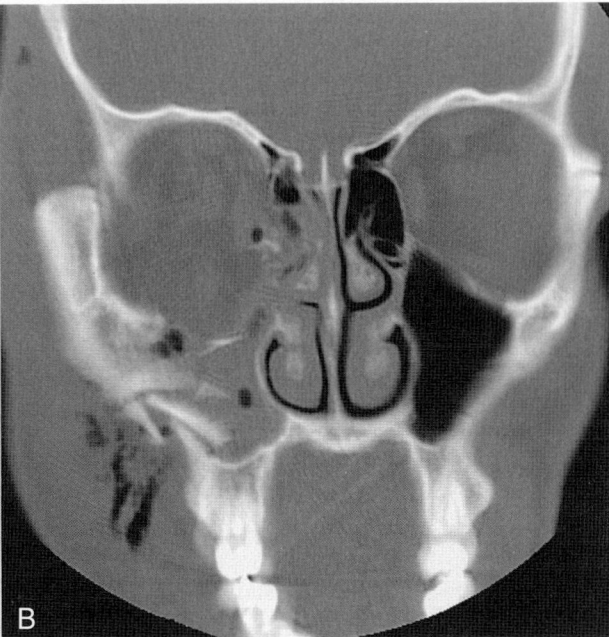

Figure 20-8 Use of computed tomography for the diagnosis of facial fractures. An axial view (**A**) and coronal view (**B**) demonstrate complex fractures involving the right maxilla, as well as the lateral, inferior, and medial walls of the right orbit. Note the opacification of the maxillary and ethmoid sinuses.

and the use of adjuncts such as stents or systemic steroids.

Pharynx and Esophagus

Injuries to the esophagus present a difficult problem. If the diagnosis is made early, primary surgical repair is generally possible. If the diagnosis is delayed for more than 12 hours, primary repair may be impractical, with diversion and drainage being the only alternative. The major morbidity and mortality associated with esophageal injuries are the result of delay in diagnosis, which underscores the necessity to aggressively exclude esophageal injury during the initial evaluation of a patient with neck injury. Any positive findings mandate operative exploration.

The basic approach to esophageal injuries is to achieve primary repair of the majority of injuries. The esophagus must be sufficiently mobilized to allow full evaluation of the wound and careful débridement of devitalized tissue. The injury should be repaired primarily if possible, either by a one-layer or two-layer technique. If the tissue loss is sufficient to preclude primary repair, cervical esophagostomy should be performed as a temporizing measure, with plans for complex reconstruction of the esophagus after the initial trauma has resolved. A drain should be left in place after all esophageal repairs.

Maxillofacial Injuries

Maxillofacial injuries are quite common and can have significant functional and cosmetic impact. Most maxillofacial injuries do not present an initial threat to life, and definitive evaluation and care are often deferred in patients with multiple injuries. Nevertheless, it is impor-

tant to carefully evaluate and appropriately treat maxillofacial injuries in timely fashion to optimize functional outcome and provide the best cosmetic result.

Resuscitative Priorities

Severe maxillofacial injuries have the potential to lead to airway obstruction, either as a direct result of anatomic derangement or secondary to the presence of blood and debris in the upper airway. These factors can make orotracheal intubation difficult or impossible, and the presence of significant midface injuries is an absolute contraindication to nasotracheal intubation. Immediate consideration must be given to the need for a surgical airway in the course of initial resuscitation. Facial fractures can lead to significant hemorrhage from the maxillary and palatine arteries, which are branches of the external carotid artery. Initial control should be obtained by anterior and posterior nasal packing, as well as direct packing of the oropharynx. Careful packing will temporarily control maxillofacial bleeding in almost all cases. A direct surgical approach is difficult, which leaves the options of angiography and selective embolization or ligation of the external carotid. In most circumstances, angiography and embolization will be the most efficacious.

The diagnosis of facial fractures is now largely done through the use of CT. CT of the face is far more accurate than plain radiographs in determining the presence and significance of fractures of the facial bones (Fig. 20-8). Obvious fractures can be seen on lower cuts of the CT scan performed for the evaluation of head trauma, and important suggestive findings such as opacification of the maxillary or ethmoid sinuses can also be seen. To fully evaluate the bony structure of the face, CT is performed

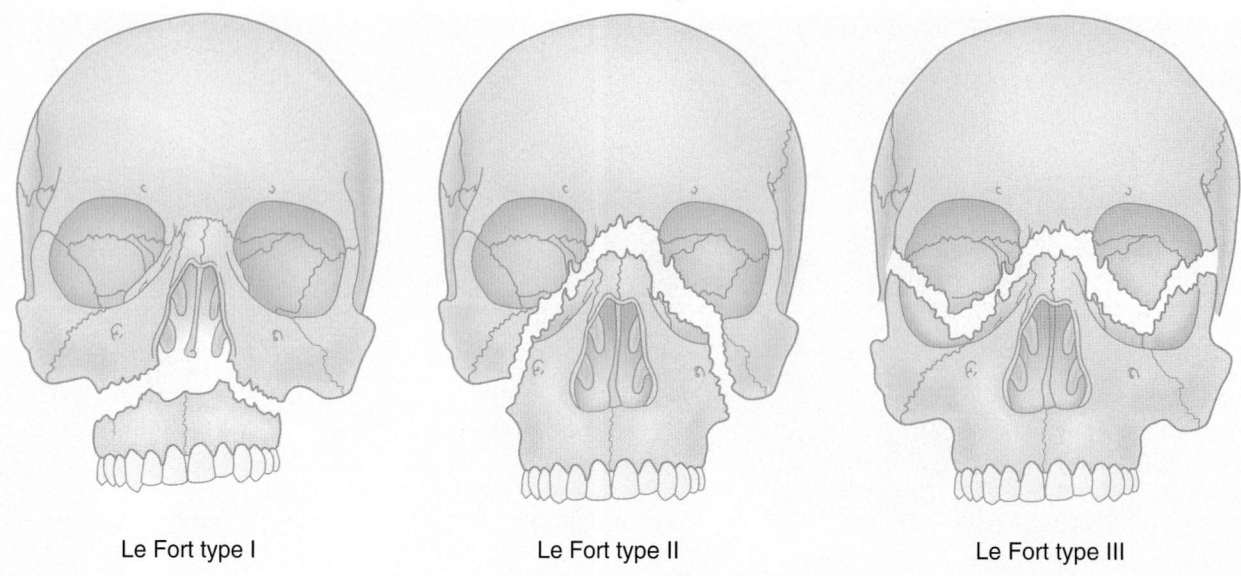

Le Fort type I

Le Fort type II

Le Fort type III

Figure 20-9 Le Forte I, II, and III fracture lines as seen in the frontal view.

in a coronal plane with 1-mm cuts. This requires that the patient be able to flex and extend the cervical spine and also requires a relatively long scanning time. Neither condition is often met in the early care of patients with significant associated injuries, and full delineation of maxillofacial fractures must often be deferred.

Fractures of the maxilla are classified according to a system proposed by Le Forte in 1901. The three types, Le Fort I, II, and III (Fig. 20-9), are determined by the type and location of fractures.

Fractures of the mandible are also classified by anatomic location (Fig. 20-10). The need for surgical intervention and its nature are determined by the type and location of the fracture, so complete radiographic evaluation is important. Imaging techniques frequently used to identify and classify mandibular fractures include plain films, panoramic tomography (Panorex), and helical CT. A recent report has demonstrated the overall superiority of helical CT over Panorex in identifying and decreasing interpretation error in patients with mandibular fractures.[22]

Reduction and fixation of mandibular fractures should be accomplished as precisely and expeditiously as possible because malocclusion is a major long-term complication. Special techniques, such as Panorex, may be valuable in the diagnosis of jaw fractures, but their superiority over plain radiographs has not been clearly demonstrated.

Definitive Care

Facial Fractures

Operative repair of facial fractures is usually undertaken for one of two indications, either to restore function or to improve cosmetic outcome. Fractures that can cause significant functional impairment are listed in Table 20-7.

The determination that a fracture must be fixed for cosmetic reasons is often an aesthetic one and sometimes cannot be made until significant facial swelling has decreased. Because there are no compelling physiologic indications, many of these operations will be undertaken late in the course, after the acute injury and swelling have decreased.

In general, facial lacerations should be carefully cleaned and gently débrided of obviously devitalized tissue. In most circumstances, primary closure is performed with deep stitches as required and fine, carefully placed sutures in the skin. These skin sutures should be removed early, usually within 3 days, to minimize cross-hatching of the scar. An alternative to sutures is the use of octyl-2-cyanoacrylate (Dermabond) for facial lacerations. This adhesive provides secure closure for the wounds, but in younger patients the cosmetic results can be less optimal than with the use of sutures.[23]

Ocular Injuries

Eye injuries have a high functional and emotional impact. The presence of ocular trauma mandates a thorough examination of the structural and functional components of the eye. Patients with maxillofacial trauma may have significant periorbital soft tissue edema. Though difficult to perform, the initial ophthalmologic examination may be the only examination performed until the edema subsides. Removal of contact lenses and debris and examination of the anterior structures of the eye may reveal proptosis, hyphema, or corneal abrasions or lacerations. The globe may be lacerated or ruptured. Compression of the optic nerve by bone fragments, retinal detachment, vitreous hemorrhage, and acute traumatic glaucoma should be identified and treated. A functional eye examination includes visual acuity, pupillary response, and assessment of extraocular eye movements.

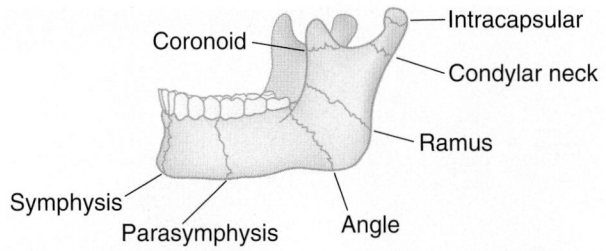

Figure 20-10 Anatomy of the mandible and common lines of fracture.

Table 20-7 Facial Fractures of Functional Significance

FRACTURE TYPE	FUNCTIONAL IMPAIRMENT
Blowout fracture of the inferior orbital floor	Entrapment of extra-ocular muscles
Maxilla, alveolar ridge	Malocclusion
Mandible	Malocclusion
Depressed zygomatic arch fracture	Entrapment of the temporalis muscle

Thoracic Trauma

Thoracic injuries account for 20% to 25% of all trauma-related deaths, and complications of chest trauma contribute to another 25% of all deaths. Considering immediate deaths after motor vehicles accidents, the most frequent injuries leading to a fatal outcome include blunt cardiac injuries with chamber disruption and injuries to the thoracic aorta. Early deaths (within the golden hour) are caused by airway obstruction, major respiratory problems such as tension pneumothorax or massive hemothorax, and cardiac tamponade. These clinical situations are easily managed if recognized promptly. Chest wall trauma is the most frequent injury after blunt thoracic trauma. The majority of thoracic injuries are managed with simple procedures such as clinical observation, thoracentesis, respiratory support, and adequate analgesia. The remaining 15% to 20% of patients sustaining chest trauma will require thoracotomy for definitive repair of major intrathoracic injuries.

Pathophysiology

The pathophysiology of chest trauma includes three factors: hypoxia, hypercapnia, and acidosis. Hypoxia can be caused by airway obstruction, changes in intrathoracic pressure, ventilation-perfusion mismatches, and hypovolemia. Hypercapnia is caused by inadequate ventilation as a result of the presence of either a collapsed lung, associated head injuries with altered mental status, or exogenous intoxication (drugs and alcohol). Acidosis is due mainly to hypoperfusion from blood loss.

Initial Evaluation

The initial evaluation of a patient sustaining chest trauma follows the same principles and guidelines outlined by the ATLS course. The first priority is maintenance of a patent airway, which may be achieved by simply repositioning the head, anteriorizing the mandible (chin lift and jaw thrust), or removing foreign bodies from the oropharynx. Some patients with more severe thoracic or head injuries will require tracheal intubation either by a nasal or oral route or by means of a surgical airway. Physical examination of the chest is extremely important in identifying life-threatening situations that require immediate attention, including tension pneumothorax, massive hemothorax, open pneumothorax, flail chest, and cardiac tamponade.

The chest radiograph is of utmost importance in thoracic trauma; however, the aforementioned life-threatening injuries preclude the necessity of a chest radiograph for diagnosis and should be identified clinically. The chest radiograph is useful to identify pneumothorax, hemothorax, rib fractures, a widened mediastinum, pneumomediastinum, and clavicular and scapular fractures. Other diagnostic modalities include ultrasonography, chest CT, esophagography, esophagoscopy, bronchoscopy, and angiography.

Ultrasound has been used less frequently for the evaluation of chest trauma than for the evaluation of abdominal trauma. However, recent reports have shown that the pleural spaces can be evaluated by ultrasound to diagnose or exclude hemothorax and pneumothorax. Two ultrasonographic signs have been used to rule out pneumothorax. One is the lung sliding sign, which is to-and-fro movement of the hyperechoic line between the chest wall and aerated lung with respiration. The other sign is so-called comet tail artifacts, which are ray-like hyperechoic reverberation artifacts that arise from the visceral pleural line and spread to the edge of the screen; this sign is indicative of the absence of pneumothorax.[24]

With the development of helical scanners, CT has been used more liberally for the evaluation of chest trauma, and some authors have recommended its routine use despite the results of plain chest films. Reformatted chest CT scans can also be used to identify thoracolumbar and sternal fractures, thus avoiding the need for plain films.

Tube Thoracostomy

Tube thoracostomy is the most common procedure performed in the management of thoracic trauma. In fact, 85% of patients sustaining chest injuries will require only clinical observation or tube thoracostomy. A large-bore (36-40 French) chest tube should be used in adolescents and adult patients. The proper site of insertion is in the fifth or sixth intercostal space in the midaxillary line. The index finger should be inserted into the pleural space before tube placement to ensure that the pleural cavity has been entered and is free of adhesions and that any intra-abdominal organs have not herniated through the diaphragm. The tube should be advanced posteriorly and superiorly in the pleural cavity. After insertion, the tube should be secured in the skin of the chest wall and connected to a collection system under suction. A chest radiograph is usually obtained after insertion of the chest tube to confirm adequate placement and positioning. General criteria for chest tube removal include absence of air leak and less than 100 mL of fluid drainage over a 24-hour period.

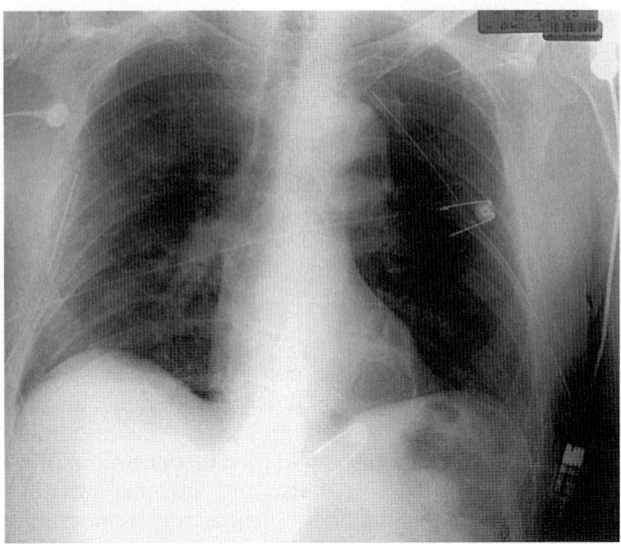

Figure 20-11 Chest film showing multiple rib fractures.

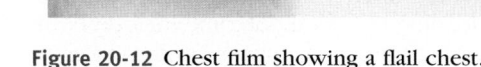

Figure 20-12 Chest film showing a flail chest.

Thoracotomy

Emergency thoracotomy is indicated after chest trauma in the following situations:

1. Cardiac arrest (resuscitative thoracotomy)
2. Massive hemothorax (>1500 mL of blood through the chest tube acutely or >200-300 mL/hr after initial drainage)
3. Penetrating injuries of the anterior aspect of the chest with cardiac tamponade
4. Large open wounds of the thoracic cage
5. Major thoracic vascular injuries in the presence of hemodynamic instability
6. Major tracheobronchial injuries
7. Evidence of esophageal perforation

Specific Injuries

Rib Fractures

Rib fractures are the most common injuries after blunt chest trauma. Ribs 4 through 10 are usually fractured. Fracture of one or two ribs without pleural or lung involvement is generally treated on an outpatient basis. However, in the elderly, because of decreased bone density, reduced chest wall compliance, and an increased incidence of underlying parenchymal disease, rib fractures may lead to a decreased ability to cough, reduced vital capacity, and infectious complications. Pain on inspiration is usually the primary clinical manifestation after rib fractures. Other clinical signs associated with rib fractures include tenderness to palpation and crepitus. Rib fractures are confirmed with a chest radiograph (Fig. 20-11).

Poor pain control significantly contributes to complications such as atelectasis and pneumonia. Pain control is attempted initially with oral or IV analgesics. Intercostal nerve blocks with bupivacaine are effective for pain control; however, such blocks are not feasible for multiple fractures and require frequent injections. Epidural analgesia is adequate for patients with multiple or bilateral fractures because it provides satisfactory pain control and appropriate pulmonary toilette, thereby decreasing the number of complications.

Flail Chest

By definition, a flail chest occurs in the presence of two or more fractures in three or more consecutive ribs and causes instability of the chest wall; however, it can also occur after costochondral separation (Fig. 20-12). Flail chest is characterized by paradoxical motion of the chest wall (inward with inspiration and outward with expiration). Fractures can be located in the anterior, lateral, or posterior chest wall. Flail chest occurs in 10% to 15% of patients sustaining major chest trauma, and the chance of having an intrathoracic injury in this situation increases severalfold. Closed head injury is the most frequently associated extrathoracic injury, and it contributes to higher morbidity and mortality rates. Isolated flail chest carries a low mortality rate in younger patients.

The paradoxical motion increases the work of breathing, and the most important consequence of flail chest is respiratory failure. Until recently it was believed that ineffective air movement between both lungs caused by paradoxical motion of the chest wall was the main cause of the respiratory distress in patients with flail chest. It is now understood that underlying pulmonary contusion and pain during inspiration are the most important components in the pathophysiology of the respiratory failure (Fig. 20-13). Sequential measurements of forced vital capacity, tidal volume, and inspiratory force are useful to predict which patients will require ventilatory support. The pathophysiologic effects may be present immediately or may progress over a period of several hours and be manifested as late respiratory decompensation.

Care should be taken to not overload these patients with fluid because respiratory function may be impaired even further. Patients without evidence of respiratory distress can be managed with only analgesia. Pain control can be provided by an intercostal nerve block or more adequately by epidural anesthesia.

If respiratory distress develops, endotracheal intubation and mechanical ventilation with peak end-expiratory pressure are usually indicated, provided that pain control is adequate. Open reduction plus internal fixation of sternal or rib fractures is rarely needed.

Sternal Fractures

Though rare, sternal fractures may occur after motor vehicle accidents. The presence of a fractured sternum implies significant trauma to the anterior chest wall with high energy transfer. Signs and symptoms include chest pain, particularly over the sternum, and crepitus. A hematoma over the sternum may be seen eventually (caused by the steering wheel) or across the chest (seat belt sign). A lateral radiograph should be obtained in these circumstances and generally confirms the diagnosis. Evidence of sternal fractures may be seen on CT scans of the chest. Sternal fractures also constitute a marker for serious associated injuries, including myocardial contusion, myocardial rupture, esophageal perforation, airway injury, and thoracic aortic rupture.

Treatment is usually conservative, although patients with significant chest wall instability and debilitating chest pain may require open reduction and internal fixation.

Pulmonary Contusion

Pulmonary contusion occurs more frequently after blunt chest trauma; however, penetrating injuries may also cause significant lung parenchymal contusions. This has been defined as a pathologic state in which hemorrhage and edema of the lung parenchyma occur without parenchymal disruption. Mortality rates vary according to age, associated injuries, and chronic underlying lung disease. The pathophysiology of pulmonary contusion involves decreased lung compliance and the development of a ventilation-perfusion mismatch leading to hypoxemia and increased work of breathing.

Respiratory failure occurs more often in patients with large contusions, in the elderly, and in those with underlying chronic lung disease aggravated by inadequate pain control. The diagnosis is confirmed by low PaO_2 and by a chest radiograph demonstrating a well-defined infiltrate underlying the contused area on the chest wall. It is important to realize, however, that radiologic findings may not be present on admission and may develop 24 to 48 hours after the initial injury. Pulmonary contusion may be confused with adult respiratory distress syndrome or may even be associated with it.

Management is directed toward maintaining good oxygenation and adequate pulmonary toilette. Judicious crystalloid infusion is important to avoid fluid overload and pulmonary edema; however, intravascular volume depletion should also be avoided to decrease the risk for global ischemia and multiple organ failure. Patients with persistently low PaO_2 who do not respond to supplemental oxygen, pulmonary toilette, and pain control should be intubated and mechanically ventilated. Correction of

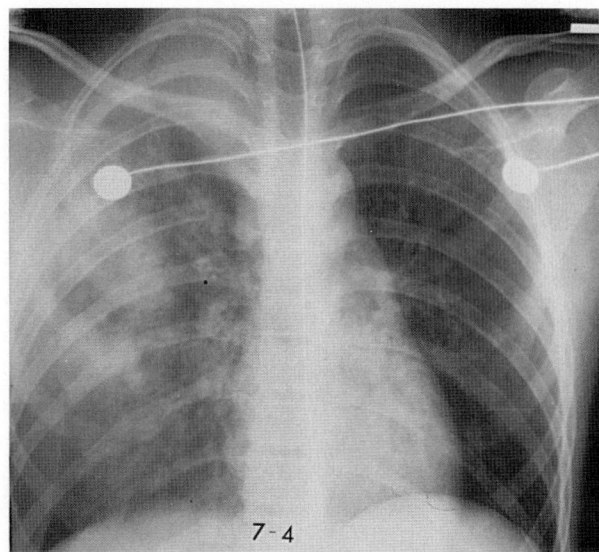

Figure 20-13 Chest film showing a pulmonary contusion.

acute anemia and coagulopathy by transfusion of packed red blood cells and blood products is important to minimize blood loss and increase oxygen-carrying capacity and delivery of oxygen to tissues. No benefits have been demonstrated with the use of prophylactic antibiotics or steroids.

Pneumonia is the most frequent complication, particularly in the elderly; it aggravates chronic lung diseases, increases ventilator days, and significantly contributes to mortality.

Lung Blast Injury

Bomb blasts have become a preferred means of attack by terrorists. Lung blast injury is one of the major causes of death and morbidity in these attacks. The increase in frequency and the potential for future massive catastrophic attacks require increased knowledge by physicians about the pathophysiology, management, and outcome of patients sustaining these injuries.

Some of the most frequent injuries that occur after bomb blasts are listed:

1. Ruptured tympanic membranes
2. Lung blast injury
3. Intestinal blast injury
4. Fractures
5. Burns

The mechanisms of injury caused by the explosion include the initial pressure wave, expelled projectiles, fire, and secondary collision of victims with surrounding stationary objects. The effect of the pressure wave depends on the distance of the victim from the explosion. Victims close to the explosion experience a sudden rise in intrathoracic pressure that causes alveolar disruption and parenchymal hemorrhage. Impalement with projectiles from the improvised explosive device (IED) and possible inhalation injuries from fires lead to severe thoracic and pulmonary injuries.

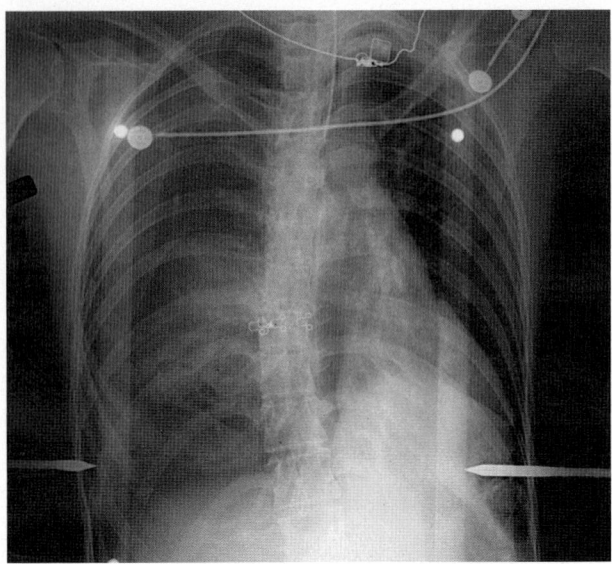

Figure 20-14 Chest film showing a right pneumothorax.

Pneumothorax and, rarely, air embolism are complications associated with mechanical ventilation in patients with lung blast injury; alveolovenous fistulas secondary to the blast have been identified as the source of air emboli.[25]

Pneumothorax

Pneumothorax occurs when air from an injured lung or airway is trapped within the pleural cavity and increases the normal negative intrapleural pressure. It may be caused by penetrating or blunt mechanisms. After blunt trauma, pneumothorax is caused by rib fractures penetrating the lung parenchyma or by lung injuries without chest wall involvement. Deceleration injuries and sudden increases in intrathoracic pressure can also cause pneumothorax.

Clinical findings suggestive of pneumothorax include decreased breath sounds, hyperresonance to percussion, and decreased expansion of the affected lung during inspiration. Pneumothorax is classified according to the volume of lung loss or collapse identified on chest radiograph or by respiratory and systemic signs.

With a small pneumothorax, the volume loss is a third of the normal lung volume. With a large pneumothorax, the lung is completely collapsed but there is no mediastinal shift or associated hypotension. A tension pneumothorax is characterized by complete lung collapse, tracheal deviation, and mediastinal shift leading to decreased venous return to the heart, hypotension, and respiratory distress. It usually occurs in patients with parenchymal lung injury managed by positive pressure ventilation (Fig. 20-14). Clinical signs and symptoms include dyspnea, tachypnea, hypotension, diaphoresis, and distended neck veins. It is diagnosed clinically and constitutes a life-threatening emergency. Chest radiographs are not necessary to confirm the diagnosis, and delays in definitive treatment significantly increase the risk for circulatory

collapse and cardiorespiratory arrest. Treatment includes chest decompression initially with a large-bore needle inserted in the second intercostal space on the midclavicular line and subsequent tube thoracostomy. Re-expansion of the lung and reapproximation of the pleural surfaces usually seal the lung defect.

Open Pneumothorax

Open pneumothorax, also known as a *sucking chest wound,* occurs when a significant defect in the chest wall (e.g., from a large-caliber gunshot wound or traumatic thoracotomy) large enough to exceed the laryngeal cross-sectional area allows air to enter from the exterior into the pleural cavity and results in lung collapse because of rapid equilibration between intrathoracic (pleural) and atmospheric pressure. The increased intrathoracic pressure also causes mediastinal shift and decreased venous return. Signs and symptoms include hypoxia, hypercapnia, hypotension, and respiratory and circulatory failure.

Management includes application of an occlusive dressing and insertion of a chest tube before closure of the chest wall defect to avoid the development of tension pneumothorax.

Hemothorax

Blood may accumulate in the pleural cavity after blunt or penetrating injuries. Depending on the nature of the injury, bleeding may vary from minor to massive. Symptoms depend on the amount of blood accumulated in the pleural space. On physical examination, breath sounds may be decreased on the side of the injury. A chest radiograph obtained in the supine position may reveal accumulations of blood greater than 200 mL; however, a supine film may demonstrate diffuse haziness or none at all. The pleural space can accumulate up to 3 L of blood. Massive hemothorax is generally the result of a major pulmonary vascular injury or major arterial wound, whereas minor lung injuries cause a small hemothorax (Fig. 20-15).

Hemothorax is initially treated by chest tube placement (36-French tube), and in approximately 85% of cases, the bleeding will stop as the lung is re-expanded because of the low pressure in the systemic circulation. A small number of patients will have continued bleeding and will require thoracotomy. These are usually injuries to systemic arteries (intercostal arteries or internal mammary artery) or veins or major pulmonary vessels or are cardiac in origin, and autotransfusion should be considered in these circumstances.

As previously described, indications for emergency thoracotomy are initial chest tube output of 1500 mL of blood or persistent drainage of 200 to 300 mL/hr.

Pulmonary Parenchymal Injury

Simple lacerations of the lung are common after penetrating injuries and rare after blunt trauma. Patients usually have variable degrees of pneumothorax and hemothorax. Management generally includes chest tube placement to drain the blood collection in the pleural space and re-expand the lung.

Occasionally, major and persistent air leaks will develop in some patients. This situation is sometimes identified immediately after chest tube placement but may be more evident when mechanical ventilation with positive pressure is started. Massive air leaks should raise suspicion for major tracheobronchial injuries.

Although less than 10% of patients with severe chest injuries will require thoracotomy and some degree of pulmonary resection, recent studies have reported better results with lung-sparing techniques (nonanatomic resection and tractotomy) than with formal lobectomy or pneumonectomy.[26,27]

Massive hemorrhage from extensive lung injuries can be treated by oversewing or stapling the wound or, more rarely, by performing wedging or lobar resections.[28] Gunshot wounds causing through-and-through injuries to the lung can be managed by opening up the missile trajectory (tractotomy) communicating with both the entrance and exit wounds to obtain hemostasis. Wedge resection of peripheral injuries to lung parenchyma that is actively bleeding can be accomplished with a stapler. Complications associated with large injuries to the lung parenchyma, as well as after tractotomy, include increased bleeding and air embolism, which may be controlled by stapling the lung parenchyma. Air embolism can be minimized by decreasing peak inspiratory pressure and cross-clamping the pulmonary hilum.

Tracheobronchial Injuries

Tracheobronchial injuries are uncommon. Most patients with these injuries die at the scene or during transport because of poor ventilation and severe associated injuries. Blunt injuries occur after direct compression of the airway with a closed glottis or after decelerating injuries causing partial or complete avulsion of the right main stem bronchus from the carina or tracheal lacerations. Penetrating wounds may cause tracheobronchial injuries at any level.

Patients with tracheobronchial injuries may have pneumothorax, massive air leak, subcutaneous emphysema, hemoptysis, pneumomediastinum, and respiratory distress. Bronchoscopy is always required if one of these signs is present and, ideally, should be performed before intubation. Minor injuries to the upper airway after blunt trauma should be treated by placing the endotracheal tube beyond the injury. If not possible, a tracheostomy should be performed.

More extensive wounds, greater than a third the circumference of the airway, are primarily repaired after the contralateral bronchus has been selectively intubated.

Small injuries usually heal spontaneously; however, late complications such as stricture formation at the injury site, recurrent pulmonary infection, and atelectasis may occur.

Blunt Cardiac Injuries

Significant trauma to the anterior chest wall may cause injury to the heart. Blunt cardiac injury encompasses a wide spectrum of injuries from contusion of the cardiac wall to cardiac chamber or valvular rupture. Most patients sustaining rupture of the cardiac chambers do not reach

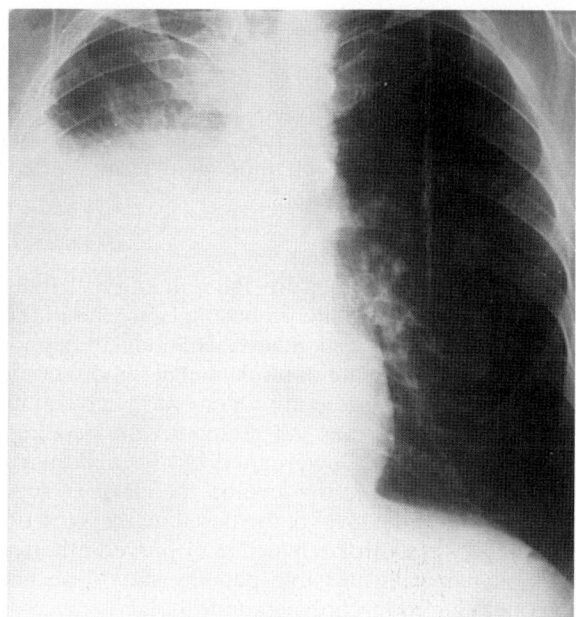

Figure 20-15 Chest film showing a right hemothorax.

the hospital alive; however, rupture should be suspected in patients sustaining severe chest trauma in whom pericardial tamponade develops. The right ventricle is most frequently involved because of its proximity to the sternum. Prompt imaging with ultrasound may identify pericardial fluid and lead to improved survival in these patients.

Myocardial contusion may occur in less severe chest trauma. Its definition, diagnosis, clinical significance, and management are still subject to debate. It has been estimated that 15% to 20% of patients sustaining severe chest trauma have some degree of cardiac involvement. Small myocardial contusions may produce wall motion abnormalities and lead to the development of arrhythmias. There are no classic findings suggestive of myocardial contusion, and there is no consensus in terms of diagnostic criteria. Increased central venous pressure in the absence of an obvious cause may indicate right ventricular dysfunction secondary to cardiac contusion, provided that the appropriate mechanism has occurred.

The electrocardiogram (ECG) is the first diagnostic test. Patients are usually monitored for a period varying from 8 to 24 hours. If the initial ECG is normal, no further workup is generally necessary. The most frequent arrhythmias are ST-segment and T-waves changes and sinus tachycardia. Right bundle branch block is common. Supraventricular and ventricular arrhythmias should be treated accordingly in an intensive care unit setting. Measurement of the MB band of creatine kinase, expressed as a percentage of total creatine kinase, has been used as a diagnostic tool. The specificity of this test is low because other muscle injuries can falsely elevate the MB band. Two-dimensional echocardiography may demonstrate a wall motion abnormality, but its clinical significance without hemodynamic instability or arrhythmias is unknown. Radionuclide scans may be more specific than the previously described methods, but such scans are impractical in clinical use.

The combination of an ECG and serum troponin I levels at admission and 8 hours after injury can rule out the diagnosis of significant blunt cardiac injury. Patients with normal results at both time points can be safely discharged from the hospital.[29]

Penetrating Cardiac Injuries

Penetrating cardiac injuries are still a great challenge for trauma surgeons. Adequate prehospital care, rapid transportation, aggressive resuscitation, immediate diagnosis, and prompt treatment are of fundamental importance and constitute the basis for the improvement in survival rates seen in the past decade. All patients with penetrating injuries within an area determined by the midclavicular line bilaterally, a line at the level of the clavicles superiorly, and a line at the level of the costal margins inferiorly potentially have a cardiac injury until proved otherwise.

Hemodynamically unstable patients should be taken to the operating room for emergency thoracotomy. Stable patients should have a chest radiograph to identify other injuries and to determine the trajectory of the missile in the case of gunshot wounds. The diagnosis is usually made by echocardiography, which can identify abnormal amounts of pericardial fluid, or more accurately by performing a subxiphoid pericardial window. If the result is positive, median sternotomy is performed for definitive cardiac repair.

Sequelae or complications after cardiac repair include valvular insufficiency and septal defects. Repair of these acquired lesions may involve valve replacement or repair or patch closure of septal lesions and should be performed at a later time.

Mortality rates vary from 8.5% to 81.3%. The presence of shock or hemodynamic instability has been cited as an important determinant of mortality. Characterization of the physiologic status of the patient on admission by using a score for quantification or even use of the Revised Trauma Score seems to be more appropriate.[30] The survival rate is greater than 70% if vital signs are present on admission.

Pericardial tamponade must be suspected in all patients sustaining penetrating injuries to the anterior aspect of the chest. Classic signs of pericardial tamponade include muffled heart tones, distended neck veins, and hypotension, also known as Beck's triad. All these signs are present in approximately 30% to 40% of patients with a cardiac injury. Neck vein distention reflects increases in central venous pressure and is the most useful clinical sign, but hypotensive patients with associated injuries may not demonstrate neck vein distention because of excessive blood loss. Volume resuscitation transiently improves cardiac output by increasing venous return; however, treatment consists of evacuating small amounts of blood (pericardiocentesis), followed by immediate repair of the underlying injury. It is generally agreed that tamponade is more frequent with stab wounds. It seems reasonable to assume that tamponade leads to "temporary" hemodynamic compensation, thus playing a role in survival.

Diaphragmatic Injuries

Diaphragmatic injuries are often caused by penetrating injuries. Patients sustaining penetrating injuries below the nipples and above the costal margins should be investigated to rule out diaphragmatic injury. Controversy exists about the best workup to exclude diaphragmatic injury, and options include contrast-enhanced CT, peritoneal lavage in those with stab wounds to the epigastrium, thoracoscopy in patients with hemothorax or pneumothorax, or laparoscopy in those with a normal chest film and an external wound in the thoracoabdominal transition. Chest and abdominal radiographs should be obtained in hemodynamically stable patients sustaining a gunshot wound in an attempt to determine the trajectory of the missile. If the bullet is in the abdomen, the patient will undergo exploratory laparotomy, and the diagnosis of a diaphragmatic injury will be made intraoperatively.

After blunt trauma, injury to the diaphragm involves both sides equally, as reported in autopsy and CT scan studies, although in clinical practice, left-sided injuries are more frequent. The diagnosis is suspected when respiratory distress develops after a severe blow to the abdomen without apparent chest injury or when an upright chest film demonstrates visceral herniation. In fact, herniation of intra-abdominal contents may not occur immediately or may not be evident on initial chest radiographs, thus delaying the diagnosis. Herniation occurs as a result of the pressure differential between the thoracic and abdominal cavity (Fig. 20-16).

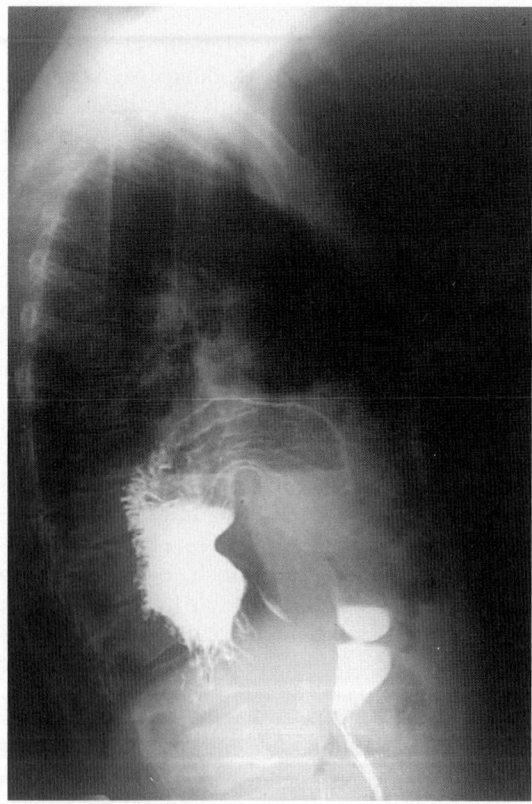

Figure 20-16 Lateral chest film showing herniation of the stomach into the left pleural cavity.

At the time of surgical exploration the entire diaphragm should be inspected. Diaphragmatic injuries are repaired with interrupted horizontal sutures. Larger defects may eventually require the use of prosthetic material.

Acute diaphragmatic rupture is generally repaired through a midline abdominal incision because of the increased incidence of associated intra-abdominal injuries. Chronic defects discovered months or years after the initial injury can be treated through a transthoracic, an abdominal, or a combined approach.

Esophageal Injuries

Most esophageal injuries are secondary to penetrating trauma and may occur at any level. The esophagus is well protected in the posterior mediastinum, and injuries after blunt trauma are rare. Sudden increases in intraesophageal pressure from a direct blow to the epigastrium may cause rupture of the distal segment of the esophagus. Associated injuries are the rule. Esophageal injury after blunt trauma should be considered in patients with a pleural effusion but no rib fractures, pain out of proportion to the clinical findings, subcutaneous emphysema or pneumomediastinum without an obvious source, and the presence of gastric contents in the chest tube. All mediastinum-traversing gunshot wounds or stab wounds near the posterior midline should be evaluated for possible esophageal injury.

The diagnosis is confirmed by esophagography and esophagoscopy. These tests have a reported sensitivity varying from 50% to 90%.

Delay in the diagnosis of traumatic esophageal injuries is accompanied by high morbidity and mortality. A recent multicenter study was carried out to define the period after which delays in the management of penetrating esophageal injuries lead to increased morbidity and mortality. Patients were divided into two groups: those operated on immediately after arrival at the trauma center and those who underwent a preoperative workup. The average length of time until arrival at the operating room was 1 hour and 13 hours, respectively. The overall incidence of complications, as well as the incidence of esophageal-related complications, was significantly higher in the preoperative workup group. The optimal time interval between admission and operative intervention in these patients remains to be defined; however, rapid assessment and early operative intervention are accompanied by decreased complications.

Treatment consists of early débridement, primary repair, and drainage if identified within 24 hours after injury. Injuries diagnosed after 24 hours with mediastinal contamination are treated by cervical esophagostomy and distal feeding access. Esophageal resection is rarely needed but may be indicated in patients with esophageal necrosis or severe mediastinitis.

Transmediastinal Gunshot Wounds

Transmediastinal gunshot wounds constitute a significant challenge for trauma surgeons. Hemodynamically unstable patients are treated by exploratory thoracotomy, and the diagnosis of specific injuries will be made during the operation. Hemodynamically stable patients can be evaluated by multiple diagnostic modalities, but significant controversy remains regarding the best methods and the most appropriate sequence of tests.

Traditionally, evaluation often includes angiography, esophagoscopy, esophagography, bronchoscopy, cardiac two-dimensional echocardiography, and pericardial window. More recently, contrast-enhanced CT has been used as a screening modality to determine the trajectory of the projectile, identify specific injuries, and determine the need for further evaluation by other diagnostic modalities.[31]

Blunt Transection of the Aorta

Victims of high-speed collisions are at risk of sustaining rupture of the thoracic aorta. This injury is the cause of death in up to 15% of motor vehicle collisions.

The most common sites of thoracic aortic rupture are the descending aorta just distal to the left subclavian artery and the ascending aorta just proximal to the innominate artery. Stresses applied to the aorta that are thought to cause the rupture include shearing, bending, twisting, and a so-called water hammer effect. These last two stress mechanisms are believed to be the cause of ascending thoracic aortic rupture. Once these severe stresses are applied to the aortic wall, the intima and media rupture, with free bleeding contained by the adventitia in surviving patients.

Blunt rupture of the thoracic aorta should be suspected in patients sustaining significant direct chest trauma or falls from great heights. An initial chest radiograph demonstrates a wide mediastinum in up to 90% of patients with a ruptured thoracic aorta. It is now widely accepted that thin-slice helical CT angiography should be used for screening patients who are stable with a wide mediastinum on chest radiography. CT angiography should also be considered in patients with a normal-appearing mediastinum but a significant mechanism of injury to rule out a ruptured thoracic aorta. Angiography should be performed if findings on CT are equivocal or other great vessel injuries are suspected.

Management of patients who are stable and found to have a ruptured thoracic aorta is evolving. In the past, prompt operative management was the standard. At present, options for treatment include operative repair, endovascular stent placement, or nonoperative management with an antihypertensive modality in high-risk patients. Repair of the thoracic aorta should proceed after other life-threatening injuries such as a ruptured spleen or bleeding from a pelvic fracture are addressed. Patients with acute pulmonary insufficiency or severe head injuries should not undergo repair of the aorta until their overall condition has improved.

Abdominal Trauma

The abdomen is frequently injured after both blunt and penetrating trauma. Approximately 25% of all trauma victims will require abdominal exploration. Clinical evaluation of the abdomen by means of physical examination is inadequate to identify intra-abdominal injuries because of the high number of patients with altered mental status secondary to head trauma, alcohol, or drugs and because of the inaccessibility of the pelvic, upper abdominal, and retroperitoneal organs to palpation. For these reasons, several diagnostic modalities have evolved during the past 3 decades, including diagnostic peritoneal lavage (DPL), ultrasound, CT, and laparoscopy, all of which have advantages, disadvantages, and limitations.

The development of more modern technology, experience, and invasiveness have been the most important determinants of the use of diagnostic methods for abdominal trauma. In modern trauma centers in the 21st century, better noninvasive technology favors the use of ultrasound and CT in the evaluation of trauma victims.

Mechanism of Injury

Blunt trauma secondary to motor vehicle accidents, motorcycle accidents, falls, assaults, and striking of pedestrians remains the most frequent mechanism of abdominal injury. Penetrating abdominal wounds are usually caused by either gunshot or stab wounds and by a significantly smaller number of shotgun wounds.

Based on the high frequency of intra-abdominal organ injury after gunshot wounds, mandatory abdominal exploration, with the rare exception of tangential and superficial wound trajectories restricted to the right upper quadrant, remains the standard form of management. Stab wounds to the abdomen, however, carry a significantly lower risk of intra-abdominal organ injury than do gunshot wounds, and several studies have recently favored a more selective approach, as opposed to mandatory exploratory laparotomy.

The impetus for nonoperative management of solid organ injury in stable blunt trauma patients has expanded to penetrating trauma as well. With improved imaging, more stable patients sustaining a single solid organ injury after stab and gunshot wounds to the abdomen will be treated conservatively.

In children, besides the aforementioned mechanisms of injury, child abuse and trauma secondary to recreational activities such as bicycling, swimming, and roller skating should also be considered.

Diagnosis

The history of the traumatic event is particularly important in determining the likelihood of an intra-abdominal organ injury. All possible information should be obtained from the prehospital personnel, including the mechanism of injury, the height of a fall, damage to the interior and exterior of a vehicle in a motor vehicle accident, other deaths at the scene, ejection, vital signs, mental status, the presence of external bleeding, the type of weapon, and other pertinent data.

On arrival at the hospital, the history and physical examination are usually accurate in determining intra-abdominal injury in an awake and responsive patient, although the limitations of physical examination are significant. Many patients with moderate intra-abdominal bleeding will be in a compensated hemodynamic condition and will not have peritoneal signs. Furthermore, retroperitoneal and pelvic injuries cannot be ruled out on the basis of only physical findings. We believe that an objective abdominal evaluation is necessary and should be performed by any of the available diagnostic modalities, in addition to the physical examination. The test of choice depends on the hemodynamic stability of the patient and the severity of associated injuries.

Hemodynamically stable patients sustaining blunt trauma are adequately evaluated by abdominal ultrasound or CT, unless other severe injuries take priority and the patient needs to go to the operating room before the objective abdominal evaluation. In such instances, DPL or focused abdominal sonography for trauma (FAST) is usually performed in the operating room to rule out intra-abdominal bleeding requiring immediate surgical exploration.

Hemodynamically stable blunt trauma patients are evaluated by ultrasound in the resuscitation room, if available, or by DPL to rule out intra-abdominal injuries as the source of blood loss and hypotension.

Hypotensive patients with isolated penetrating abdominal trauma who are hypotensive or in shock or have peritoneal signs should go to the operating room despite the mechanism of injury. Stab wound victims without peritoneal signs, evisceration, or hypotension benefit from wound exploration and DPL. Gunshot wound victims should generally undergo exploration.

Plain Radiographs

The chest radiograph is a useful test to reveal pneumoperitoneum, abdominal contents in the chest (ruptured hemidiaphragm), or lower rib fractures. This later sign increases the probability of splenic and hepatic injury.

IV pyelography (IVP) and retrograde cystography, useful tests in the past in the evaluation of a trauma patient with hematuria, have largely been substituted by contrast-enhanced CT.

With the current frequent use of CT to objectively evaluate the abdomen after blunt trauma in stable patients, the routine use of AP pelvic radiographs, as recommended by the ATLS course, has been questioned. Stable patients undergoing CT of the abdomen and pelvis do not need a pelvic radiograph. Unstable patients, however, may continue to benefit from a pelvic radiograph because other priorities may take place that will require prompt diagnosis of a pelvic fracture in the trauma resuscitation room.

Other studies suggest that clinical factors could accurately identify patients at high risk for pelvic fractures, thus making routine films unnecessary.[32]

Diagnostic Peritoneal Lavage

DPL is a rapid and accurate test used to identify intra-abdominal injuries after blunt trauma in a hypotensive or unresponsive patient without obvious indication for abdominal exploration. Standard criteria for positive DPL findings in blunt trauma include aspiration of at least 10 mL of gross blood, a bloody lavage effluent, a red blood cell count greater than 100,000/mm³, a white blood cell count greater than 500/mm³, amylase level greater than 175 IU/dL, or detection of bile, bacteria, or food fibers. The indications and contraindications for DPL are listed in Box 20-2. DPL is highly sensitive to the presence of intraperitoneal blood; however, its specificity is low, and because positive DPL findings prompt surgical exploration, a significant number of explorations will be nontherapeutic.

Significant injuries may also be missed by DPL. Diaphragmatic tears, retroperitoneal hematomas, and renal, pancreatic, duodenal, minor intestinal, and extraperitoneal bladder injuries are frequently underdiagnosed by DPL alone. Complications are infrequent and mostly related to iatrogenic injuries caused during insertion of the catheter into the abdominal cavity. A semiopen or open technique should be the preferred method to avoid or reduce the incidence of such complications.

DPL results can be misleading in the presence of a pelvic fracture. False-positive findings are expected with bleeding from the retroperitoneum into the peritoneal cavity.

Anterior abdominal and flank wounds can be accurately evaluated by DPL. False-positive results are frequent after DPL because of bleeding of the abdominal wall, thus increasing the number of negative explorations. Another potential disadvantage of DPL is its low

accuracy in the diagnosis of hollow viscus injuries. Debate still exists regarding the most appropriate positive criteria to determine the threshold for surgical exploration after stab wounds to the abdomen. If a red blood cell count of 1000/mm³ is considered, the number of negative explorations may be higher than 20%. If 100,000/mm³ is considered, the missed injury rate will approach 5%. There is no consensus on this matter, although most trauma centers use a low threshold (cell count between 1000 and 5000/mm³) for exploration.

Ultrasound

Ultrasound has been used more frequently in recent years in the United States for evaluation of blunt abdominal trauma patients. The objective of ultrasound evaluation is to search for free intraperitoneal fluid. It can be done expeditiously and is as accurate as DPL in detecting hemoperitoneum. It can also evaluate the liver and the spleen once free fluid is identified; however, this is not its main purpose. Portable machines can be used in the resuscitation area or in the emergency department in a hemodynamically unstable patient without delaying the resuscitation. Another advantage of ultrasound over DPL is its noninvasiveness. No further workup is necessary after a negative ultrasound in a stable patient. CT of the abdomen usually follows positive ultrasound findings in a stable patient. The advantages and disadvantages of abdominal ultrasound are listed in Box 20-3. Its sensitivity ranges from 85% to 99% and its specificity from 97% to 100%.[33]

Abdominal Computed Tomography

CT is the most frequently used method to evaluate a stable blunt abdominal trauma patient. The retroperitoneum is best evaluated by CT. The indications and contraindications for abdominal CT are listed in Box 20-4. The drawback of CT is the need to transport the patient to the radiology department. Additionally, it is more expensive than other tests. CT also evaluates solid organ injury, and in a stable patient with positive ultrasound findings, it is indicated to grade organ injury and to evaluate contrast extravasation. If contrast extravasation is seen, even with minor hepatic or splenic injuries,

Box 20-5 Advantages and Disadvantages of Abdominal Computed Tomography

Advantages

Adequate assessment of the retroperitoneum
Nonoperative management of solid organ injuries
Assessment of renal perfusion
Noninvasive
High specificity

Disadvantages

Specialized personnel
Hardware
Duration: Helical versus conventional
Hollow viscus injuries
Cost

ment is being considered.[34] Nonoperative management of stab wounds to the anterior aspect of the abdomen has been emphasized because of the high morbidity rate after nontherapeutic laparotomy.

Other Diagnostic Modalities

Despite the initial enthusiasm, the use of diagnostic laparoscopy in blunt trauma patients is very limited. It is an invasive and expensive method and does not seem to be superior to other methods used for decision making. Missed small bowel, splenic, and retroperitoneal injuries have been reported. It seems that laparoscopy is the best method for evaluating diaphragmatic injuries after thoracoabdominal penetrating injuries.

Angiography is used to evaluate renal artery thrombosis and to manage pelvic hemorrhage in patients with pelvic fractures and bleeding from minor hepatic and splenic injuries.

Gastric Injuries

Gastric injuries often result from penetrating trauma. Less than 1% of such wounds are due to blunt trauma secondary to motor vehicle accidents, falls, cardiopulmonary resuscitation, or interpersonal violence.

The stomach is partially protected by the rib cage, thus making blunt injuries rare and relatively difficult to diagnose. Causes of blunt gastric rupture include vigorous ventilation with inadvertent placement of an endotracheal tube in the esophagus, crushing of the stomach against the spine, cardiopulmonary resuscitation, the Heimlich maneuver, and other causes leading to a sudden increase in intraluminal pressure.

Blunt gastric trauma includes a wide range of injuries, from mucosal lacerations to full-thickness disruption and gastric necrosis secondary to avulsion of the vascular pedicles. Other intra-abdominal and extra-abdominal injuries are frequently present. DPL or CT of the abdomen may confirm the diagnosis; however, in most instances the diagnosis will be made during surgical exploration.

Any penetrating abdominal injury, particularly in the upper part of the abdomen, should be suspected of causing injury to the stomach. During initial evaluation a nasogastric tube should be inserted, and if the aspirate is positive for blood, injury to the stomach should be suspected. The intraoperative evaluation includes good visualization of the esophagogastric junction, examination of the anterior gastric wall, opening of the gastrocolic ligament, and complete visualization of the posterior gastric wall. Minor injuries may not be identified and require distention of the organ with saline or methylene blue to evaluate for leak.

Most penetrating wounds are treated by débridement of the wound edges and primary closure in layers. Injuries with major tissue loss may best be treated by gastric resection. Postoperative complications include bleeding, usually from submucosal vessels; intra-abdominal abscesses; and, more rarely, gastric fistula with peritonitis.

Because of its proximity to the diaphragm, the stomach is frequently injured after thoracoabdominal wounds. Depending on the severity of contamination from spillage

exploratory laparotomy or, more recently, angiography and embolization are indicated. Another indication for CT is in the evaluation of patients with solid organ injuries initially treated nonoperatively who have a falling hematocrit. The most important disadvantage of CT is its inability to reliably diagnose hollow viscus injury (Box 20-5). Usually, the presence of free abdominal fluid on CT without solid organ injury should raise suspicion for mesenteric, intestinal, or bladder injury, and exploratory laparotomy is often warranted.

One of the most intriguing problems regarding the objective evaluation of blunt abdominal trauma by CT is what to do when free fluid without signs of solid organ or mesenteric injury is found. Coupled with the relatively marginal sensitivity of CT to diagnose hollow viscus injury, it creates a dilemma for most trauma surgeons. The options are either to surgically explore all patients and accept a significant rate of nontherapeutic laparotomy or to observe and "act" when peritoneal signs develop while keeping in mind that a delay in the diagnosis of bowel injury may be catastrophic. A recent survey in which trauma surgeons were asked what would be the appropriate management of patients in this circumstance showed a variety of responses: 42% would perform DPL, 28% would observe the patient, 16% would surgically explore, and 12% would repeat an abdominal CT scan.

As technology evolves, diagnosis of mesenteric and hollow viscus injury by CT will be facilitated. Two- and three-dimensional reconstructions may help in the identification of bowel thickening, small bubbles of free air in the proximity of the area of injury, and small amounts of free fluid between loops of bowel or in the mesentery.

The accuracy of CT ranges from 92% to 98%, with low false-positive and false-negative rates.

Although the use of abdominal CT for the evaluation of penetrating abdominal trauma has been limited because of low sensitivity in diagnosing bowel and diaphragmatic injury, newer technology (multislice spiral CT) has been evaluated in selected cases when nonoperative manage-

of gastric contents, empyema is another frequent complication.

The role of extravasation of gastric contents in the genesis of postoperative complications is closely related to the dynamics of the gastric flora. Usually, many microorganisms originating from the nasopharynx and oropharynx reach the stomach through saliva and nasal mucus. Changes in gastric pH are frequent after eating, drinking, and ingestion of saliva, which act in an attempt to neutralize gastric acidity. When gastric pH is below 4, gastric juice has bactericidal properties that act by inhibiting bacterial enzymatic activity. In this situation, microorganisms such as *Streptococcus salivarius, Streptococcus viridans, Lactobacillus, Bacteroides, Veillonella, Micrococcus, Staphylococcus,* and *Neisseria* are found in very low concentrations, usually below 1000/mL. Inversely, when gastric pH is neutralized, the bactericidal properties of gastric juice are extremely suppressed, which leads to prompt bacterial growth. Concentrations can reach as high as 10^6/mL and remain there for approximately 1 hour before returning to normal levels. If the neutralization occurs for prolonged periods, bacteria from the lower digestive tract, such as *Bacteroides fragilis, Escherichia coli, Streptococcus faecalis,* and enterobacteria, can be found inside the stomach. This fact is especially important in trauma patients, who frequently have great amounts of food and liquid inside the stomach.

Morbidity and mortality rates after penetrating abdominal injuries associated with gastric wounds have been reported to be close to 27% and 14%, respectively, in most cases because of the presence of associated injuries, although the risk for morbidity from gastric injury itself is close to 6%.

Injuries to the Duodenum

The majority of duodenal injuries are caused by penetrating trauma; however, blunt injuries, though infrequent, are difficult to diagnose because patients may have subtle findings on admission. The incidence of duodenal injuries varies from 3% to 5%. Most duodenal injuries are accompanied by other intra-abdominal injuries because of the close anatomic relationship of the duodenum with other solid organs and major vessels.

A motor vehicle accident causing impact of the steering wheel on the epigastrium is the most common mechanism of blunt duodenal injuries. Other mechanisms such as assault and falls also cause duodenal injuries. Closed-loop compression from a direct blow to an air-filled loop can account for duodenal rupture.

The retroperitoneal location of the duodenum (second and third portions) exerts a protective effect against injuries, but it also prevents early diagnosis. Isolated injury to the duodenum is rare and does not usually cause significant clinical signs of peritonitis or hemodynamic instability. A thorough search based on the mechanism of injury is necessary to prevent delays in diagnosis. Failure to recognize this injury is associated with the development of intra-abdominal abscesses and sepsis and high mortality rates.

Hyperamylasemia occurs in about 50% of patients with blunt injury to the duodenum, and although it is not

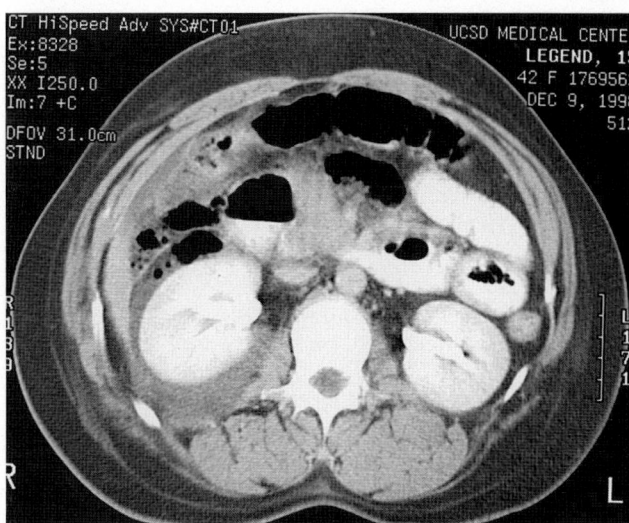

Figure 20-17 Computed tomography scan showing a blunt duodenal injury with retroperitoneal air.

diagnostic of an injury, its presence should raise suspicion and further diagnostic studies should be obtained.

Plain films of the abdomen may suggest duodenal injury by showing mild scoliosis, obliteration of the right psoas shadow, absence of air in the duodenal bulb, or air in the retroperitoneum outlining the kidney. Definitive diagnosis requires a diatrizoate meglumine (Gastrografin) upper gastrointestinal series or a CT scan of the abdomen with oral and IV contrast in hemodynamically stable patients (Fig. 20-17). Extravasation of contrast material is an absolute indication for laparotomy. The radiographic finding of a duodenal hematoma (coiled spring or stacked coin sign) is not an indication for surgical exploration. If a hematoma is causing obstruction that fails to resolve, operative management is indicated. If CT findings are equivocal, an upper gastrointestinal series with diluted barium is the test of choice.

The utility of duodenography in the diagnosis of blunt duodenal injury was recently evaluated and compared with that of abdominal CT. Duodenography in patients with CT findings suggestive of duodenal injury was found to be of minimal utility. The most important sign of duodenal perforation was retroperitoneal extraluminal air seen on CT.

Intraoperative evaluation of the duodenum requires adequate mobilization of the duodenum by means of a Kocher maneuver. The hepatic flexure of the colon is also mobilized to provide adequate exposure of the anterior wall of the second portion, and examination of the third and fourth portions of the duodenum should also be done. The presence of retroperitoneal hematomas around the duodenum should raise suspicion of an associated pancreatic injury.

Appropriate repair of duodenal injuries depends on the severity of the injury (Table 20-8) and elapsed time from injury to treatment. Approximately 80% to 85% of duodenal wounds can be repaired primarily. The remaining 15% to 20% are severe injuries that require more complex procedures.

Table 20-8 **Duodenum Injury Scale**

GRADE*	TYPE OF INJURY	DESCRIPTION OF INJURY
I	Hematoma	Involving a single portion of the duodenum
	Laceration	Partial thickness, no perforation
II	Hematoma	Involving more than one portion
	Laceration	Disruption <50% of the circumference
III	Laceration	Disruption 50%-75% of the circumference of D2
		Disruption 50%-100% of the circumference of D1, D3, D4
IV	Laceration	Disruption >75% of the circumference of D2 and involving the ampulla or distal common bile duct
V	Laceration	Massive disruption of the duodenopancreatic complex
	Vascular	Devascularization of the duodenum

*Advance one grade for multiple injuries up to grade III.

D1, first portion of the duodenum; D2, second portion of the duodenum; D3, third portion of the duodenum; D4, fourth portion of the duodenum.

From Moore EE, Cogbill TH, Malangoni MA, et al: Organ injury scaling: II. Pancreas, duodenum, small bowel, colon, and rectum. J Trauma 30:1427-1429, 1990, with permission.

For most minor injuries (grades I and II) diagnosed within 6 hours of injury, simple primary repair is suitable. After 6 hours the risk of leakage increases, and any form of duodenal decompression (transpyloric nasogastric tube, tube jejunostomy, or tube duodenostomy) is advisable.

Grade III injuries involving major disruption of the duodenal circumference are best treated by primary repair, pyloric exclusion, and drainage or, alternatively, by Roux-en-Y duodenojejunostomy.

Grade IV injuries (involving the ampulla or distal common bile duct) are difficult to repair. In this situation, primary repair of the duodenum, repair of the common bile duct, and placement of a T-tube with a long trans-papillary limb or a choledochoenteric anastomosis may be attempted when possible. If repair of the common bile duct is impossible, ligation and a second intervention for a biliary enterostomy can be done. Pancreaticoduo-denectomy, though rarely needed, is reserved for grade V injuries, including massive disruption of the duodenum and pancreatic head or massive devascularization of the duodenum.

Duodenal hematomas are expected to resolve in 10 to 15 days, and management consists of nasogastric suction until peristalsis resumes and the slow introduction of solid food. Exploration is indicated in the event of persistent duodenal obstruction.

The incidence of complications after duodenal injuries is high and ranges from 30% to more than 100%.[35] The most significant complication after duodenal injury is the development of a duodenal fistula, which occurs in 5% to 15% of patients. Duodenal fistulas are generally managed nonoperatively with nasogastric suction, IV nutritional support, and aggressive stoma care. Usually, closure will occur within 6 to 8 weeks. Abscesses develop in 10% to 20% of patients and may or may not be associated with a duodenal fistula. Abscesses are initially managed by percutaneous drainage. Surgical drainage is indicated if multiple abscesses are present or when located between small bowel loops.

Pancreatic Injuries

Pancreatic injury is rare and accounts for approximately 10% to 12% of all abdominal injuries. The great majority of such injuries are caused by penetrating mechanisms and are often associated with significant injuries involving other intra-abdominal organs. Blunt trauma to the abdomen caused by a direct blow or seat belt injury may compress the pancreas over the vertebral column and result in pancreatic disruption. Major abdominal vascular injuries are present in more than 75% of cases of penetrating pancreatic trauma, and injuries to solid organs and hollow viscera are common after blunt trauma.

Mortality rates range from 10% to 25%, mostly secondary to associated intra-abdominal injuries. Approximately 50% of the overall mortality after a pancreatic injury is caused by associated major abdominal vascular injuries. Sepsis and multiple organ failure account for most of the late deaths. The incidence of pancreatic-related mortality ranges from 2% to 5% in large urban trauma series.

Diagnosis of a pancreatic injury is made by having a high index of suspicion based on the history, mechanism of injury, and associated clinical findings. However, because of its retroperitoneal location, the pancreas is a well-protected organ, and signs and symptoms may appear late, thus delaying diagnosis. Increased levels of serum and urinary amylase after a blunt injury are not diagnostic, but a persistent elevation suggests pancreatic injury. Contrast-enhanced duodenography may reveal widening of the C-loop. DPL is not sensitive enough for the diagnosis of retroperitoneal injuries, but this test may be positive because of the high frequency of associated injures and should prompt abdominal exploration. Abdominal CT is of potential value, but its role is still unclear. The diagnosis of a pancreatic injury with the use of newer-generation CT scanners has improved significantly; however, some injuries may be identified only during follow-up scans obtained because of changes in clinical status (Fig. 20-18).

Isolated pancreatic injuries are rare. The diagnosis is difficult to make, and patients may complain of vague abdominal pain radiating to the back several hours after the incident. Frequently, mild abdominal tenderness develops, with peritoneal signs eventually developing in some patients. A delay in diagnosis correlates with an increased incidence of severe complications.

Patients are generally operated on because of intraperitoneal blood loss or peritonitis, and the diagnosis of a pancreatic injury is generally an incidental finding. However, patients with questionable CT scan findings, persistent abdominal pain, or elevated serum amylase

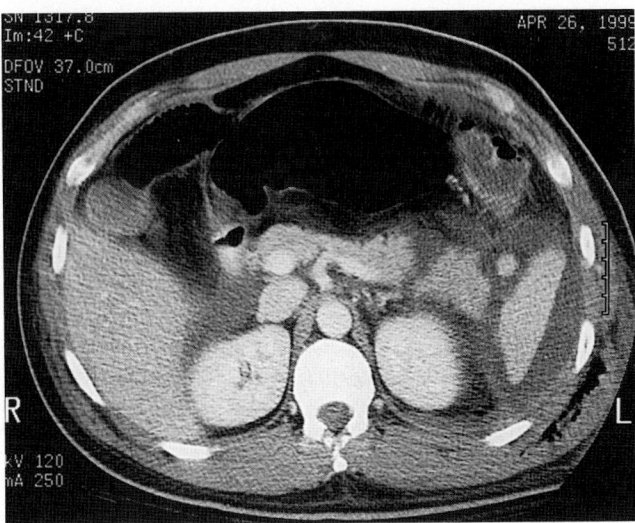

Figure 20-18 Computed tomography scan showing pancreatic transection.

Table 20-9 **Pancreas Injury Scale**

GRADE*	TYPE OF INJURY	DESCRIPTION OF INJURY
I	Hematoma	Minor contusion without duct injury
	Laceration	Superficial laceration without duct injury
II	Hematoma	Major contusion without duct injury or tissue loss
	Laceration	Major laceration without duct injury or tissue loss
III	Laceration	Distal transection or parenchymal injury with duct injury
IV	Laceration	Proximal transection or parenchymal injury involving the ampulla†
V	Laceration	Massive disruption of the pancreatic head

*Advance one grade for multiple injuries up to grade III.
†The proximal portion of the pancreas is to the patient's right of the superior mesenteric vein.

From Moore EE, Cogbill TH, Malangoni MA, et al: Organ injury scaling: II. Pancreas, duodenum, small bowel, colon, and rectum. J Trauma 30:1427-1429, 1990, with permission.

may benefit from a repeat CT scan. At laparotomy, careful examination of the pancreas should be carried out. All retroperitoneal hematomas surrounding the pancreas should be explored.

The presence of a pancreatic duct injury appears to be a key factor in postoperative morbidity.[36] There is still controversy regarding the best method to evaluate the main pancreatic duct during laparotomy. Several authors are in favor of aggressively pursuing the identification of ductal injury by performing intraoperative pancreatography. Others favor a more conservative approach and base their management on the location and surgical identification of ductal injuries. In fact, a more conservative approach to the diagnosis and management of pancreatic injuries has been advocated recently.

Pancreatic injuries are divided into proximal or distal according to the location on the right or left of the superior mesenteric vessels. Classification of pancreatic injuries according to injury severity is presented in Table 20-9.

Most distal pancreatic injuries with suspected ductal injury are treated by distal resection with or without splenectomy.

If there is any evidence that the pancreas has been contused, it should be drained independent of the location of the contusion. Complete transection of the midportion of the pancreas can theoretically be treated by pancreaticojejunostomy, but there are no data to support this approach over distal pancreatectomy.

Penetrating wounds to the right of the superior mesenteric vein should be treated by débridement and direct suture ligation of areas of bleeding. Extensive injuries to the pancreatic head or to the right of the superior mesenteric vessels are usually associated with a greater than 40% probability of a temporary pancreatic fistula. In these circumstances, drainage seems to be the best treatment option, particularly when compared with proximal pancreatectomy or a Whipple procedure, which is reserved for severe combined pancreaticoduodenal injuries. Severe

trauma to the duodenum and head of the pancreas may be treated by débridement of the pancreas, closure of the duodenal wound, and pyloric exclusion. Wide drainage is also mandatory in this situation.

The most frequent complications after pancreatic trauma are pancreatic fistula and peripancreatic abscess. These complications occur in approximately 35% to 40% of patients sustaining pancreatic injuries. Pancreatic fistulas, if well drained, will close spontaneously in the majority of patients. Somatostatin has been used to expedite the healing of pancreatic fistulas, but the results are controversial. Peripancreatic abscesses are treated by surgical débridement and drainage. The incidence of pancreatitis after a pancreatic injury is 8% to 18%. Pancreatic pseudocysts are infrequent.

Small Intestinal Injuries

The small bowel is the most frequently injured organ after penetrating injuries. After blunt trauma, the incidence of small bowel injuries ranges from 5% to 20% in patients who require surgical exploration. The postulated mechanisms involved in blunt intestinal injury include the following:

1. Crushing injury of the bowel between the vertebral bodies and the blunt object, such as a steering wheel or handlebars
2. Deceleration shearing of the small bowel at fixed points, such as the ligament of Treitz and the ileocecal valve and around the mesenteric artery
3. Closed-loop rupture caused by a sudden increase in intra-abdominal pressure

The presence of a seat belt sign should raise suspicion for enteric and mesenteric injuries. The majority of patients with blunt intestinal trauma will have signs of peritoneal irritation; however, small lacerations may be accompanied by mild abdominal pain without peritoneal signs. If peritoneal signs or hemodynamic instability are present, the patient should be taken to the operating room for surgical exploration, and the diagnosis of intestinal rupture will be made intraoperatively. Hollow viscus injuries are often characterized by a delay in diagnosis after blunt abdominal trauma. Delay in the diagnosis and management of blunt hollow viscus injuries is associated with increased morbidity and mortality, as shown by recent studies.

Several tests may help in the diagnosis of blunt intestinal trauma in patients without a clear indication for surgical exploration. Plain films of the abdomen may reveal free air; however, this finding is uncommon. DPL is not a reliable test to identify small bowel injuries, particularly small injuries with minimal leakage. CT with IV and oral contrast also carries a significant false-negative rate, and suggestive findings include free fluid in the abdomen without solid organ injury, free air, and thickening of the small bowel wall or mesentery. Negative abdominal CT results are inadequate to safely rule out a perforated small bowel injury.[37]

Occasionally, a large tear in the mesentery occurs without bowel involvement. In these instances bowel necrosis and subsequent perforation occur hours or even days after the initial injury, and the patients may have frank peritoneal signs, acidosis, and sepsis.

At laparotomy, careful examination of the entire small bowel should be performed. Bleeding should initially be controlled and clamps or sutures applied to prevent further leakage of intestinal contents into the peritoneal cavity. Penetrating injuries caused by firearms should be débrided, and small tears are usually closed primarily. If two adjacent holes are found, they can be connected across the bridge of normal bowel and closed transversely to avoid narrowing of the intestinal lumen. Extensive lacerations, devascularized segments, or multiple lacerations in a short segment of bowel are better treated by resection and reanastomosis. All mesenteric hematomas should be explored because they can hide small bowel injuries.

During the initial postoperative period, patients are usually maintained with a nasogastric tube for decompression until peristalsis resumes and feeding is started. Postoperative complications include intra-abdominal abscess and sepsis, anastomotic leakage, wound infection, enteric fistulas, and intestinal obstruction. Enteric leakage caused by suture breakdown is rare and manifested by fever, leukocytosis, leak through the surgical wounds, or peritonitis.

Short-bowel syndrome is a devastating complication after extensive resection of the small bowel. It is characterized by persistent diarrhea, loss of protein and fat in stool, and weight loss. Ileal resections are less tolerated than jejunal resections because the ileum is the site for absorption of bile salts and vitamin B_{12} and the jejunum has greater adaptive capacity. The presence of the ileal cecal valve is also of paramount importance because it slows intestinal transit time, thereby providing prolonged exposure of the intestinal mucosa to nutrients. Treatment of short-bowel syndrome includes adequate fluid intake, parenteral hyperalimentation, vitamin B_{12} replacement, cholestyramine to reduce diarrhea, H_2 blockers to reduce gastric secretion, and oral narcotics to reduce intestinal motility.

Injuries to the Colon

Colon injuries are generally the result of penetrating trauma. The colon is the second most frequently injured organ after gunshot wounds and the third after stab wounds to the abdomen. Colon injuries are relatively infrequent after blunt trauma, which accounts for only 5% of such injuries.

Recent studies have shown that morbidity rates after colonic injury vary from 20% to 35% and mortality rates range from 3% to 15%. The incidence of infectious complications after a colonic injury is related to inadequate treatment or delay in diagnosis, and several reports have confirmed that repair of a colonic injury within 2 hours dramatically reduces the incidence of infectious complications.

Physical examination is particularly useful to establish that laparotomy is necessary after a stab wound to the abdomen if peritoneal signs are present; however, a negative physical examination does not rule out the presence of a colonic injury, particularly in patients with stab wounds to the back and flanks. An objective evaluation of the abdomen is warranted after stab wounds and may include DPL or a triple-contrast (oral, IV, and rectal) CT scan. Gunshot wounds to the abdomen usually indicate the necessity for laparotomy, and with few exceptions, no further workup is necessary and the colonic injury will be diagnosed during abdominal exploration.

Laboratory studies are not generally helpful, and plain abdominal films may eventually show pneumoperitoneum. Rectal examination may show the presence of blood, which is strong evidence of colon or rectal injury. Patients undergoing abdominal exploration should receive preoperative antibiotics, an important adjunct for decreasing infectious complications.

Operative management of colonic injury is still controversial. During World War I, primary repair of colonic injuries was the treatment of choice; however, mortality rates reached 60%. During World War II, surgeons concerned about high rates of postoperative infection considered diversion of fecal contents by means of a colostomy and delayed colostomy closure to be safer than primary repair. In fact, the mortality rates reported during World War II for colonic injuries were approximately 35%. These results influenced the way that colonic injuries were treated until recent years. Recently, this concept has been challenged because colonic injuries in civilian practice are caused by low-velocity missiles and stab wounds, mechanisms different from those in military practice. This led to a resurgence of primary repair as an adequate alternative to colostomy for the treatment of most (but not all) colonic injuries.

Primary repair can be selected when known associated complicating factors have been excluded. General criteria for primary repair include early diagnosis (within 4-6 hours), absence of prolonged shock or hypotension, absence of gross contamination of the peritoneal cavity, absence of associated colonic vascular injury, less than 6 units of blood transfused, and no requirement for the use of mesh to permanently close the abdominal wall. Increased complication rates after primary repair are due to prolonged hypotension, massive intraperitoneal hemorrhage, more than two associated organs injured, significant fecal spillage, or delayed diagnosis. Most patients with low-risk penetrating colonic injuries can be treated by primary closure or resection and primary anastomosis by following these guidelines. High-risk colon injuries or those associated with severe injuries will benefit from resection and colostomy. Exteriorization of the colonic repair has been performed infrequently because of extremely high rates of failure, repair breakdown, and infectious complications. Some surgeons use different approaches to treat injuries on the right side than on the left side of the colon; however, no prospective randomized data are available to compare primary repair performed on right-sided colonic injuries with end-colostomy for left-sided injuries.

A comparison of results between primary repair and colostomy for colonic injuries should include complications that occur during or after colostomy takedown. In analyzing complications and deaths after colostomy takedown, some studies have reported an overall 10% to 50% incidence of complications.

Penetrating colon injuries requiring resection (colostomy versus primary anastomosis) were recently evaluated in a prospective multicenter study. The type of colon management was not found by multivariate analysis to be a risk factor for abdominal complications. The authors concluded that once resection is necessary, the surgical method of colon management does not affect the incidence of abdominal complications, irrespective of associated risk factors, and that primary anastomosis should be considered in all patients.[4]

The type of anastomosis used in the colon (hand sewn versus stapled) has been also the subject of controversy. A multicenter prospective study comparing stapled with hand-sewn anastomoses after penetrating colon trauma concluded that the method of colonic anastomosis does not affect the incidence of abdominal complications.

In summary, stab and low-velocity wounds to the colon with minimal contamination and hemodynamic stability can be managed by primary repair.

Postoperative complications include abscess formation, anastomotic leak, peristomal hernia, and the morbidity and mortality associated with closure of the colostomy.

Rectum

Rectal injuries are uncommon. Most rectal injuries result from gunshot wounds; however, other causes, such as a foreign body, impalement, pelvic fractures, and iatrogenic (after proctosigmoidoscopy), should be considered. Transpelvic gunshot wounds, as well as any penetrating injury to the lower part of the abdomen and buttocks, should raise suspicion for a rectal injury even if the physical examination is unremarkable. Rectal injuries can be intraperitoneal or extraperitoneal. The rectal examination may reveal blood, or an injury may be palpable. Workup of rectal injuries includes anoscopy and rigid proctosigmoidoscopy.

Primary closure of extraperitoneal rectal injuries, particularly those located in the inferior third of the rectum, should be attempted, although such closure is not always possible. A diverting colostomy, washout of the distal rectal stump, and wide presacral drainage are mandatory. Rectal stump irrigation in this setting decreases the incidence of pelvic abscess, rectal fistulas, and sepsis. Intraperitoneal rectal injuries are usually managed by primary closure and a diverting colostomy. Primary abdominal perineal resection is indicated for extensive rectal injuries.

Complications after rectal injuries include sepsis, pelvic abscesses, urinary or rectal fistulas, rectal incontinence and stricture, loss of sexual function, and urinary incontinence.

A recent study evaluated whether the use of a clinical pathway based on precise anatomic characterization of rectal injuries improves outcomes. In this study, intraperitoneal rectal injuries were treated by primary repair. Injuries to the proximal two thirds and accessible distal third of the extraperitoneal rectum were treated by repair and selective fecal diversion. Inaccessible distal rectal injuries were treated by diversion and presacral drainage. Use of a clinical pathway decreased the overall infectious complication rate from 31% to 13%. No retrorectal abscesses were found in the groups treated by using the clinical pathway. This study reinforces the importance of location and accessibility in the decision to perform diversion and presacral drainage in extraperitoneal rectal injuries.[38]

Liver Injuries

Because of its size and location in the abdominal cavity, the liver is frequently injured in both blunt and penetrating trauma. Despite progress in the management of trauma patients in the last 2 decades, mortality after hepatic trauma has remained stable.[39] Spontaneous hemostasis is observed in more than 50% of small hepatic lacerations at the time of laparotomy. In fact, most liver injuries require only documentation and no drainage. Although most liver injuries can be properly managed with simple procedures, control of profuse bleeding from deep hepatic lacerations remains a formidable challenge for trauma surgeons. The overall mortality rate ranges from 8% to 10%, and the overall morbidity rate varies from 18% to 30%, depending on the number of associated injuries and the severity of the injury. The classification of liver injuries is shown in Table 20-10. In less severe hepatic injuries (grades I-III), mortality is related to associated injuries, which are more frequently seen after blunt trauma, although in high-grade liver injuries mortality is related to the injury itself, regardless of the mechanism. The mortality rate associated with isolated liver trauma is 3%; it increases to 24% in the presence of three associated injuries.

Some small nondeep bleeding lacerations are easily controlled with simple suture or the use of hemostatic

Table 20-10   Liver Injury Scale 9 (1994 Revision)

GRADE*	TYPE OF INJURY	DESCRIPTION OF INJURY
I	Hematoma	Subcapsular, <10% surface area
	Laceration	Capsular tear, <1 cm in parenchymal depth
II	Hematoma	Subcapsular, 10%-50% surface area; intraparenchymal, <10 cm in diameter
	Laceration	Capsular tear, 1-3 cm in parenchymal depth; <10 cm in length
III	Hematoma	Subcapsular, >50% surface area of ruptured subcapsular or parenchymal hematoma; intraparenchymal hematoma, >10 cm or expanding
	Laceration	3 cm in parenchymal depth
IV	Laceration	Parenchymal disruption involving 25%-75% of the hepatic lobe or 1-3 Couinaud segments
V	Laceration	Parenchymal disruption involving >75% of the hepatic lobe or >3 Couinaud segments within a single lobe
	Vascular	Juxtahepatic venous injuries, i.e., retrohepatic vena cava/central major hepatic veins
VI	Vascular	Hepatic avulsion

*Advance one grade for multiple injuries up to grade III.
From Moore EE, Cogbill TH, Jurkovich GJ, et al: Organ injury scaling: Spleen and liver (1994 revision). J Trauma 38:323-324, 1995, with permission.

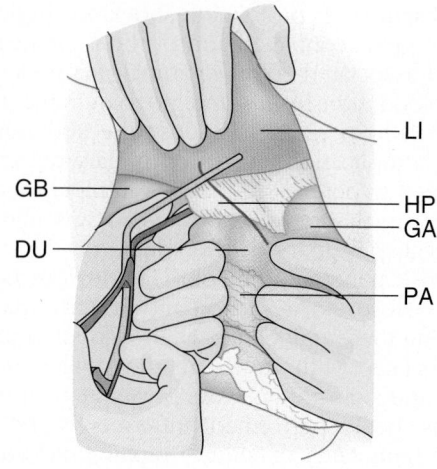

Figure 20-19 Diagram showing the Pringle maneuver. DU, duodenum; GA, gastric antrum; GB, gallbladder; HP, hepatic pedicle; LI, liver; PA, pancreas. (From Aunf B: Critical maneuvers in trauma surgery. In Editora Pedagogica e Universitaria [E. P. U.] LTDA. New York, Springer-Verlag, 1982.)

agents. More severe liver injuries require more complex procedures, including deep mattress sutures, packing, débridement, resection, mesh hepatorrhaphy, and other measures. The resurgence of packing and the emergence of damage control, as an alternative for the treatment of severe hepatic injuries in patients with shock, metabolic derangement, and coagulopathy, have been incorporated in the armamentarium of trauma surgeons in recent years. A 34% survival rate was reported when packing was used as an adjunct to other measures to control bleeding.

Injuries vary from capsular tears and nonbleeding lacerations to large fractures and lobar destruction with extensive parenchymal disruption and hepatic artery and venous injuries. The type of injury dictates the surgical management. The principles of surgical management of liver injury are the same regardless of the severity of injury. They involve control of bleeding, removal of devitalized tissue, and establishment of adequate drainage.

Simple lacerations that are not bleeding at the time of surgery do not require drainage unless they are deep into the parenchyma with the possibility of a postoperative biliary fistula. Subcapsular hematomas can simply be observed or surgically evacuated if there is no associated parenchymal injury. Lacerations that continue to bleed despite attempts at local control require a more extensive approach, usually opening the liver wound and directly approaching the bleeding vessels, a procedure known as tractotomy. Bleeding vessels and biliary radicles should be individually ligated. In the event that bleeding continues despite directly ligating small vessels, a vascular clamp or vessel loops can be placed around the porta hepatis (Pringle's maneuver) (Fig. 20-19). If the bleeding stops after clamping the portal triad, it can be assumed to be from the portal veins or hepatic artery branches. If the bleeding continues despite clamping the portal triad, an injury to the hepatic veins or the retrohepatic vena cava is suspected. The portal triad can also be intermittently clamped to allow visualization during the placement of sutures as the parenchymal vessels are ligated. If a Pringle maneuver is applied, caution regarding the duration of inflow occlusion is necessary. Hypothermic patients do not tolerate liver ischemia for prolonged periods, and significant damage to the liver parenchyma may occur as a result of ischemia. The exact length of warm ischemia time tolerated by the human liver is not known; however, some authors have reported occlusion of inflow for up to 1 hour with the use of adjuvant steroid therapy without major consequences.

Packing the liver wound is performed when the techniques just described fail to control hemorrhage. The results of temporary packing must be analyzed in light of its relation to timing. Perihepatic packing was once condemned because of the high incidence of intra-abdominal abscesses. Temporary packing has recently been used, particularly in patients with hypothermia, coagulopathy, and severe acidosis with severe injuries in other intra-abdominal organs.

Usually, these patients are taken to the intensive care unit for rewarming and resuscitation. Re-exploration for removal of the packing is performed within 48 to 72 hours after the initial operation. After hemostasis is achieved and the packs are removed, copious irrigation of the abdominal cavity is performed and closed suction drains are placed. Arteriography is a useful adjunct to locate the arterial bleeding, and embolization may be of benefit before re-exploration for removal of the packing. The incidence of intra-abdominal abscess in survivors of liver packing is generally less than 15%.

Despite the use of any method to obtain hemostasis, all necrotic tissue should be débrided before closure. If bleeding in the raw surface of the liver after resectional débridement is not significant, an omental flap can be used to cover or fill the defect in the liver parenchyma.

Deep liver lacerations should not be simply closed because of the risk for abscess formation and hemobilia. As an alternative approach for deep liver lacerations, some investigators propose extending the liver laceration to expose and directly ligate the bleeding vessel. This is achieved by performing a finger fracture hepatotomy along nonanatomic planes. This technique was used in patients with grade III to grade V liver injuries, with the remarkably low mortality rate of 10.7%. The advantage of this technique is that direct ligation of the bleeding vessels and biliary radicles is achieved; the disadvantage is that the defect in the liver parenchyma is usually bigger than the initial injury, and the technique should be performed only by experienced surgeons.

Formal hepatic resection is unusual after liver injuries and has been largely abandoned in the past decade because of high mortality and morbidity rates after this procedure and because other more conservative approaches have proved to be as effective in controlling hemorrhage, with significantly lower complication rates and mortality.

In a 5-year multi-institutional review of 1335 liver injuries, resectional débridement was performed in 36 patients (2.7%), hepatotomy and vessel ligation in 50 patients (3.7%), and segmentectomy in 18 patients (1.3%). Formal hepatic lobectomy was performed in only 12 patients (0.9%).

Another technique described recently encompasses the use of absorbable mesh, with each lobe of the liver wrapped individually and the mesh attached to the falciform ligament. This technique is useful for multiple superficial lacerations of the liver with active bleeding; however, it is not effective when major vascular injuries are present. The reported mortality rate in hepatic trauma patients managed by mesh wrapping is 25% to 37.5%.

Major hepatic injuries, including retrohepatic and juxtahepatic venous injuries, are discussed in the later section on major abdominal vascular injuries.

Ligation of the hepatic artery is also an alternative for continued bleeding; however, with the use of modern cauterization devices (electric or argon bean coagulators), topical hemostatic agents, and fibrin glue, this is seldom required. It should be reserved for the occasional stab wound or gunshot wound involving one lobe in which exposure of the wound will require extensive incision of the liver. The proper hepatic artery must never be ligated. Injudicious hepatic artery ligation may result in liver infarction, particularly if associated with portal vein injury.[40] Packing the liver is a reasonable alternative to hepatic artery ligation.

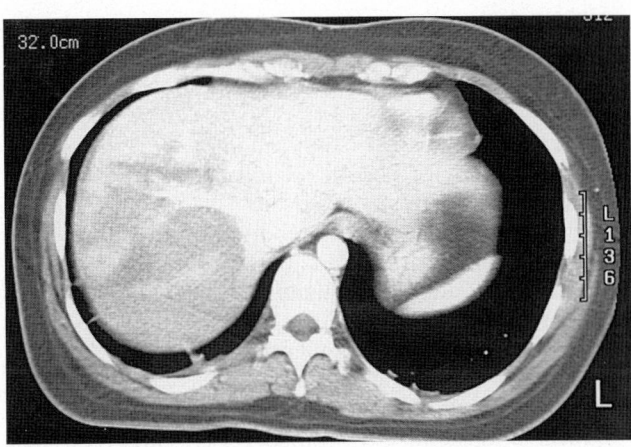

Figure 20-20 Computed tomography scan showing a grade IV liver laceration.

Nonoperative Treatment

Blunt hepatic injuries in hemodynamically stable patients without other indications for exploration are best served by a conservative, nonoperative approach.[41-43] These stable patients without peritoneal signs are better evaluated by ultrasound, and if abnormalities are found, a CT scan with contrast should be obtained (Fig. 20-20). In the absence of contrast extravasation during the arterial phase of the CT scan, most injuries can potentially be treated nonoperatively. The classic criteria for nonoperative treatment of liver injuries include hemodynamic stability, normal mental status, absence of a clear indication for laparotomy such as peritoneal signs, low-grade liver injuries (grade I-III), and transfusion requirements of less than 2 units of blood. Recently, these criteria have been challenged and a broader indication for nonoperative management has been used. It has been demonstrated that most of these patients are monitored by serial hematocrit and vital signs rather than by serial abdominal examinations, which is the reason why intact mental status is not the sine qua non for nonoperative management. Furthermore, if the hematocrit drops, most patients will undergo a repeat CT scan to evaluate and quantify the hemoperitoneum. The overall reported success of nonoperative management of blunt hepatic injuries is greater than 90% in most series. Breaking it down by injury grade, the success rate of nonoperative treatment of injury grades I to III approaches 95%, whereas for injury grades IV and V the success rate decreases to 75% to 80%. With the use of angiography and superselective embolization in patients with persistent bleeding, the success rate may in fact be higher.

Angiographic embolization has been added to the protocol for nonoperative management of liver injuries in some institutions in an attempt to decrease the necessity for blood transfusions and the number of operations.[44-46]

Patients are admitted to the intensive care unit for monitoring of vital signs and hematocrit. Usually, after 48 hours patients are transferred to an intermediate care unit, where they are started on an oral diet; however, they remain on bed rest until postinjury day 5. A repeat CT scan before discharge does not seem to be necessary. Normal physical activity resumes 3 months after injury.

A recent multicenter study attempted to determine early risk factors for hepatic-related morbidity after nonoperative management of severe (grades III-V) blunt hepatic injuries. The authors reported complication rates of 5%, 22%, and 52% for grade III, IV, and V liver injuries, respectively. Using multivariate analysis, they demonstrated that liver injury grade and 24-hour transfusion requirements predicted complications.

Currently, no single selection criterion can predict which patients will fail nonoperative management.

Croce and colleagues prospectively analyzed 112 patients treated nonoperatively over a 22-month period. They reported a failure rate of 11% (12 patients), with five failures being liver related. No relationship between injury grade and increased failure rate was observed. The authors concluded that nonoperative management is safe regardless of injury severity in hemodynamically stable patients; it carries a lower incidence of abdominal septic complications and leads to decreased transfusion requirements. They also compared 70 patients with grade III to V liver injuries treated nonoperatively with 50 patients who underwent surgical intervention. Blood transfusion at 48 hours consisted of 2.2 and 5.8 units, and mortality was 7% and 4% for nonoperative and operative controls, respectively. Although the transfusion requirement was slightly lower in the nonoperative group, no difference in mortality was demonstrated.[41]

Management of patients with contrast extravasation during the arterial phase of CT is still debatable. Fang and associates proposed a classification system based on the location and character of extravasation and pooling of contrast material from a liver laceration on CT. In type 1, there is contrast extravasation to the peritoneal cavity. All patients in this category required operative intervention.[47] Type 2 consisted of hemoperitoneum and extravasation of contrast material within the hepatic parenchyma. The authors recommend that patients in this category undergo angiography with embolization, although some will require operative intervention. Type 3 was characterized by no hemoperitoneum and extravasation of contrast material within the hepatic parenchyma. Angiography is required in this subgroup of patients, and the results are usually good.

Ciraulo and coworkers analyzed a group of 11 patients requiring continuous fluid resuscitation, with 7 requiring embolization. All embolization attempts were successful. The authors concluded that hepatic artery embolization is a viable alternative in the management of patients with severe liver injuries that require continuous fluid resuscitation, thereby bridging the therapeutic options of operative and nonoperative intervention.[44]

The most important concern of nonoperative management is the potential for missed injuries, particularly hollow viscus perforations. Delay in diagnosing a hollow viscus injury is associated with significant morbidity and increased mortality.[48]

Porta Hepatis

A recent multicenter retrospective study that included data from eight trauma centers reported an incidence of portal triad injuries of only 0.07%.[40] Penetrating trauma is the most frequent mechanism associated with porta hepatis injuries, although 30% of porta hepatis injuries in the aforementioned study followed blunt trauma. Isolated injuries to the porta hepatis are uncommon. Because of the proximity of other organs, porta hepatis injuries are usually associated with hepatic, duodenal, gastric, colonic, and other major vascular injuries. The overall mortality rate is 50%, but it increases to 80% in patients with associated injuries.

Management is difficult because of life-threatening hemorrhage and associated organ injury. If the patient survives the operation, complications such as biliary fistula, portal vein thrombosis, and hepatic ischemia may contribute to morbidity. Management of portal vein and hepatic artery injuries is discussed later under major abdominal vascular injuries.

Management of common bile duct injury is challenging. Primary repair and placement of a T-tube should be attempted for partial or minor injuries involving less than 50% of the duct's circumference. Major injuries or complete transection of the common bile duct are best managed by choledochoenteric anastomosis. This procedure significantly reduces the incidence of late postoperative complications, in particular, the development of strictures.

A closed suction drain should always be place in the vicinity of the repair to allow adequate drainage of an eventual biliary fistula. Missed extrahepatic bile duct injuries occurred in nine patients in a multicenter review, with a 75% complication rate in those who survived.[40]

Gallbladder injury is also an uncommon injury after both blunt and penetrating trauma. Cholecystectomy is the procedure of choice.

Postoperative Complications

Significant complications after liver injury include pulmonary complications, postoperative bleeding, coagulopathy, biliary fistulas, hemobilia, and subdiaphragmatic and intraparenchymal abscess formation.

Postoperative bleeding occurs in less than 10% of patients sustaining liver injuries. It may occur as a result of inappropriate hemostasis, postoperative coagulopathy, or both. If the patient is not hypothermic, coagulopathic, or acidotic, re-exploration should be undertaken. Bleeding vessels should be directly visualized and ligated, even if more extensive disruption of the hepatic parenchyma is necessary for adequate exposure. If diffuse oozing is found, packing and a planned re-exploration are performed.

Intra-abdominal abscesses have accounted for late deaths after hepatic trauma. A 7.2% incidence of perihepatic abscesses was reported in a prospective analysis of 482 injuries. The population at increased risk included patients with prolonged shock, extensive parenchymal disruption, associated hollow viscus injuries, hepatic ischemia from ligation of major vessels, and open drainage.

Several studies have criticized the use of drains after liver injury because of the risk for intraperitoneal infection. It seems that injury grades I and II do not require drain placement. However, in severe injuries, drainage, though controversial, is frequently used.[39]

The presence of nonviable hepatic tissue is also an important cause of postoperative abscess formation and points to the fact that adequate débridement of all devitalized tissue is an important step before closing the abdomen. CT is the method of choice to diagnose intra-abdominal abscesses. Percutaneous drainage is the treatment of choice for nonloculated abscesses. However, patients with peritoneal signs, persistence of fever despite percutaneous drainage, or multiple abscesses should be surgically re-explored through the same incision used for the initial operation.

The incidence of biliary fistulas after hepatic trauma varies from 7% to 10%.[9] In a recent multicenter review of hepatic injuries, an 8% incidence of biliary fistula was noted in 210 patients with grade III, IV, and V hepatic injuries. The group at risk includes patients with severe hepatic injuries (grade III and higher) and those requiring hepatic resection or extensive débridement. Usually, biliary fistulas close spontaneously after a period of 2 to 4 weeks of closed drainage.

Hemobilia is a rare complication that usually occurs after blunt intrahepatic hematomas have formed and is manifested as bleeding into the bile ducts and subsequently into the small bowel. Patients generally complain of jaundice, right upper quadrant pain, malaise, and melena. Hemobilia can be diagnosed by upper gastrointestinal endoscopy and treated by angiographic embolization. Surgery is rarely required.

Splenic Injuries

The spleen is the intra-abdominal organ most frequently injured in blunt trauma. Suspicion of a splenic injury should be raised in any patient with blunt abdominal trauma. History of a blow, fall, or sports-related injury to the left side of the chest, flank, or left upper part of the abdomen is usually associated with splenic injury. The diagnosis is confirmed by abdominal CT in a hemodynamically stable patient or during exploratory laparotomy in an unstable patient with positive DPL findings.

For several decades, splenectomy was considered the only acceptable surgical option for splenic injuries. With the significant experience in nonoperative management of splenic injuries in the pediatric population and with the recognition of overwhelming postsplenectomy syndrome as a serious postoperative threat, other options have emerged in the past decades. Initially, splenic repair and, more recently, nonoperative management in the adult population have been considered adequate options in selected patients. Pediatric surgeons initiated this more conservative approach, and their experience was later applied to the adult trauma population.

In 1952, a postsplenectomy syndrome of severe, sometimes fatal meningitis and sepsis in four of five children splenectomized before the age of 6 months for congenital hemolytic anemia was reported. The term *overwhelming*

postsplenectomy infection (OPSI) was introduced in 1969.

The true incidence of overwhelming postsplenectomy sepsis is not well defined, although a commonly used estimation of the incidence of OPSI is 0.6% in children and 0.3% in adults, which may be a low estimate. The courses of 688 patients (388 children, 300 adults) who underwent splenectomy for injury to the spleen were reviewed. Among these were 10 patients with sepsis (incidence of 1.45%), 4 of whom died, for a mortality rate of 0.58%. When combined with four deaths from sepsis after splenectomy for trauma in another series of 342 children, the incidence of mortality from sepsis is 0.78%, or 78 times the expected rate in the general population. The risk for postsplenectomy septicemia, pneumonia, and meningitis was estimated to be 8.3% in trauma patients, or 166 times the 0.05% rate expected in the general population. The longest follow-up of splenectomy patients included 740 World War II veterans who underwent splenectomy between 1939 and 1945. Six patients in this group (0.8%) died of pneumonia, whereas none of the 740 matched control patients died.

This syndrome is unlike fulminating bacteremia and septicemia in patients with normal splenic function. OPSI syndrome is distinct from septicemia in patients with normal immune function and is characterized by a sudden onset of symptoms and a rapid and fulminating course that often lasts only 12 to 18 hours. Patients usually complain of fever, nausea, vomiting, headache, and altered mental status. It is mainly caused by pneumococci, but other bacteria such as *E. coli, Haemophilus influenzae,* meningococci, *Staphylococcus,* and *Streptococcus* may also be found in decreasing frequency. The disease is complicated by shock, electrolyte imbalance, hypoglycemia, and disseminated intravascular coagulation. The overall mortality rate is as high as 50% to 80%. Because of the severity of the disease process and high mortality rates, the universal use of polyvalent pneumococcal vaccine (Pneumovax 23, Merck; Pnu-Immune, Lederle) and close follow-up after splenectomy for trauma is routine. Patients should receive the vaccine before discharge. The effectiveness of the vaccine in splenectomized patients is unclear. The use of prophylactic antibiotics in asplenic patients is also controversial; however, minor infections in this group should be treated with antibiotics.

Management

Hemodynamically stable patients now undergo ultrasound examination. If the ultrasound findings are positive for free fluid and the patient remains stable, an abdominal CT scan is obtained to identify the source of bleeding, evaluate for contrast extravasation and other intra-abdominal injuries that would require an operation, and grade the severity of the splenic injury (Fig. 20-21). The finding of contrast extravasation or contrast blush during the arterial phase of the IV contrast on abdominal CT scanning is indicative of persistent bleeding. Some authors would argue that when present in the spleen, contrast blush should prompt operative intervention, whereas others argue that there is an opportunity for angiographic

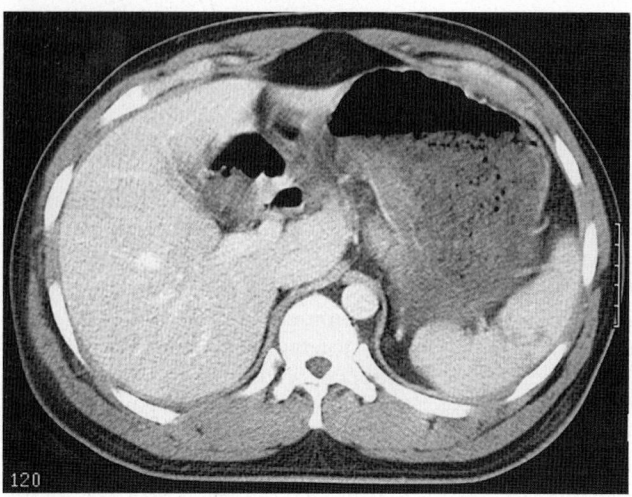

Figure 20-21 Computed tomography scan showing a splenic laceration.

embolization and continuation of nonoperative management provided that the patient remains hemodynamically stable. In a recent study the authors found contrast blush in 11% of patients with splenic injuries. No correlation between contrast blush and operative intervention was found. The authors concluded that the presence of contrast blush is not an absolute indication for operative or angiographic intervention.

Some institutions advocate more routine use of angiography, but overall splenic salvage rates are similar to those in institutions following more selective use of angiography. Prospective studies should clarify this issue in the future.[49]

More than 70% of all stable patients are currently being treated by means of a nonoperative approach. The classic criteria for nonoperative treatment include hemodynamic stability, negative abdominal examination, absence of contrast extravasation on CT, absence of other clear indications for exploratory laparotomy or associated injuries requiring surgical intervention, absence of associated health conditions that carry an increased risk for bleeding (coagulopathy, hepatic failure, use of anticoagulants, specific coagulation factor deficiency), and injury grade I to III.

Recent series have also indicated that nonoperative management should be performed in patients older than 55 years, those with a large hemoperitoneum, and patients with injury grades IV and V, which in the past have been relative contraindications.

It has been shown that inclusion of high-risk patients increases the nonoperative management rate without changing the failure rate significantly. Age older than 55 years and grade IV and V splenic injuries are predictors but do not constitute contraindications to nonoperative management of splenic injuries.

Patients are usually admitted to the intensive care unit and kept on bed rest with a nasogastric tube in place. Serial abdominal examinations and hematocrit determinations are performed during the initial 48 to 72 hours. The

necessity for blood transfusion is recorded. At 48 to 72 hours, stable patients are transferred to an intermediate care unit, start walking and eating, and are monitored clinically. A repeat CT scan is obtained in the event of a falling hematocrit, hypotension, or persistent ileus. If contrast extravasation is observed or a pseudoaneurysm found, a select group of patients benefit from angiography and selective embolization.

A repeat CT scan before discharge does not seem to be necessary. Patients are instructed to avoid intense physical activity and contact sports for 3 months. The success rate of nonoperative treatment is greater than 90%. Several reports have concluded that nonoperative treatment of splenic injuries is safe and effective.

Areas of Controversy

Currently, with the increased use of faster CT scanning, the critical question is whether a select group of patients with negative abdominal ultrasound findings should undergo CT scanning to diagnose intraparenchymal solid organ injury. There is no doubt that a small number of patients will sustain splenic (as well as liver) injuries without hemoperitoneum or with small amounts of blood in the peritoneal cavity undetectable by ultrasonography. These injuries are usually minor and their clinical relevance may be insignificant, so the cost of CT scanning is not justifiable.

Another area of controversy in nonoperative management of splenic injuries is related to the use of angiographic embolization. The definition of *extravasation* and *blush* has been inconsistent in several studies, thus adding confusion to the topic. However, it is important to state that a technically adequate abdominal CT scan with IV and oral contrast (water could substitute for oral lipid-soluble contrast) is mandatory. Images should be obtained during the arterial phase and also during the excretory phase. In this way, possible areas of contrast extravasation and blush could be confirmed by the presence of radiolucency within the parenchyma when the contrast in the vascular system has been already washed out.

Surgical treatment of a splenic injury depends on its severity (Table 20-11), the presence of shock, and associated injuries.

The spectrum of injury may vary from a simple laceration or contusion without capsular disruption to total fragmentation of the spleen. During laparotomy, the spleen is evaluated for active bleeding. If active hemorrhage is present, the surgeon must decide to perform either total splenectomy or a splenic salvage procedure. Careful adequate mobilization of the spleen is essential to prevent further injury. Ongoing bleeding from the spleen during mobilization can be controlled by digital compression. Capsular tears of the spleen can be controlled by compression only or by using topical hemostatic agents. Deeper lacerations can be controlled with horizontal absorbable mattress sutures. Major lacerations involving less than 50% of the splenic parenchyma and not extending into the hilum can be treated by segmental or partial splenic resection. Resection is indicated only if the patient is stable and no other major injuries are

Table 20-11   Spleen Injury Scale (1994 Revision)

GRADE*	TYPE OF INJURY	DESCRIPTION OF INJURY
I	Hematoma	Subcapsular, <10% surface area
	Laceration	Capsular tear, <1 cm in parenchymal depth
II	Hematoma	Subcapsular, 10%-50% surface area; intraparenchymal, <5 cm in diameter
	Laceration	Capsular tear, 1-3 cm in parenchymal depth and not involving a trabecular vessel
III	Hematoma	Subcapsular, >50% surface area or expanding, ruptured subcapsular or parenchymal hematoma; intraparenchymal hematoma, ≥5 cm or expanding
	Laceration	>3 cm in parenchymal depth or involving the trabecular vessels
IV	Laceration	Laceration involving the segmental or hilar vessels and producing major devascularization (>25% of spleen)
V	Laceration	Completely shattered spleen
	Vascular	Hilar vascular injury that devascularizes the spleen

*Advance one grade for multiple injuries up to grade III.

From Moore EE, Cogbill TH, Jurkovich GJ, et al: Organ injury scaling: Spleen and liver (1994 revision). J Trauma 38:323-324, 1995, with permission.

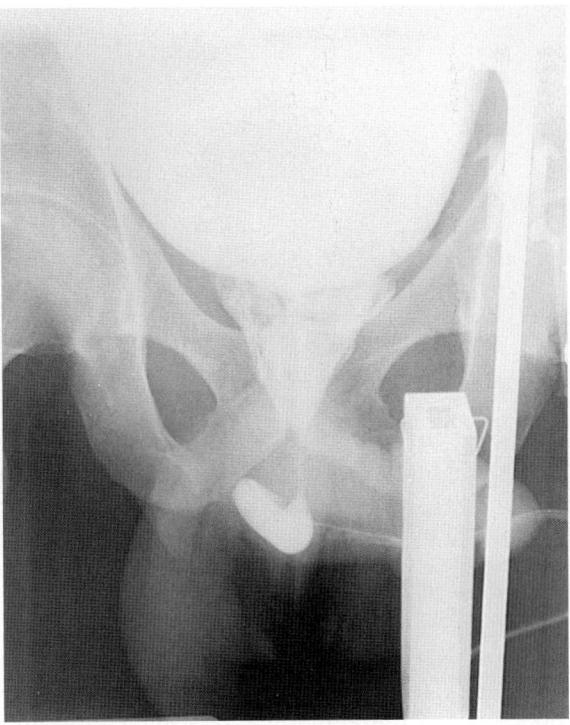

Figure 20-22 Urethrogram showing a complete urethral injury.

present. More extensive injuries involving the hilum or the central portion of the spleen may be managed by splenectomy; however, alternative procedures have been described. The technique of implanting thin splenic fragments in an omental pouch (autotransplantation) remains experimental and controversial but may provide significant long-term splenic function. The use of a Dexon or Vicryl mesh to wrap the spleen or use of the argon beam coagulator and fibrin glue has been described in selected patients. The success rate of splenic salvage procedures varies from 40% to 60%. It increases to 90% if nonoperative treatment is included.

Complications

Inadequate hemostasis, massive transfusion, or coagulopathy may cause bleeding after splenectomy or splenic salvage procedures. Other complications include transient thrombocytosis, pancreatitis, and intra-abdominal abscess.

Urinary Tract Injuries

Injuries to the genitourinary tract are often clinically unsuspected and frequently overlooked. Gross hematuria is the most frequent sign associated with urinary tract injuries. An understanding of the mechanism of injury and the forces involved is essential to identify urologic trauma and avoid missed injuries. In blunt trauma, fractures of the lower ribs or spinous processes, abdominal or pelvic crush injuries, direct blows to the back and flanks, or decelerating injuries such as with falls or motor vehicles accidents have been associated with urologic injuries. Upper urologic tract injuries are frequently accompanied by gross or microscopic hematuria. Lower urinary tract injuries are usually manifested as blood in the urethral meatus, a floating or displaced prostate on rectal examination, bladder distention, inability to void, and large perineal hematomas or other perineal injuries.

Penetrating injuries to the back or the flank have the potential to cause significant renal injury without obvious clinical manifestations.

The workup of patients with suspected urinary tract injuries depends on hemodynamic status. Patients sustaining penetrating abdominal injuries requiring immediate exploratory laparotomy may undergo one-shot IVP. Victims of blunt trauma with blood at the urethral meatus should undergo urethrocystography to rule out the presence of a urethral injury before bladder catheterization (Fig. 20-22). Once urethral injury has been ruled out, cystography is performed by injecting 250 to 300 mL of contrast medium through the Foley catheter to maximally distend the bladder. Films should be obtained after full distention and after emptying the bladder. This postvoid film is important to identify posterior extravasation of contrast that is not seen on AP films obtained when the bladder is maximally distended (Fig. 20-23). Patients with pelvic fractures involving the anterior arch are particularly likely to have an associated bladder injury.

CT is as effective as IVP for evaluating the urinary tract; however, its major advantage over IVP is its ability

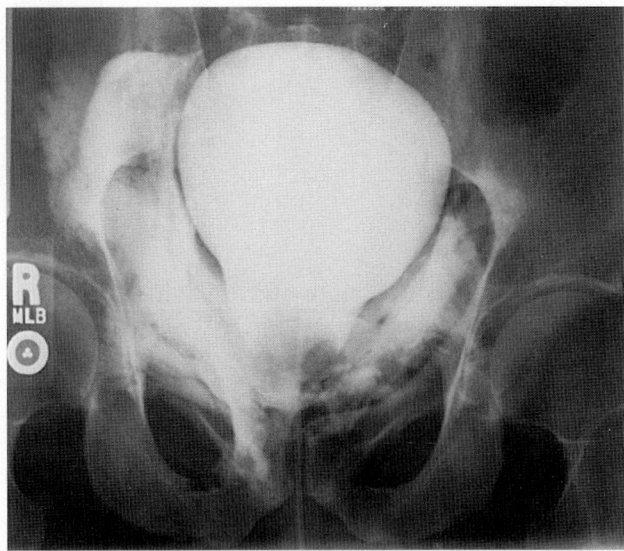

Figure 20-23 Cystogram showing a bladder injury

to evaluate potential intra-abdominal injuries and the retroperitoneum. It is also useful for staging renal injuries and evaluating renal perfusion and function. Absence of kidney perfusion is an indication for renal artery angiography.

Specific Injuries

Renal Injuries The kidney is the most commonly injured part of the urinary tract. Penetrating wounds causing small parenchymal injuries are generally treated by débridement, primary repair, and drainage. More extensive wounds may require partial or total nephrectomy. An important technical aspect to keep in mind is that in major perinephric hematomas, proximal control of the renal pedicle before opening Gerota's fascia is advisable. Injuries involving the hilum are seldom repaired primarily, and in most circumstances total nephrectomy is necessary. More than 80% of patients sustaining penetrating renal injuries have other intra-abdominal injuries.

Blunt renal injuries are generally divided into minor and major injuries (Fig. 20-24). Minor injuries account for approximately 85% of cases. A classification system for renal injuries proposed by the American Association for the Surgery of Trauma was recently validated. It found that the severity of organ injury correlates with the need for operative intervention.

Renal contusions encompass the vast majority of minor renal trauma and can almost invariably be treated nonoperatively. Major renal trauma includes deep cortical medullary lacerations with extravasation, large perinephric hematomas, and vascular injuries of the renal pedicle. These injuries should be explored because of a high incidence of complications such as bleeding, abscess formation, and hypertension, among others. At laparotomy the major problem is the decision to explore a perinephric hematoma.

It is our opinion that all perinephric hematomas caused by penetrating mechanisms that have not previously been

evaluated by IVP should be explored. If preoperative IVP shows renal pedicle injury, extensive parenchymal laceration, or urinary extravasation, surgical exploration remains the best option.

Ureteral Injuries Injury to the ureter is uncommon and occurs mostly after penetrating trauma. The presence of hematuria in ureteral injury is the exception rather than the rule. Ureteral injury is suspected preoperatively by the location of the entrance site of penetrating injuries or, in the case of blunt injury, by the presence of concomitant intra-abdominal or other genitourinary tract injuries. Nondiagnosed ureteral injuries may lead to complications such as fistulas, urinomas, and abscess formation. In the majority of cases, IVP will confirm the diagnosis. In approximately 15% to 20% of ureteral injuries, retrograde ureterography will be required to confirm the diagnosis. In hemodynamically unstable patients the diagnosis of ureteral injury may be made at the time of laparotomy by injecting 5 mL of methylene blue or indigo carmine dye IV. Extravasation of blue-stained urine confirms the presence of a ureteral injury. The principles of ureteral repair are adequate débridement, tension-free repair, spatulated anastomosis, watertight closure, ureteral stenting, and drainage. Surgical options include ureteroureterostomy for injuries located in the upper and middle thirds of the ureter. The use of a double-J stent is indicated because it seems to decrease the incidence of postoperative fistulas. More distal injuries may require ureteral reimplantation in the bladder. Percutaneous nephrostomy is indicated to divert urinary flow in cases in which primary repair is not feasible, either because of the overall clinical condition of the patient or when a long segment of the ureter has been lost. Other options in the presence of extensive ureteral injuries include transureteroureterostomy or kidney autotransplantation into the iliac fossa.

Bladder Injuries The majority of bladder injuries occur as a result of blunt trauma, and the association of bladder rupture and pelvic fractures is extremely high. In fact, approximately 70% of patients with bladder rupture have associated pelvic fractures. Hematuria is the most frequent sign and, in the presence of a pelvic fracture, should increase suspicion for bladder injury. Bladder rupture may be extraperitoneal or intraperitoneal. Extraperitoneal rupture usually results from perforation by adjacent bony fragments. Intraperitoneal rupture of the bladder results from injuries located in the dome, which occur when a full bladder sustains a direct blow. The diagnosis is made by cystography. As stated previously, a postvoid film is necessary to identify lateral or posterior injuries.

Intraperitoneal injuries are repaired primarily via a transabdominal approach, including a three-layer closure. Suprapubic cystostomy may be necessary with large wounds.

Management of extraperitoneal rupture of the bladder is primarily nonoperative and consists of leaving the Foley catheter in place for 10 to 14 days, provided that the patient has no intra-abdominal injuries requiring surgical exploration. Patients with severe pelvic fractures and massive retroperitoneal bleeding are always initially managed nonoperatively. Once the retroperitoneal bleeding is controlled and the patient is stable, delayed repair of the extraperitoneal rupture can be performed, if necessary. Complications of bladder rupture include hemorrhage, urinoma, abscess formation, and sepsis.

Injuries to the Urethra Disruption of the urethra is a rare injury in women. It is found mostly in men, frequently after either pelvic fractures or straddle injuries. Posterior urethral injuries are present in approximately 10% of pelvic fractures. Anterior urethral injuries are generally associated with straddle injuries and are often isolated lesions. Urethral injuries should be suspected on the basis of the mechanism of injury, associated pelvic fracture, perineal hematoma or perineal injury, blood at the urethral meatus, and displacement of the prostate gland. A retrograde urethrogram is essential for diagnosis. Currently, patients sustaining urethral injuries should be managed initially by bladder decompression via suprapubic cystostomy and delayed urethroplasty. Complications of urethral injuries include stricture, incontinence, and impotence with disruptions of the urethra.

Pelvic Fractures

Pelvic fractures are the prototype of severe trauma and account for less than 5% of all fractures after trauma. The most frequent mechanisms causing pelvic fractures are motor vehicle accidents, motorcycle accidents, falls, and accidents involving pedestrians. Unstable pelvic fractures are accompanied, most of the time, by major retroperitoneal hemorrhage. The incidence of associated injuries is high, particularly intra-abdominal, thoracic, and head injuries.

Mortality rates vary depending on the amount of bleeding and the number of associated injuries. The mortality rate directly attributed to pelvic fracture is less than 15% in most series.

Pain is frequently present in an awake and alert patient. Urethral injury in males is also frequent and may be manifested as urethral bleeding or inability to void with a distended bladder. Careful examination of the perineum is imperative because the mortality associated with open pelvic fractures is severalfold higher than that for closed fractures. A rectal examination should be performed carefully to identify rectal bleeding, to evaluate the position of the prostate gland, and to assess for mucosal lacerations. If the prostate is misplaced or urethral bleeding is present, a retrograde urethrogram is mandatory before Foley catheter placement.

An AP film of the pelvis usually shows the fracture and asymmetry of the pelvis if present. The radiographic evaluation in these circumstances should be complemented by inlet and outlet views of the pelvis. CT scan of the pelvis provides information on displacement of the sacroiliac joint, acetabular fractures, and sacral fractures; however it should not be performed in a hemodynamically unstable patient.

Pelvic fractures can be classified according to the resultant vector force (AP compression, lateral compression, and vertical shear), anatomy of the fracture lines, and pelvic stability.

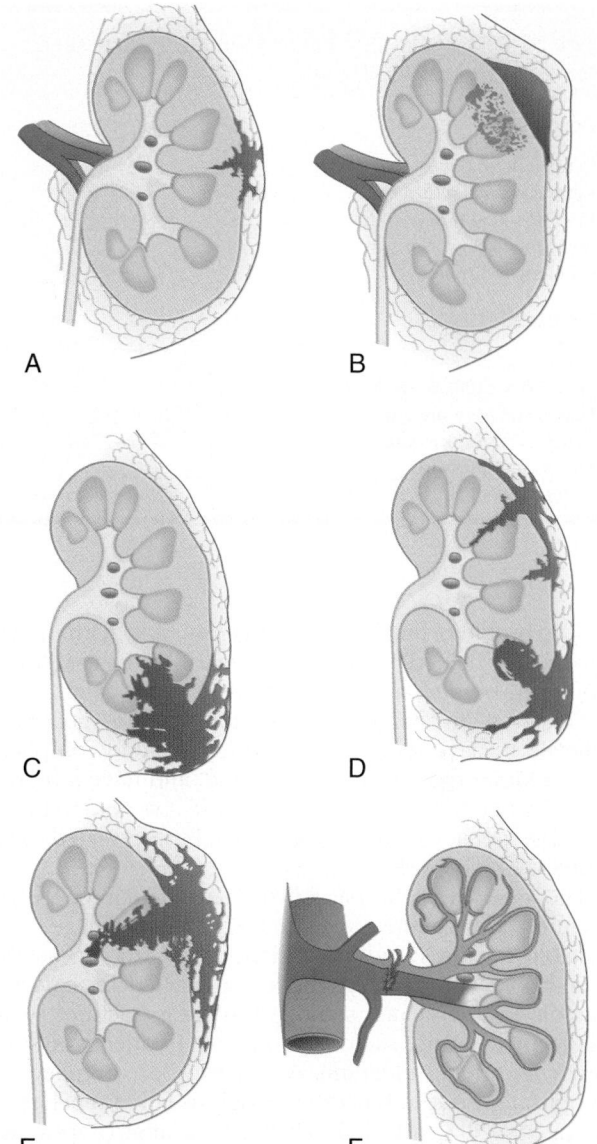

Figure 20-24 Different types of renal injury. **A,** Small renal laceration with contained subcapsular hematoma. **B,** Minor subcapsular and parenchymal hematoma. **C,** Parenchymal laceration extending through the renal cortex without involvement of the collecting system. **D,** Multiple parenchymal lacerations; the inferior one extends through the cortex and collecting system. **E,** Parenchymal laceration extending through the cortex, medulla, and collecting system, along with major subcapsular hematoma and urine extravasation. **F,** Injury to the renal vessels at the hilum. (From Peterson NE: Genitourinary trauma. In Feliciano DV, Moore EE, Mattox KL [eds]: Trauma, 3rd ed. Norwalk, CT, Appleton & Lange, 1996, p 667, with permission of the McGraw-Hill Companies.)

Box 20-6   Physiologic Consequences of Increased Intra-abdominal Pressure

Decreased

Cardiac output
Central venous return
Visceral blood flow
Renal blood flow
Glomerular filtration

Increased

Cardiac rate
Pulmonary capillary wedge pressure
Peak inspiratory pressure
Central venous pressure
Intrapleural pressure
Systemic vascular resistance

The problem that trauma surgeons face with pelvic fractures is related to retroperitoneal bleeding. Hemorrhage can be arterial, venous, or osseous in origin.

Fractures involving the posterior ring are generally believed to have more associated injuries and complications, require more resuscitation fluid, and have a higher mortality rate than is the case with pure anterior fractures. Unstable pelvic fractures are generally associated with increased blood loss.

The objectives of the initial management of pelvic fractures are directed to control of hemorrhage. For unstable fractures and particularly those known as the open-book type, this can be accomplished by external fixation in the acute setting. Posterior fractures with involvement of the sacroiliac joint are frequently associated with arterial bleeding, which can be controlled by embolization of the bleeding vessel, usually branches of the internal iliac artery. Indications for angiography are recurrent hypotension after initial resuscitation attributable to the pelvic fracture or transfusion requirements exceeding 4 to 6 units within the first 2 hours after injury. Blood infusion should be started early during resuscitation in hemodynamically unstable patients. As a temporizing measure, the abdominal component of the MAST suit can be inflated during transport or in the resuscitation room to stabilize the pelvis and control bleeding.

Because of the high incidence of associated intra-abdominal injuries, supraumbilical DPL should be performed; however there is an approximately 35% rate of false-positive results with DPL in the presence of retroperitoneal hematoma. Stable patients are best evaluated with an abdominal CT scan.

If there is a clear indication for abdominal exploration and the retroperitoneum is intact, the hematoma should not be entered because of an increased risk for uncontrolled bleeding. In this circumstance, stabilization of the pelvis and angiographic embolization should be performed. If the retroperitoneum is ruptured and active bleeding is found during exploratory laparotomy, packing the pelvis with temporary closure of the abdomen, followed by external fixation and angiographic evaluation, is appropriate.

Damage Control

The traditional approach to abdominal trauma is not applicable in devastating injuries. Repeated episodes of hypotension and organ hypoperfusion will lead to severe metabolic acidosis, coagulopathy, and hypothermia that persist during the postoperative period despite adequate surgical treatment of multiple injuries. Recently, a new approach has been proposed in these circumstances. Damage control includes an abbreviated laparotomy, temporary packing, and closure of the abdomen in an effort to blunt the physiologic response to prolonged shock and massive hemorrhage. During the initial operation, bleeding and contamination are controlled with temporary measures. The abdomen is packed and temporarily closed, and reconstruction and repair are delayed. The patient is then transferred to an intensive care unit, where further resuscitation and rewarming are performed, acidosis and coagulopathy are corrected, and full physiologic support is instituted. When the patient is stable and organ function is maintained, usually 48 to 72 hours after the initial operation, the patient is taken back to the operating room for removal of the packing, débridement of nonviable tissue, and definitive repair.[8]

Abdominal Compartment Syndrome

Abdominal compartment syndrome occurs predominantly in patients in profound shock, in patients requiring large amounts of resuscitation fluids and blood, and in those with major visceral or vascular abdominal injuries.

Abdominal compartment syndrome is characterized by a sudden increase in intra-abdominal pressure, increased peak inspiratory pressure, decreased urinary output, hypoxia, hypercapnia, and hypotension secondary to decreased venous return to the heart. The diagnosis is confirmed by measuring bladder pressure, which ultimately represents intra-abdominal pressure. Treatment includes rapid decompression of the elevated intra-abdominal pressure by opening the abdominal wound and performing a temporary closure of the abdominal wall with mesh or a plastic bag (Bogota bag). The physiologic consequences of persistent elevated intra-abdominal pressure are listed in Box 20-6.

Wound-Related Complications of Damage Control

Temporary closure of the abdomen in damage control procedures is accompanied by high rates of wound complications. Wound complications such as infection, abscess, or fistula formation occurred in 25%. Death after wound closure occurred in 12%, and deaths were directly related to the wound complication in 23%. Morbidity is associated with the timing and method of wound closure (primary closure, skin grafting or absorbable mesh [or both], and prosthetic material [absorbable mesh]) and transfusion volume, but unrelated to severity of the injury. Delayed primary closure during the first week after injury seems to be associated with lower complication rates.[50]

Selected References

Acosta JA, Yang JC, Winchell RJ, et al: Lethal injuries and time to death in a level I trauma center. J Am Coll Surg 186:528-533, 1998.

This paper describes a 10-year experience of death after injury and delineates the time to death in a level I trauma center. It serves as a good reference for assessing the outcome of injured patients and helps define the priorities for ongoing research in hemorrhage control, resuscitation, and management of head injury and multiple organ failure.

Brain Trauma Foundation, American Association of Neurological Surgeons, Joint Section on Neurotrauma and Critical Care: Guidelines for the management of severe head injury. J Neurotrauma 17:471-491, 2000.

This article represents the recommendations of the Brain Trauma Foundation based on their evidence-based assessment and development of guidelines for the management of head injury. This is the second revision of this important work and is the most complete example to date of the use of evidence-based medicine in trauma. It has changed the way in which most people approach head injury, and there is some evidence to suggest that following these guidelines improves overall outcome.

Committee on Trauma: Resources for Optimal Care of the Injured Patient: 2006. Chicago, American College of Surgeons, 2006.

This monograph, written by the Committee on Trauma, defines the resources for optimal care of an injured patient. This document is rewritten every 4 to 5 years and has evolved as the standard for trauma care in the United States and for much of the world. The monograph is written by members of the Committee on Trauma, who are all national authorities on trauma care. The current version is the basis for assessing trauma centers and verifying them against these standards.

Feliciano DV, Moore EE: Mattox KL: Trauma, 5th ed. New York, McGraw-Hill, 2005.

This text is the classic reference in trauma throughout the world. It is in its fifth edition and is written by authors who truly represent the leaders in trauma care. The book is comprehensive and covers all aspects from the history of trauma centers to the critical care of trauma patients. The chapters are current and the reference lists are excellent; this should be viewed as the standard textbook in trauma care.

Ivatury RR, Cayton CG: Textbook of Penetrating Trauma. Philadelphia, Lea & Febiger, 1996.

This is the first book devoted exclusively to the management of penetrating trauma. The authors are leading authorities throughout the country, and the text covers all aspects of trauma care for penetrating injuries.

MacKenzie EJ, Hoyt DB, Sacra JC, et al: National Inventory of Hospital Trauma Centers. JAMA 289:1515-1522, 2003.

This paper describes a national inventory of trauma centers and reflects the current status of trauma center distribution and readiness. It is an important paper that describes how far we have come since the last assessment (in the early 1990s) and how far we have to go. This is particularly important given the fact that a trauma system is the basis for an organized response to disasters.

Mullins RJ: The Skamania Conference. J Trauma 47(3):S2, 1999.

This consensus conference at Skamania evaluated the overall status of trauma system development and established a consensus regarding the efficacy of trauma systems in reducing mortality. The entire reference list raises essentially every issue. It has been effectively used to help encourage development of trauma systems nationwide.

Bonnie RJ, Fulco CE, Liverman CT (eds): Reducing the Burden of Injury: Advancing Prevention and Treatment. Washington, DC, Committee on Injury Prevention and Control, Division of Health Promotion and Disease Prevention. Institute of Medicine, National Academic Press, 1999.

This monograph is the most recent evaluation of current problems with regard to the development of trauma systems and challenges for acute care. The study was commissioned by the Institute of Medicine and represents the most current synthesis of what is known and what is left to be done in trauma care in the United States.

References

1. Acosta JA, Yang JC, Winchell RJ, et al: Lethal injuries and time to death in a level I trauma center. J Am Coll Surg 186:528-533, 1998.
2. Nathens AB, Jurkovich GJ, Maier RV, et al: Relationship between trauma center volume and outcomes. JAMA 285:1164-1171, 2001.
3. MacKenzie EJ, Hoyt DB, Sacra JC, et al: National Inventory of Hospital Trauma Centers. JAMA 289:1515-1522, 2003.
4. Demetriades D, Murray J, Chan L, et al: Penetrating colon injuries requiring resection: Diversion or primary anastomosis? AAST prospective multicenter study. J Trauma 50:765-775, 2001.
5. Accidental Death and Disability: The Neglected Disease of Modern Society. Washington, DC, National Academy of Sciences, National Research Council, 1966.
6. Shackford SR, MacKersie RC, Hoyt DB, et al: Impact of a trauma system on outcome of severely injured patients. Arch Surg 122:523-527, 1987.
7. Bickel WH, Wall MJ, Pepe PE, et al: Immediate versus delayed fluid resuscitation for hypotensive patients with penetrating torso injuries. N Engl J Med, 331:1105-1109, 1994.
8. Rotondo MF, Schwab CW, McGonigal MD, et al: "Damage control": An approach for improved survival in exsanguinating penetrating abdominal injury. J Trauma 35:375-383, 1993.
9. Holbrook TL, Anderson JP, Sieber WJ, et al: Outcome after major trauma: 12-month and 18 month follow-up results from the Trauma Recovery Project. J Trauma 46:765-773, 1999.
10. Hoyt DB, Moore EE, Shackford SR, et al: Trauma surgeon's leadership role in the development of trauma systems [editorial]. J Trauma 46:1142, 1999.
11. Bochicchio GV, Ilahi O, Joshi, M, et al: Endotracheal intubation in the field does not improve outcome in trauma patients who present without an acutely lethal traumatic brain injury. J Trauma 54:307-311, 2003.
12. Patel NY, Hoyt DB, Nakhai P, et al: Traumatic brain injury: Patterns of failure of nonoperative management. J Trauma 48:367-375, 2000.
13. Lee LA, Sharar SR, Lam AM: Perioperative head injury management in the multiply injured trauma patient. Int Anesthesiol Clin 40:31-52, 2002.
14. The Brain Trauma Foundation, The American Association of Neurological Surgeons, The Joint Section on Neurotrauma and Critical Care: Guidelines for the management of severe head injury. J Neurotrauma 17:471-491, 2000.
15. Sarrafzadeh AS, Peltonen EE, Kaisers U, et al: Secondary insults in severe head injury—do multiply injured patients do worse? Crit Care Med 29:1116-1123, 2001.
16. Bracken MB, Shepard MJ, Holford TR, et al: Administration of methylprednisolone for 24 or 48 hours or tirilazad mesylate for 48 hours in the treatment of acute spinal cord

injury—results of the Third National Acute Spinal Cord Injury Randomized Controlled Trial. JAMA 277:1597-1604, 1997.

17. Asensio JA, Valenziano CP, Falcone RE, Grosh JD: Management of penetrating neck injuries. The controversy surrounding zone II injuries. Surg Clin North Am 71:267-296, 1991

18. Mazolewski PJ, Dylan C, Browder T, Fildes J: Computerized tomographic scan can be used for surgical decision making in zone II penetrating neck injuries. J Trauma 51:315-319, 2001.

19. Schneidereit NP, Simons R, Nicolaou S, et al: Utility of screening for blunt vascular neck injuries with computed tomographic angiography. J Trauma 60:209-216, 2006.

20. Hoyt DB, Coimbra R, Potenza BM, Rappold JF: Anatomic exposures for vascular injuries. Surg Clin North Am 81:1299-1330, 2001.

21. Cothren CC, Moore EE, Ray CE Jr, et al: Carotid artery stents for blunt cerebrovascular injury: Risks exceed benefits. Arch Surg 140:480-486, 2005.

22. Roth FS, Kokoska MS, Awwad EE, et al: The identification of mandible fractures by helical computed tomography and Panorex tomography. J Craniofac Surg 16:394-399, 2005.

23. Handschel JG, Depprich RA, Dirksen D, et al: A prospective comparison of octyl-2-cyanoacrylate and suture in standardized facial wounds. Int J Oral Maxillofac Surg 35:318-323, 2005.

24. Sisley A, Rozycki G, Ballard R, et al: Rapid detection of traumatic effusion using surgeon-performed ultrasound. J Trauma 44:291-297, 1998.

25. Avidan V, Hersch M, Armon Y, et al: Blast lung injury: Clinical manifestations, treatment, and outcome. Am J Surg 190:945-950, 2005.

26. Cothren C, Moore E, Biffl WL, et al: Lung-sparing techniques are associated with improved outcome compared with anatomic resection for severe lung injuries. J Trauma 53:483-487, 2002.

27. Karmy-Jones R, Jurkovich GJ, Shatz DV, et al: Management of traumatic lung injury: A Western Trauma Association multicenter review. J Trauma 51:1049-1053, 2001.

28. Wall M, Hirshberg A, Mattox K: Pulmonary tractotomy with selective vascular ligation for penetrating injuries to the lung. Am J Surg 168:665-669, 1994.

29. Velmahos GC, Karaiskakis M, Salim A, et al: Normal electrocardiography and serum troponin I levels preclude the presence of clinically significant blunt cardiac injury. J Trauma 54:45-51, 2003.

30. Coimbra R, Pinto MCC, Razuk A, et al: Penetrating cardiac wounds: Predictive value of trauma indices and the necessity of terminology standardization. Am Surg 61:448-452, 1995.

31. Stassen NA, Lukan JK, Spain DA, et al: Reevaluation of diagnostic procedures for transmediastinal gunshot wounds. J Trauma 53:635-638, 2002.

32. Duane TM, Tan BB, Golay D, et al: Blunt trauma and the role of routine pelvic radiographs: A prospective analysis. J Trauma 53:463-468, 2002.

33. Healey MA, Simons RK, Winchell RJ, et al: A prospective evaluation of abdominal ultrasound in blunt trauma: Is it useful? J Trauma 40:875-885, 1996.

34. Velmahos GC, Constantinou C, Tillou A, et al: Abdominal computed tomographic scan for patients with gunshot wounds to the abdomen selected for non-operative management. J Trauma 59:1155-1161, 2005.

35. Ivatury RR, Nallathambi M, Gaudino J, et al: Penetrating duodenal injuries: Analysis of 100 consecutive cases. Ann Surg 202:153-158, 1985.

36. Jurkovich GJ, Carrico CJ: Pancreatic trauma. Surg Clin North Am 70:575-593, 1990.

37. Fakhry SM, Watts DD, Luchette FA, for the EAST Multi-Institutional HVI Research Group: Current diagnostic approaches lack sensitivity in the diagnosis of perforated blunt small bowel injury. An analysis from 275,557 trauma admissions from the EAST multi-institutional trial. J Trauma 54:295-306, 2003.

38. Weinberg JA, Fabian TC, Magnotti LJ, et al: Penetrating rectal trauma: Management by anatomic distinction improves outcome. J Trauma 60:508-514, 2006.

39. Cogbill TH, Moore EE, Jurkovich GJ, et al: Severe hepatic trauma: A multi-center experience with 1335 liver injuries. J Trauma 28:1433-1438, 1988.

40. Jurkovich G, Hoyt D, Moore F, et al: Portal triad injuries: A multi-institutional study. J Trauma 39:426-434, 1995.

41. Croce MA, Fabian TC, Menke PG, et al: Nonoperative management of blunt trauma is the treatment of choice for hemodynamically stable patients. Results of a prospective trial. Ann Surg 221:744-755, 1995.

42. Demetriades D, Gomez H, Chahwan S, et al: Gunshot injuries to the liver: The role of selective nonoperative management. J Am Coll Surg 188:343-348, 1999.

43. Malhotra AK, Fabian TC, Croce MA, et al: Blunt hepatic injury: A paradigm shift from operative to nonoperative management in the 1990s. Ann Surg 231:804-813, 2000.

44. Ciraulo DL, Luk S, Palter M, et al: Selective hepatic arterial embolization of grade IV and V blunt hepatic injuries: An extension of resuscitation in the non-operative management of traumatic hepatic injuries. J Trauma 45:353-359, 1998.

45. Hagiwara A, Murata A, Matsuda T, et al: The efficacy and limitations of transarterial embolization for severe hepatic injury. J Trauma 52:1091-1096, 2002.

46. Richardson JD, Franklin GA, Lukan JK, et al: Evolution in the management of hepatic trauma: A 25-year experience. Ann Surg 232:324-330, 2000.

47. Fang JF, Chen RJ, Wong YC, et al: Classification and treatment of pooling of contrast material on computed tomographic scan of blunt hepatic trauma. J Trauma 49:1083-1088, 2000.

48. Nance ML, Peden GW, Shapiro MB, et al: Solid viscus injury predicts major hollow viscus injury in blunt abdominal trauma. J Trauma 43:618-623, 1997.

49. Haan J, Scott J, Boyd-Kranis RL, et al: Admission angiography for blunt splenic injury: Advantages and pitfalls. J Trauma 51:1161-1165, 2001.

50. Miller RS, Morris JA Jr, Diaz JJ Jr, et al: Complications after 344 damage-control open celiotomies. J Trauma 59:1365-1374, 2005.

Emergency Care of Musculoskeletal Injuries

Bruce D. Browner, MD   and   Joseph P. DeAngelis, MD

- Epidemiology of Orthopedic Injuries
- Terminology
- Fixation Principles
- Patient Evaluation
- Initial Management
- Orthopedic Emergencies
- Common Long Bone Fractures
- Complications
- Postoperative Mobilization
- Summary

EPIDEMIOLOGY OF ORTHOPEDIC INJURIES

Accidents continue to be a prominent cause of death and disability throughout the world. In the first 5 decades of life, trauma accounts for more deaths than any other cause, and in all age groups, accidents are the fifth leading cause of death in the United States. In general, it is the amount of energy absorbed by a multiply injured patient that corresponds to the extent of the musculoskeletal injuries. Because high energy is frequently involved, fractures and soft tissue injuries are common. Of the more than 174,000 patient records in the Major Trauma Outcomes Study, 48.6% had one or more musculoskeletal injuries between 1982 and 1990.[1] When the disability associated with musculoskeletal injuries is tabulated, the ensuing costs are staggering; hundreds of billions of dollars are consumed by medical expenses, lost productivity, and property damage annually.

At the national and global levels, substantial improvements in both transportation safety and delivery of medical care have helped address this growing pandemic. Seat belt and helmet laws, enforcement of drunk-driving laws, mandates for improved safety features in automobiles, rapid deployment of emergency medical

teams, and establishment of trauma centers have decreased the number of accident scene fatalities. With more victims now likely to survive accidents that might have been fatal in the past, caregivers will be challenged with managing more complex fractures and soft tissue wounds. These realities demand that trauma teams be aware of the frequency and the consequences of musculoskeletal injuries in every patient. An appreciation for the unique features of skeletal injury in patients who may also have severe head, thoracic, or intra-abdominal trauma is essential. In this way, a cohesive, integrated approach to the diagnosis and treatment of musculoskeletal injuries is integral to the care of a multiply injured patient.

TERMINOLOGY

Communication among collaborating specialists is central to patient care, and the trauma and emergency department findings need to be relayed precisely to consulting specialists. This task is particularly challenging in view of the variety of anatomic locations and fracture patterns encountered in orthopedics. Although many injuries are identified by eponyms within the orthopedic community, the most practical and universally understood characterizations of injuries are those that adhere to basic anatomic and mechanical principles.

Fracture Types

A *fracture* is a disruption of the normal architecture of bone. In pediatric injuries, this disruption can include an injury to or through the cartilaginous growth plate that may not be evident radiographically. *Acute* fractures have sharp, well-defined edges of the fragments. *Chronic* fractures have a rounded and sclerotic appearance after resorption of bone has occurred at the fracture ends. This distinction can usually be made on clinical examination. Incomplete disruptions of bone are termed *greenstick fractures* in children or *infractions* in adults. Chronic, repetitive trauma can also cause microscopic disruptions when bone is stressed beyond its failure point. These injuries are termed *stress fractures* and are considered overuse injuries.

When a bone fails through an area weakened by pre-existing disease, it is termed a *pathologic fracture*. Causes may include weakness from primary bone tumors, metastatic lesions, infection, metabolic disease, and injury to an old fracture site. Though not commonly referred to in this way, fractures in osteoporotic bone are technically pathologic. However, the term *insufficiency* or *fragility fracture* is most frequently used to describe these injuries. In distinction to acute fractures in healthy bone, fragility fractures normally result from accidents with much lower energy, such as a fall from standing height. Hip fractures, compression fractures of the vertebral bodies, and distal radius fractures in the elderly are common examples.

A fracture is considered *open* when an overlying wound produces communication between the fracture site and the outside environment. These fractures can range from an inside-to-outside poke hole in the skin to severe crush injuries. High-energy fracture patterns indicate that the soft tissues, as well as the bones, have absorbed large forces. Although the skin laceration is the most obvious component, the energy of the fracture, the degree of contamination, and the soft tissue injury must all be taken into account when grading the severity of the injury. Contamination of bone can lead to the development of osteomyelitis and all of its catastrophic consequences and thus necessitates emergency treatment.

An *intra-articular* fracture extends into a joint. When there is significant cartilage damage, late degenerative changes are likely. These injuries are normally caused by a compressive, or axial, load across the joint. Displaced intra-articular fractures require urgent anatomic reduction and rigid fixation to minimize post-traumatic arthritis.

Long bone fractures are characterized by anatomic location. The *epiphysis* includes the area between the growth plate (physis), or physeal scar, and the articular surface. The *metaphysis* is located between the epiphysis and the shaft and includes the growth plate. The bone in this area is softer and more vascular because of its cancellous nature. The *diaphysis* encompasses the shaft of the bone between the proximal and distal metaphyses. Fractures can be described according to location within these three sections or location in the bone (proximal, middle, and distal). Distally, the humerus and femur flare to form their articular surfaces. These flares are termed the *epicondyles*, and fractures in these areas are referred to as *supracondylar*. The articular surfaces are known as *condyles*. Condylar fractures are intra-articular and may extend proximally. Such distinctions are important because these injuries present difficult treatment challenges.

A fracture may also be described by the pattern of cortical disruption. The orientation of the primary fracture line may be transverse, oblique, or spiral. *Transverse* and *oblique fractures* occur when a bending moment is applied. *Spiral fractures* generally result from a rotational

force about the long axis of the bone. *Comminution* is the presence of multiple fragments involved in a fracture and usually connotes a higher-energy injury or weakened bone in an elderly patient. A *butterfly fragment* is an area of comminution in one of the simple fracture patterns previously described (Fig. 21-1D).

Displacement, if present, is described from a combination of principles. These deformities may occur in any plane. When viewed on plain radiographs, all injuries will be resolved into pure coronal or sagittal displacement. However, it is important to realize that the true displacement usually occurs in a plane that is somewhere in between. *Translation* is the relationship of the proximal fracture fragment to the distal one. It is described in terms of percent overlap. A fracture with 100% translation in any plane is completely displaced. *Angulation* is simply the angle created by the displaced fracture fragments. It is described by the direction of the apex that the fracture fragments form (e.g., 20 degree apex lateral). The final component is *rotation*. To truly describe rotation, a full-length film of the limb segment involved, including the joints above and below, must be examined. A fracture may appear nondisplaced on one radiographic view yet be significantly displaced on another.

Once a fracture has been identified, it must be described in a consistent, systematic manner. All descriptions begin with whether the fracture is open and its grade. A closed fracture is assumed if no indication is given otherwise. The presence of an intra-articular fracture is then communicated. The side of the body and the injured bone are stated next. A description of the pattern followed by its location in the bone is then indicated. Finally, the displacement as described previously is related. Adherence to this scheme allows universal understanding of the fracture.

Other Injuries

Ligamentous injuries are commonly encountered in all areas of orthopedics. When a ligament is damaged but is still in continuity, it is termed a *sprain*. Sprains can range in severity from minimal injuries to moderate instability about a joint. Grade I ligamentous injuries are caused by stretching of a ligament or ligament complex. They do not normally result in instability. A simple ankle sprain is the typical example of this type of injury. Partial ruptures of ligaments can result in minor instability and are considered grade II injuries. Complete ruptures, or grade III injuries, lead to significant instability at the associated joint. Avulsion fractures at the insertion of ligamentous structures also fall into this category. Ligamentous injuries cannot be overlooked because they can produce significant joint instability and endanger the surrounding soft tissue and neurovascular structures. This detail is critical when evaluating injuries to the axial skeleton.

A *strain* is an injury to a muscle or tendon. These injuries are most commonly of an overuse nature. Further loading of the already weakened structure can compound these injuries. Rest, ice, compression, and elevation are the mainstays of treatment.

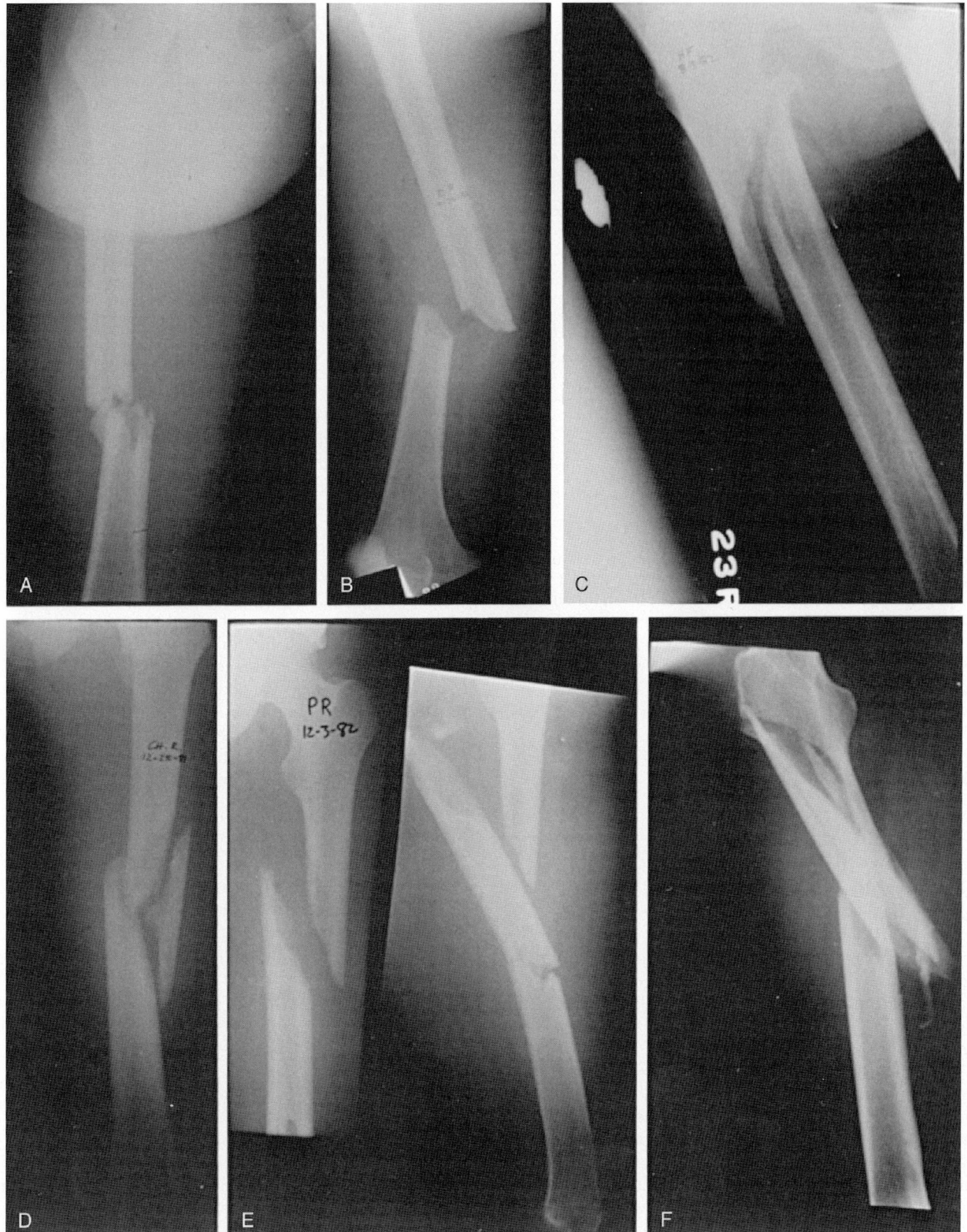

Figure 21-1 Descriptive terms used to characterize femoral shaft fractures. **A,** Transverse midshaft fracture. **B,** Short oblique fracture. **C,** Long oblique fracture. **D,** Butterfly (or wedge) fragment in a midshaft femoral fracture. **E,** Segmental fracture. **F,** Comminuted fracture. (From Wolinsky PR, Johnson KD: Femoral shaft fractures. In Browner BD, Jupiter TB, Levine AM, Trafton PG [eds]: Skeletal Trauma, 2nd ed. Philadelphia, WB Saunders, 1998.)

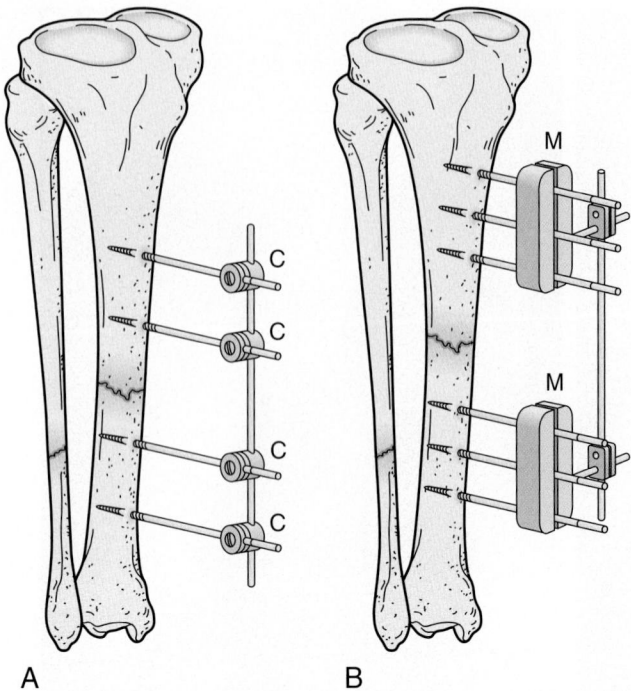

Figure 21-2 Frame types. **A,** Simple frame clamps (C) connect a single pin individually to the rod or rods. **B,** Modular frame clamps (M) connect clusters of two or three pins to the connecting rod or rods. (From Pollak AN, Ziran BH: Principles of external fixation. In Browner BD, Jupiter TB, Levine AM, Trafton PG [eds]: Skeletal Trauma, 3rd ed. Philadelphia, WB Saunders, 2003.)

FIXATION PRINCIPLES

External Fixation

External fixation provides stabilization of an injured limb segment through the use of pins or wires connected to rods via clamps or rings. With the exception of the pins or wires, the rigid construct is external to the body, as the name implies. Recent designs are more complex but are easier to apply and more stable than ever before. The addition of modularity has added to their prospective uses and has led to more adaptable and adjustable constructs.

The primary use of external fixation is for the treatment of open fractures, fractures in unstable patients who cannot tolerate significant anesthesia times or blood loss, complex fractures in which open reduction plus internal fixation (ORIF) is not warranted, and fractures with associated vascular injuries requiring stabilization and urgent vascular repair, as well as for use in specialized limb reconstruction surgery. In fractures with soft tissue injuries, placement of percutaneously inserted pins that minimize further soft tissue damage and avoid the area of contamination helps decrease the incidence of infection and delayed union. External fixators may be used for temporary stabilization or for definitive treatment in select instances. In complex fractures around joints, fixation

with implanted plates or screws may not provide adequate stability. Additionally, overlying soft tissue damage makes operative exposure dangerous. In these instances, an external fixator with the pins placed at a distance from the fracture—and the injured soft tissue—can provide the osseous stability necessary for fracture healing.

External frames are constructed from three components: pins, connectors, and rods (Fig. 21-2). Pins are either threaded or smooth and vary in both length and diameter. They serve to connect the bone to the rest of the device. Pin placement is chosen to best stabilize the fracture while not compromising the viability of the fragments. Pins are never placed through compromised or infected skin. A variety of different clamps serve as connectors and secure pins to the rods that form the external frames. Most are universal joints that allow multiple degrees of freedom. Connecting clamps have advanced to the point that they now snap in place onto the pins and the rods. They may be combined with rings or hinged rods and allow infinite permutations of frame constructs. Stabilizing rods are nearly universally radiolucent to allow radiographic examination after application. Threaded rods, bone transport rails, motorized lengthening devices, and dynamic struts represent a small sample of the types of rods that can be used to achieve specific results.

Once applied, external fixators require regular care and monitoring. Pin care is begun immediately and consists of cleansing with either normal saline or half-strength peroxide solution. Drainage from pin sites must be addressed with local care, antibiotics, pin removal and replacement, or a combination of these measures. Pins are checked regularly to ensure that they have not loosened. Depending on the fracture pattern, the fixator construct, and the goals of treatment, the weight-bearing status is adjusted.

Internal Fixation

ORIF implies that an incision is made at or near the site of injury to facilitate reduction of the fracture under direct vision (open reduction) and rigid stabilization with plates, screws, wires, or combinations thereof (internal fixation). ORIF is frequently used to treat periarticular fractures and fractures of the axial skeleton. This technique allows anatomic reduction and the creation of highly stable constructs. Multiple types of implants can be used to achieve these results.

Pins and Screws
Pins and screws are the simplest implants. They can be introduced in a variety of areas and are often placed percutaneously. Kirschner wires may be used temporarily and frequently are used for the stabilization of small fragments. They can also be used provisionally to hold the fracture reduction while more stable fixation is applied. Screws can be used for interfragmentary compression when placed with a lag technique (Fig. 21-3). This technique involves the use of a gliding hole in one fragment to allow the screw to compress one fragment against another.

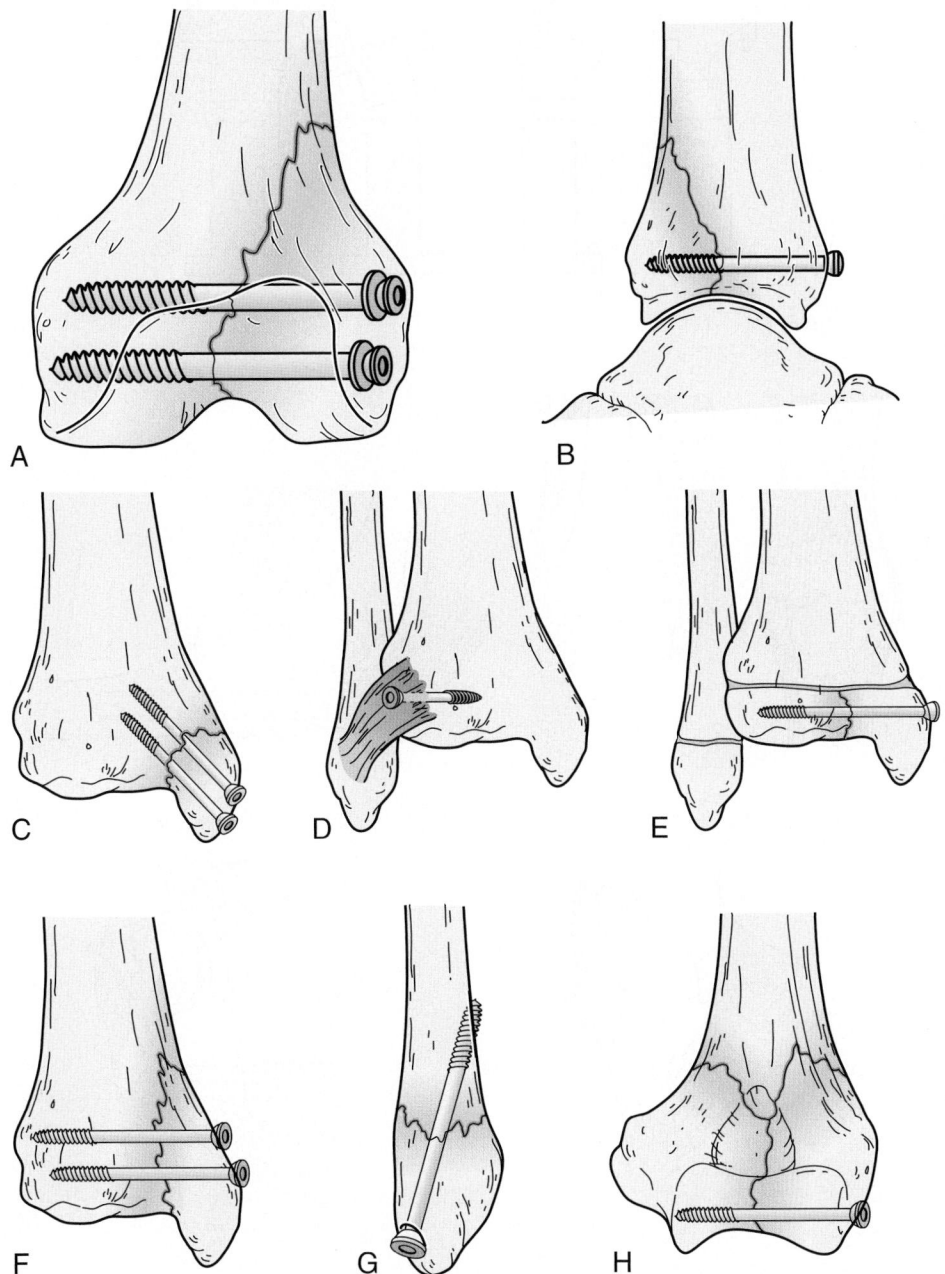

Figure 21-3 Typical indications for cancellous lag screws. **A,** Two 6.5-mm cancellous screws with a 32-mm thread, used with washers to fix a lateral femoral condyle fracture. **B,** A 4.0-mm cancellous screw inserted from front to back to fix the posterior lip fragment of the distal tibia. **C,** Two 4.0-mm cancellous screws used to fix a medial malleolus fracture. **D,** A 4.0-mm cancellous screw used to fix a fragment from the anterior aspect of the distal tibia carrying the syndesmotic ligament. **E,** A 4.0-mm cancellous screw used to fix an epiphyseal fracture of the distal tibia. **F,** Two 4.0-mm cancellous screws used to fix an oblique fracture of the medial malleolus. **G,** A malleolar screw inserted obliquely to fix a short, oblique fracture of the distal fibula. This direction of insertion allows cortical purchase with increased compression force. **H,** A 4.0-mm cancellous screw used to fix the vertical component of a supracondylar Y fracture of the distal humerus. (From Mazzocca AD, Caputo AE, Browner BD, et al: Principles of internal fixation. In Browner BD, Jupiter TB, Levine AM, Trafton PG [eds]: Skeletal Trauma, 3rd ed. Philadelphia, WB Saunders, 2003.)

Tension Bands

When the forces across a fracture site tend to displace the fractured pieces in tension, the tension band technique can be applied to convert the displacing tensile forces on one side of a fracture into a compressive force across the entire contact area (Fig. 21-4). Traditionally, wires or cables are used to create tension bands. However, nonabsorbable suture and plates can also be used. Tension bands are used most frequently for fractures of the olecranon, patella, and greater trochanter.

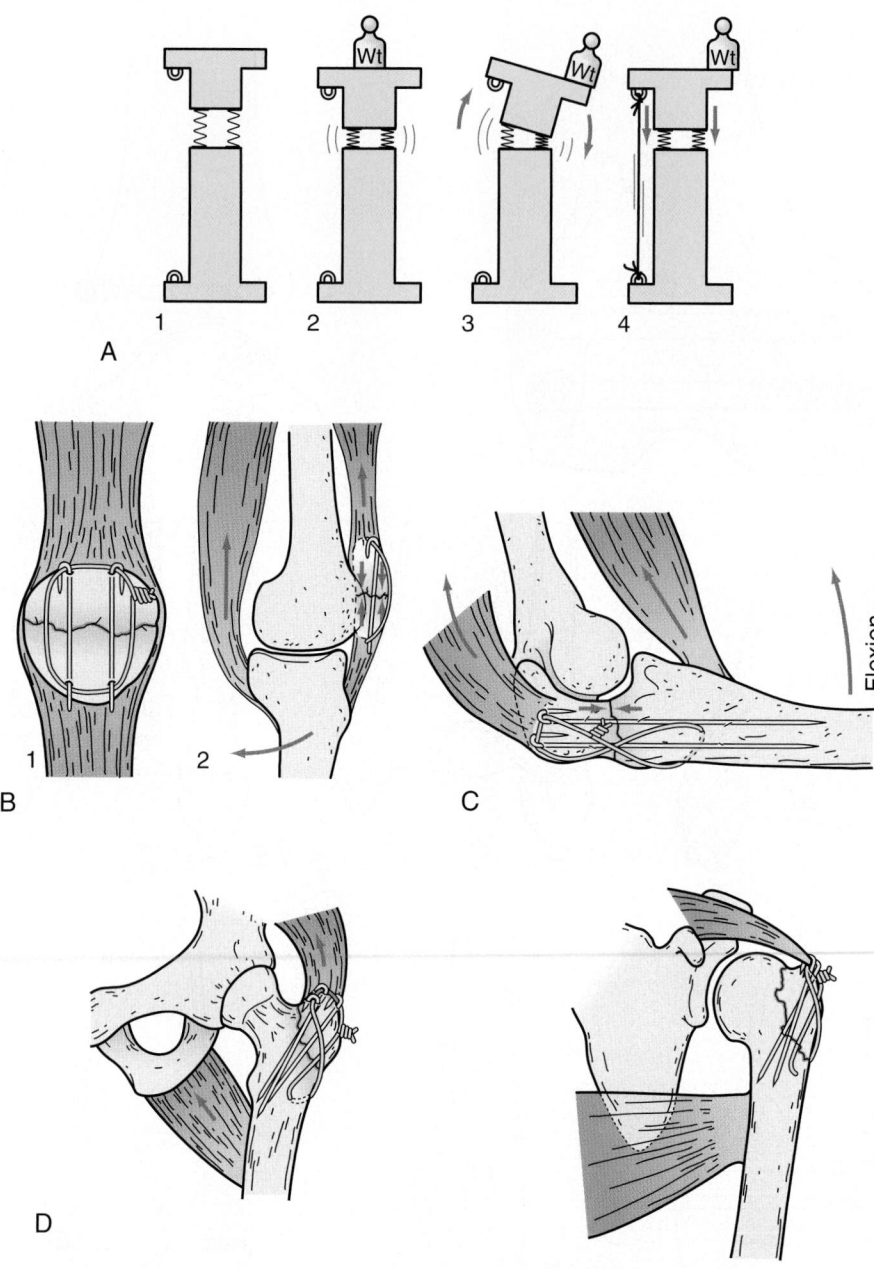

Figure 21-4 Tension band principles. **A,** (1) An interrupted I-beam connected by two springs. (2) The I-beam is loaded with a weight (Wt) placed over the central axis of the beam; there is uniform compression of both springs at the interruption. (3) When the I-beam is loaded eccentrically by placing the weight at a distance from the central axis of the beam, the spring on the same side compresses, whereas the spring on the opposite side is placed in tension and stretches. (4) If a tension band is applied before the eccentric loading, it resists the tension that would otherwise stretch the opposite spring and thus causes uniform compression of both springs. **B,** The tension band principle applied to fixation of a transverse patellar fracture. (1) The anteroposterior view shows the placement of parallel Kirschner wires and the anterior tension band. (2) The lateral view demonstrates antagonistic pull of the hamstrings and quadriceps, which causes a bending moment of the patella over the femoral trochlea. An anterior tension band transforms this eccentric loading into compression at the fracture site. **C,** The tension band principle applied to fixation of a fracture of the ulna. The antagonistic pull of the triceps and brachialis causes a bending moment of the ulna over the humeral trochlea. The dorsal tension band transforms this eccentric load into compression at the fracture site. **D,** The tension band principle applied to fixation of a fracture of the greater trochanter. With the hip as a fulcrum, the antagonistic pull of the adductors and abductors causes a bending moment in the femur. The lateral tension band transforms this eccentric load into compression at the greater trochanteric fracture site. **E,** The tension band principle applied to fixation of a fracture of the greater tuberosity of the humerus. Using the glenoid as a fulcrum, the antagonistic pull of the pectoralis major and supraspinatus causes a bending moment of the humerus. The lateral tension band transforms this eccentric load into compression at the greater tuberosity fracture site. (From Mazzocca AD, Caputo AE, Browner BD, et al: Principles of internal fixation. In Browner BD, Jupiter TB, Levine AM, Trafton PG [eds]: Skeletal Trauma, 3rd ed. Philadelphia, WB Saunders, 2003.)

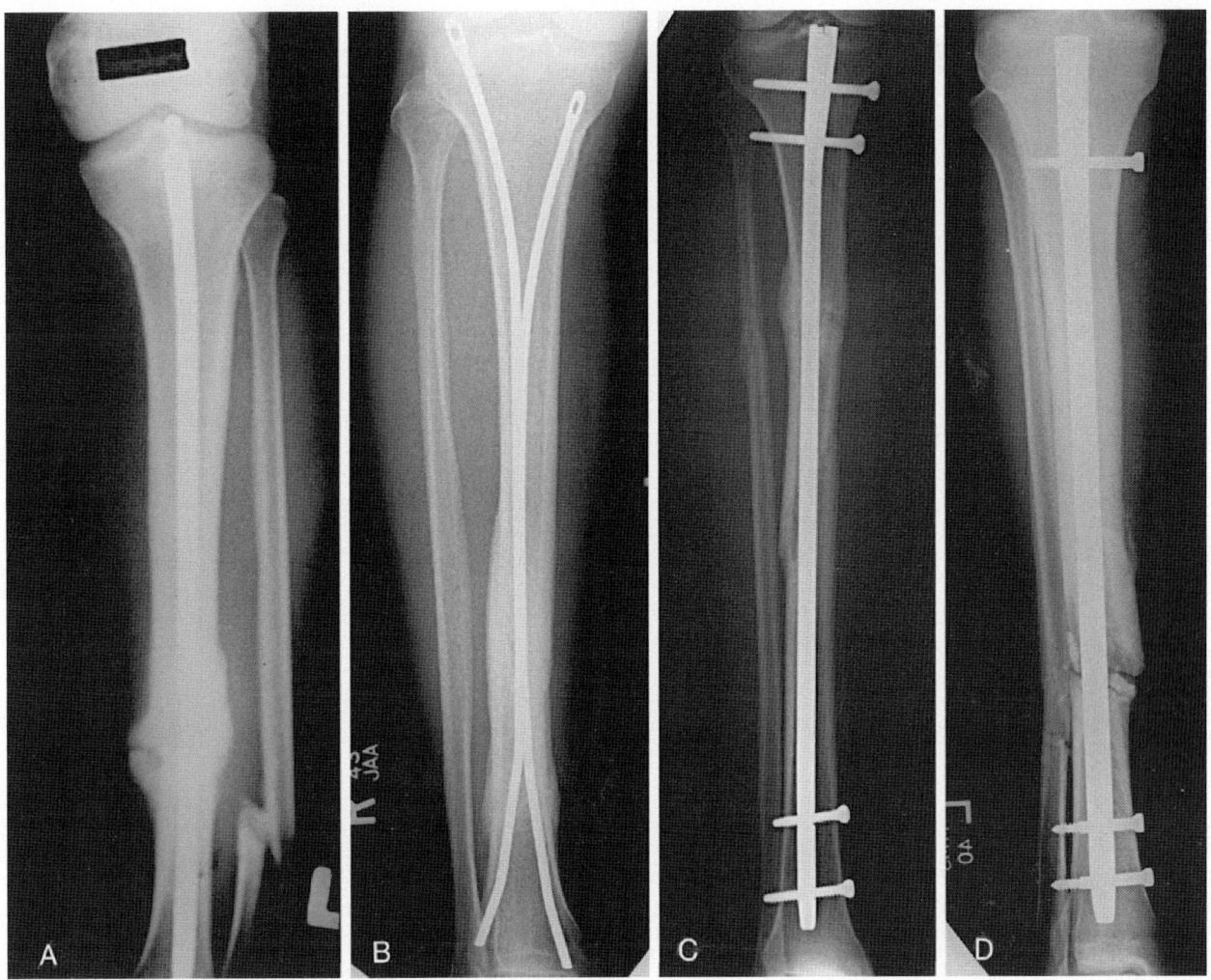

Figure 21-5 Examples of intramedullary fixation of tibial shaft fractures. **A,** Lottes nail. **B,** Ender nails in a patient with an open, comminuted injury of major severity. The wound and fracture healed benignly. The prominent lateral nail was associated with some knee pain until it was removed. **C,** Nonreamed, static, locked intramedullary nail in a patient with a healing, major comminuted injury. **D,** Reamed, locked nail in a patient with a closed injury of major severity. (From Trafton PF: Tibial shaft fractures. In Browner BD, Jupiter TB, Levine AM, Trafton PG [eds]: Skeletal Trauma, 2nd ed. Philadelphia, WB Saunders, 1998.)

Plates

Plates are used frequently for the internal fixation of fractures. They allow even distribution of force across their length and can serve a variety of biomechanical functions.

A *neutralization plate* is used to protect another form of fixation from excessive force. Often used in combination with a lag screw, these plates add stability by preventing torsion and bending. The addition of a neutralization plate allows mobilization earlier than would have been possible with less stable fixation.

Buttress plates are used to counteract forces that occur with axial loading. Longitudinal and oblique fractures near joints tend to displace along the line of the fracture when subjected to axial loads. Plates placed in longitudinal fashion can form an axilla with the intact cortex that prevents axial displacement. Some plates are specifi-

cally designed for buttressing; however, any plate can be applied in a buttress mode.

Compression plating is used to increase the stability of fixation when the two major fracture fragments can be brought into contact. This technique allows direct compression of the fracture ends. Compression plates have oval screw holes with oblique edges that allow eccentric placement of screws. When a screw is applied eccentrically, the plate (and the bone fragment fixed to it) translates as the screw tightens down against the plate to create compression at the fracture. Additionally, compression can also be achieved by overbending a plate or by introducing a tensioning device.

Highly comminuted and segmental fractures may not allow anatomic reduction and direct fixation of all the fragments. In these situations, a *bridge plate* can be used to rigidly stabilize a long bone. The proximal and distal

Table 21-1 Common Patterns and Their Associated Injuries

INJURY PATTERN/MECHANISM	ASSOCIATED INJURIES
Fall from a height	Calcaneus fracture Tibial plateau fracture Fractures around the hip (proximal femur, acetabulum) Vertebral burst fracture
Ejection from a vehicle	Closed head injury Spine fractures
"T-bone" motor vehicle accident	Lateral compression-type pelvic fracture Closed head injury Thoracic injury
Head-on motor vehicle accident	Abdominal visceral injury "Open-book" pelvic fracture Retroperitoneal bleeding
Posterior knee dislocation Supracondylar humerus fracture	Popliteal artery injury Brachial artery injury Nerve injury (median or radial)
Anterior shoulder dislocation Posterior hip dislocation	Axillary nerve injury Sciatic (peroneal division) nerve injury

fragments are rigidly fixed to each other with a plate while the fracture site is bypassed. This concept has been popularized because it allows less dissection at the fracture site, which may devitalize the comminuted and segmental fragments.

Special plates have been designed for certain fracture patterns and anatomic locations. Blade plates, dynamic condylar screws, and pelvic reconstruction plates are examples of these specialized plates.

Intramedullary Nails

In contrast to wires, plates, and screws, intramedullary (IM) nails are placed in the medullary canal of long bones. They are used to splint or bridge a fracture while still controlling axial, bending, and rotational forces. IM nailing also permits fixation of a fracture through an incision distant from the fracture site. This technique has been described as *closed nailing* because the fracture site is not opened. Nails are made of a variety of materials and can be fluted, smooth, solid, or cannulated (Fig. 21-5). When transverse screws are placed through the proximal and distal ends of the nail, the nail is "locked." Locked nails control rotation better and maintain bone length in the presence of comminution or bone loss. The locking holes in nails may be round or oval. Using a nail with an oval hole or leaving the nail unlocked at one end allows the bone fragment to slide axially along the nail and produces compression at the fracture site. Nails locked in this fashion are *dynamically locked.* When screws are inserted through round holes in both ends of the nail, no motion is allowed within the construct; they are *statically locked* (Fig. 21-6).

IM nails can be introduced in a proximal-to-distal or distal-to-proximal direction and are termed *antegrade* and *retrograde,* respectively. Nails may be inserted with or without canal preparation by reaming. *Reaming* involves passing a large drill down the medullary canal to remove the cancellous bone and effectively widen the canal. This increased width allows the insertion of a larger-diameter nail to increase the strength and stiffness of the construct. However, reaming leads to increased pressure in the medullary canal, increased temperature in the cortical bone, and embolization of marrow contents into the vascular system. In patients with severe derangement of pulmonary function or hemodynamic instability, embolization is not well tolerated. At the same time, reaming morcellizes the cancellous and cortical bone in the canal and deposits this exceptional autogenous bone graft at the fracture site.

Unreamed nails are inserted without reaming of the canal, and destruction of the cortical blood supply from the medullary system is largely avoided. In fractures in which there is a large degree of soft tissue loss or periosteal stripping, an unreamed nail is typically used.

PATIENT EVALUATION

History

Obtaining a detailed history of a skeletally injured patient is essential for accurate diagnosis and treatment and is challenging with multiply injured and elderly patients in the trauma setting. However, it is important to gather as much information as possible regarding the mechanism of injury. Descriptions from the accident or injury scene can be most helpful because common patterns of injury follow from specific mechanisms (Table 21-1).

A general history that includes demographic information, past medical history, past surgical history, and social history are obtained. Knowledge of allergies, current medications, and time since last oral intake is useful in guiding treatment. In addition, it is important to obtain information about the position of the limb before and after the injury. Ambulatory status before the injury helps determine realistic goals for functional recovery. Any transient neurologic symptoms, such as loss of consciousness, numbness, paresthesias, and spasm, must be documented. Loss of bowel or bladder control in patients with back or neck pain must also be noted. The time elapsed since injury becomes critical information in a patient with a vascular injury, an open wound, or a dislocation.

Trauma Room Evaluation

Examination of a multiply injured patient must follow advanced trauma life support protocols in a systematic fashion and must be accompanied by treatment. The first 5 minutes of trauma resuscitation is used to secure an airway, establish ventilation, and maintain circulatory support. Hemodynamically unstable patients are assumed to be in hemorrhagic shock until proved otherwise. A search for occult hemorrhage is undertaken and may include the pleural cavities, abdomen, retroperitoneum,

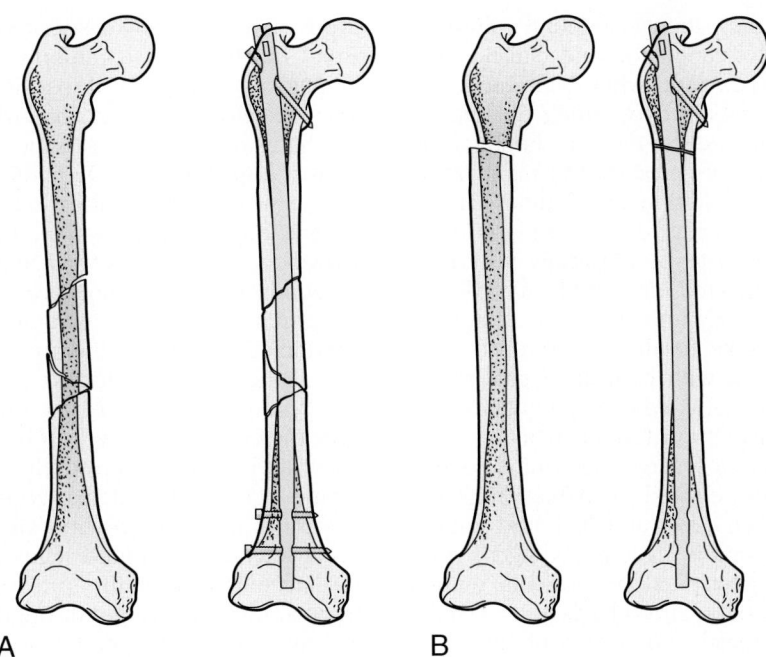

Figure 21-6 A, *Static* locked intramedullary nail fixed to *both* the proximal and the distal fragments. **B,** *Dynamic* locked intramedullary nail fixed to *either* the proximal (as shown) or the distal fragment, but not to both. (From Wolinsky PR, Johnson KD: Femoral shaft fractures. In Browner BD, Jupiter TB, Levine AM, Trafton PG [eds]: Skeletal Trauma, 2nd ed. Philadelphia, WB Saunders, 1998.)

or pelvis. Diagnostic peritoneal lavage or serial transabdominal ultrasound examinations are performed in unstable patients with suspected intra-abdominal injuries. A plain chest radiograph may quickly reveal a hemothorax. Chest tubes are placed, if necessary. The width of the mediastinum is noted, and arteriography is undertaken after life-threatening hemorrhage is controlled. Pelvic instability and the need for rapid external pelvic fixation are addressed. The patient's neurologic status is noted on admission, and the Glasgow Coma Scale score is calculated. Patients with suspected head injury need to be evaluated as soon as possible by computed tomography (CT). Peripheral vascular injuries and musculoskeletal injuries are next in priority, followed by maxillofacial injuries. All open fractures need to be treated within the first 8 hours.[2] Early trauma room management includes antibiotics, tetanus prophylaxis, splinting, and wound coverage. *Sterile dressings* placed at the scene or in the trauma room need to be left in place until the patient reaches the operating room. This practice has led to decreased infection rates when compared with routinely redressing wounds in the trauma area.[3] Urgent stabilization of fractures, vascular repair, débridement, and fasciotomy in severely injured extremities have reduced the incidence of adult respiratory distress syndrome (ARDS) and multisystem organ failure.[2,4] In less severe injuries, once the patient is stabilized, wound closure, complex joint reconstruction, and repair of maxillofacial injuries can be completed.

Severe pelvic fractures are addressed in the primary survey because of the possibility of exsanguination. Cervical spine injuries with associated neurologic compro-

mise also deserve immediate attention. These exceptions aside, examination and management of the extremities are deferred to the secondary survey after the airway has been controlled and hemodynamic stability is obtained. In a team approach, these examinations and treatments are taking place simultaneously. Throughout the resuscitation phase and the remainder of the hospital course, reexamination will ensure that no injury goes unrecognized (tertiary survey).

Evidence of pelvic fractures is assessed early in the resuscitative effort. Massive flank or buttock contusions and swelling are indicative of significant bleeding. The Morel-Lavallée lesion is an ecchymotic lesion over the greater trochanter that represents a subcutaneous degloving injury. This lesion is frequently associated with acetabular fractures. Blood at the urethral meatus, signifying injury to the genitourinary tract, may be a sign of an underlying pelvic fracture. Palpation of the symphysis pubis, as well as the sacroiliac joints, can help determine the presence of gapping. Gentle rocking and lateral compression through the anterior iliac crests can provide helpful clues to the stability of the pelvic ring. Any opening or looseness signifies instability and may represent a source of hemorrhage. Rectal and vaginal examinations are performed, with notation made of any bleeding, lacerations, bony fragments, hematomas, or masses. Wounds and palpable bony fragments found on either of these examinations are diagnostic of an open pelvic fracture, which carries a poor prognosis.

At all times, the trauma team must take steps to protect the patient from self-inflicted or iatrogenic spinal cord injury. Therefore, full spine precautions must be observed until it is confirmed that the patient's vertebral column is intact, either by physical examination and clinical findings or by radiologic confirmation when warranted.

The cervical spine is stabilized by fitting the patient with a hard cervical collar, and the thoracic, lumbar, and sacral segments of the spine are protected by maintaining the patient in the supine position at all times. If the patient is to be moved, strict log roll technique is used. At times a patient may have to be physically restrained to prevent potential self-inflicted injury by head or lower extremity movements that may impart rotational, translational, or bending moments to the vertebral column. Special care must be taken with combative patients or those with altered mental status who may have lost the ability to protect themselves from further injury.

The examiner notes the presence of deformity, edema, or ecchymosis. Tenderness elicited on palpation of the spine is recorded for each level at which the patient complains of pain. Distinction is made regarding whether the pain is midline or paraspinal. In patients with a known neurologic deficit or localized back or neck pain, perianal sensation and rectal sphincter tone must be evaluated. Deep tendon reflexes and pathologic reflexes, such as the bulbocavernosus and Babinski reflexes, are tested. The presence of sacral sparing (intact perianal sensation, rectal tone, or great toe flexion) represents at least partial continuity of the white matter long tracts. In one large series,[5] sacral sparing was predictive of the completeness of injury in 97% of patients with spinal cord injury. Radiographs of the thoracolumbar spine are indicated when the patient reports pain; when ecchymoses, abrasions, or a step-off is present; or when ejection from a vehicle or a fall from a significant height has occurred. In *all* trauma patients, anteroposterior, lateral, and odontoid radiographs of the cervical spine must be obtained. Radiographs are not considered adequate unless the entire cervical spine can be visualized from the superior tip of the dens distally to the superior end plate of the first thoracic vertebra.

Cervical spine injuries can occur by several mechanisms, which can be divided into three main categories. The first involves direct trauma to the neck itself. The second mechanism involves motion of the head relative to the axial skeleton. This injury can occur either by direct trauma to the head or by continued movement of the head relative to the fixed body, as often occurs in blunt trauma such as motor vehicle collisions when the body is restrained. In attempting to tether the head against motion, the cervical spine endures a large bending or twisting moment that results in flexion-extension injuries or rotational injuries, respectively.

A third mechanism of cervical spine injury involves a direct axial load imparted on the cranium that causes axial compression forces across the cervical vertebrae. This mechanism may result in a *burst fracture* and potential spinal cord injury, although this pattern of injury is more commonly seen in the lumbar spine. Burst fractures, by definition, involve injury to the posterior third of the vertebral body, or the middle column. These fractures are to be differentiated from *compression fractures,* which involve the anterior column only (anterior two thirds) and are rarely associated with spinal cord injury. Burst fractures are commonly found after falls from a height in which an axial load is transmitted to the upper axial skeleton when the feet strike the ground first. This mechanism results in a common pattern of calcaneal and lumbar burst fractures. Depending on the fracture pattern, treatment of spine injuries may range from observation to bracing, surgical fixation, or external halo fixation. However, treatment of all injuries begins with strict immobilization and spine precautions.

Examination of the extremities in a patient with isolated injuries or in a multitrauma patient follows a simple, systematic, and reproducible pattern. Even when an isolated extremity injury is the primary reason for evaluation, the entire skeleton must be examined. The examiner must not be distracted from the task by obvious or severe injuries. Deformity, edema, ecchymosis, crepitus, tenderness, and pain with motion are the cardinal signs of an acute fracture. Each limb segment needs to be examined for lacerations and the previously described signs of trauma. All joints are put through passive range of motion at a minimum. Active range of motion is tested whenever possible. Joint effusions are evidence of intra-articular pathology (e.g., ligament or cartilage damage or an intra-articular fracture). The joints are then manually stressed to assess the integrity of the ligamentous structures. A neurovascular examination is performed and documented. Pulses are recorded and compared with the opposite, uninvolved extremity when possible. Doppler signals are obtained when palpable pulses are not present or are weak. Motor function and sensation must be documented for the extremity dermatomes as well as the trunk in a patient with thoracic spine pain. To avoid the complications of a missed compartment syndrome, palpation of the involved compartments is performed. Any firm or tense compartments are checked for increased pressure if time and the patient's condition allow. Fasciotomies are performed urgently if pressures are elevated. Gross alignment and interim immobilization of long bone fractures are achieved before transportation of the patient from the trauma room. This intervention will facilitate transfer, reduce pain, decrease soft tissue trauma and hemorrhage, lessen the chance of turning a closed fracture into an open one, improve the quality of radiographic studies, and prevent potential neurovascular injury. Traction splints or skeletal traction is applied when indicated.

Diagnostic Imaging

Radiographic examination is used to supplement and enhance the information gathered during the primary survey, history, and physical examination. In a multiply injured patient, the advanced trauma life support protocol calls for a lateral cervical spine film and anteroposterior views of the pelvis and chest. The secondary survey then dictates which extremity radiographs are necessary. When filming long bone injuries, it is important to verify the integrity of adjacent limb segments. Therefore, the joints above and below the level of injury are always included in the films. They are filmed separately if the cassette is not large enough to accommodate the entire view. Similarly, when pathology is suspected in a joint, the long bones above and below are imaged as well. This practice helps identify commonly associated injuries to the adjacent limb segments that might otherwise be missed.

Because bone is a three-dimensional object, a single two-dimensional radiograph cannot describe a fracture. To understand the position and direction of the fracture fragments, orthogonal views (images taken at 90 degrees to one another) must be obtained. All extremities with deformity need to be rotated to the anatomic position before taking radiographs to help decrease confusion when describing the fracture.

The goal of radiographic assessment of intra-articular fractures is quantitation of articular incongruity. Orthogonal views of the joint and adjacent long bones are obtained. Radiographs made parallel to the articular surface best display any step-off that may be present. In complex intra-articular fractures, a CT scan is usually necessary to fully understand the position and displacement of all articular fragments. CT scans provide fine detail, help locate small fragments in the joint, and can further describe the extension of intra-articular fracture lines. They must not be used in lieu of acceptable plain radiographs, however. Plain radiographs are better suited to accurately describe overall fracture characteristics and limb alignment.

Additional imaging is undertaken in specific circumstances only after acceptable plain radiographs have been thoroughly reviewed. Stress radiographs are taken when ligamentous or growth plate injuries are suspected after clinical examination but are not evident on plain films. Gapping of the joint or physis while stressing the structure in question is diagnostic (Fig. 21-7). Cervical spine ligamentous injuries are often diagnosed this way with *active* flexion-extension radiographs. *Passive* flexion-extension must not be attempted. Oblique views are sometimes necessary to evaluate more complex structures such as the shoulder, proximal tibia, and acetabulum. True anteroposterior and lateral views of the shoulder must be taken in relation to the scapula because of the orientation of the joint. The most useful lateral view is an axillary radiograph. The tube is angled cephalad with the plate on the superior aspect of the abducted shoulder. This view is often difficult to obtain because of pain or instability at the proximal end of the humerus. Judet views, or 45-degree oblique views of the pelvis, are used to evaluate the acetabuli. Because of the spatial orientation of the acetabulum, these views represent orthogonal projections when the x-ray tube is canted toward or away from the affected side. Similarly, inlet and outlet views of the pelvis allow closer examination of the sacroiliac joints and the sacrum itself. The inlet view is taken with the beam angled 60 degrees caudad, thus making the beam perpendicular to the pelvic brim. The sacral ala and displacement of the sacroiliac joints in the anteroposterior plane are easily seen. The outlet view is a 30-degree oblique view with the tube angled cephalad. The sacrum is pictured *en fosse*, and the foramina are easily evaluated.

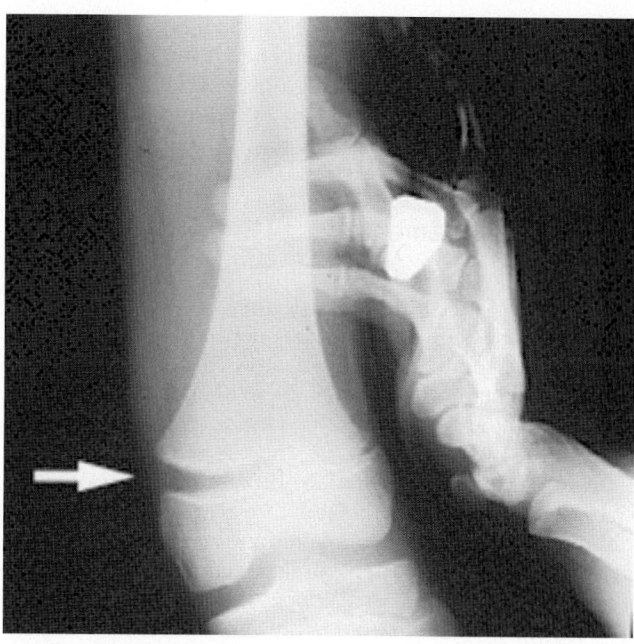

Figure 21-7 Stress radiograph of a physeal injury of the distal femur. An anteroposterior radiograph with valgus stress applied reveals unstable physeal disruption.

Magnetic resonance imaging (MRI) has become a particularly useful imaging modality. It is used to evaluate soft tissue, acute fractures, stress fractures, spinal cord injuries, and intra-articular pathology. Its role in the trauma setting has expanded as well, and it is particularly helpful in the setting of spinal cord injury. More frequently, MRI is being used in the outpatient setting to evaluate soft tissue injuries and pathologic lesions. MRI is now commonly used for the diagnosis of acute fractures when plain films are negative. In elderly patients with osteopenic femoral neck fractures, bone scans, though accurate, are unreliable within 48 hours after injury. MRI has been shown to be at least as accurate as bone scans in the diagnosis of acute fractures. Additionally, the sensitivity and specificity of MRI were the same within 24 hours of admission as later.[6] Earlier diagnosis can potentially lead to shorter hospital stays and therefore more than offsets the additional cost of MRI.

Arteriography is another important modality used for the evaluation of extremity and pelvic injuries. It is indicated any time that signs of distal ischemia are noted in an extremity. Knee dislocations are a common cause of arterial injury secondary to the proximity of the popliteal vessels. Prompt reduction of these injuries is mandatory, followed by re-evaluation of vascular status. In cases in which pulses return after reduction, arteriography is still indicated because of the probability of intimal damage to the artery and late thrombosis.

INITIAL MANAGEMENT

Care of musculoskeletal injuries often begins in the field. The extent of fracture and wound management differs with the level of training and experience of the first responders (lay people, police) and emergency medical personnel. Therefore, it is essential that the initial treating physician perform a thorough assessment and begin initial management, including splinting and wound care.

Wound Management

After a thorough physical examination, treatment is begun immediately. All sterile wound dressings placed in the field or in the emergency department are left intact until they can be removed under controlled conditions. Nontraction splints and dressings are partially removed by a single examiner using sterile technique. Superficial contamination by dirt, gravel, or grass is removed. If a significant delay is anticipated before formal operative débridement, pulsatile lavage can be performed in the trauma room. Sterile saline solution or povidone-iodine–soaked dressings are then applied. Careless wound management in the emergency department has been shown to increase the ultimate infection rate by 300% to 400%.[7] Tetanus prophylaxis and broad-spectrum intravenous (IV) antibiotics are administered. Immobilization is then undertaken in the same manner as for a closed injury. External bleeding in the extremities is controlled by direct manual pressure.

After wound care in the initial period, subsequent early débridement and reassessment of wounds with *frequent dressing changes* can prevent secondary infection and subsequent bacterial translocation. In addition, treatment of protein malnutrition can protect against gut translocation and systemic infection. Early range of motion and muscle strengthening can result in a decrease in the length of hospitalization, rehabilitative time, and long-term disability.[8,9]

Reduction and Immobilization

All displaced fractures and dislocations are gently reduced to reestablish limb alignment provisionally. If the patient's condition allows, precise reductions are performed and the extremities are splinted formally to maintain the fracture reduction. With time, the difficulty of reduction increases, as does edema and muscle spasm. Therefore, reduction needs to be attempted as soon as possible and with the patient as relaxed as possible. Often, narcotic analgesics and sedatives are necessary, particularly with large joint dislocations. Muscle spasm can obstruct atraumatic reduction of these injuries. If a joint is still dislocated after adequate sedation and relaxation, general anesthesia may be necessary.

Reduction maneuvers follow the same principles for all fracture and dislocation types. First, in-line traction is applied to the limb. If the soft tissue envelope surrounding the fracture fragments is intact, in-line traction alone may produce satisfactory alignment (Fig. 21-8). In most cases, the deformity must be recreated and exaggerated to unhook the fractured ends. Finally, the mechanism of injury is reversed and the fracture immobilized. Neurovascular status is documented before and after any reduc-

tion maneuver or splint application. Once satisfactory reduction or alignment is achieved, it must be maintained by immobilization through casting, splinting, or continuous traction. The joints above and below the fracture must be included to prevent displacement. Postreduction radiographs are required to confirm alignment and rotation.

Nondisplaced fractures are treated like displaced fractures without reduction. It is important to obtain adequate radiographs and to fully evaluate the injured limb. The same principles of immobilization apply. Most nondisplaced fractures do not require surgical treatment. Splints are placed initially and then changed to circumferential casts after the swelling subsides.

Ligamentous injuries may also require immobilization. The joint is fully evaluated as described previously, and a thorough neurovascular examination is performed on the limb. Frequently, pain, effusions, or hemarthroses occur and represent intra-articular pathology. The limb is then immobilized and re-evaluated after the acute pain and swelling decrease.

The rationale for immobilization is threefold. First, splinting, particularly with traction or compression devices, reduces bleeding. Second, additional soft tissue injury may be averted, and the chance of converting a closed to an open fracture is reduced. Third, immobilization of the fracture reduces patient discomfort and facilitates transportation and radiographic evaluation of the patient.[10] All fractures and dislocations are splinted or immobilized in the emergency department. Most frequently, splints are fashioned from padded plaster or fiberglass. Splints can be secured with a bias-cut stockinette, elastic wraps, and gauze bandage, provided that they are wrapped in a nonconstrictive fashion. The role of circumferential casting in the acute setting is questionable. Because swelling of the injured extremity increases for 48 to 72 hours, a circular cast would be too constrictive and can lead to pressure necrosis or compartment syndrome. In select cases in which a cast will be the definitive treatment, the initial circumferential cast can be applied and then cut longitudinally on two sides to allow swelling without splitting of the padding. This technique maintains a reduction more effectively than an open splint does.

Traction

Traction is used to immobilize fractures or dislocations displaced by muscle forces that cannot be adequately controlled with simple splints. The most common indications are vertical shear injuries of the pelvis, hip dislocations, acetabular fractures, and fractures of the upper two thirds of the femur. Traction may be applied through the skin or skeletally through a pin inserted distal to the injury site. Traction of greater than 8 lb through the skin for any extended period causes skin damage and therefore is practical only for geriatric hip fractures and pediatric injuries requiring limited distraction force. The Hare traction splint applies a distraction force through an ankle stirrup and can provide effective immobilization for femoral shaft fractures. It can be applied in the field and

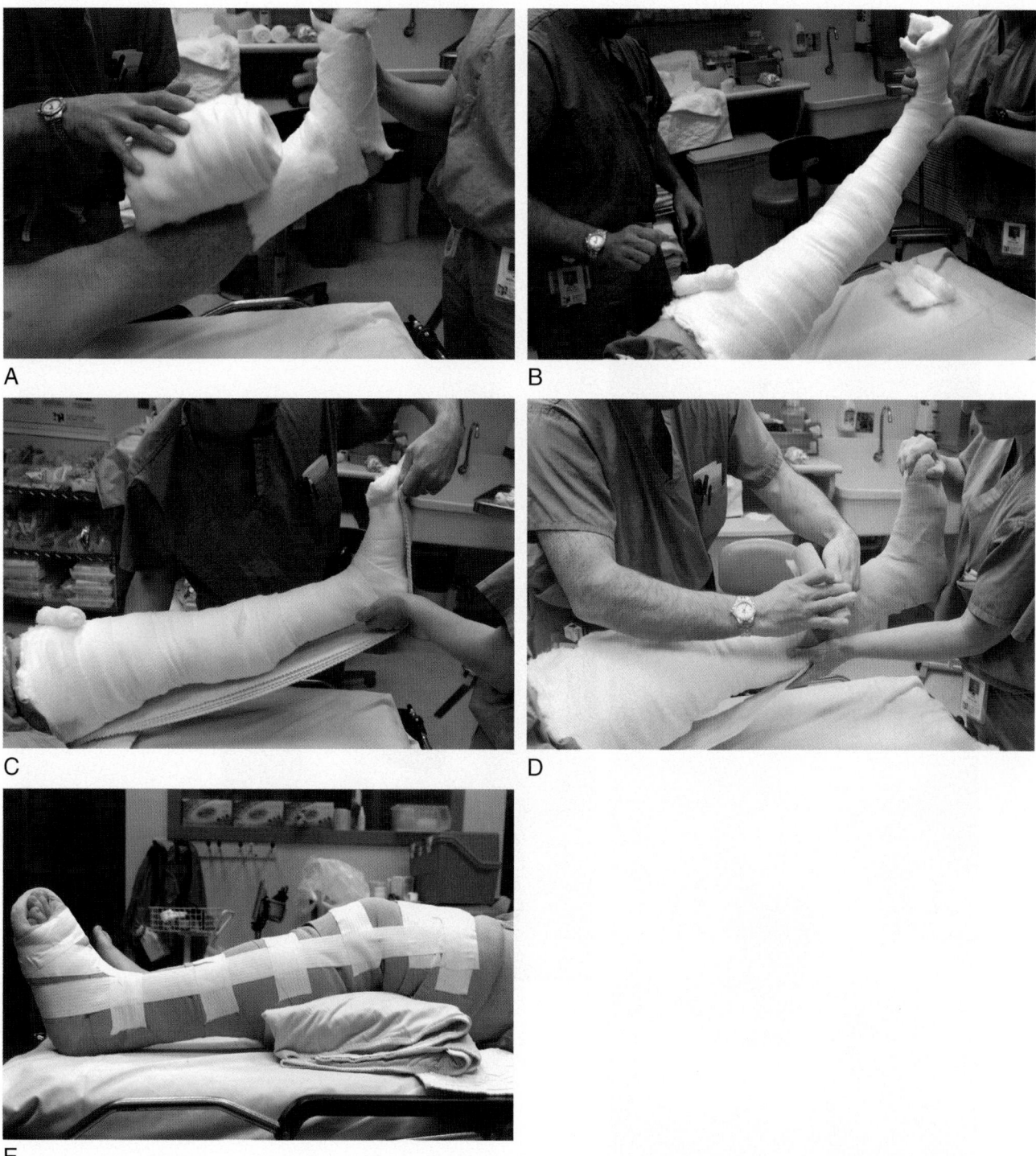

Figure 21-8 Method for provisional reduction and splint application of the lower (distal femur to foot) and upper (distal humerus to wrist) extremity. **A,** In-line (axial) traction is applied to the injured extremity and the normal overall alignment is reestablished. **B,** The limb is protected with a soft dressing (circumferential Robert Jones cotton or longitudinal sheets of cast padding). **C** and **D,** A splint (plaster or fiberglass) is measured and applied to the injured extremity with a light compression wrap (elastic bandage or bias-cut stockinette). **E,** The compressive wrap is secured with tape in a safe position. When possible, the knee is flexed and the ankle is placed in neutral position to prevent equinus contracture.

Continued

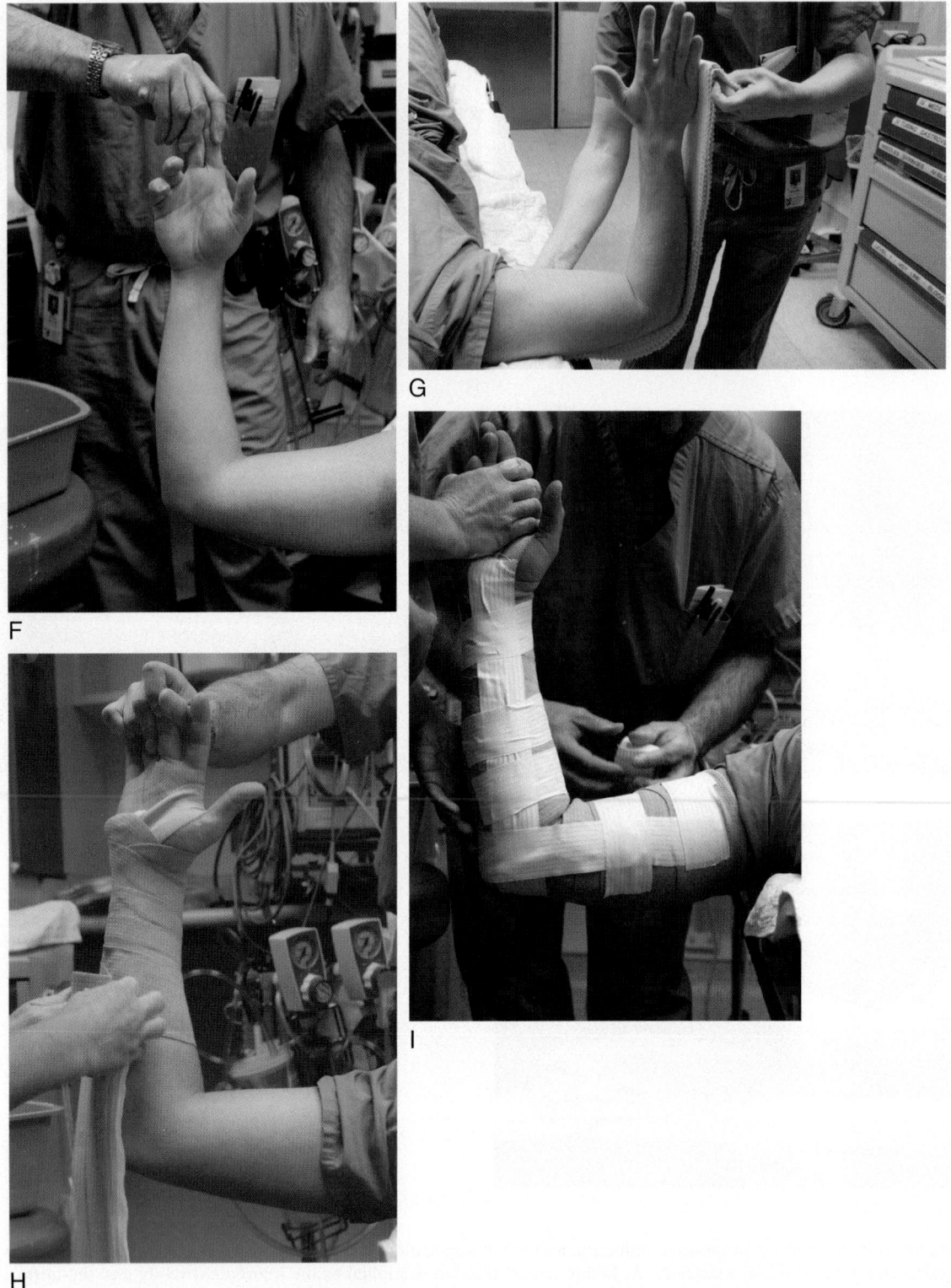

Figure 21-8, cont'd F, The injured extremity is placed in neutral position with gravity traction. **G** and **H,** A well-padded splint (plaster or fiberglass) is measured and applied to the limb with a light compression wrap (elastic bandage or bias-cut stockinette). **I,** The compressive wrap is secured with tape in a safe position.

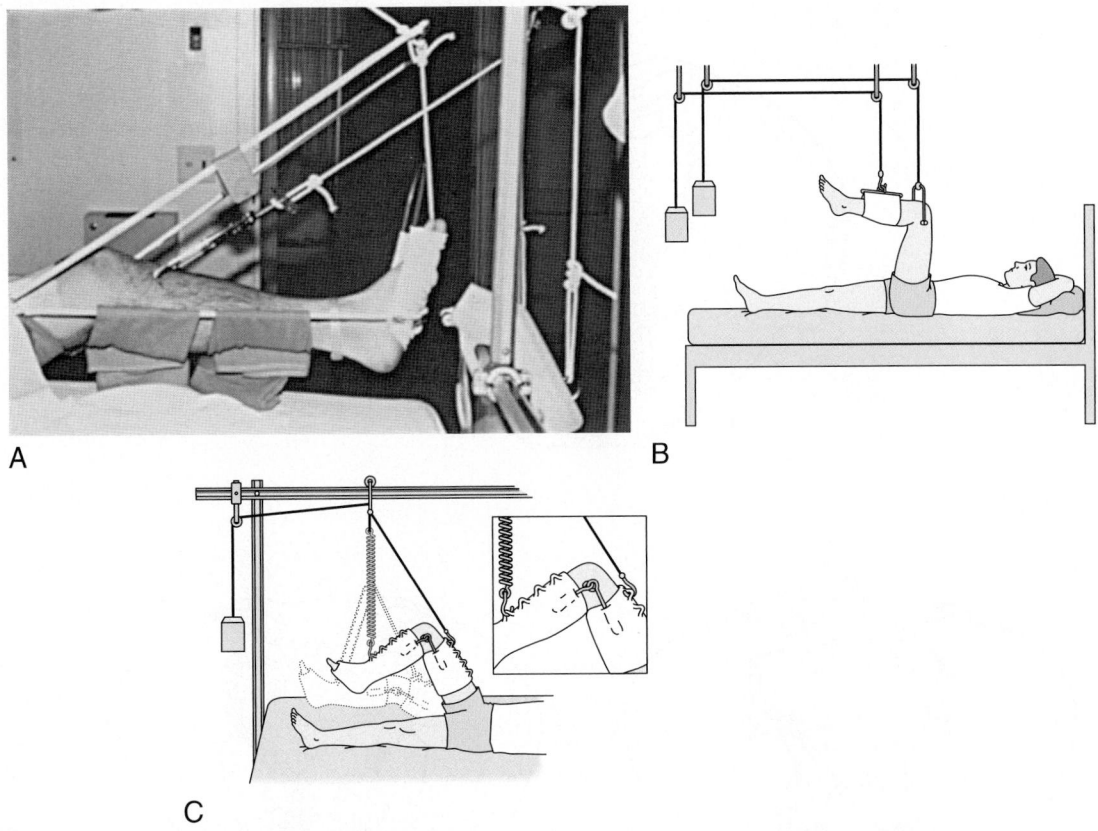

Figure 21-9 A, Skeletal traction applied to a femoral shaft fracture through a tibial pin. Balanced suspension was achieved with the use of a Thomas splint and a Pearson attachment. **B,** 90-90 skeletal traction. **C,** Roller traction, as described by Neufeld and Mooney. The fracture brace incorporates a traction pin in the tibial tubercle. (From Wolinsky PR, Johnson KD: Femoral shaft fractures. In Browner BD, Jupiter TB, Levine AM, Trafton PG [eds]: Skeletal Trauma, 2nd ed. Philadelphia, WB Saunders, 1998.)

helps facilitate transport and mobilization, but it is used only temporarily.

Skeletal traction may be maintained for longer periods with greater weight than possible with skin traction (Fig. 21-9). Neurovascular structures must be avoided during placement of the pins. Once the pins are placed, the skin is checked for tension and relieved with incisions, if necessary. The wounds are then dressed with povidone-iodine–soaked sponges. Pin tract infections are a common complication and can lead to osteomyelitis in the worst cases. For this reason, all pin sites are cleaned with a half-strength hydrogen peroxide solution and sterilely dressed every nursing shift.

Prioritization of Surgical Care

After the secondary survey is completed and necessary diagnostic studies are obtained, a multiply injured patient may be moved to the operating room. Because operative decisions are made on a continuous basis as the patient's condition evolves, the trauma surgeon serves as the coordinator of care and prioritizes all surgical procedures after consulting with the anesthesiologist, neurosurgeon, and orthopedic surgeon. Critical procedures are carried out first, and each additional intervention is reviewed as

the patient's status evolves. Intra-abdominal, thoracic, retroperitoneal, and intracranial hemorrhages are immediate surgical priorities. These injuries include acute visceral hemorrhage, aortic or caval injuries, injuries to the heart and pulmonary vessels, intracranial mass lesions, depressed skull fractures, and pelvic fractures with associated instability. In addition to hemorrhage, immediate surgery is indicated for the prevention of pulmonary failure, prevention of local and systemic infections from open or devitalized wounds, and limb salvage. Stabilization of severe open and femoral shaft fractures may be performed simultaneously or after hemodynamic stabilization of the surgical patient. Limb-threatening vascular injuries are managed on an emergency basis because limiting the warm ischemia time to 6 hours is essential for optimal recovery. Decisions regarding limb viability, compartment syndrome, and the need for amputation of a mangled extremity are made in concert with all services involved. Consideration must also be given to emergency capsulotomy and ORIF of femoral head fractures, as well as reduction of posterior hip dislocations, to prevent avascular necrosis. Definitive care of complex upper extremity fractures or intra-articular fractures is undertaken if the patient's condition permits. Spine, acetabular, and upper extremity injuries are addressed next.

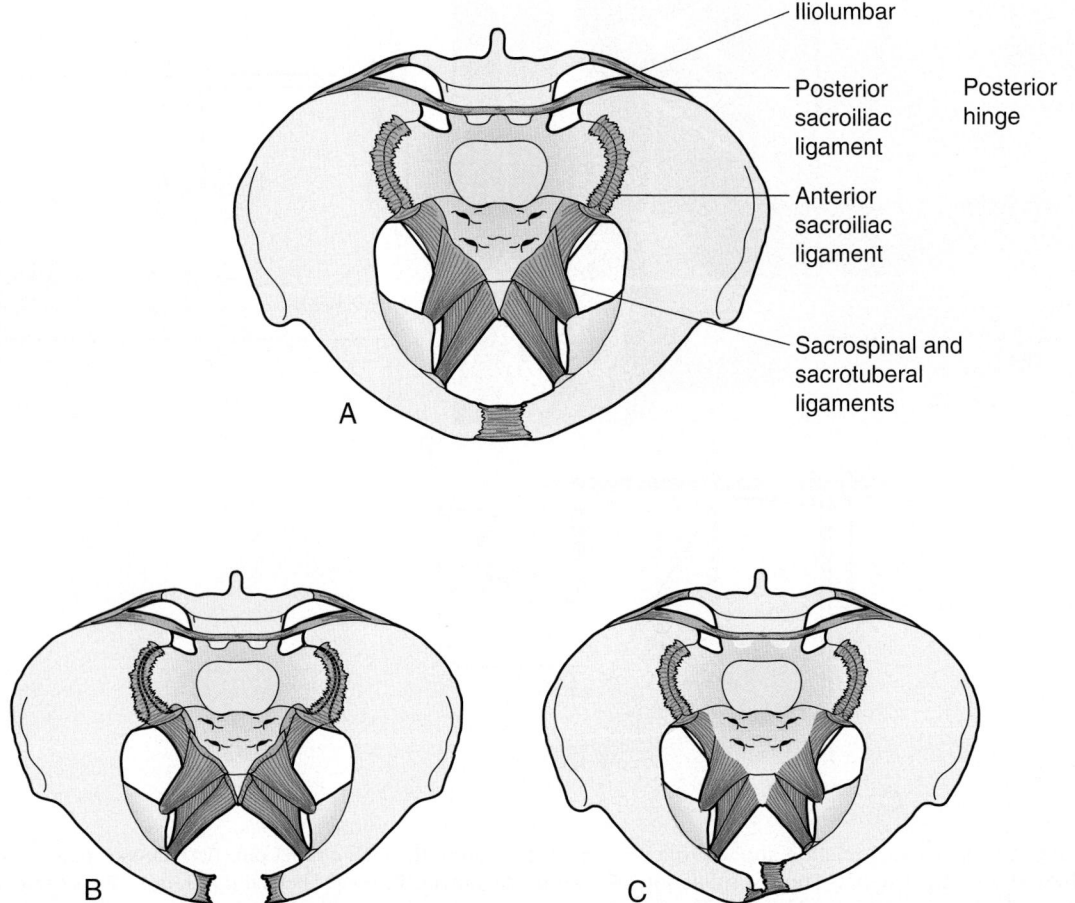

Figure 21-10 Pelvic stability. **A,** The intact ligamentous bony structures of the pelvis maintain its integrity with regard to stability. The posterior hinge, consisting of the posterior sacroiliac ligaments and the iliolumbar ligaments, is imperative to maintain vertical stability. The sacrospinous prevents rotation, and the sacrotuberous prevents vertical migration. As long as these structures, the anterior sacroiliac, and the symphysis are intact, the pelvis will remain stable. If, however, the anterior symphysis is separated or the sacrum is crushed posteriorly, as seen in **B** and **C,** the posterior hinge remains intact and the pelvis is usually stable vertically. The sacrospinous ligaments are intact, and rotatory abnormalities are thus prevented. (From Kellam JF, Mayo K: Pelvic ring disruptions. In Browner BD, Jupiter TB, Levine AM, Trafton PG [eds]: Skeletal Trauma, 3rd ed. Philadelphia, WB Saunders, 2003.)

Operative repair of maxillofacial injuries can usually be delayed for several days, depending on the status of the patient.

ORTHOPEDIC EMERGENCIES

Pelvic Ring Disruption

Pelvic ring disruption is a major cause of mortality and morbidity in multiply injured patients. Fatalities result from uncontrolled retroperitoneal hemorrhage and other associated injuries, and long-term disability such as low back pain, leg length discrepancies, dyspareunia, difficulty with childbearing, and impotence is due to anatomic disruption of the pelvic ring. Pelvic fractures can be particularly lethal when they occur in conjunction with significant injuries to other major organ systems.[11] Because of the high force necessary to disrupt the pelvic ring in young patients, it is not surprising that up to 80%

of these patients have additional musculoskeletal injuries. Mortality rates in patients with high-energy pelvic ring injuries are approximately 15% to 25%. Mortality increases nearly 13-fold when the patient is hypotensive. When combined with either a head or an abdominal injury that requires surgical intervention, mortality increases to 50%. When both procedures are necessary, mortality approaches 90%.

Classification

Orthopedic surgeons and traumatologists broadly classify pelvic ring disruption into two major groups: stable and unstable. A *stable* pelvis is defined as one that can withstand normal physiologic forces without displacing. This stability depends on integrity of the osseous and ligamentous structures (Fig. 21-10). *Instability* can be divided into rotational and vertical components (Fig. 21-11). These displacements can be appreciated on the anteroposterior radiograph in the trauma survey. Stable injuries include nondisplaced fractures of the pelvic ring and anterior

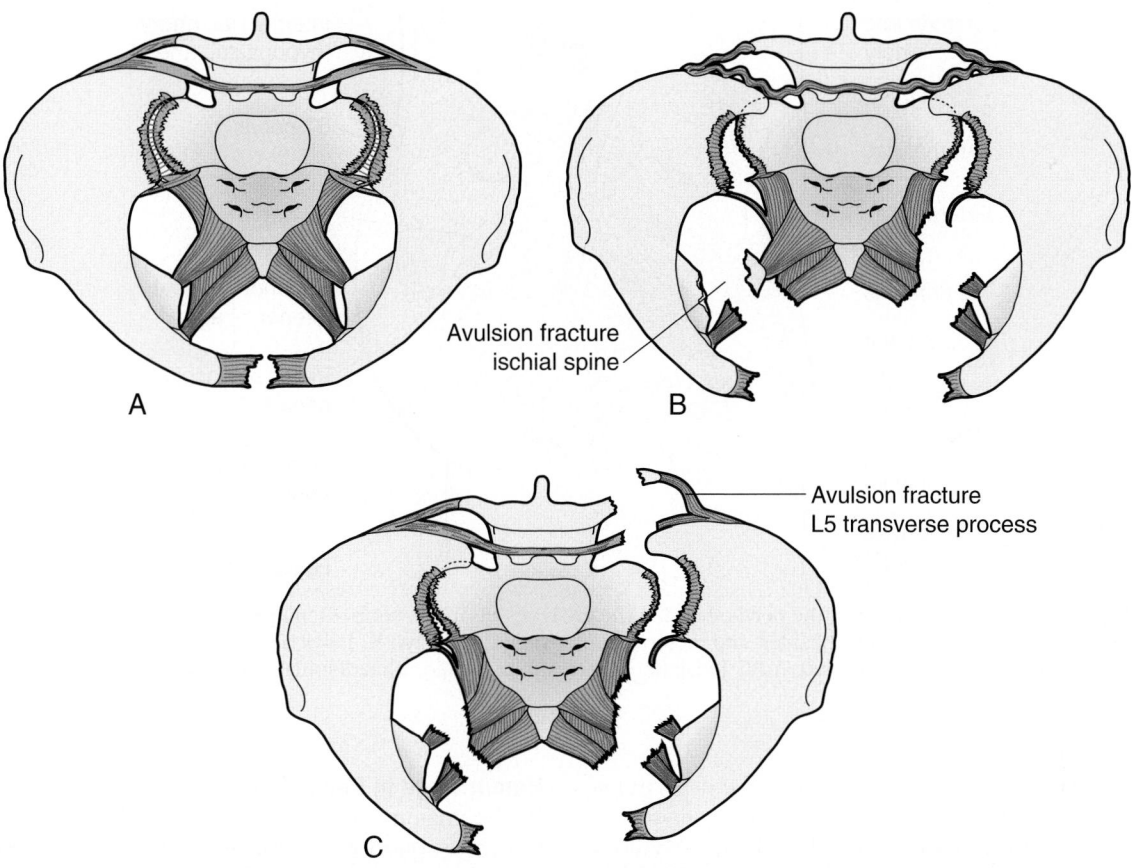

Avulsion fracture
ischial spine

Avulsion fracture
L5 transverse process

Figure 21-11 A, Division of the symphysis pubis will allow the pelvis to open to approximately 2.5 cm with no damage to any posterior ligamentous structures. **B,** Division of the anterior sacroiliac and sacrospinous ligaments, either by direct division of their fibers *(right)* or by avulsion of the tip of the ischial spine *(left),* allows the pelvis to rotate externally until the posterior superior iliac spines abut the sacrum. Note, however, that the posterior ligamentous structures (e.g., the posterior sacroiliac and iliolumbar ligaments) remain intact. Therefore, no displacement in the vertical plane is possible. **C,** Division of the posterior tension band ligaments, that is, the posterior sacroiliac, as well as the iliolumbar, depicted here on the left side, plus avulsion of the transverse process of L5 causes complete instability of the hemipelvis. Note that posterior displacement is now possible. (From Kellam JF, Mayo K: Pelvic ring disruptions. In Browner BD, Jupiter TB, Levine AM, Trafton PG [eds]: Skeletal Trauma, 3rd ed. Philadelphia, WB Saunders, 2003.)

displacements less than 2.5 cm. Rotational instability is characterized by widening of the symphysis pubis or displacement of pubic rami fractures greater than 2.5 cm. Superior translation of a hemipelvis through fractures of the sacrum or ilium plus disruption of the sacroiliac joint by more than 1 cm constitutes vertical instability. Serial sectioning studies reveal that division of the symphyseal ligaments alone leads to anterior diastasis of 2.5 cm or less and maintenance of stability.[12] Further sectioning of the anterior sacroiliac ligaments and sacrospinous and sacrotuberous ligaments (pelvic floor) imparts rotational instability. Vertical instability results only after the posterior sacroiliac ligaments are sectioned. Displaced fractures (superior and inferior pubic rami fractures, sacral or iliac wing fracture) can result in similar instability patterns. Because the pelvis is a true ring structure, significant anterior displacement must be accompanied by posterior disruption. Disruptions in the pelvic ring are usually a combination of osseous and ligamentous injury.

Early recognition of unstable pelvic rings is essential because they are associated with potentially fatal hemorrhage. Additionally, these injuries require intervention to reestablish the pelvic ring anatomy and minimize late disability. Determination of the stability of the injured hemipelvis must be established through a combination of physical examination and review of the anteroposterior radiograph. An anterior defect can sometimes be detected by palpation at the symphysis pubis. Rotational instability can be appreciated with lateral compression of the pelvis through the anterior iliac spines. Because repeated manipulation can cause iatrogenic injury, such handling needs to be performed once. Vertical instability may be appreciated when traction is applied and removed through an extended, uninjured lower extremity if it produces movement of the hemipelvis. In 90% of cases, the physical examination and anteroposterior pelvic radiograph are sufficient to assess stability and guide initial treatment. Anterior injuries are easily identified on this projection, and most unstable posterior injuries can

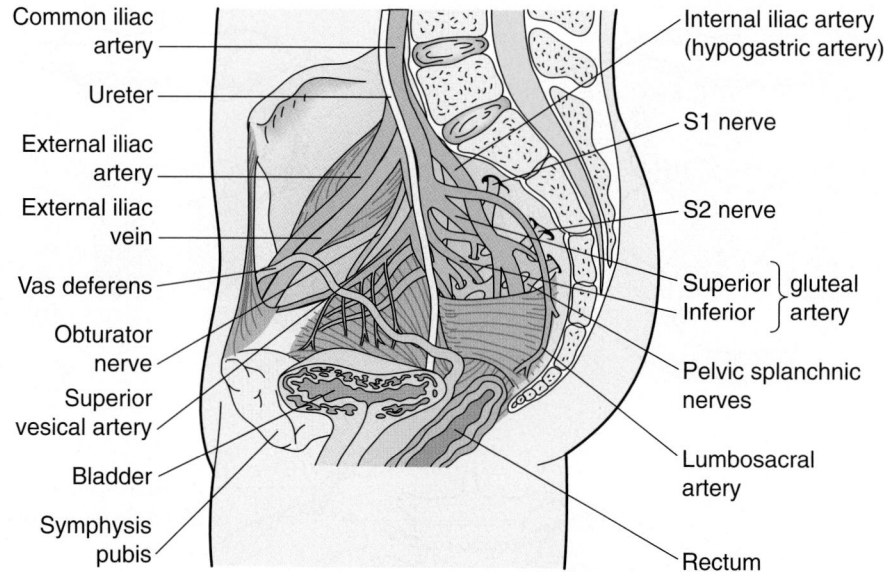

Figure 21-12 Internal aspect of the pelvis showing the great vessels in the lumbosacral plexus, as well as the pelvic floor and the pelvic contents, bladder, and rectum. (From Kellam JF, Mayo K: Pelvic ring disruptions. In Browner BD, Jupiter TB, Levine AM, Trafton PG [eds]: Skeletal Trauma, 3rd ed. Philadelphia, WB Saunders, 2003.)

also be appreciated. Avulsion fractures of the L5 transverse process and the ischial spines reflect ligamentous disruption and are usually identifiable. Large posterior displacement or superior translation of the hemipelvis more than 1 cm indicates complete posterior injury and gross instability.[12]

Detailed classification systems have been developed on the basis of the direction of force, stability of the pelvis, location of the fracture, or whether it is an open or closed injury. The Comprehensive Pelvic Disruption classification of the Arbeitsgemeinschaft fur Osteosynthe-sefragen (AO) combines the mechanism of injury with the degree of pelvic instability. Type A injuries preserve the integrity of the posterior ligamentous and bony structures. These injuries maintain a stable pelvic ring and generally require no further treatment unless neurologic injury is associated with a sacral fracture. Type B injuries represent incomplete disruption of the posterior pelvis and result in rotational instability of the pelvis. A varying degree of sacroiliac joint or sacral disruption is characteristic. These injuries occur with both anterior and lateral compression mechanisms. In type C pelvic injuries, the hemipelvis is vertically, rotationally, and posteriorly unstable.

Lateral compression– and vertical shear–type fractures are associated with intra-abdominal and head injuries. The most common cause of death in a patient with a lateral compression injury of the pelvis is associated closed head trauma.[3] Anteroposterior compression–type injuries have the greatest risk for retroperitoneal hemorrhage. Intrapelvic visceral injuries are also more common with the anteroposterior patterns. Mortality in anteroposterior compression–type injuries is related to a combination of retroperitoneal bleeding and visceral injuries.[3]

Hemorrhage in Pelvic Fracture

In the majority of pelvic fractures, hemorrhage results from disruption of the pelvic venous plexus posteriorly and bleeding cancellous bone. Pelvic bleeding from a named artery occurs in less 10% of cases (Fig. 21-12).[13-15] Bleeding from a larger artery is even less frequent. Two large series have demonstrated bleeding from the femoral or iliac vessels in 1% and 0% of patients.[16] As a result, initial treatment of hemorrhage must focus on control of venous bleeding via reduction and stabilization of the pelvic ring. Reduction leads to a decrease in pelvic volume and tamponade of the bleeding vessels through compression of the viscera and pelvic hematoma. Stabilization maintains the reduction and avoids movement of the hemipelvis, thereby reducing pain and limiting disruption of any organizing thrombus. Because reduction and stabilization alone usually control venous bleeding, patients who do not respond to these maneuvers are more likely to have arterial bleeding.

Stabilization

Reduction and stabilization of the pelvis can be achieved by a variety of mechanical means (Fig. 21-13). When field personnel detect unstable pelvic ring disruptions on physical examination, they can begin treatment by binding the pelvis with a rolled sheet or applying pneumatic antishock garments (PASGs). Like air splints applied to the extremities, the garment functions by compressing the pelvis. If applied in the field, PASGs should not be deflated until the patient is being resuscitated in the trauma room. A PASG has the advantage of ease of use, application in the field, and reusability. However, it blocks access to the patient and restricts excursion of the diaphragm, and there have been reports of gluteal and

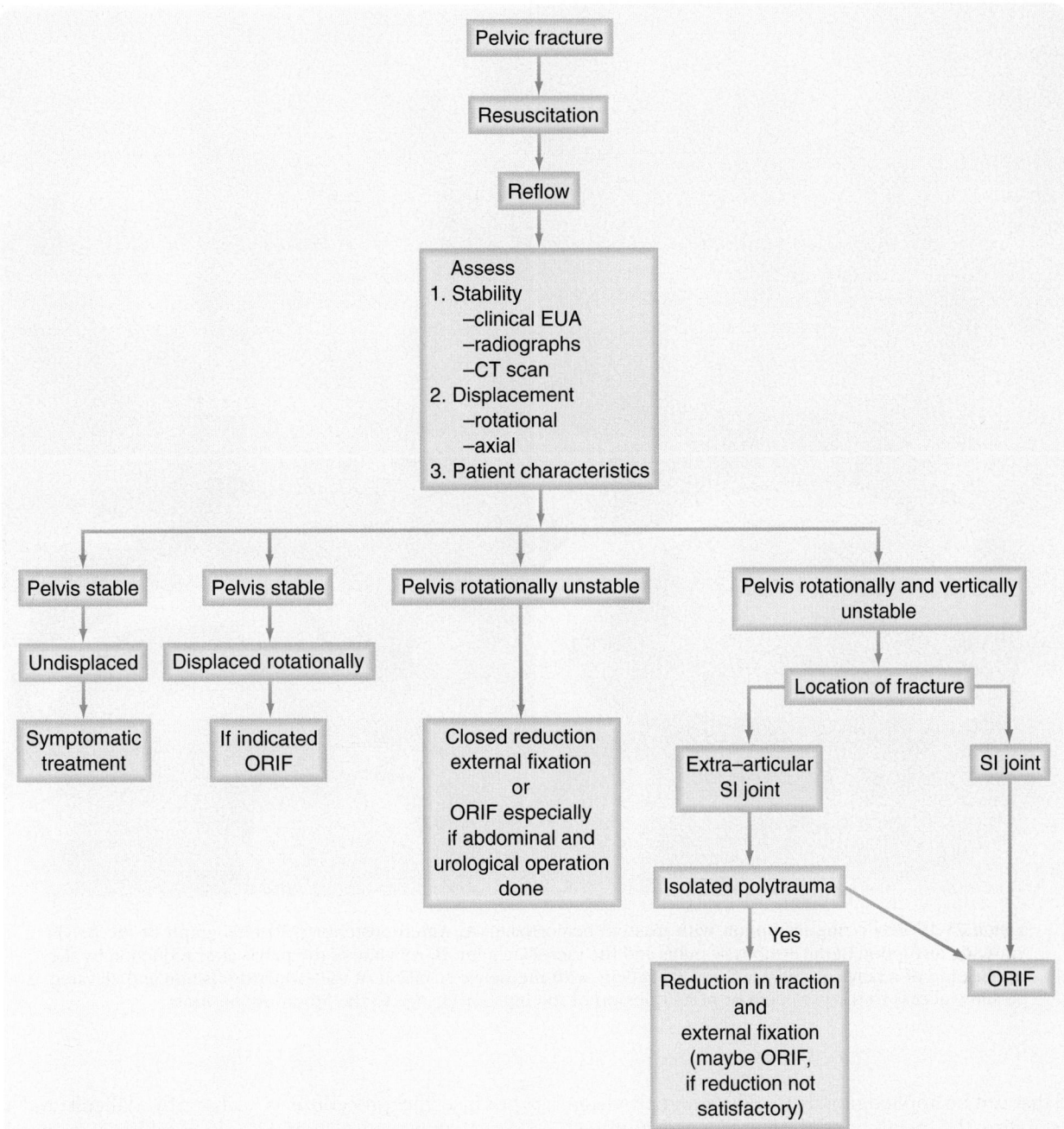

Figure 21-13 Algorithm for the management of pelvic fractures. CT, computed tomography; EUA, examination under anesthesia; ORIF, open reduction and internal fixation; SI, sacroiliac. (From Kellam JF, Mayo K: Pelvic ring disruptions. In Browner BD, Jupiter TB, Levine AM, Trafton PG [eds]: Skeletal Trauma, 3rd ed. Philadelphia, WB Saunders, 2003.)

thigh compartment syndromes developing after extended use of PASGs in hypotensive patients.

Historically, the standard method for controlling pelvic hemorrhage has been the application of an anterior external fixation frame. When applied properly, an anterior pelvic external fixator should provide stability to the pelvis and hematoma while allowing access to the abdomen for surgical procedures. Multiple studies have shown that outcomes can improve with the routine use

of such fixators.[14,15,17] Although these devices can be applied in the emergency department, placement is frequently deferred until the patient is brought to the operating suite. In these circumstances the pelvis can remain displaced for many hours with venous bleeding continuing uncontrolled.

If an external fixator cannot be applied expeditiously, another method of provisional stabilization must be used. Recently, devices called *pelvic C-clamps* have been devel-

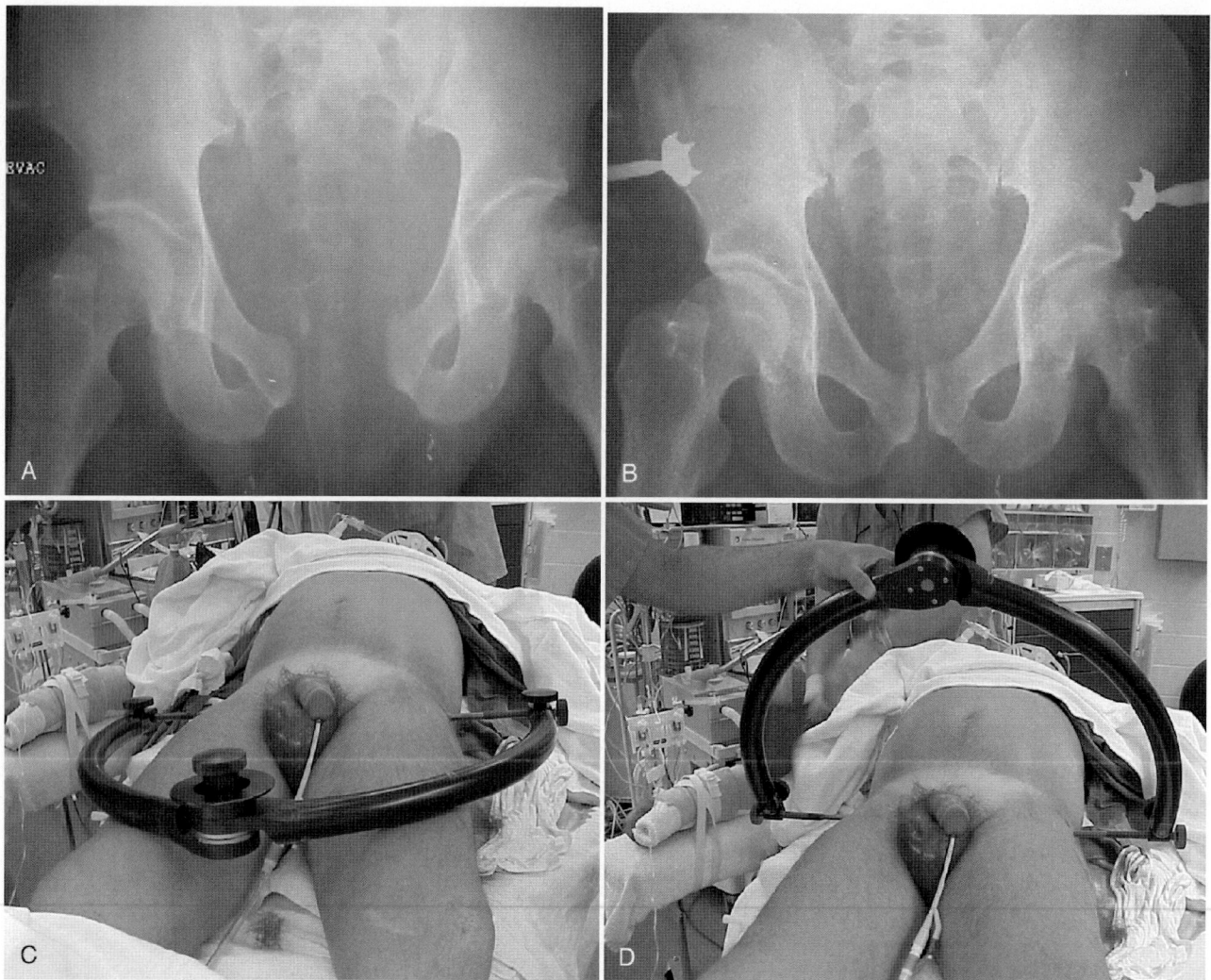

Figure 21-14 Pelvic ring disruption with massive hemorrhage. **A,** Anteroposterior (AP) radiograph of the pelvis showing disruption of the symphysis pubis and the sacroiliac joint. **B,** AP view of the pelvis after reduction by the application of a pelvic stabilizer. **C** and **D,** Patient with the pelvic stabilizer in the standard position and elevated to allow access to the perineum or permit flexion of the hips for change to the lithotomy position.

oped that can be applied rapidly to reduce and provisionally stabilize the pelvis in the emergency department. Their design allows compression of the pelvis through percutaneous pins applied to the outer surface of the ilium, and they permit easy access to the abdomen or extremities (Fig. 21-14). The C-clamps can remain in place throughout the resuscitation phase and then be replaced by definitive stabilization methods when appropriate. Care must be taken in the application of these clamps because serious complications can result from misplacement of the pins or inappropriate use. Accordingly, these devices are best applied in certain rotationally and vertically unstable pelvic ring disruptions.

The role of angiography in the diagnosis and management of pelvic hemorrhage remains controversial. The incidence of arterial hemorrhage amenable to embolization is approximately 10%, and in these cases, arteriography with embolization can be lifesaving.[13,14] However,

because the procedure is technically difficult and time consuming, its use should be reserved for cases in which all other methods of hemorrhage control have been exhausted.[13]

Management Algorithms

Algorithms for the management of a hypotensive patient with a pelvic fracture should begin with a search for the cause of the shock (Fig. 21-15). All possible causes of bleeding are to be explored. Auscultation of the chest and review of the chest radiograph can determine the presence of hemothorax and the need for thoracotomy. Once hemothorax is ruled out or controlled by chest tube placement, diagnostic peritoneal lavage or ultrasound of the abdomen is performed. Examination of the pelvis is carried out as previously described. Any wounds around the pelvis or in the perineum are noted. Bleeding from

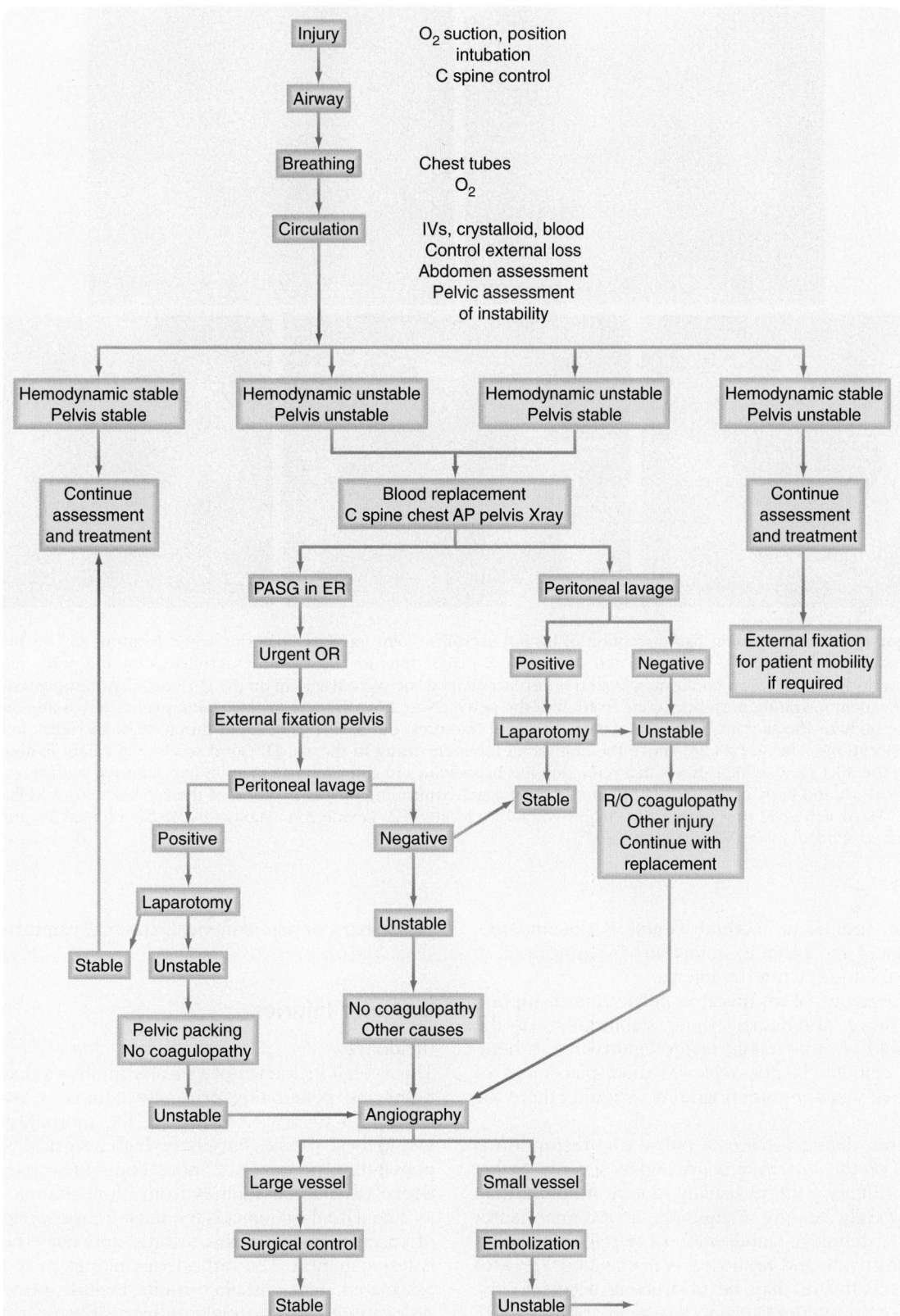

Figure 21-15 Algorithm for resuscitation after pelvic disruption. C spine, cervical spine; ER, emergency room; Fx, fracture; IVs, intravenous lines; OR, operating room; PASG, pneumatic antishock garment; RPH, retroperitoneal hematoma; R/O, rule out. (From Kellam JF, Mayo K: Pelvic ring disruptions. In Browner BD, Jupiter TB, Levine AM, Trafton PG [eds]: Skeletal Trauma, 3rd ed. Philadelphia, WB Saunders, 2003.)

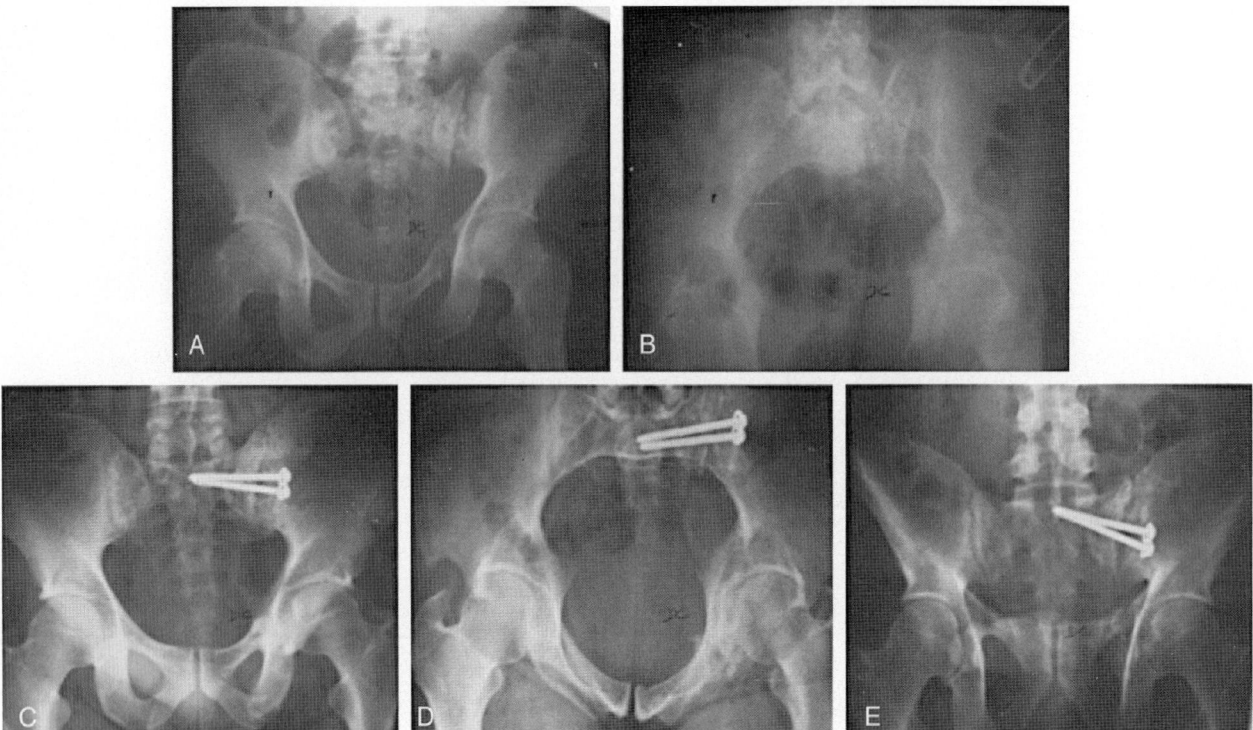

Figure 21-16 This patient had disruption of his left sacroiliac joint fixed by posterior screw fixation. **A,** This man was struck from behind by a truck and suffered a displaced fracture through the sacroiliac joint and pubic rami anteriorly. **B,** Inlet view confirming posterior displacement at the sacroiliac joint on the left side. **C,** Anteroposterior view demonstrating posterior screw fixation of the pelvis. Note how the screws have been placed across and into the body of the sacrum. This is necessary for sacral fractures, but it also gains good purchase in sacroiliac joint dislocations. The screws are above the first sacral foramen sitting in the ala. **D,** Good screw placement is noted on the inlet view, which shows that reduction has been achieved and adequate fixation has occurred with screws in the ala and body of the sacrum. **E,** Outlet view again confirming proper position of the screws. (From Kellam JF, Mayo K: Pelvic ring disruptions. In Browner BD, Jupiter TB, Levine AM, Trafton PG [eds]: Skeletal Trauma, 3rd ed. Philadelphia, WB Saunders, 2003.)

the rectum, vagina, or urethral meatus is documented. Digital vaginal and rectal examinations are performed to identify tears and fracture fragments.

In the presence of an unstable pelvic ring disruption and a positive abdominal study, stabilization of the pelvis should be undertaken *before laparotomy.* If hemodynamic stability is not achieved after placement of the external fixator, arteriography should then be performed.

Long-term, definitive care of pelvic ring disruption is dependent on the pattern of injury and its severity. Stable fractures or injury patterns usually require no more than restricted weight bearing. Frequently, an external fixator can provide definitive stabilization of unstable injuries if applied effectively and reduction is maintained. In cases in which the fixator may be obstructing access to the abdomen or an interim C-clamp has been applied, ORIF or closed reduction and percutaneous fixation may be indicated. When rotational or vertical instability is present, both the anterior and the posterior pelvis must be stabilized. Anteriorly, the symphysis is often secured with a plate and screws. Posteriorly, more options exist. The sacroiliac joint or sacral fractures can be secured with

plates, bars, or percutaneously inserted cannulated screws (Fig. 21-16).

Vascular Injuries

Incidence

The overall incidence of vascular injuries associated with blunt and penetrating extremity trauma is low, ranging from 0.2% to 1.5%.[18] However, the morbidity and limb loss in these injuries have been high historically. Although penetrating trauma is a more common cause, the incidence of vascular injuries from blunt trauma is as high as 20%. Distal ischemia is the most frequent manifestation of vascular injury in this setting, and overt hemorrhage is less common. The orthopedic injuries most frequently associated with vascular insults include posterior knee dislocations, supracondylar humerus fractures, and elbow dislocations. Vascular injuries occur in association with posterior knee dislocations 40% of the time, and delay in diagnosis or repair has led to amputation rates as high as 85%. Fractures such as supracondylar femoral, tibial plateau, or combined tibial-fibular fractures are rarely associated with vascular injury.[18] Extensive soft tissue

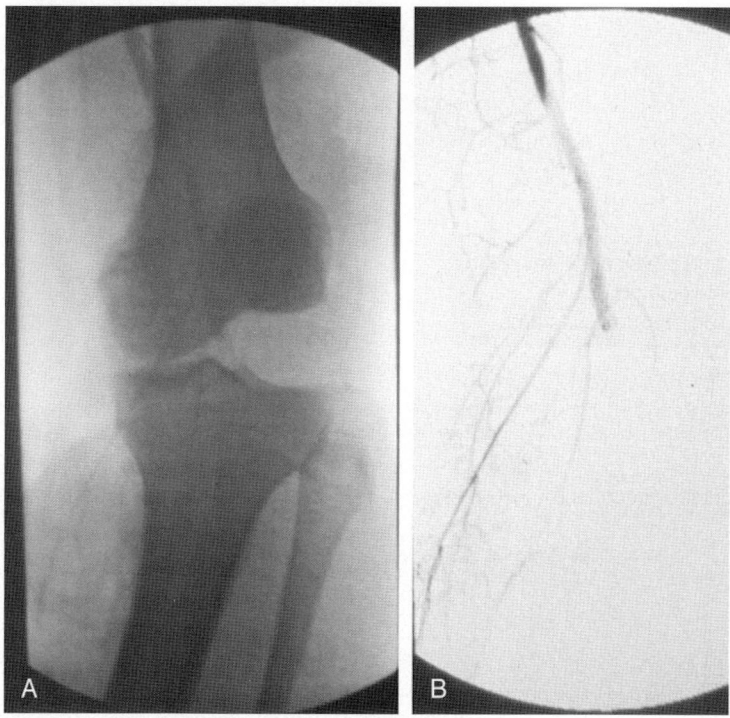

Figure 21-17 Angiogram of the lower extremity after posterior knee dislocation. **A,** The fluoroscopic image shows significant displacement after posterior knee dislocation. **B,** Disruption of popliteal blood flow at the level of the dislocation is clearly appreciated on the angiogram.

trauma is also associated with vascular abnormalities, and factors associated with a poor prognosis include extensive soft tissue and skeletal damage, warm ischemic time longer than 6 hours, a mangled extremity severity score (MESS) greater than 7, and tibial nerve injury.[19]

Although upper extremity injuries account for nearly 30% of all peripheral vascular injuries, lower extremity vascular trauma carries a poorer prognosis and is potentially more serious. In particular, the popliteal region is prone to ischemia for several reasons. Although there is abundant collateral circulation around the knee, these vessels are fragile and are easily damaged by direct trauma or adjacent swelling. The popliteal artery begins at the adductor hiatus, which restricts its movement. The soleus muscles also prevents excursion of the popliteal artery, thus making it prone to injury with knee dislocation (Fig. 21-17). In the setting of popliteal artery thrombosis, lack of high-flow collaterals may lead to end-vessel thrombosis in situ secondary to low flow. Patency of these vessels is critical in limb salvage. Injuries to the common femoral or superficial femoral artery rarely result in amputation because of the rich collateral circulation and the profunda femoris artery. Though rarely injured, injury to this vessel may be clinically silent and the diagnosis must be made by angiography.

Management
Optimal results in treating combined vascular and orthopedic injuries depend on a high index of suspicion and expeditious intervention (Fig. 21-18). A thorough vascular examination is performed in the trauma room, and all upper and lower extremity pulses are evaluated. Color, temperature, and the presence of pain or paresis are noted. Systolic pressure in the arm as well as at the ankle is recorded, and the ankle-brachial index is calculated by dividing ankle pressure by brachial pressure. In the absence of chronic peripheral vascular disease, the index should be greater than 0.95. Usually, ankle-brachial indices and pulses are symmetrical bilaterally. Audible bruits over blood vessels at affected areas may signify arterial injury or a traumatic fistula. Abnormal swelling may indicate deep vessel injury or rupture. Any pulse deficit or ankle-brachial index less than 0.90 warrants formal arteriography. Prolonged or severe ischemia mandates immediate operative exploration. Intraoperative arteriography may be useful in planning vascular reconstruction if a vascular injury is present without critical ischemia. Direct arterial exploration of suspected injuries is warranted in open fractures.

Staging of skeletal stabilization and vascular repair should be individualized. Generally, vascular reconstruction precedes fracture fixation because disruption of the vascular repair after orthopedic fixation is rare, provided that the repair is performed with limb length restored. The ipsilateral and contralateral limbs are prepared widely to allow access to distal vessels, fasciotomy, and contralateral saphenous vein harvest. Fasciotomy is performed before vascular repair if compartment syndrome is suspected. In knee dislocations, it is advisable to release the compartments of the lower part of the leg because of the chance of reperfusion injury and the development of compartment syndrome. Proximal and distal control is

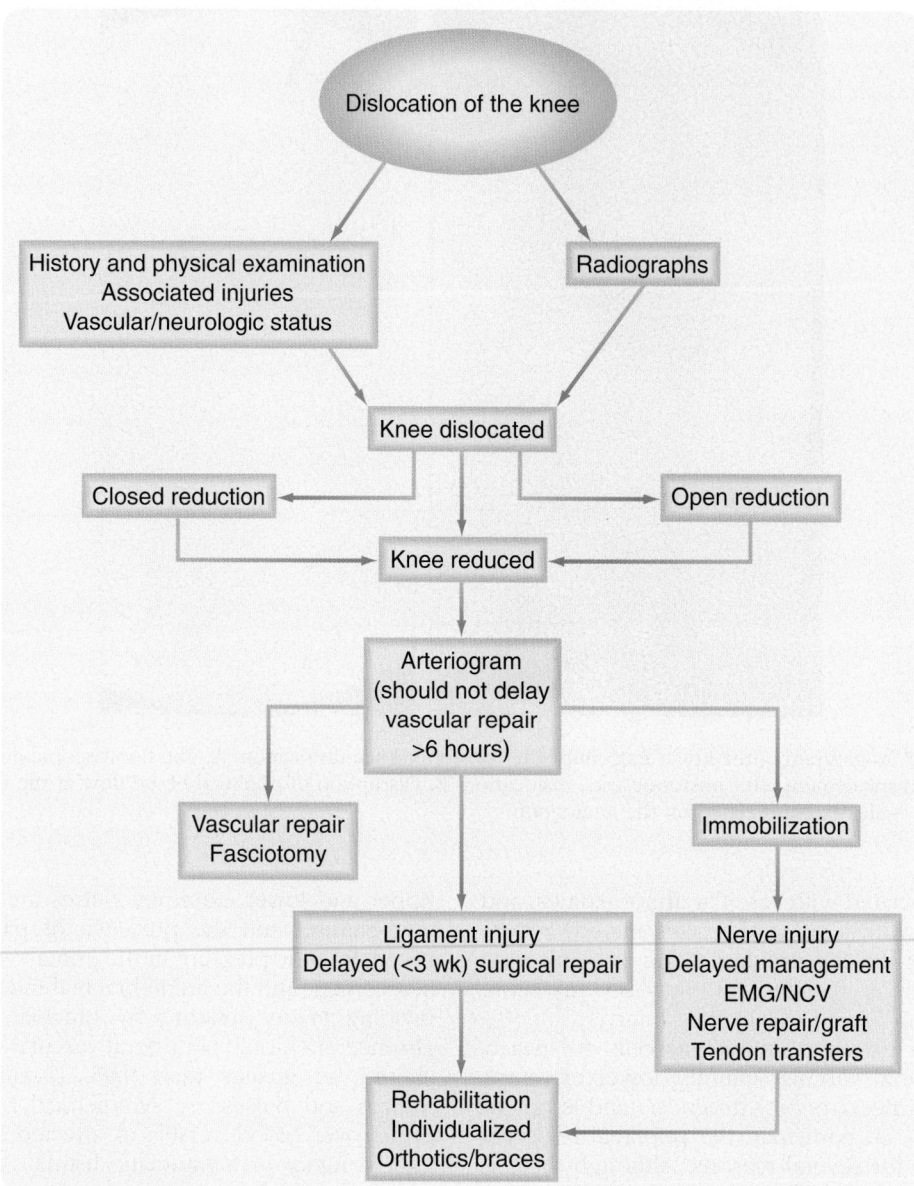

Figure 21-18 Treatment algorithm for dislocation of the knee. EMG/NCV, electromyography/nerve conduction velocity. (From Siliski JM: Dislocations and soft tissue injuries of the knee. In Browner BD, Jupiter TB, Levine AM, Trafton PG [eds]: Skeletal Trauma, 3rd ed. Philadelphia, WB Saunders, 2003.)

obtained before exploration of the hematoma. The artery and vein are carefully inspected, and an assessment of the injury is made.

The use of indwelling intraoperative shunts is appropriate for selected unstable skeletal lesions.[20] Standard carotid endarterectomy shunts are often used in this setting. Proximal and distal thrombectomy is performed before shunt placement or repair. Frequently, arterial resection is necessary to obtain acceptable margins, and a saphenous vein graft is used if primary repair without tension is not possible. A completion arteriogram is performed routinely because limb salvage depends on arterial patency. All major vein injuries are repaired to

increase the patency rate of the arterial repair and prevent the sequelae of chronic venous congestion.

Acute Compartment Syndrome

Early recognition plus treatment of compartment syndrome is critical in a trauma patient to avoid death, early amputation, and limb dysfunction. Volkmann was the first to describe the sequelae of postischemic contracture more than a century ago. He attributed permanent muscle contracture to trauma, swelling, and tight bandaging. Seddon and associates reviewed the late complications of compartment syndrome of the upper and lower extremities and stressed the importance of early recognition and fasciotomy.[21,22] Failure to diagnose and treat compartment syndrome in a trauma patient has resulted in numerous cases of preventable morbidity, as well as litigation, often resulting in settlements in favor of the plaintiff.[23]

Various compartment syndromes have been described in both the upper and lower extremities, including compartment syndromes of the shoulder, arm, forearm, hand, buttocks, thigh, lower part of the leg, and foot. The causes of compartment syndrome are numerous and include, but are not limited to, open and closed fractures, arterial injury, gunshot wounds, snake bites, extravasation at venous and arterial access sites, limb compression, burns, constrictive dressings, and tight casts. Rapid diagnosis plus management of compartment syndrome is paramount to achieve a successful clinical outcome. This section addresses the pathogenesis, diagnosis, and management of acute compartment syndrome, specifically in the forearm and lower part of the leg.

Pathogenesis

Compartment syndrome occurs secondary to increased pressure in the enclosed osseofascial space. The most common cause of compartment syndrome in an orthopedic patient is muscle edema from direct trauma to the extremity or reperfusion after vascular injury. This edema causes an increase in compartment pressure, which prevents venous outflow from the affected extremity and thus leads to backflow congestion and furthers the cycle of increasing pressure and muscle ischemia. In the case of an orthopedic trauma patient with a long bone fracture, bleeding from the fracture that produces a space-occupying hematoma exacerbates the situation. Upon reduction of the fracture, compartment pressures increase secondary to a decrease in the compartmental volume. External compressive casts or bandages further reduce the ability of the compartment to expand.

Controversy exists regarding the level of compartment pressure for which surgical intervention is required. Whitesides and Heckman recommended a fasciotomy when intracompartmental pressure approaches 20 mm Hg below diastolic pressure in the presence of worsening general condition, documented rising tissue pressure, significant tissue injury, or a history of 6 hours of total ischemia time of an extremity.[24] Mubarak and Hargens determined that absolute tissue pressure of 30 mm Hg is the critical value at which fasciotomy should be performed.[25] They concluded that because normal capillary pressure is 30 mm Hg, higher pressure will result in tissue necrosis. Finally, Matsen and associates stated that the critical compartment pressure requiring fasciotomy is 45 mm Hg.[26] They stated that as compartment pressure increases, capillary pressure must increase with the rise in venous pressure. As a result, they believed that normal baseline capillary pressure is irrelevant in determining whether compartment syndrome is present.

Although there is controversy regarding when a fasciotomy should be performed, there is little debate regarding the effect of prolonged ischemia on skeletal muscle and nerve tissue. Investigators have established that

peripheral nerves and muscles can survive for as long as 4 hours under ischemic conditions without irreversible damage. An ischemic time of 6 hours results in a variable return of function in both muscle and nerve tissue, and a total ischemic time longer than 8 hours leads to irreversible nerve and muscle injury.[24]

Diagnosis

The diagnosis of acute compartment syndrome requires a high degree of clinical suspicion, a full understanding of the mechanism of injury, and careful serial physical examinations (Fig. 21-19). Tscherne and Gotzen stated that the more severe the initial soft tissue injury, the greater the probability that soft tissue complications, including compartment syndrome, will develop.[7] The diagnosis of compartment syndrome relies on an understanding of those at risk, subjective complaints of the patients, and an appreciation of early and late physical and clinical findings.

The presence of distal pulses and the absence of pallor cannot exclude the diagnosis of compartment syndrome because tissue perfusion in a compartment is dependent on both arterial and capillary perfusion gradients. Paralysis and paresthesias are unreliable because studies have shown that peripheral nerves can conduct impulses after 1 hour or more of total ischemic time. Ischemia of muscles, however, causes pain. Patients are typically said to have "pain out of proportion to that expected for the injury." Unusual requests for frequent narcotic analgesics can be reflective of ischemic pain. Passive stretching of the ischemic muscle of the compartment in question causes exquisite pain and is the most sensitive clinical finding in a developing compartment syndrome. Clinical palpation of the compartment in question plus comparison with the contralateral limb is useful in evaluating a compartment at risk, and any evidence of increased tension or fullness of the compartment should raise clinical suspicion.

Although pain out of proportion to the injury is a cardinal clinical finding of an impending compartment syndrome, it must be emphasized that this pain will diminish as further ischemia occurs. In addition, the clinical findings may be obscured in patients medicated with narcotics, and therefore narcotic administration should be closely monitored.

Systemic hypotension, vascular injury, external limb compression, coagulopathy, and deep venous thrombosis predispose trauma patients to the development of compartment syndrome. In an uncooperative, intoxicated, intubated, or neurologically impaired patient, the diagnosis of compartment syndrome may depend more on measurement of compartment pressures.

Tissue Pressure Measurements

Five methods have been described for evaluation of compartment pressure: the wick catheter, the slit catheter, Whitesides' infusion technique, the Stic (Stryker) catheter, and the use of near-infrared spectroscopy (Fig. 21-20).[24] Although the first three techniques are still used, the most common method of measurement is the Stryker Stic device. This hand-held electronic device is easily

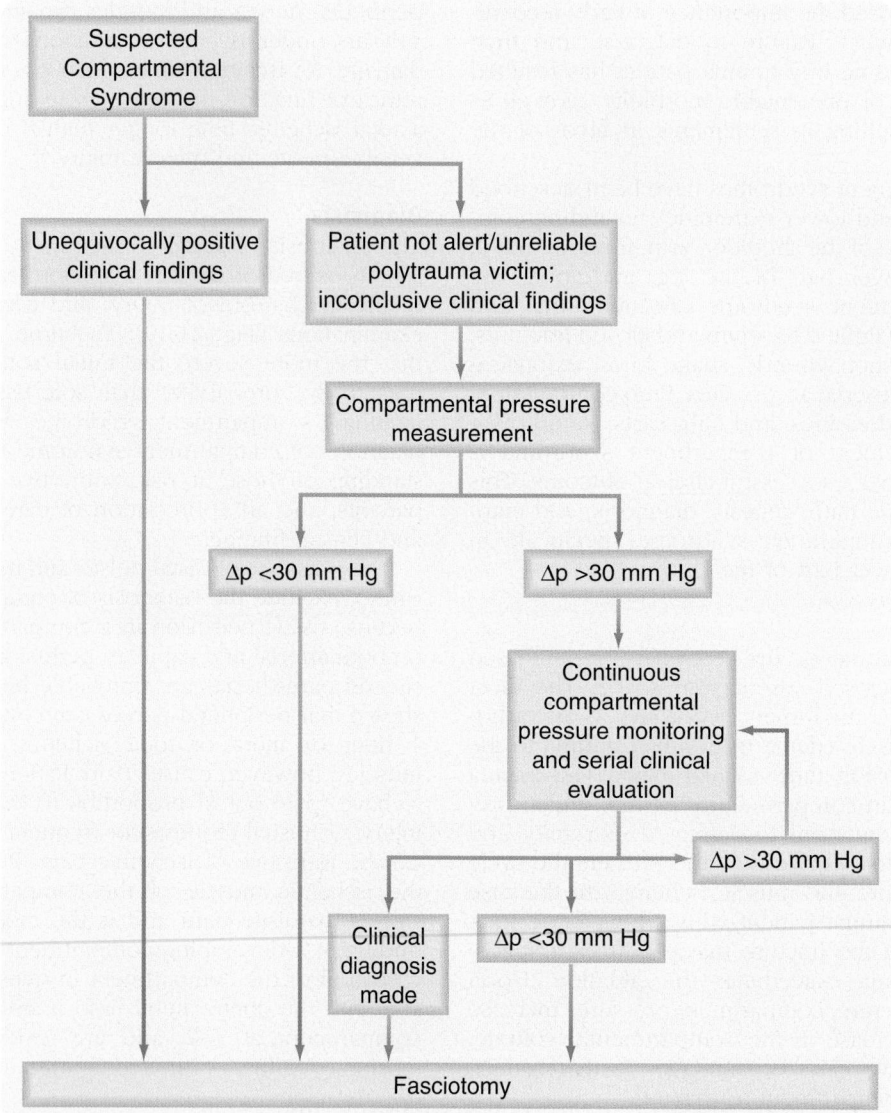

Figure 21-19 Algorithm for the management of a patient with suspected compartment syndrome. (From Amendola A, Twaddle BC: Compartment syndromes. In Browner BD, Jupiter TB, Levine AM, Trafton PG [eds]: Skeletal Trauma, 3rd ed. Philadelphia, WB Saunders, 2003.)

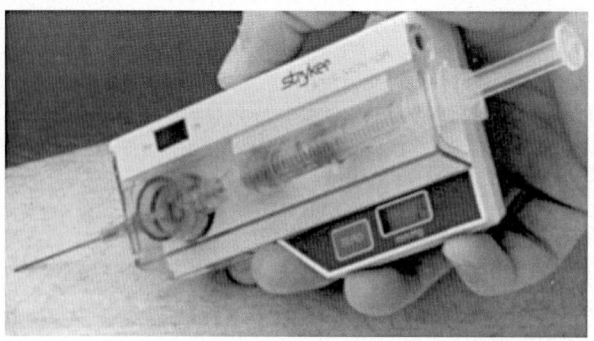

Figure 21-20 The Stic catheter. (Courtesy of Stryker, Mississauga, Ontario, Canada.)

calibrated and used. Pressures are obtained by inserting the needle into each compartment. It is generally used to make measurements at one point in time and is not an indwelling device.

Heckman and colleagues, in a prospective study of tibia fractures, reviewed the correlation between the site at which the Stic device is introduced into the compartment and the proximity of the fracture site.[27] They reported that the highest compartment pressures were usually found at the level of the fracture or within 5 cm of it. Tissue pressure decreased at an increasing distance proximal and distal to the fracture site. It is important to take this into consideration when using the Stryker Stic device to measure compartment pressure in the presence of a long bone fracture.

In place of invasive methods of measuring compartment pressure, fiberoptic devices are available in which near-infrared spectroscopy is used to measure tissue perfusion as a function of hemoglobin saturation. These devices allow continuous, transcutaneous monitoring and are becoming more widely available. By using the absorptive wavelength of venous muscle oxyhemoglobin, near-infrared spectroscopy can be used to evaluate the viability of a compartment at risk. Increased application of this technology in the diagnosis of chronic compartment syndrome has encouraged its use more routinely in the acute and subacute setting.[28]

Surgical Treatment

The two-incision approach to fasciotomy (Fig. 21-21) of the lower part of the leg is a reliable and straightforward procedure, given that the anatomy is well understood (Table 21-2). It involves making an anterolateral incision over the anterior and lateral compartments and a medial incision just posterior to the medial aspect of the tibia. The anterolateral incision is centered halfway between the fibular shaft and the tibia. Once the fascia is identified, a small transverse incision is made to identify the anterior and lateral compartments, as well as the superficial peroneal nerve traveling in the lateral compartment. It is important to release the entire compartment, including the most proximal and distal aspects, while protecting the superficial peroneal nerve. The posteromedial incision is used to decompress both the superficial and the deep posterior compartments. The incision is made approximately 2 cm posterior to the tibial shaft. Care must be taken to preserve the saphenous nerve and vein. Once the fascia is identified, a transverse incision is made to delineate the superficial and deep compartments. The superficial posterior compartment is released first, proximally and distally to the medial malleolus. In similar fashion, the deep posterior compartment is released. To completely decompress the deep compartment, the soleus muscle must be taken down off the medial side of the tibia.

Skin closure of the fasciotomy is facilitated with vessel loops laced through staples placed along the skin edges. The vessel loops can be tightened daily at the bedside as the soft tissue swelling diminishes, which may eliminate the need for skin grafting.

Open Fractures

Open fractures are surgical emergencies because the long-term complications may threaten the patient's limb and can, with systemic sepsis, threaten the patient's life. The difficulty of open fracture management has been recognized for centuries. Amputation had been the mainstay of treatment until the mid-1800s, when antiseptic technique came into use. Antisepsis, combined with débridement of all contaminated and devitalized tissue, provided the first reduction in open fracture–related mortality. Contemporaneous advances in antibiotic prophylaxis, aggressive débridement and open wound management, rotational muscle flaps, free tissue transfer, and bone grafting techniques have dramatically enhanced our capacity to treat severe open fractures resulting from motor vehicle accidents and gunshot wounds.

Classification

A fracture is considered open when the fracture site communicates with the environment. Although the laceration or skin avulsion is the most obvious component, the

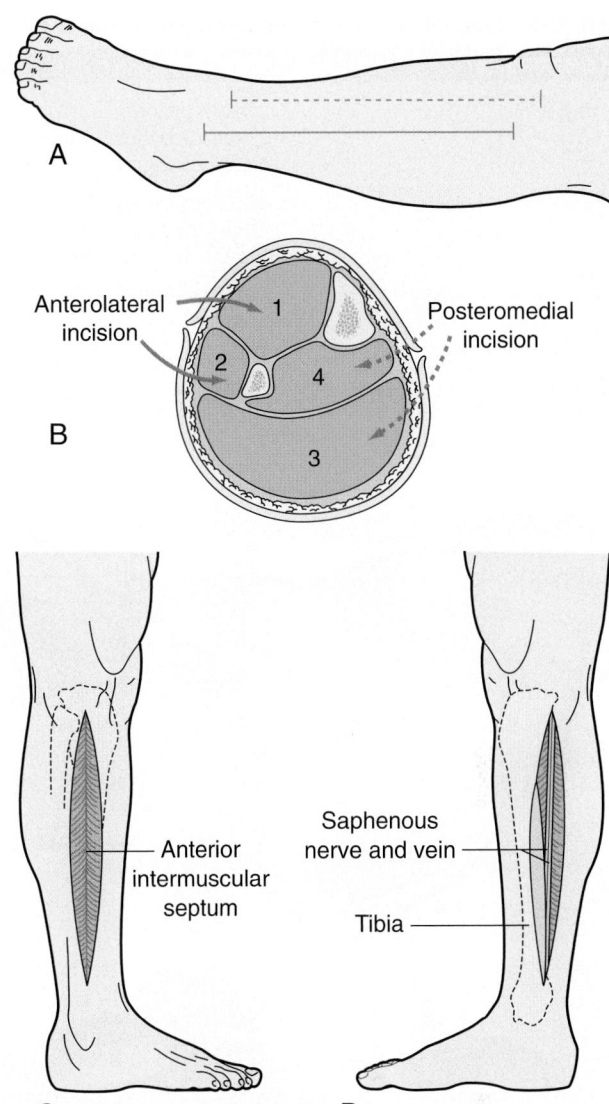

Figure 21-21 A, The double-incision technique for performing fasciotomies of all four compartments of the lower extremity. **B,** Cross section of the lower extremity showing a position of anterolateral and posteromedial incisions that allows access to the anterior and lateral compartments (1 and 2) and the superficial and deep posterior compartments (3 and 4). **C,** A vertical anterior incision is centered midway between the tibia and fibula. The anterior intermuscular septum is identified, and two fasciotomy incisions are made: one anterior and one posterior to the septum. **D,** A vertical posteromedial incision is centered 2 cm to the rear of the tibia. Care is taken to avoid injury to the saphenous vein and nerve. (Modified from Matsen FA, Bubarak SJ, Rorabeck CH: A practical approach to compartmental syndromes. In Evarts CM [ed]: AAOS Instructional Course Lectures, vol 32. St Louis, CV Mosby, 1983, pp 88-113.)

Table 21-2　Contents of Fascial Compartments in the Leg

COMPARTMENT	MUSCLES	VESSELS	NERVES
Anterior	Tibialis anterior Extensor hallucis longus Extensor digitorum communis	Anterior tibial	Deep peroneal
Deep posterior	Tibialis posterior Flexor hallucis longus Flexor digitorum longus	Posterior tibial Peroneal	Tibial
Superficial posterior	Gastrocnemius Soleus Plantaris		
Lateral	Peroneals		Superficial peroneal

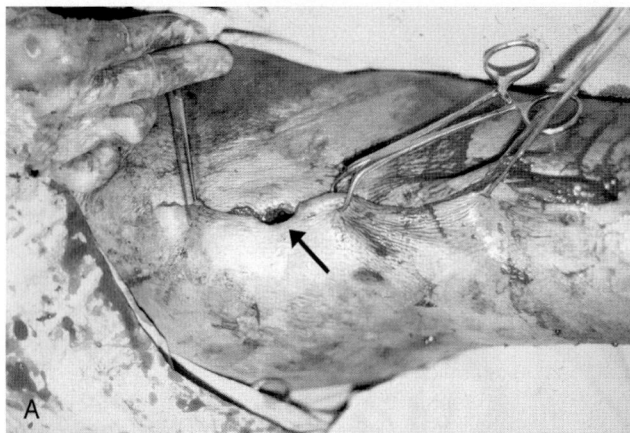

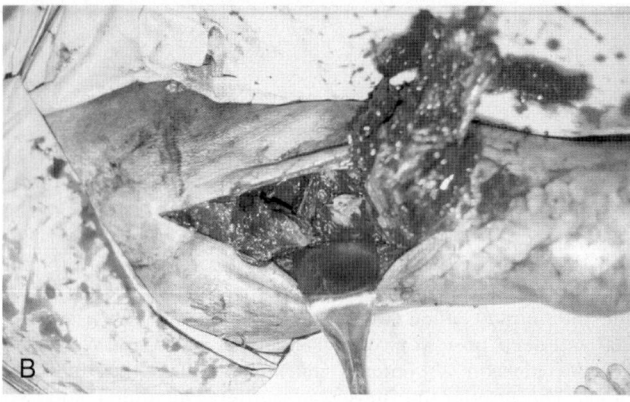

Figure 21-22 Débridement of an open wound. **A,** The small original skin wound *(arrow)* is shown in the center of a surgical incision. **B,** The full extent of underlying soft tissue damage cannot be appreciated until after exploration.

entire zone of injury must be fully appreciated at the time of surgical exploration to adequately assign a severity grade (Fig. 21-22). Gustilo and Andersen[29] devised the most commonly cited classification of fractures with soft tissue injury (Table 21-3). They divided fractures into three types and subdivided type III lesions into three subgroups based on the length of the skin opening and the degree of comminution, soft tissue injury, and con-

tamination. This classification scheme represents a continuum. Sharp divisions between groups are difficult to discern, particularly among the intermediate types; thus, interobserver variation occurs.

The Gustilo-Andersen classification provides useful information regarding the prognosis and treatment of the injured extremity. Infection rates tend to increase from type I through type III. Seven percent of type I, 11% of type II, 18% of type IIIA, and 56% of type IIIB/IIIC fractures became infected in one series. Wound cultures taken in the emergency department are positive in 60% to 70% of open fractures, with most growing saprophytic organisms.[7,30] More useful cultures can be obtained after formal irrigation and débridement of the wounds. Forty-three percent of cultures taken from type I, II, and IIIA fractures after débridement grew *Staphylococcus aureus,* and 14% grew facultative or aerobic gram-negative rods. In type IIIB and IIIC lesions, *S. aureus* was recovered only 7% of the time, whereas gram-negative rods accounted for 67% of the recovered organisms. Regardless of type, antimicrobials and tetanus prophylaxis are administered in the trauma room for any open fracture. In type I and II open fractures and in closed fractures with soft tissue injuries, a first-generation cephalosporin is preferred. In type III fractures, the addition of an aminoglycoside is recommended. For any fracture with suspected soil contamination, high-dose penicillin is added to the regimen to cover *Clostridium* species. The duration of treatment remains controversial.

The soft tissue destruction in a closed injury can be worse than that in comparable open injuries. Tscherne and Gotzen classified closed fractures (Table 21-4) by creating a spectrum similar to what was recognized in open fractures.[7] Although this system has not been critically validated with outcome measures, it provides a means to gauge the significance of associated soft tissue injury. When these tissues become necrotic or if a surgical approach is carried out through them, infection rates could potentially increase.

Initial Management

Early irrigation and débridement are the mainstays of treatment. Once the patient is in the operating room, dressings can be removed along with all loose debris.

Table 21-3 Gustilo-Andersen Classification of Open Fractures

FRACTURE TYPE	DESCRIPTION
I	Skin opening of less than 1 cm, clean; most likely inside-to-outside lesion; minimal muscle contusion; simple transverse or oblique fracture
II	Laceration greater than 1 cm with extensive soft tissue damage, flaps, or avulsion; minimal to moderate crushing; simple transverse or short oblique fracture with minimal comminution
III	Extensive soft tissue damage, including muscle, skin, and neurovascular structures; often a high-velocity injury with a severe crushing component
IIIA	Extensive laceration, adequate bone coverage; segmental fracture; gunshot injuries
IIIB	Extensive soft tissue damage with periosteal stripping and bone exposure; usually associated with massive contamination
IIIC	Vascular injury requiring repair

From Gustilo R, Mendoza R, Williams DN: Problems in the management of type III (severe) open fractures. J Trauma 24:742-746, 1984.

Table 21-4 Tscherne Classification of Fractures With Soft Tissue Injuries

FRACTURE TYPE	DESCRIPTION
0	Minimal soft tissue damage; indirect violence; simple fracture patterns; *example:* torsion fracture of the tibia in skiers
I	Superficial abrasion or contusion caused by pressure from within; mild to moderately severe fracture configuration; *example:* pronation fracture-dislocation of the ankle joint with a soft tissue lesion over the medial malleolus
II	Deep, contaminated abrasion associated with a localized skin or muscle contusion; impending compartment syndrome; severe fracture configuration; *example:* segmental "bumper" fracture of the tibia
III	Extensive skin contusion or crushing injury; underlying muscle damage may be severe; subcutaneous avulsion; decompensated compartment syndrome; associated major vascular injury; severe or comminuted fracture configuration

From Tscherne H, Oestern H: Die Klassifizierung des Weichteilschadens bei offenen und geschlossenen Frakturen. Unfallheikunde 85:111-115, 1982.

Débridement requires meticulous removal and resection of all foreign and nonviable material from the wound. The goal is reduction of the bacterial count by leaving only clearly viable tissue behind. The wound is aggressively explored because the zone of injury is always larger than initially evident. Areas in which the extent of injury is commonly misjudged include the thigh and posterior of the leg because of their considerable muscle bulk. The fascial compartments are not completely decompressed by open fractures, and therefore fasciotomies are liberally performed during débridement. Irrigation with copious amounts of saline solution is then performed. Repeat débridement is performed 48 to 72 hours later because the tissue may demarcate and necrose. Surgical incisions used to enlarge the wound for exploration are closed primarily. The original wound created by the injury is usually left open. Dressings soaked in saline solution are applied and changed one or twice daily. In contrast to temporary dressings applied for transport from the emergency department, definitive wound management dressings should not be soaked in povidone-iodine because it causes tissue destruction.

Planning for wound coverage begins with the initial débridement. Early plastic surgery consultation may be helpful and will play a key role in determining the timing and method of soft tissue reconstruction. If skin grafting or muscle flap coverage is necessary, it should be performed within the first week before secondary colonization and wound fibrosis develop.[31] The desire to avoid nosocomial infection has promoted a trend toward immediate coverage of open fracture wounds.

Limb Salvage Versus Primary Amputation

The choice between primary amputation and salvage of a severely injured extremity is a difficult one. Successful salvage depends on multiple factors, including vascular status, extent of soft tissue injury, degree of comminution and bone loss, and neurologic function.

In addition to these local factors, ultimate success depends on systemic and psychological elements. Patients with poor nutrition, multisystem injuries, or psychoses and those not able to cooperate with a lengthy reconstructive process may not be candidates for limb salvage. Several scoring systems have been devised to help assess the need for primary amputation objectively. These systems were developed retrospectively in reference to injuries involving the lower part of the leg. Severely injured upper extremities have a far greater impact on the overall functioning status of the patient, and thus indications for upper extremity amputation are significantly more limited.

Lange and colleagues described indications for primary below-knee amputation in 1985.[32] Absolute indications were defined as anatomically complete disruption of the tibial nerve in an adult and warm ischemia time longer than 6 hours in a crush injury. Relative indications are serious associated polytrauma, severe ipsilateral foot trauma, and an anticipated protracted course to achieve soft tissue coverage and bony reconstruction. The authors suggested that if either of the absolute indications or two of the three relative indications were met, amputation was indicated. Although no further studies have been performed to validate this scheme, these guidelines have

Table 21-5   Mangled Extremity Severity Score

COMPONENT	POINTS
Skeletal and Soft Tissue Injury	
Low energy (stab, simple fracture, "civilian" gunshot wound)	1
Medium energy (open or multiplex fractures, dislocation)	2
High energy (close-range shotgun or "military" gunshot wound; crush injury)	3
Very high energy (same as above plus gross contamination, soft tissue avulsion)	4
Limb Ischemia (Doubled When >6 hr)	
Pulse reduced or absent but perfusion normal	1
Pulseless; paresthesias, diminished capillary refill	2
Cool, paralyzed, insensate, numb	3
Shock	
Systolic blood pressure always >90 mm Hg	0
Hypotensive transiently	1
Persistent hypotension	2
Age (yr)	
<30	0
30-50	1
>50	2

From Johansen K, Daines M, Howey T, et al: Objective criteria accurately predict amputation following lower extremity trauma. J Trauma 30:568-573, 1990.

been adopted widely and are considered the standard of care.

The MESS is the most widely validated classification system. It is the product of a retrospective review of 25 charts of patients with severe open fractures of the lower extremity (Table 21-5).[33] Investigators found that limb salvage was related to vascular status, patient age, duration of ischemia, and absorbed energy. A score of 7 or higher consistently predicted the need for amputation, whereas all limbs with initial scores of 6 or less remained viable in the long term. This system has been validated prospectively, and subsequent studies have supported the specificity of MESS in evaluating a severely injured lower leg with near uniformity.[19]

Limb salvage has routinely been accepted as preservation of a viable extremity, with no concern given to the functional status of the limb. Few studies have compared the functional outcome of below-knee amputation with that of salvaged limbs. Those that have show that patients with below-knee amputations returned to function and work more rapidly and had high levels of satisfaction. In contrast, limb salvage requires significantly more operative procedures and more disability time. Although some patients in this group were more dysfunctional than amputees, others were extremely satisfied and highly functional.

When presented with a severely mangled extremity, it is important to document all pertinent local and systemic factors accurately. A MESS should be calculated for each patient and used as a guideline to supplement the clinical findings. Whenever possible, pictures should be taken and added to the permanent medical record. Primary amputation should be performed when injuries include complete tibial or sciatic nerve injury in an adult or irreparable osseous or arterial injury. When the indications are not absolute, it is essential that several surgeons independently evaluate the patient and document their opinion in the medical record.

Treatment

Skeletal stabilization has been shown to be crucial for soft tissue healing. When compared with cast and splints, internal or external fixation permits greater access for wound care and is more effective in controlling pain during mobilization. At the cellular level, the inflammatory response is shortened and the spread of bacteria is diminished. The decision to use one mode of fixation over another is dependent on the fracture pattern, degree of contamination, and surgeon preference.

The most widely accepted method of fixation has been external fixation. Advances in design have made these devices lighter, more stable, and easier to apply. External fixation minimizes dissection and avoids the insertion of large metallic implants. It is easily removed, replaced, and adjusted and can be combined with other means of fixation.

However, external fixators are not without their problems. Although pin tract osteomyelitis has become rare with changes in design and the technique of pin insertion, superficial infection with drainage occurs in approximately 30% of all patients. Because of their size and location, further débridement and coverage can be cumbersome. In the tibia, for instance, pin insertion through the subcutaneous anteromedial border reduces pin tract infection but often results in obstructed access for plastic and reconstructive surgery. In other cases, more extensive fracture patterns may require more complex frame constructs that further limit access. Though effective in providing skeletal stabilization during soft tissue reconstruction, external fixation is not ideal for achieving fracture union. Additional surgery, including bone grafting or conversion to internal fixation, is often necessary.

For these reasons, IM nailing appears to be an attractive option. Definitive fracture care can usually be accomplished in a single operation. Without bulky exposed hardware, mobilization and daily wound care are facilitated. However, several early series[34] reported an unacceptably high incidence of infection when reamed IM nails were used for type III open tibia fractures. For this reason, external fixation remained the standard of care for these serious fractures throughout the 1980s. Originally, the increased infection rate was believed to be due to destruction of cortical blood flow by reaming. Animal studies showed a 70% as opposed to a 30% reduction in infection when a nail is placed without reaming.[35] Although the injury itself caused periosteal stripping and significant soft tissue loss, loss of the medullary blood supply further weakened the bone's healing potential and resistance to infection.

When unreamed, small-diameter nails were used for open fracture care, rates of deep infection and nonunion

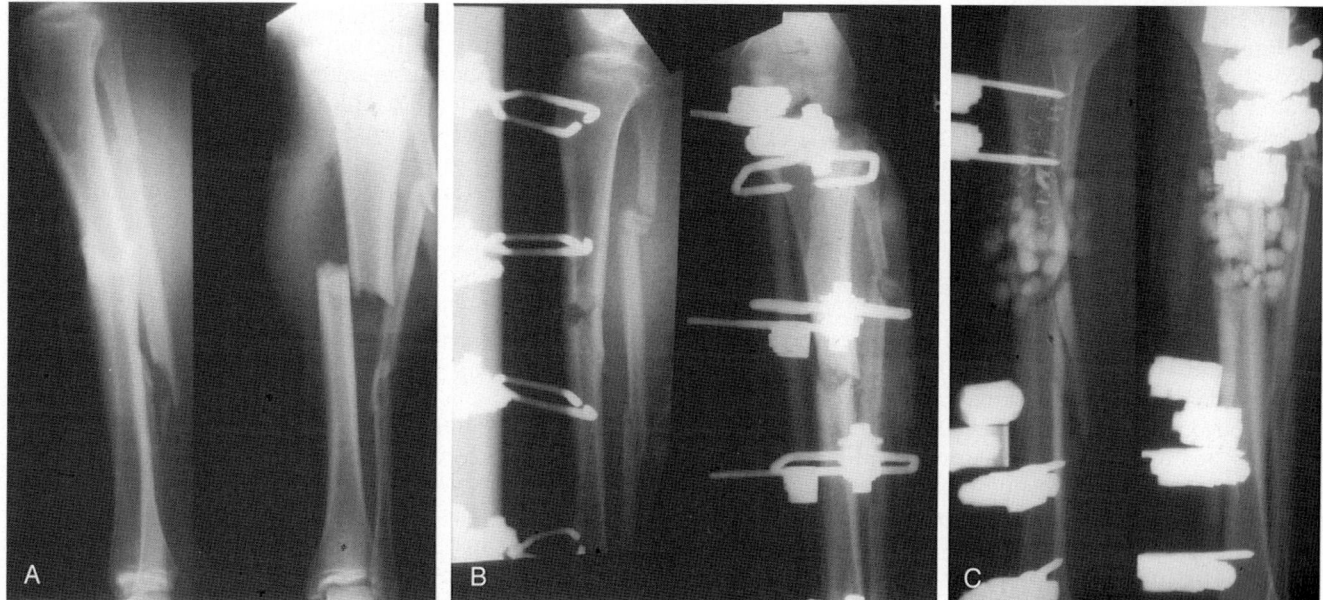

Figure 21-23 Management of open tibia/fibula fracture with external fixators. **A,** Anteroposterior and lateral views of a tibia/fibula fracture. **B,** Interim stabilization is achieved with a pinless external fixator. Note that the pins do not traverse the medullary canal. **C,** Conversion to a definitive external fixator (because of a severe open wound and significant bone loss precluding intramedullary nailing) and insertion of antibiotic-impregnated beads after débridement of necrotic bone.

were found to be the same as with external fixation. Studies have shown that with aggressive irrigation and débridement, closed unreamed nailing can be carried out immediately, even in severe type III open tibia fractures.[4,36,37]

Although the benefits of unreamed nailing have been documented, problems with their application have led to a significant reoperation rate for removal of screws, fibular osteotomy, exchange with larger-diameter reamed nails, or bone grafting. Use of small-diameter rods and cross-locking screws has led to some implant failure, particularly with premature weight bearing. Intraoperative malalignment and subsequent malunion of proximal fractures have been a continuing problem. Despite these issues, unreamed locked IM nailing has supplanted external fixation for most open tibia fractures.[4]

Another approach to the treatment of open tibia fractures has been the initial use of external fixation followed by reamed IM nailing or plating. Many investigators have reported a high incidence of infection when reamed IM nailing was attempted after a substantial period of external fixation. Osteomyelitis after IM nailing was associated with long periods of external fixation and a history of pin tract infection. If this technique is to be used, the external fixator should be left on no longer than 2 weeks.[38]

To avoid these problems, the pinless external fixator was developed. This device allows the tibial fragments to be fixed with a series of C-clamps that grasp the outer cortex without penetrating the medullary canal (Fig. 21-23). This method reduces IM contamination and provides another route for safe conversion to reamed IM nails.[39] Because the pins do not penetrate the canal, the

device may even be left in place to help maintain alignment and stability during the subsequent IM nailing. However, early investigations have shown problems with soft tissue necrosis from the current clamp design that may be eliminated by subsequent design improvements.

Despite the discussions regarding skeletal fixation, the hallmarks of successful treatment of open femoral fractures are still antibiotic prophylaxis, irrigation, débridement, compartment decompression, stabilization, and early wound coverage. Although external fixation is a safe and useful tool, its use for type I, II, and IIIA open fractures of the tibia has been replaced by unreamed IM nailing. Although evidence suggests that this is a safe practice for type IIIB fractures,[36] some are reluctant to adopt it. Until further evidence is available, some form of external fixation should be applied initially and then converted to a reamed, locked nail within 2 weeks for these difficult fractures. Coverage for all wounds is accomplished within 1 week, whenever possible. With these guidelines the amputation rate has fallen dramatically.

Dislocations

Dislocations of major joints (e.g., the shoulder, elbow, hip, knee, or ankle) are considered orthopedic emergencies. Prolonged dislocation can lead to cartilage cell death, post-traumatic arthritis, neurovascular injury, ankylosis, and avascular necrosis. These injuries, which are more likely to occur in young, active patients, can have devastating consequences.

Most dislocations have characteristic physical findings. After a dislocation, muscles around the joint typically become spasmodic, thereby limiting range of motion as the limb assumes a distinctive position. In posterior hip dislocations, the thigh is held flexed and internally rotated. The affected limb is often shortened and cannot be passively extended. An anterior shoulder dislocation causes an externally rotated and adducted arm position. Elbow and knee dislocations (most commonly posterior) result in an extremity locked in extension. As with all extremity injuries, a meticulous neurovascular examination must be performed and documented before and after manipulation.

Hip dislocations require special discussion because of the extreme consequences of failure to recognize and address them in timely fashion. Sciatic nerve injury, cartilage cell death, and avascular necrosis can result from delay in treatment of these injuries. Of these complications, avascular necrosis is the most devastating because of its propensity to cause collapse of the femoral head and the subsequent development of degenerative joint disease. This problem can lead to a need for total hip replacement or hip fusion at a young age. After these procedures, multiple major reconstructive operations are common during the patient's lifetime.

Avascular necrosis usually develops in a time-dependent fashion. In the dislocated position, tension on the capsular blood vessels restricts blood flow to the femoral head. If the hip remains dislocated for 24 hours, avascular necrosis will ensue in 100% of cases. Although irreversible damage to the blood supply may occur at the time of injury, reduction within 6 hours is generally believed to reduce the incidence of ischemic changes.

Reduction of dislocations often requires IV sedation to reduce the muscle spasm at the joint. If a joint cannot be reduced by closed methods with adequate sedation, general anesthesia is required. Attempts are made to reduce the joint by closed techniques in the operating room, with staff available for open reduction if this fails.

COMMON LONG BONE FRACTURES

To fully appreciate the nature of a musculoskeletal injury, it is important to identify not only the presence of a fracture but also the energy involved in its origin. The fracture pattern offers clues to the mechanism of injury; low-energy twisting injuries typically produce simple spiral fractures, direct impact usually induces a bending moment that results in a transverse fracture, and severe, high-energy injuries have complex segmental or comminuted patterns. Ultimately, the fracture pattern serves to identify the mechanism of injury and illuminates the amount of energy absorbed by both the fracture and the surrounding soft tissue. It is often the injury to surrounding tissue that decides the fate of the fractured bone.

Femur Fractures

Epidemiology and Significance
Femoral shaft fractures deserve special attention. Femur fractures occur at a rate of 1 per 10,000 people per year.

A closed femoral shaft fracture is considered a "major" injury when calculating the injury severity score (ISS). Therefore, another major injury in any other organ system qualifies the patient as multiply injured. With the exception of pathologic or insufficiency fractures in the elderly, these fractures are the result of a high-energy injury and, in the trauma setting, are predictive of small bowel injury. Frequently, these injuries lead to significant bleeding. Because of the geometry of the thigh, several units of blood can be hidden in the tissues with little external evidence of bleeding. Transfusion with packed red blood cells is often necessary, with 40% of patients needing 2.5 or more units.

Initial Management
All femur fractures must be immobilized before the patient is transported from the scene of the accident. Leaving a displaced fracture without a splint leads to increased edema, bleeding, and further damage to the surrounding soft tissues and neurovascular structures. Continued motion at the fracture site also results in increased fat embolization and contributes to the development of ARDS. Proper immobilization begins with in-line traction to increase the length of the thigh compartment and decrease its diameter. The soft tissues are then under tension and can tamponade bleeding at the fracture site. For patients in extremis, a posterior splint alone will suffice until formal traction or immobilization can be achieved. If time allows, a traction pin can be placed through the proximal tibia to provide skeletal traction and allow access to the distal femur. A Hare traction splint, either with skin traction through the ankle or attached to a skeletal traction pin, is quite effective in immobilizing a femur fracture temporarily (Fig. 21-24).

Definitive Stabilization
Definitive stabilization of femur fractures within the first 24 hours is essential in a polytrauma victim.[8] Some studies have shown deleterious effects when fracture fixation is delayed only 2 to 4 days.[40,41] Immediate fixation leads to earlier mobilization, prevention of deep venous thrombosis and decubitus ulcers, easier nursing care, and decreased need for analgesia. Furthermore, the magnitude of fat embolized is also decreased.[8] Taken together, these factors can significantly improve pulmonary status and decrease the incidence of ARDS. This benefit is magnified as the ISS increases. In patients with severe trauma (ISS >40), delayed fixation of femoral shaft fractures leads to a fivefold increase in the incidence of ARDS. In addition, immediate stabilization of femoral fractures significantly decreases the cost of the hospital stay.[8]

Contraindications to immediate stabilization include hypothermia, coagulopathy, excessive intracranial pressure, and high pulmonary shunting. The findings in femoral fracture studies have been broadened to support immediate fixation of all long bone fractures, but definitive studies have not yet been performed. In isolated long bone fractures, the need for immediate fixation is not evident. However, if the institution is capable of performing stabilization within 24 hours, there is no reason to

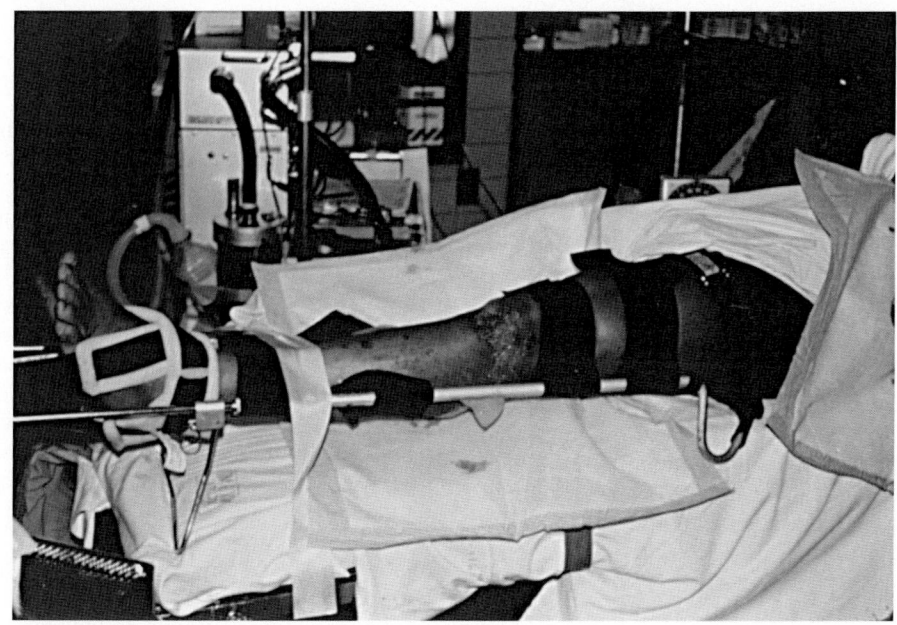

Figure 21-24 Patient in the emergency department with a Hare temporary traction splint in place to stabilize a femoral shaft fracture and aid in transport. (From Wolinsky PR, Johnson KD: Femoral shaft fractures. In Browner BD, Jupiter TB, Levine AM, Trafton PG [eds]: Skeletal Trauma, 2nd ed. Philadelphia, WB Saunders, 1998.)

delay because early fixation shortens the hospital stay, decreases overall cost, and reduces patient morbidity.

Fixation of femoral shaft fractures has become fairly uniform. The treatment of choice for closed fractures and type I through IIIA open fractures is closed, locked IM nailing. In contrast to open reduction methods, closed IM nailing reduces bleeding and soft tissue disruption at the fracture site. These minimally invasive techniques reduce perioperative stress and decrease the incidence of infection and nonunion. Treatment of type IIIB and IIIC open femoral shaft fractures is usually staged, with immediate external fixation.

Tibial Shaft Fractures

Tibial shaft fractures are among the most common musculoskeletal injuries, and the tibia is the most common diaphyseal long bone fractured. Pedestrians struck by motor vehicles and motorcyclists sustain the worst tibia fractures. Successful treatment of such fractures is fraught with difficulty because of the varying anatomic demands and fixation limitations as one moves proximally to distally.

Blood Supply

Tibia shaft fractures tend to be slow healing as a result of their tenuous blood supply and limited soft tissue envelope. A single nutrient artery that branches from the posterior tibial artery serves the entire diaphysis. It enters the medullary canal and travels proximally and distally to anastomose with metaphyseal endosteal vessels. Although there is some contribution from the penetrating branches of the periosteal arteries that supply the outer third of the cortex, a diaphyseal fracture can easily compromise the nutrient arterial blood supply. Concomitant soft tissue stripping may leave an entire segment of tibia devascularized. This fragile environment predisposes tibia shaft fractures to impaired healing and, with open fractures, to osteomyelitis.

Associated Soft Tissue Injuries

Aside from injuries to the overlying skin and muscle, tibia shaft fractures often have other associated soft tissue injuries. Ligamentous injuries causing knee instability are not uncommon and are often identified later as a source of continued morbidity.

Neurovascular injury must always be suspected and a careful examination must always be performed. Both the dorsalis pedis and posterior tibial arterial pulses are palpated and capillary refill is assessed. If injury is suspected, a Doppler probe can be used to further assess arterial blood flow. When used with a blood pressure cuff proximally, arterial pressure can be measured and compared with brachial artery pressure. This test is a sensitive and specific indicator of significant arterial injury. An ankle-brachial index less than 0.9 indicates a high probability of vessel injury.

Neurologic examination includes assessment of all four major nerves that travel distally in the leg. The deep peroneal nerve can be evaluated by testing first dorsal web space sensation and foot and toe dorsiflexion. Testing sensation along the dorsum of the foot and eversion strength can assess superficial peroneal nerve function. The tibial nerve provides sensation to the sole of the foot and motor function to the foot and toe plantar flexors. The sural nerve is a pure sensory nerve, and testing sensation to the lateral aspect of the heel can assess its function.

Management and Treatment

Management and treatment of tibia shaft fractures have evolved over the years. A closed fracture with minimal displacement can be treated by cast immobilization and functional bracing. However, almost all moderate and severe fractures benefit from surgical stabilization. Reamed IM nailing is the technique of choice when appropriate. Although there is still debate regarding the use of reamed IM nailing in open fractures, external fixation continues to be a viable option for the treatment of tibia shaft fractures, even though it is generally reserved for temporary stabilization. Plate fixation has fallen out of favor for diaphyseal fractures because of the high risk for wound-healing complications. However, ORIF remains a valuable treatment option for diaphyseal fractures that extend proximally or distally into the metaphysis, which are less amenable to IM stabilization. Newer percutaneous plating techniques have advanced the use of plate fixation by limiting surgical dissection in the zone of injury.

Humeral Shaft Fractures

Humeral shaft fractures represent 3% of all fractures. Many of them can be treated nonoperatively because of the internal splinting effects of the intermuscular septa. In addition, the mobility of the shoulder and elbow joints will tolerate 15 degrees of malrotation, 20 degrees of flexion-extension deformity, 30 degrees of varus-valgus deformity, and 3 cm of shortening without significant compromise in function or appearance.

Transverse diaphyseal fractures pose a unique problem because they are harder to control than spiral oblique fractures. With distal-third spiral fractures, the radial nerve is at risk as it courses distally in the spiral groove. For this reason, radial nerve function must be carefully assessed and documented (Holstein-Lewis fracture). In the trauma setting, right-sided humeral shaft fractures are significantly predictive of concomitant liver injury.

Treatment

Various nonoperative options exist for treating humeral shaft fractures: hanging arm casts, coaptation splints, Velpeau dressing, sling, and swathe. Typically, a coaptation splint is applied in the acute setting and subsequently replaced by a functional fracture brace after the initial painful fracture period has passed (3-7 days). Patients are then allowed free elbow flexion-extension and arm abduction to 60 degrees. Motion is encouraged to stimulate fracture healing because the hydraulic compression created by muscle contraction helps achieve fracture union.

In certain circumstances, operative intervention is indicated. Failed closed reduction, intra-articular fractures, concomitant neurologic or vascular injury, ipsilateral forearm or elbow fractures ("floating elbow"), segmental fractures, open fractures, and polytrauma patients all benefit from surgical management. Operative options include IM nailing, plate and screw fixation, and external fixation.

COMPLICATIONS

Missed Injuries

Missed musculoskeletal injuries account for a large proportion of delays in diagnosis within the first few days of care of a critically injured patient.[42] Clinical reassessment of trauma patients within 24 hours has reduced the incidence of missed injuries by nearly 40%. Patients should be reexamined as they regain consciousness and resume activity. Repeated assessment should be routinely performed in all patients, including unstable and neurologically impaired patients. The tertiary trauma survey includes a comprehensive examination and review of laboratory results and radiographs within 24 hours of initial evaluation. Specific injury patterns should be reviewed closely, especially in patients with multiple injuries and severe disability. External soft tissue trauma may be indicative of a more severe underlying injury. Missed cervical spine trauma occurs in 5% of all spine injuries and can potentially lead to paralysis and death.[9] Formal radiology rounds can facilitate greater recognition of occult injuries.[42,43]

Drug and Alcohol Use

The incidence of drug and alcohol use in patients with musculoskeletal injuries has been reported to be as high as 50%. Nearly 25% of all patients tested positive for two or more drugs. Alcohol and drug use results in more severe orthopedic injuries and more frequent injuries requiring longer hospitalization. Associated complications include those from cocaine use, such as fever, hypertension, acute myocardial ischemia, arrhythmias, and stroke. Cocaine can also facilitate cardiac arrhythmias when combined with halothane, nitrous oxide, and ketamine. Furthermore, the use of alcohol or drugs can adversely affect the administration of premedicating drugs. Proper monitoring and preparation should accompany the administration of any IV drug in the trauma setting. Prophylaxis for delirium tremens in postoperative patients should be performed when indicated. Inpatient detoxification consultation should be obtained before discharge.

Thromboembolic Complications

When compared with patients with isolated injuries, multiply injured patients have an increased incidence of thromboembolic complications, including deep venous thrombosis and pulmonary embolism.[8] The incidence of pulmonary embolism in major trauma patients ranges from 2% to 22%, and it is the third leading cause of death in these patients (Fig. 21-25).[44] Multiply injured patients represent a high-risk group for venous thromboembolism, along with patients undergoing elective neurosurgical, orthopedic, and oncologic surgery. In particular, long bone fractures, pelvic fractures, advanced age, spinal cord injuries, and surgical procedures are associated with an increased risk for deep venous thrombosis in trauma patients.[6] The use of indwelling venous catheters also leads to an increase in thromboembolic complications.

There have been few randomized trials evaluating deep venous thrombosis prophylaxis in trauma patients, and therefore no specific recommendations have been established. The most common forms of pharmacologic prophylaxis include adjusted-dose unfractionated heparin, low-molecular-weight heparin, warfarin, and aspirin. In addition, hirudin, a selective thrombin inhibitor, has been used for prophylaxis in elective hip surgery. Other forms of prophylaxis include mechanical devices, such as foot pumps and sequential calf compression pumps, and barrier devices, such as vena cava filters.

It is generally agreed that prophylaxis is critical in a high-risk trauma patient. Two controversial issues in the prevention of venous thromboembolism in a trauma patient are currently being debated. The first is the role of venous surveillance. Several authors recommend routine duplex surveillance and formal institutional protocols to detect thromboembolic events because the incidence of proximal deep venous thrombosis is higher than suspected.[45,46] The second issue is appropriate prophylaxis. No single form of anticoagulation has proved maximally efficacious in minimizing the incidence of deep venous thrombosis in trauma patients. Adjusted-dose heparin and low-molecular-weight heparin are currently the most common forms of prophylaxis. In a randomized study comparing low-dose unfractionated heparin with low-molecular-weight heparin, Geerts and coworkers documented an overall 44% incidence of deep venous thrombosis in trauma patients receiving low-dose unfractionated heparin versus 31% in those receiving enoxaparin.[47] There was a slight increase in major bleeding in the enoxaparin-treated group; however, in none of the patients did hemoglobin drop by more than 2 g/dL. Further research in this area is needed to determine the appropriate prophylaxis for trauma patients with orthopedic injuries.

Frequently, multiply injured trauma patients have multiple contraindications to the use of anticoagulation therapy, and in such cases mechanical compression devices are an alternative form of prophylaxis. Patients with significant head injury or coagulopathy or those at risk for ongoing bleeding may not be appropriate candidates for anticoagulation. Intermittent pneumatic compression devices deliver sequential rhythmic compression to the calf and thigh and can help reduce the rate of deep venous thrombosis in trauma patients. Unfortunately, a third of patients with orthopedic injuries are not candidates for intermittent pneumatic compression because of long bone fractures or open wounds. In this setting, foot compression devices are a reasonable alternative to calf compression.[48]

Vena cava filters offer prophylaxis for pulmonary embolism in high-risk patients who have failed anticoagulation, are not appropriate candidates for anticoagulation, or are at very high risk secondary to the severity of injury. These devices are not routinely placed because of potential morbidity, including migration of the filter, bleeding during or after placement, or filter thrombosis. Selected patients who may benefit from prophylactic filter placement include those with severe spinal cord injuries and neurologic deficit, multiple long bone frac-

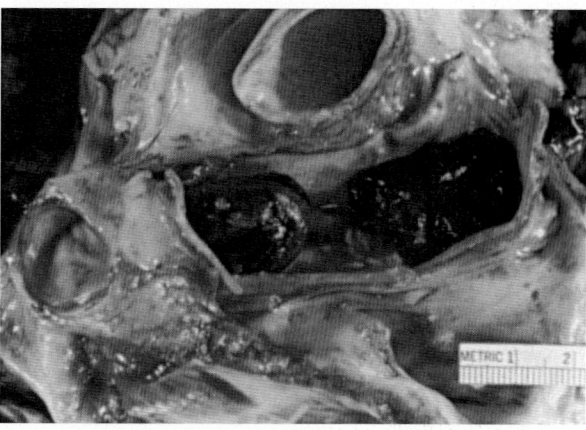

Figure 21-25 A large embolus in the pulmonary artery, which was the cause of death. (Courtesy of James E. Parker, MD, University of Louisville, Louisville, KY.)

tures, or long bone fractures associated with pelvic fractures, as well as patients with severe head injury who cannot receive anticoagulation.

Pulmonary Failure: Fat Emboli Syndrome and Adult Respiratory Distress Syndrome

Fat emboli syndrome (FES) is a condition characterized by respiratory distress, altered mental status, and skin petechiae. First described as a syndrome in 1873, it occurs in multiply injured patients, especially those with orthopedic injuries. Clinical signs are evident hours to days after an injury involving multiple long bone fractures or isolated femoral, tibial, and pelvic fractures. Although fat embolization may occur in nearly 100% of traumatized patients, the incidence of FES ranges from 1% to 17%.[49] In patients with isolated long bone fractures, the incidence is between 2% and 5%. In a multiply injured patient with long bone fractures or pelvic fractures, the incidence of FES is as high as 15%. Marrow fat from the fracture site is believed to enter the pulmonary circulation, where it causes activation of the coagulation cascade, platelet dysfunction, and subsequent release of vasoactive substances.[50] The histopathologic diagnosis of FES is difficult. The presence of lipid within alveolar macrophages obtained by bronchoalveolar lavage may help in the early diagnosis of FES.[51] Morbidity from FES may be anywhere between 0% and 20%.[49] In an autopsy study of more than 5000 individuals, FES was causative in 16% of injury-related deaths. In this way, FES may represent a subset of ARDS. ARDS is a pulmonary failure state defined as a PaO_2/FIO_2 ratio less than 200 for more than 5 consecutive days or bilateral diffuse infiltrates on chest radiographs in the absence of congestive heart failure.[52] FES may be causative in the development of ARDS, and the timing of intervention has been correlated with surgical outcomes. Early fixation has resulted in a reduction in FES and ARDS in several studies.[53,54] Johnson and associates reported a 17% incidence of ARDS with early fracture stabilization as compared with 75% after delayed fixation.[55] Both clinical and experimental studies suggest that the method of fracture fixation plays a minor role in the development of pulmonary complications.[56] The early ventilatory dependency, which occurs immediately after severe trauma, is secondary to the effects of any thoracic trauma or fluid resuscitation that may accompany such cases. ARDS occurs several days after the primary insult, and its frequency can be lessened with early fixation, débridement of necrotic soft tissue and hematoma, and maintenance of the upright position.

POSTOPERATIVE MOBILIZATION

The benefits of early fixation and mobilization of multiply injured patients have already been discussed. However, distinction between mobilization and weight bearing is essential. *Mobilization* is transfer of the patient from the supine position, either under the patient's own power or with the help of nurses and therapists. This includes turning the patient every shift by nurses, sitting up in bed, or transferring the patient to a chair. All patients should be mobilized by the second postoperative day if their general condition permits. Mobilization helps prevent the development of pulmonary and septic complications.

Weight bearing, in contrast, is transmission of load with an extremity. For a patient to be allowed to bear weight on an injured extremity, the following three conditions must be met:

1. There must be bone-to-bone contact at the fracture site, as demonstrated intraoperatively or on postreduction radiographs. Without contact of the fracture ends, the fixation devices will be subjected to all the stresses applied to the extremity, which will frequently result in failure of the fixation.
2. Stable fixation of the fracture must be achieved. By definition, stable fixation is not disrupted when subjected to normal physiologic loads. Stable fixation is dependent on multiple factors. Fixation may be less than ideal in patients with osteopenic bone or severely comminuted fractures. When excessive loads are anticipated, such as with heavy or obese patients, the typical fixation may not be adequate.
3. The patient must be able to comply with the weight-bearing status. Frequently, reliability of the patient is a significant consideration in the determination of weight-bearing status. Social, psychological, or emotional circumstances can affect a patient's ability to comply with weight-bearing restrictions.

Unless all three criteria are met, the fixation will need to be protected with restricted weight-bearing status. *Touch-down weight bearing* allows the weight of the leg to be applied with the foot flat on the floor and is often permitted in patients with injuries around the hip. Touch-down weight bearing allows extension of the hip and knee and dorsiflexion at the ankle. This natural position relaxes the hip musculature and minimizes joint reactive forces. Crutch walking with the foot off the floor (non–weight bearing) leads to a significant increase in force across the hip joint, greater than in the touch-down weight-bearing state. *Toe-touch weight bearing,* a term often used synonymously with touch-down weight bearing, is an unfortunate use of terminology. Most patients attempt to walk while touching only the toe of the injured extremity to the ground. In this position, the hip and knee are flexed and the ankle is held in equinus. When this status is maintained for any significant amount of time, contractures at the hip, knee, and ankle are common. For this reason, use of this terminology is discouraged.

Partial weight bearing is defined in terms of the percentage of body weight applied to an injured extremity. It is gradually increased as the fracture gains stability through healing. With the use of a scale the patient can learn what different amounts of body weight feel like. When a fracture and the patient are stable enough to withstand normal loads, *weight bearing as tolerated* is instituted. It is believed that reliable patients limit their own weight bearing according to their pain.

Even when weight bearing is not allowed, mobilization of affected and adjacent joints is typically performed within a few days. After surgical treatment, joints are typically immobilized briefly and then allowed either passive or active range of motion in bed if weight bearing is not prudent. Early joint mobilization decreases the likelihood of fibrosis and therefore increases early mobility. Furthermore, joint motion is necessary for the good health of articular cartilage. Cartilage is nourished from synovial fluid most efficiently when the joint is moving. Early joint mobilization has become a basic tenet of orthopedic care and has led to a decrease in the morbidity associated with musculoskeletal injuries.

SUMMARY

In all trauma settings, preservation of a patient's life takes precedent over preservation of a limb. Injuries to the extremities and axial skeleton may be life threatening in rare circumstances. However, once the critical period has passed, musculoskeletal injuries are a major cause of post-traumatic morbidity, as demonstrated by increased health care costs, lost work days, physical disability, emotional distress, and diminished quality of life. Accordingly, it is essential that a detailed and complete extremity and axial musculoskeletal survey be performed on every patient, that injuries be identified early, and that the consulting orthopedic surgical team be notified of the specifics of these injuries in timely fashion. This allows them the opportunity to make the necessary arrangements to address the specific injury. Moreover, the patient should not be transported from the trauma room, unless necessary for lifesaving interventions, until the orthopedic team has evaluated and stabilized the involved extremity to protect it against further injury and morbidity.

Selected References

Bone LB, Johnson KD, Weigelt J, et al: Early versus delayed stabilization of femoral shaft fractures: A prospective randomized study. J Bone Joint Surg Am 71:336-340, 1989.

This classic article has shaped the treatment of multiply injured patients. It was the first to clearly define the benefits of early stabilization of femoral shaft fractures prospectively.

Browner, BD, Jupiter JB, Levine AM, Trafton PG (eds): Skeletal Trauma: Fractures, Dislocations, Ligamentous Injuries, 3rd ed. Philadelphia, WB Saunders, 2003.

This is one of the premiere, comprehensive texts covering traumatic musculoskeletal injuries. This two-volume set is now in its third edition, with the most recent update in 2003. It is clearly written and visually appealing. The chapter authors are the elite orthopedic trauma surgeons in the world. It is an excellent reference for any surgical resident dealing with a multiply injured patient.

Gustilo R, Anderson J: Prevention of infection in the treatment of 1025 open fractures of long bones: Retrospective and prospective analyses. J Bone Joint Surg Am 58:453-458, 1976.

This classic article defined the classification and proposed management guidelines in patients with open fractures. It includes more than 300 cases reviewed retrospectively and another 600 prospective cases in which the new classification was applied.

Tile M (ed): Fractures of the Pelvis and Acetabulum, 2nd ed. Baltimore, Williams & Wilkins, 1988.

This text covers pelvic and acetabular trauma in depth. It is written for the orthopedic trauma surgeon but includes a clear description of the mechanisms of injuries and the classification of pelvic ring injuries.

Tscherne H, Gotzen L: Fractures with Soft Tissue Injuries. Berlin, Springer-Verlag, 1984.

This fracture textbook is comprehensive in its coverage of open and closed fractures with soft tissue injuries. It covers all classifications, immediate management, fracture care, and wound care of these injuries. It uses the team approach to dealing with these complicated injuries.

References

1. Copes W: Musculoskeletal injuries in the major trauma outcome study. Personal Communication, Trianalytics, Inc, Baltimore, 1999.
2. Committee on Trauma: ATLS Instruction Manual. Chicago, American College of Surgeons, Committee on Trauma, 1993.
3. Burgess A, Eastridge BJ, Young JW, et al: Pelvic ring disruption: Effective classification system and treatment protocols. J Trauma 30:848-856, 1990.
4. Court-Brown C, Keating J, McQueen MM: Infection after intramedullary nailing of the tibia: Incidence and protocol for management. J Bone Joint Surg Br 74:770-774, 1992.
5. Waters RL, Adkins RH, Yakura JS: Definition of complete spinal cord injury. Paraplegia 29:573-581, 1991.
6. Geerts W, Code K, Jay RM, et al: A prospective study of venous thromboembolism after major trauma. N Engl J Med 331:1601-1606, 1994.
7. Tscherne H, Gotzen L: Fractures with Soft Tissue Injuries. Berlin, Springer-Verlag, 1984.
8. Bone L, Johnson KD, Weigelt J, et al: Early versus delayed stabilization of femoral shaft fractures: A prospective randomized study. J Bone Joint Surg Am 71:336-340, 1989.
9. Latenser B, Gentilello L, Tarver AA, et al: Improved outcome with early fixation of skeletally unstable pelvic fractures. J Trauma 31:28-31, 1991.
10. Harkess J, Ramsey W, Harkess J: Principles of fractures and dislocations. In Rockwood C, Green D, Bucholz R, Heckman J (eds): Rockwood and Green's Fractures in Adults, 4th ed. Philadelphia, Lippincott-Raven, 1996.
11. Ochsner MG Jr, Hoffman AP, DiPasquale D, et al: Associated aortic rupture–pelvic fracture: An alert for orthopaedic and general surgeon. J Trauma 33:429-434, 1992.
12. Tile M: Pelvic ring fractures: Should they be fixed? J Bone Joint Surg Br 70:1-12, 1988.
13. Ben-Menachem Y: Exploratory angiography and transcatheter embolization for control of arterial hemorrhage in patients with pelvic ring disruption. Tech Orthop 9:271-274, 1995.
14. Buckle R, Browner B, Morandi M:: Emergency reduction for pelvic ring disruptions and control of associated hemorrhage using the pelvic stabilizer. Tech Orthop 9:258-266, 1995.
15. Ganz R, Krushell RJ, Jakob RP, Kuffer J: The antishock pelvic clamp. Clin Orthop Relat Res 267:71-78, 1991.
16. Klein S, Saroyan M, Baumgartner F, et al: Management strategy of vascular injuries associated with pelvic fractures. J Cardiovasc Surg 33:349-357, 1992.
17. Riemer BL, Butterfield SL, Diamond DL, et al: Acute mortality associated with injuries to the pelvic ring: The role of early patient mobilization and external fixation. J Trauma 35:671-677, 1993.
18. Breest T, Moody M: Frequency of vascular injury with blunt trauma–induced extremity injury. Am J Surg 160:226-228, 1990.
19. Helfet D, Howey T, Sanders R, et al: Limb salvage versus amputation: Preliminary results of the MESS. Clin Orthop Relat Res 256:80-86, 1990.
20. Nichols J, Svoboda J, Parks SN, et al: Use of temporary intraluminal shunts in selected peripheral arterial injuries. J Trauma 26:1094-1096, 1996.
21. Seddon HJ: Volkmann's contracture: Treatment by excision of the infarct. J Bone Joint Surg Br 38:152-174, 1956.
22. Seddon H: Volkmann's ischemia of the lower limb. J Bone Joint Surg Br 48:627-636, 1966.
23. Orthopaedic Trauma Association: Economic costs of missed compartment syndrome. Eighth Annual Orthopaedic Trauma Association Meeting, Nov. 6-10, 1992, Minneapolis, MN.
24. Whitesides T, Heckman M: Acute compartment syndrome: Update on diagnosis and treatment. J Am Acad Orthop Surg 4:209-218, 1996.
25. Mubarak S, Hargens A (eds): Compartment Syndromes and Volkmann's Contracture. Philadelphia, WB Saunders, 1981.
26. Matsen FA III, Winquist R, Krugmire RB Jr: Diagnosis and management of compartment syndromes. J Bone Joint Surg Am 62:286-291, 1980.
27. Heckman MM, Whitesides TE Jr, Grewe SR, et al: Compartment pressure in association with closed tibial fractures: The relationship between tissue pressure, compartment, and distance from the site of fracture. J Bone Joint Surg Am 76:1285-1292, 1994.
28. Garr JL, Gentilello LM, Cole PA, et al: Monitoring for compartmental syndrome using near-infrared spectroscopy: A noninvasive, continuous, transcutaneous monitoring technique. J Trauma 46:613-616, 1999.
29. Gustilo R, Anderson J: Prevention of infection in the treatment of 1025 open fractures of long bones: Retrospective and prospective analyses. J Bone Joint Surg Am 58:453-458, 1976.

30. Patzakis M: Management of open fractures. Instr Course Lect 31:62-64, 1982.

31. Patzakis M, Wilkins J, Moore TM, et al: Considerations in reducing the infection rate of open tibia fractures. Clin Orthop Relat Res 178:36-41, 1983.

32. Lange RH, Bach AW, Hansen ST, et al: Open tibial fractures with associated vascular injuries: Prognosis for limb salvage. J Trauma 25:203-208, 1985.

33. Johansen K, Daines M, Howey T, et al: Objective criteria accurately predict amputation following lower extremity trauma. J Trauma 30:568-573, 1990.

34. Jenny J, Jenny G, Kempf I: Infection after reamed intramedullary nailing of lower limb fractures: A review of 1464 cases over 15 years. Acta Orthop Scand 65:94-96, 1994.

35. Schemitsch E, Kowalski MJ, Swiontkowski MF, et al: Cortical bone blood flow in reamed and unreamed locked intramedullary nailing: A fractured tibia model in sheep. J Orthop Trauma 8:373-382, 1994.

36. Tornetta P III, Bergman M, Watnik N, et al: Treatment of type IIIB open tibial fractures: A prospective randomized comparison of external fixation and non-reamed locked nailing. J Bone Joint Surg Br 76:13-19, 1994.

37. Tu Y, Lin C, Su JI, et al: Unreamed interlocking nail versus external fixator for open type III tibia fractures. J Trauma 39:361-367, 1995.

38. Blachut P, Meek R, O'Brien PJ: External fixation and delayed intramedullary nailing of open fractures of the tibial shaft: A sequential protocol. J Bone Joint Surg Am 72:729-735, 1990.

39. Schutz M, Sudkamp N, Frigg R, et al: Pinless external fixator: Indications and preliminary result in tibial shaft fractures. Clin Orthop Relat Res 347:35-42, 1998.

40. Fakhry S, Rutledge R, Dahners LE, et al: Incidence, management, and outcome of femoral shaft fracture: Statewide population-based analysis of 2805 adult patients in a rural state. J Trauma 37:255-260, 1994.

41. Reynolds M: Is the timing of fracture fixation important for the patient with multiple trauma? Ann Surg 222:470-481, 1995.

42. Janjua K, Sugrue M, Deane SA: Prospective evaluation of early missed injuries and the role of tertiary survey. J Trauma 44:1000-1007, 1998.

43. Rizoli SB, Boulanger BR, McClellan BA, Sharkey PW: Injuries missed during initial assessment of blunt trauma. Accid Anal Prev 26:681-686, 1994.

44. O'Malley K, Ross S: Pulmonary embolism in major trauma patients. J Trauma 30:748-750, 1990.

45. Montgomery K, Geerts W, Potter HG, et al: Practical management of venous thromboembolism following pelvic fractures. Orthop Clin North Am 28:397-404, 1997.

46. Velmahos G, Nigro J, Tatevossian R, et al: Inability of an aggressive policy of thromboprophylaxis to prevent deep venous thrombosis (DVT) in critically injured patients: Are current methods of DVT prophylaxis insufficient? J Am Coll Surg 187:529-533, 1998.

47. Geerts W, Jay R, Code KI, et al: A comparison of low-dose heparin with low-dose unfractionated heparin as prophylaxis against venous thromboembolism after major trauma. N Engl J Med 335:701-707, 1996.

48. Spain D, Bergamini T, Hoffmann JF, et al: Comparison of sequential compression devices and foot pumps for prophylaxis of deep venous thrombosis in high risk trauma patients. Am Surg 64:522-525, 1998.

49. Ganong RB: Fat emboli syndrome in isolated fractures of the tibia and femur. Clin Orthop Relat Res 291:208-214, 1993.

50. Turen C, Dube M, LeCroy MC, et al: Approach to the polytraumatized patient with musculoskeletal injuries. J Am Acad Orthop Surg 7:154-165, 1999.

51. Benzer A, Offner D, Totsch M, et al: Early diagnosis of fat embolism syndrome by automated image analysis of alveolar macrophages. J Clin Monit 10:213-215, 1994.

52. Bernard G, Artigas A, Brigham KL, et al: The American-European Consensus Conference on ARDS: Definitions, mechanisms, relevant outcomes, and clinical trial coordination. Am J Respir Crit Care Med 149:818-824, 1994.

53. Pape H, Aufmkolk M, Paffrath T, et al: Primary intramedullary femur fixation in multiple trauma patients with associated lung contusion: A cause of posttraumatic ARDS? J Trauma 34:540-548, 1993.

54. Seibel R, LaDuca J, Hassett JM, et al: Blunt multiple trauma (ISS 36), femur traction, and the pulmonary-failure septic state. Ann Surg 202:283-295, 1985.

55. Johnson K, Cadambi A, Seibert GB, et al: Incidence of adult respiratory distress syndrome in patients with multiple musculoskeletal injuries: Effect of early operative stabilization of fractures. J Trauma 25:375-384, 1985.

56. Richards R: Fat embolism syndrome. Can J Surg 40:334-339, 1997.

CHAPTER 22

Burns

James J. Gallagher, MD   Steven E. Wolf, MD   and   David N. Herndon, MD

More than 1.2 million people are burned in the United States every year; most cases are minor and treated in the outpatient setting. However, approximately 50,000 burns per year in the United States are moderate to severe and require hospitalization for appropriate treatment. Of these cases, more than 3900 people die of complications related to burns *(www.cdc.gov/ncicp/ wisqars)*. The societal significance of severe burns is supported by the finding that only motor vehicle collisions cause more trauma-related deaths.

Burn deaths generally occur in a bimodal distribution, either immediately after the injury or weeks later as a result of multiorgan failure, a pattern similar to all trauma-related deaths. Two thirds of all burns occur at home and commonly involve young adult men, children younger than 15 years, and the elderly. Seventy-five percent of all burn-related deaths occur in house fires. Young adults are frequently burned with flammable liquids, whereas toddlers are often scalded by hot liquids. A significant percentage of burns in children are due to child abuse. Other risk factors include low socioeconomic class and unsafe environments. These generaliza-

tions emphasize that most of these injuries are preventable and therefore amenable to prevention strategies.

Morbidity and mortality rates associated with burns are decreasing. Recent reports have revealed a 50% decline in burn-related deaths and hospital admissions in the United States over a 20-year period. This rate of decline was similar in sample statistics for all burns above a reportable level of severity.[1] The declines were probably the consequence of prevention efforts resulting in a decreased number of patients with potentially fatal burns, as well as improved clinical management of persons sustaining severe burns.

Burn incidence rates in the developing world, however, continue to be high at four to five times the rate in the United States. Women in the developing world tend to be at greatest risk. They are engaged in cooking at floor level in unsafe kitchens. Inexpensive, poorly made kerosine or propane stoves are produced without safety features. The women wear loose-fitting, draping traditional clothing, which easily catches fire. Flame is the number one cause of burns in the developing world.[2] Improvement in the burn incidence rate in the developing world will come about through education and prevention programs.

In the West, prevention strategies have decreased the number and severity of injuries. Successful approaches have included legislation mandating nonflammable children's sleepwear, changes in the National Electrical Code producing a decrease in oral commissure burns, elevation of hot water heaters from the ground, and increased smoke alarm use. In addition, the mortality rate has improved in patients sustaining severe injuries. In 1949, Bull and Fisher from the Birmingham Burns Centre in the United Kingdom[3] first reported a 50% mortality rate in children 14 years and younger with burns involving 49% of their total body surface area (TBSA); 50% mortality was reached in patients 15 to 44 years old with 46% TBSA burns, in those aged 45 to 64 years with 27% TBSA burns, and in patients 65 years and older with 10% TBSA burns.

These dismal statistics have improved,[4] with the latest studies reporting a 50% mortality rate for 98% TBSA burns in children 14 years and younger and 75% TBSA burns in other young age groups.[5] Therefore, a healthy young patient with almost any size burn might be expected to live with the use of modern treatment techniques. Advances in treatment are based on improved understanding of resuscitation, enhanced wound coverage, better support of the hypermetabolic response to injury, more appropriate infection control, and improved treatment of inhalation injuries. Additional improvements can be made in these areas, and investigators are active in all these fields to discover means to further improve survival and outcomes.

BURN UNITS

Improvements in burn care originated in specialized units specifically dedicated to the care of burned patients. These units consist of experienced personnel with resources to maximize outcome from these devastating injuries (Box 22-1). Because of these specialized resources, burned patients are best treated in such places. Patients with the following criteria are referred to a designated burn center:

1. Partial-thickness burns greater than 10% TBSA
2. Burns involving the face, hands, feet, genitalia, perineum, or major joints
3. Any full-thickness burn
4. Electrical burns, including lightning injury
5. Chemical burns
6. Inhalation injury
7. Burns in patients with preexisting medical disorders that could complicate management, prolong recovery, or affect outcome
8. Any patient with burns and concomitant trauma (e.g., fractures) in which the burn injury poses the greater immediate risk for morbidity and mortality. In such cases, if the trauma poses the greater immediate risk, the patient may be initially stabilized in a trauma center before being transferred to a burn unit. Physician judgment is necessary in such situations, and decisions must be made in concert with the regional medical control plan and triage protocols

9. Burned children in hospitals without qualified personnel or equipment to care for children
10. Burns in patients who will require special social, emotional, or long-term rehabilitative intervention

PATHOPHYSIOLOGY OF BURNS

Local Changes

Burn causes coagulative necrosis of the epidermis and underlying tissues, with the depth depending on the temperature to which the skin is exposed and the duration of exposure. The specific heat of the causative agent also affects the depth. For example, the specific heat of fat is higher than that of water; thus, a grease burn is deeper than a scald burn from water with the same temperature and duration of exposure.

Burns are classified into five different causal categories and depths of injury (Box 22-2). Causes include injury from flame, hot liquids (scald), contact with hot or cold objects, chemical exposure, and conduction of electricity. The first three induce cellular damage primarily by the transfer of energy and lead to coagulative necrosis. Chemicals and electricity cause direct injury to cellular membranes in addition to transfer of heat.

The skin provides a robust barrier to transfer of energy to deeper tissues; therefore, much of the injury is confined to this layer. However, after the inciting focus is removed, the response of local tissues can lead to injury in the deeper layers. The area of cutaneous injury has been divided into three zones: zone of coagulation, zone of stasis, and zone of hyperemia (Fig. 22-1). The necrotic area of a burn where cells have been disrupted is termed the *zone of coagulation*. This tissue is irreversibly damaged at the time of injury. The area immediately surrounding the necrotic zone has a moderate degree of insult with decreased tissue perfusion. This area is termed the *zone of stasis* and, depending on the wound environment, can either survive or progress to coagulative necro-

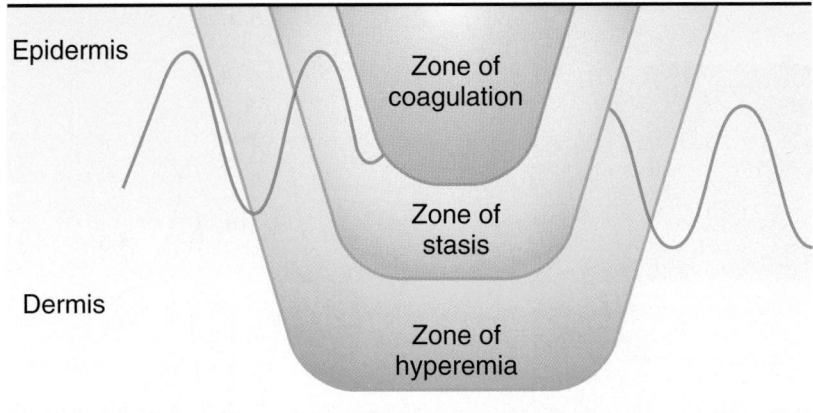

Figure 22-1 Zones of injury after a burn. The zone of coagulation is the portion irreversibly injured. The zones of stasis and hyperemia are defined in response to the injury.

sis. The zone of stasis is associated with vascular damage and vessel leakage. Thromboxane A$_2$, a potent vasoconstrictor, is present in high concentrations in burn wounds, and local application of inhibitors improves blood flow and decreases the zone of stasis.

Antioxidants, bradykinin antagonists, and subatmospheric wound pressure also improve blood flow and affect the depth of injury. Local endothelial interactions with neutrophils mediate some of the local inflammatory responses associated with the zone of stasis. Blocking leukocyte adherence with anti-CD18 or anti–intercellular adhesion molecule monoclonal antibodies improves tissue perfusion and tissue survival in animal models, thus indicating that treatment directed at the control of inflammation immediately after injury may spare the zone of stasis. The last area is termed the *zone of hyperemia,* which is characterized by vasodilation from inflammation surrounding the burn wound. This region contains clearly viable tissue from which the healing process begins and is generally not at risk for further necrosis.

Burn Depth

The depth of a burn depends on the degree of tissue damage. Burn depth is classified according to the degree of injury in the epidermis, dermis, subcutaneous fat, and underlying structures (Fig. 22-2). First-degree burns are, by definition, injuries confined to the epidermis. These burns are painful and erythematous, blanch to the touch, and have an intact epidermal barrier. Examples include sunburn or a minor scald from a kitchen accident. First-degree burns do not result in scarring, and treatment is aimed at comfort with the use of topical soothing salves, with or without aloe, and oral nonsteroidal anti-inflammatory agents.

Second-degree burns are divided into two types: superficial and deep. All second-degree burns have some degree of dermal damage, and the distinction is based on the depth of injury into this structure. Superficial dermal burns are erythematous and painful, blanch to touch, and often blister. Examples include scald injuries from overheated bathtub water and flash flame burns

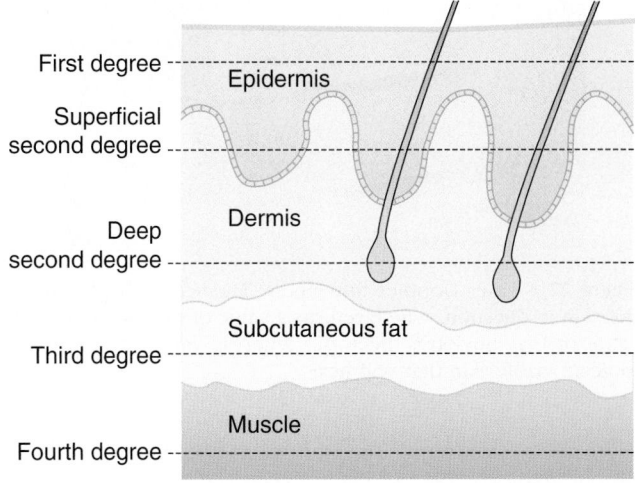

Figure 22-2 Depths of a burn. First-degree burns are confined to the epidermis. Second-degree burns extend into the dermis (dermal burns). Third-degree burns are "full thickness" through the epidermis and dermis. Fourth-degree burns involve injury to underlying tissue structures such as muscle, tendons, and bone.

from open carburetors. These wounds spontaneously re-epithelialize from retained epidermal structures in the rete ridges, hair follicles, and sweat glands in 7 to 14 days. After healing, these burns may result in some slight skin discoloration over the long term. Deep dermal burns into the reticular dermis appear more pale and mottled, do not blanch to touch, but remain painful to pinprick. These burns heal in 14 to 35 days by re-epithelialization from hair follicles and sweat gland keratinocytes, often with severe scarring as a result of the loss of dermis.

Third-degree burns are full thickness through the epidermis and dermis and are characterized by a hard, leathery eschar that is painless and black, white, or cherry red. No epidermal or dermal appendages remain; thus, these wounds must heal by re-epithelialization from the wound edges. Deep dermal and full-thickness burns

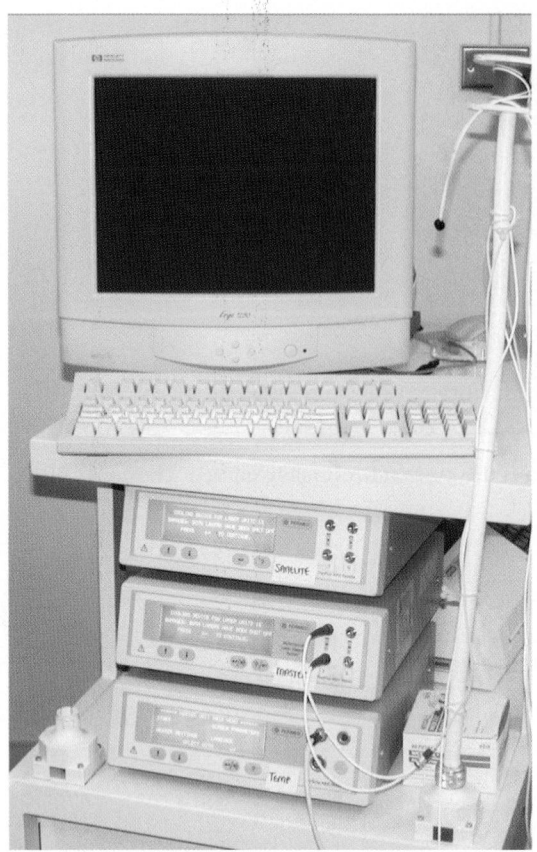

Figure 22-3 Laser Doppler flowmeter. The sensor is placed on the skin in question, which returns a value of perfusion units. A value of 0 is obviously necrotic, whereas values of about 80 indicate viable skin that will heal.

require excision with skin grafting to heal the wounds in timely fashion.

Fourth-degree burns involve other organs beneath the skin, such as muscle, bone, and brain.

Currently, burn depth is most accurately assessed by the judgment of experienced practitioners. Accurate depth determination is critical because wounds that will heal with local treatment are treated differently from those requiring operative intervention. Examination of the entire wound by the physicians ultimately responsible for their management is the gold standard used to guide further treatment decisions. New technologies, such as the multisensor heatable laser Doppler flowmeter, hold promise for quantitatively determining burn depth. Several recent reports claim superiority of this method over clinical judgment in the determination of wounds requiring skin grafting for timely healing (Fig. 22-3); this device may lead to a change in the standard of care in the near future.[6]

Burn Size
Determination of burn size estimates the extent of injury. Burn size is generally assessed by the so-called rule of nines (Fig. 22-4). In adults, each upper extremity and the head and neck are 9% of TBSA, the lower extremities and the anterior and posterior aspects of the trunk are

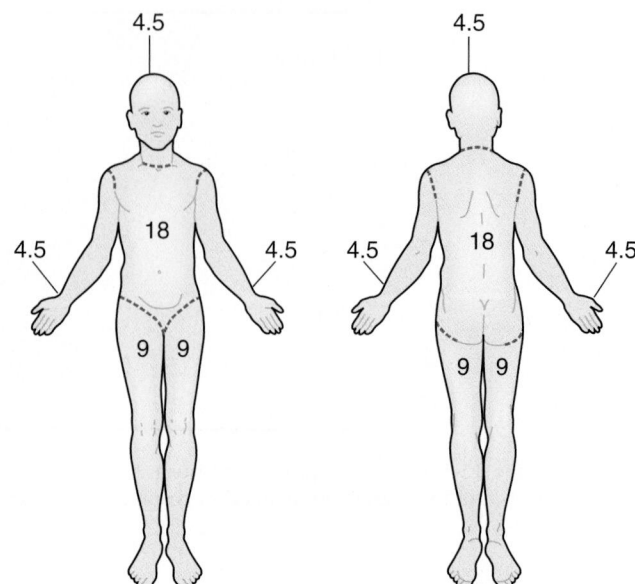

Figure 22-4 Body surface area diagram. This figure depicts the relative percentage of the total body surface area of defined anatomic areas.

18% each, and the perineum and genitalia are assumed to be 1% of TBSA. Another method of estimating smaller burns is to consider the area of the open hand (including the palm and extended fingers) of the patient to be approximately 1% of TBSA and then transpose that measurement visually onto the wound for a determination of its size. This method is helpful when evaluating splash burns and other burns of mixed distribution.

Children have a relatively larger proportion of body surface area in their head and neck, which is compensated for by a relatively smaller surface area in the lower extremities. Infants have 21% of TBSA in the head and neck and 13% in each leg, which incrementally approaches the adult proportions with increasing age. The Berkow formula is used to accurately determine burn size in children (Table 22-1).

Systemic Changes

Inflammation and Edema
Significant burns are associated with massive release of inflammatory mediators, both in the wound and in other tissues (Fig. 22-5). These mediators produce vasoconstriction and vasodilation, increased capillary permeability, and edema locally and in distant organs. The generalized edema occurs in response to changes in Starling forces in both burned and unburned skin. Initially, interstitial hydrostatic pressure decreases dramatically in the burned skin, and there is an associated slight increase in interstitial pressure in the nonburned skin. As plasma oncotic pressure decreases and interstitial oncotic pressure increases as a result of the protein loss induced by increased capillary permeability, edema forms in the burned and nonburned tissues. The edema is greater in the burned tissues because of lower interstitial pressure.

Table 22-1 **Berkow Diagram to Estimate Burn Size (%) Based on Area of Burn in an Isolated Body Part***

BODY PART	0-1 yr	1-4 yr	5-9 yr	10-14 yr	15-18 yr	ADULT
Head	19	17	13	11	9	7
Neck	2	2	2	2	2	2
Anterior trunk	13	13	13	13	13	13
Posterior trunk	13	13	13	13	13	13
Right buttock	2.5	2.5	2.5	2.5	2.5	2.5
Left buttock	2.5	2.5	2.5	2.5	2.5	2.5
Genitalia	1	1	1	1	1	1
Right upper arm	4	4	4	4	4	4
Left upper arm	4	4	4	4	4	4
Right lower arm	3	3	3	3	3	3
Left lower arm	3	3	3	3	3	3
Right hand	2.5	2.5	2.5	2.5	2.5	2.5
Left hand	2.5	2.5	2.5	2.5	2.5	2.5
Right thigh	5.5	6.5	8	8.5	9	9.5
Left thigh	5.5	6.5	8	8.5	9	9.5
Right leg	5	5	5.5	6	6.5	7
Left leg	5	5	5.5	6	6.5	7
Right foot	3.5	3.5	3.5	3.5	3.5	3.5
Left foot	3.5	3.5	3.5	3.5	3.5	3.5

*Estimates are made, recorded, and then summed to gain an accurate estimate of the body surface area burned.

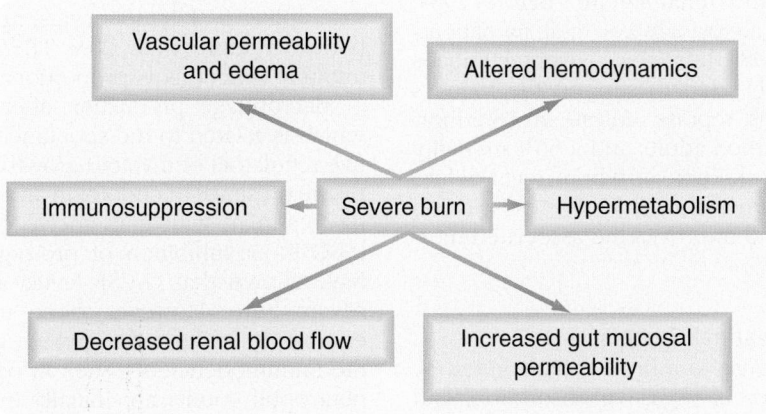

Figure 22-5 Systemic effects of a severe burn.

Many mediators have been proposed to account for the changes in permeability after a burn injury, including histamine, bradykinin, vasoactive amines, prostaglandins, leukotrienes, activated complement, and catecholamines, among others. Mast cells in the burned skin release histamine in large quantities immediately after injury, which elicits the characteristic response of increasing intercellular junction space formation in venules. The use of antihistamines in the treatment of burn edema, however, has had limited success. In addition, aggregated platelets release serotonin, which plays a major role in edema formation. This agent acts directly to increase pulmonary vascular resistance, and it indirectly aggravates the vasoconstrictive effects of various vasoactive amines. Serotonin blockade improves the cardiac index, decreases pulmonary artery pressure, and decreases oxygen consumption after a burn. When the antiserotonin agent methysergide was given to animals after scald injury, wound edema formation decreased as a result of local effects. In addition, decreases in resuscitation fluid requirements are seen in patients given high-dose vitamin C therapy immediately after a burn, presumably because of its anti-inflammatory effects.

Another mediator likely to play a role in changes in permeability and fluid shifts is thromboxane A_2. Thromboxane increases dramatically in the plasma and wounds of burned patients. This potent vasoconstrictor leads to vasoconstriction and platelet aggregation in the wound, thereby contributing to expansion of the zone of stasis. It also causes prominent mesenteric vasoconstriction and decreased gut blood flow in animal models, with compromised gut mucosal integrity and decreased gut immune function.

Microvascular changes induce cardiopulmonary alterations characterized by loss of plasma volume, increased peripheral vascular resistance, and subsequent decreased cardiac output immediately after injury.[7] Cardiac output remains depressed from the decreased blood volume and increased blood viscosity, as well as decreased cardiac contractility. Ventricular dysfunction in this period is attributed to a circulating myocardial depressant factor present in lymphatic fluid, although the specific factor has never been isolated. Cardiac output is almost completely restored with resuscitation.

Effects on the Renal System

Diminished blood volume and cardiac output result in decreased renal blood flow and glomerular filtration rate. Other stress-induced hormones and mediators such as angiotensin, aldosterone, and vasopressin further reduce renal blood flow immediately after the injury. These effects result in oliguria, which if left untreated will cause acute tubular necrosis and renal failure. Before 1984, acute renal failure was almost always fatal in patients with burn injuries; after 1984, however, newer techniques in dialysis became widely used to support the kidneys during recovery. The latest reports indicate an 88% mortality rate for severely burned adults and a 56% mortality rate for severely burned children in whom renal failure develops in the postburn period.[8] Early resuscitation decreases renal failure and improves the associated mortality rate.[5]

Effects on the Gastrointestinal System

The gastrointestinal response to a burn is highlighted by mucosal atrophy, changes in digestive absorption, and increased intestinal permeability. Atrophy of the small bowel mucosa occurs within 12 hours of injury in proportion to the burn size and is related to increased epithelial cell death by apoptosis. The cytoskeleton of the mucosal brush border undergoes atrophic changes associated with vesiculation of microvilli and disruption of the terminal web actin filaments. These findings were most pronounced 18 hours after injury, which suggests that changes in the cytoskeleton, such as those associated with cell death by apoptosis, are processes involved in the changed gut mucosa. Burn also causes reduced uptake of glucose and amino acids, decreased absorption of fatty acids, and a reduction in brush border lipase activity. These changes peak in the first several hours

after a burn and return to normal at 48 to 72 hours after injury, a timing that parallels mucosal atrophy.

Intestinal permeability to macromolecules, which are normally repelled by an intact mucosal barrier, increases after a burn. Intestinal permeability to polyethylene glycol 3350, lactulose, and mannitol increases after injury in proportion to the extent of the burn. Gut permeability increases even further when burn wounds become infected. A study using fluorescent dextrans showed that larger molecules appeared to cross the mucosa between the cells whereas smaller molecules traversed the mucosa through the epithelial cells, presumably by pinocytosis and vesiculation. Mucosal permeability also paralleled increases in gut epithelial apoptosis.

Changes in gut blood flow are related to changes in permeability. Intestinal blood flow was shown to decrease in animals, a change that was associated with increased gut permeability 5 hours after a burn. This effect was abolished at 24 hours. Systolic hypotension has been shown to occur in the hours immediately after a burn in animals with a 40% TBSA full-thickness injury. These animals showed an inverse correlation between blood flow and permeability to intact *Candida*.[9]

Effects on the Immune System

Burns cause a global depression in immune function, which is shown by prolonged allograft skin survival on burn wounds. Burned patients are then at great risk for a number of infectious complications, including bacterial wound infection, pneumonia, and fungal and viral infections. These susceptibilities and conditions are based on depressed cellular function in all parts of the immune system, including activation and activity of neutrophils, macrophages, T lymphocytes, and B lymphocytes. With burns of more than 20% TBSA, impairment of these immune functions is proportional to burn size.

Macrophage production after a burn is diminished, which is related to the spontaneous elaboration of negative regulators of myeloid growth. This effect is enhanced by the presence of endotoxin and can be partially reversed by treatment with granulocyte colony-stimulating factor (G-CSF) or inhibition of prostaglandin E_2. Investigators have shown that G-CSF levels actually increase after a severe burn. However, bone marrow G-CSF receptor expression is decreased, which may in part account for the immunodeficiency seen in patients with burns. Total neutrophil counts are initially increased after a burn, a phenomenon that is related to a decrease in cell death by apoptosis. However, the neutrophils that are present are dysfunctional in terms of diapedesis, chemotaxis, and phagocytosis. These effects are explained, in part, by a deficiency in CD11b/CD18 expression after inflammatory stimuli, decreased respiratory burst activity associated with a deficiency in p47-phox activity, and impaired actin mechanics related to neutrophil motile responses. After 48 to 72 hours, neutrophil counts decrease somewhat like macrophages, with similar causes.

The depressed helper T-cell function that occurs after a severe burn is associated with polarization from the interleukin-2 and interferon-γ cytokine–based T-helper 1 (T_H1) response toward the T_H2 response. The T_H2 response

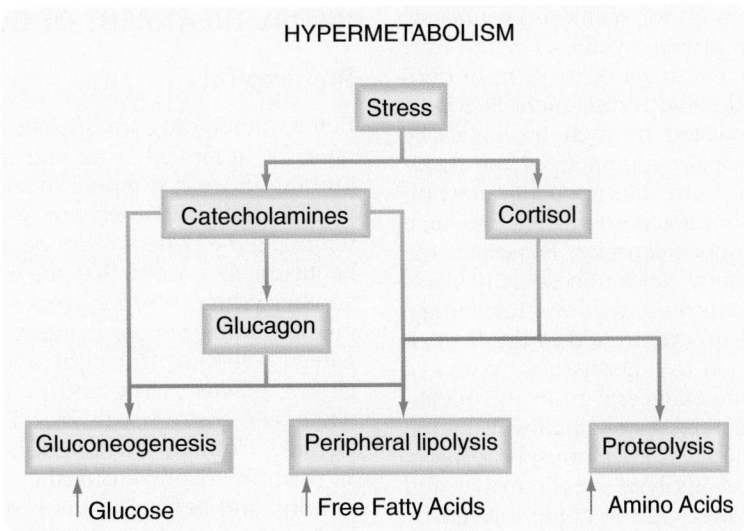

Figure 22-6 Results of hypermetabolism. A stress such as a severe burn induces the release of inflammatory hormones, which results in gluconeogenesis, lipolysis, and proteolysis.

is characterized by the production of interleukin-4 and interleukin-10. The T_H1 response is important in cell-mediated immune defense, whereas the T_H2 response is important in antibody responses to infection. As this polarization increases, so does the mortality rate. Administration of interleukin-10 antibodies and growth hormone has partially reversed this response and improved mortality after burns in animals. Burns also impair cytotoxic T-lymphocyte activity as a function of burn size, thus increasing the risk for infection, particularly from fungi and viruses. Early burn wound excision improves cytotoxic T-cell activity.

Hypermetabolism

Hypermetabolism, characterized by tachycardia, increased cardiac output, elevated energy expenditure, increased oxygen consumption, proteolysis and lipolysis, and severe nitrogen loss, develops after severe burns and resuscitation. Even though this response is seen in all major injuries, it is present in its most dramatic form in a severe burn, in which it may be sustained for months and lead to weight loss and decreased strength (particularly when strength is needed to recover from the complications associated with the injury). These alterations in metabolism are due in part to the release of catabolic hormones, which include catecholamines, glucocorticoids, and glucagon (Fig. 22-6).

Catecholamines act directly and indirectly to increase glucose availability through hepatic gluconeogenesis and glycogenolysis, as well as fatty acid availability through peripheral lipolysis. The direct effects are mediated through α- and β-adrenergic receptors on hepatocytes and lipocytes. The indirect effects are mediated through stimulation of adrenergic receptors in endocrine tissue within the pancreas, which causes a relative increase in glucagon release as compared with insulin. Normally, release of glucagon causes an increase in hepatic glucose production and peripheral lipolysis, whereas insulin has

the opposite effects of decreasing hepatic glucose production and peripheral lipolysis. Catecholamine stimulation of β-adrenergic receptors within the pancreas increases the release of both glucagon and insulin, but concurrent stimulation of α-receptors has a greater inhibitory effect on insulin than on glucagon, thereby resulting in greater net release of glucagon than insulin. The effects of catecholamine-stimulated glucagon release then outweigh the effects of insulin on glucose and fatty acid production and release. Glucocorticoid hormones, released by way of the hypothalamic-pituitary-adrenal axis, are mediated through neural stimulation. Cortisol has similar actions on energy substrates, and it induces insulin resistance, which is additive to the hyperglycemia because of the release of liver glucose. Catecholamines, when combined with glucagon and cortisol, augment glucose release, which could initially be beneficial because glucose is the principal fuel of inflammatory cells, as well as neural tissue.

Substrate supply for hepatic gluconeogenesis is produced by proteolysis and to some extent by peripheral lipolysis. Structural and constitutive proteins, degraded to amino acids:

1. Enter the tricarboxylic acid cycle for energy production
2. Circulate to the liver where they are used as substrate for gluconeogenesis
3. Are used for the synthesis of acute phase proteins

Most body protein available for this process is located in the musculature, thus depleting the muscle of its basic building blocks. Lactate and alanine are important intermediates that are released in proportion to the extent of injury. Glutamine is also released in massive quantities and can deplete muscle tissue stores to 50% of normal concentrations. After conversion to pyruvate or oxaloacetate, these amino acids form glucose with a net loss of adenosine triphosphate. Eighteen of the 20 amino acids are glucogenic and can be used for synthesis of glucose. The increased acute phase protein synthesis in the liver includes compounds such as C-reactive protein, fibrinogen, α_2-macroglobulin, and some complement factors.

Peripheral lipolysis, mediated through the catabolic hormones, is another principal component of the metabolic response to a severe burn. Elevation of catecholamine, glucagon, and cortisol levels stimulates the same or similar intracellular hormone-sensitive lipases in the adipocyte to release free fatty acids. These fatty acids circulate to the liver, where they are oxidized for energy, re-esterified to triglyceride, and deposited in the liver or further packaged for transport to other tissues by way of very-low-density lipoproteins. Glycerol from the breakdown of fat enters the gluconeogenic pathway at the glyceraldehyde 3-phosphate level after phosphorylation. In injured patients, rates of lipolysis are dramatic, and processing of lipid by the liver can be compromised by the increasing amount of circulating fat. The development of fatty liver in this situation is thought to be secondary to the overload of normal processing enzymes or perhaps to down-regulation of fatty acid handling mechanisms as a result of hormonal or cytokine manipulation associated with the injury.

The classic description of the ebb and flow phases of the response to illness and trauma deserves mention. The ebb phase is characterized by a low metabolic rate, hypothermia, and low cardiac output. It is often temporally related to the onset of disease or time of injury. After resuscitation, this state gives way to the flow phase, which is characterized by high cardiac output and oxygen consumption, increased heat production, hyperglycemia, and an elevated metabolic rate. Moore has expanded these definitions to the *catabolic* and *anabolic* portions of the flow phase of recovery.[10] The duration of the catabolic flow phase is also dependent on the type of injury and the efficacy of therapeutic interventions. In addition, the frequency and severity of complications have a bearing on the length of this phase of recovery, which in critically ill patients can last for weeks. The anabolic flow phase is characterized by a slow reaccumulation of protein and fat. This phase continues for months after injury.

Modulation of the hypermetabolic response to preserve lean body mass is an implicit goal of much of the treatment of a burned patient. Two agents have been shown to directly decrease catabolism and increase anabolism. β-Blockade blunts the response to the catecholamine surge with a decrease in physiologic thermogenesis, tachycardia, cardiac work, and resting energy expenditure. When dosed to decrease the heart rate in a burn patient by 20%, loss of lean body mass decreases from 9% to 1%.[11] Oxandrolone, an androgenic steroid, acts as an anabolic hormone similar to testosterone but with much decreased activity. At a dose of 0.1 mg/kg twice daily, oxandrolone improved muscle protein metabolism by enhancing the efficiency of protein synthesis. In addition to increasing lean body mass, in burned children oxandrolone has been shown to increase bone mineral content, synthesis of hepatic constitutive proteins such as albumin and prealbumin, and attenuate acute phase reactive protein levels.[12]

INITIAL TREATMENT OF BURNS

Prehospital

Before undergoing any specific treatment, burned patients must be removed from the source of injury and the burning process stopped. Inhalation injury is always suspected and 100% oxygen given by facemask. While removing the patient from the source of injury, care must be taken to ensure that the rescuer does not become another victim. All caregivers need to be aware that they might be injured by contact with the patient or the patient's clothing. Universal precautions including wearing gloves, gowns, mask, and protective eyewear, are used whenever contact with blood or body fluids is likely. Burning clothing is extinguished and removed as soon as possible to prevent further injury. All rings, watches, jewelry, and belts are removed because they retain heat and can produce a tourniquet-like effect. Room-temperature water can be poured on the wound within 15 minutes of injury to decrease the depth of the wound, but any subsequent measures to cool the wound are avoided to prevent hypothermia during resuscitation.

Initial Assessment

As with any trauma patient, the initial assessment of a burned patient is divided into a primary and secondary survey. In the primary survey, immediately life-threatening conditions are quickly identified and treated. In the secondary survey, a more thorough head-to-toe evaluation of the patient is undertaken.

Exposure to heated gases and smoke results in damage to the upper respiratory tract. Direct injury to the upper airway results in edema, which together with the generalized whole-body edema associated with a severe burn, may obstruct the airway. Airway injury must be suspected with facial burns, singed nasal hairs, carbonaceous sputum, and tachypnea. Because upper airway obstruction may develop rapidly, the patient's respiratory status must be continually monitored to assess the need for airway control and ventilatory support. Progressive hoarseness is a sign of impending airway obstruction, and endotracheal intubation needs to be instituted early before edema distorts the upper airway anatomy. This is especially important in patients with massive burns, who may appear to breathe without problems early in the resuscitation period until several liters of volume are given to maintain homeostasis and significant airway edema ensues.

The chest is exposed in order to assess breathing; airway patency alone does not ensure adequate ventilation. Chest expansion and equal breath sounds with CO_2 return from the endotracheal tube ensure adequate air exchange.

Blood pressure may be difficult to measure in burned patients with edematous or charred extremities. The pulse rate can be used as an indirect measure of circulation; however, most burned patients remain tachycardic even with adequate resuscitation. For the primary survey of burned patients, the presence of pulses or Doppler signals in the distal extremities may be sufficient to determine whether blood circulation is adequate until better monitors can be established, such as arterial pressure measurements and urine output.

In patients who have been in an explosion or deceleration accident, the possibility of spinal cord injury exists. Appropriate cervical spine stabilization must be accomplished by whatever means necessary, including the use of cervical collars to keep the head immobilized until the condition can be evaluated.

Wound Care

Prehospital care of a burn wound is basic and simple because it requires only protection from the environment with application of a clean dry dressing or sheet to cover the involved part. Damp dressings are not used. The patient is wrapped in a blanket to minimize heat loss and for temperature control during transport. The first step in diminishing pain is to cover the wounds to prevent contact with exposed nerve endings. Intramuscular or subcutaneous narcotic injections for pain are never used because drug absorption is decreased as a result of the peripheral vasoconstriction. This might become a problem later when the patient is resuscitated and vasodilation increases absorption of the narcotic depot with resulting apnea. Small doses of intravenous (IV) morphine may be given after complete assessment of the patient and once it is determined to be safe by an experienced practitioner.

Although prehospital management is simple, it is often difficult to enact, particularly in at-risk populations. A recent study in New Zealand showed that initial first aid treatment of burns was inadequate in 60% of patients interviewed. These authors also showed that inadequate first aid care was clearly associated with poorer outcomes. They suggested that defined education programs targeted to at-risk populations might improve these outcomes.[13]

Transport

Rapid, uncontrolled transport of a burn victim is not a priority, except when other life-threatening conditions coexist. In most incidents involving major burns, ground transportation of victims to the receiving hospital is appropriate. Helicopter transport is of greatest use when the distance between the accident and the hospital is 30 to 150 miles. For distances of more than 150 miles, transport by fixed-wing aircraft is most appropriate. Whatever the mode of transport, it needs to be of appropriate size and have emergency equipment available, along with trained personnel on board such as nurses, physicians, paramedics, or respiratory therapists who are familiar with multiply injured trauma patients.

Resuscitation

Adequate resuscitation of a burned patient depends on establishment and maintenance of reliable IV access. Increased times to initiating resuscitation of burned patients result in poorer outcomes, and delays must be minimized. Venous access is best attained through short peripheral catheters in unburned skin; however, veins in burned skin can be used and are preferable to no IV access. Superficial veins are often thrombosed in full-thickness injuries and are therefore not suitable for cannulation. Saphenous vein cut-down is useful in patients with difficult access and is used in preference to central vein cannulation because of lower complication rates. In children younger than 6 years, experienced practitioners can use intramedullary access in the proximal end of the tibia until IV access is achieved. Lactated Ringer's solution without dextrose is the fluid of choice, except in children younger than 2 years, who receive lactated Ringer's solution with 5% dextrose. The initial rate can be rapidly estimated by the TBSA burned multiplied by the patient's weight in kilograms and then dividing by 8. Thus, the rate of infusion for an 80-kg man with a 40% TBSA burn would be

$$80 \text{ kg} \times 40\% \text{ TBSA}/8 = 400 \text{ mL/hr}$$

This rate is continued until a formal calculation of resuscitation needs is performed.

Many formulas have been devised to determine the proper amount of fluid to give a burned patient, all originating from experimental studies on the pathophysiology of burn shock. Baxter[14] and others established the basis for modern fluid resuscitation protocols. They showed that edema fluid in burn wounds is isotonic and contains the same amount of protein as plasma does and that the greatest loss of fluid is into the interstitium. They used various volumes of intravascular fluid to determine the optimal amount in terms of cardiac output and extracellular volume in a canine burn model, and these data were applied to the clinical realm in the Parkland formula. Plasma volume changes were not related to the type of resuscitation fluid in the first 24 hours, but thereafter, colloid solutions could increase plasma volume by the amount infused. From these findings, they concluded that colloid solutions should not be used in the first 24 hours until capillary permeability returned closer to normal. Others have argued that normal capillary permeability is restored somewhat earlier after a burn (6-8 hours) and therefore colloids could be used earlier.

Concurrently, Pruitt and associates[7] showed the hemodynamic effects of fluid resuscitation in burns, which culminated in the Brooke formula. They found that fluid resuscitation caused an obligatory 20% decrease in both extracellular fluid and plasma volume that concluded after 24 hours. In the second 24 hours, plasma volume returned to normal with the administration of colloid. Cardiac output was low on the first day despite resuscitation, but it subsequently increased to supernormal levels as the flow phase of hypermetabolism was established. Since these studies, it has been found that much of the fluid needs are due to leaky capillaries that permit the passage of large molecules into the interstitial space, which increases extravascular colloid osmotic pressure. Intravascular volume follows the gradient to tissues, both into the burn wound and into nonburned tissues. Approximately 50% of fluid resuscitation needs are sequestered in nonburned tissues in patients with 50% TBSA burns.

Table 22-2 Resuscitation Formulas

FORMULA	CRYSTALLOID VOLUME	COLLOID VOLUME	FREE WATER
Parkland	4 mL/kg per % TBSA burn	None	None
Brooke	1.5 mL/kg per % TBSA burn	0.5 mL/kg per % TBSA burn	2.0 L
Galveston (pediatric)	5000 mL/m² burned area + 1500 mL/m² total area	None	None

These guidelines are used for the initial fluid management after a burn injury. The response to fluid resuscitation should be continuously monitored, and adjustments in the rate of fluid administration should be made accordingly.

TBSA, total body surface area.

Hypertonic saline solutions have theoretical advantages in burn resuscitation. These solutions decrease net fluid intake, reduce edema, and increase lymph flow, probably by transfer of volume from the intracellular space to the interstitium. When using these solutions, hypernatremia must be avoided, and it is recommended that serum sodium concentrations not exceed 160 mEq/dL. However, it must be noted that for patients with more than 20% TBSA burns who were randomized to either hypertonic saline or lactated Ringer's solution, there was no significant differences in volume requirements or changes in percentage of weight gain.[15] Other investigators found an increase in renal failure with hypertonic solutions, which has tempered further efforts in this area of investigation.[16] Some burn units successfully use a modified hypertonic solution of 1 ampule of sodium bicarbonate (50 mEq) in 1 L of lactated Ringer's solution. Further research needs to be done to determine the optimal formula for reducing edema formation and maintaining adequate cellular function.

Most burn units use something akin to either the Parkland or Brooke formula, which calls for administering varying amounts of crystalloid and colloid for the first 24 hours (Table 22-2). The fluids are generally changed in the second 24 hours to permit an increase in colloid use. These are guidelines to direct resuscitation of the amount of fluid necessary to maintain adequate perfusion. In fact, recent studies have shown that the Parkland formula often underestimates the volume of crystalloid received in the first 24 hours after a severe burn; this phenomenon has been termed *fluid creep* by Pruitt.[17] No clear single cause has been identified. More liberal use of opioid analgesic and positive pressure ventilation has been suggested.[18] The increased fluid volumes are not without consequence; the increased compartment pressure in the extremities, abdomen, and most recently the orbit[19] has been suggested as requiring monitoring and possible release to prevent increased morbidity and mortality. The abdominal compartment is clinically monitored with a Foley catheter. When pressure increases toward and above 30 mm Hg, complete abdominal escharotomy is performed, and paralytics are considered. If the increased abdominal pressure persists at a level greater than 30 mm Hg, improved outcome rests on the performance of decompressive laparotomy. However, patients who require this procedure have mortality rates of 60% to nearly 100%, depending on the series.[20] Therefore, monitoring of resuscitation fluids is crucial to ensure an acceptable outcome and is easily accomplished in burned patients with normal renal function by following the volume of urine output, which should be 0.5 mL/kg/hr in adults and 1.0 mL/kg/hr in children. Changes in IV fluid infusion rates are made on an hourly basis as determined by the response of the patient to the particular fluid volume administered.

For burned children, formulas modified to account for changes in the ratio of surface area to mass are commonly used. These changes are necessary because a child with a burn comparable to that in an adult requires more resuscitation fluid per kilogram. The Galveston formula uses 5000 mL/TBSA burned (in meters squared) + 1500 mL/m² total area for maintenance in the first 24 hours. This formula accounts for both maintenance needs and the increased fluid requirements of a child with a burn. All the formulas listed in Table 22-2 calculate the amount of volume given in the first 24 hours, half of which is given in the first 8 hours.

Recently, the use of albumin during IV resuscitation has come under criticism. In a meta-analysis of 31 trials, the Cochrane group showed that the risk of death was higher in burned patients who received albumin than in those who received crystalloid, with a relative risk of death of 2.40 (95% confidence interval, 1.11-5.19).[21] Another meta-analysis of all critically ill patients refuted this finding and showed no differences in relative risk between albumin-treated and crystalloid-treated groups.[22] In fact, as quality of the trials improved, the relative risks were reduced. Additional recent evidence suggests that albumin supplementation, even after resuscitation, does not affect the distribution of fluid among the intracellular/extracellular compartments.[23] What we can conclude from these trials and meta-analyses is that albumin used during resuscitation is at best equal to crystalloid and at worst detrimental to the outcome of burned patients. For these reasons, we cannot recommend the use of albumin during resuscitation.

To combat any regurgitation in patients with intestinal ileus, a nasogastric tube is inserted in all patients with major burns to decompress the stomach. This is especially important for all patients being transported in aircraft at high altitudes. Additionally, all patients are restricted from taking anything by mouth until the transfer has been completed. Decompression of the stomach is usually necessary because the apprehensive patient will swallow considerable amounts of air and distend the stomach.

Recommendations for tetanus prophylaxis are based on the condition of the wound and the patient's immunization history. All patients with burns of greater than 10% TBSA receive 0.5 mL of tetanus toxoid. If previous immunization is absent or unclear or the last booster dose was given longer than 10 years ago, 250 units of tetanus immunoglobulin is also administered.

Escharotomies

When deep second- and third-degree burn wounds encompass the circumference of an extremity, peripheral circulation to the limb can be compromised. The development of generalized edema beneath a nonyielding eschar impedes venous outflow and eventually affects arterial inflow to the distal beds. This can be recognized by numbness and tingling in the limb and increased pain in the digits. Arterial flow can be assessed by determination of Doppler signals in the digital arteries and the palmar and plantar arches in affected extremities. Capillary refill can also be assessed. Extremities at risk are identified either on clinical examination or by measurement of tissue pressures greater than 40 mm Hg. These extremities require escharotomies, which consist of release of the burn eschar at the bedside by incising the lateral and medial aspects of the extremity with a scalpel or electrocautery unit.

The entire constricting eschar must be incised longitudinally to completely relieve the impediment to blood flow. The incisions are carried down onto the thenar and hypothenar eminences and along the dorsolateral sides of the digits to completely open the hand, if it is involved (Fig. 22-7). If it is clear that the wound will require excision and grafting because of its depth, escharotomies are safest to restore perfusion to the underlying nonburned tissues until formal excision is performed. If vascular compromise has been prolonged, reperfusion after escharotomy may cause reactive hyperemia and further edema formation in the muscle, thus making continued surveillance of the distal extremities necessary. Increased muscle compartment pressures may necessitate fasciotomies. The most common complications associated with these procedures are blood loss and transient hypotension caused by the release of anaerobic metabolites. If distal perfusion does not improve with these measures, central hypotension secondary to hypovolemia is suspected and treated.

A constricting truncal eschar can cause a similar phenomenon, except that its effect is to decrease ventilation by limiting chest excursion. Any decrease in ventilation of a burned patient leads to inspection of the chest with appropriate escharotomies to relieve the constriction and allow adequate tidal volumes. This need becomes evident in a patient maintained on a volume control ventilator whose peak airway pressures increase.

INHALATION INJURY

One major factor contributing to death in burn injury patients is the presence of inhalation injury. Smoke damage adds another inflammatory focus to the burn and impedes the normal gas exchange vital for critically

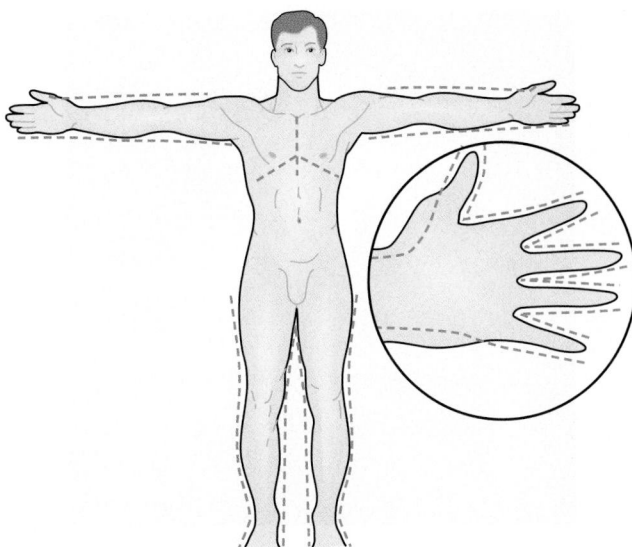

Figure 22-7 Recommended escharotomies. In limbs requiring escharotomies, the incisions are made on the medial and lateral sides of the extremity through the eschar. In the case of the hand, incisions are made on the medial and lateral digits and on the dorsum of the hand.

injured patients. Inhalation injury increases the amount of time spent on mechanical ventilation, which is a predictor of mortality.[5] Early diagnosis plus prevention of complications is necessary to decrease the morbidity and mortality associated with this condition.

With inhalation injury, damage is caused primarily by inhaled toxins. Heat is dispersed in the upper airways, whereas the cooled particles of smoke and toxins are carried distally into the bronchi. Thus, the injury to the airways is principally chemical in nature. Direct thermal damage to the lung is seldom seen because of dispersal of the heat in the pharynx. The exception is high-pressure steam inhalation, which has 4000 times the heat-carrying capacity of dry air.

The response to smoke inhalation is an immediate dramatic increase in blood flow in the bronchial arteries to the bronchi along with edema formation and increases in lung lymph flow. The lung lymph in this situation is similar to serum, thus indicating that permeability at the capillary level is markedly increased. The edema that results is associated with an increase in lung neutrophils, and it is postulated that these cells may be the primary mediators of pulmonary damage with this injury. Neutrophils release proteases and oxygen free radicals, which can produce conjugated dienes by lipid peroxidation. High concentrations of conjugated dienes are present in lung lymph and pulmonary tissue after inhalation injury, thus suggesting that the increased concentration of neutrophils is active in producing cytotoxic substances. When neutrophils are depleted before injury by nitrogen mustard, the increases in lung lymph flow and conjugated diene levels are markedly reduced.

Another hallmark of inhalation injury is separation of ciliated epithelial cells from the basement membrane, followed by the formation of exudate within the airways.

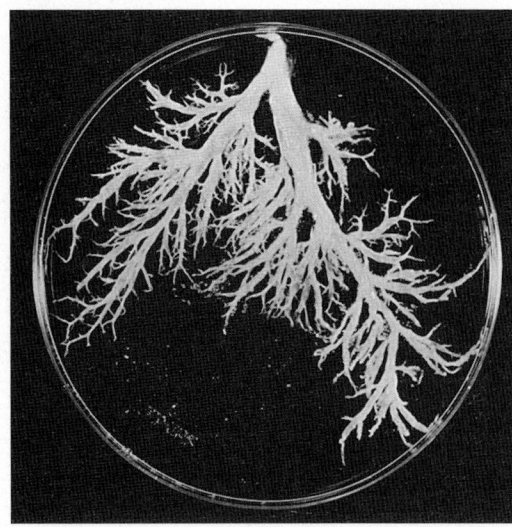

Figure 22-8 Bronchial cast found at autopsy of a patient with an inhalation injury.

Table 22-3 Clinical Indications for Intubation

CRITERIA	VALUE
PaO_2 (mm Hg)	<60
$PaCO_2$ (mm Hg)	>50 (acutely)
PaO_2/FIO_2 ratio	<200
Respiratory/ventilatory failure	Impending
Upper airway edema	Severe

The exudate consists of proteins found in the lung lymph, and eventually it coalesces to form fibrin casts (Fig. 22-8). Clinically, these fibrin casts can be difficult to clear with standard airway suction techniques, and bronchoscopic removal could therefore be required. These casts also add barotrauma to localized areas of lung by producing a so-called ball-valve effect. During inspiration, airway diameter increases and air flows past the cast into the distal airways. During expiration, airway diameter decreases and the cast effectively occludes the airway, thereby preventing the inhaled air from escaping. Increasing volume leads to localized increases in pressure that are associated with numerous complications, including pneumothorax and decreased lung compliance.

Smoke inhalation injury is often seen with a clinical history of exposure to smoke in a closed space, hoarseness, wheezing, and carbonaceous sputum. It may also be associated with facial burns and singed nasal hairs. Each of these findings has poor sensitivity and specificity; therefore, a definitive diagnosis must be established by the use of bronchoscopy or less commonly by xenon 133 ventilation scanning. Bronchoscopy can reveal early inflammatory changes such as erythema, ulceration, and prominent vasculature, in addition to infraglottic soot. The findings of airway erythema and ulceration alone are also nonspecific, and these findings must be considered in conjunction with all of the clinical manifestations to verify significant inhalation injury. Ventilation scanning with ^{133}Xe reveals areas of the lung retaining isotope 90 seconds after IV injection, thus indicating segmental airway obstruction from inhalation injury. Many of these patients require mechanical ventilation to maintain gas exchange, and repeat bronchoscopy may reveal continued ulceration of the airways with the formation of granulation tissue and exudate, inspissation of secretions, and focal edema. Eventually, the airway heals by replacement of the sloughed cuboidal ciliated epithelium with squamous cells and scar.

The clinical course of patients with inhalation injury is divided into three stages. The first is acute pulmonary insufficiency. Patients with severe lung injury may begin to show signs of pulmonary failure from the time of injury, such as asphyxia, carbon monoxide poisoning, bronchospasm, and upper airway obstruction. Clinical signs of parenchymal damage with hypoxia are not common during this phase. The second stage occurs 72 to 96 hours after injury and is associated with hypoxia and the development of diffuse lobar infiltrates. This condition is clinically similar to the adult respiratory distress syndrome (ARDS) that occurs in nonburned injured and critically ill patients. In the third stage, clinical bronchopneumonia dominates. These infections generally occur 3 to 10 days after inhalation injury and are associated with the expectoration of large mucous casts formed in the tracheobronchial tree. Differentiation of pneumonia from tracheobronchitis is difficult at this stage, and bronchoscopy with lavage may be of assistance. Early pneumonia is usually caused by penicillin-resistant *Staphylococcus* species, whereas after 5 to 7 days, the changing flora of the burn wound is reflected in the appearance of gram-negative species in the lung, especially *Pseudomonas*. Ball-valve effects and ventilator-associated barotrauma are also hallmarks of this period.

Management of inhalation injury is directed at maintaining open airways and maximizing gas exchange while the lung heals. A coughing patient with a patent airway can clear secretions effectively, and effort is made to manage patients without mechanical ventilation if possible. If respiratory failure is imminent, intubation is instituted, with frequent chest physiotherapy and suctioning performed to maintain pulmonary toilet (Table 22-3). Frequent bronchoscopy may be needed to clear inspissated secretions. Mechanical ventilation is used to provide gas exchange with as little barotrauma as possible. *Permissive hypercapnia* and the current ARDS Network ventilation protocols can be used with lower ventilatory rates and volumes to maintain arterial pH at greater than 7.25, thus minimizing positive airway pressure delivered by the ventilator.[24] Arterial oxygen tension greater than 60 mm Hg (or oxygen saturation of 92%) is also tolerated to minimize oxygen toxicity to the lungs. When the clinical condition improves to the point that the patient can be weaned from ventilatory support, the oxygen concentration, positive end-expiratory pressure, and ventilator volumes and rate are decreased in a graduated manner until the patient can be extubated. This process may take several weeks.

Inhalation treatments have been effective in improving the clearance of tracheobronchial secretions and decreasing bronchospasm (Table 22-4). IV heparin has been shown to reduce tracheobronchial cast formation, minute ventilation, and peak inspiratory pressure after smoke inhalation. When heparin was administered directly to the lungs in a nebulized form, it had similar effects on casts without causing systemic coagulopathy. When *N*-acetylcysteine treatments are added to nebulized heparin in burned children with inhalation injury, reintubation rates and mortality rates are decreased. In addition to the measures already discussed, adequate humidification plus treatment of bronchospasm with β-agonists is indicated. Steroids have not been shown to be of benefit in inhalation injury and are not given unless the patient was steroid dependent before the injury or had bronchospasm resistant to standard therapy.

In addition to conventional ventilator methods, novel ventilator therapies have been devised to minimize barotrauma, including high-frequency percussive ventilation. This method combines standard tidal volumes and respirations (ventilator rates of 6-20/min) with smaller high-frequency respirations (200-500/min) and permits adequate ventilation and oxygenation in patients who have failed conventional ventilation. One reason for the greater utility of this method is that it recruits alveoli at lower airway pressure. This ventilator method may also have a percussive effect that loosens inspissated secretions and improves pulmonary toilet. Prospective, randomized trials in which this method is being compared with conventional therapies are under way, the first of which has shown improved oxygenation in the first 3 days after inhalation injury. Liquid ventilation using perfluorocarbons and the use of inhaled nitric oxide as a selective pulmonary vasodilator are also being studied as adjuncts to current methods. Recent animal studies with perfluorocarbons, however, have had disappointing results, which has led to decreased enthusiasm for this treatment.

Several clinical studies have shown that pulmonary edema is not prevented by fluid restriction. Indeed, fluid resuscitation appropriate for the patient's other needs results in a decrease in lung water, has no adverse effect on pulmonary histology, and improves survival rates. Although overhydration could increase pulmonary edema, inadequate hydration increases the severity of pulmonary injury by sequestration of polymorphonuclear cells, which leads to an increased risk for death. In both animal and clinical studies, resuscitation was adequate if a normal cardiac index or urine output was maintained.

Prophylactic antibiotics for inhalation injury are not indicated but are clearly needed for documented lung infections. Empirical choices for treatment of pneumonia before culture results are returned include coverage of methicillin-resistant *Staphylococcus aureus* and gram-negative organisms (especially *Pseudomonas*). Systemic antibiotic regimens are based on serially monitored sputum cultures, bronchial washings, or transtracheal aspirates.

As patients recover from lung injury, they need to be extubated as soon as possible. Patients are able to clear their own airways through coughing more effectively than suction through an endotracheal tube can; therefore, patients without a need for ventilatory support are extubated. Extubation is preferably done as soon as the upper airway edema has resolved (injury days 1-2) in those who were intubated for control of the airway or for burn excision. It is our experience that patients with the same degree of inhalation injury who are extubated do better than those who are intubated. Standard extubation criteria can be used, although many patients who do not meet these criteria may also do well without mechanical ventilation. If the airway is easily accessible, a trial of extubation might be of benefit in patients with borderline weaning parameters.

WOUND CARE

After the airway is assessed and resuscitation is under way, attention must be turned to the burn wound. Treatment depends on the characteristics and size of the wound. All treatments are aimed at rapid and painless healing. Current therapy directed specifically toward burn wounds can be divided into three stages: assessment, management, and rehabilitation. Once the extent and depth of the wounds have been assessed and the wounds have been thoroughly cleaned and débrided, the management phase begins. Each wound is dressed with an appropriate covering that serves several functions. First, it protects the damaged epithelium, minimizes bacterial and fungal colonization, and provides splinting action to maintain the desired position of function. Second, the dressing is occlusive to reduce evaporative heat loss and minimize cold stress. Third, the dressing needs to provide comfort over the painful wound.

The choice of dressing is based on the characteristics of the treated wound (Table 22-5). First-degree wounds are minor with minimal loss of barrier function. These wounds require no dressing and are treated with topical salves to decrease pain and keep the skin moist. Systemic nonsteroidal anti-inflammatory agents given by mouth assist in pain control. Second-degree wounds can be treated with daily dressing changes and topical antibiotics, cotton gauze, and elastic wraps. Alternatively, the wounds can be treated with a temporary biologic or synthetic covering to close the wound. Deep second-degree and third-degree wounds require excision and

Table 22-4 Inhalation Treatments of Smoke Inhalation Injury

TREATMENT	TIME/DOSAGE
Bronchodilators (Albuterol)	q2h
Nebulized heparin	5000 to 10,000 units with 3 mL normal saline q4h
Nebulized acetylcysteine	20%, 3 mL q4h
Hypertonic saline	Induce effective coughing
Racemic epinephrine	Reduce mucosal edema

Table 22-5 **Burn Wound Dressings**

DRESSINGS	ADVANTAGES AND DISADVANTAGES
Antimicrobial Salves	
Silver sulfadiazine (Silvadene)	Broad-spectrum antimicrobial; painless and easy to use; does not penetrate eschar; may leave black tattoos from silver ion; mild inhibition of epithelialization
Mafenide acetate (Sulfamylon)	Broad-spectrum antimicrobial; penetrates eschar; may cause pain in sensate skin; wide application may cause metabolic acidosis; mild inhibition of epithelialization
Bacitracin	Ease of application; painless; antimicrobial spectrum not as wide as above agents
Neomycin	Ease of application; painless; antimicrobial spectrum not as wide
Polymyxin B	Ease of application; painless; antimicrobial spectrum not as wide
Nystatin (Mycostatin)	Effective in inhibiting most fungal growth; cannot be used in combination with mafenide acetate
Mupirocin (Bactroban)	More effective staphylococcal coverage; does not inhibit epithelialization; expensive
Antimicrobial Soaks	
0.5% Silver nitrate	Effective against all microorganisms; stains contacted areas; leaches sodium from wounds; may cause methemoglobinemia
5% Mafenide acetate	Wide antibacterial coverage; no fungal coverage; painful on application to sensate wound; wide application associated with metabolic acidosis
0.025% Sodium hypochlorite (Dakin solution)	Effective against almost all microbes, particularly gram-positive organisms; mildly inhibits epithelialization
0.25% Acetic acid	Effective against most organisms, particularly gram-negative ones; mildly inhibits epithelialization
Synthetic Coverings	
OpSite	Provides a moisture barrier; inexpensive; decreased wound pain; use complicated by accumulation of transudate and exudate requiring removal; no antimicrobial properties
Biobrane	Provides a wound barrier; associated with decreased pain; use complicated by accumulation of exudate risking invasive wound infection; no antimicrobial properties
Transcyte	Provides a wound barrier; decreased pain; accelerated wound healing; use complicated by accumulation of exudate; no antimicrobial properties
Integra	Provides complete wound closure and leaves a dermal equivalent; sporadic take rates; no antimicrobial properties
Biologic Coverings	
Xenograft (pig skin)	Completely closes the wound; provides some immunologic benefits; must be removed or allowed to slough
Allograft (homograft, cadaver skin)	Provides all the normal functions of skin; can leave a dermal equivalent; epithelium must be removed or allowed to slough

grafting for sizable burns, and the choice of initial dressing is aimed at holding bacterial proliferation in check and providing occlusion until surgery is performed.

Antimicrobials

Timely and effective use of antimicrobials has revolutionized burn care by decreasing invasive wound infections. An untreated burn wound rapidly becomes colonized with bacteria and fungi because of the loss of normal skin barrier mechanisms. As the organisms proliferate to high wound counts ($>10^5$ organisms per gram of tissue), they may penetrate into viable tissue. Organisms then invade blood vessels and cause a systemic infection that often leads to death of the patient. This scenario has become uncommon in most burn units because of the effective use of antibiotics and wound care techniques. The antimicrobials that are used can be divided into those given topically and those given systemically.

Available topical antibiotics can be divided into two classes: salves and soaks. Salves are generally applied directly to the wound with cotton dressings placed over them, and soaks are generally poured into cotton dressings on the wound. Each of these classes of antimicrobials has advantages and disadvantages. Salves may be applied once or twice a day but could lose their effectiveness between dressing changes. Frequent dressing changes can result in shearing with loss of grafts or underlying healing cells. Soaks remain effective because antibiotic solution can be added without removing the dressing; however, the underlying skin can become macerated.

Topical antibiotic salves include 11% mafenide acetate (Sulfamylon), 1% silver sulfadiazine (Silvadene), polymyxin B, neomycin, bacitracin, mupirocin, and the antifungal agent nystatin. No single agent is completely effective, and each has advantages and disadvantages. Silver sulfadiazine is the most commonly used. It has a broad spectrum of activity because its silver and sulfa moieties cover gram-positive, most gram-negative, and some fungal forms. Some *Pseudomonas* species possess plasmid-mediated resistance. Silver sulfadiazine is relatively painless on application, has high patient acceptance, and is easy to use. Occasionally, patients complain of a burning sensation after it is applied, and in a few patients, a transient leukopenia develops 3 to 5 days after its continued use. This leukopenia is generally harmless and resolves with or without cessation of treatment.

Mafenide acetate is another topical agent with a broad spectrum of activity because of its sulfa moiety. It is particularly useful against resistant *Pseudomonas* and *Enterococcus* species. It can also penetrate eschar, which silver sulfadiazine cannot. Disadvantages include painful application on skin, such as in second-degree wounds. It can also cause an allergic rash, and it has carbonic anhydrase inhibitory characteristics that can result in metabolic acidosis when applied over large surfaces. For these reasons, mafenide sulfate is typically reserved for small full-thickness injuries.

Petrolatum-based antimicrobial ointments with polymyxin B, neomycin, and bacitracin are clear on application and painless and allow easy wound observation. These agents are commonly used for the treatment of facial burns, graft sites, healing donor sites, and small partial-thickness burns. Mupirocin is a relatively new petrolatum-based ointment that has improved activity against gram-positive bacteria, particularly methicillin-resistant *S. aureus* and selected gram-negative bacteria. Nystatin either in salve or in powder form can be applied to wounds to control fungal growth. Nystatin-containing ointments can be combined with other topical agents to decrease colonization of both bacteria and fungi. The exception is the combination of nystatin and mafenide acetate; each inactivates the other.

Agents available for application as a soak include 0.5% silver nitrate solution, 0.025% sodium hypochlorite (Dakin solution), 0.25% acetic acid, and mafenide acetate as a 5% solution. Silver nitrate has the advantage of being painless on application and having complete antimicrobial effectiveness. Its disadvantages include staining of surfaces to a dull gray or black when the solution dries. This can become problematic in deciphering wound depth during excision of burns and in keeping the patient and surroundings clean of the black staining. The solution is hypotonic as well, and continuous use can cause electrolyte leaching, with rare methemoglobinemia as another complication. A new commercial dressing containing biologically potent silver ions (Acticoat) that are activated in the presence of moisture is available. This dressing holds promise to retain the effectiveness of silver nitrate without the problems of silver nitrate soaks.

Dakin solution (0.25% sodium hypochlorite) is effective against most microbes; however, it also has cytotoxic effects on the healing cells of patients' wounds. Low concentrations of sodium hypochlorite (0.025%) have less cytotoxic effects while maintaining most of the antimicrobial effects. Hypochlorite ion is inactivated by contact with protein, so the solution must be continually changed. The same is true for acetic acid solutions, which may be more effective against *Pseudomonas*. Mafenide acetate soaks have the same characteristics as mafenide acetate salve, except that they are in liquid form.

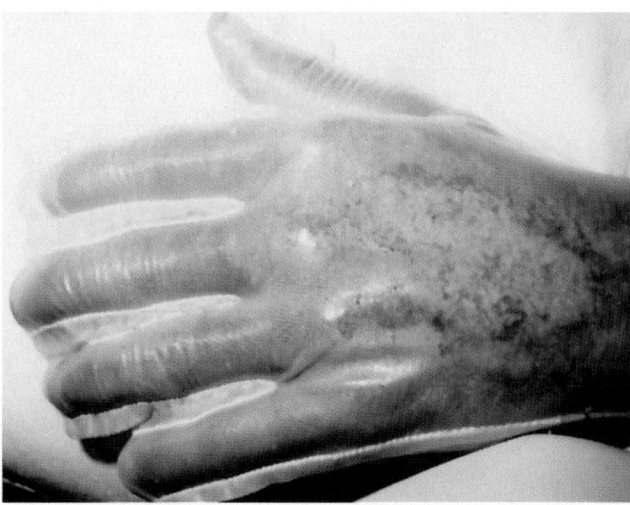

Figure 22-9 Biobrane in the form of a glove. This artificial dressing has elastic properties that form a seal with the wound. Once the wound exudate has dried to form a barrier, epithelialization takes place under the dressing in partial-thickness wounds in 1 to 2 weeks.

The use of perioperative systemic antimicrobials also has a role in decreasing burn wound sepsis until the burn wound is closed. Common organisms that must be considered when choosing a perioperative regimen include *S. aureus* and *Pseudomonas* species, which are prevalent in burn wounds.

Synthetic and Biologic Dressings

Synthetic and biologic dressings are an alternative to antimicrobial dressings. These types of dressings afford stable coverage without painful dressing changes, provide a barrier to evaporative losses, and decrease pain in the wounds. They do not inhibit epithelialization, which is a feature of most topical antimicrobials. These coverings include allograft (cadaver skin), xenograft (pig skin), Transcyte, Biobrane, and Integra. They generally are applied within 72 hours of the injury, before high bacterial colonization of the wound occurs. Most often, synthetic and biologic dressings are used to cover second-degree wounds while the underlying epithelium heals or to cover full-thickness wounds for which autograft is not yet available. Each type of dressing has its advantages and disadvantages.

Biobrane consists of collagen-coated silicone manufactured into a sheet (Fig. 22-9). It is placed on the wound and becomes adherent in 24 to 48 hours with dried wound transudate. This sheet then becomes a barrier to moisture loss, and it provides a relatively painless wound bed that does not require dressing changes. When the epithelium is complete under the Biobrane sheet, it is easily peeled off the wound. Caution must be exercised when using this product to ensure that copious exudate does not form under the Biobrane, which provides an optimum environment for bacterial proliferation and eventual invasive wound infection. Biobrane has no

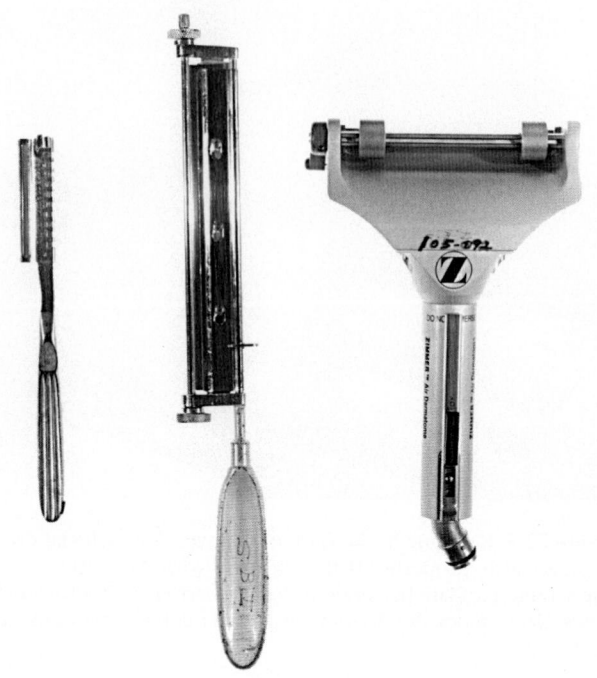

Figure 22-10 Instruments for tangential excision of burn wounds. Each of these instruments may be used to excise the burn wound in layers until viable tissue is reached. Powered dermatomes such as the Zimmer instrument shown here *(right)* require either nitrogen or electricity. The others (the Watson blade, which is the larger blade, and Weck blade) are hand instruments.

antimicrobial activities. It is used primarily for superficial second-degree burns and split-thickness skin graft donor sites.

Transcyte is a product that is similar to Biobrane, but with the addition of growth factors from lysed fibroblasts grown in culture; it has been shown to decrease hospital stay and the incidence of autografting.[25] This product has the theoretical advantages of Biobrane with the additional benefit of stimulated wound healing. Applications are the same for Transcyte and Biobrane, with the additional use of Transcyte for deeper second-degree wounds that will heal with stimulation.

Integra is a product that combines a collagen matrix (dermal substitute) with a silicone sheet outside layer (epidermal substitute). The collagen matrix engrafts into the wound, and after 2 weeks the silicone layer is removed and replaced with available autograft. The advantages of this product are that it can be used in full-thickness burns to close the wound. It also provides a dermal equivalent that has the theoretical advantage of inhibiting future scarring of the burn wound. The disadvantages are similar to those of all synthetic products in that it has no antimicrobial properties and thus its use can be complicated by invasive wound infections. Additionally, it takes two operations for wound coverage because the silicone layer simulating the epidermis must be replaced 2 to 3 weeks after application with autograft. Recent reports on the use of Integra purport acceptable take and infection rates.[26] One of the potential advantages of this product is limita-

tion of scarring because of the presence of the dermal substitute; however, this has not been borne out in the initial reports.[27] Further studies with larger numbers of patients are required to test whether decreased scarring is an additional benefit with the use of this product.

Biologic dressings include xenografts from swine and allografts from cadaver donors. These human skin equivalents are applied to wounds in the manner of skin grafts, where they engraft and perform the immunologic and barrier functions of normal skin. Thus, these biologic dressings are the optimal wound coverage in the absence of normal skin. Eventually, these biologic dressings will be rejected by usual immune mechanisms and the grafts will slough. They can then be replaced, or the open wound can be covered with autograft skin from the patient. Generally, severely burned patients are immunosuppressed, and biologic dressings that have adhered will not be rejected for several weeks. Biologic dressings can be used to cover any wound as a temporary dressing. They are particularly well suited for massive partial-thickness injuries (>50% TBSA) to close the wound and allow healing to take place underneath the dressing. Disadvantages include potential transmission of viral diseases with allograft and the possibility that a residual mesh pattern will be left from engrafted cadaver dermis if meshed allograft is used.

Excision and Grafting

Deep second- and third-degree burns do not heal in timely fashion without autografting. In fact, the practice of leaving this dead tissue serves only as a nidus for inflammation and infection that could lead to the patient's death. Early excision plus grafting of these wounds is currently done by most burn surgeons because reports have shown benefit over serial débridement in terms of survival, blood loss, incidence of sepsis, and length of hospitalization.[28] The technique of early excision and grafting has made conservative treatment of full-thickness wounds a practice to be used only in the elderly and in the infrequent cases in which anesthesia and surgery are contraindicated. Attempts are made to excise tangentially to optimize cosmetic outcome. A number of instruments are commonly used to perform these excisions (Fig. 22-10). Rarely, excision to the level of fascia is required to remove all nonviable tissue, or it may become necessary at subsequent operations for infectious complications. Excision can be performed under tourniquet control or with application of topical epinephrine and thrombin to minimize blood loss.

After a burn wound has been excised, the wound must be covered. This covering is ideally the patient's own skin. Wounds covering 20% to 30% of TBSA can usually be closed at one operation with autograft split-thickness skin taken from the patient's available donor sites. In these operations, the skin grafts are not meshed, or they are meshed with a narrow ratio (≤2:1) to maximize cosmetic outcome. In major burns, autograft skin may be limited to the extent that the wound cannot be completely closed. The availability of cadaver allograft skin has changed the course of modern burn treatment of

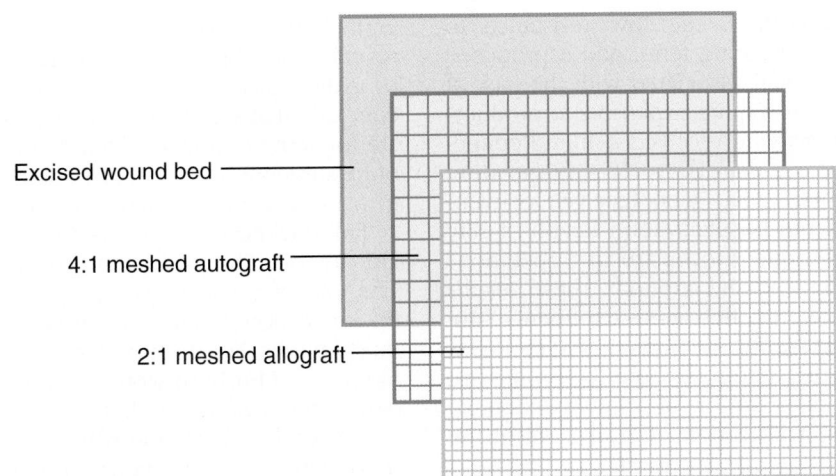

Excised wound bed

4:1 meshed autograft

2:1 meshed allograft

Figure 22-11 Diagram of skin closure using widely meshed autografts. A widely meshed autograft is placed on a freshly excised viable wound bed. The remaining open wound between the interstices of the autograft is closed with an overlying layer of allograft, which can also be meshed to allow transudate, exudate, and hematoma to escape.

these massive wounds. A typical method of treatment is to use widely expanded autografts (≥4:1) covered with cadaver allograft to completely close the wounds for which autograft is available. The 4:1 autograft skin heals underneath the cadaver skin in approximately 21 days, and the cadaver skin falls off (Fig. 22-11). The portions of the wound that cannot be covered with even widely meshed autograft are covered with allograft skin in preparation for autografting when the donor sites have healed. Ideally, areas with less cosmetic importance are covered with widely meshed skin to close most of the wound before using nonmeshed grafts at later operations for cosmetically important areas, such as the hands and face.

Most surgeons excise the burn wound in the first week, sometimes in serial operations by removing 20% of the burn wound per operation on subsequent days. Others remove the whole of the burn wound in one operative procedure; however, this can be limited by the development of hypothermia or continuing massive blood loss. It is our practice to perform the excision immediately after the patient is stabilized following a burn injury because blood loss diminishes if the operation can be done the first day after injury. This decreased blood loss may be due to the relative predominance of vasoconstrictive substances such as thromboxane and catecholamines and the natural edema planes that develop immediately after the injury. When the wound becomes hyperemic after 2 days, blood loss can be a considerable problem. The use of hemostatic agents such as epinephrine, thrombin, and tourniquets greatly aids in this approach.

Early excision is reserved for third-degree wounds. A deep second-degree burn can appear to be a third-degree wound at 24 to 48 hours after injury, particularly if it has been treated with topical antimicrobials, which combine with wound fluid to form a dense pseudoeschar. A randomized, prospective study comparing early excision

versus conservative therapy with late grafting of deep second-degree wounds showed that those excised early had more wound excised, more blood loss, and more time in the operating room. No difference in hospital length of stay or infection rate was seen.[29] Long-term scarring and functional outcome, however, have not been examined in detail.

Occasionally, split-thickness skin grafts do not adhere. Loss of skin grafts is due to one or more of the following reasons: fluid collection under the graft, shearing forces that disrupt the adhered graft, the presence of infection causing graft lysis, or inadequate excision of the wound bed with necrotic tissue remaining. Meticulous hemostasis, appropriate meshing of grafts, or rolling of sheet grafts or bolsters over appropriate areas minimizes fluid collections. Shearing is decreased by immobilization of the grafted area. Infection is controlled by the appropriate use of perioperative antibiotics and covering the grafts with topical antimicrobials at the time of surgery. Inadequate excision of wound beds is diminished by careful excision to viable tissue by experienced surgeons. Punctate bleeding or color of the dermis or fat in areas excised under tourniquet control denotes the proper level of excision. Tissues that retain a red color after excision typically do not take grafts.

One alternative to split-thickness autografts typically used for skin grafting is cultured keratinocytes from the patient's own skin. Keratinocytes can be cultured in sheets from full-thickness skin biopsy samples and the sheets then applied as autografts. This technology has been used to greatly expand the capacity of a donor site such that most of the body can be covered with grafts from a single small, full-thickness biopsy sample. Cultured epithelial autografts are of use in truly massive burns (>80% TBSA) because of the limited donor sites of these patients. The disadvantages of cultured epithelial autografts are the length of time required to grow the autografts (2-3 weeks), a 50% to 75% take rate of the grafts after initial application, the low resistance to mechanical trauma over the long term, and a proposed increase in scarring potential associated with the lack of dermis. These grafts are also quite expensive to produce. When a group of patients who received cultured epithelial autografts with greater than 80% TBSA burns were compared with a similar group who received conventional treatment, the acute hospitalization length of stay and the number of subsequent reconstructive operations were lower in the conventional group.[30] These results demonstrate that more research and experience are needed to further optimize this technique. Technologies such as cultured epithelial autografts hold the promise to radically limit donor sites, and it may be the optimal closure in combination with a dermal equivalent in the future.

The use of anabolic agents to accelerate wound healing has been investigated. The most effective agent to date has been systemically administered recombinant human growth hormone. The use of growth hormone has stimulated donor sites to heal faster, thereby allowing more frequent donor site harvest and thus less time between operations. Growth hormone decreased donor site healing time by an average of 2 days and was associated with a reduction in the length of hospital stay from 0.8 day per percent TBSA burn to 0.54 day per percent TBSA burn. This improved healing time was associated with a cost saving of 23% for a typical 80% TBSA burn, including cost of the growth hormone. This effect is thought to be due to stimulation of insulin-like growth factor-I release, as well as up-regulation of insulin-like growth factor-I receptors in the wound. It has recently been shown that insulin in pharmacologic doses may have similar effects on wound healing. Insulin given at 30 μU/kg/min for 7 days decreased donor site healing time from 6.5 ± 0.9 days to 4.7 ± 2.3 days.[31] In this study, the caloric intake necessary to maintain euglycemia during the insulin infusion was double that of the placebo time period. The effects of insulin on wound healing also seem to be potentiated with additional amino acids.[32] Studies are under way in which much lower doses are being used to determine whether a significant effect is still present at doses that would be clinically safer to use.

In all burned patients, every effort is made to maximize the long-term appearance of the wound because almost all patients will survive to bear the scars of their injury. Burn wound scarring causes both functional and cosmetic deficits associated with wound contracture. Experience has shown that full-thickness skin grafts that include the entire dermal and epidermal layer provide the best outcomes in wound coverage, with diminished contracture and superior skin appearance in comparison to split-thickness skin grafts. Split-thickness and full-thickness grafts both have a complete epidermal layer; therefore, the superior function and appearance of full-thickness grafts must lie in the uninterrupted complete dermal layer. The thickness of split-thickness skin grafts is also addressed because it is thought by extension that thicker skin grafts carrying more dermis will diminish the amount of contracture and scarring. A recent study comparing standard-thickness grafts (0.015 inch) with thick grafts (0.025 inch) applied to full-thickness hand wounds revealed no differences in range of motion, appearance, or patient satisfaction.[33] Therefore, it is reasonable to conclude that standard-thickness skin grafts are appropriate for acute coverage of burn wounds. The challenge to burn surgeons in terms of minimizing scarring, then, is to provide complete dermis during wound coverage.

Full-thickness skin grafts to supply the dermal layer are not plentiful and cannot be used more than once. The use of tissue expanders to increase available full-thickness donor skin is conceivable, but impractical for most injuries. For these reasons, these grafts are not commonly used for burn wound coverage. Engrafted cadaver dermis that has the epidermis removed by dermabrasion 1 to 2 weeks after being placed on the wound has been used with some success to provide the dermal layer. Presumably, the sparse cellular component of the dermis is removed by immunologic processes and the dermal matrix is left in place as scaffolding for the ingrowth of normal dermal cells. A commercially available product of decellularized preserved cadaver dermis (AlloDerm) has likewise been used to provide a dermal equivalent in wound coverage. As discussed earlier, the product Integra also has a dermal equivalent component to form a neodermis. All these coverings have the potential to minimize scarring contractures and to maximize the cosmetic appearance of burn scars. The long-term results with the use of these techniques are not yet known.

Recently, the use of vacuum-assisted closure of wounds has been reported. These vacuum-assisted devices have been used successfully for closure of complicated decubitus ulcers, among other uses, and have now been tried in burn wounds to secure skin grafts and improve take rates.[34] Those treated with vacuum-assisted devices versus standard bolster fastening of skin grafts had significantly improved rates of reoperation for failed skin grafts without differences in complications.

MINIMIZING COMPLICATIONS

Early, aggressive resuscitation regimens have improved survival rates dramatically. With the advent of vigorous fluid resuscitation, irreversible burn shock has been replaced by sepsis and subsequent multiorgan failure as the leading cause of death associated with burns. In our pediatric burn population with burns of more than 80% TBSA, sepsis defined by bacteremia developed in 17.5% of the children.[5] The mortality rate in the whole group was 33%; most of these deaths were attributable to multiorgan failure. Some of the patients who died were bacteremic and septic, but most were not. These findings highlight the observation that the development of multiorgan failure is often associated with infectious sepsis, but infection is by no means required for multiorgan failure to develop. What is required is an inflammatory focus, which in severe burns is the massive skin injury that requires inflammation to heal. It has been postulated that progression to multiorgan failure exists in a continuum with the systemic inflammatory response syndrome. Nearly all burned patients meet the criteria for systemic inflammatory response syndrome as defined by the consensus conference of the American College of Chest Physicians and the Society of Critical Care Medicine.[35] It is therefore not surprising that multiorgan failure is common in burned patients.

Insulin

Stress-induced hyperglycemia is ubiquitously found in the intensive care unit (ICU). Since the 2001 article by Van den Berghe and colleagues,[36] the clinical practice of maintaining tight glycemic control to decrease complication rates has been studied extensively and confirmed. The nearly 50% reduction in mortality in a mixed adult ICU population is a motivator to test the efficacy of tight glycemic control in other populations. Burn patients, though not excluded, were not a meaningful part of this landmark paper. Follow-up studies in burn patients have supported tight glycemic control. A prospective study of 30 burned children with historical controls at the same institution demonstrated a decreased sepsis rate and a fourfold increase in survival in the study group with tight glycemic control (90-120 mg/dL). At this time, tight glycemic control is recommended and further studies are ongoing to understand the full impact of such care on burn patients.[37]

Etiology and Pathophysiology

The progression from systemic inflammatory response syndrome to multiorgan failure is not well explained, although some of the mechanisms responsible are recognized and most are found in patients with inflammation from infectious sources. In a burned patient, these infectious sources most likely emanate from invasive wound infection or from lung infections (pneumonia). As organisms proliferate out of control, endotoxins are liberated from gram-negative bacterial walls, and exotoxins are released from gram-positive and gram-negative bacteria. Their release causes the initiation of a cascade of inflammatory mediators that can result, if unchecked, in organ damage and progression to organ failure. Occasionally, failure of the gut barrier with penetration of organisms into the systemic circulation may incite a similar reaction. However, this phenomenon has been demonstrated only in animal models, and it remains to be seen whether this is a cause of human disease.

Inflammation from the presence of necrotic tissue and open wounds can incite an inflammatory mediator response similar to that seen with endotoxin. The mechanism by which this occurs, however, is not well understood. Regardless, it is known that a cascade of systemic events is set in motion, either by invasive organisms or by open wounds that initiate the systemic inflammatory response syndrome, which may progress to multiorgan failure. Evidence from animal studies and clinical trials suggests that these events converge to a common pathway that results in the activation of several cascade systems. Those circulating mediators can, if secreted in excessive amounts, damage organs distant from their site of origin. Among these mediators are endotoxin, the arachidonic acid metabolites, cytokines, neutrophils and their adher-

ence molecules, nitric oxide, complement components, and oxygen free radicals.

Prevention

Because different cascade systems are involved in the pathogenesis of burn-induced multiorgan failure, it has thus far been impossible to pinpoint a single mediator that initiates the event. Accordingly, because the mechanisms of progression are not well known, prevention is currently the best solution. The current recommendations are to prevent the development of organ dysfunction and provide optimal support to avoid conditions that promote its onset.

A great reduction in mortality rates from large burns was seen with early excision and an aggressive surgical approach to the treatment of deep wounds. Early removal of devitalized tissue prevents wound infections and decreases inflammation associated with the wound. In addition, it eliminates small, colonized foci, which are a frequent source of transient bacteremia. These transient bacteremias during surgical manipulations may prime immune cells to react in an exaggerated fashion to subsequent insults and thereby lead to whole-body inflammation and remote organ damage. We recommend complete early excision of clearly full-thickness wounds within 48 hours of the injury.

Oxidative damage from reperfusion after low-flow states makes early, aggressive fluid resuscitation imperative. This is particularly important during the initial phases of treatment and operative excision with its attendant blood losses. Furthermore, the volume of fluid may not be as important as the timeliness with which it is given. In the study of children with greater than 80% TBSA burns, it was found that one of the most important contributors to survival was the time required to start IV resuscitation, regardless of the initial volume given.

Topical and systemic antimicrobial therapy has significantly diminished the incidence of invasive burn wound sepsis. Perioperative antibiotics clearly benefit patients with burns greater than 30% TBSA. Vigilant and scheduled replacement of intravascular devices minimizes the incidence of catheter-related sepsis. We recommend changing indwelling catheters every 3 days. The first can be done over a wire with sterile Seldinger technique, but the second change requires a new site. This protocol is maintained as long as IV access is required. When possible, peripheral veins are used for cannulation, even through burned tissue. The saphenous vein, however, is avoided because of the high risk for thrombophlebitis.

Pneumonia, which contributes significantly to death in burned patients, is vigilantly anticipated and aggressively treated. Every attempt is made to wean patients as early as possible from the ventilator to reduce the risk for ventilator-associated nosocomial pneumonia. Furthermore, early ambulation is an effective means of preventing respiratory complications. With sufficient analgesics, even patients maintained on continuous ventilatory support can be out of bed and in a chair.

The most common sources of sepsis are the wounds and the tracheobronchial tree; efforts to identify causative agents are concentrated there. Another potential source, however, is the gastrointestinal tract, which is a natural reservoir for bacteria. Starvation and hypovolemia shunt blood from the splanchnic bed and promote mucosal atrophy and failure of the gut barrier. Early enteral feeding reduces septic morbidity and prevents failure of the gut barrier. At our institution, patients are fed immediately through a nasogastric tube. Early enteral feeding is tolerated in burned patients, preserves mucosal integrity, and may reduce the magnitude of the hypermetabolic response to injury. Support of the gut goes along with carefully monitored hemodynamics.

Organ Failure

Even with the best efforts at prevention, the presence of the systemic inflammatory response syndrome, which is ubiquitous in burned patients, may progress to organ failure. It was recently found that severe multiorgan dysfunction will develop in approximately 28% of patients with greater than 20% TBSA burns, with severe sepsis and septic shock also developing in 14%.[38] The general development of multiorgan dysfunction begins in either the renal or the pulmonary system and can progress through the liver, gut, hematologic system, and central nervous system. The development of multiorgan failure does not predict mortality, however, and effort to support the organs until they heal is justified.

Renal Failure

With the advent of early aggressive resuscitation, the incidence of renal failure coincident with the initial phases of recovery has diminished significantly in severely burned patients. However, a second period of risk for the development of renal failure is still present 2 to 14 days after resuscitation. Renal failure is hallmarked by decreasing urine output; fluid overload; electrolyte abnormalities, including metabolic acidosis and hyperkalemia; the development of azotemia; and an increased serum creatinine level. Treatment is aimed at averting complications associated with these conditions.

Urine output greater than 1 mL/kg/hr is an adequate measure of renal perfusion in the absence of underlying renal disease. Decreasing the volume of fluid being given can alleviate volume overload in burned patients. These patients have increased insensible losses from the wounds, which can be roughly calculated as 1500 mL/m² TBSA + 3750 mL/m² TBSA burned. Further losses are accrued on airbeds (1 L/day in an adult). Decreasing the infused volume of IV fluids and enteral feeding to less than the expected insensate losses alleviates fluid overload problems. Electrolyte abnormalities can be minimized by decreasing potassium in the enteral nutrition and giving oral bicarbonate solutions such as Bicitra. Almost invariably, severely burned patients require exogenous potassium because the heightened aldosterone response results in potassium wasting; therefore, hyperkalemia is rare, even with some renal insufficiency.

If the problems listed earlier overwhelm the conservative measures, some form of dialysis may be necessary. Indications for dialysis are volume overload or electrolyte abnormalities not amenable to other treatments. Peritoneal dialysis is effective in removing volume and correcting electrolyte abnormalities in burned patients. Occasionally, hemodialysis is required. Continuous venovenous hemodialysis is often indicated in these patients because of the fluid shifts that occur. All hemodialysis techniques are performed in conjunction with experienced nephrologists who are well versed in the techniques.

After beginning dialysis, renal function may return, especially in patients who maintain some urine output. Therefore, patients needing such treatment may not require lifelong dialysis. It is a clinical observation that whatever urine output was present will decrease once dialysis is begun, but it may return in several days to weeks once the acute process of closing the burn wound nears completion.

Pulmonary Failure

Many burned patients require mechanical ventilation to protect the airway in the initial phases of their injury. We recommend that these patients be extubated as soon as possible after the risk is diminished. A trial of extubation is often warranted in the first few days after injury, and reintubation in this setting is not a failure. Performance of this technique safely, however, requires the involvement of experts in obtaining an airway. The goal is extubation as soon as possible to allow patients to clear their own airways because they can perform their own pulmonary toilet better than through an endotracheal tube or tracheostomy. The first sign of impending pulmonary failure is a decline in oxygenation. This is best monitored by continuous oximetry, and a decrease in saturation to less than 92% is indicative of failure. Increasing concentrations of inspired oxygen are necessary, and when ventilation begins to fail, as denoted by an increasing respiratory rate and hypercapnia, intubation is needed.

Some have stated that early tracheostomy (within the first week) might be indicated in those with significant burn who are likely to require long-term ventilation. In one study of severely burned children who underwent early tracheostomy, it was found that peak inspiratory pressure was lower and ventilatory volumes, pulmonary compliance, and PaO_2/FIO_2 ratios were higher.[39] No instances of tracheostomy site infection or tracheal stenosis were identified in the 28 patients studied. Another randomized study comparing severely burned patients who underwent early tracheostomy with those who did not found similar improvements in oxygenation; however, no significant differences could be found in outcome measures such as ventilator days, length of stay, incidence of pneumonia, or survival. In fact, 26% of those not undergoing tracheostomy were successfully extubated within 2 weeks of admission, thus implying that they would not have required tracheostomy at all.[40] It seems that although tracheostomy may be required in some severely burned patients maintained on ventilatory support, the advantages of early tracheostomy do not outweigh the disadvantages. Further data from other centers may change this conclusion in the future.

Hepatic Failure

The development of hepatic failure in burned patients is a challenging problem without many solutions. The liver synthesizes circulating proteins, detoxifies plasma, produces bile, and provides immunologic support. When the liver begins to fail, protein concentrations of the coagulation cascade decrease to critical levels and the patient becomes coagulopathic. Toxins are not cleared from the bloodstream, and concentrations of bilirubin increase. Complete hepatic failure is not compatible with life, but a gradation of liver failure with some decline in function is common. Efforts to prevent hepatic failure are the only effective methods of treatment.

With the development of coagulopathies, treatment is directed at replacement of factors II, VII, IX, and X until the liver recovers. Albumin replacement may also be required. Obstructive causes of hyperbilirubinemia, such as acalculous cholecystitis, need to be considered as well. Initial treatment of this condition is gallbladder drainage, which can be performed percutaneously.

Hematologic Failure

Burned patients may become coagulopathic through two mechanisms:

1. Depletion and impaired synthesis of coagulation factors
2. Thrombocytopenia

Disseminated intravascular coagulation associated with sepsis can result in depletion of coagulation factors. This process is also common with coincident head injury. With breakdown of the blood-brain barrier, brain lipids are exposed to plasma, which activates the coagulation cascade. Varying penetrance of this problem results in differing degrees of coagulopathy. Treatment of disseminated intravascular coagulation includes infusion of fresh frozen plasma and cryoprecipitate to maintain plasma levels of coagulation factors. For disseminated intravascular coagulation induced by brain injury, monitoring the concentration of fibrinogen and repleting levels with cryoprecipitate are the most specific indicators. Impaired synthesis of factors from liver failure is treated as alluded to earlier.

Thrombocytopenia is frequent in severe burns as a result of depletion of platelets during excision of the burn wound. Platelet counts lower than 50,000 are common and do not require treatment. Only when the bleeding is diffuse and is noted to occur from IV sites should administration of exogenous platelets be considered.

Paradoxically, it was found that severely burned patients are also at risk for thrombotic and embolic complications, probably related to immobilization. Complications of deep venous thrombosis were found to be associated with increasing age, weight, and TBSA burned.[41] These data intimate that prophylaxis for deep venous thrombosis would be prudent for adult patients in the absence of bleeding complications.

Central Nervous System Failure

Obtundation is one of the hallmarks of sepsis, and burn patients are no exception. A new onset of mental status changes not attributed to sedative medications in a severely burned patient incites a search for a septic source. Treatment is supportive.

NUTRITION

The response to injury known as *hypermetabolism* occurs dramatically after a severe burn. Increases in oxygen consumption, metabolic rate, urinary nitrogen excretion, lipolysis, and weight loss are directly proportional to the size of the burn. This response can be as high as 200% of the normal metabolic rate and returns to normal only with complete closure of the wound. Because the metabolic rate is so high, energy requirements are immense. These requirements are met by mobilization of carbohydrate, fat, and protein stores. Because the demands are prolonged, these energy stores are quickly depleted, and loss of active muscle tissue and malnutrition ensue. This malnutrition is associated with functional impairment of many organs, delayed and abnormal wound healing, decreased immunocompetence, and altered active transport functions of the cellular membrane. Malnutrition in patients with burns can be subverted to some extent by the delivery of adequate exogenous nutritional support. The goals of nutritional support are to maintain and improve organ function and prevent protein-calorie malnutrition.

Several formulas are used to calculate caloric requirements in burned patients. One formula multiplies the basal energy expenditure determined by the Harris-Benedict formula by 2 in burns greater than 40% TBSA, assuming a 100% increase in total energy expenditure. When total energy expenditure was measured by the doubly labeled water method, actual expenditures were found to be 1.33 times the predicted basal energy expenditure for pediatric patients with burns greater than 40% TBSA.[42] To meet the minimal needs of all the patients in this study, 1.55 times the predicted basal energy expenditure would be required; however, giving caloric loads in excess of this figure probably leads to fat accumulation without affecting lean mass accretion. This correlated to 1.4 times the measured resting energy expenditure by indirect calorimetry. These studies indicate that the calculation of 2 times the predicted basal energy expenditure might be too high.

Other commonly used calculations include the Curreri formula, which calls for 25 kcal/kg/day plus 40 kcal per percent TBSA burned per day. This formula provides for maintenance needs plus the additional caloric needs related to the burn wounds.[43] The Curreri formula was devised as a regression from nitrogen balance data in severely burned adults. In children, formulas based on body surface area are more appropriate because of the greater body surface area per kilogram of weight. We recommend formulas that depend on the child's age, as shown in Table 22-6. These formulas were determined to maintain body weight in severely burned children.[44] The formulas change with age based on the alterations in body surface area that occur with growth.

The composition of the nutritional supplement is also important. The optimal dietary composition contains 1 to 2 g/kg/day of protein, which provides a calorie-to-nitrogen ratio of around 100:1 with the caloric intake suggested earlier. This amount of protein provides for the synthetic needs of the patient, thus to some extent sparing the proteolysis occurring in active muscle tissue. Nonprotein calories can be given either as carbohydrate or as fat. Carbohydrates have the advantage of stimulating endogenous insulin production, which may have beneficial effects on muscle and burn wounds as an anabolic hormone. In addition, it was recently shown that almost all the fat transported in very-low-density lipoprotein after a severe burn is derived from peripheral lipolysis and not from de novo synthesis of fatty acids in the liver from dietary carbohydrates.[45] Consequently, provision of additional fat to deliver noncarbohydrate calories has little support.

The diet may be delivered in two forms: either enterally through enteric tubes or parenterally through IV catheters. Parenteral nutrition may be given in isotonic solutions through peripheral catheters or in hypertonic solutions through central catheters. In general, the caloric demands of burned patients prohibit the use of peripheral parenteral nutrition. Total parenteral nutrition delivered centrally in burned patients has been associated with increased complications and mortality when compared with enteral feeding. Total parenteral nutrition is reserved only for patients who cannot tolerate enteral feeding. Enteral feeding has, however, been associated with some complications that can be disastrous, including mechanical complications, enteral feeding intolerance, and diarrhea.

Recently, interest in nutritional adjunctive treatment with anabolic agents has received attention as a means of decreasing loss of lean mass after severe injury. Agents used include growth hormone, insulin-like growth factor, insulin, oxandrolone,[46] testosterone,[47] and propranolol.[48] Each of these agents has different mechanisms for stimulating protein synthesis through an increase in protein synthetic efficiency. Put simply, the free amino acids available in the cytoplasm from stimulated protein breakdown with severe injury or illness are preferentially shunted toward protein synthesis rather than export out of the cell (Fig. 22-12). Some of these agents, such as insulin and oxandrolone, have shown efficacy not only in improving protein kinetics but also in improving lean mass after a severe burn. Further research will reveal whether these biochemical and physiologic measures translate to improved function.

Table 22-6   Formulas to Predict Caloric Needs in Severely Burned Children

AGE GROUP	MAINTENANCE NEEDS	BURN WOUND NEEDS
Infants (0-12 mo)	2100 kcal/% TBSA burned/ 24 hr	1000 kcal/% TBSA burned/ 24 hr
Children (1-12 yr)	1800 kcal/% TBSA burned/ 24 hr	1300 kcal/% TBSA burned/ 24 hr
Adolescents (12-18 yr)	1500 kcal/% TBSA burned/ 24 hr	1500 kcal/% TBSA burned/ 24 hr

TBSA, total body surface area.

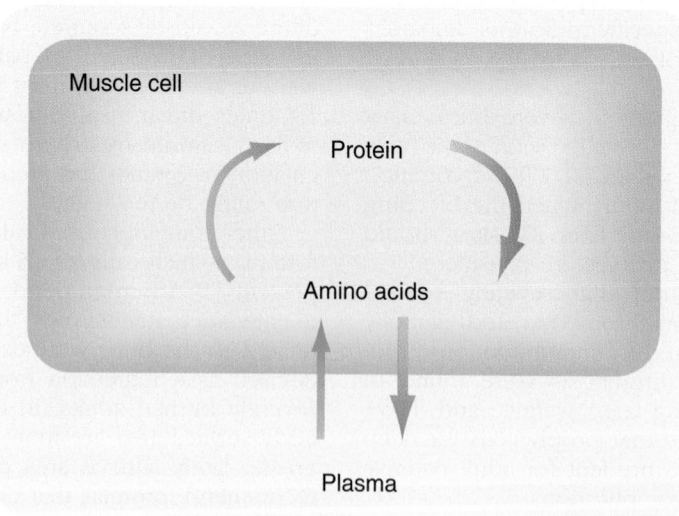

Figure 22-12 Amino acids from stimulated protein breakdown in the neurocele cell are routed out of the cell to provide substrate for recovery. Anabolic agents attenuate this action by directing these amino acids back into protein synthesis.

OUTCOMES

Many of the burn treatments are directed at improving functional, psychological, and work outcomes, which are only now being systematically studied. Authors are currently reporting new methods to evaluate outcomes through burn-specific health scales[49] and measures of adjustment. Authors have found that severely burned adult patients adjust relatively well, although clinically significant psychological disturbances develop in some patients, such as somatization and phobic anxiety. Children with severe burns were found to have similar somatization problems, as well as sleep disturbances, but in general they were well adjusted. Time off work in adult patients was found to be associated with increasing percent TBSA burned, a psychiatric history, and extremity burns with considerable job disruption.[50] These data intimate that major burns can lead to significant disturbances in psychiatric health and outcomes, but in general, these problems can be overcome.

ELECTRICAL BURNS

Initial Treatment

Three percent to 5% of all burned patients admitted are injured by contact with electricity. Electrical injury is unlike other burn injuries in that the visible areas of tissue necrosis represent only a small portion of the destroyed tissue. Electrical current enters a part of the body, such as the fingers or hand, and proceeds through tissues with the lowest resistance to current, generally the nerves, blood vessels, and muscles. The skin has relatively high resistance to electrical current and is therefore mostly spared. The current then leaves the body at a grounded area, typically the foot. Heat generated by the transfer of electrical current and passage of the current itself then injures the tissues. During this exchange, the muscle is the major tissue through which the current flows, and thus it sustains the most damage. Most muscle is in close proximity to bones. Blood vessels transmitting much of the electricity initially remain patent, but they may proceed to progressive thrombosis as the cells either die or repair themselves, thus resulting in further tissue loss from ischemia.

Injuries are divided into high- and low-voltage injuries. Low-voltage injury is similar to thermal burns without transmission to deeper tissues; zones of injury extend from the surface into the tissue. Most household current (110-220 V) produces this type of injury, which causes only local damage. The worst of these injuries are those involving the edge of the mouth (oral commissure), which are sustained when children gnaw on household electrical cords.

The syndrome of high-voltage injury consists of varying degrees of cutaneous burn at the entry and exit sites, combined with hidden destruction of deep tissue. Frequently, these patients also have cutaneous burns associated with ignition of clothing from the discharge of electrical current. Initial evaluation consists of cardiopulmonary resuscitation if ventricular fibrillation is induced. Thereafter, if the initial electrocardiographic findings are abnormal or there is a history of cardiac arrest associated with the injury, continued cardiac monitoring is necessary along with pharmacologic treatment of any arrhythmias. The most serious derangements occur in the first 24 hours after injury. If patients with electrical injuries have no cardiac arrhythmias on initial electrocardiography or no recent history of cardiac arrest, no further monitoring is necessary.

Patients with electrical injuries are at risk for other injuries, such as being thrown by the electrical jolt or falling from heights after disengaging from the electrical current. In addition, the violent tetanic muscular contractions that result from alternating current sources may cause a variety of fractures and dislocations. These patients are assessed as any other patient with blunt traumatic injuries.

The key to managing patients with an electrical injury lies in treatment of the wound. The most significant injury is within the deep tissue, and subsequent edema formation can cause vascular compromise in any area distal to the injury. Assessment includes evaluation of the circulation to distal vascular beds because immediate escharotomy and fasciotomy may be required. If the muscle compartment is extensively injured and necrotic such that the prospects for eventual function are dismal, early amputation may be necessary. We advocate early exploration of affected muscle beds and débridement of devitalized tissues, with attention directed to the deeper periosteous planes because this is the area with the most muscle tissue. Fasciotomies must be complete and may require nerve decompression, such as carpal tunnel and Guyon canal release. Tissue that has questionable viability is left in place, with planned re-exploration in 48 hours. Many such re-explorations may be required until the wound is completely débrided. Electrical damage to vessels may be delayed, and the extent of necrosis may increase after the initial débridement. After the devitalized tissues are removed, closure of the wound becomes paramount. Although skin grafts suffice as closure for most wounds, flaps may offer a better alternative, particularly with exposed bones and tendons. Even exposed and superficially infected bones and tendons can be salvaged with coverage by vascularized tissue. Early involvement by reconstructive surgeons versed in the various methods of wound closure is optimal.

Muscle damage results in the release of hemochromogens (myoglobin), which are filtered in the glomeruli and may result in obstructive nephropathy. Therefore, vigorous hydration and infusion of IV sodium bicarbonate (5% continuous infusion) and mannitol (25 g every 6 hours for adults) are indicated to solubilize the hemochromogens and maintain urine output if significant amounts are found in serum. These patients also require additional IV volumes over predicted amounts based on the wound area because most of the wound is deep and cannot be assessed by standard physical examination. In this situation, urine output is maintained at 2 mL/kg/hr.

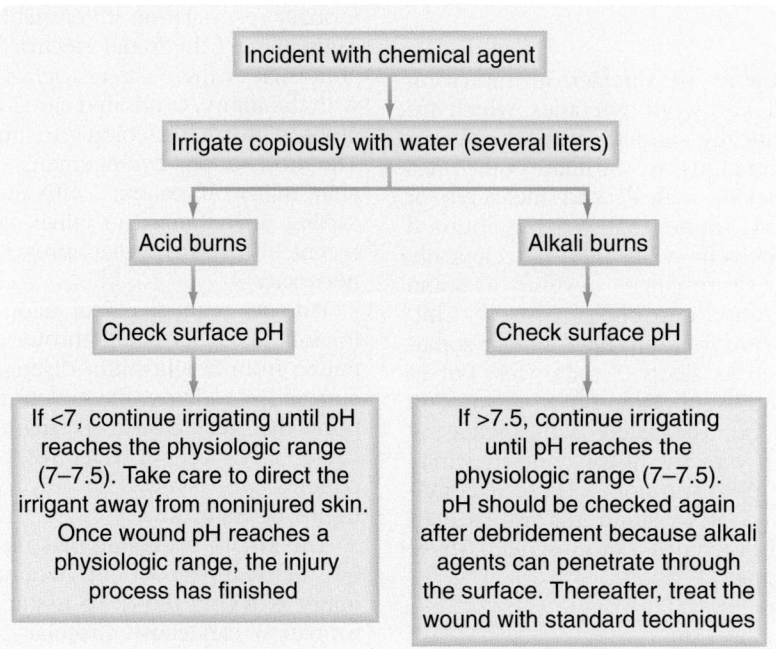

Figure 22-13 Treatment of acid and alkali burns.

Delayed Effects

Neurologic deficits may occur. Serial neurologic evaluations are performed as part of the routine examination to detect any early or late neuropathology. Central nervous system effects such as cortical encephalopathy, hemiplegia, aphasia, and brainstem dysfunction have been reported up to 9 months after injury; others report delayed peripheral nerve lesions characterized by demyelination with vacuolization and reactive gliosis. Another devastating long-term effect is the development of cataracts, which can be delayed for several years. These complications may occur in up to 30% of patients with significant high-voltage injury, and patients are made aware of their possibility even with the best treatment.

CHEMICAL BURNS

Most chemical burns are accidental and result from mishandling of household cleaners, although some of the most dramatic manifestations involve industrial exposure. Thermal burns are, in general, caused by short-term exposure to heat, but chemical injuries may be of longer duration, even for hours in the absence of appropriate treatment. The degree of tissue damage, as well as the level of toxicity, is determined by the chemical nature of the agent, the concentration of the agent, and the duration of skin contact. Chemicals cause their injury by protein destruction, with denaturation, oxidation, formation of protein esters, or desiccation of the tissue. In the United States, the composition of most household and industrial chemicals can be obtained from the poison control center in the area, which can give suggestions for treatment.

Speed is essential in the management of chemical burns. For all chemicals, lavage with copious quantities of clean water needs to be performed immediately after removing all clothing. Dry powders must be brushed from the affected areas before irrigation. Early irrigation dilutes the chemical, which is already in contact with the skin, and timeliness increases effectiveness. Several liters of irrigant may be required. For example, 10 mL of 98% sulfuric acid dissolved in 12 L of water decreases the pH to 5.0, a range that can still cause injury. If the chemical composition is known (acid or base), monitoring of the pH of the spent lavage solution gives a good indication of lavage effectiveness and completion. A good rule of thumb is to lavage with 15 to 20 L of tap water or more for significant chemical injuries. The lavage site is kept drained to remove the earlier, more concentrated effluent. Care is taken to direct the drainage away from uninjured areas to avoid further exposure.

All patients must be monitored according to the severity of their injuries. They may have metabolic disturbances, usually from pH abnormalities because of exposure to strong acids or caustics. If any respiratory difficulty is apparent, oxygen therapy and mechanical ventilation must be instituted. Resuscitation is guided by the body surface area involved (burn formulas); however, the total fluid needs may be dramatically different from the calculated volumes. Some of these injuries may be more superficial than they appear, particularly in the case of acids, and therefore require less resuscitation volume. Injuries from bases, however, may penetrate beyond what is apparent on examination and therefore require more volume. For this reason, patients with chemical injuries are observed closely for signs of adequate perfusion, such as urine output. All patients with significant chemical injuries are monitored with indwelling bladder catheters to accurately measure output.

Operative débridement, if indicated, takes place as soon as a patient is stable and resuscitated (Fig. 22-13). After adequate lavage and débridement, burn wounds are covered with antimicrobial agents or skin substitutes. Once the wounds have stabilized with the indicated treatment, they are taken care of similar to any loss of soft tissue. Skin grafting or flap coverage is performed as needed.

Alkali

Alkalis, such as lime, potassium hydroxide, bleach, and sodium hydroxide, are among the most common agents involved in chemical injury. Accidental injury frequently occurs in infants and toddlers exploring cleaning cabinets. Three factors are involved in the mechanism of alkali burns:

1. Saponification of fat causes loss of the insulation of heat formed in the chemical reaction with tissue
2. Massive extraction of water from cells causes damage because of the hygroscopic nature of alkali
3. Alkalis dissolve and unite with the proteins of tissues to form alkaline proteinates, which are soluble and contain hydroxide ions (these ions induce further chemical reactions that penetrate deeper into the tissue)

Treatment involves immediate removal of the causative agent with lavage of large volumes of fluid, usually water. Attempts to neutralize alkali agents with weak acids are not recommended because the heat released by neutralization reactions induces further injury. Particularly strong bases are treated by lavage and consideration of the addition of wound débridement in the operating room. Tangential removal of affected areas is performed until the tissues removed are at normal pH.

Cement (calcium oxide) burns are alkali in nature, occur commonly, and are usually work-related injuries. The critical substance responsible for the skin damage is the hydroxyl ion. Often, the agent has been in contact with the skin for prolonged periods, such as underneath the boots of a cement worker who seeks treatment hours after the exposure or after the cement penetrates clothing and, when combined with perspiration, induces an exothermic reaction. Treatment consists of removing all clothing and irrigating the affected area with water and soap until all the cement is removed and the effluent has a pH of less than 8. Injuries tend to be deep because of exposure times, and surgical excision and grafting of the resultant eschar may be required.

Acid

Acid injuries are treated initially like any other chemical injury: removal of all chemicals by disrobing the affected area and copious irrigation. Acids induce protein breakdown by hydrolysis, which results in a hard eschar that does not penetrate as deeply as alkalis do. These agents also induce thermal injury by generation of heat after contact with skin, thus causing additional soft tissue damage. Some acids have added effects, which are discussed here.

Formic acid injuries are relatively rare and usually involve an organic acid used for industrial descaling and as a hay preservative. Electrolyte abnormalities are of great concern in patients who have sustained extensive formic acid injuries, with metabolic acidosis, renal failure, intravascular hemolysis, and pulmonary complications (acute respiratory distress syndrome) being common. Acidemia detected by the presence of metabolic acidosis on arterial blood gas analysis is corrected with IV sodium bicarbonate. Hemodialysis may be required when extensive absorption of formic acid has occurred. Mannitol diuresis is required if severe hemolysis occurs after deep injury. A formic acid wound typically has a greenish appearance and is deeper than it initially appears to be; it is best treated by surgical excision.

Hydrofluoric acid is a toxic substance used widely in both industrial and domestic settings and is the strongest inorganic acid known. Such burns are managed differently from other acid burns in general. Hydrofluoric acid produces dehydration and corrosion of tissue by free hydrogen ions. In addition, the fluoride ion complexes with bivalent cations such as calcium and magnesium to form insoluble salts. Systemic absorption of the fluoride ion can then induce intravascular calcium chelation and hypocalcemia, which causes life-threatening arrhythmias. Beyond initial copious irrigation with clean water, the burned area is treated immediately with copious 2.5% calcium gluconate gel. These wounds are generally extremely painful because of the calcium chelation and associated potassium release. This finding can be used to determine the effectiveness of treatment. The gel is changed at 15-minute intervals until the pain subsides, an indication of removal of the active fluoride ion. If pain relief is incomplete after several applications or if symptoms recur, intradermal injection of 10% calcium gluconate ($0.5\ mL/cm^2$ affected), intra-arterial injection of calcium gluconate into the affected extremity, or both may be required to alleviate symptoms. If the burn is not treated in such a fashion, decalcification of the bone underlying the injury and extension of the soft tissue injury may occur.

All patients with hydrofluoric acid burns are admitted for cardiac monitoring, with particular attention paid to prolongation of the QT interval. A total of 20 mL of a 10% calcium gluconate solution is added to the first liter of resuscitation fluid, and serum electrolytes must be closely monitored. Any electrocardiographic changes require a rapid response consisting of IV administration of calcium chloride to maintain heart function. Several grams of calcium may be required in the end until the chemical response has run its course. Serum magnesium and potassium are also closely monitored and replaced. Speed is the key to effective treatment.

Hydrocarbons

The organic solvent properties of hydrocarbons promote cell membrane dissolution and skin necrosis. Symptoms include erythema and blistering, and the burns are typically superficial and heal spontaneously. If absorbed systemically, toxicity can produce respiratory depression and eventual hepatic injury thought to be associated with benzenes. Ignition of hydrocarbons on the skin induces a deep full-thickness injury.

SUMMARY

Treatment of burns is complex. Minor injuries can be treated in the community by knowledgeable physicians. Moderate and severe injuries, however, require treatment in dedicated facilities with resources to maximize outcomes from these often devastating events. The care of burned patients has markedly improved such that most patients survive even with massive injuries. Challenges for the future will be in the areas of scar modulation and acceleration of the healing time to result in functional and visually appealing outcomes in a prompt fashion.

Selected References

Baxter CR: Fluid volume and electrolyte changes in the early post-burn period. Clin Plast Surg 1:693-703, 1974.

This is the classic article describing development and use of the Parkland formula for resuscitation of burned patients.

Bull JP, Fisher AJ: A study in mortality in a burn unit: Standards for the evaluation for alternative methods of treatment. Ann Surg 130:160-173, 1949.

Bull and Fisher first described the incidence of burn mortality in this classic article. Mortality has significantly improved since these statistics.

Cioffi WG, DeMeules JE, Gamelli RL: The effects of burn injury and fluid resuscitation on cardiac function in vitro. J Trauma 26:638-645, 1986.

This paper describes the effect of severe burn on cardiac dynamics and explains the effects that we see on hemodynamics early in resuscitation.

Curreri PW: Nutritional support of burn patients. World J Surg 2:215-222, 1978.

This was the seminal manuscript describing the Curreri formula, which is still used in many burn units for the prescription of nutritional needs after severe burn.

Herndon DN, Parks DH: Comparison of serial débridement and autografting and early massive excision with cadaver skin overlay in the treatment of large burns in children. J Trauma 26:149-152, 1986.

This paper describes the use and superiority of early wound excision over serial débridement, a practice that is almost uniformly followed now in the treatment of severe burns.

Mozingo D, Smith A, McManus W, et al: Chemical burns. J Trauma 28:642-647, 1988.

This article describes the evaluation and modern treatment of chemical burns.

Wolf SE, Rose JK, Desai MH, et al: Mortality determinants in massive pediatric burns: An analysis of 103 children with ≥80% TBSA burns (≥70% full-thickness). Ann Surg 225:554-569, 1997.

Mortality in massive pediatric burns is described in this paper, with a formula devised to predict the children with massive burns who will survive and who will die. Treatment of massively burned children is also described.

References

1. McGwin G Jr, Cross JM, Ford JW, et al: Long-term trends in mortality according to age among adult burn patients. J Burn Care Rehabil 24:21-25, 2003.
2. Ahuja RB, Bhattacharya S: Burns in the developing world and burn disasters. BMJ 329:447-449, 2004.
3. Bull JP, Fisher AJ: A study in mortality in a burn unit: Standards for the evaluation for alternative methods of treatment. Ann Surg 130:160-173, 1949.
4. Rashid A, Khanna A, Gowar JP, et al: Revised estimates of mortality from burns in the last 20 years at the Birmingham Burns Centre. Burns 27:723-730, 2001.
5. Wolf SE, Rose JK, Desai MH, et al: Mortality determinants in massive pediatric burns: An analysis of 103 children with ≥80% TBSA burns (≥70% full-thickness). Ann Surg 225:554-569, 1997.
6. Holland AJ, Martin HC, Cass DT: Laser Doppler imaging prediction of burn wound outcome in children. Burns 28:11-17, 2002.
7. Pruitt BA Jr, Mason AD Jr, Moncrief JA: Hemodynamic changes in the early postburn patient: The influence of fluid administration and of a vasodilator (hydralazine). J Trauma 11:36-46, 1971.
8. Chrysopoulo MT, Jeschke MG, Dziewulski P, et al: Acute renal dysfunction in severely burned adults. J Trauma 46:141-144, 1999.
9. Gianotti L, Alexander JW, Fukushima R, et al: Translocation of *Candida albicans* is related to the blood flow of individual intestinal villi. Circ Shock 40:250-257, 1993.
10. Moore FD: Bodily changes during surgical convalescence. Ann Surg 137:289-295, 1953.
11. Herndon, DN, Hart DW, Wolf SE, et al: Reversal of catabolism by beta-blockade after severe burns. N Engl J Med 345:1223-1229, 2001.
12. Herndon DN, Tompkins RG: Support of the metabolic response to burn injury. Lancet 363:1895-1902, 2004.
13. Skinner A, Peat B: Burns treatment for children and adults: A study of initial burns first aid and hospital care. N Z Med J 115:U199, 2002.
14. Baxter CR: Fluid volume and electrolyte changes of the early postburn period. Clin Plast Surg 1:693-703, 1974.
15. Gunn ML, Hansbrough JF, Davis JW, et al: Prospective, randomized trial of hypertonic sodium lactate versus lactated Ringer's solution for burn shock resuscitation. J Trauma 29:1261-1267, 1989.
16. Huang PP, Stucky FS, Dimick AR, et al: Hypertonic sodium resuscitation is associated with renal failure and death. Ann Surg 221:543-557, 1995.
17. Pruitt BA Jr: Protection from excessive resuscitation: Pushing the pendulum back. J Trauma 49:567-568, 2000.
18. Sullivan SR, Friedrich JB, Engrav LH, et al: "Opioid creep" is real and may be the cause of "fluid creep." Burns 30:583-590, 2004.

19. Sullivan SR, Ahmadi AJ, Singh CN, et al: Elevated orbital pressure: Another untoward effect of massive resuscitation after burn injury. J Trauma 60:72-76, 2006.

20. Hobson KG, Young KM, Ciraulo A, et al: Release of abdominal compartment syndrome improves survival in patients with burn injury. J Trauma 53:1129-1134, 2002.

21. Alderson P, Bunn F, Lefebvre C, et al: Human albumin solution for resuscitation and volume expansion in critically ill patients. Cochrane Database Syst Rev 4:CD001208, 2002.

22. Wilkes MM, Navickis RJ: Patient survival after human albumin administration: A meta-analysis of randomized, controlled trials. Ann Intern Med 135:149-164, 2001.

23. Zdolsek HJ, Lisander B, Jones AW, et al: Albumin supplementation during the first week after a burn does not mobilize tissue oedema in humans. Intensive Care Med 27:844-852, 2001.

24. Ventilation with lower tidal volumes as compared with traditional tidal volumes for acute lung injury and the acute respiratory distress syndrome. The Acute Respiratory Distress Syndrome Network. N Engl J Med 342:1301-1308, 2000.

25. Lukish JR, Eichelberger MR, Newman KD, et al: The use of a bioactive skin substitute decreases length of stay for pediatric burn patients. J Pediatr Surg 36:1118-1121, 2001.

26. Heimbach DM, Warden GD, Luterman A, et al: Multicenter postapproval clinical trial of Integra dermal regeneration template for burn treatment. J Burn Care Rehabil 24:42-48, 2003.

27. Dantzer E, Braye FM: Reconstructive surgery using an artificial dermis (Integra): Results with 39 grafts. Br J Plast Surg 54:659-664, 2001.

28. Herndon DN, Parks DH: Comparison of serial débridement and autografting and early massive excision with cadaver skin overlay in the treatment of large burns in children. J Trauma 26:149-152, 1986.

29. Desai MH, Rutan RL, Herndon DN: Conservative treatment of scald burns is superior to early excision. J Burn Care Rehabil 12:482-484, 1991.

30. Barret JP, Wolf SE, Desai MH, et al: Cost-efficacy of cultured epidermal autografts in massive pediatric burns. Ann Surg 231:869-876, 2000.

31. Pierre EJ, Barrow RE, Hawkins HK, et al: Effects of insulin on wound healing. J Trauma 44:342-345, 1998.

32. Zhang XJ, Chinkes DL, Irtun O, et al: Anabolic action of insulin on skin wound protein is augmented by exogenous amino acids. Am J Physiol Endocrinol Metab 282:E1308-E1315, 2002.

33. Mann R, Gibran NS, Engrav LH, et al: Prospective trial of thick versus standard split-thickness skin grafts in burns of the hand. J Burn Care Rehabil 22:390-392, 2001.

34. Scherer LA, Shiver S, Chang M, et al: The vacuum-assisted closure device: A method of securing skin grafts and improving graft survival. Arch Surg 137:930-934, 2002.

35. Muckart DJ, Bhagwanjee S: American College of Chest Physicians/Society of Critical Care Medicine Consensus Conference definitions of the systemic inflammatory response syndrome and allied disorders in relation to critically injured patients. Crit Care Med 25:1789-1795, 1997.

36. Van den Berghe G, Wouters P, Weekers F, et al: Intensive insulin therapy in critically ill patients. N Engl J Med 345:1359-1367, 2001.

37. Pham TN, Warren AJ, Phan HH, et al: Impact of tight glycemic control in severely burned children. J Trauma 59:1148-1154, 2005.

38. Cumming J, Purdue GF, Hunt JL, et al: Objective estimates of the incidence and consequences of multiple organ dysfunction and sepsis after burn trauma. J Trauma 50:510-515, 2001.

39. Palmieri TL, Jackson W, Greenhalgh DG: Benefits of early tracheostomy in severely burned children. Crit Care Med 30:922-924, 2002.

40. Saffle JR, Morris SE, Edelman L: Early tracheostomy does not improve outcome in burn patients. J Burn Care Rehabil 23:431-438, 2002.

41. Harrington DT, Mozingo DW, Cancio L, et al: Thermally injured patients are at significant risk for thromboembolic complications. J Trauma 50:495-499, 2001.

42. Goran MI, Peters EJ, Herndon DN, et al: Total energy expenditure in burned children using the doubly labeled water technique. Am J Physiol 259:E576-E585, 1990.

43. Curreri PW: Nutritional support of burn patients. World J Surg 2:215-222, 1978.

44. Hildreth MA, Herndon DN, Desai MH, et al: Current treatment reduces calories required to maintain weight in pediatric patients with burns. J Burn Care Rehabil 11:405-409, 1990.

45. Aarsland A, Chinkes D, Wolfe RR, et al: Beta-blockade lowers peripheral lipolysis in burn patients receiving growth hormone: Rate of hepatic very low-density lipoprotein triglyceride secretion remains unchanged. Ann Surg 223:777-789, 1996.

46. Hart DW, Wolf SE, Ramzy PI, et al: Anabolic effects of oxandrolone after severe burn. Ann Surg 233:556-564, 2001.

47. Ferrando AA, Sheffield-Moore M, Wolf SE, et al: Testosterone administration in severe burns ameliorates muscle catabolism. Crit Care Med 29:1936-1942, 2001.

48. Herndon DN, Hart DW, Wolf SE, et al: Reversal of catabolism by beta-blockade after severe burns. N Engl J Med 345:1223-1229, 2001.

49. Kildal M, Andersson G, Fugl-Meyer AR, et al: Development of a brief version of the Burn Specific Health Scale (BSHS-B). J Trauma 51:740-746, 2001.

50. Brych SB, Engrav LH, Rivara FP, et al: Time off work and return to work rates after burns: Systematic review of the literature and a large two-center series. J Burn Care Rehabil 22:401-405, 2001.

Bites and Stings

Robert L. Norris, MD   Paul S. Auerbach, MD, MS   and   Elaine E. Nelson, MD

Snakebites
Mammalian Bites
Arthropod Bites and Stings
Marine Bites and Stings

SNAKEBITES

Epidemiology

An estimated 50,000 to 100,000 individuals worldwide die each year of venomous snakebites. Those at greatest risk include agricultural workers and hunters living in tropical countries.[1] In the United States, approximately 8000 bites by venomous snakes occur each year,[2] with around six deaths.[3] Venomous species indigenous to the United States can be found in all states except Alaska, Maine, and Hawaii. The typical victim is a young male, often intoxicated, and bitten on an extremity. Lower extremity bites tend to result from stepping near a snake, whereas purposeful handling of a snake is more likely to produce a bite on the upper extremity. Snakes are poikilothermic, which accounts for the higher incidence of bites during warmer months.[2]

Species

In the United States, snakes of the subfamily Crotalinae (pit vipers), which includes the rattlesnakes (Fig. 23-1), copperheads, and cottonmouths, are responsible for 99% of medically significant bites. Only 1% of bites are attributable to the other family of venomous snakes indigenous to the United States, the Elapidae (coral snakes).[4]

Several characteristics distinguish pit vipers from non-venomous snakes. Pit vipers tend to have relatively tri-angular heads, elliptical pupils, heat-sensing facial pits, large retractable anterior fangs, and a single row of sub-caudal scales. Nonvenomous snakes often have more rounded heads, circular pupils, no fangs, and a double row of subcaudal scales (Fig. 23-2). Coral snakes possess a red, black, and yellow-banded pattern. In the United States, the alignment of red bands next to yellow reliably differentiates coral snakes from nonvenomous mimics. There are three species of coral snakes in the United States—the eastern and Texas coral snakes (*Micrurus fulvius* and *Micrurus tener,* respectively) and the Sonoran or Arizona coral snake *(Micruroides euryxanthus).*

Toxicology

Snake venoms are complex and possess many peptides and enzymes. Peptides can damage vascular endothelium, thereby increasing permeability and leading to edema and hypovolemic shock. Enzymes include proteases and L-amino acid oxidase, which cause tissue necrosis; hyaluronidase, which facilitates the spread of venom through tissues; and phospholipase A_2, which damages erythrocytes and muscle cells. Other enzymes include endonucleases, alkaline phosphatase, acid phosphatase, and cholinesterase.[4,5] Besides causing local injury, these components also have deleterious effects on the cardiovascular, pulmonary, renal, and neurologic systems.[6] Other components of the venom profoundly affect coagulation, fibrinolysis, platelet function, and vascular integrity, sometimes producing hemorrhagic or thrombotic sequelae.[7]

Clinical Manifestations

Local

Approximately 20% of bites by pit vipers lack any venom injection ("dry bites").[8] The only findings in such cases are puncture wounds or lacerations and minimal pain.

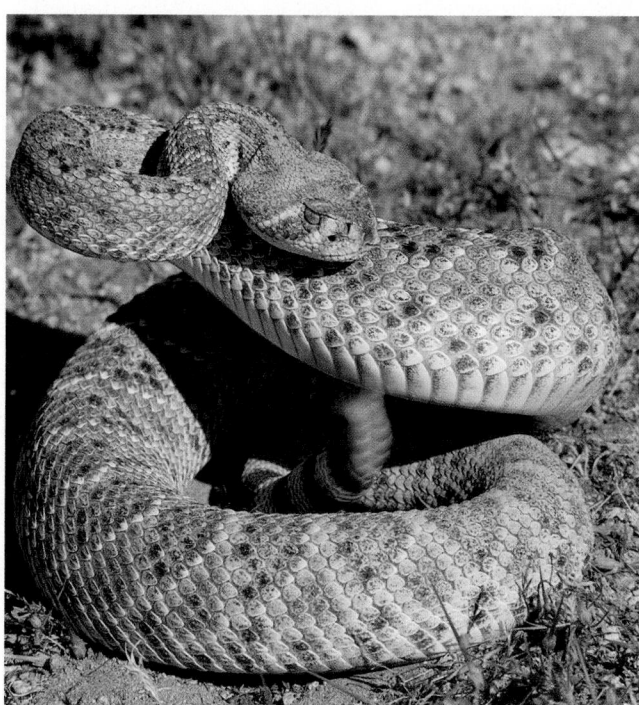

Figure 23-1 A typical North American pit viper—the western diamondback rattlesnake, *Crotalus atrox*. (Courtesy of Michael Cardwell.)

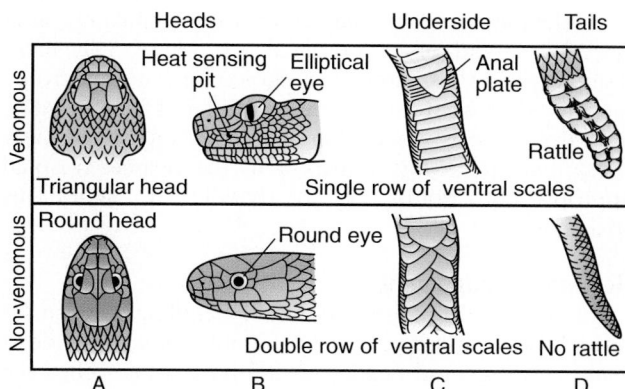

Figure 23-2 Comparison of pit vipers and nonvenomous snakes. The rattle *(D, top panel)* applies to rattlesnakes only. (From Sullivan JB, Wingert WA, Norris RL: North American venomous reptile bites. In Auerbach PS [ed]: Wilderness Medicine: Management of Wilderness and Environmental Emergencies, 3rd ed. St Louis, Mosby–Year Book, 1995, p 684.)

Actual envenomation produces burning pain within minutes, followed by edema and erythema. Swelling progresses over the next few hours, and ecchymoses and hemorrhagic bullae may appear (Fig. 23-3). Involvement of the lymphatic system is common and heralded by lymphangitis and lymphadenopathy.[4,6] With delayed or inadequate treatment, severe tissue necrosis can occur.

Systemic

Patients may complain of weakness, nausea, vomiting, perioral paresthesias, a metallic taste, and muscle twitching.[6,9] Diffuse capillary leakage leads to pulmonary edema, hypotension, and eventually, shock. In victims of severe bites, a consumptive coagulopathy can develop within an hour.[7] Such patients can spontaneously bleed from almost any anatomic site, although clinically significant bleeding is uncommon, even in the face of significantly abnormal coagulation test results. Multifactorial acute renal failure resulting from direct nephrotoxins, circulatory collapse, myoglobinuria, and consumptive coagulopathy is possible. Laboratory abnormalities may include hypofibrinogenemia, thrombocytopenia, prolonged prothrombin and partial thromboplastin times, increased fibrin split products, elevated creatinine and creatine phosphokinase, proteinuria, hematuria, and anemia or hemoconcentration.[7,9]

Unlike pit viper venoms, which tend to affect multiple organ systems, coral snake venom is primarily neurotoxic. Local injury is generally minimal or absent. Systemic signs of coral snake bites, including cranial nerve dysfunction and loss of deep tendon reflexes, may pro-

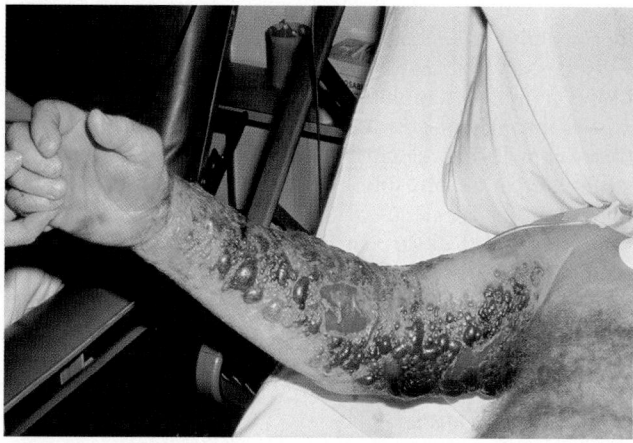

Figure 23-3 A case of severe envenomation by a western diamondback rattlesnake *(Crotalus atrox)* 4 days after the bite. Note the soft tissue swelling and hemorrhagic and serum-filled vesicles. (Courtesy of David Hardy, MD.)

gress to respiratory depression and paralysis over a period of several hours.[4] Differences in therapy make it important to distinguish between coral snake and pit viper bites.

Management

Field Treatment

The patient is removed from the vicinity of the snake and placed at rest. The wound is cleansed and immobilized at approximately heart level, if possible. Cryotherapy, suction, tourniquets, and electric shock therapy are harmful and must be avoided. Most pit viper bites in the United States pose more of a threat to local tissues than to the life of the victim, and the use of any method to restrict venom to the bite site may be ill advised. The Australian pressure immobilization technique, in which the entire bitten extremity is snugly wrapped with a bandage, beginning at the bite site, and splinted, has been demonstrated in small studies to significantly limit systemic spread of various snake venoms.[3] This technique is the field treatment of choice for a non-necrotizing bite such as from a coral snake,[10] but it may make the local necrosis worse after a pit viper bite. Field measures must not delay transport to the nearest hospital appropriately equipped to handle a venomous snakebite.

Hospital Management

Caution must be exercised when handling any snake brought in with the patient for identification. Even dead snakes and severed heads can still have a bite reflex for up to an hour.

A rapid, detailed history of the incident, type of snake, field management, and previous antivenom exposure is important. Physical assessment emphasizes vital signs, cardiopulmonary status, neurologic examination, and wound appearance and size. The bitten extremity is marked at two or three locations so that circumferences can be measured every 15 minutes to judge the progression of local findings. Such measurements continue until the swelling has clearly stabilized.

Necessary laboratory analyses include a complete blood count, coagulation studies (prothrombin time, partial thromboplastin time, fibrin degradation products, fibrinogen level), electrolytes, blood urea nitrogen, creatinine, creatine phosphokinase, and urinalysis. No laboratory studies are necessary for a coral snake bite. A chest radiograph and electrocardiogram are obtained in older patients and anyone with severe poisoning.

If the patient is completely asymptomatic 6 hours after a pit viper bite or 24 hours after a coral snake bite and all laboratory results are normal, it is unlikely that envenomation occurred, and discharge is acceptable. All envenomed patients are best observed for at least 24 hours in the hospital.

Antivenom Therapy

Deciding when to administer antivenom to a victim of a venomous snakebite requires significant clinical judgment, and consultation with a toxicologist or an envenomation specialist is prudent. The treating physician must quickly weigh the potential benefits of giving heterologous antiserum to the victim in an effort to halt the progression of envenomation against the risks inherent in the administration of such a product—anaphylactoid reaction or serum sickness. Furthermore, because snake envenomation is a dynamic process, the decision for or against antivenom must be re-evaluated as the syndrome declares its severity over time. Currently, antivenom is administered to any patient with evidence of envenomation and clear progression in severity after arrival at the hospital or without delay in any patient with clearly serious poisoning (e.g., severe swelling, hypotension, respiratory distress).

In the United States there are currently two pit viper antivenoms commercially available. Antivenom (Crotalidae) polyvalent (ACP) (Wyeth-Ayerst Laboratories, Philadelphia) has been available for more than 50 years. It can be administered as per the package insert. In 2000, the

U.S. Food and Drug Administration (FDA) approved a second pit viper antivenom for use in this country, CroFab (Protherics, Inc., London). This product, produced in sheep and purified by Fab technology, appears to be more effective and safer to use than ACP (see later).[11-13] Unlike ACP, no skin testing is recommended, and no pretreatment in an effort to reduce the risk for acute adverse reaction to the product is needed with CroFab.

CroFab is given intravenously (IV) as four to six vials in 250 mL of diluent over a period of approximately 1 hour. If, after the initial dose, the severity of venom toxicity progresses over the next hour, the loading dose is repeated. This sequence is repeated as needed until the victim has stabilized. After stabilization, to prevent recurrence of the effects of the venom, two vials of CroFab are administered IV every 6 hours for three additional doses.[13] The same dosing regimen is used for children, and pregnancy is not a contraindication to antivenom therapy. ACP is administered as per the accompanying package insert, although the manufacturer-recommended skin test for possible allergy is unreliable and should be omitted.

A separate antivenom, North American Coral Snake Antivenin, also produced by Wyeth-Ayerst, is available for eastern and Texas coral snake bites. Administration is similar to that for ACP, except that therapy is initiated in all cases in which a positively identified coral snake bite has occurred—even in the absence of local or systemic symptoms because such symptoms may be delayed many hours in onset. Once established, envenomation can be hard to reverse, even with the use of antivenom. There is no antivenom produced to treat Sonoran coral snake bites, but there have been no reported fatalities after bites by this small animal. Any currently available snakebite antivenom carries some risk for acute anaphylactoid reaction and delayed serum sickness. Informed consent is obtained for its use whenever possible, and epinephrine always must be immediately available during administration. Patients must also be warned of the symptoms of serum sickness before discharge from the hospital. Serum sickness is generally easily treated with steroids and antihistamines.

Poison control centers and zoos can provide important information regarding procurement of antivenom and management of the occasional exotic snakebite that occurs in the United States in zookeepers or private hobbyists. The University of Arizona Poison and Drug Information Center (telephone, 520-626-6016) is a useful source of information for physicians needing help in managing venomous snakebites.

Wound Care/Blood Products

The bite site is cleansed thoroughly and the extremity splinted and elevated. Good conservative wound care is indicated, with surgical débridement of clearly necrotic tissue performed as necessary after any coagulopathy has resolved. Tetanus toxoid and tetanus immune globulin are administered as needed according to the patient's immunization history. Prophylactic antibiotics are reserved for cases in which misdirected first aid included incisions into the bite site or mouth suction. Otherwise, antibiotics

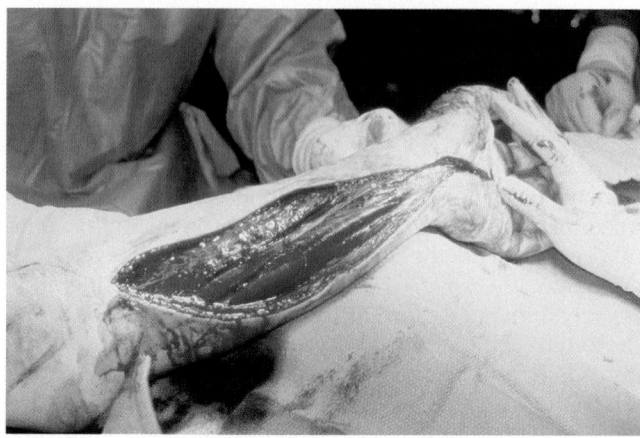

Figure 23-4 Fasciotomy of the forearm compartments in a victim of a severe rattlesnake bite on the hand. Intracompartmental pressures were documented to be exceedingly elevated in this patient despite limb elevation and large doses of antivenom. (Courtesy of Robert Norris, MD.)

are needed solely for the rare wound in which secondary infection develops.[14,15]

Blood products are needed only in the rare setting of clinically significant bleeding that is not reversed with antivenom. Patients with serious bleeding (e.g., gastrointestinal bleeding, intracranial bleeding, hemoptysis) may need packed red cells, platelets, fresh frozen plasma, or cryoprecipitate, depending on the scenario and the results of serial complete blood counts and coagulation studies. Antivenom must be started before these second-line agents are infused, however.[16] Patients in whom coagulopathy has developed while in the hospital after a pit viper bite must be warned that coagulation abnormalities can recur for up to 2 weeks after the bite, even after antivenom therapy.[17] They need to be advised to look for signs of bleeding and to avoid any elective surgery or activities with an inherent high risk of injury during this period.

Fasciotomy
Most snakebites result in subcutaneous deposition of venom. Venom that is deposited by larger snakes into muscle compartments, however, can result in an increase in intracompartmental pressure. Clinically differentiating a true compartment syndrome from the typical swollen, painful extremity seen after subcutaneous envenomation is difficult and may require measurement of compartment pressure. Fasciotomies are considered only if pressures are documented to exceed 30 to 40 mm Hg despite antivenom treatment and elevation (Fig. 23-4). In a hemodynamically stable patient, a trial of IV mannitol in addition to antivenom and elevation may obviate the need for surgery if intracompartmental pressure can be reduced within approximately 1 hour. In areas too small to measure pressure (e.g., the digits), increased pressure may be suspected when pricking the skin of the affected digit yields dark venous blood flow.[18] There is no role for routine or prophylactic fasciotomy in venomous snakebites.[19] Preliminary animal evidence suggests that

fasciotomy may actually increase the severity of local myonecrosis in snake venom–induced compartment syndrome.[20] Nevertheless, the ischemic stress to nerves in tight muscle compartments must be relieved. It is important to obtain informed consent from patients before fasciotomy.

MAMMALIAN BITES

Epidemiology

The incidence of mammalian bite injuries is unknown because most patients with minor wounds never seek medical care. Although death from animal bites is uncommon in the United States, thousands of people are killed around the world each year, primarily by large animals such as lions and tigers. Dogs are responsible for 80% to 90% of animal bites in the United States, followed by cats and humans.[21] An estimated 4.7 million dog bites occur annually in the United States and account for 1% of emergency department visits.[21,22] A majority of these bites are from a family pet or a neighborhood dog. Animal bites occur most frequently on the extremities of adults and on the head, face, and neck of children. More than 60% of reported bites occur in children, especially boys 5 to 9 years of age.[22]

Treatment
Evaluation
Humans attacked by animals are at risk for blunt and penetrating trauma. Animals produce blunt injuries by striking with their extremities, biting with their powerful jaws, and crushing with their body weight. Teeth and claws can puncture body cavities, including the cranium, and amputate extremities. Patients with serious injuries are managed in a similar fashion to other potential polytrauma victims, with special attention given to wound management. Useful laboratory tests include a hematocrit when blood loss is of concern and cultures when an infection is present. Radiographs are obtained to diagnose potential fractures, joint penetration, severe infections, and retained foreign bodies such as teeth. The patient's tetanus status needs to be updated, as necessary.

Wound Care
Local wound management reduces the risk for infection and maximizes functional and aesthetic outcomes. Early wound cleansing is the most important therapy for preventing infection and zoonotic diseases such as rabies. Intact skin surrounding dirty wounds is scrubbed with a sponge and 1% povidone-iodine solution. Copious high-pressure irrigation of the wound with normal saline or tap water via a syringe and needle or flexible catheter significantly decreases the likelihood of infection. Alternatively, a 1% povidone-iodine solution can be used for irrigation, as long as the wound is flushed afterward with normal saline or water. Scrubbing the wound surface itself can increase tissue damage and infection and thus needs to be avoided. Wounds that are dirty or contain

devitalized tissue are cleansed lightly with gauze or a porous sponge and débrided.[21]

Options for wound repair include primary, delayed primary, and secondary closure. The anatomic location of the bite, the source of the bite, and the type of injury determine the most appropriate method. Primary closure is appropriate for most bites to optimize the aesthetic and functional outcome,[21,23] especially head and neck wounds that are initially seen within 24 hours of the bite and for which aesthetic results are important and infection rates are low.[24] Primary closure can also be used for low-risk wounds to the arms, legs, and trunk if seen within 6 to 12 hours of the bite.[21] Severe human bites and avulsion injuries of the face that require flaps have been successfully repaired by primary closure; however, this technique remains controversial. Wounds prone to the development of infection (Box 23-1), such as those initially seen longer than 24 hours after the bite (or longer than 6 hours if ear or nose cartilage is involved), are covered with moist dressings and undergo delayed primary closure after 3 to 5 days.[24] Puncture wounds have an increased incidence of infection and are not sutured. Deep irrigation of small puncture wounds and wide exci-

sion have not proved beneficial. Larger puncture wounds, however, usually benefit from irrigation and débridement.[21,25] Healing by secondary intention generally produces unacceptable scars in cosmetic areas.

Bites involving the hands or feet have a much greater chance of becoming infected and are left open.[21] The primary goal in repairing bite wounds on the hand is to maximize functional outcome. Approximately a third of dog bites on the hand become infected, even with adequate therapy.[25] Healing by secondary intention is recommended for most hand lacerations.[21] After thorough exploration, irrigation, and débridement, the hand is immobilized, wrapped in a bulky dressing, and elevated.

A common human bite wound associated with high morbidity is a clenched-fist injury (fight bite) resulting from striking another person's mouth. Regardless of the history obtained, injuries over the dorsum of the metacarpophalangeal joints are treated as clenched-fist injuries. These minor-appearing wounds often result in serious injury to the extensor tendon or joint capsule and have significant oral bacterial contamination. The extensor tendon retracts when the hand is opened, so evaluation needs to be carried out with the hand in both the open and clenched positions. Minor injuries are irrigated, débrided, and left open. Potentially deeper injuries and infected bites require exploration and débridement in the operating room and administration of IV antibiotics.[26]

All bite injuries are re-evaluated in 1 or 2 days to rule out secondary infection.

Microbiology

Given the large variety and concentration of bacteria in mouths, it is not surprising that wound infection is the main complication of bites, with 3% to 18% of dog bite wounds becoming infected and approximately 50% of cat bite wounds.[27] Infected wounds contain both aerobic and anaerobic bacteria and yield an average of five isolates per culture (Box 23-2).[27] Although many wounds are infected by *Staphylococcus* and *Streptococcus* species and anaerobes, *Pasteurella* species are the most common bacterial pathogen (found in 50% of dog bites and 75% of cat bites).[27] Human bite wounds are frequently contaminated with *Eikenella corrodens* in addition to the microorganisms found after dog and cat bites.[26,28]

Systemic diseases such as rabies, cat-scratch disease, cowpox, tularemia, leptospirosis, and brucellosis can be acquired through animal bites. Human bites have transmitted hepatitis B and C, tuberculosis, syphilis, and human immunodeficiency virus (HIV).[24] Although HIV transmission from human bites is rare, seroconversion is possible when a person with an open wound, either from a bite or from a preexisting injury, is exposed to saliva containing HIV-positive blood.[29] In this scenario, baseline and 6-month postexposure HIV testing is performed and prophylactic treatment with anti-HIV drugs considered.

Antibiotics

Prophylactic antibiotics are recommended for patients with high-risk bites.[21,25] The initial antibiotic choice and route are based on the type of animal and the severity and location of the bite. Cat bites often cause puncture wounds that require antibiotics. Patients with low-risk dog and human bites do not benefit from prophylactic antibiotics unless the hand or foot is involved.[21,28] Patients seen 24 hours after a bite without signs of infection do not usually need prophylactic antibiotics. Routine cultures of uninfected wounds have not proved useful and are reserved for infected wounds.[21,25]

Initial antibiotic selection needs to cover *Staphylococcus* and *Streptococcus* species, anaerobes, *Pasteurella* species for dog and cat bites, and *E. corrodens* for human bites. Amoxicillin-clavulanate is an acceptable first-line antibiotic for most bites. Alternatives include second-generation cephalosporins, such as cefoxitin, or a combination of penicillin and a first-generation cephalosporin. Penicillin-allergic patients can receive clindamycin combined with ciprofloxacin (or combined with trimethoprim-sulfamethoxazole if the patient is pregnant or a child).[21,24] Moxifloxacin has also been suggested as monotherapy.[24] Infections developing within 24 hours of the bite are generally caused by *Pasteurella* species and are treated by antibiotics with appropriate coverage.[24] Patients with serious infections require hospital admission and parenteral antibiotics such as ampicillin-sulbactam, cefoxitin, ticarcillin-clavulanate or clindamycin combined with a fluoroquinolone or trimethoprim-sulfamethoxazole.[24]

Rabies

Annually, thousands of people die of rabies worldwide, with dog bites or scratches being the major source.[30] In the United States, rabies is primarily found in wildlife, with raccoons being the primary source, followed by skunks, bats, and foxes.[31] Cats and dogs account for less than 5% of cases since the establishment of rabies control programs. Although the number of infected animals in the United States continues to increase, with the total approaching 8000 per year, human infection rates remain constant at one to three cases annually.[31] Bats have been the main source of human rabies reported in this country during the past 20 years, although a history of bat contact is absent in most victims.[32]

Rabies is caused by a rhabdovirus found in the saliva of animals and is transmitted through bites or scratches. Acute encephalitis develops and patients almost invariably die. The disease usually begins with a prodromal phase of nonspecific complaints and paresthesias, with itching or burning at the bite site spreading to the entire bitten extremity.[33] The disease then progresses to an acute neurologic phase. This phase generally takes one of two forms. The more common encephalitic or furious form is typified by fever and hyperactivity that can be stimulated by internal or external factors such as thirst, fear, light, or noise, followed by fluctuating levels of consciousness, aerophobia or hydrophobia, inspiratory spasm, and abnormalities of the autonomic nervous system. The paralytic form of rabies is manifested by fever, progressive weakness, loss of deep tendon reflexes, and urinary incontinence. Both forms progress to paralysis, coma, circulatory collapse, and death.[33]

Adequate wound care and postexposure prophylaxis can prevent the development of rabies. Wounds are

---

Box 23-2   Common Bacteria Found in Animals' Mouths

Acinetobacter species
Actinobacillus species
Aeromonas hydrophila
Bacillus species
Bacteroides species
Bordetella species
Brucella canis
Capnocytophaga canimorsus
Clostridium perfringens
Corynebacterium species
Eikenella corrodens
Enterobacter species
Escherichia coli
Eubacterium species
Fusobacterium species
Haemophilus aphrophilus
Haemophilus haemolyticus
Klebsiella species
Leptotrichia buccalis
Micrococcus species
Moraxella species
Neisseria species
Pasteurella aerogenes
Pasteurella canis
Pasteurella dagmatis
Pasteurella multocida
Peptococcus species
Peptostreptococcus species
Propionibacterium species
Proteus mirabilis
Pseudomonas species
Serratia marcescens
Staphylococcus aureus
Staphylococcus epidermidis
Streptococcus species
Veillonella parvula

Data from Keogh S, Callaham ML: Bites and injuries inflicted by domestic animals. In Auerbach PS (ed): Wilderness Medicine: Management of Wilderness and Environmental Emergencies, 4th ed. St Louis, CV Mosby, 2001, pp 961-978.

---

washed with soap and water and irrigated with a virucidal agent such as povidone-iodine solution. If rabies exposure is strongly suspected, consider leaving the wound open. The decision to administer rabies prophylaxis after an animal bite or scratch depends on the offending species and the nature of the event. Guidelines for administering rabies prophylaxis can be obtained from local public health agencies or from a publication by the Advisory Committee on Immunization Practices.[34] Research indicates that rabies prophylaxis is not being administered according to guidelines, which results in costly overtreatment or potentially life-threatening undertreatment.[32]

Worldwide, nearly 1 million people receive rabies prophylaxis each year, 40,000 from the United States.[30,32] Unprovoked attacks are more likely to occur by rabid animals. All wild carnivores must be considered rabid, but birds and reptiles do not contract or transmit rabies.

In cases of bites by domestic animals, rodents, or lago-morphs, the local health department needs to be consulted before beginning rabies prophylaxis.[34] A bite from a healthy-appearing domestic animal does not require prophylaxis if the animal can be observed for 10 days.[34]

Rabies prophylaxis involves both passive and active immunization. Passive immunization consists of administering 20 IU/kg body weight of rabies immune globulin. As much of the dose as possible is infiltrated into and around the wound. The rest can be given intramuscularly at a site remote from where the vaccine was administered. Active immunization consists of administering 1 mL of human diploid cell vaccine, purified chick embryo cell vaccine, or rabies vaccine absorbed intramuscularly into the deltoid in adults and into the anterolateral aspect of the thigh in children on days 0, 3, 7, 14, and 28. Patients with pre-exposure immunization do not require passive immunization and need active immunization only on days 0 and 3.[33,34]

ARTHROPOD BITES AND STINGS

Black Widow Spiders

Widow spiders (genus *Latrodectus*) are found throughout the world. At least one of five species inhabits all areas of the United States except Alaska.[35] The best-known widow spider is the black widow *(Latrodectus mactans)*. The female has a leg span of 1 to 4 cm and a shiny black body with a distinctive red ventral marking (often hourglass shaped) (Fig. 23-5). Variations in color occur among other species, with some appearing brown or red and some without the ventral marking. The nonaggressive female widow spider bites in defense. Males are too small to bite through human skin.

Toxicology

Widow spiders produce neurotoxic venom with minimal local effects. The major component is α-latrotoxin, which acts at presynaptic terminals by enhancing release of neurotransmitters. The ensuing clinical picture results from excess stimulation of neuromuscular junctions, as well as the sympathetic and parasympathetic nervous systems.[36]

Clinical Manifestations

The bite itself may be painless or felt as a "pinprick." Local findings are minimal.[35,37] The patient may have systemic complaints and no history of a spider bite, thus making the diagnosis challenging. Neuromuscular symptoms may occur as early as 30 minutes after the bite and include severe pain and spasms of large muscle groups. Abdominal cramps and rigidity could mimic a surgical abdomen, but rebound is absent. Dyspnea can result from chest wall muscle tightness. Autonomic stimulation produces hypertension, diaphoresis, and tachycardia. Other symptoms include muscle twitching, nausea and vomiting, headache, paresthesias, fatigue, and salivation.[35,37] Symptoms typically peak at several hours and

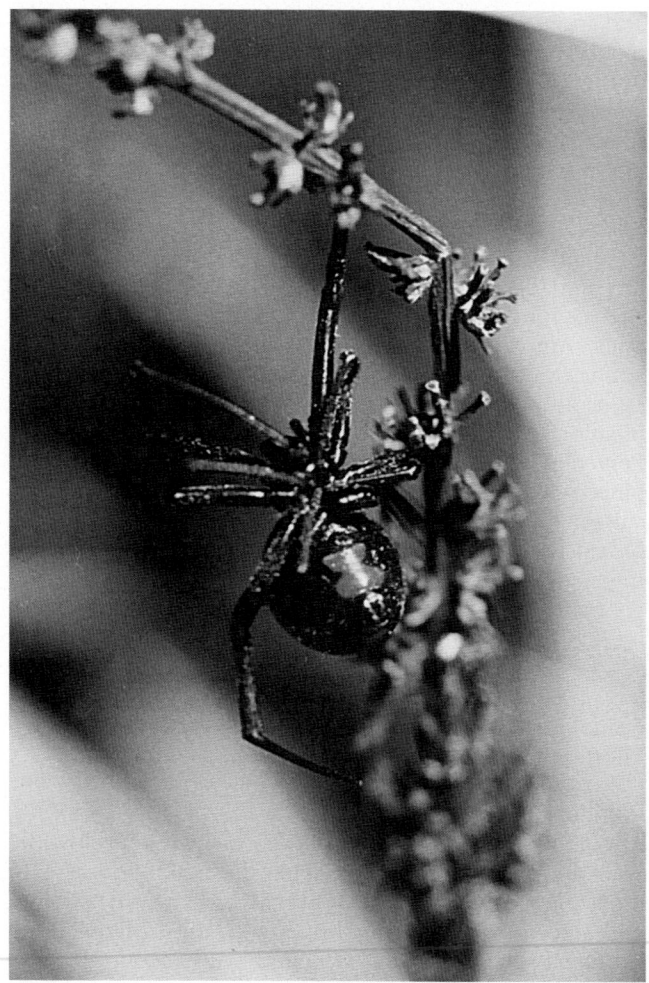

Figure 23-5 Female black widow spider *(Latrodectus mactans)* with the characteristic hourglass marking. (Courtesy of Paul Auerbach, MD.)

resolve in 1 to 2 days. Mild pain and nonspecific symptoms, primarily neurologic, can persist for several weeks. Death is an unusual result of widow spider bites.

Treatment

Mild bites are managed with local wound care—cleansing, intermittent application of ice, and tetanus prophylaxis as needed. The possibility of delayed, severe symptoms makes an observation period of several hours prudent. The optimal therapy for severe envenomation is controversial. IV calcium gluconate, previously recommended as a first-line drug to relieve muscle spasms after widow spider bites, has no significant efficacy.[35,37] Narcotics and benzodiazepines are more effective agents to relieve muscular pain.

In the United States, antivenom derived from horse serum is available (Black Widow Spider Antivenin, Merck & Co., West Point, PA). Because this antivenom can cause anaphylactoid reactions or serum sickness, however, it must be reserved for serious cases. Antivenom is currently recommended for pregnant women, children younger than 16 years, individuals older than 60 years, and patients with severe envenomation and uncontrolled hypertension or respiratory distress.[35] Skin testing for possible allergy to the U.S. antivenom is recommended by the manufacturer and is outlined in the package insert, although the reliability of such testing is low. Patients about to receive antivenom may be pretreated with antihistamines to reduce the likelihood or severity of a systemic reaction to the serum. The initial recommended dose is one vial IV or intramuscularly, repeated as necessary (although it is exceedingly rare for more than two vials to be required). Studies have demonstrated that antivenom can decrease a patient's hospital stay, with discharge occurring as early as several hours after administration.[37] A high-quality antivenom is also available in Australia for *Latrodectus* bites. It appears that any widow spider antivenom is effective regardless of which species inflicted the bite.[38,39]

Brown Recluse Spiders

Envenomation by brown spiders of the genus *Loxosceles* is termed necrotic arachnidism or loxoscelism. These arthropods primarily inhabit North and South America, Africa, and Europe. Several species of *Loxosceles* are found throughout the United States, with the greatest concentration in the Midwest. Most significant bites in the United States are by *Loxosceles reclusa*—the brown recluse. The brown spiders are varying shades of brownish gray, with a characteristic dark brown, violin-shaped marking over the cephalothorax—hence the name violin spider (Fig. 23-6). Whereas most spiders have four pairs

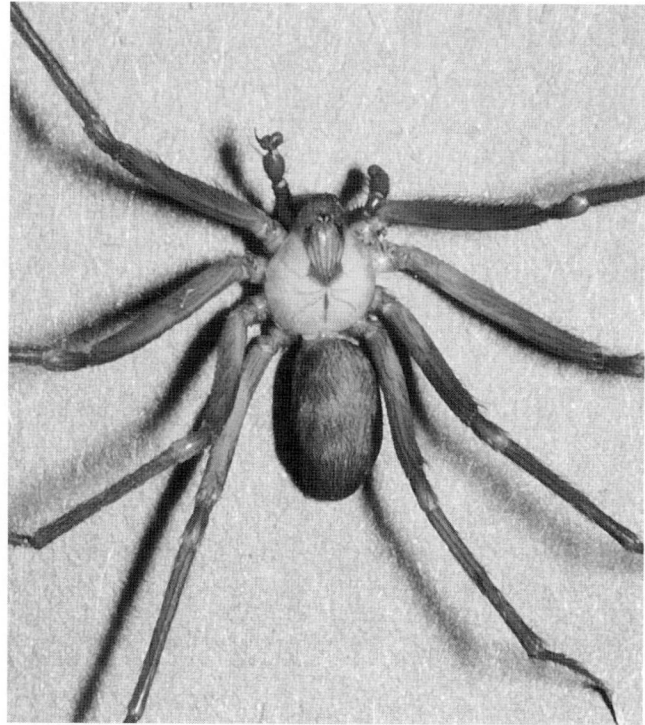

Figure 23-6 Brown recluse spider *(Loxosceles reclusa)* with a violin-shaped marking on the cephalothorax. (Courtesy of Sherman Minton, MD, Indiana University.)

of eyes, brown spiders have only three pairs. Both male and female specimens can bite and may do so when threatened.

Toxicology

Although several enzymes have been isolated from the venom, the major deleterious factor is sphingomyelinase D, which causes both dermonecrosis and hemolysis.[35,40] It is a phospholipase that interacts with the cell membranes of erythrocytes, platelets, and endothelial cells and causes hemolysis, coagulation, and platelet aggregation. Host responses have some significance in determining the severity of envenomation because functioning polymorphonuclear leukocytes and complement are necessary for the venom to have maximal effect.[40,41]

Clinical Manifestations

Local findings at the bite site range from mild irritation to severe necrosis with ulceration.[42] The patient is often completely unaware of the bite or may have felt a slight stinging. It is unusual for the victim to actually see or capture the spider. This can make the diagnosis very challenging because similar skin lesions can represent bites by other arthropods, skin infections (including methicillin-resistant *Staphylococcus aureus*), herpes zoster, dermatologic manifestation of a systemic illness, or other causes of dermatitis and vasculitis.[43] Within several hours of a *Loxosceles* bite, local tissue ischemia will develop in some patients with resulting pain, itching, swelling, and erythema. A blister may form at the site. In more severe bites, the central area turns purple as a result of microvascular thrombosis. Peripheral vasoconstriction can also create a pale border surrounding the central region of necrosis. Over the next several days, an eschar develops over the widening necrotic area. The eschar separates and leaves an ulcer that usually heals over a period of many weeks to months, but occasionally skin grafting is required.[35,44] Necrosis is most severe in fatty areas such as the abdomen and thigh.[36,44]

Systemic features can include headache, nausea and vomiting, fever, malaise, arthralgias, and maculopapular rash.[35] Additional findings may include thrombocytopenia, disseminated intravascular coagulation, hemolytic anemia, coma, and possibly death. Renal failure can result from intravascular hemolysis.[40,44]

In patients with lesions consistent with brown spider bites, a search for evidence of systemic involvement (viscerocutaneous or systemic loxoscelism) is initiated, particularly if the victim has any systemic complaints. Appropriate laboratory tests include a complete blood count (with platelet count) and a bedside urine test for blood. If the results of any of these tests are abnormal, electrolytes, liver function studies, and coagulation studies are in order, but there are no truly diagnostic studies available. Systemic loxoscelism is more common in children and can occur with minimal local findings.[35]

Treatment

Recommended management remains controversial. The bite site is splinted, elevated, and treated with cold compresses. Cold therapy inhibits venom activity and reduces inflammation and necrosis. Heat application, in contrast, enhances tissue damage and ulcer development.[35,36] Though controversial, a lipophilic, prophylactic antibiotic such as erythromycin or cephalexin can be administered in standard doses for a few days.[36] Tetanus status is updated as needed. Brown spider bites in which necrosis does not develop within 72 hours generally heal well and require no additional therapy. There is no commercial antivenom available in the United States.

Some research suggests that more severe lesions may benefit from dapsone if administered within the first few days after the bite, even though the drug is not approved for this indication.[45] Dapsone may reduce local inflammation and necrosis by inhibiting neutrophil function. The suggested adult dose is 100 mg/day. Dapsone can cause methemoglobinemia and is contraindicated in patients with glucose-6-phosphate dehydrogenase deficiency. Thus, levels of this enzyme are checked as therapy begins and dapsone discontinued if the enzyme is found to be deficient. Dapsone is not approved for use in children.

Early surgical intervention, other than simple, conservative débridement of obviously necrotic tissue, is avoided. It is difficult or impossible to predict with any certainty the extent of eventual necrosis, and early surgery is apt to be overaggressive and needlessly disfiguring.[35] Pyoderma gangrenosum, manifested as nonhealing ulcers and failure of skin grafts, occurs more often in patients undergoing early excision and débridement, possibly as a result of the rapid spread of venom.[40] After 1 to 2 weeks, when eschar margins are defined, débridement can be performed as necessary. In severe cases, wide excision and split-thickness skin grafting are necessary while dapsone therapy is continued.[36]

The efficacy of using hyperbaric oxygen therapy for *Loxosceles* bites remains controversial.[46] If a hyperbaric chamber is readily available and there is evidence of significant necrosis, such therapy can be attempted.

Steroid administration, by any route, has never been proved to be beneficial in limiting dermonecrosis. A short course (few days) of oral steroids can help stabilize red blood cell membranes and reduce hemolysis in the setting of systemic loxoscelism.

Patients with rapidly expanding, necrotic lesions or a clinical picture suggesting systemic loxoscelism are admitted for close observation and management. Patients with less serious lesions can be monitored on an outpatient basis with frequent wound checks. Visits during the first 72 hours include reassessment for any evidence of systemic involvement based on symptoms, signs, and possibly a bedside urine test for blood.

Scorpions

Significant scorpion envenomation occurs worldwide by species belonging to the family Buthidae. In this group the bark scorpion *(Centruroides exilicauda)* is the only potentially dangerous species in the United States. It is found throughout Arizona and occasionally in immediately contiguous areas of surrounding states. It is a yellow to brown crablike arthropod up to 5 cm in length.

Approximately 15,000 scorpion stings were reported during 2004 in the United States, and this is probably a significant underestimate of the total number of stings that occurred.[47] Scorpions tend to be nocturnal and sting when threatened.

Toxicology

Neurotoxic scorpion venoms, such as that produced by the bark scorpion, contain multiple low-molecular-weight basic proteins but possess very little enzymatic activity. The neurotoxins target excitable tissues and work primarily on ion channels, particularly sodium and potassium channels. They cause massive release of multiple neurotransmitters throughout the autonomic nervous system and the adrenal medulla.[48,49] Almost any organ system can be adversely affected, either by direct toxin effects or by the flood of autonomic neurotransmitters. Because of the speed of their systemic absorption, these neurotoxic scorpion venoms can cause rapid systemic toxicity and potentially death.[48]

Clinical Manifestations

Most scorpion stings in the United States result in short-lived, searing pain and mild, local irritation with slight swelling. Stings by the bark scorpion typically produce local paresthesias and burning pain. Systemic manifestations may include cranial nerve and neuromuscular hyperactivity and respiratory distress.[50,51] Signs of adrenergic stimulation, accompanied by nausea and vomiting, may also develop. Young children are at greatest risk for severe stings from the bark scorpion. Death can occur from bark scorpion stings but is rare.

Treatment

All patients receive tetanus prophylaxis if indicated, application of cold compresses to the sting site, and analgesics for pain. Victims of bark scorpion stings with signs of systemic envenomation require supportive care, with close monitoring of cardiovascular and respiratory status in an intensive care setting. Although an antivenom for this arthropod has been available in the past, production has currently ceased. The product was derived from goats (with a resultant risk for allergic sequelae), lacked FDA approval, and was available for use only within Arizona. Its use was highly controversial. There is an antivenom produced for related scorpions in Mexico that is currently being evaluated for possible use in the United States.

Ticks

Several potentially serious diseases occur from tick bites, including Rocky Mountain spotted fever, ehrlichiosis, tularemia, babesiosis, Colorado tick fever, relapsing fever, and Lyme disease. Timely and adequate removal of the tick is important to prevent disease. Common lay recommendations for tick removal, such as the application of local heat, gasoline, methylated spirits, and fingernail polish, are ineffective. Proper removal involves grasping the tick by the body as close to the skin surface as possible with an instrument and applying gradual, gentle axial traction, without twisting. Commercial tick removal devices are superior to standard tweezers for this purpose.[52] An alternative removal method involves looping a length of suture material in a simple overhand knot around the body of the tick. The loop is slipped down as close to the patient's skin surface as possible. The knot is then tightened and the tick is pulled backward and out, over its head in a "somersault" action.[53] Crushing the tick is avoided because potentially infectious secretions may be squeezed into the wound. After extraction, the wound is cleansed with alcohol or povidone-iodine. Any retained mouth parts of the tick are removed with the tip of a needle. If the tick was embedded for less than 24 hours, the risk of transmitting infection is very low. Tetanus immunization needs to be current. Occasionally, a granulomatous lesion requiring steroid injection or surgical excision may develop at the tick bite site a few weeks after the incident.[54] Patients in whom a local rash or systemic symptoms develop within 4 weeks of exposure to tick-infested areas (even in the absence of a known bite) need to be evaluated for infectious complications such as Lyme disease,[52] the most common vector-borne disease in the United States.

Lyme disease is caused by the spirochete *Borrelia burgdorferi* and may initially be seen in any of three stages—early localized (stage 1), early disseminated (stage 2), or late/persistent (stage 3). Stage 1 findings of limited infection include a rash in at least 80% of patients that develops after an incubation period of approximately 3 to 30 days.[55,56] The rash, termed erythema migrans, is typically a round or oval erythematous lesion that begins at the bite site and expands at a relatively rapid rate (up to 1 cm each day) to a median size of 15 cm in diameter.[57] As the rash expands, there may be evidence of central clearing and, less commonly, a central vesicle or necrotic eschar.[57] The rash may be accompanied by fatigue, myalgias, headache, fever, nausea, vomiting, regional lymphadenopathy, sore throat, photophobia, anorexia, and arthralgias.[55,56] Without treatment, the rash fades in approximately 4 weeks.[55] If untreated, the infection may disseminate, and between 30 and 120 days later, multiple erythema migrans lesions (generally smaller than the primary lesion) and neurologic, cardiac, or joint abnormalities may develop.[55] Neuroborreliosis occurs in approximately 15% of untreated patients and is characterized by central or peripheral findings such as lymphocytic meningitis, subtle encephalitis, cranial neuritis (especially facial nerve palsy, which may be unilateral or bilateral), cerebellar ataxia, and motor neuropathies.[58] Cardiac findings occur in approximately 5% of untreated patients and are usually manifested as atrioventricular nodal block or myocarditis.[56] Oligoarticular arthritis is a common finding in early, disseminated Lyme disease that occurs in approximately 60% of untreated victims.[56] There is a particular propensity for larger joints such as the knee, which becomes recurrently and intermittently swollen and painful.[56] Findings of early disseminated Lyme disease eventually disappear with or without treatment.[56] Over time, as much as a year after the initial tick bite, Lyme disease can progress to its chronic form manifested by chronic arthritis, chronic synovitis, neurocognitive disorders, chronic fatigue, or any combination of these findings.[55]

The diagnosis of Lyme disease is based largely on the presence of classic erythema migrans in a patient with a history of possible tick exposure in an endemic area or the presence of one or more findings of disseminated infection (nervous system, cardiovascular system, or joint involvement) and positive serology. Serologic testing is done in two stages.[59] The first test to perform is an enzyme-linked immunosorbent assay for IgM and IgG antibodies to *B. burgdorferi*. If this test is reactive or indeterminate, it needs to be confirmed with a second test, a Western blot. If the patient has been ill for longer than a month, only IgG is assayed because an isolated positive IgM antibody level is probably a false-positive finding at this stage. Patients from highly endemic areas with the classic findings of stage 1 disease (including erythema migrans) can be treated without serologic confirmation because testing may be falsely negative at this early stage.[60]

First-line treatment of early or disseminated Lyme disease, in the absence of neurologic involvement, is oral doxycycline for 14 to 21 days. The second-line agent for use in children 8 years or younger and pregnant women is amoxicillin. An equally effective third choice is cefuroxime axetil. Each of these oral agents provides a cure in better than 90% of patients.[56] If the patient has any evidence of neuroborreliosis, treatment consists of daily IV ceftriaxone for 14 to 28 days.[56] Likewise, patients with cardiac manifestations are treated via the IV route for at least part of their course and undergo cardiac monitoring if atrioventricular nodal block is significant (i.e., PR interval >0.3 second).[56] Oral antibiotics for 30 to 60 days or IV therapy for 30 days is usually effective for Lyme arthritis, although approximately 10% of patients will have persistent joint complaints after treatment.[56,57] Persistent arthritis in these nonresponders after antibiotic therapy is thought to be autoimmune mediated because the spirochete has been eradicated.[56,61] Treatment of persistent arthritis after antibiotic therapy consists of anti-inflammatory agents or arthroscopic synovectomy.[56,61]

Decisions to prophylactically treat a victim of a tick bite to prevent Lyme disease are controversial. Some authors condemn such an approach given the low (~1.4%) risk for transmission after a tick bite, even in an endemic area.[57] Research has shown, however, that a single dose of doxycycline, 200 mg orally given within 72 hours of a tick bite, can further reduce the already low risk of disease transmission.[56,62] A recent vaccine against Lyme disease has been withdrawn from the market because of adverse drug reactions. The best prevention for tick-borne diseases such as Lyme disease is the use of insect repellent and frequent body checks for ticks when traveling through their habitat.

Hymenoptera

Most arthropod envenomation occurs by species belonging to the order Hymenoptera, which includes bees, wasps, yellow jackets, hornets, and stinging ants. The winged Hymenoptera are located throughout the United States, whereas the so-called fire ants are currently limited to the southeastern and southwestern regions. The Africanized honeybee, which characteristically attacks in massive numbers, has recently migrated into the southwestern United States.

Toxicology

Hymenopterans sting humans defensively, especially if their nests are disturbed. The stingers of most hymenopterans are attached to venom sacs located on the abdomen and can be used repeatedly. Some bees, however, have barb-shaped stingers that prevent detachment from the victim and thus render the bees capable of only a single sting. Hymenoptera venom contains vasoactive compounds such as histamine and serotonin, which are responsible for the local reaction and pain. The venom also contain peptides, such as melitin, and enzymes (primarily phospholipases and hyaluronidases), which are highly allergenic and elicit an IgE-mediated response in some victims.[63] Fire ant venom consists primarily of nonallergenic alkaloids that release histamine and cause mild, local necrosis. Allergenic proteins constitute only 0.1% of fire ant venom.

Clinical Reactions

A Hymenoptera sting in a nonallergic individual produces immediate pain followed by a wheal and flare reaction. Fire ants characteristically produce multiple pustules from repetitive stings at the same site. Multiple Hymenoptera stings can produce a toxic reaction characterized by vomiting, diarrhea, generalized edema, cardiovascular collapse, and hemolysis, which can be difficult to distinguish from an acute, anaphylactic reaction.[64]

Large, exaggerated local reactions develop in approximately 17% of envenomed subjects.[63] These reactions are manifested as erythematous, edematous, painful, and pruritic areas larger than 10 cm in diameter and may last 2 to 5 days. The precise pathophysiology of such reactions remains unclear, although they may, in part, be IgE mediated.[65] Patients in whom large local reactions develop are at risk for similar episodes with future stings, but they do not appear to be at increased risk for systemic allergic reactions.[63]

Bee sting anaphylaxis develops in 0.3% to 3% of the general population and is responsible for approximately 40 reported deaths annually in the United States.[63,64] Fatalities occur most often in adults, usually within 1 hour of the sting. Symptoms generally occur within minutes and range from mild urticaria and angioedema to respiratory arrest secondary to airway edema and bronchospasm and finally cardiovascular collapse. A positive IgE-mediated skin test to Hymenoptera extract helps predict an allergic sting reaction.

Unusual reactions to Hymenoptera stings include late-onset allergic reactions (>5 hours after the sting), serum sickness, renal disease, neurologic disorders such as Guillain-Barré syndrome, and vasculitis.[66] The etiology of these reactions is thought to be immune mediated.

Treatment

If a stinger has been left behind by an offending bee, it is removed as quickly as possible to prevent continued injection of venom.[67] The sting site is cleansed and locally cooled. Topical or injected lidocaine can help decrease pain from the sting. Antihistamines administered orally or topically can decrease pruritus. Blisters and pustules (typically sterile) from fire ant stings are left intact. Tetanus status is updated as needed.

Treatment of an exaggerated, local envenomation includes the aforementioned therapy in addition to elevation of the extremity and analgesics. A 5-day course of oral prednisone (1 mg/kg/day) is also recommended.[63] Isolated local reactions (typical or exaggerated) do not require epinephrine or referral for immunotherapy.

Mild anaphylaxis can be treated with 0.01 mL/kg (up to 0.5 mL) of 1:1000 intramuscular epinephrine and an oral or parenteral antihistamine. More severe cases are also treated with steroids and may require oxygen, endotracheal intubation, IV epinephrine infusion, bronchodilators, IV fluids, or vasopressors. These patients are observed for approximately 24 hours in a monitored environment for any recurrence of severe symptoms.

Venom immunotherapy effectively prevents recurrent anaphylaxis from subsequent stings in patients with positive skin tests.[64,68] All persons with previous severe, systemic, allergic reactions to Hymenoptera stings or in whom serum sickness develops are referred for possible immunotherapy. Referral is also recommended for adults with purely generalized dermal reactions such as diffuse hives. Children with skin manifestations alone appear to be at relatively low risk for more serious anaphylaxis on subsequent stings and do not need referral.[64] Patients with a history of systemic reactions resulting from Hymenoptera stings need to carry injectable epinephrine with them at all times; they also need to wear an identification medallion identifying their medical condition.

MARINE BITES AND STINGS

Four fifths of all living creatures reside underwater.[69] Hazardous marine animals are encountered by humans primarily in temperate or tropical seas. Exposure to marine life through recreation, research, and industry leads to frequent encounters with aquatic organisms. Injuries generally occur through bites, stings, or punctures and infrequently through electrical shock from creatures such as the torpedo ray.

Initial Assessment

Injuries from marine organisms can range from mild local irritant skin reactions to systemic collapse from major trauma or severe envenomation.[70] Several environmental aspects unique to marine trauma may make treatment of these patients challenging. Immersion in cold water predisposes patients to hypothermia and near drowning. Rapid ascent after an encounter with a marine organism can cause air embolism or decompression illness in a scuba diver. Anaphylactic reaction to venom may further complicate an envenomation. Late complications include unique infections caused by a wide variety of aquatic microorganisms, as well as immune-mediated phenomena.

Microbiology

Most marine isolates are gram-negative rods.[69] *Vibrio* species are of primary concern, particularly in immunocompromised hosts. In fresh water, *Aeromonas* species can be particularly aggressive pathogens. *Staphylococcus* and *Streptococcus* species are also frequently cultured from infections. The laboratory is notified that cultures are being requested for aquatic-acquired infections to alert them of the need for appropriate culture media and conditions.

General Management

Initial management is focused on the airway, breathing, and circulation. Anaphylaxis needs to be anticipated and the victim treated accordingly. Patients with extensive blunt and penetrating injuries are managed as major trauma victims. Patients who have been envenomed receive specific intervention directed against a toxin (discussed separately, according to the marine creature), in addition to general supportive care. Antivenom can be administered if available. Antitetanus immunization is updated after a bite, cut, or sting. Radiographs are obtained to locate foreign bodies and fractures. Magnetic resonance imaging is more useful than ultrasound or computed tomography to identify small spine fragments.

Selection of antibiotics is tailored to marine bacteriology. Third-generation cephalosporins provide adequate coverage for the gram-positive and gram-negative microorganisms found in ocean water, including *Vibrio* species.[69] Ciprofloxacin, cefoperazone, gentamicin, and trimethoprim-sulfamethoxazole are acceptable antibiotics. Norfloxacin may be less efficacious against certain vibrios. Other quinolones (ofloxacin, enoxacin, pefloxacin, fleroxacin, lomefloxacin, moxifloxacin) have not been extensively tested against *Vibrio;* they may be useful alternatives, but this awaits definitive evaluation.[71,72] Outpatient regimens include ciprofloxacin, trimethoprim-sulfamethoxazole, or doxycycline.[69] Patients with large abrasions, lacerations, puncture wounds, or hand injuries, as well as immunocompromised patients, receive prophylactic antibiotics. Infected wounds are cultured. If a wound, commonly on the hand after a minor scrape or puncture, appears erysipeloid in nature, infection by *Erysipelothrix rhusiopathiae* is suspected. A suitable initial antibiotic based on this presumptive diagnosis would be penicillin, cephalexin, or ciprofloxacin.

Wound Care

Meticulous wound care is necessary to reduce the risk for infection and to optimize the aesthetic and functional outcome.[73] Wounds are irrigated with normal saline. Débridement of devitalized tissue can decrease infection and promote healing. Large wounds are explored in the operating room. The decision to close a wound primarily must balance the cosmetic result against the risk for infection. Wounds are loosely closed and drainage allowed. Primary closure is avoided with distal extremity wounds, punctures, and crush injuries. For shark wounds, postoperative management may be prolonged and complicated by acute renal failure attributed to hypovolemia and shock, massive blood transfusion, myoglobinuria, and administration of nephrotoxic antibiotics. Rehabilitation may include the creation of prosthetic devices.

Antivenom

Antivenom is available for several types of envenomation, including those from the box jellyfish, sea snake, and stonefish.[74] Patients demonstrating severe reactions to such envenomation benefit from antivenom. Skin testing to determine which patients might benefit from pretreatment with diphenhydramine or epinephrine can be performed before antivenom is administered, but it is not an absolute predictor of severe reactions. Ovine-derived antivenom (Commonwealth Serum Laboratories) to treat severe *Chironex fleckeri* (box jellyfish) envenomation has been administered intramuscularly by field rescuers for many years without report of a serious adverse reaction. Serum sickness is a complication of antivenom therapy and can be treated with corticosteroids. Regional poison control centers or major marine aquariums can sometimes assist in locating antivenom.

Injuries From Nonvenomous Aquatic Animals

Sharks

Approximately 50 to 100 shark attacks are reported annually. However, these attacks cause fewer than 10 deaths each year.[73,75] Tiger, great white, gray reef, and bull sharks are responsible for most attacks.[73] Most incidents occur at the surface of shallow water within 100 ft of shore.[58] Sharks locate prey by detecting motion, electrical fields, and sounds and by sensing body fluids through smell and taste. Most sharks bite the victim one time and then leave.[73,75] Most injuries occur to the lower extremities.

Powerful jaws and sharp teeth produce crushing, tearing injuries. Hypovolemic shock and near drowning are life-threatening consequences of an attack.[73] Other complications include soft tissue and neurovascular damage, bone fractures, and infection.[75] Most wounds require exploration and repair in the operating room (see the section on wound care). Radiographs may reveal one or more shark teeth in the wound. Occasionally, "bumping" by sharks can produce abrasions, which are treated as second-degree burns.[69]

Moray Eels

Morays are bottom dwellers that reside in holes or crevices. Eels bite defensively and produce multiple small puncture wounds and rare gaping lacerations. The hand is most frequently bitten. Occasionally, the eel remains attached to the victim, with decapitation of the animal required for release. Puncture wounds and bites on the hand from all animals, including eels, are at high risk for infection and must not be closed primarily if the capability exists for delayed primary closure.[69]

Alligators and Crocodiles

Crocodiles can attain a length of more than 20 ft and travel at speeds of 20 mph in water and on land. Like sharks, alligators and crocodiles attack primarily in shallow water. These animals can produce severe injuries by grasping victims with their powerful jaws and dragging them underwater, where they roll while crushing their prey. Injuries from alligator and crocodile attacks are treated like shark bites.

Miscellaneous

Other nonvenomous animals capable of attacking include the barracuda, giant grouper, sea lion, mantis shrimp, triggerfish, needlefish, and freshwater piranha. Except for the needlefish, which spears a human victim with its elongated snout, these animals bite. Barracuda are attracted to shiny objects and have bitten fingers, wrists, scalps, or dangling legs adorned with reflective jewelry.

Envenomation by Invertebrates

Coelenterates

The phylum Coelenterata consists of hydrozoans, which include fire coral, hydroids, and Portuguese man-of-war; scyphozoans, which include jellyfish and sea nettles; and anthozoans, which include sea anemones. Coelenterates carry specialized living stinging cells called cnidocytes that encapsulate intracytoplasmic stinging organelles called cnidae, which include nematocysts.[76]

Mild envenomation, typically inflicted by fire coral, hydroids, and anemones, produces skin irritation.[74] The victim notices immediate stinging followed by pruritus, paresthesias, and throbbing pain with proximal radiation. Edema and erythema develop in the involved area, followed by blisters and petechiae. This can progress to local infection and ulceration.

Severe envenomation is caused by anemones, sea nettles, and jellyfish.[74] Patients have systemic symptoms in addition to the local manifestations. An anaphylactic reaction to the venom may contribute to the pathophysiology of envenomation. Fever, nausea, vomiting, and malaise can develop. Any organ system can be involved, and death is attributed to hypotension and cardiorespiratory arrest. One of the most venomous sea creatures, found primarily off the coast of northern Australia, is the box jellyfish *C. fleckeri*. In the United States, *Physalia physalis*, *Chiropsalmus quadrigatus*, and *Cyanea capillata* are substantial stingers.

Therapy consists of detoxification of nematocysts and systemic support. Dilute (5%) acetic acid (vinegar) can inactivate most coelenterate toxins and is applied for 30 minutes or until the pain is relieved.[74] This is critical with the box jellyfish. If a detoxicant is not available, the wound may be rinsed in seawater and gently dried.[74] Fresh water and vigorous rubbing can cause nematocysts to discharge. For a sting from the box jellyfish, Australian authorities previously recommended the pressure immobilization technique. This is no longer recommended.[77] Instead, the envenomed limb is kept as motionless as possible and the victim promptly taken to a setting where antivenom and advanced life support are available.

To decontaminate other jellyfish stings, isopropyl alcohol is used only if vinegar is ineffective. Baking soda may be more effective than acetic acid for inactivating the toxin of U.S. eastern coastal Chesapeake Bay sea nettles.[74] Baking soda must not be applied after vinegar without a brisk saline or water rinse in between the two substances to avoid an exothermic reaction. Powdered or solubilized papain (meat tenderizer) may be more effective than other remedies for sea bather's eruption (often misnomered *sea lice*) caused by thimble jellyfishes or larval forms of certain sea anemones. Fresh lime or lemon juice, household ammonia, olive oil, or sugar may be effective, depending on the species of stinging creature.

After the skin surface has been treated, any remaining nematocysts must be removed. One method is to apply shaving cream or a flour paste and shave the area with a razor. The affected area again is irrigated, dressed, and elevated. Medical care providers need to wear gloves for self-protection. Cryotherapy, local anesthetics, antihistamines, and steroids can relieve pain after the toxin is inactivated. Prophylactic antibiotics are not usually necessary. Ocean bathers can be advised to apply Safe Sea jellyfish-safe sun block (Nidaria Technology Ltd., Jordan Valley, Israel) as a preventive measure before entering the water.

Sponges

Two syndromes occur after contact with sponges.[74] The first is an allergic plant–like contact dermatitis characterized by itching and burning within hours of contact. This dermatitis can progress to soft tissue edema, vesicle development, and joint swelling. Large areas of involvement can cause systemic toxicity with fever, nausea, and muscle cramps. The second syndrome is an irritant dermatitis after penetration of the skin with small spicules. Sponge diver's disease is actually caused by anemones that colonize the sponges rather than by the sponges themselves.

Treatment consists of washing and drying gently the affected area. Dilute (5%) acetic acid (vinegar) is applied for 30 minutes three times daily.[74] Any remaining spicules can be removed with adhesive tape. A steroid cream can be applied to the skin after decontamination. Occasionally, a systemic glucocorticoid and an antihistamine are required.

Echinodermata

Starfish, sea urchins, and sea cucumbers are members of the phylum Echinodermata. Starfish and sea cucumbers produce venom that can cause contact dermatitis.[76] Sea cucumbers occasionally feed on coelenterates and secrete nematocysts; therefore, local therapy for coelenterates also needs to be considered. Sea urchins are covered with venomous spines capable of causing local and systemic reactions similar to those from coelenterates.[76] First aid consists of soaking the wound in hot, but tolerable water. Residual spines can be located with soft tissue radiographs or magnetic resonance imaging. Purple skin discoloration at the site of entrance wounds may be indicative of dye leached from the surface of an extracted urchin spine. This temporary tattoo disappears in 48 hours, which often confirms the absence of a retained foreign body. A spine is removed only if it is easily accessible or if it is closely aligned to a joint or critical neurovascular structure. Reactive fusiform digit swelling attributed to a spine near a metacarpal bone or flexor tendon sheath may be alleviated by a high-dose glucocorticoid administered in an oral 14-day tapering schedule. Retained spines may cause the formation of granulomas that are amenable to excision or intralesional injection with triamcinolone hexacetonide (5 mg/mL).

Mollusks

Octopuses and cone snails are the primary envenoming species in the phylum Mollusca. Most harmful cone snails are found in Indo-Pacific waters. Envenomation occurs from a detachable harpoon-like dart injected via an extensible proboscis into the victim.[74,76] Blue-ringed octopuses can bite and inject tetrodotoxin, a paralytic agent. Both species can produce local symptoms such as burning and paresthesias. Systemic manifestations are primarily neurologic and include bulbar dysfunction and systemic muscular paralysis. Management of the bite site is best achieved by pressure and immobilization to contain the venom. This is accomplished by applying a circumferential wrap 15 cm wide over a gauze pad or cloth that has been placed directly over the wound. The dressing is applied at venous-lymphatic pressure with preservation of distal arterial pulses. Once the victim has been transported to a medical facility, the bandage can be released. Treatment of systemic complications is supportive.

Annelid Worms (Bristleworms)

Annelid worms (bristleworms) carry rows of soft, easily detached fiberglass-like spines capable of inflicting painful stings and irritant dermatitis. Inflammation may persist for up to a week. Visible bristles are removed with forceps and adhesive tape or a commercial facial peel. Alternatively, a thin layer of rubber cement may be used to trap the spines and then peel them away. Household vinegar, rubbing alcohol, or dilute household ammonia may provide additional relief. Local inflammation is treated with a topical or systemic glucocorticoid.

Envenomation by Vertebrates

Stingrays

Rays are bottom dwellers ranging from a few inches to 12 ft long (tip to tail). Venom is stored in whiplike caudal appendages. Stingrays react defensively by thrusting spines into a victim and producing puncture wounds and lacerations. The most common site of injury is the lower part of the leg and top of the foot. Local damage can be severe, with occasional penetration of body cavities.[78] This is worsened by the vasoconstrictive properties of the venom, which produce cyanotic-appearing wounds. The venom is often myonecrotic. Systemic complaints include weakness, nausea, diarrhea, headache, and muscle cramps. The venom can cause vasoconstriction, cardiac dysrhythmias, respiratory arrest, and seizures.[79]

The wound is irrigated and then soaked in nonscalding hot water (up to 45°C) for an hour.[79,80] Débridement, exploration, and removal of spines occur during or after hot water soaking. Immersion cryotherapy is detrimental. The wound is not closed primarily. Lacerations heal by secondary intention or are repaired by delayed closure. The wound is dressed and elevated. Pain is relieved locally or systemically. Radiographic studies are obtained to locate any remaining spines. Acute infection with aggressive pathogens is anticipated.[74] In the event of a nonhealing, draining wound, retention of a foreign body is suspected.

Miscellaneous

Other fish with spines that can produce injuries similar to those of stingrays include lionfish, scorpionfish, stonefish, catfish, and weeverfish. Each can produce envenomation, puncture wounds, and lacerations, with spines transmitting venom. Clinical manifestations and therapy are similar to those pertaining to stingrays. In the case of lionfish, vesiculations are sometimes noted. An equine-derived antivenom (Commonwealth Serum Laboratories) exists for administration in the event of significant stonefish envenomation.

Sea Snakes

Sea snakes of the family Hydrophiidae appear similar to land snakes. They inhabit the Pacific and Indian Oceans. Venom produces neurologic signs and symptoms, with possible death from paralysis and respiratory arrest. Local manifestations can be minimal or absent. Therapy is similar to that for coral snake (Elapidae) bites. The pressure immobilization technique is recommended in the field. Polyvalent sea snake antivenom is administered if any signs of envenomation develop.[79,80] The initial dose is 1 ampule, repeated as needed.

Selected References

Auerbach PS (ed): Wilderness Medicine, 5th ed. St Louis, CV Mosby, 2007.

This textbook is an in-depth review of wilderness medicine. Bites and stings by many organisms are discussed in detail by experts from each field. Many recent, pertinent studies are reviewed.

Freeman TM: Clinical practice. Hypersensitivity to Hymenoptera stings. N Engl J Med 351:1978-1984, 2004.

The reactions to Hymenoptera stings are well organized in this practical monograph. The natural history of stinging insect allergy is reviewed. Therapeutic considerations are discussed.

Gold BS, Dart RC, Barish RA: Bites of venomous snakes. N Engl J Med 347:347-356, 2002.

This article is a concise, practical review of snake venom poisoning in the United States. Proper use of the new North American antivenom is well summarized.

Isbister GK, Graudins A, White J, Warrell D: Antivenom treatment in arachnidism. J Toxicol Clin Toxicol 41:291-300, 2003.

This piece is an excellent review of the use of antivenom in spider bites around the world.

Mebs D: Venomous and Poisonous Animals. Boca Raton, FL, CRC Press, 2002.

> This book is a superbly illustrated collection of fascinating, detailed information about venoms and poisons in the animal kingdom, including marine and terrestrial animals.

Steere AC: Medical progress: Lyme disease. N Engl J Med 345:115-125, 2001.

> This manuscript is a thorough review of the current understanding of Lyme borreliosis and clearly outlines diagnosis and treatment.

Swanson DL, Vetter RS: Bites of brown recluse spiders and suspected necrotic arachnidism. N Engl J Med 352:700-707, 2005.

> This article is an excellent review of necrotic arachnidism, including the approach to diagnosis and management.

Williamson JA, Fenner PJ, Burnett JW (eds): Venomous and Poisonous Marine Animals. Sydney, Australia, University of New South Wales Press, 1996.

> This book is a superb reference with a complete discussion of all common and uncommon toxic marine animals.

References

1. Warrell DA, Fenner PJ: Venomous bites and stings. Br Med Bull 49:423-439, 1993.
2. Parrish HM: Incidence of treated snakebites in the United States. Public Health Rep 81:269-276, 1966.
3. Norris RL, Bush SP: North American venomous reptile bites. In Auerbach PS (ed): Wilderness Medicine: Management of Wilderness and Environmental Emergencies, 4th ed. St Louis, Mosby–Year Book, 2001, pp 896-926.
4. Gold BS, Wingert WA: Snake venom poisoning in the United States: A review of therapeutic practice. South Med J 87:579-589, 1994.
5. Ownby CL: Pathology of rattlesnake envenomation. In Tu AT (ed): Rattlesnake Venoms. New York, Marcel Dekker, 1982, pp 164-169.
6. Russell FE: Snake Venom Poisoning. New York, Scholium International, 1983.
7. Hutton RA, Warrell DA: Action of snake venom components on the haemostatic system. Blood Rev 7:176-189, 1993.
8. Russell FE, Carlson RW, Wainschel J, et al: Snake venom poisoning in the United States: Experiences with 550 cases. JAMA 233:341-344, 1975.
9. Wingert WA, Chan L: Rattlesnake bites in southern California and rationale for recommended treatment. West J Med 148:37-44, 1988.
10. German BT, Hack JB, Brewer K, Meggs WJ: Pressure-immobilization bandages delay toxicity in a porcine model of eastern coral snake *(Micrurus fulvius fulvius)* envenomation. Ann Emerg Med 45:603-608, 2005.
11. Consroe P, Egen NB, Russell FE, et al: Comparison of a new ovine antigen binding fragment (Fab) antivenin for United States Crotalidae with the commercial antivenin for protection against venom-induced lethality in mice. Am J Trop Med Hyg 53:507-510, 1995.
12. Dart RC, Seifert SA, Carroll L, et al: Affinity-purified, mixed monospecific crotalid antivenom ovine Fab for the treatment of crotalid venom poisoning. Ann Emerg Med 30:33-39, 1997.
13. Gold BS, Dart RC, Barish RA: Bites of venomous snakes. N Engl J Med 347:347-356, 2002.
14. Clark RF, Selden BS, Furbee B: The incidence of wound infection following crotalid envenomation. J Emerg Med 11:583-586, 1993.
15. Kerrigan KR, Mertz BL, Nelson SJ, et al: Antibiotic prophylaxis for pit viper envenomation: Prospective, controlled trial. World J Surg 21:369-373, 1997.
16. Burgess JL, Dart RC: Snake venom coagulopathy: Use and abuse of blood products in the treatment of pit viper envenomation. Ann Emerg Med 20:795-801, 1991.
17. Bogdan GM, Dart RC, Falbo SC, et al: Recurrent coagulopathy after antivenom treatment of crotalid snakebite. South Med J 93:562-566, 2000.
18. Vigasio A, Battiston B, De Filippo G, et al: Compartmental syndrome due to viper bite. Arch Orthop Trauma Surg 110:175-177, 1991.
19. Garfin SR, Castilonia RR, Mubarak SJ, et al: Role of surgical decompression in treatment of rattlesnake bites. Surg Forum 30:502-504, 1979.
20. Tanen DA, Danish DC, Grice GA, et al: Fasciotomy worsens the amount of myonecrosis in a porcine model of crotaline envenomation. Ann Emerg Med 44:99-104, 2004.
21. Keogh S, Callaham ML: Bites and injuries inflicted by domestic animals. In Auerbach PS (ed): Wilderness Medicine: Management of Wilderness and Environmental Emergencies, 4th ed. St Louis, Mosby–Year Book, 2001, pp 961-978.
22. Centers for Disease Control and Prevention (CDC): Nonfatal dog bite–related injuries treated in hospital emergency department—United States, 2001. MMWR Morb Mortal Wkly Rep 52(26):605-610, 2003.
23. Chen E, Hornig S, Shepherd SM, et al: Primary closure of mammalian bites. Acad Emerg Med 7:157-161, 2000.
24. Stefanopoulos PK, Tarantzopoulou AD: Facial bite wounds: Management update. Int J Oral Maxillofac Surg 34:464-472, 2005.
25. Callaham M: Prophylactic antibiotics in common dog bite wounds: A controlled study. Ann Emerg Med 9:410-414, 1980.
26. Perron AD, Miller MD, Brady WJ: Orthopedic pitfalls in the ED: Fight bite. Am J Emerg Med 20:114-117, 2002.
27. Talan DA, Citron DM, Abrahamian FM, et al: Bacteriologic analysis of infected dog and cat bites. Emergency Medicine Animal Bite Infection Study Group. N Engl J Med 340:85-92, 1999.
28. Broder J, Jerrard D, Olshaker J, et al: Low risk of infection in selected human bites treated without antibiotics. Am J Emerg Med 22:10-13, 2004.
29. Vidmar L, Poljak M, Tomazic J, et al: Transmission of HIV-1 by human bite. Lancet 347:1762, 1996.
30. World Health Organization: Rabies surveillance and control—The world survey of rabies No. 35 for the year 1999. Geneva, World Health Organization, 2002. Available at http://www.who.int/rabies/resources/wsr1999/en/. Accessed March 23, 2006.
31. Krebs JW, Wheeling JT, Childs JE: Rabies surveillance in the United States during 2002. J Am Vet Med Assoc 223:1736-1748, 2003.
32. Moran GJ, Talan DA, Mower W, et al: Appropriateness of rabies postexposure prophylaxis treatment for animal exposures. Emergency ID Net Study Group. JAMA 284:1001-1007, 2000.
33. Hankins DG, Rosekrans JA: Overview, prevention, and treatment of rabies. Mayo Clin Proc 79:671-676, 2004.
34. Human rabies prevention—United States, 1999. Recommendations of the Advisory Committee on Immunization Practices (ACIP). MMWR Recomm Rep 48(RR-1):1-21, 1999.

35. Boyer LV, McNally JT, Binford GJ: Spider bites. In Auerbach PS (ed): Wilderness Medicine: Management of Wilderness and Environmental Emergencies, 4th ed. St Louis, Mosby–Year Book, 2001, pp 807-838.

36. Wilson DC, King LE Jr: Spiders and spider bites. Dermatol Clin North Am 8:277-286, 1990.

37. Clark RF, Wethern-Kestner S, Vance MV, et al: Clinical presentation and treatment of black widow spider envenomation: A review of 163 cases. Ann Emerg Med 21:782-787, 1992.

38. Wong RC, Hughes SE, Voorhees JJ: Spider bites. Arch Dermatol 123:98-104, 1987.

39. Isbister GK, Graudins A, White J, Warrell D: Antivenom treatment in arachnidism. J Toxicol Clin Toxicol 41:291-300, 2003.

40. Futrell JM: Loxoscelism. Am J Med Sci 304:261-267, 1992.

41. Smith CW, Micks DW: The role of polymorphonuclear leukocytes in the lesion caused by the venom of the brown spider, *Loxosceles reclusa*. Lab Invest 22:90-93, 1970.

42. Sams HH, Dunnick CA, Smith ML, et al: Necrotic arachnidism. J Am Acad Dermatol 44:561-573; quiz 573-576, 2001.

43. Swanson DL, Vetter RS: Bites of brown recluse spiders and suspected necrotic arachnidism. N Engl J Med 352:700-707, 2005.

44. Ingber A, Trattner A, Cleper R, et al: Morbidity of brown recluse spider bites: Clinical picture, treatment, and prognosis. Acta Derm Venereol 71:337-340, 1991.

45. King LE Jr, Rees RS: Dapsone treatment of a brown recluse bite. JAMA 250:648, 1983.

46. Tutrone WD, Green KM, Norris T, et al: Brown recluse spider envenomation: Dermatologic application of hyperbaric oxygen therapy. J Drugs Dermatol 4:424-428, 2005.

47. Watson WA, Litovitz TL, Rodgers GC, et al: 2004 Annual report of the American Association of Poison Control Centers Toxic Exposure Surveillance System. Am J Emerg Med 23:589-666, 2005.

48. Simard JM, Watt DD: Venoms and toxins. In Polis GA (ed): The Biology of Scorpions. Stanford, CA, Stanford University Press, 1990, pp 414-444.

49. LoVecchio F, McBride C: Scorpion envenomations in young children in central Arizona. J Toxicol Clin Toxicol 41:937-940, 2003.

50. Connor DA, Seldon BS: Scorpion envenomations. In Auerbach PS (ed): Wilderness Medicine: Management of Wilderness and Environmental Emergencies, 3rd ed. St Louis, Mosby–Year Book, 1995, pp 831-842.

51. Gateau T, Bloom M, Clark R: Response to specific *Centruroides sculpturatus* antivenom in 151 cases of scorpion stings. J Toxicol Clin Toxicol 32:165-171, 1994.

52. Stewart RL, Burgdorfer W, Needham GR: Evaluation of three commercial tick removal tools. Wild Environ Med 9:137-142, 1998.

53. Celenza A, Rogers IR: The "knot method" of tick removal. Wild Environ Med 13:179-180, 2002.

54. Metry DW, Hebert AA: Insect and arachnid stings, bites, infestations, and repellents. Pediatr Annu 29:39-48, 2000.

55. Montiel NJ, Baumgarten JM, Sinha AA: Lyme disease: II. Clinical features and treatment. Cutis 69:443-448, 2002.

56. Steere AC: Lyme disease. N Engl J Med 345:115-125, 2001.

57. Shapiro ED, Gerber MA: Lyme disease. Clin Infect Dis 31:533-542, 2000.

58. Steere AC: A 58-year-old man with a diagnosis of chronic Lyme disease. JAMA 288:1002-1010, 2002.

59. Wilske B: Epidemiology and diagnosis of Lyme borreliosis. Ann Med 37:568-579, 2005.

60. Depietropaolo DL, Powers JH, Gill JM, Foy AJ: Diagnosis of Lyme disease. Am Fam Physician 72:297-304, 309, 2005.

61. Dinser R, Jendro MC, Schnarr S, Zeidler H: Antibiotic treatment of Lyme borreliosis: What is the evidence? Ann Rheum Dis 64:519-523, 2005.

62. Nadelman RB, Nowakowski J, Fish D, et al, for the Tick Bite Study Group: Prophylaxis with single-dose doxycycline for the prevention of Lyme disease after an *Ixodes scapularis* tick bite. N Engl J Med 345:79-84, 2001.

63. Wright DN, Lockey RF: Local reactions to stinging insects (Hymenoptera). Allergy Proc 11:23-28, 1990.

64. Reisman RE: Stinging insect allergy. Med Clin North Am 76:883-894, 1992.

65. Reisman RE: Insect stings. N Engl J Med 331:523-527, 1994.

66. Reisman RE: Unusual reactions to insect venoms. Allergy Proc 12:395-399, 1991.

67. Visscher PK, Vetter RS, Camazine S: Removing bee stings. Lancet 348:301-302, 1996.

68. Freeman TM: Clinical practice. Hypersensitivity to hymenoptera stings. N Engl J Med 351:1978-1984, 2004.

69. Auerbach PS, Halstead BW: Injuries from nonvenomous aquatic animals. In Auerbach PS (ed): Wilderness Medicine: Management of Wilderness and Environmental Emergencies, 4th ed. St Louis, Mosby–Year Book, 2001, pp 1418-1449.

70. Williamson JA, Fenner PJ, Burnett JW (eds): Venomous and Poisonous Marine Animals. Sydney, Australia, University of New South Wales Press, 1996.

71. Morris JG, Tenney JH, Drusano GL: In vitro susceptibility of pathogenic *Vibrio* species to norfloxacin and six other antimicrobial agents. Antimicrob Agents Chemother 28:442-445, 1985.

72. Qadri SM, Lee G, Brodie L: Antibacterial activity of norfloxacin against 1700 relatively resistant clinical isolates. Drugs Exp Clin Res 15:349-353, 1989.

73. Howard RJ, Burgess GH: Surgical hazards posed by marine and freshwater animals in Florida. Am J Surg 166:563-567, 1993.

74. Barber GR, Swygert JS: Necrotizing fasciitis due to *Photobacterium damsela* in a man lashed by a stingray. N Engl J Med 342:824, 2000.

75. Guidera KJ, Ogden JA, Highhouse K, et al: Shark attack: A case study of the injury and treatment. J Orthop Trauma 5:204-208, 1991.

76. McGoldrick J, Marx JA: Marine envenomations: II. Invertebrates. J Emerg Med 10:71-77, 1992.

77. Little M: Is there a role for the use of pressure immobilization bandages in the treatment of jellyfish envenomation in Australia? Emerg Med (Fremantle) 14:171-174, 2002.

78. Cooper MNK: Stone fish and stingrays—some notes on the injuries that they cause to man. J R Army Med Corps 137:136-140, 1991.

79. McGoldrick J, Marx JA: Marine envenomations: I. Vertebrates. J Emerg Med 9:497-502, 1991.

80. Auerbach PS: Envenomation by aquatic vertebrates. In Auerbach PS (ed): Wilderness Medicine: Management of Wilderness and Environmental Emergencies, 4th ed. St Louis, Mosby–Year Book, 2001, pp 1488-1505.

Surgical Critical Care

Charles A. Adams, Jr., MD   Walter L. Biffl, MD   and   William G. Cioffi, MD

Central Nervous System
Cardiovascular System
Respiratory System
Gastrointestinal System
Acute Renal Failure
Hepatic Dysfunction
Endocrine System
Hematologic System
Sepsis and Multiple Organ Failure

For most surgical patients, there is a reasonable expectation of return to their premorbid state of health and function after surgical therapy. However, in a subset of patients the illness or injury is so severe or extensive that without specialized supportive care, they would surely die. This level of care falls into the category of critical care and is typically delivered by specialized teams of trained health care providers in an intensive care unit (ICU). Although many of these ICUs are closed units or structured so that patient management decisions are made by the critical care team, it is important that surgeons remain up to date and be acquainted with the ever-changing field of critical care so that they can be a vital part of the patient's health care team, especially when critical care is being delivered by nonsurgical specialists. This chapter approaches the vast topic of critical care in an organ system fashion and highlights recent developments and concepts.

CENTRAL NERVOUS SYSTEM

Neurologic Dysfunction

The central nervous system (CNS) is the most complex and specialized organ system in the body and, as such,

is vulnerable to disturbances by a whole host of conditions and factors. The etiology of altered consciousness is so broad that a clouded sensorium is the norm in the ICU rather than the exception. The list of consciousness-altering causes includes both endogenous and exogenous factors. Some endogenous causes include sepsis, CNS infections, hypoxic-ischemic encephalopathy, tumors, trauma, and metabolic conditions, whereas exogenous causes can be due to medications, environmental settings, and toxins. Unexplained changes in a patient's level of consciousness must be evaluated aggressively. The diagnosis *ICU psychosis* is considered strictly a diagnosis of exclusion. The term *altered mental status* is nonspecific; more descriptive definitions were offered by Plum and Posner more than 25 years ago and still apply today. *Confusion* refers to bewilderment, with difficulty following commands, disturbed memory, and drowsiness or nighttime agitation. *Delirium* is "a floridly abnormal mental state characterized by disorientation, fear, irritability, misperception of sensory stimuli, and often, visual hallucinations." The presence of delirium can have far-reaching consequences and is associated with increased hospital length of stay and mortality.[1] *Obtundation* is defined as mental blunting associated with slowed psychological responses to stimulation. *Stupor* is described as "a condition of deep sleep or behaviorally similar unresponsiveness in which the patient can be aroused only by vigorous and repeated stimuli." *Coma* is "a state of unarousable psychologic unresponsiveness in which the subject lies with eyes closed and shows no psychologically understandable response to external stimuli or inner need." A *vegetative state* is a state of wakefulness but with apparent total lack of cognitive function. *Death* in the presence of cardiopulmonary function (so-called brain death) refers to the absence of function of the brain and brainstem. There are specific criteria for the diagnosis of death, but the absence of cerebral function is paramount. Cortical nonfunction must be accompanied by the loss of pupillary light and corneal stimulation reflexes, loss of the vestibulo-ocular and oropharyngeal reflexes, and apnea in the presence of so-called adequate stimulation ($PaCO_2$ >60 mm Hg for 30 seconds). Generally, two clinical examinations must be documented, separated by a defined time interval (e.g., 6 hours) and confirmed by two physicians. It is important that there be a reason sufficient to cause death and no complicating conditions (e.g., sedative or anesthetic agents, hypothermia, hypoglycemia or hyperglycemia, or severe hyponatremia or hypernatremia). If such complicating conditions preclude the completion of a clinical examination with an apnea test, additional tests are required. Electroencephalography, radioisotope brain scanning, transcranial Doppler ultrasonography, and cerebral arteriography with documentation of absent cortical flow are all helpful in defining brain death, but this diagnosis must conform to the criteria set forth by each state government.

In a patient with altered neurologic status, the assessment is thorough yet rapid, with initial management and corrective measures instituted concurrently to minimize irreversible CNS damage. The patient's level of consciousness may be described as alert, responsive to verbal stimuli, responsive to painful stimuli, or unresponsive. Acute loss of consciousness (seconds to minutes) is consistent with a cerebrovascular accident or head trauma. A subacute course (many minutes to hours) may suggest intoxication, infection, or a metabolic disturbance, whereas a more prolonged course may suggest a CNS tumor. The pupillary examination can be particularly informative. Damage to the midbrain affects the reticular activating system (and thus consciousness), as well as pupil reactivity, whereas metabolic disease may produce coma but usually leaves the light reflex intact. Small reactive pupils are the hallmark of drug (particularly opiate) intoxication and metabolic disease, whereas large unreactive pupils may be associated with anticholinergic drugs, glutethimide, anoxia, or intracranial hypertension. A unilateral, fixed dilated pupil suggests third nerve dysfunction or uncal herniation. In the absence of purposeful eye movements, spontaneous roving eye movements imply intact cortical control of the brainstem. If no spontaneous eye movement is found, the cervical ocular reflex (so-called doll's eyes maneuver) is tested after excluding a cervical cord or spinal lesion. The reflex is tested by rapidly turning the head from midline to one side. Contralateral conjugate eye movement with the eyes seemingly kept fixed on a point in space suggests an intact brainstem. The head is turned in the opposite direction to check for symmetry. Failure of this reflex in either direction implies brainstem dysfunction. If this maneuver cannot be performed, the vestibulo-ocular reflex may be assessed (cold caloric testing) instead. This reflex is tested by elevating the head to 30 degrees and rapidly instilling 50 mL of ice water into the external auditory canal, which results in reflex slow eye movement toward the stimulus. In an intact brain, the frontal eye fields attempt to override this stimulus by producing rapid saccades away from the stimulus (nystagmus). Conversely, if there is cortical damage, the eyes will maintain a fixed deviation, which implies a hemispheric lesion on the side toward which the eyes deviate. Assessment of motor function helps identify the location and severity of deficits. The motor component of the Glasgow Coma Scale appears to be the most predictive portion of the scale after head trauma. Asymmetry of motor function suggests a focal cerebral lesion contralateral to the deficit. Decorticate posturing (flexion of the arms and extension of the legs) and decerebrate posturing (extension of both the arms and legs) are poor prognostic signs.

Laboratory studies can help identify metabolic derangements such as hypothyroidism, electrolyte abnormalities, infections, and ingestion of toxic substances. Urine toxicology screening is mandatory because drug intoxication is one of the most common causes of coma of unknown etiology. Arterial blood gas (ABG) analysis is performed to rule out hypoxia, hypercapnia, or acidosis as a cause of an altered mental state. Computed tomography (CT) is indicated in any patient with coma or focal neurologic findings and patients with a depressed level of consciousness preventing adequate physical examination. A lumbar puncture is performed on any patient for whom the cause of coma is still unknown, as well as in patients in whom meningitis, encephalitis, or occult subarachnoid hemorrhage is suspected. In a post–head injury or neurosurgical postoperative patient, clinical deterioration in the absence of a new structural lesion (i.e., CT scan finding), coupled with signs of infection (fever, leukocytosis, etc.), may be a sign of CNS infection, and therefore a lumbar puncture is warranted.

Initial management begins with assurance of a patent *a*irway and adequate *b*reathing and *c*irculation (the "ABCs" as taught in the advanced trauma life support program). Comatose patients are intubated for airway protection; however, stability of the cervical spine must be ensured in trauma patients. If there is a possibility of increased intracranial pressure (ICP), lidocaine (1.5 mg/kg) or thiopental (3-5 mg/kg) is administered to blunt the spike in ICP associated with intubation. Hypotension is corrected with fluids, vasopressors, or both. A dose of 50 mL of 50% dextrose is given immediately to any patient in coma of unknown etiology. Dextrose will produce no detrimental effect on any causes of coma except Wernicke's encephalopathy (see later) and will correct the underlying problem if it is secondary to hypoglycemia. Even in patients with hyperglycemia producing coma, a marginal increase in glucose concentration will not adversely affect the patient. In alcoholic patients or others with poor general nutrition, thiamine (1 mg/kg) is administered before glucose. Administration of thiamine may avoid acute Wernicke's encephalopathy (confusion, ataxia, ophthalmoplegia) and its associated necrosis of midline gray matter. Narcotic overdose is a common cause of coma and is marked by shallow respirations, small reactive pupils, and hypotension. Naloxone (Narcan) (0.4-2 mg) is an opioid antagonist and is given to patients with suspected opiate-induced coma. Flumazenil (0.2 mg) may be administered for suspected benzodiazepine intoxication; however, care is exercised in patients taking benzodiazepines on a chronic basis or suspected of mixed ingestion because other agents may lower the seizure threshold and lead to severe seizures after the administration of flumazenil. Activated charcoal (25-50 mg) is given for the ingestion of most drugs and toxins, but its effectiveness diminishes as the interval from ingestion to administration increases. Empirical antibiotic therapy directed at suspected demographically associated pathogens is warranted if bacterial meningitis is suspected.

If increased ICP is assumed to be the cause of coma, treatment is initiated immediately by elevating the head of the bed to 30 to 45 degrees. Hyperventilation is effective in lowering ICP, but prolonged or extreme hyperventilation can lead to cerebral vasoconstriction and detrimental regional ischemia. Thus, a target $PaCO_2$ of 35 to 40 mm Hg is optimal. Vasogenic cerebral edema leads to increased ICP under the Monro-Kellie doctrine, which states that the pressure inside the head must rise if any intracranial component increases (i.e., blood, brain, or cerebrospinal fluid) because the cranial vault is a rigid, nonexpansive structure. Accordingly, the osmotic diuretic mannitol (0.5-1 g/kg) is administered and may be repeated every 4 to 6 hours as long as the serum sodium level and osmolarity remain less than 155 mEq/L and 320 mosmol/kg, respectively. Other factors involved in managing ICP include adequate sedation and suppression of fever and seizures. If the patient has refractory intracranial hypertension, second-tier therapies are used, such as ventriculostomy drainage, neuromuscular blockade, barbiturate coma, vasopressors to increase cerebral perfusion pressure, and decompressive craniectomy.

Seizure activity is often the first sign of a CNS complication. Because the majority of seizures terminate rapidly, the most important initial intervention is protecting the patient from harm. The cause of the seizures is investigated and treated. CT scanning or magnetic resonance imaging (MRI) of the brain is indicated for new-onset seizures, and electroencephalograms are obtained to exclude status epilepticus in patients who have persistent or recurrent seizures or do not awaken after seizure activity. Status epilepticus is treated with benzodiazepines, such as lorazepam (0.1 mg/kg), followed by phenytoin (1 g). If this regimen is unsuccessful in breaking the seizure activity, second-tier therapies are administered, such as high-dose benzodiazepines or barbiturates or propofol. The major systemic complications of seizures are rhabdomyolysis, hyperthermia, and cerebral edema.

Analgesia, Sedation, and Neuromuscular Blockade

Pain and anxiety are commonplace in ICU patients. Pain may be due to an underlying disease state, trauma, invasive procedures, or surgical wounds. Pain is exacerbated by nursing interventions, invasive monitoring, therapeutic devices, immobility, and mechanical ventilation. Unrelieved pain can provoke a sympathetic stress response, as well as contribute to agitation and metabolic stress. Unfortunately, the severity of pain is often underappreciated in the ICU and consequently treated suboptimally. A universal goal for practitioners is to ensure an optimal level of comfort and safety for all patients.

Pain Assessment and Management

Perception of pain is influenced by previous experiences, negative expectations, and the cognitive capacity of the patient. The patient and family need to be advised of the potential for pain and strategies to communicate pain. Patient self-reporting is the gold standard for the assessment of pain and adequacy of analgesia. Pain assessment tools such as the visual analog scale or numeric rating scale are most useful. In noncommunicative patients, assessment of behavioral (movements, facial expressions, posturing) and physiologic (heart rate [HR], blood pressure, respiratory rate) indicators is necessary.

Opiates are the mainstay of pain management in the ICU. Nonpharmacologic interventions such as a providing a comfortable environment, paying attention to positioning and the arrangement of tubing and drains, and avoiding unnecessary noise are used as adjuncts to pain management. Opiates are particularly useful in the ICU because they have a rapid onset of action, are easily titrated, lack an accumulation of parent drug or active metabolites, and are relatively inexpensive. The most commonly prescribed opiates are morphine, fentanyl, and hydromorphone. Fentanyl has a rapid onset of action and a short half-life and generates no active metabolites. It is ideal for use in hemodynamically unstable patients because it does not cause release of histamine and its resultant vasodilation, which can worsen hypotension. Continuous infusions of fentanyl have been associated with accumulation in lipid stores and thus a prolonged effect, and high doses have been associated with muscle rigidity syndromes. Morphine has a slower onset of action and longer half-life and may not be suitable for hemodynamically unstable patients because of its potential to cause release of histamine and hypotension. This histaminergic effect is also responsible for morphine's propensity to cause pruritus. An active metabolite of morphine, morphine-6-glucuronide, can accumulate in patients with renal insufficiency and lead to undesirable effects. Morphine also causes spasm of the sphincter of Oddi, which may be detrimental in patients with biliary tract disease. Hydromorphone has a half-life similar to morphine, but it generates no active metabolites and does not cause histamine release. It is typically used when high-dose morphine or fentanyl is ineffective or in patients in whom a large fluid volume is undesirable. To some extent, all opioid analgesics are associated with varying degrees of respiratory depression, hypotension, and ileus.

Preventing pain is more effective than treating established pain. Accordingly, continuous or scheduled intermittent dosing is preferable to "as needed" administration. Patient-controlled analgesia (PCA) via specialized infusion pumps is becoming extremely popular and may offer superior pain control but requires patients to be active participants in their care, which may not always be possible. PCA can decrease opioid consumption, oversedation, and other adverse effects while providing good pain control. To avoid variable absorption, analgesics are given intravenously (IV) to critically ill patients. Alternatives to opioids include acetaminophen and nonsteroidal anti-inflammatory drugs (NSAIDs). Ketorolac is the prototypical IV NSAID and is an effective analgesic agent used alone or in combination with opiates. It is primarily eliminated by renal excretion, so it is relatively contraindicated in patients with renal insufficiency, and it has been associated with bleeding complications, so its use in fresh postoperative patients must be carefully considered.

Epidural anesthesia is achieved by delivering drugs via a catheter placed in the extradural or epidural space. Many benefits of epidural anesthesia have been reported, including better suppression of surgical stress and pain, minimized hemodynamic effects, improved peripheral circulation, and reduced blood loss. A prospective, randomized study of 1021 abdominal surgery patients demonstrated that epidural opioid analgesia provides better postoperative pain relief than parenteral opioids do.[2] Furthermore, in patients undergoing abdominal aortic operations, overall morbidity and mortality were improved, and intubation time and ICU length of stay were shorter. Patient-controlled epidural anesthesia is also possible and combines many of the benefits of both PCA and epidural anesthesia.

Sedation

Inability to communicate, constant noise and light, disrupted sleep-wake cycles, and immobility contribute to increased anxiety in ICU patients, which may be compounded further by mechanical ventilation. Sedation is necessary to alleviate anxiety and provide comfort, as well as prevent the patient from removing lines, catheters, and other crucial devices. A predetermined sedation goal needs to be established, and the level of sedation is documented objectively according to a sedation scale such as the Richmond Agitation and Sedation Scale (RASS) (Table 24-1). The RASS is a rapid, simple construct that has been shown to detect changes in sedation in ICU patients over several days and facilitates the proper administration of analgesic and sedative medications.[3]

The ideal level of sedation depends on the clinical situation, but a patient who is calm and easily arousable is appropriately sedated. Benzodiazepines have both sedative and hypnotic effects, and some possess partial anterograde amnestic effects. They may potentiate opiates and moderate the pain response when used in combination with them; however, they are devoid of any analgesic properties. Diazepam, lorazepam, and midazolam are the most frequently used agents in the ICU. Diazepam has a short onset of action and short half-life, but its long-acting metabolite may accumulate after repetitive dosing. Lorazepam has a slow onset and intermediate half-life, thus making it most useful for medium- to long-term sedation. Lorazepam can accumulate in elderly patients with hepatic and renal dysfunction and result in prolonged sedation. Midazolam is a rapid-onset, short-acting drug with amnestic properties and thus is the agent of choice for acutely agitated patients. Prolonged sedation with midazolam results in accumulation of the agent and erratic effects and metabolism.

Propofol is a general anesthetic agent with significant sedative and hypnotic properties, but no analgesic effect. Propofol has a rapid onset and an ultrashort duration of action. Its phospholipid vehicle can cause hypertriglyceridemia and pancreatitis, as well as pain on injection. Propofol is most often used for the sedation of neurosurgical patients because it allows rapid awakening for

Table 24-1 Richmond Agitation Sedation Scale

SCORE	TERM	DESCRIPTION
+4	Combative	Overly combative or violent. Immediate danger to staff
+3	Very agitated	Pulls/removes tubes or catheters. Has aggressive behavior toward staff
+2	Agitated	Frequent nonpurposeful movement. Patient-ventilator dyssynchrony
+1	Restless	Anxious or apprehensive but movements not aggressive or vigorous
0	Alert and calm	
−1	Drowsy	Not fully alert, but has sustained (>10 sec) awakening with eye contact to voice
−2	Light sedation	Briefly (<10 sec) awakens with eye contact to voice
−3	Moderate sedation	Any movement (but no eye contact) to voice
−4	Deep sedation	No response to voice, but any movement to physical stimulation
−5	Unarousable	No response to voice or physical stimulation

Adapted from Ely EW, Truman B, Shintani A, et al: Monitoring sedation status over time in ICU patients: Reliability and validity of the Richmond Agitation Sedation Scale (RASS). JAMA 289:2983-2991, 2003.

neurologic assessment and may decrease cerebral metabolism and reduce ICP. The main disadvantages of prolonged use are its high cost and dose-related hypotension. Figure 24-1 is an algorithm for the provision of analgesia and sedation in the ICU.[4]

Neuromuscular Blockade

Skeletal muscle relaxation may be warranted to minimize O_2 consumption or facilitate patient-ventilator synchrony, particularly when using nonconventional modes of ventilation such as inverse ratio ventilation or prone positioning. There are two major categories of neuromuscular blockers (NMBs). Depolarizing NMBs mimic acetylcholine (ACh) by binding ACh receptors of the motor end plate and causing depolarization of the muscle, which is seen clinically as muscle fasciculations. Succinylcholine, the only depolarizing NMB available for use, is characterized by a rapid onset and a short half-life. It is most commonly used as the paralytic of choice for rapid-sequence intubation and may be useful for short invasive procedures. Succinylcholine is degraded by plasma pseudocholinesterase and has a very short half-life, but in patients with a deficiency of this enzyme, prolonged effects can occur. Side effects of succinylcholine include muscle pain, rhabdomyolysis, ocular hypertension, malignant hyperthermia, and hyperkalemia. Patients with

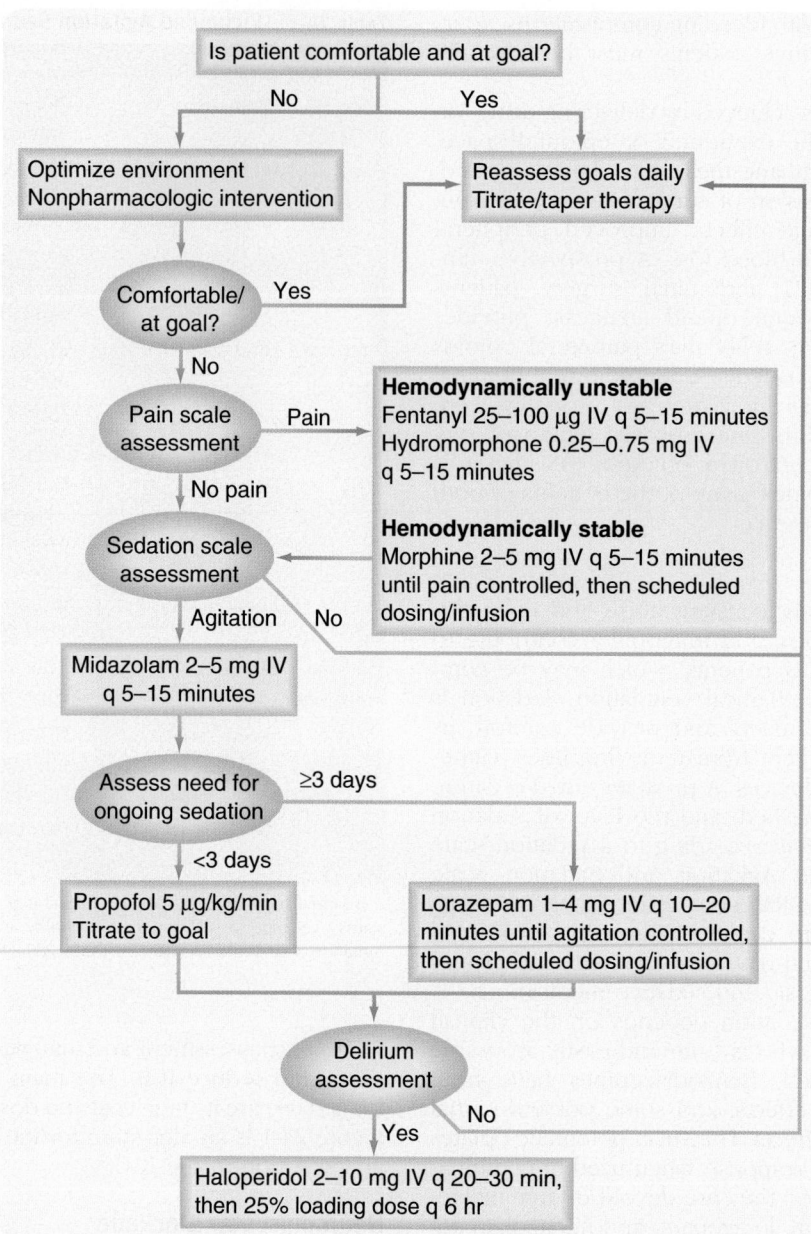

Figure 24-1 Algorithm for analgesia and sedation in the intensive care unit. (Adapted from Jacobi J, Fraser GL, Coursin DB, et al: Clinical practice guidelines for the sustained use of sedatives and analgesics in the critically ill adult. Crit Care Med 30:119-141, 2002.)

spinal cord injuries, large burns, upper and lower motor neuron disease, renal failure, or prolonged immobility are at particular risk for hyperkalemia and resultant cardiac dysrhythmias.

The nondepolarizing NMBs bind ACh receptors but do not activate them, thus blocking the receptor and inhibiting its function. There are two types of nondepolarizing NMBs: steroidal and nonsteroidal. The aminosteroidal compounds include agents such as rocuronium, vecuronium, and pancuronium. Rocuronium has a rapid onset of action and intermediate duration of action, which makes it useful for short procedures, as well as

prolonged relaxation. Vecuronium is an intermediate-acting agent; it achieves neuromuscular blockade within 1 to 2 minutes and lasts about 30 minutes, but it too can be infused continuously. Patients with renal or hepatic dysfunction may have a prolonged response because vecuronium is cleared by both the kidney and liver. Pancuronium is long acting (up to 90 minutes) and relatively contraindicated in patients with coronary artery disease because its associated vagolytic effect causes pronounced tachycardia. Like vecuronium, pancuronium is eliminated by both the kidney and liver and requires dose adjustments in the setting of renal or hepatic dys-

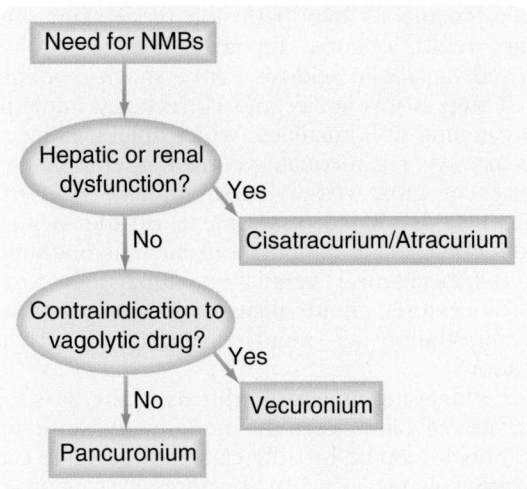

Figure 24-2 Algorithm for neuromuscular blockade (NMB) in the intensive care unit. (Adapted from Murray MJ, Cowen J, DeBlock H, et al: Clinical practice guidelines for sustained neuromuscular blockade in the adult critically ill patient. Crit Care Med 30:141-156, 2002.)

function. The nonsteroidal, nondepolarizing NMBs, or benzylisoquinolonium compounds, include atracurium, cisatracurium, tubocurarine, and mivacurium. Of these, atracurium and cisatracurium are the two agents most commonly used in the ICU. Atracurium is intermediate acting with minimal cardiovascular effects, but it does have the tendency to promote histamine release. Because it is metabolized by plasma ester hydrolysis and undergoes spontaneous degradation, it is most useful in patients with hepatic and renal dysfunction. A metabolite of atracurium may precipitate seizure activity if used at extremely high doses. Cisatracurium is an isomer of atracurium, with fewer tendencies to induce release of histamine. Like atracurium, elimination is by ester hydrolysis and Hoffman elimination. An algorithm for the provision of neuromuscular blockade in the ICU is outlined in Figure 24-2.

Monitoring of neuromuscular blockade is accomplished by train-of-four testing, with one to two twitches being considered the optimal depth. It is important to remember that in paralyzed patients, assessment of adequate analgesia and sedation is extremely difficult, and patients must be presumptively medicated. Bispectral index monitoring is a form of electroencephalomyography that helps determine the level of awareness in a paralyzed patient so that the level of sedation can be optimized. Prolonged recovery from paralysis is associated with the steroidal NMBs, and critical illness myopathy syndromes have been reported in patients receiving NMBs and corticosteroids. Though not seemingly related to specific NMB agents, prolonged exposure to NMBs appears to be the key risk factor. Consequently, patients undergo daily medication withdrawal to allow some muscle activity and reassess the need for NMBs.[5]

CARDIOVASCULAR SYSTEM

Hemodynamic Monitoring

Arterial Catheters
Placement of an arterial catheter is indicated if vasoactive drugs are being administered, continuous monitoring of systemic arterial pressure is required, or frequent ABGs or blood samples are going to be tested. The primary complications associated with arterial catheters are infections and arterial thrombosis. The risk for infection associated with an arterial catheter is much lower than with a central venous catheter, but arterial catheters must still be placed under sterile conditions. Thrombosis with distal ischemia can be minimized by placing catheters in arteries with good collateral circulation. Thus, the radial or dorsalis pedis arteries are preferred over the brachial or femoral arteries. An Allen test is performed before placement of a radial artery catheter to document adequate collateral flow from the ulnar artery.

Stiffness and resistance of a catheter and measuring system, catheter whip, and the distance from the heart all contribute to variance between the actual and measured systolic (SBP) and diastolic (DBP) blood pressure. Thus, mean arterial pressure (MAP) is the most accurate measurement obtained and can be determined by using the formula

$$MAP = DBP + \frac{1}{3}(SBP - DBP)$$

Central Venous Catheters
Placement of a central venous catheter may be indicated for long-term venous access, administration of parenteral nutrition or chemotherapeutic agents, or measurement of central venous pressure (CVP). The most common complications associated with the insertion of central venous catheters include dysrhythmias, pneumothorax (up to 5% after subclavian vein placement), arterial puncture with a resultant intimal flap, pseudoaneurysm formation, hemorrhage or arteriovenous fistulization, and air or catheter embolism. These complications represent technical errors, which emphasizes the importance of knowledge of anatomy and proper insertion techniques.

Measurement of CVP can be helpful in assessing right heart function, but it is important to remember that right-sided heart function is an unreliable predictor of left-sided heart function in critically ill patients. In mechanically ventilated patients, intracardiac pressure is increased during the inspiratory phase, whereas end-expiratory pressure is typically the lowest pressure recorded. Conversely, during spontaneous respiration, intracardiac pressure falls as negative intrathoracic pressure is generated; thus, end-expiratory pressure is typically the highest pressure recorded. Measurements are made at end expiration because it is relatively independent of ventilatory status. If more information is desired or if the patient's clinical status or response to therapy seems incongruous, a pulmonary arterial catheter (PAC) may be useful.

Pulmonary Arterial Catheters
PACs allow direct measurement of CVP, right atrial pressure, pulmonary arterial pressure, right ventricular

end-diastolic pressure, pulmonary artery wedge pressure (PAWP), and mixed venous oxygen saturation ($S\bar{v}O_2$), as well as indirect calculations of left heart filling pressure and cardiac output (CO). Insertion of a PAC is warranted in any patient with severe cardiopulmonary derangement and is most useful in guiding therapy by repeated monitoring of hemodynamic parameters rather than making a primary diagnosis. It provides information about volume status and cardiac performance and helps determine the need for volume, inotropic support, and vasoactive drugs. Complications related to PAC placement include those associated with central venous catheter placement, plus arrhythmias, conduction defects, pulmonary infarction, pulmonary artery rupture, valvular damage, and knotting or catheter entrapment. Pulmonary artery rupture, probably the most feared complication, has been reported to occur as a result of distal catheter positioning and rapid balloon inflation or in the setting of noncompliant pulmonary vessels (i.e., pulmonary hypertension). Prophylactic lidocaine may help prevent dysrhythmias in patients with irritable myocardium. Floating a PAC in a patient with left heart block can be particularly hazardous because the catheter may interfere with conduction in the right bundle and result in a complete heart block. This is particularly problematic in patients with new-onset left heart block. Atropine and a pacemaker are immediately available, and the risk-benefit ratio of PAC insertion are re-evaluated.

Placement of a PAC relies on correct interpretation of pressure tracings from the distal catheter transducer. The catheter is inserted between 15 and 20 cm and the balloon inflated. Passage into the right ventricle is usually obvious because it is accompanied by wide excursions in the pressure tracing. As the catheter is continuously advanced, exit into the pulmonary artery is heralded by much higher diastolic pressure, with gradually decreasing pressure waves during diastole and an obvious dicrotic notch. A dampened waveform usually signals the wedge position. The catheter is incrementally moved back to achieve minimum insertion and acquire a proper wedge tracing. A chest radiograph is used to confirm position of the catheter in the pulmonary arterial trunk and to look for complications of central venous access if the PAC was inserted through a freshly placed introducer sheath.

Cardiovascular Dysfunction

Shock
Shock is simply defined as perfusion that is inadequate to meet the body's metabolic needs. Management of a patient in shock is focused on the following:

1. Identifying the presence of shock
2. Searching for and treating immediately life-threatening conditions
3. Treating shock based on the underlying pathophysiology (Chapter 5)

Shock is commonly manifested as hypotension, but it is important to recognize that it can exist in patients with normal blood pressure. Other signs of shock may include tachycardia, bradycardia, tachypnea, mental status changes, cutaneous hypoperfusion (cool skin, sluggish capillary refill), oliguria, myocardial ischemia, hypoxemia, and metabolic acidosis. Once shock is identified, the first step is to identify and correct any immediately life-threatening abnormalities, which might include loss of the airway or inadequate ventilation, compression of the heart or great vessels, dysrhythmias, hemorrhage, or anaphylaxis. Rapid assessment of the ABCs can help direct lifesaving interventions such as endotracheal intubation/mechanical ventilation, tube thoracostomy, pericardiocentesis, fluid resuscitation or transfusion, or administration of antidysrhythmic or vasoactive medications.

After addressing immediate threats to life, it is important to identify and treat the underlying cause of the shock. Shock may be broadly classified into five categories: hypovolemic, cardiac compressive, neurogenic, septic, and cardiogenic. Hypovolemic shock may be due to third-spacing of fluid, gastrointestinal or insensible losses, or hemorrhage. Hypovolemic shock secondary to acute blood loss is typically called *hemorrhagic shock*. A crystalloid bolus (20 mL/kg) is administered immediately and repeated if necessary. In addition to its therapeutic benefit, the response to fluid may help confirm the assessment of hypovolemia. Glucose-containing fluids are avoided because they may stimulate osmotic diuresis. If hemorrhage is suspected and the hemodynamic response to crystalloid is not satisfactory, blood transfusion is initiated without delay and a search for the source of hemorrhage aggressively undertaken. The rapidity of resuscitation is predicated on the patient's condition: restoration of normal blood pressure, HR, skin color, mentation, and urine output signifies a reversal of hypoperfusion. The need for continued resuscitation may be estimated by additional measurements (see End Points of Resuscitation later). In the setting of hemorrhagic shock or ongoing bleeding, it is prudent to restore hemoglobin (Hb) to nearly normal levels in the acute phase.

Cardiac/great vessel compressive shock may be due to tension pneumothorax or massive hemothorax, which can impede venous return by shifting the mediastinum, or pericardial tamponade, which prohibits cardiac diastolic filling. Tube thoracostomy relieves the mediastinal shift associated with tension pneumothorax or hemothorax, and it may provide definitive management of the problem. Pericardial tamponade may be due to blood, transudative fluid, or air in the pericardium. A hemodynamically unstable patient with pericardial tamponade undergoes immediate decompression via either thoracotomy or pericardiocentesis. The latter may be performed under ultrasound guidance and a catheter left in place with a stopcock to allow intermittent drainage while transporting the patient for definitive management (thoracotomy or pericardial window). The appearance of hemodynamic stability must be interpreted with caution, however, because ongoing subendocardial ischemia may compromise long-term recovery from the insult. Thus, confirmation of pericardial tamponade calls for action (fluid resuscitation and plans for decompression) without delay. Neurogenic shock is typically seen in the setting of a spinal cord injury resulting in loss of vasomotor tone.

Treatment is judicious fluid administration, with α-adrenergic vasopressors as needed. Other causes of shock such as hemorrhage are aggressively sought because in the acute setting, neurogenic shock is considered a diagnosis of exclusion.

Septic shock represents cardiovascular collapse associated with an infectious process and is the final stage on the continuum from systemic inflammatory response syndrome (SIRS) to sepsis and septic shock. Management of septic shock involves treatment of the underlying infectious process (source control), administration of appropriate antibiotics (see Sepsis later), and volume resuscitation. Cardiogenic shock refers to primary pump failure. In contrast to the first three types of shock, inflammatory shock and cardiogenic shock more often require more than just fluid administration.

Support of the Circulation

To reverse shock, one must ensure adequate perfusion of tissues. Factors that determine perfusion are the O_2 content of blood (CaO_2), the pumping function of the heart, and the tone of the vasculature. Thus, O_2 delivery (DO_2) is the product of CaO_2 (mL O_2/100 mL blood) and CO (L/min). DO_2 is usually indexed to body surface area, so the cardiac index (CI) is used in the calculation and the result is reported in mL O_2/min/m^2:

$$DO_2 = CaO_2 \times CI \times 10$$

CaO_2 consists of the oxygen carried by Hb and that dissolved in the blood itself:

$$CaO_2 = [Hb \times SaO_2 \times 1.39] + [0.003 \times PaO_2]$$

where Hb is the concentration of hemoglobin in g/dL, SaO_2 is arterial O_2 saturation (%), and PaO_2 is the partial pressure of O_2 (mm Hg) in arterial blood. Usually, the fraction of O_2 that is dissolved in blood is inconsequential; an exceptional circumstance is a patient with a critically low Hb (e.g., a Jehovah's Witness who is profoundly anemic). To optimize DO_2 to tissues, one tries to maximize SaO_2 and provide a normal concentration of Hb. The usual guidelines for transfusion (see later) do not apply to a patient in shock. Once CaO_2 is maximized, CO must be addressed. CO is equal to stroke volume times HR and is influenced by cardiac rhythm and contractility, as well as vascular tone. The approach to augmenting CO begins with ensuring a perfusing HR and rhythm and good contractility of the heart.

Dysrhythmias

Dysrhythmias are common in the ICU, and correct interpretation of the rhythm is the key to proper treatment. In a patient with cardiopulmonary arrest, it is very helpful to diagnose the rhythm with quick-look paddles. The most recent algorithm from the American Heart Association stresses the need for nearly continuous cardiopulmonary resuscitation (CPR). A supplemental issue of *Circulation* (2005;112[Suppl 1]) deals with the revised guidelines for CPR, including advanced cardiac life support. For ventricular fibrillation or pulseless ventricular tachycardia, defibrillation with 360 J (monophasic) or 120 to 200 J (biphasic) is undertaken. If the phase type

of the defibrillator is unknown, 200 J is selected, whereas automatic external defibrillators will administer their preprogrammed electrical dose. If defibrillation is successful, amiodarone or lidocaine is initiated as a bolus, followed by a continuous infusion. If not successful, CPR continues and the following steps are taken:

1. Infuse epinephrine, 1 mg IV, or vasopressin, 40 units IV.
2. Epinephrine may be redosed every 3 to 5 minutes but is not administered for 10 minutes after a vasopressin bolus, which is typically given as a one-time dose.
3. CPR is continued throughout this process and additional shocks delivered after every five cycles of CPR.

Asystole can be verified by rotating leads, and high-quality CPR is initiated. Epinephrine (1 mg IV) or a one-time dose of vasopressin (40 units IV) is given. Atropine (1 mg IV) is given as well and repeated every 5 minutes for a total of three doses. Countershock is given only if fine ventricular tachycardia is suspected. There is no role for antiarrhythmics or defibrillation in asystolic cardiac arrest. Please see Box 24-1.

Patients without cardiac arrest are approached differently. Unstable patients with bradycardia (HR <60 beats/min) are treated promptly with transcutaneous pacing. Atropine (1 mg) and epinephrine (2 to 10 μg/min) can be adjuncts if pacing is not readily available. When approaching any patient with a cardiac dysrhythmia, a 12-lead electrocardiogram (ECG) and rhythm strip are obtained. If the QRS complex is found to be wide and rapid, cardioversion and amiodarone are indicated because the dysrhythmia is most likely ventricular in

---

Box 24-1   Guidelines for the Management of Cardiopulmonary Arrest

Ventricular Fibrillation/Pulseless Ventricular Tachycardia

Give 1 shock (monophasic, 360 J; biphasic, 100 to 200 J)
CPR, additional countershocks if shockable rhythm obtained
Epinephrine, 1 mg IV, repeat every 3 to 5 minutes, *or* vasopressin, 40 units IV (may be given to replace the first or second dose of epinephrine)
Consider amiodarone (300 mg IV), lidocaine (1-1.5 mg/kg), magnesium (1-2 g IV)
If no shockable rhythm, revert to asystole/pulseless electrical activity algorithm

Asystole/Pulseless Electrical Activity

Verify with lead rotation
Epinephrine, 1 mg IV, repeat every 3 to 5 minutes, *or* vasopressin, 40 units IV (may be given to replace the first or second dose of epinephrine)
Consider atropine (1 mg IV every 3-5 minutes, up to 3 doses)
If shockable rhythm, revert to ventricular fibrillation/ventricular tachycardia algorithm

Adapted from 2005 American Heart Association Guidelines for Cardiopulmonary Resuscitation and Emergency Care, Part 7.2: Management of Cardiac Arrest. Circulation 112(Suppl 1):IV-59, 2005.

origin. If the QRS is narrow and the patient is hemodynamically unstable, synchronized cardioversion is warranted. The differential diagnosis includes supraventricular tachycardia, atrial fibrillation, atrial flutter, multifocal atrial tachycardia, and uncertain tachycardia, all of which require different treatment. A detailed discussion of the management of these rhythm abnormalities is beyond the scope of this chapter, and expert consultation may be necessary.

Sinus tachycardia is the most common tachycardia in the ICU and is not a dysrhythmia per se, but it can be an appropriate response to fever, pain, sympathetic stimulation, hypotension, sepsis, or inflammation. Therapy is directed at the underlying cause. If the QRS width is unclear, adenosine (6 mg, repeated once) may be administered and will typically facilitate identification of the underlying rhythm. If the rate does not slow, it is treated as a wide-complex tachycardia; if it slows, it is treated as a narrow-complex tachycardia.

The most common sustained dysrhythmia is atrial fibrillation, which has a prevalence of 5% in people older than 65 years. Numerous stresses in the perioperative period may trigger new-onset atrial fibrillation or loss of rate control in a patient with chronic atrial fibrillation. Cardioversion is performed for hemodynamic instability; otherwise, rate control is attempted while the underlying cause (e.g., myocardial ischemia, fluid overload, electrolyte imbalance, hypoxemia, acidosis, pulmonary embolism [PE]) is identified and treated. IV amiodarone, calcium channel blockers, or β-blockers are usually effective in rapid conversion; digoxin takes several hours for maximal effect. A number of medications are used for conversion of atrial fibrillation to sinus rhythm, but not all are approved by the Food and Drug Administration for this indication and thus will not be discussed. In patients who have had atrial fibrillation for less than 48 hours or who are already taking warfarin, no anticoagulation is necessary. If the precise time of onset is not known, however, it is probably safest to either administer anticoagulants before cardioversion or perform cardioversion under guidance by transesophageal echocardiography. Recently, five randomized trials have addressed rate control and rate conversion in patients with atrial fibrillation, and although the groups may not have been homogeneous, it appears that conversion offers no real benefit over rate control.[6]

Pump Dysfunction

In patients with inflammatory or cardiogenic shock, cardiac pump function may be disturbed as a result of circulating myocardial depressants or ischemia. The clinical manifestations of a failing heart may include pulmonary edema (left heart failure), and peripheral edema and distended neck veins (right heart failure). Once CaO_2 has been maximized and a perfusing rhythm has been ensured, the next step is to optimize CO. The principal determinants of CO are preload, afterload, and contractility. At a minimum, CVP monitoring is instituted, and if CVP and MAP are both low, volume replacement is warranted. If CVP is high and MAP is low, however, a PAC is inserted for monitoring PAWP and CO. If PAWP and

CO are both high, the patient may have been over-resuscitated; delivery of fluids is slowed and diuretic therapy considered. Low PAWP and CO may be associated with inflammatory shock, anaphylaxis, and hepatic or autonomic dysfunction. If PAWP and CO are both low, administer fluid boluses of crystalloid to increase PAWP by 3 to 5 mm Hg and remeasure CO; if it improves, repeat until the patient stabilizes. If PAWP is high and CO is low, either an inotropic agent or an afterload-reducing agent may be warranted. If the patient is normotensive, an afterload reducer may be helpful. Sodium nitroprusside and nitroglycerin are most frequently used, but angiotensin-converting enzyme inhibitors (ACEIs) or ganglionic blocking agents (e.g., trimethaphan) may be considered. Nitroprusside (0.5 µg/kg/min) is desirable because of its rapid onset and reversibility and rare tolerance or tachyphylaxis. A by-product is cyanide, which is converted to thiocyanate and excreted by the kidneys. Cyanide toxicity may be heralded by increasing mixed venous oxygen saturation and is treated by administering 3% sodium nitrite (10 mL), followed by methylene blue (1 mg/kg). Thiocyanate levels higher than 10 mg/dL may necessitate hemodialysis. Nitroglycerin (5 µg/min, titrated up to 300 µg/min) is a good choice in patients with elevated preload as well as afterload, especially those with pulmonary edema.

Hypotensive patients may require medication to augment cardiac contractility, increase systemic arterial vasoconstriction, or both. Several agents may be used, each with a unique profile of activity on adrenergic receptors (Table 24-2). α_1-Receptors have their primary effect on systemic arterial vasoconstriction and lesser effects on systemic veins and pulmonary arteries. β_1-Receptors act primarily on the heart and increase HR, contractility, and atrioventricular conduction. β_2-Receptors increase HR and contractility, but they also exert vasodilatory effects on the systemic and pulmonary vasculature. Dopaminergic receptors modulate arterial vasodilation and, to a lesser degree, cardiac contractility, but the effects of dopamine are unpredictable and the side effects may be substantial, so enthusiasm for its use in the ICU has been waning.[7]

Three of the most commonly used medications for hypotensive patients are epinephrine, norepinephrine, and phenylephrine. Dopamine was widely used in the past, but as previously noted, interest in its use has faded in the ICU.[7] Epinephrine is a potent α- and β-adrenergic agonist and increases myocardial contractility, as well as vasoconstriction. It increases myocardial O_2 consumption and is arrhythmogenic, so its usefulness in the ICU is limited to patients with profound hypotension. Norepinephrine's primary value is to increase MAP by augmenting systemic vascular resistance via the α-adrenergic receptor. It may have deleterious effects on CO in high-afterload states such cardiogenic shock; however, it does increase HR and myocardial contractility via β-adrenergic stimulation, so it is particularly useful in patients with myocardial dysfunction and peripheral vasodilation. Phenylephrine is a pure α-adrenergic agonist and as such can be helpful in increasing systolic blood pressure through its action on the vasculature while not affecting

Table 24-2 Effects of Selected Vasoactive Agents

DRUG	DOSAGE (µg/kg/min)	RECEPTOR ACTIVITY			HEMODYNAMIC RESPONSE			
		α	β₁	β₂	HR	MAP	CO	SVR
Dopamine	3-5	(−)	++	(−)	↑	↑	↑	→
	5-20	++	++	(−)	↑↑	↑↑	↑	↑↑
Dobutamine	2-20	(−)	++	+	↑↑	↑	↑	↓
Norepinephrine	1-20 µg/min	++	+	(−)	↑	↑↑	↑	↑↑
Phenylephrine	10-100 µg/min	++	(−)	(−)	→	↑↑	↓	↑↑
Epinephrine	0.005-0.02	(−)	++	++	↑↑	↑	↑	↓
	0.01-0.1	++	++	+	↑↑	↑↑	↑	↑↑
Isoproterenol	0.03-0.15	(−)	++	+	↑↑	→	↑	↓
Amiodarone	5-10				→	→	↑↑	↓
Milrinone	0.3-1.5				→	→	↑↑	↓

CO, cardiac output; HR, heart rate; MAP mean arterial blood pressure; SVR, systemic vascular resistance.

the heart at all. It is commonly used by anesthesiologists and may be particularly useful in reversing the vasodilation caused by epidural anesthetics, but its association with tachyphylaxis limits its effectiveness.

Vasopressin is commonly used by critical care practitioners, but supporting data are limited.[8] Vasopressin is not an adrenergic drug but instead functions through a G protein–coupled receptor and thus may be useful in patients who are refractory to catecholamines. Its main function in the body appears to be regulation of water balance, but in shock it is a potent vasopressor irrespective of the level of circulating endogenous vasopressin. In septic shock it is typically administered in doses up to 0.04 U/min, which mimics physiologic levels and avoids some of the adverse effects associated with higher doses, such as myocardial ischemia.

In patients who have adequate MAP but who need help with myocardial contractility, inotropic drugs are indicated. For the most part, these drugs have vasodilatory effects, so it is important to ensure adequate preload before infusion. Dobutamine (5-15 µg/kg/min) can be very effective, but it does increase myocardial oxygen demand and may be arrhythmogenic. Isoproterenol is a powerful synthetic β-adrenergic agonist that is no longer used in clinical practice because of its associated arrhythmogenicity. The phosphodiesterase inhibitors amrinone and milrinone are thought to act by inhibiting the breakdown of cyclic adenosine monophosphate. They increase CO and reduce preload and afterload; amrinone may cause profound vasodilation, and long-term administration is associated with thrombocytopenia and gastrointestinal side effects. Milrinone is a more potent inotrope with fewer side effects, but it too is associated with vasodilation and arrhythmias as well. It causes pulmonary vascular vasodilation and may be helpful in treating myocardial dysfunction in the setting of pulmonary hypertension. The phosphodiesterase inhibitors appear to be able to increase myocardial contractility without affecting myocardial oxygen demand by reducing wall stress, which counteracts the increased oxygen requirement to support enhanced contractility. Please see Table 24-2.

Resuscitation

Fluids

Fluid resuscitation is the initial maneuver whenever a shock state is recognized. Crystalloid is typically administered to expand intravascular volume, although only about a third of the fluid will remain in the intravascular space. There may be cellular dysfunction resulting in loss of capillary integrity and massive fluid extravasation resulting in widespread tissue edema. For nearly half a century, a debate about the pros and cons of resuscitation with crystalloid versus colloid fluid has raged. Although colloids provide more effective volume expansion than crystalloid solutions do because of their ability to remain in the vascular space, prospective randomized clinical trials (PRCTs) have demonstrated that survival is no better—and possibly worse—when albumin is given instead of crystalloid. This argument is countered by meta-analyses showing that the administration of albumin reduces morbidity in acutely ill hospitalized patients and may have beneficial effects in a wide range of clinical settings. Whatever the outcome of this debate, it is apparent that many more studies will be required before a definitive conclusion to this debate is achieved. One thing is certain, however: in the case of severe hemorrhagic shock, the usual transfusion triggers and the colloid-crystalloid debate do not apply, and Hb is restored to near-normal levels.

End Points of Resuscitation

Although fluid resuscitation may normalize many clinical parameters such as HR, blood pressure, skin color, mentation, and urine output, it does not ensure that the O_2 debt has been repaid. For this reason there needs to be an objective measure of the success of resuscitation in meeting tissue metabolic needs. In the early 1990s, Bishop, Shoemaker, and colleagues[9] identified values for

CI (4.5 L/min/m^2), DO_2 (600 mL O_2/min/m^2), and O_2 consumption (VO_2) (170 mL O_2/min/m^2) above which survival could be predicted in critically ill patients. Subsequent PRCTs testing these resuscitation goals offered mixed results. Kern and Shoemaker[10] reviewed published data and suggested that if hemodynamic optimization is applied to subgroups with an expected mortality of 20% or greater, before the development of organ failure, and the goal of increased DO_2 is achieved, survival will be improved. Although it is difficult to argue that early aggressive resuscitation benefits critically ill patients, it is important to augment DO_2 whenever possible because this is the cornerstone of goal-directed resuscitation.[11] It must be recognized, however, that not all patients respond in the same way. For example, Moore and colleagues[12] reported that 38% of severely injured patients were unable to attain a VO_2 of 150 mL O_2/min/m^2 despite supranormal DO_2. This group appeared to have defective aerobic metabolism leading to a higher incidence of multiple organ failure (MOF). Thus, routine resuscitation to supranormal targets may be unnecessary when shock is readily reversed, fruitless when the patient does not respond, and even detrimental when it results in abdominal compartment syndrome (ACS).[13]

Alternative parameters that may serve as resuscitation end points include mixed venous oxygen saturation ($S\bar{v}O_2$), end-tidal carbon dioxide ($ETCO_2$), gastric intramucosal pH (pHi), base deficit, and arterial lactate. $S\bar{v}O_2$ is an indicator of O_2 extraction and is used to calculate VO_2. Continuous monitoring of $S\bar{v}O_2$ can provide early clues about inadequate perfusion (e.g., hemorrhage, myocardial ischemia, or shock) before it becomes fully manifested, but intermittent measurements are not as helpful. Fortunately, continuous $S\bar{v}O_2$-monitoring PACs are readily available and can offer valuable insight into the status of a patient's hemodynamics, provided that the clinician understands the limitations of the measurement. Furthermore, whereas a low value may be helpful in prompting clinical action, a normal or high $S\bar{v}O_2$ may be misleading. For example, in severe sepsis or preterminal shock, high $S\bar{v}O_2$ can result from significant shunting with little O_2 being delivered to tissue beds or from mitochondrial dysfunction preventing oxygen utilization. Assessment of serum lactate or base deficit in conjunction with $S\bar{v}O_2$ measurement can be particularly helpful in this setting and provides more information than either parameter alone does. In general, over-reliance on any one parameter is unwise and can result in inappropriate and harmful therapeutic interventions. A classic example is vigorous fluid administration to correct a lactic acidosis from a type B lactic acidosis, in which tissue perfusion is maintained and the acidosis is due to causes such as metformin, antiviral agents, or even acute alcohol intoxication, and pulmonary edema or congestive failure needlessly develops.

$ETCO_2$ reflects alveolar CO_2. Decreased CO or increased pulmonary dead space may decrease $ETCO_2$ and increase the arterial-$ETCO_2$ difference, which has been associated with nonsurvival. The splanchnic circulation is the first to be compromised in shock and the last to be restored. Gastric tonometry measures pHi in the stomach, which

Table 24-3 Risk Factors for Perioperative Cardiac Complications in Patients Undergoing Noncardiac Surgery

RISK FACTOR	ODDS RATIO
Diabetes mellitus	3.0 (1.3-7.1)
Renal insufficiency	3.0 (1.4-6.8)
High-risk surgery	2.8 (1.6-4.9)
Ischemic heart disease	2.4 (1.3-4.2)
Congestive heart failure	1.9 (1.1-3.5)
Poor functional status	1.8 (0.9-3.5)

reflects mesenteric tissue ischemia. A threshold of a pHi value greater than 7.3 has compared favorably with supranormal DO_2 and VO_2 (600 and 150 mL/min/m^2, respectively) as an end point.[14] The major drawbacks to the widespread use of gastric tonometry are technologic limitations, cost, and inconvenience. A number of investigators have measured transcutaneous O_2 and CO_2 levels, as well as skeletal muscle oxyhemoglobin. Early results have been encouraging, but these techniques have not gained broad acceptance. Arterial lactate and base deficit are measures of global tissue perfusion and can be particularly helpful in predicting which patients will experience an adverse outcome because the time to normalization strongly correlates with mortality and morbidity.[15] In addition to their prognostic significance, these parameters allow the degree of physiologic derangement to be quantified and they serve as targets for ongoing resuscitation, but it appears that lactate may offer improved predictive ability over base deficit.

With few exceptions, every prospective, goal-directed clinical trial that has shown a survival advantage has espoused the principles of the supranormal DO_2 strategy: volume loading with or without transfusion plus inotropic support as needed to meet a predetermined goal. Although the optimal algorithm for administration of fluids and inotropes has not yet been determined, it is clear that a defined end point is desirable. Rather than selecting a goal that simply confirms the act of resuscitation, it is more appropriate to select an end point that confirms a response to resuscitation.

Perioperative Cardiac Support

Cardiac Risk Assessment

Cardiovascular complications are all too frequent after noncardiac surgery. Nearly a decade ago it was estimated that annually, 50,000 patients will have a perioperative myocardial infarction and another million will have a cardiac complication.[16] As our population ages, cardiac complications will continue to increase, thus requiring increased vigilance in assessing and minimizing cardiac risk. In the setting of an acute surgical emergency, preoperative risk assessment is limited to vital signs, volume status, and ECG. There is no opportunity for further risk assessment or risk reduction; however, in less urgent circumstances, evaluation proceeds in accordance with the presence of risk factors (Table 24-3). If the patient has no risk factors, no further testing or treatment is necessary. One or two risk factors do not by themselves warrant additional testing, but in the presence of a past medical history consistent with coronary artery disease, noninvasive testing is prudent. Three or more risk factors mandate noninvasive testing[16]; however, the optimal noninvasive test is debatable. Exercise (stress) ECG is generally advocated as the initial test, but it is not suitable for patients who have uninterpretable ECGs or those unable to exercise. In such cases, an imaging test such as dipyridamole thallium scanning that simulates exercise is necessary. Additionally, imaging to assess myocardial viability is indicated in patients with poor myocardial function or previous revascularization. The choice of imaging, radionuclide perfusion imaging versus echocardiography, depends primarily on local expertise. An abnormal noninvasive test result mandates cardiac catheterization with coronary arteriography. Left main or three-vessel coronary artery disease may be an indication for coronary artery bypass surgery, whereas one- or two-vessel disease may be treated by coronary angioplasty. Revascularization is limited to patients with a clear need, independent of the necessity for noncardiac surgery.

Patients who will not be referred for revascularization but who harbor cardiac risk factors receive medical therapy aimed at minimizing perioperative risk. Clinical trials have not proved perioperative monitoring with a PAC to be of benefit. β-Blockers are administered to all patients who are at risk for cardiac events and are scheduled to undergo surgery.[16,17] If possible, therapy is instituted in advance, with administration of shorter-acting agents such as metoprolol and a target resting HR lower than 60 beats/min.

Heart Failure

Heart failure may be encountered in the perioperative period, particularly during emergency surgery in patients with significant medical comorbid conditions. Shock is managed as previously outlined. Less severe episodes may be manifested by tachycardia, low CO, and pulmonary (if left-sided failure) or peripheral (if right-sided failure) edema. The most common cause of heart failure in the surgical ICU is myocardial ischemia, but it may also represent decompensation of chronic heart failure. Thus, the history and physical examination is supplemented with ECG and cardiac enzyme analysis. Chest radiographs may be helpful to identify pulmonary pathology. Invasive monitoring with a PAC allows determination of right- and left-sided filling pressure, CO, and afterload and helps distinguish cardiogenic from noncardiogenic pulmonary edema. Because the PAC is less helpful in differentiating systolic from diastolic dysfunction, echocardiography may be a more useful tool in patients with acute heart failure. Echocardiography provides information on chamber size and ventricular and valvular function, indirect measurements of pressure, and identification of extracardiac problems such as pericardial effusion. Diuretics and vasodilators are the mainstays of therapy for heart failure. Diuretics improve pulmonary congestion and reduce ventricular end-diastolic volume, thereby improving myocardial Vo_2. Loop diuretics are the

class of choice in the acute setting because of reliable efficacy, short onset, and potency. Vasodilators, including ACEIs, hydralazine, and nitrates, are also used. ACEIs prevent the formation of angiotensin II, a potent vasoconstrictor and stimulus for aldosterone secretion. In addition to decreasing afterload, they augment stroke volume and thus are generally preferred, particularly in patients with a depressed (<40%) left ventricular ejection fraction. They provide symptomatic improvement, as well as a long-term survival advantage.[16] Hydralazine and nitroglycerin are second-line agents for patients who cannot tolerate ACEI therapy. The cardiac glycoside digoxin has a limited role in the treatment of acute heart failure. Inotropes may exacerbate failure in patients with diastolic failure, and treatment with agents capable of reducing myocardial wall tension may be needed. β-Blockers help attenuate the sympathetic overactivity associated with heart failure and decrease myocardial Vo_2; however, careful monitoring is required when even small doses of a β-blocker are administered. Mechanical support, including intra-aortic balloon pumps or left ventricular assist devices, may be required in postbypass cardiogenic shock patients or as a bridge to heart transplantation.

RESPIRATORY SYSTEM

Respiratory Failure

Acute respiratory failure, commonplace in surgical ICUs, can manifest as poor oxygenation without hypercapnia (hypoxemic or type I respiratory failure) or hypoxia with CO_2 retention (hypercapnic or type II respiratory failure). Causes of respiratory failure are numerous and may include preexisting cardiopulmonary or neuromuscular diseases that compromise respiratory mechanics, gas exchange, or ventilatory drive. A number of factors also affect postsurgical or critically ill patients: respiratory mechanics may be compromised by the acute disease process, the surgical intervention, or pain; gas exchange may be adversely affected by fluid shifts, lung injury, or systemic inflammation with resultant acute lung injury; and ventilatory drive or airway protection may be depressed because of analgesics or sedatives. To minimize the morbidity and mortality associated with respiratory failure, it is critically important to recognize it, ascertain the cause, and treat it.

Symptoms and signs of acute respiratory failure include shortness of breath, anxiety, altered mental status, cyanosis, the use of accessory muscles of respiration, stridor, tachypnea, tachycardia, and hypoxia. The initial evaluation includes a rapid assessment to ensure airway patency and air movement. Stridor implies impending airway obstruction and is an emergency. Vital signs, including pulse oximetry, are obtained and supplemental O_2 provided immediately as other causes of failure are sought. A chest radiograph and ABG analysis are mandatory, and other studies such as ECG, bronchoscopy, ventilation-perfusion ($\dot{V}/\dot{Q}$) scanning, and CT scanning are considered. There are several options for delivery of supplemental

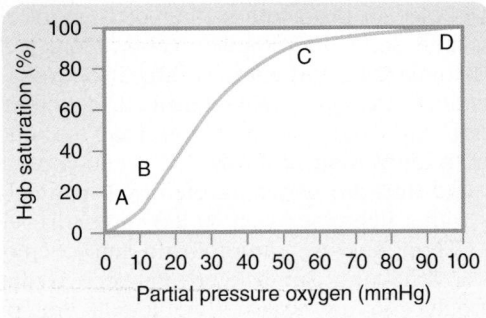

Figure 24-3 Oxygen-hemoglobin (Hgb) dissociation curve. A sigmoid-shaped curve shows maximal oxygen loading in the lung and unloading of O_2 in the periphery occurring over a very narrow range of PaO_2.

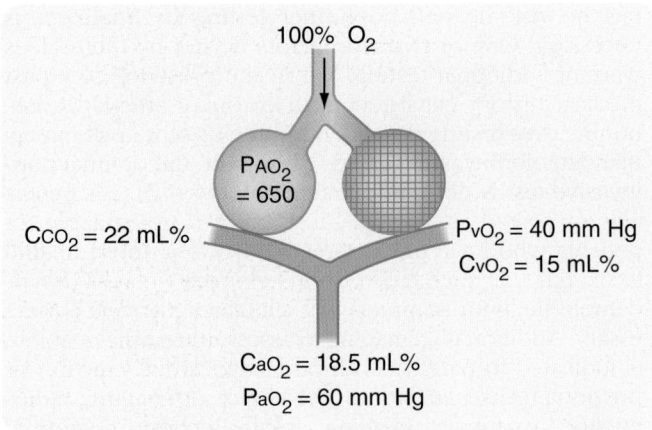

Figure 24-4 A model of the two-alveolus theory of lung function. In the presence of alveolar collapse or alveolar flooding *(hatched area)*, nonoxygenated venous blood on the right is allowed to shunt past the alveolus with no oxygen transfer, for a PaO_2 of 40 mm Hg and oxygen content of 15 mL%. Despite a normal alveolus on the left and normal oxygen content after passing by the alveolus (O_2 content, 22 mL%), the mixing of right and left blood flow gives the systemic blood a PO_2 of 60 mm Hg and a low O_2 content of 18.5 mL%. (From Hall JB, Wood LD: Acute hypoxemic respiratory failure. In Hall JB, Schmidt GA, Wood LDH [eds]: Principles of Critical Care. New York, McGraw-Hill, 1992, with permission of the McGraw-Hill Companies.)

O_2, including nasal cannula, face tent, facemask, noninvasive positive pressure systems, and endotracheal intubation with mechanical ventilation. The choice is dictated by the patient's condition and ventilatory needs. Indications for intubation and mechanical ventilation include SOAP: excessive *s*ecretions requiring pulmonary toilet, impaired *o*xygenation requiring positive pressure ventilation, *a*irway obstruction or inability to protect the airway, and compromised *p*ulmonary function (i.e., inability to generate adequate respiratory effort or to meet minute ventilatory needs).

The amount of O_2 that must be supplied is the lowest amount that provides adequate CaO_2 in blood. As discussed earlier, this is directly related to the Hb concentration and SaO_2. Therefore, as in the setting of shock, consideration is given to restoring near-normal Hb levels in patients with acute respiratory failure. Pulse oximetry and ABG analysis will yield information on SaO_2 and PaO_2, respectively. Though related, PaO_2 and SaO_2 have a complex relationship, as indicated by the Hb-O_2 dissociation curve (Fig. 24-3). At low levels of O_2 tension (point A to point B), increases in PaO_2 translate into only small increases in the percentage of O_2 bound to Hb, but during midrange O_2 tension (point B to point C), the relationship of PaO_2 to O_2-Hb binding is nearly linear, with significant increases in SaO_2 resulting from increases in PaO_2. This relationship is not linear at higher O_2 tension (point C to point D), such that continued increases in PaO_2 result in very little increase in SaO_2. The goal in acute respiratory failure is to achieve a PaO_2 that lies on the upper plateau of the curve.

Hypoxemia is affected by inspired O_2, ventilation, shunting, and $\dot{V}/\dot{Q}$ matching. $\dot{V}/\dot{Q}$ matching is the balance between ventilation and perfusion at the alveolar level. It is a continuum that ranges from a complete shunt (perfused but nonventilated space) to dead space (ventilated but nonperfused space). Alveolar collapse (e.g., atelectasis, alveolar flooding with fluid or proteinaceous debris) results in a shunt. Blood that perfuses such an alveolus returns to the left atrium with low CaO_2—essentially the same as that of mixed venous blood. Dead space ventilation occurs in the conducting airways, where perfusion is limited and essentially no gas exchange

occurs. Ultimately, PaO_2 represents the sum total of gas exchange (Fig. 24-4). Defects can be quantified as the alveolar-arterial O_2 gradient ($AaDO_2$):

$$AaDO_2 = PAO_2 - PaO_2$$

where

$$PAO_2 = [FIO_2 \times (PB - PH_2O)] - PACO_2$$

PB is atmospheric pressure (760 mm Hg at sea level and 627 mm Hg at 5280 ft); PH_2O is the vapor pressure of water (47 mm Hg); and $PACO_2$ is the alveolar pressure of CO_2, which can be calculated by dividing $PaCO_2$ by the respiratory quotient (normally 0.8). Thus, as an example, for an individual breathing room air at sea level and having a $PaCO_2$ of 40 mm Hg:

$$PAO_2 = [0.21 \times (760 - 47) - (40/0.8)$$
$$= (0.21 \times 713) - 50 = 150 - 50 = 100 \text{ mm Hg}$$

At 5280 ft, PAO_2 is 72 mm Hg, and at sea level while breathing 100% O_2, PAO_2 is 663 mm Hg. Subtracting PaO_2 from PAO_2 quantifies $AaDO_2$. In healthy individuals, ventilation and perfusion are well matched and $AaDO_2$ is low (10-25 mm Hg) because it reflects only dead space ventilation in the conducting airways and shunting of small amounts of blood via the bronchial vessels and thebesian veins. Elevated $AaDO_2$ suggests impaired gas exchange. Nonpulmonary causes of right-to-left shunting include atrial septal defects, pulmonary arteriovenous malformations, severe sepsis, and cirrhosis. There are numerous pulmonary causes of pulmonary dysfunction, including aspiration, atelectasis, pneumonia, pulmonary contusion, PE, pulmonary edema, and acute lung injury/acute respiratory distress syndrome (ARDS).

Aspiration is a common problem in the ICU and may lead to chemical pneumonitis, ventilator-associated pneumonia, and even ARDS. Aspiration is due to impaired laryngeal competence and glottic closure or gastric reflux secondary to ileus or gastric outlet obstruction, and it is facilitated by indwelling tubes that disrupt the normal protective mechanisms. If the aspiration event is significant, the initial manifestations are due to the mechanical effects of airway obstruction. Patients with diminished sensorium are at particular risk and will not cough to expel the aspirate, thereby resulting in more severe effects. Soon after, the chemical injury becomes evident, and bronchoconstriction and fluid sequestration in the alveoli take place. An inflammatory response follows, with release of leukocyte- and platelet-derived inflammatory mediators and leakage of protein-rich fluid into the alveoli. Pulmonary function progressively worsens throughout these phases. Because of immunosuppression and compromised airway defenses, bacterial pneumonia is a major risk during the clinical course. Treatment of aspiration is to mechanically clear the airways of debris, decompress the stomach to prevent further events, and provide supportive respiratory care (e.g., bronchodilators, bronchoscopy, and mechanical ventilation) as needed. There is no role for prophylactic antibiotics because they will serve only to select for bacterial resistance; however, the clinician remains vigilant for true pneumonia.

Atelectasis is most often seen in postsurgical or immobilized patients. Alveolar collapse leads to shunting with resultant hypoxemia. Additional findings are related to the degree of atelectasis and include diminished breath sounds and reduced lung volumes, elevated hemidiaphragms, or consolidation on the chest radiograph. Associated fever may be significant but usually abates with reinflation; however, collapsed alveoli are prone to bacterial colonization, which can lead to the development of pneumonia. Treatment is aimed at re-expansion of collapsed alveoli, so maintenance of airway patency and pulmonary toilet is of prime importance. Pain management is pivotal to balance pain-induced splinting with sedation and hypoventilation.

Pneumonia is common in the ICU, particularly in ventilated patients and those with direct lung injury. The clinical manifestation involves fever, leukocytosis, hypoxia, a distinct radiographic infiltrate, and purulent sputum with high numbers of bacterial organisms and neutrophils. Respiratory support, pulmonary toilet, and antibiotics are the fundamentals of treatment; however, preventive measures such as backrest elevation, good oral hygiene, daily interruption of sedation, and avoidance of aspiration are paramount.[18] Diagnosis and management of pneumonia are discussed in Chapter 14. Pulmonary contusion is associated with chest wall injury, so pulmonary dysfunction stems not only from disruption of respiratory mechanics and hypoventilation secondary to pain but also from disruption of lung tissue, with alveolar hemorrhage and fluid sequestration overwhelming the innate alveolar protective mechanisms. The initial findings vary widely, and the condition typically worsens during the ensuing 24 to 48 hours with evolution of the inflammatory response and fluid shifts resulting in so-called blossoming. Management is supportive and consists of respiratory support and pulmonary toilet, but the contusion remains fertile ground for the development of pneumonia. This is discussed further in Chapter 59.

Pulmonary edema is a potentially catastrophic event that is initially manifested by hypoxemia. Clinical signs include dyspnea, tachypnea, hypoxemia, and bilateral rhonchi/rales. Patients may have signs of hypervolemia with congestive heart failure, distended neck veins, and peripheral edema. Radiographic findings include redistribution of blood flow (cephalization), perivascular cuffing, an enlarged cardiac silhouette, and pleural effusions. The underlying cause may be either volume overload or left-sided heart failure. In patients with cardiopulmonary or renal dysfunction, invasive hemodynamic monitoring may be warranted to clarify the diagnosis and optimize therapy. Hypoxemia and hypercapnia are treated supportively, and inotropic support is provided as needed. Diuretics and nitrates may be administered to decrease preload, whereas nitroprusside or an ACEI can be used to promote afterload reduction.

Acute Lung Injury/Acute Respiratory Distress Syndrome

Acute lung injury and ARDS are clinical syndromes of pulmonary dysfunction that may result from any number of infectious, inflammatory, tissue injury, or cellular shock conditions. Criteria for the diagnosis of ARDS include acute onset, bilateral pulmonary infiltrates on chest radiograph, absence of cardiogenic pulmonary edema (i.e., PAWP <18 mm Hg), and hypoxemia (PaO_2/FIO_2 ratio <200).[19] On the same continuum, acute lung injury is a milder form, with a PaO_2/FIO_2 ratio of 201 to 300.

The mortality associated with ARDS approaches 50%, with most deaths attributed to MOF. The pathogenesis of ARDS progresses through three stages. The first stage, which coincides with the acute onset of respiratory failure, is known as the exudative phase. Disruption of the alveolar epithelium results in the influx of protein-rich edema fluid and leukocytes into the alveolus. Destruction of type II pneumocytes disrupts normal alveolar fluid transport and surfactant production, thereby contributing to alveolar flooding and collapse. Macrophages release proinflammatory cytokines that attract and activate neutrophils, which provoke the tissue injury. Some patients have an uncomplicated course with resolution of the process, whereas others progress to the fibroproliferative phase. Mesenchymal cells fill the alveolar space and initiate fibrosis, with collagen and fibronectin accumulating in the lung. In the final stage, or resolution phase, the alveolar edema is resolved as type II pneumocytes repopulate the epithelium, protein is cleared, and there is gradual remodeling of granulation tissue and fibrosis.

Treatment of ARDS is primarily supportive, and any underlying cause is identified and treated. Nutritional support is provided, along with initiation of appropriate prophylactic measures against venous thromboembolism and stress gastritis. Adequate oxygenation and ventilation must be provided, which universally requires intubation and mechanical ventilation. A number of novel adjunctive therapies have been studied for the treatment of ARDS. Preliminary clinical studies suggest that fluid management aimed at lowering filling pressures may decrease pulmonary edema; whether this measure improves outcome, however, remains to be seen. Surfactant replacement therapy has been successful in neonates but has not yet proved beneficial in adults with ARDS. Despite encouraging results in observational studies, nitric oxide and other vasodilators have not proved beneficial in improving outcomes in patients with ARDS. Corticosteroids were never found to be beneficial when administered early in ARDS; however, as the pathophysiology became better understood, this therapy was applied to the later fibroproliferative phase of ARDS. Although early results in observational studies and a small PRCT were encouraging, recent trials have shown that corticosteroids may result in increased mortality.[20] Accordingly, the role of corticosteroids in the management of ARDS remains unclear, and they must be used with caution because they predispose patients to an increased risk for infection.

Previously, a number of methods have been used to ventilate patients with ARDS, including extracorporeal membrane oxygenation, extracorporeal carbon dioxide removal, high-frequency jet or oscillatory ventilation, liquid and partial liquid ventilation, and inverse ratio ventilation. Gradually, it has become apparent that a strategy of lung protective ventilation using a tidal volume (V_T) of 6 mL/kg has been associated with a reduction in mortality.[21,22] In fact, the National Institutes of Health ARDS Network study group performed a multicenter PRCT in which patients were randomized to a V_T of 12 mL/kg versus 6 mL/kg; after enrolling 861 patients, however, the trial was stopped because interim analysis showed that in-hospital mortality was reduced from 40% to 31%.[22] In this study, plateau pressures were maintained at less than 50 and less than 30 cm H_2O, respectively, in the traditional and lung protective groups, and respiratory acidosis was treated by increasing minute ventilation and bicarbonate infusions. The results of this study, though discrepant from earlier, smaller trials, have been borne out in follow-up studies, so this approach has gained widespread acceptance as the ventilatory strategy of choice for treating ARDS.[23]

Prone positioning has been proposed as a means to improve oxygenation by increasing end-expiratory lung volume, improving $\dot{V}/\dot{Q}$ matching, and changing chest wall mechanics. In a multicenter PRCT, prone positioning improved oxygenation but not survival.[24] Although this intervention may be useful in treating severe hypoxemia for short periods, care must be exercised to minimize complications such as pressure ulceration, accidental extubation, and loss of vascular catheters and feeding/drainage tubes. Recent work has shown that prone positioning for longer periods (mean of 17 hr/day) can have added benefits, but the frequency of complications related to turns remains fairly high.[25]

Positive end-expiratory pressure (PEEP) can improve oxygenation by recruiting collapsed alveoli and increasing functional residual capacity. Conventional ventilation generally calls for the minimal PEEP necessary to provide acceptable oxygenation. However, in the setting of ARDS there may be benefit in increasing PEEP to improve oxygenation, as well as protect the lung, by preventing the repetitive recruitment/derecruitment of alveoli and thereby reducing cyclic reopening and stretch during mechanical breaths. The optimal level of PEEP may be determined by incrementally increasing PEEP to maximize the PaO_2/FIO_2 ratio; however, some argue that this practice ignores lung mechanics. A lung pressure-volume curve may be generated for a given patient and the lower inflection point (P_{FLEX}) identified; P_{FLEX} is the point at which the slope increases in steepness, and it represents the pressure at which the majority of alveolar units are open. Alternatively, PEEP may be titrated to maximal compliance, which may be easier to measure at the bedside. Available evidence seems to support the concept that higher levels of PEEP in patients with ARDS may limit stretch trauma to the lung and may have beneficial effects on outcomes.[21]

Ventilatory Support

Noninvasive Ventilatory Support
Many patients require more support than a passive O_2 delivery device. Several noninvasive ventilatory interventions can support oxygenation and ventilation and possibly obviate the need for endotracheal intubation and mechanical ventilation. Intermittent positive pressure breathing aids in clearance of secretions but is labor intensive and, because it is not continuously applied, does not permanently recruit air spaces. Continuous positive airway pressure (CPAP) applied by a tight-fitting mask can maintain and restore functional residual capacity and therefore provides a temporary salutary effect on oxygenation as the underlying cause of hypoxia is treated. This intervention has no effect on ventilation and requires a nasogastric tube because of associated aerophagia. Additionally, a decreased level of consciousness is a relative contraindication to the use of a tight-fitting mask because the patient may vomit and not be able to remove the mask, thereby resulting in aspiration. Bilevel positive airway pressure (BiPAP) also involves the use of a tight-fitting mask, but it requires the ventilator to deliver high airway pressure during spontaneous patient-initiated breaths and a lower baseline pressure during exhalation (like PEEP). It may provide enough assistance to prevent fatigue and stave off endotracheal intubation. Like CPAP, BiPAP is considered a short-term therapy that allows identification and treatment of the underlying derangement. Continued close monitoring is necessary for patients maintained on CPAP and BiPAP because their condition may deteriorate precipitously. A cautionary note must be sounded regarding the use of noninvasive ventilation to treat postextubation respiratory failure because it may be associated with higher mortality than occurs with standard therapy.[26]

Mechanical Ventilation
As outlined earlier, there are four primary indications for endotracheal intubation and mechanical ventilation: excessive secretions, impaired oxygenation, airway obstruction or inability to protect the airway, and compromised pulmonary function.[27] Once mechanical ventila-

tion is instituted, the ventilator must be programmed to meet the patient's needs. The first variable to set is the trigger, that is, the variable that will initiate inspiration. The trigger may be a time interval or a threshold rate of airflow. The second variable to set is an inspiratory limit, which may be a volume, a pressure, or a maximum airflow rate. The third variable to set is the cycle, which may be a volume, pressure, or time. Based on these variables, the ventilator will deliver one of three types of breaths: mandatory, assisted, or spontaneous. A mandatory breath is triggered, limited, and cycled by the machine. An assisted breath is triggered by the patient but is limited and cycled by the ventilator. A spontaneous breath is triggered, limited, and cycled by the patient.

Volume-Cycled Ventilation

This type of ventilation delivers a preset V_T with each breath. Advantages include delivery of a reliable minute volume and ease of use. Its major disadvantage is the potential for high airway pressure and resulting lung injury. The different modes of volume-cycled ventilation include controlled mandatory ventilation (CMV), assist/control ventilation (AC), and intermittent mandatory ventilation (IMV). With CMV, the patient receives a set number of fixed-volume breaths but is unable to increase minute ventilation by triggering additional breaths. CMV is used only in the operating room under general anesthesia. AC differs from CMV in that the patient is able to trigger additional breaths. Every triggered breath will be a full machine-cycled breath. AC is used when full ventilatory support is required, but it is not suitable for an agitated patient who is tachypneic because it may lead to severe respiratory alkalosis. IMV allows spontaneous breathing. It delivers intermittent fixed-volume breaths and allows the patient to breathe spontaneously between mechanical breaths. Synchronized IMV (SIMV) allows the mechanical breaths to be triggered by the patient's own respiratory effort and avoids stacking of breaths. Varying degrees of pressure support may be added to the spontaneous breaths to assist the patient. SIMV is a useful mode of ventilation when attempting to wean or in individuals with patient-ventilator asynchrony. In general, volume-cycled ventilation is the most uncomfortable for the patient and may result in significant patient-ventilator dyssynchrony requiring the liberal use of sedation.

Pressure-Cycled Ventilation

Pressure control ventilation is designed to protect the lung from alveolar overdistention and epithelial injury. A set pressure applied to the ventilatory circuit during each breath allows the lungs to expand on the basis of thoracic compliance. The major advantages are lower mean and peak airway pressure and an exponential decelerating flow pattern that tends to be more comfortable for the patient. The major disadvantage is fluctuating minute ventilation in the face of changing lung compliance. Pressure-cycled breaths can be delivered in an analogous fashion to volume-cycled breaths in either an AC or SIMV mode. Pressure support ventilation (PSV) is a spontaneous ventilatory mode. A negative inspiratory force created by the patient will trigger the ventilator to apply a certain pressure to the ventilator circuit. PSV is the most comfortable mode of ventilation because the patient is able to control all elements of inspiration and expiration. PSV has become the mode of choice for weaning patients from mechanical ventilation. The major disadvantage of PSV is that minute ventilation cannot be ensured and hypoventilation and apnea can occur, so patients must have an intact respiratory drive and be carefully monitored.

Difficult-to-Ventilate Patients

Patients with severe lung disease can be a challenge to oxygenate and ventilate. On volume-cycled ventilator modes, airway pressures may climb; on pressure-cycled modes, the delivered V_T may decrease. Goals include maintenance of airway pressure less than 35 to 40 cm H_2O and SaO_2 greater than 90%. Definitive recommendations for optimal ventilator strategies are not available, but a number of maneuvers can be attempted. Prone positioning, inhaled nitric oxide, and permissive hypercapnia have been discussed previously. Inverse ratio ventilation involves lengthening the inspiratory time to greater than 50% of the respiratory cycle, which increases mean airway pressure and recruits air spaces by auto-PEEP in a manner similar to applied PEEP. Inverse ratio ventilation is used with caution in patients with known severe chronic obstructive pulmonary disease and asthma, given their propensity for air trapping. Pharmacologic paralysis relaxes the chest wall musculature and allows synchronization of the ventilator and patient while decreasing VO_2 and CO_2 production. Tracheal gas insufflation provides 2 to 10 L/min of 100% O_2 delivered 1 cm above the carina. It decreases $PaCO_2$ by washing out proximal anatomic dead space. It can be useful when permissive hypercapnia is being used to attenuate respiratory acidosis. A tracheostomy may be necessary to facilitate weaning and discontinuation of mechanical ventilation is some patients because it can decrease the work of breathing. Though still controversial, it appears that early tracheostomy can significantly reduce the duration of mechanical ventilation and length of ICU stay.[28]

High-frequency ventilation typically delivers a V_T of 1 to 3 mL/kg at rates of 100 to 3000 cycles/min and allows adjustment of mean airway pressure to maintain oxygenation. Extracorporeal membrane oxygenation or CO_2 removal may offer enough lung protection to salvage critically ill patients, but expertise and availability are variable. Partial liquid ventilation, in which the lung is filled with perfluorocarbon and then subjected to standard mechanical ventilation, may be efficacious in preserving lung histology, lung compliance, and systemic oxygenation. Anecdotal success has been reported for each of these innovations, but it is unlikely that any one of them will be anything more than an interesting idea in the treatment of severe respiratory failure.

Weaning From Mechanical Ventilation

Patients who are intubated for pulmonary failure usually require a period of weaning to regain strength and prove their ability to support themselves. When considering liberation of a patient from the ventilator, it is important to first ensure that the underlying problem leading to intubation has been rectified and the patient is otherwise stable. One may then make the same SOAP assessment as in determining the need for intubation:

1. Are the secretions too much for the patient to handle?
2. Is the patient oxygenating adequately (i.e., PaO_2/FIO_2 ratio >200; which requires an FIO_2 <0.40-0.50 and PEEP <5-8 cm H_2O)?
3. Can the airway be protected by the patient?
4. Is pulmonary function adequate?

Ideally, the patient is assessed while breathing spontaneously, and a number of parameters may be obtained to evaluate pulmonary function. Negative inspiratory force (>−20−−30 cm H_2O), minute ventilation (<10-15 L/min), VT (>5 mL/kg), and respiratory rate (<30/min) are all useful indicators. Perhaps the most reliable single test is the f/VT ratio, or the rapid shallow breathing index.[27] A value higher than 105 predicts failure of extubation with a 95% likelihood, whereas a value lower than 80 predicts success in 95%. There are four primary methods of weaning. Multiple daily T-piece trials may be performed, with extubation occurring once the patient tolerates several hours. This method is labor intensive and may cause the patient undue stress, particularly if intubated with a small-diameter endotracheal tube. A single daily T-piece trial may be performed, with extubation if it is successful. If the trial is unsuccessful, the patient is rested for 24 hours, and the test is repeated the following day. IMV and PSV weaning are popular, without a proven advantage of one over the other. What is clear, however, is that trials of spontaneous breathing shorten weaning time.

Before extubating a patient, the bedside clinician systematically reviews the patient's overall condition, in addition to the previously mentioned "SOAP" assessment, with a focus on factors other than respiratory mechanics. Upper airway edema and obstruction needs to be ruled out by checking for a cuff leak. An unambiguous and objective method of doing this requires the patient to cough around the endotracheal tube with the cuff down and a finger occluding the tube's lumen. The chart and anesthesia record are reviewed to ensure that the initial intubation was straightforward in the event that the patient needs to be reintubated. Patients intubated after multiple attempts, bronchoscopically assisted or via retrograde intubation, are best extubated under controlled circumstances rather than in the middle of the night. Finally, factors necessitating increased ventilatory demand, such as acid-base disturbances, hepatic or renal failure, high fever, sepsis, and pronounced anxiety or agitation, are corrected if possible. Patients who are difficult to sedate and alternate between agitation and oversedation may benefit from the α_2-agonist dexmedetomidine, which exerts only minimal effects on hemodynamic stability or respiratory drive.[29]

GASTROINTESTINAL SYSTEM

Stress Gastritis

Stress-related mucosal lesions are the result of gastric acid acting on compromised gastric mucosa, that is, poorly perfused or immunologically incompetent mucosa, or both. These lesions have been reported to develop in 25% to 100% of ICU patients within 24 to 48 hours of admission, with clinically significant bleeding being manifested in only 5% to 10% of patients. Based on these data, routine stress ulcer prophylaxis is provided in most ICUs; however, it is probably not necessary in every ICU patient. The evolution of care in ICUs has provided earlier and better resuscitation and nutritional support, which has resulted in improved mucosal perfusion and preserved integrity. Risk factors for stress gastritis include mechanical ventilation longer than 48 hours, coagulopathy, significant burns, and head injury. Patients with risk factors receive prophylaxis until they are ingesting a gastric, enteral diet at greater than 50% of caloric intake goals because gastric feeding is one of the most effective means of preventing stress gastritis. Prophylactic agents include antacids, sucralfate, histamine-2 (H_2) receptor antagonists, and proton pump inhibitors, with the latter becoming the mainstay of therapy because of their long duration of action and efficacy. Antacids have not proved effective in ICU patients at risk and are not considered a first-line agent. Sucralfate is a sucrose-based polymer that is activated in an acidic environment; it binds to exposed gastric mucosa and ulcer craters and forms a protective barrier. It also stimulates local prostaglandin synthesis and is given as an elixir by mouth or via nasogastric tube (1 g every 6 hours). Early trials suggested a lower risk for nosocomial pneumonia than with H_2 receptor antagonists because of preservation of an acidic gastric environment and less bacterial proliferation. The major disadvantage of sucralfate is its interference with the absorption of other medications such as antibiotics, warfarin (Coumadin), and phenytoin (Dilantin). H_2 receptor antagonists have potent acid-reducing properties. Concerns regarding H_2 receptor antagonists include the development of tachyphylaxis and increased gastric bacterial colonization leading to the development of pneumonia. A large, multicenter PRCT comparing the use of sucralfate with ranitidine in ICU patients with risk factors determined that H_2 receptor antagonists were superior to sucralfate in preventing clinically important bleeding. The rate of ventilator-associated pneumonia was similar between the groups. Although proton pump inhibitors have been shown to be superior to H_2 receptor antagonists in the treatment of peptic ulcer disease, clinical trials demonstrating their superiority in preventing stress gastritis are lacking. Additionally, an association has been made between proton pump inhibitor use and community-acquired *Clostridium difficile* colitis.

Selective Digestive Decontamination

Selective digestive decontamination is a strategy aimed at reducing the bacterial load in the intestine. The concept is based on the belief that gut bacteria translocate to the systemic circulation and incite an inflammatory response that leads to MOF (see later).[30] Although the phenomenon of microbial translocation has been documented in animals and suggested in some human studies, there is no convincing evidence that translocation of bacteria is responsible for adverse clinical outcomes. In contrast, there is evidence that inflammatory mediators may traverse the gut in times of stress, aided by gut hypoperfusion and the loss of mucosal integrity, immunoglobulins, and enterocytes. Selective digestive decontamination is designed to reduce the load of gram-negative aerobic and anaerobic pathogens in the gut. A typical formulation includes a paste of polymyxin, tobramycin, and amphotericin applied to the oral mucosa, a slurry administered into the stomach, and a third-generation cephalosporin administered IV. Of numerous clinical trials in various patient populations, the only groups that seem to benefit are those with severe pancreatitis and patients who have undergone organ transplantation.[31] The topic of selective digestive decontamination remains hotly debated, and innumerable studies have yielded mixed results; however, emerging work suggests that it may be beneficial, particularly in surgical ICU patients.

Abdominal Compartment Syndrome

The abdomen is a closed space bound by the relatively nonexpansile fascia of the abdominal musculature and as such is susceptible to compartment syndrome analogous to that seen in the lower extremities. *ACS* is fundamentally defined as increased intra-abdominal pressure (IAP) associated with adverse physiologic consequences. ACS has most commonly been described in patients with massive abdominal or pelvic hemorrhage, often after damage control laparotomy, but it may be encountered in various clinical scenarios. Circumferential burn eschar, reduction of a large ventral hernia, or the use of military antishock trousers may significantly increase IAP. Bowel distention secondary to obstruction or ileus, ascites, or pneumoperitoneum may lead to ACS. Pancreatitis or surgical dissection may give rise to profound retroperitoneal edema. Edema of the bowel may result from prolonged evisceration during surgery, which elongates and narrows the mesenteric veins and lymphatics; it may also be related to ischemia-reperfusion of the bowel aggravated by resuscitation with large volumes of crystalloid solutions. *Secondary ACS* refers to ACS in the absence of abdominal or pelvic pathology and is entirely due to edema and ascites after shock and aggressive resuscitation.[32] In this setting, particularly in nontrauma patients, it may represent a state of irreversible shock, with loss of capillary integrity.

The organ systems that appear to be most affected by ACS are the cardiovascular, pulmonary, and renal systems. Cardiovascular effects of increased IAP include decreased CO as a result of diminished venous return. Ensuring adequate volume status is a key feature in the management of ACS and can be used to temporize the situation while arrangements are made for decompression. Markedly increased systemic vascular resistance has also been recognized. Increased IAP diminishes diaphragmatic excursion, decreases pulmonary compliance, and creates high airway pressure with diminishing VT and respiratory acidosis. Renal dysfunction with oliguria progressing to anuria as a result of ACS appears to be due to direct parenchymal compression and shunting of renal

plasma flow. Visceral blood flow is similarly affected, with subsequent intestinal necrosis, hepatic dysfunction, and gut anastomotic breakdown. Intracranial hypertension is also aggravated by ACS. Decompressive celiotomy can immediately reverse these changes, but untreated, ACS leads to lethal organ failure, with collective mortality rates exceeding 50%.

Recognition of ACS is not difficult once the diagnosis is considered. Those at highest risk include severely injured patients who require abdominal packing for abbreviated/staged laparotomy, particularly those with a coagulopathy secondary to core hypothermia or cirrhosis. It is prudent to screen patients at high risk for ACS, particularly those acutely resuscitated from shock, requiring vasopressors, and receiving more than 6 L of crystalloid or 6 units of packed red blood cells over a 6-hour period.[32] The findings of a tensely distended abdomen, progressive oliguria despite adequate CO, or hypoxia with increasing airway pressure are sufficient to justify abdominal decompression. Because physical findings alone may be inaccurate in a critically ill patient, bladder pressures can be measured to ascertain the presence of elevated IAP and correlate it with physiologic parameters; as a consequence, bladder pressure has become the objective measure for confirming ACS. The level of IAP at which ACS occurs is patient specific, and thus the diagnosis (and treatment) is based on the patient's physiologic response to increased IAP. Rough correlations can be made between the level of elevation in IAP and the need for decompression (Table 24-4). Although significant alterations in physiology can be demonstrated in patients with IAP between 10 and 15 mm Hg (grade I), it is doubtful that abdominal decompression is warranted at this level. With IAP between 15 and 25 mm Hg (grade II), the need for treatment is based on the patient's clinical condition; in the absence of oliguria, hypoxia, or significantly elevated airway pressure, abdominal decompression is difficult to justify. Continued monitoring is clearly indicated because signs and symptoms of intra-abdominal hypertension progress insidiously. Most patients with IAP between 25 and 35 mm Hg (grade III) ultimately require decompression. All patients with IAP greater than 35 mm Hg (grade IV) require immediate decompression because this group of patients may deteriorate to cardiac arrest at any time. Percutaneous drainage of ascitic fluid may be a temporizing maneuver, but

Table 24-4 Grading System for Abdominal Compartment Syndrome

GRADE	INTRA-ABDOMINAL PRESSURE (mm Hg)	TREATMENT
I	10-14	Normovolemic resuscitation
II	15-24	Hypovolemic resuscitation
III	25-35	Decompression
IV	>35	Emergency re-exploration

operative decompression is mandatory. At the time of decompression, an abdominal closure that affords additional intra-abdominal domain is indicated. Of the various dressings described, the most effective appears to be based on some type of vacuum, either commercially available or homemade, so that bowel edema and lateral retraction of the fascia are minimized and peritoneal fluid is controlled. Every reasonable effort is made to achieve definitive abdominal closure within 3 or 4 days because the lateral retractive forces of the broad, flat muscles of the abdominal wall can make primary closure difficult. If the abdomen cannot be closed, absorbable mesh or skin grafts are used to minimize the risk for intestinal fistulas. Interestingly, vacuum-assisted wound dressings may facilitate early definitive abdominal closure, as well as late closure many weeks after the initial operation.

Nutritional Support

The neuroendocrine response to critical illness and injury includes the release of stress hormones (epinephrine, glucagon, and cortisol) and inflammatory mediators, which culminate in a hypercatabolic state (see Chapter 4). Endogenous nutrient substrates are mobilized, with depletion of glucose and fat stores and breakdown of lean muscle mass. Subsequently, visceral proteins are eroded, and organ system and immune dysfunction ensues. At present we are unable to significantly modulate the systemic inflammatory response, so the preferred therapeutic strategy is to administer exogenous substrate in the form of nutritional support. Nutritional support is considered if the following has ocurred:

1. The patient has been without nutrition for 5 to 7 days.
2. The duration of illness is expected to exceed 10 days.
3. The patient is malnourished.

Recent unintended weight loss of 15% to 20% suggests moderate malnutrition, whereas loss greater than 20% implies severe caloric malnutrition. Serum protein levels, such as albumin or transferrin, may be measured but they are affected by severe illness. Once the decision is made to provide support, the next step is to determine the nutritional needs of the patient. A practical rule of thumb is based on weight: 30 kcal/kg/day generally is adequate for normal-weight patients, 35 kcal/kg/day may be targeted for underweight patients, and 25 kcal/kg/day for overweight patients. A more precise value of basal energy expenditure (BEE, kcal/day) may be estimated by the Harris-Benedict equations:

$$BEE = 66 + (13.7 \times Weight) + (5 \times Height) - (6.8 \times Age) \ (Males)$$

$$BEE = 665 + (9.6 \times Weight) + (1.8 \times Height) - (4.7 \times Age) \ (Females)$$

where weight is measured in kilograms, height in centimeters, and age in years. The BEE estimate is then multiplied by a "stress factor" ranging from 1.25 to 1.75, depending on the severity of illness. In stable mechanically ventilated patients in whom overfeeding or under-

feeding would be particularly detrimental, those whose energy expenditure is significantly altered from expected values, or patients who are not responding as expected to calculated regimens, indirect calorimetry can be used to calculate measured energy expenditure (MEE):

$$MEE = [(3.9 \times V_{O_2}) + 1.1 + V_{CO_2}] \times [1.44 - (2.8 \times U_{UN})]$$

where V_{O_2} and CO_2 production (V_{CO_2}) reflect a 30-minute period. The preferred ratio of nonprotein calories to nitrogen varies with the stress level. In minimally stressed patients, 200:1 to 300:1 is appropriate, but it is decreased to 150:1 in moderately stressed and to 100:1 or less in severely stressed patients. In patients with hepatic or renal failure, protein restriction may be warranted. An alternative method of determining protein needs is based on weight and stress: 1.5 for mild, 2.0 for moderate, and 2.5 g protein/kg for severe stress. Finally, measurement of urine urea nitrogen (U_{UN}) can help determine protein needs because as stress-related catabolism increases, nitrogen excretion (and U_{UN}) increases. U_{UN} represents 90% of excreted nitrogen. Calculation of protein losses (g/day) may be based on 24-hour U_{UN}:

$$Protein \ loss = U_{UN} + 4 \ g \ insensible \ loss + Nonurea \ nitrogen \ loss$$

The goal of nutritional support is to provide a positive nitrogen balance of 3 to 5 g/day, so additional protein must be added beyond the calculated requirements. To calculate the protein requirements, nitrogen requirements are multiplied by 6.25.

The optimal route and method for delivery of nutritional support remains highly controversial. In general, a patient with a functioning gastrointestinal tract is fed enterally. Enteral feeding preserves gut mucosal integrity, barrier function, IgA production, and normal flora, which may explain the reduction in septic complications and improved survival seen in enterally fed patients with severe injuries, acute pancreatitis, inflammatory bowel disease, and liver transplantation. Furthermore, the safety and feasibility of early postoperative enteral feeding have been proved. On the other hand, there are some conflicting data and absence of a clear superiority of enteral nutrition over parenteral nutrition. Parenteral delivery of nutrition can ensure adequate provision of nutrients and is used when enteral feeding is not tolerated or in the presence of a short gut or high-output/proximal gastrointestinal fistulas. In critically ill patients, postpyloric feeding is believed to be safer than gastric feeding in terms of the risk for macroaspiration; however, the incidence of microaspiration is probably similar. Although several trials have suggested that gastric feeding with the administration of promotility agents is equally safe, these studies have been underpowered to reflect the occasional catastrophic event; nonetheless, erythromycin can promote gastric emptying and facilitates enteral nutrition.

So-called immune-enhancing diets provide specific nutrients (glutamine, arginine, nucleotides, and ω-3 fatty acids) that exert favorable immunomodulatory effects. Glutamine is an oxidative fuel for enterocytes and other rapidly replicating cells and is said to be conditionally essential. Arginine promotes normal T-cell function, aids in wound healing, and is necessary for the metabolism of ammonia. Nucleotides enhance the replication of rapidly dividing cells, as well as promote immune responsiveness. The ω-3 fatty acids compete with ω-6 fatty acids (specifically, arachidonic acid) in metabolism of cyclooxygenase, thereby resulting in production of prostaglandins of the 3 series and leukotrienes of the 5 series. These eicosanoids are less inflammatory and immunosuppressive than the 2-series prostaglandins and 4-series leukotrienes produced by arachidonic acid. Although several clinical trials have suggested significant benefits with these diets, the literature remains mixed and a mortality benefit is lacking.

ACUTE RENAL FAILURE

Acute renal failure (ARF) is a deadly problem, with mortality rates exceeding 50% and increasing up to 60% to 90% if dialysis is required. Its onset is heralded by oliguria (<0.5 mL/kg/hr or <400 mL/24 hr) or a rising serum creatinine concentration, which prompts a search for its cause (prerenal, renal parenchymal, or postrenal). The first step is physical examination to look for signs of hypovolemia, heart failure, shock, obstruction, ACS, or rashes. The most common cause of oliguria in surgical patients is hypovolemia. A Foley catheter is inserted to exclude outlet obstruction and monitor urine output closely. Next, a fluid bolus (500-1000 mL, or 10% of circulating blood volume) is administered, except in patients in whom heart failure is suspected, in which case measurement of CVP or PAWP is more helpful in directing therapy. If the patient does not respond to fluid administration, a more extensive evaluation must be undertaken, and invasive hemodynamic monitoring is warranted to measure filling pressures and assess cardiac function. A spot urine sodium (U_{Na}) level may be helpful in distinguishing prerenal from renal parenchymal causes of ARF because a U_{Na} level lower than 20 mEq/L is consistent with a prerenal cause and greater than 40 mEq/L with a renal parenchymal cause. By measuring both sodium and creatinine in urine as well as plasma, fractional excretion of sodium (FE_{Na}) may be calculated:

$$FE_{Na} = [(U_{Na} \times P_{Cr})/(P_{Na} \times U_{Cr})] \times 100$$

FE_{Na} less than 1% indicates a prerenal cause of ARF, whereas FE_{Na} greater than 3% suggests a renal parenchymal or postrenal problem. The patient's medication list is reviewed for nephrotoxic agents, and renal ultrasonography can be used to identify postrenal pathology. Urinalysis can also provide clues to the underlying cause: high urine specific gravity and low pH are consistent with prerenal ARF; tubular casts are indicative of renal parenchymal dysfunction; hemoglobinuria is consistent with a transfusion reaction, vasculitis, or rhabdomyolysis; myoglobinuria is suggestive of rhabdomyolysis; and eosinophilia is associated with interstitial nephritis. These laboratory investigations are less helpful in the elderly, those with chronic renal dysfunction, or patients who have received diuretics or osmotic agents in the previous 24 hours.

Management of prerenal ARF is augmentation of renal perfusion through volume loading and inotropic support as needed. Unfortunately, renal vasoconstriction may be an unwanted side effect of inotropic agents. Formerly, low-dose (0.3-3 µg/kg/min) dopamine was touted in the treatment of ARF to dilate the renal vasculature and stimulate diuresis; however, evidence to support such treatment is lacking.[7,33] Nephrotoxic drugs, including contrast agents, are avoided, and renally excreted drugs are dose adjusted. Creatinine clearance (C_{Cr}; mL/min) can be used for adjustment of the medication dose:

$$C_{Cr} = (U_{Cr} \times V)/P_{Cr}$$

where U_{Cr} is urine creatinine concentration (mg/dL), V is urine volume (mL/min), and P_{Cr} is plasma creatinine concentration (mg/dL). A 24-hour collection is most accurate, but a 4-hour sample may be used. An immediate calculation may be made by using the Cockcroft-Gault approximation:

$$C_{Cr} = [(140 - Age) \times Weight]/(P_{Cr} \times 72)$$

where weight is measured in kilograms. In females, the value is multiplied by 0.85. Normal C_{Cr} is 95 mL/min in women and 120 mL/min in men. In cases of rhabdomyolysis and transfusion reactions, clearance of circulating myoglobin or Hb may be achieved by forcing diuresis (>100 mL/hr) with crystalloids and osmotic diuretics. Obstructing lesions are treated, comorbid conditions addressed, and nutritional support provided. Although conversion of oliguric to nonoliguric ARF may facilitate volume management, there is insufficient evidence that it improves outcomes. Diuretic use in ARF remains controversial, with some trials suggesting an increased risk for nonrecovery of renal function and mortality whereas others do not.

Renal replacement therapy (RRT) may be indicated for symptomatic fluid overload, severe electrolyte or acid-base disorders, sepsis, or uremic complications such as encephalopathy or pericarditis. Several options for RRT exist, including intermittent techniques such as peritoneal dialysis or hemodialysis. Peritoneal dialysis is appropriate in chronic renal failure patients who do not have peritonitis or have not recently undergone abdominal surgery, but it has limited applications in the ICU. Hemodialysis provides efficient removal of fluid, solutes, and some toxins, but it may be associated with hemodynamic instability and is relatively resource intensive. Continuous RRT techniques offer the advantages of improved hemodynamic stability and relatively less resource utilization, but they require some anticoagulation and have not proved superior to hemodialysis in improving outcomes, except in some limited clinical trials. Interestingly, RRT has been shown to remove cytokines and inflammatory mediators from the blood of septic patients without having a significant impact on survival. Continuous hemofiltration may be used to remove fluid and solutes in patients who suffer only from fluid overload, but continuous venovenous hemodialysis is the most commonly used method in the ICU. It involves the use of a double-lumen central venous catheter, and blood is pumped through a filter against the flow of dialysate before returning to the patient. Continuous arteriovenous hemodiafiltration is similar but requires a large-bore arterial cannula and adequate patient arterial pressure to drive the process and as such has fallen out of favor.

Given the significant morbidity and mortality associated with ARF, the ideal strategy is prevention, which involves careful attention to fluid balance and perfusion, proper dosing of medications, and avoidance of nephrotoxic drugs. Radiographic contrast material causes 10% to 15% of hospital-acquired ARF. Hydration and the use of nonionic contrast agents may help reduce this occurrence. Hydration with sodium bicarbonate before delivery of a contrast load has been shown to be an effective means of preventing ARF in patients with preexisting renal insufficiency.[34]

HEPATIC DYSFUNCTION

Liver disease is suspected in patients with a history of alcohol or IV drug abuse, blood transfusions, or the presence of tattoos. Physical stigmata of liver disease include jaundice, ascites, malnutrition, encephalopathy, gynecomastia, testicular atrophy, muscle wasting, spider angiomas, palmar erythema, fetor hepaticus, and caput medusae. Laboratory findings reveal elevated bilirubin, a prolonged prothrombin time, hypoalbuminemia, and increased or normal transaminase levels, depending on the stage of liver failure. Secondary liver failure manifested by cholestatic jaundice, impaired synthetic activity, and altered mental status may develop in critically ill patients. Treatment is directed at the underlying condition, but failure to correct this problem often results in MOF and death. Primary liver failure may represent an exacerbation of chronic liver disease or an acute problem caused by viral illness, drugs, or other toxins. In cases of acute liver failure, both the cause and extrahepatic complications (fluid, electrolyte, and coagulation abnormalities; renal, pulmonary, and immune dysfunction) are treated medically. Cerebral edema is present in 80% of patients dying of fulminant hepatic failure, so aggressive management, including early ICP monitoring, is critical. Orthotopic liver transplantation may prove lifesaving, but it must be considered before irreversible brain damage or MOF sets in.

Patients with an exacerbation of chronic liver disease usually have a complication that must be treated. Variceal hemorrhage is the most dramatic manifestation and carries higher mortality (see Chapter 52). Patients with ascites and acute physiologic decompensation undergo diagnostic paracentesis and a cell count to exclude bacterial peritonitis. A white blood cell count greater than 500/mm³ suggests bacterial peritonitis. Primary bacterial peritonitis occurs in more than 20% of cirrhotic patients with ascites. It is typically monomicrobial (pneumococcus) and is treated by antibiotic therapy alone, but its associated 1-year mortality is 50%. Polymicrobial peritonitis is indicative of an intra-abdominal abscess or perforated viscus. Patients showing signs of intra-abdominal hypertension secondary to tense ascites may require large-volume paracentesis to alleviate the symptoms. Medical management of ascites includes sodium (1-2 g/day) and water restriction and diuresis. Spironolactone is preferred because it inhibits sodium reabsorption, but furosemide may be required in addition. Large-volume paracentesis is generally well tolerated but with albumin replacement (7-9 g/L) may decrease renal insufficiency and encephalopathy. Management of hepatic encephalopathy begins with reversal of any precipitating factors, such as removing drugs with CNS effects, treating infections, and correcting fluid/electrolyte abnormalities. Ammonia formation and elimination are addressed by administering neomycin and lactulose, respectively.

Hepatorenal syndrome is a functional renal problem seen in patients with end-stage liver disease; it is due to a combination of systemic vasodilation, relative hypovolemia, and increased activity of the renin-angiotensin-aldosterone system. Hepatorenal syndrome is marked by azotemia, oliguria, extremely low urinary sodium (<10 mEq/L), and high urinary osmolality. The prognosis is dismal, but systemic vasoconstriction with terlipressin or ornipressin has shown promising results and octreotide has proved largely ineffective. Care is mainly supportive and orthotopic liver transplantation may be curative. Nutritional support limits protein to 1 to 1.2 g/kg/day and provides 25 to 35 kcal/kg/day, with 30% to 40% of nonprotein calories being in the form of fat.

ENDOCRINE SYSTEM

Adrenal Insufficiency

The hypothalamic-pituitary-adrenal axis is activated by physiologic stress, and proportional increases in corticotropin-releasing hormone, adrenocorticotropic hormone, and cortisol ensue (see Chapter 39). Stress may unmask adrenal insufficiency, with potentially devastating consequences. Patients with potential adrenal insufficiency may be identified by a history of chronic or recent steroid administration or clinical findings consistent with hypercortisolism/Cushing's syndrome (hypertension, diabetes, truncal obesity, hirsutism, buffalo hump) or primary adrenal insufficiency/Addison's disease (thin, hyperpigmented patient with constitutional complaints). In this setting, steroids are administered in accordance with the anticipated degree of stress. For minor surgical procedures, a patient receives 25 mg hydrocortisone equivalent daily (Table 24-5), and for moderate stress, 50 to 75 mg/day. In the ICU it is safe to assume higher stress, and thus the targeted dose is 100 to 150 mg daily.

An acute adrenal (addisonian) crisis may be difficult to diagnose in the ICU and is manifested by unexplained hypotension, fever, abdominal pain, or weakness. If adrenal crisis is suspected, hydrocortisone or dexamethasone is administered while awaiting confirmatory laboratory values (hyponatremia, hyperkalemia, hypoglycemia, azotemia, cortisol <20 µg/dL). Dexamethasone does not interfere with the serum cortisol assay, but hydrocortisone does. If adrenal insufficiency is present, hydrocor-

Table 24-5   Relative Potency of Corticosteroid Preparations

DRUG	EQUIVALENT DOSE (mg)	GLUCOCORTICOID POTENCY*	MINERALOCORTICOID POTENCY*	HALF-LIFE (hr)
Cortisone	25	0.8	0.8	8-12
Hydrocortisone	20	1	1	8-12
Prednisone	5	4	0.8	12-36
Prednisolone	5	4	0.8	12-36
Methylprednisolone	4	54	0	12-36
Triamcinolone	4	5	0	12-36
Betamethasone	0.80	25	0	36-54
Dexamethasone	0.67	30	0	36-54

tisone is continued at 200 to 300 mg/day in divided doses. Relative adrenal insufficiency has become an emerging problem in ICUs and is manifested as hypotension refractory to fluid or vasopressor therapy (or both). If there is a concern about adrenal insufficiency, a random (baseline) serum cortisol level is measured because critical illness is associated with loss of diurnal variation in cortisol secretion, and a cosyntropin (250 μg) stimulation test is performed. A baseline level greater than 34 μg/dL suggests normal adrenal function, and no further testing is required, whereas less than 15 μg/dL is consistent with hypoadrenalism, and corticosteroids are administered. For cortisol levels between 15 and 34 μg/dL, the response to cosyntropin stimulation defines the presence of adrenal insufficiency. Failure to increase by at least 9 μg/dL over baseline is consistent with hypoadrenalism and prompts corticosteroid therapy.[35] In patients with septic shock, hydrocortisone replacement therapy has been shown in a randomized, controlled trial to facilitate weaning from vasopressors and lower mortality in patients with relative adrenal insufficiency.[36]

Glucose Disorders

Diabetic ketoacidosis (DKA) is typically seen in patients with type 1 diabetes mellitus because of noncompliance with insulin therapy or acute illness or injury. Patients typically have symptoms of nausea, abdominal pain, excessive thirst, or fatigue; however, hemodynamic instability and an altered level of consciousness are possible. A classic finding is Kussmaul breathing (rapid, deep respirations) and an acetone or fruity breath odor. Laboratory findings include hyperglycemia (400-800 mg/dL), a high–anion gap metabolic acidosis, and ketosis. Hyperkalemia is common despite a total body potassium deficit. Mortality from DKA can approach 10% to 15%, so aggressive treatment is critical. Normal saline is infused to replace intravascular volume, along with regular insulin (0.1-0.2 U/kg bolus, followed by 0.1 U/kg/hr) and frequent glucose monitoring. Glucose is added to the fluid resuscitation once serum glucose falls below 250 mg/dL. The insulin infusion is titrated but continued until the ketoacidosis resolves. Hypokalemia and hypophosphate-

mia commonly develop during therapy and are aggressively corrected.

Hyperosmolar nonketotic dehydration (HONK) syndrome is more common in patients who have sufficient insulin to prevent ketoacidosis, but not hyperglycemia. Its precipitating factors and clinical manifestations are similar to those of DKA, but mental status changes are more common and pronounced. The hyperglycemia of HONK syndrome is more extreme, generally exceeding 800 mg/dL; however, ketoacidosis is absent. Osmotic diuresis leads to dehydration and hypernatremia, but the sodium level can be misleading because of hyperglycemic pseudohyponatremia. The free water deficit may be calculated on the basis of the corrected serum sodium level (add 1.6 mmol/L for every 100 mg/dL elevation in glucose):

$$\text{Free water deficit} = 0.6 \times \text{Weight} \times [1 - (140/\text{Serum Na})]$$

where weight is in kilograms and free water deficit in liters. Treatment of HONK is similar to that of DKA, except that fluid resuscitation needs to be more aggressive.

Hyperglycemia in the absence of a diagnosis of diabetes mellitus is quite common in critically ill patients. The phenomenon of stress-related hyperglycemia appears to be related to insulin resistance as a result of the release of counter-regulatory hormones (e.g., glucagon, epinephrine, norepinephrine, glucocorticoids, growth hormone) and cytokines (e.g., tumor necrosis factor, interleukin-1, and interleukin-6). It may be present on ICU admission and typically resolves as the catabolic illness subsides; however, ongoing metabolic dysregulation and protracted hyperglycemia may persist in some patients, particularly those with untreated infection or ongoing inflammation. The consequences of protracted hyperglycemia include increased postoperative infectious complications[37] and worse outcomes after myocardial infarction, stroke, and head injury. Insulin is now viewed as a therapeutic drug in critical illness, with prospective, randomized clinical data demonstrating improved survival associated with intensive insulin therapy (i.e., maintenance of glucose between 80 and 110 mg/dL as opposed to 180 or 200 mg/dL).[38] The benefit of tight glucose control appears to be based on maintenance of normoglycemia rather than on the dose of insulin infused.[39]

HEMATOLOGIC SYSTEM

Venous Thromboembolism

Deep Venous Thrombosis

ICU patients typically manifest all three components of Virchow's triad—stasis, endothelial injury, and hypercoagulability—and hence deep venous thrombosis (DVT) occurs in 30% of these patients.[40] Accordingly, it is prudent for every institution to have a formal prevention strategy for venous thromboembolism (VTE). High-risk factors that justify prophylaxis include major general surgery (thoracic or abdominal operations under general anesthesia that last longer than 30 minutes), neurosurgical procedures, coronary artery bypass surgery, surgery for gynecologic malignancies, major urologic surgery, multiple trauma, hip fracture, spinal cord injury, surgery or chemotherapy for malignancy, congestive heart failure, and respiratory failure. There are additional risk factors that are not sufficient to justify prophylaxis but may in combination warrant or alter prophylaxis: previous VTE, age older than 40 years, obesity, prolonged immobility, hormone replacement therapy, antiphospholipid antibody syndrome, and hereditary risk factors. Because ICU patients typically have at least one risk factor and usually more, DVT prophylaxis is considered routine. All patients have intermittent pneumatic compression devices applied. If there is no contraindication, low-molecular-weight heparin (LMWH), low-dose unfractionated heparin, adjusted-dose heparin, or oral anticoagulants are administered.[40] Fondaparinux sodium, a synthetic pentasaccharide that inhibits activated factor X, appears promising in major orthopedic surgery and possibly as therapy for heparin-induced thrombocytopenia (HIT; see later). The use of prophylactic inferior vena cava filters is controversial. In general, their use is limited to high-risk patients who have contraindications to anticoagulation or to patients with recurrent PE.

Clinical signs and symptoms (leg pain, swelling, rubor, fever) of DVT are unreliable in the ICU. Venography is considered the gold standard for diagnosis, but it is invasive and requires a contrast load. Imaging with CT or MRI is expensive and requires moving the patient. On the other hand, duplex ultrasonography is noninvasive and portable and has a sensitivity and specificity of greater than 95%, which makes it an excellent screening tool. The literature has supported use of the D-dimer assay because of its high negative predictive value; however, D-dimer is insufficient to exclude DVT in patients who have moderate to high clinical probability based on pretest assessment.[41] In contrast, the combination of a normal D-dimer concentration and a low pretest probability is probably adequate to rule out VTE.[42]

Treatment of DVT has classically consisted of IV unfractionated heparin (UFH); however, because of its more consistent and predictable response, favorable dosing, lack of need for monitoring, and equivalent efficacy with fewer bleeding complications, LMWH is now preferred. LMWH affords the option of long-term treatment, thereby obviating the need for warfarin. Treatment of VTE generally lasts for 6 months, although this remains debatable. Thrombolytic therapy is considered for limb-threatening thrombosis of the iliofemoral system, but otherwise it offers little additional benefit to offset its bleeding risk. Upper extremity DVT is treated as aggressively as lower extremity DVT because the rate of PE exceeds 10%.

Pulmonary Embolism

PE is a common and probably underdiagnosed problem. Its clinical manifestations are nonspecific, and it is likely that the majority of episodes are clinically insignificant. The most common signs of PE are tachypnea, hypoxemia, and tachyarrhythmias; however, hypotension may be seen with moderate-sized PE. If PE is clinically suspected and the clinical situation allows, UFH is administered empirically while a diagnosis is pursued. Lytic therapy is considered in moderate to severe cases. If clinical suspicion for PE is low, a noninvasive study such as D-dimer assay or duplex ultrasonography may be used, but a normal D-dimer level in this setting can obviate the need for further testing.[42] If the PE was moderate to severe, a more definitive test is needed. Pulmonary angiography is considered the gold standard, but it is invasive and requires interventional radiologic capability. V̇/Q̇ scanning, the former first-line test, is valuable only if it is either negative or high probability. Spiral CT pulmonary angiography is fairly accurate in diagnosing PE and may demonstrate additional/alternative pathology. Catastrophic PE, such as seen with a large saddle embolus, may cause sudden death. Immediate CPR is required, along with large doses of heparin or thrombolytics. Trendelenburg's procedure is an option but is rarely indicated and infrequently successful.

Heparin-Induced Thrombocytopenia

Up to 15% of patients who receive heparin experience acute thrombocytopenia that resolves spontaneously and has limited clinical sequelae. It is caused by platelet clumping or transient sequestration of platelets and is termed *HIT type I. HIT type II* is due to heparin-associated antiplatelet antibodies (platelet factor 4; PF4), which develop in 1% to 3% of patients taking UFH and 0.1% of patients taking LMWH. HIT type II leads to platelet activation and aggregation, which results in severe VTE phenomena that typically occur an average of 8 days after the beginning of heparin administration (5 days if a patient was previously sensitized). The diagnosis of HIT is suspected in patients with resistance to anticoagulation, thromboembolic events, a fall in the platelet count of greater than 30%, or an absolute platelet count less than 100,000/mm³. If HIT is suspected, all forms of heparin are stopped and the patient tested for PF4. If no antibodies are detected, heparin can be resumed; however, if anti-PF4 antibodies are found, all forms of heparin need to be discontinued and alternative anticoagulants may be necessary. Patients with PF4 antibodies who require ongoing VTE prophylaxis are usually treated with the direct thrombin inhibitors lepirudin or argatroban, which bind thrombin and block its activity. Drugs that have been used for VTE prophylaxis in PF4-positive patients include the factor Xa inhibitors fondaparinux, idraparinux, razaxaban, and other direct thrombin inhibitors; bivalirudin and ximelagatran or other agents; and danaparoid; however, these remain off-label uses at this time. Anti-PF4 antibodies tend to fade over a period of weeks to months, so patients may receive heparin in the future if retesting is negative. The role of long-term anticoagulation with warfarin remains unclear.

Blood Transfusions

Anemia secondary to injury, surgery, diagnostic tests, and decreased erythropoiesis is a widespread problem in critically ill patients that results in frequent blood transfusions. A multicenter observational study reported that 29% of patients admitted to ICUs had Hb levels lower than 10 g/dL, and 37% received transfusions during their stay. Clinical trials indicate that Hb tends to reach a kind of steady state around 8.5 g/dL in ICU patients.[43] Moderate anemia (Hb of 7-10 g/dL) is well tolerated in healthy individuals, but some ICU patients with excessive metabolic demands may not tolerate the associated decrease in DO_2. Transfusion therapy is not without risk because blood is altered during storage such that transfusion may incite electrolyte and acid-base disturbances, coagulopathy, and diminished oxygen-delivering capacity. Despite improved safety of the current blood supply, there is still the potential for viral infections, incompatibility resulting in hemolytic reactions, anaphylaxis, and febrile reactions. Blood transfusions have significant immunomodulatory properties and can improve the survival of renal allografts, but they are also associated with an increased recurrence of cancers and postoperative infections. Finally, blood transfusion has been identified as a robust independent predictor of postinjury MOF.[44] In light of these reasons, the transfusion trigger is constantly being revised as our appreciation that the risk-to-benefit ratio of blood transfusion continues to evolve.

A multicenter PRCT examined the effects of a restrictive transfusion strategy consisting of transfusion for Hb values less than 7 g/dL and maintenance of Hb at 7 to 9 g/dL versus a liberal strategy (maintaining Hb at 10-12 g/dL).[43] In-hospital mortality was lower in the restrictive strategy group. In this same group, 30-day mortality was lower in the subsets who were less acutely ill (Acute Physiology, Age, and Chronic Health Evaluation [APACHE] scores <20) and younger (<55 years), but not in those with clinically significant cardiac disease. Based on the current literature, a rational set of transfusion guidelines may be constructed (Box 24-2).

In recognition of the detrimental effects of low DO_2 and blood transfusion, alternatives to transfusion are being investigated. In elective surgery, practical alternatives include preoperative autologous blood donation, normovolemic hemodilution, induced hypotension to reduce blood loss, and red blood cell salvage systems;

> **Box 24-2 Transfusion Guidelines**
>
> **Packed Red Blood Cells**
>
> Hemoglobin <7 g/dL
> Acute blood volume loss >15%
> Greater than a 20% drop in blood pressure or blood pressure <100 mm Hg because of blood loss
> Hemoglobin <10 g/dL accompanied by symptoms (chest pain, dyspnea, fatigability, light-headedness, orthostatic hypotension) or in the presence of significant cardiac disease
> Hemoglobin <11 g/dL for patients at risk for multiple organ failure
>
> **Fresh Frozen Plasma**
>
> Prothrombin time >17 seconds
> Clotting factor deficiency (<25% of normal value)
> Massive transfusion (1 U/5 U red blood cells) or if clinically bleeding
> Severe traumatic brain injury
>
> **Platelets**
>
> Platelet count <10,000/µL
> Platelet count <10,000/µL to 20,000/µL with bleeding
> Platelet count <50,000/µL acutely after severe trauma
> Bleeding time >15 minutes
>
> **Cryoprecipitate**
>
> Fibrinogen <100 mg/dL
> Hemophilia A, von Willebrand's disease
> Severe traumatic brain injury

however, these alternatives are not feasible in the ICU. Autotransfusion involves the recovery and readministration of shed blood from body cavities, wounds, and drains. The blood is collected in a reservoir containing an anticoagulant and reinfused after washing or filtering, or both. There is virtually no risk of transmission of infectious disease, and transfusion reactions are essentially eliminated. On the other hand, shed blood recovered from body cavities is defibrinated and essentially depleted of clotting factors, so dilutional coagulopathy may result from major autotransfusion. Because the blood has been partially clotted with subsequent lysis, transfusion of these products of fibrinolysis can activate the patient's coagulation system and result in disseminated intravascular coagulation. There is also a risk of contamination of the shed blood, particularly during gastrointestinal surgery or trauma. An inability to predict who will benefit from autotransfusion and its labor intensity limit its cost-effectiveness.

The anemia of critical illness is associated with a blunted increase in circulating erythropoietin concentrations in response to physiologic stimuli. A multicenter PRCT found that weekly administration of 40,000 units of recombinant human erythropoietin increased Hb and decreased transfusions. This therapy has been shown to be effective in reducing requirements for blood transfusion, but whether this reduction is associated with a fall in transfusion-related mortality remains to be seen.

Blood Substitutes

Blood products require typing and crossmatching, have a limited shelf life, and are not immediately available in all health care facilities or clinical settings. Consequently, Hb substitutes that will provide physiologic O_2-carrying capacity and volume expansion without adverse effects or risks remain a focus of active investigation (Box 24-3). Over the past 20 years, two strategies of blood substitutes have been developed and tested clinically: perfluorocarbon emulsions and Hb solutions. Perfluorocarbons have solubility for O_2 that is 10 to 20 times that of blood, but they have no special affinity for O_2 and thus their efficacy relies on maintaining a high PaO_2. Presently, they offer no discrete benefit over crystalloid solutions and have been associated with unacceptable toxicity. Development continues with a product in phase II clinical trials in the United States and Europe.

The Hb tetramer is the active ingredient of the red blood cell and is quite durable; it functions independently to transport O_2 outside its cell membrane. Unfortunately, unmodified tetrameric Hb is unsuitable for clinical use because it dissociates into heterodimers and extravasates, with scavenging of nitric oxide resulting in unwanted vasoconstriction. Unmodified tetrameric Hb is further hindered by its low oxygen half-saturation pressure (P-50) and relatively high osmolality. Modification of Hb, therefore, has at least four major objectives:

1. Minimize toxicity
2. Prolong intravascular retention
3. Decrease O_2 affinity
4. Reduce colloid osmotic pressure

There are at least four Hb-based red blood cell substitutes that have been investigated in clinical trials. The primary differences in the Hb solutions lie in the source and the technical aspects of polymerization. Diaspirin–cross-linked Hb, derived from outdated human blood, has been one of the most widely studied solutions. Unfortunately, clinical experience has been disappointing. A multicenter randomized trial in patients with hemorrhagic shock found that mortality was higher in the study group (46%) than in a saline resuscitation comparison group (17%). The cause of the excessive death rate is not known but is theorized to be due to its negative effect on nitric oxide. Another product, *O*-raffinose–polymerized Hb, has been shown in phase II clinical trials to be potentially effective in reducing transfusions in patients undergoing coronary artery bypass grafting; however, this compound was similarly hindered by its pressor effect. A glutaraldehyde-polymerized bovine Hb

product has a reduced O_2 affinity that promotes O_2 unloading in tissues. In clinical trials it has been able to reduce the need for transfusions, but at the cost of increased systemic vascular resistance and methemoglobinemia. Finally, human Hb-based glutaraldehyde-polymerized pyridoxylated stroma-free Hb (Poly SFH-P) solution (PolyHeme, Northfield Laboratories, Chicago) has a nearly normal P-50, and essentially all unreacted tetramer is removed in a purification process. Clinical trials have demonstrated the safety and physiologic function of Poly-Heme, as well as the ability to avoid transfusions of allogeneic blood.[45] Unlike the other solutions, there is no evidence that PolyHeme increases systemic or pulmonary vascular resistance because the transfusion-related hyperinflammatory response appears to be blunted by PolyHeme. A recently completed, controversial, waiver-of-consent, phase III trial of PolyHeme did not reveal undue safety concerns, although the results of this trial are still unavailable.

SEPSIS AND MULTIPLE ORGAN FAILURE

Sepsis

The earliest reports of MOF syndrome, in the 1970s, linked the syndrome to sepsis. In the ensuing decade it became clearer that the systemic manifestations of gram-negative sepsis could result from noninfectious stimuli. To clarify terminology in this area, the American College of Chest Physicians and the Society of Critical Care Medicine published a consensus description and definition of SIRS (Box 24-4).[46] These definitions are important so that clinicians can communicate effectively and convey a true sense of a patient's illness, as well as identify patients who might be candidates for adjunctive therapies.

An epidemiologic study based on hospital discharge databases from seven states, representing 25% of the

U.S. population at that time, determined that severe sepsis affects 751,000 patients annually (2.3 per 100 hospital discharges), with 29% mortality.[11] As the U.S. population ages, it is anticipated that the incidence of sepsis will increase roughly 1.5% per year. Not every infection, however, causes sepsis. The occurrence of sepsis depends on a combination of bacterial virulence factors (e.g., adherence properties, resistance to phagocytosis or antibiotics, endotoxin from gram-negative bacteria, exotoxin from gram-positive bacteria) and host factors (immune status and immune response, epithelial barrier function, gender, genetic factors).

The fundamental strategy in managing septic patients involves fluid resuscitation and treatment of the underlying infection, or source control, plus the administration of appropriate antibiotics. Proper empirical antibiotic therapy for severe sepsis includes carbapenems, third- or fourth-generation cephalosporins with additional anaerobic coverage, or antipseudomonal penicillins. Agents with activity against methicillin-resistant *Staphylococcus aureus* are used if there is reasonable concern that this organism is present (e.g., nosocomial infections, chronic health facility residents). Source control refers to drainage of abscesses, débridement of devitalized tissue, removal of infected foreign bodies, and definitive management of the source (e.g., appendectomy, cholecystectomy). Resuscitation of patients follows the principles previously outlined. The benefits of early goal-directed therapy with a target CVP of 8 to 12 mm Hg, MAP of 65 of 90 mm Hg, and central venous SO_2 greater than 70% have been demonstrated in a prospective clinical trial.[47] In this study, in-hospital mortality was reduced in all patients, including the subgroup with severe sepsis and septic shock.

Septic shock represents an abnormal vasodilatory distribution of CO, where CO may be normal or increased. Septic shock is often refractory to catecholamines, which may be a manifestation of vasopressin deficiency. Thus, there is a role for vasopressin administration in patients with septic shock. Indeed, an early clinical trial found that 14 of 16 patients with catecholamine-refractory septic shock had an immediate and sustained increase in MAP associated with vasopressin infusion. The increased recognition of adrenal insufficiency in critically ill patients has prompted resurgence of glucocorticoid therapy for sepsis, as well as for critical care in general, as noted earlier. In the seminal study of steroids in septic shock, steroids were shown to reverse shock, reduce vasopressor requirements, moderate organ dysfunction scores, and improve survival.[36]

A number of adjunctive therapies have shown promise in preclinical studies or small clinical trials, but large multicenter PRCTs have not demonstrated survival benefits. Agents used include ibuprofen, prostaglandin E_1, pentoxifylline, *N*-acetylcysteine, selenium, antithrombin III, IV immunoglobulins, hemofiltration, recombinant tissue factor pathway inhibitor, p55–tumor necrosis factor (TNF) receptor fusion protein, and antibodies to TNF-α and endotoxin. Only recombinant human activated protein C (APC) has been shown to improve survival in patients with severe sepsis. APC is an endogenous protein that promotes fibrinolysis and inhibits thrombosis and

inflammation, and it is an important modulator of the coagulation and inflammation associated with severe sepsis. In a multicenter PRCT involving 1690 randomized patients with severe sepsis, APC reduced mortality from 31% to 25%.[48] The only significant adverse effect was an increase in bleeding complications in the APC group (3.5% versus 2.0%, *P* = .06).

Multiple Organ Failure

MOF has been called a *syndrome of surgical progress* because its emergence was the result of advances in treating circulatory shock, renal failure, and pulmonary insufficiency. The description of MOF as a distinct entity dates back to the 1970s, when a number of groups reported the progressive failure of organ systems with a sequential pattern.[49] Mortality associated with MOF ranges from 40% to 100% and is related directly to the number and duration of organ systems that fail. Unfortunately, neither the incidence nor the mortality of the syndrome has improved significantly in recent years, and it remains a leading cause of death in the ICU.

Early reports of MOF implicated infection as the primary etiologic factor,[50] but subsequent studies have emphasized that overt clinical infections were not a requisite for MOF. Indeed, about a third of patient dying of MOF will have positive blood cultures with no identifiable source. The current thought is that MOF represents the culmination of a generalized and excessive neuroendocrine, immune, and inflammatory response. The cascade may be precipitated by a wide variety of insults, broadly classified as tissue injury, cellular shock, inflammation, and infection. Burgeoning evidence supports the concept that multiple insults are probably responsible for MOF. In the two-event model of MOF (Fig. 24-5), the

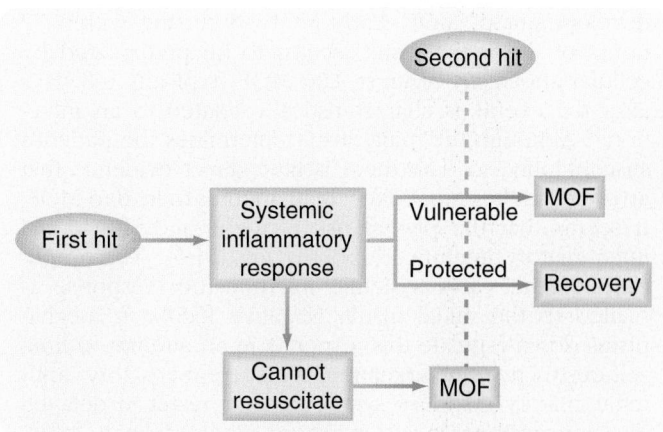

Figure 24-5 The two-event model of multiple organ failure (MOF). An initial insult results in systemic hyperinflammation. If either the insult or the inflammatory response is exaggerated or perpetuated, overt MOF may develop. More commonly, the host endures multiple sequential insults. A second insult during a vulnerable period amplifies the systemic inflammatory response to produce MOF.

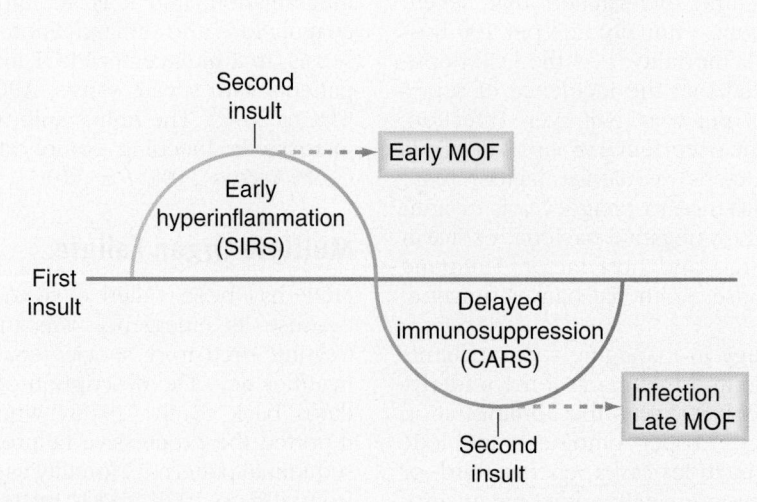

Figure 24-6 A dysfunctional inflammatory/immune response leads to multiple organ failure (MOF). The amplitude of the early systemic inflammatory response syndrome (SIRS) is related to the initial insult. A compensatory anti-inflammatory response (CARS) may result in delayed immunosuppression. Sequential insults superimposed on either the hyperinflammatory state or the immunosuppressed state may result in MOF.

host experiences sequential insults such that the subsequent systemic inflammatory response exceeds the typical response elicited by either insult alone. The initial insult primes the inflammatory response, and patients enter a state of systemic hyperinflammation (i.e., SIRS). If the insult or the inflammatory response is exaggerated or perpetuated, patients enter a state of malignant systemic hyperinflammation (severe SIRS) that can evolve into overt MOF, independent of other factors. The more common scenario involves multiple sequential insults. A second insult during a vulnerable period amplifies SIRS to produce MOF. The progression appears to be dependent on the type of insult, with a bimodal pattern of the development of MOF. Early MOF (occurring within 72 hours of the initial insult) seems to be precipitated by cellular shock. In contrast, late MOF (typically 6-8 days after the event) is characteristically related to an infection.[50] Although the initial insult determines the patient's susceptibility, to date there is little direct evidence that any one insult is more likely than another to lead to MOF. It seems that the pivotal risk factor is a dysfunctional inflammatory/immune response (Fig. 24-6). The amplitude of the early systemic inflammatory response is related to the initial insult. Negative feedback mechanisms down-regulate this response in an attempt to limit self-destructive inflammation. This compensatory anti-inflammatory response syndrome may result in delayed immunosuppression and increased susceptibility to infection. In this paradigm, a second hit during either early hyperinflammation or delayed immunosuppression will have the same net effect, deterioration into MOF.

Despite nearly 3 decades of clinical and basic science research and a whole host of failed antimediators, mortality rates for patients with MOF remain largely unchanged. This fact, along with our inability to significantly modify

the syndrome, points to the overriding importance of adopting strategies to prevent the development of MOF. Avoiding so-called second hits can be accomplished in three distinct areas: resuscitation, operative interventions, and critical care. Resuscitation end points such as clearance of lactate and base deficit represent repayment of the oxygen debt and may minimize the cellular injury resulting from shock. Even the choice of resuscitation fluid is important. Hypertonic saline appears to have favorable immunomodulatory properties, whereas transfusion of banked blood may serve as a second hit.

In one of the seminal articles describing MOF,[49] more than half the cases of MOF were due to an intraoperative error or perioperative mistake. Meticulous surgical technique in which tissue trauma is minimized, avoidance of hematomas and blood loss requiring transfusion, adequate débridement of necrotic tissue, timely and appropriate antibiotic therapy, and embracing the concept of damage control surgery are all ways that operative management can lessen the incidence of MOF. Avoidance plus timely treatment of ACS is key because it represents one of the only reversible forms of MOF. Finally, maintaining a high index of suspicion for missed injuries and intra-abdominal catastrophes in the postoperative period and remaining amenable to exploring hostile abdomens are additional ways that the risk for MOF can be lessened.

The purpose of this chapter was to give readers a brief but focused overview of surgical critical care so that they can continue to take effective care of their patients. Part of this efficacy is embracing management strategies that have been shown to have a real impact on morbidity and mortality, such as tight glucose control, lung protective ventilation, early and adequate nutrition, restrictive blood transfusion practices, and DVT and stress gastritis prophylaxis. This list is by no means all-inclusive but is part of the strategy to minimize the development of complications and reduce the potential for development of MOF.

Selected References

Annane D, Sebille V, Charpentier C, et al: Effect of treatment with low doses of hydrocortisone and fludrocortisone on mortality in patients with septic shock. JAMA 288:862-871, 2002.

Key article showing a reduction in mortality with physiologic corticosteroid replacement therapy in patients in septic shock and relative adrenal insufficiency.

Bernard GR, Vincent JL, Laterre PF, et al: Efficacy and safety of recombinant human activated protein C for severe sepsis. N Engl J Med 344:699-709, 2001.

First article dealing with the benefits of recombinant activated protein C in patients with severe sepsis.

Davis JW, Kaups KL, Parks SN: Base deficit is superior to pH in evaluating clearance of acidosis after traumatic shock. J Trauma 44:114-118, 1998.

Classic reference illustrating the predictive power of clearance of acidosis in survivors and nonsurvivors after major trauma.

Debaveye YA, Van den Berghe GH: Is there still a place for dopamine in the modern intensive care unit? Anesth Analg 98:461-468, 2004.

A critical review of the role of dopamine in critically ill patients highlighting its dubious efficacy and potential to cause unwanted effects.

Fleisher LA, Beckman JA, Brown KA, et al: ACC/AHA 2006 guideline update on perioperative cardiovascular evaluation for noncardiac surgery: Focused update on perioperative beta blocker therapy: A report of the American College of Cardiology/American Heart Association Task Force on Practice Guidelines (Writing Committee to Update the 2002 Guidelines on Perioperative Cardiovascular Evaluation for Noncardiac Surgery): Developed in collaboration with the American Society of Echocardiography, American Society of Nuclear Cardiology, Heart Rhythm Society, Society of Cardiovascular Anesthesiologists, Society for Cardiovascular Angiography and Interventions, and Society for Vascular Medicine and Biology. Circulation 113:2662-2674, 2006.

State-of-the art review and consensus paper establishing the role of β-adrenergic blockade as a means of reducing cardiac events in patients undergoing noncardiac surgical procedures.

Merten GJ, Burgess WP, Gray LV, et al: Prevention of contrast-induced nephropathy with sodium bicarbonate: A randomized controlled trial. JAMA 291:2328-2334, 2004.

Prospective trial documenting bicarbonate infusions as a means of minimizing contrast nephropathy in patients with preexisting renal insufficiency.

Tobin MJ: Advances in mechanical ventilation. N Engl J Med 344:1986-1996, 2001.

Classic review of ventilator strategies and weaning from mechanical ventilation.

The Acute Respiratory Distress Network: Ventilation with lower tidal volumes as compared with traditional tidal volumes for acute lung injury and the acute respiratory distress syndrome. N Engl J Med 341:1301-1308, 2000.

Seminal article establishing the benefit of lung-protective ventilation in patients with ARDS.

Van den Berghe G, Wouters P, Weekers F, et al: Intensive insulin therapy in critically ill patients. N Engl J Med 345:1359-1367, 2001.

Seminal article listing the beneficial effects of keeping a patient's blood glucose level less than 110 mg/dL in the ICU.

Vincent JL: Vasopressin in hypotensive and shock states. Crit Care Clin 22:187-197, 2006.

A review of clinical and basic science data examining the effect of vasopressin therapy in hemorrhagic and septic shock states. The author emphasizes that vasopressin has shown positive effects on blood pressure and urine output, but a mortality benefit remains to be proved.

References

1. Ely EW, Shintani A, Truman B, et al: Delirium as a predictor of mortality in mechanically ventilated patients in the intensive care unit. JAMA 291:1753-1762, 2004.
2. Park WY, Thompson JS, Lee KK: Effect of epidural anesthesia and analgesia on perioperative outcome: A randomized, controlled Veterans Affairs cooperative study. Ann Surg 234:560-569; discussion 569-571, 2001.
3. Ely EW, Truman B, Shintani A, et al: Monitoring sedation status over time in ICU patients: Reliability and validity of the Richmond Agitation-Sedation Scale (RASS). JAMA 289:2983-2991, 2003.
4. Jacobi J, Fraser GL, Coursin DB, et al: Clinical practice guidelines for the sustained use of sedatives and analgesics in the critically ill adult. Crit Care Med 30:119-141, 2002.
5. Murray MJ, Cowen J, DeBlock H, et al: Clinical practice guidelines for sustained neuromuscular blockade in the adult critically ill patient. Crit Care Med 30:142-156, 2002.
6. Crijns HJ: Rate versus rhythm control in patients with atrial fibrillation: What the trials really say. Drugs 65:1651-1667, 2005.
7. Debaveye YA, Van den Berghe GH: Is there still a place for dopamine in the modern intensive care unit? Anesth Analg 98:461-468, 2004.
8. Vincent JL: Vasopressin in hypotensive and shock states. Crit Care Clin 22:187-197, v, 2006.
9. Bishop MH, Shoemaker WC, Appel PL, et al: Relationship between supranormal circulatory values, time delays, and outcome in severely traumatized patients. Crit Care Med 21:56-63, 1993.
10. Kern JW, Shoemaker WC: Meta-analysis of hemodynamic optimization in high-risk patients. Crit Care Med 30:1686-1692, 2002.
11. Angus DC, Linde-Zwirble WT, Lidicker J, et al: Epidemiology of severe sepsis in the United States: Analysis of incidence, outcome, and associated costs of care. Crit Care Med 29:1303-1310, 2001.
12. Moore FA, Haenel JB, Moore EE: Incommensurate oxygen consumption in response to maximal oxygen availability predicts postinjury multiple organ failure. J Trauma 33:58-66, 2005.
13. Balogh Z, McKinley BA, Cocanour CS: Supranormal resuscitation causes more cases of abdominal compartment syndrome. Arch Surg 138:637-643, 2003.
14. Ivatury RR, Simon RJ, Islam S, et al: A prospective randomized study of end points of resuscitation after major trauma: Global oxygen transport indices versus organ-specific gastric mucosal pH. J Am Coll Surg 183:145-154, 1996.

15. Davis JW, Kaups KL, Parks SN: Base deficit is superior to pH in evaluating clearance of acidosis after traumatic shock. J Trauma 44:114-118, 1998.

16. Fleisher LA, Eagle KA: Lowering cardiac risk in noncardiac surgery. N Engl J Med 345:1677-1682, 2001.

17. Fleisher LA, Beckman JA, Brown KA, et al: ACC/AHA 2006 guideline update on perioperative cardiovascular evaluation for noncardiac surgery: Focused update on perioperative beta-blocker therapy: A report of the American College of Cardiology/American Heart Association Task Force on Practice Guidelines (Writing Committee to Update the 2002 Guidelines on Perioperative Cardiovascular Evaluation for Noncardiac Surgery): Developed in collaboration with the American Society of Echocardiography, American Society of Nuclear Cardiology, Heart Rhythm Society, Society of Cardiovascular Anesthesiologists, Society for Cardiovascular Angiography and Interventions, and Society for Vascular Medicine and Biology. Circulation 113:2662-2674, 2006.

18. Ferrer R, Artigas A: Clinical review: Non-antibiotic strategies for preventing ventilator-associated pneumonia. Crit Care 6:45-51, 2002.

19. Bernard GR, Artigas A, Brigham KL: The America-European Consensus Conference on ARDS. Definitions, mechanisms, relevant outcomes, and clinical trial coordination. Am J Respir Crit Care Med 149:818-824, 1994.

20. Steinberg KP, Hudson LD, Goodman RB, et al: Efficacy and safety of corticosteroids for persistent acute respiratory distress syndrome. N Engl J Med 354:1671-1684, 2006.

21. Amato MB, Barbas CS, Medeiros DM, et al: Effect of a protective-ventilation strategy on mortality in the acute respiratory distress syndrome. N Engl J Med 338:347-354, 1998.

22. The Acute Respiratory Distress Network: Ventilation with lower tidal volumes as compared with traditional tidal volumes for acute lung injury and the acute respiratory distress syndrome. The Acute Respiratory Distress Syndrome Network. N Engl J Med 342:1301-1308, 2000.

23. Petrucci N, Iacovelli W: Ventilation with lower tidal volumes versus traditional tidal volumes in adults for acute lung injury and acute respiratory distress syndrome. Cochrane Database Syst Rev 2:CD003844, 2004.

24. Gattinoni L, Tognoni G, Pesenti A, et al: Effect of prone positioning on the survival of patients with acute respiratory failure. N Engl J Med 345:568-573, 2001.

25. Mancebo J, Fernandez R, Blanch L, et al: A multicenter trial of prolonged prone ventilation in severe acute respiratory distress syndrome. Am J Respir Crit Care Med 173:1233-1239, 2006.

26. Esteban A, Frutos-Vivar F, Ferguson ND, et al: Noninvasive positive-pressure ventilation for respiratory failure after extubation. N Engl J Med 350:2452-2460, 2004.

27. Tobin MJ: Advances in mechanical ventilation. N Engl J Med 344:1986-1996, 2001.

28. Freeman BD, Borecki IB, Coopersmith CM, et al: Relationship between tracheostomy timing and duration of mechanical ventilation in critically ill patients. Crit Care Med 33:2513-2520, 2005.

29. Siobal MS, Kallet RH, Kivett VA, et al: Use of dexmedetomidine to facilitate extubation in surgical intensive-care-unit patients who failed previous weaning attempts following prolonged mechanical ventilation: A pilot study. Respir Care 51:492-496, 2006.

30. Deitch EA, Xu D, Kaise VL: Role of the gut in the development of injury- and shock-induced SIRS and MODS: The gut-lymph hypothesis, a review. Front Biosci 11:520-528, 2006.

31. Ramsay G, van Saene RH: Selective gut decontamination in intensive care and surgical practice: Where are we? World J Surg 22:164-170, 1998.

32. Biffl WL, Moore EE, Burch JM, et al: Secondary abdominal compartment syndrome is a highly lethal event. Am J Surg 182:645-648, 2001.

33. Friedrich JO, Adhikari N, Herridge MS, et al: Meta-analysis: Low-dose dopamine increases urine output but does not prevent renal dysfunction or death. Ann Intern Med 142:510-524, 2005.

34. Merten GJ, Burgess WP, Gray LV, et al: Prevention of contrast-induced nephropathy with sodium bicarbonate: A randomized controlled trial. JAMA 291:2328-2334, 2004.

35. Cooper MS, Stewart PM: Corticosteroid insufficiency in acutely ill patients. N Engl J Med 348:727-734, 2003.

36. Annane D, Sebille V, Charpentier C, et al: Effect of treatment with low doses of hydrocortisone and fludrocortisone on mortality in patients with septic shock. JAMA 288:862-871, 2002.

37. Golden SH, Peart-Vigilance C, Kao WH, et al: Perioperative glycemic control and the risk of infectious complications in a cohort of adults with diabetes. Diabetes Care 22:1408-1414, 1999.

38. Van den Berghe G, Wouters P, Weekers F, et al: Intensive insulin therapy in critically ill patients. N Engl J Med 345:1359-1367, 2001.

39. Van den Berghe G, Wouters PJ, Bouillon R, et al: Outcome benefit of intensive insulin therapy in the critically ill: Insulin dose versus glycemic control. Crit Care Med 31:359-366, 2003.

40. Geerts WH, Heit JA, Clagett GP, et al: Prevention of venous thromboembolism. Chest 119:132S-175S, 2001.

41. American College of Emergency Physicians (ACEP) Clinical Policies Committee; ACEP Clinical Policies Subcommittee on Suspected Lower-Extremity Deep Venous Thrombosis: Clinical policy: Critical issues in the evaluation and management of adult patients presenting with suspected lower-extremity deep venous thrombosis. Ann Emerg Med 42:124-135, 2003.

42. Kearon C, Ginsberg JS, Douketis J, et al: An evaluation of D-dimer in the diagnosis of pulmonary embolism: A randomized trial. Ann Intern Med 144:812-821, 2006.

43. Hebert PC, Wells G, Blajchman MA, et al: A multicenter, randomized, controlled clinical trial of transfusion requirements in critical care. Transfusion Requirements in Critical Care Investigators, Canadian Critical Care Trials Group. N Engl J Med 340:409-417, 1999.

44. Moore FA, Moore EE, Sauaia A: Blood transfusion. An independent risk factor for postinjury multiple organ failure. Arch Surg 132:620-624; discussion 624-625, 1997.

45. Gould SA, Moore EE, Hoyt DB, et al: The life-sustaining capacity of human polymerized hemoglobin when red cells might be unavailable. J Am Coll Surg 195:445-452; discussion 452-445, 2002.

46. American College of Chest Physicians/Society of Critical Care Medicine Consensus Conference: Definitions for sepsis and organ failure and guidelines for the use of innovative therapies in sepsis. Crit Care Med 20:864-874, 1992.

47. Rivers E, Nguyen B, Havstad S, et al: Early goal-directed therapy in the treatment of severe sepsis and septic shock. N Engl J Med 345:1368-1377, 2001.

48. Bernard GR, Vincent JL, Laterre PF, et al: Efficacy and safety of recombinant human activated protein C for severe sepsis. N Engl J Med 344:699-709, 2001.

49. Eiseman B, Beart R, Norton L: Multiple organ failure. Surg Gynecol Obstet 144:323-326, 1997.

50. Fry DE, Pearlstein L, Fulton RL, et al: Multiple system organ failure: The role of uncontrolled infection. Arch Surg 115:136-140, 1980.

CHAPTER 25

Bedside Surgical Procedures

Addison K. May, MD   and   Jose J. Diaz, MD

Safety Practices for Bedside Surgical Procedures

Selection of Patients for Bedside Surgical Procedures

Bedside Laparotomy

Tracheostomy

Percutaneous Endoscopic Gastrostomy

Bronchoscopy

Over approximately the last decade several factors have combined to increase the frequency and appropriateness of operative procedures performed at the bedside in the intensive care unit (ICU) for critically ill surgical patients. Such factors include the increasing severity of illness in critically ill surgical patients; acceptance of staged and damage control management strategies for severe abdominal, soft tissue, and orthopedic pathology; advances in endoscopic and percutaneous techniques; increasing competition for operating room space; difficulty associated with transporting severely critically ill patients; and cost of repetitive operative procedures.

For abdominal procedures in particular, introduction of the open abdominal approach for the management of abdominal catastrophes and abdominal compartment syndrome (ACS) has created the need for frequent and repetitive abdominal procedures that can be done safely and efficiently at the bedside. Additionally, acceptance of the utility of early tracheostomy by many surgeons and the introduction of percutaneous tracheostomy and endoscopically guided feeding access have resulted in a number of procedures being performed at the bedside in the ICU that historically had been performed in the operating theater. As an example, over the 56-month period between July 2001 and February 2006, our Division of Trauma and Surgical Critical Care performed more than 4500 bedside surgical procedures, including more than 1400 tracheostomies, placement of over 800 gastros-

tomy or gastrojejunostomy tubes, more than 1700 bronchoscopy procedures, and 480 laparotomies. Our monthly bedside laparotomy rate has increased from 1.9 per month during the years 1996 to 2000 to 8.7 per month during the years 2001 to 2006. During these two periods, the indication for laparotomy shifted significantly toward the elective and semielective indications of washout or closure; 27% of laparotomies were performed for these indications during the earlier period, whereas 75% were performed for such indications in the later period.[1,2]

Documenting the safety and cost-effectiveness of bedside surgical procedures is made difficult by the breadth of procedures, diverse populations, and variable indications for these procedures. However, for the common procedures, sufficient data support both safety and cost-effectiveness. Early reports of combined analysis of common bedside procedures, including percutaneous dilational tracheostomy (PDT), placement of percutaneous endoscopic gastrostomy (PEG) tubes, placement of inferior vena cava (IVC) filters, and laparotomies, demonstrated complication rates similar to those performed in the operating theater, but with a significant reduction in cost.[3,4] Additionally, more recent reports examining PDT, PEG, and bedside laparotomy individually have also demonstrated these procedures to be both safe and more cost-effective than the same procedures performed in the operating room.[1,2,5-8] Additionally, bedside procedures avoid the risk and difficulties introduced by transportation of the patient for procedures performed in the operating room. Although progress has been made in the safe transport of critically ill, high-risk patients, serious adverse events and death can occur.[9] A small group of patients are simply not transportable because of either the severity of pulmonary dysfunction or the rapidity with which the underlying process must be addressed. In this population, rapidly performed bedside procedures can be lifesaving.

Even though bedside operative procedures can be performed safely with complication rates equal to those in the operating room suite, doing so mandates that patients be appropriately selected and that appropriate safety practices be consistently implemented. The ICU is a complex environment in which to perform complicated processes and procedures. Recognition of the numerous potentials for errors and adverse events in such settings is important. Based on the experience of high-reliability organizations, prevention of errors and adverse events requires standardization of processes and elimination of variability.[10] Protocols and safety practices specifically designed for bedside operative procedures must be in place to ensure the ability to perform these procedures safely, with low infection rates, and with the assurance of comfort and amnesia. This chapter discusses the following:

1. Systematic safety methodologies and practices to ensure safe performance of bedside procedures
2. Selection of patients for bedside surgical procedures
3. Specific considerations for common bedside procedures
   - Bedside laparotomy
   - Percutaneous tracheostomy
   - Placement of percutaneous endoscopic feeding tubes
   - Bronchoscopy

SAFETY PRACTICES FOR BEDSIDE SURGICAL PROCEDURES

To ensure the safety of operative procedures performed at the bedside, systematic measures are undertaken for the following reasons:

1. To ensure the appropriate selection of patients
2. To ensure adequate expertise of supporting personnel
3. To reduce procedural variability
4. To prevent communication errors

Numerous tools and techniques are available, and typically a number of complementary measures are used to achieve a high level of safe performance. In our ICUs, we use several to ensure safety, including the following:

- Specifically trained, procedure support personnel
- Management guidelines and standard operating procedure documents to ensure standardization of personnel, equipment, and performance
- Preprocedure time-out and procedural checklists to ensure the application of appropriate practices
- Compliance monitoring, event reporting, and outcome review for quality assurance and process improvement

Each of these safety mechanisms are discussed in more detail in the following text.

The use of specifically trained procedure support personnel to perform bedside operative procedures within the ICU greatly facilitates reduction in variability, compliance with standard operative procedures, reduction in communication errors, and maintenance of appropriate

skill sets. Depending on the volume of procedures, these personnel can be unit or service specific or be used to support bedside procedures on numerous services in multiple ICUs. Limiting this procedure support role to a small number of personnel allows a greater degree of expertise to be developed and has, in our experience, been extremely valuable in maintaining procedural safety, particularly in handling the airway and endotracheal tube during percutaneous tracheostomies. Additionally, these personnel are charged with developing and monitoring safety practices and ensuring their application during all procedures.

Management guidelines, protocols, and standard operating procedures need to be in place before the routine performance of bedside operative procedures. They must be in line with those developed for the operating theater and be easily accessible and monitored for compliance. Because of variations in specific personnel and practice patterns in various ICUs, our documents are customized to each location to ensure appropriate application during bedside operative procedures. These documents need to address the selection of appropriate patients and mandatory personnel, equipment, medications, monitoring, and other requirements. An example of our bedside operative guideline is provided in Box 25-1.[2] All patients have blood pressure, electrocardiography, pulse oximetry, and ventilation routinely monitored throughout the procedures. Adequate personnel must be present to allow performance of the procedure, monitoring of sedation/anesthesia, administration of medication, manipulation of ventilation if required, and documentation. The actual number of personnel required depends on the procedure and the particular expertise of the personnel. Both analgesia and sedation must be ensured with appropriate medications under the direction of the critical care faculty. Additionally, guidelines and protocols include standards for adequate preparation, equipment, and accounting of instruments.

The use of a preprocedure time-out and procedural checklists aids in ensuring appropriate safety practices. Use of these tools helps limit communication errors, facilitates compliance with standard operating procedures, and can aid in documentation and monitoring of compliance. Again, these tools are consistent with practices used in the operating room to reduce variability when appropriate. Figure 25-1 provides an example of such a procedural checklist. Ideally, these tools can be combined with forms for documentation and the information used for analysis of quality and performance.

Ensuring a high degree of safety of bedside operative procedures and providing documentation of such when required mandate that mechanisms for tracking performance of procedures, monitoring compliance, and reviewing and reporting adverse events be developed. They must be applicable locally to facilitate consistent, nonvariable performance and interface with global hospital safety mechanisms and initiatives. The development of process-mapping flow charts and diagrams facilitates the integration of unit-specific, departmental, and hospital-wide processes and helps delineate lines of communication and authority.

SELECTION OF PATIENTS FOR BEDSIDE SURGICAL PROCEDURES

As noted previously, bedside operative procedures can be performed with a similar risk for complications as when performed in the operating room, at lower cost, and without transportation risks if selected appropriately.[1,2,4,7-9,11] Unfortunately, no randomized studies and few retrospective reviews have evaluated the safety of bedside operative procedures or delineated the appropriate patient populations and operative procedures. Additionally, both the safety and efficacy of bedside procedures depend on the local experience and application of safety practices. As experience is gained, indications may broaden and the frequency increase. When making a decision to perform an operative procedure at the bedside, one needs to consider the difficulty and risk associated with transport, the complexity of the operation, the ability to achieve timely operating room space, and the safety, ease, and cost savings of performing the procedure at the bedside. The vast majority of major operative procedures are performed in the operating room, and in general, indications for bedside operative procedures fall into two categories: (1) the patient is too unstable for transport to the operating room and the procedure is a required, lifesaving intervention, or (2) the procedure is modest enough that the difficulties of transport, scheduling, and cost of the operating room seem unjustified.[12]

Factors that generally favor performance of procedures in the operating room include complex procedures, risk of bleeding from major vascular structures, need for insertion of prosthetic materials, significant lighting requirements, and lengthy procedures. Commonly performed bedside procedures include percutaneous and open tracheostomy, placement of PEG or percutaneous endoscopic gastrojejunostomy (PEGJ) tubes, bronchoscopy, soft tissue débridement, decompressive laparotomy for abdominal hypertension, washout and removal of packing after damage control laparotomy, placement of IVC filters, and damage control orthopedic procedures. On occasion, very critically ill patients can be temporized at the bedside by the performance of a bedside operative procedure, with subsequent definitive operations performed in the operating room.

BESIDE LAPAROTOMY

Bedside laparotomy was initially a procedure of last resort in patients too sick to proceed to the operating room. A heroic attempt was made to identify reversible intra-abdominal pathology as the patient was near death.[2] However, recognition of ACS as a frequent complication of the resuscitation of acutely ill patients plus acceptance of the damage control approach to the management of acutely ill patients with intra-abdominal pathology has resulted in a dramatic increase in the application of bedside laparotomy in more controlled settings.[1,2,12-14] Both damage control and management of ACS involve

---

Box 25-1   Bedside Surgery Protocol

Indications

Decompressive celiotomy for abdominal compartment syndrome

Exploratory celiotomy for intra-abdominal hemorrhage after damage control and packing

Re-exploration of a previously open abdomen for washout or closure

Exploratory celiotomy to rule out intra-abdominal sepsis in a patient with ventilatory requirements prohibitive of safe transport to the operating room

Bedside Surgery Protocol

The intensive care unit attending and the operating surgeon will be present for the entire surgical procedure

Informed consent obtained (if possible)

Preprocedure checklist to be reviewed by the bedside nurse

The bedside nurse and a respiratory therapist will monitor the patient and record the procedure (conscious sedation sheet)

Indications to proceed to the operating room (level 1):
    Surgical bleeding
    Dead bowel
    Need to open another body cavity
    Surgeon preference

For laparotomies:
    A sterile perimeter will be set up in the patient's room. All individuals must wear a surgical head covering and mask
    The intensive care unit attending will oversee anesthetic management of the patient
    General anesthesia—narcotics, benzodiazepines, propofol, paralytics, and ventilator management
    A sterile hand wash is performed by the operating team
    Preoperative antibiotics are indicated only if a new surgical wound is to be made (cefazolin [Ancef], 1 g IV).
    A povidone-iodine (Betadine)/chlorhexidine abdominal preparation will be used
    A standard Bovie will be set up (when indicated)
    Wall suction canisters set up
    Four-liter warm irrigation with normal saline
    A standard bedside celiotomy tray will be set up with suture on a sterile field

Adapted from Emergency General Surgery Protocols at Vanderbilt University Medical Center: Bedside Surgery Protocol, 2006. Available at http://www.mc.vanderbilt.edu/surgery/trauma/egs/protocols.htm. Accessed December 1, 2006.

---

the use of an open abdominal approach in which the fascia remains open and various temporary abdominal closure techniques are used. Indications for bedside laparotomy can be classified as emergency or semielective.

Common emergency indications follow:

1. Decompressive laparotomy for ACS
2. Control and packing for recurrent bleeding after a previous damage control laparotomy
3. Suspicion of intra-abdominal infection in patients too critical to be transported to the operating room

Common semielective indications follow:

1. Removal of packing after damage control laparotomy

SICU Procedure "TIMEOUT" Check List		
Complete this form (a) just prior to beginning the procedure and (b) at the location where the procedure is to be performed		
Patient's Name: _____ Medical record number: _____		
Procedure Type: ☐ Planned non-emergent ☐ Not planned non-emergent ☐ Emergent		
VERIFICATION		
1. Invasive procedure to be performed:		
	Circle one	
2. H&P completed if patient admitted within past 24 hours	Yes	No
3. Informed consent obtained? (Verified by Bedside RN and Procedure RN)	Yes	No
4. Correct patient identity? ☐ Arm Band ☐ MRN ☐ Consent If procedure is emergent, Bedside RN, Procedure RN, and Physician performing procedure need to verify patient ID and initial this form.	Yes	No
5. Agreement on procedure (Agreement b/w Physician performing procedure and Procedure RN)	Yes	No
6. Correct side/site verified and marked? ☐ NA ☐ Right ☐ Left ☐ Site: (Verified and marked by Physician performing procedure and Procedure RN)	Yes	No
7. Correct equipment available? (Verified by Physician performing procedure and Procedure RN)	Yes	No
8. Required resources available? (Verified by Physician performing procedure and Procedure RN)	Yes	No
9. Ready to setup procedure? (Verified by Procedure RN)	Yes	No
9. Ready to proceed with procedure? (Verified by Procedure RN)	Yes	No
TIMEOUT: All individuals performing and assisting with the procedure are to review the checklist and sign below		
Physician performing procedure:		
Procedure RN name:		
Bedside RN name:		
Other:	Other:	Other:
Staff calling "TIMEOUT": (Title and signature)		

Figure 25-1 Surgical intensive care unit procedure time-out checklist.

2. Irrigation and débridement of the open abdomen
3. Source control for sepsis secondary to intra-abdominal pathology
4. Management of traumatic abdominal defects

The most common emergency indication for bedside laparotomy is decompression of abdominal hypertension. Recognition and understanding of the pathophysiology of increased intra-abdominal pressure leading to organ system dysfunction, termed *ACS*, have increased significantly since Kron and colleagues first described measurement of intra-abdominal pressure as an indication for abdominal re-exploration.[13,15-18] ACS can be classified as either primary, attributable to intra-abdominal processes, or secondary, caused by bowel edema and intra-abdominal fluid as a result of resuscitation and treatment of extra-abdominal pathology. Increasing intra-abdominal pressure leads to alterations in abdominal perfusion pressure, restricted venous return, and a reduction in pulmonary compliance. These alterations can, in turn, lead to cardiac failure, pulmonary decompensation, and oliguria.

Severe elevations in abdominal pressure can result in organ hypoperfusion and ischemia, although the pressure at which this complication occurs may vary, depending on mean arterial pressure. Grading systems for the degree of abdominal hypertension have been proposed, with grades III (21-25 mm Hg) and IV (>25 mm Hg) considered to be significantly elevated and indicative of ACS.[18] Management of ACS may involve solely measures to ensure adequate abdominal perfusion at lower pressure, but as intra-abdominal pressure increases, abdominal decompression by laparotomy is indicated. Appropriate treatment requires recognition of development of this syndrome. Thus, routine monitoring of bladder pressure is essential in patients requiring significant resuscitation after abdominal procedures and those being resuscitated from significant shock (base deficit >10) who receive 6 L or more of crystalloid or 6 or more units of packed red blood cells in a 6-hour period.[13]

Acceptance of damage control, or an abbreviated laparotomy performed to salvage trauma patients with exsanguination before correction of the patient's systemic pathophysiology, has led to increased application of bedside laparotomy for control of recurrent bleeding within the abdomen and for removal of abdominal packs, irrigation, and debridement.[19] Bedside laparotomy is commonly performed in most level I trauma centers, where damage control and temporary abdominal closure for patients in extremis are frequently necessary. Numerous methods of temporary abdominal closure have been described, and they continue to evolve. The authors prefer the use of negative pressure systems, and facility with the application of these systems is required for patient management.

The open abdominal approach is also applied to the general surgery population, most commonly for the management of necrotizing pancreatitis, necrotizing soft tissue infection of the abdominal wall, diffuse peritonitis in patients at high risk for failure of source control, and mesenteric ischemia.[2,12] Damage control techniques with staged gastrointestinal reconstruction, serial abdominal washout for source control, and delayed abdominal wall closure can be used in the management of these very complex patients. Controlled trials of these techniques are limited, and the indications and settings in which the open abdominal approach is most appropriate have not been fully determined.

TRACHEOSTOMY

Both open tracheostomy and PDT can be performed safely at the bedside in the ICU.[7,8,20,21] The ease and convenience of bedside tracheostomy and the acceptance of early tracheostomy in critically ill surgical patients have probably led to a dramatic increase in their performance at the bedside. Indications for tracheostomy in surgical patients include the following:

1. The presence of pathologic conditions predicting prolonged mechanical intubation or an inability to protect the airway (or both)
2. Airway edema and a high-risk airway after maxillofacial surgery and trauma
3. A high-risk airway secondary to cervical immobilization for fracture fixation
4. Need for a surgical airway because of inability to intubate the patient.

However, identification of all these indications is not straightforward, and clinical decision making remains difficult. Nonetheless, perioperative mortality related to PDT appears to be less than 0.2% in randomized studies.[5,7,8,20-22] Thus, if the risk of death from failed extubation or loss of the airway is estimated to be higher than 0.2%, PDT is performed. When tracheostomy is being considered for the indication of predicted prolonged mechanical ventilation, the timing of tracheostomy remains somewhat controversial. Recent studies support early tracheostomy (up to 7 days) versus delayed tracheostomy (after 7 days) because of shorter ICU stays and less mechanical ventilation but no difference in mortality in both trauma and nontrauma populations.[22,23] However, one recent randomized study of medical ICU patients demonstrated a significant reduction in mortality (32% versus 62%), pneumonia (5% versus 25%), and accidental extubation (0% versus 6%) when early tracheostomy (48 hours) was compared with delayed tracheostomy (14-16 days) in patients predicted to require 14 days of mechanical ventilation.[24] The early group also spent significantly less time in the ICU and required less mechanical ventilation.

PDT has become the procedure of choice for elective tracheostomy in critically ill adult patients. Ciaglia first described elective PDT in 1985,[25] and since that time numerous modifications have been made in the technique. When PDT was compared with standard surgical tracheostomy performed in the operating room, PDT demonstrated decreased wound infection, clinically relevant bleeding, and mortality.[7,20] Percutaneous tracheostomy has also been shown to be more cost-effective in critically ill ICU patients.[5,8,21] However, long-term complications have not been adequately studied in randomized trials to draw conclusions.

The most commonly used commercial percutaneous tracheostomy kit is the Ciaglia Blue Rhino (Cook Critical Care, Bloomington, IL), which is practical, easy to use, and safe.[26] Reported perioperative complications of percutaneous tracheostomy follow:

1. Peristomal bleeding from injury to the anterior jugular veins or thyroid isthmus
2. Injury to the esophagus by entry through the back wall of the trachea
3. Extraluminal placement by creating a false tract during insertion of the tracheostomy tube
4. Loss of the airway

Major perioperative complications can be minimized by using the safety measures outlined in earlier sections. The authors find that management of the airway by specifically trained support personnel is particularly helpful in limiting airway mishaps. Additionally, one of two techniques is used to ensure proper positioning of the tracheostomy tube and minimize the risk for loss of the airway by inadvertent extubation during the procedure: (1) bronchoscopic guidance or (2) a semiopen technique with blunt anterior tracheal dissection.[27,28] However, bronchoscopic guidance does not eliminate severe tracheal injuries, and involvement of experienced personnel is important to prevent these complications. PDT can be performed safely in morbidly obese patients, but care is taken when selecting the size and length of the tracheostomy tube.[29] Because no studies have appropriately described methods of selecting the proper length of tracheostomy tube, the authors routinely place long, rather than standard-length, tubes in patients with a body mass index greater than 35 and those who are massively edematous.

The long-term incidence of serious tracheal stenosis after percutaneous tracheostomy is low, with reports as low as 6%,[30,31] and the stenosis usually occurs high in the subglottic area. Subclinical tracheal stenosis is found in 40% of patients.[32]

PERCUTANEOUS ENDOSCOPIC GASTROSTOMY

Drs. Gauderer and Ponsky first described PEG in 1980 for access to the stomach to deliver enteral feeding with the use of a pull technique.[33] Various other techniques have since been described. The principle of sutureless approximation of the stomach to the anterior abdominal wall has allowed the pull technique to become the most popular method used. The other two most commonly used techniques are the push and introducer techniques, both of which require the use of stay sutures to approximate the stomach to the anterior abdominal wall. Newer PEGJ tubes combine both gastric and jejunal ports to allow distal feeding and proximal decompression.

The primary indications for PEG or PEGJ include an inability to swallow, high risk for aspiration, severe facial trauma, and need for mechanical ventilation for longer than 4 weeks.[6,34] Other indications include PEG/PEGJ use

in debilitated and demented patients suffering from severe malnutrition. PEG tubes have been associated with reduced overall hospital cost.[35]

A number of gastrostomy and gastrojejunostomy tubes are commercially available. Most allow simple gastrostomy access with or without a valve. Some are inserted flush with the skin, and only during feeding is attachment of a tube required. For critical care patients with an increased risk for aspiration, a percutaneous endoscopic transgastric jejunostomy tube with three lumens is available. The tube allows drainage of the stomach and proximal jejunal feeding. A balloon maintains the tube in place.[36] Although feeding can be started on the same day as PEG tube placement, feeding is not initiated in most critically ill patients for 24 hours.[37] A number of contraindications to PEG tube placement exist:

1. No endoscopic access
2. Severe coagulopathy
3. Gastric outlet obstruction
4. Anticipated survival of less than 4 weeks
5. Inability to approximate the gastric wall to the abdominal wall

There are a few relative contraindications, such as inability to transilluminate in an obese patient. Anterior wall inflammation or infection is treated before the procedure. Ascites can be drained before the procedure and is not be an absolute contraindication.[38] A PEG tube is not placed at the same setting as a ventriculoperitoneal shunt or a dialysis catheter, but separated by 1 to 2 weeks.[39,40] A history of previous or recent laparotomy is not a contraindication to PEG.[41]

PEG is thought to be a safe procedure, whether performed in the gastrointestinal laboratory, in the operating room, or at the bedside in the ICU. PEG is commonly performed in sick, debilitated patients who do not tolerate complications and have high mortality.[42] Complications of PEG tube placement are divided into early and late. Free air after PEG tube placement is common and can persist for as long as 4 weeks.[43] Infection can occur as an early complication of PEG tube placement. An adequate skin incision and preprocedure antibiotics are indicated because they have been demonstrated to decrease PEG site infections, especially with the pull technique.[44,45] Rarely, the PEG tube can become dislodged from the stomach during the initial 10 to 14 days, before the development of a fibrous tract; this is a surgical emergency because gastric contents would spill into the abdominal cavity. Operative closure of the tract is required.

BRONCHOSCOPY

Fiberoptic bronchoscopy is used for diagnostic and therapeutic purposes in surgical patients. Among potential therapeutic indications, bronchoscopy can be used to insert an endotracheal tube, remove foreign bodies inadvertently aspirated and mucous plugs, reverse atelectasis in mechanically ventilated patients, suction thick tenacious secretions, and diagnose obstructive pneumonia.[46]

Diagnostic bronchoscopy is most commonly used to obtain pulmonary specimens for the diagnosis and management of pneumonia.[47] Quantitative cultures obtained by fiberoptic bronchoscopy have been demonstrated to eliminate the diagnosis of pneumonia in nearly 50% of patients with clinical signs of pneumonia, decrease inappropriate antibiotic use, and improve mortality when compared with nonquantitative techniques. Culture techniques need to be standardized.[48]

The risk associated with bronchoscopy is related more to the need for conscious sedation and the medications used if performed in a nonintubated patient. It could possibly result in depressed mental status progressing to hypoventilation, airway vulnerability, and risk for aspiration. Risks associated with the procedure itself are pneumothorax, hypoxia, airway hyperreactivity, pulmonary hemorrhage, and systemic hypotension or hypertension.

Selected References

Byhahn C, Wilke HJ, Halbig S, et al: Percutaneous tracheostomy: Ciaglia blue rhino versus the basic Ciaglia technique of percutaneous dilational tracheostomy. Anesth Analg 91:882-886, 2000.

Primary article describing the most common technique currently used for percutaneous dilational tracheostomy.

Delaney A, Bagshaw SM, Nalos M: Percutaneous dilatational tracheostomy versus surgical tracheostomy in critically ill patients: A systematic review and meta-analysis. Crit Care 10: R55, 2006.

This most current meta-analysis of PDT versus standard open surgical tracheostomy supports the benefits of PDT.

Diaz JJ Jr, Mejia V, Subhawong AP, et al: Protocol for bedside laparotomy in trauma and emergency general surgery: A low return to the operating room. Am Surg 71:986-991, 2005.

Primary article examining outcomes of bedside laparotomy with a protocol for indications and support.

Fagon JY: Diagnosis and treatment of ventilator-associated pneumonia: Fiberoptic bronchoscopy with bronchoalveolar lavage is essential. Semin Respir Crit Care Med 27:34-44, 2006.

Review of the indications, benefits, and performance of bronchoscopy for the diagnosis of pneumonia.

Griffiths J, Barber VS, Morgan L, Young JD: Systematic review and meta-analysis of studies of the timing of tracheostomy in adult patients undergoing artificial ventilation. BMJ 330:1243, 2005.

Meta-analysis of studies evaluating the timing of tracheostomy. Early tracheostomy was defined as less than 7 days.

Meduri GU, Chastre J: The standardization of bronchoscopic techniques for ventilator-associated pneumonia. Chest 102(Suppl 1):557S-564S, 1992.

Extensive review of the techniques and limitations of quantitative culture in diagnosing pneumonia.

Moore AF, Hargest R, Martin M, Delicata RJ: Intra-abdominal hypertension and the abdominal compartment syndrome. Br J Surg 91:1102-1110, 2004.

Review of the pathophysiology and treatment of abdominal compartment syndrome.

Rumbak MJ, Newton M, Truncale T, et al: A prospective, randomized, study comparing early percutaneous dilational tracheotomy to prolonged translaryngeal intubation (delayed tracheotomy) in critically ill medical patients. Crit Care Med 32:1689-1694, 2004.

Primary article examining the benefit of tracheostomy at 48 hours versus 14 days. This study demonstrated a significant reduction in complications and mortality when performed early.

Shapiro MB, Jenkins DH, Schwab CW, Rotondo MF: Damage control: Collective review. J Trauma 49:969-978, 2000.

Collective review of the history, indications, and performance of damage control laparotomy.

Van Natta TL, Morris JA Jr, Eddy VA, et al: Elective bedside surgery in critically injured patients is safe and cost-effective. Ann Surg 227:618-624, 1998.

First report of the safety and effectiveness of bedside surgical procedures.

References

1. Diaz JJ Jr, Mauer A, May AK, et al: Bedside laparotomy for trauma: Are there risks? Surg Infect (Larchmt) 5:15-20, 2004.
2. Diaz JJ Jr, Mejia V, Subhawong AP, et al: Protocol for bedside laparotomy in trauma and emergency general surgery: A low return to the operating room. Am Surg 71:986-991, 2005.
3. Porter JM, Ivatury RR, Kavarana M, et al: The surgical intensive care unit as a cost-efficient substitute for an operating room at a level I trauma center. Am Surg 65:328-330, 1999.
4. Van Natta TL, Morris JA Jr, Eddy VA, et al: Elective bedside surgery in critically injured patients is safe and cost-effective. Ann Surg 227:618-624, 1998.
5. Bowen CP, Whitney LR, Truwit JD, et al: Comparison of safety and cost of percutaneous versus surgical tracheostomy. Am Surg 67:54-60, 2001.
6. Carrillo EH, Heniford BT, Osborne DL, et al: Bedside percutaneous endoscopic gastrostomy. A safe alternative for early nutritional support in critically ill trauma patients. Surg Endosc 11:1068-1071, 1997.
7. Freeman BD, Isabella K, Lin N, et al: A meta-analysis of prospective trials comparing percutaneous and surgical tracheostomy in critically ill patients. Chest 118:1412-1418, 2000.
8. Freeman BD, Isabella K, Cobb JP, et al: A prospective, randomized study comparing percutaneous with surgical tracheostomy in critically ill patients. Crit Care Med 29:926-930, 2001.
9. Beckmann U, Gillies DM, Berenholtz SM, et al: Incidents relating to the intra-hospital transfer of critically ill patients. An analysis of the reports submitted to the Australian Incident Monitoring Study in Intensive Care. Intensive Care Med 30:1579-1585, 2004.
10. Pronovost PJ, Thompson DA: Reducing defects in the use of interventions. Intensive Care Med 30:1505-1507, 2004.
11. Porter JM, Ivatury RR, Kavarana M, et al: The surgical intensive care unit as a cost efficient substitute for an operating room at a level I trauma center. Am Surg 65:328-330, 1999.
12. Mayberry JC: Bedside open abdominal surgery. Utility and wound management. Crit Care Clin 16:151-172, 2000.

13. Biffl WL, Moore EE, Burch JM, et al: Secondary abdominal compartment syndrome is highly lethal event. Am J Surg 182:645-648, 2001.

14. Miller RS, Morris JA Jr, Diaz JJ, et al: Complications after 344 damage-control open celiotomies. J Trauma 59:1365-1371, 2005.

15. Kirkpatrick AW, Balogh Z, Ball CG, et al: The secondary abdominal compartment syndrome: Iatrogenic or unavoidable? J Am Coll Surg 202:668-679, 2006.

16. Leppaniemi A, Kemppainen E: Recent advances in the surgical management of necrotizing pancreatitis. Curr Opin Crit Care 11:349-352, 2005.

17. Moore AF, Hargest R, Martin M, et al: Intra-abdominal hypertension and the abdominal compartment syndrome. Br J Surg 91:1102-1110, 2004.

18. Sugrue M: Abdominal compartment syndrome. Curr Opin Crit Care 11:333-338, 2005.

19. Shapiro MB, Jenkins DH, Schwab CW, et al: Damage control: Collective review. J Trauma 49:969-978, 2000.

20. Delaney A, Bagshaw SM, Nalos M: Percutaneous dilatational tracheostomy versus surgical tracheostomy in critically ill patients: A systematic review and meta-analysis. Crit Care 10:R55, 2006.

21. Heikkinen M, Aarnio P, Hannukainen J: Percutaneous dilational tracheostomy or conventional surgical tracheostomy? Crit Care Med 28:1399-1402, 2000.

22. Griffiths J, Barber VS, Morgan L, et al: Systematic review and meta-analysis of studies of the timing of tracheostomy in adult patients undergoing artificial ventilation. BMJ 330:1243, 2005.

23. Arabi Y, Haddad S, Shirawi N, et al: Early tracheostomy in intensive care trauma patients improves resource utilization: A cohort study and literature review. Crit Care 8:R347-R352, 2004.

24. Rumbak MJ, Newton M, Truncale T, et al: A prospective, randomized, study comparing early percutaneous dilational tracheotomy to prolonged translaryngeal intubation (delayed tracheotomy) in critically ill medical patients. Crit Care Med 32:1689-1694, 2004.

25. Ciaglia P, Firsching R, Syniec C: Elective percutaneous dilatational tracheostomy. A new simple bedside procedure; preliminary report. Chest 87:715-719, 1985.

26. Byhahn C, Wilke HJ, Halbig S, et al: Percutaneous tracheostomy: Ciaglia blue rhino versus the basic Ciaglia technique of percutaneous dilational tracheostomy. Anesth Analg 91:882-886, 2000.

27. Paran H, Butnaru G, Hass I, et al: Evaluation of a modified percutaneous tracheostomy technique without bronchoscopic guidance. Chest 126:868-871, 2004.

28. Polderman KH, Spijkstra JJ, de Bree R, et al: Percutaneous dilatational tracheostomy in the ICU: Optimal organization, low complication rates, and description of a new complication. Chest 123:1595-1602, 2003.

29. Heyrosa MG, Melniczek DM, Rovito P, et al: Percutaneous tracheostomy: A safe procedure in the morbidly obese. J Am Coll Surg 202:618-622, 2006.

30. Fikkers BG, Briede IS, Verwiel JM, et al: Percutaneous tracheostomy with the Blue Rhino technique: Presentation of 100 consecutive patients. Anaesthesia 57:1094-1097, 2002.

31. Norwood S, Vallina VL, Short K, et al: Incidence of tracheal stenosis and other late complications after percutaneous tracheostomy. Ann Surg 232:233-241, 2000.

32. Walz MK, Peitgen K, Thurauf N, et al: Percutaneous dilatational tracheostomy—early results and long-term outcome of 326 critically ill patients. Intensive Care Med 24:685-690, 1998.

33. Gauderer MW, Ponsky JL, Izant RJ Jr: Gastrostomy without laparotomy: A percutaneous endoscopic technique. J Pediatr Surg 15:872-875, 1980.

34. Adams GF, Guest DP, Ciraulo DL, et al: Maximizing tolerance of enteral nutrition in severely injured trauma patients: A comparison of enteral feedings by means of percutaneous endoscopic gastrostomy versus percutaneous endoscopic gastrojejunostomy. J Trauma 48:459-464, 2000.

35. Harbrecht BG, Moraca RJ, Saul M, et al: Percutaneous endoscopic gastrostomy reduces total hospital costs in head-injured patients. Am J Surg 176:311-314, 1998.

36. Shang E, Kahler G, Meier-Hellmann A, et al: Advantages of endoscopic therapy of gastrojejunal dissociation in critical care patients. Intensive Care Med 25:162-165, 1999.

37. Stein J, Schulte-Bockholt A, Sabin M, et al: A randomized prospective trial of immediate vs. next-day feeding after percutaneous endoscopic gastrostomy in intensive care patients. Intensive Care Med 28:1656-1660, 2002.

38. Wejda BU, Deppe H, Huchzermeyer H, et al: PEG placement in patients with ascites: A new approach. Gastrointest Endosc 61:178-180, 2005.

39. Schulman AS, Sawyer RG: The safety of percutaneous endoscopic gastrostomy tube placement in patients with existing ventriculoperitoneal shunts. JPEN J Parenter Enteral Nutr 29:442-444, 2005.

40. Taylor AL, Carroll TA, Jakubowski J, et al: Percutaneous endoscopic gastrostomy in patients with ventriculoperitoneal shunts. Br J Surg 88:724-727, 2001.

41. Eleftheriadis E, Kotzampassi K: Percutaneous endoscopic gastrostomy after abdominal surgery. Surg Endosc 15:213-216, 2001.

42. Lockett MA, Templeton ML, Byrne TK, et al: Percutaneous endoscopic gastrostomy complications in a tertiary-care center. Am Surg 68:117-120, 2002.

43. Dulabon GR, Abrams JE, Rutherford EJ: The incidence and significance of free air after percutaneous endoscopic gastrostomy. Am Surg 68:590-593, 2002.

44. Ahmad I, Mouncher A, Abdoolah A, et al: Antibiotic prophylaxis for percutaneous endoscopic gastrostomy—a prospective, randomised, double-blind trial. Aliment Pharmacol Ther 18:209-215, 2003.

45. Sharma VK, Howden CW: Meta-analysis of randomized, controlled trials of antibiotic prophylaxis before percutaneous endoscopic gastrostomy. Am J Gastroenterol 95:3133-3136, 2000.

46. Labbe A, Meyer F, Albertini M: Bronchoscopy in intensive care units. Paediatr Respir Rev 5(Suppl A):S15-S19, 2004.

47. Fagon JY: Diagnosis and treatment of ventilator-associated pneumonia: Fiberoptic bronchoscopy with bronchoalveolar lavage is essential. Semin Respir Crit Care Med 27:34-44, 2006.

48. Meduri GU, Chastre J: The standardization of bronchoscopic techniques for ventilator-associated pneumonia. Chest 102(Suppl 1):557S-564S, 1992.

CHAPTER 26

The Surgeon's Role in Unconventional Civilian Disasters

Eric R. Frykberg, MD

General Principles of Disaster Management
Disaster Response
Medical Care
Terrorist Weapons of Mass Destruction
Summary

Disasters and mass casualty events that result from intentional or unintentional infliction of injury and death in civilian populations and that lead to disruption and destruction of the infrastructure of society are occurring with increasing frequency around the world. Many of these events are due to acts of terrorism, which is defined as the unlawful exercise of random and ruthless violence against people and property in order to intimidate governments or societies for political or ideologic purposes.[1] Some of these events involve industrial accidents, with the widespread release of hazardous materials, whereas others result from natural disasters. All threaten the welfare of a largely unsuspecting and unprotected civilian population.

Medical providers are responsible for the daunting challenges posed by the care of disaster casualties. From a medical perspective, the defining characteristic of a true mass casualty event or disaster is the adverse imbalance between the need for medical resources and their availability. This imbalance is most often caused by such a large number of casualties and perhaps by such a severe and unusual spectrum of injuries that local resources and personnel are overwhelmed and full care of each casualty is prevented.[2-5] This situation differs from the more common *multiple casualty* event or *limited mass casualty* event, such as a busy night in an emergency room, when resources are strained but all patients can still be fully treated.[6] Rationing of care therefore becomes necessary to most efficiently use the limited resources to provide the *greatest good for the greatest number* rather than the

optimal care of each individual. The population rather than the individual must become the focus of medical care.

A successful medical response to a mass casualty disaster requires special education and training, precisely because it must be different from routine medical care. Disasters are rarely encountered by the medical community, and the unique principles required for their successful medical management are not taught in medical school or residency training. Furthermore, many of these principles are antithetic to the standard values and moral precepts of medical providers.[2,4,7,8]

Surgeons and other acute care providers who facilitate surgical capability (i.e., emergency medicine physicians; emergency, critical care, operating room, and trauma nurses; anesthesiologists; and prehospital emergency medical services [EMS] providers) are likely to be the *first receivers* of mass casualties from most types of disasters. Because physical trauma must be anticipated in all disasters, surgeons play an important role in disaster planning and management. Furthermore, trauma centers that specialize in the care of injured patients serve as the foundation of any disaster response. These institutions deal with large numbers of injured patients on a regular basis and maintain liaisons with entities that are essential in any disaster response (i.e., prehospital EMS, public health department, medical examiner, transportation assets, fire department, law enforcement, government and military assets). It is therefore incumbent on surgeons to understand how to care for surgical problems in the unique context of mass casualty events, in which the casualty load and nature of injuries may be quite different from their normal experience. Additional education and training are necessary in the evaluation and care of injuries from weapons of mass destruction (i.e., biologic, chemical, radiologic, explosive), the principles of disaster planning, and the structure of a disaster response in order to maximize the salvage of casualties and the success of the medical response.[7,8]

GENERAL PRINCIPLES OF DISASTER MANAGEMENT

Disaster Planning and Pitfalls

True mass casualty disasters occur rarely, randomly, and unpredictably, which makes it essential that advance preparation be in place if the response is to be successful. Furthermore, the magnitude of disasters, in terms of the large casualty loads and disruption of the infrastructure, requires a response that is far more organized, rapid, comprehensive, extensive, and multidisciplinary than is the case in the routine EMS approach to emergency care. Because many disparate personnel and agencies that normally do not work together must respond to and manage a disaster, a detailed plan is required to define their roles and working relationships in advance.[2,9-11]

All communities and hospitals must have written plans for internal and external disasters that specify personnel roles, who is in charge, and how medical care is organized, among many other issues. Because the location of a disaster is never known in advance, all locales must be prepared. All disasters are ultimately local, which mandates that all hospitals and communities be prepared to function on their own for several days before outside help arrives.[2,12] The Joint Commission for Accreditation of Healthcare Organizations (JCAHO) requires that all hospitals have a plan for disasters of all types, termed the *all-hazards approach*.[13]

There is a tendency for written disaster plans to be unrealistic, overly comprehensive, and unworkable in real scenarios, a pitfall known as the *paper plan syndrome*.[3] It is not uncommon for a plan to be discarded within the first few minutes of a disaster because of its inadequacy.[14] To be useful, any plan must be based on a realistic appraisal of the most likely threats in a given locale, which is be determined by *hazards vulnerability analysis*. The plan must also take an all-hazards approach that incorporates the many known patterns of injury, casualty flow, and response behavior that most disasters have in common while maintaining the flexibility to allow it to adapt to the unique circumstances of any specific disaster (Box 26-1).[3]

In many ways the disaster planning *process* is more important than the actual plan. This process must include a review of the most likely threats to a particular community or region and must involve all stakeholders who will be affected by and be a necessary part of any disaster response (Box 26-2). Through participation in the planning process, a realistic appreciation of the challenges and solutions to a successful disaster response can best be achieved.

Knowledge of the lessons learned from past disasters is a necessary factor in disaster planning. Such knowledge paves the way for creating a plan that anticipates and encompasses the patterns of behavior and injuries, as well as the impediments, encountered in most events.[14,15] The most common barriers to an effective disaster response are well documented to include communications failures, failure to designate authority and responsibility, security problems at the disaster scene and at the hospital, ineffective systems of medical care, and poor control and disposition of medical personnel, who typically inundate the casualty treatment areas in a misguided desire to help.[14,16-20] The fact that these problems are so consistent in past reports indicates how poorly we learn from past mistakes, even though the information needed to improve future responses is widely published.

Box 26-1   Essential Elements of a Disaster Plan

- Based on valid assumptions of what happens in a disaster
- Based on the most likely threats in a specific area
- Interorganizational approach that specifies roles and relationships
- Includes the resources of time, money, space, personnel, and supplies that are necessary to execute the plan
- Includes effective education and training to ensure that those involved understand the plan
- Those who must execute the plan must be involved in its development and testing

From Auf der Heide E: Disaster Response: Principles of Preparation and Coordination. St Louis, CV Mosby, 1989.

Box 26-2   Stakeholders and Participants in Disaster Planning

Hospital Assets

Medical and nursing staff
Administration
Security
Food services
Hospital emergency incident command system (HEICS)
Volunteer pool
Blood bank/laboratory
Imaging services
Operating room staff
Intensive care unit staff
Public information office
Chaplains
Rehabilitation services

Community Assets

Emergency operations center
Public health department
Prehospital emergency medical services
Law enforcement
Fire department
Search and rescue
Media
Transportation/evacuation services
Area blood banks/Red Cross
Area hospital representatives
Mental health services
Local medical society
Civil engineers

Thus, all disaster plans need to include multiple backup contingencies for communications, specific delineation of who is in charge, procedures for establishing scene and hospital security, a system of rapid evaluation and treatment of mass casualties, and restrictions on access to treatment areas. Protection of medical personnel must be a major priority of disaster plans, with adequate decontamination of casualties required before reaching the hospital and medical providers prevented from leaving the hospital or going to the scene. Computer modeling studies have shown that effective planning improves the ability of hospitals to deliver optimal medical care and to manage the flow of casualties in a mass casualty event.[21]

An essential part of disaster planning is testing of the written plan through hospital drills and community exercises with simulated mass casualty events. These *dress rehearsals* of disaster preparedness are the only way to honestly determine the feasibility of a plan in the absence of an actual event and are best done before such an event occurs. All leaders and designated personnel who are assigned roles in a disaster response must participate in these drills and exercises if they are to be of any value in identifying and improving the weaknesses and vulnerabilities of the written plan as applied to real scenarios. These drills must be realistic if their benefit is to be maximized, and therefore they require interruption of the daily activity of a hospital or community, the use of simulated victims and actual equipment, and the use of real-time simulation of all actions.[22] At the completion of these drills and exercises, it is essential that all participants meet to conduct an honest and objective debriefing and critique of the response and use the lessons learned to revise the disaster plan accordingly.[3,4,10,11,17,23-25]

It is important that surgeons actively participate in disaster planning in order to understand their role and how they must interact with other elements of a disaster response. Most disasters involve large numbers of casualties with physical trauma that requires rapid decision making, which surgeons do commonly. Only by becoming involved at the planning stages can surgeons provide proper input regarding their most appropriate disposition and function in an actual disaster.[2,7,26,27]

Disaster Triage

Sorting plus prioritizing disaster casualties according to the urgency of their treatment needs is termed *triage,* which is one of the most important processes in the medical response to a mass casualty event. In the routine management of injured patients, triage is seldom practiced to any significant extent in developed countries, essentially because of unlimited resources that allow each casualty maximal care. If choices must be made, they are based on the extent and severity of injury and the urgency of need for treatment, with those most severely injured being prioritized for immediate care. However, in a true mass casualty scenario, in which medical resources are limited and overwhelmed by the number of casualties, triage assumes critical importance in rationing these resources to only those who will most benefit from them.

The challenge of triage here is to rapidly identify the minority of casualties who require immediate care from among the great majority with non–life-threatening injuries.[17] One additional factor that must be considered in mass casualty scenarios is the *salvageability* of casualties and the extent of resources that must be applied to one and taken away from others who may be more likely to survive. In fact, in a mass casualty event, the *most* severely injured may have the *lowest* priority and actually be denied care that would normally be provided so that the survival of the whole population is maximized to achieve the ultimate goal of the greatest good for the greatest number.[4,7,23,24,28,29]

There are five standard triage categories. The *immediate* category represents the first priority for treatment and consists of casualties with urgent life-threatening injuries who have a good chance of survival with minimal resource utilization (e.g., hypotension with torso trauma). The *delayed* category includes casualties who require hospital treatment that can be delayed without much impact on outcome (e.g., open extremity fractures, penetrating torso wounds with normal vital signs). *Minimal* casualties are those that require no treatment beyond first aid and do not use hospital resources. The *expectant* category consists of casualties who are alive and under normal conditions may survive with extensive and time-consuming resource utilization but, in a mass casualty setting, must be denied care because they would divert the limited resources away from the care of many more salvageable casualties and therefore jeopardize more lives (e.g., unresponsive with an open skull fracture, multisystem injuries with hypotension, respiratory failure, toxic chemical contamination). This category represents the essential difference of mass casualty care from routine emergency care and is the hardest for medical providers to apply because it is antithetic to the moral and ethical principles of patient care. These casualties are provided only comfort care during the period of acute casualty influx and could be reassessed for treatment once casualty influx abates and the remaining resources have been inventoried. The *dead* category is important to recognize early so that the unnecessary use of resources for evaluation and resuscitation is avoided. Any unresponsive patient without a pulse is considered dead. These casualties are segregated to allow later autopsy and identification.[7,28,30]

The accuracy of triage clearly has an impact on casualty outcome because it determines how rapidly care is provided to critically injured casualties who most need it. Minimizing both *under-triage,* or assignment of critical casualties to delayed care, and *over-triage,* or assignment of noncritical casualties to immediate care, is necessary to most accurately match casualty needs with the proper resources and thus optimize their survival. Over-triage tends to be the most common error of triage in mass casualty events, as has been shown for major terrorist bombings (Table 26-1). In this setting, over-triage has been directly correlated with mortality in critically injured casualties *(critical mortality rate),* presumably because of the difficulty of quickly sorting the minority of critical casualties who need immediate care from the large

Table 26-1 **Profile of Critical Injuries, Over-Triage, and Critical Mortality in Survivors of 12 Terrorist Bombing Events**

EVENT	YEAR	NO. SURVIVORS	NO. CRITICALLY INJURED (%)*	NO. OVERTRIAGE (%)[†]	NO. CRITICAL MORTALITY (%)[‡]
Cu Chi	1969	34	3 (9)	9 (75)	1 (33)
Craigavon	1970s	339	113 (33)	29 (20)	5 (4)
Old Bailey	1973	160	4 (2.5)	15 (79)	1 (25)
Guildford	1974	64	22 (34)	2 (8.3)	0
Birmingham	1974	119	9 (8)	12 (57)	2 (22)
Tower of London	1974	37	10 (27)	9 (47)	1 (10)
Bologna	1980	218	48 (22)	133 (73.5)	11 (23)
Beirut	1983	112	19 (17)	77 (80)	7 (37)
AMIA	1994	200	14 (7)	47 (56)	4 (29)
Oklahoma City	1995	597	52 (9)	31 (37)	5 (10)
NYC 9/11[§]	2001	30	7 (23)	23 (77)	2 (29)
Madrid[¶]	2004	312	29 (9)	62 (68)	5 (17)
Total		**2222**	**330 (15)**	**449 (58)**	**44 (13.3)**

*Percentage of total survivors.
[†]Number of noncritical survivors triaged to immediate care as a percentage of all casualties triaged to immediate care.
[‡]Number and percentage of all critically injured survivors who died.
[§]Casualties received at Bellevue Hospital in New York City, September 11, 2001, after the World Trade Center terrorist attacks.
[¶]Casualties received at Gregorio Maranon University Hospital after the Madrid train bombings, March 11, 2004.
Adapted from: Frykberg ER: Triage: Principles and practice. Scand J Surg 94:272-278, 2005.

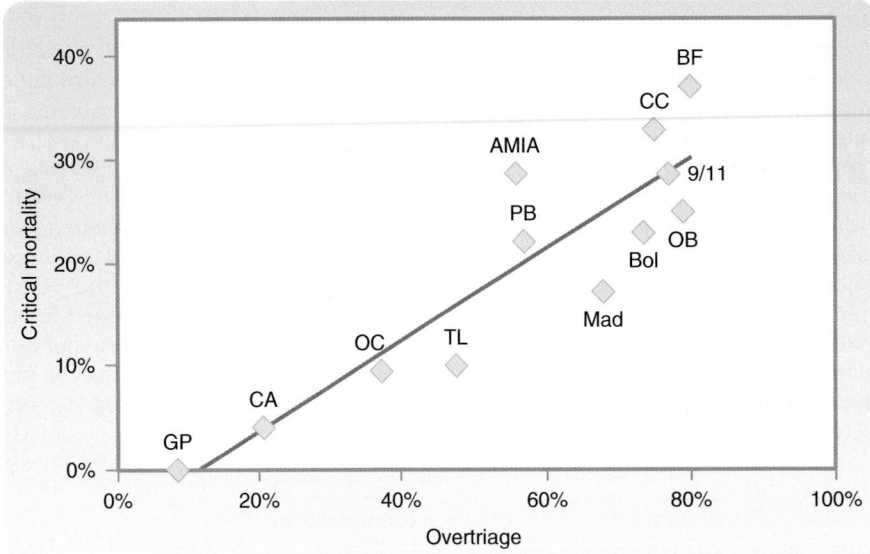

Figure 26-1 Relationship between the over-triage rate and the critical mortality rate in casualties of 12 major terrorist bombing events from 1969 to 2004, derived from data in Table 26-1. The linear correlation coefficient (r) = 0.92. AMIA, Buenos Aires, Argentina; BE, Beirut, Lebanon; Bol, Bologna, Italy; BP, Birmingham pubs, UK; CA, Craigavon, Northern Ireland; CC, Cu Chi, Vietnam; GP, Guildford pubs, UK; Mad, Madrid, Spain; OB, Old Bailey, UK; OC, Oklahoma City, US; TL, Tower of London, UK; 9/11, New York, US. (Adapted from Frykberg ER: Triage: Principles and Practice. Scand J Surg 94:272-278, 2005.)

majority of noncritical casualties who do not (Fig. 26-1).[7,24,28,30] Computer modeling has shown a similar finding of more rapid deterioration in the quality of hospital care to mass casualties with increasing rates of over-triage.[21]

The triage officer who performs mass casualty triage thus has a major responsibility that may affect casualty survival. This person must have considerable expertise in the types of injuries that a disaster causes and must additionally understand how to prioritize these injuries in a mass casualty setting to minimize triage errors. The triage officer must have absolute authority to make these critical decisions, which requires qualities of leadership

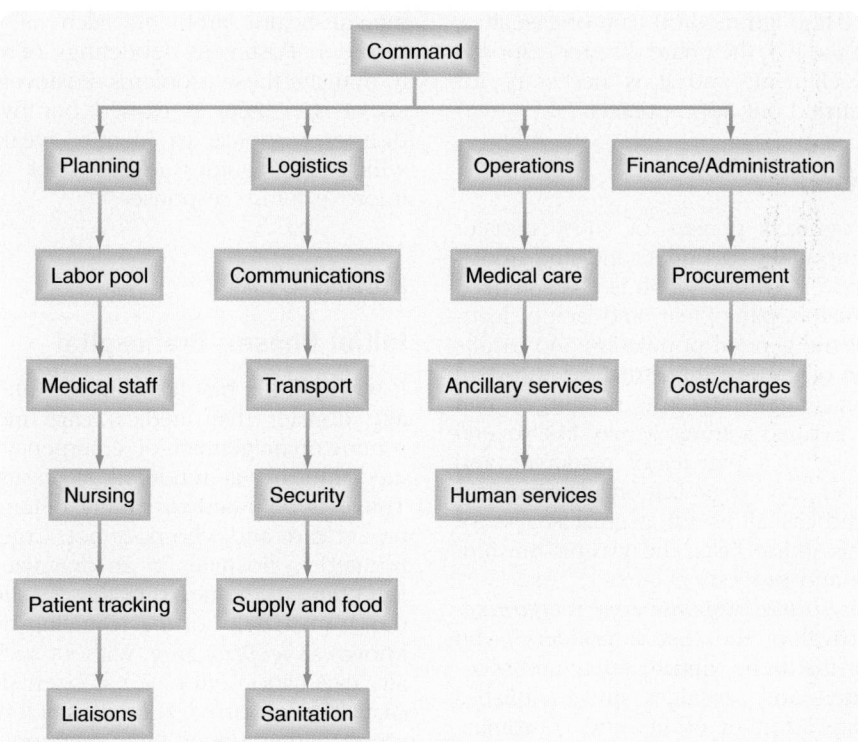

Figure 26-2 Organizational structure of the incident command system.

and respect. This position requires a keen sense of *situational awareness* of all relevant aspects of the ongoing disaster response, such as casualty numbers and available hospital resources. Once designated as a triage officer, this person cannot function in any other role. Although surgeons would make excellent triage officers in events involving such surgical issues as burns and physical trauma, they are also an important resource for the evaluation and possible operative treatment of these injuries. The nature of the event and the availability of resources must be considered when assigning an individual to perform triage.

Although effort is made to minimize triage errors, they will always occur to some extent in the chaotic and unpredictable environment of most mass casualty disasters. The most successful hospital response to a disaster is one that incorporates *error tolerance,* with a system in place to mitigate the consequences of errors that must be anticipated to occur. The potentially life-threatening consequences of under-triage can be mitigated by monitoring casualties assigned to delayed care so that any deterioration can be recognized early and the casualty quickly reassigned to a more appropriate treatment category. The adverse effects of over-triage can be mitigated by establishing multiple triage stations to allow progressively more discrimination and elimination of casualties from hospital admission who do not require urgent care so that only urgent casualties consume the limited resources without interference.[17,30]

DISASTER RESPONSE

Organization

Surgeons and other acute care medical personnel, who are most likely the first receivers of casualties after disasters, must understand all elements of a full disaster response because this response involves much more than medical care. Disaster management requires a close working relationship among several disparate agencies, organizations, and personnel that do not normally work together, ranging from hospitals to prehospital EMS, law enforcement, transportation, communications, and sanitation assets. This requires extensive planning, as well as a unified command structure, to allow effective coordination of all elements so that the common goals of establishing order out of chaos and maximizing casualty survival are achieved. The incident command system (ICS) has been widely adopted as a successful organizational framework for the management of major emergencies and disasters. It consists of five functional elements under a single command, and its modular design allows flexibility and adaptation to disasters of all sizes and types (Fig. 26-2). It is applicable to individual hospitals, as well as to communities, regions, and the nation as a whole, depending on the magnitude of a disaster. The National Incident Management System (NIMS) is the designated command structure of the National Response Plan (NRP) for any national disaster in the United States and is based on the ICS structure. Although medical care of casualties is only a small part of the ICS, the entire disaster response centers around this element, and it is necessary for medical care to be carried out appropriately.[31,32]

Phases of Response

There are four recognized phases of most disaster responses that are important to understand and anticipate.[17,32] The first phase is *chaos,* which is characterized by disorganized confusion, panic, fear, and lack of leadership or direction of the general population and results from major disruption of societal infrastructure. In urban environments, this phase generally lasts no longer than 1 hour, but in more isolated settings it may last several hours or days because of a paucity of resources and personnel to establish any organization. During this phase, critically injured casualties are at greatest risk for death. The longer this phase lasts, the greater the tendency for loss of life and property.

The second phase, *initial response and reorganization,* begins with arrival of the first responders, who establish control over the scene, initiate safety and security for both responders and casualties, and establish a command post to direct further efforts and coordinate with the central command at the emergency operations center. The nature of the event and any further hazards (i.e., structural instability, hazardous material contamination) is assessed at this time.[4]

The third response phase, *site clearing,* involves the development of response planning, including removal of debris, recovery of casualties for transport to hospitals, and initiation of medical care (search and rescue). The command structure is established and begins to organize response efforts. Identified scene hazards are addressed to protect personnel. Triage and decontamination of casualties begin as casualty collection points are established. Generally, after 24 hours there is little chance of further survivors, and these efforts change to search and recovery of the dead. Security is instituted at the scene area to restrict access to only those trained to handle the many dangers of the scene. Many disaster scenes are also crime scenes and thus require law enforcement to become involved for the purpose of preserving forensic evidence.

The final response phase of *recovery* involves long-term efforts at definitive medical care of casualties, rebuilding and restoration of destroyed property and infrastructure, and recognition and management of psychoemotional consequences among the afflicted population. These are all attempts to return life to some semblance of predisaster normalcy. Help from outside the disaster area generally arrives after a period of 3 to 5 days or longer, depending on the location and magnitude of disruption, and includes such federal assets as the National Disaster Medical System (NDMS) and government relief agencies (e.g., Federal Emergency Management Agency [FEMA]), the military (e.g., National Guard), and private relief organizations (e.g., the American Red Cross). An organized program must be developed to monitor the population and first responders for

mental health problems such as post-traumatic stress disorder. Postevent debriefings of workers are planned to mitigate these problems. Postevent critique and analysis of the event is carried out by participants in the disaster response to identify weaknesses and pitfalls, which then guides revisions of the disaster plan to improve future responses.[8,23]

MEDICAL CARE

Initial Phase—Prehospital

It is within the first few minutes after a major mass casualty disaster that medical care most differs from the routine management of emergency patients. Very little medical care is rendered to casualties in this phase. Triage is confined to simply determining who requires urgent care and who does not. Urgent casualties are distributed to hospitals in an organized sequential fashion according to the needs of the casualties and the capabilities and capacity of the receiving hospitals in a process known as *leapfrogging.* Without such an organized casualty evacuation effort, it has been shown that 75% of all casualties will arrive at the hospital nearest to the disaster scene, either under their own power or sent by EMS units. This common *geographic effect* must be minimized by an effective scene response because the inundation of casualties will overwhelm the resources of the one hospital and impair its ability to properly care for all casualties.[3,9,12,17]

The major effort in this prehospital phase of casualty care revolves around removal of casualties from the dangerous scene and transporting them to one or more *casualty collection points.*[4] These areas are visible and familiar to all prehospital personnel, easily accessible, and uphill and upwind from any biologic, chemical, or radiation hazards to prevent ongoing contamination. At these points the casualties can be more fully evaluated, triaged, and transported to hospitals for continuing care. Any decontamination deemed necessary must be carried out at this time before arrival at the hospital. Once again, *minimal acceptable care* is provided, in addition to urgent lifesaving interventions, to facilitate the rapid outflow of casualties so that room is made for those incoming.[17]

Initial Phase—Hospital

The hospital must clear its major spaces in the emergency department (ED), operating rooms (ORs), intensive care units (ICUs), and general wards of existing patients to the extent possible to accommodate incoming casualties. Extra personnel, equipment, and supplies must be mobilized to allow at least a 90% level of optimal care to be delivered to these casualties, which is termed *surge capacity.* It is generally recommended that a 20% expansion of existing beds and resources be achieved for adequate surge capacity, which is most appropriately expressed in dynamic terms such as a *casualty arrival rate* rather than simply as a number of beds. Once this arrival rate exceeds the existing spaces and resources, the quality of care must decline. Over-triage and poor planning and preparation tend to reduce surge capacity, whereas good planning and preparation allow rapid mobilization of adequate resources and increase surge capacity.[21]

Casualties undergo *secondary triage* on arrival at the hospital in order to restrict admission to this limited and valuable resource to only those who require it for the management of life-threatening injuries, thus minimizing over-triage and potential loss of life. It is essential that all casualties undergo decontamination before hospital entry. In the hospital, rapid triage is again performed to determine the destinations of casualties according to their needs, either to the general wards, OR, or ICU. The standard of *minimal acceptable care* is still applied to all but the most critical casualties to allow diversion of the limited resources to where they can be most effectively applied to maximize casualty salvage. Reports from major terrorist bombing events in Israel document that 60% of hospitalized casualties required emergency operative intervention within 90 minutes, and 36% of these casualties were transported directly from the ED to the OR. The initial operations were multidisciplinary abdominal, thoracic, and vascular procedures, whereas later procedures were for orthopedic, neurosurgical, and plastic surgery problems. One third of the casualties were admitted to an ICU, 31% directly from the ED.[25] These data emphasize the importance of immediate surgical capability and the advantage of trauma centers being the major receiving hospitals for optimal casualty outcomes.[24]

Unidirectional forward movement of casualties must be maintained in the hospital to avoid backups, which will foster chaos and impair the ability to optimally care for all casualties. Rapid evaluation, minimal acceptable care, rapid transport to assigned treatment areas, and avoidance of all imaging and laboratory testing are necessary during the period of acute casualty influx. Focused abdominal sonography for trauma (FAST) is one of the few acceptable diagnostic modalities in this setting in view of its simplicity, accuracy, and rapidity.[17,33] The OR must be conserved as a critical resource and be used only for the most life-threatening injuries that can be stabilized in a short time. Medical controllers must be assigned to the ED, OR, and ICU to enforce the rigid standards of rapid evaluation, unidirectional flow, minimal acceptable care, appropriateness of assignment to that space, and rapid room turnover in the OR through the use of *damage control procedures*.[17,33] These standards must be maintained as long as casualty influx persists. Because of communications failures, the hospital typically never knows how many casualties are coming or how long this casualty flow will last. Therefore, continued conservation of hospital resources is essential until this flow stops.

The geographic effect of inundation of the nearest hospital in mass casualty events may be mitigated by conversion of this hospital to a *triage hospital,* otherwise termed an *evacuation* or *ground zero* hospital. Triage hospitals do not render care but simply act as another casualty collection point, from which all casualties are distributed to area hospitals according to their triage assignments. This simply moves the triage and distribution of casualties away from the scene to the nearest hospital and thus exploits rather than fights this tendency to inundate the nearest hospital.[3,17]

Definitive Phase

Once casualty arrival at the hospital abates, all casualties can be re-evaluated and more thoroughly treated in accordance with the remaining resources. Casualties assigned to expectant care may be reassessed for initiation of treatment if resources and the needs of other casualties permit.

Casualties with less urgent injuries may now undergo surgery for specialty care, such as burns, skeletal fractures, soft tissue injuries, head injuries, and ocular injuries. Diagnostic imaging with modalities such as computed tomography, magnetic resonance imaging, and angiography may be more liberally used to fully assess casualty needs. Some casualties may be transported to other hospitals to more evenly distribute the casualty load and expedite definitive care in a process known as secondary casualty distribution.[12,17,18]

An essential component of hospital care in a mass casualty disaster is accurate and complete documentation of the triage and treatment rendered to each casualty, which is the only means of ensuring continuity of care in a chaotic setting in which casualties are moved to successive echelons of care from different providers. It allows tracking of casualties so that they are not lost. Concise records move with each casualty and contain identifiers and information on the injuries, triage assignment, treatment rendered, what further treatment is needed, and where the casualty needs to go. The forms are the same as those normally used by providers in their routine practice to minimize confusion. Another value of these records is to enable critical analysis of the medical response after the event to determine weaknesses and errors and how they affected casualty outcomes. These lessons can be applied to improving the disaster plan and future responses. Inadequate documentation leads to loss of all these important lessons.[7,14,28]

TERRORIST WEAPONS OF MASS DESTRUCTION

Four major categories of unconventional weapons have been used or have the potential to be used for acts of terrorism or result from industrial accidents: explosive agents, biologic agents, chemical agents, and radiologic or nuclear agents. With each of these threats, surgeons are confronted with major challenges in decision making and management because their effects and manifestations are unusual and not generally taught in medical education or training. A successful medical response to disasters caused by these agents requires an understanding of their pathophysiology and management.

Explosions and Blast Injuries

The magnitude of force, the innovative methods of delivery, and the many thousands of casualties that have been achieved by terrorist bombings over the past 3 decades

Table 26-2   Major Explosive Disasters Involving Ammonium Nitrate (Fertilizer) Detonations

EVENT	YEAR	NO. CASUALTIES	NO. DEAD
Texas City, Texas accidental ship explosion	1946	2000	600
*U.S. Marine barracks terrorist suicide truck bombing—Beirut, Lebanon	1983	346	241
*Israeli embassy terrorist bombing—Buenos Aires, Argentina	1994	286	86
*Murrah Building terrorist bombing—Oklahoma City, Oklahoma	1995	759	168
*UN Headquarters terrorist suicide bombing—Baghdad, Iraq	2003	100	17
Train explosion—Ryongchon, North Korea	2004	1249	54

*Associated with major building collapse.

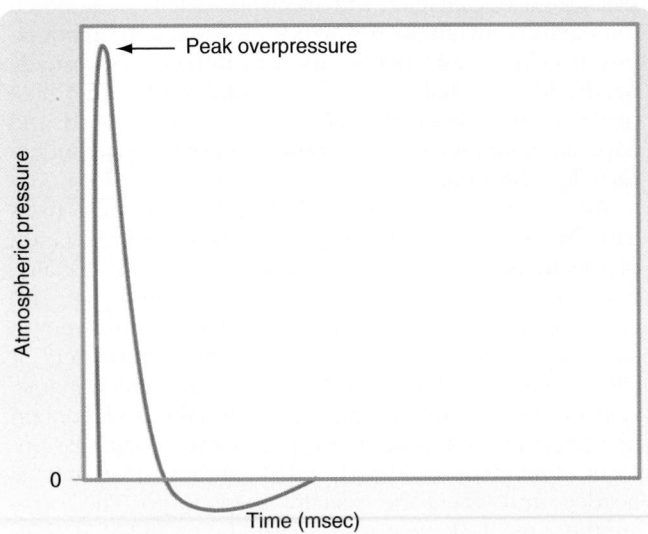

Figure 26-3 Pressure characteristics of a blast wave over time after an explosion.

clearly justify their inclusion as weapons of mass destruction. Furthermore, bombings have been the most common weapons of terrorism historically and therefore remain the most prominent and most likely threat for which surgeons must be prepared (see Table 26-1). Bombings are the most effective means of achieving the terrorist goals of maximal casualty generation and lethality with little cost or training. An understanding of the physics and pathophysiology of blasts is necessary to properly plan for the management of their medical consequences.[7,17,34,35]

Blast Physics and Pathophysiology
Explosions cause a sudden compression of surrounding air that creates a *peak overpressure* within a fraction of a second, with the magnitude being dependent on the blast force. A pressure wave is created and propagates out radially from the blast at speeds of 3000 to 8000 m/sec after high-energy explosions. The leading edge of this *blast wave* is called the *blast front*. The peak overpressure is followed by a more gradual ebbing of pressure that lasts 10-fold longer and falls below ambient pressure in

a negative pressure phase before returning to atmospheric pressure (Fig. 26-3). The blast wave dissipates rapidly in air according to the cube of the distance such that moving three times further away from the blast reduces the blast force by 27-fold. Underwater blasts are more powerful because of the greater density of water; such blasts propagate at three times the speed and distance than blasts do in air. However, within confined spaces the blast wave is magnified rather than dissipated by reflecting off walls, floors, and ceilings, and much greater destruction and injury are created.[35] This is why terrorists try to place bombs within buildings, buses, or other confined spaces to maximize the generation of casualties.[23,24] One of the most common and most effective agents used to generate massive explosions, both intentionally and unintentionally, has been ammonium nitrate (fertilizer) soaked in diesel oil and constructed as a fuel-air explosive (Table 26-2).[7,10,36]

There are four major categories of blast injury that derive from the physical characteristics of explosions. *Primary blast injury* is the tissue damage caused by passage of the blast wave through the body. It mainly affects air-containing organs such as the lungs and bowels and disrupts tissue at air-liquid interfaces in a process termed *spalling*. *Secondary blast injury* causes physical trauma from the impact of objects and debris set in motion by the blast. *Tertiary blast injury* is trauma caused by the body being thrown into other objects. *Quaternary, or miscellaneous, blast injury* includes a variety of injuries indirectly related to an explosion, such as burns, crush injuries from structural collapse, inhalational injuries from dust and toxic chemicals, and biologic, chemical, and radiologic contamination disseminated by *dirty bombs*. Complex penetrating wounds from the shrapnel that is increasingly being used in bombs are also included in this category.[16] Primary blast injury is highly lethal, and most survivors of explosive events suffer body trauma from secondary and tertiary blast injuries, thus emphasizing the importance of immediate surgical capability for these casualties.[16,24,34,35]

Patterns of Injury and Mortality
The abundant published literature on explosive disasters reveals definite patterns of injury and mortality that are in fact similar to most other forms of mass casualty events. This permits an anticipation of what to expect

Table 26-3 Effect of Building Collapse on Casualty Outcome in Oklahoma City Terrorist Bombing, 1995*

CASUALTY LOCATION	NO. CASUALTIES	NO. DEAD (%)	NO. SURVIVORS	NO. SURVIVORS HOSPITALIZED (%)
Collapsed	175	153 (87)	22	18 (82)
Uncollapsed	186	10 (5)	176	32 (18)
Total	361	163 (45)	198	50 (25)

*Includes only 361 casualties inside the Murrah Federal Building at the time of the explosion, stratified according to the portion of the building in which they were located.

Adapted from data in Mallonee S, Shariat S, Stennies G, et al: Physical injuries and fatalities resulting from the Oklahoma City bombing. JAMA 276:382-387, 1996.

and therefore the opportunity to plan and prepare for disasters. Terrorist bombings may thus be considered a universal model for disaster management.

The immediate mortality rate after high-energy explosions is typically high (30%-70%), with fatal head and torso injuries, traumatic amputation, and primary blast injuries of the lung with cerebral and coronary air embolism being the major causes of immediate death. An indoor location, especially when associated with building collapse, increases immediate mortality to as high as 99% of all casualties (Table 26-3).[10,23,24,28]

Most survivors of explosive disasters are *not* critically injured, primarily because of the fact that most critical injuries cause immediate death.[7,10,28,36] Only 10% to 25% of survivors have critical injuries that require immediate lifesaving interventions, with non–life-threatening skeletal and soft tissue injuries from secondary and tertiary blast effects predominating in this group. The major challenge of medical care in this setting is to rapidly identify and triage the minority of critical injuries from among the great majority of casualties who do not require immediate care. The greater the inundation of noncritical casualties (i.e., over-triage), the more difficult and error prone the triage process (see Fig. 26-1). External markers of severity that correlate with underlying critical injuries and therefore facilitate accurate triage among blast survivors include perforated eardrums, penetrating chest and abdominal trauma, soft tissue shrapnel wounds, primary blast lung injury, traumatic amputation, open skull fractures, and burns involving more than 30% of total body surface area.[37,38] The most important prognostic factors for casualties of major explosive disasters can be derived from an understanding of the physics and injury patterns of blasts discussed earlier (Box 26-3).

The so-called second-hit phenomenon is a pattern of a delayed blast that follows an initial one and additionally injures or kills all curious onlookers and first responders lured in initially. This is a common and effective terrorist tactic in bombing events, but variations of this phenomenon can occur in most other forms of disasters as well (i.e., delayed structural collapse, as occurred with the World Trade Center towers after the initial airliner crashes on 9/11 or resulting from aftershocks following an earthquake, delayed explosion of combustible cargo after a vehicle crash and fire). This emphasizes the dangers of any disaster scene, the importance of restricting access to the scene to only those trained for the hazards, and

---

Box 26-3   Prognostic Factors for Casualty Outcome After Explosive Disasters

Magnitude of the blast force
Distance from the explosion
Time interval to treatment
Casualty management factors:
   Rapidity of evaluation and flow
   Triage accuracy
   Presence of surgical capability
Environmental factors:
   Building collapse
   Confined-space versus open-air location
   Urban versus isolated setting
Anatomic markers of injury severity:
   Blast lung injury
   Traumatic amputation
   Torso trauma
   Toxic or radiologic contamination
   Severe head injury
   Multisystem injuries

---

the need to protect first responders and medical personnel as the top priority of any disaster response.[7,17,28]

Biologic Agents

Bioterrorism refers to the use of microorganisms, or toxins derived from them, to intentionally inflict disease and death on large populations. The most unique and dangerous feature that distinguishes biologic weapons from all other weapons of mass destruction is the delay in their clinical manifestations. A large number of casualties may occur before the medical community is first aware of an attack and able to institute containment measures. The effectiveness of biologic agents as weapons depends on the type of agent, its virulence, the susceptibility of the population to the infectious or toxic effects, the mode of dissemination, and the concentration of the population exposed. Frontline health care providers must know the clinical manifestations of these agents and have a high index of suspicion for their deliberate use to contain an attack as early as possible. They must also practice strict protective measures to avoid becoming casualties themselves (Table 26-4). The U.S. Centers for Disease Control and Prevention designates category A

Table 26-4 **Infection Control Measures Required for Bioterrorism Agents**

BIOAGENT	TYPE OF ISOLATION REQUIRED	PATIENT PLACEMENT	PROVIDER MEASURES
Anthrax Botulism Tularemia	Standard precautions	Private room only if noncompliant in maintaining appropriate hygiene or environmental control	Hand washing, gloving; if sprays of body fluids possible, then masks, goggles, or face shields
Infectious diarrheas (e.g., cholera)	Contact precautions	Private room or room with patients who have active infection with the same microorganism but no other infection (cohorting)	Gown and gloves Goggles or face shield per standard precautions
Plague	Droplet precautions	Private room or room with patients who have active infection with the same microorganism but no other infection (cohorting)	Wear a surgical mask when working within 3 ft of the patient When patient contact is likely, use contact precautions: gown and gloves
Smallpox Tuberculosis	Airborne precautions	Private room that has negative air pressure with 6 to 12 air changes per hour and high-efficiency filtration of room air before discharge to other areas in the hospital	Standard precautions plus N95 respirator When patient contact is likely, use contact precautions: gown and gloves Use goggles or face shield per standard precautions
Hemorrhagic fevers (e.g., Ebola, Lassa, Marburg)	Airborne, contact, and droplet precautions	Private room that has negative air pressure with 6 to 12 air changes per hour and high-efficiency filtration of room air before discharge to other areas in the hospital	Standard precautions and wear N95 respirator, gown, gloves, and goggles Treat all body fluid–stained material as infective

Adapted from Centers for Disease Control and Prevention. Department of Health and Human Services. CDC Public Health Emergency Preparedness & Response Site. Available from http://www.bt.cdc.gov. Accessed June 29, 2003.

biologic agents as those with the most favorable characteristics for use as terrorist weapons. Such agents include anthrax, plague, botulinum toxin, tularemia, smallpox, and organisms causing viral hemorrhagic fever.[39]

Anthrax is considered the most likely agent to be used in this setting because it is virtually always fatal if untreated. Its spores can easily be produced in large quantities with little training, they can be stored for years without loss of potency, and the spores are easily spread in air by delivery mechanisms such as sprayers, bombs, and missiles. When inhaled, anthrax has a high fatality rate. One report estimates that aerosolized release of 100 kg of spores could result in up to 3 million deaths in the Washington, DC, area. The incubation rate of anthrax is between 2 and 60 days, and it has three clinical forms—cutaneous, gastrointestinal, and pulmonary. The cutaneous form occurs naturally, has a 20% fatality rate, and is the most common form in developed countries. The gastrointestinal form requires the ingestion of contaminated meat and is manifested as nonspecific gastrointestinal symptoms that may progress to bleeding and peritonitis if untreated. The pulmonary form is 100% fatal if untreated and 80% fatal if treatment is initiated after the onset of symptoms; it is considered the most likely to result from a terrorist attack. Penicillin is the treatment of choice. Prophylaxis of personnel at high risk of exposure is carried out with a combination of antibiotics and vaccination.[40]

Botulinum toxin, a neurotoxin and one of the most poisonous substances known, causes neuromuscular blockade that leads to respiratory failure. Though most commonly caused by the ingestion of contaminated food, the likely method of deliberate attack would be through an aerosolized form, which can result in widespread disease very quickly because it is tasteless, colorless, and odorless. Treatment is supportive care and antitoxin.

Bubonic plague and tularemia are bacterial infections, and smallpox is a virulent viral disease; all three have high infectious potential and lethality and an established history of causing millions of deaths. Viral hemorrhagic fever is a clinical syndrome of fever, myalgia, headache, and malaise that quickly progresses to shock, hemorrhage from mucous membranes, and death; included in this category are Ebola and Marburg viruses and such diseases as Lassa fever, Rift Valley fever, yellow fever, and dengue. All can be transmitted by airborne contamination, all have actually been prepared and in some instances used as biologic weapons intended to decimate large populations, and all are considered major threats as bioterrorist agents.

The process of *syndromic surveillance,* or a system of recognition of illness patterns over a wide area, is essential to allow early determination of pandemic disease and terrorist-related attacks. Personal protection measures must be initiated among health care providers in these settings to protect against the further spread of infection through mucosal surfaces, the respiratory system, and skin. Public health officials and infectious disease experts are integrally involved in the response to bioterrorist disasters.[41,42]

Chemical Agents

Toxic chemicals have a proven capability to cause severe and widespread morbidity and mortality in large populations, as well as spread panic, which in itself could lead to societal disruption, and thus pose a major threat from the intentional use of such agents by terrorists. These agents can exert their deadly effects through the inhalation of aerosolized or gaseous forms, ingestion of poisoned foods, and direct contact with the skin and eyes. Poison gases have been used extensively in warfare, especially in the 20th century, with as many as 1 million casualties caused by these agents in World War I. The worst chemical disaster in history occurred in Bhopal, India, in 1984, when the accidental release of 40 tons of gaseous methyl isocyanate led to 6000 deaths and 400,000 injuries, thus demonstrating the potential of these agents as effective terrorist weapons. The bomb that exploded in the World Trade Center in 1993 in New York City contained enough cyanide to contaminate the entire building, but it was destroyed by the blast. In 1995, the first terrorist use of the nerve agent sarin on a civilian population occurred in Tokyo, Japan, and led to 12 deaths and 5000 injuries.[43,44] The major categories of chemical poisons and their treatment are shown in Table 26-5.

The initial phase of management of clinical attacks requires early detection, which is often difficult without a high index of suspicion. Patterns that involve large numbers of patients with similar symptom clusters must be recognized, and thus knowledge of the signs and symptoms associated with chemical toxicity is required. The source of contamination must be identified and neutralized, victims must be evacuated to prevent further contamination, and effective treatment must be initiated. The classic symptoms that heighten awareness of chemical poisoning include coughing and choking, dry mouth and mucus membranes, seizures, eye irritation, and cholinergic symptoms of organophosphate exposure as described by the DUMBBELS mnemonic (diarrhea, urination, miosis, bronchospasm or bronchorrhea, emesis, lacrimation, salivation).[45,46]

Health care workers must wear personal protective equipment to prevent them from inhaling any off-gassing that may emanate from victims, as well as equipment to avoid skin and eye exposure. Triage and decontamination must be established outside the hospital to prevent any disabling contamination that will prevent treatment of victims and potentially shut down the hospital. All victims must undergo decontamination as early as possible. Simply removing clothing plus showering with soap and water can remove up to 90% of all contaminating agents and is called *gross decontamination*. More intensive *technical decontamination* can then follow for specific forms of exposure, such as hypochlorite washing for mustard agents and copious eye irrigation with saline solutions for any agents that contaminate the eyes. Poison control centers, public health officials, pharmacologists, and toxicologists are important resources and personnel who need to be involved in the planning and management of chemical disasters.[45]

Table 26-5 Potential Chemical Terrorism Agents

CATEGORY	AGENTS	TREATMENT
Blood agents	Cyanide	Decontamination 100% oxygen Amyl nitrite
Vesicants (blistering)	Lewisite Phosgene oxime	Hypochlorite (bleach) Dimercaprol
Pulmonary irritants	Chlorine Ammonia Mace	Water cleansing Bronchodilators Mechanical ventilation
Incapacitating agents (anticholinergics)	BZ	Intravenous hydration Physostigmine
Nerve agents	Tabun, sarin, soman, VX	Atropine Pralidoxime (2-PAM) Diazepam Airway management Decontamination

Nuclear/Radiologic Agents

Ionizing radiation damages living tissue, especially in the gastrointestinal tract and bone marrow, through its direct energy, as well as through indirect effects from the creation of unstable, toxic superoxide molecules. The two major forms of ionizing radiation are electromagnetic (gamma rays, x-rays, which have high penetration and cause the most damage), and particle (alpha and beta particles, which have very low penetration and cause harm only if ingested, and neutrons, which have high penetration and destructive energy). Exposure to radiation does not make a person radioactive. The major factors that determine the severity of biologic effects are time, distance, and shielding. The absorbed dose decreases rapidly with the square of the distance from the source, so doubling the distance reduces the dose rate to a fourth the original level.[45,47]

Dispersal of radioactive substances poses a major potential for a terrorist attack because of the theoretical damage that could be inflicted on large populations, although a deliberate attack on civilian populations outside of war has never occurred. These agents also carry the potential for large-scale psychosocial effects and panic because of the mystique that is associated with radiation among the general population, which is far out of proportion to many of the actual dangers. Radiation exposure from a terrorist attack is generally easier to manage than biologic and chemical attacks because of easy detection methods with various forms of dose rate meters and Geiger counters, the large number of hospital and government personnel who regularly deal with radiation, and the well-known clinical effects, which can be monitored with simple laboratory tests.[47-50]

The two major forms that a terrorist radiologic attack could take are the dispersal of common radioactive materials used in industry and medicine (e.g., cobalt 60,

Table 26-6   Clinical Manifestations After Different Doses of Radiation Exposure

	AMOUNT OF RADIATION DOSE				
	1-2 Gy	**2-4 Gy**	**4-6 Gy**	**6-8 Gy**	**>8 Gy**
Temperature control Frequency	Normal	Febrile (1-3 hr) 50-80%	Febrile (1-2 hr) 80-100%	High fever 100%	High fever 100%
Skin Timing	None	Hair loss ≥15 days	Hair loss 11-21 days	Complete hair loss ≤11-15 days	Complete hair loss <10 days
Vomiting Incidence	At 2 hr <50%	1-2 hr 70-90%	<1 hr 100%	<30 min 100%	<10 min 100%
Diarrhea Timing	None	None	Mild 3-8 hr	Severe 1-3 hr	Severe <1 hr
Headache Timing	Slight	Mild	Moderate 4-24 hr	Severe 3-4 hr	Severe 1-2 hr
Mental status	Normal	Normal	Normal	Altered	Unconscious
Granulocytes (3-6 days) (10^9 cells/L)	>2.0	1.5-2.0	1.0-1.5	≤0.5	≤0.1
Lymphocytes (3-6 days) (10^9 cells/L)	0.8-1.5	0.5-0.8	0.3-0.5	0.1-0.3	<0.1
Platelets (3-6 days) (10^9 cells/L) Incidence	60-100 10%-25%	30-60 25%-40%	25-35 40%-80%	15-25 60%-80%	<20 80%-100%
Mortality rates Timing	0	<50% 6-8 wk	20-70% 4-8 wk	50-100% 1-2 wk	100% 1-2 wk

Adapted from Guskova AK: Radiation sickness classification. In Gusev IA, Guskova AK, Mettler FA (eds): Medical Management of Radiation Accidents. Boca Raton, FL, CRC Press, 2001, pp 23-31.

cesium 137, iridium 192), most likely through explosions *(dirty bombs),* and the atmospheric release of large amounts of intense ionizing radiation through the sabotage of nuclear power plants or detonation of nuclear weapons. Dirty bombs are easy to construct with little training. They could spread contamination over a few city blocks at most and also cause body injuries from the blast, as well as fear and panic in the affected population. The actual damage to property and individuals is unlikely to be extensive, and the relatively small area of contamination can easily be monitored and contained for long-term cleanup. Terrorist nuclear events, on the other hand, are considered relatively low risk because they require significant technical expertise and money to carry out. However, these weapons pose the threat of substantial destruction to property and people over a range of hundreds of miles because of the physical effects of the air blast, the thermal and blinding effects of the ensuing fireball, and the intense ionizing radiation thrown into the atmosphere that can spread lethal levels of radioactive fallout over large areas.

Medical treatment of radiologic casualties is largely supportive and consists of symptomatic care and isolation for the gastrointestinal (nausea, vomiting, diarrhea, bleeding) and hematopoietic (bone marrow depression) manifestations that make up *acute radiation syndrome.* Evaluation and triage of radiologic casualties are facilitated by the close relationship between the onset and timing of symptoms and the absorbed dose and prognosis (Table 26-6). Acute doses of less than 1.0 Gy (equivalent to 100 rad) result only in the long-term effect of possible malignancies. Local effects from low-penetration alpha- and beta-particle contamination include thermal burns with erythema, desquamation, and blistering. The effects of whole-body exposure from highly penetrating gamma rays, x-rays, and neutrons are dependent on the dose and duration; they do not cause contamination and thus do not require decontamination. Ten gray is considered the highest survivable dose exposure with maximal medical therapy and is marked by the most severe gastrointestinal symptoms and blood cell count depression as monitored by lymphocyte counts. With doses greater than 10 Gy, symptoms develop within minutes, and doses in excess of 30 Gy produce cardiovascular and nervous system collapse and lead to death in 24 to 72 hours.[45,50]

Internal contamination through inhalation, ingestion, or skin absorption can be treated by dilution, blockage, displacement by nonradioactive materials, administration of agents to minimize absorption, mobilization of renal and gastrointestinal elimination, and chelation. These measures, as well as bone marrow and stem cell transplantation, have little if any demonstrated effectiveness. There is no antiradiation drug. Potassium iodide effectively blocks thyroid uptake of radioactive iodine, which is found after nuclear explosions or spills, but only if given within 4 hours of exposure; it has substantial clinical utility solely in children. This drug has no effect on the symptoms of acute radiation syndrome, only on the long-term development of thyroid cancer.[49,50]

External contamination is easily managed by removing clothing and showering with soap and water, which remove more than 90% of the contamination (gross decontamination). More thorough technical decontamination involves further scrubbing of the body, washing and shaving of hair, and cleansing of open wounds to minimize ongoing exposure and contain contamination. The clothing, hair, and runoff fluids are bagged and properly disposed. Open wounds that have been exposed to doses in excess of 1.0 Gy or contaminated are gently washed and débrided and then closed as soon as possible to prevent them from becoming portals for lethal internal contamination. Wound excision is considered for contamination with long-lived radionuclides (i.e., alpha emitters). External radiologic contamination does not constitute the medical emergency for victims or medical personnel that chemical contamination does and needs to be considered much the same as dirt—something that is preferably cleaned off by gross decontamination before treatment but should not delay lifesaving interventions or lead to suboptimal care in any way. Medical personnel need to adhere to standard universal precautions and are not at risk for any significant radiation exposure, even with the highest levels of contamination and exposure of casualties.[47-50]

Management of a radiologic disaster involves proper planning and preparation through training and education of personnel, accurate scene and hospital triage, and contact with national government resources for guidance in the recognition and management of radiation exposure. Severely injured victims with radiation exposure/contamination are transported to different facilities for definitive management than those who are not seriously injured to facilitate containment of radiation spread. Radiologic exposure or contamination cannot alter the priorities of medical care. Procedures for dealing with the stress and psychosocial effects that are inevitable in victims, medical personnel, and the overall population must be established.[45,47-50]

SUMMARY

The medical response to a mass casualty disaster requires education and training in the principles and organization of disaster response and in the unique approach to medical care that is necessary to maximize casualty survival. A thorough understanding by medical providers of evaluation and treatment of the unusual injuries that current unconventional disaster threats pose, as well as how this treatment must interdigitate with the demands of a mass casualty event, is essential for successful medical management of these events. In view of their training and experience in rapid decision making for multiple casualties and given the physical trauma that needs to be anticipated in casualties of most forms of disasters, surgeons must actively participate and lead in the planning, rehearsal, and management of mass casualty disasters.

References

1. U.S. Department of State: International Terrorism, Selected Documents, No. 24. Washington, DC, US Government Printing Office, 1986.
2. Berry FB: The medical management of mass casualties: The Scudder Oration on Trauma 1955. Bull Am Coll Surg 41:60-66, 1956.
3. Auf der Heide E: Disaster Response: Principles of Preparation and Coordination. St Louis, CV Mosby, 1989.
4. Waeckerle JF: Disaster planning and response. N Engl J Med 324:815-821, 1991.
5. Hogan DE, Burstein JL: Basic physics of disasters. In Hogan DE, Burstein JL (eds): Disaster Medicine. Philadelphia, Lippincott Williams & Wilkins, 2002, pp 3-9.
6. American College of Surgeons Committee on Trauma: Disaster management. In Resources for Optimal Care of the Injured Patient. Chicago, American College of Surgeons, 1998, pp 87-91.
7. Frykberg ER: Medical management of disasters and mass casualties from terrorist bombings: How can we cope? J Trauma 53:201-212, 2002.
8. Ciraulo DL, Barie PS, Briggs SM, et al: An update on the surgeons scope and depth of practice to all hazards emergency response. J Trauma 60:1267-1274, 2006.
9. Jacobs LM, Goody MM, Sinclair A: The role of a trauma center in disaster management. J Trauma 23:697-701, 1983.
10. Mallonee S, Shariat S, Stennies G, et al: Physical injuries and fatalities resulting from the Oklahoma City bombing. JAMA 276:382-387, 1996.
11. Halpern P, Tsai M-C, Arnold JL, et al: Mass-casualty, terrorist bombings: Implications for emergency department and hospital emergency response. Prehosp Disas Med 18:235-241, 2003.
12. Einav S, Feigenberg Z, Weissman C, et al: Evacuation priorities in mass casualty terror-related events—implications for contingency planning. Ann Surg 239:304-310, 2004.
13. Joint Commission on Accreditation of Healthcare Organizations: Emergency Management Standard. Oak Brook Terrace, IL, Joint Commission on Accreditation of Healthcare Organizations, 2001.
14. Klein JS, Weigelt JA: Disaster management: Lessons learned. Surg Clin North Am 71:257-266 1991.
15. Quarantelli EL: Delivery of Emergency Medical Services in Disasters: Assumptions and Realities. New York, Irvington, 1983.
16. Feliciano DV, Anderson GV, Rozycki GS, et al: Management of casualties from the bombing at the Centennial Olympics. Am J Surg 176:538-543, 1998.
17. Stein M, Hirshberg A: Medical consequences of terrorism: The conventional weapons threat. Surg Clin North Am 79:1537-1552, 1999.
18. Millie M, Senkowski C, Stuart L, et al: Tornado disaster in rural Georgia: Triage response, injury patterns, lessons learned. Am Surg 66:223-228, 2000.
19. Cocanour CS, Allen SJ, Mazabob J, et al: Lessons learned from the evacuation of an urban teaching hospital. Arch Surg 137:1141-1145, 2002.
20. Shamir MY, Weiss YG, Willner D, et al: Multiple casualty terror events: The anesthesiologist's perspective. Anesth Analg 98:1746-1752, 2004.
21. Hirshberg A, Scott BG, Granchi T, et al: How does casualty load affect trauma care in urban bombing incidents? A quantitative analysis. J Trauma 58:686-695, 2005.
22. Lennquist S: Education and training in disaster medicine. Scand J Surg 94:300-310, 2005.
23. Kluger Y: Bomb explosions in acts of terrorism—detonation, wound ballistics, triage and medical concerns. Isr Med Assoc J 5:235-240, 2003.
24. Almogy G, Rivkind AI: Surgical lessons learned from suicide bombing attacks. J Am Coll Surg 202:313-319, 2006.

25. Einav S, Aharonson-Daniel L, Weissman C, et al: In-hospital resource utilization during multiple casualty incidents. Ann Surg 243:533-540, 2006.

26. Frykberg ER: Disaster and mass casualty management: A commentary on the American College of Surgeons position statement. J Am Coll Surg 197:857-859, 2003.

27. Frykberg ER: Principles of mass casualty management following terrorist disasters. Ann Surg 239:319-321, 2004.

28. Frykberg ER, Tepas JJ: Terrorist bombings: Lessons learned from Belfast to Beirut. Ann Surg 208:569-576, 1988.

29. Almogy G, Belzberg H, Rivkind AI: Suicide bombing attacks: Updates and modifications to the protocol. Ann Surg 239:295-303, 2004.

30. Frykberg ER: Triage: Principles and practice. Scand J Surg 94:272-278, 2005.

31. Irwin RL: The incident command system (ICS). In Auf der Heide E (ed): Disaster Response: Principles of Preparation and Coordination. St Louis, CV Mosby, 1989, pp 133-163.

32. O'Neill PA: The ABC's of disaster response. Scand J Surg 94:259-266, 2005.

33. Hirshberg A, Stein M, Walden R: Surgical resource utilization in urban terrorist bombing: A computer simulation. J Trauma 47:545-550, 1999.

34. Ciraulo DL, Frykberg ER, Feliciano DV, et al: A survey assessment of preparedness for domestic terrorism and mass casualty incidents among Eastern Association for the Surgery of Trauma members. J Trauma 56:1033-1041, 2004.

35. DePalma RG, Burris DG, Champion HR, et al: Blast injuries. N Engl J Med 352:1335-1342, 2005.

36. Born CT: Blast trauma: The fourth weapon of mass destruction. Scand J Surg 94:279-285, 2005.

37. Almogy G, Luria T, Richter E, et al: Can external signs of trauma guide management? Lessons learned from suicide bombing attacks in Israel. Arch Surg 140:390-393, 2005.

38. Almogy G, Mintz Y, Zamir G, et al: Suicide bombing attacks: Can external signs predict internal injuries? Ann Surg 243:541-546, 2006.

39. Eachempati SR, Flomenbaum N, Barie PS: Biological warfare: Current concerns for the health care provider. J Trauma 52:179-186, 2002.

40. Inglesby TV, Henderson DA, Bartlett JG, et al: Anthrax as a biological weapon. JAMA 281:1735-1745, 1999.

41. Fry DE, Schecter WP, Parker JS, et al: The surgeon and acts of civilian terrorism: Biologic agents. J Am Coll Surg 200:291-302, 2005.

42. Green MS, Kaufman Z: Syndromic surveillance for early detection and monitoring of infectious disease outbreaks associated with bioterrorism. In Shemer J, Shoenfield Y (eds): Terror and Medicine: Medical Aspects of Biological, Chemical and Radiological Terrorism. Lengerich, Germany, Pabst Science Publishers, 2003, pp 81-95.

43. Jenkins BM: Understanding the link between motives and methods. In Roberts B (ed): Terrorism with Chemical and Biological Weapons: Calibrating Risks and Responses. Alexandria, VA, Chemical and Biological Arms Control Institute, 1997, pp 43-52.

44. Keim M: Intentional chemical disasters. In Hogan DE, Burstein JL (eds): Disaster Medicine. Philadelphia, Lippincott Williams & Wilkins, 2002, pp 340-349.

45. Grey MR, Spaeth KR: The Bioterrorism Sourcebook. New York, McGraw-Hill, 2006.

46. Schecter WP, Fry DE: The surgeon and acts of civilian terrorism: Chemical agents. J Am Coll Surg 200:128-135, 2005.

47. Fry DE, Schecter WP, Hartshorne MF: The surgeon and acts of civilian terrorism: Radiation exposure and injury. J Am Coll Surg 202:146-154, 2006.

48. Mettler FA, Voelz GL: Major radiation exposure—What to expect and how to respond. N Engl J Med 346:1554-1560, 2002.

49. Fong FH: Medical management of radiation accidents. In Hogan DE, Burstein JL (eds): Disaster Medicine. Philadelphia, Lippincott Williams & Wilkins, 2002, pp 237-257.

50. Yehezkelli J, Lehavi O, Dushnitsky T, et al: Radiation terrorism—the medical challenge. In Shemer J, Shoenfield Y (eds): Terror and Medicine—Medical Aspects of Biological, Chemical and Radiological Terrorism. Lengerich, Germany, Pabst Science Publishers, 2003, pp 335-346.

TRANSPLANTATION AND IMMUNOLOGY

CHAPTER 27

Transplantation Immunology and Immunosuppression

Darla K. Granger, MD   and   Suzanne T. Ildstad, MD

Transplantation of solid organs has become the treatment of choice for end-stage renal, hepatic, cardiac, and pulmonary disease. The field has progressed rapidly in the past 5 decades, primarily because of the development of safer and more effective immunosuppressive agents.

After Carrel described a reliable technique for vascular anastomoses in the early 1900s, the technical problems confronting surgeons seeking to replace diseased kidneys and other solid organs were largely resolved. However, the crucial advance that made clinical organ transplantation feasible between unrelated individuals was the development of immunosuppressive drugs to prevent or control rejection.

The combination of azathioprine with corticosteroids, introduced in 1962, was the first effective clinical immunosuppressive regimen. The introduction of cyclosporine in 1978, a specific and nonmyelotoxic immunosuppressant, changed heart and liver transplantation from research to service procedures and dramatically increased the success rates of renal transplantation. Continued improvements in the control of rejection at both the cellular and molecular level have been possible as a result of increased understanding of the complexity of the immune system and the events that constitute the rejection process. Because outcomes may vary with the type of graft and

the patient's clinical history, the choice of immunosuppression depends on complete understanding of the interrelationship between the host and graft. In the past decade a diverse armamentarium of immunosuppressive agents targeting various aspects of the immune system has emerged and allowed a significant reduction in the toxicity of immunosuppression.

CONCEPTUAL APPROACHES TO IMMUNOSUPPRESSIVE THERAPY

The key components of the immune system are lymphocytes, antigen-presenting cells (APCs), and effector cells (Fig. 27-1). Each plays a specific role in generating an immune response to foreign invaders, most notably pathogens. Unfortunately, the immune system cannot discriminate good invaders (organ transplants) from bad invaders (pathogens).

Lymphocytes have an essential, central role in the immune response and mediate its specificity.[1] The rejection reaction begins when T lymphocytes recognize foreign histocompatibility antigens on cells of the transplanted tissue. The foreign antigen is thought to be presented directly to host lymphocytes by APCs, most notably dendritic cells and macrophages, which phagocytose and then display the processed antigenic epitope on their surface. The ability to differentiate *self* from *nonself* resides with lymphocytes.[1] Early in the development of the body's immune system, groups or clones of lymphocytes are formed that have discrete target specificity. A lymphocyte can therefore recognize only one or a few closely related antigens. The range of possible antigen configurations is matched by a panoply of lymphocyte clones arrayed against them. Immune specificity is acquired during early development, and it is postulated that fully competent clones of small resting lymphocytes await immunologic stimulation by foreign tissue antigens (Fig. 27-2). Among the vast variety of antigens that can

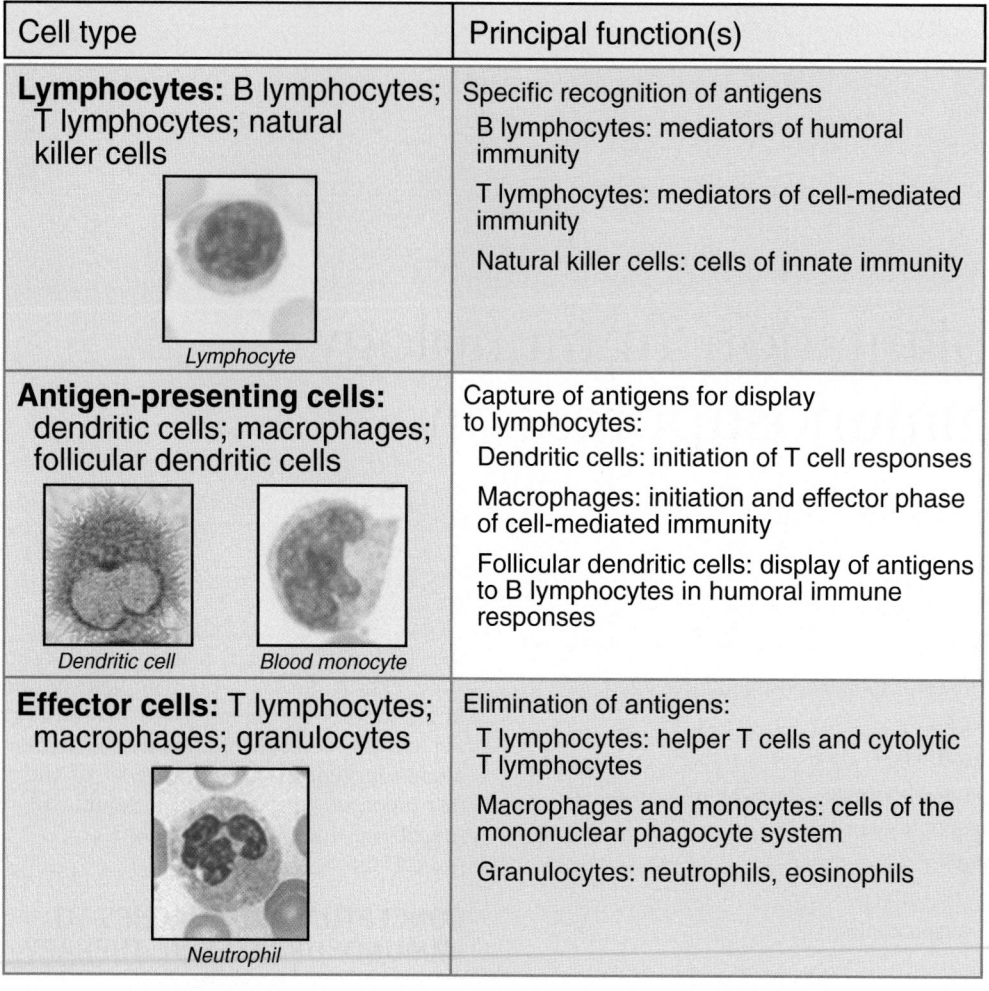

Cell type	Principal function(s)
Lymphocytes: B lymphocytes; T lymphocytes; natural killer cells *Lymphocyte*	Specific recognition of antigens B lymphocytes: mediators of humoral immunity T lymphocytes: mediators of cell-mediated immunity Natural killer cells: cells of innate immunity
Antigen-presenting cells: dendritic cells; macrophages; follicular dendritic cells *Dendritic cell* *Blood monocyte*	Capture of antigens for display to lymphocytes: Dendritic cells: initiation of T cell responses Macrophages: initiation and effector phase of cell-mediated immunity Follicular dendritic cells: display of antigens to B lymphocytes in humoral immune responses
Effector cells: T lymphocytes; macrophages; granulocytes *Neutrophil*	Elimination of antigens: T lymphocytes: helper T cells and cytolytic T lymphocytes Macrophages and monocytes: cells of the mononuclear phagocyte system Granulocytes: neutrophils, eosinophils

Figure 27-1 Principal cells of the immune system. The major cell types involved in immune responses and their functions are shown. Micrographs in the *left panels* illustrate the morphology of some of the cells of each type. (From Introduction to the immune system. In Abbas A, Lichtman AH: Basic Immunology: Functions and Disorders of the Immune System, Updated Edition 2006-2007, 2nd ed. Philadelphia, Elsevier, 2006.)

be recognized are foreign antigens, which are governed by the major histocompatibility complex (MHC).[1]

Stimulation of a resting lymphocyte by the antigen for which it is specific causes it to transform into a large active cell that secretes chemical communicators called *cytokines*. These soluble proteins or glycoproteins (Table 27-1) are effective across short distances and, in turn, amplify the response and activate other cells.[1] Before the antigen is disposed of, however, a series of cellular and subcellular events ensue. Interference with this complex series of events at one or more stages offers many opportunities for therapeutic intervention to suppress the rejection response.[2] For transplant patients, encounter of the APC and the T lymphocyte is generally considered to be the first point of possible immunosuppressive attack. Once the lymphocyte has responded to a foreign antigen and becomes activated (Fig. 27-3), immunosuppressive therapy is less effective. Many cells and molecules are involved. Specific effectors, such as preformed antibodies and activated killer (cytotoxic) lymphocytes, as well as nonspecific agents such as platelets, neutrophils, complement, and coagulation factors, are difficult

to suppress. Suppression of only one or two effectors is ineffective.[3]

In the early days of organ transplantation, the major problem was suppression of allograft rejection. Even though such suppression can be achieved, its consequences and potential dangers are apparent. Immunosuppressive agents act largely in a broad, *nonspecific manner* to suppress the entire immune response. As a result, there is increased risk for opportunistic infections and malignancy. Effective general immunosuppression can cripple the host's response to infections or suppress other proliferating cells (e.g., bone marrow and intestinal mucosal cells). Infections with agents such as cytomegalovirus (CMV) and *Pneumocystis carinii,* which are not life threatening to normal individuals, frequently become lethal to a transplant recipient. As our understanding of the immune responses has evolved, more specific targeting of immune system activation has become possible.

At present, clinical immunosuppression relies on three general approaches. The first is to simply deplete circulating lymphocytes by destroying them. The second is to use an inhibitor of lymphocyte activation (cyclosporine

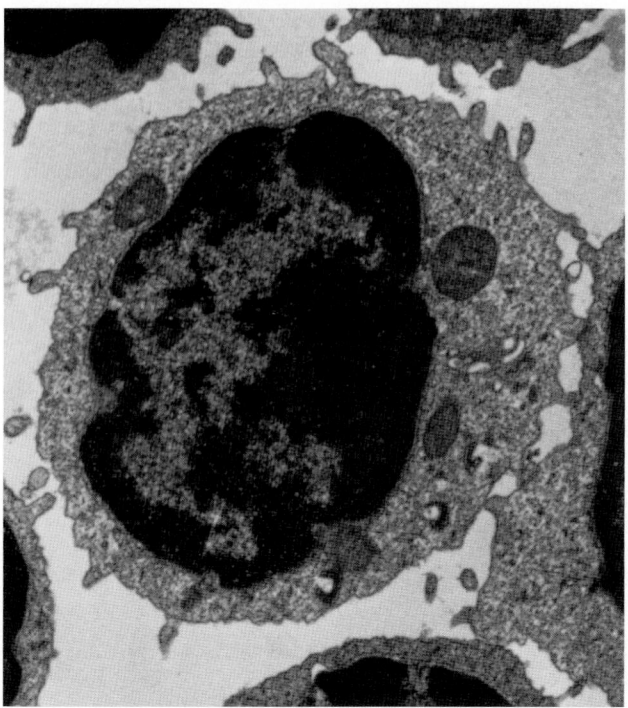

Figure 27-2 The morphology of this small lymphocyte is typical of mammalian peripheral small lymphocytes from the blood, thoracic duct, lymph nodes, or spleen. The dense, inactive nucleus occupies much of the intracellular space, with occasional mitochondria. The small lymphocytes are resting cells that are awaiting immunologic stimulation to transform them into large active cells. If resting lymphocytes do not encounter antigen, they probably die within a few days or weeks (×12,000).

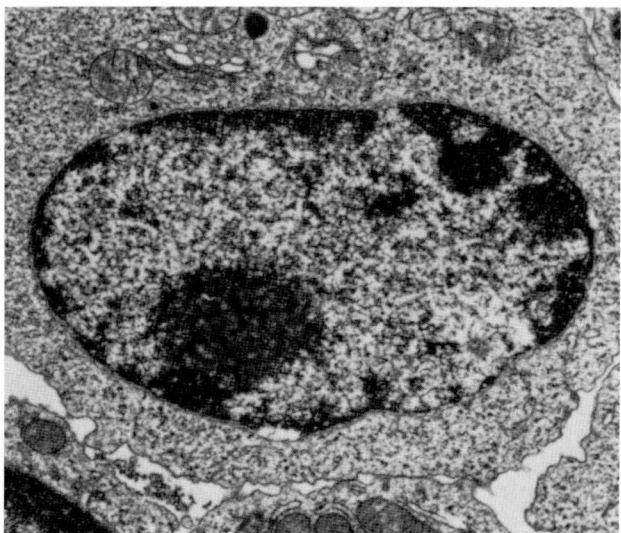

Figure 27-3 The transformed lymphocyte, 24 hours after stimulation, is a much larger, more active cell. The open nucleus is the site of increased RNA synthesis, and the enlarged cytoplasm contains abundant polysomes and mitochondria. Many subcellular changes take place in the conversion from resting to active lymphocytes. These biosynthetic events are vulnerable to the antimetabolites used to prevent allograft rejection. In addition, these cells begin to synthesize DNA at this time, thereby increasing their susceptibility to antimetabolites, alkylating agents, and radiation (×12,000).

or tacrolimus [formerly FK-506]) to interrupt the early events of antigen-induced T-lymphocyte activation and cytokine production crucial for the subsequent cascade of immunologic events leading to graft rejection. The third is to use various metabolic inhibitors (e.g., azathioprine, mycophenolate mofetil [MMF]) to interfere with the lymphocyte proliferation essential for amplification of the response. These agents are biochemically specific but do not distinguish between dividing lymphocytes and other proliferating cells.[3,4]

Future progress in immunosuppressive therapy involves the successful implementation of an *antigen-specific approach* in which the goal is to induce long-lasting *donor-specific unresponsiveness* (immunologic tolerance) in the host while preserving general immunocompetence.[5] The full promise of transplantation will not be fulfilled until graft rejection can be specifically and safely prevented while the integrity of the immune system as a whole is maintained. Such tolerance of the recipient to allografted organs without the requirement for non-specific immunosuppression is the ultimate goal in clinical transplantation.[5] Approaches to achieve tolerance are discussed later. Finally, because the number of individuals who can benefit from a transplant far exceeds the number of donors available, xenotransplantation and stem cell–mediated regeneration of damaged tissues are considered by some to hold promise for the future.

THE CELLS INVOLVED

Key Components of the Immune System

The immune system is composed of *innate* and *adaptive* immune responses (Fig. 27-4). *Innate,* or natural, immunity is a powerful early defense mechanism that is immediate and precedes the adaptive immune response. Phagocytes, natural killer (NK) cells, and complement are the critical components of innate immunity. *Adaptive* immune responses entail sequential, genetically programmed phases involving recognition of antigen by *lymphocytes;* activation, differentiation, and proliferation of the lymphocytes; and an effector phase to eliminate the antigen. T and B lymphocytes are the only cells with specific receptors for recognizing antigen. However, innate immune responses also influence the development of adaptive immune responses. The two components cross-regulate each other by bidirectional cellular cross-talk (Fig. 27-5).

Development of the lymphoid system begins with pluripotential stem cells in the liver of the fetus. As the fetus matures, the bone marrow becomes the primary site for lymphopoiesis. The pre–T cells migrate to the thymus, which becomes the primary lymphoid organ wherein CD3+ T lymphocytes mature and become educated to self. Mature T cells are then released to populate peripheral lymphoid tissues, including the lymph nodes, spleen, and gut. In the thymus, T cells acquire their cell surface antigen-specific receptors (T-cell receptors [TCRs]) (Table 27-2), which in turn confer specificity to the immune

Table 27-1 Summary of Cytokines and Their Associated Functions*

CYTOKINE		CELL SOURCE	FUNCTIONS
Interleukin-1	IL-1	Mononuclear phagocytes, T and B cells, NK, cells fibroblasts, neutrophils, smooth muscle cells	Proliferation of T and B cells; fever, inflammation; endothelial cell activation; increases liver protein synthesis. Binds to CD121
Interleukin-2	IL-2	Activated T cells	T-cell growth factor, cytotoxic T-cell generation; B-cell proliferation/differentiation; growth/activation of NK cells. Binds to CD122
Interleukin-4	IL-4	CD4$^+$ T cells, mast cells	B-cell activation/differentiation, T- and mast cell growth factor. Binds to CDw124
Interleukin-5	IL-5	T cell	Eosinophil proliferation/activation. Binds to CD125
Interleukin-6	IL-6	Mononuclear phagocyte, T cell, endothelial cells	B-cell proliferation/differentiation; T-cell activation; increases liver acute phase reactants; fever, inflammation. Binds to CD126
Interleukin-7	IL-7	Bone marrow, thymic stromal cells, spleen cells	Stimulates growth of progenitor B cells and T cells and mature T cells
Interleukin-8	IL-8	Lymphocytes, monocytes, multiple other cell types	Stimulates granulocyte activity, chemotactic activity; potent angiogenic factor
Interleukin-9	IL-9	Activated T$_H$2 lymphocytes	Enhances proliferation of T cells, mast cell lines, erythroid precursors, and megakaryoblastic cell lines
Interleukin-10	IL-10	Mononuclear phagocyte, T cells	B-cell activation/differentiation, inhibition, mononuclear phagocyte
Interleukin-11	IL-11	Fibroblasts, bone marrow stromal cell lines	Stimulates growth of hematopoietic multipotential and committed megakaryocytic and macrophage progenitors, stimulates growth of plasmacytomas, inhibits adipogenesis
Interleukin-12	IL-12	Mononuclear phagocyte, dendritic cell	IFN-γ synthesis, T-cell cytolytic function, CD4$^+$ T-cell differentiation
Interleukin-13	IL-13	Activated T cells	Inhibits cytokine and nitric oxide production by activated macrophages, induces B-cell proliferation, stimulates IgE and IgG isotype switching
Interleukin-14	IL-14	T cells and some B-cell tumors	Enhances proliferation of activated B cells, inhibits immunoglobulin synthesis
Interleukin-15	IL-15	Mononuclear phagocyte, others	NK and T-cell proliferation
Interferon-γ	IFN-γ	NK and T cells	Increased expression of class I and class II MHC, activates macrophages and endothelial cells, augments NK activity, antiviral. Binds to CDw119
Interferon-α, β	IFN-α, β	Mononuclear phagocyte—α Fibroblast—β	Mononuclear phagocyte increases class I MHC expression, antiviral, NK-cell activation. Binds to CD118
Tumor necrosis factor-α, β	TNF-α, β	NK and T cells, mononuclear phagocyte	B-cell growth/differentiation, enhances T-cell function, macrophage activator, neutrophil activator. Binds to CD120
Transforming growth factor-β	TGF-β	T cells, mononuclear phagocyte	T-cell inhibition
Lymphotoxin		T cell	Neutrophil activator, endothelial activation

*Cytokines are secreted polypeptides that mediate *autocrine* (act on self) and *paracrine* (nearby) cellular communication but do not bind antigen. They include compounds previously termed interleukins and lymphokines.

MHC, major histocompatibility complex; NK, natural killer.

Adapted from Abbas AK, Lichtman AH, Pober JS: Cellular and Molecular Immunology, 4th ed. Philadelphia, WB Saunders, 2000.

system and immune responses.[1] Another lymphocyte subpopulation produced by the hematopoietic stem cell is the B cell. B cells derive their name from the primary lymphoid organ that produces B cells in birds, the bursa of Fabricius. In humans and other mammals, bone marrow is the primary site of B-cell development.[1]

T cells, B cells, NK cells, and APCs have unique roles in orchestrating the immune response. It is a very tightly controlled network, with most communication mediated by cytokines. B cells have the unique capacity to synthesize antibody. A behavioral difference between B and T cells reflects their functional abilities. B cells are special-

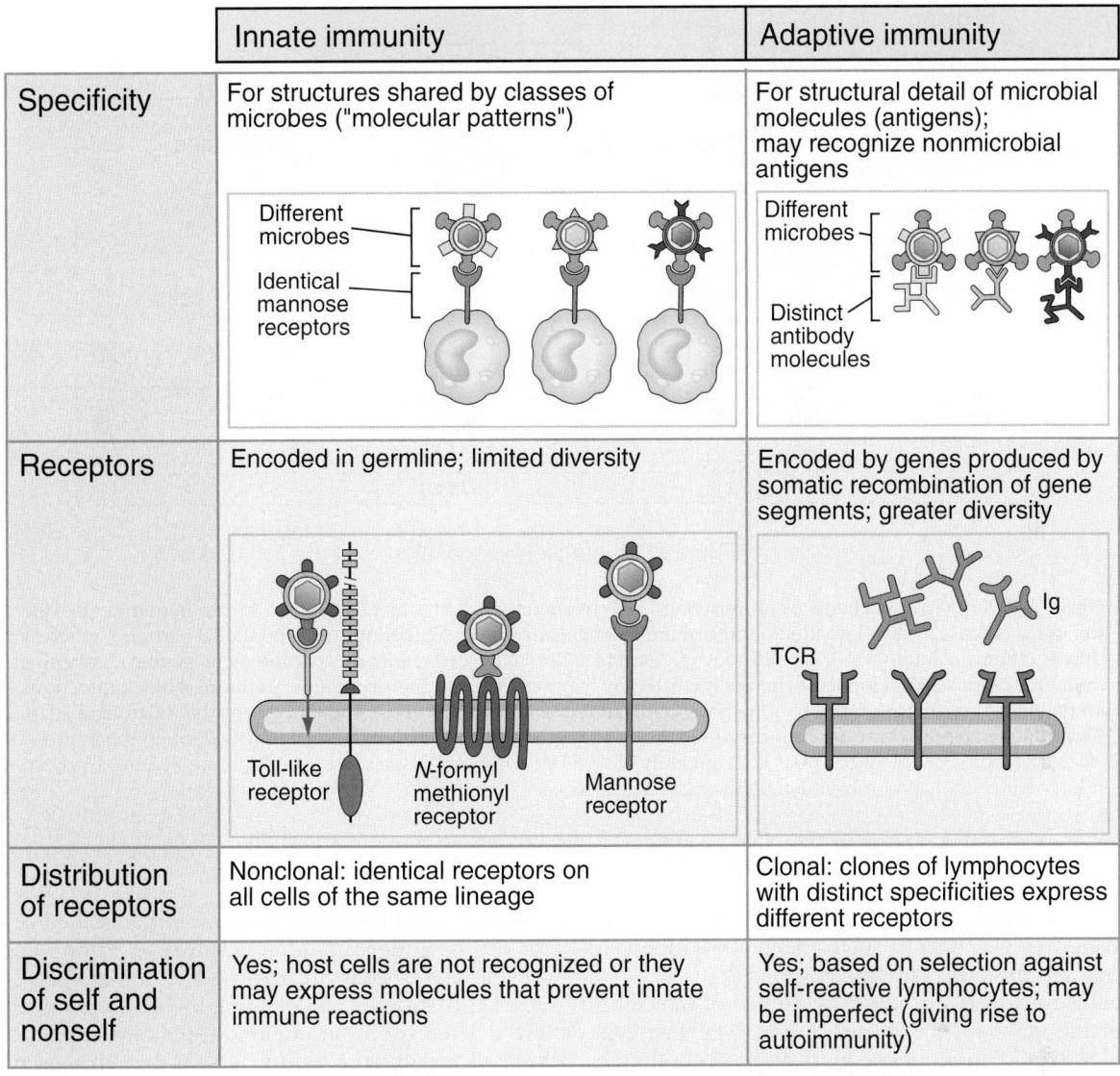

	Innate immunity	Adaptive immunity
Specificity	For structures shared by classes of microbes ("molecular patterns")	For structural detail of microbial molecules (antigens); may recognize nonmicrobial antigens
Receptors	Encoded in germline; limited diversity	Encoded by genes produced by somatic recombination of gene segments; greater diversity
Distribution of receptors	Nonclonal: identical receptors on all cells of the same lineage	Clonal: clones of lymphocytes with distinct specificities express different receptors
Discrimination of self and nonself	Yes; host cells are not recognized or they may express molecules that prevent innate immune reactions	Yes; based on selection against self-reactive lymphocytes; may be imperfect (giving rise to autoimmunity)

Figure 27-4 Specificity of innate immunity and adaptive immunity. The important features of the specificity and receptors of innate and adaptive immunity are summarized, with selected examples, some of which are illustrated in the *boxed panels*. (From Introduction to the immune system. In Abbas A, Lichtman AH: Basic Immunology: Functions and Disorders of the Immune System, Updated Edition 2006-2007, 2nd ed. Philadelphia, Elsevier, 2006.)

ized to respond to whole antigen by synthesizing and secreting antibody that can interact with antigen at distant sites. The T cells that are responsible for cell-mediated immunity must migrate to the periphery to neutralize or eliminate foreign antigens. From the peripheral blood, T cells enter the lymph nodes or spleen through highly specialized regions in the postcapillary venules. After exiting the lymphoid tissue through the efferent lymph, they percolate through the thoracic duct and return to the blood to begin recirculation in quest of antigen. When an organ is transplanted, responsive clones of T cells are activated in the organ itself. In addition, donor dendritic cells leave the graft, home to host lymph nodes, and stimulate both host T cells and B cells therein. Activated T cells leave the lymph nodes and can augment

the cellular response in the graft. B cells send out antibody molecules that bind to antigens in the graft within a few days, thereby mediating destructive reactions.[1]

Considerable progress has been made in dissecting the mechanisms of T-cell maturation in the thymus. Precursor T cells migrate to the thymus, where they undergo a series of preprogrammed maturational changes. All T cells express on their surface an antigen-specific TCR that is the site for antigen binding. The majority of T cells are αβ-TCR+. A smaller subpopulation, which primarily resides in the gut, is γδ-TCR+. There are also transmembrane proteins (CD3) with the TCR. Collectively, these complexes compose the TCR complex and provide the signaling molecules needed to respond to foreign antigens. As the components and mechanism of T-cell activa-

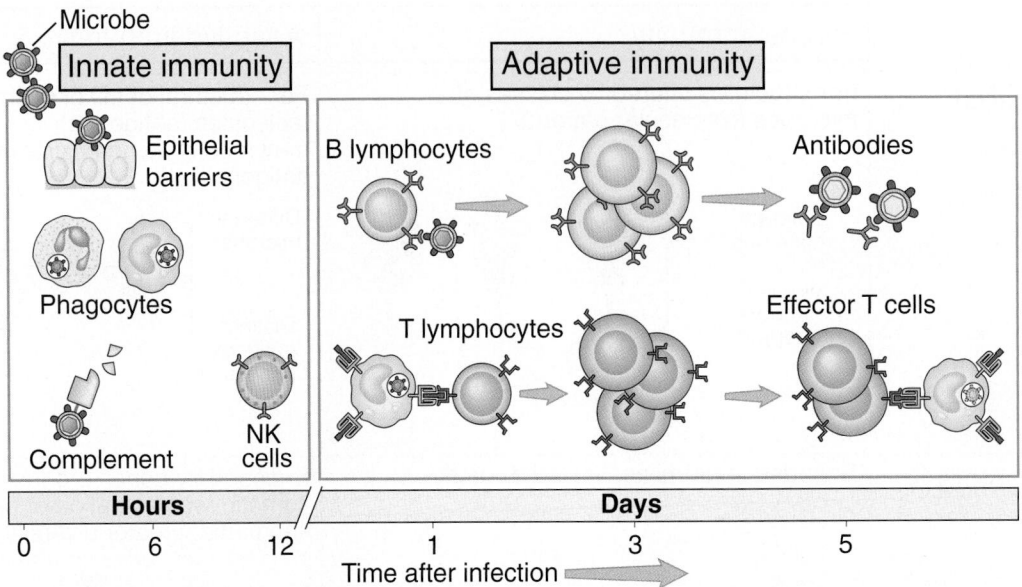

Figure 27-5 Principal mechanisms of innate and adaptive immunity. The mechanisms of innate immunity provide the initial defense against infections. Some of the mechanisms prevent infections (e.g., epithelial barriers), whereas others eliminate microbes (e.g., phagocytes, natural killer [NK] cells, and the complement system). Adaptive immune responses develop later and are mediated by lymphocytes and their products. Antibodies block infections and eliminate microbes, and T lymphocytes eradicate intracellular microbes. The kinetics of the innate and adaptive immune responses are approximations and may vary in different infections. (From Introduction to the immune system. In Abbas A, Lichtman AH: Basic Immunology: Functions and Disorders of the Immune System, Updated Edition 2006-2007, 2nd ed. Philadelphia, Elsevier, 2006.)

tion have been defined, new, more specific immunosuppressive agents have been developed to selectively suppress the rejection response.

Thymic stromal cells produce two types of molecules that are important for T-cell maturation. The first type consists of thymic hormones (e.g., thymopoietin, thymosin) and the cytokine interleukin-7 (IL-7), which regulate functional differentiation of the peripheral T-cell system. The second type consists of MHC molecules, which are important for selection of the T-cell repertoire. Fundamental properties of a mature T-cell repertoire include (1) restriction to self-MHC and (2) tolerance to self-antigens.[1]

The development of self-tolerance occurs through both central and peripheral mechanisms. Each of these mechanisms is vital for discrimination of self from nonself. Central tolerance is achieved through clonal deletion occurring in the thymus.[3] Acquisition of the TCR complex is mediated through a series of genetically programmed maturational steps. Pre–T cells, not yet expressing CD4 or CD8 molecules, enter the thymus and proliferate to an intermediate stage of development, where they become double-positive (CD4+ and CD8+) cells. These cells are educated by self-MHC class I or class II complexes (present on host stromal cells). T cells expressing TCR molecules that interact at an intermediate affinity with self-MHC are selected to survive, whereas those with too low or too high affinity for MHC do not. This phenomenon is termed *positive selection*. Cells that do not

bind to class I or class II undergo programmed cell death or death by neglect. After positive selection occurs, the developing T cells are exposed to self-antigens. If they react too strongly to self-antigen–MHC complexes, they are deleted from the immune repertoire, a phenomenon termed *negative selection* (Fig. 27-6).[3] This occurs by a process called *apoptosis*.

Programmed Cell Death

Apoptosis is a form of regulated cell death whereby the nucleus of the cell condenses and becomes fragmented, the plasma membrane becomes vesiculated, and the dead cell is rapidly phagocytosed. There is subsequently no release of the cellular contents, and an inflammatory response does not occur. This programmed cell death is an important homeostatic mechanism that limits the lymphoid pool so that it remains relatively constant throughout a lifetime.

Activation-induced cell death is an apoptotic pathway that is important for maintenance of self-tolerance in the periphery. The hallmark of this system is Fas (CD95)/FasL (CD95 ligand) interactions. The physiologic importance of this system is to prevent uncontrolled T-cell activation and resulting autoimmune disease. The importance of Fas/FasL to peripheral tolerance was first discovered in two mouse strains: *lpr* and *gld*. The *lpr* mutation occurs in the gene that encodes Fas and results in lack of Fas expression. The *gld* mutation results in a defective FasL

Table 27-2   Summary of Cell Surface CD Markers

MARKER	MAIN CELLULAR EXPRESSION	FUNCTION
T Cell Associated		
CD3	T cells, thymocytes	Cell surface expression and signal transduction with TCR; ε is required for both expression and signal transduction
CD4	Class II–restricted T cells, thymocyte subsets, monocytes, macrophages	Adhesion molecule, binds to class II MHC; signal transduction; thymocyte development; primary receptor for HIV retroviruses
CD5	T cells, B-cell subset	Ligand for CD72
CD8	Class I–restricted T cells, thymocyte subsets	Adhesion molecule, binds to class I MHC; signal transduction, thymocyte development
CD28	T cells (most CD4$^+$, some CD8$^+$)	T-cell receptor for the co-stimulatory molecules CD80 (B7-1) and CD86 (B7-2)
CD152	Activated T lymphocytes	Inhibitory signaling in T cells, binds CD80 (B7-1) and CD86 (B7-2) on antigen-presenting cells
CD154	Activated CD4$^+$ T cells	Activates B cells, macrophages, and endothelial cells; ligand for CD40
B Cell Associated		
CD10	Immature and some mature B cells, granulocytes	Cell surface metallopeptidase
CD19	Most B cells	B-cell activation, forms coreceptor with CD21 and CD81 to synergize with signals from B-cell antigen receptor complexes
CD20	Most or all B cells	? B-cell activation or regulation, calcium ion channel
CD21	Mature B cells, follicular dendritic cells	B-cell activation; receptor for C3d, forms a coreceptor with CD19 and CD81 to deliver activated signals in B cells; EBV receptor
CD40	B cells, macrophages, dendritic cells, endothelial cells, epithelial cells	Role in B-cell activation by T-cell contact; receptor for CD154 (CD40 ligand); macrophage, dendritic cell, and endothelial cell activation
CD80 (B7-1)	Dendritic cells, activated B cells, macrophages	Co-stimulator for T-cell activation, ligand for CD28 and CD152 (CTLA-4)
CD86 (B7-2)	B cells, monocytes	Co-stimulator for T-cell activation, ligand for CD28 and CD152 (CTLA-4)
Myeloid Cell Associated		
CD11a	Leukocytes	Adhesion, binds to CD54 (ICAM-1), CD102 (ICAM-2), CD50 (ICAM-3)
CD11b	Granulocytes, monocytes, NK cells	Adhesion, phagocytosis of iC3b-coated particles
CD11c	Granulocytes, monocytes, NK cells, dendritic cells	Similar to CD11b; major CD11, CD18 integrin on macrophages and dendritic cells
NK Cell Associated		
CD16a	Macrophages, NK cells	Low-affinity Fc receptor; activation of NK cells, ADCC
CD16b	Neutrophils	Immune complex–mediated neutrophil activation
CD57	NK cells, subset of T cells	? Adhesion
Platelet Associated		
CD31	Platelets, monocytes, granulocytes, B cells, endothelial cells, T cells	Adhesion molecule in leukocyte diapedesis
CD41	Platelets, megakaryocytes	Platelet aggregation and activation, binds to fibrinogen
Miscellaneous		
CD25	Activated T cells and B cells	Complexes with IL-2R, high-affinity IL-2 receptor
CD34	Precursors of hematopoietic cells	Ligand for L-selectin, cell-to-cell adhesion
CD55	Broad	Regulation of complement activation; binds C3b, C4b
CD58	Broad	Adhesion, ligand for CD2
CD59	Broad	Inhibits formation of complement MAC
CDw70	Activated T and B cells, macrophages	Binds CD27, co-stimulatory signals
CD95	Multiple cell types	Binds Fas ligand, mediates activation-induced cell death
CD102 (ICAM-2)	Endothelial cells, monocytes, other leukocytes	Ligand for CD11a CD18 (LFA-1), cell-cell adhesion
CD105	Endothelial cells, activated macrophages	Binds TGF-β, modulates cell response to TGF-β

ADCC, antibody-dependent cellular cytotoxicity; EBV, Epstein-Barr virus; HIV, human immunodeficiency virus; ICAM, intracellular adhesion molecule; IL, interleukin; LFA, leukocyte function associated; MAC, membrane attack complex; MHC, major histocompatibility complex; NK, natural killer; TCR, T-cell receptor; TGF, transforming growth factor.
Adapted from Abbas AK, Lichtman AH, Pober JS: Cellular and Molecular Immunology, 4th ed. Philadelphia, WB Saunders, 2000.

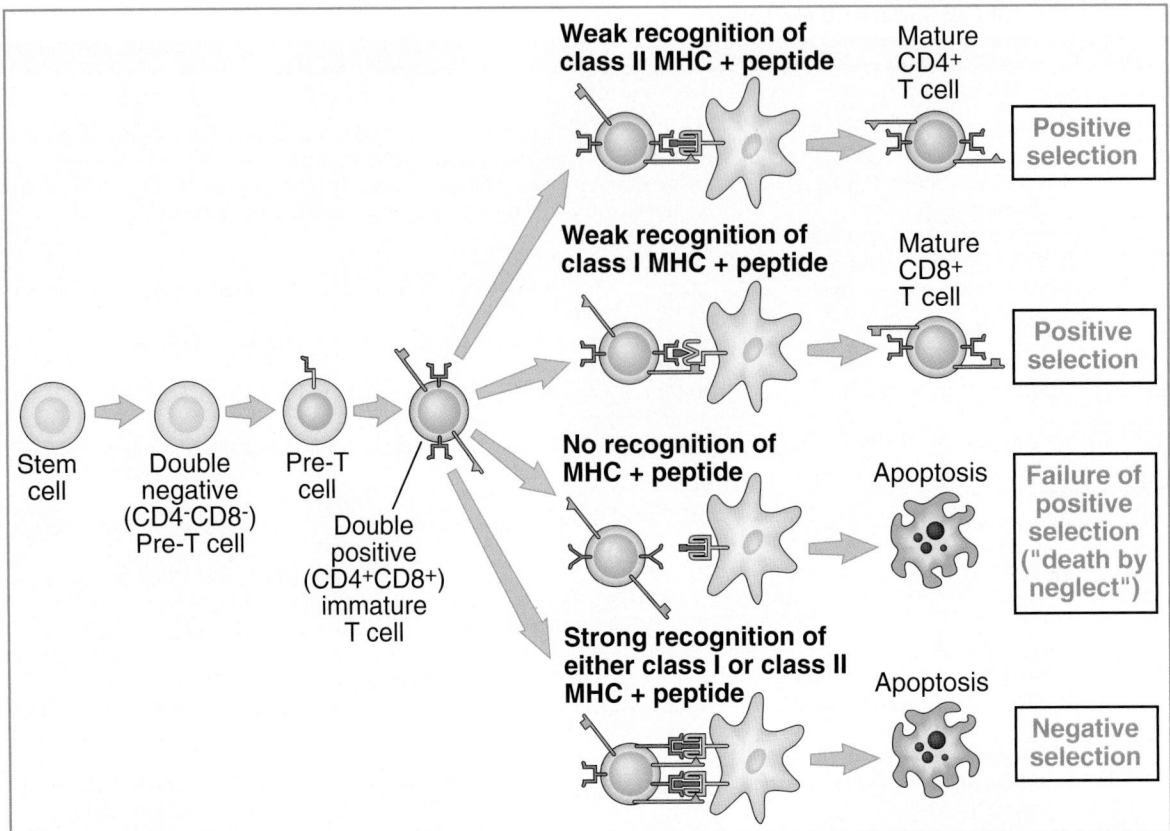

Figure 27-6 Steps in the maturation and selection of major histocompatibility complex (MHC)-restricted T lymphocytes. Maturation of T lymphocytes in the thymus proceeds through sequential steps that are often defined by expression of the CD4 and CD8 coreceptors. The T-cell receptor (TCR) β chain is first expressed at the double-negative pre–T-cell stage, and the complete TCR is expressed in double-positive cells. Maturation culminates in the development of CD4$^+$ and CD8$^+$ single-positive T cells. As in B cells, failure to express antigen receptors at any stage leads to death of the cells by apoptosis. (From Introduction to the immune system. In Abbas A, Lichtman AH: Basic Immunology: Functions and Disorders of the Immune System, Updated Edition 2006-2007, 2nd ed. Philadelphia, Elsevier, 2006.)

protein that lacks the ability to bind to the Fas receptor. Either of these mutations results in severe, accelerated autoimmune disease.[6]

Fas is a surface receptor expressed on activated T cells. Expression of FasL occurs in response to increased levels of IL-2 secreted by activated T cells. This expression of Fas and FasL leads to cell death through apoptosis.[6] The Fas/FasL system is believed to be one mechanism for keeping immune responses from being too robust. Binding of FasL to Fas results in the activation of intracellular cysteine proteases, which ultimately results in the fragmentation of nucleoproteins and apoptotic cell death. CD4$^+$ T cells appear to be more sensitive to the Fas/FasL interaction than CD8$^+$ T cells are.

CELL-TO-CELL INTERACTIONS

Once confronted with an antigen, the response of lymphocytes is complex. Multiple cell-to-cell interactions are required to produce the immune response.[1] T cells, B cells, APCs, and cytokines all play a role. Critical to this response are professional APCs—dendritic cells and mac-

rophages—which bind antigen and present it to T and B cells. Protein antigens need to be digested by phagocytic cells before the antigenic information can be presented to the lymphocyte for self and nonself recognition by the MHC. In addition, activated macrophages produce and secrete IL-1, a cytokine that further amplifies the response and stimulates T- and B-lymphocyte activation.[1] For a productive immune response to be generated, the TCR complex must bind to the antigen presented on the MHC on an APC (signal 1), be stabilized by co-stimulatory molecules (signal 2), and result in intracellular signaling leading to activation of the lymphocyte and production of cytokines (signal 3).

T-Lymphocyte Activation

T-cell activation is an elegant series of events that are continuously being further delineated (see Fig. 27-6). Antigen recognition by T cells is the initiating stimulus for their activation and proliferation, cytokine production, and performance of regulatory or cytolytic effector functions. The TCR is composed of membrane proteins expressed only on T lymphocytes. The TCR does not recognize soluble antigens; rather, it must recognize antigen in the context of peptide (6-13 amino acids in length)-MHC complexes on the surface of APCs. Associated with the TCR is the CD3 molecule. Together they make up the *TCR complex.*[1]

Most TCRs are heterodimers that consist of two transmembrane polypeptide chains designated α and β, which are bonded covalently as previously mentioned; other TCRs are composed of $\alpha\alpha$ chains. All TCRs have a variable region that confers antigen specificity. The $\alpha\beta$-TCR is noncovalently associated with CD3. This highly conserved complex of proteins is responsible for providing the signaling components to the antigen-binding TCR heterodimer. Binding of a foreign antigen results in conformational change in the complex. The associated CD3 molecules transduce the intracellular signals after antigen binding occurs. The development of monoclonal antibodies directed against CD3, such as OKT3, which interfere with T-cell function by altering or inhibiting intracellular signaling, have played a significant clinical role as focused immunosuppressive agents in organ transplantation.[1,7]

Both MHC molecules and $\alpha\beta$-TCR are expressed on resting T cells; however, the IL-2 receptor (IL-2R) is expressed at only very low levels. When T-cell activation occurs, there is a decrease in the number of TCRs expressed on the T cell, accompanied by an increase in IL-2R expression. Activated T cells produce and secrete IL-2, thereby exerting an *autocrine* (acting on self) and *paracrine* (acting on cells nearby) response. Only T cells that have been activated by their specific antigen and express the high-affinity IL-2R can respond to IL-2. After IL-2R binds IL-2, T-cell proliferation begins. Once the antigenic stimulus is removed, the number of surface IL-2Rs starts to decrease, and the TCR complex is re-expressed on the cell surface. This inverse relationship between TCR and IL-2R suggests a negative feedback mechanism. This is an elegant system that is reactive only in the presence of an antigen and ceases to function as the antigen is removed.

Molecular signaling via the TCR-CD3 complex and its relationship with IL-2 production and IL-2R expression have been characterized. Antigen binding initiates the activation of two signal transduction pathways through a conformational change in the TCR complex. The β chain of the complex is phosphorylated via a CD4- or CD8-associated tyrosine kinase–dependent pathway. The activated TCR complex is coupled via a G-binding protein to phospholipase C. Activation of phospholipase C results in the hydrolysis of phosphatidylinositol 4,5-biphosphate to produce diacylglycerol and inositol 1,4,5-triphosphate. These are the second messengers responsible for the mobilization of intracellular and extracellular Ca^{+2} that activates protein kinase C. The result of these changes is the transcription of early-activation genes (*NFAT* and *c-fos*) and the production of mRNA for IL-2 and its receptor (Fig. 27-7).[1]

Co-stimulatory Pathways

Two signals are required for T-cell activation: an antigen-specific signal via TCR (signal 1) and a co-stimulatory signal (signal 2). The co-stimulatory pathways present on APC surface molecules provide the second signal for T-cell activation. If these co-stimulatory pathways are interrupted or blocked, such as with monoclonal antibodies directed at the receptors, the result of signal 1 alone is *clonal anergy* (specific nonresponsiveness). Co-stimulatory molecules on the T-cell surface specifically interact with molecules on the APC surface. One of the most well characterized important co-stimulatory pathway involves the T-cell surface molecule CD28. CD28 binds to B7 molecules found on APCs (dendritic cells, monocytes, B cells). Signaling through CD28 enhances the T-cell response to antigens (Fig. 27-8). To balance the enhancing response, another T-cell surface molecule is present that inhibits T-cell activation, CD152 (CTLA-4). CD28 is constitutively expressed on all $CD4^+$ T cells and on about 50% of $CD8^+$ T cells. CD28 is up-regulated after the T cell receives signal 1. In contrast, CD152 is not expressed on any resting T cells but is induced after T-cell activation; its highest concentrations are reached 48 hours after stimulation. The postulated mechanism for this inhibitory function is through abrogation of the tyrosine kinase activity required for TCR signaling.[1,8]

The mechanism by which CD28 promotes T-cell activation has not been fully defined. Proposed mechanisms include CD28-mediated expression of IL-2 by the T cell. This expression is enhanced at the level of mRNA production and results in increased production. Another mechanism involving CD28 is protection of T cells from programmed cell death, or apoptosis. CD28 is associated with increased expression of Bcl-x_L, a survival protein. Expression of this gene results in resistance to T-cell death by apoptosis.[1]

Closely related to this CD28/CD152 pathway is the CD40/CD154 (also known as CD40 ligand) pathway. CD40 is a surface molecule constitutively expressed on B cells. After antigen recognition by B cells, there is up-regulation of CD80 (B7-1) and CD86 (B7-2); these molecules interact with T-cell CD28 and cause increased expression of CD154 by the activated T cell, which binds to the CD40 receptor on B cells. This CD40/CD154 interaction provides the stimulus for B cells to continue activation and proliferation.[8] Co-stimulatory blockade with anti-CD154 monoclonal antibodies is very effective in inducing anergic and regulatory T cells. This further emphasizes the importance of the CD40/CD154 pathway in providing co-stimulation and up-regulating the effects of CD28/B7 pathway. Manipulation of both of these important pathways is under investigation in clinical transplantation protocols in an attempt to induce antigen-specific tolerance.

T-Cell Effector Functions

In addition to acquiring the TCR complex during thymic maturation, T cells also acquire differentiation receptors called *cluster of differentiation (CD) antigens.* CD4 and CD8 are the best-known CD markers. Other frequently occurring CD markers can be found in Table 27-2. The subpopulations of T cells have several different functional activities. T cells bearing the CD8 molecule interact

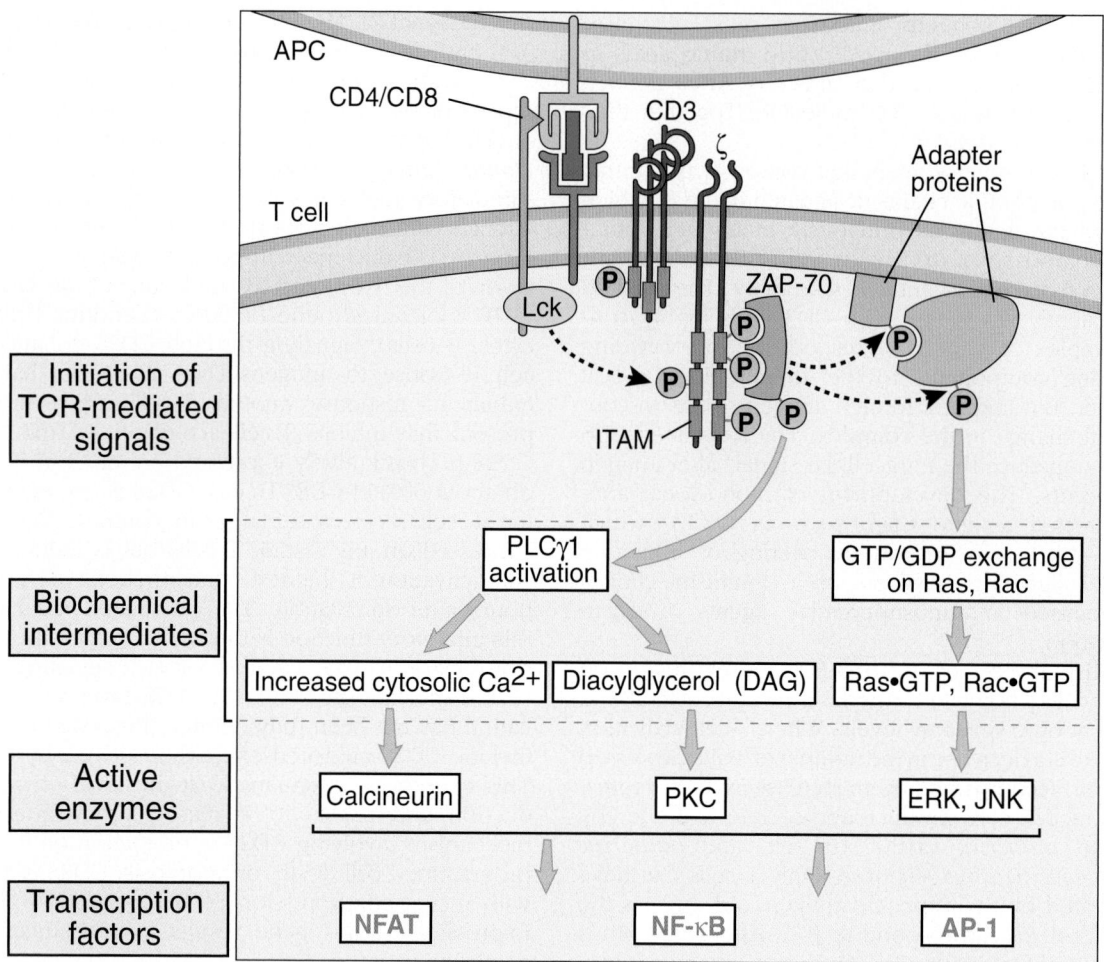

Figure 27-7 Signal transduction pathways in T lymphocytes. Antigen recognition by T cells induces early signaling events, which include tyrosine phosphorylation of molecules of the T-cell receptor (TCR) complex and recruitment of adapter proteins to the site of T-cell antigen recognition. These early events lead to activation of several biochemical intermediates, which in turn activate transcription factors that stimulate the transcription of genes whose products mediate the responses of T cells. The possible effects of co-stimulation on these signaling pathways are not shown. PLCγ1 refers to the γ1 isoform of phosphatidylinositol-specific phospholipase C. AP-1, activator protein-1; ERK, extracellular signal–regulated kinase; GDP, guanosine diphosphate; GTP, guanosine triphosphate; ITAM, immunoreceptor tyrosine activation motif; JNK, Jun N-terminal kinase; NFAT, nuclear factor of activated T cells; NF-κB, nuclear factor κB; PKC, protein kinase C. (From Introduction to the immune system. In Abbas A, Lichtman AH: Basic Immunology: Functions and Disorders of the Immune System, Updated Edition 2006-2007, 2nd ed. Philadelphia, Elsevier, 2006.)

with MHC class I–peptide complexes and can directly lyse a foreign or tumor cell on activation. These activated CD8[+] T cells are the cytotoxic T lymphocytes (CTLs). In contrast, CD4[+] T cells recognize antigen in the context of MHC class II molecules. CD4[+] T cells become T helper (T_H) cells after activation and primarily function through the secretion of distinct cytokines to induce either a cell-mediated response (T_H1) or a humoral response (T_H2).[1]

Even the recognition of foreign cells is a complex process. The initial responding and proliferating T cells do not destroy foreign grafts; rather, they serve as helper T cells (CD4[+] T_H) that activate another group of T cells (CTLs), which in turn damage the graft (Fig. 27-9). T_H-cell proliferation is an important step in amplification of the immune response, and these actively dividing cells are particularly vulnerable to antimetabolites. The activity of

CD4[+] T_H cells is thus one of the major targets of clinical immunosuppression with drugs or monoclonal antibodies.[2] T_H cells have a central role in response to alloantigen. Once antigen has been processed and presented in the context of cell surface MHC class II molecules on an APC, the T_H cell proliferates.

The two distinct T_H populations (T_H1 and T_H2 subsets) differ in their pattern of cytokine synthesis (see Fig. 27-9).[9] In T_H1 responses, the main cytokine is interferon-γ (IFN-γ). These cytokines in turn enhance macrophage activation and cell-mediated immunity. The T_H1 response is balanced by the T_H2 response. The T_H2 response results in the production of IL-4 and IL-5. The effect of T_H2 cells is to inhibit macrophage activation. An important feature of these CD4[+] T_H cells is the ability of one subset to regulate the activity of the other. Thus,

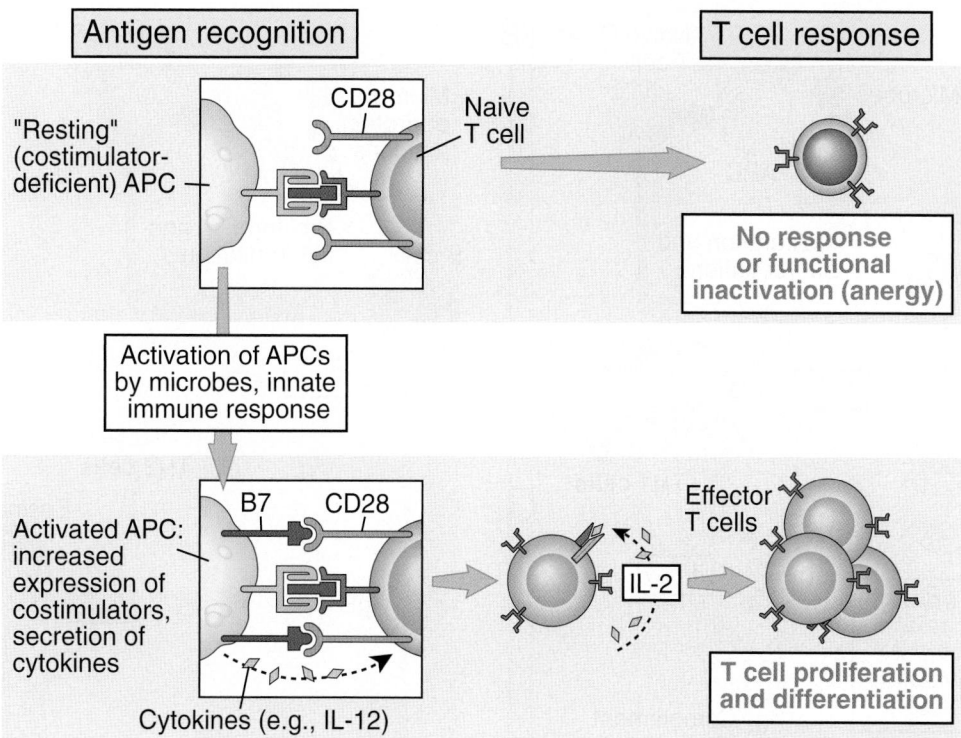

Figure 27-8 The role of co-stimulation in T-cell activation. Resting antigen-presenting cells (APCs) that have not been exposed to microbes or adjuvants may present peptide antigens but do not express co-stimulators and are unable to activate naïve T cells. Naïve T cells that have recognized antigen without co-stimulation may become unresponsive to subsequent exposure to antigen, even if co-stimulators are present, and this state of unresponsiveness is called *anergy*. Microbes, as well as cytokines produced during innate immune responses to microbes, induce the expression of co-stimulators, such as B7 molecules, on APCs. The B7 co-stimulators are recognized by the CD28 receptor on naïve T cells, thereby providing signal 2, and in conjunction with antigen recognition (signal 1), T-cell responses are initiated. IL-2, interleukin-2. (From Introduction to the immune system. In Abbas A, Lichtman AH: Basic Immunology: Functions and Disorders of the Immune System, Updated Edition 2006-2007, 2nd ed. Philadelphia, Elsevier, 2006.)

IFN-γ directly inhibits the proliferation of T_H2 cells, whereas IL-5 inhibits cytokine production by T_H1 cells. This cross-regulation occurs at the level of the effector cells triggered by these subsets. IFN-γ inhibits IL-4–induced B-cell activation, whereas IL-4 suppresses IL-2–induced T- and B-cell proliferation. The current theory postulates that differentiation of naïve CD4+ T cells, down either pathway, is directly related to the neighboring cells and the cytokines that these neighboring cells produce.[9]

Regulatory T cells (T_{reg}) have received a great deal of attention recently and may hold significant promise for strategies to achieve antigen-specific tolerance in the clinic.[10] T_{reg} are defined by their function: suppression of alloreactivity in vitro (a state reversed by exogenous IL-2) and down-regulation of the proliferation of other T-cell populations via IL-10. Initially, they are cell (antigen) contact dependent but, on maturation, become contact independent to amplify the response. The most important T_{reg} subset is *CD4+/CD25+*.[5] CD4+/CD25+ T_{reg} are characterized by the transcriptional factor Fox-3. In animal models, T_{reg} have been shown to play a role in the maintenance of self-tolerance and prevention of graft-versus-host

(GVH) disease after marrow transplantation.[10] In autoimmune type 1 diabetes, the T_{reg} are dysfunctional, which results in a breakdown in self-tolerance.[11] Clinical protocols using T_{reg} in transplant recipients are currently being developed.

B Lymphocytes

Similar to all other cells in the immune system, B cells are derived from pluripotent bone marrow stem cells. IL-7, produced by bone marrow stromal cells, is a growth factor for pre–B cells. IL-4, IL-5, and IL-6 are cytokines that stimulate the maturation and proliferation of mature primed B cells.[1] B cells are responsible for the humoral or antibody-mediated immune response against foreign antigen (Fig. 27-10). Antibodies prevent infection by blocking the ability of microbes to enter the host cell. B cells express immunoglobulin (antibody) on their cell surface. These membrane-bound immunoglobulins are the B-cell antigen receptors and allow specific antigen recognition. Only one antigen-specific antibody is produced by each mature B cell. Each antibody is composed of two heavy chains and two light chains. Both heavy

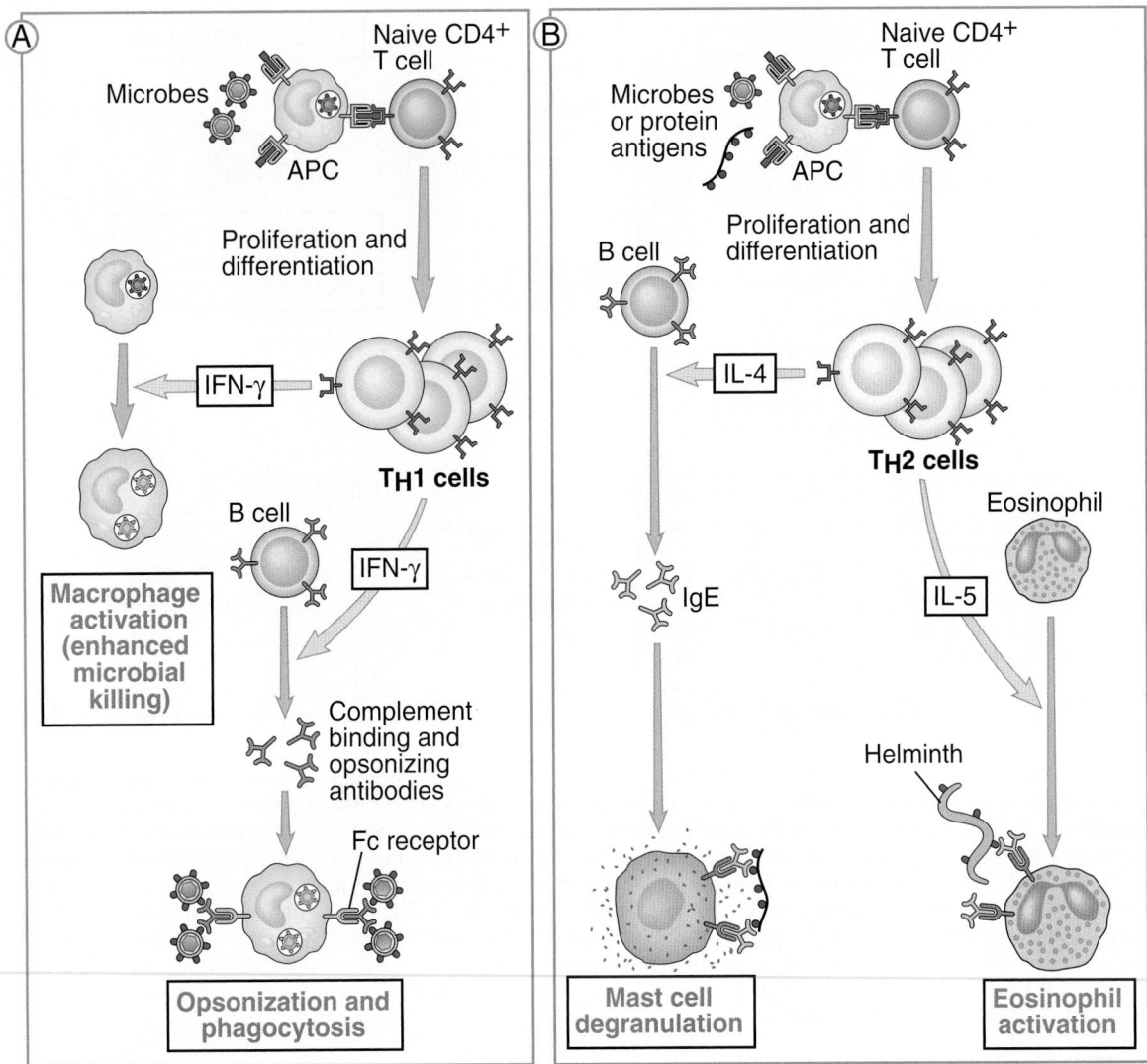

Figure 27-9 Functions of the T_H1 and T_H2 subsets of CD4$^+$ helper T lymphocytes. **A,** T_H1 cells produce the cytokine interferon-γ (IFN-γ), which activates phagocytes to kill ingested microbes and stimulates the production of antibodies that promote the ingestion of microbes by phagocytes. **B,** T_H2 cells specific for microbial or nonmicrobial protein antigens produce the cytokines interleukin-4 (IL-4), which stimulates the production of IgE antibody, and IL-5, which activates eosinophils. IgE participates in the activation of mast cells by protein antigens and coats helminths for destruction by eosinophils.

and light chains have a constant region (Fc), as well as a variable, antigen-binding region (Fab). The antibody-binding site is composed of both the heavy- and light-chain variable regions.[1] The ability of antibody to neutralize microbes is entirely a function of the antigen-binding region.

In humans there are nine different immunoglobulin subclasses: IgM, IgD, IgG1, IgG2, IgG3, IgG4, IgA1, IgA2, and IgE. Resting naïve B cells express IgD and IgM on their cell surface. On antigen stimulation and with the help of CD4$^+$ T cells, B cells undergo isotype switching. Distinct immune effector functions are assigned to each isotype. IgM and IgG antibodies provide a pivotal role in the endogenous or intravascular immune response. IgA is secreted into the lumen of the gastrointestinal and respiratory tracts and is responsible for *mucosal immunity*. The first isotype produced in response to a foreign

antigen is IgM, which is very efficient at binding complement to facilitate phagocytosis or cell lysis. B cells undergo isotype switching with the maturation of the immune response against a specific antigen. This results in a decrease in IgM titer with a concomitant rise in IgG titer (see Fig. 27-10).[1] A primed B cell may undergo further mutation within the variable regions that leads to increased affinity of antibody, termed *somatic hypermutation.*

Monocytes

Mononuclear phagocytes, which also have an integral role in the immune response, are derived from bone marrow. This cell type initially emerges as a monocyte while in peripheral blood. Monocytes are recruited to the site of tissue inflammation, where they mature to become

© Property	T$_H$1 subset	T$_H$2 subset
Cytokines produced IFN-γ, IL-2, TNF IL-4, IL-5, IL-13 IL-10 IL-3, GM-CSF	+++ - +/- ++	- +++ ++ ++
Cytokine receptor expression IL-12R β chain IL-18R	++ ++	- -
Chemokine receptor expression CCR3, CCR4 CXCR3, CCR5	+/- ++	++ +/-
Ligands for E- and P- selectin	++	+/-
Antibody isotypes stimulated	IgG2a (mouse)	IgE; IgG1 (mouse)/ IgG4 (humans)
Macrophage activation	+++	-

Figure 27-9, cont'd C, The main differences between the T$_H$1 and T$_H$2 subsets of helper T cells are summarized. Note that many helper T cells are not readily classified into these distinct and polarized subsets. The chemokine receptors are called CCR or CXCR because they bind chemokines classified as CC or CXC according to whether key cysteines are adjacent or separated by one amino acid. Different chemokine receptors control the migration of different types of cells. These, in combination with selectins, determine whether T$_H$1 or T$_H$2 cells dominate in different inflammatory reactions in various tissues. APC, antigen-presenting cell; GM-CSF, granulocyte-macrophage colony-stimulating factor; IFN-γ, interferon-γ; IL-12R, interleukin-12 receptor. (From Introduction to the immune system. In Abbas A, Lichtman AH: Basic Immunology: Functions and Disorders of the Immune System, Updated Edition 2006-2007, 2nd ed. Philadelphia, Elsevier, 2006.)

macrophages or *histiocytes*. The main function of monocytes and macrophages is phagocytosis of foreign antigen. After phagocytosis, they process antigen, present the antigen to lymphocytes, and produce various cytokines (see Table 27-1) that regulate the immune response.[12]

Dendritic Cells

The most potent APCs are dendritic cells, which are distributed ubiquitously throughout the lymphoid and nonlymphoid tissues of the body. Different types of dendritic cells serve distinct functions in inducing and regulating T-cell as well as B-cell immune responses (Fig. 27-11). Immature dendritic cells are located along the gut mucosa, skin, and other sites of antigen entry.

On contact with antigen, dendritic cells are activated to mature, and expression of both MHC class II and co-stimulatory molecules (e.g., CD40, CD80, and CD86) is increased. As dendritic cells mature, they migrate to peripheral lymphoid tissue, where they can activate T cells to respond to antigen. Dendritic cells provide signals that initiate clonal expansion of T cells, as well as provide signals to promote naïve T cells to either a T$_H$1 or T$_H$2 response.[13] A number of subsets of dendritic cells have

been described. For example, myeloid dendritic cells (DC1) are more immunogenic, whereas plasmacytoid dendritic cells (pDC) are more tolerogenic. Antigen presentation by immature dendritic cells leads to TCR signaling without co-stimulation and induces T-cell anergy. Recent data in animals suggest that pDC, under specific conditions, can be potently tolerogenic in vivo and may therefore in the future provide cell-based therapies to induce tolerance to transplanted grafts.

Natural Killer Cells

NK cells are a critical component of innate immunity. NK cells express cell receptors that are distinct from the TCR complex. Functionally, these cells are defined by their ability to lyse target cells without requiring priming. NK cells lyse cell targets that lack expression of self-MHC class I. NK cells produce the cytokine IFN-γ, which in turn activates macrophages to kill host cells infected by intracellular microbes. NK cells also play an important role in immune defenses, especially after hematopoietic stem cell and organ transplantation. In addition, they contribute to the defense against virus-infected cells, graft rejection, and neoplasia and participate in the regulation

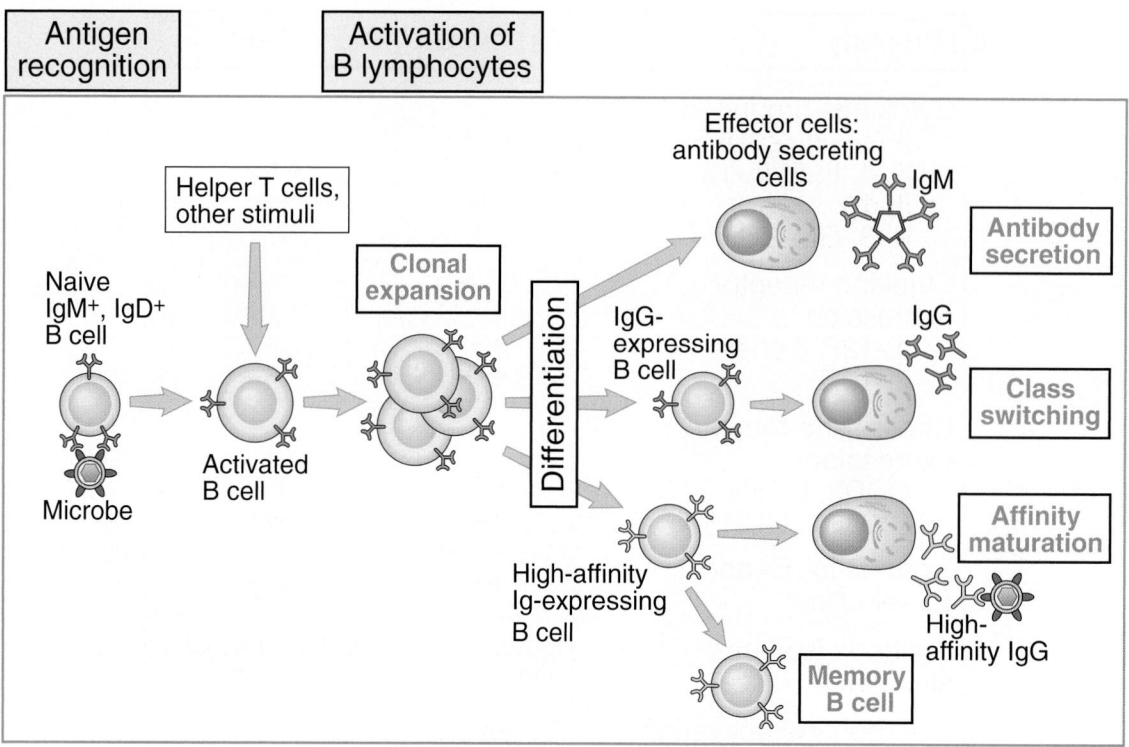

Figure 27-10 Phases of humoral immune responses. Naïve B lymphocytes recognize antigens, and under the influence of helper T cells and other stimuli (not shown), the B cells are activated to proliferate, thereby giving rise to clonal expansion, and to differentiate into antibody-secreting effector cells. Some of the activated B cells undergo heavy-chain class switching and affinity maturation, and some become long-lived memory cells. (From Introduction to the immune system. In Abbas A, Lichtman AH: Basic Immunology: Functions and Disorders of the Immune System, Updated Edition 2006-2007, 2nd ed. Philadelphia, Elsevier, 2006.)

of hematopoiesis through cytokine production and cell-to-cell interaction. NK cells also mediate rejection in xenotransplantation.[14]

MAJOR HISTOCOMPATIBILITY LOCUS: TRANSPLANTATION ANTIGENS

The MHC is a region of highly conserved polymorphic genes. The products of these genes are expressed on the cell surface of a wide array of cell types. MHC genes play a pivotal role in the immune response. The MHC is so important because antigen-specific T lymphocytes do not recognize antigens in the free form or in soluble form, only as small peptides, products of protein digestion, that are bound to MHC molecules. There are two types of cell surface MHC molecules: class I and class II (Fig. 27-12). Any lymphocyte is restricted to one of these two classes. Antigens associated with class I are recognized by CD8+ T cells; antigens associated with class II are recognized by CD4+ T cells.[1]

Human Histocompatibility Complex

The strongest antigens present in transplantation are the MHC molecules and the peptides that they hold. The MHC in humans is located on chromosome 6. The gene products of the MHC molecules in humans are called *human leukocyte antigens* (HLA). Class I molecules important to transplantation in humans are expressions of HLA-A, HLA-B, and HLA-C genes. HLA-E, HLA-F, and HLA-G are more conserved but may later demonstrate importance in transplantation. The class II molecules are expressions of HLA-DR, HLA-DQ, HLA-DP, and HLA-DM genes.[1] There are class III molecules, but they are not cell surface proteins involved in antigen recognition. Instead, class III molecules contain mainly soluble mediators of immune function and include tumor necrosis factor-α (TNF-α) and TNF-β, complement components, heat shock protein, and nuclear transcription factor-β.

Class I and class II molecules were previously considered antigens. They are, however, vital to T-cell and B-cell interactions. HLA class I molecules are present on all nucleated cells. In contrast, class II molecules are found almost exclusively on cells associated with the immune system (macrophages, dendritic cells, B cells, and activated T cells). Resting T cells do not express class II molecules. Both class I and class II MHC molecules are similar in their structures. These structures have been elucidated by x-ray crystallography. This important advance added much to the understanding of antigen recognition (Fig. 27-13). MHC molecules are composed of four domains: a peptide-binding domain, an immunoglobulin (Ig)-like domain, a transmembrane domain, and a cytoplasmic domain. The Ig-like domain has limited

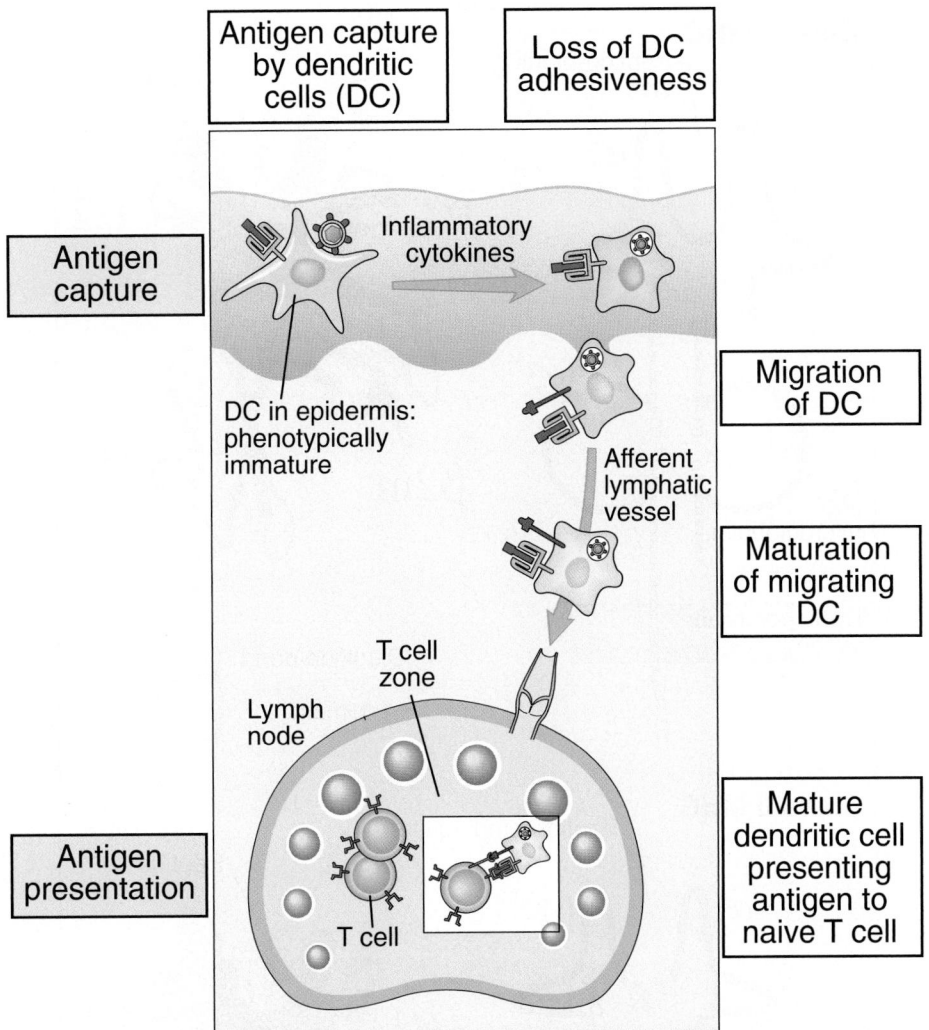

Figure 27-11 Capture and presentation of protein antigens by dendritic cells. Immature dendritic cells in the epithelium (skin, in the example shown, where the dendritic cells are called *Langerhans cells*) capture microbial antigens and leave the epithelium. The dendritic cells migrate to draining lymph nodes after being attracted there by chemokines produced in the nodes. During their migration and probably in response to the microbe, the dendritic cells mature, and in the lymph nodes, the dendritic cells present antigens to naïve T lymphocytes. Dendritic cells at different stages of maturation may express different membrane proteins. Immature dendritic cells express surface receptors that capture microbial antigens, whereas mature dendritic cells express high levels of major histocompatibility complex molecules and co-stimulators, which function to stimulate T cells. (From Introduction to the immune system. In Abbas A, Lichtman AH: Basic Immunology: Functions and Disorders of the Immune System, Updated Edition 2006-2007, 2nd ed. Philadelphia, Elsevier, 2006.)

polymorphism and contains the interaction region for CD8/class I and CD4/class II molecules. The considerable homology between class I and class II molecules suggests a common evolutionary origin.[1]

Class I MHC

Class I molecules in humans are expressions of HLA-A, HLA-B, HLA-C genes, which are recognized by cytotoxic CD8+ T cells. The class I molecules are composed of a 44-kd transmembrane glycoprotein in a noncovalent complex with a nonpolymorphic 12-kd polypeptide called *β₂-microglobulin*. The peptide-binding region of class I, composed of the first and second domains

of a protein, forms a binding cleft. The α3 Ig-like domain, which is the domain closest to the membrane and interacts with CD8, demonstrates limited polymorphism and contains conserved interactions restricted to CD8+ T cells. Class I molecules are expressed on nearly all cells in adults; however, this expression can be increased by cytokines, which is important as an amplification mechanism. Interferons (IFN-α, IFN-β, IFN-γ) induce an increase in the expression of class I molecules by increasing levels of gene transcription.[1] Interestingly, the areas specific for antigen binding are not conserved, whereas the non–antigen-binding regions are conserved.

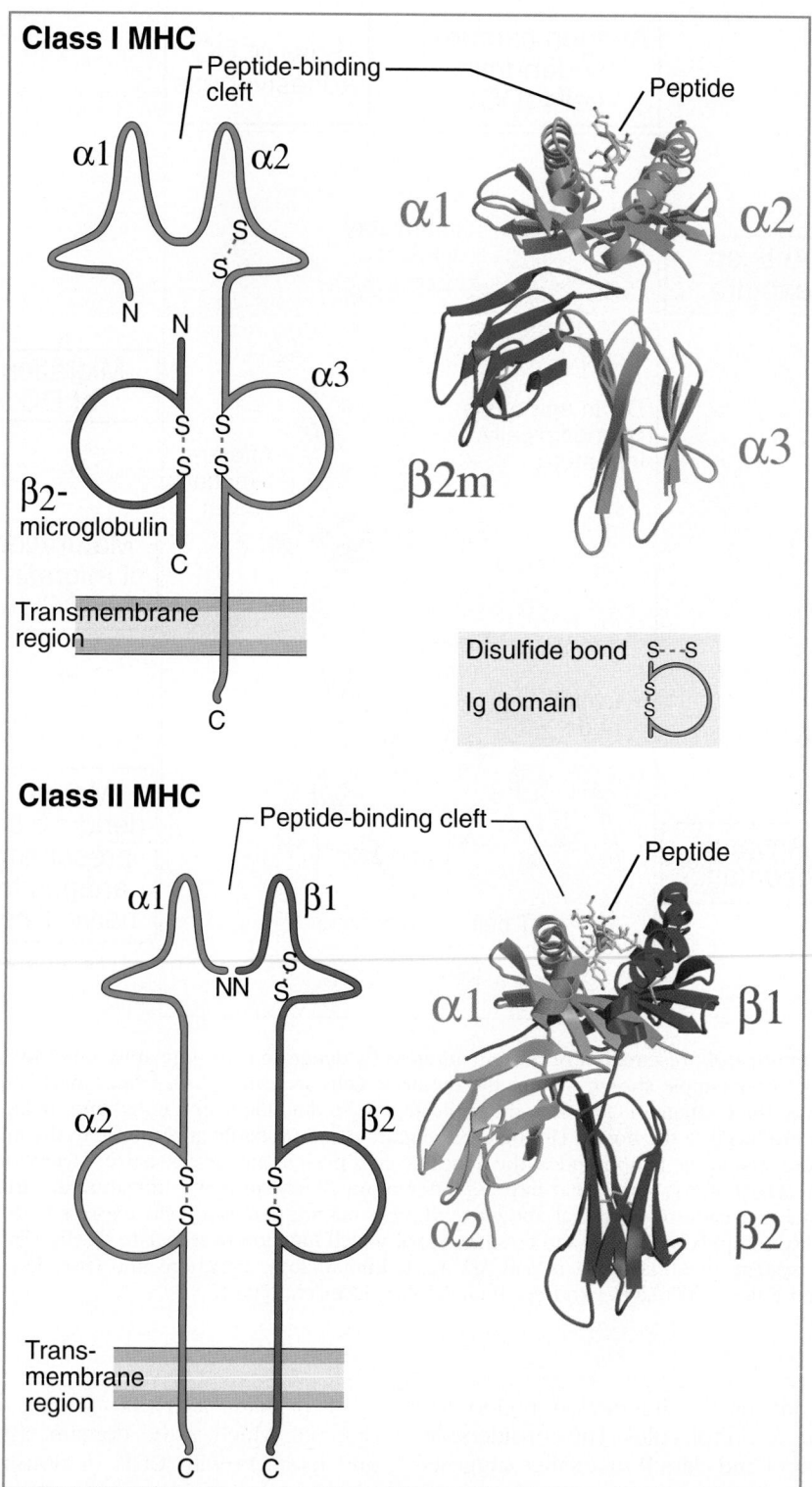

Figure 27-12 Structure of class I major histocompatibility complex (MHC) and class II MHC molecules. The schematic diagrams and models of the crystal structures of class I and class II MHC molecules illustrate the domains of the molecules and the fundamental similarities between them. Both types of MHC molecules contain peptide-binding clefts and invariant portions that bind CD8 (the α3 domain of class I) or CD4 (the β2 domain of class II). β2m, β$_2$-microglobulin. (From Introduction to the immune system. In Abbas A, Lichtman AH: Basic Immunology: Functions and Disorders of the Immune System, Updated Edition 2006-2007, 2nd ed. Philadelphia, Elsevier, 2006. Crystal structures courtesy of Dr. P. Bjorkman, California Institute of Technology, Pasadena.)

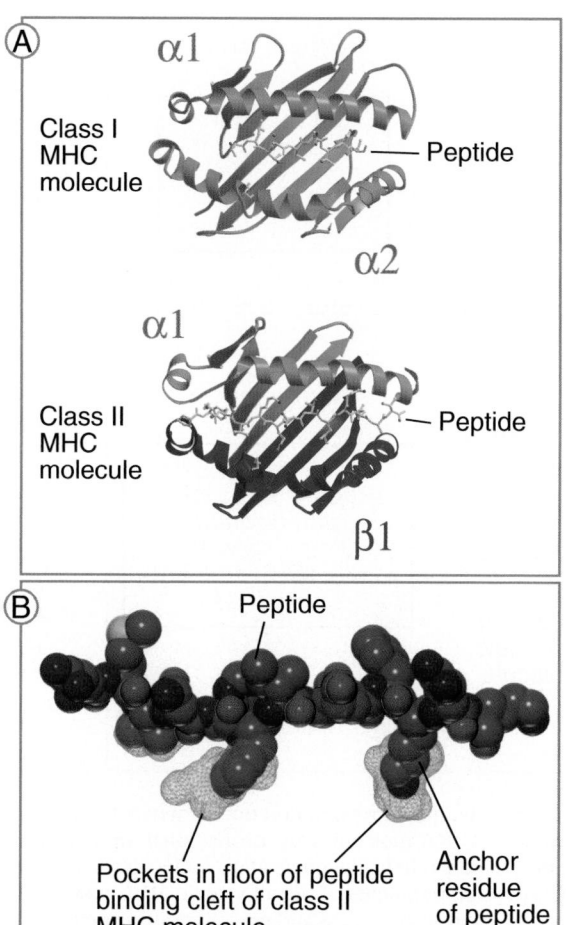

Figure 27-13 Binding of peptides to major histocompatibility complex (MHC) molecules. **A,** These top views of the crystal structures of MHC molecules show how peptides (in yellow) lie on the floors of the peptide-binding clefts and are available for recognition by T cells. (Courtesy of Dr. P. Bjorkman, California Institute of Technology, Pasadena.) **B,** A side view of a cut-out of a peptide bound to a class II MHC molecule shows how anchor residues of the peptide hold it in the pockets in the cleft of the MHC molecule. (Adapted from Scott CA, Peterson PA, Teyton L, Wilson IA: Crystal structures of two I-A^d-peptide complexes reveal that high affinity can be achieved without large anchor residues. Immunity 8:319-329, 1998. © Cell Press; with permission. From Introduction to the immune system. In Abbas A, Lichtman AH: Basic Immunology: Functions and Disorders of the Immune System, Updated Edition 2006-2007, 2nd ed. Philadelphia, Elsevier, 2006.)

Class II MHC

Class II molecules are expressions of the HLA-DR, HLA-DQ, HLA-DP, and HLA-DM genes. Class II molecules contain two MHC-encoded polymorphic chains, one approximately 32 kd and the other approximately 30 kd. The peptide-binding region is composed of the α1 and β1 domains. The Ig-like domain is composed of the α2 and β2 segments. Similar to the class I Ig-like domain, there is limited polymorphism, and interactions are restricted to CD4$^+$ T cells. Class II molecules are constitutively expressed on professional APCs, including dendritic cells, B lymphocytes, and macrophages.[1] Exposure

of these APCs to antigen or inflammation causes increased expression of class II and is associated with activation and maturation of the APC. Expression can be induced on endothelial cells with cytokine stimulation and on other cells in certain disease states, such as bile duct epithelium in primary sclerosing cholangitis and beta islet cells in diabetes.

Expression of MHC Molecules

MHC molecules are essential for recognizing interactions between cells. They are the primary determinant of whether T lymphocytes can interact with foreign antigens. For the most part, class I molecules contain peptides that originate inside the cell, whereas class II molecules hold peptides that were outside the cell, have been internalized, and were degraded in lysozymes. Importantly, in the regulation of cytotoxic effector cell function, neither class I nor class II molecules can be expressed on the cell surface without a bound peptide. Therefore, the peptide-binding groove is always occupied with either self or foreign peptides.

The class I and class II genes can generally be expressed in one of several states in a particular cell. First, the genes can be constitutively expressed and further up-regulation can occur with the presence of cytokines. Second, the genes are not expressed but rather are induced by cytokines. Third, the genes are not expressed and not inducible. These states are of tremendous importance in clinical transplantation and in determining the antigenicity of the transplanted allograft. Expression of MHC molecules is important in T-cell–mediated rejection because of recognition of nonself.

Antigen Presentation: Direct Versus Indirect Recognition

In conventional antigen recognition, the foreign antigen is ingested by the host APC, digested into small peptides, and presented to T cells that recognize the antigen, as well as class I or class II of the APC. This process is termed *indirect antigen presentation* or *indirect recognition*. In addition, when a solid organ is transplanted, the professional (dendritic cells, macrophages) and nonprofessional (activated vascular endothelial cells) APCs of the donor present themselves. This process is termed *direct recognition* (Fig. 27-14). In solid organ transplantation, both pathways play an important role. Recent studies in knockout mice show that induction of tolerance through mechanisms of co-stimulatory blockade may be selective for the indirect pathway because elimination of direct antigen presentation alone does not induce tolerance when combined with co-stimulatory blockade. Graft prolongation is relatively easily achieved by blockade of the CD28/B7 or CD154/CD40 co-stimulatory pathways (signal 2) in mice.[15]

HLA Typing: Prevention and Rejection

Organ transplantation in a recipient with a fully functional immune system may result in rejection. To minimize rejection, approaches that make the graft less antigenic to the host can be applied. The major strategy

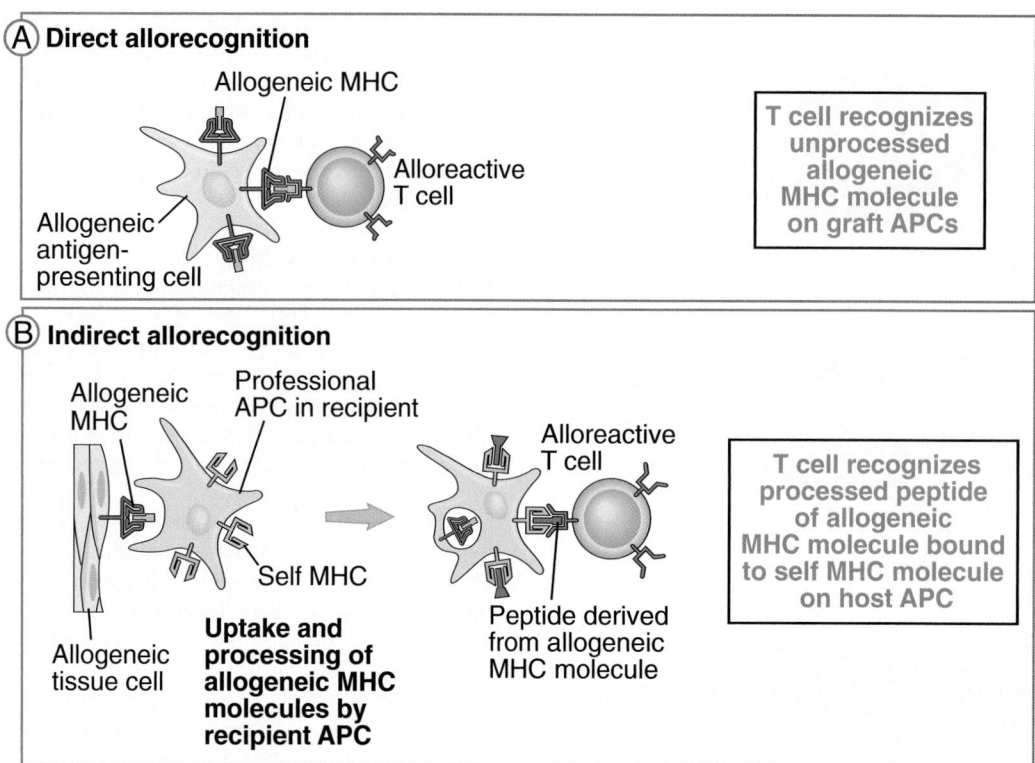

Figure 27-14 Direct and indirect recognition of alloantigens. **A,** Direct alloantigen recognition occurs when T cells bind directly to intact allogeneic major histocompatibility complex (MHC) molecules on professional antigen-presenting cells (APCs) in a graft. **B,** Indirect alloantigen recognition occurs when allogeneic MHC molecules from graft cells are taken up and processed by recipient APCs and then peptide fragments of the allogeneic MHC molecules are presented by recipient (self) MHC molecules. Recipient APCs may also process and present graft proteins other than allogeneic MHC molecules. (From Introduction to the immune system. In Abbas A, Lichtman AH: Basic Immunology: Functions and Disorders of the Immune System, Updated Edition 2006-2007, 2nd ed. Philadelphia, Elsevier, 2006.)

in achieving this objective is to minimize alloantigen differences between the donor and host. ABO compatibility is determined to avoid hyperacute rejection of renal allografts. Another determining factor is HLA typing or *tissue typing*. Potential donors and recipients are typed for HLA-A, HLA-B, and HLA-DR molecules. On close examination of graft survival, HLA matching is the best means of prolonging allograft survival. The larger the number of HLA-A, HLA-B, and HLA-DR alleles that are matched between both donor and recipient, the better the survival rate, particularly in the first year after transplantation.[1] Current immunosuppressive regimens negate much of the impact of matching, however. Humans have two different HLA-A, HLA-B, and HLA-DR alleles (one from each parent, six alleles in total). Large, single-center trials have shown significant survival benefit for only six of six antigen matches. Matching remains controversial in the transplant community. It may be that previously imprecise tissue typing led to the contradictory results of some studies.

Historically, serologic testing with the microcytotoxicity technique was used for both crossmatching and antibody testing. A gradual transition to molecular typing has occurred because of its greater accuracy. Poor HLA class II resolution, limitations in cell viability, and broad cross-reactivity for different cross-reactive antigens limit the

utility of serologic testing, especially for bone marrow transplantation. The serologic method uses an antigen-specific serum that binds to cells expressing that particular antigen. The functional method measures the reactivity of the lymphocytes of a potential recipient to a donor. When antigens are recognized as foreign, lymphocyte proliferation results.[1]

Molecular techniques for performing HLA typing that use polymerase chain reaction (PCR) have been developed and are now commonly used. PCR permits more complete typing of class II loci (HLA-DR, HLA-DQ, and HLA-DP subsets), as well as precise typing of HLA-A and HLA-B. This DNA typing has become the predominant method because it better defines the crucial sequence of amino acids around the peptide-binding groove. Studies have been conducted to compare HLA-DR typing with the traditional serologic method versus PCR methods. Serologic typing will probably be abandoned over time.

In clinical transplantation, crossmatching is performed with microcytotoxicity or flow cytometric techniques. Crossmatching differs from tissue typing. In crossmatching, serum from the recipient is tested for preformed antibodies against donor cells to exclude the possibility of hyperacute rejection. Despite excellent histocompatibility matching, hyperacute rejection can still occur if preformed antibodies are present.[1] Preservation time is more severely limited in heart, lung, and liver transplantation; therefore, in these organs, crossmatching is performed before organ recovery for recipients with known antibody titers only.

Rejection

Graft rejection requires the participation of various combinations of immunologically specific and nonspecific cells. Three types of graft rejection occur (Fig. 27-15). *Hyperacute rejection* occurs within minutes to days after transplantation and is mediated primarily by preformed antibody. This type of rejection is prevented by screening the recipient for preformed antibodies, not by classic antirejection pharmaceuticals. *Acute rejection* is mediated primarily by T lymphocytes and first occurs between 1 and 3 weeks after solid organ transplantation without immunosuppression. Acute rejection episodes are most common in the first 3 to 6 months after transplantation but can occur at any time. Acute rejection can quickly destroy a graft if left untreated. The new immunosuppressive agents have made acute rejection increasingly less common. *Chronic rejection* occurs over a span of months to years and is the most common cause of graft loss after 1 year. From an immunologic standpoint, chronic rejection is mediated by both T- and B-cell responses.[1]

Hyperacute rejection is mediated by preformed antibodies that bind to endothelium and subsequently activate complement. This rejection is characterized by rapid thrombotic occlusion of the vasculature of the transplanted allograft. The thrombotic response occurs within minutes to hours after host blood vessels are anastomosed to donor vessels. Hyperacute rejection is mediated predominantly by IgG antibodies directed toward foreign protein molecules, such as MHC molecules. These IgG antibodies are the result of previous exposure to alloantigens from blood transfusions, pregnancy, or previous transplantation.[1]

There are two forms of acute rejection: acute vascular rejection and acute cellular rejection. *Acute vascular rejection* is the more severe form, with greater potential for long-term complications for the graft. In the setting of acute vascular rejection, the response is mediated by IgG antibodies that develop in response to the graft against the endothelial antigens and involves the activation of complement. T cells contribute to the acute vascular rejection episode by responding to the foreign antigen. This response leads to direct lysis of the endothelial cells or the production of cytokines that further recruit and activate inflammatory cells. The end result is endothelial necrosis. This process occurs within the first week of allograft transplantation in the absence of immunosuppression.[1]

In the setting of *acute cellular rejection,* necrosis of parenchymal cells occurs as a result of infiltration of T cells and macrophages. The exact mechanism that underlies this process has not been fully delineated. The effector mechanism in macrophage-mediated lysis is similar to a delayed-type hypersensitivity response. The T-cell effector mechanism is mediated by CTL-induced lysis. Much of the evidence emerging has implicated the alloreactive CD8+ CTL. The CD8+ CTL recognizes and lyses foreign cells. To support this mechanism, the cellular infiltrate present in acute rejection is enriched for CD8+ CTL.[1]

The mechanism of *chronic rejection* is less clearly defined and is an area of intense study. Chronic rejection appears as fibrosis and scarring in all organs currently transplanted, although the specific histopathologic lesions vary with the organ. Chronic rejection is manifested as accelerated atherosclerosis in heart recipients, as bronchiolitis obliterans in lung recipients, as so-called vanishing bile duct syndrome in liver recipients, and as fibrosis and glomerulopathy in kidney recipients. It is unlikely that chronic rejection is strictly an immunologic phenomenon—ischemia and inflammation, among other processes, also play a role. Risk factors for development of the lesions of chronic rejection include the following:

1. Previous acute rejection episodes, with increased severity and an increased number of episodes further increasing the risk for chronic rejection
2. Inadequate immunosuppression, including patient noncompliance
3. Initial delayed graft function
4. Donor issues such as age and hypertension
5. Organ recovery–related issues, including preservation and reperfusion injury
6. Recipient diabetes, hypertension, or post-transplant infections

In essence, almost any injury to the organ in the donor or after transplantation can contribute to the development of chronic rejection.[16] Therefore, given the multifactorial basis of chronic rejection, the transplant is not completely protected with currently available immunosuppression. Episodes of acute rejection are a very significant risk factor, however, for the subsequent development of chronic rejection.[16] To the extent that immunosuppressive agents prevent acute rejection episodes, the drugs do clearly decrease chronic rejection. New immunosuppressive drugs are evaluated not only by their ability to prevent acute rejection episodes and their safety profiles but also by their ability to prevent chronic rejection and improve recipient quality of life. Improved side effect profiles may enhance recipient compliance with immunosuppressive regimens.

The preceding, abbreviated description of the development of allograft immunity discloses many processes that may potentially be manipulated to suppress the immune response:

1. Destroying the immunocompetent cells that would otherwise react to donor antigen *before* transplantation
2. Minimizing histoincompatibility or altering the antigen to make it unrecognizable or even toxic to the reactive lymphocyte clones
3. Interfering with antigen processing and presentation by the recipient cells
4. Inhibiting antigen recognition by lymphocytes
5. Inhibiting production or release by macrophages or lymphocytes of the signal substances or cytokines involved in differentiating lymphocytes into cytotoxic or antibody-synthesizing cells

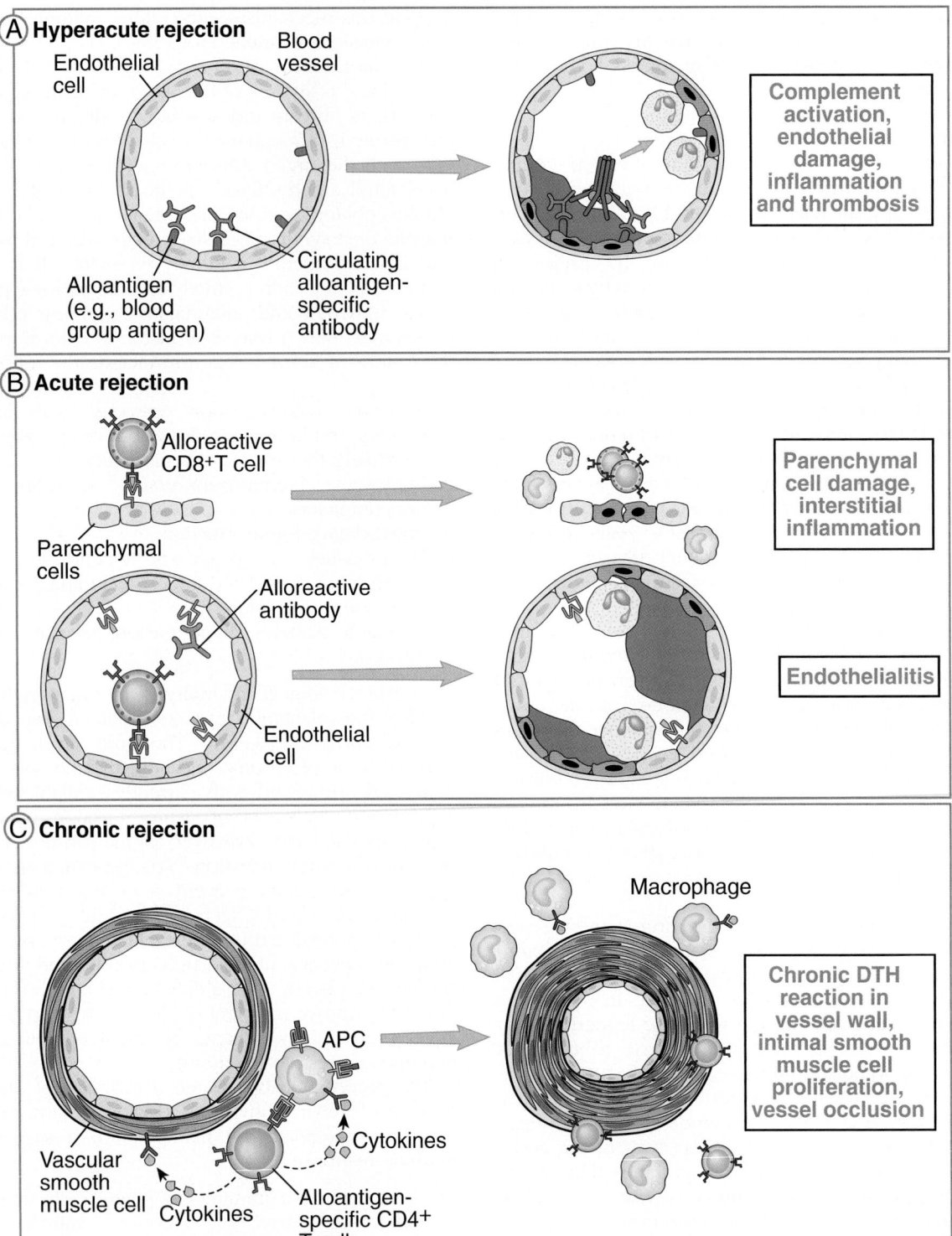

Figure 27-15 Mechanisms of graft rejection. A, In hyperacute rejection, preformed antibodies react with alloantigens on the vascular endothelium of the graft, activate complement, and trigger rapid intravascular thrombosis and necrosis of the vessel wall. **B,** In acute cellular rejection, CD8$^+$ T lymphocytes reactive with alloantigens on graft endothelial cells and parenchymal cells cause damage to these cell types. Inflammation of the endothelium is sometimes called *endothelialitis*. Alloreactive antibodies may also contribute to vascular injury. **C,** In chronic rejection with graft arteriosclerosis, T cells reactive with graft alloantigens may produce cytokines that induce proliferation of endothelial cells and intimal smooth muscle cells, thereby leading to luminal occlusion. This type of rejection is probably a chronic delayed-type hypersensitivity (DTH) reaction to alloantigens in the vessel wall. APC, antigen-presenting cell. (From Introduction to the immune system. In Abbas A, Lichtman AH: Basic Immunology: Functions and Disorders of the Immune System, Updated Edition 2006-2007, 2nd ed. Philadelphia, Elsevier, 2006.)

6. Suppressing clonal expansion of lymphocytes
7. Activating sufficient numbers of suppressor lymphocytes
8. Interfering with the binding of immunoglobulins to graft target antigens
9. Preventing tissue damage by the nonspecific cells and molecules that are activated by sensitized cells or antigen-antibody complexes
10. Inducing donor-specific transplantation tolerance[5]

Potential sites for regulation are discussed in detail later.

CLINICAL IMMUNOSUPPRESSION

Immunosuppressive agents are, for the most part, essential to graft survival. It is rare for a transplant recipient to become drug free, even over a prolonged period. Shortly after cardiac transplantation, recipients must orchestrate taking approximately 60 pills per day. Over time, fewer numbers of medications are required, but the medication regimen still takes its toll. It is estimated that it costs at least $15,000 per year to prevent graft rejection and treat the complications of nonspecific immunosuppression in transplant recipients.

The relatively nonspecific mechanism of action with the currently available immunosuppressive agents is associated with an increased rate of infections (particularly viral infections) and malignancy. In addition, the individual agents themselves have specific toxicities. The overall risks associated with immunosuppression, the individual agents used in modern-day immunosuppression, and possible immunosuppressive drug regimens will each be discussed separately. As the effector mechanisms responsible for graft rejection have been increasingly well defined, strategies to develop immunosuppressive agents with increasingly specific actions have emerged. Although tolerance remains the unattained goal of research in transplantation, significant improvements in immunosuppressive medication regimens have occurred in the past few years as newer agents and newer protocols have been developed.

Overall Risks Associated With Immunosuppression

Risk for Infection

Prevention of rejection in any recipient is possible, but prevention itself is achieved at a high cost in terms of increased risk for infections and malignancies as a result of increased immunosuppression. Immunosuppressive drugs do not specifically block alloreactivity, and a certain degree of increased susceptibility to opportunistic infection plagues all transplant recipients (Fig. 27-16). This increased risk is caused not only by environmental pathogens but also by reactivation of previously controlled internal pathogens. An important example of the latter is CMV infection, which can result in pneumonia, hepatitis, pancreatitis, and gastrointestinal side effects in transplant recipients (Fig. 27-17). CMV has been implicated in the lesions of heart transplant recipients with chronic rejection. The risk for reactivation is highest approximately 6 to 12 weeks after transplantation and again after periods of increased immunosuppression for rejection episodes.[17]

Prophylaxis has been successfully used to prevent post-transplant infections. Transplant programs use various prophylactic regimens, depending on the organs transplanted. Many regimens include pneumococcal vaccine; hepatitis B vaccine; trimethoprim-sulfamethoxazole for *Pneumocystis* pneumonia and urinary tract infections (pentamidine nebulizers may be substituted in those allergic to sulfa); acyclovir, ganciclovir, or valganciclovir for CMV; and clotrimazole troche or nystatin for oral and esophageal fungal infections. Hyper-CMV immunoglobulins are also used to prevent Ebstein-Barr virus (EBV)-derived lymphomas in some high-risk populations.

Although outcomes have significantly improved, infections remain a major problem in transplantation despite prophylaxis.[17] Recent attention has focused on the potential role of BK virus in the development of renal allograft dysfunction. Studies have previously reported the role of the virus in ureteral stenosis. BK virus–associated nephropathy is diagnosed by the presence of viral inclusion bodies on biopsy, along with urine and plasma PCR testing. Sixty percent to 80% of the adult population is seropositive for BK virus, so determining the true role of the virus as a pathogen may be difficult. The nephropathy has reportedly improved with decreases in immunosuppression. Low doses of cidofovir and intravenous (IV) immunoglobulin[18] (IVIG) have been used to eradicate the virus.

Risk for Malignancy

Malignancy is also a complication of chronic immunosuppressive therapy.[19] The rate of malignancy is increased approximately 10-fold over controls.[19] Most post-transplant malignancies are easily treatable in situ carcinomas of the cervix or low-grade skin tumors. Virus-mediated tumors occur with greater frequency in transplant recipients, similar to those found in patients with acquired immunodeficiency syndrome. Human papillomavirus is associated with cancer of the cervix, hepatitis B and C virus with hepatoma, and human herpesvirus 8 with Kaposi's sarcoma. Lymphomas, particularly those associated with EBV, have an increased incidence in immunosuppressed transplant patients. Recipients treated repeatedly for acute rejection are at increased risk, as are young recipients of liver and small bowel transplants.

The EBV-associated lymphomas are often referred to as post-transplant lymphoproliferative disorders (PTLDs) to better distinguish the differences in etiology and treatment from lymphomas in nonimmunocompromised populations. PTLD varies from asymptomatic to life threatening, and treatment varies from no treatment, to reduction or withdrawal of immunosuppression in non-lifesaving transplants, to treatment with antiviral agents, to traditional chemotherapy.[19] Rituximab (anti-CD20), a monoclonal antibody that depletes B cells, has been successfully used in the treatment of EBV-associated PTLD in solid organ transplant recipients.[20] Hyper-CMV immu-

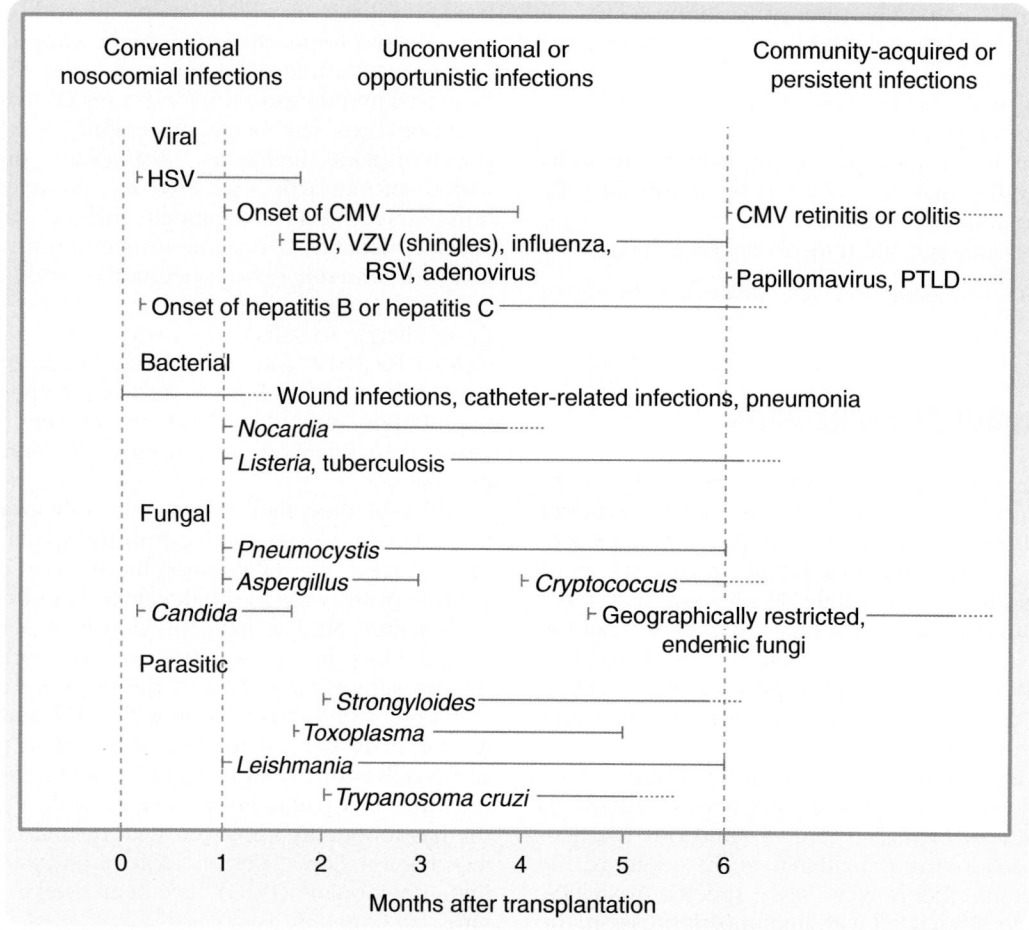

Figure 27-16 Usual sequence of infections after organ transplantation. Exceptions to the usual sequence of infections after transplantation suggest the presence of unusual epidemiologic exposure or excessive immuno-suppression. CMV, cytomegalovirus; EBV, Epstein-Barr virus; HSV, herpes simplex virus; PTLD, post-transplant lymphoproliferative disorder; RSV, respiratory syncytial virus; VZV, varicella-zoster virus. *Zero* indicates the time of transplantation, *solid lines* indicate the most common period for the onset of infection, and *dotted lines* indicate periods of continued risk at reduced levels. (Reprinted from Am J Med, Vol 70, Rubin RH, Wolfson JS, Cosimi AB, Tolkoff-Rubin NE: Infection in the renal transplant patient, pp. 405-411, Copyright 1981, with permission from Excerpta Medica, Inc.)

noglobulin has also been used as prophylaxis in high-risk recipient groups.

Risk for Cardiovascular Disease

Cardiovascular disease remains a significant cause of morbidity and mortality in transplant recipients. After the first year, the most common causes of death in transplant recipients are (1) allograft loss from chronic rejection and (2) death of the patient with a functioning graft secondary to cardiovascular death, disease, or infection.

Atherosclerotic disease in heart transplant recipients is multifactorial. It can be related to chronic rejection, CMV infection, or classic hyperlipidemia. Pancreas allograft recipients suffer from the increased cardiovascular risk factors associated with diabetes, and renal allograft recipients are at increased risk for cardiovascular events as a result of underlying diseases, including diabetes and hypertension with concomitant left ventricular hypertrophy.

These pretransplant risk factors are amplified by post-transplant immunosuppression. Cyclosporine and corticosteroids, in particular, are associated with increased coronary artery disease. Adequate pretransplant assessment for coronary artery disease, including liberal use of coronary angiography, can help identify patients at risk. Post-transplant manipulation of immunosuppression in high-risk recipients needs to be undertaken. For instance, switching from cyclosporine to tacrolimus is considered, as well as avoidance or withdrawal of steroids in selected patients. 3-Hydroxy-3-methylglutaryl coenzyme A (HMG-CoA) reductase inhibitors may lower lipid levels in transplant recipients, in addition to protecting the graft. Exercise and smoking cessation are also emphasized.[21]

Induction Agents

Immunosuppressive drugs are divided into two groups—agents used for *induction therapy* immediately after

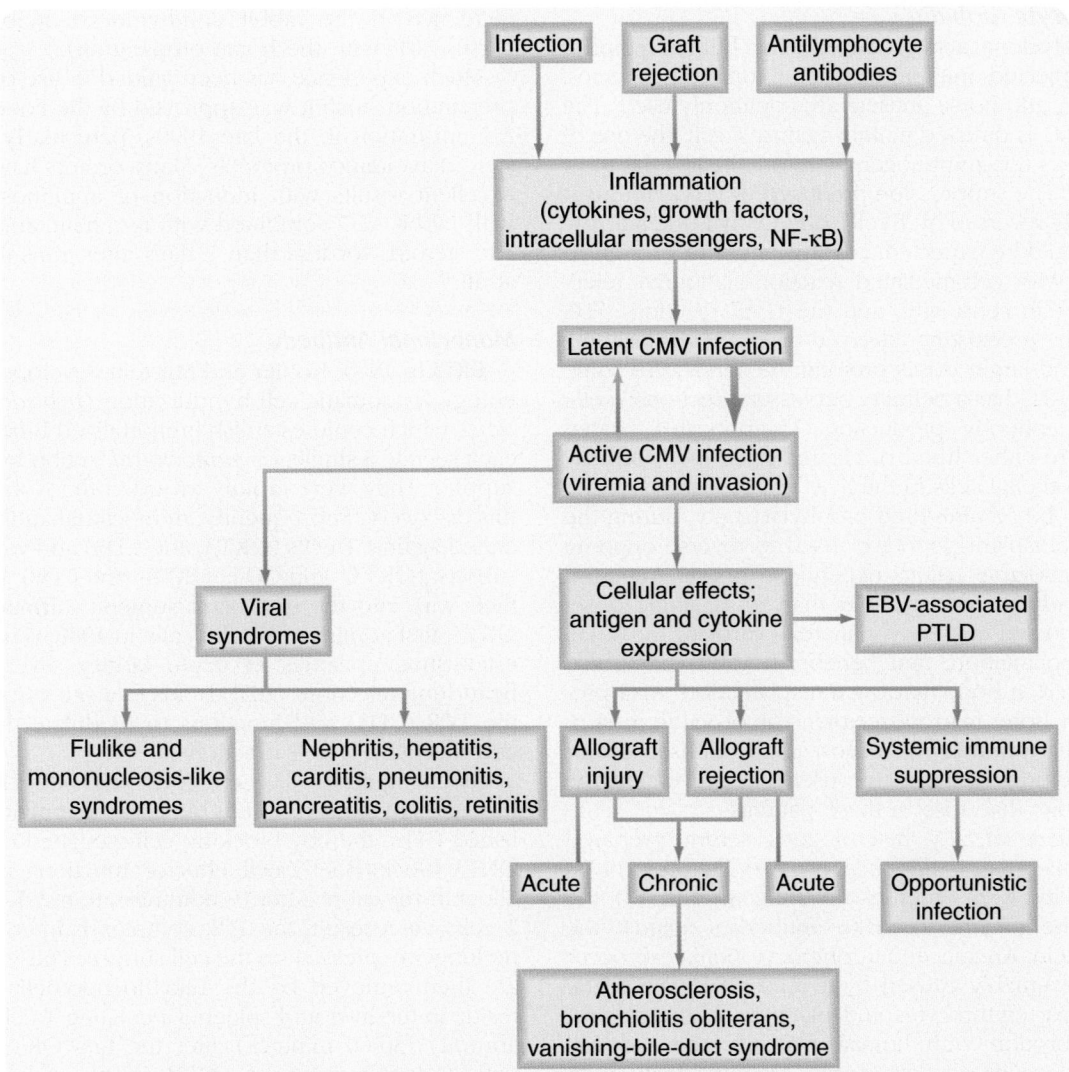

Figure 27-17 Role of cytomegalovirus (CMV) infection in transplant recipients. Mediators of systemic inflammation link the activation of CMV infection to allograft injury and rejection, to infection with opportunistic pathogens, and to the development of cancer in organ transplant recipients. EBV, Epstein-Barr virus; PTLD, post-transplant lymphoproliferative disorder. (From Fishman JA, Rubin RH: Infection in organ transplant recipients. N Engl J Med 338:1741-1751, 1998. Copyright © 1998 Massachusetts Medical Society. All rights reserved.)

transplantation and drugs used for *maintenance therapy*. Major advances in tailoring immunosuppression have occurred in the past decade as a result of advances in research on the immunology of transplantation. Induction therapy primarily includes various antibody preparations directed at lymphocyte populations.

Currently, five commercially available agents are used primarily for induction:

- Two polyclonal antilymphocyte agents
- Two monoclonal antibodies against IL-2R
- One monoclonal antibody against CD3 cells

Three other agents are also being tested experimentally in the perioperative period:

- Anti-CD20 monoclonal antibody
- Anti-CD52 monoclonal antibody
- IVIG

The induction therapy agents also are often used to treat acute rejection episodes. These types are each discussed in the following text.

Lymphocyte Depletion Measures

Many clinically important immunosuppressive agents are effective because they deplete the host of lymphocytes. As the mechanism of action of these agents becomes better understood, a more sophisticated classification system may evolve, but for the present, antilymphocyte globulin (ALG) and traditional monoclonal antibody therapy appear to act by relatively nonselective lymphocyte depletion or inactivation.[5] The profound immunosuppression resulting from the use of ALG or OKT3 increases the recipient's risk for opportunistic infection or lymphoma. Because of these risks, the use of ALG or OKT3 is generally limited to less than 3 weeks.

Antilymphocyte Globulin

ALGs are polyclonal sera produced when human lymphocytes are injected into animals of a different species. Rabbit, goat, and horse antisera are commonly used. The action of ALG is directed mainly against T cell; the use of thymocytes as the immunogen therefore creates the most potent sera. The suppression produced by ALG can be at least partially reversed by T cells, but not by bone marrow cells. As would be expected, administration of ALG interferes most with cell-mediated reactions: allograft rejection, tuberculin sensitivity, and the GVH reaction. ALG can abolish preexisting delayed-type hypersensitivity reactions, and larger doses prolong the survival of some xenografts. ALG has a definite, but lesser effect on T-cell–dependent antibody production. Lymphocytes coated with ALG are either lysed or cleared from the blood by reticuloendothelial cells in the liver and spleen.

ALG may be administered prophylactically, during the early post-transplant period, or used to reverse ongoing rejection. Favorable results depend on potent ALG and prolonged administration rather than on a single dose. ALG is often used in kidney, pancreas, cardiac, and small bowel transplantation, and beneficial results have also been reported in bone marrow transplantation. ALG pretreatment of bone marrow recipients is of value in suppressing the response of the host to the infused donor cells. In addition, ALG may be useful in preventing the GVH reactions that arise in these patients.

The toxicity of any heterologous serum prepared against human tissue depends on two factors: (1) its cross-reactivity with other tissue antigens and (2) the ability of the patient to make antibodies against the foreign protein. Anemia and thrombocytopenia can occur and are presumably caused by a reaction between the ALG and host erythrocytes and platelets. Although preceding absorption with human platelets and red cell stroma reduces its severity, some cross-reactivity with these cells persists in all ALG preparations.

Allergic reactions to the antiserum itself are the most common clinical problems associated with the use of ALG. Urticaria, anaphylactoid reactions, and serum sickness, including joint pain, fever, and malaise, all follow the development of immunity to the heterologous globulin. These reactions are reduced, however, in the presence of the other immunosuppressive drugs used in transplantation.

Currently, two ALGs are commercially available. The first is a horse antithymocyte globulin and the second is a rabbit antithymocyte globulin, which is the most commonly used. Clinical trials have demonstrated that the rabbit antithymocyte globulin has greater efficacy in preventing acute rejection episodes after transplantation. The rabbit antithymocyte globulin has antibodies against CD2, CD3, CD4, CD8, CD11a, CD18, CD25, HLA-DR, and HLA class I. Both the horse and rabbit preparations have been effective in preventing and reversing acute rejection episodes. The results of a multicenter trial demonstrated that the rabbit antithymocyte globulin had a higher rejection reversal rate than the horse preparation did (88% versus 76%) and that it was associated with a lower incidence of recurrent rejection within 90 days after therapy (17%

incidence in the rabbit antithymocyte globulin group versus 36% with the horse preparation).[22]

Much experience has been gained in use of the rabbit preparation since it was approved by the Food and Drug Administration in the late 1990s, particularly as part of steroid avoidance protocols. Many centers have achieved excellent results with induction of immunosuppression with rabbit ALG combined with two maintenance agents and steroids for less than 7 days after transplantation, if at all.[21]

Monoclonal Antibody

OKT3 In 1975, Kohler and Milstein developed the technology for somatic cell hybridization *(hybridoma formation),* which could establish immortalized B-cell lines that each secrete a single, or *monoclonal,* antibody in limitless supply.[1] They were rapidly awarded the Nobel Prize for this discovery. Subsequently, monoclonal antibodies generated against T cells (OKT3, anti-CD3) and various T-cell subsets (OKT4, anti-CD4; OKT8, anti-CD8) have made their way into the transplant surgeon's armamentarium. OKT3, first administered clinically in 1980, is used to treat established episodes of acute kidney, liver, heart, or heart-lung rejection. OKT3 binds to a site associated with the TCR (CD3) and functions to modulate the receptor and inactivate T-cell function.[7]

By engaging the TCR complex, OKT3 blocks not only the function of naïve T cells but also the function of established CTLs, thereby blocking cell-mediated cytotoxicity. OKT3 blocks the T-cell effector functions involved in allograft rejection. After IV administration, OKT3 binds to T cells. As a result, the TCR complex is internalized and no longer expressed on the cell surface. These key T cells are then removed by the reticuloendothelial cells that reside in the liver and spleen. Circulating T cells decrease abruptly (30-60 minutes) after the first OKT3 injection. Once administration of OKT3 is stopped, CD3+ cells rapidly return to their normal levels, probably because of re-expression of the TCR complex on the cell surface.

The major limitation to the use of OKT3 is that it is immunogenic and can elicit immune reactions.[7] After prolonged use, OKT3 becomes less effective as a result of the production of human antimouse antibodies that bind to the circulating OKT3. An acute cytokine release syndrome can also be seen, usually with the first or second dose of the drug. Concomitant administration of steroids or indomethacin can ameliorate this problem. Because of these problems, rabbit antithymocyte globulin has essentially replaced the use of OKT3 at many centers.

Interleukin-2 Receptor Inhibitors The IL-2R is a complex of several transmembrane polypeptide chains. Three IL-2R binding chains, α (CD25, 55 kd), β (75 kd), and γ (64 kd), have been characterized. Noncovalent association of these chains forms the high-affinity binding site for IL-2. The α chain (IL-2Ra) is present only on activated T cells and a subset of activated B cells and APCs. Thus, anti-CD25 monoclonal antibody treatment targets the population of lymphocytes enriched for antigen-activated T cells. Two agents became available in 1998 that share as their mechanism of action binding of the α chain of IL-2R. These monoclonal antibodies, basiliximab and daclizumab, are thought to decrease rejection by binding to IL-2R without activating it, thus leaving the cell with no free receptors for IL-2 to bind. The two agents differ in that daclizumab is a humanized anti-CD25 monoclonal antibody whereas basiliximab is a chimeric anti-CD25 monoclonal antibody.

The immunogenicity of these molecules, as measured by in vivo circulating half-life and by the appearance of antibodies against the agents, is significantly reduced when compared with strictly murine anti-CD25 monoclonal antibodies. Early studies using these agents demonstrated a decrease in acute rejection episodes without a concomitant increase in infections or malignancy. Both these agents are well tolerated and can be administered through a peripheral IV line. Neither agent results in the type of cytokine release syndrome occasionally found with OKT3 administration, nor in the serum sickness seen with ALGs.[23,24] Neither agent provides adequate immunosuppression on its own to prevent rejection because T-cell proliferation can occur by other pathways. Therefore, both agents must be used in conjunction with other immunosuppressive drugs.

Anti-CD20 Monoclonal Antibody (Rituximab) Rituximab, as mentioned earlier, has been used as an anti-PTLD agent because of its depleting effect on B cells. CD20 is a surface molecule expressed on B cells. The antibody has also been used in some centers to decrease antibody production in recipients with high panel-reactive antibody (PRA) or as part of positive crossmatch protocols. Additionally, rituximab has been used to treat humoral rejection in cardiac recipients.

Anti-CD52 Monoclonal Antibody (Alemtuzumab [Campath 1H]) Alemtuzumab is a humanized monoclonal antibody against CD52, which is expressed on B cells, T cells, monocytes, and macrophages. Administration of the agent results in a dramatic, prolonged depletion of lymphocytes that lasts 2 to 6 months. Alemtuzumab has been used in the treatment of lymphoid malignancies, rheumatoid arthritis, and multiple sclerosis. It has prevented rejection in renal allograft recipients in conjunction with tacrolimus and MMF, as well as with various monotherapy agents.[25] Alemtuzumab has also been used to treat lung transplant rejection and as an induction agent in small bowel transplantation. Longer-term results are beginning to come available, and the benefits of this type of protocol are exciting in terms of both efficacy and decreased cost.[25] The benefit of lymphodepletion is that it is often steroid sparing. Characteristics of the T-lymphocyte recovery have been studied; interestingly, many alemtuzumab-treated recipients remain unresponsive to donor antigen even after their T lymphocytes return.[25]

Intravenous Immunoglobulin

IVIG is made from the pooled plasma of thousands of screened donors and contains all the antibodies normally found in humans. IVIG works through many mechanisms to modulate the immune system, including neutralization of circulating autoantibodies by anti-idiotypes and selective down-regulation of antibody production. The preparation can also regulate the production of T-cell cytokines, inhibit lymphocyte proliferation, and regulate apoptosis.

The use of IVIG has increased dramatically in transplantation over the last few years for the desensitization of sensitized recipients with high PRA titers, as well as for positive crossmatch and ABO-incompatible protocols. It is often used in combination with plasmapheresis. Additionally, IVIG has successfully treated humoral rejection in all types of organ transplants, including some rejection episodes resistant to steroids and antithymocyte globulin.[26]

Maintenance Agents

A general rule in the management of immunosuppression is that the greatest amount of drug is required early after transplantation. Usually, dosages can be slowly tapered after the graft has been in place for a period. However, it is highly unusual for a transplant recipient to become drug free. The mainstay of human organ transplantation is daily immunosuppression with oral pharmaceuticals, although maintenance immunosuppression with monthly or bimonthly parenteral medications is now under study. Prednisone and azathioprine have been used for many years. In those early years of transplantation, though, severe complications with steroid therapy were common when very high doses were used. Multidrug therapy with immunosuppressive agents that have a nonoverlapping mechanism of action is used in most organ recipients to decrease the side effects associated with any individual drug administered in doses large enough to adequately prevent rejection (Box 27-1). The new approach to induction therapy followed by maintenance immunosuppression has allowed the need for steroids to often be overcome.

Adrenal Corticosteroids

Adrenal corticosteroids have been widely used as immunosuppressive agents.[27] Glucocorticoids have many diverse anti-inflammatory actions, which make them potent immunosuppressants. A major effect of corticosteroids appears to be inhibition of cytokine gene transcription in macrophages, as well as inhibition of cytokine secretion (IL-1, IL-6, TNF). Corticosteroids also suppress

---

Box 27-1　Maintenance Agents

Adrenal Corticosteroid

Prednisone

Antiproliferative Agents

Azathioprine
Mycophenolate mofetil
Leflunomide

T-Cell–Directed Immunosuppressants

Calcineurin inhibitors: cyclosporine, tacrolimus
Cell cycle arrest: sirolimus

Lymphocyte Sequestration

FTY720

the production and effect of T-cell cytokines, which amplify the responses of lymphocytes and macrophages. Thus, IL-2 production and binding of IL-2 to its receptor are inhibited by glucocorticoids. Moreover, the ability of macrophages to respond to lymphocyte-derived signals such as migration inhibition factor and macrophage activation factor is blocked by corticosteroids. This may underlie the marked inhibition of delayed-type hypersensitivity reactions observed with the use of these agents. An additional effect is suppression of prostaglandin synthesis. Corticosteroids have little net effect on antibody production.

Some of the molecular mechanisms by which glucocorticoids exert their effect have been elucidated. Much activity is initiated at the subcellular level by means of hormone receptors. Unlike polypeptide mediators with receptors on the cell surface, steroids move freely through the cell membrane to bind receptors in the cytoplasm and produce a steroid-receptor complex. This complex then moves into the nucleus, where it attaches to DNA. There, it acts on gene promoters to either depress or activate part of the genome and cause transcription of specific messenger RNA. Thus, some protein synthesis is down-regulated and other proteins are synthesized. These changes are the presumed effectors of glucocorticoid action.

Specific intracytoplasmic receptors for glucocorticoids have been identified in normal human lymphocytes, monocytes, neutrophils, and eosinophils. In addition, varying degrees of receptor density have been demonstrated in different lymphoid cell subpopulations. Presumably, the sensitivity of a particular subpopulation of lymphocytes relates to the relative density of the intracytoplasmic receptors for the corticosteroids. These messengers can inhibit DNA, RNA, and protein synthesis. Glucose and amino acid transport can also be affected.

The effectiveness of cortisone in suppressing allograft rejection was first recognized in the 1950s in research showing that it prolonged skin graft survival in rabbits. In organ allografts, corticosteroids are not effective by themselves, but they have proved valuable when combined with other agents. Steroids, in high doses, are especially effective at interrupting ongoing rejection reactions in clinical practice, but prolonged use leads to unacceptable side effects such as hypertension, weight gain, peptic ulcers and gastrointestinal bleeding, euphoric personality changes, cataract formation, hyperglycemia that could progress to diabetes, pancreatitis, muscle wasting, and osteoporosis with avascular necrosis of the femoral head and other bones. Susceptibility to pyogenic and opportunistic infections is a direct result of the suppression of phagocytic microbial killing by macrophages and neutrophils. Cushingoid features are the external signs of these dangerous processes. These significant side effects have led many centers to develop steroid avoidance protocols. Earlier attempts at steroid withdrawal resulted in unacceptably high rejection rates. Current protocols, many using rabbit antithymocyte globulin or anti-CD52, or both, for induction and less than 7 days of steroids, have had much better results. A possible explanation for the success of steroid avoidance over steroid

withdrawal may be prevention of up-regulation of steroid receptors in the avoidance protocols; however, this hypothesis remains just conjecture at this point.[21]

Antiproliferative Agents

Antiproliferative agents inhibit full expression of the immune response by preventing differentiation and division of immunocompetent lymphocytes after their encounter with antigen. They either structurally resemble essential metabolites or combine with certain cellular components, such as DNA, and thereby interfere with molecular function.

Antimetabolites, the former group, either inhibit enzymes that regulate a particular metabolic pathway or are incorporated during synthesis to produce *faulty* molecules. They include purine, pyrimidine, and folic acid analogues and are most effective against proliferating and differentiating cells. These drugs are given at the time of transplantation when the immunocompetent cells are first stimulated and for the life of the graft to inhibit the continuing response of the immune system.

Azathioprine

Until the mid-1990s, the purine analogue azathioprine was the most widely used immunosuppressive drug in clinical organ transplantation. In fact, Hitchings and Elion were awarded the Nobel Prize for a simple modification that made the drug safe for use in transplantation. Azathioprine is 6-mercaptopurine (6-MP) plus a side chain to protect the labile sulfhydryl group. In the liver, the side chain is split off to form the active compound 6-MP. The mechanism of action of these two compounds is similar, although azathioprine appears to have the advantage of slightly lower toxicity.

Full metabolic activity occurs in the cell with the addition of ribose-S6-phosphate from phosphoribosyl pyrophosphate to form 6-MP ribonucleotide. The structural resemblance of this molecule to inosine monophosphate is obvious, and 6-MP ribonucleotide inhibits the enzymes that begin to convert inosine nucleotide to adenosine and guanosine monophosphate. In addition, the presence of 6-MP ribonucleotides slows the entire purine biosynthetic pathway by fraudulent feedback inhibition of an early step. The steric similarity to either adenosine or guanine nucleotides is not sufficient to allow significant incorporation into DNA or RNA and synthesis of faulty molecules. The result of inhibiting these several enzymes, however, is to block the synthesis of cellular DNA, RNA, certain cofactors, and other active nucleotides.

The biologic activity of azathioprine and 6-MP is greatest when nucleic acid synthesis is most required. These agents thus strongly inhibit the development of both humoral and cellular immunity by interfering with differentiation and proliferation of the responding lymphocytes. When the expansion of fully immunocompetent cells is complete, nucleic acid synthesis is less important and the drug is less effective. An additional benefit of azathioprine is that it can also reduce neutrophil production and macrophage activation, effects that suppress the nonspecific inflammatory components of the immune reaction.

The toxicity of azathioprine derives from the same antimetabolite action. The primary effect is bone marrow suppression leading to leukopenia. Liver toxicity may also occur, possibly because of the high rate of RNA synthesis by hepatocytes. Because hepatic dysfunction does not appear to be dose related, the mechanism is unclear.

Mycophenolate Mofetil

MMF is a newer immunosuppressive agent that functions by inhibition of purine metabolism. It inhibits inosine monophosphate dehydrogenase and blocks the proliferation of lymphocytes. MMF blocks proliferation late in the cell cycle. It has almost completely replaced azathioprine as part of traditional triple-therapy immunosuppression. The U.S. Renal Transplant Mycophenolate Mofetil study demonstrated that in primary renal transplant recipients randomized to azathioprine, MMF 2 g/day, or MMF 3 g/day, the incidence of rejection decreased from 38% in the first group to 19.8% in the 2 g/day group and to 17.5% in the 3 g/day group. The 3 g/day group, however, had significant gastrointestinal side effects. Most recipients currently receive 2 g/day. The major clinical side effects of this medication are leukopenia and gastrointestinal upset, particularly diarrhea.[4] An enteric-coated formulation of mycophenolic acid is also now available.

Leflunomide

Approved for use in the United States for the treatment of rheumatoid arthritis, leflunomide has been used experimentally and clinically in solid organ transplantation. The drug reversibly blocks dihydroorotate dehydrogenase, an enzyme necessary for de novo pyrimidine synthesis in lymphocytes. Experimentally, the drug demonstrates synergy with calcineurin inhibitors and inhibits herpesvirus (including ganciclovir-resistant CMV). Major toxicities appear to vary by organ transplant type. Liver transplant recipients have had significant increases in transaminases, whereas renal transplant recipients have suffered gastrointestinal upset and anemia. Because of sizable patient-to-patient variations in rates of metabolism, drug levels need to be monitored. Not enough experience with leflunomide has been gained to determine whether the successes reported experimentally in preventing chronic rejection will translate into the clinical arena.[3] FK-778, an analogue of the active metabolite of leflunomide, is in clinical trials in renal transplant recipients.[28]

T-Cell–Directed Immunosuppressants

Cyclosporine

Borel's discovery in 1972 of the immunosuppressive properties of cyclosporine, a fungal metabolite extracted from *Tolypocladium inflatum* Gams, contributed enormously to the rapid and successful growth of the field of clinical organ transplantation, especially liver and heart transplantation.[29] It represented a completely new class of clinically important immunosuppressive agents. Many of its selective, suppressive effects on T cells appear to be related to its selective inhibition of TCR-mediated activation events (Fig. 27-18). It inhibits cytokine production by T_H cells in vitro and impairs the development of mature CD4+ and CD8+ T cells in the thymus. Cyclosporine is a cyclic peptide (11 amino acids; molecular weight, 1202 d).

Cyclosporine was discovered to be immunosuppressive by its ability to suppress antibody production in mice. Other in vivo properties include inhibition of antibody plaque-forming cell production, GVH disease, skin graft rejection, delayed solid organ allograft rejection, and delayed-type hypersensitivity reactions. Absence of myelosuppression was a major advance over other immunosuppressive agents and indicated that the mechanism of action was relatively specific for lymphocytes.[29] Other inflammatory cells are much less sensitive to its inhibitory effects. Clinically, prophylactic administration of cyclosporine suppresses allograft rejection and GVH disease.

Analysis of the effect of cyclosporine on T lymphocytes has shown the following:

1. Inhibition of both IL-2–producing T lymphocytes and CTLs
2. Inhibition of IL-2 gene expression by activated T lymphocytes
3. No inhibition of activated T lymphocytes in response to exogenous IL-2
4. Inhibition of resting T-lymphocyte activation in response to alloantigen and exogenous lymphokine
5. Inhibition of IL-1 production
6. Inhibition of mitogen (concanavalin A) activation of IL-2–producing T lymphocytes

These T-lymphocyte responses involve both CD4+ (T_H) and CD8+ (T cytotoxic/suppressor) lymphocytes, and the inhibition appears to occur at the level of activation, and perhaps even maturation, of the resting cell. In mice, maturation of T cells in the thymus is significantly suppressed by cyclosporine, thus enriching a population of immature and less responsive T cells.

Cyclosporine induces potent immunosuppression without myelosuppression. The addition of steroids to cyclosporine permitted lowering of the cyclosporine dosage and decreased nephrotoxicity (the principal clinical side effect of the drug). The introduction of cyclosporine into clinical use in 1983 led to substantial improvement in the outcome of cadaveric renal transplantation and permitted the widespread practice of heart and liver grafting.

Cyclosporine is metabolized in the liver by cytochrome P-450 enzymes. Medications that increase or decrease cytochrome P-450 function can dramatically increase or decrease cyclosporine or tacrolimus levels. The narrow therapeutic windows of these immunosuppressants require care in prescribing practices. Antibiotics, seizure medications, and some calcium channel blockers are major culprits, but interactions need to be verified before prescribing any new medication to a transplant recipient.

The potential adverse effects of cyclosporine include nephrotoxicity, hypertension, hyperkalemia, hirsutism, gingival hyperplasia, tremor and other neurotoxicities,

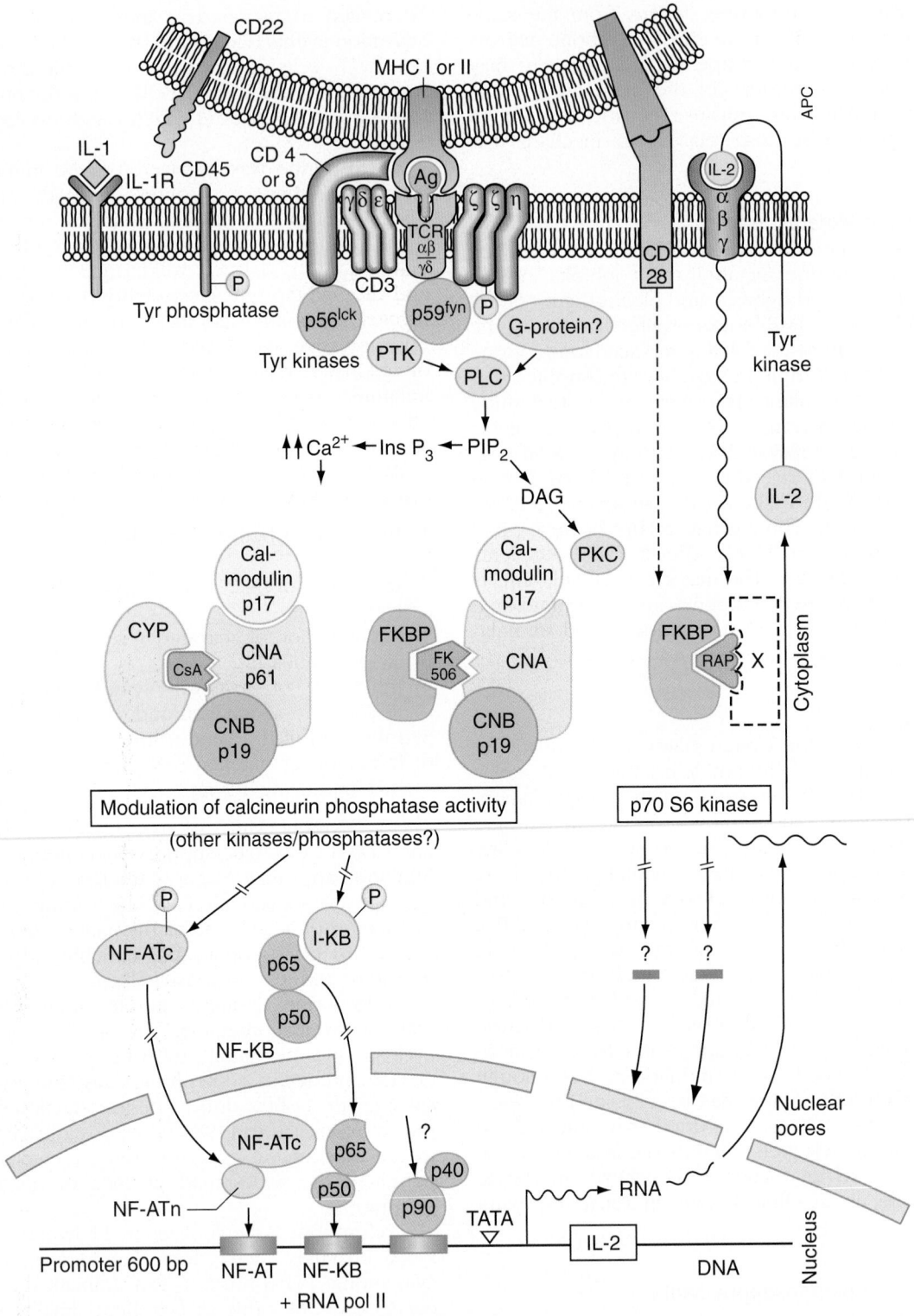

Figure 27-18 Signal transduction in activated T cells and the sites (*center* of figure) at which cyclosporine (CsA), tacrolimus (FK-506), and sirolimus (rapamycin [RAP]) are believed to act. CsA or FK-506 bound to their respective immunophilins (cyclophilin [CYP]) or to FK-506–binding protein (FKBP) forms pentameric complexes with calmodulin and calcineurin A (CNA) and B. Inhibition of the phosphatase activity of calcineurin is believed to inhibit translocation to the nucleus of the cytoplasmic component of the nuclear factor of activated T cells (NF-ATc), which is required for activation of the interleukin-2 (IL-2) gene. RAP, which also binds to FKBP, inhibits phosphorylation and activation of a 70-kd, ribosomal S6 protein kinase (p70S6), which normally occurs within minutes of cell activation by cytokine receptors. RAP also targets other kinases (not shown) that are essential for cell cycle progression. *"X"* refers to target of rapamycin. (From Schreier M, Quesniaux VFJ, Baumann G, et al: Moleculear basis of immunosuppression. Transplant Sci 3:185, 1993.)

diabetogenicity, and hepatotoxicity. As with other immunosuppressive agents, cyclosporine therapy increases the risk for infection and malignancy, but by reducing steroid requirements, an overall general decrease in infection rates is seen in comparison to historic immunotherapy.

Tacrolimus

Tacrolimus (formerly known as FK-506) is a potent immunosuppressive agent that was isolated in 1984 in Japan from the soil fungus *Streptomyces tsukubaensis*. It is a macrocyclic lactone with a molecular weight of 822 d. Though structurally distinct from cyclosporine, it exhibits a very similar molecular action. Both drugs are regarded as *prodrugs*. Their antilymphocytic effects result from the formation of active complexes between the drug and its respective intracellular binding protein *immunophilin* (cyclophilin or FK-506–binding protein [FKBP]) (see Fig. 27-18).[29] The drug-immunophilin complex blocks the phosphatase activity of calcineurin, which is important in regulation of IL-2 gene transcription. The activity of tacrolimus in vitro, however, is approximately 100 times greater than that of cyclosporine.

Like cyclosporine, tacrolimus functions to inhibit the following:

1. IL-2 gene expression and IL-2 production
2. Mixed lymphocyte culture cellular proliferation, which is mediated by T_H cells
3. The generation of CTLs
4. The appearance of IL-2R on human lymphocytes

In vivo, tacrolimus prolongs the survival of MHC-disparate skin, as well as cardiac, renal, hepatic, and small bowel allografts. Tacrolimus has been approved for the treatment of liver allograft rejection. It also has efficacy in rescue therapy for recurrent acute allograft rejection in renal allograft recipients. The side effects of cyclosporine and tacrolimus are similar, but tacrolimus does not cause hirsutism or gum hypertrophy. It does, however, cause alopecia and is associated with an increased incidence of post-transplant diabetes when compared with cyclosporine, particularly at higher doses. Drug levels must be monitored.

Sirolimus

Similar to tacrolimus, the immunosuppressant sirolimus (also known as rapamycin) is a macrolide antibiotic. It is a close structural analogue of tacrolimus and binds to the same cytoplasmic receptor (FKBP). Unlike tacrolimus or cyclosporine, however, sirolimus does not block T-cell cytokine gene expression but instead inhibits transduction of signals from IL-2R to the nucleus.[29] Binding of sirolimus to FKBP inhibits p70S6 protein kinase activity, which is essential for ribosomal phosphorylation and cell cycle progression (see Fig. 27-18). Sirolimus potently inhibits allograft rejection. This drug acts synergistically with cyclosporine both by increasing its efficacy in preventing rejection and by increasing the nephrotoxicity of the calcineurin inhibitor. Sirolimus has been combined with cyclosporine, tacrolimus, or MMF in attempts to decrease or avoid calcineurin inhibitors with their

associated nephrotoxicity. Trials are ongoing to assess its impact on chronic allograft dysfunction in renal allograft recipients. Sirolimus is also being used as a coating in cardiac stents to prevent restenosis. Clinical trials have demonstrated that sirolimus is not significantly nephrotoxic; however, it has been demonstrated to increase triglycerides and decrease platelets and hemoglobin in some recipients. An increased incidence of lymphoceles and delays in wound healing have also been reported with the use of sirolimus.[30] More recently, studies have reported an increase in proteinuria in recipients administered sirolimus. Current recommendations are to avoid sirolimus in recipients with proteinuria greater than 2 g/day.[31]

Co-stimulation Blockade

An interesting new paradigm is developing in the area of maintenance immunosuppression; studies using parenteral immunosuppression for maintenance therapy are now under way. Orally bioavailable compounds are the mainstay of long-term immunosuppression, but new studies have focused on injectable forms that could be administered every month or two. Compliance with multidrug regimens has always been problematic, with late rejection episodes often being associated with noncompliance with immunosuppression. Parenteral administration at the transplant center would allow physicians to be assured that medications had been received.

Belatacept is a selective co-stimulation blockade agent currently in phase III clinical trials. It is a fusion protein of the extracellular portion of CTLA-4 and the constant region fragment of human IgG1.[32] It has demonstrated efficacy equivalent to that of cyclosporine in renal transplant recipients receiving MMF and steroids when administered monthly or bimonthly. Also under more preliminary study is the use of monoclonal antibodies against IL-2R as maintenance therapy.

Local Immunosuppression

One approach to reducing the drug-specific and general adverse consequences of systemic immunosuppression is the use of local drug administration systems to establish a more selective presence of immunosuppressive agents in the transplanted organ. Experimental drug-targeting approaches include intra-arterial drug infusion, implantable infusion pumps, controlled-release matrices, drug-impregnated polymer rods, liposomes, topical application (skin or cornea), and aerosol inhalation (lung). Details on this topic are reviewed elsewhere.[33] Currently, this approach is used only in composite tissue allotransplant recipients in whom topical immunosuppression is added to systemic immunosuppression to boost levels to the skin.[33,34]

Sensitized Recipients

Previous transfusion, pregnancy, ventricular assist devices, and prior transplantation can sensitize individuals.[25,26] Transplant outcomes are significantly inferior in sensitized recipients.[35] Left ventricular assist devices can also result in high PRA titers in potential heart recipients.

These preformed antibodies can result in hyperacute rejection of transplanted organs. In the case of sensitized potential kidney recipients, such people may languish on the lists for years while waiting for a match.

New protocols using various combinations of plasmapheresis, IVIG, splenectomy, and anti-CD20 monoclonal antibodies, combined with conventional immunosuppression, have been developed to allow successful transplantation in these otherwise untransplantable individuals. These protocols have been successful, particularly for recipients with living donors, in allowing pretreatment before a scheduled transplant. Antibody levels can be measured and transplantation undertaken when antibody levels decrease appropriately. A few potential recipients will not decrease their antibody levels, however, and will remain untransplantable.[26]

Individualized Immunosuppressive Regimens

In the past, immunosuppression was a "one-size-fits-all" approach. Most allograft recipients received an induction agent consisting of either ALG or OKT3, followed by cyclosporine, azathioprine, and prednisone as triple-drug maintenance therapy. The new agents now available have allowed many more options and thus some tailoring of immunosuppression to the recipient's situation.

Although tolerance, or a drug-free state, remains the long-term goal in transplantation, the addition of new agents to the pharmacologic armamentarium has reduced the incidence of acute allograft rejection while decreasing the side effects in individual recipients. Decreasing side effects increases the likelihood that a recipient will actually continue the immunosuppressive medications. Noncompliance with medications remains a significant issue in long-term graft survival. A young woman with severe hirsutism may think twice about continuing her cyclosporine therapy; switching treatment to tacrolimus may be a more appropriate option in such cases. A recipient with inadequate financial resources may more appropriately continue taking prednisone and azathioprine than the more costly MMF.

Recipients who prove to be difficult compliance problems may benefit from the experimental injectable drug regimens. In this way transplant centers will definitely know whether a recipient received the drug. We are beginning to reach an era in transplantation in which we can "custom fit" immunosuppression to the recipient based on donor and recipient factors, as well as the organ transplanted. Greater emphasis is also being placed on avoidance of corticosteroids in all organs.[21] From experimental "tolerizing" protocols using alemtuzumab or rabbit antithymocyte globulin, followed by low-dose monotherapy with tacrolimus, cyclosporine, or sirolimus, to more traditional triple-therapy regimens with or without induction agents, to steroid avoidance—no standard protocols exist today.

Treatment of Acute Rejection

Although there is debate about the most appropriate agents and the duration of therapy in the treatment of acute rejection, there is little debate over the importance of a prompt and accurate diagnosis, which usually requires biopsy. Most often, therapy is tailored to the degree of rejection. Mild rejections are usually treated with high-dose methylprednisolone with or without a subsequent oral prednisone taper. Mild liver allograft rejection is often treated with increased tacrolimus doses. Moderate to severe rejection is treated with either rabbit antithymocyte globulin or the monoclonal antibody OKT3; failing that, alemtuzumab, rituximab, and IVIG have all been used with some success.[7,22,26] CMV prophylaxis with ganciclovir or valganciclovir is generally administered concurrently with therapy for acute rejection. Repeated treatments of acute rejection increase the risk for both infection and malignant complications, particularly PTLD.

Antirejection therapy is achieved at a high cost to the recipient, both financially and physically. Complete treatment of rejection is critically important, however, because inadequately treated acute rejection is a leading cause of chronic rejection and subsequent graft loss.[16] Chronic rejection remains the primary cause of late graft loss.[36] Even with perfect patient compliance there is a fixed rate of graft loss for all transplanted organs. For example, whereas some graft loss is due to technical problems or patient death, only 72% of hearts transplanted function at 5 years, 67% of kidneys, and 67% of livers (OPTN/SRTR 2005 Annual Report, available at http://www.ustransplant.org.) It has become clear that the immunosuppressive agents that are so effective at controlling acute rejection are not as effective at controlling chronic rejection.

XENOTRANSPLANTATION

There is a critical shortage of organs available for transplantation. More than 90,000 potential recipients are currently listed and awaiting organ transplantation. Many more patients could benefit from transplantation but, given the current shortage of organs, are not even considered for transplantation. Many experts in the field have concluded that the supply of human donors will never meet the demand. Currently, about 6000 deceased donors are recovered each year (United Network for Organ Sharing [UNOS] data). This number has increased somewhat over the years as older donors have been included, but organ donation in the United States has reached a plateau. This shortage forces continued interest in xenotransplantation, although it remains hotly debated.

A possibility for expansion of the donor pool includes the use of nonhuman sources as donors. However, the mechanisms of xenoreactivity differ from those of alloreactivity, and the resulting rejection is vigorous. The principal barrier to the widespread use of xenotransplantation is the presence of natural antibodies. Similar to ABO blood groupings, natural IgM antibodies develop against nonself carbohydrate moieties. These naturally occurring antibodies are reduced in number as the species are more closely related, such as with humans and chimpanzees. Naturally occurring antibodies mediate the hyperacute rejection typically found with transplantation across species. The majority of naturally occurring antibodies are directed against the carbohydrate moiety α-galactose.[5,37] The preferred xenogeneic species for human clinical transplantation is the pig because of size and availability.

Xenogeneic hyperacute rejection has many features similar to the allogenic hyperacute rejection seen immediately after the transplantation of ABO-incompatible organs. This reaction is dependent on complement with the generation of procoagulants and platelet-aggregating substances. Unlike the situation with allogeneic organ transplantation, in xenotransplantation the ability to limit or control the complement cascade is lost. In humans, a decay factor (CD55) is present that limits the complement-induced injury. In pig cells, CD55 is not expressed. Strategies are emerging in which soluble factors such as human CD55 and complement receptors are administered to limit the extent of the hyperacute rejection.[1] Transgenic pigs that express human CD55 have been developed. Additionally, pigs have been cloned that do not produce the galactosyltransferase enzyme.[37]

On inhibition of the soluble agents to eliminate the complement-mediated hyperacute rejection, the next problem is with delayed xenograft rejection. Research models that inhibit the complement system have made delayed xenograft rejection available for study. This form of rejection involves both NK cells and macrophages as mediators of the inflammatory process. NK cell activities are initiated, and because of lack of the self-MHC molecules that normally provide inhibitory signals for NK cells, NK function remains unopposed. These activated NK cells secrete cytokines, such as TNF and IFN-γ, that both recruit and activate macrophages.[1,5,14]

TOLERANCE

Historical Background

The cherished goal of the transplant scientist and clinician is to induce donor-specific tolerance and eliminate the need for exogenous immunosuppression.[38] Although tolerance has been achieved in numerous species, including humans, widespread clinical application depends on improving the safety and reducing the risk of such an approach. Nevertheless, there are rare instances of establishment of drug-free unresponsiveness to organ allografts in humans who have discontinued immunosuppressive therapy for various reasons. Moreover, some humans have been rendered drug free for acceptance of kidney allografts after a bone marrow transplant from the same donor for leukemia.[39] Contemporary developments in our understanding of cellular and molecular immunology and the basis of experimental tolerance induction hold promise for the development of clinically effective approaches. Authentic transplantation tolerance is antigen specific. It is induced as the result of previous exposure to antigen and does not depend on the continuous administration of exogenous antigen-nonspecific immunosuppressive agents.

In 1953 in a seminal study, Billingham, Brent, and Medawar[40] were among the first to demonstrate actively acquired donor-specific tolerance. They performed historic experiments in which they exchanged reciprocal skin grafts between freemartin cattle twins. Freemartin cattle are genetically different cattle twins that share a common placenta. Billingham, Brent, and Medawar predicted that the cattle would reject these grafts because they were genetically different. However, the grafts were accepted. This result was explained by Owen's observation that freemartin cattle share a common placenta; they are actually red blood cell chimeras.[41] With this observation, the researchers returned to the laboratory and demonstrated that when they transplanted bone marrow–derived cells from a donor into a fetal mouse, they could actively transfer acquired tolerance to the recipient. If a skin graft from the same bone marrow donor was transplanted, the graft was permanently accepted. The tolerance was donor specific because when a third-party skin graft was transplanted, the graft was rejected.[40] An important lesson learned from this experiment was that the acquired tolerance was due to the immunologic incompetence of the graft recipient and not to any alteration in the grafted tissue itself. Similar mixed chimerism plus tolerance was established in adult mice with the addition of conditioning.[42]

Mechanisms

Reliable, nontoxic methods of inducing transplantation tolerance are needed to overcome the problems of chronic organ graft rejection and immunosuppression-related toxicity. Potential approaches for induction of tolerance in *adults* include the following:

1. Cell depletion protocols using total body irradiation, total lymphoid irradiation, or depleting monoclonal antibodies
2. Reconstitution protocols using allogeneic bone marrow
3. A combination of approaches 1 and 2
4. Cell surface molecule–targeted therapy (e.g., use of anti-CD4 or anti–intercellular adhesion molecule monoclonal antibodies)
5. Immunosuppressive drugs (e.g., cyclosporine, sirolimus)
6. Donor-specific blood transfusion combined with drug or monoclonal antibody therapy
7. Manipulation of specific cell populations (i.e., tolerogenic dendritic cells and regulatory T cells)

The principal hypotheses proposed for the cellular basis of transplantation tolerance are *clonal deletion* (cell death of donor-reactive T cells) and *clonal anergy* (functional inactivation without cell death). Clonal deletion of antigen-reactive lymphocytes occurs either in the thymus or peripherally. Clonal anergy of lymphocytes is caused by delivery of the antigenic signal alone (signal 1) without co-stimulatory signals (signal 2) or by suppressor mechanisms. Suppressor mechanisms involve regulatory cells directed against the TCR idiotype of the responsive T lymphocytes, *veto* cells, or suppressor cytokines such as tumor growth factor-β. It has yet to be definitely established whether clonal deletion and clonal anergy are stages along a continuum in the T-cell interactions or whether these are two independent pathways produced by exposure to different tolerogens under different conditions. An individual's immune system may develop unresponsiveness to a particular antigen despite the presence of normally responsive lymphocytes. The normally responsive cells may be inhibited by other mechanisms such as suppressor cells. Thus, any combination of deletion or inactivation of T cells and B cells could result in failure of the immune system to respond to an antigen.

Monoclonal Antibodies

One of the major goals in therapeutic immunosuppression has been to achieve a long-term benefit from a short-term therapy. A variety of monoclonal antibodies to cell surface molecules, in particular, anti-CD4 used alone or in combination with other immunosuppressive modalities such as cyclosporine or total lymphoid irradiation, induce tolerance in rodents.[2] The development of CD4 monoclonal antibodies that can induce immunologic tolerance without depleting CD4[+] T cells has reawakened interest in the use of nondepleting monoclonal antibodies for reprogramming the immune system in autoimmunity and transplantation. The mechanisms involved in induction of tolerance and its maintenance are under debate.

In a number of allogeneic transplant models (heart, skin, bone marrow), anti-CD4 (+CD8) antibodies block the rejection process by selectively promoting the development of CD4[+]/CD25[+] regulatory T cells. As a result, linked suppression or infectious tolerance occurs via these potent regulatory cells. This promotion of CD4[+] T cells provides a link between suppression and tolerance. In these models, T cells that have never been exposed to CD4 antibodies become tolerant to grafted antigens when exposed to antigen in the microenvironment of regulatory T cells.[2] In addition to anti-CD4 monoclonal antibodies, antibodies targeting adhesion molecules, other molecules on T cells, or other molecules on APCs have emerged as important approaches to promoting induction of tolerance. Therapy with combinations of anti-CD154, anti-CD80, and anti-CD86 monoclonal antibodies, all of which are co-stimulatory molecules, has been used in attempts at inducing tolerance in primates.[43]

Donor Bone Marrow

Donor bone marrow has been shown to have a strong regulatory effect. Induction of unresponsiveness with a combination of antilymphocyte serum and donor bone marrow has been achieved in mice, dogs, and monkeys. It is thought that under these circumstances, a naturally occurring regulatory cell (veto or suppressor cell) induces tolerance within the bone marrow inoculum. The development of these cells may be facilitated by appropriate growth factors such as granulocyte-macrophage colony-stimulating factor and IL-3. Bone marrow infusion has been shown to have a beneficial effect on the long-term survival of solid organ allografts. Ciancio and colleagues

have demonstrated a significant decrease in the incidence of chronic rejection in human deceased donor renal recipients receiving donor bone marrow at the time of renal transplantation.[44] Acute rejection episodes were similar in the group receiving bone marrow infusion and controls. However, in 6 years of follow-up, biopsy-proven chronic rejection developed in only 2 of 63 recipients receiving bone marrow as compared with 41 of 219 control recipients. Immunosuppressive drug therapy was identical in both groups. Similar improved graft outcomes have been observed in long-term lung transplant recipients who received bone marrow infusion and in renal allograft recipients, with less severe chronic rejection in this cohort.

Starzl and colleagues[45] have reported long-lasting donor cell chimerism in conventionally immunosuppressed human organ allograft recipients. Augmentation of this *natural chimerism* by infusion of donor bone marrow at the time of organ transplantation is being performed in patients who do not receive any form of cytoreductive therapy. The procedure has been shown to be safe and effective in augmenting chimerism, but the chimerism is not yet accompanied by donor-specific tolerance.[44]

Suppressor Cells and Induction of Tolerance

Suppressor cells have been implicated in a number of experimental models of tolerance induction.[1] The existence of suppressor T cells generated in the presence of cyclosporine can be demonstrated by the adoptive transfer of tolerance from cyclosporine-treated allograft recipients. It has not been possible, however, to show that cyclosporine can induce authentic tolerance in human organ transplantation. In experimental animals, donor-specific blood transfusion before transplantation induces antigen-specific unresponsiveness associated with dysregulation of IL-2 production and the generation of suppressor cells. Donor-specific blood transfusion with cyclosporine has been shown clinically to reduce sensitization and improve renal allograft outcome.

Hematopoietic Stem Cell Chimerism and Tolerance

The most robust form of donor-specific tolerance is that associated with hematopoietic stem cell chimerism. The first association between chimerism and tolerance was observed in the 1940s when Dr. Owen reported that freemartin cattle were red blood cell chimeras.[41] The common placenta that they shared allowed exchange of hematopoietic stem cells. Though genetically disparate, these cattle accepted skin grafts from the other twin. Billingham, Brent, and Medawar[40] demonstrated that this active transfer of tolerance to donor antigens was due to bone marrow hematopoietic stem cells from the sibling donor. Subsequently, chimerism has been demonstrated to be associated with tolerance in mice, rats, pigs, nonhuman primates, and humans.

Until recently, the risk associated with conventional bone marrow transplantation was too great to accept in clinical attempts to induce tolerance. However, a number of advances have made the clinical application of hematopoietic stem cell chimerism to induce tolerance a clinical reality. Reconstitution of mice with mixtures of T-cell–depleted syngeneic and allogeneic bone marrow (pioneered by Ildstad and Sachs) produces mixed hematopoietic bone marrow chimerism and donor-specific tolerance to skin grafts. Most importantly, 1% donor chimerism is sufficient to provide robust deletional tolerance, thereby opening the door to nonmyeloablative partial conditioning strategies to establish mixed chimerism. These nonmyeloablative approaches using anti–T-cell monoclonal antibodies, cyclophosphamide, ALG, and tacrolimus, in addition to sublethal total body irradiation plus donor bone marrow, have been shown to induce tolerance in mice. Recent improvements in bone marrow processing and graft engineering to decrease the toxicity associated with GVH disease may increase interest in this approach.

Mixed lymphopoietic chimerism has induced tolerance in humans treated by nonmyeloablative bone marrow transplantation for myeloma who also received a renal allograft. Both were myeloma and rejection free after receiving a nonmyeloablative conditioning regimen of cyclophosphamide, horse antithymocyte globulin, thymic irradiation with donor bone marrow infusion, kidney transplantation, and a 12-day course of cyclosporine. Chimerism was maintained for approximately 100 days before it became undetectable. Lack of durability of the chimerism did not have an impact on the result; both recipients remain free of rejection without immunosuppressive drugs.[39] Protocols are active in the clinic to intentionally establish low levels of donor chimerism in kidney and cardiac allograft recipients.

Manipulation of Dendritic Cells

Recent work has focused on specific cell populations that may be used for induction of tolerance. Evidence is mounting that specific immune cells may play a role in the development of donor-specific tolerance. In a recent review, Coates and Thomson emphasized the potential role of dendritic cells as mediators of allorecognition and as a potential target to induce donor-specific tolerance.[46] Dendritic cells are an excellent population to use for cell-based antirejection therapy in transplantation because they specifically target to the T-cell–rich regions of draining lymph nodes. Immature dendritic cells, the best known of which are precursor plasmacytoid dendritic cells, can be driven to produce immunoregulatory properties by presentation of donor antigen in the absence of a second signal, thereby inducing anergy in donor-specific recipient T cells.[46] In the clinic, mobilization of hematopoietic stem cells with granulocyte colony-stimulating factor also mobilizes higher concentrations of precursor tolerogenic (plasmacytoid) dendritic cells. Studies to analyze the effect of these populations on induction of tolerance in the clinic are in progress.[46]

Additionally, another new and potentially important immune-modulating strategy is conversion of the anti-donor response from a T_H1 to a T_H2 response. The vast majority of aggressive rejection immune responses are associated with a T_H1 phenotype, whereas animals with demonstrated allograft acceptance generally have T cells with a predominantly T_H2 phenotype. It is thought that dendritic cells may promote immune deviation from a T_H1 rejection profile by selective activation of T_H2 T cells.

NEW AREAS OF TRANSPLANTATION

Composite Tissue Allotransplantation

Composite tissue transplantation could benefit millions worldwide with lost limbs and extensive tissue defects. Since the first hand transplant was performed in Lyon, France, in September 1998, a total of 24 hand transplants have been performed within 8 years; 12 patients received single hand transplants and 4 received double hand transplants. All have had good functional recovery, but the first recipient required amputation after he elected to stop immunosuppression. The longest surviving hand recipient received his transplant in Louisville, Kentucky, in January 1999. His current abilities include tying his shoes, dialing his cell phone, turning doorknobs, throwing a ball, and sensitivity to hot and cold.[33]

Hand transplantation combines two well-established procedures—hand reimplantation and immunosuppressive therapy (Figs. 27-19 and 27-20). These transplant recipients have been maintained on standard immunosuppressive regimens of tacrolimus, MMF, and prednisone. Tacrolimus speeds nerve regeneration in animal models, which also seems to be the case in the hand transplant recipients, in whom nerve regeneration has proceeded more rapidly than would be expected from replant experience.[33] Despite the transplantation of vascularized bone marrow with the hand transplant, no evidence of donor chimerism or GVH disease has been observed in the recipients.[47] The success with hand transplantation has spurred research into other composite tissue allografts. Larynx transplantation successfully restored the voice of a 40-year-old man 20 years after a laryngeal crush injury.[48] Currently, vascularized knee, maxillofacial, and abdominal wall transplants are being performed throughout the world.

In 2005, plastic and transplant surgeons in France successfully transplanted a partial face to repair an extensive defect left by a dog mauling. The allograft provided excellent tissue coverage of the defect, as shown in Figure 27-21. The transplant represents an important change in philosophy; it is the first time that surgeons purposely chose to repair a facial injury with an allograft. No primary repair was attempted at the time of the injury to ensure maximal success with the subsequent transplant. The patient wore a surgical mask to cover the defect until a donor became available months later (personal communication with Professor Jean-Michel Dubernard). If success is seen with tolerance protocols, further use of composite tissue allotransplants in areas of reconstructive surgery can be expected.

Islet Cell Transplantation

Nowhere in the field of transplantation are the advances in immunosuppression clearer than in the area of islet cell transplantation. Attempts at islet transplantation uni-

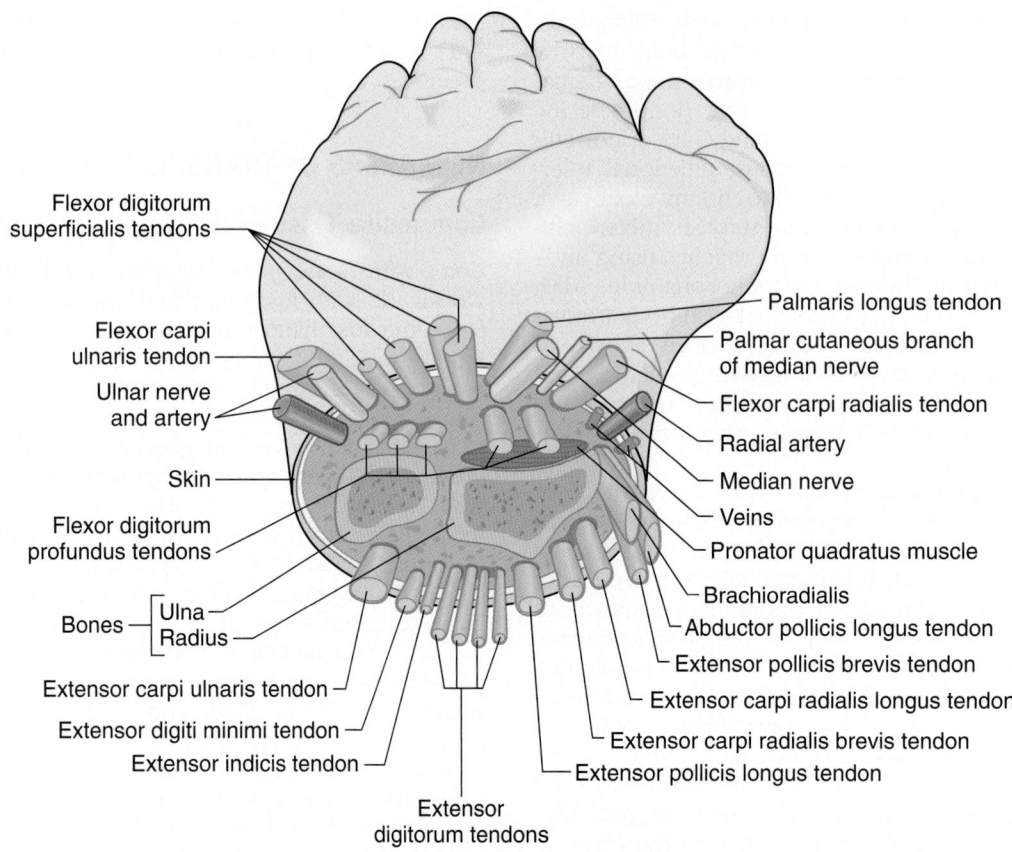

Flexor digitorum
superficialis tendons

Flexor carpi
ulnaris tendon

Ulnar nerve
and artery

Skin

Flexor digitorum
profundus tendons

Bones ⎡ Ulna
        ⎣ Radius

Extensor carpi ulnaris tendon

Extensor digiti minimi tendon

Extensor indicis tendon

Extensor
digitorum tendons

Palmaris longus tendon

Palmar cutaneous branch
of median nerve

Flexor carpi radialis tendon

Radial artery

Median nerve

Veins

Pronator quadratus muscle

Brachioradialis

Abductor pollicis longus tendon

Extensor pollicis brevis tendon

Extensor carpi radialis longus tendon

Extensor carpi radialis brevis tendon

Extensor pollicis longus tendon

Figure 27-19 Schematic of a hand transplant drawn by Elaine Bammerlin.

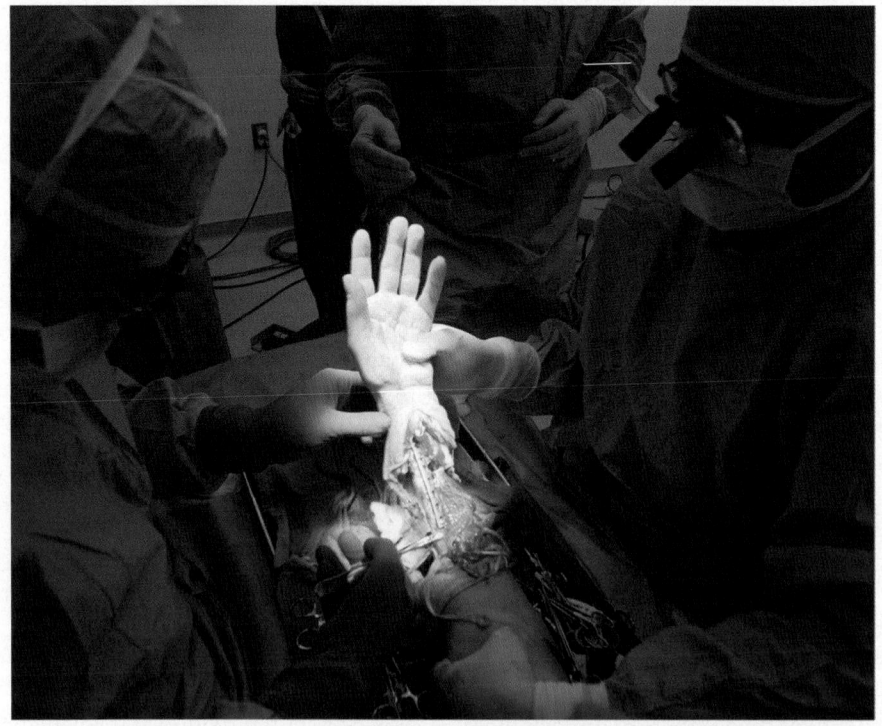

Figure 27-20 Dr. Warren Breidenbach and colleagues begin to attach the hand transplant. (Photo by Patrick Pfister, Jewish Hospital, Louisville, KY.)

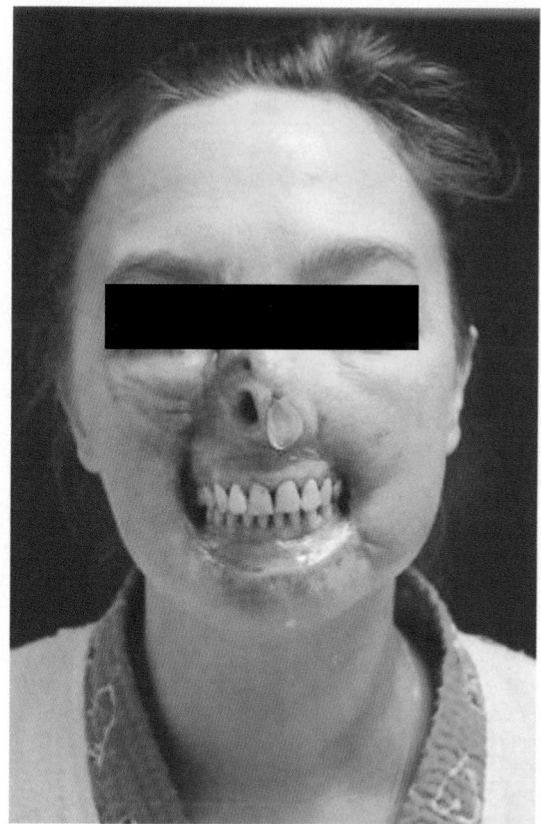

A

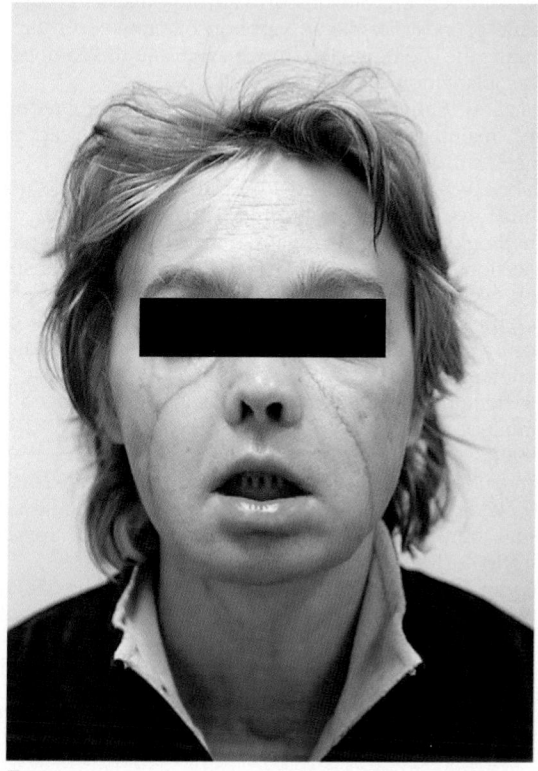

B

Figure 27-21 Pretransplant and post-transplant views of the world's first partial face transplant. (Courtesy of Professor Jean Michel Dubernard.)

formly failed until development of the so-called Edmonton protocol. A group in Edmonton, Alberta, reported their success in rendering recipients free of the necessity of taking insulin by using an immunosuppressive protocol of daclizumab, low-dose tacrolimus, and sirolimus. Steroids and high doses of tacrolimus were avoided because both are known to be toxic to islets.[49]

Initially, islets from between two and four pancreata were needed to achieve insulin independence in these recipients. Approximately 9000 islet equivalents per kilogram of recipient body weight have been necessary to attain insulin independence.[49] Success with the Edmonton protocol has focused interest in steroid avoidance regimens in other organ transplants.[21]

Tissue Engineering and Regenerative Medicine

The ultimate goal of transplantation resides in the ability to restore living cells to maintain or even enhance existing tissue function. This goal is emerging through the process of tissue engineering. Initial discoveries in engineered tissues were made in the mid-1980s with skin-based products. By developing replacement tissues with bioactive properties that remain intact after implantation and retain physiologic functions, as well as provide structure to the tissue or organ damaged by disease or trauma, tissue engineering could provide an alternative. Skin replacement products are the most advanced, with several tissue-engineered wound care materials currently on the market worldwide. The potential impact of this field is endless, and it offers unique solutions to the medical field for tissue and organ replacement. Tissue engineering may eventually be applied to the regeneration of diverse tissues such as the liver, small intestine, cardiovascular structures, nerve, and cartilage. Work on bioartificial liver devices has been under way for several years. Bladder tissue has been successfully grown from an initial bladder biopsy specimen and implanted.[50]

The sources of cells required for tissue engineering are summarized by three categories: autologous cells (from the patient), allogeneic cells (from a donor, but not immunologically identical), and xenogeneic cells (donor from a different species). Each category may be further delineated in terms of stem cells (adult or embryonic) or differentiated cells obtained from tissue in which the cell population obtained from tissue dissociation consists of a mixture of cells at different maturation stages and includes rare stem and progenitor cells. Recent discoveries have indicated that stem cells can repair damaged tissue (e.g., hematopoietic stem cells home to infarcted myocardium and repair the tissue). Tissue engineering will remain an area of intense research. Advances in the areas of growth factors, stromal matrices, gene encapsulation, and gene delivery will all play a role.

CONCLUSION

The field of transplantation is an excellent example of the impact that research, both basic and clinical observation, can have on progress in a field. The concept of replacing damaged with functioning tissue has become a reality, and through research we will continue to improve the quality of life of transplant recipients and the afflictions that can be treated. Progress continues in the areas of immunosuppressive therapy, xenotransplantation, induction of transplant tolerance, tissue engineering, and our overall understanding of how the immune system functions on a cellular and subcellular level. Much remains to be learned, however, before patients with end-organ failure can live free of the risks and expenses now associated with solid organ transplantation. Still, it is an exciting time to be involved in transplantation—the so-called Holy Grail of transplantation, namely, transplantation tolerance, does appear to be much closer but still remains out of our grasp.[38]

Acknowledgment

The authors wish to acknowledge the technical assistance of Carolyn DeLautre in preparation of the manuscript.

Selected References

Abbas AK, Lichtman AH, Pober JS: Cellular and Molecular Immunology, 5th ed. Philadelphia, WB Saunders, 2005.

Concise, well-illustrated textbook of immunology.

Kaufman DB, Leventhal JR, Gallon LG, Parker MA: Alemtuzumab induction and prednisone-free maintenance immunotherapy in simultaneous pancreas-kidney transplantation comparison with rabbit antithymocyte globulin induction—long-term results. Am J Transplant 6:331-339, 2006.

Large single-center experience with steroid-sparing immunosuppression.

Newell KA, Larsen CP, Kirk AD: Transplant tolerance: Converging on a moving target. Transplantation 81:1-6, 2006.

Excellent review of issues preventing the development of tolerance in humans, including the issues of testing for tolerance.

Wood KJ, Sakaguchi S: Regulatory T cells in transplantation tolerance. Nat Rev Immunol 3:199-210, 2003.

Review of regulatory T cells and their mechanism of action.

References

1. Abbas AK, Lichtman AH, Pober JS: Cellular and Molecular Immunology, 5th ed. Philadelphia, WB Saunders, 2005.
2. Waldmann H, Cobbold S: How do monoclonal antibodies induce tolerance? A role for infectious tolerance? Annu Rev Immunol 16:619-644, 1998.
3. Kappler JW, Roehm N, Marrack P: T cell tolerance by clonal elimination in the thymus. Cell 49:273-280, 1987.
4. Sollinger HW: Mycophenolate mofetil for the prevention of acute rejection in primary cadaveric renal allograft recipients. U.S. Renal Transplant Mycophenolate Mofetil Study Group. Transplantation 60:225-232, 1995.
5. Brouha PC, Ildstad ST: Mixed allogeneic chimerism. Past, present, and prospects for the future. Transplantation 72:S36-S42, 2001.
6. Nagata S, Suda T: Fas and Fas ligand: lpr and gld mutations. Immunol Today 16:39-43, 1995.
7. de Mattos AM, Norman DJ: OKT3 for treatment of rejection in renal transplantation 72:S36-S42, 1993.
8. Greenfield EA, Nguyen KA, Kuchroo VK: CD28/B7 costimulation: A review. Crit Rev Immunol 18:389-418, 1998.
9. Romagnani S: The Th1/Th2 paradigm. Immunol Today 18:263-266, 1997.
10. Wood KJ, Sakaguchi S: Regulatory T cells in transplantation tolerance. Nat Rev Immunol 3:199-210, 2003.
11. Filippi C, Bresson D, von Herrath M: Antigen-specific induction of regulatory T cells for type 1 diabetes therapy. Int Rev Immunol 24:341-360, 2005.
12. van Furth R: Human monocytes and cytokines. Res Immunol 149:719-720, 1998.
13. Rissoan MC, Soumelis V, Kadowaki N, et al: Reciprocal control of T helper cell and dendritic cell differentiation. Science 283:1183-1186, 1999.
14. Manilay JO, Sykes M: Natural killer cells and their role in graft rejection. Curr Opin Immunol 10:532-538, 1998.
15. Rulifson IC, Szot GL, Palmer E, et al: Inability to induce tolerance through direct antigen presentation. Am J Transplant 2:510-519, 2002.
16. Halloran PF, Melk A, Barth C: Rethinking chronic allograft nephropathy: The concept of accelerated senescence. J Am Soc Nephrol 10:167-181, 1999.
17. Fishman JA, Rubin RH: Infection in organ-transplant recipients. N Engl J Med 338:1741-1751, 1998.
18. Sener A, House AA, Jevnikar AM, et al: Intravenous immunoglobulin as a treatment for BK virus associated nephropathy: One-year follow-up of renal allograft recipients. Transplantation 81:117-120, 2006.
19. Penn I: Posttransplant malignancies. Transplant Proc 31:1260-1262, 1999.
20. Verschuuren EA, Stevens SJ, van Imhoff GW, et al: Treatment of posttransplant lymphoproliferative disease with rituximab: The remission, the relapse, and the complication. Transplantation 73:100-104, 2002.
21. Matas AJ, Kandaswamy R, Gillingham KJ, et al: Prednisone-free maintenance immunosuppression—a 5-year experience. Am J Transplant 5:2473-2478, 2005.
22. Gaber AO, First MR, Tesi RJ, et al: Results of the double-blind, randomized, multicenter, phase III clinical trial of Thymoglobulin versus Atgam in the treatment of acute graft rejection episodes after renal transplantation. Transplantation 66:29-37, 1998.
23. Kahan BD, Rajagopalan PR, Hall M: Reduction of the occurrence of acute cellular rejection among renal allograft recipients treated with basiliximab, a chimeric anti–interleukin-2-receptor monoclonal antibody. United States Simulect Renal Study Group. Transplantation 67:276-284, 1999.
24. Vincenti F, Kirkman R, Light S, et al: Interleukin-2-receptor blockade with daclizumab to prevent acute rejection in renal transplantation. Daclizumab Triple Therapy Study Group. N Engl J Med 338:161-165, 1998.
25. Bloom DD, Hu H, Fechner JH, et al: T-lymphocyte allo-responses of Campath-1H–treated kidney transplant patients. Transplantation 81:81-87, 2006.
26. Jordan SC, Vo AA, Peng A, et al: Intravenous gammaglobulin (IVIG): A novel approach to improve transplant rates and outcomes in highly HLA-sensitized patients. Am J Transplant 6:459-466, 2006.
27. Gruber SA, Chan GLC, Canafax DM, et al: Immunosuppression in renal transplantation: II. Corticosteroids, antilymphocyte globulin, and OKT3. Clin Transplant 5:219-232, 1991.
28. Vanrenterghem Y, van Hooff JP, Klinger M, et al: The effects of FK778 in combination with tacrolimus and steroids: A

phase II multicenter study in renal transplant patients. Transplantation 78:9-14, 2004.

29. Sigal NH, Dumont FJ: Cyclosporin A, FK-506, and rapamycin: Pharmacologic probes of lymphocyte signal transduction. Annu Rev Immunol 10:519-560, 1992.

30. Langer RM, Kahan BD: Incidence, therapy, and consequences of lymphocele after sirolimus-cyclosporine-prednisone immunosuppression in renal transplant recipients. Transplantation 74:804-808, 2002.

31. Straathof-Galema L, Wetzels JF, Dijkman HB, et al: Sirolimus-associated heavy proteinuria in a renal transplant recipient: Evidence for a tubular mechanism. Am J Transplant 6:429-433, 2006.

32. Vincenti F, Larsen C, Durrbach A, et al: Costimulation blockade with belatacept in renal transplantation. N Engl J Med 353:770-781, 2005.

33. Jones JW, Gruber SA, Barker JH, et al: Successful hand transplantation. One-year follow-up. Louisville Hand Transplant Team. N Engl J Med 343:468-473, 2000.

34. Schneeberger S, Ninkovic M, Piza-Katzer H, et al: Status 5 years after bilateral hand transplantation. Am J Transplant 6:834-841, 2006.

35. Xu H, Chilton PM, Tanner MK, et al: Humoral immunity is the dominant barrier for allogeneic bone marrow engraftment in sensitized recipients. Blood 108:3611-3619, 2006.

36. Cecka JM, Terasaki PI: Clinical Transplants 2005, UCLA Immunogenetics Centers, Los Angeles, Regents of the University of California, 2006.

37. Dorling A: Clinical xenotransplantation: Pigs might fly? Am J Transplant 2:695-700, 2002.

38. Newell KA, Larsen CP, Kirk AD: Transplant tolerance: Converging on a moving target. Transplantation 81:1-6, 2006.

39. Buhler LH, Spitzer TR, Sykes M, et al: Induction of kidney allograft tolerance after transient lymphohematopoietic chimerism in patients with multiple myeloma and end-stage renal disease. Transplantation 74:1405-1409, 2002.

40. Billingham RE, Brent L, Medawar PB: Actively acquired tolerance of foreign cells. Nature 172:603-606, 1953.

41. Owen RD: Immunogenetic consequences of vascular anastomoses between bovine twins. Science 102:400-401, 1945.

42. Ildstad ST, Sachs DH: Reconstitution with syngeneic plus allogeneic or xenogeneic bone marrow leads to specific acceptance of allografts or xenografts. Nature 307:168-170, 1984.

43. Montgomery SP, Xu H, Tadaki DK, et al: Combination induction therapy with monoclonal antibodies specific for CD80, CD86, and CD154 in nonhuman primate renal transplantation. Transplantation 74:1365-1369, 2002.

44. Ciancio G, Miller J, Garcia-Morales RO, et al: Six-year clinical effect of donor bone marrow infusions in renal transplant patients. Transplantation 71:827-835, 2001.

45. Starzl TE, Demetris AJ, Murase N, et al: Cell migration, chimerism, and graft acceptance. Lancet 339:1579-1582, 1992.

46. Coates PT, Thomson AW: Dendritic cells, tolerance induction and transplant outcome. Am J Transplant 2:299-307, 2002.

47. Granger DK, Briedenbach WC, Pidwell DJ, et al: Lack of donor hyporesponsiveness and donor chimerism after clinical transplantation of the hand. Transplantation 74:1624-1630, 2002.

48. Birchall MA, Lorenz RR, Berke GS, et al: Laryngeal transplantation in 2005: A review. Am J Transplant 6:20-26, 2006.

49. Ryan EA, Lakey JR, Paty BW, et al: Successful islet transplantation: Continued insulin reserve provides long-term glycemic control. Diabetes 51:2148-2157, 2002.

50. Atala A, Bauer SB, Soker S, et al: Tissue-engineered autologous bladders for patients needing cystoplasty. Lancet 367:1241-1246, 2006.

Transplantation of Abdominal Organs

James F. Markmann, MD, PhD   Heidi Yeh, MD   Ali Naji, MD, PhD   Kim M. Olthoff, MD

Abraham Shaked, MD, PhD   and   Clyde F. Barker, MD

Renal Transplantation

Liver Transplantation

Pancreatic Transplantation

Transplantation of Isolated Pancreatic Islets

Intestinal Transplantation

Ethical Considerations

The earliest attempts at human organ transplantation were made in the early 1900s from animal donors. Because the grafts functioned either briefly or not at all, these efforts soon stopped. During the same period, Alexis Carrel successfully transplanted kidneys and other organs in animals and developed techniques of modern vascular surgery that resulted in being awarded a Nobel Prize in 1912. In the early 1950s, Medawar and colleagues described rejection and its prevention in mice (Nobel Prize, 1960), which stimulated surgeons to resume human renal transplantation. In 1954, Murray performed the first successful transplant in Boston by using identical twins as a donor/recipient pair and, later, whole-body irradiation to prevent rejection of allografts in a few instances (Nobel Prize, 1990). Immunosuppressive drugs finally became available in the early 1960s and allowed Starzl and others to achieve more consistent success. Progress in histocompatibility typing, immunosuppressive therapy, and organ preservation and accumulation of clinical experience gradually resulted in further improvement in transplantation that allowed successful replacement of not only failing kidneys but other vital organs as well.

This chapter describes kidney, liver, pancreas, small bowel, and isolated pancreatic islet transplantation. Because the kidney was the first organ to be transplanted extensively, experience acquired in renal transplantation has formed the basis of much of the current management of other organ transplants as well. Therefore, renal trans-

plantation is considered first; contained in this section are discussions on several topics that are also relevant to all other organs: histocompatibility, immunosuppression, management of cadaveric donors, and the possibilities of xenotransplantation.

RENAL TRANSPLANTATION

Indications

Renal transplantation offers better quality of life than dialysis does and is projected to provide a 10-year extension in life. Long-term mortality (3-4 years) is 68% lower in transplant recipients than in those who remain on the waitlist, the largest benefit occurring in patients 20 to 39 years of age, including diabetics.[1] In 1999, mortality was higher in transplant recipients for the first 106 days than in dialysis patients, presumably because of operative complications, but by 10 months after transplantation the mortality rate was lower for transplant recipients. Because 1-year mortality after transplantation has decreased by at least 10% since then, the survival benefit probably continues to increase.

The three most common causes of renal failure treated by kidney transplantation are diabetes mellitus (27%), glomerular diseases (21%), and hypertension (20%), which account for 68% of total transplants. In African Americans, hypertensive nephrosclerosis is the most common cause of renal failure. Other important causes include polycystic kidney disease (7.6%), Alport's syndrome, IgA nephropathy, systemic lupus erythematosus, interstitial nephritis (4.2%), pyelonephritis, and obstructive nephropathy. Even patients whose transplanted kidneys may be damaged by recurrent disease (e.g., lupus erythematosus, cystinosis, amyloidosis, diabetes, and some forms of glomerulonephritis) are often better palliated by transplantation than by dialysis. Unfortunately, the insufficient number of donors keeps many

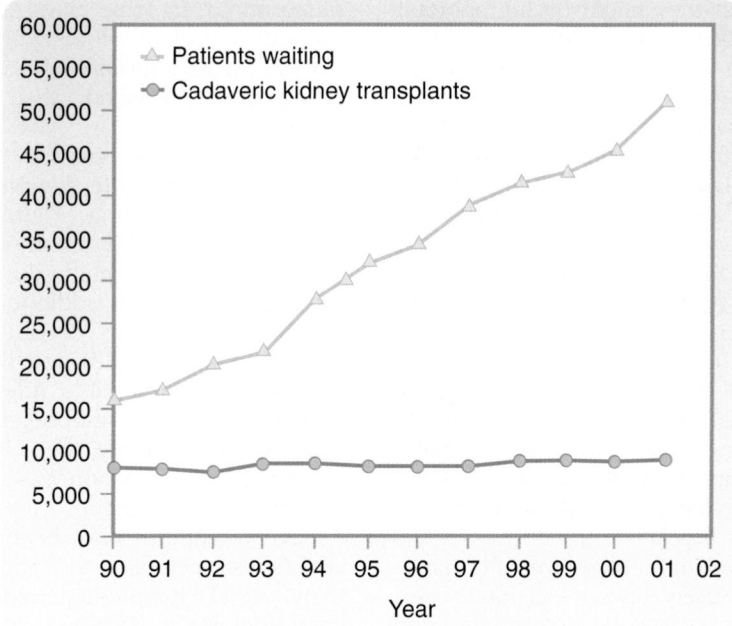

Figure 28-1 Managing the waitlist.

appropriate transplant candidates on chronic dialysis. In 2004 there were 57,910 patients on the waitlist, but only 15,671 kidneys were transplanted.[2] By the end of 2005, there were 65,859 patients on the waitlist (Fig. 28-1). The median time to transplantation for patients registered in 2001 was 39.2 months; in 1995, it was only 30.6 months.[3]

Recipient Evaluation and Preparation

The best recipients are young individuals who do not have a systemic disease that will damage the transplanted kidney or result in death of the recipient from extrarenal causes. In addition to a standard medical workup, evaluation of all transplant candidates includes a cytomegalovirus (CMV) antibody titer; creatinine clearance; serologic tests for syphilis, human immunodeficiency virus (HIV), hepatitis B virus (HBV), and hepatitis C virus (HCV); parathyroid evaluation; coagulation profile; Papanicolaou smear; ABO and HLA typing; urologic evaluation (including a voiding cystourethrogram in select patients to assess obstruction and reflux); gastrointestinal evaluation (including routine colonoscopy); and psychiatric assessment. Infection or malignancy that cannot be eradicated remains an absolute contraindication to transplantation.

After successful treatment of cancer, at least 2 years without evidence of disease is usually required before transplantation. However, cancer sometimes recurs in recipients who were tumor-free for more than 5 years before transplantation. Noncompliance, prevalent in teen-age recipients, is another contraindication because careful adherence to immunosuppression is necessary. Because cardiovascular complications are as common as infection as a cause of post-transplant mortality, the patient's cardiovascular status is carefully evaluated and

optimized. In older patients and diabetics, stress testing, cardiac catheterization, or even pretransplant coronary artery bypass may be required. Unreconstructible aortoiliac disease may make it technically impossible to adequately vascularize a transplanted kidney. Age alone is no longer a criterion for determining candidacy. In fact, the greatest percent increase in waitlist registrations in 2004 (20%) occurred in patients older than 65, and the 50- to 64-year-old age group had the next highest increase (15%).[2]

Patients become eligible to be listed for a cadaveric kidney when their renal function has declined to a glomerular filtration rate (GFR) of less than 20 mL/min. This decline often occurs before institution of dialysis. Preemptive transplantation before dialysis is psychologically preferable and results in superior outcomes, but the proper timing of transplantation is sometimes difficult to determine because renal dysfunction progresses unpredictably. Thus, transplantation performed too early is not only accompanied by the risks associated with surgery and immunosuppression but also starts the clock on the finite half-life of the successfully transplanted kidney. In contrast, advanced uremic symptoms such as pericarditis, cardiac failure, severe anemia, osteodystrophy, and neuropathy can be life threatening and obviously needs to be avoided when possible by early transplantation. Even when a donor is available, pretransplant dialysis may be necessary to optimize the patient's general condition (nutrition, electrolyte balance, and coagulation status).

Blood Group Typing and Histocompatibility and Crossmatching

Because the major blood group antigens are not expressed by human leukocytes, it was assumed in the early days of renal transplantation that they might be unimportant in transplant rejection. However, it was soon noted that ABO incompatibility often led to acute or hyperacute rejection. More recently, because of the organ shortage and reports of ABO-incompatible liver and heart allografts, attempts have been made to breach the ABO barrier for kidneys. Successful transplantation is possible in blood group O or B recipients of kidneys from A_2 donors, who have a lower number of A antigenic determinants on their cells than A_1 donors do. Successful ABO-incompatible transplantation has also been reported in recipients whose antibodies have been removed by plasmapheresis or immunoadsorption. Antibodies eventually reappear, so most centers use only blood group–compatible organs. However, considering such protocols is theoretically attractive because they may allow the use of ABO-incompatible family donors. One report of 67 ABO-incompatible kidney donor transplants indicated that 75% of such grafts survive after 6 years.[3]

HLA antigens are encoded on the short arm of chromosome 6 in humans. Six closely linked loci have been defined, and the existence of several others has been deduced from family studies and immunochemical findings. The extreme polymorphism of HLA alleles plays a pivotal role in the immune response. The gene products of the A, B, and C loci of HLA are referred to as class I major histocompatibility complex (MHC) antigens, and products of the HLA-DP, HLA-DQ, and HLA-DR regions are class II MHC antigens. Class I MHC antigens are expressed on all nucleated cells. Class II MHC antigens are important in antigen presentation and are expressed on B lymphocytes, dendritic cells, endothelium, and activated T cells. HLA antigens are inherited as codominant alleles, and because of their relatively low recombinant frequency, the HLA genes are generally inherited en bloc from each parent. Any two siblings have a 25% chance of being HLA identical, that is, of having inherited the same chromosome 6 (haplotype) from each parent, a 50% chance of sharing one haplotype, and a 25% chance of sharing neither haplotype. Parent-to-child donation always involves a one-haplotype identity. Although the significance of various levels of HLA matching among unrelated donors is equivocal, an HLA-identical kidney from a sibling or a zero antigen–mismatch kidney from a cadaveric donor is associated with a superior outcome.

Sensitization to HLA, as indicated by the presence of lymphocytotoxic antibodies in the recipient's serum, may occur as a result of pregnancy, blood transfusions, or previous transplantation. The presence of donor-reactive antibodies, detected by incubation of recipient serum with donor cells in the presence of complement (positive crossmatch), is a contraindication to renal transplantation because of its strong association with hyperacute rejection. Serum from patients awaiting cadaveric renal transplantation is periodically screened against a panel of randomly selected, HLA-typed lymphocyte donors (panel-reactive antibody [PRA]) or, more recently, by flow cytometry using a panel of beads coated with a panel of defined HLA antigens. The greater the percentage of the panel that a patient's serum reacts with (high PRA), the lower the likelihood of being crossmatch-compatible

with a donor. In some patients, titers of lymphocytotoxic antibodies decline or disappear with time. A positive crossmatch with the use of peak reactive serum may be disregarded, provided that the current serum is negative.

Not all positive crossmatches portend hyperacute rejection. For example, lymphocytotoxic autoantibodies do not cause rejection. There is also controversy over sensitive crossmatching methods such as flow cytometry because they may exclude donors who might have been used successfully. In addition, the clinical relevance of positive crossmatches to B lymphocytes (especially if performed in the cold) and those caused only by IgM antibodies is questionable. Attempts have also been made to define the role of antibodies against minor (non-HLA) antigens. For example, there is evidence that antibodies against determinants on vascular endothelial cells can damage renal allografts.

Several methods have been used to remove cytotoxic antibodies, including thoracic duct drainage, splenectomy, total lymphoid irradiation, intravenous (IV) immunoglobulin (IVIG), B cell–depleting agents, and plasmapheresis. In a limited number of patients, the combination of IVIG and plasmapheresis reduced levels of antibody in highly sensitized patients, thus increasing the likelihood of finding a crossmatch-negative donor and allowing successful transplantation. Adjuvant therapy with anti-CD20 to help prevent antibody recurrence is currently being explored systematically. Because none of these maneuvers has yet gained wide acceptance, sensitization remains a huge problem for potential recipients. The wait time with a PRA greater than 10% is 80% longer than with a PRA less than 10%. Although the percentage of patients with a PRA greater than 10% went from 51% in 1995 to 40% in 2004, this represents a significant increase in the actual number of sensitized patients because the waitlist doubled in size during that time.[2]

Attempts to Induce Specific Unresponsiveness

Blood Transfusions

In the first 2 decades of renal transplantation, transfusions were avoided to minimize the formation of lymphocytotoxic antibodies. However, in 1973, Opelz and colleagues observed in a multi-institutional survey that renal allograft survival was actually 10% to 15% better in transfused than in nontransfused recipients. This resulted in a worldwide policy of deliberate pretransplant blood transfusion, which was subsequently credited with a substantial improvement in the outcome of renal transplantation over the next decade. Reasons for this beneficial so-called transfusion effect were unclear. Transfusions may prevent high-responder patients from undergoing transplantation by making them crossmatch positive, thereby resulting in transplantation being performed only in low-responder patients who remain crossmatch negative despite exposure to antigens and thus less likely to reject a kidney for host factors unrelated to transfusion. Transfusion may also have a true immunosuppressive effect mediated by induction of regulatory T lymphocytes or enhancing alloantibodies. When overall graft survival improved with the use of cyclosporine in 1984, the previously observed benefit of transfusion was no longer seen. Because of the risks of transmitting infection (HIV and hepatitis) and sensitizing patients to prospective donors for no apparent benefit, pretransplant transfusions have been abandoned.

Bone Marrow Conditioning

There still remains interest in conditioning recipients with donor bone marrow because the self-replicating ability of bone marrow raises the potential for persistent chimerism. Animal experiments have shown that administration of donor bone marrow is an effective method of conditioning transplant recipients. In 1987, Barber and colleagues initiated a randomized study in which cryopreserved donor bone marrow was administered 10 to 14 days after kidney transplantation to recipients who received antilymphocyte serum (ALS) and other standard immunosuppressive agents. The incidence of acute rejection was decreased, but there was little improvement in long-term patient and graft survival, and chronic rejection was not prevented. More recently, patients with renal failure secondary to multiple myeloma have been treated by combined kidney/nonmyeloablative bone marrow transplantation (cyclophosphamide, thymic irradiation, and antithymocyte globulin) from HLA-identical donors. Four of six patients were successfully withdrawn from immunosuppression entirely, although one had a rejection episode requiring treatment and transient reinstitution of immunosuppression. The remaining two patients continued taking chronic steroids with or without mycophenolate mofetil (MMF) for graft-versus-host disease (GVHD) and did not have any rejection episodes.[4] Three patients who did not have multiple myeloma have undergone combined kidney/nonmyeloablative bone marrow transplantation protocols with non–HLA-matched donors; long-term results are not yet available.

Pretransplant Operations

Any necessary urinary tract reconstructions must be carried out before transplantation (e.g., lysis of posterior urethral valves, transurethral resection for obstructing prostatic hypertrophy). The patient's own bladder is used for ureteroneocystostomy, even if bladder reconstruction or augmentation of a small bladder by ileocecocystoplasty is necessary. Careful intermittent catheterization of a neurogenic bladder three or four times daily after transplantation is preferable to the use of an intestinal conduit. In the absence of an alternative strategy, ileal conduits are constructed at least 6 weeks before the transplant operation to avoid the risk of infection. Bilateral native nephrectomy was once routine, the rationale being that previously pyelonephritic kidneys could be a continued focus of infection and glomerulonephritic kidneys were a stimulus for autoimmune destruction of the allograft. Over time, this concern has not been substantiated, so nephrectomies are now performed only for special indications, such as recalcitrant urinary tract infections (especially in the presence of stones, reflux, or obstruction), uncontrolled hypertension, massive proteinuria, bilateral

renal tumors, or polycystic kidneys with recurrent bleeding, infection, or symptoms caused by large size.

Splenectomy was at one time performed empirically for its nonspecific immunosuppressive effect, but a large randomized study has shown that the procedure only modestly improves early, but not late, graft survival.

Selection and Management of Living Donors

For the recipient, a well-timed living donor transplant obviates the discomfort, expense, and risks associated with prolonged dialysis while awaiting a cadaver kidney, as well as decreases the chance of post-transplant acute tubular necrosis (ATN). Graft survival is better with living donor kidneys (95% and 80% 1- and 5-year survival rates) than with standard criteria cadaveric kidneys (91% and 69%). Patient survival rates at 1 and 5 years are 96% and 84% after standard criteria cadaveric transplants and 98% and 91% after living donor transplants. The superiority of results with living donor kidneys is based on several factors. Living donor kidneys are generally in better condition.

In addition, the timing of transplantation and the medical status of the recipient can be optimized, the cold ischemia time can be kept to a minimum, and there is potential for better HLA matching. Living donor kidneys account for about 40% of all kidney transplants. There are presently more living kidney donors than cadaveric kidney donors, but only one kidney transplant is available per living donor, whereas there are usually two per cadaveric donor. In the past, unrelated volunteers were excluded from donation because the major benefit of living donor transplantation was thought to arise from closer HLA matching. However, living unrelated transplants have been proved to exhibit graft survival as good at 5 and 10 years as those from living related donors, except for transplants between HLA-identical siblings, which have significantly better outcomes than those of cadaveric kidneys. Genetically unrelated but emotionally related donors (especially spouses) now account for about 36% of living donor transplants.[2]

Despite the major advantages of living donor kidneys, their use is justified only if the risks to the donor are minimal, and it is important to present these risks frankly to potential donors. Overall mortality for living kidney donation is 0.03%, and complications such as bleeding, readmission for nausea/vomiting, wound infections, chronic pain syndromes, deep venous thrombosis/pulmonary embolism, and rhabdomyolysis occur in less than 5% of donors.[5] A traditional policy has been to accept as donors only individuals in excellent health, aged 18 to 60 years. Although acceptable donor age limits are now becoming extended, it is remains important to avoid excessive risk. Ablation of renal tissue in an experimental rat model leads to hyperfiltration by the remaining kidney tissue and eventual sclerosis. For possibly similar reasons, proteinuria and hypertension develop in some human donors within 10 years after nephrectomy, and a small number even progress to renal failure, but in the largest single-center study with more than 20 years' follow-up, this number did not differ from the control population.[6]

Therefore, nearly normal renal function and life expectancy are anticipated as a result of compensatory hypertrophy of the remaining kidney after unilateral nephrectomy. It is important that potential candidates be protected from pressure to donate against their will, especially if they are minors. However, most family members willingly donate and experience profound psychological benefit from doing so.

Obviously, the living donor must have two normal kidneys, as confirmed by standard renal function tests, IV pyelography, and imaging of the renal vessels. Magnetic resonance or computed tomographic (CT) angiography is now substituted for contrast arteriography at many centers. This minimizes the risk of the procedure to the donor, although small accessory renal arteries may not be as well defined. The left kidney is preferred because the longer renal vein facilitates implantation. If preoperative imaging reveals multiple renal arteries on one side, the kidney with a single artery is usually selected to facilitate the anastomosis.

Techniques of Living Donor Nephrectomy

Open living donor nephrectomy is performed through an oblique flank incision. After incising Gerota's fascia, the lateral border and upper pole of the kidney are mobilized, and then the hilar structures are exposed. On the left side, the adrenal and gonadal veins are divided so that the full length of the renal vein can be used. Traction on the renal artery is carefully avoided because it causes spasm and decreased kidney perfusion, possibly compromising early function. The ureter is mobilized with its blood supply and a generous amount of periureteric tissue. It is divided close to the bladder after ligating the distal end. Mannitol and furosemide are useful in promoting diuresis and may help minimize ischemia-reperfusion injury through antioxidant effects and decreasing metabolic activity of the kidney. Once the recipient iliac vessels are prepared, the donor renal artery and vein are clamped and divided, in that order. Heparinized preservative solution cooled to 4°C is flushed through the artery while the kidney is immersed in a basin of cold solution. The donor blood vessels are oversewn, and the incision is closed without drainage. A recent series including over 5000 open donor nephrectomies had no deaths to report and a complication rate of just under 2%.[6]

More than 50% of living donor kidneys are now removed laparoscopically, a procedure that is associated with a shorter hospital stay, less discomfort, and earlier return to work. The mortality rate for laparoscopic donor nephrectomy is 0.06%, with a complication rate of about 4%. Most of these complications involve bleeding requiring transfusion or reoperation, or gastrointestinal complaints.[7] The stapling devices used to transect vessels shorten them by 1 to 1.5 cm, and some centers have reported earlier ureteral complications and early graft dysfunction in kidneys removed laparoscopically, but this has not had an adverse impact on long-term results. Hand-assisted laparoscopic nephrectomy results in fewer complications than non–hand-assisted laparoscopy does.

Selection and Management of Cadaveric Donors

In most countries, acceptance of the concept of brain death allows removal of viable organs from heart-beating donors. Treatment of potential donors before death and the definition or declaration of death are the responsibility of the patient's primary physician or a neurologic consultant. To avoid any conflict of interest, the transplant team must never be involved in care of the donor or in decisions regarding prognosis or therapy. Commonly accepted criteria for brain death include two in-hospital examinations at least 12 hours apart by a neurologist or neurosurgeon in which loss of function of the entire brain is documented.

Loss of cerebral function is documented by lack of response to painful stimuli or absence of movement, except for spinal reflexes. Loss of brainstem function is documented by fixed pupils; absence of corneal, oculo-vestibular, and oculocephalic reflexes; loss of the gag reflex; and absence of movement or spontaneous respiration off the respirator for 3 minutes, a test that is done only after other criteria indicate no brain function. The declaration of brain death may be accelerated by 6 hours if a confirmatory test such as a brain scan or an electroencephalogram is performed. The diagnosis of brain death cannot be made in the presence of severe hypothermia, marked hypovolemia, or toxic levels of depressant drugs such as barbiturates. It is important that primary physicians, neurosurgeons, and intensive care nurses identify potential donors. Procurement personnel (usually part of a regional team) are then available to help obtain permission from the family and coordinate removal and distribution of viable organs. There has also been increasing use of donors after cardiac death or patients whose families have decided to withdraw care because they have irreversible brain injury without meeting the criteria for brain death.

The Uniform Anatomical Gift Act has been adopted in all 50 states, but transplant surgeons have been reluctant to proceed with organ recovery on the basis of donor cards alone without permission from the next of kin. In fact, organs are recovered from only about 40% of the 20,000 potentially acceptable donors because of lack of consent from relatives of the deceased for a variety of cultural and personal reasons. This situation is terribly unfortunate because on average, an organ donor provides 30.8 life-years to 2.9 recipients (generally some combination of liver and kidney transplants). A donor who contributes all seven organs (two lungs, two kidneys, pancreas, heart, liver) provides 55.8 life-years.[7] The optimal cadaveric renal donors are previously healthy subjects between 3 and 60 years of age who have been declared brain dead from any of a variety of causes. Donors older than 60 years or those between 50 and 60 years who died of stroke or who have diabetes, hypertension, or an elevated creatinine level are designated *expanded criteria donors* (ECDs), and transplants from these donors have been shown to have an inferior, but still acceptable outcome.

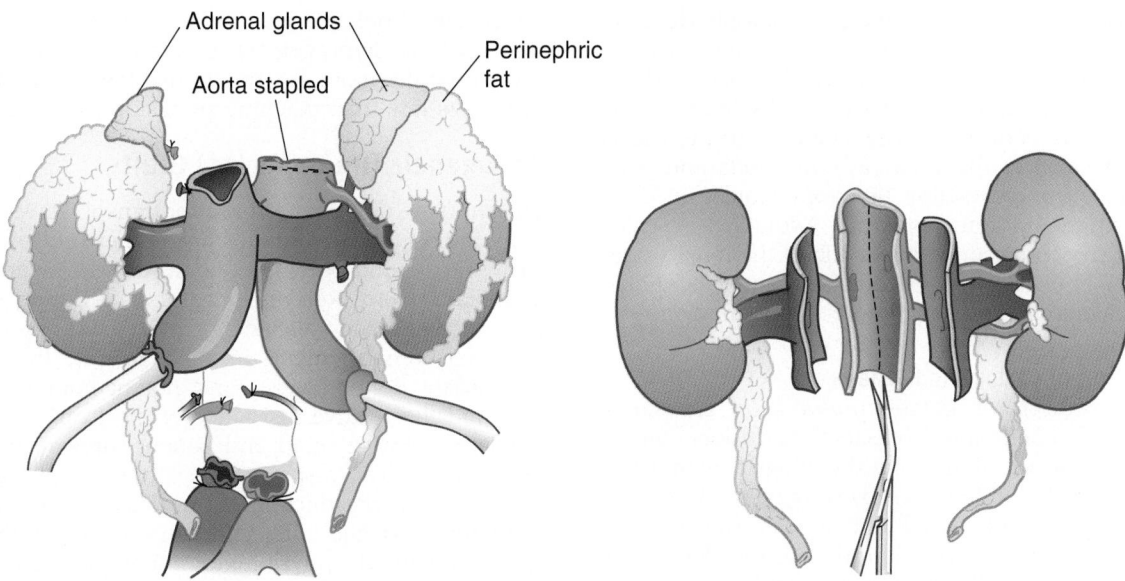

Figure 28-2 Kidney recovery.

A careful history, physical examination, and laboratory surveys are carried out to uncover factors that are contraindications to organ donation, such as the presence of generalized infections with no effective therapy (e.g., HIV, active herpes simplex virus [HSV] encephalitis, human T-lymphotropic virus type 1 [HTLV-1], HTLV-2), high-risk social behavior (e.g., use of IV drugs), known renal disease, and malignancy other than nonmetastasizing brain tumors. ECD kidneys routinely undergo biopsy, even if serum markers of kidney function are acceptable. Donors even older than 70 years may sometimes be suitable, but special care must be taken during anatomic evaluation for the presence of severe atherosclerotic disease. Transplantation of both kidneys from an older cadaveric donor with reduced nephron mass to a single recipient has been proposed for the salvage of organs that would otherwise be discarded. Transplantation of both kidneys from infant donors is also performed but is associated with a higher incidence of technical complications.

Donor Pretreatment
There have been attempts to pretreat cadaveric donors with immunosuppressive drugs such as methylprednisolone, cyclophosphamide, and cyclosporine in an effort to eradicate cells of hematopoietic origin in the transplant organ (passenger cells), which may act as antigen-presenting cells (APCs). Results have been conflicting, and since Starzl and Zinkernagel observed that some transplant recipients of many years' standing have persistent donor lymphoid cells (especially dendritic cells) in the skin, thymus, and brain, some have postulated that passenger cells are actually helpful.[8]

HLA Considerations in Cadaver Donor Selection
The benefit of zero antigen–mismatched cadaveric kidney transplants is uncontested, and they are therefore mandated to be shared on a national basis. The importance of lesser degrees of matching remains controversial, and the United Network of Organ Sharing (UNOS) is considering changing the point system for cadaveric kidney allocation, which currently emphasizes HLA matching.

Operative Technique for Cadaveric Donors
After declaration of brain death, the donor is brought to the operating room and optimal respiration and circulation are maintained throughout the procedure. Before and during the operation it is often necessary to administer large volumes of IV fluids because of diabetes insipidus or to restore any intravascular volume that may have been depleted during attempts to decrease brain swelling before death. For non–heart-beating donors, the recovery team must be in the operating room ready to start the procedure as soon as death is pronounced on the basis of cessation of cardiac function.

The following technique of in situ perfusion and en bloc dissection has evolved as the standard (Fig. 28-2). The peritoneal cavity is entered through a midline incision, usually extended to the suprasternal notch to facilitate heart, lung, and liver donation. After exploration for unsuspected neoplasia or infection, a right medial visceral rotation is performed to expose the aorta and inferior vena cava. After dissection of the vascular structures of the extrarenal organs to be concomitantly recovered (liver, pancreas, heart, lung), heparin is administered. A large-bore cannula is inserted into the aorta just above the bifurcation for retrograde in situ perfusion. The aorta is clamped proximally above the celiac axis at the diaphragm, and infusion of cold (4°C) preservation solution via the aortic cannula is initiated along with simultaneous decompression via the inferior vena cava as it enters the right atrium. The kidneys, which rapidly become pale and cold, are then mobilized while avoiding damage to the hilar structures or ureters. The distal aorta and vena cava are divided at the bifurcation and sharply dissected off the spine and back muscles. The entire block of kidneys, ureters, aorta, and vena cava is transferred to a basin of cold solution, where careful dissection of the renal vessels is performed. The kidneys are then separated by division of the vena cava and aorta and packaged for cold storage to allow time for recipient selection, tissue typing, and transportation. Additional so-called bench surgery for accurate dissection of the renal vessels and ureter is usually carried out later under continued hypothermic conditions just before transplantation.

Preservation of Cadaveric Kidneys

The two methods of kidney preservation are simple cooling and continuous pulsatile perfusion. Simple cooling is achieved by flushing the allograft with a cold preservation solution followed by storage at 4°C to 10°C. The most commonly used solution is University of Wisconsin (UW) solution, introduced by Belzer and Southard in 1987. UW solution's cationic composition (high K^+, low Na^+) mimics intracellular levels to minimize diffusion down electrochemical gradients. It contains lactobionate, which suppresses hypothermia-induced cell swelling by virtue of being an osmotic agent, inhibits calcium-dependent enzymes that can autodigest cells by chelating calcium, and minimizes oxidative damage during reperfusion by chelating iron. Phosphate buffers are included to counteract the accumulation of acids. In pulsatile perfusion, either cryoprecipitated homologous plasma or a preservation solution is circulated through the kidney. For preservation times shorter than 24 hours, pulsatile perfusion has little advantage. For longer preservation times, however, kidneys have a significantly lower rate of delayed graft function with pulsatile perfusion, but no improvement in graft survival has been shown. Furthermore, temporary dialysis after transplantation costs less than machine perfusion.

Xenogeneic (Interspecies) Grafts

The shortage of human organs for transplantation has led to an interest in using organs from other species, particularly primate and porcine donors. About 40 whole-organ xenografts were performed in humans during the 20th century. Starzl and colleagues transplanted baboon livers into two human patients in 1992. Despite the use of a concordant donor species and potent immunosuppression and the relative resistance of the liver to antibody-mediated damage, graft and patient survival were short (25 and 70 days, respectively). Moreover, the development of graft dysfunction in the absence of significant histologic evidence of rejection raised concern that some as-yet-undefined physiologic incompatibility existed between the graft and recipient. In any case, primates are in short supply and difficult to breed, and the ethics of sacrificing them for organ donation has been questioned.

The temporary success of transplanted porcine organs in nonhuman primates has suggested that these discordant donors might be used successfully in humans. The α1,3-galactosyltransferase (Gal) epitopes on the cell surface are the major xenoantigens responsible for hyperacute rejection in pig-to-primate transplants and may be involved in acute vascular rejection as well. Previous gene therapy approaches involved transducing porcine cells with regulators of complement activation so that they could avoid the consequences of antibody binding. More promising has been the generation of Gal-knockout pigs whose hearts have been transplanted into baboons; survival was 2 to 6 months.[9] Porcine islet endocrine cells have also garnered special attention because they do not express the Gal epitope and their associated endothelial cells do not survive pretransplant culture.[10] Two groups have reported porcine islet survival of longer than 100 days in macaques with various immunosuppression regimens.[10,11] Zoonoses are a concern, particularly with regard to the porcine endogenous retrovirus (PERV), which is present in all pigs and has been shown to infect human cells in vitro. The macaques that received porcine islets in the liver were polymerase chain reaction (PCR) positive for PERV sequences but had no evidence of systemic dissemination, and in a survey of 160 patients treated with living porcine tissue (skin, cells, heart valves), there has been no evidence of virus transmission.[12]

The Recipient Operation

General anesthesia is typically used. Excessive administration of muscle relaxants (especially succinylcholine) is avoided because the low cholinesterase levels in dialysis patients may lead to prolonged apnea. Atracurium has a short half-life and its degradation is independent of renal and hepatic function.

The retroperitoneum is entered through an oblique incision just above the inguinal ligament (Fig. 28-3). The

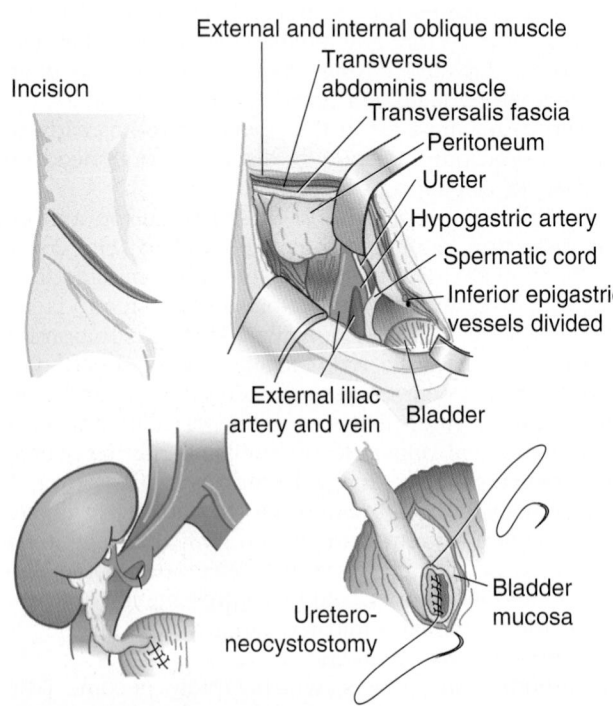

Incision

External and internal oblique muscle
Transversus abdominis muscle
Transversalis fascia
Peritoneum
Ureter
Hypogastric artery
Spermatic cord
Inferior epigastric vessels divided

External iliac artery and vein
Bladder

Uretero-neocystostomy
Bladder mucosa

Figure 28-3 Recipient kidney operation.

dissection is slightly easier on the right, but a more important consideration is avoiding sites of previous transplants, other operations (e.g., appendectomy, herniorrhaphy, or bladder or ureteral operations), or peritoneal dialysis catheters. The lymphatics are divided between ties to prevent prolonged lymph drainage or lymphocele formation. Exposure of the bladder is facilitated by dividing the inferior epigastric vessels and, in females, the round ligament. Division of the spermatic cord is avoided because this may cause epididymitis, testicular ischemia, and atrophy.

Historically, the arterial anastomosis was performed in end-to-end fashion between the donor renal artery and the proximal end of the recipient's divided internal iliac artery. Most surgeons now routinely perform an end-to-side anastomosis to the external iliac artery because exposure of the external iliac artery requires less dissection and there is less chance for anastomotic narrowing, especially if a Carrel patch of donor aorta is used. An end-to-side anastomosis between the end of the donor renal vein and the side of the external iliac vein is standard.

If there are multiple donor renal arteries without an aortic cuff, we favor anastomosis of the end of the smaller renal arteries to the side of the largest renal artery. These anastomoses are performed while the ex vivo kidney is protected by immersion in a basin of cold preservative solution. Revascularization in the recipient can then be accomplished rapidly with a single anastomosis. Sacrificing these end arteries will cause renal infarcts, and preservation of accessory arteries to the lower portion of the kidney is especially important because they may constitute the blood supply to the ureter and ligation of them may lead to necrosis and urinary fistula formation. In 470 living related donors studied at the University of Pennsylvania, multiple renal arteries were found to be present in one kidney in 30% and bilaterally in 9%. In 42 patients in whom the type of ex vivo anastomosis described previously was performed for multiple arteries, only one kidney was lost, as a result of a technical complication, and the 1-year survival rate of 76% was no different from that of single-artery kidneys in the precyclosporine period. The venous collateral circulation is almost always adequate, so in instances of multiple renal veins (which are even more common than multiple arteries), only one large vein need be saved for anastomosis. If a large adult kidney is to be transplanted into a small child, a transperitoneal approach is used to provide adequate room for the kidney, which is revascularized via the aorta and vena cava.

Urinary tract continuity is usually established by ureteroneocystostomy. The ureter passes beneath the spermatic cord to avoid obstruction. Ureteropyelostomy, or anastomosis of the recipient's ureter to the pelvis of the donor kidney, is an alternative procedure that is used when the donor ureter has been devascularized or damaged. A few surgeons prefer this procedure to ureteroneocystostomy, but it is associated with a higher incidence of urinary fistula.

Meticulous technique and hemostasis are particularly important because of uremic coagulopathy and immuno-suppression. We prefer to close the wound without drains, but if hemostasis is suboptimal, closed suction catheters may be used.

Post-transplant Management

If the transplanted kidney has not suffered ischemic damage, brisk diuresis is likely to begin within minutes of revascularization. Urine output may reach 1000 mL/hr because of blood urea nitrogen acting as an osmotic agent; chronic fluid and electrolyte overload secondary to underdialysis, in addition to fluid loading in the operating room; and mild proximal tubular damage from allograft ischemia. For the first 12 to 24 hours, urine output is encouraged by replacement of urine volume milliliter for milliliter and, if necessary, by administration of diuretics. Hypovolemia cannot be allowed to become an issue and delay the diagnosis of vascular occlusion, urinary obstruction, or early rejection as a cause of oliguria. Severe electrolyte abnormalities, particularly hyponatremia, can result from massive diuresis, especially in children, and serum levels may need to be checked more often than once a day. A 0.45% saline solution with 30 mEq/L sodium bicarbonate is recommended as the replacement fluid. If the transplant is not producing urine, dialysis may be required for hypervolemia and hyperkalemia.

Because of the retroperitoneal approach, medications and fluids can generally be given by mouth within 12 to 24 hours. Ambulation on the first postoperative day is beneficial. The Foley catheter can be removed within the first few days. Hypertension, which is common, is managed conventionally with β-blockers, hydralazine, and calcium channel blockers. Antacids are given to prevent ulcers, and nystatin (Mycostatin) is used for prophylaxis against oral candidal infections. Perioperative antibiotics (which are given for <48 hours) decrease the incidence of wound infection. Trimethoprim-sulfamethoxazole is used routinely by most centers for prophylaxis against urinary tract infections and *Pneumocystis carinii*. If rejection and other postoperative complications do not occur, subsequent care is relatively simple because restoration of renal function is associated with rapid return to normal health in patients previously suffering from single-organ system failure.

Immunosuppression

Prevention of human renal allograft rejection by whole-body irradiation was first attempted in the 1950s. Although one irradiated patient retained his allograft for 25 years without ever receiving immunosuppressive drugs, 11 others died of infections secondary to the profound immunodepression caused by this treatment. The development of pharmacologic agents allowed safer, reversible, and more predictable immunosuppression.

Steroids

Historically, steroids were administered chronically to all kidney recipients as part of their maintenance regimen, with high-dose pulses being given for induction or for treatment of acute rejection. Corticosteroids intervene at many points in the immune system. They inhibit DNA and RNA production, and after forming complexes with intracellular receptors, they impair the transcription of cytokines such as interleukin-1 (IL-1), IL-2, IL-6, interferon-γ (IFN-γ), and tumor necrosis factor-α (TNF-α). In addition, they act in an anti-inflammatory fashion by inhibiting margination of lymphocytes, decreasing chemotaxis, and impairing the function of macrophages and granulocytes. Long-term administration of corticosteroids is associated with multiple side effects, including hypertension, hyperlipidemia, hyperglycemia, cataract formation, osteoporosis, psychosis, pancreatitis, gastrointestinal tract bleeding, ulceration and perforation, poor wound healing, and growth retardation. Because of these adverse effects, newer protocols for select patients may include steroid withdrawal within a week to months of transplantation. Steroid dosing is generally standardized across adults without adjustment for body weight or metabolic rate.

Calcineurin Inhibitors

Calcineurin is a Ca^{2+}-dependent serine/threonine phosphatase that dephosphorylates a number of DNA transcription factors, including NFAT (nuclear factor of activated T cells). After dephosphorylation, NFAT localizes to the nucleus and binds to the promoter region of the IL-2 gene, thereby resulting in up-regulation of IL-2 expression. Cyclosporine (Neoral/Sandimmune), a cyclic peptide drug derived from a fungus, binds to cyclophilin-A, a peptidyl-prolyl isomerase that normally facilitates cellular protein folding. The cyclosporine-cyclophilin complex inhibits the phosphatase activity of calcineurin, which results in failure of IL-2 production. The introduction of cyclosporine in the early 1980s revolutionized transplantation by facilitating successful extrarenal transplants and improving cadaveric kidney graft survival. It is useful as maintenance therapy, but it is not effective in the treatment of acute rejection. One of the notable complications of cyclosporine use is *nephrotoxicity* from a combination of vasoconstriction and interstitial nephritis, and it may occur even at subtherapeutic levels or after a prolonged, stable dosage. Long-term use leads to the development of interstitial fibrosis in the kidney.

Other side effects include gingival hyperplasia, hypertension, and hyperkalemia. Cyclosporine is metabolized by the cytochrome P-450 system in the liver, and its dosing must be adjusted when given with other drugs that either compete for the P-450 system or up-regulate its activity (e.g., erythromycin, cimetidine, phenytoin, phenobarbital, diltiazem, fluconazole, and ketoconazole). Dosing is determined by trough levels in whole blood, which are maintained at 100 to 200 μg/L (as determined by high-performance liquid chromatography), although goal levels can be decreased as the recipient is further removed from transplantation. Tacrolimus (FK-506/Prograf) binds to a cellular protein named FK-506 binding protein (FKBP). The FK-506–FKBP complex inhibits calcineurin activity, ultimately inhibiting IL-2 expression, much as cyclosporine does. FK-506 also inhibits the production of IL-3, IL-4, and IFN-γ and expression of the IL-2 receptor. Like cyclosporine, FK-506 can cause sig-

nificant nephrotoxicity, hypertension, and hyperkalemia at high serum levels.

Other electrolyte abnormalities include hypomagnesemia. FK-506–induced central nervous system (CNS) toxicity can be manifested as headaches, tremors, mental status changes, or even seizures. Another serious side effect of FK-506 is diabetes, which seems to be related to inhibition of insulin gene transcription, as well as some degree of beta cell toxicity, rather than insulin resistance, although preexisting insulin resistance increases the patient's risk for requiring insulin. FK-506–associated diabetes is sometimes reversible after discontinuation of the drug. Tacrolimus is about 100 times more potent than cyclosporine as an anti–T-cell agent (on a per-milligram basis), and prospective randomized trials indicate that patient and graft survival is the same or better with tacrolimus than with cyclosporine, but the incidence of acute rejection is significantly lower with tacrolimus. Tacrolimus has therefore replaced cyclosporine at most centers.

Cell Cycle Inhibitors

Sirolimus (rapamycin/Rapamune) is a macrocyclic antibiotic produced by *Streptomyces hygroscopicus* that also binds to FKBP but does not exert its immunosuppressive activity via the calcineurin pathway. Rather, the sirolimus-FKBP complex binds to and inhibits a kinase named FRAP (FKBP-rapamycin/sirolimus–associated protein), which is variably known as *target of Rapamune* (TOR). FRAP/TOR kinase activity is required to activate the cyclin-dependent kinases necessary for T cells to progress from the G_1 to the S phase during the proliferative response to IL-2 and IL-6. Sirolimus has much less nephrotoxicity but is associated with hyperlipidemia, thrombocytopenia, pneumonitis, rash, and profound delays in wound healing by interfering with fibroblast activity. There has been increased interest in sirolimus because of the nephrotoxicity and neurotoxicity of calcineurin inhibitors. Unfortunately, sirolimus potentiates the nephrotoxicity of calcineurin inhibitors and may slow recovery from ATN.

Co-stimulation Blockade

Belatacept (LEA29Y) is a human fusion protein combining the extracellular portion of CTLA-4 (cytotoxic T-lymphocyte–associated antigen 4) with two amino acid substitutions to increase its binding affinity and the Fc portion of IgG. It blocks CD80 and CD86, ligands on APCs that normally bind CD28 on T cells to deliver the co-stimulatory signal necessary for full T-cell activation. Failure to deliver this second signal results in anergy and apoptosis of T cells. Trials using belatacept to replace calcineurin inhibitors as maintenance therapy showed rates of acute rejection (diagnosed by biopsy) and infection at 6 months similar to those of cyclosporine, but a higher GFR and less chronic allograft nephropathy at 12 months.[13] It is, however, administered only by IV infusion and is not available in an oral preparation.

Antimetabolites

Mycophenolate mofetil (CellCept/Myfortic) is a prodrug that is hydrolyzed to mycophenolic acid (MPA), the active form of MMF. MPA inhibits the activity of inosine monophosphate dehydrogenase, an enzyme in the de novo guanine synthesis pathway. B and T cells are dependent on de novo guanine synthesis for proliferation because they lack the salvage pathway on which other rapidly dividing cells frequently depend. As a result, MPA inhibits leukocyte proliferation, without the skin, hair, and gastrointestinal side effects that other antimetabolites cause. MPA also blocks glycosylation of adhesion molecules, thereby inhibiting leukocyte recruitment and adhesion to endothelial cells. Although MMF is not associated with renal toxicity, it does cause bone marrow suppression and gastrointestinal symptoms such as nausea, diarrhea, and vague abdominal pain. It is contraindicated in pregnancy. Absorption of MMF is reduced with magnesium and aluminum hydroxide. Trials combining MMF with cyclosporine have indicated that the risk for biopsy-proven acute rejection declined to less than 20% and the frequency of resistant rejection was markedly decreased. As a result, MMF has virtually replaced azathioprine at many transplant centers. Unfortunately, MMF has not altered the rate of chronic graft rejection.

In 1988, the Nobel Prize was awarded to Gertrude Elion and George Hitchings for the development of azathioprine (Imuran), and together with steroids, it was the mainstay of immunosuppression before the introduction of cyclosporine in 1983. Azathioprine contains an imidazole linked to 6-mercaptopurine, which is converted to its active form 6-thioguanine in the liver by hypoxanthine-guanine phosphoribosyltransferase. The substituted purine resembles a real purine sufficiently to get incorporated into DNA, but not enough to allow DNA replication and RNA transcription. Its preferential uptake into B and T lymphocytes and hence its selective inhibition of DNA and RNA synthesis in leukocytes are not well understood. Adverse effects include an increased risk for malignancy, hepatitis, myelosuppression (especially leukopenia), cholestasis, alopecia, and pancreatitis. The dosage of azathioprine must be decreased if given with allopurinol because allopurinol inhibits one of the enzymes that degrade azathioprine to its inactive metabolite. Azathioprine is also contraindicated in pregnancy. It is not used with angiotensin-converting enzyme inhibitors because the combination can result in severe anemia and pancytopenia. At most centers azathioprine is now used only in patients who are intolerant of MMF.

Antilymphocyte Antibodies
Polyclonal and monoclonal antibodies directed toward cell surface proteins on T lymphocytes are used as part of induction therapies or for the treatment of steroid-resistant acute rejection. Thymoglobulin is a polyclonal preparation purified from the serum of rabbits that have been repeatedly inoculated with human thymocytes. Atgam is similar to Thymoglobulin, except that it is isolated from horses. Once T cells are bound by antibody, they are depleted from the circulation through opsonization and complement-assisted, antibody-dependent cell-mediated cytotoxicity (ADCC). Damaged T cells are cleared by the lymphoreticular system. *OKT3* (muromonab-CD3) is a monoclonal murine IgG2a antibody against the T-cell receptor–CD3 complex. Administration of OKT3 results first in transient activation of T cells and massive release of cytokines. This is called the *cytokine release syndrome* and is characterized by severe flulike symptoms (fevers, chills, dyspnea, bronchospasm), flash pulmonary edema, and CNS complications. Antibody-bound T cells are then removed from the circulation by opsonization in the liver and spleen and cytolysis via ADCC. Although T cells will reappear, they are CD3 negative as a result of receptor down-regulation and are not able to be activated. Large doses or prolonged therapy with antilymphocytic antibodies leads to leukopenia, thrombocytopenia, and serious infections, especially of viral origin (e.g., herpesvirus, CMV, varicella-zoster). In addition, patients form antibodies to the heterologous protein, thus limiting further use. Consequently, these agents are used for induction and steroid-resistant rejection rather than for maintenance therapy. Concomitant administration of azathioprine and corticosteroids may delay the production of new lymphocytes and prolong the immunosuppressive effect of antilymphocytic antibodies. T-cell populations can be measured to monitor the effectiveness of antilymphocytic antibodies in the absence of a good clinical response.

Rituximab is a human/murine chimeric antibody with the human IgG1 Fc regions fused to the murine variable light- and heavy-chain regions that recognize CD20, a surface marker found on B cells. Through binding of complement to the Fc portion, rituximab eliminates B cells via complement and ADCC. Frequently used to treat non-Hodgkin's B-cell lymphoma, its use has recently entered the transplant arena mainly for the treatment of steroid-resistant antibody-mediated rejection or rejection with evidence of vasculitis, especially in patients with peritubular C4d-positive immunohistochemical staining as a marker for humoral rejection. It is also used for the treatment of post-transplant lymphoproliferative disorder (see later). As with other antibody treatments, production of antirituximab antibodies results in poor efficacy because the agent is cleared from the circulation before it can bind CD20 and activate complement. In addition, plasma cells do not express high levels of CD20 and are therefore not good targets.

Alemtuzumab (Campath 1H) is a depleting, humanized, monoclonal rat antibody directed against CD52, a membrane protein of unknown function expressed on T cells, B cells, natural killer cells, monocytes, macrophages, and dendritic cells, but not on plasma cells or memory cells. After administration, it takes 3 to 12 months for repopulation of B cells and monocytes and more than 3 years for reconstitution of T cells. It has been used in induction regimens with low-dose calcineurin inhibitor maintenance monotherapy and has produced either better or similar rates of short-term graft survival and early rejection and no increase in infectious or malignant complications (1-3–year follow-up). Higher rates of late acute rejection episodes were noted and may be related to very low calcineurin inhibitor levels.[14] When used with rapamycin monotherapy, patients had almost twice the average rate of humoral rejection seen with standard regimens; one patient lost his graft because of acute rejection, and many patients with acute rejection had to return to triple-agent maintenance therapy. There is very limited experience with the use of alemtuzumab for acute rejection.

Basiliximab (Simulect) is a chimeric murine/human IgG1 produced by a genetically engineered mouse myeloma cell line. It expresses plasmids encoding the human heavy- and light-chain constant regions fused to the mouse heavy- and light-chain variable regions that encode an antibody that binds to the IL-2 receptor α chain. Also known as CD25, this component of the high-affinity IL-2 receptor is expressed preferentially on activated T lymphocytes. Simulect binds but does not activate the IL-2 receptor and thus functions as a competitive inhibitor for endogenous IL-2. *Daclizumab* (Zenapax) is another construct that has been humanized to a greater degree (90% human versus 70%) and has a murine variable region that binds to a different epitope of the IL-2 high-affinity receptor. These agents are used for induction, but not for the treatment of rejection. Both are primarily used as induction agents. Daclizumab saturates the IL-2 receptor for up to 120 days, whereas basiliximab works for only 59 days.

Rejection

Hyperacute Rejection

Hyperacute rejection results from preformed antibodies against the donor organ. Within minutes of revascularization, the kidney turns blue and soon undergoes vascular thrombosis. Histologically, extensive intravascular deposits of fibrin and platelets and intraglomerular accumulation of polymorphonuclear leukocytes, fibrin, platelets, and red blood cells occur along with accumulation of leukocytes in the peritubular and glomerular capillaries. The classic form of hyperacute rejection is rare because crossmatching is fairly reliable at identifying recipients with such antibodies. Post-transplant immunosuppression and anticoagulation are not effective in reversing the process, although certain pretransplant desensitization protocols are likely to prevent hyperacute rejection by converting a recipient from being crossmatch positive to being compatible, as discussed previously.

Acute Cellular Rejection

Acute cellular rejection occurs in 10% to 20% of patients during the first few weeks to months after transplantation, although it may occasionally occur years later. Classic signs and symptoms include malaise, fever, oliguria, hypertension, tenderness, and swelling of the allograft, but elevated creatinine is generally the only signal. In these circumstances we usually obtain a radioisotope renal perfusion scan or renal ultrasound, which cannot provide specific evidence of rejection but can exclude mechanical problems such as vascular occlusion, ureteral obstruction, or urinary leak. Urinalysis is also performed to rule out a urinary tract infection.

A biopsy is often performed when rejection is suspected. This procedure may be performed percutaneously with little risk. The interstitium, tubules, and vessels are then evaluated for lymphocytic infiltration, fibrosis,

and thrombosis and categorized according to the Banff criteria. In acute cellular rejection there are five grades: IA, greater than 25% interstitial infiltration and 5 to 10 mononuclear cells per tubular cross section; IB, greater than 25% interstitial infiltration and more than 10 mononuclear cells per tubular cross section; IIA, up to 25% of the luminal area involved with intimal arteritis; IIB, intimal arteritis involving greater than 25% of the luminal area; and III, transmural arteritis, fibrinoid change, or necrosis of the medial smooth muscle. The diagnosis of antibody-mediated rejection includes documentation of donor-specific antibodies in the recipient and positive immunohistochemical staining for the complement split product C4d. Humoral rejection is divided into three grades: I, ATN-like (minimal inflammation); II, capillary (polymorphonuclear or mononuclear leukocytes, or both, in peritubular capillaries); and III, arterial (transmural inflammation/fibrinoid change).

However, biopsies are subject to sampling error, and variable degrees of lymphocytic infiltration have been observed in patients with ATN and calcineurin inhibitor toxicity. High drug levels, reversal of dysfunction within a few days after dose reduction, and arteriolar hyalinosis suggest drug toxicity rather than rejection. Sometimes, empirical antirejection therapy is used for both diagnosis and treatment of suspected rejection. Sixty-five percent of acute rejections respond to three to five doses of IV high-dose corticosteroids (0.5-1.0 g methylprednisolone). Five to seven doses of antilymphocyte antibodies are used for steroid-resistant rejection. Antibody-mediated rejection requires some combination of IVIG, plasmapheresis, and rituximab and is often resistant to treatment.

Chronic Allograft Nephropathy

The term *chronic allograft nephropathy* refers to the fibrotic changes that occur in a transplanted kidney from a variety of ill-defined causes, including immune injury (humoral and cellular), calcineurin inhibitor use, and other nephrotoxic agents and events. Clinically, these entities are manifested by proteinuria, microscopic hematuria, and slowly deteriorating function.

Chronic allograft nephropathy often begins after years of stable function but may be accelerated in allografts that have had multiple or incompletely treated episodes of acute rejection. It is divided by the Banff criteria into grade I (mild), mild interstitial fibrosis and tubular atrophy without (a) or with (b) specific changes suggesting chronic rejection; grade II (moderate), moderate interstitial fibrosis and tubular atrophy (a) or (b); and grade III (severe), severe interstitial fibrosis and tubular loss (a) or (b). Antirejection therapy is ineffective and leads only to opportunistic infections or other serious sequelae. Abrupt cessation of immunosuppression is not recommended because progression to end-stage renal failure may be slow and a significant period of transplant function may remain. Immunosuppression is gradually reduced because calcineurin inhibitors are nephrotoxic and uremia is an immunosuppressant. It is important to remember that acute cellular rejection is also occasionally encountered after years of stable transplant function, sometimes as a result of discontinuation of immunosuppression by a careless or noncompliant patient. Late cellular rejection (unlike chronic allograft nephropathy) can sometimes be reversed if treated before severe damage occurs.

Complications of Renal Transplantation

Vascular Complications

Arterial or venous obstruction in the early postoperative period, though uncommon, is a surgical emergency and needs to be excluded if an established diuresis suddenly ceases. Although radioisotopic scanning and ultrasound will confirm vascular occlusion, immediate reoperation is the sole chance for salvaging such a graft because only a few minutes of total ischemia can be tolerated. Arterial occlusion may occur as a result of injury to a diseased artery, anastomotic problems, hypercoagulability, or unfortunate positioning of the allograft. Renal vein occlusion can result from technical errors, kinking, hypercoagulability, or compression. Iliofemoral venous thrombosis occasionally follows renal transplantation, presumably because of clamping of the vein or compression by the transplant. Such thrombus rarely extends into the renal vein, and standard anticoagulant treatment is generally effective, although urokinase and surgical thrombectomy have been used for clots occluding the renal vein. If pulmonary embolism occurs despite adequate anticoagulation, a vena cava filter is placed; such filters rarely compromise transplant function.

Imperfect operative hemostasis in the setting of uremic coagulopathy or anticoagulation during hemodialysis is the usual cause of early postoperative bleeding. Fracture and frank rupture of the transplanted kidney are unusual but may occur from rapid swelling of the transplant during acute rejection. Rupture is more common in kidneys from infant or child donors because a small organ is sometimes unable to tolerate adult levels of blood pressure and flow. Bleeding from the arterial suture line, except in the early hours postoperatively, raises suspicion of infection. Resuturing of an infected suture line is futile because of recurrent disruption. The kidney needs to be removed. If the hypogastric artery was used for vascularization of the transplant, it is securely ligated. If the anastomosis is at the common or external iliac artery, the suture line closing the iliac arteriotomy becomes a potential site of arterial disruption, and ligation of the iliac artery and extra-anatomic bypass (femorofemoral or axillofemoral) may be necessary.

Between 3 months and 2 years (peaking at 6 months) after transplantation, renal transplant artery stenosis (RTAS) may result in refractory hypertension and elevated creatinine. When 100 consecutive transplant patients underwent routine postoperative arteriography by Lacombe,[15] RTAS was found in 23%, but only 4% to 12% of patients had symptomatic RTAS. About 70% of such lesions occur at the anastomotic site. Because 20% of stenoses are distal to the anastomosis in the transplant renal artery proper, use of a Carrel patch does not preclude this complication. It can occur as a result of improper anastomosis, injury to the intima of the renal artery, kinking from redundancy or twisting of the arteries, or arteriosclerotic lesions of the donor or recipient vessels, especially transplants

performed in older patients and with organs from older donors. Since the intimal proliferation and subintimal fibrotic changes seen in RTAS are similar to small vessel changes caused by rejection, there may also be an immune component. Because surgical treatment is difficult and no more successful than percutaneous transluminal angioplasty, surgery is generally reserved for persistent or recurrent stenoses. Preserved cadaveric iliac artery may be useful in the operative repair.

Urinary Complications

The most common cause of sudden cessation of urinary output in the immediate postoperative period is the presence of a blood clot in the bladder or urethral catheter, which can be relieved by irrigation. A ureteroneocystostomy may become occluded by a hematoma at the site of the submucosal tunnel in the bladder or by a technically unsatisfactory anastomosis. An adynamic ureter or edema at the orifice of the bladder can also cause temporary partial obstruction. Devascularization of the ureter during donor nephrectomy is a more serious problem that may lead to ureteral necrosis and fistula formation within the first few days or weeks. Fluid obtained from wound drains or needle aspiration can be identified as urine by a urea content severalfold higher than that of serum or lymph.

Ultrasound, nuclear scans, and cystograms can be helpful in identifying urinomas, urinary obstruction, or extravasation of urine. Treatment may consist of drainage or stenting (or both) but more frequently involves redoing the ureteroneocystostomy or ureteropyelostomy. Further out from transplantation, ureteral strictures from mild ischemia, infection with BK virus, or technical errors usually require temporary percutaneous nephrostomies and uterography. These strictures can often be treated by dilation and stenting but occasionally require surgical reconstruction.

Acute Tubular Necrosis–Reperfusion Injury

Ischemia-reperfusion injury results in ATN or delayed graft function requiring dialysis in less than 5% of living donor transplants, but in cadaver transplants, the incidence is higher than 20%. In the absence of vascular or ureteral problems, initially nonfunctional cadaver kidneys may be assumed to suffer from ATN, especially if nuclear scans demonstrate good blood flow and poor tubular function. Oliguria in the early transplant period is treated with aliquots of fluid and colloid to exclude hypovolemia while care is taken to not overload the patient with fluid.

IV mannitol, 12.5 to 25 g, and furosemide, 100 to 200 mg, may increase urine output without altering the course of ATN, but a good response to fluid loading and diuretics rules out catastrophes such as vascular occlusion. Some kidneys that never produce urine (termed *primary nonfunction*) may be lost if ATN is compounded by unrecognized rejection such that antirejection therapy is delayed until the immunologic damage has become irreversible. In an attempt to avoid this quandary, many centers use polyclonal anti–T-cell antibody therapy for induction. Because there is no specific treatment of ATN, return of function (usually within 1 to 4 weeks) must be patiently awaited while adequate immunosuppression and a good general condition are maintained. If there is reasonable clinical confidence in the diagnosis of ATN, it is best to minimize the use of invasive studies. Serial renal scans to identify decreases in blood flow may be helpful in making the difficult diagnosis of rejection during ATN, but biopsy is often necessary for confirmation. Even in the absence of rejection, management of immunosuppression is difficult during ATN because of the nephrotoxic potential of calcineurin inhibitors.

Lymphoceles

Extensive mobilization of the iliac vessels during the transplant operation or failure to ligate the lymphatics crossing them can result in lymphoceles, which occur in 0.6% to 18% of transplants. Symptoms may not occur until weeks later and consist of swelling of the wound; edema of the scrotum, labia, and lower extremity; or urinary obstruction from pressure on the collecting system or ureter. Ultrasound easily identifies a perinephric fluid collection. Aspiration is of only temporary benefit because lymph reaccumulates rapidly. Percutaneous drainage via a catheter can be successful, although the cavity may require chemical sclerosis for obliteration. Fenestration of the cyst into the peritoneal cavity is definitive but requires another operation, which can often be accomplished laparoscopically.

Infections

Thirty percent to 60% of patients suffer some type of infection during the first transplant year, and in half of the deaths that occur during the first year, infection is an important contributing factor. During the first month after transplantation, conventional bacterial infections are the most common, and the urinary tract, respiratory system, and wound are the most prevalent sites. These infections generally respond to conventional antibiotic therapy if instituted promptly. Acute bacterial infections may have a clinical manifestation that can be confused with rejection: fever, malaise, edema, decreased urine output, or even a rising creatinine level. It is obviously important to exclude the possibility of infection before instituting antirejection therapy. The 1% to 10% incidence of wound infections is reduced by preoperative or intraoperative antibiotic prophylaxis, but more important is meticulous surgical technique. Transplant recipients are subject to the usual respiratory infections that occur in normal or hospitalized individuals, and bacterial pneumonia is potentially lethal. Urinary tract infections, which are the most common bacterial infections in transplant recipients, can be decreased by 50% by using trimethoprim-sulfamethoxazole for the first 6 months after transplantation. This drug combination is also helpful in decreasing the incidence of *P. carinii* infection.

The first 180 days after transplantation is the period of most intense immunosuppression and is also the most common time for opportunistic infections that rarely cause significant illness in the general population. Viral infections are especially important. CMV, a ubiquitous member of the herpesvirus family, has infected most people at some point. In healthy individuals, CMV infections are either clinically silent or mild, but latent virus and seropositivity persist for life. With immunosuppression, previously infected patients excrete CMV and exhibit elevated antibody titers and, in 20%, symptomatic illness. Nonetheless, the course is usually mild, presumably because previous exposure and immunity confer protection. However, 60% of seronegative recipients who receive a kidney from a seropositive donor will have symptomatic illness, and 25% of these recipients have severe disease in the form of a debilitating syndrome marked by leukopenia, hepatitis, interstitial pneumonia, arthritis, CNS changes including coma, gastrointestinal ulceration and bleeding, renal insufficiency, and even death. Rapid diagnosis can be made by checking antigenemia levels, performing PCR assays of blood, or finding histologic evidence of virus on biopsy. Although CMV can cause direct damage (so-called glomerulopathy), infections are also associated with rejection, probably because of decreasing immunosuppression and the generalized inflammatory state. The decision to treat rejection must be weighed against the potential for lethal superinfection. Fortunately, both the incidence and the severity of CMV disease can be diminished by prophylactic antivirals (acyclovir, ganciclovir, or valganciclovir). In established clinical CMV disease, IV ganciclovir is required for 2 to 4 weeks; viremia needs to be cleared before discontinuance of therapy. Passive immunization with immune globulin has also been used effectively by some centers.

Primary infections with polyomavirus (type BK) occur in up to 90% of the population, typically without specific signs or symptoms. This virus persists in the kidney, where reactivation and shedding into urine may be detected in 0.5% to 20% of healthy individuals, depending on the sensitivity of the assay (PCR versus detection of so-called decoy cells containing viral inclusions on urinary cytology). Before 1996, BK virus nephropathy was virtually unreported. It now appears that up to 5% of renal allograft recipients are affected. It is unclear whether the increasing prevalence is a function of more potent immunosuppressive agents, more virulent viral genotypes, or simply greater awareness. Urinary cytology is suggestive, but definitive diagnosis requires allograft biopsy to demonstrate nuclear inclusions in tubular epithelial cells and the absence of rejection or drug toxicity. Progression from inflammation to fibrosis to sclerosis and irreversible allograft failure occurs in as many as 45% of affected cases. Current management is based on judicious decreases in immunosuppression to allow clearance of virus. In a few instances the antiviral agent cidofovir has been used with success.

Other opportunistic infections such as aspergillosis, blastomycosis, nocardiosis, toxoplasmosis, and cryptococcosis are particularly likely to occur in transplant patients. The protozoan *P. carinii*, which has infected most individuals by 10 years of age, is pathogenic only in immunosuppressed patients. It is the most common organism causing fatal pneumonia in this group, but it is treatable and preventable with trimethoprim-sulfamethoxazole. Aggressive measures such as bronchoscopic alveolar lavage and brushings and percutaneous transbronchoscopic or open lung biopsy is considered for the diagnosis of atypical pulmonary infections because effective treatment requires identification of the organism. Mycobacterial infections are unusual, even in transplant patients, but they are always kept in mind because of their potentially lethal nature.

Gastrointestinal Complications

Ulceration and perforation of the stomach, duodenum, and small and large intestine may be accompanied by minimal signs and symptoms in immunosuppressed patients. Minor signs of peritoneal irritation, persistent fevers, and vague gastrointestinal complaints merit very close attention and workup. Colonic diverticulitis is the most common cause of perforation (36%), followed by ischemic colitis (24%). Pancreatitis is another recognized complication of both azathioprine and corticosteroid therapy and can be fatal. Infections such as *Candida* stomatitis and esophagitis, pseudomembranous colitis, and CMV ulceration are also common.

Hyperparathyroidism

Secondary hyperparathyroidism from chronic renal failure usually subsides after successful transplantation. However, tertiary hyperparathyroidism has been reported in 2% to 3% of patients. When hypercalcemia and elevated parathyroid hormone levels persist for more than 12 months in the setting of normal renal function, we advocate total parathyroidectomy and autotransplantation of fragments from a portion of one gland into the muscle of the forearm, where they are accessible for further resection without neck exploration should hypercalcemia persist or recur. Some authors note that single or double parathyroid adenomas may be responsible for up to 30% of tertiary hyperparathyroidism. They advocate preoperative imaging and intraoperative monitoring of parathyroid hormone to spare these patients from total parathyroidectomy. Most sequelae of hyperparathyroidism, such as renal calculi, bone pain, and muscle weakness, resolve after parathyroidectomy. In some unfortunate patients, diffuse cutaneous vascular calcification (calciphylaxis) leads to extensive ulceration and gangrene. Xerography shows extensive small and medium vessel calcification. These lesions frequently fail to heal even after parathyroidectomy and may eventually lead to sepsis and death.

Tumors

The increased risk for neoplasia in transplant patients has been attributed to suppression of the immunologic surveillance mechanisms that would normally destroy malignant cells expressing mutant proteins or viral oncogenes and the direct carcinogenic effect of immunosuppressive drugs. The risk for cancer in transplant patients is 3 to 14 times that in the general population. Viral-associated neoplasms, such as cervical cancer (associated with various subtypes of human papillomavirus [HPV]), carcinoma of the vulva and perineum (HSV), squamous cell carcinoma of the skin and lip (HPV), Kaposi's sarcoma (Epstein-Barr virus [EBV]), hepatocellular carcinoma (HBV, HCV), and non-Hodgkin's lymphomas (EBV and HTLV-1), are especially prevalent. The incidence of the more common cancers, such as lung, breast, prostate, and colon, is not increased in transplant recipients. The most frequent types of tumors are lymphomas (post-transplant lymphoproliferative disorder [PTLD]) and squamous cell carcinomas, and their incidence is related to the intensity and duration of immunosuppression, particularly antilymphocyte antibody therapy. Renal cancer and various sarcomas are also more prevalent in transplant patients.

Eighty-five percent of the time, PTLD represents a spectrum of EBV-related proliferation ranging from polyclonal B-cell hyperplasia to monoclonal B-cell lymphomas, most often within 1 year after transplantation and especially in children (15% of post-transplant T-cell lymphomas are usually related to HTLV-1 and tend to develop longer than 5 years after transplantation). All levels of clonality and histology can be found at different sites in the same patient. Although the epithelial cells of the upper respiratory tract are the initial site of EBV infection, B lymphocytes become secondarily infected as they travel through the lymphoid tissues of the oropharynx; more than 90% of adults are seropositive for EBV and harbor latently infected B lymphocytes. Proteins expressed from the viral genome inactivate the cellular transcription inhibitors that normally promote terminal differentiation and apoptosis and prevent proliferation. Activity of the nuclear factor NFκB is up-regulated, which leads to the production of inflammatory cytokines, thus further promoting uncontrolled proliferation. Activation of *RAG* genes promotes chromosomal rearrangements leading to chromosomal instability, thereby increasing the likelihood of malignant transformation. PTLD can be manifested as unexplained fevers, a mononucleosis-like syndrome, hepatitis, bleeding mesenteric masses or intestinal obstruction, or CNS symptoms such as seizures, altered mental status, or focal neurologic dysfunction as a consequence of neurologic tumor burden. The absence of adenopathy on radiologic imaging does not rule out PTLD because the disease can be totally extranodal. The diagnosis is made by tissue biopsy.

The mainstay of treatment of PTLD is to decrease the level of immunosuppression. Up to 86% of patients have regression of PTLD with reduction of immunosuppression alone; however, this is not effective if PTLD has progressed to a true monoclonal B-cell lymphoma. Acyclovir, ganciclovir, and foscarnet have also been used as prophylaxis or in early PTLD, but reports of their success are anecdotal; tumor cells are latently infected and do not express thymidine kinase, so there is no reason to expect PTLD to respond to antiviral agents. CHOP (cyclophosphamide, hydroxydaunomycin, Oncovin [vincristine], and prednisone) chemotherapy has been used, and there have been promising results with the anti–B-cell monoclonal antibody rituximab. Occasionally, patients will undergo surgical reduction or radiation therapy for debulking of massive local disease.

In the early days of transplantation it was found that using donors with cancer risked transmission of the tumor. The overall rate of transmission of cancer from a

Table 28-1   Graft Survival After Kidney Transplantation

TRANSPLANT TYPE	SURVIVAL	
	1 Year	5 Years
All deceased donor	89%	67%
Non-ECD	90%	70%
Non-ECD, age 11-34	93%	73%-75%
Non-ECD, age >50	88%	62%
ECD	81%	53%
All living donor (LD)	95%	80%
HLA-identical LD	98%	87%
Total mismatch LD	95%	79%
0-Ag mismatch, non-ECD	93%	74%
Non-ECD, PRA <10%	90%	70%
Non-ECD, PRA 10%-79%	90%	65%
Non-ECD, PRA >80%	90%	63%
ECD, PRA <10%	81%	54%
ECD, PRA 10%-79%	76%	43%
ECD, PRA >80%	76%	43%
LD, PRA <10%	95%	80%
LD, PRA 10%-79%	94%	77%
LD, PRA >80%	90%	74%
Non-ECD, no DGF	94%	74%
Non-ECD, with DGF	79%	54%
ECD, no DGF	88%	59%
ECD, with DGF	69%	41%
LD, no DGF	97%	82%
LD, with DGF	65%	50%

Ag, antigen; DGF, delayed graft function; ECD, expanded criteria donor; PRA, panel-reactive antibody.

donor to recipient was found to be about 50%, and that for melanoma approached 80%. For transmission to occur the transplanted organ need not be one that is a typical site of metastasis for the donor's tumor. Cessation of immunosuppression is sometimes followed by rejection of not only the transplanted kidney but also the alloge-neic tumor, but once the transplanted tumor becomes well established, it may continue to flourish and cause death even in the absence of immunosuppression.

Recurrent Disease in Transplanted Kidneys

Because transplantation does not reverse the extrarenal aspects of diseases that cause renal failure, it is not sur-prising that the transplanted kidney sometimes becomes a target for destruction by the original disease process, especially in autoimmune or metabolic diseases.

Glomerulonephritis

Of 30 twin grafts performed in the 1950s, 8 failed as a result of recurrent glomerulonephritis, thus making a strong case for the use of mild immunosuppression even in recipients of twin grafts. Recurrent disease is less common in allografts, but its clinical manifestations and even histologic changes are similar to those of chronic rejection. Rates of allograft loss from recurrent glomeru-lonephritis range from 2% to 4% for the first several years and at 10 years are no higher than rates in patients with other causes of renal failure. Recurrent disease is most likely to develop in patients who had a rapid initial

course of disease, high PRA, mesangiocapillary type I glomerulonephritis, focal segmental membranous nephropathy, IgA nephropathy, and immune crescentic glomerulonephritis. It appears to be most likely in twins and next most likely in recipients of closely matched, related donor allografts. However, the other advantages of related living donors appear to override the risks of recurrent glomerulonephritis, and their graft survival remains superior to that of mismatched cadaveric grafts.

Collagen Diseases

Collagen vascular diseases such as systemic lupus erythe-matosus rarely cause recurrent damage and are often well palliated by transplantation.

Metabolic Diseases

Cystinosis causes intracellular deposition of cysteine crys-tals in various organs and usually leads to end-stage renal disease by 10 years of age. Although recurrent renal deposition may occur after transplantation, its effects appear to be mild.

Oxalosis is likely to reappear and destroy transplanted kidneys very rapidly. Simultaneous hepatic transplanta-tion reverses the metabolic defect and is ideal in patients with systemic oxalate damage.

Diabetes has become one of the most common indica-tions for renal transplantation. Kimmelstiel-Wilson lesions may be found in the transplanted kidney within 2 years. However, it is 10 to 20 years before functional deteriora-tion is likely and transplantation still gives diabetics a better chance of survival than chronic dialysis does. Simultaneous pancreas transplantation may prevent dia-betic changes in the transplanted kidney.

Results of Renal Transplantation

Overall, deceased donor transplanted kidneys have 1-, 5-, and 10-year survival rates of 89%, 67%, and 40%. Considered separately, 1- and 5-year graft survival rates for non-ECD kidneys (83% of deceased donor trans-plants) are 90% and 70%, and for ECD kidneys (17% of deceased donor transplants), they drop to 81% and 53% (Table 28-1). Because of the inferior outcome of ECD kidneys, a recent analysis suggests that only patients who are older than 40 years and are either diabetic or are listed in an organ procurement organization with a wait time longer than 44 months derive any life span benefit from accepting an ECD kidney,[16] but this study did not take into consideration quality-of-life issues.

Among non-ECD kidneys, donors aged 11 to 34 years (38% of all deceased donors) resulted in the best outcome, with 1- and 5-year graft survival rates of 93% and 75%, which drop to 88% and 62% for donors older than 50 (28% of all deceased donors). In contrast, living donor kidneys have 1-, 5-, and 10-year survival rates of 95%, 80%, and 56%. One-year and 5-year graft survival rates for HLA-identical living donor kidneys are 98% and 87%, but even totally mismatched living donor kidneys (95% and 79%) have better graft survival than zero antigen–mismatch non-ECD kidneys (93% and 74%). Delayed

Table 28-2   Indications for Liver Transplantation

ADULTS	%	CHILDREN	%
Noncholestatic cirrhosis	65	Biliary atresia	58
Viral hepatitis B		Inborn errors of	
and C		metabolism	11
Alcoholic*		Cholestatic	9
Cryptogenic		Primary sclerosing	
		cholangitis	
Cholestatic	14	Alagille's syndrome	
Primary biliary		Autoimmune	4
cirrhosis			
Primary sclerosing		Viral hepatitis	2
cholangitis			
Autoimmune	5	Miscellaneous	16
Malignant neoplasm	2		
Miscellaneous	14		

*Most alcoholic patients are coinfected with hepatitis C virus.

Table 28-3   Child-Turcote-Pugh Score of the Severity of Liver Disease*

	POINTS		
	1	2	3
Encephalopathy	None	1-2	3-4
Ascites	Absent	Slight	Moderate
Bilirubin (mg/dL)	<2	2-3	>3
For PBC/PSC	<4	4-10	>10
Albumin (g/dL)	>3.5	2.8-3.5	<2.8
PT (INR)	<1.7	1.7-2.3	>2.3

*A patient can be placed on the transplant waiting list when the score is higher than 7. Higher status is assigned when the score is greater than 10 or when severe life-threatening complications related to liver failure are developing.

INR, international normalized ratio; PBC, primary biliary cirrhosis; PSC, primary sclerosing cholangitis; PT, prothrombin time.

graft function, or the need for dialysis in the first week after transplantation, is associated with a poor prognosis: graft survival rates are 15% to 20% lower after deceased donor transplants and over 30% lower after living donor transplants.

For ECD transplants, previous kidney transplantation and high PRA (>10%) resulted in 1- and 5-year survival rates that were 5% and 11% less, but these factors had less effect on non-ECD and living donor kidney survival. The use of kidneys from non–heart-beating donors was expected to result in inferior outcomes; although the incidence of delayed graft function was nearly double that of heart-beating brain-dead donors (43% versus 22%), 1- and 5-year survival rates were the same, perhaps because these donors were selected more carefully for other criteria, such as age. Late graft loss was twice as frequent in African Americans as in other recipients, regardless of whether the donor was living or cadaveric. Matching at the B locus for allocation of cadaveric donor organs was recently discontinued because racially associated histocompatibility differences have put African Americans at a disadvantage for allocation of cadaveric kidneys, the majority of which come from white donors.

LIVER TRANSPLANTATION

Indications for Liver Transplantation

Liver transplantation is the procedure of choice for a wide range of diseases that result in acute or chronic end-stage liver disease, as well as for several diseases in which a genetic defect affects production of an essential protein by the liver. It may also be considered as treatment for a limited number of carefully selected patients who have liver tumors resectable only by total hepatectomy that have not metastasized outside the liver.

Indications for liver transplantation in adults and children are summarized in Table 28-2. Despite differences in the etiology of these diseases, their shared pathophysiology leads to a common set of symptoms and signs typical of end-stage liver failure. The Child-Turcote-Pugh (CTP) score was established in an attempt to standardize the severity of chronic liver failure by using a reliable set of criteria that reflect the residual function of the liver (Table 28-3). A combination of clinical symptoms and laboratory data are used to provide insight into the severity of the disease and residual function of the liver. In the absence of more reliable methods, the CTP scoring system was adopted as the standard method for placement of patients suffering from end-stage liver disease on the transplant waiting list. Because categorization based on the CTP score was not a continuous scale, waiting time on the list was used to stratify patients within a CTP score group.

In 2002, UNOS put in place a new system for allocation that did not suffer from emphasis on waiting time and subjective clinical parameters (e.g., the degree of ascites or encephalopathy) integral to the CTP system. The overall goal of this major revision to liver allocation was to assign priority to the sickest patients by using a system based on objective variables. To accomplish this, a statistical model for end-stage liver disease (MELD) was used for adult patients that had been shown to have high predictive capacity in identifying patients with end-stage liver disease who were at greatest risk for mortality within 3 months.[17] The MELD score was based on three laboratory values—total bilirubin, international normalized ratio, and creatinine value—and demonstrated better correlation with 3-month survival than the CTP score did (Table 28-4). A similar approach was developed for pediatric patients, although the relevant variables differ slightly (PELD score).

This approach is not applied to urgent patients with fulminant liver failure (status 1 patients) but appears to work well for those with chronic liver disease. It is modified for certain conditions that express unique variables, such as small and potentially curable but nonresectable hepatocellular carcinomas and inborn errors of

Table 28-4 Concordance With 3-Month Mortality: MELD and CTP

SCORE	CONCORDANCE (%)	95% CONFIDENCE INTERVAL (%)
Model for End-Stage Liver Disease (MELD)	0.88	0.85-0.90
Child-Turcote-Pugh (CTP)	0.79	0.75-0.83

metabolism. The system is also adjusted to meet the special needs of children whose liver disease may be characterized by failure to thrive or recurrent cholangitis. It is recognized that no scoring system is perfect at identifying those at greatest risk; however, multiple laboratory tests such as serum levels of hyaluronate and amino-terminal propeptide collagen type III, indocyanine green clearance, or galactose elimination proved no better in quantitation of hepatocyte function or in correlation with the progression of liver disease.

Specific exclusion criteria for liver transplantation have not been formally established, although it is generally agreed that active sepsis and extrahepatic malignancy are absolute contraindications. Still controversial are conditions such as HIV infection in the absence of acquired immunodeficiency syndrome, large-size hepatocellular cancer (>5 cm), or cholangiocarcinoma. Several other entities once considered contraindications to transplantation, such as portal vein thrombosis, are no longer so categorized.

It is essential for the general surgeon to recognize the dynamics of chronic liver disease and to be able to assess residual liver function in the presence of chronic liver disease. It is not uncommon for minor surgical procedures to exhaust the residual reserve and precipitate the development of acute on chronic failure. Management of these complications is extremely difficult. If liver transplantation must be performed during such circumstances, it is associated with higher morbidity and mortality.

Diseases Treated by Liver Transplantation

Conditions that result in end-stage acute or chronic liver failure are different in the pediatric and adult populations. Whereas the incidence of most liver diseases has remained relatively constant over recent times, the prevalence of liver failure from viral hepatitis is increasing as a result of the increased rate of infection in the past 2 decades. It is expected that the relatively recent availability of hepatitis B vaccine and the ability to detect HCV in donated blood will lower the rate of new infections and the number of individuals in whom chronic disease subsequently develops.

Hepatitis B

HBV belongs to a family of closely related DNA viruses called the *hepadnaviruses*. Chronic HBV infection afflicts 1.25 million people in the United States and is characterized serologically by the persistent presence of HBV

DNA and usually HBV antigen in serum. Treatment with recombinant interferon alfa-2b leads to remission in 40% of patients.[18] Persistent infection is associated with a continuous host immune attack against HBV proteins expressed on the surface of the hepatocyte and results in the development of cirrhosis. HBV infection is also a risk factor for hepatocellular carcinoma. As with other forms of liver cancer, tumors associated with hepatitis B result from chronic inflammation and repeated cellular regeneration, typically occurring only after 25 to 30 years of infection. If untreated, most patients with chronic hepatitis B undergoing liver transplantation will reinfect the hepatic graft, and some experience rapidly progressive liver failure. Fortunately, prophylaxis consisting of high-titer hepatitis B immune globulin or antiviral therapy (or both) is highly effective in the control of viral replication and recurrent disease after transplantation.

Hepatitis C

HCV is an RNA virus of the flavivirus family that leads to chronic inflammation of the liver in about 85% of infected individuals. It is detected by the persistence of anti-HCV antibodies, serum viral proteins, and HCV RNA. Histologic features of chronic hepatitis develop in virtually all patients with chronic HCV infection, and cirrhosis develops in as many as 20% of patients within 10 to 20 years of HCV infection. The typical complications of chronic liver disease develop, including portal hypertension, hepatocellular failure, and hepatic encephalopathy. Hepatocellular carcinoma may ensue in 1% to 4% of chronic active hepatitis C patients per year with established cirrhosis.[19] Serial liver biopsies every few years may be an important tool for monitoring the course of chronic hepatitis C because they demonstrate the degree of inflammation and the amount of fibrosis present.

For patients with advanced liver disease, liver transplantation is often the only therapeutic option. The initial results of transplantation are good, with patient and graft survival rates of 85% and 90%, respectively, at 1 year. However, virtually all patients become reinfected with HCV after transplantation, and histologic evidence of chronic hepatitis develops in about half of them within a few months. There is growing concern regarding the eventual recurrence of liver failure in these patients 5 to 10 years after transplantation, and recent evidence indicates that the long-term survival of patients who undergo transplantation for HCV may be significantly inferior to transplantation for other causes of liver disease.[20]

Alcoholic Liver Disease

Alcoholic liver injury results from the toxic effects of ethanol on hepatocytes, accumulation of fatty acids within the cells, and subsequent degeneration and necrosis. The intensity of the inflammatory process is directly related to the amount of alcohol consumed and is associated with fibrosis and subsequent cirrhosis. The coexistence of HCV infection accelerates the liver injury in most cases. Discontinuation of alcohol consumption may arrest hepatocyte destruction and allow regeneration and relatively compensated cirrhosis. Continued deterioration of liver function in the absence of alcohol ingestion plus an appropriate CTP score is an indication for transplantation, just as in other liver diseases. Transplant candidates with alcoholic cirrhosis undergo careful psychosocial evaluation in an attempt to document their sobriety for at least 6 months and the likelihood of post-transplant recidivism. Careful selection results in a low rate of recidivism in most centers. Outcomes of the transplant procedure are similar to those in other disease processes.

Primary Biliary Cirrhosis and Primary Sclerosing Cholangitis

Primary biliary cirrhosis (PBC) and primary sclerosing cholangitis (PSC) share many clinical, biochemical, and pathologic features. Clinically, both give rise to characteristic symptoms and signs of chronic biliary tract disease (e.g., pruritus and jaundice). In both conditions the most characteristic biochemical abnormality is an increased serum alkaline phosphatase level. Central to the pathologic changes in both PBC and PSC is damage to bile ducts; in the case of PBC, the smaller intrahepatic ducts are mainly involved, whereas in PSC, large ducts outside the liver are also affected, as well as the gallbladder and even pancreatic ducts. Unique to PSC is its association with inflammatory bowel disease, which occurs in 70% of the patients. There is an increased incidence of cholangiocarcinoma in PSC patients. Liver failure in both diseases is manifested by hyperbilirubinemia. Transplantation is highly successful in both groups and leads to long-term survival rates higher than 90% and an insignificant incidence of recurrence.

Hepatocellular Carcinoma

The rationale for liver transplantation in patients with nonresectable hepatocellular carcinoma is based on the logical potential of complete removal of disease that is confined to the liver. Unfortunately, it has become evident that in many cases the tumor recurs. However, the procedure can provide significant benefit in a specific subpopulation of patients identified by the following characteristics: histologic grading of G1 to G2, tumor size less than 5 cm, and limited multifocally. The initial workup in all transplant candidates must exclude extrahepatic metastases and macrovascular invasion of the liver on imaging. The results of transplantation in this selected group are variable, but they have been reported to have a disease-free survival rate of 60% to 85% at 3 years. It is yet to be determined whether the addition of pre-transplant measures to gain local tumor regression (e.g., radiofrequency ablation of transcatheter arterial chemoembolization) or the addition of adjuvant chemotherapy after transplantation will improve the control of tumor recurrence.

Biliary Atresia

Extrahepatic biliary atresia is an obliterative cholangiopathy that affects all or part of the extrahepatic biliary tree. The condition occurs in 1 in 10,000 neonates. The diagnosis is suggested in neonates who remain jaundiced for 6 weeks or more after birth and have pale stools and dark urine. By then, the liver is enlarged and firm or hard, a reflection of the presence of underlying portal fibrosis. The Kasai procedure (hepatic portoenterostomy with resection of the obliterated bile ducts and reestablishment of biliary drainage to the intestine) can increase survival rates at the early stage. However, progressive intrahepatic bile duct destruction by chronic inflammation, fibrosis, and cirrhosis commonly occurs. Failure of the Kasai procedure is manifested by failure to thrive, recurrent cholangitis, and typical signs of end-stage liver disease, which are indications for transplantation.

Failure of a Previous Liver Graft

An important and increasingly common indication for transplantation is failure of a previous graft. It occurs in the acute setting immediately after transplantation and is caused by technical failures discussed later or chronically as a result of chronic rejection or disease recurrence. Retransplantation can be particularly complex in the chronic setting because of the usual factors associated with reoperative surgery. Overall, the results of retransplantation are inferior to those achieved with primary grafts, and each subsequent transplant is associated with an additional decrement in survival.

Patient Selection and Preoperative Consideration

Patients who experience progressive deterioration or acute decompensation of preexisting chronic liver disease or previously normal patients in whom fulminant liver failure suddenly develops are candidates for transplantation and need to be referred promptly to a transplant center for evaluation. An extensive workup is performed to assess the degree of liver disease and the potential for recovery, as well as to determine the existence of other extrahepatic conditions that might compromise the outcome of a transplant.

Comprehensive medical assessment is mandatory to establish the candidate's ability to withstand complex major surgery and to determine the potential for long-term survival. Only a few specific contradictions totally preclude transplantation in high-risk candidates (i.e., extrahepatic malignancy, irreversible CNS damage, severe cardiopulmonary failure, or uncontrollable sepsis). In patients with liver failure, deterioration of the kidneys (hepatorenal) and deterioration of the lungs (hepatopulmonary) are well-defined syndromes that may be reversible in the presence of a functioning liver and should not exclude candidates from liver transplantation. Irreversible kidney damage can be managed successfully by combined liver-kidney transplantation.

Assessment of Acute Liver Failure

The hallmarks of fulminant liver failure include the development of encephalopathy, coagulopathy, and hypoglycemia. Careful neurologic evaluation must determine the stage of hepatic coma. Progression from a state of confusion to one of unresponsiveness is associated with an increased likelihood that the brain damage is irreversible. At this stage, assessment must include brain imaging with CT or magnetic resonance imaging, and monitoring of intracranial pressure (ICP) is considered. An attempt is made to help promote cerebral perfusion (>60 mm Hg) by reducing ICP and maintaining high mean arterial pressure. Irreversible injury is associated with persistent elevation of ICP, which leads to the development of severe brain edema and herniation. Other variables that define the extent of liver injury and predict the chance of recovery relate to changes in prothrombin time, levels of factor V, phosphorus levels, and persistence of hypoglycemia. Coagulopathy may be resistant to correction but is best treated by transfusion of fresh frozen plasma. Plasmapheresis may be beneficial in small children, in whom administration of large fluid volumes is problematic. Severe hypoglycemia is usually controlled by dextrose infusion. Interestingly, changes in liver transaminases are not reliable indicators of the potential for recovery.

Superimposed acute liver failure in patients with chronic liver disease may have a clinical manifestation similar to that of fulminant liver failure in previously normal patients. In most cases the precipitating factor is related to acute bleeding or infection. Management is directed toward resuscitation and control of the bleeding or infection. Ideally, successful stabilization and clinical improvement are followed by urgent transplantation. However, these candidates are at higher risk for morbidity and mortality, mostly because of the development of bacterial and fungal infections. The surgeon must use clinical judgment to determine the presence of irreversible multiorgan system failure and avoid unnecessary or futile transplantation.

In the absence of definitive therapy for most types of liver disease, it must be expected that the natural course of decompensated liver disease will lead to worsening of the patient's general condition and the development of life-threatening complications, including variceal bleeding, hepatic encephalopathy, spontaneous bacterial peritonitis, and hepatorenal syndrome. Unfortunately, there are few effective means to prevent such complications. Thus, patients who are judged to be at risk for decompensation are given priority for urgent transplantation.

Donor Assessment

A major limitation to clinical transplantation is the availability of organ donors. Appropriate management of brain-dead donors and avoidance of damage to the graft during the procurement procedure are essential in securing optimal function of the transplant. It is important to establish aggressive donor management protocols to minimize the adverse physiologic consequences of brain death. These protocols include respiratory and hemodynamic support, adequate fluid resuscitation, and the initiation of hormone replacement. Brain death is associated with significant instability, and minute-to-minute management by experienced personnel in the intensive care unit (ICU) is necessary to ensure adequate perfusion of all organs. Simultaneously, the donor's liver function must be determined. Rapid screening and serial follow-up of liver enzymes and synthetic function are performed to determine the degree of liver injury and predict the potential for recovery. Routine assessment for diseases that might be transmitted by the liver graft must include hepatitis screening, as well as any history of the use of toxic substances such as long-standing alcohol consumption.

The donor shortage has led to more frequent use of livers that would have been discarded in the past. The terms *marginal donor* and *expanded criteria donor* have evolved as transplant programs have been forced to consider suboptimal donors, including older donors, hepatitis C– and hepatitis B core antibody–positive donors, and livers with a moderate amount of steatosis (up to 30%). Although donor age has been shown to have an adverse impact on outcome, most programs now consider the use of donors up to 75 or 80 years of age. This approach has been necessary because of the desperate need for lifesaving organs and is supported by scientific evidence of a relatively slow aging process occurring within the liver parenchyma. It also appears that grafts from donors with serology positive for a pathogen present in the recipient (i.e., hepatitis B or C) can be used with results equal to those of transplantation with uninfected grafts, as long as the liver does not have established severe hepatitis or fibrosis.[20] Severe steatosis in liver grafts is associated with a high degree of primary nonfunction, but acceptable results can be obtained if the steatosis is mild to moderate (10%-30%). Whenever a marginal graft is used, controllable variables, such as cold ischemic time, need to be kept to a minimum.

Donor and recipient matching are based on ABO blood group compatibility and size. However, these barriers may be crossed when transplantation is urgent. Most surgeons try to match donor-recipient age for pediatric recipients because variation may have an impact on long-term graft survival.

Donor Operation

Liver procurement is almost always part of a multiteam approach aiming to maximize the number of transplantable organs that can be recovered from a single donor. A midline incision extending from the suprasternal notch to the symphysis pubis allows access to the thoracic and abdominal organs. The round ligament is ligated and divided, the falciform ligament is incised, and the left lateral segment is freed from the diaphragm. Inspection of the gastrohepatic ligament will reveal a replaced left hepatic artery. Medial reflection of the right colon and small bowel allows exposure of the infrahepatic vena cava and renal veins, control of the distal aorta, and identification of the inferior mesenteric vein.

Attention is then turned to the hepatoduodenal ligament, where a variable order of dissection is performed with the aim of identifying one or more of the structures, including the common hepatic artery, common bile duct, and portal vein. Attention must be directed toward preservation of aberrant or accessory arteries to the liver, or both. Technique varies between procurement surgeons, with some preferring to perform the majority of the dissection while the heart is still beating and others first identifying the basic anatomy and then completing the dissection after cold perfusion. After all teams complete the dissection of all organs, the donor is heparinized, followed by perfusion with cold preservation solution via cannulas inserted in the distal aorta and a branch of the portal vein and placement of topical ice. The liver is then removed with the entire length of the celiac artery or any other accessory or replaced arteries, a significant length of the portal vein, the common bile duct, and the entire retrohepatic vena cava (Fig. 28-4). Further preparation of the graft before transplantation is done on the bench while the liver is kept immersed in ice. Such preparation usually includes removal of the diaphragm and excess tissue around the blood vessels and, if necessary, reconstruction of the replaced hepatic arteries to one common trunk.

The tolerance of liver grafts to extended periods of cold ischemia depends on the composition of the preservation solution, donor age, the presence of steatosis, and hemodynamic stability before procurement. In theory, UW preservation solution may extend the cold ischemia time up to 24 hours before revascularization. However, most experienced surgeons prefer to minimize the length of cold ischemia to less than 10 hours.

Recipient Operation

The unpredictable nature of organ availability dictates that most liver transplants be done without extensive preoperative preparation of the recipient. Most patients do not need complete bowel preparation, but they receive preoperative prophylaxis with antibiotics to cover grampositive and gram-negative bacteria. Administration of immunosuppressive agents before transplantation is dictated by the specific protocol being used.

Anesthesia management in most cases begins by preparation for continuous monitoring of arterial blood pressure, pulmonary artery pressure, and cardiac output. Large-bore IV cannulas and a rapid infuser may be inserted in anticipation of possible major blood loss. Correction of coagulopathy and replacement of blood lost is initiated early in the operation before any possible extensive bleeding or the development of significant circulatory compromise.

Orthotopic liver transplantation is a three-step surgical procedure, with each step presenting different unique challenges for surgeons and anesthesiologists.

Recipient Hepatectomy

The abdominal cavity is entered via a bilateral subcostal incision with a midline extension toward the xiphoid. The round ligament is clamped, divided, and ligated. Exploration of the abdominal cavity is performed, and any accumulated ascites is removed. The falciform ligament is divided down to the suprahepatic vena cava. Placement of an appropriate mechanical retractor allows adequate exposure of the liver and its attachments. At this stage the left lateral segment is separated from the diaphragm and the hepatogastric ligament is divided. The rest of the dissection is done on the hepatoduodenal ligament. The right and left branches of the hepatic artery are then ligated and divided at the hilum. Similarly, the common bile and cystic ducts are ligated and divided. At this stage the portal vein is skeletonized. The rest of the

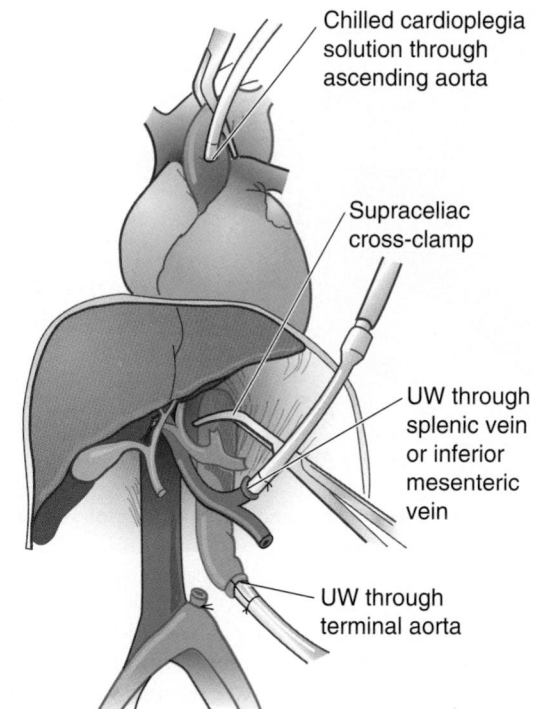

Figure 28-4 Liver cadaveric donor operation. UW, University of Wisconsin solution.

Chilled cardioplegia solution through ascending aorta

Supraceliac cross-clamp

UW through splenic vein or inferior mesenteric vein

UW through terminal aorta

dissection includes detachment of the liver from the retroperitoneum (bare area) and exposure of the infrahepatic and suprahepatic vena cava. Clamps are then placed on the portal vein and suprahepatic vena cava, and the liver is removed. To keep blood loss to a minimum, the majority of the dissection is carried out with electrocautery, and hemostasis is achieved with the argon beam coagulator.

This standard technique is slightly modified in some centers, specifically with regard to the surgeon's preference for the use of venovenous bypass. The reduction of venous blood return from the portal system and the infrahepatic inferior vena cava may result in hemodynamic instability and portal venous congestion. This problem can be avoided by inflow cannulation of the portal and femoral/iliac veins (by either percutaneous or cutdown techniques) and outflow via a cannula in the internal jugular vein to allow return of more than 2.5 L/min. Additional important advantages of this technique include control of body temperature with the use of a warming circuit and the potential for ultrafiltration with attached filters. Many surgeons do not advocate routine use of venovenous bypass and contend that most patients can tolerate clamping of the portal vein and that the entire vena cava may be preserved without interrupting blood flow.

Anhepatic Phase

After hemostasis, the retroperitoneum may be reapproximated to cover the bare area. The suprahepatic vena caval cuff is prepared by opening the orifice of the right, middle, and left hepatic veins and oversewing the phrenic

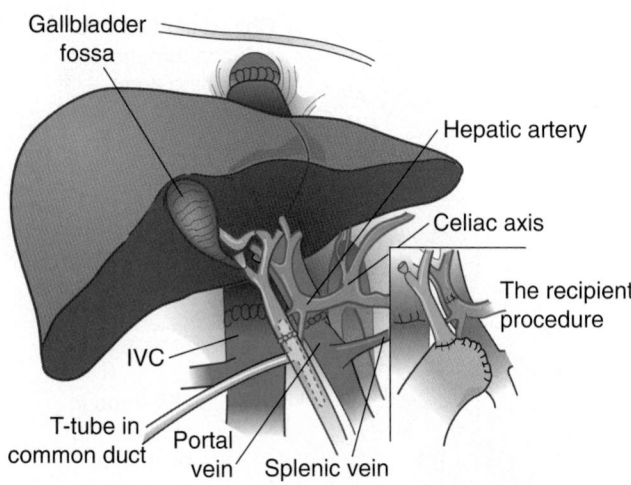

Figure 28-5 Liver recipient operation. IVC, inferior vena cava.

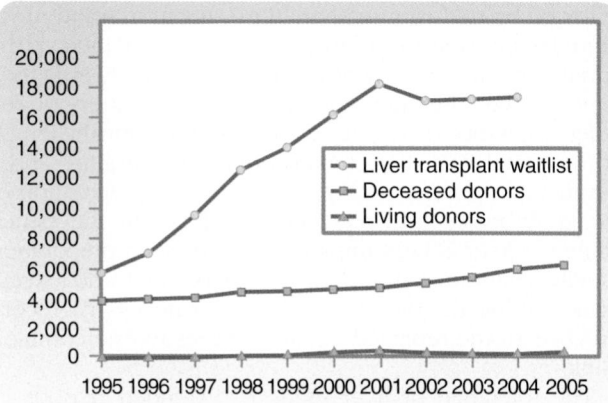

Figure 28-6 Growth in liver transplantation.

branches. Transplantation is done by end-to-end anastomosis of the donor and recipient suprahepatic venae cava, followed by similar end-to-end anastomosis of the infrahepatic venae cavae. Alternatively, an end-to-side anastomosis of the vena cavae may be performed in a piggyback fashion in which the recipient's entire vena cava is left intact. The preservation solution is next flushed out with lactated Ringer's solution, the portal bypass cannula is removed, and portal vein anastomosis is carried out via a continuous suture with the use of a growth factor to prevent stenosis at this anastomosis. The clamps are then released, and the liver is reperfused with portal blood. This part of the procedure is critical and is characterized by varying degrees of *reperfusion syndrome,* which is manifested by hypotension, bradycardia, arrhythmias, and rarely, cardiac arrest because of a sudden influx of cold, hyperkalemic, acidotic blood into the heart.

Arterial Revascularization and Biliary Reconstruction

After hemostasis and reperfusion, the recipient hepatic artery is freed from surrounding tissue. The preferred method for reconstruction is an end-to-end anastomosis using an aortic Carrel patch of the donor celiac artery and a branch patch of the recipient artery at the level of the gastroduodenal bifurcation. This method allows the creation of a relatively wide anastomosis and minimizes the potential for hepatic artery thrombosis. In most cases, biliary drainage can be achieved with a duct-to-duct anastomosis with or without placement of a T tube. Alternatively, pathology of the bile duct, such as the presence of PSC or biliary atresia, requires biliary drainage via a choledochojejunostomy. Completion of this phase is demonstrated in Figure 28-5. After adequate hemostasis, three drains are placed around the liver, and the abdominal cavity is closed.

Segmental and Lobar Liver Transplantation

The necessity to maximize the number of liver grafts has led to several surgical innovations, including transplanta-

tion of so-called split livers from cadaveric and living donors. These procedures are possible by virtue of the unique segmental anatomy of the liver and its regenerative capacity. For pediatric recipients, transplantation of left lateral segments split from cadaveric donors or a living donor has become standard practice. Especially for very young children, for whom cadaveric grafts of the appropriate size are rare, the availability of these options in addition to whole cadaveric grafts has led to a significant reduction in waiting time for pediatric patients and a reduction in waiting list mortality.

Translating this experience to benefit adults awaiting transplantation required the development of new approaches. The limitation of segmental liver graft transplantation for larger adult recipients is related to the minimum liver mass necessary for adequate support of the recipient in the immediate post-transplant period. It is generally accepted that a graft–to–body weight ratio of greater than 1% would allow adequate physiologic function. For this reason, right lobe grafts have recently been favored for live donor transplantation in adults.[21] Removal of up to 60% of the donor's liver mass is naturally associated with greater potential for morbidity and mortality than is a left lateral segmentectomy used for small children. This had led to cautious application of the procedure at experienced centers to target patients who are at risk for waiting list mortality before a cadaveric donor liver becomes available. Thus, frequent recipients in this group have been patients with hepatocellular carcinoma and those in whom the MELD score is thought to underestimate the patient's risk for mortality. This approach is reflected in the fact that the average MELD score of living donor liver recipients is less than 20 whereas in those receiving cadaveric grafts it is nearly 25. Because of the continuously increasing number of patients awaiting transplantation, there has been an increase in living donor liver transplantation that peaked at 519 such procedures in 2002 but fell to approximately 300 to 350 per year since implementation of the MELD-based allocation system in 2002. In 2005, 321 living donor liver transplants were performed (Fig. 28-6).

Recent analysis of recipients of living donor right lobe grafts has documented that a massive amount of regeneration occurs in the first 1 to 2 weeks. Recipients of partial grafts have rapid proliferation of liver mass, with the majority reaching a calculated standard liver volume by 1 month. The donors, however, do not reach their complete starting volume, even by 1 year. This is contrary to what was believed and different from rodent models and remains to be studied in detail in the human setting. It also became apparent that the graft-to-recipient size ratio was critical inasmuch as grafts that were too small had decreased survival. These findings correlated with clinical experience in that small-for-size grafts regenerate to an appropriate size for the recipient; however, there was significant functional impairment of grafts that were less than 50% of expected weight, as demonstrated by prolonged cholestasis and histologic changes consistent with ischemic injury. Liver grafts with a graft weight/standard liver volume of less than 40% have poor graft survival and prolonged hyperbilirubinemia.

Removal of a segment from a living donor, or an attempt to split a cadaveric liver for use in two recipients, is a complex procedure that requires precise knowledge of the hepatic anatomy of the donor. In the case of a living donor, the surgeon's primary responsibility is to remove the donated segment without harming the donor. Similarly, splitting a cadaveric liver needs to be done without compromising either segment. Preoperative assessment of the live or cadaveric donor is similar to that described previously. In addition, it is helpful to perform imaging studies in a living donor before surgery to determine the volume of the donated segment and its vascular supply.

The living donor operation is begun before the recipient hepatectomy and includes isolation of the individual branches of the hepatic artery, portal vein, and bile duct leading to the donated segment. The liver is separated from the vena cava, which is left intact, and all small hepatic vein branches are ligated. Further preparation includes isolation of the main hepatic vein, which provides the outflow tract. Completion of hepatic parenchymal division is done via careful dissection along anatomic planes by using the finger fracture technique, the harmonic scalpel, or the Cavitron ultrasonic aspirator (Fig. 28-7). It is important to preserve intact blood flow to the segment until after transection of the hepatic parenchyma, at which point the vessels are clamped and transected and the segment is flushed with cold preservation solution. To minimize cold ischemia time, the recipient operation is started once the donor anatomy is clearly identified to be favorable and the parenchyma is dissected. The diseased liver is then completely removed from the recipient when the donated segment is available for transplantation.

Transplantation of the donated lobe is performed by techniques similar to those developed for whole liver grafts, with a few modifications: the entire length of the recipient vena cava is preserved, and the lobe is transplanted in piggyback fashion. The graft is placed in the usual anatomic position to allow anastomoses of the portal vein and the hepatic artery without the need for interposition grafts. In most cases, bile duct reconstruction is done via hepaticojejunostomy.

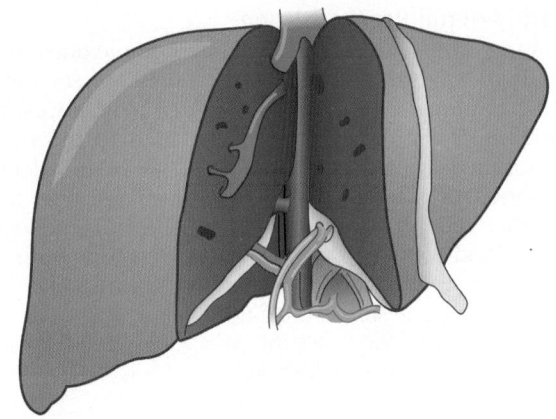

Figure 28-7 Living donor right lobe procedure.

Safety issues are of the highest priority for a living donor. Careful selection of the candidate, combined with fastidious surgical technique, minimize any potential complications. Early data regarding donor morbidity and mortality in adult-to-adult cases suggest that the procedure can be performed with a high degree of safety. Nonetheless, donor mortality from the procedure has been reported. In addition, the recipient of these grafts may have an increased risk for postoperative complications such as bleeding or bile leakage from the cut surface and potential short- and long-term problems with the biliary-enteric anastomosis. This reinforces the notion that living donor transplantation for adult recipients is reserved for those who are unlikely to undergo transplantation in time with conventional cadaveric transplantation.

Operative Complexities and Complications

Operative Bleeding

Excessive bleeding from portal hypertension may occur during hepatectomy and is likely to be accentuated by coagulopathy or adhesions from previous surgery. Removal of the cirrhotic organ, transplantation of a graft with normal function, and correction of coagulopathy by the appropriate use of platelets and fresh frozen plasma best control bleeding during hepatectomy and after reperfusion.

Thrombosis of the Portal Vein

Dissection may be more complex in the presence of a partially or totally thrombosed portal vein. In most cases the thrombosed portion extends to the bifurcation of the splenic/superior mesenteric vein confluence, and the thrombus can be removed by endarterectomy techniques while preserving an intact main portal vein. Rarely, a vein graft to the superior mesenteric vein may be necessary. Complete occlusion of the portal venous system is not an absolute contraindication to transplantation because the infrahepatic vena cava can be anastomosed to the donor portal vein to provide adequate venous flow. At times, a large collateral vein such as the coronary may be used for inflow.

Hepatic Arterial Reconstruction

The surgeon is faced with arterial complexities more often than venous abnormalities. Intimal dissection or other pathology of the hepatic artery may necessitate placement of an allogeneic vascular graft to the recipient's supraceliac or infrarenal aorta. The potential need for venous or arterial grafts for revascularization mandates that the procuring team always obtain adequate donor blood vessels for potential extension grafts. In addition, any unused blood vessel grafts must be kept refrigerated under sterile conditions for a few days after transplantation in the event of emergency need for subsequent vascular reconstruction.

Post-transplant Management

Liver transplant recipients may require a short stay in the ICU after surgery. This period is used to observe recovery of the graft and ensure hemodynamic and respiratory stability, as well as adequate kidney function. The principles of care are similar to those for other critically ill patients in the ICU setting but are rendered more complex by the necessity for immunosuppressive therapy. Common complications encountered in the early postoperative period are related to initial graft function, technical misadventures, infections, and rejection. Treatment with antirejection drugs may be associated with the development of several serious side effects such as metabolic encephalopathy, hypertension, and diabetes.

Common Complications

Primary Nonfunction

The mechanisms of immediate graft failure after successful revascularization of the transplanted liver are not completely understood but may relate to donor variables, inadequate preservation, prolonged cold ischemia time, or the humoral immune response. This problem is encountered in 2% to 5% of liver grafts. It is characterized by clinical and laboratory findings indicating poor synthetic function and severe hepatocyte injury. Postoperatively, the recipient may exhibit progressive hemodynamic instability, multiorgan system failure, and encephalopathy. Laboratory findings demonstrate worsening acidosis, coagulopathy, and extremely elevated liver enzymes (lactate dehydrogenase, aspartate aminotransferase, and alanine aminotransferase). The development of primary nonfunction is a surgical emergency that can be successfully treated by early retransplantation. Failure to find a suitable graft within 7 days is associated with higher morbidity and mortality. Delayed nonfunction of the graft is characterized by failure of all liver functions, which leads to persistent coagulopathy and progressive hyperbilirubinemia. In these circumstances vital organs fail or infection ensues (or both), in most cases rapidly leading to death from bacterial or fungal sepsis.

Intra-abdominal Bleeding

Persistence of immediate post-transplant coagulopathy, fibrinolysis, and the presence of multiple vascular anastomoses place these patients at high risk for postoperative bleeding. However, the coagulopathy spontaneously corrects in the presence of recovering liver graft function and with infusion of platelets. A persistent drop in hemoglobin and a need for transfusion of more than 6 units of packed red blood cells are usually indications for re-exploration and evacuation of the hematoma. In most cases, removal of the clot will be sufficient to arrest further fibrinolysis and will stop the bleeding. Occasionally, it will be necessary to repair the bleeding sites.

Vascular Thrombosis

Vascular complications after liver transplantation are more common in the pediatric population and are directly related to the small size of the vessels used for reconstruction. The most frequent complication is hepatic artery thrombosis, which can be manifested as rapid or indolent worsening of graft function or as necrosis of the bile duct and dehiscence of the biliary-enteric anastomosis. Early recognition and successful thrombectomy may salvage the graft. However, deteriorating liver function and bile duct necrosis indicate the need for immediate retransplantation.

Biliary Leak

Reconstruction of the biliary system by either duct-to-duct anastomosis or choledochojejunostomy may be complicated by a bile leak, usually secondary to a technical error or ischemia of the donor duct. Early leakage can be diagnosed by the appearance of bile in the drains and is confirmed by T-tube cholangiography, hepato-iminodiacetic acid (HIDA) scanning, or endoscopic retrograde cholangiopancreatography (ERCP). Surgical exploration and revision of the anastomosis or stenting of the anastomosis by ERCP are mandatory and will solve the problem in most cases. However, a leak secondary to ischemic bile duct injury as a result of early hepatic artery thrombosis is an indication for urgent retransplantation.

Infections

Infections remain the most significant complications in liver transplantation and are responsible for most of the mortality in the early postoperative period. There seems to be a direct correlation between the preoperative status of the recipient, the pattern of recovery after transplantation, and the incidence of bacterial and fungal infections. The probability for the development of such complications is highest in patients who await a transplant in an ICU. These chronically ill and malnourished patients are unusually susceptible to resistant hospital flora before surgery and are then placed at further risk for infection by high-dose immunosuppression after the procedure. The development of organ system failure or graft malfunction further contributes to the morbid outcome. The spectrum of infection is evolving to more frequent infection by resistant gram-positive bacteria (enterococci and staphylococci) than by gram-negative bacteria. The deliberate use of broad-spectrum antibiotics in immunosuppressed patients contributes in part to the development of systemic fungal infection (*Candida, Aspergillus*). It is wise to begin antibiotic therapy for common bacteria as soon as a patient's clinical status suggests the presence of infection. The treatment can then be modified when and if results of culture and sensitivity studies dictate a change.

Immunologic Aspects of Liver Transplantation

The relatively low immunogenicity of liver allografts and the unique ability of the liver to regenerate are probably the main reasons for the excellent long-term outcome. Good results are achieved when graft and recipient are ABO blood group compatible. Preoperative HLA matching does not appear to be necessary and has not been shown to afford any benefit. Most recipients are treated with combination therapy that includes a calcineurin inhibitor (cyclosporine or tacrolimus), along with prednisone, with or without azathioprine or MMF. Protocols are adjusted for rapid taper of corticosteroids within the first 3 to 6 months after surgery and a significant reduction in the dose of the calcineurin inhibitor. Long-term maintenance of immunosuppression seems to be necessary in most recipients because complete cessation of immunosuppression carries significant risk for the development of acute and chronic rejection.

Acute Rejection

T-cell–mediated acute rejection is seen at a rate of 30% to 50% within the first 6 months after transplantation, most often within the first 10 days. The clinical findings are variable and may include the development of fever, abdominal pain, and elevated liver enzymes and bilirubin. Patients with a T-tube may manifest a decrease in quantity and a change in the character of bile. The diagnosis is confirmed by a liver biopsy demonstrating the presence of a periportal lymphocytic infiltrate that extends into the liver parenchyma, as well as invasion of inflammatory cells into the vascular endothelium. Most rejection episodes are responsive to the administration of high-dose corticosteroids. More potent monoclonal or polyclonal anti–T-cell antibodies are effective against corticosteroid-resistant rejection and lead to reversal of the acute episode in more than 90% of recipients. Rejection seems to be less responsive if an acute episode occurs long after transplantation or in the case of chronic rejection.

Chronic Rejection

This type of rejection is seen months or years after transplantation. It is manifested by poor synthetic liver function and hyperbilirubinemia. Chronic rejection is usually characterized histologically by paucity of the bile ducts and is thus often described as *vanishing bile duct syndrome*. The etiology of this phenomenon is not well understood and may be related to a humoral reaction involving antibodies and fibrogenic cytokines. Treatment of chronic rejection is limited, and some of these patients may be considered candidates for retransplantation.

Recurrent Disease

Replacement of the liver may not permanently cure recipients of their original disease. Recurrence of viral hepatitis is likely within a short time after transplantation in infected recipients. Control of active HBV infection is possible in most patients with lamivudine, which inhibits viral DNA polymerase, as well as with hepatitis B immune globulin. In contrast, interferon alfa or ribavirin, or both, are less effective in HCV infection. Reinfection of the liver graft may be mild and in many cases will not result in liver failure. Retransplantation for recurrent hepatitis B or C remains controversial. The obvious recurrence of viral hepatitis contrasts with reports describing the pattern of early pathologic findings seen in patients who undergo transplantation for PBC and PSC. The significance of these findings is not clear because they rarely result in liver failure necessitating retransplantation.

Most liver transplant recipients who survive the immediate post-transplant period enjoy full functional recovery. However, restoration of a fully functional status depends on the patient's preoperative condition, an appropriate support system, and the patient's attitude toward rehabilitation.

Long-Term Results

The number of cadaveric liver transplants performed has steadily risen from about 5000 in 2002 to more than 6000 in 2005. At the end of 2005, over 17,000 patients were listed for liver transplantation. UNOS registry data on more than 78,000 liver transplants performed since 1988 demonstrate impressive long-term survival. At 5 years, adult patient survival rates exceed 70%. The results in children are even better, with more than 80% surviving at 5 years (Fig. 28-8).

Morbidity and mortality after orthotopic liver transplantation directly correlate with the recipient's preoperative status and immediate function of the liver allograft. Higher mortality has been reported in recipients whose UNOS status was categorized as urgent and those who

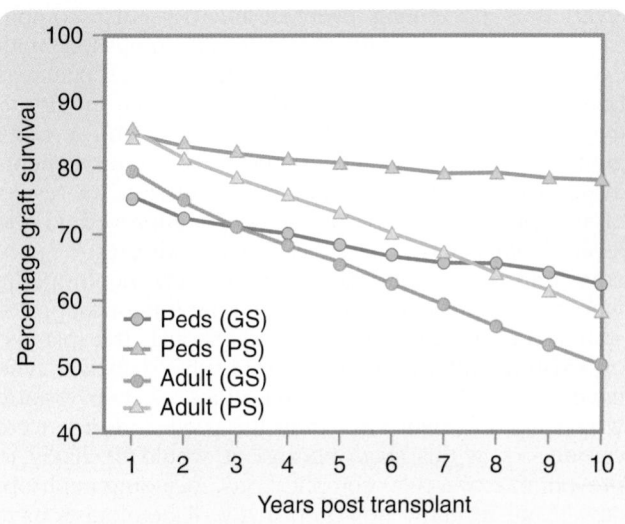

Figure 28-8 Pediatric (Peds) versus adult liver transplant survival. GS, graft survival; PS, patient survival.

had multiorgan system failure. Other variables associated with decreased survival include older age, ventilator dependency, pretransplant need for dialysis, and retransplantation. It is controversial whether scarce livers should be used in these circumstances because there would be greater chance of long-term function in patients who are less seriously ill. Stratification of recipients by MELD score also correlates with observed post-transplant survival. If the MELD score is higher than 25, the 1-year survival rate is less (85%) than in groups with lower scores (MELD score of 19-24, 88% at 1 year; MELD score <19, 90% at 1 year). However, the rationale for continuing to perform transplantation in the sickest patients is their unquestionably poor outcome without a transplant. In fact, a variety of analyses suggest that transplantation in patients even at the highest MELD scores results in the greatest gain based on the total number of life-years saved.

Overall, long-term survival after liver transplantation is excellent; however, recipients may suffer from significant side effects of the immunosuppressive drugs. Physical and psychosocial growth may be inhibited in the pediatric group. In contrast, most adults will experience an average gain in weight of 15 to 20 lb. Recognized outcomes of corticosteroid and calcineurin inhibitors include renal failure, osteoporosis, hypertension, hyperglycemia, and hyperlipidemia. Recipients have an increased incidence of malignancy, particularly PTLD. This condition can often be resolved by a reduction or complete withdrawal of corticosteroids and a significant reduction in cyclosporine or tacrolimus. However, attempts to stop all immunosuppression usually result in the development of acute or chronic rejection, or both.

PANCREATIC TRANSPLANTATION

The purpose of pancreas transplantation is complete normalization of the diabetic recipient's blood glucose level, thus preventing eventual microvascular complications, a result unlikely to be accomplished with exogenous insulin therapy. The outcome of pancreas transplantation in the 1960s and 1970s was far inferior to that with other organs (frequent fatalities and a <20% graft survival rate). However, because of improvements in surgical technique and immunosuppression, the results of the procedure have progressively improved to the level of other transplants. The usual candidates for pancreas transplants are patients with diabetic nephropathy who are obligated to undergo chronic immunosuppression to prevent rejection of a simultaneously transplanted or existing kidney allograft. Ironically, diabetics who have no renal or other complications of their disease would likely benefit most from the procedure if it were carried out at this stage because it would be likely to prevent microvascular complications, including nephropathy. Until recently, however, many diabetologists have been reluctant to recommend pancreatic transplantation in nonuremic diabetics because it would expose them to the risks associated with chronic immunosuppression.

Indications for Pancreas Transplantation and Patient Selection

Because insulin is effective therapy for most diabetics (except for its failure to prevent eventual microvascular complications), pancreas transplantation is not considered a lifesaving procedure unless the patient is experiencing episodes of severe hypoglycemic unawareness. Thus, in considering pancreas transplantation, the requisite dangers of a major operation and lifelong immunosuppression must be balanced against the possible benefits.

The evidence is now convincing that minimizing hyperglycemia by optimizing exogenous insulin therapy favorably influences the progression of microvascular complications. That successful pancreas transplantation would also do so is based on softer evidence, although the assumption seems quite safe that the even better control of hyperglycemia associated with this method would provide optimal protection from complications. Microvascular sequelae, such as ocular, neurologic, and renal disabilities, will eventually occur in more than 50% of diabetics receiving insulin therapy. Thus, the possibility of achieving glucose homeostasis by pancreas transplantation and avoiding microvascular complications is very attractive to patients, including many with advanced complications in whom objective analysis of the risks and benefits does not support its use. It is important for patients to understand that advanced complications (e.g., blindness, pregangrenous extremities, end-stage nephropathy) will not be reversed. Transplant surgeons are the best positioned to understand the risks and benefits and, along with their diabetologist colleagues, serve as patients' advisors and advocates in considering transplantation. Because of the poor results of transplantation in the precyclosporine era, most clinicians then considered the risk unacceptable. Even now that success is more common, only a relatively small proportion of the world's many diabetics are appropriate candidates for pancreatic transplantation.

Because of the prevalence of microvascular disease in diabetics, especially in the coronary arteries, evaluation of the risks associated with major surgery is especially important. Indeed, one of the most common causes of pancreas transplant failure is death from myocardial infarction. Therefore, if substantial coronary artery disease is identified, it may need to be corrected before transplantation is undertaken.

Uremic type 1 diabetics who are candidates for cadaver donor kidney transplants account for the majority of patients to be considered for pancreas transplantation, which is most often carried out simultaneously with kidney transplantation. Also appropriate for pancreas transplantation are diabetics who harbor a previously transplanted, functioning kidney allograft because they are already committed to immunosuppression. In nonuremic diabetics who either do not need a kidney transplant or have not previously had one, the indications for pancreas transplantation are controversial. However, extremely labile diabetics who are at substantial risk from repeated episodes of dangerous hypoglycemia are considered for transplantation even if they are not uremic.

In patients with seemingly early diabetic nephropathy, the presence of macroalbuminemia or microalbuminuria indicates that significant renal disease exists and that it will eventually progress to end-stage disease if they remain diabetic. In these cases it seems likely that progression of the nephropathy could be halted, or at least slowed, by successful pancreas transplantation, although actual evidence for this effect is scarce because the procedure has been uncommon in this early stage. According to the International Pancreas Transplant Registry, between 1988 and 2004 more than 15,000 pancreas transplants were performed in the United States; about 78% were simultaneous pancreas-kidney (SPK) transplants, 16% were pancreas-after-kidney (PAK) transplants, and only 7% were pancreas transplants alone (PTA). The proportion of PAK and PTA grafts has steadily increased; in 2003 these categories combined represented 33% of all pancreas transplants.

Donor Selection and Management

Selection of acceptable cadaveric donors of pancreas allografts is based on standard criteria, with avoidance of donors who are aged, infected, hemodynamically unstable, or afflicted with malignancies. Hyperglycemia occurring after brain death is not necessarily a deterrent because this finding may be the result of an insulin-resistant state that often develops after head trauma. Serum amylase levels are not particularly helpful in evaluating prospective donors. Inspection of the pancreas by an experienced observer at the time of organ recovery is probably the best indicator of whether the pancreas is suitable for transplantation. The outcome of the transplant also appears to be strongly influenced by the care and expertise with which the donor operation is conducted.

The Donor Operation

Whenever possible, multiorgan en bloc excision is performed so that several transplantable organs can be obtained from the same donor. Through a midline abdominal incision (extended from the midline thoracic incision usually made for removal of the heart or lungs), the abdominal viscera are inspected. The blood supply to the liver is evaluated because anomalies in its arterial circulation occasionally preclude use of both the pancreas and the liver. If both organs cannot be used safely, priority must be granted to the liver because it is a life-saving organ.

Once the decision is made that both the pancreas and liver can be recovered, the gastrocolic ligament is divided to expose the anterior surface of the pancreas. The transverse colon is mobilized to allow the pancreas to be freed from the surrounding retroperitoneal tissues. The short gastric vessels are ligated and divided. The left gastric vessels are ligated and divided near the stomach to preserve the blood supply to the liver via the celiac axis. After a povidone-iodine/amphotericin/antibiotic solution

is instilled into the duodenal segment through a nasogastric tube, the duodenum is divided just distal to the pylorus.

Division of the lienophrenic ligament allows mobilization of the pancreaticoduodenal allograft. The pancreas is freed from its posterior attachments to the left kidney and the left adrenal gland. The spleen is left in continuity with the pancreas to serve as a handle to minimize manipulation of the pancreas. The celiac axis and superior mesenteric and splenic arteries are dissected from the surrounding lymphatic tissue and celiac ganglion. The infrahepatic inferior vena cava is exposed above the renal veins to facilitate division of the inferior vena cava after in situ irrigation of the donor organs with a cooled preservation solution. If both the liver and pancreas are to be used, the gastroduodenal artery is ligated and divided. If only the pancreas is to be transplanted, this artery is left intact. The common bile duct is ligated and divided close to the pancreas. Through an opening in the gallbladder, the biliary ducts are irrigated with normal saline solution until clear of bile. A Kocher maneuver is performed to mobilize the head of the pancreas. The hepatic artery is freed from the surrounding lymphatics, and the proximal 1 to 2 cm of the splenic artery is dissected to complete exposure of the portal triad structures.

The donor is then systemically heparinized. The jejunum at the level of the ligament of Treitz is divided with a GIA stapler. The abdominal aorta is ligated at its bifurcation and cannulated for perfusion. The supraceliac aorta is then clamped and the portal vein divided about 1 cm cephalad to the superior margin of the pancreas. An in situ arterial flush with UW solution cooled to 4°C is begun, and the suprahepatic vena cava is divided. The liver can also be flushed through the open end of the portal vein (Fig. 28-9). Topical cooling of the liver and pancreas is also carried out. If the liver and pancreas are

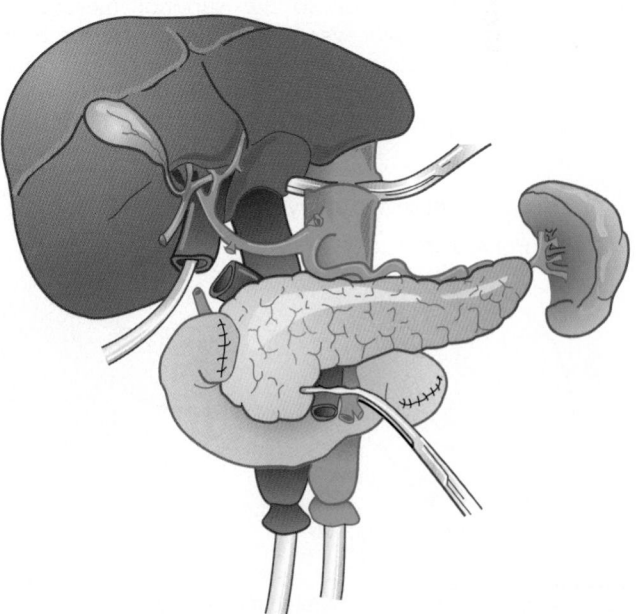

Figure 28-9 En bloc liver-pancreas recovery.

procured en bloc, the portal vein is not divided in situ and the portal circulation can be flushed through the inferior mesenteric vein.

The pancreas and the liver can be separated in situ or ex vivo. If the liver is to be used, the celiac axis is usually left in continuity with the hepatic artery. The splenic artery is divided about 0.5 cm beyond its origin from the celiac trunk. The mesentery of the small intestine, which courses through the parenchyma of the pancreas, is divided inferior to the pancreas either by individual ligature of the mesenteric vessels or by en mass occlusion with a TA90 stapler. This completes the pancreas dissection. Long segments of the common, internal, and external iliac arteries and veins are also removed for use as vascular extension grafts if necessary.

Ex Vivo Preparation of the Donor Pancreas for Transplantation

The pancreaticoduodenal graft is submerged in a basin of cold UW solution for further preparation. The splenic hilar vessels are ligated and the spleen removed while avoiding injury to the tail of the pancreas. About 5 cm of duodenum beyond the ampulla of Vater are retained with the graft. It is important to be sure that the proximal duodenum was divided distal to the pylorus and that no gastric mucosa is transplanted with the graft. If the mesenteric axis was divided with staples, the staple line is reinforced with running suture.

Commonly, an arterial extension Y graft is used to facilitate the transplant operation so that only one arterial anastomosis will be required in the recipient. The external iliac artery of the extension graft is anastomosed to the superior mesenteric artery of the pancreas graft, and the internal iliac artery of the extension graft is anastomosed to the stump of the splenic artery of the pancreas graft (Fig. 28-10). If there is sufficient length of both arteries, the splenic artery of the pancreas graft can be anastomosed end to side to the superior mesenteric artery. If the donor liver was not procured or if the liver team allowed the celiac axis to remain with the pancreas graft, a patch of aorta, including the origins of the celiac axis and the superior mesenteric artery, is available for

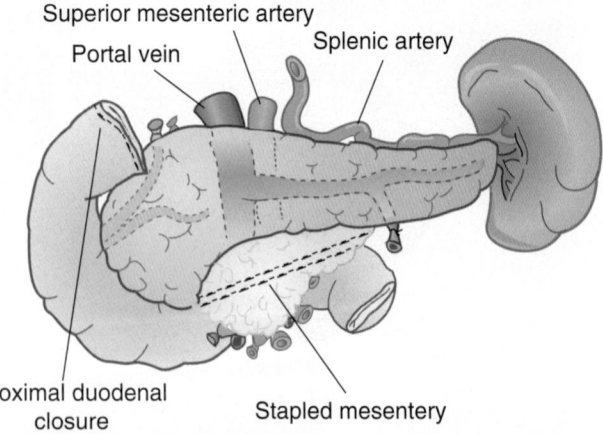

Superior mesenteric artery

Portal vein

Splenic artery

Proximal duodenal closure

Stapled mesentery

Figure 28-10 Pancreatic allograft.

anastomosis directly to the recipient's vessels. An extension of the portal vein can be fashioned from the external iliac vein of the donor, but this is rarely necessary and may be associated with an increased risk for thrombosis of the portal vein.

The Recipient Operation

Although segmental grafts (consisting of only the pancreatic body and tail) were once common, the entire pancreas and its associated duodenal segment are now almost always transplanted (unless a living donor is used). Ligation or obliteration of the pancreatic duct was also once commonly practiced, but these techniques have also been abandoned. Instead, the pancreatic exocrine secretions are drained internally into either the small intestine or the bladder. Until recently, most centers used only the bladder drainage technique, but since the late 1990s, enteric drainage has become the most common method in SPK grafts. The kidney and pancreas grafts can both be placed within the peritoneal cavity through a midline incision. However, we have sometimes used two lateral incisions because they provide easier access to the iliac vessels and allow the kidney to be transplanted to its usual extraperitoneal location more easily. To avoid the consequences of fluid collection around the pancreas, the pancreas graft is placed intraperitoneally.

If a combined kidney-pancreas transplant is performed, the pancreas is usually transplanted first to minimize ischemia time for the pancreas. However, if two teams are operating, the kidney can be transplanted while the pancreas is prepared for transplantation on a separate back table. This approach also affords the advantage that a well-functioning kidney with vigorous diuresis will help minimize edema of the pancreas after reperfusion.

The external iliac arteries and veins are mobilized, preferably on the right side. The anatomic relationship of the vessels, as well as the presence of the colon, makes placement of a pancreas graft on the left more difficult and can result in a higher incidence of vascular thrombosis. Some surgeons advocate systemic heparinization, although others believe that it is not necessary in uremic recipients, whose clotting mechanisms are impaired. The arterial anastomosis is performed end to side to the external iliac artery by using either the aortic patch (containing the ostia of the celiac axis and superior mesenteric artery) or the common iliac artery portion of the Y-graft extension or the superior mesenteric artery if the splenic artery was anastomosed to it. The portal vein of the graft is anastomosed to the side of the external iliac vein of the recipient. Venous anastomosis is facilitated by complete mobilization of the common and external iliac veins with ligation of all venous branches; alternatively, the graft can be implanted to the aorta and vena cava and oriented with the head facing cephalad. The latter orientation may promote enteric drainage. Portal venous drainage can also be accomplished by anastomosing the portal vein of the pancreatic allograft to the superior mesenteric vein.

For bladder drainage of pancreaticoduodenal secretions, a horizontal cystotomy is made on the posterosu-

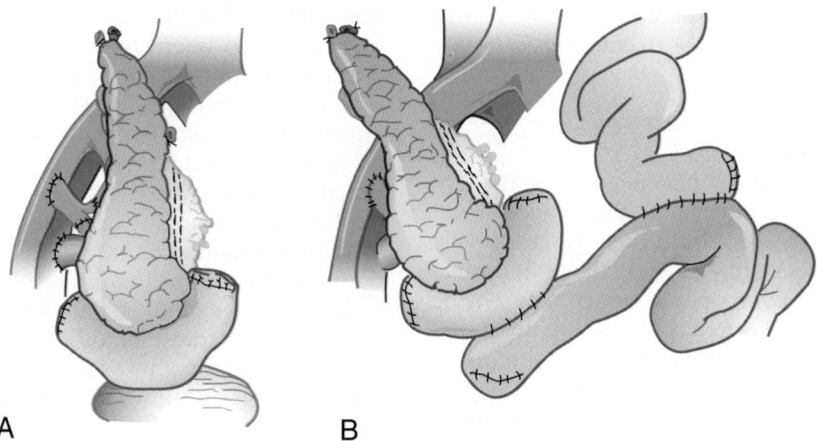

Figure 28-11 A and **B,** Pancreas recipient procedure.

perior aspect of the bladder and a two-layer anastomosis is constructed between the bladder and duodenum (Fig. 28-11A). Absorbable sutures are used for the inner layer to avoid leaving a nidus for stone formation. If enteric drainage is chosen, it can be performed as a simple side-to-side anastomosis of the donor duodenal segment to a convenient loop of small bowel or to a Roux-en-Y loop (see Fig. 28-11B). Because the procedure involves opening the intestine, the wound is irrigated with antibacterial and antifungal agents. Drains are generally unnecessary. If bladder drainage has been performed, a Foley catheter is left in the bladder for 5 to 7 days.

An additional technical factor of possible importance is whether venous drainage should be systemic (via the iliac vein) or through the portal system. Portal venous drainage prevents the hyperinsulinemia resulting from systemic venous drainage, but whether normal serum insulin and the somewhat more physiologic lipoprotein profile seen in patients with portal vein–drained grafts have meaningful benefits is uncertain. In view of the well-documented but subtle immunologic advantage of portal vein drainage of allografts in rodent models, it is intriguing that in a larger retrospective study at the University of Maryland, portal vein–drained pancreas grafts had fewer acute rejection episodes and better survival than those drained systemically.[23] Although these results remain unconfirmed by other centers, interest in these findings resulted in 23% to 44% of all U.S. pancreas transplants between 2000 and 2004 being performed with portal drainage, depending on the type of graft (23% SPK, 27% PAK, 44% PTA). However, the 1-year survival of these grafts was similar to those with systemic venous drainage, and there was no difference in technical failure rates.[22]

Biologic Factors Influencing the Outcome of Pancreas Transplantation

Histocompatibility Matching
That donor-recipient histocompatibility is advantageous for pancreas transplants has been shown by the some-

what superior outcome of the 142 living related donor pancreas transplants that had been reported as of October 2001 as compared with cadaveric pancreas grafts. Despite this immunologic advantage of related donors, they have been used in only 0.8% of pancreas transplants because of the potential risks to the donor, including not only the morbidity of the operation itself but also the possibility of impairing the donor's glucose metabolism.[24] In addition, there is a theoretical concern that a pancreas transplanted from an HLA-matched related donor may be subject to increased susceptibility to the development of recurrent autoimmune diabetes in the graft, a risk analogous to that for the development of recurrent autoimmune glomerulonephritis in kidney transplants from identical twin or HLA-identical sibling donors.

Most of the information regarding living donor transplants comes from the University of Minnesota, where 120 such transplants have been performed, or 8.5% of that institution's pancreas transplants.[24] The graft survival rate of living donor transplants was 6% to 11% better at 1 year than that of cadaveric transplants done at the same institution.

For cadaveric transplants, the advantage of matching is subtle. Analysis of International Pancreas Transplant Registry results from 2000 to 2004 indicated significant benefit of HLA matching only for zero antigen–mismatched PTA grafts.[22]

Immunosuppression
The immunosuppressive therapy used for pancreas transplant recipients is very similar to that used for other solid organ transplant recipients. In the late 1980s and early 1990s, cyclosporine, in combination with azathioprine and prednisone, was used in most centers. Between 2000 and 2004, more than 80% of recipients were treated with a tacrolimus and MMF–based maintenance regimen.[22] More recently, sirolimus has been used in some patients. Most centers also continue to use corticosteroids, although because of their known diabetogenic effect some groups have tried to withdraw or do entirely without them. Anti–T-cell antibodies are also commonly used for induc-

tion immunosuppression because of the prevalence of early rejection and the difficulty of diagnosing it.

Rejection

Prevalence and Severity

Whether human vascularized pancreas allografts are more or less vulnerable to rejection than vascularized allografts of other organs is a difficult question, especially since the pancreas is a composite organ with distinct exocrine and endocrine components, which may not be equally subject to rejection. Rejection of a kidney and pancreas transplanted simultaneously from the same donor is often manifested at the same time. However, either organ may undergo earlier or more severe rejection. In patients who receive pancreas and kidney transplants, rejection episodes tend to be more frequent than in those receiving only a kidney. Yet pancreatic graft loss from rejection is more frequent if the pancreas alone is transplanted than if both the kidney and pancreas are transplanted.

Diagnosis of Rejection

Early diagnosis of pancreatic allograft rejection is particularly important because physiologic evidence of islet damage (hyperglycemia) is a late indicator of rejection. Once islet damage is advanced, it is often difficult or impossible to reverse it by intensifying immunosuppression. The importance of identifying early rejection has led to exploration of a number of methods, such as imaging techniques and blood and urine tests, none of which have proved to be very reliable. Thus, in an effort to recognize early rejection, a combination of nonspecific indicators are used, including increases in serum amylase, lipase, and anodal trypsinogen; decreases in urinary amylase (in the case of bladder-drained allografts); impaired function of a concomitantly transplanted kidney allograft; biopsy of the kidney or pancreas allograft; and finally, hyperglycemia.

Histologic evidence of rejection is, of course, the most definitive indicator of rejection. Biopsy of the concomitantly transplanted kidney or the duodenum associated with the pancreas may be helpful, but most specific of all is biopsy of the pancreatic allograft itself, which can be performed by ultrasound-guided transcutaneous or transcystoscopic techniques. If necessary, open biopsies can also be performed safely.

Treatment of Rejection Episodes

Although early initiation of antirejection therapy is more important in pancreas than in kidney transplantation, treatment of rejection episodes is similar to that for kidney allograft rejection: high-dose corticosteroids and anti–T-cell antibodies. Early rejection episodes can usually be reversed, but if extensive islet damage is allowed to occur, there is much less chance of rescue than in the case of kidney or liver transplants. Because corticosteroids, cyclosporine, tacrolimus, and OKT3 all have a propensity for islet damage, increasing antirejection or heavy-maintenance immunosuppression needs to be avoided if possible.

Autoimmune Recurrence

In addition to rejection, an immunologic threat to pancreas transplants is the autoimmune response to islets that was responsible for elimination of the native pancreatic beta cells. In the case of kidney transplants, an analogous vulnerability of transplanted kidneys was noted in the early 1960s when patients with glomerulonephritis were found to be subject to autoimmune damage of the transplanted kidney even if rejection was avoided by using an identical twin donor.

In 1979, we demonstrated that autoimmunity alone would destroy transplanted pancreatic islets in spontaneously diabetic rats, an experimental model in which the autoimmune response to transplanted islets could be examined independently of allograft rejection. Several years after the demonstration that recurrent autoimmunity in animals could rapidly destroy transplanted islets in the absence of allogeneic rejection, Sutherland and colleagues found that an analogous process in humans could damage the islets of whole-organ pancreatic grafts transplanted from identical twin donors. However, in these patients islet destruction occurred only after many weeks. This suggested that a vascularized pancreas graft might differ in its immunologic vulnerability from that of isolated islets, a question we also studied in spontaneously diabetic rats. Whereas isolated islet grafts were routinely destroyed by autoimmunity within a few days, only a minority of whole-organ recipients became diabetic within 100 days, thus indicating that recurrent autoimmunity, though a substantial threat to isolated islet transplants, might be easy to overcome with immunosuppression in the case of a vascularized pancreas.

The unique experience at the University of Minnesota with identical twin donor pancreas transplants provides definitive information on this issue.[25] Seven technically successful identical twin segmental pancreas transplants have been performed there. The first three recipients underwent transplantation before the risks of recurrent disease were recognized. They received no immunosuppression. Biopsy-proven recurrent disease occurred in 1 to 4 months. The fourth patient received only azathioprine and suffered recurrence 5 years after transplantation. More recent twins received standard immunosuppression and did not experience graft loss as a result of recurrent autoimmunity.

Recurrence of autoimmune diabetes with selective beta cell destruction has also been observed in pancreas transplants from living related HLA-identical donors. Until recently it was thought that it would be unlikely to occur in HLA-mismatched cadaveric transplants, either because the disease was MHC restricted or because the more intensive immunosuppression routinely used to prevent rejection of mismatched allografts would easily prevent autoimmune islet damage. However, in several recipients of cadaveric pancreas transplants, failures have been reported in which histologic evidence indicated that autoimmunity rather than rejection was the cause. The transplanted pancreas in these patients exhibited selective destruction of beta cells with preservation of alpha and delta cells, a pattern characteristic of patients with insulin-dependent diabetes.

Complications of Pancreas Transplantation

Pancreas transplant patients are susceptible to the complications common to all immunosuppressed patients (e.g., infection, malignancy, corticosteroid-induced osteonecrosis). In addition, they are subject to several nonimmunologic complications specific to this type of transplant.

Vascular Thrombosis

The most common nonimmunologic cause of pancreas allograft failure is vascular thrombosis. This complication is most frequent during the first 7 days after transplantation. It almost always results in loss of the graft and is responsible for about 70% of technical failures. The reported incidence of this complication in transplants performed between 2000 and 2004 is about 7%. Its etiology appears to be the relatively sluggish blood flow to the pancreas, estimated as only 1% of cardiac output, in comparison to the rapid blood flow through kidney, heart, or liver transplants. Risk factors were analyzed in a large experience (438 patients) at the University of Minnesota, where at various times most of the technical variations have been evaluated with regard to duct management, vascular reconstruction, and segmental versus whole-organ transplants. Their overall thrombosis rate was 12% (5% arterial, 7% venous). There were no instances of obvious technical problems such as faulty vascular anastomoses. Thromboses did not appear to be caused by mechanical obstruction of the major vessels of the allograft but instead by abnormalities or changes in the microcirculation of the pancreas. Therefore, it is not surprising that strategies devised to increase blood flow in the major vessels (e.g., arteriovenous fistulas) have failed to decrease the incidence of thrombosis.

Other findings of the Minnesota study were that the risk for thrombosis was highest in PAK transplant patients. Segmental grafts also had a propensity for thrombosis. Other risk factors identified were advanced donor age, cardiocerebral cause of donor death, prolonged preservation time, portal vein extension grafts, allograft pancreatitis, and transplantation of the pancreas graft to the left rather than the right iliac fossa. Although some centers advocate the use of anticoagulants, this remains of unproven benefit and is associated with bleeding complications in the perioperative period.

Allograft Pancreatitis

Allograft pancreatitis in the early post-transplant period occurs in 10% to 20% of recipients. Predisposing factors are donor abnormalities (hemodynamic instability, vasopressor administration), procurement injury, perfusion injury (excessive pressure or volume), ischemic damage during preservation, and reperfusion injury.

In severe pancreatitis, compromised pancreatic microcirculation causes necrosis and then arterial thrombosis. Mild edematous pancreatitis may be obvious at the time of allograft revascularization, but the diagnosis of significant pancreatitis and determination of its severity and progression are difficult. Serum amylase levels may not accurately reflect the degree of pancreatitis. Allograft pancreatitis may be difficult to differentiate from rejection or other complications such as extravasation of pancreatic juice, urine, or enteric contents. All of these complications can be manifested as abdominal pain and tenderness, leukocytosis, hyperamylasemia, and CT abnormalities demonstrating graft edema. Unlike major leaks, however, graft pancreatitis is treated nonsurgically, with Foley catheter drainage for bladder-drained grafts and, perhaps, with octreotide.

Fistula and Abscess

Extravasation of pancreatic juice from the pancreatic anastomosis is a more serious complication in enteric-drained than in bladder-drained allografts. During the era of more dangerous immunosuppression from 1987 to 1992, this accounted for a substantial difference in survival between the two methods (for bladder-drained pancreas transplants the survival rate was 75% as compared with only 54% for those enterically drained).[26] However, as immunosuppression and patient management have improved, this difference has become minimal, and from 2000 to 2004, enteric-drained and bladder-drained success was similar as judged by 1-year graft survival rates (85% versus 87%) and patient survival rates (96% versus 94%), respectively.[22]

Urologic Complications

Urologic complications, such as urethritis, urethral disruption, hematuria, and recurrent urinary tract infections, are quite common in bladder-drained recipients. These problems and bicarbonate loss are the major disadvantages of this technique. Urethritis often resolves after a period of Foley catheter drainage, but if not, enteric conversion is required to prevent scarring or disruption of the urethra. Hematuria may sometimes respond to simple bladder irrigation. If it persists, fulguration of the bleeding site may be effective; if not, enteric conversion is necessary.

Results of Pancreas Transplantation

Impact on Metabolic Defects of Diabetes

Successful pancreatic transplantation restores normoglycemia and normal levels of hemoglobin A_{1c}. The response to a glucose challenge and to IV arginine and secretin is also normalized. Counter-regulation of glucose, which occurs in instances of insulin-induced hypoglycemia, is also improved by pancreatic transplantation.

Successful recipients exhibit hyperinsulinemia because of systemic venous drainage of the allograft and insulin resistance secondary to corticosteroid therapy. These abnormalities cause no symptoms. Their long-term significance is unknown, although hyperinsulinemia can elevate triglyceride levels, which could accelerate atherosclerosis. However, pancreas transplantation generally has a beneficial impact on the abnormal lipid profiles of diabetics. Even though systemic venous drainage of the graft via the donor's iliac vein has been the standard method, several groups have evaluated the alternative of directing the venous effluent into the recipient's portal vein. Because this is the physiologic route, there has been

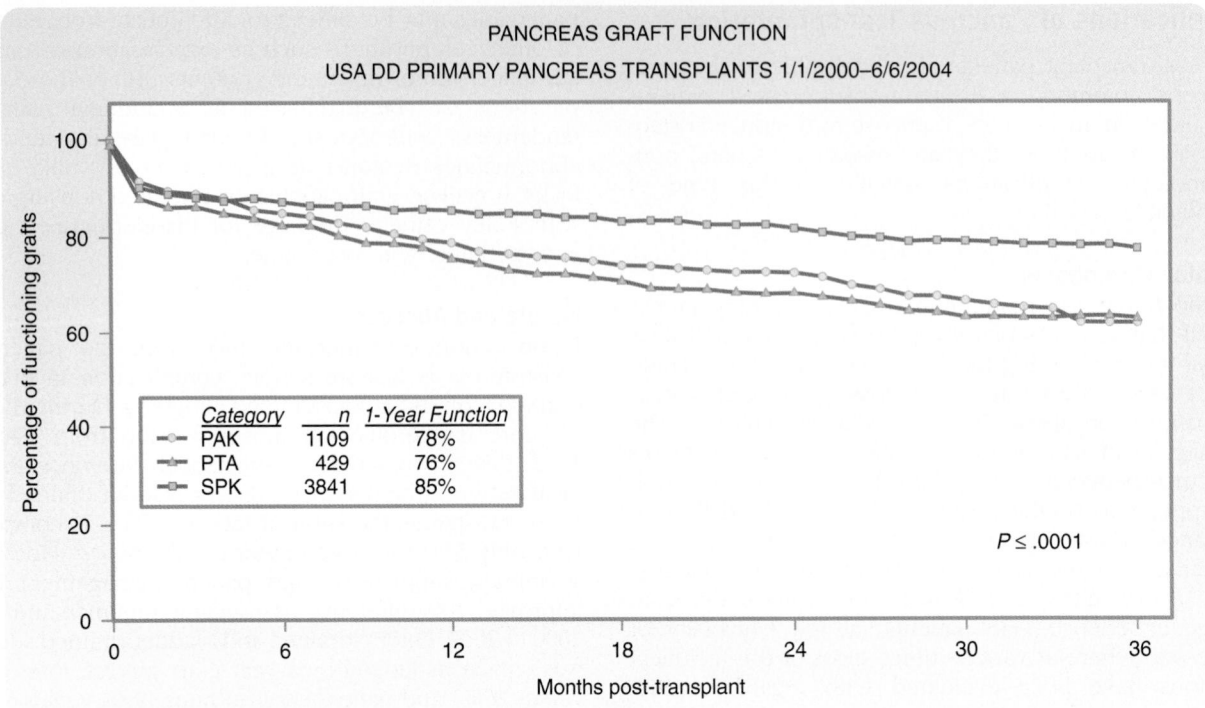

PANCREAS GRAFT FUNCTION

USA DD PRIMARY PANCREAS TRANSPLANTS 1/1/2000–6/6/2004

Category	n	1-Year Function
PAK	1109	78%
PTA	429	76%
SPK	3841	85%

$P \leq .0001$

Months post-transplant

Figure 28-12 Pancreas graft survival. DD, deceased donor; PAK, pancreas after kidney (transplantation); PTA, pancreas transplantation alone; SPK, simultaneous pancreas-kidney (transplantation).

speculation that it would have a metabolic advantage. It does, in fact, prevent hyperinsulinemia. However, the procedure is more complex and there is little evidence that it has a meaningful advantage.

Graft Survival

After disappointing outcomes during the early years of pancreas transplantation, patient and graft survival rates for the procedure now approach those of other solid organ transplants. As of the end of 2004, 23,043 pancreas transplants had been reported to the International Pancreas Transplant Registry, including 17,127 performed in the United States.[22] For cases performed between 2000 and 2004, patient survival rates were higher than 95% at 1 year and higher than 88% at 3 years. Graft survival rates in the same cohort at 1 year were 85% for SPK, 78% for PAK, and 76% for PTA (Fig. 28-12).[22]

Impact of Duct Management Technique

In the United States, bladder drainage was until recently by far the most common technique for duct management because it was relatively safe and facilitated early diagnosis of rejection by serial measurement of urinary amylase, which decreases if the graft suffers immunologic damage. From 1987 to 1996, more than 90% of transplants were done by this method. Unfortunately, the bladder drainage technique carries its own urologic and metabolic morbidities, including cystitis, urethritis, and chronic acidosis from bicarbonate loss. In fact, in 15% of bladder-drained transplants, these problems are serious enough to warrant enteric conversion within 3 years.

Because of these issues the use of enteric drainage has now become the preferred method. Whereas in 1988 only 2% of U.S. transplants were performed by the enteric method, in 1997 48% of SPK transplants were drained enterically, and between 2002 and 2003, 82% of SPK transplants were performed by this method.

Although in earlier years bladder drainage grafts fared substantially better, from 2000 to 2004 the 1-year graft survival rate of SPK transplants was nearly the same for bladder-drained (87%) and enteric-drained (85%) transplants. Interestingly, when early graft losses from technical problems were avoided, the subsequent loss of pancreas transplants was surprisingly low. In 2978 technically successful SPK cases, the pancreas graft failure rate from immunologic causes was only 2% at 1 year. In SPK grafts, the immunologic risk of failure did not differ according to the duct management technique. However, for technically successful PAK and PTA cases, immunologic graft loss was higher (5% and 7%, respectively).

Impact of Pancreas Transplantation on Microvascular Complications

Evaluating the impact of successful pancreas transplantation on the secondary complications of diabetes is difficult because randomized controlled studies are lacking. Defining appropriate control groups is also complicated because in SPK recipients, uremia and diabetes are corrected at the same time. Some complications of diabetes such as neuropathy are likely to be improved by kidney transplantation alone. Thus, uremic diabetics who receive only a kidney transplant are a necessary control group for assessing the benefits of pancreas transplantation on microvascular complications.

Neuropathy

In nonuremic diabetic PTA recipients at the University of Minnesota Hospital, improvement in nerve conduction velocity was documented after 1 year.[27] Evoked muscle and nerve action potentials and amplitudes remained stable or improved in patients with long-standing pancreas grafts, whereas amplitudes continued to decrease in diabetic recipients whose pancreas transplants failed early.[28] Thus, in the Minnesota patients, restoration of normoglycemia by successful pancreas transplantation appeared to halt the progression of diabetic neuropathy fairly promptly. However, other investigators believe that improvement in neuropathy, including autonomic neuropathy, is delayed by as much as 2 years.[29]

Retinopathy

Several investigators have reported improvement in retinopathy in uremic diabetic patients after a successful pancreas transplant, but most of these studies have been poorly controlled. In nonuremic patients at the University of Minnesota Hospital, the retinas of successful pancreas recipients were compared over a 5-year period with those of patients who experienced early graft failure.[30] In the first 3 post-transplant years, the probability of progression of retinopathy was the same (30%) in both groups. However, after 3 years, retinopathy appeared to stabilize in patients with successful pancreas transplants, but it continued to worsen in those with failed grafts. After 5 years, 55% of patients with failed grafts had progressed to a more severe state of retinopathy, whereas in successful recipients, similar progression in retinopathy had occurred in only 30%. In contrast to these patients with mild retinopathy, it seems unlikely that a pancreas transplant will benefit those with advanced retinal changes.

Nephropathy

Microscopic lesions of diabetic nephropathy commonly appear within 1 to 2 years in kidneys from normal donors transplanted to diabetic patients who are treated only with insulin. However, in recipients of successful SPK transplants in the Minnesota study, the development of diabetic nephropathy in the transplanted kidney was generally prevented, presumably because the blood glucose level was normalized.[31] The Minnesota group has also contended that a PAK transplant may halt the progression of lesions that evolved in the renal graft before pancreas transplantation was performed.[31] In patients whose kidneys were sampled an average of 8 years after transplantation, the mean glomerular mesangial volume was significantly less in patients who had a successful pancreas transplant than in those who did not.

Whether restoration of normoglycemia with a pancreas transplant can influence the course of early lesions of diabetic nephropathy in the native kidneys of nonuremic, diabetic patients remains controversial. In a preliminary report from the University of Minnesota, native kidneys were sampled in seven nonuremic pancreas recipients who experienced early to moderately advanced diabetic nephropathy (albuminuria was present in all; mean creatinine clearance was 90 ± 20 mL/min) 2 years after a successful pancreas transplant. Mean glomerular mesangial volume was significantly reduced after transplantation when compared with pretransplant biopsies. However, despite this histologic improvement, creatinine clearance had deteriorated in these pancreas transplant patients from 90 ± 15 to 60 ± 14 mL/min over the same 2-year period. The nephrotoxic effect of cyclosporine may explain this apparent paradox. The lesions of diabetic nephropathy in the patient's native kidneys were not ameliorated by pancreas transplantation, even after 5 years of normoglycemia. However, neither of these studies proves that restoring normoglycemia after a pancreas transplant cannot prevent or retard progression of diabetic nephropathy.

Several other PTA recipients have been observed to progress to a uremic state despite a successful pancreas graft,[27,32] but in most nonuremic diabetic PTA recipients, serum creatinine and creatinine clearance values at 1 to 5 years after transplantation did not deteriorate from those obtained 6 months post-transplant. In summary, in all three categories of diabetic pancreas graft recipients (SPK, PAK, and PTA), there is encouraging histologic evidence that restoring euglycemia can prevent or halt the progression of diabetic nephropathy. Whether this benefit is sufficient to offset the nephrotoxic effect of immunosuppressive agents such as cyclosporine or tacrolimus is a critical question.

Although these studies strongly suggest that pancreas transplantation may improve diabetic retinopathy, nephropathy, and neuropathy, no controlled or randomized studies have yet confirmed these results. Whether transplantation can also prevent diabetic complications in otherwise unaffected patients, as tight insulin control has been shown to do, has not been investigated because pancreas transplantation, before the onset of any complications, is rarely performed. Therefore, the potential benefits of pancreas transplantation over other forms of intensive diabetic treatment cannot be fully assessed at this time, although it seems likely that the optimal control of blood glucose possible from a pancreas transplant would be the optimal prophylaxis for microvascular complications.

Conclusion

The results of pancreas transplantation have improved remarkably since the mid-1980s, and the likelihood of success now approaches that of other solid organ transplants.[27] Because pancreas transplants are not immediately lifesaving, except in patients with profound hyperglycemic unawareness, the serious side effects of lifelong immunosuppression must be weighed against the somewhat unpredictable sequelae of insulin-managed diabetes. Currently, transplantation is limited at most centers to diabetics who require a kidney transplant or have already had one. Prevention of the microvascular complications of diabetes by pancreas transplantation seems likely but has not been proved by randomized studies. Advanced complications are much less likely to be stabilized or reversed.

Recent reports indicate that a successful kidney-pancreas transplant is associated with improved long-term patient survival relative to successful renal transplantation alone.[33] A 10-year follow-up of 13,467 diabetics on the UNOS waiting list indicated that despite earlier complications and deaths in pancreas recipients, the calculated life expectancy was 23.4 years for kidney-pancreas recipients versus 20.9 years for related kidney-alone recipients and 12.6 years for cadaveric kidney-alone recipients.

The morbidity and monetary expense associated with conventional insulin therapy, along with its complicating factors, must also be compared with those of successful transplantation and immunosuppression to determine the eventual place of pancreatic and islet transplantation. Possibly as important a consideration as the impact of a pancreas transplant on microvascular complications is its potential for improving quality of life. Recipients of successful pancreatic allografts usually report increased vitality, greater capability for self-care, and general improvement in quality of life.

TRANSPLANTATION OF ISOLATED PANCREATIC ISLETS

The advantage of transplanting isolated pancreatic islets rather than the pancreas is avoidance of the complex vascular reconstruction required with whole-pancreas transplantation and elimination of the unnecessary transplantation of the associated exocrine component of the gland. In the early 1970s, the initial descriptions of partial and complete reversal of experimental diabetes in animals by transplantation of isolated islets of Langerhans excited considerable interest because the risks associated with this procedure seemed minimal and human pancreatic transplants of that era were dangerous and rarely successful. It was also theorized that because some other endocrine tissues were known to have minimal immunogenicity, islet allografts might succeed without immunosuppression. However, initial human islet transplants during the 1970s all failed, probably from technical difficulty in producing preparations with adequate islet yield or purity or because of immune destruction. Although considerable knowledge has been accumulated since then, both in the techniques of islet isolation and in preventing damage to the transplant by rejection or autoimmunity, much of the progress has been in experimental models. Until very recently, successful human islet transplantation has been exceedingly rare.

With the report in the year 2000 of seven consecutive successful human islet transplants by investigators in Edmonton, Alberta, a new era commenced for this field.[34] Within 5 years of this report, almost 500 islet transplants had been performed worldwide with 1-year islet graft survival rates in many of the approximately 30 centers performing them comparable to those of pancreas transplantation. Disappointingly, however, most of the islet recipients subsequently needed to resume insulin therapy within 5 years. Briefly summarized in the following text

are the history of islet transplantation, the barriers that remain, and recent clinical results.

Lessons Learned From Experimental Islet Transplantation

Techniques of Islet Preparation

Separation of islets from the pancreas is begun by distending the pancreas via infusion of a collagenase enzyme solution into the pancreatic duct. After mechanical disruption, islets are separated from acinar, ductal, lymph nodal, and vascular elements by handpicking under magnification or by density gradient centrifugation. Although most nonislet tissue is thus eliminated, many islets are destroyed or discarded in the process.

Sites of Islet Transplantation

A potentially important advantage of a free graft, such as isolated islet grafts, is the flexibility that exists in selecting a site for transplantation. Surprisingly, unlike the situation with other free grafts of endocrine tissue, only a few transplant sites will support engraftment and adequate function of transplanted islets. The peritoneal cavity is advantageous because any remaining exocrine tissue that has not been separated from the islets can be tolerated there, but this transplant site is also relatively inefficient in that large numbers of islets are required for reversal of diabetes. For reasons not completely understood, the most easily accessible sites (subcutaneous or intramuscular) have not proved successful unless extremely large numbers of islets from multiple donors were transplanted. The spleen has been used successfully as a transplant site; however, the risk of splenic injury and bleeding is a deterrent. Thus, somewhat surprisingly, the liver via portal vein embolization has become the most commonly used transplant site. The liver's dual vascular supply allows embolized islets to completely occlude portal venules without infarcting the transplant site, which remains nourished by hepatic arterial blood (Fig. 28-13).

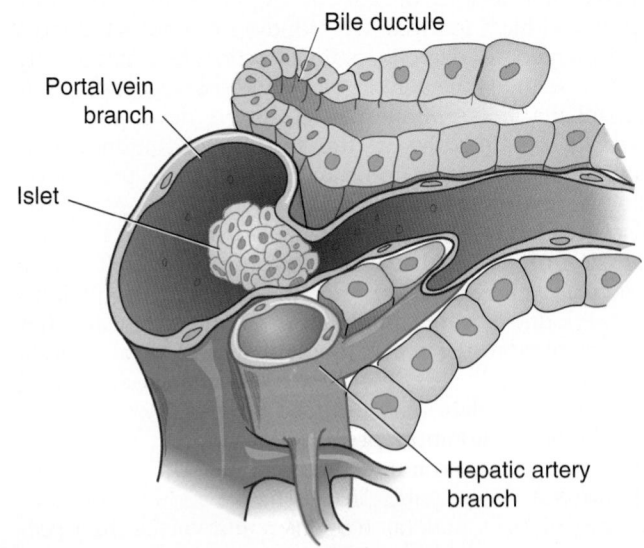

Figure 28-13 Islet transplant in the liver.

The renal subcapsular space is another excellent islet transplant site in rodents, but it has rarely been used in humans. A surgically constructed omental pouch is another site currently being tested that has achieved some success in animal models.

A number of immunologically privileged transplantation sites have been evaluated, including the anterior chamber of the eye, the brain, the pregnant uterus, the placenta, the testis, and the thymus. Several of these sites have been shown to provide at least partial sanctuary for allogeneic islets while allowing normal physiologic function. However, the technical considerations and potential morbidity of engraftment into these sites discourage their clinical use.

In animal models, genetic alteration of islets to delete important alloantigens has allowed successful transplantation without immunosuppression.[35] Genetic modifications of islet allografts have also been attempted in an effort to create a protective environment that would be similar to a privileged site. An example of this strategy would be to induce the transplanted islets to produce immunosuppressive cytokines such as IL-10 and transforming growth factor. To test this method, Min transfected isolated murine islets with the genes encoding these factors.[36] When the transfected islets were transplanted to allogeneic hosts, their survival was significantly prolonged.

Islet Allograft Immunogenicity

Contrary to the early hope that islet tissue would be immunologically privileged like certain other endocrine tissues (e.g., the parathyroid), the earliest reversal of experimental diabetes by islet transplantation indicated that unless the donor was genetically identical to the recipient, rejection was prompt. Subsequent experiments indicated that rejection could be overcome by immunosuppression and also identified several other unusual strategies by which rejection could be avoided. For example, pretransplant storage of islets in tissue culture was found to reduce their immunogenicity, sometimes allowing successful transplantation without immunosuppression. This outcome was found to depend on depleting the islets of passenger leukocytes, especially class II MHC APCs such as macrophages and dendritic cells, which may be important triggers of rejection.[37] Prolonged pretransplant tissue culture of islets (1-2 weeks) allowed selective survival of endocrine cells but not the antigen-presenting lymphoid cells. Other methods that deplete or render APCs from islets nonfunctional include ultraviolet irradiation, gamma irradiation, and treatment with antibodies directed against APCs along with complement. Thus far, these methods have been shown to be effective only in rodent models.

Immunosuppression

In animal models, conventional pharmacologic immunosuppressive agents, such as cyclosporine and tacrolimus, are somewhat less effective in prolonging islet allograft survival; dangerously higher doses are required to prolong islet survival beyond what is necessary for surgically vascularized solid organ allografts. In addition, cyclosporine, tacrolimus, and corticosteroids have been found to have toxic effects on islets. Antilymphocytic antibodies and specific anti–T-cell agents such as anti-CD4 have proved far more successful in preventing islet allograft rejection.

Co-stimulatory blockade has also been applied to islet transplants, with encouraging results. Kenyon and colleagues[38] reported the results of anti-CD154 treatment on the survival of isolated islet allografts in rhesus monkeys. Each of six monkeys treated with anti-CD154 antibody monotherapy demonstrated prolonged restoration of normoglycemia.

Tolerance

Classic immunologic tolerance induced by neonatal IV administration of allogeneic lymphoid cells from a prospective donor strain was shown many years ago to prevent skin allograft rejection. Only donor lymphoid cells, not other cell types such as kidney cells, which cannot migrate to host lymphoid organs, proved effective as tolerogens. Knowledge that the thymus serves as the primary site for initiation of self-tolerance led Posselt and associates to investigate whether nonlymphoid donor cells such as islets might also possess tolerogenic properties if introduced directly into the thymus.[39] They injected allogeneic islets into the thymus of adult rats that were briefly immunosuppressed with a single dose of ALS to delete their mature T cells. Not only did these islets survive in the thymus, but they also allowed a second islet allograft from the same donor strain to be successfully transplanted under the kidney capsule 100 to 200 days later without any additional immunosuppression. Attempts to induce tolerance by this method in larger animal models have not been as encouraging.

Autoimmune Recipients

Successful islet transplantation in human type 1 diabetics requires avoidance of not only rejection but also damage by the autoimmune process, which causes failure of native islets in this disease. Insight into the possible importance of autoimmune recurrence in transplant islet failure has been provided by studies in two rodent models of spontaneous autoimmune diabetes: the BioBreeding (BB) rat and the nonobese diabetic (NOD) mouse. These animals are similar to human type 1 diabetics in many ways, including abrupt disease onset in early adulthood and the presence of both cellular and humoral immune responses directed specifically against the beta cells of the islets. Without insulin therapy, ketoacidosis and death are inevitable. Thus, NOD mice and BB rats are suitable models for determining the vulnerability of transplanted islets in autoimmune recipients and possible methods of avoiding it. Studies in BB rats demonstrated that islets are more vulnerable to autoimmune recurrence after transplantation when they are isolated than they are if transplanted as part of a whole pancreas.

Xenografts

Even if the technical and immunologic difficulties of islet transplantation were overcome, the donor shortage would leave millions of diabetics waiting for a transplant. An often discussed solution to a demand of this magnitude would be the use of xenogeneic tissues.

Porcine insulin is effective in the treatment of human diabetics, which suggests that the pig may be a promising source of islet tissue for xenotransplantation. Preformed antibodies against porcine histocompatibility antigens are present in humans, and these antibodies have been shown to bind islets and activate complement. However, unlike the situation for vascularized xenografts, there is apparently no hyperacute rejection of islets. Instead, the problems of cellular immunity seem to play a more prominent role in islet xenograft rejection. Encouraging progress in islet xenotransplantation has been reported with porcine donors in which the major target of humoral immunity has been genetically eliminated.[6-8]

Clinical Islet Transplantation

In theory, islet transplantation is the ideal treatment for patients with insulin-dependent diabetes because it has the potential to completely normalize blood glucose without the substantial risks associated with the operation of whole-pancreas transplantation. In rodent models, the technical and immunologic problems of islet transplantation have been overcome, thus routinely allowing consistent success. Recent improvement in the success of clinical islet transplantation suggests that islet transplantation could eventually replace both insulin therapy and whole-pancreas transplantation as the optimal treatment of type 1 diabetes.[40]

Isolation Methods

Digestion of the compact fibrous pancreas and isolation of viable islets are more difficult in humans than in rodents. In addition, the hemodynamic instability and hyperglycemia of cadaveric human donors and the prolonged pancreatic ischemia before initiation of the separation process have compromised efforts to obtain islet preparations of high quality. The fact that pancreata from the best donors are likely to be used for whole-organ grafts further reduces the likelihood of optimal islet recovery. Most centers now use an automated method of islet isolation described by Ricordi and coworkers.[41]

The pancreas is digested enzymatically by collagenase in a chamber. During a period of agitation, islets and small fragments of the contaminating exocrine tissue remaining in the bottom of the chamber fall through a screen and are collected. After the collagenase solution is washed from the islets, they are separated from the acinar fragments and ductal elements by centrifugation through density gradients. Islets account for about 2% of the mass of an intact pancreas. Current islet separation methods are sometimes capable of yielding preparations composed of 90% pure islets, whereas at other times the same procedure may yield a preparation of less than 50% purity. The more manipulation carried out in an effort to reduce acinar tissue contamination, the more islets are lost. Even with the best techniques, many islets are lost or damaged. An important variable that contributes to inconsistency in the isolation process is the collagenase enzyme used to digest the pancreas. Recent refinement

of the enzyme preparation has led to marked improvement in isolation yield, purity, and number.

Another important technical achievement is islet preservation. Short-term preservation (days to several weeks) can be achieved by in vitro tissue culture. Islet culture has been shown to diminish the immunogenicity of islets in animal experiments, but this has not been evaluated in humans. Although even short-term culture (12-24 hours) also helps decrease the acinar tissue contaminating islet preparations, it occurs at the expense of substantial loss of viable islets. Frozen islets can probably be stored permanently and, after thawing by appropriate techniques, appear to have virtually normal function. Cryopreservation allows islet preparations from multiple donors to be pooled so that a sufficient number of islets for reversal of diabetes could be used for every transplant, thereby obviating the possibility of performing a transplant with an inadequate number of islets from a single donor.[41]

Surgical Technique and Complications

In human transplants, the islets have usually been transplanted by embolization to the liver via the portal vein. Other transplant sites, proven effective in animals, such as the peritoneal cavity and the renal subcapsular space, have rarely been used in humans. Islets can be inoculated into the portal venous system by cannulating the umbilical vein via a minilaparotomy or by transcutaneous, transhepatic cannulation of the portal vein itself. Islets are suspended in a heparinized solution for portal vein infusion. Portal venous pressure is monitored during islet infusion because the development of portal hypertension may be an indication of intravascular clotting. Although most patients tolerate the inoculation of intraportal islets, severe complications have been reported in a few, including portal vein thrombosis and disseminated intravascular coagulation.[42] These complications are probably related to rapid infusion of insufficiently pure islet preparations containing large amounts of enzymatically rich acinar tissue. With islet preparations of high purity, these sequelae have been rare. However, the procedure is not without other risks. Even in the recent experience, a death has been reported as a result of hepatic arterial injury during transhepatic portal vein cannulation.

Metabolic Factors Influencing Success

During islet engraftment in the immediate post-transplant period, it is believed that maintenance of normal blood glucose levels is important to avoid islet damage. During the early post-transplant period, to avoid even brief episodes of hyperglycemia, patients are treated with continuous IV infusions of insulin. In most cases, after several days this regimen is converted to subcutaneous insulin therapy, which may be maintained for several more weeks, even if the transplanted islets appear to be capable of maintaining normoglycemia. This intensive early insulin therapy is thought to be critical because islets traumatized by recent isolation may be particularly sensitive to increases in metabolic demand. Hyperglycemia might damage the beta cells by stimulating them to produce insulin until they become exhausted. However, no randomized studies to support this theory have been conducted, and it should also be noted that successful islet engraftment in rodents does not require concomitant insulin therapy.

Islet Autotransplantation

Modern human islet transplantation began in 1977 when Sutherland and colleagues at the University of Minnesota performed intraportal autotransplantation of islets in a patient who was undergoing nearly total pancreatectomy for the persistent pain of chronic pancreatitis.[43] This patient remained insulin independent for 6 years after transplantation, thus proving that transplanted islets could function in humans. The largest experience has been at the University of Minnesota, where between 1977 and 2006 more than 150 patients with chronic pancreatitis were subjected to total or nearly total pancreatectomy for relief of pain.

Islets isolated from the excised organ were transplanted into the pancreatectomized patient's liver via the portal vein to prevent the otherwise inevitable diabetes.[44] Because the exocrine pancreas in such patients is almost always atrophic, purification of the digested pancreas is unnecessary. Because the islets were autologous, rejection was not a possibility, and because these patients were not type 1 diabetics, there was no concern over recurrent autoimmune damage. In an early report of this series of patients, the incidence of insulin independence after 2 years was 34%. Since they adopted the automated islet isolation method of Ricordi to increase their islet yield, the Minnesota group has increased their success rate to 55%. Furthermore, of the autograft recipients in whom at least 300,000 islets were transplanted, 74% were insulin independent after 2 years. Importantly, stable insulin independence has been documented with follow-up of patients for up to 13 years. As discussed later, this result differs significantly from the experience with islet allografts.

Islet Allografts After Total Pancreatectomy in Patients With Malignant Disease

Before the Edmonton report in 2000,[34] the most consistent success with pancreatic islet allografts may have been in patients at the University of Pittsburgh who had their pancreas and liver removed as part of upper abdominal exenteration for malignant disease.[45] Eleven such patients were treated with combined liver and islet allotransplantation. Six of them exhibited sustained insulin independence after the procedure. Although they all eventually died of recurrence of their malignancy, one remained insulin independent for 58 months and had normal insulin–C-peptide levels at 18, 30, and 57 months after transplantation and, at autopsy, had histologically normal intrahepatic islets. In these cases the transplanted islets were from the same cadaveric donor as the liver (although several of them additionally received islets from third-party donors). The substantially better result of islet transplantation in these patients than in other islet transplants of that era has two possible explanations that are not mutually exclusive: (1) the recipients were not type 1 diabetics and thus autoimmune damage of the

transplanted islets was not a threat, and (2) successful liver allografts are known to have a protective influence that can prevent rejection of allografts of other tissues transplanted from the same donor.

Islet Allografts for Insulin-Dependent Diabetes

By far the largest number of candidates for allogeneic transplantation are type 1 diabetics. Ironically, it is in such patients that a successful outcome has until recently been so difficult to achieve. Between 1990 and 2000, more than 300 type 1 diabetics worldwide received islet transplants at 35 institutions, but insulin independence was noted in less than 10% at 1 year.[46] A multivariate analysis of all islet transplants reported to the International Transplant Registry identified four characteristics that were associated with *success* (defined as achievement of insulin independence or at least some evidence of islet engraftment):

1. Preservation of the donor pancreas for less than 8 hours before islet isolation
2. Transplantation of at least 6000 islets per kilogram of body weight
3. Choice of the liver via the portal vein as the transplant site
4. The use of antilymphocyte or antithymocyte globulin for induction immunosuppression

In cases in which all four of these positive predictive parameters were present, 70% of patients had some evidence of transplant islet function, 83% had normal hemoglobin A_{1c} levels, and 20% were insulin independent 1 year after transplantation.[46] Although this analysis is based on a small number of successful cases, it provided a framework for the design of further trials of islet transplantation, including the landmark 2000 report by the Edmonton workers.[34]

A problem in devising optimal immunosuppressive protocols for islet transplantation is the known diabetogenic nature of the commonly used immunosuppressive drugs. Prednisone may cause insulin resistance and hyperglycemia, whereas both cyclosporine and tacrolimus suppress insulin secretion. The diabetogenic effect of these drugs may in part explain the requirement for a larger than anticipated number of islets for successful allografts and the longer than expected time to engraftment. That induction immunosuppression with anti–T-cell antibodies has a positive correlation with islet allograft success may be explained by the lack of islet toxicity of these agents.

In the setting of the usual failure of islet transplantation even in the 1990s, the report in 2000 by the Edmonton group of seven consecutive successes gained much attention.[34] Investigators who had become pessimistic regarding islet transplantation expressed renewed interest in the procedure. The Edmonton workers attributed their success to several innovations. First, corticosteroids, the mainstay of traditional immunosuppressive regimens, were completely avoided because of their known diabetogenic properties. Also novel was the immunosuppressive regimen selected, which included induction therapy with anti–IL-2 receptor antibody and mainte-

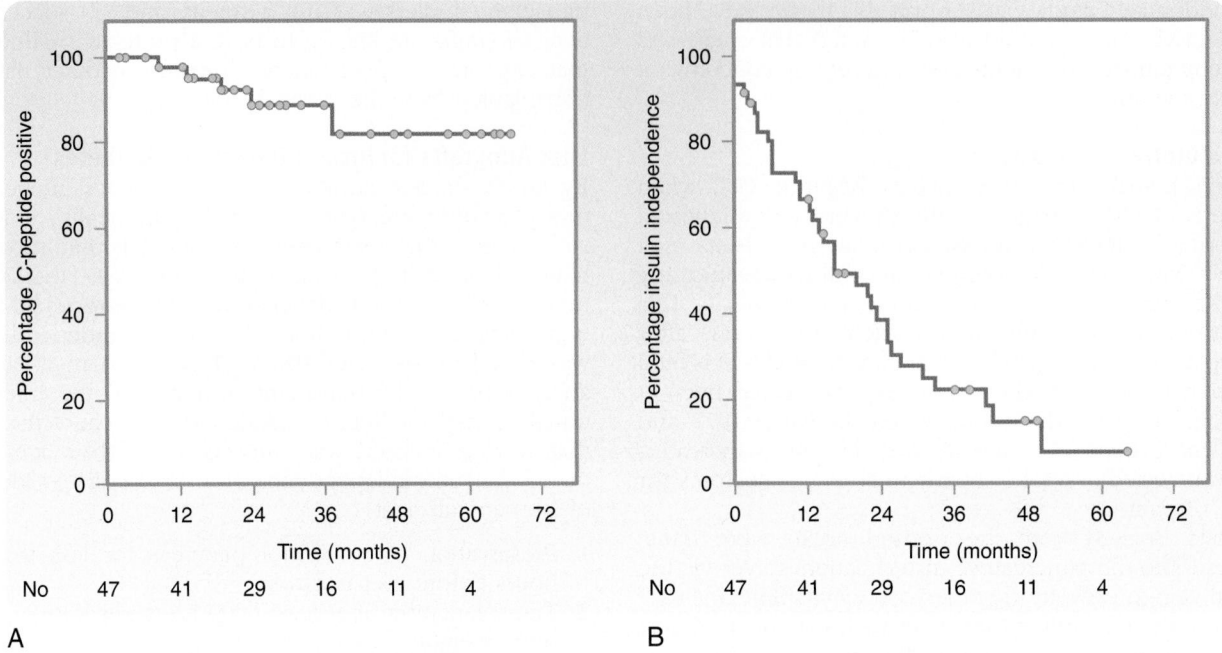

Figure 28-14 A and **B,** Islet allograft survival versus insulin independence. (From Ryan EA, Paty BQ, Senior PA, et al: Five year follow-up after clinical islet transplantation. Diabetes 54:2060-2069, 2005.)

nance therapy with a combination of low-dose tacrolimus and sirolimus.

Although these innovations may have played a role in their success, the subsequent experience of other investigators using different immunosuppressive regimens, including low-dose steroids, makes it seem more likely that the crucial factor in the success of the *Edmonton protocol* was that larger numbers of islets were transplanted by repeated islet infusions. Whereas many previous investigators had achieved evidence of some islet transplant function by detectable C-peptide after transplanting islets from a single donor, unless their patients became insulin independent, they usually considered the transplant a failure and discontinued immunosuppression. These earlier patients were not maintained on immunosuppression and regrafted with more islets. Shapiro and colleagues, in contrast, maintained the immunosuppression and administered second and even third doses of islets from additional donors until insulin independence was achieved.[34] As in the rodent experiments detailed earlier, the inefficiencies of the isolation process and engraftment in the recipient often make the islet yield obtained from a single donor insufficient to completely reverse hyperglycemia.

Based on the encouraging results in Edmonton, numerous centers in the United States and abroad have initiated islet transplant programs, usually copying the Edmonton approach to the immunosuppressive protocol and retransplantation. Many, but not all of these centers have achieved success comparable to that of the Edmonton group, who have now reported more than 70 islet transplants with a 90% success rate in achieving insulin independence.[40] Unfortunately, even in the Edmonton experience islet function gradually diminishes for

unknown reasons, possibly including chronic rejection, recurrence of autoimmune damage, or islet exhaustion. Insulin independence after 5 years is seen in only 10% of patients, even though evidence of islet survival is seen in up to 80% of patients (Fig. 28-14).[40]

Despite the encouraging recent successes in islet transplantation, several obstacles must be overcome before the procedure can be widely used, including the need for multiple infusions from multiple cadaveric donors, the limited duration of insulin independence, the expense of the procedure ($80,000 per recipient), and the donor shortage. At present, only about 6000 cadaveric donors are available each year in the United States, of which approximately 1500 pancreata are used for whole-organ transplantation. Even if the remainder were suitable for islet isolation, this would allow only 2000 diabetics to be successfully treated if two organs are needed for each recipient. Because there are nearly 1.5 million type 1 diabetics in the United States, other sources of transplantable beta cells would be necessary for transplantation to have its full impact in the treatment of type 1 diabetes.

Several possible alternative sources of beta cells have been suggested, including xenogeneic donors, genetically altered tissues, stem cells, and living donors. None of these sources are immediately at hand, except living donors who volunteer to donate part of their pancreas. Living donors have been used successfully for segmental pancreatic grafts, and recently a group from Japan reported successful transplantation of a diabetic child with islets recovered from the distal pancreas of the patient's mother.[47]

Fetal Islet Allografts and Xenografts

It is believed that more than 5000 transplants of fetal islets have been performed, mostly in Russia and China.

Apparently, most of these patients either received no immunosuppression or were treated with agents of unknown immunosuppressive activity (e.g., Chinese traditional medicines). Information of any sort is available on fewer than 200 of these procedures. Thus far, it is doubtful that insulin independence has been achieved in any of the recipients who were type 1 diabetics, although increases in C-peptide levels have been reported.

Lafferty and associates performed 16 human fetal pancreas allografts in type 1 diabetic patients who were receiving simultaneous renal transplants.[47] They cultured fetal pancreatic fragments (1 mm^3) for 5 to 10 days before transplantation under the renal subcapsule of the kidney transplant. They obtained histologic evidence that the grafted fetal pancreas became revascularized within 14 days and had differentiated into islets by 3 months after implantation. Eight patients received tissue from a single fetal donor, and eight others received tissue from two to four donors. The latter group exhibited some reduction in their insulin requirements in comparison to a control group of diabetics who received a kidney transplant alone. One patient had a 65% reduction in insulin requirement, measurable serum C-peptide levels, and a normal hemoglobin A$_{1c}$ level 2 years after transplantation. Evidence of meaningful islet function was never evident sooner than 3 to 6 months after transplantation. Even if insulin independence could be achieved with fetal pancreas allografts, the political and ethical issues surrounding the use of human fetal tissues remain a substantial barrier to widespread use of this method.

The use of animal donors for fetal islet transplants might circumvent ethical issues, an interesting possibility that has been explored by Groth and coworkers.[48] They transplanted fetal porcine islets into 10 type 1 diabetic patients. In eight patients with functional renal transplants, the grafts were placed in the liver, and two patients had the fetal islets placed in the renal subcapsular space of a concomitantly transplanted kidney. The presence of preformed antibodies to this discordant xenogeneic tissue, as well as strong cellular rejection, would be expected to cause rapid destruction of these transplants. Surprisingly, porcine C-peptide was detectable in the urine of four patients from 200 to 400 days after transplantation; however, no change was observed in the insulin requirement of these patients.

Postoperative Monitoring for Rejection

A management problem nearly unique to islet transplantation is the lack of a reliable marker for early graft rejection. Hyperglycemia is likely to be a late indication of rejection that becomes apparent when the graft is not salvageable by antirejection therapy. More sensitive measures of insulin reserve, such as Sustacal stimulation tests or arginine-induced insulin release assays, are cumbersome and not practical for serial monitoring of graft function.

Immune markers of graft dysfunction have been sought. Olack and colleagues[49] reported a rise in PRA in patients with islet graft dysfunction. Islet grafts in this series were from multiple donors, which may have been responsible for the marked increases in PRA that were

observed. Elevations in islet autoantibodies have also been reported after transplantation, and their presence before transplantation may correlate with poorer graft survival.[50] Whether either alloreactive or autoreactive humoral responses have an important role in islet graft destruction is unknown but would not be surprising given the liver's potential for antibody-dependent cytotoxicity with its large population of resident phagocytes. However, it is unlikely that serologic markers are of promise for routine graft monitoring.

INTESTINAL TRANSPLANTATION

The introduction of IV hyperalimentation by Dudrick and associates in 1968 allowed long-term survival of patients with complete intestinal failure who would previously have died rapidly. However, total parenteral nutrition (TPN) severely affects quality of life and may be associated with a number of highly morbid and sometimes fatal complications.

An alternative to lifelong IV nutrition is restoration of enteral absorptive function by intestinal replacement. The earliest experimental transplants of the intestine performed by Lillehei in the 1960s indicated that success of intestinal grafts would be more difficult to achieve than that reported for other solid organ grafts.[51] In fact, it was not until the availability of cyclosporine that even occasional success was achieved. However, since then the results have greatly improved. Three varieties of intestinal transplantation have been reported:

1. Small bowel with or without a portion of the colon (SI)
2. Combined liver–small bowel grafts (LI)
3. Multivisceral grafts in which up to five organs are transplanted simultaneously (MV)

Nearly equal numbers of SI and LI grafts have been reported, whereas only a few MV grafts have been performed (~10% of the total). It is speculated that a concomitantly transplanted liver graft from the same donor would provide immunologic protection to the more immunogenic intestinal graft, as shown in some animal models. Although the issue is far from resolved, recent clinical results indicate that in humans, this protective effect is minor if present at all. This and the fact that failure of a small bowel graft alone may be successfully treated by removal of the graft and reinstitution of TPN whereas a failed liver graft is fatal without urgent liver retransplantation cause most groups to perform combined transplants only if both organs are failing. Selection of an isolated small intestinal graft would allow the possibility of using a living related donor, a procedure with considerable technical and immunologic advantages.[52]

The most frequent cause of intestinal failure is the short-gut syndrome, which follows extensive resection for intestinal ischemia or disease. At present, the most common indication for intestinal replacement is inability to sustain successful TPN because of lack of IV access sites or severe complications from chronic TPN, such as liver failure. That successful intestinal transplantation allows resumption of normal oral intake would make intestinal transplantation the preferred method of therapy for intestinal failure if the risks of this relatively new procedure can be decreased further.

The principal barrier to widespread application of intestinal replacement at present is the unusually vigorous rejection response elicited by intestinal grafts. The reasons for this difference are not entirely clear, but it is assumed that the large amount of gut-associated lymphoid tissue is responsible. Which of the transferred lymphoid cells may be most important in this regard or the antigenic characteristic of these cells has not been elucidated.

A uniquely dangerous consequence of intestinal transplant rejection is loss of the protective mucosal barrier of the gut, consequent bacterial translocation, and systemic sepsis in an immunocompromised host. Thus, it is not surprising that the most common cause of death after small bowel transplantation is sepsis and multiorgan failure. Early diagnosis of rejection is therefore crucial. Unfortunately, intestinal rejection is associated with only nonspecific clinical signs and symptoms such as fever, anorexia, abdominal pain, and changes in the output and character of intestinal contents (often observable as output from an ostium). Even endoscopic biopsies are not entirely reliable in diagnosing rejection because the histologic manifestations of rejection can be patchy, with some areas of the graft appearing entirely normal.

Because the intestine is the largest lymphoid organ in the human body, an intestinal graft can mount a formidable immune response against the host, GVHD. In the simplest manifestation of GVHD, the immune cells and antibody produced by blood group–compatible but nonidentical grafts mediate a severe hemolytic reaction by targeting foreign blood group antigens on the host's red blood cells. A more severe form of GVHD occurs when T cells of the graft respond to foreign histocompatibility antigens of diverse host tissues, thereby leading to a spectrum of pathology, the most fulminant form including destruction of host hematopoiesis. Interestingly, despite the outcome predicted by animal experiments, GVHD has not been a severe problem in most clinical cases. Perhaps the potent immunosuppressive regimens administered to human patients are especially effective in preventing GVHD. If so, development of tolerogenic protocols to obviate heavy immunosuppression would ironically be counterproductive for intestinal grafting because in experimental bowel transplant models, induction of tolerance leads to dramatically more severe GVHD.

Results

Data from the most recent International Intestinal Transplant Registry accumulated from 61 programs indicate that from April 1985 to May 2003, 989 transplants were performed in 923 patients.[53] About 60% of these grafts were performed in recipients younger than 18 years, and about half were isolated bowel (SI) and half included a simultaneous liver graft (LI). Only 17% of grafts were MV. For grafts transplanted since 1999, 1-year graft survival

rates were nearly equivalent in all three groups (SI, 65%; LI, 59%; MV, 61%), as was patient survival.[54] Overall, there has been a marked and steady improvement in short-term graft and patient survival over the past decade. The 1-year graft survival rate in 1995 was 56.8% versus 76.8% in 2003. It is hoped that this will translate into improved intermediate- and long-term benefit because the 5-year graft survival of patients who received transplants in 1999 was relatively disappointing (34%).

Factors associated with better graft survival included patients transplanted from home versus those hospitalized (68% versus 50% at 1 year) and the use of induction antibody treatment (75% versus 46% at 1 year). With antithymocyte globulin induction and tacrolimus maintenance immunosuppression, patient survival rates of 80% at 1 year have been reported, a rate nearly equivalent to that observed in high-risk liver transplant recipients. These dramatically improved results have been hailed as a new era in intestinal transplantation but will probably await longer-term follow-up before the procedure is accepted as the preferred therapy for patients with intestinal failure.

ETHICAL CONSIDERATIONS

Public interest in transplantation during the 1980s led to appointment of a national task force to address issues such as the donor shortage, establishment of standards, and provision of transplant services to all citizens. As a result, the National Organ Transplant Act was passed by Congress, which mandated a national Organ Procurement and Transplantation Network. In 1986, a government contract to provide these services was awarded to UNOS, a private nonprofit organization that had been formed by representatives of the majority of transplant centers in anticipation of these governmental actions.

The board of directors of UNOS includes representatives of the 11 regions that have been established in the United States and is composed of transplant surgeons and physicians, nurses, representatives of voluntary health organizations, transplant recipient families, lawyers, ethicists, theologians, and health care financing representatives. UNOS has established criteria for accreditation of transplantation centers, histocompatibility laboratories, and local organ procurement organizations. All patients awaiting transplants must now be registered with UNOS. A central computer and a point system based on medical criteria determine the assignment of cadaveric donor organs, which local organ procurement organizations distribute first locally, then regionally, and then nationally. Because hospitals performing transplantation must be members of UNOS to be eligible for Medicare funding, the organization has assumed a powerful role. Each center must now submit outcome data on every transplant performed, and these data are published regularly.

The severe donor shortage, which limits the application of transplantation as a lifesaving treatment, causes an ethical dilemma. Criteria for distribution of cadaveric organs are the subject of continuing debate. By law, age, race, and socioeconomic status can play no role. Should scarce organs go to high-risk patients, such as older, highly sensitized individuals whose need might be more pressing but who are unlikely to experience long-term benefit because of rejection or death? Alternatively, should younger, better-risk patients whose need is less acute receive transplants because they will have a more lasting benefit? An additional related issue is whether organ allocation should be based on national or regional listing of patients.

The sale of human organs has been condemned by the (International) Transplantation Society and is forbidden by law in most Western countries. It remains an issue because needy individuals in many parts of the world are sometimes willing to sell one of their kidneys for the high price that it will bring. Of additional concern are reports of the use of organs from executed criminals in China. These tarnish the image of transplantation.

The number of patients dying while awaiting an organ transplant grows every year. This increase in mortality is the result of an expanding number of candidates listed for organ transplants, coupled with a continuing shortage of donor organs. In the United States, obtaining organs from a cadaver donor relies on voluntary consent of a family to donate the organs of a deceased relative or, less commonly, the documented intent of the deceased. In the past 10 years the number of cadaveric organs recovered has increased by only 10%, clearly inadequate to meet the demand. The inadequacy of the current system is based on a decrease in the number of dying individuals suitable for organ donation and the low rate of family consent for donation from suitable donors (40%-60%).

A panel of ethicists, organ procurement organization executives, physicians, and surgeons was recently convened by the American Society of Transplant Surgeons to consider whether to recommend a pilot trial to provide a financial incentive for a family to consent to organ donation from a deceased relative. Currently, financial compensation for donation of organs is against the law in the United States. Another concern is that an offer of payment for donated organs might be offensive to some families and decrease their inclination to make an altruistic donation. The panel was unanimously opposed to the exchange of money for donor organs because it would violate the standard of altruism and commercialize the value of human life. However, a majority of the panel supported reimbursement for funeral expenses or a charitable contribution as an ethically permissible approach. The concept of a pilot project of this sort has been supported by the UNOS Board of Directors and the American Medical Association, but it remains controversial, as shown by the opposition of others, including the American College of Surgeons.

The evolution of transplantation from an experimental curiosity to a highly successful therapy represents one of the remarkable achievements of 20th century medicine. Terminal diseases of the kidney, liver, and other organs were uniformly fatal until the 1960s but can now be treated with greater success than most cancers. Because many victims of these diseases are relatively young and productive, the achievement of a successful transplant is one of the most gratifying of all surgical therapies.

Selected References

Bussutil RW, Klintman GB (eds): Transplantation of the Liver. Philadelphia, Elsevier Saunders, 2005.

> Second edition of the standard text on this topic.

Grant D, Abu-Elmagd KA, Reyes J, et al: 2003 report of the intestine transplant registry—a new era has dawned. Ann Surg 241:607-613, 2005.

> Review and analysis of intestine transplantation.

http://www.optn.org/data.

> National databank of cadaveric and living donor transplants in the United States.

Malinchoc M, Kamath PS, Gordon FD, et al: A model to predict survival in patients undergoing transjugular intrahepatic portosystemic shunts. Hepatology 31:864-871, 2000.

> Landmark study that resulted in complete overhaul of the liver allocation policy.

Morris PJ (ed): Kidney Transplantation: Principles and Practice. Philadelphia, WB Saunders, 2001.

> The fifth edition is the most comprehensive work on the subject.

Ryan EA, Paty BQ, Senior PA, et al: Five year follow-up after clinical islet transplantation. Diabetes 54:2060-2069, 2005.

> Update on the status of islet transplantation.

Schnitzler MA, Whiting JF, Brennan DC, et al: The life years saved by a deceased organ donor. Transplantation 5:2289-2296, 2005.

> Important analysis of the survival benefit provided by cadaveric organ transplants.

References

1. Davis CL, Delmonico FL: Living donor kidney transplantation: A review of the current practices for the live donor. J Am Soc Nephrol 16:2098-2110, 2005.
2. Matas AJ, Bartlett ST, Leichtman AB, Delmonico FL: Morbidity and mortality after living kidney donation, 1999-2001: Survey of United States transplant centers. Am J Transplant 3:830-834, 2003.
3. Tanabe K, Takahashi K, Sonda K, et al: Long-term results of ABO-incompatible living kidney transplantation: A single-center experience. Transplantation 65:224-228, 1998.
4. Fudaba Y, Spitzer TR, Shaffer J, et al: Myeloma responses and tolerance following combined kidney and nonmyeloablative marrow transplantation: In vivo and in vitro analyses. Am J Transplant 6:2121-2133, 2006.
5. Matas AJ, Bartlett ST, Leichtman AB, Delmonico FL: Morbidity and mortality after living kidney donation, 1999-2000: Survey of United States transplant centers. Am J Transplant 3:830-834, 2003.
6. Davis CL, Delmonico FL: Living donor kidney transplantation: A review of the current practices for the live donor. J Am Soc Nephrol 16:2098-2110, 2005.
7. Schnitzler MA, Whiting JF, Brennan DC, et al: The life years saved by a deceased organ donor. Transplantation 5:2289-2296, 2005.

8. Starzl TE, Zinkernagel RM: Antigen localization and migration in immunity and tolerance. N Engl J Med 339:1905-1913, 1998.

9. Tseng Y, Kuwaki K, Dor FJMF, et al: Alpha 1, 3-galactosyl-transferase gene–knockout pig heart transplantation in baboons with survival approaching 6 months. Transplantation 80:1493-1500, 2005.

10. Hering BJ, Wijkstrom M, Graham ML, et al: Prolonged diabetes reversal after intraportal xenotransplantation of wild-type porcine islets in immunosuppressed nonhuman primates. Nat Med 12:301-303, 2006.

11. Cardona K, Dorbutt GS, Milas Z, et al: Long-term survival of neonatal porcine islets in nonhuman primates by targeting costimulation pathways. Nat Med 12:304-306, 2006.

12. Paradis K, Langford G, Long Z, et al: Search for cross-species transmission of porcine endogenous retrovirus in patients treated with living pig tissue. The XEN 111 Study Group. Science 285:1236-1241, 1999.

13. Vincenti F, Larsen C, Durrbach A, et al: Costimulation blockade with belatacept in renal transplantation. N Engl J Med 35:770-781, 2005.

14. Knechtle SJ, Fernandez LA, Pirsch JD, et al: Campath-1H in renal transplantation: The University of Wisconsin experience. Surgery 136:754-760, 2004.

15. Lacombe M: Arterial stenosis complicating renal allotransplantation in man: A study of 38 cases. Ann Surg 181:283-288, 1975.

16. Knechtle SJ, Pirsch JD, Fechner JH Jr, et al: Campath-1H induction plus rapamycin monotherapy for renal transplantation: Results of a pilot study. Am J Transplant 3:722-730, 2003.

17. Malinchoc M, Kamath PS, Gordon FD, et al: A model to predict poor survival in patients undergoing transjugular intrahepatic portosystemic shunts. Hepatology 31:864-871, 2000.

18. Hoofnagle JH, Di Bisceglie AM: The treatment of chronic viral hepatitis. N Engl J Med 336:347-356, 1997.

19. Di Bisceglie AM: Hepatitis C and hepatocellular carcinoma. Hepatology 26:34S-38S, 1997.

20. Velidedeoglu E, Desai NM, Campos L, et al: The outcome of liver grafts procured from hepatitis C–positive donors. Transplantation 73:582-587, 2002.

21. Wachs ME, Bak TE, Karrer FM, et al: Adult living donor liver transplantation using a right hepatic lobe. Transplantation 66:1313-1316, 1998.

22. Sutherland DE, Gruessner A, Bland B, et al: International Pancreas Transplant Registry (IPTR) Annual Report for 2004. Available at http://www.med.umn.edu/IPTR/annual_reports/2004_annual_report.html.

23. Philosophe B, Farney AC, Schweitzer EJ, et al: Superiority of portal venous drainage over systemic venous drainage in pancreas transplantation: A retrospective study. Ann Surg 234:689-696, 2001.

24. Gruessner RW, Sutherland DE: Living donor pancreas transplantation. Transplant Rev 16:108-119, 2002.

25. Sutherland DE, Sibley R, Xu XZ, et al: Twin-to-twin pancreas transplantation: Reversal and reenactment of the pathogenesis of type I diabetes. Trans Assoc Am Physicians 97:80-87, 1984.

26. Sutherland DE, Gruessner RW, Gores PF, et al: Pancreas transplantation: An update. Diabetes Metab Rev 11:337-363, 1995.

27. Sutherland DE: Effect of pancreas transplants on secondary complications of diabetes: Review of observations at a single institution. Transplant Proc 24:859-860, 1992.

28. Kennedy WR, Navarro X, Goetz FC, et al: Effects of pancreatic transplantation on diabetic neuropathy. N Engl J Med 322:1031-1037, 1990.

29. Solders G, Tyden G, Tibell A, et al: Improvement in nerve conduction 8 years after combined pancreatic and renal transplantation. Transplant Proc 27:3091, 1995.

30. Ramsay RC, Goetz FC, Sutherland DE, et al: Progression of diabetic retinopathy after pancreas transplantation for insulin-dependent diabetes mellitus. N Engl J Med 318:208-214, 1988.

31. Bilous RW, Mauer SM, Sutherland DE, et al: Glomerular structure and function following successful pancreas transplantation for insulin-dependent diabetes mellitus. Diabetes 36:43A, 1987.

32. Morel P, Sutherland DE, Almond PS, et al: Assessment of renal function in type I diabetic patients after kidney, pancreas, or combined kidney-pancreas transplantation. Transplantation 51:1184-1189, 1991.

33. Ojo AO, Meier-Kriesche HU, Hanson JA, et al: The impact of simultaneous pancreas-kidney transplantation on long-term patient survival. Transplantation 71:82-90, 2001.

34. Shapiro AM, Lakey JR, Ryan EA, et al: Islet transplantation in seven patients with type 1 diabetes mellitus using a glucocorticoid-free immunosuppressive regimen. N Engl J Med 343:230-238, 2000.

35. Markmann JF, Bassiri H, Desai NM, et al: Indefinite survival of MHC class 1–deficient murine pancreatic islet allografts. Transplantation 54:1085-1089, 1992.

36. Min JK: Adenoviral mediated gene transfer of TGF-beta 1 and vlL promotes long-term survival of islet allografts. Surg Forum 46:438-440, 1995.

37. Lafferty KJ, Prowse SJ, Simeonovic CJ, et al: Immunobiology of tissue transplantation: A return to the passenger leukocyte concept. Annu Rev Immunol 1:143-173, 1983.

38. Kenyon NS, Chatzipetrou M, Masetti M, et al: Long-term survival and function of intrahepatic islet allografts in rhesus monkeys treated with humanized anti-CD154. Proc Natl Acad Sci U S A 96:8132-8137, 1999.

39. Posselt AM, Barker CF, Tomaszewski JE, et al: Induction of donor-specific unresponsiveness by intrathymic islet transplantation. Science 249:1293-1295, 1990.

40. Ryan EA, Paty BW, Senior PA, et al: Five year follow-up after clinical islet transplantation. Diabetes 54:2060-2069, 2005.

41. Ricordi C, Lacy PE, Finke EH, et al: Automated method for isolation of human pancreatic islets. Diabetes 37:413-420, 1988.

42. Mehigan DG, Bell WR, Zuidema GD, et al: Disseminated intravascular coagulation and portal hypertension following pancreatic islet autotransplantation. Ann Surg 191:287-293, 1980.

43. Robertson RP, Lanz KJ, Sutherland ER, Kendall DM: Prevention of diabetes for up to 13 years by autoislet transplantation after pancreatectomy for chronic pancreatitis. Diabetes 50:47-50, 2001.

44. Wahoff DC, Papalois BE, Najarian JS, et al: Autologous islet transplantation to prevent diabetes after pancreatic resection. Ann Surg 222:562-579, 1995.

45. Rilo HL, Carroll PB, Tzakis A, et al: Insulin independence for 58 months following pancreatic islet cell transplantation in a patient undergoing upper abdominal exenteration. Transplant Proc 27:3164-3165, 1995.

46. Hering BJ, Ricordi C: Graft islet transplantation for patients with type I diabetes. Graft 2:12-27, 1999.

47. Lafferty KJ, Hao L, Babcock SK, et al: Is there a future for fetal pancreas transplantation? Transplant Proc 21:2611-2613, 1989.

48. Groth CG, Korsgren O, Tibell A, et al: Transplantation of porcine fetal pancreas to diabetic patients. Lancet 344:1402-1404, 1994.

49. Olack BJ, Swanson CJ, Flavin KS, et al: Sensitization to HLA antigens in islet recipients with failing transplants. Transplant Proc 29:2268-2269, 1997.

50. Jaeger C, Brendel MD, Hering BJ, et al: Progressive islet graft failure occurs significantly earlier in autoantibody-positive than in autoantibody-negative IDDM recipients of intrahepatic islet allografts. Diabetes 46:1907-1910, 1997.

51. Khan FA, Tzakis AG: Intestinal and multivisceral transplantation. In Ginns LC, Cosimi AB, Morris PJ (eds): Transplantation. Malden, MA, Blackwell, 1999, pp 422-437.

52. Gruessner RW, Sharp HL: Living-related intestinal transplantation: First report of a standardized surgical technique. Transplantation 64:1605-1607, 1997.

53. Grant D, Abu-Elmagd KA, Reyes J, et al: 2003 report of the intestine transplant registry—a new era has dawned. Ann Surg 241:607-613, 2005.

54. McDonald JC: The National Organ Procurement and Transplantation Network. JAMA 259:725-726, 1988.

SURGICAL ONCOLOGY

CHAPTER 29

Tumor Biology and Tumor Markers

Marcus C. B. Tan, MBBS (Hons)   Peter S. Goedegebuure, PhD
and   Timothy J. Eberlein, MD

Epidemiology
Tumor Biology
Carcinogenesis
Tumor Markers

Neoplasia (literally meaning "new growth") is the uncontrolled proliferation of transformed cells. The term *tumor,* which was originally used to describe the swelling caused by inflammation, is now used interchangeably with *neoplasm.* Transformation is the multistep process in which normal cells acquire malignant characteristics. Each step reflects a genetic alteration that confers a growth advantage over normal cells. There are a number of essential alterations in cell physiology that collectively enable malignant growth[1,2]: self-sufficiency in growth signals, evasion of programmed cell death (apoptosis), avoidance of immune detection and destruction, limitless replicative potential, sustained angiogenesis, and tissue invasion and metastasis. These characteristics are shared by most, if not all, human tumors.

EPIDEMIOLOGY

Incidence is the number of new cases within a specified time frame and is usually expressed as cases per 100,000 people per year. *Prevalence* is the number of patients with the disease in the population. A person's risk of contracting or dying of cancer is usually expressed in terms of *lifetime risk* (risk over the course of a lifetime) or, when describing the relationship of specific risk factors with a particular cancer, as *relative risk* (in comparison to those with or without a certain exposure or trait).

About 1.4 million new cases of cancer are expected to be diagnosed in 2006, apart from the more than a million new cases of basal and squamous cell cancer (Fig. 29-1). In men, the most common cancers involve the prostate, lung, colorectum, and urinary bladder (Table 29-1). In women, the most common cancers are breast, lung, colorectal, and uterine (cervical and endometrial).

Cancer is the second most common cause of death in the United States and accounts for one in every four deaths (Fig. 29-2). In 2006, about 564,800 Americans will die of cancer.

Global Burden of Cancer

Worldwide, cancer is responsible for one in eight deaths. By 2020, 70% of all cancer-related deaths will occur in developing countries, where survival rates (20%-30%) are barely half that of developed countries.[3] Indeed, 80% to 90% of people in whom cancer is diagnosed in developing countries are initially found to have late-stage, terminal cancer.[3] It can therefore be seen that the vast majority of cancer deaths will occur in the countries least equipped to handle the burden.

Aging and Cancer

Cancer disproportionately affects people 65 years and older. In the United States, this age group accounts for 56% of all newly diagnosed cancer patients and 71% of all cancer deaths.[4] The median age at death for cancers common to both males and females (including lung, colorectal, pancreas, stomach, and urinary bladder) ranges from 71 to 77 years.[4] The number of people in this age group will double to 70 million (or 1 in 5 people) over the next 25 years, driven by the so-called baby boom cohort born between 1946 and 1964.[4] This is a recognized trend throughout the developed world.

With an increasingly older population, the incidence of cancer will increase, thereby increasing the overall cancer burden on society. Additionally, cancer care will be of increasingly greater complexity. Reasons for this include older people having more comorbid conditions of greater severity in the setting of declining physiologic

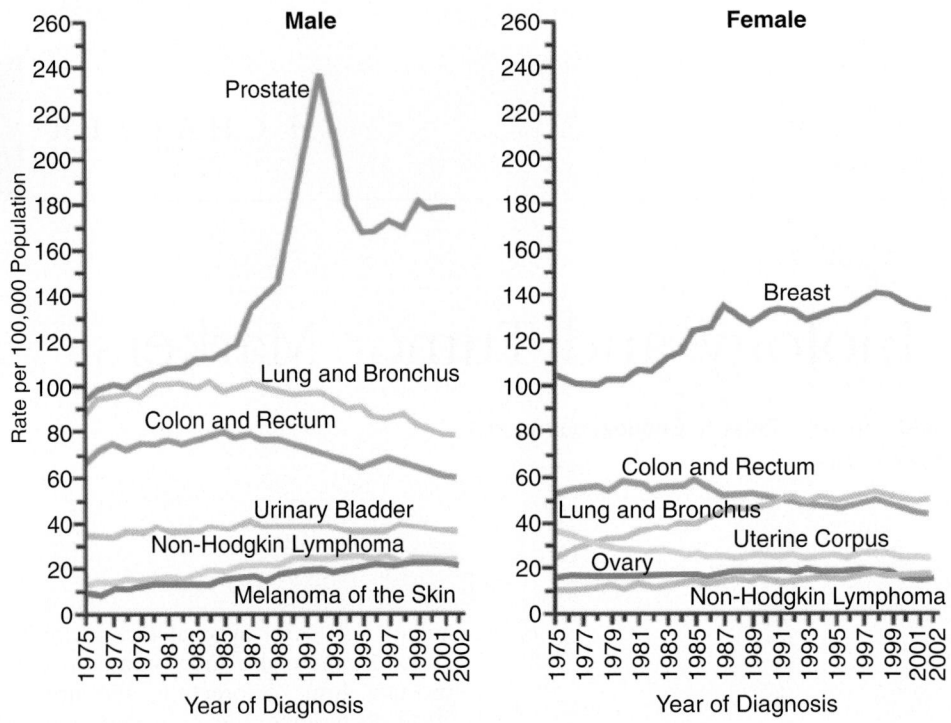

Figure 29-1 Annual age-adjusted cancer incidence rates for males and females for selected cancers in the United States, 1975 to 2002. (From Jemal A, Siegel R, Ward E, et al: Cancer statistics, 2006. CA Cancer J Clin 56:106-130, 2006, with permission.)

reserve, difficulty with access to care, and lack of social support.

Cancer treatment in the elderly is less well studied, and it has been shown that the elderly population is underrepresented in clinical trials.[5-7] There have been a number of reports of the underuse of adjuvant therapy, both chemotherapy and radiotherapy, in the aging population. O'Connell and colleagues[8] studied the Surveillance, Epidemiology, and End Results (SEER) database (1988-1997) and found that although elderly patients with colorectal or breast cancer had excellent rates of receiving cancer-directed surgery, rates were variable for many other neoplasms, including lung, esophagus, stomach, liver, and pancreas cancer. Surgical intervention being "not recommended" was the most common reason. Clearly, the surgeon must more carefully weigh the individual's operative risk in the context of the difficulty, length, and morbidity of the procedure and give greater consideration to quality of life and functional status, beyond just postoperative morbidity and mortality and long-term survival.

Obesity and Cancer

The prevalence of overweight (body mass index [BMI] of 25-30) and obesity (BMI >30) in most developed countries (and in urban areas of many less developed countries) has been increasing markedly over the past 2 decades. In the United States, approximately a third of the population is now classified as obese. Although obesity has long been recognized as an important cause of diabetes and cardiovascular disease, the relationship

between obesity and cancer has received less attention. Epidemiologic studies indicate that adiposity contributes to an increased incidence or death (or both) from cancers of the colon, breast (in postmenopausal women), endometrium, kidney (renal cell), esophagus (adenocarcinoma), gastric cardia, pancreas, gallbladder, and liver (hepatocellular carcinoma [HCC]). It has been estimated that 15% to 20% of all cancer deaths in the United States can be attributed to overweight and obesity.[9]

The mechanisms by which obesity increases cancer risk appear to involve the metabolic and endocrine effects of obesity via their alterations in levels of peptide and steroid hormones. For example, greater amounts of adipose tissue lead to increased circulating levels of free fatty acids, which in turn causes liver, muscle, and other tissues to increase their use of fats for energy production, thereby reducing their need for uptake and metabolism of glucose. Hyperglycemia results. This functional insulin resistance forces an increase in pancreatic insulin secretion. Epidemiologic and experimental evidence suggests that chronic hyperinsulinemia increases the risk for cancer of the colon and endometrium and probably other tumors as well (e.g., those of the pancreas and kidney).

Circulating levels of estrogens are strongly related to adiposity. For cancers of the breast (in postmenopausal women) and endometrium, the effects of overweight and obesity on cancer risk are largely mediated by increased estrogen levels. For patients with breast cancer, adiposity has been associated with both poorer survival and an increased likelihood of recurrence, an effect that persisted after adjustment for tumor stage and grade, hormone receptor status, and adjuvant therapy.

Table 29-1 The 10 Leading Cancer Types for Men and Women by Incidence and Mortality*

ESTIMATED NEW CASES			
Men		**Women**	
Prostate	33%	Breast	31%
Lung and bronchus	13%	Lung and bronchus	12%
Colon and rectum	10%	Colon and rectum	11%
Urinary bladder	6%	Uterine corpus	6%
Melanoma of the skin	5%	Non-Hodgkin's lymphoma	4%
Non-Hodgkin's lymphoma	4%	Melanoma of the skin	4%
Kidney and renal pelvis	3%	Thyroid	3%
Oral cavity and pharynx	3%	Ovary	3%
Leukemia	3%	Urinary bladder	2%
Pancreas	2%	Pancreas	2%
All other sites	18%	All other sites	22%
ESTIMATED DEATHS			
Men		**Women**	
Lung and Bronchus	31%	Lung and bronchus	26%
Colon and rectum	10%	Breast	15%
Prostate	9%	Colon and rectum	10%
Pancreas	6%	Pancreas	6%
Leukemia	4%	Ovary	6%
Liver and intrahepatic bile duct	4%	Leukemia	4%
Esophagus	4%	Non-Hodgkin's lymphoma	3%
Non-Hodgkin's lymphoma	3%	Uterine corpus	3%
Urinary bladder	3%	Multiple myeloma	2%
Kidney	3%	Brain and other nervous system	2%
All other sites	23%	All other sites	23%

*Excluding basal and squamous cell skin cancers and in situ carcinomas except those of the urinary bladder.

Modified with permission from Jemal A, Siegel R, Ward E, et al: Cancer statistics, 2006. CA Cancer J Clin 56:106-130, 2006.

TUMOR BIOLOGY

Much has been learned about the multistep process of tumorigenesis. A well-documented example of tumor development is presented in Table 29-2. The transformation of melanocytes into malignant melanoma can be divided histopathologically and clinically into five major identifiable steps. Successive genetic changes each confer a growth advantage leading to progressive conversion of normal cells to cancer cells. This process is associated with a number of distinct changes in cell physiology, in particular, self-sufficiency in growth signals, insensitivity to inhibitory growth signals, evasion of programmed cell death, limitless replicative potential, sustained angiogenesis, tissue invasion and metastasis, and immunoediting (Fig. 29-3).[1,2] Although the underlying genetic alterations may differ from tumor to tumor, these physiologic changes are common to the vast majority of cancers. Each of these traits is further discussed in the following sections.

Self-sufficiency in Growth Signals

Cells within normal tissues are largely instructed to grow by neighboring cells (paracrine signals) or via systemic (endocrine) signals. Likewise, cell-to-cell growth signaling occurs in the vast majority of tumors as well. The immediate tumor environment (the stroma) contains residing nonmalignant cells such as parenchymal cells, epithelial cells, fibroblasts, endothelial cells, and mast cells. In addition, most tumors are characterized by infiltrating immune cells such as lymphocytes, polymorphonuclear cells, and macrophages.

In some tumors these cooperating cells may eventually transform themselves and co-evolve with the tumor cells

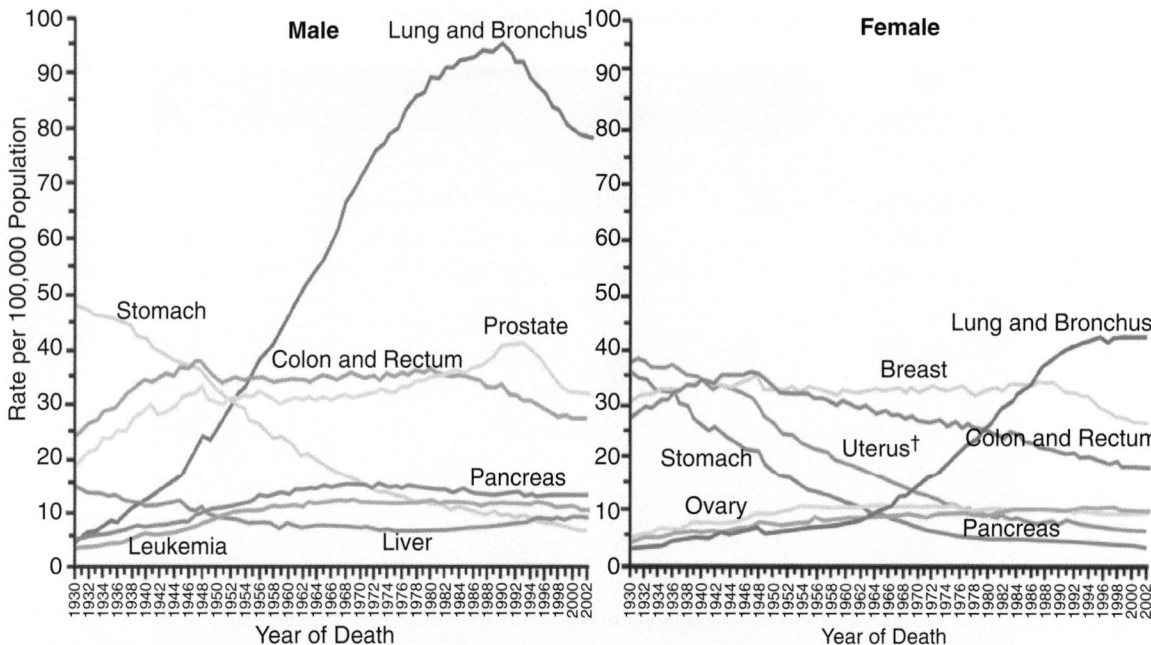

Figure 29-2 Annual age-adjusted cancer mortality rates for males and females with selected cancers in the United States, 1930 to 2002. Rates are age-adjusted to the 2000 U.S. standard population. (From Jemal A, Siegel R, Ward E, et al: Cancer statistics, 2006. CA Cancer J Clin 56:106-130, 2006, with permission.)

Table 29-2 Stepwise Progression From Melanocyte to Metastatic Melanoma

STEP*	CHARACTERISTICS
1	Common melanocytic nevus
2	Dysplastic nevus
3	Radial growth phase of melanoma
4	Vertical growth phase of melanoma
5	Metastatic melanoma

*Common acquired and congenital nevi without cytologic atypia (step 1) may progress to dysplastic nevi with clear atypical histologic and cytologic features (step 2). Most of these lesions are stable, but a few may progress to a malignant melanoma that tends to grow outward along the radius of the plaque (step 3). Within the plaque, a nodule of fast-growing cells develops and expands in a vertical direction, where it invades the dermis and elevates the epidermis (step 4). Finally, the tumor metastasizes (step 5).

Adapted from Clark WH: A study of tumor progression: The precursor lesions of superficial spreading and nodular melanoma. Hum Pathol 15:1147, 1984.

to sustain growth of the latter. Finally, basement membranes form the extracellular matrix (ECM) that provides a scaffold for the proliferation of fibroblast and endothelial cells. Together, tumor cells and stroma produce factors (autocrine and paracrine factors) that in cell-bound, matrix-bound, or soluble form, directly or indirectly influence tumor development. Autocrine factors secreted by tumor cells promote the growth of tumor cells but may also stimulate neighboring cells. In addition, tumor cells secrete paracrine factors that act on host cells or ECM to generate a supportive microenvironment. For example, transforming growth factor-β (TGF-β) may induce angiogenesis, production of ECM molecules, and elaboration of other cytokines by fibroblasts and endothelial cells. Simplified, tumor growth is dependent on the response of tumor cells to paracrine and autocrine factors (Fig. 29-4). Such factors include angiogenesis factors, growth factors, chemokines (polypeptide signaling molecules originally characterized by their ability to induce chemotaxis), cytokines, hormones, enzymes, cytolytic factors, and so forth, which may promote or reduce tumor growth (Table 29-3).

During the evolution of a tumor, its responsiveness to growth signals changes. Paracrine growth mechanisms are dominant during the early development of a tumor. Tumors become resistant to paracrine growth inhibitors and gain responsiveness to paracrine growth promoters. However, autocrine growth mechanisms become more prominent as tumors develop further. The observation that in late-stage tumors, metastatic tumor cells tend to spread more randomly through the body suggests that autocrine growth mechanisms may be more dominant than paracrine growth mechanisms. Advanced breast cancers, for example, lose hormone responsiveness. It is even possible for a tumor to grow completely autonomously (acrine state) and to be independent of growth factors and inhibitors (Fig. 29-5).

To achieve growth self-sufficiency, growth signaling pathways are altered. This process involves alteration of extracellular growth signals, transmembrane transducers of these signals, or intracellular signaling pathways that translate these signals into action. Growth factor receptors are overexpressed in many cancers. Receptor over-

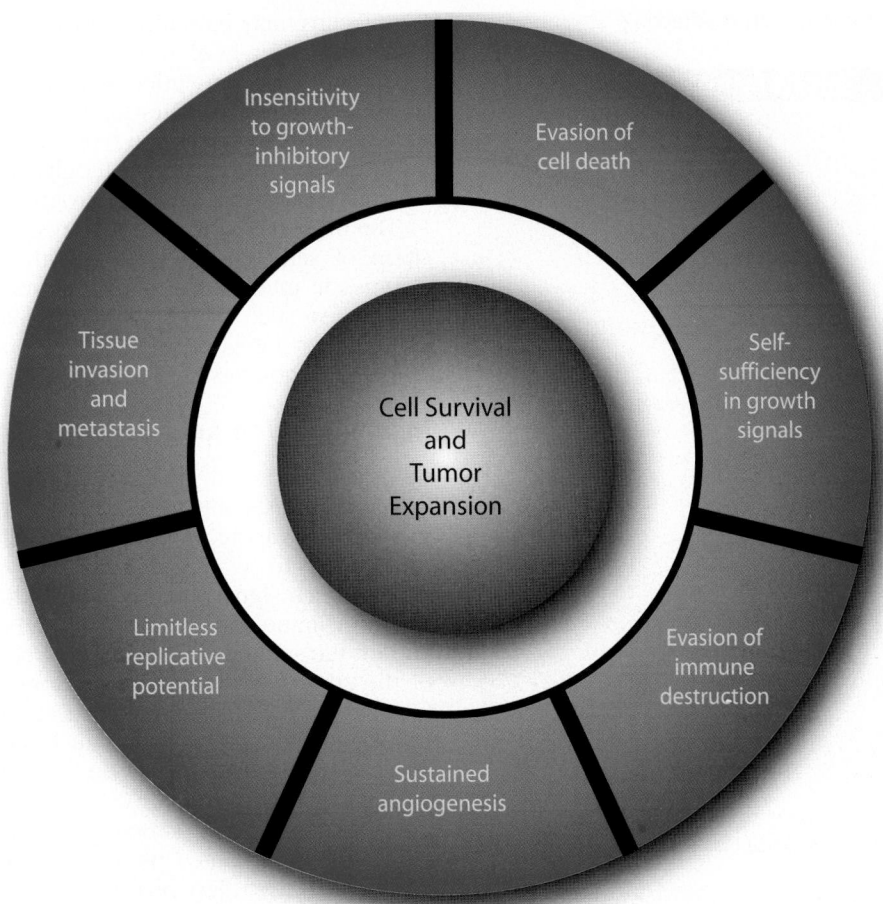

Figure 29-3 Changes in cell physiology associated with progressive conversion of normal cells to tumor cells. The indicated traits are common to the vast majority of human cancers and together confer cell survival or tumor expansion, or both. (Adapted from Hanahan D, Weinberg RA: Hallmarks of cancer. Cell 100:57-70, 2000.)

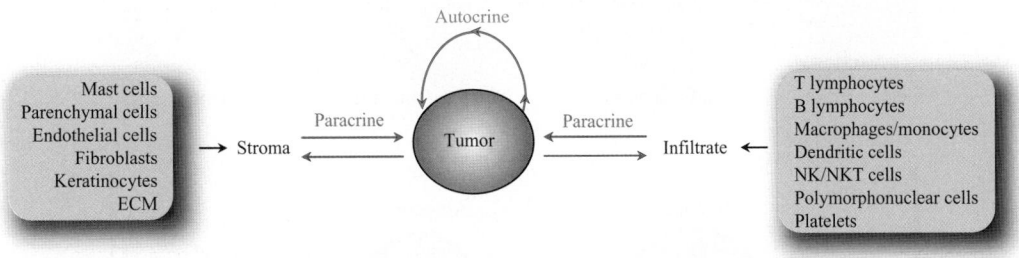

Figure 29-4 Paracrine and autocrine growth mechanisms. Both stromal cells and infiltrate secrete paracrine factors that affect tumor development. Additionally, tumor cells secrete autocrine as well as paracrine factors, which in turn act on stromal cells and infiltrating cells. ECM, extracellular matrix; NK, natural killer.

expression may enable the cancer cell to respond to low levels of growth factor that would not normally trigger proliferation. For example, the epidermal growth factor receptor (EGFR) and the Her2/neu receptor are overexpressed in breast and other epithelial cancers. Additionally, gross overexpression of growth factor receptors can elicit growth factor–independent signaling. The latter can also be achieved through structural alteration of

receptors, such as truncated versions of the EGFR that lack much of its cytoplasmic domain and are constitutively activated.

Cancer cells can also modulate their stromal environment, including the ECM, through secretion of factors such as basic fibroblast growth factor (bFGF), platelet-derived growth factor, TGF-β, and others. ECM components, such as collagens, fibronectins, laminins, and

Table 29-3   Cells and Soluble Factors Affecting Tumor Development*

CELLS	SOLUBLE FACTORS
Stroma	
Parenchymal cells	Growth factors, growth inhibitors,
Endothelial cells	nutritional factors, hormones,
Fibroblasts	degradative enzymes, cytokines,
Mast cells	angiogenesis factors
Extracellular matrix	
Keratinocytes	
Infiltrate	
T lymphocytes	Cytokines, chemokines, cytolytic
B lymphocytes	factors, angiogenesis factors,
Natural killer cells	growth (inhibitory) factors,
Natural killer T	degradative enzymes, cytostatic
(NKT) cells	factors, antibodies
Macrophages/	
monocytes	
Dendritic cells	
Polymorphonuclear	
cells	
Platelets	
Tumor	Chemokines, cytokines,
	angiogenesis factors, degradative
	enzymes, growth (inhibitory)
	factors

*The list of cells and soluble factors is not meant to be complete but to illustrate the complexity of factors affecting tumor development.

vitronectins, may bind to two or more receptors and may also bind other ECM molecules. The matrix molecule–receptor interaction induces signals that influence cell behavior, including entrance into the active cell cycle. Cancer cells can switch the types of ECM receptors (integrins and heparan sulfate proteoglycans) that they express and favor ones that transmit progrowth signals.

The third and most complex mechanism for the acquisition of self-sufficiency in growth signals stems from changes in intracellular signaling pathways. Many of the oncogenes, such as *ras,* mimic normal growth signaling and induce mitogenic signals without stimulation from upstream regulators.

Insensitivity to Antigrowth Signals

Cell division is an ordered, tightly regulated process involving both stimulatory and inhibitory signals. Thus, in addition to acquiring stimulatory growth signals, tumor cells need to overcome/neutralize inhibitory growth signals. Such signals include both soluble growth inhibitors and immobilized inhibitors embedded in the ECM and on the surfaces of neighboring cells. Similar to many of the stimulatory signals, inhibitory growth signals are transduced by transmembrane receptors coupled to intracellular signaling pathways that target genes regulating the cell cycle. The cell cycle can be divided into an interphase and a mitotic (M) phase (Fig. 29-6).[10] The interphase is further subdivided into two gap phases (G_1 and G_2), separated by a phase of DNA synthesis (S phase). The two gap phases involve crucial regulatory

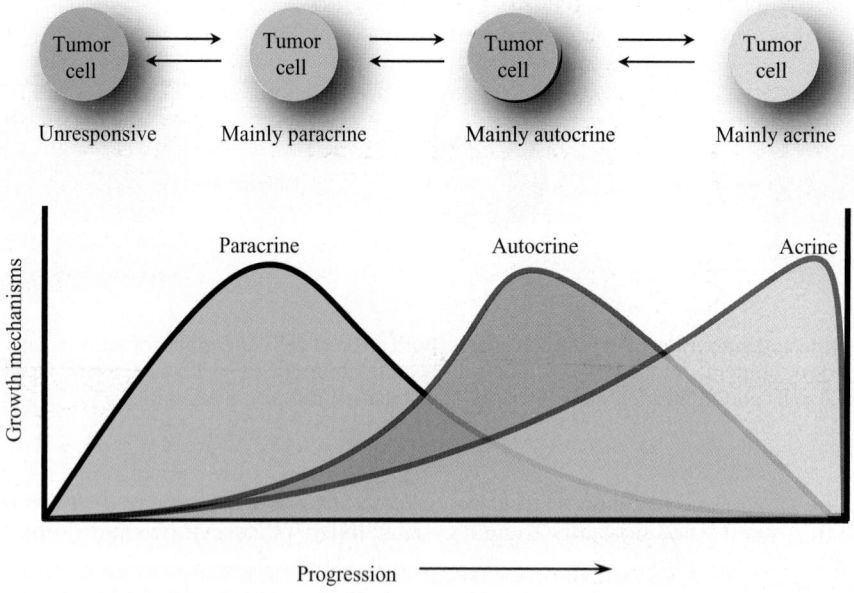

Figure 29-5 Changes in contribution of growth mechanisms to tumor development. During tumor progression, the contribution of paracrine growth mechanisms decreases, and the tumor becomes more dependent on autocrine growth mechanisms. At later stages, the tumor may even become independent of growth mechanisms (acrine state).

events that prepare the cell for DNA replication and mitosis. Central to cell cycle progression are the cyclin-dependent kinases (cdks) that bind to cyclin proteins. These proteins are regulated by numerous other proteins, including tumor suppressors and oncogenes that induce stimulatory or inhibitory signals. Antigrowth signals can block cell division by two distinct mechanisms. Cells may be forced to exit the cell cycle into a quiescent (G_0) state (see Fig. 29-6).

Alternatively, cells may be induced to enter a postmitotic state, usually associated with terminal differentiation. Many of the signaling pathways that enable normal cells to respond to antigrowth signals are associated with the cell cycle block, specifically with components governing the restriction point in the G_1 phase of the cell cycle. The restriction point marks the transition from early to late G_1 phase and represents an irreversible commitment to undergo one cell division. Cells monitor their external environment during this period and, on the basis of sensed signals, decide whether to proliferate, be quiescent, or enter into a postmitotic state. At the molecular level, many and perhaps all antiproliferative signals involve the retinoblastoma protein (pRb) and its two family members p107 and p130.[10] pRb is a key negative regulator at the restriction point. When in a hypophosphorylated state, pRb blocks cell division by binding E2F transcription factors that control the expression of many genes essential for progression from G_1 to S phase (see Fig. 29-6).

In contrast, unphosphorylated pRb in G_0 does not bind E2F factors and is considered inactive. Likewise, disruption of the pRb pathway liberates E2F and thus allows

cell proliferation; cells are rendered insensitive to the antigrowth factors that normally operate along this pathway to block advance through the G_1 phase of the cell cycle. For example, TGF-β prevents the phosphorylation of pRb that inactivates pRb and thereby blocks advance through G_1. In some tumors such as breast, colon, liver, and pancreas cancer, TGF-β responsiveness is lost through down-regulation of TGF-β receptors or through expression of mutant, dysfunctional receptors. In other tumors such as colon, lung, and liver cancer, the cytoplasmic Smad4 protein, which transduces signals from ligand-activated TGF-β receptors to downstream targets, may be eliminated through mutation of its encoding gene. Alternatively, in cervical carcinomas induced by human papillomavirus (HPV), the viral oncoprotein E7 binds pRb and thereby induces dissociation of E2F and subsequent transcription of the genes necessary for cell cycle progression. In addition, cancer cells can also turn off the expression of integrins and other cell adhesion molecules (CAMs) that send antigrowth signals. In summary, the antigrowth signaling pathways converging onto Rb and the cell cycle are disrupted in a majority of human cancers.

Cyclin-cdk complexes, essential for cell cycle progression, are regulated by two families of cyclin-cdk inhibitors in normal cells. However, in tumor cells, regulatory proteins such as the p16 member of the INK4 family are frequently deleted, thereby allowing tumor cells to bypass cell cycle arrest.

In addition to avoiding antigrowth signals, tumor cells may also avoid terminal differentiation, such as through overexpression of the oncogene c-*myc*, which encodes

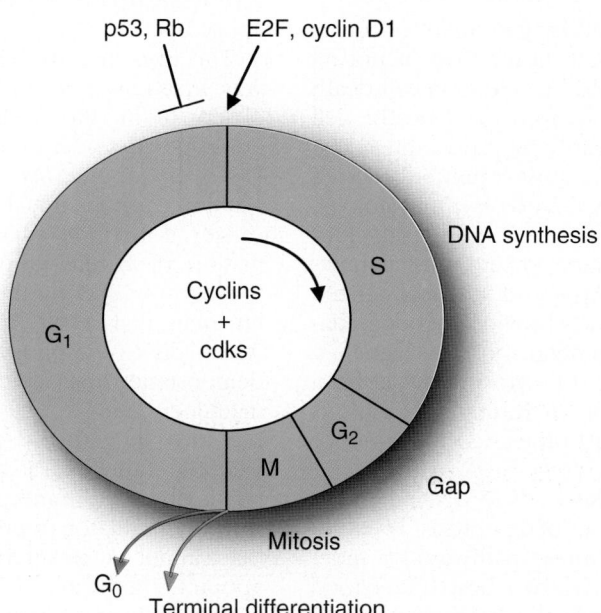

Figure 29-6 Schematic overview of the cell cycle. Cell division is governed by cyclin proteins and cyclin-dependent kinases (cdks). After mitosis, a cell can terminally differentiate, enter a quiescent state, or reenter the cell cycle. A critical point in cell cycle control is the transition from G_1 to S. After passing this checkpoint, the cell is committed to division. Tumor suppressor genes such as the retinoblastoma *(Rb)* gene and *p53* block the G_1-to-S transition, whereas oncogenes such as *cyclin D1* and *E2F* promote transition.

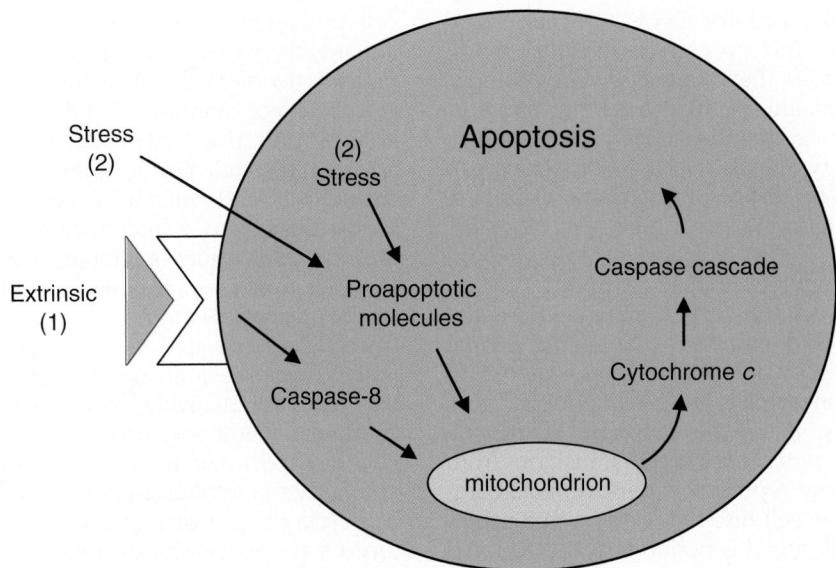

Figure 29-7 Apoptotic pathways. Extracellular and intracellular stress can induce apoptosis in tumor cells. Extracellular triggering can occur through a receptor-dependent (1) or receptor-independent (2) pathway. Both pathways induce the release of cytochrome *c* from mitochondria, which triggers the activation of various caspases in sequence and ultimately leads to apoptosis.

a transcription factor regulating expression of cyclins and cdks, or through up-regulation of Id (inhibitor of differentiation) family members. Likewise, during human colon carcinogenesis, inactivation of the adenomatous polyposis coli (APC)/β-catenin pathway serves to block the egress of enterocytes in the colonic crypts into a differentiated, postmitotic state.

Evasion of Cell Death

Growth of tumors is determined by the ability of tumor cells to proliferate, offset by cell death. Most, if not all types of tumors are characterized by defects in cell death signaling pathways and are resistant to cell death. Cell death in tumors is caused primarily by programmed cell death, or apoptosis, which is the most common and well defined form of cell death.[11] Apoptosis is a physiologic cell suicide program essential for embryonic development, functioning of the immune system, and maintenance of tissue homeostasis. Apoptosis is characterized by disruption of membranes and chromosomal degradation in a matter of hours. The general apoptosis signaling pathway involves the release of cytochrome *c* from mitochondria and subsequent activation of various caspases (a family of at least 10 proteases) in sequence (Fig. 29-7).

Activation of caspase cascades leads to DNA fragmentation and apoptosis. Induction of apoptosis is either death receptor dependent (extrinsic pathway) or independent (intrinsic pathway). The two best understood death receptor pathways include the Fas receptor and the death receptor (DR-5), which bind the extracellular Fas ligand and TRAIL (tumor necrosis factor [TNF]-related apoptosis-inducing factor), respectively. Binding of the ligands triggers the activation of caspase 8 and promotes the cascade of procaspase activation leading to release

of cytochrome *c* from mitochondria and eventually apoptosis. The intrinsic pathway is triggered by various extracellular and intracellular stresses, such as growth factor withdrawal, hypoxia, DNA damage, and oncogene induction. Receptor-independent pathways involve the translocation of proapoptotic molecules from the cytoplasm to the mitochondria, where they cause mitochondrial damage and release of cytochrome *c*. Cytochrome *c* is directly involved in the activation of caspase 9, which activates caspase 3; activation of caspase 3 then leads to apoptosis.

The idea that apoptosis forms a constraint to cancer was first raised in 1972 when massive apoptosis was observed in the cells populating rapidly growing, hormone-dependent tumors after hormone withdrawal.[12] Discovery of the *bcl*-2 oncogene having antiapoptotic activity opened up the investigation of apoptosis in cancer at the molecular level.[13,14] *bcl*-2 promotes the formation of B-cell lymphomas through a chromosomal translocation linking the *bcl*-2 gene to an immunoglobulin locus that results in constitutive activation of *bcl*-2, which drives lymphocyte survival. Further research has demonstrated that altering components of the apoptotic machinery allows a cell to resist death signals and thus provides it with a selective growth advantage. For example, functional inactivation of the tumor suppressor p53 is observed in more than 50% of human cancers. p53 is a key regulator of apoptosis by sensing DNA damage that cannot be repaired and subsequently activating the apoptotic pathway.

Other abnormalities such as hypoxia and oncogene overexpression are also channeled in part via p53 to the apoptotic machinery and fail to elicit apoptosis when p53 function is lost. Additionally, alterations in cell survival pathways can suppress or alter apoptosis. For example, the phosphatidylinositol-3'-kinase (PI3-kinase)-AKT pathway, which transmits antiapoptotic survival signals, is probably involved in inhibiting apoptosis in many human tumors. This signaling pathway can be activated by extracellular factors such as insulin-like growth factor I/II (IGF-I/II) or interleukin-3 (IL-3), by intracellular signals from Ras, or by loss of the pTEN tumor suppressor that negatively regulates the PI3-kinase–AKT pathway. A final example is the discovery of a nonsignaling decoy receptor for Fas ligand in a high fraction of lung and colon carcinoma cell lines. Expression of this decoy receptor dilutes the death signal mediated through Fas.

Nonapoptotic types of cell death include necrosis, autophagy, and mitotic catastrophe. Necrosis is normally induced by pathophysiologic conditions such as infection, inflammation, or ischemia. Necrosis is characterized by unregulated cell destruction. Autophagy, on the other hand, is characterized by proteolysis of long-lived proteins and organelle components in lysosomes.[15] Cells that undergo excessive autophagy undergo apoptosis. Autophagy is triggered by growth factor withdrawal, differentiation, and developmental triggers.[11,15] Finally, aberrant mitosis caused by failure of the G_2 checkpoint to block mitosis when DNA is damaged can lead to cell death and is known as mitotic catastrophe. The signaling pathways involved in these types of nonapoptotic cell death are less well defined than those that regulate apoptosis, but it is clear that defects in nonapoptotic cell death pathways have been linked to cancer. For example, amplification of the *MDM2* oncogene, which negatively regulates expression of p53, results in inadequate expression of p53 and thereby loss of tumor suppressor function. Another example is deletion of the autophagy-regulating gene *becklin-1* in a high percentage of ovarian, breast, and prostate cancer. In addition to cell death, cells can undergo permanent growth arrest, called *senescence,* when repair of damaged DNA fails. Senescent cells lose their clonogenicity, but defects in the senescent program contribute to tumor development.

Limitless Replication Potential

Acquired disruption of cell-to-cell signaling by itself does not ensure expansive tumor growth on its own. This is due to the intrinsic programmed decline in replication potential that limits the multiplication of normal somatic cells. This program must be disrupted for a clone of cells to develop into a macroscopic tumor. Normal cells have a finite replicative potential. Once a cell has progressed through a certain number of doublings, it stops growing—a process termed *senescence.*

With the exception of stem cells, activated lymphocytes, and germline cells, normal cells have limited replicative potential. Stem cells give rise to progenitor cells that can progress through a certain number of doublings with an increasing degree of differentiation. Fully differentiated cells do not have replicative potential. The number of doublings is controlled by telomers, the ends of chromosomes that are composed of several thousand repeats of a short 6–base pair (bp) sequence element.[16] Telomeres prevent end-to-end chromosomal fusion. However, each DNA replication is associated with the

loss of 50 to 100 bp of telomeric DNA from the ends of every chromosome. This progressive shortening of telomeres through successive cycles of replication eventually causes them to lose their ability to protect the ends of chromosomal DNA. When the critical length is bridged, the unprotected chromosomal ends participate in end-to-end chromosomal fusion to yield a karyotype disarray that almost inevitably results in death of the affected cell.[16] Telomeric attrition is negated by the enzyme telomerase, which elongates telomeric DNA. Telomerase activity is high during embryonic development and in certain cell populations such as stem cells in adults. However, many tumors are characterized by elevated telomerase activity. Alternatively, telomeres are maintained through recombination-based interchromosomal exchange of sequence information. Thus, by maintaining a telomere length above a critical threshold, tumor cells have unlimited proliferative potential and are considered immortal.

Recently, evidence has been obtained for the existence of cancer stem cells that give rise to tissue-specific progenitor cells and phenotypically diverse cancer cells with limited replicative potential.[17] For example, in breast and brain tumors, a small population of cancer stem cells have the ability to replicate, whereas the majority of cancer cells have no or a limited ability to proliferate. The most likely origin of cancer stem cells is normal adult stem cells that replace short-lived mature cells in tissues such as skin, gut, and blood.[18] When normal stem cells divide, one of the daughter cells inherits stem cell capabilities, whereas the other cell is launched along the differentiation pathway. In cancer stem cells, genes regulating self-renewal, such as *Bmi*-1, are overexpressed, thereby suppressing the default pathway of differentiation.

Sustained Angiogenesis

Based on the observation that many individuals who died of non–cancer-related causes had in situ tumors at the time of autopsy, physicians and scientists concluded that these microscopic tumors were in a dormant state. The reason for tumor dormancy is that the body blocks the tumor from recruiting its own blood supply to provide tumor cells with the required oxygen and nutrients. The growth of new blood vessels, or angiogenesis, is a highly regulated process to ensure supply to all cells within an organ. Surprisingly, the microscopic tumors lack the ability to induce angiogenesis, and only an estimated 1 in 600 acquire angiogenic activity. Research pioneered by Judah Folkman has demonstrated that naturally occurring endogenous angiogenesis inhibitors prevent tumors from expanding.[19] The angiogenesis inhibitors keep the tumors in check by counterbalancing the angiogenic signals. These signals are mediated by soluble factors and their receptors on endothelial cells, as well as by integrins and adhesion molecules mediating cell-matrix and cell-cell interactions. Angiogenic activity is induced by growth factors such as vascular endothelial growth factor (VEGF), bFGF and acidic FGF (aFGF), and platelet-derived growth factor. Each binds to transmembrane tyrosine kinase receptors on endothelial cells that are connected to intracellular signaling pathways. Angiogenesis inhibitors are associated with specific tissues or circulate in blood. The first inhibitor, interferon-α (IFN-α), was reported in 1980, and an additional 26 endogenous inhibitors have been identified since then,[19] including thrombospondin, tumstatin, canstatin, endostatin, and angiostatin. Evidence for the importance of inducing and sustaining angiogenesis in tumors is overwhelming. Most telling are the results of clinical studies with the anti-VEGF antibody bevacizumab (Avastin), the first angiogenesis inhibitor approved by the Food and Drug Administration for the treatment of colon cancer. Avastin significantly prolongs the survival of patients with advanced cancer. Similarly, a dominant interfering version of the VEGF receptor 2 proved to impair neovascularization and growth of subcutaneous tumors in mice.

The ability to induce and sustain angiogenesis seems to be acquired in a discrete step (or steps) during tumor development via a switch to the angiogenic phenotype.[19,20] Tumors appear to activate the angiogenic switch by changing the balance between total angiogenic stimulation and total angiogenic inhibition.[21] This occurs in most cases when angiogenesis stimulators overwhelm angiogenesis inhibitors. In some tumors these changes may be linked. It is likely that such disruption in angiogenic balance is under control of the genetic makeup of the individual tumor cell and its microenvironment. Angiogenesis inducers and inhibitors may be genetically controlled by tumor suppressor genes such as *p53*, whereas oncogenes such as *ras* may down-regulate transcription of endogenous inhibitors or activate inducers. For example, activation of *bcl-2* leads to significantly increased expression of VEGF and angiogenesis. Another dimension of regulation is through proteases, which can control the bioavailability of angiogenic activators and inhibitors. Thus, a variety of proteases can release bFGF stored in the ECM, whereas plasmin, a proangiogenic component of the clotting system, can cleave itself into an angiogenesis inhibitor form called *angiostatin*. Another angiogenesis inhibitor, endostatin, is an internal fragment of the basement membrane collagen XVIII. The coordinated expression of proangiogenic and antiangiogenic signaling molecules and their modulation by proteolysis appear to reflect the complex homeostatic regulation of normal tissue angiogenesis and vascular integrity. Different types of tumors use distinct molecular strategies to activate the angiogenic switch.

Tissue Invasion and Metastasis

Progressing tumors give rise to distant metastases, which are the cause of 90% of human cancer deaths.[22] The formation of tumor metastases is characterized by detachment of some tumor cells from the primary tumor and infiltration into the bloodstream or lymphatics (intravasation). The reciprocal process occurs at other locations in the body (extravasation). Both intravasation and extravasation are characterized by changes in ECMs and their interactions with tumor cells. The cell-cell and cell-matrix interactions are mediated through CAMs, primarily by members of the immunoglobulin and calcium-dependent

cadherin families,[23] the hyaluronan receptor CD44, and integrins,[24] which link cells to ECM substrates. Recent studies have shown that the molecules mediating adhesion are also capable of signal transduction. As such, changes in expression of adhesion molecules will alter signaling pathways, and, conversely, signaling molecules can directly affect the function of adhesion molecules.

Epithelial (E)-cadherin is the prototype cadherin responsible for cell polarity and organization of the epithelium. E-cadherin function is lost in most epithelial tumors during progression to tumor malignancy and may in fact be a prerequisite for tumor cell invasion and metastasis. In normal cells, extracellular domains of E-cadherin on opposing cells couple and form cell-cell junctions (Fig. 29-8). The cytoplasmic cell adhesion complex is linked to the actin cytoskeleton through catenins (α, β, and γ). Certain mechanisms, including mutational inactivation of the E-cadherin or β-catenin genes, transcriptional repression, or proteases of the extracellular cadherin domain, induce loss of E-cadherin function.[23] This prevents catenins from binding and leads to their accumulation in cytoplasm. Inactivation of nonsequestered β- and γ-catenin is dependent on the presence of the tumor suppressor gene *APC* and an inactive Wnt signaling pathway (see Fig. 29-8). However, when APC function is lost, as is the case in many colon cancers or in the case of Wnt activation, β-catenin is not degraded but instead translocates to the nucleus, where transcription of genes involved in cell proliferation and tumor progression, such as c-*myc*, cyclin D1, CD44, and others, is activated.

Changes in expression of CAMs in the immunoglobulin superfamily also appear to play critical roles in the processes of invasion and metastasis.[2,23] Neuronal CAM (N-CAM), for example, undergoes a switch in expression from a highly adhesive isoform to poorly adhesive (or even repulsive) forms in Wilms' tumor, neuroblastoma, and small cell lung cancer. In invasive pancreatic cancer and colorectal cancers, the overall expression of N-CAM is reduced.

Changes in integrin expression are also evident in invasive and metastatic cells. For invading and metastasizing cells to be successful, they need to adapt to changing tissue microenvironments, which is accomplished through shifts in the spectrum of integrin α and β subunits displayed by the migrating cells that bind ECM molecules such as collagens, laminin, and fibronectin. Each integrin molecule consists of an α subunit and a β subunit, but a particular β subunit can dimerize with several different α subunits. These novel permutations result in different integrin subtypes (of which there are more than 22) having distinct substrate preferences. Thus, carcinoma cells facilitate invasion by shifting their expression of integrins from those that favor the ECM present in normal epithelium to other integrins that preferentially bind the degraded stromal components produced by extracellular proteases.[2] For example, expression of $\alpha_4\beta_1$, which binds fibronectin, correlates with progression of melanoma. The changes are incompletely understood because of the large number of distinct integrin genes, the even larger number of heterodimeric receptors result-

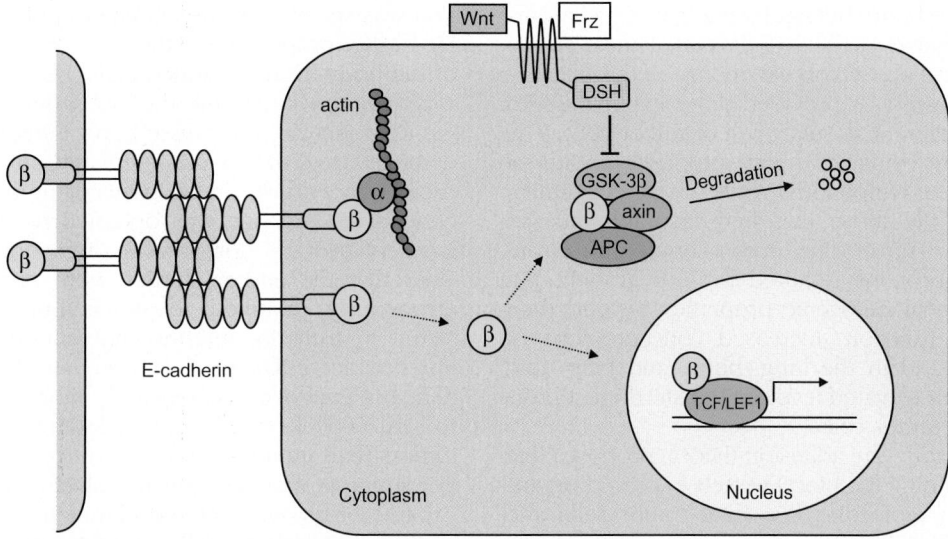

Figure 29-8 Loss of E-cadherin permits tumor progression. Functional loss of E-cadherin to sequester β-catenin leads to the accumulation of β-catenin in cytoplasm. Likewise, Wnt signaling inactivates GSK-3β, which leads to stabilization of β-catenin instead of its degradation. In addition, loss of APC function may result in the accumulation of β-catenin in cytoplasm. This leads to translocation of β-catenin to the nucleus, where it binds the T-cell–specific transcription factor/lymphoid enhancer factor-1 (TCF/LEF-1) and induces a genetic program that leads to tumor progression. α, α-catenin; APC, adenomatous polyposis coli; β, β-catenin; Frz, frizzled (transmembrane receptor for Wnt growth factors); DSH, disheveled; GSK-3β, glycogen synthase kinase 3β.

ing from combinatorial expression of various α and β receptor subunits, and the increasing evidence of complex signals emitted by the cytoplasmic domains of these receptors. Changes in integrin expression may also be essential for expansion of the tumor stem cell compartment by inhibiting differentiation or apoptosis.[25]

The second general parameter of invasive and metastatic capability involves extracellular proteases that regulate ECM turnover. It has become clear that tumor progression may involve increased expression of proteases, decreased expression of protease inhibitors, and inactive zymogen forms of proteases converted into active enzymes. Expression of the protease tenascin, which neutralizes adhesion to fibronectin, is increased 10-fold in invasive breast carcinoma as compared with normal breast tissue. Matrix metalloproteinases are overexpressed in melanoma, invasive breast carcinoma, and invasive squamous cell carcinoma. Matrix-degrading proteases are characteristically associated with the cell surface by synthesis with a transmembrane domain, by binding to specific protease receptors, or by association with integrins. One imagines that docking of active proteases on the cell surface can facilitate invasion by cancer cells into nearby stroma, across blood vessel walls, and through normal epithelial cell layers. That notion notwithstanding, it is difficult to unambiguously ascribe the functions of particular proteases solely to this capability, given their evident roles in other hallmark capabilities, including angiogenesis and growth signaling, which in turn contribute directly or indirectly to invasive/metastatic capability. A further complexity derives from the multiple cell types involved in protease expression and display, including stromal and inflammatory cells.

Activation of extracellular proteases and the altered binding specificities of cadherins, CAMs, and integrins are clearly central to the acquisition of invasiveness and metastatic potential. The clonal and genetic diversity of tumors permits adhesion and detachment from the same matrix. Some tumor cells within a primary tumor may have the correct genotype and phenotype to permit both detachment from the surrounding tissue and entry into blood or lymphatic vessels. Likewise, extravasation may be mediated by a few tumor cells that express the required receptors for certain ECM molecules. In general, mutations that confer escape from homeostatic control mechanisms in the host or that give the tumor cell a growth advantage over others are favorably selected. Thus, tumor clones that best complement the environment with expression of particular ECM receptors may thrive because this provides an advantage over other clones. However, the regulatory pathways and molecular mechanisms that govern these changes are incompletely understood and appear to differ from one tissue environment to another.

Outgrowth at Preferred Sites

Invasion and metastatic spread of tumor cells do not appear to be random processes. Paget observed in 1889 that breast carcinoma often metastasized to the liver, lungs, bone, adrenals, or brain. He hypothesized that tumor cells (the "seed") would grow only in selective environments (the "soil") where conditions supported tumor growth, hence the so-called seed-and-soil hypothesis. Since then, additional studies have confirmed this hypothesis. For example, malignant melanoma metastasizes to the brain, but ocular malignant melanoma frequently metastasizes to the liver. Prostate cancer metastasizes to the bone and colon carcinoma to the liver.

Molecular analysis has provided three major theories to explain the preferential outgrowth of tumor cells. The first theory, the growth factor theory, proposes that tumor cells in the blood or lymphatics invade organs at a similar frequency, but only those that find favorable growth factors multiply. Transferrins, for example, are iron-transferring ferroproteins required for cell growth, but they have additional mitogenic properties beyond their iron-transporting function. Increased concentrations of transferrin are found in the lung, bone, and brain and are associated with elevated levels of transferrin receptors on metastasizing tumor cells.

The second theory, the adhesion theory, proposes that endothelial cells lining the blood vessels in certain organs express adhesion molecules that bind tumor cells and permit extravasation. The third theory is that chemokines secreted by the target organ can enter the circulation and selectively attract tumor cells that express receptors for the chemokines. Evidence for the importance of chemokines in tumor progression was recently obtained for breast cancer cells preferentially metastasizing in bone marrow, liver, lymph nodes, and lung.[26] These organs were found to secrete CXCL12, the ligand for the chemokine receptor CXCR4, which is enriched on breast cancer cells as opposed to normal breast epithelial cells. A similar phenomenon was observed for melanoma cells, which were found to express elevated levels of the receptors CXCR4, CCR7, and CCR10 in comparison to normal melanocytes.[26] Lymph nodes, lung, liver, bone marrow, and skin express the highest levels of ligands for these receptors and are the preferred sites for metastatic spread of melanomas. Because chemokines are now known to affect angiogenesis and expression of cytokines, adhesion molecules, and proteases, in addition to inducing migration, it appears that chemokines and their receptors play an essential role in the successful outgrowth of tumors at preferential sites.

Central to the mechanisms dictating metastatic predisposition is bone marrow–derived progenitor cells expressing the VEGF receptor 1 (VEGFR1) and VLA-4, which are prompted by the primary tumor to establish premetastatic niches before the arrival of metastatic tumor cells.[27] Tumor-secreted humoral factors induce expression of fibronectin (a VLA-4 ligand) on fibroblasts and fibroblast-like cells in specific distant organs. Simultaneously, the VEGFR1+, VLA-4+ cells leave the bone marrow and migrate to the premetastatic niche, where they form cellular clusters that permit the development of metastases.

Immunosurveillance and Immunoediting

In the early 1900s it was proposed by Paul Ehrlich that the frequency of cancerous transformation would be very high if it were not for the defense system of the host. This concept was later substantiated in the 1950s and 1960s, and the term *immunosurveillance* was introduced by Burnet in 1970. Burnet hypothesized that the development of T-lymphocyte–mediated immunity during evolu-

tion was specific for the elimination of transformed cells. He further proposed that there is continuous surveillance of the body for transformed cells, hence the term *immunosurveillance*. During the subsequent years, experiments in immunosuppressed and immunodeficient mice demonstrated that T-cell–mediated immunity provides protection against virally induced tumors. However, no conclusive evidence was obtained for immune surveillance of cancer. More recent discoveries have made it clear that the earlier studies were performed in mice erroneously assumed to be immunodeficient. When tested in truly immunoincompetent mice, evidence of immune surveillance of cancer was obtained: immunodeficient mice were significantly more susceptible to the formation of chemically induced tumors and spontaneous tumors than immunocompetent mice were.[1] This discovery suggests that the unmanipulated immune system is capable of recognizing and eliminating primary tumors.

Does immune surveillance of cancer exist in humans? Evaluation of long-term studies in transplant patients who were immunosuppressed and individuals with immunodeficiencies showed an increased incidence of virally induced tumors such as non-Hodgkin's lymphoma, Kaposi's sarcoma, and carcinomas of the genitourinary and anogenital regions. However, they also showed a higher incidence of tumors with no apparent viral etiology, such as malignant melanoma, lung cancer, pancreatic cancer, colon cancer, and kidney cancer. More conclusive are observations from patients with paraneoplastic neurologic degeneration (PND).[28] Patients with PND are susceptible to autoimmune neurologic disease in discrete regions of the nervous system, mediated through antibodies and cytotoxic T cells against neuronal antigens. Clinical examination reveals systemic malignancies, most commonly breast or ovarian adenocarcinoma or small cell lung cancer, that are generally small, show limited spread, and are sensitive to treatment. Importantly, the presence of antineuronal T cells and antibodies in all PND patients studied is associated with clinical and pathologic evidence of suppression of tumor growth. Some cancer patients mount a PND immune response but do not contract neurologic disease. These patients have smaller tumors and survive longer than those without such immune responses. The data from mouse and human studies combined suggest that immune surveillance of cancer does exist and is mediated through immune cells and soluble factors. Although the immune system may eliminate most transformed cells, some cells manage to escape and may develop into tumors.

The continuous pressure of the immune system in an immunocompetent host to a great degree determines whether and how tumors evolve, a process called *immunoediting* (Fig. 29-9).[1] In this process the immune system plays a dual role in the interactions between tumor and the host. On one hand, the immune system effectively eliminates highly immunogenic tumor cells. At the same time, however, the immune system permits tumor cells with reduced immunogenicity to develop, thereby selecting for tumor variants that are poorly recognized by the immune system or that have acquired immune evasion mechanisms. Over time, this selection leads to the out-

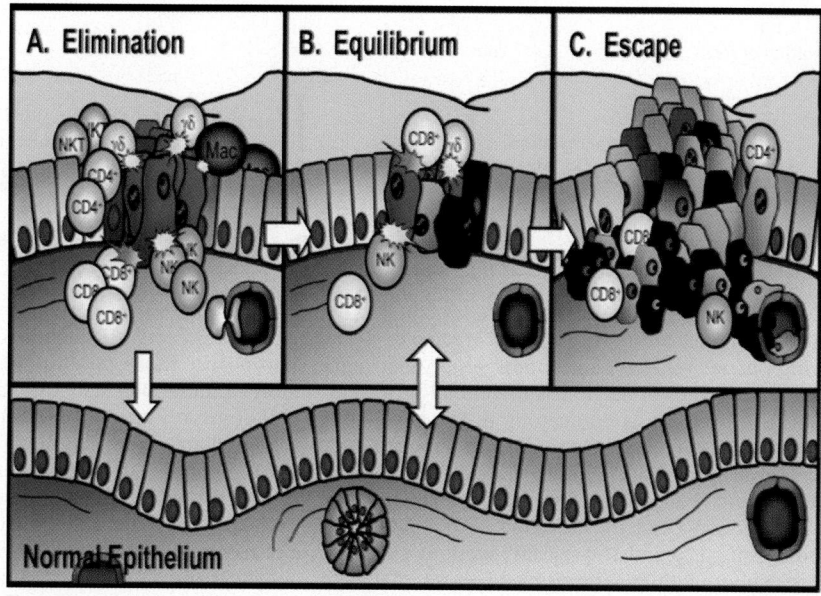

Figure 29-9 Schematic overview of immunoediting. When developing tumors disrupt local tissue structures, proinflammatory cytokines are released and, together with secreted chemokines, attract innate immune cells such as macrophages, natural killer (NK) cells, and NKT cells. Innate immune cells can directly recognize and lyse tumor cells, but they can also induce an adaptive immune response mediated by T and B lymphocytes. Whereas most tumor cells are eliminated (elimination phase, *A*), tumor cell variants may survive and expand. However, the activated immune system keeps the tumor in check by eliminating tumor cells that are sufficiently immunogenic (equilibrium phase, *B*). The immunologic pressure may cause selection toward tumor cell variants with reduced immunogenicity that are capable of escaping immune recognition (escape phase, *C*). These variants can expand in an immunologically intact environment. (Reprinted, with permission, from the *Annual Review of Immonology*, Volume 22 © 2004 by Annual Reviews www.annualreviews.org.)

growth of tumor cells that fail to induce an effective immune response. As such, the interactions between an intact immune system and tumor cells evolve through three phases, referred to as the elimination phase, the equilibrium phase, and the escape phase. Recognition along with elimination of transformed cells is a concerted effort between innate and adaptive immunity, representing the two arms of the immune system. The local disruption of tissue that occurs as a result of the expansion of transformed cells is associated with the release of chemokines and proinflammatory cytokines that trigger innate immunity, such as IFNs, IL-1, IL-6, and TNF-α.

The innate immune system represents the first line of defense against transformed cells (and microorganisms). The most important outcome of these initial events is the production of IFN-γ by activated innate immune cells. IFN-γ has direct antitumor effects and further boosts tumor cell lysis by innate immune cells. The resulting availability of tumor antigen triggers an adaptive immune response. Key in this process is the uptake of antigen by antigen-presenting cells, primarily dendritic cells. The dendritic cells migrate to tumor-draining lymph nodes and stimulate T and B lymphocytes. The development of adaptive immunity represents the second line of defense against tumors and, together with innate immunity, could completely eliminate the tumor. However, elimination does not always occur and may lead to what is referred to as the equilibrium phase. This phase is characterized by a balance between tumor growth and tumor elimination, as the name suggests. Antitumor immunity leads to

destruction of immunogenic tumor cells, whereas tumor cells with reduced immunity go unnoticed.

Over time, genetic instability and heterogeneity of the tumor cells may give rise to tumor variants better able to withstand the immunologic pressure. Once this point has been reached, referred to as the escape phase, the immune system can no longer contain the tumor, and the tumor grows progressively. During the past decade, multiple mechanisms have been identified through which tumors escape elimination by the immune system. These mechanisms include host-related factors, tumor-related factors, or a combination of both. Among host-related factors are treatment-related immunosuppression, acquired or inherited immunodeficiency, and aging. The list of tumor-related escape mechanisms includes loss of major histocompatibility complex (MHC) alleles, reduced antigen processing or presentation (or both), decreased expression of co-stimulatory molecules required for T-cell recognition, secretion of immunosuppressive factors (TGF-β, IL-10), stimulation of suppressor cells, and mechanisms that actively induce tolerance or apoptosis.

CARCINOGENESIS

Cancer Genetics

As stated earlier, malignant transformation is the process by which a clonal population of cells acquires alterations that confer a growth advantage over normal cells. Many

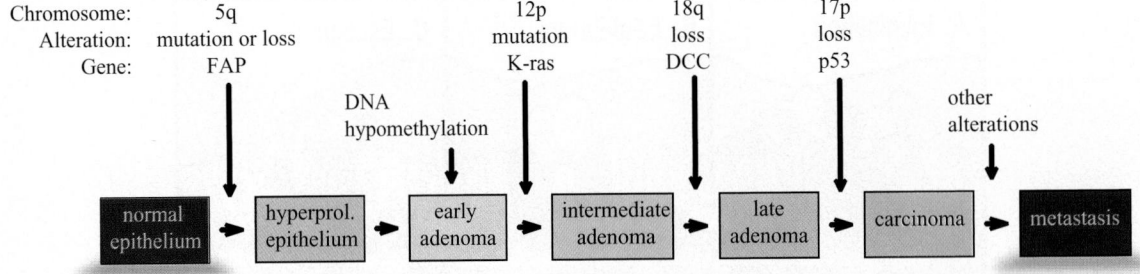

Figure 29-10 A genetic model for colorectal tumorigenesis. Tumorigenesis proceeds through a series of genetic alterations involving oncogenes *(ras)* and tumor suppressor genes (particularly those on chromosomes 5q, 12p, 17p, and 18q). The three stages of adenomas in general represent tumors of increasing size, dysplasia, and villous content. In patients with familial adenomatous polyposis (FAP), a mutation on chromosome 5q *(APC* gene) is inherited. This alteration may be responsible for the hypoproliferative epithelium present in these patients. Hypomethylation is present in very small adenomas in patients with or without polyposis, and this alteration may lead to aneuploidy and result in the loss of suppressor gene alleles. The *ras* gene mutation appears to occur in one cell of a preexisting small adenoma and, through clonal expansion, produces a larger and more dysplastic tumor. Allelic deletions of chromosomes 17p and 18q usually occur at a later stage of tumorigenesis than do deletions of chromosome 5q or *ras* gene mutations. The order of these changes is not invariant, however, and accumulation of these changes, rather than their order with respect to one another, seems to be most important. Tumors continue to progress once carcinomas have formed, and the accumulated loss of suppressor genes on additional chromosomes correlates with the ability of the carcinomas to metastasize and cause death. (From Fearon ER: A genetic model for colorectal tumorigenesis. Cell 61:759, 1990.)

of these alterations occur at the genetic level and involve gain of function by oncogenes or loss of function by tumor suppressor genes. A multistep model for colorectal tumorigenesis has been described (Fig. 29-10). Designation as an oncogene or tumor suppressor gene relates to the directionality of effect, without implications about molecular detail. Indeed, the original name for what came to be known as tumor suppressor genes was in fact *anti-oncogenes.*

Genetic mutations that are inherited from one's parents and are present in all cells of the body are called *germline* (or constitutional) mutations; in contrast, *somatic* mutations are acquired during an individual's lifetime and cannot be passed to one's children. Somatic mutations, which account for most mutations in cancer, may be caused by exposure to carcinogens in the form of radiation, chemicals, or chronic inflammation (see later).

A tumor that arises in an individual may be classified as either hereditary or sporadic. In hereditary cases, a germline mutation is responsible for the predisposition to neoplasia. The index case, or *proband,* is the individual in whom the syndrome is first diagnosed, even if earlier generations are later recognized as also having the syndrome. If the patient with a tumor does not have an inherited predisposition and the tumor's genetic mutations are all somatic, the tumor is classified as sporadic. In some hereditary cancer syndromes, the germline mutation causes a tendency for the cell to accumulate somatic mutations.

Although hereditary cancer syndromes are rare, their study has provided powerful insights into more common forms of cancer (Table 29-4). Key germline mutations in hereditary cancers are often the same as somatic muta-

tions present in sporadic cancers. *p53* is the most commonly mutated gene in human cancer and, if inherited in a mutant form, causes Li-Fraumeni syndrome. Familial adenomatous polyposis (FAP) is caused by a germline mutation in the *APC* gene. More than 80% of *sporadic* colorectal cancers also have a somatic mutation of this same gene. Similarly, mutation in the *ret* proto-oncogene is responsible for the predisposition to development of the familial form of medullary thyroid cancer (MTC). Somatic mutations of *ret* are found in about 50% of sporadic MTCs.

Predisposition in familial cancer syndromes is generally inherited in an autosomal dominant fashion. Exceptions include ataxia-telangiectasia and xeroderma pigmentosa, which are transmitted in an autosomal recessive manner. Not all the inherited genetic mutations have complete penetrance. There is close to complete penetrance of colorectal cancer in FAP and of MTC in multiple endocrine neoplasia type 2 (MEN 2). In contrast, penetrance is less than 50% for pheochromocytoma in neurofibromatosis. Penetrance can also vary considerably for different characteristics of the same syndrome. However, the factors determining penetrance remain largely unknown.

A number of features of hereditary cancers distinguish them phenotypically from their sporadic counterparts. The former tend to cause the development of multifocal, bilateral cancer at an early age, whereas in the latter, cancer occurs later and is usually unilateral. Hereditary cancers will display clustering of the same cancer type in relatives and may be associated with other conditions such as mental retardation and pathognomonic skin lesions.

Table 29-4 Familial Cancer Syndromes

SYNDROME	GENES	LOCATIONS	CANCER SITES AND ASSOCIATED TRAITS
Breast/ovarian syndrome	*BRCA1* *BRCA2*	17q21 13q12.3	Cancer of the breast, ovary, colon, prostate Cancer of the breast, ovary, colon, prostate, gallbladder and biliary tree, pancreas, stomach; melanoma
Cowden's disease	*PTEN*	10q23.3	Cancer of the breast, endometrium, thyroid
Familial adenomatous polyposis (FAP)	*APC*	17q21	Colorectal carcinoma, duodenal and gastric neoplasms, medulloblastomas, osteomas
Familial melanoma	*p16* *CDK4*	9p21 12q14	Melanoma, pancreatic cancer, dysplastic nevi, atypical moles
Hereditary diffuse gastric cancer	*CDH1*	16q22	Gastric cancer
Hereditary nonpolyposis colorectal cancer	*hMLH1* *hMSH2* *hMSH6* *hPMS1* *hPMS2*	3p21 2p22-21 2p16 2q31.1 7p22.2	Colorectal cancer, endometrial cancer, transitional cell carcinoma of the ureter and renal pelvis, carcinomas of the stomach, small bowel, pancreas, ovary
Hereditary papillary renal cell carcinoma	*MET*	7q31	Renal cell cancer
Hereditary paraganglioma and pheochromocytoma	*SDHB* *SDHC* *SDHD*	1p36.1-p35 1q21 11q23	Paraganglioma, pheochromocytoma
Juvenile polyposis coli	*BMPRIA* *SMAD4/DPC4*	10q21-q22 18q21.1	Juvenile polyps of the gastrointestinal tract, gastrointestinal malignancies
Li-Fraumeni	*p53* *hCHK2*	17p13 22q12.1	Breast cancer, soft tissue sarcoma, osteosarcoma, brain tumors, adrenocortical carcinoma, Wilms' tumor, phyllodes tumor (breast), pancreatic cancer, leukemia, neuroblastoma
Multiple endocrine neoplasia type 1 (MEN 1)	*MEN1*	11q13	Pancreatic islet cell tumors, parathyroid hyperplasia, pituitary adenomas
Multiple endocrine neoplasia type 2 (MEN 2)	*RET*	10q11.2	Medullary thyroid cancer, pheochromocytoma, parathyroid hyperplasia
MYH-associated adenomatous polyposis	*MYH*	1p34.3-p32.1	Cancer of the colon, rectum, breast, stomach
Neurofibromatosis type I	*NF1*	17q11	Neurofibromas, neurofibrosarcoma, acute myelogenous leukemia, brain tumors
Neurofibromatosis type II	*NF2*	22q12	Acoustic neuromas, meningiomas, gliomas, ependymomas
Nevoid basal cell carcinoma	*PTC*	9q22.3	Basal cell carcinoma
Peutz-Jeghers syndrome	*STK11*	19p13.3	Gastrointestinal carcinomas, breast cancer, testicular cancer, pancreatic cancer, benign pigmentation of the skin and mucosa
Retinoblastoma	*RB*	13q14	Retinoblastoma, sarcomas, melanoma, malignant neoplasms of the brain and meninges
Tuberous sclerosis	*TSC1* *TSC2*	9q34 16p13	Multiple hamartomas, renal cell carcinoma, astrocytoma
von Hippel-Lindau syndrome	*VHL*	3p25	Renal cell carcinoma, hemangioblastomas of the retina and central nervous system, pheochromocytoma
Wilms' tumor	*WT*	11p13	Wilms' tumor, aniridia, genitourinary abnormalities, mental retardation

From Marsh DJ, Zori RT. Genetic insights into familial cancers—update and recent discoveries. Cancer Lett 181:125-164, 2002, with permission.

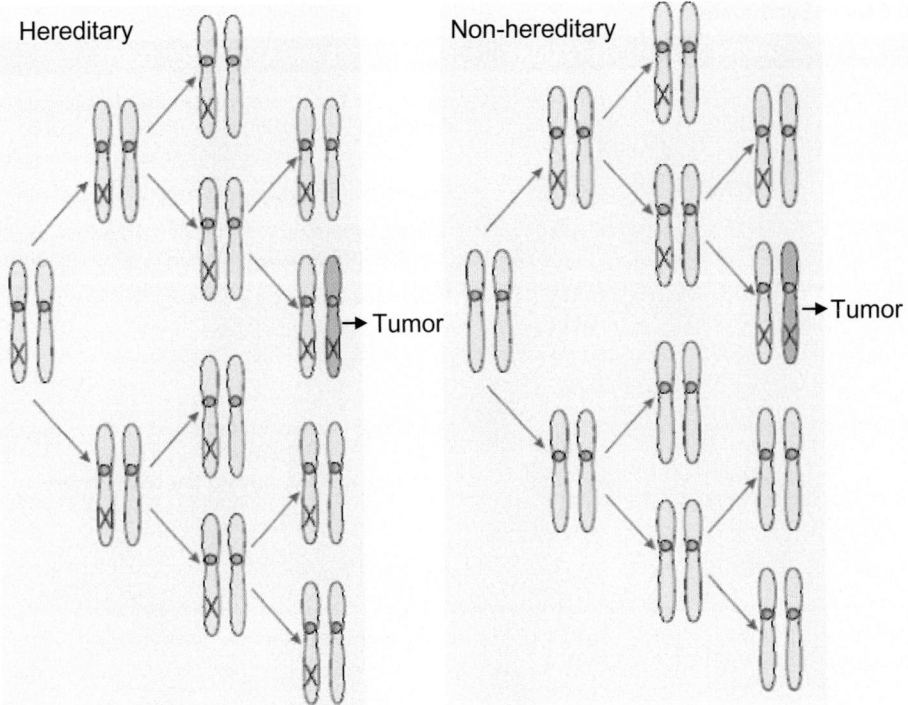

Hereditary

Non-hereditary

→ Tumor

→ Tumor

Figure 29-11 Two genetic hits to cancer. In hereditary retinoblastoma, all retinoblasts are heterozygous for the mutant allele (indicated by X)—all have already sustained one hit. In contrast, the preneoplastic clone in nonhereditary retinoblastoma must acquire this mutation before sustaining the so-called second hit to complete malignant transformation. (Modified from Knudson AG: Two genetic hits [more or less] to cancer. Nat Rev Cancer 1:57-62, 2001, with permission.)

Selected Familial Cancer Syndromes

Retinoblastoma

Retinoblastoma is a pediatric retinal tumor that holds an important place in the history of cancer genetics because the causative gene, *RB1*, was the first tumor suppressor gene to be cloned. Most cases are detected by 7 years of age, but bilateral disease occurs earlier, usually within the first year of life. It is associated with extraocular malignancies, including sarcomas, melanomas, and tumors of the central nervous system. Distinct sporadic and hereditary forms of retinoblastoma have long been recognized, with predisposition conferred by a germline mutation in approximately 40% of cases. Knudson reasoned that the germline mutation is necessary but not by itself sufficient for tumorigenesis because some children with an affected parent do not develop a tumor but later produce an affected child, thus indicating that they are carriers of the germline mutation. In most affected children with an affected parent, tumors develop bilaterally. He further hypothesized that hereditary retinoblastoma requires two mutations, one of which is germline and the other somatic. In children with unilateral disease and no family history, both mutations are somatic. The hereditary and nonhereditary forms of the tumor require the same number of events—the so-called two-hit hypothesis (Fig. 29-11). The RB1 protein product is a key regulator of the cell cycle, and its loss results in failure of retinoblasts to differentiate properly.

Li-Fraumeni Syndrome

In 1969, Li and Fraumeni reported a new familial syndrome involving sarcomas (of both soft tissue and bone), breast cancers (the most common malignancy in this syndrome), and cerebral neoplasms, as well as a variety of other cancers. The syndrome that now bears their names has been defined in several ways:

1. As a proband in which sarcoma is diagnosed before the age of 45 years
2. With a first-degree relative with any cancer diagnosed before the age of 45 years
3. As an additional first- or second-degree relative either with a sarcoma at any age or with any cancer when younger than 45 years

Fifty percent of Li-Fraumeni kindreds have mutations in the *TP53* gene, which produces the protein p53. The syndrome is inherited in an autosomal dominant fashion. Penetrance is 50% by 30 years of age. Patients exhibit increased sensitivity to radiation—the irradiated field is susceptible to the development of new malignancies. For kindreds who lack germline *TP53* mutations, a number of candidate genes have been proposed, including the cell cycle checkpoint kinase gene *hChk2*, which directly phosphorylates p53. It is likely that other such causative genes serve tumor suppressive functions similar to p53 or are involved in the regulation of p53.

Familial Adenomatous Polyposis

FAP accounts for 1% of the total colorectal cancer burden. It is an autosomal dominant condition caused by mutation in the *APC* gene located on chromosome 5q21. Penetrance is extremely high, with colorectal cancer developing in more than 90% of affected individuals. It is characterized clinically by the development of several hundred to more than a thousand adenomatous polyps that carpet the colon. The first clear FAP kindreds were described in 1925 by the surgeon Lockhart-Mummery. The phenotype usually emerges during the second and third decades of life. The polyps are indistinguishable (macroscopically and microscopically) from sporadic adenomatous polyps, and each individual polyp does not have a greater propensity to undergo malignant degeneration than sporadic polyps do. Rather, it is the sheer number of polyps that makes the collective risk for malignancy so high. Untreated individuals typically contract colorectal cancer at 35 to 40 years of age, around 30 years earlier than the median age for sporadic colorectal cancer. Extracolonic manifestations of FAP include upper gastrointestinal polyps, desmoid tumors (15%), and thyroid cancer (1%-2%; usually papillary). Polyps of the stomach and duodenum are present in more than 90% of patients by 70 years of age, with two thirds of duodenal polyps located in the periampullary region. Indeed, duodenal adenocarcinoma is the third leading cause of death in FAP, after metastatic colorectal carcinoma and desmoid tumors. Desmoid tumors are locally invasive fibromatoses that occur within the abdomen or abdominal wall. Patients with FAP have a relative risk for the development of desmoid disease that is 850 times that of the general population.

The *APC* gene was first localized in 1987 and then cloned in 1991 after mutation analyses of FAP kindreds. It encodes a 300-kd protein, expressed in a variety of cell types, whose major function is as a scaffolding protein, and it affects cell adhesion and migration. It is part of a protein complex, modulated by the Wnt signaling pathway, that regulates the phosphorylation and degradation of β-catenin. When *APC* is mutated, β-catenin is not phosphorylated and accumulates in the cytoplasm, where it binds to the Tcf family of transcription factors and alters the expression of various genes involved in cell proliferation, migration, differentiation, and apoptosis. More than 700 disease-causing mutations in the *APC* gene have been reported, the most common of which involve a frameshift mutation (68%), a nonsense mutation (30%), or a large deletion (2%). Most of these mutations are located in what is referred to as the *mutation cluster region,* at the 5′ end of exon 15.

The location of the mutation plays a role in determining the phenotype. Mutations between 976 and 1067 are associated with a threefold to fourfold increased risk for the development of duodenal adenomas. Congenital hypertrophy of the retinal pigment epithelium (CHRPE) is associated with mutations between codons 463 and 1387. Gardner's syndrome is associated with mutations between codons 1403 and 1578[29] and, in addition to colorectal cancer, is characterized by osteomas of the mandible or skull, epidermal cysts, and multiple skin and soft tissue tumors, especially desmoids and thyroid tumors. Attenuated FAP is a phenotypically distinct variant of FAP in which the following is true:

1. Affected individuals have fewer than 100 adenomas.
2. The polyps are more proximally distributed in the colon
3. The onset of colorectal cancer occurs about 15 years later than in patients with FAP.

Mutations responsible for this variant occur in the extreme proximal or distal portions of the *APC* gene.

MYH-associated polyposis (MAP) is a recently described syndrome caused by mutations in the human MutY homologue *(MYH)* gene. It accounts for the same percentage of cases of colorectal cancer as FAP does, but unlike FAP, MAP is inherited in an autosomal *recessive* manner. Phenotypically, MAP-associated colorectal cancer is indistinguishable from classic or attenuated FAP, although it occurs later, around the age of 50 years. The polyps are distributed throughout the colon, but there are conflicting data about right- and left-sided tumor predominance. Extracolonic manifestations include breast cancer (18%) and upper gastrointestinal polyps (a third).[30] The *MYH* gene encodes a DNA glycosylase involved in the base excision repair (BER) pathway, which is important in preventing mutations secondary to oxidative damage. *Y165C* and *G382D* mutations account for more than 80% of all mutations discovered thus far. Penetrance is estimated at 50%.[30] Homozygotes or compound heterozygotes for germline mutations of the *MYH* gene have a 93-fold increased risk for colorectal cancer.[31] Mutation leads to chromosomal instability in which there is an accelerated rate of chromosomal misaggregation during cell division. This leads to aneuploidy, which has been recognized as an early genetic change in the stepwise carcinogenesis of both FAP and MAP tumors. Polyps bearing *MYH* mutations have twice the overall incidence of aneuploidy as those in patients with FAP. Current evidence suggests that carriers of single mutated alleles are unlikely to have more than a 50% increased risk for colorectal cancer.

Hereditary Nonpolyposis Colorectal Cancer

Also known as Lynch's syndrome, hereditary nonpolyposis colorectal cancer (HNPCC) accounts for 5% to 10% of all colorectal cancers. It is an autosomal dominant condition caused by mutations in DNA mismatch repair genes. When originally described by Lynch, kindreds were subclassified into types I and II based on whether only colorectal cancer developed (type I) or whether extracolonic cancers were present (type II). Penetrance is high. The broad phenotype of HNPCC is right-sided predominance of colonic cancers (70% proximal to the splenic flexure) that appear at an earlier age (median age at diagnosis, 44 years), with an increased likelihood of synchronous and metachronous cancers. Extracolonic malignancies occur, especially in the endometrium and ovary. Although the actual incidence of adenomatous polyps is the same as for those in whom sporadic colorectal cancer develops, once a tumor develops, there is an increased rate of tumor progression because the rate of genetic mutation in HNPCC cells is two to three times higher than in normal cells. A colonic adenoma may progress to carcinoma within 2 to 3 years, in contrast to the 8 to 10 years typical of sporadic cases.

Mutations in DNA mismatch repair genes cause microsatellite instability. Microsatellites are genomic regions in which short DNA sequences are repeated. During replication of these sequences, slippage of the DNA polymerase complex can occur and result in the formation of daughter strands that contain too many or too few copies of these sequences. Mutations may occur when these microsatellites are misaligned. The mutations then persist when the DNA mismatch repair proteins fail to correct the errors. Mutations in a number of DNA mismatch repair genes have been identified in patients with HNPCC. Mutations in *hMSH2* and *hMLH1* account for about two thirds of cases. *MSH6* mutations are responsible for a further 10% of cases. Other mismatch repair genes in which mutations lead to HNPCC include *PMS1* and *PMS2*. Note that 15% of sporadic colorectal cancers have microsatellite instability, but it occurs through methylation silencing of the *hMLH1* gene rather than through mutation as in HNPCC.

BRCA1 and BRCA2

About 5% to 10% of all breast cancers are hereditary and attributable to mutations in high-penetrance susceptibility genes. However, only two of these genes have been identified: *BRCA1* and *BRCA2*. One quarter of high-risk kindreds have mutations in either of these genes. Although the estimated risk for breast cancer is 80% in a 70-year-old woman with a germline mutation in *BRCA1* or *BRCA2*, different mutations vary in their risk for malignancy.

Carriers are at risk for other cancers, especially those of the ovary. The risk for ovarian cancer in a patient who is a carrier for *BRCA1* or *BRCA2* is 60% and 27%, respectively. Approximately 5% of all ovarian cancers are attributed to *BRCA1* germline mutations. The risk for ovarian cancer in patients with *BRCA2* mutations is lower, around 15% to 20%. Male carriers are at greater risk for prostate cancer.

The *BRCA1* gene is located on the long arm of chromosome 17. It is a large gene of some 100,000 nucleic acids, and more than 250 different mutations have been reported. The sheer number of mutations makes the task of identifying the specific mutation in a new kindred very difficult. The *BRCA2* gene is an even larger gene than *BRCA1*, and about 100 mutations have been reported. As for *BRCA1*, the vast majority of alterations are frameshift or nonsense mutations that produce a truncated protein. Both *BRCA1* and *BRCA2* are tumor suppressor genes—they are nonfunctional in malignant cells as a result of a combined germline mutation followed by inactivation of the second allele in the tumor (the Knudson two-hit hypothesis). These genes have key roles in DNA damage repair, regulation of gene expression, and cell cycle control.

Multiple Endocrine Neoplasia Type 1

MEN 1 is an autosomal dominant condition characterized phenotypically by tumors of the parathyroid gland leading to hyperparathyroidism, pancreatic islet cell tumors, and tumors of the pituitary gland.

Lipomas, adenomas of the adrenal and thyroid glands, cutaneous angiofibromas, and carcinoid tumors can also develop in affected individuals.

Mutations in the tumor suppressor gene called *MEN1*, located on chromosome 11q13, are responsible for this syndrome. Eighty percent of mutations identified result in loss of function of the gene product, called *menin*. Menin is a 67-kd protein predominantly found in the nucleus. It binds with a variety of proteins that have roles in the regulation of transcription, DNA repair, and organization of the cytoskeleton. None of these menin pathways have yet been found to be critical in *MEN1* tumorigenesis, although a number of candidates such as JunD have been proposed.

Multiple Endocrine Neoplasia Type 2

MTC develops in all affected individuals with MEN 2. It is subclassified into type A and type B. MEN 2A is manifested as pheochromocytoma (50%) and hyperparathyroidism (25%). In addition to MTC and pheochromocytoma, MEN 2B is characterized by mucosal neuromas on the tongue, lips, and subconjunctival areas; intestinal ganglioneuromatosis; and a marfanoid body habitus. The majority of cases of MEN 2B are the result of spontaneous new *ret* mutations, not inherited from either parent.

Both types are caused by germline mutations in the *ret* (*re*arranged during *t*ransfection) proto-oncogene located on chromosome 10q11. It encodes a transmembrane tyrosine kinase receptor that is expressed on a wide variety of neuroendocrine and neural cells, including thyroid C cells, adrenal medullary cells, and autonomic ganglion cells. Once mutated, the receptor constitutively activates various signaling pathways, including the p38/MAPK and JNK pathways.

von Hippel-Lindau Syndrome

von Hippel-Lindau syndrome is a rare, autosomal dominant condition characterized by the development of highly vascularized tumors in multiple organs. Such tumors include hemangioblastomas of the retina and central nervous system, renal cysts that develop into clear cell renal cell cancer, and pheochromocytomas. It is caused by mutations in the *VHL* gene. Penetrance is 90% by 65 years of age, with the mean age at diagnosis being 26. Since discovery of the role of the *VHL* gene in this syndrome, mutations of this same gene have been found in the majority of sporadic clear cell renal cell carcinomas. That loss of *VHL* function is a critical event during renal cell carcinogenesis is supported by experiments in which the introduction of wild-type *VHL* into *VHL*-deficient renal cancer cell lines resulted in suppression of tumor growth.

The protein product of the *VHL* gene, pVHL, functions as a tumor suppressor. It is part of the cell's response mechanism to hypoxia. Under conditions of low cellular oxygen tension, hypoxia inducible factor-1 (HIF-1) and HIF-2 regulate genes involved in metabolism, angiogenesis, erythropoiesis, and cell proliferation. pVHL targets the α subunit of HIF for oxygen-dependent proteolysis.

Therefore, lack of pVHL results in persistence of the HIF complex, with increased HIF transcriptional activity and up-regulation of HIF target genes, including *VEGF, GLUT-1,* and *erythropoietin,* independent of cellular oxygen levels. pVHL also has roles in regulating ECM turnover and microtubule stability.

Cancer Epigenetics

Epigenetic inheritance is defined as cellular information, other than the nucleotide sequence, that is heritable during cell division. There are three main interrelated forms: DNA methylation, genomic imprinting, and histone modification. These epigenetic templates control gene expression and can be transmitted to daughter cells independently of the DNA sequence.

One of the best studied types of epigenetic changes is cytosine methylation at CpG dinucleotides. CpG islands (CGIs) are approximately 1-kb stretches of DNA containing clusters of CpG dinucleotides that are usually unmethylated in normal cells and are often located near the 5′ ends of genes. Methylation of promoter CpG islands is associated with a closed chromatin structure and transcriptional silencing of the associated gene. This has been shown to be a common event in carcinogenesis. Tumor suppressor genes such as *CDKN2A, RB, VHL,* and *BRCA1* are inactivated by hypermethylation of their promoter CGIs.

Conversely, genes that are hypomethylated, leading to increased transcription, have been identified. For example, promoter CpG demethylation has been shown to result in overexpression of cyclin D2 and maspin in gastric cancer.[32] DNA hypomethylation has also been associated with genomic instability. Loss of methylation is particularly severe in pericentromeric satellite sequences, and cancers of the ovary and breast frequently contain unbalanced chromosomal translocations with breakpoints in the pericentromeric regions of chromosomes 1 and 16. Demethylation of these satellite sequences may predispose to their breakage and recombination.

Genomic imprinting refers to conditioning of the maternal and paternal genomes during gametogenesis such that a specific parental allele is more abundantly (or exclusively) expressed in the offspring. In Wilms' tumors, loss of imprinting has been demonstrated to lead to pathologic biallelic expression of *IGF2*. This appears to occur in combination with hypermethylation of regions of the reciprocally imprinted *H19* gene. These two phenomena are the earliest detectable genetic changes in this cancer and strongly suggest a gatekeeper role for epigenetic alterations in cancer.

CGI methylation is associated with a condensed chromatin structure that blocks the access of transcription factors to DNA promoter sites and thereby leads to transcriptional silencing. Modification of histones, such as by acetylation, methylation, or phosphorylation, is important in compaction of the chromatin structure. Recent work in colorectal cancer suggests that the combination of DNA hypermethylation and histone modification plays a critical role in the maintenance of gene silencing.[33] This is an emerging area of research.

Carcinogens

Any agent that can contribute to tumor formation is referred to as a carcinogen, and it can be chemical, physical or biologic. The International Agency for Research on Cancer (IARC) maintains a registry of human carcinogens that is available on the Internet (www.iarc.fr). The compounds are categorized into five groups based on epidemiologic studies, animal models, and short-term mutagenesis tests. Group 1 contains what are considered to be proven human carcinogens. Group 2A agents are probable human carcinogens; there is limited evidence of carcinogenicity in humans but sufficient evidence to prove carcinogenicity in experimental animals. The group 2B category includes agents that are possibly carcinogenic to humans, but there is limited evidence of carcinogenicity in humans and less than sufficient evidence of carcinogenicity in experimental animals. For agents included in group 3, there is inadequate evidence for carcinogenicity in humans or experimental animals. Group 4 agents are probably not carcinogenic to humans.

Chemical

Chemicals that initiate carcinogenesis are extremely diverse in structure and function and include both natural and synthetic products (Tables 29-5 and 29-6). They fall into one of two categories: (1) direct-acting compounds, which do not require chemical transformation for their carcinogenicity, and (2) indirect-acting compounds, or procarcinogens, which require metabolic conversion in vivo for their carcinogenic effects. All these compounds, or their active metabolites in the latter category, share the essential property of being highly reactive electrophiles (having electron-deficient atoms) that can react with nucleophilic (electron-rich) sites in the cell. These reactions are nonenzymatic and result in the formation of covalent adducts between the chemical carcinogens and (almost always) DNA.

The vast majority of chemical carcinogens require metabolic activation for their carcinogenic effects. The metabolic pathway that produces the active metabolite may be just one of a number of metabolic pathways for degradation of the parent compound. Thus, the carcinogenic potency of the carcinogen is determined not just by the reactivity of the electrophilic derivative or derivatives but also by the balance between the metabolic activation and inactivation reactions. Most of the known carcinogens are metabolized by cytochrome P-450–dependent mono-oxygenases. Because these enzymes are essential for the activation of procarcinogens, individual susceptibility to carcinogenesis is regulated in part by polymorphisms in the genes that encode these enzymes. For example, a product of the P-450 gene, CYP1A1, metabolizes polycyclic aromatic hydrocarbons such as benzo(a)pyrene. About 10% of the white population has a highly inducible form of this enzyme that is associated with an increased risk for lung cancer in smokers. Light smokers with the susceptible genotype of CYP1Q1 have a sevenfold higher risk for the development of lung cancer than do smokers without the permis-

Table 29-5   Selected IARC Group I Chemical Carcinogens

CHEMICAL CARCINOGEN	MEANS OF EXPOSURE	PREDOMINANT TUMOR TYPE
Aflatoxins	Ingestion of contaminated maize and peanuts grown in hot, humid climates	Hepatocellular carcinoma
Arsenic	Ingestion; also inhalation by smelter workers	Skin cancer
Asbestos	Inhalation	Mesothelioma, lung cancer
Benzene	Inhalation, especially in gasoline-related industries or in the production of other chemicals from benzene	Leukemia
Benzidine	Inhalation by workers in the dye industry	Cancer of the urinary bladder
Beryllium	Inhalation by workers in metal refining and production of beryllium-containing products; also those in the aircraft, aerospace, electronics, and nuclear industries	Lung cancer
Cadmium	Inhalation by workers in cadmium production and refining, nickel-cadmium battery manufacturing, other cadmium-related industries	Lung cancer
Chromium compounds	Inhalation during chromium plating, chromate production, welding	Lung cancer
Coal tars	Inhalation, transcutaneous absorption in a variety of industrial settings	Skin cancer, scrotal cancer
Ethylene oxide	Inhalation during the production of various industrial chemicals, e.g., ethylene glycol	Leukemia, lymphoma
Nickel	Inhalation, ingestion, or skin contact in nickel or nickel alloy production plants, welding, or electroplating operations	Lung cancer, nasal cancer
Radon	Inhalation in underground mines	Lung cancer
Tobacco smoke	Inhalation	Lung cancer, oral cancer, pharyngeal cancer, laryngeal cancer, esophageal cancer
Vinyl chloride	Inhalation during production of polyvinyl chloride	Hepatic angiosarcoma, hepatocellular carcinoma, brain tumors, lung cancer, hematopoietic malignancies

Based on information from IARC Monographs on the Evaluation of Carcinogenic Risks to Humans. International Agency for Research on Cancer (IARC), 2004. Available at http://monographs.iarc.fr/ENG/Monographs/allmonos90.php.

Table 29-6   Selected IARC Group 1 Pharmaceutical Carcinogens

PHARMACEUTICAL CARCINOGENS	PREDOMINANT TUMOR TYPE
Azathioprine	Non-Hodgkin's lymphoma, squamous cell cancer of the skin, hepatocellular carcinoma, cholangiocarcinoma
Cyclophosphamide	Cancer of the urinary bladder, leukemia
Chlorambucil	Leukemia
Tamoxifen	Endometrial cancer
Estrogens (OCP, HRT)	Cancer of the breast and endometrium

HRT, hormone replacement therapy; OCP, oral contraceptive pill.
Based on information from IARC Monographs on the Evaluation of Carcinogenic Risks to Humans. International Agency for Research on Cancer (IARC), 2004. Available at http://monographs.iarc.fr/ENG/Monographs/allmonos90.php.

sive genotype. Age, sex, and nutritional status also have an effect on the metabolism of carcinogens and thus their probability of inducing malignancy.

DNA is the primary target of chemical carcinogens. The ability of these compounds to induce mutations is termed *mutagenic potential*. The Ames test is the most common method for evaluating mutagenic potential and measures the ability of a chemical to induce mutations in the bacterium *Salmonella typhimurium*. The vast majority of known chemical carcinogens score positive on the Ames test, so it is useful for screening. However, not all compounds with mutagenic potential in vitro also have in vivo effects. Although no single mutation is unique to all chemical carcinogens, individual compounds have been found to induce characteristic changes in DNA. For example, aflatoxin B1 induces a $G:C \rightarrow T:A$ transconversion in codon 249 of the *TP53* gene (249^{ser} *p53* mutation). In individuals from areas with a high level of exposure to aflatoxin B1, HCC develops in those with this characteristic mutation. This mutation is an otherwise uncommon occurrence in HCC caused by other agents such as hepatitis B virus (HBV).

The carcinogenicity of some chemicals is augmented by the subsequent administration of other agents called *promoters* that are by themselves nontumorigenic. Such chemicals include phorbol esters, hormones, and phenols. Their fundamental characteristic is an ability to induce cell proliferation. Promotion may involve multiple compounds acting as promoters on different regulatory pathways. The end result is the clonal expansion of initiated cells.

Radiation Carcinogenesis

The two most important forms of radiation causing malignant change in humans are ultraviolet (UV) and ionizing radiation. Whereas the latter has been found to cause a variety of cancers, the former is principally implicated in the causation of skin cancer. There is typically a long latency period between radiant exposure and the clinical development of cancer.

UV radiation is a known risk factor for squamous cell carcinoma, basal cell carcinoma, and possibly malignant melanoma. The degree of risk depends on the type of UV rays, the intensity of exposure, and the quantity of melanin present in the individual's skin. The UV portion of the electromagnetic spectrum can be divided into three wavelength ranges: UVA (320-400 nm), UVB (280-320 nm), and UVC (200-280 nm). Of these, UVB is the most important. UVC, also a potent mutagen, is filtered out by the planetary ozone layer. The carcinogenicity of UVB is due to its formation of pyrimidine dimers in DNA. This damage may be repaired by the nucleotide excision repair (NER) pathway. This is a multistep process involving recognition of the damaged DNA strands, incision and removal of these strands, and synthesis of a patch containing the correct nucleotide sequence, which is then annealed to the DNA structure. With excessive sun exposure, it is postulated that the capacity of this pathway is overwhelmed and some DNA damage remains unrepaired. Xeroderma pigmentosa, a family of autosomal recessive disorders characterized by extreme photosensitivity and a 2000-fold increased risk for skin cancer, is caused by mutations in the genes involved in NER. Mutations in the *ras* and *p53* genes occur early in skin cancers, mainly at dipyrimidine sequences.

Ionizing radiation includes both electromagnetic (x-rays, gamma rays) and particulate (alpha particles, beta particles, protons, neutrons) forms. Ionizing radiation is both a carcinogen and a therapeutic agent—low-dose exposure can increase an individual's risk for development of cancer, but when given at high doses, it can slow or stop tumor growth. Ionizing radiation has a multitude of effects on tissues and affects both cells and their microenvironment. It leads to rapid, global, and persistent activation of the microenvironment. Inflammation results in the production of reactive oxygen species or reactive nitrogen species (or both) by tissue macrophages or neutrophils. Long-term sublethal exposure to these inflammatory products may cause genomic instability in parenchymal cells, eventually leading to chromosomal abnormalities, gene mutations, or both. In addition, it is becoming apparent that irradiated stroma has a persistent "activated" phenotype. Irradiated stroma has been shown

Table 29-7   Selected IARC Group 1 Infectious Carcinogens

INFECTIOUS CARCINOGENS	PREDOMINANT TUMOR TYPE
Epstein-Barr virus (EBV)	Burkitt's lymphoma, Hodgkin's disease, immunosuppression-related lymphoma, nasopharyngeal carcinoma
Hepatitis B	Hepatocellular carcinoma
Hepatitis C	Hepatocellular carcinoma
Human immunodeficiency virus (HIV) type 1	Kaposi's sarcoma
Human papillomavirus (HPV) types 16 and 18	Cervical cancer, anal cancer
Human T-cell lymphotropic virus type I (HTLV-1)	Adult T-cell leukemia
Helicobacter pylori	Gastric adenocarcinoma
Opisthorchis viverrini	Cholangiocarcinoma, hepatocellular carcinoma
Schistosoma haematobium	Cancer of the urinary bladder

Based on information from IARC Monographs on the Evaluation of Carcinogenic Risks to Humans. International Agency for Research on Cancer (IARC), 2004. Available at http://monographs.iarc.fr/ENG/Monographs/allmonos90.php.

to contribute to the selection and proliferation of malignant clones in animal models.

In survivors of the atomic bombs dropped on Hiroshima and Nagasaki, leukemias developed after an average latency period of 7 years, but these survivors have also suffered an increased incidence of solid organ tumors (e.g., breast, colon, thyroid, lung). Irradiation of the head and neck in childhood has been associated with a high incidence of thyroid cancer in adulthood.

There is a defined vulnerability of different tissues to radiation-induced carcinogenesis. Most vulnerable is the hematopoietic cell line, in which exposure to radiation causes leukemias (except chronic lymphocytic leukemia), followed by the thyroid gland. In the intermediate category are the breast, lung, and salivary glands. Skin, bone, and the gastrointestinal tract are relatively radioresistant.

Infectious Carcinogens

One of the first observations that cancer may be caused by transmissible agents was by Peyton Rous in 1911, when he demonstrated that cell-free extracts from sarcomas in chickens could transmit sarcomas to other animals injected with these extracts. This was subsequently discovered to represent viral transmission of cancer by the Rous sarcoma virus.

Infectious agents (Table 29-7) may cause or increase the risk for malignancy by a number of mechanisms, including direct transformation, expression of oncogenes that interfere with cell cycle checkpoints or DNA repair,

---

Box 29-1   Tenets of Viral Carcinogenesis

Viruses can cause neoplasia in animals and humans.

Tumor viruses frequently establish persistent infections in natural hosts.

Viral infections are more common than virus-related tumor formation.

Long latent periods usually elapse between initial viral infection and tumor appearance.

Host factors are important determinants of virus-induced tumorigenesis.

Viruses may be either direct- or indirect-acting carcinogenic agents.

Viruses are seldom complete carcinogens.

Viral strains may differ in oncogenic potential.

Oncogenic viruses modulate growth control pathways in cells.

In tumors affected by viral carcinogenesis, viral markers are usually present in neoplastic cells.

One virus may be associated with more than one type of neoplasia.

Modified from Butel JS: Viral carcinogenesis: Revelation of molecular mechanisms and etiology of human disease. Carcinogenesis 21:405-426, 2000.

---

expression of cytokines or other growth factors, and alteration of the immune system.

Viral Carcinogenesis

Approximately 15% of all human tumors worldwide are caused by viruses. This number reflects predominantly two malignancies: cervical cancer caused by HPV and HCC caused by HBV and hepatitis C virus (HCV).

Tenets of Viral Carcinogenesis Human tumor viruses display different mechanisms of cell transformation and fall into both direct- and indirect-acting categories (Box 29-1). Direct-acting viruses carry one or more oncogenes, whereas indirect-acting agents do not appear to possess an oncogene. Both types establish long-term persistent infections in their target cell types.

Small DNA Tumor Viruses As a result of their limited genetic content, small DNA tumor viruses such as HPV are dependent on host cell machinery to replicate their viral genome. Virus-encoded nonstructural proteins stimulate resting cells to enter S phase to provide the enzymes and environment conducive to viral DNA replication. Because of this ability to usurp cell cycle control, such proteins are also responsible for cell transformation. Binding of viral oncoproteins to the cellular tumor suppressor proteins p53 and pRb is fundamental to the effects of the small DNA tumor viruses on host cells. For example, the E6 oncoprotein of HPV forms a complex with p53, after which it is targeted for ubiquitin-mediated degradation.

Hepatitis B Virus (a DNA Virus) The development of HCC after HBV infection probably involves a combination of indirect and direct mechanisms. Chronic liver injury secondary to persistent viral infection leads to necrosis, inflammation, and hepatocyte regeneration. The constitutive induction of liver cell progression into the cell cycle overwhelms DNA repair mechanisms in the presence of

mutational events. This may induce fixed DNA mutations and chromosomal rearrangements, which are major determinants of cell transformation; concurrently, fibrosis disrupts the normal lobular structure and modifies cell-cell and cell-ECM interactions, with further loss of control over cell growth. The HBV X protein (HBx) may also act as a potential viral oncoprotein. As a transcription factor, it acts on a number of viral and cellular promoters. It influences signal transduction pathways both in the cytoplasm and in the mitochondrion. HBx also binds p53 and inhibits several critical p53-mediated processes, including DNA sequence–specific binding, transcriptional transactivation, and apoptosis. Integration of HBV DNA into the host genome occurs in 90% of HBV-related HCC and has been postulated to be an early event in chronic viral infection. Neither the HBV DNA sequences inserted nor the chromosomal sites of insertion are uniform. It is postulated that the integrated sequences could alter tumor suppressor genes or activate proto-oncogenes by alteration of their regulating elements.

RNA Viruses (Human T-Cell Lymphotropic Virus 1, Hepatitis C Virus) After viral infection, the single-stranded RNA viral genome is transcribed into a double-stranded DNA copy, which is then integrated into the chromosomal DNA of the cell. Retroviral infection is permanent. Oncogenic retroviruses carry oncogenes derived from cellular genes that for the most part are involved in mitogenic signaling and growth control. Examples of such proto-oncogenes are protein kinases, G proteins, growth factors, and transcription factors. Alternatively, retroviruses that do not possess oncogenes may cause tumors during integration into the cellular genome. If this occurs near normal cellular proto-oncogenes, the strong promoter and enhancer sequences of the provirus (which allow viral replication) will also affect the expression of proto-oncogenes. This mechanism is termed *proviral insertional mutagenesis.*

Hepatitis C Virus (an RNA Flavivirus) The mechanistic role of HCV in the development of HCC appears to be indirect, that is, by induction of chronic hepatocellular injury, coupled with inflammation and liver cell regeneration. A number of HCV proteins have been implicated in its carcinogenic activity.[34] Both the HCV core protein and NS3 protein modulate expression of the cyclin-dependent inhibitor p21WAF1 and affect the activity of p53. NS5A protein acts as a transcription factor and interacts with cellular signaling pathways and various cell cycle regulatory kinases to block the apoptotic cellular response to persistent HCV infection. Unlike retroviruses, HCV (a flavivirus) does not appear to cause integration of its DNA into the cellular genome.[35]

Helicobacter pylori

H. pylori infection is the most important risk factor for the development of gastric cancer. It was the first bacterium linked to human cancer and was classified as a group 1 carcinogen by the IARC in 1996. The mechanisms by which *H. pylori* causes cancer remain largely unknown but are thought to involve both host and bacterial characteristics. The chronic inflammatory response to the infection elicited by *H. pylori* is thought to be an important mechanism by which infection may eventually lead to neoplasia. However, it is unknown why and how the infection and resulting inflammation select certain individuals and which individuals do not enter the neoplastic cascade. The gastric microenvironment, such as acid secretion, may play a key role. IL-1β is a very potent inhibitor of acid secretion. Polymorphisms of the gene encoding this cytokine and also the gene encoding the IL-1β receptor antagonist gene, part of the same gene cluster, have been associated with increased risk for gastric cancer.

Infection with strains of *H. pylori* that carry the cytotoxin-associated antigen A *(cagA)* gene is associated with gastric carcinoma. The *cagA* gene product CagA is delivered into gastric epithelial cells by the bacterial type IV secretion system, in essence, a molecular syringe. Once intracellular, CagA is tyrosine phosphorylated by SRC family kinases and is then able to specifically bind and activate the cellular oncoprotein SHP2. Thus, it can be seen that CagA deregulation of SHP2 mimics a situation in which SHP2 acquires a gain-of-function mutation. CagA is thought to be important during the early phases of gastric carcinogenesis, in particular, progression from superficial gastritis to atrophic gastritis to intestinal metaplasia. However, the presence of CagA alone is not sufficient for transformation of gastric epithelial cells to a malignant phenotype.

Chronic Inflammation

Chronic inflammation in the absence of infection has long been linked with the development of cancer. Examples include the development of squamous cell carcinoma of the skin in areas of chronic ulceration (Marjolin's ulcer) and the high risk for colorectal cancer in patients with ulcerative colitis. However, the exact mechanistic changes occurring during chronic inflammation that lead to malignant transformation are just beginning to be elucidated. For example, in ulcerative colitis–associated colorectal cancer, a dual mechanism has been proposed. Ulceration of the epithelium exposes underlying cell layers to the contents of the bowel lumen. The intestinal flora triggers the nuclear factor NF-κB pathway in macrophages and causes them to release proinflammatory agents such as prostaglandins, chemokines, and interleukins that indirectly promote the survival of transformed epithelial cells. Independently, the intestinal flora directly triggers the survival NF-κB pathway through toll-like receptors (TLRs) on the transformed cell.

TUMOR MARKERS

Tumor markers are indicators of cellular, biochemical, molecular, or genetic alterations by which neoplasia can be recognized. These surrogate measures of the biology of the cancer provide insight into the clinical behavior of the tumor. This is particularly useful when the cancer is not clinically detectable. The information provided may

- Be diagnostic and distinguish benign from malignant disease

---

> **Box 29-2   Potential Nonprotein Tumor Markers**
>
> **RNA-Based Markers**
>
> Overexpressed/underexpressed transcripts
> Regulatory RNA (e.g., micro-RNA)
>
> **DNA-Based Markers**
>
> Single-nucleotide polymorphisms (SNPs)
> Chromosomal translocations—*bcr-abl* (Philadelphia)
> Changes in DNA copy number
> Microsatellite instability
> Epigenetic changes (e.g., differential promoter region methylation)
>
> From Ludwig JA, Weinstein JN: Biomarkers in cancer staging, prognosis and treatment selection. Nat Rev Cancer 5:845-856, 2005.

- Correlate with the amount of tumor present (so-called tumor burden)
- Allow subtype classification to more accurately stage patients
- Be prognostic, either by the presence or absence of the marker or by its concentration
- Guide choice of therapy and predict response to therapy

The ideal tumor marker has three defining characteristics:

1. The marker is expressed exclusively by the particular tumor
2. Collection of the specimen for the tumor marker assay is easy.
3. The assay itself is reproducible, rapid, and inexpensive.

Currently, there is no one marker that fulfills all these criteria for any cancer, nor is there any specific cancer in which there are biomarkers that completely describe its behavior.

Tumor markers fall into three broad categories—proteins, genetic mutations, and epigenetic changes (Box 29-2). All three may be found in the tumor tissue itself. Tumor markers found in body fluids, particularly blood and urine, have the greatest potential for clinical application because of the ease of access to these fluids for analysis and because repeated sampling allows in vivo monitoring of the malignancy for such features as disease progression or recurrence, metastasis, and response to therapy.

Rather than provide an exhaustive review of all tumor markers, this section outlines the major categories of tumor markers and focuses on evidence for the tumor markers currently in clinical use.

Protein Tumor Markers

Proteins were the first type of tumor marker identified and hence are considered the so-called classic tumor markers. However, despite decades of research, few are in clinical use. Those routinely used are in general limited by poor sensitivity and specificity. Their concentrations in serum or plasma generally correlate with tumor burden inasmuch as they are shed from the expanding neoplasm.

Carcinoembryonic Antigen

Carcinoembryonic antigen (CEA) is probably the most studied cancer tumor marker and is predominantly used clinically in patients with cancer of the colon and rectum. It is an oncofetal protein that is normally present during fetal life but can be seen in low concentration in healthy adults. Structurally, it is a glycoprotein with a molecular weight of 200 kd and is a component of the glycocalyx, located on the luminal side of the cell membrane of normal epithelial intestinal cells. CEA is a member of a large family of proteins that are related to the immunoglobulin gene superfamily. The molecule itself is secreted into the circulation and is also found in the mucous secretions of the stomach, small intestine, and biliary tree. Although its exact function is unknown, CEA has been shown to be involved in cell adhesion and is able to inhibit apoptosis induced by loss of anchorage to the ECM.

Testing

Immunoassay kits allow determination of serum CEA levels accurately, reproducibly, and relatively inexpensively. Normal serum levels are less than 2.5 ng/mL, borderline if 2.5 to 5.0 ng/mL, and elevated if greater than 5.0 ng/mL. Borderline levels occur with benign disorders such as inflammatory bowel disease, pancreatitis, cirrhosis, and chronic obstructive pulmonary disease, and smoking can also increase CEA—the upper limit of normal in smokers is considered 5 ng/mL.

Screening

CEA is not useful as a screening test because of its low sensitivity in early-stage disease—elevated CEA levels occur in only 5% to 40% of patients with localized disease.

Prognosis

Elevated CEA levels reflect the burden of tumor present. The degree of CEA elevation correlates with increasing stage of disease, and therefore CEA levels have prognostic value. Preoperative serum CEA is an independent predictor of survival—the higher the preoperative serum level, the poorer the prognosis. This effect persists even after patients are stratified for resectability and extent of local tumor invasion. Five-year survival is significantly worse in patients with elevated preoperative CEA levels than in those with a normal preoperative CEA level. Furthermore, 5-year survival is higher in patients whose elevated preoperative CEA normalized postoperatively. Finally, patients with elevated preoperative CEA levels have higher recurrence rates than do those with normal CEA levels.

Monitoring

The most common application of CEA is to monitor patients for recurrent disease. CEA is most sensitive for hepatic or retroperitoneal metastasis and relatively insensitive for local, pulmonary, or peritoneal involvement.

About 75% of patients with recurrent colorectal cancer have an elevated serum CEA level before the development of symptoms. However, the pattern or magnitude of the rise in CEA levels is of no value in distinguishing localized recurrence from distant disease. Because elevations of CEA may be transient, repeat measurement is performed as confirmation of the trend. A confirmed rising trend in CEA prompts evaluation for recurrent disease.

Because CEA reflects tumor burden, it is useful in monitoring response to chemotherapy in patients with metastatic cancer. An elevated CEA level is an independent factor associated with poor survival and progression on 5-fluorouracil chemotherapy in patients with metastatic colorectal cancer. Patients with advanced cancer whose CEA levels fall during chemotherapy survive significantly longer than do patients whose CEA levels do not change or increase.

α-Fetoprotein

α-Fetoprotein (AFP) is used for the detection and management of HCC. It is an oncofetal antigen that consists of a single-chain polypeptide with a molecular weight of 700 kd. Levels are elevated in the fetus, decrease sharply after birth, and are increased during pregnancy. It is synthesized by hepatocytes and endodermally derived gastrointestinal tissues.

Testing

AFP is measured with immunoassay kits, either enzyme-linked immunoassays or radioimmunoassays. The upper limit of normal for a healthy, nonpregnant adult is less than 25 ng/mL. Ten percent to 20% of HCCs do not have detectable levels of AFP. Levels are also raised in nonseminomatous testicular cancer, for which it is a valuable tumor marker (see discussion later). Twenty percent of patients with gastric or pancreatic cancer and 5% of patients with colorectal or lung cancer have significant elevations (>5 ng/mL) in serum AFP levels. Elevated levels are also seen in hepatitis, inflammatory bowel disease, and cirrhosis.

Screening

AFP has an estimated sensitivity of 25% to 75%, a specificity of 76% to 94%, and a positive predictive value of 9% to 50%. However, note that the sensitivity and specificity vary with the cutoff value chosen. If the cutoff is set at 20 ng/mL, the sensitivity and specificity are 30% and 87%, respectively, but if raised to 100 and 400 ng/mL, the sensitivity and specificity vary from 72% to 56% and 70% to 94%, respectively.

The combination of AFP and ultrasound improves the efficacy of screening. One surveillance study of 1125 patients with HCV reported a sensitivity of 100% with a combination of AFP and ultrasound versus a sensitivity of 75% for AFP alone and 87% for ultrasound alone.[36] Cost-effectiveness analysis is used to calculate the cost of each additional life year gained in terms of quality-adjusted life years (QALYs). A QALY less than $50,000 is considered cost-effective. In the United States, recent studies suggest that surveillance of patients with HCV-related cirrhosis with a combination of AFP and an imaging modality (either ultrasound or computed tomography) would gain QALYs at acceptable cost.[37-39]

Prognosis
The AFP concentration reflects tumor size, with levels higher than 400 ng/mL being associated with larger tumors. As a result, it has been shown that AFP correlates with stage and prognosis. The rate of increase, expressed as AFP doubling time, has also been associated with poorer prognosis.

Monitoring
AFP has been shown to decline after resection or ablation. After complete resection, AFP levels should drop and remain at less than 10 ng/mL. Shirabe and colleagues[40] found that in patients with HCC whose preoperative AFP level was higher than 100 ng/mL and postoperative AFP did not fall below 20 ng/mL, early recurrence within the first postoperative year should be strongly suspected. In patients whose AFP levels do normalize postoperatively, a subsequent rise in AFP over the course of serial serum measurements has been found to be the best indicator of recurrent disease. It was the first measured abnormality in 34% of these patients. However, in some patients who had elevated serum levels of AFP with their original HCC, postoperative levels of AFP were unreliable in detecting recurrence. Five (12%) patients did not have elevated serum levels despite the presence of recurrent disease.

Tumor regrowth after chemoembolization does not correlate with rate of increase in AFP or tumor burden.

AFP levels usually decline in response to effective chemotherapy. Monitoring of AFP therefore avoids prolonged use of ineffective and potentially toxic chemotherapy.

Carbohydrate Antigen 19-9
Carbohydrate antigen 19-9 (CA 19-9) is widely used as a serum marker for pancreas cancer, but its use is limited to monitoring response to therapy, not as a diagnostic marker. It is a mucin-type glycoprotein expressed on the surface of pancreatic cancer cells and was initially detected by monoclonal antibodies raised against colon cancer cell lines in a mouse model. The CA 19-9 epitope is normally present within the biliary tree. Biliary tract disease, both acute and chronic, can elevate serum CA 19-9 levels.

Testing
CA 19-9 is detected with an immunoassay, and the upper limit of normal for a healthy adult is 37 U/mL. Sensitivities of CA 19-9 in the diagnosis of pancreatic cancer range from 67% to 92%, with specificities ranging from 68% to 92%. The utility of CA 19-9 as a diagnostic marker is limited in a number of ways. First, patients with negative Lewis[a] blood group antigen cannot synthesize CA 19-9, and therefore it is not used as a serologic marker in these individuals, who make up about 10% of the population. Second, patients with benign biliary tract disease can have levels up to 400 U/mL, with 87% having concentrations higher than 70 U/mL. Significant numbers of patients

with pancreatitis, either acute or chronic, also have elevated levels. Third, besides pancreatic cancer, CA 19-9 levels are also elevated in patients with other cancers, including those of the biliary tree (95%), stomach (5%), colon (15%), liver (HCC, 7%) and lung (13%). For colorectal cancer, CA 19-9 levels add little clinically useful information to determination of CEA levels.

Screening
CA 19-9 is not useful as a screening modality because of its low sensitivity in early-stage disease. With increasing levels of CA 19-9, the diagnosis of pancreatic cancer becomes more accurate. When a cutoff level of 100 U/mL is used, a number of studies have demonstrated that although sensitivity ranges from 60% to 84%, specificity for pancreas cancer is 95% or greater. Levels higher than 1000 U/mL are almost diagnostic of pancreatic cancer. Because of its frequent elevation in benign biliary tract disease, CA 19-9 is not useful in distinguishing benign from malignant distal common bile duct strictures.

Prognosis
In patients with pancreatic cancer who have CA 19-9 detectable in their serum, the level has been shown to correlate with tumor burden. For example, higher CA 19-9 levels typically correlate with higher tumor stage, and more than 95% of patients with unresectable disease have levels higher than 1000 U/mL. Of patients who undergo curative resection, those whose CA 19-9 levels returned to normal survived longer than those whose levels fell but never normalized.

Monitoring
Serial measurement of CA 19-9 is used to monitor response to therapy. A rise in CA 19-9 after curative resection has been shown to precede clinical or computed tomographic evidence of recurrence by 2 to 9 months. In patients with unresectable/metastatic disease, failure of CA 19-9 levels to fall with chemotherapy reflects poor tumor response. However, in both settings, the lack of alternative effective therapies limits the utility of serial monitoring of CA 19-9.

Prostate-Specific Antigen
Prostate-specific antigen (PSA) is a serine protease that is formed in the prostatic epithelium and secreted into the prostatic ducts. Its function is to digest the gel that is formed in seminal fluid after ejaculation. Under normal circumstances, only small amounts of PSA leak into the circulation. With enlargement of the gland (e.g., in patients with benign prostatic hyperplasia [BPH]) or distortion of its architecture, serum PSA levels increase. Thus, PSA is considered a tissue-specific rather than a prostate cancer–specific marker—patients who have undergone curative radical prostatectomy, as well as females, have no detectable PSA.

Testing
PSA is detected with an immunoassay. Besides BPH, other instances in which serum PSA levels may be elevated include prostatitis, prostatic massage, prostatic

biopsy, and digital rectal examination. Initial studies set the upper limit of normal for PSA at 4 ng/mL, with levels greater than 10 ng/mL being suspicious for malignancy and levels of 4 to 10 ng/mL being indeterminate. Since then, it has been found that the upper limit of the normal range of PSA increases with age. The limit is 2.5 ng/mL for men aged 40 to 49 years, 3.5 ng/mL for those 50 to 59, 4.5 ng/mL for those 60 to 69, and 6.5 ng/mL for men 70 years and older. The rate of increase in PSA in a normal 60-year-old is 0.04 ng/mL/yr.

Expressing PSA relative to prostatic volume and time has also helped discriminate cancer from benign conditions in which the PSA level is less than 10 ng/mL but greater than the upper limit of normal for the patient's age. PSA density is defined as the ratio of PSA to prostatic volume, as measured by transrectal ultrasound or magnetic resonance imaging. Higher PSA densities are more suggestive of malignancy than BPH because the amount of PSA released per gram of prostate cancer is significantly greater than that released from normal prostatic tissue.

The ratio of free to total PSA has also been found to improve the specificity of prostate cancer diagnosis in the PSA range of 4 to 10 ng/mL. The PSA slope (also known as PSA velocity) is the rate of change in the concentration of PSA over time. For individuals with initial levels lower than 4.0 ng/mL, a PSA slope of greater than 0.75 ng/mL/yr is considered significant; for patients whose baseline level is higher than 4.0 ng/mL, a slope greater than 0.4 ng/mL/yr is considered significant.

Screening

PSA is widely used as a screening tool for prostate cancer because it enables early detection and diagnosis of this disease. At present, two large randomized trials for prostate cancer, one in Europe (The European Randomized Study of Screening for Prostate Cancer) and the other in the United States (The Prostate, Lung, Colorectal and Ovary Cancer), are aiming to answer the question of whether screening reduces mortality. Results are expected in 2008.

Screening detects prostate cancer earlier. However, much concern has been raised about the risk of overdiagnosis. Autopsy studies have found that prostate cancer can be found in 55% of men in their 5th decade of life and 64% in their 7th decade, thus indicating that a significant proportion of these cancers are not lethal. Only one in eight screening-detected cancers is likely to kill its host if left untreated.

Monitoring Response to Therapy

After operative resection, the PSA level is expected to normalize after 2 to 3 weeks. In patients whose PSA level remained elevated 6 months after radical prostatectomy, recurrent disease eventually developed. In contrast, it takes 3 to 5 months for PSA to normalize after radiotherapy. However, failure of the PSA level to normalize after radiotherapy also predicts relapse. A rise in serum PSA is usually the first sign of either local recurrence or metastatic progression. In patients with advanced disease, PSA levels are also used to monitor response to systemic therapy.

Carbohydrate Antigen 125

Carbohydrate antigen 125 (CA 125) is a carbohydrate epitope on a glycoprotein carcinoma antigen. It is present in the fetus and in derivatives of the coelomic epithelium, including the peritoneum, pleura, pericardium, and amnion. In healthy adults, CA 125 has been detected by immunohistochemistry in the epithelium of the fallopian tubes, endometrium, and endocervix. However, neither adult nor fetal ovarian epithelium expresses CA 125.

Testing

CA 125 levels are measured with an immunoassay, with the upper limit of normal set at 35 U/mL. Elevated levels are detected in 80% of patients with ovarian cancer. In patients with ovarian masses, an elevated CA 125 level has a sensitivity of 75% and a specificity of approximately 90% for malignancy. It is also detectable in a high percentage of patients with cancer of the fallopian tube, endometrium, and cervix, as well as in nongynecologic malignancies of the pancreas, colon, lung, and liver. Benign conditions in which CA 125 is elevated include endometriosis, adenomyosis, uterine fibroids, pelvic inflammatory disease, cirrhosis, and ascites. As for CA 19-9 in patients with pancreatic cancer, CA 125 is an adjunct to diagnosis rather than being diagnostic by itself.

Screening

Alone, CA 125 is not useful as a screening tool for ovarian cancer because of its poor specificity. However, the United Kingdom Collaborative Trial of Ovarian Cancer Screening is evaluating the effectiveness of CA 125 in postmenopausal women. In this study, women classified as high risk according to their CA 125 level are further screened with transvaginal ultrasound.

Prognosis

Patients with elevated CA 125 levels at the time of diagnosis have a worse prognosis than patients with normal levels do. Absolute levels of CA 125 do not clearly correlate with tumor stage, although with increasing stage, greater percentages of patients have elevated CA 125 levels—50% of stage I patients, 70% of stage II patients, 90% of stage III patients, and 98% of stage IV patients.

Monitoring Response to Therapy

CA 125 is of value in monitoring the disease course. Partial or complete response to therapy is associated with a decrease in CA 125 levels in more than 95% of patients. Increasing levels of CA 125 correlate with disease recurrence and precede clinical or imaging evidence of recurrence by a median of 3 months. When rising CA 125 levels are used as an indication for second-look laparotomy, recurrent disease is found approximately 90% of the time.

CA 125 levels in peritoneal fluid may be more sensitive than serum levels. Thus, in patients whose serum CA 125 level normalizes during therapy, peritoneal fluid CA 125 levels may better be able to distinguish patients with residual disease from those without. The upper limit of normal for peritoneal fluid CA 125 is 200 U/mL.

α-Fetoprotein and Human Chorionic Gonadotropin in Testicular Germ Cell Tumors

Nonseminomatous testicular cancers comprise several different histologic types, including embryonal carcinoma, syncytiotrophoblasts (choriocarcinoma), yolk sac tumors, and teratomas. Marker expression can be predicted on the basis of the predominant histologic type—human chorionic gonadotropin (HCG) is detected in more than 90% of choriocarcinomas, whereas AFP is expressed by 90% to 95% of yolk sac tumors, 20% of teratomas, and 10% of embryonal carcinomas.

Diagnosis

Of patients with proven nonseminomatous testicular germ cell tumors, about 50% will have elevated serum levels of HCG and 60% will have elevated AFP, with either marker being elevated in 90% of cases. Determination of both marker levels is very important because nearly half these tumors secrete only one of these substances. In addition to the high rate of marker positivity, there have been very few cases of spuriously elevated serum levels of HCG or AFP in patients without testicular cancer. The presence of a testicular tumor in combination with an elevated level of AFP or HCG is suggestive of testicular cancer, without being diagnostic. Elevated levels of these markers in a man younger than 40 years without signs of a testicular tumor may indicate extratesticular germ cell cancer.

Prognosis

An absolute AFP concentration greater than 500 ng/mL or an HCG level higher than 1000 ng/mL is predictive of a poor prognosis. These tumor markers are useful in identifying biologically distinct categories of morphologically similar tumors. In one study considering pretreatment levels of AFP and HCG, 92% of patients with normal levels of both markers achieved complete remission as compared with just 26% of those with elevated AFP only, 46% of those with elevated HCG only, and 35% of those with elevations in both. Similarly, when comparing groups of patients with similar disease burdens, those with elevated marker levels have a worse prognosis than do those with normal marker levels.[41]

Monitoring

In the majority of patients with nonseminomatous germ cell tumors, tumor marker levels correlate with response to chemotherapy. The rate of marker decline (half-life), calculated from weekly determinations after initiation of chemotherapy, can be used for early identification of patients who will respond poorly to chemotherapy. Half-lives longer than 3.5 days for HCG or longer than 7 days for AFP suggest that very aggressive therapy is required, such as high-dose chemotherapy in combination with stem cell transplantation. However, there is a significant percentage of patients whose levels of tumor markers fall despite failure of their tumors to regress with therapy.

After completion of primary therapy, increasing marker concentrations, even in the absence of other features of recurrence, may lead to salvage chemotherapy. Therefore, it is important to exclude false-positive results. The

HCG level needs to be measured in urine, where the concentration is generally similar to that in serum; however, interfering substances are not excreted into urine. Intensive chemotherapy may induce hypogonadism with associated HCG levels of up to 5 to 10 IU/L. It can be differentiated from relapse by measurement of luteinizing hormone and follicle-stimulating hormone—similar to the postmenopausal state in women, levels higher than 30 to 50 IU/L indicate that HCG is derived from the pituitary.

DNA-Based Markers

Specific mutations in oncogenes, tumor-suppressor genes, and mismatch repair genes can serve as biomarkers. These mutations may be germline, such as the *ret* proto-oncogene of MEN 2 and the *APC* gene of FAP, or somatic mutations, such as the occurrence of *p53* mutations in a wide variety of tumors. Chromosomal abnormalities such as the 9:22 translocation that creates the *bcr-abl* oncogene are also useful biomarkers. Specific single-nucleotide polymorphisms have been identified that are associated with increased risk for specific cancers, and haplotype assessment has been shown to predict susceptibility to several cancers, including prostate, breast, lung, and colon cancer. Paik and coworkers[42] described an algorithm to predict the likelihood of distant recurrence in patients with node-negative, tamoxifen-treated breast cancer based on the expression of 21 genes in tumor tissue.

Epigenetic Changes

Testing for epigenetic changes is still at an early discovery stage and has not yet reached the clinic. However, it has great potential for a number of reasons. First, DNA assays for aberrant methylation are easier and more sensitive than those for point mutations. Second, cancer-specific DNA methylation patterns can be detected in tumor-derived free DNA in the bloodstream and in epithelial tumor cells shed into the lumen. This ease of access to sample medium may facilitate efforts at detection and monitoring of cancer. Third, DNA-methylation profiles are more chemically and biologically stable than RNA or most proteins. As a result, they may be more reliably detected in diverse biologic fluids.

Methylation biomarker studies have been performed in a variety of cancers, including breast, esophageal, gastric, colorectal, and prostate cancer. Sources of the DNA have included plasma/serum, urine, sputum, and saliva. A number of general observations have been made. Targeted biologic fluid sources of DNA, such as urine for bladder cancer, tended to give higher clinical sensitivities than serum or plasma analysis did. In contrast, the specificity of plasma or serum detection of tumor-specific markers was found to be extremely high—approximately 100%. Combining DNA methylation assays may complement existing screening methods with high sensitivity but low specificity, such as PSA in prostate cancer. The use of panels of methylation targets in these studies improved the clinical sensitivity of the assay.

Potential Applications

1. Early detection. Although abnormal epigenetic silencing of genes can occur at any time during carcinogenesis, it appears to occur most frequently early in the transformation process. Aberrant crypt foci that contain preneoplastic hyperplastic colonic epithelial cells have been found to demonstrate abnormal methylation in promoter regions of genes involved in abnormal activation of the Wnt signaling pathway.[43] Detection of abnormal methylation patterns in histologically normal cells may emerge as a useful marker for assessment of cancer risk.

2. Predict response to therapy. Methylation of specific genes can be linked to the biologic behavior of the tumor. A number of studies have reported associations between DNA methylation markers and response to chemotherapy. The most extensive work has been done on CpG hypermethylation of the O^6-methylguanine DNA methyltransferase *(MGMT)* gene, which appears to confer sensitivity to various alkylating chemotherapeutic agents. *MGMT* methylation was associated with prolonged survival in glioma patients treated with carmustine and in patients with large diffuse B-cell lymphoma who were treated with cyclophosphamide as part of multidrug regimens.[44] Widschwendter and associates[45] studied the correlation between methylation profiles and hormone receptor status in breast cancer. In particular, they found that methylation of the *ESR1* gene and the *PGR* gene was the best predictor of progesterone and estrogen receptor status, respectively. Furthermore, *ESR1* methylation outperformed hormone receptor status as a predictor of clinical response in patients treated with tamoxifen. Individual methylation markers, such as the E-cadherin promoter, have also been linked to breast cancer metastasis.

3. Prognostication. Abnormal methylation of combinations of genes has been associated with a poor outcome.

On an opposite note, loss of methylation is increasingly being recognized as an important event in carcinogenesis.[32] Hypomethylated CpG islands have been associated with the activation of nearby genes. For example, hypomethylation of the promoter for the cancer/testis antigen CAGE correlates with increased expression of the gene and is found in premalignant lesions of the stomach.[46] Similar instances of demethylated promoters activating their downstream genes have been found in numerous other cancers, including those of the colon, pancreas, liver, uterus, lung, and cervix.[32] In a recent study of ovarian carcinogenesis, hypomethylation of centromeric and juxtacentromeric satellite DNA was found to be increased in tumors of advanced stage or high grade, and this strong hypomethylation was an independent marker of poor prognosis.[47] Furthermore, genome-wide hypomethylation has also been detected in cancer cells and may contribute to genomic instability.[43]

DNA-methylation profiles in which both hypermethylation and hypomethylation are examined may provide greater insight into tumor behavior than possible with either profile alone.

RNA-Based Markers

RNA-based markers have been identified in the context of global mRNA expression by high-throughput technologies. These microarrays ("gene chips") allow us to measure the expression of 30,000 to 40,000 human genes in a single experiment. Statistical modeling then allows selection of groups of genes, or so-called fingerprints, that best distinguish disease states. For example, a variety of studies have used gene expression profiles in breast cancer cells to identify previously unrecognized molecular subtypes associated with differences in survival,[48] more accurately predict outcome,[49] and predict response to neoadjuvant therapy.[50] The level of expression of genes responsible for the metabolism of chemotherapeutic agents has been used to predict clinical response to these agents in lung and colon cancer. Similar methods have been applied to many other cancers. Though very promising, these assays will require extensive multi-institutional validation before they can be used in routine practice.

Proteomic Profiling

Proteomics is the study of all the proteins expressed by the genome. Ultimately, genetic mutations are manifested at the protein level and involve derangements in protein function and communication within diseased cells and within their microenvironment. Execution of the disease process occurs through altered protein function. Protein tumor biomarkers are thought to be low-abundance proteins (concentrations in the nanomolar range) that are shed from tumor cells or from the tumor-host interface into the circulation. Detection and measurement of these proteins provide information about the clinical behavior of the cancer. Proteomic profiling using mass spectrometry technologies generates complex fingerprints of ion peaks corresponding to protein concentrations, which can be correlated with disease states. Numerous studies using samples of blood (plasma or serum), urine, and pancreatic juice have demonstrated the feasibility of this technology for discovery of biomarkers and early detection of ovarian, breast, prostate, and pancreatic cancer. Identification of reproducible protein signatures of specific diseases has the potential to achieve much higher diagnostic sensitivity and specificity than possible with currently available biomarkers. Proteomic profiling lacks a standardized methodology and remains time and labor intensive. For the moment, these technologies are not ready for routine clinical use. Their principal role is in discovery of protein biomarkers. Candidate biomarkers discovered through this process can be validated with standard immunometric techniques after the development of specific antibodies.

Clearly, the future holds great promise for the greater use of biomarkers in the clinical management of patients with cancer (Table 29-8). We expect that combinations of tumor markers, including combinations of different types of tumor markers, will be developed and then

Table 29-8 Biomarkers and Biologically Targeted Therapies

CANCER	BIOMARKER	THERAPY
Breast	Estrogen receptor, progesterone receptor	Tamoxifen/ aromatase inhibitors
Lymphoma	CD20	Rituximab
Chronic myelogenous leukemia (CML)	*bcr-abl*	Imatinib
Gastrointestinal stromal tumor (GIST)	*c-kit*	Imatinib
Non–small cell lung cancer	EGFR mutation	Gefitinib
Breast	*HER2/neu*	Trastuzumab

Biomarker expression is increasingly being used, independent of formal staging criteria, to decide which patients receive biologically targeted therapies.

EGFR, epidermal growth factor receptor.

From Ludwig JA, Weinstein JN: Biomarkers in cancer staging, prognosis and treatment selection. Nat Rev Cancer 5:845-856, 2005.

incorporated into formal staging criteria. There will also be further delineation of the role of tumor markers in predicting the response to biologic and other types of therapy.

Acknowledgment

The authors thank Justin W. Larson for his help with the illustrations.

Selected References

Clark WH Jr, Elder DE, Guerry DT, et al: A study of tumor progression: The precursor lesions of superficial spreading and nodular melanoma. Hum Pathol 15:1147-1165, 1984.

This paper summarizes observations of tumor progression and defines the series of proliferative lesions that constitute the progression from melanocytic neoplasia to malignant melanoma. Based on their observations, the authors provide a paradigm for the development of neoplasia in general and provide a list of six lesional steps.

Dunn GP, Old LJ, Schreiber RD: The immunobiology of cancer immunosurveillance and immunoediting. Immunity 21:137-148, 2004.

This paper reviews the evidence for immune surveillance of cancer.

Fearon ER, Vogelstein B: A genetic model for colorectal tumorigenesis. Cell 61:759-767, 1990.

The first genetic model for tumorigenesis involving a series of genetic mutations, including mutational activation of oncogenes and inactivation of tumor suppressor genes.

Feinberg AP, Tycko B: The history of cancer epigenetics. Nat Rev Cancer 4:143-153, 2004.

Excellent overview of the development and progress of the emerging field of cancer epigenetics with a discussion of hypomethylation, hypermethylation, loss of imprinting, and chromatin modification.

Hanahan D, Folkman J: Patterns and emerging mechanisms of the angiogenic switch during tumorigenesis. Cell 86:353-364, 1996.

A review of the scientific evidence that tumors acquire the ability to induce angiogenesis.

Hanahan D, Weinberg RA: The hallmarks of cancer. Cell 100:57-70, 2000.

The authors provide a comprehensive overview of the common physiologic and molecular characteristics of cancer.

Knudson AG: Two genetic hits (more or less) to cancer. Nat Rev Cancer 1:157-162, 2001.

This paper provides a perspective on the number of genetic mutations that lead to cancer by using retinoblastoma as a model.

Korsmeyer SJ: Chromosomal translocations in lymphoid malignancies reveal novel proto-oncogenes. Annu Rev Immunol 10:785-807, 1992.

Review of chromosomal translocations in lymphoid tumors that led to the discovery of novel proto-oncogenes, including the family of oncogenes regulating programmed cell death and the first discovered family member, *bcl-2*.

Paik S, Shak S, Tang G, et al: A multigene assay to predict recurrence of tamoxifen-treated, node-negative breast cancer. N Engl J Med 351:2817-2826, 2004.

The expression of 21 genes in breast tumor tissue was used to define an algorithm allowing quantitative prediction of clinical outcome.

References

1. Dunn GP, Old LJ, Schreiber RD: The immunobiology of cancer immunosurveillance and immunoediting. Immunity 21:137-148, 2004.
2. Hanahan D, Weinberg RA: The hallmarks of cancer. Cell 100:57-70, 2000.
3. Sener SF, Grey N: The global burden of cancer. J Surg Oncol 92:1-3, 2005.
4. Yancik R: Population aging and cancer: A cross-national concern. Cancer J 11:437-441, 2005.
5. Hutchins LF, Unger JM, Crowley JJ, et al: Underrepresentation of patients 65 years of age or older in cancer-treatment trials. N Engl J Med 341:2061-2067, 1999.
6. Lewis JH, Kilgore ML, Goldman DP, et al: Participation of patients 65 years of age or older in cancer clinical trials. J Clin Oncol 21:1383-1389, 2003.
7. Trimble EL, Carter CL, Cain D, et al: Representation of older patients in cancer treatment trials. Cancer 74:2208-2214, 1994.
8. O'Connell JB, Maggard MA, Ko CY: Cancer-directed surgery for localized disease: Decreased use in the elderly. Ann Surg Oncol 11:962-969, 2004.
9. Calle EE, Rodriguez C, Walker-Thurmond K, et al: Overweight, obesity, and mortality from cancer in a prospectively studied cohort of U.S. adults. N Engl J Med 348:1625-1638, 2003.
10. Ho A, Dowdy SF: Regulation of G_1 cell-cycle progression by oncogenes and tumor suppressor genes. Curr Opin Genet Dev 12:47-52, 2002.
11. Okada H, Mak TW: Pathways of apoptotic and non-apoptotic death in tumour cells. Nat Rev Cancer 4:592-603, 2004.
12. Kerr JF, Wyllie AH, Currie AR: Apoptosis: A basic biological phenomenon with wide-ranging implications in tissue kinetics. Br J Cancer 26:239-257, 1972.

13. Korsmeyer SJ: Chromosomal translocations in lymphoid malignancies reveal novel proto-oncogenes. Annu Rev Immunol 10:785-807, 1992.

14. Vaux DL, Cory S, Adams JM: Bcl-2 gene promotes haemopoietic cell survival and cooperates with c-myc to immortalize pre-B cells. Nature 335:440-442, 1988.

15. Kelekar A: Autophagy. Ann N Y Acad Sci 1066:259-271, 2006.

16. Shin JS, Hong A, Solomon MJ, et al: The role of telomeres and telomerase in the pathology of human cancer and aging. Pathology 38:103-113, 2006.

17. Clarke MF, Fuller M: Stem cells and cancer: Two faces of Eve. Cell 124:1111-1115, 2006.

18. Bjerkvig R, Tysnes BB, Aboody KS, et al: Opinion: The origin of the cancer stem cell: Current controversies and new insights. Nat Rev Cancer 5:899-904, 2005.

19. Folkman J: Angiogenesis. Annu Rev Med 57:1-18, 2006.

20. Folkman J, Kalluri R: Cancer without disease. Nature 427:787, 2004.

21. Hanahan D, Folkman J: Patterns and emerging mechanisms of the angiogenic switch during tumorigenesis. Cell 86:353-364, 1996.

22. Sporn MB: The war on cancer. Lancet 347:1377-1381, 1996.

23. Cavallaro U, Christofori G: Cell adhesion and signaling by cadherins and Ig-CAMs in cancer. Nat Rev Cancer 4:118-132, 2004.

24. Schwartz MA: Integrin signaling revisited. Trends Cell Biol 11:466-470, 2001.

25. Janes SM, Watt FM: New roles for integrins in squamous-cell carcinoma. Nat Rev Cancer 6:175-183, 2006.

26. Zlotnik A: Chemokines and cancer. Int J Cancer 119:2026-2029, 2006.

27. Kaplan RN, Riba RD, Zacharoulis S, et al: VEGFR1-positive haematopoietic bone marrow progenitors initiate the pre-metastatic niche. Nature 438:820-827, 2005.

28. Darnell RB, Posner JB: Observing the invisible: Successful tumor immunity in humans. Nat Immunol 4:201, 2003.

29. Fearon ER: Human cancer syndromes: Clues to the origin and nature of cancer. Science 278:1043-1050, 1997.

30. Nielsen M, Franken PF, Reinards TH, et al: Multiplicity in polyp count and extracolonic manifestations in 40 Dutch patients with MYH associated polyposis coli (MAP). J Med Genet 42:e54, 2005.

31. Galiatsatos P, Foulkes WD: Familial adenomatous polyposis. Am J Gastroenterol 101:385-398, 2006.

32. Feinberg AP, Tycko B: The history of cancer epigenetics. Nat Rev Cancer 4:143-153, 2004.

33. Kondo Y, Shen L, Issa JP: Critical role of histone methylation in tumor suppressor gene silencing in colorectal cancer. Mol Cell Biol 23:206-215, 2003.

34. Anzola M: Hepatocellular carcinoma: Role of hepatitis B and hepatitis C viruses proteins in hepatocarcinogenesis. J Viral Hepat 11:383-393, 2004.

35. Butel JS: Viral carcinogenesis: Revelation of molecular mechanisms and etiology of human disease. Carcinogenesis 21:405-426, 2000.

36. Izzo F, Cremona F, Ruffolo F, et al: Outcome of 67 patients with hepatocellular cancer detected during screening of 1125 patients with chronic hepatitis. Ann Surg 227:513-518, 1998.

37. Arguedas MR, Chen VK, Eloubeidi MA, et al: Screening for hepatocellular carcinoma in patients with hepatitis C cirrhosis: A cost-utility analysis. Am J Gastroenterol 98:679-690, 2003.

38. Lin OS, Keeffe EB, Sanders GD, et al: Cost-effectiveness of screening for hepatocellular carcinoma in patients with cirrhosis due to chronic hepatitis C. Aliment Pharmacol Ther 19:1159-1172, 2004.

39. Saab S, Ly D, Nieto J, et al: Hepatocellular carcinoma screening in patients waiting for liver transplantation: A decision analytic model. Liver Transpl 9:672-681, 2003.

40. Shirabe K, Takenaka K, Gion T, et al: Significance of alpha-fetoprotein levels for detection of early recurrence of hepatocellular carcinoma after hepatic resection. J Surg Oncol 64:143-146, 1997.

41. Birch R, Williams S, Cone A, et al: Prognostic factors for favorable outcome in disseminated germ cell tumors. J Clin Oncol 4:400-407, 1986.

42. Paik S, Shak S, Tang G, et al: A multigene assay to predict recurrence of tamoxifen-treated, node-negative breast cancer. N Engl J Med 351:2817-2826, 2004.

43. Baylin SB, Ohm JE: Epigenetic gene silencing in cancer—a mechanism for early oncogenic pathway addiction? Nat Rev Cancer 6:107-116, 2006.

44. Laird PW: The power and the promise of DNA methylation markers. Nat Rev Cancer 3:253-266, 2003.

45. Widschwendter M, Siegmund KD, Muller HM, et al: Association of breast cancer DNA methylation profiles with hormone receptor status and response to tamoxifen. Cancer Res 64:3807-3813, 2004.

46. Cho B, Lee H, Jeong S, et al: Promoter hypomethylation of a novel cancer/testis antigen gene CAGE is correlated with its aberrant expression and is seen in premalignant stage of gastric carcinoma. Biochem Biophys Res Commun 307:52-63, 2003.

47. Widschwendter M, Jiang G, Woods C, et al: DNA hypomethylation and ovarian cancer biology. Cancer Res 64:4472-4480, 2004.

48. Perou CM, Sorlie T, Eisen MB, et al: Molecular portraits of human breast tumours. Nature 406:747-752, 2000.

49. van't Veer LJ, Dai H, van de Vijver MJ, et al: Gene expression profiling predicts clinical outcome of breast cancer. Nature 415:530-536, 2002.

50. Chang JC, Wooten EC, Tsimelzon A, et al: Gene expression profiling for the prediction of therapeutic response to docetaxel in patients with breast cancer. Lancet 362:362-369, 2003.

CHAPTER 30

Melanoma and Cutaneous Malignancies

Marshall M. Urist, MD   and   Seng-jaw Soong, PhD

Skin cancers account for more than 40% of all malignancies in the United States, and the incidence continues to rise. This increase is attributed to environmental exposure, principally sunlight. The majority of skin cancers are basal cell carcinoma (BCC), squamous cell carcinoma (SCC), and melanoma, which account for more than 95% of the total. This chapter focuses on these three major types and briefly discusses the identification and management of less common cutaneous malignancies.

MELANOMA

Melanocytes are cells of neural crest origin that migrate during fetal development to multiple sites in the body, principally the skin. Positioned along the basement membrane at the dermoepidermal junction, these cells are exposed to carcinogenic stimuli that result in malignant transformation to become melanoma. This event is relatively rare when compared with the transformation rate for the neighboring basal keratinocytes that become SCC and BCC. Melanoma accounts for only 4% to 5% of all skin cancers but causes the majority of deaths from skin malignancies. It is the eighth most common cancer in the United States, and the incidence is rising faster than any other type of cancer. It is estimated that there will be 62,190 new cases diagnosed and 7910 deaths from melanoma in 2006.[1] The lifetime probability of melanoma developing is 1 in 57 for males and 1 in 81 for females. In whites, the 5-year relative survival rate has risen from 80% in 1974 to 1976 to 89% in 1992 to 1998.[2] This impressive progress has resulted from increased public awareness and education programs.

Epidemiology and Etiology

The incidence and outcome of melanoma are related to multiple factors. Melanoma is principally a disease of whites, particularly those of Celtic ancestry. The disease occurs much less commonly in Asian and black populations. It is estimated that melanoma develops 20 times more frequently in whites than in blacks. The reason for this difference is unknown. The disease occurs slightly more often in men than women, and the prognosis is slightly better for women when other prognostic factors are taken into account. The anatomic distribution of melanoma varies between the two genders. Melanomas arise more commonly on the lower extremity in women and more often on the trunk and head and neck in men. These differences in distribution are not accounted for by sun exposure alone. Melanoma can occur at any age from birth to advanced age. The median age at diagnosis is in the range of 45 to 55 years. Tumors rarely develop before the age of puberty; however, there is a significant incidence in the third and fourth decades of life.

It is well established that exposure to sunlight, specifically, solar ultraviolet (UV) radiation, increases the risk for development of melanoma in susceptible populations. UVA and UVB cause different patterns of effect in the skin; however, both are considered to be carcinogenic. UVB induces the effects of sunburn, increases melanin production, and is the most carcinogenic part of the UV spectrum. UVA has a deeper level of penetration that results in dermal connective tissue damage, loss of elasticity, and skin wrinkling. It is not clear whether it is the total amount of UV exposure or the pattern in which individuals receive UV irradiation that leads to the development of melanoma. It is reported that people incurring severe burns in childhood appear to be at higher risk for the development of melanoma years later. In contrast, those who receive exposure on a regular basis may not be at as high a risk. There is also a role for skin type inasmuch as individuals who tan easily are not at as high a risk for the development of melanoma, even with prolonged exposure. The highest-risk population appears to be individuals with a fair complexion who receive intermittent doses of radiation that result in severe sunburns.

Additional factors that increase the risk for development of melanoma include dysplastic nevus (DN) syndrome, xeroderma pigmentosum, a history of nonmelanoma skin cancer (NMSC), and a family history of melanoma.

The risk for melanoma increases with age; however, the role of aging is not clear. With increasing age there is more opportunity for the initiation of new tumors, either through exposure to carcinogens (UV irradiation) or through the decreasing ability of individual cells to repair DNA damage.

Precursor Lesions and Risk Factors

Congenital nevi, DNs, Spitz nevi, and familial patterns all raise the risk for development of melanoma. Individuals with congenital nevi have an increased risk that is proportional to the size and number of nevi. Small congenital nevi represent a low risk and are therefore observed unless local changes appear. Giant congenital nevi are rare (1 in 20,000 newborns) and carry an increased risk for the development of melanoma within the nevi (Fig. 30-1). This lifetime risk has been estimated to be in the range of 5% to 8%, which has led some authors to recommend complete excision if possible. At minimum, these patients need to be examined regularly throughout life.

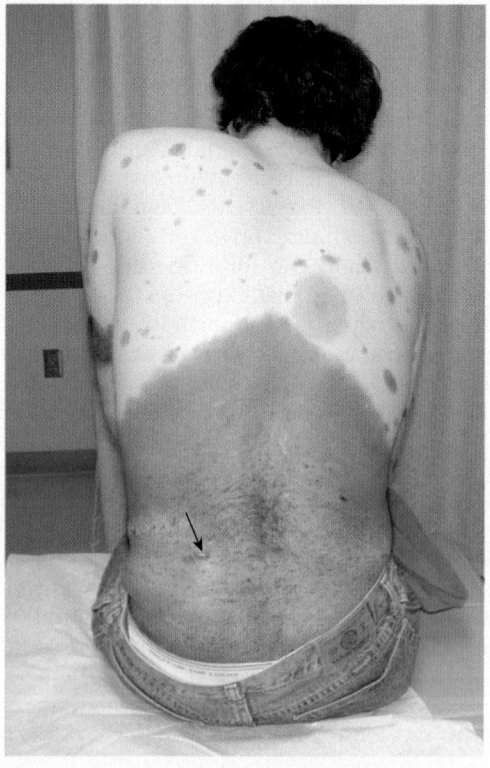

Figure 30-1 Giant congenital nevus of the trunk with a melanoma *(arrow)* arising on the lower part of the back.

In general, a DN is a large (6-15 mm) pigmented flat skin lesion with indistinct margins and variable color. This simple definition belies the difficulty in making the diagnosis because precise criteria may vary both clinically and histologically. DNs may occur sporadically or in a familial pattern. Individuals with DNs and a family history of melanoma have an extremely high risk for the development of melanoma. Patients with DN syndrome (B-K mole syndrome, familial atypical mole–malignant melanoma syndrome) have multiple nevi (>100) that present a great challenge to the patient and physician. There is a lack of consensus regarding the management of DNs because it may be difficult to monitor changes in multiple nevi over time and most DNs will not become melanoma. Excision of all nevi might be reassuring for the patient and physician, but surveillance for the appearance of new lesions is still required. In most instances, physician examinations are scheduled at 3- to 6-month intervals, in addition to monthly patient self-examination. When multiple nevi are present, reference photographs provide an excellent way to compare the appearance of nevi over time.[3]

Spitz nevi (juvenile melanoma, spindle cell melanoma, epithelioid cell melanoma) are rapidly growing, pink or brown benign skin lesions arising most often in children and adolescents, although adult skin lesions may also have spitzoid features. They may be difficult to distinguish histologically from melanoma. Consultation with an experienced pathologist is often required to accurately diagnose these lesions. Complete local excision is the treatment of choice. In borderline cases, it may be necessary to excise the areas as if a melanoma to ensure adequate treatment.[4] Sentinel lymph node (SLN) biopsy has been proposed as a mechanism to clarify the malignant potential in indeterminate cases.[5] If the diagnosis of *melanoma arising within a Spitz nevus* is made, treatment is based on the same criteria as for other types of melanoma.

Familial Melanoma

Approximately 5% to 10% of melanoma patients have a family history of the disease. When compared with patients who have sporadic melanoma, the age of onset is earlier, the incidence of DNs is higher, and multiple primary melanomas are more common. Chromosome mapping studies have shown evidence of linkage and heterogeneity to chromosomes 1p and 9p. Chromosome 1p contributes to both sporadic and familial melanoma, whereas 9p contributes more to sporadic melanoma alone. All reported kindreds are white.

Clinical Features

Cutaneous Melanoma

Melanoma commonly develops as a changing, pigmented skin lesion. Patients typically describe a flat lesion that spreads over the surface of the skin and later becomes elevated. If the lesion is allowed to progress, itching, bleeding, and ulceration will follow. In some instances, melanomas arise in preexisting nevi; however, the majority arise de novo. The most important aspect of the history is change. Even experienced clinicians may not recognize a melanoma; therefore, physicians need to have a low threshold for performing a diagnostic biopsy on any changing lesion. Several other pigmented benign skin lesions can mimic the appearance of melanoma: nevi (congenital and acquired), blue nevus, solar lentigo, keratosis, hemangioma, and pyogenic granuloma. The common features of melanoma are summarized in the mnemonic ABCDE: *a*symmetric outline, changing irregular *b*orders, variation in *c*olor, *d*iameter greater than 6 mm, and *e*levation. In early melanoma, the changes may be limited to two or three features.

Not all melanomas are pigmented. Amelanotic lesions appear as raised papules that can be pink, red, purple, or normal skin colors. Their atypical appearance frequently leads to a delay in diagnosis and therefore a poorer prognosis. Desmoplastic melanoma is a specific type of amelanotic melanoma that commonly arises on the face and can be associated with lentigo maligna melanoma (LMM). Desmoplastic melanomas exhibit neurotropism, which is also a poor prognostic factor. The prognosis appears to be worse because they are thicker lesions than nondesmoplastic tumors; however, the specific histologic type, "pure" versus "mixed," is also important to determine.[6]

In summary, any changing skin lesion needs to be evaluated carefully, and clinicians need to have a low threshold to perform a diagnostic biopsy, especially in individuals who have multiple pigmented lesions, a history of atypical or dysplastic lesions, or a family history of skin cancer.

Unknown Primary Melanoma

Nodal or distant metastasis may be the first evidence of melanoma. This occurs in less than 2% of all melanoma cases and in less than 5% of all patients with metastatic melanoma.[7] In these circumstances the prognosis may be as good or better than if the primary were known. A thorough search for the primary lesion includes a histologic review of all previously removed skin lesions; questions regarding skin lesions that resolved without treatment; and inspection of areas that may have been missed at the initial examination, including the scalp, external auditory canal, oral and nasal mucosa, nail beds, genitalia, anal canal, perianal skin, and the eye. In the case of lymph node metastasis, completion regional lymph node dissection is performed on the assumption that it is a regional node and therefore represents stage III rather than stage IV disease. Such patients may have a better prognosis than those with known primary sites.[8] The patient is then evaluated for adjuvant therapy, especially for participation in investigational protocols. For metastases at other sites, see Surgical Considerations for Metastases, later in this chapter.

Noncutaneous Melanoma

In embryogenesis, melanocytes arise in the neural crest area and migrate to many sites other than the skin. Less than 10% of melanomas arise in these areas, which include the eye, mucosal surfaces, and unknown primary sites. A review from the National Cancer Database from 1985 to 1994 reported on a population of patients with more than 80,000 melanomas; 91% were found in the skin, 5.2% occurred in the eye, 1.3% developed on mucosal surfaces, and 2.2% were considered to be unknown primary origin.[7] Although melanoma has been reported to arise from many tissues and organs throughout the body, there is often the possibility that these lesions are actually metastases from an unknown primary site on the skin. One exception may be in the esophagus, where melanocytic atypia and melanoma in situ have been shown to occur.

Ocular melanoma is the most common malignancy arising in the eye. Within the eye, melanocytes are found in the retina and uveal tract (iris, ciliary body, and choroids). Options for treatment are photocoagulation, partial resection, radiation, or enucleation. Although ocular and cutaneous melanomas have several common histologic features, their clinical course is quite different. Ocular melanoma rarely metastasizes to lymph nodes because the uveal tract has no lymphatic vessels. The most common site of distant metastases is the liver, which may be the first detected site of disease in patients with retinal melanoma.

The most common sites of origin for melanomas arising on the mucous membranes are the head and neck (oral cavity, oropharynx, nasopharynx, and paranasal sinuses), anal canal, rectum, and female genitalia. When compared with melanomas arising on the skin, mucosal melanomas are more advanced and have a poorer prognosis. These tumors are excised to negative margins. Extensive local resections do not affect survival, although locoregional control may be improved.[9] In general, lymph node dissections are not indicated unless patients have clinically evident lymphadenopathy. The one exception involves patients with vulvar melanoma—SLN biopsy is now being performed for this group of patients.[10] The overall prognosis for patients with mucosal melanomas is poor, with less than 10% surviving 5 years.

Clinical Management

Choice of Biopsy

Clinical management of melanoma begins with an accurate diagnosis. The classic signs of melanoma include a skin lesion with changing characteristics such as irregular borders, varying degrees of pigmentation, an irregular surface, bleeding, itching, and ulceration. The decision to perform a biopsy is frequently based on clinical experience; however, even senior dermatologists and surgeons may underdiagnose melanoma. Concern on the part of either the physician or the patient is a valid indication for biopsy. The specific method of biopsy depends on the size of the lesion and its anatomic location. Regardless of the method, biopsy specimens are full thickness into subcutaneous tissue. For small lesions, an excisional biopsy is commonly performed that includes a narrow (1-2 mm) margin of surrounding skin. The biopsy area is not enlarged to permit a better cosmetic appearance because this may lead to unnecessary expansion of the final wide excision. Although shave biopsies are commonly performed for benign-appearing lesions,

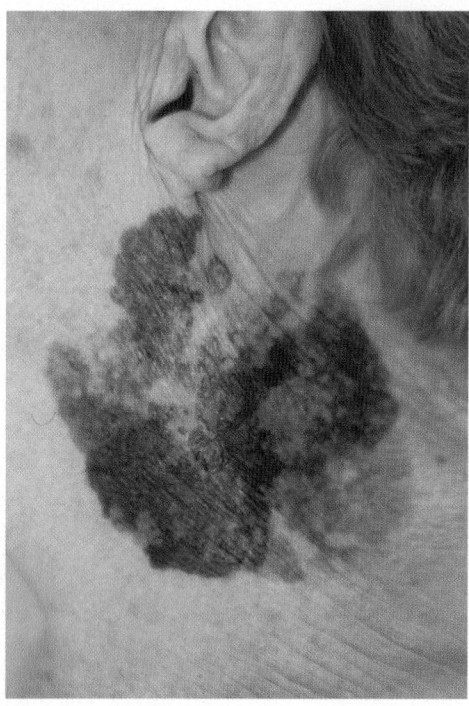

Figure 30-2 Lentigo maligna melanoma covering the left side of the neck. Despite a long history of growth, tumor thickness remained less than 1 mm.

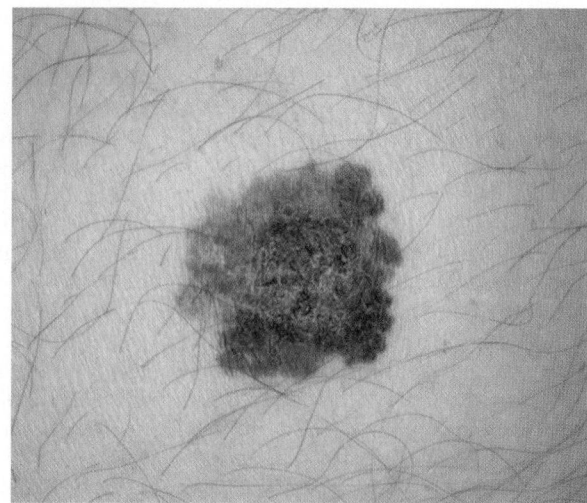

Figure 30-3 Superficial spreading melanoma. This 2-cm diameter melanoma developed over a 2-year period.

this technique must not be used when melanoma is suspected. A shave biopsy may lead to a pathology report showing extension of tumor to the deep margins of excision. In these circumstances the most important prognostic factor, tumor thickness, will not be accurate and could lead to incorrect decisions regarding wide local excision (WLE), SLN biopsy, and adjuvant therapy. The clinical appearance of melanoma may be deceptively benign, which is why the use of cautery or cryoablation may lead to a delay in the diagnosis of melanoma. If a skin lesion reappears at the site of a previously cauterized or frozen skin lesion, excisional biopsy and histopathologic analysis are required.

The technique of performing a surgical biopsy is straightforward. The biopsy removes the full thickness of skin, including a layer of the underlying fatty tissue and the entire visible tumor. Care must be taken to not crush or otherwise traumatize the specimen so that histologic interpretation is not compromised. These biopsies are performed under local anesthesia in the office or outpatient setting. The wound is closed in one or two layers in an orientation that is consistent with a possible wider excision. There may be circumstances in which complete surgical excision is not appropriate, for example, because of a large primary lesion or proximity of the lesion to important structures such as the eye, nose, or ear. In these circumstances, punch biopsy or excision of a segment of the lesion is appropriate. Again, the biopsy is a full-thickness specimen and includes a margin of adjacent normal skin if possible. When biopsy of a large lesion is performed, at least one punch is placed through the most elevated portion to accurately classify its thickness.

When performing diagnostic biopsy, orientation of the biopsy closure may affect options for closure of the WLE. For this reason, biopsy excisions on the extremities are closed longitudinally to maximize the possibility for primary wound closure and decrease the need for skin grafts. Larger tissue defects may be closed with local rotational/advancement skin flaps or a skin graft.

Histologic Features of Cutaneous Melanoma

Histologically, melanoma is divided into four major types based on growth pattern and location: LMM, superficial spreading melanoma (SSM), acral lentiginous melanoma (ALM), and nodular melanoma (NM). Melanomas arise as proliferations of melanocytes in the basal layer of the skin. As they multiply, these cells expand radially in the epidermis and superficial dermal layer. With time, growth begins in a vertical direction and the skin lesion may become palpable. NMs are an exception to this pattern in that the vertical growth phase is present from an early point in tumor development. It is the vertical growth phase more than any other histologic parameter of the primary tumor that determines prognosis.

LMM (~10%) has distinctive clinical and histologic features. It occurs most commonly in older individuals with sun-damaged skin and appears as a flat, darkly pigmented lesion with irregular borders and a history of slow development. It is not uncommon to see LMMs that are several centimeters in diameter, thereby resulting in an inability of the patient to detect slow progress of the lesion (Fig. 30-2). Overall, the prognosis of LMM is better than that for other histopathologic types; however, this better prognosis is primarily related to the superficial nature of these lesions.

The most common histologic type is SSM (~70%). It is not necessarily associated with sun-exposed skin. As the name SSM suggests, these lesions initially appear as a flat, pigmented lesion growing in a radial pattern (Fig. 30-3).

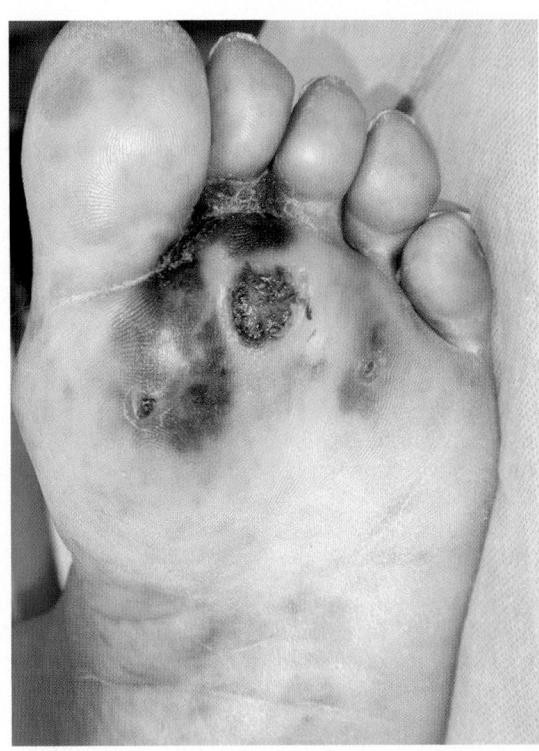

Figure 30-4 Acral lentiginous melanoma. The extensively pigmented areas on the sole were predominately melanoma in situ. The single invasive area was ulcerated.

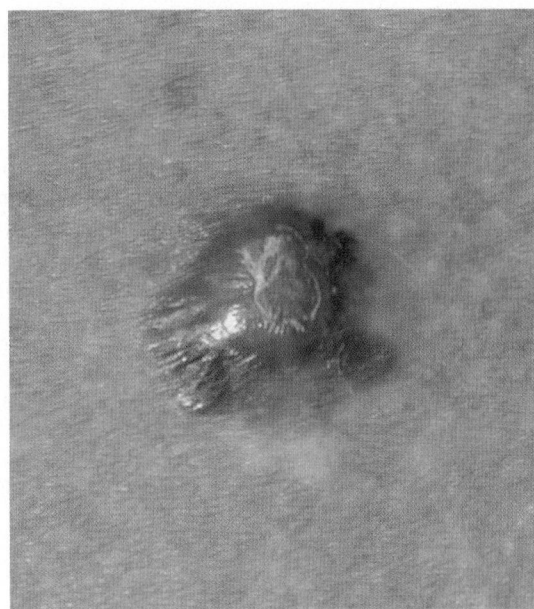

Figure 30-5 Nodular melanoma. This raised lesion had no radial growth phase.

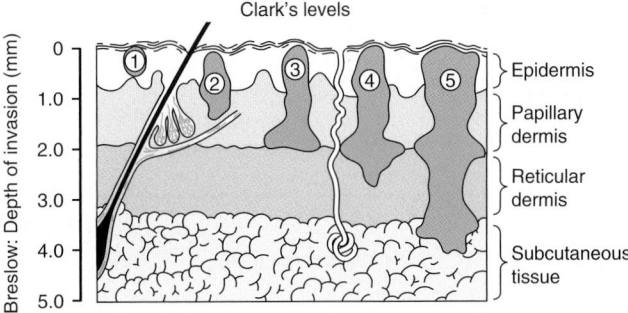

Figure 30-6 Schematic representation of Clark's levels of tumor penetration in relation to the normal layers of skin.

If left in place, the lesion begins to thicken as the vertical growth phase develops.

ALM (~5%) is classified principally by its anatomic site of origin, although it does have a characteristic histologic appearance. These tumors are confined to the subungual areas and the glabrous skin of the palms and soles (Fig. 30-4). ALM is the most common histologic variant arising in blacks, and the diagnosis is often delayed because of the common appearance of irregular benign pigmentation on the surfaces. For this reason, the overall prognosis is poor. Melanomas arising in subungual areas are also frequently ignored because of their similar appearance to subungual hematomas secondary to trauma. The histologic appearance of ALM is similar to that of melanomas arising on mucous membranes.

A vertical growth pattern develops early in the history of NMs (~15%), and they may be devoid of junctional changes (Fig. 30-5). Melanomas in this group have the worst prognosis because of a higher average tumor thickness.

Historically, classification of melanoma into various histologic types had a role in clinical management. With improved understanding of prognostic factors, management is based primarily on thickness and ulceration.

Prognostic Factors

Until the 1960s, invasive melanoma was considered to be a high-risk disease that required extensive local excision for *all* tumors. In 1969, Clark and associates[11] described a classification of melanoma based on the extent of tumor invasion relative to the anatomic layers of the skin and showed that the level of invasion was related to survival (Fig. 30-6). Level 1 tumors are limited to the epidermis, are in situ, and theoretically have no risk for metastasis. Level 2 lesions extend into the papillary dermis and also have an excellent prognosis. Clark level 3 tumors fill the papillary dermis and are associated with a significant risk for metastasis. Extension into the reticular dermis defines a Clark 4 lesion, and growth into subcutaneous fat characterizes Clark level 5, both of which impart high risk for mortality. In some cases, determining the Clark level was found to be difficult, and readings of the same slides could differ between pathologists (especially in the level 3 to 4 range). In 1970, Breslow described a more straightforward system based on measuring the vertical thickness of the tumor in millimeters.[12] This method was found to be accurately reproducible between pathologists, and there was excellent correlation with 5-year survival. The prognosis worsens with increasing thickness as a continuous logarithmic function without stair-step areas or natural breakpoints (Fig. 30-7). The mortality rate begins to plateau at about 8 mm and never reaches 100%. Comparison of the two systems showed that the Clark level added little to prognosis as determined by the Breslow thickness.

In melanoma, analysis of factors contributing to prognosis has led to a remarkably accurate prediction of outcome. Balch and collaborators from 13 institutions[13] collected a complete data set on 17,600 patients to form the American Joint Committee on Cancer (AJCC) melanoma database. In an analysis of 13,581 patients with localized melanoma, they defined the relative contribution of multiple known prognostic factors, including age, gender, level, site, thickness, and ulceration. The findings of their multifactorial analysis are summarized in Table 30-1. As in all previous studies, tumor thickness was found to be the strongest predictor of outcome. Mela-

noma thickness is also associated with an increasing risk for local recurrence, regional metastases, distant metastases, and survival. The findings were the same at participating institutions in Australia, Europe, and North America and have been confirmed in a population-based study using Surveillance, Epidemiology, and End Results (SEER) data, which suggest that population-based survival rates may be higher than AJCC outcomes.[14]

Based on the findings just discussed, a complete pathologic report of cutaneous melanoma includes the following: Breslow thickness, presence or absence of ulceration, Clark level, status of the surgical margins, histologic type, presence or absence of satellitosis, and presence or absence of regression. The report may also describe tumor-infiltrating lymphocytes, lymphovascular invasion, vertical growth phase, neurotropism, and mitotic rate.[15]

Staging

Staging for melanoma uses the tumor-node-metastasis (TNM) system of classification as defined by the AJCC staging system for cutaneous melanoma (Tables 30-2 and 30-3). The sixth edition (2002) of the *AJCC Cancer Staging Manual* contains important changes from the 1977 edition.[16] These changes are based on the in-depth analysis of prognostic factors cited earlier (see Table 30-1).[14]

As is true for other malignancies, a patient with melanoma undergoes a systematic evaluation for metastatic disease. Such evaluation begins with a history focused on constitutional, central nervous system, pulmonary, gastrointestinal, and soft tissue symptoms. A standard physical examination includes a detailed inspection and palpation of the skin and subcutaneous tissue to detect satellites, in-transit metastases, other primary tumors, and lymph node enlargement. When present, all symptoms and signs of metastasis require further radiologic evaluation. Patients with clinical stage 0 and I do not require any further tests. Patients with stage II and III may have a chest radiograph and serum lactate dehydrogenase level determined; however, findings are rarely abnormal in asymptomatic patients.

This 2002 version of the AJCC staging system provides excellent separation of prognostic groups by stage, as

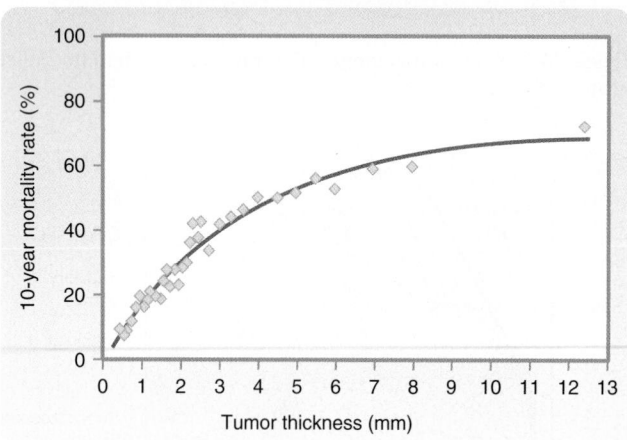

Figure 30-7 Observed *(diamonds)* and predicted *(solid line)* 10-year mortality rate for patients with clinically localized melanoma. This is based on a mathematical model derived from the American Joint Committee on Cancer melanoma database of 15,230 patients. (From Balch CM, Soong S-j, Gerschenwald JE, et al: Prognostic factors analysis of 17,600 melanoma patients: Validation of the American Joint Committee on Cancer melanoma staging system. J Clin Oncol 19:3622-3634, 2001.)

Table 30-1 Cox Regression Analysis for 13,581 Patients With Melanoma Without Evidence of Nodal or Distant Metastases

VARIABLE	DF	CHI-SQUARE VALUE	P	RISK RATIO	95% CL
Thickness	1	244.3	<.00001	1.558	1.473-1.647
Ulceration	1	189.5	<.00001	1.901	1.735-1.083
Age	1	45.6	<.00001	1.101	1.071-1.132
Site	1	41.0	<.00001	1.338	1.224-1.463
Level	1	32.7	<.00001	1.214	1.136-1.297
Gender	1	15.1	.001	0.836	0.764-0.915

CL, confidence limits; DF, degrees of freedom.
Revised from Balch CM, Soong S-j, Gerschenwald JE, et al: Prognostic factors analysis of 17,600 melanoma patients: Validation of the American Joint Committee on Cancer Melanoma Staging System. J Clin Oncol 19:3622-3634, 2001.

Table 30-2 **American Joint Committee on Cancer TNM Melanoma Classification—2002**

Primary Tumor (T)

TX	Primary tumor cannot be assessed (e.g., shave biopsy or regressed melanoma)
T0	No evidence of primary tumor
Tis	Melanoma in situ
T1	Melanoma ≤1.0 mm in thickness, with or without ulceration
T1a	Melanoma ≤1.0 mm in thickness and level II or III, no ulceration
T1b	Melanoma ≤1.0 mm in thickness and level IV or V or with ulceration
T2	Melanoma 1.01-2.0 mm in thickness, with or without ulceration
T2a	Melanoma 1.01-2.0 mm in thickness, no ulceration
T2b	Melanoma 1.01-2.0 mm in thickness, with ulceration
T3	Melanoma 2.01-4.0 mm in thickness, with or without ulceration
T3a	Melanoma 2.01-4.0 mm in thickness, no ulceration
T3b	Melanoma 2.01-4.0 mm in thickness, with ulceration
T4	Melanoma >4.0 mm in thickness, with or without ulceration
T4a	Melanoma >4.0 mm in thickness, no ulceration
T4b	Melanoma >4.0 mm in thickness, with ulceration

Regional Lymph Nodes (N)

NX	Regional lymph nodes cannot be assessed
N0	No regional lymph node metastasis
N1	Metastasis in one lymph node
N1a	Clinically occult (microscopic) metastasis
N1b	Clinically apparent (macroscopic) metastasis
N2	Metastasis in two or three regional nodes or intralymphatic regional metastasis without nodal metastases
N2a	Clinically occult (microscopic) metastasis
N2b	Clinically apparent (macroscopic) metastasis
N2c	Satellite or in-transit metastasis without nodal metastasis
N3	Metastasis in four or more regional nodes, matted metastatic nodes, in-transit metastasis, or satellites with metastasis in regional node(s)

Distant Metastasis (M)

MX	Distant metastasis cannot be assessed
M0	No distant metastasis
M1	Distant metastasis
M1a	Metastasis to skin, subcutaneous tissue, or distant lymph nodes
M1b	Metastasis to lung
M1c	Metastasis to all other visceral sites or distant metastasis at any site associated with elevated serum lactate dehydrogenase

Table 30-3 **American Joint Committee on Cancer Melanoma Stage Classification**

PATHOLOGIC STAGE	GROUPING		
	Tumor	Node	Metastasis
0	Tis	N0	M0
IA	T1a	N0	M0
IB	T1b	N0	M0
	T2a	N0	M0
IIA	T2b	N0	M0
	T3a	N0	M0
IIB	T3b	N0	M0
	T4a	N0	M0
IIC	T4b	N0	M0
IIIA	T1-4a	N1a	M0
	T1-4a	N2a	M0
IIIB	T1-4b	N1a	M0
	T1-4b	N2a	M0
	T1-4a	N1b	M0
	T1-4a	N2b	M0
	T1-4a/b	N2c	M0
IIIC	T1-4b	N1b	M0
	T1-4b	N2b	M0
	Any T	N3	M0
IV	Any T	Any N	M1

Table 30-4 **Ten-Year Survival Rates for Stage I and II Melanomas**

STAGE	TUMOR ULCERATION	T STAGE	APPROXIMATE 10-YEAR SURVIVAL (%)
IA	No	T1a	90
IB	Yes	T1b	80
	No	T2a	80
IIA	Yes	T2b	65
	No	T3a	65
IIB	Yes	T3b	50
	No	T4a	55
IIC	Yes	T4b	35

shown in Figure 30-8. The presence of ulceration indicates a significantly worse prognosis and can result in a change in stage (Table 30-4). The new system also provides useful substaging within the N category based on the number of positive lymph nodes and the presence or absence of ulceration, as shown in Table 30-5.

Surgical Management of the Primary Lesion

The fundamental principle in the management of primary melanoma is to resect the tumor and minimize the risk for local recurrence. Historically, resection of the primary site and surrounding skin was based on recommendations proffered by William Sampson Handley in 1907. From observations made on the autopsy of a single patient with locally advanced melanoma, he recommended WLE and regional lymph node dissection. This became the standard treatment except in anatomic locations where major adjacent structures (especially the head and neck) were spared. With the insightful contributions of Wallace Clark[11] and Alexander Breslow[12] in the late 1960s, the natural history of melanoma became better understood. From many retrospective studies it was clear that the risk for local recurrence and overall survival rates were related to tumor thickness. Five randomized studies have been carried out to test whether narrow margins of excision could achieve the same results as wide margins. The current guidelines for WLE (Table 30-6) are based on these studies. These trials confirm that melanomas measuring 1 mm or less in thickness can be resected with a 1-cm margin with a low subsequent risk for local recurrence. Melanomas between 1 and 2 mm in thickness have an equally low risk for local recurrence when a 2-cm margin is used. These margins may be lowered to 1 cm when primary closure of the wound would be facilitated. A narrower margin may result in a small increase in the number of patients in whom local recurrence develops; however, no statistically significant difference in survival has been observed. The factor that most closely correlated with local recurrence was primary tumor ulceration. When melanomas are greater than 4 mm in thickness, recommendations for management are based on retrospective analyses in which there does not appear to be any advantage to extending the resection beyond 2 cm.

Members of the Melanoma Committee of the National Comprehensive Cancer Network, a consortium of oncologists from National Cancer Institute–designated cancer centers, annually update their consensus-based guidelines for the treatment of cancer. Guidelines for the management of primary melanoma are summarized in Figure 30-9. (The complete guideline algorithm is available on-line.[17])

Table 30-5 Five-Year Survival Rates for Stage III Melanoma Patients

STAGE	TUMOR ULCERATION	N STAGE	APPROXIMATE 5-YEAR SURVIVAL (%)
IIIA	No	N1a	70
	No	N2a	60
IIIB	Yes	N1a	55
	Yes	N2a	50
	No	N1b	55
	No	N2b	45
IIIC	Yes	N1b	30
	Yes	N2b	25
	Yes or No	N3	30

Table 30-6 Recommended Margins for Surgical Resection of Primary Melanoma

TUMOR THICKNESS (mm)	MARGIN RADIUS (cm)*
In situ	0.5
<1.0	1.0
1-2	1.0-2.0
>2.0	≥2.0

*Recommended margins may be adjusted to accommodate anatomic or cosmetic circumstances.

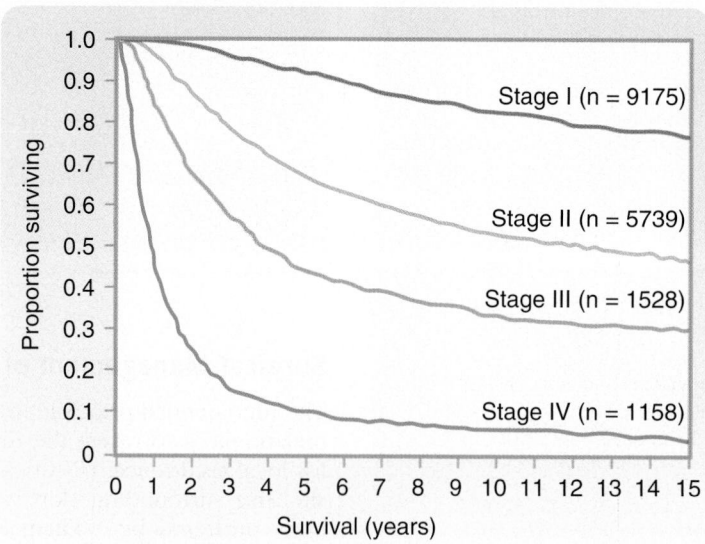

Figure 30-8 Fifteen-year survival curves for the melanoma staging system in which localized melanoma (stages I and II), regional metastases (stage III), and distant metastases (stage IV) were compared. The numbers in parentheses are the numbers of patients from the American Joint Committee on Cancer melanoma staging database used to calculate the survival rates. Differences between the curves are highly significant ($P < .0001$). (From Balch CM, Buzaid AC, Soong S-j, et al: Final version of the American Joint Committee on Cancer Staging System for cutaneous melanoma. J Clin Oncol 19:3635-3648, 2001.)

The operative procedure of WLE is often performed under local anesthesia with intravenous sedation if necessary. In most cases the margin for WLE is measured from the edges of the biopsy scar, which again emphasizes the importance of minimal excision for the original biopsy to limit the size of the final resection. The incision is made through the skin and subcutaneous tissue to the level of the superficial fascia. The specimen is oriented for the pathologist and submitted for permanent section. In many cases the resulting wound can be closed by elevation and advancement of the skin edges or the use of local skin flaps. Skin grafts may be required on the hands, feet, and distal ends of the extremities. Tumors arising in proximity to structures such as the nose, eye, and ear may require a compromise in the conventional margins to avoid deformities or disabilities. Subungual melanomas are treated by amputation of the distal digit to provide 1 cm of margin from the tumor. For fingers, amputation commonly involves only the distal phalanx; ray amputations are unnecessary. In all cases, resection reaches histologically normal margins.

Local extension of mucosal melanomas commonly occurs before they become symptomatic. Oral cavity melanomas are an exception to this rule because they may be discovered during routine dental examination. Nonetheless, diagnosis of melanomas in this area can be delayed because of similarities to amalgam stains. Tumors are resected with histologically clear margins; however, there is no evidence that WLE increases the chance for cure. Anorectal melanomas are excised to clear margins. For extensive tumors, abdominoperineal resection may be necessary. Abdominoperineal resection reduces the incidence of local and regional recurrence but does not result in an improvement in overall survival.

Melanoma and Pregnancy

Early reports suggested an adverse relationship between pregnancy and outcome in patients with melanoma. This was reinforced by the finding of estrogen receptors in some melanoma tumors. More recent comprehensive analyses have not confirmed any difference in the course of the disease in gravid versus nongravid patients when all relevant prognostic factors are taken into account. Unfortunately, recommendations derived from these early reports included early termination of pregnancy when the diagnosis was made and delaying pregnancy for 2 years after treatment of melanoma. The decision regarding pregnancy is no different for melanoma than for other malignancies. These decisions are made between the patient and her physicians after an in-depth discussion of prognosis and options for treatment.

Management of Regional Lymph Nodes

After WLE of the primary tumor, the most common sites of first recurrence are regional (lymph nodes, in-transit metastases, and local recurrences). Nodal metastases generally appear in the basin or basins draining from the primary site. This is a predictable pattern for extremity melanomas; however, truncal and head and neck melanomas may drain to more than one site. Lines of drainage for truncal melanomas are divided by the midline and the line of Sappey, which extends from the umbilicus across the iliac crest and around to the spine at the level of L2. This sequence of recurrences led surgeons to conclude that resection of nodal basins containing occult metastases could provide an increase in survival. This procedure, termed *elective lymph node dissection* (ELND), was commonly practiced but was often accompanied by

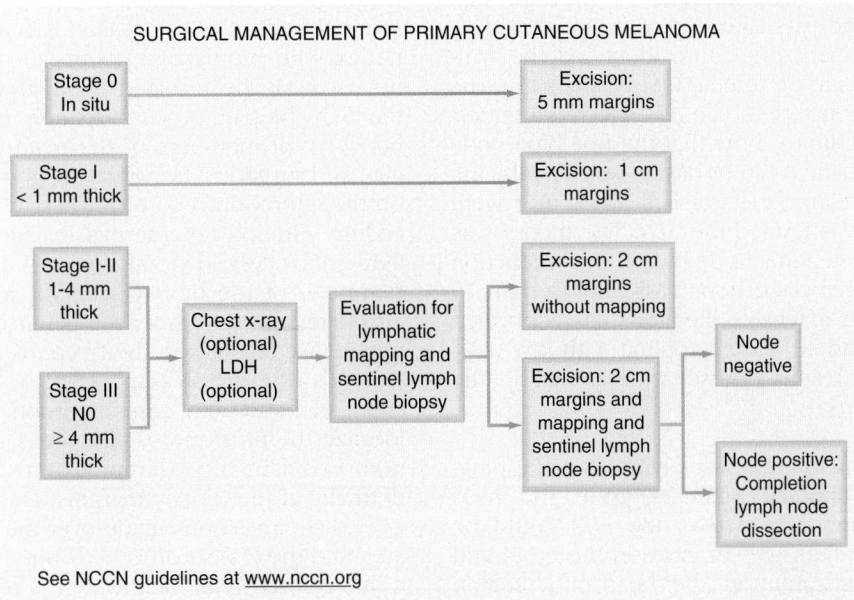

Figure 30-9 Management algorithm for primary cutaneous melanoma derived from the National Comprehensive Cancer Network (NCCN) guidelines (available at www.nccn.org). LDH, lactate dehydrogenase.

significant morbidity, including lymphedema, muscle weakness, and restricted range of motion.

As prognostic factors became better understood, it was postulated that patients with thin tumors (<1 mm in thickness) would have a low risk of metastases at any site and patients with thick tumors (>4 mm in thickness) would have a high risk of distant as well as regional metastases. In contrast, patients with intermediate-thickness melanoma (1-4 mm) would have an elevated risk for nodal metastases without a high risk for distant disease. The intermediate-thickness group formed the population of patients who would, in theory, benefit from ELND. Early retrospective analyses supported this hypothesis and provided the rationale for prospective, randomized trials comparing WLE alone versus WLE with ELND. Subsequent larger retrospective series reported no benefit. Four phase III prospective, randomized trials have failed to provide convincing evidence to support ELND. Two early trials were criticized for being underpowered and uncontrolled for important prognostic factors. Subsequently, the Intergroup Melanoma Trial and the World Health Organization Melanoma Programme Trial were designed and powered to answer the question, but neither showed a survival benefit for ELND.

Development of the SLN concept ended one debate over ELND, changed clinical management, and opened a new series of questions about the tumor biology of melanoma. In the mid-1970s, Dr. Donald Morton and colleagues described a radionuclide mapping technique to define the lymphatic drainage area from any primary site on the skin. This technique was designed to define a perplexing problem for surgeons planning elective lymphadenectomy to resect occult metastases, specifically, the location of at-risk lymph nodes. Primary sites, especially on the trunk and on the head and neck, could potentially drain to multiple lymphatic basins. In this mapping technique, technetium 99m–labeled colloid was injected intradermally at the primary site, flowed through lymphatic vessels, and was taken up in regional nodes.

This simple outpatient procedure identified the lymphatic basin or basins to be resected. More than 15 years later, Dr. Morton's group used blue dye injected intradermally at the primary site to show that the first blue node in the regional lymphatic basin or basins was actually the node that would contain a metastasis if any tumor were present. This node was termed the *SLN*. The theory was tested by performing sentinel node biopsy in conjunction with complete regional dissection.[18] After more than 10 years' experience, an extensive literature has confirmed that this technique can be widely applied with low morbidity and accurate results. These reports include the following observations:

1. By using a combination of isotope lymphatic mapping, an intraoperative hand-held gamma probe, and intraoperative injection of blue dye, the SLN could be identified in more than 95% of cases in the groin and axilla, with identification in the head/neck region being slightly lower (85%).
2. There was great anatomic variation resulting in drainage to multiple or uncommon sites.[19-21]

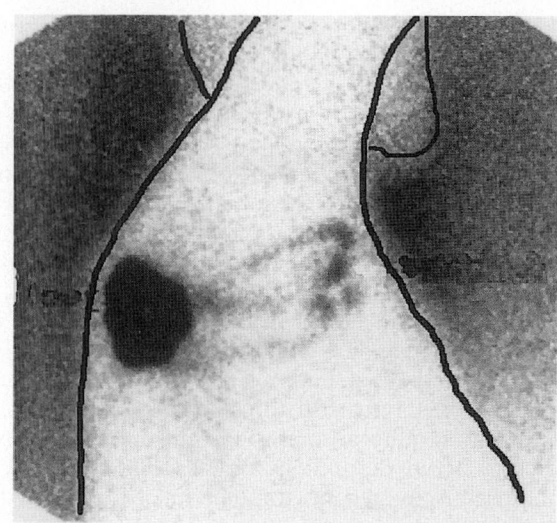

Figure 30-10 Lymphoscintigram showing the lateral view of a patient with a primary melanoma of the back. Note the three parallel lymphatic vascular pathways leading to the axillary sentinel lymph nodes.

3. Detailed pathologic analysis of the sentinel nodes via step sections enabled detection of micrometastases that could be missed by standard techniques.[22]
4. The probability of finding a positive sentinel node can be predicted by using a nomogram derived from multifactorial analysis.[23]
5. In most cases a positive sentinel node was the only positive node.[24]
6. No prognostic factors were found that accurately identified a subpopulation of SLN-positive patients at zero risk of harboring other positive nodes.[25,26]

Additional studies have confirmed that the hottest lymph node (most radioactive) is not always the positive sentinel node. For this reason it is recommended that all nodes with radioactive counts greater than 10% of the hottest node be resected for analysis.[27,28] The details of the SLN biopsy process require close communication between all members of the team (radiologist, pathologist, and surgeon). Lymphoscintigraphy can be scheduled on the afternoon before or the day of the operative procedure. Multiple intradermal injections of technetium Tc 99m sulfur colloid (total dose, ~1 mCi) are made at the perimeter of the biopsy scar. All regional node-bearing areas are scanned under the gamma camera, and sites of uptake are labeled on the lymphoscintigram (and on the patient's skin if necessary) (Fig. 30-10). In the operating room, a hand-held gamma probe is used to precisely localize the most radioactive areas. Before skin preparation, isosulfan blue (lymphazurin) dye is injected intradermally at the biopsy margins. During the procedure, a 2- to 4-cm incision is made over the previously identified area and the dissection is performed by blunt means until a dye-colored lymphatic vessel is seen (Fig. 30-11). This vessel is traced down to the blue node, which is removed. By using a combination of inspection and the gamma probe, the wound is examined for all blue or hot nodes

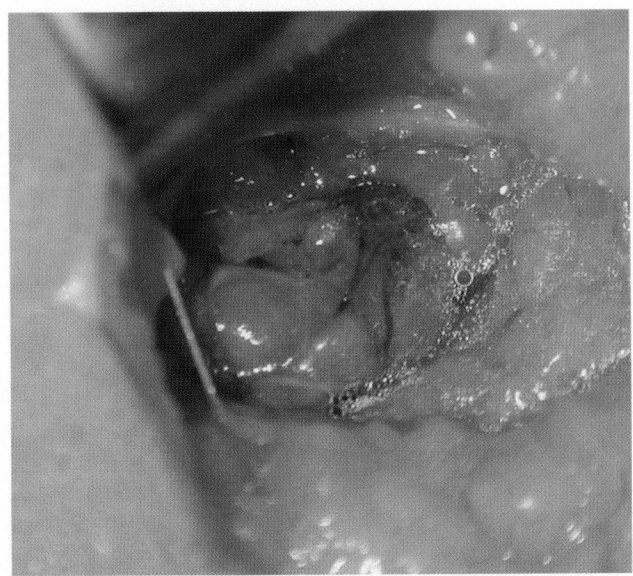

Figure 30-11 Operative view of a sentinel lymph node stained with isosulfan blue dye. Note the two parallel afferent vessels leading to the sentinel node.

(or both). The wound is also palpated because nodes obliterated by tumor may not take up blue dye or radioisotope.

SLN biopsy has rapidly become a standard procedure for patients with tumors greater than 1 mm in thickness to accurately stage the disease and provide guidance for treatment planning (see Fig. 30-9).[29] In a retrospective analysis, SLN biopsy appeared to provide a survival benefit when compared with WLE alone.[30] This therapeutic benefit is now being evaluated in the Multicenter Selective Lymphadenectomy Trial (MSLT-I), in which patients with melanomas greater than 1 mm in thickness were randomized to undergo WLE alone or WLE plus SLN biopsy. Patients with positive SLNs then underwent completion lymph node dissection. This trial addresses one of the oldest questions in surgical oncology: is there a therapeutic benefit from diagnosis and resection of early lymphatic metastases? Accessions to this trial were closed at the end of March 2002 after 2001 patients were enrolled. The primary outcome is melanoma-related death, with secondary outcomes being disease-free survival and local, regional, and distant recurrence rates. The procedure was found to be safe, with low morbidity, and surgeon performance improved with experience.[31]

In an interim analysis after a median follow-up of 59.5 months, there was no statistically significant difference in survival between the two groups. Interestingly, 15.9% of patients were found to have a positive sentinel node, and in the same percentage of patients a clinically positive node developed in follow-up after WLE alone. The average number of positive nodes after SLN biopsy and completion lymph node dissection was 1.4 versus an average of 3.6 positive nodes after resection of palpable nodes. The SLN-positive group had a significant 5-year survival advantage over the therapeutic dissection group, 71.2% versus 53.4%, respectively.[32] The absence of an

improvement in overall survival and the lack of effective adjuvant therapy for node-positive patients have caused some investigators to question the value of SLN biopsy. Proponents of the technique point to the value of accurate nodal staging and the eligibility of patients for prospective adjuvant therapy trials. The MSLT investigators have initiated a second trial to test the value of completion lymph node dissection in patients who are SLN positive.

A second large trial currently examining the value of SLN biopsy is the Sunbelt Melanoma Trial. In this ongoing study, all patients with melanoma greater than 1 mm in thickness undergo SLN biopsy. Patients whose SLN is positive for metastasis by hematoxylin/eosin staining, immunohistochemistry (S-100 and HMB-45), or reverse transcriptase polymerase chain reaction (tyrosinase, MAGE1, MART3, gp100) may participate in further randomization to surgery (completion lymph node dissection) or adjuvant interferon therapy, or both. The role of interferon in stage III patients with melanoma remains controversial. The Sunbelt Melanoma Trial will determine whether interferon has a beneficial role to play in the treatment of stage III patients with a minimal burden of metastatic disease.

Monitoring of Patients After Surgical Therapy

After primary treatment of melanoma, prediction of the pattern of recurrence can be based on the same factors used to estimate survival (tumor thickness, ulceration, and lymph node status). The risk of the first metastasis being at a distant site increases with thick primary tumors and resected regional positive nodes. Follow-up examinations focus on detection of treatable metastases. The most common sites of initial recurrence are local and regional. Patients are informed about the common symptoms and signs of recurrence so that they can report important changes arising between scheduled examinations. Such changes include local swelling, itching, new lesions in and beneath the skin, enlargement of lymph nodes, central nervous system changes, and pulmonary and gastrointestinal symptoms.

The physical examination is the most important aspect of the return visit. A complete skin examination is performed with inspection and palpation of the primary site and skin surfaces leading to regional nodal basins. In-transit metastases may be palpable but not visible.

The follow-up examination schedule reflects the risk for recurrence. Initially, patients are seen at 3- to 6-month intervals until they have reached the 3-year anniversary. By this time, 75% of patients in whom a metastasis would ever develop would have had that event occur. Annual examinations are scheduled thereafter. Patients with early melanoma, stage IA, are monitored without radiologic or laboratory studies. For asymptomatic patients, a chest radiograph and serum lactate dehydrogenase assay may be performed at 6- to 12-month intervals, although there is no evidence that the routine use of these follow-up tests results in a survival benefit. The routine use of screening computed tomography (CT), magnetic resonance imaging, or positron emission tomography (PET) has not been shown to be cost-effective and remains a subject of investigation.[33] In stage III patients, PET scan results change treatment decisions in up to 20% of cases; however, the rate is very low in patients with a single microscopic nodal metastasis. Scans and other tests may be required for patients participating in clinical protocols.

Surgical Considerations for Metastases

Approximately 80% of patients who are treated for melanoma are cured of their disease. Recurrent disease appears locally, regionally, systemically, or in a combination of these sites.

Regional Nodal Recurrence

Regional nodal metastases are the most common site of first recurrence in patients who undergo WLE alone. When palpable lymph nodes develop, the diagnosis is most rapidly made by fine-needle aspiration (FNA) performed during the office visit. If positive, complete resection of the nodal basin will control regional disease in a large proportion of patients. If FNA is negative or insufficient, excisional biopsy is performed to verify the diagnosis. If nodes are positive, long-term survival is unfortunately low. Even with a single palpable nodal metastasis, the 5-year survival rate is 40% to 50% (see Table 30-5).

Before complete regional lymphadenectomy, a full metastatic workup is performed, including CT scans of the head, chest, abdomen, and pelvis, although these scans are normal in the majority of patients who are otherwise asymptomatic. The risk for further locoregional recurrence after complete lymph node basin dissection is increased in the presence of multiple positive nodes, especially those containing extracapsular extension. Postoperative irradiation of the involved areas has been advocated in some centers as a way to further reduce recurrences; however, such radiotherapy has not been tested in a prospective, randomized trial.[34]

Local and Regional Recurrences

True local recurrence (N2c, stage III) is defined as tumor appearing in skin or subcutaneous tissue within a 5-cm radius of the primary wide excision site (Fig. 30-12). Factors that predict local recurrence are the same as those predicting overall survival. The risk for local recurrence has been reported to be 0.2% for primary tumors less than 0.76 mm, 2% for those 0.76 to 1.49 mm, 6% for lesions 1.5 to 3.99 mm, and 13% for melanomas thicker than 4 mm. Local recurrence is a poor prognostic sign: less than 20% of patients survive long-term after local recurrence.

Local recurrence is treated by surgical resection to attain histologically clear margins. WLE guidelines for primary tumors do not apply to local recurrences.

Amputation for extensive local-regional recurrence is seldom indicated. These patients have a high risk of having other distant metastases, and therefore long-term disease-free survival is not achieved by resection. Occasionally, patients have indolent locoregional disease for

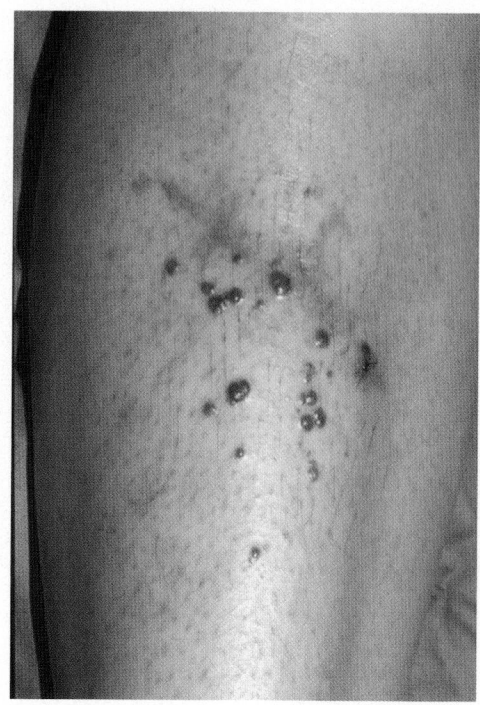

Figure 30-12 Multiple local recurrences growing around the scar on the leg of a patient who had undergone wide local excision 4 years earlier.

which amputation is indicated only after other attempts at locoregional tumor control have been unsuccessful.

Patients with multiple recurrences on the limbs may be candidates for isolated hyperthermic limb perfusion (IHLP). This technique, introduced in the 1950s, involves the use of cannulation of the principal extremity artery and vein, a tourniquet, and hyperthermic perfusion (~40°C) with L-phenylalanine mustard. Interleukin-2, tumor necrosis factor, and multiple other chemotherapeutic agents have also been used. Response rates exceed 80%, and complete responses are seen in 10% to 15% of patients. Unfortunately, many of these complete responses are short-lived. Reperfusion of extremities can be performed in patients who have an excellent initial response. Based on encouraging results with therapeutic IHLP, a randomized trial was designed to test the value of prophylactic perfusion in patients with high-risk melanoma (>1.5 mm in thickness). After more than 6 years' median follow-up, there was no improvement in overall survival.[35] Therefore, IHLP is recommended only for patients with established multiple in-transit metastases.

Distant Metastases

The most common sites of initial distant metastases are the brain, lung, and liver and less commonly the skin, bone, and other gastrointestinal tract sites. The prognosis varies significantly with the site of first metastases (Table 30-7). In the majority of cases, metastases appear at multiple sites simultaneously. In such circumstances, systemic therapy is indicated for palliation. Occasionally, metastases develop that are apparently isolated to a single site. These patients are evaluated for surgical resec-

Table 30-7 One-Year Survival Rates for Patients With Distant Metastases

STAGE	METASTATIC SITE(S)	APPROXIMATE 1-YEAR SURVIVAL (%)
M1a	Skin, subcutaneous tissues, lymph nodes	60
M1b	Lung	55
M1c	Other visceral sites	40

tion because the long-term disease-free survival rate after metastasectomy is reported to range from 10% to 20%.[36] Patients being considered for resection of visceral metastases undergo complete staging, including CT and PET scans. In general, the prognosis for metastases to distant sites is related to the number of metastases and the disease-free interval between primary therapy and recurrent disease. Highly selected patients may undergo excision of multiple intra-abdominal metastases with a favorable outcome.

For patients with isolated lung metastases, a period of observation (which may include chemotherapy or investigational protocols) has been recommended to determine whether additional metastases might appear in a short period (4-6 weeks). Pulmonary resection is then indicated for patients with no evidence of further recurrence. Melanoma is one of the most frequent tumors that metastasizes to the gastrointestinal tract. These metastases are commonly intramural lesions that may grow to form an intussusception and subsequent obstruction. Isolated metastases may appear in the adrenal glands, which if stable, are also appropriately treated by resection. Complete surgical excision of distant metastases, when possible, is associated with improved survival in comparison to systemic therapies.[37]

Symptomatic skeletal metastases can be effectively palliated with radiation. Metastases resulting in fractures of weight-bearing bones require internal fixation before radiation therapy.

Melanoma patients can also have central nervous system metastases, which are commonly multiple lesions at the time of diagnosis. At autopsy, the majority of patients have central nervous system metastases. When single-brain metastases cause symptoms, long-term favorable results have been obtained with surgical resection followed by irradiation. The most successful form of radiation therapy is a stereotactic program (gamma knife).[38]

Systemic Treatment of Melanoma

Most of the increase in the incidence of melanoma is attributable to thin melanomas with an excellent prognosis. Unfortunately, the number of deaths from melanoma is also rising. Although melanoma has been reported to metastasize to almost any tissue site, the most common areas are the lung, liver, bone, and brain. The most frequently used drug for systemic therapy is dacarbazine,

which has a response rate of 15% to 30%; however, complete responses are rare. A large number of clinical trials have investigated combinations of chemotherapy in an attempt to improve response rates and prolong survival. A doubling of the response rate has been observed with CVD (cisplatin, vinblastine, dacarbazine) combined with interferon alfa, interleukin-2, or a combination of these two biologicals. Unfortunately, the increases in survival have been either nonsignificant or less than 6 months. A randomized trial comparing CVD with dacarbazine indicated a doubling of the response rate and no effect on overall survival. The combination of CVD, interferon, and interleukin-2 (frequently called *biochemotherapy*) has a response rate of 50% and a complete response rate of 15%; however, several trials of this combination have not shown significant prolongation of survival. Temozolomide is also being used in combination with other drugs. Current recommendations for chemotherapy are summarized in the National Comprehensive Cancer Network guidelines.

Stage IV patients are also candidates for investigational protocols involving the use of immunotherapy. Despite an extensive history of immunotherapy for melanoma, this modality remains investigational.[39,40] It is postulated that stage IV patients who can undergo resection of all detectable disease will be a group of patients who will benefit from systemic therapies such as immunotherapy.

Adjuvant Systemic Therapy

Adjuvant systemic therapy has proved to be a distinct advance in the treatment of common cancers such as those arising in the breast and colon. Clinical investigators have been attempting to identify an effective adjuvant therapy for melanoma for more than 40 years, but no treatment regimen has shown a conclusive benefit. In the mid-1990s the U.S. Food and Drug Administration approved interferon alfa-2b as adjuvant therapy for patients with nodal metastases or thick melanomas in whom the expected survival rate is less than 50%. This approval was based on results from a single trial showing a significant increase in disease-free and overall survival. Subsequent randomized trials of interferon therapy have failed to confirm the initial observation. Updated analyses of randomized trials[41,42] do not show a consistent benefit for interferon adjuvant therapy. At the present time, stage IIc and III patients are evaluated for and invited to participate in randomized clinical trials of adjuvant therapy, when available.

CUTANEOUS MALIGNANCIES: NONMELANOMA SKIN CANCER

SCC and BCC are the most common types of malignant neoplasms in the world. Just as in melanoma, the incidence of these cancers is rising each year. Current predictions are that this disease will develop in one in five Americans during their lifetime. Fortunately, mortality rates for NMSC are falling, and this decrease is attributed to early detection and effective treatment. Patients in

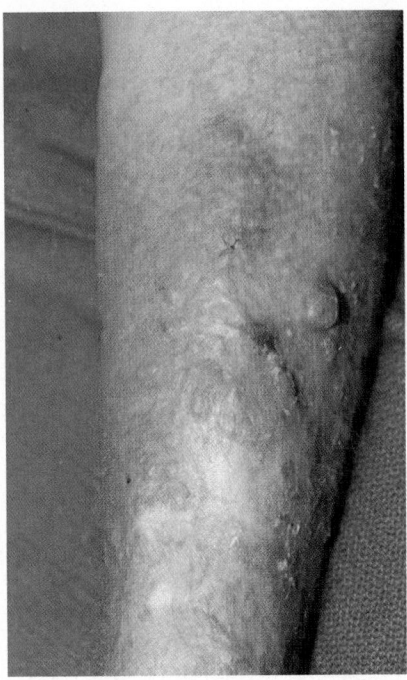

Figure 30-13 Multiple squamous cell carcinomas on the upper extremity of a patient 11 years after kidney transplantation.

whom any type of skin cancer develops undergo long-term periodic surveillance. After the initial diagnosis of BCC or SCC, the risk for development of an additional skin cancer is estimated to be 35% in 3 years and 50% in 5 years. In addition, there is a risk for other common malignancies such as lung cancer.

Squamous Cell Carcinoma

Epidemiology and Etiology

By some estimates, NMSC develops in more than 1 million people annually; however, accurate statistics are problematic for a disease that is often treated without a histologic diagnosis. Although BCC is the most common type of NMSC, SCC has a higher mortality rate. As is true with other types of skin cancer, the incidence of SCC is increasing. There is a disproportionate increasing risk for women as opposed to men.

Causes of SCC include the following: sunlight, susceptible phenotype, and compromised immunity, in addition to environmental conditions and diseases. Sunlight is thought to be the major causative factor because most SCCs occur on sun-exposed surfaces of the head and neck. In susceptible individuals (fair skin, blonde hair, blue eyes), increasing sun exposure carries a growing risk for the development of SCC. Individuals with dark complexions have a lower risk, even with prolonged sun exposure. Specifically, UVB is thought to be the form of UV radiation causing this disease. Most of the evidence for UV radiation comes from population-based studies in Australia, where individuals of Celtic origin moved to a geographic area in which they were subjected to higher sun exposure. The pattern of skin cancer appearing in

this population indicated that exposure to UV radiation earlier in life was a major risk factor because individuals who moved to Australia after adolescence had a lower incidence of skin cancer than did those who moved in childhood. The risk for skin cancer increases with occupational or recreational sun exposure, advancing age, and proximity to the equator. The amount of sun exposure is also proportional to the incidence of precursor skin changes for SCC, namely, nevi, atrophy, and actinic keratosis.

It is postulated that UV radiation affects the skin in two ways that result in an increased incidence of SCC. First, there is a direct carcinogenic effect on frequently dividing keratinocytes in the basilar layer of the epidermis. Unrepaired mutations result in tumor promotion and growth. The second mechanism relates to depression of the cutaneous immune surveillance response, which in turn inhibits tumor rejection. The *p53* tumor suppressor gene is mutated in more than 90% of SCCs.

Occupational and environmental exposure to arsenic, organic hydrocarbon, ionizing radiation, and cigarette smoke has been associated with increasing risk for SCCs. Genetic disorders, including xeroderma pigmentosum and albinism, are associated with increased risk for many types of skin cancer. Chronic conditions of the skin such as burn scars (Marjolin's ulcer), draining sinuses, infections, and ulcers can predate the development of SCCs. Previously healed wounds that break down or chronic wounds that will not heal undergo biopsy for the presence of SCC.

Impaired immunity, especially cell-mediated immunity, is a well-established cause of SCCs of the skin. The largest population of chronically immunosuppressed patients are those who underwent organ transplantation (Fig. 30-13). Immunosuppressive drugs such as azathioprine, cyclosporine, and prednisone have been linked to a greater than 50% increase in the risk for SCC. Both the intensity of immunosuppression and the duration of therapy are associated with the risk for development of malignancies. After 10 years of immunosuppression, malignancies develop in 10% of patients, and this figure increases to 40% after 20 years.[43] Conditions associated with acquired impaired cell-mediated immunity, including lymphomas, leukemias, and autoimmune diseases, all increase the risk for SCCs. Human papillomavirus, an infection associated with immunosuppression, is proposed as a causative factor for the development of SCCs.

Most SCCs begin with a proliferation of keratin cells in the basal layer of the epidermis that appear as red or pink areas, clinically termed *actinic keratoses* (solar keratoses).[44] Local symptoms may wax and wane over a period of many months. Lesions are scaling with an uneven surface and an erythematous base. Individual lesions are usually less than 1 cm in diameter and appear in chronically sun-damaged skin. The diagnosis is both clinical and histologic because actinic keratoses have many features in common with SCC in situ microscopically. The overall risk for malignant conversion to invasive SCC is low and estimated to be in the range of 1 in 1000 lesions per year. When the reddened area begins

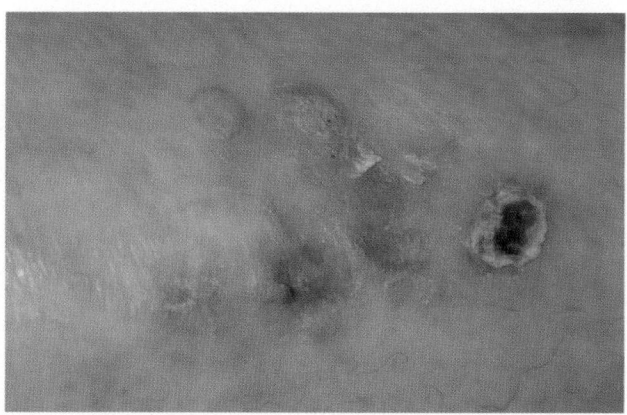

Figure 30-14 Squamous cell carcinoma appearing as areas of thickened, red, scaling skin.

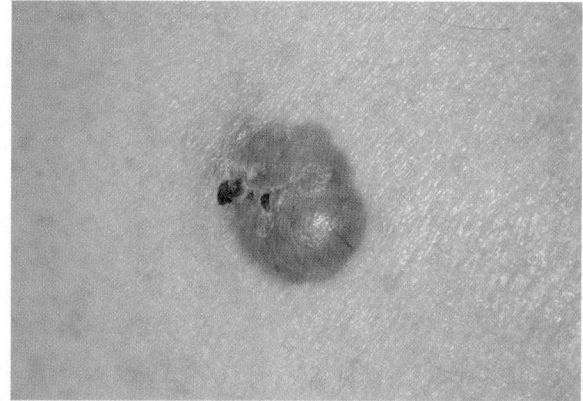

Figure 30-15 Nodular basal cell carcinoma.

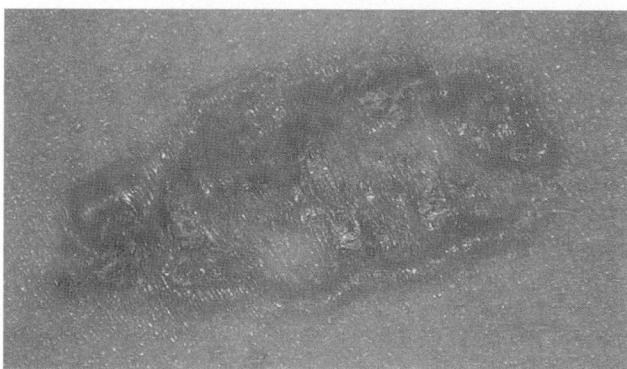

Figure 30-16 Basal cell carcinoma simulating the appearance of psoriasis.

to develop a plaque-like thickening, it is termed *Bowen's disease,* which appears histologically as SCC in situ and may vary from small lesions less than 1 cm to large areas of the anogluteal region.

Invasive SCCs are palpable scaling lesions that become ulcerated centrally and have elevated edges (Fig. 30-14). They may be confused with keratoacanthoma, a benign lesion that can also thicken and ulcerate. Biopsy may be required to differentiate between these two conditions.

Most SCCs can be treated locally with excellent results (see the later section on treatment options). Recurrence is associated with tumor size, degree of differentiation, depth of invasion, perineural involvement, immune status of the patient, and anatomic site. Local recurrence is associated with increased risk for regional and distant metastases. The first site of metastasis is usually the regional lymph nodes.

Basal Cell Carcinoma

In contrast to SCCs and actinic keratoses, there is no precursor skin lesion for BCCs. These lesions may have an appearance that varies from nodules in the skin to a large nonhealing sore with drainage and crusting. In comparison to SCCs, they have a slow growth rate, which can lead to a delay in diagnosis.[45]

BCCs grow in distinct patterns described as nodular, pigmented, cystic, and superficial. The nodular growth pattern is characterized by a well-defined, elevated lesion with a waxy appearance (Fig. 30-15). As the lesion grows, pearly opalescent nodules develop along the margins. A central depression with umbilication is a classic sign. Distinct blood vessels (telangiectasia) may be seen across the surface of the tumor mass. Although most BCCs are pink or skin colored, they may also have shades of brown or black pigmentation, thereby mimicking a benign mole or melanoma. Cystic BCCs are less common but have a distinctive appearance. Their surface is translucent and they may appear blue or gray and be confused with a blue nevus. Superficial BCCs (20%) are more macular than other growth patterns and may extend over the surface of the skin in a multicentric pattern (Fig.

30-16). The center can ulcerate and the margins become ill defined. These lesions may appear very similar to psoriasis, tinea, or eczema. They may also be multiple, pink or red, small, slightly elevated lesions that pepper the skin. This more aggressive growth pattern is associated with extension well beyond visible changes in the skin surface, and lesions can penetrate deep into the underlying subdermis. The white scarring varieties of this growth pattern are termed *morpheaform.*

BCCs commonly infiltrate locally but rarely metastasize. Metastases are associated with advanced patient age and neglected large lesions. The primary site has often been resected on multiple occasions before metastases appear. The median survival time for patients with metastatic disease is less than 1 year.

Treatment Options for Squamous and Basal Cell Carcinoma

NMSC is staged by different criteria than melanoma. The T stage is determined by the largest diameter of the lesion on the skin surface and by invasion of extradermal structures (Table 30-8).[16] The overall favorable prognosis and the fact that multiple primary skin cancers develop in many patients make this staging system less useful in planning treatment than the melanoma staging system.

Table 30-8   American Joint Committee on Cancer System for Classification and Staging of Carcinomas of the Skin—2002

Primary Tumor (T)	
TX	Primary tumor cannot be assessed
T0	No evidence of primary tumor
Tis	Carcinoma in situ
T1	Tumor ≤2 cm in greatest dimension
T2	Tumor >2 cm, but not >5 cm, in greatest dimension
T3	Tumor >5 cm in greatest dimension
T4	Tumor invades deep extradermal structures (i.e., cartilage, skeletal muscle, or bone)

Regional Lymph Nodes (N)	
NX	Regional lymph nodes cannot be assessed
N0	No regional lymph node metastasis
N1	Regional lymph node metastasis

Distant Metastasis (M)	
MX	Distant metastasis cannot be assessed
M0	No distant metastasis
M1	Distant metastasis

Stage Grouping			
Stage 0	Tis	N0	M0
Stage I	T1	N0	M0
Stage II	T2	N0	M0
	T3	N0	M0
Stage III	T4	N0	M0
	Any T	N1	M0
Stage IV	Any T	Any N	M1

Table 30-9   Nonmelanoma Skin Cancer: Risk Factors for Local Recurrence Based on Characteristics of the Primary Tumor

FACTOR	LOW RISK	HIGH RISK
Location		
Trunk and extremities	<20 mm	≥20 mm
Forehead and neck	<10 mm	≥10 mm
Central part of the face	<6 mm	≥6 mm
Borders	Well defined	Poorly defined
Incidence	Primary	Recurrent
Immunosuppression	Negative	Positive
Previous radiation therapy/chronic inflammation	Negative	Positive
Rapid growth rate	Negative	Positive
Neurologic symptoms	Negative	Positive
Differentiation	Well	Moderate or poorly
Perineural/vascular invasion	Negative	Positive

Modified from National Comprehensive Cancer Network Practice Guidelines in Oncology. Available at www.nccn.org.

Actinic keratoses and the precursor lesions of SCC are most often treated with cryotherapy; however, alternative treatments include topical 5-fluorouracil, electrodessication and curettage, CO_2 laser, dermabrasion, and chemical peel. Tissue biopsy is indicated when the actinic keratosis is raised or recurrent after topical therapy.

Because multiple techniques are available, the strategy for surgical treatment of SCCs and BCCs begins with an assessment for high-risk factors (Table 30-9). Considerations include size, location, primary versus recurrent, histology, and individual patient factors. All appropriate options are reviewed with the patient, in addition to making a specific recommendation. Surgical resection techniques include histopathologic analysis to define the margins of resection. In contrast, field therapies treat a generalized area but do not define the status of margins. Such approaches include radiation therapy, cryosurgery, curettage, and electrodessication.

Standard surgical excision is the preferred treatment of the majority of SCCs and BCCs. This procedure is usually performed under local anesthesia. The width of the margin for resection is not as well defined as in the treatment of melanoma. A minimum acceptable margin is one that is found to be histologically free of carcinoma, commonly a 3- to 4-mm area of normal-appearing skin. The risk for local recurrence is less when wider margins are obtained, especially in the presence of micronodular, infiltrative, and morpheaform histologic patterns. With these methods, the local cure rate is greater than 90%. An alternative surgical approach is the use of Mohs' micrographic excision (MME), which has a high rate of local tumor control with the use of horizontal frozen sections. The high success rate of MME is attributed to examination of a greater proportion of the margin of excision, in addition to mapping the precise location of any margins found to be positive. Excisions in positive areas continue until clear margins are obtained. MME is ideal under high-risk conditions and for anatomic areas in which it is important to preserve as much tissue as possible, such as around the eye, nose, mouth, and ear.[46]

Although field therapy techniques (cryotherapy, topical fluorouracil, electrodessication) do not histologically define the margins of treatment, they may still be effective in local tumor control. Cryotherapy is best suited for small superficial lesions and can be expected to achieve local control rates of greater than 90%. Treated areas may heal slowly by secondary intention and leave pale scars.

Radiation therapy is highly effective in the treatment of BCC and SCC, especially for preserving wide areas of skin in the head and neck region. Radiation is also useful in treating areas that are at high risk for recurrence after extensive surgical excision.

Uncommon Cutaneous Malignancies

Among the hundreds of specific types of skin conditions and tumors, four uncommon skin malignancies are important for the general surgeon to understand and be prepared to manage.

Cutaneous angiosarcoma is a rare, aggressive soft tissue sarcoma derived from blood or lymphatic vessel endothelium. It is most often seen on the face and scalp of older white men. In addition, angiosarcoma has been observed as a consequence of chronic lymphedema after axillary dissection for breast cancer (Stewart-Treves syndrome). Angiosarcoma may also arise in irradiated tissues after intervals of 10 to 20 years. The typical finding is a flat, painless, often pruritic macule or plaque with a red, blue, or purple color that develops into a mass and ulcerates if left in place. Histologically, angiosarcomas are high grade and often multifocal with skip areas of normal-appearing skin. When compared with other sarcomas, there is a high incidence of lymph node metastasis (~15%). Treatment consists of resection with histologically negative margins and irradiation of the involved field. Lymph node dissection is indicated if adenopathy appears before distant metastases are identified. There is no consensus about the role of adjuvant chemotherapy. The 5-year survival rate is less than 40%.

Dermatofibrosarcoma protuberans is a low-grade sarcoma arising from dermal fibroblasts. The lesion appears as a smooth nodule in or immediately beneath the skin (trunk, 40%; head/neck, 40%) in midadult life. Because of their slow growth, lesions are commonly 1 to 2 cm at diagnosis. Their external appearance belies their true character because tumor cells frequently invade the underlying soft tissues, thereby leading to incomplete excision and local recurrence. Treatment consists of WLE with 3- to 4-cm margins. Specimen orientation and pathologic analysis of margins are required. Distant metastases are uncommon and are preceded by two or more local recurrences. Radiation therapy has been used effectively after resection of recurrences.

Extramammary Paget's disease (EMPD) is a rare form of adenocarcinoma that arises from apocrine glands of the skin, most commonly in the perianal area, vulva, and scrotum. The clinical appearance is that of an erythematous plaque, but white or depigmented areas with crusts and scaling may also be present. The size is variable, from less than 1 cm to an entire area in the anogenital region. Because EMPD can have many clinical characteristics in common with eczema, bacterial and fungal infections, and nonspecific dermatitis, the diagnosis is often made by biopsy of lesions not responding to standard therapies. In the majority of cases EMPD is confined to the epidermis and is well controlled with excision. When invasion of the deeper structures occurs, the disease becomes increasingly difficult to control and the mortality rate increases to about 50%. Because EMPD is also associated with an increased risk for simultaneous internal malignancies in the genitourinary and gastrointestinal tracts (~40%), a complete workup includes a survey of these locations. Standard treatment is surgical resection extending to histologically clear margins, which may require multiple procedures because the histologic changes are best seen on permanent section. Patients require close clinical follow-up because local recurrences are common.[47] Radiation therapy has been reported to reduce the incidence of local recurrence after excision.

Kaposi's sarcoma, a low-grade soft tissue malignancy, arises from lymphatic vascular endothelial cells in the skin. The incidence is rising because it is most often seen in patients with acquired immunodeficiency syndrome (AIDS) and other immunosuppressed states such as organ transplantation. In patients infected with human immunodeficiency virus, human herpesvirus-8 has been identified as the causative agent of Kaposi's sarcoma. There is also a classic variant seen on the lower extremities of older men of Eastern European and Mediterranean descent. The clinical picture is variable; asymptomatic purple to brown bruises develop and progress to spots, plaques, or nodules on both lower extremities. Local symptoms appear late as the tumors become advanced. In AIDS patients, skin changes respond best to aggressive antiretroviral therapy. Symptomatic skin lesions can be treated with radiation therapy, intralesional injection of chemotherapeutic agents, cryotherapy, or excision.

Merkel cell carcinoma, derived from neuroendocrine cells, is histologically indistinguishable from small cell carcinoma arising in the lung or any other site. The initial workup includes a chest radiograph to rule out a pulmonary primary. From any site of origin, small cell carcinoma is a highly malignant tumor with a propensity to spread locally and regionally to nodes and distant sites. In the skin it appears as a rapidly growing red-blue nodule most frequently in the head and neck area of elderly individuals. The diagnosis is confirmed by biopsy, and the primary treatment is WLE (2-3 cm) with histologically confirmed negative margins. SLN biopsy has been used successfully to identify patients with occult regional lymphatic metastases (10%-30%), but there is no evidence that patients benefit other than by improved regional tumor control. SLN biopsy–negative patients do have significantly better survival than biopsy-positive patients do.[48] Involved-field irradiation has been shown to reduce the local recurrence rate, and some reports have suggested a survival benefit; however, all studies are too small and uncontrolled to draw definitive conclusions.[49] Although metastases may be responsive to chemotherapy, there is little evidence to support adjuvant systemic therapy. Overall, the prognosis is poor, with variable mortality rates of 55% to 79%.[50]

Many other cutaneous lesions and conditions are associated with malignancy but are beyond the scope of this chapter; however, the important principles in the management of these entities are the same as reviewed earlier:

1. Clinicians must have a low threshold for biopsy of new or changing skin lesions.
2. The diagnosis is made by biopsy and histologic analysis.
3. If appropriate, surgical excision is performed with histologically defined negative margins.
4. Further treatment and follow-up schedules will be determined by the specific diagnosis.

Selected References

Allen PJ, Coit DG: The surgical management of metastatic melanoma. Ann Surg Oncol 9:762-770, 2002.

In selected patients, surgical resection of distant melanoma metastases will result in long-term disease-free survival. This is a comprehensive review of indications and results.

Gimotty PA, Botbyl J, Soong S-j, et al: A population-based validation of the American Joint Committee on Cancer melanoma staging system. J Clin Oncol 23:8065-8075, 2005.

This detailed analysis of a large population-based melanoma database confirms the AJCC database and supports the changes in the 2002 melanoma staging system.

Grunhagen DJ, deWilt JH, ten Hagen TL, et al: Isolated limb perfusion for melanoma patients—a review of its indications and the role of tumour necrosis factor-alpha. Eur J Surg Oncol 32:371-380, 2006.

With standardization of techniques, isolated limb perfusion has become an effective tool in the management of metastatic melanoma in the small number of patients with disease limited to an extremity.

Kirkwood JM: Building upon the standard of care in adjuvant therapy of high-risk melanoma. J Clin Oncol 23:8559-8563, 2005.

Dr. Kirkwood has been the leading investigator in adjuvant trials and he provides an excellent perspective for this challenging aspect of melanoma patient care.

Morton DL, Cochran AJ, Thompson JF, et al: Sentinel node biopsy for early-stage melanoma. Accuracy and morbidity in MSLT-I, an international multicenter trial. Ann Surg 242:302-313, 2005.

This paper reports the initial results from the MSLT-I trial, which is testing the therapeutic value of sentinel lymph node biopsy.

National Comprehensive Cancer Network (NCCN) Practice Guidelines in Oncology. Available at www.nccn.org.

The NCCN updates these on-line consensus-based guidelines annually or more often, whenever major clinical information becomes available to change practice recommendations. Guidelines are described for all major types of malignancies. A CD-ROM can be ordered free of charge from the NCCN. The guidelines for melanoma and nonmelanoma skin cancer apply to this chapter.

Rubin AI, Chen EH, Ratner D: Current concepts: Basal cell carcinoma. N Engl J Med 353:2262-2269, 2005.

This is a well-balanced discussion of the biology and management of this common problem.

Thompson JF, Shaw HM: The prognosis of patients with thick primary melanomas: Is regional lymph node status relevant and does removing positive regional nodes influence outcome [editorial]? Ann Surg Oncol 9:719-722, 2002.

Drs. Thompson and Shaw from the Sydney Melanoma Unit present a well-balanced discussion about the role of lymphatic metastases in patients with high risk for disease.

References

1. Jemal A, Siegel R, Ward E, et al: Cancer Statistics, 2003. CA Cancer J Clin 56:106-130, 2006.
2. Rigel DS, Carucci JA: Malignant melanoma: Prevention, early detection, and treatment in the 21st century. CA Cancer J Clin 50:215-236, 2000.
3. Tucker MA, Fraser MC, Goldstein AM, et al: A natural history of melanomas and dysplastic nevi: An atlas of lesions in melanoma-prone families. Cancer 94:3192-3209, 2002.
4. Murphy ME, Boyer JD, Stashower ME, et al: The surgical management of Spitz nevi. Dermatol Surg 28:1065-1069, 2002.
5. Su LD, Fullen DR, Sondak VK, et al: Sentinel lymph node biopsy for patients with problematic spitzoid melanocytic lesions. Cancer 97:499-507, 2003.
6. Hawkins WG, Busam KJ, Ben-Porat L, et al: Desmoplastic melanoma: A pathologically and clinically distinct form of cutaneous melanoma. Ann Surg Oncol 12:207-213, 2005.
7. Chang AE, Karnell LH, Menck HR: The National Cancer Data Base report on cutaneous and noncutaneous melanoma: A summary of 84,836 cases from the past decade. Cancer 83:1664-1678, 1998.
8. Cormier JN, Xing Y, Feng L, et al: Metastatic melanoma to lymph nodes in patients with unknown primary sites. Cancer 106:2012-2020 2006.
9. Droesch JT, Flum DR, Mann GN: Wide local excision or abdominoperineal resection as the initial treatment for anorectal melanoma? Am J Surg 189:446-449, 2005.
10. Wechter ME, Reynolds RK, Haefner HK, et al: Vulvar melanoma: Review of diagnosis, staging, and therapy. J Low Genit Tract Dis 8:58-69, 2004.
11. Clark WH Jr, From L, Bernadino EA, et al: The histogenesis and biologic behavior of primary human malignant melanomas of the skin. Cancer Res 29:705-727, 1969.
12. Breslow A: Thickness, cross-sectional areas and depth of invasion in the prognosis of cutaneous melanoma. Ann Surg 172:902-908, 1970.
13. Balch CM, Soong S-j, Gerschenwald JE, et al: Prognostic factors analysis of 17,600 melanoma patients: Validation of the American Joint Committee on Cancer melanoma staging system. J Clin Oncol 19:3622-3634, 2001.
14. Gimotty PA, Botbyl J, Soong S-j, Guerry D: A population-based validation of the American Joint Committee on Cancer melanoma staging system. J Clin Oncol 23:8065-8075, 2005.
15. Crowson AN, Magro CM, Mihm MC: Prognosticators of melanoma, the melanoma report, and the sentinel lymph node. Mod Pathol 19(Suppl) 2:S71-S87, 2006.
16. Greene FL, Page DL, Fleming ID, et al (eds): AJCC Cancer Staging Manual, 6th ed. New York, Springer-Verlag, 2002.
17. National Comprehensive Cancer Network Practice Guidelines in Oncology. Available at www.nccn.org.
18. Kelley MC, Ollila DW, Morton DL: Lymphatic mapping and sentinel lymphadenectomy for melanoma. Semin Surg Oncol 14:283-290, 1998.
19. Thompson JF, Uren RF, Shaw HM, et al: Location of sentinel lymph nodes in patients with cutaneous melanoma: New insights into lymphatic anatomy. J Am Coll Surg 189:195-206, 1999.
20. Schmalbach CE, Nussenbaum F, Rees RS, et al: Reliability of sentinel lymph node mapping with biopsy for head and neck cutaneous melanoma. Arch Otolaryngol Head Neck Surg 129:61-65, 2003.
21. Chao C, Wong SL, Edwards MJ, et al: Sentinel lymph node biopsy for head and neck melanomas. Ann Surg Oncol 10:21-26, 2003.
22. Clary BM, Brady MS, Lewis JJ, et al: Sentinel lymph node biopsy in the management of patients with primary cutaneous melanoma: Review of a large single-institutional experience with an emphasis on recurrence. Ann Surg 233:250-258, 2001.
23. Wong SL, Kattan MW, McMasters KM, et al: A nomogram that predicts the presence of sentinel node metastasis in melanoma with better discrimination than the American

Joint Committee on Cancer staging system. Ann Surg Oncol 12:282-288, 2005.

24. Chao C, Wong SL, Ross MI, et al: Patterns of early recurrence after sentinel lymph node biopsy for melanoma. Am J Surg 184:520-524, 2002.

25. McMasters KM, Wong SL, Edwards MJ, et al: Frequency of non-sentinel lymph node metastasis in melanoma. Ann Surg Oncol 9:137-141, 2002.

26. Reeves ME, Delgado R, Busam KJ, et al: Prediction of non-sentinel lymph node status in melanoma. Ann Surg Oncol 10:27-31, 2003.

27. McMasters KM, Reintgen DS, Ross MI, et al: Sentinel lymph node biopsy for melanoma: How many radioactive nodes should be removed? Ann Surg Oncol 8:192-197, 2001.

28. McMasters KM, Reintgen DS, Ross MI, et al: Sentinel lymph node biopsy for melanoma: Controversy despite widespread agreement. J Clin Oncol 19:2851-2855, 2001.

29. Thompson JF, Shaw HM: The prognosis of patients with thick primary melanomas: Is regional lymph node status relevant, and does removing positive regional nodes influence outcome [editorial]? Ann Surg Oncol 9:719-722, 2002.

30. Dessureault S, Soong SJ, Ross MI, et al: Improved staging of node-negative patients with intermediate to thick melanomas (>1 mm) with the use of lymphatic mapping and sentinel lymph node biopsy. Ann Surg Oncol 8:766-770, 2001.

31. Morton DL, Cochran AJ, Thompson JF, et al: Sentinel node biopsy for early-stage melanoma. Accuracy and morbidity in MSLT-I, an international multicenter trial. Ann Surg 242:302-313, 2005.

32. Thompson JF, Shaw HM: Benefits of sentinel node biopsy for melanoma: A review based on interim results of the first multicenter selective lymphadenectomy trial. Aust N Z J Surg 76:100-103, 2006.

33. Juweid ME, Cheson BD: Positron-emission tomography and assessment of cancer therapy. N Engl J Med 354:496-507, 2006.

34. Ballo MT, Ross MI, Cormier JN, et al: Combined-modality therapy for patients with regional nodal metastases from melanoma. Int J Radiat Oncol Biol Phys 1:106-113, 2006.

35. Grunhagen DJ, deWilt JH, ten Hagen TL, et al: Isolated limb perfusion for melanoma patients—a review of its indications and the role of tumour necrosis factor-alpha. Eur J Surg Oncol 32:371-380, 2006.

36. Allen PJ, Coit DG: The surgical management of metastatic melanoma. Ann Surg Oncol 9:762-770, 2002.

37. Essner R, Lee JH, Wanek LS: Contemporary surgical treatment of advanced-stage melanoma. Arch Surg 139:961-967, 2004.

38. Douglas JG, Margolin K: The treatment of brain metastases from malignant melanoma. Semin Oncol 29:518-524, 2002.

39. Dudley ME, Wunderlich JR, Robbins PF, et al: Cancer regression and autoimmunity in patients after clonal repopulation with antitumor lymphocytes. Science 298:850-854, 2002.

40. Sondak VK, Sabel MS, Mule JJ: Allogeneic and autologous melanoma vaccines: Where have we been and where are we going? Clin Cancer Res 12:2337-2341, 2006.

41. Verma S, Quirt I, McCready D, et al: Systematic review of systemic adjuvant therapy for patients at high risk for recurrent melanoma. Cancer 106:1431-1442, 2006.

42. Kirkwood JM: Building upon the standard of care in adjuvant therapy of high-risk melanoma. J Clin Oncol 23:8559-8563, 2005.

43. Euvrard S, Kanitakis J, Claudy A: Skin cancers after organ transplantation. N Engl J Med 348:1681-1691, 2003.

44. Fu W, Cockerell CJ: The actinic (solar) keratosis. Arch Dermatol 139:66-70, 2003.

45. Rubin AI, Chen EH, Ratner D: Current concepts: Basal cell carcinoma. N Engl J Med 353:2262-2269, 2005.

46. Kuijpers DI, Thissen MR, Neumann MH: Basal cell carcinoma: Treatment options and prognosis, a scientific approach to a common malignancy. Am J Clin Dermatol 3:247-259, 2002.

47. Pierie JP, Choudry U, Muzikansky A, et al: Prognosis and management of extramammary Paget's disease and the association with secondary malignancies. J Am Coll Surg 196:45-50, 2003.

48. Allen PH, Bowne WB, Brennen MF, et al: Merkel cell carcinoma: Prognosis and treatment of patients from a single institution. J Clin Oncol 23:2300-2309, 2005.

49. Medina-Franco H, Urist MM, Fiveash J, et al: Multimodality treatment of Merkel cell carcinoma: Case series and literature review of 1024 cases. Ann Surg Oncol 8:204-208, 2001.

50. Goessling W, McKee PH, Mayer RJ: Merkel cell carcinoma. J Clin Oncol 20:588-598, 2002.

Soft Tissue Sarcomas

Samuel Singer, MD

Predisposing Factors and Molecular Genetics

Pathologic Evaluation

Clinical Evaluation and Diagnosis

Evaluation of Extent of Disease

Staging

Management

Treatment of Recurrent Disease

Prognostic Factors and Results

Long-Term Follow-up

Summary

Soft tissue sarcomas are rare and unusual neoplasms that account for about 1% of adult human cancers and 15% of pediatric malignancies. However, sarcomas continue to carry biologic and clinical interest and significance disproportionate to their clinical frequency because of the often clearly defined molecular genetic basis and the challenges that they pose in diagnosis and management. Although these tumors may develop in any anatomic site, 43% occur in the extremities, with two thirds of extremity lesions occurring in the lower limb, followed in order of frequency by visceral (19%), retroperitoneal (15%), trunk/thoracic (10%), and other locations (13%).[1] This section focuses on the biology and management of soft tissue sarcomas in adults (>16 years).

PREDISPOSING FACTORS AND MOLECULAR GENETICS

In most patients no specific etiologic agent is found. Multiple predisposing factors have been identified (Box 31-1). Genetic syndromes such as neurofibromatosis, familial adenomatous polyposis, and Li-Fraumeni syndrome have all been shown to be associated with the development of soft tissue sarcoma.[2,3] Ionizing radiation

and lymphedema are well-established, but uncommon antecedents to the development of soft tissue sarcoma.[1] The association with trauma is uncertain as a true causal factor. Chemical carcinogens have also been widely implicated, but data to support their association are not well founded.[4]

Genetic alterations that play a role in the development of soft tissue sarcoma segregate into two major types. The first type consists of sarcomas with specific genetic alterations that result in simple karyotypes, including fusion genes secondary to reciprocal translocations and specific point mutations such as *KIT* mutations in gastrointestinal stromal tumors (GISTs) and *APC*/β-catenin mutations in desmoid tumors. The second type consists of sarcomas with nonspecific genetic alterations and typically complex unbalanced karyotypes representing numerous genetic losses and gains. A significant subset of soft tissue sarcoma, as well as most types of adipocyte tumors, are characterized by specific chromosomal aberrations, most commonly reciprocal translocations, that can be diagnostically[5] and occasionally prognostically useful (Table 31-1).[6,7]

The fusion gene translocations include 11 different gene fusions involving the *EWS* gene or *EWS* family members (*TLS, TAF2N*) found in five different sarcomas and 10 other types of fusions found in seven other sarcoma types.[8] If conventional cytogenetics is not available, molecular genetic techniques (e.g., reverse transcription polymerase chain reaction and fluorescence in situ hybridization) are useful as diagnostic adjuncts. In addition, investigation of molecular changes in genes at sites of chromosomal alterations has led to the identification of novel genes and characterization of their mechanisms of deregulation. The tumor suppressor genes best studied in sarcoma are *p53* and *RB1*. Inactivation of both genes is involved in the tumorigenesis of several sarcomas. The relevance of the *p53* gene to sarcoma tumorigenesis is underscored by the frequent occurrence of soft tissue sarcomas in Li-Fraumeni syndrome; all families studied have *p53* germline mutations.

Box 31-1   Predisposing Factors for Sarcomas

Genetic Predisposition

Neurofibromatosis (von Recklinghausen's disease)
Li-Fraumeni syndrome
Retinoblastoma
Gardner's syndrome (familial adenomatous polyposis)

Radiation Exposure

Therapeutic radiation in the orthovoltage and megavoltage range

Lymphedema

Postsurgical
Postirradiation status
Parasitic infection (filariasis)

Trauma

Postparturition status
Extremity

Chemical

2,3,7,8-Tetrachlorodibenzodioxin (TCDD)
Polyvinyl chloride
Hemochromatosis
Arsenic

Major mechanisms of inactivation of the *p53* pathway in sarcomas include *p53* point mutations, homozygous deletion of *CDKN2A*, which encodes both *p14ARF* and *p16*, and *MDM2* amplification. In sarcomas with specific reciprocal translocations, alteration of the *p53* pathway is a rare event but, when present, is a strong prognostic factor associated with significantly decreased survival in patients with synovial sarcoma,[9,10] myxoid liposarcoma,[11] and Ewing's sarcoma/peripheral neuroectodermal tumor (PNET).[12] Decreased survival in Ewing's sarcoma/PNET was associated with deletion of *CDKN2A*, which represents a type of alteration of the *p53* pathway caused by loss of the *CDKN2A* alternative product p14ARF.[13,14] In contrast, in sarcomas with nonspecific genetic alterations and complex karyotypes, alteration of the *p53* pathway is more common and has weaker prognostic value, with large numbers of patients often required to achieve statistical significance, as demonstrated in several studies of mixed adult soft tissue sarcoma. Its high prevalence in this class of sarcomas may account for its limited ability to define distinct clinical prognostic subsets in these tumors.

In addition to serving as very specific and powerful diagnostic markers, fusion genes resulting from translocations encode chimeric proteins that are important determinants of tumor biology by acting as abnormal

Table 31-1   Cytogenetic and Molecular Abnormalities in Sarcomas

HISTOLOGIC TYPE	CYTOGENETIC CHANGES	GENE REARRANGEMENT/MOLECULAR ABNORMALITY
Synovial sarcoma	t(X;18)(p11.2;q11.2)	*SYT-SSX1* fusion *SYT-SSX2* fusion
Myxoid/round cell liposarcoma	t(12;16)(q13;q11) t(12;22)(q13;q11-12)	*CHOP-TLS* fusion *CHOP-EWS* fusion
Ewing's sarcoma	t(11;22)(q24;q12) t(21;22)(q22;q12) t(7;22)(p22;q12) t(17;22)(q12;q12) t(2;22)(q33;q12)	*FLI1-EWS* fusion *ERG-EWS* fusion *ETV1-EWS* fusion *EIAF-EWS* fusion *FEV-EWS* fusion
Alveolar rhabdomyosarcoma	t(2;13)(q35;q14) t(1;13)(p36;q14)	*PAX3-FKHR* fusion *PAX7-FKHR* fusion
Extraskeletal myxoid chondrosarcoma	t(9;22)(q22;q12)	*TEC-EWS* fusion
Dermatofibrosarcoma protuberans	t(17;22)(q22;q13)	*PDGFB-COL1A1* fusion
Desmoplastic small round cell tumor	t(11;22)(p13;q12)	*WT1-EWS* fusion
Clear cell sarcoma	t(12;22)(q13;q12)	*ATF1-EWS* fusion
Infantile fibrosarcoma	t(12;15)(p13;q25)	*ETV6-NTRK3* fusion
Alveolar soft part sarcoma	17q25 rearrangement	Unknown
Atypical lipomatous tumor/well-differentiated liposarcoma	12q rings and giant markers	*HMGI-C*, *CDK4*, and *MDM2* amplification
Leiomyosarcoma	Complex	*RB1* point mutations or deletions
Malignant fibrous histiocytoma	Complex	*p53* point mutations or deletions
Malignant peripheral nerve sheath tumor	Complex	*NF1*

transcription factors that alter the transcription of multiple downstream genes and pathways.[15] The structure of these chimeric proteins plays a prominent role in the pathogenesis of sarcoma, as evidenced by the impact of relatively minor cytogenetic variability, as a result of variant molecular breakpoints, on tumor phenotype and clinical behavior.[7,16] A recent analysis of synovial sarcoma has clearly identified a characteristic *SYT-SSX* fusion gene resulting from the chromosomal translocation t(x;18)(p11;q11) that is detectable in almost all synovial sarcomas. Translocation fuses the *SYT* gene from chromosome 18 to either of two highly homologous genes at Xp11, SSX1, or SSX2. *SYT-SSX1* and *SYT-SSX2* are thought to function in aberrant transcriptional regulation. Recent analysis has suggested that these fusion products may influence outcome. It does appear that all biphasic synovial sarcomas have an *SYT-SSX1* fusion transcript, and tumors that were positive for *SYT-SSX2* were monophasic. Conversely, monophasic sarcomas may have either transcript.[6]

PATHOLOGIC EVALUATION

More than 50 histologic subtypes of soft tissue sarcoma are recognized, many of which are associated with distinctive clinical, therapeutic, or prognostic features. Detailed descriptions of the histopathologic classification and guidelines for histologic reporting of soft tissue sarcoma have been published elsewhere.[17] To summarize, the most commonly found are liposarcoma, malignant fibrous histiocytoma (MFH), and leiomyosarcoma (Fig. 31-1). Histopathology is dependent on the anatomic site: the common subtypes in the extremity are liposarcoma and MFH; in the retroperitoneal–intra-abdominal location, liposarcoma and leiomyosarcoma are the most common histiotypes; and in the visceral location, GISTs and leiomyosarcoma are found almost exclusively (Fig. 31-2). Liposarcoma is further classified into five histologic subtypes based on strict morphologic features and cytogenetic aberrations: well differentiated, dedifferentiated, myxoid, round cell, and pleomorphic.[17] The well-differentiated and dedifferentiated subtypes account for 43% and 16% of liposarcomas, respectively, and are more commonly found in the retroperitoneal location (Fig. 31-3). The myxoid/round cell and pleomorphic subtypes account for 29% and 12% of liposarcomas, respectively, and are usually located in the extremity (see Fig. 31-3).

Age is also a factor in histopathology. Embryonal rhabdomyosarcoma is most common in childhood, synovial sarcoma is more likely to be seen in young adults (<35 years), and there is an even distribution of liposarcoma and MFH as the predominant types in the older population (Fig. 31-4). The designation MFH is currently being re-evaluated, with many of these tumors being reclassified as myofibrosarcoma, pleomorphic sarcoma, or dedifferentiated liposarcoma. Sarcoma histiotype and liposarcoma subtype are generally important determinants of prognosis and a predictor of distinctive patterns of behavior because none of the existing grading systems is ideal and applicable to all tumor types. Biologic behav-

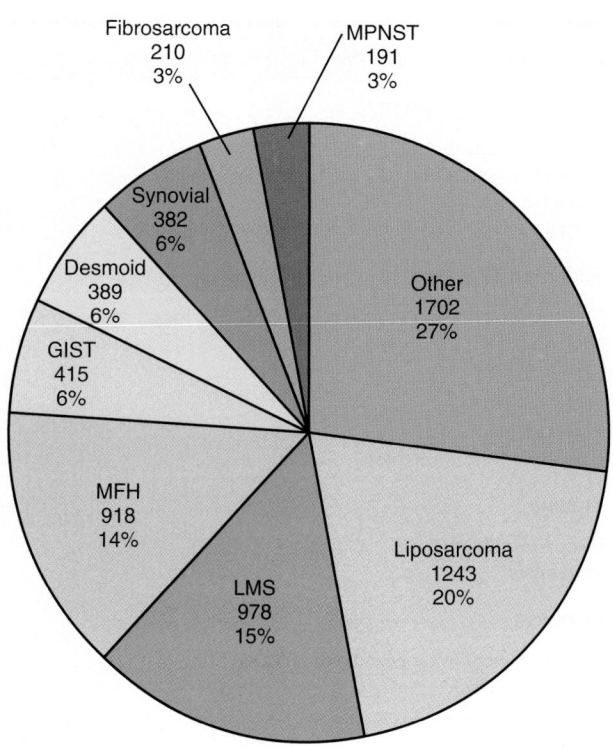

Figure 31-1 Histologic distribution in 6486 patients with soft tissue sarcoma treated at Memorial Sloan-Kettering Cancer Center from July 1, 1982, through June 30, 2005. These data include extremity, trunk, visceral, and retroperitoneal tumors. GIST, gastrointestinal stromal tumor; LMS, leiomyosarcoma; MFH, malignant fibrous histiocytoma; MPNST, malignant peripheral nerve sheath tumor.

ior is currently best predicted on the basis of histologic type, histologic grade, tumor size, and depth.

Although many published series have combined all the histologic types of sarcoma, the significance of such subtyping is exemplified by liposarcoma, in which the five subsets (well differentiated, dedifferentiated, myxoid, round cell, and pleomorphic) have totally different biology and patterns of behavior.[17-20] A further clear demonstration is the importance of myogenic differentiation in pleomorphic sarcomas, which is associated with a substantially increased risk for metastasis.[21] In a postoperative nomogram based on a database of 2136 adult patients from Memorial Sloan-Kettering Cancer Center (MSKCC), histologic type was found to be one of the most important predictors of sarcoma-specific death, with malignant peripheral nerve sheath tumors having the highest risk for mortality.[22] A more recent liposarcoma-based nomogram further highlights the importance of histologic subtype.[23]

CLINICAL EVALUATION AND DIAGNOSIS

Patients with extremity sarcoma usually have a painless mass, although in up to 33% of patients pain is noted at initial evaluation. The diagnosis is frequently delayed, with hematoma or a pulled muscle being the most

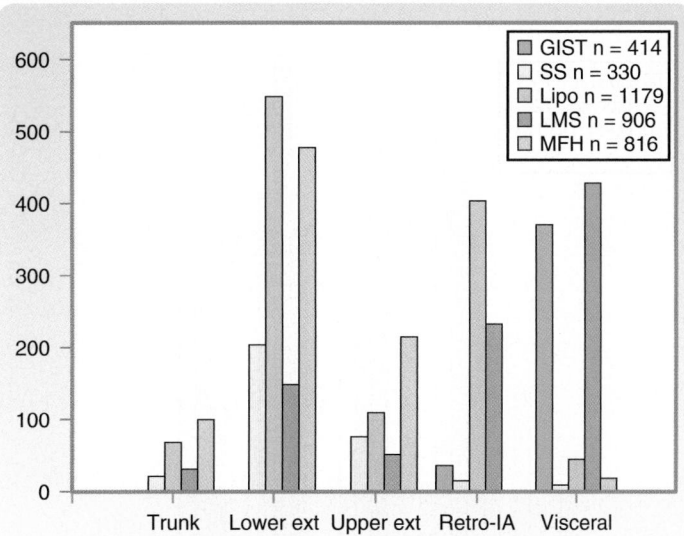

Figure 31-2 Site-specific histologic distribution in 3706 patients with soft tissue sarcoma treated at Memorial Sloan-Kettering Cancer Center from July 1, 1982, through June 30, 2005. GIST, gastrointestinal stromal tumor; Lipo, liposarcoma; LMS, leiomyosarcoma; MFH, malignant fibrous histiocytoma; Retro-IA, retroperitoneal–intra-abdominal; SS, synovial sarcoma.

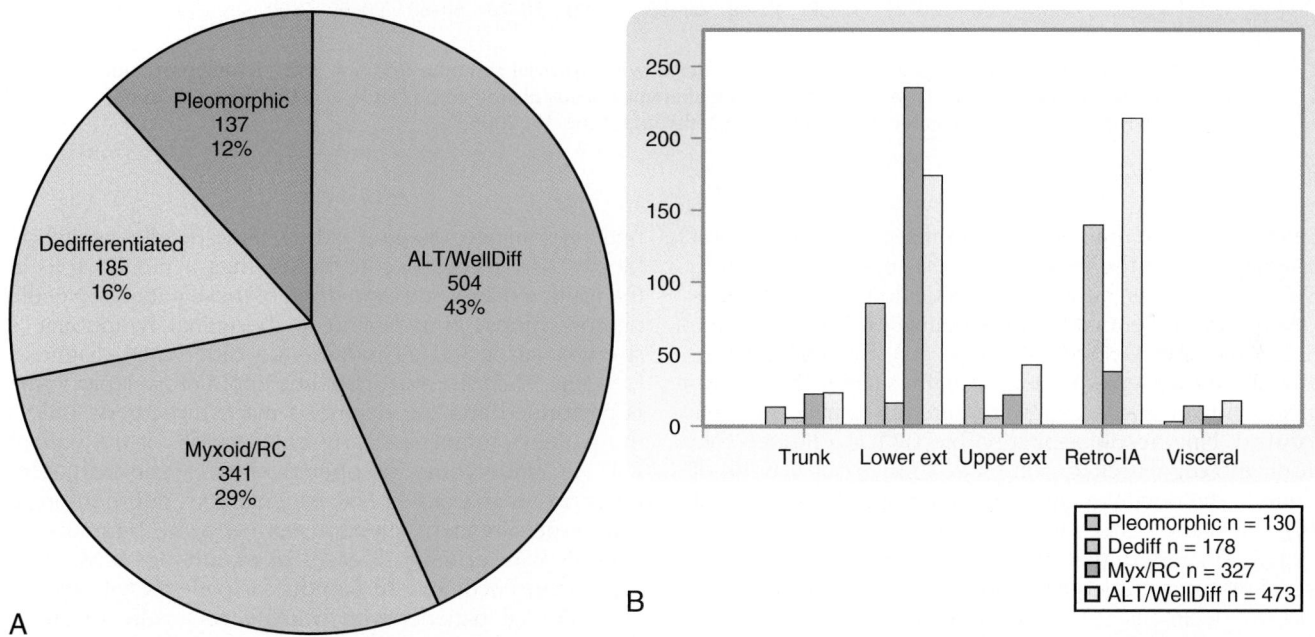

Figure 31-3 A, Histologic subtype distribution in 1125 patients with liposarcoma treated at Memorial Sloan-Kettering Cancer Center from July 1, 1982, through June 30, 2005. These data include extremity, trunk, visceral, and retroperitoneal tumors. **B,** Site-specific histologic subtype distribution in 1125 patients with liposarcoma treated at Memorial Sloan-Kettering Cancer Center from July 1, 1982, through June 30, 2005. ALT, atypical lipomatous tumor; RC, round cell; Retro-IA, retroperitoneal–intra-abdominal.

common condition in the differential diagnosis for extremity and trunk lesions. Physical examination includes assessment of the size of the mass and its relationship to neurovascular and bony structures. Generally, any soft tissue mass in an adult that is symptomatic or enlarging, any mass that is larger than 5 cm, or any new mass that persists beyond 4 weeks is sampled. Biopsy technique is important. For most soft tissue masses an incisional or

core biopsy is usually preferred. Ideally, the initial diagnostic procedure is performed at the center where the patient will be treated. This facilitates proper placement of the biopsy site (or incision) and also avoids the complications and diagnostic difficulties that can arise if such biopsy samples are handled infrequently.

Limb masses are generally best sampled through a longitudinal incision so that the entire biopsy tract can

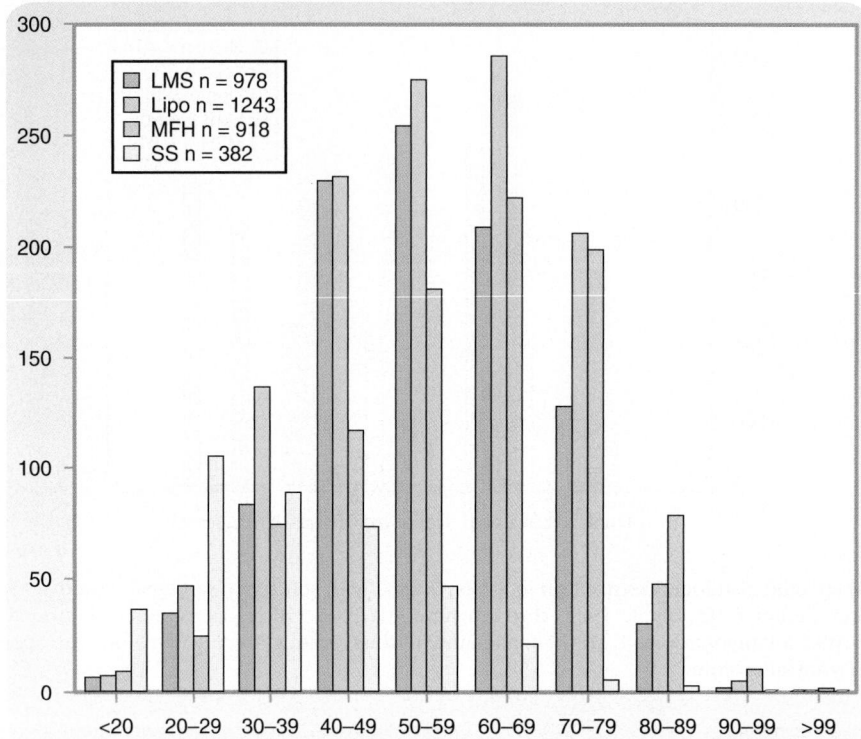

Figure 31-4 Distribution by age and diagnosis of patients with synovial sarcoma (SS; $n = 382$), leiomyosarcoma (LMS; $n = 978$), liposarcoma (Lipo; $n = 1262$), and malignant fibrous histiocytoma (MFH; $n = 960$) seen at Memorial Sloan-Kettering Cancer Center from July 1, 1982, through June 30, 2005.

be excised at the time of definitive resection. The incision is centered over the mass in its most superficial location. No tissue flap is raised, and meticulous hemostasis is ensured to prevent cellular dissemination by hematoma. Excisional biopsy is recommended only for small cutaneous or subcutaneous tumors, usually smaller than 3 cm, in which wide re-excision (if required) is usually straightforward. Fine-needle aspiration biopsy has a limited role in diagnosing extremity soft tissue tumors but may be of value in the documentation of recurrence. An analysis of 164 soft tissue masses to determine the value of Tru-cut biopsy suggested that 83% of specimens obtained at initial biopsy are adequate for diagnosis. Of the adequate biopsy specimens, 95% correlated with the final resection diagnosis for malignancy, 88% for histologic grade, and 75% for histologic subtype. Tru-cut biopsy can thus be advocated as the first step in the diagnostic armamentarium. The ease of performance, low cost, and low complication rate make this technique attractive. Should tissue be inadequate or there be any indecision, an open, linearly placed incisional biopsy is indicated. Biopsy is indicated only if the actual treatment will be altered by a definitive diagnosis. Tumor type and grade are correctly identified in most patients.

Patients with intra-abdominal or retroperitoneal sarcomas often experience nonspecific abdominal discomfort and gastrointestinal symptoms before diagnosis. The diagnosis is usually suspected on finding a soft tissue mass on abdominal computed tomography (CT) or mag-

netic resonance imaging (MRI). Fine-needle aspiration biopsy or CT-guided core biopsy has a limited role in the routine diagnostic evaluation of these patients. Needle or core biopsy is indicated if abdominal lymphoma is strongly suspected as part of the differential diagnosis (see Fig. 31-7). In most patients, exploratory laparotomy is performed and the diagnosis made at surgery, unless the patient's tumor is clearly unresectable or the patient will be undergoing preoperative investigational treatment. In an analysis of 500 patients with retroperitoneal soft tissue sarcoma,[24] median survival was 72 months for patients with primary disease, 28 months for those with local recurrence, and 10 months for patients with metastasis. For all patients with primary or locally recurrent tumors, complete resection was the most favorable factor in outcome.

EVALUATION OF EXTENT OF DISEASE

All patients require a thorough history and physical examination. MRI is generally the preferred procedure for imaging extremity soft tissue masses. MRI enhances the contrast between tumor and adjacent structures and provides excellent three-dimensional definition of fascial planes. The relative value of MRI over CT has been the subject of a national study, the results of which showed no statistically significant difference between CT and MRI in determining tumor involvement of muscle, bone, joints, or neurovascular structures. Combined interpretation of CT and MRI did not significantly improve accuracy.[25] Once the diagnosis and grade are known, evaluation for sites of potential metastasis can be performed. Lymph node metastases occur in less than 3% of adult soft tissue sarcomas.[26] For extremity lesions, the lung is the principal site for metastasis of high-grade lesions; for visceral lesions, the liver is the principal site.[27] Thus, patients with low-grade extremity lesions require a chest radiograph, and the majority of those with high-grade lesions require chest CT. Patients with visceral lesions have their liver imaged as part of the initial abdominal CT or MRI examination. The author does not generally perform angiography because it adds little that will change the management strategy.

STAGING

Current staging systems focus on the histologic grade of the tumor, the size of the primary tumor, and the presence or absence of metastasis.[28] The present 2002 staging system takes into account the relative infrequency of high-grade, large, superficial sarcomas[28] and simplifies the category of stage III tumors so that they represent only large, deep, high-grade sarcomas. Histologic grade is a major prognostic determinant and is based on the degree of mitosis, cellularity, necrosis, differentiation, and stromal content. Various grading systems exist, all of which are considered categories in a histologic spectrum. For therapeutic planning, the broad categories of low (I or II) and high (III or IV) grade suffice. Clearly, such arbitrary decisions may be difficult to make, but they facilitate practical management of the patient. Low-grade lesions are assumed to have a low (<15%) risk for subsequent metastasis, and high-grade lesions have a high (>50%) risk for subsequent metastasis.

Size has historically been considered a less important determinant of biologic behavior, but large lesions can be associated with late recurrence. Unequivocal characterization of grade is difficult in large lesions, especially in tumors that can reach 2 or 3 kg. Conversely, very small, high-grade lesions less than 5 cm in maximal diameter have limited risk for metastatic disease if treated appropriately at the first encounter. The current staging system for soft tissue sarcoma, updated in 1992 and 1997, has been further updated more recently (Table 31-2). The new staging system[29] addresses the issue of depth and size as independent variables. However, the staging system continues to undergo evolution. Analysis of the primary extremity soft tissue sarcomas seen at MSKCC from July 1, 1982, to June 30, 2002, suggests that the probability of metastasis by stage is better discriminated in the new American Joint Committee on Cancer (AJCC) 2002 staging system (Table 31-3). The large, low-grade, and deep tumors in stage 2A of the 1997 AJCC system are now considered stage 1 disease in the AJCC 2002 staging system. Figure 31-5 shows the excellent discrimination by stage for distant recurrence-free survival with use of the AJCC 2002 system. It is important to emphasize that staging systems (1) apply to risk for metastasis or to

Table 31-2 Current Staging System for Soft Tissue Sarcoma

G, Histologic Grade

GX	Grade cannot be assessed
G1	Well differentiated
G2	Moderately differentiated
G3	Poorly differentiated
G4	Undifferentiated

T, Primary Tumor Size

TX	Primary size cannot be assessed
T0	No evidence of primary tumor
T1	Tumor less than 5 cm
T1a	Superficial tumor
T1b	Deep tumor
T2	Tumor 5 cm or greater
T2a	Superficial tumor
T2b	Deep tumor

N, Regional Nodes

NX	Regional nodes cannot be assessed
N0	No regional lymph node metastasis
N1	Regional lymph node metastasis

M, Distant Metastasis

MX	Presence of distant metastasis cannot be assessed
M0	No distant metastasis
M1	Distant metastasis present

Staging	Grouping			
Stage I	G1-2	T1a, 1b, 2a, 2b	N0	M0
Stage II	G3-4	T1a, 1b, 2a	N0	M0
Stage III	G3-4	T2b	N0	M0
Stage IV	Any G	Any T	N1	M0
	Any G	Any T	N0	M1

From Greene F, Page D, Fleming I, et al (eds): AJCC Cancer Staging Manual, 6th ed. Heidelberg, Springer-Verlag, 2002.

Table 31-3 Primary Extremity Soft Tissue Sarcoma: Distant Metastases by Stage (N = 1410)*

	TOTAL (N)	DISTANT METASTASES (%)
Old AJCC Staging System (1992)		
1A	136	2 (1%)
1B	252	31 (12%)
3A	362	72 (20%)
3B	660	274 (42%)
AJCC Staging System (1997)		
1A	136	2 (1%)
1B	28	3 (11%)
2A	224	28 (13%)
2B	362	72 (20%)
2C	33	13 (40%)
3A	302	105 (35%)
3B	325	156 (48%)
AJCC Staging System (2002)		
1	388	33 (9%)
2	395	85 (22%)
3	627	261 (42%)

*From Memorial Sloan-Kettering Cancer Center, July 1, 1982, to June 30, 2002. Excludes desmoid and dermatofibrosarcoma protuberans.
AJCC, American Joint Committee on Cancer.

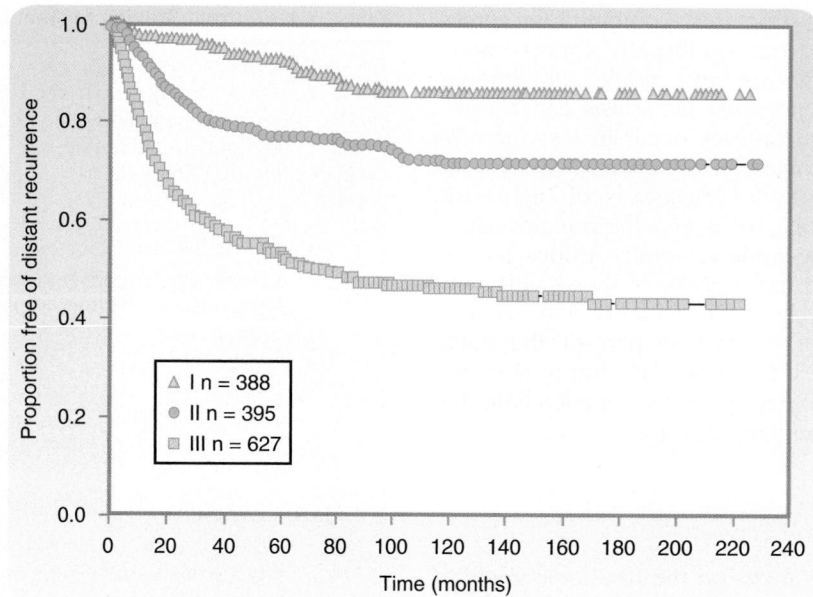

Figure 31-5 Distant recurrence-free survival in patients with primary extremity soft tissue sarcoma (*N* = 1410) by American Joint Committee on Cancer 2002 stage seen at Memorial Sloan-Kettering Cancer Center from July 1, 1982, through June 30, 2002 (excludes desmoid and dermatofibrosarcoma protuberans).

disease-specific or overall survival and (2) are almost exclusively confined to extremity lesions. There is as yet no adequate staging system for retroperitoneal and visceral lesions.

MANAGEMENT

Extremity and Superficial Trunk Sarcoma

Although surgery remains the principal therapeutic modality for soft tissue sarcoma, the extent of surgery required, along with the optimum combination of radiotherapy and chemotherapy, remains controversial. The important clinical and pathologic prognostic variables are used by the surgeon to design the most effective treatment plan for the individual patient based on the predicted patterns of spread of certain sarcoma histologic types with the aim of minimizing local recurrence, maximizing function, and improving overall survival. An algorithm for the management of soft tissue sarcomas of the extremity and trunk is presented in Figure 31-6. Surgical excision remains the dominant modality of curative therapy. Whenever possible, function- and limb-sparing procedures are performed. As long as the entire tumor is removed, less radical procedures have not been demonstrated to adversely affect local recurrence or outcome.[30]

The surgical objective is complete removal of the tumor with negative margins and maximal preservation of function. When possible, tumors are excised with 1 to 2 cm of normal tissue because of the propensity for local, unappreciated spread. Conversely, deliberate sacrifice of major neurovascular structures can generally be avoided,

provided that the surgeon pays meticulous attention to dissection.[30] Resection of bone is rarely required given the very low incidence of direct bone invasion by soft tissue sarcoma. For sarcomas that closely approximate bone, the periosteum, if removed intact, can serve as a sufficient fascial margin. The most extensive resection is clearly amputation. This is only rarely indicated for soft tissue sarcomas at the present time because limb-sparing operations are possible in 95% of patients. Experience over the past 25 years at MSKCC indicates that the 50% amputation rate in the late 1960s is now less than 5%. Amputations are reserved, in the main, for patients who have tumors that are not able to be resected by any other means, who are without evidence of metastatic disease, and who have the propensity for good long-term functional rehabilitation. Frequently, these patients have large, low-grade tumors causing considerable cosmetic and functional deformity and can be rendered symptom-free by a major amputation.

The effectiveness of adjuvant radiation therapy in improving local control has clearly been shown not only through retrospective data but also through three prospective randomized trials that have compared surgery alone with surgery and radiation therapy,[30-32] including either brachytherapy for high-grade lesions or external beam radiation therapy for large (>5 cm) high- or low-grade lesions.[31,32] For subcutaneous or intramuscular high-grade sarcomas smaller than 5 cm or any size low-grade sarcoma, surgery alone is considered if adequate wide excision with a good 1- to 2-cm cuff of surrounding fat and muscle can be achieved. If the excision margin is close, particularly with extramuscular involvement, or if local recurrence would result in the sacrifice of a major neurovascular bundle or amputation, adjuvant radiation

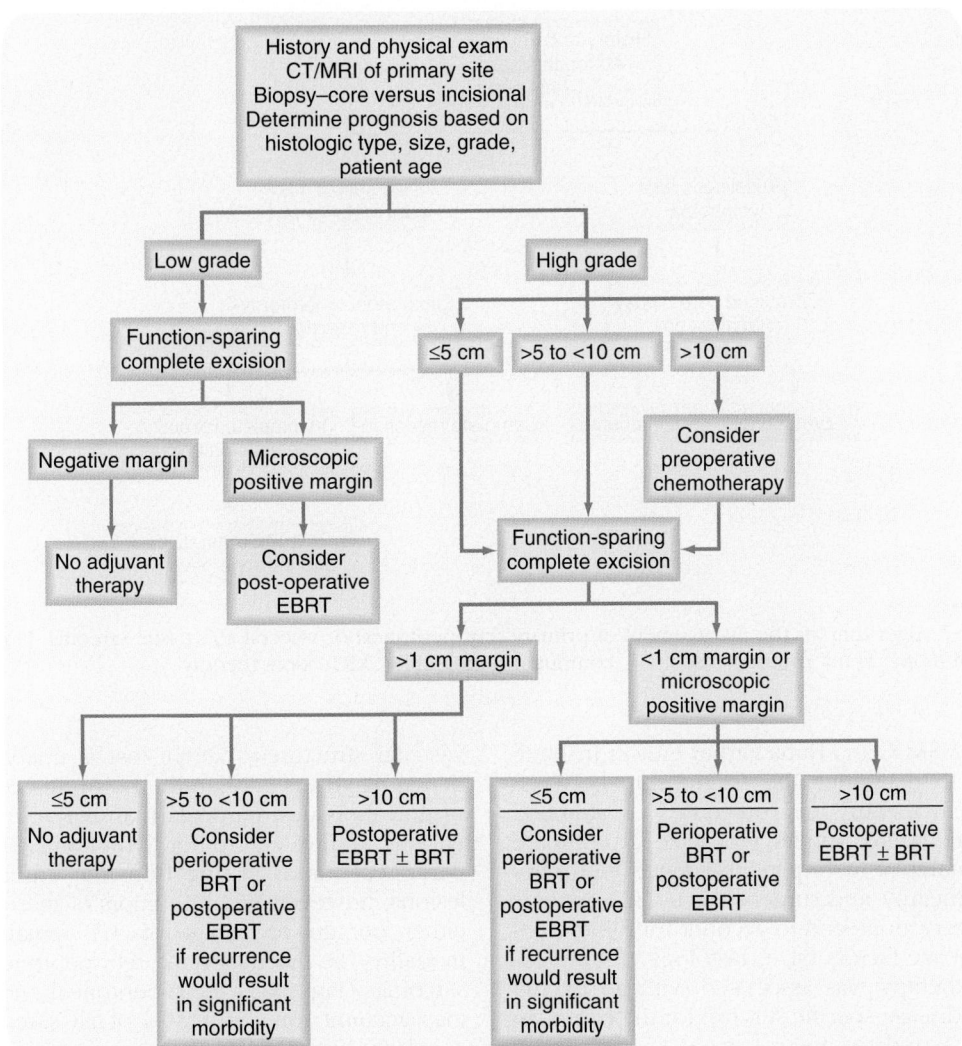

Figure 31-6 Algorithm for the management of primary (with no metastases) extremity or trunk soft tissue sarcoma based on a biologic rationale (i.e., size and grade of tumor). BRT, brachytherapy; CT, computed tomography; EBRT, external beam radiation therapy; MRI, magnetic resonance imaging.

therapy is added to the surgical resection to reduce the probability of local failure.[31] Particular histologic types such as myxofibrosarcoma (formally MFH) are often multifocal and deserve increased consideration for treatment with radiation. However, irrespective of grade, the author believes that postoperative irradiation is probably used more than strictly necessary. In fact, several studies have shown that a significant subset of subcutaneous and intramuscular sarcomas can be treated by wide excision alone, with a local recurrence rate of 5% to 10%.[33,34]

The value of chemotherapy depends on the histologic type of sarcoma. Neoadjuvant chemotherapy is usually indicated for the treatment of Ewing's sarcoma (PNET) and rhabdomyosarcoma because of the high risk for microscopic metastasis at diagnosis and high response rate with such therapy.[35,36] The potential for cure is inversely proportional to the volume and spread of disease. For other histologic subtypes of sarcoma, the role of chemotherapy remains controversial. Adjuvant

chemotherapy has not made any measurable impact on overall survival, with a small 10% to 15% improvement in disease-free survival.[37] Thus, adjuvant chemotherapy for soft tissue sarcoma is regarded as investigational and is rarely indicated, except in a clinical trial. The preoperative use of neoadjuvant combination chemotherapy (usually with doxorubicin [Adriamycin] and ifosfamide) for adult soft tissue sarcoma has several potential advantages:

1. It can make subsequent surgery easier.
2. It may treat micrometastatic disease early before the acquisition of resistance.
3. It leaves the vasculature intact for improved drug delivery.
4. It enables assessment of therapeutic response or resistance to therapy.

A retrospective analysis of patients with high-grade extremity sarcoma from prospectively acquired databases

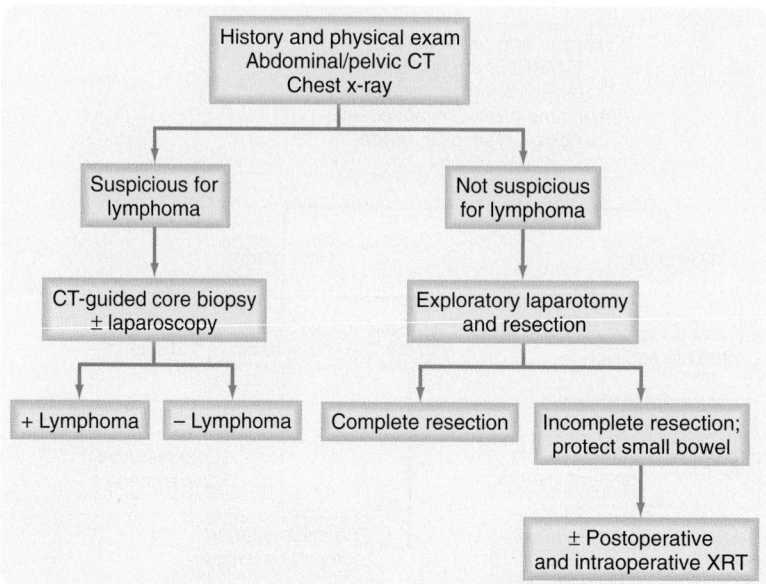

Figure 31-7 Algorithm for the management of primary retroperitoneal or visceral soft tissue sarcoma. Fine-needle aspiration biopsy is not routinely used. CT, computed tomography; XRT, x-ray therapy.

of patients from MSKCC and Dana Farber Cancer Institute was performed to determine the relationship between neoadjuvant chemotherapy and outcome.[38] A stratified Cox proportional hazards model was used to compare disease-specific survival in 74 patients treated with neo-adjuvant chemotherapy and surgery versus 282 patients treated with surgery alone and to account for differences in known prognostic factors (size, histology, age). Neo-adjuvant chemotherapy was associated with an overall improvement in disease-specific survival for the complete cohort of patients, and this improvement appears to be driven by the benefit of neoadjuvant chemotherapy in patients with extremity sarcomas larger than 10 cm. In this high-risk group there was a 21% improvement in disease-specific survival at 3 years.

Conversely, no association was seen between neoad-juvant chemotherapy and improved disease-specific sur-vival in patients with extremity sarcomas between 5 and 10 cm. There was also a trend toward improvement in recurrence-free survival in patients with tumors larger than 10 cm treated with neoadjuvant chemotherapy. Recently, Adriamycin-ifosfamide–based chemotherapy has been associated with improved disease-specific sur-vival in patients with large, high-grade extremity liposar-coma[39] and synovial sarcoma.[40] Taken together, these results suggest that neoadjuvant chemotherapy may be justified in carefully selected high-risk patients with large, high-grade tumors.

Retroperitoneal and Visceral Sarcoma

Most patients have an asymptomatic abdominal mass when initially seen, although on occasion pain is present. Less common symptoms include gastrointestinal bleed-ing, incomplete obstruction, and neurologic symptoms related to retroperitoneal invasion or pressure on neuro-

vascular structures. Weight loss is uncommon and inci-dental diagnosis is often the norm. Important differential diagnostic issues, particularly in the young, are the pres-ence of a germ cell tumor, lymphoma, or primary retro-peritoneal tumor arising from the adrenal gland. Most lesions, however, will be tumors of mesenchymal origin, either benign or malignant. CT remains the primary modality for evaluation of retroperitoneal and visceral sarcomas (Fig. 31-7). Retroperitoneal and visceral sarco-mas account for about 34% of all sarcomas. The most common histopathologic types in the retroperitoneum are liposarcoma (40%), leiomyosarcoma (25%), malignant peripheral nerve sheath tumor, and fibrosarcoma. In the visceral location, GIST, leiomyosarcoma, and desmoid are the most common histologic types (see Fig. 31-2). About 55% of retroperitoneal liposarcomas will be well differ-entiated and low grade, with roughly 40% of patients showing dedifferentiated, high-grade histology at initial evaluation.

Surgery remains the dominant method of therapy for retroperitoneal and visceral lesions,[18,24] and completeness of resection and grade are the most important prognostic factors for survival. Preoperative bowel preparation is important because resection of the intestine is frequently needed for technical reasons to achieve complete removal of all sarcoma. Although resection of adjacent organs is common,[18,24] proof that more extensive resection of adja-cent organs has an impact on long-term survival seems very limited. It is very clear that complete surgical resec-tion is the primary factor in outcome (Fig. 31-8). Once complete resection is accounted for, the predominant factor in outcome is the grade of the lesion. Despite an aggressive surgical approach, local control is still a major problem, and multifocal, unresectable tumors recur in many patients, particularly those with liposarcoma. The role of radiation therapy for retroperitoneal sarcoma is

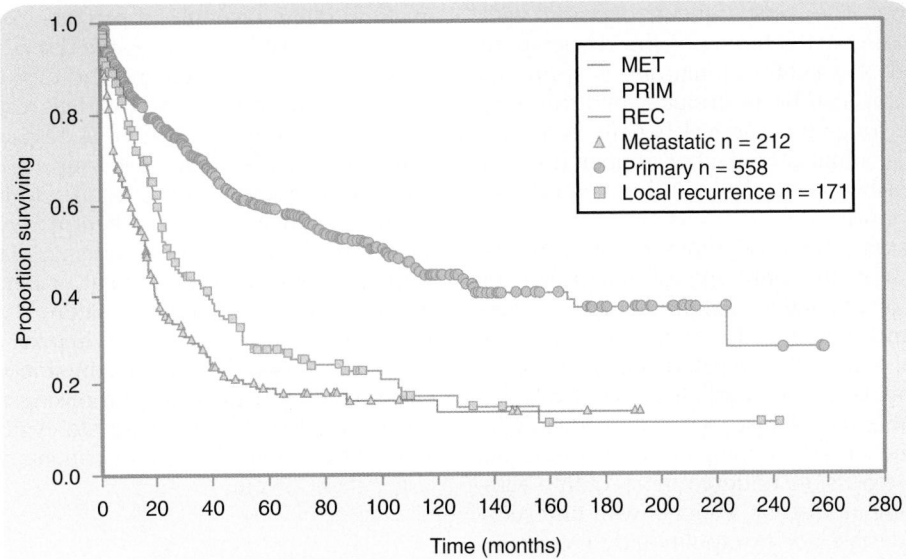

Figure 31-8 Disease-specific survival for patients with retroperitoneal–intra-abdominal soft tissue sarcoma grouped by status at initial evaluation. Of the 1002 patients, 590 (59%) had primary disease (PRIM), 184 (18%) had local recurrence (REC), and 228 (23%) had metastasis (MET). Median survival was 86 months in those with primary disease, 23 months in those with local recurrence, and 12 months in those with metastasis. Patients were seen at Memorial Sloan-Kettering Cancer Center from July 1, 1982, to June 30, 2005.

not well defined and is in need of further investigation.[41] In theory, preoperative or postoperative irradiation of this site is desirable, but in reality it is often not possible to deliver full-dose radiation therapy (60-66 Gy) to areas at risk because the dose is limited by the large treatment volume required and the sensitivities of adjacent normal tissues, such as the bowel, kidney, liver, and spinal cord. Brachytherapy or intraoperative radiation therapy at the time of surgical resection may be used to treat a localized area at high risk for microscopic or gross residual disease when further surgical excision is not possible. However, care must be taken to avoid the excessive morbidity and mortality that may result from aggressive brachytherapy, particularly when combined with external beam radiation therapy.[42] Therefore, the ideal radiation approach is one that could dose-escalate preoperative radiation therapy.

With conventional radiation it is impossible to escalate preoperative radiation therapy beyond 5040 cGy without incurring excessive toxicity. However, with a dose-painting preoperative intensity-modulated radiation therapy (IMRT) approach, targeted dose escalation to areas at highest risk is achievable. The whole tumor volume will receive 5040 cGy, thus respecting the tolerance of tissues, while at the same time the posterior structures, where there are no intestines, will receive 6000 cGy. A recent report from the University of Alabama showed the feasibility of such an approach to give a boost within the field. In that study 14 patients were treated with 4500 cGy preoperative radiation to the whole target volume. The area that was judged to be at risk for a positive margin at the time of resection then received an additional boost with IMRT to bring the total dose to 5750 cGy. Only one patient experienced grade 3 nausea and vomiting. Eleven patients had complete resection with negative margins. At a median follow-up of 12 months, there was no late toxicity related to the radiation therapy. Further dosimetric studies showed the technical feasibility of delivering doses as high as 7520 to 8280 cGy with this technique.[43] Trials of preoperative radiation therapy with or without intraoperative irradiation are under way. It remains to be determined whether preoperative IMRT in addition to resection improves local control and hence survival in comparison to resection alone in patients with primary retroperitoneal sarcoma.

TREATMENT OF RECURRENT DISEASE

Despite optimum multimodality limb-sparing treatment of extremity soft tissue sarcoma, distant metastasis continues to develop in a significant number of patients. In an analysis of 994 patients with primary extremity soft tissue sarcomas and a median follow-up of 33 months, distant metastasis developed in 230 patients (23%). Median survival after the development of metastasis was 11.6 months, and in 73% of these patients the lungs were the first metastatic site. Multivariate analysis suggests that the extent of metastatic disease, length of disease-free interval, presence of a preceding local recurrence, and older age were all significant predictors of postmetastasis survival. Local extremity recurrence is manifested as a nodular mass or series of nodules arising in the surgical scar. Patients with retroperitoneal recurrence usually have nonspecific symptoms, often only after the lesion has reached substantial size. After workup to determine the extent of disease, patients with isolated local recurrence undergo re-resection. The most difficult decision with retroperitoneal liposarcoma is timing of the reoperation; frequently, a period of watchful monitoring is appropriate. When re-resection can be performed, two thirds of patients experience long-term survival benefit. Adjuvant radiation therapy is administered after reoperation on the extremity, if feasible, depending on the method and extent of previous irradiation.

For extremity lesions, the most common site of metastasis is the lung. It is the only site of recurrence in approximately half of all patients. Extrapulmonary metastasis is relatively uncommon and generally occurs as a late manifestation of widely disseminated disease. Patients whose primary tumors are controlled or controllable, who have no extrathoracic disease, who are medically fit for thoracotomy, and in whom complete resection of all lung disease appears possible undergo thoracotomy with the intent of resecting all disease. Patients with unresectable pulmonary metastases or extrapulmonary metastatic sarcoma in more than a single site have a uniformly poor prognosis and are best treated with systemic chemotherapy. The role of chemotherapy in advanced sarcoma is controversial, and at present, treatment of metastatic sarcoma represents palliative, not curative therapy. Current active drugs that have significant response rates include doxorubicin, ifosfamide, and dacarbazine, but none has had a major impact on long-term survival.[44] The combination of mesna, Adriamycin, ifosfamide, and dacarbazine (MAID) has been demonstrated to have a 47% response rate and a 10% complete response rate. In randomized prospective clinical trials, combination chemotherapy regimens such as MAID and other ifosfamide-doxorubicin combinations with cytokine support have been shown to yield statistically improved rates of antitumor response.[44] However, these improved responses do not translate into improvements in survival and come at the cost of increased toxicity and a decrease in quality of life.

Given the limitations and toxicities associated with cytotoxic chemotherapy, emphasis has been placed on developing novel drugs against rational drug targets such as the KIT receptor tyrosine kinase, which is constitutively activated in most GISTs. GISTs are mesenchymal neoplasms showing differentiation toward the interstitial cells of Cajal and are typically characterized by expression of the receptor tyrosine kinase KIT (CD117).[45] Recent studies have established that activating mutations of *KIT* are present in up to 92% of GISTs and probably play a key role in the development of these tumors.[46,47] Along with mitotic activity, histologic subtype, and size, the type and the location of the *KIT* mutation are prognostic of survival in patients with GIST.[48] Imatinib is a competitive inhibitor of BCR-ABL, KIT, and PDGFR tyrosine kinases. In preclinical studies, imatinib was active against mutant isoforms of KIT commonly found in GIST.[49] A recently completed phase II trial has shown substantial response rates, as well as clinical benefit, with the use of imatinib in patients with advanced and metastatic GIST,[50] a group typically highly resistant to conventional doxorubicin/ifosfamide-based chemotherapy. A total of 147 patients were randomly assigned to receive 400 or 600 mg of imatinib daily. Overall, 79 patients (53.7%) had a partial response, 41 (27.9%) had stable disease, and for technical reasons, response could not be evaluated in 7 patients (4.8%). No patient had a complete response to the treatment. The median duration of response had not been reached after a median follow-up of 24 weeks after the onset of response. Early resistance to imatinib was noted in 20 patients (13.6%). Therapy was well tolerated, although mild to moderate edema, diarrhea, and fatigue were common. Gastrointestinal or intra-abdominal hemorrhage occurred in approximately 5% of patients. There were no significant differences in toxic effects or response between the two doses. Thus, inhibition of the KIT signal transduction pathway is a promising treatment of GIST. Trials are presently under way to evaluate the efficacy of adjuvant imatinib therapy in patients with primary GIST larger than 2.5 cm.

PROGNOSTIC FACTORS AND RESULTS

A prospectively collected series of more than 1000 patients has characterized the risk factors for outcome in patients with extremity soft tissue sarcoma. The overall 5-year survival rate for this cohort of patients was 76% at a median follow-up of 4 years. Significant independent adverse prognostic factors are outlined in Table 31-4. The important prognostic factors for local recurrence were age older than 50 years, signs and symptoms of recurrent disease, microscopically positive surgical margins, and the histologic subtypes fibrosarcoma and malignant peripheral nerve tumor.

For distant recurrence, large tumor size, deep location, high histologic grade, the presence of signs and symptoms of recurrent disease, and leiomyosarcoma and nonliposarcoma histology were all independent adverse prognostic factors. For disease-specific survival, large tumor size, high grade, deep location, signs and symptoms of recurrent disease, the histologic subtypes leiomyosarcoma and malignant peripheral nerve tumor, and microscopically positive margins were all adverse prognostic factors. This emphasizes that there are numerous independent adverse prognostic factors for distant recurrence and disease-specific survival and that they are clearly different from those involved in local recurrence.

For retroperitoneal soft tissue sarcoma, an analysis of 500 patients treated and monitored at a single institution has been reported.[24] Two hundred seventy-eight of these patients had a primary tumor, and 222, or 44%, had recurrent disease at a median follow-up of 28 months (1-172 months with a 40-month follow-up for all survivors); this suggests a median survival of 72 months for patients with primary disease, 28 months for those with local recurrence, and 10 months for those with metastasis. Patients with locally recurrent tumors, unresectable disease, or incomplete resection and high-grade tumors all had diminished survival time. Both for primary and for locally recurrent tumors, the ability to completely resect the tumor was a predominant factor in outcome. After complete resection, the presence of a low-grade tumor was

Table 31-4 Multivariate Analysis of Prognostic Factors for Outcome in 1041 Patients With Extremity Soft Tissue Sarcoma Managed at a Single Institution

	LOCAL RECURRENCE	DISTANT RECURRENCE	DISEASE-SPECIFIC SURVIVAL
Age >50 yr	0.001		
Recurrence manifestations	0.0001	0.015	0.003
Size >10 cm		0.03	0.0001
Size >5 cm		0.0001	
Deep location		0.0007	0.0002
High grade		0.0001	0.0001
Histology			
Fibrosarcoma	0.006		
Not liposarcoma		0.003	
Leiomyosarcoma		0.024	0.012
Malignant peripheral nerve tumor	0.001		0.008
Positive margin	0.0001		0.011

Modified from Pisters P, Leung D, Woodruff J, et al: Analysis of prognostic factors in 1041 patients with localized soft tissue sarcomas of the extremity. J Clin Oncol 14:1679, 1996.

a favorable factor for outcome. Disease-specific survival is illustrated in Figure 31-8. It was of value to re-resect sarcoma in patients who experienced recurrence, but the complete resectability rate fell with progressive recurrence, and few tumors were ever able to be completely resected after a third or subsequent recurrence.

An analysis of 200 patients identified as having GIST morphologically but not by expression of KIT by immunohistochemistry has suggested that complete surgical resection is the only factor that provides a significant outcome benefit for the patient.[27] Size but not microscopic margin appears to be a factor in predicting survival. A more recent analysis of 49 patients with GIST,[48] all confirmed by significant immunohistochemical expression of KIT, has demonstrated the prognostic importance of both mitotic activity and GIST mutation type in predicting sarcoma-specific survival in a group of patients with GIST before the availability of imatinib therapy. In contradistinction to retroperitoneal sarcomas, recurrence occurs equally both locally throughout the peritoneal cavity and systemically in the liver. Unfortunately, almost half of all patients will be found to have metastasis, usually to the liver. If complete surgical resection of gross disease in patients with primary sarcoma can be achieved, these patients will have a 5-year actuarial survival rate of 54%.

LONG-TERM FOLLOW-UP

It is essential to emphasize that long-term follow-up of all patients with soft tissue sarcoma is important. A recent analysis of long-term follow-up in patients monitored for more than 5 years showed that approximately 9% of patients who were disease-free at the end of 5 years would eventually experience further recurrence of the primary extremity sarcoma.

SUMMARY

Soft tissue sarcomas are relatively rare, with an annual incidence of 10,000 to 10,500 in the United States. Primary therapy is predicated on surgical resection with an adequate margin of normal tissue. For high-risk patients, local control is improved with postoperative adjuvant radiation therapy. Local recurrence rates vary, depending on the anatomic site. In extremity lesions, locally recurrent disease develops in a third of patients, with a median disease-free interval of 18 months. Treatment results for localized extremity recurrence may approach those for primary disease. Isolated pulmonary metastases may be resected, with 3-year survival rates of 20% to 30% after complete resection. In patients with retroperitoneal and visceral sarcoma, complete resection remains the dominant factor in outcome. As opposed to extremity sites, local recurrence in this site is a common cause of death. Patients with unresectable pulmonary metastases or extrapulmonary metastatic sarcoma have a uniformly poor prognosis and are best treated with systemic chemotherapy, with surgical resection reserved for meaningful palliation.

Selected References

Baldini EH, Goldberg J, Jenner C, et al: Long-term outcomes after function-sparing surgery without radiotherapy for soft tissue sarcoma of the extremities and trunk. J Clin Oncol 17:3252-3259, 1999.

This study suggests that there may be a select subset of patients with soft tissue sarcoma in whom carefully performed function-sparing surgery may serve as definitive therapy and in whom adjuvant radiotherapy may not be necessary.

Brennan MF, Lewis JJ: Diagnosis and Management of Soft Tissue Sarcoma. London, Martin Dunitz, 2002.

Brennan MF, Singer S, Maki RG, O'Sullivan B: Sarcomas of the soft tissues and bone. In DeVita VT, Hellman S, Rosenberg SA (eds): Cancer Principles and Practice of Oncology. Philadelphia, Lippincott Williams & Wilkins, 2005, p 1584.

Singer S, Demetri GD, Baldini EH, Fletcher CDM: Management of soft-tissue sarcomas: An overview and update. Lancet Oncol 1:75-85, 2000.

These reviews summarize the subject in a single monograph/book.

Antonescu CR, Besmer P, Guo T, et al: Acquired resistance to imatinib in gastrointestinal stromal tumor occurs through secondary gene mutation. Clin Cancer Res 11:4182-4190, 2005.

Demetri GD, von Mehren M, Blanke CD, et al: Efficacy and safety of imatinib mesylate in advanced gastrointestinal stromal tumors. N Engl J Med 347:472-480, 2002.

Heinrich MC, Corless, CL, Demetri, GD, et al: Kinase mutations and imatinib response in patients with metastatic gastrointestinal stromal tumor. J Clin Oncol 21:4342-4349, 2003.

Singer S, Rubin BP, Lux ML, et al: Prognostic value of *KIT* mutation type, mitotic activity, and histologic subtype in gastrointestinal stromal tumors. J Clin Oncol 20:3898-3905, 2002.

These studies demonstrate the importance of KIT activation and mutations in GIST pathogenesis and the rationale and application of KIT tyrosine kinase inhibitors for targeted treatment of GIST. The importance of KIT mutation type for predicting response to imatinib and the development of secondary mutations as a mechanism for acquired resistance to imatinib is described in the Antonescu and Heinrich references.

Ladanyi M, Bridge JA: Contribution of molecular genetic data to the classification of sarcomas. Hum Pathol 31:532-538, 2000.

This thorough review details the significant progress made in recent years in characterizing chromosomal changes associated with soft tissue sarcomas. In addition, recent molecular analyses of several sarcoma-associated translocations and the identification of novel genes and mechanisms of dysregulation are discussed. The role of cytogenetics and molecular changes is discussed in the context of diagnosis and future investigation.

Lewis JJ, Leung D, Woodruff JM, Brennan MF: Retroperitoneal soft tissue sarcoma: Analysis of 500 patients treated and followed at a single institution. Ann Surg 228:355-365, 1998.

Singer S, Antonescu CR, Riedel E, Brennan MF: Histologic subtype and margin of resection predict pattern of recurrence and survival for retroperitoneal liposarcoma. Ann Surg 238:358-370, 2003.

These manuscripts provide an extensive description of outcome in patients with retroperitoneal sarcoma and retroperitoneal liposarcoma.

Pisters P, Leung D, Woodruff J, et al: Analysis of prognostic factors in 1041 patients with localized soft tissue sarcomas of the extremity. J Clin Oncol 14:1679-1689, 1996.

This manuscript provides data on prognostic factors for extremity soft tissue sarcoma from a large single-institution series.

Pisters PWT, Harrison LB, Leung DH, et al: Long-term results of a prospective randomized trial evaluating the role of adjuvant brachytherapy in soft tissue sarcoma. J Clin Oncol 14:859-868, 1996.

Yang JC, Chang AE, Baker AR, et al: Randomized prospective study of the benefit of adjuvant radiation therapy in the treatment of soft tissue sarcomas of the extremity. J Clin Oncol 16:197-203, 1998.

These studies confirm the benefit of adjuvant radiation therapy in patients with completely resected localized extremity sarcoma.

References

1. Brennan MF, Singer S, Maki RG, et al: Sarcomas of the soft tissues and bone. In DeVita VT, Hellman S, Rosenberg SA (eds): Cancer Principles and Practice of Oncology. Philadelphia, Lippincott Williams & Wilkins, 2005, p 1584.
2. Li FP, Fraumeni JF Jr: Soft-tissue sarcomas, breast cancer, and other neoplasms. A familial syndrome? Ann Intern Med 71:747-752, 1969.
3. Sorensen SA, Mulvihill JJ, Nielsen A: Long-term follow-up of von Recklinghausen neurofibromatosis. Survival and malignant neoplasms. N Engl J Med 314:1010-1015, 1986.
4. Mundt KA, Dell LD, Austin RP, et al: Historical cohort study of 10 109 men in the North American vinyl chloride industry, 1942-72: Update of cancer mortality to 31 December 1995. Occup Environ Med 57:774-781, 2000.
5. Meis-Kindblom JM, Sjogren H, Kindblom LG, et al: Cytogenetic and molecular genetic analyses of liposarcoma and its soft tissue simulators: Recognition of new variants and differential diagnosis. Virchows Arch 439:141-151, 2001.
6. Kawai A, Woodruff J, Healey JH, et al: SYT-SSX gene fusion as a determinant of morphology and prognosis in synovial sarcoma. N Engl J Med 338:153-160, 1998.
7. Ladanyi M, Antonescu CR, Leung DH, et al: Impact of SYT-SSX fusion type on the clinical behavior of synovial sarcoma: A multi-institutional retrospective study of 243 patients. Cancer Res 62:135-140, 2002.
8. Bennicelli JL, Barr FG: Chromosomal translocations and sarcomas. Curr Opin Oncol 14:412-419, 2002.
9. Antonescu CR, Leung DH, Dudas M, et al: Alterations of cell cycle regulators in localized synovial sarcoma: A multifactorial study with prognostic implications. Am J Pathol 156:977-983, 2000.
10. Oda Y, Sakamoto A, Satio T, et al: Molecular abnormalities of p53, MDM2, and H-ras in synovial sarcoma. Mod Pathol 13:994-1004, 2000.
11. Antonescu CR, Tschernyavsky SJ, Decuseara R, et al: Prognostic impact of P53 status, TLS-CHOP fusion transcript structure, and histological grade in myxoid liposarcoma: A molecular and clinicopathologic study of 82 cases. Clin Cancer Res 7:3977-3987, 2001.
12. de Alava E, Antonescu CR, Panizo A, et al: Prognostic impact of P53 status in Ewing sarcoma. Cancer 89:783-792, 2000.
13. Wei G, Antonescu CR, de Alava E, et al: Prognostic impact of INK4A deletion in Ewing sarcoma. Cancer 89:793-799, 2000.
14. Lopez-Guerrero JA, Pellin A, Noguera R, et al: Molecular analysis of the 9p21 locus and p53 genes in Ewing family tumors. Lab Invest 81:803-814, 2001.
15. Ladanyi M, Bridge JA: Contribution of molecular genetic data to the classification of sarcomas. Hum Pathol 31:532-538, 2000.
16. Sorensen PH, Lynch JC, Qualman SJ, et al: PAX3-FKHR and PAX7-FKHR gene fusions are prognostic indicators in alveolar rhabdomyosarcoma: A report from the Children's Oncology Group. J Clin Oncol 20:2672-2679, 2002.
17. Fletcher CD, Unni KK, Mertens F: Pathology and genetics of tumors of soft tissue and bone. In Kleihues P, Sobin LH (eds): World Health Organization Classification of Tumors, vol 1. Lyon, France, IARC Press, 2002.
18. Singer S, Antonescu CR, Riedel E, et al: Histologic subtype and margin of resection predict pattern of recurrence and

survival for retroperitoneal liposarcoma. Ann Surg 238:358-370, discussion 370-351, 2003.

19. Kooby DA, Antonescu CR, Brennan MF, et al: Atypical lipomatous tumor/well-differentiated liposarcoma of the extremity and trunk wall: Importance of histological subtype with treatment recommendations. Ann Surg Oncol 11:78-84, 2004.

20. Eilber FC, Eilber FR, Eckardt J, et al: The impact of chemotherapy on the survival of patients with high-grade primary extremity liposarcoma. Ann Surg 240:686-695, discussion 695-687, 2004.

21. Brown FM, Fletcher CD: Problems in grading soft tissue sarcomas. Am J Clin Pathol 114(Suppl):S82-S89, 2000.

22. Kattan MW, Leung DH, Brennan MF: Postoperative nomogram for 12-year sarcoma-specific death. J Clin Oncol 20:791-796, 2002.

23. Dalal KM, Kattan MW, Antonescu CR, et al: Subtype-specific prognostic nomogram for patients with primary liposarcoma of the retroperitoneum, extremity, or trunk. Ann Surg 244:381-391, 2006.

24. Lewis JJ, Leung D, Woodruff JM, et al: Retroperitoneal soft-tissue sarcoma: Analysis of 500 patients treated and followed at a single institution. Ann Surg 228:355-365, 1998.

25. Panicek DM, Gatsonis C, Rosenthal DI, et al: CT and MR imaging in the local staging of primary malignant musculoskeletal neoplasms: Report of the Radiology Diagnostic Oncology Group. Radiology 202:237-246, 1997.

26. Fong Y, Coit DG, Woodruff JM, et al: Lymph node metastasis from soft tissue sarcoma in adults. Analysis of data from a prospective database of 1772 sarcoma patients. Ann Surg 217:72-77, 1993.

27. DeMatteo RP, Lewis JJ, Leung D, et al: Two hundred gastrointestinal stromal tumors: Recurrence patterns and prognostic factors for survival. Ann Surg 231:51-58, 2000.

28. Brennan MF: Staging of soft tissue sarcomas. Ann Surg Oncol 6:8-9, 1999.

29. Greene F, Page D, Fleming I, Fritz A, et al (eds): AJCC Cancer Staging Manual, 6th ed. Heidelberg, Germany, Springer-Verlag, 2002.

30. Rosenberg SA, Tepper J, Glatstein E, et al: The treatment of soft-tissue sarcomas of the extremities: Prospective randomized evaluations of (1) limb-sparing surgery plus radiation therapy compared with amputation and (2) the role of adjuvant chemotherapy. Ann Surg 196:305-315, 1982.

31. Yang JC, Chang AE, Baker AR, et al: Randomized prospective study of the benefit of adjuvant radiation therapy in the treatment of soft tissue sarcomas of the extremity. J Clin Oncol 16:197-203, 1998.

32. Pisters PW, Harrison LB, Leung DH, et al: Long-term results of a prospective randomized trial of adjuvant brachytherapy in soft tissue sarcoma. J Clin Oncol 14:859-868, 1996.

33. Baldini EH, Goldberg J, Jenner C, et al: Long-term outcomes after function-sparing surgery without radiotherapy for soft tissue sarcoma of the extremities and trunk. J Clin Oncol 17:3252-3259, 1999.

34. Alektiar KM, Leung D, Zelefsky MJ, et al: Adjuvant radiation for stage II-B soft tissue sarcoma of the extremity. J Clin Oncol 20:1643-1650, 2002.

35. Baldini EH, Demetri GD, Fletcher CD, et al: Adults with Ewing's sarcoma/primitive neuroectodermal tumor: Adverse effect of older age and primary extraosseous disease on outcome. Ann Surg 230:79-86, 1999.

36. Esnaola NF, Rubin BP, Baldini EH, et al: Response to chemotherapy and predictors of survival in adult rhabdomyosarcoma. Ann Surg 234:215-223, 2001.

37. Tierney JF, Stewart LA, Parmar MKB, et al: Adjuvant chemotherapy for localised resectable soft-tissue sarcoma of adults: Meta-analysis of individual data. Sarcoma Meta-analysis Collaboration. Lancet 350:1647-1654, 1997.

38. Grobmyer SR, Maki RG, Demetri GD, et al: Neo-adjuvant chemotherapy for primary high-grade extremity soft tissue sarcoma. Ann Oncol 15:1667-1672, 2004.

39. Eilber FC, Eilber FR, Eckardt J, et al: The impact of chemotherapy on the survival of patients with high-grade primary extremity liposarcoma. Ann Surg 240:686-695, discussion 695-687, 2004.

40. Eilber FC, Brennan MF, Eilber FR, et al: Chemotherapy is associated with improved survival in adult patients with primary extremity synovial sarcoma. Ann Surg 246:105-113, 2007.

41. Brennan MF: Retroperitoneal sarcoma: Time for a national trial? Ann Surg Oncol 9:324-325, 2002.

42. Alektiar KM, Hu K, Anderson L, et al: High-dose-rate intraoperative radiation therapy (HDR-IORT) for retroperitoneal sarcomas. Int J Radiat Oncol Biol Phys 47:157-163, 2000.

43. Popple RA, Prellop PB, Spencer SA, et al: Simultaneous optimization of sequential IMRT plans. Med Phys 32:3257-3266, 2005.

44. Antman K, Crowley J, Balcerzak SP, et al: An intergroup phase III randomized study of doxorubicin and dacarbazine with or without ifosfamide and mesna in advanced soft tissue and bone sarcomas. J Clin Oncol 11:1276-1285, 1993.

45. Fletcher CD, Berman JJ, Corless C, et al: Diagnosis of gastrointestinal stromal tumors: A consensus approach. Hum Pathol 33:459-465, 2002.

46. Hirota S, Isozaki K, Moriyama Y, et al: Gain-of-function mutations of c-*kit* in human gastrointestinal stromal tumors. Science 279:577-580, 1998.

47. Rubin BP, Singer S, Tsao C, et al: KIT activation is a ubiquitous feature of gastrointestinal stromal tumors. Cancer Res 61:8118-8121, 2001.

48. Singer S, Rubin BP, Lux ML, et al: Prognostic value of KIT mutation type, mitotic activity, and histologic subtype in gastrointestinal stromal tumors. J Clin Oncol 20:3898-3905, 2002.

49. Tuveson DA, Willis NA, Jacks T, et al: STI571 inactivation of the gastrointestinal stromal tumor c-KIT oncoprotein: Biological and clinical implications. Oncogene 20:5054-5058, 2001.

50. Demetri GD, von Mehren M, Blanke CD, et al: Efficacy and safety of imatinib mesylate in advanced gastrointestinal stromal tumors. N Engl J Med 347:472-480, 2002.

Bone Tumors

Ginger E. Holt, MD   and   Herbert S. Schwartz, MD

Orthopedic oncology is a complex surgical discipline that involves the care and management of individuals with both primary and secondary neoplasms of the musculoskeletal system. The neoplasms may be benign or malignant. This chapter deals with bone tumors only.

Management of bone tumors is more difficult than treatment of neoplasms in other organ sites because of the need for skeletal reconstruction. Adequate oncologic resection is only half the battle. The other half involves skeletal reconstruction and restoration of function. The process of reconstruction is facilitated by the very nature of the skeletal system. Bone has the unique property of regenerating, even in adults.

There is nothing more important than establishing a tissue diagnosis when dealing with human cancer. This is extremely important not only in the initial diagnosis but also in subsequent staging procedures as the disease evolves. A radiographic diagnosis is not sufficient in the majority of cases. There are many tumor simulators that occur in the skeleton. Cartilaginous anlage, hemangiomas, and bone islands are just some of the simulators that remain scintigraphically active and may mimic the radiographic appearance of a bone tumor late in adult life.

Biopsy is a complex cognitive skill in the skeleton. Fine-needle, core, or scalpel biopsy tracts harbor malig-

nant cells. Therefore, definitive surgical resection of cancer requires removing the biopsy tract, all iatrogenic contamination, and the bone tumor in an en bloc resection. This requires extensive exposure with wide flaps and mobilization of neurovascular structures. Inappropriately placed biopsy or needle puncture sites can complicate placement of the definitive surgical incision or require multiple incisions, thereby jeopardizing limb salvage. Key structures may be contaminated by the biopsy tract. It has been conclusively shown in several studies that inexperienced musculoskeletal oncologic surgeons have a three to four times increased rate of complications from a poorly placed biopsy site.[1-3] Unfortunately, this results in unnecessary surgery, unnecessarily complex surgery, and in some instances, amputation instead of limb salvage.

Staging of skeletal sarcomas is straightforward and has remained relatively unchanged since its original description by Enneking and colleagues.[4] Roman numeral one (I) refers to a low-grade skeletal sarcoma as interpreted by the pathologist. Roman numeral two (II) is high grade. Roman numeral three (III) signifies metastasis, whether it be regional or distant. The letter "A" refers to intracompartmental tumor localization, whereas the letter "B" refers to extracompartmental growth of the primary skeletal sarcoma. A bone tumor that begins in the femur and grows into the quadriceps musculature is extracompartmental because it has grown out of its original compartment into another. Pathologic fractures can be thought of as extracompartmental tumors. The Enneking system has five stages: IA, IB, IIA, IIB, and III. Stage IIB tumors are high risk. Stage III represents metastases of any type. The staging system of the American Joint Committee on Cancer has not been universally adopted for skeletal sarcomas.

Bone tumor management can be schematically represented by the points of a triangle. Point 1 is the adequacy of oncologic resection. Point 2 is the type and extent of skeletal reconstruction. Point 3 is the functional outcome anticipated by the specific type of skeletal reconstruction.

All three factors must be weighed and discussed with the patient and caregivers to decide on the optimal management for any particular individual. Adequacy of the surgical oncologic margin is not always the prime consideration; surgical resection for palliation is often important.

ONCOLOGIC RESECTION

There are four and only four types of surgical resection. They are defined by the margin. The margin represents the surgical dissection plane relative to the pseudocapsule and the neoplasm itself. *Intralesional* resections are exemplified by curettage. The surgical dissection plane goes through the tumor itself and potentially leaves gross tumor behind. *Marginal* resections generate a dissection plane at the periphery of the tumor through its pseudocapsule. An example may be subperiosteal long bone dissection. Theoretically, microscopic tumor may be left behind. *Wide* surgical margins have a dissection plane through a cuff of normal tissue. The cuff of normal tissue may be 1 cm or 1 m distant to the tumor. Theoretically, only satellite malignant cells may be left behind. With *radical* resection margins, the entire compartment that the tumor resides in is resected. For example, a tumor that originates in the distal end of the femur would undergo radical resection if the entire femur were removed from the hip joint to the knee joint. Local recurrence rates are inversely proportional to the radicality of the surgical procedure. There are only two ways to achieve any one of the four surgical margins: amputation and limb salvage. It is common for a limb salvage procedure to achieve a more radical margin than amputation. For example, limb salvage resection of a distal femoral sarcoma can achieve a wide surgical margin that spares the popliteal vessels and most of the extensor mechanism and calf musculature. In contrast, an amputation that goes through the tumor of a distal femoral sarcoma achieves only an intralesional resection margin.

SKELETAL RECONSTRUCTION

The skeleton is a dynamic organ that receives 20% of the cardiac output and can heal itself in the majority of instances. Surgical care and preparation of the resection bed optimize the chance for skeletal regeneration. Children regenerate bone at a greater rate than their adult counterparts do. Small bone defects on the order of 5 cm or less are often bone grafted with autogenous bone obtained from the iliac crest, allograft bone obtained from bone banks, or a combination. Recently, growth factors such as bone morphogenetic protein 2 (BMP2) and BMP7 are being used to potentiate osteoinduction. Demineralized bone matrix is a commercially derived allograft product that retains the noncellular protein constituents of normal bone and may facilitate osteogenesis.

Larger skeletal defects require more complex reconstruction strategies. If a joint is nearby, reconstruction often involves the use of an arthroplasty or arthrodesis.

These two options frequently require the application of a metal or structural bone allograft spacer. Occasionally, a vascularized autograft such as a fibula may be used by itself or in conjunction with another biologic or metal spacer. An intercalary segmental defect involves the shaft of a long bone and does not require joint reconstruction. In these instances, structural bone allografts and metal spacers are used along with internal fixation such as intramedullary rods or plates and screws.

FUNCTION

The long-term functional outcome after skeletal reconstruction is directly related to the durability of the implant. Metallic implants offer good immediate function, but they suffer from metal fatigue after millions of repetitive loading cycles, and long-term failure eventually occurs. In contrast, bone autografts or allografts provide short-term partial stability (protected weight bearing) but have the potential long-term advantage of permanent osteogenic ingrowth along with revascularization leading to intact viable bone. The weight-bearing needs of the lower extremities are different from those of the high-demand, non–weight-bearing functions of the upper extremities. The axial skeleton has a mixture of high-demand and load-bearing requirements. Skeletal reconstruction in children requires calculation for limb growth. Growing prostheses and limb lengthening need to be explained to the patient and their families. The more complicated the reconstruction, the higher the infection rate. Infections of metallic endoprostheses or large structural allografts can often be devastating and result in amputation. Terminal cancer patients who require skeletal reconstruction have different functional needs: immediate functional use with inconsequential long-term demands.

GENETICS

Alterations in DNA by inheritance, carcinogen exposure, sporadic replication or housekeeping error, mutation, chromosomal rearrangement, amplification, deletion, or change in expression can be oncogenic. Neoplastic cells that acquire such genetic change may begin a multistep process that confers a potential growth advantage. Further genetic change leads to more mutations and the creation of clones of cells that acquire malignant characteristics.

Benign and malignant skeletal neoplasms have a host of DNA alterations catalogued by the absence or presence of suppressor genes, oncogenes, translocations, and chromosome gains or losses. Table 32-1 lists these genetic alterations for some selected bone tumors.[5] This table is meant to be a summary rather than an exhaustive list.

In contrast, skeletal metastases (e.g., carcinomas) manipulate the normal bone microenvironment to create osteolytic bone destruction while promoting the growth and spread of cancer cells.[6,7] Cell adhesion molecules are used for both cell-to-cell and cell-to-matrix binding. Deregulation of matrix metalloproteinases disrupts the delicate balance of matrix homeostasis by increasing

Table 32-1 Genetic Alterations for Selected Bone Tumors

SKELETAL TUMOR	NEOPLASIA			DNA ALTERATIONS		
	Suppressor Gene	Oncogene	Translocations	Chromosome Loss	Chromosome Gain	Protein Change
Osteosarcoma	*RB, p53, INK4A, INK2A*	*CDK4, FOS, cMYC, MDM2, MET*		6q, 13q, 15q, 17p, 18q	1q, 5p, 6p, 7q, 8q, 12q, 17p, 19q, 7p, 12q, 21q	
Ewing's sarcoma	*KCMF1*	*CD99*	t(11;22)(q24;q12) *EWS-FLI1* t(21;22)(q22;q12) *EWS-ERG*			
Chondrosarcoma				1p, 5q, 6p, 9p, 14q, 22q	7p, 12q, 21q	
Osteochondroma	*EXT1, EXT2*					
Enchondroma					12q	IHH-PTHrP (Indian hedgehog–parathyroid hormone–related protein)
Aneurysmal bone cyst			t(16;17)(q22;p13) *CDH11-USP6*			
Fibrous dysplasia		*GNAS1*		20q		GS
Giant cell tumor		*TPX2*	Telomeric fusions		20q	RANKL

proteolytic activity. Degradation of the extracellular matrix results in cancer cell invasion. Angiogenesis stimulators such as vascular endothelial growth factor, fibroblast growth factor, and transforming growth factor-α are triggered by cancer cells to promote their own growth. Parathyroid hormone–related protein is released by certain tumor cells acting on the same receptors for parathyroid hormones to promote osteoclast-mediated bone resorption. Osteoclastogenesis is also promoted by interleukin-6, interleukin-8, and RANKL (receptor activator of nuclear factor κB ligand). There is a complex interaction between many cell receptors, cytokines, growth factors, and proteases in the metastatic bone microenvironment.

BENIGN BONE TUMORS

Incidence

The incidence of benign bone tumors far exceeds that of skeletal sarcomas. In these authors' clinical experience there are at least five benign bone tumors for every primary malignant bone neoplasm. In the most current edition of *Dahlin's Bone Tumors,* approximately 54% of benign bone tumors are chondrogenic.[8] Osteochondroma and enchondroma are the most common benign tumors. Both can be polyostotic. Osteochondromas are surface neoplasms of bone, whereas enchondromas are located intraosseously. The true prevalence of these tumors

is unknown because many go undetected and unreported.

Overview

The significance of benign bone tumors is that they occur more frequently in the pediatric population than in adults. Fractures are often the initial mode of expression. A pathologic fracture may occur during running or other activities, with pain being the initial symptom. Frequently, benign bone tumors are detected in the pediatric or adult population as an incidental radiographic discovery. A patient with rotator cuff tendonitis may complain of shoulder pain and a plain radiograph identifies an abnormality in the proximal humeral metaphysis, which by itself is asymptomatic. Benign bone tumors grow with the child and generally stop growing when the child reaches skeletal maturity. Surgical indications include deformity (angular or limb length inequality), pain, pathologic fracture, or malignant transformation.

Surgical Oncology

Most benign bone tumors can be resected safely with an intralesional resection margin. The goal is a local recurrence rate of less than 10%. These procedures typically consist of curettage. Careful attention must be directed to not injuring the physis.

Reconstruction of benign bone tumors after curettage is often accomplished with a combination of bone graft-

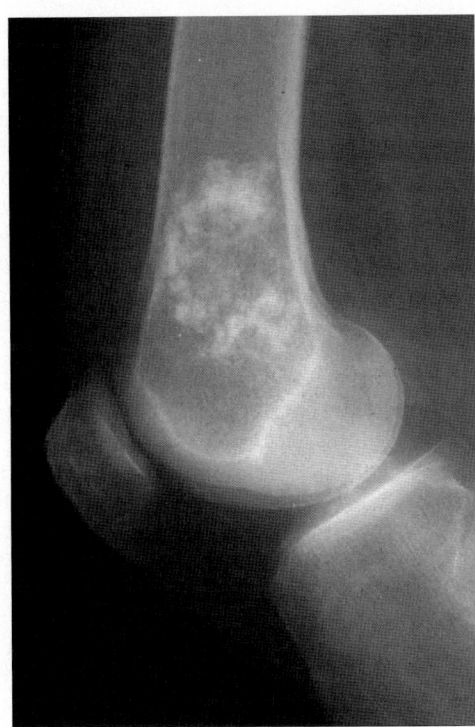

Figure 32-1 Plain radiograph, lateral projection, of an enchondroma of the distal end of the femur. Note the heavy calcification of the benign chondroid matrix.

ing and stabilization of impending fractures. Bone grafting can be performed with either autogenous bone or allograft. Many allograft preparations are commercially available, including demineralized bone matrix from an American Association of Tissue Banks–approved bone bank.[9] Adequate curettage demands a large bone portal to access the intraosseous cavity, which, however, severely compromises the biomechanical integrity of the bone and requires operative stabilization. Stabilization can be done extracorporally, such as a with cast or splint. Internal bone stabilization can be accomplished with a combination of rods, plates, pins, or screws. The goal is to achieve osteogenesis, preserve skeletal growth, and gain strength in a few months.

Function

The functional outcome after bone grafting, especially in a child, is excellent. Limb length inequalities, especially overgrowth, may occur when the procedure is performed in a young child. The younger the child, the more conservative the internal fixation techniques are. Casting is preferred because joint stiffness is seldom a problem in this patient population.

Examples

1. Enchondroma (Fig. 32-1) is a benign proliferation of hyaline cartilage typically found in long bones, but it may occur in the axial skeleton as well. Cartilage anlage or islands retain chondroid features and continue to grow until skeletal maturity, when they begin

to undergo calcification. Their long-term physiologic activity is the reason that they remain scintigraphically active decades later. An enchondroma typically begins in the metaphysis and extends into the diaphysis. It seldom occurs in the epiphysis of long bones. Polyostotic syndromes may occur, often with unilateral predominance. Ollier's disease is the eponym associated with multiple skeletal enchondromas. Maffucci's syndrome is Ollier's disease associated with multiple subcutaneous hemangiomas. In the pediatric population, management revolves around maintaining a strong, straight, and symmetrical bone of appropriate length. After skeletal maturity, malignant transformation is rare. However, the greater the tumor burden, the greater the late malignant transformation rate. Therefore, patients with Ollier's disease often have a higher incidence of chondrosarcoma formation than do individuals with solitary disease. The more axial located tumors of the pelvis, spine, and scapula have the worst prognosis. Interestingly, individuals with Maffucci's syndrome have the same elevated incidence of chondrosarcoma formation; however, this unique patient population frequently succumbs to the development of occult carcinomas.[10]

Treatment of enchondromas remains conservative. Intralesional curettage and bone grafting often result in excellent outcomes. Enchondromas are particularly common in the small bones of the hands and feet. Histopathologic interpretation of benign cartilage tumors is difficult because it is extremely dependent on the clinical findings and plain radiographic appearance of the tumor. Rarely, cytogenetic abnormalities are identified in enchondromas. It appears that abnormalities in 12q13-15 appear to be common in both benign and malignant cartilaginous neoplasms.[5]

2. Fibrous dysplasia (Fig. 32-2) is not a true neoplasm but represents dysplasia in the fibro-osseous proliferation of bone. It may be monostotic or polyostotic. The cause appears to be a postfertilization mutation in the gene encoding the α-activating subunit of the G (guanine nucleotide binding) protein that participates in guanosine triphosphatase activity. The mutation occurs on chromosome 20 at location 20q13.2. It appears to be a missense point mutation at the arginine 201 amino acid that leads to constitutive activation of the formation of cyclic adenosine monophosphate.[11,12] Fibrous dysplasia may be monostotic, polyostotic, or associated with an endocrinopathy syndrome called *McCune-Albright*. This syndrome occurs more often in females and is characterized by the triad of polyostotic fibrous dysplasia predominating on one side, precocious puberty (may be manifested as vaginal bleeding within the first few months of life), and large macules often overlying the involved bone. Treatment mimics that of other benign bone tumors; however, it is important to realize that complete extirpation of the tumor is not necessary. The bone is biomechanically weak, and therefore treatment is aimed at structural stabilization. Rarely, late sarcomatous transformation occurs. The incidence of fibrous dysplasia parallels that of giant cell tumor.

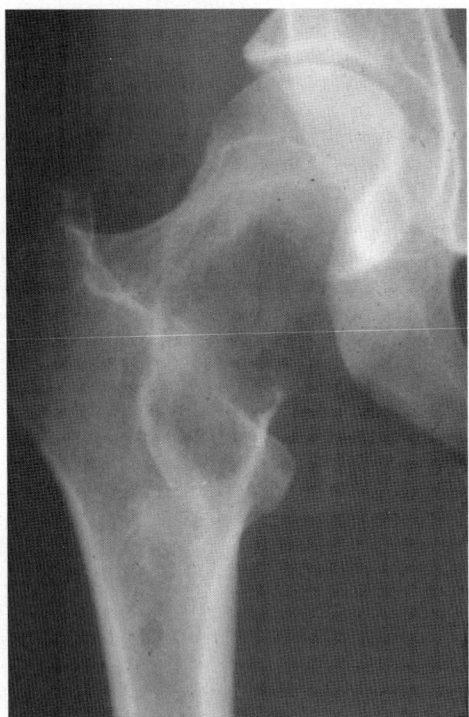

Figure 32-2 Fibrous dysplasia shown on a plain anteroposterior radiograph of the right hip. Note the partially ossified matrix of the tumor with loss of normal bone trabeculae.

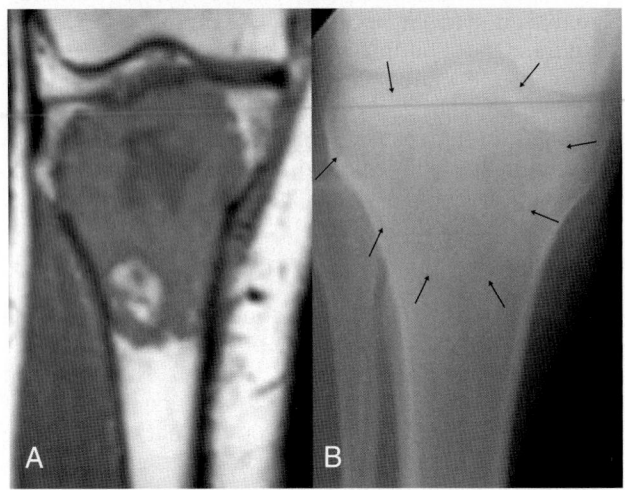

Figure 32-3 A and **B,** Giant cell tumor of bone involving the proximal tibia, seen on MRI scan (**A**) and indicated by arrows on plain radiography (**B**).

3. Giant cell tumor (Fig. 32-3) occurs in approximately 20% of benign bone tumors. It perhaps represents the most aggressive benign tumor and threatens the true definition of a benign cancer because benign pulmonary metastases develop in approximately 1% to 2% of giant cell tumors.[13] In these cases, the metastatic focus in the lung does not histopathologically meet the criteria for malignancy and is identical in appearance to the benign bone tumor in the skeleton. Survival rates are approximately 80% with aggressive treatment. Local recurrence rates after treatment of

giant cell tumor in a bone can be as high as 40% but have been halved through aggressive surgical treatment, often with the use of local adjuvants,[14] including high-speed turbine burring, polymethylmethacrylate bone cement, liquid nitrogen, phenol, and argon beam laser. This tumor typically develops in the epiphysis of long bones, although it may occur in the flat bones of the pelvis, often between the ages of 20 and 40, and is manifested as an intra-articular displaced pathologic fracture. Management involves radiographic pulmonary examination, aggressive local treatment with a large surgical approach and exposure of the bone cavity, and aggressive local intralesional resection, with or without adjuvant therapy. Reconstruction demands stability, and bone grafting alone is frequently not adequate. Cement provides immediate stability but is associated with the potential for late arthritic development in the adjacent joint. The tumor often extends to subchondral bone under the articular cartilage. The spectrum of biologic behavior of this capricious tumor is not well understood. The cytogenetics of giant cell tumor is fascinating but does not belie its true biologic potential. The presence of telomere-to-telomere chromosomal translocations (telomeric associations) in giant cell tumor is a rarely reported cytogenetic phenomenon in human neoplasia.[15] Giant cell tumor also has the unique ability to grow in a variety of microenvironments and therefore represents a challenge to the surgeon inasmuch as iatrogenic implantation and metastases are distinctly common occurrences. Patients require long-term follow-up because recurrences may develop several years postoperatively. Giant cell tumors in the spine, sacrum, and pelvis present greater surgical challenges. Oftentimes, preoperative embolization is required because intraoperative tumor hemorrhage is significant. Radiation treatment may have a role in primary giant cell tumors of the axial skeleton or in recurrent refractory giant cell tumors in a long bone. There is strong evidence, however, that irradiation of giant cell tumors increases the chance for malignant transformation to a frank giant cell sarcoma decades later.[16]

SKELETAL SARCOMAS

Incidence

Approximately 2300 skeletal sarcomas occur each year in the United States.[17] This incidence translates into approximately one new case per 100,000 population per year. Osteosarcoma is the most common primary malignant neoplasm of bone; it represents a third of cases and often occurs in teenagers. Chondrosarcoma accounts for 25% of skeletal sarcomas, followed by Ewing's sarcoma at 16%. The incidence of skeletal sarcomas is approximately equal in the pediatric and adult populations.

Overview

The need for complex skeletal reconstruction, often using large metallic endoprosthetic implants or structural allografts (or both), ushered in the era of neoadjuvant chemotherapy and limb salvage (Fig. 32-4). Many skeletal sarcomas are sensitive to chemotherapy. In the 1970s, intensive chemotherapy was administered to many teenagers with nonmetastatic osteosarcoma of the extremities after biopsy.[18] While a custom endoprosthesis was being fabricated, treatment continued with systemic cytotoxic chemotherapy. After several months the tumor was surgically removed and the implant inserted to preserve the limb. The resected bone tumor was then examined histopathologically for the necrotic effect of preoperative or neoadjuvant chemotherapy.

Surgical Oncology

Wide surgical margins are preferred for the treatment of skeletal sarcomas. For many skeletal sarcomas, resection follows neoadjuvant chemotherapy. Chemotherapy facilitates limb salvage by allowing easier dissection and mobilization of critical neurovascular structures. The surgical goal is a local recurrence rate of less than 10%. Early studies by Simon,[19] Link,[20] and their colleagues documented equivalent local recurrence and survival rates with limb salvage and amputation for distal femoral osteosarcoma. Cure rates are approximately 67% for extremity sarcomas, whereas axial tumors in the pelvis or spine have a worse prognosis (33%) for a similar tissue type.[21,22]

Reconstruction of large skeletal defects, frequently greater than 15 cm, requires the use of metallic endoprostheses, structural allografts, or combinations of allograft-prosthesis composites. Reconstruction strategies are more complicated in the pediatric population because it is difficult to manufacture a growing prosthesis.

Function

It has been demonstrated that limb salvage is more cost-effective over a period of decades than immediate amputation in the teenage population.[23] Implant survival is complicated in the short term by infection (allografts) and in the long term by aseptic loosening (metal).[24] Ten-year implant survival rates for metallic prostheses range from 50% to 80% in the proximal tibia, distal femur, and proximal femur, respectively.[25] Wound healing, especially while administering chemotherapy, is enhanced with healthy local flaps. This is especially true around the knee, where gastrocnemius flaps are necessary to cover the prosthesis and restore function to the extensor mechanism.

Examples

1. Osteosarcoma, or osteogenic sarcoma (Fig. 32-5) is defined as a malignant tumor that produces neoplastic osteoid. Neoplastic cartilage or fibrous tissue may be present. There are many types of osteosarcoma and they vary by location (intraosseous, surface, or diaphyseal), grade, or etiology. Spontaneous osteosarcomas are most common, but many osteosarcomas occur in the genetic syndromes of Li-Fraumeni and hereditary retinoblastoma and in postradiation scenarios.[26-28]

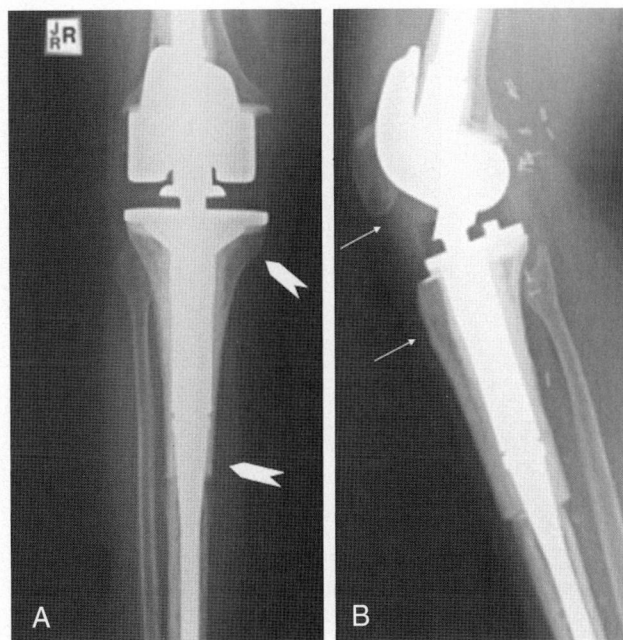

Figure 32-4 A and **B,** Limb salvage resection and reconstruction with allograft tibia and prosthetic knee arthroplasty.

There is a bimodal age of tumor occurrence. Conventional osteosarcomas occur in the first 2 decades of life, whereas post-treatment or secondary (malignant transformation) osteosarcomas occur much later. Post-radiation skeletal sarcomas of the chest wall are becoming increasingly more common with the gaining popularity of lumpectomy and radiation treatment of mammary carcinoma.[29] Survival is best predicted by the degree of chemotherapy-induced necrosis.[30] Nonmetastatic extremity osteosarcoma with greater than 90% chemotherapy-induced necrosis has survival rates of 80% at 5 years. Pelvic osteosarcoma with less than 90% chemotherapy-induced necrosis has a survival rate of approximately 30%.[21,22]

2. Ewing's sarcoma (Fig. 32-6) and primitive neuroectodermal tumor are small blue cell (microscopic appearance) malignancies of bone that cytogenetically represent the same entity. They share a common translocation, t(11;22)(q24;q12), in 85% of cases. Molecular cloning of the translocation reveals fusion between the 5′ end of the *EWS* gene from the 22q12 chromosome and the 3′ end of the 11q24 *FLI1* gene.[31-33] This tumor is exquisitely sensitive to chemotherapy and radiation treatment. Neither modality alone or in combination is sufficient to maximize the cure rate, however. Surgical extirpation in conjunction with chemotherapy is the preferred treatment. Reconstruction options follow those of other skeletal sarcomas.

3. Chondrosarcoma (Fig. 32-7) is a malignant skeletal neoplasm that produces hyaline cartilage. Several rarer pathologic subtypes exist in which the neoplastic cells produce unusual matrices. Histopathology alone does

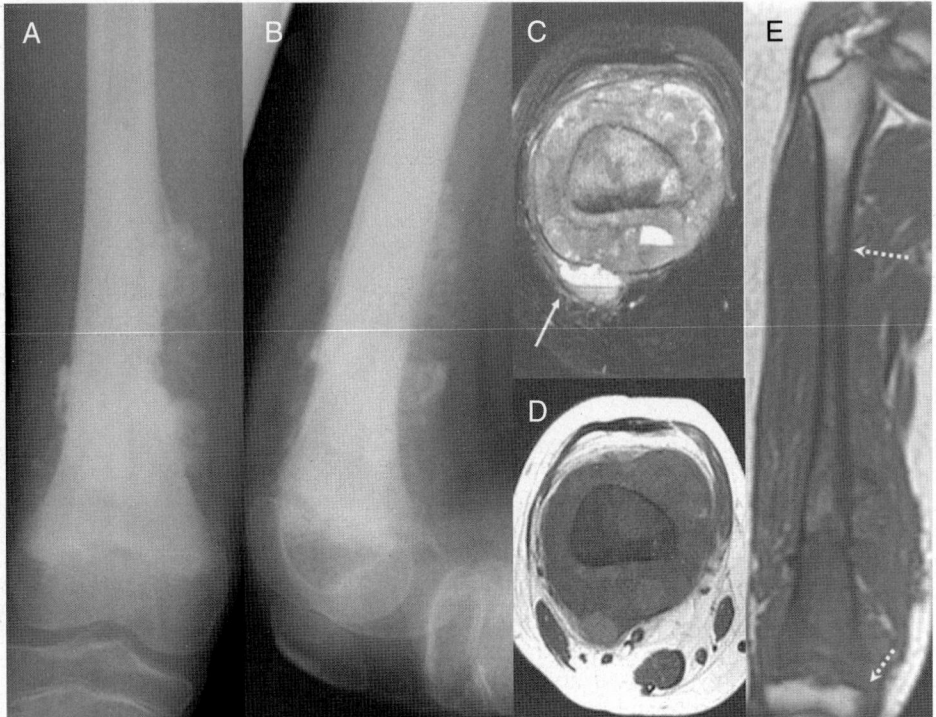

Figure 32-5 Osteosarcoma. Anterioposterior (**A**) and lateral (**B**) radiographs show malignant intramedullary and extramedullary bone formation. T$_2$ (**C**) and T$_1$ (**D**) weighted MRI scans demonstrate a large circumferential soft tissue mass with extension into the posterior compartment (*arrow*). **E,** Coronal MRI scan shows tumor extending from the diaphysial femur to the distal physis (*arrows*).

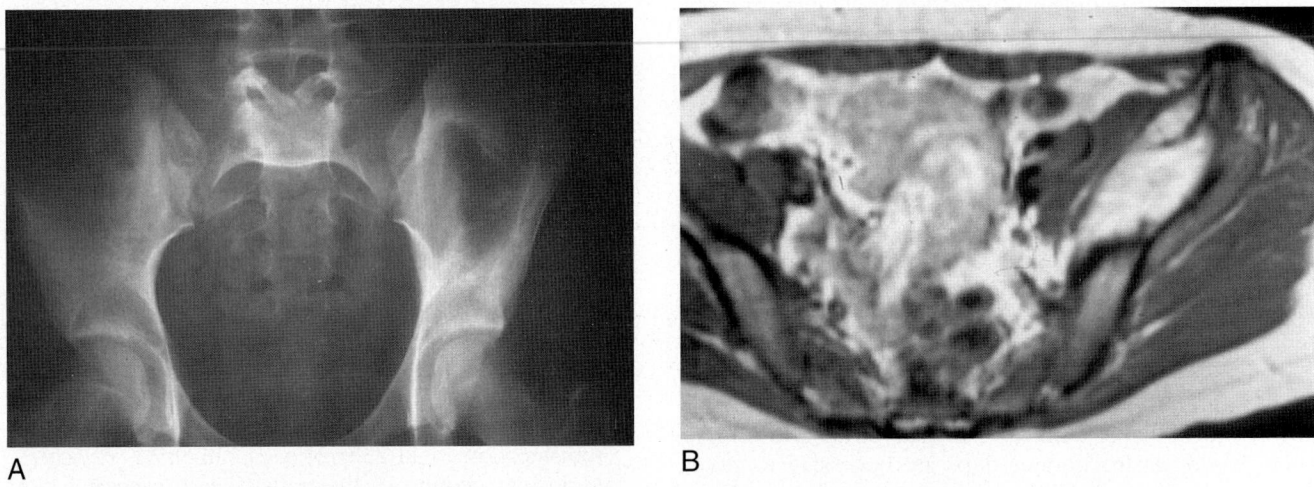

Figure 32-6 Ewing's sarcoma. **A,** Anteroposterior plain radiograph of the pelvis. Note the destructive and permeative changes in the left pelvis (ilium). **B,** Axial T2-weighted magnetic resonance image demonstrating the white tumor infiltrating the left ilium and breaking out into the musculature as an extraosseous soft tissue mass.

not predict biologic behavior. Rather, a combination of histopathology, age, location, and radiographic appearance yields the best predictor of tumor aggressiveness. A low-grade cartilage tumor of the phalanx may have the same microscopic appearance as a pelvic chondrosarcoma. Essentially no one will die of a phalanx cartilage tumor; however, local control is notoriously difficult to achieve in pelvic chondrosar-

comas, and long-term cure rates require massive resection. Secondary chondrosarcomas are frequent and occur after malignant transformation of a benign cartilage tumor such as enchondroma or osteochondroma.[34] There is increasing molecular evidence that growth plate chondrocyte signaling pathways are recapitulated in cartilage neoplasia (Indian hedgehog–parathyroid hormone–related protein axis).

SKELETAL METASTASES

Incidence

Skeletal metastases are approximately 500 times more common than skeletal sarcomas.[17] Approximately 1.2 million new cases of carcinoma are diagnosed each year in the United States. Osteophiles include prostate, thyroid, breast, lung, and kidney cancer.

Overview

Adults are more commonly afflicted with skeletal metastases than children are. The prevalence of individuals with skeletal metastases continues to rise as cancer therapies improve with time. Pathologic fractures and impending pathologic fractures represent common problems for the orthopedic oncologist. The workup for a metastatic skeletal carcinoma of unknown primary origin consists of only a computed axial tomographic scan of the chest, abdomen, and pelvis; a bone scan; serum protein electrophoresis; and assay for prostate-specific antigen.[35] Physical examination of the breast and prostate is mandatory. Bisphosphonate therapy diminishes osteoclast resorption of bone and preserves the biomechanical integrity of the skeleton.

Surgical Oncology

Intralesional resection after tissue confirmation of the diagnosis minimizes the chance of local recurrence. Treatment goals include whole-bone prophylaxis with long, intramedullary locked nails. Postoperative radiation therapy must include delivery to the entire bone from joint to joint. A surgical goal of a local recurrence rate less than 10% is preferred. Isolated metastases such as from renal cell carcinoma or melanoma can be treated aggressively if they are indeed isolated and occur after a long hiatus (several years) after the primary. Cures, in such instances, are not rare.

Reconstructive goals consist of choosing an implant durable enough to outlive the patient. The bone cannot be expected to heal after tumor resection and chemoradiation therapy. Therefore, cement and metal must be used to preserve biomechanical integrity, especially in weight-bearing joints (Fig. 32-8) and the spine.

A variety of surgical techniques are used to reconstruct a skeleton that is symptomatic and has metastatic carcinoma. Examples requiring different techniques include a weight-bearing long bone such as the femur, a non–weight-bearing long bone such as the humerus, and a flat bone such as the pelvis (see the illustrations). Aggressive surgical management of premyelopathic isolated spinal metastases in conjunction with radiotherapy is preferred over radiation therapy alone.[36]

Function

Palliative relief of pain and maximization of function are the goals of surgery. The idea is to keep the patient pain-free, mobile, and independent. Bisphosphonates significantly diminish osteoclast function and therefore bone

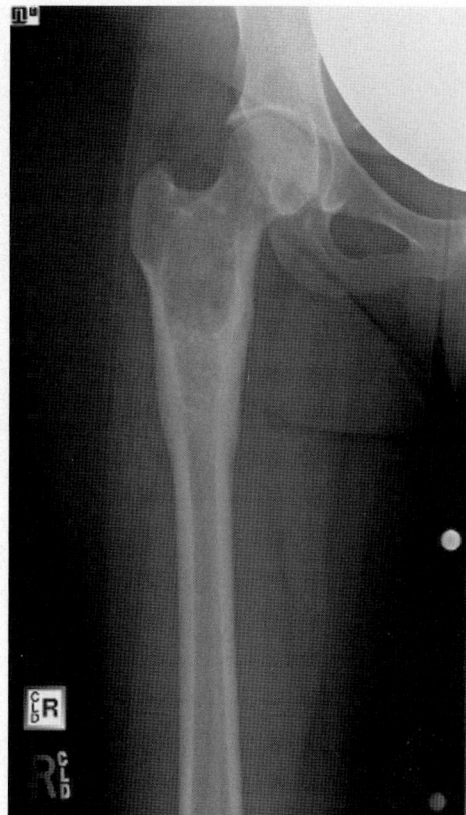

A

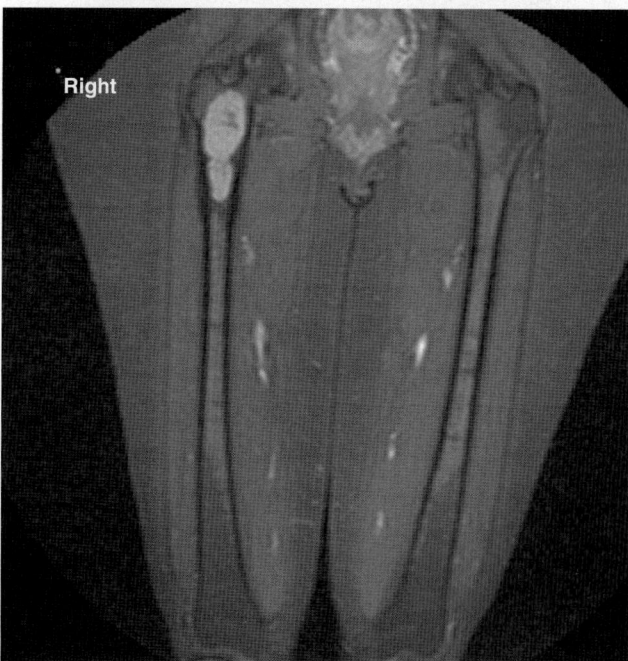

B

Figure 32-7 Chondrosarcoma. **A,** Anteroposterior plain radiograph of the right proximal femur showing expansion of the bone from the poorly mineralized malignant chondroid matrix. **B,** Coronal magnetic resonance image demonstrating the extent of the tumor into the intramedullary space.

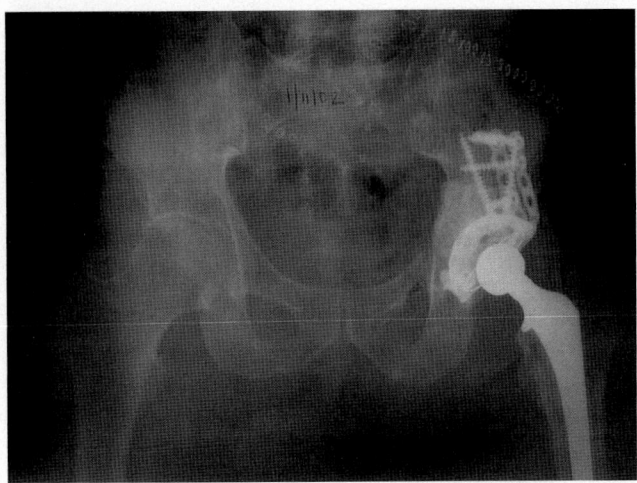

Figure 32-8 Carcinoma metastatic to the left acetabulum. After resection, reconstruction was accomplished with cement, screws, and total hip arthroplasty.

resorption. They have become an important tool in preventing pathologic fractures in patients with metastatic disease and preserving function.

FUTURE

Advances in the treatment of skeletal malignancies will require better understanding of the molecular causes of the disease. Implants will improve, but material and biomechanical principles are at a plateau in development. In contrast, knowledge of the genetic causes of sarcomas and the microenvironment surrounding them is growing rapidly. Identifying skeletal sarcoma biomarkers of high-risk biologic behavior may someday stratify patients by metastatic potential early in the cancer treatment course. Examining the microenvironment of bone may identify molecular triggers of matrix lysis and endothelial invasion. Targeted therapies that downgrade the growth and invasive potential of cancers offer the hope of prolonged survival through new treatment paradigms.

References

1. Mankin HJ, Mankin CJ, Simon MA: The methods of biopsy revisited. J Bone Joint Surg Am 78:656-663, 1996.
2. Randall RL, Bruckner JD, Papenhausen MD, et al: Errors in diagnosis and margin determination of soft tissue sarcoma initially treated at non-tertiary centers. Orthopedics 27:209-212, 2004.
3. Trovik CK: Scandinavian Sarcoma Group Project. Acta Orthop Scand Suppl 300:1-31, 2001.
4. Enneking WF, Spanier SS, Goodman MA: A system for the staging of musculoskeletal sarcoma. Clin Orthop Relat Res 153:106-120, 1980.
5. Sandberg AA, Bridge JA: Updates on the cytogenetics and molecular genetics of bone and soft tissue tumors: Osteosarcomas and related tumors. Cancer Genet Cytogenet 145:1-30, 2003.
6. Roodman GD: Mechanisms of bone metastasis. N Engl J Med 350:1655-1664, 2004.
7. Kang Y, Siegel PM, Shu W, et al: A multigenic program mediating breast cancer metastasis to bone. Cancer Cell 3:537-549, 2003.
8. Unni KK: Dahlin's Bone Tumors: General Aspects and Data on 11,087 Cases, 5th ed. Philadelphia, Lippincott-Raven, 1996.
9. Joyce MJ: Safety and FDA regulations for musculoskeletal allografts. Clin Orthop Relat Res 435:22-30, 2005.
10. Schwartz HS, Zimmerman NB, Simon MA, et al: The malignant potential of enchondromatosis. J Bone Joint Surg Am 69:269-274, 1987.
11. Ding C, Deng Z, Levine MA: A highly sensitive PCR method detects activating mutations of the GNAS1 gene in peripheral blood cells of patients with McCune-Albright syndrome or isolated fibrous dysplasia. J Bone Miner Res 16(Suppl 1): S417-S422, 2001.
12. Weinstein LS, Shenker A, Gejman PV, et al: Activating mutations of the stimulating G protein in the McCune-Albright syndrome. N Engl J Med 325:1688-1695, 1991.
13. Siebenrock KA, Unni KK, Rock MG: Giant cell tumor of bone metastasizing to the lungs. J Bone Joint Surg Br 80:43-47, 1998.
14. Zhen W, Yaotian H, Songjian L, et al: Giant-cell tumor of bone. J Bone Joint Surg Br 86:212-216, 2004.
15. Schwartz HS, Jenkins RB, Dahl RJ, Dewald GW: Cytogenetic analyses on giant cell tumor of bone. Clin Orthop Relat Res 240:250-260, 1989.
16. Rock MG, Sim FH, Unni KK: Secondary malignant giant cell tumor of bone. J Bone Joint Surg Am 68:1073-1079, 1986.
17. Jemal A, Murray T, Ward E, et al: Cancer statistics, 2005. CA Cancer J Clin 55:10-30, 2005.
18. Rosen G, Marcove RC, Caparros B, et al: Primary osteogenic sarcoma: The rationale for preoperative chemotherapy and delayed surgery. Cancer 42:2163-2177, 1979.
19. Simon MA, Aschliman MA, Thomas N, Mankin HJ: Limb-salvage treatment versus amputation for osteosarcoma of the distal end of the femur. J Bone Joint Surg Am 68:1331-1337, 1986.
20. Link MP, Goorin AM, Miser AW, et al: The effect of adjuvant chemotherapy on relapse-free survival in patients with osteosarcoma of the extremity. N Engl J Med 314:1600-1606, 1986.
21. Bacci G, Ferrari S, Bertoni F, et al: Long term outcome of patients with nonmetastatic osteosarcoma of extremity. J Clin Oncol 18:4016-4027, 2000.
22. Goorin AM, Schwartzentruber DJ, Devidas M, et al: Pediatric Oncology Group. Presurgical chemotherapy combined with immediate surgery and adjuvant chemotherapy for nonmetastatic osteosarcoma. POG 8651. J Clin Oncol 21:1574-1580, 2003.
23. Grimer RJ, Carter SR, Pynsent PB: The cost-effectiveness of limb salvage for bone tumors. J Bone Joint Surg Br 79:558-561, 1997.
24. Mankin HJ, Hornicek FJ, Raskin KA: Infection in massive bone allografts. Clin Orthop Relat Res 432:210-216, 2005.
25. Unwin PS, Cannon SR, Grimer RJ, et al: Aseptic loosening in cemented custom-made prosthetic replacements for bone tumours of the lower limb. J Bone Joint Surg Br 78:5-13, 1996.
26. Li FP, Fraumeni JF, Mulvihill JJ, et al: A cancer family syndrome in 24 kindreds. Cancer Res 48:5358-5362, 1988.
27. Draper GJ, Sanders BM, Kingston JE: Second primary neoplasms in patients with retinoblastoma. Br J Cancer 53:661-671, 1986.

28. Yap J, Chuba PJ, Thomas R, et al: Sarcoma as a second malignancy after treatment for breast cancer. Int J Radiat Oncol Biol Phys 52:1231-1237, 2002.
29. Holt, GE, Thomson AB, Griffin AM, et al: Multifocality and post-radiation sarcomas. Clin Orthop Relat Res 450:67-75, 2006.
30. Picci P, Bacci G, Campanacci M, et al: Histologic evaluation of necrosis in osteosarcoma induced by chemotherapy. Regional mapping of viable and nonviable tumor. Cancer 56:1515-1521, 1985.
31. Aurias A, Rimbaut C, Buffe D, et al: Chromosomal translocations in Ewing's sarcoma. N Engl J Med 309:496-497, 1983.
32. deAlava E, Gerald WL: Molecular biology of the Ewing's sarcoma/primitive neuroectodermal tumor family. J Clin Oncol 18:204-213, 2000.
33. Hu-Lieskovan S, Zhang J, Wu L, et al: EWS-FLI1 fusion protein up-regulates critical genes in neural crest development and is responsible for the observed phenotype of Ewing's family of tumors. Cancer Res 65:4633-4644, 2005.
34. Bovee JVMG, Cleton-Jansen A, Taminiau AHM, Hogendoorn PCW: Emerging pathways in the development of chondrosarcoma of bone and implications for targeted treatment. Lancet 6:599-607, 2005.
35. Rougraff BT, Kneisl JS, Simon MA: Skeletal metastasis of unknown origin: A prospective study of a diagnosis strategy. J Bone Joint Surg Am 75:1276-1281, 1993 .
36. Patchell RA, Tibbs PA, Regine WF, et al: Direct decompressive surgical resection in the treatment of spinal cord compression caused by metastatic cancer: A randomized trial. Lancet 366:643-648, 2005.

HEAD AND NECK

CHAPTER 33

Head and Neck

Robert R. Lorenz, MD   James L. Netterville, MD   and   Brian B. Burkey, MD

NORMAL HISTOLOGY

The normal histology of the upper aerodigestive tract varies within each site.[1] A review of the thyroid and parathyroid glands is beyond the scope of this chapter. The nasal vestibule is considered a cutaneous structure and is lined by keratinizing squamous epithelium. The limen nasi, or mucocutaneous junction, is where the epithelium changes to a ciliated pseudostratified columnar (respiratory) epithelium to line the nasal cavities. The exception is the olfactory epithelium at the roof of the nasal cavity, which is composed of bipolar, spindle-shaped olfactory neural cells with surrounding supporting cells. The paranasal sinuses are also lined by respiratory epithelium, but it tends to be thinner and less vascular than that of the nasal cavity. The nasopharyngeal lining varies from squamous to respiratory epithelium in an inconsistent manner. The adenoidal pad is composed of lymphoid tissue containing germinal centers without capsules or sinusoids. The oral cavity is lined by non-keratinized stratified squamous epithelium with minor salivary glands throughout the submucosa and within the muscular tissue of the tongue. Although the oropharynx

is lined by squamous epithelium, Waldeyer's ring is formed by lymphoid tissues of the palatine tonsils, adenoids, lingual tonsils, and the adjacent submucosal lymphatics. The tonsils contain germinal centers without capsules or sinusoids, but unlike the adenoids, the tonsils have crypts lined by stratified squamous epithelium.

The hypopharynx is lined by nonkeratinizing, stratified squamous epithelium. Seromucous glands are found throughout the submucosa of the hypopharynx, in the lower two thirds of the epiglottis, and in the potential space between the true and false vocal folds known as the *ventricle*. Nonkeratinizing stratified squamous epithelium lines the epiglottis and true vocal fold. Pseudostratified, ciliated respiratory epithelium lines the false vocal fold, ventricle, and subglottis. The thyroid, cricoid, and arytenoid cartilages are composed of hyaline cartilage, whereas the epiglottis, cuneiform, and corniculate cartilages are composed of elastic-type cartilage. The external ear is a cutaneous structure lined with keratinizing squamous epithelium and associated adnexal structures. The external third of the external auditory canal is unique in that it contains modified apocrine glands that produce cerumen. The middle ear is lined with respiratory epithelium.

Numerous noncancerous changes in squamous epithelium can be seen in the upper aerodigestive tract. Leukoplakia, which describes any white mucosal lesion, and erythroplasia, which describes any red mucosal lesion, are both clinical descriptions and should not be used as diagnostic terms (Fig. 33-1). Erythroplakia is more often indicative of an underlying malignant lesion. *Hyperplasia* refers to thickening of the epithelium secondary to an increase in the total number of cells. *Parakeratosis* is an abnormal presence of nuclei in the keratin layers, whereas *dyskeratosis* refers to any abnormal keratinization of epithelial cells and is found in dysplastic lesions. *Koilocytosis* is a descriptive term for vacuolization of squamous cells and is suggestive of viral infection, especially human papillomavirus.

EPIDEMIOLOGY

The American Joint Committee on Cancer (AJCC) staging system divides sites of malignancy originating in the head and neck into six major groups: lip and oral cavity, pharynx, larynx, nasal cavity and paranasal sinuses, major salivary glands, and thyroid.[2] Of the sites arising from the aerodigestive tract, laryngeal cancer remains the most common cause of death (Table 33-1). Although there clearly remains a male preponderance in aerodigestive tract malignancies, the male-to-female ratio has been steadily decreasing because of the direct association between tobacco as a causative agent and the increased incidence of female smokers. Tobacco abuse increases the odds ratio for the development of laryngeal cancer by 15.1, whereas alcohol abuse carries an odds ratio of 2.11. Combined abuse of alcohol and tobacco is not additive in terms of the odds ratio but multiplicative. Worldwide, 400,000 new cases of head and neck cancer are expected in 2005, with two thirds occurring in developing countries, usually in association with alcohol and tobacco use.[3] The highest incidence rates in males exceed 30 per 100,000 in areas of France, Hong Kong, India, Spain, Italy, and Brazil, as well as in U.S. blacks, with recent dramatic increases in oral cancer being seen in Central and Eastern Europe.[4] The highest female rates are greater than 10 per 100,000 and are found in India, where chewing of betel quid and tobacco is common. Although aggregate rates are slowly declining in select areas such as India, Hong Kong, and Brazil, as well as in U.S. whites, rates are increasing in most other regions of the world. In addition to alcohol and tobacco consumption as causative factors, other risk factors include human papillomavirus and Epstein-Barr virus infection, Plummer-Vinson syndrome, metabolic polymorphisms, malnutrition, and occupational exposure to mutagenic agents. According to the National Cancer Data Base, squamous cell carcinoma (SCC) is the most common head and neck malignant diagnosis (55.8%), followed by adenocarcinoma (19.4%) and lymphoma (15.1%).[5]

CARCINOGENESIS

Carcinogenesis is a multistep process consisting of sequential accumulation of genetic alterations. These alterations, or mutations, are expressed phenotypically in the cancer cells as clonal outgrowth, increased proliferative capacity, immortality, cell motility, and invasion. Additionally, tumor cells induce changes in nontumor host cells to create paracrine growth feedback loops, inhibit host immunity, and cause neovascularization. Direct damage to DNA can be caused by either exogenous factors, such as radiation, chemical carcinogens, oxidative stress, and viral insertions, or intrinsic factors, such as spontaneous deletions, missense mutations, insertions, and chromosomal translocations. It is estimated that between 3 (early-onset nasal cancer) and 11 (laryngeal cancer) separate mutations are required to allow a head and neck tumor to develop. Mutations then affect the two types of genes involved in carcinogenesis: proto-oncogenes and tumor suppressor genes.

Proto-oncogenes normally encode for proteins involved in cell regulatory function, but when mutated, they cause malignant characteristics such as increased proliferation, decreased apoptosis, and increased angiogenesis. The proto-oncogenes studied in association with head and neck SCC (HNSCC) include cyclin D1 (PRAD1), vascular endothelial growth factor (VEGF), transforming growth factor-α (TGF-α), TGF-β, and epidermal growth factor receptor (EGFR). VEGF is an endothelial cell mitogen that

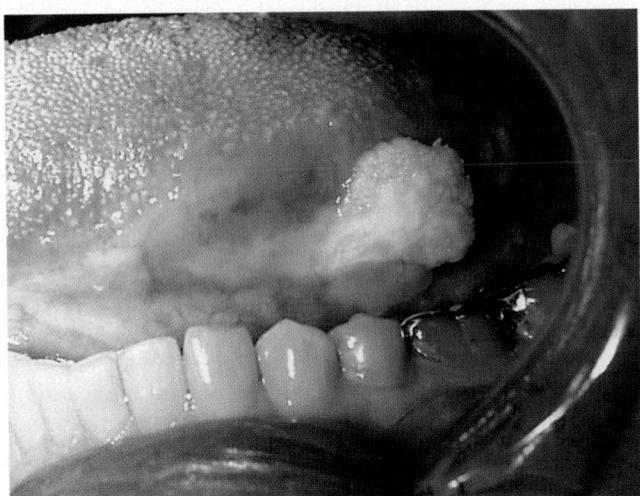

Figure 33-1 Leukoplakic lesion on the left mobile tongue. This lesion was determined to be hyperkeratosis without invasive cancer on biopsy.

Table 33-1 **Head and Neck Cancer, 2002 Statistics: Upper Aerodigestive Tract**

	ESTIMATED INCIDENCE			ESTIMATED DEATHS		
SITE	Both Sexes	Male	Female	Both Sexes	Male	Female
Tongue	7100	4700	2400	1700	1100	600
Mouth	9800	5200	4600	2000	1100	900
Pharynx	8600	6500	2100	2100	1500	600
Other oral cavity	3400	2500	900	1600	1200	400
Larynx	8900	6900	2000	3700	2900	800

From Jemal A, Thomas A, Murray T, et al: Cancer statistics, 2002. CA Cancer J Clin 52:23-47, 2002.

also promotes cell mobility and penetration of the endothelium. In a study of 77 patients with either oral or oropharyngeal carcinoma, VEGF was found in 41% of tumors, and its presence was the most significant predictor of poor patient prognosis.[6] The cyclin family of proteins is responsible for driving cellular proliferation. Cyclin D1 is encoded at the 11q13 chromosomal locus and is overexpressed in approximately 68% of tongue cancers. Although some studies are contradictory, increased expression of cyclin D1 has been shown to be an independent prognostic indicator of recurrence. EGFR overexpression or increased activation is ubiquitous in HNSCC and has also been shown to correlate with poor survival and resistance to radiation therapy.[7]

Tumor suppressor genes normally encode for proteins that inhibit tumor development. Typically, tumorigenesis occurs only with the loss of both alleles, but p53 is the exception to this rule. As the most commonly altered tumor suppressor in human tumors, p53 is also the most studied tumor suppressor gene. Because mutated p53 is not degraded as rapidly as wild-type p53, overexpression is actually a signal that p53 has been altered and is nonfunctional. A steady increase in the number of p53 abnormalities occurs during the progression of HNSCC, with p53 being overexpressed in 19% of normal epithelia, 29% of hyperplastic lesions, 45% of dysplastic lesions, and 58% of invasive cancers.[8] p53 mutations also are correlated with tobacco and alcohol abuse. In analyses of different HNSCCs, 58% of tumors in patients who abused both alcohol and tobacco contained p53 mutations as compared with 33% of lesions in patients who abused tobacco alone and 17% in patients who abused neither alcohol nor tobacco. p53 has been shown to be inactivated not only by mutation and deletion but also by the protein products of both Epstein-Barr virus (associated with the majority of nasopharyngeal carcinomas) and human papillomavirus (associated with 50% of oropharyngeal SCCs). In addition to being inactivated by viral proteins, deletions, and mutations, p53 is also intimately connected with the tumor suppressor gene that is most frequently altered in HNSCC, the *p16-ARF* gene. The p16-ARF gene locus uniquely encodes two proteins translated in different reading frames, p16 and ARF. p16 is an inhibitor of cyclin-dependent kinase and can therefore be considered an activator of retinoblastoma, with the biologic effect of stopping cellular proliferation. ARF, the other protein encoded by this gene locus, is an activator of p53 and can cause either cell cycle arrest or apoptosis. The p16-ARF gene locus is altered in more than 50% of HNSCCs, thus suggesting that inactivation of both retinoblastoma and p53 is important for the formation of these tumors.

The ultimate clinical goal of deciphering the molecular abnormalities that result in head and neck cancer is to aid in the development of targeted molecular therapy. The recent success of imatinib mesylate (Gleevec), an inhibitor of abl tyrosine kinase, in the treatment of chronic myelogenous leukemia and gastrointestinal stromal tumors has advanced the cause of biologic therapy. The concept is that seemingly homogeneous head and neck cancers differ in their gene and protein expression profiles and will therefore differ in their response to biologic therapy. A chimeric form of the monoclonal antibody against EGFR (IMC-C225, cetuximab; Imclone Systems), when combined with cisplatin, causes increased tumor regression in a small number of patients, and phase II/III trials are under way in which IMC-C225 is being combined with cisplatin or radiation therapy.[7] The ability to identify patients who might benefit from EGFR antibody is a major challenge, and there is surprisingly no correlation between expression of EGFR and the efficacy of the EGFR inhibitors.

Carcinogenesis in HNSCC also includes the development of second primary tumors, with patients having a 3% to 7% yearly incidence of secondary lesions in the upper aerodigestive tract, esophagus, or lung. A synchronous second primary lesion is defined as a tumor detected within 6 months of the index tumor. The occurrence of a second primary lesion more than 6 months after the initial lesion is referred to as *metachronous*. There is debate regarding whether second lesions represent reseeding of the primary tumor or genetically separate lesions caused by the so-called field cancerization effect resulting from exposure to carcinogens. When analyzing p53 mutations in patients with second primary tumors, up to 100% of p53 changes are different between the primary lesion and the secondary cancer, thus strongly suggesting that these lesions arise as independent events. Conversely, when analyzing synchronous oral carcinomas, both identical alterations (60%) and discordant alterations (40%) have been identified, which suggests that synchronous lesions can be of independent origin in some patients but may be of clonal origin in others.[9] A second primary will develop in the aerodigestive tract of 14% of patients with HNSCC over the course of their lifetime, with more than half these lesions occurring within the first 2 years of the index tumor. Because of the incidence of either second lung primaries or metastatic lung lesions, both posteroanterior and lateral chest radiographs are obtained at the time of diagnosis and annually for the patient's post-treatment cancer surveillance.

STAGING

Staging of head and neck cancer follows the TNM classification established by the AJCC.[2] The T classification refers to the extent of the primary tumor and is specific to each of the six sites of origin, with subclassifications within each site. The N classification refers to the pattern of lymphatic spread within the neck nodes and is the same for most head and neck sites, except nasopharynx and thyroid (Table 33-2). Clinical staging of the neck is based primarily on palpation, although radiographic studies, including computed tomography (CT) and magnetic resonance imaging (MRI), have been shown to be accurate in detecting positive nodes. If the CT criteria of nodes with central necrosis or size greater than 1.0 cm is used to determine positivity, only 7% of pathologically positive lymph nodes would be missed, and these smaller nodes are most often found in necks with more extensive disease.[9] Metastatic disease is reported simply as Mx

Table 33-2 **Regional Lymph Node Metastatic Staging**

CLASSIFICATION	DESCRIPTION
NX	Regional lymph nodes cannot be assessed
N0	No regional lymph node metastasis
N1	Metastasis in a single ipsilateral lymph node, ≤3 cm in greatest dimension
N2	Metastasis in a single ipsilateral lymph node, >3 cm but not >6 cm in greatest dimension; or in multiple ipsilateral lymph nodes, none >6 cm in greatest dimension; or in bilateral or contralateral lymph nodes, none >6 cm in greatest dimension
N2a	Metastasis in a single ipsilateral lymph node >3 cm but not >6 cm in greatest dimension
N2b	Metastasis in multiple ipsilateral lymph nodes, none >6 cm in greatest dimension
N2c	Metastasis in bilateral or contralateral lymph nodes, none >6 cm in greatest dimension
N3	Metastasis in a lymph node >6 cm in greatest dimension

From Greene FL, Page DL, Fleming ID, et al (eds): AJCC Cancer Staging Manual, 6th ed. New York, Springer-Verlag, 2002.

(cannot be assessed), M0 (no distant metastases are present), or M1 (metastases present). The most common sites of distant spread are the lungs and bones, whereas hepatic and brain metastases occur less frequently. The risk for distant metastases is more dependent on nodal staging than on primary tumor size.

After complete resection of the primary and nodal disease, pathologic staging may be reported. This is designated by a preceding "p," as in pTNM. It must be remembered when measuring a pathologic mucosal specimen that tumor size may decrease up to 30% after resection. Although clinical T staging is of primary concern, pathologic N staging allows detection of occult microscopic disease and is useful in determining prognosis. Site-specific staging systems are discussed according to the primary site. The major change in the 2002 edition of the AJCC staging system for HNSCC sites is the staging of T4 disease, which has been divided into T4a (resectable) and T4b (unresectable), leading to the division of stage IVA (advanced resectable), stage IVB (advanced unresectable), and stage IVC (advanced distant metastatic disease).

CLINICAL OVERVIEW

Evaluation

Proper treatment of HNSCC requires careful evaluation and accurate staging, both clinically and radiographically.

Patients with HNSCC are initially evaluated in a similar manner regardless of the site of tumor. Patient histories focus on symptomatology of the tumor, including the duration of symptoms, detection of masses, location of pain, and the presence of referred pain. Special attention is paid to numbness, cranial nerve weakness, dysphagia, odynophagia, hoarseness, disarticulation, airway compromise, trismus, nasal obstruction, epistaxis, and hemoptysis. Alcohol and tobacco use histories are elicited. Office examination includes nasopharyngeal and laryngeal visualization with either a mirror or fiberoptic endoscopy. The examiner should be especially vigilant for second primary tumors and not be preoccupied by the obvious primary lesion. Contrast-enhanced CT and MRI of the head and neck may be performed for evaluation of the tumor and detection of occult lymphadenopathy. CT scanning is best at evaluating bony destruction, whereas MRI can determine soft tissue involvement and is excellent at evaluating parotid and parapharyngeal space tumors. Chest radiography or chest CT is performed to rule out synchronous lung lesions. Serum tumor markers such as alkaline phosphatase and calcium may be determined, but such tests are not standard.

Direct laryngoscopy and examination under anesthesia are commonly performed as part of the evaluation of HNSCC. These procedures allow the physician to evaluate tumors without patient discomfort and with muscle paralysis, as well as evaluate the oropharynx, hypopharynx, and larynx and obtain biopsy samples. Pathologic confirmation of cancer is mandatory before initiating treatment. Concurrent bronchoscopy and esophagoscopy have historically been recommended for detection of synchronous second primaries of the aerodigestive tract, which occur in 4% to 8% of patients who have one head and neck malignancy. In the face of a normal chest radiograph or CT scan, bronchoscopy has a low yield for discovering bronchial tree second primaries. A barium esophagogram may substitute for esophagoscopy in patients at low risk for the development of esophageal tumors.

Positron Emission Tomography

Fluorodeoxyglucose F 18 is a glucose analogue that is preferentially absorbed by neoplastic cells and can be detected by positron emission tomography (PET). Recently, the role of PET has been investigated in the initial evaluation of patients with HNSCC.[10] PET is more sensitive than CT in identifying the primary lesion, but it is not able to detect unknown primary tumors with more than 50% sensitivity. More than a third of patients have a change in their TNM score based on PET findings, and 14% of patients are assigned a different stage when it is added to the diagnostic workup. PET evaluates neck metastases with a sensitivity equal to that of CT but with fewer false-positive results. PET is able to detect a higher percentage of lung metastases than chest radiography, bronchoscopy, or CT is, but the specificity ranges from 50% to 80%, and how to treat a patient with a positive PET and an otherwise negative lung workup is still in question. In approximately 10% of patients, a synchro-

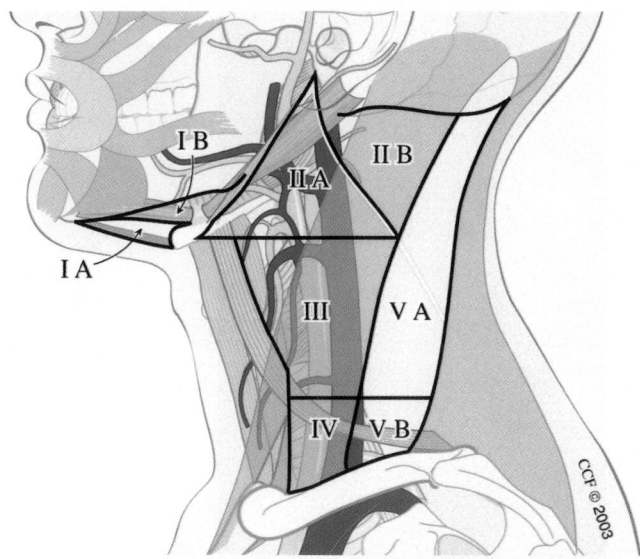

Figure 33-2 Diagram of cervical lymph node levels I through V. Level II is divided into regions A and B by the spinal accessory nerve. (© Cleveland Clinic Foundation, 2003.)

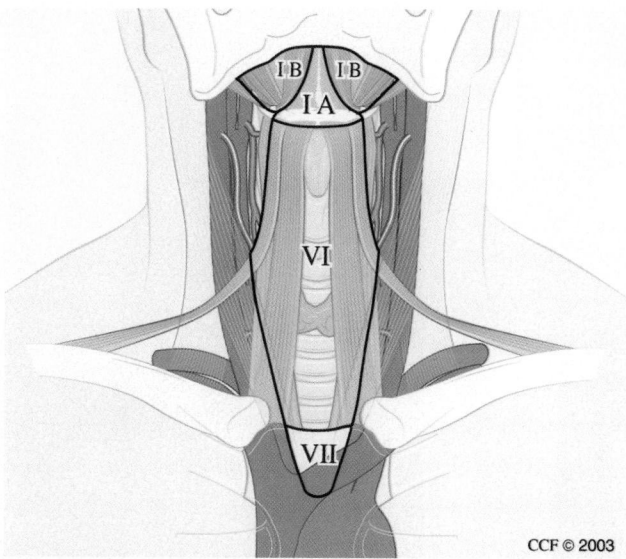

Figure 33-3 Diagram of anterior lymph node levels I, VI, and VII. Though large in area, the majority of level VI lymph nodes are confined to the paratracheal region. (© Cleveland Clinic Foundation, 2003.)

nous second primary cancer is detected in various sites, including the stomach, pancreas, colon, and thyroid.[11] Patients with tumors that demonstrate high uptake on PET have a worse prognosis than do patients with less avid tumors and also have less response to radiation therapy. The exact role of PET in the initial evaluation of HNSCC is still under investigation, and its use is becoming more routine, but it is not within the current standard of care.

Lymphatic Spread

The cervical lymphatic nodal basins contain between 50 and 70 lymph nodes per side and are divided into seven levels (Figs. 33-2 and 33-3).

1. Level I is subdivided.
   - Level IA is bounded by the anterior belly of the digastric muscle, the hyoid bone, and the midline.
   - Level IB is bounded by the anterior and posterior bellies of the digastric muscle and the inferior border of the mandible. Level IB contains the submandibular gland.
2. Level II is bounded superiorly by the skull base, anteriorly by the stylohyoid muscle, inferiorly by a horizontal plane extending posteriorly from the hyoid bone, and posteriorly by the posterior edge of the sternocleidomastoid muscle. Level II is further subdivided.
   - Level IIA is anterior to the spinal accessory nerve.
   - Level IIB, or the so-called submuscular triangle, is posterior to the nerve.
3. Level III begins at the inferior edge of level II and is bounded by the laryngeal strap muscles anteriorly, by the posterior border of the sternocleidomastoid muscle posteriorly, and by a horizontal plane extending posteriorly from the inferior border of the cricoid cartilage.

4. Level IV begins at the inferior border of level III and is bounded anteriorly by the strap muscles, posteriorly by the posterior edge of the sternocleidomastoid muscle, and inferiorly by the clavicle.
5. Level V is posterior to the posterior edge of the sternocleidomastoid muscle, anterior to the trapezius muscle, superior to the clavicle, and inferior to the base of skull (Fig. 33-4).
6. Level VI is bounded by the hyoid bone superiorly, the common carotid arteries laterally, and the sternum inferiorly. Although level VI is large in area, the few lymph nodes that it contains are mostly in the paratracheal regions near the thyroid gland.
7. Level VII (superior mediastinum) lies between the common carotid arteries and is superior to the aortic arch and inferior to the upper border of the sternum.

Lymphatic drainage usually occurs in a superior-to-inferior direction and follows predictable patterns based on the primary site. Primary tumors of the lip and oral cavity generally metastasize to nodes in levels I, II, and III, although skip metastases may occur in lower levels. The upper lip primarily metastasizes ipsilaterally, whereas the lower lip has both ipsilateral and contralateral drainage. Tumors in the oropharynx, hypopharynx, and larynx most commonly metastasize to levels II, III, and IV. Tumors of the nasopharynx spread to the retropharyngeal and parapharyngeal lymph nodes, as well as to levels II through V. Other sites that metastasize to the retropharyngeal lymph nodes are the soft palate, posterior and lateral oropharynx, and hypopharynx. Tumors of the subglottis, thyroid, hypopharynx, and cervical esophagus spread to levels VI and VII. In addition to the lower lip, the supraglottis, base of the tongue, and soft palate have a high incidence of bilateral metastases.

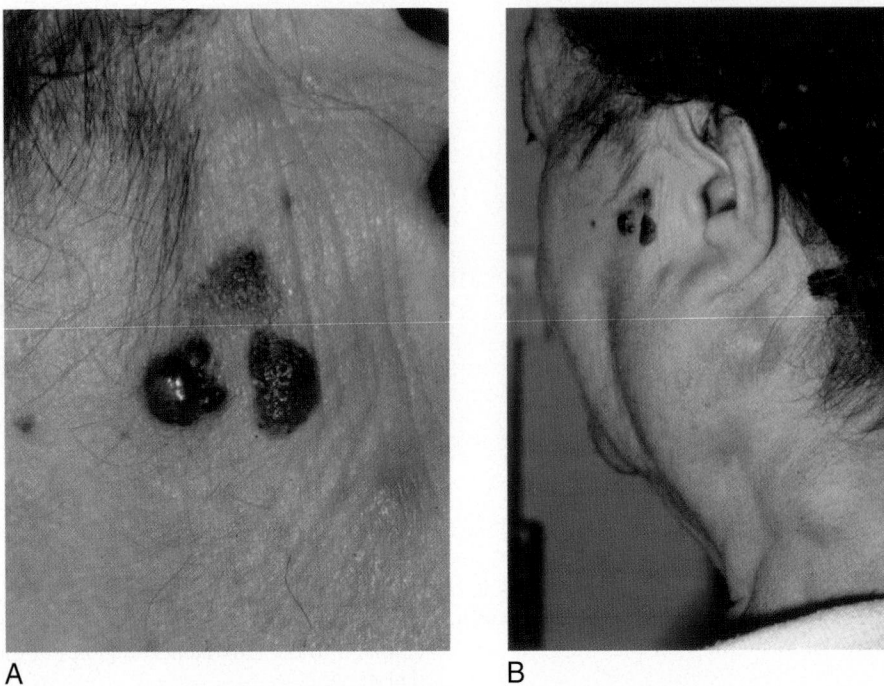

A   B

Figure 33-4 A, Cutaneous melanoma arising in the preauricular area. **B,** Multiple cervical metastases visible in the nodal basins that drain the site of the primary malignancy.

Therapeutic Options

Therapeutic options for patients with HNSCC include surgery, radiation therapy, chemotherapy, and combination regimens. In general, early-stage disease (stage I or II) is treated by either surgery or radiation therapy. Late-stage disease (stage III or IV) is best treated by a combination of either surgery and radiation therapy or chemotherapy and radiation therapy, or all three modalities, depending on the site of the primary. Because surgery was the first therapeutic option available to physicians, it has the longest track record of the three and established the head and neck surgeon as the leader of the treatment team for HNSCC. Photon irradiation is superior to surgery in eradicating microscopic disease and is an excellent alternative to surgery for early lesions. Tonsil, tongue base, and nasopharyngeal primary tumors are especially responsive to photon irradiation. Neutron and proton irradiation is used much less often in the head and neck, although experience is growing with their role in salivary gland malignancies and skull base cancers, respectively. Electrons are not commonly used in the head and neck for noncutaneous tumors. With the advent of intensity-modulated radiation therapy, which is able to reduce the photon dosage to surrounding normal tissue through computer three-dimensional planning, the dogma that patients may not receive greater than 7200 cGy to tissue of the head and neck is being called into question. Hyperfractionation is the practice of administering radiation more than once per day, and recent results of the European Organization for Research and Treatment of Cancer have determined that hyperfractionation for HNSCC produces greater locoregional control than conventional once-a-day regimens do.[12] Radiation therapy is not as effective in treating large-volume, low-grade neoplasms or tumors in close proximity to the mandible because of the risk for osteoradionecrosis. The loss of salivary function with irradiation of the oral and oropharyngeal cavity can be quite disabling to patients, and its impact should not be minimized in the decision-making process.

The most heralded chemotherapy trial for HNSCC was the Veterans Affairs (VA) larynx trial, published in 1991.[13] Although chemotherapy alone is not curative in HNSCC, its role as a radiation sensitizer was established in this study. Two thirds of the patients treated with both radiation therapy and chemotherapy were able to keep their larynx, and survival was equal to that of patients treated with laryngectomy and radiation therapy. Recurrences after radiation therapy have been shown to be multifocal in the bed of the original tumor, and the salvage surgeon should be familiar with the original tumor location and volume. Chemotherapy is commonly used in the treatment of incurable HNSCC, such as unresectable and metastatic disease, and can provide excellent symptom control in these patients.

Recent data from two large-scale, independent trials examined the benefit of adding chemotherapy to postoperative irradiation for HNSCC.[14,15] Both the European Organization for Research and Treatment of Cancer Trial and the Radiation Therapy Oncology Group 9501/Intergroup treated advanced-stage, high-risk patients with cisplatin concurrently with postoperative radiation therapy and compared the outcomes with those of patients undergoing postoperative irradiation alone. In the Radiation Therapy Oncology Group, the 2-year locoregional control rate was 82% for the group receiving chemoradiation therapy versus 72% for the radiation therapy–alone group.

Disease-free survival was significantly longer in the chemoradiation therapy patients, although overall survival was not significantly different between the groups. Not unexpectedly, significantly more toxicity and treatment morbidity were seen in the combined-treatment group, and further prognostic indicators about which patients are at high risk for failure are needed to predict what groups warrant this more intensive adjuvant therapy.

The neck should be treated when there are clinically positive nodes or the risk for occult disease is greater than 20% based on the location and stage of the primary lesion. The decision to perform neck dissection or irradiate the neck is related to treatment of the primary lesion. If the index tumor is being treated with radiation and the neck is N0 (no clinically detectable disease) or N1, the nodes are usually treated with irradiation. For surgically treated primary lesions, N0 or N1 neck disease may be treated surgically as well. Negative prognostic factors such as extracapsular spread of tumor, perineural invasion, vascular invasion, fixation to surrounding structures, and multiple positive nodes are indicators for postoperative adjuvant radiation therapy. For N2 or N3 neck disease, neck dissection with planned postoperative radiation therapy is performed. When chemoradiation therapy protocols are used in treating the primary lesion and there is a complete response in both the primary tumor and an N2 or N3 neck, planned neck dissection 8 weeks after chemoradiation therapy will contain cancer in up to a third of specimens.[16] If the neck mass persists, the percentage of residual disease increases to two thirds. When patients have advanced neck disease that involves the carotid artery or the deep neck musculature, radiation or chemoradiation therapy is given preoperatively in the hope that the tumor reduces in size and becomes resectable. CT scans notoriously carry a high false-positive rate for determining carotid encasement. When carotid resection is necessary, the associated morbidity is high (major neurologic injury in 17%), with a 22% 2-year survival rate, and the decision to resect should be weighed carefully.

Radical neck dissection (RND) was described by Crile in 1906 and was considered the gold standard for removal of nodal metastases. Through close reading of Crile's later surgical notes, it has been revealed that he had begun to modify his surgical technique to remove only selected regions of the neck, depending on the site of the primary tumor. Today, this has become common surgical practice for HNSCC. All modifications of neck dissection are described in relation to the standard RND, which removes nodal levels I through V, the sternocleidomastoid muscle, the internal jugular vein, cranial nerve XI, the cervical plexus, and the submandibular gland. Preservation of the sternocleidomastoid muscle, internal jugular vein, or cranial nerve XI in any combination is referred to as a *modified radical neck dissection* (MRND), and the structures preserved are specified for nomenclature. A modified neck dissection may also be referred to as a Bocca neck dissection after the surgeon who demonstrated that not only is MRND equally as effective in controlling neck disease as RND when structures are preserved that are not directly involved in tumor but the functional out-

comes of patients after MRND are also superior to those after RND.[17] Although resection of the sternocleidomastoid muscle or one internal jugular vein is relatively nonmorbid, loss of cranial nerve XI leaves a denervated trapezius muscle, which can cause a painful chronic frozen shoulder.

Either RND or MRND can be performed for removal of detectable nodal disease. Preservation of any of levels I through V during neck dissection is referred to as *selective neck dissection* (SND) and is based on knowledge of the patterns of spread to neck regions. SND is performed on a clinically negative (N0) neck with preservation of nodal groups carrying less than a 20% chance of being involved with metastatic disease. Regional control has been shown to be as effective after SND as after MRND in patients with a clinically negative neck. Recent studies evaluating treatment of an N0 neck have investigated the use of sentinel lymph node biopsy, which attempts to predict the disease status of the neck based on the first echelon of nodes that drain the tumor. Although sentinel lymph node biopsy has been used extensively with melanoma, its use in HNSCC has come about more gradually. Early results using isosulfan blue dye alone suggested that this technique could not consistently identify the sentinel node in HNSCC. More recent results using a gamma probe have been more encouraging, although there appears to be a learning curve in the ability to identify the node identified as the primary drainage pathway, and sentinel lymph node mapping is not currently considered the standard of care.[18]

ANATOMIC SITES

Lip

Anatomically, the lip is considered a subsite of the oral cavity. The lip begins at the junction of the vermilion border and the skin and is composed of the vermilion surface, which refers to the mucosa that contacts the opposing lip. It is divided into the upper lip, lower lip, and oral commissures. Most lip cancers occur on the lower lip (90%-95%) and less often on the upper lip (2%-7%) and commissures (1%). White men 50 to 80 years of age are the most common group in which lip cancer develops. Sun exposure and pipe smoking are associated with lip cancer. Although SCC is the most common lip cancer (90%), the most common cancer of the upper lip is basal cell carcinoma. Other lip cancers include variants of SCC, such as spindle cell and adenoid squamous carcinoma, as well as malignant melanoma and minor salivary gland cancers.

The most common clinical manifestation of lip cancer is an ulcerative lesion on the vermilion or skin surface. Palpation is necessary to determine the submucosal extent of the lesion and possible fixation to underlying bone. Sensation of the chin should be tested to determine involvement of the mental nerve. Poor prognostic indicators include nerve involvement, fixation to the maxilla or mandible, cancer arising on the upper lip or commissure, positive nodal disease, and age younger than 40 years at diagnosis. The most frequently involved nodal basins are the submental and submandibular levels. A depth of tumor invasion of 4 to 5 mm has been shown to be a cutoff above which the incidence of cervical nodal disease is significantly increased.[19]

Like the rest of the oral cavity, staging of lip cancer is based on size at initial evaluation. Early-stage disease may be treated by surgery or radiation therapy with equal success. Local surgery (wide local excision) with negative margin control of at least 3 mm is the preferred treatment, with supraomohyoid neck dissection performed for tumors with clinically negative necks but deeper primary invasion or size greater than 3 cm. Neck dissection with postoperative radiation therapy for patients with clinically evident neck disease has an acceptable 91% regional control rate in the neck.[20] The overall 5-year cure rate of 90% drops to 50% in the presence of neck metastases. Postoperative irradiation is also indicated for advanced-stage primary disease, tumors with perineural involvement, or close or positive margins at the time of resection.

The goals of lip reconstruction include reinstitution of oral competence, cosmesis, and maintenance of *dynamic* function while allowing adequate access for oral hygiene. Fortunately, the surgeon is able to remove up to half of the lip and still close the defect primarily, particularly defects in the lower lip, which contains more excess tissue than the upper lip. A lower lip wedge excision should not be carried below the mental crease unless the tumor dictates its excision. Care is taken to achieve close approximation of the white line on either side of the defect at the vermilion border because the eye is drawn to any mismatch that exists at this critical aesthetic location.

Defects encompassing between half and two thirds of the lip require augmentation. The Estlander and Abbé flaps are lip switch flaps based on the sublabial or superior labial artery. The Estlander flap is used when the defect involves the commissure, whereas the Abbé flap is used for more midline defects and requires second-stage division of the pedicle (Fig. 33-5). The Karapandžić flap consists of circumoral incisions with circular rotation of the skin flaps while maintaining innervation of the orbicularis oris musculature. This one-stage procedure is used for defects involving more than two thirds of the lip. Microstomia is a potential complication from these types of flap reconstructions, and denture use may not be possible. For defects greater than two thirds, the Webster, Gillies, or Bernard types of repairs may also be used.

Oral Cavity

Because the oral cavity begins at the skin-vermilion junction, the lips are considered part of the oral cavity for staging purposes. Other subsites within the oral cavity include the buccal mucosa, the upper and lower alveolar ridges, the retromolar trigone, the floor of mouth, the hard palate, and the oral tongue. The tongue is divided into the oral tongue (two thirds of the tongue volume), anterior to the circumvallate papillae, and the base of tongue, which is not considered part of the oral cavity but rather the oropharynx. Staging of the oral cavity is based on size: T1, 0 to 2 cm; T2, 2 to 4 cm; T3, 4 to 6 cm; and T4, tumors greater than 6 cm or invading adjacent structures, including bone (cortical bone of the mandible or maxilla, not superficial erosion or tooth sockets), the deep tongue musculature, or facial skin. SCC accounts for 90% of tumors located in these subsites, with a male preponderance in the fifth and sixth decades of life. There is a close association with alcohol and tobacco abuse.

Oral Tongue

The oral tongue begins at the junction between the tongue and the floor of mouth and extends posteriorly to the circumvallate papillae. Tumors appear as exophytic, ulcerative, or submucosal masses that may be associated with tenderness or irritation with mastication. Benign tumors tend to be submucosal and include leiomyomas, neurofibromas, and granular cell tumors. Although granular cell tumors can arise in the larynx, they occur more frequently in the tongue and can be confused with SCC because of overlying pseudoepitheliomatous hyperplasia. Complete excision is curative, but histologic borders are notorious for extending beyond gross disease, and negative intraoperative margins are mandatory.

SCC is by far the most common type of malignancy, but leiomyosarcomas and rhabdomyosarcomas are also encountered rarely. Neurotropic malignancies may involve the lingual or hypoglossal nerves, so tongue deviation or loss of sensation should be examined closely. Treatment of oral tongue cancer is primarily surgical, with wide local excision and negative margin control. The development of cervical metastases is related to the depth of invasion, perineural spread, advanced T stage, and tumor differentiation. Infiltration of more than 4 to 5 mm into the tongue musculature increases the incidence of occult cervical metastases. Metastases from the anterior of the tongue most frequently spread to the submental and submandibular regions. Tumors more posterior often metastasize to levels II and III. Indications for postoperative radiation therapy include evidence of perineural or angiolymphatic spread or positive nodal disease.

Small tumors may be removed by wide local excision and primary closure or closure by secondary intention. Excision of larger tumors requires partial glossectomy or hemiglossectomy. Extirpation may result in significant dysfunction in terms of disarticulation and dysphagia from an inability to contact the palate, sense oral contents, or manipulate the tongue against the alveolus or lips. Reconstructive efforts should focus on maintaining tongue mobility without excess bulk. Split-thickness skin grafts, primary closure, or healing by secondary intention of larger tongue defects often results in tongue tethering. Thin, pliable, fasciocutaneous flaps (e.g., the radial forearm free flap) are the preferred reconstructive technique for such defects. A palatal augmentation prosthesis may assist in maintaining palatal contact, important in both speech and posterior propulsion of food boluses.

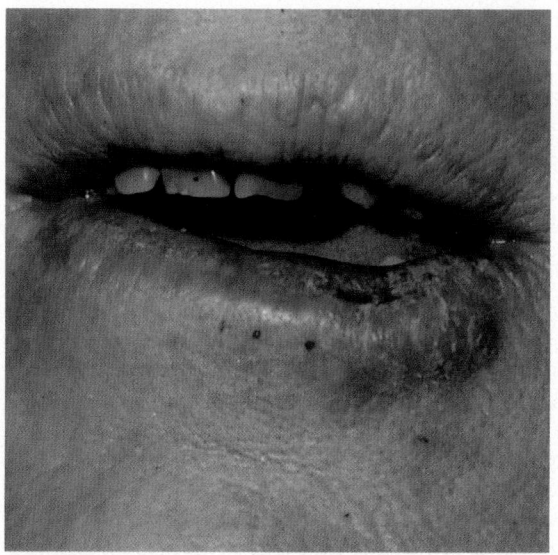

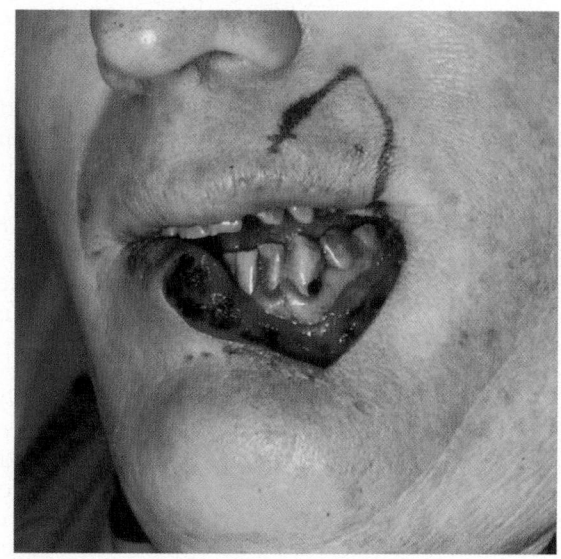

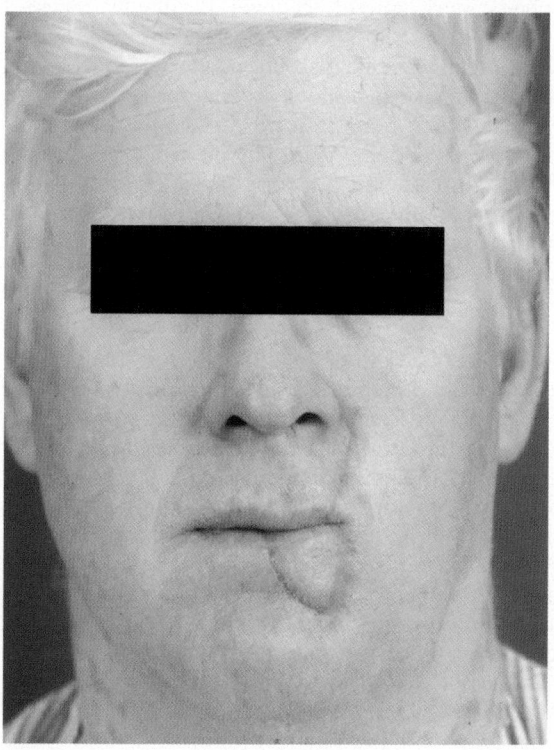

Figure 33-5 A, Squamous cell carcinoma involving the lower lip and encroaching on the oral commissure. **B,** Full-thickness excision and an outlined Estlander flap for reconstruction based on the contralateral superior labial artery. **C,** Reconstructive result 3 months postoperatively.

Floor of the Mouth

The floor of mouth extends from the inner surface of the mandible medially to the ventral surface of the tongue and from the anterior-most frenulum posteriorly to the anterior tonsillar pillars. The mucosa of the floor of the mouth contains the openings of the sublingual gland and submandibular gland (via Wharton's ducts). The muscular floor is composed of the genioglossus, mylohyoid, and hyoglossus muscles, with the lingual nerve located immediately submucosally.

Bimanual palpation can often determine fixation of tumors of the floor of the mouth to the mandible. CT

demonstrates the depth of mandibular bony invasion, and widening of the cranial neural foramen, such as the foramen ovale, suggests neurotropic intracranial spread in advanced tumors. Determining mandibular invasion is of utmost importance in preoperative planning (Fig. 33-6). Invasion into the tongue musculature necessitates partial glossectomy concurrently with removal of the lesion on the floor of the mouth.

Treatment of lesions on the floor of the mouth is primarily surgical, with excision of involved tongue or mandible as necessary to obtain negative margins. Removal of bone with soft tissue in continuity is commonly referred

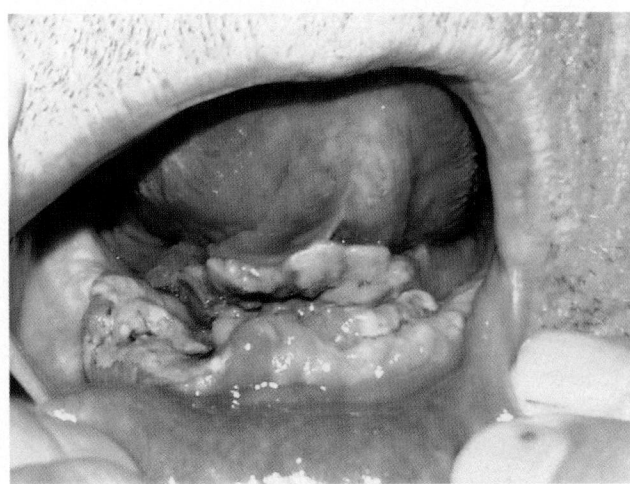

Figure 33-6 A 62-year-old man with squamous cell carcinoma of the anterior floor of mouth invading the mandible.

to as a *commando* or *composite resection*. Involvement of the neck may occur either by direct extension of tumor through the floor of the mouth musculature or by lymphatic spread. The primary lesion and neck specimen should be taken in continuity such that accompanying lymphatic channels are resected. Adjuvant radiation therapy has similar indications as in oral tongue cancers. The primary goal of reconstruction is separation of the oral cavity from the neck by creating a water-tight oral closure. This prevents orocutaneous salivary fistula formation. Secondary goals are maintaining tongue mobility, creating a lingual-alveolar sulcus, and preserving mandibular continuity. Local flaps for soft tissue reconstruction include the platysmal and submental myocutaneous pedicled flaps. Larger defects, including mandibular resection, require complex reconstruction, which is most often performed with free flaps.

Alveolus

The alveolus and its accompanying gingiva constitute the dental surfaces of the maxilla and mandible and extend from the gingivobuccal sulcus laterally to the floor of the mouth and hard palate medially. Posteriorly, the alveolus extends to the pterygopalatine arch and the ascending ramus of the mandible (also referred to as the *retromolar trigone*). Because of the tight attachment between the mucosa and underlying bone, treatment of alveolar SCC often involves treatment of the maxilla or mandible. Seventy percent of gingival carcinomas occur on the lower gum. The periosteum of the mandible is a strong tumor barrier, and tumors that abut the bone may often be resected along with the adjacent periosteum only. Tumors adherent to the periosteum should undergo excision with marginal mandibulectomy, which involves resection of the superior or inner cortical portions of the mandible with preservation of a continuous rim. Even superficial tumors that invade the outermost part of the mandible may be resected with a marginal mandibulectomy, although this is not oncologically sound if the

tumor is a recurrence after radiation therapy. Segmental mandibulectomy entails excision of the full thickness of the mandible, thus interrupting mandibular continuity, and is indicated in patients with gross bone invasion by tumor. Primary radiation therapy for mandibular tumors is not a viable option for treatment because of the high likelihood of osteoradionecrosis and the poor response of involved bone to radiation therapy.

Buccal Mucosa

The buccal mucosa extends from the inner surface of the opposing surfaces of the lips to the alveolar ridges and pterygomandibular raphe. Buccal cancer is uncommon and represents 5% of all oral cavity carcinomas. Smoking, alcohol abuse, lichen planus, dental trauma, snuff dipping, and tobacco chewing are etiologic agents associated with buccal cancer. Approximately 65% of patients with buccal cancer are initially found to have extension beyond the cheek mucosa. Lymphatic drainage is to the submandibular lymph nodes; however, tumors in the posterior aspect of the cheek may spread to level II initially. Stage I cancers have historically been treated by surgery and did not involve elective neck dissection because of the low rate of occult metastases. More recent studies, however, have suggested high rates of local recurrence for lesions treated by surgery alone, and adjuvant radiation therapy has been suggested even for early-stage lesions.[21] Deep invasion may require through-and-through excision of cheek skin, thus necessitating both internal and external lining, usually with a fasciocutaneous free flap.

Palate

The hard palate is defined as the area medial to the maxillary alveolar ridges and extending posterior to the edge of the palatine bone. Chronic inflammatory lesions such as viral lesions, zoster, and pemphigoid can mimic neoplasms, and biopsy is indicated for persistent lesions. Necrotizing sialometaplasia is a benign, self-limited process of the minor salivary glands that has a predilection for the palate and can clinically mimic malignancy. The most common intraoral site for Kaposi's sarcoma is the palate in immunosuppressed patients. Torus palatinus is benign exostosis of the midline hard palate and may require surgery if it interferes with denture wearing.

Minor salivary gland tumors, along with SCC, make up the majority of hard palate tumors. Adenoid cystic carcinoma, mucoepidermoid carcinoma, adenocarcinoma, and polymorphous low-grade adenocarcinoma are common malignancies of salivary gland origin that tend to arise at the junction of the hard and soft palate. Malignancies of the hard palate are treated by local excision if early, but most commonly require resection of bone because of close adherence of the mucosa to the palate. Inferior maxillectomy, subtotal maxillectomy, or total maxillectomy is indicated for progressively destructive tumors extending into the maxillary antrum. Adjuvant radiation therapy is given for advanced lesions. Reconstruction may be accomplished with soft tissue flaps for small defects, obturation with a dental prosthesis for defects with some remaining hard palate, or bony free tissue transfer for extensive palatal resections.

Oropharynx

The borders of the oropharynx include the circumvallate papillae anteriorly, the plane of the superior surface of the soft palate superiorly, the plane of the hyoid bone inferiorly, the pharyngeal constrictors laterally and posteriorly, and the medial aspect of the mandible laterally. The oropharynx includes the base of the tongue, the inferior surface of the soft palate and uvula, the anterior and posterior tonsillar pillars, the glossotonsillar sulci, the pharyngeal tonsils, and the lateral and posterior pharyngeal walls. Similar to the oral cavity, T staging in the oropharynx is dependent on size. T4 tumors may extend out of the oropharynx posteriorly into the parapharyngeal space, inferiorly into the larynx, or laterally into the mandible.

Ninety percent of tumors of the oropharynx are SCC. Other tumors include lymphoma of the tonsils or tongue base or salivary gland neoplasms arising from minor salivary glands in the soft palate or tongue base. Initial symptoms include sore throat, bleeding, dysphagia and odynophagia, referred otalgia, and voice changes, including a muffled quality or hot potato voice. Trismus suggests involvement of the pterygoid musculature. Imaging studies should focus on invasion through the pharyngeal constrictors, bony involvement of the pterygoid plates or mandible, invasion of the parapharyngeal space or carotid artery, involvement of the prevertebral fascia, and extension into the larynx. Lymph node metastases generally occur in the upper jugular chain (levels II-IV), although lesions may skip to lower levels and spread to level V; such lesions are more common with oropharyngeal tumors than with tumors of the oral cavity. Bilateral metastases are more common with tongue base and soft palate lesions, especially those with midline lesions.

Treatment of oropharyngeal SCC has focused increasingly on conservation therapy with chemotherapy and radiation therapy. Many tumors of the oropharynx are poorly differentiated and respond well to radiation. Chemotherapy has been used as a radiation sensitizer in numerous recent studies, and the local control rate achieved has been 90%, even in stage IV disease, although overall survival has not improved over more traditional surgery and radiation therapy.[22] Surgery is necessary for primary disease that involves the mandible and for resectable recurrent disease and has a role in very early, superficial tumors that do not justify a full course of radiation therapy. Extensive surgery of the tongue base significantly alters a patient's ability to swallow. Reconstruction of the tongue with preservation of the larynx requires surgical techniques that maintain tongue mobility and suspend the larynx and neotongue to prevent aspiration.

Resection or contracture after irradiation of the soft palate may result in velopharyngeal insufficiency, which is manifested clinically as nasal regurgitation of liquids and solids and hypernasal speech. Augmentation of the soft palate may be performed surgically or via palatal obturation. Although a palatal obturator requires cleaning and is not permanent, patients are able to remove it for sleep. With surgical augmentation of the palate, a balance between reducing velopharyngeal insufficiency and causing obstructive sleep apnea is difficult to achieve. After tongue base resection, an inferiorly directed palatal obturator assists in achieving the contact at the tongue base that is necessary for projection of food posteriorly during the oral and pharyngeal phases of swallowing.

Hypopharynx

The hypopharynx is the portion of the pharynx that extends inferiorly from the horizontal plane of the top of the hyoid bone to a horizontal plane extending posteriorly from the inferior border of the cricoid cartilage. The hypopharynx includes both piriform sinuses, the lateral and posterior hypopharyngeal walls, and the postcricoid region. The postcricoid area extends inferiorly from the two arytenoid cartilages to the inferior border of the cricoid cartilage, thereby connecting the piriform sinuses and forming the anterior hypopharyngeal wall. The piriform sinuses are inverted, pyramid-shaped potential spaces medial to the thyroid lamina; they begin at the pharyngoepiglottic folds and extend to the cervical esophagus at the inferior border of the cricoid cartilage.

Hypopharyngeal cancer is more common in men 55 to 70 years of age with a history of alcohol abuse and smoking. The exception is in the postcricoid area, in which cancers are more common worldwide in women. This is directly related to Plummer-Vinson syndrome, a combination of dysphagia, hypopharyngeal and esophageal webs, weight loss, and iron deficiency anemia, usually occurring in middle-aged women. In patients who fail to undergo treatment consisting of dilation, iron replacement, and vitamin therapy, postcricoid carcinoma may develop just proximal to the web.

Hypopharyngeal tumors are manifested as a chronic sore throat, dysphagia, referred otalgia, and a foreign body sensation in the throat. A high index of suspicion should be maintained because similar symptoms may be seen with the more common gastroesophageal reflux disease. In advanced disease, hoarseness may develop from direct involvement of the arytenoid, the recurrent laryngeal nerve, or the paraglottic space. The rich lymphatics that drain the hypopharyngeal region contribute to the fact that 70% of patients with hypopharyngeal cancer are initially seen with palpable lymphadenopathy. Patients with hypopharyngeal cancer have the highest rate of synchronous malignancies and the highest rate of development of second HNSCC primaries of any of the head and neck sites. Staging for hypopharyngeal cancer is based on either the number of involved subsites or the size of the tumor.

Physical examination for hypopharyngeal lesions includes fiberoptic endoscopy. Having the patient blow against closed lips and pinching the nose closed will inflate the potential spaces of the piriforms and assist in visualization of the tumor. Palpation of the larynx may demonstrate loss of laryngeal crepitus. A fixed larynx suggests posterior extension into the prevertebral fascia and unresectability. Barium swallow may demonstrate mucosal abnormalities associated with an exophytic tumor and is useful in determining involvement of the cervical esophagus. It also assists in determining the presence and amount of aspiration present. CT can be used to determine the presence of thyroid cartilage invasion, direct extension into the neck, and pathologic lymphadenopathy. Biopsy of the hypopharynx usually requires direct laryngoscopy under general anesthesia.

The most common area for lymphatic spread is the upper jugular nodes, even with inferior tumors. Other regions include the paratracheal and retropharyngeal nodes. The presence of contralateral cervical metastases or level V involvement is a grave prognostic indicator. Treatment of hypopharyngeal cancer yields poor results in comparison to other sites in the head and neck, presumably because of the late stage of the disease at diagnosis. For early lesions confined to the medial wall of the piriform or posterior pharyngeal wall, radiation or chemoradiation therapy is effective as a primary treatment modality. Seldom is laryngeal-sparing partial pharyngectomy possible. Small tumors of the medial piriform wall or pharyngoepiglottic fold may be amenable to conservation surgery, but they must not involve the piriform apex and the patient must have mobile vocal cords and adequate pulmonary reserve.

The most common treatment of hypopharyngeal cancer is laryngopharyngectomy and bilateral neck dissection, including the paratracheal compartments, along with adjuvant radiation therapy. Trials of neoadjuvant chemotherapy followed by concomitant chemotherapy and radiation therapy have shown promise in organ preservation in hypopharyngeal cancer.[23] The estimated 5-year laryngeal preservation rate is 35%, and induction chemotherapy appears to decrease the rate of death from distant metastases.

After total laryngectomy and partial pharyngectomy, primary closure may be possible if at least 4 cm of viable pharyngeal mucosa remains. Primary closure using less than 4 cm of mucosa generally leads to stricture and an inability to swallow effectively. A pedicled cutaneous flap such as a pectoralis myocutaneous flap can be used to augment any remaining mucosa in these cases. When total laryngopharyngectomy with esophagectomy has been performed, a gastric pull-up may be used for reconstruction. More recently, free flap reconstruction with enteric flaps or tubed cutaneous flaps, such as radial forearm or anterolateral thigh flaps, has been used to reconstruct the total pharyngectomy defect.

Larynx

The three-dimensional boundaries of the larynx are complex, and exacting definitions are necessary before understanding pathologic conditions affecting this organ system. The anterior border of the larynx is composed of the lingual surface of the epiglottis, the thyrohyoid membrane, the anterior commissure, and the anterior wall of the subglottis, which consists of the thyroid cartilage, the cricothyroid membrane, and the anterior arch of the cricoid cartilage. The posterior and lateral limits of the larynx are the arytenoids and the interarytenoid region, the aryepiglottic folds, and the posterior wall of

the subglottis, which is composed of the mucosa covering the cricoid cartilage. The superior limits are the tip and lateral borders of the epiglottis. The inferior limit is made up of the plane passing through the inferior edge of the cricoid cartilage.

For staging purposes, the larynx is divided into three regions: the supraglottis, the glottis, and the subglottis. The supraglottis is composed of the epiglottis, the laryngeal surfaces of the aryepiglottic folds, the arytenoids, and the false vocal folds. In addition to these supraglottic subsites, the epiglottis is divided into the suprahyoid and infrahyoid epiglottis, for a total of five supraglottic subsites. The inferior limit of the supraglottis is a horizontal plane through the ventricles, which is the lateral recess between the true and false vocal folds. This plane is also the superior border of the glottis, which is composed of the superior and inferior surfaces of the true vocal folds and extends inferiorly from the true vocal folds 1 cm in thickness. Also included in the glottis are the anterior and posterior commissures. The subglottis extends from the lower border of the glottis to the lower margin of the cricoid cartilage.

Innervation of the larynx includes the superior laryngeal nerve, which supplies the cricothyroid and inferior constrictor muscles and contains afferent sensory fibers from the mucosa of the false vocal folds and piriform sinuses. The recurrent laryngeal nerve supplies motor innervation to all the intrinsic muscles of the larynx, as well as sensation to the mucosa of the true vocal folds, the subglottic region, and the adjacent esophageal mucosa. The normal functions of the larynx are to provide airway patency, protect the tracheobronchial tree from aspiration, provide resistance for Valsalva maneuvers and coughing, and facilitate phonation. Tumors that involve the larynx impair these functions to a variable degree, depending on location, size, and depth of invasion.

Glottic tumors are often manifested early as hoarseness because the vibratory edge of the true vocal fold is normally responsible for the quality of voice and is sensitive to even small lesions. Signs of airway compromise occur later in disease progression when tumor bulk obstructs the glottic opening. Impaired movement of the vocal fold may cause hoarseness, aspiration, impaired cough, or obstructive symptoms. Impaired movement is caused by tumor bulk, direct invasion of the thyroarytenoid muscle, invasion of the cricoarytenoid joint, or invasion of the recurrent nerve. Hemoptysis occurs with hemorrhagic lesions.

When compared with glottic tumors, supraglottic lesions are relatively indolent and are initially seen at a later stage of disease (Fig. 33-7). Patients often complain of sore throat or odynophagia. Referred otalgia is caused by Arnold's nerve, the vagal branch that supplies part of ear sensation. Bulky tumors of the epiglottis are often associated with a hot potato or muffled voice quality because of airway compromise. Dysphagia may cause weight loss and malnutrition. Subglottic tumors are rare and most often manifested as airway obstruction, vocal fold immobility, or pain.

The respiratory and squamous epithelia of the larynx are most often the cause of laryngeal neoplasms, both

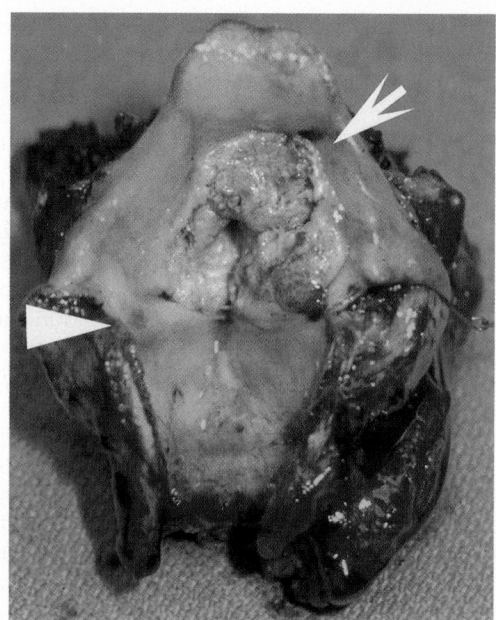

Figure 33-7 A pathologic specimen of supraglottic squamous cell carcinoma. The tumor's epicenter is in the region of the infrahyoid epiglottis and petiole *(arrow)* and is superior to the level of the true vocal folds *(arrowhead).*

and functional impairment. Stroboscopic laryngoscopy can detect subtle impairment of true fold mucosal waves that suggest significant tumor penetration. Direct laryngoscopy under anesthesia allows examination of all laryngeal subsites along with the ability to perform biopsy. Specific sites that are important to examine in supraglottic tumors include the ventricle, anterior commissure, vallecula, base of the tongue, piriform sinus, and the pre-epiglottic space. Key areas of glottic involvement include the false vocal fold, the ventricle, the anterior commissure, the arytenoids, the subglottis, and the posterior commissure or postcricoid mucosa. Under general anesthesia, paralysis of the vocal fold is differentiated from arytenoid fixation by palpation of the vocal process portion of the arytenoid.

CT is routinely performed for laryngeal lesions and images the pre-epiglottic and paraglottic regions and the extent of cartilage involvement, as well as determines direct extension into the deep neck structures. For the natural barriers and pathways of direct tumor spread, the reader is referred to the landmark histopathologic work of Kirchner.[24] CT examination should be performed with contrast agents and thin (1.5-mm) cuts through the larynx. Lymph node metastases are identified on CT as well. The lymphatic drainage of the larynx differs in the supraglottic and glottic regions. Supraglottic epidermoid cancers metastasize early, with up to 50% of lesions having positive nodes. Contralateral and bilateral nodal metastases are common with supraglottic lesions because of the embryologic development of the supraglottis as a midline structure. Lymphatic drainage exits along the course of the superior laryngeal neurovascular pedicle and pierces the thyrohyoid membrane to drain to the subdigastric and superior jugular groups of nodes (levels II and III). Lymphatic drainage of tumors in the glottic and subglottic areas exits via the cricothyroid ligament and drains to the prelaryngeal (Delphian) node, the paratracheal nodes, and the deep cervical nodes in the region of the inferior thyroid artery. Tumors confined to the glottis are only rarely associated with regional disease (4%), and positive nodes, when present, are most often ipsilateral.

Decision making in the treatment of laryngeal cancer is governed by tumor location and characteristics of tumor aggressiveness, as well as the patient's overall constitution and lifestyle. Poor prognostic factors include size, nodal metastasis, perineural invasion, and extracapsular spread. Low-grade epidermoid lesions of the larynx such as dysplasia and carcinoma in situ can be managed with local excision such as microscopic excision of the mucosa. Concurrent denuding of the mucosa of both vocal folds near the anterior commissure can lead to the formation of an anterior web, which reduces voice quality and is a difficult complication to correct. Successful treatment of low-grade lesions includes close follow-up with repeat office or operative laryngoscopy, as well as strict smoking cessation. For invasive disease, multiple treatment options are available, including both conservation surgery and aggressive surgery, radiation therapy, and chemoradiation therapy. In general, conservation of the larynx in early-stage disease is key and can be accomplished with either laryngeal preservation surgery or

benign and malignant. Laryngeal papillomatosis is a benign, exophytic growth of squamous epithelium with a tendency to recur despite surgical excision. It has a bimodal distribution, referred to as the *juvenile type* and the *adult type.* Granular cell tumors are also benign but may be confused with SCC because of a characteristic pseudoepitheliomatous hyperplasia that overlies this subepithelial lesion. Less frequent benign lesions include chondromas and rhabdomyomas. Non-neoplastic lesions of the larynx include vocal fold nodules and polyps, contact ulcers, subglottic stenosis, amyloidosis, and sarcoidosis. Finally, with exposure to carcinogens (tobacco), the epithelium of the larynx may undergo a series of precancerous changes, clinically referred to as *leukoplakia* (any white lesion of the mucosa) or erythroplakia (a red lesion), that consist of either hyperplasia, metaplasia, or variable degrees of dysplasia.

The most common malignant lesion of the larynx is SCC, which is often classified as SCC in situ, microinvasive SCC, or invasive SCC. Spindle cell carcinoma and basaloid SCC are rare and represent more aggressive variants of SCC. Verrucous carcinoma is a highly differentiated variant of SCC that is locally destructive but does not metastasize and should respond to complete surgical excision. The nonepithelial components of the larynx may also undergo malignant transformation leading to tumors of salivary origin such as adenocarcinoma, adenoid cystic carcinoma, and mucoepidermoid carcinoma. Other tumors include neuroendocrine carcinoma, adenosquamous carcinoma, chondrosarcoma, synovial sarcoma, and distant metastases from other organ systems.

The staging system for laryngeal cancers is based on subsite involvement and vocal fold mobility. Office examination includes flexible laryngoscopy to assess location

radiation therapy. Later-stage disease that is still confined to the larynx is more commonly treated by chemoradiation therapy, with total laryngectomy used for salvage.

Laryngeal preservation surgery includes endoscopic surgery with cold steel endoscopic laser resection and open surgery with preservation of some portion of the larynx to maintain the ability to talk. Transoral laser microsurgery, promoted by Steiner and colleagues in Germany, has been used to treat not only all stages of laryngeal cancer but also oropharyngeal and hypopharyngeal tumors. Challenging the dogma that non–en bloc resection of tumors promotes locoregional recurrence, these authors have demonstrated comparable cancer survival while decreasing perioperative morbidity. In supraglottic cancers, this group reported 100% 5-year control rates for T1 and 89% for T2, with excellent functional outcomes, including minimal aspiration and short recovery periods.[25]

In recurrent glottic tumors after failure of radiation therapy, transoral laser microsurgery demonstrated an overall 3-year survival rate of 74%, comparable to that of total laryngectomy.[26] Although laser microsurgery requires significant technical expertise, acceptance of this oncologic technique is increasing and changing the approach to upper aerodigestive tract malignancies.

Open conservation laryngeal surgery entails maintaining a conduit for airflow through the remnant of larynx to permit the ability to talk without aspiration. When deciding whether a patient is a candidate for laryngeal preservation surgery, factors such as pulmonary function and cardiovascular status must be examined because these patients will often have to tolerate some amount of aspiration or airway compromise.

Pulmonary function testing such as spirometry and arterial blood gas analysis is performed preoperatively. An excellent functional test is to have the patient climb two flights of stairs successively without becoming short of breath. The least invasive of the open procedures is open cordectomy, which is indicated for small midfold lesions and for which 100% and 97% 5-year control rates for T1 and T2 lesions, respectively, have been reported.[27] Reconstruction is performed with a false vocal fold flap. For lesions involving the anterior commissure with less than 10 mm of inferior extension, an anterior frontal partial laryngectomy may be performed.

Conservation surgery options for more extensive tumors include vertical partial laryngectomy, supracricoid laryngectomy, and supraglottic laryngectomy. For T1 or T2 glottic lesions, vertical partial laryngectomy plus reconstruction with a false vocal cord pull-down or local muscle flap is indicated, as long as the cartilage is not involved. For T3 lesions not involving the pre-epiglottic space or arytenoid cartilage, supracricoid laryngectomy with cricohyoidopexy or cricohyoidoepiglottopexy is possible (Fig. 33-8). Excellent disease control has been achieved with this technique, largely because of removal of the paraglottic space and thyroid cartilage. Naudo and coworkers have shown that removal of feeding tubes and respiration without a tracheotomy can be achieved in 98% of patients.[28] The standard supraglottic laryngectomy preserves both true vocal folds, both arytenoids, the tongue base, and the hyoid bone (Fig. 33-9). Because there are numerous extensions of this operation in which more than the standard structures are resected, cure rates are difficult to compare, but in general, T1 and T2 local control rates range from 85% to 100%, with decreased control for higher-stage lesions.

If a decision has been made to undergo nonsurgical therapy, the patient must be able to complete the full course of radiation therapy, which usually includes 5 to 7 weeks of continuous daily therapy visits. Previous irradiation is a contraindication to further radiation therapy. Finally, the patient must be reliable in adhering to follow-up for years to come because recurrences may be indolent and difficult to detect.

For neoadjuvant or concurrent chemotherapy, the patient must have sufficient constitutional health to withstand the chemotherapeutic agents. For early laryngeal cancer (T1 or T2), irradiation provides excellent disease control with good to excellent post-therapy voice quality. For professional voice users with early lesions, irradiation is most often the choice of therapy.

The combination of chemotherapy and radiation therapy for advanced-stage disease (stages III and IV) was first brought into the mainstream with the VA larynx trial in 1991.[13] Induction chemotherapy followed by radiation therapy was found to provide 2-year survival equal to that after total laryngectomy with postoperative radiation therapy, in addition to being able to preserve the larynx in 64% of patients. More recently, trials with concurrent chemotherapy and radiation therapy have demonstrated even better local control of advanced laryngeal cancers.

In patients who have disease extending outside the larynx, who fail conservative therapy (although some failures may still be amenable to conservation surgery), or who are not otherwise candidates for organ-preserving strategies, total laryngectomy is still commonly performed. It involves a permanent tracheostoma and loss of the voice with permanent separation of the upper respiratory and digestive tracts.

Patients may experience a period of depression or social withdrawal after becoming aphonic. Speech and swallowing rehabilitation has become an integral part of laryngeal cancer treatment and should begin preoperatively. Speech rehabilitation options include speech with an electrolarynx, esophageal speech, and tracheoesophageal puncture. The electrolarynx is considered the easiest of the three methods to use and consists of a vibratory sound wave generator that is usually placed directly on either the submandibular area or the cheek. The patient mouths words to produce a monotone, electronic-sounding speech. Becoming understandable can take considerable time and patience.

Esophageal speech is produced by swallowing air into the esophagus and expulsing the air back through the pharynx, which vibrates as the air passes. The ability to master esophageal speech takes a motivated patient to be able to control the release of air through the upper esophageal sphincter and occurs in only 20% of laryngectomized patients.

Finally, tracheoesophageal puncture is a surgically created conduit between the tracheal stoma and the

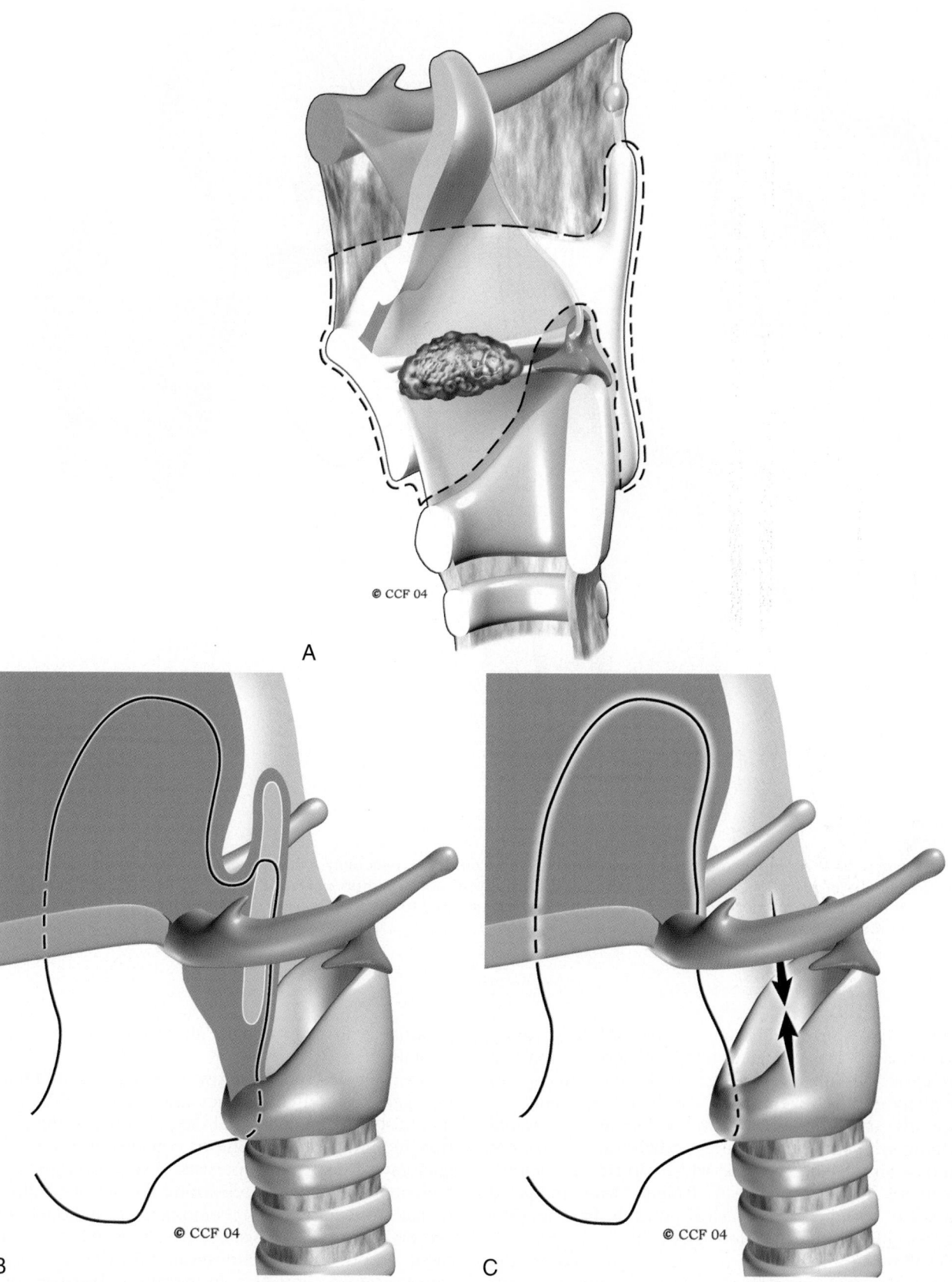

A

B

C

Figure 33-8 A, Lesion of the glottis deemed removable by supracricoid laryngectomy. The *dotted line* demonstrates resection of the true vocal fold to the arytenoid cartilages, including the entire laryngeal cartilage and paraglottic spaces laterally. **B,** Reconstruction by cricohyoidoepiglottopexy with the cricoid cartilage sutured directly to the epiglottic remnant and hyoid bone or **(C)** cricohyoidopexy with the cricoid sutured to the hyoid bone head tongue base directly. (© Cleveland Clinic Foundation, 2004.)

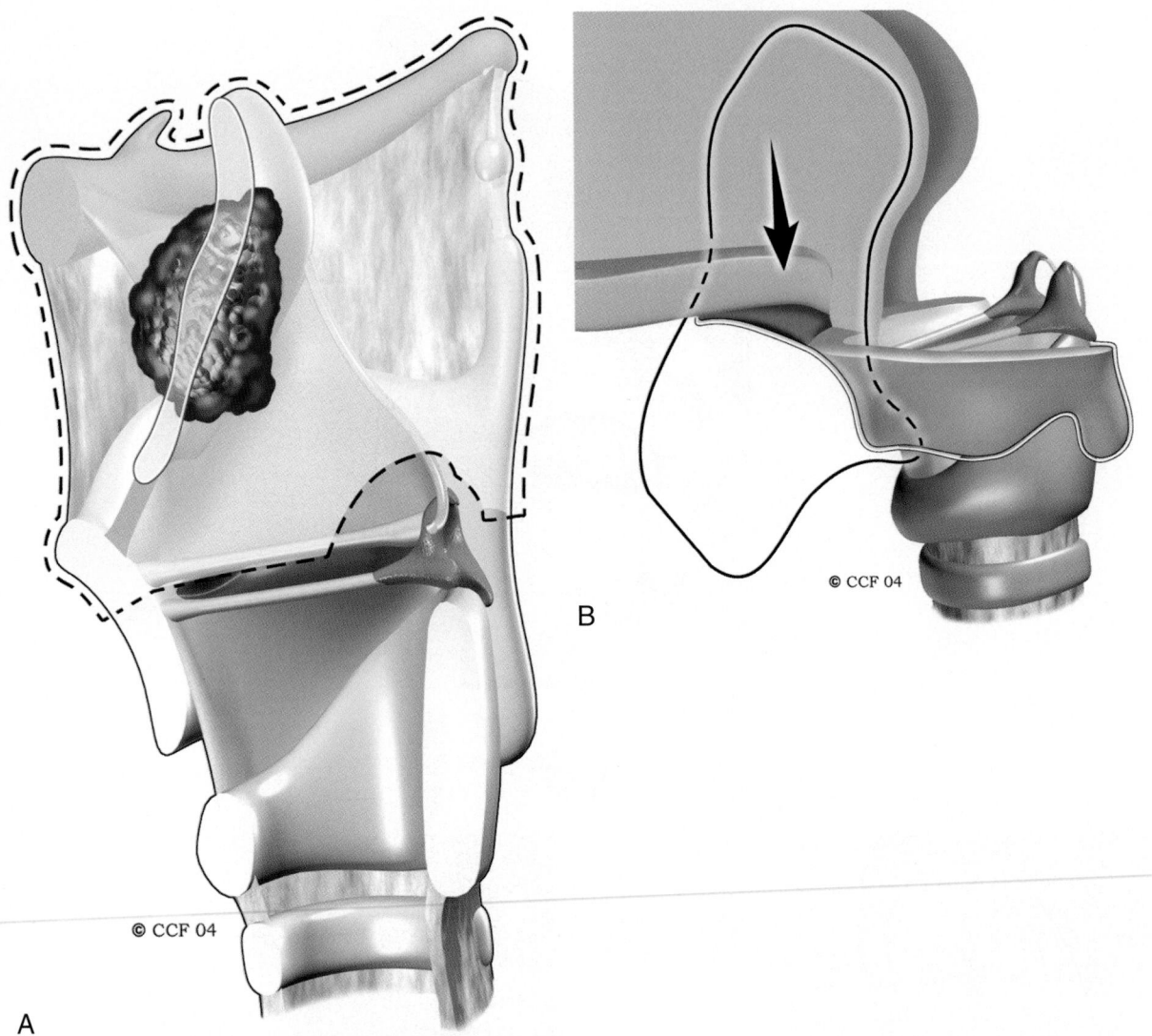

Figure 33-9 A, Supraglottic lesion, resectable by supraglottic laryngectomy, with the *dotted line* demonstrating borders of resection, including the false vocal folds, hyoid bone, and pre-epiglottic space. **B,** Reconstruction of the remaining inferior segment of the thyroid cartilage sutured to the tongue base. (© Cleveland Clinic Foundation, 2004.)

pharynx that is made either at the time of laryngectomy or secondarily. This conduit is fitted with a one-way valve that allows passage of air posteriorly from the trachea to the pharynx but prevents food and liquid from entering anteriorly into the airway. By occluding the stomal opening with the thumb during exhalation, the patient can pass air into the pharynx, which vibrates and allows remarkable clarity of speech. Patients who are good candidates for tracheoesophageal puncture have an 80% success rate of achieving fluent speech.

Swallowing rehabilitation is a second role of the speech therapist in rehabilitating a laryngeal cancer patient, whether treated surgically or nonsurgically. Partial laryngectomy patients may have impaired pharyngeal movement and sensation, impaired vocal fold movement, decreased laryngeal elevation, and decreased subglottic

pressure with poor cough, all contributing to possible aspiration.

Specially designed swallowing maneuvers and training in regard to food consistency are offered by the speech therapist to maintain an oral diet, although some patients may require gastric feeding or conversion to total laryngectomy if aspiration persists. Even laryngectomized patients have difficulty relearning the act of swallowing. Radiation therapy and chemotherapy, although organ preserving, cause fibrosis, decreased sensation and movement, and decreased lubrication, which have a negative impact on swallowing. Furthermore, because of the exposed circumferential ulcerated mucosa of the pharynx that occurs with chemoradiation therapy, pharyngeal stenosis may develop during the recovery phase and necessitate dilation and even pharyngeal augmentation surgery with healthy, nonirradiated tissue. Thus, the speech therapist and surgeon must work as a team to rehabilitate a larynx cancer patient.

Nasal Cavity and Paranasal Sinuses

The nasal cavity consists of the nares, vestibule, septum, lateral nasal wall, and roof. The paranasal sinuses include the frontal sinuses, maxillary sinuses, ethmoid sinuses, and the sphenoid sinus. The lateral nasal wall includes the highly vascular inferior, middle, superior, and occasionally the supreme turbinates, as well as the ostiomeatal complex and nasolacrimal duct and orifice. The frontal sinuses are two asymmetric air cavities within the frontal bone that drain into the nasal cavity via the frontal recesses. The ethmoid sinuses are a complex bony labyrinth directly beneath the anterior cranial fossa. The lamina papyracea is the paper-thin lateral wall of the ethmoid sinus that constitutes the medial wall of the orbit. The anterior ethmoids drain into the middle meatus (inferior to the middle turbinate), whereas the posterior ethmoids drain via the sphenoethmoidal recess. The sphenoid sinus lies in the middle of the sphenoid bone and also drains via the sphenoethmoidal recess. The vital structures of the optic nerves, carotid arteries, and cavernous sinuses are contained within the lateral walls of the sphenoid sinus, whereas the sella turcica and optic chiasm lie superiorly within the roof. The maxillary sinuses drain into the middle meatus and are bound posteriorly by the pterygopalatine and infratemporal fossae.

Tumors of the nasal cavity and paranasal sinuses tend to initially be seen at a late stage because their symptoms are often attributed to more mundane causes. Symptoms include epistaxis, nasal congestion, headache, and facial pain. Orbital involvement produces proptosis, orbital pain, diplopia, epiphora, and even vision loss. Nerve involvement is heralded by numbness in the distribution of the infraorbital nerve. A variety of benign tumors occur in the nasal region. Sinonasal papilloma (or schneiderian papilloma) is classified into three groups:

1. *Septal papillomas* (50%) arise on the septum. They are exophytic and not associated with malignant degeneration.
2. *Inverted papilloma* (47%) and
3. *Cylindrical cell papillomas* (3%) arise on the lateral nasal wall or from the paranasal sinuses and are associated with malignant degeneration (10%-15%), usually into SCC.

Previously thought to call for radical extirpation, sinonasal papillomas require only local surgical excision with negative margins.

Other benign nasal lesions include hemangioma, benign fibrous histiocytoma, fibromatosis, leiomyoma, ameloblastoma, myxoma, hemangiopericytoma (a benign, aggressive lesion with a tendency to metastasize), fibromyxoma, and fibro-osseous and osseous lesions such as fibrous dysplasia, ossifying fibroma, and osteoma. Intracranial tissues may extend into the nasal area and give rise to encephaloceles, meningoceles, and pituitary tumors. CT and MRI demonstrate the intracranial connection, and

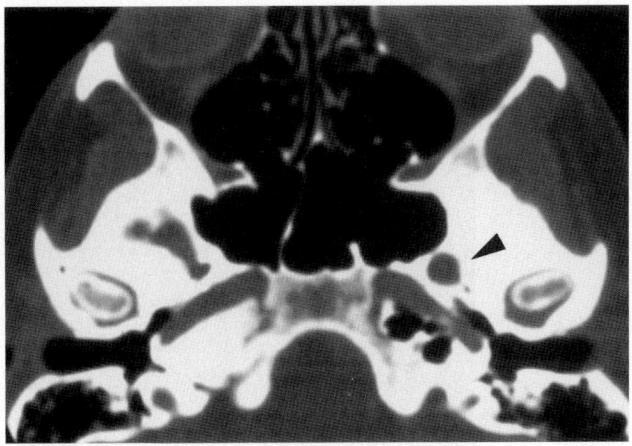

Figure 33-10 A 38-year-old woman with adenoid cystic carcinoma demonstrating perineural spread along V3 and widening of the foramen ovale on CT *(arrowhead).*

biopsy without previous imaging is unwarranted because of the risk for cerebrospinal fluid (CSF) leakage or uncontrollable bleeding from vascular tumors.

Malignancies of the sinonasal tract represent only 1% of all cancers or 3% of upper respiratory tract malignancies and have a 2:1 male-to-female ratio. Because respiratory epithelium can differentiate into squamous or glandular histology, SCC and adenocarcinoma represent two of the most common sinonasal cancers.[29] Sinonasal carcinoma is related to exposure to nickel, Thorotrast, and softwood dust. Chronic exposure to hardwood dust or leatherworking has been associated with adenocarcinoma of the sinonasal tract. Other malignancies include olfactory neuroblastoma, malignant fibrous histiocytoma, midline malignant reticulosis (also known as lethal midline granuloma or polymorphic reticulosis), osteosarcoma, chondrosarcoma, mucosal melanoma, lymphoma, fibrosarcoma, leiomyosarcoma, angiosarcoma, teratocarcinoma, and metastases from other organ systems, especially renal cell carcinoma.

Staging of sinonasal tumors has recently been altered in the 2002 AJCC staging manual. The nasal cavity and ethmoid sinuses are now considered separate primary sites in addition to the maxillary sinus. The staging system is only for carcinomatous malignancies and does not include the frontal or sphenoid sinuses as separate sites because of the rarity of tumors arising in these sites. Staging is partly dependent on local spread of tumor. Ohngren's line extends from the medial canthus to the mandibular angle. Maxillary tumors superior to Ohngren's line have a poorer prognosis than do those inferior to the line because of the proximity to the orbit and cranial cavity. Local spread of tumors may occur along nerves or vessels or directly through bone. Advanced tumors of the maxillary sinuses commonly involve the pterygopalatine and infratemporal fossae. Widening of the foramen rotundum (V2) or foramen ovale (V3) on imaging suggests neural spread with intracranial involvement (Fig. 33-10). Because olfactory neuroblastomas are thought to arise from the olfactory neuroepithelium, these tumors commonly involve the cribriform plate and spread intra-

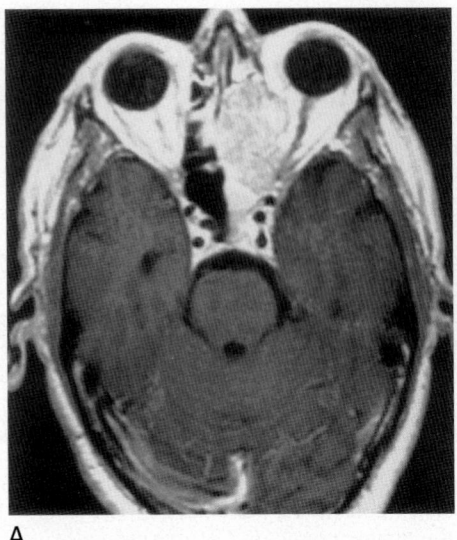
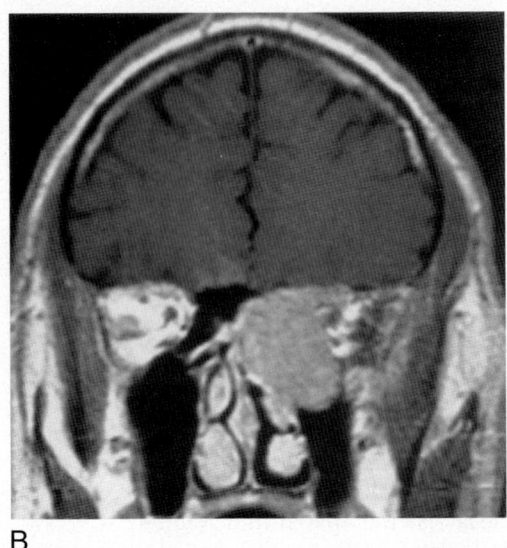

Figure 33-11 A, Axial MRI of a patient with adenosquamous carcinoma of the ethmoids involving the orbital fat. Orbital exenteration was necessary. **B,** Coronal MRI of the same patient demonstrating tumor extension to the floor of the anterior cranial fossa.

cranially toward the frontal lobes. Sphenoidal tumors may include extension to the cavernous sinuses, carotid arteries, optic nerves, or the ophthalmic or maxillary branches of the trigeminal nerves. Lymph node metastases are in general uncommon (15%), and elective neck dissection or irradiation of a clinically negative neck is most often unwarranted. Involved nodal groups include the retropharyngeal, parapharyngeal, submental, and upper jugulodigastric nodes.

The standard treatment of sinonasal malignancies is surgical resection, with postoperative radiation or chemoradiation therapy used for high-grade histology or advanced local disease. Because these cancers can involve the dentition, orbits, or brain, treatment requires a multidisciplinary team, including a head and neck surgeon, neurosurgeon, ophthalmologist, prosthodontist, oral surgeon, and reconstructive surgeon. After a preoperative workup consisting of imaging, endoscopy, and biopsy, a tumor map and operative plan are formulated. Vascular tumors are embolized by an interventional radiologist, preferably within 24 hours of surgery. Patients with tumors requiring skull base exploration may need a lumbar drain to decompress the dura from the cranium and reduce the risk for postoperative CSF leakage. Routine prophylactic use of tracheotomies for craniofacial surgery to reduce the risk for postoperative pneumocephalus is controversial.

Low-grade tumors limited to the lateral nasal wall, ethmoid sinuses, or septum are increasingly being removed with endoscopic techniques. A lateral rhinotomy incision is the classic open approach for a medial maxillectomy and entails removal of the lateral nasal wall. If the tumor involves the inferior maxilla, an inferior maxillectomy, including removal of the hard palate and the medial, lateral, and posterior maxillary sinus walls, is performed. For tumors more superior in the maxillary sinus, a total maxillectomy, including excision of the roof, is performed. If the bone of the floor of the orbit is involved, removal with postoperative reconstruction is indicated. If the orbital periosteum is involved with tumor, it may be resected with preservation of the orbit, although more extensive involvement of fat or muscle necessitates orbital exenteration (Fig. 33-11).[30]

If the anterior cranial floor is involved with tumor, as it often is in olfactory neuroblastomas, craniofacial resection is indicated. This procedure combines a craniotomy approach with a transfacial approach. Surgical disruption of the cribriform region causes postoperative anosmia. Reconstruction of the anterior cranial fossa requires separation of the cranial vault from the nasal cavity with either a pericranial flap, temporoparietal fascial flap, fascia lata free graft, or, when extensive resection has been performed, a microvascular free flap.[31] Unresectable lesions include those with brain involvement, carotid artery encasement, or bilateral optic nerve involvement.

Radiation therapy and chemotherapy for sinonasal malignancies are being used with increasing frequency. Sinonasal undifferentiated carcinoma, rhabdomyosarcoma, and midline reticulocytosis are examples of aggressive cancers in which neoadjuvant chemotherapy and radiation therapy play an integral role. Combining chemotherapy with radiation therapy and surgery for treatment of advanced sinonasal SCC has met with variable success.

Nasopharynx

The nasopharynx begins at the posterior nasal choana and ends at the horizontal plane between the posterior edge of the hard palate and the posterior pharyngeal wall. The nasopharynx includes the vault; the lateral walls, which contain the eustachian tube orifices and the fossae of Rosenmüller; the roof, which is made up of the sphenoid rostrum; and the posterior wall, which consists of the basiocciput or clivus. Both malignant and benign tumors of the nasopharynx are usually related to the normal histology, which includes squamous and respiratory epithelium; the lymphoid tissues of the adenoids; and deeper tissues, including fascia, cartilage, bone, and muscle. Benign tumors of the nasopharynx are rare and include fibromyxomatous polyps, papillomas, teratomas, and pedunculated fibromas. Angiofibroma, a benign tumor that affects young males, is the most common benign tumor of the nasopharynx. Rathke's pouch cysts arise high in the nasopharynx at the sphenovomerian junction. The cyst develops from a remnant of ectoderm that normally invaginates to form the anterior pituitary and may become infected later in life. Thornwaldt's bursa is located more inferiorly and arises from a remnant of the caudal notochord; it can contain a jelly-like material. It too may become infected in later life, and marsupialization is most often all that is required to treat both it and Rathke's pouch cysts. Craniopharyngiomas, extracranial meningiomas, encephaloceles, hemangiomas, paragangliomas, chordomas (which can cause extensive destruction), and antral-choanal polyps can also be seen in the nasopharynx.

The clinical findings in patients with nasopharyngeal tumors include symptoms of nasal obstruction, serous otitis with effusion and associated conductive hearing loss, epistaxis, and nasal drainage. Findings such as a cervical mass, headache, otalgia, trismus, and cranial nerve involvement suggest malignancy. Examination of the nasopharynx was historically performed with a mirror and has greatly been improved with the use of either rigid or flexible nasopharyngoscopes in the office. CT scanning is excellent for determining bony destruction and widening of foramina. MRI is used to assess soft tissue involvement and intracranial extension, as well as nerve, cavernous sinus, and carotid involvement.

Angiofibromas are vascular lesions found exclusively in males, usually develop during puberty, and are commonly referred to as *juvenile nasopharyngeal angiofibromas*. Although they are benign tumors, angiofibromas often erode bone and cause significant structural and functional dysfunction, as well as bleeding. CT findings of a nasopharyngeal mass, anterior bowing of the posterior wall of the antrum, erosion of the sphenoid bone, erosion of the hard palate, erosion of the medial wall of the maxillary sinus, and displacement of the nasal septum in an adolescent male are highly suggestive of angiofibroma (Fig. 33-12). Surgery after embolization is the primary treatment modality, and understanding the location of origin is critical for complete tumor extirpation. Tumors originate at the posterolateral wall of the roof of the nasal cavity, at the sphenopalatine foramen. Whether performed endoscopically or via an open approach such as lateral rhinotomy or the Caldwell-Luc operation, complete removal of all tumor and bone in the sphenopalatine region is crucial to decrease the possibility of recurrence. Radiation has been successfully used as treatment of these tumors but, given the young age at diagnosis and the lifelong risks associated with radiation exposure, is usually reserved for unresectable angiofibromas and recurrences.

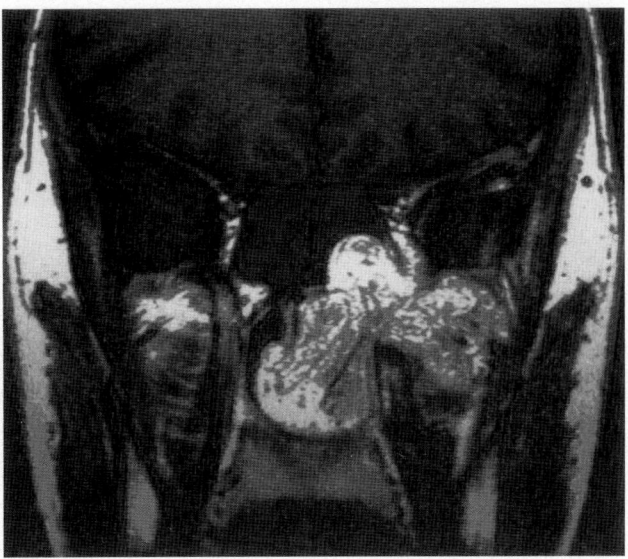

Figure 33-12 MRI of a 16-year-old boy with a left-sided juvenile angiofibroma. The tumor arises in the pterygomaxillary region and has extended into the nasopharynx and infratemporal fossa.

Possible malignancies include nasopharyngeal carcinoma, low-grade nasopharyngeal papillary adenocarcinoma, lymphoma, rhabdomyosarcoma, malignant schwannoma, liposarcoma, and aggressive chordoma. The staging system of malignant tumors of the nasopharynx is for epithelial tumors only and is based on confinement to the nasopharynx or spread to surrounding structures. Although nasopharyngeal carcinoma accounts for only 0.25% of all cancers in North America, it represents approximately 18% of all malignancies in China. There is a strong correlation with Epstein-Barr virus, which has been demonstrated in all histologic subtypes of nasopharyngeal carcinoma.[32] The World Health Organization has divided nasopharyngeal carcinoma into three histologic variants—keratinizing (25%), nonkeratinizing (15%), and undifferentiated (60%)—although more recent classifications combine nonkeratinizing and undifferentiated tumors. The most common initial sign is neck node metastases, especially to the posterior cervical triangle, and inferiorly positioned positive nodes predict poor outcomes. Treatment is based on radiation therapy both to the primary site and bilaterally in the neck. With the addition of cisplatin and 5-fluorouracil, the rate of distant metastases decreases and both disease-free and overall survival increases.[33] Intracavitary irradiation is used to provide a boost at the primary site for advanced tumors and is used in cases of re-irradiation. Surgery is reserved for persistent neck disease or for selected cases of local recurrence. It is unique that the risk for recurrence with nonkeratinizing and undifferentiated carcinoma appears to be chronic and does not level off at 5 years as it does with most other cancers. Rhabdomyosarcoma is the most frequent soft tissue sarcoma in the pediatric population and is the most common sarcoma occurring in the head and neck. Excluding the orbit, the most common site in the head and neck is the nasopharynx. Treatment is

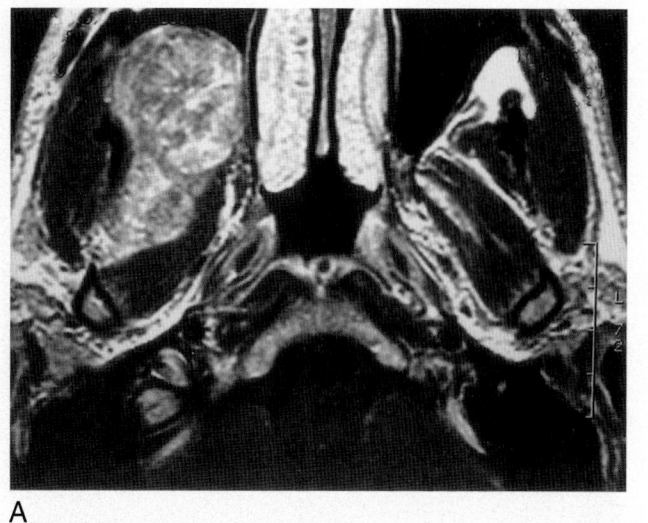

A

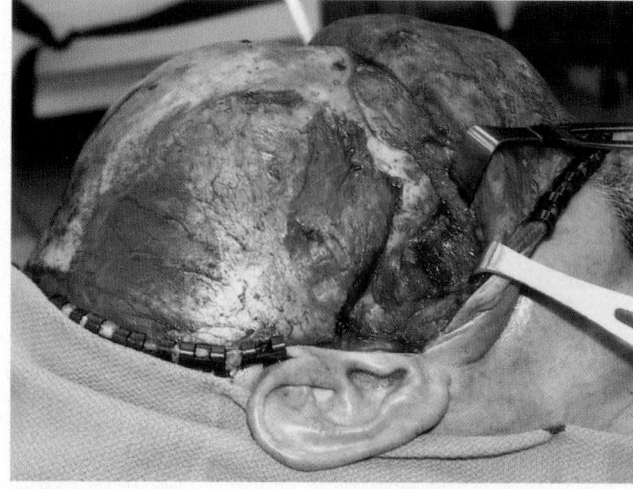

B

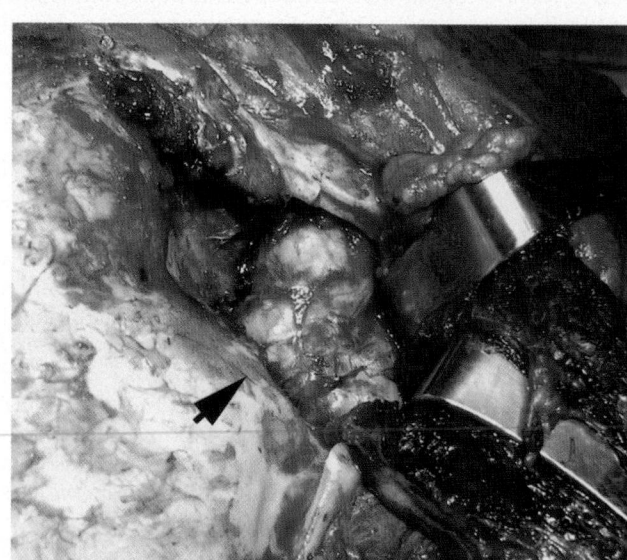

C

Figure 33-13 A, MRI of a 60-year-old man with a right-sided neuroma of V3 extending into the infratemporal fossa and parapharyngeal space. **B,** A bicoronal incision with a transzygomatic approach is used to access the tumor **(C),** which is visualized (after reflecting the temporalis muscle) emanating from the foramen ovale region *(arrow).*

based on multimodality therapy consisting of nonradical surgery and radiotherapy plus multiagent chemotherapy.

Although surgery of the nasopharynx is used primarily for benign pathologies, multiple approaches have been described, both endoscopic and open, to the surrounding skull base region. Little has been reported regarding the use of endoscopic removal of nasopharyngeal and medial skull base neoplasms.[34] Endoscopic techniques not only avoid facial incisions but also allow shorter hospital stays. The most commonly described tumor removed via transnasal techniques is an inverting papilloma, which is excised in piecemeal fashion. Success has also been reported with the endoscopic removal of mucoceles. Numerous open surgical approaches have been described to obtain access to the central skull base. For tumors of the nasopharynx, the transpalatal approach offers excellent visualization. The transfacial approach of lateral rhinotomy with unilateral or bilateral medial maxillectomy creates a facial incision but offers greater lateral expo-

sure. The midfacial degloving procedure allows excellent bilateral exposure of the maxillae, paranasal sinuses, and the nasopharynx without facial incisions. The posterior wall of the maxillary sinus may be removed to allow access to the pterygomaxillary fossa and deeper infratemporal fossa. For disease located more laterally, the transmastoid, transcochlear, and translabyrinthine approaches described by Fisch are used alone or in combination with more anterior approaches. More extensive approaches include the lateral facial split and mandibular swing, the frontal-orbital or frontal-orbital-zygomatic approach, and the maxillary swing, and for disease of the high nasopharynx, the subfrontal approach affords excellent medial exposure (Fig. 33-13).

Pituitary Surgery

Although neurosurgery maintains the discipline responsible for the comprehensive management of hypophyseal disease, a recent collaboration between otolaryngologists with endoscopic sinus surgery skills and neurosurgeons has resulted in the development of minimally invasive pituitary surgery. The endoscopic transnasal transsphenoidal approach provides excellent visualization of the operative field and avoids intraoral or anterior nasal incisions, nasal packing, and postoperative complications such as septal deviation and lip anesthesia. Length of hospital stay, use of lumbar drains, and the need for nasal packing have been demonstrated to be significantly reduced with minimally invasive pituitary surgery as compared with open traditional approaches.[34] Reconstruction of the sella by minimally invasive endoscopic repair has demonstrated that normal sphenoidal function can be maintained while obtaining excellent results in terms of a low incidence of CSF leakage and harvest site morbidity (Fig. 33-14).[35]

Ear and Temporal Bone

When referring to tumors of the ear, the structures commonly involved include the external ear, the middle ear, and the inner ear. The external ear consists of the auricle or pinna and the external auditory canal to the tympanic membrane. The middle ear contains the tympanic cavity proper, the ossicles, the eustachian tube, the epitympanic recess, and the mastoid cavity. The borders of the middle ear include the tympanic membrane and the squamous portion of the temporal bone laterally, the petrous temporal bone medially, the tegmen tympani or roof superiorly, the carotid canal anteriorly, the mastoid posteriorly, and the floor of the tympanic bone inferiorly. The inner ear is contained within the petrous portion of the temporal bone and consists of the membranous and osseous labyrinth and the internal auditory canal.

Evaluation of ear and temporal bone neoplasms requires appropriate physical examination and audiologic and vestibular testing, as well as radiologic assessment. Findings of hearing loss, vertigo, eustachian tube dysfunction with serous otitis media, cranial nerve deficits, pulsatile tinnitus, drainage, and deep boring pain are often associated with tumors and must be thoroughly evaluated. CT plays a crucial role in evaluating the temporal bone because of the complex anatomy contained within bony confines. MRI with gadolinium contrast is complementary and used to define soft tissue anatomy (Fig. 33-15).

Neoplasms of the pinna are most often related to sun exposure and include basal cell carcinoma and SCC. Keratoacanthoma is a benign tumor characterized by rapid growth and spontaneous involution and may be confused with SCC. In the external auditory canal, ceruminal gland adenocarcinomas, adenoid cystic carcinoma, and atypical fibroxanthomas may arise. Within the temporal bone, benign neoplasms include adenoma, paraganglioma (both at the tympanic membrane and at the jugular bulb), acoustic neuroma, and meningioma. SCC is the most common cancer of the temporal bone; others include adenocarcinoma of either middle ear or endolymphatic sac origin. In the pediatric population, soft tissue sarcomas such as rhabdomyosarcoma predomi-

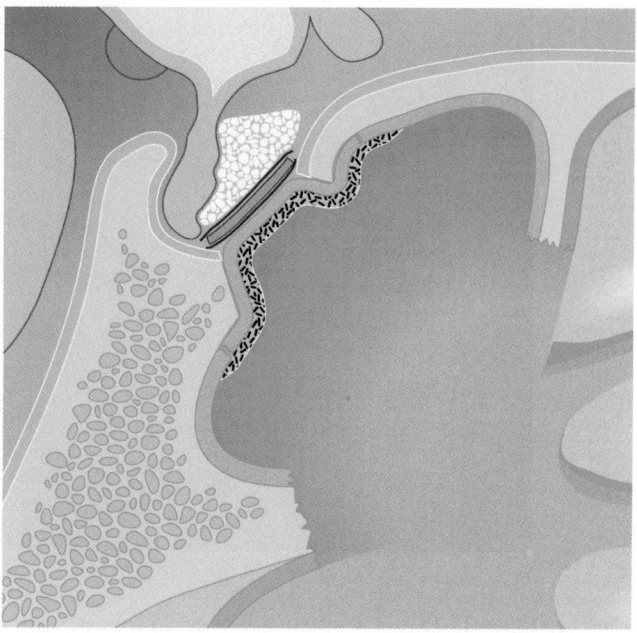

Figure 33-14 After endoscopically opening the sphenoid sinus in the minimally invasive hypophysectomy technique and resecting the pituitary tumor, sellar reconstruction is performed in layered fashion. The sellar defect is partially filled with Gelfoam or fat, followed by layers of acellular human dermis, cartilage, acellular human dermis, mucosa, and fibrin glue. (With permission, from Lorenz RR, Dean RL, Chuang J, Citardi MJ: Endoscopic reconstruction of anterior and middle cranial fossa defects using acellular dermal allograft. *Laryngoscope* 113:496-501, 2003.)

nate. Metastases are an under-recognized cause of petrous bone tumors.

Malignancies of the pinna are treated similarly to skin cancers elsewhere on the face. Mohs microsurgery with frozen section control of margins minimizes the amount of normal tissue resected with the cutaneous malignancy. Involvement of underlying cartilage leads to more disseminated growth necessitating partial or total auriculectomy. If the extent of disease is great, lateral temporal bone resection may be indicated with attempted preservation of the facial nerve and inner ear. When the facial nerve or parotid gland is involved, lateral temporal bone resection with parotidectomy is performed. Radiation therapy may be used uncommonly for primary treatment or more commonly for adjuvant treatment in the case of perineural spread or poorly differentiated tumors.

Treatment of tumors involving the middle ear and bony canal consists of en bloc resection of structures at risk for involvement. Rarely, when the tumor involves only the external canal without bony destruction, sleeve resection of the canal can be performed. Lateral temporal bone resection removes the bony and cartilaginous canal, tympanic membrane, and ossicles. Subtotal temporal bone resection involves removal of the ear canal, middle ear, petrous bone, temporomandibular joint, and facial nerve. Involvement of the petrous apex necessitates total temporal bone resection with removal of the carotid artery. SCC within the petrous apex is considered incur-

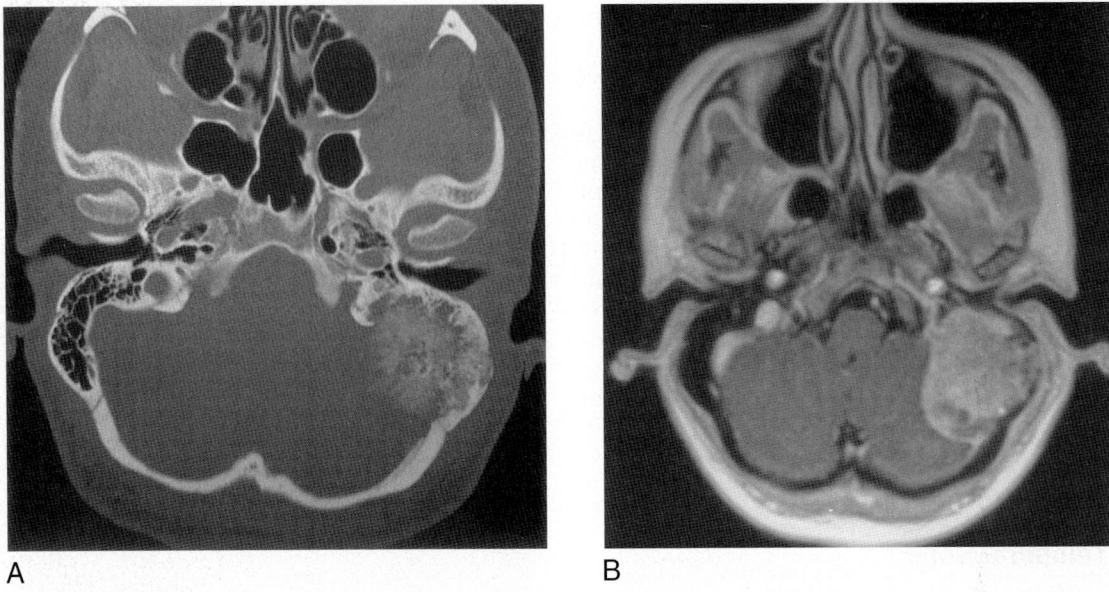

Figure 33-15 **A,** CT scan of a 19-year-old woman with osteosarcoma of the left temporal bone and bony destruction of the mastoid. **B,** MRI is useful in determining the extent of the tumor and the lack of brain invasion.

able, although adenoid cystic carcinoma and select low-grade sarcomas may be excised with total temporal bone resection. The goals of reconstruction of temporal bone defects are protection from CSF leaks and coverage of vital structures and remaining bone to prepare for postoperative radiation therapy. Facial nerve rehabilitation is covered in salivary gland malignancies. Pedicled myocutaneous flaps, such as the lower trapezius flap, have been used to accomplish these goals and provide bulk to restore some cosmesis to the area.[36] A prosthetic ear provides acceptable rehabilitation when total auriculectomy has been performed.

Salivary Gland Neoplasms

The major salivary glands include the parotid glands, the submandibular glands, and the sublingual glands. There are also approximately 750 minor salivary glands scattered throughout the submucosa of the oral cavity, oropharynx, hypopharynx, larynx, parapharyngeal space, and nasopharynx. Salivary gland neoplasms are rare and constitute 3% to 4% of head and neck neoplasms. The majority of neoplasms arise in the parotid gland (70%), whereas tumors of the submandibular gland (22%) and sublingual and minor salivary glands (8%) are less common. The ratio of malignant to benign tumors varies by site as well: parotid gland, 80% benign and 20% malignant; submandibular gland and sublingual gland, 50% benign and 50% malignant; and minor salivary glands, 25% benign and 75% malignant.

The parotid gland is the largest salivary gland and is divided into the superficial lobe and deep lobe by the facial nerve. On imaging, the lobes can be differentiated by the retromandibular vein, which is commonly found at the division of the lobes. Deep lobe tumors lie within

the parapharyngeal space. Stensen's duct is approximately 5 cm long; it pierces the buccal fat pad and opens in the oral cavity opposite the second maxillary molar. The submandibular glands are closely associated with the lingual nerve in the submandibular triangle and empty via Wharton's duct into the papilla just lateral to the frenulum. The sublingual gland lies on the inner table of the mandible and secretes via tiny openings (ducts of Rivinus) directly into the floor of the mouth or via several ducts that unite to form the common sublingual duct (Bartholin), which then merges with Wharton's duct.

Numerous non-neoplastic diseases commonly affect the salivary glands. Sialadenitis is an acute, subacute, or chronic inflammation of a salivary gland. Acute sialadenitis commonly affects the parotid and submandibular glands and can be caused by bacterial (most frequently *Staphylococcus aureus*) or viral (mumps) infection. Chronic sialadenitis results from granulomatous inflammation of the glands and is commonly associated with sarcoidosis, actinomycosis, tuberculosis, and cat-scratch disease. Sialolithiasis is the accumulation of obstructive calcifications within the glandular ductal system, more common in the submandibular gland (90%) than the parotid (10%). When the calculi become obstructive, stasis of saliva may cause infection and create a painful, acutely swollen gland. Benign lymphoepithelial lesions of the salivary glands are non-neoplastic glandular enlargements associated with autoimmune diseases such as Sjögren's syndrome.

Salivary gland neoplasms are most often manifested as slow-growing, well-circumscribed masses. Symptoms such as pain, rapid growth, nerve weakness, and paresthesias and signs of cervical lymphadenopathy and fixation to skin or underlying muscles suggest malignancy. When the initial symptom is complete unilateral facial paralysis, Bell's palsy may be misdiagnosed as the cause, and it is important to remember that all patients with Bell's palsy will show some improvement in facial movement within 6 months of the onset of weakness. Trismus is associated with involvement of the pterygoid musculature by deep parotid lobe malignancies. Bimanual palpation of submandibular masses assists in determining fixation to surrounding structures. CT and MRI tend to show irregular tumor borders and obliteration of fat planes in the parapharyngeal space with deep parotid lobe cancers. The accuracy of fine-needle aspiration cytology of the salivary glands has been well established. The sensitivity, specificity, and accuracy of parotid gland aspirates in one series were 92%, 100%, and 98%, respectively.[37] Excision of the gland is used to confirm the final diagnosis.

Benign tumors of the salivary glands include pleomorphic adenomas, a variety of monomorphic adenomas (including Warthins's tumors, oncocytomas, basal cell adenomas, canalicular adenomas, and myoepitheliomas), a variety of ductal papillomas, and capillary hemangiomas. Pleomorphic adenomas account for 40% to 70% of all tumors of the salivary glands and most commonly occur in the tail of the parotid. Like all benign parotid tumors, the treatment of choice is surgical excision with a margin of normal tissue (e.g., superficial parotidectomy). In the parotid gland, if excision is possible without complete removal of the affected lobe, the postoperative cosmetic appearance will be superior to that in patients in whom a complete lobe is removed. Shelling out of pleomorphic adenomas is to be avoided because it has been shown to correlate with increased rates of recurrence.[38] The facial nerve should not be sacrificed when removing a benign lesion (Fig. 33-16). Warthin's tumor, or papillary cystadenoma lymphomatosum, is the second most common benign parotid tumor and occurs most often in older white men. Because of the high mitochondrial content within oncocytes, the oncocyte-rich Warthin tumor and oncocytomas will incorporate technetium Tc 99m and appear as hot spots on radionuclide scans. If fine-needle aspiration suggests a slow-growing Warthin tumor with confirmatory technetium scanning in a patient with contraindications to surgery, the tumor may be closely monitored because it has no malignant potential.

Malignant salivary tumors are staged according to size: T1 is less than 2 cm, T2 is 2 to 4 cm, T3 is greater than 4 cm or any tumor with macroscopic extraparenchymal extension, and T4 involves invasion of surrounding tissues. Malignant salivary tumors are listed in Box 33-1. Mucoepidermoid carcinoma is the most common malignant tumor of the parotid gland and can be divided into low-grade and high-grade tumors. High-grade lesions have a propensity for both regional and distant metastases and corresponding shorter survival rates than low-grade mucoepidermoid carcinomas. Adenoid cystic carcinoma constitutes 10% of all salivary neoplasms, with two thirds occurring in the minor salivary glands. The histologic types of adenoid cystic carcinoma are tubular, cribriform, and solid, listed from best prognosis to worst.

Box 33-1 Tumors of the Major and Minor Salivary Glands

Benign

Pleomorphic adenoma
Warthin's tumor
Capillary hemangioma
Oncocytoma
Basal cell adenoma
Canalicular adenoma
Myoepithelioma
Sialadenoma papilliferum
Intraductal papilloma
Inverted ductal papilloma

Malignant

Acinic cell carcinoma
Mucoepidermoid carcinoma
Adenoid cystic carcinoma
Polymorphous low-grade adenocarcinoma
Epithelial-myoepithelial carcinoma
Basal cell adenocarcinoma
Sebaceous carcinoma
Papillary cystadenocarcinoma
Mucinous adenocarcinoma
Oncocytic carcinoma
Salivary duct carcinoma
Adenocarcinoma
Myoepithelial carcinoma
Malignant mixed tumor
Squamous cell carcinoma
Small cell carcinoma
Lymphoma
Metastatic carcinoma
Carcinoma ex pleomorphic adenoma

An indolent growth pattern and a relentless propensity for perineural invasion characterize adenoid cystic carcinoma. Regional lymphatic spread is uncommon, although distant metastases occur within the first 5 years after diagnosis and may remain asymptomatic for decades. Malignant mixed tumors include both cancers originating from pleomorphic adenomas, termed *carcinoma ex pleomorphic adenoma,* and de novo malignant mixed tumors. The risk for malignant transformation of benign pleomorphic adenomas is 1.5% within the first 5 years but increases to 9.5% once the benign tumor has been present for more than 15 years.[39] Most salivary gland lymphomas are of the non-Hodgkin's variety (85%). The risk for malignant lymphoma in patients with Sjögren's syndrome is 44-fold higher than in the normal population. Metastatic tumors are most often derived from cutaneous carcinomas and melanomas from the scalp, temporal area, and ear. Distant metastatic tumors are rare but may arise from the lung, kidneys, and breasts.

Treatment of salivary gland malignancies is en bloc surgical excision. Radiation therapy is administered postoperatively for high-grade malignancies demonstrating extraglandular disease, perineural invasion, direct invasion of surrounding tissue, or regional metastases. For

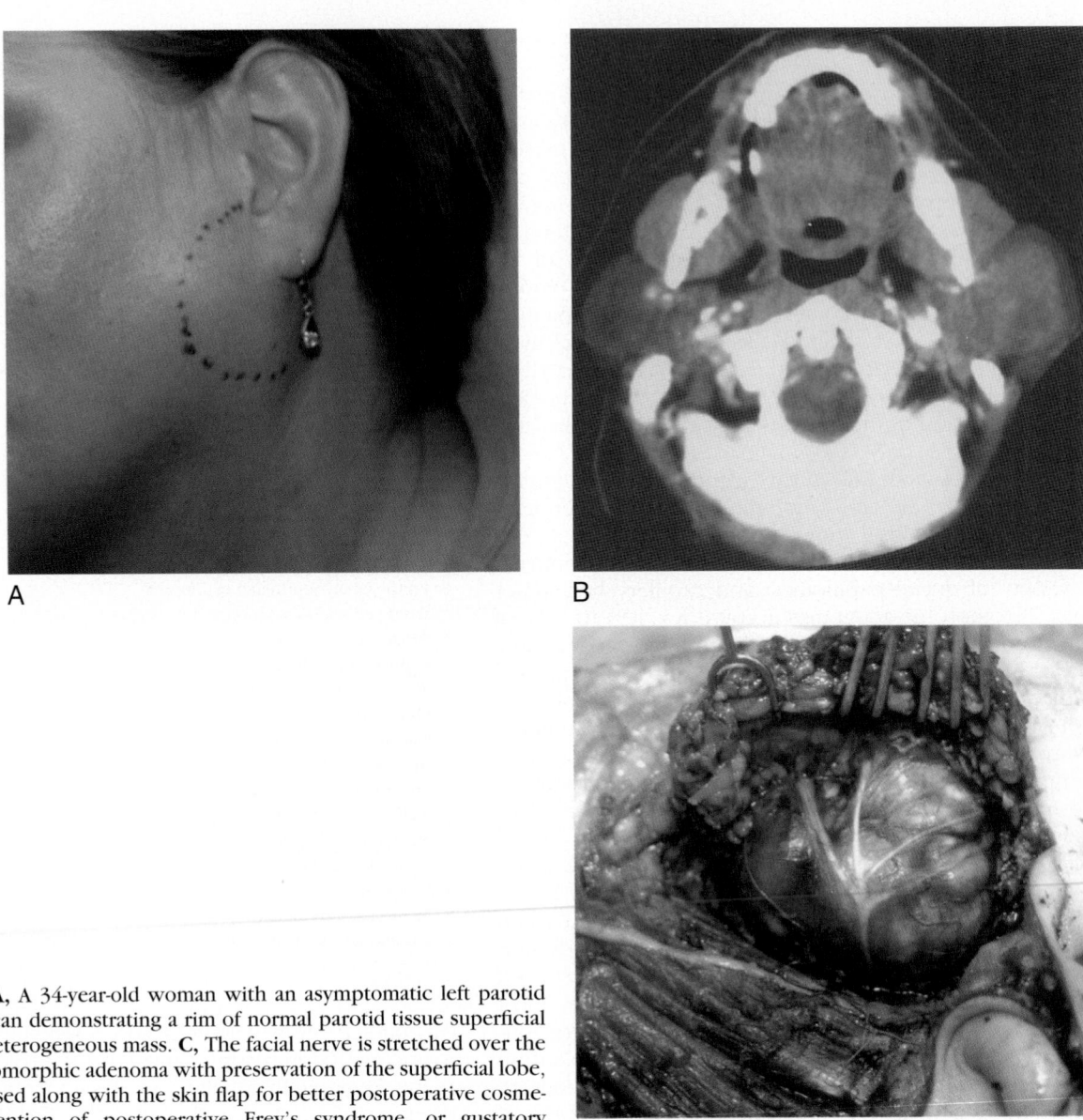

Figure 33-16 A, A 34-year-old woman with an asymptomatic left parotid mass. **B,** CT scan demonstrating a rim of normal parotid tissue superficial to a deeper, heterogeneous mass. **C,** The facial nerve is stretched over the deep-lobe pleomorphic adenoma with preservation of the superficial lobe, which was raised along with the skin flap for better postoperative cosmesis and prevention of postoperative Frey's syndrome, or gustatory sweating.

tumors confined to the superficial lobe of the parotid gland, lateral lobectomy with preservation of the facial nerve may be performed. Gross tumor should not be left in situ, but if the facial nerve is able to be preserved by peeling tumor off the nerve, the nerve should be preserved and radiation therapy given for microscopic residual disease. For cancers of the deep lobe, total parotidectomy is performed. Elective neck dissections are performed for high-grade malignancies such as high-grade mucoepidermoid carcinoma. In patients with gross facial nerve involvement, temporal bone resection is performed and the nerve is sacrificed proximally to obtain a negative margin. When the facial nerve is removed, rehabilitation with a simultaneous nerve graft may be performed in the hope of producing facial muscular tone. Although the primary goal of facial nerve rehabilitation

is protection of the cornea from chronic exposure, other concerns include oral competency, nasal valve maintenance, and cosmesis. Upper lid gold weights, lateral tarsorrhaphies, static fascial slings, dynamic muscular slings, and delayed reinnervation procedures are also used for facial rehabilitation. Submandibular gland and minor salivary gland malignancies are treated similarly to parotid gland cancers, by en bloc resection. Submandibular gland malignancies are removed with level I contents and accompanying MRND. Gross involvement of the hypoglossal or lingual nerves requires sacrificing them and obtaining a negative margin by following the nerves toward the skull base. Adenoid cystic cancers are highly neurotropic, and treatment consists of removal of gross tumor with radiation therapy for the microscopic disease that is assumed to exist at the periphery of the tumor.

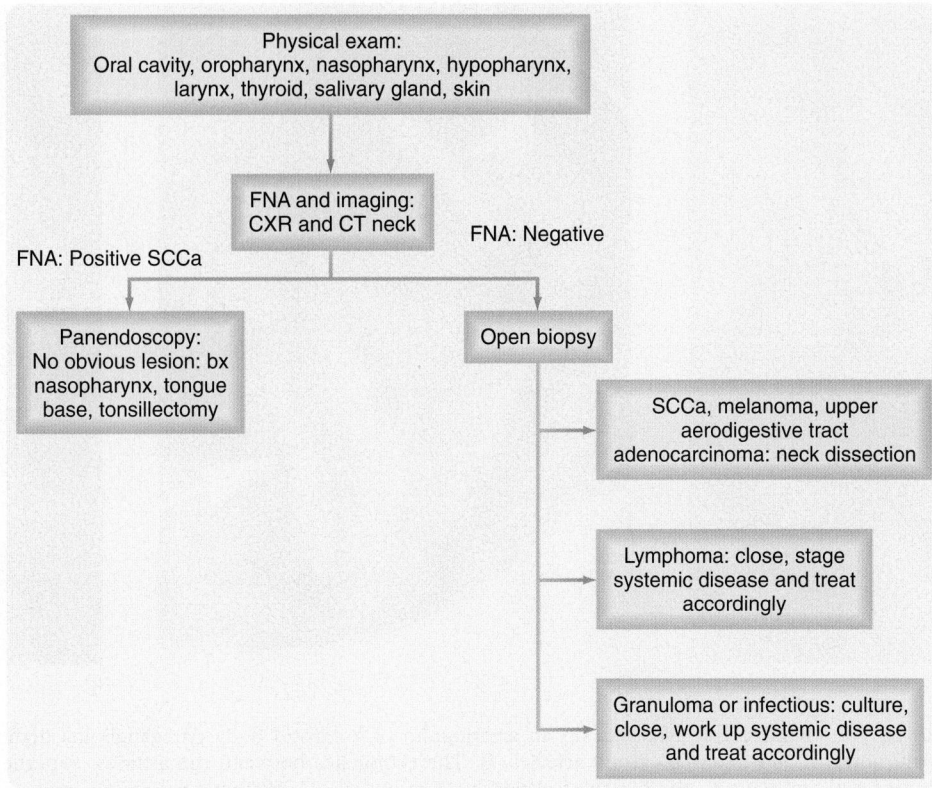

Figure 33-17 Workup of an asymptomatic, unilateral neck mass in adults. CT, computed tomography; CXR, chest x-ray; FNA, fine-needle aspiration; SCCa, squamous cell carcinoma.

Neck and Unknown Primary

The workup of a neck mass is different in children than it is in adults because of differing causes. Cervical masses are common in children and most often represent inflammatory processes or congenital abnormalities. Of pediatric neck masses that are persistent, 2% to 15% that are removed will be malignant. Pediatric evaluation requires thorough head and neck examination, including endoscopy of the nasopharynx and larynx. The most common cause of cervical adenopathy is viral upper respiratory tract infections. The associated lymphadenopathy generally subsides within 2 weeks, although mononucleosis-related lymphadenopathy may persist for 4 to 6 weeks. The location of the mass, as well as its character, most often leads to the diagnosis. Lymphadenopathy not attributable to viral infections may represent a less common infectious process. Bacterial cervical adenitis is most often caused by group A β-hemolytic streptococci or *S. aureus*. Scrofula is cervical adenitis secondary to tuberculosis and is relatively uncommon in industrialized countries, although atypical mycobacteria may also cause cervical adenitis. Cat-scratch disease should be suspected if there is a history of cat contact, and indirect fluorescence antibody testing for *Bartonella henselae* should be performed. Midline masses include thyroglossal duct cysts, enlarged lymph nodes, dermoid cysts, hemangiomas, or pyramidal lobes of the thyroid. Nonlymphoid masses anterior to the sternocleidomastoid muscle are most commonly branchial cleft cysts.

A soft, compressible mass of the posterior triangle may represent a lymphangioma (or cystic hygroma), which usually develops before the age of 2 years. Cervical teratomas are present at birth and may involve compression of the airway or esophagus. Malignancies most commonly encountered in pediatric neck masses include sarcomas, lymphomas, and metastatic thyroid carcinoma.

In adults, neck masses represent malignancies more often than in children. *Persistent masses larger than 2 cm represent cancer in 80% of cases.* In addition to head and neck examination, CT scanning assists in evaluating not only the masses but also potential primary sites. Fine-needle aspiration (<22 gauge) is performed as one of the initial steps in the workup of neck masses; it has an overall accuracy of 95% for benign neck masses and 87% for malignant masses (Fig. 33-17).[40] As in children, the location of the mass has a bearing on the likelihood of diagnosis: midline masses may represent thyroglossal duct cysts, dermoid tumors, Delphian nodes, thyroid masses, lipomas, or sebaceous cysts. Thyroglossal duct cysts represent the vestigial tract of descent that the thyroid followed from the foramen cecum to its normal location below the cricoid. The cyst may become enlarged later in life concurrent with an upper respiratory tract infection. Surgical excision should include the central portion of the hyoid bone (Sistrunk's procedure), or recurrence is more likely.

Persistent lateral neck masses in adults may represent enlarged benign or malignant lymph nodes, neuromas or

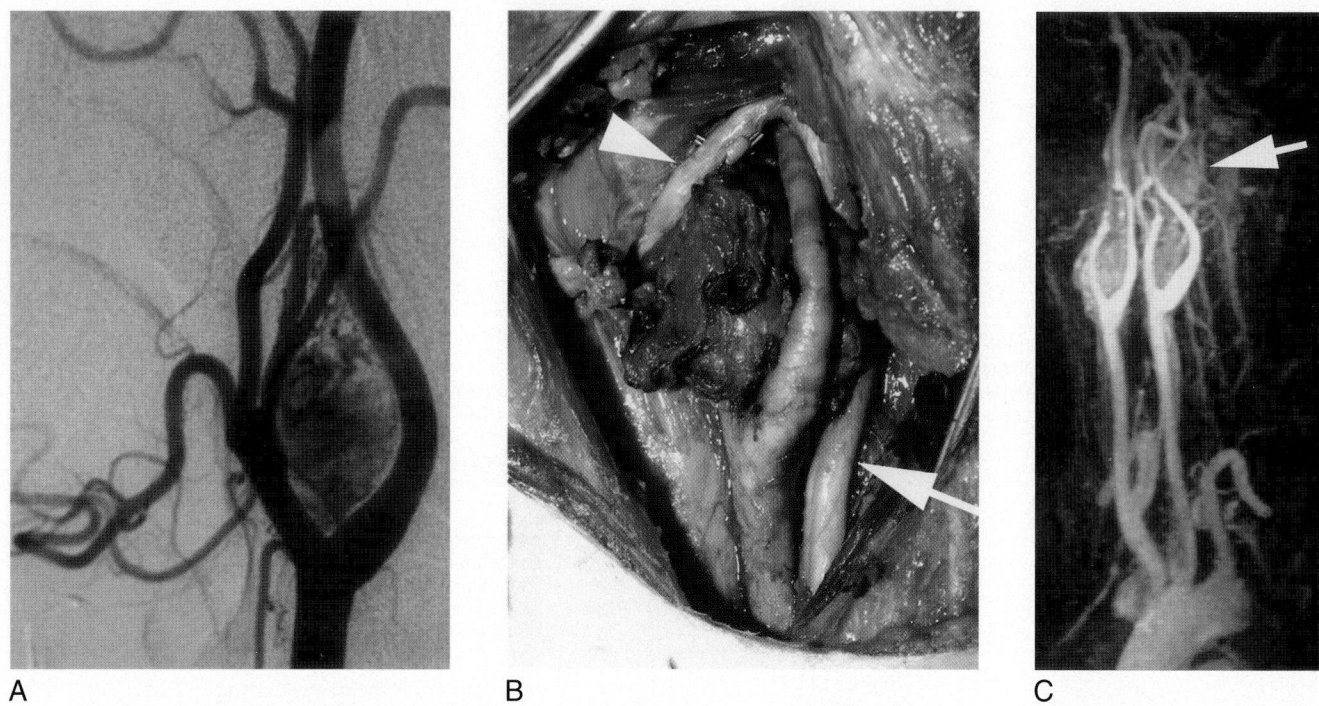

A   B   C

Figure 33-18 A, The characteristic lyre sign on an arteriogram of a carotid body paraganglioma demonstrating splaying of the internal and external carotid arteries. **B,** The tumor lies between the arteries, superficial to the vagus nerve *(arrow)* and deep to the hypoglossal nerve *(arrowhead)*. **C,** Magnetic resonance angiography of a different patient demonstrating bilateral carotid body tumors, in addition to a separate, more superior left vagal paraganglioma *(arrow)*.

neurofibromas, carotid body tumors, branchial cleft cysts, lipomas, sebaceous cysts, parathyroid cysts, or a primary soft tissue tumor. Enlarged lymph nodes may be due to an infectious cause, similar to those in the pediatric population; lymphoma; regional metastases from SCC, melanoma, thyroid carcinoma, or salivary gland tumors; or distant metastases. Most commonly, lymphadenopathy in an adult is indicative of metastatic HNSCC, with lymphoma being less likely. Metastatic SCC is most frequently from the nasopharynx, oropharynx, or hypopharynx, and its presence is a negative prognostic indicator. In all cases of metastases to the neck, lymphadenectomy as treatment is valuable only in cases of SCC, salivary gland tumors, melanoma, and thyroid carcinoma. Otherwise, removal of metastatic lymph nodes is indicated for diagnosis only, and systemic treatment must be initiated. In cases of multiple lymph node enlargement, a diagnosis of human immunodeficiency virus infection, toxoplasmosis, or fungal infection should be investigated.

Less frequently, benign neck masses can develop in adults. The branchial cleft apparatus that persists after birth may give rise to a number of neck masses. First branchial cleft cysts develop in the preauricular or submandibular areas, are intimately associated with the external auditory canal and parotid gland, and may require dissection of the facial nerve during excision. Second and third branchial cleft cysts and tracts develop anterior to the sternocleidomastoid muscle and often

become symptomatic after upper respiratory tract infections. Although the second branchial cleft communicates with the ipsilateral tonsillar fossa, the third communicates with the piriform sinus. Removal of the cyst and tract necessitates dissection along the course of embryologic descent. Second branchial cleft tracts course between the internal and external carotid arteries. Third branchial cleft tracts course posterior to both branches of the carotid artery. Occasionally, a carcinoma may be found within the cyst. Debate continues about whether the carcinoma represents a cystic metastasis from the tongue base or tonsil or whether cancer may occur de novo within a branchial cleft cyst.[41]

Carotid body tumors or chemodectomas are more properly referred to as *paragangliomas* and arise from the branchiomeric paraganglia at the carotid body. These tumors are usually benign, unifocal, and nonhereditary; they are manifested as a nonpainful mass at the carotid bifurcation and have a characteristic lyre sign on carotid arteriography (Fig. 33-18). Because of their highly vascular nature, biopsy is contraindicated. Preoperative embolization is performed for tumors larger than 3 cm. The most frequent sequela from resection is cranial nerve injury, most commonly of the superior laryngeal nerve, but also the vagal nerve or hypoglossal nerve with large tumors. Tumors larger than 5 cm are associated with a need for concurrent carotid artery replacement.[42] *First-bite syndrome* has been coined to describe the phenom-

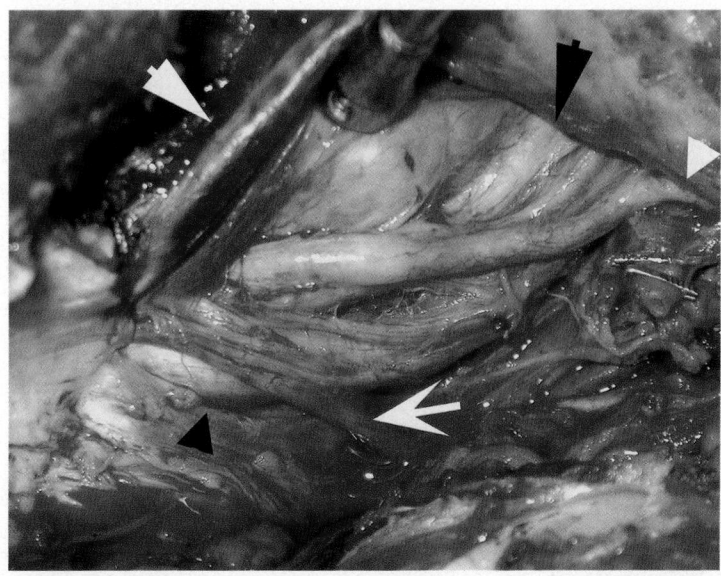

Figure 33-19 Left poststyloid space after removal of a parapharyngeal space tumor and lateral temporal bone resection. The carotid is seen anteriorly *(black arrowhead)* where it enters the skull base, whereas the internal jugular vein *(large white arrowhead)* is retracted posteriorly. The vagus nerve *(large black arrowhead)* is intimately associated with the hypoglossal nerve *(small white arrowhead),* and separation of the two nerves at this level often leads to vocal cord paralysis. The glossopharyngeal nerve is seen anteriorly *(large white arrow).*

enon of pain with the initiation of mastication; it is thought to be due to removal of the sympathetic nerves surrounding the carotid bifurcation and reinnervation of the parotid secretory glands by parasympathetic fibers. Excision of bilateral carotid body tumors may lead to baroreceptor failure with wide fluctuations in blood pressure.

Tumors of the parapharyngeal space are distinguished by their location: either prestyloid, usually of salivary gland origin, or poststyloid, usually vascular or neurogenic in origin. Initial symptoms may consist of a superior neck mass, fullness of the parotid gland or tonsillar fossa, trismus, dysphagia, Horner's syndrome, or cranial nerve impairment. Tumors include paraganglioma, salivary gland neoplasms, schwannoma or neurilemoma, lipoma, sarcoma, or lymphadenopathy. Access to these tumors is most commonly performed transcervically, and care must be taken to preserve uninvolved structures such as the carotid artery and major cranial nerves (Fig. 33-19). Rarely is a mandibulotomy approach required.

TRACHEOTOMY

Tracheotomy is most commonly used today in patients requiring prolonged mechanical ventilation to reduce the risk of damage to the larynx, assist ventilation and pulmonary hygiene, and improve patient comfort and oral care. There is no hard rule about how long a translaryngeal endotracheal tube can be left in place. Some laryngologists recommend conversion to a tracheotomy after 3 days of intubation, although most use 2 to 3 weeks as

a limit. Other common reasons for tracheotomy include chronic aspiration, acute airway obstruction secondary to facial or laryngeal trauma or oral or deep neck space infections, or perioperatively during radical cancer ablation.

The term *tracheotomy* implies formation of an opening that will close spontaneously once the tracheotomy tube is decannulated. Closure via secondary intention generally occurs over a period of 5 to 7 days, and the healing process should not be hastened by suturing the overlying skin closed or an abscess may form in this highly contaminated wound. The term *tracheostomy* implies the formation of a permanent opening that remains open after removal of the tube. The surgeon can form a tracheostomy by suturing an inferiorly based tracheal ring flap to the skin at the time of surgery. Although this flap allows safer replacement of the tracheal tube should it become accidentally decannulated, once the mucocutaneous junction forms, a surgical procedure with rotational skin flaps is required to close the tracheostomy. A permanent tracheostomy should be considered in cases of extended mechanical ventilation, chronic aspiration, obstructive sleep apnea, and uncorrectable upper airway obstruction.

Preoperative assessment should include a history of previous tracheotomy or neck surgery, laryngeal pathology, bleeding difficulties, or cervical spine injuries. Perioperative complications of tracheotomy include bleeding, aspiration, pneumothorax and pneumomediastinum, recurrent laryngeal nerve injury, and hypoxia. Long-term problems include the formation of granulation tissue both at the skin and within the trachea, collapse of tracheal

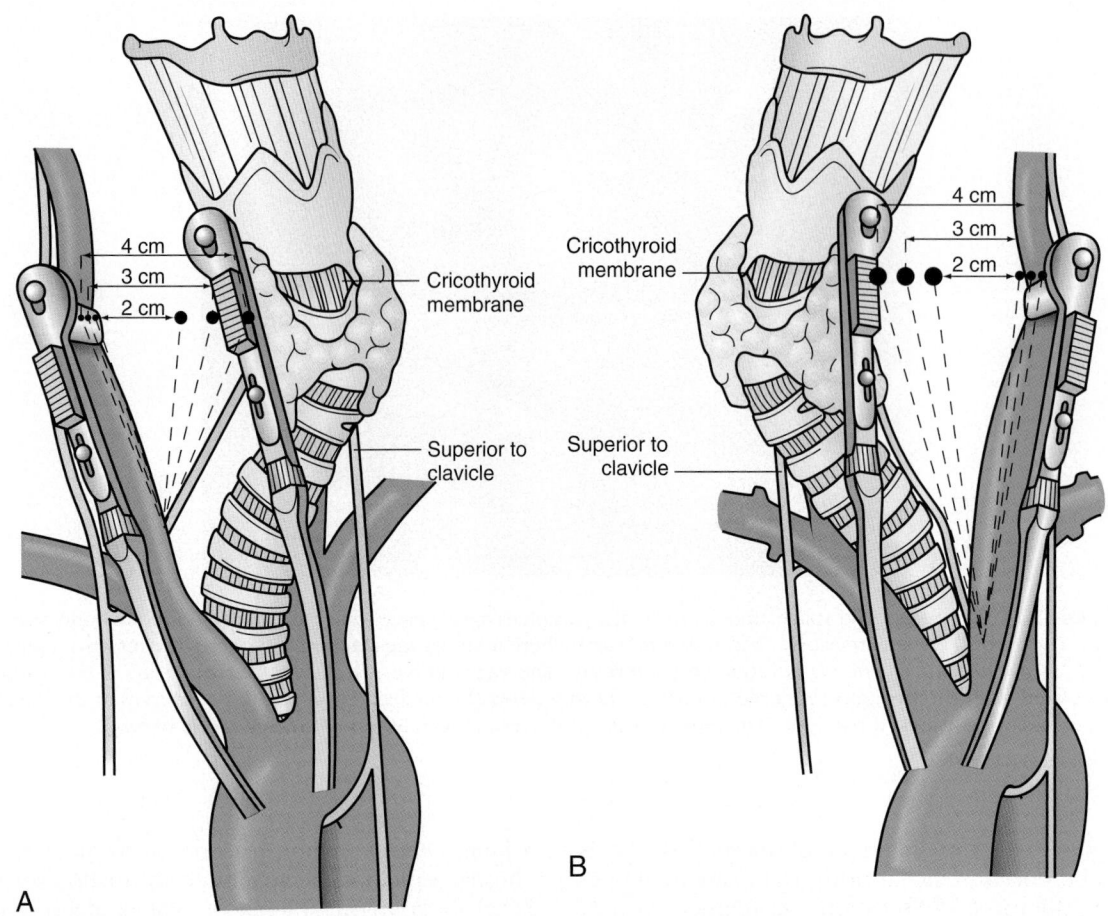

Figure 33-20 Anatomy of the right **(A)** and left **(B)** recurrent laryngeal nerve. The more diagonal course on the right side predisposes patients to traction injury during anterior cervical neck surgery. (With permission, from Netterville JL, Koriwchak MJ, Winkle M, et al: Vocal fold paralysis following the anterior approach to the cervical spine. Ann Otol Rhinol Laryngol 105:85-91, 1996.)

cartilage and airway obstruction, and tracheoinnominate artery and tracheoesophageal fistulas.

Although the traditional open tracheotomy technique is still primarily used and preferred, percutaneous tracheotomy has recently been gaining in use. There are reports of both increased and decreased complication rates with the percutaneous technique versus the open technique.[43,44] Although one might suspect that the trauma from dilating the tracheal rings in the percutaneous technique may be associated with a substantial increase in long-term tracheal stenosis, such does not always seem to be the case, and percutaneous tracheotomies have become common in many intensive care units in patients with favorable anatomy and supportive clinical settings.

VOCAL CORD PARALYSIS

More appropriately termed *vocal fold immobility,* loss of vocal cord function remains a common occurrence. The recurrent laryngeal nerve supplies all the laryngeal musculature except for the cricothyroid muscle, which is supplied by the superior laryngeal nerve. Paralysis of the laryngeal muscles may occur from a lesion in the central nervous system or, more commonly, with peripheral nerve involvement (90%). Once the vagus nerve exits the jugular foramen, the superior laryngeal nerve divides superiorly in the parapharyngeal space and passes deep to the carotid artery. On the left side, the recurrent laryngeal nerve separates from the vagus nerve in the thorax, passes around the aortic arch at the ductus arteriosus, and travels superiorly in the tracheoesophageal groove to the cricothyroid joint. Probably as a result of the left recurrent nerve's longer course, left vocal cord paralysis is more common than on the right. The right recurrent nerve separates from the vagus and passes around the right subclavian artery and back to the larynx (Fig 33-20). A nonrecurrent recurrent laryngeal nerve is a rare finding (0.5%-1.0%) on the right side; when present, the nerve separates from the vagus before descending into the chest, passes directly to the larynx, and is associated with a retroesophageal right subclavian artery. Approaches to the cervical spine should generally be performed from the left to reduce traction injury on the recurrent nerve because right-sided approaches have been associated with a higher rate of laryngeal nerve injury.[45]

Dysfunction of the superior laryngeal nerve most commonly occurs after thyroidectomy because the nerve is in close proximity to the superior thyroid vascular pedicle, and affected patients may have difficulty achieving precision in pitch, noticeable most commonly in professional voice users. Injury to the recurrent laryngeal nerve results in vocal fold paresis or paralysis. Patients with unilateral vocal cord immobility may have hoarseness, ineffective cough, dysphagia, aspiration, or airway compromise or may be completely asymptomatic because of their ability to compensate. Definitive diagnosis is made via laryngoscopy, and subtle weakness may require stroboscopic examination. Causes of paralysis include surgical trauma (most commonly thyroidectomy); malignancies of the thyroid, mediastinum, esophagus, or larynx; mediastinal compression; viral neuropathy; collagen vascular disease; sarcoidosis; diabetic neuropathy; and a multitude of other reported causes. The etiology remains unknown in 20% of patients. Because re-creating volitional abduction and adduction of the vocal cord is not currently feasible, the goal of treatment entails creating sufficient medialization of the involved vocal cord to allow efficient voicing and cough, as well as reduce hoarseness and aspiration. Medialization may be accomplished with intracordal injection of a variety of substances, including fat, Gelfoam, and human cadaveric collagen preparations. Because of the risk for granuloma formation, Teflon injection is rarely used today. Medialization thyroplasty, with or without concurrent arytenoid adduction, consists of a surgically created window in the thyroid cartilage with the insertion of Silastic, hydroxyapatite, or Gore-Tex and has shown excellent results. Laryngeal reinnervation via an ansa cervicalis–recurrent laryngeal nerve anastomosis provides medialization with tone to the paralyzed cord but takes several months to become effective. Bilateral vocal fold paralysis is an uncommon scenario manifested by both vocal folds remaining near the midline position. Patients maintain a strong voice because the vocal folds continue to vibrate, but they might suffer life-threatening airway obstruction and stridor and require immediate reintubation or tracheotomy.

RECONSTRUCTION

Perhaps the area of head and neck surgery that has undergone the most advancement in the past 25 years is reconstruction, fueled largely by the advent of microvascular free flaps. Today, there is almost no defect that cannot be repaired, and this has afforded the ablative surgeon more leeway in obtaining tumor-free margins. The head and neck region is unique in the intricacy of its form and function, and careful reconstruction is needed to return patients back to their premorbid condition. Speech, swallowing, and cosmesis are most commonly focused on when considering rehabilitative goals. Swallowing may be impaired by resection of local tissues of the oral cavity, oropharynx, hypopharynx, larynx, and cervical esophagus. Loss of innervation, either sensory or motor, locally or at the skull base, can severely impair

swallowing. Irradiation leads to fibrosis of local tissues, as well as loss of saliva and taste, and may cause stenosis years after treatment is finished. Rehabilitation of speech is covered in the larynx section. Because of the proximity and complexity of the airway and digestive tracts at the oral cavity, oropharynx, larynx, and hypopharynx, the ability to maintain the two functions is closely related. Frequently, aspiration occurs when the swallowing process is impeded. Although a tracheotomy tube helps protect the airway somewhat from aspiration and allows increased pulmonary suctioning, it also tethers the larynx to the skin and often exacerbates dysphagia. Once dysfunction has occurred, the physician is hampered by trying to maintain balance between airway, speech, and swallowing, and one function may have to be further impaired to improve another. In a severely dysfunctional upper airway, total sacrifice of one function may have to be accepted, and laryngectomy or a permanent gastric tube may be required.

Cosmetic deformities are most obvious in the head and neck area. Functional deficits not only occur in speech and swallowing but also affect eyelid function, oral competence, and maintenance of a nasal and oral airway. General principles of facial restoration include reconstructing the underlying bony framework, replacing skin with skin of matching quality, minimizing scar visibility and contracture, and reconstructing in zones of facial units. Skin should be matched by color, thickness, and hair-bearing units when possible. The aesthetic facial units include the forehead, eyes and periorbital area, midface, nose (which itself contains several subunits), and the lips and mentum. A spectrum of reconstructive options exist, with healing by secondary intention and primary closure at one end and extensive reconstruction such as microvascular free flaps at the other. Which option is selected depends on the location and severity of the defect, the overall health of the patient, the available donor sites for flaps, the status of the tissue adjacent to the defect (irradiated, infected, previously operated), and the functionality of the area to be reconstructed. Not only must the reconstructive surgeon choose which option is best for a given defect, but secondary and tertiary options should be also planned in the event of flap failure or recurrent disease.

Healing by secondary intention is an excellent option in several clinical scenarios. Mucosal defects with an underlying layer of vascularized muscle or bone that will not contract to the point of impeding function may be left to close by secondary intention. Examples include small tonsillectomy defects, tongue resections, and some laryngeal mucosal defects. Primary closure is likely to be the most commonly used option for closure of cutaneous defects. Attempts should be made to keep incisions within the lines of relaxed skin tension. These lines are caused by muscular insertion into the skin and form when mimetic motion occurs. Incisions that parallel the lines of relaxed skin tension not only respect the aesthetic units of the face but also have the least amount of tension along them, which decreases scarring. A Z-plasty may be used to reorient an unfavorable line of closure into a relaxed skin tension line.

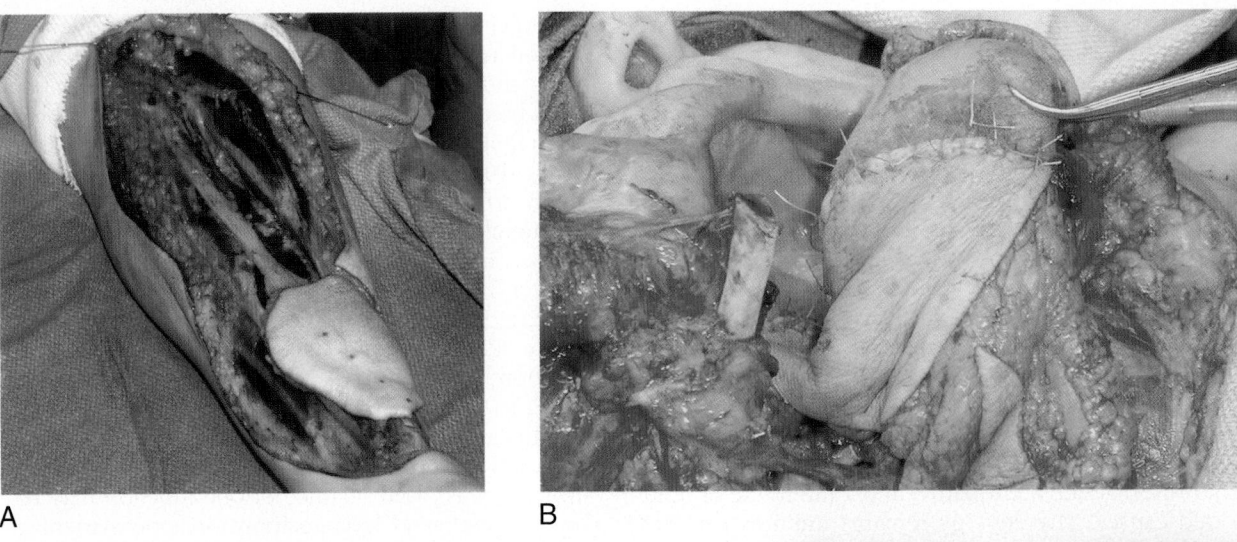

A

B

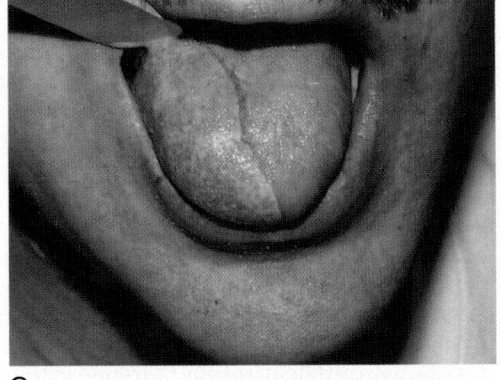

C

Figure 33-21 A, Harvest of a radial forearm fasciocutaneous free flap based on the radial artery. **B,** Right hemiglossectomy for squamous cell carcinoma of the right mobile tongue reconstructed with a radial forearm flap. **C,** Postoperative result 1 year later demonstrating excellent contour and tongue mobility.

Skin grafts are most commonly used for oral cavity, ear, or maxillectomy defects, as well as for coverage of donor sites, such as the radial forearm and fibular free flaps and the deltopectoral flap. Skin grafts are completely dependent for nutrition on the tissue over which they are placed and can heal well over muscle, perichondrium, and periosteum. They do not take well over bone or cartilage, nor on tissue that has been irradiated or infected or is hypovascular. Split-thickness skin grafts contain the epidermis and a portion of the dermis and are harvested with a dermatome at approximately $^{12}/_{1000}$- to $^{18}/_{1000}$-inch thickness. Thinner grafts require less nutrients to remain viable but will also contract more when healing. Grafts may be meshed to allow greater surface coverage, but these types of grafts are generally restricted to the scalp or over muscle because of a less cosmetic result. A nonadherent antibiotic-impregnated bolster is commonly used to maintain stability between the split-thickness skin graft and the recipient bed for 5 days to allow transmission of nutrients and capillary ingrowth while healing. Harvest sites include the anterior and lateral aspects of the thighs and buttocks.

Full-thickness skin grafts are characterized by a better color match, texture, and contour and less contracture but decreased success rates than with split-thickness skin grafts. Commonly used donor sites include the postau-

ricular, upper eyelid, and supraclavicular fossa skin. Composite grafts are occasionally needed for cartilage and skin reconstruction of the nasal ala and may be harvested from the conchal bowl without significantly affecting the appearance of the pinna. Acellular cadaveric human dermis that has been prepared by removing immunogenic cells while leaving intact the collagen matrix has recently been growing in popularity as a skin graft substitute and avoids the need for a donor site.

Local skin flaps have an excellent tissue match because of their proximity to the defect. Commonly used designs include advancement, rotation, transposition, rhomboid, and bilobed flaps. Similar to primary closure, local flaps should be designed to be incorporated into the lines of relaxed skin tension. Although local flaps depend on the subdermal plexus of capillaries, regional flaps have an axial blood supply. This latter vascular pedicle is necessary for flap viability because greater distances are spanned by the flap and it is contained either within the subcutaneous fascia, as in a fasciocutaneous flap, or within an underlying muscle, as in a myocutaneous flap. The deltopectoral or Bakamjian flap was one of the early regional flaps and was used extensively in head and neck reconstruction. Based on the intercostal perforating branches from the internal mammary artery, the flap is based medially and designed over the upper pectoralis

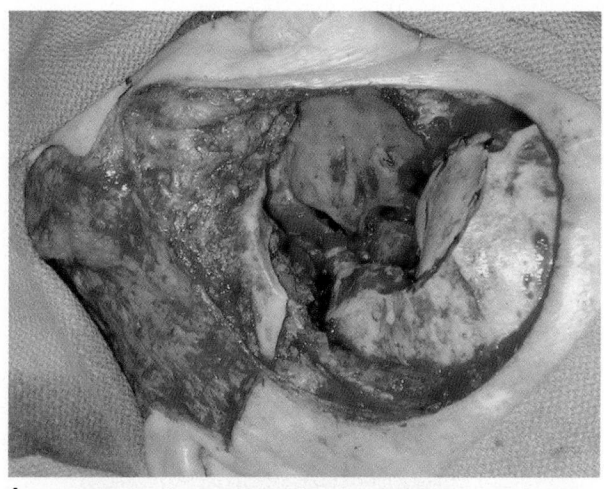

A

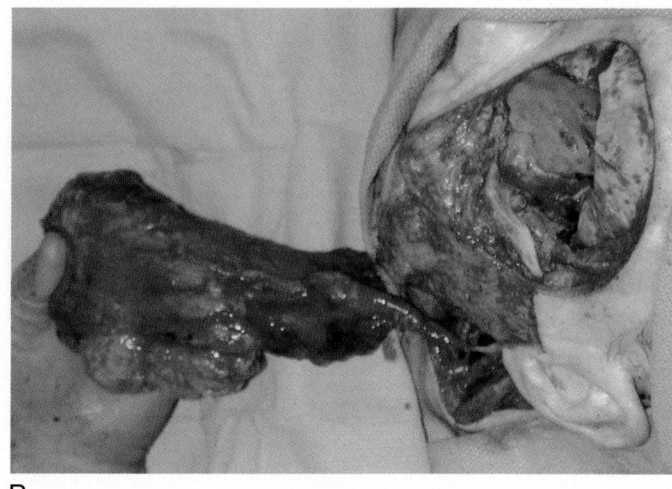

B

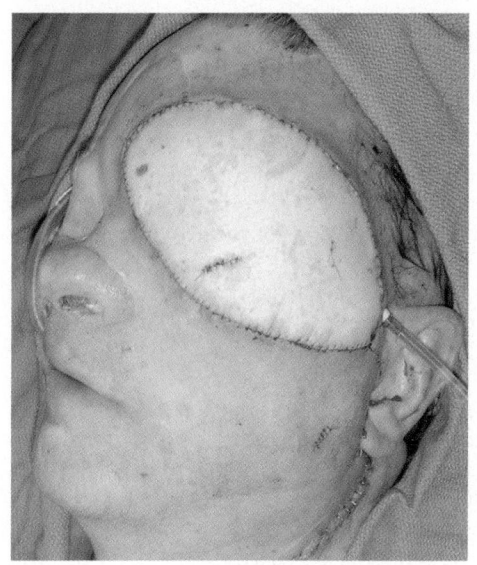

C

Figure 33-22 A, Resection of a recurrent skin squamous cell carcinoma invading the left orbit, paranasal sinuses, and frontal lobe dura. **B,** A rectus abdominis myocutaneous free flap has been revascularized with microvascular techniques into the recipient vessels of the neck, with the flap inset into place **(C)** for cutaneous and skull base reconstruction.

and deltoid regions. Because of the pliability of the transferred skin, it can be swung upward for skin defects or pharyngeal reconstruction. Perhaps the development with the most significant impact on head and neck reconstruction was introduction of the pectoralis myocutaneous flap in 1978. Based on the pectoral branch of the thoracoacromial artery, the artery pierces the pectoralis muscle from the deep surface. A skin paddle designed over the muscle, or simply the muscle itself, may be transferred to reconstruct defects up to the nasopharynx. Historically, the pectoralis muscle is tunneled under the intervening skin to preserve the ipsilateral deltopectoral flap in the event that it is needed for future coverage. Division of the pectoral nerve branches ensures atrophy of the muscle and reduces the bulge over the clavicle. In addition to reconstruction of mucosal defects with the vascularized skin, coverage of an exposed carotid artery is an excellent use of the myogenous flap. The trapezius muscle offers multiple soft tissue flaps that may be rotated into head and neck defects. The lower trapezius myocutaneous flap, based on the dorsal scapular artery, has

already been referred to as an excellent choice for lateral temporal bone defects.[36] Finally, the submental and platysmal flaps are based on the facial artery and provide excellent local flap coverage for oral and oropharyngeal defects.

A free flap entails removal of composite tissue from a distant site along with its blood supply and reimplantation of the vasculature in the reconstructive field. Although the first successful human microvasculature transfer was a jejunal interposition flap in 1959, the modern era of microvasculature reconstruction did not arise until the 1970s with improvements in instrumentation and technique. Today's selection of donor sites allows the benefit of choosing between sites with large-caliber, long vascular pedicles that are anatomically consistent. In addition to favorable vascularity, optimal donor sites allow a simultaneous two-team approach of ablation and harvesting, the possibility of a sensate flap, the composite transfer of bone stock capable of accepting osseointegrated implants, the transfer of secretory mucosa, or any combinations of these options. Patient selection for free flap

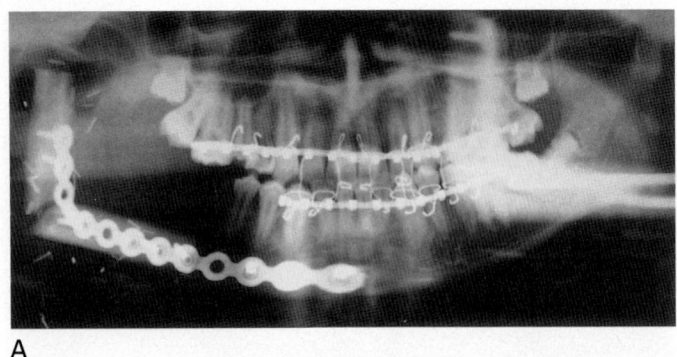

A

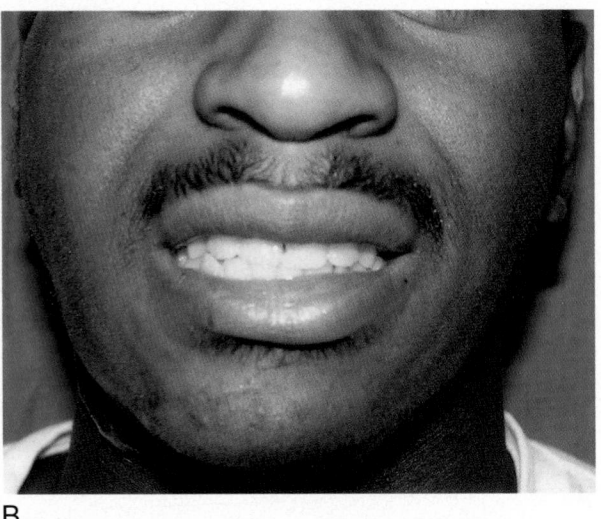

B

Figure 33-23 A, Immediate postoperative radiograph of a 35-year-old man after resection of an osteosarcoma of the mandibular ramus and reconstruction with a fibular osseocutaneous free flap. **B,** Six months postoperatively, the patient's dental occlusion has been preserved along with excellent facial contour.

reconstruction is of critical importance. Advanced age is not a contraindication to microvascular reconstruction, although previous recipient bed irradiation, contraction of tissues after secondary reconstruction, or previous free flap failure should raise concern in the reconstructive surgeon. Complete loss of a free tissue transfer should occur in less than 5% of cases.

The radial aspect of the forearm has emerged as the workhorse of soft tissue free flaps in head and neck reconstruction. A fasciocutaneous flap with sensate capabilities, the radial forearm flap is based on the radial artery and its venae comitantes or cephalic vein (or both) for drainage. Variations of the flap include harvest of partial radius bone or palmaris longus tendon for bony or suspensory reconstruction, respectively. The main advantage of the radial forearm flap is the thinness and pliability of the harvested skin, which makes it ideal not only for external cutaneous defects but also for reconstruction of the floor of the mouth or tongue (Fig. 33-21), soft palate and oropharyngeal wall, and pharynx, as well as skull base reconstruction.[46] Although the donor site is more cosmetically obvious than other donor sites, long-term morbidity of the harvest is minimal. Other soft tissue flaps include the lateral arm flap, anterolateral thigh and lateral thigh flaps, latissimus dorsi flap, and rectus abdominis flap. The lateral arm flap is an excellent alternative to the radial forearm flap when the patient exhibits a dominant radial artery supply to the hand, which is a contraindication to use of the forearm site. The lateral arm flap is based on the posterior branches of the radial collateral vessels. It offers slightly more bulk than the radial forearm flap does but is compromised to some extent by vessels that are smaller in caliber. Experience with the thigh flaps has shown excellent results in tubed reconstruction of the pharynx. Both the latissimus dorsi and rectus abdominis flaps can be transferred as myogenous or myocutaneous flaps. Although skin match is not ideal, these flaps are best suited to large defects, including skull base repair or maxillectomy defects with orbital exenteration (Fig. 33-22). Harvest of the rectus abdominis may lead to the complication of postoperative hernia formation.

Enteric flaps include the gastro-omental flap and the jejunal flap. Disadvantages of these donor sites includes the need for a laparotomy, which may preclude a two-team approach. In addition, the acceptable ischemia time is shortest with the enteric flaps because of their high tissue oxygen and nutrient demand. Unlike other donor sites, the pedicle of these flaps cannot be divided even years postoperatively because the flap tissues do not incorporate blood supply from the surrounding tissue bed. The main advantages of enteric flaps are their pliability and ability to continue secreting mucus. In an irradiated patient who suffers from xerostomia, enteric reconstruction of recurrent oral or oropharyngeal tumors affords the opportunity to significantly improve quality of life. The omentum of the gastro-omental flap may be draped into the neck to provide contour and bulk to a neck that has previously been dissected.

The most commonly used osseous free flaps include the fibula, scapula, and iliac crest. The fibular free flap is based on the peroneal artery and vein, and the blood supply to the foot should be investigated before harvesting this flap.[47] Up to 25 cm of fibula may be harvested for mandibular or maxillary reconstruction with an osseous or osteocutaneous graft, and donor site morbidity is minimal (Fig. 33-23). The bone stock of the fibula is sufficient to allow osseointegrated implantation for dentition or prosthetic anchors. The iliac crest osteocutaneous free flap allows even greater bone stock and is naturally shaped to approximate the mandibular angle. Like the rectus abdominis flap, the iliac crest is hampered by the potential for postoperative hernias and has a relatively short vascular pedicle. Although the scapular free flap has the least bone stock of the three osseous flaps, it offers the advantage of simultaneous muscular, cutane-

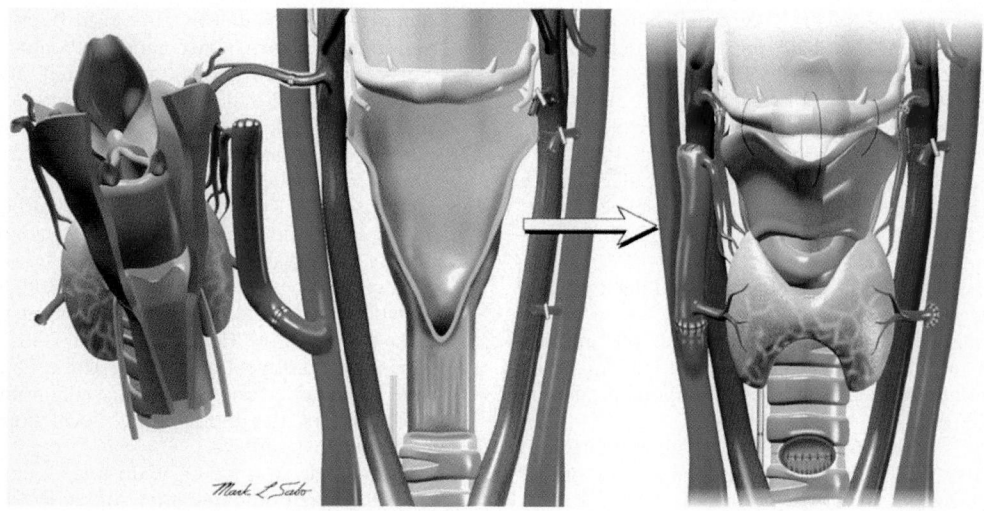

Figure 33-24 Schematic of the first successful laryngeal transplantation, performed in 1998. Not only was the larynx transplanted, but the thyroid, parathyroids, pharynx, and five rings of trachea accompanied the vascularized and innervated organ. (From Strome M, Stein J, Esclamado R, et al: Laryngeal transplantation and 48-month follow-up. N Engl J Med 344:1676-1679, 2001.)

ous, and bony reconstruction based on separate pedicles, thus allowing tremendous versatility in flap orientation. The mega-flap includes the lateral border of the scapula based on the angular artery or the periosteal branch of the circumflex scapular artery, the scapular or parascapular skin paddle based on cutaneous branches of the circumflex scapular artery, and the latissimus dorsi and serratus anterior muscles supplied by the thoracodorsal artery. All arterial branches lead to the subscapular artery where it branches from the axillary artery, and revascularization of all segments may be accomplished with a single arterial anastomosis.

Perhaps the ultimate in head and neck reconstruction lies in the possibility of replacing ablated tissue with identical cadaveric donor tissue. In 1998, the first successful human laryngeal transplantation was performed with microvascular reconstruction (Fig. 33-24).[48] Not only the larynx but also the pharynx, thyroid, parathyroids, and trachea were transplanted. Although work continues in creating immunosuppressive regimens with minimal comorbidity, transplantation of nonvital organs is probably not going to become commonplace until nontoxic immunosuppressive drugs and protection against fostering tumor recurrence have been developed.

Selected References

Bocca E, Pignataro: A conservation technique in radical neck dissection. Ann Otol Rhinol Laryngol 76:975-987, 1967.

A landmark paper demonstrating equal control of metastatic neck disease with radical neck dissection and modified radical neck dissection while avoiding the morbidity of unnecessary removal of neck structures.

Cooper JS, Pajak TF, Forastiere AA, et al: Postoperative concurrent radiotherapy and chemotherapy for high-risk squamous cell carcinoma of the head and neck. N Engl J Med 350:1937-1944, 2004.

A prospective trial demonstrating an advantage to administering postoperative chemoradiation therapy versus radiation therapy alone.

Naudo P, Laccourreye O, Weinstein G, et al: Complications and functional outcome after supracricoid partial laryngectomy with cricohyoidoepiglottopexy. Otolaryngol Head Neck Surg 118:124-129, 1998.

This paper describes the outstanding functional results of supracricoid laryngectomy in terms of speech and swallowing while obtaining excellent local control of disease.

Netterville JL, Koriwchak MJ, Winkle M, et al: Vocal fold paralysis following the anterior approach to the cervical spine. Ann Otol Rhinol Laryngol 105:85-91, 1996.

A practice-changing paper reporting a higher incidence of vocal cord paralysis after right-sided cervical spine approaches and describing the anatomic rationale for approaching the cervical spine from the left side.

The Department of Veterans Affairs Laryngeal Cancer Study Group: Induction chemotherapy plus radiation compared with surgery plus radiation in patients with advanced laryngeal cancer. N Engl J Med 324:1685-1690, 1991.

This multi-institutional, randomized trial demonstrated equal success between chemoradiation therapy and surgery with irradiation for laryngeal carcinoma while allowing patients who responded to the conservation treatment to keep their larynx.

References

1. Wenig BM: Atlas of Head and Neck Pathology. Philadelphia, WB Saunders, 1993.
2. Greene FL, Page DL, Fleming ID, et al (eds): AJCC Cancer Staging Manual, 6th ed. New York, Springer-Verlag, 2002.
3. Dobrossy L: Epidemiology of head and neck cancer: Magnitude of the problem. Cancer Metastasis Rev 24:9-17, 2005.

4. Sankaranarayanan R, Masuyer E, Swaminathan R, et al: Head and neck cancer: A global perspective on epidemiology and prognosis. Anticancer Res 18:4779-4786, 1998.

5. Hoffman HT, Karnell LH, Funk GF, et al: The National Cancer Data Base report on cancer of the head and neck. Arch Otolaryngol Head Neck Surg 124:951-962, 1998.

6. Smith BD, Smith GL, Carter D, et al: Prognostic significance of vascular endothelial growth factor protein levels in oral and oropharyngeal squamous cell carcinoma. J Clin Oncol 18:2046-2052, 2000.

7. Modjtahedi H: Molecular therapy of head and neck cancer. Cancer Metastasis Rev 24:129-146, 2005.

8. Shin DM, Charuruks N, Lippman SM, et al: p53 protein accumulation and genomic instability in head and neck multistep tumorigenesis. Cancer Epidemiol Biomarkers Prev 10:603-609, 2001.

9. Scholes AGM, Woolgar JA, Boyle MA, et al: Synchronous oral carcinomas: Independent or common clonal origin? Cancer Res 58:2003-2006, 1998.

10. Kutler DI, Wong RJ, Kraus DH: Functional imaging in head and neck cancer. Curr Oncol Rep 7:137-144, 2005.

11. Nishiyama Y, Yamamoto Y, Yokoe K, et al: FDG PET as a procedure for detecting simultaneous tumours in head and neck cancer patients. Nucl Med Commun 26:239-244, 2005.

12. Bourhis J, Wibault P, Lusinchi A, et al: Status of accelerated fractionation radiotherapy in head and neck squamous cell carcinomas. Curr Opin Oncol 9:262-266, 1997.

13. The Department of Veterans Affairs Laryngeal Cancer Study Group: Induction chemotherapy plus radiation compared with surgery plus radiation in patients with advanced laryngeal cancer. N Engl J Med 324:1685-1690, 1991.

14. Bernier J, Domenge C, Ozashin M, et al: Postoperative irradiation with or without concurrent chemotherapy for locally advanced head and neck cancer. N Engl J Med 350:1945-1952, 2004.

15. Cooper JS, Pajak TF, Forastiere AA, et al: Postoperative concurrent radiotherapy and chemotherapy for high-risk squamous cell carcinoma of the head and neck. N Engl J Med 350:1937-1944, 2004.

16. Roy S, Tibesar RJ, Daly K, et al: Role of planned neck dissection for advanced metastatic disease in tongue base or tonsil squamous cell carcinoma treated with radiotherapy. Head Neck 24:474-481, 2002.

17. Bocca E, Pignataro O: A conservation technique in radical neck dissection. Ann Otol Rhinol Laryngol 76:975-987, 1967.

18. Ross GL, Shoaib T, Soutar DS, et al: The First International Conference on Sentinel Node Biopsy in Mucosal Head and Neck Cancer and adoption of a multicenter trial protocol. Ann Surg Oncol 9:406-410, 2002.

19. Onercl M, Yilmaz T, Gedikolu G: Tumor thickness as a predictor of cervical lymph node metastasis in squamous cell carcinoma of the lower lip. Otolaryngol Head Neck Surg 122:139-142, 2000.

20. Gooris PJ, Vermey A, de Visscher JG, et al: Supraomohyoid neck dissection in the management of cervical lymph node metastases of squamous cell carcinoma of the lower lip. Head Neck 24:678-683, 2002.

21. Strome SE, To W, Strawderman M, et al: Squamous cell carcinoma of the buccal mucosa. Otolaryngol Head Neck Surg 120:375-379, 1999.

22. Adelstein DJ, Saxton JP, Rybicki LA, et al: Multiagent concurrent chemoradiotherapy for locoregionally advanced squamous cell head and neck cancer: Mature results from a single institution. J Clin Oncol 24:1064-1071, 2006.

23. Lefebvre JL, Chevalier D, Luboinski B, et al: Larynx preservation in piriform sinus cancer: Preliminary results of a European Organization for Research and Treatment of Cancer phase III trial. EORTC Head and Neck Cancer Cooperative Group. J Natl Cancer Inst 88:890-899, 1996.

24. Kirchner JA: Vocal Fold Histopathology: A Symposium. San Diego, CA, College-Hill Press, 1986.

25. Ambrosch P, Kron M, Steiner W: Carbon dioxide laser microsurgery for early supraglottic carcinoma. Ann Otol Rhinol Laryngol 107:680-688, 1998.

26. Steiner W, Vogt P, Ambrosch P, Kron M: Transoral carbon dioxide laser microsurgery for recurrent glottic carcinoma after radiotherapy. Head Neck 26:477-484, 2004.

27. Muscatello L, Laccourreye O, Biacabe B, et al: Laryngofissure and cordectomy for glottic carcinoma limited to the mid third of the mobile true vocal cord. Laryngoscope 107:1507-1510, 1997.

28. Naudo P, Laccourreye O, Weinstein G, et al: Complications and functional outcome after supracricoid partial laryngectomy with cricohyoidoepiglottopexy. Otolaryngol Head Neck Surg 118:124-129, 1998.

29. Myers LL, Nussenbaum B, Bradford CR, et al: Paranasal sinus malignancies: An 18-year single-institutional experience. Laryngoscope 112:1964-1969, 2002.

30. Imola MJ, Schramm VL: Orbital preservation in surgical management of sinonasal malignancy. Laryngoscope 112:1357-1365, 2002.

31. Teknos TN, Smith JC, Day TA, et al: Microvascular free tissue transfer in reconstructing skull base defects: Lessons learned. Laryngoscope 112:1871-1876, 2002.

32. Vasef MA, Ferlito A, Weiss LM: Clinicopathological consultation: Nasopharyngeal carcinoma, with emphasis on its relationship to Epstein-Barr virus. Ann Otol Rhinol Laryngol 106:348-356, 1997.

33. Al-Sarraf M, LeBlanc M, Giri PB, et al: Chemoradiotherapy versus radiotherapy in patients with advanced nasopharyngeal cancer: Phase III randomized Intergroup Study 0099. J Clin Oncol 16:1310-1317, 1998.

34. White DR, Sonnenburg RE, Ewend MG, Senior BA: Safety of minimally invasive pituitary surgery (MIPS) compared with a traditional approach. Laryngoscope 114:1945-1948, 2004.

35. Lorenz RR, Dean RL, Chuang J, Citardi MJ: Endoscopic reconstruction of anterior and middle cranial fossa defects using acellular dermal allograft. Laryngoscope 113:496-501, 2003.

36. Netterville JL, Wood DE: The lower trapezius flap: Vascular anatomy and surgical technique. Arch Otolaryngol Head Neck Surg 117:73-76, 1991.

37. Stewart CJ, MacKenzie K, McGarry GW, et al: Fine-needle aspiration cytology of salivary gland: A review of 341 cases. Diagn Cytopathol 22:139-146, 2000.

38. Witt RL: The significance of the margin in parotid surgery for pleomorphic adenoma. Laryngoscope 112:2141-2154, 2002.

39. Seifert G: Histopathology of malignant salivary gland tumours. Eur J Cancer B Oral Oncol 28B:49-52, 1992.

40. Amedee RG, Dhurandhar NR: Fine-needle aspiration biopsy. Laryngoscope 111:1551-1557, 2001.

41. Zimmermann CE, von Domarus H, Moubayed P: Carcinoma in situ in a lateral cervical cyst. Head Neck 24:965-969, 2002.

42. Netterville JL, Reilly KM, Robertson D, et al: Carotid body tumors: A review of 30 patients with 46 tumors. Laryngoscope 105:115-126, 1995.

43. van Heurn LW, Goei R, de Ploeg I, et al: Late complications of percutaneous dilatational tracheotomy. Chest 110:1572-1576, 1996.

44. Kost KM: Endoscopic percutaneous dilatational tracheotomy: A prospective evaluation of 500 consecutive cases. Laryngoscope 115:1-30, 2005.
45. Netterville JL, Koriwchak MJ, Winkle M, et al: Vocal fold paralysis following the anterior approach to the cervical spine. Ann Otol Rhinol Laryngol 105:85-91, 1996.
46. Burkey BB, Gerek M, Day T: Repair of the persistent cerebrospinal fluid leak with the radial forearm free fascial flap. Laryngoscope 109:1003-1006, 1999.
47. Lorenz RR, Esclamado R: Preoperative magnetic resonance angiography in fibular free flap reconstruction of head and neck defects. Head Neck 23:844-850, 2001.
48. Strome M, Stein J, Esclamado R, et al: Laryngeal transplantation and 40-month follow-up. N Engl J Med 344:1676-1679, 2001.

BREAST

CHAPTER 34

Diseases of the Breast

J. Dirk Iglehart, MD   and   Barbara L. Smith, MD, PhD

ANATOMY

The mature breast lies in adipose tissue between the subcutaneous fat layer and the superficial pectoral fascia (Fig. 34-1). Between the breast and the pectoralis major muscle lies the retromammary space, a thin layer of loose areolar tissue that contains lymphatics and small vessels. During removal of the breast, the breast is separated from the pectoral muscle in the plane of the retromammary space over the muscle.

Located deep to the pectoralis major muscle, the pectoralis minor muscle is enclosed in the clavipectoral fascia, which extends laterally to fuse with the axillary fascia. Dissection along the lateral border of the pectoralis minor muscle divides the axillary fascia and exposes the contents of the axilla. Within the loose areolar fat of the axilla are a variable number of lymph nodes, grouped as shown in Figure 34-2. The number of lymph nodes found in the axilla depends on the extent of dissection; the upper limit was determined by examination of

Halsted-type radical mastectomy specimens to be about 50 nodes.

To standardize the extent of axillary dissection, the axillary nodes are arbitrarily divided into three levels. Level I nodes are located lateral to the lateral border of the pectoralis minor muscle. Level II nodes are in the central axillary group and are located under the pectoralis minor muscle. Level III nodes include the subclavicular nodes medial to the pectoralis minor muscle and are difficult to visualize and remove unless the pectoralis minor muscle is sacrificed or divided. The apex of the axilla is defined by the costoclavicular ligament (Halsted's ligament), at which point the axillary vein passes into the thorax and becomes the subclavian vein. Lymph nodes in the space between the pectoralis major and minor muscles are known as the *interpectoral group,* or *Rotter's nodes,* as described by Grossman and Rotter. Unless this group is specifically exposed, they are not encompassed in surgical procedures that preserve the pectoral muscles.

Lymphatic channels are abundant in the breast parenchyma and dermis. Specialized lymphatic channels collect under the nipple and areola and form Sappey's plexus, named for the anatomist who described them in 1885. Lymph flows from the skin to the subareolar plexus and then into the interlobular lymphatics of the breast parenchyma. Appreciation of lymphatic flow is important for performing successful sentinel node biopsy, described later. Seventy-five percent of lymphatic flow from the breast is into the axillary lymph nodes, and a minor amount goes through the pectoralis muscle and into more medial lymph node groups, as shown in Figure 34-2. A major route of breast cancer metastasis is through lymphatic channels, and the anatomy of the lymphatic system determines the favored locations for regional spread of cancer.

Coursing close to the chest wall on the medial side of the axilla is the long thoracic nerve, or the external respiratory nerve of Bell, which innervates the serratus anterior muscle. This muscle is important for fixing the

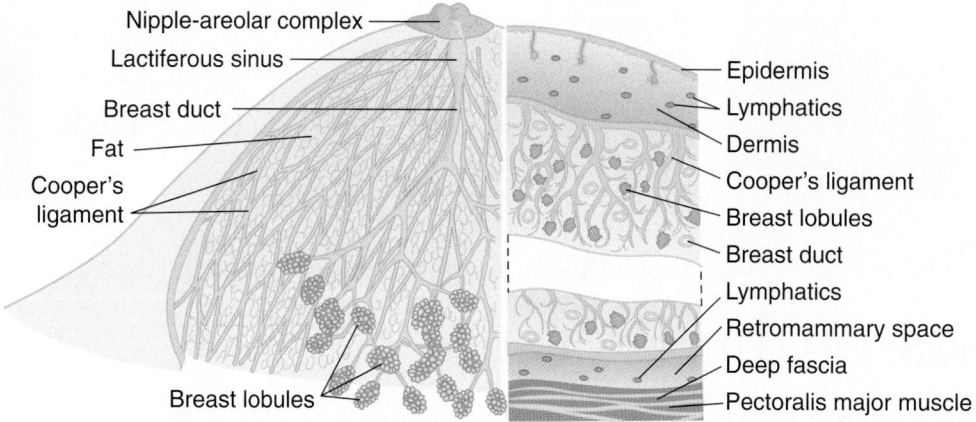

Figure 34-1 Cut-away diagram of a mature resting breast. The breast lies cushioned in fat between the overlying skin and the pectoralis major muscle. Both the skin and the retromammary space under the breast are rich with lymphatic channels. Cooper's ligaments, the suspensory ligaments of the breast, fuse with the overlying superficial fascia just under the dermis, coalesce as the interlobular fascia in the breast parenchyma, and then join with the deep fascia of breast over the pectoralis muscle. The system of ducts in the breast is configured like an inverted tree, with the largest ducts just under the nipple and successively smaller ducts in the periphery. After several branching generations, small ducts at the periphery enter the breast lobule, which is the milk-forming glandular unit of the breast.

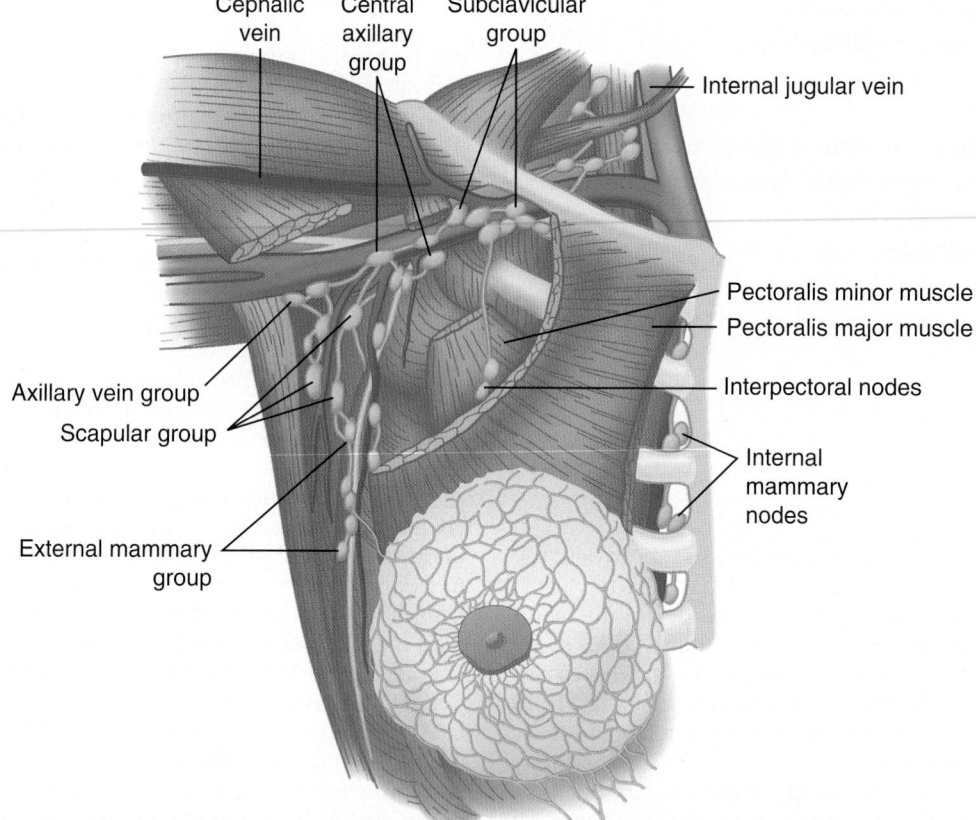

Figure 34-2 Contents of the axilla. In this diagram there are five named and contiguous groupings of lymph nodes in the full axilla. Complete axillary dissection, as done in the historical radical mastectomy, removes all these nodes. However, note that the subclavicular nodes in the axilla are continuous with the supraclavicular nodes in the neck and nodes between the pectoralis major and minor muscles, called the *interpectoral nodes* in this diagram and also named *Rotter's lymph nodes.* The internal mammary nodes probably drain independently from the breast. The sentinel lymph node, located in modern sentinel biopsy, is functionally the first and lowest node in the axillary chain and anatomically is usually found in the external mammary group. (From Donegan WL, Spratt JS: Cancer of the Breast, 3rd ed. Philadelphia, WB Saunders, 1988, p 19.)

scapula to the chest wall during adduction of the shoulder and extension of the arm, and division of the nerve may result in the winged scapula deformity. For this reason the long thoracic nerve is preserved during standard axillary dissection. The second major nerve trunk encountered during axillary dissection is the thoracodorsal nerve to the latissimus dorsi muscle at the lateral border of the axilla. This nerve arises from the posterior cord of the brachial plexus and enters the axillary space under the axillary vein, close to the entrance of the long thoracic nerve. It then crosses the axilla to the medial surface of the latissimus dorsi muscle. The thoracodorsal nerve is usually preserved during dissection of the axillary nodes. The medial pectoral nerves innervate the pectoralis major muscle and are in a neurovascular bundle that wraps around the lateral border of the pectoralis minor muscle. The pectoral neurovascular bundle is a good landmark in that it indicates the position of the axillary vein just above and deep (superior and posterior) to the bundle. This neurovascular bundle needs to be preserved during standard axillary dissection.

The large sensory intercostal brachial or brachial cutaneous nerves span the axillary space and supply sensation to the undersurface of the upper part of the arm and skin of the chest wall along the posterior margin of the axilla. Cutting these nerves causes cutaneous anesthesia in these areas, which is described to patients before axillary dissection. Denervation of the areas supplied by these sensory nerves can cause chronic and uncomfortable pain syndromes in a small percentage of patients. Preservation of the superior-most nerve leaves sensation to the posterior aspect of the upper part of the arm intact without compromising the axillary dissection in most patients.

MICROSCOPIC ANATOMY

A mature breast is composed of three principal tissue types: (1) glandular epithelium, (2) fibrous stroma and supporting structures, and (3) fat. Infiltrating cells, including lymphocytes and macrophages, are also found within the breast. In youth, the predominant tissues are epithelium and stroma, which may be replaced by fat in postmenopausal women as they age. However, there is great variability among individual women of any age. Mammography in women younger than 30 years, whose breast tissue is dense with stroma and epithelium, may produce an image without much definition. Fat absorbs relatively little radiation and provides a contrasting background that favors detection of small lesions in older patients. Throughout the fat of the breast, coursing from the overlying skin to the underlying deep fascia, strands of dense connective tissue called *Cooper's ligaments* provide shape to the breast. Because they are anchored into the skin, tethering of these ligaments by a small scirrhous (scarring) carcinoma commonly produces a dimple or subtle deformity on the otherwise smooth surface of the breast.

The glandular apparatus of the breast is composed of a branching system of ducts, roughly organized in a radial

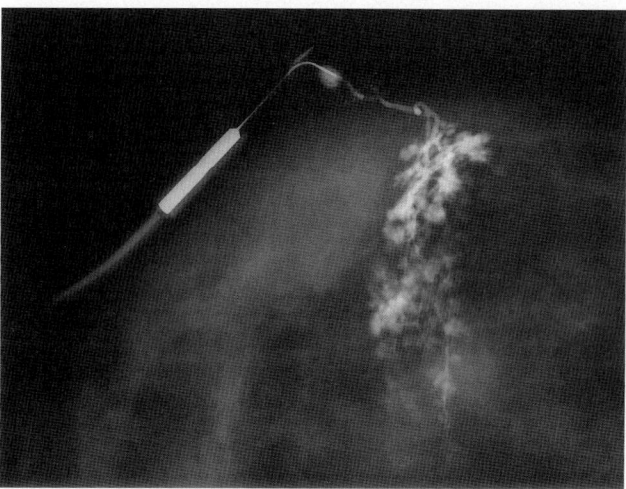

Figure 34-3 Injection of contrast into a single ductal system (ductogram). Occasionally used to evaluate surgically significant nipple discharge, ductography is performed by cannulation of an individual duct orifice and injection of contrast material. This ductogram opacifies the entire ductal tree from the retroareolar duct to the lobules at the end of the tree. This picture also demonstrates the functional independence of each duct system; there is no cross-communication between independent systems.

pattern spreading outward and downward from the nipple-areolar complex (see Fig. 34-1). It is possible to cannulate individual ducts and visualize the lactiferous ducts with contrast agents. Figure 34-3 shows such an image and demonstrates the arborizing tree of branching ducts, which end in terminal lobules. The contrast dye opacifies only a single ductal system and does not enter adjacent and intertwined branches from functionally independent ductal trees. At the summit of the arborizing ductal system, the subareolar ducts widen to form the lactiferous sinuses, which then exit through 10 to 15 orifices on the nipple. These large ducts close to the nipple are lined with a low columnar or cuboidal epithelium that abruptly meets the squamous epithelium of the nipple surface and invades the duct for a short distance.

At the opposite end of the ductal system and after progressive generations of branching, the ducts end blindly in clusters of spaces called *terminal ductules* or *acini* (Fig. 34-4). These are the milk-forming glands of the lactating breast and, together with their small efferent ducts or ductules, are known as *lobular units* or *lobules*. As shown in Figure 34-4, the terminal ductules are invested in a specialized loose connective tissue that contains capillaries, lymphocytes, and other migratory mononuclear cells. This intralobular stroma is clearly distinguished from the denser and less cellular interlobular stroma and from the fat within the breast.

Under the luminal epithelium, the entire ductal system is surrounded by specialized myoepithelial cells that have contractile properties and serve to propel milk formed in the lobules toward the nipple. Outside the epithelial and myoepithelial layers, the ducts of the breast are

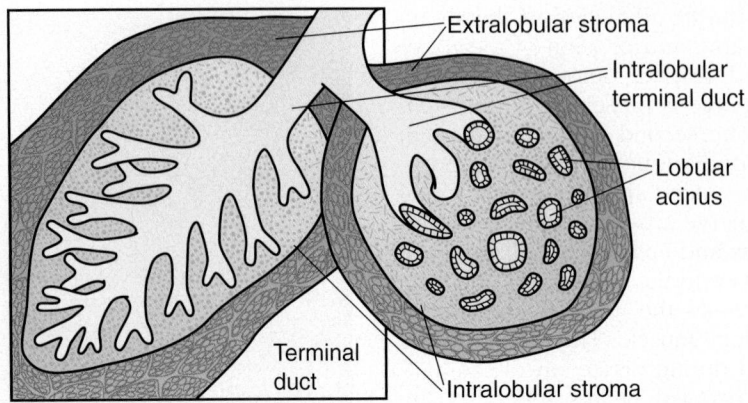

Figure 34-4 The mature resting lobular unit. At the distal end of the ductal system is the lobule. This structure is formed by multiple branching events at the end of terminal ducts, each ending in a blind sac or acini, and is invested with specialized stroma. The lobule is a three-dimensional structure but is seen in two dimensions in a histologic thin section, shown in the lower right. The intralobular terminal ductule and the acini are invested in loose connective tissue containing a modest number of infiltrating lymphocytes and plasma cells. The lobule is distinct from the denser interlobular stroma, which contains larger breast ducts, blood vessels, and fat.

surrounded by a continuous basement membrane containing laminin, type IV collagen, and proteoglycans. The basement membrane layer is extremely important in differentiating in situ from invasive breast cancer. Continuity of this layer around proliferations of ductal cells identifies ductal carcinoma in situ (DCIS) or noninvasive breast cancer (discussed later in the section Pathology of Breast Cancer).

BREAST DEVELOPMENT AND PHYSIOLOGY

Normal Development and Physiology

During prepuberty, the breast is composed primarily of dense fibrous stroma and scattered ducts lined with epithelium. In the United States, puberty, as measured by breast development and the growth of pubic hair, begins between the ages of 9 and 12, and menarche (onset of menstrual cycles) begins about 12 to 13 years of age. These events are initiated by low-amplitude pulses of pituitary gonadotropins, which raise serum estradiol concentrations. In the breast, this hormone-dependent maturation *(thelarche)* entails increased deposition of fat, the formation of new ducts by branching and elongation, and the first appearance of lobular units. This process of remarkable growth and cell division is under the control of estrogen, progesterone, adrenal hormones, pituitary hormones, and the trophic effects of insulin and thyroid hormone. There is evidence that local growth factor networks are also important. The exact timing of these events and the coordinated development of both breast buds may vary from the average in individual patients. The term *prepubertal gynecomastia* refers to symmetrical enlargement and projection of the breast bud in a young girl before the average age of 12 years, unaccompanied by the other changes of puberty. This process, which may be unilateral, should not be confused with neoplastic growth and is not an indication for biopsy.[1-4]

The postpubertal mature or *resting* breast contains fat, stroma, lactiferous ducts, and lobular units. During phases of the menstrual cycle or in response to exogenous hormones, the breast epithelium and lobular stroma undergo cyclic stimulation. It appears that the dominant process is hypertrophy and alteration of morphology rather than hyperplasia. In the late luteal (premenstrual) phase, there is an accumulation of fluid and intralobular edema. It is probable that this edema produces both pain and breast engorgement.

On physical examination and by mammography, this accumulation of fluid leads to increased nodularity and may be mistaken for a dominant tumor. Ill-defined masses in premenopausal women are correctly observed through the course of one or two menstrual cycles. With pregnancy, there is diminution of the fibrous stroma and the formation of new acini or lobules, termed the *adenosis of pregnancy*. After birth there is a sudden loss of placental hormones, which combined with continued high levels of prolactin, is the principal trigger for lactation. The actual expulsion of milk is under hormonal control and is caused by contraction of the myoepithelial cells that surround the breast ducts and terminal ductules. There is no evidence for innervation of these myoepithelial cells; their contraction appears to occur in response to the pituitary-derived peptide oxytocin. Stimulation of the nipple appears to be the physiologic signal for both continued pituitary secretion of prolactin and acute release of oxytocin. When breast-feeding ceases, there is a fall in prolactin and no stimulus for release of oxytocin. The breast then returns to a resting state and to the cyclic changes induced when menstruation begins again.

Menopause is defined by cessation in menstrual flow for 1 year; in the United States it usually occurs between the ages of 40 and 55, with a median age of 51 years. Menopause may be accompanied by constitutional systems such as diaphoresis, vaginal dryness, urinary tract infections, and cognitive impairment (possibly secondary to interruption of sleep by hot flashes). Menopause results in involution and a general decrease in the epithelial elements of the resting breast. These changes include increased fat deposition, diminished connective tissue, and the disappearance of lobular units. The persistence of lobules, hyperplasia of the ductal epithelium, and even cyst formation can all occur under the influence of exogenous ovarian hormones, usually in the form of postmenopausal hormone replacement therapy (HRT). Physicians need to inquire about the menstrual history, establish the cessation of menses in postmenopausal women, and record the use of HRT. A history of hormone use is important to the radiologist looking at a mammogram and to the pathologist evaluating a breast biopsy specimen.

Fibrocystic Changes and Breast Pain

The fibrocystic condition (FCC), previously referred to as *fibrocystic disease,* represents a spectrum of clinical, mammographic, and histologic findings and is common during the forth and fifth decades of life, generally until the approximate age of menopause. FCC appears to represent an exaggerated response of breast stroma and epithelium to a variety of circulating and locally produced hormones and growth factors and is frequently characterized by the constellation of breast pain, tenderness, and nodularity. Symptomatically, the condition is manifested as premenstrual cyclic mastalgia with pain and tenderness to touch. Breast pain is not a symptom of breast cancer. Haagensen carefully recorded the symptoms of women with breast carcinoma and found pain as an unprompted symptom in 5.4% of patients. In women with breast pain and an associated palpable mass, the presence of the mass is the focus of evaluation and treatment. Normal ovarian hormonal influences on breast glandular elements frequently produce *cyclic mastalgia,* generally pain in phase with the menstrual cycle. *Noncyclic mastalgia* is more likely idiopathic and difficult to treat. Women 30 years and older with noncyclic mastalgia probably need to undergo mammography. The exception to this rule is when clinical breast examination reveals a mass, which becomes the focus of subsequent evaluation. Occasionally, a simple cyst may cause noncyclic breast pain, and aspiration of the cyst ends the evaluation.[5]

Patients with fibrocystic change have clinical breast findings that range from mild alterations in texture to dense, firm breast tissue with palpable lumps. The appearance of gross or palpable cysts completes the picture. Mammographically, FCC is usually seen as diffuse or focal radiologically dense tissue. By ultrasound, cysts exist in up to a third of all women 35 to 50 years of age, with most of them being nonpalpable. However, palpable cysts or multiple small cysts are typical of FCC. Cysts, with or without FCC, are uncommon in women older than 60 and younger than 30 years.

Histologically, in addition to macrocysts and microcysts, identified solid elements include adenosis, sclerosis, apocrine metaplasia, stromal fibrosis, and epithelial metaplasia and hyperplasia. Depending on the presence of epithelial hyperplasia, FCC is classified as nonprolifera-

tive, proliferative without atypia, or proliferative with atypia. All three alterations can occur alone or in combination and to a variable degree, and in the absence of epithelial atypia, they represent the histologic spectrum of normal breast tissue. However, atypical epithelial hyperplasia (atypical ductal hyperplasia [ADH]) may display some features of more advanced in situ neoplasia and is a risk factor for the development of breast cancer. As discussed later, atypical proliferations of ductal epithelial cells confer increased risk for breast cancer. However, FCC is not itself a risk factor for the development of breast malignancy.

ABNORMAL DEVELOPMENT AND PHYSIOLOGY

Absent or Accessory Breast Tissue

Absence of breast tissue *(amastia)* and absence of the nipple *(athelia)* are rare anomalies. Unilateral rudimentary breast development is much more common, as is adolescent hypertrophy of one breast with lesser development of the other. In contrast, accessory breast tissue *(polymastia)* and accessory nipples (supernumerary nipples) are both common. Supernumerary nipples are usually rudimentary and occur along the milk line from the axilla to the pubis in both males and females. They may be mistaken for a small mole. However, accessory nipples are removed only for cosmetic reasons. *True polythelia* refers to more than one nipple serving a single breast, which is rare. *Accessory breast tissue* is commonly located above the breast in the axilla. Rudimentary nipple development may be present, and lactation is possible with more complete development. Accessory breast tissue may be seen as an enlarging mass in the axilla during pregnancy and persists as excess tissue in the axilla after lactation is complete. The accessory mammary tissue may be removed surgically if it is large or cosmetically deforming or to prevent enlargement during future pregnancy.[3]

Gynecomastia

Hypertrophy of breast tissue in men is a common clinical entity for which there is frequently no identifiable cause. *Pubertal hypertrophy* occurs in boys between the ages of 13 and early adulthood, and *senescent hypertrophy* is diagnosed in men older than 50 years. Gynecomastia in teenage boys is common and may be either bilateral or unilateral. Unless it is unilateral or painful, it may pass unnoticed and regress with adulthood. Pubertal hypertrophy is generally treated by reassurance without surgery. Surgical excision may be discussed if the enlargement is unilateral, fails to regress, or is cosmetically unacceptable. Hypertrophy in older men is also common. The enlargement is frequently unilateral, although the contralateral breast may enlarge with time. A number of commonly used medications, such as digoxin, thiazides, estrogens, phenothiazines, and theophylline, may exacerbate senescent gynecomastia. In addition, gynecomastia may be a systemic manifestation of hepatic cirrhosis, renal failure, and malnutrition. In both ages the mass is smooth, firm, and symmetrically distributed beneath the areola. It is frequently tender and the reason for seeking medical attention. Both pubertal and senescent gynecomastia may be left untreated and do not require biopsy. There is little confusion with carcinoma occurring in the male breast. Carcinoma is not usually tender, it is asymmetrically located either beneath or beside the areola, and it may be fixed to the overlying dermis or to the deep fascia. A dominant mass suspected of being carcinoma is sampled or carefully observed.

Nipple Discharge

The appearance of a discharge from the nipple of a nonlactating woman is frightening out of proportion to its medical significance. Nipple discharge is common and is rarely associated with an underlying carcinoma. In one review of 270 subareolar biopsies for discharge coming from one identifiable duct and without an associated breast mass, carcinoma was found in only 16 patients (5.9%). In each of these cases the fluid either was bloody or tested strongly positive for occult hemoglobin. In another series of 249 patients, breast carcinoma was found in 10 (4%). In 8 of these patients a mass lesion coexisted with the discharge. In the absence of a palpable mass or a suspicious mammogram, discharge is rarely associated with cancer.

It is important to establish whether the discharge comes from one breast or from both breasts, whether it comes from multiple duct orifices or from just one, and whether the discharge is grossly bloody or contains blood. A milky discharge from both breasts is termed *galactorrhea*. In the absence of lactation or a history of recent lactation, galactorrhea may be associated with increased production of prolactin. Radioimmunoassay for serum prolactin is diagnostic. However, true galactorrhea is rare and is diagnosed only when the discharge is milky (contains lactose, fat, and milk-specific proteins). Unilateral, nonmilky discharge coming from one duct orifice is surgically significant and warrants special attention (Fig. 34-5). However, the underlying cause is rarely a breast malignancy.

The most common cause of spontaneous nipple discharge from a single duct is a solitary intraductal papilloma in one of the large subareolar ducts under the nipple. Subareolar duct ectasia producing inflammation and dilation of large collecting ducts under the nipple is common and usually involves discharge from multiple ducts. Cancer is a very unusual cause of discharge in the absence of other signs. In summary, nipple discharge that is bilateral and comes from multiple ducts is not usually a surgical problem. Bloody discharge from a single duct, as depicted in Figure 34-5, does require surgical biopsy to establish a diagnosis. Intraductal papilloma is found in most of these cases.

Galactocele

A galactocele is a milk-filled cyst that is round, well circumscribed, and easily movable within the breast. It generally occurs after the cessation of lactation or when feeding frequency has curtailed significantly. Haagensen states that galactoceles may occur up to 6 to 10 months after breast-feeding has stopped. The pathogenesis of galactocele is not known, but it is thought that inspissated milk within ducts is responsible. The tumor is usually located in the central portion of the breast or under the nipple. Needle aspiration produces thick, creamy material that may be tinged dark green or brown. Although it appears purulent, the fluid is sterile. Treatment is needle aspiration, and withdrawal of thick milky secretion confirms the diagnosis; surgery is reserved for cysts that cannot be aspirated or those that become infected.

DIAGNOSIS OF BREAST DISEASE

History

The examiner determines the patient's age and obtains a reproductive history, including age at menarche, menstrual irregularities, and age at menopause. Ask about previous breast surgery, particularly breast biopsies and their pathologic findings. Determine whether a hysterectomy has been performed and, because hysterectomy is a common procedure, whether the ovaries were removed. If a hysterectomy has been performed, it may be useful to inquire about menopausal symptoms. In younger (premenopausal) women, a recent history of pregnancy and lactation are recorded. A drug history is elicited and attention paid to HRT or the use of hormones for contraception. The family history is directed to cancer of the breast and ovaries in primary relatives (parents, siblings, and offspring).[5]

In questioning the patient about the specific breast problem, it is worthwhile to inquire about breast pain, nipple discharge, and new masses in the breast. If a mass is present, it helps to know how it was found, how long it has been present, what has happened since its discovery, and whether it changes with the menstrual cycle. If cancer is likely, inquiry about constitutional symptoms, bone pain, weight loss, respiratory changes, and similar clinical indications of metastatic disease may occasionally reveal unsuspected distant spread.

Physical Examination

The examination begins with the patient in the upright sitting position with careful visual inspection for obvious masses, asymmetries, and skin changes. The nipples are inspected and compared for the presence of retraction, nipple inversion, or excoriation of the superficial epidermis in Paget's disease (see Fig. 34-5). The use of indirect lighting can unmask subtle dimpling of the skin or nipple caused by a carcinoma placing Cooper's ligaments under tension (see Fig. 34-5). Simple maneuvers such as stretching the arms high above the head or tensing the pectoralis muscles may accentuate asymmetries and dimpling. If carefully sought, dimpling of the skin or nipple retraction is a sensitive and specific sign of underlying cancer.

Edema of the skin, frequently accompanied by erythema, produces a clinical sign known as *peau d'orange*

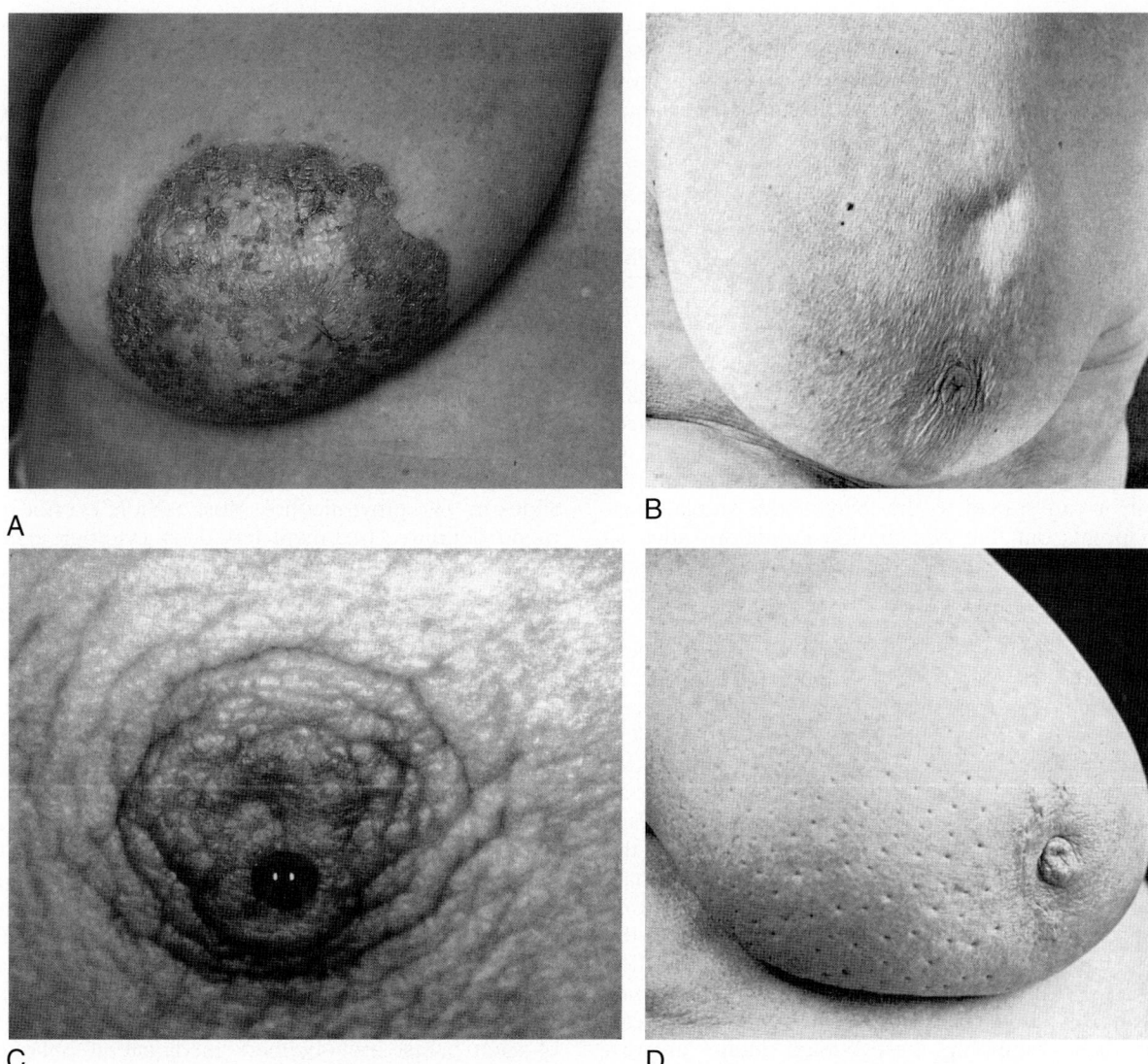

Figure 34-5 Common physical findings during breast examination. **A,** Paget's disease of the nipple. Malignant ductal cells invade the epidermis without traversing the basement membrane of either the subareolar duct or the epidermis. The disease appears as a psoriatic rash that begins on the nipple and spreads off onto the areola and into the skin of the breast. **B,** Skin dimpling. Traction on Cooper's ligaments by a scirrhous tumor is distorting the surface of the breast and producing a dimple best seen with angled indirect lighting during abduction of the arms upward. **C,** Nipple discharge. Discharge from multiple ducts or bilateral discharge is a common finding in healthy breasts. In this case the discharge is from a single duct orifice and may signify underlying disease in the discharging duct. In this patient a papilloma was the source of her symptoms. **D,** Peau d'orange (skin of the orange) or edema of the skin of the breast. This finding may be due to dependency of the breast, lymphatic blockage (from surgery or radiation), or mastitis. The most feared cause is inflammatory carcinoma, in which malignant cells plug the dermal lymphatics (the pathologic hallmark of the disease).

(see Fig. 34-5). When combined with tenderness and warmth, these signs and symptoms are the hallmark of *inflammatory carcinoma* and may be mistaken for acute mastitis. The inflammatory changes and edema are caused by obstruction of dermal lymphatic channels with emboli of carcinoma cells. Occasionally, a bulky tumor may produce obstruction of lymph channels that results in overlying skin edema. This is not, strictly speaking, an inflammatory carcinoma, in which the visible signs are out of proportion to the palpable mass. In 40 patients with inflammatory carcinoma who underwent treatment

with Haagensen, erythema and edema of the skin were present in all cases, a palpable mass or localized induration was noted in 19, and in 21 patients no localized tumor was present.

Involvement of the nipple and areola is common in breast carcinoma. Direct involvement may accompany tumors originating in breast tissue under the areola and may result in retraction of the nipple. Flattening or actual inversion of the nipple can be caused by fibrosis in certain benign conditions, especially subareolar duct ectasia. In these cases the finding is frequently bilateral and the history confirms that the condition has been present for many years. Unilateral retraction or retraction that develops over a period of weeks or months is more suggestive of carcinoma. Centrally located tumors may directly invade and ulcerate the skin of the areola or nipple. Peripheral tumors may distort the normal symmetry of the nipples by traction on Cooper's ligaments.

The second clinical feature of carcinoma that directly involves the nipple was described by Sir James Paget in 1874 and named *Paget's disease.* Histologically, this disease is produced by intraductal carcinoma in the large sinuses just under the nipple (see Fig. 34-5). Carcinoma cells invade across the junction of epidermal and ductal epithelial cells and enter the epidermal layer of the skin of the nipple. Clinically, this histologic variant produces a dermatitis that may appear eczematoid and moist or dry and psoriatic. It is usually confined to the nipple, although it can spread to the skin of the areola. Haagensen points out that benign skin conditions such as eczema frequently begin on the areola whereas Paget's disease originates on the nipple and secondarily involves the areola.

Palpation follows visual inspection. While the patient is still in the sitting position, the examiner supports the patient's arm and palpates each axilla to detect the presence of enlarged axillary lymph nodes. The supraclavicular and infraclavicular spaces are similarly palpated for enlarged nodes. Palpation of the breast is always done with the patient lying supine on a solid examining surface with the arm stretched above the head. Palpation of the breast while the patient is sitting is insensitive and inaccurate. The breast is compressed against the chest wall, with palpation of each quadrant and the tissue under the areola. Masses found are characterized according to their size, shape, consistency, and location. Benign tumors, such as fibroadenomas and cysts, can be as firm as carcinoma; most commonly, these benign entities are distinct, well circumscribed, and movable. Carcinoma is typically firm but less circumscribed, and moving it produces a drag of adjacent tissue. Neither benign nor malignant tumors are usually tender; tenderness is rarely a helpful diagnostic sign. Generally, 75% of palpable masses are self-discovered by patients during casual or intentional self-examination.

Fine-Needle Aspiration

Fine-needle aspiration (FNA) has become a routine part of the physical diagnosis of breast masses. It can be done with a 22-gauge needle, an appropriate-size syringe, and an alcohol preparation pad. The main utility of FNA is differentiation of solid from cystic masses, but it may be done whenever a new dominant, unexplained mass is found in the breast. This simple procedure is postponed only if mammography is necessary and might confuse the radiographic evaluation. Cyst fluid is usually turbid and dark green or amber and can be discarded if the mass totally disappears and the fluid is not bloody. By using FNA in routine examination of the breast, unnecessary open biopsy of cystic change is avoided. As a result of adding FNA to the routine examination of breast

masses, restating of the criteria for open biopsy is helpful. Carcinoma will not be missed if a surgical biopsy is done when (1) needle aspiration produces no cyst fluid and a solid mass is diagnosed, (2) the cyst fluid produced is thick and blood tinged, and (3) fluid is produced but the mass fails to resolve completely. Other surgeons have added frequent reappearance of the cyst in the same location and rapid reaccumulation of fluid after initial aspiration (within a few days).

If the mass is solid and the clinical situation is consistent with carcinoma, cytologic examination of the aspirated material is performed. The needle is repeatedly inserted into the mass while constant negative pressure is applied to the syringe. Suction is released and the needle is withdrawn. The scanty fluid and cellular material within the needle are either submitted in physiologically buffered saline (Normosol) or fixed immediately on slides in 95% ethyl alcohol. Most authors do not recommend definitive treatment based on cytologic examination. In addition, the presence of carcinoma cells on FNA does not differentiate between in situ and invasive breast cancer. However, a positive result allows informed discussions with the patient, definite plans for treatment, and appropriate consultations or second opinions.

BREAST IMAGING

Breast imaging techniques are used to detect small, nonpalpable breast abnormalities, evaluate clinical findings, and guide diagnostic procedures. *Mammography* is the primary imaging modality for screening asymptomatic women. During mammography the breast is compressed between Plexiglas plates to reduce the thickness of the tissue through which the radiation must pass, separate adjacent structures, and improve resolution. Two views of each breast are obtained: mediolateral oblique and craniocaudal. Additional magnification and compression views are used to provide additional detail. Mammographic sensitivity is limited by breast density, with as many as 10% to 15% of clinically evident breast cancers having no associated mammographic abnormality. *Digital mammography* acquires digital images and stores them electronically, thereby allowing manipulation and enhancement of images to facilitate interpretation. Digital mammography appears to be superior to traditional film-screen mammography for detecting cancer in younger women and those with dense breasts. *Ultrasonography* is useful in determining whether a lesion detected by other modalities is solid or cystic and in determining contour and internal properties of a lesion, but it is not a useful screening modality.[6-8]

Magnetic resonance imaging (MRI) is increasingly being used for the evaluation of breast abnormalities. It is useful in finding the primary breast lesion in patients with malignant axillary nodes but no palpable or mammographic evidence of a primary breast tumor. MRI may be more accurate than mammography in assessing the extent of the primary tumor, particularly in young women with dense breast tissue, and in diagnosing invasive lobular cancer, and it may help determine eligibility for

Table 34-1   Prospective, Randomized Trials of Screening Mammography*

STUDY	YEARS CONDUCTED	AGE (yr)	MEDIAN FOLLOW-UP (yr)	SCREENING INTERVAL (mo)	MAMMOGRAPH VIEWS (N)	RR FOR DEATH FROM BREAST CANCER (95% CI)	ABSOLUTE RISK REDUCTION PER 1000 WOMEN	WOMEN INVITED (N)	CONTROL (N)
Mammography Alone									
Stockholm	1981-1986	40-64	13.8	24-28	1	0.91 (0.65-1.27)	0.288	40,318	19,943
Gothenburg	1983-1988	39-59	12.8	18	1, 2	0.76 (0.56-1.04)	0.878	20,724	28,809
Malmö	1977-1990	45-70	17.1	18-24	1, 2	0.82 (0.67-1.00)	1.712	21,088	21,195
Swedish Two-County Trial[†]	1977-1989	40-74	17	24-33	1	0.68 (0.59-0.80)	1.809	77,080	55,985
Mammography Plus Clinical Breast Examination									
CNBSS-1	1980-1985	40-49	13	12	2	0.97 (0.74-1.27)	0.12	25,214	25,216
CNBSS-2	1980-1985	50-59	13	12	2	1.02 (0.78-1.33)	0.097	19,711	19,694
HIP	1963-1966	40-64	16	12	2	0.79	1.438	30,239	30,256
Edinburgh	1978-1985	45-64	13	24	1, 2	0.79 (0.60-1.02)	1.020	28,628	26,015

*Results of eight randomized trials summarized in the National Institutes of Health Consensus Development Panel. National Institutes of Health Consensus Development Conference Statement: Breast cancer screening for women ages 40-49, January 21-23, 1997. J Natl Cancer Inst Monogr 22:vii-xii, 1997, and updated in Humphrey LL, Helfand M, Chan BK, et al: Breast cancer screening: A summary of the evidence for the U.S. Preventive Services Task Force. Ann Intern Med 137:347, 2002.

[†]The Swedish Two-County Trial combines data from Ostergotland and Kopparberg.

CI, confidence interval; CNBSS, Canadian National Breast Screening Study; HIP, Health Insurance Plan of New York; RR, relative risk.

breast conservation. The utility of MRI as a screening tool is under investigation, although it appears promising for early detection of malignancy in patients with *BRCA* gene mutations. The sensitivity of MRI for invasive cancer is greater than 90%, but it is only 60% or less for DCIS. The specificity of MRI is only moderate, with significant overlap in the appearance of benign and malignant lesions.

Screening Mammography

Screening mammography is performed in asymptomatic women with the goal of detecting breast cancer that is not yet clinically evident. This approach assumes that breast cancers identified through screening will be smaller, have a better prognosis, and require less aggressive treatment than cancers identified by palpation. These potential benefits of screening are weighed against the cost of screening and the number of false-positive studies that prompt additional workup, biopsies, and patient anxiety.[9,10]

Eight prospective randomized trials of screening mammography, which together randomized nearly 500,000 women, are summarized in Table 34-1. In response to periodic controversies, the results from randomized trials have undergone additional analysis. In 2002, the U.S. Preventive Service Task Force reviewed the eight trials and performed a meta-analysis using a bayesian random effects model to evaluate the effectiveness of screening mammography after 14 years of observation. In the analysis of all age groups, screening mammography reduced the risk for breast cancer death by 16% (relative risk [RR], 0.84; confidence interval [CI], 0.77-0.91). In women 50 years and older, the reduction in risk was 15% (RR, 0.85; CI, 0.73-0.99) with inclusion of the Canadian trial and

22% (RR, 0.78; CI, 0.67-0.96) with exclusion of this study. For women aged 40 to 49, screening mammography reduced the risk for breast cancer by 15% (RR, 0.85; CI, 0.73-0.99).

At present, screening mammography is offered annually to women 50 years and older and at least biennially to women 40 to 49 years of age, with the screening interval determined on an individual basis after consideration of the risk factors for breast cancer. Younger women with a significant family history, histologic risk factors, or a history of previous breast cancer are offered annual screening. Although none of the randomized trials enrolled women older than 74 years, breast cancer risk increases with advancing age, and the sensitivity and specificity of mammography are highest in older women, whose breast tissue has usually been replaced by fat. It is reasonable to continue mammographic screening in older women who are in sufficiently good health to tolerate wide excision of any cancer detected on mammography.

Nonpalpable Mammographic Abnormalities

Mammographic abnormalities that cannot be detected by physical examination include clustered microcalcifications and areas of abnormal density (masses, architectural distortions, and asymmetries) that have not produced a palpable finding (Fig. 34-6). The Breast Imaging Reporting and Data System (BI-RADS) is used to categorize the degree of suspicion of malignancy for a mammographic abnormality (Table 34-2). To avoid unnecessary biopsies for low-suspicion mammographic findings, probably benign lesions are designated BI-RADS 3 and are monitored with a schedule of short-interval mammograms

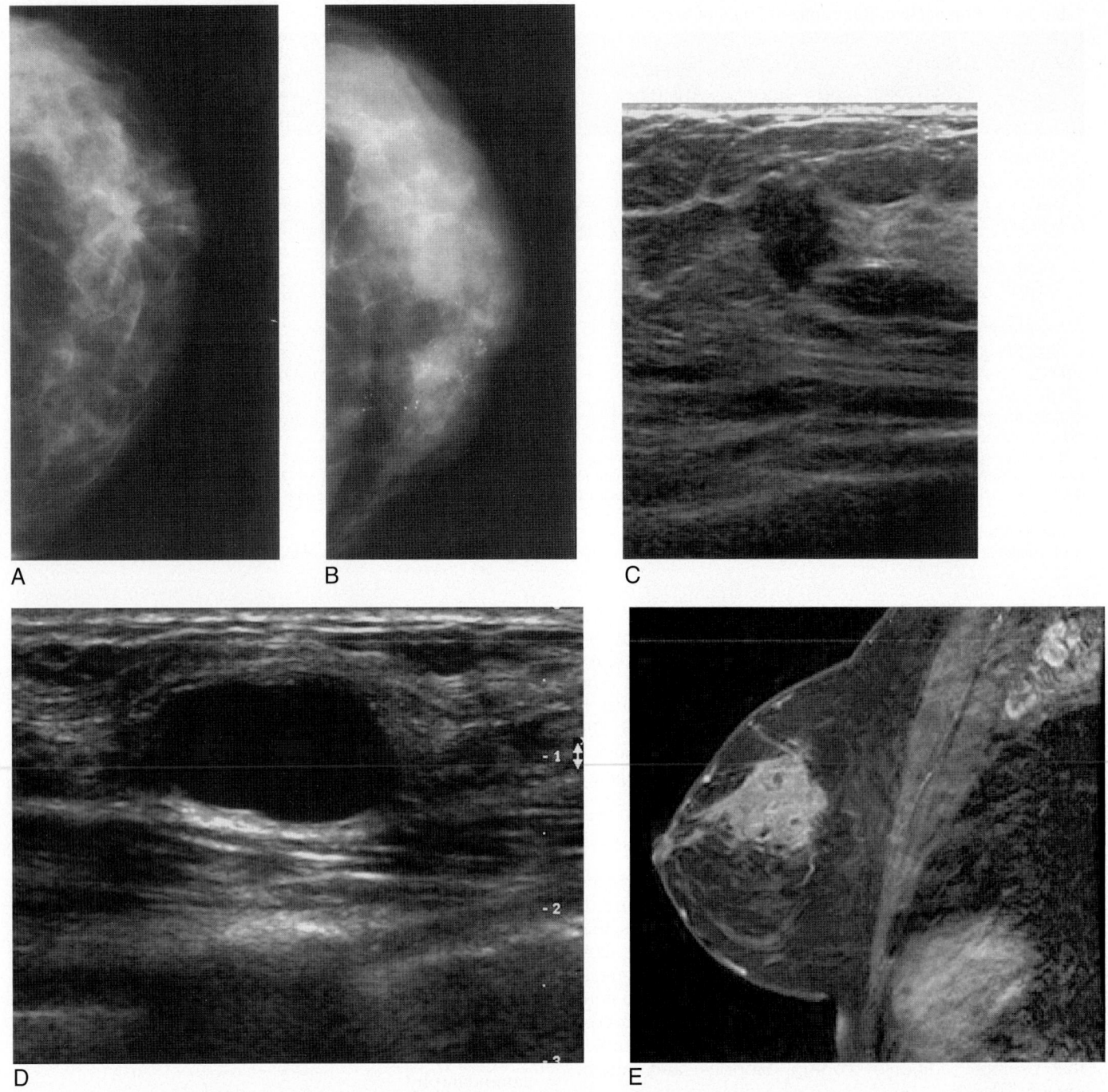

Figure 34-6 Mammographic, ultrasonographic, and MRI findings in breast disease. **A,** Stellate mass in the breast. The combination of a density with spiculated borders and distortion of surrounding breast architecture suggests a malignancy. **B,** Clustered microcalcifications. Fine, pleomorphic, and linear calcifications that cluster together suggest the diagnosis of ductal carcinoma in situ. **C,** Ultrasound image of breast cancer. The mass is solid, contains internal echoes, and displays an irregular border. Most malignant lesions are taller than they are wide. **D,** Ultrasound image of a simple cyst. By ultrasound, the cyst is round with smooth borders, there is a paucity of internal sound echoes, and there is increased through-transmission of sound with enhanced posterior echoes. **E,** Breast MRI showing gadolinium enhancement of a breast cancer. Rapid and intense gadolinium enhancement reflects increased tumor vascularity. Lesion contour and size may also be assessed by MRI.

over a 2-year period. Biopsy is performed only for lesions that progress during follow-up.

Diagnostic biopsy of a nonpalpable mammographic lesion may be performed by image-guided core needle biopsy or image-guided wire localization (to mark the area of the lesion) and surgical excision. Because 75% to 80% of patients for whom biopsy is recommended will have benign findings, the less invasive and less costly image-guided core needle biopsy approach is preferred whenever feasible.

Table 34-2 Breast Imaging Reporting and Data System (BI-RADS): Final Assessment Category

CATEGORY	DEFINITION
0	Incomplete assessment; need additional imaging evaluation
1	Negative; routine mammogram in 1 year recommended
2	Benign finding; routine mammogram in 1 year recommended
3	Probably benign finding; short-term follow-up suggested
4	Suspicious abnormality; biopsy should be considered
5	Highly suggestive of malignancy; appropriate action should be taken

Adapted from Liberman L, Abramson AF, Squires FB, et al: The Breast Imaging Reporting and Data System: Positive predictive values of mammographic feature and final assessment categories. AJR Am J Roentgenol 171:35, 1998; and Liberman L, Menell JH: Breast imaging reporting and data systems (BI-RADS). Radiol Clin North Am 40:409, 2002.

Wire-Localized Surgical Excision

Nonpalpable breast lesions may require excision for diagnosis or as part of breast-conserving treatment of a known cancer. Immediately before surgery, a localizing wire is placed adjacent to the lesion under mammographic or ultrasound guidance. The wire is placed though an introducer needle and has a hook that engages to hold it in position after the introducer is withdrawn. Images with the wire in place are made available in the operating room to guide the surgeon. Proper surgical technique will place the incision directly over the lesion to be excised and not necessarily at the wire entry site. After excision, the specimen is sent directly to the breast imaging suite and an image of the specimen taken to confirm that the targeted lesion has been excised.

Image-Guided Core Needle Biopsy

Core needle biopsy is now the method of choice to sample nonpalpable mammographic abnormalities. This technique is also useful for minimally invasive diagnosis of palpable lesions that can be visualized on mammography or ultrasound.[11]

Core needle biopsy can be performed under mammographic (stereotactic), ultrasound, or MRI guidance. Lesions visualized on ultrasound can be sampled under ultrasound guidance; calcifications and densities, seen best on mammography, are sampled under stereotactic guidance. In stereotactic core needle biopsy the breast is compressed, most often with the patient lying prone on the stereotactic core biopsy table. After local anesthetic is injected, a 3-mm skin incision is made, and an 11-gauge core biopsy needle with vacuum assistance is inserted into the lesion to obtain the tissue sample. A robotic arm and biopsy device are positioned by computed analysis of triangulated mammographic images.

Multiple core samples are obtained and a clip placed to mark the site of the lesion, particularly for small lesions that may be difficult to find after extensive sampling. A similar approach is used for MRI-guided biopsy of lesions visualized only on MRI.

Specimen radiography of excised cores is performed to confirm that the targeted lesion has been sampled, and a postbiopsy mammogram confirms that a defect has been created within the target lesion and that the marking clip is in the correct position. Wire localization and surgical excision are required if the lesion cannot be adequately sampled by core biopsy approaches.

Interpretation of Core Needle Biopsy Results: Caveats

The limited sample size obtained by core biopsy techniques requires proper interpretation of the pathology results obtained. The majority of patients undergoing core biopsy will have a definitive benign finding and may return to routine screening with no other intervention required. If a malignancy is diagnosed, histologic and receptor data may be determined on the core biopsy sample, and the patient may proceed to definitive treatment of the cancer. Surgeons need to be aware that approximately 10% of patients noted to have DCIS on core biopsy will be found to have some associated invasive carcinoma at definitive surgery.[12]

Approximately 10% of patients who undergo core biopsy will have inconclusive results and require wire-localized surgical biopsy for definitive diagnosis. Biopsy results that are not concordant with the targeted lesion (e.g., a spiculated mass on imaging and normal breast tissue on core biopsy) require surgical excision. When ADH is found on core biopsy, surgical excision will reveal DCIS or invasive carcinoma in 20% or more of cases because of difficulty distinguishing ADH and DCIS in a limited tissue sample. A finding of a cellular fibroadenoma on core biopsy requires excision to rule out a phyllodes tumor.

IDENTIFICATION AND MANAGEMENT OF HIGH-RISK PATIENTS

Risk Factors for Breast Cancer

Identification of factors responsible for increasing the chance of breast cancer developing is important in daily clinical practice for clinicians who care for women. Risk factors are broadly divided into those useful in clinical practice, that is, significantly influencing the odds of contracting breast cancer in individual women, and those very important in large public health trends in populations. A partial list of these factors is presented in Box 34-1.

Age and Gender

Age is probably the most important risk factor that clinicians use in everyday clinical practice. The age-adjusted incidence of breast cancer continues to increase with advancing age of the female population. Breast cancer is rare in persons younger than 20 years, and cases in

Box 34-1 Risk Factors for Breast Cancer

Factors Important in Populations

Age at menarche and menopause
Parity
Age at first birth
Breast-feeding
Exogenous hormone use or exposure
Alcohol consumption

Factors Important in Individual Patients

Gender (female >> male)
Age (steady increase with age)
Family history (mothers, sisters, daughters)
History of previous breast cancer (noninvasive or invasive, ipsilateral or contralateral)

Histologic Risk Factors

Proliferative breast disease
Atypical ductal hyperplasia (ADH)
Atypical lobular hyperplasia (ALH)
Lobular carcinoma in situ (LCIS)

---

women younger than 30 constitute less than 2% of the total cases. Thereafter, the incidence increases to 1 in 93 by age 40, 1 in 50 by age 50, 1 in 24 by age 60, 1 in 14 by age 70, and 1 in 10 by age 80. Alternatively stated, the annual frequency of breast cancer in the eighth decade of life is greater than 300 cases per 100,000. Gender is also an important risk factor. Males are at risk for breast cancer, although the incidence in males is less than 1% of the incidence in females, with 1720 cases of invasive breast cancer anticipated in 2006 (out of a total burden of 215,000 estimated cases). Lumps in the male breast are much more likely to be benign and the result of gynecomastia (discussed earlier) or other noncancerous tumors.[13]

Lobular Carcinoma In Situ and Personal History

Histologic abnormalities diagnosed by breast biopsy represent an important category of breast cancer risk factors. A history of mammary cancer in one breast increases the likelihood of a second primary cancer in the contralateral breast. In many studies, the RR (ratio of observed cases over expected cases) for contralateral breast cancer ranges between 3 and 4 after breast cancer in one breast. The magnitude of RR depends on the age at diagnosis of the first primary cancer. In patients younger than 45, the risk for the cancer in the remaining breast is five or six times that of the general population. In older patients, this risk decreases to a twofold or less increased risk. In absolute terms, the actual risk varies between 1% per year in young patients to 0.2% in older patients.[3,14]

Lobular carcinoma in situ (LCIS) is a relatively uncommon condition that is observed predominantly in younger, premenopausal women. It is typically an incidental finding at biopsy for another condition and does not itself form a palpable mass, nor is LCIS commonly manifested as calcifications mammographically. Haagensen has col-

lected the largest series of patients with LCIS, all of whom were identified by review of biopsy material. In this review, LCIS was found in 3.6% of more than 5000 biopsies performed for benign disease. In his review of 297 patients with LCIS treated by biopsy and careful observation, Haagensen determined that the actuarial probability of carcinoma developing at the end of 35 years was 21.4%. When compared with the Connecticut Tumor Registry data, a risk ratio (ratio of observed to expected cases) of 7:1 was calculated. Significantly, 40% of the carcinomas that subsequently developed were purely in situ lesions, the invasive cancers that developed were predominantly ductal and not lobular in histology, and half of the carcinomas occurred in the contralateral breast. Thus, LCIS is not a breast cancer but rather a histologic marker for increased breast cancer susceptibility, which is estimated at slightly less than 1% per year longitudinally.

Although no direct survey of surgical practice has been done, a conservative approach rather than mastectomy is more commonly taken with LCIS patients. Certainly, a policy of close observation with or without tamoxifen chemoprevention is widely recognized as standard care. Patients are informed that LCIS predisposes to subsequent carcinoma and that the risk is lifelong and increases with time. Because the risk for subsequent breast cancer is equal for both breasts, biopsy of the opposite breast adds little useful information. A 5-year course of tamoxifen provides a 56% reduction in breast cancer risk (see later). For those who elect surgery in preference to observation, bilateral total mastectomy remains the procedure of choice. Subcutaneous mastectomy, with preservation of the nipple-areolar complex, retains breast glandular cells in the nipple and behind the areola and therefore is not an appropriate method of cancer prevention.

Other Histologic Risk Factors

Benign breast disease, including FCC, is an important risk factor for the eventual development of breast cancer. Benign disease produces a spectrum of histologic changes, and FCC is broadly divided into histologic lesions that display *proliferative* epithelial alterations and those that display *nonproliferative* alterations. Nonproliferative changes include mild to moderate hyperplasia of luminal cells within breast ducts, and these changes do not appear to significantly increase a women's lifetime risk for breast cancer. The excess risk for breast cancer is concentrated in women whose specimens show proliferative changes within breast ducts. Dupont and Page divided proliferative lesions into those with atypical epithelial hyperplasia and those without atypia (sometimes proliferative lesions without atypia are called *severe hyperplasia*).

Subsequent studies have adhered to this classification scheme, which in summary consists of nonproliferative lesions, proliferation of breast epithelium without atypia (severe hyperplasia), and proliferation with atypia. The latter category includes *ADH* and *atypical lobular hyperplasia (ALH)*. The RR for cancer in women with either ADH or ALH is between four and five times the risk for development of breast cancer in a control population of

Table 34-3   Histologic Risk Factors for Breast Cancer*

HISTOLOGIC DIAGNOSIS	RELATIVE RISK ESTIMATES†
Nonproliferative disease‡	1.0
Proliferative disease without atypia§	1.3-1.9
Proliferative disease with atypia¶	3.7-4.2
and a strong family history	4-9
and premenopausal or age ≥50	5-7
Lobular carcinoma in situ (LCIS)	>7

*Estimates have been compiled from several sources, including (1) Hartmann LC, Sellers TA, Frost MH, et al: Benign breast disease and the risk of breast cancer. N Engl J Med 353:229, 2005; (2) London SJ, Connolly JL, Schnitt SJ, Colditz GA: A prospective study of benign breast disease and the risk of breast cancer. JAMA 267:1780, 1992; (3) Dupont WD, Parl FF, Hartmann WH, et al: Breast cancer risk associated with proliferative breast disease and atypical hyperplasia. Cancer 71:1258, 1993.

†Ratio of observed incidence over the incidence in women without proliferative disease.

‡Fibrocystic change with no, usual, or mild hyperplasia.

§Fibrocystic change with hyperplasia greater than mild or usual, papilloma, papillomatosis, sclerosing adenosis, radial scar, and other findings.

¶Any diagnosis of atypical ductal or lobular hyperplasia, or both.

women. Coexistence of a positive family history with atypical hyperplasia increases the risk to nearly nine times that of the general population. Thus, the annual risk for development of breast cancer in a woman with LCIS is slightly less than 1% per year, and with either ADH or ALH it is between 0.5% and 1% per year. These estimates are influenced by age at diagnosis, menopausal status, and family history. An overview of histologic risk factors is presented in Table 34-3.[15]

Family History and Genetic Risk Factors

Many studies have examined the relationship of family history and the risk for breast cancer. These studies can be summarized as follows:

1. First-degree relatives (mothers, sisters, and daughters) of patients with breast cancer have a twofold to threefold excess risk for the disease.
2. Risk decreases quickly in women with distant relatives affected with breast cancer (cousins, aunts, grandmothers).
3. Risk is much higher if affected first-degree relatives had premenopausal onset and bilateral breast cancer.

In families with multiple affected members, particularly with bilateral and early-onset cancer, the absolute risk in first-degree relatives approaches 50%, consistent with an autosomal dominant mode of inheritance in these families.[16]

Genetic factors are estimated to cause 5% to 10% of all breast cancer cases, but they may account for 25% of cases in women younger than 30 years. In 1990 a group led by Mary-Claire King identified a region on the long arm of chromosome 17 (17q21) that contained a cancer susceptibility gene. The gene, *BRCA1,* was finally discov-

ered in 1994 and accounts for up to 40% of familial breast cancer. One year later a second susceptibility gene, *BRCA2,* was discovered. In addition to increased breast cancer risk, women with mutations in either *BRCA1* or *BRCA2* are at increased risk for ovarian cancer (45% lifetime risk for *BRCA1* carriers).

Deleterious mutations in *BRCA1* or *BRCA2* are rare in the general population. The frequency of mutations is about 1 in 1000 people (0.1%) in the American population. Certain relatively closed populations may have higher prevalence rates and show preference for certain mutations, called *founder mutations,* including the 185delAG and 5382insC mutations in *BRCA1,* which are found in up to 1.0% of the Ashkenazi Jewish population (Jews of Eastern European descent), and the C4446T mutation in French Canadian families. *BRCA1* is a large gene with 22 coding exons and more than 500 mutations, many unique and limited to a given family, which makes genetic testing a technically difficult procedure. *BRCA1* is a tumor suppressor gene with disease susceptibility inherited in autosomal dominant fashion. Germline mutation inactivates a single inherited allele of *BRCA1* in every cell and precedes a somatic event in breast epithelial cells that eliminates the remaining allele and causes the cancer. The gene product may provide negative regulation of cell growth or perhaps is involved in recognition and repair of genetic damage or spontaneous mutation.

BRCA2 is located on chromosome 13 and accounts for up to 30% of familial breast cancer; unlike *BRCA1,* it is associated with increased breast cancer risk in males. Women with a mutation in *BRCA2* also have a 20% to 30% lifelong risk for ovarian cancer. Founder mutations of *BRCA2* include the 617delT mutation present in 1.4% of the Ashkenazi population, the 8765delAG mutation in the French Canadian population, and the 999del15 mutation in the Icelandic population. In Iceland, 7% of unselected female breast cancer patients and 0.6% of the general population carry the 999del15 mutation.

Penetrance of *BRCA1* and *BRCA2* refers to the chance that carriers of mutations in these genes will actually develop breast cancer. The initial estimates of this chance were high, but a more recent estimate places the penetrance of *BRCA1* and *BRCA2* mutations at 56%, with a 95% confidence interval between 40% and 73%. It is reasonable to quote lifelong rates of breast cancer between 50% and 70% for carriers of *BRCA1* or *BRCA2* mutations.

The histopathology of *BRCA1*-associated cancer is unfavorable when compared with *BRCA2*-associated cancer and includes tumors that are high grade, hormone receptor negative, and aneuploid with an increased S-phase fraction. There is a strong association between the so-called basal-like breast cancer and *BRCA1* mutation. Women who carry a *BRCA1* mutation and contract breast cancer are highly likely to have a basal-like tumor, and up to 10% of tumors that are basal-like arise in women found to have a mutation. The same is not true for *BRCA2*-associated cancers. *BRCA2* tumors are commonly hormone receptor positive. Overall mortality rates in patients with *BRCA1*- or *BRCA2*-associated cancer are probably similar to those in women with sporadic breast cancer. Because the risk for breast cancer is high in carriers of a mutation, the question of increased screening versus chemoprevention, as well as these strategies versus prophylactic mastectomy, is discussed in detail in the subsequent sections.

Reproductive Risk Factors

Reproductive milestones that increase a woman's lifetime estrogen exposure are thought to increase her breast cancer risk and include menarche before 12 years of age, first live childbirth after age 30, nulliparity, and menopause after age 55. There is a 10% reduction in breast cancer risk for each 2-year delay in menarche. The risk doubles with menopause after age 55. Those having a full-term first pregnancy before age 18 have half the risk for development of breast cancer than do women whose first pregnancy is after age 30. There is no known increase or decrease in breast cancer risk associated with induced abortion. When compared with gender, age, histologic risk factors, and genetics, reproductive risk factors are relatively mild (RR from 0.5 to 2.0). However, these factors (unlike family history or histologic factors) affect everyone and have a large influence on breast cancer prevalence in populations.[15]

Exogenous Hormone Use

Therapeutic or supplemental estrogen and progesterone are taken for a variety of conditions. The two most common scenarios are oral contraceptives in premenopausal women and postmenopausal HRT; other indications are for menstrual irregularities, polycystic ovaries, fertility treatment, or hormone insufficiency states. There is no apparent increased risk for breast cancer in current or past users of oral contraceptives (RR of close to 1.0 for both current and past users).[4,17]

The use of HRT was studied by the Women's Health Initiative, a prospective, randomized controlled trial in which healthy postmenopausal women 50 to 79 years of age received various dietary and vitamin supplements and postmenopausal HRT. The study assessed the benefits and risks associated with HRT, a low-fat diet, and calcium and vitamin D supplementation and their effect on rates of cancer, cardiovascular disease, and osteoporosis-related fractures. A total of 16,608 women were randomized to receive combined conjugated equine estrogens (e.g., Premarin, 0.625 mg/day) plus medroxyprogesterone acetate (2.5 mg/day) or placebo from 1993 to 1998 at 40 centers in the United States. Screening mammography and clinical breast examinations were performed at baseline and yearly thereafter. The study reached a stopping rule at 5.2 years of follow-up. There were 245 cases of breast cancer (invasive and noninvasive) in the combined HRT group versus 185 cases in the placebo group (RR = 1.24; $P < .001$). There was a suggestion that tumors in women taking combined HRT were larger and more likely to be node positive. Women who had a hysterectomy were randomized to estrogen only versus placebo, and this part of the study was reported in 2006.

The finding for estrogen-only supplementation was quite different. After 7 years of follow-up, 10,739 women receiving conjugated equine estrogens (e.g., Premarin) at a dose of 0.625 mg daily or an identical-appearing placebo had equivalent rates of breast cancer (RR = 0.88; 95% CI, 0.62-1.04). The only difference that was statistically significant between the treatment and control groups was the need for short-interval mammographic follow-up examinations, which was higher in the hormone group (36.2% versus 28.1%) over the life of the trial. Therefore, women receiving combination HRT with both estrogen and progesterone for 5 years have approximately a 20% increased risk for breast cancer. Women who can take estrogen-only formulations (because of previous hysterectomy) do not appear to suffer an increased incidence of breast cancer.

Risk Assessment Tools

A model for breast cancer risk was developed from case-control data in the Breast Cancer Detection Demonstration Project by Gail and coworkers. These investigators determined that age, race, age at menarche, age at first live birth, number of previous breast biopsies, presence of proliferative disease with atypia, and number of first-degree female relatives with breast cancer influenced the risk for breast cancer. This model is available for clinical use at http://cancer.gov/bcrisktool. The model does not include detailed information about genetic factors and may underestimate the risk for a *BRCA1* or *BRCA2* mutation carrier and overestimate the risk in a noncarrier. The Gail model for breast cancer risk was used in the design of the Breast Cancer Prevention Trial, which randomly assigned women at high risk to receive tamoxifen or a placebo, and in the ongoing Study of Tamoxifen and Raloxifene (STAR), which randomly assigned women at high risk to receive tamoxifen or raloxifene.

Management of High-Risk Patients

In practice, clinicians prioritize risk factors and consider those that are important to individual patients in making recommendations about screening and intervention. For instance, as discussed earlier, reproductive factors are important for breast cancer incidence in populations but generally insufficient to base a recommendation for medical or surgical intervention. Box 34-1 lists many of the breast cancer risk factors commonly asked about in everyday practice and divides them by their priority for populations or individual women. For women harboring individual risk factors for breast cancer, options include close surveillance with clinical breast examination, mammography, and possibly breast MRI. Interventions include chemoprevention with tamoxifen or raloxifene or bilateral prophylactic mastectomy.

Close Surveillance

Surveillance guidelines for individuals at high risk for breast cancer were established in 2002 by the National Comprehensive Cancer Network and the Cancer Genetics Studies Consortium. These guidelines are based primarily on expert opinion; screening guidelines for high-risk individuals are not established by prospective trials.

Recommendations for women in a family with a breast and ovarian cancer syndrome include monthly breast self-examination beginning at 18 to 20 years of age, semiannual clinical breast examination beginning at age 25, and annual mammography beginning at age 25, or 10 years before the earliest age at onset of breast cancer in a family member. Nonetheless, studies of women with known *BRCA1* or *BRCA2* mutations find that half the detected breast cancers were diagnosed as interval cancers; that is, they occurred between screening episodes and not during the course of routine screening. This observation has prompted many groups to add annual screening MRI to mammography, with some doing both simultaneously and others staggering the two examinations. If not done previously, genetic counseling is offered to those with a strong family history of early-onset breast and ovarian cancer, including a discussion of genetic testing for *BRCA1* and *BRCA2* mutations.

Chemoprevention for Breast Cancer

The only drug currently approved for reducing breast cancer risk is tamoxifen. Tamoxifen is an estrogen antagonist with proven benefit for the treatment of estrogen receptor (ER)-positive breast cancer. Furthermore, tamoxifen reduces the incidence of a second primary breast cancer in the contralateral breast of women who received the drug as adjuvant therapy for a first breast cancer. In the Early Breast Cancer Trialists' Collaborative Group (EBCTCG), adjuvant tamoxifen reduced the risk for a second breast cancer in the unaffected breast by 47%. Four prospective, randomized trials of preventive tamoxifen were initiated in healthy women, and the National Cancer Institute (NCI) and the National Surgical Adjuvant Breast and Bowel Project (NSABP) recently announced findings of the STAR trial of tamoxifen versus raloxifene (another selective estrogen receptor modulator [SERM], see later).[18]

The U.S. trial of tamoxifen versus placebo was performed by the NSABP and randomized 13,388 women aged 35 to 59 with a diagnosis of LCIS, women whose risk for breast cancer was moderately increased (RR of 1.66 over a 5-year period), and women 60 years or older. The risk estimates were based on the Gail model of risk (http://cancer.gov/bcrisktool; see earlier). In this study, tamoxifen reduced the risk for invasive breast cancer by 49% through 69 months of follow-up, with a risk reduction of 59% in the subgroup with LCIS and 86% in those with atypical ductal or lobular hyperplasia. The reduction in risk was noted only for ER-positive cancers. Tamoxifen treatment for 5 years was not devoid of complications. In the tamoxifen treatment arm, endometrial cancers resulting from estrogen-like effects of the drug on the endometrium were increased by a factor of about 2.5. Pulmonary embolism (RR of 3) and deep venous thrombosis (RR of 1.7) were also more common. Data on the efficacy of tamoxifen for reduction of breast cancer risk in *BRCA1* and *BRCA2* mutation carriers are currently too limited to quantify.

The second prevention trial conducted by the NSABP is the STAR trial, in which tamoxifen was compared with raloxifene. This comparison was based on analysis of more than 10,000 women who participated in placebo-controlled trials to evaluate the efficacy of raloxifene for prevention and treatment of osteoporosis. At an average 3 years of follow-up there was a 54% reduction in the incidence of breast cancer and no increase in uterine cancer. STAR enrolled 19,747 women at increased risk for breast cancer, who received either tamoxifen or raloxifene. Both drugs reduced the risk for invasive breast cancer by about 50%. In favor of raloxifene, the number of uterine cancers was reduced by 36%, women taking raloxifene had 29% fewer episodes of venous thrombosis, and pulmonary embolism developed in fewer women (http://www.cancer.gov/star).

Prophylactic Mastectomy

To summarize the accumulating evidence, prophylactic mastectomy probably reduces the chance of contracting breast cancer in high-risk women by 90%. However, women who are screened by mammograms annually have an overall 80% chance of surviving the occurrence of breast cancer. Coupled with penetrance figures in the range of 50% to 60% for mutation carriers, the chance of dying of breast cancer for carriers of *BRCA1* or *BRCA2* mutations is approximately 10% without undergoing preventive mastectomy.[19]

In a retrospective study by Hartmann, 639 women with a family history of breast cancer underwent prophylactic mastectomy. Based on family pedigrees, the women were divided into high-risk (*n* = 214) and moderate-risk (*n* = 425) groups, with high-risk patients defined as those with a family history suggestive of an autosomal dominant predisposition to breast cancer. For women of moderate risk, the number of expected breast cancers was calculated according to the Gail model. Based on this model, 37.4 breast cancers were expected to have developed and 4 cancers actually did, for an incidence risk reduction of 89%. For women in the high-risk cohort, the Gail model would underestimate the risk for development of breast cancer. Thus, the expected number of breast cancers was calculated by using three different statistical models from a control study of the high-risk probands (sisters). Three breast cancers developed after prophylactic mastectomy, for an incident risk reduction of at least 90%.

Two groups have reported prospective results in *BRCA1* and *BRCA2* mutation carriers after prophylactic mastectomy versus surveillance. Meijers-Heijboer reported that at 2.9 years of follow-up, breast cancer had not developed in any of 76 mutation carriers who underwent preventive mastectomy whereas it did in 8 of 63 women choosing surveillance. Scheuer reported that at 24.2 months of follow-up, none of 29 women who underwent mastectomy contracted breast cancer as opposed to 12 of 165 high-risk women not choosing preventive mastectomy. There is an underlying assumption that a reduction in the risk for breast cancer will translate into survival benefits, although this is currently unproven.

Summary: Risk Assessment and Management

Risk factors for disease provide clues to pathogenesis and identify patients likely to benefit from surveillance and

Table 34-4 **Significant Risk Factors for Breast Cancer in Women: Assessment and Recommendations**

RISK FACTORS	MAMMOGRAPHY SCREENING RECOMMENDATIONS	PREVENTIVE OPTIONS
Factors Conferring Moderate to High Risk		
Age >60 yr	Annual	Not usually recommended
Atypical hyperplasia (ductal or lobular)	Annual after diagnosis	Tamoxifen, 20 mg/day × 5 yr
LCIS	Annual after diagnosis	Tamoxifen, 20 mg/day × 5 yr
Personal history of either DCIS or invasive cancer, age >40 yr	Annual after diagnosis	No specific preventive recommended*
Family history of breast cancer (1st-degree relative, age <50 yr; two relatives on same side of family)	Annual after age 40	Referral for genetic counseling
Factors Conferring Very High Risk		
Therapeutic thoracic radiation (age <30 yr)	Annual at 10 yr after radiotherapy	No specific preventive recommended*
Personal history of DCIS or invasive cancer, age <40 yr	Annual after diagnosis	No specific preventive recommended*
Family history of breast cancer (two 1st-degree relatives, age <50)	Annual after age 35-40	Referral for genetic counseling
Family history of breast and ovarian cancer (1st-degree relatives)	Annual after age 35-40	Referral for genetic counseling
Known carrier of a mutation in *BRCA1* or *BRCA2* or a 1st-degree relative with a mutation	Annual after age 25; consider annual MRI	Genetic testing for relatives; discuss prophylactic mastectomy or oophorectomy for carriers

*No specific recommendations made for prevention after standard therapy.
DCIS, ductal carcinoma in situ; LCIS, lobular carcinoma in situ; MRI, magnetic resonance imaging.

risk reduction interventions. Although breast cancer can develop in both sexes, women are at greatly increased risk and breast cancer in males is uncommon. Age is a useful risk factor applied everyday in clinical practice; breast cancer is rare in women younger than 30 and very common in women older than 60. Family history is most significant when breast cancer affects young first-degree relatives (mothers, sisters, and daughters) and when cases of ovarian cancer are found within the same side of the family. Histologic risk factors most concerning are ADH, ALH, and LCIS. A personal history of breast cancer predisposes to contralateral breast cancer in women undergoing mastectomy and to bilateral breast cancer in women undergoing breast conservation with wide excision and radiation. These factors are summarized in Table 34-4, which includes suggestions for management. These suggestions are meant only to guide discussions with patients; women's preferences and the specific clinical situation are often more complicated.

BENIGN BREAST TUMORS AND RELATED DISEASES

Breast Cysts

Cysts within the breast are fluid-filled, epithelium-lined cavities that may vary in size from microscopic to large, palpable masses containing as much as 20 to 30 mL of fluid. A palpable cyst develops in at least 1 in every 14 women, and 50% of cysts are multiple or recurrent. The pathogenesis of cyst formation is not well understood; however, cysts appear to arise from destruction and dilation of lobules and terminal ductules. Microscopic studies

have shown that fibrosis at or near the lobule, combined with continued secretion, results in unfolding of the lobule and expansion of an epithelium-lined cavity containing fluid.[3,20,21]

Cysts are influenced by ovarian hormones, a fact that explains their variation with the menstrual cycle. Most cysts occur in women older than 35. The incidence of cyst development steadily increases until menopause and sharply declines thereafter. New cyst formation in older women is generally associated with exogenous hormone replacement.

Intracystic carcinoma is exceedingly rare. Rosemond was able to report only three cancers in more than 3000 cyst aspirations (0.1%). Other investigators have confirmed this exceedingly low incidence. There is no evidence of increased risk for breast cancer associated with cyst formation.

A palpable mass can be confirmed to be a cyst by aspiration or ultrasound. Cyst fluid can be straw colored, opaque, or dark green and may contain flecks of debris. Given the low risk for malignancy within a cyst, if the palpable mass disappears completely after aspiration and the cyst contents are not grossly bloody, the fluid need not be sent for cytologic analysis. If the cyst recurs multiple times (more than two times is a reasonable rule), cytology is justified. Surgical removal of a cyst is usually indicated if the cytologic findings are suspicious or the cyst recurs multiple times.

Fibroadenoma and Related Tumors

Fibroadenomas are benign solid tumors composed of stromal and epithelial elements. After carcinoma, fibroadenoma is the second most common tumor in the breast and is the most common tumor in women younger than 30 years. In contrast to cysts, fibroadenomas appear in teenage girls and women during their early reproductive years; they are rarely seen as new masses in women after the age of 40 or 45. Clinically, they are firm tumors that may increase in size over a period of several months. They slip easily under the examining fingers and may be lobulated. On excision, fibroadenomas are well-encapsulated masses that may detach easily from surrounding breast tissue. Mammography is of little help in distinguishing between cysts and fibroadenomas; however, ultrasound usually clearly shows the cavity of a cyst.

Fibroadenomas do not have malignant potential, although neoplasia may develop in the epithelial elements within them, just as in epithelium elsewhere in the breast. Cancer in a newly discovered fibroadenoma is exceedingly rare. Half the neoplasias that involve fibroadenomas are LCIS, 35% are infiltrating carcinomas, and 15% are intraductal carcinoma.

Treatment of fibroadenoma follows that for any unexplained solid mass within the breast. A tissue diagnosis is required to rule out malignancy and may be accomplished by image-guided core needle biopsy or excisional biopsy.

Two subtypes of fibroadenoma are recognized. *Giant fibroadenoma* is a descriptive term applied to a fibroadenoma that attains an unusually large size, typically greater than 5 cm. *Juvenile fibroadenoma* refers to the occasional large fibroadenoma that occurs in adolescents and young adults and histologically is more cellular than the usual fibroadenoma. Although these lesions may display remarkably rapid growth, surgical removal is curative.

Hamartoma and Adenoma

These lesions are benign proliferations of variable amounts of epithelium and stromal supporting tissue. A hamartoma is a discrete nodule that contains closely packed lobules and prominent, ectatic extralobular ducts. On physical examination, mammography, and gross inspection, a hamartoma is indistinguishable from fibroadenoma. Excision is curative. Page and Anderson describe an adenoma or tubular adenoma as a benign cellular neoplasm of ductules packed closely together such that they form a sheet of tiny glands without supporting stroma. During pregnancy and lactation, these tumors may increase in size, and histologic examination shows secretory differentiation. Biopsy is required to establish the diagnosis.

Breast Abscess and Infections

Infections of the breast fall into two general categories, lactational infections and chronic subareolar infections associated with duct ectasia.

Lactational infections are thought to arise from entry of bacteria through the nipple into the duct system and are characterized by fever, leukocytosis, erythema, and tenderness. Infections are most often due to *Staphylococcus aureus* and may be manifested as cellulitis, termed *mastitis,* or as abscesses. Treatment requires antibiotics

and frequent emptying of the breast. True abscesses require surgical drainage because they are generally multiloculated.

In women who are not lactating, a chronic relapsing form of infection may develop in the subareolar ducts of the breast that is variously known as periductal mastitis or duct ectasia. This condition appears to be associated with smoking and diabetes. The infections that arise are most often mixed infections that include both aerobic and anaerobic skin flora. A series of infections with resulting inflammatory changes and scarring may lead to retraction or inversion of the nipple, masses in the subareolar area, and occasionally, a chronic fistula from the subareolar ducts to the periareolar skin. Palpable masses and mammographic changes that mimic carcinoma may result.

Subareolar infections may initially be manifested as subareolar pain and mild erythema. If treated at this stage, warm soaks and oral antibiotics may be effective. Antibiotic treatment is often unsuccessful unless both aerobic and anaerobic coverage is included. If an abscess has developed, acute treatment requires incision and drainage with antibiotics. Repeated infections are treated by excision of the entire subareolar duct complex after the acute infection has resolved completely, together with intravenous antibiotic coverage. Rare patients will have recurrent infections requiring excision of the nipple and areola.

A presumed infection of the breast generally clears promptly and completely with antibiotic therapy. If erythema or edema persists, inflammatory carcinoma is considered.

Papillomas and Papillomatosis

Solitary intraductal papillomas are true polyps of epithelium-lined breast ducts. Solitary papillomas are most often located close to the areola but may be present in peripheral locations. Most papillomas are less than 1 cm but can grow to as large as 4 or 5 cm. Larger papillomas may appear to arise within a cystic structure, probably representing a greatly expanded duct. Papillomas are not associated with an increased risk for breast cancer.

Papillomas are often accompanied by bloody nipple discharge. Less frequently, they are discovered as a palpable mass under the areola or as a density lesion on a mammogram. Treatment is excision through a circumareolar incision. For peripheral papillomas, the differential diagnosis is between papilloma and invasive papillary carcinoma.

It is important to distinguish *papillomatosis* from solitary or multiple papillomas. Papillomatosis refers to epithelial hyperplasia, which commonly occurs in younger women or is associated with fibrocystic change. This lesion is not composed of true papillomas. The hyperplastic epithelium in papillomatosis may fill individual ducts like a true polyp but has no stalk of fibrovascular tissue.

Sclerosing Adenosis

Adenosis refers to an increased number of small terminal ductules or acini. It is frequently associated with a proliferation of stromal tissue producing a histologic lesion, sclerosing adenosis, that can simulate carcinoma both grossly and histologically. There may be deposition of calcium, which can be seen on mammography in a pattern indistinguishable from the microcalcifications of intraductal carcinoma. Sclerosing adenosis is the most common pathologic diagnosis in patients undergoing needle-directed biopsy of microcalcifications in many series. Sclerosing adenosis is frequently listed as one of the component lesions of fibrocystic disease; it is quite common and has no malignant potential.

Radial Scar

Radial scars belong to a group of abnormalities known as complex sclerosing lesions. They can simulate carcinoma mammographically and on physical examination. These lesions contain microcysts, epithelial hyperplasia, adenosis, and a prominent display of central sclerosis. The gross abnormality is rarely more than 1 cm in diameter. Larger lesions form palpable tumors and appear as a spiculated mass with prominent architectural distortion on mammography. These tumors can even result in skin dimpling by producing traction on surrounding tissues. Radial scars are associated with a modestly increased risk for breast cancer.

Fat Necrosis

Fat necrosis can mimic cancer by producing a palpable mass or a density on mammography that may contain calcifications. Fat necrosis may follow an episode of trauma to the breast, but frequently there is no history of trauma. Histologically, the lesion is composed of lipid-laden macrophages, scar tissue, and chronic inflammatory cells. This lesion has no malignant potential.

PATHOLOGY OF BREAST CANCER

Each year, more than 211,000 cases of invasive breast cancer and more than 58,000 cases of in situ breast cancer are diagnosed in the United States, and approximately 40,000 women die of breast cancer. More than a million cases of breast cancer are diagnosed worldwide each year. The overall incidence of breast cancer has been rising because of increases in the average life span, lifestyle changes that increase risk for breast cancer, and improved survival from other diseases. Despite an increasing incidence, mortality from breast cancer has continued to fall, thought to be the result of both earlier detection via mammographic screening and improvements in therapy. Current treatment of breast cancer is guided by recent insights into breast cancer biology, an increasing ability to define disease biology and status in individual patients, and the availability of improved treatments.[20-22]

Noninvasive Breast Cancer

Noninvasive neoplasms are broadly divided into two major types: LCIS and DCIS (or intraductal carcinoma) (Box 34-2). Histology and nomenclature do not always

---

Box 34-2 Classification of Primary Breast Cancer

Noninvasive Epithelial Cancers

Lobular carcinoma in situ (LCIS)
Ductal carcinoma in situ (DCIS) or intraductal carcinoma
    Papillary, cribriform, solid, and comedo types

Invasive Epithelial Cancers (Percentage of Total)

Invasive lobular carcinoma (10%-15%)
Invasive ductal carcinoma
    Invasive ductal carcinoma, NOS (50%-70%)
    Tubular carcinoma (2%-3%)
    Mucinous or colloid carcinoma (2%-3%)
    Medullary carcinoma (5%)
    Invasive cribriform carcinoma (1%-3%)
    Invasive papillary carcinoma (1%-2%)
    Adenoid cystic carcinoma (1%)
    Metaplastic carcinoma (1%)

Mixed Connective and Epithelial Tumors

Phyllodes tumors, benign and malignant
Carcinosarcoma
Angiosarcoma

NOS, not otherwise specified.

---

accurately reflect biology. LCIS, once considered a malignant lesion, is now regarded more as a risk factor for the development of breast cancer. LCIS is recognized by its conformity to the outline of the normal lobule, with expanded and filled acini (Fig. 34-7). DCIS is a more heterogeneous lesion morphologically, and pathologists recognize four broad categories: papillary, cribriform, solid, and comedo, the latter three types being shown in Figure 34-7. DCIS is recognized as discrete spaces surrounded by basement membrane that are filled with malignant cells and usually with a recognizable, basally located cell layer made up of presumably normal myoepithelial cells. The four morphologic categories are prototypes of pure lesions, but in reality these appearances blend into one another. However, the papillary and cribriform types of DCIS probably transform to invasive cancer over a longer time frame and are of lower grade. The solid and comedo types of DCIS are generally higher-grade lesions and probably invade over a shortened natural history.

As the cells inside the ductal membrane grow, they have a tendency to undergo central necrosis, perhaps because the blood supply to these cells is located outside the basement membrane. The necrotic debris in the center of the duct undergoes coagulation and finally calcification, thereby leading to the tiny, pleomorphic, and frequently linear forms seen on high-quality mammograms. In some patients an entire ductal tree seems to be involved in the malignancy, and the mammogram shows typical calcifications from the nipple extending posteriorly into the interior of the breast (termed *segmental calcifications*). For reasons not understood, DCIS transforms into an invasive cancer, usually recapitulating the morphology of the cells inside the duct. In other

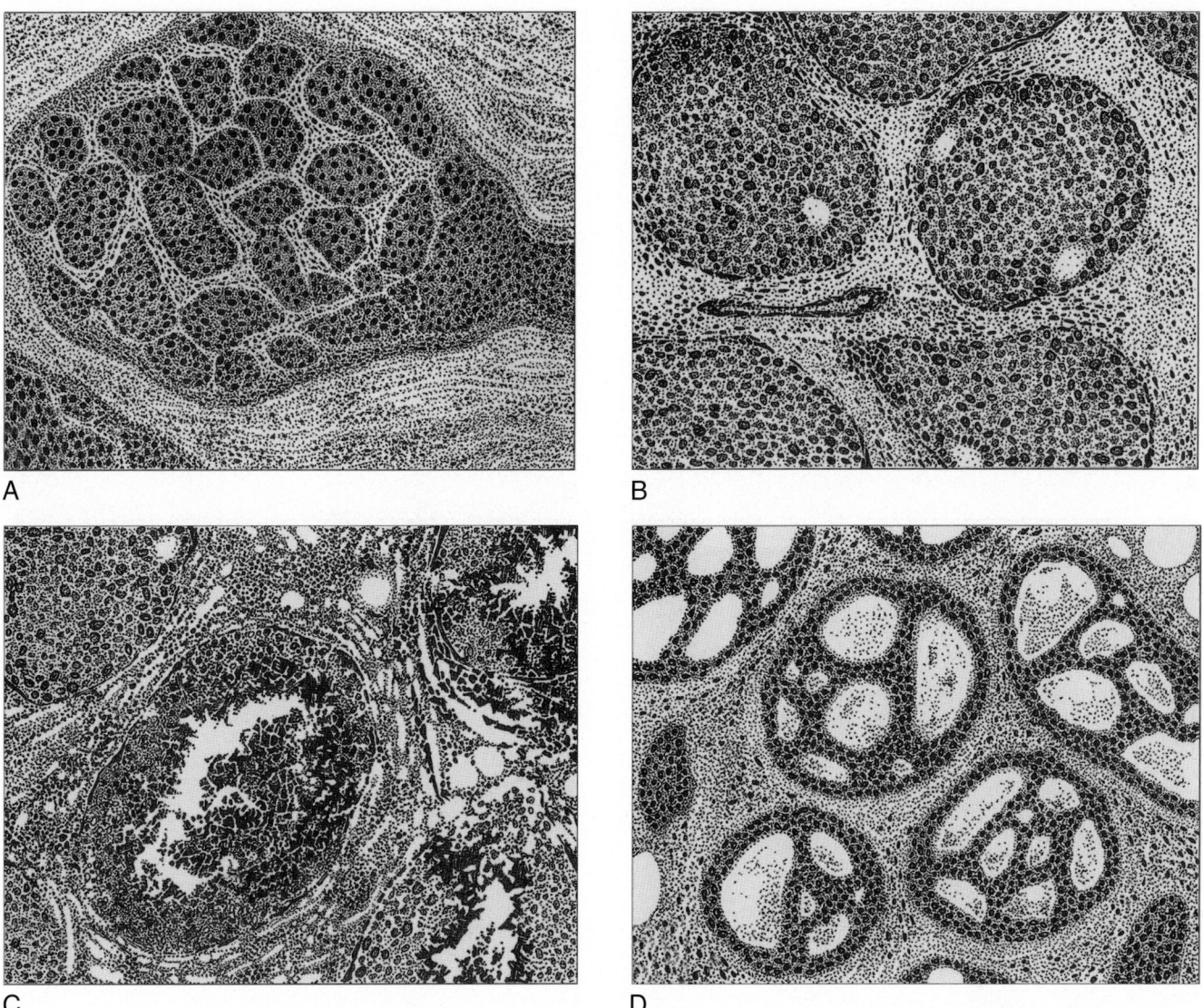

A

B

C

D

Figure 34-7 Noninvasive breast cancer. **A,** Lobular carcinoma in situ (LCIS). The neoplastic cells are small with compact, bland nuclei and are distending the acini but preserving the cross-sectional architecture of the lobular unit. **B,** Ductal carcinoma in situ (DCIS), solid type. The cells are larger than in LCIS and are filling the ductal rather than the lobular spaces. However, the cells are contained within the basement membrane of the duct and do not invade the breast stroma. **C,** DCIS, comedo type. In comedo DCIS, the malignant cells in the center undergo necrosis, coagulation, and calcification. **D,** DCIS, cribriform type. In this type, bridges of tumor cells span the ductal space and leave round, punched-out spaces.

words, low-grade cribriform DCIS tends to invade as a low-grade lesion retaining some cribriform features. There is not, as may be thought, a tendency for the grade to advance with invasion. Finally, DCIS frequently coexists with otherwise invasive cancers, and again the two phases of the malignancy are in step with each other morphologically.

Invasive Breast Cancer

Invasive cancers are recognized by their lack of overall architecture, by the infiltration of cells haphazardly into a variable amount of stroma, or by the formation of sheets of continuous and monotonous cells without respect for form and function of a glandular organ. Clinicians and pathologists broadly divide invasive breast cancer into *lobular* and *ductal* histology, which probably does not reflect histogenesis and only imperfectly predicts clinical behavior. However, invasive lobular cancer tends to permeate the breast in a single-file nature, which explains why it remains clinically occult and escapes detection on mammography or physical examination until the total extent of the disease is large. Likewise, ductal cancers tend to grow as a more coherent mass; they form discrete abnormalities on mammograms and appear sooner as a lump in the breast. The growth

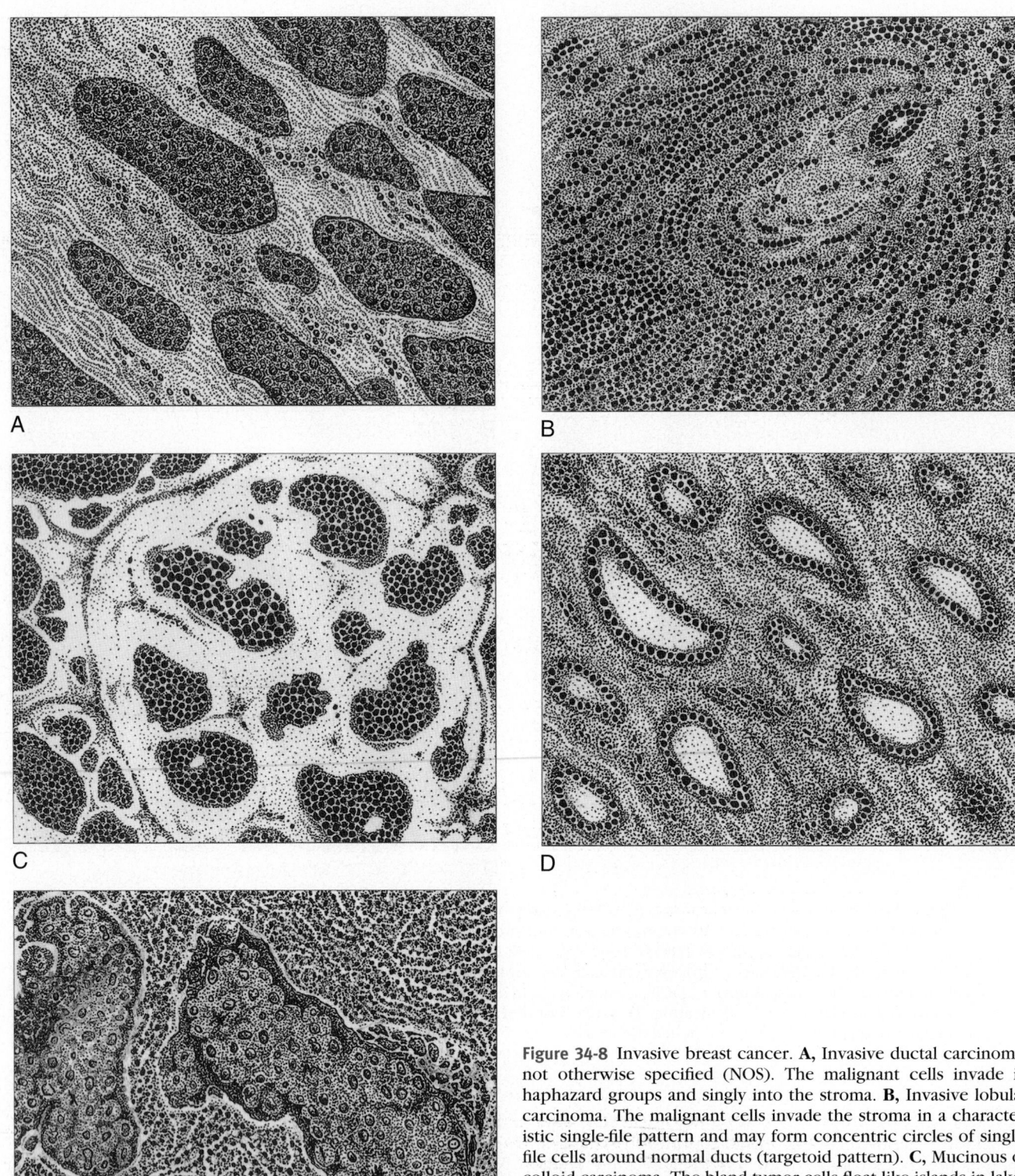

Figure 34-8 Invasive breast cancer. **A,** Invasive ductal carcinoma, not otherwise specified (NOS). The malignant cells invade in haphazard groups and singly into the stroma. **B,** Invasive lobular carcinoma. The malignant cells invade the stroma in a characteristic single-file pattern and may form concentric circles of single-file cells around normal ducts (targetoid pattern). **C,** Mucinous or colloid carcinoma. The bland tumor cells float like islands in lakes of mucin. **D,** Invasive tubular carcinoma. The cancer invades as small tubules, lined by a single layer of well-differentiated cells. **E,** Medullary carcinoma. The tumor cells are large, very undifferentiated with pleomorphic nuclei. The distinctive features of this tumor are the infiltrate of lymphocytes and the syncytial-appearing sheets of tumor cells.

pattern of these lesions is shown in Figure 34-8, with invasive ductal cancer in panel A and invasive lobular cancer in panel B.

Invasive ductal cancer, or infiltrating ductal carcinoma, is the most common form of breast cancer and accounts for 50% to 70% of invasive breast cancers. When this cancer does not take on special features, it is called *infiltrating ductal carcinoma, NOS* (which is an abbreviation for *not otherwise specified*). Invasive lobular carcinoma accounts for 10% to 15% of breast cancer, and mixed ductal and lobular cancers are increasingly being recognized and described in pathology reports. When infiltrating ductal carcinomas take on differentiated features, they are named according to the features that they display. If the infiltrating cells form small glands lined by a single row of bland epithelium, they are called *infiltrating tubular carcinoma* (see Fig. 34-8D). The infiltrating cells may secrete copious amounts of mucinous material and appear to float in this material. These lesions are called *mucinous* or *colloid tumors*. Both tubular and mucinous tumors are low-grade (grade I) lesions and represent about 2% or 3% each of invasive ductal carcinomas.

In contrast, bizarre invasive cells with high-grade nuclear features, many mitoses, and lack of an in situ component characterize *medullary cancer*. The malignancy forms sheets of cells in an almost syncytial fashion, surrounded by an infiltrate of small mononuclear lymphocytes. The borders of the tumor push into the surrounding breast rather than infiltrate or permeate the stroma. This tumor is shown in Figure 34-8E, which shows the bizarre and pleomorphic nuclear features of the cells. In its pure form it accounts for only about 5% of breast cancers; however, various pathologists describe a so-called medullary variant that has some features of the pure form of the cancer. These tumors are uniformly high grade, ER and progesterone receptor (PR) negative, and negative for the HER-2 cell surface receptor, and in recognition of their lack of receptor expression, they may be called *triple-negative* breast cancers. Newer microarray analysis of breast cancer has found that these tumors are distinctly different from other ductal breast cancers and express molecular markers found in basal or myoepithelial cells, hence the term *basal-like* breast cancer. Newer classification schemes favor the term *basal-like* over the older nomenclature.

It is commonly held that infiltrating ductal carcinoma, NOS, is the most common form of breast cancer and its prognosis is variable, modified by histologic grade and expression of molecular markers (see later). Basal-like cancer, or medullary cancer in older classifications, is also an aggressive form of breast cancer. Because it is triple negative, there are no targeted treatments for this form of cancer. Infiltrating lobular breast cancers carry an intermediate prognosis, whereas tubular and mucinous cancers are the least clinically aggressive cancers. However, these generalizations are useful only in context of tumor size, grade, and receptor status and are subject to many exceptions to these rules. Modern classification schemes are replacing these older morphologic descriptions with the determination of molecular markers (ER and HER-2, see later).

Other Primary Tumors of the Breast

Phyllodes Tumors

Tumors of mixed connective tissue and epithelium constitute an important group of unusual primary breast cancers. On one extreme, these tumors are exemplified by the benign fibroadenoma, which is characterized by a proliferation of connective tissue and a variable component of ductal elements that may appear compressed by the swirls of fibroblastic growth. More perplexing are the intermediate neoplastic growths comprising phyllodes tumors, which contain a biphasic proliferation of stroma and mammary epithelium. First called *cystosarcoma phyllodes,* the name has been changed to *phyllodes tumor* in recognition of its usually benign course. However, with increasing cellularity, an invasive margin, and truly sarcomatous appearance, these tumors may be classified as malignant phyllodes tumors. Benign phyllodes tumors are recognized as firm, lobulated masses between 2 and up to 40 cm in size, with an average size of about 5 cm (larger than average fibroadenomas). Histologically, these tumors are similar to fibroadenomas, but the whorled stroma forms larger clefts lined by epithelium that resemble clusters of leaflike structures. The stroma is more cellular than a fibroadenoma, but the fibroblastic cells are bland and mitoses are infrequent.

Mammographically, these lesions are seen as round densities with smooth borders and are indistinguishable from fibroadenomas. Ultrasound may reveal a discrete structure with cystic spaces. The diagnosis is suggested by the larger size, a history of rapid growth, and occurrence in older patients. Cytologic analysis is unreliable in differentiating a low-grade phyllodes tumor from a fibroadenoma. In one series of core needle biopsies, the correct diagnosis was rendered in only 50% of cases. Thus, the diagnosis is best made by excisional biopsy followed by careful pathologic review.

Local excision of a benign phyllodes tumor is curative, and clearly benign tumors are treated like a fibroadenoma. There is a group of intermediate tumors, so-called borderline phyllodes tumors, in which it is difficult to assign a benign label. These tumors are treated by excision with margins of at least 1 cm. Affected patients are at some risk for local recurrence, most often within the first 2 years after excision, and close follow-up with examination and imaging allows early detection of recurrence. Finally, at the other end of the spectrum are frankly malignant stromal sarcomas. Malignant phyllodes tumors are treated like sarcomas on the trunk or extremities. En bloc surgical excision of the entire affected part is advised, in this case total mastectomy. As with sarcomas in general, regional lymph node dissection is not required.

Metastases from malignant phyllodes tumors occur via hematogenous spread, with common sites including lung, bone, abdominal viscera, and mediastinum. There are no reports of long-term survivors. The optimal palliative treatment of metastatic phyllodes tumors has not been determined. The systemic therapeutic agents used for sarcomas have resulted in minimal success.

Angiosarcoma

This vascular tumor may occur de novo in the breast, but the clinically important manifestation is in the dermis after breast irradiation or in the lymphedematous upper extremity, historically after radical mastectomy. Angiosarcoma arising in the absence of previous radiation therapy or surgery may form a mass within the parenchyma of the breast, in contrast to radiation-induced angiosarcoma, which arises in irradiated skin. Vascular proliferations in the skin are common after exposure of any part of the body to radiation, and the differential diagnosis is frequently between malignant angiosarcoma and atypical vascular proliferations in irradiated skin. Histologically, the tumor is composed of an anastomosing tangle of blood vessels in the dermis and superficial subcutaneous fat. The atypical and crowded vessels invade through the dermis and into subcutaneous fat. These cancers are graded by the appearance and behavior of the associated endothelial cells. Pleomorphic nuclei, frequent mitoses, and stacking of the endothelial cells lining neoplastic vessels are features seen in higher-grade lesions. Rarely seen in hemangiomas, necrosis is common in high-grade angiosarcomas. Clinically, radiation-induced angiosarcoma is identified as a reddish brown to purple raised rash within the radiation portals and on the skin of the breast. As the disease progresses or with high-grade sarcomas, tumors protruding from the surface of the skin may predominate.

Mammography is unrevealing in a third of cases. In the absence of metastatic disease at initial evaluation, surgery is required to secure negative skin margins and most commonly involves simple or radical mastectomy and frequently a split-thickness skin graft or myocutaneous flap. Metastasis to regional nodes is extraordinarily rare and axillary dissection is not required.

Patients remain at high risk for local recurrence after resection. Because radiation therapy is of benefit in the treatment of related sarcomas in other body sites, some authors recommend postoperative radiation therapy to the chest wall for the treatment of primary angiosarcoma. Metastatic spread occurs hematogenously, most commonly to the lungs and bone and less frequently to abdominal viscera, brain, and even the contralateral breast. Chemotherapy has provided minimal improvement in the outcome of angiosarcoma. For those free of metastatic disease at initial evaluation, the median time to recurrence after mastectomy is 8 months and the median survival is 2 years.

STAGING OF BREAST CANCER

Breast cancer stage is determined by the results of surgical resection and imaging studies. Breast cancer is classified with the TNM classification system, which groups different patterns of breast, nodal, and distant tumor involvement into tumor stages that reflect prognosis. The most widely used system is that of the American Joint Committee on Cancer (AJCC). This system is based on description of the primary tumor (T), the status of regional lymph nodes (N), and the presence of distant metastases (M). It is regularly updated to reflect current understanding of tumor behavior. The most recent updates have incorporated the use of sentinel node biopsy and include classification of the size of metastatic deposits in sentinel nodes, as well as the number and location of regional node metastases. Table 34-5 presents the TNM working

Table 34-5 American Joint Committee on Cancer Staging System for Breast Cancer, 2002

(p)T (Primary Tumor)	
Tis	Carcinoma in situ (lobular or ductal)
T1	Tumor ≤2 cm
T1a	Tumor ≥0.1 cm, ≤0.5 cm
T1b	Tumor >0.5 cm, ≤1 cm
T1c	Tumor >1 cm, ≤2 cm
T2	Tumor >2 cm, ≤5 cm
T3	Tumor >5 cm
T4	Tumor any size with extension to the chest wall or skin
T4a	Tumor extending to the chest wall (excluding the pectoralis)
T4b	Tumor extending to the skin with ulceration, edema, satellite nodules
T4c	Both T4a and T4b
T4d	Inflammatory carcinoma

(p)N (Nodes)	
N0	No regional node involvement, no special studies
N0 (i⁻)	No regional node involvement, negative IHC
N0 (i⁺)	Node(s) with isolated tumor cells spanning <0.2 mm
N0 (mol⁻)	Negative node(s) histologically, negative PCR
N0 (mol⁺)	Negative node(s) histologically, positive PCR
N1	Metastasis to 1-3 axillary nodes *and/or* int. mammary positive by biopsy
N1(mic)	Micrometastasis (>0.2 mm, none >2.0 mm)
N1a	Metastasis to 1-3 axillary nodes
N1b	Metastasis in int. mammary by sentinel biopsy
N1c	Metastasis to 1-3 axillary nodes *and* int. mammary by biopsy
N2	Metastasis to 4-9 axillary nodes *or* int. mammary clinically positive, without axillary metastasis
N2a	Metastasis to 4-9 axillary nodes, at least 1 >2.0 mm
N2b	Int. mammary clinically apparent, negative axillary nodes
N3	Metastasis to ≥10 axillary nodes *or* combination of axillary and int. mammary metastasis
N3a	≥10 axillary nodes (>2.0 mm), or infraclavicular nodes
N3b	Positive int. mammary clinically with ≥1 axillary nodes *or* >3 positive axillary nodes with int. mammary positive by biopsy
N3c	Metastasis to ipsilateral supraclavicular nodes

M (Metastasis)	
M0	No distant metastasis
M1	Distant metastasis

IHC, immunohistochemistry; int. mammary, internal mammary lymph nodes; (p), pathologic staging of the tumor or axillary nodes; PCR, polymerase chain reaction.

Table 34-6 American Joint Committee on Cancer Stage Grouping

STAGE	TNM	5-YEAR RELATIVE SURVIVAL RATE (%)*
0	Tis, N0, M0	100
I	T1, N0, M0	100
IIA	T0, N1, M0 T1, N1, M0 T2, N0, M0	92
IIB	T2, N1, M0 T3, N0, M0	81
IIIA	T0, N2, M0 T1, N2, M0 T2, N2, M0 T3, N1, M0 T3, N2, M0	67
IIIB	T4, N0, M0 T4, N1, M0 T4, N2, M0	54
IIIC	Any T, N3, M0	†
IV	Any T, any N, M1	20

*Breast Cancer Survival by Stage: American College of Surgeons National Cancer Data Base.

†These numbers are based on patients in whom cancer was diagnosed from 1995 to 1998. Five-year survival rates are not yet available for stage IIIC breast cancer because this stage was defined only recently.

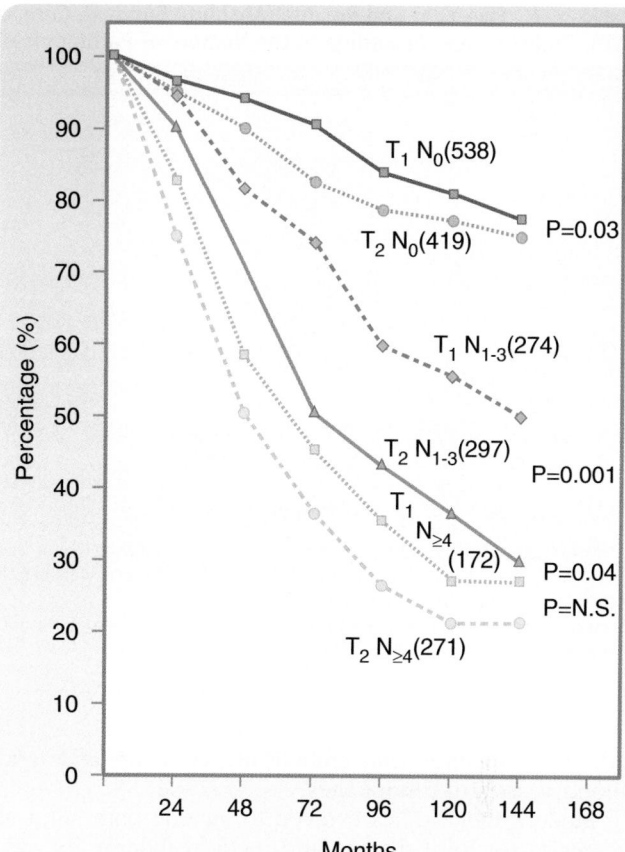

Figure 34-9 Survival by nodal status and by tumor size. These data are from a natural history database of 1971 patients treated at three large centers in the United States and Europe. None of these patients received postoperative systemic therapy (hormones or chemotherapy), and these results serve as a reference for comparison to modern trials, presented later in the chapter. (From Moon TE: Development of a natural history data base of breast cancer studies. In Jones SE, Salmon SE [eds]: Adjuvant Therapy of Cancer IV. Orlando, FL, Grune & Stratton, 1984.)

guide. Stage groupings and their 5-year survival rates are shown in Table 34-6.

Older survival data from the prechemotherapy era have been used to assess survival after surgery alone and serve to identify patients at high enough risk for recurrence to justify the use of systemic therapy. The natural history of breast cancer of differing size and nodal status treated by radical mastectomy alone is illustrated in Figure 34-9. Metastasis to ipsilateral axillary nodes predicts outcome after surgical treatment more powerfully than tumor size does. A 1980 American College of Surgeons survey of patients treated by surgery alone revealed an almost linear decrement in survival rate with increasing nodal involvement (Table 34-7).

SURGICAL TREATMENT OF BREAST CANCER

Modern Surgical Management: Historical Perspective

Through the mid-20th century, breast cancer was thought to arise in the breast and progress to other sites largely via centrifugal spread. In this model, more extensive surgical procedures were expected to reduce mortality. This model was supported by the success of the Halsted radical mastectomy in improving breast cancer survival relative to the local excision of tumors that had been used previously. Introduced in the 1890s, radical mastectomy included excision of the breast, overlying skin, and

underlying pectoralis muscles in continuity with the regional lymph nodes along the axillary vein to the costoclavicular ligament. This procedure often required a skin graft to close the large skin defect created. This approach was well suited to breast cancer biology of the time, when most tumors were locally advanced, frequently with chest wall or skin involvement and extensive axillary nodal disease. Radical mastectomy provided greatly improved local control of tumor and led to an increasing population of long-term survivors. Radical mastectomy remained the mainstay of surgical therapy into the 1970s.

Unfortunately, a large number of women continued to die of metastatic breast cancer after radical mastectomy. Even more extensive surgical procedures, including en bloc resection of the internal mammary and supraclavicular nodes, failed to improve survival. This led to recognition that breast cancer spreads both centrifugally to

Table 34-7 Five-Year End Results (Absolute Survival, Cure, and Recurrence Rates) in 20,547 Patients With Breast Cancer According to the Number of Pathologically Positive Axillary Nodes*

POSITIVE AXILLARY LYMPH NODES (N)	TOTAL OBSERVED	SURVIVAL (%)	CURE (%)	RECURRENCE (%)
0	12,299	71.8	59.7	19.4
1	2012	63.1	48.4	32.9
2	1338	62.2	45.4	39.9
3	842	58.8	39.3	43.0
4	615	51.9	38.4	43.9
5	478	46.9	29.1	54.2
6-10	1261	40.7	23.0	63.4
11-15	562	29.4	14.8	71.5
16-20	301	28.9	13.3	75.1
21+	225	22.2	9.8	82.2
All nodes or some nodes positive	614	40.4	26.9	58.6
Total, positive nodes	**8248**	**50.9**	**35.0**	**49.2**

*Excluding cases with distant metastasis.

From Nemoto T, Vana J, Bedwani RN, et al: Management and survival of female breast cancer: Results of a national survey by the American College of Surgeons. Cancer 45:2917-2924, 1980.

adjacent structures *and* embolically via lymphatics and blood vessels to distant sites.

Modern therapy has evolved to include both surgical resection for local disease and medical therapy for systemic disease. Randomized trials demonstrated the equivalence of modified radical mastectomy and radical mastectomy, which led to abandonment of the more radical mastectomy and its greater morbidity. The use of radiation therapy in conjunction with surgery has allowed dramatic reductions in the extent of surgery required for local control of breast cancer, with a majority of patients now eligible for breast-conserving surgery. It is recognized that breast cancer is a heterogeneous disease. Current treatment strategies take into account properties of the individual patient's tumor cells, as well as the size and location of tumor, to guide treatment.

Insights From Older Surgical Trials of Local Therapy for Operable Breast Cancer

Radical Mastectomy Versus Simple Mastectomy With or Without Axillary Radiation Therapy

The NSABP B-04 trial randomized patients with clinically negative nodes to one of three treatment regimens: radical mastectomy, total mastectomy with irradiation of the ipsilateral nodes, or total mastectomy alone with delayed axillary dissection if nodes became clinically enlarged. At 25 years of follow-up, overall survival and disease-free survival were equivalent in all three treatment arms. Axillary recurrence rates approached 18% in patients undergoing total mastectomy without dissection or radiation therapy, but these patients had equivalent survival with delayed axillary dissection. The results of this trial led to the conclusion that the mode and time of treatment of axillary nodes do not alter disease-free survival or overall survival. Immediate removal, delayed

removal, or irradiation produced equivalent clinical results.[23]

Clinical Trials Comparing Breast Conservation With Mastectomy

Six prospective clinical trials have randomized more than 4500 patients to various surgical strategies, all of which included a mastectomy arm and a breast-preserving arm (Table 34-8). In all these trials there was no survival advantage for mastectomy over breast preservation. Ipsilateral breast recurrence rates were higher in patients undergoing breast-conserving surgery, but local recurrences could be salvaged by mastectomy at the time of recurrence, with no significant detriment in survival. Data from these trials have served to define predictors of local recurrence after lumpectomy and have led to modifications in surgical and radiation techniques to reduce local recurrence. Results of these trials are summarized in the following paragraphs.

NSABP B-06: Mastectomy, Lumpectomy, and Lumpectomy With Irradiation

A total of 1851 patients with tumors up to 4 cm in diameter and clinically negative lymph nodes were randomized to receive modified radical mastectomy, lumpectomy alone, or lumpectomy with postoperative irradiation of the breast but without an extra boost to the lumpectomy site. All patients with histologically positive axillary nodes received chemotherapy. With 25 years of follow-up, overall survival and disease-free survival were the same in all three treatment arms (Fig. 34-10).

NSABP B-06 provided valuable information about rates of ipsilateral breast cancer recurrence after lumpectomy, with or without breast irradiation. At 20 years of follow-up, local recurrence rates were 14.3% in women

Table 34-8 Prospective Trials Comparing Mastectomy With Lumpectomy Plus or Minus Radiation Therapy

SURGICAL TRIAL	NO. OF PATIENTS (N)	MAXIMUM TUMOR SIZE (cm)	SYSTEMIC THERAPY	FOLLOW-UP (yr)	SURVIVAL (%) Lumpectomy and Radiation Therapy	Mastectomy	LOCAL RECURRENCE (RADIATION THERAPY) (%)
NSABP B-06[1]	1851	4	Yes	20	47	46	14*
Milan Cancer Institute[2]	701	2	Yes	20	44	43	8.8*
Institute Gustave-Roussy[3]	179	2	No		73	65	13
National Cancer Institute, USA[4]	237	5	Yes	10	77	75	16
European Organization for Research and Treatment of Cancer (EORTC)[5]	868	5	Yes	10	65	66	17.6
Danish Breast Cancer Group[6]	905	None	Yes	6	79	82	3

[1]Data from Fisher B, Anderson S, Bryant J, et al: Twenty-year follow-up of a randomized trial comparing total mastectomy, lumpectomy, and lumpectomy plus irradiation for the treatment of invasive breast cancer. N Engl J Med 347:1233, 2002.

[2]Data from Veronesi U, Cascinelli N, Mariani L, et al: Twenty-year follow-up of a randomized study comparing breast-conserving surgery with radical mastectomy for early breast cancer. N Engl J Med 347:1227, 2002.

[3]Data from Arriagada R, Le M, Rochard F, et al: Conservative treatment versus mastectomy in early breast cancer: Patterns of failure with 15 years of follow-up data. J Clin Oncol 14:1558, 1996.

[4]Data from Jacobson J, Danforth D, Cowan K, et al: Ten-year results of a comparison of conservation with mastectomy in the treatment of stage I and II breast cancer. N Engl J Med 332:907, 1995.

[5]Data from van Dongen J, Voogd A, Fentiman I, et al: Long-term results of a randomized trial comparing breast-conserving therapy with mastectomy: European Organization for Research and Treatment of Cancer 10801 Trial. J Natl Cancer Inst 92:1143, 2000.

[6]Data from Blichert-Toft M, Rose C, Andersen J, et al: Danish randomized trial comparing breast conservation therapy with mastectomy: Six years of life-table analysis. Danish Breast Cancer Cooperative Group. J Natl Cancer Inst Monogr 11:19, 1992.

*Includes only women whose excision margins were negative.

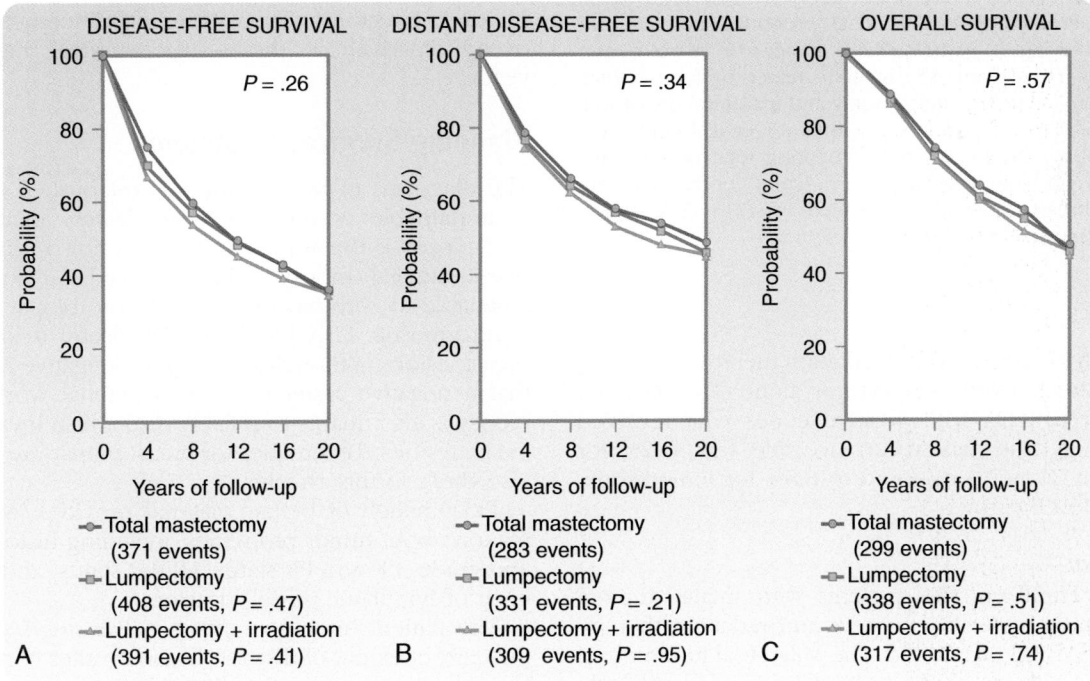

Figure 34-10 Disease-free survival **(A)**, distant disease-free survival **(B)**, and overall survival **(C)** after 20 years of follow-up in the NSABP Protocol B-06. There were no significant differences in the three randomized arms of this trial. (From Fisher B, Anderson S, Bryant J, et al: Twenty-year follow-up of a randomized trial comparing total mastectomy, lumpectomy, and lumpectomy plus irradiation for the treatment of invasive breast cancer. N Engl J Med 347:1237, 2002. Copyright 2002 Massachusetts Medical Society.)

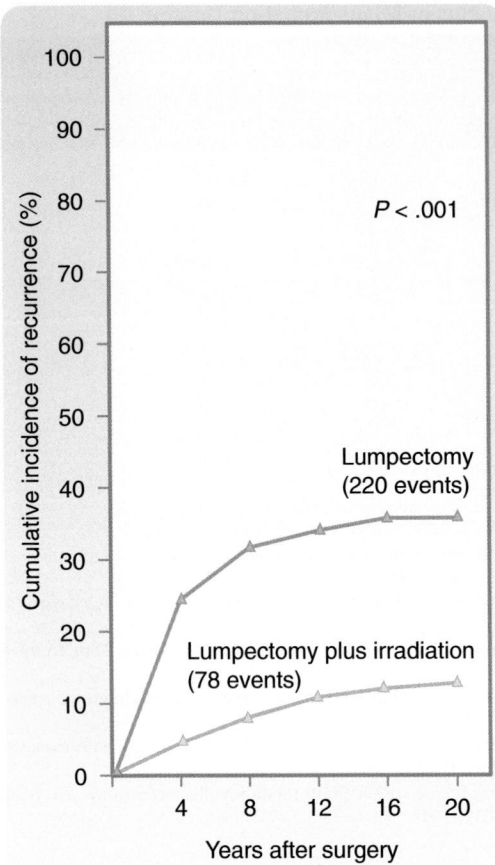

Figure 34-11 Cumulative incidence of a first recurrence of cancer in the treated, conserved breast during 20 years of follow-up in the NSABP Protocol B-06. The data presented here are for patients achieving a pathologically tumor-free margin after lumpectomy. There were 570 women treated by lumpectomy alone and 567 treated by lumpectomy and ipsilateral breast irradiation. (From Fisher B, Anderson S, Bryant J, et al: Twenty-year follow-up of a randomized trial comparing total mastectomy, lumpectomy, and lumpectomy plus irradiation for the treatment of invasive breast cancer. N Engl J Med 347:1233, 2002. Copyright 2002 Massachusetts Medical Society.)

treated with lumpectomy and radiation therapy and 39.2% in women treated with lumpectomy alone ($P = .001$, Fig. 34-11). For patients with positive nodes who received chemotherapy, the local recurrence rate was 44.2% for lumpectomy alone as opposed to 8.8% for lumpectomy plus radiation therapy.

Milan I Trial

The Milan I trial enrolled patients with smaller tumors and used more extensive surgery and radiation therapy than the NSABP B-06 trial did. The Milan trial randomized 701 women with tumors up to 2 cm in size and clinically negative nodes to receive radical mastectomy versus quadrantectomy, axillary dissection, and postoperative irradiation. Pathologically node-positive patients received chemotherapy. Overall survival at 20 years was no different in the two groups.

Local failure on the chest wall after radical mastectomy occurred in 2.3% of women. The local failure rate after quadrantectomy and radiation therapy was 8.8% over a 20-year period. Contralateral breast cancer rates were identical at about 0.66% per year for all women, thus contradicting the hypothesis that irradiation increases the incidence of contralateral cancer. Local failure rates were higher in younger women after quadrantectomy, with rates of 1% per year in women younger than 45 and only 0.5% per year in older women.

Other Trials

Three other randomized trials found no survival benefit of mastectomy over breast-conserving therapy. The European Organization for Research and Treatment of Cancer (EORTC) Trial 10801 randomized 868 women to modified radical mastectomy or lumpectomy and irradiation and found no difference in survival at 10 years. Importantly, this trial included tumors up to 5 cm, and 80% of women enrolled had tumors larger than 2.0 cm. Positive margins were allowed, and the results showed lower rates of local recurrence with clear versus involved margins.

The Institut Gustave-Roussy Trial randomized 179 women with tumors smaller than 2 cm to modified radical mastectomy versus lumpectomy with a 2-cm margin of normal tissue around the cancer. No differences were observed between the two surgical groups in risk for death, metastases, contralateral breast cancer, or local-regional recurrence at 15 years of follow-up.

The NCI (United States) trial randomized 237 women with tumors 5 cm or smaller to compare lumpectomy, axillary dissection, and radiation therapy versus modified radical mastectomy. There were no differences seen in overall survival or disease-free survival rates at 10 years.

Planning Surgical Treatments

The diagnosis of breast cancer is established by biopsy of a palpable or image-detected lesion. Image-guided core biopsy is the approach of choice for diagnosis, with open surgical biopsy being reserved for lesions not amenable to core biopsy or when core biopsy has been nondiagnostic. FNA biopsy is also useful in diagnosing breast lesions, although its high false-negative rate means that a negative result requires additional workup. FNA biopsy is also unable to reliably distinguish invasive from in situ lesions. Techniques for breast biopsy are described elsewhere in this chapter.

Examination of biopsy material provides initial information about tumor properties, including histologic type and grade, ER and PR status, HER-2 status, and the presence of lymphatic vessel invasion.

The patient undergoes *preoperative staging* to assess the current extent of disease. Common sites of metastases from breast cancer—the liver, lungs and bones—are assessed in all patients by chest radiographs and liver function tests. Computed tomography scans, bone scans, and other imaging studies are reserved for patients with abnormalities on blood tests or chest radiographs and for patients with large or clinically node-positive tumors.

Thorough imaging of the contralateral breast is performed to look for additional areas of concern, and breast MRI may be used in selected cases to define the extent of tumor and to look for additional breast lesions.

In the absence of metastatic disease, the first intervention is surgery to excise tumor and surgically stage the axilla when appropriate. Pathology results from the tumor and axillary nodes define the patient's *pathologic stage* and provide an estimate of the prognosis to inform systemic therapy decisions. Patients with locally advanced tumors may receive systemic therapy before surgery to shrink their tumor and facilitate surgery (see the section on neoadjuvant systemic therapy).

Selection of surgical procedures takes into account patient characteristics, as well as the properties of the tumor and its stage. Patient characteristics, including age, risk factors, family history, menopausal status, and overall health, are assessed. Some patients may undergo genetic testing for risk gene mutations at the time of diagnosis if they might consider bilateral mastectomy for treatment and prevention. The location of tumor within the breast and tumor size relative to breast size are evaluated. Patient preferences for breast preservation versus mastectomy are determined. For patients considering mastectomy, options for immediate reconstruction are discussed.

Eligibility for Breast Conservation
Randomized trials demonstrated the efficacy of breast-conserving surgery for a wide variety of breast cancers and have defined eligibility for breast conservation. With these criteria and current surgical and radiation approaches, local recurrence rates after lumpectomy and radiation therapy are now less than 5% at 10 years in many large centers.

Tumor Size
Tumors up to 5 cm in size, tumors with clinically positive nodes, and tumors with both lobular and ductal histology were included in the randomized trials. In current practice, lumpectomy is considered in cases in which the tumor can be excised to clear margins and leave an acceptable cosmetic result.

Margins
Local recurrence rates are reduced when 2 to 3 mm of microscopically clear margin is obtained on all aspects of the lumpectomy specimen. Margins must be clear for both invasive cancer and DCIS.

Histology
Invasive lobular cancers and cancers with an extensive intraductal component are eligible for lumpectomy if clear margins are achieved. Atypical hyperplasia and LCIS at resection margins do not increase local recurrence rates.

Patient Age
Local recurrence rates are somewhat higher for younger versus older women. Local recurrence rates are reduced in patients of all ages with the use of radiation therapy.

A radiation boost to the tumor bed has been shown to reduce local failures after lumpectomy, particularly in younger women.

Indications for Mastectomy
Certain tumors still require mastectomy, including those that are large relative to breast size, those with extensive calcifications on mammography, tumors for which clear margins cannot be obtained on wide local excision, and patients with contraindications to breast irradiation. Contraindications include previous breast or chest wall irradiation, active lupus or scleroderma, and pregnancy (although many patients pregnant at diagnosis can complete their pregnancy and receive radiation therapy after delivery). Patient preference for mastectomy or a desire to avoid radiation is also a valid indication for mastectomy.

Breast Reconstruction
Breast reconstruction may be performed as *immediate reconstruction,* that is, the same day as mastectomy, or as *delayed reconstruction,* months or years later. Immediate reconstruction has the advantages of preserving the maximum amount of breast skin for use in reconstruction, combining the recovery period for both procedures, and avoiding a period of time without reconstruction. Immediate reconstruction does not have a detrimental effect on long-term survival or local recurrence rates. Reconstruction may be delayed in patients who might require postmastectomy radiation therapy and is usually delayed in patients with locally advanced cancer. Reconstruction options include tissue expander and implant reconstructions and autologous tissue reconstructions, most often with transverse rectus abdominis muscle (TRAM) flaps, latissimus dorsi flaps, and more recently, muscle-preserving perforator abdominal flaps.

Surgical Procedures for Breast Cancer
Simple and Modified Radical Mastectomy
Simple or *total mastectomy* refers to complete removal of the mammary gland, including the nipple and areola. Sentinel node biopsy may be added for axillary staging and may be performed through the mastectomy incision or through a separate axillary incision. *Modified radical mastectomy* refers to removal of the mammary gland, nipple, and areola with the addition of axillary dissection (Fig. 34-12).[2,24]

An elliptical skin incision is made, as shown in Figure 34-12A. Skin flaps are raised to separate the underlying gland from the overlying skin, as shown in Figure 34-12B and C. If immediate reconstruction is not to be performed, sufficient skin is taken to allow smooth closure of skin flaps without redundant skin folds to facilitate comfortable use of a breast prosthesis. If immediate reconstruction is planned, a skin-sparing mastectomy may be performed in which only the nipple-areola complex is removed and the maximum amount of skin is left for use in the reconstruction.

Breast tissue is separated from the underlying pectoralis muscle, and the pectoral fascia is taken with the

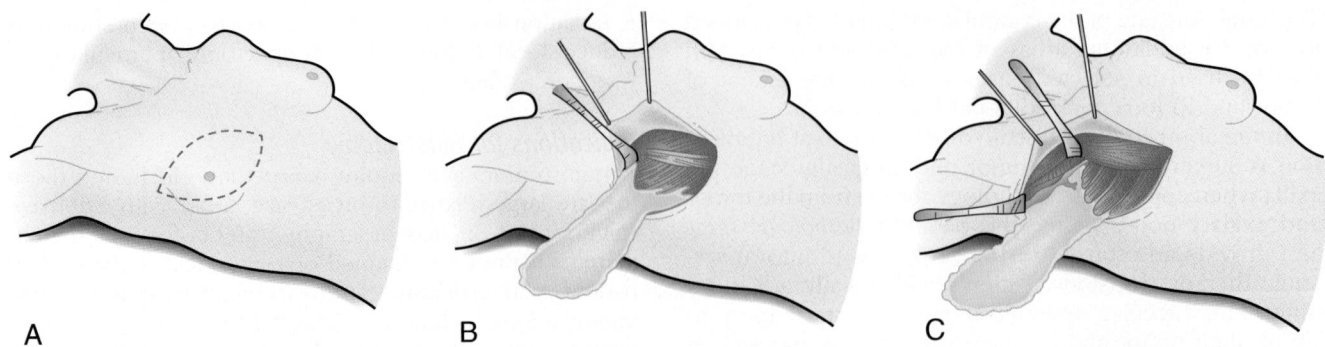

A B C

Figure 34-12 Total mastectomy with and without axillary dissection. **A,** Skin incisions are generally transverse and surround the central breast and nipple-areolar complex. **B,** Skin flaps are raised sharply to separate the gland from the overlying skin and then the gland from the underlying muscle. Simple mastectomy divides the breast from the axillary contents and stops at the clavipectoral fascia. **C,** In modified radical mastectomy, dissection continues into the axilla and generally extends up to the axillary vein, with removal of level I or level I and II nodes. Division of a branch of the axillary vein is shown in this panel, with separation of the node-bearing axillary fat from the axillary vein at the superior aspect of the dissection.

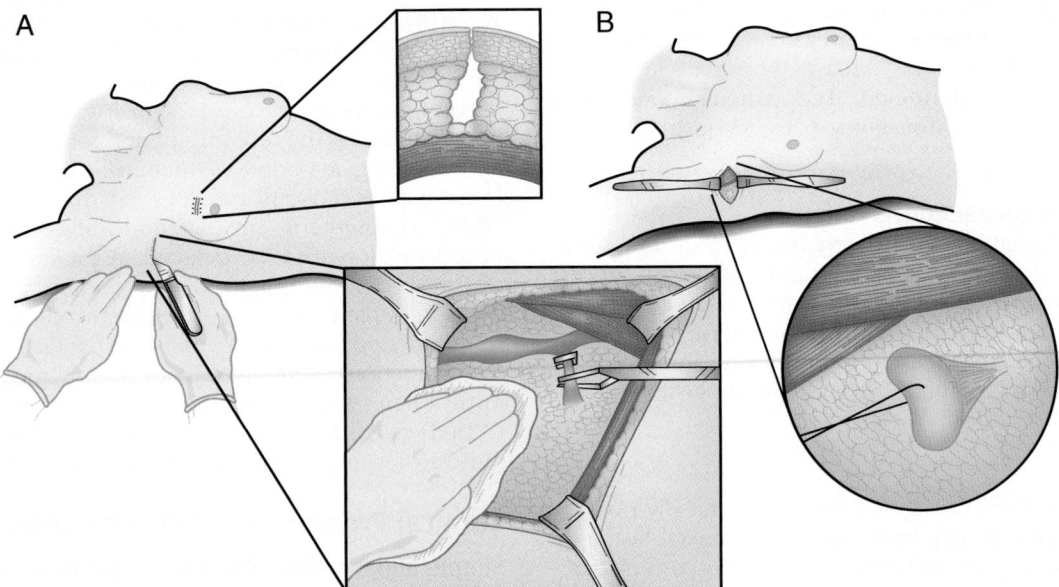

A B

Figure 34-13 Breast-conserving surgery. **A,** Incisions to remove malignant tumors are placed directly over the tumor, without tunneling. A transverse incision in the low axillary region is used for either sentinel node biopsy or axillary dissection. The axillary dissection is identical to the procedure for a modified radical mastectomy. The boundaries of the operation are the axillary vein superiorly, the latissimus dorsi muscle laterally, and the chest wall medially. The inferior dissection enters the tail of Spence (the axillary tail of the breast). The *inset* shows the excision cavity of the lumpectomy; no attempt is made to approximate the sides of the cavity, which fills with serous fluid and gradually shrinks. **B,** In sentinel node biopsy, a similar transverse incision is made (it may be located by percutaneous mapping with the gamma probe if radiolabeled colloid is used) and extended through the clavipectoral fascia, and the true axilla is entered. The sentinel node is located by virtue of its staining with dye or radioactivity, or both, and dissected free as a single specimen.

breast specimen. In a simple mastectomy, Figure 34-12B, breast tissue is separated from the axillary contents, and all breast tissue superficial to the fascia of the axilla is removed. For a modified radical mastectomy, level I and II axillary nodal tissue is taken with axillary breast tissue (see Fig. 34-12C). Level I nodes are those inferior to the axillary vein and lateral to the pectoralis minor muscle, and level II nodes are those under the pectoralis minor.

Wide Local Excision and Radiation Therapy

Excision of the primary tumor with preservation of the breast has been referred to by many names, including *lumpectomy, partial mastectomy,* and *segmentectomy. Wide local excision* seems to be the most descriptive term for the procedure, which removes the malignancy with a surrounding rim of grossly normal breast parenchyma. This procedure is depicted in Figure 34-13, which shows the completed lumpectomy and the skin incision for the axillary component of the procedure. A more extensive local procedure, *quadrantectomy,* used in early European trials of breast conservation, removes 2 to 3 cm of adjacent breast and skin over the tumor. These more extensive margins and skin excision have not been shown to improve survival and are not used in current breast conservation.

The specimen that is removed is oriented and its edges inked before sectioning. If a histologically positive margin is found, re-excision to remove more tissue will frequently achieve a clear margin and allow conservation of the breast. Orientation of the surgical specimen allows focal re-excision of involved margins rather than global re-excision and improves the cosmetic result.

The surgical defect created after lumpectomy is closed in cosmetic fashion. There is increasing interest in the use of advancement flap closure and other oncoplastic surgical techniques to maximize the cosmetic result.

Surgical staging of the axilla is performed through a separate incision in the majority of patients undergoing breast conservation. Sentinel node biopsy (see Fig. 34-13B) has largely replaced anatomic axillary node dissection in patients with clinically negative axillary nodes. For patients who require axillary dissection, the extent of the dissection is identical to the axillary component of the modified radical mastectomy (see Fig. 34-13A).

Surgical Staging of the Axilla

The pathologic status of the axillary lymph nodes is a key prognostic factor in patients with breast cancer. Identification of metastatic tumor deposits in the axillary nodes indicates a poorer prognosis and often prompts a recommendation for more aggressive systemic and local therapy.[24-26]

Surgical staging of the axilla has long been a routine component of breast cancer treatment. In the past it was accomplished though axillary dissection and clearance of node-bearing tissue between the pectoralis major and latissimus dorsi muscles from the edge of the breast tissue in the low axillary region to the axillary vein and underneath the pectoralis minor muscle. Axillary dissection provides prognostic information about axillary node status and also plays a therapeutic role in removing axillary tumor in patients with positive nodes.

Unfortunately, axillary dissection is often the main source of morbidity in patients with early-stage breast cancer. Immediate problems include acute pain, the need for hospital stay, reduced range of motion, and the need for a drain in the surgical bed for a week or more. Long-term problems resulting from axillary dissection include permanent lymphedema of the ipsilateral arm, numbness, chronic pain, and reduced range of motion.

The technique of sentinel node biopsy was developed with the goal of reducing the morbidity associated with surgical staging of the axilla in patients with no palpable axillary nodes. Identification of the first, or sentinel, nodes draining the affected breast with technetium-radio-labeled sulfur colloid particles or blue dye has allowed selective and minimally traumatic excision of only the most informative axillary nodes. In sentinel node mapping, tracer particles injected into breast tissue, either at the site of the tumor or in the subareolar area, pass through the breast lymphatics to the axilla and accumulate in the first node encountered. The sentinel node is identified as a blue or radioactive node (or both). If pathologic analysis of the sentinel node shows no evidence of metastasis, the likelihood of other nodes being involved is sufficiently low that therapeutic axillary dissection is not required.

Morbidity rates are substantially lower with sentinel node biopsy than with axillary dissection. Sentinel node biopsy is an outpatient procedure that does not require a drain, allows rapid return to full mobility, and permits return to work weeks sooner than after axillary dissection. Longer term morbidity, including lymphedema, numbness, and chronic pain, is greatly reduced.

Sentinel node biopsy has been shown to provide reliable pathologic staging of the axilla with false-negative rates generally lower than 5% in experienced hands. Axillary recurrence rates have been shown to be extremely low after a negative sentinel node biopsy without axillary dissection. A negative sentinel node biopsy is now widely accepted as sufficient to establish a patient as node negative, with no further axillary treatment required.

When the sentinel node contains metastatic disease, the likelihood of additional involved nodes is directly proportional to the size of the breast primary, the presence of lymphatic vascular invasion, and the size of the lymph node metastasis. In approximately half of patients with positive sentinel nodes, the sentinel node is the only positive node (Table 34-9). In the presence of a positive sentinel node, current medical practice dictates additional treatment of the axilla. This is most commonly achieved with a completion level I to II axillary dissection, although clinical trials are addressing options of systemic therapy or axillary radiation therapy, or both, as an alternative to dissection.

Axillary dissection remains the standard of care for patients with palpable axillary nodes and those with locally advanced or inflammatory breast cancer.

Ductal Carcinoma In Situ, or Intraductal Carcinoma

DCIS, or intraductal cancer, currently accounts for 20% to 25% of all newly diagnosed breast cancers, with more than 55,000 new cases expected in 2006. Most DCIS is characterized by an area of clustered calcifications on a screening mammogram, without an associated palpable abnormality. Rarely, DCIS will be manifested as a palpable mass or as unilateral, single-duct nipple discharge.

Mammographic findings in DCIS include clustered calcifications without an associated density in 75% of patients, calcifications coexisting with an associated density in 15%, and a density alone in 10%. The calcifications seen on a mammogram are deposited within the central necrotic debris in the involved duct. DCIS calcifications tend to cluster closely together, are pleomorphic, and may be linear or branching, thus suggesting their ductal origin.

Table 34-9 **Sentinel Node Biopsy Positive: Additional Affected Nodes**

STUDY	YEAR	SITE OF STUDY	NO. WITH POSITIVE SENTINEL NODE	NO. WITH POSITIVE NONSENTINEL NODE
Sachdev[1]	2002	Mt. Sinai	55	21 (38%)
Weiser[2]	2001	Memorial	206	66 (32%)
Abdessabum[3]	2001	Ohio State	100	40 (40%)
Tafra[4]	2001	Annapolis	326	204 (63%)
Wong[5]	2001	U. Louisville	389	144 (37%)
Chua[6]	2001	Australia	51	24 (47%)
Cox[7]	2000	Moffitt	315	125 (40%)
Haigh[8]	2000	John Wayne	90	38 (42%)
Hill[9]	1999	Memorial	114	45 (39%)
Kollias[10]	1999	Australia	31	18 (58%)
Reynolds[11]	1999	Mayo	60	28 (47%)
Veronesi[12]	1999	Milan	168	95 (57%)
Borgstein[13]	1998	Amsterdam	44	18 (41%)
Krag[14]	1998	Multicenter	101	41 (41%)
Total				**873/2046 (43%)**

[1]Data from Sachdev U, Murphy K, Derzie A, et al: Predictors of nonsentinel lymph node metastasis in breast cancer patients. Am J Surg 183:213, 2002.

[2]Data from Weiser MR, Montgomery LL, Tan LK, et al: Lymphovascular invasion enhances the prediction of non-sentinel node metastases in breast cancer patients with positive sentinel nodes. Ann Surg Oncol 8:145, 2001.

[3]Data from Abdessalam SF, Zervos EE, Prasad M, et al: Predictors of positive axillary lymph nodes after sentinel lymph node biopsy in breast cancer. Am J Surg 182:316, 2001.

[4]Data from Tafra L, Lannin DR, Swanson MS, et al: Multicenter trial of sentinel node biopsy for breast cancer using both technetium sulfur colloid and isosulfan blue dye. Ann Surg 233:51, 2001.

[5]Data from Wong SL, Edwards MJ, Chao C, et al: Predicting the status of the nonsentinel axillary nodes. Arch Surg 136:563, 2001.

[6]Data from Chua B, Ung O, Taylor R, et al: Treatment implications of a positive sentinel lymph node biopsy for patients with early-stage breast carcinoma. Cancer 92:1769, 2001.

[7]Data from Cox CE, Bass SS, McCann CR, et al: Lymphatic mapping and sentinel lymph node biopsy in patients with breast cancer. Annu Rev Med 51:525, 2000.

[8]Data from Haigh PI, Hansen NM, Qi K, et al: Biopsy method and excision volume do not affect success rate of subsequent sentinel lymph node dissection in breast cancer. Ann Surg Oncol 7:21, 2000.

[9]Data from Hill AD, Tran KN, Akhurst T, et al: Lessons learned from 500 cases of lymphatic mapping for breast cancer. Ann Surg 229:528, 1999.

[10]Data from Kollias J, Gill PG, Chatterton BE, et al: Reliability of sentinel node status in predicting axillary lymph node involvement in breast cancer. Med J Aust 171:461, 1999.

[11]Data from Reynolds C, Mick R, Donohue JH, et al: Sentinel lymph node biopsy with metastasis: Can axillary dissections be avoided in some patients with breast cancer? J Clin Oncol 17:1720, 1999.

[12]Data from Veronesi U, Paganelli G, Viale G, et al: Sentinel lymph node biopsy and axillary dissection in breast cancer: Results in a large series. J Natl Cancer Inst 91:368, 1999.

[13]Data from Borgstein PJ, Pijpers R, Comans EF, et al: Sentinel lymph node biopsy in breast cancer: Guidelines and pitfalls of lymphoscintigraphy and gamma probe detection. J Am Coll Surg 186:275, 1998.

[14]Data from Krag D, Weaver D, Ashikaga T, et al: The sentinel node in breast cancer: A multicenter validation study. N Engl J Med 339:941, 1998.

DCIS is viewed as a precursor of invasive ductal cancer, and treatment aims to remove the DCIS to prevent progression to invasive disease. Because the risk for metastatic disease in patients with DCIS but no invasion is 1%, systemic chemotherapy is not required. Hormonal therapy may be used for prevention of new primary tumors and to improve local control after breast-conserving therapy (see later).

Treatment recommendations for an individual patient with DCIS are based on the extent of disease within the breast, its histologic grade, ER status, and the presence of microinvasion, as well as patient age and interest in breast conservation. Treatment options for DCIS include mastectomy, wide excision with irradiation, and wide excision alone. With the choice of breast conservation,

there is also the option of adjuvant hormonal therapy with tamoxifen or other agents.[27-30]

Mastectomy in DCIS

Breast cancer mortality after treatment of DCIS by total or simple mastectomy is 1%, which is the standard against which breast-conserving approaches are compared (Table 34-10). Local recurrences are rare and suggest malignant transformation of residual glandular tissue. Metastatic recurrences are suggestive of either a histologically unrecognized invasive carcinoma in the mastectomy specimen or the development of a contralateral primary.

In current practice, reasons to select total mastectomy for treatment of DCIS include the following:

Table 34-10 Recurrence and Mortality Rates After Mastectomy for Ductal Carcinoma In Situ

STUDY	DATES	NO. OF PATIENTS	FOLLOW-UP (yr)	NONCLINICAL (%)	NO. OF RECURRENCES	NO. DEAD OF DISEASE
Farrow[1]	1949-1967	181	5-20	0	6	4
Brown[2]	1952-1975	39	1-15	10	0	0
Carter[3]	1960-1975	28	1-14 (6.2)	—	1	1
Sunshine[4]	1960-1980	73	10-yr minimum	0	4	3
Von Rueden[5]	1960-1981	45	Not stated	8	1	0
Ashikari[6]	1960-1969	92	11-yr maximum	40	0	0
Schuh[7]	1965-1984	49	5.5 mean	33	1	1
Kinne[8]	1970-1976	101	11.5 median	58	1	1
Lagios[9]	1975-1980	42	Not stated	—	0	0
Fisher[10]	1976-1984	27	5	—	1	1
Arnesson[11]	1978-1984	28	6.4 median	100	0	0
Ward[12]	1979-1983	123	10	11	1	?
Silverstein[13]	1979-1990	98	4.9 median	62	1	0
Total		**926**			**17 (2%)**	**11 (1%)**

[1]Data from Farrow JH: Current concepts in the detection and treatment of the earliest of the early breast cancers. Cancer 25:468, 1970.

[2]Data from Brown PW, Silverman J, Owens E, et al: Intraductal "noninfiltrating" carcinoma of the breast. Arch Surg 111:1063, 1976.

[3]Data from Carter D, Smith RL: Carcinoma in situ of the breast. Cancer 40:1189, 1977.

[4]Data from Sunshine JA, Moseley MS, Fletcher WS, et al: Breast carcinoma in situ: A retrospective review of 112 cases with a minimum 10-year follow-up. Am J Surg 150:44, 1985.

[5]Data from Von Rueden DG, Wilson RE: Intraductal carcinoma of the breast. Surg Gynecol Obstet 158:105, 1984.

[6]Data from Ashikari R, Hajdu SI, Robbins GF: Intraductal carcinoma of the breast (1960-1969). Cancer 28:1182, 1971.

[7]Data from Schuh ME, Nemoto T, Penetrante R, et al: Intraductal carcinoma: Analysis of presentation, pathologic findings, and outcome of disease. Arch Surg 121:1303, 1986.

[8]Data from Kinne DW, Petrek JA, Osborne MP, et al: Breast carcinoma in situ. Arch Surg 124:33, 1989.

[9]Data from Lagios MD, Westdahl PR, Margolin FR, et al: Duct carcinoma in situ: Relationship of extent of noninvasive disease to the frequency of occult invasion, multicentricity, lymph node metastases, and short-term treatment failures. Cancer 50:1309, 1982.

[10]Data from Fisher ER, Sass R, Fisher B, et al: Pathologic findings from the National Surgical Adjuvant Breast Project (Protocol 6), I: Intraductal carcinoma (DCIS). Cancer 57:197, 1986.

[11]Data from Arnesson LG, Smeds S, Fagerberg G, et al: Follow-up of two treatment modalities for ductal cancer in situ of the breast. Br J Surg 76:672, 1989.

[12]Data from Ward BA, McKhann CF, Ravikumar TS: Ten-year follow-up of breast carcinoma in situ in Connecticut. Arch Surg 127:1392, 1992.

[13]Data from Silverstein MJ (ed): Ductal Carcinoma In Situ of the Breast. Baltimore, Williams & Wilkins, 1997, p 443.

1. Diffuse suspicious mammographic calcifications suggestive of extensive disease
2. Inability to obtain clear margins on wide excision
3. Likelihood of a poor cosmetic result after wide excision of involved tissue
4. Patient not motivated to preserve her breast
5. Contraindications to radiation therapy and a lesion not eligible for wide excision alone.

Contraindications to breast irradiation include the following:

1. Previous irradiation of the breast or chest wall
2. Presence of collagen vascular disease (scleroderma or active lupus)
3. First- or second-trimester pregnancy

Breast Conservation in DCIS

As is the case for invasive breast cancer, breast conservation for DCIS requires resection to microscopically clear margins. The use of radiation therapy markedly decreases the risk for local recurrence and reduces the proportion of recurrences that contain invasive histology. The use of hormonal therapy in ER-positive DCIS can further decrease the risk for local recurrence and also reduces the risk for development of new contralateral and ipsilateral breast cancers.

Three prospective, randomized trials have evaluated the efficacy of breast-conserving surgery with and without radiation therapy for the treatment of DCIS. NSABP B-06 randomized 1855 women with *invasive* breast cancer to mastectomy versus lumpectomy with radiation therapy versus lumpectomy alone. During subsequent pathology review, 76 specimens were identified as having DCIS only, without an invasive breast cancer component. At 10 years of follow-up, the local recurrence rate was 0% (0 of 28) in those who underwent mastectomy, 7% (2 of 27) in those who underwent lumpectomy with irradiation, and 43% (9 of 21) in those who underwent lumpectomy alone.

The NSABP B-17 protocol randomized 818 women with DCIS to lumpectomy alone versus lumpectomy plus 50 Gy of postoperative irradiation. Twelve-year actuarial recurrence data showed that the addition of radiation decreased the ipsilateral recurrence rate from 30.8% in

Table 34-11   Randomized Trials of Lumpectomy for Ductal Carcinoma In Situ: Impact of Radiation Therapy and Tamoxifen

	NO. OF PATIENTS	FOLLOW-UP (yr)	LOCAL RECURRENCE RATE (%)			P VALUE
			Lumpectomy	Lumpectomy + XRT	Lumpectomy + XRT + Tamoxifen	
NSABP B-17[1]	818	12	30.8	14.9		<.000005
EORTC 10853[2]	1010	4.25	16	9		<.005
NSABP B-24[3]	1804	7		9	6	.04

[1]Data from Fisher B, Dignam J, Wolmark N, et al: Lumpectomy and radiation therapy for the treatment of intraductal breast cancer: Findings from National Surgical Adjuvant Breast and Bowel Project B-17. J Clin Oncol 16:441, 1998.

[2]Data from Julien JP, Bijker N, Fentiman IS, et al: Radiotherapy in breast-conserving treatment for ductal carcinoma in situ: First results of the EORTC randomised phase III trial 10853. EORTC Breast Cancer Cooperative Group and EORTC Radiotherapy Group. Lancet 355:528, 2000.

[3]Fisher B, Land S, Mamounas E, et al: Prevention of invasive breast cancer in women with ductal carcinoma in situ: An update of the National Surgical Adjuvant Breast and Bowel Project experience. Semin Oncol 28:400, 2001.

XRT, x-ray therapy.

patients undergoing excision alone to 14.9% in patients undergoing excision with irradiation ($P < .000005$). Use of radiation therapy resulted in a decrease in the incidence of invasive breast cancer (16.4% versus 7.1%, $P < .00001$), with a smaller decrease in the incidence of in situ recurrence (14.1% versus 7.8%, $P < .001$) (Table 34-11).

The EORTC 10853 trial randomized 1010 women with DCIS to lumpectomy alone versus lumpectomy plus 50 Gy of radiation therapy. The 4.25-year actuarial ipsilateral recurrence rate was 16% in patients undergoing excision alone and 9% in patients undergoing excision with radiation therapy ($P < .005$). This decrease was statistically significant for the reduction in occurrence of invasive breast cancer (8% versus 4%, $P < .04$) but was not statistically significant for the reduction in in situ recurrence (8% versus 4%, $P < .06$) (see Table 34-11).

Pathologic findings from the NSABP B-17 study found that uncertain or involved specimen margins and the presence of comedo necrosis were associated with an increased risk for ipsilateral breast tumor recurrence. The EORTC 10853 study found that involved surgical margins and solid and cribriform histology were associated with increased risk for local recurrence. Solin and colleagues reported 15-year results of treatment of DCIS by surgical excision and irradiation. With 5 years of follow-up, only 2% of the noncomedo lesions had an in-breast recurrence as compared with 11% of comedo lesions. After 15 years of follow-up, the in-breast recurrence rate for noncomedo lesions was 15% and that for comedo lesions was 17%. These data suggest that the histologic subtype has an impact on short-term recurrence rates but does not change long-term recurrence rates.

These prospective trials all confirm that the use of radiation therapy after excision reduces the risk for local recurrence of intraductal carcinoma by approximately 50% when compared with excision alone. Radiation therapy also reduces the proportion of local recurrences that include invasive histology. The chance of metastatic disease developing when breast conservation is chosen for treatment of DCIS is estimated to be between 0% and 3%. These infrequent distant recurrences are thought to arise from invasive cancers that develop during recurrence of DCIS.

Attempts have been made to identify subsets of DCIS for which wide excision without irradiation would provide sufficient local control. Silverstein and colleagues derived the Van Nuys criteria from a series of DCIS patients treated by wide excision with and without radiation therapy and proposed a system to identify patients who do not need radiation therapy based on DCIS nuclear grade, size of the lesion, and width of the surgical margin. In a prospective trial testing this approach, Wong and associates enrolled 158 patients from the most favorable Van Nuys subset (low- or intermediate-grade DCIS measuring less than 2.5 cm with a minimum 1-cm margin on excision) to follow-up without radiation therapy. The annual local recurrence rate was 2.4% with an actuarial 12% risk for local recurrence at 5 years, thus suggesting that even this favorable subset of DCIS lesions has a substantial local recurrence rate without radiation therapy.

Role of Tamoxifen in DCIS

The use of tamoxifen has been shown to reduce the risk for new breast cancer in high-risk women, including those with previous breast cancer (see the earlier section Chemoprevention for Breast Cancer). To evaluate the benefit of tamoxifen for DCIS, the NSABP B-24 protocol randomized 1804 women who underwent lumpectomy and radiation therapy for DCIS to 5 years of tamoxifen versus placebo. Study criteria allowed enrollment of patients with positive margins, and ER measurements were not performed. At 7 years of follow-up, the addition of tamoxifen to lumpectomy and radiation therapy decreased the incidence of recurrent ipsilateral breast cancer from 9% to 6%, and the risk for a new contralateral breast cancer was reduced by 47% (an absolute reduction of 2%) (see Table 34-11).

Combining the results of NSABP B-17 and NSABP B-24 at 7 years of follow-up, the total ipsilateral and contralateral breast cancer recurrence rate was 30% for excision alone, 17% for excision with radiation therapy, and 10% for excision, irradiation, and tamoxifen. Subsequent analysis demonstrated that benefit from tamoxifen is seen only in women whose DCIS is ER positive. Patients at highest risk for local recurrence, and therefore those most likely to benefit from tamoxifen, were patients with positive margins, comedo necrosis, a mass on physical examination, and age younger than 50 years. For individual patients, the benefits of tamoxifen are weighed against its side effects, including risk for endometrial carcinoma, thromboembolic events, hot flashes, and cataracts.

Sentinel Node Biopsy in DCIS

DCIS, by definition, represents breast cancer contained within an intact basement membrane and without access to lymphatic or vascular channels. However, when axillary dissection is performed during mastectomy for intraductal disease, positive nodes can be seen in up to 3.6% of cases, as identified in a review of more than 10,000 patients in the National Cancer Database. These positive nodes probably result from the presence of microinvasion not detected on routine pathologic analysis.

To assess the risk for invasion in DCIS lesions of different size, Lagios and coworkers performed extensive pathologic processing of 111 specimens of intraductal carcinoma. For DCIS lesions 45 mm or smaller ($n = 80$), there were no cases of microscopic invasion. For DCIS measuring 46 to 55 mm ($n = 6$), 17% harbored occult microscopic disease. In 25 patients with DCIS measuring 56 mm or greater, 12 (48%) had evidence of microscopic invasion, and 2 of these patients had cancer in axillary nodes. The extent of the primary DCIS in these two patients was 68 and 160 mm.

These data suggest that patients with a small mammographically detected area of DCIS have very low rates of occult invasion and therefore surgical staging of the axilla is not necessary. However, in women undergoing breast-conserving surgery for larger areas of DCIS, particularly those with high-grade histology or when suspicion for microinvasion is high, sentinel node mapping to evaluate the lymph nodes may be considered.

Sentinel node biopsy is currently recommended when mastectomy is performed for DCIS because up to 10% of patients with DCIS on a diagnostic biopsy will be found to have invasive cancer in their mastectomy specimen. The addition of sentinel node biopsy to mastectomy adds minimal morbidity and, because sentinel node mapping is no longer possible after mastectomy, avoids the need for axillary dissection if invasive cancer is identified.

Radiation Therapy After Breast-Conserving Surgery

In modern practice, wide local excision is part of a multidisciplinary approach that nearly always includes postoperative radiation therapy. Radiation is most often delivered to the entire breast as *whole-breast irradiation.* For whole-breast radiation, doses of 4500 to 5000 cGy are administered to the entire breast, often with an additional boost of 1000 to 1200 cGy delivered to the region of the tumor bed.[31-33]

More recently, there has been exploration of *partial-breast irradiation* for early-stage breast cancer, a technique that delivers radiation only to breast tissue around the tumor bed, usually over a period of 4 to 5 days, in contrast to the 6- to 7-week course required for whole-breast irradiation. Partial-breast irradiation may be performed with brachytherapy catheters, balloon catheters, or external beam radiation. Clinical trials of these methods are in progress.

In selected cases, radiation therapy can be extended to include the axillary nodes in women not undergoing axillary dissection and full regional nodal irradiation for women with high-risk nodal metastases.

Postmastectomy Radiation Therapy

In most patients who undergo mastectomy for early-stage breast cancer, mastectomy provides effective local control, and radiation therapy is not required. However, certain subsets remain at increased risk for local and regional recurrence and benefit from radiation's ability to control any microscopic residual tumor that may remain in the skin flaps, in axillary tissue not removed with axillary dissection, and in other regional nodes not removed by mastectomy (level III axillary, supraclavicular, and internal mammary nodes).

Three prospective randomized trials have addressed the role of postmastectomy irradiation. In the Danish Trials, premenopausal women with stage II or III breast cancer were randomized to chemotherapy alone or chemotherapy plus chest wall and nodal irradiation (protocol 82b), and postmenopausal women were randomized to tamoxifen alone or tamoxifen plus radiation therapy (protocol 82c). In the British Columbia study, premenopausal women with node-positive breast cancer were randomized to chemotherapy alone or chemotherapy plus chest wall and nodal irradiation. In addition to the expected benefit in reducing local-regional recurrences, postmastectomy irradiation also resulted in a significant improvement in overall survival in all three trials (Table 34-12).

Although the design and execution of these three studies raised some question about the general applicability of their results, meta-analyses from the EBCTCG and McMaster University found that postmastectomy irradiation reduced the risk for local or regional recurrence by approximately two thirds and reduced breast cancer–specific mortality. Although the McMaster University analysis showed a survival advantage with radiation therapy after mastectomy (odds ratio of 0.83), in the ECBTCG analysis, decreased breast cancer mortality was offset by deaths from other causes, in particular, vascular events thought to be related to radiation therapy.

Most centers now recommend chest wall and nodal irradiation after mastectomy for patients at increased risk for local and regional recurrence, including those with multiple positive nodes (more than four positive nodes), for patients with large cancers or very aggressive histology (e.g., diffuse vascular invasion), and for extranodal extension of breast cancer. Some centers will recommend postmastectomy irradiation for patients with any positive axillary nodes.

Treatment of Locally Advanced and Inflammatory Breast Cancer

Patients with locally advanced breast cancer include those with large primary tumors (>5 cm), tumors involv-

Table 34-12 Trials of Systemic Therapy With or Without Irradiation After Mastectomy

RADIATION TRIALS	NO. OF PATIENTS			LOCAL RECURRENCE RATE (%)			OVERALL SURVIVAL (%)		
	Systemic + Radiation	Systemic Alone	Total	Systemic + Radiation	Systemic Alone	P Value	Systemic + Radiation	Systemic Alone	P Value
DBCG 82b Trial (chemotherapy)[1]	852	856	1708	9	32	<.001	54	45	<.001
DBCG 82c Trial (tamoxifen)[2]	686	689	1375	8	35	<.001	45	38	.03
British Columbia Trial[3]	164	154	318	13	25	.003*	64	54	.003*

[1]Data from Overgaard M, Hansen Per S, Overgaard J, et al: Postoperative radiotherapy in high-risk premenopausal women with breast cancer who receive adjuvant chemotherapy. N Engl J Med 337:949, 1997.

[2]Data from Overgaard M, Jensen M-B, Overgaard J, et al: Postoperative radiotherapy in high-risk postmenopausal breast cancer patients given adjuvant tamoxifen: Danish Breast Cancer Cooperative Group DBCG 82c randomized trial. Lancet 353:1641, 1999.

[3]Data from Ragaz J, Jackson S, Le N, et al: Adjuvant radiotherapy and chemotherapy in node-positive premenopausal women with breast cancer. N Engl J Med 337:956, 1997.

*Aggregate *P* value for comparisons at various follow-up intervals; this is the 10-year result.

ing the chest wall, skin involvement, ulceration or satellite skin nodules, inflammatory carcinoma, bulky or fixed axillary nodes, or clinically apparent internal mammary or supraclavicular nodal involvement. Such cancers span stages IIB, IIIA, and IIIB disease. Central to treatment is the concept that the disease is advanced on the chest wall or in regional lymph nodes (or both), with no evidence of metastasis to distant sites. Such patients are recognized to be at significant risk for the development of subsequent metastases, and treatment must address the risk for both local and systemic relapse.

Experience before the 1970s demonstrated that surgery alone provided poor local control, with local relapse rates in the range of 30% to 50% and mortality rates of 70%. Similar results were reported when radiation therapy was the sole modality of treatment. Current management includes surgery, radiation therapy, and systemic therapy, with the sequence and extent of treatment determined by specifics of the individual patient's circumstance.

Neoadjuvant Systemic Therapy for Operable Breast Cancer

Administration of systemic chemotherapy or hormonal therapy before surgery can result in a significant reduction in tumor size in 50% to 80% of patients with locally advanced breast cancer. This preoperative, or neoadjuvant, therapy can convert inoperable tumors to operable ones, can convert tumors that would require mastectomy to eligibility for lumpectomy, and can shrink larger tumors to allow a more cosmetic lumpectomy. This approach also allows study of tumor biology via serial analysis of tumor tissue before, during, and after treatment and has been used to study the efficacy and mechanism of action of systemic therapy agents.[34]

Several prospective, randomized trials have evaluated the efficacy of chemotherapy and hormonal therapy administered before (neoadjuvant) versus after (adjuvant) definitive surgery. These studies all demonstrated increased rates of breast conservation with the use of systemic therapy before surgery. The NSABP B-18 trial included 1523 patients and found no survival advantage (or detriment) in patients who received preoperative doxorubicin and cyclophosphamide chemotherapy versus the same regimen delivered postoperatively. The breast conservation rate was higher in women completing preoperative chemotherapy, and in-breast recurrence after preoperative therapy was not significantly different from that in women who underwent lumpectomy before adjuvant chemotherapy. Response to preoperative therapy was found to correlate with prognosis. At 9 years of follow-up, the disease-free survival rate in patients achieving a complete pathologic response in the preoperative arm (no evidence of tumor at surgery) was 75% as opposed to 58% in patients who had any residual invasive disease left after chemotherapy.

In practice, the neoadjuvant approach is used routinely for patients with inoperable locally advanced breast cancer, including those with inflammatory breast cancer, those with large, fixed or erosive lesions not amenable to mastectomy, and those with advanced nodal disease that is fixed, bulky, or causing arm edema. Most of these patients will then undergo mastectomy, radiation therapy, and additional systemic therapy.

The neoadjuvant approach is also used for operable patients who would require mastectomy but could become candidates for breast conservation if their primary tumor size could be reduced before surgery. By the end of systemic therapy, 10% to 15% of such patients will have complete resolution of their tumors by clinical examination and imaging but may have microscopic residual disease. Consequently, a metallic clip is placed in the tumor under image guidance before initiating chemotherapy to allow identification of the original tumor site for excision.

Management of the axilla in patients undergoing neoadjuvant therapy is in transition. Some centers perform sentinel node biopsy before neoadjuvant therapy in patients with clinically negative nodes to inform systemic and radiation therapy decisions. Advocates of sentinel node biopsy before neoadjuvant chemotherapy cite concerns about lower rates of successful mapping and higher false-negative rates after neoadjuvant therapy. Other centers favor sentinel node biopsy after neoadjuvant therapy for any patient whose axilla is clinically negative after therapy to obtain more information about the status of the nodes *after* neoadjuvant therapy because they have found that the response of disease in the axilla correlates with survival. Other centers continue to advocate complete axillary dissection for all patients receiving neoadjuvant therapy.

Inflammatory Breast Cancer

Inflammatory breast cancer is an ominous clinical category of breast cancer associated with diffuse tumor involvement of the lymphatic channels within the breast and overlying skin. It is clinically manifested as erythema, edema, and warmth of the breast as a result of lymphatic obstruction. There may be no mammographic abnormality beyond skin thickening, and a palpable mass is not required for the diagnosis. *Peau d'orange* is the term used to describe the orange peel appearance of the skin resulting from edema and dimpling at sites of hair follicles (see Fig. 34-5).

Inflammatory cancer is a clinical diagnosis and can occur with tumors of either ductal or lobular histology. The pathologic hallmark of inflammatory cancer is the presence of tumor cells within dermal lymphatics. Axillary nodal metastases are common, and there is a significant risk for distant metastases.

Current treatment approaches emphasize aggressive use of combined-modality treatment, including neoadjuvant chemotherapy, mastectomy, and radiation therapy, with hormonal therapy in estrogen-responsive tumors. The results of such multimodality treatment now show relapse-free survival rates of 50% or higher at 5 years as compared with a single-institution historical series showing a 7% 5-year survival rate in patients receiving lesser treatment.

Treatment of Special Conditions

Breast Cancer in the Elderly

Several studies have explored options that reduce the extent of surgery and radiation therapy for elderly women with breast cancer. Two recent trials randomized older women to lumpectomy with or without irradiation. In the Cancer and Leukemia Group B (CALGB) 9343 trial, 647 women 70 years or older with ER-positive tumors 2 cm or less in size and clinically negative nodes received lumpectomy and tamoxifen and were randomized to irradiation or no irradiation. At 5 years' follow-up, survival was identical, and the in-breast recurrence rate was only 4% in the no-radiation arm versus 1% in the radiation arm. The death rate from breast cancer was 1% at 5 years in this population, with a 17% death rate from other causes.[35,36]

Fyles and coauthors reported the results of a Canadian trial with more inclusive eligibility criteria in which 769

women aged 50 years or older with tumors up to 5 cm and positive or negative ER status were enrolled. All patients underwent wide excision, received tamoxifen, and were randomized to irradiation or no irradiation. Recurrence rates were significantly higher overall in patients who did not receive radiation therapy. However, in an unplanned subset of 193 women older than 60, the local recurrence rate was only 1.2% without radiation versus no recurrences with radiation therapy.

These low rates of local recurrence and the significant rates of death from other comorbid conditions have led to acceptance of wide excision and hormonal therapy without irradiation for selected elderly patients with small ER-positive tumors and clinically negative axillary nodes. Axillary surgery is routinely omitted in such patients.

Paget's Disease

Paget's disease accounts for 1% or less of breast malignancies. It is characterized clinically by nipple erythema and irritation with associated itching and may progress to nipple crusting and ulceration. The condition may spread outward off the nipple and onto the areola and surrounding skin of the breast (see Fig. 34-5). The clinical differential diagnosis of scaling skin and erythema of the nipple-areola complex includes eczema, contact dermatitis, postradiation dermatitis, and Paget's disease. A skin specimen containing Paget cells secures the diagnosis and can be obtained by nipple scrape cytology or biopsy.[37]

Pathologically, a Paget cell is a large, pale-staining cell with round or oval nuclei and large nucleoli located between the normal keratinocytes of the nipple epidermis. The Paget cells spread into the lactiferous sinuses under the nipple and upward to invade the overlying epidermis of the nipple. Paget cells do not invade through the dermal basement membrane and therefore are a form of carcinoma in situ.

More than 97% of patients with Paget's disease have an underlying breast carcinoma. Paget's disease may (54%) or may not (46%) be accompanied by a mass. Invasive breast cancer coexists with Paget's disease in 93% of patients with a mass and in 38% of patients without a mass.

Treatment of Paget's disease includes mastectomy with axillary staging or wide excision of the nipple and areola to achieve clear margins, axillary staging, and radiation therapy. For many patients, lumpectomy and irradiation will give a very acceptable cosmetic appearance and avoid the more extensive surgery of mastectomy and reconstruction. For patients considering lumpectomy, thorough preoperative evaluation is required to rule out occult multicentric disease.

Male Breast Cancer

Breast cancer occurring in the mammary gland of men is infrequent; it accounts for 0.8% of all breast cancers, less than 1% of all newly diagnosed male cancers, and 0.2% of male cancer deaths. Annually in the United States, 1500 new cases and 400 deaths are reported. The median age at diagnosis is 68 years, 5 years older than in women.[2,38]

Risk factors include increasing age, radiation exposure, and factors related to abnormalities in estrogen and androgen balance, including testicular disease, infertility, obesity, and cirrhosis. Risk factors related to a genetic predisposition include Klinefelter's syndrome (47,XXY karyotype), family history, and *BRCA* gene mutations, particularly *BRCA2* mutations. Gynecomastia is not a risk factor.

Histologically, 90% of male breast cancers are invasive ductal carcinomas. Approximately 80% are ER positive, 75% are PR positive, and 35% overexpress HER-2/neu. The remaining 10% are DCIS. Given the absence of terminal lobules in the normal male breast, lobular carcinoma, both invasive and in situ, is rarely seen.

The majority of men with breast cancer have a breast mass, and the differential diagnosis includes gynecomastia, primary breast carcinoma, metastatic carcinoma to the breast, sarcoma, and breast abscess. In addition to local pain and axillary adenopathy, other initial symptoms may include nipple retraction, ulceration, bleeding, and discharge. Evaluation includes breast imaging studies and diagnostic needle or surgical biopsy.

Prognostic factors in male breast cancer are the same as in female breast cancer and include nodal involvement, tumor size, histologic grade, and hormone receptor status. When matched for age and stage, survival is similar to that in women.

Treatment of carcinoma in the male breast depends on the stage and local extent of the tumor, with treatment choices similar to those for women. Small tumors may be treated by local excision and irradiation or by mastectomy. Sentinel node biopsy has been shown to be effective for staging male breast cancer. Breast tumors in men more commonly involve the pectoralis major muscle, probably because breast tissue in men is scant. If the underlying pectoral muscle is involved, modified radical mastectomy with excision of the involved portion of muscle is adequate treatment and may be combined with postoperative radiation therapy.

Adjuvant systemic therapy for male breast cancer is used as for female breast cancer. Most male breast cancers are hormone sensitive. Adjuvant hormonal therapy with tamoxifen or aromatase inhibitors is indicated for node-positive and high-risk node-negative patients. Adjuvant chemotherapy is used in men at substantial risk for metastatic disease.

CHEMOTHERAPY AND HORMONE THERAPY FOR BREAST CANCER

As radical local surgery gave way to less invasive surgical procedures, the concept of cancer as spreading sequentially from primary site to more and more distant sites was challenged by newer theories of cancer metastasis. Current thinking places the metastatic event early in the progression of breast cancer, probably before initial clinical evaluation in the majority of patients. This concept argues for a systemic approach to breast cancer, administered in concert with local treatment. The missing link is the ability to accurately detect occult metastatic disease

and select appropriate patients to receive systemic treatment.

Metastatic disease is the principal cause of death from breast cancer. Patients who benefit from chemotherapy or hormonal therapy do so because metastasis is prevented, cured, or delayed. The first prospective trials of systemic treatment combined oophorectomy, to deprive patients of estrogens, with radical mastectomy. Since these early trials, hundreds of prospective studies have involved thousands of women. The literature on systemic adjuvant treatment of breast cancer is now more than 25 years old. A comprehensive analysis of systemic therapy after surgery for early-stage breast cancer is updated continuously by the EBCTCG. Centered in England, the EBCTCG has conducted meta-analyses of randomized clinical trials for 25 years. The 2005 update on chemotherapy and tamoxifen included 100,000 women enrolled worldwide in randomized trials of surgery with or without systemic therapy.

Interpreting Results of Clinical Trials

Survival curves are the most familiar method of comparing groups of patients in randomized trials involving different therapies. To estimate the survival curve for any group of people, investigators use the life-table method (also called the *actuarial method*). Kaplan and Meier proposed a popular modification of these general methods that suits clinical trials, and the resulting curves are often called *Kaplan-Meier curves*. This method tabulates the number of patients surviving as a proportion of the total number of patients reaching the interval of time in question after entering the trial. Plotting data for each time interval generates the familiar curves. Survival or death is only one outcome that can be expressed in actuarial terms. Disease-free survival, event-free survival, and freedom from local failure (just to list a few) can all be expressed in actuarial terms.

Comparisons between groups (e.g., treated versus control) can be described in several ways, each of which has limitations and ambiguities. As shown in Figure 34-14, the simplest way is to measure the absolute difference between the curves at any specified interval of time during follow-up, as demonstrated by the vertical dashed lines between the Kaplan-Meier curves. Alternatively, for any specific proportion of patients, there is a different time until relapse or death between the two curves, as shown by the horizontal dashed line in Figure 34-14. For instance, the median survival time is the length of survival free of relapse or death for 50% of the patients. Differences in median survival times between treated and control patients may be significant even though absolute differences are small. For most treatment comparisons, there are three groups to consider. Some patients will remain free of recurrence or death with the control treatment, shown as the area under the lower curve (C). Other patients are destined to fail both the experimental and control treatments, shown as the area above the experimental curve (upper curve [A]). It is only the patients falling between the two curves (B) who benefit (or are harmed) by the experimental treatment. The concept of

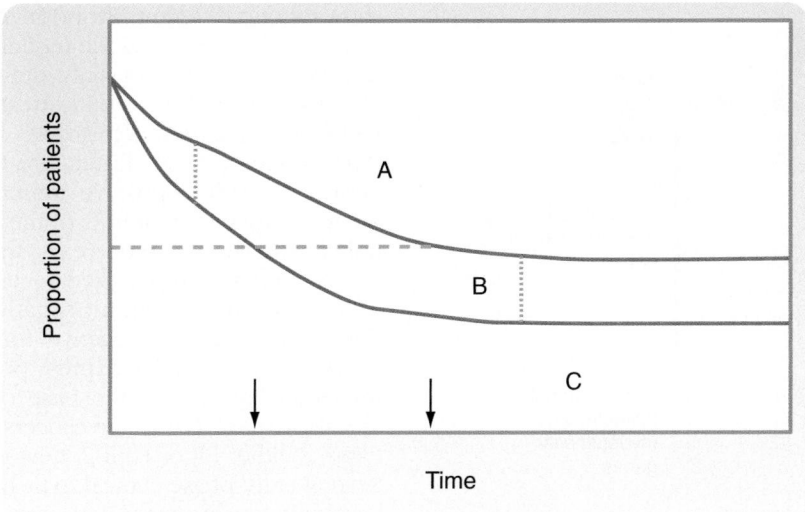

Figure 34-14 Interpretation of actuarial curves used in clinical trials comparing two groups of patients. Refer to the text for an explanation of the annotations.

proportional benefit is important when evaluating adjuvant chemotherapy or hormonal therapy for breast cancer; only a small proportion of treated patients benefit from receiving postoperative adjuvant treatments.

A popular way to express the difference between control and experimental groups is to cite the proportional reduction in treatment failures. For instance, the proportional reduction in mortality is the difference in survival between the two groups at an interval divided by the percentage of patients dead in the control group in the same interval. For the same proportional reduction in mortality, the absolute difference in survival varies greatly and is generally larger for groups of patients with a higher risk of dying (e.g., node-positive versus node-negative patients). To calculate the proportional increase in survival, the absolute difference between the control and experimental curves in a specified interval is divided by the total surviving in the experimental group (assuming that it is larger). For groups with poor survival, small absolute differences lead to larger estimates of the percent increase in survival.

Modern Concept of Breast Cancer Classification: Molecular Markers

Before discovery of the ER, all breast cancers were considered potentially sensitive to endocrine therapy. Gradually, clinical trials and laboratory research established that only cancers containing ER (ER-positive cancers) respond to endocrine treatments, either additive or ablative. In 1985, a second important growth factor receptor was discovered, the HER-2 or erb-B2/neu protein. This protein is the product of the *erb-B2* gene and is amplified in about 20% of human breast cancers. The extracellular domain of the receptor is present on the surface of breast cancer cells, and an intracellular tyrosine kinase enzyme links the receptor to the internal machinery of the cell. There are three binding partners of the HER-2 protein,

including HER-1, or the epidermal growth factor receptor (EGFR), HER-3, and HER-4. The tyrosine kinase of HER-2 is activated by growth factors binding to these partners and cross-stimulating the HER-2 kinase. Amplification leads to protein overexpression, generally measured clinically by immunohistochemistry and scored on a scale from 0 to 3+. Alternatively, fluorescent in situ hybridization (FISH) directly detects the quantity of HER-2 gene copies, with the normal copy number being two. Research showed that inhibition of the function of the HER-2 receptor–like protein slowed the growth of HER-2–amplified tumors both in laboratory models and in clinical trials. Trastuzumab is a humanized antibody directed against the extracellular domain of the surface receptor and is effective treatment of HER-positive breast cancer (see later).[39,40]

A logical classification scheme for invasive breast cancer is based on expression of ER status and HER-2 proteins and has the advantage of directing treatment choices. ER-positive tumors receive endocrine therapies and HER-2–positive cancers are treated with inhibitors of HER-2. However, breast cancer is a heterogeneous disease, and different breast cancers behave in very different ways. For instance, some ER-positive tumors are indolent and not terribly life threatening, whereas other ER-positive tumors are very aggressive cancers. In an attempt to further subclassify the disease, investigators are turning to global assessment of gene expression by using microarrays composed of oligonucleotide probes to virtually every known expressed sequence of DNA in the human genome. Similar technologies based on single-nucleotide polymorphisms (SNPs) in the cancer DNA and profiles of expressed proteins are being developed for the purpose of subclassifying cancers and directing treatment.

A typical microarray experiment is shown in Figure 34-15, popularly called a *heat map,* where colors indicate levels of gene expression. Such portrayal of the disease

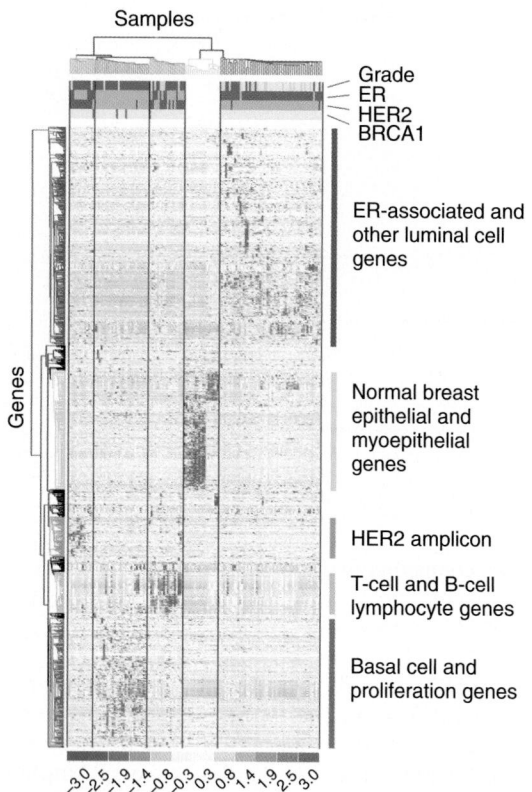

Samples

Grade
ER
HER2
BRCA1

ER-associated and
other luminal cell
genes

Genes

Normal breast
epithelial and
myoepithelial
genes

HER2 amplicon

T-cell and B-cell
lymphocyte genes

Basal cell and
proliferation genes

-3.0 -2.5 -1.9 -1.4 -0.8 -0.3 0.3 0.8 1.4 1.9 2.5 3.0

Figure 34-15 Microarray representation of human breast cancer. This portrayal of global gene expression is called a *heat map,* with shades of red indicating high gene expression and shades of blue indicating low gene expression relative to a mean across tissue samples. Tissue samples are present across the top in columns and individual genes in rows down the side; the intersection is an individual gene in a particular sample. A computer clustering algorithm aligns samples with similar gene expression and genes with similar expression patterns in the samples (two-way clustering). This illustration provides an unbiased look at breast cancer according to gene expression. The dendrogram at the top depicts the degree of similarity of the tissue samples: yellow, normal breast epithelium; blue, predominantly estrogen receptor (ER)-positive cancers; red, basal-like or triple-negative cancers; and green, HER-2–positive cancers (in two clusters defined by the degree of lymphocytic infiltrate). The *stripes* at the top indicate grade (shades of darker purple are higher grades), ER expression (purple is positive; green is negative), and HER-2 (purple is positive; green is negative). *BRCA1* mutation was determined for other reasons in this experiment. (Provided by Andrea Richardson, MD, PhD, Department of Pathology, Brigham and Women's Hospital.)

shows how different ER-positive is from ER-negative cancer and underscores the modern concept that subclassification needs to not only define different groups of breast cancer but also guide treatment. In Figure 34-15, HER-2–positive tumors form two clusters (in green at the top), although these clusters are fused together in many depictions. HER-2–positive tumors cluster similarly and are responsive to inhibitors of the HER-2 tyrosine kinase–linked surface receptor (e.g., trastuzumab). An unexpected finding, emphasized recently, is the uniqueness of tumors that are both ER negative and HER-2 negative. These cancers, also negative for PR, are called *triple-negative* cancers. They express proteins in common with myoepithelial cells at the base of mammary ducts and are also called *basal-like* cancers. Because they do not express either ER or HER-2, new treatments are required. Several early-phase clinical trials have begun to target the basal-like breast cancer with new approaches and drugs. Interestingly, women who carry a disease-associated mutation in *BRCA1* (but not *BRCA2*) are much more likely to contract a basal-like cancer than other subtypes. In summary, categorizing breast cancer according to the expression of molecular targets of treatments is practical and appears to agree with nonbiased classifications based on gene expression. Classification schemes reflect biology and predict treatment efficacy. The classification scheme proposed in Table 34-13 lists treatment strategies currently being used for these biologically different diseases.

In addition to classification, molecular markers are used to select patients for systemic treatment (chemotherapy or endocrine therapy) and to predict the response of patients to these drug treatments. The simplest example is the use of ER or HER-2 status to predict the response to endocrine treatment or trastuzumab. Multiple gene products may be used in combination for these determinations. Microarray experiments use thousands of gene transcripts (mRNAs) to provide a snapshot of an individual cancer's molecular phenotype. To adapt this technology for clinical application, investigators have selected critical assemblies of gene products that provide the same predictive ability as a nonbiased, genome-wide analysis. The most advanced is a 21-gene test that can be used on paraffin-embedded tumor material from breast surgical specimens. Originally designed to predict the recurrence of ER-positive, node-negative breast cancer treated with adjuvant endocrine therapy, the 21-gene test provides a recurrence score for ER-positive breast cancer that is used clinically to guide whether women with high-risk ER-

Table 34-13   Breast Cancer Classification Based on Molecular Markers

MARKER CATEGORY	DESIGNATION	TREATMENT (STANDARD TREATMENT PLUS . . .)
ER positive/HER-2 negative	ER positive*	Endocrine treatment
ER positive/HER-2 positive	HER-2 positive	HER-2–directed treatment (e.g., trastuzumab); endocrine treatment for ER-positive cancers
ER negative/HER-2 positive		
ER negative/HER-2 negative	Basal-like	Unknown

*Histologic grade subdivides estrogen receptor (ER)-positive tumors into high-grade ER-positive and low-grade ER-positive cancers.

positive breast cancer should receive adjuvant chemotherapy in addition to tamoxifen (an endocrine therapy, see later). It is likely that tests based on critical combinations of genes will increasingly be used to assist clinical decision making in treating breast cancer.

Adjuvant Chemotherapy for Operable Breast Cancer

The first trials of prolonged postoperative chemotherapy for operable breast cancer were started by the NSABP in 1972 and by the NCI of Italy (NCI-Milan) in 1973. Only patients with positive axillary nodes were chosen for study. NSABP B-05 compared oral L-phenylalanine mustard (L-PAM, melphalan) with placebo in patients undergoing radical mastectomy. The NCI-Milan trial studied a combination of cyclophosphamide, methotrexate, and 5-fluorouracil (CMF) versus no treatment after either radical mastectomy or extended radical mastectomy. The results from these two trials are similar and convincingly positive for women undergoing chemotherapy who are younger than 50 years. In both studies, the magnitude of difference in this subgroup was relatively large and statistically significant. Twenty-year follow-up of the NCI-Milan CMF combination has shown very few complications. Since these two trials, there have been more than 200 prospective randomized trials of chemotherapy given before or after curative operations for breast cancer in patients who are younger or older than 50 years and in node-positive and node-negative women.[41]

Meta-analysis of Adjuvant Chemotherapy for Breast Cancer

Surgical treatment of breast cancer can eradicate disease that is found in the breast or regional lymph nodes. However, deposits of undetected breast cancer may already be present either on the chest wall near the breast or at sites elsewhere in the body. Adjuvant chemotherapy refers to the administration of generally cytotoxic drugs to women after surgical eradication of breast cancer in the hope of eliminating distant deposits of disease that cannot be detected clinically in a patient seemingly disease free. Substantial improvements in recurrence and survival have been attributed to adjuvant chemotherapy in virtually all categories of women with invasive breast cancer. This brief overview will summarize an international collaboration that collected data from high-quality randomized clinical trials opened before 1995 and including women randomized before 2000. There were 33,000 women who participated in more than 100 clinical trials worldwide. Results are published on a 5-year cycle and were last summarized in 2005. Because this consortium was started in 1985, 15-year follow-up is available from many clinical trials completed in the early 1990s.[42]

Strategies tested in this overview include no chemotherapy (the control group), single-agent chemotherapy, polychemotherapy, and polychemotherapy containing an anthracycline (doxorubicin or epirubicin). The overview analysis also looked at shorter (<6 months) or longer (>6 months) durations of chemotherapy. The most popular combinations were CMF and FAC (5-fluorouracil, Adriamycin [doxorubicin], and cyclophosphamide). In the United States, a combination of Adriamycin (doxorubicin) and cyclophosphamide (AC) or AC plus a taxane (docetaxel, paclitaxel) are likely to be used as polychemotherapy; single-agent treatment is rarely used in adjuvant therapy. These trials were conducted before the widespread use of taxanes and hence do not report the results of adding taxanes to polychemotherapy regimens. In addition, trials using trastuzumab for patients with HER-2–positive breast cancer were not reported. For HER-2–positive breast cancer, adding trastuzumab to polychemotherapy is approved for use as a surgical adjuvant.

Overall, treatment of women with an anthracycline-based chemotherapy combination reduces the estimated breast cancer death rate by about 38% (±5%) when used in women younger than 50 years and by 31% (±3%) when used after surgery in women between 50 and 69 years of age. This proportional reduction is seen in virtually all subtypes of breast cancer based on node status, ER status, and characteristics of the tumor. Anthracycline-containing combinations were significantly better than no treatment, single-agent treatment, or CMF. Figure 34-16 shows the probability of recurrence in patients receiving chemotherapy combinations that include any two agents used together; results using anthracycline-based combinations would produce slightly better outcomes. The figure includes women younger than 50 or between 50 and 69 years of age, both axillary node negative and node positive. Table 34-14 shows the observed versus expected recurrence rates and the calculated proportional reduction in recurrence provided by treatment in several subgroups of patients (stratified by age) and tumor characteristics.

The principle of a constant proportional reduction in recurrence rates with treatment is useful, and it helps patients and physicians make decisions about adjuvant treatment. If the odds of recurrence are high, a proportional reduction of 30% to 40% is very significant (e.g., reducing a recurrence rate of 50%-30% or 35%). These absolute gains far exceed the risks assumed by treatment, which may include bone marrow suppression, infection, cardiac toxicity, and neurotoxicity. Serious and life-threatening complications of modern adjuvant chemotherapy are very rare. In contrast, if the risk for recurrence is 10%, the absolute benefit is only 3% or 4%. In this case, the risks and perceived side effects of chemotherapy may exceed its benefits, and the patient or her doctor may decide against treatment. This is particularly an issue in patients whose breast cancer is lymph node negative. In patients with node-negative cancer, certain groups may suffer higher relapse rates, and the absolute benefits of chemotherapy are greater. Poor prognostic signs follow:

1. Tumor size >2 cm
2. Poor histologic and nuclear grade
3. Absent hormone receptors
4. High proliferative fraction (S phase)
5. Content of certain oncogenes such as *erb-B2 (HER-2/neu)*

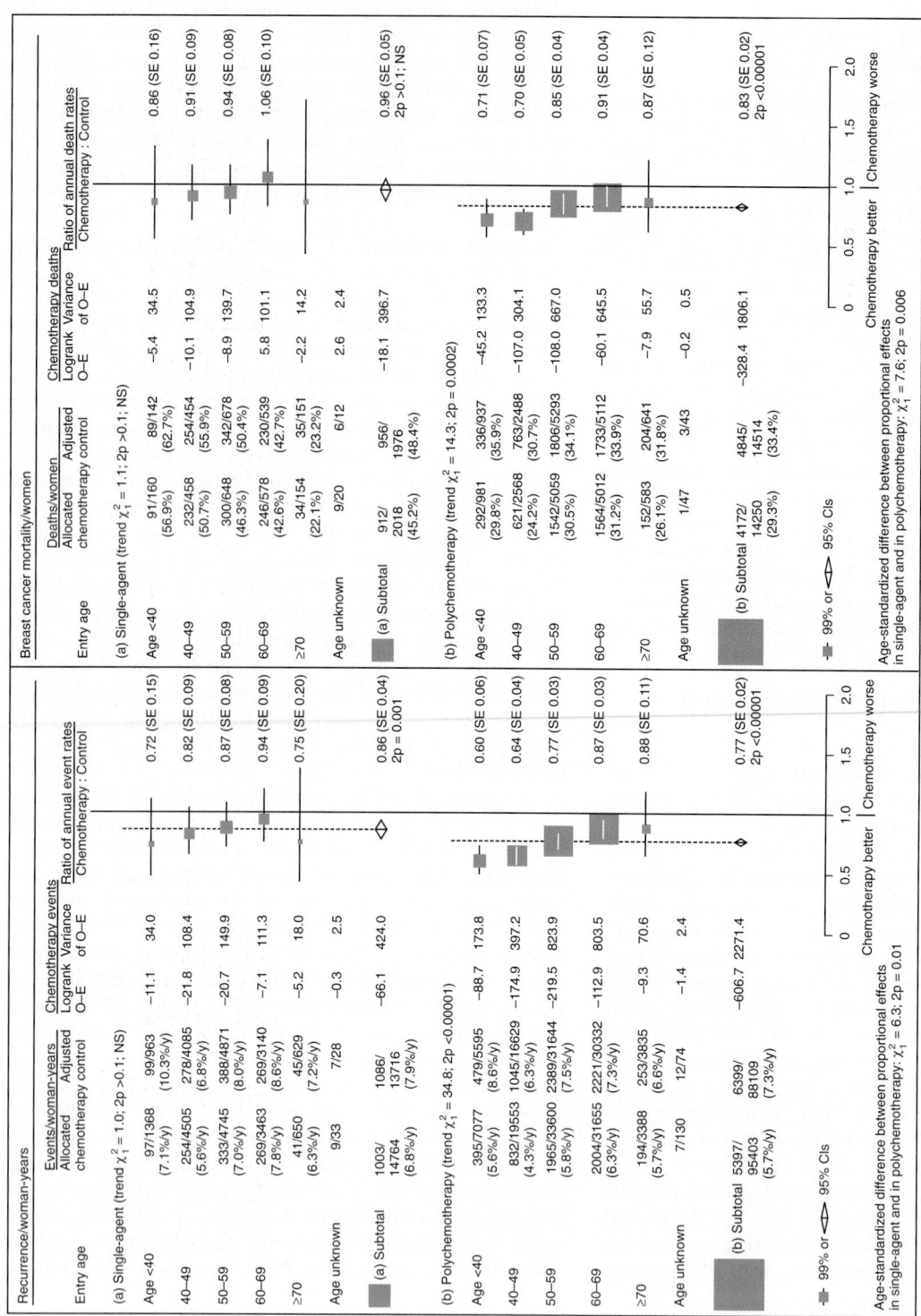

Figure 34-16 Risk reductions in the international overview of adjuvant chemotherapy after surgery for operable breast cancer. In this figure, the results of adjuvant polychemotherapy are presented at 5 years but persist at 15 years of follow-up. Polychemotherapy generally consisted of either cyclophosphamide, methotrexate, and 5-fluorouracil (CMF) or combinations based on an anthracycline (e.g., doxorubicin). All patients were treated by adequate local treatment (surgery, radiation therapy, or both) and were randomized to receive postoperative adjuvant chemotherapy or no postoperative treatment (control in this figure). The four panels show the results in younger patients (top two panels) and are divided into lymph node–positive and node-negative women. The bottom two panels show results for women between 50 and 69 years of age, again divided by node status. The biggest reduction in the odds of recurrence were seen in younger women treated with chemotherapy; node-negative women 50 years of age and older received the smallest proportion benefit. O–E number of observed events–number of expected events. (From Early Breast Cancer Trialists' Collaborative Group: Effects of chemotherapy and hormonal therapy for early breast cancer on recurrence and 15-year survival: An overview of the randomised trials. Lancet 365:1687-1717, 2005.)

Table 34-14   **Cancer Recurrence After No Treatment or Polychemotherapy Adjuvant Treatment***

PATIENT OR TUMOR CHARACTERISTICS	RECURRENCE RATE (%)		PROPORTIONAL REDUCTION IN RECURRENCE (%)
	No Treatment	Polychemotherapy	
Node Status and Age			
Node positive, age <50	55.2	40.6	26.4
Node positive, age 50-69	42.6	36.7	13.5
Node negative, age <50	27.4	17.5	36
Node negative, age 50-69	19.6	14.3	27
ER Status and Age			
ER poor, age <50	38.8	25.5	34.2
ER poor, age 50-69	42.9	33.3	22.3
ER positive, age <50[†]	21.6	14.0	35.2
ER positive, age 50-69[†]	28.9	24.0	17

*Five-year data from the Early Breast Cancer Trialists' Collaborative Group (EBCTCG): Effects of chemotherapy and hormonal therapy for early breast cancer on recurrence and 15-year survival: An overview of the randomised trials. Lancet 365:1687-1717, 2005.
[†]Estrogen receptor (ER)-positive patients received tamoxifen, and the comparison is between tamoxifen alone versus polychemotherapy plus tamoxifen.

Newer Approaches in Chemotherapy for Breast Cancer

Dose Intensity

Dose intensity is defined as the amount of drug given over an interval of time (milligrams of delivered dose per meter squared per unit of time); more intense regimens give a higher dose in a shorter interval than less intense regimens do. The hypothesis that dose intensity is an important determinant of response has been tested in national cooperative trials. The first was a randomized trial of different dose levels of chemotherapy given to women with node-positive (stage II) breast cancer after curative surgery (mastectomy or conservation with radiation therapy). Three arms in this study received escalating dose intensity (by varying both the duration and total dose) of chemotherapy. Women given either high- or moderate-dose intense chemotherapy had a significantly longer disease-free and a better overall survival rate than did the low-dose (and low-intensity) arm. Subsequent studies of further increasing doses of cyclophosphamide (NSABP B-22 and B-25) or doxorubicin (CALGB 9344) have not shown additional benefit in patients with node-positive breast cancer. There may be an optimal dose intensity that must be reached for a given drug but exceeding that level does not add benefit.[43]

The benefit of very-high-dose chemotherapy was addressed in the CALGB 9082 trial. In this study, women with 10 or more positive lymph nodes received standard doxorubicin-based chemotherapy followed by randomization to high-dose chemotherapy with bone marrow transplantation versus moderate-dose chemotherapy. To date, this trial shows a modest disease-free survival advantage, but no overall survival advantage, with high-dose therapy. Even though these results may improve with time, data from other randomized trials currently do not support the use of high-dose chemotherapy given with infusions of hematopoietic cells.

The concept of dose density has been tested in recent clinical trials. The U.S. Intergroup tested dose-dense versus conventionally scheduled combination chemotherapy in women with positive axillary lymph nodes as an adjuvant to surgery. In this study, patients were randomly assigned to multiple schedules of three chemotherapy drugs (doxorubicin, cyclophosphamide, and paclitaxel). Although it was a complicated study, the women receiving compressed schedules of the three drugs at higher doses were better off during follow-up than their counterparts who received so-called less dense treatment (disease-free survival rate at 4 years of 82% for the dose-dense group versus 75% for the other groups). In practice, the duration of adjuvant treatment for breast cancer may be shortened to even less than the usual 4 to 6 months.

New Agents

Trastuzumab (Herceptin) is a humanized murine monoclonal antibody raised against the erb-B2 or HER-2 surface receptor. Cancers with high-level expression (3+ by immunohistochemistry) or amplification by FISH may respond to trastuzumab. Three recent studies have evaluated the addition of trastuzumab to conventional chemotherapy in women with operable breast cancer (as a surgical adjuvant) and in women with metastatic disease that is HER-2 positive. The outcomes of each study are remarkably similar and show about a 50% reduction in either recurrence (for adjuvant treatment) or time to progression (for trials in metastatic disease). A number of small-molecule inhibitors of tyrosine kinase enzyme activity linked to either or both erb-B1 (EGFR) and erb-B2 (HER-2) are entering clinical trials. Agents that specifically target EGFR include erlotinib and gefitinib and the monoclonal antibody cetuximab. These drugs have found most use in non–small cell lung, pancreatic, and colorectal cancer. Because breast cancer does not harbor EGFR amplification or mutation, it is generally less responsive to EGFR-directed treatment. However, dual inhibitors of both EGFR and HER-2 have been developed and are finding their way into the treatment of breast cancer (e.g., lapatinib, a dual inhibitor of both enzymes).[44,45]

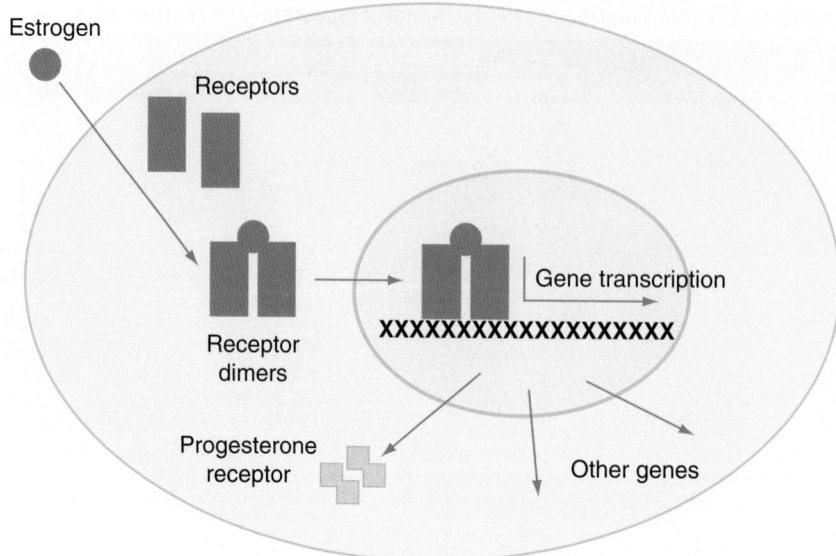

Figure 34-17 Physiology of estrogen and the estrogen receptor, shown schematically. Estrogen binds to estrogen receptors, either in the cytoplasm or in the nucleus, and the ligand-activated receptor interacts with promoter elements in target genes. This interaction results in gene transcription of estrogen response genes, such as the progesterone receptor. Other genes induced directly or indirectly by the estrogen receptor influence cell growth and differentiation.

Hormonal Therapy for Breast Cancer

The effect of steroid hormones and inhibitors on sensitive tissues is the basis for effective treatment of breast cancer. Beatson, a surgeon at the Glasgow Cancer Hospital, was the first to demonstrate that bilateral oophorectomy can lead to regression of metastatic breast cancer. Surgically induced menopause became the first effective means of controlling advanced breast cancer; it produced a beneficial regression in 25% to 40% of premenopausal patients. Huggins re-emphasized oophorectomy and demonstrated the effectiveness of adrenalectomy in the treatment of postmenopausal metastatic breast cancer patients. Endocrine organ ablation has been replaced by antiestrogen therapy in most patients. The drug tamoxifen is an estrogen agonist-antagonist and currently the first-line treatment of estrogen-sensitive breast cancer. However, there has been a renaissance in the development and use of hormonally active drugs; many new agents and treatment approaches will be tested in the coming years.[42]

Steroid Hormone Receptors

Reproductive and certain other sensitive tissues possess high-affinity protein receptors for estrogen and progesterone (ER and PR). Specific receptors for both hormones may be present in tumor tissue of mammary origin. These receptor proteins are activated when occupied by their specific hormone ligand. Activation of ER leads to the induction of numerous cellular genes, including those that may encode critical enzymes and secreted peptide growth factors (Fig. 34-17). Clinically, the most important protein induced by ER is the receptor for progesterone. Therefore, PR may serve as an indicator for the presence of a functional ER, which may explain why PR-positive

Table 34-15 Distribution of Steroid Receptors in Tumor Biopsy Specimens According to Patient Endocrine Status*

RECEPTOR STATUS OF TUMOR BIOPSY SPECIMEN	ENDOCRINE STATUS OF PATIENT	
	Premenopausal (%)	Postmenopausal (%)
ER⁺, PR⁺	222 (45)	520 (63)
ER⁺, PR⁻	58 (12)	128 (15)
ER⁻, PR⁻	136 (28)	137 (17)
ER⁻, PR⁺	72 (15)	41 (5)
Total	488 (44)	826 (44)

*Fifty-five years of age was chosen as an age at which virtually every woman may be considered postmenopausal.

ER, estrogen receptor; PR, progesterone receptor.

From Wittlift JL: Steroid hormone receptors in breast cancer. Cancer 53(Suppl):630-643, 1984.

breast cancers display intermediate responsiveness to hormonal treatments, even if the measured value of ER is very low or zero. Newer assay formats for ER and PR are based on immunohistochemistry and detection of the receptors by antibodies. These slide-based assays may be done on either frozen or paraffin-embedded tumor sections. In general, if greater than 10% of tumor cells stain positive for the nuclear receptor, the assay is reported as positive and a response to hormonal treatment is likely. About 60% of human breast tumors contain detectable amounts of either ER or PR or both, and the likelihood that a patient's tumor is hormone sensitive increases with advancing age at diagnosis, as shown in Table 34-15. Male breast cancer is almost always ER positive.[2,41]

The presence of ER predicts clinical response to all types of endocrine therapy, both additive and ablative. Furthermore, because progesterone expression is induced by binding of estrogen to its receptor, the presence of progesterone correlates with response to endocrine therapy. The presence of both receptors in a tumor is associated with almost an 80% chance of favorably responding to hormone addition or blockade (Table 34-16).

Hormonal Agents for Breast Cancer

Targeting the estrogen/ER pathway is both selective for breast cancer cells that express ER and relatively nontoxic (when compared with many cytotoxic agents). Novel drugs developed in the past 3 decades target the production of estrogen, its interaction with ER, and the receptor itself. These drugs fall into several classes, and each class of compound or mechanism of action has several competing new agents available for clinical use. Some of these agents and their clinical use are summarized in Table 34-17.[46,47]

The SERMs are exemplified by tamoxifen. Tamoxifen is a weak estrogen agonist. In molar excess, tamoxifen acts like a competitive antagonist of estrogen activity in the breast but not in other estrogen-sensitive tissues. Both the beneficial and unfavorable actions of tamoxifen in tissues other than the breast are due to its estrogen-like actions. Tamoxifen can replace oophorectomy in premenopausal women with ER-positive metastatic cancer, and it is considered the drug of first choice in both premenopausal and postmenopausal patients with ER-positive breast cancer. As noted in Table 34-16, response rates in metastatic disease are high when the tumor is ER or PR positive and decrease to 10% or less for receptor-negative tumors. Newer SERMS are listed in Table 34-17. The ideal SERM blocks the ER in breast cancer tissue, is neutral or inhibitory in the endometrium, lacks the procoagulant activity of estrogen and tamoxifen, and acts like estrogen in the skeletal, cardiovascular, and central nervous systems.

Aromatase inhibitors block the conversion of androstenedione to estrone, the last step in conversion of steroid to active hormones. The first inhibitor and prototype of this class is aminoglutethimide. However, this compound inhibits upstream enzymes and interferes with the synthesis of cortisone. Selective aromatase inhibitors (SAIs) were developed that inhibit only the last enzymatic step in the formation of estrone. SAIs include nonsteroidal compounds that are reversible inhibitors (letrozole and anastrozole) and steroid-based compounds that are irreversible (suicide) inhibitors (exemestane and formestane) of aromatase. The SAI group of drugs is used in postmenopausal women and completely suppresses the production of estrogen from extragonadal, nonovarian peripheral sites (principally in adipose tissue). In premenopausal women, SAIs cause reflex pituitary release of gonadotropins, the development of polycystic ovaries, and excessive androgen production. However, these drugs may find application in premenopausal patients when combined with luteinizing hormone–releasing hormone agonists (LHRH-As) (see later).

As noted earlier, the SERMs are agents with both agonist and antagonist activity. Pure antiestrogens have been developed. The first of these agents in clinical use is fulvestrant, a steroid that binds with high affinity to the ER and blocks ER dimerization and DNA binding; it also leads to rapid degradation of the receptor protein. This

Table 34-16 Relationship Between Steroid Receptor Status of Breast Tumor and Patients' Objective Response to Endocrine Therapy

STEROID RECEPTOR STATUS*			
ER⁺, PR⁺	ER⁺, PR⁻	ER⁻, PR⁻	ER⁻, PR⁺
137/174	55/164	17/165	5/11
(79%)	(34%)	(10%)	(45%)

*Number of patients responding to treatment/number of women with receptor status designated.

Based on a collective paper presented at the National Institutes of Health (NIH) Consensus Development Conference on Steroid Receptors in Breast Cancer (Proceedings of the NIH Consensus Development Conference, 1980).

ER, estrogen receptor; PR, progesterone receptor.

From Donegan WL, Spratt JS (eds): Cancer of the Breast. Philadelphia, WB Saunders, 1988.

Table 34-17 Endocrine-Active Agents Used in the Treatment of Breast Cancer

CLASS	COMMON EXAMPLES	CLINICAL USE
Selective estrogen receptor modulators (SERMS)	Tamoxifen, raloxifene, toremifene	Adjuvant therapy for metastatic disease
Aromatase inhibitors (AIs)	Anastrozole, letrozole, exemestane	Adjuvant therapy for metastatic disease
Pure antiestrogens	Fulvestrant	Second-line therapy for metastatic disease
Luteinizing hormone–releasing hormone (LHRH) agonists	Goserelin, leuprolide	Adjuvant therapy* for metastatic disease
Progestational agents	Megestrol	Second-line agent for metastatic disease
Androgens	Fluoxymesterone	Third-line agent for metastatic disease
High-dose estrogens	Diethylstilbestrol	Third-line agent for metastatic disease

*Selectively used as an adjuvant in premenopausal women with estrogen receptor–positive disease.

Table 34-18 Recommendations for Adjuvant Treatment of Operable Breast Cancer, Stratified by Patient Categories and by Risk for Recurrence

PATIENT CATEGORY	TREATMENT STRATIFIED BY RISK PROFILE		
	Low	Intermediate	High
Premenopausal, receptor positive*	± Hormone†	Hormone ± chemotherapy	Chemotherapy + hormone
Premenopausal, receptor negative	No recommendations	Chemotherapy	Chemotherapy
Postmenopausal, receptor positive	± Hormone	Hormone	Chemotherapy + hormone
Postmenopausal, receptor negative	± Chemotherapy	± Chemotherapy	Chemotherapy
Elderly with comorbid conditions	± Hormone	± Hormone	± Hormone

Risk definitions—Low risk: T ≤1 cm, ER or PR positive, age ≥35 (has all factors); intermediate risk: T = 1 to 2 cm, ER or PR positive, grade 1 to 2 (has all factors); high risk: T ≥2 cm, ER and PR negative, grade 2 to 3, age ≤35 (has at least one factor).
*Either estrogen receptor (ER) or progesterone receptor (PR) positive.
†Hormone generally refers to tamoxifen for 5 years. In postmenopausal women, use of an aromatase inhibitor in place of tamoxifen, or sequentially, is suggested by some.
Adapted from multiple sources.

compound has reached phase III testing in postmenopausal women with ER-negative metastatic breast cancer whose disease has progressed after tamoxifen treatment. Fulvestrant is probably as effective as the SAI group of drugs in these women. This compound is given as a single intramuscular injection every month, thus making it a convenient agent to use.

Though not new, estrogen levels can be reduced in premenopausal women with functioning ovaries by the use of LHRH-As. The LHRH-As are superagonists that cause early, massive release of pituitary gonadotropins, followed by paralysis of the pituitary and resistance to normal LHRH. Gonadotropin levels fall and result in rapidly declining estrogen levels and suppression of ovarian hormonal function. LHRH-As are peptide analogues of the normal releasing hormone and are 50 to 100 times as potent. Two are in clinical use for the treatment of breast cancer (goserelin and leuprolide). Included in Table 34-17 are progestational agents (PR agonists), androgens, and high-dose estrogens, all of which are used clinically and thus emphasize the complexity of endocrine therapy.

Adjuvant Hormonal Therapy for Operable Breast Cancer

Early trials of endocrine manipulation after breast cancer surgery involved the use of ovarian irradiation or surgical oophorectomy. The first modern trial of adjuvant tamoxifen was begun in 1975 and followed by two others in 1977 (the NATO trial) and 1978 (the Scottish trial). These early experiments randomized women after surgery for breast cancer and included all patients regardless of their ER status. In fact, only about half the tumors from patients in these trials were assayed for ER content.

However, both trials were positive and demonstrated a reduction in both recurrence and fatality rates in the tamoxifen-treated patients. For instance, the Scottish trial demonstrated a reduction in recurrence rates from 38% to 24% (proportional reduction of 37%, similar in magnitude to the reduction after chemotherapy) and survival rates from 23% in the control arm to 18% in the tamoxifen-treated arm. These findings have been con-

firmed in more than 20 trials in which a tamoxifen treatment arm was compared with a no-treatment control, and they were combined into a large meta-analysis by the EBCTCG. By the 1980s, routine determination of ER status was common, and later trials showed that all benefit from endocrine treatment occurs in women with ER-positive disease; in ER-negative disease, there is no benefit from receiving tamoxifen or other hormonal treatments (with the possible exception of PR-positive but ER-poor tumors).

Meta-analysis of Adjuvant Tamoxifen for Breast Cancer

More than 60 randomized trials compared 1 to 2 years of tamoxifen with no treatment, 5 years with no treatment, or shorter versus longer treatment. All recent trials were conducted in women with ER-positive breast cancer. The results are strikingly positive, and all groups of women with ER-positive tumors benefited with tamoxifen. Five years of treatment was better than 1 to 2 years. Remarkably, these proportional reductions were largely unaffected by age, menopausal status, nodal status, or concomitant treatment. The only significant predictor was ER status, which clearly showed that benefit from tamoxifen was limited to patients with ER-positive tumors. In women with ER-positive breast cancer, 5 years of tamoxifen after surgical treatment nearly halved their recurrence rate and reduced breast cancer mortality by a third (Fig. 34-18). For premenopausal women with ER-positive disease, the combination of sequential anthracycline-based chemotherapy and tamoxifen administration was estimated to reduce overall mortality by nearly 50% in the overview analysis of trials in this group.[42,47]

Adjuvant Ovarian Suppression or Ablation

Ovarian ablation refers to the removal of both ovaries by surgery or the obliteration of ovarian endocrine function by external radiation. Ovarian suppression is accomplished with LHRH-As. As with tamoxifen, both ablation and suppression are effective only in women with ER-positive breast cancer. The ovaries produce estrogen only between puberty and menopause, and ovarian ablation or suppression is effective solely in premenopausal

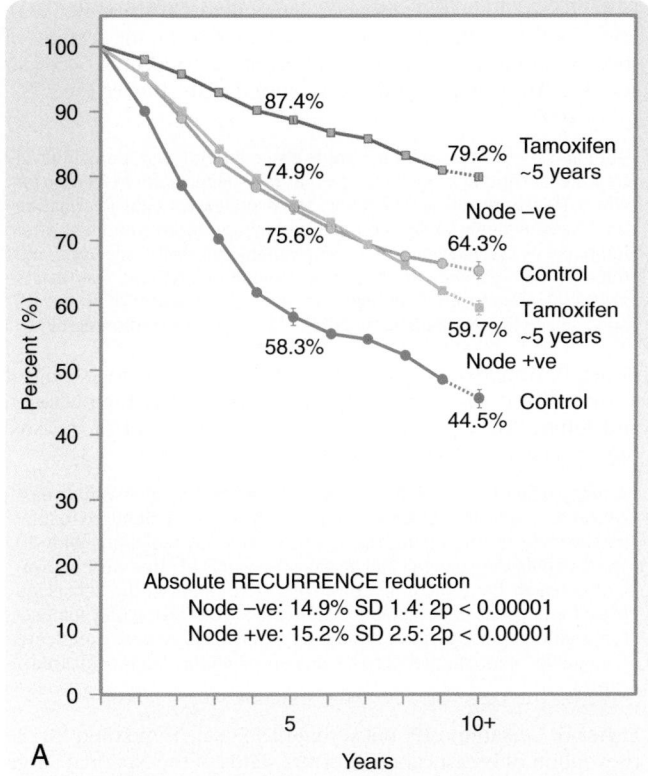

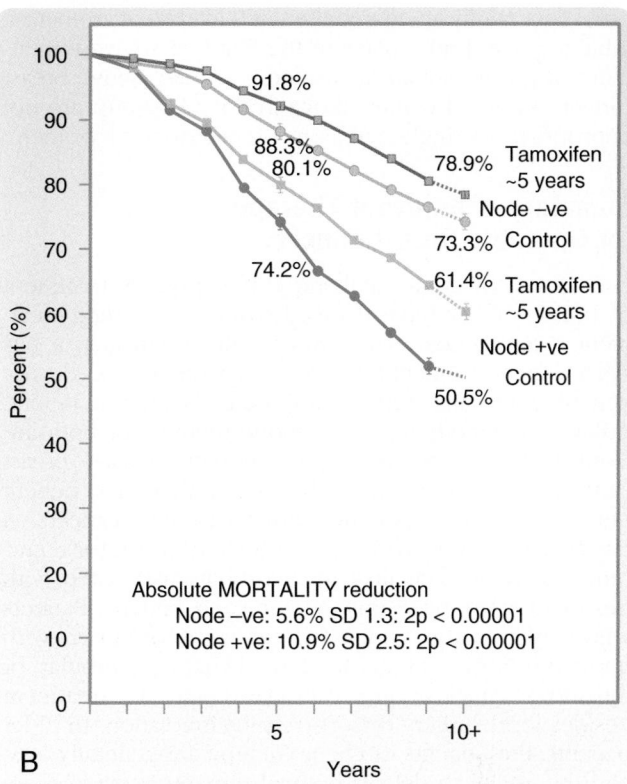

Figure 34-18 Results of the international overview of randomized trials comparing tamoxifen-treated patients with control subjects after either mastectomy or breast-conserving surgery for operable breast cancer. The figure divides randomized patients according to the content of estrogen receptor (ER) in their breast tumor, either ER positive or ER poor, and shows results for 1 to 2 years of treatment *(top)* and for 5 years of treatment *(bottom)*. In **A,** the results are for recurrence, and in **B,** the results are for breast cancer mortality. The position of the *squares* relative to the center line represents the ratio of events (recurrence and mortality) for tamoxifen-treated versus control groups. The lines through the *boxes* represent 95% confidence limits, and the area of each *square* represents the amount of information available for each comparison. In patients with ER-positive but not ER-negative cancer, tamoxifen decreased both recurrence and mortality (annual event rates in the figure). Five years of tamoxifen was superior to treatments for lesser periods. (From Effects of chemotherapy and hormonal therapy for early breast cancer on recurrence and 15-year survival: An overview of the randomised trials. Early Breast Cancer Trialists' Collaborative Group [EBCTCG]. Lancet 365:1687-1717, 2005.)

women. The overview by the EBCTCG found significant effects of both suppression and ablation on recurrence and mortality in premenopausal women. However, in the modern environment of many competing and effective systemic treatments, the magnitude of the effect was not greater than that with tamoxifen. Many medical oncologists reserve ovarian suppression and occasionally surgical oophorectomy for young women with ER-positive cancer, positive axillary nodes, or large primary tumors.[42]

Aromatase Inhibitors as Adjuvant Therapy

Several clinical trials are introducing SAIs into adjuvant therapy and comparing these agents with tamoxifen, the current standard for adjuvant therapy for ER-positive breast cancer after local treatment. One of the oldest and largest trials directly compared 5 years of tamoxifen with 5 years of the SAI anastrozole and added a third arm that combined tamoxifen with anastrozole. The so-called ATAC trial is a large, multinational, prospective, double-blinded study that accrued 9366 women from 381 centers in 21 countries. Postmenopausal women with invasive breast cancer were eligible after surgical treatment or after completion of chemotherapy. Women with ER-positive, ER-negative, or unknown receptor status were eligible, and these subsets were analyzed individually after unmasking the randomization and analyzing the results.[46,48,49]

Results at 4 years of follow-up in the ATAC trial favor the use of anastrozole over either tamoxifen or the combination of anastrozole and tamoxifen. Disease-free survival and time to recurrence were prolonged with the use of anastrozole as a single agent, with a 14% reduction in the risk for recurrence and a small absolute benefit of 2.4%. However, the benefits were larger in women with ER-positive breast cancers, and there was no difference among the three treatment arms for women with ER-negative breast cancer, as expected. At least six trials have opened with various strategies; all are comparing aromatase inhibitors with tamoxifen or adding aromatase inhibitors sequentially after tamoxifen. It is likely that aromatase inhibitors will find a place in the first-line adjuvant treatment of postmenopausal women with ER-positive breast cancer. As noted earlier, drugs in the SAI group are not appropriate as single agents in premenopausal women.

Summary of Adjuvant Therapy for Operable Breast Cancer

Guidelines for adjuvant therapy after primary treatment of breast cancer have evolved toward extending treatment recommendations to more patients. In fact, it has been difficult to identify a group of women who do not benefit from some form of adjuvant systemic treatment. Adjuvant chemotherapy, endocrine therapy, or both are likely to benefit nearly all patients with invasive breast cancer, although adjuvant hormonal therapies benefit only breast cancer patients with ER-positive cancers. A risk-benefit ratio in which the reduction in risk for recurrence is weighed against the morbidity associated with treatment must be estimated for each patient. Patients with very favorable tumors (≤1 cm in size or tumors with good histology and up to 2 or 3 cm, e.g., tubular or mucinous cancers) are candidates for no treatment besides local surgery or surgery plus irradiation. In older patients, the benefits of chemotherapy are generally less, and the ability to deliver optimal therapy is made more difficult by the presence of other impairments. In elderly patients, the decision to administer adjuvant chemotherapy is made on an individual basis.[50]

Adjuvant tamoxifen is recommended for ER-positive or PR-positive cancers, and treatment is continued for 5 years. Though remarkably free of toxicity, a slightly increased incidence of endometrial cancer and venous thrombosis are the major complications of tamoxifen. Therapy for more than 5 years or doses larger than 20 mg/day are not recommended. Aromatase inhibitors may play a role in the adjuvant treatment of breast cancer, but tamoxifen probably remains the current standard. These recommendations are summarized in Table 34-18, which has been adapted from consensus panels on the treatment of primary breast cancer. These recommendations change as ongoing trials mature, toxicities improve, and new therapies reach clinical application.

Selected References

Early Breast Cancer Trialists' Collaborative Group (EBCTCG): Effects of chemotherapy and hormonal therapy for early breast cancer on recurrence and 15-year survival: An overview of the randomised trials. Lancet 365:1687-1717, 2005.

> Summarizes the results of 194 randomized trials of adjuvant chemotherapy or hormonal therapy that were initiated before 1995 and includes more than 110,000 participating patients with early-stage breast cancer. The overview focuses on adjuvant chemotherapy and compares regimens containing anthracyclines with the more standard CMF regimens. The analysis also reports results from adjuvant endocrine therapy with a focus on trials comparing tamoxifen and placebo and methods of ovarian suppression. These results form the basis for recommending adjuvant therapy for breast cancer. Because the overview stresses 15-year follow-up, it does not contain information about trastuzumab and aromatase inhibitors.

Early Breast Cancer Trialists' Collaborative Group (EBCTCG): Effects of radiotherapy and of differences in the extent of surgery for early breast cancer on local recurrence and 15-year survival: An overview of the randomised trials. Lancet 366:2087-2106, 2005.

> Summarizes the results of clinical trials comparing variations in local treatment of operable breast cancer that were begun before 1995 and for which 15-year results are available. The overview contains information on 42,000 women randomized to radiotherapy or no treatment after lumpectomy, 23,500 women receiving variable surgical procedures, and 9300 women receiving more surgery versus radiotherapy. The results stress the adverse effect of higher rates of local recurrence on overall survival and the requirement for adequate surgery and radiotherapy.

Fisher B, Anderson S, Bryant J, et al: Twenty-year follow-up of a randomized trial comparing total mastectomy, lumpectomy, and lumpectomy plus irradiation for the treatment of invasive breast cancer. N Engl J Med 347:1233-1241, 2002.

> A prospective three-arm trial of more than 1800 women with breast cancer and clinically negative axillary lymph nodes, randomized to total mastectomy versus lumpectomy with or without radiation. With 20 years of follow-up, overall and disease-free survival rates were equivalent between the three arms. However, local failure in the conserved breast group was unacceptably high in the arm receiving only lumpectomy without postoperative radiation therapy. This 20-year experience is valuable for its comprehensive summary of modern surgery for breast cancer.

Fisher B, Costantino JP, Wickerham DL, et al: Tamoxifen for the prevention of breast cancer: Current status of the National Surgical Adjuvant Breast and Bowel Project P-1 study. J Natl Cancer Inst 97:1652-1662, 2005.

> This paper summarized results of the prospective randomized trial of tamoxifen versus placebo in 13,388 women at increased risk for breast cancer. Use of tamoxifen reduced the incidence of breast cancer by approximately 50%, but in older women, it also added to the risk for endometrial cancer and thromboembolic events. This was the first demonstration of breast cancer prevention through the use of hormonal therapy.

Fisher B, Jeong J-H, Anderson S, et al: Twenty-five-year follow-up of a randomized trial comparing radical mastectomy, total mastectomy, and total mastectomy followed by irradiation. N Engl J Med 347:567-575, 2002.

> This is the 25-year summary of a prospective trial of more than 1079 women with breast cancer and both clinically negative and positive axillary nodes. Node-negative patients were randomized to radical mastectomy, simple mastectomy, or simple mastectomy with axillary radiation therapy. Node-positive patients were randomized to radical mastectomy or to simple mastectomy, leaving the involved nodes, and irradiating the nodes. With 25 years of follow-up, overall and disease-free survival rates were equivalent between node-negative patients randomized to three different treatments and node-positive patients randomized to two treatment arms. Published accounts of NSABP B-04 provide a sound basis for understanding the principles behind the surgical approach to the axillary nodes in patients with breast cancer. B-04 can also be studied for the insight it provides regarding the mechanism and timing of breast cancer metastasis.

Gail MH, Brinton LA, Byar DP, et al: Projecting individualized probabilities of developing breast cancer for white females who are being examined annually. J Natl Cancer Inst 81:1879-1886, 1989.

> The Gail model calculates actuarial estimates of future breast cancer risk based on race, age, reproductive risk factors, maternal family history, and previous breast biopsy status. However, the Gail model may underestimate the risk in those with a strong paternal family history of breast cancer, those with a history of breast and ovarian cancer, and individuals who carry a *BRCA1* or *BRCA2* mutation.

Hartmann LC, Schaid DJ, Woods JE, et al: Efficacy of bilateral prophylactic mastectomy in women with a family history of breast cancer. N Engl J Med 340:77-84, 1999.

In this retrospective study, 639 women with a family history of breast cancer underwent prophylactic mastectomy. Based on family pedigrees, the women were divided into high-risk (n = 214) and moderate-risk (n = 425) groups, with high-risk patients defined as those with a family history suggestive of an autosomal dominant predisposition to breast cancer. For women of moderate risk, the number of expected breast cancers was calculated with the Gail model and yielded an incident risk reduction of 89%. For women in the high-risk cohort, the expected number of breast cancers was calculated with three different statistical models and yielded an incident risk reduction of at least 90%.

Narod SA, Offit K: Prevention and management of hereditary breast cancer. J Clin Oncol 23:1656-1663, 2005.

Mutations in BRCA1 and BRCA2 genes confer a markedly increased risk for breast and ovarian cancer. Patients who carry such risk gene mutations require different breast cancer screening strategies, and the use of preventive agents and prophylactic surgery to lower their risk may be considered. This review covers genetic testing, screening, and prevention in high-risk patients and addresses management of a new breast cancer diagnosis in the setting of a risk gene mutation.

Perou CM, Sorlie T, Eisen MB, et al: Molecular portraits of human breast tumors. Nature 406:747-752, 2000.

This paper has become a classic recent work on the heterogeneity of breast cancer and the use of microarray technology to resolve the genetic diversity of human breast cancer. This work emphasized the group of breast cancers that are both HER2 negative and hormone receptor negative and were deemed basal-like on the basis of their similarity to the myoepithelial cells (basal cells) that line the walls of breast ducts and acini.

Rossouw JE, Anderson GL, Prentice RL, et al: Risks and benefits of estrogen plus progestin in healthy postmenopausal women: Principal results from the Women's Health Initiative randomized controlled trial. JAMA 288:321-333, 2002.
Stefanick ML, Anderson GL, Margolis KL, et al: Effects of conjugated equine estrogens on breast cancer and mammography screening in postmenopausal women with hysterectomy. JAMA 295:1647-1657, 2006.

These prospective, randomized controlled trials from the Women's Health Initiative (WHI) enrolled 16,608 healthy postmenopausal women aged 50 to 79. The study assessed the benefits and risks associated with hormone replacement therapy, a low-fat diet, and calcium and vitamin D supplementation on rates of cancer, cardiovascular disease, and osteoporosis-related fractures. Results from the WHI have influenced thinking about hormone replacement, diet, and vitamin supplements.

References

1. Bennett S, Kaelin CM: Benign breast disease. In Branch WT (ed): Office Practice of Medicine, 4th ed. Philadelphia, WB Saunders, 2003.
2. Donegan WL, Spratt JS: Cancer of the Breast, 5th ed. Philadelphia, WB Saunders, 2002.
3. Haagensen CD: Diseases of the Breast, 3rd ed. Philadelphia, WB Saunders, 1986.
4. Rossouw JE, Anderson GL, Prentice RL, et al: Risks and benefits of estrogen plus progestin in healthy postmenopausal women: Principal results from the Women's Health Initiative randomized controlled trial. JAMA 288:321-333, 2002.
5. Lind DS, Smith BL, Souba WW: 5 Breast Complaints. 2 Breast, Skin, Soft Tissue, and Neck. ACS Surgery Online. In Souba WW, Fink MP, Jurkovich GJ et al (eds): WebMD. New York, 2004.
6. Pisano ED, Gatsonis C, Hendrick E, et al: Digital Mammographic Imaging Screening Trial (DMIST) Investigators Group. Diagnostic performance of digital versus film mammography for breast-cancer screening. N Engl J Med 353:1773-1783, 2005.
7. Silverstein MJ, Lagios MD, Recht A, et al: Image-detected breast cancer: State of the art diagnosis and treatment. J Am Coll Surg 201:586-597, 2005.
8. Hylton N: Magnetic resonance imaging of the breast: Opportunities to improve breast cancer management. J Clin Oncol 23:1678-1684, 2005.
9. Elmore JG, Armstrong K, Lehman CD, Fletcher SW: Screening for breast cancer. JAMA 293:1245-1256, 2005.
10. Berry DA, Cronin KA, Plevritis SK, et al: Effect of screening and adjuvant therapy on mortality from breast cancer. N Engl J Med 353:1784-1792, 2005.
11. Meyer JE, Smith DN, Lester SC, et al: Large-core needle biopsy of nonpalpable breast lesions. JAMA 281:1638-1641, 1999.
12. Darling ML, Smith DN, Lester SC, et al: Atypical ductal hyperplasia and ductal carcinoma in situ as revealed by large-core needle breast biopsy: Results of surgical excision. AJR Am J Roentgenol 175:1341-1346, 2000.
13. Willett WC, Rockhill B, Hankinson SE, et al: Nongenetic factors in the causation of breast cancer. In Harris JR, Lippman ME, Morrow M, Osborne CK (eds): Diseases of the Breast, 3rd ed. Philadelphia, Lippincott Williams & Wilkins, 2004, pp 223-276.
14. Rosen PR: Rosen's Breast Pathology, 2nd ed. Philadelphia, Lippincott Williams & Wilkins, 2001.
15. Hartmann LC, Sellers TA, Frost MH, et al: Benign breast disease and the risk of breast cancer. N Engl J Med 353:229-237, 2005.
16. Domchek S, Weber BL: Inherited genetic factors and breast cancer. In Harris JR, Lippman ME, Morrow M, Osborne CK (eds): Diseases of the Breast, 3rd ed. Philadelphia, Lippincott Williams & Wilkins, 2004, pp 276-313.
17. Stefanick ML, Anderson GL, Margolis KL, et al: Effects of conjugated equine estrogens on breast cancer and mammography screening in postmenopausal women with hysterectomy. JAMA 295:1647-1657, 2006.
18. Powels TJ: Anti-oestrogenic prevention of breast cancer—the make or break point. Nat Rev Cancer 2:787-794, 2002.
19. Hartmann LC, Schaid DJ, Woods JE, et al: Efficacy of bilateral prophylactic mastectomy in women with a family history of breast cancer. N Engl J Med 340:77-84, 1999.
20. Elston CW, Ellis IO: Systemic Pathology: The Breast, 3rd ed. Edinburgh, Churchill Livingstone, 1998.
21. Rosen PR: Rosen's Breast Pathology, 2nd ed. Philadelphia, Lippincott Williams & Wilkins, 2001.
22. Jemal A, Siegel R, Ward E, et al: Cancer statistics, 2006. CA Cancer J Clin 56:106-130, 2006.
23. Fisher B, Jeong JH, Anderson S, et al: Twenty-five-year follow-up of a randomized trial comparing radical mastectomy, total mastectomy, and total mastectomy followed by irradiation. N Engl J Med 347:567-575, 2002.
24. Smith BL, Souba WW: Breast Procedures, American College of Surgeons Surgery: Principles and Practice. In Wilmore DW, Cheung LY (eds): WebMD. New York, 2002, pp 606-619.
25. Lyman GH, Giuliano AE, Somerfield MR, et al: American Society of Clinical Oncology guideline recommendations for sentinel lymph node biopsy in early-stage breast cancer. J Clin Oncol 23:7703-7720, 2005.

26. Naik AM, Fey J, Gemignani M, et al: The risk of axillary relapse after sentinel lymph node biopsy for breast cancer is comparable with that of axillary lymph node dissection: A follow-up study of 4008 procedures. Ann Surg 240:462-468, 2004.

27. Fisher B, Dignam J, Wolmark N, et al: Tamoxifen in treatment of intraductal breast cancer: National Surgical Adjuvant Breast and Bowel Project B-24 randomised controlled trial. Lancet 353:1993-2000, 1999.

28. Fisher B, Dignam J, Wolmark N, et al: Lumpectomy and radiation therapy for the treatment of intraductal breast cancer: Findings from National Surgical Adjuvant Breast and Bowel Project B-17. J Clin Oncol 16:441-452, 1998.

29. Wong JS, Kaelin CM, Troyan SL, et al: A prospective study of wide excision alone for ductal carcinoma in situ (DCIS) of the breast. J Clin Oncol 24:1031-1036, 2006.

30. Silverstein MJ, Lagios MD, Craig PH, et al: A prognostic index for ductal carcinoma in situ of the breast. Cancer 77:2267-2274, 1996.

31. Early Breast Cancer Trialists' Collaborative Group: Favourable and unfavourable effects on long-term survival of radiotherapy for early breast cancer: An overview of the randomised trials. Lancet 355:1757-1770, 2000.

32. Arthur DW, Vicini FA: Accelerated partial breast irradiation as a part of breast conservation therapy. J Clin Oncol 23:1726-1735, 2005.

33. Taghian A, Jeong JH, Mamounas E, et al: Patterns of locoregional failure in patients with operable breast cancer treated by mastectomy and adjuvant chemotherapy with or without tamoxifen and without radiotherapy: Results from five NSABP randomized clinical trials. J Clin Oncol 22:4247-4254, 2004.

34. Wolmark N, Wang J, Mamounas E, et al: Preoperative chemotherapy in patients with operable breast cancer: Nine-year results from National Surgical Adjuvant Breast and Bowel Project B-18. J Natl Cancer Inst Monogr 30:96-102, 2001.

35. Hughes KS, Schnaper L, Berry D, et al: Comparison of lumpectomy plus tamoxifen with and without radiotherapy (rt) in women 70 years of age or older who have clinical stage I, estrogen receptor–positive breast carcinoma. N Engl J Med 351:971-977, 2004.

36. Fyles AW, McCready DR, Manchul LA, et al: Tamoxifen with or without breast irradiation in women 50 years of age or older with early breast cancer. N Engl J Med 351:963-970, 2004.

37. Smith BL: Advanced Therapy of Breast Disease, Paget's Disease. Hamilton, Ontario, BC Decker, 2000.

38. Giordano SH, Buzdar AU, Hortobagyi GN: Breast cancer in men. Ann Intern Med 137:678-687, 2002.

39. Perou CM, Sorlie T, Eisen MB, et al: Molecular portraits of human breast tumors. Nature 406:747-752, 2000.

40. Paik S, Tang G, Shak S, et al: Gene expression and benefit of chemotherapy in women with node-negative, estrogen receptor–positive breast cancer. J Clin Oncol 24:3726-3734, 2006.

41. Harris JR, Lippman ME, Morrow M, Osborne CK (eds): Diseases of the Breast, 3rd ed. Philadelphia, Lippincott Williams & Wilkins, 2004.

42. Early Breast Cancer Trialists' Collaborative Group: Effects of chemotherapy and hormonal therapy for early breast cancer on recurrence and 15-year survival: An overview of the randomised trials. Lancet 365:1687-1717, 2005.

43. Citron ML, Berry DA, Cirrincione C, et al: Randomized trial of dose-dense versus conventionally scheduled and sequential versus concurrent combination chemotherapy as postoperative adjuvant treatment of node-positive primary breast cancer: First report of Intergroup Trial C9741/Cancer and Leukemia Group B Trial 9741. J Clin Oncol 21:1431-1439, 2003.

44. Romond EH, Perez EA, Bryant J, et al: Trastuzumab plus adjuvant chemotherapy for operable HER2-positive breast cancer. N Engl J Med 353:1673-1684, 2005.

45. Joensuu H, Kellokumpu-Lehtinen P-L, Bono P, et al: Adjuvant docetaxel or vinorelbine with or without trastuzumab for breast cancer. N Engl J Med 354:809-820, 2006.

46. Goss PE, Strasser K: Aromatase inhibitors in the treatment and prevention of breast cancer. J Clin Oncol 19:881-894, 2001.

47. Early Breast Cancer Trialists' Collaborative Group: Tamoxifen for early breast cancer: An overview of the randomised trials. Lancet 351:1451-1467, 1998.

48. Mouridsen HT, Robert NJ: The role of aromatase inhibitors as adjuvant therapy for early breast cancer in postmenopausal women. Eur J Cancer 41:1678-1689, 2005.

49. Winer EP, Hudis C, Burstein HJ, et al: American Society of Clinical Oncology technology assessment on the use of aromatase inhibitors as adjuvant therapy for women with hormone receptor–positive breast cancer: Status report 2002. J Clin Oncol 20:3317-3327, 2002.

50. Goldhirsch A, Glick JH, Gelber RD, et al: Meeting highlights: International expert consensus on the primary therapy of early breast cancer 2005. Ann Oncol 16:1569-1583, 2005.

CHAPTER 35

Breast Reconstruction

Bradon J. Wilhelmi, MD   and   Linda G. Phillips, MD

THE ROLE OF THE GENERAL SURGEON IN BREAST RECONSTRUCTION

Breast cancer is an extremely emotional topic by virtue of its anatomic location and the importance of the female breast in today's society. Therefore, it is imperative for surgeons performing breast surgery to have a basic understanding of which patients are candidates for breast reconstruction and what the reconstructive options are. Most patients start their inquiry about breast reconstruction with the surgeon who will be performing the mastectomy. They may ask, "What will it look like when you are done?" or "Will I have to live without a breast?" It is at this point that general surgeons greatly influence a woman's decision to pursue breast reconstruction.

Although the reconstructive surgeon goes into detail about the surgical options, risks, and expected outcomes, ablative surgeons must be prepared for at least a basic discussion with patients. Whether breast implants versus autogenous tissue will be used, where the scars will be, and how long the recovery will take are all questions that most patients want answered. Whether they undergo breast reconstruction or not can be influenced by the bias of ablative surgeons. Oncologic surgeons are trained to place priority on ablation of the tumor; however, care standards now dictate that we also be sensitive to the resulting deformity. Only through a close alliance between the surgical oncologist and reconstructive surgeon can the patient's emotional, physical, and oncologic needs be addressed.

HISTORY

In the late 1800s, the prognosis of patients with breast cancer was poor. Such notable surgeons as Volkmann, Czerny, and Billroth reported local recurrence rates ranging from 52% to 85%. Within 2 decades of these reports, William Halsted presented his successful treatment of breast cancer with only a 6% recurrence rate. The halstedian theory of breast cancer treatment would remain the mainstay of breast cancer surgery for the next 60 years. He believed that "the slightest inattention to detail and or attempts to hasten convalescence by such plastic operations as are feasible only when a restricted amount of skin is removed may sacrifice his patient to the disease." So, concerned with the possibility of inadequate skin excision, Halsted went on to say: "To attempt to close the breast wound more or less regularly by any plastic method is hazardous, and in my opinion, to be vigorously discounted." Therefore, true attempts at breast reconstruction would have to wait for almost 50 years.

Despite Halsted's condemnation of reconstructive procedures, it was recognized that the sizable defects left after this radical surgery did need to be closed. Although primary closure was often used, skin grafting of larger wounds was acceptable. Even though plastic procedures had been reported by Legueu and Graeve of France and J. Collins Warren of the United States, these were merely chest wall closure techniques and not true breast mound reconstructions.

Table 35-1 Operative Risk Factors for Breast Reconstruction With the TRAM Flap

Obesity	
Moderate: <25% above ideal body weight	1
Severe: >25% over ideal body weight	5
Small Vessel Disease	
Light to moderate smoking (1+ pack/day for 2-10 yr)	1
Chronic heavy smoking (10-20 pack-years)	2
Chronic heavy smoking (20-30 pack-years)	5
Autoimmune disease (e.g., scleroderma, Raynaud's)	8
Diabetes mellitus: non–insulin dependent	5
Diabetes mellitus: insulin dependent	10
Psychosocial Problems	
Unstable emotional state (life crisis)	2
Personality disorder	3
Substance abuse	5
Abdominal Scars	
If "planned out" of flap design	0.5
Disruption of vascular perforators: transection of superior epigastric vessels (e.g., chevron incision, abdominoplasty)	10
Patient's Attitude	
Patient unwilling or unable to invest the time required for healing or objects to an abdominal scar	10
Surgeon's Inexperience	
<10 TRAM flaps	1
Major System Disease Process	
Chronic lung disease	10
Severe cardiovascular disease	10

TRAM, transverse rectus abdominis myocutaneous.

Adapted from Hartrampf CR Jr: The transverse abdominal island flap for breast reconstruction: A 7-year experience. Clin Plast Surg 15:703-716, 1988.

The first attempt at true breast reconstruction occurred in 1895, when Vincent Czerny transplanted a large lipoma from his patient's flank to the mastectomy site. In a recount of this case by Dr. Robert Goldwyn, it was noted that 1 year after surgery the patient was doing well and had good breast symmetry. In this particular case, the mastectomy was performed for fibrocystic disease and not cancer. Tansini described the first use of the latissimus dorsi myocutaneous flap in 1906. Unfortunately, this remarkable operation would not gain acceptance for another 70 years.

In 1942, Sir Harold Gillies of England started using a tubed pedicle technique of breast reconstruction. In this operation he would "waltz" a flap from the abdomen to the chest to reconstruct the breast. Although this technique was very successful, the multiple procedures and prolonged treatment course precluded its widespread application.

Since about 1970, many advances in reconstructive surgery have occurred and been applied to breast recon-

struction. The development of breast implants was the first of these revolutions. In 1963, the silicone breast implant was introduced for breast augmentation and was quickly adopted for breast reconstruction. In 1963, Cronin and Gerow presented a series of patients who received implants for reconstruction of mastectomy defects.[1] For the first time the plastic surgeon had a procedure that could simulate the missing breast without the need for multiple procedures and a prolonged treatment course. In many ways it was the simplicity and safety of breast implants that ignited interest in breast reconstruction. By the later 1970s, reconstruction was being performed immediately after breast ablation.[2-4]

The development of muscle, musculocutaneous, and fasciocutaneous flaps and microsurgical transplantation has had a tremendous impact on breast reconstruction. The ideal material to reconstruct any defect is like-tissue. Up until the early 1970s, such tissue was available only in limited quantities for breast reconstruction. The landmark work by Manchot[5] on vascular territories of the body was rediscovered, and surgeons were then able to exploit this basic knowledge to design flaps based on the axial patterns of named blood vessels. These technical developments allowed surgeons to reliably rearrange tissues and more precisely reconstruct all types of defects, including those of the breast.[6]

PATIENT SELECTION

Opinions about which patients should undergo breast reconstruction are as varied as the surgeons who perform the procedures. In general, young healthy patients with early-stage disease are the best candidates for reconstruction, and consequently, older patients with advanced disease are poorer candidates. However, because of the multitude of different reconstructive options available, all women at least need to be presented with the options before being excluded.[7]

With the increasing popularity of autogenous breast reconstruction, more stringent guidelines may be needed for the selection of potential reconstructive candidates. With regard to mastectomy alone, the greater surgical trauma, increased operative time, increased blood loss, and prolonged recovery mandate that all patients, regardless of their desire for reconstruction, be thoroughly evaluated both physically and psychologically.

Although designed to help select candidates for transverse rectus abdominis myocutaneous (TRAM) flap reconstruction, the risk factor severity score devised by Carl Hartrampf can be applied to most patients, regardless of the technique used. Each risk is given a numerical weight. The total is added to derive a numerical score. Any patient with a score greater than 5 or with three or more risk factors is a poor candidate for TRAM reconstruction but may also be a poor candidate for the other procedures. Those with two risk factors are considered marginal candidates (Table 35-1). Of the risk factors listed, advanced age, obesity, smoking, concomitant disease, and the patient's psychological/emotional state are the most important to consider (Box 35-1).

TIMING

The timing of breast reconstruction after mastectomy has progressed from delayed to immediate because of advances and refinements in breast reconstructive techniques and recognition of beneficial psychological effects.[8-10] Because studies have shown a psychological benefit, cost-effectiveness, cosmetic advantage, and no increased risk for complications or oncologic risk with immediate breast reconstruction, it has become the preferred timing of reconstruction. In 1990, the American Society of Plastic and Reconstructive Surgeons reported that members performed 38% immediate versus 62% delayed reconstructions.[11] In a more recent study, 75% of reconstructions were performed immediately.[12]

Physician support for immediate reconstruction is based on the absence of medical contraindications and the anticipation of significant benefits to the woman. Early reconstruction after mastectomy reduces the emotional impact of mastectomy. Patients who underwent immediate breast reconstruction did not experience the loss of femininity, self-esteem, body image, and sexuality that patients did who had a delay in reconstruction.[13] Another study confirmed that patients who underwent immediate breast reconstruction experienced less depression than those who underwent reconstruction later.[14]

Immediate reconstruction is more cost-effective because it requires only one major operation, anesthetic, and hospitalization. Delayed breast reconstruction is 62% more expensive.[15] Moreover, immediate breast reconstruction less frequently results in the need for a secondary symmetry procedure.[16] Interruption of lifestyle occurs once, not twice.

Better breast symmetry can be achieved with immediate breast reconstruction because the skin flaps are pliable and not contracted to the chest wall. This improved symmetry with immediate reconstruction was confirmed by a recent study in which 67% (462 of 689) of delayed reconstructions required a symmetry procedure versus only 22% (155 of 705) of immediate reconstructions.[17] With immediate breast reconstruction using autologous tissue, more of the original breast skin that is sensate can be preserved, whereas with delayed breast reconstruction, much of the reconstructed breast skin is insensate. The skin-sparing mastectomy technique can be used with immediate breast reconstruction to maximize the sensate breast skin and confine the scar to the region around the areola (Fig. 35-1). With immediate reconstruction it is easier to preserve the inframammary crease than to reestablish it at a later date.[18]

Studies have demonstrated no statistically significant difference in complication rates after intermediate versus delayed breast reconstruction.[19,20] Furthermore, there is no increased oncologic risk for immediate breast reconstruction.[20] Clinical trials have shown that there is no increased risk for cancer recurrence and no increased difficulty with surveillance for recurrence of breast cancer after immediate reconstruction.[19] Because breast cancer recurrence in reconstructed breasts is usually seen in skin or subcutaneous tissue, the diagnosis is not generally delayed by immediate reconstruction. When breast cancer recurs in the chest wall, it is highly associated with metastatic disease, and the survival rate is not likely to have been influenced by earlier detection.[21] Studies have shown that immediate breast reconstruction does not delay postoperative administration of chemotherapy and radiotherapy.[22]

SURGICAL PLANNING

For the ideal breast reconstruction, the patient's native chest skin is preserved, and the reconstructive surgeon merely fills a skin brassiere. Unfortunately, this is not always possible, but ablative surgical planning as early as the breast biopsy can improve the reconstructive outcome. In most patients the surgical approach for biopsy or the insertion site for needle core biopsy can be made in or very near the nipple-areola complex. If the scars are placed around the areolar-cutaneous junction, the most favorable scar can be achieved. If the results of the biopsy are positive for cancer, re-excision of the first scar with a limited amount of skin prepares the patient for the most favorable reconstruction.

Contrary to previous teaching, large amounts of skin do not need to be removed to effectively treat breast cancer. Therefore, skin-sparing mastectomy can be performed whenever feasible. Skin-sparing mastectomy spares the breast skin by removing the breast tissue through a small opening only around the areola. Depend-

Box 35-1   Factors Affecting Choice of Reconstruction Procedures

Patient Factors

Age
Medical conditions
  Previous abdominal or thoracic surgery
  Coronary artery disease
  Chronic obstructive pulmonary disease
  Medications
  Chronic corticosteroid use
  Obesity
Body morphology
Occupation
Social activities
Financial resources
Support systems
Expectations/desires

Disease Factors

Stage of disease
Type of tumor
Need for adjuvant therapy

Miscellaneous Factors

Experience of the surgeon
Availability of equipment (e.g., microscope)
Religious beliefs regarding blood transfusion
Blood banking facilities

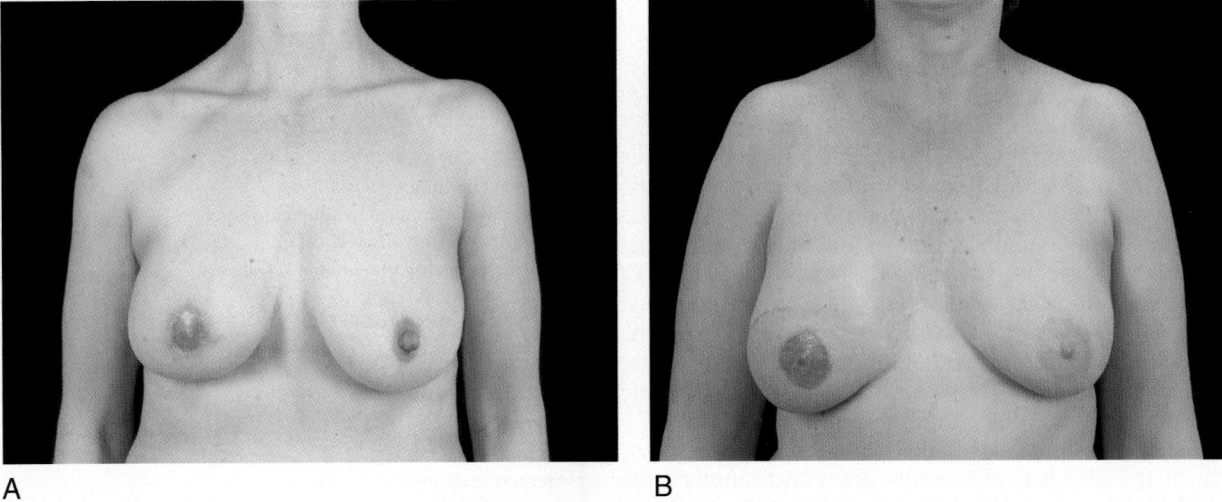

A   B

Figure 35-1 A, Patient who underwent immediate breast reconstruction of a skin-sparing mastectomy with a pedi-cled TRAM flap and later nipple-areolar reconstruction. **B,** This patient underwent delayed breast reconstruction 5 years after modified radical mastectomy. A pedicled TRAM flap was used for her breast reconstruction. Notice the much larger skin paddle on the delayed breast reconstruction versus the skin paddle confined to the areola in the immediate reconstruction.

ing on the size and location of the lesion, only the nipple-areola complex may need to be excised.[23] Additional incisions can be added to help with the dissection, such as a lateral extension of the periareolar incision for access to a large mammary gland or a separate incision in the axillary crease for lymphadenectomy (Fig. 35-2).

The nipple and areola are removed because of the oncologic risk of involvement, which has been shown to be around 10.4% to 10.6%.[24,25] Moreover, there is minimal aesthetic advantage to preservation of the areola because of the risk for not only areolar skin sloughing and necro-sis but also loss of sensation (57%), delayed wound healing (29%), asymmetry (50%), recurrence (27%), and still a frequent need for a secondary procedure (36%).[26] In addition, a recent study demonstrated no improvement for nipple-sparing mastectomy over skin-sparing mastectomy.[27]

Skin-sparing mastectomy can provide superior aes-thetic results by confining the scar to the area around the skin paddle of the flap, which will ultimately be camou-flaged as the rim around the reconstructed nipple-areolar complex. Skin-sparing mastectomy is oncologically safe. Studies have demonstrated no increased risk for local recurrence and no increased risk for distant metastasis or spread of cancer, and disease-free survival for skin-sparing mastectomy is the same as for traditional mastec-tomy, as long as the mastectomy flaps are not too thick.[28,29] However, it is critical that the mastectomy skin not be too thin because blood flow to this skin will be compro-mised. A recent study demonstrated that residual disease was found in 9.5% of the women and was associated with skin flaps greater than 5 mm thick.[30]

Shaving the skin flaps too thin leads to tissue necrosis of the mastectomy flap skin over the viable flap. Perfu-sion of this skin can be assessed with a fluorescein test. If the mastectomy skin has questionable viability, it can be discarded and the skin paddle on the flap made larger;

alternatively, the reconstruction may have to be delayed. Care needs to be taken to avoid disrupting the inframam-mary crease. Although a small amount of breast tissue is present below the level of this crease, it does not usually need to be excised in a standard mastectomy. Preopera-tive marking of the inframammary crease helps remind the surgeon to avoid releasing this important surface landmark.[31] With the patient supine, the breast can be lifted. The natural crease is evident by the indentation made by the dermal fascial attachments. The crease can be marked with methylene blue, a permanent marker, or staples. Other surgeons have advocated placing sutures at the inframammary crease that are palpable during dis-section of the inferior breast tissue.

In large or very ptotic breasts with lesions in the middle or lower third of the breast mound, alternative skin incisions can be planned with the reconstructive surgeon. A breast reduction type of skin incision using the keyhole-type pattern provides the ablative surgeon with excellent exposure of the breast mound and ade-quate exposure for axillary dissection (Fig. 35-3). If the patient is undergoing a contralateral breast reduction or mastopexy, the standard elliptical mastectomy incision provides less symmetry. The keyhole (pattern of Wise) incision design affords skin excision in the horizontal and vertical planes, which results in a less ptotic, more conical breast mound that is easier to shape.

SURGICAL OPTIONS

Breast reconstruction is a process that involves more than just creation of a mound on a woman's chest. Even the most perfectly shaped breast will leave a patient unhappy if it is not matched to the other side. It is often said that asymmetry is worse than ugliness and that symmetry is ultimately more important to a successful outcome than

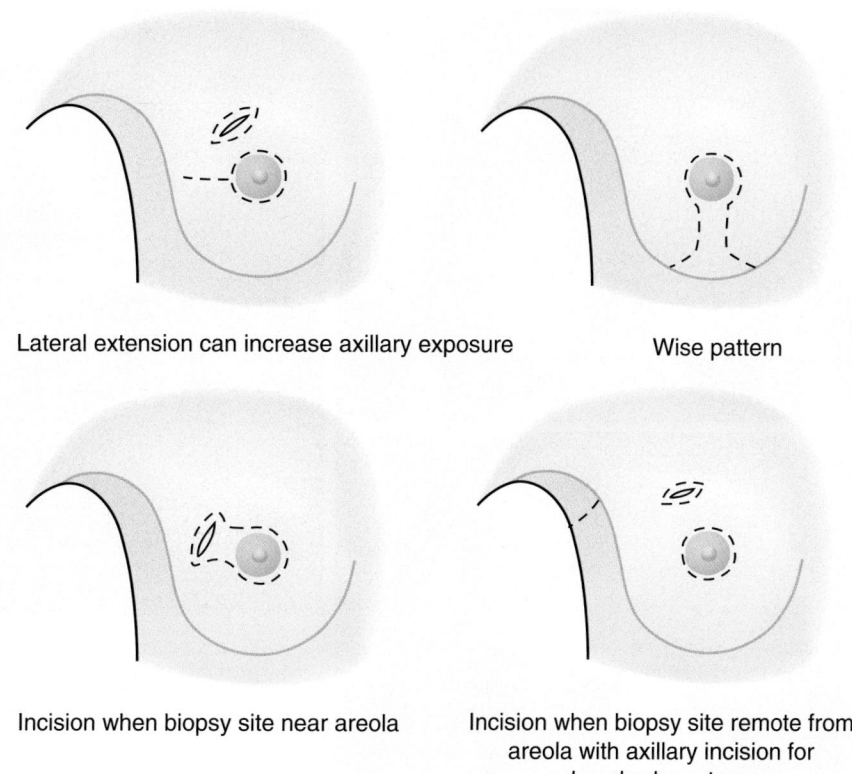

Lateral extension can increase axillary exposure

Wise pattern

Incision when biopsy site near areola

Incision when biopsy site remote from areola with axillary incision for lymphadenectomy

Figure 35-2 Diagrams of options for placement of incisions in patients undergoing skin-sparing mastectomy. The more native chest skin that can be spared, the more natural the reconstruction tends to be. If possible, the biopsy incision is placed periareolarly to avoid making multiple incisions or increasing the amount of tissue excised from the breast.

anything else. Therefore, the reconstructive plan must accommodate not only the size and shape of the opposite breast but also the position on the chest wall; the location of the inframammary crease; the height, size, and color of the nipple-areolar complex; and the amount of breast ptosis.

Reconstructive options can be divided into two main types: those that use autogenous tissue and those that require alloplastic material. In general, autogenous tissue will usually provide better symmetry than an implant. Only 35% of TRAM flap reconstructions required a symmetry procedure versus 55% of implant reconstructions in one study.[32] The choice of procedure for a given patient is affected by her age, health, contralateral breast size and shape, and personal preference and the expertise of the reconstructive surgeon (Box 35-2).

Complications can occur with any type of breast reconstruction. The most significant effect is delay of initiation of adjuvant therapy. Partial or complete flap loss, wound breakdown, and infection are all reasons why chemotherapy or radiation therapy would be delayed. Complication rates are higher in patients who require radiotherapy postoperatively. In patients who require postoperative radiotherapy, TRAM reconstructions can provide better cosmetic outcomes and lower complication rates than implant reconstructions can.[33] Because postoperative radiotherapy has been recognized to worsen the outcome of an immediate TRAM recon-

struction, there has been a movement to delay reconstruction in patients who are expected to need postoperative radiotherapy.[34] However, the just-stated advantages of immediate reconstruction outweigh the risk for late complications seen with irradiated immediate TRAM reconstructions. In general, radiotherapy after mastectomy and immediate TRAM flap reconstruction is well tolerated and not associated with an increased rate of acute complications or interruption of radiation therapy. Although survival in patients who have undergone reconstruction is no different from that in patients who have undergone mastectomy alone, the anxiety associated with delays in treatment can be significant to patients and waiting oncologists.[33]

Another concern to patients is blood loss. The average blood loss from reconstructive procedures ranges from 300 to 575 mL, depending on the pedicle technique used. It may be advisable for patients to autodonate 2 units of blood before surgery to minimize the need for allotransfusion. Other surgeons, to prevent delay of the ablative procedure, will proceed without autodonation in the knowledge that a relatively healthy patient can sustain blood loss of 600 mL without becoming symptomatic.

Breast Reconstruction With Implants

Of the several methods of breast reconstruction available, breast implants can provide a technically simple means

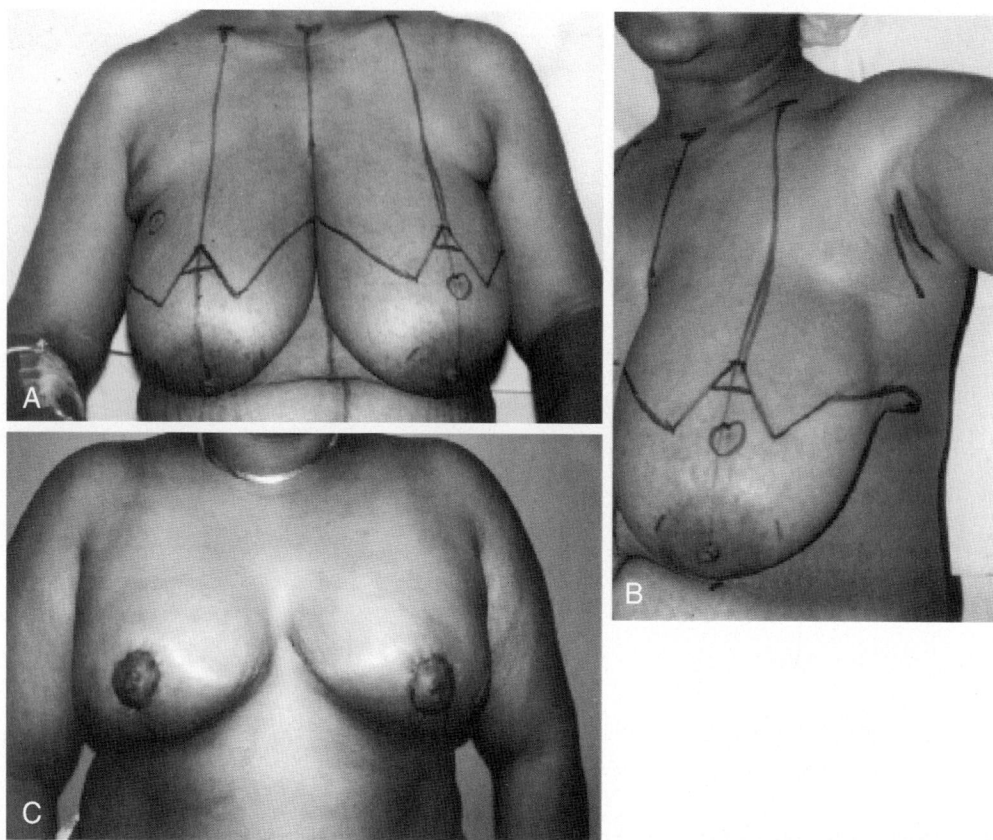

Figure 35-3 A, View of a patient marked for a Wise-pattern breast reduction incision. *Circles* show previous biopsy sites. The left breast biopsy was positive for carcinoma. The patient was otherwise a candidate for lumpectomy but requested breast reduction in conjunction with ablative surgery. Right breast biopsy and subsequent pathology failed to demonstrate carcinoma. **B,** Marking for breast reduction, as well as a separate axillary incision for axillary node sampling. **C,** Photograph of the postoperative results after breast reduction. The patient started adjunctive therapy 5 weeks after surgery.

of achieving breast symmetry and they pose minimal risk in properly selected patients. This approach to breast reconstruction is appropriate for patients requiring bilateral breast reconstruction. Through the use of bilateral, identical implants, excellent symmetry can be achieved (Fig. 35-4). Unilateral mastectomy patients with small breasts and minimal ptosis can also benefit from this technique. Though initially popularized for breast augmentation, use of the silicone implant was extended to breast reconstruction after mastectomy procedures.[1,35] In the original description, the implant was inserted into the subcutaneous breast wound. The use of saline-filled implants precludes subcutaneous placement because these implants visibly ripple the skin. Placement of the implant in a submuscular plane beneath the pectoralis major, superior portion of the rectus abdominis, and serratus anterior muscles provides better protection against implant extrusion, as well as decreased risk for capsular contracture and implant displacement (Fig. 35-5). Many surgeons now avoid sub–rectus abdominis placement because the tight fascial amalgamation can flatten the implant inferiorly and displace it supariorly. Some surgeons place expenders or implants in the subpectoral plane, without elevation of the serratus muscle, by adding

a sheet of acellular dermis that is sutured in place between the inframammary fold and the edge of the pectoralis major.[36,37] In approximating the pectoralis major to the serratus anterior muscles, preservation of the clavipectoral fascia, when possible, facilitates prevention of the suture pulling through muscle and ripping muscle fibers.[38]

In women with a large contralateral breast, a larger implant may be required for symmetrical reconstruction than can be placed submuscularly in the immediate setting. For these patients, permanent or temporary tissue expanders are used (Fig. 35-6). These expanders are silicone envelopes with an integrated or remote port for episodic injection of saline in the outpatient setting.[39,40] Most surgeons overinflate past the desired size. Overinflation affords a larger skin envelope that gives some ptosis in the end result. Waiting at least 6 weeks from the last expansion to implant exchange is believed to limit the rapid shrinkage of expanded skin. At a secondary procedure, the expander is exchanged for a permanent implant. In women with very large breasts, a Wise-pattern incision can be used for the mastectomy. The complication of implant exposure caused by separation of the inverted-T wound can be avoided by preserving and de-

Box 35-2 Options for Breast Reconstruction

Autogenous
  Abdominal-based flaps
    TRAM
    Single pedicle
    Double pedicle
    Free flap*
    Deep inferior epigastric perforator flap*
  Upper abdominal horizontal flap
  Vertical abdominal flap
  Tubed abdominal flap
Latissimus dorsi musculocutaneous flap
Gluteal flap*
  Superiorly based
  Inferiorly based
Rubens flap*
Thoracoepigastric flap
Lateral thigh flap*
Breast-splitting procedure[†]
Alloplastic
  Silicone gel implant
  Silicone implant with saline fill
    Smooth wall
    Textured wall
    Round shaped
    Anatomic shaped
  Silicone injection[†]
Combination procedures
  Latissimus dorsi flap with implant
  TRAM flap with implant

TRAM, transverse rectus abdominis myocutaneous.

*Requires microsurgical procedure.

[†]Historical note only.

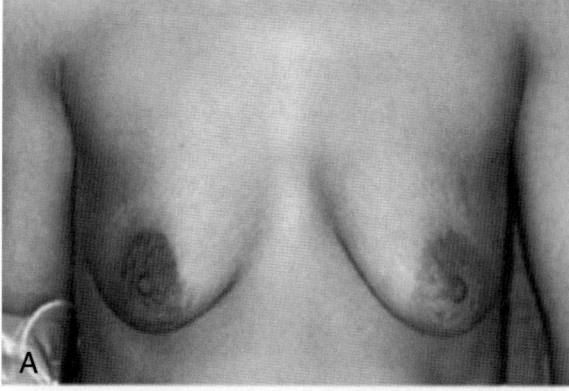
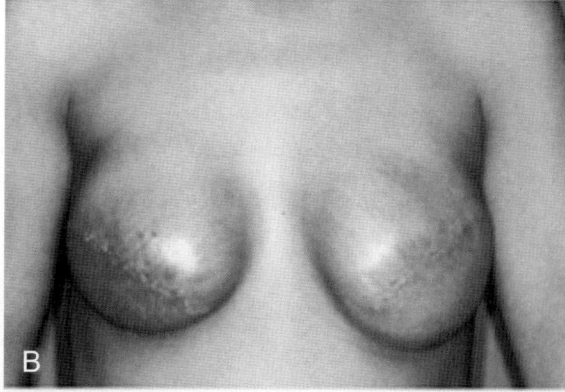
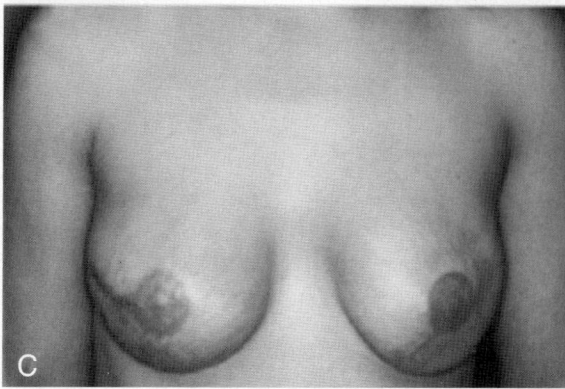

Figure 35-4 A, A 37-year-old woman with right breast carcinoma and a significant family history of breast cancer elected bilateral mastectomy and implant reconstruction. **B,** First stage of reconstruction with bilateral implants in place after mastectomy. **C,** Completed reconstruction, including secondary nipple reconstruction with local flaps and areola reconstruction with tattooed pigment.

epithelializing the inferior breast skin and repairing the cephalic edge of this de-epithelialized inferior breast skin to the caudal edge of the pectoralis major muscle to protect the implant (Fig. 35-7).[41]

An alternative technique involves the use of a permanent Becker silicone/saline implant expander with a remote port. This implant expander is filled to the desired breast size over the course of several weeks postoperatively. Later, the port can be taken out as an outpatient procedure.

Complications associated with the use of breast implants can occur in the immediate perioperative period or years later.[42] Such complications include exposure, extrusion, or infection of the implants.[20] Careful attention when closing the submuscular pocket and skin can help avoid these problems. Longer term problems also include asymmetry, capsular contracture, malposition of the implant, rupture, and pain.[34,43,44]

Several studies have demonstrated the risk for capsular contracture to be significantly elevated in patients who undergo radiation therapy: a 15% risk without radiation and 42% with radiation.[43,44] Furthermore, symmetry after breast implant reconstruction is better if radiation therapy can be avoided.[44] A breast implant may be used for thin patients who have inadequate abdominal and back soft

tissue for use with TRAM or latissimus dorsi myocutaneous flaps. A breast implant may also be used in conjunction with a myocutaneous flap to provide coverage and protection. The complication of capsule contracture in women with implants who undergo radiation therapy can be lessened with muscle flap coverage of the implant.[44] Certain abdominal (subcostal and transverse) or chest (lateral thoracotomy) scars represent previous transection of flap muscle and blood supply and serve as absolute contraindications to the use of modes of autogenous reconstruction, thus requiring the use of a breast implant

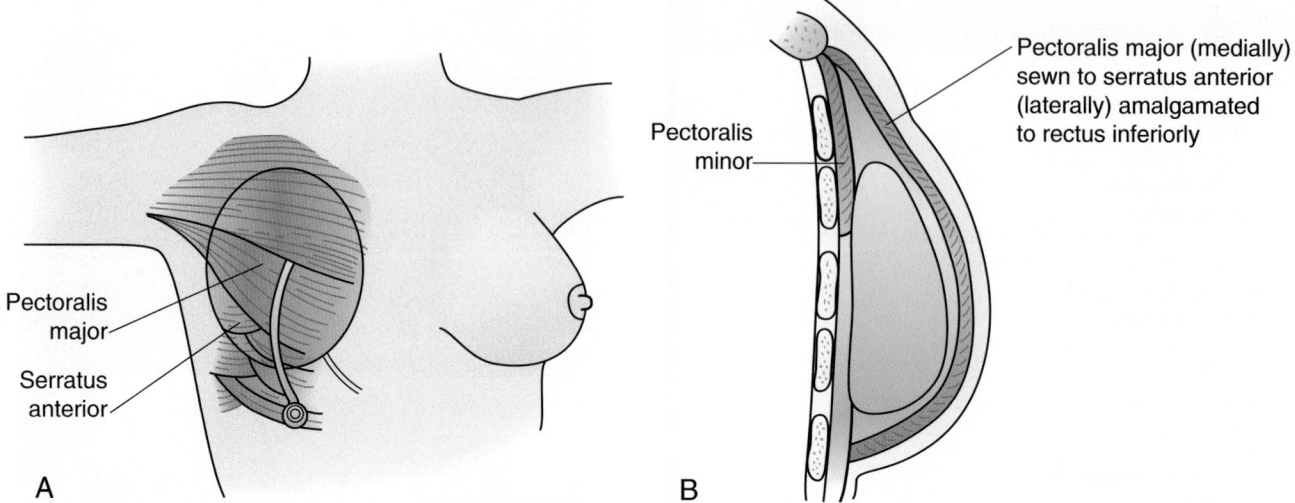

Pectoralis major (medially) sewn to serratus anterior (laterally) amalgamated to rectus inferiorly

Pectoralis minor

Pectoralis major

Serratus anterior

A

B

Figure 35-5 A, Proper placement of a tissue expander underneath the pectoralis major/serratus anterior muscle. **B,** Sagittal cut demonstrating the pectoralis major/serratus anterior muscle anteriorly. A complete muscular pocket was created to protect the implant from exposure through the thin remaining mastectomy flaps; this technique is also used to help re-create the inframammary fold.

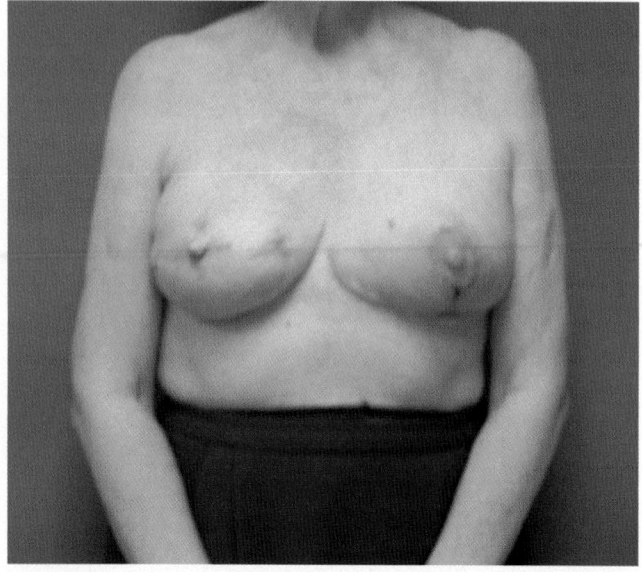

Figure 35-6 This patient underwent immediate breast reconstruction with an expander that was later replaced with a permanent breast implant.

for reconstruction of the breast. Women expected to receive radiotherapy have a relative contraindication to reconstruction with implants because of increased risk for capsular contracture and inelastic skin impeding tissue expansion (Box 35-3). In patients who unexpectedly require postoperative radiation therapy, reconstruction with a myocutaneous flap technique may be required to salvage a firm, contracted implant reconstruction.[45]

Latissimus Dorsi Myocutaneous Flap

By the early 1970s, breast reconstruction with implants was widely accepted as a simple and safe means of reconstruction, but there were some significant limitations. One of the main problems plaguing implant recon-

struction was—and still is—the lack of tissue on the chest wall after mastectomy. If a moderate-sized to large breast is being matched or if there is any degree of breast ptosis, there is never enough skin to cover the needed implant. In an effort to improve outcome, plastic surgeons worked toward developing single-stage operations for breast reconstruction that would supply the necessary additional skin to the chest wall and provide bulk to create a larger breast mound. The latissimus dorsi myocutaneous flap was the first to be widely applied in breast reconstruction.

Though first described by Professor Iginio Tansini for chest wall coverage in 1906, the latissimus dorsi myocutaneous flap was not commonly used until the 1970s.[46,47] The latissimus dorsi is a flat, triangular muscle that originates from the spines of the lumbar and sacral vertebrae and inserts into the intertubular groove of the humerus. Its blood supply comes from the thoracodorsal artery and from multiple segmental perforators off the lumbar intercostal arteries.[48,49] These arteries provide musculocutaneous perforating vessels that penetrate the subcutaneous tissue to supply a territory of skin directly overlying the muscle (Fig. 35-8). This flap is so hardy that it can be safely elevated even if the thoracodorsal artery is cut because it receives retrograde blood flow from a branch to the serratus anterior muscle. Nevertheless, if this flap is the planned method of reconstruction, care is taken to not injure the thoracodorsal artery and vein during axillary dissection. The skin donor site on the back can, in most cases, be closed primarily and, if planned properly, will be hidden by the patient's bra line.

This flap is ideally suited for single-stage reconstruction in women with small breasts and a moderate degree of breast ptosis. In some women who do not require a modified radical mastectomy and in whom the resultant segmental resection excision is enough to cause significant breast deformity, the latissimus dorsi flap can be

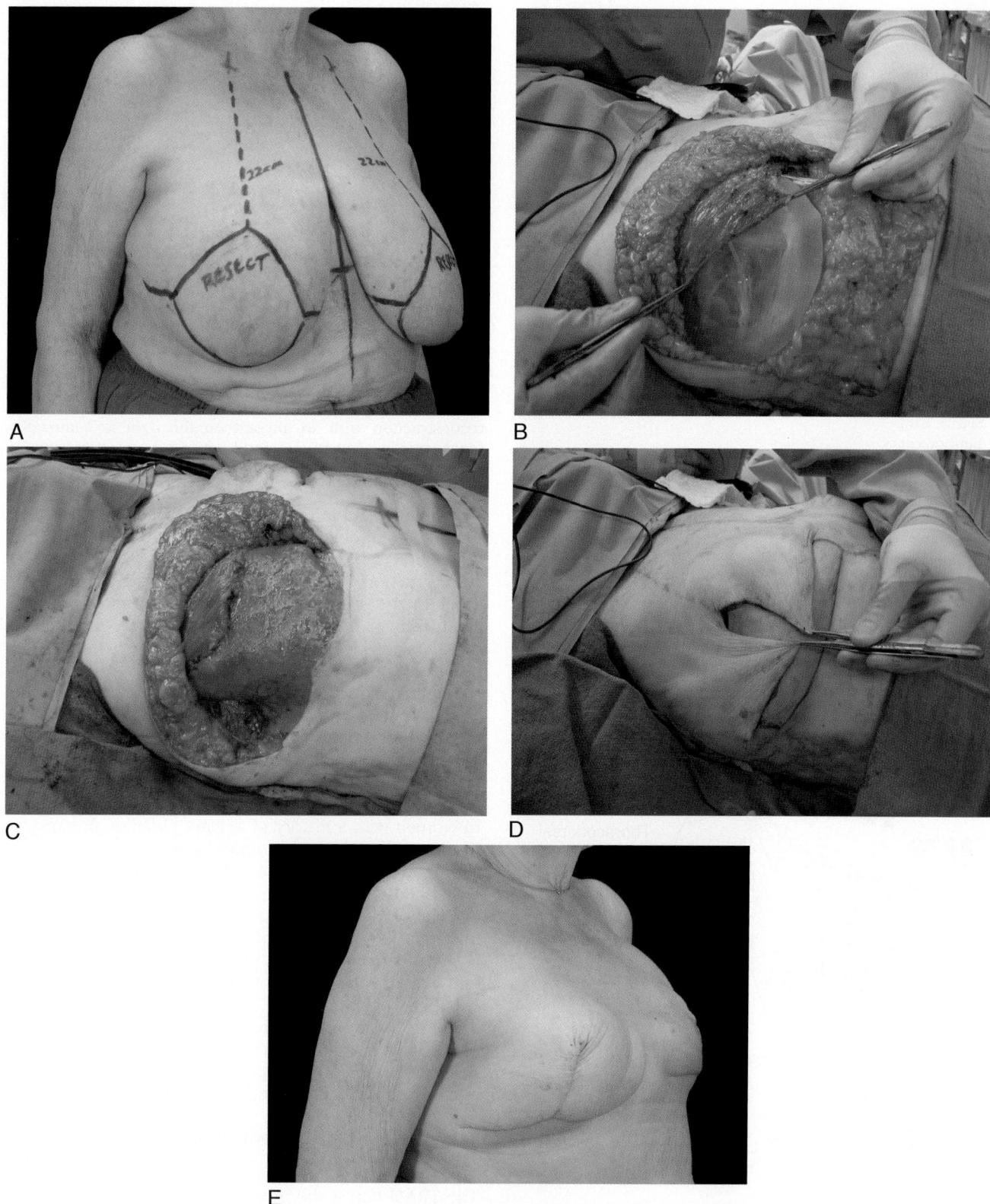

Figure 35-7 A to **E,** This patient underwent immediate breast reconstruction with implants through a Wise-pattern breast reduction incision protected by a de-epithelialized inferior skin flap. This inferior-based skin flap is repaired to the lower edge of the pectoralis major muscle to fully cover the implant should the Wise-pattern skin incision break down.

Box 35-3 Implant Reconstruction

Indications

Bilateral reconstruction
Patient requesting augmentation in addition to reconstruction
Patient not suited for long surgery
Lack of adequate abdominal tissue
Patient unwilling to have additional scars on either her back or abdomen
Small breast mound with minimal ptosis

Relative Contraindications

Young age (may need an implant replaced multiple times)
Patient unwilling to adhere to follow-up
Very large breast
Very ptotic breast

Contraindications

Silicon allergy
Implant fear
Previous failed implants
Need for adjuvant radiation therapy

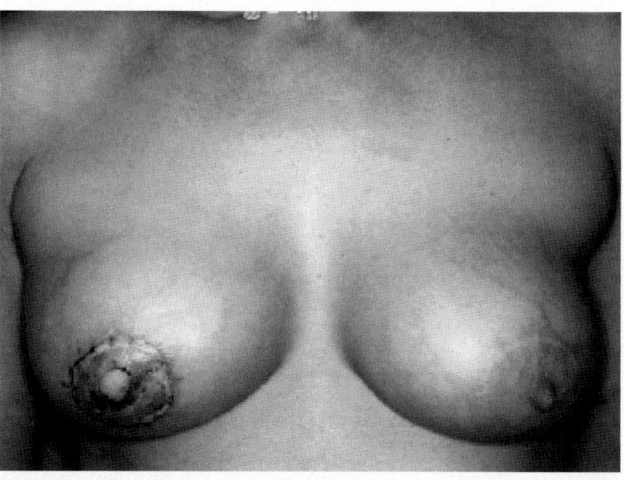

Figure 35-9 Woman undergoing right-sided simple mastectomy for chronic mastitis who elected to undergo latissimus dorsi reconstruction with an implant on the right and immediate nipple-areola reconstruction and left mastopexy augmentation. She was seen 3 weeks after her single-stage surgery.

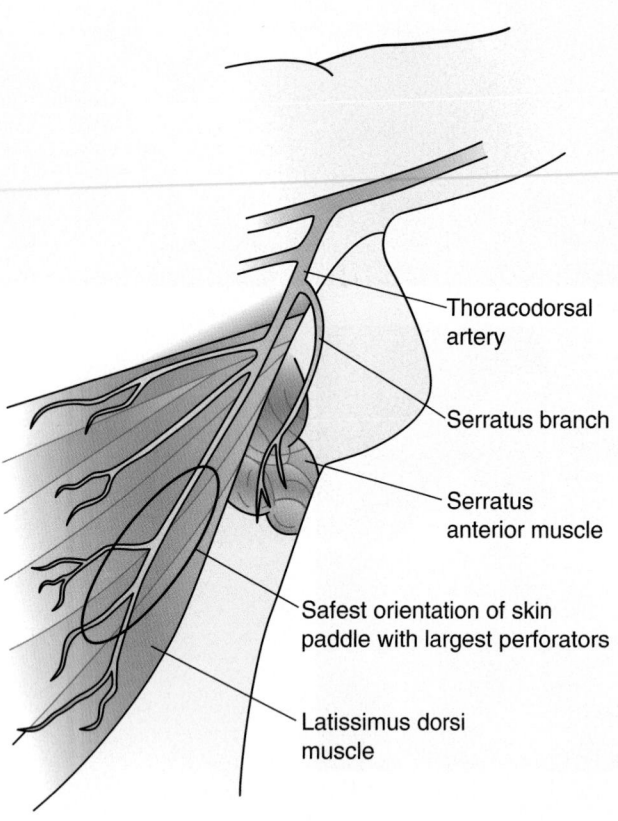

Figure 35-8 Pertinent anatomy in latissimus dorsi muscle reconstruction, including the latissimus dorsi muscle subscapular axis with thoracodorsal vessels, as well as communication with the serratus anterior muscle via the serratus anterior communicating branch.

extremely useful in restoring breast contour. If the breast volume requirements exceed the available tissue from this region, a breast implant can be used to augment the reconstruction (Fig. 35-9). However, if a large or very ptotic breast is needed, this technique would be discouraged in favor of the TRAM flap to provide a larger and bulkier skin envelope.

Despite the popularity of the latissimus dorsi flap in breast reconstruction, not all patients are candidates (Box 35-4). Women with large breast volume requirements are not ideal candidates. Patients who have previously undergone back or axillary surgery (lateral thoracotomies) usually have had their latissimus muscle divided and are discouraged from undergoing this form of reconstruction. In women with a history of axillary radiation therapy, the resultant fibrosis and arteritis may impair the blood supply to this flap, and use of the latissimus dorsi flap is prohibited.

One of the disadvantages of this technique is that simultaneous harvesting of the flap while the mastectomy is being performed is not possible. Although the mastectomy can be performed with the patient in the lateral decubitus position, inset of the flap necessitates repositioning the patient before breast shaping and closure. This results in mild inconvenience to the operating staff, delays the operation, and raises the theoretical consideration of contamination and increased rates of infection.

Transverse Rectus Abdominis Myocutaneous Flap

The TRAM flap is the most commonly performed autogenous reconstructive procedure. The abdomen has always been seen as a potential source of donor tissue, especially for breast reconstruction. The skin and adipose composition of the breast and abdomen are very similar. Sir Harold Gillies[50] reported the initial use of tubed pedicle flaps of abdominal tissue more than 70 years ago. Unfortunately, his operation allowed only a limited amount of tissue to be transposed, required multiple procedures, and left significant scars along the way. With each step of the transfer, more fat necrosed, which left a firm scar and a smaller flap volume. Further use of this technique was abandoned with the growing application of axial-pattern flaps.

Though first suggested in 1979 by Robbins, the TRAM flap was popularized in 1982 by Hartrampf and coworkers.[28] In its original description, an ellipse of skin from the upper part of the abdomen was used. This skin paddle design was later modified to be placed over the lower part of the abdomen to take advantage of the larger amount of adipose tissue available, the more favorable scar location, and the longer pedicle for ease in transposition (Box 35-5). Anatomic studies by Moon and Taylor[51] confirmed the rich supply of perforating vessels of the abdominal wall. The flap is divided into four regions on the basis of entrance of the perforating vessels (Fig. 35-10). The most reliable zones are either directly over the muscle (zone I) or directly adjacent to this zone (zones II, III). Zone IV is the contralateral tissue farthest away from the musculocutaneous perforators and, in most cases, must be discarded, especially in obese patients and smokers. Perfusion studies have further delineated that zone III, which has an axial blood supply, has more reliable perfusion than zone II, which is supplied across the midline and therefore random.[52]

One of the advantages of this technique over other forms of breast reconstruction is the diversity of configurations available to the surgeon. This flap can be harvested as a single- or double-pedicle flap based on the deep superior epigastric blood supply. It may also be harvested as a free flap based on the deep inferior epigastric vessels anastomosed to the thoracodorsal or internal mammary artery and vein. The inferior epigastric artery is the dominant blood supply to the abdominal skin. In patients who are obese, have larger tissue requirements, or have upper abdominal scars, use of the free inferiorly based TRAM flap is considered more reliable. The free TRAM flap is also advocated for patients who smoke because the relatively increased blood supply through the deep inferior epigastric artery protects against the nicotine-induced vasospasm that these patients have.

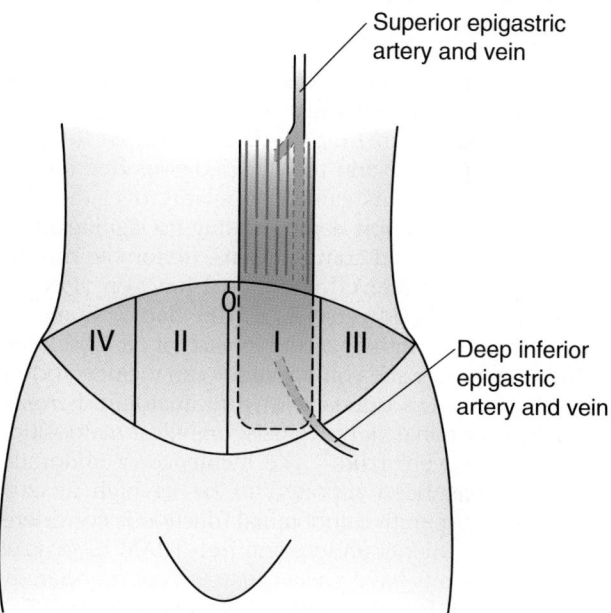

Figure 35-10 Vascular territories of the abdominal wall provided by a unilateral TRAM flap. Studies by Moon and Taylor[51] show the most reliable cutaneous portion to be directly overlying the muscle (zone I), followed by zones III, II, and IV, respectively.

Preparation of the artery for microanastomosis results in stripping of the sympathetic nerves in the adventitia, thereby protecting against vasospasm. Recently, the free flap has been based only on perforators from the deep inferior epigastric vessels with preservation of the entire rectus abdominis muscle; this is called the *deep inferior epigastric perforator* (DIEP) *flap*. The disadvantage of the perforator TRAM flap (DIEP) is the reported increased risk for fat necrosis from a less reliable blood supply than with the standard free TRAM flap.[53,54]

Another modification of the deep perforator flap includes basing the flap on the superficial inferior epigastric vessels. However, one study found that the TRAM

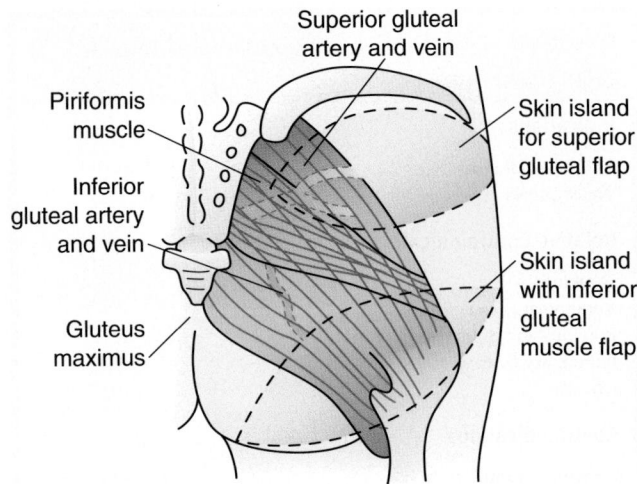

Figure 35-11 Pertinent anatomy and outline for a free gluteal flap. Either a superior- or inferior-based skin paddle can be designed on the respective inferior/superior gluteal artery and vein. Cosmesis is considered good and is best suited in patients with slight buttock ptosis.

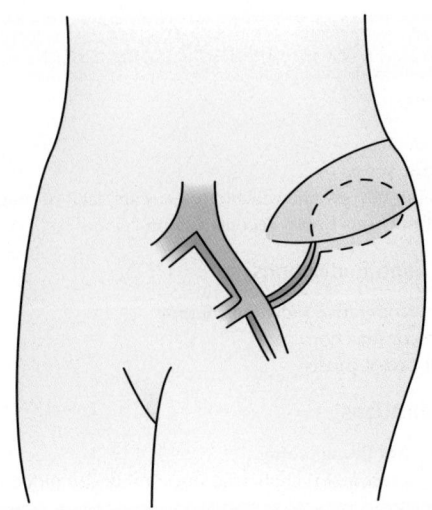

Figure 35-12 Diagram of the Rubens flap as described by Hartrampf and coworkers[65] in 1994. This flap is based on the circumflex iliac artery and is best suited in women who are not candidates for TRAM flaps and have adequate soft tissue in their hip region. Symmetry procedures usually need to be performed, with excision of a similar amount of tissue from the contralateral hip.

flap could not be routinely based on the superficial inferior epigastric pedicle because it was not available (48%) or too small, less than 1 mm in diameter (20%). Recently, the technically easier and more expeditious free muscle-sparing TRAM flap has gained popularity over the DIEP flap because of a report demonstrating no significant difference in flap-related complications, donor site morbidity, and patient-perceived abdominal function after free muscle-sparing TRAM versus free DIEP flaps.[55] Complications may occur either at the breast or at abdominal donor sites. Donor site complications can include abdominal wall laxity (as opposed to true anatomic hernias), diastasis, abdominal skin necrosis, umbilical malposition, seroma, and severe pain.[56] The incidence of abdominal wall laxity has been reported to be as high as 20%. Although postoperative abdominal function is considered to be best in patients undergoing free TRAM reconstruction, most patients have greater than 95% of preoperative abdominal wall function within 1 year of surgery.[57-59]

Many surgeons use mesh to close the abdominal wall defect caused by elevation of the muscle flap. Others close the defect by approximating the fascia. Studies have demonstrated that primary closure of the fascia and the use of onlay mesh result in lower hernia and bulge rates.[60,61] Preserving the anterior and posterior fascia below the semilunar line of Douglas allows primary closure of the fascia. For subsequent abdominal procedures, it is helpful to obtain a plastic surgery consultation, perhaps even for opening and closing the abdominal cavity.

Breast complications include partial or complete flap loss. Most large series report less than a 4% flap failure rate and up to a 20% rate of partial flap loss. Although the total flap loss rate is greater with free TRAM flaps (8%), partial loss is greatest with pedicle flaps (13%-20%). There is an indication that the ipsilateral pedicled TRAM flap may have a lower rate of partial necrosis than the contralateral design.[38] Fat necrosis is a late complication

that affects about 7% of pedicled TRAM flaps and 1% to 2% of free TRAM flaps.[44] Frequently, patients and oncologists are concerned about a firm nodule in the reconstructed breast. Biopsy may be needed to make the final diagnosis and to satisfy both the patient and oncologist.

Complications of TRAM breast reconstructions, such as wound infection, mastectomy flap necrosis, abdominal flap necrosis, and fat necrosis, are well documented to be increased with smoking.[53,62] This risk has been lowered with cessation of smoking 4 weeks before surgery.[63]

Other Options for Autologous Breast Reconstructions

When autologous breast reconstruction is desired but TRAM and latissimus flaps are not available, other flaps have been described for postmastectomy reconstruction. The free gluteal flap has been used for breast reconstruction as a myocutaneous flap based on either the inferior or the superior vessels (Fig. 35-11).[64] Because of the technical complexity of the procedure and complications, including sciatica, seroma, unfavorable scar location, and asymmetric buttock contour, this option is a secondary choice for breast reconstruction. The vascular pedicle is quite short, so either vein interposition or removal of costochondral cartilage is required to permit anastomosis to the internal mammary vessels.

The Rubens flap is based on the circumflex iliac vessels.[65] This option is most applicable for women who have an excess of soft tissue over the hips, as accentuated in women painted by Rubens during the Renaissance. The flap is elevated with a full thickness of tissue over the hip and underlying musculature, including the oblique and transverse muscles (Fig. 35-12). Because this recon-

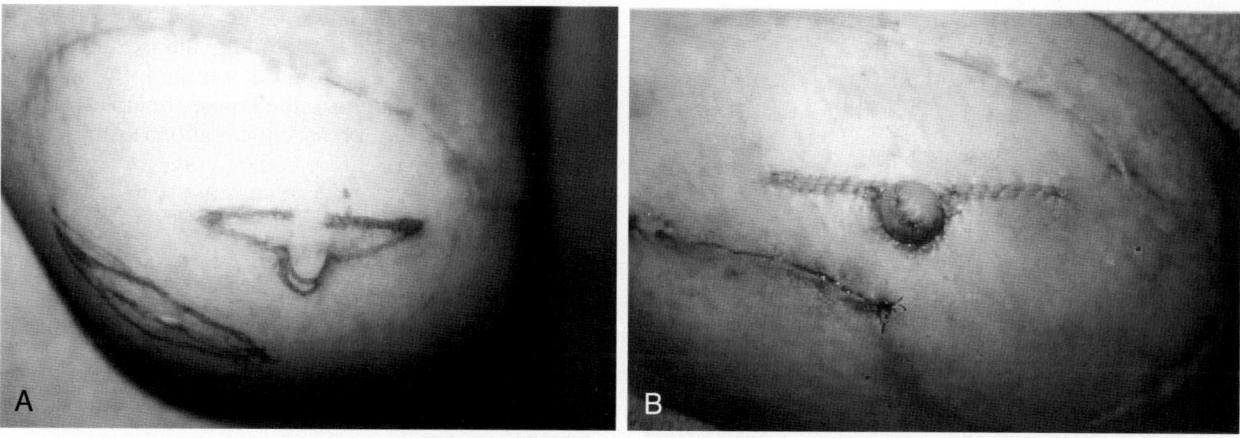

Figure 35-13 A, Basic design of a modified star flap on a left breast before elevation. Additional markings show area of minor revision. This procedure was performed with the patient under local anesthesia in the office. **B,** Completed and closed nipple reconstruction.

structive procedure is limited in bulk and skin envelope and often requires a balancing procedure on the contralateral hip, it is not generally considered as a first option.

Reconstruction of a Partial Mastectomy

Recent literature supports immediate reconstruction after partial mastectomy to reduce the overall number of operations that a patient may need. Although all of the previously discussed options for total breast reconstruction can be used for reconstructing a partial mastectomy wound, common options for partial mastectomy wounds include a latissimus dorsi muscle flap or local rearrangement of breast tissue. The primary goal of oncologic resection is to achieve tumor ablation. The resection must not be compromised by a surgeon striving for an aesthetic result. The disadvantage of immediate reconstruction after partial mastectomy is the risk for a positive margin reported days later on routine pathologic evaluation, which could require sacrifice of the entire breast and flap. Additional risks associated with immediate partial breast reconstruction include fat necrosis and nipple necrosis. The rate of fat necrosis could be worsened by radiotherapy.

Nipple-Areola Reconstruction

The first stage of breast reconstruction centers solely on reconstruction of the breast mound. For some patients, merely having a breast mound is all the reconstruction that they desire. They are able to appear symmetrical in their clothes, including bathing suits. If patients desire reconstruction of the nipple-areola complex, it is performed as a second stage. If the patient is to receive adjunctive chemotherapy or radiation therapy, most surgeons prefer to wait until after completion of such therapy. Changes in breast mound shape and position on the chest wall are expected after surgery and in response to radiation. Therefore, proper position of the nipple may not be able to be determined until 2 to 3 months after the initial surgery.

The nipple is created from local flaps on the breast mound. Numerous different techniques have been described, but all have similar limitations. Within 12 months, most undergo at least a 50% reduction in projection. Therefore, at the initial surgery the nipple is made larger than desired (Fig. 35-13). The pigmented areola was originally reconstructed with split-thickness skin grafts from the hyperpigmented upper medial aspect of the thigh, labia majora, or retroauricular regions. This has been replaced with medical tattooing. Pigment is matched to the native nipple areola from the other side. Tattooing is performed 3 to 6 weeks after creation of the nipple. In most cases the pigment fades over time and should be tattooed darker than desired. Because of fading of the areolar tattoo and flattening of the nipple flap, others have attempted cryopreservation of the nipple, which has produced only mediocre results because of tissue injury with the freezing process. Moreover, as mentioned earlier, preservation of the nipple-areolar complex poses an oncologic risk.

OUTCOME

In the past, the concerns of immediate breast reconstruction have been possible compromise of the ablative procedure, increased risks associated with surgery, altered survival, and impaired detection of locally recurrent disease. Therefore, surgeons have been reluctant to suggest reconstruction to their patients. One of the main concerns expressed by surgeons who perform mastectomies is whether a reconstructed breast can be adequately monitored for recurrence. These concerns are only increased as more and more surgeons are performing skin-sparing mastectomies in conjunction with immediate reconstruction. To date, no study has been able to demonstrate any difference in survival between patients undergoing breast reconstruction and those undergoing mastectomy alone. Even in cases of advanced disease, reconstruction has not adversely affected outcomes. Some studies have even stated that the complications of seroma and mastectomy skin flap necrosis are significantly

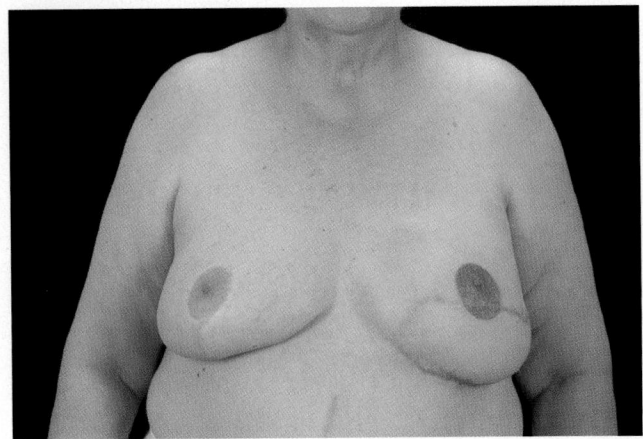

Figure 35-14 This patient underwent delayed breast reconstruction with a pedicled TRAM flap on her left breast and a breast reduction symmetry procedure on the right breast.

decreased. Therefore, based on oncologic concerns alone, breast reconstruction is not excluded from the treatment of breast cancer.

MANAGEMENT OF THE CONTRALATERAL BREAST

The challenge of breast reconstruction requires not only creating a natural-appearing breast but also achieving breast symmetry. Accordingly, on occasion, breast reconstruction requires an additional procedure on the contralateral breast. Occasionally, the mastectomy affords the patient the opportunity to obtain the breast size or shape modification that she had long desired previously. In reconstructing postmastectomy breasts, matching preexisting ptosis and larger contralateral breast size is a difficult task. In the absence of medical contraindications, a reduction mammoplasty, mastopexy, or insertion of an implant may be required to optimize the breast reconstruction to achieve optimal symmetry (Fig. 35-14). Although the risk for development of cancer in the contralateral breast is low (~4%), in reconstructing the contralateral breast, results are best if done with the same reconstructive option. *BRCA*-positive patients require additional counseling to discuss their ultimate risk for a metachronous cancer in the contralateral breast, and such women may opt for simultaneous, bilateral mastectomy with reconstruction.

SURVEILLANCE

Reconstructed breasts can be monitored clinically for evidence of recurrence. If a firm subcutaneous mass or cobblestoning of the skin develops, fine-needle biopsy or core biopsy is performed.[66] This firm mass is usually fat necrosis, which is very common after radiotherapy. Routine mammographic screening of a TRAM flap breast reconstruction for surveillance is not recommended.

Several other tools have been used to evaluate for recurrent breast cancer, including ultrasound, magnetic resonance imaging, computed tomography, and scintimammography. Overall, the most reliable means of diagnosing recurrent breast cancer after TRAM flap reconstruction has been fine-needle, core, or open biopsy when indicated.[66] Cancer recurrence can be effectively managed with surgical excision of the involved tissues, chemotherapy, or radiation therapy, or any combination of these treatments. Removal of the flap was necessary only in the setting of mulitfocal recurrence or involvement of the flap pedicle with disease.[67]

CONCLUSION

Breast reconstruction may be one of the most significant female surgeries of this era and may reverse the dread that has been associated with the loss of one's breast. Breast reconstruction may even lessen the fear that contributes to women's avoidance of medical evaluation of breast problems. Immediate breast reconstruction is favored because studies have demonstrated no increased oncologic risk, no delay in adjuvant therapy, better aesthetic outcomes, less depression, and more cost-effectiveness. Skin-sparing mastectomy can provide a better outcome at no increased risk for local recurrence, distant spread, or decreased disease-free survival. The planning and options for breast reconstruction must be individualized for each patient to minimize the risk for complications. The use of autogenous tissue can provide superior results but at the cost of a donor site. With the advent of tissue engineering, it may some day be possible to reconstruct a patient's breast with her own cultured adipocytes harvested by liposuction with minimal risk of donor site complications.

Selected References

Grotting JC, Urist MM, Maddox WA, Vasconez LO: Conventional TRAM flap versus free microsurgical TRAM flap for immediate breast reconstruction. Plast Reconstr Surg 83:828-844, 1989.

The authors described use of the lower abdomen skin paddle and rectus abdominis muscle as a free flap for microvascular tissue transfer in breast reconstruction with several advantages over the pedicled TRAM flap.

Hartrampf CR, Scheflan M, Black PW: Breast reconstruction with a transverse abdominal island flap. Plast Reconstr Surg 69:216-225, 1982.

The authors redescribed reconstruction of mastectomy defects with a transversely oriented skin paddle based on perforators from the rectus abdominis muscle.

Khoo A, Kross SS, Reece GP, et al: A comparison of resource costs of immediate and delayed breast reconstruction. Plast Reconstr Surg 101:964-970, 1998.

This report evaluated the cost of delayed versus immediate breast reconstruction in 276 patients and concluded that mastectomy with immediate breast reconstruction is significantly less expensive than mastectomy followed by delayed reconstruction.

Shaw WW: Breast reconstruction by superior gluteal microvascular free flaps without silicone implants. Plast Reconstr Surg 72:490-501, 1983.

> The author described his successful experience in reconstructing mastectomy defects with the free superior gluteal flap in 10 patients.

Singletary SE: Skin-sparing mastectomy with immediate breast reconstruction: The M. D. Anderson Cancer Center experience. Ann Surg Oncol 3:411-416, 1996.

> This report on 545 patients undergoing skin-sparing mastectomies and immediate breast reconstruction demonstrated a low regional recurrence rate of 2.6%. This recurrence was found to be a function of tumor biology and disease stage, not use of immediate breast reconstruction or skin-sparing mastectomy.

Stevens LA, McGrath MH, Druss GD, et al: The psychological impact of immediate breast reconstruction for women with early breast cancer. Plast Reconstr Surg 73:619-628, 1984.

> This prospective study evaluated the psychological effects of immediate versus delayed breast reconstruction. Patients' mood, body image, sexuality, femininity, and social and occupational functioning were found to be superior in the group who underwent immediate breast reconstruction.

References

1. Cronin TD, Gerow FJ: Augmentation mammaplasty: A new natural feel prosthesis. In Transactions of the Third International Congress of Plastic Surgery. Amsterdam, Excerpta Medica, 1963.
2. Mandel MA: Subcutaneous mastectomy with immediate reconstruction of the large breast. Surg Gynecol Obstet 146:90-92, 1978.
3. Pontes R: Single stage reconstruction of the missing breast. Br J Plast Surg 26:377-380, 1973.
4. Snyderman RK, Guthrie RH: Reconstruction of the female breast following radical mastectomy. Plast Reconstr Surg 47:565-567, 1971.
5. Manchot C: Die Hautarterien des Menschlichen Korpers. Leipzig, Vogel, 1889.
6. Ryan JJ: A lower thoracic advancement flap in breast reconstruction after mastectomy. Plast Reconstr Surg 70:153-160, 1982.
7. Dowden RV: Selection criteria for successful immediate breast reconstruction. Plast Reconstr Surg 88:628-634, 1991.
8. Brandberg Y, Malm M, Blomqvist L: A prospective and randomized study, "SVEA," comparing effects of three methods for delayed breast reconstruction on quality of life, patient-defined problem areas of life, and cosmetic result. Plast Reconstr Surg 105:66-76, 2000.
9. Schain WS, Wellisch DK, Pasnau RO, et al: The sooner the better: A study of psychological factors in women undergoing immediate versus delayed breast reconstruction. Am J Psychiatry 142:40-46, 1985.
10. Schain WS, Jacobs E, Wellisch DK: Psychosocial issues in breast reconstruction: Intrapsychic, interpersonal, and practical concerns. Clin Plast Surg 11:237-251, 1984.
11. Rowland JH: Psychological impact of treatments for breast cancer. In Spear SL (ed): Surgery of the Breast: Principles and Art. Philadelphia, Lippincott-Raven, 1998, pp 295-313.
12. Rowland J, Meyerowitz B, Ganz PA, et al: Body image and sexual functioning following reconstructive surgery in breast cancer survivors. Proc Am Soc Clin Oncol 15:124, 1996.
13. Stevens LA, McGrath MH, Druss RG, et al: The psychological impact of immediate breast reconstruction for women with early breast cancer. Plast Reconstr Surg 73:619-628, 1984.
14. Wellisch DK, Schain WS, Noone RB, et al: Psychosocial correlates of immediate versus delayed reconstruction of the breast. Plast Reconstr Surg 76:713-718, 1985.
15. Khoo A, Kroll SS, Reece GP, et al: A comparison of resource costs of immediate and delayed breast reconstruction. Plast Reconstr Surg 101:964-970, 1998.
16. Losken A, Carlson GW, Bostwick J III, et al: Trends in unilateral breast reconstruction and management of the contralateral breast: The Emory experience. Plast Reconstr Surg 110:89-97, 2002.
17. Losken A, Elwood ET, Styblo TM, et al: The role of reduction mammaplasty in reconstructing partial mastectomy defects. Plast Reconstr Surg 109:968-977, 2002.
18. English JM, Tittle BJ, Barton FE: Breast cancer, cancer prophylaxis and breast reconstruction: Selected readings. Plast Surg 7:11, 1994.
19. Trabulsy PP, Anthony JP, Mathes SJ: Changing trends in postmastectomy breast reconstruction: A 13-year experience. Plast Reconstr Surg 93:1418-1427, 1994.
20. Salhab M, Al Sarakbi W, Joseph A, et al: Skin-sparing mastectomy and immediate breast reconstruction: Patient satisfaction and clinical outcome. Int J Clin Oncol 11:51-54, 2006.
21. Langstein HN, Cheng MH, Singletary SE, et al: Breast cancer recurrence after immediate reconstruction: Patterns and significance. Plast Reconstr Surg 111:712-722, 2003.
22. Allweis TM, Boisvert ME, Otero SE, et al: Immediate reconstruction after mastectomy for breast cancer does not prolong the time to starting adjuvant chemotherapy. Am J Surg 183:218-221, 2002.
23. Singletary SE: Skin-sparing mastectomy with immediate breast reconstruction: The M. D. Anderson Cancer Center experience. Ann Surg Oncol 3:411-416, 1996.
24. Simmons RM, Brennan M, Christos P, et al: Analysis of nipple/areolar involvement with mastectomy: Can the areola be preserved? Ann Surg Oncol 9:165-168, 2002.
25. Petit JY, Veronesi U, Orecchia R, et al: Nipple-sparing mastectomy in association with intra operative radiotherapy: A new type of mastectomy for breast cancer treatment. Breast Cancer Res Treat 96:47-51, 2006.
26. Nahabedian MY, Tsangaris TN: Breast reconstruction following subcutaneous mastectomy for cancer: A critical appraisal of the nipple-areola complex. Plast Reconstr Surg 117:1083-1090, 2006.
27. Mori H, Umeda T, Osanai T, Hata Y: Esthetic evaluation of immediate breast reconstruction after nipple-sparing or skin-sparing mastectomy. Breast Cancer 12:299-303, 2005.
28. Hartrampf CR, Scheflan M, Black PW: Breast reconstruction with a transverse abdominal island flap. Plast Reconstr Surg 69:216-225, 1982.
29. Kroll SS, Schusterman MA, Tadjalli HE, et al: Risk of recurrence after treatment of early breast cancer with skin-sparing mastectomy. Ann Surg Oncol 4:193-197, 1997.
30. Torresan RZ, dos Santos CC, Okamura H, Alvarenga M: Evaluation of residual glandular tissue after skin-sparing mastectomies. Ann Surg Oncol 12:1037-1044, 2005.
31. Pennisi VR: Making a definite inframammary fold under a reconstructed breast. Plast Reconstr Surg 60:523-525, 1977.
32. Giacalone PL, Bricout N, Dantas MJ, et al: Achieving symmetry in unilateral breast reconstruction: 17 years experience with 683 patients. Aesthetic Plast Surg 26:299-302, 2002.

33. Chawla AK, Kachnic LA, Taghian AG, et al: Radiotherapy and breast reconstruction: Complications and cosmesis with TRAM versus tissue expander/implant. Int J Radiat Oncol Biol Phys 54:520-526, 2002.

34. Javaid M, Song F, Leinster S, et al: Radiation effects on the cosmetic outcomes of immediate and delayed autologous breast reconstruction: An argument about timing. J Plast Reconstr Aesthet Surg 59:16-26, 2006.

35. Gruber RP: Nipple-areola reconstruction: A review of techniques. Clin Plast Surg 6:71-83, 1979.

36. Gamboa-Bobadilla GM: Implant breast reconstruction using acellular dermal matrix. Ann Plast Surg 56:22-25, 2006.

37. Breuing KH, Warren SM: Immediate bilateral breast reconstruction with implants and inferolateral AlloDerm slings. Ann Plast Surg 55:232-239, 2005.

38. Clugston PA, Gingrass MK, Azurin D, et al: Ipsilateral pedicled TRAM flaps: The safer alternative? Plast Reconstr Surg 105:77-82, 2000.

39. Gibney J: Use of a permanent tissue expander for breast reconstruction. Plast Reconstr Surg 84:607-620, 1989.

40. Radovan C: Breast reconstruction after mastectomy using the temporary expander. Plast Reconstr Surg 69:195-208, 1982.

41. Hammond DC, Capraro PA, Ozolins EB, et al: Use of a skin-sparing reduction pattern to create a combination skin-muscle flap pocket in immediate breast reconstruction. Plast Reconstr Surg 110:206-211, 2002.

42. Shaikh N, LaTrenta G, Swistel A, et al: Detection of recurrent breast cancer after TRAM flap reconstruction. Ann Plast Surg 47:602-607, 2001.

43. Benediktsson K, Perbeck L: Capsular contracture around saline-filled and textured subcutaneously-placed implants in irradiated and non-irradiated breast cancer patients: Five years of monitoring of a prospective trial. J Plast Reconstr Aesthet Surg 59:27-34, 2006.

44. Ascherman JA, Hanasono MM, Newman MI, Hughes DB: Immediate breast reconstruction in breast cancer patients treated with radiation therapy. Plast Reconstr Surg 117:359-365, 2006.

45. Spear SL, Onyewu C: Staged breast reconstruction with saline-filled implants in the irradiated breast: Recent trends and therapeutic implications. Plast Reconstr Surg 105:930-942, 2000.

46. Bostwick J III, Scheflan M: The latissimus dorsi musculocutaneous flap: A one-stage breast reconstruction. Clin Plast Surg 7:71-78, 1980.

47. Biggs TM, Cronin ED: Technical aspects of the latissimus dorsi myocutaneous flap in breast reconstruction. Ann Plast Surg 6:381-388, 1981.

48. Cohen BE, Cronin ED: Breast reconstruction with the latissimus dorsi musculocutaneous flap. Clin Plast Surg 11:287-302, 1984.

49. Maxwell GP, McGibbon BM, Hoopes JE: Vascular considerations in the use of a latissimus dorsi myocutaneous flap after a mastectomy with an axillary dissection. Plast Reconstr Surg 64:771-780, 1979.

50. Gillies HD: Design of direct pedicle flaps. BMJ 2:1008, 1932.

51. Moon HK, Taylor GI: The vascular anatomy of rectus abdominis musculocutaneous flaps based on the deep superior epigastric system. Plast Reconstr Surg 82:815-832, 1988.

52. Holm C, Mayr M, Hofter E, Ninkovic M: Perfusion zones of the DIEP flap revisited: A clinical study. Plast Recontr Surg 117:37-43, 2006.

53. Kroll SS: Fat necrosis in free transverse rectus abdominis myocutaneous and deep inferior epigastric perforator flaps. Plast Reconstr Surg 106:576-583, 2000.

54. Scheer AS, Novak CB, Neligan PC, Lipa JE: Complications associated with breast reconstruction using a perforator flap compared with a free TRAM flap. Ann Plast Surg 56:355-358, 2006.

55. Bajaj AK, Chevray PM, Chang DW: Comparison of donor-site complications and functional outcomes in free muscle-sparing TRAM flap and free DIEP flap breast reconstruction. Plast Reconstr Surg 117:737-746, 2006.

56. Kroll SS, Netscher DT: Complications of TRAM flap breast reconstruction in obese patients. Plast Reconstr Surg 84:886-892, 1989.

57. Lejour M, Dome M: Abdominal wall function after rectus abdominis transfer. Plast Reconstr Surg 87:1054-1068, 1991.

58. Grotting JC, Urist MM, Maddox WA, et al: Conventional TRAM flap versus free microsurgical TRAM flap for immediate breast reconstruction. Plast Reconstr Surg 83:828-844, 1989.

59. Hartrampf CR Jr: Abdominal wall competence in transverse abdominal island flap operations. Ann Plast Surg 12:139-146, 1984.

60. Paterson P, Sterne GD, Fatah F: Mesh assisted direct closure of bilateral TRAM flap donor sites. Br J Plast Surg 2005, Dec 11 [Epub ahead of print].

61. Zienowicz RJ, May JW Jr: Hernia prevention and aesthetic contouring of the abdomen following TRAM flap breast reconstruction by the use of poly polypropylene mesh. Plast Reconstr Surg 96:1346-1350, 1995.

62. Selber JC, Kurichi JE, Vega SJ, et al: Risk factors and complications in free TRAM flap breast reconstruction. Ann Plast Surg 56:492-497, 2006.

63. Spear SL, Ducic I, Cuoco F, Hannan C: The effect of smoking on flap and donor-site complications in pedicled TRAM breast reconstruction. Plast Reconstr Surg 116:1873-1880, 2005.

64. Shaw WW: Breast reconstruction by superior gluteal microvascular free flaps without silicone implants. Plast Reconstr Surg 72:490-501, 1983.

65. Hartrampf CR Jr, Noel RT, Drazan L, et al: Rubens' fat pad for breast reconstruction: A peri-iliac soft-tissue free flap. Plast Reconstr Surg 93:402-407, 1994.

66. Ulasal BG, Cheng MH, Wei FC, et al: Breast reconstruction using the entire transverse abdominal adipocutaneous flap based on unilateral superficial or deep inferior epigastric vessls. Plast Reconstr Surg 117:1395-1403, 2006.

67. Howard MA, Polo K, Pusic AL, et al: Breast cancer local recurrence after mastectomy and TRAM flap reconstruction: Incidence and treatment options. Plast Reconstr Surg 15:1381-1386, 2006.

ENDOCRINE

CHAPTER 36

Thyroid

John B. Hanks, MD   and   Leslie J. Salomone, MD

Historical Perspective
Anatomy
Physiology of the Thyroid Gland
Disorders of Thyroid Metabolism—Benign Thyroid Disease
Workup and Diagnosis of a Solitary Thyroid Nodule
Thyroid Malignancies
Surgical Approaches to the Thyroid Gland and Adjacent Structures

HISTORICAL PERSPECTIVE

The name thyroid is derived from the Greek description of a shield-shaped gland in the anterior aspect of the neck *(thyreoides)*. Classic anatomic descriptions of the thyroid were available in the 16th and 17th centuries, but the function of the gland was not well understood. By the 19th century, pathologic enlargement of the thyroid, or goiter, was described. Iodine-rich seaweed was used to treat this condition. Direct surgical approaches to thyroid masses had frighteningly high complication and mortality rates.

In the late 19th century, two surgeon-physiologists revolutionized treatment of thyroid diseases. Theodor Billroth and Emil Theodor Kocher established large clinics in Europe and, through development of skilled surgical techniques combined with newer anesthetic and antiseptic principles, provided surgical results that proved the safety and efficacy of thyroid surgery for benign and malignant problems. As a result of his pioneering developments in the understanding of thyroid physiology, Kocher received the Nobel Prize in 1909.

The 20th century started with the contributions of Kocher and Billroth. In rapid succession, the understand-ing of altered physiology, including hypothyroidism, hyperthyroidism, and thyroid cancer, and advances in imaging, epidemiology, and most recently, minimally invasive diagnostic and surgical techniques have taken place. These advances have allowed the diagnosis and treatment of thyroid diseases to become rapid, cost-effective, low-morbidity procedures.

ANATOMY

Embryology

The tissue bud that ultimately becomes the thyroid gland arises initially as a midline diverticulum in the floor of the pharynx. This tissue originates in the primitive alimentary tract and consists of cells of endodermal origin. The main portion of this cellular structure descends into the neck and develops into a bilobar solid organ. The original attachment in the pharynx is in the buccal cavity at the foramen cecum. This structure becomes the thyroglossal duct, which is usually reabsorbed after 6 weeks of age. The very distal end of this remnant may occasionally be retained and mature as a pyramidal lobe in the adult thyroid.

Microscopic thyroid follicles first appear as the lateral lobes develop. When the embryo is about 6 cm in length, these follicles begin to develop colloid. In the third month the follicular cells first demonstrate iodine trapping, and thyroid hormone secretion initially begins. Calcitonin-producing C cells arise from the fourth pharyngeal pouch and migrate from the neural crest into the lateral lobes of the thyroid. These cells migrate into the lateral and posterior upper two thirds of the thyroid lobes and are distributed among the follicles. In adults, they remain limited to the upper and middle areas of the gland, usually in the posterior and medial aspects. These C cells are the only component of the adult gland not of endodermal origin.

Knowledge of basic embryology is essential for understanding certain embryologic congenital malformations, including thyroglossal duct cysts and fistulas, which result from retained tissue along the thyroglossal duct. Most thyroglossal duct cysts are found immediately beneath the hyoid bone and are noted in early childhood or infancy. These cysts are almost always in the midline and can be found from the base of the tongue to the suprasternal notch. They usually occur as a mass found in the midline on physical examination or when a localized infection occurs within that mass. A chronically infected or draining thyroglossal duct cyst can lead to a chronic draining fistula. For this reason, all thyroglossal duct cysts, on diagnosis, are treated surgically and excised because of their potential for infection. The thyroglossal duct commonly passes through the center of the hyoid bone, thus requiring removal of the central portion of the structure. Occasionally, papillary cancer can occur in the thyroid tissue within the thyroglossal duct cyst, and complete removal of the tract is required.

When the median thyroid anlage does not descend in normal fashion, a lingual thyroid can result. In most of these cases this may be the only thyroid tissue that remains. Enlargement of a lingual thyroid can cause airway obstruction, dysphagia, or bleeding. Most lingual thyroid glands can be suppressed with thyroid hormone administration. In particularly resistant lingual thyroids, radioactive iodine treatment may represent another alternative.

In unusual circumstances, ectopic thyroid tissue can be found in the central compartment of the neck. Small amounts of ectopic tissue may be located under the lower poles of a normal thyroid and occasionally in the anterior mediastinum. Historically, the thyroid tissue described in lateral neck compartments was known as lateral aberrant thyroid tissue and was explained as an embryologic variation. This concept has essentially been disproved, and it is thought that any thyroid tissue found in the lateral aspect of the neck, including around the vascular structures of the neck, may represent metastatic deposits from well-differentiated thyroid carcinoma.

Adult Surgical Anatomy

A normally developed adult thyroid is a bilobed structure that lies next to the thyroid cartilage in a position anterior and lateral to the junction of the larynx and trachea. In this position the thyroid encircles about 75% of the diameter of the junction of the larynx and the upper part of the trachea. The two lateral lobes are joined at the midline by an isthmus, whose superior edge is situated at or just below the cricoid cartilage. The pyramidal lobe represents the most distal portion of the thyroglossal duct and in an adult may be a prominent structure that can extend from the midline of the isthmus as far cephalad as the hyoid bone.

A thin layer of connective tissue surrounds the thyroid. This tissue is part of the fascial layer that invests the trachea. This fascia is different from the thyroid capsule, and during surgery it can easily be separated from the capsule, whereas the true capsule of the thyroid cannot.

This fascia coalesces with the thyroid capsule posteriorly and laterally to form a suspensory ligament known as the ligament of Berry. The ligament of Berry is closely attached to the cricoid cartilage and has important surgical implications because of its relationship to the recurrent laryngeal nerve.

Recurrent Laryngeal Nerve

The recurrent laryngeal nerves ascend on either side of the trachea, and each lies just lateral to the ligament of Berry as they enter the larynx. There are a number of important variations. In about 25% of patients the recurrent laryngeal nerve is contained within the ligament as it enters the larynx. On the right side, the recurrent laryngeal nerve separates from the vagus as it crosses the subclavian artery; it then passes posteriorly and ascends in a lateral position to the trachea along the tracheoesophageal groove. The right recurrent laryngeal nerve can usually be found no further than 1 cm lateral to or within the tracheoesophageal groove at the level of the lower border of the thyroid. As it ascends to the midportion of the thyroid, however, the nerve assumes its position within the tracheoesophageal groove. At this location the nerve might divide into one, two, or more branches as it enters the first or second ring of the trachea, with the most important branch disappearing beneath the inferior border of the cricothyroid muscle. The nerve can usually be found immediately anterior or posterior to a main arterial trunk of the inferior thyroid artery at this level. Unusually, a nonrecurrent right laryngeal nerve can arise directly from the vagus and course medially into the larynx. This nonrecurrent anatomy is found in 0.5% to 1.5% of patients. Even more infrequently, patients may have both a recurrent and a nonrecurrent laryngeal nerve on the right. These two nerves usually join in a position beneath the lower border of the thyroid.[1]

On the left side, the recurrent laryngeal nerve separates from the vagus as that nerve traverses over the arch of the aorta. The left recurrent laryngeal nerve then passes inferior and medial to the aorta and begins to ascend toward the larynx, where it finds its way into the tracheoesophageal groove as it ascends to the level of the lower lobe of the thyroid. Both recurrent laryngeal nerves are consistently found within the tracheoesophageal groove when they are within 2.5 cm of their entrance into the larynx. These nerves pass either inferior or posterior to an arterial branch of the inferior thyroid artery and eventually enter the larynx at the level of the cricothyroid articulation on the caudal border of the cricothyroid muscle. Here the nerve is immediately adjacent to the superior parathyroid, the inferior thyroid artery, and the most posterior aspect of the thyroid. Great care is needed during surgical dissection in this area because the nerve is essentially tethered as it dives beneath the cricothyroid muscle and can be stretched by overly vigorous dissection (Fig. 36-1).

The recurrent laryngeal nerve has mixed motor, sensate, and autonomic functions. Damage to a recurrent laryngeal nerve results in mixed pathology, the most important of which is paralysis of the vocal cord on the side affected. Such damage might result in a cord that

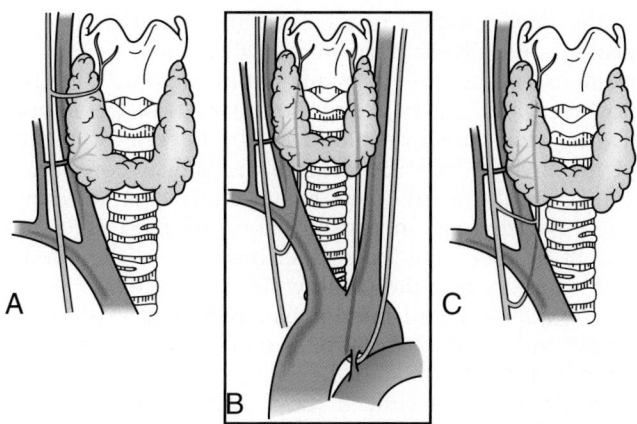

Figure 36-1 Anomalous variations in the course of the right recurrent laryngeal nerve. **A,** A nonrecurrent laryngeal nerve arises from the vagus. **B,** The normal course of the recurrent laryngeal nerve arises from the vagus after it passes beneath the subclavian artery. **C,** The unusual nonrecurrent nerve and the recurrent laryngeal nerve join to form a common distal nerve. (From Greenfield LJ [ed]: Surgery: Scientific Principles and Practice, 2nd ed. Philadelphia, Lippincott-Raven, 1997, p 1165.)

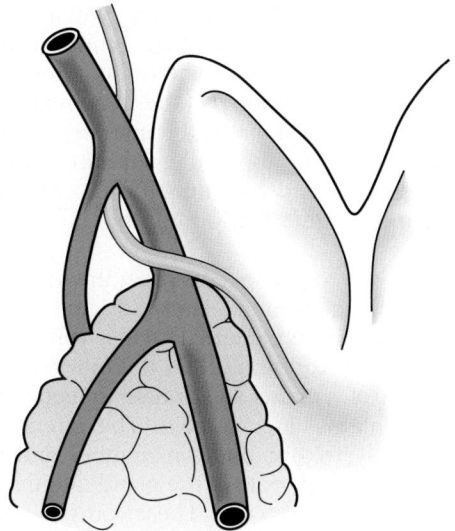

Figure 36-2 Relationship between the external branch of the superior laryngeal nerve (*yellow*) and the superior thyroid artery. The nerve can course inferiorly and medially and may run partly along with or around the artery or branches of the artery as they enter the superior lobe of the thyroid. (From Duh QY: Surgical anatomy and embryology of the thyroid and parathyroid glands and recurrent and external laryngeal nerves. In Clark OH, Duh QY [eds]: Textbook of Endocrine Surgery. Philadelphia, WB Saunders, 1997, p 11.)

remains in a medial position or just lateral to the midline. A normal voice, albeit weakened, can occur if the remaining functioning contralateral cord is able to approximate the paralyzed cord. If the vocal cord remains paralyzed in an abducted position and closure cannot occur, a severely impaired voice and ineffective cough can result. If the recurrent laryngeal nerves are damaged bilaterally, complete loss of voice or airway obstruction may occur and possibly require emergency intubation and tracheostomy. Occasionally, bilateral damage can result in cords taking an abducted position, which although allowing airway movement, may result in upper respiratory infection because of ineffective cough.[1]

Superior Laryngeal Nerve

The superior laryngeal nerve separates from the vagus nerve at the base of the skull and descends toward the superior pole of the thyroid along the internal carotid artery. At the level of the hyoid cornu it divides into two branches. The larger internal branch has sensory function and enters the thyrohyoid membrane, where it innervates the larynx. The smaller external branch continues to travel along the lateral surface of the inferior pharyngeal constrictor muscle and usually descends anteriorly and medially along with the superior thyroid artery. Within 1 cm of the entrance of the superior thyroid artery into the thyroid capsule, the nerve generally takes a medial course and enters the cricothyroid muscle (Fig. 36-2). This relationship is extremely important because during thyroid lobectomy, the external branch is not usually visualized since it has already entered the inferior pharyngeal muscle fascia. This nerve is at risk of being severed or entrapped, however, if the superior pole vessels are ligated at too great a distance above the superior pole of the thyroid. Damage to the external

branch can result in severe loss of voice quality or strength. Although such loss may not be as clinically devastating as recurrent laryngeal nerve damage, it is extremely bothersome to patients whose occupation demands good voice quality.[1]

Blood Supply

The arterial supply to the thyroid gland consists of four main arteries, two superior and two inferior. The superior thyroid artery is the first branch of the external carotid artery and arises immediately above the bifurcation of the common carotid artery. The superior thyroid artery courses medially onto the surface of the inferior pharyngeal constrictor muscle and enters the apex of the superior pole. As the superior thyroid artery proceeds medially, it is adjacent to the external branch of the superior laryngeal nerve, and thus care must be taken to not damage it when controlling the artery.

The inferior thyroid artery takes its origin from the thyrocervical trunk. This artery ascends into the neck on either side behind the carotid sheath and then arches medially and enters the thyroid gland posteriorly, usually near the ligament of Berry. There is generally no direct arterial supply to the thyroid inferiorly. However, a thyroidea ima artery may be present in less than 5% of patients and usually arise directly from the innominate artery or from the aorta.

The inferior thyroid artery has important anatomic relationships. The recurrent laryngeal nerve is usually directly adjacent (in either an anterior or posterior position) to the inferior thyroid artery, within 1 cm of its entrance into the larynx. Careful dissection of the artery in this case is mandatory and cannot be completed until knowledge of the position of the recurrent laryngeal nerve is absolute. Additionally, the inferior thyroid artery almost always supplies both the superior and inferior parathyroid glands, and care must be taken to evaluate the parathyroids after division of the inferior thyroid artery.

Three pairs of venous systems drain the thyroid. Superior venous drainage is immediately adjacent to the superior arteries and joins the internal jugular vein at the level of the carotid bifurcation. Middle thyroid veins exist in more than half of patients and course immediately laterally into the internal jugular vein. The inferior thyroid veins are usually two or three in number and descend directly from the lower pole of the gland into the innominate and brachiocephalic veins. These veins often descend into the tail of the thymus gland.

Lymphatic System

The relationship of the thyroid gland to its lymphatic drainage is most important when considering surgical treatment of thyroid carcinoma. The thyroid gland and its neighboring structures have a rich lymphatic supply that drains the thyroid in almost every direction. Within the gland, lymphatic channels are present immediately beneath the capsule and communicate between lobes through the isthmus. This drainage connects to structures directly adjacent to the thyroid, with numerous lymphatic channels into the regional lymph nodes. These regional lymph nodes occupy a pretracheal position immediately superior to the isthmus; paratracheal nodes; tracheo-esophageal groove lymph nodes; mediastinal nodes in the anterior and superior position; jugular lymph nodes in the upper, middle, and lower distribution; and retropharyngeal and esophageal lymph nodes. Laterally, cervical lymph nodes within the posterior triangle may be involved in patients with widespread thyroid cancer. Additionally, lymph nodes within the submaxillary triangle may be involved in metastatic activity.

Papillary carcinoma of the thyroid is commonly associated with adjacent nodal metastasis. Medullary carcinoma has a strong predilection for metastatic lymphatic involvement, generally within the central compartment (the space between the internal jugular veins). For this reason, central compartment lymph node dissection is indicated at the time of total thyroidectomy for medullary carcinoma.

Parathyroid Glands

The thyroid sheath encases the lateral and posterior portion of each thyroid lobe and, as such, frequently provides a covering for the superior parathyroid gland. When the superior portion of the thyroid lobe is dissected and rolled medially, an area containing fat beneath this fascia is apparent. The superior parathyroid gland almost always lies within this fat beneath the thyroid sheath in a posterior position relative to the superior part of the thyroid lobe. The inferior parathyroid gland may also be located within the thyroid sheath on the posterior aspect

of the lower portion of the lobe and, like the superior gland, is usually encased in a small amount of fat. The position of the inferior parathyroid is more variable, however, and can be along the branches of the inferior thyroid vein lateral or inferior to the lowermost portion of the thyroid lobe. Because of the similar consistency and color of the parathyroids and the fat that surrounds them, parathyroids in both positions are most efficiently sought by following the smaller branches of the inferior thyroid artery into the parathyroid substance.

The superior and inferior parathyroid glands have a single end artery that supplies them medially from the inferior thyroid artery. If the main trunk of the inferior thyroid artery is sacrificed for dissection, both parathyroids on that side become devascularized because there is no collateral blood supply to maintain viability. Careful dissection attempts to divide only the branches of the inferior thyroid entering the thyroid capsule during excision. With careful technique it is possible to maintain good vascular supply to the superior and inferior parathyroid even when total thyroidectomy is performed.

PHYSIOLOGY OF THE THYROID GLAND

The thyroid gland weighs 10 to 20 g in normal adults and is responsible for the production of two families of metabolic hormones: the thyroid hormones thyroxine (T_4) and triiodothyronine (T_3) and the calcium-regulating hormone calcitonin. The spherical thyroid follicular unit is the important site of thyroid hormone production. The thyroid follicle is made up of a single layer of cuboidal follicular cells that encompass a central depository of colloid filled mostly with thyroglobulin (Tg), the protein within which T_4 and T_3 are synthesized and stored.[2] Each follicle is surrounded by a rich network of capillaries that interdigitate among the multiple follicular units contained within normal thyroid matrix.

C cells, derived from the neural crest, migrate into the thyroid during embryologic development. These cells rest in a parafollicular position, predominantly in the upper lobe of each thyroid. C cells are responsible for production of the hormone calcitonin, which has important regulatory properties on calcium metabolism.

Iodine Metabolism

Iodine is essential for normal thyroid function. It can be efficiently absorbed from the gastrointestinal tract in the form of inorganic iodide and rapidly enters the extracellular iodide pool. The thyroid gland is responsible for storing 90% of total body iodide at any given time, with less than 10% existing in the extracellular pool. The extracellular pool consists of freshly absorbed iodide, as well as the total derived from the breakdown of previously formed thyroid hormone. Within the thyroid, iodide is stored either as preformed thyroid hormone or as iodinated amino acids.

Iodide is transported from the extracellular space into the follicular cells against a chemical and electrical gradient. The transporter is an intrinsic transmembrane protein

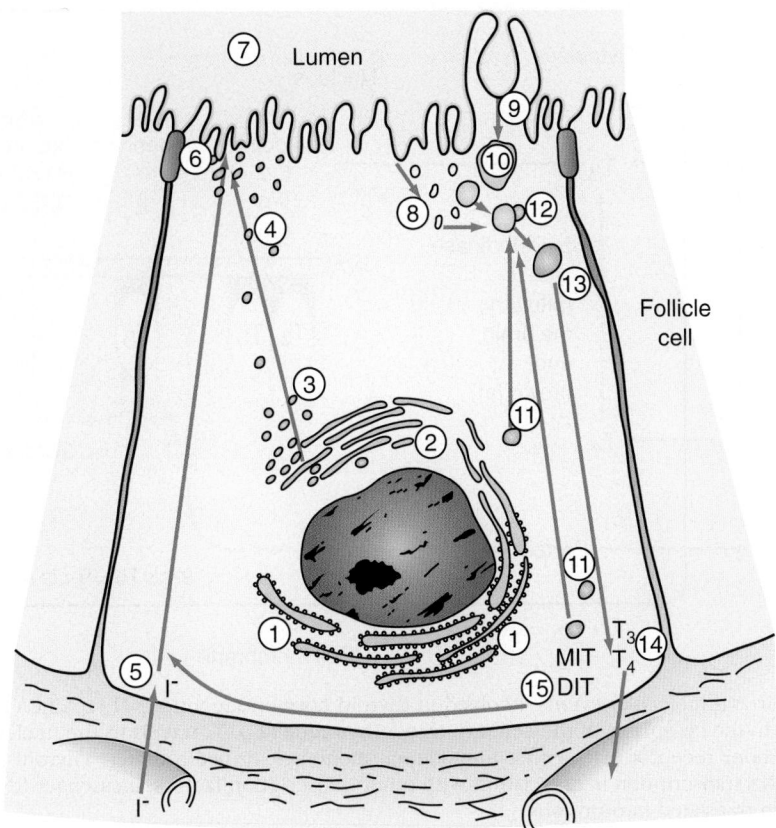

Figure 36-3 Diagrammatic scheme of thyroid hormone formation and secretion. 1, Thyroglobulin (Tg) and protein synthesis in the rough endoplasmic reticulum. 2, Coupling of the Tg carbohydrate units in the smooth endoplasmic reticulum and Golgi apparatus. 3, Formation of exocytotic vesicles. 4, Transport of exocytotic vesicles with non-iodinated Tg to the apical surface of the follicle cell and into the follicular lumen. 5, Iodide transport at the basal cell membrane. 6, Iodide oxidation, Tg iodination, and coupling of iodotyrosyl to iodothyronyl residues. 7, Storage of iodinated Tg in the follicular lumen. 8, Endocytosis by micropinocytosis. 9, Endocytosis by macropinocytosis (pseudopods). 10, Colloid droplets. 11, Lysosome migrating to the apical pole. 12, Fusion of lysosomes with colloid droplets. 13, Phagolysosomes with Tg hydrolysis. 14, Triiodothyronine (T_3) and thyroxine (T_4) secretion. 15, Monoidotyrosine (MIT) and diiodotyrosine (DIT) deiodination.

located in the basolateral membrane of the thyroid follicular cells.[3] Once inside the cells, iodide rapidly diffuses to the apical surface, where it is quickly moved to exocytic vesicles. Here it is rapidly oxidized and bound to Tg. Transport of iodide into follicular cells is regulated by thyroid-stimulating hormone (TSH) from the pituitary gland, as well as by the follicular content of iodide.

The relationship between iodine ingestion and thyroid disease has been known for more than 100 years. At the turn of the 20th century, the practice of iodine supplementation of food and water came as a result of careful study in areas where iodine insufficiency was demonstrated and linked to endemic goiter. Significant iodine deficiency still occurs in various undeveloped parts of the world. Surprisingly, recent evaluation of urinary iodine excretion in the U.S. population indicates that a substantial number of people are currently iodine deficient here as well.[4] Iodine deficiency can result in nodular goiter, hypothyroidism and cretinism, and possibly the development of follicular thyroid carcinoma (FTC). The World Health Organization has been involved in provid-

ing dietary iodine supplementation to treat entire populations in certain areas of the world. In situations in which iodine excess occurs, processes such as Graves' disease and Hashimoto's thyroiditis can occur.

Thyroid Hormone Synthesis

Once organic iodide is efficiently oxidized and bound, it couples to Tg with tyrosine moieties to form iodotyrosines in either a single conformation (monoiodotyrosine [MIT]) or a coupled conformation (diiodotyrosine [DIT]) (Fig. 36-3). The formation of DIT and MIT is dependent on an important intracellular catalytic agent, thyroid peroxidase, which has been well characterized and is an integral part of the initial process of organification and storage of inorganic iodide. This enzyme is localized to the apical portion of the follicular cell, where it reacts at the cell-colloid interface.

MIT and DIT are biologically inert. Coupling of these two residues gives rise to the two biologically active thyroid hormones T_4 and T_3. T_4 is formed by coupling of two molecules of DIT, whereas T_3 is formed by coupling

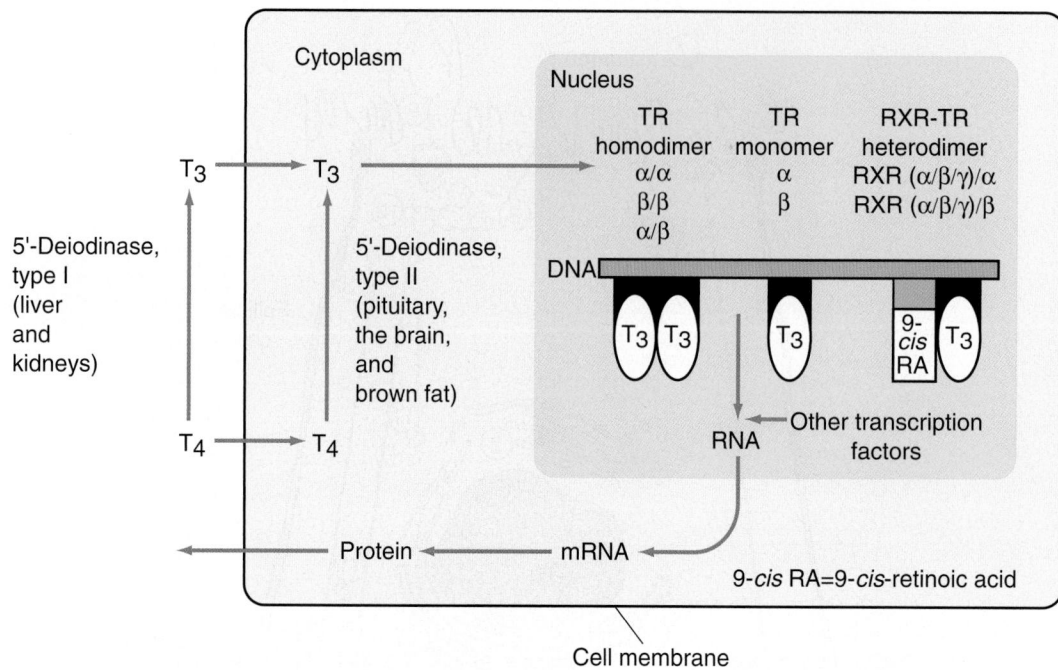

Cell membrane

Figure 36-4 Cellular and molecular events involved in thyroid hormone function. Thyroxine (T_4) is converted in the periphery and in the cytoplasm of the cell into triiodothyronine (T_3). T_3 travels to the nucleus, where it binds to the thyroid hormone receptor (TR), either homodimer, monomer, or heterodimer. Thyroid hormone receptor binding leads to RNA transcription in association with other transcription factors; messenger RNA is subsequently expressed and then translated into protein.

of a molecule of MIT with a molecule of DIT. In normal circumstances, formation of T_4 is the major pathway. Both T_3 and T_4 are bound to Tg and stored within the colloid in the center of the follicular unit, which allows quicker secretion of the hormones than if they had to be synthesized. This rapid and metabolically active process results in the storage of about 2 weeks' worth of thyroid hormone within the organism under normal circumstances.[5] The majority of thyroid hormone released from the thyroid gland is T_4, which is deiodinated in peripheral extrathyroidal tissues and converted to T_3.

Release of T_4 and T_3 is regulated by the apical membrane of the follicular cell via lysosomal hydrolysis of the colloid that contains the Tg-bound hormones. The apical membrane of the thyroid cell forms multiple pseudopodia and incorporates Tg into small vesicles, which are then brought within the cell apparatus. Within the vesicles, lysosomal hydrolysis results in reduction of the disulfide bonds, and both T_3 and T_4 are then free to pass through the basement membrane and be absorbed into the circulation, where more than 99% of each of the hormones is bound to serum proteins.[6] This metabolic process is efficient in releasing T_3 and T_4 while maintaining the storage components Tg and colloid within the follicular apparatus. Although sensitive assays of peripheral blood can measure Tg, peripheral Tg represents an extremely small fraction of total body stores. Residual iodotyrosines undergo peripheral breakdown, deiodination, and recycling and can then be added to the recently absorbed iodide stores and become available for the synthesis of new thyroid hormone (Fig. 36-4).[5]

Regulation of Thyroid Hormone Secretion

Triiodothyronine and Thyroxine

The hypothalamic-pituitary-thyroid axis regulates thyroid hormone production and release in a classic endocrine feedback system. The major regulator of thyroid gland activity is the glycoprotein TSH, which is a major growth factor for the thyroid. TSH stimulates thyroid cell growth and differentiation, as well as iodine uptake and organification and release of T_3 and T_4 from Tg. Additionally, TSH has been shown to stimulate the growth and invasive characteristics of some well-differentiated thyroid cancer cell lines in vitro.

TSH is a 28-kd glycoprotein that is secreted in a pulsatile fashion by the anterior pituitary gland. It has two components. The α subunit is common to other anterior pituitary hormones. However, the β subunit is unique to TSH and determines the hormone's biologic specificity. TSH has specific activity through a receptor on the surface of the thyroid cell. Once the receptor is activated, it interacts with a guanine nucleotide–binding protein (G protein). This interaction stimulates the production of cyclic adenosine monophosphate (AMP). It is through this cyclic AMP pathway that the synthesis of thyroid hormones is mediated. The G-protein, cyclic AMP signal transduction pathway is an important hormone-synthesizing event. Receptors that are coupled with G proteins have seven transmembrane-spanning domains with cytoplasmic and extracellular loops. The first three of these cytoplasmic loops have important relationships in mediating the TSH-dependent increase in cyclic AMP production and therefore in stimulating thyroid hormone production. The receptors that respond to TSH have been identified and cloned. Specific mutations in the genetics of this system have been identified and associated with follicular thyroid neoplasms.[7]

The feedback loop is an important regulator of TSH secretion. Increased thyrotropin-releasing hormone (TRH) from the paraventricular nucleus of the hypothalamus and reduced levels of T_3 stimulate release of TSH from the anterior pituitary. TRH is a three–amino acid peptide that passes through the hypothalamic portal system into the median eminence and through the pituitary stalk to the anterior pituitary. Peripheral thyroid hormone levels may, in addition to stimulating release of TSH from the anterior pituitary, enhance TRH secretion.

Negative feedback through increased peripheral levels of T_3 and T_4 can affect TSH secretion. Peripheral T_4 is locally deiodinated in the pituitary and converted to T_3, which then directly inhibits the release and synthesis of TSH. It may be that T_3 results in this process by down-regulating TRH receptors on the surface of anterior pituitary cells, thereby decreasing local responsiveness to TRH. Other metabolic events also appear to affect the synthesis and secretion of thyroid hormone. Catechol-amines, especially epinephrine, may have a direct stimulatory effect on thyroid hormone release and production. Human chorionic gonadotropin stimulates thyroid hormone production, and thus synthesis of thyroid hormone is increased during pregnancy. Occasional gynecologic malignancies, including hydatidiform moles with resultant elevated human chorionic gonadotropin levels, may result in elevated thyroid hormone levels. Glucocorticoids decrease thyroid hormone production through suppression of pituitary TSH secretion. A wide variety of disorders, including severe illness, lead to reduced levels of peripheral thyroid hormone without a resultant rise in TSH (nonthyroidal illness syndrome). Chronic hyperthermia and chronic starvation are associated with markedly reduced levels of both T_4 and T_3 without compensatory elevations in TSH.

Intrinsic autoregulatory mechanisms are alternative routes by which the thyroid can control intraglandular stores of thyroid hormones. In areas where dietary iodide is excessive, the thyroid gland has an autoregulated process that inhibits uptake of iodide into follicular cells. The reverse is true in iodide deficiency. Excessively large doses of iodide have interesting and complex effects, including an initial increase in organification followed by suppressive effects, a syndrome known as the Wolff-Chaikoff effect.

Thyroglobulin

Tg is a 660-kd glycoprotein that is the primary component of the colloid matrix contained within the follicle. Tg facilitates the conversion of MIT and DIT into T_3 and T_4. This process is accompanied by escape of Tg into the peripheral bloodstream, where it can be assayed. TSH enhances the whole process of endocytosis, proteolysis, and release through an adenylate cyclase system. Excess peripheral levels of iodine inhibit further release by enhancing Tg resistance to proteolysis.

Peripheral Tg can be measured to evaluate benign or malignant thyroid neoplasms. Measurement of peripheral Tg has predictive value for recurrence of well-differentiated thyroid carcinoma either locally or in metastatic deposits after initial total thyroidectomy.[8]

Calcitonin

Calcitonin is a 32–amino acid polypeptide that is secreted by the parafollicular cells, or C cells, located superolaterally in each thyroid lobe. Calcitonin acts principally to inhibit calcium absorption by osteoclasts and thereby to lower peripheral serum calcium levels. Increased peripheral levels of serum calcium stimulate calcitonin secretion. Calcitonin secretion can be stimulated clinically by infusion of calcium, pentagastrin, and alcohol.

The specific action of calcitonin takes place on the surface receptors of osteoclasts. However, its effect does not result in a marked decrease in calcium levels. In fact, patients with clinical calcitonin excess syndromes, such as medullary carcinoma of the thyroid (MCT), have little alteration in peripheral calcium metabolism. Basal or stimulated calcitonin levels are sensitive markers for primary or recurrent MCT. Whether calcitonin should be evaluated routinely for all thyroid masses in an attempt to detect the unusual sporadic medullary carcinoma is not universally agreed on.

Peripheral Action of Thyroid Hormones

In the periphery, T_3 is much more potent than T_4. T_4 has low affinity for peripheral nuclear thyroid hormone receptors (TRs) in comparison to T_3, most likely because T_4 is converted to the active form T_3 to gain the most efficient use of thyroid hormone release. As a result, the action of thyroid hormones in the periphery consists predominantly of interaction of T_3 with the nuclear TR, which then binds to regulatory regions in various gene-regulated processes. TR belongs to the steroid hormone receptor family. Two genes regulate TR production and activity, the α and β forms, which are located on chromosomes 17 and 3 (see Fig. 36-4). The receptors modulate specific patterns of expression within the tissue that contains them. The β form of TR is contained within the liver; the central nervous system contains predominantly an α form of TR. Expression of TR may be regulated by peripheral thyroid hormone concentrations; low peripheral serum thyroid hormone concentrations appear to result in an increase in TR numbers as a compensatory response. TR is directly responsible for the clinical manifestation of hormone action. The clinical result of thyroid hormone action is regulated through TR and its effect on various genes, expressions of which are then regulated in the nucleus via production of polypeptides. For example, T_3 acts on the pituitary by regulating transcription of the genes for both the α and β subunits of TSH, which results in TSH secretion. T_3 affects cardiac contractility by regulating the transcription of myosin heavy-chain production in cardiac muscle.[2]

Eighty percent of circulating T_3 and T_4 is bound to thyroxine-binding globulin in the periphery. Additionally, T_4 is bound to prealbumin, thyroxine-binding protein, and albumin. In pregnancy and other clinical situations with elevated estrogen levels (oral contraceptive pill use), thyroxine-binding globulin levels are significantly increased, thereby resulting in higher levels of bound T_4 (total) in the periphery. Such states are clinically euthyroid, however, because free T_4 levels are not altered.

Most T_3 and T_4 are bound to the extent that free T_4 constitutes less than 1% of peripheral hormone. The bound form of thyroid hormones is unable to pass from the extracellular space and must be in the free form to diffuse into extracellular tissues to affect major metabolic activity. T_3 is especially important in this regard. The process whereby T_3 and T_4 dissociate from binding protein and diffuse into extracellular tissues is an efficient process that allows tight control of peripheral metabolic activities. Most T_3 is peripherally derived by conversion from T_4. This conversion occurs as a result of deiodination, which takes place largely in the plasma and liver. Other deiodination processes are found in the central nervous system, especially the pituitary gland and brain tissues, as well as in brown adipose tissue. Peripheral conversion of T_4 to T_3 can be impaired in many clinical circumstances, such as overwhelming sepsis and malnutrition. High-dose steroid therapy can result in functional hypothyroidism as well.

The half-life of T_3 is about 8 to 12 hours, and free levels disappear rapidly from the peripheral circulation. In adults, the half-life of T_4 is about 7 days because of the efficient and significant degree of binding to carrier proteins. Therefore, thyroid hormones generally have a slow turnover time in the peripheral circulation, and the body is ensured of at least a 7- to 10-day supply of T_4 that is available for peripheral metabolism.

Inhibition of Thyroid Synthesis

Drugs

Antithyroid medications are an option for the treatment of thyroid excess states. The thionamide class of antithyroid drugs includes propylthiouracil (PTU) and methimazole (Tapazole). This class of drugs acts by inhibiting the organification and oxidation of inorganic iodine, as well as by inhibiting linkage of the initial iodotyrosine molecules MIT and DIT. In addition to these effects, PTU inhibits the peripheral conversion of T_4 to T_3. Because of this added capability, PTU is a popular choice for the rapid treatment of hyperthyroid conditions. Methimazole has longer activity and requires a single daily dose; however, it has the capability of crossing the placenta and can affect fetal development in pregnant patients. Both drugs can cause agranulocytosis; however, this occurs in less than 1% of cases. Other side effects include rash, arthralgias, neuritis, and liver dysfunction.

Iodine

Iodine, given in large doses after the administration of an antithyroid medication, can inhibit thyroid hormone release by altering the organic binding process (Wolff-Chaikoff effect). This stunning effect is transient; however, iodine supplementation can be used to treat hyperactivity of the gland in preparation for surgery.

Corticosteroids

Exogenous glucocorticoids can effectively suppress the pituitary-thyroid axis. Additionally, they can act in the periphery to inhibit peripheral conversion of T_4 to T_3. This effectively lowers serum T_3 levels, thus allowing steroids to be used as a rapid inhibitory agent in hyperthyroid conditions. Steroids can also lower serum TSH. The rapid action of steroids makes them a potentially important primary treatment of severe, previously untreated or resistant hyperthyroidism; however, they are not without potential side effects.

β-Blockers

Patients with thyrotoxicosis have increased adrenergic stimulation. Although β-blockers do not directly inhibit thyroid hormone synthesis per se, they are valuable in controlling peripheral sensitivity to catecholamines by blocking their effects. Therefore, cardiovascular symptoms such as an increased pulse rate, tremor, and anxiousness can be improved, but the hypermetabolic state can remain or progress with this treatment alone.

Tests of Thyroid Function

Evaluation of the Pituitary-Thyroid Feedback Loop

Evaluation of serum TSH is an important screening test for the diagnosis of thyroid dysfunction. TSH is measured by an ultrasensitive radioimmunometric assay, which has greatly improved clinical diagnosis. This assay is especially important in the delineation of hypothyroid from euthyroid states. Additionally, clinically euthyroid patients may have suppressed TSH levels (subclinical hyperthyroidism), and the assay can therefore demonstrate hyperthyroidism before it becomes clinically manifested. The sensitivity of the TSH assay is less affected by nonthyroidal disease processes and remains unaffected by changes in thyroid hormone–binding proteins.

More elaborate tests of the functional status of the hypothalamic-pituitary axis may require the use of a TRH stimulation test. An intravenous (IV) dose of TRH is given, for which a normal response is an elevation in TSH that peaks within 15 to 35 minutes. Patients with pituitary insufficiency then demonstrate a subnormal response to TRH, whereas those with primary hypothyroidism demonstrate enhanced TSH release from the anterior pituitary.

Serum Triiodothyronine and Thyroxine Levels

Thyroid production is initially screened by measuring serum free T_4. Total T_4, which measures both free and protein-bound hormone, can be affected by changes in hormone production or hormone binding to serum proteins; therefore, accurate evaluation of thyroid function requires measurement of free T_4 levels. However, if a direct free T_4 assay is unavailable, indirect methods suffice. The T_3 resin uptake test is one of the most common indirect measurements of the proportion of T_4 that is not protein bound. This test involves the addition of radiolabeled T_3 to the individual patient's serum. The mixture is incubated with an ion exchange resin, which allows competition for the serum-binding proteins for thyroid hormone. At higher levels of free T_4, the availability of unoccupied binding sites diminishes, and a lesser percentage of the radiolabeled T_3 is attached to the resin. If the absolute concentration of free T_4 is low, more radiolabeled T_3 is bound, and resin uptake is therefore high. The percentage of tracer bound varies inversely with the concentration and the affinity of unoccupied binding sites on the serum T_4-binding proteins. The product of the percentage of uptake and the total serum T_4 concentration is used to calculate the free T_4 index. This value reflects the absolute concentration of serum T_4. These measures are not generally used for routine screening but are helpful in the diagnosis of T_3 thyrotoxicosis.

Calcitonin

In patients with thyroid masses and in whom multiple endocrine neoplasia type 2 (MEN 2) syndrome or isolated medullary carcinoma is suspected, a baseline calcitonin level can be calculated. If there is doubt about the diagnosis, pentagastrin- or calcium-stimulated calcitonin evaluation, a 4- to 5-hour test, can be performed. Additionally, calcitonin can be used as a screening test in families with MEN 2 syndrome to document clinically inapparent disease. Use of calcitonin screening in patients with a thyroid mass, however, is not cost-efficient or necessary.

Radioactive Iodine Uptake

The radioactive iodine uptake test is becoming less widely used because of more precise biochemical measurements of T_3, T_4, and TSH. This test has in the past involved oral administration of iodine 123 (^{123}I) and calculated its uptake with radioscintigraphy. A normal result is 15% to 30% uptake of the radionuclide after about 24 hours. Use of ^{123}I is preferable because of a shorter half-life and lesser radiation exposure than with ^{131}I, which is used to radioablate thyroid neoplasms.

Thyroid Autoantibody Levels

Thyroid antigens are produced in autoimmune thyroid disorders (thyroid-stimulating immunoglobulin, antimicrosomal antibodies), including Graves' disease and Hashimoto's thyroiditis. Detection of autoantibodies can be extremely important if either of these autoimmune conditions is suspected. About 95% of patients with Hashimoto's thyroiditis and 80% with Graves' disease have detectable antimicrosomal antibodies. In Graves' disease, circulating antibodies have high affinity for TSH receptor (TSH-R) on thyroid follicular cells. Newer assays have greater sensitivity and may allow earlier detection of Graves' disease and more accurate monitoring of the effects of thyroid medication.

DISORDERS OF THYROID METABOLISM— BENIGN THYROID DISEASE

Hypothyroidism

A delicate balance between central production and peripheral action of T_3 and T_4 is required for a euthyroid state in the periphery. Clinical hypothyroidism is usually associated with decreased production in the thyroid gland, although states of limited activity in the periphery can also occur. In many underdeveloped countries, lack of sufficient iodine intake explains a large proportion of hypothyroid conditions. In more developed countries, most cases of adult hypothyroidism are caused by Hashimoto's thyroiditis, radioactive iodine therapy, or surgical removal. Another cause of hypothyroidism that is becoming increasingly relevant is drug-related altered thyroid function, particularly in the case of the cardiac antiarrhythmic drug amiodarone. Other rarer causes of hypothyroidism include inherited defects in thyroid hormone synthesis, such as defects in thyroid peroxidase and Tg production. Additionally, congenital aberrant thyroid development can occur in children, including thyroid agenesis and thyroid hypoplasia. Central nervous system abnormalities resulting in either anterior pituitary gland disease or hypothalamic disorders can give rise to centrally based hypothyroidism secondary to lack of either TSH or TRH secretion. Finally, peripheral tissue resistance to the action of thyroid hormone, possibly through an altered receptor mechanism, has been described.[7]

Endemic Goiter

Iodine deficiency can lead to a preventable disease referred to as endemic goiter, which in its severest form results in endemic cretinism. As many as a third of the world's population, specifically in underdeveloped countries, are at risk for iodine deficiency, and about 12 million people may suffer from endemic cretinism. Although countries in Southeast Asia, including India, Indonesia, and China, account for most of the total population of the world at risk for iodine deficiency, mild to moderate iodine deficiency can still be seen in a number of European countries, including Italy, Spain, Hungary, Poland, and Yugoslavia. In areas with the most severe iodine deficiency, clinical signs and symptoms of goiter appear at an earlier age. The prevalence increases dramatically in the later childhood years, with the peak attained at puberty. The appearance of goiter decreases during adulthood but remains slightly greater in women.[9]

Metabolic Consequences of Iodine Deficiency

The chronic physiologic changes that result from a lifetime of iodine deficiency involve anatomic and metabolic alterations of varying significance. As a result of chronic deficient iodine intake, production of T_4 and T_3 is decreased, thereby resulting in gradually increasing thyroid clearance of iodine and decreased renal excretion. Chronic preferential production of T_3 rather than T_4 occurs, as well as enhanced peripheral conversion of T_4 to T_3. By making production of T_3 and clearance of the metabolically active hormone as efficient as possible, clinical hypothyroidism is largely avoided by a biochemical pattern of low serum T_4 with elevated TSH and normal or above-normal levels of T_3. In the severest cases, serum T_3 and T_4 concentrations are low and serum TSH is elevated. In these situations, endemic cretinism is often found. Accompanying the physiologic changes in response to iodine deficiency, diffuse enlargement of the thyroid gland often occurs. The thyroid follicles demonstrate a hypertrophic response with a reduction in follicular spaces. As the iodine deficiency becomes more severe, follicles can become inactive and distended with colloid. Focal areas of nodular hyperplasia may develop and form nodules, some of which may become hot nodules and have autonomous function. Others become inactive and inert. Necrosis, scarring, and hemorrhage can occur and result in fibrous ingrowth; all these disorders are accompanied by marked enlargement of the gland, often in an asymmetric pattern.[9]

Postirradiation Hypothyroidism

Planned clinical hypothyroidism can be the result of treatment of certain disorders with [131]I. This treatment has become increasingly popular for patients with hyperthyroid conditions, especially Graves' disease. Between 50% and 70% of patients who receive greater than 10 mCi are at risk of becoming clinically hypothyroid. For patients undergoing this type of treatment, continued thyroid monitoring is necessary, at least on an annual basis.

External beam irradiation for lymphomatous disease of the mediastinum or for head and neck cancer is associated with subclinical hypothyroidism. This becomes particularly important in patients who have previously undergone thyroid resection for either benign or malignant disease processes.

Postsurgical Hypothyroidism

In the event that ^{131}I therapy is not available for patients with hyperthyroidism or Graves' disease, subtotal or total thyroidectomy effectively produces hypothyroidism. The incidence of permanent postoperative hypothyroidism varies with the skill of the operating surgeon and the amount of thyroid that is truly ablated. The rate of complications, however, such as recurrent laryngeal nerve damage and hypocalcemia, is increased with more aggressive surgical ablation. Other factors affecting postoperative development of hypothyroidism include antithyroid drug administration, dietary iodine availability, and lymphocytic infiltration of the remaining tissue.

Pharmacologic Hypothyroidism

Antithyroid Drugs

Common antithyroid drugs (methimazole and PTU) can, if given in sufficient quantity, result in hypothyroidism. Careful monitoring of patients taking these drugs and understanding the disease process for which they are given are mandatory in managing these patients.

Amiodarone

Amiodarone is an antiarrhythmic drug that is efficacious in treating arrhythmias. This drug contains a significant amount of iodine, and a standard dosage can aggravate thyroid dysfunction. Prolonged administration can result in thyroiditis and subsequent hyperthyroidism, followed by transient hypothyroidism. This thyroiditis is often associated with an increase in serum interleukin-6 levels, thus suggesting a cytokine inflammatory response. Severe

thyroid dysfunction can occur in patients taking amiodarone, especially those with previously documented Hashimoto's thyroiditis.

Lithium

Manic-depressive disorders rely on lithium for treatment. Lithium has the capability of inhibiting the cyclic AMP–dependent pathway of hormone formation and may, by this mechanism, inhibit the formation of thyroid hormone. Hypothyroidism in patients taking lithium is usually seen more frequently in those with underlying Hashimoto's thyroiditis, although it can occur in patients with normal thyroid function.

Cytokines

The effects of cytokines in thyroiditis may well be responsible for generation and aggravation of the disease process. The exact nature of the effects of cytokines on the development of Hashimoto's thyroiditis is unclear. It is known that hypothyroidism can develop in patients undergoing treatment with interferon alfa or interleukin-2 for certain malignant diseases; in such cases the hypothyroidism is reversible with discontinuation of these drugs. This point is particularly important in patients with underlying Hashimoto's thyroiditis, and careful history taking is essential in these patients.

Clinical Features and Diagnosis of Hypothyroidism

The developing fetus and newborn are usually protected from hypothyroidism by the transplacental passage of T_4. After birth, failure of thyroid function, if prolonged, can result in significant and sometimes irreversible changes in development leading to poor growth, mental retardation, and dwarfism. This syndrome is referred to as cretinism. During the later childhood years, hypothyroidism can result in decreased intellectual capacity but not necessarily mental retardation. Physical signs such as rectal prolapse, abdominal distention, and umbilical hernia may be present. During adolescence this condition is known as juvenile hypothyroidism.

In adults, spontaneous hypothyroidism is usually manifested in females (80%) and is a more insidious process associated with slow, progressive failure of function. In the majority of cases, this process is due to a lymphocytic thyroiditis. The classic symptoms are fatigue, headache, weight gain, dry skin, brittle hair, and muscle cramps. Severe progression of disease can result in cardiovascular symptoms, including hypertension, pericardial effusion, bradycardia, and pleural effusions. Abdominal distention with bowel edema and constipation is a sign of severe hypothyroidism. Anemia may occur in 12% of cases.

Diagnosis

In the workup of a patient with subjective symptoms of fatigue or constipation or in the workup of cardiac abnormalities, evaluation of thyroid function cannot be forgotten. Classic laboratory tests for hypothyroidism demonstrate decreased T_4 and T_3 values with increased TSH and cholesterol levels.

Treatment

Levothyroxine is a safe and effective treatment once the diagnosis is made. It is available in oral, intramuscular, and IV preparations. The vast majority of patients can be treated with oral medication. The dose is calculated according to the patient's weight. Patients with severe clinical hypothyroidism are monitored closely and gradually started on increasing doses because of sensitivity to the hormone as a result of chronic depletion of catecholamines in the myocardium.

Thyroiditis

Acute Suppurative Thyroiditis

Acute suppurative thyroiditis is extremely rare and usually the result of a severe pyogenic infection of the upper airway. The process results in severe localized pain and is generally unilateral. Abscess drainage followed by the administration of antibiotics is effective, and long-term deleterious effects on thyroid function rarely result.

Hashimoto's Thyroiditis

The major cause of hypothyroidism in the adult population is Hashimoto's thyroiditis. A complex immunologic phenomenon results in the formation of immune complexes and complement in the basement membrane of follicular cells. This leads to alterations in thyroid cell function that impair T_3 and T_4 production. These cellular reactions ultimately result in infiltration of lymphocytes and resultant fibrosis, which decreases the number and efficiency of individual follicles. As this immune phenomenon continues, the presence of TSH-blocking antibodies can be detected. Thyroid microsomal antibodies are produced that are most likely key mediators in the initial complement fixation process. As the immune process continues, changes in thyroid function can be altered by levels of these antibodies. Ultimately, a clinical hypothyroid state can occur in patients with persistent TSH-blocking antibodies.

Subacute Thyroiditis

Subacute thyroiditis occurs predominantly in females (2:1) in the United States, England, and Japan. The mean age of patients is in the 40s in most series. The exact cause is not known, although it is thought to have a viral or autoimmune origin. In the vast majority of patients, a history of an upper respiratory infection before the onset of thyroiditis can be elicited. Patients have diffuse swelling in the cervical area and a sudden increase in pain. Approximately two thirds of patients demonstrate fever, weight loss, and severe fatigue. Fine-needle aspiration (FNA) can be diagnostic if it demonstrates giant cells of an epithelioid foreign body type, which characterizes the lesion. Microscopic pathology shows large follicles infiltrated by mononuclear cells, neutrophils, and lymphocytes.

Treatment with corticosteroids or nonsteroidal anti-inflammatory drugs is effective in relieving symptoms. However, the disease process generally continues, unaffected by these medications.

Riedel's Struma

Riedel's thyroiditis (struma) is a rare entity characterized by a firm thyroid secondary to a chronic inflammatory process involving the entire gland. Symptoms of severe discomfort can occur and are due to extension into the trachea, esophagus, and laryngeal nerve. As a result, patients may have impending airway obstruction or dysphagia. Unilateral involvement of symptoms may suggest a malignancy and lead to surgical intervention. The findings at surgery can also be impressive because the process can extend into the trachea and esophagus with obliteration of anatomic planes and landmarks. Surgical pathology reveals dense fibrous tissue and nearly total obliteration of normal follicular architecture. Grossly, direct involvement of the process can result in severe tracheal and esophageal obstruction.

Treatment with thyroid hormone replacement is effective. Immediate tracheal or esophageal obstruction may require a surgical approach to relieve symptoms. Such surgery should be performed by an experienced thyroid surgeon. Only the constricting portion of the thyroid is removed.

Hyperthyroidism

Disease processes associated with increased thyroid secretion result in a predictable hypermetabolic state. Increased thyroid secretion can be caused by primary alterations within the gland (Graves' disease, toxic nodular goiter, toxic thyroid adenoma) or central nervous system disorders and increased TSH-produced stimulation of the thyroid. Most hyperthyroid states occur because of primary malfunction. Even more unusual hyperthyroid states can result from mismanaged exogenous thyroid ingestion, molar pregnancy with increased release of human chorionic gonadotropin, and unusually, thyroid malignancy with overproduction of thyroid hormone.

Graves' Disease

Grave's disease is the most common cause of hyperthyroidism (diffuse toxic goiter). This disease entity was originally described by an Irish physician, Dr. Robert Graves, in 1835. Women between the ages of 20 and 40 years are most commonly affected. The hyperthyroidism in Grave's disease is caused by stimulatory autoantibodies to TSH-R. Although several theories about the stimulus that initiates production of these antibodies have been proposed, there is no universal agreement about the etiology of the process. Genetic susceptibility to this disease is possible as evidenced by the increased probability of Grave's disease in monozygotic twins.[10]

Pathology

On microscopic examination, the follicles are small with hyperplastic columnar epithelium. Hyperplasia of these cells is exhibited by rapidly dividing nuclei and papillary projections of the follicular epithelium within the central follicles. Increased deposition of lymphoid tissue is also demonstrable in many patients with Graves' disease.

Clinical Features

A patient with classic Graves' disease usually has a visibly enlarged neck mass consistent with a goiter that may

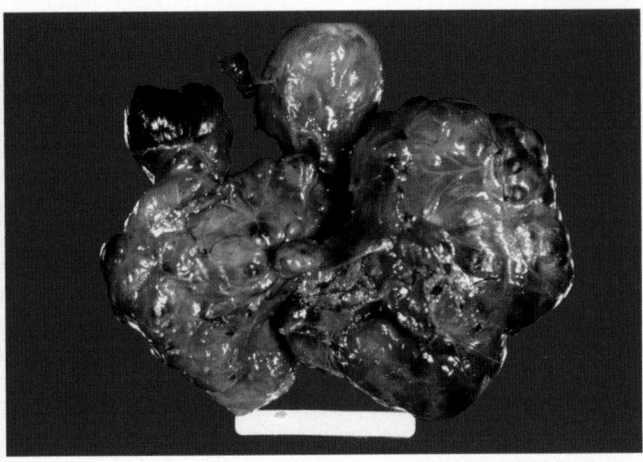

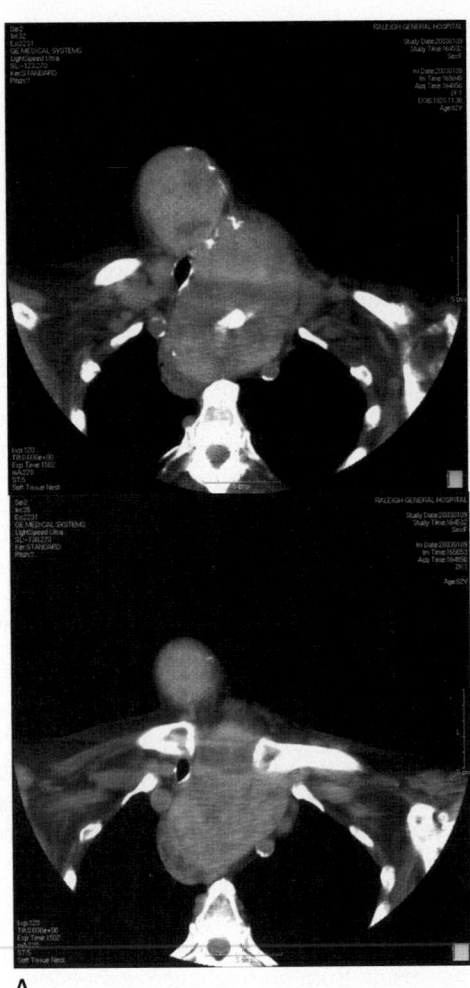

Figure 36-5 A, Computed tomography scan at the level of the thoracic inlet demonstrating a heterogeneous, large thyroid mass that has involved both lobes of the thyroid and displaced the trachea. It has extended into the anterior mediastinum. This patient ultimately proved to have a large multinodular goiter. **B,** Gross picture of the resected multinodular goiter.

demonstrate an audible bruit secondary to increased vascular flow. Clinical thyrotoxicosis and exophthalmos complete the classic triad of the disease. Hair loss, myxedema, gynecomastia, and splenomegaly can accompany the clinical findings. Tracheal compression can result in symptoms of airway obstruction, although acute compression with respiratory distress is exceedingly rare.

The ocular consequences of prolonged and untreated thyrotoxicosis, such as proptosis, supraorbital and infraorbital swelling, and conjunctival swelling and edema, can be severe. The ophthalmopathy is thought to be due to stimulation of the overexpressed TSH-R in the retroorbital tissues of Grave's patients.[11] In its most severe form, spasm of the upper eyelid resulting in retraction and visualization of a larger amount of sclera than normal can lead to lid lag and exacerbation of the already swollen conjunctiva. All these pressure-related phenomena can progress to decreased oculomuscular movements, ophthalmoplegia, and diplopia. Optic nerve damage and blindness can be a long-term consequence if the underlying condition is not corrected. However, this is rarely seen currently with improved screening assays that detect Grave's disease at early stages. Sustained hyperthyroidism is treated aggressively to remove the stimulus to the retro-orbital tissues.

The hypermetabolic state of hyperthyroidism is clinically manifested as sweating, weight loss, heat intolerance, and thirst. Cardiovascular stress can be demonstrated by high-output cardiac failure, congestive heart failure with peripheral edema, and arrhythmias such as ventricular tachycardia or atrial fibrillation. Gastrointestinal signs may include diarrhea and electrolyte wasting. The menstrual cycle can be altered to the point of amenorrhea. Psychiatric signs may include altered sleep patterns, emotional mood swings, fatigue, excitability, and agitation.

Diagnosis

An enlarged smooth thyroid mass and signs and symptoms of thyrotoxicosis suggest the diagnosis. A cost-effective workup can include an extensive history, physical examination, and thyroid function tests. In addition to elevated levels of T_3 and T_4, a decreased or undetectable level of TSH is demonstrated. Thyroid antibodies are usually detected in elevated quantities. An ^{123}I radionuclide scan demonstrates diffuse uptake throughout an enlarged gland. Ultrasound or computed tomography (CT) of the neck can be used to evaluate clinical landmarks (Fig. 36-5). However, the absolute requirement of CT and ultrasound for preoperative assessment is not universally agreed on.[12]

Treatment

When a diagnosis of Graves' disease has been made, therapy is initiated rapidly to ameliorate symptoms and decrease thyroid hormone synthesis. This is particularly crucial for patients with vision-threatening exophthalmos. The former is accomplished with β-blocker therapy, which is started immediately, and the latter with thionamide, radioactive iodine ablation, or surgery, each of which is equally effective in normalizing serum thyroid hormone levels within 6 weeks.[13] Clearly, patients with Grave's disease need to be educated regarding appropriate choices, the risks associated with each treatment, and the expectation of complete success.

Radionuclide Therapy Radioiodide ablation with ^{131}I is the therapy of choice in the United States. It ablates the thyroid within 6 to 18 weeks.[14] Patients with mild, well-tolerated hyperthyroidism can safely proceed to radioactive iodine ablation immediately. However, those who are elderly or severely thyrotoxic may require pretreatment with a thionamide. The overall cure rate with radioactive iodine is 90%. Hypothyroidism will develop in cured individuals, hence the need for careful measurement of thyroid hormone and TSH levels at regular intervals after therapy. Most patients are candidates for radioactive iodine; exceptions include women who are pregnant or lactating or those with a suspicious nodule.

Advantages of ^{131}I therapy include avoidance of surgery and the associated risks of recurrent laryngeal nerve damage, hypothyroidism, or postsurgical recurrence. It may be that ^{131}I therapy is more cost-effective in the long run; however, the financial advantage is not as clear if repeated ^{131}I therapy is needed. Additional disadvantages include exacerbation of cardiac arrhythmias, particularly in elderly patients, possible fetal damage in pregnant women, worsening ophthalmic problems, and rare, but possibly life-threatening thyroid storm.

Antithyroid Medication PTU and methimazole inhibit the organification of intrathyroid iodine, as well as the coupling of iodotyrosine molecules to form T_3 and T_4. PTU has the additive effect of blocking peripheral conversion of T_4 to T_3. This is important because peripheral access to T_3 and T_4 has multiple hyperdynamic and hypermetabolic effects. Additionally, the peripheral adrenergic effects of thyrotoxicosis can be modulated by the use of β-blocking agents such as propranolol. Corticosteroids in combination with β-blockers can help gain rapid control of the hypermetabolic effects of increased peripheral T_4 and T_3. Patients may choose a trial of antithyroid medication over radioactive iodine therapy. The goal of this therapy is to attain euthyroidism; however, hypothyroidism may result and necessitate thyroid hormone replacement. Antithyroid medication is effective in gaining rapid control of thyrotoxicosis, but the relapse rate after discontinuation of medication may approach 50% 12 to 18 months after cessation. Additionally, patients need to be monitored for side effects of the drugs, which may include granulocytopenia and, in rare instances, aplastic anemia. Other side effects include fever, polyarteritis, and rash.[13]

Thyroid Resection Surgery is advocated by a minority of thyroid specialists in the United States. It is primarily indicated for patients who have an obstructive goiter, have a fear of radioactivity, are noncompliant, or have had an adverse effect with thionamide drugs. Additional candidates are pregnant patients or those with a suspicious nodule. Advantages of surgical ablation of the thyroid include rapid, effective treatment of thyrotoxicosis without the necessity for medications and their accompanying side effects. The amount of residual tissue is a subject of debate. Complete ablation of thyroid tissue requires total thyroidectomy, which is associated with the highest rates of hypoparathyroidism and recurrent laryngeal nerve damage. Some groups have reported that total thyroidectomy is the most effective way to treat patients with severe Graves' disease because it offers the lowest rate of relapse. It may be that patients, particularly those with ophthalmopathy, are stabilized most successfully by total thyroidectomy. Removal of the entire antigenic focus may be the most likely explanation for this observation. Other subtotal resections include near-total thyroidectomy or subtotal thyroidectomy.

Careful documentation of euthyroid status before surgery in all hyperthyroid patients is mandatory. If the patient is not properly treated preoperatively, thyroid storm can be life threatening. Fortunately, this complication is rarely encountered if appropriately anticipated. Thyroid storm is manifested by severe tachycardia, fever, confusion, vomiting to the point of dehydration, and adrenergic overstimulation to the point of mania and coma after thyroid resection in an uncontrolled hyperthyroid patient. The best way to treat thyroid storm is preoperative anticipation and preparation. Additionally, all patients undergoing general anesthesia are checked for undiagnosed hyperthyroidism, if clinically suspected. Treatment of a patient with overt thyroid storm includes rapid fluid replacement and institution of antithyroid drugs, β-blockers, iodine solutions, and steroids. In life-threatening circumstances, peritoneal dialysis or hemodialysis may be effective in lowering T_4 and T_3 levels.

Toxic Nodular Goiter/Toxic Adenoma

Toxic nodular goiter, also known as Plummer's disease, refers to a nodule contained within an otherwise goitrous thyroid gland that has autonomous function. It usually occurs in the setting of a patient with endemic goiter. Increased thyroid hormone production occurs independent of TSH control. Such patients generally have a milder course and are older than those with Graves' disease. The thyroid in these patients may be diffusely enlarged or associated with retrosternal goiters. Initial symptoms are mild, peripheral thyroid hormone levels are elevated, and TSH levels are suppressed. Antithyroid antibody levels are usually decreased. The diagnosis is generally confirmed after clinical suspicion, and an ^{131}I radionuclide scan is performed that localizes one or two autonomous areas of function while the rest of the gland is suppressed (Fig. 36-6).[12] Toxic nodular goiter can be treated with thionamides, radioiodine therapy, or surgery; however, the latter two are preferred because these nodules rarely resolve with prolonged thionamide therapy. Radioiodine is widely used for patients with toxic adenomas, although it is not as effective as in Grave's disease.[14] Most patients are euthyroid after radioiodine therapy because the radio-

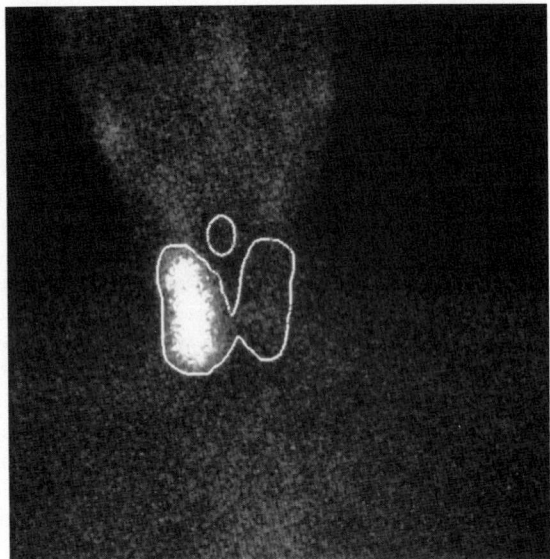

Figure 36-6 ^{131}I scan demonstrating an area of increased uptake in the right lobe of a 32-year-old woman with increased thyroid function test values and a palpable nodule. This scan is consistent with a toxic or hyperfunctioning nodule.

iodine preferentially accumulates in hyperfunctioning nodules. The surgical approach is lobectomy or near-total thyroidectomy, particularly when clinical symptoms are pronounced. In the case of a single, hyperfunctioning adenoma, lobectomy is generally curative.

Nontoxic Goiter

Multinodular Goiter

Multinodular goiter describes an enlarged, diffusely heterogeneous thyroid gland. Initial findings may include diffuse enlargement, but asymmetric nodularity of the mass often develops. The cause of this mass is usually iodine deficiency. Initially the mass is euthyroid, but with increasing size, elevations in T_3 and T_4 can occur and gradually progress to clinical hyperthyroidism. Workup and diagnosis involve evaluation of thyroid function tests. Ultrasound and radioisotopic scanning demonstrate heterogeneous thyroid substance. Nodules with poor uptake can appear as lesions suggestive of malignancy. The incidence of carcinoma in multinodular goiter has been reported to be 5% to 10%. Therefore, FNA for diagnosis and resection for suspicious lesions is considered.[15]

Substernal Goiter

A substernal goiter is an unusual manifestation of intrathoracic extension of an enlarged thyroid that generally occurs as a result of multinodular goiter. Most intrathoracic or substernal goiters are labeled *secondary* because they are enlargements or extensions of multinodular goiters based on the inferior thyroid vasculature. They expand downward into the anterior mediastinum. The extremely rare (~1%) *primary* substernal goiter arises as aberrant thyroid tissue within the anterior or posterior mediastinum and is based on the intrathoracic vasculature and not supplied by the inferior thyroid artery.

Special Considerations for Patients With Goiter

Patients with an enlarged thyroid mass (>5 cm) can have a spectrum of symptoms ranging from none to severe dysphagia, choking, and pain. Occasionally, the diagnosis is suggested by the presence of an anterior mediastinal mass on chest radiography. In 10% to 20% of cases, an asymptomatic patient may have no palpable abnormality in the cervical area and a completely intrathoracic lesion.

CT is the preferred imaging study, and all regions from the mandible to the upper part of the abdomen are included in the scan (see Fig. 36-5). The lesion itself is scrutinized. Benign goiters have rounded, smooth borders. Thyroid malignancies generally have more ill-defined borders. CT also allows evaluation of regional lymph nodes and metastasis. If the patient has a history of cervical pain and night sweats, a diagnosis of lymphoma is considered. The use of FNA with CT guidance is important to secure a tissue diagnosis. Magnetic resonance imaging (MRI) does not usually add significant information to a well-performed CT scan. For patients with an intrathoracic lesion and a history of coughing, preoperative bronchoscopy can give important information about vocal cord status and possible luminal invasion by a malignancy.

Almost all goiters and other thyroid masses are initially approached surgically through a cervical incision. Goiters are usually mobilized easily, even when they are substernal. The blood supply is generally based on the inferior thyroid artery, which is in its normal position and allows even large substernal masses to be gently mobilized into the neck. Careful attention must be directed to the location of the esophagus, trachea, and recurrent laryngeal nerve. The esophagus can be injured by overaggressive manipulation of the thyroid mass. The recurrent laryngeal nerve is usually displaced posteriorly and inferiorly; however, it can be draped anteriorly over the mass and damaged in that position. Great care must be exercised in mobilization of the mass until the nerve is identified. The cervical incision is extended to a median sternotomy if there is significant bleeding from the anterior mediastinum, if the anatomy and location of the recurrent laryngeal nerve are in doubt, or if the mass cannot be mobilized through the surgical field.

WORKUP AND DIAGNOSIS OF A SOLITARY THYROID NODULE

Management and the ultimate decision to proceed to surgical intervention after detection of a solitary nodule depend on the findings of a cost-effective workup and the prognosis (Fig. 36-7). The majority of patients with a solitary thyroid nodule will have a benign lesion; however, thyroid cancer is a definite possibility in all patients. Deciding between conservative management or surgical therapy relies on careful analysis of the clinical findings, assessment of images, and interventional diagnostic methods.[12,16,17]

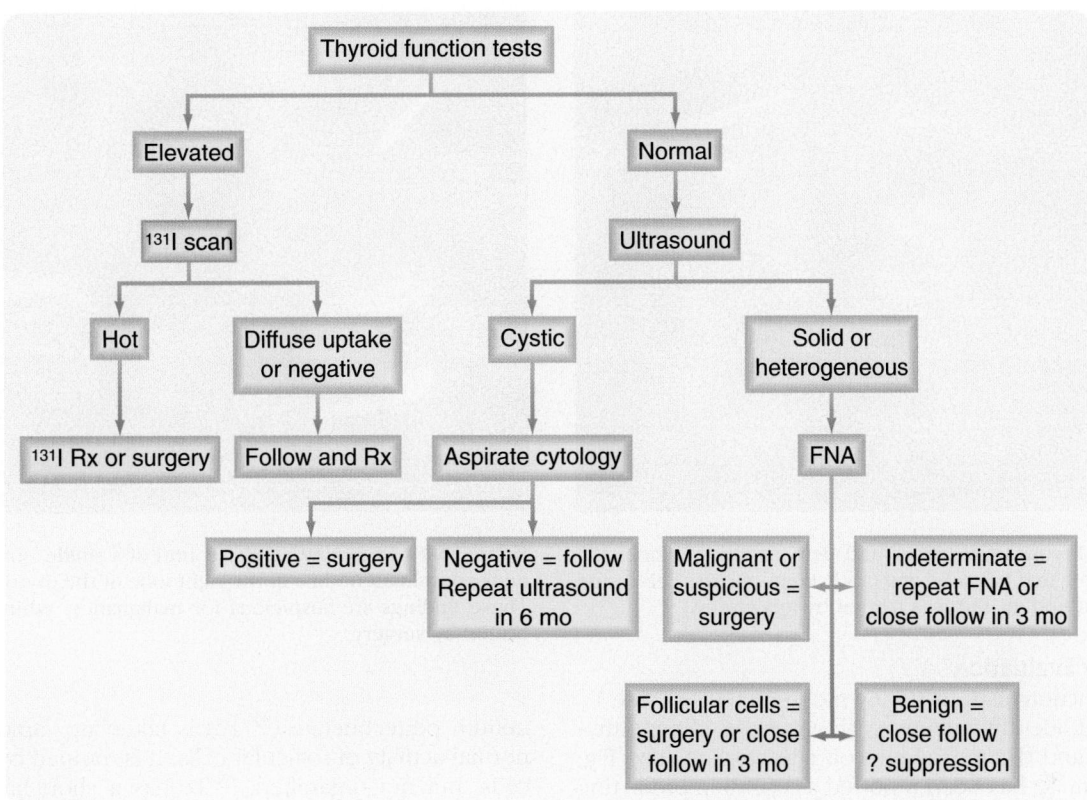

Figure 36-7 Workup of a solitary thyroid nodule. FNA, fine-needle aspiration; Rx, therapy.

Clinical Features

Increasing numbers of thyroid nodules are being found incidentally, possibly because of the increasing availability and sophistication of imaging techniques. The frequency of palpable and nonpalpable thyroid nodules rises with age. Solitary palpable nodules are about four times more prevalent in women than in men. Several different disorders can cause a thyroid nodule. It is important to exclude thyroid cancer in any clinical setting. Rapid growth and signs of possible invasion, such as pain or hoarseness, are most suggestive, but not conclusive of malignancy (Fig. 36-8).[12]

Diagnosis

The workup of a patient with a solitary nodule begins with a careful history and physical examination. Clinical groups with the highest risk for malignancy in a thyroid nodule are children, males, adults younger than 30 or older than 60 years, and those exposed to radiation therapy, especially during childhood. A careful history includes any exposure to radiation, either through occupational sources or through irradiation of the head or neck, particularly in childhood. Additionally, a thorough history of specific endocrine disorders, including medullary carcinoma, MEN 2, or papillary thyroid cancer (PTC), or a history of familial polyposis, including Gardner's syndrome, is warranted.

On physical examination it is important to include thorough palpation of the thyroid, as well as the anterior

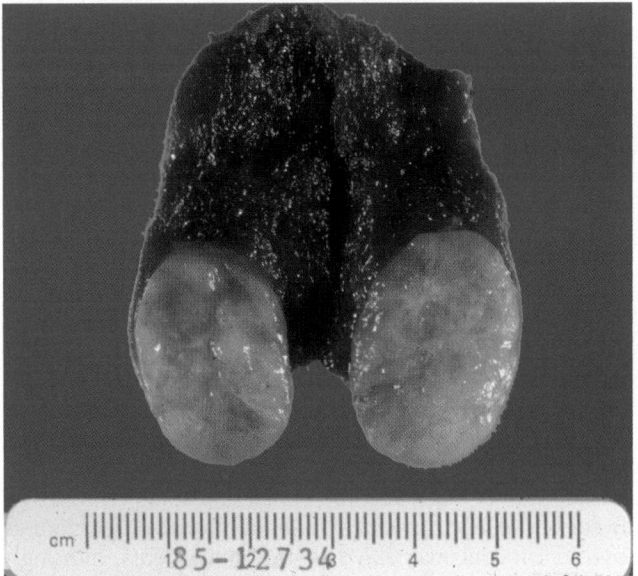

Figure 36-8 This solid 2 × 2.5-cm solid nodule was confirmed as a benign follicular adenoma on permanent section pathology.

and posterior cervical triangles. Determining the size and consistency of the nodule is important. Multiple nodules or diffuse nodularity is associated with a more benign diagnosis. A firm solitary nodule, particularly in older men, is suggestive of a malignant diagnosis.

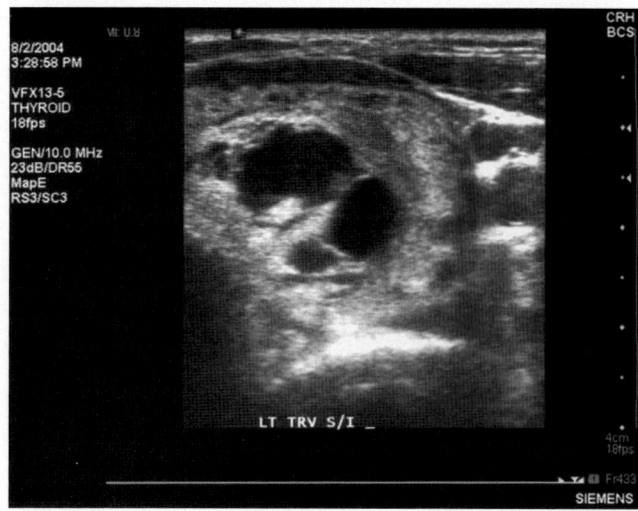

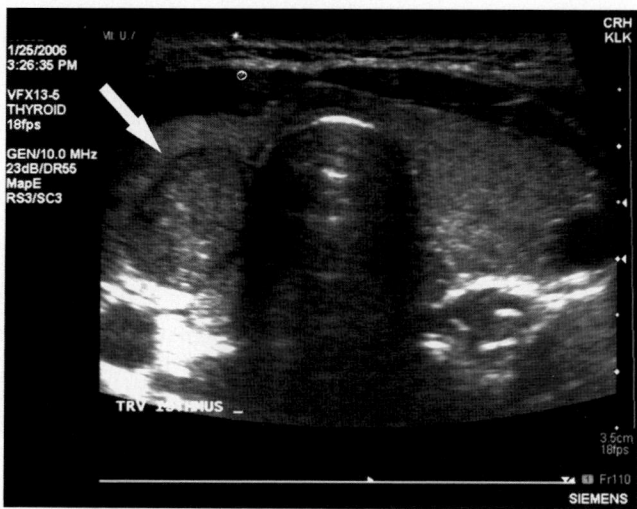

Figure 36-9 Preoperative ultrasound demonstrating a large left thyroid nodule that has solid and cystic components. This lesion was a colloid nodule and was treated by lobectomy.

Figure 36-10 Preoperative ultrasound of a single, solid homogeneous dominant nodule in the right lobe of the thyroid (*arrow*). These findings are suspicious for malignancy, which was confirmed by surgery.

Laboratory Evaluation

Thyroid function tests, including measurements of free T_4, T_3, and TSH, identify patients with unsuspected hyperthyroid states and dictate the appropriate workup (see Fig. 36-7). Serum Tg has been reported as useful in predicting a well-differentiated carcinoma; however, its standard use is not universally agreed on. When there is clinical suspicion of medullary carcinoma, either by family history or by FNA, the serum calcitonin level can be measured. The routine use of serum calcitonin measurement for thyroid masses is not likely to be helpful.[16]

Thyroid Imaging

Ultrasound

Ultrasound is helpful in assessing a thyroid nodule. Its advantages include portability, cost-effectiveness, and lack of ionizing radiation. It is extremely useful in patients who are being managed conservatively because it can easily determine whether a nodule has increased in size. Ultrasound is used routinely in the office setting and is also available for intraoperative evaluation. It has proved highly effective in determining the location and characteristics (cystic versus solid) of nodules but is unable to accurately predict the diagnosis of solid nodules (Figs. 36-9 and 36-10). The finding of a cystic lesion may be reassuring, but such lesions represent a small minority of thyroid nodules (1%-5%). Additionally, well-differentiated thyroid cancers may have cystic components, although this is very unusual.

Ultrasound uses a high-frequency probe in the 7.5- to 12-MHz range. Ultrasound devices have become portable enough to allow use in the clinic and the operating room. B-mode ultrasonography can be used preoperatively or intraoperatively. It is increasingly being used to assist in FNA.[18]

Radioisotope Scanning

Whereas ultrasound allows anatomic evaluation, radionuclide scans allow assessment of thyroid function. Tech-netium pertechnetate (^{99m}Tc) is taken up rapidly by the normal activity of follicular cells. It is trapped by follicular cells, but not organified. ^{99m}Tc has a short half-life and low radiation dose. Its rapid absorption allows quick evaluation of increased uptake (so-called hot) or hypofunctioning (so-called cold) areas of the thyroid. Because screening with ^{99m}Tc shows uptake in the salivary glands and major vascular structures, interpretation of thyroid pathology requires a higher level of expertise.

^{123}I and ^{131}I iodine scintigraphy is also used to evaluate the functional status of the gland (see Fig. 36-6). Both are trapped by active follicular cells and organified. ^{123}I has a shorter half-life (12-13 hours) and allows a quicker image. Advantages of scanning with ^{123}I include a low dose of radiation (30 mrad) and short half-life. ^{123}I is a good choice for evaluating suspected lingual thyroids or substernal goiters.

^{131}I has a longer half-life (8 days) and emits higher levels of β-radiation. ^{131}I is optimal for imaging thyroid carcinoma.[19] It is the screening modality of choice for the evaluation of distant metastasis.

Radionuclide scanning demonstrates the function of thyroid nodules as *hot* (excess uptake) or *cold* (no uptake) in comparison to surrounding tissue. Malignancy has been shown to occur in 15% to 20% of cold nodules and, additionally, in 5% to 9% of nodules with uptake that is warm or hot, thus mandating a continued aggressive approach to clinically suspicious nodules, even if they are not cold.

Positron emission tomography (PET) with ^{18}F-fluorodeoxyglucose can be used to provide three-dimensional reconstruction images. There is increasing enthusiasm for its use in detecting primary and metastatic thyroid cancer. Interestingly, PET scans identify occasional so-called thyroid incidentalomas when evaluating other solid malignancies. The majority of these findings, however, are not malignant. The appropriateness of PET in the workup or follow-up of thyroid nodules remains to be firmly established or agreed on.[20]

CT and MRI

It is fairly well agreed that CT and MRI do not add significantly to the workup of uncomplicated thyroid nodules. Either modality, however, may be of help in evaluating for local extension in more advanced stages of thyroid cancer. CT or MRI is particularly appropriate for a suspicious mass (or biopsy-proven cancer) with palpable cervical lymph nodes. Additionally, either can be used for postoperative follow-up, particularly for suspicion of recurrent disease. Preoperative CT or MRI is advisable for larger thyroid masses that show significant tracheal deviation suggestive of a substernal goiter on chest radiographs.

CT and MRI are both equally sensitive and specific for the evaluation of thyroid masses. Consideration must be given to the use of IV contrast for CT evaluation of a possible cancer. The iodine load may interfere with postoperative plans for ^{131}I scanning.[17]

Fine-Needle Aspiration

FNA of the thyroid with a small-gauge needle has become increasingly popular and is now one of the initial diagnostic modalities in patients with thyroid nodules. Use of a smaller-gauge needle has allowed a marked drop in the complication rate associated with the use of large-bore or core needle biopsies while maintaining diagnostic accuracy. In a series of 561 patients, FNA was found to have a sensitivity of 86% and a specificity of 91%. Accurate diagnosis of benign lesions has significantly decreased rates of surgery in patients with thyroid nodules. Additionally, preoperative FNA is replacing the use of intraoperative frozen section pathologic analysis.[21] Despite the widespread use of ultrasound-guided FNA, this modality is also associated with a significant rate of initial nondiagnostic cytology approaching 20% to 25%.[18] The finding of a malignant diagnosis on FNA is associated with a high rate of accuracy approaching 100%. Certain discrete cytologic characteristics of papillary carcinoma allow the use of FNA to be extremely accurate in diagnosis (Fig. 36-11).

The diagnosis of follicular carcinoma cannot be made with FNA. FNA diagnosis of medullary or anaplastic carcinoma is somewhat more difficult but can be accomplished by experienced cytopathologists. When FNA reveals follicular cells, an important decision must be made. Although most of these cases are benign (follicular adenoma), this diagnosis cannot be secure and ultimately depends on complete histologic examination of the resected specimen. Large series show malignancy in 6% to 20% of thyroid lesions when follicular cells are demonstrated on FNA.[22]

The presence of colloid and macrophages within the aspirate strongly suggests a benign lesion. In this circumstance, a safe diagnosis of a colloid nodule or benign process can be made. The patient must understand, however, that this diagnosis depends only on the aspirated material. Tissue immediately adjacent to or contained within another part of the nodule may harbor malignant cells. The false-negative rate of FNA has been

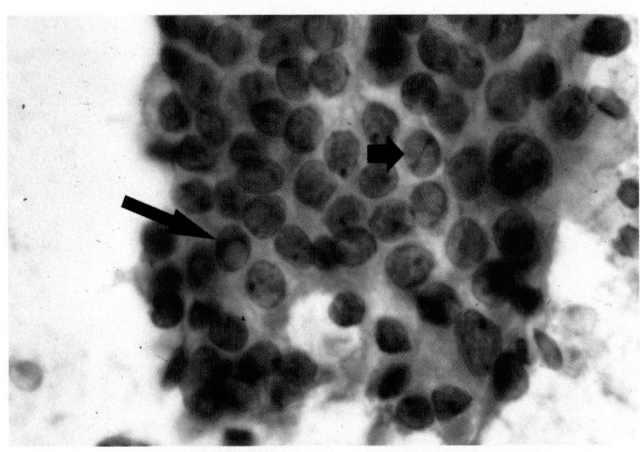

Figure 36-11 Fine-needle aspiration of a thyroid mass allows determination of individual cellular morphology. Cells in this aspirate demonstrate intranuclear grooving *(fat arrow)*, as well as ground-glass cytoplasmic inclusions *(thin arrow)* (so-called Orphan Annie eyes). These cellular features are consistent with a diagnosis of papillary carcinoma of the thyroid.

reported to be between 1% and 6%.[16] Therefore, benign nodules diagnosed by FNA are monitored sequentially with ultrasound to ensure that their characteristics do not change. If FNA leads to a diagnosis that is "suspicious but not confirmatory," an aggressive workup continues for the possibility of malignancy. Certain series state that more than half of such FNA results are associated with malignant cells. If the FNA findings are indeterminate, either repeat aspiration or close conservative follow-up of the nodule is undertaken.[12]

FNA can also be used for lesions that are determined to be cystic by ultrasound. A larger-bore needle can be used to aspirate the cystic fluid. Examination of most cystic fluid results in benign cytologic findings; however, an occasional papillary carcinoma can be manifested as a cyst and diagnosed by cytologic examination of cystic fluid.

Decision Making and Treatment

Decision making about thyroid nodules depends on interpretation and the judicious use of thyroid function tests, imaging, and FNA (Table 36-1; also see Fig. 36-7). All patients with a thyroid nodule undergo thyroid function tests (including T_4, TSH, and T_3 resin uptake). If the patient is hyperthyroid, a technetium scan is used to confirm a hot nodule. If such is the case, the patient is carefully monitored with thyroid suppression and is seen again after 6 months for confirmation of successful suppression and reevaluation. If suppressive therapy fails, surgery (usually lobectomy) is highly effective but not generally required (see Toxic Nodular Goiter/Toxic Adenoma).

In a patient with a thyroid nodule and normal thyroid function test results, ultrasound is performed. Cystic lesions on ultrasound are usually benign; however, cystic papillary carcinomas, though rare, do occur. Cystic lesions are aspirated (bloody or suspicious aspirates can be sent for cytologic examination). After aspiration, these patients are seen again in 6 months. Patients with recurrent cysts are considered surgical candidates.

Table 36-1 **Thyroid Nodules**

DIAGNOSIS	FACTORS ASSOCIATED WITH DIAGNOSIS	FACTORS THAT CONFIRM THE DIAGNOSIS	FACTORS ASSOCIATED WITH A WORSE PROGNOSIS
Benign			
Colloid	Multinodular goiter FNA shows colloid and macrophages	Surgery	—
Hyperfunctioning nodule	Hyperthyroidism	^{131}I scan	—
Malignant			
Papillary carcinoma	Radiation exposure Previous surgery for papillary carcinoma	FNA or surgery	Male gender, age >40 yr, size >3 cm, tall-cell variant
Follicular carcinoma	"Follicular cells" by FNA	Permanent section pathology	Male gender, age >40 yr, size >3 cm, poorly differentiated cell type
Medullary carcinoma	MEN 2A and 2B Elevated calcitonin level	Surgery, FNA Calcitonin levels *ret* oncogene	MEN 2B and sporadic
Anaplastic carcinoma	Rapid progression of tumor mass Pain, hoarseness	FNA Surgery	Diagnosis

FNA, fine-needle aspiration; MEN, multiple endocrine neoplasia.

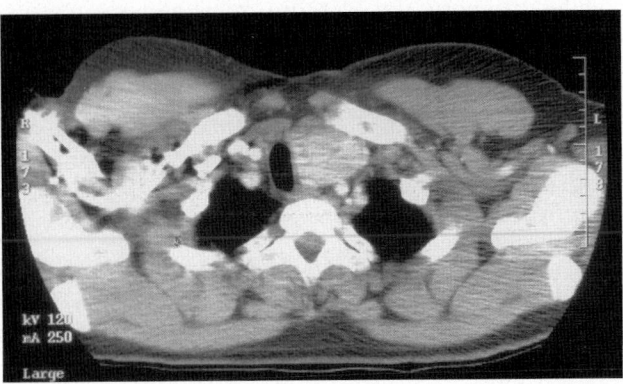

Figure 36-12 Computed tomographic findings of a 4-cm mass in the left lobe of a 40-year-old man suggesting an infraclavicular or substernal location. The mass ultimately proved to be papillary carcinoma.

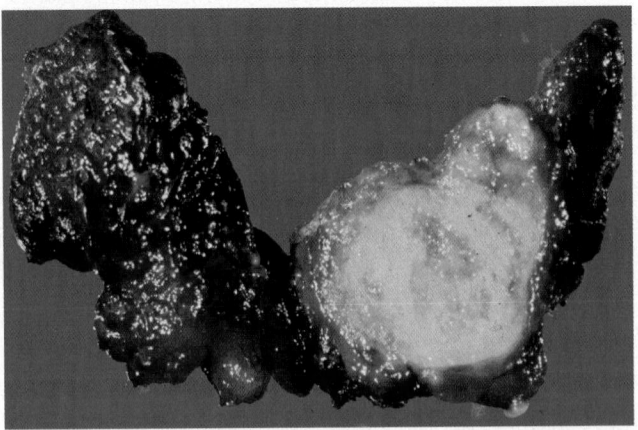

Figure 36-13 This 4- to 5-cm right lobe mass was removed as part of total thyroidectomy. Permanent section pathology revealed papillary carcinoma.

For patients whose nodules on ultrasound are solid or have mixed solid-cystic components, decision making depends on additional information. If these patients have other risks factors mentioned earlier, the likelihood of having a malignancy in a thyroid nodule is increased. They are counseled to consider a surgical option. In the remainder of patients, the option of FNA exists. FNA can be used to diagnose papillary cancer and is strongly suggestive of medullary cancer or anaplastic cancer. It cannot confirm follicular cancer, nor can it confirm a completely benign diagnosis. Patients with follicular cells seen on FNA have a 6% to 20% incidence of malignancy. Therefore, risk assessment is crucial in advising patients with a solid nodule for whom the diagnosis is not secure with FNA. Colloid nodules are usually suggested by a mixed solid-cystic appearance on ultrasound, and FNA shows colloid and macrophages. If not otherwise suspicious, these lesions can be monitored closely with serial ultrasonography every 6 months to establish stability. Alterations in appearance of the suspicious lesion indicate a need for surgery (Figs. 36-12 and 36-13).[12,16]

The increased availability of ultrasound appears to have affected the incidence of small thyroid cancers in the United States. The majority seem to be asymptomatic papillary carcinomas less than 1 cm in size. The fact that these lesions are highly curable and associated with virtually nonexistent mortality needs to be taken into account when deciding whether to perform FNA and proceed to surgery.[23]

THYROID MALIGNANCIES

Thyroid cancer represents less than 1% of all malignancies in the United States, with about 40 developing per 1 million people per year. Six deaths per 1 million people occur annually. Ninety percent to 95% of thyroid cancers

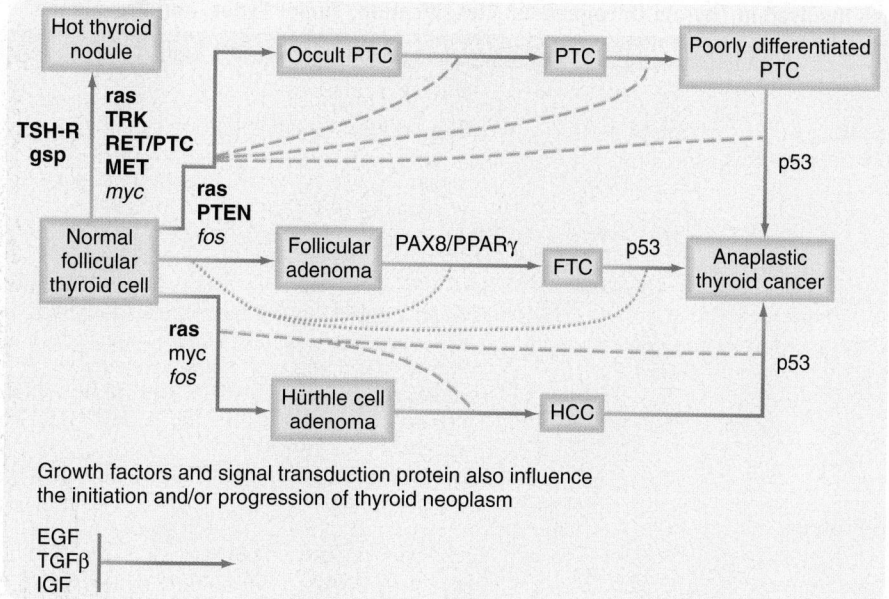

Figure 36-14 Genetic events that occur in thyroid oncogenesis (the main genetic events are in bold). The *dashed lines* for each histologic type of thyroid cancer indicate that an adenoma-to-carcinoma progression is not necessarily always the sequence of progression in carcinogenesis. EGF, epidermal growth factor; FTC, follicular thyroid carcinoma; HCC, Hürthle cell carcinoma; IGF, insulin-like growth factor; PPARγ, peroxisome proliferator–activated receptor-γ; PTC, papillary thyroid carcinoma; TGFβ, transforming growth factor-β; TSH-R, thyroid-simulating hormone receptor. (From Kebebew E: Thyroid oncogenesis. In Clark OH [ed]: Textbook of Endocrine Surgery, 2nd ed. Philadelphia, Elsevier Saunders, 2005, pp 289.)

are categorized as well-differentiated tumors arising from the follicular cells. Papillary, follicular, and Hürthle cell carcinomas are included in this category. MCT accounts for about 6% of thyroid cancers (~20%-30% of which occur on a familial basis, MEN 2A and 2B). Anaplastic carcinoma is an aggressive malignancy that is responsible for less than 1% of thyroid carcinomas in the United States. These cases occur primarily in iodine-deficient areas.

Thyroid Oncogenesis

Genetic processes that lead to thyroid neoplasia include two important possibilities: mutated proto-oncogenes, which result in altered protein production and thus in accelerated growth, and alterations in growth suppression genes, which when initiated, allow unregulated cell growth. Several known oncogenes have been associated with thyroid tumors, but few are limited to specific thyroid malignancies. Examples include *ras,* c-*myc,* and c-*fos.* The *PTC/RET* proto-oncogene has received perhaps the most attention in thyroid tumorigenesis studies.[24]

Oncogenes in Well-Differentiated Cancer

The association of the *RET* proto-oncogene and MCT has been well characterized. The working model for oncogenes causing papillary and follicular cancer is not so well understood. It appears that at least three gene categories of locations or actions are important (Fig. 36-14; Table 36-2).

Receptor Proteins

This group includes TSH-R, which is a member of the G protein–coupled receptor family. TSH activation mutations appear to be associated with growth of adenoma, but not malignancy. A larger group of receptor proteins includes the tyrosine kinase receptors. Activation of tyrosine kinase receptors results in a cascade of events that through phosphorylation activate downstream signaling pathways with multiple metabolic results. Several different tyrosine kinase receptor groups (RET, trk, and met) have been implicated in the development of thyroid cancer.[25]

RET Proto-Oncogene

The *PTC/RET* proto-oncogene encodes for a tyrosine kinase receptor on the cell membrane. This proto-oncogene may well be involved in the differentiation of neuronal cells. Cells of neural crest origin appear to have increased expression of this oncogene because it has been found in neuroblastoma, pheochromocytoma, and MCT tissue. Alterations in this system have been shown to result in developmental abnormalities in a number of other neuronal tissues, as well as in patients with Hirschsprung's disease. Expression of the *RET* oncogene is predominantly found only in malignant tissue. It has not been detected to any substantial degree in nonmalignant thyroid disease processes. Rearrangement of the *PTC/RET* oncogene has been demonstrated in the development of PTC. It may also be that patients with the oncogene may have a predilection for distant metastasis.

Table 36-2   Main Genes Involved in Thyroid Oncogenesis: Classification, Tumor Types, and Prevalence

GENES	HISTOLOGIC TYPE	PREVALENCE	COMMENT
Receptor			
TSH	Autonomous follicular adenoma	3%-82%	TSH activation mutations are not oncogenic
TRK	PTC	6%-20%	Tyrosine kinase receptor, somatic mutation absent in benign thyroid neoplasms
RET/PTC	PTC	2.5%-85%, higher with radiation exposure	Tyrosine kinase receptor, somatic mutation Higher prevalence with radiation exposure Possibly associated with more aggressive tumors Five chimeric subtypes have been identified
Met	PTC, FTC	~75% PTC ~25% FTC	Tyrosine kinase receptor, somatic mutation Possibly associated with aggressive tumors Overexpressed mostly in PTC and poorly differentiated DTC
c-erb-2	PTC	~50% PTC	Tyrosine kinase activity, similar to epidermal growth factor receptor Though overexpressed in PTC, the oncogene is not overamplified
Signal Transduction Proteins			
ras	PTC, FTC, HCC, autonomous follicular adenoma	7%-92% (~30% overall)	Early event in carcinogenesis May be associated with aggressive PTC
gsp	Autonomous follicular adenoma	7%-28%	Early event in carcinogenesis Similar frequency in benign and malignant thyroid neoplasms Coexisting *ras* and *gsp* mutations in same tumor may be associated with aggressive DTC
Tumor Suppressor Genes and Nuclear Oncogenes			
PAX8/PPARγ	FTC	75%	The presence of this fusion oncoprotein may be used to differentiate follicular adenoma from carcinoma
p53	Poorly DTC, ATC	~75%	p53 immunohistochemistry may be predictive of tumor aggressiveness Thought to occur as a late genetic event in thyroid carcinogenesis
PTEN	Benign follicular adenoma, infrequently in DTC	26% of benign, 6% of malignant	Higher rate in benign than malignant tumor questions the presence of a strict adenoma-to-carcinoma sequence

ATC, anaplastic thyroid cancer; DTC, differentiated thyroid cancer; FTC, follicular thyroid cancer; HCC, Hürthle cell carcinoma; PTC, papillary thyroid cancer; TSH, thyroid-stimulating hormone.

From Kebebew E: Thyroid oncogenesis. In Clark OH (ed): Textbook of Endocrine Surgery, 2nd ed. Philadelphia, Elsevier Saunders, 2005, p 289.

In addition, the *RET* proto-oncogene is associated with a high frequency of missense mutations in patients with MEN 2A. Genetic analysis for this mutation allows a secure diagnosis in children before the clinical appearance of MCT.

Signal Transduction Proteins

ras Gene Family

The *ras* gene family encodes signal transduction G proteins. Mutational activation of this oncogene results in the production of an inactive form of an enzyme (guanosine triphosphatase) that is ineffective in inactivating protein degradation. Thus, continued protein accumulation is allowed because of a failed enzymatic process. It appears that as many as 40% of thyroid tumors may have one of three *ras* gene point mutations (H-*ras*, K-*ras*, or N-*ras*). Additionally, *ras* mutations may occur in benign and malignant neoplasms. Patients who live in iodine-deficient areas may have an incidence of *ras* mutations that is slightly decreased in comparison to those in iodine-sufficient areas. K-*ras* mutations appear more frequently in radiation-induced papillary cancers. As knowledge is gained about this particular oncogene family, it appears that tumor oncogenesis may be related not only to the prevalence of certain mutations but also to other genetic factors, as well as environmental factors such as iodine availability.[25]

gsp Oncogene

The stimulating guanosine triphosphate–binding protein activates adenyl cyclase via the TSH signal transduction pathway. The *gsp* oncogene has been detected mostly in hot nodules and very infrequently in thyroid malignancies. *gsp* mutations in combination with *ras* mutations have been found in more aggressive papillary and follicular cancers.

Tumor Suppressor Genes and Nuclear Oncogenes

This family of genes allows deregulated cell growth as a result of specific mutations. The *p53* tumor suppressor gene is one of the most common genetic alterations seen in human cancer. It may be sensitive to radiation exposure. Increased p53 activity appears to be associated with more aggressive papillary and follicular cancers.

PTEN is a tyrosine phosphatase protein that inhibits phosphatidylinositol-3 kinase activity. It is associated with Cowden's syndrome, which in itself is associated with thyroid malignancy. However, PTEN has been demonstrated largely in benign thyroid nodules and much less so in malignant tissue, thus casting doubt on a possible primary role in malignant degeneration.[26]

The nuclear proto-oncogenes c-*myc* and c-*fos* appear to be overexpressed in certain thyroid cancers; c-*myc* may correlate with tumor aggressiveness. Almost all Hürthle cell cancers are positive for N-myc protein by immunohistochemistry. The exact role that c-*myc* and c-*fos* play in thyroid tumorigenesis is unclear.[26]

Papillary Carcinoma

Papillary carcinoma is the most common of the thyroid neoplasms and is usually associated with an excellent prognosis, particularly in female patients younger than 40 years. About 70% to 80% of patients in the United States in whom thyroid carcinoma is newly diagnosed have papillary carcinoma. Several studies have shown that the incidence of well-differentiated thyroid carcinoma has increased perhaps as much as 50% since 1990. Whether this increase is due to enhanced sophistication in screening and diagnostic techniques or possible exposure to environmental factors such as radiation or environmental mutagenic chemicals is not clear.

The association of irradiation and thyroid cancer has been known for years. The use of external beam irradiation in children and young adults in the 1950s and 1960s for acne and tonsillitis has been shown to result in an increased incidence of well-differentiated carcinoma (usually papillary) at any time, generally 5 years after exposure. Additionally, patients who have received external irradiation for soft tissue malignancy, such as Hodgkin's lymphoma, have an increased incidence of thyroid nodules and cancer (as many as 30%-35% of those exposed). Areas near known nuclear fallout contamination, such as Chernobyl in the former Soviet Union and areas of the southwest United States, have increased incidence rates of well-differentiated thyroid carcinoma.[27]

Pathologic Classification

The pathologic diagnosis of papillary carcinoma depends on the cytologic findings of well-recognized papillary cytomorphology. The neoplasm may form well-defined follicles with only minimal papillary architecture. The latter group can be classified as the follicular variant of papillary carcinoma. Classic papillary carcinoma and the follicular variant of papillary carcinoma have much the same prognostic implications. Individual cellular morphology may be used to make the diagnosis of papillary carcinoma. Intranuclear inclusion bodies and cellular grooving allow the diagnosis of papillary carcinoma on inspection of individual cellular components obtained by

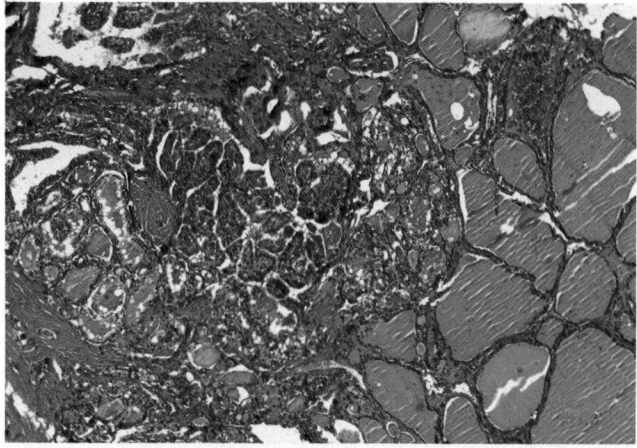

A

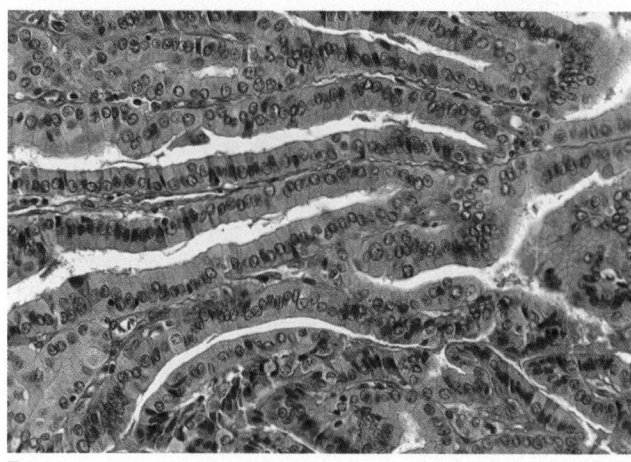

B

Figure 36-15 A, Hematoxylin and eosin (H&E) staining of a thyroid mass reveals papillary projections consistent with papillary carcinoma. **B,** H&E staining of a papillary carcinoma shows cells with an increased height-to-width ratio in a single row of cells. This is the so-called tall cell variant of papillary carcinoma, which is associated with a poorer prognosis than well-differentiated papillary cancer.

FNA, which is a minimally invasive technique with important diagnostic capability (see Fig. 36-11). Additionally, the finding of calcified clumps of cells, known as psammoma bodies and most likely caused by sloughed papillary projections, is diagnostic of papillary cancer.

Other subtypes of papillary carcinoma are more unpredictably aggressive in their biologic behavior. Insular, columnar, and tall cell carcinomas represent these forms of papillary carcinoma. Although these subtypes are rare, they tend to occur in older patients, and the prognosis is less favorable. These latter groups represent perhaps less than 1% of all papillary carcinomas (Fig. 36-15).[28]

Clinical Features

Thyroid masses may occur in either males or females at almost any age. Solitary masses that are painless and firm are regarded with particular suspicion. Occasionally, a mass in the lateral aspect of the neck is manifested as a

Table 36-3 **Prognostic Risk Classification for Patients With Well-Differentiated Thyroid Cancer (AMES or AGES)**

	LOW RISK	HIGH RISK
Age	<40 years	>40 years
Sex	Female	Male
Extent	No local extension, intrathyroidal, no capsular invasion	Capsular invasion, extrathyroidal extension
Metastasis	None	Regional or distant
Size	<2 cm	>4 cm
Grade	Well differentiated	Poorly differentiated

AGES, age, pathologic grade of tumor, and extent and size of the primary tumor; AMES, age, distant metastasis, extent of the primary tumor, and size of the primary tumor.

painless entity and FNA biopsy confirms a metastatic thyroid malignancy, even with a normal thyroid examination. Thorough head and neck examination, often aided by office-based ultrasound, allows characterization of the mass.

Most patients with papillary carcinoma can expect an excellent prognosis, with the 10-year survival rate approaching 95% for the most favorable stages. Various factors in the clinical findings and pathologic staging, however, may alter the excellent prognosis (Table 36-3). In 1979, Cady and associates[29] first evaluated a clinical scoring system and reported a 30-year study of a group of patients in which the investigators attempted to place the patients into risk stratification groups. These studies described the AMES clinical scoring system, which is based on age, distant metastasis, extent of the primary tumor, and size of the primary tumor. Hay[30] reported the Mayo Clinic experience and developed his own scoring scale, the AGES clinical scoring system, which was based on age, pathologic grade of tumor, and extent and size of the primary tumor. Both the AMES and the AGES clinical scoring systems have proved beneficial in predicting the prognosis of papillary and follicular cancer. Age at diagnosis turns out to be the most important factor; diagnosis at an age younger than 40 years is associated with excellent survival. In women this age benefit is extended to 50 years. Absence of distant metastasis at the time of initial treatment and size less than 4 cm are likewise important positive predictors. Tumor size greater than 4 cm and extension of the primary tumor through the capsule of the lesion increase the risk for mortality. The AGES system describes a scoring system for presence or absence of these factors. A score of less than 4 is associated with a 20-year mortality rate of less than 1%. The more advanced stages have 5-year survival rates approaching 50%.

Study of DNA ploidy has been used to evaluate clinical prognosis. Increased nuclear DNA (aneuploidy) has been thought to increase the risk for mortality. Universal agreement about this concept does not exist, however. Information on DNA ploidy may have some implication

for prognosis but has had no definite impact on therapeutics.

Papillary carcinoma may be found incidentally in a thyroid sample resected for a benign process. These carcinomas are usually less than 5 mm in size and are not generally associated with clinically apparent cervical or distant metastatic activity.

Detection of a solitary palpable thyroid mass (1-2 cm) strongly suggests a malignant diagnosis. Confirmation of the diagnosis may be initiated by ultrasound, which determines multinodularity and whether the nodule is solid or cystic. FNA of a palpable solid lesion is the next step. PTC can be diagnosed by this technique because the individual cellular architecture can be evaluated and a secure diagnosis made. Multicentricity can be anticipated in as many as 70% of patients with the diagnosis of papillary cancer. Additionally, cervical lymph node metastasis must be anticipated. Palpable lymphadenopathy leads to FNA of suspected lesions. Younger patients have been shown to have a high rate of lymph node metastasis; however, this does not appreciably affect mortality. The presence of lymph node metastasis in patients with completely contained intrathyroidal primary papillary carcinoma also does not affect long-term survival. If the final pathology demonstrates extension of a primary papillary carcinoma through the thyroid capsule, a poor prognosis and possibly a higher rate of lymph node metastasis may be anticipated.[31,32]

Treatment

The primary treatment of PTC is surgical ablation. For lesions smaller than 1 cm, there is general agreement in the literature that lobectomy plus isthmectomy is appropriate, particularly for incidentally found papillary carcinomas.

Several factors enter into surgical decision making. Younger patients, especially those 15 years or younger, have a high rate of cervical metastasis to the extent that perhaps 90% of children with papillary carcinoma may have documented metastatic activity within the lymph nodes. Therefore, there is consensus that patients in this age group undergo total thyroidectomy and lymph node dissection in the presence of palpable cervical lymph nodes.[17] Additionally, in older patients with a history of neck irradiation, a more aggressive approach may be taken, including total thyroidectomy and modified neck dissection in those with palpable cervical lymph nodes. There appears to be no survival benefit with prophylactic lymph node dissection for nonpalpable nodes.[33]

Controversy exists about the use of total thyroidectomy versus lobectomy and isthmectomy in adults with a 1- to 2-cm PTC. The advantages of total thyroidectomy include the efficient use of radioiodine postoperative treatment. Radioablation is much less effective and requires a larger dosage if residual thyroid exists. Advantages of the lesser procedure are decreased rates of bilateral recurrent laryngeal nerve damage and hypoparathyroidism. A recent study evaluated papillary microcarcinomas 5 mm to 1.5 cm in size. Their conclusions were that total thyroidectomy needs to be considered for these lesions because of the local aggressiveness of residual multicentric tumor deposits.[17,34] However, other studies show no increase in mortality rates for small, incidentally found papillary cancers.[23]

If papillary carcinoma is manifested as a palpable lesion larger than 2 cm, total thyroidectomy is definitely considered. A diligent search for multicentricity within the thyroid, as well as for regional lymph node metastasis, may be undertaken with the use of ultrasound or neck CT. Distant metastatic activity may be evaluated with chest radiographs, radionuclide scanning, CT, and other techniques as guided by clinical suspicion. In patients after total thyroidectomy, postoperative Tg levels may be followed to monitor for recurrence.[8,27]

For patients with lower-stage disease (by AMES or AGES), surgical resection generally results in excellent 5- to 10-year survival rates exceeding 90%. With larger lesions, survival may decrease, especially in older men, and postoperative ^{131}I therapy has been advocated.[27] Recurrence in local or regional lymph nodes after initial surgery is treated by completion thyroidectomy, if residual tissue exists, plus regional lymph node dissection. Radioiodine therapy is used as adjunctive therapy. Distant metastases are rare but have a poor prognosis (Fig. 36-16). The Mayo Clinic has published a follow-up series of patients with papillary cancer dating back to 1940.[35] In the first 10 years of the study (1940-1949), lobectomy was the primary procedure and was performed in nearly 70% of cases. Since 1950, near-total or total thyroidectomy has essentially been the standard procedure and has led to significantly improved survival in comparison to the earlier group. Cause-specific mortality and local recurrence rates have remained stable since then and over the last 50 years of the study, despite the more frequent use of postoperative irradiation.

Follicular Carcinoma

FTC is the second category of well-differentiated thyroid cancer. All types of papillary, follicular, and mixed papillary-follicular cancer account for about 90% of thyroid cancer. Pure FTC represents the minority of these cancers and constitutes about 10% of all thyroid malignancies. FTC is a disease of an older population, often 50 years or older. It has a predilection for women, with a ratio of about 3:1. A subtype of FTC, known as Hürthle cell carcinoma, consists of oxyphilic cells and tends to occur in older patients, usually 60 to 75 years of age.[27,32] There appears to be an increased incidence of FTC in geographic distributions associated with iodine deficiency.

Pathologic Classification

FTC is a malignant neoplasm of the thyroid epithelium that can have a wide spectrum of microscopic changes anywhere from virtually normal follicular architecture and function to severely altered cellular architecture. In large series, 10% to 15% of patients with thyroid cancer have FTC.[27] Histologic diagnosis of FTC depends on the demonstration of normal-appearing follicular cells occupying abnormal positions, including capsular, lymphatic, or vascular invasion (Fig. 36-17). If these structures do not contain follicular cells, a diagnosis of a benign fol-

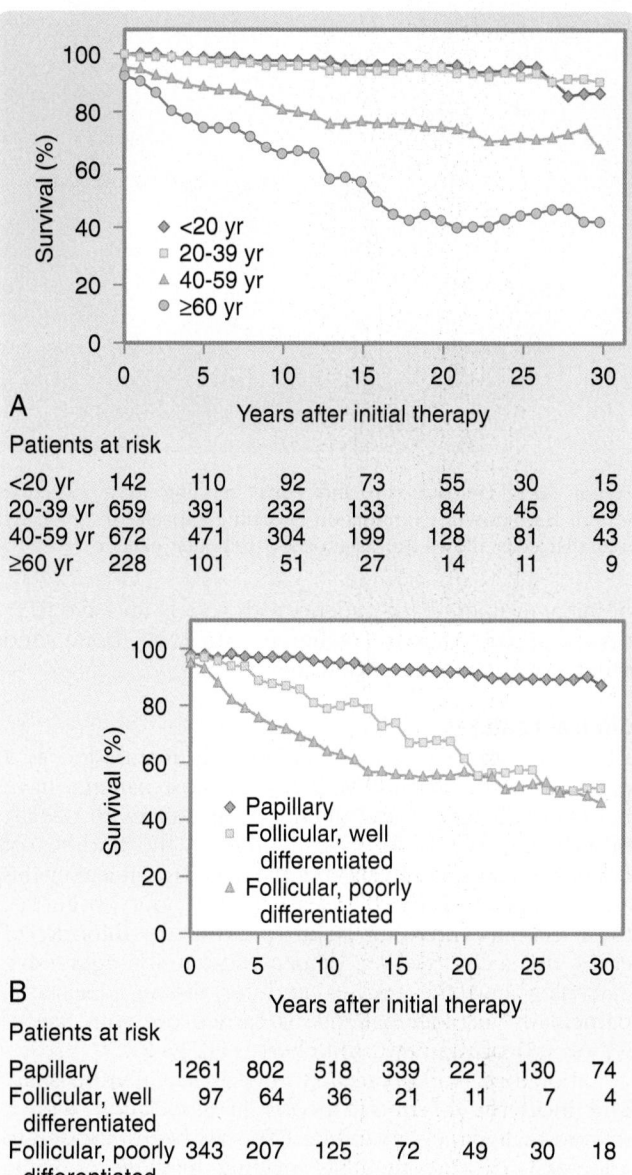

Figure 36-16 Survival rates of 1701 patients with papillary or follicular carcinoma (no distant metastasis at time of diagnosis). Overall survival rates were 82% at 10 years, 72% at 20 years, and 60% at 30 years. Patients were followed at the Institut Gustav-Roussy in France. **A,** Effect of age at diagnosis on mortality for combined groups. **B,** Survival rate according to histologic subtype. (From Schlumberger ML: Medical progress: Papillary and follicular thyroid carcinoma. N Engl J Med 338:300, 1998. Copyright © 1998 Massachusetts Medical Society. All rights reserved.)

licular adenoma is made. Using these criteria, two types of follicular carcinoma are usually described: minimally invasive and widely invasive. There is increasing evidence that microscopic angioinvasion is an important prognostic finding.[36] Lymph node involvement is unusual and occurs in less than 10% of cases. This is in contradistinction to papillary carcinoma, which is characterized by a higher rate of lymph node involvement at the time

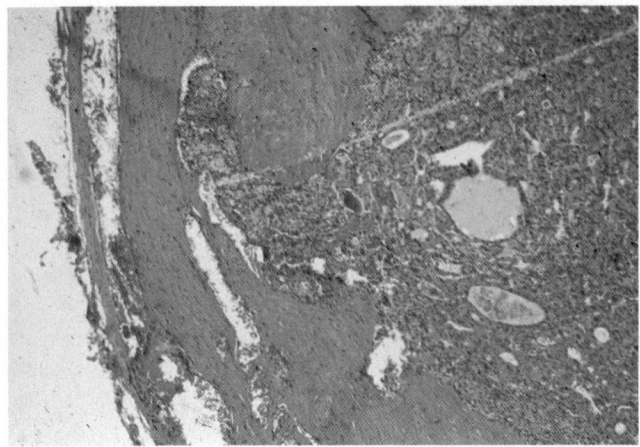

Figure 36-17 Hematoxylin and eosin staining of a follicular lesion. High-power examination revealing capsular invasion by follicular cells allows the diagnosis of follicular cancer.

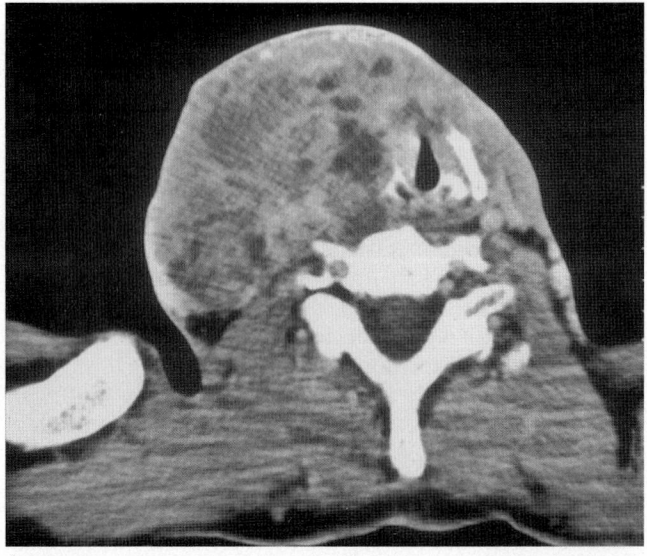

A

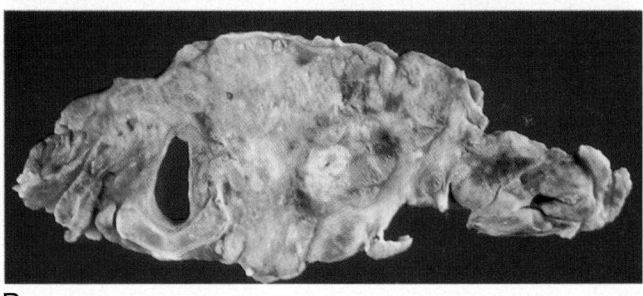

B

Figure 36-18 A and **B,** Rapidly enlarging thyroid mass in a 70-year-old man. Computed tomography demonstrates displacement of the larynx and lateral involvement of both jugular veins. This patient died within 6 months of rapidly progressing follicular cancer.

of initial evaluation. In patients with widely invasive FTC, distant spread is more common, and lung, bone, and other solid organs are often involved.[36]

Clinical Features

FTC, like papillary cancer, is classically manifested as a painless thyroid mass. Even though most patients have benign disease, FTC and multinodular goiter can coexist in as many as 10% of cases. Although the findings of hoarseness and firm fixation of the mass on clinical evaluation suggest advanced disease and a poor prognosis, these circumstances are again found in the minority of cases. In such cases, a diligent search for aggressive extension into the trachea and for distant metastasis, particularly in older patients, is carried out with use of CT or MRI of the neck and chest (Fig. 36-18).[31]

Laboratory workup usually reveals a euthyroid state. The incidence of thyrotoxicosis in association with a thyroid malignancy, including FTC, has been reported to approach 2%. Preoperative imaging may be of some assistance in assessing the extent of a palpable mass. Ultrasound can determine the size and multicentricity of the malignancy; however, FTC is usually manifested as a solitary mass. Radionuclide scanning can determine whether a mass is functioning or is cold, although a minority of cold nodules actually prove to be malignant.

The use of FNA cytology has limited value in the preoperative diagnosis of FTC. Diagnosis of FTC requires demonstration of cellular invasion of the capsule or vascular or lymphatic channels. Invasion cannot be determined with the preoperative use of FNA. Additionally, intraoperative frozen section has been notoriously ineffective in making a definitive diagnosis.[21,22]

Treatment

Treatment of follicular carcinoma is primarily surgical. The diagnosis of the carcinoma cannot be determined by preoperative FNA or intraoperative frozen section diagnosis of a follicular lesion. The surgeon is left to select the most efficacious treatment of a "follicular lesion,"

which, lacking the obvious gross characteristics of malignancy and widely invasive FTC, is most likely a benign lesion. If the lesion is 2 cm or smaller and well contained within one thyroid lobe, an argument may be made for thyroid lobectomy and isthmectomy. If the lesion is larger than 2 cm, the surgeon may well proceed with total thyroidectomy. If the follicular lesion is larger than 4 cm, the risk for cancer is greater than 50%, and total thyroidectomy is an obvious choice. Lymph node dissection is not necessary in the absence of palpable lymph nodes and adds nothing to survival data.[27]

The prognosis after treatment of FTC depends on age. Patients younger than 40 years have the best prognosis, with survival rates approaching 95% at 5 and 10 years. Series comparing FTC with PTC have shown a poorer prognosis for FTC, although this disparity is more prominent after 10 to 15 years. Poorly differentiated FTC and well-differentiated FTC have 60% and 80% 10-year survival rates, respectively (see Fig. 36-16).[31]

A particularly vexing problem occurs when thyroid lobectomy has been performed for a presumed benign thyroid adenoma but the final pathologic diagnosis is follicular carcinoma. Two considerations must then take place. After determining an AMES or AGES score, a decision needs to be made regarding whether the lesion is low risk (small lesion in a younger patient), in which case the patient might be watched closely with ultrasound evaluations every 6 months. Alternatively, the lesion might be higher risk (>2 cm in a patient >60 years) and require surgery followed by radioablation. Reoperation mandates completion thyroidectomy, which is associated with increased technical difficulty and the possibility of complications.

Postoperative Treatment

Accepted postsurgical management of PTC and FTC involves the use of radioiodine ablation and long-term monitoring of Tg. [131]I contains both high energy (gamma rays) and medium energy (beta particles), which enhances the therapeutic effect. Patients are usually withheld from thyroid replacement therapy so that TSH levels may become elevated and thus maximize the effect of [131]I. Several studies suggest that ^{131}I ablation reduces disease-specific mortality in patients with primary tumors measuring at least 1 cm.[27]

If a patient has undergone complete thyroid ablation, postoperative Tg levels should be undetectable. The recent development of human recombinant TSH has redefined the efficacy of monitoring stimulated Tg levels as evidence of recurrence. It may be that the use of human recombinant TSH can detect tumor recurrence at an earlier time and thus allow earlier treatment. Despite these advances, the use of Tg to monitor tumor recurrence remains imperfect.[8] As many as 15% to 30% of patients with thyroid carcinoma have anti-Tg antibodies, which seriously compromises the use of Tg as a tumor marker.[37]

Hürthle Cell Carcinoma

Hürthle cell carcinoma is a subtype of follicular carcinoma that closely resembles FTC both grossly and on microscopic examination. The tumor contains an abundance of oxyphilic cells, or oncocytes. These cells are derived from follicular cells and have abundant granular acidophilic cytoplasm. Some studies have suggested that Hürthle cell carcinoma may have a worse clinical prognosis than standard FTC; however, there is no uniform agreement on these findings. It appears in an older age group and is very unusual in children. Unlike papillary and follicular cancer, spread to local lymph nodes is a poor prognostic event associated with nearly 70% mortality.[38]

Prognosis and Treatment

Hürthle cell carcinoma is manifested in much the same fashion as follicular cell neoplasms. The use of preoperative FNA raises many of the same issues; the finding of Hürthle cells leaves open the question of invasiveness and the diagnosis of malignancy. Treatment is surgical, following the same principles as for the workup of a follicular neoplasm.[38]

Medullary Carcinoma

MCT accounts for 5% to 10% of thyroid cancers. The malignancy involves the parafollicular cell, or C cell,

derived from the neural crest. MCT is associated with the secretion of a biologic marker, calcitonin. Excess secretion of calcitonin has been demonstrated to be an effective marker for the presence of MCT. Calcitonin excess is not associated with hypocalcemia.

Medullary carcinoma can occur in a sporadic form or as part of MEN 2A or 2B. The MEN syndromes are covered in more detail in Chapter 40. MEN 2A usually has a more favorable long-term outcome than MEN 2B or sporadic MCT does.[27]

Clinical Features

A patient with a sporadic medullary carcinoma may have either of two manifestations: a palpable mass for which a diagnosis can be made with FNA or the finding of an elevated calcitonin level. In sporadic MCT, the tumors are usually single and have no familial predisposition. The presence of both a mass and an elevated calcitonin level is virtually diagnostic of MCT, whereas the finding of an elevated basal calcitonin level in the absence of a thyroid mass might require further workup, including repeat basal calcitonin measurement and a calcium-stimulated or gastrin-stimulated test. Family members of patients with MEN 2 ideally are screened for the *RET* proto-oncogene. The workup of these patients includes a detailed and in-depth family history to inquire about the characteristics of MEN 2 in the patient and family members (Fig. 36-19). If MCT is suspected, serum calcium and urinary catecholamines must be determined to evaluate for hyperparathyroidism and possible pheochromocytoma.

Treatment

The surgical approach to sporadic medullary carcinoma involves at least total thyroidectomy with or without central lymph node dissection. Total thyroidectomy allows complete removal of the gland and a search for multicentricity. In sporadic MCT, the lesion is generally contained within one lobe, whereas in MEN 2, the malignancy involves the upper halves of both lobes. Dissection of the central lymph node compartment allows appropriate staging of this process. Any palpable lymph nodes in lateral areas require a modified radical neck dissection. A successful operation with a good prognosis is predicted for patients with smaller masses and in whom calcitonin levels are undetectable after surgery. Radioactive scanning may be used to ablate any residual thyroid. The literature describes the use of basal and stimulated calcitonin tests to monitor for recurrence because stimulated calcitonin values may rise before basal calcitonin levels do. Unfortunately, documentation of recurrent MCT by biochemical means is often associated with unresectable recurrence in distant metastatic locations, including the lung and liver.[27]

Anaplastic Thyroid Cancer

Anaplastic thyroid carcinoma represents less than 1% of all thyroid malignancies. It is the most aggressive form of thyroid cancer. A typical manifestation is an older patient with dysphagia, cervical tenderness, and a painful, rapidly enlarging neck mass. Superior vena cava

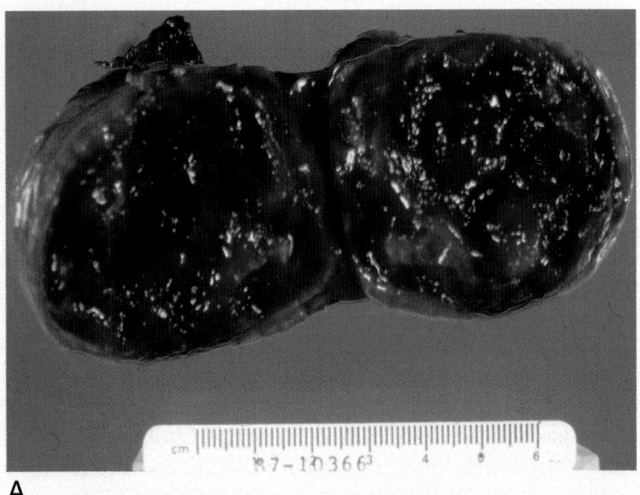

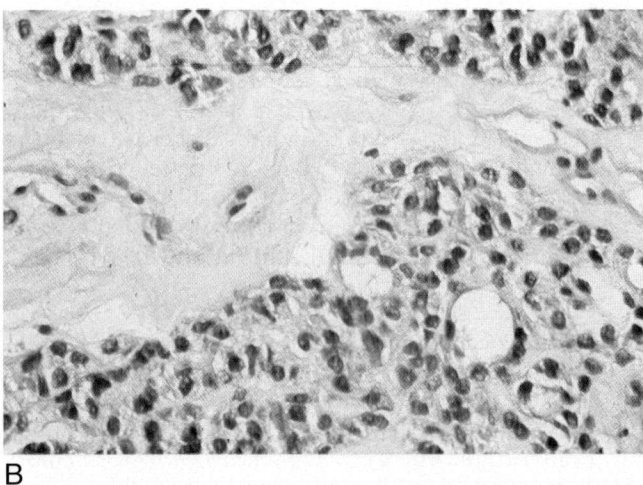

A

B

Figure 36-19 A, This 4-cm solitary mass in a thyroid lobe was removed by total thyroidectomy. **B,** Hematoxylin and eosin staining of this mass demonstrated cells consistent with medullary carcinoma with amyloid infiltrate.

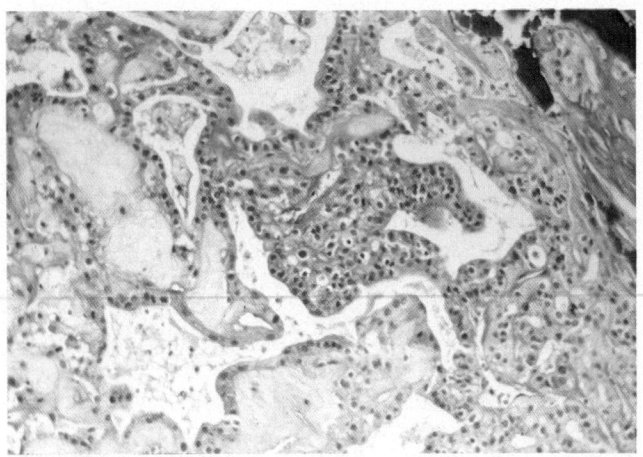

Figure 36-20 Hematoxylin and eosin staining of a thyroid mass reveals a population of poorly differentiated cells, many of which are multinucleated. This is consistent with anaplastic carcinoma of the thyroid.

syndrome can also be part of the findings. The clinical situation deteriorates rapidly into tracheal obstruction and rapid local invasion of surrounding structures.

Pathology

Grossly, the tumor is locally invasive, with a firm, whitish appearance. On microscopic evaluation, giant cells with intranuclear cytoplasmic invaginations can be seen. There is a wide variety of cell types ranging from moderately differentiated to extremely poorly differentiated cells (Fig. 36-20). Occasionally, squamous cell elements or islands of more recognizable differentiated thyroid carcinoma, such as papillary carcinoma, can be identified within the locus of the tumor. This has led to speculation that anaplastic carcinoma might arise from more well-differentiated carcinoma; however, there has been no solid proof of this theory.[27]

Treatment

The results of any surgical treatment of anaplastic thyroid carcinoma are tempered by its rapidly progressive clinical course. Most reports of resection are not optimistic. FNA is accurate in 90% of cases, thus making open biopsy a less needed option. Three types of cell populations have been classified: small spindle cell, giant cell, and squamous. All have a poor prognosis. *p53* mutations are found in 15% of tumors, a much higher rate than noted with well-differentiated cancers. Postoperative external beam irradiation or adjunctive chemotherapy adds little to the overall prognosis.[39]

It appears that if anaplastic carcinoma is initially confirmed to be resectable, some small improvement in survival may be seen. The finding of distant metastasis or invasion into locally unresectable structures, such as the trachea or vasculature of the anterior mediastinum, leads to a more conservative surgical approach such as tracheostomy.

Lymphoma

Primary thyroid lymphoma, though rare, is being recognized more often. The diagnosis is considered in patients with a goiter, especially one that has apparently grown significantly in a short period. Other initial symptoms include hoarseness, dysphagia, and fever. There is also an increased association between lymphoma and Hashimoto's thyroiditis.

Workup and Diagnosis

Patients with lymphoma undergo the standard workup for a thyroid mass or goiter. Suspicious signs are rapid enlargement and diffuse pain. Ultrasound may demonstrate a classic pseudocystic pattern. FNA can be diagnostic in this situation. The use of flow cytometry for monoclonality can confirm the diagnosis. If FNA is nondiagnostic, core needle biopsy or open biopsy can be considered. If the diagnosis is either confirmed or highly suspicious, additional preoperative evaluation includes neck, chest, and abdominal CT or MRI to assess for extrathyroidal spread. Most thyroid lymphomas are B cell in origin. A subgroup of mucosa-associated lymphoid tissue (MALT) lymphomas occur in 6% to 27% of patients in some series.[40]

Treatment

Treatment philosophies differ with regard to preoperative chemotherapy or surgical ablation. Use of the CHOP regimen (cyclophosphamide, hydroxydaunomycin [doxorubicin], vincristine, and prednisolone) has been associated with excellent survival. Surgical resection, including near-total or total thyroidectomy, is thought to enhance these results, particularly for MALT lymphomas. There can be a significant amount of pericapsular edema and swelling with loss of normal tissue planes. MALT lymphomas are usually diagnosed at an earlier stage and have an indolent course. Diffuse and mixed large cell lymphomas behave more aggressively and are often initially found to have widespread involvement. Five-year survival rates for MALT lymphomas approach 100%, whereas rates for large cell and mixed large cell lymphoma are 71% and 78%, respectively.[39]

Molecular Markers for Thyroid Cancer

Despite advances in imaging technology and treatment of thyroid cancer, recurrence or distant metastasis (or both) can occur in as many as 20% of cases. No highly dependable, specific means of detection of malignant tissue, either as primary tumor or recurrent disease, is available. Molecular detection of tissue or tumor-specific DNA or RNA either in peripheral blood or in FNA samples holds great promise but is currently under investigation. These techniques hold particular promise for two difficult situations in thyroid cancer—FNA cytology of a follicular thyroid nodule and postoperative surveillance.[41]

Analysis of Fine-Needle Aspirates

Currently, a specific molecular marker for thyroid cancer has not been found that would allow accurate diagnosis of specimens obtained from FNA. Evaluation of genetic alterations in DNA or RNA appears to hold promise, especially *ras* point mutations or *PAX8-PPARγ* rearrangement for follicular carcinoma and methylation of TSH-R for well-differentiated thyroid cancer.[42] However, these studies are evolving and are by no means established.

Galectin-3

Galectin-3 (GAL-3) is a β-galactosyl–binding protein with cell-cell and cell-matrix interaction. The galectins have been thought to be associated with initiation of cell growth and malignant transformation.[43] There has been enthusiasm for GAL-3 as a marker of malignancy in FNA and surgical specimens; however, it may also appear in Hashimoto's thyroiditis.[44] If Hashimoto's thyroiditis is excluded, GAL-3 may be an important marker for malignancy.

RET/PTC Rearrangements

Chromosome 10q11-2 is the locus of the *RET* proto-oncogene. *RET* activation has been documented in PTC cells and is therefore known as RET/PTC. As many as five variants of RET/PTC have been described. A recent study has reported that three of the most common of these variants (RET/PTC 1, 2, and 3) have been found in FNA samples of PTC with no false positives.[45] Despite enthusiasm for its diagnostic possibility, other reports have shown RET/PTC rearrangements in benign tissue as well.

CD44

The CD44 family of membrane glycoproteins is associated with adhesion, lymphocyte activation, and tumor growth and metastasis. A number of variant isoforms (CD44v), especially v6 through v10, have been shown to be overexpressed in PTC.[46] CD44 has been reported in aspirates of PTC samples. However, others have found CD44 in benign tissue.[47] FNA detection of the combination of GAL-3 and CD44 variants in RNA holds great promise for more accurate preoperative diagnosis. Given the established excellent specificity of conventional FNA samples for PTC, the additional value of CD44v6 or other isoforms in FNA-derived tissue needs to be developed further.

BRAF Mutation

The Ras/Raf mitogen-activated protein kinase (MAPK) signaling pathway is an important constituent of cell growth, proliferation, and division. Of all the isoforms of this RAF kinase, the B type (BRAF) is apparently the most potent stimulator of MAPK signaling. It appears that activating mutations of *BRAF* induce the MAPK pathway and initiate malignant transformation. Several groups report that *BRAF* mutations are found in as many as 70% of operative specimens. Cohen and colleagues[48] found a 94% concordance in evaluating preoperative FNA specimens with the postoperative result in documented PTC cases. Xing and coworkers[49] found that the *BRAF* gene was associated with an increased likelihood of postoperative tumor recurrence.

Analysis of Peripheral Blood

A second area of the potential usefulness of molecular markers would be the finding of a reliable diagnostic predictor of recurrence obtained via a peripheral blood sample. Detection of a circulating thyroid-specific mRNA of recurrent thyroid cancer was reported almost 10 years ago.[50] However, subsequent studies evaluating Tg mRNA have yielded mixed findings, with positive results being found in benign situations as well.[51] More sophisticated developments in Tg mRNA analysis may lead to discovery of a marker of recurrence that can be detected by peripheral blood analysis. However, its current reliability is not well established.

Molecular Profiling

Because no single gene or tumor marker appears to be definitive in the initial diagnosis of malignancy, the fascinating concept of molecular profiling has been advanced. Microarray analysis can evaluate expression profiles of a large number of genes and determine whether groups of genes are preferentially expressed in

Table 36-4 Indications for Interventional Procedures

PROCEDURE	ADVANTAGE	DISADVANTAGE OR COMPLICATIONS	INDICATION
Fine-needle aspiration (FNA)	Accurate diagnosis of malignancy	Cannot confirm benign diagnosis Capsular hemorrhage	Tissue diagnosis of ultrasound-determined solid nodule Previous "nondiagnostic" result
Open biopsy	Direct visualization	Requires an operating room, possibly general anesthesia	Complex case in which FNA has failed to give a diagnosis
"Nodulectomy" (less than a lobectomy)	None	Difficult second operation to complete the lobectomy if a diagnosis of cancer is made	None
Lobectomy (with isthmectomy)	Lower rates of hypocalcemia and nerve damage	May require completion thyroidectomy if a diagnosis of cancer is made	Strong suspicion of benign disease Well-differentiated cancer <1 cm
Near-total thyroidectomy	Lower rates of hypocalcemia and nerve damage	Possible recurrence in residual thyroid tissue	Benign multinodular disease <2-cm nodule on the complete lobectomy side Hyperthyroidism
Total thyroidectomy	Use of postoperative ^{131}I is most efficacious Use of post-thyroglobulin levels for recurrence	Higher rate of hypocalcemia and nerve damage	Extensive multinodular disease Hyperthyroidism >2-cm thyroid cancer (nonpalpable lymph nodes)
Modified radical lymph node dissection	Decreased rate of recurrence	Cranial nerve XII damage Loss of sensation over the ear and lateral cervical area (Left) Thoracic duct leak and lymphocele Horner's syndrome	Palpable adenopathy with a diagnosis of papillary, follicular, or medullary cancer
Median sternotomy	Exposure of mediastinal contents	Bleeding Nonunion of the sternum (if complete sternotomy) Increased hospital stay	Extension of the malignancy into the anterior mediastinum Inability to mobilize a large substernal goiter
Central lymph node dissection	Decreased risk for recurrence	Increased risk for hypocalcemia and nerve damage	Medullary carcinoma requires removal of lymph nodes in the central cervical compartment (medial to the jugular veins)

certain types of thyroid neoplasms. Finley and associates[52] analyzed 62 samples of thyroid resections (including 26 benign nodules). The sensitivity and specificity of diagnosing malignancy were 92% and 96%, respectively. The cancer gene group included cancer-associated genes such as GAL-3, as well as several previously unrecognized genes. This group offers the exciting possibility that future efficiency in diagnostic techniques might lie with cluster analysis of groups of genes rather than finding a single marker.

SURGICAL APPROACHES TO THE THYROID GLAND AND ADJACENT STRUCTURES
(Table 36-4)

Cervical Approach

Before any cervical exploration the patient must be appropriately positioned with the neck extended. We favor full muscle relaxation, which allows optimal positioning. After positioning, and before skin preparation, an excellent opportunity to perform neck ultrasound is available. A transverse incision is made about two fingerbreadths above the clavicular heads. The incision is placed in a way that provides a direct approach to the thyroid gland and its adjacent structures while allowing optimal postoperative cosmetic results. If possible, the incision incorporates normal skin lines to aid in optimal cosmetic healing. The lateral borders of the incision can approach the medial borders of the sternocleidomastoid muscle but can be lengthened if the lateral aspect of the neck is to be investigated. The skin incision is carried through subcutaneous fat and the platysmal muscle, and superior and inferior flaps are dissected in a bloodless plane beneath the platysmal layer. The anterior jugular veins are identified, and any that are crossing or running along the midline can be divided (Fig. 36-21).

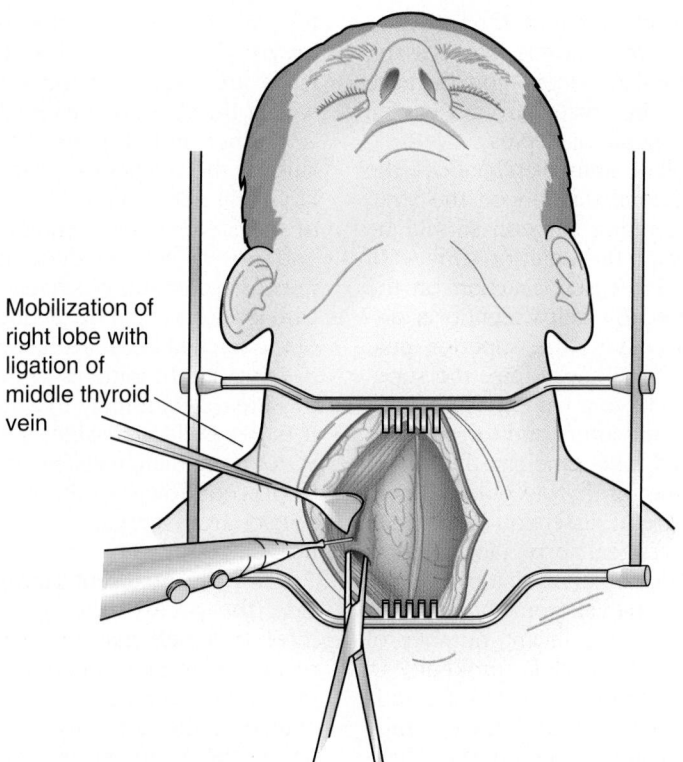

Mobilization of right lobe with ligation of middle thyroid vein

Figure 36-21 A Mahorner retractor is inserted, and towels (not shown) are placed so that only the incision is exposed. The strap muscles (sternohyoid and sternothyroid) are then separated by dividing the tissues in the avascular midline plane from the thyroid cartilage to the suprasternal notch. The thyroid lobe is exposed by mobilizing the strap muscles away from the lobe by means of lateral retraction on the muscles. The middle vein is exposed, divided, and ligated. (From Sabiston DC Jr [ed]: Atlas of General Surgery. Philadelphia, WB Saunders, 1995.)

The midline raphe can be identified between the sternohyoid muscles, and this raphe is divided in a bloodless plane from the thyroid cartilage superiorly to the sternal notch inferiorly. As the plane immediately beneath the sternohyoid muscles is entered, one encounters the isthmus of the thyroid in the midline and each of the lobes laterally. Above and below the isthmus are the cartilaginous rings of the trachea. Blunt finger dissection can separate the sternohyoid muscle from the thyroid capsule medially and identify the sternothyroid muscles in a deep and lateral position. The sternothyroid muscles do not meet in the midline and must be separated off the thyroid capsule to gain lateral exposure to the thyroid. In patients who have previously undergone FNA, it may be that the planes under the sternothyroid muscle are obliterated by recent hemorrhage or scarring. If the patient has previously had thyroid surgery, these muscle groups will be densely adherent to the trachea and perhaps the tracheoesophageal groove. Great care must be used in this circumstance to identify the parathyroids and recurrent laryngeal nerve.

When the recurrent laryngeal nerve has been identified on either side, it is mandatory to track it through any scar tissue or thyroid carcinoma. Every effort must be made to avoid sacrificing the nerve. In rare situations, such as anaplastic thyroid carcinoma, aggressive well-differentiated carcinoma, or obvious involvement with other head and neck tumors, the nerve may be sacrificed. If a recurrent laryngeal nerve is found to have been injured during the course of an otherwise uncomplicated operation, every attempt is made to repair it initially with microscope-aided visualization and microvascular technique (8-0 or 9-0 monofilament sutures).

Dissection between the sternohyoid and the sternothyroid muscles gains exposure to the lateral and deeper structures. Exposure of these lateral structures is enhanced by placing medial traction on the thyroid lobe on the side being dissected. Care must be taken to divide the middle thyroid vein before it is placed under excessive traction by this maneuver. With lateral retraction of the muscles and medial retraction of the thyroid lobe, the common carotid is quickly defined. On the left side, the esophagus is more prominent because of its more lateral position at this level in the neck. Definition of this area can be enhanced by placement of an esophageal stethoscope, which allows easier palpation of the esophagus.

In the case of complicated lateral thyroid masses, lymphadenopathy, or previous surgery, it may be necessary to gain exposure laterally by dividing the sternohyoid and sternothyroid muscles. It is rarely necessary to divide these two muscles, however, because lateral traction generally provides good exposure. If transection of the sternohyoid or sternothyroid muscle is necessary, it is done superiorly to minimize denervation because both these muscle groups are innervated from a caudal direction through the ansa hypoglossi nerves.

By gaining access to the plane immediately above the thyroid sheath and placing lateral traction on the strap muscles of the neck, the operating surgeon should be able to visualize the entirety of the anterior surface of the thyroid, even in reoperative cases. Traction on the thyroid lobes in a medial direction helps identify a dissection plane for gaining access to the superior pole vessels (Figs. 36-22 and 36-23). To skeletonize the superior pole vessels, one needs to have good exposure laterally between the common carotid artery and the superior aspect of the ipsilateral thyroid lobe. One can then enter behind or posterior to the superior thyroid pole adjacent to the cricothyroid muscle. Careful dissection in this area avoids injury to the external laryngeal nerve. Most patients (75%-80%) have external laryngeal nerves that run on the cricothyroid muscle and are separate from the superior vessels; however, this leaves a significant number of patients in whom the nerve runs in close proximity to the superior pole vessels and could be divided if care is not exercised. After the superior pole vessels are carefully dissected and identified, they can be double-ligated adjacent to their entrance into the thyroid lobe. After the superior thyroid vessels and middle thyroid veins have been divided, continued medial retraction of the thyroid

lobe allows the posterior aspect of the thyroid lobe to be visualized. It is in this area that the superior parathyroids are usually found lying in small deposits of fat within the thyroid sheath (Figs. 36-24 and 36-25).

Further mobilization of the thyroid lobe allows exposure of the tracheoesophageal groove and the recurrent laryngeal nerve (Figs. 36-26 to 36-30). Minimal dissection of the lower vessels entering the thyroid is undertaken, and no division is done until the recurrent laryngeal nerve is seen and positively identified. On the right side, care is taken when dissecting in the posterolateral aspects of the trachea because the esophagus is not well palpated in this area. In patients undergoing thyroid reoperations, this area is extremely treacherous because of scar tissue. It is generally advisable, if the recurrent laryngeal nerve is not immediately visible at the level of the thyroid lobe, to proceed lower in the neck tissue in previously undissected areas to gain access to the recurrent laryngeal nerve.

After the recurrent laryngeal nerve is seen on either side, the pace of the operation may be increased; the inferior vessels may be divided while the course of the recurrent laryngeal nerve is directly visualized. Continued medial traction on the lobe then identifies the cephalad course of the nerve to the point at which it disappears under the ligament of Berry or into its final destination, the caudal border of the cricothyroid muscle. The ligament of Berry is in a position just anterior and slightly medial to the nerve's entrance underneath the

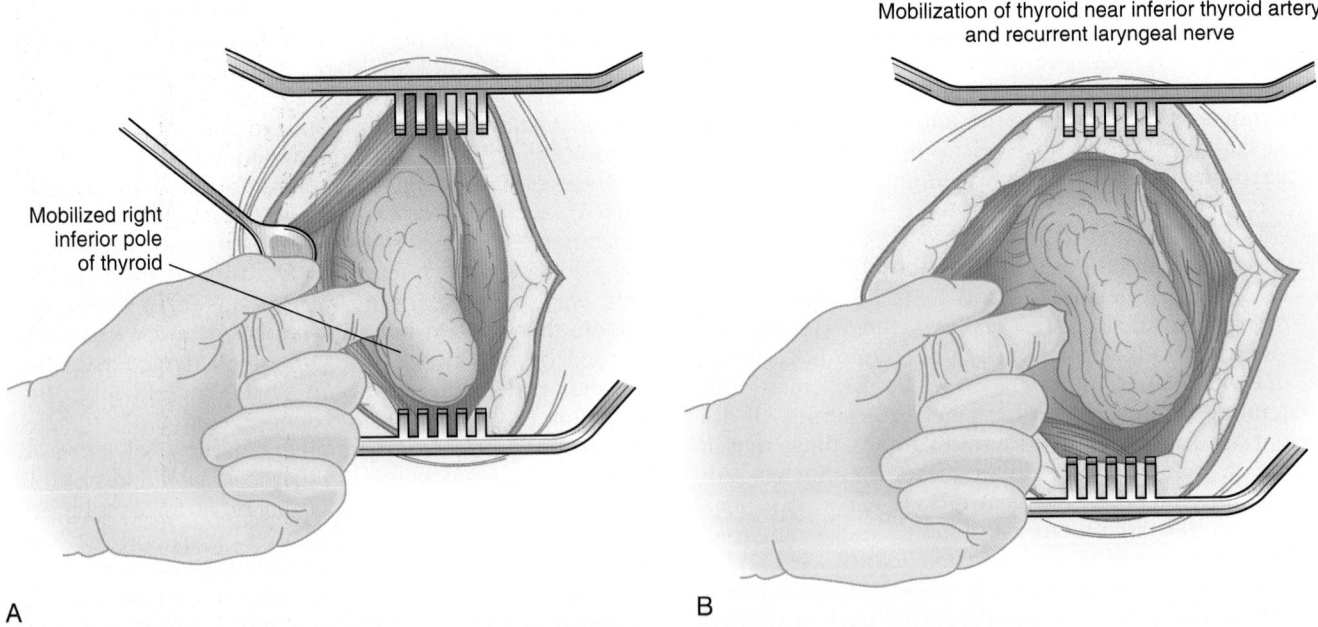

Figure 36-22 A and **B,** The thyroid lobe is retracted medially to expose the area where the parathyroid glands and recurrent laryngeal nerve are located. (From Sabiston DC Jr [ed]: Atlas of General Surgery. Philadelphia, WB Saunders, 1995.)

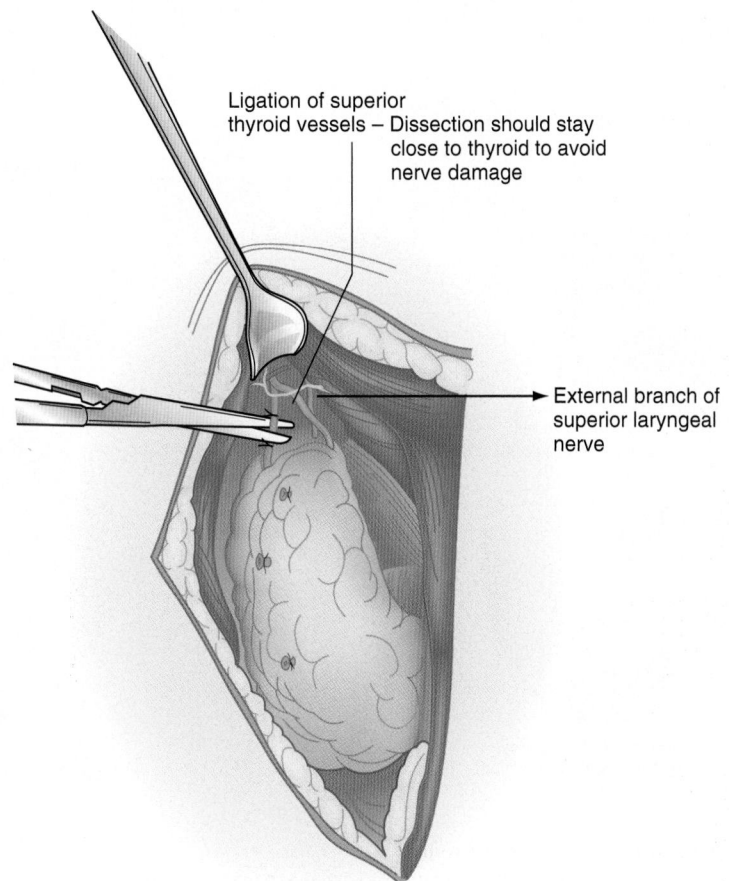

Ligation of superior
thyroid vessels – Dissection should stay
close to thyroid to avoid
nerve damage

External branch of
superior laryngeal
nerve

Figure 36-23 Downward traction exposes the superior pole vessels, including branches of the superior thyroid artery. The external laryngeal nerve courses along the cricothyroid muscle just medial to the superior pole vessels. To avoid injury to this nerve, which controls tension of the vocal cords, the superior pole vessels are divided individually as close as possible to the point where they enter the thyroid gland. (From Sabiston DC Jr [ed]: Atlas of General Surgery. Philadelphia, WB Saunders, 1995.)

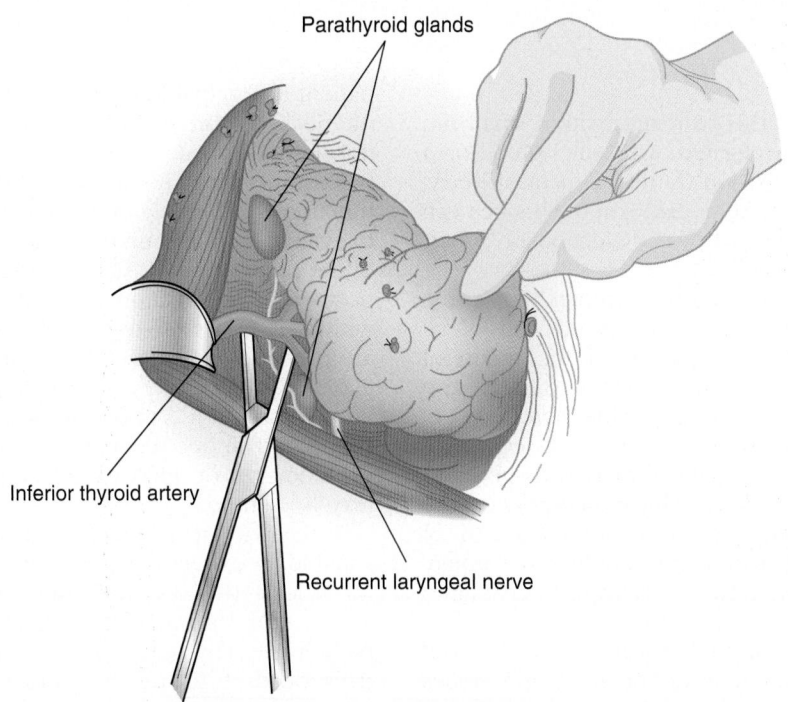

Parathyroid glands

Inferior thyroid artery

Recurrent laryngeal nerve

Figure 36-24 As the thyroid is retracted medially, gentle dissection is used to expose the parathyroid glands, inferior thyroid artery, and recurrent laryngeal nerve. The recurrent nerve usually passes behind the inferior thyroid but occasionally lies anterior to it. It is best found by careful dissection just inferior to the artery. The nerve can then be traced upward, and its position in relation to the thyroid can be determined. Parathyroid glands that lie on the thyroid surface can be mobilized with their vascular supply and thus preserved. (From Sabiston DC Jr [ed]: Atlas of General Surgery. Philadelphia, WB Saunders, 1995.)

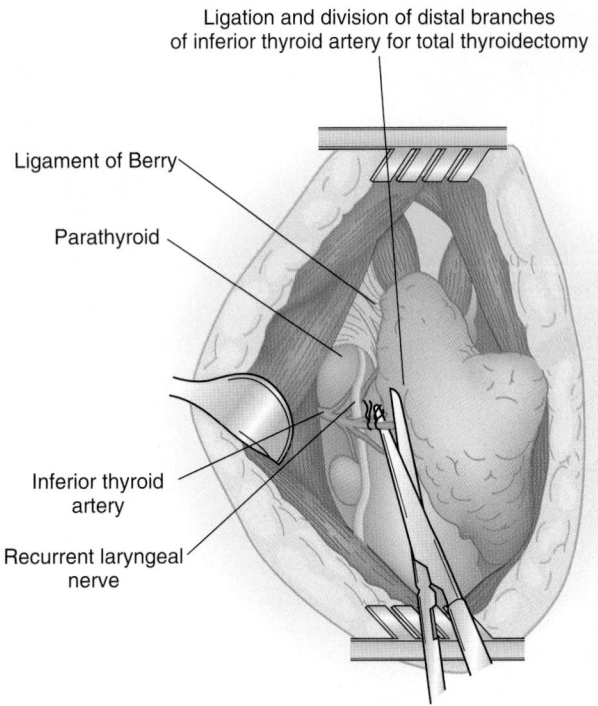

Ligation and division of distal branches
of inferior thyroid artery for total thyroidectomy

Ligament of Berry

Parathyroid

Inferior thyroid
artery

Recurrent laryngeal
nerve

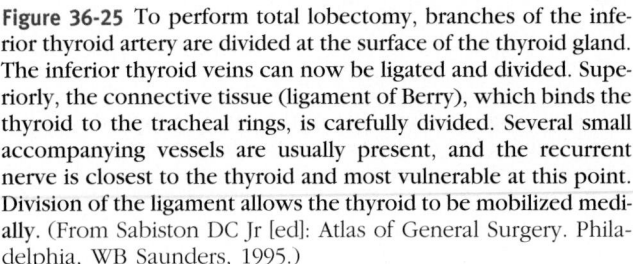

Figure 36-25 To perform total lobectomy, branches of the inferior thyroid artery are divided at the surface of the thyroid gland. The inferior thyroid veins can now be ligated and divided. Superiorly, the connective tissue (ligament of Berry), which binds the thyroid to the tracheal rings, is carefully divided. Several small accompanying vessels are usually present, and the recurrent nerve is closest to the thyroid and most vulnerable at this point. Division of the ligament allows the thyroid to be mobilized medially. (From Sabiston DC Jr [ed]: Atlas of General Surgery. Philadelphia, WB Saunders, 1995.)

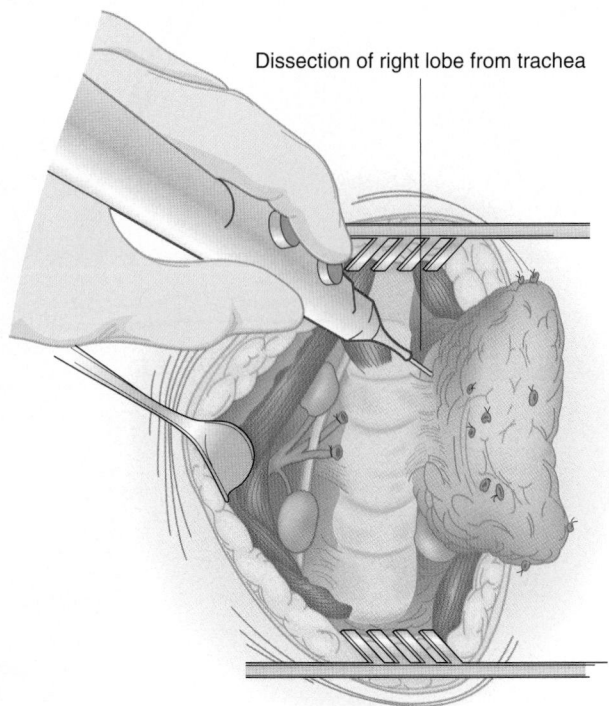

Dissection of right lobe from trachea

Figure 36-26 Dissection of the thyroid from the trachea can be performed with the cautery by division of the loose connective tissue between these structures. Dissection is extended under the isthmus, and the specimen is divided so that the isthmus is included with the resected lobe. The pyramidal lobe is also included if present. (From Sabiston DC Jr [ed]: Atlas of General Surgery. Philadelphia, WB Saunders, 1995.)

cricothyroid muscle, and this structure, with a small rim of thyroid tissue, can be ligated with silk suture or a harmonic scalpel. After division of the ligament of Berry, the attachment of the thyroid medially on the trachea can be divided with low-energy Bovie dissection or a harmonic scalpel (see Fig. 36-26).

Terminology for thyroid surgery is inconsistent in the literature. Total thyroidectomy involves division of all thyroid tissue between the entrance of the recurrent laryngeal nerves bilaterally at the ligament of Berry, and it results in complete removal of all visible thyroid tissue. Near-total thyroidectomy involves complete dissection on one side while leaving a remnant of thyroid tissue laterally on the contralateral side, which incorporates the parathyroids. Subtotal thyroidectomy leaves a rim of thyroid tissue bilaterally to ensure parathyroid viability and avoid entrance of the recurrent laryngeal nerves into the larynx (see Figs. 36-25 to 36-29).

Central lymph node dissection can be carried out under direct vision, with removal of all lymph nodes immediately adjacent to the thyroid, especially in the tracheoesophageal groove in patients with well-differentiated carcinoma. This dissection proceeds laterally to and includes the lymph nodes within the carotid sheath. If a

patient has palpable lymph nodes in the lateral aspect of the neck, a more complete modified radical neck dissection is performed.

Postoperative monitoring of thyroid and parathyroid function is extremely important. The surgeon is obligated to evaluate and inform the patient and referring physician of the details of the resection and its expected impact on postoperative function. A calcium assay is performed within 24 hours of surgery. If no signs of hypocalcemia are present, particularly if the surgeon has visualized the glands during surgery, no calcium supplementation may be necessary. If symptoms occur or if the surgeon is concerned about the patient's parathyroid status, daily supplements of 1500 to 3000 mg of elemental calcium may be started.

If the patient was euthyroid before surgery, it is reasonable to expect that replacement may not be needed for at least 10 days, even after total thyroidectomy. This allows time for complete evaluation of the specimen by pathology. Thyroid replacement generally requires a daily dose of 100 µg of levothyroxine (Synthroid) for a person of normal weight. Most endocrinologists believe that the levothyroxine dose needs to be adjusted to keep TSH levels at low normal values after resection for cancer or suppressive therapy.

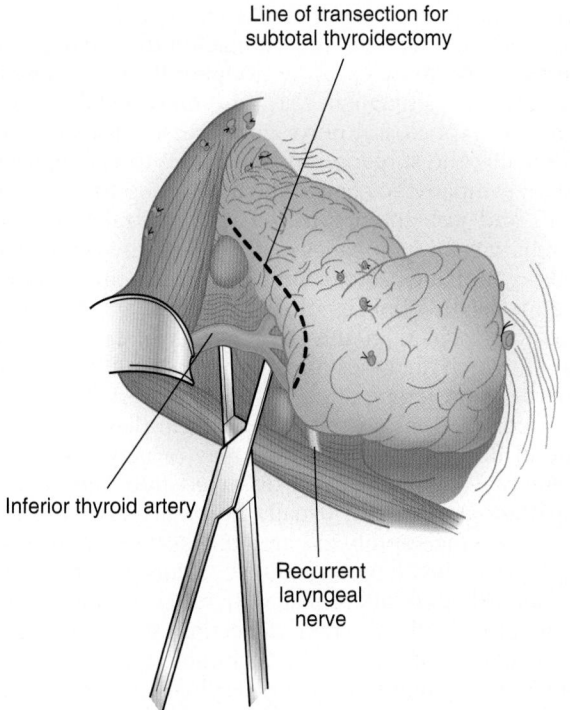

Figure 36-27 Subtotal lobectomy necessitates identification of the parathyroid glands, inferior thyroid artery, and recurrent laryngeal nerve, as previously described. The line of resection is selected to preserve the parathyroid glands and their blood supply and to protect the recurrent laryngeal nerve. It is based on the inferior thyroid artery or its major branches. (From Sabiston DC Jr [ed]: Atlas of General Surgery. Philadelphia, WB Saunders, 1995.)

Modified Radical Neck Dissection

Although there is some controversy about when to perform a modified radical neck dissection for thyroid carcinoma, it is safe to say that this operation is most widely performed in patients with documented disease in whom obvious and palpable lymphadenopathy lateral to the carotid sheath exists at the time of the original diagnosis or occurs after preceding thyroid surgery. There appear to be limited data on the use of prophylactic neck dissection in patients with well-differentiated thyroid carcinoma who do not have palpable lymph nodes.

In the case of papillary carcinoma, concern about multicentricity and microscopic lymph node involvement appears to fuel this controversy. For larger tumors and palpable nodes in this area, most authors advocate total thyroidectomy and, at a minimum, central lymph node dissection. In the case of microscopic lymph node involvement in the absence of palpable lateral lymph nodes, the use of radioactive iodine before proceeding with prophylactic lateral lymph node dissection has been advocated but not overwhelmingly accepted. Radioactive iodine appears to be beneficial in this circumstance but is much less effective in ablating palpable regional metastatic lymph node involvement. The use of selected removal of palpable nodes in the lateral compartment (so-called cherry picking) has largely been abandoned. Therefore, modified radical neck dissection is primarily reserved for patients with thyroid carcinoma and clinically palpable cervical lymph node metastases. This can be accomplished with an en bloc dissection that removes all the lymphatic and adipose tissue in the lateral neck compartment while avoiding the cosmetic or functional

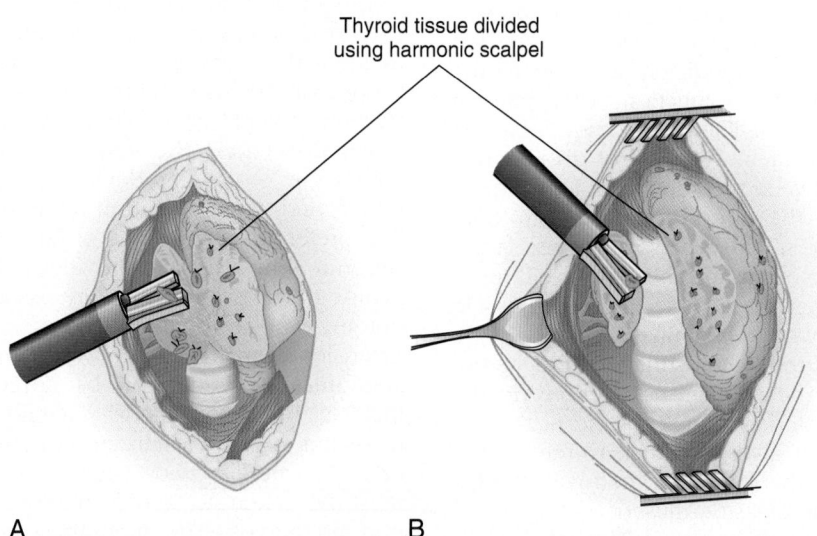

Figure 36-28 **A** and **B,** The thyroid gland is divided with a harmonic scalpel. (From Sabiston DC Jr [ed]: Atlas of General Surgery. Philadelphia, WB Saunders, 1995.)

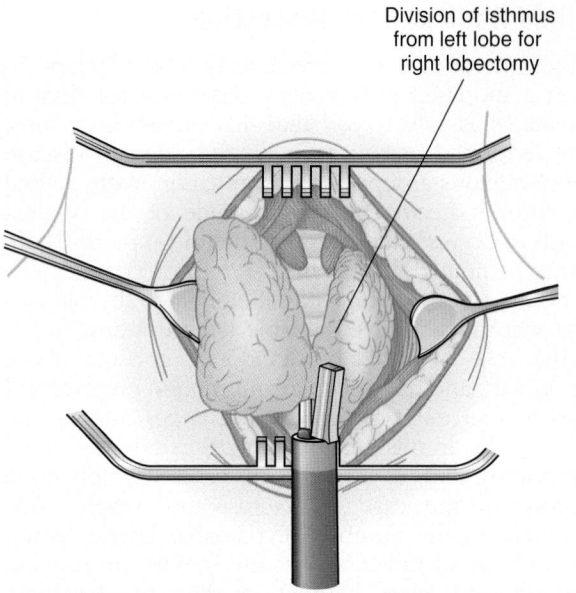

Division of isthmus
from left lobe for
right lobectomy

Figure 36-29 The thyroid can now be divided with the harmonic scalpel so that the isthmus is included in the specimen. (From Sabiston DC Jr [ed]: Atlas of General Surgery. Philadelphia, WB Saunders, 1995.)

abnormality associated with removal of muscle groups that is used in the classic radical neck dissection. The sternocleidomastoid muscle and spinal accessory nerve are spared.[53]

A cervical skin incision is used for the operation, which is standard for most thyroid operations. It is extended laterally and superiorly along the border of the sternocleidomastoid muscle. Occasionally, it is necessary to make a higher incision parallel to the previous surgical incision if higher lymph nodes are palpable. In initiating the neck dissection, the surgeon must gain access deep to the sternocleidomastoid muscle and remain anterior to the carotid sheath above the clavicle. Laterally, the phrenic nerve is identified and preserved in the prevertebral fascia on the anterior scalene muscle. On the left side, the phrenic nerve is immediately adjacent to the thoracic duct at the level of the junction of the internal jugular and subclavian veins. The dissection begins just above the clavicle in this area. The goal of dissection is removal of all tissue between the superficial and prevertebral fascia, except for the carotid artery, jugular vein, vagus, and phrenic and spinal accessory nerves. Additionally, the sympathetic chain and the sternocleidomastoid muscle must be preserved. Dissection continues in the cephalad direction, where the spinal accessory nerve is identified at the deep and lateral surface of the sternocleidomastoid muscle. The nerve runs inferiorly in the lateral aspect of the posterior triangle of the neck. The nerve can be traced as it gives a branch to the sternocleidomastoid muscle at this level and then passes adjacent and posterior to the digastric muscle.

As the dissection proceeds in a more cephalad direction, the hypoglossal nerve is encountered; it crosses anteriorly to the internal carotid artery and internal jugular

vein yet deep to the anterior facial vein. It follows the stylohyoid muscle into the submandibular triangle and innervates the muscles of the tongue. If one chooses to ligate the internal jugular vein, care must be taken to not injure the hypoglossal nerve as it crosses in this area.

Medially, the surgeon must take care to not injure the cervical sympathetic chain, which lies deep to the carotid sheath and just anterior to the prevertebral fascia. The retropharyngeal lymphatics connect with the cervical and jugular lymphatics across the chain in this area and may have metastatic deposits of thyroid cancer. Injury to the sympathetic chain in this area results in Horner's syndrome, which includes ptosis, miosis, anhidrosis, and increased skin temperature on the involved side.

On completion of a modified radical dissection, a triangle of fibrofatty tissue, which may or may not include the internal jugular vein, is dissected free and oriented for pathology. It is not usually necessary to extend dissection into the suprahyoid area unless there is extensive lymph node involvement, which occurs in only a few patients with well-differentiated thyroid carcinoma (~1%). Great care is taken when dissecting structures in the lateral aspect of the neck, including the sympathetic chain and recurrent laryngeal and spinal accessory nerves, unless they are obviously and grossly involved with tumor.

Median Sternotomy

Exploration of the anterior mediastinal space is within the armamentarium of an experienced thyroid surgeon. Nearly every benign and malignant thyroid tumor can be removed through cervical exploration. Occasionally, a median sternotomy may be necessary in patients who need a reoperation, have large invasive tumors, have low-lying thyroid glands and a large tumor, or have previously undergone radioiodine ablation or external beam irradiation.

Initial exploration usually involves a cervical incision. If a median sternotomy is then required, a midline incision is made from the middle of the cervical wound and extended inferiorly and onto the manubrium. Before dividing the sternum, access is gained on the superior border of the manubrium and all tissues deep to the sternum swept away bluntly with cotton sponges or finger dissection. The midline sternal incision is made with a saw or splitting device and carried to the level of the second, third, or fourth intercostal space as needed. We prefer a sternal split of the cephalad half of the sternum, which usually provides excellent exposure and avoids the possible instability associated with full sternotomy. Substernal thyroid masses, including goiters or extension of malignancies, as well as ectopic parathyroid adenomatous tissue, can be approached through this incision. The anteromedial fat pad and thymus can be dissected to gain visualization of the pericardium superiorly. As one proceeds laterally in this dissection, care must be taken to avoid injuring the pleura and the phrenic nerves. The innominate vein is deep to the thymus. Virtually all low-lying thyroid masses can be approached through this incision.

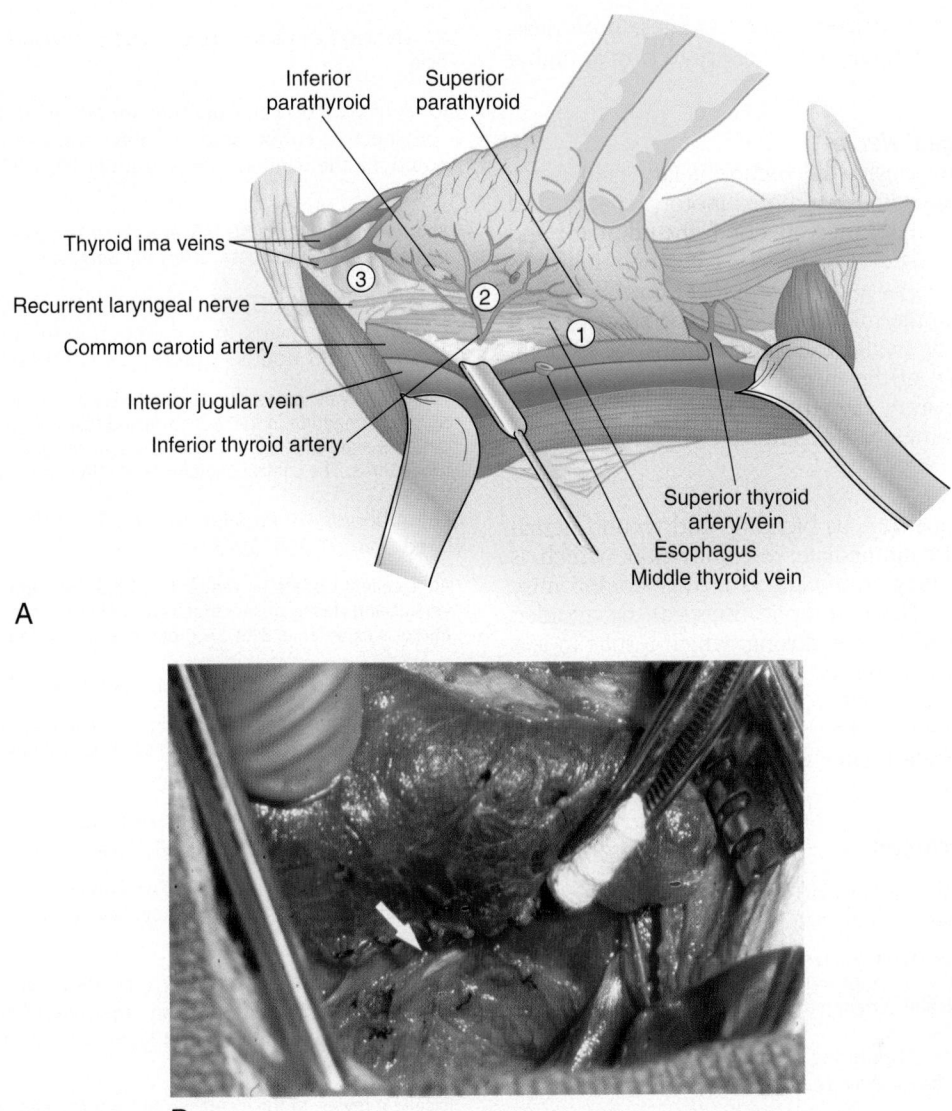

Inferior parathyroid
Superior parathyroid
Thyroid ima veins
Recurrent laryngeal nerve
Common carotid artery
Interior jugular vein
Inferior thyroid artery
③
②
①
Superior thyroid artery/vein
Esophagus
Middle thyroid vein

A

B

Figure 36-30 A, During thyroidectomy, the recurrent laryngeal nerve is at greatest risk for injury (*1*) at the ligament of Berry, (*2*) during ligation of branches of the inferior thyroid artery, and (*3*) at the thoracic inlet. **B,** Intraoperative photo of the recurrent laryngeal nerve in the tracheoesophageal groove *(white arrow).* (**A,** From Kahky MP, Weber RS: Intraoperative problems: Complications of surgery of the thyroid and parathyroid glands. Surg Clin North Am 73:307, 1993.)

Complications of Surgery

The advantage of complete removal of disease-bearing tissue and efficient subsequent application of postprocedure radioiodine ablation after total thyroidectomy must be weighed against lesser procedures such as lobectomy in terms of surgical complications. The most important complications are postprocedure hypocalcemia secondary to devascularization of the parathyroid and significant hoarseness caused by recurrent laryngeal nerve injury induced by either traction or division (see Fig. 36-30).

Hypocalcemia

Rates of postprocedure hypocalcemia are about 5%, and it resolves in 80% of cases in about 12 months.[54] Therefore, every effort is made to evaluate the parathyroid

tissue intraoperatively. For glands that appear to be devascularized, the use of immediate parathyroid autotransplantation of 1-mm fragments of saline-chilled tissue into pockets made in the sternocleidomastoid muscle or, more commonly, the brachioradialis muscle is extremely effective in avoiding hypocalcemia.

Nerve Injury

Superior Laryngeal Nerve

The superior laryngeal nerve has two branches—an internal one that supplies sensory fibers to the larynx and an external one that supplies motor fibers to the cricothyroid muscles and tenses the vocal cords. The external branch can run closely adherent to the superior thyroid artery, and care must be exercised during dissection in this area.

Injury to the branch causes voice changes, huskiness, poor volume voice fatigue, and inability to sing at higher ranges.[1,55]

Recurrent Laryngeal Nerve

As mentioned previously, the recurrent laryngeal nerve arises from the vagus and is a mixed motor, sensory, and autonomous nerve that innervates both the adductor and abductor muscles (see Fig. 36-30). Unilateral injury is classically described as a paralyzed vocal cord with loss of movement from the midline. A wide spectrum of injuries to the voice or swallowing mechanisms, or to both, can occur because of the mixed fibers contained within the nerve.[1] Temporary or permanent voice change can result and is extremely distressing to the patient.

Bleeding

Other complications such as bleeding and wound hematomas may require immediate re-exploration, which is done in the operating room unless airway compromise dictates otherwise. These complications can be avoided by meticulous hemostasis at closing, which results in less than a 1% rate of occurrence.[55]

Complication rates appear to be affected by surgeon experience. A study in Maryland of 5860 patients reported the lowest complication rates in patients of surgeons who performed more than 100 neck explorations annually.[56]

Selected References

Bojaunga J, Zeuzem S: Molecular detection of thyroid cancer: An update. Clin Endocrinol 61:523-530, 2004.

An excellent update on new molecular biologic techniques for detection of thyroid cancer by FNA or peripheral blood markers. Good discussion of promising research and current pitfalls.

Castro MR, Gharib H: Continuing controversies in the management of thyroid nodules. Ann Intern Med 142:926-931, 2005.

Good update that includes a discussion of micro nodules and markers for malignancy.

Hartl DM, Travagli JP, Leboulleux S, et al: Clinical review: Current concepts in the management of unilateral recurrent laryngeal nerve paralysis after thyroid surgery. J Clin Endocrinol Metab 90:3084-3088, 2005.

An excellent discussion of the pathophysiology of surgically induced damage to the external branch of the superior laryngeal and recurrent laryngeal nerves. Must reading for any thyroid surgeon.

Hay ID, Thompson GB, Grant CS et al: Papillary thyroid carcinoma managed at the Mayo Clinic during six decades (1940-1999): Temporal trends in initial therapy and long-term outcome in 2444 consecutively treated patients. World J Surg 26:879-885, 2002.

Another excellent Mayo Clinic contribution in the area of thyroid cancer that possibly represents the longest study of this cancer. It confirms the use of more extensive resection and postoperative radioablation and substantiates their data with 50 years of follow-up.

Hermus AR, Huysmans DA: Treatment of benign nodular thyroid disease. N Engl J Med 338:1438-1447, 1998.

An excellent update on the diagnosis and treatment of solitary nodules, multinodular goiter, and nontoxic and toxic nodules. This paper has

77 references and is based on the authors' extensive experience in the field.

Hundahl SA, Cady B, Cunningham MP, et al: Initial results from a prospective cohort study of 5583 cases of thyroid carcinoma treated in the United States during 1996. Cancer 89:202-217, 2000.

An excellent update of the U.S. experience compiled by the Commission on Cancer of the American College of Surgeons.

Sabel MS, Staren ED, Gianakakis LM, et al: Use of fine-needle aspiration biopsy and frozen section in the management of the solitary thyroid nodule. Surgery 122:1021-1027, 1997.

This study was presented at the American Association of Endocrine Surgeons meeting in 1997. It reviewed FNA and frozen section in 561 patients and assessed the accuracy, sensitivity, and specificity of both procedures. The clinical usefulness of FNA was documented.

Schlumberger MJ: Papillary and follicular thyroid cancer. N Engl J Med 338:297-306, 1998.

An excellent update on the topic, with 93 references. Modern controversies and classic observations are well discussed and presented. The author's experience with 1700 patients is included in the discussion.

Sherma SI: Thyroid carcinoma. Lancet 361:501-511, 2003.

An excellent seminar on the diagnosis, treatment, and follow-up monitoring of all four cancer groups. This review includes 168 references and excellent discussion.

Wong CKM, Wheeler MH: Thyroid nodules: Rational management. World J Surg 24:934-941, 2000.

A good review and discussion of workup and management strategies from an internationally known surgical group from Wales, United Kingdom.

Zarnegar R, Brunaud L, Clark OH: Prevention, evaluation and management of complication following thyroidectomy for thyroid carcinoma. Endocrinol Metab Clin North Am 32:483-502, 2003.

Excellent review of the incidence and management of complications of thyroid surgery

References

1. Hartl DM, Travagli JP, Leboulleux S, et al: Clinical review: Current concepts in the management of unilateral recurrent laryngeal nerve paralysis after thyroid surgery. J Clin Endocrinol Metab 90:3084-3088, 2005.
2. Brent GA: The molecular basis of thyroid hormone action. N Engl J Med 331:847-853, 1994.
3. Spitzweg C, Heufelder AE, Morris JC: Thyroid iodine transport. Thyroid 10:321-330, 2000.
4. Hollowell JG, Staehling NW, Hannon WH, et al: Iodine nutrition in the United States. Trends and public health implications: Iodine excretion data from National Health and Nutrition Examination Surveys I and III (1971-1974 and 1988-1994). J Clin Endocrinol Metab 83:3401-3408, 1998.
5. Chopra IJ: Nature, source, and relative significance of circulating thyroid hormones. In Braverman LE, Utiger RE (eds): Werner and Ingbar's The Thyroid, 7th ed. Philadelphia, Lippincott-Raven, 1996, pp 111-124.
6. Robins J: Thyroid hormone transplant proteins and the physiology of hormone binding in the thyroid. In Braverman LE, Utiger RD (eds): The Thyroid: A Fundamental and

Clinical Text, 8th ed. Philadelphia, Lippincott Williams & Wilkins, 2000, p 105.

7. Duh QY, Grossman RF: Thyroid growth factors, signal transduction pathways, and oncogenes. Surg Clin North Am 75:421-437, 1995.

8. Mazzaferri EL, Robbins RJ, Spencer CA, et al: A consensus report of the role of serum Tg as a monitoring method for low-risk patients with papillary thyroid carcinoma. J Clin Endocrinol Metab 88:1433-1441, 2003.

9. Cheung P: Medical and surgical treatment of endemic goiter. In Clark OH, Duh QY (eds): Textbook of Endocrine Surgery. Philadelphia, WB Saunders, 1997, pp 15-21.

10. Tomer Y, Barbesino G, Greenberg DA, et al: Mapping the major susceptibility loci for familial Graves' and Hashimoto's diseases: Evidence for genetic heterogeneity and gene interactions. J Clin Endocrinol Metab 84:4656-4664, 1999.

11. Bahn RS, Dutton CM, Joba W, et al: Thyrotropin receptor expression in cultured Graves' orbital preadipocyte fibroblasts is stimulated by thyrotropin. Thyroid 8:193-196, 1998.

12. Wong CK, Wheeler MH: Thyroid nodules: Rational management. World J Surg 24:934-941, 2000.

13. Torring O, Tallstedt L, Wallin G, et al: Graves' hyperthyroidism: Treatment with antithyroid drugs, surgery, or radioiodine—a prospective, randomized study. Thyroid Study Group. J Clin Endocrinol Metab 81:2986-2993, 1996.

14. Franklyn JA: The management of hyperthyroidism. N Engl J Med 330:1731-1738, 1994.

15. Hermus AR, Huysmans DA: Treatment of benign nodular thyroid disease. N Engl J Med 338:1438-1447, 1998.

16. Castro MR, Gharib H: Continuing controversies in the management of thyroid nodules. Ann Intern Med 142:926-931, 2005.

17. Cooper DS, Doherty GM, Haugen BR, et al: Management guidelines for patients with thyroid nodules and differentiated thyroid cancer. Thyroid 16:109-142, 2006.

18. Alexander EK, Heering JP, Benson CB, et al: Assessment of nondiagnostic ultrasound-guided fine needle aspirations of thyroid nodules. J Clin Endocrinol Metab 87:4924-4927, 2002.

19. Noguchi S: Localization tests in patients with thyroid cancer. In Clark OH (ed): Textbook of Endocrine Surgery, 2nd ed. Philadelphia, Elsevier Saunders, 2005, pp 142-150.

20. Crippa F, Alessi A, Gerali A, et al: FDG-PET in thyroid cancer. Tumori 89:540-543, 2003.

21. Sabel MS, Staren ED, Gianakakis LM, et al: User of fine-needle aspiration biopsy and frozen section in the management of the solitary thyroid nodule. Surgery 122:1021-1026, discussion 1026-1027, 1997.

22. Boyd LA, Earnhardt RC, Dunn JT, et al: Preoperative evaluation and predictive value of fine-needle aspiration and frozen section of thyroid nodules. J Am Coll Surg 187:494-502, 1998.

23. Davies L, Welch HG: Increasing incidence of thyroid cancer in the United States, 1973-2002. JAMA 295:2164-2167, 2006.

24. Kim DS, McCabe CJ, Buchanan MA, et al: Oncogenes in thyroid cancer. Clin Otolaryngol Allied Sci 28:386-395, 2003.

25. Goretzki PE, Gorelev V, Simon D, Rocher H: Oncogenes in thyroid tumors. In Clark OH (ed): Textbook of Endocrine Surgery, 2nd ed. Philadelphia, Elsevier Saunders, 2005, pp 280-287.

26. Kebebew E: Thyroid oncogenesis. In Clark OH (ed): Textbook of Endocrine Surgery, 2nd ed. Philadelphia, Elsevier Saunders, 2005, pp 288-294.

27. Sherman SI: Thyroid carcinoma. Lancet 361:501-511, 2003.

28. Cornetta AJ, Burchard AE, Pribitkin EA, et al: Insular carcinoma of the thyroid. Ear Nose Throat J 82:384-386, 388-389, 2003.

29. Cady B, Sedgwick CE, Meissner WA, et al: Risk factor analysis in differentiated thyroid cancer. Cancer 43:810-820, 1979.

30. Hay ID: Prognostic factors in thyroid carcinoma. Thyroid Today 12:1-9, 1989.

31. Schlumberger MJ: Papillary and follicular thyroid carcinoma. N Engl J Med 338:297-306, 1998.

32. Hundahl SA, Cady B, Cunningham MP, et al: Initial results from a prospective cohort study of 5583 cases of thyroid carcinoma treated in the United States during 1996. U.S. and German Thyroid Cancer Study Group. An American College of Surgeons Commission on Cancer Patient Care Evaluation study. Cancer 89:202-217, 2000.

33. Wada N, Duh QY, Sugino K, et al: Lymph node metastasis from 259 papillary thyroid microcarcinomas: Frequency, pattern of occurrence and recurrence, and optimal strategy for neck dissection. Ann Surg 237:399-407, 2003.

34. Pellegriti G, Scollo C, Lumera G, et al: Clinical behavior and outcome of papillary thyroid cancers smaller than 1.5 cm in diameter: Study of 299 cases. J Clin Endocrinol Metab 89:3713-3720, 2004.

35. Hay ID, Thompson GB, Grant CS, et al: Papillary thyroid carcinoma managed at the Mayo Clinic during six decades (1940-1999): Temporal trends in initial therapy and long-term outcome in 2444 consecutively treated patients. World J Surg 26:879-885, 2002.

36. D'Avanzo A, Treseler P, Ituarte PH, et al: Follicular thyroid carcinoma: Histology and prognosis. Cancer 100:1123-1129, 2004.

37. Kinder BK: Well differentiated thyroid cancer. Curr Opin Oncol 15:71-77, 2003.

38. Kushchayeva Y, Duh QY, Kebebew E, et al: Prognostic indications for Hürthle cell cancer. World J Surg 28:1266-1270, 2004.

39. Pasieka JL: Anaplastic thyroid cancer. Curr Opin Oncol 15:78-83, 2003.

40. Widder S, Pasieka JL: Primary thyroid lymphomas. Curr Treat Options Oncol 5:307-313, 2004.

41. Bojunga J, Zeuzem S: Molecular detection of thyroid cancer: An update. Clin Endocrinol (Oxf) 61:523-530, 2004.

42. Nikiforova MN, Lynch RA, Biddinger PW, et al: RAS point mutations and PAX8-PPAR gamma rearrangement in thyroid tumors: Evidence for distinct molecular pathways in thyroid follicular carcinoma. J Clin Endocrinol Metab 88:2318-2326, 2003.

43. Fernandez PL, Merino MJ, Gomez M, et al: Galectin-3 and laminin expression in neoplastic and non-neoplastic thyroid tissue. J Pathol 181:80-86, 1997.

44. Niedziela M, Maceluch J, Korman E: Galectin-3 is not an universal marker of malignancy in thyroid nodular disease in children and adolescents. J Clin Endocrinol Metab 87:4411-4415, 2002.

45. Cheung CC, Carydis B, Ezzat S, et al: Analysis of ret/PTC gene rearrangements refines the fine needle aspiration diagnosis of thyroid cancer. J Clin Endocrinol Metab 86:2187-2190, 2001.

46. Chhieng DC, Ross JS, McKenna BJ: CD44 immunostaining of thyroid fine-needle aspirates differentiates thyroid papillary carcinoma from other lesions with nuclear grooves and inclusions. Cancer 81:157-162, 1997.

47. Aogi K, Kitahara K, Urquidi V, et al: Comparison of telomerase and CD44 expression as diagnostic tumor markers in lesions of the thyroid. Clin Cancer Res 5:2790-2797, 1999.

48. Cohen Y, Rosenbaum E, Clark DP, et al: Mutational analysis of BRAF in fine needle aspiration biopsies of the thyroid: A potential application for the preoperative assessment of thyroid nodules. Clin Cancer Res 10:2761-2765, 2004.

49. Xing M, Westra WH, Tufano RP, et al: BRAF mutation predicts a poorer clinical prognosis for papillary thyroid cancer. J Clin Endocrinol Metab 90:6373-6379, 2005.

50. Ditkoff BA, Marvin MR, Yemul S, et al: Detection of circulating thyroid cells in peripheral blood. Surgery 120:959-964, discussion 964-955, 1996.

51. Elisei R, Vivaldi A, Agate L, et al: Low specificity of blood Tg messenger ribonucleic acid assay prevents its use in the follow-up of differentiated thyroid cancer patients. J Clin Endocrinol Metab 89:33-39, 2004.

52. Finley DJ, Zhu B, Barden CB, et al: Discrimination of benign and malignant thyroid nodules by molecular profiling. Ann Surg 240:425-436, discussion 436-427, 2004.

53. Attie JN: Modified neck dissection in treatment of thyroid cancer: A safe procedure. Eur J Cancer Clin Oncol 24:315-324, 1988.

54. Mazzaferri EL, Kloos RT: Clinical review 128: Current approaches to primary therapy for papillary and follicular thyroid cancer. J Clin Endocrinol Metab 86:1447-1463, 2001.

55. Zarnegar R, Brunaud L, Clark OH: Prevention, evaluation, and management of complications following thyroidectomy for thyroid carcinoma. Endocrinol Metab Clin North Am 32:483-502, 2003.

56. Sosa JA, Bowman HM, Tielsch JM, et al: The importance of surgeon experience for clinical and economic outcomes from thyroidectomy. Ann Surg 228:320-330, 1998.

CHAPTER 37

The Parathyroid Glands

Julie Ann Sosa, MA, MD   and   Robert Udelsman, MD, MBA

The clinical features, diagnosis, and treatment of parathyroid disease have changed radically over the past 25 years as a result of technologic advances in the fields of laboratory medicine, radiology, medicine, and surgery. In particular, there have been many technical advances in the surgical management of primary hyperparathyroidism (HPT).

HISTORY

Advances in parathyroid surgery have been colorful and international. Although the Swedish medical student Ivar Sandstrom is credited with first describing the "glandularae parathyrtreoidae" in 1880,[1] Sir Richard Owen made the original description in 1850.[2] Understanding of parathyroid function predated appreciation of the glands themselves; tetany was described in 1879 in a patient who underwent thyroidectomy (and incidental parathyroidectomy),[3] and the connection between the parathyroids and tetany was identified in 1891.[4] Famous patients with HPT include Albert Gahne, a Viennese tram car conductor who underwent two separate parathyroid resections in the 1920s by Felix Mandl for what was most likely parathyroid carcinoma,[5] and Captain Charles Martell, a Merchant Marine captain who underwent seven operations and was eventually found to have a mediastinal parathyroid adenoma.[6] Both men succumbed to their disease and the consequences of its treatment.

The relationship between chronic renal disease and HPT was first suggested by Albright and colleagues in 1934.[7] Castleman and Mallory described the pathologic finding of parathyroid hyperplasia of chief cells with marked gland enlargement.[8] Stanbury and associates described renal rickets, azotemic osteomalacia, and azotemic HPT and also performed the first subtotal parathyroidectomy as definitive therapy for renal osteitis fibrosa.[9] Rasmussen and Craig and, independently, Aurbach extracted a stable homogeneous parathyroid polypeptide and demonstrated that hypercalcemia and phosphaturic properties reside in parathyroid hormone (PTH).[10] Berson and Yalow won the Nobel prize in 1977 for developing an immunoassay for the measurement of PTH,[11] and Reiss and Canterbury developed an assay to measure the C-terminal and later the mid-molecule portion of PTH.[12]

Introduction of the serum channel autoanalyzer in the mid-1960s ushered in a new era of parathyroid surgery in that it facilitated earlier diagnosis of primary HPT. There was an increase in incidence of the disease, and asymptomatic patients became commonplace. Additional technical advances have included improved preoperative localization with sestamibi scans, often using single-photon emission computed tomography (SPECT), the rapid intraoperative PTH assay, and the use of minimally invasive parathyroidectomy (MIP) with unilateral neck exploration through a small incision and regional anesthesia in the ambulatory setting.

Table 37-1 Actions of Major Calcium-Regulating Hormones

	BONE	KIDNEY	INTESTINE
Parathyroid hormone	Stimulates resorption of calcium and phosphate	Stimulates resorption of calcium and conversion of 25(OH)D$_3$; inhibits resorption of phosphate and bicarbonate	No direct effects
Vitamin D	Stimulates transport of calcium	Inhibits resorption of calcium	Stimulates calcium and phosphate absorption
Calcitonin	Inhibits resorption of calcium and phosphate	Inhibits resorption of calcium and phosphate	No direct effects

From Gauger PG, Doherty GM: Parathyroid gland. In Townsend CM, Beauchamp RD, Evers BM, Mattox KL (eds): Sabiston Textbook of Surgery. Philadelphia, Elsevier Saunders, 2004, p 987.

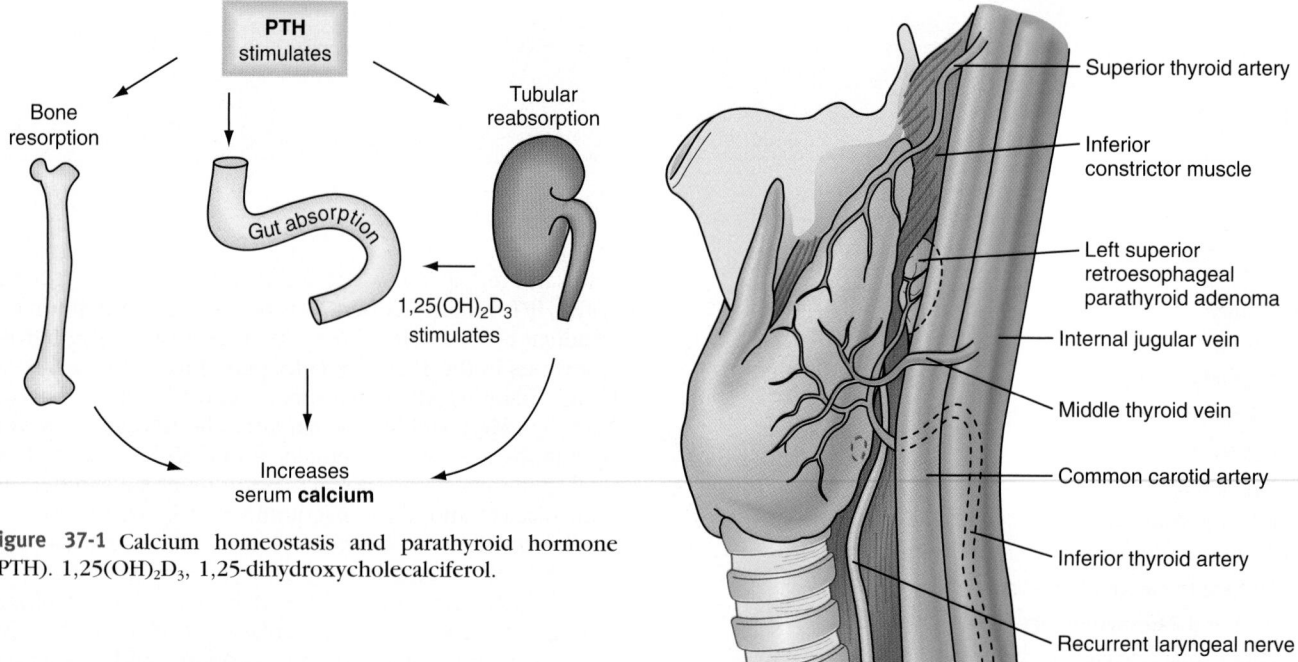

Figure 37-1 Calcium homeostasis and parathyroid hormone (PTH). 1,25(OH)$_2$D$_3$, 1,25-dihydroxycholecalciferol.

Figure 37-2 Anatomic relationship of a left superior parathyroid adenoma to nearby structures, including the recurrent laryngeal nerve, the carotid sheath, and its blood supply from the inferior thyroid artery. Aberrantly located parathyroid glands can be found behind the esophagus, as well as within the carotid sheath, the thymus, and the mediastinum.

CALCIUM PHYSIOLOGY

Calcium exists in extracellular plasma in a free ionized state, as well as bound to other molecules. So-called normal plasma levels of total calcium vary between laboratories, but the range of (bound and unbound) calcium is usually between 8.5 and 10.2 mg/dL (2.2 and 2.5 mmol/L). The biologically inert bound fraction (55% of the total) binds to proteins. Changes in albumin alter total calcium levels significantly because the majority of protein-bound calcium associates with albumin (80%). A small percentage of calcium is associated with other proteins, such as β-globulins, or with nonprotein molecules, such as phosphate and citrate. Mathematical formulas correcting for disparate albumin levels (e.g., corrected calcium = 0.8-mg/dL decrease for every 1.0 mg/dL decrease in albumin; [total calcium+0.025] × [40−albumin]) are notoriously inaccurate.[13] Consequently, ionized calcium levels are measured when required. Forty-five percent of the total calcium is biologically active and exists in the ionized form, with a normal level of 4.5 to 5.0 mg/dL. Ionized calcium levels are inversely affected by the pH of blood; a 1-unit rise in pH will decrease the ionized calcium level

by 0.36 mmol/L.[14] Accordingly, patients who are hypocalcemic and hyperventilate can enhance their hypocalcemic symptoms, including perioral paresthesia, tingling in the fingers and toes, muscle cramping, and seizures.

Levels of calcium are highly modulated through a delicate interplay between PTH, calcitonin, and vitamin D acting on target organs such as bone, kidney, and the gastrointestinal tract[15] (Table 37-1 and Fig. 37-1). Chief cells in the parathyroid glands secrete PTH, an 84–amino acid protein, whenever serum calcium levels fall. PTH binds to its peripheral receptors and stimulates osteoclasts to increase bone resorption, the kidney to increase calcium resorption and renal production of 1,25-

dihydroxyvitamin D_3 (1,25[OH]$_2$D$_3$), and the intestine to increase absorption of calcium and phosphate. Together, these processes raise the serum calcium level. The recently cloned calcium-sensing receptors (CaSRs) in the parathyroid glands detect changes in calcium levels, which results in a negative feedback loop that decreases PTH production.

Calcitonin is a 32–amino acid protein secreted by the parafollicular cells of the thyroid gland in response to high calcium levels. Its actions oppose those of PTH. Calcitonin rapidly inhibits bone resorption, thereby leading to a transient decrease in serum calcium levels. Although calcitonin plays a significant homeostatic function in other species, its effects on calcium metabolism in humans is not significant when the individual is exposed to chronically elevated calcitonin levels. Accordingly, patients with extensive medullary carcinoma of the thyroid who have extraordinarily high serum calcitonin levels are usually eucalcemic.

Vitamin D is ingested or synthesized in precursor form, which then undergoes two hydroxylation steps before becoming biologically active. The first hydroxylation at carbon 25 occurs in the liver, and the second hydroxylation at carbon 1 occurs in the kidney in response to increased PTH levels. 1,25(OH)$_2$D$_3$ increases calcium and phosphate resorption from the gastrointestinal tract and stimulates bone resorption, which raises calcium levels. As a result, patients who are deficient in 1,25(OH)$_2$D$_3$ have an impaired ability to absorb calcium from their gastrointestinal tract.

ANATOMY

There are usually four parathyroid glands, which lie on the posterior surface of the thyroid. The superior glands are normally located on the posteromedial aspect of the thyroid near the tracheoesophageal groove, whereas the inferior parathyroids are more widely distributed in the region below the inferior thyroid artery (Fig. 37-2). Common sites for ectopic parathyroids are the thyrothymic ligament, superior thyroid poles, tracheoesophageal groove, retroesophageal space, and carotid sheath (Fig. 37-3).[16] The percentage of individuals with supernumerary glands varies in published series from 2.5% to 22%.[17] The average weight of a normal parathyroid gland is 35 to 40 mg, and in adults its color turns to yellow as the fat content increases. The inferior parathyroids originate from the third branchial pouch, whereas the superior parathyroids descend from the fourth branchial pouch. Both the superior and inferior parathyroid glands receive their blood supply from the inferior thyroid artery in 80% of cases. Each parathyroid gland generally receives a single end-artery blood supply that is vulnerable to injury during surgical manipulation. The glands are made up of chief and oxyphil cells, as well as fibrovascular stroma and adipose tissue.

Primary HPT can be produced by three different pathologic lesions. A parathyroid adenoma is a benign encapsulated neoplasm that is responsible for 80% to 90% of cases. It usually affects a single gland, but 2% to 5% of patients with primary HPT have adenomas in two

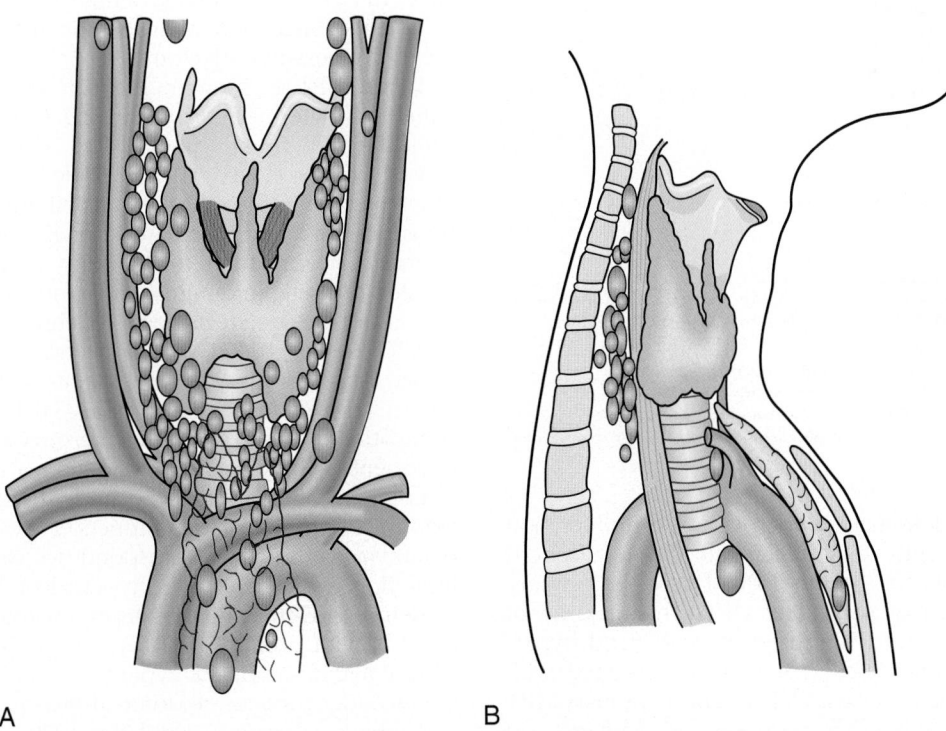

A   B

Figure 37-3 Possible locations of enlarged parathyroid glands in the neck and superior mediastinum with the use of an anteroposterior projection (**A**) and a lateral projection (**B**). (From Udelsman R, Donovan PI: Remedial parathyroid surgery: Changing trends in 130 consecutive cases. Ann Surg 244:471-479, 2006.)

Box 37-1 Differential Diagnosis of Hypercalcemia

Parathyroid

Primary hyperparathyroidism
  Sporadic
  Familial

Nonparathyroid Endocrine

Thyrotoxicosis
Pheochromocytoma
Acute adrenal insufficiency
Vasointestinal polypeptide hormone–producing tumor (VIPoma)

Malignancy

Solid tumors
Lytic bone metastases
Lymphoma and leukemia
Parathyroid hormone–related peptide (PTHrP)
Excess production of $1,25(OH)_2D_3$
Other factors (cytokines, growth factors)

Granulomatous Diseases

Sarcoidosis
Tuberculosis
Histoplasmosis
Coccidiomycosis
Leprosy

Medications

Calcium supplementation
Thiazide diuretics
Lithium
Estrogens/antiestrogens, testosterone in breast cancer
Vitamin A or D intoxication

Other

Benign familial hypocalciuric hypercalcemia (BFHH)
Milk-alkali syndrome
Immobilization
Paget's disease
Acute and chronic renal insufficiency
Aluminum excess
Parenteral nutrition

Malignancy is the most common cause of hypercalcemia in the inpatient setting; primary hyperparathyroidism is the most common cause in the outpatient setting.

Adapted from Mulder JE, Bilezikian JP: Acute management of hypercalcemia. In Bilezikian JP, Marcus R, Levine MA (eds): The Parathyroids, 2nd ed. San Diego, CA, Academic Press, 2001, p 730.

glands (double adenomas). Hyperplasia is a proliferation of parenchymal cells that affects all the parathyroid glands; it accounts for 10% to 15% of cases of primary HPT and all cases of secondary HPT. The majority of patients with primary HPT caused by multigland hyperplasia have sporadic disease. It is also associated with multiple endocrine neoplasia (MEN) type 1 (primary HPT combined with lesions of the pancreas and pituitary) and type 2A (primary HPT, medullary thyroid cancer, and pheochromocytoma) syndromes. Parathyroid carcinoma is a slow-growing, invasive neoplasm of parenchymal

cells that is responsible for less than 1% of cases of primary HPT. Although fibrosis and mitotic activity are common, they are not specific for malignancy. The diagnosis of carcinoma is restricted to tumors that show invasion of blood vessels, perineural spaces, soft tissues, the thyroid gland or other adjacent structures, or to tumors with documented metastases. It is often difficult for the pathologist to make this diagnosis, especially if there is only a frozen section analysis of a resected parathyroid gland.

DIAGNOSIS AND CLINICAL FEATURES

Primary HPT is the third most common endocrine disorder, after diabetes mellitus and thyroid disease. Middle-aged and elderly women are most commonly affected by the disease. It is characterized by hypersecretion of PTH leading to hypercalcemia. Box 37-1 lists the differential diagnosis for hypercalcemia. The diagnosis is made by demonstrating elevated serum calcium and intact PTH (iPTH) levels and normal or increased urinary calcium in the setting of normal renal function. In up to 15% of patients, serum PTH levels fall within the upper normal range, but these levels are inappropriate relative to the elevated serum calcium levels. A 24-hour urine collection can help exclude the diagnosis of benign familial hypocalciuric hypercalcemia (BFHH), which results in increased blood calcium and iPTH levels but low urinary calcium. Whereas the calcium-creatinine (Ca/Cr) clearance ratio is typically less than 0.01 in patients with BFHH, the ratio is usually greater than 0.02 in primary HPT. BFHH is a generally benign condition transmitted in an autosomal dominant fashion that cannot be corrected by parathyroidectomy.

When HPT is seen in the setting of chronic renal failure, it is termed *secondary HPT*. This is a discrete clinical entity from primary HPT. Other less common causes of secondary HPT include malabsorptive and other metabolic disorders. Renal failure leads to hyperphosphatemia and decreased renal conversion of 25-hydroxycholecalciferol to 1,25-dihydroxycholecalciferol, thereby resulting in diminished intestinal calcium absorption. Both these effects lead to chronic hypocalcemia, which stimulates PTH secretion and parathyroid hyperplasia. As many as 90% of patients with chronic renal failure have evidence of secondary HPT. With prolonged stimulation of the parathyroids, *tertiary HPT* can develop in patients with chronic renal failure or those with long-standing secondary HPT who undergo kidney transplantation. Autonomous hyperfunction develops and the parathyroids no longer respond to calcium feedback inhibition, which results in hypercalcemia.

Before advent of the serum channel autoanalyzer, patients with primary HPT were typically seen with the clinical manifestations of hypercalcemia, including painful bones, kidney stones, abdominal groans, psychic moans, and fatigue overtones. Until the 1970s, 75% of patients initially presented with nephrolithiasis. Today, however, a biochemical diagnosis is usually made before the appearance of symptoms, and many patients are asymptomatic or minimally symptomatic.[18] Less than 20% of primary HPT patients have renal symptoms, and less than 5% have evidence of osteitis fibrosis cystica. Bone turnover is increased in up to 80% of patients with primary HPT, and serial measurements demonstrate a rapid fall in bone resorption within 2 weeks of parathyroidectomy.

Most contemporary series, however, demonstrate that at least half the patients today have a nonrenal, nonosseous manifestation, and several series have demonstrated than 30% to 40% of patients are asymptomatic. Nonspecific complaints such as fatigue, lethargy, and depression are most commonly cited. Hypertension has been noted in approximately a third of patients with HPT, and a significant inverse relationship between mean arterial pressure and the glomerular filtration rate has been noted in these patients.

HYPERCALCEMIC CRISIS

Occasionally, patients with primary HPT are initially seen after symptoms and extremely high serum calcium levels have developed. Management of a so-called hypercalcemic crisis involves urgent medical and surgical strategies. Pharmacologic agents associated with or adversely affected by hypercalcemia need to be discontinued; specifically, digoxin potentiates arrhythmias in the setting of hypercalcemia. These patients are almost always severely dehydrated, and initial management requires hydration with normal saline. Medical management promotes the renal excretion of calcium. Once a patient with primary HPT is stabilized and serum calcium levels have been reduced to levels acceptable for induction of anesthesia (either general or locoregional, if a minimally invasive surgical technique is anticipated), expedient efforts are made to localize the parathyroid disease in anticipation of urgent parathyroidectomy.

Intravenous (IV) fluids, preferably normal saline, are administered at a rapid rate (200-300 mL/hr) to reverse the intravascular volume contraction and promote renal excretion of calcium. Bedside vigilance to prevent fluid overload is essential. Loop diuretics are added to the regimen to reduce the risk for volume overload and inhibit calcium resorption in the loop of Henle. Patients with renal failure often cannot tolerate such large-volume resuscitation; instead, they undergo dialysis with a low-calcium dialysate.

Glucocorticoids lower calcium by inhibiting the effects of vitamin D. They also have been shown to decrease intestinal absorption of calcium, increase renal calcium excretion, and inhibit osteoclast-activating factor. Glucocorticoids are particularly effective in the setting of hypercalcemia secondary to granulomatous disease, where the hypercalcemia stems from vitamin D toxicity. The initial dose of hydrocortisone is 200 to 400 mg/day IV for 3 to 5 days. Steroids are ineffective in most cases of hypercalcemia associated with malignancy.

Hypercalcemia of malignancy occurs by two mechanisms: (1) as a direct result of extensive osseous metastases and (2) indirectly by release of parathyroid hormone–related peptide (PTHrP) by the tumor. Treatment of hypercalcemia of malignancy includes surgery, chemotherapy, or radiation therapy (or any combination of these therapies) to treat the underlying cancer, as well as the administration of pharmacologic agents. Gallium nitrate, a compound that inhibits osteoclast resorption and lowers calcium levels, can be used at 200 mg/m^2 daily IV for 5 days. In this setting, gallium nitrate and pamidronate, a bisphosphonate (see later), have been equivalent in controlling hypercalcemia in small studies.

Calcitonin acts quickly (within 24-48 hours) to lower serum calcium levels and is more effective when used in combination with glucocorticoids. In a small, double-blind randomized trial of 50 cancer patients, however, calcitonin (up to 8 IU/kg subcutaneously [SC]/intramuscularly for 5 days) was less effective than gallium nitrate. Because preparations of calcitonin are manufactured from salmon, patients with preformed antibodies or those with previous exposure to calcitonin can demonstrate an allergic reaction consisting of respiratory distress, flushing, nausea, vomiting, and tingling in the extremities.

Bisphosphonates are pyrophosphate analogues that have high affinity for hydroxyapatite in bone. They potently inhibit osteoclast activity for up to a month. In hypercalcemia of malignancy, pamidronate (90 mg IV) or zoledronic acid (4 mg IV as initial treatment, 8 mg on re-treatment) normalizes calcium levels in most patients. Although a single dose of pamidronate lowers calcium levels, recent evidence suggests that zoledronic acid might become the bisphosphonate of choice because of its rapid onset of action and ability to lengthen the time to relapse by twofold. However, zoledronic acid also has been associated with compromised renal function.

HYPOPARATHYROIDISM

Hypoparathyroidism is an endocrine disorder in which hypocalcemia and hyperphosphatemia are the result of a deficiency in PTH secretion or action. The most common cause of hypoparathyroidism is damage to the parathyroid glands during thyroidectomy, but it also can occur after parathyroid exploration (see Postoperative Complications, later). The signs and symptoms of hypocalcemia are caused by neuromuscular excitability from reduced plasma ionized calcium. Early manifestations include perioral numbness and tingling in the fingers. Anxiety or confusion can follow, and it is important for the surgical team to reassure patients early to reduce psychiatric and neurocognitive symptoms. Anxiety often results in hyperventilation, which can then lead to respiratory alkalosis and a further reduction in the serum calcium level. Tetany, marked by carpopedal spasm, convulsions, or laryngospasm (or any combination of the three), may follow and can be fatal. Physical examination includes testing for a *Chvostek sign,* which is contraction of the facial muscles after tapping on the facial nerve anterior to the ear. Approximately 15% of normal individuals have a positive Chvostek sign, however.

Box 37-2   Criteria for Surgical Referral From the 2002 National Institutes of Health Workshop on Asymptomatic Primary Hyperparathyroidism

Serum calcium concentration >1 mg/dL above the upper limits of normal

24-hour urinary calcium >400 mg

Creatinine clearance reduced by >30% in comparison to age-matched subjects

Bone density at the lumbar spine, hip, or distal end of the radius that is >2 standard deviations below peak bone mass (T-score <−2.5)

All individuals with primary hyperparathyroidism and <50 years are referred for surgery

Patients for whom medical surveillance is either undesirable or impossible

---

There are also inherited forms of hypoparathyroidism.[19] It can occur as part of a multiglandular endocrine deficiency syndrome (type 1) characterized most commonly by hypoparathyroidism, adrenal insufficiency, and mucocutaneous candidiasis. This syndrome usually develops in childhood, and not all patients express the classic triad. Idiopathic hypoparathyroidism also occurs sporadically in adults and is associated with antiparathyroid antibodies. Some cases might be related to incomplete penetrance of familial multiglandular syndrome type 1.

Disorders in which there is abnormal or absent formation of the parathyroid glands are associated with hypocalcemia. For example, DiGeorge's syndrome occurs when the third and fourth branchial pouches develop abnormally. Transient neonatal hypocalcemia, a self-limited disorder, is more common than the genetic disorders that lead to permanent hypoparathyroidism. Parathyroid gland function can be impaired by infiltrative involvement of the glands in diseases such as hemochromatosis, Wilson's disease, sarcoidosis, tuberculosis, or amyloidosis. Exposure to external radiation or very large doses of ^{131}I for Graves' disease or well-differentiated thyroid cancer has rarely been associated with hypocalcemia. Finally, abnormalities in magnesium levels are associated with a reversible abnormality of PTH secretion.

Pseudohypoparathyroidism is an uncommon metabolic disorder characterized by biochemical hypoparathyroidism, increased PTH secretion, and target tissue unresponsiveness to the biologic action of PTH. In addition to functional hypoparathyroidism, many of these patients exhibit a distinctive constellation of developmental and skeletal defects collectively termed *Albright's hereditary osteodystrophy,* including a round face, short stature, obesity, brachydactyly, heterotopic ossification, and mental retardation. Several forms of pseudohypoparathyroidism have been described, and a diagnostic classification system has been developed (types 1a to 1c and 2).

PRIMARY HYPERPARATHYROIDISM

Effects of Surgery

Even though a National Institutes of Health (NIH) consensus conference was conducted in 1990 and another workshop was held in 2002 on the management of asymptomatic primary HPT, there is still no consensus among endocrinologists and endocrine surgeons about whether to administer nonoperative medical therapy and monitor patients or to refer them for early parathyroidectomy. Criteria for surgery have been established according to the best evidence to date (Box 37-2).[20] To some extent, the role of parathyroidectomy in asymptomatic patients with mild to moderate hypercalcemia is debated because the natural history of the disease is still not well understood. Overall, rapid increases in the serum calcium level or progression of symptoms of complications, or both, are uncommon in patients with borderline hypercalcemia.

Neuromuscular symptoms of primary HPT vary in expression and response to parathyroidectomy from series to series. However, proximal muscle weakness detected by examination of the isokinetic strength of knee extension and flexion appears to have a higher prevalence and good response to parathyroidectomy, as does respiratory muscle capacity. Psychiatric symptoms such as mental dullness, confusion, and depression are a focus of ongoing investigation. In a recent study by Roman and coworkers, 55 patients with primary HPT and benign euthyroid thyroid disease referred for surgery were evaluated preoperatively and postoperatively with validated psychometric and neurocognitive instruments.[21] Patients with primary HPT reported more symptoms of depression preoperatively that improved postoperatively. Preoperatively, patients with primary HPT also showed greater delays in spatial learning. All subjects learned across the neurocognitive trials, but primary HPT patients were more delayed. After surgery, primary HPT patients improved and functioned at a level equivalent to that of patients with thyroid disease. The authors concluded that primary HPT may be associated with a deficit in spatial learning and processing that improves after parathyroidectomy.

Significant increases in bone mineral density in the lumbar spine and hip occur after parathyroidectomy, and these improvements are durable. Changes in bone remodeling and density are apparent within 6 months of surgery. No effect of successful surgery has been noted on either hypertension or renal impairment. Urinary calcium excretion and the incidence of nephrolithiasis are reduced by surgery. In the end, there are still no convincing data proving that surgical cure increases life expectancy. A Swedish case-control study conducted retrospectively demonstrated that 23 patients who underwent parathyroidectomy had a hazard ratio for death of 0.89 in comparison to matched controls in the normal population, but the numbers were too small to achieve statistical significance.[22]

Noninvasive Preoperative Localization

One of the major advances over the past few years has been improvement in imaging techniques. This has led to the development of more localized surgery, with the opportunity for short operation times, the use of local or regional anesthesia, and limited or no hospital stay. There

Table 37-2　Preoperative Imaging in Patients With Primary Hyperparathyroidism

	SENSITIVITY	SPECIFICITY	COST	SAFETY
Noninvasive				
Sestamibi	Moderate	Moderate	Moderate	Safe
Sestamibi SPECT	High	High	Moderate	Safe
Ultrasound	Moderate	Moderate	Low	Safe
CT	Low	Moderate	Moderate	Radiation
MRI	Low	Moderate	Moderate	Safe
PET-CT	?	?	High	Radiation
Invasive				
Angiography	Moderate	Moderate	Very high	Hematoma, CVA, nephropathy*
Venous localization	High	High	Very high	Hematoma, nephropathy*
Ultrasound, biopsy	High	High	Moderate	Hematoma, infection

*Intravenous contrast nephropathy.

CT, computed tomography; CVA, cerebrovascular accident (stroke); MRI, magnetic resonance imaging; PET, positron emission tomography; SPECT, single-photon emission computed tomography.

is now consensus—as marked by the recommendation of the 2002 NIH workshop—that preoperative localization is imperative before primary exploration if unilateral exploration is desired. This marks a change since the 1990 NIH consensus conference.[20] Localization continues to be essential before all remedial parathyroidectomies (Table 37-2).

Several noninvasive preoperative localization modalities are available, including technetium Tc 99m sestamibi scintigraphy, ultrasonography, computed tomography (CT), magnetic resonance imaging (MRI), and thallous chloride Tl 201–technetium Tc 99m pertechnetate subtraction scanning. Most recently, four-dimensional CT and positron emission tomography (PET)-CT fusion studies have also been used with success for parathyroid localization. There is general consensus that the single best study is sestamibi, especially when combined with SPECT, and it is now the most common nuclear medicine study performed. In 1989, Coakley and colleagues reported that the agent ^{99m}Tc used for cardiac imaging also was avidly taken up by parathyroid tissue.[23] The study works by mitochondrial uptake of ^{99m}Tc-sestamibi, and parathyroid cells typically have a large number of mitochondria. Sestamibi, a monovalent lipophilic cation, diffuses passively across cell membranes and concentrates in mitochondria. Hence, it preferentially is concentrated in adenomatous and hyperplastic parathyroid tissue because of increased blood supply, higher metabolic activity, and absence of P-glycoprotein on the cell membrane (Fig. 37-4). Sestamibi imaging can be performed preoperatively for planning of MIP or on the morning of surgery in the operating room in conjunction with the use of a gamma probe to guide the surgeon during surgery.

A meta-analysis of the sensitivity and specificity of sestamibi scanning in 6331 cases demonstrated values of 91% and 99%, respectively, and suggested that 87% of patients with sporadic primary HPT would be candidates for unilateral exploration.[24] Routine preoperative screening becomes cost-effective when more than 51% of patients are suitable for a unilateral operation. The sen-

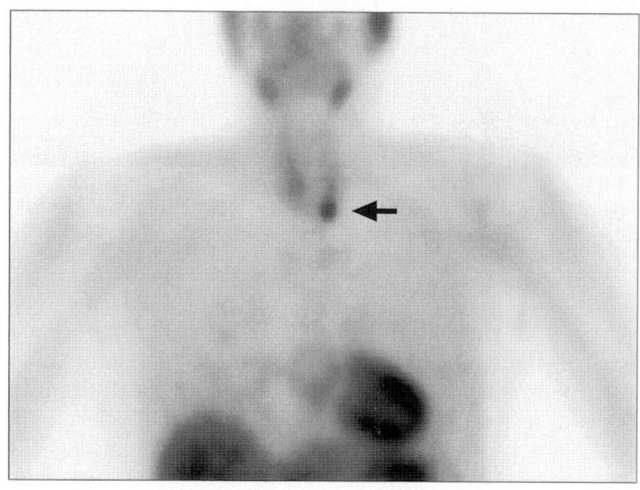

Figure 37-4 Sestamibi scan demonstrating a left inferior parathyroid adenoma (*arrow*). Physiologic areas of increased tracer uptake include the thyroid, salivary glands, heart, and liver.

sitivity of sestamibi is limited in multiglandular disease. In one large study, scintigraphy localized at least one gland in all patients, but only 62% of the total number of hyperplastic glands.[25] SPECT, which allows localization of structures in the anterior-posterior plane, is particularly helpful in detecting smaller lesions and adenomas located behind the thyroid. The overall sensitivity for localizing adenomas smaller than 500 mg ranges considerably from 53% to 92%.

A significant limitation of sestamibi scans is related to the coexistence of thyroid pathology or other metabolically active tissue (e.g., lymph nodes, diffuse hyperplasia, and metastatic thyroid cancer) that can mimic parathyroid adenomas by causing false-positive results on sestamibi scans. This limitation can be overcome in part by using the double-tracer subtraction technique of sestamibi, in

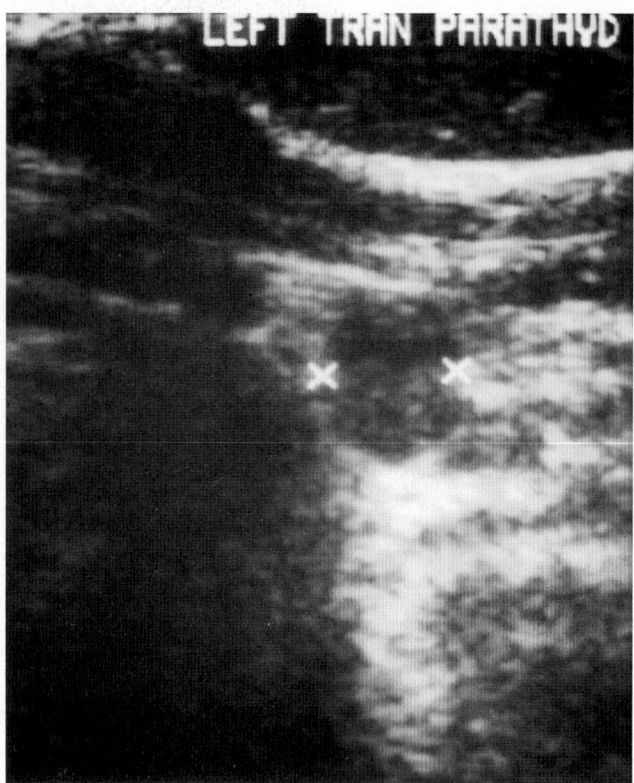

Figure 37-5 Ultrasound image of a hypoechoic parathyroid adenoma (with tumor perimeter marked).

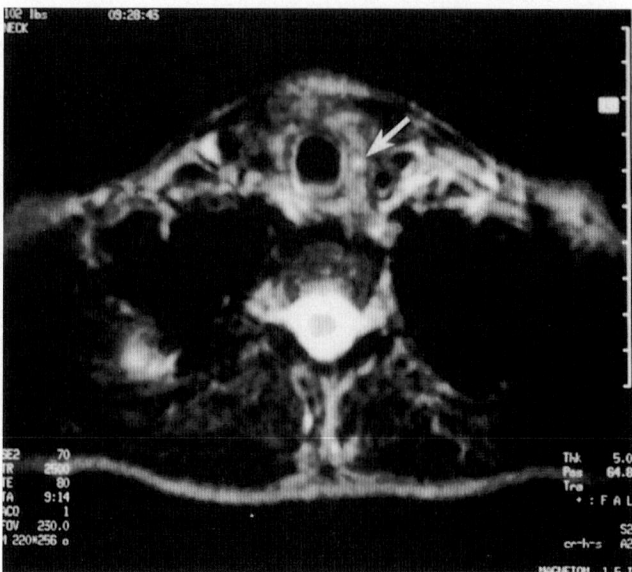

Figure 37-6 MRI showing a bright signal in the left side of the neck consistent with a parathyroid adenoma (*arrow*).

which both thyroid and parathyroid nodular abnormalities can be diagnosed simultaneously, or in combination with neck ultrasonography to preoperatively distinguish thyroid lesions and parathyroid adenomas. Sestamibi scans are now being performed with simultaneous CT imaging to yield correlative functional and anatomic localization.

Ultrasound is effective, noninvasive, and inexpensive, but its limitations include operator dependency and restriction to application in the neck because it cannot image mediastinal parathyroid lesions (Fig. 37-5). It has a 48% to 74% true-positive rate. Ultrasound often is used in combination with sestamibi, in which case the combined true-positive rate rises to 90%. CT and MRI provide cross-sectional imaging and are useful for visualizing mediastinal tumors and glands within the tracheoesophageal groove. MRI does not involve the use of radiation, and parathyroid adenomas appear intense on T2-weighted images (Fig. 37-6). CT is less expensive and has a sensitivity of 70% and a specificity of nearly 100%. In a study of 42 surgical patients with primary HPT in which alternative preoperative localization strategies were compared, sensitivity was highest for sestamibi using the ^{99m}Tc subtraction technique (95%), followed by ^{201}Tl/^{99m}Tc subtraction (86%), CT (83%), and ultrasound (81%).[26]

Invasive Preoperative Localization

A subset of patients who require re-exploration will have negative, discordant, or nonconvincing noninvasive local-

ization studies. Current guidelines recommend that these patients undergo invasive localization in the form of selective arteriography in conjunction with venous sampling for PTH (Fig. 37-7). This technique requires catheterization of multiple veins in the neck and mediastinum, from which blood samples are obtained. In the past, samples were collected, stored on ice, and sent to the laboratory, and the serum later was analyzed by immunoradiometric assay (IRMA) for iPTH. Rapid PTH measurement is now being performed in the angiography suite.[27] Results are available quickly, so interventional radiologists can obtain additional samples from a region in which a subtle, but potentially significant PTH gradient is detected. Because parathyroid adenomas have increased vascularity, they have a characteristic blush on arteriography. Although these studies have a sensitivity of only 60%, they yield few false-positive results. This use of interventional radiology rarely causes serious complications such as visual field defects or other cerebrovascular events, but such studies are time consuming and expensive and must be performed only at centers with expertise.

In the remedial setting, ultrasound localization can be used to guide fine-needle aspiration of a lesion suspicious for a parathyroid adenoma. This technique can be used with rapid PTH measurement of the parathyroid aspirate in the ultrasound suite to give ultrasonographers immediate feedback so that they can continue searching for an abnormal parathyroid gland if the aspirate of the suspicious lesion is negative.

Intraoperative Localization

The rapid intraoperative PTH assay can be used to confirm adequate removal of hypersecreting parathyroids and predict a curative procedure. Its use is associated with reduced operating time. The first reported applica-

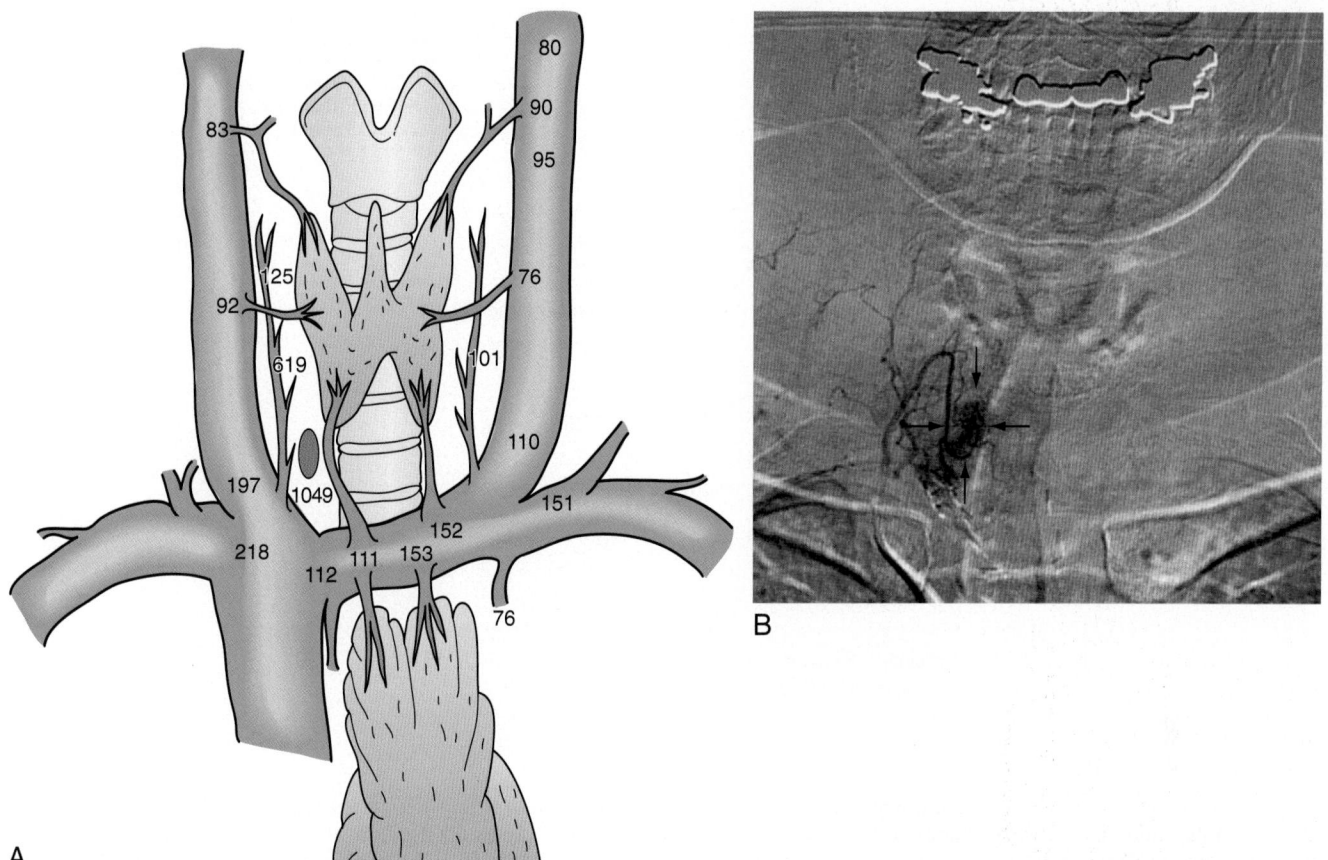

A

B

Figure 37-7 A, Venous localization mapping parathyroid hormone levels at different cervical sampling sites. The 1049 level is consistent with a right posterior parathyroid adenoma. **B,** Corresponding angiogram showing the adenoma as a classic blush in the right posterior position (*arrows*). (From Udelsman R, Aruny JE, Donovan PI, et al: Rapid parathyroid hormone analysis during venous localization. Ann Surg 237:714-719, 2003.)

tion of the assay was in 1988, but it has been refined since then, largely because of the work of George Irvin in Miami.[28] The rapid PTH assay is an immunometric assay that uses chemiluminescent acridinium esters as a label. In the presence of hydrogen peroxide and sodium hydroxide triggers, the acridinium esters are oxidized to an excited state, and subsequent return to the ground state causes an emission of light that is quantified. The amount of bound labeled antibody is directly proportional to the concentration of PTH in the sample. A certified clinical laboratory technician ideally performs the assay either inside the operating room or in its proximity; results of the assay are available in as little as 9 minutes.

A peripheral blood specimen is obtained immediately before surgery. Repeated blood samples are then drawn intraoperatively after resection of the enlarged gland or glands (to capture a potential hormone spike caused by manipulation of the gland during manipulation) and then 5 and 10 minutes after excision (Fig. 37-8). These protocols have been designed to account for the half-life of PTH, which is approximately $3\frac{1}{2}$ to 4 minutes. A 50% reduction in the PTH value from baseline is used as an indication that the exploration has been successful, and

this has proved to be predictive of cure in 96% of cases.[29]

The rapid PTH assay is especially helpful when the surgeon has difficulty distinguishing between thyroid tissue, lymph nodes, or a parathyroid adenoma. Aspiration of parathyroid tissue yields substantially higher hormone values than the upper limit of the standard curve; values greater than 1500 pg/mL secure the tissue diagnosis. Intraoperative ex vivo PTH aspiration has become a useful alternative to frozen section for identification of the parathyroid gland. It is also much faster and less expensive.

Operative failure rates for initial and remedial parathyroidectomy appear to have decreased significantly in centers that use this intraoperative adjunct. Irvin demonstrated that operative failure rates from initial parathyroidectomy have decreased significantly with use of the rapid PTH assay, from 6% to 1.5%.[30] Although experience seems to vary, even in the more difficult field of reoperation, the use of intraoperative PTH testing has been reported to increase success rates from 76% to 94%.[31] Critics emphasize that false-negative predictions from the test lead to unnecessary exploration and that surgeons who depend on hormone measurement for intraopera-

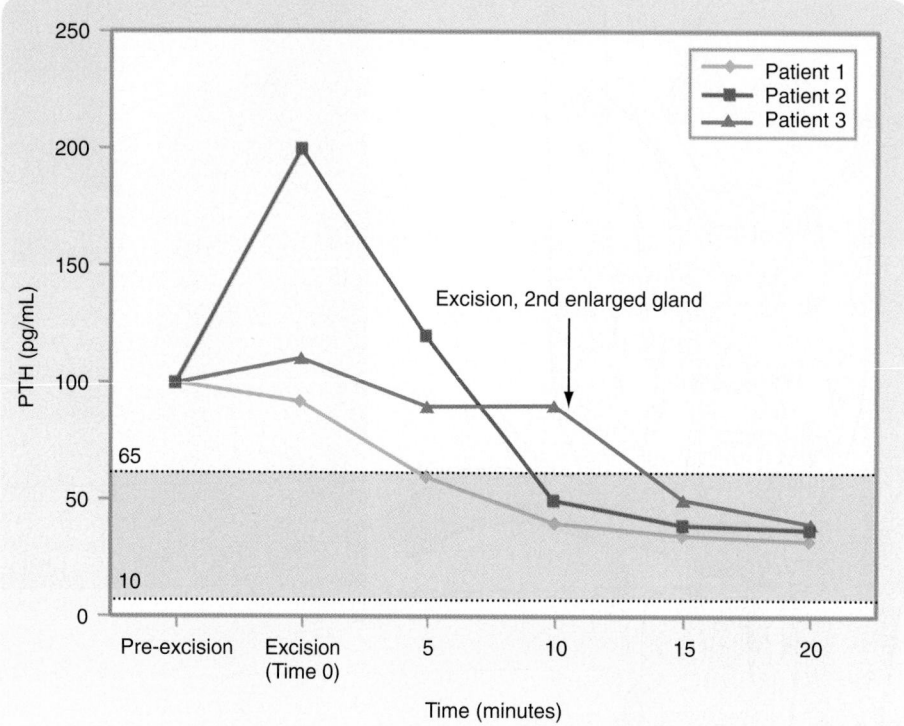

Figure 37-8 Intraoperative parathyroid hormone (PTH) values of patients with primary hyperparathyroidism undergoing minimally invasive parathyroidectomy. Patient 1 demonstrates classic PTH degradation, patient 2 shows a spike in PTH at excision as a result of surgical manipulation of the adenoma, and patient 3 shows failure of PTH to decline after excision of the first gland and adequate decline after excision of the second adenoma (double adenoma). The *lavender* region represents the normal range of the rapid PTH assay (10-65 pg/mL).

tive decisions cease to be cost-effective.[32] Although there continues to be some controversy, the largest endocrine surgery centers overall use the assay as an important adjunct to MIP. In patients with multigland disease in particular, intraoperative PTH testing has been shown to be essential; in a recent review of 519 patients, the assay changed operative management in 17% of all patients and in 82% of patients who had incorrect or negative preoperative imaging.[33]

In radioguided parathyroidectomy, developed in 1996, 20 mCi of ^{99m}Tc-sestamibi is injected IV 2 to 4 hours before surgery, and the adenoma is localized intraoperatively with a hand-held quantitative gamma counter with a 9- to 14-mm probe.[34] Gamma counts are obtained at the start of the operation in all four quadrants of the neck, through the skin, and after the incision under the strap muscles. Care is taken to not interpret radioactivity emitted by the heart. Exploration where counts are highest focuses surgery and reduces operative time. The activity of the removed parathyroid is checked with the gamma probe to confirm cure. The excised adenoma emits radioactivity at least 20% and often 50% in excess of the postexcision background. Finally, the postexcision radioactivity in all four quadrants of the neck should equalize.

Theoretically, use of the gamma probe can expedite some of the intraoperative decision making associated with routine parathyroidectomy by providing functional feedback to the surgeon. This has been shown to be particularly helpful in the setting of false-positive sestamibi scans, ectopic parathyroid adenomas, and remedial parathyroidectomy in which attempts at localization have been suboptimal. Still, intraoperative use of the gamma probe has not been embraced by most experienced endocrine surgeons because it yields little additional information over that obtained by adequate preoperative localization and the intraoperative PTH assay.

Bilateral Neck Exploration

The classic approach to the surgical management of primary HPT traditionally has been bilateral neck exploration under general anesthesia with intraoperative histopathologic frozen-section examination of excised parathyroid tissue. Ideally, parathyroid glands are identified, and the surgeon removes the pathologically enlarged gland or glands. Historically, patients were admitted to the hospital for 1 or 2 days, and failure rates in the best series were consistently less than 3% to 5%. Standard bilateral neck exploration is still considered an excellent operation with a complication rate in the 1% to 2% range and a *cure rate* (defined as normocalcemia 6 months postoperatively) of greater than 95%.

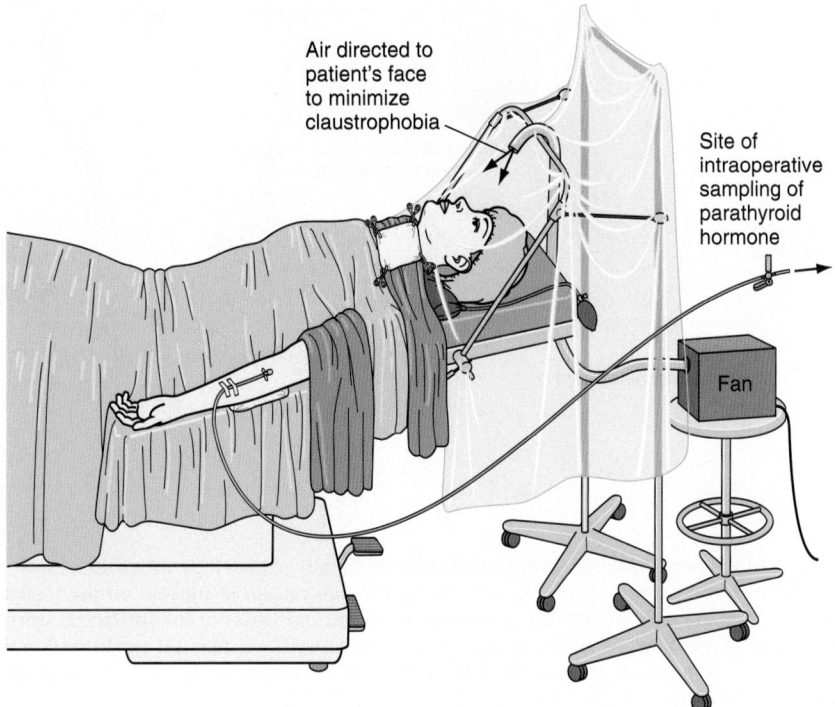

Air directed to
patient's face
to minimize
claustrophobia

Site of
intraoperative
sampling of
parathyroid
hormone

Fan

Figure 37-9 Organization of an ambulatory operating room used for minimally invasive parathyroidectomy. A large-bore IV line facilitates sedation and performance of the rapid parathyroid hormone assay. At the head of the bed, cool air blows over the patient to minimize claustrophobia. (From Udelsman R: Unilateral neck exploration under local or regional anesthesia. In Gagner M, Inabnet W [eds]: Textbook of Minimally Invasive Endocrine Surgery. Philadelphia, JB Lippincott, 2002.)

Minimally Invasive Parathyroidectomy

Because 85% of primary HPT results from a single adenoma and is cured by excision of the culprit gland, directed surgery after accurate preoperative localization is being used with increased frequency. MIP involves the use of unilateral neck exploration under regional or local anesthesia in the ambulatory setting.

The initial approach to unilateral surgery for primary HPT was advocated by Roth and colleagues in 1975, with selection of the side to be explored based on palpation or imaging, including esophagography, venography, or angiography.[35] If an enlarged and normal gland were found on the initial side, contralateral exploration was deferred. Intraoperative staining with Sudan black was performed. Wang advocated a similar approach and argued that bilateral exploration increased the risk, cost, and morbidity associated with parathyroidectomy for primary HPT.[36] Tibblin and associates in 1982 advocated *unilateral parathyroidectomy,* which they defined as removal of both the adenoma and normal gland from one side.[37] Excised tissue stained with oil red O, which stains fat droplets, was studied under the microscope during surgery, and the decision to stop the operation was based on demonstration of a reduction in intracytoplasmic fat droplets in the excised adenomatous parathyroid tissue. Both techniques would fail, however, in the setting of double adenomas on the contralateral side if the random choice of which side to explore was in error.

Recently, Tibblin reported the results of a prospective randomized controlled trial comparing unilateral with bilateral neck exploration.[38] In this study of 91 patients, comparison was made between patients assigned to preoperative sestamibi localization, unilateral neck exploration, and use of the rapid PTH assay (cases) and patients assigned to bilateral neck exploration (controls). Patients who underwent unilateral neck exploration had a lower incidence of early postoperative hypocalcemia requiring the administration of supplemental calcium. There were no statistical differences between complication rates, cost, and operative time between the two treatment groups. The study was not blinded, and it was flawed by a high crossover rate; only 62% of patients assigned to unilateral neck exploration in fact underwent the assigned operation. The balance underwent bilateral neck exploration, probably because sestamibi had a sensitivity of only 71% in the study.

Today, MIP requires preoperative localization (typically with sestamibi combined with SPECT) followed by limited exploration, often using cervical block anesthesia and the intraoperative PTH assay to confirm the adequacy of resection (Fig. 37-9). Patients with known multigland hyperplasia are not generally offered MIP. However, if such a patient is encountered during MIP, bilateral neck exploration can often be accomplished with the technique, or the procedure can be converted to general anesthesia if necessary. The vast majority of patients undergoing MIP are discharged on the day of

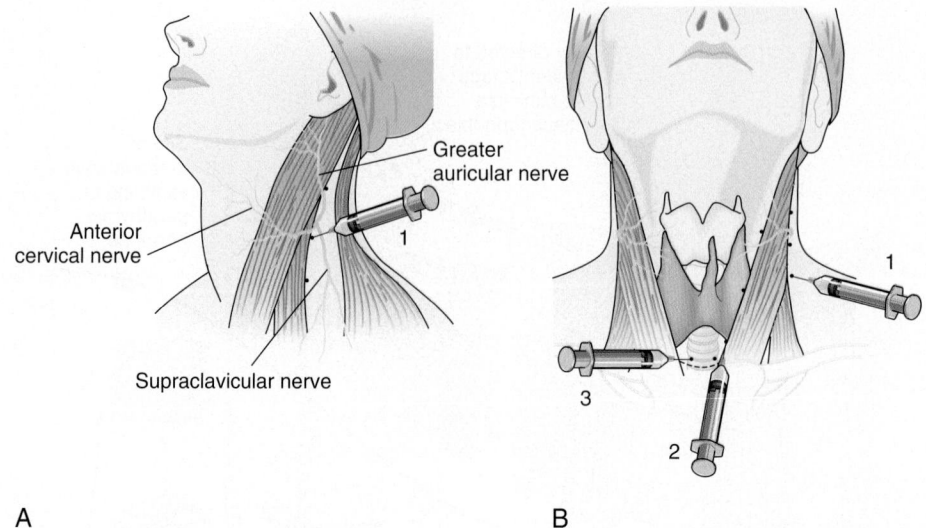

Greater
auricular nerve

Anterior
cervical nerve

Supraclavicular nerve

A

B

Figure 37-10 Cervical block performed by a surgeon during minimally invasive parathyroidectomy. **A,** A superficial cervical block is administered posterior and deep to the sternocleidomastoid muscle on the ipsilateral side of the parathyroid adenoma. **B,** Local anesthetic infiltrated along the anterior border of the ipsilateral sternocleidomastoid muscle, along with a field block at the incision site. (From Udelsman R: Unilateral neck exploration under local or regional anesthesia. In Gagner M, Inabnet W [eds]: Textbook of Minimally Invasive Endocrine Surgery. Philadelphia, JB Lippincott, 2002, p 97.)

surgery. They are monitored carefully as outpatients, and serum calcium and iPTH levels are measured within the first week of follow-up.

The skin incision is small, typically 2 to 4 cm. A superficial cervical block is administered posterior and deep to the sternocleidomastoid muscle on the ipsilateral side of the sestamibi-localized adenoma (Fig 37-10A and B). In most patients, 1% lidocaine containing 1:100,000 epinephrine is used; it can be supplemented if required during the operation. Care is always taken to aspirate before delivering the anesthetic to avoid intravascular administration. We have found that by also infiltrating along the anterior border of the sternocleidomastoid muscle, as well as performing a local field block, excellent analgesia is obtained in virtually all cases. The total volume of lidocaine required is typically 18 to 25 mL.

The regional block is performed in the operating room, and IV supplementation is administered by the anesthesia staff. Propofol is discontinued at least 5 minutes before PTH sampling because it may interfere with the PTH assay. Sedation with fentanyl or midazolam, or both, is used to minimize patient anxiety while maintaining an awake, conscious patient who can phonate. Lo Gerfo has shown that bilateral neck exploration under regional anesthesia can be performed safely and effectively in patients with coexisting thyroid disease and a nonlocalized adenoma.[39] In a series of 236 patients undergoing MIP, 62% had a nonlocalizing sestamibi scan preoperatively or no scan at all, but only 4 required conversion to general anesthesia. A simultaneous procedure was performed in 23%, and 85% underwent bilateral neck exploration. The average operating time in the series was 43 minutes for parathyroid procedures and 66 minutes for combined parathyroid/thyroid procedures.

A focused exploration is performed according to the results of the preoperative imaging study, and the intraoperative PTH assay is used to confirm the adequacy of resection in the operating room (Fig. 37-11). The success of MIP has been confirmed by evidence of cure and complication rates that are at least as good as those achieved with conventional bilateral exploration. Specifically, in a series of 656 consecutive parathyroidectomies (401 of which were performed in standard fashion and 255 with MIP) between 1990 and 2001, there were no significant differences in complication rates (3% and 1.2%, respectively) or cure rates (97% and 99%, respectively).[40] MIP was associated with a 50% reduction in operating time (1.3 hours for MIP versus 2.4 hours for the standard operation), a sevenfold reduction in length of hospital stay (0.24 versus 1.64 days, respectively), and a mean savings of $2693 per procedure, which represents a reduction in total hospital charges by nearly half.

Video-Assisted Parathyroidectomy

The technique of video-assisted parathyroidectomy was introduced and pioneered by Paolo Miccoli.[41] It does not require steady gas flow, but rather a brief insufflation of carbon dioxide to establish the operative space, which is then maintained by external retraction. Preoperative localization is essential and general anesthesia is typically used, although local anesthesia might be feasible.

A 15-mm skin incision is created 1 cm above the sternal notch to accommodate tactile assessment, suction irrigation, and dissection and retraction equipment. The incision can be moved, depending on the location of the adenoma. Another 10-mm trocar site is made vertically

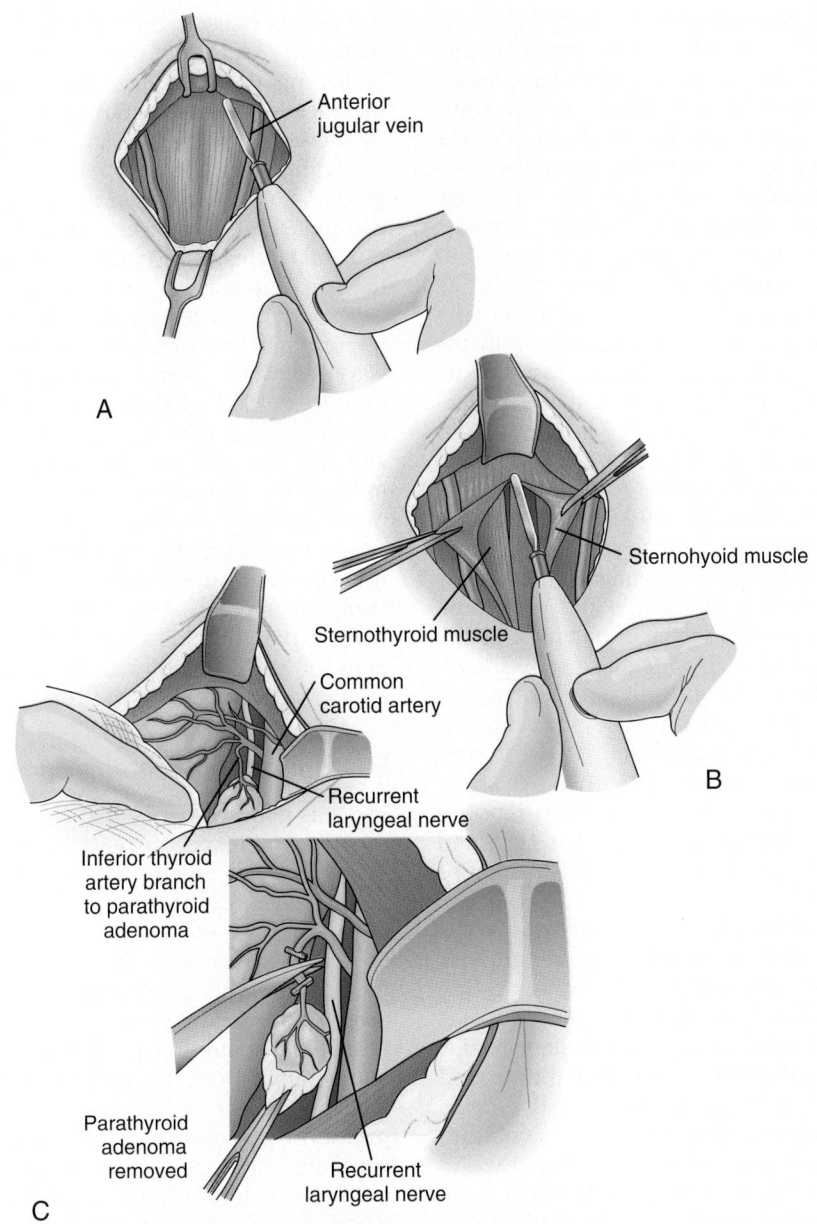

Figure 37-11 Technique of minimally invasive parathyroidectomy. **A,** A small transverse cervical skin incision is made, the platysma is divided, and the anterior jugular veins are preserved. **B,** The raphe between the strap muscles is divided in the midline. **C,** The parathyroid adenoma is excised, with care taken to preserve the recurrent laryngeal nerve and minimize manipulation of the tumor during ligation of the end artery. (From Udelsman R: Unilateral neck exploration under local or regional anesthesia. In Gagner M, Inabnet W [eds]: Textbook of Minimally Invasive Endocrine Surgery. Philadelphia, JB Lippincott, 2002.)

in the midline below the strap muscles and above the thyroid gland on the ipsilateral side of the suspected adenoma to accommodate the insufflator at the start of the case; a 30-degree, 5-mm endoscope is then inserted with two retractors for moving the thyroid medially and the strap muscles laterally. Suction irrigation is feasible because continuous insufflation is not required.

A multi-institution series from Italy, Germany, the United States, and Turkey included 123 patients enrolled between 1997 and 1999 who were successfully evaluated with preoperative localization studies and did not have evidence of multiglandular disease, thyroid malignancy,

a large thyroid mass, or previous neck surgery or irradiation.[42] The rapid PTH assay was used as an adjunct. All patients were cured by the video-assisted technique. Conversion to open parathyroidectomy occurred in 11% of patients, and two patients experienced recurrent laryngeal nerve palsy. The operating time was 55 minutes on average, with a median hospital stay of 1.5 days.

Endoscopic Parathyroidectomy

Advances in laparoscopy and endoscopy have been applied to parathyroidectomy. The first report of endoscopic removal of a parathyroid tumor was by Prinz and associates in 1994, who described four patients with persistent primary HPT who were found to have mediastinal parathyroid adenomas.[43] After preoperative imaging localized the disease to the mediastinum, the patients were placed in the right lateral decubitus position, and parathyroidectomies were performed through three thoracoscopic ports in less than $3\frac{1}{2}$ hours with no morbidity. One patient's tumor recurred, however.

The first endoscopic removal of a parathyroid in the neck was reported by Gagner in 1996.[44] In a patient with familial hypercalcemia, the neck was explored with the use of four 5-mm ports and carbon dioxide insufflation. Three and a half glands were excised, and the patient was cured. However, the operation took 5 hours and was complicated by intraoperative hypercapnia and postoperative subcutaneous emphysema.

Endoscopic parathyroidectomy has since been modified. It is generally reserved for patients with single-gland disease and requires preoperative imaging to localize the culprit parathyroid adenoma and guide the operation. Generally, access for the endoscope is obtained at the manubrium, and two additional ports are inserted laterally in the neck, anterior to the sternocleidomastoid muscle and ipsilateral to the parathyroid tumor. In this way, it is similar to the lateral approach used for conventional remedial neck exploration. The operative space is created between the platysma and the strap muscles by using insufflation at low pressure (5-8 mm Hg), and the strap muscles and thyroid are mobilized to expose the parathyroid.

Variations on this technique exist. Henry suggested that all three trocars can be inserted along the anterior border of the sternocleidomastoid muscle on the ipsilateral side of the adenoma, thus reducing the need for constant insufflation. Dulucq described excellent results with insertion of the endoscope at the manubrium and the other two trocars on opposite sides of the neck. Regardless of the technique used, there is a significant learning curve associated with endoscopic parathyroidectomy. Even with low insufflation pressure there can still be problems with small amounts of blood obscuring the field of view, metabolic disturbances from carbon dioxide absorption, and subcutaneous emphysema. Finally, the operative space can be lost during suction, and there is no opportunity for tactile assessment.

Remedial Parathyroidectomy

Remedial parathyroidectomy is indicated for persistent and recurrent HPT. Persistent HPT is defined by an inability to achieve normalization of the serum calcium level after initial exploration and represents an immediate technical failure. Recurrent disease is defined by initial normalization of the serum calcium level but then delayed hypercalcemia after 6 months of eucalcemia.

Preoperative localization and use of the rapid intraoperative PTH assay are important adjuncts for enhancing success rates during remedial parathyroid surgery. Reoperative neck exploration is more difficult because of scar tissue and distortion of normal tissue planes. It is more dangerous because of a greater chance of injury to the recurrent and superior laryngeal nerves. Therefore, reviewing the data from the initial exploration (noting the location of the parathyroids encountered, biopsied, or excised from the operative and pathology reports) and obtaining adequate preoperative imaging are essential for guided surgical exploration. In cases of re-exploration, it can be useful to have cryopreservation available because the only remaining parathyroid tissue might in fact be the site of persistent or recurrent disease.

Experience with parathyroid surgery is still the most important predictor of success in reoperative parathyroidectomy.[15] The lateral approach to parathyroidectomy described first by Feind—specifically, dissection between the anterior border of the sternocleidomastoid muscle and the posterior border of the strap muscles—can be invaluable. This approach provides a dissection plane more likely to be free of scar tissue from the previous exploration than the traditional anterior approach does. It is sometimes necessary to perform a partial or (rarely) complete median sternotomy at the time of re-exploration for parathyroids located in the mediastinum. Success rates of 85% to 95% can be achieved by experienced endocrine surgeons in the remedial setting.

Postoperative Complications

There is good evidence that clinical outcomes are related to the experience of the surgeon performing the parathyroidectomy, such that high-volume endocrine surgeons have higher cure rates and lower complication rates. The rate of persistent HPT can be as high as 30% in less experienced hands. Operative complications include injury to the recurrent laryngeal nerve or nerves, leading to hoarseness or frank airway compromise if both nerves are injured (Fig. 37-12). Reported rates of nerve injury range from 1% to 10%. Superior laryngeal nerve injury results in subtle voice changes, which can have profound deleterious effects in professional singers or speakers. Hematoma and wound infection are uncommon. The risk for these complications is theoretically less when exploration is confined to one side of the neck.

Hypoparathyroidism from injury to or removal/devascularization of the remaining parathyroids can occur and result in hypocalcemia (see Hypoparathyroidism earlier). Transient postoperative hypocalcemia is not uncommon. Risk factors for the development of hypocalcemia after parathyroidectomy include subtotal or three and a half gland parathyroidectomy, bilateral neck exploration, removal of the parathyroids together with the thyroid gland, or a history of previous neck dissection. For such patients, a calcium gluconate drip needs to be available to facilitate rapid administration. The drip is prepared by diluting 10 ampules of calcium gluconate in 1 L of normal saline. The initial rate of infusion is 30 mL/hr, which needs to be titrated according to symptoms and serial serum calcium levels. Coincident electrolyte abnormalities, such as hypomagnesemia, need to be corrected to facilitate correction of the hypocalcemia. Oral calcium and vitamin D analogues are used for long-term management.

Treatment Controversies

The optimal clinical treatment of patients with asymptomatic primary HPT has not yet been established. The principal debate is whether patients should be treated with early surgery or whether surveillance or medical therapy can be used safely until symptoms develop. Although consensus-based recommendations have existed for more than a decade regarding optimal management of the disease, there continues to be substantial variation in the practice patterns of endocrine surgeons and endocrinologists. A cross-sectional survey of North American members of the American Association of Endocrine Surgeons demonstrated that even among a group of highly experienced surgeons, criteria for parathyroidectomy vary widely and appear to be associated with surgeon experience.[45] High-volume surgeons (>50 cases per year) had significantly lower thresholds for surgery with respect to abnormalities in preoperative creatinine clearance, bone densitometry changes, and levels of iPTH and urinary calcium than did their low-volume colleagues (1-15 cases per year). In addition, their criteria for surgery diverged from NIH guidelines. It is interesting to note that there was a statistically significant association between several self-reported surgical outcomes and surgeon volume, a finding that has been shown with administrative data for several complex procedures.

A national survey of endocrinologists in the United States was conducted in 1998 to examine the treatment of patients with primary HPT and awareness of NIH recommendations.[46] Data regarding practice demographics and annual primary HPT case volume were also collected. High-volume physicians were more aware of the NIH guidelines than low-volume physicians were. Marked variation in treatment was noted, with 7% of all physicians referring more than 90% of their asymptomatic patients for surgery and 31% referring less than 10%. Adherence to monitoring recommendations for nonoperatively treated patients ranged widely, depending on the indication. Surgical referral practices varied as well, with 25% of endocrinologists referring patients because of mild abnormalities in hypercalcemia, 39% because of moderate hypercalcemia, 31% because of severe hypercalcemia, and 4% reporting that hypercalcemia by itself was not a sufficient reason to refer for parathyroidectomy. These results challenged the endocrine community to examine the evidential basis for decisions made in the treatment of primary HPT.

Medical Alternatives

There are no long-term medical therapies for which data are convincing regarding either their efficacy or safety in the treatment of primary HPT. Three relatively new classes of agents—bisphosphonates, selective estrogen receptor modulators, and calcimimetics—have shown preliminary efficacy on surrogate markers of severity of disease, including serum calcium and bone density, but these effects have not been verified based on clinical outcomes.

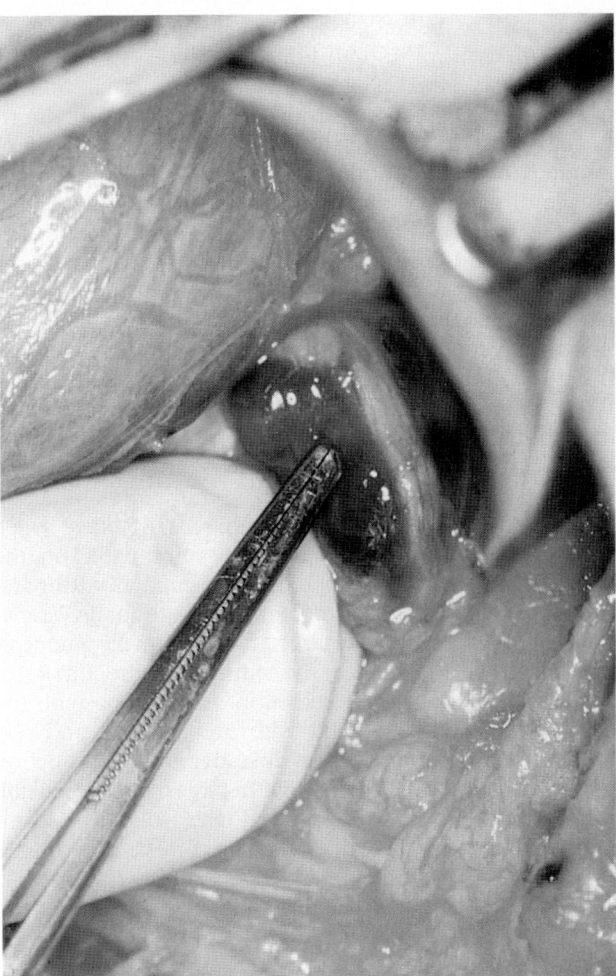

Figure 37-12 Parathyroid adenoma with the thyroid gland above and the recurrent laryngeal nerve splayed around it (tip of the forceps).

Bisphosphonates such as etidronate, alendronate, and pamidronate have been used in the treatment of Paget's disease, osteoporosis, and hypercalcemia of malignancy (see earlier). IV pamidronate appears to be the most effective in the acute treatment of hypercalcemia associated with primary HPT. Limitations of long-term treatment include poor gastrointestinal drug absorption, a rise in PTH levels with increased renal tubular resorption and gastrointestinal absorption of calcium, and their expense.

Bone mineral density has been a primary end point in studies of hormonal therapy in patients with primary HPT. The risk-benefit equation for determining the utility of hormone replacement therapy is complex, however, because estrogen-replacement therapy does not reduce PTH concentrations in patients with primary HPT. In addition, unopposed estrogen increases the risk for endometrial hyperplasia and carcinoma, as well as the risk for venous thromboembolism, and it may cause vaginal bleeding or increase the risk for breast cancer. As a result, selective estrogen receptor inhibitors such as raloxifene and tamoxifen have been used in a preliminary fashion. In one report of 11 postmenopausal women with mild primary HPT, the mean serum calcium level declined 0.7 mg/dL over a 7-month follow-up.

Discovery of the CaSR and its molecular role in mineral metabolism represents a major scientific advance during the past decade. The CaSR is a low-affinity, G protein–coupled receptor found in high concentrations on the surface of parathyroid cells, as well as on thyroid C cells secreting calcitonin and in the nephron, brain, bone, and other tissues. Activation of the CaSR by small changes in extracellular ionized calcium accounts for the steep inverse relationship between PTH and small changes in blood calcium, as well as the sharp pursuant rise in urinary calcium. Alterations of the receptor are responsible for BFHH, severe infantile HPT, and hereditary forms of hypoparathyroidism. Acquired alterations in CaSR might play a role in the pathophysiologic features of primary HPT and secondary HPT. Parathyroids obtained from uremic patients with secondary HPT have been shown to exhibit reduced expression of CaSR on the surface of parathyroid cells; data from patients with parathyroid adenomas or carcinomas are more inconsistent.

The CaSR became the target for the development of compounds that enhance the affinity of the CaSR for calcium and reduce PTH secretion. Experience with the compound R-568 in patients with primary HPT and secondary HPT demonstrated a dose-dependent reduction in PTH and blood calcium, with larger doses causing more sustained effects. The long-term role of calcimimetic agents such as cinacalcet has yet to be determined for the treatment of primary HPT, but it has rapidly become established as a mainstay in the management of secondary HPT (see later).

SECONDARY HYPERPARATHYROIDISM IN RENAL FAILURE

Pathogenesis

Although renal osteodystrophy was recognized for many years, Slatopolsky and Brickers first postulated in 1973 that uremic hyperphosphatemia leads to hypocalcemia, which in turn leads to HPT. This then becomes a compensatory mechanism serving to maintain phosphate balance in uremia. The trade-off was normalization of calcium and phosphate levels at the cost of sustained high PTH levels. It is now believed that the pathogenesis of secondary HPT has multiple contributing factors, including possible genetic mutations, altered vitamin D metabolism and resistance, impaired calcemic response to PTH, retention of phosphorus, and altered metabolism of PTH. In all cases of secondary HPT, the failing kidney is unable to hydroxylate vitamin D_2 to active vitamin D_3 (calcitriol).

The pathways leading to secondary HPT seem to have different predominating factors, depending on the severity of the renal failure. In early renal failure, possible mutations in CaSR and a generalized defect in calcitriol receptors could lead to incipient secondary HPT. Subtle changes in calcitriol levels and serum phosphate levels and the direct action of phosphate on the parathyroids may further potentiate HPT. Altered calcitriol levels and receptor binding seem to begin to alter PTH secretion.

In progressing renal failure, calcitriol deficiency becomes more important and phosphate retention plays a major role in worsening secondary HPT. Changes in calcium set points, increasing skeletal resistance to PTH, and decreased metabolic clearance of PTH contribute to the clinical syndrome of secondary HPT.

Indications for Surgery

Although secondary HPT is typically managed initially with nonoperative strategies, there are pathophysiologic sequelae of chronic renal failure that serve as indications for parathyroidectomy. *Renal osteodystrophy* is a term used to describe the multiple skeletal complications of end-stage renal disease (ESRD), including osteitis fibrosa cystica, osteomalacia, and adynamic bone disease. It is a disorder of bone remodeling and is affected by HPT. Osteitis fibrosa cystica is marked by marrow fibrosis with increased bone remodeling as a result of the increased number and activity of osteoclasts, as well as higher rates of bone formation. It is associated with osteopenia, bone cysts, brown tumors, and decreased bone strength resulting in long bone fractures because of dystrophic bone formation. High levels of PTH coupled with increased cytokine production and low calcitriol levels cause the condition. Osteomalacia is characterized by lower bone turnover, mineralization deficiency, and accumulation of unmineralized osteoid. Deposition of aluminum and other heavy metals associated with ESRD leads to defective mineralization. The incidence has been declining, although the disease has not disappeared completely. Osteomalacia is marked by skeletal deformity, fractures, and pain. It is refractory to vitamin D administration. Adynamic bone disease is characterized by hypocellular bone surfaces with little or no evidence of remodeling, and it is common in patients with normal or low PTH or severe diabetes and aluminum intoxication. It has been associated with long-term peritoneal dialysis. It can cause fractures and microfractures leading to bone pain.

The diagnosis of bone complications from secondary HPT can be established by bone biopsy, along with measurement of serum alkaline phosphatase, PTH, and serum aluminum concentrations, as well as bone scintigraphy. Radiographic examination of the hands, skull, and long bones will show osteopenia, periosteal bone resorption, and occasionally cysts. Medical control of osteodystrophy includes a low-phosphate diet, addition of calcium-based phosphate binders, and limitation of magnesium intake because magnesium inhibits mineralization. Maintaining positive calcium balance and aiming for a serum concentration on the high end of normal to suppress overactivity of the parathyroids are also beneficial.

Administration of vitamin D analogues has been used to treat secondary HPT and to correct the endogenous deficiency of chronic renal failure. The calcimimetic agents (e.g., cinacalcet) have revolutionized the medical management of secondary HPT in chronic renal failure patients undergoing dialysis. The drugs directly lower PTH levels by increasing the sensitivity of the CaSR to extracellular calcium. The starting dose of the drug is

30 mg/day, and it is titrated every 2 to 4 weeks to a maximum of 180 mg/day in divided doses to achieve a target PTH level.

Uremic pruritus, or severe itching with end-stage renal failure, has been postulated to occur as a result of increased calcium salt deposition in the dermis without visible skin lesions. Parathyroidectomy appears to relieve these symptoms within a few days. General weakness is common in uremic patients, particularly in those with secondary HPT. Chou and coworkers described a series of 56 patients with ESRD and secondary HPT who were evaluated by muscle strength flexion and extension, as well as overall activity.[47] Patients then underwent parathyroidectomy with resolution of the secondary HPT. At 3 months all patients showed an increase in muscle force measurements and improvement in physical activity. Finally, anemia is common in uremic patients. It is believed that PTH may directly inhibit renal and extrarenal production of erythropoietin. Excess PTH secretion in secondary HPT can lead to marrow fibrosis, thereby potentiating anemia. There are more complex effects mediated by PTH that affect hemoglobin levels, including intracellular and extracellular calcium and phosphate levels, osteoclast resorption, and erythropoietic progenitor cell response to exogenous erythropoietin. Improvements in anemia have been reported after parathyroidectomy.

Calciphylaxis is a rare, severe complication of secondary HPT characterized by calcification of the media of small to medium-sized arteries; it results in ischemic damage in dermal and epidermal structures. Calcification can lead to nonhealing ulcers, gangrene, sepsis, and death. Women maintained on hemodialysis are almost three times as likely to contract the disease as men. The diagnosis of calciphylaxis is usually based on clinical findings of characteristic skin lesions and can be supported by microscopic examination of skin biopsy samples. Lesions are mottled and painful and advance to hard, tender plaques that develop central ulceration and then eschar. Serum calcium and PTH can be normal or slightly elevated. Parathyroidectomy is effective in some patients in slowing progression of the disease and allowing eventual healing of the wounds with intensive local therapy. Overall, calciphylaxis involving the trunk, shoulder, buttock, or thigh has a poorer prognosis than in patients with distal extremity disease.

Surgical Strategies

Generally, preoperative imaging before initial parathyroidectomy for secondary HPT is not indicated because bilateral neck exploration is required for identification of all glands, given that the underlying pathology is parathyroid hyperplasia. Imaging techniques are indicated for reoperative parathyroidectomy when heterotopic or supernumerary glands cannot be identified despite adequate first-time surgical exploration. The sensitivity and specificity of imaging are limited in patients with ESRD, perhaps because of variations in size and function among the different glands despite increased metabolic activity overall.

After the first successful surgical intervention by Stanbury in 1960, subtotal parathyroidectomy became the standard operative strategy. In 1975, with the demonstration by PTH assay of parathyroid autograft function after forearm autotransplantation, total parathyroidectomy with heterotopic autotransplantation became popular.[48] Total parathyroidectomy without autotransplantation has been described but is not widely used because it appears to have long-term detrimental effects on bone. The debate over which procedure is better has been long-standing. Both approaches require thorough neck exploration through a cervical incision. When performing subtotal parathyroidectomy, it is well advised to choose the most easily accessible gland for the vascularized remnant. Most often this will be an inferior gland because of its more anterior location. If the remnant appears ischemic, a second gland is chosen. Surgery consists of removal of three (or more, if supernumerary glands are identified) glands in toto and 50% to 75% removal of one gland with preservation of a viable, histologically confirmed remnant. Marking the remnant with a titanium clip enables later identification if recurrence develops in the remnant. Use of intraoperative PTH measurements can help ensure that adequate tissue has been resected. Cervical thymectomy is considered in all patients undergoing surgery for secondary HPT because supernumerary, intrathymic parathyroid glands are a common cause of persistent or recurrent disease.

Subtotal parathyroidectomy has several advantages. A well-vascularized eutopic gland will maintain function, in contrast to an autotransplanted gland, which would need to undergo neovascularization. This might be particularly important in a noncompliant patient less likely to faithfully take calcium and vitamin D supplementation postoperatively. Choosing an accessible gland and marking it with a clip for potential identification make re-exploration easier. Finally, avoiding an arm incision allows easier hemodialysis access. Its disadvantages are that a second neck surgery is necessary if HPT recurs, and hypoparathyroidism with significant hypocalcemia may develop if the remnant is not well vascularized. However, because it is advantageous to avoid remedial cervical exploration, heterotopic parathyroid transplantation is attractive.

Total parathyroidectomy with autotransplantation removes all identified glands and uses an easily accessible area, most commonly the forearm or the sternocleidomastoid muscle, as the site for implantation. The gland to be transplanted is minced into 1-mm pieces, and 12 to 18 pieces are embedded in well-vascularized muscle and marked with a stitch or clip. Some groups use a technique of injection into subcutaneous tissue. Neovascularization occurs over a period of several weeks. The principal advantage of this technique is that residual parathyroid function is easily monitored, and recurrences can be treated by partial resection under local anesthesia without the need for cervical re-exploration. There are several disadvantages. More aggressive medical treatment is necessary postoperatively to maintain adequate serum calcium levels and avoid serious hypocalcemic complications. Autograft failure can lead to hypoparathyroidism, which can be profound. Retrieval of all small grafts may be difficult at reoperation. Implantation into muscle may interfere with hemodialysis access in the future, and invasive growth of autografts into muscle and adjacent tissue requiring radical resection has been described. Finally, supernumerary glands may still be present in the neck, thereby resulting in two potential sites of recurrence.

Subtotal parathyroidectomy seems to be the preferred surgical approach in most, but not all patients. The recurrence rate of secondary HPT varies from 5% to 17%, and the incidence is directly related to the length of patient survival. The residual parathyroid tissue in the neck or forearm will grow and cause recurrent disease if survival is prolonged and patients do not receive a renal transplant. Nodular proliferation in glands seems to predispose to recurrence more often than homogeneous gland hyperplasia does. Cryopreservation of excised tissue (if available) is a good strategy when total parathyroidectomy with autotransplantation is planned in the event that the autograft is nonfunctional.

TERTIARY HYPERPARATHYROIDISM

Tertiary HPT occurs in two settings. The first is in a subset of patients with secondary HPT in which the parathyroid glands become autonomous and hypercalcemia develops. The second was first recognized by St. Goar, who described how secondary HPT can persist even after patients underwent renal transplantation; he postulated that the parathyroids became autonomous. Theoretically, reversal of parathyroid hyperplasia should be expected after successful renal transplantation. Nevertheless, studies show that hypercalcemia can persist in 8.5% to 53% of transplant recipients. Of these, less than 1% require parathyroidectomy for tertiary HPT. Transplant patients may have additional factors that can contribute to persistent tertiary HPT; glucocorticoids, cyclosporine, thiazide diuretics, and alterations in the glomerular filtration rate as a result of tubular injury or rejection episodes can influence parathyroid function and bone response. Accordingly, patients with severe secondary HPT should not undergo renal transplantation until their secondary HPT has been treated.

It is known that severe hypercalcemia may adversely affect renal graft function. Therefore, calcium levels higher than 11 mg/dL may need to be addressed more aggressively. Patients with symptomatic bone disease or other serious sequelae of uremic HPT may benefit from surgery. Otherwise, given the finding that in most cases HPT will resolve after transplantation, medical treatment may be indicated. Surgical treatment of tertiary HPT after renal transplantation is not common and is reserved for patients without resolution of symptoms, patients with hormonal and chemical abnormalities such as elevated or increasing iPTH levels and an increase in serum calcium to greater than 12.0 mg/dL that persists more than 1 year after transplantation, and patients with acute hypercalcemia (calcium level >12.5 mg/dL) in the immediate post-transplant period.

INHERITED PARATHYROID DISEASE

Surgical management of HPT in the setting of inherited parathyroid disease differs depending on the specific syndromes, and the complexity is magnified by patients' predisposition to persistent or recurrent HPT. The basic principles of surgery are to achieve and maintain normocalcemia for as long as possible, avoid iatrogenic hypocalcemia and other perioperative complications, and facilitate future surgery, should it be indicated.[49]

Multiple Endocrine Neoplasia Type 1

MEN 1 syndrome consists of primary HPT resulting from parathyroid hyperplasia associated with lesions of the pancreas and pituitary. HPT is the most common and usually the first glandular manifestation, and it typically occurs in the third to fifth decades of life. The parathyroid glands are asymmetrically enlarged, and there is a high incidence of supernumerary glands (up to 20%). Parathyroid surgery in patients with MEN 1 is thought of as a debulking or palliative procedure because recurrence is inevitable if survival is unlimited; it is indicated to treat and prevent the complications of HPT. Controversy exists regarding timing of the procedure. Although early parathyroidectomy may reduce the exposure to long-term HPT and the associated osteopenia, it also might predispose to an earlier recurrence of HPT and the possibility of difficult reoperations.

The initial surgical procedure of choice in a patient with MEN 1 and HPT is either subtotal parathyroidectomy or total parathyroidectomy with heterotopic autotransplantation of resected parathyroid tissue; transcervical thymectomy is performed as well at the initial operation. Subtotal parathyroidectomy requires identification of all parathyroids, and a remnant the size of a normal parathyroid is left in situ and marked with a surgical clip to facilitate remedial surgery. Total parathyroidectomy is accompanied by heterotopic transplantation of 12 to 18 1-mm pieces of fresh parathyroid into individual pockets typically created in the brachioradialis muscle of the nondominant forearm. Reoperative debulking surgery of the forearm graft can then be performed when necessary under local anesthesia. Because parathyroid remnants can become ischemic or necrose and result in permanent hypoparathyroidism, cryopreservation of parathyroid tissue is performed at the time of total parathyroidectomy whenever possible.

Multiple Endocrine Neoplasia Type 2

MEN 2A is marked by the findings of medullary thyroid cancer, pheochromocytoma, and primary HPT. HPT in MEN 2A is the least common manifestation and occurs in 20% to 30% of patients. HPT in MEN 2A differs from MEN 1 in several important features, and the indications for parathyroidectomy and diagnostic criteria are more similar to those of sporadic primary HPT. When compared with HPT in MEN 1, HPT in MEN 2A tends to be milder and more often asymptomatic because of a single adenoma, although multiglandular hyperplasia does occur. Therefore, curative resection can be less aggressive. Enlarged parathyroids encountered during thyroidectomy for medullary thyroid cancer in a normocalcemic patient are resected. Most, but not all endocrine surgeons leave normal-appearing parathyroids in situ, although total parathyroidectomy with autotransplantation to the forearm has been advocated by some.

Familial Hyperparathyroidism

Other, less common forms of familial HPT include the HPT–jaw tumor syndrome (HPT-JT); familial isolated hyperparathyroidism (FIHPT); and a number of syndromes marked by mutations in CaSR, including autosomal dominant mild HPT (ADMH), or familial hypercalcemia with hypercalciuria, and neonatal severe HPT (NSHPT). Recommendations for parathyroid surgery in these settings are still evolving, although some general principles exist. HPT is the most common feature of HPT-JT and is associated with a high incidence of severe hypercalcemia and a risk for parathyroid carcinoma. In general, HPT may be treated similar to MEN 2A, with resection of grossly enlarged parathyroids unless parathyroid cancer is suspected. An alternative strategy is total parathyroidectomy to achieve a theoretically lower risk for carcinoma.

In FIHPT, if uniglandular disease is encountered, adenoma resection can be performed, whereas multiglandular hyperplasia is treated by subtotal parathyroidectomy. In this setting, the rapid intraoperative PTH assay can be helpful to ensure that an adequate resection is performed. Parathyroid surgery for syndromes associated with CaSR abnormalities is variable. NSHPT is manifested in neonates as severe hypercalcemia and is typically lethal unless total parathyroidectomy is performed in the first months of life. For patients with ADMH, radical subtotal parathyroid resection or total parathyroidectomy with autotransplantation can be performed. Diffuse to nodular neoplasia was found on pathologic examination, and persistent hypercalcemia was noted in 60% of patients undergoing the less radical procedure in one study.

PARATHYROID CARCINOMA

Parathyroid carcinoma is rare. It tends to occur a decade earlier than adenomas, and the gender ratio approaches equality, in contrast to the female preponderance of adenomas.[50] A history of previous neck irradiation is a risk factor for the development of parathyroid adenomas, but the role of radiation in the development of parathyroid carcinoma is less clear. Parathyroid carcinoma has also been reported rarely in patients with secondary HPT; in most of these cases, patients had received hemodialysis.

Most patients with carcinomas have marked hypercalcemia (>14 mg/dL) and are more likely to have associated bone and renal disease than those with adenomas. Hypercalcemia is usually manifested as muscle weakness,

fatigue, depression, nausea, and polyuria. Suspicion also is raised by an extremely high iPTH, a palpable neck mass on physical examination, significant uptake on sestamibi scan, or ultrasound evidence of invasion with loss of planes between the parathyroid and the thyroid, occasionally with lymphadenopathy.

If a large, gray-white, locally invasive parathyroid carcinoma is suspected on exploration, an initial aggressive surgical approach involving en bloc tumor resection, ipsilateral thyroid lobectomy, and resection of adjacent soft tissues is performed because this is the only potentially curative treatment. If the procedure is being performed with a minimally invasive technique, the surgery is converted to general anesthesia if necessary to facilitate a thorough oncologic operation. A frozen-section biopsy is not performed before resection because it could lead to capsular rupture and potentially spread tumor cells within the neck.

En bloc resection is associated with an 8% local recurrence rate and an overall survival rate of 89% (mean follow-up, 69 months).[51] Simple parathyroidectomy, in contrast, is associated with a 51% local recurrence rate and a 53% long-term survival rate (mean follow-up, 62 months). Overall adverse prognostic factors for survival are simple parathyroidectomy alone, the presence of nodal or distant metastases at initial evaluation, and nonfunctional status of the tumor. Parathyroid carcinomas tend to recur locally after incomplete excision. Distant metastases generally develop in the lungs, liver, and bone; they can occasionally be treated by resection of individual tumor deposits. Generally, control of hypercalcemia by surgical resection of metastases is more effective than medical treatment. There are no effective chemotherapeutic agents, although cinacalcet (the calcimimetic agent described earlier) is approved by the Food and Drug Administration for symptomatic control of hypercalcemia. In selected patients, adjuvant external beam radiation appears to decrease the rate of local recurrence and may improve disease-free survival, particularly in high-risk patients. Most patients with metastatic or locally unresectable disease die of the metabolic effects of uncontrolled hypercalcemia. At present, there are no generally accepted staging systems for parathyroid carcinoma.

Selected References

Akerström G, Malmaeus J, Bergström R: Surgical anatomy of human parathyroid glands. Surgery 95:14-21, 1984.

> This large autopsy study increased understanding of the most common eutopic and ectopic locations of parathyroid glands.

Bilezikian JP, Potts JT Jr, Fuleihan EH, et al: Summary statement from a workshop on asymptomatic primary hyperparathyroidism: A perspective for the 21st century. J Clin Endocrinol Metab 87:5353-5361, 2002.

> This recent revision of the management principles for patients with asymptomatic primary hyperparathyroidism represents the combined opinions of many medical and surgical leaders in the treatment of primary hyperparathyroidism, as well as a synthesis of published medical evidence.

Boggs JE, Irvin GL, Molinari AS, et al: Intraoperative parathyroid hormone monitoring as an adjunct to parathyroidectomy. Surgery 120:954-958, 1996.

> In this landmark article, 89 patients with hyperparathyroidism had plasma samples measured for iPTH levels during parathyroidectomy. Prediction of postoperative calcium levels by means of the rapid PTH assay had a sensitivity of 97%, specificity of 100%, and overall accuracy of 97%, which led the authors to conclude that the assay should be considered as a routine intraoperative adjunct.

Roman SA, Sosa JA, Mayes L, et al: Parathyroidectomy improves neurocognitive deficits in patients with primary hyperparathyroidism, Surgery 138:1121-1129, 2005.

> This prospective study compares patients with primary hyperparathyroidism undergoing parathyroidectomy and patients with benign euthyroid disease undergoing thyroidectomy. It shows that primary hyperparathyroidism appears to be associated with a spatial learning and processing deficit that improves after surgery and raises the question of whether neurocognitive symptoms should be considered as criteria for parathyroidectomy.

Udelsman R, Donovan P: Remedial parathyroid surgery: Changing trends in 130 consecutive cases. Ann Surg 244:471-479, 2006.

> This large recent clinical series demonstrates that remedial parathyroidectomy can be performed safely with a cure rate of greater than 94% when done by an experienced endocrine surgeon. Novel preoperative imaging techniques are useful, and minimally invasive parathyroidectomy can be used in a subset of these patients.

References

1. Sandstrom IV: On a new gland in man and several mammals. Bull Inst Hist Med 6:192-222, 1938.
2. Owen R: On the anatomy of the Indian rhinoceros (Rh. Unicornis, L). Tran Zool Soc Lond 4:31-58, 1862.
3. Organ CH Jr: The history of parathyroid surgery, 1850-1996: The Excelsior Surgical Society 1998 Edward D. Churchill lecture. J Am Coll Surg 191:284-299, 2000.
4. Gley ME: Sur les functions du corps thyroide. CR Soc Biol 43:841-843, 1891.
5. Mandl F: Attempt to treat generalized fibrous osteitis by extirpation of parathyroid tumor. Zentralbl Chir 53:260-264, 1926.
6. Bauer W, Albright F, Aub JC: A case of osteitis fibrosa cystica (osteomalacia?) with evidence of hyperactivity of the parathyroid bodies: A metabolic study. J Clin Invest 8:228-248, 1930.
7. Albright F, Baird PC, Cope O, et al: Studies on the physiology of parathyroid glands—renal complications of hyperparathyroidism. Am J Med Sci 187:49-65, 1934.
8. Castleman B, Mallory TB: Parathyroid hyperplasia in chronic renal insufficiency. Am J Pathol 13:553-558, 1937.
9. Stanbury WS, Lumb GA, Nicholson WF: Elective subtotal parathyroidectomy for renal hyperparathyroidism. Lancet 1:793, 1960.
10. Rasmussen H, Craig LC: Purification of parathyroid hormone by use of countercurrent distribution. J Am Chem Soc 81:5003, 1959.
11. Berson SA, Yalow RS, Aurbach GD, et al: Immunoassay of bovine and human parathyroid hormone. Proc Natl Acad Sci USA 49:613-617, 1963.
12. Reiss E, Canterbury JA: A radioimmunoassay for parathyroid hormone in man. Proc Soc Exp Biol Med 128:501-504, 1968.
13. Slomp J, van der Voort PH, Gerritsen RT, et al: Albumin-adjusted calcium is not suitable for diagnosis of hyper- and hypocalcemia in the critically ill. Crit Care Med 31:1389-1393, 2003.
14. Wang S: pH effects on measurements of ionized calcium and ionized magnesium in blood. Arch Pathol Lab Med 126:947-950, 2002.
15. Edis AJ, Grant CS, Egdahl RH (eds): Manual of Endocrine Surgery, 2nd ed. New York, Springer-Verlag, 1984.
16. Udelsman R, Donovan PI: Remedial parathyroid surgery: Changing trends in 130 consecutive cases. Ann Surg 244:471-479, 2006.
17. Akerström G, Malmaeus J, Bergström R: Surgical anatomy of human parathyroid glands. Surgery 95:14-21, 1984.
18. Silverberg SJ, Bilezikian JP, Bone HG, et al: To treat or not to treat: Conclusions from the NIH consensus conference. J Clin Endocrinol Metab 84:2275-2278, 1999.
19. Downs RW: Hypoparathyroidism in the differential diagnosis of hypocalcemia. In Bilezikian JP, Marcus R, Levine MA (eds): The Parathyroids: Basic and Clinical Concepts, 2nd ed. San Diego, CA, Academic Press, 2001.
20. Bilezikian JP, Potts JT Jr, Fuleihan EH, et al: Summary statement from a workshop on asymptomatic primary hyperparathyroidism: A perspective for the 21st century. J Clin Endocrinol Metab 87:5353-5361, 2002.
21. Roman SA, Sosa JA, Mayes L, et al: Parathyroidectomy improves neurocognitive deficits in patients with primary hyperparathyroidism, Surgery 138:1121-1129, 2005.
22. Lundgren E, Lind L, Palmer Jakobsson S, et al: Increased cardiovascular mortality and normalized serum calcium in patients with mild hypercalcemia followed up for 25 years. Surgery 130:978-985, 2001.
23. Coakley AJ, Kettle AG, Wells CP: ^{99m}Tc sestamibi: A new agent for parathyroid imaging. Nucl Med Commun 10:791-794, 1989.
24. Denham DW, Norman J: Cost effectiveness of preoperative sestamibi scan for primary hyperparathyroidism is dependent solely upon the surgeon's choice of operative procedure. J Am Coll Surg 186:293-305, 1998.
25. Blanco I, Carril JM, Banzo I, et al: Double-phase Tc-99m sestamibi scintigraphy in the preoperative localization of lesions causing hyperparathyroidism. Clin Nucl Med 23:291-297, 1998.
26. Geatti O, Shapiro B, Orsolon PG, et al: Localization of parathyroid enlargement: Experience with technetium-99m methoxyisobutylisonitrile and thallium-201 scintigraphy, ultrasonography and computed tomography. Eur J Nucl Med 21:17-22, 1994.
27. Udelsman R, Aruny JE, Donovan P, et al: Rapid parathyroid hormone analysis during venous localization. Ann Surg 237:714-719, discussion 719-721, 2003.
28. Boggs JE, Irvin GL, Molinari AS, et al: Intraoperative parathyroid hormone monitoring as an adjunct to parathyroidectomy. Surgery 120:954-958, 1996.
29. Garner SC, Leight GS Jr: Initial experience with intraoperative PTH determinations in the surgical management of 130 cases of primary hyperparathyroidism. Surgery 126:1132-1137, 1999.
30. Boggs JE, Carneiro DM, Irvin GL: The evolution of parathyroidectomy failures. Surgery 126:998-1003, 1999.
31. Irvin GL, Molinari AS, Fegueroa C, et al: Improved success rate in reoperative parathyroidectomy with intraoperative PTH assay. Ann Surg 229:874-878, 1999.
32. Mozzon M, Mortier PE, Jacob PM, et al: Surgical management of primary hyperparathyroidism: The case for giving up quick intraoperative PTH assay in favor of routine PTH measurement the morning after. Ann Surg 240:949-953, 2004.

33. Carneiro-Pla DM, Solorzano CC, Irvin GL: Consequences of targeted parathyroidectomy guided by localization studies without intraoperative parathyroid hormone monitoring. J Am Coll Surg 202:715-722, 2006.

34. Goldstein RE, Blevins L, Delbeke D, et al: Effect of minimally invasive radioguided parathyroidectomy on efficacy, length of stay, and costs in the management of primary hyperparathyroidism. Ann Surg 231:732-742, 2000.

35. Roth SI, Wang CA, Potts JT Jr: The team approach to primary hyperparathyroidism. Hum Pathol 6:645-658, 1975.

36. Wang CA: Surgical management of primary hyperparathyroidism. Curr Probl Surg 22:1-50, 1985.

37. Tibblin S, Bondeson AG, Ljungber O: Unilateral parathyroidectomy in hyperparathyroidism due to single adenoma. Ann Surg 195:245-252, 1982.

38. Bergenfelz A, Lindblom P, Tibblin S, et al: Unilateral vs. bilateral neck exploration for primary hyperparathyroidism: A prospective randomized controlled trial. Ann Surg 236:543-551, 2002.

39. Lo Gerfo P: Bilateral neck exploration for parathyroidectomy under local anesthesia: A viable technique for patients with coexisting thyroid disease with or without sestamibi scanning. Surgery 126:1011-1014, discussion 1014-1015, 1999.

40. Udelsman R: Six hundred fifty-six consecutive explorations for primary hyperparathyroidism. Ann Surg 235:665-672, 2002.

41. Miccoli P, Bendinelli C, Conte M, et al: Endoscopic parathyroidectomy by a gasless approach. J Laparoendosc Adv Surg Tech A 8:189-194, 1998.

42. Lorenz K, Miccoli P, Monchik JM, et al: Minimally invasive video-assisted parathyroidectomy: A multi-institutional study. World J Surg 25:704-707, 2001.

43. Prinz RA, Lonchyna V, Carnaille B, et al: Thoracoscopic excision of enlarged mediastinal parathyroid glands. Surgery 116:999-1004, 1994.

44. Gagner M: Endoscopic parathyroidectomy [letter]. Br J Surg 83:875, 1996.

45. Sosa JA, Powe NR, Levine MA, et al: Cost implications of different surgical management strategies for primary hyperparathyroidism. Surgery 124:1028-1036, 1998.

46. Mahadevia PJ, Sosa JA, Levine MA, et al: Clinical management of primary hyperparathyroidism and thresholds for surgical referral: A national study examining concordance between practice patterns and consensus panel recommendations. Endocr Pract 9:494-501, 2003.

47. Chou FF, Chiang HL, Chen JB: General weakness as an indication for parathyroid surgery in patients with secondary hyperparathyroidism. Arch Surg 134:1108-1111, 1999.

48. Wells SA, Gunnells JC, Shelburne JD: Transplantation of the parathyroid glands in man: Clinical indications and results. Surgery 78:34-44, 1975.

49. Carling T, Udelsman R: Parathyroid surgery in familial hyperparathyroid disorders. J Intern Med 257:27-37, 2005.

50. DeLellis RA: Parathyroid carcinoma: An overview. Adv Anat Pathol 12:53-61, 2005.

51. Koea JB, Shaw JH: Parathyroid cancer: Biology and management. Surg Oncol 8:155-165, 1999.

Endocrine Pancreas

James C. Thompson, MD   and   Courtney M. Townsend, Jr., MD

| History |
| Embryology |
| Histomorphology of Islets |
| Endocrine Physiology |
| Islet Cell Tumors |
| Medical Therapy for Islet Cell Tumors |
| What's Next? |

HISTORY

Endocrine cells are diffusely scattered in small clumps throughout the pancreas. While a medical student in 1869, Paul Langerhans described collections of pale-staining cells within the pancreas, the islets that now bear his name. In 1889, Minkowski, after learning that the urine of a pancreatectomized dog attracted flies, analyzed the urine and found glycosuria. Eugene Opie detected hyaline changes in the islets of diabetic patients in 1901 and is generally credited with establishing the association between diabetes and islet pathology. In 1908, A. G. Nichols reported a patient with a simple adenoma of islet tissue. Frederick Banting, an orthopedist, and Charles Best, a medical student in Toronto, discovered insulin in 1922, and soon thereafter, insulin became available for the treatment of diabetes. The relationship between hyperinsulinism and an unresectable pancreatic islet cell carcinoma was established by W. J. Mayo, and the first surgical cure of insulinoma syndrome was achieved by Roscoe Graham in Toronto in 1929. In 1935, Whipple and Frantz[1] described a diagnostic triad for insulinoma: symptoms of hypoglycemia, low concentrations of blood glucose, and relief of symptoms by the administration of glucose.

Endocrine cells of the pancreas reside in islets, and the adult human pancreatic islet contains multiple types (Table 38-1): the A (alpha) cell secretes glucagon, the B (beta) cell secretes insulin, the D (delta) cell secretes somatostatin, the D_2 (delta-2) cell secretes vasoactive intestinal peptide (VIP), and the PP (or F) cell secretes pancreatic polypeptide (PP). Ghrelin, the peptide that stimulates appetite and comes mainly from the stomach, is also present in the pancreas; the cell of origin is unknown. Enterochromaffin cells (EC) are quite rare. Gastrin cells are normally present only in the fetal pancreas. Ectopic gastrin cells may give rise to gastrinomas in the pancreas, duodenum, or adjacent structures. Tumors of any of these cells may in fact secrete multiple peptides, serially or simultaneously. The syndromes produced are named for the peptide whose symptoms predominate. Thus, the endocrine pancreas may produce insulinomas, glucagonomas, somatostatinomas, VIPomas, PPomas, or gastrinomas. The characteristics of each islet cell tumor syndrome are summarized in Table 38-1.

In 1955, Robert M. Zollinger and Edwin H. Ellison at the Ohio State University Hospital reported on two patients on whom they had operated, both of whom had a fulminant peptic ulcer diathesis, massive acid hypersecretion, and a non-beta islet cell tumor of the pancreas. Mort Grossman and Rod Gregory determined that the secretagogue was gastrin, and we know that gastrinomas cause the Zollinger-Ellison syndrome (ZES) (see Selected References).

In 1958, J. V. Verner and A. B. Morrison[2] reported two patients who died of watery diarrhea and hypokalemia, both of whom had been found at autopsy to have benign islet cell tumors. Bloom and colleagues[3] measured high levels of circulating VIP in patients with this watery diarrhea, hypokalemia, and achlorhydria syndrome and proposed VIP to be the agent responsible. In 1942, Becker and colleagues[4] reported a patient with a severe dermatitis (later determined to be necrolytic migratory

CELLS	CONTENT	% ISLET CELLS	SECRETORY GRANULE SIZE (nm)	TUMOR SYNDROMES	CLINICAL FEATURES	DIAGNOSTIC HORMONE LEVELS	% MALIGNANT	% MULTIPLE	MEN 1	AT SURGERY: % IDENTIFIED/ %RESECTABLE
A	Glucagon, glicentin (TRH, CCK, endorphin, PYY, pancreastatin)	15	225	Glucagonoma	Necrolytic migratory erythema, diabetes, anemia	Normal=<150 pg/mL Tumor=200-2000 pg/mL	Nearly all	Rare	Few	98/35
B	Insulin (TRH, CGRP, amylin, pancreastatin, prolactin)	65	300	Insulinoma	Hypoglycemic symptoms (catecholamine release) plus mental confusion	>5 μU/mL in the face of hypoglycemia	10	10	10%	80-100/>90
D	Somatostatin (met-encephalon)	5	200-235	Somatostatinoma	Diabetes, gallstones, steatorrhea	Normal=10-25 pg/mL Tumor=100-400 pg/mL	Nearly all	0	—	100/60
D₂	VIP	<1	120	VIPoma (watery diarrhea, hypokalemia, achlorhydria [WDHA] [Verner-Morrison])	High-volume secretory diarrhea, hypokalemia, metabolic acidosis, hypochlorhydria	Normal=<200 pg/mL Tumor=225-2000 pg/mL	50	Rare	Few	100/70
EC	Substance P and serotonin	<1	325	?	—	—	—	—	—	—
G*	Gastrin (ACTH-related peptides)	—	300	Gastrinoma (Zollinger-Ellison syndrome)	Abdominal pain with ulcer disease, massive gastric hypersecretion, secretory diarrhea that can be halted by nasogastric aspiration	Normal=<100 pg/mL Suspicious=>1000 pg/mL With secretin test, >200 pg/mL diagnostic	70	—	25%	50-85/79 Of the 70%: pancreatic, <20 duodenal, all ectopic, 80
PP (F)	Pancreatic polypeptide (met-enkephalin, PHI)	15	140	Tumors (PPomas) are without endocrine symptoms	—	—	—	—	Frequent	—
Prob B	Ghrelin†	?	?	None known	N/A	—	—	—	—	—

*Gastrin is present in fetal but not in normal adult pancreatic islets.

†Broglio F, Gottero C, Benso A, et al: Ghrelin and the Endocrine Pancreas. Endocrine 22:19-24:2003.

ACTH, adrenocorticotropic hormone; CCK, cholecystokinin; CGRP, calcitonin gene-related peptide; MEN 1, multiple endocrine neoplasia type 1; PHI, peptide histidine isoleucine; PYY, peptide YY; TRH, thyrotropin-releasing hormone; VIP, vasoactive intestinal peptide.

Modified from Bonner-Weir S: Anatomy of the islet of Langerhans. In Samols E (ed): The Endocrine Pancreas. New York, Raven Press, 1991, p 16; and Marx M, Newman JB, Guice KS, et al: Clinical significance of gastrointestinal hormones. In Thompson JC, Greeley GH Jr, Rayford PL, Townsend CM Jr (eds): Gastrointestinal Endocrinology. New York, McGraw-Hill, 1987, p 416.

Table 38-2   Efficacy of Localization of Endocrine Tumors of the Pancreas and Duodenum

MODALITY	TRUE POSITIVES (%)
Noninvasive	
Ultrasonography	23
Octreotide radioimaging (SRS)*	86
CT	43
MRI	26
Invasive	
Endoscopic ultrasonography	82
Selective angiography	56
Portal venous sampling	76
Provocative angiography†	65

*Rarely for melanoma.
†Calcium for insulinoma; secretin for gastrinoma.
SRS, somatostatin receptor scintigraphy.
Modified from Norton JA: Neuroendocrine tumors of the pancreas and duodenum. Curr Probl Surg 31:97, 1994.

erythema), anemia, and diabetes. She was found to have an islet cell carcinoma of the pancreas, but it was not until 1966 that McGavran and associates[5] identified glucagon from an alpha cell carcinoma of the pancreas as the agent responsible. The syndrome produced is not specific but is usually characterized by diabetes, gallstones, steatorrhea, and hypochlorhydria. The tumor is often discovered at cholecystectomy, and preoperative diagnosis is extraordinarily rare. Many endocrine tumors produce PP, and its chief usefulness is as a marker for endocrine tumors of the pancreas; co-elevations of PP and Ca^{2+} signal multiple endocrine neoplasia (MEN) type 1 syndrome. Pancreatic islet tumors have been found on rare occasion to produce growth hormone–releasing factor (GRF), adrenocorticotropic hormone (ACTH), and parathyroid hormone–related peptide (PTHrP). The development of radioimmunoassay by Berson and associates in 1956[6] allowed measurements of circulating concentrations of peptides, which has greatly facilitated the diagnosis of islet cell tumor syndromes. The efficacy of various imaging and sampling techniques for localization of islet cell tumors of the pancreas and duodenum is shown in Table 38-2.

Surgical management of these tumors has undergone serial evolution. First, all pancreatic endocrine tumors are rare (estimated at ~5 cases per 1 million population per year), so time is required for the evolution of logical strategies for treatment. We attempt to briefly cover the major points that the reader would like to know about the endocrine pancreas, and we focus on clinical identification of tumors, their preoperative localization and operative management, the usefulness of palliation, and the outcomes that can be expected.

EMBRYOLOGY

The pancreas originates from two diverticular buds of the foregut that give rise to a ventral and a dorsal pancreas. With rotation of the foregut, the two masses fuse in human embryos during the fifth and sixth weeks of fetal development. In humans, the first islets of endocrine tissue appear in the early fetal period (~10 weeks); islets appear initially and in greater number in the tail of the pancreas. The *origin* of the endocrine cells of the pancreas has been a subject of hot debate. Gittes and Rutter[7] studied the patterns of genetic expression of hormonal messenger RNA and concluded that both endocrine and exocrine cells of the pancreas arise from embryonic foregut endoderm (not from the neural crest), a view now generally accepted. Islets of Langerhans cells have been grown from adult pancreatic stem cells, which may provide autogenous islets in the future for clinical implants.[8]

The development of human fetal islets has been divided into three stages: in the first phase (weeks 14-16), the islet cells bud off of ductules; in the second phase (weeks 17-20), beta cells appear in the center of the islets, with non-beta cells on the periphery; in phase 3 (weeks 21-26), beta and non-beta cells become positioned throughout the islet. Some exceptions to this orderly arrangement persist: 10% of total islet cells consist of beta cells outside discrete pancreatic islets. In rat embryos, specific insulin, glucagon, and cholecystokinin (CCK) cells can be identified at the beginning of the second half of gestation (day 12), and somatostatin cells appear 3 to 4 days later. Glucagon cells have been found in human embryos at 3 weeks. An example of the genetic mechanisms controlling the appearance of peptide hormones is that the upstream promoter element of the glucagon gene, *G1,* has been shown to restrict glucagon gene expression to alpha cells; though widely expressed at several embryonic stages, expression of the insulin gene in adults is restricted to islet beta cells.

HISTOMORPHOLOGY OF ISLETS

Islets account for less than 2% of the adult pancreatic mass and thus in humans weigh about 1 g. In the fetus, islets represent nearly a third of the pancreatic mass, but after birth, this percentage is greatly diluted by the accelerated growth of exocrine tissue. The adult human pancreas contains about 10^6 islets scattered throughout the parenchyma. The average adult human islet contains about 3000 cells, but islets vary greatly in size (40-400 μm in diameter). A scanning electron micrograph of an isolated islet is shown in Figure 38-1. Most islets are small, but the largest 15% of islets make up 60% of total islet volume. Adult islets are composed of four major cell types (A, B, D, and PP) and two or more minor types (see Table 38-1). The location of cells within the islet itself is tightly regulated: beta cells occupy the center, and the peripheral mantle is composed of A, D, and PP cells.[9] A cells are columnar and well supplied with granules measuring 200 to 250 nm in diameter. B cells are polyhedral, truncated pyramids with secretory granules measuring 250 to 300 nm. D cells are smaller than A and B cells and are often dendritic. PP cells are the most variable: in humans the granules are elongated, electron dense, and 120 to 160 nm, whereas in other species they

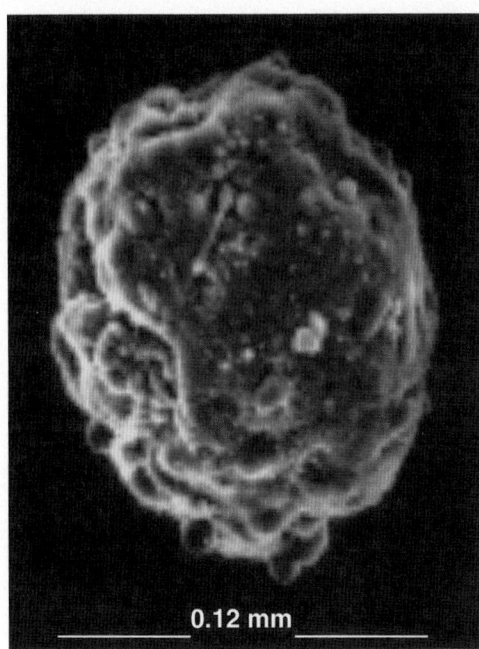

0.12 mm

Figure 38-1 Scanning electron micrograph of an isolated islet of **Langerhans.** (From Orci L: Macro- and micro-domains in the endocrine pancreas. Diabetes 31:563, 1982.)

are spherical and much larger. Any single cell may secrete more than one peptide; for example, the A cell may secrete CCK, and the B cell may secrete thyrotropin-releasing hormone and amylin (see Table 38-1). Glucagon-producing A cells and PP-producing PP cells have mutually exclusive domains that follow a regional distribution: islets in the head and uncinate process are rich in PP cells but poor in A cells, whereas islets in the body and tail show the opposite predominance; B and D cells are evenly distributed. The physiologic significance of these quirks of distribution is unknown but sometimes important; for example, a Whipple resection removes nearly all PP cells but spares almost all glucagon-producing A cells.

Great interest has been focused on the microcirculation of islets and its putative significance in endocrine-to-endocrine cell signaling. A popular concept holds that arterioles pierce the islet through short discontinuities in the mantle of non-beta cells and enter directly into the B-cell core.[10] Efferent capillaries coalesce at the edge of the islets and pass through the mantle of non-beta cells. This has given rise to the concept that there is a simple B to A to D cell order of cellular perfusion, with resultant control of glucagon secretion, for example, depending on insulin output. This concept has been challenged in a study on rat islet microcirculation in which the supplying arteriole was found to deliver blood first to capillaries in the mantle of the islet and then to the core, thus suggesting a more complex pattern and casting doubt on the circulating progression from B to A to D cells. This is not a matter solely of academic interest because the core-to-mantle interislet portal microcirculation has been held responsible for major abnormalities in glucagon secretion in diabetes.[10]

Studies on a possible portovenous connection between endocrine islets and exocrine acini have been reviewed[11]; insulin stimulates exocrine pancreatic secretion, transport of amino acids, and synthesis of proteins and enzymes. Glucagon inhibits pancreatic secretion and enzyme synthesis. Insulin and glucagon act antagonistically on the exocrine pancreas, but the role of somatostatin is controversial; it may act via its inhibitory effect on islet B cells, although acinar cells themselves possess receptors for somatostatin.

ENDOCRINE PHYSIOLOGY

The chief physiologic function of the endocrine pancreas might be starkly summarized as regulation of body energy (a role largely achieved by hormonal control of carbohydrate metabolism). Simply stated, insulin is the hormone of energy storage and glucagon the hormone of energy release. Insulin stores energy by decreasing blood glucose levels, increasing protein synthesis, decreasing glycogenolysis, decreasing lipolysis, and increasing glucose transport into cells (except beta cells, hepatocytes, and central nervous system cells). Glucagon releases energy by increasing blood glucose levels via stimulation of glycogenolysis, gluconeogenesis, and lipolysis. Chief attention in this chapter is directed to the physiology of insulin and glucagon and their interactions with somatostatin.

Insulin

The insulin molecule contains 56 amino acids and is arranged into A and B chains connected by two disulfide bridges. In newly synthesized insulin, these chains are joined by means of a connecting (C) peptide (Fig. 38-2). This proinsulin, which is synthesized in the endoplasmic reticulum, travels on stimulation to the Golgi complex of the beta cell, where the C peptide is cleaved and insulin is moved via microtubules into secretory granules to be released into the bloodstream by extrusion of the 6-kd polypeptide through the cell membrane (exocytosis). Patients with type 1 (insulin-dependent) diabetes have undergone loss of beta cells and have an absolute insulin deficiency. In common with structures that are truly vital, there is a great backup supply of beta cells; the development of diabetes requires destruction of more than 80% of the beta cells. Insulin secretion is regulated by circulating levels of glucose and by humoral and neural factors. The glucose-sensing mechanism of the beta cell is highly alert and, on detecting a high blood glucose level, reacts with an immediate output of stored insulin that lasts about 5 minutes, followed by a longer sustained secretion that appears to be newly synthesized insulin.

Oral ingestion of glucose in humans and other species has been shown repeatedly to cause release of pancreatic insulin in an amount greater than the insulin response to an identical dose of glucose given intravenously (IV), even though blood levels of glucose may be the same. Several peptides released from the proximal portion of the gut in response to a normal meal have the capacity

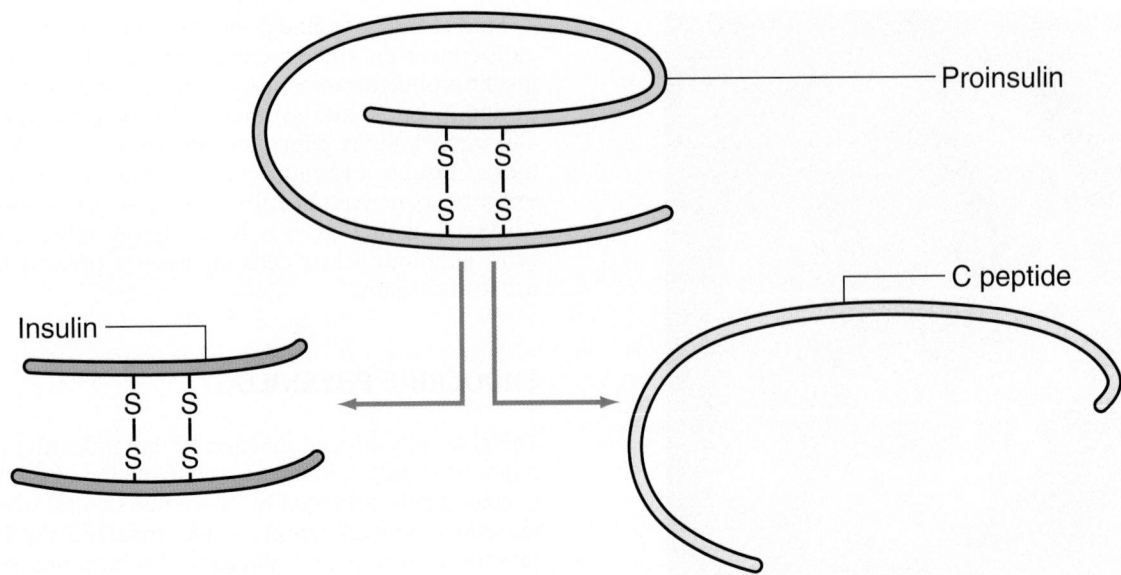

Figure 38-2 Diagram of insulin synthesis. Proinsulin, synthesized by the endoplasmic reticulum, is packaged within secretory granules of the beta cell, where it is cleaved to insulin and C peptide. Equimolar amounts of insulin and C peptide are secreted into the bloodstream. (From Andersen DK, Brunicardi FC: Pancreatic anatomy and physiology. In Greenfield LJ, Mulholland MW, Oldham KT, et al [eds]: Surgery: Scientific Principles and Practice, 2nd ed. Philadelphia, Lippincott-Raven, 1997, p 869.)

to augment nutrient-induced release of insulin. These insulinotropic factors apparently act directly on beta cells and are called *incretins*. Gastric inhibitory peptide (GIP) is by far the best candidate for physiologic incretin action, with CCK a distant second. Humoral inhibitors of insulin release include somatostatin, pancreastatin, amylin, and the fatty tissue hormone leptin.

Neural control of insulin release can be simplistically summarized by stating that the vagus nerve stimulates release of insulin and the sympathetic nervous system inhibits it. However, further study shows a more complex picture: α-sympathetic fibers strongly inhibit insulin secretion, but β-fibers stimulate it. The nerve fibers release peptides, and these peptidergic influences react with circulating regulatory peptides to modulate secretion by both alpha and beta cells. Insulin release is stimulated by the peptidergic nerve release of gastrin-releasing peptide (GRP), CCK, gastrin, enkephalin, and VIP, whereas insulin release is inhibited by peptidergic nerve release of neurotensin, substance P, and somatostatin.

Secreted insulin is transported rapidly to the portovenous system, and slightly more than half is cleared by hepatocytes on first transit through the liver; insulin has a half-life of 7 to 10 minutes. All cells except cerebrocytes and red blood cells take up insulin. Renal excretion is scant. A major role of insulin is promotion of glucose transport into cells, and such transport may be enhanced by regulation of membrane-bound glucose transporter peptides. Insulin binds to a specific membrane receptor, a glycoprotein with a molecular weight of 300 kd. Peripheral resistance to insulin may result from either a diminished number of receptors or decreased receptor affinity for insulin. Type 2 diabetes is caused, at least in part, by receptor defects leading to insulin resistance. The complexity of control of insulin metabolism has been demonstrated repeatedly in normal individuals and in diabetic patients. In one study in patients with hepatic resistance to insulin after resection of the head of the pancreas for trauma, infusion of PP corrected hepatic resistance to insulin, evidence that provides support for a role of PP as a glucose regulatory hormone.

Glucagon

Glucagon, secreted by A cells of the islet, is a straight-chain, 29–amino acid polypeptide with a molecular weight of 3.5 kd, the main function of which is to promote conversion of hepatic glycogen to glucose. As with insulin, glucagon secretion is controlled by a complex interaction of neural, hormonal, and nutrient factors. Also as with insulin, the primary regulator of glucagon release is circulating glucose, high levels of which inhibit glucagon secretion. Glucagon and insulin exercise a yin-yang reciprocal control of carbohydrate metabolism. Failure of glucagon secretion can cause hypoglycemia, and excess glucagon may bring about hyperglycemia. Insulin and somatostatin suppress glucagon release, probably via the islet portovenous system. Neural control of glucagon output is similar to that of insulin, but sympathetic neural transmitters and the neural hormone epinephrine stimulate A cells, whereas they inhibit B cells. The putative hormone-hormone interrelationship (B to A to D) among islet cells as mediated by portovenous islet flow is discussed earlier in the section on insulin. Another item of uncertainty is whether the hormone-hormone interrelationships are all carried out via the interislet circulation or whether some may be simply cell-to-cell paracrine effects.

Somatostatin

Somatostatin, which its codiscoverer Roger Guillemin proposed to be a universal hormonal "off switch," is a small, straight-chain, 14–amino acid (1.6-kd) polypeptide that is secreted by acinar D cells. Although it is attractive and logical to consider that somatostatin has a modulating influence on the secretion of other islet hormones, its actual function within the pancreas is unknown. In addition, if it does influence other cells, techniques are not yet available to reveal whether this occurs through transport via the islet portovenous system or by simple paracrine leakage. The full molecule has a short half-life, but the octapeptide analogue octreotide has a longer life in circulation and has been used to treat secretory diarrhea, bowel fistulas, and endocrine hypersecretory syndromes.

Pancreatic Polypeptide

PP is a 36–amino acid, 4.2-kd, straight-chain molecule secreted by PP (or F) cells located primarily in the uncinate process and the head of the pancreas. The physiologic actions of PP are unknown, and its clinical usefulness is limited to a role as a marker for other endocrine tumors of the pancreas. Absence of PP may play a role in the diabetes seen after pancreatic resection or after chronic atrophic pancreatitis.

Other Peptides

VIP is a 28–amino acid, 3.3-kd polypeptide secreted by D_2 cells of the pancreas. It stimulates insulin and inhibits gastric secretion. It is found throughout the gastrointestinal tract, and its major function appears to be vasodilation and bronchodilation. Amylin is a 36–amino acid polypeptide secreted by the B cell that inhibits insulin secretion and uptake. Pancreastatin is part of a larger ubiquitous molecule, chromogranin A, found in the envelope of secretory granules. Pancreastatin inhibits insulin secretion. Gastrin cells are present in fetal but not normal adult islets. Other peptides (glicentin, thyrotropin-releasing hormone, CCK, endorphin, peptide YY, GRF, calcitonin gene–related peptide, prolactin, met-enkephalin, ACTH, peptide histidine isoleucine, and PTHrP) have been reported in normal islets and in islet cell tumors. Ghrelin is a 28–amino acid peptide produced primarily by the stomach but also in lower amounts by other tissues, including the pancreas. Ghrelin secretion is increased in anorexia but reduced in obesity. Beta cells may contain ghrelin and nerve growth factor.

ISLET CELL TUMORS

In 1935, Whipple and Frantz reported the association of hyperinsulinism with adenomas of pancreatic islet cells, thereby establishing a functional connection between islet cell tumors and endocrine syndromes. Later, syndromes were described for islet tumors producing gastrin, glucagon, somatostatin, VIP, and other peptides. To repeat, these tumors are rare. The annual incidence in this country has been estimated at between 5 and 10 cases per 1 million population per year. The autopsy rate is said to be 1%, or expressed another way, these tumors are 1000 to 2000 times more common in autopsy statistics than in annual clinical practice; most are clearly nonfunctional and benign.

The incidence of malignancy in these tumors varies greatly, from about 10% in insulinomas to nearly all glucagonomas and somatostatinomas (see Table 38-1). In a manner reminiscent of stage-by-stage progression of normal gut epithelium to eventual malignancy, tumorigenesis of neuroendocrine cells appears to involve multiple genetic events (mutational activation or inactivation of oncogenes or tumor suppressor genes) (Fig. 38-3).[12] For these tumors, the criterion of malignancy is simple: if they metastasize, they are malignant. On hematoxylin and eosin–stained sections, all pancreatic endocrine tumors, including carcinoid tumors of the bowel, look alike. Immunostaining with antibodies to specific hormones allows identification of the endocrine content of cells. By ordinary light microscopy, there are no characteristics that separate benign from malignant tumors. Region-specific antibodies to chromogranin A may be helpful in differentiating between benign and malignant tumors. Some large aggressive tumors may invade adjacent structures and by such action proclaim their malignancy, but most tumors larger than 2 cm are malignant anyway. Mixed exocrine-endocrine tumors are rare; when present, the endocrine cells are inactive, except in pancreaticoblastomas.

Endocrine tumors of the pancreas vary greatly in mode of onset and severity of symptoms, location, and malignant potential.[13] With time, they may vary greatly in secretion and biologic aggressiveness. So great is the variation even within specific tumor syndromes that any generalization may not apply to a particular patient. One accurate generalization is that even though multiple hormones may be produced by a single tumor (or even by a single cell within that tumor), the syndrome is recognized and named by the clinical signs associated with the predominant endocrine agent. As many as 40% of patients with islet cell neoplasms may have elevated levels of multiple hormones, not all of which produce symptoms. We treated a young woman several years ago with ZES who did well after total gastrectomy until a virulent syndrome of hypertension, muscle weakness, and anorexia developed. She was found to have high levels of ACTH and died in steroid crisis as we were preparing her for adrenalectomy. Her ACTH levels were more than 200 times normal, and she was asymptomatic from remaining gastrinoma tissue (the tumor cell line was established in nude mice).[14] Moertel[15] wondered whether this phenomenon represents multiple clones of tumor cells or a common stem cell with multiple potential for hormone production.

Although the tumor syndromes are classically ascribed to *pancreatic* islet tumors, tumors are often found in extrapancreatic locations, especially in the duodenum and peripancreatic areas above, below, and to the right of the duodenum. Nearly all insulinomas, glucagonomas, and VIPomas occur within the pancreas itself, whereas

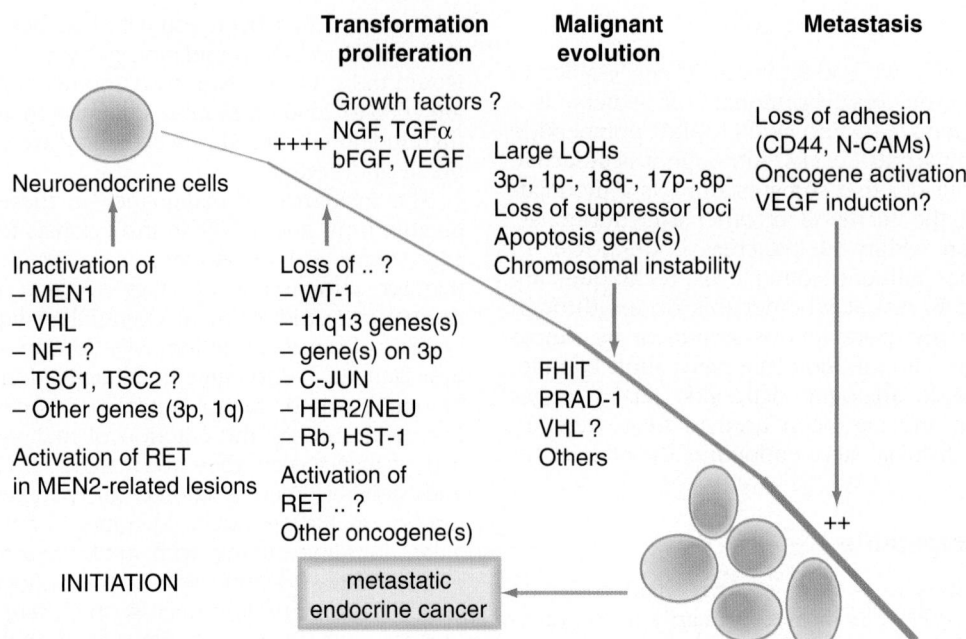

Figure 38-3 Diagram summarizing the major events involved in tumor initiation, progression, and pathogenic mechanisms involved in metastasis. bFGF, basic fibroblast growth factor; FHIT, fragile histidine triad; MEN1, multiple endocrine neoplasia type 1; NF1, neurofibromatosis type 1 (neurofibromin); NGF, nerve growth factor; PRAD-1, parathyroid adenoma–related protein; TGF, transforming growth factor; TSC1 and TSC2, tuberous sclerosis genes; VEGF, vasculoendothelial growth factor; VHL, von Hippel-Lindau genes. (From Calender A: Molecular genetics of neuroendocrine tumors. Digestion 62[Suppl 1]:3-18, 2000.)

most gastrinomas occur in the duodenum, with the pancreas second. Somatostatinomas are divided equally between the pancreas and the proximal part of the small bowel. Patients with von Recklinghausen's disease may have somatostatinomas or gastrinomas in the duodenum.

Tumors may demonstrate an anatomic preference for bimodal distribution. An analysis of several reported series suggests that gastrinomas, PPomas, and somatostatinomas show a 75% preference for an anatomic location to the right of the superior mesenteric arteries in peripancreatic tissue, in the duodenum, and in the head of the pancreas. By contrast, about 75% of insulinomas and glucagonomas were located in the body and tail of the pancreas to the left of the superior mesenteric artery. Further review of these findings suggested that the distribution of glucagonomas, insulinomas, and PPomas corresponded to the normal distribution of these endocrine cell types within the pancreas.

Pancreatic endocrine tumors may occur sporadically or in conjunction with the MEN 1 syndrome. MEN 1 is characterized by tumors of the parathyroid, pituitary, and pancreas and occasionally the adrenal gland. MEN 1 is genetically associated with a defect on chromosome 11 and is inherited in an autosomal dominant fashion. Because islet cell tumors in patients with MEN 1 are always multiple, preoperative recognition of MEN 1 status is necessary. About 25% of patients with gastrinomas, 10% of those with insulinomas, and lesser percentages of patients with glucagonomas and VIPomas have MEN

syndrome. Of all MEN 1 patients, more than half have gastrinomas, and one in five has an insulinoma. Most (70%-90%) patients with MEN 1 manifest hyperparathyroidism, usually caused by hyperplasia of all four glands. A series of 107 patients with MEN 1 and ZES monitored prospectively at the National Institutes of Health (NIH) were compared with more than 1000 cases from the literature. The NIH patients more frequently had pituitary (60%), adrenal (45%), and carcinoid tumors (30%), but as in other series, hyperparathyroidism was far more frequent (94%). Twenty-five percent of patients had no family history of MEN.[16] Calcium levels need to be measured in any patient with a pancreatic endocrine tumor syndrome, and if elevated, the parathyroids and the pituitary must be studied. A general principle is that in MEN 1 patients with islet tumors, the hyperparathyroidism is surgically managed first, preferably by removing all four glands with an immediate autograft.

From a clinical viewpoint, the most important aspects of dealing with patients with endocrine tumors of the pancreas are the means of localization and the proper operative treatment. In a meta-analysis of a dozen individual reports, the efficacy of true-positive tumor localization has been summarized (see Table 38-2). Techniques of both localization and surgical excision have undergone radical changes in the past decade and are still in the process of evolution. The following sections offer a brief review of current methods of diagnosis, localization, and surgical techniques. Each is discussed in detail under the appropriate tumor heading.

Insulinoma

Insulinoma is the most common functioning tumor of the pancreas, and affected patients have a tableau of symptoms referable to hypoglycemia (symptoms of catecholamine release), mental confusion and obtundation, or both. Many patients have symptoms for years. Some have been greatly troubled by emotional instability and fits of rage, often followed by somnolence. A review of the world literature from 1914 to 1957 reported 356 cases of hyperinsulinism secondary to benign islet cell adenomas.[17]

Clinical Features and Diagnosis

The diagnostic hallmark of the syndrome is the so-called Whipple triad, namely, symptoms of hypoglycemia (catecholamine release) and low blood glucose (40-50 mg/dL) and relief of symptoms after the IV administration of glucose. The triad is not entirely diagnostic because it may be emulated by factitious administration of hypoglycemic agents, by rare soft tissue tumors, or occasionally by reactive hypoglycemia. The clinical syndrome of hyperinsulinism may follow one of two patterns or sometimes a combination of both. The symptom complex may be due to autonomic nervous overactivity, as expressed by fatigue, weakness, fearfulness, hunger, tremor, sweating, and tachycardia, or alternatively, a central nervous system disturbance with apathy (or irritability or anxiety), confusion, excitement, loss of orientation, blurring of vision, delirium, stupor, coma, or convulsions.

The pathognomonic finding is an inappropriately high (>5 μU/mL) level of serum insulin during symptomatic hypoglycemia. A possible mechanism for this high level of insulin in the face of hypoglycemia may be overexpression of the insulin splice variant. A diagnostic ratio of blood insulin (in microunits per milliliter) to glucose (in milligrams per deciliter) of greater than 0.4 or C peptide levels higher than 2 nmol/L have proved valuable in diagnosis. The best way to induce hypoglycemia is with fasting: two thirds of patients will experience hypoglycemic symptoms in 24 hours, and nearly all other patients experience symptoms by 72 hours of fasting. Provocative tests, usually involving tolbutamide or glucagon, have been used, but they may cause dangerously profound hypoglycemia and are not generally necessary. Because cerebrocytes metabolize only glucose, prolonged profound hypoglycemia may cause permanent brain damage. Clinicians need to be alert to this problem when attempting to induce hypoglycemia by fasting. Most important, preoperative fasting orders *must* be accompanied by IV administration of glucose.

A particularly troubling cause of the clinical picture of hyperinsulinemia is brought about by factitious administration of insulin or a hypoglycemic agent such as sulfonylurea. Individuals so involved are usually workers in health care who have access to insulin or other hypoglycemic agents. Their motives are obscure but are clearly aimed at securing attention. Self-administration of insulin can be detected because these patients do not have the usual consonant concentrations of C peptide or proinsulin (see Fig. 38-2); sulfonylurea may be detected, with

difficulty, in blood (and more important, insulin levels are not inappropriately high).

As soon as a patient with insulinoma is identified, care must be taken to prevent severe hypoglycemia with possible loss of cerebrocytes. The diet is modified to include frequent meals, even awakening at night to eat. The standard drug is diazoxide, which is helpful in about two thirds of patients but discontinued at least a week before surgery because it may cause intraoperative hypotension. The long-acting somatostatin analogue octreotide, though helpful in children with nesidioblastosis, has been effective only rarely in adults.

Localization

Insulinomas are small (usually <1.5 cm), usually single (only 10% are multiple and those are usually associated with MEN 1 syndrome), usually benign (only 5%-10% are malignant), and generally hard to find. Success in localization often parallels the degree of invasiveness of the study (see Table 38-2). Plain abdominal radiographic and ultrasound studies are rarely helpful, but contrast-augmented computed tomography (CT) and magnetic resonance imaging (MRI) locate 50% to 60% of tumors. Because few insulinomas have many somatostatin receptors, somatostatin receptor scintigraphy (SRS) is not highly successful. Success in localization by selective arteriography varies with the size of the tumor; 90% accuracy rates have been reported with insulinomas. Demonstration of islet tumors by enhanced CT, enhanced MRI, or arteriography (Fig. 38-4) depends, of course, on the relatively rich blood supply to islet tumors as compared with the rest of the pancreatic parenchyma. Also helpful has been selective portovenous sampling for measurement of insulin levels in pancreatic venous tributaries (Fig. 38-5), a method that does not absolutely localize the site of the tumor but, in about 75% of cases, does provide accurate information on the region of the pancreas from which high levels of insulin are released. The method has a relatively high incidence of problems with bleeding into the peritoneal cavity or biliary tree. It is expensive and requires skill.

Calcium is known to release insulin, and taking a page from the intra-arterial secretin test for gastrinoma, a highly promising test has been developed for localizing insulinomas by means of selective intra-arterial injection of calcium (into the gastroduodenal, superior mesentery, right hepatic, or splenic arteries) and obtaining samples for radioimmunoassay of insulin from the right hepatic vein. A study from the NIH compared the accuracy of several techniques in the localization of insulinomas in 36 patients: the accuracy of CT was 24%; MRI, 45%; SRS, 17%; abdominal ultrasound, 13%; selective angiography, 43%; and intra-arterial calcium stimulation, 94%. By combinations of these studies, all tumors were identified before surgery; a surgeon unaware of the preoperative localization study was successful in identifying the tumor by intraoperative ultrasound in 12 (86%) of 14 patients.

Surgery

Treatment of insulinoma is surgical and performed by either open or laparoscopic approaches. In open

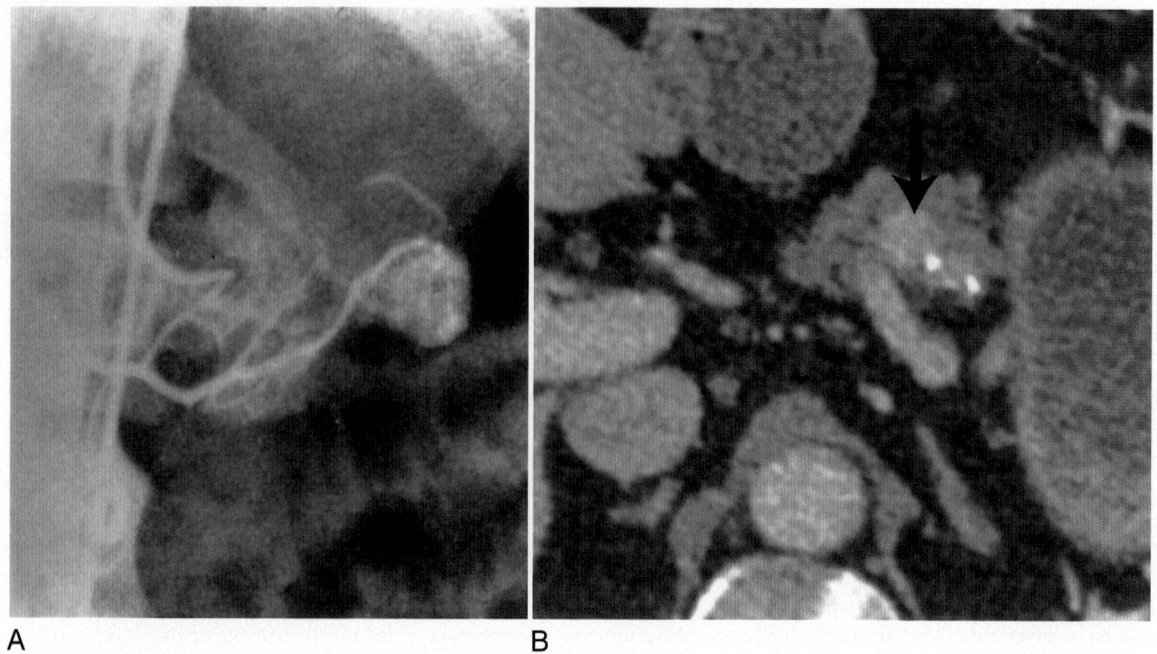

A   B

Figure 38-4 Arteriographic demonstration of an insulinoma. **A,** Selective injection into the specific dorsal pancreatic artery demonstrates the tumor precisely. **B,** Insulinoma with triphasic enhancement on CT. The mass in the pancreatic body (*arrow*) demonstrates early and prolonged enhancement with washout during the portal venous phase; note that the maximal difference in enhancement between the tumor and normal pancreas occurs during the pancreatic phase (shown). (**A,** From Edis AJ, McIlrath DC, Van Heerden JA, et al: Insulinoma: Current diagnosis and surgical management. Curr Probl Surg 13:1-45, 1976; **B,** from Ros PR, Mortele KJ: Imaging features of pancreatic neoplasms. JBR-BTR 84:239-249, 2001.)

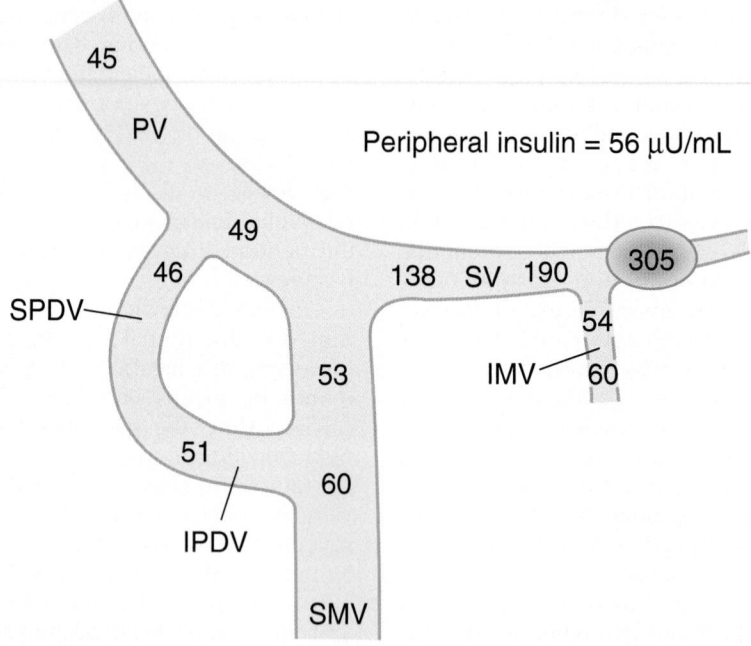

Figure 38-5 Transhepatic selective venous sampling of the portal vein and its tributaries for insulin. Venous insulin levels are greatly elevated in the distal splenic vein (*shaded circle*). Intraoperative ultrasound and palpation of the pancreas failed to reveal an insulinoma. Distal pancreatectomy was performed on the basis of the portovenous sampling gradient shown here, and the pathologists confirmed the presence of a 1-cm insulinoma. IMV, inferior mesenteric vein; IPDV, inferior pancreaticoduodenal vein; PV, portal vein; SMV, superior mesenteric vein; SPDV, superior pancreaticoduodenal vein; SV, splenic vein. Insulin concentrations are given in microunits per milliliter. (From Norton JA, Shawker TH, Doppman JL, et al: Localization and surgical treatment of occult insulinomas. Ann Surg 212:615-620, 1990.)

procedures, the incision is dictated by operator preference, either a midline incision from the xiphoid to below the umbilicus or a bilateral subcostal incision. Exposure needs to be generous, and mechanical ring retractors are an asset. The entire abdomen must be explored, with particular attention paid to possible liver metastases. Next, the pancreas is mobilized by dividing the gastrocolic ligament from left to right, incising the posterior lining of the lesser sac along the inferior and superior margins of the pancreas, and performing generous medial mobilization of the C-loop of the duodenum by incising the peritoneum along the right border (Kocher maneuver). The head of the pancreas is palpated carefully and examined anteriorly and posteriorly; the body and tail of the pancreas are palpated, any ligamentous attachments to the spleen divided, the spleen delivered into the wound, and the tail rotated anteriorly to allow palpation and visualization.

Several articles[18,19] have shown the applicability of laparoscopy to endocrine pancreatic tumors, especially insulinomas and nonfunctioning adenomas. The technique is standard (Fig. 38-6)[18] and is particularly applicable to small solitary benign islet tumors in the body and tail. As with open resection, the chief complication seems to be pancreatic fistula, most often seen after enucleation. The use of laparoscopic ultrasound is vital and allows selection of the most efficient resection (Fig. 38-7).

Anyone operating on patients with islet adenomas must be familiar with the techniques and limitations of intraoperative ultrasonography. Higher resolution (7.5-10 MHz) transducers are used in the pancreas; because of its greater depth of penetration, a 5-MHz transducer is better for the liver. Islet tumors are detected as sonolucent masses, generally of uniform consistency. Several reports attest to the high degree of accuracy of intraoperative ultrasound. The color Doppler attachment allows detection of adjacent vessels and aids in identification of the pancreatic ductal system, which shows up as a lucent tube without flow. A fair conclusion is that intra-arterial calcium infusion is the most sensitive study for preoperative localization of insulinomas and intraoperative ultrasound is essential for intraoperative detection of them.[20]

In the previous edition we concluded that careful review of the literature suggested that nearly all syndromes of hyperinsulinism were due to insulinoma and that blind resection was not indicated.[21] Recent revival of interest in adult nesidioblastosis[22] has suggested a so-called noninsulinoma pancreatogenous hypoglycemia syndrome. These rare cases appear to resemble nesidioblastosis in neonates. The number of confirmed cases is low, but in rare instances, surgeons may need to consider empirical distal pancreatectomy.

Most insulinomas are benign and can be enucleated. Nutrient vessels in the bed of the adenoma need to be cauterized. Care needs to be taken during enucleation to avoid injury to ductal structures, and if a duct is injured, it is sutured and drained. If malignant, the tumor is resected in a cancer-type operation, and if metastatic, it is worthwhile to try to remove all primary and metastatic tumor tissue in an effort to minimize persistent hyperinsulinism.

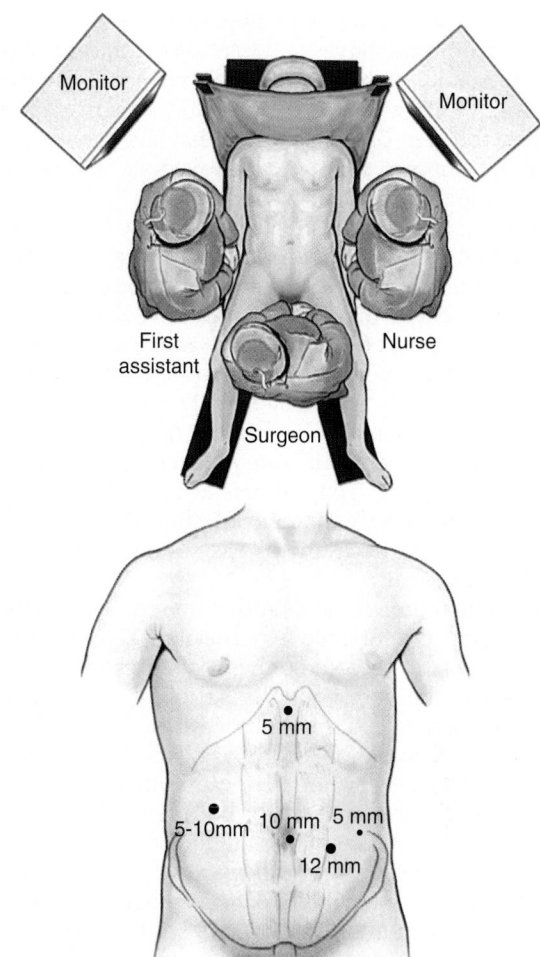

Figure 38-6 Room layout and port placement for laparoscopic surgical treatment of endocrine pancreatic tumors. (With kind permission of Springer Science and Business Media. From Figure 1 and 2 of: Assalia A, Gagner M: Laparoscopic Pancreatic Surgery for Islet Cell Tumors of the Pancreas. World J Surg 28:1239-1247, 2004.)

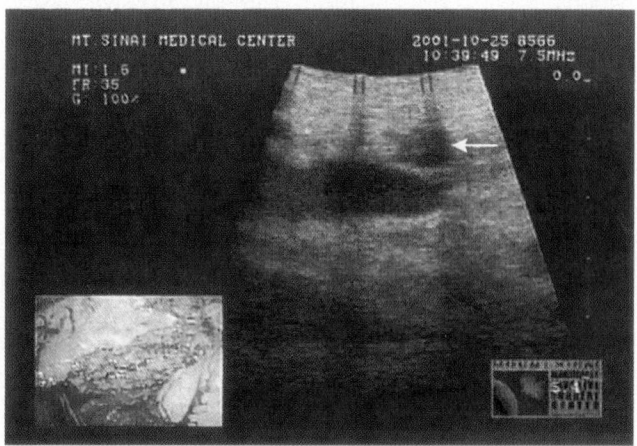

Figure 38-7 Laparoscopic ultrasonography scan showing a pancreatic islet tumor. (With kind permission of Springer Science and Business Media. From Figure 4 of: Assalia A, Gagner M: Laparoscopic Pancreatic Surgery for Islet Cell Tumors of the Pancreas. World J Surg 28: 1239-1247, 2004.)

The 10% of patients with hyperinsulinism who have MEN 1 syndrome have multiple islet tumors, one of which is usually dominant and responsible for the excessive insulin output. These are probably best managed by resecting the area of the pancreas that shows the highest insulin output on selective portovenous sampling or selective intra-arterial calcium challenge.

Persistent hyperinsulinemia after surgery for metastatic islet cell tumors may be managed by hepatic artery tumor embolization, by diazoxide, or by streptozotocin plus fluorouracil. The usual dose of diazoxide is 100 mg three times a day; side effects are rare and are chiefly fluid retention and hirsutism. The usual dose of streptozotocin is 500 mg/m^2 of body surface daily for 5 consecutive days, plus fluorouracil, 400 mg/m^2 daily over a 5-day period. White blood cell and platelet counts must be monitored carefully. Ten patients at the NIH with metastatic insulinoma had a variety of clinical findings from hepatic to lymph node metastases. Nine of the 10 had prolonged survival.[23]

Insulinomas are rare in infants; a review of 160 patients with neonatal and infantile hyperinsulinism found adenomas in only 4.[24] The commonly ascribed cause of hyperinsulinism in the very young is nesidioblastosis, literally a nestlike increase in islet cells. The problem with this concept is that nesidioblastosis appears to be a normal phase of fetal islet development rather than a pathologic entity. The best explanation for hyperinsulinism appears to be a regulatory defect in insulin synthesis, storage, or release. The problem is serious because prolonged hypoglycemia leads to mental retardation in many and perhaps most of these children. Near-total (95%-98%) pancreatectomy appears to offer the best results, with octreotide therapy reserved for preoperative preparation and those few children not rendered euglycemic after surgery.

Zollinger-Ellison Syndrome (Gastrinoma)

The initial 1955 report by Zollinger and Ellison of two patients with a virulent ulcer diathesis, massive gastric acid hypersecretion, and an islet tumor of the pancreas introduced a new disease.[25] Presciently, they ascribed the acid secretory symptoms to a hormone elaborated by the tumor. This hormone was later shown to be gastrin, and we now know that a gastrinoma is the hallmark of ZES. In the less than half century since the original description of ZES, gradual accumulation of experience has changed and greatly improved diagnostic and therapeutic approaches.[26] All interested parties have witnessed the disease in evolution, and we describe it here as it is best known in the early years of this century. Gastrinoma is the second most common islet cell tumor and is the most common symptomatic, malignant endocrine tumor of the pancreas. Having said that, current information is that gastrinomas in the duodenum are 3 to 10 times more common than in the pancreas, and although up to 70% of duodenal gastrinomas have lymph node metastases, only 5% have liver metastases.[26] Rare pulmonary, acoustic neuroma, and colon tumors may produce gastrin without causing hypergastrinemia, but outside the area of the pancreas and duodenum, only ovarian cancers can process progastrin to gastrin to bring about ZES.

Clinical Features and Diagnosis

In 75% of patients with ZES, the gastrinoma is sporadic, whereas 25% have an associated MEN 1 syndrome. In the sporadic form there is a slight (60%) male preponderance; the average age at onset is 50 years. With MEN 1, onset is usually 5 to 10 years earlier. The main symptoms are those caused by peptic acid hypersecretion, with abdominal pain being the chief complaint in about 75% of patients. Nearly two thirds of patients have diarrhea, and 10% to 20% of patients have diarrhea as the sole symptom. A unique characteristic of this diarrhea is that it is halted by nasogastric aspiration of gastric secretions, a feature that separates it from *all other* secretory diarrheas. Most patients have peptic ulcers; duodenal are the most common, but jejunal ulceration may be found (both patients in the original report by Zollinger and Ellison had jejunal ulcers). The most common complications of peptic ulcer are nausea and vomiting (in 30%), bleeding (in 10%), and perforation (in 7%). About a third of patients have signs and symptoms of gastroesophageal reflux disease, and this number appears to be increasing.

Of all MEN 1 patients, the organ most commonly involved is the parathyroid, and 70% to 95% of patients demonstrate hypercalcemia (albumin corrected). The next most common syndrome is ZES (54%), followed by insulinoma (21%), glucagonoma (3%), and VIPoma (1%). Nonfunctioning PPoma occurs in more than 80%.[27] Pituitary adenomas are common, most of which are nonfunctioning, with prolactinomas being the next most common.

As is true with any new disease, the most flagrant examples are those seen first, and with time, early and less severe cases become evident. The prescient hypothesis that gastrinoma may take either an aggressive or relatively benign clinical course has been borne out. The aggressive form, seen in about a quarter of all patients, is more frequent in women and those with MEN 1 syndrome. It is associated with larger pancreatic tumors, liver metastases, and a long-term survival rate of 30% as compared with 96% for the nonaggressive form.[24] Ninety percent of aggressive tumors are located in the pancreas, and their 10-year survival rate of 30% is starkly contrasted to a 96% survival rate with the nonaggressive form. The salient factors influencing prognosis in these aggressive tumors are liver metastases, incomplete resection, and DNA flow cytometry showing a high index of aneuploidy, among other factors.[26]

ZES must be excluded in all patients with intractable peptic ulcers, severe esophagitis, or persistent secretory diarrhea. The diagnosis depends on the presence of hypergastrinemia in the face of increased secretion of gastric acid. Most laboratories have an upper limit of normal of 100 pg/mL for fasting levels of gastrin. Levels of 100 to 1000 pg/mL are occasionally seen in non-ZES patients, and levels higher than 1000 are nearly diagnostic for ZES, provided that the patient makes gastric acid (some pernicious anemia patients have very high gastrin

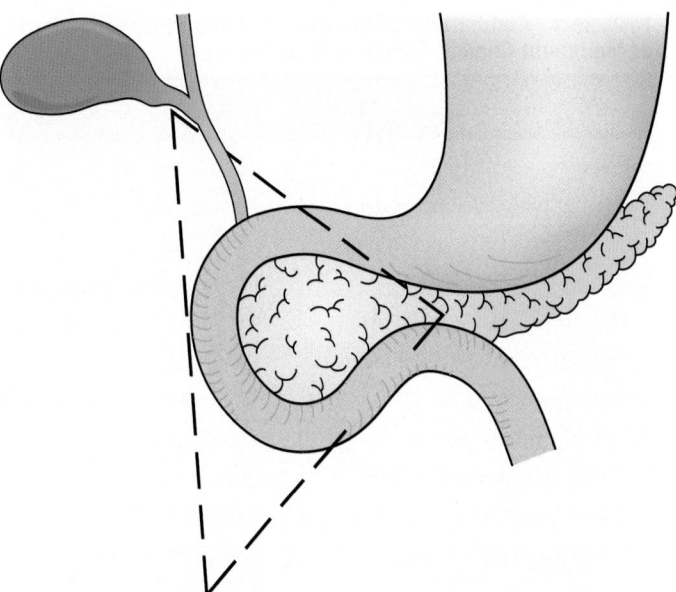

Figure 38-8 The anatomic triangle in which approximately 90% of gastrinomas are found. (From Stabile BE, Morrow DJ, Passaro E Jr: The gastrinoma triangle: Operative implications. Am J Surg 147:25-31, 1984.)

appropriate dose (60-120 mg/day; usual dose, 80 mg/day). These drugs have proved safe and effective, and enough needs to be given to curtail gastric acid output to less than 5 mEq/hr.

Pathology

Gastrinomas were originally assumed to arise in the pancreas, but most subsequent series have shown that the majority originate in the duodenum. Sixty percent to 90% are found in the so-called gastrinoma triangle,[28] an area in the upper part of the abdomen with its superior point at the junction of the cystic and common bile ducts, its inferior point at the junction of the inferior margin of the second and third parts of the duodenum, and its left lateral point at the junction of the head and neck of the pancreas (Fig. 38-8). The duodenum is the site of gastrinomas in more than 60% of patients, and there is a pronounced proximal-to-distal gradient within the duodenum (i.e., most are in the first part, none in the fourth). Gastrinomas have been reported in the renal capsule and in ovarian cancers. Histologic criteria for malignancy are either absent or unreliable. Again, if the tumors metastasize, they are malignant. In early series, 60% to 90% of tumors were malignant, whereas most subsequent studies report that only about a third are malignant, which suggests that with time, all tumors may become malignant. The cell of origin is certainly not clear because the normal postembryonic pancreas and duodenum contain no gastrin cells. Candidates would be a nest of embryonal cells or an undifferentiated line of stem cells. Gastrinomas in the duodenum and pancreas may have a different embryologic origin; that is, gastrinomas in the duodenum and pancreatic head may arise from the ventral pancreatic anlage, and tumors of the body and tail may arise

levels but make no gastric acid; the same is true to a lesser degree in patients taking proton pump inhibitors [e.g., omeprazole]). An elevated serum level of gastrin coupled with a pH less than 2 in the gastric aspirate is virtually diagnostic of ZES. Other causes of hypergastrinemia must be ruled out (Box 38-1). If the diagnosis is in doubt, the secretin provocation test is highly useful. In this test, the fasting gastrin level is measured before secretin (2 CU/kg) is administered IV, and further samples for determination of gastrin are obtained 2, 5, 10, and 20 minutes after administration of secretin. An increase of more than 200 pg/mL in the gastrin value after administration of secretin is found in 87% of patients, with no false-positive results. False-negative results may be due to *Helicobacter pylori*.

Current clinical clues to patients with ZES are the following:

- A virulent peptic ulcer or gastroesophageal reflux disease diathesis
- Absence of *H. pylori* or failure of the peptic ulcer to heal after either anti–*H. pylori* therapy or H_2 blockade
- A secretory diarrhea that persists (especially if the diarrhea is halted by nasogastric suction)
- Signs or symptoms of MEN 1 syndrome (elevated serum calcium and parathyroid hormone levels, pituitary tumor)

Once the diagnosis is established, acid secretion needs to be controlled to prevent complications and to afford symptomatic relief. The best results are achieved with proton pump inhibitor drugs, which are given in an

Table 38-3 Comparison of Clinical and Laboratory Characteristics of Patients With a Benign or Malignant Clinical Course of Gastrinoma

	CLINICAL COURSE (% ALL PATIENTS)	
CHARACTERISTICS*	Benign† (n = 140)	Malignant† (n = 45)
Percentage of patients	76	24
Initially with liver metastases	0	19
Liver metastases developing later	0	5
Gender	Predominantly male (68)	Predominantly female (67)
MEN 1 at initial evaluation	21	Uncommon (6)
Time from onset to diagnosis	Long (mean, 5.9 yr)	Short (mean, 2.7 yr)
Serum gastrin level‡	Moderately elevated (mean, 1711 pg/mL)	Very elevated (mean, 5157 pg/mL)
Size of primary tumor	Small (≤1 cm)	Large (>3 cm)
Location of primary tumor	Primarily duodenum (66)	Primarily pancreatic (92)
Survival at 10 yr	Excellent (96)	Poor (30)
Flow cytometry of tumor	Low S phase (mean, 3.3)	High S phase (mean, 5.1)
	High percentage of nontetraploid aneuploid (32)	Low percentage of nontetraploid aneuploid
	Multiple stem line aneuploid rare	Multiple stem line aneuploid frequent

*All characteristics were significantly different (*P* < .0001) between the two groups.
†The benign or nonaggressive course was not associated with the development of liver metastases (*n*=140), whereas patients in whom the gastrinoma pursued a malignant or aggressive course had liver metastases either at the initial evaluation (*n*=36) or later during follow-up (*n*=9).
‡Normal serum gastrin level less than 100 pg/mL.
MEN 1, multiple endocrine neoplasia type 1.
From Jensen RT: Gastrin-producing tumors. Cancer Treat Res 89:304, 1997.

from the dorsal anlage. ZES patients with MEN 1 syndrome have multiple tumors, often microadenomas, scattered throughout the pancreas and duodenum. Sixty percent to 80% of these MEN 1 patients have duodenal gastrinomas, which usually metastasize to local nodes (85% have lymph node metastases). In general, metastases to the liver occur from large (>3 cm) sporadic pancreatic tumors, whereas lymph node metastases do not appear to be dependent on size or location of the primary tumor (duodenal and pancreatic gastrinomas seem to be equally malignant, with about 50% of the metastases going to lymph nodes). Whether all these lymph nodes containing gastrinoma tissue are true metastases is questionable because long-standing cures have, on occasion, resulted from excision of only the lymph nodes.[26,29] More sporadic cases of ZES are initially found to have liver metastases than those with ZES plus MEN 1 syndrome, but survival without metastases (95% versus 96% at 5 years) is not different. Because of these early liver metastases, the sporadic form of ZES is more virulent than ZES plus MEN 1. An NIH study of patients with sporadic ZES at a mean follow-up of 12.5 years showed liver metastases to be the dominant factor in survival; for instance, the 10-year survival rate in patients with hepatic metastases was 30%, and that in patients without hepatic metastases was 90%. Surprisingly, the presence or absence of lymph node metastases did not affect survival.[30,31] All of this suggests that there is an initial biologic division into either a benign or a malignant clinical syndrome (Table 38-3).

Gastrinomas are usually slow growing, and some patients may live for years with metastatic disease. Zollinger and Ellison's second patient (JM) was found to have lymph node metastases at the time of her total gastrectomy in 1954. Forty years later, she underwent parathyroidectomy and was alive and well in 1999 (C. Ellison, personal communication, 1999). Patients with unresectable liver metastases have a 5-year survival rate of 20% to 40% and a 10-year survival rate of between 0% and 30%. A 10-year prospective study of 73 patients with ZES who had no radiographic evidence of liver metastases showed that long-term survival was excellent when compared with the survival of patients with distant spread, even when no tumor was found and even when resection was not curative (Fig. 38-9).

Gastrin is a potent growth factor for parietal cells, and patients with ZES have greatly increased numbers of parietal cells (from a normal value of 1×10^9 to $\sim 5 \times 10^9$ parietal cells in ZES patients). In addition to the physiologically active G17 and G34 forms, gastrinomas release smaller and larger forms of gastrin, fragments of gastrin, and glycine-extended forms. All ZES patients have an elevated level of chromogranin A (present in the wall of the secretory granule).

Localization

Attempts to localize gastrinomas by means of ultrasonography, arteriography, and enhanced CT and MRI have been only partly successful. The highly invasive technique of selective portovenous sampling has proved to

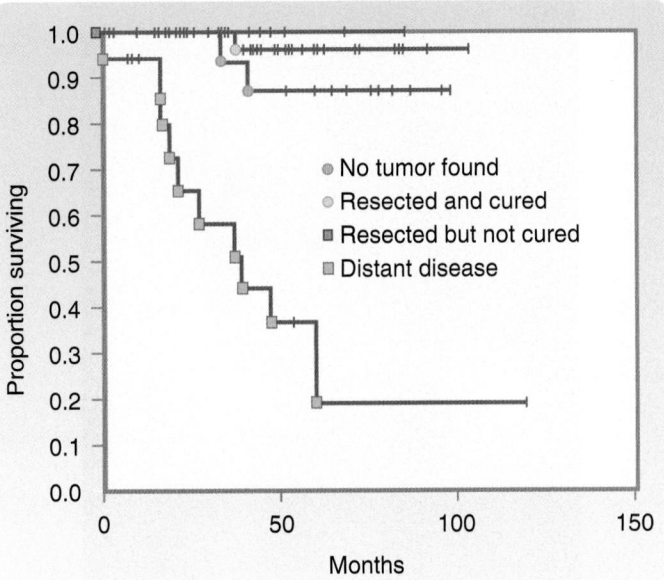

Figure 38-9 Proportion of patients surviving with Zollinger-Ellison syndrome from the day of diagnosis. Patients were divided into four groups on the basis of preoperative evaluation, operative findings, and initial postoperative evaluation: 18 patients who had distant metastatic disease at diagnosis (included as controls), 16 patients who had no tumor found at surgery, 42 patients who had tumor resected and were disease-free (cured), and 15 patients who had all of the tumor resected but were not disease-free. There were no differences among the three groups with respect to localized gastrinoma, but the group with distant disease had a significantly shorter survival time (*P* < .001). (From Norton JA, Doppman JL, Jensen RT: Curative resection in Zollinger-Ellison syndrome: Results of a 10-year prospective study. Ann Surg 215:8-18, 1992.)

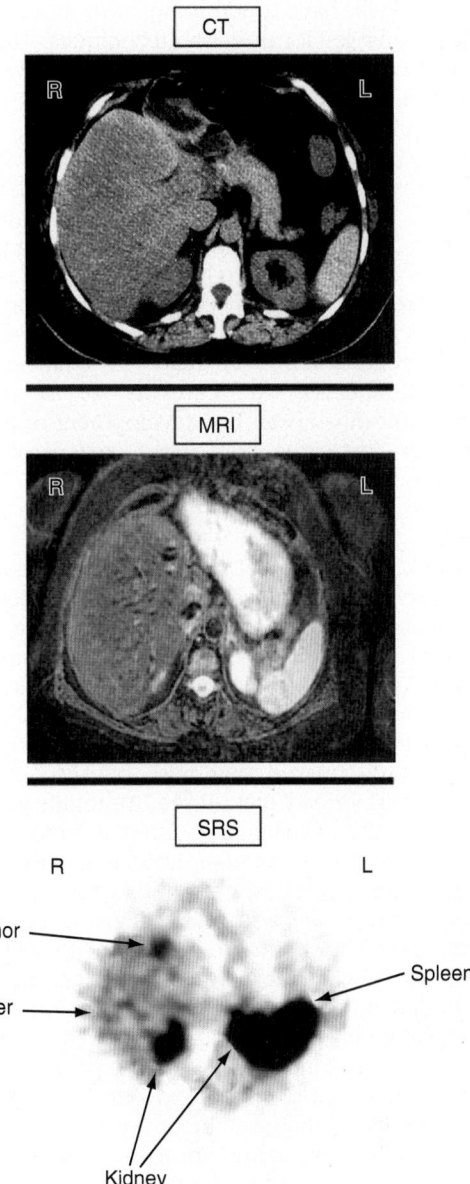

Figure 38-10 Comparison of CT, MRI, and SRS in a patient with Zollinger-Ellison syndrome. Neither the CT scan (*top*) nor MRI (*middle*) localized a gastrinoma. SRS, however, showed a focus in the left lobe of the liver. At surgery the patient had two 1-cm left lobe liver metastases and a small duodenal tumor (0.3-cm gastrinoma plus an adjacent lymph node). This result demonstrates the enhanced sensitivity of SRS but also shows that it frequently misses small tumors. (With permission from Norton JA, Jensen RT: Resolved and unresolved controversies in the surgical management of patients with Zollinger-Ellison syndrome. Ann Surg 240:757-773, 2004.)

be less helpful with gastrinomas than with insulinomas. An improvement was achieved by selective intra-arterial injection of secretin with sampling from the right hepatic vein. If, for example, venous gastrin levels spiked after injection of secretin into, say, the dorsal pancreatic artery, the gastrinoma would presumably reside within the distribution of that artery.

The most promising current method is SRS, which involves radionuclide scanning after the injection of radiolabeled octreotide.[32] Because more than 90% of gastrinomas have receptors for somatostatin, SRS is particularly sensitive in imaging both primary and metastatic gastrinoma tissue. In this technique, 6 mCi of ^{111}In-labeled octreotide is given IV, and body images are obtained with a gamma camera at 4 and 24 hours (Fig. 38-10). A study from the NIH compared tumor localization in 80 ZES patients with use of ultrasonography, CT, MRI, selective angiography, and bone scanning with SRS and found SRS to be the most sensitive method for detection of either primary or metastatic liver gastrinomas.[33] The most recent recommendations are that the initial studies should be SRS and a CT scan with contrast. These studies generally identify most primaries and distant disease.

Should these studies be negative, further investigation include selective intra-arterial injection of secretin with sampling from the right hepatic vein. Direct endoscopy and, to a lesser extent, endoscopic ultrasonography are probably the best means of detecting duodenal gastrinomas.[26] All localizing studies have overlapping sensitivities, and most patients with gastrinomas, either primary or metastatic, will have undergone two, three, or more of the available localization techniques (ultrasound, enhanced CT and MRI, arteriography, selective portovenous sampling, selective intra-arterial secretin with hepatic vein sampling, endoscopic ultrasonography, and SRS) (see Table 38-2). The percentage of patients with a positive diagnosis but with a nonlocalized tumor has steadily decreased, but it is not yet always possible to localize the tumor before surgery. Because of the complications associated with the procedure and because of often equivocal results, one study concluded that portal venous sampling for gastrin is no longer indicated: we agree.

Great progress has been made in localizing tumors, but the number of true cures is still disappointing. Improvement must await the development of techniques for earlier detection or more extensive surgical procedures.

Surgery

Pharmacologic control of acid secretion has rendered total gastrectomy unnecessary. The role of lesser acid-reducing surgical procedures (e.g., selective proximal vagotomy) in patients with unresectable gastrinomas is unclear but doubtful. Omeprazole therapy is so effective that we now operate only for tumor removal, and every patient with ZES is a candidate for a tumor removal operation until proved otherwise because of systemic illness or widespread metastases. Although gastrinomas have a high rate of malignancy, they are more apt to be cured than cancer of any other abdominal viscera. Efforts at surgical cure are clearly justified.

Every attempt is made to localize the tumor before surgery, and CT and MRI are effective with larger tumors and especially with hepatic metastases. Gastric secretion is controlled during the perioperative period with either oral or parenteral proton pump inhibitors.

The abdominal incision is either a vertical midline or a bilateral subcostal one, and exposure needs to be generous. Exploration includes the entire abdomen, from the undersurface of the diaphragm to the pelvic floor, with particular attention paid to the liver, the right subhepatic and paraduodenal area, and the pelvic cul-de-sac and ovaries. The entire small bowel and colon is examined carefully, with the surgeon looking for lymph nodes in the mesentery or attached to the wall of the bowel.

We have found small primary gastrinomas free in the small bowel mesentery, adjacent to the duodenum, in the wall of the stomach, above the confluence of the right and left hepatic ducts, and as a cystic tumor attached to the lesser curvature of the stomach.[29] Gastrinomas have been reported in the ovary and colon. Any suspicious nodules are excised and sent for frozen-section biopsy. The liver is mobilized freely and carefully visualized and palpated. Any superficial mass is excised and undergoes biopsy; specimens of deep masses may be obtained by fine needle aspiration. When asked why he robbed banks, Willie Sutton said, "That's where the money is"; the highest yield in the search for gastrinomas is in the gastrinoma triangle, especially the pancreas and duodenum (see Fig. 38-8). The pancreas is mobilized by incising its retroperitoneal attachments superiorly and

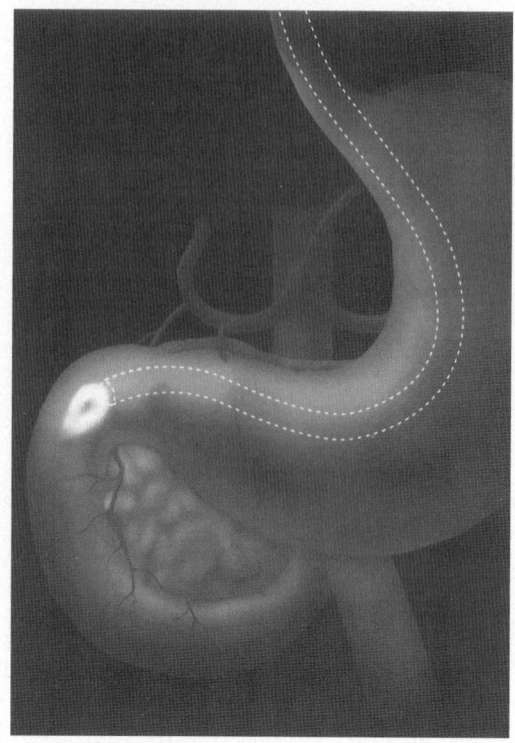

Figure 38-11 Duodenal gastrinoma demonstrated by transmural endoscopic illumination. The operating room lights must be turned off to see these small tumors, which are most common in the first part of the duodenum. (Modified from Thompson JC: Atlas of Surgery of the Stomach, Duodenum, and Small Bowel. St. Louis, Mosby–Year Book, 1992, p 301.)

inferiorly, the spleen mobilized to allow visualization and palpation of the back of the tail of the pancreas, the head of the pancreas mobilized with a wide Kocher maneuver, and care taken to maintain hemostasis in all efforts at mobilization. Gastrinomas are often firm, reddish tan masses (others have been said to be bluish red).

We carefully palpate the pancreas time and again, fore and aft, as well as possible, and then flood the abdomen with saline to facilitate intraoperative ultrasonography. Higher-resolution transducers (7.5-10 MHz) are used for the pancreas and a 5-MHz transducer for the liver. Intraoperative ultrasonography plus palpation is effective in localizing 90% to 98% of pancreatic gastrinomas.

Finding tumors in the pancreas may be difficult, but finding duodenal tumors is more difficult. Intraoperative endoscopy with transillumination of the duodenal wall facilitates visualization of many duodenal tumors (Fig. 38-11). Some are large enough to be seen directly through the endoscope itself. Palpation occasionally localizes larger tumors, but duodenotomy is essential for identification of duodenal gastrinomas, which are much more common proximally than distally (70% are in the first portion, 20% in the second, 10% in the third, and none in the fourth). Transillumination allows placement of the duodenotomy incision so that tumor tissue is avoided; the duodenotomy also must avoid injury to the papilla. Tumors are excised with a full-thickness elliptical incision, and again, the papilla must be protected. If a paraduodenal lymph node shows tumor on frozen section, the primary lesion is almost always within the duodenum.

Tumors within the pancreas are enucleated if at all possible. If they are adjacent to a duct, care must be taken to not injure the duct, but if the duct is injured, it is fine-sutured and a drain placed. Large tumors located distally can be excised by distal pancreatectomy. Tumors within the head are enucleated if at all possible. Because the mortality associated with a Whipple resection has diminished greatly in the past decade, there are several relatively enthusiastic reports of successful removal of gastrinomas of the head of the pancreas that were otherwise not susceptible to enucleation. The pros and cons of the Whipple resection for ZES have recently been evaluated with the salient difficulty of comparing long-term survival because the 10-year survival rate of sporadic ZES is 95% and that of ZES/MEN 1 is 86%.[26]

Tumors to the left of the superior mesenteric artery have a higher incidence of hepatic metastases and show more aggressive tumor behavior. If all apparent tumor is removed, immediate cure rates now approach 90%. Unfortunately, with long follow-up, nearly half the patients initially free of disease show symptomatic or biochemical (i.e., a positive secretin test result) recurrence by 5 years. An abnormal secretin test antedates recurrent symptoms. Early reports show that with careful exploration of the duodenum, mortality greatly diminishes. Routine addition of duodenotomy yields improved detection of tumors.

Treatment of metastatic disease has undergone serial changes but is still unsatisfactory. Radiation therapy and chemotherapy are largely ineffective. The combination of doxorubicin, streptozotocin, and 5-fluorouracil has a low, temporary response rate, but it is highly toxic and has no impact on survival. Similarly, octreotide and interferon alfa are associated with few temporary and partial responses. Surgical treatment of distant metastases by cytoreduction procedures (debulking) appears to be useful, and some patients with solitary localized metastatic disease have prolonged postoperative disease-free survival. In patients with unresectable metastases, the question of whether to resect the primary tumor is not settled.

No consensus has yet been reached in the treatment of patients with ZES and MEN 1, who often have multiple pancreatic and duodenal islet cell tumors.[34] A study from the Mayo Clinic suggested that because no patients were cured and few tumors are malignant, surgery was not indicated. Some surgical reports of short-term cures contradict this wait-and-see attitude,[35] but in one small, tightly controlled series, a biochemical cure (i.e., a negative secretin test) was not achieved in any of 10 patients.[36] One review concluded that because the interval required to pronounce a patient cured is long and variable, this argument will not be settled for years. The cure rate without a Whipple resection is very low (0%-10%). The infrequent appearance of aggressive gastric carcinoid tumors in patients with ZES/MEN 1 may require total gastrectomy.[26] Certainly, all ZES/MEN 1 patients with hyperparathyroidism undergo parathyroidectomy. Because missed duodenal wall gastrinomas may account for the previous inability to cure patients with combined MEN 1 and ZES, we believe that in the absence of widespread disease, laparotomy is indicated to delay progression of these gastrin-producing tumors.

In a report of 151 patients operated on between 1981 and 1998, 123 of whom had sporadic gastrinomas and 28 had ZES/MEN 1, gastrinomas were found in 93% of patients and in 100% of the last 81 patients operated on.[37] Gastrinomas were located in the duodenum in 49% of patients, in the pancreas in 24%, in lymph nodes in 11%, and in other locations in 9% of patients, with 16% having unknown primaries. The overall 10-year survival rate was 94%, and 34% of patients with sporadic gastrinomas were free of disease at 10 years, whereas none of the ZES/MEN 1 patients were free of disease. The authors of this NIH series concluded that all patients with the sporadic form of the ZES without metastatic disease need to be offered surgical exploration. The role of surgery in patients with the ZES/MEN 1 syndrome remains unclear.

Verner-Morrison Syndrome (VIPoma)

VIPomas are endocrine tumors usually arising from pancreatic islets that secrete VIP and cause a syndrome of profound watery diarrhea, hypokalemia, and achlorhydria. The diarrhea persists despite fasting (which qualifies it as a secretory diarrhea) and despite nasogastric aspiration (which differentiates it from the diarrhea of ZES). The condition was first described in 1958 in a report of two fatal cases, autopsy of which revealed a pancreatic islet cell adenoma in both.[2] The etiologic agent was found to be a VIP-producing tumor in 1973,[3] and a later report indicated that some VIPomas may be ectopic.[38] There is actually some argument about whether VIP is a normal islet hormone; some ascribe it to the D_2 cell, whereas others state that like gastrin, it occurs only in islet tumors. Verner-Morrison syndrome is highly variable. Constant features are diarrhea, hypovolemia, hypokalemia, and acidosis; variable features are achlorhydria or hypochlorhydria, hypercalcemia, hyperglycemia, and flushing with rash.[39] The tumor is rare, but one recent study reviewed 31 cases in China.[40] Another recent study reported 11 patients aged 2 to 83 years.[41]

The diagnostic triad in Verner-Morrison syndrome is a secretory diarrhea, high levels of circulating VIP, and a pancreatic tumor. Diarrhea volumes are often massive, 3 to 5 L/day, and the diagnosis of VIPoma is unlikely if stool volume is less than 700 mL/day. Conditions to be considered in the differential diagnosis are laxative abuse, bacterial and parasitic diarrhea, carcinoid syndrome (which has an elevated level of 5-hydroxyindole acetic acid in urine), and ZES (which has an elevated serum gastrin level). Of these, VIPomas alone show elevated levels of VIP; normal levels are lower than 200 pg/mL, and VIPoma patients have levels ranging from 225 to 2000 pg/mL.

The best localization is achieved either by SRS or by endoscopic ultrasound. SRS detected 91% of primary tumors and 75% of metastases.[41] Most tumors are large

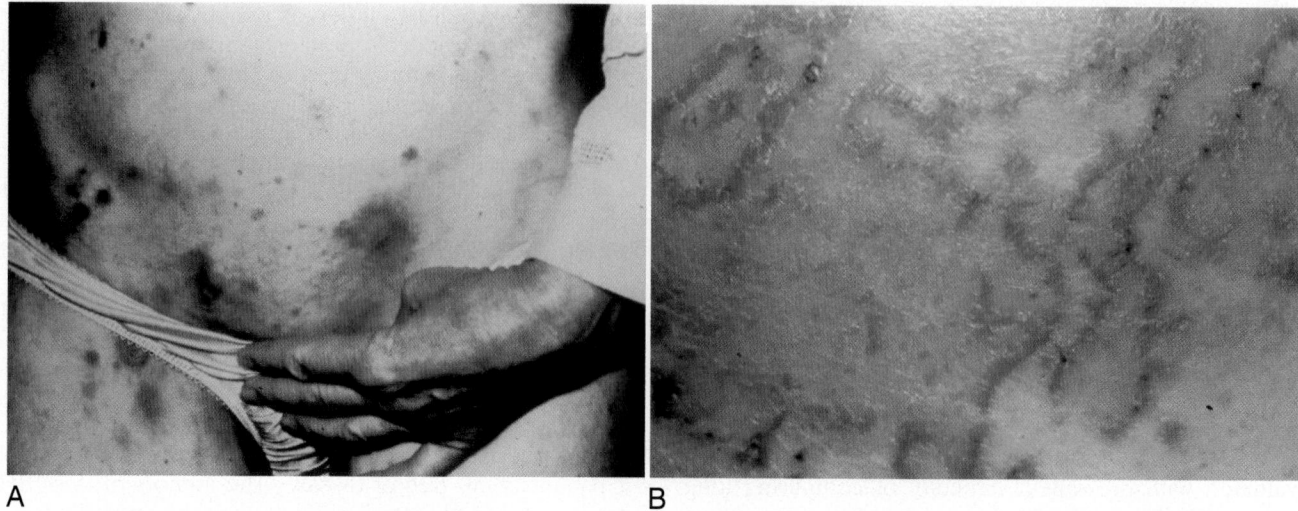

A   B

Figure 38-12 The characteristic necrolytic migrating erythematous dermatitis of the glucagonoma syndrome. **A,** Confluent patches with superficial necrosis. **B,** Close-up showing serpiginous margins. (Courtesy of Hugo V. Villar, MD.)

by the time that the syndrome is apparent, and localization is often achieved with enhanced CT or MRI or with arteriography. About 50% of patients have metastatic spread by the time of diagnosis. If abdominal studies fail to locate the tumor, thoracic CT is performed because as many as 10% of the tumors are intrathoracic. As soon as the diagnosis is established, treatment with the long-acting somatostatin analogue octreotide is used to control fluid loss.

Surgical removal of VIPoma is attempted in all patients. Most VIPomas can be excised by distal pancreatectomy. The adrenals and retroperitoneal tissue are carefully examined if no pancreatic tumor is found. In the 50% of patients with metastatic disease, local excision of as much tumor as can be safely removed (debulking) is indicated. Partial pancreatectomy plus resection of liver metastases has been reported to bring about resolution of recurrent Verner-Morrison syndrome. In patients with nonresectable tumors, chemotherapy is rarely effective, but octreotide is helpful in the control of diarrhea.

Glucagonoma

A tumor of islet alpha cells, glucagonoma causes a syndrome of a characteristic rash, diabetes mellitus, anemia, weight loss, and elevated circulating levels of glucagon. The syndrome was first described in 1942 by dermatologists who noted the relationship between pancreatic tumor and severe, unrelenting dermatitis.[4] The characteristic skin lesion, a necrolytic migrating erythema (Fig. 38-12), was reported to be associated with a glucagon-secreting alpha cell carcinoma of the pancreas.[5] The syndrome is rare (the largest single series reported until 1995 consisted of 18 patients), and most patients are initially recognized by their skin lesions and referred to surgeons by dermatologists. Glucagonoma was found to be associated with anemia, glossitis, and most importantly, a low level of amino acids; parenteral administration of amino acids was found to bring about disappearance of the skin lesions.[42] Diabetes is usually mild.

A pseudoglucagonoma syndrome has been described in patients who have necrolytic migratory erythema without a pancreatic tumor; the cause is unknown, but the condition is associated with several chronic illnesses, and only a few patients show elevated levels of glucagon.[43]

The diagnosis of glucagonoma is made from the characteristic skin lesion, elevated levels of glucagon (whose release can be provoked by secretin, if necessary), and a pancreatic tumor. The upper limit of normal for glucagon is 150 to 190 pg/mL; glucagonoma patients have levels of 200 to 2000 pg/mL. The islet tumor may be demonstrated by enhanced CT or MRI or by selective angiography.

Once the diagnosis is made, the patient is prepared by the administration of total parenteral nutrition containing amino acids, along with simultaneous octreotide for symptomatic relief. Tumors are best localized by CT, MRI, and intraoperative ultrasonography.[44] Because a third of these patients have been reported to have thrombotic complications after surgery, perioperative heparin is indicated.

Treatment is surgical excision of the tumor, which usually lies in the body or tail of the pancreas. Nearly all glucagonomas are malignant, but an aggressive approach to removal of the primary and metastatic tumor is warranted. Even so, the cure rate appears to be only 30%, and long-term chemotherapy has proved disappointing for metastatic disease. Symptomatic relief can be achieved with octreotide.

Somatostatinoma

All endocrine tumors of the pancreas are rare; somatostatinomas are exceedingly rare, and fewer than 60 cases have been reported. The tumor syndrome was first described in 1977 in separate reports on two individuals, and the full syndrome (steatorrhea, diabetes mellitus, hypochlorhydria, and gallstones) was characterized 2 years later.[45] The features of the syndrome are variable and do not always coincide with the predictable effects of high circulating levels of somatostatin. Most patients have mild diabetes, but 10% have symptoms of hypoglycemia. This illustrates the unpredictability of hormone-hormone interactions: in the case of diabetes, the suppressive effect of somatostatin on insulin release predominates; in hypoglycemic patients, the predominant inhibition affects glucagon.

The clinical findings are unpredictable; obstructive jaundice caused by pressure on the common bile duct by tumor has developed in some patients, whereas initial findings in other patients have been diarrhea and gallstones. Some duodenal somatostatinomas have been associated with von Recklinghausen's neurofibromatosis. Tumors can be localized by CT, MRI, arteriography, and even SRS because somatostatinomas do possess functioning somatostatin receptors.

Treatment is surgical. Seventy percent to 90% of tumors have been reported to be malignant. Most tumors are located in the tail of the pancreas, and caudal pancreatectomy is indicated. Localization is rarely a problem because the tumors are generally large. Hepatic metastases are common, and debulking of metastatic tumor tissue is indicated. The large size and frequency of malignancy dictate resection rather than enucleation of the pancreatic tumor. Metastases are, of course, excluded before consideration is given to a Whipple resection of the head of the pancreas. Small duodenal tumors can be treated by local excision. At surgery, cholecystectomy is performed regardless of whether the patient has gallstones because if they are not present, they will probably occur.

Still-Rarer Tumors

Various functional tumors of the endocrine pancreas have been reported, with some secreting GRF, neurotensin, PTHrP, PP, or ACTH, with the appropriate resultant endocrine syndrome. GRFomas are invariably associated with MEN 1 syndrome; 30% of GRF tumors originate in the pancreas, 50% in the lung, and 10% in the small bowel. Forty percent of patients with GRFoma have ZES, and 40% have Cushing's syndrome. Patients with ACTH-secreting tumors usually have other endocrine syndromes, most frequently ZES. They have classic symptoms of Cushing's syndrome (which occurs in 5% of all ZES patients and in 20% of patients with both ZES and MEN 1). Neurotensinomas cause hypokalemia, weight loss, hypotension, cyanosis, flushing, and diabetes. They are usually malignant. PPomas are associated with high circulating PP levels and no characteristic symptoms, although patients with PPomas have been reported with watery diarrhea and rash. PPomas are almost always large and, except when associated with MEN 1 syndrome, are usually solitary and in the head of the pancreas. Elevated levels of PP are often seen with other islet cell tumor syndromes.

Nonfunctioning Endocrine Tumors

Patients with nonfunctioning islet tumors are late in seeking help and do so finally because of symptoms of tumor progression. The incidence of nonfunctioning tumors varies between 15% and 50% in clinical series. Most such tumors are malignant and have metastasized by the time of diagnosis. A recent series of 18 patients with nonfunctioning tumors (10 of which were malignant) provides options for surgical treatment (e.g., enucleation of solitary benign tumors, as well as the role of radical surgery in patients with malignant tumors, with or without metastases).[46] Abdominal pain and jaundice are common initial complaints that result from mechanical or mass effects of the tumor. Surgical resection is attempted for cure when possible. More than 60% of tumors are metastatic at the time of diagnosis, but most appear to grow slowly, and prolonged survival is possible even with incurable disease (44% at 5 years).

MEDICAL THERAPY FOR ISLET CELL TUMORS

The best agent for pharmacologic control of hyperinsulinemia is diazoxide, which is widely used in preparing patients for surgery and in maintenance therapy for patients with unresectable metastatic insulinoma. Octreotide therapy has also been effective, although its response rate in comparison to diazoxide is not yet clear. Streptozocin combined with fluorouracil has proved effective in the treatment of advanced islet cell carcinoma, both functioning and nonfunctioning, with some long-term, symptom-free intervals.

In ZES patients, achievement of pharmacologic control of gastric acid secretion with proton pump inhibitors has revolutionized therapy. By defusing the risk for hypersecretory catastrophes, these drugs have virtually eliminated most of the urgent problems (bleeding, perforation, diarrhea, and fluid imbalance).

Proton pump inhibitors have been particularly effective and have proved to be safe despite early concerns about the potential risk of causing gastric carcinoids or other enterochromaffin cell tumors. There is a question of whether persistent hypergastrinemia in patients with MEN 1 will lead to the development of gastric carcinoids that could become malignant, a potential that appears less likely. The dosage is adjusted to achieve gastric acid secretion of less than 10 mEq/hr for the hour before the next dose of drug (in patients with severe gastroesophageal reflux disease, a reduction in acid secretion to <1 mEq/hr may be required).[34] In patients with unresectable metastatic disease, long-term antisecretory therapy with proton pump inhibitor drugs has proved more effective and more reliable than treatment with H_2 receptor antagonists or with octreotide, the long-acting somatostatin analogue.

Long-term use of octreotide has its greatest success in the long-term treatment of VIPoma symptoms, especially diarrhea. Several attempts have been made to demonstrate an antitumor effect, but significant decreases were found only in rare patients with VIPoma or GRFoma.

When metastatic disease is contained within lymph nodes and the liver, various chemotherapeutic regimens, cytoreduction (debulking) surgery, hepatic artery embolization, or combinations of these treatments are useful. However, when metastases to bone occur, only chemotherapy, interferon treatment, or the use of octreotide may be helpful. Because these tumors are rare and chemotherapeutic success unusual, accurate assessment of the role of chemotherapy will await multi-institutional trials.

All islet cell tumors except insulinomas (10%) and GRFomas (30%) have a malignancy rate of greater than 60%.[47] Response to chemotherapy has been variable: in a review of more than 700 patients with metastatic islet tumors, various agents (streptozocin, chlorozotocin, 5-fluorouracil, interferon alfa, doxorubicin, and octreotide, alone and in combination) yielded objective responses in 0% to 26% of patients. In control studies, cytoreductive operations appear to be effective. Hepatic artery embolization is recommended for patients with hepatic metastases but without extensive extrahepatic disease and may be a valuable palliative procedure, but it does not seem to prolong life.

WHAT'S NEXT?

Imaging

Great improvements in CT, nuclear scanning with labeled antibodies, and especially MRI will improve tumor localization.

Immunotherapy and Transplantation

Future advances in immune therapy, molecular biology, and genetics offer great hope in the management of pancreatic endocrinopathies.

Immune treatment of diabetes is under way, and patients with early-onset type 1 diabetes appear to respond to cyclosporine. Immunization with selected T-cell receptor peptides may lead to the generation of antibodies against clones of T cells reacting to beta cells.[48] The current best hope for surgical treatment of diabetes, of course, is to transplant islet tissue by means of either pancreatic organ transplantation or embolization of isolated islets (usually into the portal vein). The first pancreas transplantation was performed in 1966 by Kelly and colleagues.[49] By the end of 1989, nearly 2300 transplants had been performed worldwide, and the actuarial survival rate between 1985 and 1989 was 87% for patients and 56% for grafts. There are several problems: where should the pancreatic duct be drained, what type of venous anastomosis (portal or systemic) should be used, how should rejection be detected, and most important, what are the life-threatening consequences of leaks and rejection?

Transplantation of isolated islets has been performed in animals since 1972 and in humans since 1980. In most of these procedures, islets are isolated by collagenase digestion of cadaveric pancreas. They are selected for viability by means of vital staining, and viable islets are injected into the portal circulation (other sites, e.g., the spleen and the kidney, have also been used). Between 200,000 and 500,000 islets are required to achieve euglycemia, which in most instances has been transient. A few moderately long-term successes are enticing.[50] Isolated islet transplantation, though promising, has the following limitations:

1. Shortage of donor islet
2. Lack of demonstrated renewal or persistence of these islet cells with the consequent requirement for multiple transplantations
3. Need for lifelong immunosuppressive therapy[51]

A promising possibility is that multipotent stem cells may be induced to differentiate into functioning islets of Langerhans. Other possibilities are expansion of the beta cell mass by genetic regulation of beta cell growth and differentiation.[51,52] The use of fetal tissue for islet transplantation appears to offer promise. Whole-organ transplantation is cumbersome and complicated and carries significant risk, but it has a success rate that is considerably higher than that of isolated islet grafts. Current experimental efforts are in progress to modify xenogeneic (pig, cow) islets to genetically engineer human/nonhuman insulin-producing cells that will be suitable for grafting within special immunoisolation barrier membranes.

Experimental Oncology and Molecular Genetics

Experimental oncology is one of the richest fields in all of biomedical research, and we cover here only a few examples that may prove clinically useful in patients with endocrine tumors of the pancreas. Recent genomic studies have accelerated studies in the molecular genetics of these tumors. Genetic studies of endocrine tumors of the pancreas have suggested novel loci for the tumor suppressor genes *3p25*, *3p27*, and *11p13*, among others. Loss of alleles in these regions may serve as markers for malignant endocrine tumors of the pancreas. The cyclin-dependent kinase inhibitor p27[kip1] was found to be abundant in well-differentiated tumors and to be low or absent in aggressive tumors.

More than 90% of these tumors show silencing of the tumor suppressor gene *p16/MTSI*. p53 protein is prominent in exocrine tumors of the pancreas but appears to be surprisingly absent in endocrine tumors. Chromosome 3 is often deleted in sporadic malignant endocrine tumors of the pancreas, and studies suggest that chromosome 3q27-qter may contain a tumor suppressor gene. Evers and colleagues[53] have shown that gastrinomas amplify the proto-oncogene HER-2/*neu,* but not *p53* or *ras.* Others report an increase in HER-2/*neu* only in aggressive tumors.[54] Studies of insulinomas have shown that the G protein $G_{s\alpha}$ has a threefold greater expression in insulinoma than in normal islet cells, thus suggesting that it may be involved in unregulated insulin secretion or in tumorigenesis. Progression of malignant insulinomas has been shown to be accompanied by progressive accumulation of multiple genetic lesions; activation of *myc*, transforming growth factor-α, and *ras* genes may be early events in the development of insulinoma. Loss of the sex chromosome (X in women and Y in men) is frequent in endocrine tumors of the pancreas and appears to be associated with metastases and local invasion. Cytometry of benign and malignant endocrine tumors of the pancreas has shown that hypertriploid tumors have a statistically worse prognosis than diploid, triploid, and hypotriploid tumors do.

Selected References

Doherty GM, Doppman JL, Shawker TH, et al: Results of a prospective strategy to diagnose, localize, and resect insulinomas. Surgery 110:989-997, 1991.

This report from the NIH provided clear evidence that transhepatic selective portal venous sampling for insulin was the best single method for localizing insulinomas, and the authors found that intraoperative ultrasound located tumors in seven patients who did not have a palpable lesion.

Ellison EC, Sparks J, Verducci JS, et al: 50-year appraisal of gastrinoma: Recommendations for staging and treatment. J Am Coll Surg 202:897-905, 2006.

This review of 106 patients with gastrinoma seen over a 50-year period at Ohio State University Hospital (where ZES was first described) reiterates the conclusion that survival is influenced by tumor size and distant (chiefly hepatic) metastases, but not by lymph node spread.

Hirshberg B, Cochran C, Skarulis MC, et al: Malignant insulinoma: Spectrum of unusual clinical features. Cancer 104:264-272, 2005.

The authors report 10 patients with malignant insulinoma seen at the NIH. Four had lymph node metastases, and after excision all had prolonged survival free of tumor. In four other patients, hepatic spread developed years after presumed surgical cure. Nine of the 10 patients had prolonged survival, with short-term benefits provided by tumor embolization and diazoxide.

Jensen RT: Gastrin-producing tumors. Cancer Treat Res 89:293-334, 1997.

In 41 tightly packed pages, Jensen provides a scholarly précis of whatever was known about gastrinoma up to 1997. He discusses growth factors, oncogenes, and tumor suppressor genes as they affect the growth of gastrinoma. Particularly helpful are discussions on pathology (especially of duodenal gastrinoma), tumor biology, and techniques of localization, as well as a plan for patients with ZES and MEN 1. The concept of two separate clinical forms of ZES, one benign and one malignant, is strongly substantiated.

Norton JA: Neuroendocrine tumors of the pancreas and duodenum. Curr Probl Surg 31:77-156, 1994.

This review of the immense NIH experience in the surgical management of endocrine tumors of the pancreas and duodenum provides a vade mecum for students of these syndromes. Especially helpful are discussions of localization methods for insulinomas and gastrinomas and the variabilities brought about by MEN 1 syndrome. Norton concludes that nearly all these tumors can be located and that aggressive surgical management is highly beneficial. Localizing plus removing duodenal gastrinomas is of paramount import in achieving improved rates of cure of ZES.

Norton JA, Jensen RT: Resolved and unresolved controversies in the surgical management of patients with the Zollinger-Ellison syndrome. Ann Surg 240:757-773, 2004.

In this extensive review, two of the leading authorities on ZES evaluate the signal controversies in surgical management. They report that the cure rate in patients with ZES and MEN 1 is low without resort to pancreaticoduodenectomy but that the final role for this resection is not yet clear. In patients with the sporadic form of ZES, cure rates of 34% at 10 years for local resection favor an aggressive approach. They confirm division of ZES into benign and malignant (24%) forms, with long-term survival rates of 30% in the malignant form (usually associated with hepatic spread) to 96% for the nonaggressive group. They note that total gastrectomy should be reserved only for some patients with aggressive gastric carcinoid tumors.

Orci L: Macro- and micro-domains in the endocrine pancreas. Diabetes 31:538-565, 1982.

In this 1981 Banting lecture, Orci summarizes 2 decades of his work on the histomorphology and cytomorphology of islets in which he details the subcellular organization of the beta cell in the biosynthesis and release of insulin, the cellular environment of beta cells, and the cross-talk between beta and neighboring islet cells. The illustrations alone invite the reader into a new world, with electron micrographs showing freeze-fracture replicas across the Golgi apparatus of a B cell, as well as other gifts.

Stabile BE, Morrow DJ, Passaro E Jr: The gastrinoma triangle: Operative implications. Am J Surg 147:25-31, 1984.

Early efforts at operative localization of gastrinomas involved random searches of the pancreas, the subhepatic space, the retrogastric area, and the liver. Stabile and colleagues provide us with a treasure map showing where gastrinomas are likely to be found. The duodenum, which is one wall of that triangle, has been shown to contain about half of all gastrinomas.

Zollinger RM, Ellison EH: Primary peptic ulcerations of the jejunum associated with islet cell tumors of the pancreas. Ann Surg 142:709-723, 1955.

At the 1955 meeting of the American Surgical Association in Philadelphia, Zollinger and Ellison discussed their experience with two patients, and that discussion led to introduction of the entire clinical field of gastrointestinal endocrinopathies. Isolated observations of endocrine tumors in patients with gut dysfunction had been made, but Zollinger and Ellison made the prescient observation that the pancreatic tumor elaborated a secretagogue that caused the ulcer diathesis. Citation indices reveal that thousands of papers have recounted the experience of other scholars with ZES. This paper was the "can opener" for that vast picnic.

References

1. Whipple AO, Frantz VK: Adenoma of islet cells with hyperinsulinism: A review. Ann Surg 101:1299-1335, 1935.
2. Verner JV, Morrison AB: Islet cell tumor and a syndrome of refractory watery diarrhea and hypokalemia. Am J Med 25:374-380, 1958.
3. Bloom SR, Polak JM, Pearse AG: Vasoactive intestinal peptide and watery-diarrhea syndrome. Lancet 2:14-16, 1973.
4. Becker SW, Kahn D, Rothman S: Cutaneous manifestations of internal malignant tumors. Arch Dermatol Syphilol 45:1069-1080, 1942.
5. McGavran MH, Unger RH, Recant L, et al: A glucagon-secreting alpha-cell carcinoma of the pancreas. N Engl J Med 274:1408-1413, 1966.
6. Berson SA, Yalow RS, Bauman A, et al: Insulin-I[131] metabolism in human subjects: Demonstration of insulin binding globulin in the circulation of insulin treated subjects. J Clin Invest 35:170-190, 1956.
7. Gittes GK, Rutter WJ: Onset of cell-specific gene expression in the developing mouse pancreas. Proc Natl Acad Sci U S A 89:1128-1132, 1992.
8. Peck AB, Cornelius JG, Schatz D, et al: Generation of islet of Langerhans from adult pancreatic stem cells. J Hepatobiliary Pancreat Surg 9:704-709, 2002.
9. Orci L: Macro- and micro-domains in the endocrine pancreas. Diabetes 31:538-565, 1982.
10. Samols E, Stagner JI: Intraislet and islet-acinar portal systems and their significance. In Samols E (ed): The Endocrine Pancreas. New York, Raven, 1991, pp 93-124.

11. vön Schonfeld J, Goebell H, Müller MK: The islet-acinar axis of the pancreas. Int J Pancreatol 16:131-140, 1994.

12. Calender A: Molecular genetics of neuroendocrine tumors. Digestion 62(Suppl 1):3-18, 2000.

13. Norton JA: Neuroendocrine tumors of the pancreas and duodenum. Curr Probl Surg 31:77-156, 1994.

14. Evers BM, Townsend CM Jr, Thompson JC: Zollinger-Ellison syndrome. Probl Gen Surg 14:119-131, 1997.

15. Moertel CG: Karnofsky Memorial Lecture. An odyssey in the land of small tumors. J Clin Oncol 5:1502-1522, 1987.

16. Gibril F, Schumann M, Pace A, et al: Multiple endocrine neoplasia type 1 and Zollinger-Ellison syndrome: A prospective study of 107 cases and comparison with 1009 cases from the literature. Medicine (Baltimore) 83:43-83, 2004.

17. Moss NH, Rhoads JE: Hyperinsulinism and islet cell tumors of the pancreas. In Howard JM, Jordon GL Jr (eds): Surgical Diseases of the Pancreas. Philadelphia, JB Lippincott, 1960, pp 321-370.

18. Assalia A, Gagner M: Laparoscopic pancreatic surgery for islet cell tumors of the pancreas. World J Surg 28:1239-1247, 2004.

19. Jaroszewski DE, Schlinkert RT, Thompson GB, et al: Laparoscopic localization and resection of insulinomas. Arch Surg 139:270-274, 2004.

20. Doherty GM, Doppman JL, Shawker TH, et al: Results of a prospective strategy to diagnose, localize, and resect insulinomas. Surgery 110:989-997, 1991.

21. Hirshberg B, Libutti SK, Alexander HR, et al: Blind distal pancreatectomy for occult insulinoma, an inadvisable procedure. J Am Coll Surg 194:761-764, 2002.

22. Anlauf M, Wieben D, Perren A, et al: Persistent hyperinsulinemic hypoglycemia in 15 adults with diffuse nesidioblastosis: Diagnostic criteria, incidence, and characterization of beta-cell changes. Am J Surg Pathol 29:524-533, 2005.

23. Hirshberg B, Cochran C, Skarulis MC, et al: Malignant insulinoma: Spectrum of unusual clinical features. Cancer 104:264-272, 2005.

24. Thomas CG Jr, Cuenca RE, Azizkhan RG, et al: Changing concepts of islet cell dysplasia in neonatal and infantile hyperinsulinism. World J Surg 12:598-609, 1988.

25. Zollinger RM, Ellison EH: Primary peptic ulcerations of the jejunum associated with islet cell tumors of the pancreas. Ann Surg 142:709-723, 1955.

26. Norton JA, Jensen RT: Resolved and unresolved controversies in the surgical management of patients with Zollinger-Ellison syndrome. Ann Surg 240:757-773, 2004.

27. Farrow B, Thompson JC, Townsend CM Jr, et al: Endocrine tumors of the pancreas. In Zinner MJ, Ashley SW (eds): Maingot's Abdominal Operations, 11th ed. New York, McGraw-Hill, 2007, pp 1055-1071.

28. Stabile BE, Morrow DJ, Passaro E Jr: The gastrinoma triangle: Operative implications. Am J Surg 147:25-31, 1984.

29. Thompson JC, Lewis BG, Wiener I, et al: The role of surgery in the Zollinger-Ellison syndrome. Ann Surg 197:594-607, 1983.

30. Weber HC, Venzon DJ, Lin JT, et al: Determinants of metastatic rate and survival in patients with Zollinger-Ellison syndrome: A prospective long-term study. Gastroenterology 108:1637-1649, 1995.

31. Ellison EC, Sparks J, Verducci JS, et al: 50-year appraisal of gastrinoma: Recommendations for staging and treatment. J Am Coll Surg 202:897-905, 2006.

32. Alexander HR, Fraker DL, Norton JA, et al: Prospective study of somatostatin receptor scintigraphy and its effect on operative outcome in patients with Zollinger-Ellison syndrome. Ann Surg 228:228-238, 1998.

33. Gibril F, Reynolds JC, Doppman JL, et al: Somatostatin receptor scintigraphy: Its sensitivity compared with that of other imaging methods in detecting primary and metastatic gastrinomas: A prospective study. Ann Intern Med 125:26-34, 1996.

34. Jensen RT: Gastrin-producing tumors. Cancer Treat Res 89:293-334, 1997.

35. Thompson NW, Pasieka J, Fukuuchi A: Duodenal gastrinomas, duodenotomy, and duodenal exploration in the surgical management of Zollinger-Ellison syndrome. World J Surg 17:455-462, 1993.

36. MacFarlane MP, Fraker DL, Alexander HR, et al: Prospective study of surgical resection of duodenal and pancreatic gastrinomas in multiple endocrine neoplasia type 1. Surgery 118:973-980, 1995.

37. Norton JA, Fraker DL, Alexander HR, et al: Surgery to cure the Zollinger-Ellison syndrome. N Engl J Med 341:635-644, 1999.

38. Said SI, Faloona GR: Elevated plasma and tissue levels of vasoactive intestinal polypeptide in the watery-diarrhea syndrome due to pancreatic, bronchogenic, and other tumors. N Engl J Med 293:155-160, 1975.

39. Krejs GJ: VIPoma syndrome. Am J Med 82:37-48, 1987.

40. Peng SY, Li JR, Liu YB, et al: Diagnosis and treatment of VIPoma in China: (case report and 31 cases review) Diagnosis and treatment of VIPoma. Pancreas 28:93-97, 2004.

41. Nikou GC, Toubanakis C, Nikolaou P, et al: VIPomas: An update in diagnosis and management in a series of 11 patients. Hepatogastroenterology 52:1259-1265, 2005.

42. Norton JA, Kahn CR, Schiebinger R, et al: Amino acid deficiency and the skin rash associated with glucagonoma. Ann Intern Med 91:213-215, 1979.

43. Schwartz RA: Glucagonoma and pseudoglucagonoma syndromes. Int J Dermatol 36:81-89, 1997.

44. Zhang M, Xu X, Shen Y, et al: Clinical experience in diagnosis and treatment of glucagonoma syndrome. Hepatobiliary Pancreat Dis Int 3:473-475, 2004.

45. Krejs GJ, Orci L, Conlon JM, et al: Somatostatinoma syndrome. Biochemical, morphologic, and clinical features. N Engl J Med 301:285-292, 1979.

46. Dralle H, Krohn SL, Karges W, et al: Surgery of resectable nonfunctioning neuroendocrine pancreatic tumors. World J Surg 28:1248-1260, 2004.

47. Gibril F, Doppman JL, Jensen RT: Recent advances in the treatment of metastatic pancreatic endocrine tumors. Semin Gastrointest Dis 6:114-121, 1995.

48. Eisenbarth GS: Type I diabetes mellitus. A chronic autoimmune disease. N Engl J Med 314:1360-1368, 1986.

49. Kelly WD, Lillehei RC, Merkel FK, et al: Allotransplantation of the pancreas and duodenum along with the kidney in diabetic nephropathy. Surgery 61:827-837, 1967.

50. Shapiro AM, Lakey JR, Ryan EA, et al: Islet transplantation in seven patients with type 1 diabetes mellitus using a glucocorticoid-free immunosuppressive regimen. N Engl J Med 343:230-238, 2000.

51. Kim SK: Pancreatic islet cell replacement: Successes and opportunities. Ann N Y Acad Sci 961:41-43, 2002.

52. Yamaoka T: Regeneration therapy of pancreatic beta cells: Towards a cure for diabetes? Biochem Biophys Res Commun 296:1039-1043, 2002.

53. Evers BM, Rady PL, Sandoval K, et al: Gastrinomas demonstrate amplification of the HER-2/*neu* proto-oncogene. Ann Surg 219:596-604, 1994.

54. Goebel SU, Iwamoto M, Raffeld M, et al: HER-2/*neu* expression and gene amplification in gastrinomas: Correlations with tumor biology, growth, and aggressiveness. Cancer Res 62:3702-3710, 2002.

CHAPTER 39

The Adrenal Glands

Quan-Yang Duh, MD and Michael W. Yeh, MD

HISTORY

The adrenal glands were first described by the Italian anatomist Bartolomeo Eustachi in 1563. The German comparative anatomist Albert von Kölliker (1817-1905), who noted the presence of adrenals in a number of vertebrate species, is credited with first identifying two distinct portions of the adrenal gland, namely, the cortex and medulla. Although Thomas Addison described the clinical features of primary adrenal failure in 1855, it was not until nearly a century later that the adrenal hormones were fully isolated and characterized. Adrenaline (or epinephrine) was first isolated from adrenal extract at the turn of the century.

Steroid hormones were crystallized from cortical extract (cortin) by Swiss and American investigators in the 1930s, but their highly similar chemical structures made isolation of the individual compounds challenging. Edward Kendall, Tadeus Reichstein, and Philip Hench jointly received the 1950 Nobel Prize in Physiology or Medicine for their groundbreaking work on the adrenocortical hormones. The Austrian-born endocrinologist Hans Selye first described the stress response in mammals in 1936 and made major contributions to understanding of the hypothalamic-pituitary-adrenal (HPA) axis. Roger Guillemin, Andrew Schally, and Rosalyn Yalow were awarded the Nobel Prize in 1977 for characterizing the peptide hormones of the brain that underlie the HPA axis as we now understand it.[1,2]

ANATOMY AND EMBRYOLOGY

General and Developmental Aspects

The adrenal glands are paired, mustard-colored structures that are positioned superior and slightly medial to the kidneys in the retroperitoneal space (Fig. 39-1). They are flattened and roughly pyramidal (right) or crescent shaped (left) and weigh approximately 4 g each. The adrenals are among the most highly perfused organs in the body, with blood flow of 2000 mL/kg/min, behind only the kidney and the thyroid. In most respects the cortex and medulla can be considered two completely distinct organs that happen to colocalize during development. The two portions have disparate embryologic origins. The primordial cortex arises from the coelomic mesodermal tissue near the cephalic end of the mesonephros during the fourth to fifth week of gestation. Biosynthetic activity can be detected as early as the seventh week. The cortical cell mass dominates the fetal adrenal at 4 months of development, and steroidogenesis reaches its maximum during the third trimester. The adrenal medulla arises from ectodermal tissues of the embryonic neural crest. It develops in parallel with the sympathetic nervous system, beginning in the fifth to sixth week of gestation. From their original position adjacent to the neural tube, neural crest cells migrate ventrally to assume a para-aortic position near the developing adrenal cortex. There, they

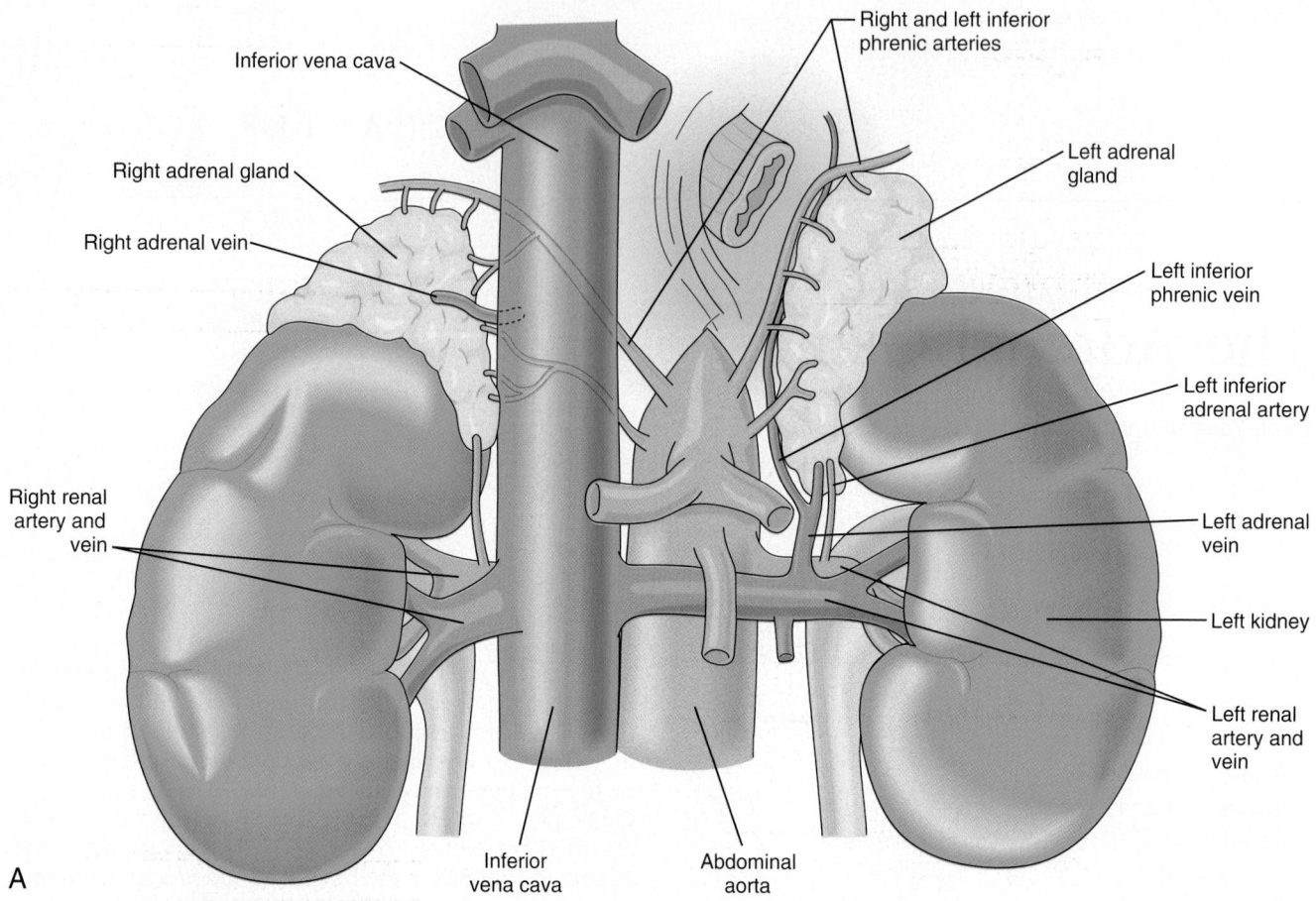

Inferior vena cava

Right adrenal gland

Right adrenal vein

Right renal artery and vein

Right and left inferior phrenic arteries

Left adrenal gland

Left inferior phrenic vein

Left inferior adrenal artery

Left adrenal vein

Left kidney

Left renal artery and vein

A

Inferior vena cava

Abdominal aorta

Figure 39-1 Anatomy of the adrenal glands. **A,** Left and right adrenal glands in situ.

differentiate into the chromaffin cells that make up the adrenal medulla.[3]

This course of embryologic development yields certain surgically relevant sequelae. Both cortical and medullary tissue can be found at extra-adrenal sites (Fig. 39-2). The range of potential sites is wider for chromaffin tissue than for cortical tissue, presumably because of the longer path of migration for the former. Pheochromocytomas may arise in extra-adrenal sites more commonly than previously thought (see later). When extra-adrenal, pheochromocytomas are also called *paragangliomas.*

Relationships

The right adrenal gland abuts the posterolateral surface of the retrohepatic vena cava. The right adrenal fossa is bounded by the right kidney inferolaterally, the diaphragm posteriorly, and the bare area of the liver anterosuperiorly. The left adrenal gland lies between the left kidney and aorta, with its inferior limb extending farther caudad toward the renal hilum than the right adrenal. The other relationships of the left adrenal gland are the diaphragm posteriorly and the tail of the pancreas and splenic hilum anteriorly. Each adrenal gland is enveloped

by its proper capsule, in addition to sharing Gerota's fascia with the kidneys. The adrenal capsules are immediately associated with the perirenal fat.

Vasculature

Knowledge of the macroscopic vascular anatomy of the adrenal glands is essential for proper surgical management. It is important to conceptualize that although the arterial supply is *diffuse,* the venous drainage of each gland is usually *solitary.* The arterial supply arises from three distinct vessels: the superior adrenal arteries from the inferior phrenic arteries, the small middle adrenal arteries from the juxtaceliac aorta, and the inferior adrenal arteries from the renal arteries. Of these, the inferior is the most prominent and is commonly a single identifiable vessel. The left adrenal vein is approximately 2 cm long and drains into the left renal vein after joining the inferior phrenic vein. The right adrenal vein is typically as short as it is wide (0.5 cm) and drains directly into the vena cava. This configuration presents a surgical challenge that will be revisited in the technical section of this chapter. In up to 20% of individuals, the right adrenal vein may drain into an accessory right hepatic vein or into the vena

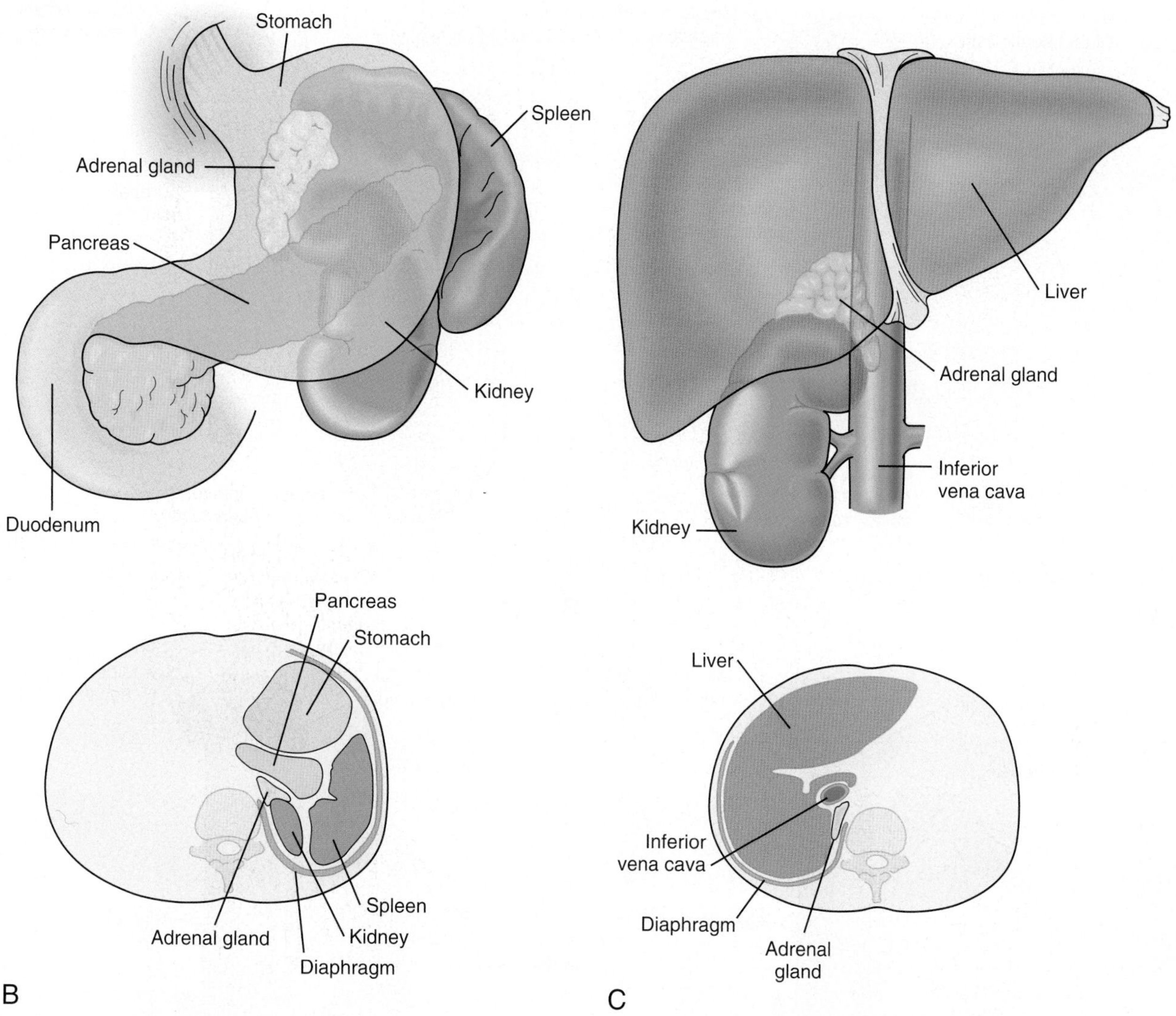

Stomach

Spleen

Adrenal gland

Pancreas

Liver

Kidney

Adrenal gland

Inferior
vena cava

Duodenum

Kidney

Pancreas

Stomach

Liver

Adrenal gland

Kidney

Spleen

Inferior
vena cava

Diaphragm

Diaphragm

Adrenal
gland

B

C

Figure 39-1, cont'd B, Relationships of the left adrenal gland. **C,** Relationships of the right adrenal gland.

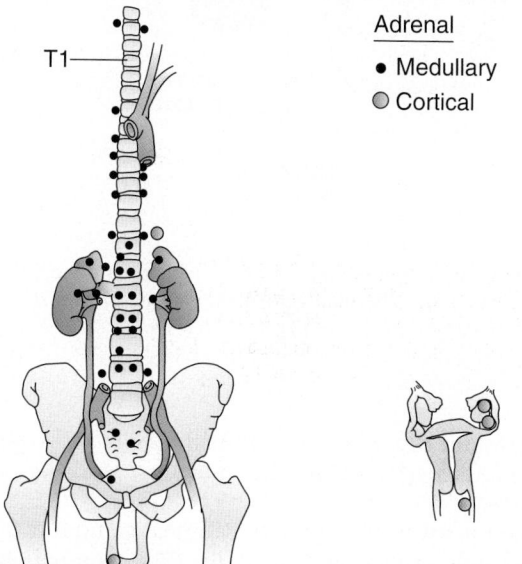

Adrenal

● Medullary
○ Cortical

T1

Figure 39-2 Sites of extra-adrenal cortical and medullary tissue.

cava at or near the confluence of such a vein.[4] Vigilance toward this variant and others (Fig. 39-3) may reduce the likelihood of intraoperative venous hemorrhage during right adrenalectomy.

NORMAL HISTOPATHOLOGY

The cortex is approximately 2 mm thick and accounts for greater than 80% of the mass of the gland. It is made up of three layers (Fig. 39-4). The outer *zona glomerulosa* is a thin layer of relatively small cells with moderately eosinophilic, lipid-poor cytoplasm. It has an undulating inner border and normally does not form a complete circumferential layer. The majority of the adrenal cortex is formed by the *zona fasciculata,* a middle layer composed of long radial columns of large, clear, lipid-laden cells. The inner *zona reticularis* is made up of small nests of compact, eosinophilic cells. The adrenal medulla con-

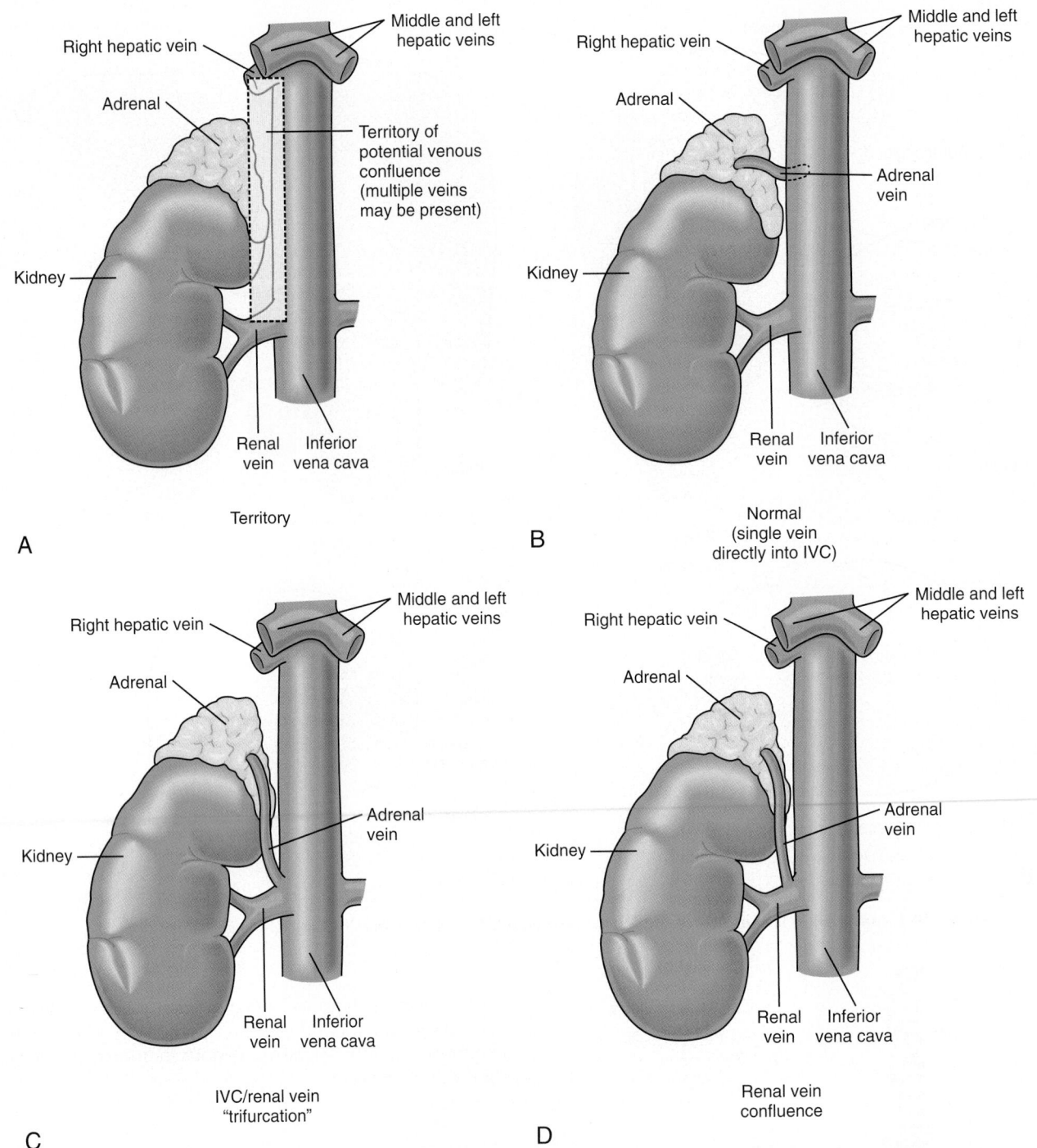

Figure 39-3 Variations in right adrenal vein anatomy. **A,** Territory of potential right adrenal vein confluence. **B,** Normal (>80%)—single vein directly into the inferior vena cava (IVC). **C,** IVC/renal vein "trifurcation." **D,** Renal vein confluence.

sists of clusters and short cords of chromaffin cells, which are large, polyhedral, and packed with basophilic secretory granules. Catecholamines within these granules yield a brown-colored reaction when treated with chromium salts, thus giving the cells their name. In contrast to the cortex, the adrenal medulla is richly endowed with autonomic nerve fibers and ganglion cells. Sympathetic fibers synapse directly with the chromaffin cells and constitute an interface between the nervous and endocrine systems.[5]

The microvasculature of the adrenal gland functionally unifies the cortex and medulla. The adrenal arteries arborize extensively before entering the capsule to form a subcapsular plexus. Blood flows centripetally through

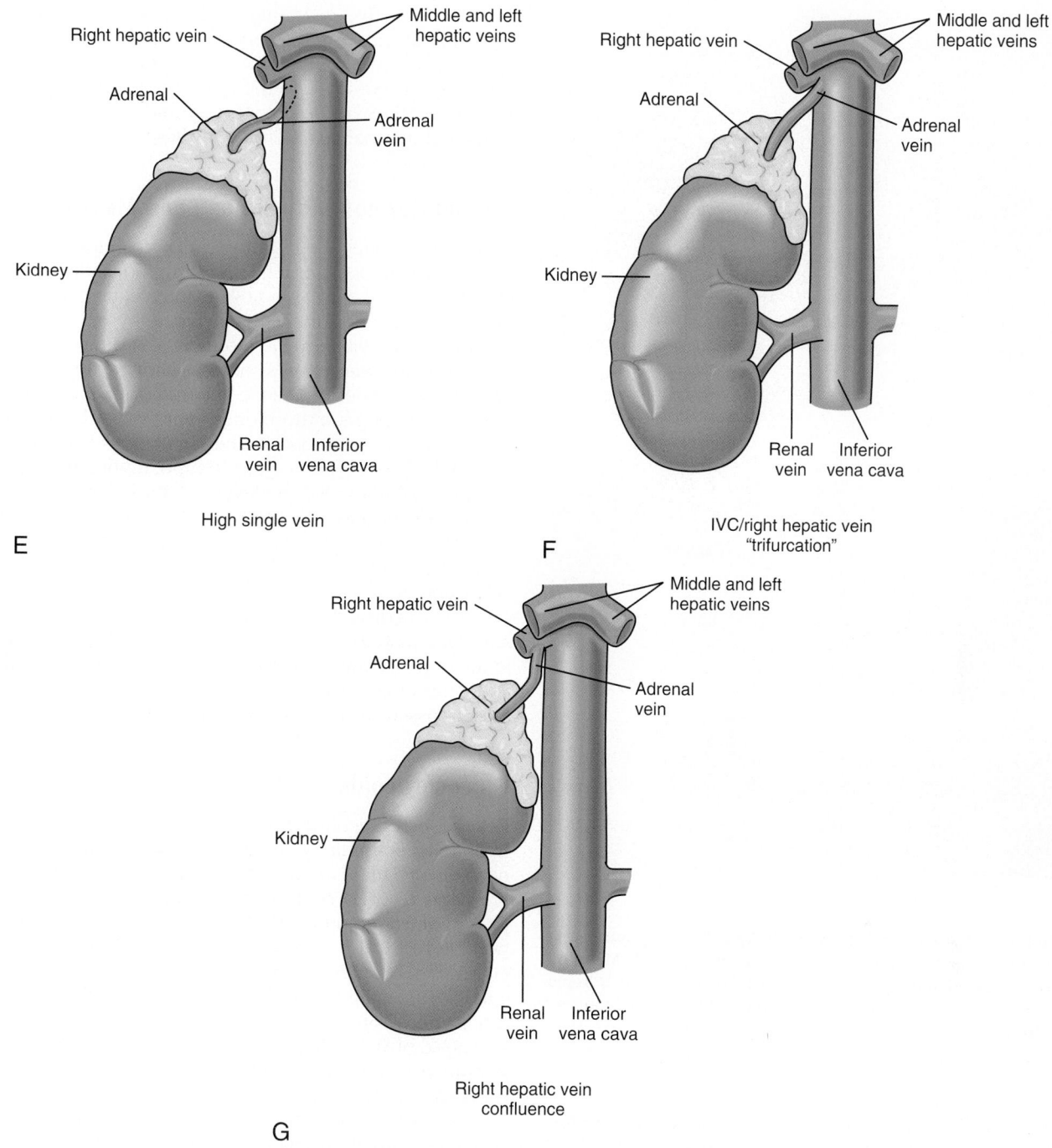

Figure 39-3, cont'd E, High single vein into the IVC. **F,** IVC/right hepatic vein "trifurcation." **G,** Right hepatic vein confluence.

capillaries in the *zona glomerulosa* and *zona fasciculata* before forming a deep plexus within the *zona reticularis.* From there, steroid-enriched postcapillary blood enters the medulla, where cortisol drives expression of phenylethanolamine-*N*-methyltransferase (PNMT). PNMT is responsible for conversion of norepinephrine to epinephrine. This microvascular arrangement is essentially a portal system between the cortex and the medulla.

BIOCHEMISTRY AND PHYSIOLOGY

Adrenal Steroid Biosynthesis

Adrenal steroid biosynthesis begins with transport of cholesterol to the inner mitochondrial membrane by the steroidogenic acute regulatory protein (StAR) (Fig. 39-5).[6] Cholesterol then undergoes a series of oxidative reac-

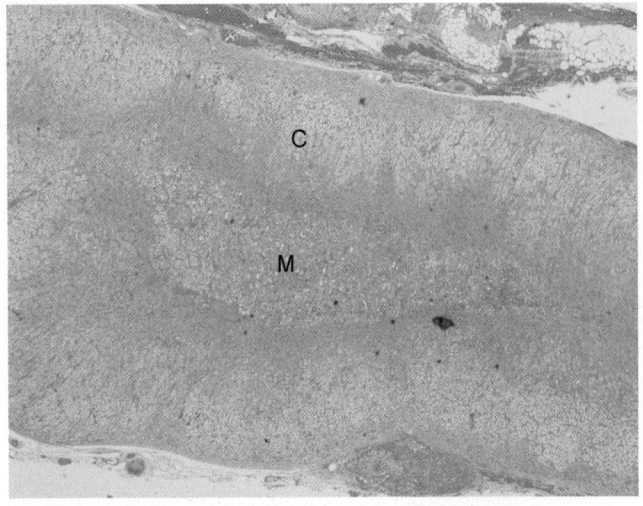

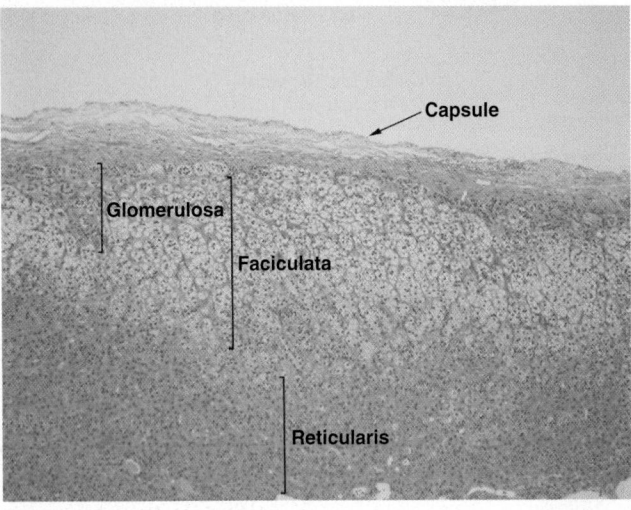

Figure 39-4 Normal adrenal histopathology. **A,** Low-power view showing the adrenal cortex (C) and medulla (M). **B,** Medium-power view demonstrating individual layers of the adrenal cortex. The thickness of the zona glomerulosa varies along its length. (Photomicrographs courtesy of Anthony Gill, MD).

tions catalyzed predominantly by membrane-associated enzymes belonging to the cytochrome P-450 (CYP) family. Cleavage of the cholesterol side chain yields the hormonally inactive compound pregnenolone, the immediate precursor to adrenal steroid hormones. Serial oxidation by CYP17 (moving "rightward" on the chart) converts pregnenolone and progesterone into the major adrenal sex steroids dehydroepiandrosterone (DHEA) and androstenedione. Additional enzymatic steps confined to the gonads (not shown) generate testosterone, estrone, and estradiol from androstenedione. Oxidation of pregnenolone and 17-hydroxypregnenolone at the carbon 3 position by 3β-hydroxysteroid dehydrogenase, followed by the action of CYP21A2 and CYP11B1 (moving "downward" on the diagram), yields the major mammalian glucocorticoids corticosterone and cortisol, with only the

latter being active in humans. Aldosterone is generated by oxidation of corticosterone at the carbon 18 position by CYP11B2 localized to the *zona glomerulosa*. CYP17 expression is confined to the *zona fasciculata* and *zona reticularis,* thus accounting for synthesis of glucocorticoids and adrenal sex steroids in these regions.

Steroid Hormone Physiology and Metabolism

Steroid hormones belong to a general class of low-molecular-weight, lipophilic signaling molecules that act by entering cells and binding to intracellular receptors. This group of hormones also includes thyroid hormone, retinoids, and vitamin D. Hormone binding results in alterations in gene expression that show a delayed and prolonged response when compared with the changes induced by peptide hormones, which act by binding to cell surface receptors. In the circulation, endogenous steroid hormones are largely bound to highly specific binding globulins. Serum levels of these proteins (and hence free hormone levels) can be altered by certain physiologic and disease states such as pregnancy, nephrotic syndrome, and cirrhosis. Metabolism of both endogenous and pharmacologic steroids generally proceeds via hydroxylation, sulfonation, or conjugation (or any combination of these processes) to glucuronic acid in the liver, followed by urinary excretion. The regulation and physiologic actions of individual steroid hormones are discussed in the following sections.

Glucocorticoids

Release of corticotropin-releasing factor (CRF) into the hypothalamic-pituitary portal system by hypothalamic neurons results in secretion of adrenocorticotropic hormone (ACTH) by the anterior pituitary. Synthesis of pro-opiomelanocortin (POMC), the large precursor peptide to ACTH, is also up-regulated. ACTH binds to a G protein–coupled receptor on the adrenocortical cell surface and stimulates glucocorticoid secretion, among other effects. Steroidogenesis is acutely up-regulated via increased StAR-mediated cholesterol transport and pregnenolone synthesis by CYP11A1 (cholesterol side chain cleavage enzyme). Chronically, ACTH increases transcription of all steroidogenic enzymes and supports maintenance of normal adrenal cell mass. ACTH is released in a pulsatile fashion that normally displays a circadian rhythm. The highest levels of ACTH, and thus cortisol, are generally detected on waking, with levels gradually declining through the day to reach a nadir in the early evening. This pattern must be considered when evaluating patients for glucocorticoid deficiency or excess. Negative feedback by glucocorticoids occurs at both the hypothalamic and pituitary levels.

Glucocorticoid hormones have broad-ranging effects on almost all organ systems in the body. As a rule, they generate a catabolic state that characterizes the body's response to stress. The hormones are so named because they cause alterations in carbohydrate, protein, and lipid metabolism that have the net effect of increasing blood

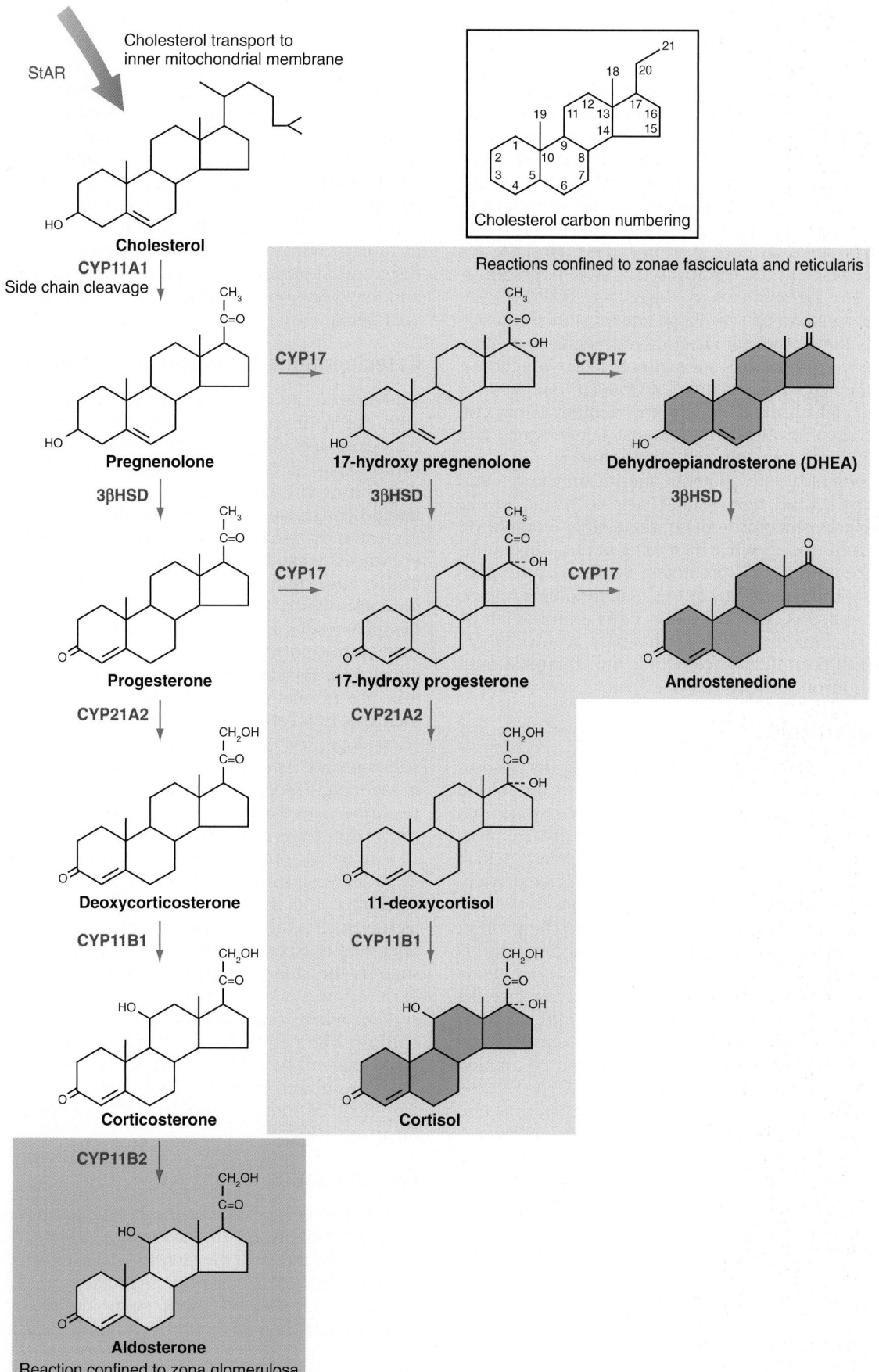

Figure 39-5 Adrenal steroid biosynthesis. Reactions confined to the zone glomerulosa are shaded *turquoise;* those confined to the zonae fasciculata and reticularis are shaded *orange.* Human mineralocorticoids are indicated in *yellow,* glucocorticoids in *green,* sex steroids in *blue.*

glucose concentrations. Hepatic glucose output is elevated by up-regulation of gluconeogenesis, and net glycogen deposition occurs. Glucose uptake by peripheral tissues is directly inhibited. Glucocorticoids stimulate lipolysis with the release of free fatty acids into the circulation, and a general state of insulin resistance is induced that results in protein catabolism. Fatty acids and amino acids serve as energy sources and substrate for gluconeogenesis. In the cardiovascular system, glucocorticoids exert a permissive and enhancing effect on catecholamine signaling by sensitizing arterial smooth muscle cells to β-adrenergic stimulation and increasing catecholamine concentrations in neuromuscular junctions.[7] Cardiac contractility and peripheral vascular tone are thus maintained, which explains why the hemodynamic collapse that accompanies acute adrenal insufficiency can be remedied by glucocorticoid administration.

Glucocorticoids are potent anti-inflammatory and immunosuppressive agents that act at many levels. Acutely, glucocorticoids reduce circulating lymphocyte and eosinophil counts while increasing neutrophil counts. Lymphocyte apoptosis is promoted, cytokine and immunoglobulin production is decreased, and histamine release is suppressed. Glucocorticoids also reduce prostaglandin synthesis via inhibition of phospholipase A_2. Additional pathologic effects of glucocorticoids are discussed later in the section on glucocorticoid excess.

Mineralocorticoids

Release of aldosterone from the *zona glomerulosa* is principally regulated by angiotensin II and the blood potassium level. The renin-angiotensin-aldosterone axis is responsive to delivery of sodium to the distal convoluted tubule of the kidney. Low sodium delivery, which occurs in states such as hypovolemia, shock, renal artery vasoconstriction, and hyponatremia, stimulates the release of renin from the juxtaglomerular apparatus. The prohormone angiotensinogen is synthesized by the liver and is cleaved to inactive angiotensin I by renin. Further cleavage of angiotensin I by angiotensin-converting enzyme in the lungs and elsewhere yields angiotensin II, a potent vasoconstrictor and stimulator of aldosterone release. Aldosterone release is also highly sensitive to minute changes in the blood potassium level. Hypokalemia reduces aldosterone release by suppressing renin secretion and also by acting directly at the *zona glomerulosa*. Hyperkalemia has the opposite effect.

Aldosterone regulates circulating fluid volume and electrolyte balance by promoting sodium and chloride retention in the distal tubule. Potassium and hydrogen ions are secreted into urine. Acutely, expansion of extracellular fluid volume and a rise in blood pressure are observed after aldosterone infusion. Negative feedback occurs primarily via an increase in sodium delivery to the distal tubule, which suppresses release of renin.

Adrenal Sex Steroids

Secretion of the adrenal androgens androstenedione, DHEA, and DHEA-S (the sulfonated derivative of DHEA, synthesized in both the adrenal and liver) is regulated by ACTH and other incompletely understood mechanisms. Of the three, androstenedione is produced in the smallest quantities. The physiologic effects of adrenal sex steroids are generally weak in comparison to the gonadal sex steroids, particularly in males. In females, peripheral conversion of DHEA and DHEA-S to more potent androgens, including androstenedione, testosterone, and dihydrotestosterone, supports normal pubic and axillary hair growth and may play a role in maintaining libido and a sense of well-being.

Catecholamine Biosynthesis and Physiology

Synthesis of catecholamines in the adrenal medulla begins with the hydroxylation of tyrosine, a rate-limiting step that generates dihydroxyphenylalanine (L-dopa) in the cytosol (Fig. 39-6). Decarboxylation of L-dopa generates dopamine, which is taken up by neurosecretory granules and β-hydroxylated to form norepinephrine. Epinephrine is created by the action of PNMT, which unlike the other enzymes involved in catecholamine synthesis, is localized to the chromaffin cells of the adrenal medulla and organ of Zuckerkandl. Sympathetic stimulation of the adrenal medulla results in depolarization of the chromaffin cell membrane and release of stored catecholamines into the circulation. Basal levels of adrenal catecholamine secretion are normally low, although large (up to 50-fold) increases in levels may be observed in response to major physiologic or psychological stressors. Target tissue responses are mediated by α- and β-adrenergic receptors. α-Adrenergic receptors display greater affinity for norepinephrine than for epinephrine, and the opposite is true for β-adrenergic receptors.

Stimulation of β_1-receptors in the myocardium results in an increase in heart rate and contractility. Stimulation of β_2-receptors results in smooth muscle relaxation in tissues such as the uterus, bronchi, and skeletal muscle arterioles. α_1-Receptors mediate vasoconstriction in tissues such as the skin and gastrointestinal tract. α_2-Receptors exist in presynaptic locations in the central nervous system, where they mediate attenuation of sympathetic outflow. The net effect of adrenal catecholamine release is to augment blood flow and delivery of oxygen to the brain, heart, and skeletal muscle (which are essential for the "fight or flight" response) at the expense of other organ systems.

Catecholamine Clearance

Catecholamines are potent, short-acting compounds with a plasma half-life on the order of 1 minute. Their presence in synapses and the circulation is controlled by tight negative regulation via both reuptake and degradation. Degradation pathways merit some discussion because they generate the metabolites commonly measured in the biochemical evaluation of pheochromocytoma (discussed later). Epinephrine and norepinephrine are inactivated by one or both of the following enzymes: monoamine oxidase (MAO) and catechol-*O*-methyltransferase (COMT) (see Fig. 39-6). Initial methylation by COMT yields meta-

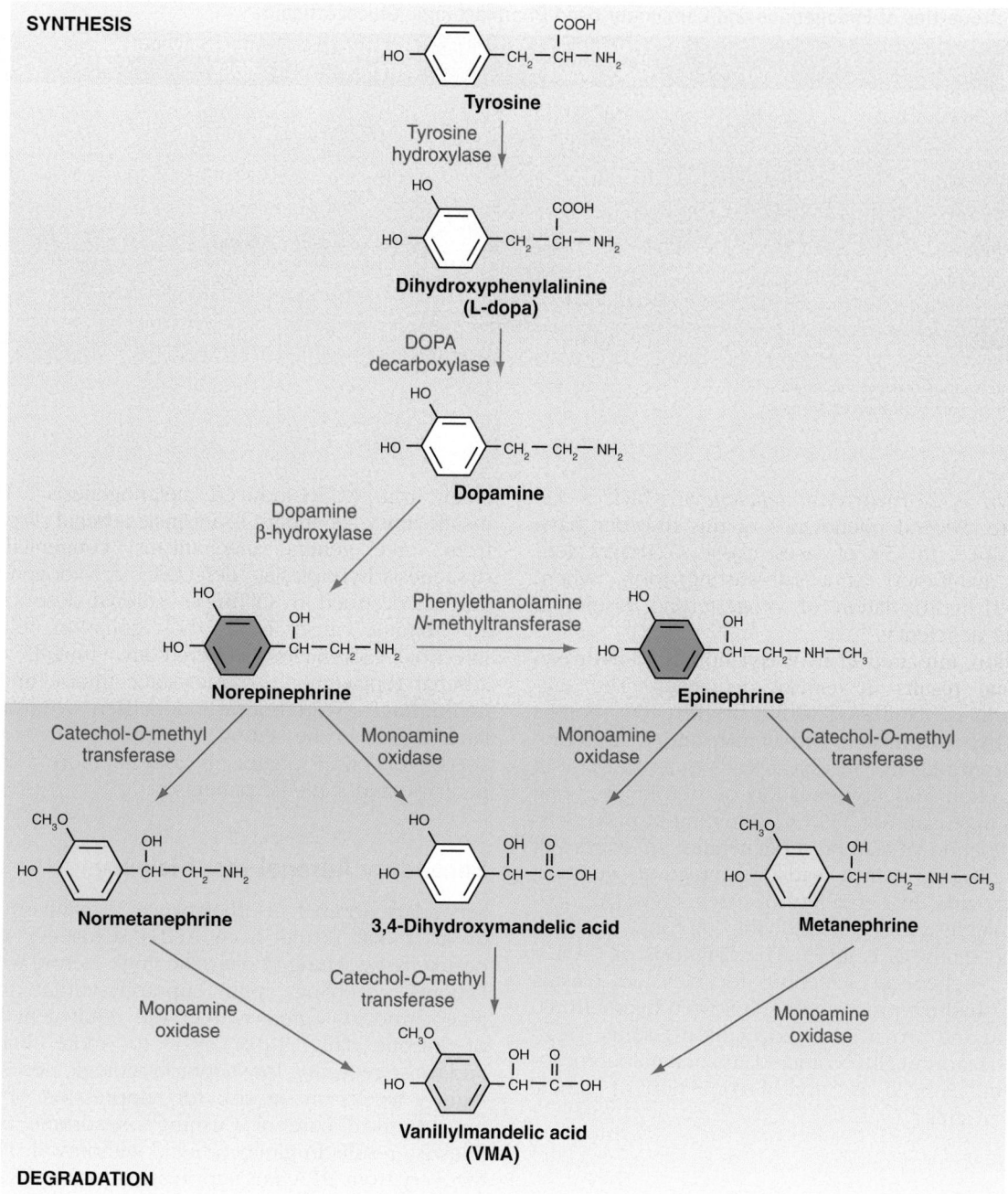

SYNTHESIS

DEGRADATION

Figure 39-6 Catecholamine biosynthesis and metabolism. Synthetic steps are shaded orange; degradative steps are shaded *turquoise*. Major catecholamines are indicated in *green,* major metabolites in *yellow.*

nephrine and normetanephrine, which can be detected in both plasma and urine. Their relatively stable plasma levels, which contrast with the high-amplitude fluctuations seen in plasma epinephrine and norepinephrine levels, make them attractive diagnostic markers.[8] The sequential action of MAO and COMT generates the major final product vanillylmandelic acid. Catecholamine metabolites are excreted in urine, sometimes after sulfonation or conjugation to glucuronic acid in the liver.

INBORN ERRORS OF METABOLISM: CONGENITAL ADRENAL HYPERPLASIA

Congenital adrenal hyperplasia (CAH) is a relatively common inherited disorder that provides insight into mechanisms of steroid biosynthesis and negative feedback. Although six enzyme defects are known to cause CAH, more than 90% are caused by CYP21A2 deficiency

Table 39-1 Properties of Endogenous and Commonly Used Pharmacologic Glucocorticoids

COMPOUND	IV/PO*	COMMON TRADE NAME	RELATIVE POTENCY	DAILY PHYSIOLOGIC DOSE	DOSING INTERVAL
Cortisol=hydrocortisone	Both	Cortef (PO) Solu-Cortef (IV)	1×	20 mg	q8-12h
Cortisone	PO	—	0.8×	25 mg	q8-12h
Prednisone	PO	—	4×	5 mg	q24h
Prednisolone	PO	—	4×	5 mg	q24h
Methylprednisolone	Both	Medrol (PO) Solu-Medrol (IV)	5×	4 mg	q24h
Dexamethasone†	Both	Decadron	25×	1 mg	q24h

*Oral and intravenous dosages are similar.
†Does not cross-react with the cortisol assay.

(also known as *21-hydroxlase deficiency*), which is discussed here. Several phenotypes of this disorder have been described. In 75% of cases, classic CYP21A2 deficiency is manifested as a salt-wasting form, where impaired 21-hydroxylation of progesterone results in aldosterone deficiency.

In addition, impaired 21-hydroxylation of 17-hydroxyprogesterone results in cortisol deficiency. The salt-wasting form is manifested within the first few months of life as hypovolemia, hyperkalemia, and hyperreninemia. Reduced negative feedback leads to an increase in ACTH secretion and accumulation of steroid hormone precursors upstream of CYP21A2. Shunting of precursors toward oxidation at carbon 17 generates an excess of adrenal androgens, which leads to ambiguous genitalia in newborn girls. In a minority of cases, CYP21A2 deficiency is manifested as a simple virilizing form, in which aldosterone synthesis is intact. The diagnosis of CAH is made by biochemical screening for elevated plasma levels of 17-hydroxyprogesterone, followed by confirmatory genetic and provocative biochemical testing. Treatment centers around glucocorticoid and mineralocorticoid replacement, as well as surgical correction of genital anomalies in girls.[9]

ADRENAL INSUFFICIENCY

Primary Adrenal Insufficiency (Addison's Disease)

Addison originally described 10 patients with "anemia . . . feebleness of the heart action . . . [and] a peculiar change of color in the skin" associated principally with tuberculous destruction of the adrenal glands. This rare disease is most commonly manifested as weakness and fatigue, anorexia, nausea or vomiting, weight loss, hyperpigmentation, hypotension, and electrolyte disturbances (hyponatremia and hyperkalemia).

Hyperpigmentation, previously thought to be caused by elevated levels of POMC and its cleavage product α-melanocyte–stimulating hormone, is now believed to result from ACTH-induced melanogenesis.[10] Hormonal insufficiency secondary to intrinsic adrenal disease arises from three general mechanisms: congenital adrenal dysgenesis/hypoplasia, defective steroidogenesis, and adrenal destruction. Of these, adrenal destruction from autoimmune causes is the most common, followed by infectious adrenalitis (tuberculous, fungal, or viral), adrenal replacement by metastatic tumor, and adrenal hemorrhage (Waterhouse-Friderichsen syndrome). The latter occurs in the setting of septicemia from meningococcus or other organisms and is more common in pediatric and asplenic patients.[11]

Secondary Adrenal Insufficiency

Secondary adrenal insufficiency is a relatively common disorder that results from ACTH deficiency and often occurs in the setting of pharmacologic steroid withdrawal. Patients receiving high supraphysiologic doses of glucocorticoids (greater than the equivalent of 20 mg prednisone daily, Table 39-1) for more than 5 days and those receiving low supraphysiologic doses for more than 3 weeks are at risk for suppression of the HPA axis. Surgical cure of Cushing's syndrome (see later) likewise results in glucocorticoid withdrawal. The rate of recovery from HPA axis suppression varies in accordance with the duration and severity of the previous glucocorticoid excess, and the need for glucocorticoid supplementation may last several years.[12] Other less common causes of secondary adrenal insufficiency include panhypopituitarism secondary to neoplastic or infiltrative replacement, granulomatous disease, and pituitary hemorrhage/infarction. Pituitary infarction may occur in the setting of severe postpartum hemorrhage (Sheehan's syndrome).

Adrenal Insufficiency in the Critically Ill

A growing body of literature suggests that critically ill patients with sepsis or systemic inflammatory response syndrome may be affected by acute reversible dysfunction of the HPA axis. The incidence of the disorder is approximately 30% in critically ill patients, although this figure may be higher in those with septic shock. Whether these patients incur increased mortality because of adrenal insufficiency remains to be defined. Proposed mechanisms of reversible HPA axis dysfunction include adrenal ACTH resistance and decreased responsiveness of target tissues to glucocorticoids. Glucocorticoid supplementation in septic patients has been the topic of at least 14 randomized, controlled trials.

In these studies there appears to be an inverse relationship between survival benefit and glucocorticoid dose, with physiologic (i.e., replacement) doses yielding a median relative survival benefit of 1.33 and high supraphysiologic doses demonstrating significant harm. Although the data remain controversial, the most recent evidence suggests that patients with vasopressor-dependent septic shock may benefit from 5- to 7-day courses of glucocorticoids in the dose range of 400 mg/day or less of hydrocortisone or equivalent.[13]

Adrenal Crisis

Acute adrenal insufficiency, or adrenal crisis, is a life-threatening condition that typically occurs in individuals with already marginal adrenocortical function who are subjected to a significant acute physiologic stressor such as infection or trauma. Sudden complete loss of adrenal function, as occurs with Waterhouse-Friderichsen syndrome and certain hypercoagulable states, can also occur with adrenal crisis. Clinical findings include shock, abdominal pain, fever, nausea and vomiting, electrolyte disturbances, and occasionally, hypoglycemia. Mineralocorticoid deficiency resulting in an inability to maintain sodium and intravascular volume is the primary pathogenetic mechanism, although diminished cardiovascular responsiveness to catecholamines secondary to glucocorticoid deficiency also plays a role. Treatment of adrenal crisis centers around large-volume (>2 L) intravenous (IV) resuscitation with isotonic saline and glucocorticoid administration in the form of either hydrocortisone (100 mg IV every 6-8 hours) or dexamethasone (4 mg IV every 24 hours). Dexamethasone is long acting and carries the advantage of not interfering with biochemical assays of endogenous glucocorticoid production. Ironically, mineralocorticoid replacement is not an early priority because the sodium- and fluid-retentive effects of mineralocorticoids do not occur until several days after administration. Fluid and electrolyte balance can be rapidly achieved by saline infusion.[14]

Diagnosis and Treatment of Adrenal Insufficiency

As is true for most endocrine disorders, diagnosis of adrenal insufficiency depends on maintaining sufficient clinical suspicion for the disease. The clinical manifestations are discussed earlier. Surgeons are most likely to encounter patients with adrenal insufficiency in the intensive care unit, the trauma suite, or the operating room when treating patients with steroid-dependent

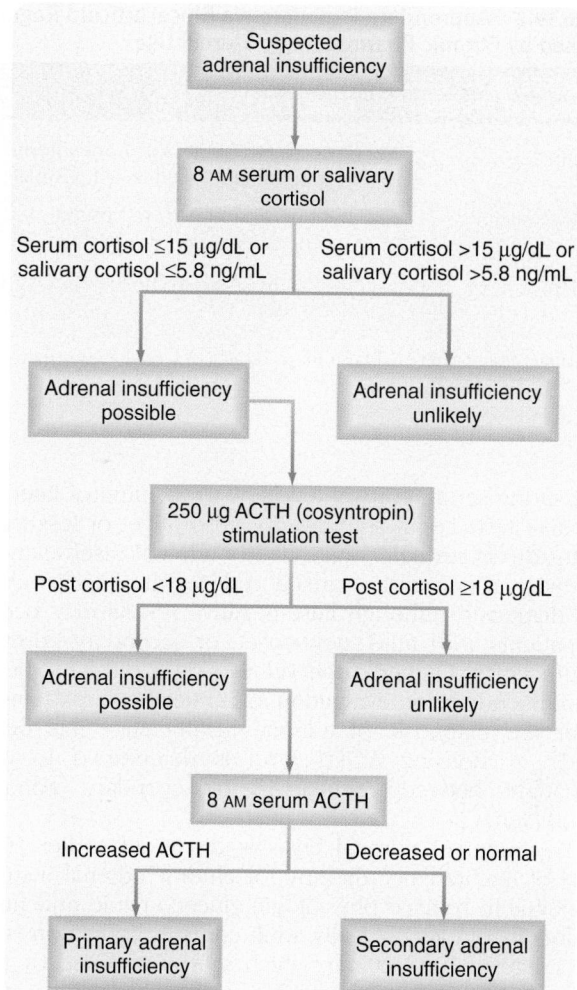

Figure 39-7 Algorithm for the diagnosis of adrenal insufficiency. The adequacy of cortisol production is initially assessed with morning cortisol measurement. Patients with low or borderline values undergo provocative adrenocorticotropic hormone (ACTH) stimulation testing, with serum cortisol being measured before and 30 to 60 minutes after the administration of ACTH. Failure to mount a adequate response to ACTH establishes the diagnosis of adrenal insufficiency in most cases. The cause of adrenal insufficiency is then investigated with morning ACTH measurement.

chronic illnesses. Routine and provocative biochemical testing is necessary to confirm the diagnosis (Fig. 39-7).

The first step is to document inadequate cortisol production, which can be done by measuring morning levels of cortisol in serum or saliva. In most patients, a morning serum cortisol concentration greater than 15 µg/dL or a morning salivary cortisol concentration greater than 5.8 ng/mL effectively excludes adrenal insufficiency. These cutoff values are deliberately set high to maximize sensitivity at the expense of specificity for this screening test. Patients whose values fall below these thresholds undergo provocative testing with exogenous ACTH (cosyntropin). A high-dose cosyntropin stimulation test is performed by administering 250 µg of cosyntropin and

Table 39-2 Appropriate Perioperative Glucocorticoid Regimens for Patients With Secondary Adrenal Insufficiency Caused by Chronic Pharmacologic Steroid Use

DEGREE OF SURGICAL STRESS	EXAMPLES	DAILY GLUCOCORTICOID DOSE
Minor	Procedures under local anesthesia, most outpatient procedures, inguinal hernia repair	Hydrocortisone, 25 mg or equivalent
Moderate	Routine abdominal, peripheral, vascular, or orthopedic surgery	Hydrocortisone, 50-75 mg or equivalent
Major	Resection of gastrointestinal cancer, cardiopulmonary bypass	Hydrocortisone, 100-150 mg or equivalent

Adapted from Salem M, Tainsh RE Jr, Bromberg J, et al: Perioperative glucocorticoid coverage. A reassessment 42 years after emergence of a problem. Ann Surg 219:416-425, 1994.

measuring serum cortisol levels 30 to 60 minutes later. A positive test (i.e., a stimulated cortisol level of less than 18 μg/dL) is strongly suggestive of adrenal insufficiency. Likewise, a normal test greatly reduces the likelihood of the diagnosis, although false-negative results may occur in patients with mild, new-onset, or secondary adrenal insufficiency. Higher cutoff values (25 μg/dL) have been recommended for evaluation of critically ill patients.[15] After the diagnosis of adrenal insufficiency has been made, a morning ACTH level is determined to differentiate between primary and secondary adrenal insufficiency.

Treatment of adrenal crisis is discussed earlier. The goal of maintenance therapy for chronic adrenal insufficiency is to replace physiologic glucocorticoid and mineralocorticoid levels. Daily adult cortisol production is in the range of 10 to 20 mg, which can be replaced by the long-acting, orally bioavailable agent prednisone at a dose of 5 mg/day. Typical mineralocorticoid replacement consists of fludrocortisone, 0.1 mg/day. Commensurate increased dosages of glucocorticoids are needed during periods of minor and major physiologic stress, such as mild infections (minor), as well as trauma, significant infections, burns, or elective surgery (major).

Perioperative Steroid Administration

Recommendations concerning glucocorticoid administration during elective surgery have been based primarily on uncontrolled, retrospective studies. The need for supraphysiologic doses of glucocorticoids in this setting has generally been overstated. Patients with secondary adrenal insufficiency as a result of chronic glucocorticoid treatment of autoimmune or inflammatory conditions have a 1% to 2% risk for hypotensive crisis without perioperative glucocorticoid coverage. To prevent this rare but hazardous complication, chronic glucocorticoid users are, at the least, maintained on their usual glucocorticoid dosage throughout the perioperative period. Supplementation above this level is given in short courses according to the guidelines listed in Table 39-2.[16] Patients undergoing unilateral adrenalectomy are given supplemental glucocorticoids only if the underlying diagnosis is Cushing's syndrome.

DISEASES OF THE ADRENAL CORTEX

Primary Hyperaldosteronism

Epidemiology and Clinical Features

Primary hyperaldosteronism, or unregulated release of excess aldosterone from one or both adrenal glands, was first described by Jerome Conn, an endocrinologist at the University of Michigan, in 1954. Primary hyperaldosteronism is classically manifested as resistant hypertension and hypokalemia, although recent reports have revealed that the majority of patients may be normokalemic, depending on the population screened. Hypokalemia is probably a manifestation of severe or late-stage disease. The prevalence of primary hyperaldosteronism has been the topic of considerable debate. Until recently it was generally believed to affect roughly 1% of patients with hypertension. Widespread application of the aldosterone-renin ratio, discussed later, as a screening test in certain centers led to reports of a 10% to 40% prevalence of primary hyperaldosteronism among hypertensives.[17] There is some consensus that these higher figures reflect strong referral bias and that the actual prevalence in unselected hypertensive patients is probably 7% or less. Nonselective use of the aldosterone-renin ratio to identify patients with primary hyperaldosteronism is known to significantly decrease the fraction of patients with surgically correctable disease (unilateral aldosteronoma), although the absolute number of surgically treatable cases increases.[18]

The mean age at diagnosis of primary hyperaldosteronism is roughly 50, and the disease has a mild male predilection. Most patients are asymptomatic, although those with significant hypokalemia may complain of muscle cramps, weakness, or paresthesias. Patients typically have moderate to severe hypertension that is refractory to medical therapy. It is common for them to require two to four antihypertensive medications. Responsiveness to spironolactone may be seen, a feature that is predictive of a good response to surgical treatment.

Primary hyperaldosteronism is a potentially curable cause of significant cardiovascular disease. A recent study comparing 124 subjects with biochemically confirmed primary hyperaldosteronism and hypertensive controls matched for age and systolic blood pressure revealed

Table 39-3 Causes of Primary Hyperaldosteronism*

	SELECTIVE SCREENING	NONSELECTIVE SCREENING
Aldosterone-producing adenoma	60%	30%
Bilateral adrenal hyperplasia (idiopathic hyperaldosteronism)	35%	65%
Aldosterone-producing adrenocortical carcinoma	<1%	<1%
Familial hyperaldosteronism		
Type 1 (glucocorticoid-remediable aldosteronism)	<1%	<1%
Type 2 (non–glucocorticoid-remediable aldosteronism)	<1%	<1%

*Rates of specific pathologies are highly dependent on the pattern of screening (selective versus nonselective).

that primary hyperaldosteronism is associated with a significantly increased risk for stroke, myocardial infarction, atrial fibrillation, and left ventricular hypertrophy.[19] These data add to existing evidence that the adverse cardiovascular sequelae of primary hyperaldosteronism are greater than those caused by blood pressure elevation alone. Successful removal of an aldosteronoma leads to regression of many of these adverse physiologic changes.

The most common causes of primary hyperaldosteronism are unilateral aldosterone-producing adenoma (aldosteronoma) and bilateral adrenal hyperplasia (also termed *idiopathic hyperaldosteronism,* Table 39-3). In the past, aldosteronoma was present in more than 60% of cases, but that figure has decreased substantially as nonselective screening with the aldosterone-renin ratio has been applied. This phenomenon may reflect increased detection of hyperplasia, which is characterized by milder biochemical abnormalities than occurs with aldosteronoma.

Biochemical Diagnosis and Localization

The goal of diagnostic testing is to identify and lateralize aldosteronomas. There is some consensus that biochemical screening should be performed in all patients with hypertension and unexplained hypokalemia, as well as those with hypertension sufficiently resistant to medical therapy to warrant investigation for secondary hypertension. Establishing the diagnosis of primary hyperaldosteronism begins with determining the ratio of plasma aldosterone to plasma renin activity (expressed here as ng/dL divided by ng/mL·h, Fig. 39-8). This test is performed after discontinuation of interfering medications such as spironolactone, angiotensin-converting enzyme inhibitors, diuretics, and β-adrenergic blockers. Variable cutoff values have been used in the literature, but a cutoff of 30 yields a sensitivity of approximately 90%.[20] A subset of patients with essential hypertension will have suppressed renin levels, which may result in false elevations of the aldosterone-renin ratio. Thus, inclusion of an absolute aldosterone concentration of greater than 15 mg/dL increases the specificity of initial screening. Patients who test positive and are younger than 30 years are genetically screened for glucocorticoid-remediable aldosteronism (familial hyperaldosteronism type 1), especially if they have a family history of early-onset hypertension. This

rare autosomal dominant condition results in abnormal regulation of aldosterone synthesis by ACTH and can be treated medically.

Confirmatory biochemical testing is aimed at demonstrating inappropriately high (nonsuppressible) aldosterone levels by creating a state of hypervolemia/sodium excess. This is done with IV saline loading (2-3 L of isotonic saline given over a 4- to 6-hour period, followed by measurement of plasma aldosterone) or oral salt loading (200 mEq=5000 mg sodium daily over a 3-day period, followed by measurement of 24-hour urine aldosterone excretion). Some centers administer high-dose fludrocortisone (0.1 mg every 6 hours) during oral salt loading to increase the specificity of suppression testing, but this method has not been widely adopted.

After the diagnosis has been confirmed, localization is performed with anatomic imaging, selective venous sampling, and sometimes functional scanning. The fact that most aldosteronomas are smaller than 15 mm in maximum dimension poses some challenge to localization. Thin-cut (3 mm) adrenal computed tomography (CT) is the preferred initial localization test (Fig. 39-9). In patients younger than 40 years, the finding of a solitary adrenal mass 1 cm or greater in size and a normal contralateral adrenal gland is sufficient to proceed to surgery. Unilateral adrenalectomy yields successful clinical outcomes in approximately 95% of such cases.

The next step in the localization algorithm is selective adrenal venous sampling. This test relies on simultaneous measurement of cortisol and aldosterone levels in the peripheral circulation, as well as the left and right adrenal veins (Fig. 39-10). Greater than a fivefold elevation in cortisol concentration in a sample relative to peripheral blood indicates successful cannulation of an adrenal vein (positive control). Lateralization is indicated by an unbalanced ratio of aldosterone to cortisol in the left and right adrenal veins, with a fourfold greater ratio on one side than on the other identifying the culprit gland. Considerable controversy exists over which patients undergo this study, an invasive procedure with a 90% technical success rate in experienced hands.[21] There is consensus that adrenal venous sampling should be applied in all cases in which the biochemical diagnosis of primary hyperaldosteronism has been confirmed and thin-cut adrenal CT reveals either no abnormalities or bilateral abnormalities. Of the remaining patients who have a unilateral mass on CT, a small but not insignificant fraction (2%-10%) will

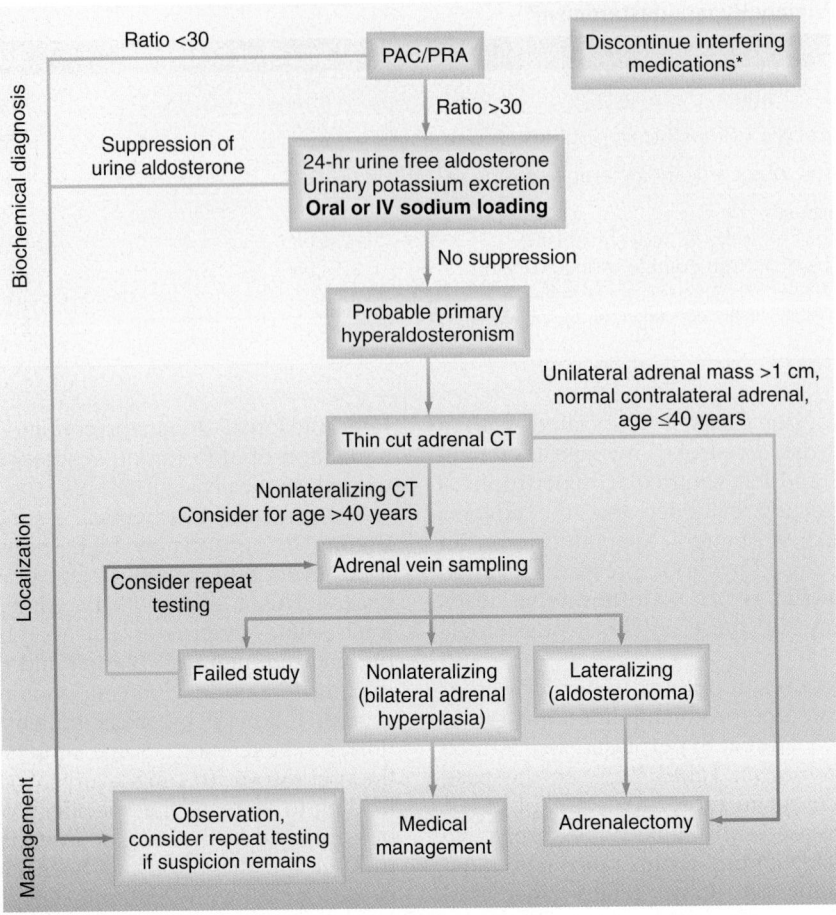

*Including spironolactone, ACE inhibitors, diuretics, β-blockers.

Figure 39-8 Algorithm for diagnosis, localization, and management of primary hyperaldosteronism. PAC, plasma aldosterone concentration in ng/dL; PRA, plasma renin activity in ng/mL·h. Initial screening with the PRA/PAC ratio is performed, followed by confirmatory testing with sodium loading. After the biochemical diagnosis has been established, noninvasive localization is attempted with CT. Patients with clear CT evidence of a unilateral abnormality can proceed to adrenalectomy with a greater than 90% cure rate. Adrenal vein sampling is performed in patients with equivocal CT findings and older patients, especially those older than 60, because nonfunctional cortical adenomas are found in 4% or more of this population and can cause false-positive CT localization.

represent false-positive localization and have persistent hyperaldosteronism after unilateral adrenalectomy. In these patients the adrenal mass represents a nonfunctioning cortical adenoma and the true underlying diagnosis is either a contralateral microaldosteronoma or bilateral adrenal hyperplasia, the latter of which is not surgically remediable.

Because patients 40 years or older are more likely to have nonfunctioning adrenal cortical adenomas, some authors have advocated adrenal venous sampling in all older patients. Yet others have recommended universal application of this test in the workup of primary hyperaldosteronism. Practically speaking, approximately 20% to 30% of patients being evaluated for primary hyperaldosteronism undergo adrenal venous sampling when it is applied to select patients. The utility of the test is limited by its low success rate in most reports (40%-80%), with the most common reason for incomplete adrenal venous sampling being failure to cannulate the right adrenal vein. Frequently, however, sufficient lateralizing information is provided during adrenal venous sampling to guide surgical treatment, even when the study is not bilaterally selective.[22] Functional scanning with radiolabeled ^{131}I-6-β-iodomethylnorcholesterol (NP-59) may be considered as a third-line localization test for patients without conclusive lateralizing information on either CT or adrenal venous sampling. The sensitivity of NP-59 scanning is low in small tumors. Most aldosteronomas are small to begin with, and those with negative CT scans represent the smallest subset of tumors. For these reasons, NP-59 scanning does not generally aid management in primary hyperaldosteronism.

Surgical Management and Outcomes

Laparoscopic adrenalectomy is the preferred procedure for the management of aldosteronoma and most other adrenal tumors.[23] Cure of primary hyperaldosteronism is defined by clinical and biochemical end points. Reductions in blood pressure, antihypertensive medication requirements, and plasma/urine aldosterone levels and resolution of hypokalemia (if previously present) are observed as soon as 24 hours after successful surgery. Overall cure rates range from 75% to 95% at subspecialty centers, depending on the specific criteria for cure that are used. In general, more than 80% of patients can expect either normalization of blood pressure or a significant reduction in antihypertensive medication requirements (typically from three to four medications down to one). In some patients, depending on the degree of preoperative sodium overload, blood pressure may take several weeks to improve. Our practice is to stop all antihypertensive medications immediately after surgery, with the exception of β-blockers, which must be tapered to avoid a rebound phenomenon. In patients who continue to be hypertensive in the short term, medications may be added back temporarily as needed until blood pressure gradually reaches a new equilibrium over time.

A subset of patients with the following preoperative features demonstrates reduced benefit from surgical treatment: male, age older than 45 years, family history of hypertension, long-standing hypertension, and no response to spironolactone.[24] These characteristics indicate a component of essential hypertension and, in some cases, irreversible cardiovascular alterations resulting from chronic disease. Based on these features, patients need to be counseled about what they can expect to gain from surgery.

Cushing's Syndrome

Epidemiology and Clinical Features

The clinical features of glucocorticoid excess were first documented by Harvey Cushing in 1912. He described a young woman of "extraordinary appearance" in whom obesity, hirsutism, amenorrhea, easy bruising, and extreme muscle weakness developed. The principal differential diagnosis to be considered when evaluating patients for Cushing's syndrome is obesity, an increasingly common condition. A subset of signs and symptoms, including easy bruising, muscle weakness, hypertension, plethora (a red facial appearance caused by thinning of the skin), and hirsutism, may allow discrimination between Cushing's syndrome and obesity based on clinical features (Fig. 39-11). The most common cause of Cushing's syndrome is pharmacologic glucocorticoid use for the treatment of inflammatory disorders. Endogenous Cushing's syndrome is rare, with 5 to 10 individuals affected per million. Of these, the majority of affected individuals (75%) will have Cushing's *disease,* that is, glucocorticoid excess caused by an ACTH-hypersecreting pituitary adenoma. The remainder will be split between primary adrenal Cushing's syndrome (15%) and ectopic ACTH syndrome (<10%), the latter of which most

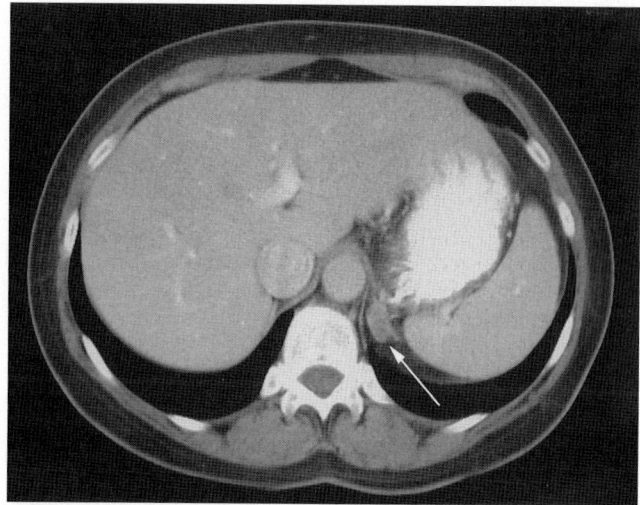

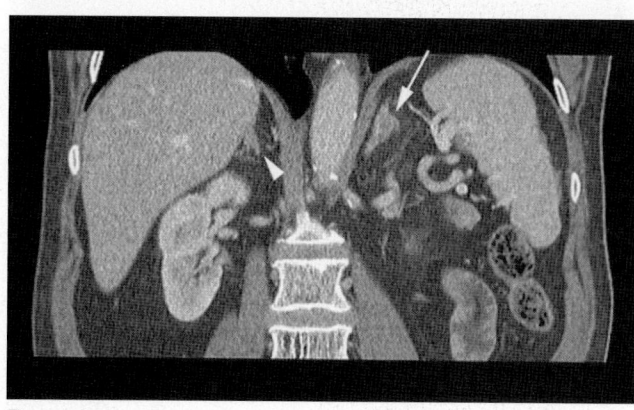

Figure 39-9 Appearance of aldosteronoma on anatomic imaging. **A,** Venous phase, contrast-enhanced CT demonstrating a 2-cm left aldosteronoma. **B,** Late arterial phase, coronal CT demonstrating a 1.7-cm left aldosteronoma (*arrow*) and a normal right adrenal gland (*arrowhead*).

commonly arises from either neuroendocrine tumors or bronchogenic malignancies in the thorax.

Cushing's syndrome is a lethal disease. The physiologic derangements resulting from glucocorticoid excess, including hypertension (present in >70% of cases), hyperglycemia, and truncal obesity, ultimately yield a fivefold excess in mortality, primarily secondary to cardiovascular complications.[25] Thus, all efforts need to be made to identify and appropriately treat patients with Cushing's syndrome.

Biochemical Diagnosis and Localization

Diagnosis of Cushing's syndrome relies on demonstration of inappropriate cortisol secretion or loss of physiologic negative feedback. Normally, cortisol release follows a predictable circadian rhythm, with the peak reached approximately 1 hour after waking and the nadir around midnight. Thus, inappropriate cortisol secretion can be detected as either elevated cortisol release over a 24-hour period or a higher than expected level in the late evening.

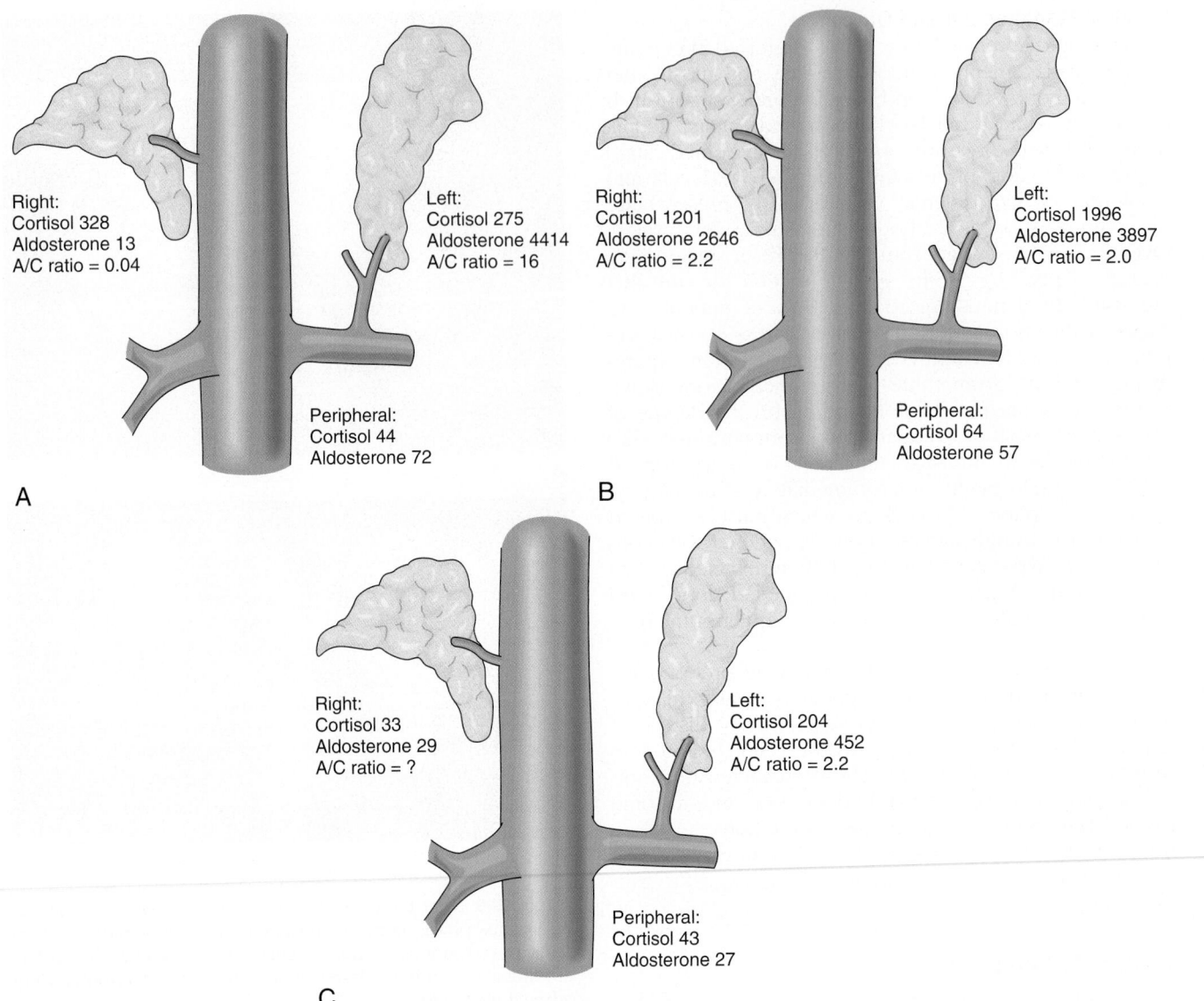

Figure 39-10 Possible outcomes of adrenal vein sampling for primary hyperaldosteronism. Aldosterone is expressed in ng/dL, cortisol in μg/dL. **A,** Successful study lateralizing strongly to the left adrenal. **B,** Successful study, non-lateralizing. Stimulation with adrenocorticotropic hormone yielded high adrenal vein cortisol levels. **C,** Failed study. The right adrenal vein was not cannulated.

Traditionally, lack of negative feedback has been assessed by dexamethasone suppression testing and other types of provocative tests, many of which are cumbersome and require inpatient hospitalization. The recent advent of late evening salivary cortisol testing has provided an attractive and feasible alternative to suppression testing.

More than 90% of circulating cortisol is bound to plasma proteins. Unbound cortisol can be detected in urine and saliva, and assessment of these body fluids forms the basis of biochemical screening for Cushing's syndrome (Fig. 39-12). Twenty-four-hour urine collection for determination of urinary free cortisol is performed at least twice for initial screening. Unequivocally elevated levels prompt immediate further testing to determine the cause/subtype of Cushing's syndrome (i.e., primary adrenal cause versus a pituitary cause versus ectopic ACTH syndrome). Patients with moderately elevated 24-hour urinary cortisol levels undergo confirmatory testing with two late evening (bedtime) cortisol measurements. A high cutoff value of 550 ng/mL carries a sensitivity of 93% and a specificity of 100%.[26]

Primary adrenal Cushing's syndrome, also termed *ACTH-independent Cushing's syndrome,* is caused by autonomous adrenal cortisol production and is therefore generally associated with an undetectable ACTH level (<5 pg/mL) because of feedback inhibition. The underlying pathology is variable, with a solitary adrenal adenoma found in approximately 90% of cases, adrenocortical carcinoma in less than 10%, and bilateral micronodular or macronodular hyperplasia in less than 1%. Nearly all

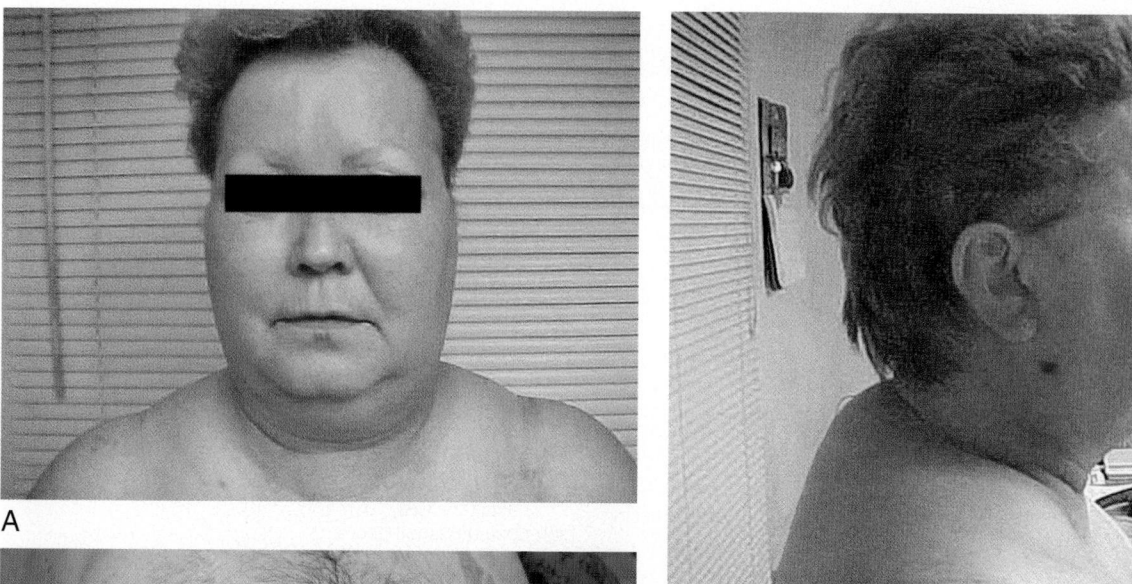

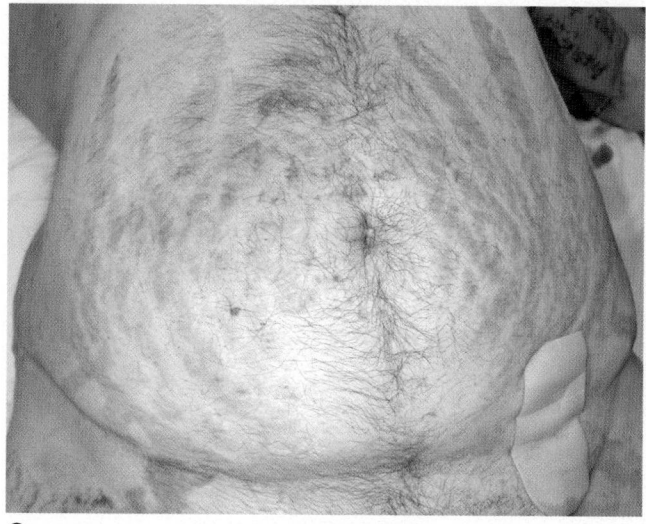

Figure 39-11 Clinical manifestations of Cushing's syndrome. **A,** Moon facies, plethora, and excess supraclavicular fat in a woman with Cushing's syndrome. **B,** Buffalo hump in a woman with Cushing's syndrome. **C,** Purple abdominal striae in a man with Cushing's syndrome.

these lesions, except micronodular hyperplasia, are readily apparent on CT.[27]

Hypercortisolemia associated with normal or elevated ACTH levels is indicative of ACTH-dependent Cushing's syndrome, which is most commonly caused by a pituitary corticotroph microadenoma (Cushing's *disease*). Suspicion of ACTH-dependent Cushing's syndrome prompts pituitary imaging and high-dose dexamethasone suppression testing (i.e., serum or urine cortisol measurement after the administration of 2 mg of dexamethasone every 6 hours over a 48-hour period). Dexamethasone is chosen because it does not cross-react with present biochemical assays for cortisol. Corticotroph adenomas are commonly suppressed in response to high-dose dexamethasone administration, whereas ectopic ACTH sources are completely lacking in feedback inhibition. Slightly more than half of corticotroph microadenomas are visible on pituitary magnetic resonance imaging (MRI). Detection of a

pituitary mass larger than 6 mm in diameter in a patient with ACTH-dependent Cushing's syndrome that is suppressed with high-dose dexamethasone justifies proceeding to pituitary surgery.[28] In the absence of a demonstrable mass, bilateral inferior petrosal sinus ACTH sampling with CRF stimulation is pursued. Demonstration of a central-to-peripheral ACTH gradient in a study performed by a skilled practitioner is sufficient to diagnose Cushing's disease. Absence of a clear gradient prompts CT imaging of the chest/abdomen and occasionally somatostatin receptor scintigraphy to identify an ectopic ACTH source.

Surgical Management and Outcomes

Perioperative and postoperative glucocorticoid administration is obviously essential in the care of patients with Cushing's syndrome. For patients undergoing adrenalectomy for Cushing's syndrome, perioperative "stress dose"

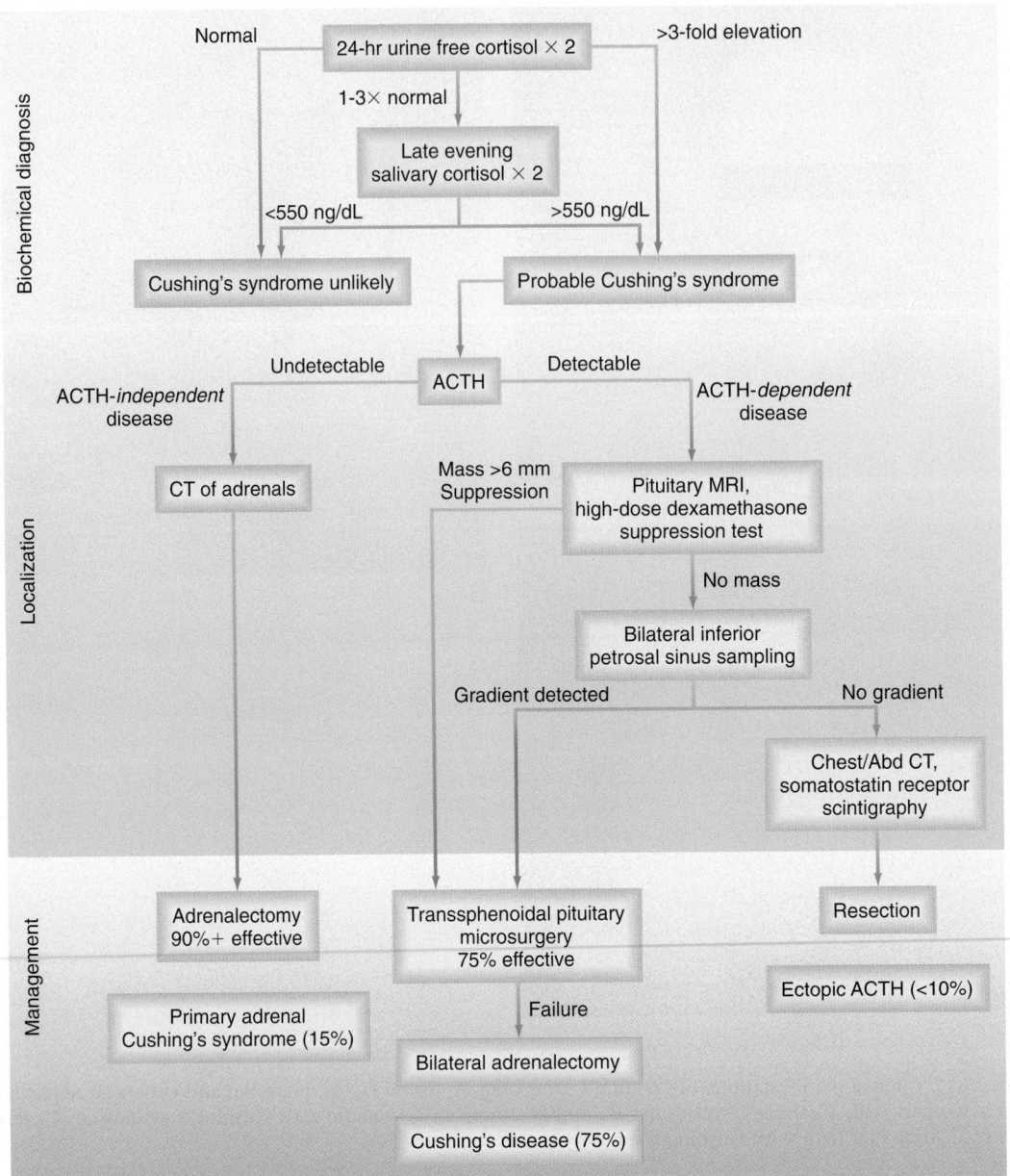

Figure 39-12 Algorithm for the diagnosis, localization, and management of endogenous Cushing's syndrome. A biochemical diagnosis can be established with either an unequivocally elevated 24-hour urine free cortisol level (greater than a threefold elevation) or an elevated late evening salivary cortisol. Most cases of Cushing's syndrome are caused by Cushing's *disease* (pituitary corticotroph microadenoma), in which plasma adrenocorticotropic hormone (ACTH) is elevated. An undetectable ACTH level establishes the diagnosis of ACTH-independent Cushing's syndrome and prompts adrenal imaging. Bilateral adrenalectomy is considered for patient's with Cushing's disease not cured by transsphenoidal surgery.

steroids (hydrocortisone, 100 mg IV every 8 hours for 24 hours) are recommended. In the most common scenario of resection of a solitary adrenal Cushing's adenoma, steroids can usually be tapered to physiologic replacement levels over the course of several weeks. However, a subset of patients with Cushing's syndrome of greater duration and severity will have lasting HPA axis suppression that requires glucocorticoid supplementation for longer periods, sometimes for more than 1 year. It is our

practice to routinely administer perioperative antibiotics for 24 hours to patients undergoing adrenalectomy for Cushing's syndrome because of their elevated risk for surgical site infection.

Management of patients who undergo pituitary surgery for Cushing's disease is variable. In some centers, glucocorticoids are withheld during the immediate postoperative period to provide a window during which early remission may be assessed.[29] A subnormal morning cortisol level on postoperative day 1 or 2 is indicative of cure. Glucocorticoid supplementation is then resumed, usually for at least 6 months, until the HPA axis recovers. Because of the significant risk for postoperative adrenal crisis in patients with Cushing's syndrome of all subtypes, glucocorticoid supplementation is ideally managed in conjunction with an experienced endocrinologist.

Adrenalectomy is more than 90% effective in the treatment of primary adrenal Cushing's syndrome. Failures may result from local and occasionally distant tumor recurrence in the case of malignant disease. Pituitary microsurgery for Cushing's disease, typically performed via a transnasal transsphenoidal approach, is approximately 75% successful in experienced hands. Remission rates may be improved by reoperation or pituitary irradiation in patients whose basal cortisol levels do not fall appropriately after initial surgery. Laparoscopic bilateral adrenalectomy is considered for patients in whom pituitary surgery has failed.[30]

Special Case: Subclinical Cushing's Syndrome

The term *subclinical Cushing's syndrome* has been used to describe patients with incidentally discovered adrenal masses (see The Incidentally Discovered Adrenal Mass, later) who display biochemical evidence of cortisol hypersecretion without overt signs or symptoms of Cushing's syndrome. This disease entity has been incompletely characterized with respect to its physiologic consequences and natural history. Clear-cut definitions for the diagnosis of subclinical Cushing's syndrome, such as cutoff values for biochemical tests and objective assessment guidelines for the presence or absence of clinical features, are lacking.

Some reports indicate that hypertension, dyslipidemia, and impaired glucose tolerance are highly prevalent in individuals with subclinical Cushing's syndrome.[31] However, adrenalectomy for this entity has not been consistently demonstrated to yield health benefits. Progression to overt Cushing's syndrome occurs in less than 10% of cases. Thus, at present, patients found to have subclinical hypercortisolism are monitored for the development of adverse cardiovascular and metabolic features. Therapy is primarily medical and directed at the subset of patients with progressive disease. However, lower biochemical thresholds for surgical treatment need to be considered for larger tumors (i.e., those 3-4 cm in diameter).

Sex Steroid Excess

Adrenal tumors causing clinical features of sex steroid excess are rare. The majority of such tumors are virilizing (as opposed to feminizing), and they may initially be seen at a late stage in association with an advanced adrenal malignancy. Virtually all feminizing tumors are malignant, whereas approximately a third of virilizing tumors are malignant. Of adrenocortical carcinomas, 20% cause virilization, with the majority of these cases occurring in children. An additional 24% of adrenocortical carcinomas will display mixed features of Cushing's syndrome and virilization.[32] Virilizing tumors may be

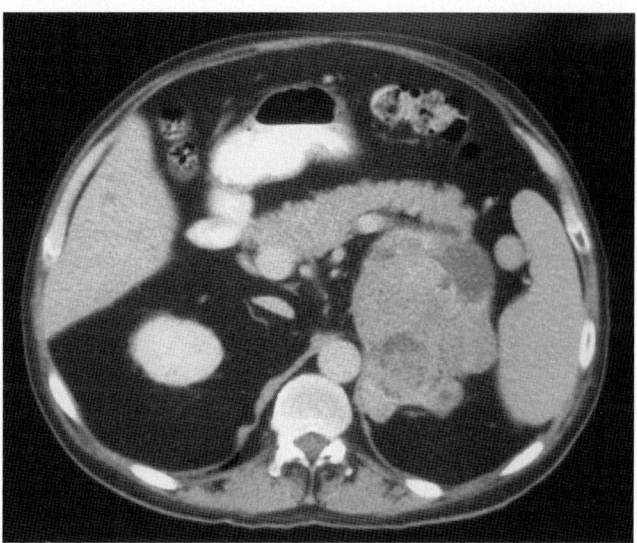

Figure 39-13 CT demonstrating a 10-cm left adrenocortical carcinoma. Note the areas of central necrosis.

biochemically detected by measurement of 24-hour urine testosterone, DHEA, and DHEA-S. Although laparoscopic adrenalectomy remains the preferred procedure for the majority of sex steroid–secreting tumors, the high probability of malignancy merits close radiographic and intraoperative inspection for evidence of invasion or metastasis, or both. Open adrenalectomy is performed for malignant tumors.

Adrenocortical Carcinoma

Adrenocortical carcinoma is a rare tumor with an annual incidence of approximately one per million. Almost all cases occur in patients 40 to 50 years of age, although there is a minor peak in children younger than 5. Adrenocortical carcinomas demonstrate no significant gender predilection. They are frequently very large at initial evaluation (mean tumor size, 9-12 cm), and they generally carry a poor prognosis. Historically, 5-year survival rates have been in the 15% to 20% range, although improved survival rates of 25% to 60% have been reported during the past several years.[33] More than half of adrenocortical carcinomas are functional. Cushing's syndrome is most commonly seen, followed by virilization. Radiographic evaluation is primarily performed with CT, which typically reveals a heterogeneous mass with irregular/indistinct borders, central necrosis, and invasion of adjacent structures (Fig. 39-13). Metastases to the lymph nodes, liver, and lungs may be found.

Treatment of adrenocortical carcinoma centers around radical open surgery. Complete resection can be achieved in up to 70% of patients in experienced hands. Management frequently involves en bloc resection of adjacent organs or regional lymphadenectomy (or both). Particular care must be taken when dealing with right-sided adrenocortical carcinomas larger than 9 cm because direct tumor extension into the inferior vena cava and sometimes the right heart may be observed. Tumors demonstrating intravascular extension may need to be resected while the patient is on cardiopulmonary bypass to reduce the likelihood of lethal intraoperative tumor embolization.

Patients who undergo incomplete resection of adrenocortical carcinomas have extremely limited life expectancy (median survival, <1 year). Even those who undergo successful surgery are prone to the development of local recurrence and metastases, which typically occur within 2 years. The principal chemotherapeutic agent for the treatment of adrenocortical carcinoma is mitotane (*o,p*-DDD, or 1,1-dichloro-2-[*o*-chlorophenyl]-2-[*p*-chloro-phenyl] ethane), a derivative of the insecticide DDT that is a direct adrenocortical toxin. Mitotane has been used clinically both as an adjuvant to surgery and as primary therapy in individuals with unresectable or metastatic disease. The rarity of adrenocortical carcinomas has made systematic assessment of mitotane's efficacy difficult. On balance, mitotane treatment does not appear to improve survival in patients who have undergone complete resection, but it may offer a moderate survival advantage in patients with unresectable or metastatic disease.[34] Its use is limited by significant gastrointestinal and neurologic toxicity. Conventional cytotoxic chemotherapy and external beam radiation therapy currently play little role in the management of adrenocortical carcinoma, although some efficacy has been demonstrated with cisplatin-based regimens.

DISEASES OF THE ADRENAL MEDULLA

Pheochromocytoma

Epidemiology and Clinical Features

The first account of pheochromocytoma was published in 1886 by Felix Frankel, who described a young woman suffering from intermittent attacks of palpitations, anxiety, vertigo, and headache. Autopsy revealed bilateral adrenal tumors that stained brown when treated with chromium salts. The characteristic positive chromaffin reaction lends these adrenomedullary tumors the name *pheochromocytoma* ("dusky-colored tumor" from the Greek *phaios,* or dusky). Successful surgical management of pheochromocytoma was initially described in 1926 by both César Roux and Charles Mayo.[35]

Pheochromocytoma affects approximately 0.2% of hypertensive individuals. Males and females are affected equally. The peak incidence in sporadic cases lies between the ages of 40 and 50, whereas familial cases tend to be manifested earlier. A subset of patients have the classic triad of headache, diaphoresis, and palpitations, although almost all patients will display at least one of these symptoms. Hypertension is present in 90% of cases and may be episodic or sustained. The principal challenge in making the diagnosis of pheochromocytoma arises from the fact that essential hypertension is common and the clinical features suggestive of pheochromocytoma are nonspecific. In fact, only 0.5% of patients with hypertension *and suggestive features* will ultimately prove

to have the disease.[36] The differential diagnosis of pheochromocytoma is extensive and encompasses such diverse processes as hyperthyroidism, hypoglycemia, coronary artery disease, heart failure, stroke, drug-related effects, and panic disorder. Pheochromocytoma has been described as a "biologic time bomb" because of the potentially lethal cardiovascular effects of the bioactive compounds secreted by these tumors. Thus, despite the challenges in diagnosis, clinicians need to aggressively screen for this disease and seek appropriate treatment for affected patients.

Previously, pheochromocytoma was dubbed the "10% tumor" for the reason that 10% are bilateral, 10% malignant, 10% extra-adrenal, and 10% familial. Recent discoveries regarding the genetic underpinnings of pheochromocytoma have challenged these old axioms.[37]

Biochemical Diagnosis and Localization

Establishment of a biochemical diagnosis of pheochromocytoma rests on detection of elevated levels of catecholamines and their metabolites in body fluids. Measurement of 24-hour urine levels of these compounds has long been the cornerstone of biochemical testing, and they remain the most reliable tests available today. In 2002, measurement of free (unconjugated) metanephrines in plasma was introduced as an alternative screening tool for pheochromocytoma.[8] Plasma free metanephrine testing carries an extremely high sensitivity that approaches 99% and, being a one-time blood test, is more convenient than 24-hour urine testing. However, the specificity of plasma free metanephrine testing is 89% at best, with specificities at most laboratories likely to lie in the 85% range or below. Given that pheochromocytoma is a rare diagnosis that is sought within a large pool of hypertensive individuals, false-positive test results are a major problem. In fact, it is estimated that false-positive tests outnumber true-positive tests as much as 30 to 1 when plasma free metanephrine testing is used as a principal screening tool.[38]

Therefore, the primary utility of plasma free metanephrine testing is to exclude pheochromocytoma when the test is negative (Fig. 39-14). When positive, confirmatory testing with 24-hour urinary levels of catecholamines and their metabolites is required. Many drugs and conditions, including sympathomimetics (present in many cold remedies), phenoxybenzamine (frequently initiated when suspicion of pheochromocytoma is raised), acetaminophen (which interferes with the plasma free metanephrine assay), many psychotropic drugs (notably tricyclic antidepressants), and major physical or psychological stressors, are capable of confounding catecholamine-based testing, thus further contributing to the problem of false-positive results. Tests performed during episodes of acute pain, critical illness, or urgent hospitalization may be misleading. The presence of confounding factors, including manifestations or treatment of competing diagnoses, is extremely common in the population being screened. Clearly, biochemical testing is ideally performed when the patient is as free as practically possible of all confounding factors.

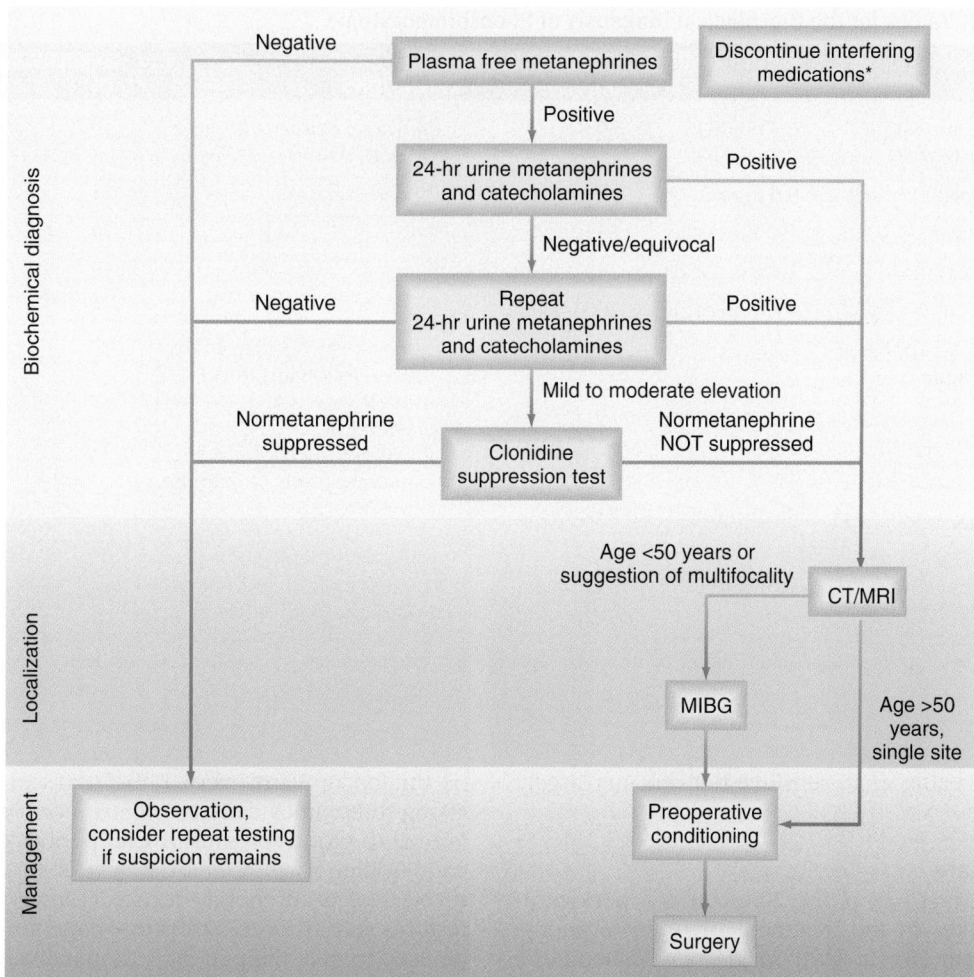

Figure 39-14 Algorithm for the diagnosis, localization, and management of pheochromocytoma. Initial plasma free metanephrine testing can effectively exclude the diagnosis if negative. Twenty-four-hour urine collection for catecholamines and their metabolites is generally performed twice, with cutoffs approximately twice the upper limit of normal being criteria for positivity (see Table 39-4). Clonidine suppression testing can be used for the small fraction of patients in whom the diagnosis remains uncertain after urine testing. Localization with CT or MRI follows biochemical confirmation of the diagnosis, with MIBG performed for younger patients and those otherwise at risk for multifocal disease. Phenoxybenzamine is given in escalating doses for at least 2 weeks before surgery.

The operating characteristics of catecholamine-based plasma and urine tests are listed along with corresponding cutoff values in Table 39-4. Cutoff values for 24-hour urine tests are deliberately set high to maximize specificity; in fact, these values are approximately *double* the upper 95% reference range in most laboratories. A urine collection may be considered positive if total metanephrines or any single catecholamine fraction (epinephrine, norepinephrine, or dopamine) is elevated above its cutoff value. This approach maintains high specificity and yields an acceptable sensitivity of 88%.[38] Importantly, it takes into account the fact that pheochromocytomas both synthesize and metabolize catecholamines and that tumors may possess heterogeneous secretory "profiles," depending on their relative expression of synthetic and degradative enzymes (see Fig. 39-6).

Two 24-hour urine collections for catecholamines and their metabolites are sufficient to make (or exclude) the diagnosis of pheochromocytoma in almost all cases. Clonidine suppression testing, or measurement of plasma free normetanephrine levels after the oral administration of 0.3 mg of clonidine, may help clarify equivocal test results. Anatomic localization may be performed with MRI or CT. MRI is slightly more sensitive, but CT often yields better anatomic definition for operative planning (Fig. 39-15). Scintigraphy with [131]I- or ^{123}I-labeled metaiodobenzylguanidine (MIBG, Fig. 39-16) is performed in select patients in whom multifocal disease is suspected. MIBG scanning is highly specific for pheochromocytoma but carries a sensitivity of only 77% to 90%. Positron-emission tomography (PET) with the use of novel ^{18}F-labeled catecholamine

Table 39-4 Cutoff Values for the Biochemical Diagnosis of Pheochromocytoma

TEST*	CUTOFF VALUE (mol)	CUTOFF VALUE (g)	DEFINITIONS	SENSITIVITY (%)	SPECIFICITY (%)
Plasma free metanephrine Plasma free normetanephrine	0.3 nmol/L 0.6 nmol/L	59 µg/L 110 µg/L	Paired test, positive if either or both values are elevated	99	85-89
Urinary total metanephrines	6.6 µmol/day	1.3 mg/day		71	99.6
Urinary epinephrine	191 nmol/day	35 µg/day		29	99.6
Urinary norepinephrine	1005 nmol/day	170 µg/day		50	99.6
Urinary dopamine	4571 nmol/day	700 µg/day		8	100
Urinary total metanephrines **and** catecholamines	—		Grouped test, positive if any one of following three urinary values are elevated: total metanephrines, epinephrine, norepinephrine, dopamine	88	99
Urinary vanillylmandelic acid	40 µmol/day	7.9 mg/day		64	95
Clonidine suppression test Plasma free normetanephrine	0.61 nmol/L	112 µg/L	Positive result=elevated level after clonidine and fall of less than 40	96	100

*When performed twice, 24-hour urine testing of urinary total metanephrines and catecholamines (grouped test) is both highly sensitive and highly specific.

analogues is probably more sensitive but remains largely investigational.[39]

Perioperative Care

Throughout the first half of the 20th century, perioperative mortality rates in the treatment of pheochromocytoma ranged from 26% to 50%. At the new millennium, the mortality rate in most specialty centers is approximately 2%. This dramatic improvement can largely be ascribed to advances in pharmacology, physiology, anesthesia, and perioperative medical care. The adverse perioperative hemodynamic changes that are most commonly observed with pheochromocytoma are intraoperative hypertension and postoperative hypotension. Intraoperative hypertension may be caused by stimulation of catecholamine release by anesthetic induction agents, as well as direct manipulation of the tumor. Postoperative hypotension may be profound. It results from a state of hypovolemia created by the presence of excess circulating catecholamines. Sudden withdrawal of this stimulus after tumor removal leads to peripheral arteriolar vasodilation, in addition to a dramatic increase in venous capacitance, which together may precipitate cardiovascular collapse. In their early report of a large, successful case series, investigators at the Mayo Clinic described the use of intraoperative α-adrenergic blockade, followed by aggressive volume repletion and administration of α-adrenergic agonists in the immediate postoperative period.[40]

The principles of contemporary perioperative care remain much the same. As soon as the biochemical diagnosis of pheochromocytoma has been confirmed, α-adrenergic blockade is initiated to protect against hemodynamic lability. Our practice is to start with phenoxybenzamine, 10 mg twice daily. The dosage can be titrated upward every 2 to 3 days to a maximum of 40 mg three times daily to achieve normalization of heart rate and blood pressure. The period of preoperative conditioning lasts at least 2 weeks to allow adequate reversal of α-adrenergic receptor down-regulation. This restores sensitivity to vasopressor agents, which can then be used to treat the patient postoperatively. Phenoxybenzamine is a nonspecific, noncompetitive (irreversible), long-acting (half-life of 24 hours) α-adrenergic antagonist. Although its use is associated with the side effects of postural hypotension and significant nasal congestion, it is generally favored over α_1-selective agents such as prazosin and doxazosin. Nasal congestion can actually serve as a useful indicator of adequate blockade. Furthermore, phenoxybenzamine provides the most complete α-blockade among available agents, and its pharmacokinetics permits serum drug levels to decay in parallel with catecholamine levels postoperatively.

β-Blockers may be administered *after* adequate α-blockade has been achieved in the subset of patients with persistent tachycardia. β-Blockers are never the first agent administered because a decrease in peripheral vasodilatory β-receptor stimulation results in unopposed α-adrenergic tone, which may exacerbate hypertension. Preoperative volume expansion with isotonic fluids has been advocated in the past. However, in our experience the need for volume expansion is significantly reduced when aggressive preoperative α-blockade has been achieved because the resultant increase in venous capacitance restores euvolemia. Clinical suspicion of hypovolemia needs to remain high in the postoperative period, and patients need to be aggressively resuscitated if they become hypotensive or oliguric. Some patients may require vasopressors after tumor removal, especially if preoperative α-blockade is incomplete.

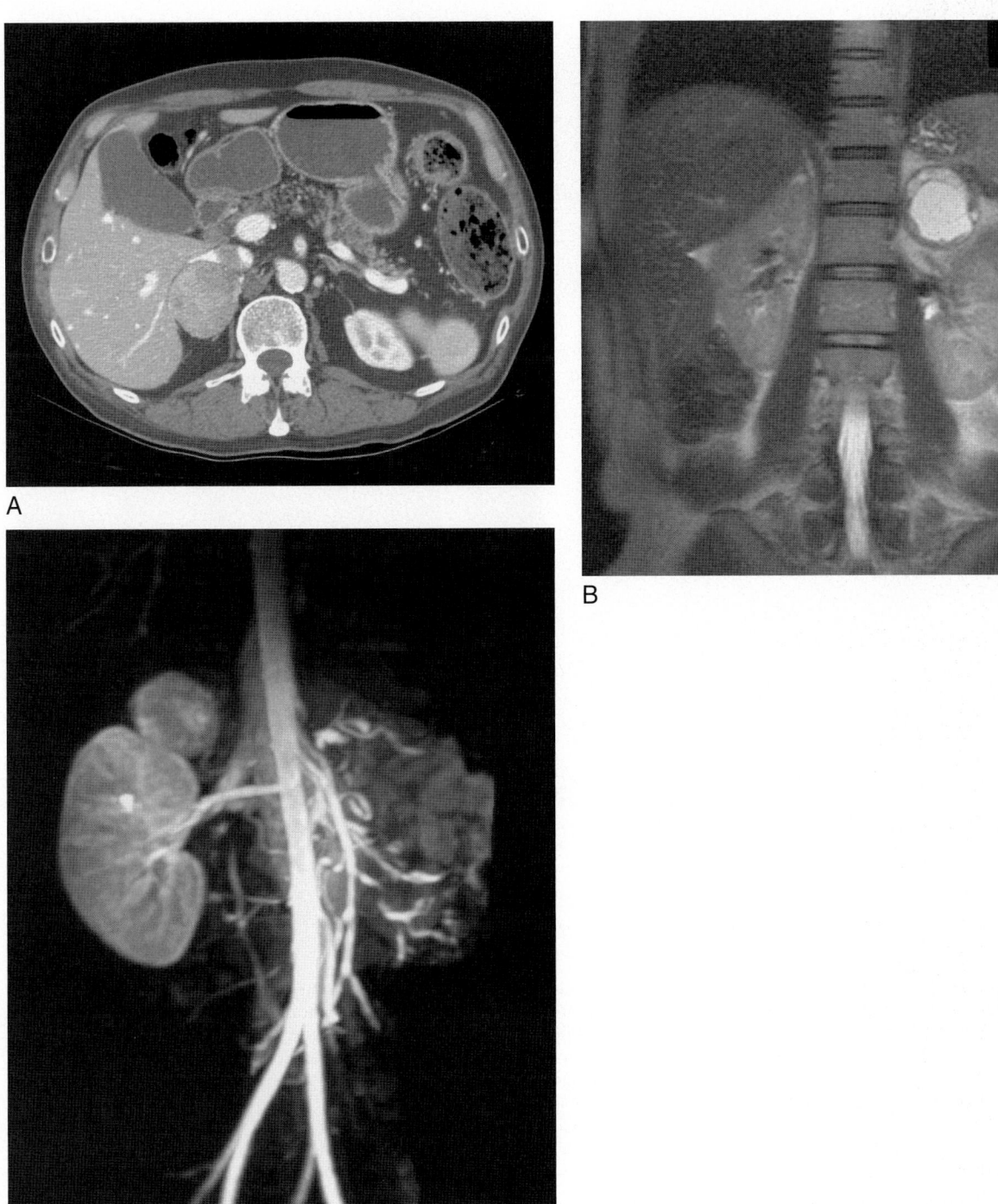

Figure 39-15 Appearance of pheochromocytoma on anatomic imaging. **A,** Venous phase, contrast-enhanced CT scan demonstrating a right adrenal pheochromocytoma. The heterogeneity in the inferior vena cava represents swirling of contrast, not tumor thrombus or invasion. **B,** Coronal T2-weighted MRI demonstrating a left adrenal pheochromocytoma with central cystic change. **C,** Left anterior oblique magnetic resonance angiographic reconstruction demonstrating a right adrenal pheochromocytoma.

Surgical Management and Outcomes

Successful operative treatment of pheochromocytoma is dependent on close communication between the surgeon and anesthesiologist. Needless to say, invasive hemodynamic monitoring is required, and fluid management must be meticulous. Manipulation of the tumor needs to be minimized, and the anesthetic team must be prepared to administer supplemental IV α- and β-blockers, as well as vasopressors, when necessary.

Surgery is curative in greater than 90% of pheochromocytoma cases. Although these tumors are highly vascular and tend to adhere to adjacent structures (Fig.

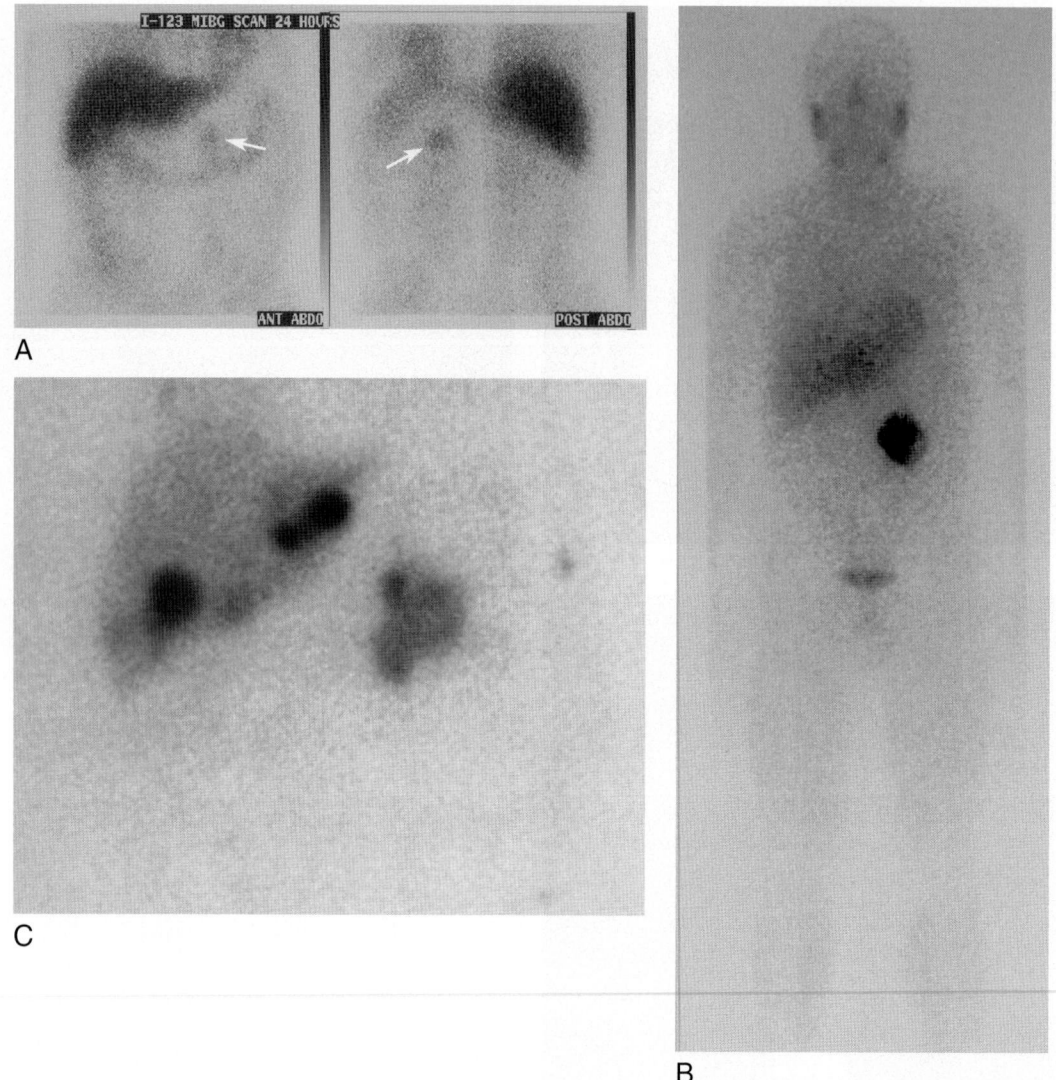

Figure 39-16 Appearance of pheochromocytoma on functional imaging (MIBG scanning). **A,** ^{123}I-MIBG scan of the abdomen demonstrating an isolated left adrenal pheochromocytoma. Physiologic radiotracer uptake is noted in the liver, right colon, and transverse colon. **B,** Whole-body ^{131}I-MIBG scan demonstrating a large left para-aortic extra-adrenal pheochromocytoma. Physiologic radiotracer uptake is noted in the liver, salivary glands, and bladder. **C,** ^{131}I-MIBG scan of the abdomen demonstrating malignant pheochromocytoma with local recurrence in the left adrenal bed and liver metastases.

39-17), the great majority of them can be removed successfully via a laparoscopic approach. Laparoscopic resection is contraindicated when preoperative imaging demonstrates local invasion. Advances in surgical technique have resulted in reduced operative complication rates. Specifically, functional image-guided focused exploration has replaced bilateral adrenal and retroperitoneal exploration and has led to diminished rates of solid organ injury.[41]

Molecular Genetics of Pheochromocytoma

A number of recent reports describing novel germline mutations have demonstrated that familial pheochromocytoma is much more common than previously thought. Before the year 2000, pheochromocytoma was known to be associated with multiple endocrine neoplasia type 2

syndromes (40%-50% penetrant), von Hippel-Lindau syndrome (10%-20% penetrant), and neurofibromatosis type 1 (1%-5% penetrant). The discovery that neuroendocrine cells of the carotid body proliferate in response to hypoxic stimuli led to the identification of mutations in the succinate dehydrogenase gene family in kindreds affected with pheochromocytoma/paraganglioma. Succinate dehydrogenase, which is made up of four subunits, is localized to the mitochondria and catalyzes essential steps in oxidative phosphorylation.

Germline mutations in the B and D subunits, which are inherited in an autosomal dominant fashion, have been identified in approximately 10% of apparently sporadic pheochromocytoma cases.[42] Thus, there is new consensus that 21% to 30% of pheochromocytomas are familial. Familial cases occur at an earlier age and are

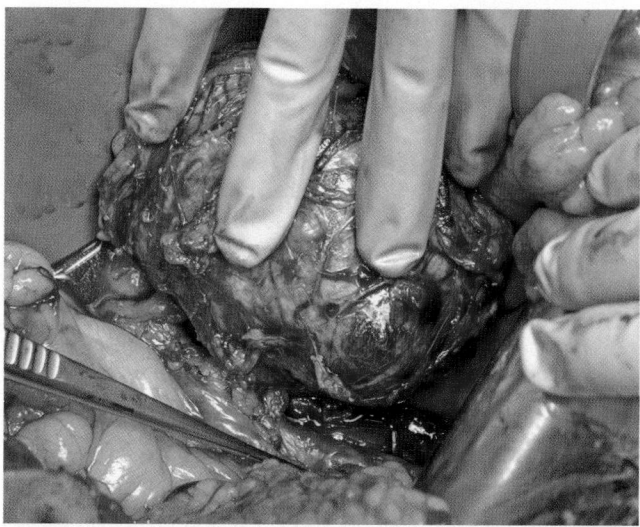

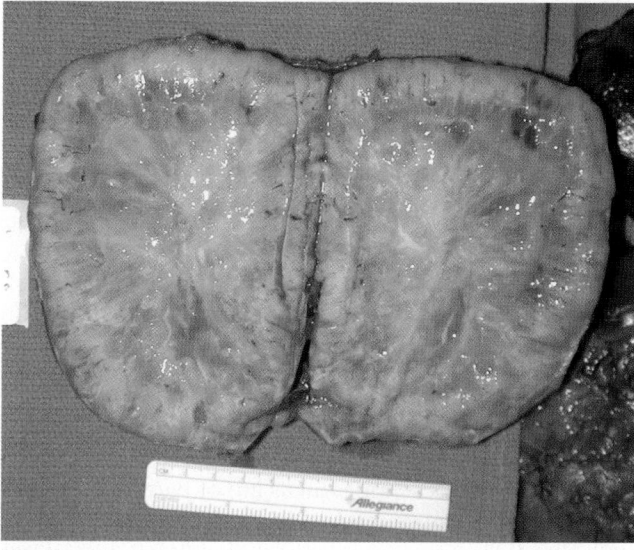

Figure 39-17 Gross appearance of pheochromocytoma. **A,** Open resection of a left para-aortic extra-adrenal pheochromocytoma (depicted in Fig. 39-16B) via an infracolic approach. The patient's head is to the right. The tumor is being rotated medially by the surgeon's hand to reveal the left ureter, indicated by forceps. **B,** Left adrenal pheochromocytoma. (**A,** Courtesy of Stan Sidhu, PhD.)

more likely to be multifocal. Succinate dehydrogenase B mutation carriers have high rates of extra-adrenal (abdominal or thoracic) pheochromocytomas and malignant disease, whereas succinate dehydrogenase D carriers tend to have multiple tumors and hormonally inactive paragangliomas of the head and neck. The lifetime penetrance of succinate dehydrogenase mutations is estimated to be greater than 75%.[43] Genetic counseling and testing is encouraged for patients in whom pheochromocytoma is diagnosed before the age of 50.

Malignant Pheochromocytoma

Depending on the underlying genotype, anywhere from 2.5% to 40% of pheochromocytomas are malignant. Sur-

vival rates at 5 years range from 20% to 45%. No histopathologic criteria for determining malignancy have demonstrated the ability to accurately predict the clinical course. Thus, malignancy is defined by the development of metastases (i.e., tumor implants distant from the primary mass in locations where neuroectodermal tissue is not normally found). The latter criterion distinguishes metastatic disease from possible multifocal primary disease.

The most common sites of metastasis are the axial skeleton, lymph nodes, liver, lung, and kidney. Treatment of both primary and recurrent disease centers on surgical resection, which even in the absence of cure has significant palliative benefits.[44] Malignant pheochromocytomas are minimally responsive to radiotherapy and chemotherapy. High-dose ^{131}I-MIBG radionuclide therapy has been used to treat malignant and metastatic pheochromocytoma. Moderate initial response has been observed, but long-term benefit is uncommon. Chronic medical management of catecholamine excess is performed with α_1-selective blockers because of their favorable side effect profile.

THE INCIDENTALLY DISCOVERED ADRENAL MASS ("INCIDENTALOMA")

Epidemiology and Differential Diagnosis

Incidentally discovered adrenal masses, also termed clinically inapparent adrenal masses or "incidentalomas," are discovered through imaging performed for unrelated/nonadrenal disease. Their existence as a clinical entity is a by-product of advanced medical imaging. Incidentalomas were first described in the early 1980s, when CT scanners became more prevalent in developed nations, and they have become a common clinical problem as the use of CT and MRI has become widespread. Incidentalomas are found in 2.1% of autopsies and 1% to 4% of abdominal imaging studies.[45] The prevalence rises to greater than 4% in patients older than 60 years.

The differential diagnosis of an adrenal mass is extensive and includes both secreting and nonsecreting neoplasms (Fig. 39-18). In patients with a history of malignancy, metastatic disease is the most likely cause of adrenal masses, particularly when bilateral (see Metastases to the Adrenal Gland, later). In those without a clear history of malignancy, at least 80% of incidentalomas will turn out to be nonfunctioning cortical adenomas or other benign lesions that do not require surgical management. Thus, in most patients, the most important aspect of management is to distinguish the subset of adrenal masses that are likely to have a clinical impact from the large proportion that will not.

Clinical Evaluation and Surgical Management

The workup for adrenal incidentaloma integrates hormonal evaluation with size criteria. The principles and methods of hormonal evaluation are discussed earlier in the tumor-specific sections and are generally applicable to incidentalomas. However, one conceptual difference

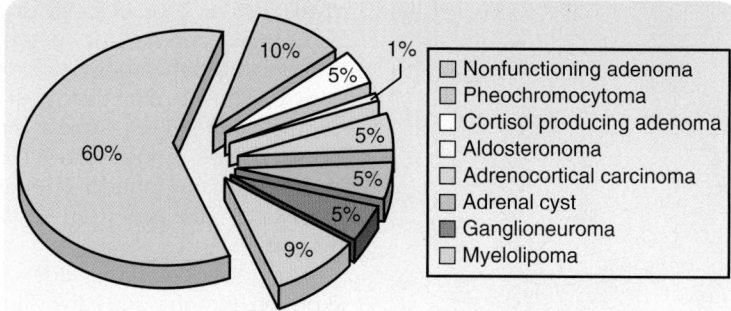

10% 1%
5%
60% 5%
5%
5%
9%

- ☐ Nonfunctioning adenoma
- ☐ Pheochromocytoma
- ☐ Cortisol producing adenoma
- ☐ Aldosteronoma
- ☐ Adrenocortical carcinoma
- ☐ Adrenal cyst
- ☐ Ganglioneuroma
- ☐ Myelolipoma

Figure 39-18 Differential diagnosis of adrenal incidentaloma in patients without a history of malignancy. Approximate proportions of the various pathologies are shown.

is that the biochemical thresholds that prompt operative treatment are somewhat lower in patients with an initial *radiographic* manifestation (incidentalomas) than in those with an initial clinical manifestation. This results from the fact that tumor size, which correlates strongly with risk for malignancy, contributes an additive effect in favor of surgical management.

Evaluation begins with history taking, with a focus on previous malignancy, hypertension, and symptoms of glucocorticoid or sex steroid excess. Biochemical investigations for hormonally active tumors are followed by consideration of size criteria (Fig. 39-19). In a general sense, surgery is recommended for hormonally active tumors and those that carry a significant risk for malignancy. Adrenocortical carcinomas represent less than 2% of adrenal tumors measuring 4 cm or less and roughly 6% of those measuring 4 to 6 cm. Tumors larger than 6 cm carry a greater than 25% risk for malignancy. Because studies have consistently found that CT and MRI underestimate adrenal tumor size by approximately 20% (an effect that is exaggerated in smaller tumors), our practice is to remove all incidentalomas measuring 5 cm or greater and to strongly consider removal of those measuring 3 to 5 cm.[46] Factors that need to be considered in surgical decision making for this latter group include suspicious imaging characteristics (heterogeneity, high attenuation, or irregular margins), the patient's age and surgical risk, growth on interval imaging, and patient preference. If observation is chosen, patients undergo repeat imaging in 6 to 12 months given the fact that 5% to 25% of adrenal masses may increase in size.

CT-guided fine-needle aspiration is rarely helpful in the evaluation of adrenal masses and may be hazardous. The diagnosis of primary adrenal malignancy cannot be reliably based on cytologic criteria alone. Therefore, the use of fine-needle aspiration is generally confined to patients with a history of extra-adrenal malignancy in whom the clinician seeks to establish the diagnosis of metastatic disease. In all cases, pheochromocytoma must be excluded before attempting such a procedure to avoid precipitating potentially fatal hypertensive crisis.

As with the other disease processes that have been discussed, most adrenal incidentalomas can be removed laparoscopically, except for those displaying obvious malignant features on imaging. No upper size limit to this approach has been established, and tumors measuring 15 cm have been successfully removed laparoscopically by experienced surgeons.

METASTASES TO THE ADRENAL GLAND

Epidemiology and Clinical Features

The adrenal glands are common sites of metastasis because of their rich vascular supply. In fact, autopsy studies reveal that adrenal involvement eventually develops in approximately 25% of patients with carcinoma. In half these cases, the metastatic disease is bilateral. The primary cancers that most often spread to the adrenals are those of the lung, gastrointestinal tract, breast, kidney, pancreas, and skin (melanoma).[47] Patients with *isolated* adrenal metastases represent a very small subset of the total. However, these individuals are of particular interest to the surgeon and oncologist because growing evidence indicates that resection of isolated adrenal metastases may improve survival. The principal determinant of survival in these patients is the disease-free interval. Patients in whom metachronous isolated adrenal metastases develop more than 6 months after the initial cancer have better survival rates than those with synchronous adrenal metastases.

Clinical Evaluation and Surgical Management

Evaluation of patients with isolated adrenal metastases must involve careful exclusion of extra-adrenal disease with CT or MRI (including the head in cases of breast cancer or melanoma and triphasic contrast-enhanced CT evaluation of the liver plus 3-mm slices through the lungs for gastrointestinal malignancies), as well as bone scan and PET when appropriate. Patients with isolated *bilateral* adrenal metastases (Fig. 39-20) must be evaluated for adrenal insufficiency secondary to replacement of all normal adrenal tissue with tumor, which may occur in up to 30% of such patients. This is best done by measurement of morning cortisol and ACTH. Cortisol insufficiency must be adequately treated before surgery to avoid perioperative adrenal crisis.

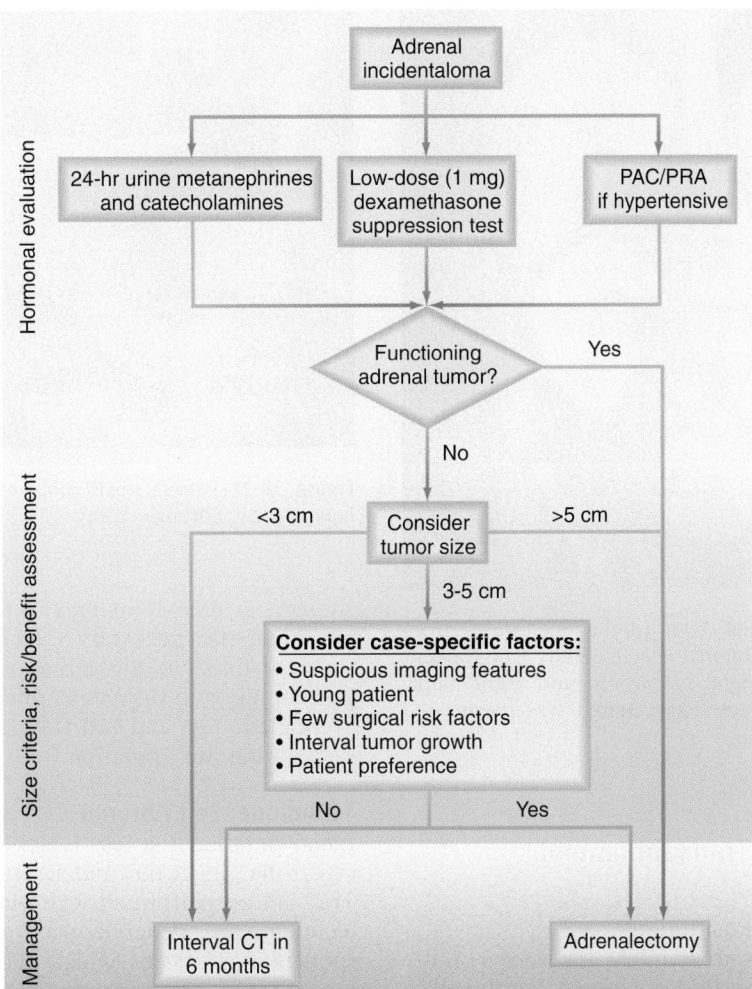

Figure 39-19 Algorithm for management of an adrenal incidentaloma. Adrenalectomy is recommended for all patients with functional tumors. For nonfunctioning tumors, the risk for malignancy is assessed according to size. Tumors larger than 5 cm on CT carry a greater than 25% risk for malignancy and need to be removed. Those smaller than 3 cm can be safely observed. Case-specific factors must be considered for intermediate-sized tumors. PAC, plasma aldosterone concentration; PRA, plasma renin activity.

The great majority of adrenal metastases are well encapsulated and thus amenable to laparoscopic resection. Complete adrenal metastasectomy has yielded a mean survival of 20 to 30 months in most series,[48] as compared with 12 months for patients with incomplete resection and 6 months for patients not undergoing surgical therapy.

TECHNICAL ASPECTS OF ADRENALECTOMY

Choice of Operative Approach

In our practice, approximately 90% of adrenalectomies are performed laparoscopically. Laparoscopic adrenalectomy affords many advantages over conventional open surgery, including reduced length of hospitalization, reduced pain, decreased operative blood loss, and a lower rate of postoperative complications.[49] Similar degrees of benefit are observed with transabdominal and

posterior retroperitoneal laparoscopic approaches. Because of the wider operative field and greater versatility afforded by the lateral transabdominal technique, it is our favored approach and is discussed in greater detail later. The lateral transabdominal approach can be used to handle very large tumors, and previous abdominal surgery does not alter the success rate significantly when the procedure is performed by an experienced surgeon. The overall conversion rate to open adrenalectomy is less than 5% in large series.

As discussed earlier, open adrenalectomy is performed for primary adrenal tumors demonstrating features suggestive of malignancy, such as large size (>8 cm), clinical feminization, hypersecretion of multiple steroid hormones, or any of the following imaging attributes: local/vascular invasion, regional adenopathy, and metastases. For open adrenalectomy, we also prefer a transabdominal approach, which is performed via a subcostal incision as discussed later.

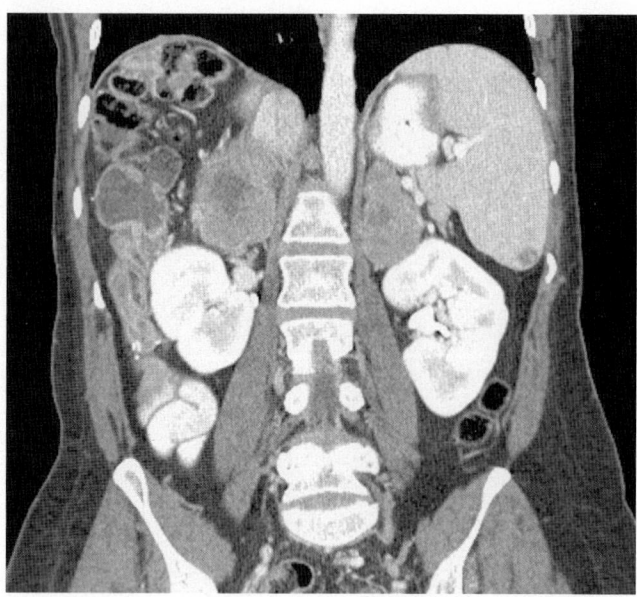

Figure 39-20 Isolated bilateral 7-cm adrenal metastases from colorectal cancer causing adrenal insufficiency. The patient had undergone previous right colectomy and right hepatectomy. Bilateral adrenal metastasectomy was performed laparoscopically.

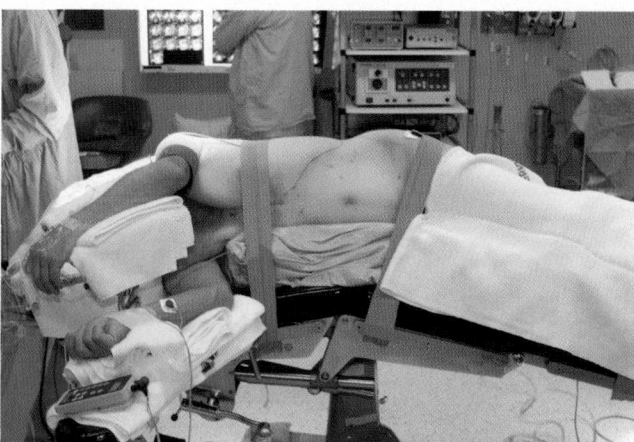

Figure 39-21 Patient positioning for left lateral transabdominal laparoscopic adrenalectomy.

Laparoscopic Lateral Transabdominal Adrenalectomy

Patient Preparation and Positioning

Draw sheets and a full-length beanbag are placed on the operating table in advance. It is important that the table be capable of flexion and have a kidney rest that can be elevated. The patient is initially positioned supine for induction of anesthesia and placement of a urinary catheter. Intermittent pneumatic compression devices are applied to the legs. Placement of an orogastric or nasogastric tube for gastric decompression is frequently helpful, particularly when treating left-sided lesions. The patient is then turned on the side (80-degree lateral decubitus position), with the side bearing the lesion facing upward (Fig. 39-21). At this point the patient is carefully positioned in the cephalocaudal dimension such that the 10th rib is directly over the breakpoint in the table. The table is flexed and the beanbag rigidified in a position that supports the buttocks and back while leaving the umbilicus (an important surface landmark) exposed. Flexing the table and raising the kidney rest serve to widen the space between the costal margin and the iliac crest and to drop the iliac crest away from the plane of the laparoscopic instruments. Wide cloth tape is used to secure the patient to the table at the chest, hips, and lower extremities. Great care must taken to protect bony prominences and points of potential peripheral nerve compression in the extremities. The surgical preparation is carried from the nipple line to the pubis and from the umbilicus to the midline of the back.

Careful positioning is essential for technical success in laparoscopic adrenalectomy. As discussed later, the

surgeon is reliant on gravity to serve as a retractor in providing the necessary exposure. Having the patient securely fixed to the table permits the often extreme positioning with respect to pitch (Trendelenburg/reverse Trendelenburg) and roll (tilting left/right) that is necessary during the operation.

Technique: Left Adrenal

Initial peritoneal access is achieved 2 cm inferior to the costal margin in the midclavicular line (Palmer's point). This can be performed with either the Veress or Hasson technique. We generally use four 11-mm radially dilating (noncutting) trocars, which allows free exchange of the laparoscope, fan retractor, dissecting devices, and clip applier as needed. The ports are equally distributed along the costal margin, with the posterior port placed as far lateral/posterior as permitted by the position of the colon (Fig. 39-22). It is advisable to leave at least 5 cm (4 fingerbreadths) between each port to minimize external interference of the laparoscopic instruments. For tissue dissection, we use the hook monopolar cautery and an energy-based tissue sealing/dividing device.

The lateral attachments of the spleen are taken down first, with the goal of rotating the left upper quadrant viscera anteromedially. Splenic mobilization is continued until the greater curvature of stomach becomes visible at its apex, at which point the spleen and tail of the pancreas are allowed to fall anteriorly with rightward tilting of the table and gentle use of the fan retractor. In many patients, the splenic flexure of the colon must be mobilized caudally by dividing the splenocolic ligament. We use an "open book" technique that involves developing the cleftlike plane just medial to the adrenal gland and lateral to the aorta (Fig. 39-23). The left-hand page of the book is composed of the spleen, tail of the pancreas, and greater curvature of the stomach. The right-hand page of the book consists of the kidney and adrenal tumor. The left crus of the diaphragm is a useful landmark that leads the surgeon to the left inferior phrenic vein. As mentioned in the anatomy section of this chapter, the left inferior phrenic vein courses along the medial aspect of

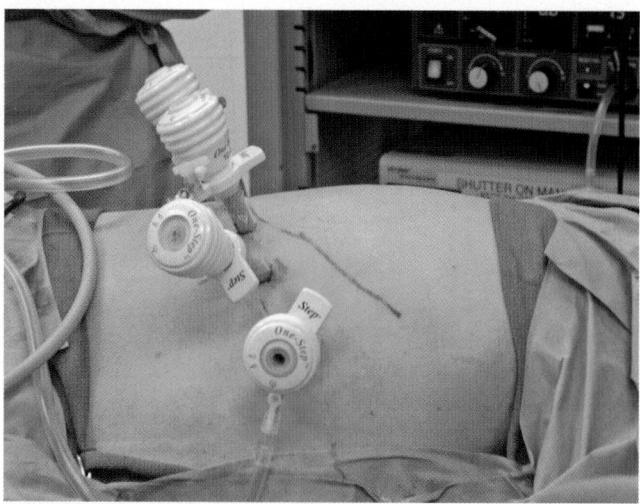

Figure 39-22 Port placement for right laparoscopic adrenalectomy. In this figure the patient is lying right-side up with the head toward the right. The *marked line* denotes the costal margin. Ports are placed approximately 2 cm inferior to the costal margin, spaced about 4 fingerbreadths apart.

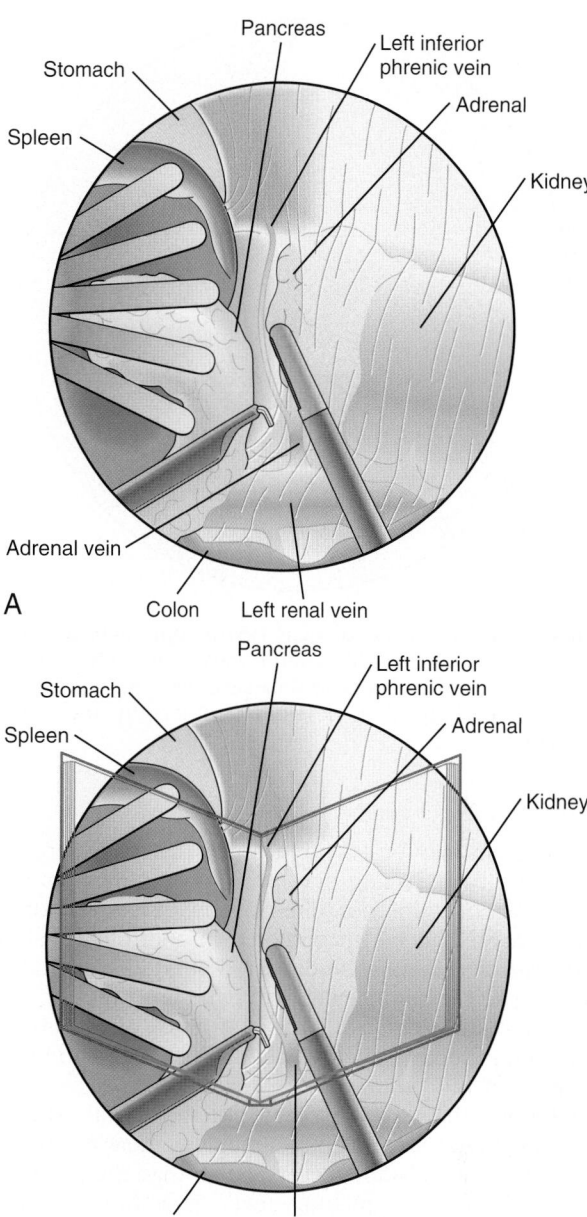

Figure 39-23 Technique of left laparoscopic adrenalectomy. The spleen and pancreatic tail have been mobilized and retracted anteromedially to expose the adrenal gland. The cleft of the "open book" is developed in a superior-to-inferior direction to identify the inferior phrenic vein and adrenal vein.

the left adrenal gland before joining with the left adrenal vein. By developing the cleft of the open book, moving in a superior-to-inferior direction, the adrenal vein is encountered at the inferomedial aspect of the adrenal gland. The small adrenal arteries that lie within this plane can be handled with energy-based coagulation. The left adrenal vein is carefully dissected out, clipped (leaving two clips on the patient side), and divided. The inferior tip of the left adrenal gland may extend quite low and approach the renal hilum within millimeters. However, because the left adrenal vein is rather long (2 cm), it is not generally necessary to expose the renal vasculature during left adrenalectomy.

The adrenal gland is liberated by completing the dissection circumferentially and posteriorly and taking the specimen off the superior pole of the kidney and posterior abdominal wall. These attachments are deliberately divided last because they aid in suspending the adrenal gland on the lateral/superior wall of the operative field, thereby providing exposure of the medial vascular plane during the critical initial portion of the procedure. The tumor is placed in a resilient catchment device, morcellated, and extracted. If noncutting trocars are used, only the skin need be closed.

Technique: Right Adrenal

Laparoscopic right adrenalectomy is, in some respects, a mirror image of the procedure just described. During right adrenalectomy, the left-hand page of the open book is made up of the kidney and adrenal tumor, and the right-hand page consists of the bare area of the liver (Fig. 39-24). To gain access to the appropriate plane, the right triangular ligament of the liver must first be completely mobilized and the liver allowed to rotate anteromedially. On the right side, the colon usually lies well inferior to the operative field. When developing the space between

the adrenal gland and inferior vena cava superiorly to inferiorly, the surgeon must be mindful of adrenal vein variants, as illustrated in the anatomy section of this chapter (see Fig. 39-3). The right adrenal vein is a potentially perilous structure to manage because it is short, wide, variable, and confluent with thin-walled, large capacitance vessels (the inferior vena cava in >80% of cases, followed by the renal vein and uncommonly the right hepatic vein) that can bleed briskly if directly injured (e.g., by cautery), lacerated from undue traction on adjacent structures, or sheared by clips. A significant second

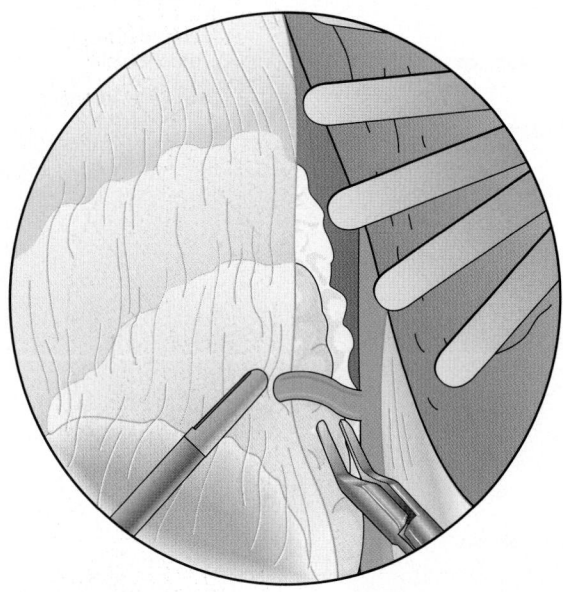

Figure 39-24 Technique of right laparoscopic adrenalectomy. The liver has been mobilized and retracted medially to expose the adrenal gland and inferior vena cava. The space just medial to the adrenal gland is developed to identify the adrenal vasculature.

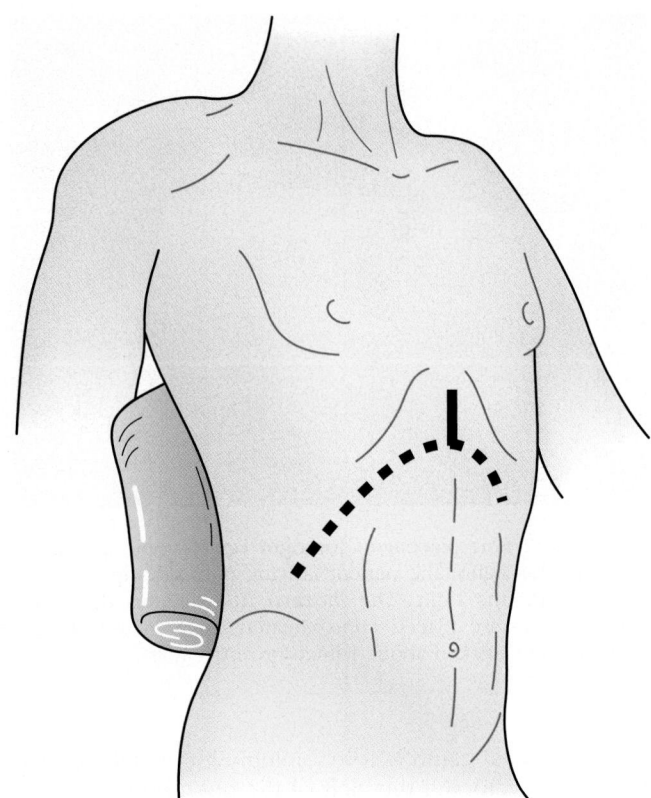

Figure 39-25 Patient positioning for open right adrenalectomy.

adrenal vein may be found in up to 10% of patients. By methodically dissecting one layer at a time and moving in a superior-to-inferior direction, all potential adrenal vein variants can be encountered in controlled fashion. The adrenal vein must be dissected out delicately, definitively ligated (again usually with two clips on the patient side), and then divided. Loss of control of the adrenal vein stump needs to be avoided; if it occurs, conversion to an open procedure may be necessary.

Of note, the junction of the inferior vena cava and right renal vein is frequently difficult to identify. In vivo, the transition is a gradual curve rather than the 90-degree takeoff depicted in anatomy texts. Therefore, it cannot be used as a reliable anatomic landmark for identification of the adrenal vein.

Complications and Postoperative Care

Potential technical complications include venous hemorrhage and bleeding from solid organ capsular injuries. Small amounts of bleeding can often be managed by coagulation or direct pressure with rolled Kittner gauze. Hollow viscus injuries are uncommon but may be associated with procedures performed in patients who have previously undergone major abdominal surgery. Pancreatic injuries and fistulas have been reported with left-sided procedures but are rare complications, as are port site hernias and port site metastases in cases of malignancy. Patients undergoing laparoscopic adrenalectomy for Cushing's syndrome are at risk for surgical site infections, including port site infections in 5% to 10% of cases and, rarely, subphrenic abscesses requiring catheter drainage, as a result of their catabolic and immunosuppressed state.

Patients who undergo laparoscopic adrenalectomy recover rapidly. Most patients, including approximately half of those treated for pheochromocytoma, are able to leave the hospital on the first postoperative day. In the treatment of adrenal tumors, successful outcomes hinge on excellent perioperative *medical* management as much as technical skill, particularly in cases of pheochromocytoma and Cushing's syndrome. These considerations are discussed earlier in the disease-specific sections.

Open Anterior Transabdominal Adrenalectomy

Patient Preparation and Positioning

Neuraxial blockade (use of an epidural catheter) is routinely used for intraoperative and postoperative anesthetic/analgesic management. The patient is positioned supine, with the ipsilateral side slightly elevated on a bolster (Fig. 39-25). A urinary catheter, orogastric or nasogastric tube, and intermittent pneumatic compression devices are placed. The surgical preparation is carried from the nipple line to the pubis and down to the table on either side.

Technique: Left Adrenal

We prefer to use a subcostal incision, which may be extended across the midline (chevron) with or without a vertical upper midline extension to achieve wide exposure. The left adrenal can be exposed by entering the lesser sac through the gastrocolic ligament and incising

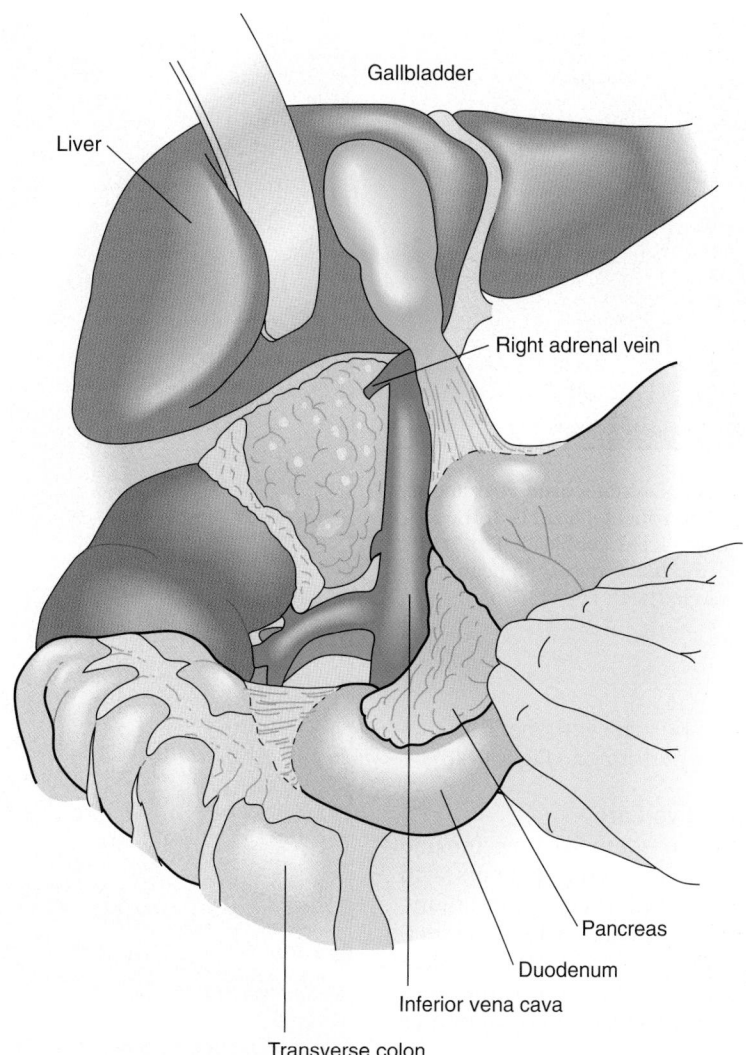

Gallbladder

Liver

Right adrenal vein

Pancreas

Duodenum

Inferior vena cava

Transverse colon

Figure 39-26 Open right adrenalectomy. The right lobe of the liver and the hepatic flexure of the colon have been completely mobilized. The retroperitoneum is entered and the duodenum and head of the pancreas reflected medially (Kocher maneuver) to expose the adrenal gland and inferior vena cava.

the retroperitoneum inferior to the tail of the pancreas or by rotating the spleen, pancreatic tail, and stomach anteromedially as described in the section on laparoscopic adrenalectomy. The latter approach is used in our practice. The splenic flexure of the colon is mobilized inferiorly and the plane medial to the adrenal gland developed. The adrenal vein is isolated, tied in continuity, and divided. The small adrenal arteries can be ligated or electrocoagulated and the specimen removed after circumferential dissection is completed.

Technique: Right Adrenal

Open right adrenalectomy begins with complete mobilization of the right lobe of the liver, including the lateral attachments and the falciform ligament. The adrenal can be exposed by rotating the liver medially or, more commonly, retracting the inferoposterior segments cephalad with long, padded retractors (liver, renal vein, Deaver, or Harrington types). The retroperitoneum is entered by

performing a Kocher maneuver (Fig. 39-26) and the inferior vena cava exposed by medial reflection of the duodenum. The plane between the adrenal gland and inferior vena cava is developed first. Vascular structures, which may be numerous in highly angiogenic tumors, are ligated sequentially. The adrenal vein is isolated, securely tied, and divided. Loss of control of the adrenal vein stump may be managed with the application of a side-biting (Satinsky) vascular clamp. As discussed earlier, open adrenalectomy is generally performed in cases of suspected or known malignancy. Locally invasive right-sided adrenal tumors can be challenging to manage given their frequent invasion of adjacent venous structures (Fig. 39-27). It is our practice to involve an experienced vascular or liver surgeon in the management of tumors with extensive venous invasion. Locally invaded organs, most commonly the kidney, are resected en bloc with the primary mass. Complete radical resection is a critical determinant of survival in patients with malignant adrenal

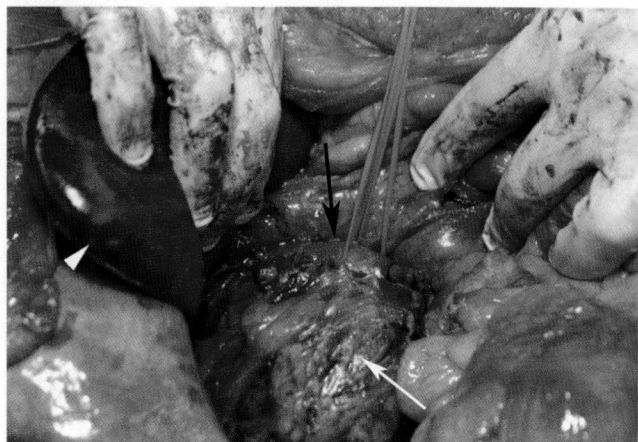

Figure 39-27 Open resection of a right adrenocortical carcinoma invading the inferior vena cava. The patient's head is to the left. The liver (*white arrowhead*) is retracted cephalad. The *white arrow* indicates the tumor and the *black arrow* indicates the inferior vena cava, which is encircled with vessel loops.

tumors; in some cases this can be achieved only if immediate venous reconstruction is performed (Fig. 39-28).

Complications and Postoperative Care

Technical complications of open adrenalectomy include venous hemorrhage, tumor embolization in patients with intravascular tumor extension, and solid organ injury. Postoperative complications are similar to those associated with other major abdominal procedures. Most patients experience return of bowel function within 3 to 4 days and are able to leave the hospital on postoperative day 5 to 7.

Selected References

Axelrod L: Perioperative management of patients treated with glucocorticoids. Endocrinol Metab Clin North Am 32:367-383, 2003.

> A thorough review of existing nonsystematic studies on steroid use that provides clear guidelines and the rationale behind them.

Gifford RW Jr, Kvale WF, Maher FT, et al: Clinical features, diagnosis and treatment of pheochromocytoma: A review of 76 cases. Mayo Clin Proc 39:281-302, 1964.

> A landmark account of the biochemical, pharmacologic, and physiologic advances that allowed collaborators at the Mayo Clinic to treat 76 patients with pheochromocytoma while experiencing only one death.

Grumbach MM, Biller BM, Braunstein GD, et al: Management of the clinically inapparent adrenal mass ("incidentaloma"). Ann Intern Med 138:424-429, 2003.

> A summary statement from the National Institutes of Health Consensus Development Program with recommendations on incidentaloma workup and indications for surgery.

Kudva YC, Sawka AM, Young WF Jr: Clinical review 164: The laboratory diagnosis of adrenal pheochromocytoma: The Mayo Clinic experience. J Clin Endocrinol Metab 88:4533-4539, 2003.

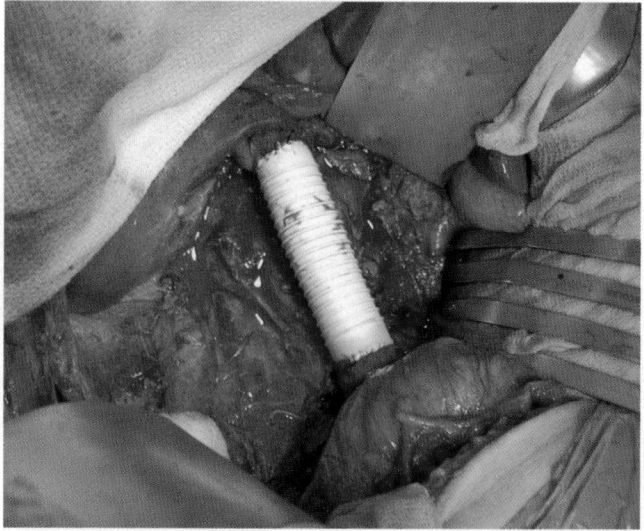

A

B

Figure 39-28 Open resection of a right adrenocortical carcinoma necessitating vascular reconstruction. **A,** The infrahepatic inferior vena cava has been replaced with a polytetrafluoroethylene graft. The liver can be seen superiorly and the colon inferiorly. **B,** Ex vivo specimen consisting of the right adrenal tumor with the kidney resected en bloc. The renal vein is indicated by the *arrow*. Forceps have been placed through the resected segment of inferior vena cava.

> A critical analysis of biochemical test operating characteristics in the diagnosis of pheochromocytoma.

Lindholm J, Juul S, Jorgensen JO, et al: Incidence and late prognosis of Cushing's syndrome: A population-based study. J Clin Endocrinol Metab 86:117-123, 2001.

> Documents the excess mortality associated with Cushing's syndrome.

Milliez P, Girerd X, Plouin PF, et al: Evidence for an increased rate of cardiovascular events in patients with primary aldosteronism. J Am Coll Cardiol 45:1243-1248, 2005.

> A compelling report on the adverse effects of primary aldosteronism in which affected patients are compared with controls matched for systolic blood pressure.

Minneci PC, Deans KJ, Banks SM, et al: Meta-analysis: The effect of steroids on survival and shock during sepsis depends on the dose. Ann Intern Med 141:47-56, 2004.

A useful analysis of various steroid regimens in the treatment of critically ill patients with relative adrenal insufficiency.

Neumann HP, Bausch B, McWhinney SR, et al: Germ-line mutations in nonsyndromic pheochromocytoma. N Engl J Med 346:1459-1466, 2002.

A landmark report documenting a surprisingly high rate of familial pheochromocytoma and calling attention to the significance of succinate dehydrogenase mutations.

Ng L, Libertino JM: Adrenocortical carcinoma: Diagnosis, evaluation and treatment. J Urol 169:5-11, 2003.

A multi-institutional descriptive report on this rare disease.

Nobel Lectures, Physiology or Medicine 1942-1962. Amsterdam, Elsevier, 1964.

An account of the clinical discoveries and advances in organic chemistry that led to identification, isolation, and artificial synthesis of adrenal cortical hormones. A full transcript can be found at http://nobelprize.org.

Nobel Lectures, Physiology or Medicine 1971-1980. Amsterdam, Elsevier, 1992.

Documents the formidable challenges surmounted in the identification of peptide hormones, found in such minute concentrations, and development of the radioimmunoassay necessary for their detection. A full transcript can be found at http://nobelprize.org.

Plouin PF, Duclos JM, Soppelsa F, et al: Factors associated with perioperative morbidity and mortality in patients with pheochromocytoma: Analysis of 165 operations at a single center. J Clin Endocrinol Metab 86:1480-1486, 2001.

One of the largest single-institution series on surgical management of pheochromocytoma documents the evolution in clinical care over more than 2 decades.

Welbourn RB: Early surgical history of phaeochromocytoma. Br J Surg 74:594-596, 1987.

Describes the initial achievements of American and European surgeons in the successful treatment of pheochromocytoma.

Young WF, Stanson AW, Thompson GB, et al: Role for adrenal venous sampling in primary aldosteronism. Surgery 136:1227-1235, 2004.

A large single-institution series documenting the unreliability of CT alone in localizing aldosteronomas. The discussion that follows the main text is particularly informative.

References

1. Nobel Lectures, Physiology or Medicine 1942-1962. Amsterdam, Elsevier, 1964.
2. Nobel Lectures, Physiology or Medicine 1971-1980. Amsterdam, Elsevier, 1992.
3. Mihai R, Farndon JR: Surgical embryology and anatomy of the adrenal glands. In Clark OH, Duh QY, Kebebew E (eds): Textbook of Endocrine Surgery, 2nd ed. Philadelphia, Elsevier Saunders, 2005.
4. MacGillivray DC, Khwaja K, Shickman SJ: Confluence of the right adrenal vein with the accessory right hepatic veins. A potential hazard in laparoscopic right adrenalectomy. Surg Endosc 10:1095-1096, 1996.
5. Lack EE: Tumors of the adrenal gland and extra-adrenal paraganglia. In Rosai J (ed): Atlas of Tumor Pathology, vol 19. Washington, DC, Armed Forced Institute of Pathology, 1997.
6. Stocco DM: StAR protein and the regulation of steroid hormone biosynthesis. Annu Rev Physiol 63:193-213, 2001.
7. Sapolsky RM, Romero LM, Munck AU: How do glucocorticoids influence stress responses? Integrating permissive, suppressive, stimulatory, and preparative actions. Endocr Rev 21:55-89, 2000.
8. Lenders JW, Pacak K, Walther MM, et al: Biochemical diagnosis of pheochromocytoma: Which test is best? JAMA 287:1427-1434, 2002.
9. Speiser PW, White PC: Congenital adrenal hyperplasia. N Engl J Med 349:776-788, 2003.
10. Nieman LK, Chanco Turner ML: Addison's disease. Clin Dermatol 24:276-280, 2006.
11. Ten S, New M, Maclaren N: Clinical review 130: Addison's disease 2001. J Clin Endocrinol Metab 86:2909-2922, 2001.
12. Shen WT, Kebebew E, Clark OH, et al: Selective use of steroid replacement after adrenalectomy: Lessons from 331 consecutive cases. Arch Surg 141:771-774, discussion 774-776, 2006.
13. Minneci PC, Deans KJ, Banks SM, et al: Meta-analysis: The effect of steroids on survival and shock during sepsis depends on the dose. Ann Intern Med 141:47-56, 2004.
14. de Herder WW, van der Lely AJ: Addisonian crisis and relative adrenal failure. Rev Endocr Metab Disord 4:143-147, 2003.
15. Dorin RI, Qualls CR, Crapo LM: Diagnosis of adrenal insufficiency. Ann Intern Med 139:194-204, 2003.
16. Axelrod L: Perioperative management of patients treated with glucocorticoids. Endocrinol Metab Clin North Am 32:367-383, 2003.
17. Kaplan NM: The current epidemic of primary aldosteronism: Causes and consequences. J Hypertens 22:863-869, 2004.
18. Mulatero P, Stowasser M, Loh KC, et al: Increased diagnosis of primary aldosteronism, including surgically correctable forms, in centers from five continents. J Clin Endocrinol Metab 89:1045-1050, 2004.
19. Milliez P, Girerd X, Plouin PF, et al: Evidence for an increased rate of cardiovascular events in patients with primary aldosteronism. J Am Coll Cardiol 45:1243-1248, 2005.
20. Doi SA, Abalkhail S, Al-Qudhaiby MM, et al: Optimal use and interpretation of the aldosterone renin ratio to detect aldosterone excess in hypertension. J Hum Hypertens 20:482-489, 2006.
21. Young WF, Stanson AW, Thompson GB, et al: Role for adrenal venous sampling in primary aldosteronism. Surgery 136:1227-1235, 2004.
22. Harvey A, Kline G, Pasieka JL: Adrenal venous sampling in primary hyperaldosteronism: Comparison of radiological with biochemical success and the clinical decision making with "less than ideal" testing. Surgery 140:847-853, discussion 853-855, 2006.
23. Lal G, Duh QY: Laparoscopic adrenalectomy—indications and technique. Surg Oncol 12:105-123, 2003.
24. Tan YY, Ogilvie JB, Triponez F, et al: Selective use of adrenal venous sampling in the lateralization of aldosterone-producing adenomas. World J Surg 30:879-885, discussion 886-877, 2006.
25. Lindholm J, Juul S, Jorgensen JO, et al: Incidence and late prognosis of Cushing's syndrome: A population-based study. J Clin Endocrinol Metab 86:117-123, 2001.

26. Papanicolaou DA, Mullen N, Kyrou I, et al: Nighttime salivary cortisol: A useful test for the diagnosis of Cushing's syndrome. J Clin Endocrinol Metab 87:4515-4521, 2002.

27. Rockall AG, Babar SA, Sohaib SA, et al: CT and MR imaging of the adrenal glands in ACTH-independent Cushing syndrome. Radiographics 24:435-452, 2004.

28. Newell-Price J, Bertagna X, Grossman AB, et al: Cushing's syndrome. Lancet 367:1605-1617, 2006.

29. Esposito F, Dusick JR, Cohan P, et al: Clinical review: Early morning cortisol levels as a predictor of remission after transsphenoidal surgery for Cushing's disease. J Clin Endocrinol Metab 91:7-13, 2006.

30. Findling JW, Raff H: Cushing's syndrome: Important issues in diagnosis and management. J Clin Endocrinol Metab 91:3746-3753, 2006.

31. Tauchmanova L, Rossi R, Biondi B, et al: Patients with subclinical Cushing's syndrome due to adrenal adenoma have increased cardiovascular risk. J Clin Endocrinol Metab 87:4872-4878, 2002.

32. Ng L, Libertino JM: Adrenocortical carcinoma: Diagnosis, evaluation and treatment. J Urol 169:5-11, 2003.

33. Icard P, Goudet P, Charpenay C, et al: Adrenocortical carcinomas: Surgical trends and results of a 253-patient series from the French Association of Endocrine Surgeons study group. World J Surg 25:891-897, 2001.

34. Dackiw AP, Lee JE, Gagel RF, et al: Adrenal cortical carcinoma. World J Surg 25:914-926, 2001.

35. Welbourn RB: Early surgical history of phaeochromocytoma. Br J Surg 74:594-596, 1987.

36. Pacak K, Linehan WM, Eisenhofer G, et al: Recent advances in genetics, diagnosis, localization, and treatment of pheochromocytoma. Ann Intern Med 134:315-329, 2001.

37. Dluhy RG: Pheochromocytoma—death of an axiom. N Engl J Med 346:1486-1488, 2002.

38. Kudva YC, Sawka AM, Young WF Jr: Clinical review 164: The laboratory diagnosis of adrenal pheochromocytoma: The Mayo Clinic experience. J Clin Endocrinol Metab 88:4533-4539, 2003.

39. Ilias I, Pacak K: Current approaches and recommended algorithm for the diagnostic localization of pheochromocytoma. J Clin Endocrinol Metab 89:479-491, 2004.

40. Gifford RW Jr, Kvale WF, Maher FT, et al: Clinical features, diagnosis and treatment of pheochromocytoma: A review of 76 cases. Mayo Clin Proc 39:281-302, 1964.

41. Plouin PF, Duclos JM, Soppelsa F, et al: Factors associated with perioperative morbidity and mortality in patients with pheochromocytoma: Analysis of 165 operations at a single center. J Clin Endocrinol Metab 86:1480-1486, 2001.

42. Neumann HP, Bausch B, McWhinney SR, et al: Germ-line mutations in nonsyndromic pheochromocytoma. N Engl J Med 346:1459-1466, 2002.

43. Benn DE, Gimenez-Roqueplo AP, Reilly JR, et al: Clinical presentation and penetrance of pheochromocytoma/paraganglioma syndromes. J Clin Endocrinol Metab 91:827-836, 2006.

44. Edstrom Elder E, Hjelm Skog AL, Hoog A, et al: The management of benign and malignant pheochromocytoma and abdominal paraganglioma. Eur J Surg Oncol 29:278-283, 2003.

45. Grumbach MM, Biller BM, Braunstein GD, et al: Management of the clinically inapparent adrenal mass ("incidentaloma"). Ann Intern Med 138:424-429, 2003.

46. Sturgeon C, Kebebew E: Laparoscopic adrenalectomy for malignancy. Surg Clin North Am 84:755-774, 2004.

47. Lam KY, Lo CY: Metastatic tumours of the adrenal glands: A 30-year experience in a teaching hospital. Clin Endocrinol (Oxf) 56:95-101, 2002.

48. Sebag F, Calzolari F, Harding J, et al: Isolated adrenal metastasis: The role of laparoscopic surgery. World J Surg 30:888-892, 2006.

49. Shen WT, Kebebew E, Clark OH, et al: Reasons for conversion from laparoscopic to open or hand-assisted adrenalectomy: Review of 261 laparoscopic adrenalectomies from 1993 to 2003. World J Surg 28:1176-1179, 2004.

CHAPTER 40

The Multiple Endocrine Neoplasia Syndromes

Terry C. Lairmore, MD   and   Jeffrey F. Moley, MD

> Multiple Endocrine Neoplasia Type 1
> Multiple Endocrine Neoplasia Type 2 Syndromes

Genetic changes in a tumor suppressor gene and a proto-oncogene result in the multiple endocrine neoplasia (MEN) types 1 and 2 syndromes, respectively. These hereditary cancer syndromes are characterized by neoplastic transformation in multiple target endocrine tissues, as well as pathologic involvement of nonendocrine tissues. The associated endocrine tumors may be benign or malignant and may develop either synchronously or metachronously. Within an affected endocrine target tissue, a diffuse preneoplastic hyperplasia typically precedes the development of microscopic invasion or grossly evident multifocal carcinoma. In the MEN syndromes, the genetic predisposition to multiple endocrine neoplasms with malignant potential is conferred on otherwise healthy, young individuals. Importantly, the recent discovery of the specific genetic basis for the MEN 1 and 2 syndromes has allowed the development of strategies for direct genetic testing and early surgical intervention. Early thyroidectomy is indicated for patients with a genetic diagnosis of MEN 2, with the aim of preventing the subsequent development of regional or distant medullary thyroid carcinoma (MTC) metastases. The optimal early surgical intervention to prevent metastatic spread of the potentially malignant neuroendocrine tumors (NETs) in patients with a genetic diagnosis of MEN 1 is currently more controversial.

The MEN syndromes are characterized by differing patterns of involvement. In its full expression, MEN 1 is characterized by the development of multiple parathyroid tumors, NETs of the pancreas and duodenum, adenomas of the anterior pituitary gland, foregut and thymic carcinoids, and other associated neoplasms. The MEN 2A syndrome is characterized by the development of MTC, pheochromocytomas, and parathyroid tumors, whereas MEN 2B consists of MTC, pheochromocytomas, mucosal neuromas, skeletal abnormalities, ganglioneuromatosis of the gastrointestinal tract, and a distinctive *marfanoid habitus*.

MULTIPLE ENDOCRINE NEOPLASIA TYPE 1

Genetic Studies and Pathogenesis

The *MEN1* gene was originally mapped to chromosome 11q13 by a combination of genetic linkage studies and tumor deletion mapping[1] and was ultimately identified by positional cloning in 1997.[2] *MEN1* is a putative tumor suppressor gene, whose protein product is presumed to function as a negative influence or brake on cellular growth and proliferation, such that complete elimination of its function would be expected to result in unregulated cell growth or neoplastic transformation. According to the "two-hit" model, the first event is a mutation inherited in the germline that confers susceptibility to neoplastic change in the involved tissues. Elimination of the remaining functional copy of the gene in a single cell through a chance somatic mutational event, or *second hit* (e.g., a gene deletion), results in clonal expansion and cancer development. The occurrence of individual second hits in several target organ cells explains the multifocal involvement characteristically observed in affected endocrine tissues. Somatic mutations in the *MEN1* gene occur frequently in sporadic parathyroid adenomas, insulinomas and gastrinomas, pituitary tumors, and bronchial carcinoids, indicating that loss of the *MEN1* gene contributes to the development of a subset of nonhereditary endocrine tumors.

The *MEN1* gene consists of 10 exons spanning 9 kb of genomic DNA and encodes a 610–amino acid protein product termed *menin*.[2] Menin is ubiquitously expressed in both endocrine and nonendocrine tissues. Other than the presence of nuclear localization signals, database analysis of the menin protein sequence reveals no significant homology to other known protein families. The menin protein sequence is highly conserved evolutionarily, with the murine *Men1* gene demonstrating 98% homology. Knockout of both *Men1* alleles in mice results in embryonic lethality,[3] suggesting that menin is essential for early development and may have a broader role in the regulation of cell growth that is not limited to the endocrine tissues affected in MEN 1. Heterozygous *Men1*[+/−] mice demonstrate somatic loss of the wild type *Men1* allele in tumors[3] and develop a constellation of endocrine tumors remarkably similar to the human MEN 1 syndrome.

Menin is predominately a nuclear protein that binds to JunD, a member of the AP-1 transcription factor family, and represses JunD-mediated transcription. In addition, menin has been shown to physically interact with a diverse variety of other proteins that comprise transcription factors, DNA processing factors, DNA repair proteins, and cytoskeletal proteins (Smad3, NF-κB, nm23, Pem, FANCD2, RPA2, ASK, and others).[4,5] The combination of findings from all current studies has not yielded a clear picture of the mechanisms of menin's tumor suppressor activity or the specific role for menin in endocrine tumorigenesis, although its diverse interactions suggest possible pivotal roles in transcriptional regulation, DNA processing and repair, and cytoskeletal integrity.

Overexpression of menin has been shown to diminish the tumorigenic phenotype of Ras-transformed NIH-3T3 cells, consistent with its putative tumor suppressor function. In addition, studies have suggested a possible role for menin in repressing telomerase activity in somatic cells, perhaps explaining in part its tumor suppressor properties. Menin has most recently been shown to regulate transcription in differentiated cells by associating with and modulating the histone methyltransferase activity of a nuclear protein complex to activate specific gene expression, including the cyclin-dependent kinase (CDK) inhibitors $p27^{Kip1}$ and $p18^{Ink4c}$,[6,7] as well as other cell cycle regulators. Several recent studies suggest that by promoting histone modifications within specific gene promotors, menin promotes the maintenance of transcription of critical cell cycle regulators essential for normal endocrine cell growth control. These findings suggest that menin may mediate its tumor suppressor action by regulating histone methylation in promoters of *HOX* genes and $p18^{Ink4c}$, $p27^{Kip1}$, and possibly other CDK inhibitors.

The MLL (mixed-lineage leukemia) protein is a histone methyltransferase mutated in subsets of acute leukemia. Evidence has been provided that the menin tumor suppressor protein is an essential oncogenic cofactor for MLL-associated leukemogenesis.[8,9] There is an unexpected paradox in these interactions between menin, the protein product of a tumor suppressor gene, and MLL, the product of a proto-oncogene. In hematopoietic cells, menin cooperates (acts as an essential oncogenic cofactor) with mutant MLL to result in leukemogenesis. In neuroendocrine cells, wild-type menin interacts with MLL to promote expression of antiproliferative (*p18, p27*) CDK inhibitors, possibly representing a central role in

menin's tumor suppressor activity. Using genome-wide chromatin immunoprecipitation coupled with microarray analysis, it has also been recently demonstrated that menin frequently colocalizes with a protein complex that modifies chromatin structure, and may also bind to many other promotors by an alternative mechanism.[10] Loss of the murine *Men1* tumor suppressor in vitro in mouse embryonic fibroblasts accelerates cell cycle G_0/G_1- to S-phase transition and, in vivo in a model in which floxed *Men1* alleles can be excised in a temporally controlled manner, directly enhances pancreatic islet cell proliferation.[11] Despite these recent findings, the specific role of menin as a tumor suppressor is complex and has not been completely elucidated.

More than 300 independent mutations have been described in the *MEN1* gene (reviewed in reference 12). Therefore, there are almost as many unique mutations as there are genetically independent families. The diverse array of *MEN1* mutations that has been reported includes nonsense, missense, frameshift, deletions, and RNA splicing defects. The mutations are scattered throughout the coding sequence and intron-exon junctions of the gene (Fig. 40-1). About two thirds of the reported mutations in the *MEN1* gene result in premature termination of translation and truncation of the C-terminal portion of the menin protein. No clear genotype-phenotype correlation has been established for MEN 1, although phenotypic variants (isolated hyperparathyroidism, frequent prolactinomas) have been described.

Genetic testing is currently available in selected centers with certain limitations. The detection of a disease-associated mutation in a family with a previously defined specific genetic change is straightforward. However, in a novel family for which the specific mutation is not known in advance, a comprehensive search of the coding sequence and intron-exon junctions is necessary to look for all possible mutations. Formal genetic counseling and informed consent, including disclosures relevant to privacy of medical information and the potential impact of the genetic information on treatment, are essential to a comprehensive program of genetic testing.

Clinical Features and Management

The principal feature that develops in essentially all individuals inheriting an *MEN1* mutation is hypercalcemia due to multiglandular parathyroid tumors. Patients may also develop NETs of the pancreas and duodenum, bronchial and thymic carcinoids, and adenomas of the anterior pituitary. In addition, bronchial and thymic carcinoids, thyroid nodules, adrenocortical nodular hyperplasia, lipomas, ependymomas, and cutaneous angiofibromas occur with increased frequency in patients with MEN 1. Clinically, *MEN 1* is defined as the occurrence of neoplasms in at least two target endocrine tissues (parathyroid, endocrine pancreas, pituitary) in an individual, and *familial MEN 1* is defined as the additional occurrence of at least one tumor type in a first-degree relative.

Males and females are affected equally by MEN 1, as predicted by the autosomal dominant inheritance pattern. MEN 1 has been described in many geographic regions

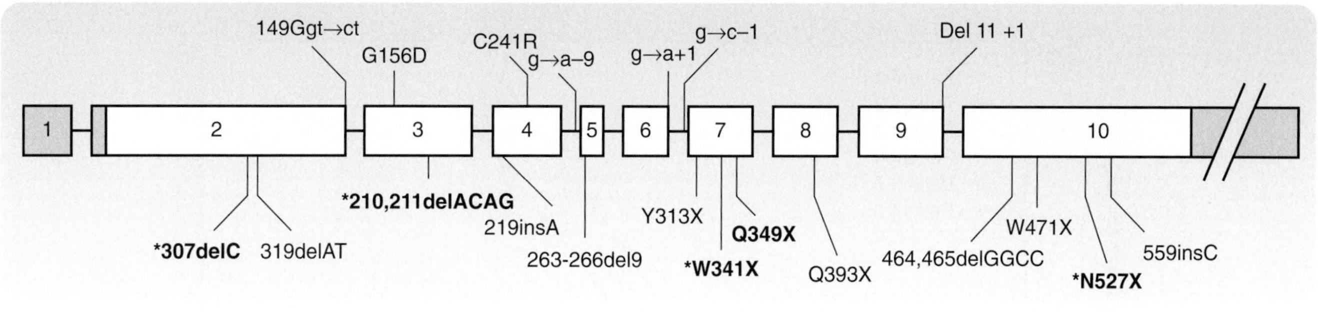

GERMLINE *MEN1* MUTATIONS

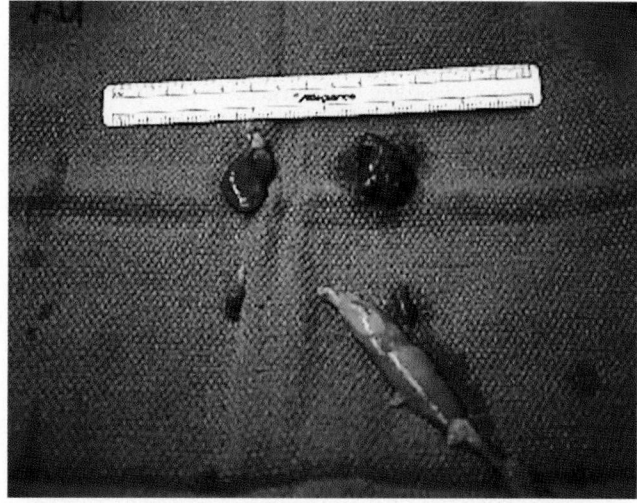

Figure 40-1 Germline mutations in the *MEN1* gene in a set of 25 independent kindreds. The mutations are distributed throughout the nine coding exons of the gene. The genetic alterations may include missense, nonsense, frame-shift, and RNA-splicing defects that may occur anywhere throughout the coding exons and immediately flanking intron sequences. Five splicing defects and two missense mutations are depicted above the *MEN1* gene, and seven nonsense and six frameshift mutations are depicted below the *MEN1* gene. (From Mutch MG, Dilley WG, Sanjurjo F, et al: Germline mutations in the multiple endocrine neoplasia type 1 gene: Evidence for frequent splicing defects. Hum Mutat 13:175-185, 1999.)

and in many ethnic groups, and no racial predilection has been demonstrated. The MEN 1 trait is transmitted with essentially 100% penetrance, but with variable expressivity, such that each affected person may exhibit some, but not necessarily all, of the components of the syndrome. The most common abnormality in MEN 1 is multiple parathyroid tumors, which eventually develop in 98% to 100% of affected individuals. Duodenopancreatic NETs (which carry a malignant potential) occur in about 30% to 80% of patients, whereas pituitary tumors become clinically evident in about 15% to 50% of affected patients. At autopsy, pathologic involvement in all three endocrine tissues has been described in essentially all patients. When compared with sporadic endocrine tumors, the endocrine tumors arising in association with the familial MEN 1 syndrome are characterized by an earlier age of onset, multifocal involvement within a target endocrine tissue, and the development of concurrent neoplasms in multiple endocrine tissues.

The clinical manifestations of patients with MEN 1 depend on the endocrine tissue involved, the specific hormone overproduced, or the local mass effect and malignant progression of the neoplasm. Previously, complications related to hormone excess, such as severe ulcer disease or hypoglycemia, were the most frequent presenting complaints. Currently, the principal cause of mortality in patients with MEN 1 is malignant progression of duodenopancreatic neuroendocrine cancers, or intrathoracic malignant carcinoids.

Parathyroid Glands

The most common endocrine abnormality (>98% of affected individuals) in MEN 1 is multiglandular parathyroid tumors. The parathyroid tumors in MEN 1 are clonal, resulting from inactivation of both alleles of the *MEN1* tumor suppressor gene by two separate events, and are therefore multiple adenomas from a strict genetic standpoint.[13] In contrast, fewer than 15% of patients with sporadic primary hyperparathyroidism have multiglandular involvement. The typical enlargement of parathyroid

Figure 40-2 Photograph of four parathyroid glands resected from a patient with MEN 1 syndrome, arranged according to location within the neck. Note the asymmetric involvement of parathyroid tumors with two markedly enlarged upper glands, and more modestly enlarged lower glands. The left inferior parathyroid was located within the cranial horn of the thymus.

glands in MEN 1 patients is asymmetric (Fig. 40-2) at any one time of intervention.[13]

Hypercalcemia is usually the first biochemical abnormality detected in patients with MEN 1 and may precede the clinical onset of a pancreatic NET or pituitary neoplasm by several years. Asymptomatic hypercalcemia may be present in many patients over a long period of observation. Renal lithiasis and skeletal complications of hyperparathyroidism occur but are uncommon. In general, hyperparathyroidism in patients with MEN 1 has an earlier age of onset and usually causes a milder hypercalcemia than that observed in primary sporadic hyperparathyroidism. Demonstrating an elevated serum calcium level in association with an inappropriately elevated parathyroid hormone (PTH) level makes the diagnosis.

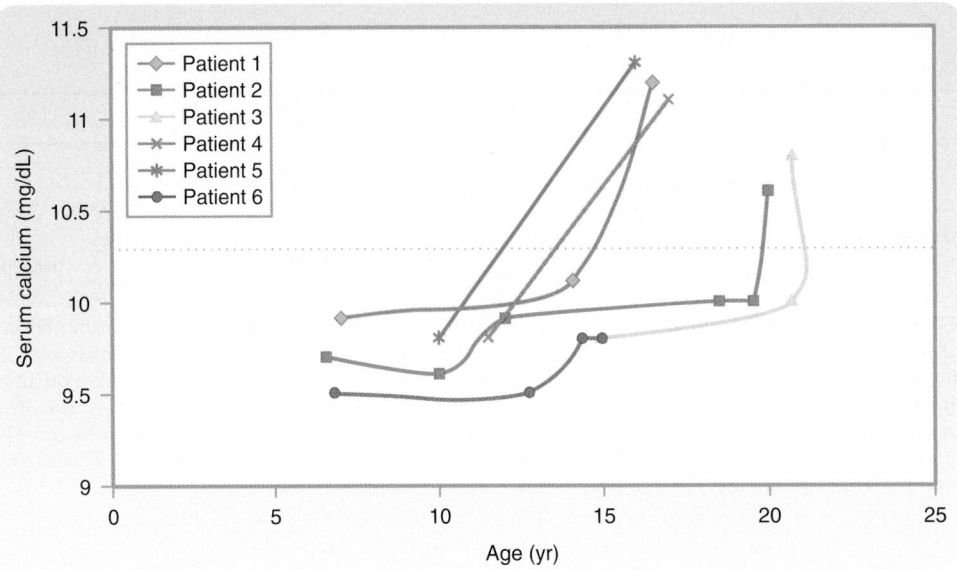

SERUM CALCIUM LEVELS VERSUS AGE IN GENETICALLY POSITIVE PATIENTS

Figure 40-3 Serum calcium levels versus age in six patients genetically positive for MEN 1. The data were obtained prospectively based on genetic diagnosis. Each patient's curve is represented by a different color and data point symbol according to the legend in the upper left corner. Serum calcium level (mg/dL) is plotted as a function of age (yr). The upper limit of normal for calcium is indicated by the *dotted line*. In this selected subset of genetically positive patients followed prospectively, a rapid rise in calcium levels is evident between the ages of 10 and **15 years.** (From Lairmore TC, Piersall LD, DeBenedetti MK, et al: Clinical genetic testing and early surgical intervention in patients with multiple endocrine neoplasia type 1 [MEN1]. Ann Surg 239:637-647, 2004.)

Patients with MEN 1 typically have a markedly elevated 24-hour urine calcium excretion. When prospective biochemical screening of known genetically positive individuals is performed, the onset of hypercalcemia in patients with an *MEN1* mutation occurs as early as 11 to 14 years of age[14] (Fig. 40-3).

The aim of surgical treatment for hyperparathyroidism in patients with MEN 1 is to achieve the lowest incidence of recurrent hypercalcemia while minimizing the complication of permanent hypoparathyroidism. Because patients with MEN 1 develop multiglandular disease, there is a significantly higher rate of recurrent or persistent hyperparathyroidism after parathyroidectomy when compared with the results for the treatment of sporadic parathyroid adenomas. Two currently accepted surgical procedures for patients with MEN 1 are either three-and-one-half gland (subtotal) parathyroidectomy leaving the parathyroid tissue remnant in situ in the neck, or total four-gland parathyroidectomy with intramuscular autotransplantation of parathyroid tissue into the forearm muscle. A transcervical, partial thymectomy also needs to be performed owing to the possibility of an ectopic or supernumerary parathyroid gland within the cranial horns of the thymus. In general, preoperative imaging tests are not necessary for patients with MEN 1 undergoing initial neck exploration because appropriate treatment requires bilateral neck exploration and identification of all four glands. Noninvasive imaging tests, such as parathyroid nuclear medicine (sestamibi) scanning and ultrasound, may be useful for parathyroid localization before reoperative surgery.

Debate continues regarding the optimal surgical procedure for hyperparathyroidism in patients with MEN 1. The incidence of recurrent hyperparathyroidism following any surgical treatment for the multiglandular disease in MEN 1 is about 30% to 40% 5 years after operation, reflecting the genetic first-hit predisposition in every parathyroid cell. A potential advantage of total parathyroidectomy and heterotopic autotransplantation to the forearm is the ability to manage recurrent hyperparathyroidism, should it develop, by excision of a portion of the grafted parathyroid tissue under local anesthesia (obviating the morbidity of repeat neck exploration). Subtotal resection is believed by many authors to achieve equivalent results without a purported higher risk for permanent hypocalcemia from autograft failure.[15,16] Currently, both treatments appear to provide essentially equivalent results, and the answer to this question awaits a randomized, prospective clinical trial. Delayed transplantation of cryopreserved autologous parathyroid tissue can salvage a proportion of patients with permanent postoperative hypocalcemia following either procedure. In a recent study,[17] about 60% of delayed, cryopreserved parathyroid autografts showed evidence of graft function based on venous PTH gradients between the grafted and nongrafted arms, and 40% of autografts achieved full competency off supplements.

Pancreas and Duodenum

The second most frequent component of MEN 1 is the development of NETs of the duodenum or pancreas. Depending on the method of study, 30% to 80% of

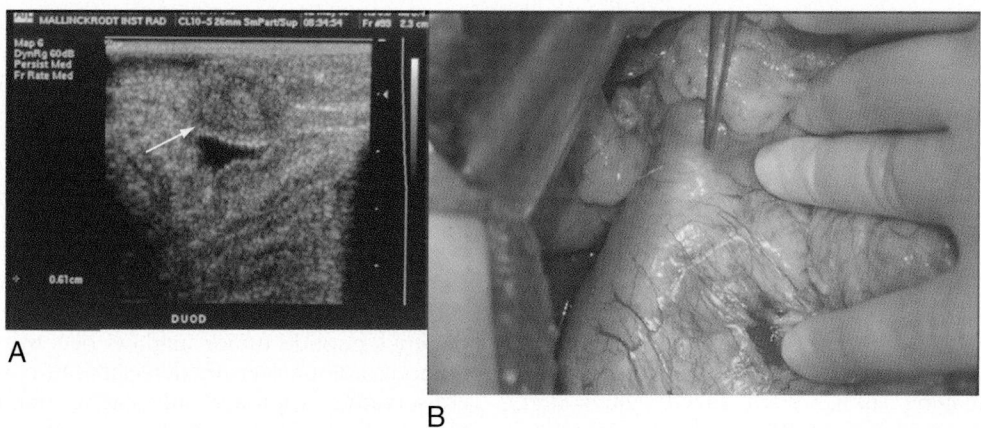

Figure 40-4 Gastrinoma in the duodenal wall from patient with MEN 1. **A,** An image from intraoperative ultrasound demonstrating a circumscribed, hypoechoic tumor in the submucosa of the duodenal wall, shown just superior to the duodenal lumen. **B,** The gross appearance of the duodenal wall tumor from the serosal surface is demonstrated.

patients with MEN 1 develop clinically evident tumors. These tumors, along with the intrathoracic carcinoids, carry a significant malignant potential and result in the majority of the MEN 1 disease-related morbidity and mortality. The pathologic change is typically multifocal, and diffuse islet cell hyperplasia and microadenoma formation may be present in areas of the pancreas distant from grossly evident tumor. Gastrinomas frequently occur within the wall of the duodenum or in extrapancreatic sites. The pancreaticoduodenal tumors in patients with MEN 1 cause symptoms due to either hormone oversecretion or the mass effects from tumor growth itself and are characterized by a high malignant potential.

Pancreatic NETs that are nonfunctioning or that secrete pancreatic polypeptide are probably the most frequent NETs that occur in patients with MEN 1. The most common *functional* NET in patients with MEN 1 is gastrinoma. The presenting signs and symptoms in patients with hypergastrinemia, or the Zollinger-Ellison syndrome (ZES), include epigastric pain, reflux esophagitis, secretory diarrhea, and weight loss. In the current era with highly effective proton pump inhibitors for medical therapy, active peptic ulcer disease is present in less than 20% of patients at the time of diagnosis. Patients may infrequently present with a severe ulcer diathesis as well as stricture or perforation of the esophagus due to severe reflux esophagitis. Gastrinoma is diagnosed by the documentation of gastric acid hypersecretion (>15 mEq/L in patients without operation, or >5 mEq/L in patients with prior ulcer surgery), associated with elevated fasting levels of serum gastrin (>100 pg/mL). The diagnosis can be confirmed by an abnormal secretin test.

Gastrinomas that develop in patients with MEN 1 are usually malignant (~80%), as indicated by the presence of regional lymph node or distant metastases. Gastrinomas were previously thought to be located predominantly in the head of the pancreas within the gastrinoma triangle. More recent data suggest that gastrinomas in patients with MEN 1 occur most frequently within the wall of the duodenum[18,19] (Fig. 40-4). Owing to the small size of these neoplasms, the primary gastrinoma may not be localized preoperatively by computed tomography (CT) scanning or angiography. Endoscopic ultrasound has been utilized successfully to localize gastrinomas within the wall of the duodenum or head of the pancreas. There is controversy about the development of primary gastrinoma within lymph nodes. Although occasional patients have been biochemically cured after resection of gastrinoma within lymph nodes,[20] it is unclear whether an occult gastrinoma primary was missed within the pancreas or wall of the duodenum.

The value of surgical resection for intended cure of gastrinoma in patients with MEN 1 is controversial. Although most evidence indicates that patients with ZES and MEN 1 rarely demonstrate long-term biochemical cure after operation,[21,22] localized resection of a potentially malignant NET is indicated in an attempt to control the tumoral process and prevent subsequent malignant dissemination. The recognition that primary gastrinomas occur frequently in the duodenal wall, combined with efforts to perform an extensive regional lymphadenectomy or even pancreaticoduodenectomy, may improve the success rate of surgery for ZES in the setting of MEN 1. Newer strategies, including rapid intraoperative gastrin determinations, are also being employed[23] in the surgical management of gastrinoma. Total gastrectomy is rarely indicated for patients with gastrinoma because medical therapy effectively prevents most of the symptoms or complications resulting from the acid hypersecretion. The availability of proton pump inhibitors allows effective medical therapy for patients with unresectable gastrinoma or extensive metastatic disease. However, careful observation of the stomach by repeated endoscopy is necessary because long-term administration of proton pump inhibitors to patients with MEN 1 and ZES has been associated with the development of gastric carcinoid tumors.[24] Patients with primary hyperparathyroidism undergo parathyroidectomy because normalization of the serum calcium level improves the ZES.

The second most common clinically evident pancreatic neuroendocrine neoplasm in patients with MEN 1 is insulinoma. These tumors are usually small (<2 cm) and occur with even distribution throughout the pancreas. Patients typically present with recurrent symptoms of neuroglycopenia: sweating, dizziness, confusion, or syncope. Documenting symptomatic hypoglycemia in association with inappropriately elevated plasma levels of insulin and C-peptide during a supervised 72-hour fast makes the diagnosis of insulinoma. Insulinomas may be occult and are infrequently localized by conventional preoperative imaging studies such as CT, ultrasound, magnetic resonance imaging (MRI), or angiography.

There is no ideal medical therapy for insulinoma; therefore, the preferred treatment is accurate localization and surgical resection of the functioning tumor to correct life-threatening hyperinsulinemia. Patients with MEN 1 characteristically develop multiple NETs, a fact that may complicate identification of the specific functional tumor responsible for the hyperinsulinism. Preoperative regional localization of the functioning tumor within the pancreas may be provided by selective catheterization of the arteries supplying the pancreas, followed by injection of an insulin secretagogue (calcium gluconate) and measurement of insulin gradients in the hepatic veins.[25] The operative approach includes complete mobilization of the pancreas and careful examination of the gland by inspection and palpation. Intraoperative ultrasound is essential for the identification of small tumors, especially within the pancreatic head or uncinate process. Small, benign insulinomas are amenable to enucleation. Partial pancreatectomy may be required for multiple or potentially malignant tumors.[26] In the event the insulinoma is not identified despite an exhaustive intraoperative search, blind subtotal pancreatectomy is not recommended.

About 10% of insulinomas occurring in patients with MEN 1 are malignant. Patients with malignant insulinoma and disseminated metastases may respond to treatment with streptozocin, and some control of hypoglycemia may be achieved by the administration of either diazoxide or octreotide.

Other functional NETs of the pancreas, such as glucagonoma, somatostatinoma, and tumors secreting vasoactive intestinal peptide or pancreatic polypeptide, occur rarely in association with MEN 1.

Controversy exists regarding the optimal timing and most appropriate operation to perform for NETs of the pancreas and duodenum in patients with MEN 1. The controversy reflects uncertainty in the natural history of small, potentially benign or nonfunctional tumors, which must be weighed against the risks of early and repeat major pancreatic interventions carrying significant risk for morbidity. Some are reluctant to advocate routine or early pancreatic exploration in young, otherwise healthy patients for small nonfunctional tumors, which are potentially clinically insignificant. On the other hand, these tumors have a malignant potential, and delay in diagnosis and effective treatment carries the risk for local or distant metastasis. It is obviously desirable to intervene early to prevent malignant dissemination, while minimizing morbidity and mortality (from either cancer or surgery). Complicating factors include the lack of genotype-phenotype correlation in MEN 1 (that might otherwise allow genetic stratification of those at higher risk for malignant progression) and failure of recent studies to identify a clear relationship between size of the tumor and risk for regional lymph node or distant metastases.[27]

The spectrum of clinical strategies proposed ranges from the most aggressive approach consisting of early surgical exploration and resection of tumors when the patient's peptide tumor markers become elevated (even without radiographically detectable tumors)[28] to the most conservative approach advocating operation only for tumors exceeding about 1 cm in size on radiographic imaging or demonstrating hormone hyperfunction.[26,29,30] The malignant potential of these neoplasms is clear, with up to 50% of patients eventually developing regional lymph node or distant metastases.[26,27] Many groups now recommend early operation and excision of these tumors to prevent malignant progression.[23,26,27,29] One recent, large retrospective study suggested improved overall survival in patients undergoing operation, especially younger patients with localized tumors, and in those with hormonally functional tumors.[27] The operative strategy for NET in patients with MEN 1 must be aimed at extirpation of all grossly evident tumors with preservation of pancreatic exocrine and endocrine function and avoiding excessive operative morbidity. These factors are complex and must be individualized to the patient.

Pituitary Gland

Adenomas of the anterior pituitary gland occur in a variable proportion of patients with MEN 1. The most frequent pituitary tumor in patients with MEN 1 is a prolactinoma. Pituitary tumors cause symptoms either by hypersecretion of hormones or by compression of adjacent structures. Large adenomas may cause visual field defects by pressure on the optic chiasm, or manifestations of hypopituitarism through compression of the adjacent normal gland. Prolactin-secreting tumors result in amenorrhea and galactorrhea in women or hypogonadism in men. MEN 1 patients with pituitary tumors may exhibit acromegaly resulting from growth hormone overproduction or Cushing's disease due to an adrenocorticotropic hormone–producing pituitary tumor.

Medical treatment with a dopamine agonist such as bromocriptine or cabergoline is effective in controlling the hyperprolactinemia in most patients. Trans-sphenoidal pituitary microsurgery and radiation therapy are indicated infrequently for rapidly enlarging macroadenomas that are unresponsive to medical therapy or result in local compressive symptoms owing to their mass effect.

Other Tumors

Bronchial and thymic carcinoids, benign thyroid tumors, benign and malignant adrenocortical tumors, lipomas, ependymomas of the central nervous system, and facial cutaneous angiofibromas and collagenomas occur with increased frequency in patients with MEN 1.

Table 40-1 Clinical Features of Sporadic MTC, MEN 2A, MEN 2B, and FMTC

CLINICAL SETTING	FEATURES OF MTC	INHERITANCE PATTERN	ASSOCIATED ABNORMALITIES	GENETIC DEFECT
Sporadic MTC	Unifocal	None	None	Somatic *RET* mutations in >20% of tumors
MEN 2A	Multifocal, bilateral	Autosomal dominant	Pheochromocytomas, hyperparathyroidism	Germline missense mutations in extracellular cysteine codons of *RET*
MEN 2B	Multifocal, bilateral	Autosomal dominant	Pheochromocytomas, mucosal neuromas, megacolon, skeletal abnormalities	Germline missense mutation in tyrosine kinase domain of *RET*
FMTC	Multifocal, bilateral	Autosomal dominant	None	Germline missense mutations in extracellular or intracellular cysteine codons of *RET*

FMTC, familial non-MEN medullary thyroid carcinoma; MEN, multiple endocrine neoplasia; MTC; medullary thyroid carcinoma.
Adapted from Moley JF, Lairmore TC, Phay JE: Hereditary endocrinopathies. Curr Probl Surg 36:653-764, 1999.

MULTIPLE ENDOCRINE NEOPLASIA TYPE 2 SYNDROMES

Epidemiology and Clinical Features

The MEN 2 syndromes include MEN 2A, MEN 2B, and familial non-MEN medullary thyroid carcinoma (FMTC). These autosomal dominant–inherited syndromes are caused by germline mutations in the *RET* gene on chromosome 10.[31] The hallmark of these syndromes is MTC, which is multifocal and bilateral and occurs at a young age. In patients affected by MEN 2A, MEN 2B, or FMTC, there is complete penetrance of MTC; all persons who inherit the disease allele develop MTC. Other features of the syndromes are variably expressed, with incomplete penetrance. These features are summarized in Table 40-1.

Twenty-five percent of all MTC cases are hereditary and occur in the setting of MEN 2A, MEN 2B, or FMTC. In MEN 2A, patients develop multifocal, bilateral MTC, associated with C-cell hyperplasia. About 42% of affected patients develop pheochromocytomas, which may also be multifocal and bilateral and are associated with adrenal medullary hyperplasia. Hyperparathyroidism develops in 10% to 35% of patients and is due to hyperplasia, which may be asymmetrical, with one or more glands becoming enlarged. Cutaneous lichen amyloidosis has been described in some patients with MEN 2A. In this entity, macular amyloidosis presents as brownish plaques of multiple tiny papules, usually in the interscapular area. Microscopically, these lesions demonstrate hyperplastic epidermis, acanthosis, lymphocytic infiltrate, and amyloid goblets. Lastly, Hirschsprung's disease is infrequently associated with MEN 2A.[31] This disease is characterized by absence of autonomic ganglion cells within the distal colonic parasympathetic plexus, resulting in obstruction and megacolon.

In MEN 2B, as in MEN 2A, all patients develop MTC. All MEN 2B individuals have mucosal neuromas, and 40% to 50% of patients develop pheochromocytomas. MEN 2B patients do not develop hyperparathyroidism. MTC in MEN 2B presents at a very young age (in infancy) and appears to be the most aggressive form of hereditary MTC. Once it presents clinically, MTC in patients with MEN 2B is rarely curable.[32] These patients often have a distinct physical appearance with a prominent mid-upper lip, everted eyebrows, multiple tongue nodules, and marfanoid body habitus, with long limbs (Fig. 40-5). The mucosal neuromas are un-encapsulated, thickened proliferations of nerves that occur principally on the lips and tongue but can also be found on the gingiva, buccal mucosa, nasal mucosa, vocal cords, and conjunctiva. MEN 2B patients also develop ganglioneuromas of the intestine in the submucosal and myenteric plexus. All MEN 2B patients have a megacolon and usually have chronic bowel problems. Intestinal dysfunction may manifest early in life with poor feeding, failure to thrive, constipation, or pseudo-obstruction. Adults with this disorder may have dysphagia from esophageal dysmotility. Rarely, a patient can present with toxic megacolon. MEN 2B patients, however, do not develop Hirschsprung's disease, as do some patients with MEN 2A.

FMTC is characterized by the occurrence of MTC without any other endocrinopathies. MTC in these patients has a later age of onset and a more indolent clinical course than MTC in patients with MEN 2A and MEN 2B. Occasional patients with FMTC never manifest clinical evidence of MTC (symptoms or a palpable neck mass), although biochemical testing and histologic evaluation of the thyroid demonstrates MTC.

Genetics

MEN 2 is inherited in an autosomal dominant mendelian fashion. Mutations in the *RET* proto-oncogene are responsible for MEN 2A, MEN 2B, and FMTC. This gene encodes a transmembrane protein tyrosine kinase. The mutations that cause the MEN 2 syndromes are activating, gain-of-function mutations that cause constitutive activation of the protein. This is unusual among hereditary cancer syndromes, which are most often caused by loss-of-function mutations in the predisposition gene (e.g., familial polyposis, *BRCA1*- and *BRCA2*-associated breast cancer, von Hippel-Lindau disease, and MEN 1). More than 30 missense mutations have been described in patients

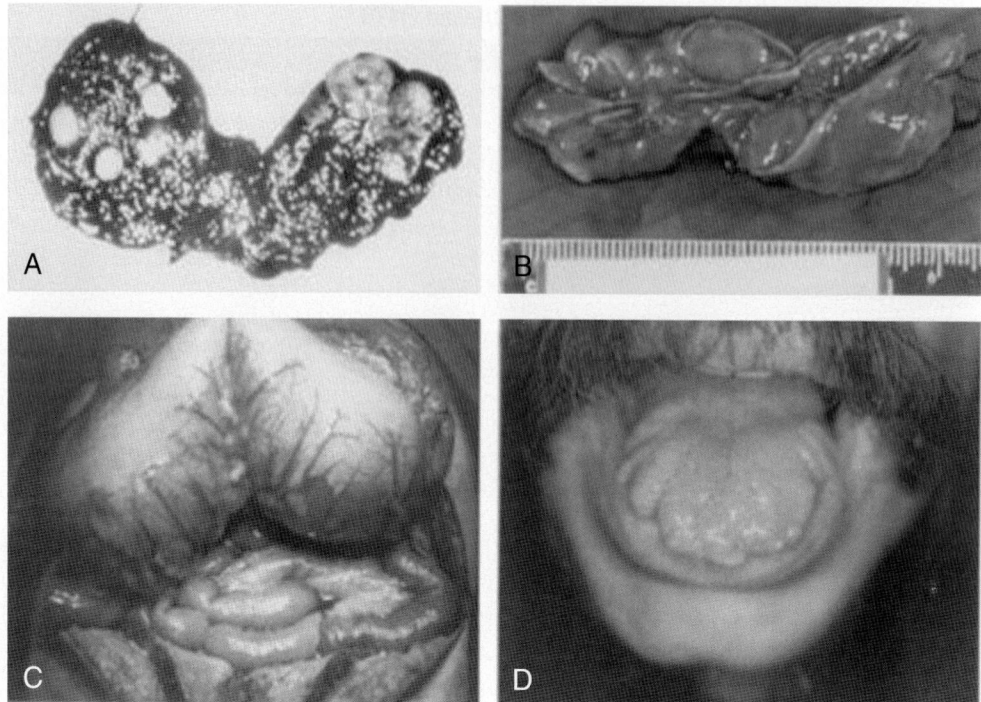

Figure 40-5 Features of patients with hereditary medullary thyroid carcinoma (MTC). **A,** Bisected thyroid gland from a patient with MEN 2A showing multicentric, bilateral foci of MTC. **B,** Adrenalectomy specimen from patient with MEN 2B demonstrating pheochromocytoma. **C,** Megacolon in patient with MEN 2B. **D,** Midface and tongue of patient with MEN 2B showing characteristic tongue notching secondary to plexiform neuromas. (**A,** Courtesy of Dr. S. A. Wells. **B-D,** Courtesy of Dr. R. Thompson. From Moley JF: Medullary thyroid cancer. In Clark OH, Duh Q-Y [eds]: Textbook of Endocrine Surgery. Philadelphia, WB Saunders, 1997.)

Table 40-2   Missense Mutations in MEN 2 Syndromes

SYNDROME	EXON	INVOLVED CODON
MEN 2A	11	635, 637
MEN 2A and FMTC	10	609, 611, 618, 620
	11	630, 634*
	13	790, 791
	14	804
	15	891
FMTC	8	532, 533
	10	600, 603, 606
	11	649
	13	768, 778, 781
	14	806, 852, 844†
	16	912
MEN 2B	14	V804M+Y806C, V804M+S904C
	15	883
	16	918‡

RET mutations in hereditary medullary thyroid carcinoma.
†Clinical features not yet characterized.
‡Most common MEN 2B mutation.
FMTC, familial non-MEN medullary thyroid carcinoma; MEN, multiple endocrine neoplasia; MTC; medullary thyroid carcinoma.

affected by the MEN 2 syndromes[31,33] (Table 40-2). Within an affected kindred, a single *RET* mutation is present, and the specific type of mutation is related to the phenotypic expression of the disease within that kindred. The aggressiveness of MTC and the probability of developing pheochromocytoma and parathyroid disease are influenced by the specific *RET* mutation in a kindred.

Patients with MEN 2B most commonly have a germline mutation in codon 918 of *RET* (ATG→ACG), which is in the tyrosine kinase domain. Other mutations have been described (codon 883 and 922). In contrast to MEN 2A and FMTC, 50% of mutations in MEN 2B patients arise de novo and are not present in the parents. In almost all of these cases, the mutation occurred in the patient's paternal allele. In offspring of the patients with de novo mutations, the disease is transmitted in an autosomal dominant fashion. The rate of de novo cases of MEN 2A and FMTC is extremely low.

In MEN 2A, codon 634 and 618 mutations are the most common, although mutations at other codons (see Table 40-2) are observed, and there is overlap in the mutations that give rise to MEN 2A and FMTC. FMTC patients have the most indolent form of MTC. The most common FMTC mutations occur in codons 609, 611, 618, 620, although mutations of other codons have also been identified (see Table 40-2). Many patients with FMTC are cured by thyroidectomy alone, and those with persistent elevation of calcitonin levels do well for many years. Occasional patients survive into the seventh or eighth decades without any treatment for or symptoms of MTC, although pathologic examination of the thyroid reveals MTC or C-cell hyperplasia.

The exon 16 mutation common in MEN 2B patients has also been identified in greater than 20% of sporadic MTC tumors, where it is assumed to be a somatic, rather than an inherited, mutation in the tumor cells only.[31]

Medullary Thyroid Carcinoma

MTC originates from the parafollicular cells, or C cells, of the thyroid. These cells comprise 1% of the total thyroid mass and are dispersed throughout the gland, with the highest concentration in the upper poles. The C cells produce, store, and secrete the hormone calcitonin. In the MEN 2 syndromes, MTC is associated with C-cell hyperplasia, which is presumed to be a precursor lesion. Histologically, MTC can be identified by calcitonin staining and by the presence of amyloid in the tumors. Hereditary MTC is often multifocal and bilateral. Basal and stimulated serum calcitonin levels correlate with tumor burden and are always elevated in patients with palpable MTC thyroid tumors. MTCs may secrete other hormones, including carcinoembryonic antigen (CEA). Secretory diarrhea and flushing, most often attributed to elevated calcitonin, are the main paraneoplastic manifestations of advanced MTC.

Early diagnosis in hereditary MTC is critical because metastases occur in the early stages of disease. Lymph node metastases are rarely present in patients in whom genetic testing establishes the diagnosis of MEN 2A or FMTC in childhood and thyroidectomy is performed before the occurrence of a thyroid mass or elevation of calcitonin level.[34] In contrast, most cases of sporadic MTC (and cases of hereditary MTC that are not detected by genetic screening) present as a neck mass detected on physical exam. Diagnosis is made by biopsy (fine-needle aspiration cytology) and measurement of calcitonin levels. Lymph node metastases are usually present in these patients by the time the diagnosis is made.

MTC spreads within the central compartment to perithyroidal and paratracheal lymph nodes (level VI nodes)[35] (Fig. 40-6). The central compartment includes tissue on the trachea, extending laterally to the carotid sheath, and from the hyoid bone superiorly to the innominate vein inferiorly. Within this compartment, spread is commonly bilateral. Upper mediastinal nodes (level VII nodes) are also frequently involved. Further lymphatic spread can also occur to the lateral neck compartment, including jugular (levels II, III, and IV nodes), posterior triangle (level V nodes), and supraclavicular nodes. The outcome of patients with involvement of lower tracheobronchial lymph nodes is equivalent to that of patients with distant metastases. The incidence of nodal metastases in palpable, established MTC is quite high. In a series from Washington University, we found that the incidence of central (levels VI and VII) node involvement was extremely high (80%), regardless of the size of the primary palpable tumor. There was also frequent involvement of ipsilateral (75%) and contralateral (47%) level II, III, and IV nodes[35] (Table 40-3).

MTC may involve adjacent structures by direct invasion or compression. Structures most commonly affected include the trachea, recurrent laryngeal nerve, jugular veins, and carotid arteries. Invasion of these structures may result in stridor, upper airway obstruction, hoarseness, dysphagia, and bleeding or arterial stenosis or occlusion. MTC in the thyroid or in cervical metastases may cause localized pain and tenderness.

Distant metastases occur in liver, lung, bone and other soft tissues, including breast (Fig. 40-7). In a study from a Swedish registry, it was noted that MTC patients with a palpable mass in the neck had distant metastatic disease in 20% of cases, regardless of heritability.[36] Occult remote metastases are the likely cause of persistent hypercalcitoninemia after thyroidectomy and extensive lymph node dissection.

Diagnosis

The prognosis of MTC is associated with disease stage at the time of diagnosis. Numerous studies of patients with MEN 2A have shown a direct correlation between early diagnosis and cure of MTC.[37] Patients with MEN 2A and FMTC have a completely normal outward appearance. In these patients, the diagnosis of MTC has been made through screening efforts (measurement of calcitonin levels or *RET* gene mutation testing) undertaken because of other affected family members, or by detection of a thyroid nodule on physical examination. More than 50% of patients with MEN 2B have normal parents, and the diagnosis in these de novo cases is not usually made until a mass is discovered in the neck. Very rarely, the diagnosis is made earlier by an astute clinician, who notes the characteristic phenotype. Most index cases of MEN 2A, MEN 2B, and FMTC present with a thyroid mass that is identified as MTC by biopsy. Palpable cervical adenopathy is present in more than 50% of patients who present with palpable MTC, and lymph node metastases are present histologically in up to 80%. Respiratory complaints, hoarseness, and dysphagia can be seen in about 13% of patients. About 12% of patients with palpable MTC present with evidence of distant metastatic disease. Occasional index cases of MEN 2 present with clinical pheochromocytoma, Hirschsprung's disease, or hyperparathyroidism before the diagnosis of MTC is made.

About 25% of all patients with MTC have MEN 2A, 2B, or FMTC. Genetic testing for the relevant mutations in the *RET* gene is widely available and is very accurate and reliable. Because of this, we feel that genetic testing needs to be considered in all patients who present with MTC. This is preceded by formal consultation with a genetic counselor who can apprise the individual of the risks and benefits of genetic testing. An in-depth family history with close attention to any relatives with hypertension, hyperparathyroidism, Hirschsprung's disease, or thyroid and adrenal tumors is essential. A careful review of systems to identify any evidence of symptomatic pheochromocytoma or hyperparathyroidism must be conducted. The caregiver also needs to note any phenotypic

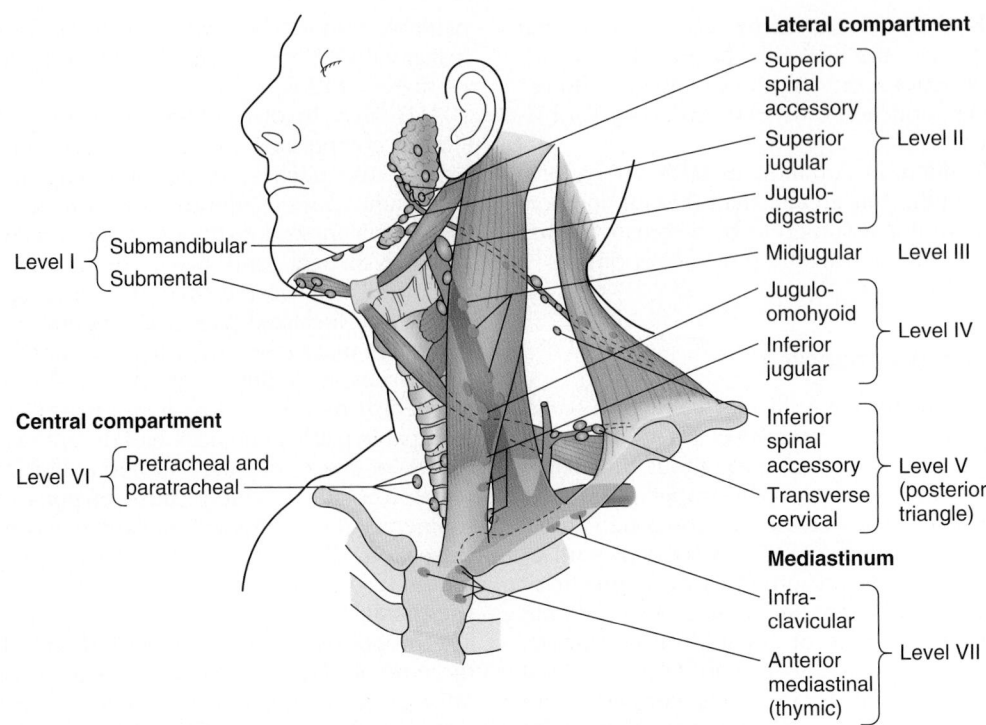

Figure 40-6 Schematic representation of the anatomic landmarks and lymph node compartments in the neck and upper mediastinum encountered in surgical reinterventions in medullary thyroid carcinoma. The central compartment is delimited inferiorly by the innominate vein, superiorly by the hyoid bone, laterally by the carotid sheaths, and dorsally by the prevertebral fascia. It comprises lymphatic and soft tissues around the esophagus as well as pretracheal and paratracheal lymph nodes, which drain the thyroid bed (level VI). The submandibular nodal group (level I) is subsumed in the central compartment by some classifications. The lateral compartments span the area between the carotid sheath, the sternocleidomastoid muscle, and the trapezius muscle. The inferior border is defined by the subclavian vein, and the hypoglossal nerve determines the superior boundary. The lymph node chain adjacent to the jugular vein is divided cranially to caudally into superior jugular nodes (level II), midjugular nodes (level III), and inferior jugular nodes (level IV). Lymph nodes situated in the posterior triangle between the dorsolateral sternocleidomastoid muscle, the trapezius muscle, and the subclavian vein are classified as level V nodes. Mediastinal lymphatic tissue is referred to as level VII lymph nodes. (Adapted from Musholt TJ, Moley JF: Management of recurrent medullary thyroid carcinoma after total thyroidectomy. Probl Gen Surg 14:89-110, 1997).

Table 40-3   Lymph Node Metastases in Palpable Medullary Thyroid Carcinoma

TUMOR SIZE (cm)	NO. OF PATIENTS	CENTRAL METASTASIS	IPSILATERAL METASTASIS	CONTRALATERAL METASTASIS
0-0.9	16	11/16	12/16	5/16
1-1.9	16	13/16	14/16	7/16
2-2.9	13	11/13	7/13	8/13
3-3.9	12	9/12	10/12	8/12
4+	16	14/16	12/16	6/16
TOTAL	73	58/73 (80%)	55/73 (75%)	34/73 (47%)

From Moley JF, DeBenedetti MK: Patterns of nodal metastases in palpable medullary thyroid carcinoma: Recommendations for extent of node dissection. Ann Surg 229:880-887; discussion 887-888, 1999.

physical characteristics that might suggest MEN 2B. If a *RET* mutation is found on genetic screening, first-degree relatives are counseled and tested for the same mutation. Patients found to have a mutation in the *RET* proto-oncogene have biochemical testing for pheochromocytoma before thyroidectomy. Failure to identify a

pheochromocytoma in a patient who undergoes thyroid surgery can have disastrous consequences because induction of anesthesia may cause a catechol surge with resultant malignant hypertension.

Thyroid C cells and MTC cells secrete calcitonin, which is an invaluable serum marker for the presence of disease in screening and follow-up settings. CEA level is also elevated in more than 50% of patients with MTC. Calcitonin is a more useful tumor marker for MTC than CEA because of its shorter half-life (days compared to months) and because many MTCs do not secrete CEA. Blood levels of calcitonin may be measured in the basal state or after the administration of the secretagogues calcium and, if available, pentagastrin.[34]

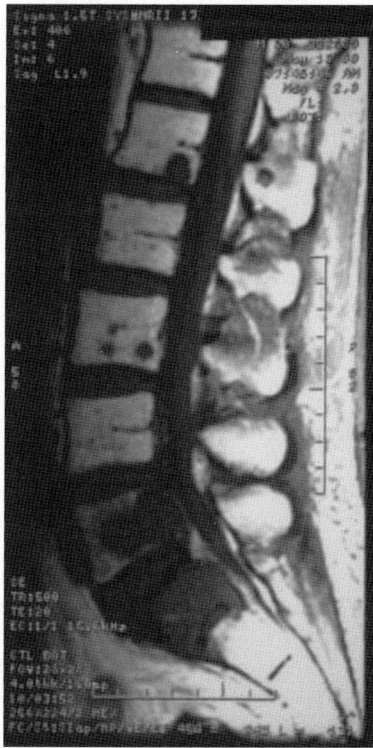

Figure 40-7 Spinal metastases from medullary thyroid carcinoma in a patient with MEN 2A.

Treatment

Recommended surgical treatment of MTC is influenced by several factors. First, the clinical course of MTC is usually more aggressive than that of differentiated thyroid cancer, with higher recurrence and mortality rates. Second, MTC cells do not take up radioactive iodine, and radiation therapy and chemotherapy are ineffective. Third, MTC is multicentric in 90% of patients with the hereditary forms of the disease. Fourth, in patients with palpable disease, more than 70% have nodal metastases. Lastly, the ability to measure postoperative stimulated calcitonin levels has allowed assessment of the adequacy of surgical extirpation. Screening for pheochromocytoma is done before performing thyroid surgery. If patients are found to have evidence of pheochromocytoma, adrenal surgery with perioperative α-blockade precedes other procedures (Fig. 40-8).

Preventive Surgery

The best chance of cure in familial MTC is provided by complete surgical resection before malignant transformation or before spread beyond the thyroid gland. Data from the EUROMEN study group suggested that the codon 634 mutation (found in 62.8% of 207 study patients) was associated with an average interval of 6.6 years for progression from primary tumor to nodal metastases.[38] Preventive thyroidectomy is the goal in patients who are identified by genetic testing to have hereditary MTC but who do not yet display clinical evidence of disease. The extent and timing of surgical resection may be guided by the genotype-phenotype correlations. Patients with MEN 2B, who demonstrate the highest risk, have a total thyroidectomy performed as early as possible—before 6 months of age and preferably within the first months of life.[39] These procedures are best performed by surgeons experienced in thyroid surgery in children.

Finding the parathyroids in infants can be extremely difficult because these parathyroids are small and translucent.[34,40] Patients with mutations with MEN2A have thyroidectomy before 5 to 6 years of age. Management

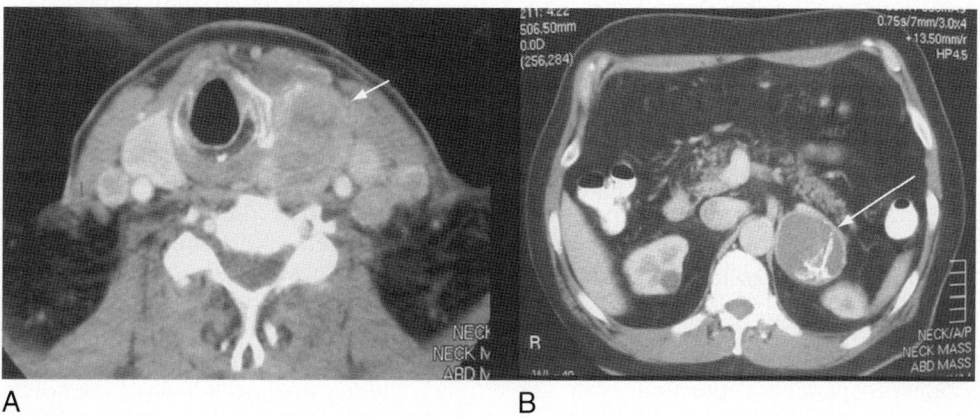

Figure 40-8 A, CT scan of the neck in a patient with MEN 2A and untreated medullary thyroid carcinoma (*arrow*) with adenopathy. **B,** Abdominal computed tomography scan of the same patient showing cystic left pheochromocytoma (*arrow*).

of central neck nodes and parathyroids is guided by calcitonin levels and type of mutation.[39] Management of patients with FMTC is more controversial, given the more indolent disease course. Recommendations include thyroidectomy before 5 to 10 years of age or on an individual basis depending on calcitonin levels.[39,41]

Some have felt that in patients with codon 13 and 14 *RET* mutations, observation and yearly calcitonin testing are acceptable, with thyroidectomy only if stimulated calcitonin levels become elevated.[42] Our general practice, however, is to recommend preventive thyroidectomy in childhood or earlier if indicated by elevated calcitonin levels. Until recently, recommendations also included central neck dissection and parathyroidectomy with autotransplantation to ensure adequate resection. Recent studies and personal experience, however, have demonstrated extremely low likelihood of nodal metastases in patients younger than 8 years with MEN 2A or FMTC and in patients with a normal calcitonin level.[34]

Our current strategy is to leave the parathyroids in situ in these patients if possible. Often, however, the desired complete removal of thyroid tissue results in compromise of parathyroid blood supply. In these situations, autotransplantation of devascularized parathyroids is required. We routinely remove and autotransplant parathyroids when a central node dissection is done. In parathyroid autotransplantation, parathyroid glands are sliced into 1×3-mm fragments and autotransplanted into individual muscle pockets in the muscle of the nondominant forearm (in patients with MEN 2A) or the sternocleidomastoid muscle (in patients with FMTC or MEN 2B). Patients are maintained on calcium and vitamin D supplementation for 4 to 8 weeks postoperatively. In a recent series of thyroidectomies performed in 50 patients with MEN 2A identified by genetic screening, total thyroidectomy and central node dissection with parathyroidectomy and parathyroid autografting was performed in all patients.[34] All autografts functioned, but supplemental calcium was required in four patients. The percentage of patients requiring calcium supplementation after parathyroidectomy with parathyroid autografting is reported to range from 0% to 18%. Parathyroidectomy with autotransplantation is done in all patients with gross parathyroid enlargement or biochemical evidence of parathyroid disease at the time of operation for MTC. The operating surgeon should be expert at preserving parathyroid function.

Surgery for Palpable Disease

In patients with MEN2 who present with a palpable thyroid mass, the risk for more extensive nodal metastatic disease is increased (see Fig. 40-8). Overall, persistent disease, evidenced by elevation of calcitonin levels, is present in more than 50% of patients after surgery for palpable MTC. In the absence of effective adjuvant therapy, there is a need to better define or predict the extent of spread of these tumors at the time of diagnosis, so that appropriate operative resection can be performed.

Metastatic involvement of cervical lymph nodes is present in more than 75% of patients with palpable MTC

tumors.[35] Surgery is the only effective therapeutic modality for MTC at the present time. Our recommendation for patients who present with palpable MTC is total thyroidectomy, parathyroidectomy with autotransplantation, central neck dissection (right and left levels VI and VII), and ipsilateral level II to V node dissection. Bilateral level II to V node dissections may be done, depending on the extent of nodal involvement apparent at operation. The central node dissection encompasses all tissue from the level of the hyoid bone superiorly to the innominate vessels inferiorly, and laterally to the carotid sheaths. Nodal tissue on the anterior surface of the trachea is removed, exposing the superior surface of the innominate vein behind the sternal notch. Fatty and nodal tissue between the carotid artery and the trachea is removed, including paratracheal nodes along the recurrent nerves. On the right, the junction of the innominate and right carotid arteries is exposed, and on the left, nodal tissue is removed to a comparable level behind the head of the left clavicle. A systematic approach to the removal of all nodal tissue in these patients has been reported to improve recurrence and survival rates when compared retrospectively to procedures in which only grossly involved nodes were removed.

Persistent or Recurrent Disease

Patients who present with palpable MTC often have elevated calcitonin levels following primary surgery, indicating residual or recurrent MTC. Currently, there is no defined role for chemotherapy or radiation therapy in these patients. Reoperation for patients with recurrent disease can be done with curative or palliative intent. Evidence of distant metastases is a contraindication to surgery unless some palliative benefit can be identified. Two such indications are to prevent invasion or compression of the airway and to debulk large tumors that cause profuse, intractable diarrhea secondary to hormone secretion. If no evidence of distant metastases is found in a patient who has not had previous cervical node dissections, re-exploration of the neck with completion of node dissection is an option for patients with persistent or recurrent elevations of calcitonin.[43] Metastatic workup consists of neck, chest, and abdominal CT or MRI scanning. We have not found octreotide, technetium, thallium, or fluorodeoxyglucose positron emission tomography scanning to be more sensitive than CT, ultrasound, or MRI,[44] although there are reports that describe positive experience with these modalities.

Diagnostic laparoscopy with direct examination of the liver is extremely useful in detecting distant metastases in these patients before reoperation on the neck. In one series, liver metastases were identified by laparoscopy in 25% of patients with persistent elevation of calcitonin levels despite negative CT or MRI scanning of the liver.[45] If distant metastases are identified, observation of the clinically negative neck is recommended, and neck reoperation is recommended if the patient develops gross cervical recurrence. If laparoscopy and imaging studies show no evidence of metastatic disease, re-exploration of the neck is considered to remove residual nodal tissue. Continued observation may be considered as well. The operative strategy in these reoperations is to remove all residual thyroid and nodal tissue in at-risk areas that was not removed at the previous operation, guided by the previous operative records, pathology reports, and imaging studies. Reoperation resulted in normalization of the calcitonin level in one third of patients in a study from our institution, although the survival advantage of such procedures has not been proved.[43]

Pheochromocytoma

Pheochromocytomas occur in 40% to 50% of MEN 2A and MEN 2B patients, with the incidence increasing with age. Pheochromocytomas arise in adrenal medullary, or chromaffin, cells that synthesize, store, and secrete catecholamines. These tumors often present with classic signs and symptoms of excess catechol secretion, that is, hypertension, headache, heart palpitations, anxiety, and tremulousness. Complications of unrecognized disease include malignant hypertension, stroke, myocardial infarction, and cardiac arrhythmias. There are frequent reports of sudden death in patients with known or unsuspected pheochromocytomas who have undergone unrelated surgical procedures, biopsies, or childbirth.

Pheochromocytomas rarely precede the development of C-cell abnormalities in MEN 2 syndrome. Adrenal medullary cells undergo predictable morphologic changes, including diffuse hyperplasia, nodular hyperplasia, and pheochromocytoma. In MEN 2, pheochromocytomas are often multifocal, with bilateral tumors occurring in more than half of these patients. As opposed to the sporadic form of the disease, malignant and extra-adrenal pheochromocytomas are very rare within MEN 2 populations. The frequency of development of pheochromocytomas varies among MEN 2 kindreds, with some kindreds displaying the tumor as the dominant characteristic. Pheochromocytomas may be clinically silent in up to 60% of MEN 2 cases, where they are detected by biochemical testing.

Diagnosis

Biochemical screening for pheochromocytoma is best done by measurement of plasma or 24-hour urine catecholamines and metanephrines.[46] This test is done on an annual basis. If testing is negative, no further workup is necessary until the next year. If the test is positive or borderline, imaging is needed to determine whether a pheochromocytoma is present. As mentioned, most MEN 2A and MEN 2B patients have some degree of adrenal medullary hyperplasia and may have borderline elevations of urinary catechols and thickening of the adrenals without a definite pheochromocytoma.

Adrenal CT or MRI can detect tumors 1 cm or larger. Opposed-phase chemical-shift MRI may distinguish a pheochromocytoma from an adrenal adenoma, which occurs in up to 9% of normal patients. Iodine-131 metaiodobenzylguanidine scanning is generally not useful in these patients because extra-adrenal pheochromocytomas are extremely rare in patients with MEN 2A and MEN 2B.

Treatment

Partial or complete adrenalectomy is recommended in patients with MEN 2A and MEN 2B who are found to have a pheochromocytoma. It is important to medically stabilize the patient before surgery to avoid any perioperative events due to excessive catechol secretion. Preoperative α-blockade is achieved by administration of phenoxybenzamine (40-200 mg/day) for 5 days to 2 weeks before surgery. The dose is titrated to the lowest blood pressure tolerated by these patients without symptomatic relative hypotension. Should tachycardia or cardiac arrhythmia result from treatment with phenoxybenzamine, a β-blocker is added to the treatment regimen. After medical stabilization, the patient is taken for operation. During the procedure, it may be necessary to control intraoperative paroxysmal hypertension with short-acting antihypertensives such as sodium nitroprusside or phentolamine.

Traditionally, controversy has existed as to whether unilateral or bilateral adrenalectomy should be performed for unilateral tumors. In a series at our institution, the results of unilateral and bilateral adrenalectomies were compared.[47] Nearly one fourth of patients undergoing bilateral adrenalectomy experienced at least one episode of acute adrenal insufficiency requiring hospitalization. Two of these patients died from episodes of adrenal insufficiency. Of the patients who had unilateral adrenalectomies, 52% developed contralateral pheochromocytomas after a mean interval of 12 years. Conversely, 48% of patients remained disease free by biochemical and symptomatic standards during a mean interval of 5 years. Based on these results, it is our practice to perform resection of the involved adrenal only and to maintain yearly biochemical screening thereafter.

Patients with MEN 2A and MEN 2B are ideally suited to laparoscopic adrenalectomy because the pheochromocytomas arising in these syndromes are rarely malignant and almost never extra-adrenal. Pheochromocytomas may be successfully removed by unilateral or bilateral laparoscopic adrenalectomy provided the adrenal tumors are small, confined to the adrenal glands, and accurately localized preoperatively by high-resolution CT or MRI, and the patient is adequately prepared pharmacologically. Laparoscopic adrenalectomy is associated with shorter hospital stay, decreased postoperative pain, and more rapid recovery when compared with open adrenalectomy.[47] Contraindications to the laparoscopic approach include large tumors (>8-10 cm), malignant pheochromocytomas, and existing contraindications to laparoscopy.

Parathyroid Disease

Hyperparathyroidism occurs in 10% to 35% of patients with MEN 2A. Unlike MEN 1, hyperparathyroidism is rarely the initial presenting problem in patients with MEN 2A. Hyperparathyroidism in MEN 2A is characterized by multiglandular hyperplasia. Fewer than one in five patients has a single parathyroid adenoma. Parathyroid hyperplasia is not found in patients with sporadic MTC or in patients with MTC in MEN 2B syndrome. Parathyroid hyperplasia, in the absence of hyperparathyroidism, is common in MEN 2A.

Diagnosis

All known MEN 2A carriers need to be screened annually for the presence of hyperparathyroidism by serum calcium measurements. PTH levels are measured if the serum calcium is high or borderline.

Treatment

The need for isolated parathyroidectomy in MEN 2 patients is rare. As discussed earlier, we usually perform routine total parathyroidectomy with autotransplantation at the time of thyroidectomy, regardless of gross appearance of the parathyroid glands. Should hyperparathyroidism occur at a later time in these patients with forearm grafts, surgical removal of all or a portion of the graft can be done. If, at the time of the initial neck exploration, the parathyroids are left in situ, subsequent development of hyperparathyroidism requires re-exploration of the neck.

Complications and Postoperative Care

The complications and immediate postoperative care in surgery for the various endocrinopathies in MEN 2 are similar to those described in more detail in the previous chapters dealing with each specific disease. In thyroidectomy for MEN 2–related MTC, complications include injury to the recurrent laryngeal nerve, hypocalcemia secondary to parathyroid damage, and compromise of the airway secondary to hematoma formation. These complications are very unusual in the hands of an experienced thyroid surgeon. Complications of central neck dissection include hypoparathyroidism and recurrent nerve injury. If the central neck dissection results in exposure of the innominate artery in the upper mediastinum, care must be taken to avoid bilateral recurrent nerve dysfunction because this may result in the need for tracheostomy, and a tracheostomy in proximity to an exposed innominate artery may result in arteritis and innominate artery rupture or tracheo-innominate fistula. Complications of lateral neck dissection are well described and include bleeding, infection, thoracic duct leak, nerve injury (including phrenic, vagus, sympathetic chain, spinal accessory, marginal mandibular, hypoglossal, and great auricular), and shoulder dysfunction.

After total thyroidectomy with parathyroid autotransplantation, it is necessary to supplement calcium, vitamin D, and thyroid hormone. Calcium and vitamin D supplementation is withdrawn 4 to 8 weeks after surgery as the parathyroid grafts begin to function. Lifelong thyroid replacement is required.

The long-term postoperative care for MEN 2 patients demands a close and lifelong relationship between the care provider and the patient. Yearly screenings for MTC recurrences and other manifestations of the syndrome must still be conducted. After thyroidectomy for MTC,

calcitonin levels are documented in the immediate postoperative period and are followed closely. If a patient is found to have persistent or elevated calcitonin level after surgery, an extensive physical examination and imaging workup for focal and metastatic disease must be conducted, as outlined in the previous section.

In patients with MEN 2A, routine yearly plasma or 24-hour urine screens must be performed to rule out a pheochromocytoma.[48] If catecholamines or metanephrines become elevated, MRI or CT are repeated to localize the tumor.

MEN 2A patients must have lifelong screening for evidence of hyperparathyroidism. Graft-dependant hyperparathyroidism may occur in patients with parathyroid autografts, and in these cases, debulking of the parathyroid autografts is performed. Intraoperative PTH assays are helpful in determining the adequacy of these procedures.

Prognosis

MTC in the MEN 2 syndromes is usually indolent and slow-growing, but it is lethal in many patients with distant metastases. Patients with MEN 2A and FMTC have a better long-term outcome than patients with MEN 2B or sporadic tumors. Within these clinical settings, however, there is variation. In the MEN 2 population, with the relatively recent widespread use of genetic screening modalities and related changes in treatment for patients identified by these methods, long-term prognosis has yet to be established. Before the use of these screening techniques, average life expectancy was 50 years for patients with MEN 2A and 30 years for patients with MEN 2B. As more kindreds are followed by genetic and biochemical screening, the long-term prognosis for MEN 2 patients in the modern era of treatment should become clearer.

Improved understanding of the molecular pathogenesis of MTC (mutations of the RET receptor protein), has led to the testing of targeted molecular therapies. Imatinib mesylate (Gleevec) is the best known tyrosine kinase inhibitor already in clinical use against chronic myelogenous leukemia and gastrointestinal stromal tumors, targeting specific tyrosine kinases. A tyrosine kinase inhibitor with specific activity against the RET protein is known as ZD6474 (Zactima).[48] The efficacy of these drugs is currently being tested in patients with locally advanced or metastatic MTC, in phase II trials. There are currently at least 12 clinical trials for novel systemic agents against thyroid carcinoma. This is a significant increase over the situation as recently as 2000.

Conclusions

The identification of mutations in the RET protooncogene associated with MEN 2A, MEN 2B, and FMTC has led to a new paradigm in surgery: the performance of an operation based on the result of a genetic test. Prophylactic thyroidectomy based on direct mutation analysis appears to be curative in MEN 2A and FMTC patients when they are screened at a young age. The application of meticulous reoperative strategies for persistent hypercalcitoninemia, combined with more accurate staging studies, have led to better patient selection for surgery and improved outcome. Testing of new agents with activity against the RET protein will lead to more effective systemic therapies for metastatic MTC.

Selected References

Chandrasekharappa SC, Guru SC, Manickamp P, et al: Positional cloning of the gene for multiple endocrine neoplasia-type 1. Science 276:404, 1997.

Original article reporting the successful positional cloning of the *MEN1* gene.

Larsson C, Skogseid B, Oberg K, et al: Multiple endocrine neoplasia type 1 gene maps to chromosome 11 and is lost in insulinoma. Nature 332:85, 1988.

This is the original report that maps the *MEN1* gene to chromosome 11 by genetic studies. Important observations of allelic loss on chromosome 11 in tumor DNA from a pair of brothers with MEN 1 and insulinoma also demonstrate that oncogenesis in MEN 1 is consistent with a two-hit model that involves inactivation of both copies of a tumor-suppressor gene.

Skinner MA, Moley JF, Dilley WG, et al: Prophylactic thyroidectomy in multiple endocrine neoplasia type 2A. N Engl J Med 353:1105-1113, 2005.

This article reports 50 consecutive preventive thyroidectomies with parathyroid autotransplantation and central neck dissection in patients with MEN 2A with greater than 5-year follow-up.

References

1. Larsson C, Skogseid B, Oberg K, et al: Multiple endocrine neoplasia type 1 gene maps to chromosome 11 and is lost in insulinoma. Nature 332:85-87, 1988.
2. Chandrasekharappa SC, Guru SC, Manickam P, et al: Positional cloning of the gene for multiple endocrine neoplasia-type 1. Science 276:404-407, 1997.
3. Crabtree JS, Scacheri PC, Ward JM, et al: A mouse model of multiple endocrine neoplasia, type 1, develops multiple endocrine tumors. Proc Natl Acad Sci U S A 98:1118-1123, 2001.
4. Agarwal SK, Kennedy PA, Scacheri PC, et al: Menin molecular interactions: Insights into normal functions and tumorigenesis. Horm Metab Res 37:369-374, 2005.
5. Schnepp RW, Hou Z, Wang H, et al: Functional interaction between tumor suppressor menin and activator of S-phase kinase. Cancer Res 64:6791-6796, 2004.
6. Karnik SK, Hughes CM, Gu X, et al: Menin regulates pancreatic islet growth by promoting histone methylation and expression of genes encoding p27Kip1 and p18INK4c. Proc Natl Acad Sci U S A 102:14659-14664, 2005.
7. Milne TA, Hughes CM, Lloyd R, et al: Menin and MLL cooperatively regulate expression of cyclin-dependent kinase inhibitors. Proc Natl Acad Sci U S A 102:749-754, 2005.
8. Yokoyama A, Somervaille TC, Smith KS, et al: The menin tumor suppressor protein is an essential oncogenic cofactor for MLL-associated leukemogenesis. Cell 123:207-218, 2005.
9. Chen YX, Yan J, Keeshan K, et al: The tumor suppressor menin regulates hematopoiesis and myeloid transformation by influencing Hox gene expression. Proc Natl Acad Sci U S A 103:1018-1023, 2006.
10. Scacheri PC, Davis S, Odom DT, et al: Genome-wide analysis of menin binding provides insights into MEN1 tumorigenesis. PLoS Genet 2:e51, 2006.
11. Schnepp RW, Chen YX, Wang H, et al: Mutation of tumor suppressor gene Men1 acutely enhances proliferation of pancreatic islet cells. Cancer Res 66:5707-5715, 2006.
12. Schussheim DH, Skarulis MC, Agarwal SK, et al: Multiple endocrine neoplasia type 1: New clinical and basic findings. Trends Endocrinol Metab 12:173-178, 2001.
13. Doherty GM, Lairmore TC, DeBenedetti MK: Multiple endocrine neoplasia type 1 parathyroid adenoma development over time. World J Surg 28:1139-1142, 2004.
14. Lairmore TC, Piersall LD, DeBenedetti MK, et al: Clinical genetic testing and early surgical intervention in patients with multiple endocrine neoplasia type 1 (MEN 1). Ann Surg 239:637-645; discussion 645-637, 2004.
15. Hubbard JG, Sebag F, Maweja S, et al: Subtotal parathyroidectomy as an adequate treatment for primary hyperparathyroidism in multiple endocrine neoplasia type 1. Arch Surg 141:235-239, 2006.
16. Lambert LA, Shapiro SE, Lee JE, et al: Surgical treatment of hyperparathyroidism in patients with multiple endocrine neoplasia type 1. Arch Surg 140:374-382, 2005.
17. Cohen MS, Dilley WG, Wells SA Jr, et al: Long-term functionality of cryopreserved parathyroid autografts: A 13-year prospective analysis. Surgery 138:1033-1040; discussion 1040-1031, 2005.
18. Thompson NW, Vinik AI, Eckhauser FE: Microgastrinomas of the duodenum: A cause of failed operations for the Zollinger-Ellison syndrome. Ann Surg 209:396-404, 1989.
19. Norton JA, Doppman JL, Jensen RT: Curative resection in Zollinger-Ellison syndrome: Results of a 10-year prospective study. Ann Surg 215:8-18, 1992.
20. Norton JA, Alexander HR, Fraker DL, et al: Possible primary lymph node gastrinoma: Occurrence, natural history, and predictive factors. A prospective study. Ann Surg 237:650-657; discussion 657-659, 2003.
21. Wolfe MM, Jensen RT: Zollinger-Ellison syndrome: Current concepts in diagnosis and management. N Engl J Med 317:1200-1209, 1987.
22. Norton JA, Fraker DL, Alexander HR, et al: Surgery to cure the Zollinger-Ellison syndrome. N Engl J Med 341:635-644, 1999.
23. Tonelli F, Fratini G, Nesi G, et al: Pancreatectomy in multiple endocrine neoplasia type 1–related gastrinomas and pancreatic endocrine neoplasias. Ann Surg 244:61-70, 2006.
24. Norton JA, Melcher ML, Gibril F, et al: Gastric carcinoid tumors in multiple endocrine neoplasia-1 patients with Zollinger-Ellison syndrome can be symptomatic, demonstrate aggressive growth, and require surgical treatment. Surgery 136:1267-1274, 2004.
25. Cohen MS, Picus D, Lairmore TC, et al: Prospective study of provocative angiograms to localize functional islet cell tumors of the pancreas. Surgery 122:1091-1100, 1997.
26. Lairmore TC, Chen VY, DeBenedetti MK, et al: Duodenopancreatic resections in patients with multiple endocrine neoplasia type 1. Ann Surg 231:909-918, 2000.
27. Kouvaraki MA, Shapiro SE, Cote GJ, et al: Management of pancreatic endocrine tumors in multiple endocrine neoplasia type 1. World J Surg 30:643-653, 2006.
28. Skogseid B, Oberg K, Eriksson B, et al: Surgery for asymptomatic pancreatic lesion in multiple endocrine neoplasia type I. World J Surg 20:872-876; discussion 877, 1996.
29. Bartsch DK, Fendrich V, Langer P, et al: Outcome of duodenopancreatic resections in patients with multiple endo-

crine neoplasia type 1. Ann Surg 242:757-764, discussion 764-756, 2005.

30. Thompson NW: Management of pancreatic endocrine tumors in patients with multiple endocrine neoplasia type 1. Surg Oncol Clin N Am 7:881-891, 1998.

31. Eng C, Mulligan LM: Mutations of the RET proto-oncogene in the multiple endocrine neoplasia type 2 syndromes, related sporadic tumours, and Hirschsprung disease. Hum Mutat 9:97-109, 1997.

32. Yip L, Cote GJ, Shapiro SE, et al: Multiple endocrine neoplasia type 2: Evaluation of the genotype-phenotype relationship. Arch Surg 138:409-416; discussion 416, 2003.

33. Mulligan LM, Eng C, Healey CS, et al: Specific mutations of the RET proto-oncogene are related to disease phenotype in MEN 2A and FMTC. Nat Genet 6:70-74, 1994.

34. Skinner MA, Moley JA, Dilley WG, et al: Prophylactic thyroidectomy in multiple endocrine neoplasia type 2A. N Engl J Med 353:1105-1113, 2005.

35. Moley JF, DeBenedetti MK: Patterns of nodal metastases in palpable medullary thyroid carcinoma: Recommendations for extent of node dissection. Ann Surg 229:880-887; discussion 887-888, 1999.

36. Bergholm U, Adami HO, Bergstrom R, et al: Clinical characteristics in sporadic and familial medullary thyroid carcinoma: A nationwide study of 249 patients in Sweden from 1959 through 1981. Cancer 63:1196-1204, 1989.

37. Wells SA Jr, Chi DD, Toshima K, et al: Predictive DNA testing and prophylactic thyroidectomy in patients at risk for multiple endocrine neoplasia type 2A. Ann Surg 220:237-247; discussion 247-250, 1994.

38. Machens A, Niccoli-Sire P, Hoegel J, et al: Early malignant progression of hereditary medullary thyroid cancer. N Engl J Med 349:1517-1525, 2003.

39. Brandi ML, Gagel RF, Angeli A, et al: Guidelines for diagnosis and therapy of MEN type 1 and type 2. J Clin Endocrinol Metab 86:5658-5671, 2001.

40. Moley JF, Lairmore TC, Phay JE: Hereditary endocrinopathies. Curr Probl Surg 36:653-762, 1999.

41. Kouvaraki MA, Shapiro SE, Perrier ND, et al: RET proto-oncogene: A review and update of genotype-phenotype correlations in hereditary medullary thyroid cancer and associated endocrine tumors. Thyroid 15:531-544, 2005.

42. Libroa I: Familial Medullary Thyroid Carcinoma, Clinical Management. Seventh International Workshop on Multiple Endocrine Neoplasia. Gubbio, Italy, 1999, pp. 113-118.

43. Moley JF, Dilley WG, DeBenedetti MK: Improved results of cervical reoperation for medullary thyroid carcinoma. Ann Surg 225:734-740; discussion 740-733, 1997.

44. Musholt TJ, Musholt PB, Dehdashti F, et al: Evaluation of fluorodeoxyglucose-positron emission tomographic scanning and its association with glucose transporter expression in medullary thyroid carcinoma and pheochromocytoma: a clinical and molecular study. Surgery 122:1049-1060; discussion 1060-1041, 1997.

45. Tung WS, Vesely TM, Moley JF: Laparoscopic detection of hepatic metastases in patients with residual or recurrent medullary thyroid cancer. Surgery 118:1024-1029; discussion 1029-1030, 1995.

46. Eisenhofer G, Lenders JW, Linehan WM, et al: Plasma normetanephrine and metanephrine for detecting pheochromocytoma in von Hippel-Lindau disease and multiple endocrine neoplasia type 2. N Engl J Med 340:1872-1879, 1999.

47. Brunt LM, Lairmore TC, Doherty GM, et al: Adrenalectomy for familial pheochromocytoma in the laparoscopic era. Ann Surg 235:713-720; discussion 720-721, 2002.

48. Carlomagno F, Vitagliano D, Guida T, et al: ZD6474, an orally available inhibitor of KDR tyrosine kinase activity, efficiently blocks oncogenic RET kinases. Cancer Res 62:7284-7290, 2002.

ESOPHAGUS

Esophagus

Mary Maish, MD

Welcome to the esophagus: the only organ that unobtrusively navigates through three body cavities while giving way to structures of greater vitality. From a distance, the esophagus appears primitive and not highly evolved, even replaceable at times. However, upon harsher scrutiny, it is clear that this magnificent organ stands tall as it bridges two diverse environments. Much like the engineering feats of the steel and concrete structures we trust to walk and drive across, the esophagus has evolved with discrete reliability. This masterfully engineered organ performs a multitude of complex functions with conservative grace in a neighborhood of histrionic, albeit vital, organs. As we struggle to overcome its anatomic and physiologic challenges, its deceptively simple form and functions become ever more apparent. Our understanding remains dampened, and our search for knowledge continues on with enthusiasm, curiosity, and great anticipation.

HISTORY AND EDUCATION

The history of esophageal surgery tells a story of the many courageous surgeons who have pioneered their efforts in uncharted anatomic territory. The story also demonstrates the evolution of the lapses that are now present in esophageal education. Secluded in the posterior mediastinum, many of the needs of the esophagus remain unattended to by physicians. Until the cries for help are dramatic or even devastating, the symptoms are treated impetuously, with nominal attention. Emslie provided an insightful perspective when he stated: "The history of esophageal surgery is the tale of men repeatedly losing to a stronger adversary yet persisting in this unequal struggle until the nature of the problems became apparent and the war [is] won."

The earliest record of esophageal disorders dates back to the Egyptian times (3000-2500 BC). The Smith Surgical Papyrus, discovered in 1862 by Edwin Smith, describes the successful treatment of "a gaping wound of the throat penetrating the gullet." At the turn of the century there were significant improvements in anesthesia that allowed for the growth of surgery in many arenas, including surgery of the esophagus. In 1901, Dr. Dobromysslow performed the first intrathoracic segmental esophageal resection and primary anastomosis, but it was Franz Torek who pioneered the first subtotal esophagogastrectomy in 1913. The use of the stomach to replace the esophagus was first attempted by Leipzin in 1920 and successfully accomplished by Oshava in 1933. A number of modifications occurred over the next 40 years, including changes in approach, anastomosis, and conduits. Ivor Lewis (1946) modified the approach by entering the right chest, and K. C. McKewon placed the anastomosis in the neck to eliminate intrathoracic leaks. Although the transhiatal approach had been attempted, it was not well established until 1978 when Orringer and Sloan[1] resurrected and perfected this operation that had been tried by many before them.

A number of other esophageal surgeries have evolved in a similar time frame, including those for achalasia, reflux, diverticula, and more. These procedures bear the names of historically famous surgeons such as Dor, Heller, Toupet, Belsey, and Nissen. Alongside the surgeons whose nimble fingers and brave hearts have established

EARLY ESOPHAGEAL EMBRYOLOGICAL DEVELOPMENT

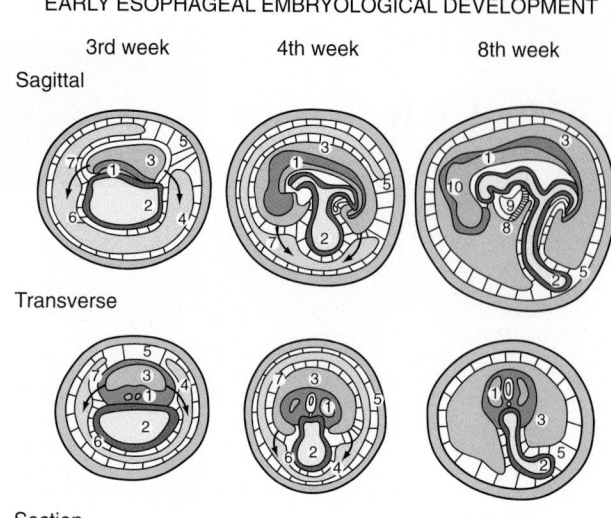

Figure 41-1 Early embryologic development. (Modified from Pearson FG, Cooper JD, Deslauriers J, et al: Esophageal Surgery, 2nd ed. New York, Churchill Livingstone, 2002, p 20.)

DEVELOPING GUT

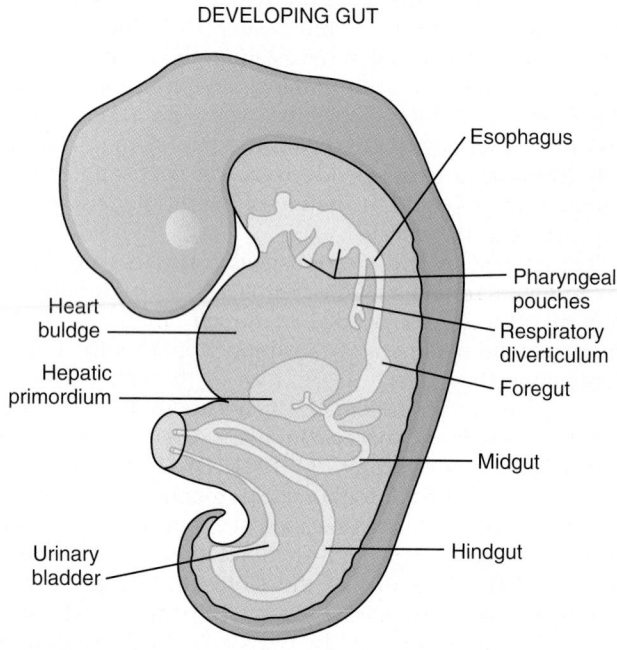

Figure 41-2 The developing gut.

their places in the archives of esophageal surgery are the physicians whose keen observations and critical minds have identified esophageal disorders that now bear their names. Boerhaave, Zenker, and Barrett are among the many physicians whose contributions also have been historically noteworthy. Many others, whose names are cast in the shadows of the greats, have contributed significantly toward gaining an understanding of the challenges that befall those whose professional passions lie within the walls of the esophagus.

The struggles with surgery of the esophagus that have been documented over the years are reflected in the

social and professional image of the esophagus. Unlike some other organs that have gone through their glamorous phase, the esophagus has not yet had its day in the sun, its era of discovery, or its position on the Surgeon General's agenda, receiving attention only for dysfunction and disorder. There are few educational tools to help understand the esophagus, and a notable lacking in esophageal education has resulted in a gross lack of understanding among most physicians. As the rise in the incidence of adenocarcinoma of the esophagus heads toward epidemic proportions, well-educated esophagologists and surgeons will be in great demand. It will be up to the academic physicians of the 21st century to carry on from where history has left off and establish the esophagus, with its medical and surgical challenges, on the forefront of the national medical agenda.

EMBRYOLOGY

Overview

Evolutionary biologists, creationists, and proponents of the theory of intelligent design alike would all agree that the process of human development is amazingly intricate and well executed. The development of the esophagus is among those remarkable feats, and a few arduous moments to appreciate the product of years of precise development will establish a sound basis from which normal and abnormal esophageal form and function can be understood. The development of the esophagus begins in the 3rd week of gestation, and by the 14th week the fetus takes its first swallow. To give life to the esophagus, there are several aspects of esophageal development that must be executed carefully: initial formation of the gut tube, molecular regulation of the gut tube, differentiation of the endoderm (the lining of the esophagus), and derivation of the muscular layers from the mesoderm.

Formation of the Gut Tube

During the embryonic period of development, cephalocaudal (Fig. 41-1) and lateral folding of the embryo occurs. As a result, a portion of the endoderm-lined yolk sac cavity is incorporated into the embryo to form the primitive gut. The primitive gut forms a blind-ending tube consisting of the foregut, the midgut, and the hindgut (Fig. 41-2). The foregut gives rise to the esophagus. It extends from the pharyngeal tube as far caudally as the liver outgrowth. By the end of the 3rd week of development, the primitive foregut develops a ventral diverticulum from which the tracheobronchial tree develops. The tracheoesophageal septum gradually partitions this diverticulum from the dorsal portion of the foregut, resulting in a ventral respiratory primordium and a dorsal esophagus (Fig. 41-3). During the 4th and 5th weeks of development, the rapid growth of the heart and liver allows the esophagus to stretch. As it elongates, the esophageal lumen is near completely obliterated at the level of the carina. The dorsal esophageal "embracement" of the trachea results in close approximation of the tracheal bifurcation to the front wall of the esophagus, further narrowing the esophageal lumen.

Molecular Regulation of the Gut Tube

Differentiation of various regions of the gut and its derivatives is dependent on a reciprocal interaction between the endoderm (epithelium) of the gut tube and surrounding splanchnic mesoderm. The mesoderm dictates the type of structure that will form, such as the esophagus forming from the foregut, through an HOX code. The induction of the HOX code is a result of sonic hedgehog (SHH) that is expressed throughout the gut endoderm. In the foregut, expression of SHH in the endoderm promotes the expression of the HOX code in the mesoderm. Once specified by this code, the mesoderm instructs the endoderm to form the various components of the foregut.[2]

Differentiation of the Endoderm

Early in gestation the mesoderm is HOX coded to instruct the endoderm to form the epithelial lining of the digestive tract. At the end of the embryonic period, from the 6th to 8th weeks of gestation, the epithelium becomes two to five cells thick and remains stratified columnar epithelium. During the 10th week of development, stratified columnar epithelium becomes ciliated. By the 12th week, the epithelium is completely ciliated, and growth is taking place only at the basal level. During the 4th and 5th months of gestation, stratified squamous epithelium replaces the ciliated columnar epithelium.

Muscular Development From the Mesoderm

The remainder of the esophagus is formed from the mesoderm. By the 6th week of gestational development, the esophagus is surrounded by a layer of undifferentiated mesoderm and a circular layer of myoblasts. Longitudinal muscle fibers appear in the lower esophagus as the circular layer of muscle becomes well established. The smooth muscle that forms the lower two thirds of the esophagus arises from the splanchnic mesoderm and is innervated by the splanchnic plexus. The striated muscle of the upper esophagus is derived from the caudal branchial arches and appears from the 12th to 15th weeks. It will eventually be innervated by the vagus nerve. Muscular proliferation peaks during the 11th and 12th weeks, so that by the 12th week of gestation, the longitudinal muscle is well defined. Ganglion cells also appear in the myenteric plexus, whereas the longitudinal muscle becomes well defined between the 10th and 12th weeks of gestation. Furthermore, the muscularis mucosa becomes well defined, and typical mucosal folds formed by longitudinal mesenchymal ridges can be appreciated.

Growth of the esophagus continues at a slower pace after morphologic changes conclude. On a functional level, swallowing first appears at the 14th week and is well established by the end of the 4th month of gestation. To be sure, not even the foundation of a house is completed within the first 3 months of construction, let alone

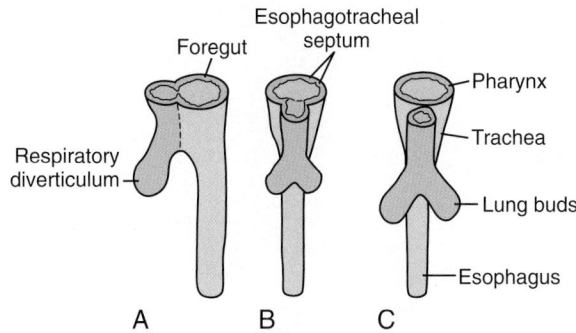

Figure 41-3 Partitioning of the foregut. (Modified from Sadler TW: Medical Embryology. Philadelphia, Lippincott Williams & Wilkins, 2003, p 290.)

a kitchen well equipped to feed a single mouth. And with this engaging story, the esophagus is born.

ANATOMY

Overview

The esophagus is a two-layered mucosa-lined muscular tube that journeys through the neck, chest, and abdomen and rests unobtrusively in the posterior mediastinum. It commences at the base of the pharynx at C6 and terminates in the abdomen, where it joins the cardia of the stomach at T11 (Fig. 41-4). Along its 25- to 30-cm course, it winds its way through a path yielding to structures of more vital efforts. The cervical esophagus begins as a midline structure that deviates slightly to the left of the trachea as it passes through the neck into the thoracic inlet. At the level of the carina, it deviates to the right to accommodate the arch of the aorta. It then winds its way back under the left main-stem bronchus and remains slightly deviated to the left as it enters the diaphragm through the esophageal hiatus at the level of the 11th thoracic vertebra. In the neck and upper thorax, the esophagus is secured between the vertebral column, posteriorly, and the trachea, anteriorly. At the level of the carina, the heart and pericardium lie directly anterior to the thoracic esophagus. Immediately before entering the abdomen, the esophagus is pushed anteriorly by the descending thoracic aorta that accompanies the esophagus through the diaphragm into the abdomen separated by the median arcuate ligament.

The journey through the muscular esophagus begins and ends with two distinct high-pressure zones: the upper (UES) and lower esophageal sphincter (LES). After passing through the UES, four esophageal segments are encountered: the pharyngeal, cervical, thoracic, and abdominal esophagus. The LES is the outlet through which passage into the stomach is then facilitated.

Esophageal Inlet

The high-pressure zone at the inlet of the esophagus is understood to be the UES and anatomically marks the

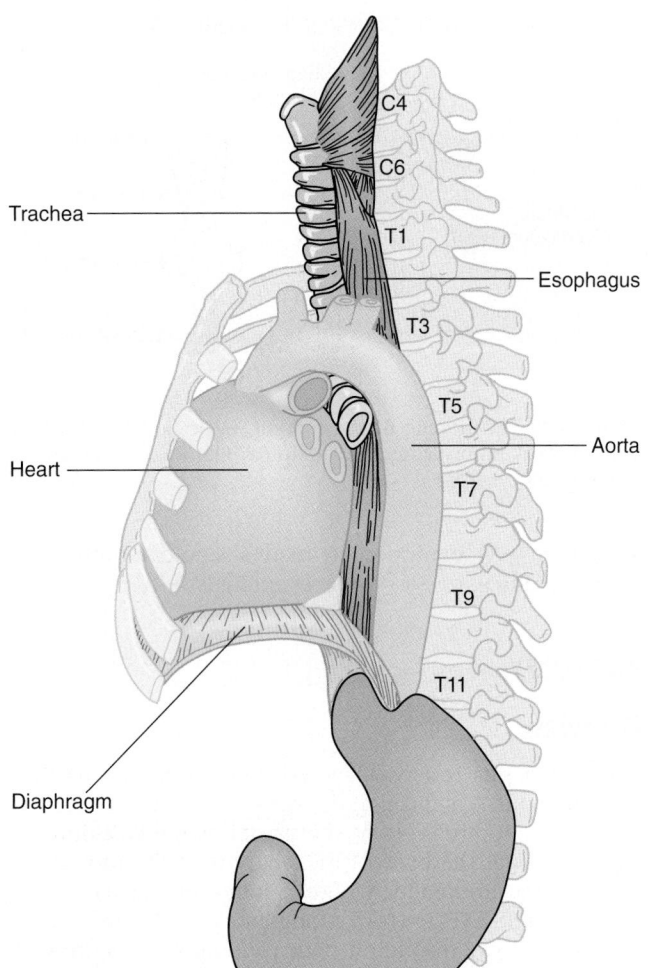

Figure 41-4 The course of the esophagus.

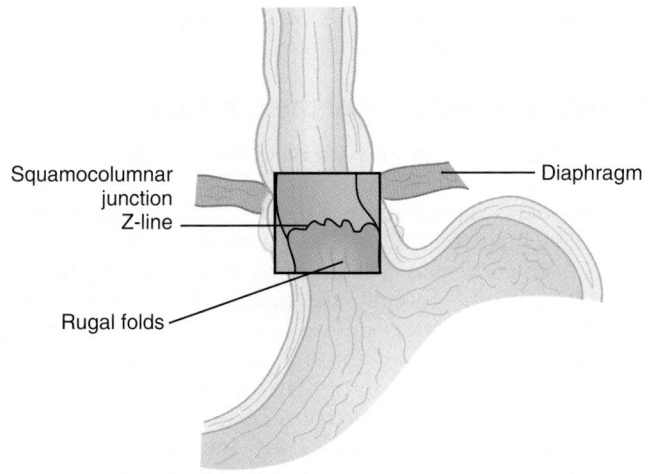

Figure 41-5 The Z-line.

end of a complex configuration of muscles that begins in the larynx and posterior pharynx and ends in the neck. The pharyngeal constrictor muscles are three consecutive muscles that begin at the base of the palate and end at the crest of the esophagus. The superior and middle pharyngeal constrictor muscles, as well as the oblique, transverse, and posterior cricoarytenoid muscles, are immediately proximal to the UES and serve to anchor the pharynx and the larynx to structures in the mouth and palate. These muscles also aid in deglutition and speech, but are not responsible for the high pressures noted in the UES. The inferior pharyngeal constrictor muscle is the final bridge between the pharyngeal and esophageal musculature.

Inserting into the median pharyngeal raphe, the inferior pharyngeal constrictor muscle is composed of two consecutive muscle beds—the thyropharyngeus and the cricopharyngeus muscles—that originate bilaterally from the lateral portions of the thyroid and cricoid cartilages, respectively. The transition between the oblique fibers of the thyropharyngeus muscle and the horizontal fibers of the cricopharyngeus muscle creates a point of potential weakness, known as *Killian's triangle* (site of a Zenker's diverticulum). The cricopharyngeus muscle is responsible

for generating a high-pressure zone that marks the position of the UES and the esophageal introitus. Its distinctive bowing array of muscle fibers is unique and serves to transition into the circular esophageal musculature. This point of transition is flanked by the longitudinal esophageal muscles that extend superiorly to attach to the midportion of the posterior surface of the cricoid cartilage and form the V-shaped area of Laimer.

Esophageal Layers

The esophagus is comprised of two proper layers: the mucosa and the muscularis propria. It is distinguished from the other layers of the alimentary tract by its lack of a serosa. The mucosa is the innermost layer and consists of squamous epithelium for most of its course. The distal 1 to 2 cm of esophageal mucosa transitions to cardiac mucosa or junctional columnar epithelium at a point known as the *Z-line* (Fig. 41-5). Within the mucosa, there are four distinct layers: the epithelium, the basement membrane, the lamina propria, and the muscularis mucosae. Deep to the muscularis mucosae lays the submucosa (Fig. 41-6). Cached within is a plush network of lymphatic and vascular structures as well as mucous glands and Meissner's neural plexus. It is the red carpet on which every esophageal cancer cell aspires to win its Oscar and seize an opportunity for successful growth and invasion!

Enveloping the mucosa, directly abutting the submucosa, is the muscularis propria. Below the cricopharyngeus muscle, the esophagus is composed of two concentric muscle bundles: an inner circular and outer longitudinal (Fig. 41-7). Both layers of the upper third of the esophagus are striated, whereas the layers of the lower two thirds are smooth muscle. The circular muscles are an extension of the cricopharyngeus muscle and traverse through the thoracic cavity into the abdomen, where they become the middle circular muscles of the lesser curvature of the stomach. The collar of Helvetius marks the transition of the circular muscles of the esophagus to oblique muscles of the stomach at the incisura (cardiac notch). Between the layers of esophageal muscle

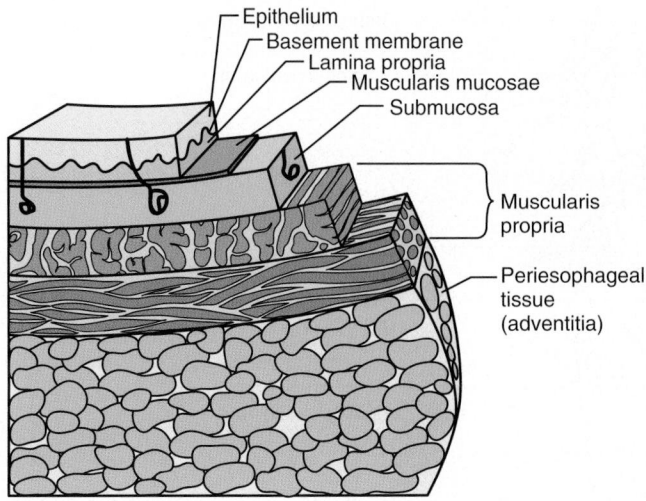

Figure 41-6 Layers of the esophagus. (Modified from Pearson FG, Cooper JD, Deslauriers J, et al: Esophageal Surgery, 2nd ed. New York, Churchill Livingstone, 2002, p 124.)

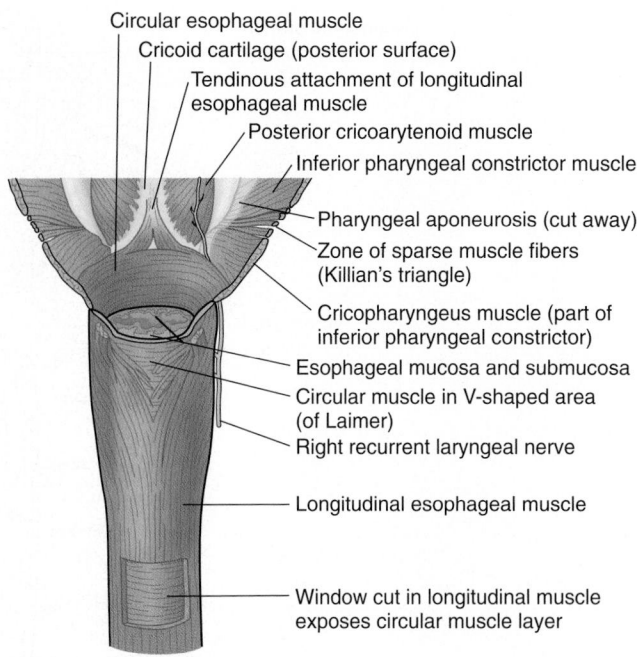

Posterior view with pharynx opened and mucosa removed

Figure 41-7 Muscles of the esophagus.

is a thin septum comprising connective tissue, blood vessels, and an interconnected network of ganglia known as *Auerbach's plexus.* Enshrouding the inner circular layer, the longitudinal muscles of the esophagus begin at the cricoid cartilage and extend into the abdomen, where they join the longitudinal musculature of the cardia of the stomach. The esophagus is then wrapped by a layer of fibroalveolar adventitia.

Anatomic Narrowing

The esophageal silhouette resembles an hourglass. There are three distinct areas of narrowing that contribute to its shape. Measuring 14 mm in diameter, the cricopharyngeus muscle is the narrowest point of the gastrointestinal tract and marks the superior-most portion of the hourglass-shaped esophagus. Occurring just below the carina, where the left main-stem bronchus and aorta abut the esophagus, the bronchoaortic constriction at the level of the 4th thoracic vertebra creates the center narrowing and measures 15 to 17 mm. Finally, the diaphragmatic constriction, measuring 16 to 19 mm, marks the inferior portion of the hourglass and occurs where the esophagus passes through the diaphragm. Between these three distinct areas of anatomic constriction are two areas of dilation known as the *superior* and *inferior dilations*. Within these areas, the esophagus resumes the normal diameter for an adult and measures about 2.5 cm.

Gastroesophageal Junction

The UES and LES mark the entrance and exit to the esophagus, respectively. These sphincters are defined by a high-pressure zone but can be difficult to identify anatomically. The UES corresponds reliably to the cricopharyngeus muscle, but the LES is more complex to discern. There are four anatomic points that identify the gastroesophageal junction (GEJ): two endoscopic and two external. Endoscopically, there are two anatomic consid-

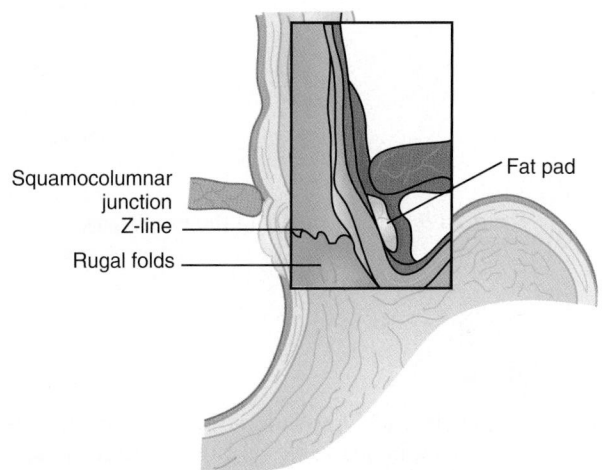

Figure 41-8 Identifiers of the gastroesophageal junction.

erations that may be used to identify the GEJ. The squamocolumnar epithelial junction (Z-line) may mark the GEJ provided the patient does not have a distal esophagus replaced by columnar-lined epithelium as seen with Barrett's esophagus. The transition from the smooth esophageal lining to the rugal folds of the stomach may also accurately identify the GEJ. Externally, the collar of Helvetius (or loop of Willis), where the circular muscular fibers of the esophagus join the oblique fibers of the stomach, and the gastroesophageal fat pad are consistent identifiers of the GEJ (Fig. 41-8).

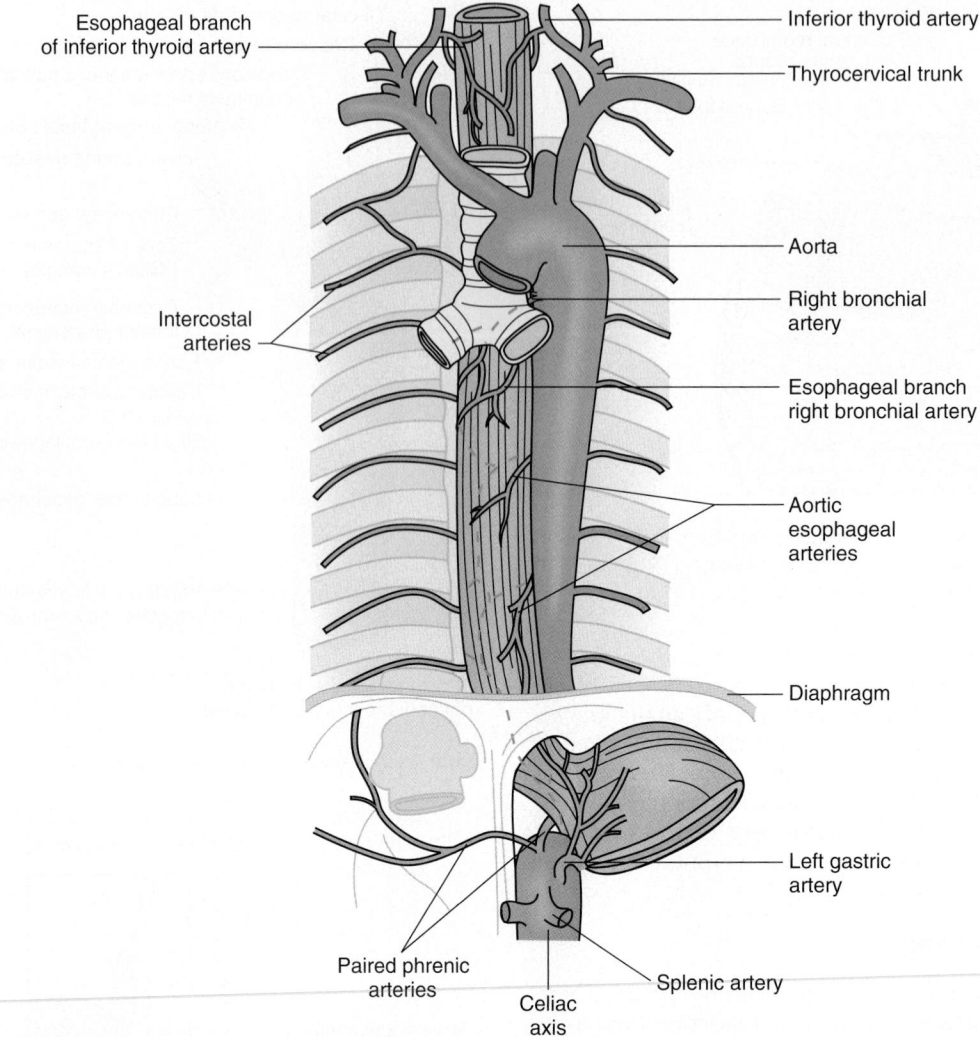

Esophageal branch
of inferior thyroid artery

Inferior thyroid artery

Thyrocervical trunk

Aorta

Right bronchial
artery

Intercostal
arteries

Esophageal branch
right bronchial artery

Aortic
esophageal
arteries

Diaphragm

Left gastric
artery

Paired phrenic
arteries

Splenic artery

Celiac
axis

Figure 41-9 Arterial supply to the esophagus.

Vasculature

The rich vascular and lymphatic structures that nourish and drain the esophagus serve as both a surgical safety net and a highway for metastases. The vasculature is divided into three segments: cervical, thoracic, and abdominal. The cervical esophagus receives most of its blood supply from the inferior thyroid arteries, which branch off of the thyrocervical trunk on the left and the subclavian artery on the right (Fig. 41-9). The cricopharyngeus muscle, which marks the inlet of the esophagus, is supplied by the superior thyroid artery. The thoracic esophagus receives its blood supply directly from four to six esophageal arteries coming off the aorta as well as esophageal branches off the right and left bronchial arteries. It is supplemented by descending branches off the inferior thyroid arteries, intercostal arteries, and ascending branches of the paired inferior phrenic arteries. The abdominal esophagus receives its blood supply from both the left gastric artery and the paired inferior phrenic arteries. All the arteries that supply blood to the esophagus terminate in a fine capillary network before they penetrate the muscular wall of the esophagus. After penetrating and supplying the muscular layers, the capillary network continues the length of the esophagus within the submucosal layer.

The venous drainage parallels the arterial vasculature, and is just as complex. In all parts of the esophagus, the rich submucosal venous plexus is the first basin for venous drainage of the esophagus. In the cervical esophagus, the submucosal venous plexus drains into the inferior thyroid veins, which are tributaries of the left subclavian vein and the right brachiocephalic vein (Fig. 41-10). The drainage of the thoracic esophagus is more intricate. The submucosal venous plexus of the thoracic esophagus joins with the more superficial esophageal venous plexus and the venae comitantes that envelop the esophagus at this level. This plexus in turn drains into the azygos and hemiazygos veins on the right and the

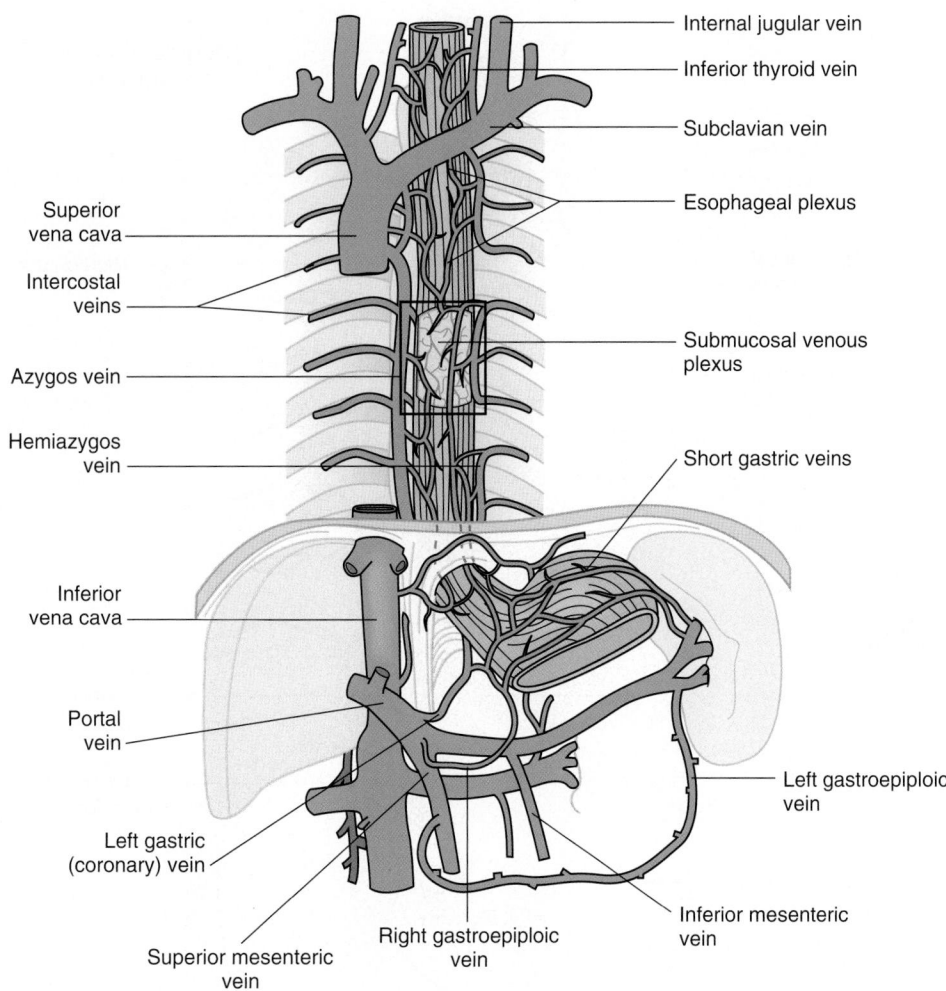

Internal jugular vein
Inferior thyroid vein
Subclavian vein
Esophageal plexus
Superior vena cava
Intercostal veins
Submucosal venous plexus
Azygos vein
Hemiazygos vein
Short gastric veins
Inferior vena cava
Portal vein
Left gastroepiploic vein
Left gastric (coronary) vein
Inferior mesenteric vein
Superior mesenteric vein
Right gastroepiploic vein

Figure 41-10 Venous drainage of the esophagus.

left side of the chest, respectively. The intercostal veins also drain into the azygos venous system. The abdominal esophagus drains into both the systemic and portal venous systems through the left and right phrenic veins, and the left gastric (coronary) vein and the short gastric veins, respectively.

Lymphatics

The lymphatic drainage of the esophagus is extensive and consists of two interconnecting lymphatic plexuses arising from the submucosa and muscularis layers. The submucosal lymphatics penetrate the muscularis propria and drain into the plexus that runs longitudinally in the esophageal wall. They then egress and drain into regional lymph node beds. In the upper two thirds of the esophagus, lymphatic flow is upward, whereas in the distal third, flow tends to be downward. Esophageal lymphatics begin in the neck with drainage to both the paratracheal lymph nodes anteriorly and the deep lateral cervical and internal jugular nodes laterally and posteriorly. Once inside the chest, the lymphatics form a matrix of interconnecting channels that drain into the mediastinal lymph nodes and thoracic duct. Anteriorly, the paratracheal

and subcarinal lymph nodes, as well as paraesophageal, retrocardiac, and infracardiac nodes, all drain the esophagus.

Other mediastinal stations, such as para-aortic and inferior pulmonary ligament nodes, also can receive drainage from the thoracic esophagus. Posteriorly, nodes along the esophagus and azygos veins are the primary sites of drainage (Fig. 41-11). The intricate lymphatic network of the esophagus allows for rapid spread of infection and tumor into three body cavities. It stands to reason that the rich arterial supply to the esophagus makes it one of the more durable organs in the body with respect to surgical manipulation, whereas its comprehensive venous and lymphatic drainage creates an oncologic challenge to controlling cellular migration. These anatomic complexities create surgical challenges when treating esophageal cancer and other esophageal diseases.

Innervation

The innervation to the esophagus is both sympathetic and parasympathetic (Fig. 41-12). The cervical sympathetic trunk arises from the superior ganglion in the neck.

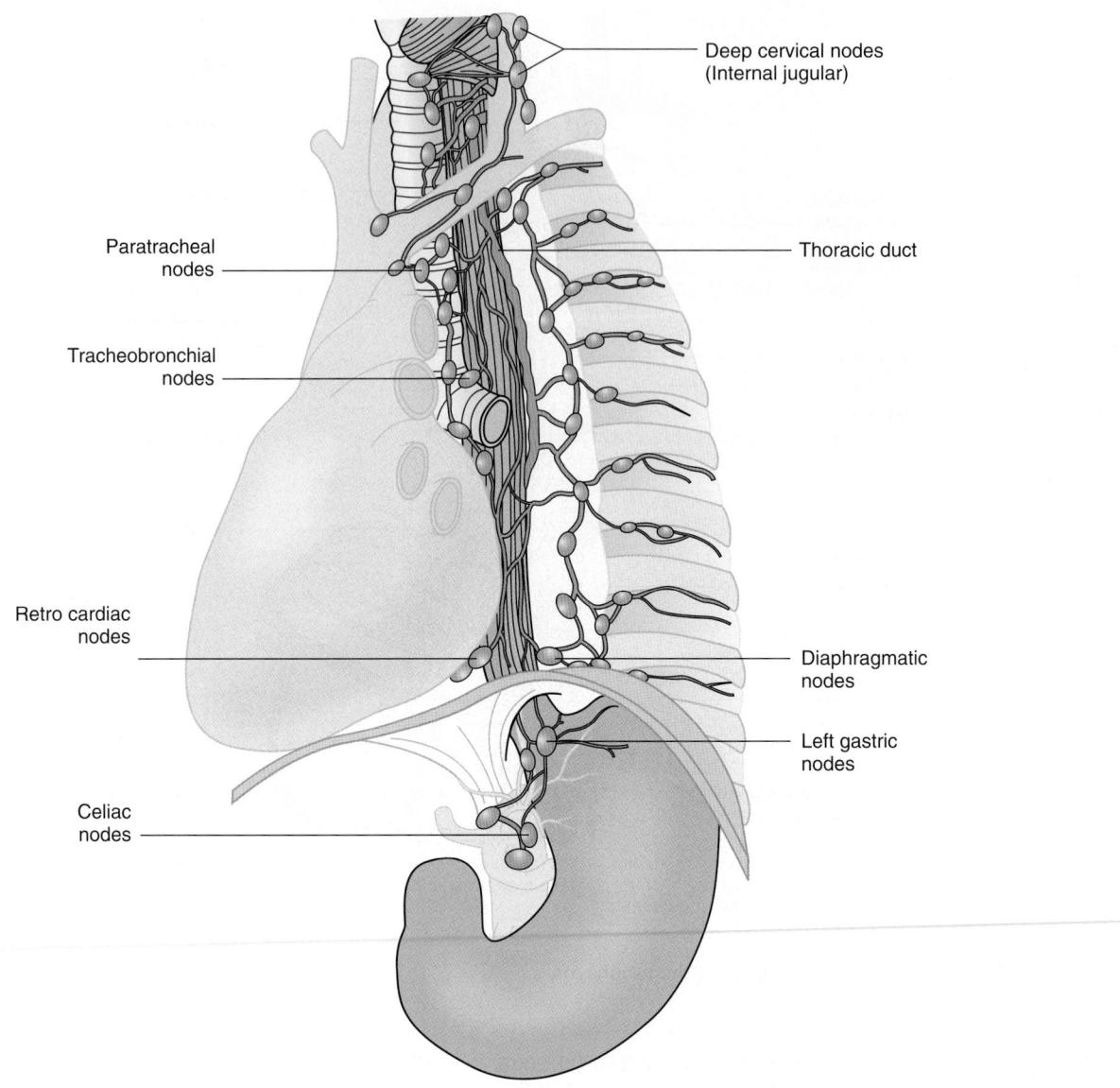

Figure 41-11 Lymphatic drainage of the esophagus.

It extends alongside the esophagus into the thoracic cavity, where it terminates in the cervicothoracic (stellate) ganglion. Along the way, it gives off branches to the cervical esophagus. The thoracic sympathetic trunk continues on from the stellate ganglion, giving off branches to the esophageal plexus that envelops the thoracic esophagus anteriorly and posteriorly. Inferiorly, the greater and lesser splanchnic nerves innervate the distal thoracic esophagus. In the abdomen, the sympathetic fibers lay posteriorly alongside the left gastric artery.

The parasympathetic fibers arise from the vagus nerve, which gives rise to the superior laryngeal nerve and the recurrent laryngeal nerve. The superior laryngeal nerve branches into the external and internal laryngeal nerves that supply motor innervation to the inferior pharyngeal constrictor muscle and cricothyroid muscle, and sensory innervation to the larynx, respectively (Fig. 41-13). The

right and left recurrent laryngeal nerves come off the vagus nerve and loop underneath the right subclavian artery and aortic arch, respectively. They then travel upward in the tracheoesophageal groove to enter the larynx laterally underneath the inferior pharyngeal constrictor muscle. Along their way, they provide innervation to the cervical esophagus, including the cricopharyngeus muscle. Unilateral injury to the superior or recurrent laryngeal nerve results in hoarseness and aspiration from laryngeal and UES dysfunction. In the thorax, the vagus nerve sends fibers to the striated muscle as well as parasympathetic preganglionic fibers to the smooth muscle of the esophagus. A weblike nervous plexus envelops the esophagus throughout its thoracic extent. These sympathetic and parasympathetic fibers penetrate through the muscular wall forming these networks between the muscle layers to become Auerbach's plexus and within

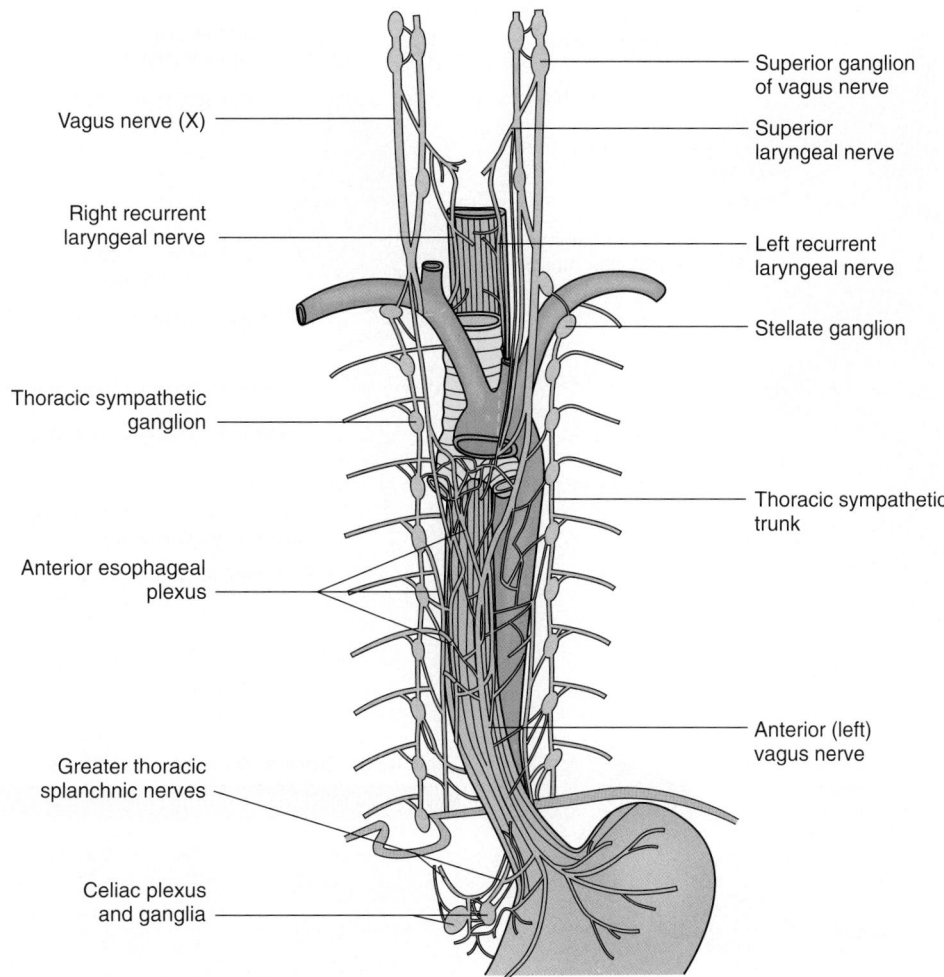

Vagus nerve (X)

Right recurrent
laryngeal nerve

Thoracic sympathetic
ganglion

Anterior esophageal
plexus

Greater thoracic
splanchnic nerves

Celiac plexus
and ganglia

Superior ganglion
of vagus nerve

Superior
laryngeal nerve

Left recurrent
laryngeal nerve

Stellate ganglion

Thoracic sympathetic
trunk

Anterior (left)
vagus nerve

Figure 41-12 Innervation of the esophagus.

the submucosal layer to become Meissner's plexus (Fig. 41-14). They provide an intrinsic autonomic nervous system within the esophageal wall that is responsible for peristalsis. Two centimeters above the diaphragm, the parasympathetic fibers coalesce into the left (anterior) and right (posterior) vagus nerves, which descend anteriorly onto the fundus and lesser curvature, and posteriorly onto the celiac plexus, respectively.

PHYSIOLOGY

Overview

Chicago architect Louis Sullivan is well known for his progressive philosophy that form should follow function. In anatomy, this is demonstrated often, and there is no better illustration of this principle in the human body than the esophagus. The primary function of the esophagus is to transport material from the pharynx to the stomach. Secondarily, the esophagus needs to constrain the amount of air that is swallowed and the amount of material that is refluxed. Its form has evolved nicely to enable its seamless functions. The esophagus measures a usual 30 cm extending from the pharynx down onto the cardia of the stomach. Under ideal physiologic conditions, the concentric muscular configuration permits effortless unidirectional flow of material from the top to the bottom of the esophagus. The UES, measuring 4 to 5 cm in length, remains in a constant state of tone (mean, 60 mm Hg), preventing a steady flow of air into the esophagus, whereas the tone in the LES (mean, 24 mm Hg) remains elevated just enough to prevent excessive material from refluxing back up into the esophagus (Table 41-1). Transportation of a food bolus from the mouth through the esophagus into the stomach begins with swallowing and ends with postrelaxation contraction of the LES, requiring coordinated peristaltic contractions in transit. It is a free ride for the material in transit as the esophageal neuromuscular form provides all functions

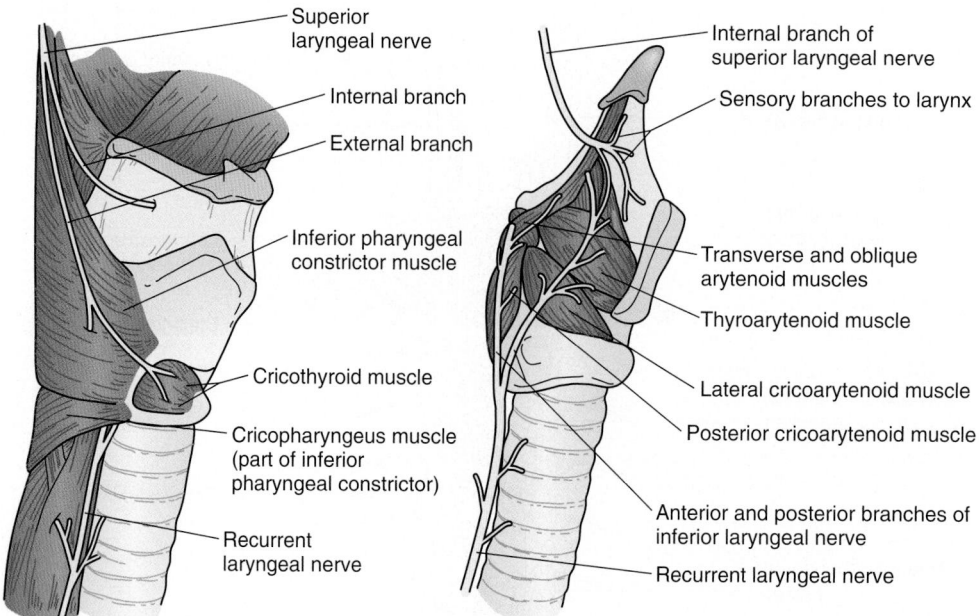

Figure 41-13 Innervation of the larynx.

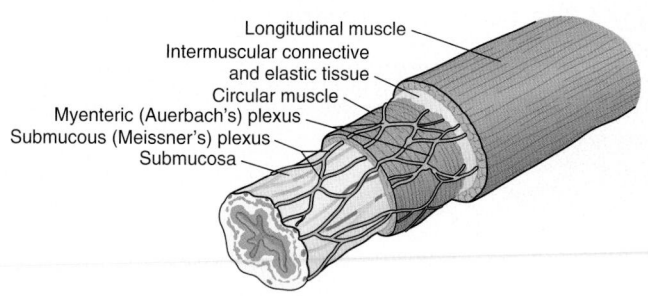

Figure 41-14 Intrinsic esophageal innervation.

Table 41-1 Normal Manometric Values

UPPER ESOPHAGEAL SPHINCTER	VALUES
Total length	4.0-5.0 cm
Resting pressure	60.0 mm Hg
Relaxation time	0.58 sec
Residual pressure	0.7-3.7 mm Hg
LOWER ESOPHAGEAL SPHINCTER	**VALUES**
Total length	3-5 cm
Abdominal length	2-4 cm
Resting pressure	6-26 mm Hg
Relaxation time	8.4 sec
Residual pressure	3 mm Hg
ESOPHAGEAL BODY CONTRACTIONS	**VALUES**
Amplitude	40-80 mm Hg
Duration	2.3-3.6 sec

necessary to power the food bolus through three body cavities.

Swallowing

There are three phases to swallowing: oral, pharyngeal, and esophageal. Six events occur during the oropharyngeal phase of swallowing (Fig. 41-15). These rapid series of events last about 1.5 seconds and, once initiated, are completely reflexive.

1. *Elevation of the Tongue.* Food is taken into the mouth and mixed with saliva to prepare a soft bolus for transport. The tongue pushes the bolus into the posterior oropharynx.
2. *Posterior Movement of the Tongue.* The tongue moves posteriorly and thrusts the food bolus into the hypopharynx.
3. *Elevation of the Soft Palate.* Simultaneously, as the tongue moves the food bolus into the hypopharynx, the soft palate is elevated to close off the passage into the nasopharynx.

4. *Elevation of the Hyoid.* To help bring the epiglottis under the tongue, the hyoid bone moves anteriorly and upward.
5. *Elevation of the Larynx.* The change in position of the hyoid elevates the larynx and opens up the retrolaryngeal space, further facilitating the movement of the epiglottis under the tongue.
6. *Tilting of the Epiglottis.* Finally, the epiglottis tilts back, covering the opening of the larynx to prevent aspiration.

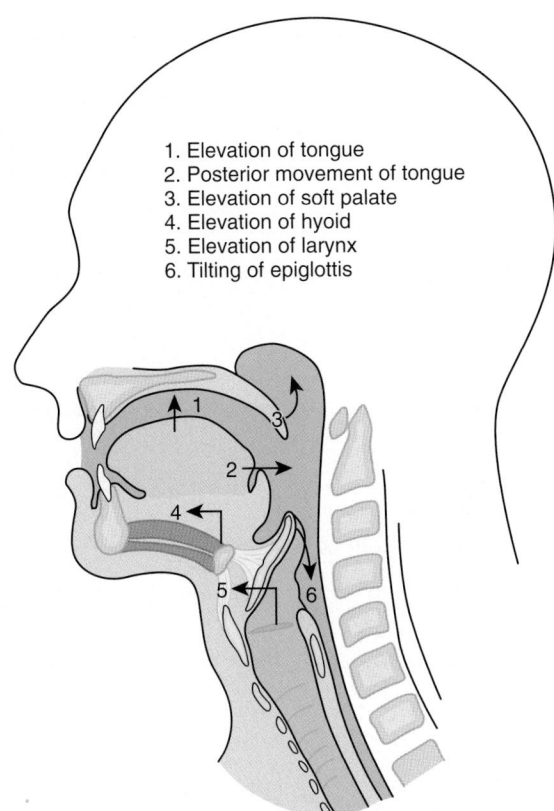

Figure 41-15 Phases of oropharyngeal swallowing. (Modified from Zuidema GD, Orringer MB: Shackelford's Surgery of the Alimentary Tract, 3rd ed. Philadelphia, WB Saunders, 1991, p 95.)

1. Elevation of tongue
2. Posterior movement of tongue
3. Elevation of soft palate
4. Elevation of hyoid
5. Elevation of larynx
6. Tilting of epiglottis

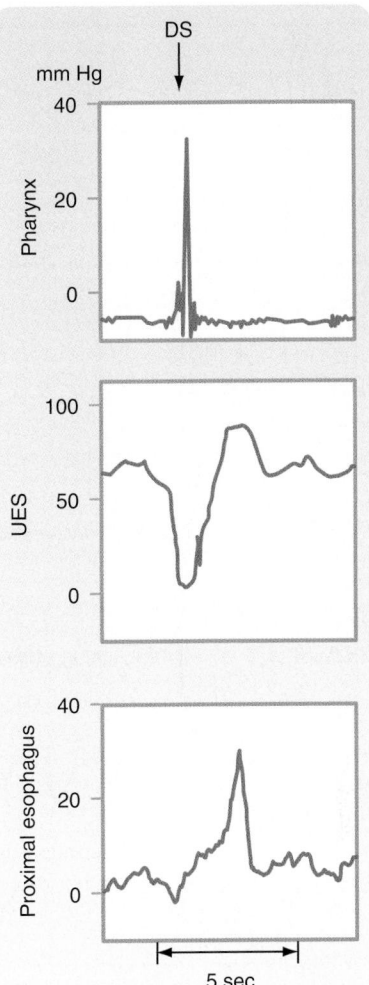

Figure 41-16 Manometry of the upper esophageal sphincter. (Modified from Pearson FG, Cooper JD, Deslauriers J, et al: Esophageal Surgery, 2nd ed. New York, Churchill Livingstone, 2002, p 480.)

Upper Esophageal Sphincter

The esophageal phase of swallowing is initiated by the activities during the pharyngeal phase. To allow passage of the food bolus, the UES relaxes, and the peristaltic contractions of the posterior pharyngeal constrictors propel the bolus into the esophagus. The pressure differential that is generated between the positive pressure in the cervical esophagus and the negative intrathoracic pressure sucks the bolus into the thoracic esophagus. Within 0.5 second of the initiation of swallowing, the UES closes, reaching close to 90 mm Hg. This postrelaxation contraction lasts 2 to 5 milliseconds and initiates peristalsis and prevents reflux of the bolus back into the pharynx. The UES pressure returns to resting pressure (60 mm Hg) as the wave travels into the midesophagus (Fig. 41-16).

Peristalsis

There are three types of esophageal contractions: primary, secondary, and tertiary. Primary peristaltic contractions are progressive and move down the esophagus at rate of 2 to 4 cm/sec and reach the LES about 9 seconds after the initiation of swallowing (Fig. 41-17). They generate an intraluminal pressure from 40 to 80 mm Hg. Successive swallows will follow with a similar peristaltic wave unless swallowing is repeated rapidly, at which time the esophagus will remain relaxed until the last swallow

occurs and peristalsis will follow. Secondary peristaltic contractions are also progressive but are generated from distention or irritation of the esophagus, rather than voluntary swallowing. They can occur as an independent local reflex to clear the esophagus of material that was left behind after the progression of the primary peristaltic wave. Tertiary contractions are nonprogressive, nonperistaltic, monophasic or multiphasic, simultaneous waves that can occur either after voluntary swallowing or spontaneously between swallows throughout the esophagus. They represent uncoordinated contractions of the smooth muscle that are responsible for esophageal spasm.

Lower Esophageal Sphincter

The final phase of esophageal bolus transit occurs through the LES. Although this is not a true sphincter, there is a distinct high-pressure zone that measures 2 to 5 cm in length and generates a resting pressure of 6 to 26 mm Hg. The LES is located both in the chest and the abdomen. A minimum total length of 2 cm, with at least 1 cm of

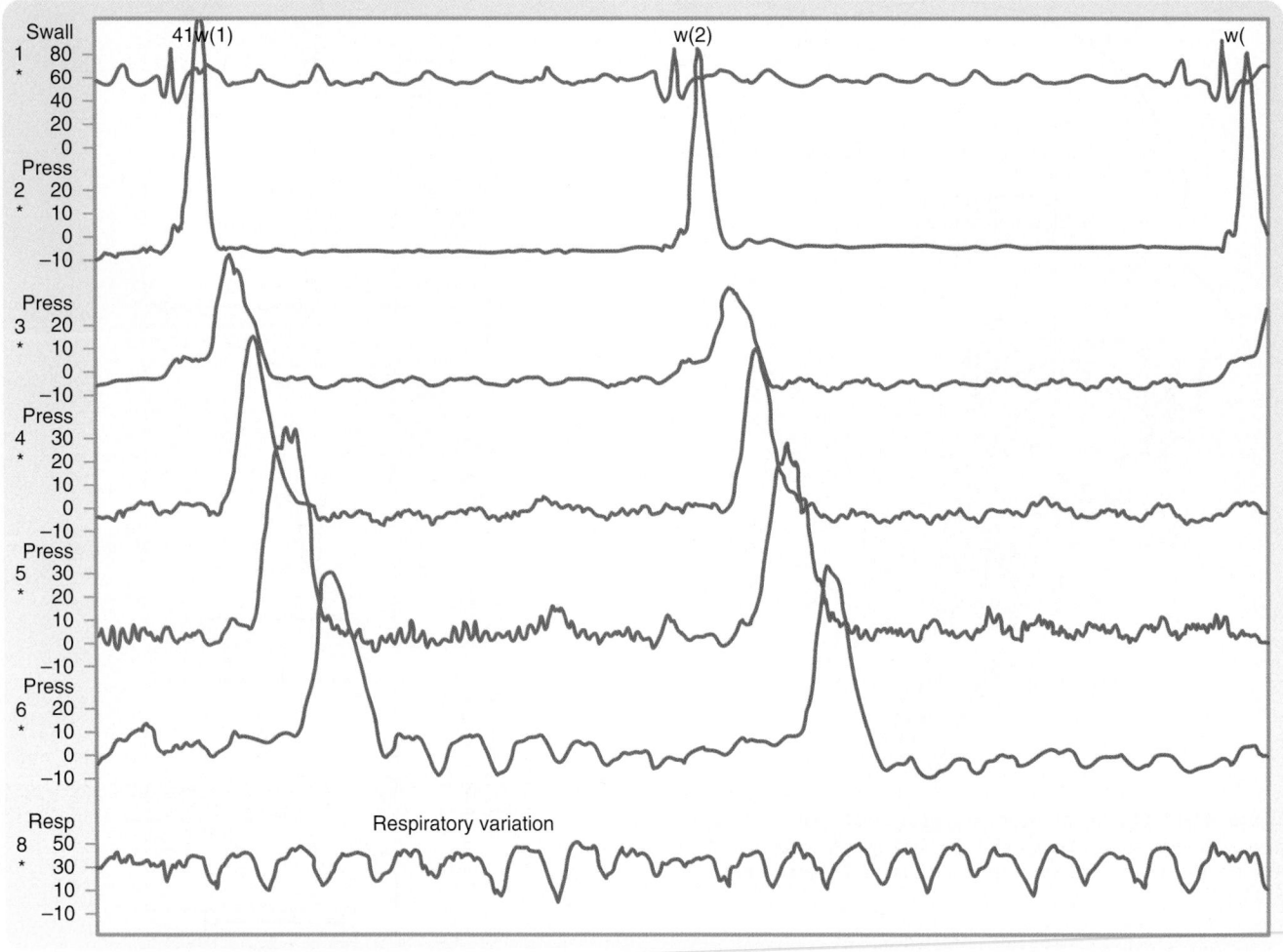

Figure 41-17 Normal esophageal peristalsis. (From Bremner CG, DeMeester TR, Bremner RM, Mason RJ: Esophageal Motility Testing Made Easy. St Louis, Quality Medical Publishing, 2001, p 35.)

intra-abdominal length, is required for normal LES function. The transition from the intrathoracic to the intraabdominal sphincter is noted on a manometric tracing and known as the *respiratory inversion point* (RIP) (Fig. 41-18). At this point, the pressure of the esophagus changes from negative to positive with inspiration and positive to negative with expiration.

Peristaltic contractions alone do not generate enough force to open up the LES. Vagal-mediated relaxation of the LES occurs 1.5 to 2.5 seconds after pharyngeal swallowing and lasts 4 to 6 seconds. This flawlessly timed relaxation is needed to allow efficient transport of a food bolus out of the esophagus and into the stomach. A postrelaxation contraction of the LES occurs after the peristaltic wave has passed through the esophagus, allowing the LES to return to its baseline pressure (Fig. 41-19), reestablishing a barrier to reflux.

Reflux Mechanism

Not all reflux is abnormal. Healthy individuals have occasional episodes of gastroesophageal reflux that is a result of spontaneous opening of the LES. The competence of the LES and its ability to establish a barrier to reflux depends on several factors: adequate pressure and length, radial symmetry, and motility of the esophagus and stomach. A competent sphincter is at least 2 cm and carries a pressure between 6 and 26 mm Hg. Radial asymmetry and abnormal peristalsis prevent proper closure and allow free refluxing of gastric material into the distal esophagus. Abnormal esophageal motility and poor gastric emptying result in inadequate esophageal clearance that also encourages reflux. Finally, neurotransmitters, hormones, and peptides that regulate the LES can increase or decrease tone. All these anatomic and physiologic disruptions can result in reflux through the LES and are implicated in the development of gastroesophageal reflux disease (GERD).

NEUROMUSCULAR DISORDERS OF THE ESOPHAGUS

Diverticula

Overview

Historically, esophageal diverticula were thought to be a primary disorder that resulted in motility abnormalities.

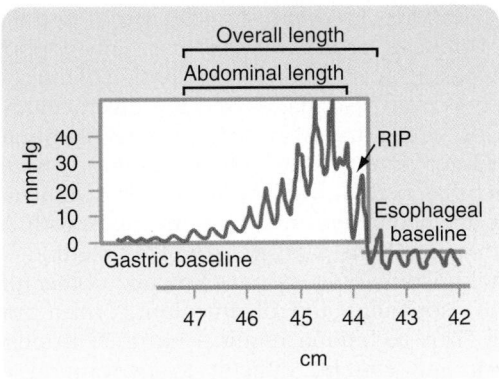

Figure 41-18 Normal lower esophageal sphincter. (From Bremner CG, DeMeester TR, Bremner RM, Mason RJ: Esophageal Motility Testing Made Easy. St Louis, Quality Medical Publishing, 2001, p 15.)

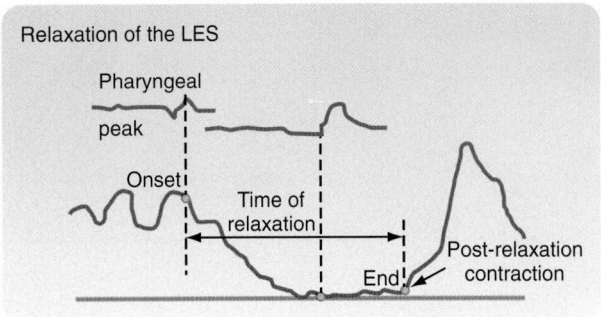

Figure 41-19 Relaxation of the lower esophageal sphincter. (From Bremner CG, DeMeester TR, Bremner RM, Mason RJ: Esophageal Motility Testing Made Easy. St Louis, Quality Medical Publishing, 2001, p 24.)

It is now well established that most diverticula are a result of a primary motor disturbance or an abnormality of the UES or LES. Early on, diverticula were classified according to their location, and as a convention, they are classifications to which we still adhere. Esophageal diverticula can occur in several places along the esophagus. The three most common sites of occurrence are pharyngoesophageal (Zenker's), parabronchial (midesophageal), and epiphrenic (supradiaphragmatic). True diverticula involve all layers of the esophageal wall, including mucosa, submucosa, and muscularis. A false diverticulum consists of mucosa and submucosa only. Pulsion diverticula are false diverticula that occur because of elevated intraluminal pressures generated from abnormal motility disorders. These forces cause the mucosa and submucosa to herniate through the esophageal musculature. Both a Zenker's diverticulum and an epiphrenic diverticulum fall under the category of false, pulsion diverticula. Traction, or true, diverticula result from external inflammatory mediastinal lymph nodes adhering to the esophagus as they heal and contract, pulling the esophagus during the process. Over time, the esophageal wall herniates, forming an outpouching, and a diverticulum ensues.

Pharyngoesophageal (Zenker's) Diverticulum

Background

Originally described by Drs. Zenker and Von Ziemssen, the pharyngoesophageal diverticulum (Zenker's diverticulum) is the most common esophageal diverticulum found today. It usually presents in older patients in the 7th decade of life and has been postulated to be a result of loss of tissue elasticity and muscle tone with age. It is specifically found herniating into Killian's triangle, between the oblique fibers of the thyropharyngeus muscle and the horizontal fibers of the cricopharyngeus muscle (Fig. 41-20). As the diverticulum enlarges, the mucosal and submucosal layers dissect down the left side of the esophagus into the superior mediastinum, posteriorly along the prevertebral space. Zenker's diverticulum is often referred to as *cricopharyngeal achalasia* and is managed accordingly.

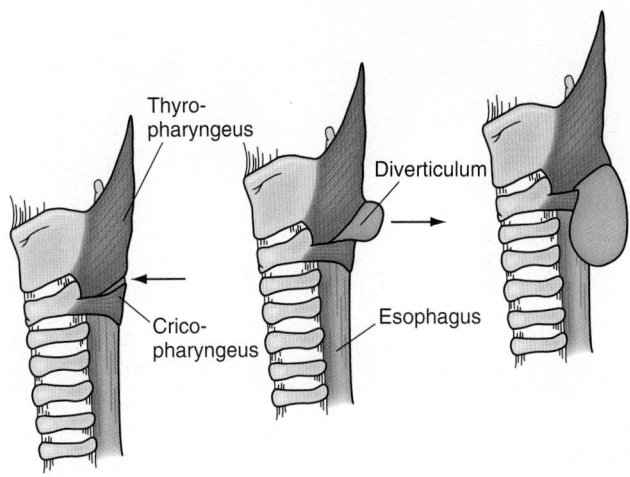

Figure 41-20 Zenker's diverticulum.

Symptoms and Diagnosis

Until the Zenker's diverticulum begins to enlarge, patients are often initially asymptomatic. Commonly, patients complain of a sticking in the throat. A nagging cough, excessive salivation, and intermittent dysphagia often are signs of progressive disease. As the sac increases in size, regurgitation of foul-smelling, undigested material is common. Halitosis, voice changes, retrosternal pain, and respiratory infections are especially common in the elderly population. Patients learn to compensate for the difficulties by avoiding social situations. The most serious complication from an untreated Zenker's diverticulum is aspiration pneumonia or lung abscess. In the elderly population, this can be morbid and sometimes fatal.

Diagnosis is made by barium esophagram (Fig. 41-21). At the level of the cricothyroid cartilage, the diverticulum can be seen filled with barium resting posteriorly alongside the esophagus. Lateral views are critical to obtain because this is usually a posterior structure. Neither esophageal manometry nor endoscopy is needed to make a diagnosis of Zenker's diverticulum.

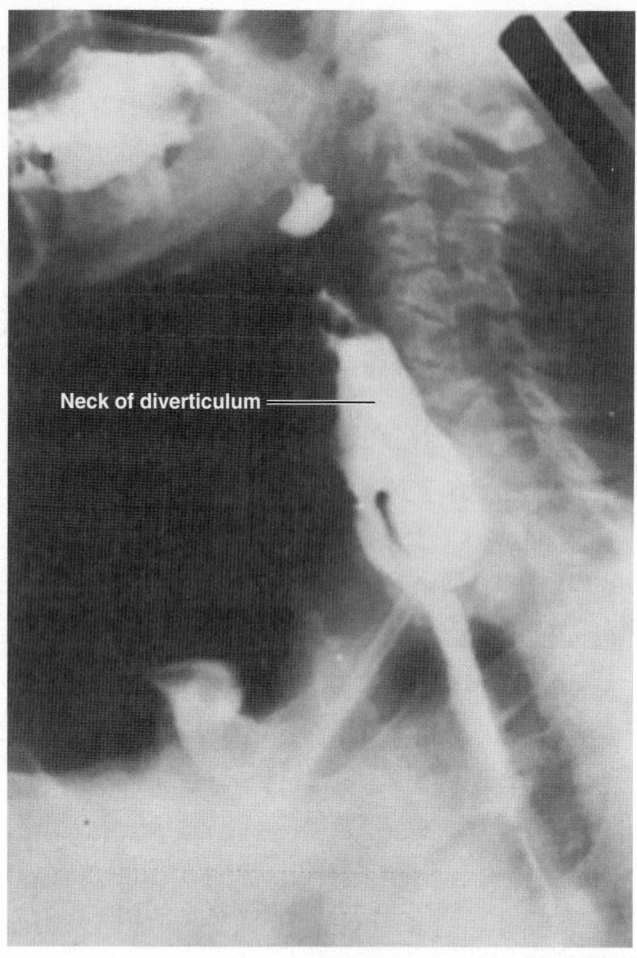

Neck of diverticulum ——————

Figure 41-21 Barium swallow showing Zenker's diverticulum. (Modified from Trastek VF, Deschamps C: Esophageal diverticula. In Shields TW, Locicero J III, Ponn RB [eds]: General Thoracic Surgery, 5th ed. Philadelphia, Lippincott Williams & Wilkins, p 1841.)

Treatment

Surgical or endoscopic repair of a Zenker's diverticulum is the gold standard of treatment. Traditionally, an open repair through the left neck was advocated. However, in recent years, endoscopic exclusion has gained popularity in many centers throughout the United States. Two types of open repair are performed: resection and pexy of the diverticulum. Both the diverticulectomy and the diverticulopexy are performed through an incision in the left neck. Under general anesthesia, they both require about 1 hour to complete. In all cases, a myotomy is performed of the proximal and distal thyropharyngeus and cricopharyngeus muscles. In cases of a small diverticulum (<2 cm), a myotomy alone is often sufficient. In frail patients who may be subject to a higher rate of cervical esophageal leak, a diverticulopexy, without resection, may be performed and will prevent symptoms from recurring.[3] In most patients with good tissue or a large sac (>5 cm), excision of the sac is indicated. The postoperative stay is about 2 to 3 days, during which the patient remains unable to eat or drink.

An alternative to open surgical repair is the endoscopic Dohlman procedure that has gained popularity over the past 10 years. Endoscopic division of the common wall between the esophagus and the diverticulum using a laser or stapler has also been successful. Because of the configuration of the inline stapling device, this approach has been advocated for larger diverticula. The risk for an incomplete myotomy increases with smaller diverticula less than 3 cm in size. This method divides the distal cricopharyngeus muscle while obliterating the sac. The esophagus and diverticulum form a common channel. This technique requires maximal extension of the neck and can be difficult to perform in elderly patients with cervical stenosis. It is done transorally under general anesthesia in about 1 hour. The postoperative course is slightly shorter, with patients taking liquids the following day and requiring only a single overnight hospital stay. For these reasons, this technique has gained favor and is advocated in patients with diverticula between 2 and 5 cm.

The results of open repair versus endoscopic repair have been well studied. For diverticula 3 cm or less in size, surgical repair is superior to endoscopic repair in eliminating symptoms. For any diverticulum greater than 3 cm, the results are the same.[4] Both the hospital stay and the length of inanition are shorter with an endoscopic procedure. Regardless of the method of repair, patients do very well, and the results are excellent.

Midesophageal Diverticula

Background

Midesophageal diverticula were first described in the 19th century. Historically, inflamed mediastinal lymph nodes from an infection with tuberculosis accounted for most cases (Fig. 41-22). More recently, infections with histoplasmosis and resultant fibrosing mediastinitis have become more common. Inflammation of the lymph nodes exerts traction on the wall of the esophagus and leads to the formation of a true diverticulum in the midesophagus. This continues to be an important mechanism for these traction diverticula; however, it is now believed that some may also be caused by a primary motility disorder such as achalasia, diffuse esophageal spasm (DES), or a nonspecific esophageal motility (NEM) disorder.

Symptoms and Diagnosis

Most patients with a midesophageal diverticulum are asymptomatic. They are often incidentally found during a workup for some other complaint. Dysphagia, chest pain, and regurgitation can be present and are usually indicative of an underlying primary motility disorder. Patients presenting with a chronic cough are under suspicion for development of a bronchoesophageal fistula. Rarely, hemoptysis can be a presenting symptom, indicating infectious erosion of lymph nodes into major vasculature and the bronchial tree. In this instance, the diverticulum is an incidental finding of lesser importance.

The diagnosis of the anatomic structure, as well as the size and location of an esophageal diverticulum, is made through a barium esophagram. Lateral views are needed to determine from which side of the esophagus the diverticulum is protruding. Midesophageal diverticula typically present on the right owing to the overabundance of structures in the midthoracic region of the left chest. It is also helpful to make a diagnosis of a concomitant fistula. A computed tomography (CT) scan is helpful to identify any mediastinal lymphadenopathy and may help to lateralize the sac. Endoscopy is important to rule out mucosal abnormalities, including cancer, that may be inconspicuously hidden in the sac. In addition, endoscopy aids in identifying a fistula. Manometric studies are undertaken in all patients, symptomatic or not, to identify a primary motor disorder. Patients presenting with dysphagia, chest pain, or regurgitation especially are manometrically evaluated. Treatment is guided by the results of the manometric findings.

Treatment

Determining the etiology for midesophageal diverticula is critical to guiding treatment. In asymptomatic patients who have inflamed mediastinal lymph nodes from tuberculosis or histoplasmosis, medical treatment with antituberculin or antifungal agents is indicated. If the diverticulum is smaller than 2 cm, it can be observed. If patients progress to become symptomatic or if the diverticulum is 2 cm or larger, surgical intervention is indicated. Usually, midesophageal diverticula have a wide mouth and rest close to the spine. For these reasons, a diverticulopexy can be performed where the diverticulum is suspended from the thoracic vertebral fascia. In patients with severe chest pain or dysphagia and a documented motor abnormality, a long esophagomyotomy is also indicated.

Epiphrenic Diverticula

Background

Epiphrenic diverticula are found adjacent to the diaphragm in the distal third of the esophagus, within 10 cm of the GEJ. They are most often related to thickened distal esophageal musculature or increased intraluminal pressure. They are pulsion, or false, diverticula that are often associated with DES, achalasia, and most commonly NEM disorders. In patients in whom a motility abnormality cannot be identified, a congenital (Ehlers-Danlos syndrome) or traumatic cause is considered. As with midesophageal diverticula, epiphrenic diverticula are more common on the right side and tend to be widemouthed.

Symptoms and Diagnosis

Most patients with epiphrenic diverticula present asymptomatically. They may present with dysphagia or chest pain, which is indicative of a motility disturbance. The diagnosis is often made during the workup for a motility disorder, and the diverticulum is found incidentally. Other symptoms, such as regurgitation, epigastric pain, anorexia, weight loss, chronic cough, and halitosis, are indicative of an advanced motility abnormality resulting in a sizable epiphrenic diverticulum.

MIDESOPHAGEAL TRACTION DIVERTICULUM

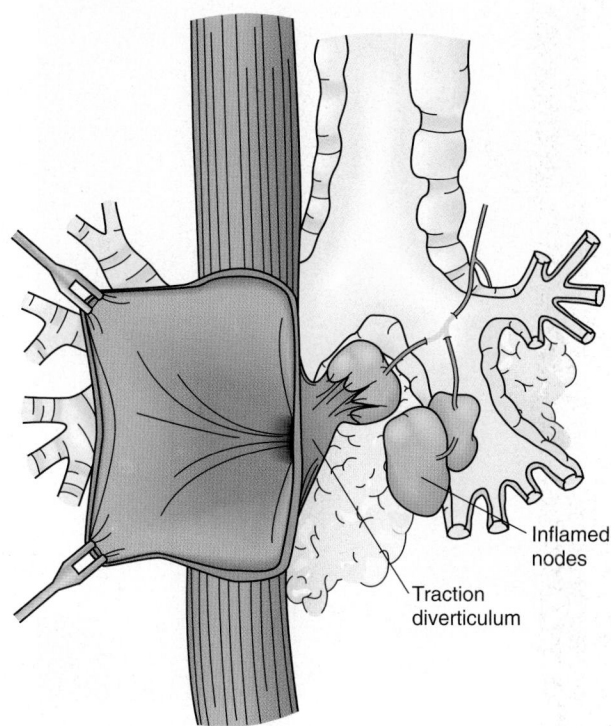

Inflamed nodes

Traction diverticulum

Figure 41-22 Midesophageal diverticulum. (Modified from Peters JH, DeMeester TR: Esophagus and diaphragmatic hernia. In Schwartz SI, Shires TG, Spencer FC [eds]: Principles of Surgery, 7th ed. New York, McGraw-Hill Professional, p 1130.)

A barium esophagram is the best diagnostic tool to detect the presence of an epiphrenic diverticulum (Fig. 41-23). The size, position, and proximity of the diverticulum to the diaphragm can all be clearly delineated. The underlying motility disorder is often identified as well; however, manometric studies need to be undertaken to evaluate the overall motility of the esophageal body and LES. An endoscopy is performed to evaluate for mucosal lesions, including esophagitis, Barrett's esophagus, and cancer.

Treatment

The treatment of an epiphrenic diverticulum is similar to that of a midesophageal diverticulum. These types of diverticula also have a wide mouth and rest close to the spine. Small (<2 cm) diverticula can be suspended from the vertebral fascia and need not be excised. In patients with severe chest pain, dysphagia, or a documented motor abnormality, a long esophagomyotomy is indicated. If a diverticulopexy is performed, the myotomy is begun at the neck of the diverticulum and extended onto the LES. If a diverticulectomy is pursued, a vertical stapling device is placed across the neck, and the diverticulum is excised. The muscle is closed over the excision site, and a long myotomy is performed on the opposite esophageal wall, extending from the level of the diverticulum onto the LES. If a large hiatal hernia is also present, the diverticulum is excised, a myotomy performed, and the hiatal hernia repaired. Failure to repair

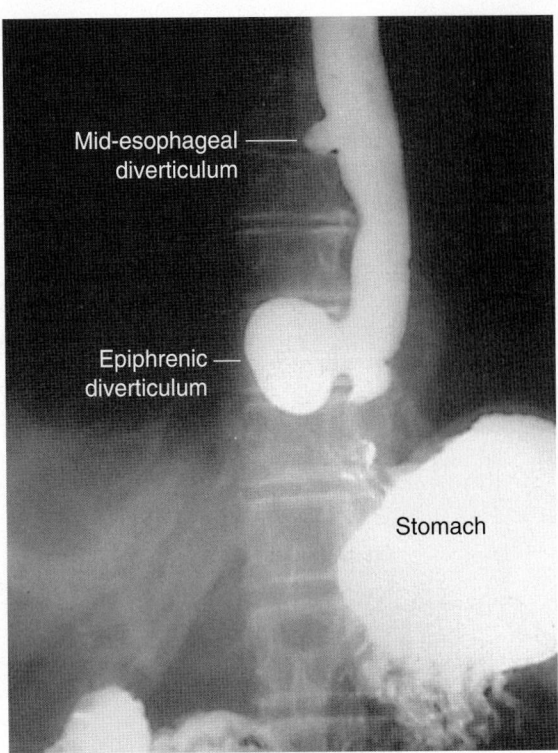

Figure 41-23 Barium swallow showing mid- and distal esophageal diverticula. (Modified from Pearson FG, Cooper JD, Deslauriers J, et al: Esophageal Surgery, 2nd ed. New York, Churchill Livingstone, 2002, p 508.)

the hernia results in a high incidence of postoperative reflux.

Motor Disorders

Overview

Motility disorders of the esophagus run on a continuum from hypomotile to hypermotile dysfunction, with intermediate types in between. There are both primary and secondary motor disorders of the esophagus. Most esophageal motility disorders fall into one of five primary motor disorders: achalasia, DES, nutcracker esophagus, hypertensive LES, and ineffective esophageal motility (IEM) (Table 41-2). The use of esophageal manometry has demonstrated a number of nonspecific abnormalities that reflect a spectrum of various stages of destruction of esophageal motor function that do not fit into a specific classification. Secondary motor disorders of the esophagus result from progression of other diseases such as collagen vascular and neuromuscular diseases and result in NEM disorders. Although the underlying pathologies are different, the presenting symptoms of primary and secondary motility disorders may be similar. A careful assessment must be done to ensure an accurate diagnosis and an appropriate treatment plan.

Achalasia

Background The literal meaning of *achalasia* is "failure to relax," which is said of any sphincter that remains in

a constant state of tone with periods of relaxation. It is the best understood of all esophageal motility disorders. The incidence is 6 per 100,000 persons per year and is seen in young women and middle-aged men and women alike. Its pathogenesis is presumed to be idiopathic or infectious neurogenic degeneration.[5] Severe emotional stress, trauma, drastic weight reduction, and Chagas' disease (parasitic infection with *Trypanosoma cruzi*) have also been implicated. Regardless of the etiology, both the muscle of the esophagus and the LES are affected. Prevailing theories support the model that the destruction of the nerves to the LES is the primary pathology and that degeneration of the neuromuscular function of the body of the esophagus is secondary. This degeneration results in both hypertension of the LES and failure of the LES to relax on pharyngeal swallowing, as well as pressurization of the esophagus, esophageal dilation, and a resultant loss of progressive peristalsis.

Vigorous achalasia is seen in a subset of patients presenting with dysphagia. In these patients, the LES is hypertensive and fails to relax, as seen in achalasia. Furthermore, the contractions of the esophageal body continue to be simultaneous and nonperistaltic. However, the amplitude of the contractions in response to swallowing is normal or high, which is inconsistent with classic achalasia. It is postulated that patients in the early development of achalasia may not have abnormalities in the esophageal body that are seen in later stages of the disease. Patients presenting with vigorous achalasia may be in this early phase and will go on to develop abnormal esophageal body contractions.

Achalasia is also known to be a premalignant condition of the esophagus. Over a 20-year period, a patient will have up to an 8% chance of developing carcinoma. Squamous cell carcinoma is the most common type identified and is thought to be the result of long-standing air-fluid levels in the body of the esophagus causing mucosal irritation and inducing metaplasia. Adenocarcinoma tends to appear in the middle third of the esophagus, below the air-fluid level where the mucosal irritation is the greatest. No specific surveillance program has yet to be initiated in patients with treated achalasia.

Symptoms and Diagnosis The classic triad of presenting symptoms consists of dysphagia, regurgitation, and weight loss. However, heartburn, postprandial choking, and nocturnal coughing are seen commonly. The dysphagia that patients experience begins with liquids and progresses to solids. Most patients describe eating as a laborious process during which they must pay special attention to the process. They eat slowly and use large volumes of water to help wash the food down into the stomach. As the water builds up pressure, retrosternal chest pain is experienced and can be quite severe until the LES opens and is quickly relieving. Regurgitation of undigested, foul-smelling foods is common, and with progressive disease, aspiration can become life-threatening. Pneumonia, lung abscess, and bronchiectasis often result from long-standing achalasia. The dysphagia progresses slowly over years, and patients adapt their lifestyle to accommodate the inconveniences that accompany this disease. Patients often do not seek medical attention

Table 41-2 Manometric Features of Primary and Nonspecific Esophageal Motility Disorders

	NORMAL	ACHALASIA	VIGOROUS ACHALASIA	HYPERTENSIVE LOWER ESOPHAGEAL SPHINCTER (LES)	DIFFUSE ESOPHAGEAL SPASM	NUTCRACKER ESOPHAGUS	INEFFECTIVE ESOPHAGEAL MOTILITY	NONSPECIFIC ESOPHAGEAL MOTILITY DISORDER
Symptoms	None	Dysphagia Chest pressure Regurgitation	Dysphagia Chest pain	Dysphagia	Chest pain Dysphagia	Dysphagia Chest pain	Dysphagia Heartburn Chest pain	Dysphagia Chest pain
Esophagram	Normal	Bird's beak Dilated esophagus	Abnormal	Distal obstruction	Corkscrew esophagus	Normal progressive contractions	Slow transit Incomplete emptying	Slow transit Incomplete emptying
Endoscopy	Normal	Patulous esophagus	Normal	Normal	Hyperperistalsis	Hyperperistalsis	Nonspecific	Nonspecific
LES Pressure	15-25 mm Hg	Hypertensive (>26 mm Hg)	Normal or hypertensive	Hypertensive (>26 mm Hg)	Normal or slightly elevated	Normal	Normal or low	Normal
LES Relaxation	Follows swallowing	Incomplete Residual pressure (>5 mm Hg)	Partial or absent	Normal	Normal	Normal	Normal	Incomplete (>90%) Residual pressure (>5 mm Hg)
Amplitude Pressure	50-120 mm Hg	Decreased (<40 mm Hg)	Normal	Normal	Normal	Hypertensive (>180 mm Hg) (>400 mm Hg)	Decreased (<30 mm Hg)	Decreased (<35 mm Hg)
Contraction Waves	Progressive	Simultaneous Mirrored Pressurized	Simultaneous Repetitive	Normal	Simultaneous Repetitive	Long duration (>6 sec)	Nontransmitted (>30%)	Nontransmitted (>20%) Triple-peaked, retrograde Prolonged (>6 sec)
Peristalsis	Normal	None	None	Normal	None	Hypertensive peristalsis	Abnormal	Abnormal

LES, lower esophageal sphincter.

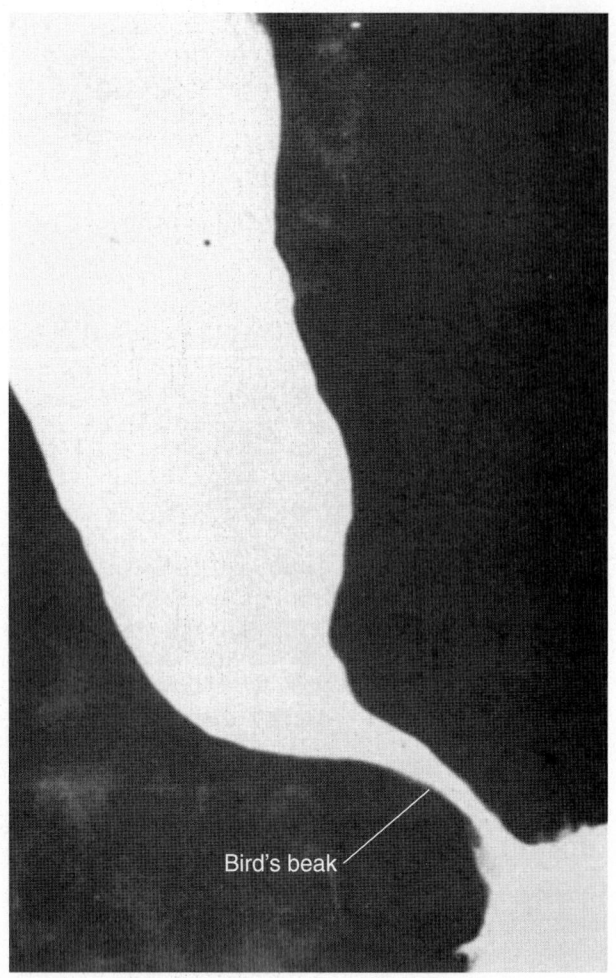

Bird's beak

Figure 41-24 Barium swallow showing achalasia. (Modified from Dalton CB: Esophageal motility disorders. In Pearson FG, Cooper JD, Deslauriers J, et al [eds]: Esophageal Surgery, 2nd ed. New York, Churchill Livingstone, 2002, p 519.)

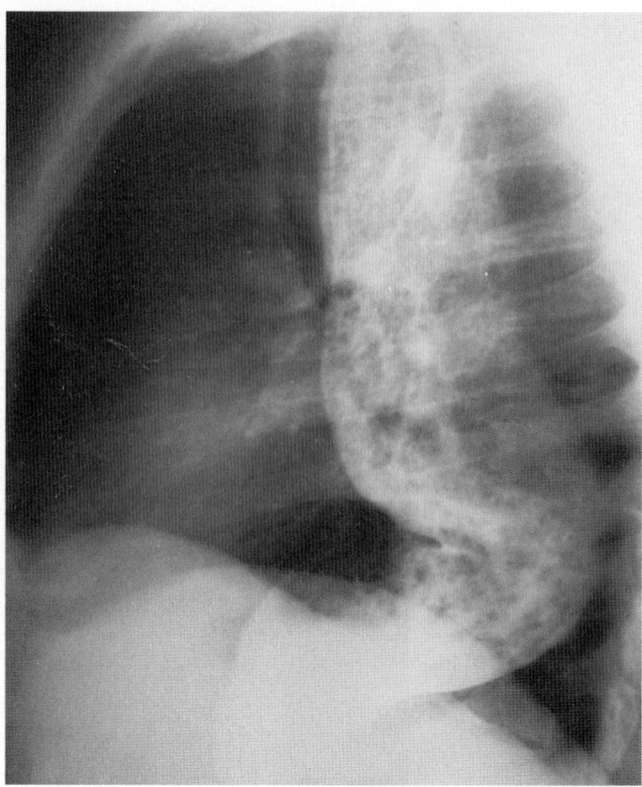

Figure 41-25 Barium swallow showing megaesophagus. (From Orringer MB: Disorders of esophageal motility. In Sabiston DC [ed]: Textbook of Surgery, The Biological Basis of Modern Surgical Practice, 15th ed. Philadelphia, WB Saunders, 1997, p 719.)

until their symptoms are quite advanced and will present with marked distension of the esophagus.

The diagnosis of achalasia is usually made from an esophagram and a motility study. The findings may vary some depending on the advanced nature of the disease. The esophagram will show a dilated esophagus with a distal narrowing referred to as the classic "bird's beak" appearance of the barium-filled esophagus (Fig. 41-24). Sphincter spasm and delayed emptying through the LES, as well as dilation of the esophageal body, are observed. A lack of peristaltic waves in the body and failure of relaxation of the LES are observed. Lack of a gastric air bubble is a common finding on the upright portion of the esophagram and is a result of the tight LES not allowing air to pass easily into the stomach. In the more advanced stage of disease, massive esophageal dilation, tortuosity, and a sigmoidal esophagus (megaesophagus) are seen (Fig. 41-25).

Manometry is the gold standard test for diagnosis and will help eliminate other potential esophageal motility disorders. In typical achalasia, the manometry tracings show five classic findings: two abnormalities of the LES and three of the esophageal body. The LES will be hypertensive with pressures usually above 35 mm Hg, but more importantly, it will fail to relax with deglutition (Fig. 41-26). The body of the esophagus will have a pressure above baseline (pressurization of the esophagus) from incomplete air evacuation, simultaneous mirrored contractions with no evidence of progressive peristalsis, and low-amplitude waveforms indicating a lack of muscular tone (Fig. 41-27). These five findings provide a diagnosis of achalasia. An endoscopy is performed to evaluate the mucosa for evidence of esophagitis or cancer. It otherwise contributes little to the diagnosis of achalasia.

Treatment There are both surgical and nonsurgical treatment options for patients with achalasia; all are directed toward relieving the obstruction caused by the LES. Because none of them addresses the issue of decreased motility in the esophageal body, they are all palliative treatments. Nonsurgical treatment options include medications and endoscopic interventions but usually are only a short-term solution to a lifelong problem. In the early stage of the disease, medical treatment with sublingual nitroglycerin, nitrates, or calcium channel blockers may offer hours of relief of chest pressure before or after a meal.[6] Bougie dilation up to 54 French may offer several months of relief but requires

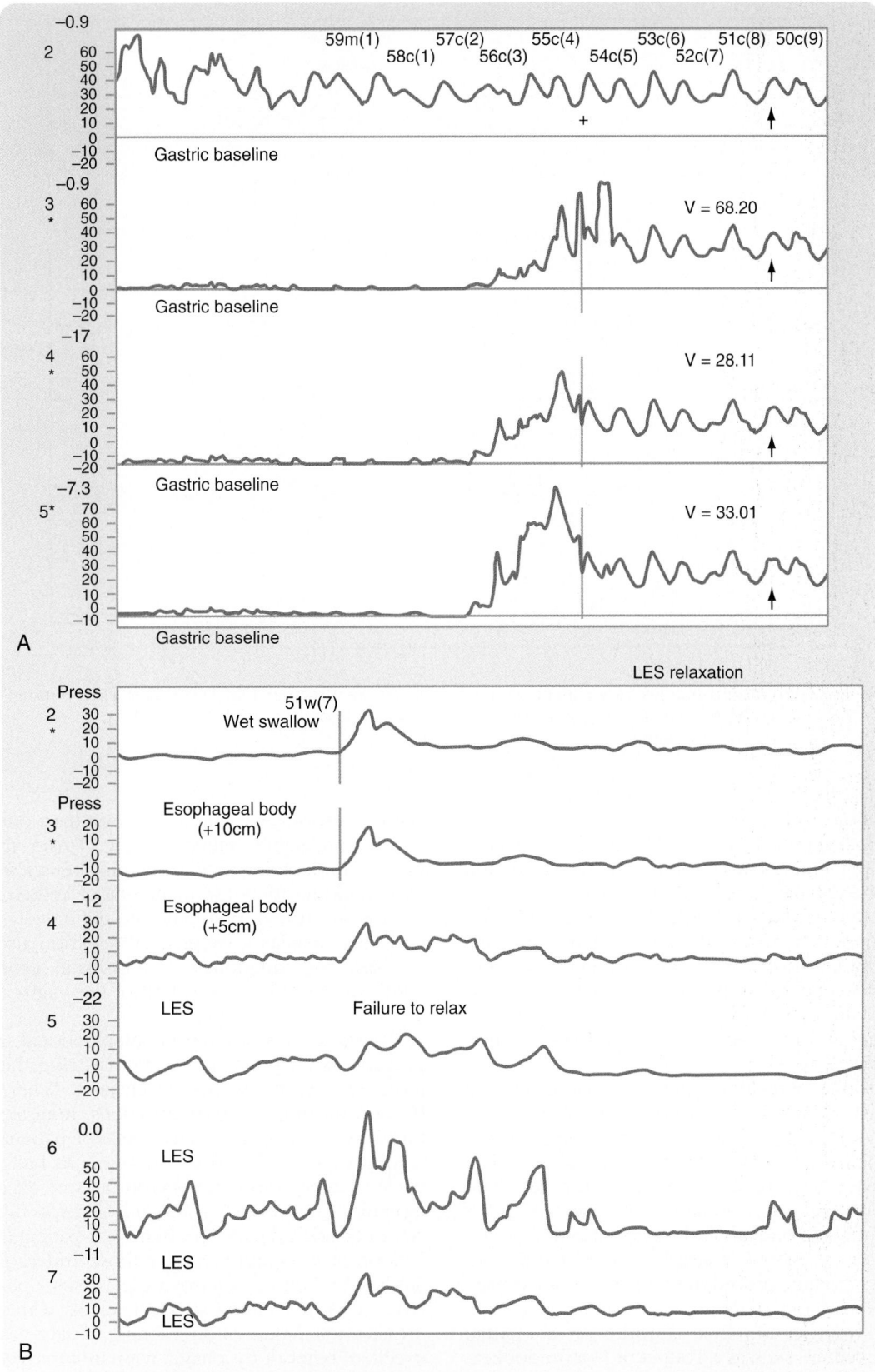

Figure 41-26 Motility of the lower esophageal sphincter in a patient with achalasia. (Modified from Pearson FG, Cooper JD, Deslauriers J, et al [eds]: Esophageal Surgery, 2nd ed. New York, Churchill Livingstone, 2002, p 520.)

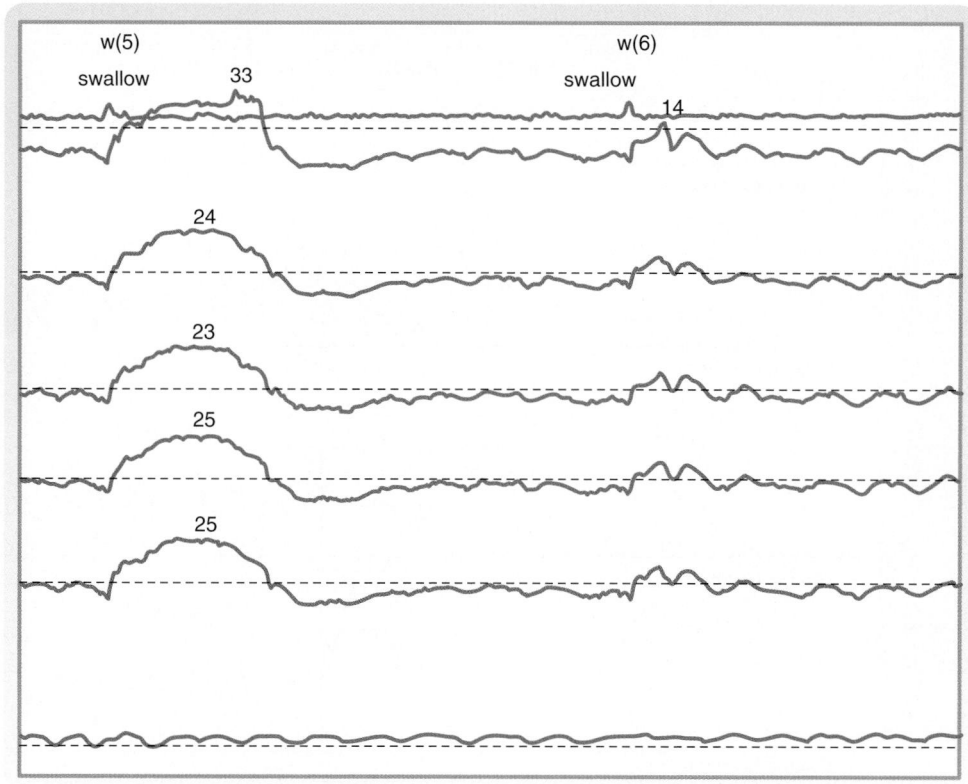

Figure 41-27 Esophageal motility in a patient with achalasia. (From Bremner CG, DeMeester TR, Bremner RM, Mason RJ: Esophageal Motility Testing Made Easy. St Louis, Quality Medical Publishing, 2001, p 75.)

repeated dilations to be sustainable. Injections of botulinum toxin (Botox) directly into the LES blocks acetylcholine release, preventing smooth muscle contraction, and effectively relaxes the LES. With repeated treatments, Botox may offer symptomatic relief for years, but symptoms recur more than 50% of the time within 6 months.[6] Dilation with a Gruntzig-type (volume-limited, pressure-control) balloon is effective in 60% of patients and has a risk for perforation less than 4%; however, perforation is life-threatening and must be weighed carefully in otherwise unhealthy patients.

Surgical esophagomyotomy offers superior results and is less traumatic than balloon dilation.[7] The current technique is a modification of the Heller myotomy that was described originally by a laparotomy in 1913.[8] A variety of changes have been made to the originally described operation; however, the modified laparoscopic Heller myotomy is now the operation of choice. It is done open or with video or robotic assistance. The decision to perform an antireflux procedure remains controversial. Most patients who have undergone a myotomy will experience some symptoms of reflux. The addition of a partial antireflux procedure, such as a Toupet or Dor fundoplication, will restore a barrier to reflux and decrease postoperative symptoms. This is especially true in patients whose esophageal clearance is greatly impaired.[9]

Esophagectomy is considered in any symptomatic patient with tortuous esophagus (megaesophagus), sigmoid esophagus, failure of more than one myotomy, or an undilatable reflux stricture. Fewer than 60% of patients undergoing repeat myotomy benefit from surgery, and fundoplication for treatment of reflux strictures is even more dismal. In addition to definitively treating the end-stage achalasia, esophageal resection also eliminates the risk for carcinoma. A transhiatal esophagectomy with[10] or without preservation of the vagus nerve offers a good long-term result.

Results Results of medical, interventional, and surgical procedures all point to surgery as being the safest and most effective treatment of achalasia. When comparing balloon dilation to Botox injections, remission of symptoms occurred in 89% versus 38% of patients at 1 year, respectively. Studies done to compare balloon dilation versus surgery show perforation rates of 4% and 1% and mortality rates of 0.5% and 0.2%, respectively. Results were considered excellent in 60% of patients undergoing balloon dilation and in 85% of those undergoing surgery. Studies looking at laparoscopic versus open myotomy have all demonstrated superior results with a minimally invasive technique. Shorter length of stay, less pain, and excellent relief of dysphagia with an improved heartburn score have all been documented with a laparoscopic approach. Furthermore, laparoscopic myotomy appears to be safe and effective even after treatment with Botox or balloon dilation, or with a massively dilated esophagus. Although most patients present fairly early in their disease process, end-stage achalasia is still found in a small percentage of patients. In these late presentations, a surgical myotomy is not likely to be effective.

Diffuse Esophageal Spasm

Background DES is a poorly understood hypermotility disorder of the esophagus. Although it presents in a similar fashion to achalasia, it is five times less common. It is seen most often in women and is often found in patients with multiple complaints. The etiology of the neuromuscular physiology is unclear. The basic pathology is related to a motor abnormality of the esophageal body that is most notable in the lower two thirds of the esophagus. Muscular hypertrophy and degeneration of the branches of the vagus nerve in the esophagus have been observed. As a result, the esophageal contractions are repetitive, simultaneous, and of high amplitude.

Symptoms and Diagnosis The clinical presentation of DES is typically that of chest pain and dysphagia. These symptoms may be related to eating or exertion and may mimic angina. Patients will complain of a squeezing pressure in the chest that may radiate to the jaw, arms, and upper back. The symptoms are often pronounced during times of heightened emotional stress. Regurgitation of esophageal contents and saliva is common, but acid reflux is not. However, acid reflux can aggravate the symptoms, as can cold liquids. Other functional gastrointestinal complaints, such as irritable bowel syndrome and pyloric spasm, may accompany DES, whereas other gastrointestinal problems, such as gallstones, peptic ulcer disease, and pancreatitis, all trigger DES.

The diagnosis of DES is made by an esophagram and manometric studies. The classic picture of the corkscrew esophagus or pseudodiverticulosis on an esophagram is due to the presence of tertiary contractions and indicative of advanced disease (Fig. 41-28). A distal bird-beak narrowing of the esophagus and normal peristalsis can also be noted. The classic manometry findings in DES are simultaneous, multipeaked contractions of high amplitude (>120 mm Hg) or long duration (>2.5 sec) (Fig. 41-29). These erratic contractions occur after more than 10% of wet swallows. Because of the spontaneous contractions and intermittent normal peristalsis, a standard manometry may not be enough to identify DES. An ambulatory motility record has been identified as being able to diagnose this disease with a sensitivity of 90% and a specificity of 100% based on an identified set of abnormalities. Correlation of subjective complaints with evidence of spasm (induced by a vagomimetic drug, bethanechol) on manometric tracings is also convincing evidence of this capricious disease.

Treatment The treatment for DES is far from ideal. Today the mainstay of treatment for DES is nonsurgical, and pharmacologic or endoscopic intervention is preferred. Surgery is reserved for patients with recurrent incapacitating episodes of dysphagia and chest pain who do not respond to medical treatment. All patients are evaluated for psychiatric conditions, including depression, psychosomatic complaints, and anxiety. Control of these disorders and reassurance of the esophageal nature of the chest pain they are experiencing is often thera-

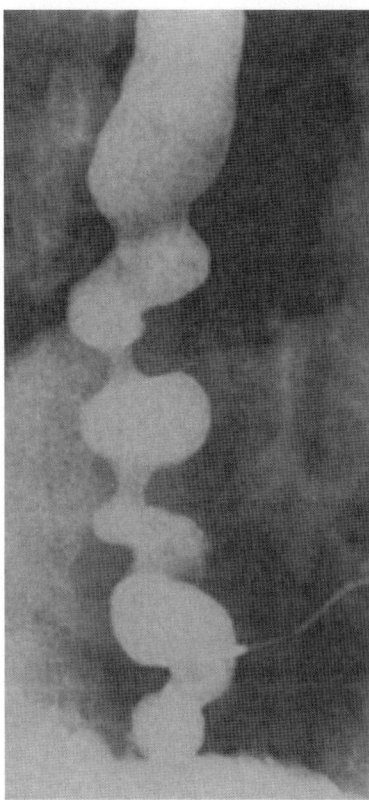

Figure 41-28 Barium esophagram of diffuse esophageal spasm. (Modified from Peters JH, DeMeester TR: Esophagus and diaphragmatic hernia. In Schwartz SI, Shires TG, Spencer FC [eds]: Principles of Surgery, 7th ed. New York, McGraw-Hill Professional, p 1129.)

peutic in and of itself. If dysphagia is a component of a patient's symptoms, steps must be taken to eliminate trigger foods or drinks from the diet. Similarly, if reflux is a component, acid suppression medications are helpful. Nitrates, calcium channel blockers, sedatives, and anticholinergics may be effective in some cases, but the relative efficacy of these medicines is not known. Peppermint may also provide temporary symptomatic relief.[11] Bougie dilation of the esophagus up to 50 or 60 French provides relief for severe dysphagia and is 70% to 80% effective. Botulinum toxin injections have also been tried with some success, but the results are not sustainable.

Surgery is indicated in patients with incapacitating chest pain or dysphagia who have failed medical and endoscopic therapy, or in the presence of a pulsion diverticulum of the thoracic esophagus. A long esophagomyotomy is performed through a left thoracotomy or a left video-assisted technique. Esophageal manometry is a useful guide to determine the extent of the myotomy. Some surgeons advocate extending the myotomy up into the thoracic inlet, but most agree that the proximal extent generally should be high enough to encompass the entire length of the abnormal motility, as determined by manometric measurements. The distal extent of the myotomy is extended down onto the LES, but the need to include the stomach is not agreed on uniformly. A Dor fundoplication is recommended to prevent healing of the myotomy

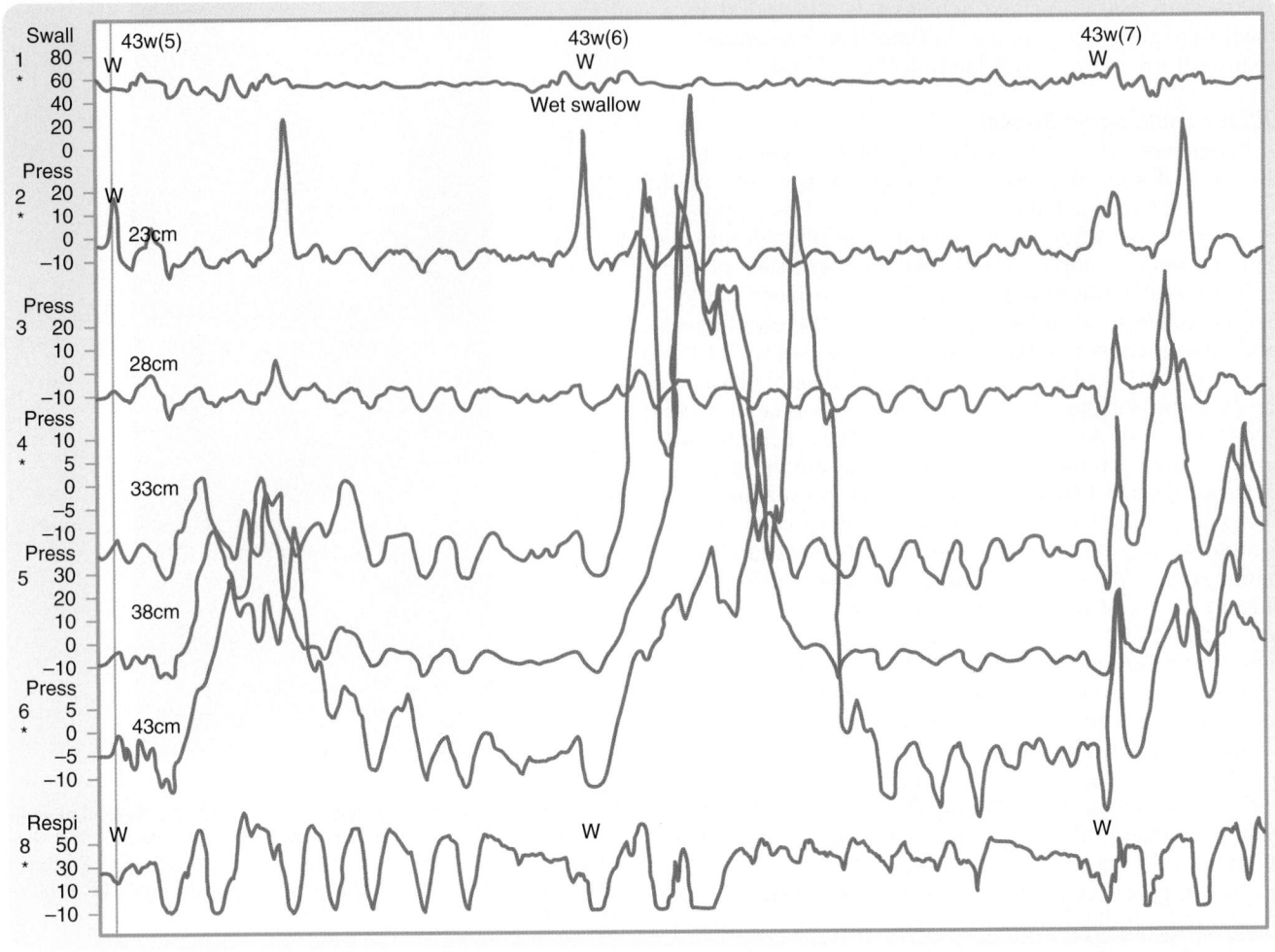

Figure 41-29 Manometry findings in diffuse esophageal spasm. (From Bremner CG, DeMeester TR, Bremner RM, Mason RJ: Esophageal Motility Testing Made Easy. St Louis, Quality Medical Publishing, 2001, p 83.)

site and provide reflux protection. Results of the long esophagomyotomy for DES are variable, but it can provide relief of symptoms up to 80% of the time.

Nutcracker Esophagus

Background Recognized in the late 1970s as an entity unto its own, nutcracker esophagus is a hypermotility disorder also known as supersqueeze esophagus. It is described as an esophagus with hypertensive peristalsis or high-amplitude peristaltic contractions. It is seen in patients of all ages with equal gender predilection and is the most common of all esophageal hypermotility disorders. Like DES, the pathophysiology is not well understood. It is associated with hypertrophic musculature that results in high-amplitude contractions of the esophagus and is the most painful of all esophageal motility disorders.

Symptoms and Diagnosis Patients present in a similar fashion to patients with DES with chest pain and dysphagia. Odynophagia is also noted, but regurgitation and reflux are uncommon. An esophagram may or may not reveal any abnormalities. The gold standard of diagnosis

is the subjective complaint of chest pain with simultaneous objective evidence of peristaltic esophageal contractions 2 standard deviations above the normal values on manometric tracings. Amplitudes of more than 400 mm Hg are common (Fig. 41-30). The LES pressure is normal, and relaxation occurs with each wet swallow. Ambulatory monitoring can help distinguish this disorder from DES. This is of critical importance because a subset of DES patients with dysphagia can be helped with esophagomyotomy, but surgery is of questionable value in patients with a nutcracker esophagus.

Treatment The treatment of nutcracker esophagus is medical. Calcium channel blockers, nitrates, and antispasmodics may offer temporary relief during acute spasms. Bougie dilation may offer some temporary relief of severe discomfort but has no long-term benefits. Patients with nutcracker esophagus may have triggers and are counseled to avoid caffeine, cold, and hot foods.

Hypertensive LES

Background The condition known as hypertensive LES was first described as a separate entity by Code and

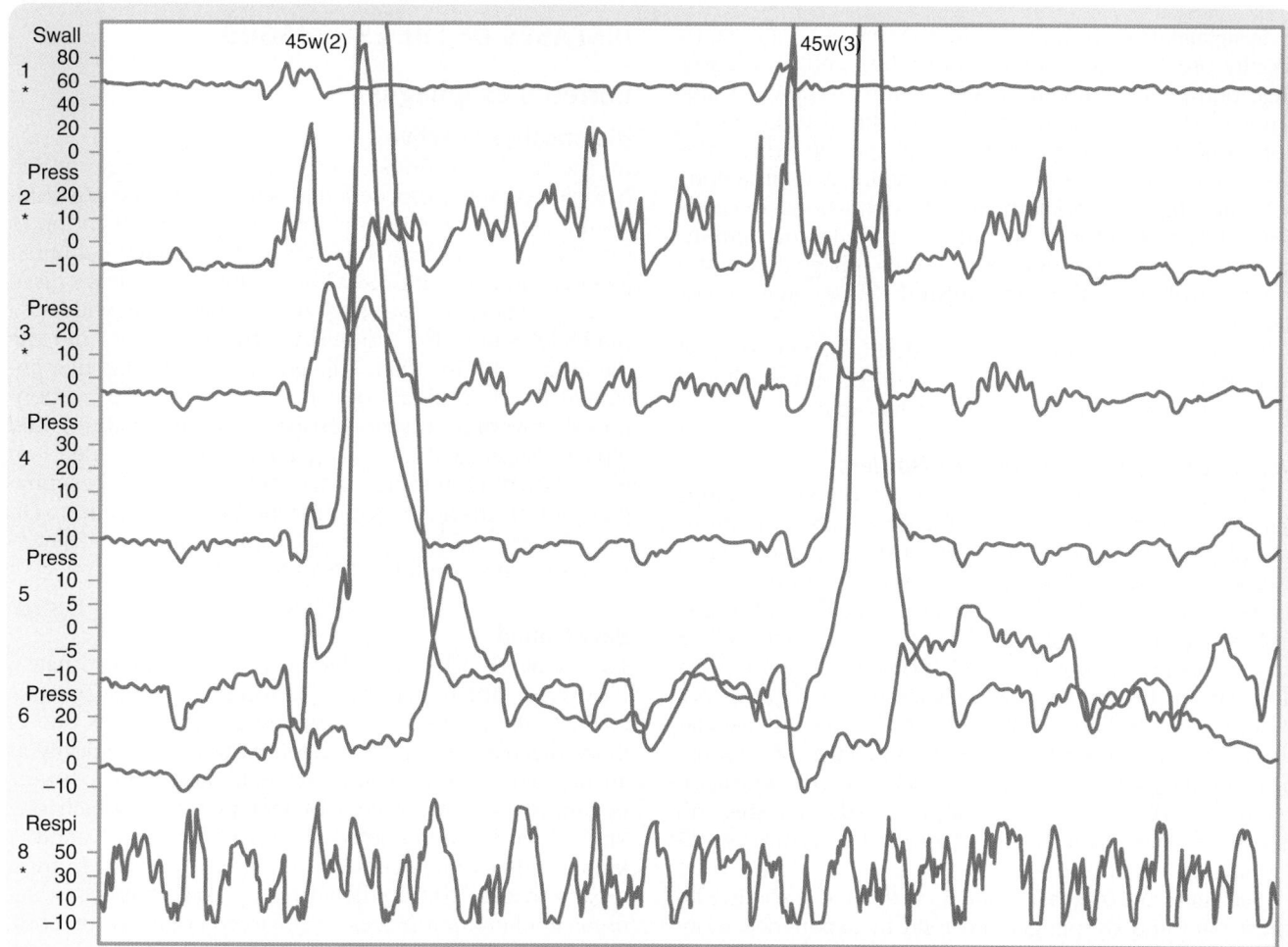

Figure 41-30 Manometry findings in nutcracker esophagus. (From Bremner CG, DeMeester TR, Bremner RM, Mason RJ: Esophageal Motility Testing Made Easy. St Louis, Quality Medical Publishing, 2001, p 85.)

colleagues.[11A] It was observed in patients presenting with dysphagia, chest pain, and manometric findings of an elevated LES. However, the manometric findings are not consistent with achalasia. The LES pressure is above normal, and relaxation will be incomplete but may not be consistently abnormal. The motility of the esophageal body may be hyperperistaltic or normal. The pathogenesis is not well understood, but it has been theorized that it may be a similar process to achalasia in evolution.

Symptoms and Diagnosis Patients with hypertensive LES present with chest pain or dysphagia. Acid reflux and regurgitation are experienced less commonly. Diagnosis is made by manometry. An esophagram may show narrowing at the GEJ with delayed flow as well as abnormalities of esophageal contraction; however, these are nonspecific findings. Manometry tracings demonstrate elevated LES pressure (>26 mm Hg) and normal relaxation of the LES. About half of the time, peristalsis in the esophageal body is normal. In the remainder, abnormal contractions are noted to be hypertensive peristaltic or simultaneous waveforms.

Treatment The treatment of hypertensive LES is with endoscopic and surgical intervention. Botox injections alleviate symptoms temporarily, and hydrostatic balloon dilation may provide long-term symptomatic relief. Surgery is indicated in patients who fail interventional treatments and those with significant symptoms. A laparoscopic modified Heller esophagomyotomy is the operation of choice. In patients with normal esophageal motility, a partial antireflux procedure (e.g., a Dor or Toupet fundoplication) is added.

Ineffective Esophageal Motility

Background IEM was first recognized as a separate motility disturbance by Castell in 2000.[12] It is defined as a contraction abnormality of the distal esophagus and most often is associated with GERD. It may be secondary to inflammatory injury of the esophageal body owing to increased exposure to gastric contents. Dampened motility of the esophageal body leads to poor acid clearance in the lower esophagus. Once altered motility is present, the condition appears to be irreversible.

Symptoms The symptoms of IEM are mixed, but patients usually present with symptoms of reflux and dysphagia. Heartburn, chest pain, and regurgitation are noted. Diagnosis is made by manometry. IEM is defined as a contraction abnormality of the distal esophagus in which the sum total of the number of low-amplitude contractions (<30 mm Hg) and nontransmitted contractions exceeds 30% of wet swallows. A barium esophagram demonstrates nonspecific abnormalities of esophageal contraction but will not further distinguish IEM from other motor disorders.

Treatment The best treatment of IEM is prevention and surrounds effective treatment of GERD. Once altered motility occurs, it appears to be irreversible.

Nonspecific Esophageal Motor Disorders

Background Those patients with manometric findings that do not fit into one of the five classic patterns are placed in the category of nonspecific esophageal motor disorders (NEM). These non-specific abnormalities support the understanding that esophageal motility disorders are a spectrum of abnormalities which reflect various stages of destruction of esophageal motor function. The pathogenesis of NEM is multifaceted and is not of any single isolated etiology. Several collagen vascular disorders are known to cause abnormalities of esophageal motility. Amongst them are scleroderma, dermatomyositis, polymyositis, and lupus erythematosus. All affect the neuromuscular esophageal architecture resulting in poor esophageal motility.

Symptoms and Diagnosis Patients with NEM present with chest pain and dysphagia and tend to experience more reflux symptoms and regurgitation than patients with other defined disorders. Diagnostic tests include barium esophagram and manometric studies. An esophagram is helpful to rule out disorders with defined abnormalities, and identifies abnormal esophageal body contractions as well as abnormalities of the LES. Manometry is critical to determine the nature of the motor abnormalities that the patient is experiencing. The LES can be normal or hypertensive, but incomplete relaxation (residual >5 mm Hg) is noted. Contractions of the esophageal body will follow one or more of the following patterns: non-transmitted, triple-peaked, retrograde, low-amplitude (<35 mm Hg) or prolonged duration (>6 sec). Interruption of normal peristalsis at various esophageal levels is also common. Some patients will have characteristic wave forms that can be ascribed to an underlying collagen vascular disorder. Patients with scleroderma will have low amplitude, simultaneous contractions of the esophageal body similar to those seen with achalasia, but the LES is noted to have normal or low pressure.

Treatment Treatment of NEM is difficult because a primary diagnosis is evasive. Those with collagen vascular or neuromuscular disorders are treated for their primary medical conditions, which often results in improved esophageal motility. For those whose underlying condition remains undiagnosed, combination therapy including medications and therapeutic interventions can be applied, as guided by the prevailing manometric findings.

DISEASES OF THE ESOPHAGUS

Barrett's Esophagus

Historical Perspective

In the 1950s, a British surgeon by the name of Dr. Norman Barrett proposed that sections of the gastrointestinal tract are defined by their mucosa. He went on to say that the esophagus ended at the squamocolumnar junction and that ulcers within columnar mucosa distal to the squamous esophageal mucosa were within "a pouch of stomach . . . drawn up by scar tissue into the mediastinum." In 1953, Allison and Johnstone demonstrated that this distal "pouch of stomach" had no peritoneal covering, normal esophageal musculature, and typical esophageal mucous glands. They concluded that this segment represented a columnar-lined distal esophagus, not stomach. Agreeing with their declaration, Dr. Barrett retracted his opinion. Despite his initial misinterpretation, this condition bears his name.

Background

To adapt to the ever-changing environments that it encounters, the human body has built in mechanisms that facilitate the necessary adjustments. Metaplasia is one of those mechanisms and has been viewed teleologically as an attempt to protect vulnerable tissues from a hostile environment. The process of metaplasia, in which one kind of fully differentiated (adult) cell replaces another kind of adult cell, occurs in a number of organs. In most organs that exhibit epithelial metaplasia, stratified squamous epithelium replaces an inflamed columnar mucosa. In contrast, Barrett's esophagus is a condition whereby an intestinal, columnar epithelium replaces the stratified squamous epithelium that normally lines the distal esophagus. Chronic gastroesophageal reflux is the factor that both injures the squamous epithelium and promotes repair through columnar metaplasia. Although these metaplastic cells may be more resistant to injury from reflux, they also are more prone to malignancy. Ten percent of patients with GERD develop Barrett's esophagus. Even more unsettling is the 40-fold increase in risk for developing esophageal carcinoma in patients with Barrett's esophagus. Prospectively following 100 patients with Barrett's esophagus for 1 year will result in 1 patient developing adenocarcinoma, a rate of 1% per year.[13] This is a similar risk to that of patients with a 20-pack-year smoking history developing lung cancer.

The incomplete intestinal metaplasia that occurs in Barrett's esophagus includes gastric surface cells, intestinal goblet cells, and intestinal absorptive cells with a rudimentary brush border (Fig. 41-31). With continued exposure to the reflux-related hostile environment of the lower esophagus, metaplastic cells undergo cellular transformation to low- and high-grade dysplasia. This may be due to a failed mechanism intrinsic to the metaplastic cell or an adaptive mechanism to its environment. In either event, left unprotected, these dysplastic cells may evolve to cancer. The exact pathophysiologic mechanism continues to be investigated; however, many investigators believe that, once metaplasia is there, it is exposure to

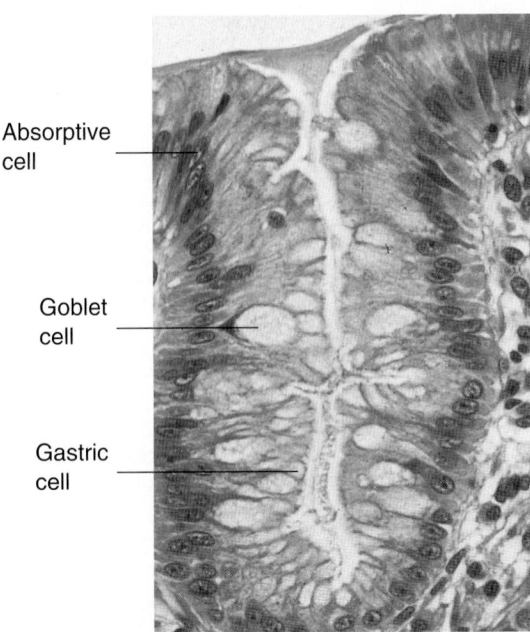

Absorptive cell

Goblet cell

Gastric cell

Figure 41-31 Histology of Barrett's esophagus. (Modified from Pearson FG, Cooper JD, Deslauriers J, et al: Esophageal Surgery, 2nd ed. New York, Churchill Livingstone, 2002, p 286.)

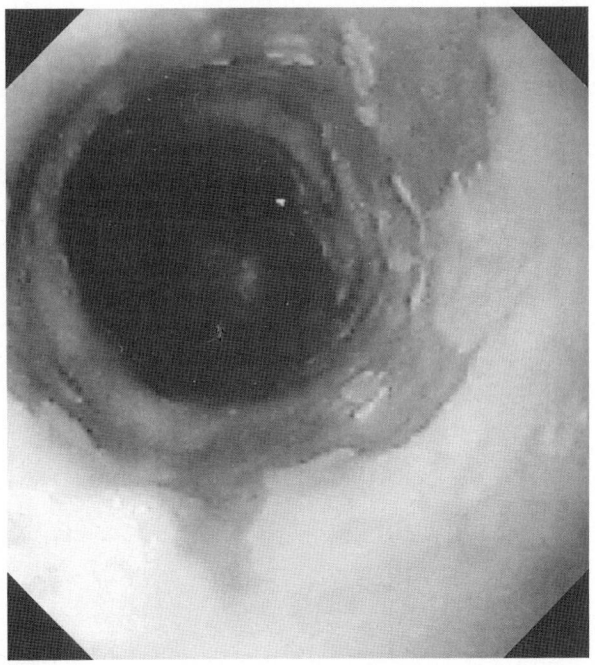

Figure 41-32 Endoscopic appearance of Barrett's esophagus. (Modified from Pearson FG, Cooper JD, Deslauriers J, et al: Esophageal Surgery, 2nd ed. New York, Churchill Livingstone, 2002, p 151.)

bile and other reflux related materials, not necessarily acid, that encourages the progression of dysplasia to cancer. In vitro studies demonstrate cellular and molecular changes in cells of all types when exposed to bile salts. Furthermore, it has been shown that patients with adenocarcinoma of the distal esophagus are three times more likely to have been taking acid suppression medications. In time, the exact role that both acid and bile exposure play in the metaplastic intestinalization of the lower esophagus will be well understood.

A number of other etiologies have been investigated in the development of Barrett's esophagus. Infectious causes, such as *Helicobacter pylori,* have been investigated, although it has not been shown to be associated with an increase in esophageal metaplasia of the esophagus. Genetic abnormalities play a role that is not well defined. An incompetent LES with or without a hiatal hernia plays an important role in the development of GERD and Barrett's esophagus. Factors that have been implicated in the pathophysiology of the LES are age, obesity, stress, caffeinated products, alcohol, tobacco, and a number of foods, including spicy, fatty, and acidic foods. Once the LES is rendered incompetent, esophagitis may appear within 1 year of symptoms of GERD, but several years of exposure to acid and bile need to occur before metaplastic changes.

Although Barrett's esophagus is found in men and women of all races, more than 70% of patients are men aged 55 to 63 years. White men predominate (up to 20:1) over African American men.[14] Men have a 15-fold increased incidence over women of adenocarcinoma of the esophagus, but women with Barrett's esophagus are increasing in number as the differences in the Western lifestyle between men and women diminish. Many Asian cultures have a high rate of squamous cell carcinoma of the esophagus, not related to Barrett's esophagus, and a very low rate of adenocarcinoma in which Barrett's esophagus has been implicated. This strongly suggests that cultural lifestyles play an important role in the evolution of Barrett's esophagus.

Symptoms and Diagnosis

Many patients harboring intestinal metaplasia in their distal esophagus are asymptomatic. Most patients present with symptoms of GERD. Heartburn, regurgitation, acid or bitter taste in the mouth, excessive belching, and indigestion are some of the common symptoms associated with GERD. Recurrent respiratory infections, adult asthma, and infections in the head and neck also are common complaints. The diagnosis of Barrett's esophagus is made by endoscopy and pathology. The presence of any endoscopically visible segment of columnar mucosa within the esophagus (Fig. 41-32) that on pathology identifies intestinal metaplasia defines Barrett's esophagus. Most patients are found to have intestinal metaplasia on a routine endoscopy done for GERD. Other diagnostic tests, such as manometry and barium esophagram, are useful in determining adjunctive esophageal pathology but offer little to obtaining a diagnosis of intestinal metaplasia.

Treatment

Until the pathophysiologic mechanisms of Barrett's esophagus are well understood, the treatment of this disease will remain controversial. Currently, treatment

BARRETT'S ESOPHAGUS: GRADE OF DYSPLASIA AND PROPOSED FOLLOW-UP

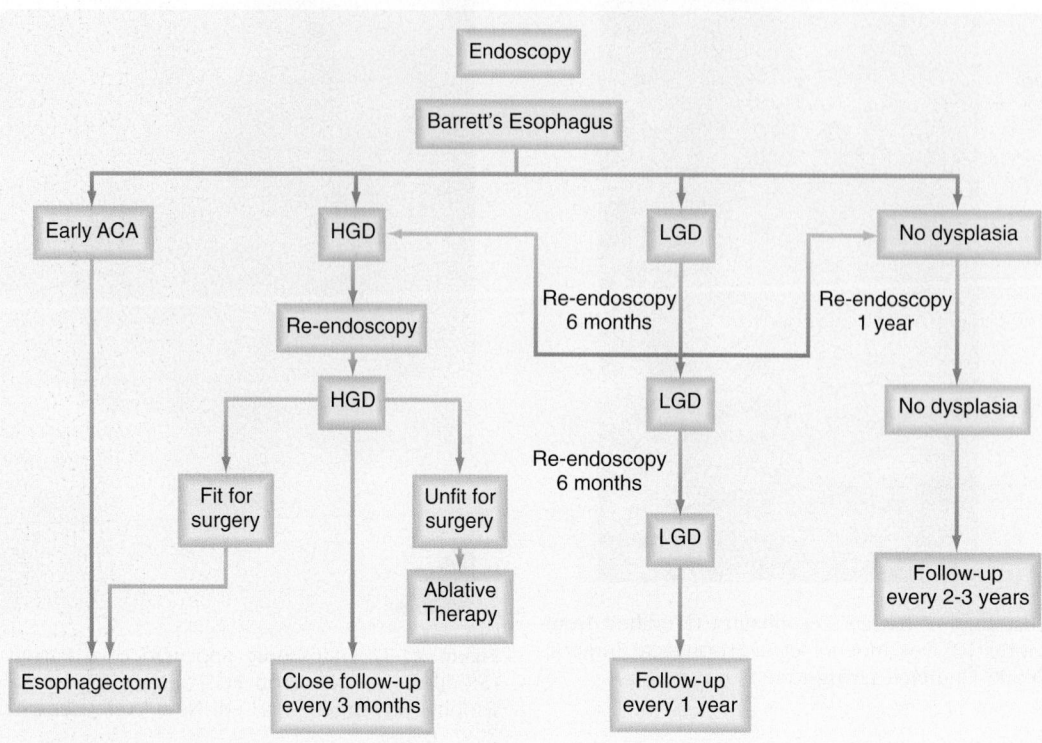

Figure 41-33 Grade of dysplasia and proposed follow-up algorithm for the treatment of Barrett's esophagus. ACA, adenocarcinoma; HGD, high-grade dysplasia; LGD, low-grade dysplasia. (Modified from Pearson FG, Cooper JD, Deslauriers J, et al [eds]: Esophageal Surgery, 2nd ed. New York, Churchill Livingstone, 2002, p 742.)

hinders on the interest and educational bias of the diagnosing physician and is greatly lacking in continuity and sound scientific data. There are several accepted treatment options: surveillance endoscopy, antireflux surgery with or without continued surveillance endoscopy, ablative therapy, endoscopic mucosal resection, and esophageal resection. In general, gastroenterologists advocate aggressive surveillance programs with high-dose acid suppression, and surgeons advocate antireflux surgery to correct the dysfunctional LES. It is quite likely that there is role for each and that a cohesive treatment plan will be established with time.

Yearly surveillance endoscopy is recommended in all patients with a diagnosis of Barrett's esophagus, regardless of the length of the segment. Practice guidelines put out by the American College of Gastroenterology suggest that surveillance be extended to every 2 to 3 years for individuals in whom there is no evidence of dysplasia on two consecutive yearly endoscopic exams (Fig. 41-33). For patients with low-grade dysplasia, surveillance endoscopy is performed at 6-month intervals for the first year and then yearly thereafter if there has been no change. Patients undergoing surveillance are placed on acid suppression medication and monitored for changes in their reflux symptoms.

Controversy surrounds the benefits of antireflux surgery in patients with Barrett's esophagus. Those in favor of surgery argue that medical therapy and endoscopic sur-

veillance may treat the symptoms but fail to address the problem. The problem is the functional impairment of the LES that leads to chronic reflux and metaplastic transformation of the lower esophageal mucosa. Surgery renders the LES competent and restores the barrier to reflux. Studies have demonstrated regression of metaplasia to normal mucosa up to 57% of the time[15] in patients who have undergone antireflux surgery. Furthermore, antireflux surgery encourages regression of low-grade dysplasia to intestinal metaplasia, or Barrett's esophagus.[15] Those who oppose surgery argue that adequate surveillance is not possible after a fundoplication, placing patients at risk for developing cancer in a hidden segment of Barrett's esophagus.

Ablative therapy for Barrett's esophagus is an additional treatment option that has gained favor in few centers in the United States. It is has been proposed mostly for patients with high-grade dysplasia. Photodynamic therapy (PDT) is the most common ablative method used. Complications include persistent metaplasia in more than 50%[16] as well as esophageal strictures in up to 34% of patients. Combined ablative therapies with PDT and laser therapy also have been tried but have gained limited acceptance. Endoscopic mucosal resection (EMR) is gaining favor for the treatment of Barrett's esophagus with low-grade dysplasia. Additionally, it is being used as a diagnostic tool to rule out cancer in a focus of Barrett's esophagus with high-grade dysplasia. Because of an increase in stricture rate with larger resections, it is not advocated for long-segment Barrett's esophagus. It is acceptable in patients with high-grade dysplasia who are not acceptable candidates for esophageal resection and useful in patients who have an isolated focus of Barrett's with dysplasia.

Esophageal resection for Barrett's esophagus is recommended only for patients in whom high-grade dysplasia is found. Pathologic data on surgical specimens demonstrate a 40% risk for adenocarcinoma within a focus of high-grade dysplasia. A patient is evaluated for operative risk and, if acceptable, undergoes an esophageal resection. Near-total esophagectomy through a transhiatal approach is recommended in most patients. Minimally invasive, as well as vagal-sparing, techniques have gained popularity in some centers throughout the United States. Transthoracic and transabdominal esophageal resections used in an attempt to preserve esophageal length are not advocated. These two approaches leave behind a vulnerable esophagus to vicious reflux induced by both the resection of the LES and a vagotomy that renders the pylorus incompetent. Resection of the diseased esophagus and replacement with a short jejunal interposition graft has been investigated on a limited basis and may offer a less morbid alternative to esophageal resection.[17]

Despite the rising incidence of GERD, Barrett's esophagus, and esophageal cancer, no cost-effective screening measures have been instituted on a national level. Judicious evaluation of each patient presenting with GERD needs to be done to identify patients at risk so that appropriate treatments, including surveillance endoscopy and surgery, can be initiated. Incidence of GERD, Barrett's esophagus, and adenocarcinoma of the esophagus continue to rise, and without serious consideration, these diseases will result in an epidemic in the years ahead.

Rings, Slings, and Webs

Overview
So many of the diseases that affect the esophagus are morbid and lead to devastating consequences. Vascular and esophageal rings, pulmonary artery slings, and esophageal webs are challenging but rewarding conditions for the surgical acrobat to treat, lending some levity to an otherwise fairly morbid cohort of diseases. All these abnormalities cause compression of the esophagus either by extrinsic compression, as with vascular rings and pulmonary artery slings, or intrinsic compression, as with esophageal webs and Schatzki's rings.

Vascular Rings and Pulmonary Artery Slings

Background
Vascular rings and pulmonary slings occur as a result of developmental abnormalities of the great vessels that cause compression of the esophagus. The most common aortic arch anomaly that creates an incomplete vascular ring is when the right subclavian artery arises from the descending aorta and travels behind the esophagus to complete its course to the right upper extremity (Fig. 41-34). Although it does not form a complete vascular

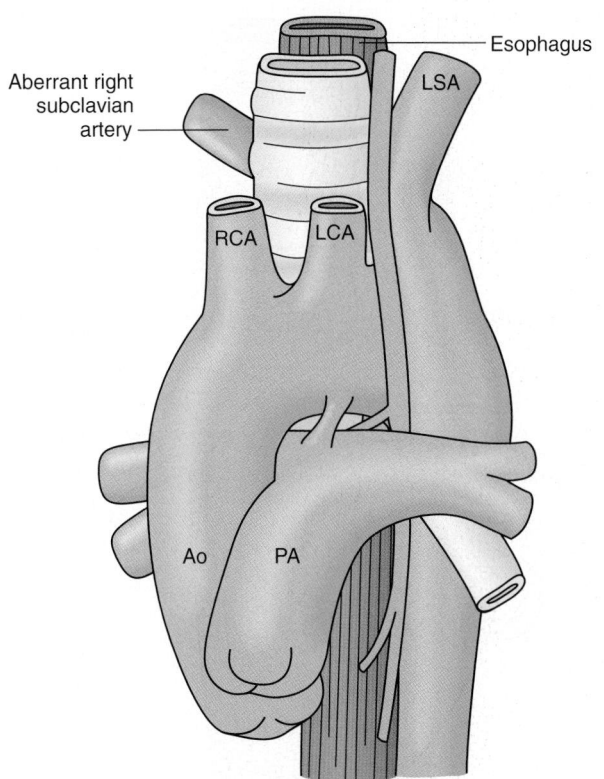

Figure 41-34 Left aortic arch with right subclavian artery. (Modified from Lamberti JL, Mainwaring RD: Tracheoesophageal compressive syndromes of vascular origins: Rings and slings. In Baue A, Geha AS, Hammond GL, et al [eds]: Glenn's Thoracic and Cardiovascular Surgery, 6th ed, Vol 2. Stamford, CT, Appleton & Lange, 1996, p 1096.)

ring, it may cause significant posterior compression of the esophagus. Anomalous formation of a right aortic arch with a left ligamentum arteriosum and a resultant retroesophageal left subclavian artery will form a complete ring that will also cause posterior esophageal compression. A pulmonary artery sling is an anomaly of the pulmonary arterial trunk whereby the left pulmonary artery arises from the right pulmonary artery instead of from the main pulmonary artery trunk (Fig. 41-35). To complete its course to the left lung, it traverses between the trachea and the esophagus and causes significant anterior compression of the esophagus. Pulmonary artery slings are commonly associated with intracardiac defects and other developmental abnormalities of the foregut.

Symptoms and Diagnosis
Both vascular rings and pulmonary artery slings cause dysphagia. Recurrent respiratory infections and difficulty breathing are also common symptoms. The tightness of the ring or sling will determine the age of clinical presentation and severity of symptoms. Aberrant right subclavian anomalies cause mild dysphagia to solids but not liquids. The term *dysphagia lusoria* (a Latin term meaning a "sport of nature") describes the error of ascribing dysphagia to the radiologic finding of this anomaly. Nevertheless, it can be found in children and adults of all ages

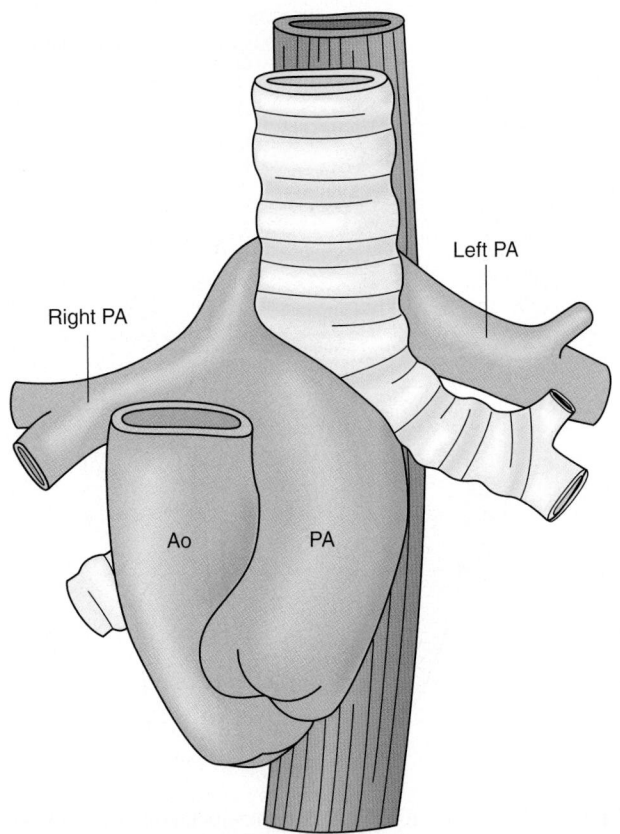

Figure 41-35 Pulmonary artery sling. (Modified from Lamberti JL, Mainwaring RD: Tracheoesophageal compressive syndromes of vascular origins: Rings and slings. In Baue A, Geha AS, Hammond GL, et al [eds]: Glenn's Thoracic and Cardiovascular Surgery, 6th ed, Vol 2. Stamford, CT, Appleton & Lange, 1996, p 1098.)

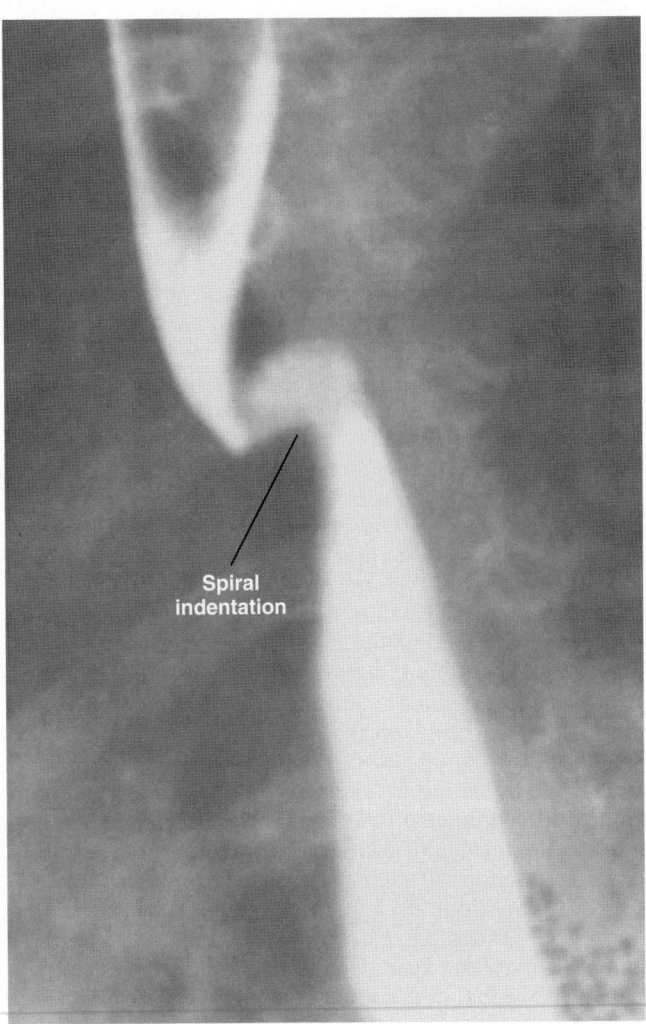

Figure 41-36 Barium esophagram in a patient with an aberrant right subclavian artery showing anterior compression of the esophagus. (Modified from Lamberti JL, Mainwaring RD: Tracheoesophageal compressive syndromes of vascular origins: Rings and slings. In Baue A, Geha AS, Hammond GL, et al [eds]: Glenn's Thoracic and Cardiovascular Surgery, 6th ed, Vol 2. Stamford, CT, Appleton & Lange, 1996, 1099.)

and needs to be considered in the differential diagnosis of dysphagia. Pulmonary artery slings may also cause dysphagia and are more often accompanied by significant respiratory problems.

Any patient presenting with dysphagia undergoes a barium esophagram. This radiographic study will reveal extrinsic anterior (Fig. 41-36) or posterior compression of the esophagus. This can be followed with angiography or high-resolution contrast CT (HRCT) to identify the anomalous anatomy.

Treatment

In symptomatic patients, both vascular rings and pulmonary artery slings are repaired. Patients with aberrant right subclavian artery anomalies may be asymptomatic and need not undergo repair in these instances. Pulmonary artery slings all require repair so as to avoid narrowing of the left pulmonary artery and tracheal stenosis that develop with time. Open sternotomy with cardiopulmonary bypass is required, and anatomic repositioning of the great vessels is performed. The results are usually good, and the dysphagia resolves nearly 100% of the time.

Esophageal Rings

Background

Esophageal rings were first described by Schatzki and Gary in 1945. Despite the lack of recognition he may have suffered, Gary, along with his colleague Schatzki, made a significant contribution to medical science by describing this acquired anomaly. Lying precisely at the squamocolumnar mucosal GEJ, this ring consists of a concentric symmetric narrowing representing an area of restricted distensibility of the lower esophagus. It consists of esophageal mucosa above and gastric mucosa below, with variable amounts of muscularis mucosae, connective tissue, and submucosal fibrosis in between (Fig. 41-37). It does not have a component of true esophageal muscle, nor is it associated with esophagitis.

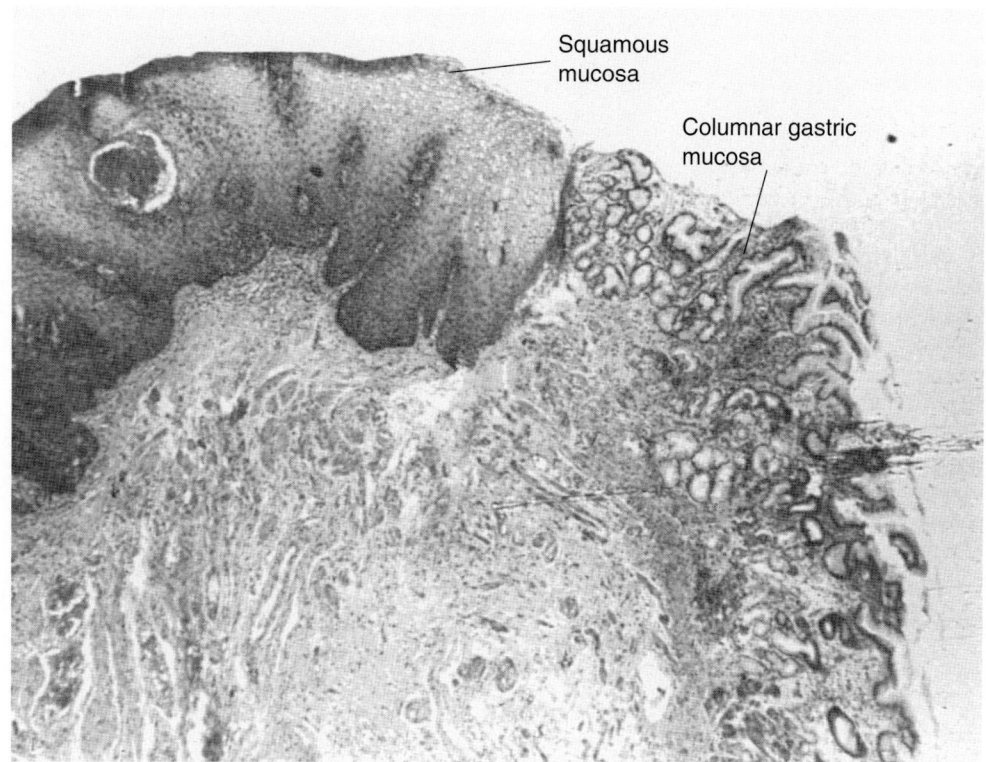

Squamous
mucosa

Columnar gastric
mucosa

Figure 41-37 Histology of a Schatzki's ring. (Modified from Wilkins EW Jr: Rings and webs. In Pearson FG, Cooper JD, Deslauriers J, et al [eds]: Esophageal Surgery, 2nd ed. New York, Churchill Livingstone, 2002, p 300.)

The etiology of Schatzki's ring is not well understood. It is often accompanied by a small hiatal hernia, and some have advocated that it is a result of reflux esophagitis. Another theory is that overcontractility of circular esophageal musculature at the level of the inferior esophageal sphincter, combined with the sliding gastric mucosa of the hiatal hernia, results in persistent apposition of the two mucosal layers and fibrosis of the submucosal layer below.

Symptoms and Diagnosis

Most patients with Schatzki's rings present with dysphagia. The dysphagia is usually to solid foods only and comes on abruptly with nearly complete obstruction. The term *episodic aphagia* is often ascribed to patients with Schatzki's ring, describing the intermittent obstruction of the nondistensible ring by large pieces of meat. Lower retrosternal pressure and pain accompany an acute obstruction and are followed by salivation and the secretion of copious, thick mucus from the esophagus. Patients are unable to eat or drink anything, and there is little a patient can do to relieve the obstruction. Forced vomiting may cause esophageal rupture, and spontaneous passage of the food bolus into the stomach usually occurs within a few minutes.

Diagnosis of a Schatzki's ring is made with a barium esophagram (Fig. 41-38). The patient is placed into the prone position, turned slightly onto the right side, and asked to take in a large breath just as the bolus of barium is reaching the esophagogastric junction. In this position, the ring is well visualized, but it may be missed in the upright position. An endoscopy is indicated if the patient presents with foreign body obstruction or if the barium esophagram is equivocal. Upper endoscopy is performed with placement of an overtube to facilitate complete evacuation of the esophagus.

Treatment

Asymptomatic patients incidentally found to have a Schatzki's ring require no treatment. Patients presenting with acute obstruction require immediate attention. The administration of oral papain in a 2.5% solution is useful for proteolytic digestion of impacted protein food. It is administered in aliquots of 5 mL every 30 minutes for a total of four doses. Intravenous (IV) meperidine (25-50 mg) may also be used in small doses to encourage spontaneous dislodgment of the impacted food bolus. Esophagoscopy, either rigid or flexible, with the use of an overtube facilitates safe extraction. General anesthesia may be desirable to adequately protect the airway. A variety of instruments are used to extract the food. Pushing the food into the stomach can result in perforation and is only done if the distal lumen is noted at the time of endoscopy. After the food is dislodged, a complete evaluation of the esophageal mucosa is done. If there is any question of the integrity of the mucosa, an esophagram is performed.

In a patient presenting with symptoms of dysphagia in which Schatzki's ring is found, treatment is disruption of the ring by oral dilation. A 50-French tapered Maloney

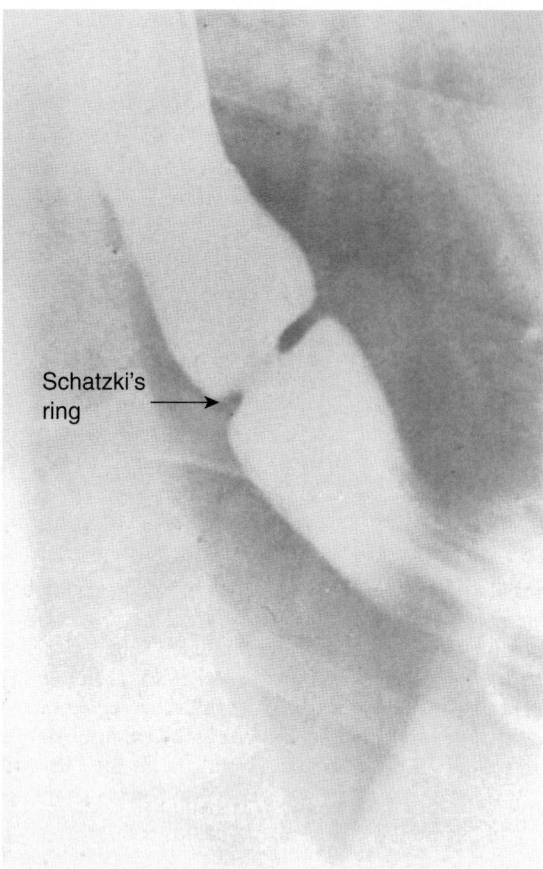

Figure 41-38 Barium esophagram of a Schatzki's ring. (Modified from Wilkins EW Jr: Rings and webs. In Pearson FG, Cooper JD, Deslauriers J, et al [eds]: Esophageal Surgery, 2nd ed. New York, Churchill Livingstone, 2002, p 298.)

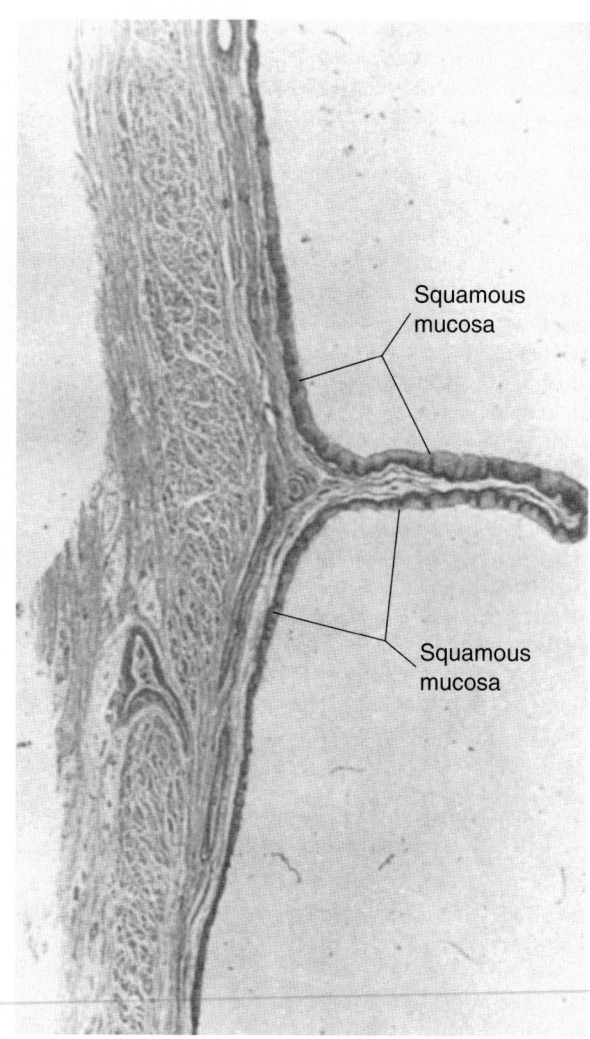

Figure 41-39 Histology of an esophageal web. (Modified from Wilkins EW Jr: Rings and webs. In Pearson FG, Cooper JD, Deslauriers J, et al [eds]: Esophageal Surgery, 2nd ed. New York, Churchill Livingstone, 2002, p 302.)

bougie is used. Symptoms are relieved for up to 18 months. Sequential bougienage dilation is carried out as symptoms recur. Surgery is not indicated for treatment of Schatzki's ring and can cause devastating esophageal strictures that are much more difficult to manage. Surgical intervention is reserved for patients who fail bougienage or have intractable reflux. In these few circumstances, intraoperative bougienage followed by a Nissen fundoplication is recommended, but excision of the ring is not indicated.

Esophageal Webs

Background
Esophageal webs are thin, membranous structures that partially or completely compromise the esophageal lumen. They usually only involve the mucosa and part of the submucosa and are composed of squamous cell epithelium above and below the web (Fig. 41-39). This distinguishes the web from a Schatzki's ring, which is composed of esophageal epithelium above and gastric epithelium below the ring. Esophageal webs are not involved in any motility disorder, although a similar radiographic appearance may be noted to accompany some motility abnormalities with no corresponding mucosal abnormality.

Webs may be congenital or acquired and present throughout the esophagus in men and women of all ages. Congenital webs are rare and are found in young children. They may occur at any level but more commonly are found in the lower two thirds of the esophagus. They are thought to be the result of a failure of coalescence of esophageal vacuoles, which normally leads to complete luminal patency between 25 and 31 days of embryologic development. The congenital web is more likely to be circumferential or eccentric and may be thick and rough rather than thin and diaphanous in nature. Any esophageal web that is found later in life needs to have been accompanied by a significant history of dysphagia throughout childhood; otherwise, it is considered an acquired condition.

Acquired esophageal webs are more common than congenital webs and are usually found in the anterior cervical esophagus causing focal narrowing in the postcricoid area. They are covered on both sides with squa-

Table 41-3 Three Phases of Tissue Injury From Alkali Ingestion

PHASE	TISSUE INJURY	ONSET	DURATION	INFLAMMATORY RESPONSE
1	Acute necrosis	1-4 days	1-4 days	Coagulation of intracellular proteins Inflammation
2	Ulceration and granulation	3-5 days	3-12 days	Tissue sloughing Granulation of ulcerated tissue bed
3	Cicatrization and scarring	3 weeks	1-6 months	Adhesion formation Scarring

mous epithelium and are usually a thin mucosal fold that protrudes into the lumen. These webs are seen in patients with Plummer-Vinson syndrome (edentulous, middle-aged, malnourished women with atrophic oral mucosa, glossitis, spoon-shaped fingernails, and iron deficiency anemia), pemphigoid, and ulcerative colitis. They are also associated with a slight increase in squamous cell cancer of the esophagus.

Symptoms and Diagnosis

In children, symptoms of poor feeding may not begin until the child is taking in solid foods. Congenital webs often are imperforate, allowing liquids to pass easily through. Nearly complete luminal obstruction results in regurgitation of nonbilious feeds in early infancy. Most adults with acquired esophageal webs are asymptomatic. Symptoms of solid-food dysphagia, especially with meat or bread, are otherwise common. The swallowing difficulty may come and go and be aggravated by specific foods. An evaluation for dysphagia always begins with a barium esophagram. This dynamic study will accurately identify an esophageal web and is useful to rule out other obstructing lesions. Endoscopy may be performed; however, the blind passage of the endoscope may take the instrument past the web without ever seeing it.

Treatment

The management of an esophageal web depends on the nature of the web. Thin webs are treated with membranous disruption through an endoscope or bougie. Piecemeal excision with a biopsy forceps or laser lysis is also an option, but not routinely performed. Balloon dilation is advocated by some and has good results. Similar to angioplasty, this technique involves the use of fluoroscopically guided balloon dilators that are inflated with water-soluble contrast material under carefully monitored pressure. The membrane is disrupted under controlled circumstances so that perforation is avoided. Results are favorable, but the technique has not been widely supported. Laser lysis has gained popularity in the recent decade and may prove to be the treatment of choice in the future. Surgical mucosal resection is reserved for patients with thick rings that are refractory to bougienage. A transcervical or transthoracic approach to the esophagus is used. A longitudinal myotomy and circumferential excision of the web is performed. Circumferential reapproximation of the mucosa is performed with interrupted absorbable sutures followed by longitudinal closure of the muscle. Treatments of all types result in good long-

term results with few recurrences of dysphagia. If recurrent dysphagia becomes a problem, repeated bougienage is usually adequate to relieve the persistent symptoms.

ACQUIRED ESOPHAGEAL CONDITIONS

Caustic Injury

Background

Caustic injuries of the esophagus can have devastating consequences, and the best cure for this condition is an ounce of prevention. In children, ingestion of caustic materials is accidental and tends to be in small quantities. In teenagers and adults, however, ingestion usually is deliberate during suicide attempts, and much larger quantities of caustic liquids are consumed. Alkali ingestion is more common than acid ingestion because of its lack of immediate symptoms. Acids cause an immediate burning sensation in the mouth, whereas alkali does not. The consequences of alkali ingestion are much more devastating and almost always lead to significant destruction of the esophagus, resulting in long-term dysfunction.

There are both acute and chronic phases to caustic esophageal injuries. The acute phase is dependent on the severity and location of the injury and on the type of substance ingested (acid versus alkali), the form of the substance (liquid versus solid), the quantity and concentration of the substance ingested, the amount of residual food in the stomach, and the duration of tissue contact. The chronic phase of caustic ingestion focuses on subsequent strictures and disruption of the swallowing mechanism that become significant problems several months down the line. There are several sites that are prone to injury because of a relative delay in transit through the esophagus. These correlate to the anatomic narrowings and can be seen in the proximal esophagus at the level of the UES, the midesophagus where the aorta abuts the left main-stem bronchus, and the distal esophagus just proximal to the LES.

Alkali Ingestion

Alkaline substances dissolve tissues by liquefactive necrosis, deeply penetrating the tissues they touch. There are three phases of tissue injury from alkali ingestion (Table 41-3):

1. *Phase 1:* The acute necrotic phase lasts 1 to 4 days after injury, during which coagulation of intracellular

Table 41-4   Endoscopic Grading and Treatment of Corrosive Esophageal and Gastric Burns

DEGREE OF BURN	ENDOSCOPIC EVALUATION	TREATMENT
First degree	Mucosal hyperemia Edema	48-hr observation Acid suppression
Second degree	Limited hemorrhage Exudates Ulceration Pseudomembrane formation	Aggressive IV resuscitation IV antibiotics Acid suppression
Third degree	Mucosal sloughing Deep ulcerations Massive hemorrhage Complete luminal obstruction Charring Perforation	Inhaled steroids Fiberoptic intubation (if needed)

proteins results in cell necrosis. The surrounding tissues develop an intense inflammatory reaction.

2. *Phase 2:* The ulceration and granulation phase is next and starts 3 to 5 days after injury and lasts about 3 to 12 days. It is during this time that the tissues slough and granulation tissue begins to fill in the ulcerated base left behind. The esophagus is at its weakest point during this second phase.

3. *Phase 3:* In the third phase, cicatrization and scarring begin, and the newly formed connective tissue begins to contract, resulting in esophageal narrowing. This occurs 3 weeks after the initial injury. Adhesions form between areas of granulation resulting in bands that significantly constrict the esophagus. During this time, efforts are aimed at reducing stricture formation.

Acid Ingestion

Ingestion of acid is difficult because it gives an immediate burning in the mouth. When compared with lye ingestions, the quantity and concentrations are quite modest. Acid substances cause coagulative necrosis, forming an eschar that limits tissue penetration. In some cases, acid burns result in full-thickness injury, although in most, it is limited. Within 48 hours, the extent to which the acid will injure the esophagus is already determined. These injuries tend to be less severe and relatively spare the esophagus over the stomach.

Symptoms and Diagnosis

Symptoms of caustic burns to the esophagus are determined by the severity of the burn and parallel the stages of tissue injury. During phase one, patients may complain of oral and substernal pain, hypersalivation, odynophagia and dysphagia, hematemesis, and vomiting. During stage two, these symptoms may disappear only to see dysphagia reappear as fibrosis and scarring begin to narrow the esophagus throughout stage three. A fever is usually an indicator that esophageal injury is present. Symptoms of respiratory distress, such as hoarseness, stridor, and dyspnea, suggest upper airway edema and are usually worse with acid ingestion. Pain in the back and chest may indicate a perforation of the mediastinal esophagus,

whereas abdominal pain may indicate abdominal visceral perforation. Studies have demonstrated that asymptomatic patients tend to have minimal injury to the esophagus, whereas symptomatic patients, especially presenting with three or more symptoms, hematemesis or respiratory distress are likely to have severe injury.[18]

Diagnosis is initiated with a physical exam specifically evaluating the mouth, airway, chest, and abdomen. Careful inspection of the lips, palate, pharynx, and larynx is done. Auscultation of the lungs is critical to determining the degree of upper airway involvement. The abdomen is examined for signs of perforation. Early endoscopy is recommended 12 to 24 hours after ingestion to identify the grade of the burn (Table 41-4). Radiographic examination in adults is not a useful tool at initial presentation but is helpful in later stages to assess stricture formation. Serial chest and abdominal radiographs are indicated to follow patients with questionable chest and abdominal exams. A CT scan is indicated in a patient with an equivocal endoscopic exam in whom there is a strong index of suspicion for a perforation.

Treatment

The treatment of caustic lesions of the esophagus is determined by the extent of the injury and addresses the injuries that occur both in the acute and chronic phase.

Acute Phase

Management of the acute phase is aimed at limiting and identifying the extent of the injury. It begins with neutralization of the ingested substance. If a patient presents within the first hour of ingestion, neutralization is attempted. Alkalis (including lye) are neutralized with half-strength vinegar or citrus juice. Acids are neutralized with milk, egg whites, or antacids. Emetics and sodium bicarbonate need to be avoided because they can increase the chance of perforation. Further treatment is guided by the extent of injury endoscopically identified and the patient's underlying condition.

No Evidence of Burn   Early observation is safe in those asymptomatic patients whose physical exam and initial

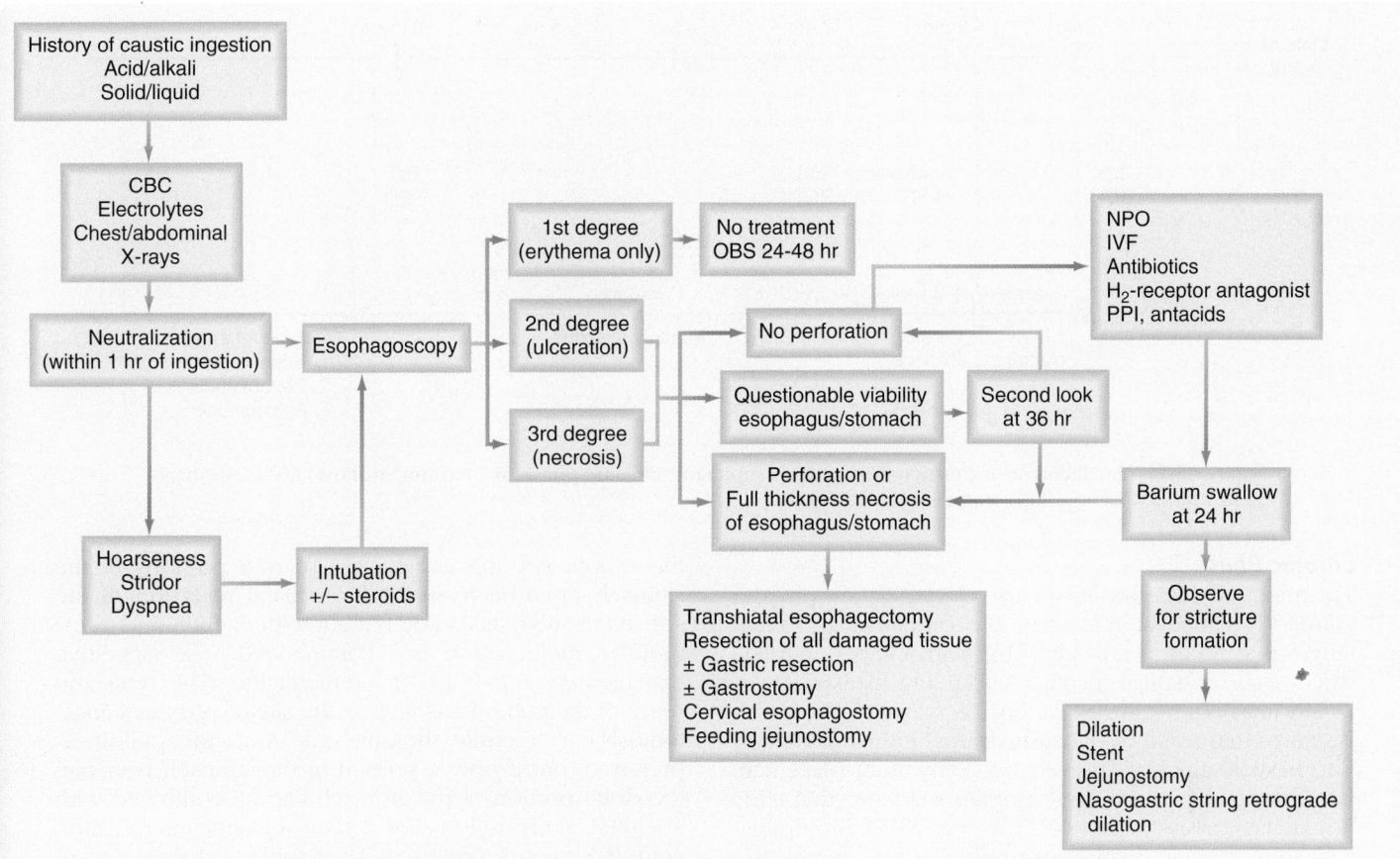

Figure 41-40 Management of caustic injury of the esophagus: acute phase. IVF, intravenous fluids; OBS, observe; PPI, proton pump inhibitor. (Modified from Zwischenberger JB, Savage C, Bidani A: Surgical aspects of esophageal disease. Am J Respir Crit Care Med 164:1037-1040, 2001.)

endoscopy are negative. Oral nutrition may be resumed when a patient can painlessly swallow saliva.

First-Degree Burn In patients with endoscopically identified first-degree burns, 48 hours of observation is indicated. Oral nutrition can be resumed when a patient can painlessly swallow saliva. A repeat endoscopy and barium esophagram are done in follow-up at intervals of 1, 2, and 8 months, at which time 60%, 80%, and nearly 100% of strictures will have developed, respectively.

Second- and Third-Degree Burns Patients with second- and third-degree burns to the esophagus are triaged similar to burn patients. Massive fluid shifts, renal failure, and sepsis can occur rapidly, and underestimation of extent of injury can lead to fatal outcomes. Resuscitation is aggressively pursued. The patient is monitored in the intensive care unit (ICU) and kept nil per os (NPO) with IV fluids. IV antibiotics and a proton pump inhibitor are started. In patients with evidence of acute airway involvement, aerosolized steroids may be used to relieve airway obstruction. Fiberoptic intubation may be needed and must be available. The use of steroids to prevent stricture formation is controversial. The largest series to date suggests that although steroids will decrease the rate of stricture formation, they will also mask symptoms of peritonitis.

The management of second- and third-degree burns of the esophagus is multifaceted and has several acceptable options. Aggressive resuscitation and placement of an esophageal stent are one option. Oral nutrition is resumed when a patient can painlessly swallow saliva. Alternatively, a feeding tube or central venous catheter is placed, and the patient is kept NPO until oral pain subsides. If the diagnosis is not secured with endoscopy, an exploratory laparoscopy (in stable patients) or laparotomy (in unstable patients) is performed. A viable stomach and esophagus are left in situ, a feeding jejunostomy tube is placed, and an esophageal stent is placed endoscopically in the operating room. A questionable esophagus and stomach are left in situ, and a second-look operation is planned for 36 hours. Management at 36 hours is dictated by the findings at that time. If full-thickness necrosis or perforation of the esophagus or stomach is found at any time, an emergent exploratory laparotomy is indicated. The esophagus and stomach and all affected surrounding organs and tissues are resected, an end-cervical esophagostomy is performed, and a feeding jejunostomy is placed (Fig. 41-40). Postoperatively, the patient is monitored in an ICU and aggressively managed.

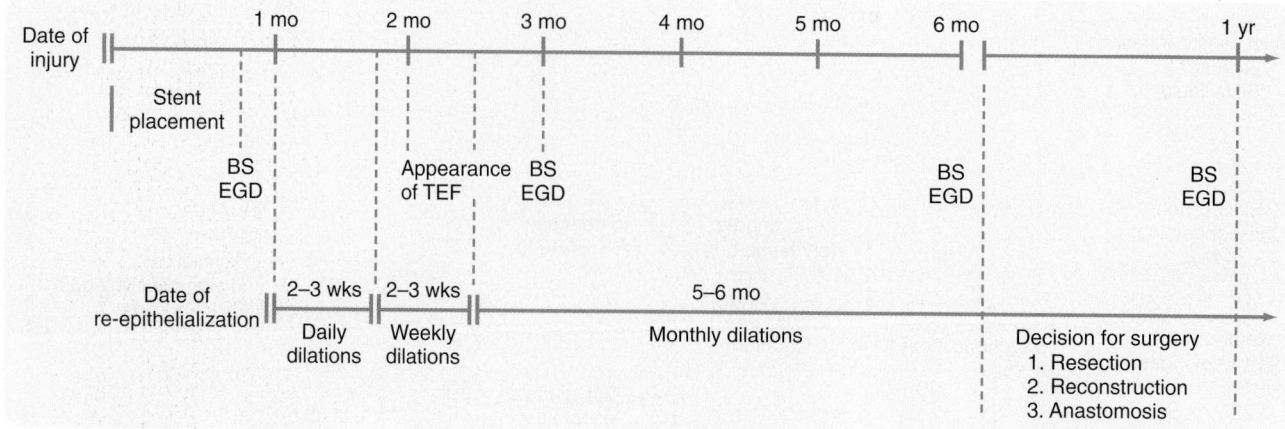

Figure 41-41 Management of caustic injury of the esophagus: chronic phase. BS, barium swallow; EGD, esophago-gastroduodenoscopy; TEF, transesophageal fistula.

Chronic Phase

Treatment in the chronic phase of caustic esophageal injuries is aimed at managing the problems and challenges that occur as a result of the burn injury, including strictures, esophageal reconstruction, and fistulas.

Strictures There are a variety of ways to deal with strictures that result from caustic burns of the esophagus. The best treatment is prevention. Early stent placement is advocated by most. There is some evidence that early bougienage is also effective. However, before re-epithelialization, bougie dilation may add insult to injury. If a stent is placed during the acute phase, it is left in place for 21 days, at which time it is removed. At 3 weeks, 3 months, and 6 months, a barium esophagram is performed to evaluate for stricture formation, gastric outlet obstruction, and linitis plastica appearance. An endoscopy is performed to appraise the extent of re-epithelialization. After re-epithelialization has occurred, patients with strictures are aggressively treated with bougie dilations. Patients with esophageal strictures undergo bougie dilation regardless of their symptoms. Waiting until symptoms arise results in long-term strictures that often fail bougie dilation and ultimately require esophageal resection. Dilations are performed daily for 2 to 3 weeks, then every other day for 2 to 3 weeks, then weekly for months. An adequate lumen needs to be reestablished within 6 months to 1 year, lengthening the intervals between dilations as time passes. Retrograde dilation may also be successful in the event that antegrade dilation is not. If endoscopic dilation fails to reestablish an adequate lumen (40 French), surgical intervention is necessary (Fig. 41-41).

Reconstruction Restoration of the alimentary tract is delayed until 6 months to 1 year. By this time, the patient is recovered from the acute insult, scar formation is by and large complete, and failed endoscopic treatment of strictures is terminated. In patients whose esophagus and stomach remain in situ, resection of the damaged organs is recommended. The incidence of esophageal cancer in patients with caustic injury is 1000-fold greater than in the general population. Unless there is prohibitive risk, the esophagus and excessively scarred portions of the stomach must be resected. Transhiatal resection of the scarred esophagus can be fraught with danger, and transthoracic mobilization is recommended. The operative management needs to be premeditated. The type and route of the conduit, as well as the site of proximal anastomosis, is carefully thought out. A gastric pull-up is preferred, but if only a portion of the stomach is viable, the distal portion of the stomach can be combined with a jejunal interposition. For a long-segment interposition graft, the colon is preferred. The esophageal replacement graft is placed in the posterior mediastinal space if possible and in the retrosternal position when the posterior mediastinum is excessively scarred. The site of the proximal anastomosis is determined by the extent of the injury to the hypopharynx and proximal esophagus.

Esophageal Perforation

Background

Perforation of the esophagus is a surgical emergency. Early detection and surgical repair within the first 24 hours results in 80% to 90% survival; after 24 hours, survival decreases to less than 50%. Upon presentation, patients suspected of having a perforation based on initial history and physical exam are evaluated quickly so that surgical intervention may be initiated promptly. Perforation from forceful vomiting (Boerhaave's syndrome), foreign body ingestion, or trauma accounts for 15%, 14%, and 10% of cases, respectively. Most esophageal perforations occur after endoscopic instrumentation for a diagnostic or therapeutic procedure, including dilation, stent placement, and laser fulguration. Other iatrogenic causes that have been noted include difficult endotracheal intubation, blind insertion of a mini-tracheostomy, and inadvertent injury during dissections in the neck, chest and abdomen.

Boerhaave's Syndrome

Professor Hermann Boerhaave first described this syndrome after performing an autopsy on Baron Jan van

Wassenaer. After relieving postprandial discomfort by self-induced vomiting, the Baron succumbed to his death from a distal esophageal perforation that was later noted at his autopsy. It has since been elucidated that recurrent emesis disrupts the normal vomiting reflex that enables sphincter relaxation, resulting in an increase in intrathoracic esophageal pressure and perforation. Postemetic rupture of the esophagus, now known as *Boerhaave's syndrome,* is only one of many causes of esophageal rupture. Similar findings are noted with blunt thoracic trauma, epileptic seizures, defecation, and childbirth, all of which are associated with increased intra-abdominal pressure. A tear in the esophageal mucosa, known as a Mallory-Weiss tear, also occurs after persistent retching, but is not associated with perforation.

Symptoms and Diagnosis

Symptoms of neck, substernal, or epigastric pain are consistently associated with esophageal perforation and generate a high index of suspicion. Vomiting, hematemesis, or dysphagia also may accompany them. In addition, a history of trauma, advanced esophageal cancer, violent wretching as seen in Boerhaave's syndrome, swallowing of a foreign body, or recent instrumentation must raise the question of esophageal perforation. Cervical perforations may present with neck ache and stiffness due to contamination of the prevertebral space. Thoracic perforations present with shortness of breath and retrosternal chest pain lateralizing to the side of perforation. Abdominal perforations present with epigastric pain that radiates to the back if the perforation is posterior. Signs of perforation change as time progresses. Early on, a patient may present with tachypnea, tachycardia, and a low-grade fever but have no other overt signs of perforation. With increased mediastinal and pleural contamination, patients progress toward hemodynamic instability and shock. On exam, subcutaneous air in the neck or chest, shallow decreased breath sounds, or a tender abdomen are all suggestive of perforation. Laboratory values of significance are an elevated white blood cell count and an elevated salivary amylase in the blood or pleural fluid.

Diagnosis of an esophageal perforation may be made radiographically. A chest roentgenogram may demonstrate a hydropneumothorax. A contrast esophagram is done using barium for a suspected thoracic perforation and Gastrografin for an abdominal perforation. Barium is inert in the chest but causes peritonitis in the abdomen, whereas aspirated Gastrografin can cause life-threatening pneumonitis. Most perforations are found above the GEJ on the left lateral wall of the esophagus (Fig. 41-42), which results in a 10% false-negative rate in the contrast esophagram if the patient is not placed in the lateral decubitus position. Chest CT shows mediastinal air and fluid at the site of perforation (Fig. 41-43). A surgical endoscopy needs to be performed if the esophagram is negative or if operative intervention is planned. Mucosal injury is suggested if blood, mucosal hematoma, or a flap is seen or if the esophagus is difficult to insufflate.

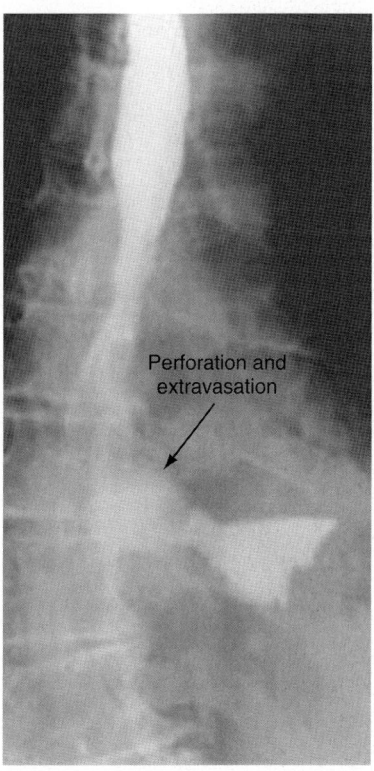

Figure 41-42 Barium esophagram of a perforated esophagus. Note the extravasation of contrast into the left chest. (Modified from Duranceau A: Perforation of the esophagus. In Sabiston DC [ed]: Textbook of Surgery, The Biological Basis of Modern Surgical Practice, 15th ed. Philadelphia, WB Saunders, 1997, p 761.)

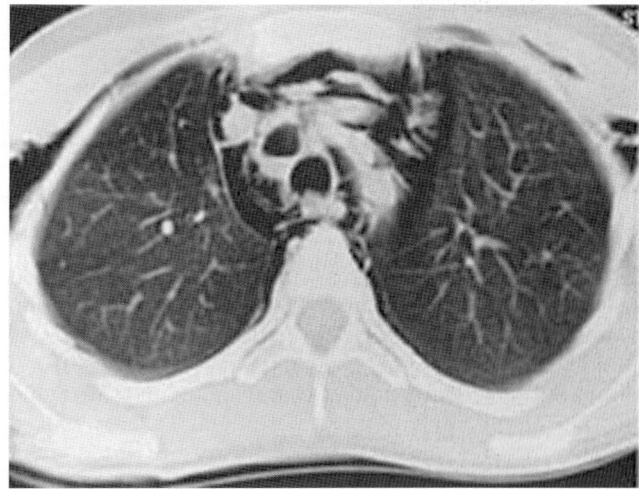

Figure 41-43 CT scan of a perforated esophagus. Note the air and fluid in the mediastinum. (Modified from Duranceau A: Perforation of the esophagus. In Sabiston DC [ed]: Textbook of Surgery, The Biological Basis of Modern Surgical Practice, 15th ed. Philadelphia, WB Saunders, 1997, p 761.)

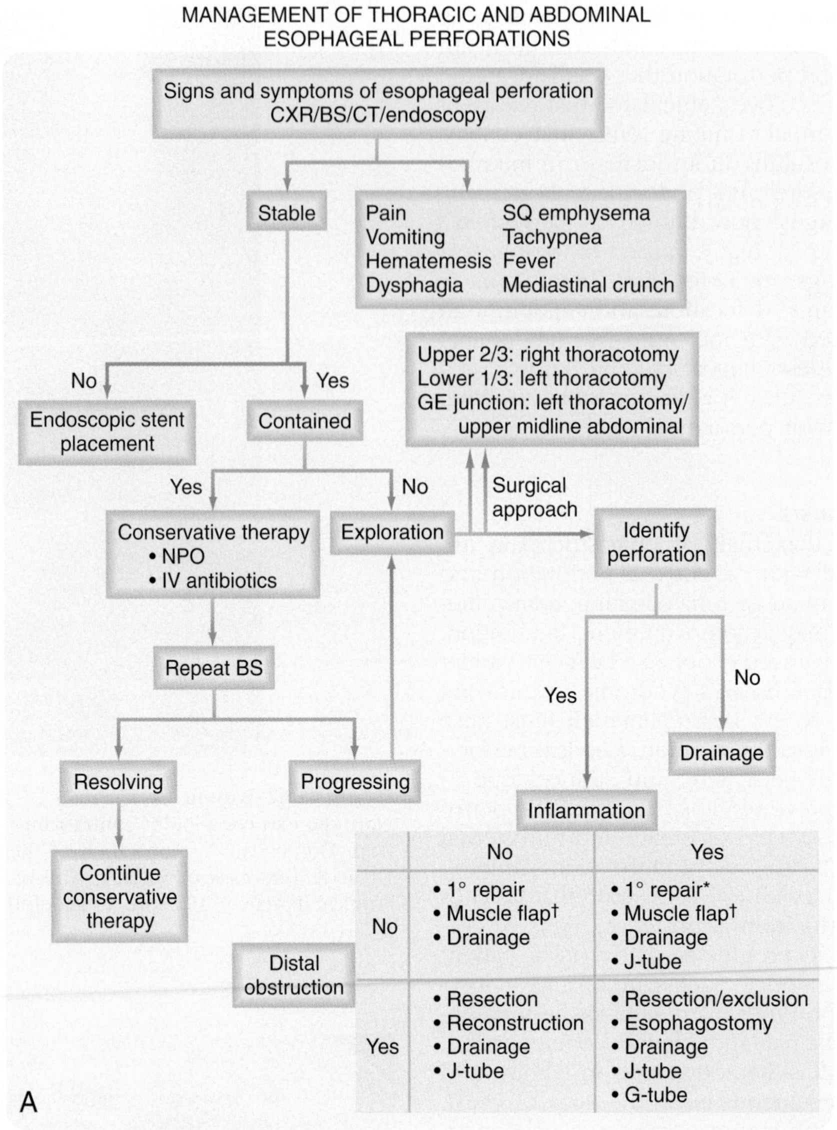

MANAGEMENT OF THORACIC AND ABDOMINAL
ESOPHAGEAL PERFORATIONS

Figure 41-44 Management of perforations of the esophagus. **A,** Thoracic and abdominal. BS, barium swallow.
*Assess ability to do primary repair.
†Gastric fundoplication used in the abdomen in place of a flap.

Treatment

The management of patients with esophageal perforation takes place in both the ICU and in the operating room. Patients with an esophageal perforation can progress rapidly to hemodynamic instability and shock. If perforation is suspected, appropriate resuscitation measures with the placement of large-bore peripheral IV catheters, a urinary catheter, and a secured airway are undertaken before the patient is sent for diagnostic testing. IV fluids and broad-spectrum antibiotics are started immediately, and the patient is monitored in an ICU. The patient is kept NPO, and nutritional access needs are assessed. A nasogastric tube is placed only after management decisions are made. These conservative measures are often lifesaving, and in patients who do not undergo surgery, they are life-sustaining.

Surgery is not indicated for every patient with a perforation of the esophagus, and management is dependent on several variables: stability of the patient, extent of contamination, degree of inflammation, underlying esophageal disease, and location of perforation (Fig. 41-44A). A stable patient will have a plethora of treatment options based on other variables. An unstable patient will need rapid assessment and expeditious treatment depending on the degree of contamination. In patients who remain clinically stable with no signs of progressive sepsis, a contained perforation may be treated conservatively. The patient is kept NPO, and nutrition is maintained by enteral access. A temporary endoluminal stent may be placed endoscopically and removed after 6 to 12 weeks. Interval esophagram or esophagoscopy is done to determine when the perforation is healed. Partial resolution of the perforation is treated with continuation of conservative therapy. Persistence or progression of the perforation without evidence of healing is treated with surgical intervention in the stable patient. During the

MANAGEMENT OF CERVICAL ESOPHAGEAL PERFORATIONS

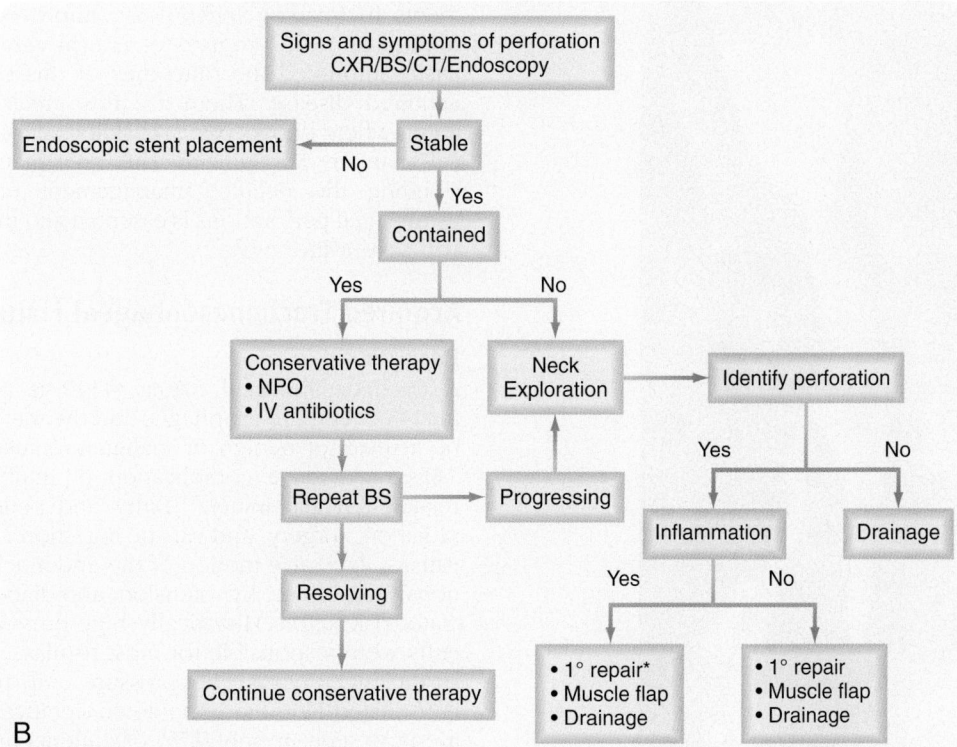

Figure 41-44, cont'd B, Management of cervical perforations of the esophagus. BS, barium swallow. *Assess ability to do a primary repair.

course of conservative management, if a patient's clinical condition deteriorates or the perforation is no longer contained, surgical intervention is advised. In an unstable patient with a contained perforation, a temporary stent may be placed and conservative measures initiated. In an unstable patient with a free perforation, surgical intervention with débridement of devitalized tissue, esophageal diversion or resection, creation of an esophagostomy, wide drainage, placement of a gastrostomy, and feeding jejunostomy is indicated.

The most critical variable that determines the surgical management of an esophageal perforation is the degree of inflammation surrounding the perforation. When patients present within 24 hours of perforation, inflammation is generally minimal, and primary surgical repair is recommended. With time, inflammation progresses, and tissues become friable and may not be amenable to primary repair. The so-called golden period for primary closure of an esophageal perforation is within the first 24 hours. Although primary repair is usually possible within this time period, it is by no means a magical cut-off time. If a healthy bed of tissue is encountered during surgical exploration, primary repair of the perforation is acceptable at any time. If a severe inflammatory reaction or mediastinitis is present and the tissues are not amenable to primary repair, a muscle flap is performed. All repairs are buttressed with healthy tissue flaps and widely drained. If primary repair or muscle flap fails, resection or exclusion of the esophagus with a cervical esophagos-

tomy, gastrostomy, feeding jejunostomy, and delayed reconstruction is recommended. Resection is recommended for patients with mid- to high-level perforations. Exclusion is recommended for low perforations in which esophageal salvage is possible or in any unstable patient in whom resection would not be tolerated.

There are four underlying conditions of the esophagus that affect that management of a free perforation of the esophagus: resectable carcinoma, megaesophagus from end-stage achalasia, severe peptic strictures, or a history of caustic ingestion. If any of these disease states is a factor, primary repair, even in the presence of a healthy tissue bed, is not recommended. Each of these entities is associated with distal narrowing and obstruction. Repair of a perforation without resolution of a distal obstruction results in fistula formation. In these circumstances, resection of the esophagus with immediate reconstruction is preferred if the patient is stable. In an unstable patient, esophageal resection with cervical esophagostomy, gastrostomy, and feeding jejunostomy with delayed reconstruction is recommended. In a patient with unresectable cancer, an esophageal stent is placed. If this does not contain the leak, then esophageal exclusion and diversion with placement of a gastrostomy and jejunostomy is indicated.

The final variable to consider in the surgical management of esophageal perforations is the location of the perforation. Cervical perforations are approached through a neck incision on the same side of the perforation

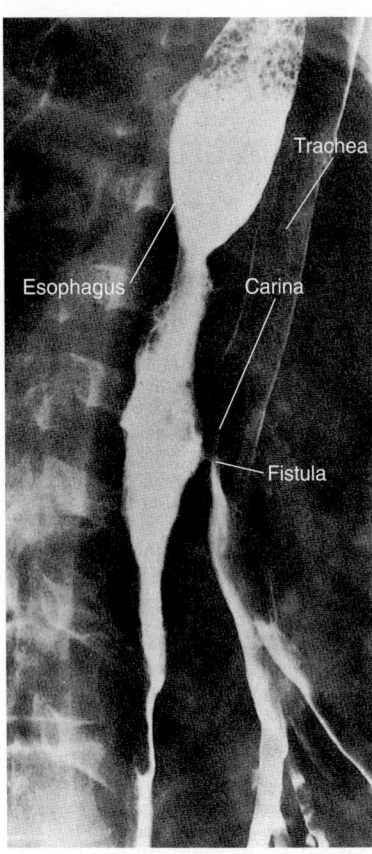

Figure 41-45 Barium esophagram of a tracheoesophageal fistula. (Modified from Little AG: Esophageal bypass. In Pearson FG, Cooper JD, Deslauriers J, et al [eds]: Esophageal Surgery, 2nd ed. New York, Churchill Livingstone, 2002, p 896.)

(see Fig. 41-44B). Small perforations may be difficult to find, and drainage without primary closure often is adequate. If primary repair is performed, a muscle flap is usually not required, but the placement of soft drains is necessary. In the event of a large perforation that is attempted to be closed primarily, a flap from a rotated strap muscle may be used to buttress the repair.

Thoracic perforations are approached from the right chest for the upper two thirds of the esophagus and the left chest for the lower third. The intercostal space is chosen based on the location of the perforation: right 4th intercostal space if the perforation is at or above the level of the carina, right 6th intercostal space for midesophageal perforations, and left 7th intercostal space for perforations of the lower third of the esophagus. Abdominal perforations are approached from either the left chest or the abdomen. If the perforation is freely contaminating the peritoneal space and is truly intra-abdominal with no intrathoracic component, an abdominal approach is used. However, this is rare circumstance, and most perforations of the abdominal esophagus are approached through a left thoracotomy. Muscle flaps are not easily accessible in this area, and instead a primary repair in this location is buttressed with a pleural patch or a fundoplication.

Perforations of the esophagus are challenging to manage. Traditionally, the mortality rate was close to 80%

in patients presenting with free perforation. Advancements in imaging technology, improved surgical techniques, and the progress of critical care medicine have vastly improved the outcomes of this once devastating acquired disease. There are few areas in the surgical arena where knowledge and skill coalesce in such a critical manner. Recognizing the presentation and understanding the detailed management of patients with esophageal perforations is essential and in many instances will save a life.

Acquired Tracheoesophageal Fistulas

Background

A tracheoesophageal fistula (TEF) is an epithelialized tract between the esophagus and the trachea. Fistulas can be a result of benign or malignant causes. Most benign TEFs occur as a complication of intubation and cuff-related tracheal injury.[19] Blunt and penetrating trauma, radiation, surgery, and caustic ingestion are also common causes. Excessive motion of the endotracheal tube, infections, steroid use, hypotension, and diabetes are all associated risk factors. Historically, high-pressure tracheostomy cuffs were responsible for most fistulas. Since the advent of the high-volume low-pressure cuff, the incidence of cuff-related TEFs has gone down significantly, and fistulas are now seen in only 0.5% of patients undergoing a tracheostomy. Fistulas can also occur as a result of erosion of tumor from the esophagus into the trachea or from the trachea into the esophagus. Management and outcomes vary with the etiology of the fistula.

Symptoms and Diagnosis

Regardless of the size and location of the TEF, most patients present with similar symptoms. Persistent coughing with meals and the production of bile-stained mucus are the prevailing complaints. Frequent respiratory infections, including pneumonia, are common with larger fistulas. Fevers suggest gross contamination of the lungs. Diagnosis is made by endoscopy, bronchoscopy, and barium esophagram. The experienced surgical endoscopist is best at identifying a TEF. Both endoscopy and bronchoscopy are performed at the same setting. The size of the fistula and the location with respect to the carina, the vocal cords, and the UES and LES is noted clearly. A barium esophagram is helpful to identify laterality and is essential in situations in which an experienced endoscopist is not available. The radiograph will demonstrate brisk opacification of the esophagus with faint opacification of the airway at and below the level of the fistula (Fig. 41-45). The absence of barium in the airway above the level of the fistula eliminates the possibility of aspiration as the cause of opacification of the airway. HRCT has also gained favor in the detection of tracheoesophageal fistulas. Recent advances have allowed sagittal, coronal, and three-dimensional reconstructions that can help to identify small fistulous tracts.[20]

Treatment

The treatment of a TEF occurs in two stages. The first stage involves preventing further contamination of the lungs. The patient is kept NPO, and a feeding tube (gastrostomy or jejunostomy) is placed. A course of IV antibiotics is given to help clean up the infection that is usually harbored in the lung. A temporary esophageal stent is placed if the fistula is large and there is evidence of gross contamination. Protection of the airway may include intubation with placement of the cuff below the fistula to help isolate the distal airway from enteric contamination. The second stage involves obliterating the fistulous tract and may be done endoscopically or surgically. Endoscopic ablation requires repeated interventions, every 3 to 4 weeks, over a 3-month period during which time the patient remains NPO. It is a reasonable option in patients with small fistulas or in patients too debilitated to undergo an operation. The application of biologic glues to obliterate a small fistulous tract also may be done with some success.[21] In most cases, surgical repair is necessary. Although surgical repair is much more extensive, most patients recover quickly and are able to begin eating within a week of the operation. Every attempt is made to wean the patient from mechanical ventilation before definitive intervention because postoperative positive-pressure ventilation increases the rate of dehiscence of the repair.

Surgical repair of a TEF takes place in three stages. The first stage is exposure of the fistulous tract through a cervical or thoracotomy incision. Stage two is segmental resection of the trachea and primary repair of the esophagus. Stage three is harvesting an appropriate muscle flap and placing it between the trachea and the esophagus to encourage healing, contain leaks, and prevent future fistulization. Although it may not be necessary to resect a segment of the trachea associated with the fistulous tract, it has been noted that in the case of repair of a postintubation TEF, tracheal resection and primary anastomosis decreases the rate of tracheal stenosis even in the absence of obvious tracheal damage.[22]

Other Esophageal Fistulas

Other types of fistulas involving the esophagus can occur after surgical manipulation. Fistulas from the esophagus or replacement grafts, such as the stomach or the colon, can form to any part of the airway, pleural space, or mediastinum. Breakdown of anastomotic sites or gastric staple lines can cause localized infections that erode into the airway or mediastinum. Although most esophageal fistulas to the airway occur at the level of the trachea, fistulas to the bronchi and distal airways can also arise. Traction diverticula, localized mediastinal infections, and ischemic perforations of esophageal replacement conduits all can lead to the formation of fistulas to the distal airways. Patients present with symptoms of a TEF, and treatment is similar to the management of patients presenting with esophageal perforations.

BENIGN TUMORS AND CYSTS

Benign tumors of the esophagus are unusual and constitute less than 1% of all esophageal neoplasms. They can be found in the muscular wall or in the lumen of the esophagus and are identified as solid tumors, cysts, or fibrovascular polyps (Table 41-5). About 60% of benign esophageal lesions are leiomyomas, 20% are cysts, 5% are polyps, and the remaining 5% are a potpourri of neoplasms. Intramural lesions are either solid tumors or cysts and are made up of smooth muscle and fibrous tissue in variable proportions. Leiomyomas are by far the most common, whereas the others (papillomas, fibromas, myomas, lipomas, neurofibromas, hemangiomas, adenomas, and glomus tumors) are all rare.

Leiomyoma

Background

Leiomyomas constitute 60% of all benign esophageal tumors. They are found in men slightly more often than women and tend to present in the 4th and 5th decades. They originate from the mesenchymal layer of embryologic development and are found in the distal two thirds of the esophagus more than 80% of the time. They are usually solitary and remain intramural, causing symptoms as they enlarge. Recently, they have been classified as a gastrointestinal stromal tumor (GIST). GIST tumors are the most common mesenchymal tumors of the gastrointestinal tract and can be benign or malignant. Nearly all GIST tumors occur from mutations of the c-*KIT* oncogene, which codes for the expression of c-*KIT* (CD117). Identification of this molecular marker is considered the most specific criterion for this diagnosis.[23] The true leiomyoma, or the non-GIST (c-*KIT*–negative) tumor, is actually quite rare. All leiomyomas are benign with malignant transformation being rare.

Symptoms and Diagnosis

Many leiomyomas are asymptomatic, and it is thought that most go undetected over a lifetime. Dysphagia and pain are the most common symptoms and can result from even the smallest tumors. Location and size tend not to correlate consistently with symptoms; however, tumors nestled between the spine and the airway often will cause dysphagia even when the tumor is just 1 cm in size. A chest radiograph is not usually helpful to diagnose a leiomyoma, but on barium esophagram, a leiomyoma has a characteristic appearance. A smooth, well-defined, noncircumferential mass with distinct borders is seen (Fig. 41-46). During endoscopy, extrinsic compression is seen, and the overlying mucosa is noted to be intact. Despite this compression, the scope is passed distally with ease as the esophagus accommodates. Diagnosis also can be made by an endoscopic ultrasound (EUS), which will demonstrate a hypoechoic mass in the submucosa or muscularis propria. Endoscopic biopsy is avoided because subsequent mucosal adherence to the mass increases the chance of a mucosal perforation during surgical resection.

Treatment

Leiomyomas are slow-growing tumors with rare malignant potential that will continue to grow and become progressively symptomatic with time. Although observation is acceptable in patients with small (<2 cm)

Table 41-5 Histogenetic Classification of Benign Esophageal Tumors

ESOPHAGEAL WALL TISSUE OF ORIGIN	TUMOR TYPE	TISSUE TYPE
Mucosa		
Epithelial lining		
Normal stratified squamous epithelium	Squamous cell papilloma	Epithelial
Acquired metaplastic columnar epithelium	True adenoma (rare) or adenomatous hyperplasia	Epithelial
Lamina propria		
Simple esophageal cardiac mucous gland	Mucus retention cyst	Epithelial
	True adenoma (rare)	Epithelial
Epithelial lining plus lamina propria	Inflammatory pseudotumor	Mesenchymal
	Fibrovascular polyp	Mesenchymal
Muscularis mucosae	Leiomyoma	Nonepithelial
Inflamed gastric mucosal fold at gastroesophageal junction	Inflammatory reflux polyp	Reflux polyp–fold complex
Submucosa		
Esophageal mucous gland proper	Mucus retention cyst	Epithelial
	Adenoma	Epithelial
Vascular connective tissue	Fibrovascular polyp (fibrolipoma, fibromyxoma)	Mesenchymal
Blood vessel	Hemangioma	Mesenchymal
Schwann cell	Granular cell tumor	Mesenchymal
	Neurilemoma	Mesenchymal
Muscularis Propria		
Striated muscle (upper one third)	Rhabdomyoma	Mesenchymal
Smooth muscle (lower two thirds)	Leiomyoma	Mesenchymal
Nerve fiber	Neurofibroma	Mesenchymal
Schwann cell	Granular cell tumor	Mesenchymal
	Neurilemoma	Mesenchymal
Tunica Adventitia		
Connective tissue	Fibroma	Mesenchymal
Nerve plexus	Schwannoma (neurilemoma)	Mesenchymal
Ectopic Tissues		
Sebaceous gland	Adenoma	Epithelial
Tracheobronchial rests	Choristoma	Mixed tissues

From Shamji F, Todd TRJ: Benign tumors. In Pearson FG, Cooper JF, Deslauriers J, et al (eds): Esophageal Surgery, 2nd ed. Philadelphia, Churchill Livingstone, 2002, p 639.

asymptomatic tumors or other significant comorbid conditions, in most patients, surgical resection is advocated. There are no known medical treatments for esophageal leiomyomas; however, imatinib (a tyrosine kinase inhibitor) is targeted therapy used on other GIST tumors that may have some benefit for esophageal leiomyomas. Surgical enucleation of the tumor remains the standard of care and is performed through a thoracotomy or with video or robotic assistance. Lesions of the proximal and midesophagus are removed through the right chest; those of distal origin are removed through the left chest. Morbidity is low, less than 5%, and includes inadvertent mucosal injury and pneumonia. The mortality rate is less than 2%, and success in relieving dysphagia approaches 100%.[24]

Esophageal Cysts

Background

Esophageal cysts are the second most common benign lesion of the esophagus. They can be congenital or acquired. Congenital cysts arise from persistent vacuoles in the wall of the foregut during embryologic development. They are lined with simple columnar, pseudostratified ciliated columnar, or stratified squamous epithelium. They are found within or in close proximity to the esophageal wall. Over time, they fill with mucus and increase in size, causing symptoms of obstruction. Most congenital cysts will present within the first year of life and are found in the upper third of the esophagus. Cysts of the lower two thirds present in childhood. Acquired cysts are probably a result of obstruction of the excretory ducts of esophageal glands. They are found in the lower esophagus and tend to present later in life.

Symptoms and Diagnosis

Most cysts, congenital or acquired, remain asymptomatic until they are large enough to obstruct the esophageal lumen. Symptoms of dysphagia or recurrent respiratory infections from aspiration of cystic fluid or a fistulous tract to the airway are common. Large cysts may impinge on the airway causing symptoms of shortness of breath and dyspnea on exertion. Diagnosis is made with a barium esophagram or CT scan (Fig. 41-47). A smooth oval mass will appear to be obstructing the lumen of the esophagus similar to that seen with a leiomyoma. EUS is helpful to distinguish a cyst from a solid mass and aids in cyst aspiration for diagnosis.

Treatment

Left untreated, an esophageal cyst will increase in size, resulting in obstruction, infection, or rupture. Cyst aspiration alone is not adequate because fluid will reaccumulate. Surgical resection of the cyst needs to be considered in all patients whenever possible. Extramucosal resection or enucleation is preferred and is done through a neck incision or thoracotomy. A fistulous tract to the airway may be present and must be sought. If one is found, it is ligated and divided.

Fibrovascular Polyps

Background

Fibrovascular polyps are uncommon tumors of the esophagus and are found in men aged 60 to 70 years. Most (85%) are located in the cervical esophagus below the cricopharyngeus muscle. They are composed of edematous connective tissue containing blood vessels and fatty tissue. They begin as small mucosal tumors and elongate over time. Some can grow to a substantial size and have extremely long pedicles. The pedicle can be very thin or thick and extremely vascular. The overlying mucosa may be ulcerated from trauma and infection. Although they are benign lesions, some polyps may harbor carcinoma and need to be thoroughly evaluated.

Symptoms and Diagnosis

Pedunculated polyps are usually asymptomatic until they grow large enough to cause dysphagia from obstruction of the esophageal lumen. Bleeding from mucosal ulcerations may occur and result in a slow gastrointestinal bleed. Diagnosis is made on endoscopy or barium esophagram. Endoscopic evaluation may miss small lesions because the polyp surface appears similar to normal esophageal mucosa. The thickness of the pedicle and the size of the tumor mass is noted. Biopsies of the overlying mucosa are undertaken to rule out cancer. A barium esophagram demonstrates an irregular filling defect of the esophagus with distal narrowing (Fig. 41-48A), and CT identifies the intraluminal mass within the esophagus (see Fig. 41-48B).

Treatment

All fibrovascular polyps are removed. Left untreated, they will continue to grow and obstruct the esophageal lumen. Endoscopic removal by electrocautery ligation is indicated if the mass is small (<2 cm) or if the pedicle is not richly vascular. Larger polyps can be removed endoscopically; however, they are difficult to pull through the esophagus past the cricopharyngeus muscle. There is a risk for airway obstruction with endoscopic removal of large polyps that do not easily pass through the pharynx. Surgical resection is recommended for all masses that are

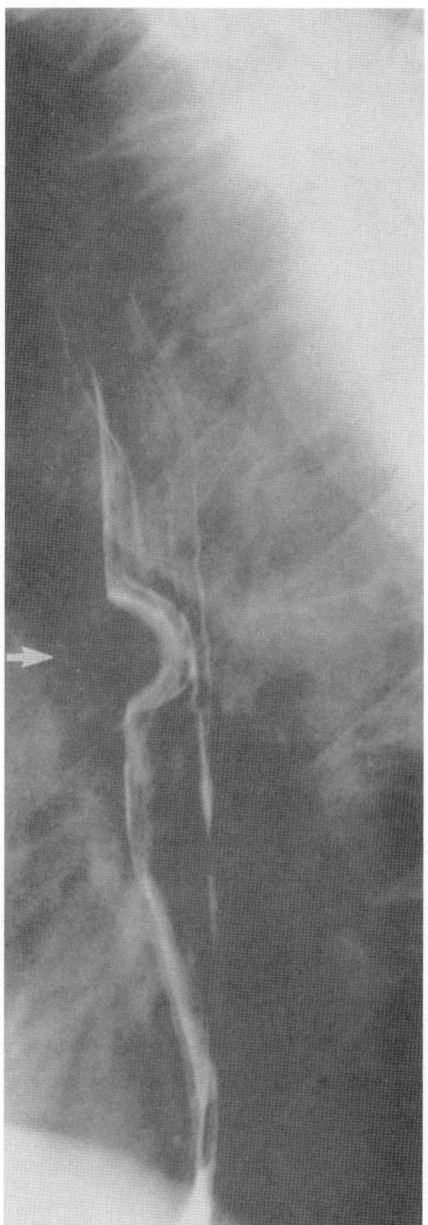

Figure 41-46 Barium esophagram showing a leiomyoma. Note the characteristic smooth, distinct borders of the mass. (From Shamji F, Todd TR: Benign tumors. In Pearson FG, Cooper JD, Deslauriers J, et al [eds]: Esophageal Surgery, 2nd ed. New York, Churchill Livingstone, 2002, p 640.)

greater than 8 cm in length or have a richly vascularized pedicle (see Fig. 41-48C). Depending on the location of the mass, resection is approached through a cervical incision or a thoracotomy.

CARCINOMA OF THE ESOPHAGUS

Background

Esophageal cancer is the fastest growing cancer in the United States. It remains the sixth most common malig-

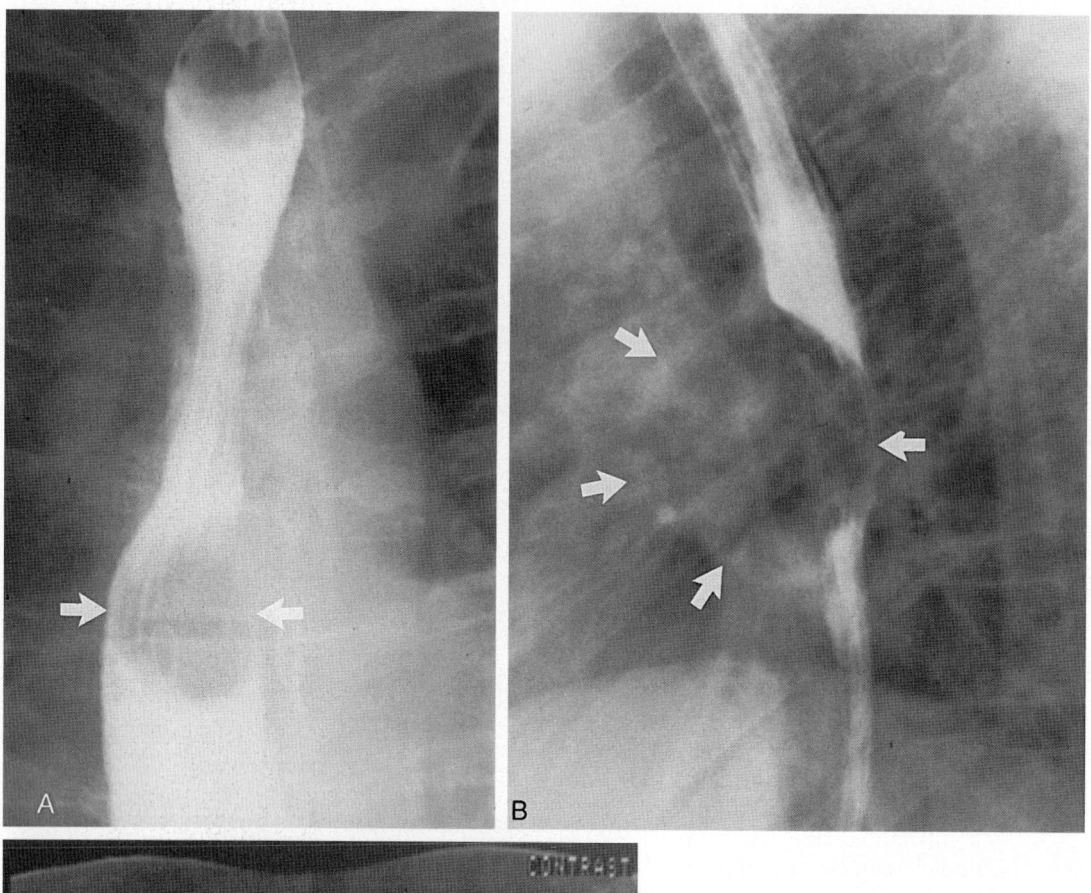

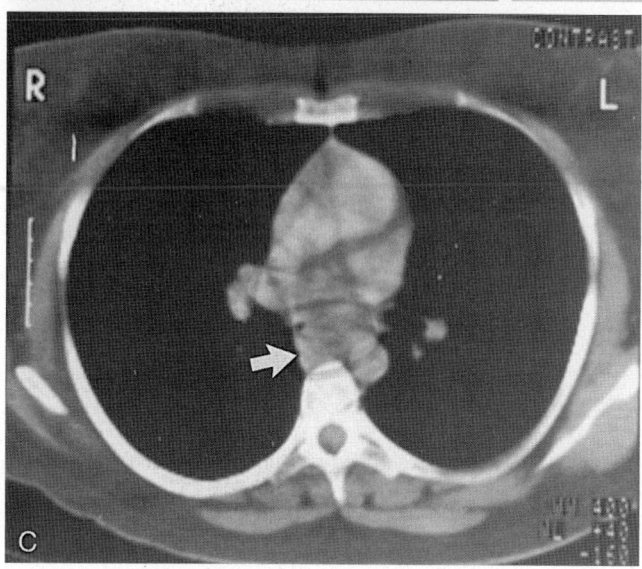

Figure 41-47 Barium esophagram and CT scan of an esophageal cyst. (Modified from Orringer MB: Tumors of the esophagus. In Sabiston DC [ed]: Textbook of Surgery, The Biological Basis of Modern Surgical Practice, 15th ed. Philadelphia, WB Saunders, 1997, p 746.)

nancy with an incidence of 20 per 100,000 and represents 4% of newly diagnosed cancers in North America. Worldwide, esophageal cancer is even more prevalent, reaching an incidence of 160 per 100,000 in parts of South Africa and China and 540 per 100,000 in Kazakhstan. Squamous cell carcinoma still accounts for most esophageal cancers diagnosed. However, in the United States, esophageal adenocarcinoma is noted in up to 70% of patients presenting with esophageal cancer. The distribu-

tion of esophageal cancer across gender, age, and race is affected by the cell type. The male-to-female ratio for squamous cell cancer is 3:1; in contrast, the ratio for adenocarcinoma is 15:1 in the fifth decade of life. Squamous cell cancer is seen rarely before the age of 30 years, with the highest mortality rates seen among men between ages 60 and 70 years. Adenocarcinoma is seen infrequently before the age of 40 years and increases in incidence with age. Racial discrepancies are observed.

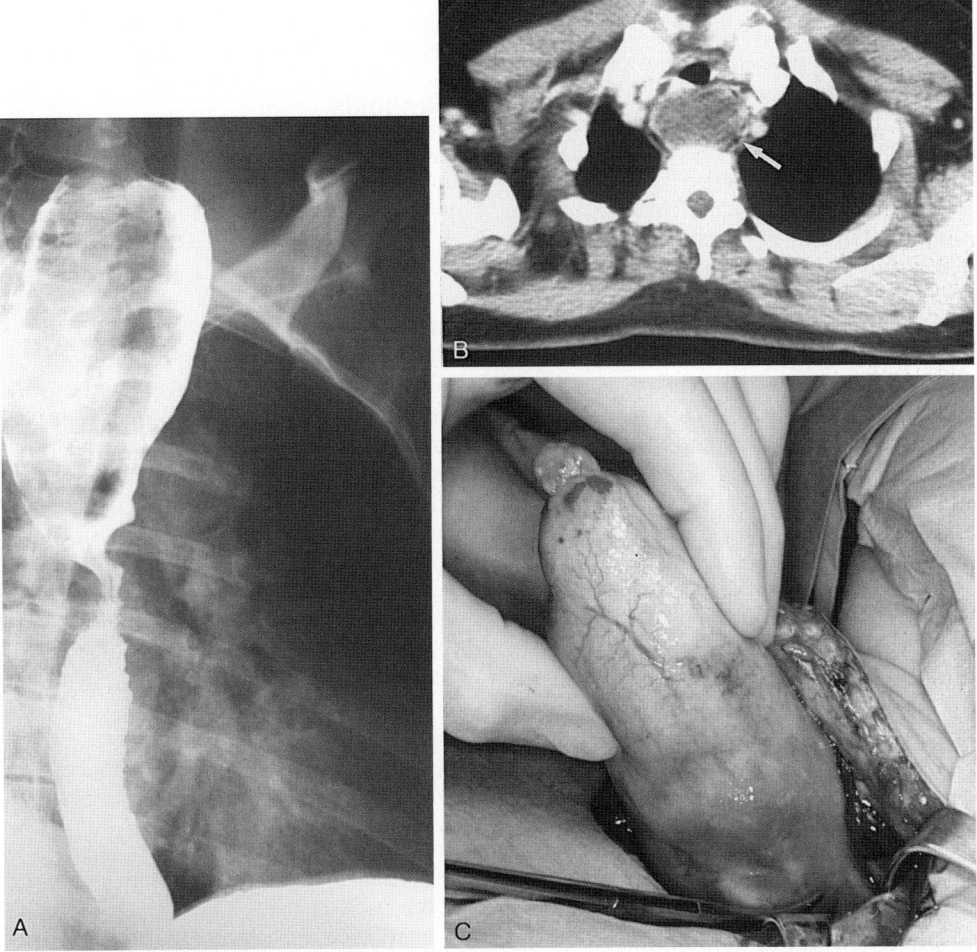

Figure 41-48 Barium esophagram (**A**) and CT scan (**B**) of an esophageal polyp. **C,** Resection of a large esophageal polyp. (Modified from Orringer MB: Tumors of the esophagus. In Sabiston DC [ed]: Textbook of Surgery, The Biological Basis of Modern Surgical Practice, 15th ed. Philadelphia, WB Saunders, 1997, p 747.)

Adenocarcinoma is a disease affecting white men, whereas squamous cell carcinoma predominantly affects African American men.

Squamous cell carcinomas arise from the squamous mucosa that is native to the esophagus and is found in the upper and middle third of the esophagus 70% of the time. This type of cancer is due to exposure to environmental factors. Smoking and alcohol both increase the risk for foregut cancers by 5-fold. Combined, the risk increases from 25- to 100-fold. Food additives, including nitrosamines found in pickled and smoked foods, long-term ingestion of hot liquids, and vitamin (vitamin A) and mineral deficiencies (zinc and molybdenum) have been implicated. Other disorders that expose the esophagus to mucosal trauma including caustic ingestion, achalasia, bulimia, tylosis (an inherited autosomal dominant trait), Plummer-Vinson syndrome, external-beam radiation, and esophageal diverticula all have known associations with squamous cell cancer. The 5-year survival rate varies but can be as good as 70% with polypoid lesions and as poor as 15% with advanced tumors.

Once a relatively unusual disease, esophageal adenocarcinoma now accounts for nearly 70% of all esophageal carcinomas diagnosed in the United States and Western countries. There are a number of factors that are responsible for this shift in cell type:

1. Increasing incidence of GERD
2. Western diet
3. Increased use of acid-suppression medications

Intake of caffeine, fats, and acidic and spicy foods all lead to decreased tone in the LES and an increase in reflux. As an adaptive measure, the squamous-lined distal esophagus changes to become lined with metaplastic columnar epithelium (Barrett's esophagus). Progressive changes from metaplastic (Barrett's esophagus) to dysplastic cells may lead to the development of esophageal adenocarcinoma. Histologically, esophageal adenocarcinoma arises from one of three places:

1. Submucosal glands of the esophagus
2. Heterotopic islands of columnar epithelium

3. Malignant degeneration of metaplastic columnar epithelium (Barrett's esophagus)

There are several intrinsic diseases of the esophagus that are considered premalignant. Patients with Plummer-Vinson syndrome, a disease of iron and vitamin deficiency that results in atrophy of the oropharyngeal and esophageal mucosa, have an increased risk for developing squamous cell cancers of the cervical esophagus. Tylosis, an uncommon familial syndrome characterized by thickening of the skin of the soles and palms, has an estimated 40% increased risk for developing squamous cell carcinoma that appears to be genetically linked. Achalasia, a disorder of esophageal motility is associated with a 16-fold increased risk for squamous cell cancer in late-stage disease. Both esophageal strictures and diverticula have been reported to be associated with a small but increased risk for esophageal cancers. Patients with aerodigestive tract cancers are also at an increased risk for developing esophageal squamous tumors. Barrett's esophagus, or metaplastic columnar epithelium in the esophagus, is associated with a 40-fold increased risk for adenocarcinoma of the esophagus. No specific infectious agents have been identified as a cause of esophageal cancer, but many remain under investigation. Genetic alterations accounting for cellular and molecular changes (as in the *p53* gene) have been associated with an increased risk for esophageal cancer.

Regardless of the cell type, esophageal cancer asserts aggressive biologic behavior. With only two layers to the esophageal wall, tumors rapidly infiltrate through the muscular wall into surrounding structures. The rich vascular and lymphatic supply facilitates spread to regional lymph nodes. Advanced disease is common at the time of presentation and contributes to the high mortality rate. Spread of disease follows lymphatic drainage patterns so that drainage tends to be to local, regional, and then to distant lymph node beds.

Symptoms

The symptoms of esophageal cancer vary with the stage of the disease. Early-stage cancers may be asymptomatic or mimic symptoms of GERD. Heartburn, regurgitation, and indigestion are symptoms of reflux, but cancer may be lurking within. Most patients with esophageal cancer present with dysphagia and weight loss. These symptoms usually indicate advanced disease. Because of the distensibility of the esophagus, a mass can obstruct two thirds of the lumen before symptoms of dysphagia are noted. Furthermore, the symptoms of dysphagia and weight loss may be slowly progressive and well compensated for over a period of months. It is not until the esophageal lumen is narrowed from an average of 24 mm to 12 mm that dysphagia is noted. Many patients will be symptomatic before narrowing occurs to this degree, but medical treatment is often not sought until the symptoms are disabling. Effortless weight loss is welcomed by most, although its true significance goes unappreciated.

Choking, coughing, and aspiration from a tracheoesophageal fistula, as well as hoarseness and vocal cord paralysis from direct invasion into the recurrent laryngeal nerve, are ominous signs of advanced disease. Systemic metastases to liver, bone, and lung can present with jaundice, excessive pain, and respiratory symptoms.

Diagnosis

There are a plethora of modalities available to diagnose and stage esophageal cancer. Radiologic tests, endoscopic procedures, and minimally invasive surgical techniques all add value to a solid staging workup in a patient with esophageal cancer.

Esophagram

A barium esophagram is recommended for any patient presenting with dysphagia. The esophagram gives an overview of anatomy and function. It is able to differentiate intraluminal from intramural lesions and to discriminate between intrinsic (from a mass protruding into the lumen) and extrinsic (from compression of a structures outside the esophagus) compression. The classic finding of an apple-core lesion in patients with esophageal cancer is recognized easily (Fig. 41-49). Although the esophagram will not be specific for cancer, it is a good first test to perform in patients presenting with dysphagia and a suspicion of esophageal cancer.

Endoscopy

The diagnosis of esophageal cancer is made best from an endoscopic biopsy. During endoscopy, it is critical to document the following:

1. Location of the lesion (with respect to distance from the incisors)
2. Nature of the lesion (friable, firm, polypoid)
3. Proximal and distal extent of the lesion
4. Relationship of the lesion to the cricopharyngeus muscle, the GEJ, and the gastric cardia
5. Distensibility of the stomach

Each of these points is important in the management of esophageal cancer and helps to guide surgical therapy. Incontrovertibly, any patient undergoing surgery for esophageal cancer must have an endoscopy performed by the operating surgeon before entering the operating room for a definitive resection.

Computed Tomography

There are additional diagnostic modalities that are used for accurate staging. A CT scan of the chest and abdomen is important to assess the length of the tumor, thickness of the esophagus and stomach, regional lymph node status (including cervical, mediastinal, and celiac lymph nodes), and distant disease to the liver and lungs. It is also helpful in determining T4 lesions where the lesion is invading surrounding structures. It may identify a fistula or other anatomic variations such as a deviated trachea. Although a CT scan is helpful, its accuracy is only 57% for T staging, 74% for N staging, and 83% for M staging.[25] Many unresectable tumors by CT scan are deemed resectable at the time of surgery. It is an important piece of the diagnostic workup, but its findings must be interpreted judiciously and only as a part of the total picture.

Positron Emission Tomography

A positron emission tomography (PET) scan evaluates the primary mass, regional lymph nodes, and distant disease (Fig. 41-50). Its sensitivity and specificity slightly exceed those of CT; however, they remain low for definitive staging. The sensitivity and specificity of PET for evaluating metastatic disease are as high as 88% and 93%, respectively. For evaluation of lymph node disease, PET has a sensitivity (72%), specificity (86%), and accuracy (76%) on par with what CT can offer.[26] As with CT, the ability of PET to evaluate local and regional lymph node disease is dependent on the location of the tumor, the size of the lymph node, and technique of the scanner. Although its role is evolving, PET appears to be an important piece of the diagnostic workup but is not reliable enough as a single diagnostic modality.

Magnetic Resonance Imaging

Magnetic resonance imaging (MRI) is not performed routinely and adds to the staging of esophageal cancer in few circumstances. To identify involvement of vascular and neural tissues, MRI is helpful. It can accurately detect T4 lesions and metastatic lesions in the liver; however, it overstages T and N status with only 74% accuracy.

Endoscopic Ultrasound

EUS is the most critical component of esophageal cancer staging. The information obtained from EUS will help guide both medical and surgical therapy. The experienced endoscopic ultrasonographer can identify the depth of the tumor, the length of the tumor, the degree of luminal compromise, the status of regional lymph nodes, and involvement of adjacent structures. In addition, biopsy samples can be obtained of the mass and lymph nodes in the paratracheal, subcarinal, paraesophageal, celiac, lesser curvature, and gastrohepatic regions. EUS tends to overstage T status and understage N status. The accuracy of EUS for T staging correlates directly with increasing T stage. For T1 lesions, EUS is 84% accurate, and it approaches 95% accuracy in estimating T4 lesions. Size and location of the lymph node influence the accuracy, so that lymph nodes smaller than 1 cm tend to be less accurately evaluated. The overall sensitivity (78%) and specificity (60%) of EUS for evaluating lymph nodes are poor but improve dramatically for evaluating celiac lymph nodes, for which the sensitivity and specificity are 72% and 97%, respectively.

Endoscopic Mucosal Resection

EMR is performed with a double-channel endoscope that is fashioned with a soft plastic cap at its tip. The cap is placed over the top of the lesion, suction is applied, and a snare is brought down over the top of the lesion. A biopsy specimen of 1 to 1.5 cm will contain mucosa and submucosa. In skilled hands, EMR provides essential staging information that guides treatment. It may also be used as a therapeutic modality for premalignant and early malignant conditions. An additional diagnostic and therapeutic tool is being explored by the Japanese and Germans. Endoscopic submucosal dissection (ESD) is a technique that uses hook cautery and scissors to resect

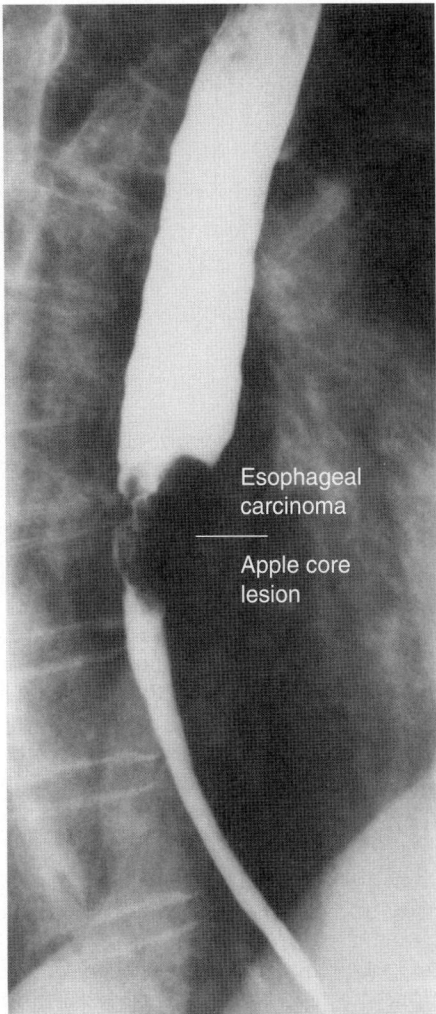

Esophageal carcinoma

Apple core lesion

Figure 41-49 Carcinoma of the esophagus. Note the appearance of an "apple core" lesion. (From Jaffer NM, Chia SH: Radiology, computed tomography and magnetic resonance imaging. In Pearson FG, Cooper JD, Deslauriers J, et al [eds]: Esophageal Surgery, 2nd ed. New York, Churchill Livingstone, 2002, p 88.)

a lesion down to the level of the muscularis propria. This is a new technique that has not yet gained enough experience worldwide; however, the future is promising.

Minimally Invasive Surgical Modalities

Bronchoscopy, mediastinoscopy, thoracoscopy, and laparoscopy are all useful staging tools. Bronchoscopy is performed in any patient presenting with a cough or evidence of a cervical esophageal cancer. It is helpful to rule out a tracheoesophageal fistula or growth of tumors into the trachea. Mediastinoscopy is still an available tool used in the workup for esophageal cancer. It is used to biopsy suspicious lymph nodes that may indicate advanced disease and that are not amenable to endo-ultrasonographic biopsy. Using video-assisted thoracoscopic surgery technology, lymph nodes in the thoracic inlet, mediastinum (including paratracheal, subcarinal, and paraesophageal lymph nodes), and along the tho-

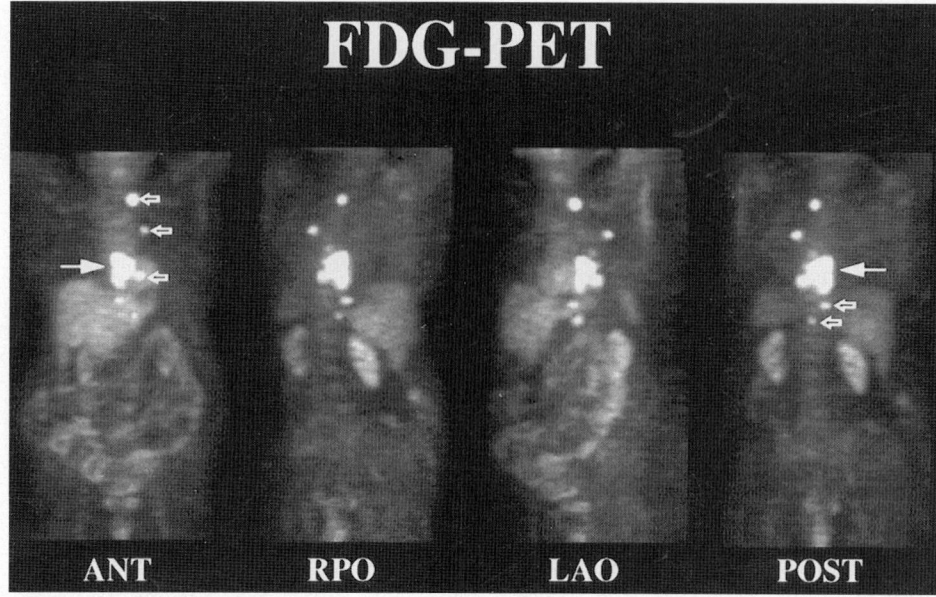

Figure 41-50 Positron emission tomography scan of an esophageal cancer. ANT, anterior; LAO, left anterior oblique; POST, posterior; RPO, right posterior oblique. (From Dehdashti F, Siegel BA: Positron emission tomography. In Pearson FG, Cooper JD, Deslauriers J, et al [eds]: Esophageal Surgery, 2nd ed. New York, Churchill Livingstone, 2002, p 117.)

racic duct and into the diaphragmatic hiatus can be evaluated. Metastatic lesions in the lung or extension of tumor into the pericardium, aorta, azygos vein, trachea, or diaphragm are noted with an accuracy of 93%.[27] Laparoscopy also has some utility in staging esophageal cancer. Extent of tumor and biopsies of the celiac axis, perihepatic, and GEJ lymph nodes can be performed. The addition of a laparoscopic ultrasound probe allows visualization of nodes as small as 3 mm in diameter, similar to that of EUS. Complementary to thoracoscopy, laparoscopy is an additional method for providing accurate staging information, with low risk to the patient.

Staging

The most critical aspect of treating a patient with esophageal cancer is procuring an accurate clinical stage. The data obtained in the process of staging the patient are more important than the stage within which the patient falls. Precise staging at the time of presentation allows for the most appropriate treatment and results in the best chance for long-term survival.

The staging of esophageal cancer has morphed through a variety of systems and remains controversial. The American Joint Committee on Cancer (AJCC) staging criteria were instituted in 1988 and are currently the most widely adopted staging system (Table 41-6). However, recognizing the flaws in the AJCC system, in 1997 Ellis proposed a staging system based on the criteria defined by Skinner that restructures the T status (Table 41-7). The AJCC classification uses the TNM (tumor, lymph node, metastasis) system to stratify patients and estimate prognosis, whereas the Ellis classification uses the WNM (wall penetration, lymph node, metastasis) system. In the AJCC system, the T represents the depth of the tumor (T1, submucosal; T2,

muscularis propria; T3, adventitia; T4, surrounding structures), the N represents involvement of lymph nodes (N0, none; N1, any), and the M represents metastatic disease to nonregional lymph nodes or distant sites (M0, none; M1a, regional lymph nodes; M1b, distant lymph nodes). In the Ellis classification, the W represents the depth of wall penetration (W0, muscularis mucosae; W1, submucosa and muscularis propria; W2, adventitia), N represents the number of positive lymph nodes (N0, none; N1, 1-4; N2, >4), and M represents distant disease (M0, none; M1, any) (Fig. 41-51). In both systems, the depth of invasion and the extent of local and regional lymph node involvement affect prognosis. However, the Ellis classification emphasizes not only that the depth of invasion is important but also that the number of lymph nodes affects survival. A comparison between the two systems is outlined in Table 41-8 and Figure 41-52.

The Japanese have further classified the T1 status.[28] In this staging system, the mucosa and submucosal layers are subdivided to identify tumors with extension into the epithelium, lamina propria, muscularis mucosae, and superficial, middle, and deep submucosal layers. These investigators have shown that depth of tumor directly relates to lymph node involvement. Tumors confined to the epithelial layer have no associated lymph node involvement. Lesions penetrating the lamina propria and muscularis mucosae are associated with lymph node involvement 5% and 18% of the time, respectively. Superficial and deep submucosal lesions have an associated 50% and 55% lymph node involvement, respectively.

Treatment

Traditionally, staging systems have been used to guide therapy and assess long-term outcomes (Fig. 41-53). As

Table 41-6 Tumor-Node-Metastasis (TNM) Staging of Esophageal Carcinoma

T: Primary Tumor	
Tx	Tumor cannot be assessed
T0	No evidence of tumor
Tis	High-grade dysplasia
T1	Tumor invades the lamina propria, muscularis mucosae, or submucosa; does not breach the submucosa
T2	Tumor invades into but not beyond the muscularis propria
T3	Tumor invades the paraesophageal tissue but does not invade adjacent structures
T4	Tumor invades adjacent structures

N: Regional Lymph Nodes	
Nx	Regional lymph nodes cannot be assessed
N0	No regional lymph node metastases
N1	Regional lymph nodes metastases

M: Distant Metastases	
Mx	Distant metastases cannot be assessed
M1a	Upper thoracic esophageal lesion metastatic to cervical lymph nodes
	Midthoracic esophageal lesion metastatic to mediastinal lymph nodes
	Lower thoracic esophageal lesion metastatic to celiac lymph nodes
M1b	Upper thoracic esophageal lesion metastatic to mediastinal or celiac lymph nodes
	Midthoracic esophageal lesion metastatic to cervical or celiac lymph nodes
	Lower thoracic esophageal lesion metastatic to cervical or upper mediastinal lymph nodes

STAGE GROUPINGS	T	N	M
Stage 0	Tis	N0	M0
Stage I	T1	N0	M0
Stage IIA	T2	N0	M0
	T3	N0	M0
Stage IIB	T1	N1	M0
	T2	N1	M0
Stage III	T3	N1	M0
	T4	Any N	M0
Stage IVA	Any T	Any N	M1a
Stage IVB	Any T	Any N	M1b

Table 41-7 Wall Penetration-Node-Metastasis (WNM) Staging of Esophageal Carcinoma

W: Wall Penetration	
W0	Intramucosal mucosa penetration
W1	Intramural mucosa penetration
W2	Transmural mucosa penetration

N: Regional Lymph Nodes	
Nx	Regional lymph nodes cannot be assessed
N0	No regional lymph node metastases
N1	Four lymph nodes metastases or fewer
N2	Greater than four lymph node metastases

M: Distant Metastases	
Mx	Distant metastases cannot be assessed
M0	No distant metastases
M1	Distant metastases present

STAGE GROUPING	W	N	M
Stage 0	W0	N0	M0
Stage I	W0	N1	M0
	W1	N0	M0
Stage II	W1	N1	M0
	W2	N0	M0
Stage III	W2	N1	M0
	W1	N2	M0
	W0	N2	M0
Stage IV	Any W	Any N	M1a

These variables guide management and help to form appropriate treatment plans that may include chemotherapy, radiotherapy, endoscopic procedures, and surgical resection. Although treatment is controversial at all stages and varies between oncologists, radiation oncologists, gastroenterologists, and surgeons as well as among surgeons themselves, multimodality therapy with chemotherapy, radiation therapy, endoscopic procedures, and surgical resection is appropriate for most patients presenting with esophageal cancer (Fig. 41-54).

Histology, Location, and Local Extent of the Primary Tumor

There are two predominant cells types of esophageal cancer: adenocarcinoma and squamous cell carcinoma. Adenocarcinoma represents more than 70% of esophageal cancers in the United States, but worldwide, squamous cell cancers dominate. The histology of the tumor is important because it guides treatment in two ways: (1) squamous cell tumors are more sensitive to chemoradiotherapy and are treated aggressively with nonsurgical therapy; (2) adenocarcinomas are not as sensitive to chemoradiotherapy and are often imbedded in long segments of Barrett's esophagus, necessitating a more aggressive surgical approach. Patients with squamous cell tumors may achieve a complete response to chemoradiotherapy, making the need for surgical intervention uncertain and not very compelling. However, most of the literature supports multimodality therapy for treatment of squamous cell tumors. Surgery is strongly advocated for most patients

technology, medical therapy, and knowledge of the biology of tumors continue to advance, staging systems are changing and becoming less functional. When a patient presents with esophageal cancer, the following variables are considered (Table 41-9):

1. Histology, location, and local extent (depth of invasion) of the primary tumor
2. Status of the local and regional lymph nodes
3. Presence of distant lymph nodes or systemic disease
4. Overall condition of the patient (including nutritional status and ability to swallow)
5. Intended goal of treatment—curative or palliative

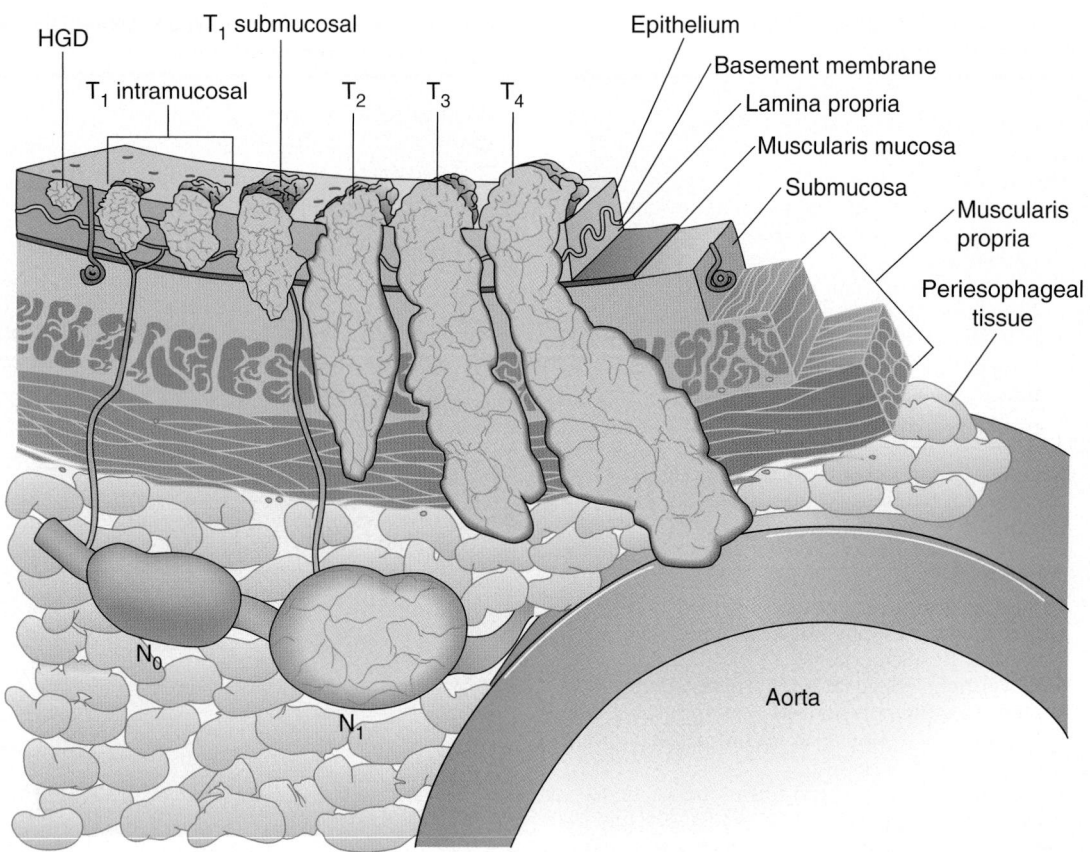

Figure 41-51 Primary tumor status (T) is defined by depth of invasion. Regional lymph node (N) is defined by the absence (N0) or presence (N1) of regional nodal metastases. HGD, high-grade dysplasia. (From Rice WR: Diagnosis and staging of esophageal carcinoma. In Pearson FG, Cooper JD, Deslauriers J, et al [eds]: Esophageal Surgery, 2nd ed. New York, Churchill Livingstone, 2002, p 687.)

Table 41-8 Comparison Between WNM and TNM Classification Systems

WNM 5-YEAR SURVIVAL (%)	WNM STAGE	WNM CLASS	TNM CLASS	TNM STAGE	TNM 5-YEAR SURVIVAL (%)
88	0	W0 N0 M0	Tis N0 M0	0	100
			T1 N0 M0	1	79
50	1	W0 N1 M0	NE	NE	NE
50	1	W1 N0 M0	T1 N0 M0	1	79
			T2 N0 M0	2A	38
23	2	W1 N1 M0	T1 N1 M0	2B	27
			T2 N1 M0		
23	2	W2 N0 M0	T3 N0 M0	2A	38
			T4 N0 M0		
11	3	W2 N1 M0	T3 N1 M0	3	14
			T4 N1 M0		
11	3	W1 N2 M0	T1 N1 M0	2B	27
			T2 N1 M0		
11	3	W0 N2 M0	NE	NE	NE
0	4	Wx Nx M1	Tx Nx M1	4	0

NE, no equivalent.

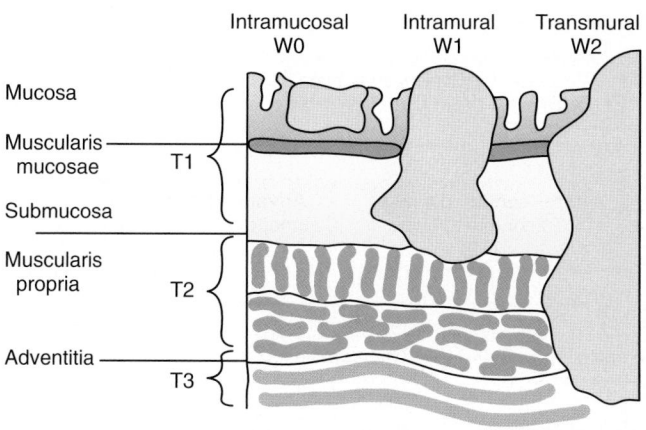

Figure 41-52 A comparison between the TNM and WNM staging systems. (Modified from DeMeester TR, Attwood SEA, Smyrk TC, et al: Surgical therapy in Barrett's esophagus. Ann Surg 212:530, 1990.)

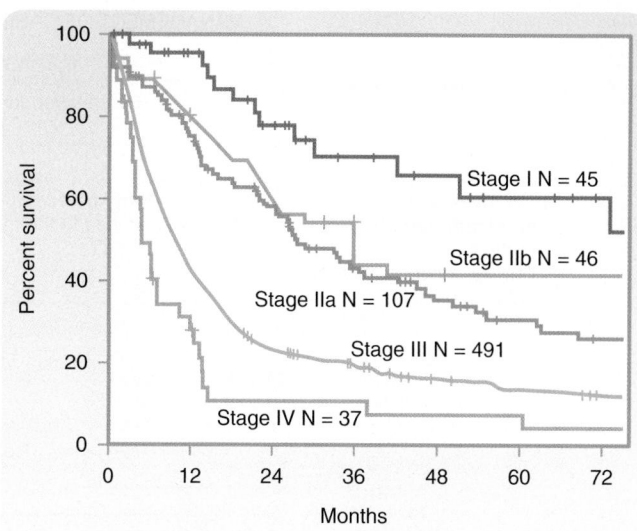

Figure 41-53 Cumulative survival curves. (From Law SYW, Wong J: Management of squamous cell carcinoma of the esophagus. In Pearson FG, Cooper JD, Deslauriers J, et al [eds]: Esophageal Surgery, 2nd ed. New York, Churchill Livingstone, 2002, p 719.)

Table 41-9 Variables to Consider in the Management of Esophageal Cancer

PRIMARY TUMOR	LYMPH NODES	DISTANT DISEASE	PATIENT CONDITION	GOALS

Histology
  Squamous cell
  Adenocarcinoma
Location
  Cervical
  Upper thoracic
  Midthoracic
  Distal thoracic/cardia
Local extent/depth
  of invasion
T1
  A: Intramucosal
  B: Submucosal
T2
  Muscularis propria
T3
  Adventitia
T4
  Adjacent structures
	Local
	  Adjacent to the primary
	    tumor
	Regional
	  One nodal basin away
	    from the primary
	    tumor
		Lymph nodes
		  More than one nodal
		    basin away from the
		    primary tumor
		Organ
		  Lung
		  Liver
		  Other
		Systemic
			Good
			  Age <75 yr
			  Comorbidities <3
			  Good pulmonary
			    function tests
			  Cardiac reserve
			  Weight loss <10%
			
			  Nutrition: serum
			    albumin >3.4 g/dL
			  No dysphagia
			Fair
			  Age >75 yr
			  Comorbidities ≥3
			  Poor pulmonary
			    function tests
			  No cardiac reserve
			  Weight loss >10%
			  Nutrition: serum
			    albumin <3.4 g/dL
			  Dysphagia
				Curative
				Palliative

with adenocarcinoma because a complete response to chemotherapy is seen only 25% of the time in this cell type. Little is known about the biology of esophageal tumors, but as knowledge is forthcoming, future medical therapies will be targeted at the biology, not the histology, of the tumor. This is already well established in other malignancies, such as breast cancer.

The location of the tumor also directs the management of esophageal cancer. Eight percent of all esophageal

tumors present in the cervical esophagus and are almost always squamous cell cancers. These tumors may be locally aggressive and are managed with chemoradiotherapy followed by segmental resection of the cervical esophagus. Upper and mid thoracic tumors account for 3% and 32% of esophageal tumors, respectively, and may be either squamous cell cancers or adenocarcinomas. Near-total esophagectomy through a thoracotomy is usually required to remove all the disease in this part of

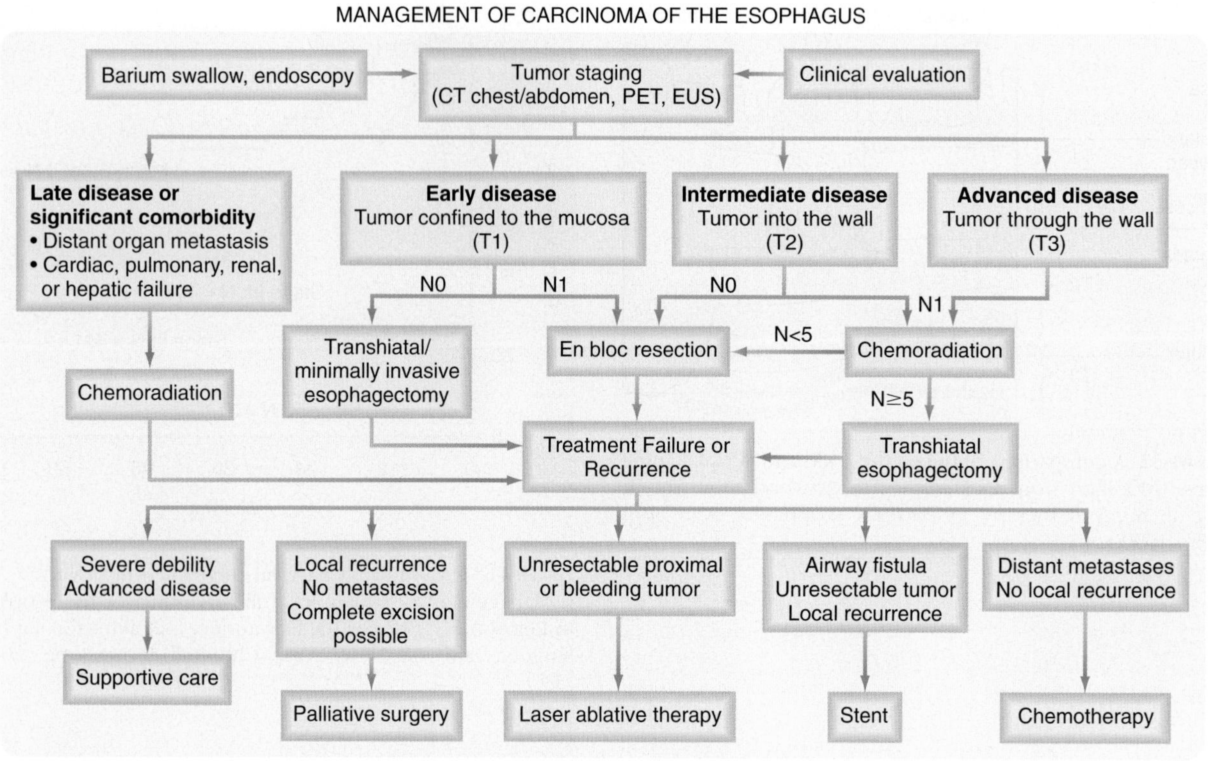

MANAGEMENT OF CARCINOMA OF THE ESOPHAGUS

Figure 41-54 Algorithm for the management of esophageal cancer.

the esophagus. The remaining tumors are found in the lower esophagus (25%) and the cardia of the stomach (32%) and tend to be adenocarcinomas. Distal esophagectomy (through a transabdominal or transthoracic approach) in patients with no known Barrett's esophagus or total gastrectomy in those with Barrett's esophagus is appropriate for early disease. Near-total esophagectomy (through a transhiatal or transthoracic approach) is recommended for patients who have tumors within segments of Barrett's esophagus or tumors of considerable length.

The depth of invasion of a tumor, the T status, is another important variable in determining stage and treatment of esophageal cancer. T1 lesions are divided into intramucosal and submucosal lesions that are associated with lymph node metastasis 18% and 50% of the time, respectively. Conservative esophageal resections, such as vagal-sparing, transhiatal, or minimally invasive esophagectomy, are recommended for any T1 lesion. For localized intramucosal tumors of limited extent, both EMR[29] and ESD are acceptable alternatives to esophagectomy. There is almost no role for chemoradiotherapy in the treatment of T1 lesions. Surgical or endoscopic resection alone carries a good long-term survival, as high as 88% in some series.

Treatment of lesions that extend into the muscularis propria, T2 lesions, remains controversial. The rate of lymph node metastasis is up to 60%, making the need for chemoradiotherapy or a radical lymphadenectomy actively debated. Aggressive surgical resection stands

alone well, but outcomes may improve if chemoradiotherapy is added. Neither approach is supported over the other in the literature. Advocates of the en bloc esophagectomy argue that a wide envelope of tissue surrounding the lesion improves long-term outcomes. Advocates of a less invasive resection for T2 lesions argue that the transhiatal resection obtains an adequate radial margin with less morbidity. A scientific comparison between the en bloc and other surgical approaches for T2 lesions has not been done to fully substantiate either argument. In combination with neoadjuvant chemoradiotherapy, a minimally invasive (thoracoscopic, laparoscopic) esophagectomy for T2 lesions results in a 5-year survival of 70%.[30]

Treatment of lesions that extend into the adventitia, T3 lesions, usually includes chemoradiotherapy and surgery. Radiation therapy controls the primary tumor and may reduce the extent of surgical resection margins. Chemotherapy controls tumor spread to local and regional lymph nodes that occurs up to 80% of the time with T3 lesions. Neoadjuvant chemoradiotherapy followed by surgery may improve survival for T3 lesions with known lymph node involvement but adversely affects surgical morbidity and mortality. The need for neoadjuvant therapy or aggressive surgical resection and radical lymphadenectomy for T3 lesions remains debated.

Lesions that extend beyond the adventitia, T4 lesions, require aggressive multimodality therapy. Neoadjuvant chemoradiotherapy followed by surgical resection removing all tissues involved with tumor is recommended.

Lesions with any known lymph node disease are not considered for surgical resection and are treated definitively with chemoradiotherapy.

Status of the Local and Regional Lymph Nodes

The status of local and regional lymph nodes is critical information needed to guide treatment for esophageal cancer. Despite the use of advanced diagnostic techniques, lymph node staging is still fairly inaccurate, and understanding patterns of lymphatic drainage is important. There are two factors that influence the probability of involved local and regional lymph nodes: location of the tumor within the esophagus and depth of tumor penetration (T stage). Lesions located in the cervical esophagus most often drain to cervical and mediastinal lymph nodes (46% of the time) and less often to abdominal lymph nodes (12% of the time). In contrast, mid-esophageal tumors drain most often to mediastinal lymph nodes (53% of the time) and abdominal lymph nodes (40% of the time) and less often to cervical lymph nodes (29% of the time). Not surprisingly, lower esophageal and cardia tumors most often drain into abdominal and mediastinal lymph nodes (74% and 58% of the time, respectively) and less often to cervical lymph nodes (27% of the time). Involved lymph nodes that reside next to the primary tumor are considered local, whereas those that reside one nodal basin away from the primary tumor are considered regional lymph nodes. Patients known to have involved local or regional lymph nodes remain acceptable surgical candidates but also need chemotherapy to address involved lymph nodes.

The depth of tumor penetration (T stage) affects lymph node involvement (LNI) in the following manner: intramucosal T1 lesions (18% LNI), submucosal T1 lesions (55% LNI), T2 lesions (60% LNI), and T3 lesions (80% LNI). Patients who are at low risk (<50% LNI) for regional lymph node involvement are not given chemotherapy and are not likely to benefit from a radical lymphadenectomy. Conservative esophageal resections such as the vagal-sparing, transhiatal, or minimally invasive esophagectomy with a limited lymph node dissection are adequate for these patients. If the surgical specimen reveals involvement of lymph nodes, adjuvant chemotherapy is given in an attempt to treat regional and possible distant lymph nodes that may be involved. Patients who are at risk (>50% LNI) for regional lymph node involvement are given neoadjuvant chemotherapy followed by esophageal resection. The need for a radical lymphadenectomy in these patients is hotly debated. Advocates of aggressive surgical resection with en bloc esophagectomy and radical lymphadenectomy argue that patients at risk for regional or distant lymph node metastasis can be cured with surgery alone and do not require adjuvant chemotherapy. Advocates of neoadjuvant therapy and conservative esophageal resection without a radical lymphadenectomy argue that even with meticulous surgical technique, it is not possible to remove every last lymph node. Instead, chemotherapy for treatment of nodal disease is recommended, not radical lymphadenectomy. Although it remains controversial, it is very likely

that both treatment options may play a role, but this remains to be established.

There have been several studies evaluating the role that the number and size of involved lymph nodes play in determining the need for adjuvant chemotherapy. The WNM staging system suggests a significant difference in 5-year survival between patients with negative nodes and those with five or more involved lymph nodes (22.5% versus 10.7%). A more recent study suggests that after neoadjuvant therapy, patients who have one positive lymph node have the same rate of 5-year survival as those who have all negative lymph nodes (34% versus 36%), whereas patients with two or more involved lymph nodes do considerably worse (6%). The study also suggests that size of the involved lymph node significantly affects long-term survival so that lymph nodes smaller than 4 mm carry a better prognosis than lymph nodes of greater size.[33] As science continues to evolve, the best treatment for patients with positive local and regional lymph nodes will be clear. Until that time, the crude guidelines that are set before us need to be interpreted judiciously, recognizing that it is often more than just science that motivates and guides the dogmas and decisions of physicians.

Evidence of Distant Lymph Node or Systemic Disease

A lymph node that is more than one nodal basin away from the primary tumor is considered a distant lymph node. If a distant lymph node is involved with tumor the patient is considered to have advanced disease. Patients presenting with involved distant lymph nodes or metastatic disease are treated with definitive chemoradiotherapy. If advanced disease is found at the time of surgery, resection is aborted, and a feeding jejunostomy tube is placed. Palliative resection may be considered if a patient with complete obstruction desires alimentary continuity to facilitate eating.

Condition of the Patient

It is well established that age, comorbidities, and nutritional status affect the ability of many patients to tolerate treatment for esophageal cancer. Although age alone is not a barrier to treatment, in the face of advanced disease, it may alter the choice of therapy. Patients older than 75 years have a higher operative risk and a shorter life expectancy, so that aggressive surgical intervention is rarely indicated. Regardless of age, patients must be carefully evaluated for underlying cardiac, pulmonary, endocrinologic, hepatic, and renal conditions that can affect their ability to undergo surgical resection. Preoperative tests to assess cardiopulmonary status, including a pulmonary function test (PFT) and a cardiac stress test, are imperative. There are no absolute contraindications to surgical resection; however, it is reserved for those in a reasonable state of health.

Many patients presenting with esophageal cancer have been nutritionally depleted for some time. More than a 10% weight loss is associated with a significant increase in operative morbidity and usually correlates well with the advanced nature of the disease. Patients presenting with a serum albumin of less than 3.4 g/dL have an increased risk for surgical complications, including anastomotic breakdown. In patients who are otherwise fit and eligible to undergo surgical resection, efforts are directed toward improving nutritional status before surgery by placing a stent or feeding jejunostomy tube. Preoperative efforts toward improving nutrition will be rewarded.

Treatment Intended to Be Curative or Palliative

Determining the appropriate treatment for a patient with esophageal cancer is multidimensional and complex. Upon evaluating the variables as outlined in this section, the final decision to make is whether or not a curative or palliative treatment program is in the patient's best interest. To properly inform and help guide patients in this difficult decision-making process, all consultants need to provide expert opinions if indicated before a surgical recommendation is made. Pulling all the pieces together—depth, location and type of tumor, lymph node and distant organ involvement, nutritional status, and underlying medical condition of the patient—a curative or palliative treatment plan can be created.

Treatment for Cure

Fewer than half of patients presenting with esophageal cancer are eligible for surgical resection. In patients for whom a cure is possible, treatment may include chemotherapy, radiation therapy, surgical resection, or a combination of these modalities. In patients with local tumor that does not involve other vital structures, who bear no evidence of distant disease, and whose clinical and nutritional status are adequate, curative treatment is implemented. Those patients with significant comorbidities, evidence of advanced or distant disease, or poor nutritional status are considered for palliation. Using the AJCC staging system, surgery is considered for any patient presenting in stage 1 through stage 3. Patients with stage 4 cancer are recommended to undergo definitive treatment with chemoradiotherapy.

Although controversy surrounds both the medical and surgical treatment of esophageal cancer, there are some general guidelines upon which most physicians will agree. The treatment for patients presenting with stage I cancer, T1 N0, is surgical resection only. If the surgical specimen reveals more advanced disease, adjuvant chemotherapy is considered. The treatment of patients presenting with stage II disease (T2 Nx, T3 N0) is the most controversial. Surgical resection is indicated, but opinions vary as to the type of surgical resection that is best and if there is a need for chemotherapy. If chemotherapy is recommended, it is given in the neoadjuvant setting. Treatment of patients presenting with stage III disease (T3 N1, T4 N0) is also debated, but a little less so. Most physicians agree that multimodality therapy is needed, but the timing and type of surgical resection remains unresolved. Advocates of aggressive surgical resection (three-field en bloc esophagectomy with a radical thoracic and abdominal lymphadenectomy) stand in opposition to those who advocate multimodal therapy with neoadjuvant chemoradiotherapy followed by a more conservative surgical approach (transhiatal or transthoracic

esophagectomy). Scientific evidence supporting the benefit of one over the other is lacking.

Chemotherapy

Although a complete understanding of tumor biology is far from our grasp, the concept that tumors begin in a particular location and spread by vascular and lymphatic channels is accepted. Although this may be an overly simplistic view of the true nature of malignancy, it is nevertheless the premise on which we have established management of esophageal cancer. In the earliest days of treatment, the only chance for cure was surgical excision of the primary tumor and regional tissues that may be involved. With the advent of chemotherapy, the management of cancer has changed dramatically, with surgery playing a less aggressive role. However, in the case of many cancers for which surgery is no longer a central theme, the chemotherapy that is available to treat those tumors is effective and able to control and often eradicate both local and distant tumor. Unfortunately, in esophageal and gastric tumors, this is not the case. Although some improvements have been made, chemotherapy for gastric and esophageal cancers remains poor for control of both local and distant disease. The best complete response rate for adenocarcinomas is 25% when chemotherapy is given in combination with radiation. Squamous cell cancers respond more favorably than adenocarcinomas, but without surgery or radiation therapy, chemotherapy is limited in its ability to achieve a cure.

Studies have shown that there is limited benefit to giving chemotherapy in combination with surgery with or without the addition of radiation. Although there is a trend toward improved survival with neoadjuvant chemotherapy, there is nothing to suggest that adjuvant chemotherapy is of any added benefit. However, the addition of radiotherapy to a neoadjuvant chemotherapeutic regimen has shown a slight improvement in long-term survival. The type of chemotherapy used is dependent on a number of factors: mechanism of action, drug side effects, and drug cost all play a role. There are six major categories of chemotherapeutic agents as defined by their mechanism of action that are used in esophageal cancers. The response to single-agent therapy (20%-30%) is lower than with combination therapy (45%-55%), and the response of metastatic disease (25%-35%) is lower than that of locoregional disease (45%-75%).

Since its introduction in 1980, cisplatin has emerged as the cornerstone of combination therapy in esophageal cancer. As a single agent, it has a response rate of 25% to 30%. Given in combination with 5-fluorouracil, a response rate of 50% may be achieved, and this is an established chemotherapeutic regimen for esophageal cancer. Administered once a week over a period of 2 to 10 weeks, up to eight cycles of chemotherapy are infused. Neoadjuvant treatment is usually limited to four cycles, whereas definitive therapy can be administered up to 3 months if the patient tolerates the side effects. The addition of a third agent, including (but not limited to) mitomycin C,[34] etoposide, or paclitaxel, is gaining favor and

Table 41-10   Compilation of Randomized Controlled Trials of Neoadjuvant Therapy Plus Surgery Versus Surgery Alone

AUTHOR	NO. OF PATIENTS Surgery Versus XRT + Surgery	OPERATIVE MORTALITY (%) Surgery Versus XRT + Surgery	SURVIVAL (%) Surgery Versus XRT + Surgery
5-Year Survival			
Arnott et al (1998)	86 vs 90	8 vs 10	16 vs 9
Nygaard et al (1992)	50 vs 58	12 vs 12	10 vs 21
Wang et al (1989)	102 vs 104	5 vs 5	37 vs 33
Launois et al (1981)	57 vs 67	11 vs 13	11 vs 10
Gignoux et al (1987)	106 vs 102	18 vs 24	10 vs 9
Total	401 vs 421	11 vs 13	18 vs 17
	Surgery Versus CRT + Surgery	Surgery Versus CRT + Surgery	Surgery Versus CRT + Surgery
3-Year Survival			
Nygaard et al (1992)	38 vs 34	13 vs 24	11 vs 18
Walsh et al (1996)	55 vs 58	2 vs 7	7 vs 3
Bosset et al (1997)	139 vs 143	4 vs 13	41 vs 43
Total	232 vs 235	5 vs 13	28 vs 37

CRT, chemoradiotherapy; XRT, radiation therapy.

showing some improvement in locoregional control and short-term survival. The use of new drugs and different combination therapy is encouraged, but patients need to be counseled as to survival with established versus non-established therapy. There is a fine line between offering hope and taking advantage of the trusting naiveté of an emotionally fragile patient.

Radiation Therapy

Radiation therapy is used to control the tumor locally but is rarely administered alone. Given as definitive treatment, a total dose of 6000 to 6400 cGy in 180 to 200 cGy fractions is given 5 days a week for a period of 6 to 7 weeks. Studies have demonstrated that there is no survival benefit to neoadjuvant radiotherapy alone; however, in combination with chemotherapy, a trend toward improved survival is noted (Table 41-10). A neoadjuvant regimen that is showing some promise is induction cisplatin and paclitaxel followed by combination chemoradiotherapy with 5-fluorouracil, cisplatin, and paclitaxel and 4500 cGy of external-beam radiation.[35] When followed by surgical resection, the 2-year survival approaches 76% for stage II and III esophageal adenocarcinomas. Neoadjuvant radiation must be limited to 4500 cGy to avoid the surgical morbidity associated with extensively radiated tissue beds. Injury to the airway and great vessels and poor tissue healing are associated with high-dose radiation. Preserving the gastric conduit for replacement of the esophagus is critical and is kept in consideration as the radiation field is prepared. Eradication of the primary tumor is not necessary and is not the goal of neoadjuvant radiation. A balance between control of disease until the time of surgery and preservation of the gastric conduit and adjacent structures is critical and often difficult to achieve.

Surgical Resection

There are a plethora of esophageal resections that are used to treat esophageal cancer, and no one technique has established dominance. In contrast, with better understanding of tumor biology, improved chemotherapy, and advanced technology, more surgical techniques are emerging. There are no prospective trials randomizing surgical resection options. All the data used to guide surgical therapy come from retrospective reviews or clinical bias. A lack of patients and financial resources to perform randomized surgical trials results in training and institutional biases that drive the polarized surgical dogmas and individual passions for particular surgical techniques. There are several factors that affect surgical decision making and subsequent operative and long-term outcomes (Table 41-11):

1. Location of the tumor
2. Surgical approach
3. Location of the anastomosis
4. Anastomotic technique
5. Type of replacement conduit
6. Position of the conduit

Location of the Tumor

Approach to Cervical Tumors   Most tumors of the upper esophagus above the level of the carina are squamous cell carcinomas. Surgical excision with immediate reconstruction significantly improves survival over radiation therapy alone for patients with upper esophageal tumors. Every attempt is made to stage these tumors properly because invasion into the trachea, vocal cords, or recurrent laryngeal nerves or positive surgical margins significantly alter outcomes. Tumors that do not invade the trachea, spine, larynx, or vessels are resected primarily.

Table 41-11 Factors Affecting Surgical Decision Making for Esophageal Cancer

TUMOR LOCATION	SURGICAL APPROACH	ANASTOMOTIC LOCATION	ANASTOMOTIC TECHNIQUE	TYPE OF CONDUIT	POSITION OF CONDUIT
Cervical	THE	Cervical	Hand sewn	Gastric	Posterior
Upper	TTE	Intrathoracic	Stapled	Free jejunum	mediastinum
thoracic	EBE	Intra-abdominal		Supercharged jejunum	Pleural space
Midthoracic	VSE	(lower mediastinal)		Colon	Substernally
Distal/cardia	MIE			Forearm free graft	Subcutaneous

EBE, en bloc esophagectomy; MIE, minimally invasive esophagectomy; THE, transhiatal esophagectomy; TTE, transthoracic esophagectomy; VSE, vagal-sparing esophagectomy.

Tumors adjacent to the cricopharyngeus muscle or the larynx are treated with two to three cycles of chemotherapy and up to 3500 cGy before surgical resection. To be sure that the tumor is resectable, surgery is initiated with endoscopy, bronchoscopy, and cervical exploration. Interval resection of tumor and esophagus with forearm free-graft reconstruction or transhiatal esophagectomy with a gastric pull-up may then be performed. Lesions that extend into the thoracic inlet are treated with a near-total esophageal resection through the transhiatal or transthoracic approach to ensure a safe and complete resection. Under these circumstances, a gastric conduit is used. In circumstances in which it is not available or offers inadequate length, alternative conduits are considered.

Approach to Thoracic and Cardia Tumors There are a variety of surgical resections for tumors of the thoracic esophagus and cardia. The transhiatal esophagectomy (THE), the transthoracic esophagectomy (TTE), the three-field en bloc esophagectomy (EBE), the vagal-sparing esophagectomy (VSE), and the minimally invasive esophagectomy (MIE) are all applied. They vary with regards to size and number of incisions, location of the anastomosis, extent of lymphadenectomy, need for a pyloroplasty and preservation of the vagus nerves (Table 41-12). They each have distinct advantages and disadvantages and the risks and benefits remain aggressively debated.

Surgical Approach

Transhiatal Esophagectomy The transhiatal esophagectomy has gained popularity in the past 20 years. It was developed to reduce the morbidity from respiratory failure and intrathoracic leak that is associated with transthoracic esophageal resections. The transhiatal resection requires two incisions: left neck and abdomen. The stomach and esophagus are mobilized through an upper midline abdominal incision, avoiding a thoracotomy. Mobilization of the esophagus is done blindly with manual manipulation through a widened hiatus. The stomach is tubularized and gently passed through the posterior mediastinum, and a cervical esophagogastric anastomosis is performed. Accessible lymph nodes in the neck, lower chest, and abdomen are removed, but there is no additional attempt to perform an extensive lymphadenectomy.

There are several distinct advantages and disadvantages to THE. Advantages include a decreased anastomotic leak rate to 3% using the stapled technique,[36] a less morbid cervical leak if a leak does occur, and a mortality rate of 4% that compares favorably against the higher rates seen with both the TTE and EBE. Reduced operative times, less blood loss, and fewer cardiorespiratory complications have all been reported with THE. Disadvantages include a higher rate of postoperative strictures, injury to great vessels, and airway structures secondary to a blind transhiatal dissection, and an inability to perform a complete lymph node dissection.

Despite these disadvantages, the literature supports that THE remains the safest esophageal resection.

Transthoracic Esophagectomy TTE was the first operation designed to resect the diseased esophagus with the intent of curing cancer. The procedure requires two incisions: right chest and abdomen. Surgery is initiated through an upper midline laparotomy incision. After the stomach and lower esophagus are mobilized, a feeding jejunostomy tube is placed, and the patient is repositioned on the left side. A thoracotomy incision is made, and the esophagus is mobilized. The esophagus is transected at the level of the azygos vein, and an intrathoracic esophagogastric anastomosis is performed. No additional attempt is made to perform a radical lymphadenectomy or preserve an additional envelope of tissue around the tumor bed.

The risks and benefits of the transthoracic resection are well established. The overall morbidity and mortality rates are slightly higher than seen with THE, but no more than seen with EBE. The mortality rate is just under 10%, and the morbidity rate approaches 30% and includes pneumonia, effusions, respiratory failure, atrial fibrillation, and myocardial ischemia. Because of the improved blood supply to the midstomach where the anastomosis is placed, the rate of anastomotic leak is the lowest of all esophageal resections and is 3% to 4% in most centers. When an anastomotic leak does occur, it may be difficult to control and lead to an intrathoracic infection, sepsis, and death. Significant reflux may occur in patients that have undergone a transthoracic resection and in the face of Barrett's esophagus may lead to the development of recurrent disease and metachronous cancers. Despite these shortcomings, advocates of the Ivor-Lewis transthoracic esophagectomy continue to demonstrate good operative and long-term results.

Table 41-12 Comparison of Esophageal Resection Techniques

	EBE	TTE	THE	VSE	MIE
Incisions	Neck Chest Abdomen	Chest Abdomen	Neck Abdomen	Neck Abdomen	Neck (Chest) (Abdomen)
Anastomosis	Neck	Chest	Neck	Neck	Neck
Lymphadenectomy	Radical thoracic, abdominal	Available thoracic, abdominal	Available lower mediastinal, abdominal	None	Available thoracic, abdominal
Pyloroplasty	Yes	Yes	Yes	No	Yes
Preservation of Vagus Nerves	No	No	No	Yes	No

EBE, en bloc esophagectomy; MIE, minimally invasive; THU, transhiatal esophagectomy; TTE, transthoracic esophagectomy; VSE, vagal-sparing esophagectomy.

En Bloc Esophagectomy EBE is an aggressive resection that aims to achieve an R0 resection. The key components of the EBE that separate it from the other esophageal resections are the addition of a radical thoracic and abdominal lymphadenectomy and a wide local resection of tissues enveloping the tumor. It is the most extensive of all esophageal resections and requires three incisions: left neck, right chest, and abdomen. Surgery is initiated through a right thoracotomy incision. The healthy tissues surrounding the esophagus are mobilized so that the tumor bed is not disturbed. The venous and lymphatic vessels, including the azygos, hemiazygos, and intercostal veins, are ligated and divided and removed en bloc with the specimen. A radical thoracic lymphadenectomy is performed, and all mediastinal (including the right paratracheal, subcarinal, paraesophageal, and right and left inferior pulmonary ligament nodes) and diaphragmatic lymph nodes, as well as the lymphatic tissues associated with the thoracic duct, are removed. An upper midline abdominal incision is made, and the stomach is mobilized. A radical abdominal lymphadenectomy is performed that includes removal of paracardial, left gastric, portal, common hepatic, celiac, splenic, and lesser and greater curvature lymph nodes. The gastric conduit is brought up through the posterior mediastinal space, and a cervical esophagogastric anastomosis is performed.

The benefits of the en bloc esophagectomy are debated by many who prefer a conservative surgical approach. Advocates of EBE are committed to the concept that an aggressive R0 resection is essential to establish locoregional control and should be considered as the primary treatment modality for patients with esophageal cancer.[37] They argue that chemotherapy alone is not effective in treating nodal disease and should be considered only for patients with more extensive disease found at the time of surgical resection. Retrospective reviews done in centers that advocate this approach show an increase in 5-year survival in patients with early-stage disease who undergo EBE as compared with THE. They have also demonstrated that for patients with fewer than nine involved lymph nodes, EBE has an improved 2-year survival when compared with THE (40% versus 32%), but

that if nine or more lymph nodes are involved, there is no added benefit to the en bloc resection.[31]

Although the advantages of EBE are disputed, the additional risks associated with this operation are not. In centers that perform this radical resection routinely, a mortality rate of 4.5% and a morbidity rate of 51% are noted.[37] Most postoperative complications are pulmonary. The anastomotic leak rate of 8% is consistent with a cervical esophagogastric anastomosis. Although there are no reports of an increase in graft failure, it is known to be a significant problem among surgeons who perform this valiant operation. EBE remains a significant approach to resection of esophageal cancer; however, it is performed in few centers and is avidly contested by those who do not perform radical resections routinely. To determine the real benefit of one esophageal resection over another, a prospective randomized trial is needed. With few patients, resources, and centers willing and able to support a radical resection, this trial will be difficult to initiate and complete. While the world waits for the surgical egos to calm and collaborate, improvements in chemotherapy and nonsurgical therapies are likely to render the radical and perhaps even more conservative surgical esophageal resections unnecessary, as they have in many other cancer arenas.

Vagal-Sparing Esophagectomy VSE is gaining favor in a few centers in the United States. It is similar to the transhiatal resection facilitating a limited nodal dissection and is advocated for treatment of intramucosal tumors. The technique varies from THE only in the method of removing the esophagus without severing the vagus nerves. The esophageal resection is performed by stripping the esophagus away from the vagus nerves, performing a highly selective vagotomy, and preserving the function of the pylorus so that a pyloroplasty is not needed. It can be done using minimally invasive techniques. Results show improved gastric function over esophageal resections that include a vagotomy and pyloroplasty.[10] Incomplete resection of the esophagus is a concern, especially if multiple biopsies have been performed and scarring or tethering to surrounding structures has occurred. The morbidity and mortality are otherwise comparable to THE.

Minimally Invasive Esophagectomy In the past 10 years, MIE has gained popularity. Thoracoscopy or transcervical mediastinoscopy are substituted for a thoracotomy, whereas laparoscopy is substituted for a laparotomy. The short-term outcomes have shown that the thoracoscopic-laparoscopic technique is safe and effective and offers comparable results to THE dissection with the benefits of less pain and a shorter hospital stay.[38] Although these minimally invasive approaches are not aimed at achieving a radical resection, a recent study demonstrated the attempt of a hand-assisted minimally invasive approach to a radical thoracic lymphadenectomy.[39] As these techniques are refined and taught in surgical training programs, the learning curves will fade, and the long-term outcomes will be established.

Location of the Anastomosis

Although the location of the anastomosis is determined by the type of surgical resection performed, the success of the anastomosis is not. As with any gastrointestinal anastomosis, good blood supply and a tension-free repair will result in success. In esophageal surgery, this is often difficult to ensure. Patients who have comorbid conditions such as diabetes, hypertension, or a history of tobacco abuse have compromised microvascular circulation that may affect the viability of the gastric conduit. In addition, radiation injury induces vascular changes that prevent proper tissue healing. An intrathoracic esophagogastric anastomosis has a slightly better chance of healing. The cervical gastroesophageal anastomosis, on the other hand, is fraught with the dangers of necrosis of the tip of the tubularized stomach due to compromised blood flow from compression of the conduit in the mediastinum. Anastomotic leaks that occur before 48 hours are due to graft ischemia as a consequence of inadequate arterial blood supply to the graft. Leaks that occur from 7 to 9 days are due to graft ischemia as a consequence of venous compromise. A reduction of cervical anastomotic leaks has occurred with newer anastomotic and reconstructive techniques.

Anastomotic Technique

There are two techniques for performing an anastomosis: hand sewn and stapled. A hand-sewn anastomosis is performed using a single-layer of interrupted 4-0 absorbable suture. The stapled anastomosis uses a linear stapling device to create the posterior layer and a hand-sewn or stapled technique to complete the anterior layer. The stapled technique has been shown to reduce the rate of postoperative strictures and cervical anastomotic leaks from 13% to 3%. If an intrathoracic anastomosis is required, an end-to-end anastomosis may be accomplished by a hand-sewn technique or a stapled technique (using an EEA stapling device) with equivalent postoperative results.

Replacement Conduits

There are several methods for reestablishing gastrointestinal continuity after esophageal resection for cancer. In most cases, the stomach can be used and is the conduit of choice. Short interpositions can be accomplished with either a free jejunal flap or a free forearm graft. The vascularity of the free flap is maintained with a microvascular anastomosis to the internal mammary artery and vein or available cervical vessels. For longer segments, a supercharged jejunal (pedical flap with an additional microvascular anastomosis) and colonic interposition are both good alternatives. Over time, long segments of jejunum or colon may assume a sigmoidal shape in the distal portions of the graft and result in obstructions that often require surgical revision. With the exception of the gastric pull-up, all conduits require an additional enteroenteric anastomosis, which increases the risk for leaks and subsequent morbidity.

Conduit Position

There are several routes along which the replacement graft may be placed: subcutaneously, substernally, in the right pleural space, or in the posterior mediastinum. The posterior mediastinal space is the shortest route between the stomach and the cervical esophagus, but it is often inaccessible. Patients undergoing resection of the esophagus with immediate reconstruction will have an opened posterior mediastinal space, which should be amenable to placement of any type of replacement conduit. A substernal route is preferred if there is evidence of fibrosis or tumor in the posterior mediastinum. It is a slightly longer route, and there is a small decrease in function over the posterior mediastinal route, but overall, a conduit in the substernal position has good functional results. The subcutaneous route is also an option, although it is cosmetically unappealing and functionally challenged. It also requires a slightly longer conduit and is used only as a last resort. A gastric pull-up in the posterior mediastinal position has the best functional result, and every effort is made to preserve and use this successful combination.

Treatment for Palliation

Palliative measures include chemotherapy, radiation therapy, photodynamic therapy, laser therapy, esophageal stenting, feeding gastrostomy or jejunostomy, and esophagectomy. These measures are aimed at either reducing tumor burden or restoring nutritional access and should be considered in any patient who either has no chance for cure or would not withstand the rigors of treatment for cure. Chemotherapy will treat systemic disease and help reduce the overall tumor burden. However, it usually needs to be given in combination with radiation therapy so that control of the local tumor is obtained. PDT is an alternative palliative treatment that provides relief from dysphagia for an average of 9.5 months.[40] Endoscopic laser therapy is an additional palliative measure that may be employed. It is effective in restoring luminal patency with low morbidity and mortality rates (<5%). Endoscopy with dilation and stent placement maintains patency of the lumen enough to handle swallowed saliva.[41] The patient is counseled for an esophagectomy before dilation because perforation occurs up to 10% of the time. A feeding tube may still be needed to restore nutritional access. The average survival after placement of a palliative stent is less than 6 months.

Many patients are interested in nontraditional treatment options such as herbal medicines, acupuncture, and chelation therapy. Some, such as acupuncture, may offer some palliation to pain, whereas others, such as herbal remedies, help to abate side effects from conventional medical treatment. There is limited scientific understanding of the plethora of alternatives that are available, and their use must be encouraged with caution.

UNUSUAL MALIGNANT ESOPHAGEAL TUMORS

Overview

Most malignant tumors in the esophagus are either squamous cell carcinomas or adenocarcinomas. These two cell types account for 98% of all malignancies of the esophagus. The remaining 2% comprises a variety of unusual tumors that can arise from different layers and structures within the esophagus, including the mucosa, submucosa, muscularis propria, and adventitia. Among them, neuroendocrine tumors, carcinosarcomas, melanomas, and sarcomas are the most common. They each have distinct locations and characteristic patterns of spread. In general, epithelial tumors tend to be located in the mid and distal esophagus, whereas tumors arising from the deeper layers of the esophageal wall are noted to be more evenly distributed throughout. These tumors have varying biologic behavior that is reflected in their metastatic patterns. Regardless of the cell type, these malignant tumors have the potential to spread through one of the following four mechanisms:

1. Intraesophageal spread
2. Wall penetration with invasion of adjacent structures
3. Lymphatic spread to regional and distant lymph nodes
4. Hematogenous spread

Background

Neuroendocrine Tumors

Neuroendocrine tumors are small cell tumors that originate from the argyrophilic or argentaffinic cells of the esophageal mucosa or carcinoid tumors that arise from cells of the amine uptake and decarboxylation (APUD) system. Small cell tumors are the most common of the unusual malignant tumors found in the esophagus. Both types of tumors are found primarily in the distal esophagus and carry a poor prognosis.

Carcinosarcomas

Carcinosarcomas are rare entities that are composed of carcinomatous and sarcomatous elements. The exact etiology is not yet elucidated, but a number of theories prevail:

1. Collision theory, whereby two separate tumors collide and become one
2. Stem cell theory, whereby both types of cells originate from same stem cell with dedifferentiation of the carcinomatous cells into sarcomatous cells

3. Idea that the sarcomatous portion represents reactive hyperplasia, not malignancy

These lesions are often polypoid, are found in the lower two thirds of the esophagus, and carry a prognosis similar to their individual elements.

Malignant Melanomas

Malignant melanomas arise from malignant transformation of melanocytes in the mucosa superficial to the lamina propria. Although uncommonly found in the esophagus, they account for 17% of all unusual esophageal tumors. They usually manifest as a polypoid, ulcerated, pigmented mass in the lower two thirds of the esophagus. Satellite lesions may also be present. More than half of patients present with metastatic disease at the time of diagnosis. They are most commonly found in the distal two thirds of the esophagus and carry a poor prognosis if there is evidence of disease outside of the esophagus.

Sarcomas

Sarcomas are a heterogeneous group of tumors consisting of leiomyosarcomas, Kaposi's, sarcoma and others. They constitute less then 1% of all unusual tumors. Leiomyosarcomas are the most common among them and arise from the smooth muscle in the muscularis mucosa and the muscularis propria. They are found with equal distribution within the esophagus.

Symptoms and Diagnosis

These patients present with dysphagia and weight loss. Barium swallow and endoscopy are the primary diagnostic modalities and identify an obstructing mass in the esophagus. Endoscopic biopsy is difficult and is associated with a poor diagnostic yield but must be pursued when possible.

Treatment

The rarity of these tumors and the lack of available information regarding treatment and survival make it difficult to establish educated therapeutic decisions. Surgical excision by esophageal resection is the treatment of choice for tumors that are clearly confined to the esophagus. The approach is guided by the location of the tumor. Adjuvant chemotherapy may be advocated for small cell tumors and atypical carcinoids. Unlike patients with other cancers of the esophagus, patients with esophageal leiomyosarcomas who have distant metastatic disease can experience long-term survival after resection if the following factors are noted:

1. Complete surgical resection
2. Early stage
3. Low grade
4. Polypoid growth pattern
5. Thoracic rather than cervical tumor

With improvements in medicine and technology, treatment of these tumors may change, and endoscopic resection with adjuvant chemotherapy may start to play a role in the overall management of these unusual tumors.

CONCLUSION

History is a story that offers guidance to the future: science is a method that guides the integrity of our work. The history of esophageal surgery, its successes and failures, offers guidance to those whose practice is dedicated to understanding the function and dysfunction of the esophagus. The practice of surgical science guides our consciences to make safe and effective therapeutic decisions in our surgical practices. It is up to the esophageal surgeons of the 21st century to create public awareness, educate malleable and well-established medical minds alike, and explore the details of this gastrointestinal territory that our surgical forefathers have courageously placed on the map. It is in our best interest to let science, not personal or institutional bias, determine the surgical dogmas of our time.

The challenges that lie ahead will stoke our curiosities and fuel our quest for knowledge as we struggle to define the complexities that lurk within the esophagus. Let us learn from history and proceed confidently and courageously as a cohesive group of well-educated surgeons dedicated to understanding the function and dysfunction of this seemingly simplistic organ. It is time for the esophagus to have its day in the sun, its era of discovery, before the Surgeon General makes the statement that "eating is hazardous to your health!"

Selected References

Banki F, Mason RJ, DeMeester SR: Vagal-sparing esophagectomy: A more physiologic alternative. Ann Surg 236:324-335, 2002.

This was the first paper to describe the technique of vagal-sparing esophagectomy and document the physiologic outcomes in detail.

Gu Y, Swisher SG, Ajani JA, et al: The number of lymph nodes with metastasis predicts survival in patients with esophageal cancer or esophagogastric junction adenocarcinoma who receive preoperative chemoradiotherapy. Cancer 106:1017-1025, 2006.

This paper discusses the notion that in addition to location and response to neoadjuvant therapy, number of lymph nodes may be one of the most significant predictors of outcome.

Orringer MB, Sloan H: Esophagectomy without thoracotomy. J Thorac Cardiovasc Surg 76:643, 1978.

This landmark paper was the first to describe the transhiatal esophagectomy and document the outcomes in detail.

Park W, Vaezi MF: Etiology and pathogenesis of achalasia: The current understanding. Am J Gastroenterol 101:202-203, 2006.

This concise review of achalasia gives a thorough overview of the evolution of the etiology and pathogenesis of this disease.

Yammamoto S, Kawahara K, Maekawa T: Minimally invasive esophagectomy for stage I and II esophageal cancer. Ann Thorac Surg 80:2070-2075, 2005.

This is one of the largest series of esophageal cancer patients undergoing a minimally invasive procedure to treat early-stage disease. It has become an important study suggesting that minimally invasive surgery may be viable option in these patients.

References

1. Orringer MB, Sloan H: Esophagectomy without thoracotomy. J Thorac Cardiovasc Surg 76:643, 1978.
2. Sadler TW: Digestive system. In Sadler TW (ed): Langman's Medical Embryology, 9th ed. Philadelphia, Lippincott Williams & Wilkins, 2003.
3. Gutschow CA, Hamoir M, Rombaux P, et al: Management of pharyngoesophageal (Zenker's) diverticulum: Which technique? Ann Thorac Surg 74:1677-1683, 2002.
4. Colombo-Benkmann M, Unruh V, Krieglstein C, et al: Cricopharyngeal myotomy in the treatment of Zenker's diverticulum. J Am Coll Surg 196:370-378, 2003.
5. Park W, Vaezi MF: Etiology and pathogenesis of achalasia: The current understanding. Am J Gastroenterol 101:202-203, 2006.
6. Richter JE: Modern management of achalasia. Curr Treat Options Gastroenterol 8:275-283, 2005.
7. Abir F, Modlin I, Kidd M, Bell R: Surgical treatment of achalasia: Current status and controversies. Digest Surg 21:165-176, 2004.
8. Deb S, Deschamps C, Allen MS, et al: Laparoscopic esophageal myotomy for achalasia: Factors affecting functional results. Ann Thorac Surg 80:1191-1194, 2005.
9. St Peter SD, Swain JM: Achalasia: A comprehensive review. Surg Laparosc Endosc Percutan Tech 13:227-240, 2003.
10. Banki F, Mason RJ, DeMeester SR: Vagal-sparing esophagectomy: A more physiologic alternative. Ann Surg 236:324-335, 2002.
11. Pimentel MM, Bonorris G, Chow EJ, Lin HC: Peppermint oil improves the manometric findings in diffuse esophageal spasm. J Clin Gastroenterol 33:27-31, 2001.
11A. Code CF, Schlegel JF, Kelley ML, et al: Hypertensive gastroesophageal sphinter. Mayo Clin Proc 35:391-399, 1960.
12. Castell DO: Hypocontractile esophagus: Ineffective esophageal motility (IEM) and hypotensive LES. In Castell DO, Diederich LL, Castell JA (eds): Esophageal Motility and pH Testing: Technique and Interpretation, 3rd ed. Highlands Ranch, CO, Sandhill Scientific, 2000.
13. Spechler SJ: Barrett's esophagus: An overrated cancer risk factor. Gastroenterology 119:587-589, 2000.
14. Pera M: Epidemiology of esophageal cancer, especially adenocarcinoma of the esophagus and esophagogastric junction. Recent Results Cancer Res 155:1-14, 2000.
15. Oelschlager BK, Barreca M, Chang L: Clinical and pathologic response of Barrett's esophagus to laparoscopic anti-reflux surgery. Ann Surg 238:458-464, 2003.
16. Rossi M, Barreca M, de Bortoli N: Efficacy of Nissen fundoplication versus medical therapy in the regression of low-grade dysplasia in patients with Barrett esophagus: A prospective study. Ann Surg 243:58-63, 2006.
17. Stein HJ, Feith M, Siewert JR: Distal esophageal resection and jejunum interposition for early Barrett carcinoma. Zentralbl Chir 126(Suppl 1):9-13, 2001.
18. Lamireau T, Rebouissoux L, Denis D, et al: Accidental caustic ingestion in children: Is endoscopy always mandatory? J Pediatr Gastroenterol Nutr 33:81-84, 2001.
19. Reed MF, Mathisen DJ: Tracheoesophageal fistula. Chest Surg Clin N Am 13:271-289, 2003.
20. Islam S, Cavanaugh E, Honeke R, et al: Diagnosis of a proximal tracheoesophageal fistula using three-dimensional CT scan: A case report. J Pediatr Surg 39:100-102, 2004.
21. Tzifa KT, Maxwell EL, Chait P, et al: Endoscopic treatment of congenital H-type and recurrent tracheoesophageal fistula with electrocautery and histoacryl glue. Int J Pediatr Otorhinolaryngol 70:925-930, 2006.

22. Macchiarini P, Verhoye JP, Chapelier A, et al: Evaluation and outcome of different surgical techniques for postintubation tracheoesophageal fistulas. J Thorac Cardiovasc Surg 119:268-276, 2000.

23. Logrono R, Jones DV, Faruqi S: Recent advances in cell biology, diagnosis, and therapy of gastrointestinal stromal tumor (GIST). Cancer Biol Ther 3:251-258, 2004.

24. Mutrie CJ, Donahue DM, Wain JC: Esophageal leiomyoma: A 40-year experience. Ann Thorac Surg 79:1122-1125, 2005.

25. Kumbasar B: Carcinoma of esophagus: Radiologic diagnosis and staging. Eur J Radiol 42:170-180, 2002.

26. Wren SM, Stijns P, Srinivas S: Positron emission tomography in the initial staging of esophageal cancer. Arch Surg 137:1001-1007, 2002.

27. Krasna MJ, Reed CE, Medzwiecki D, et al: CALGB 9380: A prospective trial of the feasibility of thoracoscopy/laparoscopy in staging esophageal cancer. Ann Thorac Surg 71:1073-1079, 2001.

28. Eguchi T, Nakanishi Y, Shimoda T: Histopathological criteria for additional treatment after endoscopic mucosal resection for esophageal cancer: Analysis of 464 surgically resected cases. Mod Pathol 19:475-480, 2006.

29. Maish MS, DeMeester SR: Endoscopic mucosal resection as a staging technique to determine the depth of invasion of esophageal adenocarcinoma. Ann Thorac Surg 78:1777-1782, 2004.

30. Yammamoto S, Kawahara K, Maekawa T: Minimally invasive esophagectomy for stage I and II esophageal cancer. Ann Thorac Surg 80:2070-2075, 2005.

31. Yusuf TE, Harewood GC, Clain JE: Clinical implications of the extent of invasion of T3 esophageal cancer by endoscopic ultrasound. J Gastroenterol Hepatol 20:1880-1885, 2005.

32. Johansson J, DeMeester TR, Hagen JA: En bloc vs transhiatal esophagectomy for stage T3N1 adenocarcinoma of the distal esophagus. Arch Surg 139:627-631, 2004.

33. Gu Y, Swisher SG, Ajani JA, et al: The number of lymph nodes with metastasis predicts survival in patients with esophageal cancer or esophagogastric junction adenocarcinoma who receive preoperative chemoradiotherapy. Cancer 106:1017-1025, 2006.

34. Geh JI, Bond SJ, Bentzen SM: Systematic overview of preoperative (neoadjuvant) chemoradiotherapy trials in oesophageal cancer: Evidence of a radiation and chemotherapy dose response. Radiother Oncol 78:236-244, 2006.

35. Henry LR, Goldberg M, Scott W: Induction cisplatin and paclitaxel followed by combination chemoradiotherapy with 5-flouorouracil, cisplatin, and paclitaxel before resection in localized esophageal cancer: A phase II report. Ann Surg Oncol 13:214-220, 2006.

36. Orringer MB, Marshall B, Iannettoni MD: Eliminating the cervical esophagogastric anastomotic leak with a side-to-side stapled anastomosis. J Thorac Cardiovasc Surg 119:277-288, 2000.

37. Portale G, Hagen JA, Peters JH: Modern 5-year survival of resectable esophageal adenocarcinoma: Single institution experience with 263 patients. J Am Coll Surg 202:588-596, 2001.

38. Luketich JD, Alvelo-Rivera M, Buenaventura PO: Minimally invasive esophagectomy: Outcomes in 222 patients. Ann Surg 238:486-494, 2003.

39. Suzuki Y, Urashima M, Ishibashi Y: Hand-assisted laparoscopic and thoracoscopic surgery (HALTS) in radical esophagectomy with three-field lymphadenectomy for thoracic esophageal cancer. Eur J Oncol 31:1166-1174, 2005.

40. Moghissi K, Dixon K: Photodynamic therapy (PDT) in esophageal cancer: A surgical view of its indications based on 14 years experience. Technol Cancer Res Treat 2:319-326, 2003.

41. Bartelsman JF, Bruno MJ, Jensema AJ: Palliation of patients esophagogastric neoplasms by insertion of a covered expandable modified Gianturco-Z endoprosthesis: Experiences in 153 patients. Gastrointest Endosc 51:134-138, 2000.

Hiatal Hernia and Gastroesophageal Reflux Disease

Brant K. Oelschlager, MD   Thomas R. Eubanks, DO   and   Carlos A. Pellegrini, MD

Gastroesophageal Reflux Disease
Paraesophageal Hernias
Summary

The role of operative treatment for hiatal hernias changed dramatically during the 1990s. Once a relatively uncommon event, antireflux operations are now performed in large numbers at many institutions around the world. The driving force behind increased surgical referral for treatment was the popularity of minimally invasive surgery. Although the techniques of antireflux operations have not changed, the approach to the surgery has become more palatable to the patient and the referring physician. More and more surgeons are called on to treat gastroesophageal reflux disease (GERD) and paraesophageal hernias. Thus, the surgeon must be familiar with all aspects of evaluating and treating both entities because he or she is ultimately responsible for the successful outcome of the patient.

GASTROESOPHAGEAL REFLUX DISEASE

Pathophysiology

The lower esophageal sphincter (LES) has the primary role of preventing reflux of the gastric contents into the esophagus. The sphincter is a unique physiologic entity, as opposed to an anatomic structure, that is located just cephalad to the gastroesophageal junction and is clearly identifiable as a zone of high pressure during manometric evaluation as the sensing device passes from the stomach into the esophagus.

Several factors contribute to the high-pressure zone. The first is the intrinsic musculature of the distal esophagus. These muscle fibers differ from those in other areas of the esophagus in that they are in a state of tonic con-

traction. They normally relax with initiation of a swallow and then return to a state of tonic contraction. The second contributing factor to LES pressure is the sling fibers of the cardia. These fibers are at the same anatomic depth as the circular muscle fibers of the esophagus but are oriented in a different direction. They run diagonally from the cardia-fundus junction to the lesser curve (Fig. 42-1). These fibers are responsible for a significant percentage of the lower esophageal high-pressure zone. The third contributing factor to the maintenance of the high-pressure zone in the distal esophagus is the diaphragm. As the esophagus passes from the chest to the abdomen, it is surrounded by the crura of the diaphragm. During inspiration, the anteroposterior diameter of the crural opening is decreased, compressing the esophagus and increasing the measured pressure at the LES. This concept is particularly important for the interpretation of esophageal manometry tracings. By convention, assess the LES pressure at mid or end expiration, thereby providing reliable, reproducible pressure measurements. The last component of the pressure generated at the lower esophageal high-pressure zone is the transmitted pressure of the abdominal cavity. The abdominal compartment has a relatively higher pressure than does the thoracic cavity. A gastroesophageal junction that is firmly anchored in the abdominal cavity will be exposed to a greater transmural pressure than one that is in the posterior mediastinum.

Gastroesophageal reflux may occur when the pressure of the high-pressure zone in the distal esophagus is too low to prevent gastric contents from entering the esophagus or when a sphincter with normal pressure undergoes spontaneous relaxation, not associated with a peristaltic wave in the body of the esophagus.[1] Although both conditions may lead to abnormal amounts of reflux, some degree of reflux is present in most individuals. Thus, the distinction between GERD and gastroesophageal reflux must be made by considering all aspects of the patient's presentation and evaluation.

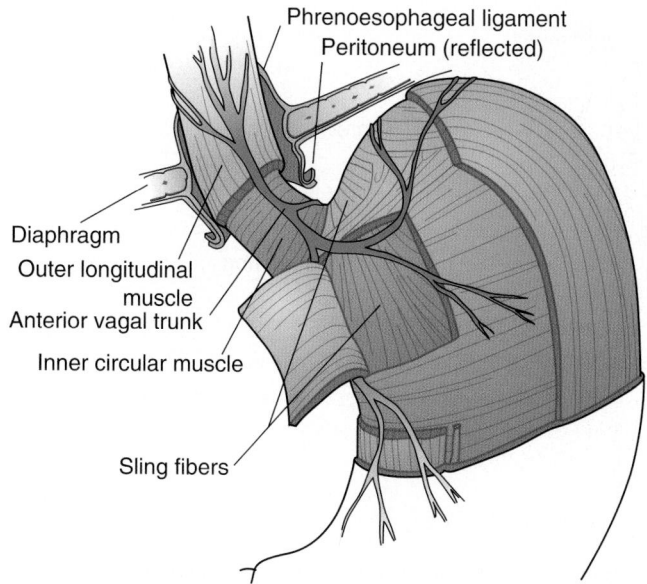

Phrenoesophageal ligament
Peritoneum (reflected)

Diaphragm
Outer longitudinal
muscle
Anterior vagal trunk

Inner circular muscle

Sling fibers

Figure 42-1 Schematic drawing of the muscle layers of the esophagogastric region. The intrinsic muscle of the esophagus, the diaphragm, and the sling fibers contribute to the lower esophageal sphincter pressure. The circular muscle fibers of the esophagus are at the same depth as the sling fibers of the cardia.

GERD is often associated with a hiatal hernia. Although any type of hiatal hernia may give rise to the classic symptoms of reflux, the most common is the type I hernia (Fig. 42-2A), also called a *sliding hiatal hernia*. A type I hernia is present when the gastroesophageal junction is not maintained in the abdominal cavity by the phrenoesophageal ligament (membrane). Thus, the cardia is allowed to migrate back and forth between the posterior mediastinum and the peritoneal cavity. The phrenoesophageal ligament is a continuation of the endoabdominal fascia, which reflects onto the esophagus at the hiatus. It lies just superficial to the peritoneal reflection at the hiatus and continues into the mediastinum (Fig. 42-3). Although the presence of a small sliding hernia does not necessarily imply an incompetent cardia, the larger its size, the greater the risk for abnormal gastroesophageal reflux.

Hiatal hernias are classified by their anatomy into three types (I-III). Type II and III hiatal hernias are often referred to as *paraesophageal hernias* and, although they may be associated with GERD, are also larger, more difficult hernias to treat and may be associated with acute or chronic obstructive symptoms. A type II hernia (see Fig. 42-2B), also called a *rolling* or *paraesophageal hernia,* occurs when the gastroesophageal junction is anchored in the abdomen but the hiatal defect, which is

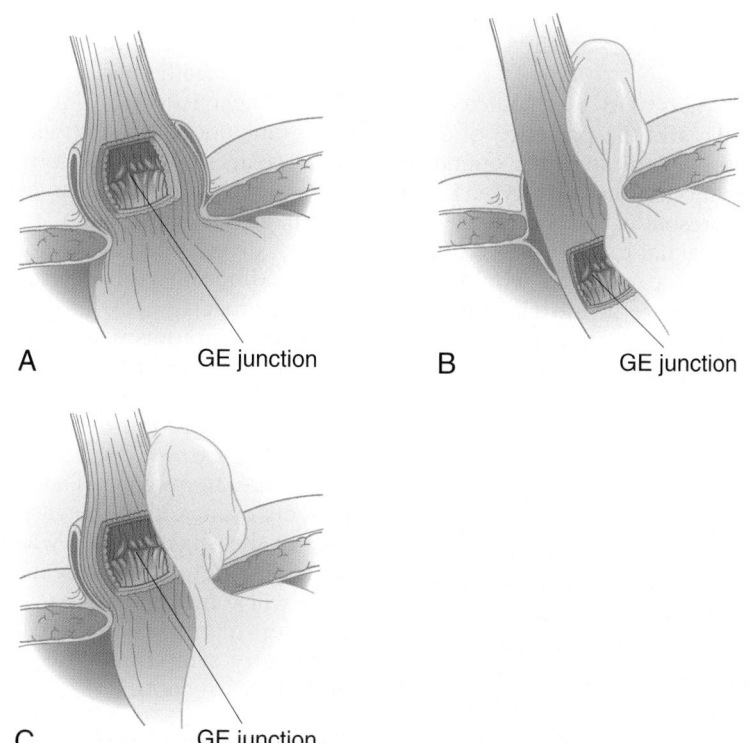

A   GE junction

B   GE junction

C   GE junction

Figure 42-2 The three types of hiatal hernia. **A,** Type I is also called a *sliding hernia*. **B,** Type II is known as a *rolling hernia*. **C,** Type III is referred to as a *mixed hernia*. GE, gastroesophageal.

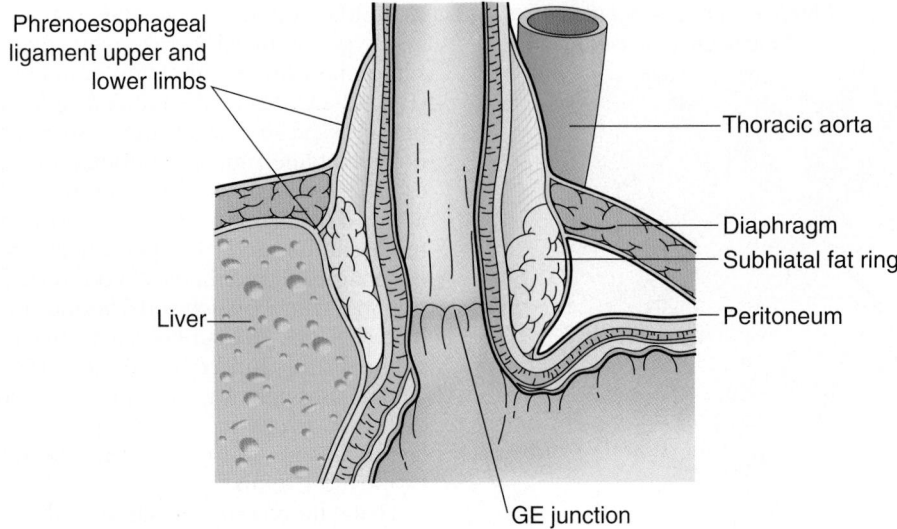

Figure 42-3 Section of the gastroesophageal (GE) junction demonstrates the relationship of the peritoneum to the phrenoesophageal membrane. The phrenoesophageal membrane continues as a separate structure into the posterior mediastinum. The parietal peritoneum continues as the visceral peritoneum as it reflects onto the stomach.

usually large, provides space for viscera to migrate into the mediastinum. The relatively negative pressure in the thorax facilitates visceral migration. Most commonly, the fundus of the stomach migrates into the mediastinum; however, the colon and spleen are also occasionally identified. This is discussed in more detail in the second part of this chapter in the discussion of paraesophageal hernias. A type III hernia (see Fig. 42-2C) is a combination of the first two, in which the gastroesophageal junction and the fundus (or other viscera) are free to move into the mediastinum.

A hiatal hernia is neither necessary nor sufficient to make the diagnosis of GERD, and the presence of such a hernia does not constitute an indication for operative correction. The theoretical implications of a type I and type III hiatal hernia being present is that the cardia and distal esophagus have the potential to be exposed to the negative pressure of the thoracic cavity. This would have the effect of lowering the pressure at the LES, thereby allowing reflux to occur more readily. Many patients with hiatal hernias do not have symptoms and do not require treatment.

Symptoms

The most common presentation of patients with GERD includes a long-standing history of heartburn and a shorter history of regurgitation. Heartburn, when typical, is a very reliable symptom. Heartburn is confined to the epigastric and retrosternal areas. It is identified as a caustic or stinging sensation. It does not radiate to the back and is not characteristically described as a pressure sensation. It is best to ask the patient to describe in detail the sensation he or she is experiencing. Sometimes the symptoms will be more characteristic of peptic ulcer disease, cholelithiasis, or coronary artery disease.

The presence of regurgitation indicates progression of the disease. Some patients will be unable to bend over without experiencing the unpleasant event. A distinction between regurgitation of undigested and digested food needs to be made. Undigested food in the regurgitant is indicative of a different pathologic process, such as an esophageal diverticulum or achalasia.

In addition to heartburn and regurgitation, dysphagia is an important symptom to elicit. Most commonly, dysphagia represents a mechanical obstruction and is more pronounced with solid food ingestion than with liquids. If dysphagia for both liquids and solids occurs at the same time and is present with the same intensity, a neuromuscular disorder is suspected. When a patient is found to have dysphagia, peptic stricture of the distal esophagus is most likely to be the cause. However, tumor, diverticula, and motor disorders need to be excluded because this determination will affect the operative approach.

Other symptoms may be present in patients with gastroesophageal reflux. Most of them arise from the gastrointestinal tract; however, many patients will have symptoms involving the respiratory tract as well. These are called *extraesophageal* (or *supraesophageal*) *symptoms*. The frequency of symptoms in more than 1000 patients evaluated at the gastrointestinal function laboratory of the University of Washington is shown in Table 42-1. Although many patients with gastrointestinal symptoms will complain of extraesophageal symptoms as well, it is less common for a patient to present with only respiratory symptoms. This is discussed in detail at the end of this section.

Physical Examination

The physical examination of patients with GERD rarely contributes to confirmation of the diagnosis. In patients

Table 42-1 Prevalence of Symptoms in >1000 Patients Evaluated for Gastroesophageal Reflux Disease*

SYMPTOM	PREDOMINANCE (%)
Heartburn	80
Regurgitation	54
Abdominal pain	29
Cough	27
Dysphagia for solids	23
Hoarseness	21
Belching	15
Bloating	15
Aspiration	14
Wheezing	7
Globus	4

*Symptoms reported occurred more frequently than once a week.

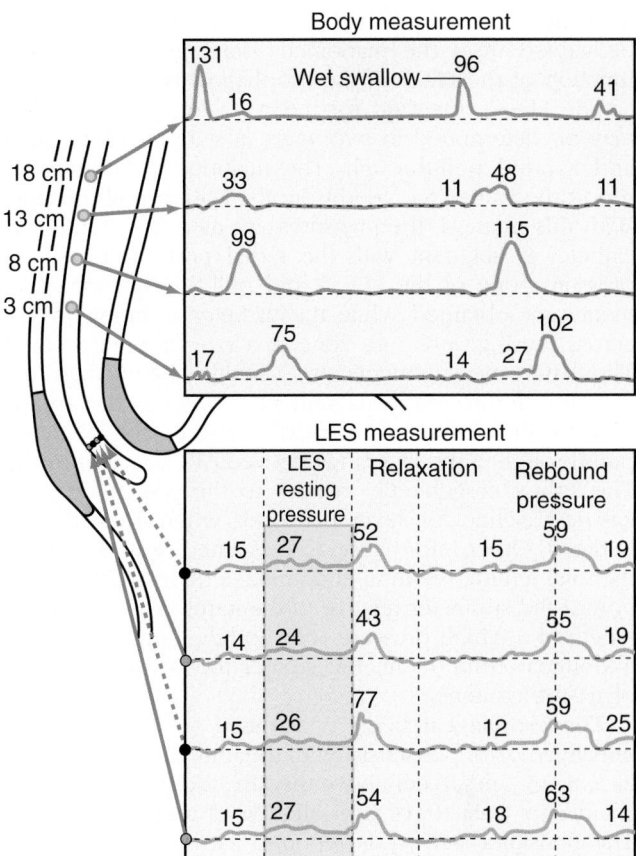

Figure 42-4 Representative tracings from the body of the esophagus and the lower esophageal sphincter (LES) show the relative positions of the pressure-sensing channels during the study. Peristalsis is seen after a wet swallow in the body, whereas the LES is seen to relax to gastric baseline levels during the same interval.

with advanced disease, several observations may help identify the source of the patient's discomfort. A patient who constantly drinks water during the interview is facilitating esophageal clearance, which may be indicative of continual reflux or distal obstruction. Other patients with advanced disease will sit leaning forward and carry out the interview with their lungs inflated to near vital capacity. This is an attempt to keep the diaphragm flattened, the anteroposterior diameter of the hiatus narrowed, and, thus, the LES pressure elevated. Patients who have severe proximal reflux with regurgitation of gastric contents into their mouth may have erosion of their dentition (revealing yellow teeth due to the loss of dentin), injected oropharyngeal mucosa, or signs of chronic sinusitis.

The physical examination may be helpful in determining the presence of other pathologic entities. The presence of abnormal supraclavicular lymph nodes in a patient with heartburn and dysphagia may suggest esophageal or gastric cancer. If the patient's retrosternal pain is reproducible with palpation, a somatic cause is likely.

Short of these extreme presentations, the physical examination is generally not helpful in confirming or excluding gastroesophageal reflux as a pathologic entity.

Preoperative Evaluation

The preoperative workup in a patient being considered for operative treatment will help confirm the diagnosis, exclude other pathologic entities, and direct the operative intervention.

Endoscopy

Endoscopy is an essential step in the evaluation of patients with GERD who are being considered for operative intervention. The value of the study is in its ability to exclude other diseases, especially a tumor, and to document the presence of peptic esophageal injury. The

degree of injury can be measured using a scoring system such as the Savary-Miller interpretation (1 indicates erythema; 2, linear ulceration; 3, confluent ulceration; and 4, stricture). The extreme of mucosal injury is Barrett's esophagus. Biopsy samples are taken to confirm the metaplastic transformation and to exclude dysplasia.

The endoscope has been used to grade the so-called flap valve.[2] This is interpreted on a retroflexed view of the gastroesophageal junction. The flap valve is graded from 1 to 4, with 4 being a completely patulous junction with the lumen of the esophagus in full view from the body of the stomach.

Manometry

A significant amount of information about the function of the esophageal body and the LES may be obtained from stationary esophageal manometry. The manometry catheter is a flexible tube with pressure-sensing devices (water perfused or solid state) arranged at 5-cm intervals (Fig. 42-4). The upper esophageal sphincter is notoriously difficult to analyze because it migrates during the cervical phase of swallowing. Fortunately, the characteristics of the upper esophageal sphincter are infrequently relevant to clinical practice. The pertinent information to be gained from the manometry tracings concerns the function of the LES and the esophageal body.

The LES is analyzed for mean resting pressure. This may be determined in two ways: a station pull-through and a rapid pull-through. The majority of laboratories report the values recorded from the station pull-through. With this method, the pressures are measured while the catheter is stagnant with the radial ports at the high-pressure zone of the LES. Rapid pull-through measurements are obtained while the catheter is being pulled across the high-pressure zone at a rate of 1 cm/second. The latter measurements are usually higher than the station pull-through measurements, owing to the artifact of catheter movement. Normal pressures for a station pull-through at the LES range between 12 and 30 mm Hg. The sphincter generally relaxes to the pressure of the gastric baseline for several seconds when a swallow is initiated. Other information to be gained from the LES is the total length, the intra-abdominal length, and the location of the sphincter relative to the nares. The longer the length of the high-pressure zone and the longer the intra-abdominal component, the greater the barrier to reflux of gastric contents.

The esophageal body is assessed to determine the effectiveness of peristalsis. With the four channels located at 3, 8, 13, and 18 cm above the LES, the patient is given a series (at least 10) of 5-mL aliquots of water to swallow. The peristaltic activity is reported as the percentage of initiated swallows that are transmitted to each channel successfully. Normally, a patient has greater than 80% peristalsis. The second characteristic of clinical importance is the amplitude of the peristaltic wave. The amplitude is simply the average of the pressures generated in the distal esophagus during effectively transmitted peristaltic waves. Ineffective esophageal motility (IEM) is defined as less than 60% peristalsis or distal esophageal amplitudes of less than 30 mm Hg and is often associated with significant GERD. It was traditionally thought that a 360-degree fundoplication is likely to cause an insurmountable obstruction to swallowing and to result in dysphagia, but this idea has been challenged recently. This is discussed further in the section "Surgical Therapy."

pH Monitoring

The gold standard for diagnosing and quantifying acid reflux is the 24-hour pH test.[3] The study is performed by placing a thin catheter containing one or more solid-state electrodes in the esophagus. The electrodes are spaced 5 to 10 cm apart and are capable of sensing fluctuations in the pH between 2 and 7. The electrodes are connected to a data recorder that the patient wears for the period of observation. There is a digital clock displayed on the recorder. When the patient has an event (e.g., heartburn, chest pain, eructation), he or she is to record the event in a diary, noting the time on the recorder (Fig. 42-5).

A large amount of information may be gleaned from the study: total number of reflux episodes (pH < 4), longest episode of reflux, number of episodes lasting longer than 5 minutes, extent of reflux in the upright position, and extent of reflux in the supine position. An overall score is obtained with the use of a formula that assigns a weight to each item according to its capacity to cause esophageal injury. This value, known as the *DeMeester score,* needs to be less than 14.7. A simpler way to determine whether abnormal reflux is occurring is to estimate the total percent time the pH is below 4 in the proximal and distal channels. The total percent time is calculated by dividing the time the pH was less than 4 by the total time of the study and multiplying by 100. In the proximal esophagus (15 cm above the LES), acid exposure normally occurs less than 1% of the time; in the distal esophagus (5 cm above the LES), it normally occurs less than 4%.

The patient's symptom diary needs to be correlated with episodes of reflux. The correlation of heartburn or chest pain with a drop in the pH has significant clinical value because it helps to confirm a cause-and-effect relationship. When interpreting these studies, keep in mind that patients often do not proceed with their normal activities and eating patterns when they have the catheter in place. Thus, their symptoms may not be as prevalent during the study period. If there is symptom correlation with low pH measurements, the suspicion of reflux-induced disease may be confirmed, even if the total acid exposure is normal.

Esophagogram

The esophagogram provides valuable information in the evaluation of patients with symptoms of GERD when an operation is contemplated or when the symptoms do not respond as expected. Often, spontaneous reflux during the examination will be demonstrated. Although reflux may be induced in patients who do not have the disease, the occurrence of spontaneous reflux lends support to the diagnosis of abnormal gastroesophageal reflux. The true value of the study is to determine the external anatomy of the esophagus and the proximal stomach. The presence and size of a hiatal hernia may be characterized (Fig. 42-6). Although this neither confirms nor refutes the presence of disease, it is extremely beneficial in planning the operation. A mediastinal gastroesophageal junction that does not reduce into the peritoneal cavity during the study is a predictor of a more difficult operation that may require an esophageal lengthening procedure. Peptic esophageal strictures may also be found on an esophageal contrast study. The presence of a stricture will taint the interpretation of the 24-hour pH study, especially if it is tight enough to prevent reflux. Other anatomic abnormalities, such as diverticula, tumors, and unexpected paraesophageal hernias, will be discovered during an esophagogram.

Other Tests

In unique circumstances, other diagnostic tests may be valuable. Occasionally, a patient will not be able to tolerate nasoesophageal intubation. A scintigraphic study to evaluate esophageal clearance and reflux may provide evidence of motility disorder and gastroesophageal reflux.[4] Gastric distention resulting from delayed emptying may also be diagnosed with a scintigraphic study.

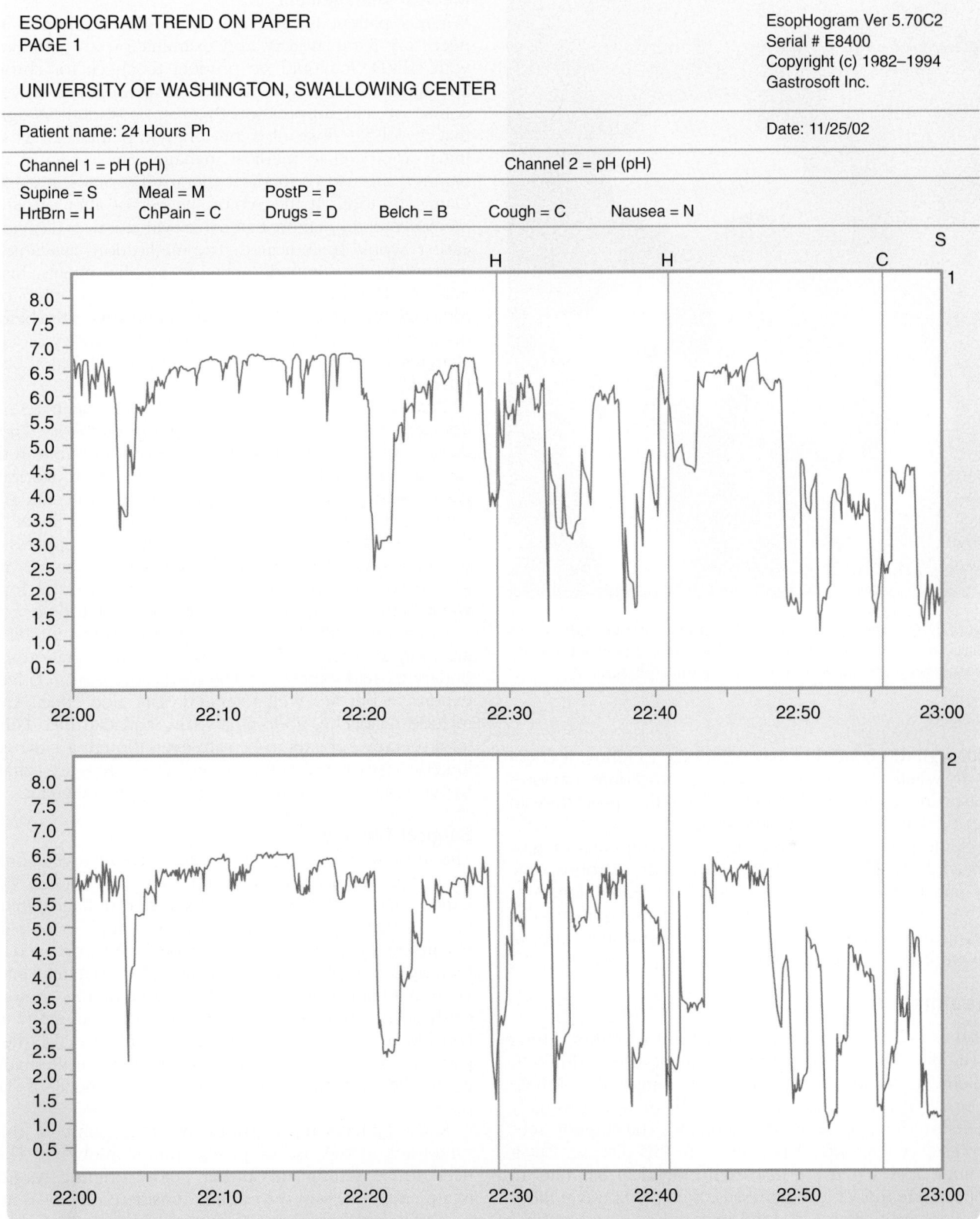

Figure 42-5 Compressed tracing of a 24-hour pH study. Time is marked on the x-axis, and pH is marked on the y-axis. Symptom events are marked along the top of the tracing. (H, heartburn; B, belching; S, supine position; and so on, as noted along the top). (Courtesy of the University of Washington Swallowing Center.)

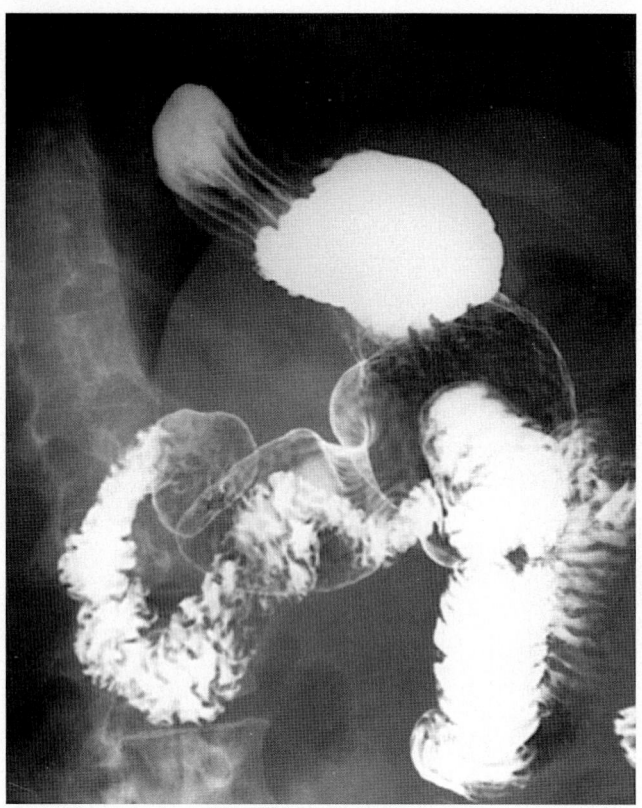

Figure 42-6 Upper gastrointestinal contrast material study shows a large hiatal hernia with the rugal folds of the stomach clearly transgressing the shadow of the left hemidiaphragm.

Although this condition may contribute to reflux, it is not clear whether a gastric emptying procedure (pyloroplasty) needs to be added to an antireflux procedure in a patient with delayed gastric emptying.

Some patients will have laryngeal symptoms of gastroesophageal reflux. Laryngoscopy and stroboscopic examinations will help provide objective evidence of extraesophageal reflux; findings include inflammation of laryngeal mucosa, muscle tension abnormalities, and, in severe cases, subglottic stenosis.

Treatment

Most people will experience symptoms of reflux during their life. A smaller percentage will proceed with self-treatment. Those with persistent symptoms will seek help from a physician, and a fraction of them will eventually be referred to a surgeon for evaluation. The surgeon sees a preselected group of patients with this disease, but it is imperative to ensure that each individual has had an appropriate trial of less aggressive therapy. Lifestyle modifications are certainly helpful in avoiding gastroesophageal reflux. Cessation of smoking, decreased caffeine intake, and avoidance of large meals before lying down will help decrease transient episodes of LES relaxation. Elevation of the head of the bed and avoidance of constricting clothing will help prevent unfavorable pressure gradients across the gastroesophageal junction.

Medical Management

When a patient is first seen, a lengthy workup is not necessary if the history and examination are consistent with GERD. It would be prudent to check for chronic anemia in such a patient and to prescribe a 6-week course of acid suppression therapy. Most authors agree that a double dose of a proton pump inhibitor is the initial approach to medical management. Given in this manner, the use of medical therapy becomes in itself a diagnostic tool.[5] If the symptoms persist after a trial of medical therapy, a more extensive evaluation, as described earlier, would be indicated. The medications available to treat acid reflux include antacids, motility agents, histamine-2 (H_2) blockers, and proton pump inhibitors. Although lifestyle modification has been advocated before or as an adjunct to medical therapy, the efficacy of such changes in the treatment of esophagitis has not been proved.[6]

Pharmacologic treatment of GERD has been revolutionized by the advent of proton pump inhibitors. These drugs act by irreversibly binding the proton pump in the parietal cells of the stomach, thus effectively stopping gastric acid production. The maximal effect occurs after about 4 days of therapy, and the effects will linger for the life of the parietal cell. Thus, the acid suppression will persist for 4 to 5 days after therapy has ended. For this reason, the patient needs to be off therapy for 1 week before being evaluated with pH monitoring.

Compared with H_2 blockers, proton pump inhibitors are more effective at healing esophageal ulceration secondary to acid exposure.[7] The medications are relatively expensive but are well tolerated. The side effects may include headache, abdominal pain, and diarrhea. Long-term therapy appears to be safe even though it has been linked to gastric polyp formation.[8] The polyps are usually hyperplastic and do not appear to be premalignant.

Surgical Therapy

The indications for surgical therapy have changed somewhat with the advent of proton pump inhibitors. Certainly, patients with evidence of severe esophageal injury (ulcer, stricture, or Barrett's mucosa) and incomplete resolution of symptoms or relapses while on medical therapy are appropriate to consider for operative intervention. Other patients with a long duration of symptoms or those in whom symptoms persist at a young age are considered for operative treatment initially. In these patients, operative therapy is considered an alternative to medical therapy rather than a treatment of last resort.

Some patients have absolutely no response of their symptoms to the use of proton pump inhibitors. They need to be scrutinized further before offering surgical treatment, as opposed to being considered medical failures who need operative treatment. Because the proton pump inhibitors are so effective at decreasing the acid production of the stomach, the diagnosis of GERD in such patients is questioned and must be demonstrated with objective testing.

Since the application of minimally invasive techniques to the treatment of GERD, the cost of the operative treat-

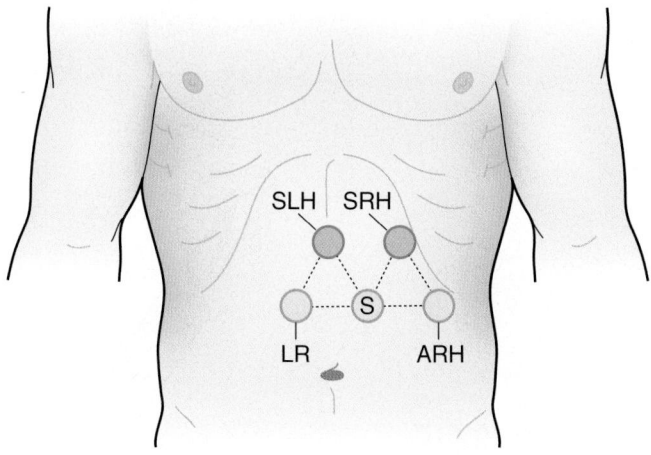

Figure 42-7 Port placement for a laparoscopic approach to the hiatus. The apices of the two triangles denote the surgeon's right (SRH) and left (SLH) hand working ports. The base port sites of the two triangles are for the liver retractor (LR), the videoendoscope (S), and the assistant's right hand (ARH).

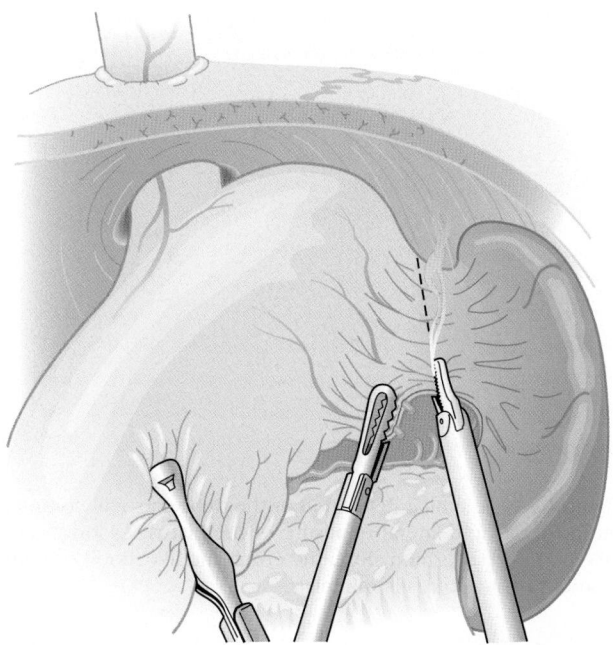

Figure 42-8 Left crus approach shows early mobilization of the fundus of the stomach. The spleen is in plain view during dissection, which helps to prevent injury.

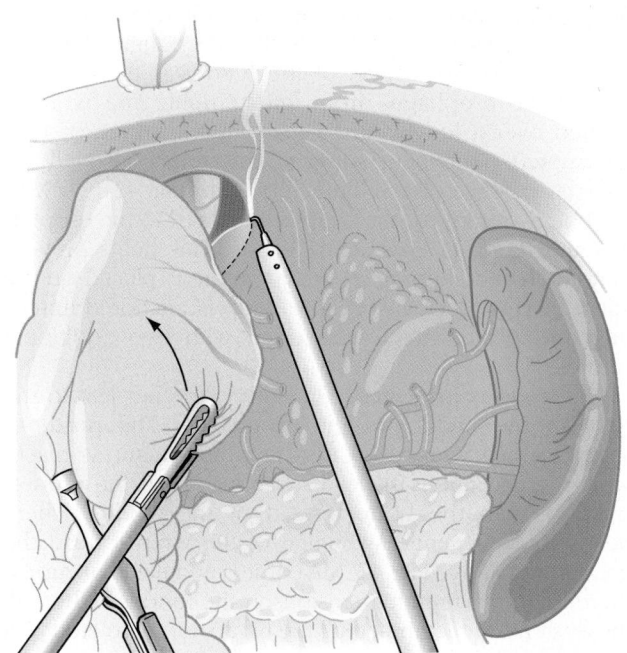

Figure 42-9 After the fundus has been mobilized, the peritoneal reflection at the hiatus and the phrenoesophageal membrane are incised anterior to the left crus to avoid injury to the esophagus and posterior vagus.

ment has decreased. This has changed the way in which surgical treatment is viewed. Considering the cost of proton pump inhibitor use and the cost of operative treatment with its accepted success rate, the length of time required for medical therapy to become more expensive than the operation is about 10 years.[9] This assumes the patient uses the lowest dose of the medication. Therefore, in patients who have more than 10 years of life expectancy and are in need of lifelong therapy due to a mechanically defective sphincter, surgical therapy may be considered the treatment of choice.

360-Degree Wrap (Left Crus Approach)

The technique described here is the left crus approach to a 360-degree wrap (*Nissen fundoplication*), which is the procedure of choice for most patients. The left crus approach provides the advantage of a direct and early view of the short gastric vessels and the spleen. After this obstacle is negotiated, there is little chance of injuring the spleen during the remainder of the procedure.

The patient is placed in a low lithotomy position. The surgeon stands between the patient's legs, with the assistant on the left side of the patient. The five trocars are placed so that two equilateral triangles sharing a common medial angle are created (Fig. 42-7). The surgeon operates through the two most cephalad ports. The assistant operates through the two closest caudad ports. The right-sided caudad port is used for the liver retractor.

With the assistant first retracting the greater curve and then the omentum, the left crus and the greater curve are dissected by the surgeon. The short gastric vessels are taken early to mobilize the fundus (Fig. 42-8). With the fundus mobilized, the phrenoesophageal membrane over the left crus may be dissected until the crural fibers are identified. The entire length of the left crus is mobilized at this time (Fig. 42-9).

Right crural dissection is then performed by opening the lesser omentum and mobilizing this to the phreno-esophageal membrane on the right. Anterior and posterior dissection of the right crus will reveal the previously dissected left crus. Care is taken to preserve the anterior and posterior vagi during this mobilization (Fig. 42-10). Both will be contained by the wrap. A Penrose drain is

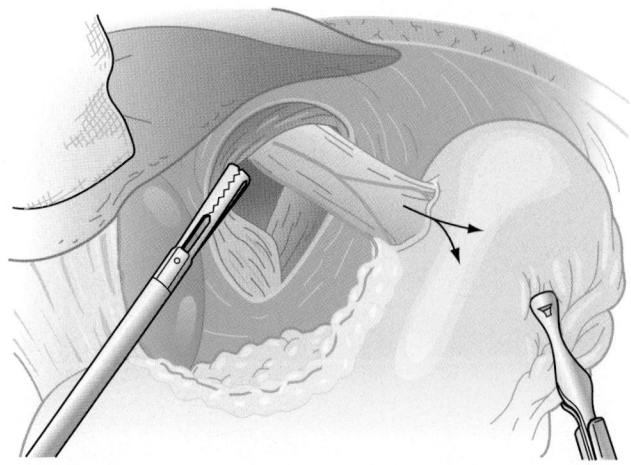

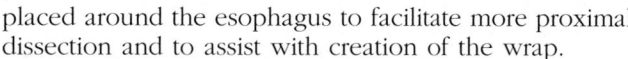

Figure 42-10 A similar dissection of the right crus will complete the posterior and lateral exposure of the hiatus. As long as the dissection is performed along the crura, the likelihood of injury to adjacent structures is minimal.

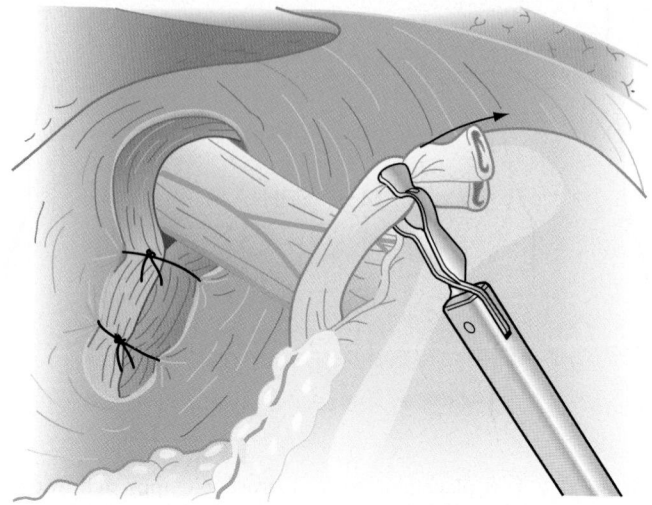

Figure 42-11 Posterior crural closure is performed with heavy permanent suture. Note how the peritoneum and, thus, the phrenoesophageal membrane are incorporated into the closure. The exposure is facilitated by displacement of the esophagus to the left and anterior.

placed around the esophagus to facilitate more proximal dissection and to assist with creation of the wrap.

After the esophagus is mobilized, the crura are reapproximated posteriorly with heavy permanent sutures to allow the easy passage of a 52-French bougie (Fig. 42-11). The posterior aspect of the fundus is then passed behind the esophagus from left to right. The wrap is created over a length of 2.5 to 3 cm with three or four interrupted permanent sutures. This repair also allows the easy passage of a 52-French bougie (Fig. 42-12). With the bougie removed, the wrap is anchored to the esophagus and the right crus at the hiatus. This helps prevent herniation and slipping. A similar suture is placed on the left (see Fig. 42-12, inset). The wrap is anchored anteriorly and posteriorly to the crura with two additional sutures.

The wrap is inspected. The suture line lies just to the right of the middle of the esophagus. The posterior aspect of the wrap does not have redundant stomach, which would imply the wrap was made too far inferior, possibly with the body instead of the fundus. There needs to be a gentle sweeping of the wrap toward the greater curvature (Fig. 42-13A). If it is angulated abruptly, there may be too much tension on the fundus. When all these steps are completed, the wrap is completed. All trocar sites larger than 5 mm have fascial closure.

Partial Fundoplication

When esophageal motility is poor, a partial fundoplication may be considered to prevent obstruction to bolus propagation in the esophagus. Although this was thought mandatory in all patients with IEM (peristalsis <60% or distal esophageal amplitudes <30 mm Hg), this practice has been questioned in recent years. Our experience is that a total fundoplication can be performed in most patients with IEM (except perhaps those with absent peristalsis), without an increase in development of dys-

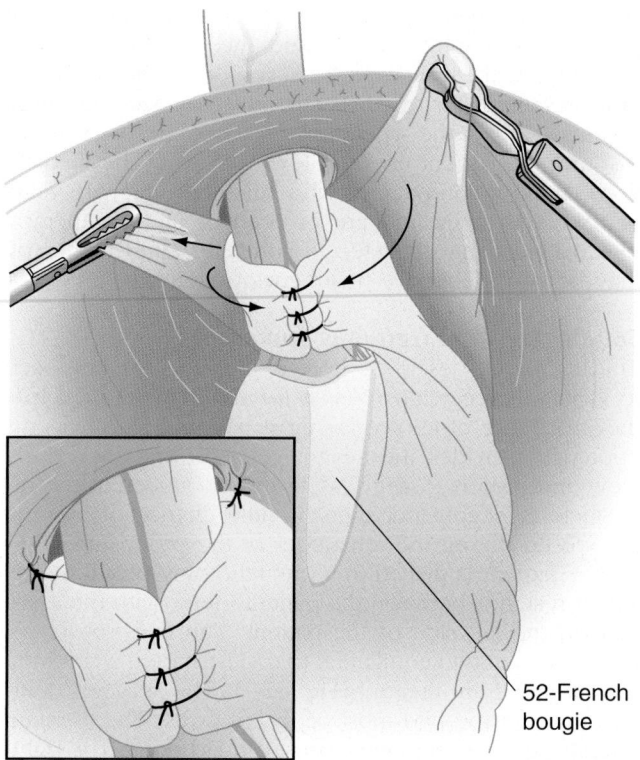

52-French bougie

Figure 42-12 The wrap is fashioned with fundus over a length of 2.5 to 3 cm. The bougie is placed after the first suture of wrap is secured to ensure a so-called floppy fundoplication. The wrap is secured to the diaphragm with right and left coronal sutures (*inset*).

phagia.[10] In fact, effective control of reflux with a total fundoplication usually improves premorbid dysphagia and often improves the esophageal motility. When needed, there are many types of partial fundoplications.

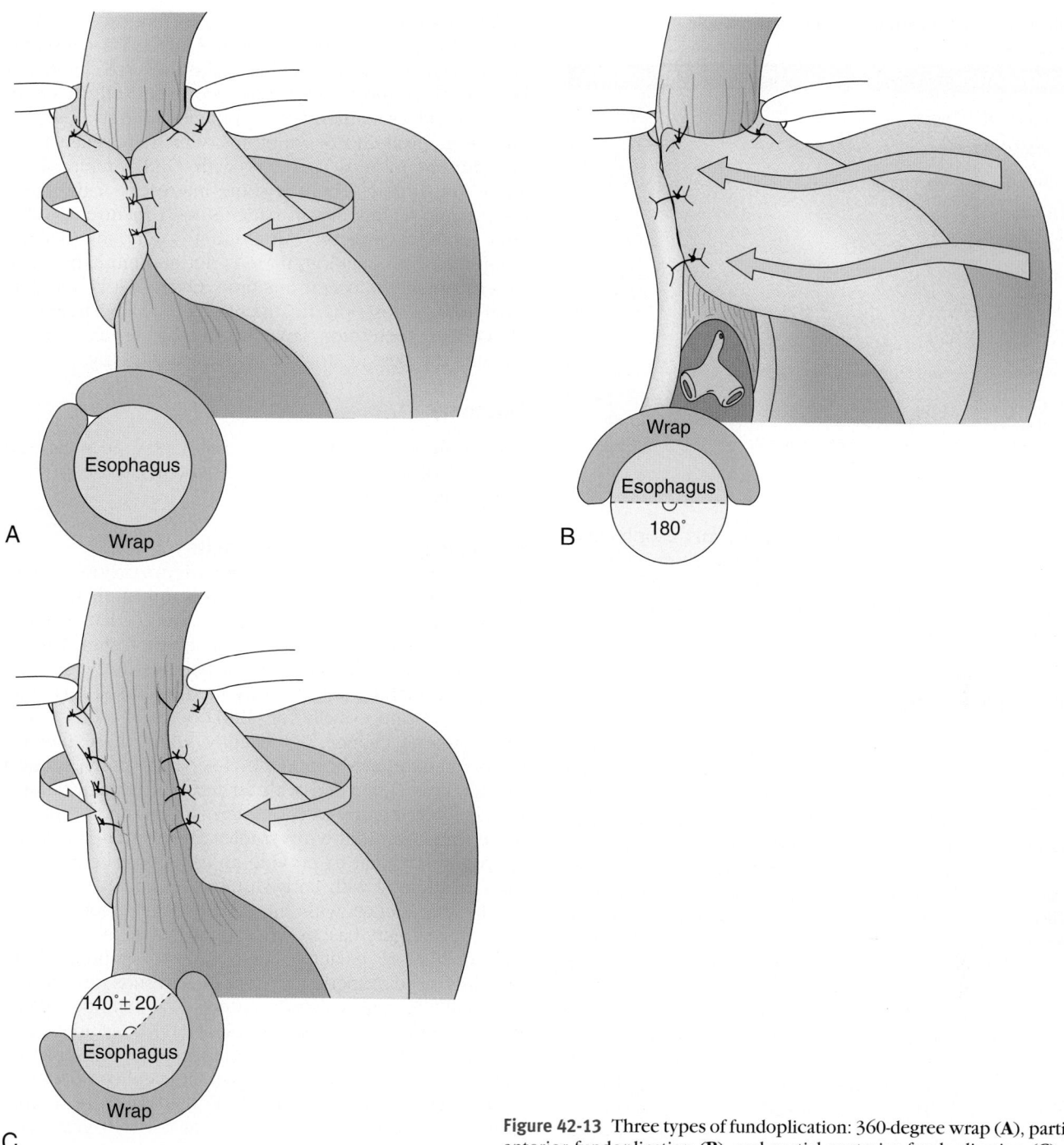

Figure 42-13 Three types of fundoplication: 360-degree wrap (**A**), partial anterior fundoplication (**B**), and partial posterior fundoplication (**C**).

Regardless of the type used, the initial dissection of the esophagus is the same.

If an anterior wrap (e.g., Thal, Dor) is to be performed, there is no need to disrupt the posterior attachments of the esophagus (see Fig. 42-13B). The Dor and Thal fundoplications are created with the fundus folded over the anterior aspect of the esophagus. They are anchored to the hiatus and esophagus as in the 360-degree wrap. The experience with these repairs is limited in patients being treated for gastroesophageal reflux. They are more commonly used in patients with achalasia after an anterior myotomy has been performed.

If a posterior wrap (Toupet) is to be performed, the entire esophageal dissection is the same as for a 360-degree wrap, and the crura are reapproximated as well. The reconstruction of the posterior fundoplication is initiated by passing the posterior fundus behind the esophagus from left to right. The fundoplication is created by anchoring the posterior fundus to the crura and the esophagus. The most cephalad sutures of the wrap

Table 42-2 Complications in 400 Laparoscopic Antireflux Procedures

COMPLICATION	NO. (%)
Postoperative ileus	28 (7)
Pneumothorax	13 (3)
Urinary retention	9 (2)
Dysphagia	9 (2)
Other minor complications	8 (2)
Liver trauma	2 (0.5)
Acute herniation	1 (0.25)
Perforated viscus	1 (0.25)
Death	1 (0.25)
Total	**72 (17.25)**

*Symptoms reported occurred more frequently than once a week.

incorporate all three structures (fundus, crus, esophagus). The wrap is anchored posteriorly to the crura with two or three sutures. The fundus is then sutured to the esophagus along the anterolateral aspects, creating a 220- to 250-degree wrap (see Fig. 42-13C).

Endoscopic Therapy

Recently, several endoscopic techniques have been developed for the treatment of GERD. These procedures have sparked significant interest because they each promise a mechanical treatment for reflux with less invasion than a fundoplication. These techniques attempt to augment the LES by suturing (EndoCinch, Bard, Billerica, MA; Full-Thickness Plicator, NDO Surgical, Mansfield, MA; ESD, Wilson-Cook Medical, Winston-Salem, NC), radiofrequency energy (Stretta, Curon Medical, Fremont, CA), Plexiglas injection (Gatekeeper, Medtronic, Minneapolis, MN), or biocompatible polymer injection (Enteryx, Boston Scientific, Marlborough, MA).

At the time of this writing, three of the devices have been removed from the market (ESD, Gatekeeper, and Enteryx). A lack of durability has limited the effectiveness of the EndoCinch, with 90% of the sutures being lost in the first year.[11] The Stretta procedure has been investigated the most and has the most published data. A treatment versus sham trial was performed using the Stretta, demonstrating a clear treatment effect on symptoms and quality of life. However, there was little change in the objective reflux control, as measured by pH monitoring, and minor differences in medication use.[12] Still, the modest treatment effects appear to be durable in small case-control studies with 2- to 3-year follow-up.[13] The most substantial control of reflux among these endoscopic procedures was demonstrated by the Full-Thickness Plicator (NDO). Whereas the EndoCinch places sutures through the mucosa, this device places a suture device at least through the muscularis of the cardia. In the initial open label trial, the Full-Thickness Plicator normalized acid exposure in 30% of patients.[14]

Although interest in the concept of endoscopic treatments of GERD remains, the modest affects on symptoms and objective control of reflux make their role limited at best. None of the devices have been used effectively in patients with hiatal hernias, esophagitis, Barrett's esophagus, or atypical GERD symptoms, which are characteristics present in most patients with GERD referred for antireflux surgery. There is some interest in using these endoscopic techniques in patients with recurrent GERD after antireflux surgery.[15] Although it is tempting to avoid complicated reoperation, there is not enough experience to recommend its use at this time. Overall, it is not clear what role endoscopic treatments have in the treatment of GERD; therefore, laparoscopic antireflux surgery remains the best alternative to medical therapy.

Outcome

The results of operative intervention may be measured by relief of symptoms, improvement in acid exposure, complications, and failures.

Symptomatic and Objective Results

Two randomized trials with long-term follow-up are available comparing medical and surgical therapy for GERD. Spechler and colleagues found that surgical therapy conferred good symptom control after 10-year follow-up.[16] Interestingly, 62% of patients in the surgical group were taking antisecretory medications at this time, although not necessarily for GERD because reflux symptoms did not change significantly when these patients stopped taking medications. In a separate study, surgical therapy was associated with far fewer treatment failures than medical therapy with long-term follow-up.[17] Although more long-term follow-up studies are needed, antireflux procedures appear to provide an excellent alternative to medical therapy with fairly durable results.

The experience with the laparoscopic approach for antireflux surgery has grown, especially because it makes surgery a more palatable alternative for patients. With this increased experience, reported results are better, especially in high-volume centers. For example, some groups report persistent control of GERD symptoms in 80% to 90% of patients and resumption of antisecretory medications in 10% to 20% of patients between 5 and 10 years after surgery.[18] Recently, the first report of a large group (100 patients) followed for at least 10 years was published.[19] After 5 years, 93% of patients were without GERD-related symptoms, and 90% remained symptom-free after 10 years. These results confirm that a laparoscopic fundoplication can provide excellent, durable relief of GERD.

Complications

In general, complications have been reported in 3% to 10% of patients.[20,21] Many of the complications are minor and are related to surgical intervention in general (urinary retention, wound infection, venous thrombosis, and ileus). Others are related specifically to the procedure or the approach (splenic injury, hollow viscus perforation, dysphagia, and pneumothorax). All complications in patients at the University of Washington are shown in Table 42-2. The complications may be divided into those identified at the time of the procedure and those identified in the postoperative period.

Operative

Pneumothorax is one of the most common intraoperative complications, occurring in 5% to 8% of patients. The actual incidence of pneumothorax is unknown because routine postoperative chest radiographs are generally not performed. Because the pneumothorax results from a violation of the pleural space by carbon dioxide, there is no need to evacuate the gas. Because carbon dioxide is absorbed rapidly and no underlying lung injury exists, the lung will reexpand without incident. If a pneumothorax is identified, the patient is maintained on oxygen therapy, and the chest radiograph is repeated 2 hours after the operation. The pneumothorax is resolved by this time.

Gastric and esophageal injuries are far less common and usually result from overaggressive tissue manipulation or from passage of the bougie. Although usually reported as less than 1%, population-based studies suggest the incidence may be as high as 1.7% in inexperienced hands.[22] The injuries can be repaired with suture or an automatic stapler without sequelae if identified at the time of operation. If the injury is not seen at surgery, the patient will likely need a second operation to repair the viscus, unless the leak is small and contained.

Major liver injury is reported rarely, and the incidence of splenic injury is about 2.3% in population-based studies.[22] Careful retraction of the left lobe of the liver will prevent significant lacerations and subcapsular hematomas. The use of a fixed retractor decreases the likelihood of liver injury. Splenic injury may result from dissection of the fundus and greater curve; avoid excessive traction on the lienogastric ligament. In more than 1500 laparoscopic antireflux operations performed at the University of Washington, splenectomy has not occurred.

Postoperative

Early postoperative complaints of bloating may occur in up to 30% of patients; however, fewer than 4% of patients have the symptom after 2 months.[23] There are at least three reasons for bloating. First, the patient may have more difficulty belching owing to the wrap. Second, vagal trauma may contribute to delayed gastric emptying. Third, the patients will still have a tendency to swallow saliva (an unconscious effort to relieve symptoms of reflux) and with it a significant amount of air. Few patients require nasogastric tube decompression after the surgery.

Postoperative dysphagia may occur in up to 20% of patients initially. A smaller percentage of patients require dilation for this problem.[23] Because the dissection of the hiatus and handling of the esophagus will cause some edema, dysphagia due to this will be short lived. When placing the wrap sutures, hematomas of the stomach or esophageal wall may result, resulting in dysphagia. If the

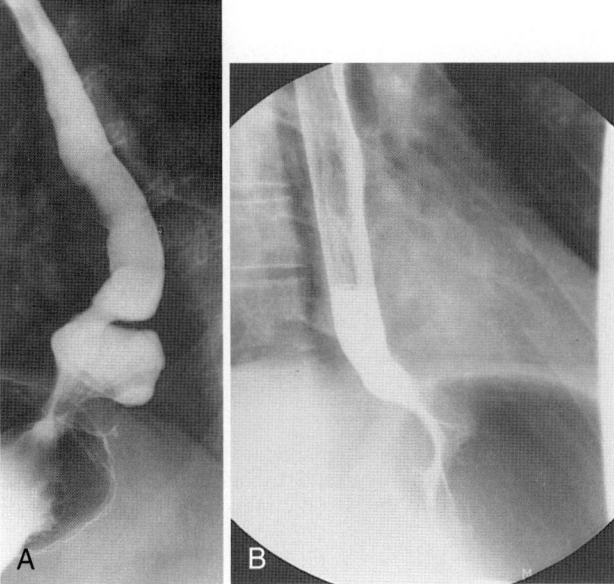

Figure 42-14 Contrast material studies are invaluable in the assessment of persistent or recurrent postoperative symptoms. **A,** Patient with a herniated (into mediastinum) and slipped (wraparound stomach) 360-degree fundoplication. **B,** Normal anatomic appearance of 360-degree wrap. Note the smooth tapering of the distal esophagus, the fluid level in the distal esophagus, and the air in the distended fundus above the wrap.

wrap is too tight, the dysphagia is unlikely to resolve without dilation. The use of a graduated diet over the course of 4 to 6 weeks after the operation will limit the amount of dysphagia from the first two causes.

Death is uncommon with this operation and is less than 0.5% in our experience. Mortality does increase when age reaches 60 years, and patients older than 80 years have an 8.3% mortality rate.[22] This must be considered with the severity of GERD when deciding to perform an antireflux procedure.

Failures

Operative failures are patients who have persistent symptoms and physiologic evidence of continued acid exposure. The incidence is about 5%. Most of these patients can be treated with acid suppression therapy with good results. All patients who present with recurrent or persistent symptoms are evaluated with manometry and pH studies. If acid exposure is documented or if symptoms are severe, an esophagogram is obtained. The presence of an anatomic abnormality of the wrap, particularly a sizable herniation, is almost always best treated with surgery (Fig. 42-14A). If the esophagogram reveals good location of the wrap and the absence of a recurrent hernia, an attempt may be made to treat the patient medically (see Fig. 42-14B). We have found, however, that in some instances reoperation will relieve symptoms even in patients with normal-appearing wraps on esophagogram.

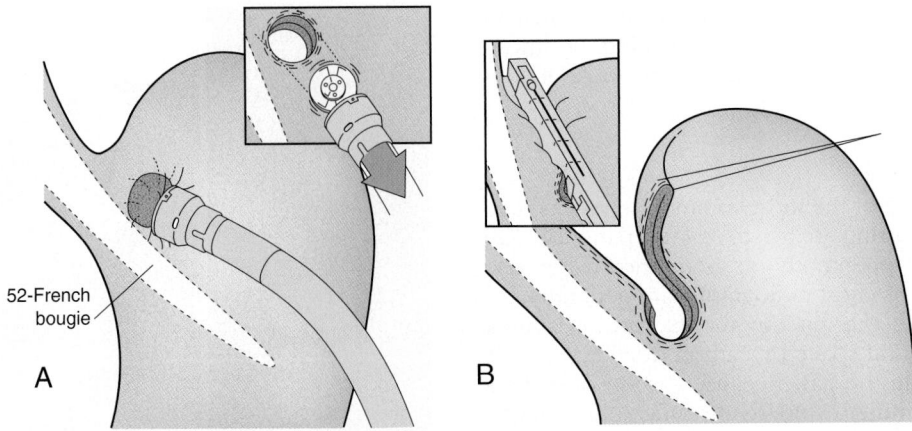

52-French bougie

A

B

Figure 42-15 Double-staple technique for esophageal lengthening. **A,** A circular stapling and cutting device is used to create a through-and-through opening of the cardia-fundus junction. **B,** A linear stapling and cutting device is then used to transect the remaining stomach toward the gastroesophageal junction.

Special Cases

Within the purview of GERD, there are several entities that have received special attention. The surgeon needs to be aware of these variations and the considerations that arise from them.

Strictures

Strictures pose a serious problem for the patient with GERD, although with better medical therapy, this is a fairly rare complication today. Dysphagia, a most troublesome symptom, often results from stricture formation. Furthermore, strictures are a manifestation of acute and chronic inflammation, which not only decreases the diameter of the esophagus but also shortens the esophagus, making operative intervention more difficult. The evaluation of these patients may be more difficult because the presence of a tight stricture may prevent reflux on the 24-hour pH study. The study would be ideally performed after dilation. Other causes of stricture (tumor or caustic injury) must be excluded before operative intervention. Strictures resulting from GERD are indicative of long-standing disease and may be associated with a shortened esophagus or Barrett's esophagus.

The most effective therapy for peptic stricture of the esophagus is an antireflux procedure. Although there is evidence to support effective symptom control with endoscopic dilation and proton pump inhibitor maintenance therapy, operative treatment results in fewer dilations per patient. Of 27 patients treated at the University of Washington for refractory peptic stricture, 21 proceeded with operative control of reflux. In these patients, the average number of dilations per patient was 2.8 preoperatively and 0.33 postoperatively. This compares favorably with the 6 patients who continued on medical therapy; they required an average of 9 dilations per patient throughout the course of treatment.

Barrett's Esophagus

In some patients, prolonged acid and perhaps alkaline injury leads to a change in the esophageal mucosa from its usual squamous epithelium to a columnar configuration (*Barrett's esophagus*). The cells almost always extend proximally from the squamocolumnar junction in a contiguous pattern. If Barrett's esophagus is found, multiple biopsies are necessary to exclude dysplasia, which may indicate a tendency toward the development of adenocarcinoma. Although the incidence of adenocarcinoma in patients with Barrett's esophagus is about 40 times greater than that in the general population (Barrett's studies with increased incidence), the incidence of cancer in these patients is still very low.

Because Barrett's esophagus arises from gastroesophageal reflux injury (of acid or bile), an antireflux procedure might be expected to decrease the rate of dysplasia and cancer. This issue is not resolved; the evidence in the literature is not conclusive.[24] Two recent series report the regression of intestinal metaplasia in 14% to 42% of patients after antireflux surgery.[25,26] Our own experience at the University of Washington supports this, having seen regression in 55% of patients with short-segment Barrett's esophagus (<3 cm). Just as important, patients with Barrett's experienced excellent long-term clinical relief of GERD symptoms.[27] Regardless of the impact of an antireflux procedure on the evolution of Barrett's esophagus, patients are examined endoscopically for surveillance of metaplasia after the operation is performed.

Short Esophagus

As a result of repeated injury, the esophagus narrows (*stricture*) and shortens. The real challenge in these patients comes in the operative approach.

By mobilizing the esophagus well into the mediastinum, a 2- to 3-cm segment of esophagus can usually be placed into the abdomen without tension. However, if this cannot be accomplished, a Collis gastroplasty may be performed. A double-staple technique may be used to create the neoesophagus (Fig. 42-15) after the dissection has been performed.

Unfortunately, the postoperative physiologic testing on these patients reveals an abnormal acid exposure in

50% of patients.[28] One reason for this is that the lengthening procedure often leaves parietal cells in the neoesophagus above the wrap.

Extraesophageal Symptoms

A relatively new area of study in GERD is the involvement of the respiratory tract. Symptoms of hoarseness, laryngitis, cough, wheezing, and aspiration may occur when patients have high proximal reflux. Pulmonary fibrosis has also been associated with high gastroesophageal reflux.[29]

About 30% of patients with typical symptoms of reflux have some type of extraesophageal symptom; however, about 10% of patients have only extraesophageal symptoms when they present for evaluation. Of the patients who present with primary laryngeal symptoms, fewer than half have typical manifestations of heartburn or regurgitation.[30] Unfortunately, standard diagnostic testing for GERD has diminished sensitivity and specificity in this group of patients. Often, the initial pH study shows abnormal acid exposure in the upper esophagus,[31] but this is not necessary for the diagnosis. The detection of acid in the pharynx on pH monitoring improves the diagnostic rates of laryngeal reflux.[32] Furthermore, pharyngeal reflux is a better predictor of response to medical[33] and surgical therapy[34] than standard esophageal measurements. Still, the measurement of pharyngeal reflux has poor sensitivity, likely because the mechanism of extraesophageal disease is by vagal stimulation from esophageal acid exposure. The diagnosis may also be supported by a stroboscopic examination of the vocal cords showing evidence of inflammation and injury,[34] although these findings are too nonspecific by themselves to reliably diagnose reflux as the culprit.

Both medical and surgical therapies have been used to treat the extraesophageal manifestations of GERD. Resolution of symptoms, increased exercise, and cessation of corticosteroid use have all been observed. The rate of symptom response to therapy is less than that of heartburn and regurgitation (75%-80%),[35] possibly owing to the selection of patients. With further evaluation of this unique group of patients, selection criteria may improve the results of both medical and operative intervention.

PARAESOPHAGEAL HERNIAS

Paraesophageal hernias, type II or type III (see Fig. 42-2B and C), are less commonly encountered in surgical practice than is GERD. The operative approach has varied considerably for several decades. The central issues have remained the same in the era of videoendoscopic surgery: the need to operate on asymptomatic patients, whether to add an antireflux procedure, whether to anchor the stomach to the abdominal wall, and the need to remove the hernia sac. The repair of a paraesophageal hernia is another procedure that is ideally suited for a laparoscopic approach.

Pathophysiology

The most common structure to herniate through the esophageal hiatus is the fundus of the stomach. Occasionally, the fundus of the stomach will rotate toward the right pleural cavity along the organoaxial axis defined by the phrenoesophageal membrane at the hiatus and the retroperitoneal attachment of the first portion of the duodenum. This results in what has been referred to as an *upside-down stomach*. Other structures that may be located in the hernia sac include the spleen, colon, and omentum. After repeated episodes of the viscera entering the hernia sac, adhesions between the wall of the sac and the structures may form, thus preventing the structures from returning to their position in the peritoneal cavity. The natural history of these large hernias is a matter of debate. Rarely, the herniated contents will become strangulated, causing an emergent condition that requires immediate operative intervention. Because of these risks and early reports of Belsey and Hill,[36,37] most for decades have recommended repair of these hernias when detected regardless of symptoms. Recent evidence, however, suggests that the risk for acute strangulation is about 1% per year.[38] Therefore we, and many others, recommend surgical intervention only for younger patients (<60 years) and those with significant symptoms.

Symptoms

The most common symptoms include intermittent dysphagia for solids, which results from episodes of acute gastric or esophageal obstruction; abdominal and chest pain secondary to visceral torsion; gastrointestinal bleeding from mucosal ischemia; and heartburn. This profile varies considerably from that of GERD. The symptoms are often nonspecific and do not lead the clinician to the diagnosis. Often, a diagnosis of paraesophageal hernia is made only after a contrast study or endoscopy is performed for proximal gastrointestinal tract complaints.

In the series of patients at the University of Washington, symptoms of heartburn were present in 50% of patients. Episodic attacks of abdominal pain and dysphagia were also present in 50% of patients. Other symptoms occurred with varying frequency. Regurgitation is likely to occur in patients with large hiatal defects and a type III hernia, which allows the gastroesophageal junction to migrate into the chest, thus promoting a pressure gradient and encouraging reflux. Episodic attacks of pain are thought to arise from transient distention and ischemia of the hernia contents. Spontaneous reduction provides relief. Dysphagia will occur if the gastroesophageal junction is angled such that a food bolus may not enter the stomach after a swallow is initiated. Gastrointestinal bleeding is caused by ulceration of the mucosa at an area where the stomach folds back onto itself, and is often the cause of iron deficiency anemia. In cases of anemia in the setting of a paraesophageal hernia, especially without another source, repair of the hernia results in resolution of the anemia.[39] Thirty-four percent of patients presenting to the University of Washington were found to have a gastrointestinal source of blood loss.

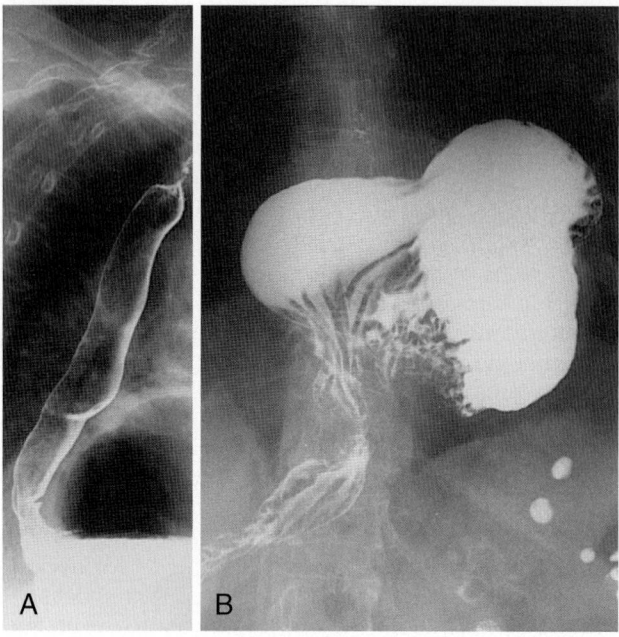

Figure 42-16 Upper gastrointestinal contrast material study is essential in the evaluation of a paraesophageal hernia. **A,** Oblique view shows the stomach with an air-fluid level anterior to the esophagus and well into the mediastinum. **B,** An anteroposterior view of a patient with complete organoaxial volvulus, with the entire stomach in the mediastinum and the pylorus at the hiatus.

Preoperative Evaluation

The evaluation of patients with paraesophageal hernias is similar to that of patients undergoing workup for GERD. A contrast esophagogram, however, in these patients is the most important diagnostic test (Fig. 42-16). Endoscopy helps to identify mucosal erosions as a source of gastrointestinal blood loss. Manometry is needed to determine the motor function of the esophageal body. The pH testing can be avoided if an antireflux procedure is performed as part of the operative repair. However, if an antireflux procedure is not planned, the extent of gastroesophageal reflux is evaluated.

In patients with large paraesophageal hernias, it may be very difficult to complete the manometry, and pH studies can be difficult. When the fundus of the stomach is angled such that the distal esophagus and gastroesophageal junction may not be negotiated with the catheters, the studies may be incomplete. It is important to obtain some idea of the degree of peristalsis in the body of the esophagus before proceeding with the operation. This can be accomplished even if the stomach and distal esophagus cannot be cannulated.

Treatment

After the introduction of laparoscopic techniques for the treatment of sliding hiatal hernias, their use in the repair of paraesophageal hernias naturally followed. Although technically more difficult, laparoscopic paraesophageal hernia repair is safe, feasible, and generally associated with less perioperative morbidity than open approaches.

However, there are recent reports suggesting recurrence rates as high as 30% to 40% (although recurrence rates are likely 15% to 20% with open approaches).[40,41] Although most of these recurrences are asymptomatic and found only on barium studies, they are of concern, and techniques to reduce recurrences are needed. Unfortunately, synthetic mesh, which is used for most other hernia repairs, is associated with occasional esophageal erosion, limiting its practical use.[42]

The operative approach through laparoscopy, our preferred approach, is similar to that of gastroesophageal reflux procedures described previously with respect to patient positioning and port placement. Several variations in the technique must be made to accommodate the unique operative findings in paraesophageal hernias.

The initial dissection for paraesophageal hernias begins with mobilization of the greater curve and fundus. Because the left crus is usually obscured by the lienogastric ligament and the short gastric vessels, crural dissection may be hazardous at the beginning of the operation. By mobilizing the fundus and dividing the short gastric vessels with ultrasonic transection, the left crus may be exposed safely.

After the crural fibers are exposed on the left, the hernia sac will, by necessity, have been divided. At this point, the peritoneal sac may be divided anteriorly with minimal risk. Further dissection of the sac from its mediastinal attachments will free the stomach and allow it to be delivered into the peritoneal cavity. After the hernia contents are returned to the peritoneal cavity, the hernia sac must be transected circumferentially at the hiatus. The technically challenging aspect of the dissection is encountered during the posterior sac dissection. The esophagus and the anterior vagus nerve are intimately associated with the sac posteriorly. Often, a lighted bougie is useful to identify the exact location of the esophagus. After the sac is freed at the hiatus, a concerted effort is made to remove as much of the hernia sac from the mediastinum as possible. It is unnecessary to remove the whole sac, and considering that the pleura, esophagus, and inferior pulmonary veins may be injured during the dissection, the desire to remove the entire sac must be tempered by the possible injury to vital structures.

After the dissection is completed, the crura are reapproximated with interrupted nonabsorbable suture, as with any antireflux procedure. An antireflux procedure is added to the procedure to prevent postoperative reflux after the extensive hiatal dissection. Although the need for an antireflux procedure is controversial, about 60% of patients with paraesophageal hernias have abnormal reflux and a hypotensive LES; thus, we consider a fundoplication appropriate.[43] The fundoplication will also act to seal the hiatus, preventing access by other viscera. As with fundoplication for GERD, the type of wrap is dictated by the preoperative manometry. Postoperative management of the patient is the same as for operations performed for type I hernias and GERD.

Outcome

Operative treatment of paraesophageal hernias is effective in the control of symptoms in 90% to 100% of patients.[44,45]

In the past, paraesophageal hernias were repaired by thoracotomy or laparotomy with a morbidity rate of about 20% and a mortality rate of 2%.[46] More recently, with the popularization of laparoscopic antireflux operations, similar (laparoscopic) approaches were used for the treatment of paraesophageal hernias. Laparoscopy has some of the benefits of thoracotomy (i.e., the hiatus can be accessed easier, the esophagus can be dissected under direct vision, and high mobilization of the esophagus is possible) and some of the advantages of the laparotomy (i.e., less morbidity, no need to collapse the lung, no need for postoperative chest tube). In fact, most paraesophageal hernias are currently repaired using a laparoscopic approach. The laparoscopic approach, as with many operations, is associated with lower rates of morbidity, less pain, and faster recovery.[47] This may be even more important in this patient population because most patients with paraesophageal hernias are older and likely to have associated medical comorbidities.

However, Hashemi and colleagues reported in 2000 that patients who had undergone laparoscopic repair of a paraesophageal hernia had a higher recurrence rate than those operated on by means of thoracotomy and laparotomy.[40] Although another study comparing open and laparoscopic repair revealed a higher incidence of recurrence in the open repair group (8% versus 0%),[47] it was based on symptomatic recurrences. Although the debate continues about whether the approach affects the recurrence rate, what is clear is that the anatomic recurrence of a hiatal hernia after these repairs is relatively high, even if many patients with a recurrence are minimally symptomatic or asymptomatic.

Use of Mesh

With the development and application of mesh materials for tension-free repair of inguinal and ventral hernias, many surgeons have begun to apply the technique of tension-free closure with a mesh to the hiatal hernia. Two randomized trials have demonstrated a significant reduction in recurrence rates by using synthetic mesh in large hiatal hernia repairs.[48,49]

However, there are potential problems introduced by using synthetic mesh at the dynamic hiatus, such as mesh erosion, ulceration, stricture, and dysphagia.[50,51] For this reason, we have employed the use of a new class of absorbable biologic mesh. A pilot study using small intestinal submucosa (SIS; Surgisis, Indianapolis, IN) for paraesophageal hernia repair suggested that it is safe and possibly effective in reducing recurrence.[52] We recently completed a multicentered randomized trial confirming that the use of SIS is associated with a lower rate of recurrence (24% versus 9%), at least in the short term (6 months). Although long-term follow-up is required, there appears to be sufficient evidence to consider the use of biologic mesh material in these difficult repairs.

Strangulation of Hernia Contents

The clinical finding of persistent thoracic or epigastric pain, fever, or sepsis in a patient known to have a paraesophageal hernia is a surgical emergency. The mortality rate for ischemic stomach in the mediastinum is high. Although the consequences of this clinical situation are grave, it is a relatively rare occurrence in patients with paraesophageal hernias. Of 31 patients with complicated paraesophageal hernias, only 2 were found to have gastric necrosis and perforation.[53] Of the initial 42 patients operated on at the University of Washington, only 1 required an emergent repair. Interestingly, 11 patients were found to have gastric volvulus at the time of the operation. Thus, 25% of the patients had the potential to develop vascular compromise, and only 1 (2%) did. Emergent reduction of a paraesophageal hernia may be approached laparoscopically, but a low threshold for conversion is maintained.

SUMMARY

Operative treatment of GERD and paraesophageal hernias has become more common in the era of laparoscopic procedures. Careful patient selection based on symptom assessment, response to medical therapy, and preoperative testing will optimize chances for successful surgical treatment. Scrupulous operative technique will allow for resolution of symptoms in almost all patients. Complications of the laparoscopic approach to these diseases are uncommon.

Selected References

Branton SA, Hinder RA, Floch NR, et al: Surgical treatment of gastroesophageal reflux disease. In Castell DO, Richter JE (eds): The Esophagus, 3rd ed. Philadelphia, Lippincott Williams & Wilkins, 1999, pp 511-525.

An excellent review of pathophysiology, workup, and surgical treatment of GERD. Excellent diagrams and technical explanations.

Duranceau A, Ferraro P, Jamieson GG: Evidence-based investigation for reflux disease. Chest Surg Clin North Am 11:495-506, 2001.

A comprehensive review of the workup of GERD, which is the cornerstone of treating the disease appropriately.

Oelschlager BK, Pellegrini CA: Paraesophageal hernias: Open, laparoscopic, or thoracic repair? Chest Surg Clin North Am 11:589-603, 2001.

This review covers the presentation, management, and controversies surrounding the repair of paraesophageal hernias.

References

1. Galmiche JP, Janssens J: The pathophysiology of gastro-oesophageal reflux disease: An overview. Scand J Gastroenterol Suppl 211:7-18, 1995.
2. Hill LD, Kozarek RA, Kraemer SJ, et al: The gastroesophageal flap valve: In vitro and in vivo observations. Gastrointest Endosc 44:541-547, 1996.
3. Demeester TR, Johnson LF, Joseph GJ, et al: Patterns of gastroesophageal reflux in health and disease. Ann Surg 184:459-470, 1976.
4. Stacher G, Bergmann H: Scintigraphic quantitation of gastrointestinal motor activity and transport: Oesophagus and stomach. Eur J Nucl Med 19:815-823, 1992.

5. Schenk BE, Kuipers EJ, Klinkenberg-Knol EC, et al: Omeprazole as a diagnostic tool in gastroesophageal reflux disease. Am J Gastroenterol 92:1997-2000, 1997.

6. Dent J: Long-term aims of treatment of reflux disease, and the role of non-drug measures. Digestion 51(Suppl 1):30-34, 1992.

7. Skoutakis VA, Joe RH, Hara DS: Comparative role of omeprazole in the treatment of gastroesophageal reflux disease. Ann Pharmacother 29:1252-1262, 1995.

8. Freston JW: Long-term acid control and proton pump inhibitors: Interactions and safety issues in perspective. Am J Gastroenterol 92:51S-57S, 1997.

9. Heudebert GR, Marks R, Wilcox CM, et al: Choice of long-term strategy for the management of patients with severe esophagitis: A cost-utility analysis. Gastroenterology 112:1078-1086, 1997.

10. Oleynikov D, Eubanks TR, Oelschlager BK, et al: Total fundoplication is the operation of choice for patients with gastroesophageal reflux and defective peristalsis. Surg Endosc 16:909-913, 2002.

11. Abou-Rebych H, Hoepffner N, Rosch T, et al: Long-term failure of endoscopic suturing in treatment of gastroesophageal reflux: A prospective follow-up study. Endoscopy 37:213-216, 2005.

12. Corley DA, Katz P, Wo JM, et al: Improvement of gastroesophageal reflux symptoms after radiofrequency energy: A randomized, sham-controlled trial. Gastroenterology 125:668-676, 2003.

13. Torquati A, Houston HL, Kaiser J, et al: Long-term follow-up study of the Stretta procedure for the treatment of gastroesophageal reflux disease. Surg Endosc 18:1475-1479, 2004.

14. Pleskow D, Rothstein R, Lo S, et al: Endoscopic full-thickness plication for the treatment of GERD: 12-month follow-up for the North American open-label trial. Gastrointest Endosc 61:643-649, 2005.

15. Islam S, Geiger JD, Coran AG, et al: Use of radiofrequency ablation of the lower esophageal sphincter to treat recurrent gastroesophageal reflux disease. J Pediatr Surg 39:282-286, 2004.

16. Spechler SJ, Lee E, Ahnen D, et al: Long-term outcome of medical and surgical therapies for gastroesophageal reflux disease: Follow-up of a randomized controlled trial. JAMA 285:2331-2338, 2001.

17. Lundell L, Miettinen P, Myrvold HE, et al: Continued (5-year) followup of a randomized clinical study comparing antireflux surgery and omeprazole in gastroesophageal reflux disease. J Am Coll Surg 192:172-181, 2001.

18. Rice S, Watson DI, Lally CJ, et al: Laparoscopic anterior 180° partial fundoplication: Five-year results and beyond. Arch Surg 141:271-275, 2006.

19. Dallemagne B, Weerts J, Markiewicz S, et al: Clinical results of laparoscopic fundoplication at ten years after surgery. Surg Endosc 20:159-165, 2006.

20. Cadiere GB, Himpens J, Rajan A, et al: Laparoscopic Nissen fundoplication: Laparoscopic dissection technique and results. Hepatogastroenterology 44:4-10, 1997.

21. Anvari M, Allen C, Borm A: Laparoscopic Nissen fundoplication is a satisfactory alternative to long-term omeprazole therapy. Br J Surg 82:938-942, 1995.

22. Flum DR, Koepsell T, Heagerty P, et al: The nationwide frequency of major adverse outcomes in antireflux surgery and the role of surgeon experience, 1992-1997. J Am Coll Surg 195:611-618, 2002.

23. Horgan S, Pellegrini CA: Surgical treatment of gastroesophageal reflux disease. Surg Clin North Am 77:1063-1082, 1997.

24. DeMeester SR, Campos GM, DeMeester TR, et al: The impact of an antireflux procedure on intestinal metaplasia of the cardia. Ann Surg 228:547-556, 1998.

25. Hofstetter WL, Peters JH, DeMeester TR, et al: Long-term outcome of antireflux surgery in patients with Barrett's esophagus. Ann Surg 234:532-539, 2001.

26. Bowers SP, Mattar SG, Smith CD, et al: Clinical and histologic follow-up after antireflux surgery for Barrett's esophagus. J Gastrointest Surg 6:532-539, 2002.

27. Oelschlager BK, Barreca M, Chang L, et al: Clinical and pathologic response of Barrett's esophagus to laparoscopic antireflux surgery. Ann Surg 238:458-466, 2003.

28. Jobe BA, Horvath KD, Swanstrom LL: Postoperative function following laparoscopic Collis gastroplasty for shortened esophagus. Arch Surg 133:867-874, 1998.

29. Mays EE, Dubois JJ, Hamilton GB: Pulmonary fibrosis associated with tracheobronchial aspiration: A study of the frequency of hiatal hernia and gastroesophageal reflux in interstitial pulmonary fibrosis of obscure etiology. Chest 69:512-515, 1976.

30. Koufman JA: The otolaryngologic manifestations of gastroesophageal reflux disease (GERD): A clinical investigation of 225 patients using ambulatory 24-hour pH monitoring and an experimental investigation of the role of acid and pepsin in the development of laryngeal injury. Laryngoscope 101:1-78, 1991.

31. Patti MG, Debas HT, Pellegrini CA: Clinical and functional characterization of high gastroesophageal reflux. Am J Surg 165:163-168, 1993.

32. Cote DN, Miller RH: The association of gastroesophageal reflux and otolaryngologic disorders. Compr Ther 21:80-84, 1995.

33. Eubanks TR, Omelanczuk P, Hillel A, et al: Pharyngeal pH measurements in patients with respiratory symptoms before and during proton pump inhibitor therapy. Am J Surg 181:466-470, 2001.

34. Oelschlager BK, Eubanks TR, Oleynikov D, et al: Symptomatic and physiologic outcomes after operative treatment for extraesophageal reflux. Surg Endosc 16:1032-1036, 2002.

35. Johnson WE, Hagen JA, DeMeester TR, et al: Outcome of respiratory symptoms after antireflux surgery on patients with gastroesophageal reflux disease. Arch Surg 131:489-492, 1996.

36. Hill LD: Incarcerated paraesophageal hernia: A surgical emergency. Am J Surg 126:286-291, 1973.

37. Skinner DB, Belsey RH: Surgical management of esophageal reflux and hiatus hernia: Long-term results with 1,030 patients. J Thorac Cardiovasc Surg 53:33-54, 1967.

38. Stylopoulos N, Gazelle GS, Rattner DW: Paraesophageal hernias: Operation or observation? Ann Surg 236:492-501, 2002.

39. Hayden JD, Jamieson GG: Effect on iron deficiency anemia of laparoscopic repair of large paraesophageal hernias. Dis Esophagus 18:329-331, 2005.

40. Hashemi M, Peters JH, DeMeester TR, et al: Laparoscopic repair of large type III hiatal hernia: Objective follow-up reveals high recurrence rate. J Am Coll Surg 190:554-561, 2000.

41. Mattar SG, Bowers SP, Galloway KD, et al: Long-term outcome of laparoscopic repair of paraesophageal hernia. Surg Endosc 16:745-749, 2002.

42. Carlson MA, Condon RE, Ludwig KA, et al: Management of intrathoracic stomach with polypropylene mesh prosthesis reinforced transabdominal hiatus hernia repair. J Am Coll Surg 187:227-230, 1998.

43. Walther B, DeMeester TR, Lafontaine E, et al: Effect of paraesophageal hernia on sphincter function and its implication on surgical therapy. Am J Surg 147:111-116, 1984.
44. Casabella F, Sinanan M, Horgan S, et al: Systematic use of gastric fundoplication in laparoscopic repair of paraesophageal hernias. Am J Surg 171:485-489, 1996.
45. Perdikis G, Hinder RA, Filipi CJ, et al: Laparoscopic paraesophageal hernia repair. Arch Surg 132:586-591, 1997.
46. Ellis FH, Crozier RE, Shea JA: Paraesophageal hiatus hernia. Arch Surg 121:416-420, 1986.
47. Schauer PR, Ikramuddin S, McLaughlin MD, et al: Comparison of laparoscopic versus open repair of paraesophageal hernia. Am J Surg 176:659-665, 1998.
48. Frantzides CT, Madan AK, Carlson MA, et al: A prospective, randomized trial of laparoscopic polytetrafluoroethylene (PTFE) patch repair vs simple cruroplasty for large hiatal hernia. Arch Surg 137:649-652, 2002.
49. Granderath FA, Schweiger UM, Kamolz T, et al: Laparoscopic Nissen fundoplication with prosthetic hiatal closure reduces postoperative intrathoracic wrap herniation: Preliminary results of a prospective randomized functional and clinical study. Arch Surg 140:40-48, 2005.
50. Paul MG, DeRosa RP, Petrucci PE, et al: Laparoscopic tension-free repair of large paraesophageal hernias. Surg Endosc 11:303-307, 1997.
51. Trus TL, Bax T, Richardson WS, et al: Complications of laparoscopic paraesophageal hernia repair. J Gastrointest Surg 1:221-228, 1997.
52. Oelschlager BK, Barreca M, Chang L, et al: The use of small intestine submucosa in the repair of paraesophageal hernias: Initial observations of a new technique. Am J Surg 186:4-8, 2003.
53. Ozdemir IA, Burke WA, Ikins PM: Paraesophageal hernia: A life-threatening disease. Ann Thorac Surg 16:547-554, 1973.

ABDOMEN

Abdominal Wall, Umbilicus, Peritoneum, Mesenteries, Omentum, and Retroperitoneum

Richard H. Turnage, MD   Kathryn A. Richardson, MD   Benjamin D. Li, MD
and   John C. McDonald, MD

Abdominal Wall and Umbilicus
Peritoneum and Peritoneal Cavity
Mesentery and Omentum
Retroperitoneum

ABDOMINAL WALL AND UMBILICUS

Embryology

The abdominal wall begins to develop in the earliest stages of embryonic differentiation from the lateral plate of the embryonic mesoderm. At this stage, the embryo consists of three principal layers: an outer protective layer termed *ectoderm,* an inner nutritive layer termed *endoderm,* and the *mesoderm.*

The mesoderm becomes divided by clefts on each side of the lateral plate, which ultimately develop into somatic and splanchnic layers. The splanchnic layer with its underlying endoderm contributes to the formation of the viscera by differentiating into muscle, blood vessels, lymphatics, and connective tissues of the alimentary tract. The somatic layer contributes to the development of the abdominal wall. Proliferation of mesodermal cells in the embryonic abdominal wall results in the formation of an inverted U-shaped tube that in its early stages communicates freely with the extraembryonic coelom.

As the embryo enlarges and the abdominal wall components grow toward one another, the ventral open area, bounded by the edge of the amnion, becomes smaller. This results in the development of the umbilical cord as a tubular structure containing the omphalomesenteric duct, allantois, and fetal blood vessels, which pass to and from the placenta. By the end of the third month of gestation, the body wall has closed, except at the umbilical ring. Because the alimentary tract increases in length more rapidly than the coelomic cavity increases in volume, much of the developing gut protrudes through the umbilical ring to lie within the umbilical cord. As the coelomic cavity enlarges to accommodate the intestine, the latter returns to the peritoneal cavity such that only the omphalomesenteric duct, the allantois, and the fetal blood vessels pass through the shrinking umbilical ring. At birth, blood no longer courses through the umbilical vessels, and the omphalomesenteric duct has been reduced to a fibrous cord that no longer communicates with the intestine. After division of the umbilical cord, the umbilical ring heals rapidly by scarring.

Anatomy

There are nine layers to the abdominal wall: skin, subcutaneous tissue, superficial fascia, external oblique muscle, internal oblique muscle, transversus abdominis muscle, transversalis fascia, preperitoneal adipose and areolar tissue, and peritoneum (Fig. 43-1).

Subcutaneous Tissues
The subcutaneous tissue consists of Camper's and Scarpa's fascia. *Camper's fascia* is the superficial layer that contains the bulk of the subcutaneous fat; *Scarpa's fascia* is a denser layer of fibrous connective tissue contiguous with the fascia lata of the thigh. Approximation of Scarpa's fascia aids in the alignment of the skin after surgical incisions in the lower abdomen.

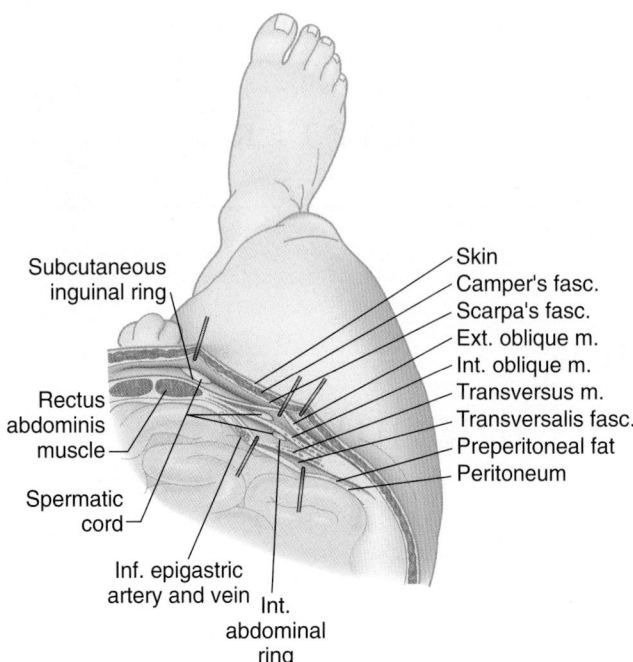

Figure 43-1 The nine layers of the anterolateral abdominal wall. (From Thorek P: Anatomy in Surgery, 2nd ed. Philadelphia, JB Lippincott, 1962, p 358.)

Muscle and Investing Fascias

The muscles of the anterolateral abdominal wall include the external and internal oblique and the transversus abdominis. These flat muscles enclose much of the circumference of the torso and give rise anteriorly to a broad, flat aponeurosis investing the rectus abdominis muscles, that is, rectus sheath. The external oblique muscles are the largest and the thickest of the flat abdominal wall muscles. They originate from the lower seven ribs and course in a superolateral to inferomedial direction. The most posterior of the fibers run vertically downward to insert into the anterior half of the iliac crest. At the midclavicular line, the muscle fibers give rise to a flat, strong aponeurosis that passes anteriorly to the rectus sheath to insert medially into the linea alba (Fig. 43-2). The lower portion of the external oblique aponeurosis is rolled posteriorly and superiorly on itself to form a groove on which the spermatic cord lies. This portion of the external oblique aponeurosis extends from the anterior superior iliac spine to the pubic tubercle and is termed the *inguinal* or *Poupart's ligament.* The inguinal ligament is the lower, free edge of the external oblique aponeurosis posterior to which pass the femoral artery, vein, and nerve and the iliacus, psoas major, and pectineus muscles. A femoral hernia passes posterior to the inguinal ligament, whereas an inguinal hernia passes

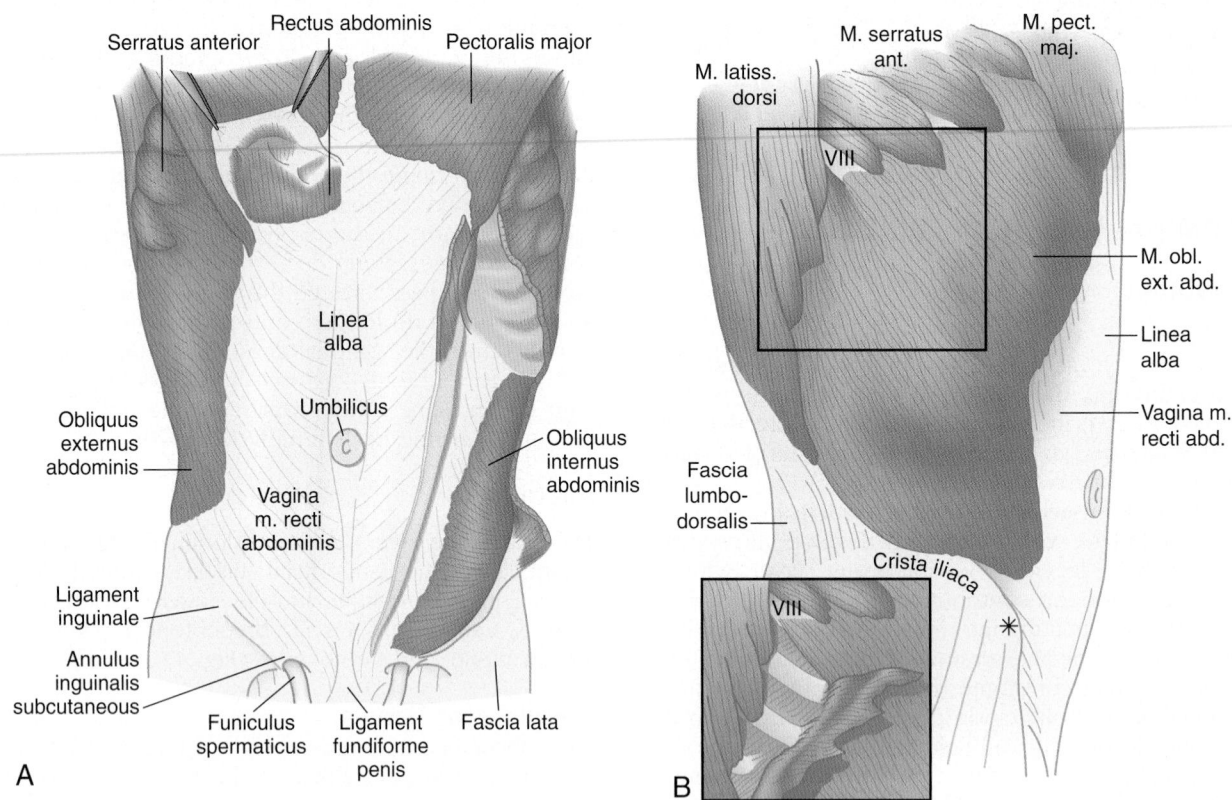

Figure 43-2 A, The external oblique, internal oblique, and rectus abdominis muscles and the anterior rectus sheath. **B,** A lateral view of the external oblique muscle and its aponeurosis as it enters the anterior rectus sheath. The *inset* shows the origin of the external oblique muscle fibers from the lower ribs and their costal cartilages. (From McVay C: Anson and McVay's Surgical Anatomy, 6th ed. Philadelphia, WB Saunders, 1984, pp 477 and 478).

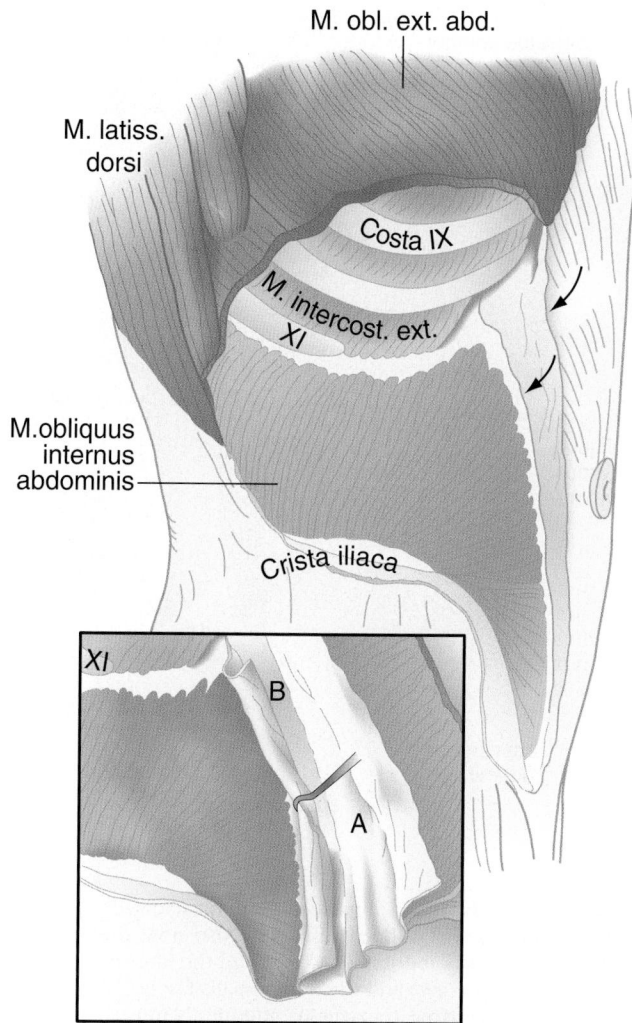

Figure 43-3 A lateral view of the internal oblique muscle. The external oblique muscle has been removed to show the underlying internal oblique muscle originating from the lower ribs and costal cartilages. (From McVay C: Anson and McVay's Surgical Anatomy, 6th ed. Philadelphia, WB Saunders, 1984, p 479.)

anterior and superior to this ligament. The shelving edge of the inguinal ligament is used in various repairs of inguinal hernia, including the Bassini and the Lichtenstein tension-free repair (see Chapter 44).

The internal oblique muscle originates from the iliopsoas fascia beneath the lateral half of the inguinal ligament, from the anterior two thirds of the iliac crest and the lumbodorsal fascia. Its fibers course in a direction opposite to those of the external oblique, that is, inferolateral to superomedial. The upper most fibers insert into the lower five ribs and their cartilages (Fig. 43-3; see Fig. 43-2A). The central fibers form an aponeurosis at the semilunar line, which, above the semicircular line (of Douglas), is divided into an anterior and posterior lamella that envelopes the rectus abdominis muscle. Below the semicircular line, the aponeurosis of the internal oblique muscle courses anteriorly to the rectus abdominis muscle as a part of the anterior rectus sheath. The lowermost

fibers of the internal oblique muscle pursue an inferomedial course paralleling that of the spermatic cord to insert between the symphysis pubis and the pubic tubercle. Some of the lower muscle fascicles accompany the spermatic cord into the scrotum as the cremasteric muscle.

The transversus abdominis muscle is the smallest of the muscles of the anterolateral abdominal wall. It arises from the lower six costal cartilages, the spines of the lumbar vertebra, the iliac crest, and the iliopsoas fascia beneath the lateral third of the inguinal ligament. The fibers course transversely to give rise to a flat aponeurotic sheet that passes posterior to the rectus abdominis muscle above the semicircular line and anterior to this muscle below it (Fig. 43-4). The inferior-most fibers of the transversus abdominis originating from the iliopsoas fascia pass inferomedially along with the lower fibers of the internal oblique muscle. These fibers form the aponeurotic arch of the transversus abdominis muscle, which lies superior to Hesselbach's triangle and is an important anatomic landmark in the repair of inguinal hernias, particularly Bassini's operation and Cooper's ligament repairs. Hesselbach's triangle is the site of direct inguinal hernias and is bordered by the inguinal ligament inferiorly, the lateral margin the rectus sheath medially, and the inferior epigastric vessels laterally. The floor of this triangle is composed of transversalis fascia.

The transversalis fascia covers the deep surface of the transversus abdominis muscle and with its various extensions forms a complete fascial envelope around the abdominal cavity (Fig. 43-5). This fascial layer is regionally named for the muscles that it covers, for example, the iliopsoas fascia, obturator fascia, and inferior fascia of the respiratory diaphragm. The transversalis fascia binds together the muscle and aponeurotic fascicles into a continuous layer and reinforces weak areas where the aponeurotic fibers are sparse. This layer is responsible for the structural integrity of the abdominal wall, and by definition, a hernia results from a defect in the transversalis fascia.

The rectus abdominis muscles are paired muscles that appear as long, flat triangular ribbons wider at their origin on the anterior surfaces of the fifth, sixth, and seventh costal cartilages and the xiphoid process than at their insertion on the pubic crest and pubic symphysis. Each muscle is composed of long, parallel fascicles interrupted by three to five tendinous inscriptions (see Fig. 43-5), which attach the rectus abdominis muscle to the anterior rectus sheath. There is no similar attachment to the posterior rectus sheath. These muscles lie adjacent to each other, being separated only by the linea alba. In addition to supporting the abdominal wall and protecting its contents, contraction of these powerful muscles flexes the vertebral column.

The rectus abdominis muscles are contained within the rectus sheath, which is derived from the aponeuroses of the three flat abdominal muscles. Superior to the semicircular line, this fascial sheath completely envelopes the rectus abdominis muscle with the external oblique and the anterior lamella of the internal oblique aponeuroses passing anterior to the rectus abdominis and with the

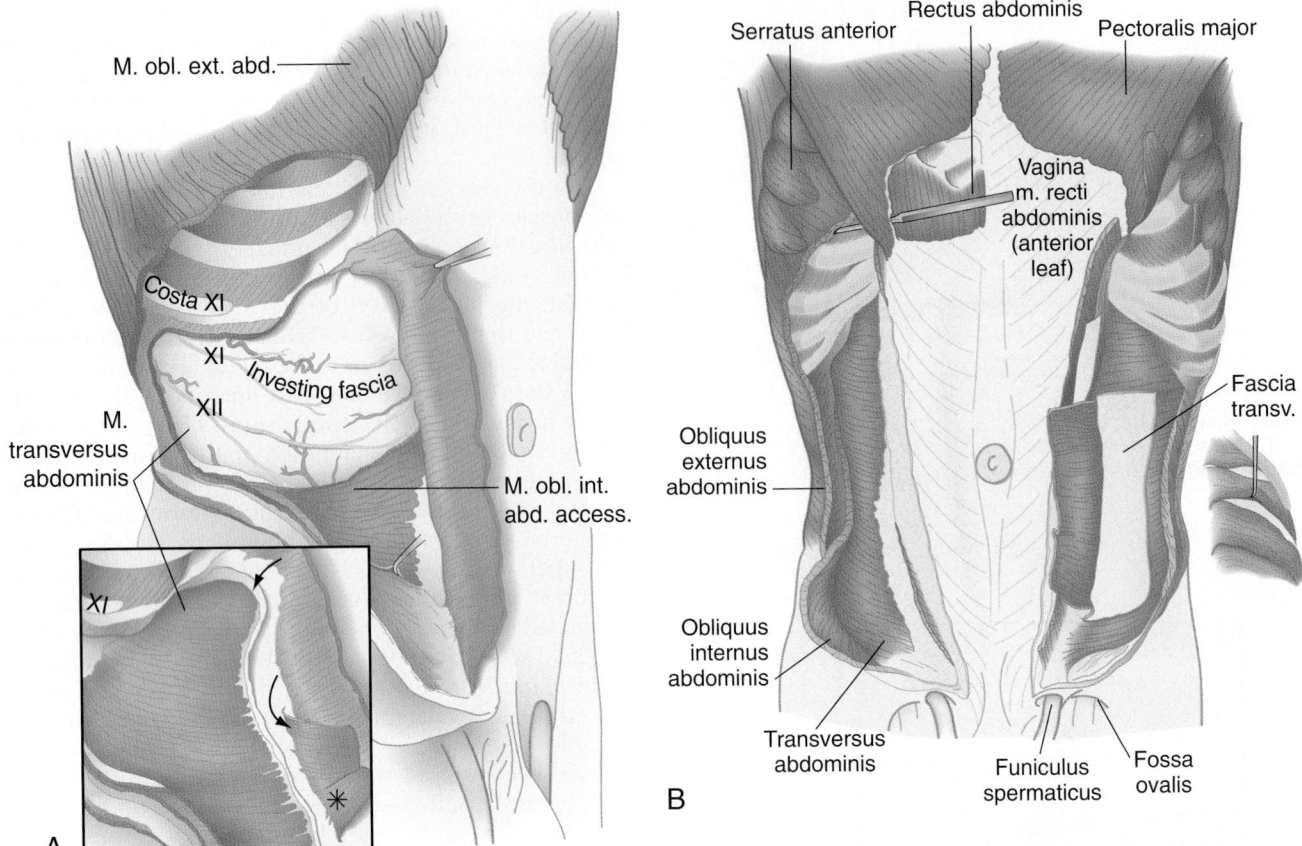

Figure 43-4 A, Anterolateral view of the investing fascia of the transversus abdominis muscle and the muscle itself with the fascia removed (*inset*). The external and internal oblique muscles have been removed. Also note the appearance of the intercostal nerves lying between the fascia of the transversus abdominis muscle and the internal oblique muscle. **B,** Anterior view of the transversus abdominis muscle (*on the left*) and the transversalis fascia (*on the right*). Note that the transversalis fascia is shown by reflecting the overlying transversus abdominis muscle medially. (From McVay C: Anson and McVay's Surgical Anatomy, 6th ed. Philadelphia, WB Saunders, 1984, pp 480 and 481.)

aponeuroses from the posterior lamella of the internal oblique muscle, the transversus abdominis muscle, and the transversalis fascia passing posterior to the rectus muscle. Below the semicircular line, all these fascial layers pass anterior to the rectus abdominis muscle except the transversalis fascia. In this location, the posterior aspect of the rectus abdominis muscle is covered only by transversalis fascia, preperitoneal areolar tissue, and peritoneum.

The rectus abdominis muscles are held closely in apposition near the anterior midline by the linea alba. The linea alba consists of a band of dense, crisscross fibers of the aponeuroses of the broad abdominal muscles that extends from the xiphoid to the pubic symphysis. It is much wider above the umbilicus than below, thus facilitating the placement of surgical incisions in the midline without entering either the right or left rectus sheath.

Preperitoneal Space and Peritoneum

The preperitoneal space lies between the transversalis fascia and the parietal peritoneum and contains adipose and areolar tissue. Coursing through the preperitoneal space are the following structures:

1. Inferior epigastric artery and vein
2. Medial umbilical ligaments (which are the vestiges of the fetal umbilical arteries)
3. Median umbilical ligament (which is a midline fibrous remnant of the fetal allantoic stalk or urachus)
4. Falciform ligament of the liver extending from the umbilicus to the liver.

The round ligament, or ligamentum teres, is contained within the free margin of the falciform ligament and represents the obliterated umbilical vein coursing from the umbilicus to the left branch of the portal vein (Fig. 43-6). The parietal peritoneum is the innermost layer of the abdominal wall. It consists of a thin layer of dense, irregular connective tissue covered on its inner surface by a single layer of squamous mesothelium.

Vessels and Nerves of the Abdominal Wall

Vascular Supply

The anterolateral abdominal wall receives its arterial supply from the last six intercostals and four lumbar arteries, the superior and inferior epigastric arteries, and the deep circumflex iliac arteries (Fig. 43-7). The trunks

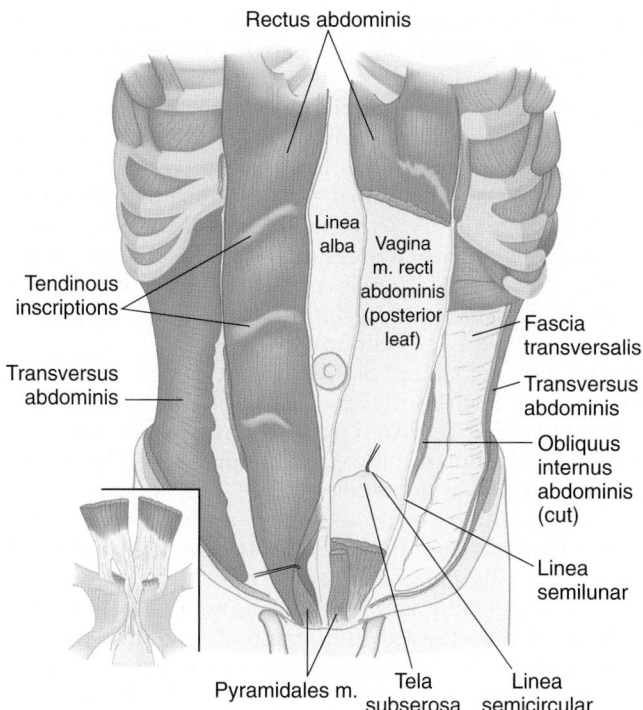

Figure 43-5 The rectus abdominis muscle and the contents of the rectus sheath. Note the semicircular line below which the posterior rectus sheath is absent and the rectus abdominis muscle overlies the transversalis fascia, preperitoneal areolar tissue, and peritoneum. (From McVay C: Anson and McVay's Surgical Anatomy, 6th ed. Philadelphia, WB Saunders, 1984, p 482.)

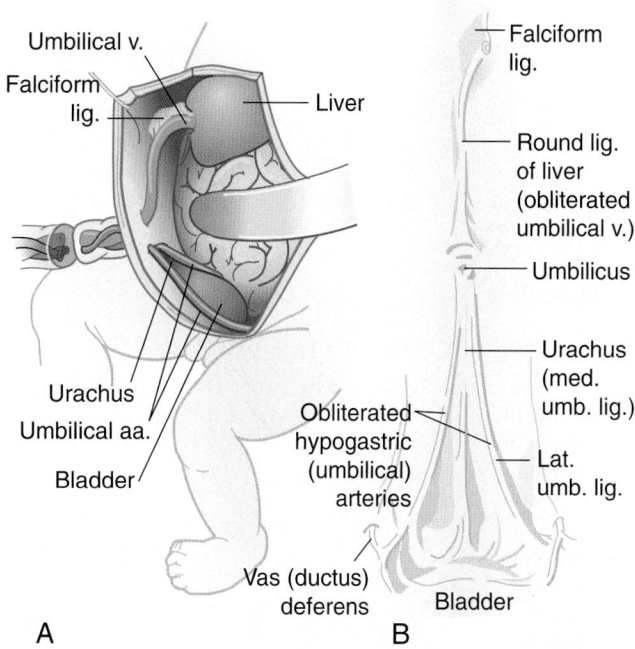

Figure 43-6 The umbilicus. **A,** In the fetus, the umbilical vein superiorly and the two umbilical arteries and urachus inferiorly radiate from the umbilicus. **B,** A view of the umbilicus from within the peritoneal cavity showing the round ligament of the liver (derived from the obliterated umbilical vein) superiorly and the median umbilical ligament (derived from the obliterated urachus) and medial umbilical ligaments (also called the *lateral umbilical ligaments;* derived from the obliterated umbilical arteries). (From Thorek P: Anatomy in Surgery, 2nd ed. Philadelphia, JB Lippincott, 1962, p 375.)

of the intercostal and lumbar arteries, together with the intercostal, iliohypogastric, and ilioinguinal nerves, course between the transversus abdominis and the internal oblique muscles. The distal-most extensions of these vessels pierce the lateral margins of the rectus sheath at various levels and communicate freely with branches of the superior and inferior epigastric arteries. The superior epigastric artery, one of the terminal branches of the internal mammary artery, reaches the posterior surface of the rectus abdominis muscle through the costoxiphoid space in the diaphragm. It descends within the rectus sheath to anastomose with branches of the inferior epigastric artery. The inferior epigastric artery, derived from the external iliac artery just proximal to the inguinal ligament, courses through the preperitoneal areolar tissue to enter the lateral rectus sheath at the semilunar line of Douglas. The deep circumflex iliac artery, arising from the lateral aspect of the external iliac artery near the origin of the inferior epigastric artery, gives rise to an ascending branch, which penetrates the abdominal wall musculature just above the iliac crest, near the anterior superior iliac spine.

The venous drainage of the anterior abdominal wall follows a relatively simple pattern in which the superficial veins above the umbilicus empty into the superior vena cava by way of the internal mammary, intercostal, and long thoracic veins. The veins inferior to the umbilicus,

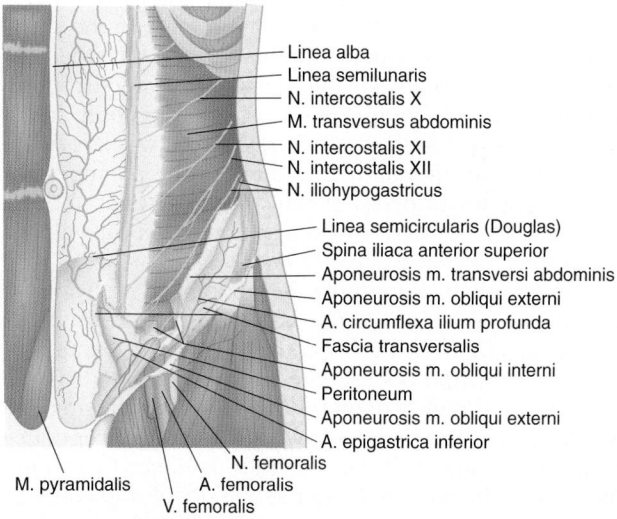

Figure 43-7 The arteries and nerves of the anterolateral abdominal wall. (From McVay C: Anson and McVay's Surgical Anatomy, 6th ed. Philadelphia, WB Saunders, 1984, p 501.)

that is, the superficial epigastric, circumflex iliac, and pudendal veins, converge toward the saphenous opening in the groin to enter the saphenous vein and become tributary to the inferior vena cava (Fig. 43-8). The numerous anastomoses between the infraumbilical and supra-

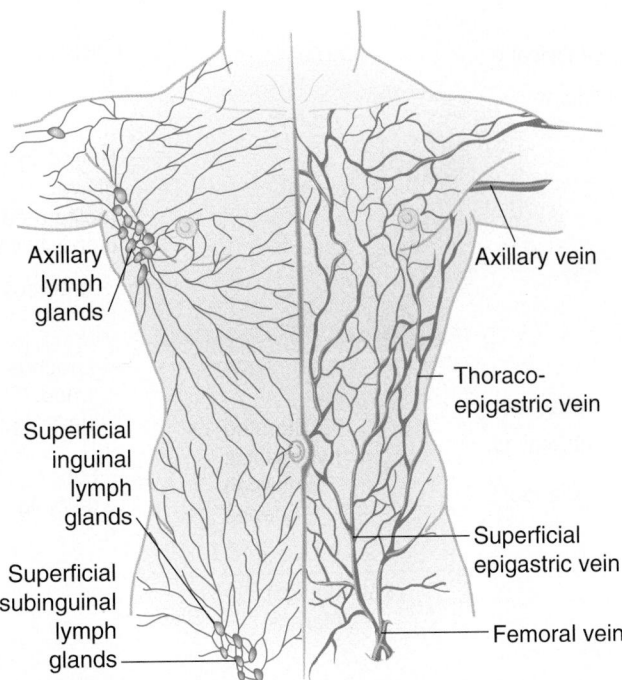

Figure 43-8 The venous and lymphatic drainage of the anterolateral abdominal wall. (From Thorek P: Anatomy in Surgery, 2nd ed. Philadelphia, JB Lippincott, 1962, p 345.)

umbilical venous systems provide collateral pathways by which venous return to the heart may bypass an obstruction of either the superior or inferior vena cava. The paraumbilical vein, which passes from the left branch of the portal vein along the ligamentum teres to the umbilicus, provides important communication between the veins of the superficial abdominal wall and the portal system in patients with portal venous obstruction. In this setting, portal blood flow is diverted away from the higher pressure portal system through the paraumbilical veins to the lower pressure veins of the anterior abdominal wall. The dilated superficial paraumbilical veins in this setting are termed *caput medusae.*

The lymphatic supply of the abdominal wall follows a pattern similar to the venous drainage. Those lymphatic vessels arising from the supraumbilical region drain into the axillary lymph nodes, whereas those arising from the infraumbilical region drain toward the superficial inguinal lymph nodes. The lymphatic vessels from the liver course along the ligamentum teres to the umbilicus to communicate with the lymphatics of the anterior abdominal wall. It is from this pathway that carcinoma in the liver may spread to involve the anterior abdominal wall at the umbilicus (Sister Mary Joseph's node).

Innervation

The anterior rami of the thoracic nerves follow a curvilinear course forward in the intercostal spaces toward the midline of the body (see Fig. 43-7). The upper six thoracic nerves end near the sternum as anterior cutaneous sensory branches. Thoracic nerves 7 to 12 pass behind the costal cartilages and lower ribs to enter a plane between the internal oblique muscle and the transversus abdominis. The 7th and 8th nerves course slightly upward or horizontally to reach the epigastrium, whereas the lower nerves have an increasingly caudal trajectory. As these nerves course medially, they provide motor branches to the abdominal wall musculature. Medially, they perforate the rectus sheath to provide sensory innervation to the anterior abdominal wall. The anterior ramus of the 10th thoracic nerve reaches the skin at the level of the umbilicus, and the 12th thoracic nerve innervates the skin of the hypogastrium.

The ilioinguinal and iliohypogastric nerves often arise in common from the anterior rami of the 12th thoracic and first lumbar nerves to provide sensory innervation to the hypogastrium and lower abdominal wall. The iliohypogastric nerve runs parallel to the 12th thoracic nerve to pierce the transversus abdominis muscle near the iliac crest. After coursing between the transversus abdominis muscle and the internal oblique for a short distance, the nerve pierces the latter to travel under the external oblique fascia toward the external inguinal ring. It emerges through the superior crus of the external inguinal ring to provide sensory innervation to the anterior abdominal wall in the hypogastrium. The ilioinguinal nerve courses parallel to the iliohypogastric but closer to the inguinal ligament. Unlike the iliohypogastric, the ilioinguinal nerve courses with the spermatic cord to emerge from the external inguinal ring, with its terminal branches providing sensory innervation to the skin of the inguinal region and the scrotum or labium. The ilioinguinal nerve, iliohypogastric nerve, and genital branch of the genitofemoral nerve are commonly encountered during the performance of inguinal herniorrhaphy.

Congenital Abnormalities

Umbilical Hernias
Umbilical hernias may be classified into three distinct forms:

1. Omphalocele and gastroschisis
2. Infantile umbilical hernia
3. Acquired umbilical hernia

Omphalocele
An omphalocele is a funnel-shaped defect in the central abdomen through which the viscera protrude into the base of the umbilical cord. It is caused by failure of the abdominal wall musculature to unite in the midline during fetal development. The umbilical vessels may be splayed over the viscera or pushed to one side. In larger defects, the liver and spleen may lie within the cord along with a major portion of the bowel. There is no skin covering these defects, only peritoneum and, more superficially, amnion. The presence of an omphalocele is associated with a 50% to 60% incidence of concomitant congenital anomalies of the skeleton, gastrointestinal tract, nervous system, genitourinary system, and cardiopulmonary system.

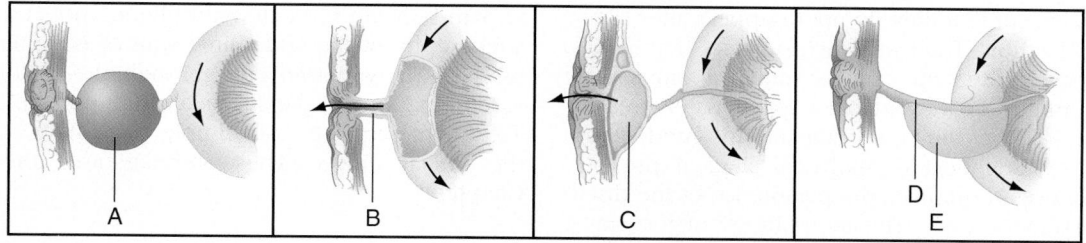

Figure 43-9 Abnormalities resulting from persistence of the omphalomesenteric duct. **A,** Omphalomesenteric duct cyst. **B,** Persistent omphalomesenteric duct with an enterocutaneous fistula. **C,** Omphalomesenteric duct cyst and sinus. **D,** Fibrous cord between the small intestine and the posterior surface of the umbilicus. **E,** Meckel's diverticulum. (From McVay C: Anson and McVay's Surgical Anatomy, 6th ed. Philadelphia, WB Saunders, 1984, p 576.)

Gastroschisis

Gastroschisis is another defect of the abdominal wall presenting at birth in which the umbilical membrane has ruptured in utero, allowing the intestine to herniate outside the abdominal cavity. The defect is nearly always to the right of the umbilical cord and the intestine is not covered with skin or amnion. Typically, the intestine has not undergone complete mesenteric rotation and fixation, and hence the infant is at risk for mesenteric volvulus with resultant intestinal ischemia and necrosis. Concomitant congenital anomalies occur in about 10% of these patients. Both omphalocele and gastroschisis are discussed in greater detail in Chapter 71.

Infantile Umbilical Hernia

Infantile umbilical hernias appear within a few days or weeks after the stump of the umbilical cord has sloughed. It is caused by a weakness in the adhesion between the scarred remnants of the umbilical cord and the umbilical ring. In contrast to omphalocele, the infantile umbilical hernia is covered by skin. Generally, these small hernias occur in the superior margin of the umbilical ring. They are easily reducible and become prominent when the infant cries. Most of these hernias resolve within the first 24 months of life, and complications such as strangulation are rare. Operative repair is indicated for those children in whom the hernia has persisted beyond the age of 3 or 4 years. This condition and its management are further discussed in Chapters 44 and 71.

Acquired Umbilical Hernia

In this condition, an umbilical hernia develops at a time remote from closure of the umbilical ring. This hernia occurs most commonly at the upper margin of the umbilicus and results from weakening of the cicatricial tissue that normally closes the umbilical ring. This may be due to excessive stretching of the abdominal wall, which may occur with pregnancy, vigorous labor, or ascites. In contrast to infantile umbilical hernias, acquired umbilical hernias do not spontaneously resolve but instead gradually increase in size. The dense fibrous ring at the neck of this hernia makes strangulation of herniated intestine or omentum an important complication.

Abnormalities Resulting From Persistence of the Omphalomesenteric Duct

During fetal development, the midgut communicates widely with the yolk sac through the vitelline or omphalomesenteric duct. As the abdominal wall components approximate one another, the omphalomesenteric duct narrows and comes to lie within the umbilical cord. Over time, communication between the yolk sac and the intestine becomes obliterated, and the intestine resides free within the peritoneal cavity. Persistence of part or all of the omphalomesenteric duct results in a variety of abnormalities related to the intestine and abdominal wall (Fig. 43-9).

Persistence of the intestinal end of the omphalomesenteric duct results in Meckel's diverticulum. These congenital, true diverticula arise from the antimesenteric border of the small intestine, most often the ileum. A "rule of two's" is often applied to lesions in that they are found in about 2% of the population, are within 2 feet of the ileocecal valve, are often 2 inches in length, and contain two types of ectopic mucosa (gastric and pancreatic). These lesions may be complicated by inflammation, perforation, hemorrhage, or obstruction. Gastrointestinal bleeding is caused by peptic ulceration of adjacent intestinal mucosa from hydrochloric acid secreted by ectopic parietal cells within the diverticulum. Intestinal obstruction associated with Meckel's diverticulum is usually due to intussusception or to volvulus around an abnormal fibrous connection between the diverticulum and the posterior aspect of the umbilicus. These lesions are discussed in Chapter 48.

The omphalomesenteric duct may remain patent throughout its course, producing an enterocutaneous fistula between the distal small intestine and the umbilicus. This condition presents with the passage of meconium and mucus from the umbilicus in the first few days of life. Because of the risk for mesenteric volvulus around a persistent omphalomesenteric duct, these lesions are promptly treated with laparotomy and excision of the fistulous tract. Persistence of the distal end of the omphalomesenteric duct results in an umbilical polyp, which is a small excrescence of omphalomesenteric ductal mucosa at the umbilicus. Such polyps resemble umbilical granulomas except that they do not disappear after silver nitrate cauterization. Their presence suggests that a persistent omphalomesenteric duct or umbilical sinus may be present, and hence they are most appropriately treated by excision of the mucosal remnant and underlying omphalomesenteric duct or umbilical sinus if present. Umbilical sinuses result from the persistence of the distal omphalomesenteric duct. The morphology of the sinus tract will be delineated by a sinogram. Treatment involves excision of the sinus. Lastly, the accumulation of mucus in a portion of a persistent omphalomesenteric duct may result in the formation of a cyst, which may be associated with either the intestine or the umbilicus by a fibrous band. Treatment consists of excision of the cyst and the associated persistent omphalomesenteric duct.

Abnormalities Resulting From Persistence of the Allantois

The allantois is the cranial-most component of the embryologic ventral cloaca. The intra-abdominal portion is termed the *urachus* and connects the urinary bladder with the umbilicus, whereas the extra-abdominal allantois is contained within the umbilical cord. At the end of gestation, the urachus is converted into a fibrous cord that courses between the extraperitoneal urinary bladder and the umbilicus as the median umbilical ligament. Persistence of a part or all of the urachus may result in the formation of a vesicocutaneous fistula with the appearance of urine at the umbilicus, an extraperitoneal urachal cyst presenting as a lower abdominal mass, or an urachal sinus with the drainage of a small amount of mucus. Treatment is excision of the urachal remnant with closure of the bladder, if necessary.

Acquired Abnormalities of the Abdominal Wall

Diastasis Recti

Diastasis recti refers to a thinning of the linea alba in the epigastrium and is manifested as a midline protrusion of the anterior abdominal wall. The transversalis fascia is intact, and hence this is not a hernia. There are no identifiable fascial margins and no risk for intestinal strangulation. The presence of diastasis recti may be particularly noticeable to the patient upon straining or upon lifting the head from the pillow. Appropriate management consists of reassurance of the patient and family regarding the innocuous nature of this condition.

Anterior Abdominal Wall Hernias

Epigastric hernias occur at sites through which vessels and nerves perforate the linea alba to course into the subcutaneum. Through these openings, extraperitoneal areolar tissue and, at times, peritoneum may herniate into the subcutaneous tissue. Although these hernias are often small, they may produce significant localized pain and tenderness due to direct pressure of the hernia sac and its contents on the nerves emerging through the same fascial opening. *Spigelian hernias* occur through the fascia in the region of the semilunar line and present with localized pain and tenderness. The hernia sac is only rarely palpable because it is often small and tends to

remain beneath the external oblique aponeurosis. Ultrasonography of the abdominal wall or computed tomography (CT) with thin cuts through the abdomen, after careful marking of the suspected site, may be diagnostic. Treatment consists of simple operative closure of the fascial defect. These hernias are considered in Chapter 44.

Rectus Sheath Hematoma

Rectus sheath hematoma is an uncommon condition characterized by acute abdominal pain and the appearance of an abdominal wall mass. It is more common in women than men and in older than younger individuals. A review of 126 patients with rectus sheath hematomas treated at the Mayo Clinic found that nearly 70% were receiving anticoagulants at the time of diagnosis. A history of nonsurgical abdominal wall trauma or injury is common (48%), as is the presence of a cough (29%).[1] In young women, rectus sheath hematomas have been associated with pregnancy.

The most common symptom associated with rectus sheath hematomas is the sudden onset of abdominal pain, which may be severe and is often exacerbated by movements requiring contraction of the abdominal wall. Physical examination will demonstrate tenderness over the rectus sheath, often with voluntary guarding. An abdominal wall mass may be noted in some patients, 63% in the Mayo Clinic series.[1] Abdominal wall ecchymosis, including periumbilical ecchymosis (Cullen's sign) and blue discoloration in the flanks (Grey Turner's sign), may be present if there is a delay from the onset of symptoms to presentation. The pain and tenderness associated with this process may be severe enough to suggest peritonitis. In those cases in which the hematoma expands into the perivesical and preperitoneal space, the hematocrit may fall, although hemodynamic instability is uncommon.

Ultrasonography or CT will confirm the presence of the hematoma and localize it to the abdominal wall in nearly all cases. In most instances, patients with rectus sheath hematomas may be successfully managed with rest and analgesics and, if necessary, blood transfusion. In the Mayo Clinic series, nearly 90% of patients were managed successfully in this manner.[1] In general, coagulopathies are corrected; however, continued anticoagulation of selected patients may be prudent depending on the indications for anticoagulation and the seriousness of the bleeding. Progression of the hematoma necessitates angiographic embolization of the bleeding vessel or, uncommonly, operative evacuation of the hematoma and hemostasis.

Malignancies of the Abdominal Wall

The most common primary malignancies of the abdominal wall are desmoid tumors and sarcomas. Metastatic disease may also occur in the abdominal wall, although this is generally a late event in the natural history of that disease. An exception is the transperitoneal seeding of the abdominal wall by intra-abdominal malignancies, which may complicate transabdominal biopsies or operative procedures.

Desmoid Tumor

Desmoid tumor, also known as *aggressive fibromatosis*, is an uncommon neoplasm that occurs sporadically or as part of an inherited syndrome, most notably, familial adenomatous polyposis (FAP). The tumor may arise from fascia or muscle and has been classified as superficial (fascial) or deep (musculoaponeurotic). The superficial disease, also known as *Dupuytren's fibromatosis*, is slow growing, is small in size, and rarely involves deeper structures. Deep fibromatosis has a relatively rapid growth rate, often attains a large size, has a high rate of local recurrence, and involves the musculature of the trunk and extremities. Desmoid tumors are also classified as extra-abdominal (e.g., shoulder girdle), abdominal wall, and intra-abdominal (mesenteric and pelvic desmoid). Most spontaneous desmoid tumors occur at the shoulder girdle or the abdominal wall, whereas intra-abdominal desmoids, especially mesenteric desmoids, are more common in patients with FAP.[2,3]

In the general population, desmoid tumors occur with a frequency of 2.4 to 4.3 cases per million people[4]; this risk is increased 1000-fold in patients with FAP.[3] Typically, sporadic abdominal wall desmoid tumors occur in young women during gestation or, more frequently, within a year of childbirth. Oral contraceptive use has also been associated with the occurrence of these tumors. These associations, combined with the detection of estrogen receptors within the tumor, suggest a regulatory role for estrogen in this disease. There is also often a temporal association between the development of this neoplasm and an antecedent history of abdominal trauma or operation.[4]

Patients with desmoid tumors present with a painless enlarging mass. Local symptoms may arise from compression of adjacent organs or neurovascular structures. Magnetic resonance imaging (MRI) provides information regarding the extent of the disease and its relationship to intra-abdominal organs. These tumors appear homogeneous and isointense to muscle on T1-weighted images; T2-weighted images demonstrate greater heterogeneity with a signal slightly less intense than fat. After MRI, an incisional biopsy or a core needle biopsy is performed, which will demonstrate a tumor composed of interwoven bundles of spindle cells and variable amounts of collagen. The center of the tumor is often acellular, whereas the periphery has diffuse cellularity suggesting a low-grade fibrosarcoma. Unlike sarcoma, the fibroblasts are highly differentiated and lack mitotic activity. Despite this benign histologic appearance, desmoids are diffusely infiltrative and tend to recur locally, even after complete resection. In contrast, systemic metastases are extremely unusual.[2]

The treatment of abdominal wall desmoids is complete resection with a tumor-free margin. Unfortunately, even with complete resection, the local recurrence rate is as high as 40%.[2] Multiple local recurrences of the tumor are common, and re-resection is indicated even in those instances in which tumor-free margins may not be possible. In one study of 203 patients with desmoid tumors, the presence of microscopic disease did not necessarily affect long-term disease-free survival.[5] The role of radiation therapy in the management of these tumors, either as an adjunct to surgery or as primary treatment, continues to be defined. In a review of 22 reports, Nuyttens and colleagues[6] found that local control rates were 61% for surgery alone and 75% for surgery plus radiation therapy. More importantly, the combination of radiation therapy and resection reduced local failure rates in patients after incomplete resection, particularly in those patients with close or microscopically positive margins, from about 80% to 90% to 50% to 60%. Although reports of radiation therapy alone for the treatment of desmoid tumor exist in the literature, this is generally reserved for patients with tumors deemed unresectable.

Antiproliferative agents and cytotoxic chemotherapy have been used to palliate these tumors with variable results.[4,7] The two most widely used groups of noncytotoxic drugs are nonsteroidal anti-inflammatory drugs (NSAIDs) and antiestrogens. The objective response rate for each of these agents is about 50%.[7] Chemotherapy has generally been reserved for unresectable, symptomatic, and clinically aggressive disease. Partial responses have been observed after treatment with doxorubicin, actinomycin C, dacarbazine, or carboplatin, although toxicity has been relatively high.[4]

Abdominal Wall Sarcoma

Truncal sarcomas (including both chest and abdominal wall) account for about 10% of sarcomas. Histologic subtypes include liposarcoma, fibrosarcoma, leiomyosarcoma, rhabdomyosarcoma, and malignant fibrous histiocytoma. The clinical behavior of these tumors is determined more by anatomic site, grade, and size than by specific histologic pattern. Similar to desmoid tumors, abdominal wall sarcomas present as a painless mass. The differential diagnosis includes many common conditions such as ventral hernias, benign soft tissue tumors, and inflammatory processes, such as needle site granulomas in diabetics. Following is a list of clinical characteristics that suggest an abdominal wall malignancy:

1. Nonreducible lesions arising from below the superficial fascia
2. Size greater than 5 cm
3. Recent increase in size
4. Fixation to the abdominal wall
5. Fixation to organs in the abdomen

MRI will provide information regarding the location and extent of the tumor as well as involvement of contiguous structures. Definitive diagnosis requires biopsy, which may be performed with a core needle or by incision. If an incisional biopsy is performed, the incision is oriented in the same plane as the underlying muscle to minimize unnecessary tissue loss at the definitive procedure and ease reconstructive efforts. No attempt is made to develop tissue flaps around the lesion, and hemostasis is meticulous to avoid dissemination of the tumor along the tissue planes by a postoperative hematoma. Treatment of these malignancies is resection with a tumor-free margin. Reconstruction of the abdominal wall defect may be accomplished primarily, with myocutaneous flaps, or with prosthetic meshes, depending on the site and extent of resection.

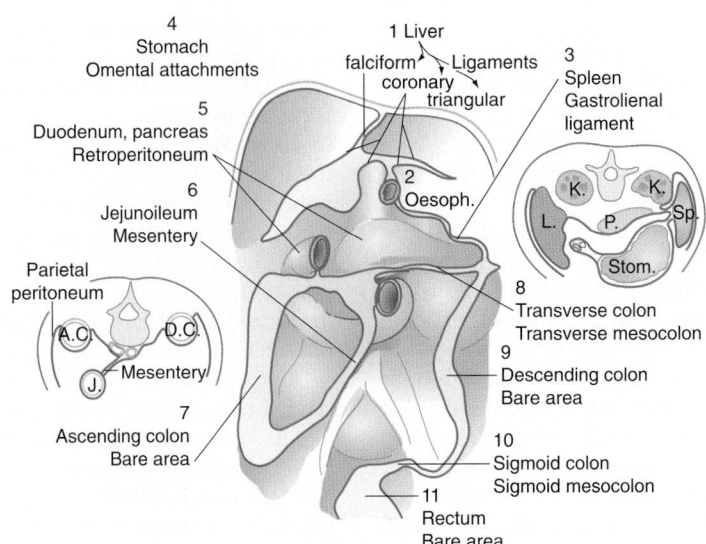

Figure 43-10 Peritoneal ligaments and mesenteric reflections in the adult. These attachments partition the abdomen into nine potential spaces: right and left subphrenic, subhepatic, supramesenteric and inframesenteric spaces, right and left paracolic gutters, pelvis, and omental bursa (shown in *inset on right*). (From McVay C: Anson and McVay's Surgical Anatomy, 6th ed. Philadelphia, WB Saunders, 1984, p 589.)

Symptoms of Intra-abdominal Diseases Referred to the Abdominal Wall

Abdominal pain may be categorized as visceral, somato-parietal, and referred. Visceral pain is caused by stimulation of visceral nociceptors by inflammation, distention, or ischemia. The pain is dull in nature and poorly localized to the epigastrium, periumbilical regions, or hypogastrium, depending on the embryonic origin of the organ involved. Inflammation of the stomach, duodenum, and biliary tract (derivatives of the embryonic foregut) localizes visceral pain to the epigastrium. Stimulation of nociceptors in midgut-derived organs (i.e., small intestine, appendix, and right colon) causes the sensation of pain in the periumbilical region, whereas inflammation or distention of hindgut-derived organs (left colon and rectum) causes hypogastric pain. The pain is felt in the midline because these organs transmit sympathetic sensory afferents to both sides of the spinal cord. The pain is poorly localized because the innervation of most viscera is multisegmental and contains fewer nerve receptors than highly sensitive organs such as the skin. The pain is often characterized as cramping, burning, or gnawing and may be accompanied by secondary autonomic effects such as sweating, restlessness, nausea, vomiting, perspiration, and pallor.

Somatoparietal pain arises from inflammation of the parietal peritoneum and is more intense and more precisely localized than visceral pain. The nerve impulses mediating parietal pain travel within the somatosensory spinal nerves and reach the spinal cord in the peripheral nerves corresponding to the cutaneous dermatomes from the sixth thoracic to the first lumbar region. Lateralization of parietal pain is possible because only one side of the nervous system innervates a given part of the parietal peritoneum.

The difference between visceral and somatoparietal pain is well illustrated by the pain associated with acute appendicitis in which the early vague periumbilical visceral pain is followed by the localized somatoparietal pain at the McBurney point. The visceral pain is produced by distention and inflammation of the appendix, whereas the localized somatoparietal pain in the right lower quadrant of the abdomen is due to extension of the inflammation to the parietal peritoneum.

Referred pain is felt in anatomic regions remote from the diseased organ. This phenomenon is caused by convergence of visceral afferent neurons innervating an injured or inflamed organ with somatic afferent fibers arising from another anatomic region. This occurs within the spinal cord at the level of second-order neurons. Well-known examples of referred pain include shoulder pain upon irritation of the diaphragm, scapular pain associated with acute biliary tract disease, or testicular or labial pain caused by retroperitoneal inflammation.

PERITONEUM AND PERITONEAL CAVITY

Anatomy

The peritoneum consists of a single sheet of simple squamous epithelium of mesodermal origin, termed *mesothelium,* lying on a thin connective tissue stroma. The surface area is 1.0 to 1.7 m^2, about that of the total body surface area. In males, the peritoneal cavity is sealed, whereas in females, it is open to the exterior through the ostia of the fallopian tubes. The peritoneal membrane is divided into parietal and visceral components. The parietal peritoneum covers the anterior, lateral, and posterior abdominal wall surfaces as well as the inferior surface of the diaphragm and the pelvis. The visceral peritoneum covers most of the surface of the intraperitoneal organs (i.e., the stomach, jejunum, ileum, transverse colon, liver, and spleen) and the anterior aspect of the retroperitoneal organs (i.e., the duodenum, left and right colon, pancreas, kidneys, and adrenal glands).

The peritoneal cavity is subdivided into interconnected compartments or spaces by 11 ligaments and mesenteries. The peritoneal ligaments or mesenteries include the coronary, gastrohepatic, hepatoduodenal, falciform, gastrocolic, duodenocolic, gastrosplenic, splenorenal, and phrenicocolic ligaments and the transverse mesocolon and small bowel mesentery (Fig. 43-10). These structures partition the abdomen into nine potential spaces: right and left subphrenic, subhepatic, supramesenteric and inframesenteric, right and left paracolic gutters, pelvis, and lesser space. These ligaments, mesenteries, and peritoneal spaces direct the circulation of fluid in the peritoneal cavity and thus may be useful in predicting the route of spread of infectious and malignant diseases. For example, perforation of the duodenum from peptic ulcer disease may result in the movement of fluid (and the development of abscesses) in the subhepatic space, the right paracolic gutter, and the pelvis. The blood supply to the visceral peritoneum is derived from the splanchnic blood vessels, whereas the parietal peritoneum is supplied by branches of the intercostals, subcostal, lumbar, and iliac vessels. The innervation of the visceral and parietal peritoneum is discussed earlier.

Physiology

The peritoneum is a bidirectional, semipermeable membrane that controls the amount of fluid within the peritoneal cavity, promotes the sequestration and removal of bacteria from the peritoneal cavity, and facilitates the migration of inflammatory cells from the microvasculature into the peritoneal cavity. Normally, the peritoneal cavity contains less than 100 mL of sterile serous fluid. Microvilli on the apical surface of the peritoneal mesothelium markedly increase the surface area and promote the rapid absorption of fluid from the peritoneal cavity into the lymphatics and the portal and systemic circulation. The amount of fluid within the peritoneal cavity may increase to many liters in various diseases such as cirrhosis, nephrotic syndrome, and peritoneal carcinomatosis.

The circulation of fluid within the peritoneal cavity is driven in part by the movement of the diaphragm. Intercellular pores in the peritoneum covering the inferior surface of the diaphragm (termed *stomata*) communicate with lymphatic pools within the diaphragm. Lymph flows from these diaphragmatic lymphatic channels through subpleural lymphatics to the regional lymph nodes and ultimately the thoracic duct. Relaxation of the diaphragm during exhalation opens the stomata, and the negative intrathoracic pressure draws fluid and particles, including bacteria, into the stomata. Contraction of the diaphragm during inhalation propels the lymph through the mediastinal lymphatic channels into the thoracic duct. It is postulated that this so-called diaphragmatic pump drives the movement of peritoneal fluid in a cephalad direction

toward the diaphragm and into the thoracic lymphatic vessels. This circulatory pattern of peritoneal fluid toward the diaphragm and into the central lymphatic channels is consistent with the rapid appearance of sepsis in patients with generalized intra-abdominal infections as well as the perihepatitis of Fitz-Hugh–Curtis syndrome in patients with acute salpingitis.

The peritoneum and peritoneal cavity respond to infection in five ways:

1. Bacteria are rapidly removed from the peritoneal cavity through the diaphragmatic stomata and lymphatics, as described in the preceding paragraph.
2. Peritoneal macrophages release proinflammatory mediators that promote the migration of leukocytes into the peritoneal cavity from the surrounding microvasculature.
3. Degranulation of peritoneal mast cells releases histamine and other vasoactive products, causing local vasodilation and the extravasation of protein-rich fluid containing complement and immunoglobulins into the peritoneal space.
4. Protein within the peritoneal fluid opsonizes bacteria, which, along with activation of the complement cascade, promotes neutrophil- and macrophage-mediated bacterial phagocytosis and destruction.
5. Bacteria become sequestered within fibrin matrices, thereby promoting abscess formation and limiting the generalized spread of the infection.

Ascites

Pathophysiology and Etiology

Ascites is the pathologic accumulation of fluid within the peritoneal cavity. The principal causes of ascites formation and their pathophysiologic basis are listed in Table 43-1. Cirrhosis is the most common cause of ascites in the United States, accounting for about 85% of cases. Ascites is the most common complication of cirrhosis, with about 50% of compensated cirrhotic patients developing ascites within 10 years of diagnosis.[8] The onset of ascites is an important and poor prognostic factor for patients with cirrhosis because it is associated with the occurrence of spontaneous bacterial peritonitis, renal failure, a worsened quality of life and an increased likelihood of death within the subsequent 2 to 5 years.[9,10]

The two principal factors underlying the formation of ascites in cirrhotic patients are renal sodium and water retention and portal hypertension. Renal sodium retention is driven by activation of renin-angiotensin-aldosterone and sympathetic nervous systems, which cause proximal and distal renal tubule sodium reabsorption. It is postulated that the abnormal release of nitric oxide within the splanchnic circulation causes vasodilation and a decrease in the effective circulating blood volume. Renin, aldosterone, and other hormones are generated as a counter-regulatory mechanism to restore the effective circulating blood volume to normal. Portal hypertension is produced by postsinusoidal vascular obstruction from the deposition of collagen in the cirrhotic liver. Increased hydrostatic pressure within the hepatic sinusoids and the splanchnic vasculature drives the extravasa-

Table 43-1 Principal Causes of Ascites Formation Categorized According to Their Underlying Pathophysiology

Portal Hypertension

Cirrhosis
Noncirrhotic
    Prehepatic portal venous obstruction
        Chronic mesenteric venous thrombosis
        Multiple hepatic metastases
    Posthepatic venous obstruction
        Budd-Chiari syndrome

Cardiac

Congestive heart failure
Chronic pericardial tamponade
Constrictive pericarditis

Malignancy

Peritoneal carcinomatosis
    Primary peritoneal malignancies
        Primary peritoneal mesothelioma
        Serous carcinoma
    Metastatic carcinoma
        Gastrointestinal carcinomas, e.g., gastric, colonic, and pancreatic cancer
        Genitourinary carcinomas, e.g., ovarian cancer
Retroperitoneal obstruction of lymphatic channels
    Lymphoma
    Lymph node metastases, e.g., testicular cancer, melanoma
Obstruction of the lymphatic channels at the base of the mesentery
    Gastrointestinal carcinoid tumors

Miscellaneous

Bile ascites
    Iatrogenic after operations of the liver or biliary tract
    Traumatic after injuries to the liver or biliary tract
Pancreatic ascites
    Acute pancreatitis
    Pancreatic pseudocyst
Chylous ascites
    Disruptions of retroperitoneal lymphatic channels
        Iatrogenic during retroperitoneal dissections
            Retroperitoneal lymphadenectomy
            Abdominal aortic aneurysmorrhaphy
        Blunt or penetrating trauma
    Malignancy
        Obstruction of retroperitoneal lymphatic channels
        Obstruction of lymphatic channels at the base of the mesentery
    Congenital lymphatic abnormalities
        Primary lymphatic hypoplasia
Peritoneal infections
    Tuberculous peritonitis
    Myxedema
    Nephrotic syndrome
    Serositis in connective tissue disease

tion of fluid from the microvasculature into the extracellular compartment. Ascites results when the capacity of the lymphatic system to return this fluid to the systemic circulation is overwhelmed.[9,11]

Obstruction of the portal or hepatic venous blood flow in the absence of cirrhosis (e.g., portal vein thrombosis or Budd-Chiari syndrome, respectively) also promotes

ascites formation by increasing hydrostatic pressure within the microvasculature. A similar pressure-based mechanism contributes to ascites formation in patients with heart failure, although the release of vasopressin and renin-angiotensin-aldosterone also promote sodium and water retention in these patients.

Patients with malignancies develop ascites by one of three mechanisms:

1. Multiple hepatic metastases cause portal hypertension by narrowing or occluding branches of the portal venous system.
2. Malignant cells scattered throughout the peritoneal cavity release protein-rich fluid into the peritoneal cavity, as in carcinomatosis.
3. Obstruction of retroperitoneal lymphatics by a tumor, such as lymphoma, causes rupture of major lymphatic channels and the leakage of chyle into the peritoneal cavity.

Lastly, ascites may result from the leakage of pancreatic juice, bile, or lymph into the peritoneal cavity after iatrogenic or inflammatory disruption of a major pancreatic, bile, or lymphatic duct.

Clinical Presentation

The diagnosis of ascites is made on the basis of the medical history and the appearance of the abdomen. Obviously, risk factors for hepatitis or cirrhosis are sought, as is evidence of cardiac or renal disease or malignancy. A full, bulging abdomen with dullness of the flanks upon percussion is suggestive of the presence of ascites. About 1.5 liters of fluid must be present before dullness can be detected by percussion.[12] Physical evidence of cirrhosis is also sought, such as palmar erythema, dilated abdominal wall collateral veins, and multiple spider angiomas. Patients with cardiac ascites have impressive jugular venous distention and other evidence of congestive heart failure.

Ascitic Fluid Analysis

Paracentesis with ascitic fluid analysis is the most rapid and cost-effective method of determining the etiology of ascites and hence is performed in all patients with new-onset ascites. Another important indication for early paracentesis in a patient with ascites is the occurrence of signs and symptoms of infection, such as abdominal pain or tenderness, fever, encephalopathy, hypotension, renal failure, acidosis, or leukocytosis. Paracentesis can be performed safely in most patients, including those with cirrhosis and mild coagulopathy. It is most commonly performed in the lower abdomen, with the left lower quadrant preferred over the right. Ultrasound guidance may be useful in obese patients and in those with a history of laparotomy. Runyon[8] suggests that only ongoing disseminated intravascular coagulation or clinically evident fibrinolysis is a contraindication to paracentesis in patients with ascites. He reported no cases of hemoperitoneum, deaths, or infections after more than 229 paracenteses performed in 125 cirrhotic patients; abdominal hematomas occurred in 2% of cases, with only half of these requiring blood transfusion.

Examination of the ascitic fluid begins with its gross appearance. Normal ascitic fluid is slightly yellow and transparent. The presence of more than 5000 leukocytes/mm³ will cause the fluid to be cloudy, whereas ascitic fluid specimens with fewer than 1000 cells/mm³ are nearly clear. Blood within the ascitic fluid may be due to a traumatic tap, in which case the fluid may be blood streaked and will often clot unless immediately transferred to a tube containing an anticoagulant. Nontraumatic blood-tinged ascitic fluid does not clot because the required factors have been depleted by previous clotting within the peritoneal cavity. Lipid within the ascitic fluid, such as that which accompanies chylous ascites, causes the fluid to appear opalescent, ranging from cloudy to completely opaque. If placed in the refrigerator for 48 to 72 hours, the lipids usually layer out.

The most valuable laboratory tests on ascitic fluid are the cell count and differential and the ascitic fluid albumin and total protein concentrations. The leukocyte count in uncomplicated cirrhotic ascites is usually less than 500 cells/mm³, and about half of these cells are neutrophils. More than 250 neutrophils/mm³ of ascitic fluid suggests an acute inflammatory process, the most common of which is spontaneous bacterial peritonitis. In this instance, both the total white blood cell count and the absolute neutrophil count are elevated, and neutrophils usually account for more than 70% of the total cell count.

The serum-ascites albumin gradient (SAAG) is the most reliable method to categorize the various causes of ascites. The SAAG is calculated by measuring the albumin concentration of serum and ascitic fluid specimens and subtracting the ascitic fluid value from the serum value. If the SAAG is greater than or equal to 1.1 g/dL, the patient has portal hypertension; an SAAG of less than 1.1 g/dL is consistent with the absence of portal hypertension. Examples of high- and low-gradient causes of ascites are shown in Table 43-2. The accuracy of this measurement in predicting the presence or absence of portal hypertension is about 97%.[13]

Table 43-2 Classification of Ascites by Serum-Ascites Albumin Gradient

HIGH GRADIENT (≥1.1 g/dL)	LOW GRADIENT (<1.1 g/dL)
Cirrhosis	Peritoneal carcinomatosis
Alcoholic hepatitis	Tuberculous peritonitis
Cardiac ascites	Pancreatic ascites
Massive liver metastases	Biliary ascites
Fulminant hepatic failure	Nephrotic syndrome
Budd-Chiari syndrome	Postoperative lymphatic leak
Portal vein thrombosis	Serositis in connective tissue diseases
Myxedema	

From Runyon B: Ascites; spontaneous bacterial peritonitis. In Sleisenger MH, Feldman M, Friedman LS (eds): Sleisenger and Fordtran's Gastrointestinal and Liver Disease: Pathophysiology/Diagnosis/Management, 7th ed. Philadelphia, WB Saunders, p 1523.

Management of Ascites in Cirrhotic Patients

The standard treatment protocol for patients with ascites due to cirrhosis is a stepwise approach beginning with sodium restriction, diuretic therapy, and paracentesis.[9,11,14] The initial goal of medical therapy is to induce a state in which renal sodium excretion exceeds sodium intake, a situation that will reduce the extracellular volume and improve ascites. A reasonable dietary sodium restriction for most cirrhotic patients with ascites is 2 g/day. Patient compliance may be assessed by measuring the 24-hour urinary sodium excretion. Patients who are compliant with their dietary restriction and excrete more than 78 mmol/day of sodium in their urine lose weight. If the weight is increasing despite urinary sodium losses greater than 78 mmol/day, one can assume that the patient is consuming more sodium than is prescribed. Spironolactone and furosemide, when given in a dosing ratio of 100:40, will promote natriuresis while maintaining normokalemia. In general, spironolactone (100 mg/day) and furosemide (40 mg/day) are begun initially. If this regimen is ineffective in both increasing urinary sodium and decreasing body weight, the doses of these drugs may be increased while maintaining the 100:40 ratio.

Large-volume paracentesis, in which more than 5 liters of ascites fluid is removed from the peritoneal cavity, may be useful for patients with ascites that has been unresponsive to sodium restriction and diuretic treatment; this occurs in less than 10% of patients. The intravenous (IV) infusion of albumin (6-8 g/L of ascitic fluid removed) at the time of paracentesis will minimize the symptoms of intravascular volume depletion and renal insufficiency, which may accompany the removal of large volumes of ascitic fluid. The continuation of diuretics and salt restriction will prevent or delay the reaccumulation of ascites after paracentesis. Others have suggested that weekly albumin administration, independent of large-volume paracentesis, may be a useful adjunct to salt restriction and diuretic therapy in patients with refractory ascites.[15] Transjugular intrahepatic portosystemic shunt, peritoneovenous shunts, and, ultimately, hepatic transplantation have been used to manage ascites refractory to simpler, less invasive options. These modalities are discussed in Chapter 53.

Chylous Ascites

Chylous ascites is the collection of chyle in the peritoneal cavity and may result from one of three principal mechanisms:

1. Obstruction of the major lymphatic channels at the base of the mesentery or the cisterna chyli, with exudation of chyle from dilated mesenteric lymphatics
2. Direct leakage of chyle through a lymphoperitoneal fistula due to abnormal or injured retroperitoneal lymphatic vessels
3. Exudation of chyle through the walls of retroperitoneal megalymphatics without a visible fistula or thoracic duct obstruction

In adults, the most common cause of chylous ascites is an intra-abdominal malignancy obstructing the lymphatic channels at the base of the mesentery or in the retroperitoneum. Lymphoma is the most common malignancy associated with chylous ascites, although chylous ascites has also been associated with ovarian, colon, renal, prostate, pancreatic, and gastric malignancies. Carcinoid tumors may cause chylous ascites by obstructing the lymphatics at the base of the mesentery through direct invasion and the dense fibrosis characteristic of this neoplasm. Chylous ascites may also result from injury of the retroperitoneal lymphatics during surgical procedures such as operations on the abdominal aorta and retroperitoneal lymph node dissections. Blunt and penetrating traumatic injuries are also important causes of chylous ascites, particularly in children. Chylous ascites in children may be due to congenital lymphatic abnormalities, such as primary lymphatic hypoplasia, resulting in lower extremity lymphedema, chylothorax, and chylous ascites.

Patients with chylous ascites most often present with painless abdominal distention. Malnutrition and dyspnea occur in about 50% of cases. Paracentesis yields a characteristic milky fluid with a high protein and fat content. The SAAG will be less than 1.1 mg/dL, and the triglyceride level will be greater than that of plasma, often two to eight times that of plasma. CT, lymphoscintigraphy, and lymphangiography may provide information regarding the site of obstruction, although the latter two modalities are rarely available.

Management of patients with chylous ascites includes the maintenance or improvement of nutrition, reduction in the rate of chyle formation, and correction of the underlying disease process. A low-fat, medium-chain triglyceride diet, combined with diuretics, has been used successfully to treat adults with chylous ascites complicating retroperitoneal lymph node dissections.[16] It is postulated that reducing long-chain triglyceride intake will reduce the rate of chyle flow because their metabolites are transported through the splanchnic lymphatics as chylomicrons. In contrast, medium-chain triglycerides are directly absorbed by enterocytes and transported to the liver through the splanchnic blood vessels as free fatty acids and glycerol. Fasting with total parenteral nutrition, either alone or in combination with somatostatin, has also been used successfully to manage patients with retroperitoneal lymphatic leak.[17,18] Paracentesis may temporarily relieve the dyspnea and abdominal discomfort associated with chylous ascites; however, repeated paracentesis leads to hypoproteinemia and malnutrition. Experience with peritoneovenous shunts to treat chylous ascites has generally been disappointing. Surgical exploration of the abdomen and the retroperitoneum is generally reserved for those patients failing to improve with nonoperative management.

Peritonitis

Peritonitis is inflammation of the peritoneum and peritoneal cavity and is most commonly due to a localized or generalized infection. Primary peritonitis results from bacterial, chlamydial, fungal, or mycobacterial infection in the absence of perforation of the gastrointestinal tract, whereas secondary peritonitis occurs in the setting of gastrointestinal perforation. Frequent causes of secondary bacterial peritonitis include peptic ulcer disease, acute appendicitis, colonic diverticulitis, and pelvic inflammatory disease.

Spontaneous Bacterial Peritonitis

Spontaneous bacterial peritonitis (SBP) is defined as a bacterial infection of ascitic fluid in the absence of an intra-abdominal, surgically treatable source of infection. Although most commonly associated with cirrhosis, SBP may also occur in patients with nephrotic syndrome and, less commonly, congestive heart failure. It is extremely rare for patients with ascitic fluid containing a high protein concentration to develop SBP, such as those with peritoneal carcinomatosis.[19] The most common pathogens in adults with SBP are the aerobic enteric flora *Escherichia coli* and *Klebsiella pneumoniae*. In children with nephrogenic or hepatogenic ascites, group A streptococcus, *Staphylococcus aureus*, and *Streptococcus pneumonia* are common isolates. The pathogenesis of SBP remains unclear; however, several lines of evidence suggest that bacterial translocation from the gastrointestinal tract plays an important role in the development of this infection.[20] It is postulated that local and systemic immune dysfunction in cirrhotic patients prevents effective opsonization, phagocytosis, and killing of translocated bacteria. Gomez and associates[21] reported impaired Fc gamma receptors on the surface of macrophages of cirrhotic patients, which may prevent effective phagocytosis. Others have suggested that a low ascitic fluid opsonic activity also prevents effective uptake and killing of bacteria by both macrophages and neutrophils.[22,23]

The diagnosis of SBP is made initially by demonstrating more than 250 neutrophils/mm^3 of ascitic fluid in a clinical setting consistent with this diagnosis, that is, abdominal pain, fever, or leukocytosis in a patient with low-protein ascites.[19] It is very unusual to document bacterascites on Gram stain of ascitic fluid, and delay of appropriate antibiotic management until the ascitic fluid cultures grow bacterial isolates risks the development of overwhelming infection and death.

Broad-spectrum antibiotics, such as a third-generation cephalosporin, are started immediately in patients suspected of having ascitic fluid infection. These agents cover about 95% of the flora most commonly associated with SBP. The spectrum of the antibiotic coverage may be narrowed once the results of antibiotic sensitivity tests are known. Repeat paracentesis with ascitic fluid analysis is not needed in the usual case in which there is rapid improvement in response to antibiotic therapy. If the setting, symptoms, ascitic fluid analysis, or response to therapy are atypical, repeat paracentesis may be helpful in detecting secondary peritonitis. Multiple bacterial isolates, particularly of gram-negative enteric organisms, combined with a poor response to antibiotic therapy, suggests the presence of secondary peritonitis.

The immediate mortality risk due to SBP is low, particularly if recognized and treated expeditiously. However, the development of other complications of hepatic failure, including gastrointestinal hemorrhage or hepatorenal syndrome, contributes to the death of many of these patients during the hospitalization in which SBP is detected. The occurrence of SBP is an important landmark in the natural history of cirrhosis, with 1- and 2-year survival rates of about 30% and 20%, respectively.[19] Several recent studies, including a randomized controlled trial, have shown that plasma expansion with albumin improves circulatory function and reduces the risk for hepatorenal syndrome and hospital mortality in patients with SBP.[24,25]

Tuberculous Peritonitis

Tuberculosis is common in impoverished areas of the world and is encountered with increasing frequency in the United States and other developed countries. Since 1985, the number of cases of tuberculosis in the United States and European nations has increased dramatically as the number of immigrants, refugees, and individuals with acquired immunodeficiency syndrome (AIDS) has increased. Others have described an association between peritoneal tuberculosis and alcoholic cirrhosis and chronic renal failure.[26,27] Peritoneal tuberculosis is the sixth most common site of extrapulmonary tuberculosis after lymphatic, genitourinary, bone and joint, miliary, and meningeal. Most cases of tuberculous peritonitis result from reactivation of latent peritoneal disease that had been previously established hematogenously from a primary pulmonary focus. About one-sixth of cases are associated with active pulmonary disease.

The illness often presents insidiously, with patients having had symptoms for several weeks to months at the time of presentation. Abdominal swelling due to ascites formation is the most common symptom, occurring in more that 80% of instances. Similarly, most patients complain of a nonlocalized, vague abdominal pain. Constitutional symptoms such as low-grade fever and night sweats, weight loss, anorexia, and malaise are reported in about 60% of patients. The concomitant presence of other chronic conditions such as uremia, cirrhosis, and AIDS makes these symptoms difficult to quantify. Abdominal tenderness is present upon palpation in about half of patients with peritoneal tuberculosis.[26] A positive tuberculin skin test is present in most cases, whereas only about half of these patients will have an abnormal chest radiograph. The ascitic fluid SAAG is less than 1.1 g/dL, consistent with a high protein concentration within the ascitic fluid. Microscopic examination of the ascites shows erythrocytes and an increased number of leukocytes, most of which are lymphocytes.

Abdominal imaging with ultrasound or CT may suggest the diagnosis but lacks the sensitivity and specificity to be diagnostic. Ultrasound may demonstrate the presence of echogenic material within the ascitic fluid, seen as fine mobile strands or particulate matter. CT will demonstrate the thickened and nodular mesentery with mesenteric lymphadenopathy and omental thickening.

The diagnosis is made by laparoscopy with directed biopsy of the peritoneum. In more than 90% of cases, laparoscopy demonstrates multiple whitish nodules (<5 mm) scattered over the visceral and parietal peritoneum; histologic examination of these nodules demonstrates caseating granulomas. Multiple adhesions are

commonly present between the abdominal organs and the parietal peritoneum. The gross appearance of the peritoneal cavity is similar to that of peritoneal carcinomatosis, sarcoidosis, and Crohn's disease, thus reiterating the importance of biopsy. Blind percutaneous peritoneal biopsy has a much lower yield than directed biopsy, and laparotomy with peritoneal biopsy is reserved for those cases in which laparoscopy has been nondiagnostic or cannot be safely performed. Microscopic examination of ascitic fluid for acid-fast bacilli identifies the organism in less than 3% of cases, and culture results are positive in less than 20% of cases. Furthermore, the diagnostic usefulness of mycobacterial cultures is further limited by the time it may take for the cultures to yield definitive information (up to 8 weeks).

Treatment of peritoneal tuberculosis includes antituberculous drugs. Drug regimens useful in treating pulmonary tuberculosis are also effective for peritoneal disease, with isoniazid and rifampin daily for 9 months being a commonly used and effective regimen.

Peritonitis Associated With Chronic Ambulatory Peritoneal Dialysis

In the United States, about 8% of patients with chronic renal failure undergo peritoneal dialysis. Peritonitis is one of the most common complications of chronic ambulatory peritoneal dialysis, occurring with an incidence of about one episode every 1 to 3 years. A recent study of all patients undergoing peritoneal dialysis in Scotland between 1999 and 2002 found that one episode of peritonitis occurred in every 19.2 months of peritoneal dialysis. Importantly, refractory or recurrent peritonitis was the most common cause of technical failure, accounting for 43% of all cases of technique failure.[28]

Patients present with abdominal pain, fever, and cloudy peritoneal dialysate containing more than 100 leukocytes/mm^3, with more than 50% of the cells being neutrophils. Gram stain detects organisms in only about 10% to 40% of cases. About 75% of infections are due to gram-positive organisms, with *Staphylococcus epidermidis* accounting for 30% to 50% of cases. *S. aureus,* gram-negative bacilli, and fungi are also important causes of dialysis-associated peritonitis.[28]

Peritoneal dialysis–associated peritonitis is treated by the intraperitoneal administration of antibiotics, most commonly a first-generation cephalosporin. Overall, 75% of infections are cured by culture-directed antibiotic therapy. The cure rate for peritonitis due to coagulase-negative staphylococcus is nearly 90%, compared with the rates for peritonitis due to *S. aureus,* gram-negative bacilli, or fungi of 66%, 56%, and 0%, respectively.[28] Recurrent or persistent peritonitis requires removal of the dialysis catheter and resumption of hemodialysis.

Malignant Neoplasms of the Peritoneum

Malignant neoplasms of the peritoneum may be classified as primary or secondary depending on the site of origin of the tumor. Primary malignancies of the peritoneum are rare and include malignant mesothelioma and sarcomas.

Most malignancies of the peritoneum are transperitoneal metastases from a carcinoma of the gastrointestinal tract (especially the stomach, colon, and pancreas), the genitourinary tract (most commonly, ovarian), or more rarely, an extra-abdominal site (e.g., breast). When metastatic cancer deposits diffusely coat the visceral and parietal peritoneum, these peritoneal metastases are referred to as *carcinomatosis.*

Malignant Peritoneal Mesothelioma

The most common primary malignant peritoneal neoplasm is malignant mesothelioma. The median survival rate for patients with this rare tumor is 4 to 12 months. At least in part, this poor prognosis is due to the very advanced stage of the disease at the time of presentation. Patients present with abdominal pain, ascites, and weight loss. Fifty to 70 percent of patients have a history of asbestos exposure.[29] The omentum may be diffusely involved with tumor and present as an epigastric mass. CT demonstrates mesenteric thickening, peritoneal studding, hemorrhage within the tumor, and ascites. At laparotomy, the ascitic fluid ranges from a serous transudate to a viscous fluid rich in mucopolysaccharides. The neoplasm tends to involve all peritoneal surfaces, producing large masses of tumor. In contrast to pseudomyxoma peritonei, local invasion of intra-abdominal organs, such as the liver, intestine, bladder, and abdominal wall, is common.

It may be difficult to differentiate a malignant peritoneal mesothelioma from diffuse peritoneal carcinomatosis arising from an intra-abdominal organ such as the stomach, pancreas, colon, or ovary. Careful intraoperative examination of the pattern of spread and biopsy with histologic examination allow this distinction to be made. Furthermore, malignant peritoneal mesothelioma generally remains confined to the abdomen, whereas advanced-stage intra-abdominal carcinomas frequently have pulmonary and other extra-abdominal metastases. Extension of the mesothelioma into one or both pleural cavities is more likely than hematogenous dissemination.

Complete surgical resection is technically challenging and requires peritonectomy with resection of involved organs. Combined-modality approaches using surgery and chemotherapy hint of a brighter future. In one retrospective review of 15 patients treated with cytoreductive surgery and chemotherapy, Eltabbakh and colleagues[30] reported a median survival time of 29 months. Radiation therapy alone, whether using open-field techniques, intraperitoneal instillation of radioactive agents, or external-beam irradiation, has had very limited success and substantial associated morbidity. Intraperitoneal chemotherapy, including the use of cisplatin and mitomycin C, has been reported but with very limited success. Even in those patients with complete response, relapse is generally rapid. Park and associates[31] reported that cytoreductive surgery, followed by hyperthermic peritoneal perfusion with cisplatin, led to a median progression-free survival time of 26 months and an overall 2-year survival rate of 80%. Loggie and associates[29] combined cytoreductive surgery with intraperitoneal hyperthermic perfusion with mitomycin C in 12 patients for whom the median

survival time was 34.2 months with follow-up to 45 months.

Pseudomyxoma Peritonei

Pseudomyxoma peritonei is a rare malignant process of the peritoneal cavity that characteristically arises from a ruptured ovarian or appendiceal adenocarcinoma. In this disease, the peritoneum becomes coated with a mucus-secreting tumor that fills the peritoneal cavity with tenacious, semisolid mucus and large loculated cystic masses. Pseudomyxoma peritonei is most prevalent in women between 50 and 70 years of age. It is often asymptomatic until very late in its course, and patients often experience a global deterioration in their health long before the diagnosis of pseudomyxoma peritonei is made. Symptoms include abdominal pain and distention as well as numerous nonspecific symptoms. Physical examination reveals a distended abdomen with nonshifting dullness. On occasion, a palpable abdominal mass may be present, especially in tumors of appendiceal origin. CT may demonstrate posterior displacement of the small intestine, loculated collections of fluid-density material, and scalloping of intra-abdominal organs due to extrinsic compression by adjacent peritoneal implants. At laparotomy, liters of yellowish gray mucoid material is present on the omental and peritoneal surfaces.

The management of these patients includes drainage of the mucus and intraperitoneal fluid and cytoreduction of the primary and secondary tumor implants, including peritonectomy and omentectomy. For those tumors originating from an appendiceal adenocarcinoma, a right colectomy is also performed. Ovarian malignancies are treated with total abdominal hysterectomy and bilateral salpingo-oophorectomy as well as cytoreduction. In the setting of an indeterminate site of origin, a right colectomy and resection of the omentum along with bilateral oophorectomy and cytoreduction surgery are performed. Postoperative adjuvant therapy has included the use of intraperitoneal 5-fluorouracil, mitomycin C, and oxiliplatin, as well as intraperitoneal mucolytics, such as dextran sulfate and plasminogen activator (urokinase). Although the tumor recurs in about two thirds of patients, the slow progression of the disease results in 5- and 10-year survival rates of 50% and 20%, respectively.[32] In some reports, aggressive cytoreductive surgery combined with intraperitoneal 5-fluorouracil and mitomycin C resulted in a 10-year survival rate of 80%.[33]

MESENTERY AND OMENTUM

Embryology and Anatomy

The greater and lesser omenta are complex peritoneal folds that pass from the stomach to the liver, transverse colon, spleen, bile duct, pancreas, and diaphragm. They originate from the dorsal and ventral midline mesenteries of the embryonic gut. In the very early stages of development, the alimentary canal traverses the future coelomic cavity as a straight tube suspended posteriorly by an uninterrupted dorsal mesentery and anteriorly by a ventral mesentery in the cranial portion of its extent. The embryonic stomach rotates 90 degrees on its longitudinal axis such that the lesser curvature faces to the right and the greater curvature to the left. Much of the embryonic ventral mesentery is resorbed; however, the portion extending from the fissure of the ligamentum venosum and the porta hepatis to the proximal duodenum and the lesser curvature of the stomach (gastrohepatic ligament) persists as the lesser omentum. The right border of the lesser omentum is a free edge that forms the anterior border of the opening into the lesser sac, termed the *foramen of Winslow.* Between the layers of the lesser omentum and at its right border are the common hepatic duct, the portal vein, and the hepatic artery.

The embryonic dorsal mesogastrium grows as a sheet of peritoneum extending from the greater curvature of the stomach over the anterior surface of the small intestine. After passing inferiorly almost to the pelvis, the peritoneal membrane turns up on itself to pass upward to a line of attachment on the transverse colon slightly above that of the transverse mesocolon. Fat is laid down in this omental apron and provides an insulating layer of protection of the abdominal viscera.

Early in its development, the small intestine elongates to form an anteriorly oriented intestinal loop, which then rotates counterclockwise such that the cecum and the ascending colon move to the right side of the peritoneal cavity and the descending colon assumes a vertical position on the left wall of the peritoneal cavity. The jejunum and ileum are supported by the peritoneum-covered dorsal mesentery carrying the mesenteric blood vessels and lymphatics. The posterior line of attachment of the mesentery extends obliquely from the duodenojejunal junction at the left side of the second lumbar vertebra toward the right iliac fossa to terminate anterior to the sacroiliac articulation.

Physiology

The omentum and the intestinal mesentery are rich in lymphatics and blood vessels. The omentum contains areas with high concentrations of macrophages, which may aid in the removal of foreign material and bacteria. Furthermore, the omentum becomes densely adherent to intraperitoneal sites of inflammation, often preventing diffuse peritonitis during instances of intestinal gangrene or perforation, such as acute diverticulitis or acute appendicitis.

Diseases of the Omentum

Omental Cysts

Omental cysts are unilocular or multilocular cysts containing serous fluid that are thought to arise from congenital or acquired obstruction of omental lymphatic channels. They are lined by a lymphatic endothelium similar to that of cystic lymphangiomas. These lesions are most common in children or young adults, in whom small cysts are usually asymptomatic and discovered incidentally, whereas larger cysts present as a palpable abdominal mass. Uncomplicated cysts usually lie in the lower mid abdomen and are freely moveable, smooth,

and nontender. Complications are more common in children and include torsion, infection, and rupture.

Plain radiographs of the abdomen may show a well-circumscribed soft tissue density in the mid abdomen, and contrast studies of the intestine may show displacement of intestinal loops and extrinsic compression on adjacent bowel. Ultrasound or CT will show a fluid-filled, complex, cystic mass with internal septations. The differential diagnosis of these lesions includes cysts and solid tumors of the mesentery, peritoneum, and retroperitoneum, including desmoid tumors. Ultimately, the diagnosis is made by excision of the cyst and histologic examination of the wall. Local excision is curative; recently, laparoscopic resection of these lesions has been reported.

Omental Torsion and Infarction

Torsion of the greater omentum is defined as the axial twisting of the omentum along its long axis. If the twist is tight enough (or the venous obstruction is of sufficient duration), arterial inflow will become compromised, leading to infarction and necrosis. Omental torsion is classified as primary when no coexisting causative condition is identified or secondary when the torsion occurs in association with a causative condition such as a hernia, tumor, or adhesion. Primary omental torsion most commonly involves the right side of the omentum.

Omental torsion occurs twice as often in men as women and is most frequent in patients in their fourth or fifth decade of life. Patients present with the acute onset of severe abdominal pain that is localized to the right side of the abdomen in 80% of patients. Nausea and vomiting may be present but are not predominant findings. The patient's temperature is usually normal, and palpation of the abdomen demonstrates localized abdominal tenderness with guarding, suggesting peritonitis. A mass may be palpable if the involved omentum is sufficiently large.

The differential diagnosis includes any disease associated with right-sided abdominal pain and tenderness, most notably acute appendicitis, acute cholecystitis, and torsion of an ovarian cyst. CT often demonstrates an omental mass with signs of inflammation. Usually, the patient's clinical presentation justifies laparotomy or laparoscopy, at which time a segment of the omentum appears congested and acutely inflamed. Serosanguineous fluid often is present in the peritoneal cavity. Treatment consists of resection of the involved omentum and correction of any related condition.

Omental Neoplasms

Primary malignancies of the omentum are extremely rare and are usually of soft tissue origin. More commonly, the omentum is invaded by metastatic tumor that has spread transperitoneally from an intra-abdominal carcinoma.

Omental Grafts and Transpositions

The arterial and venous blood supply to the greater omentum are derived from omental branches of the right and left gastroepiploic arteries, which course along the greater curvature of the stomach. Division of the right or

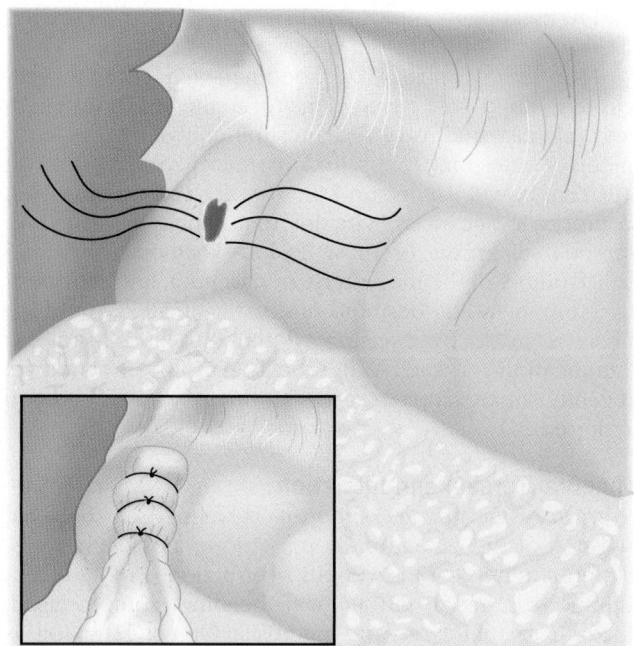

Figure 43-11 Closure of a perforated duodenal ulcer with an omental (Graham) patch. (From Graham RR: The treatment of perforated duodenal ulcers. Surg Gynecol Obstet 64:235-238, 1937.)

left gastroepiploic artery and the vasa recta along the greater curvature of the stomach with mobilization of the omentum from the transverse colon allows the development of a vascularized omental pedicle flap. This graft may be used to cover chest and mediastinal wounds after chest wall resections and to prevent the small intestine from entering the pelvis after abdominal perineal resection (thus preventing radiation enteritis during radiation therapy for rectal carcinoma). Lastly, the formation of dense adhesions between the omentum and sites of perforation or inflammation facilitates its use as a patch for duodenal perforations from ulcer disease (termed a *Graham patch,* Fig. 43-11).

Diseases of the Mesentery

Mesenteric Cysts

The most common non-neoplastic mesenteric cysts are termed *mesothelial cysts* based on the ultrastructure of the cells lining the cyst. The cysts contain either chyle or a clear serous fluid and may occur in the mesentery of either the small intestine (60%) or the colon (40%). These cysts occur most commonly in adults with a mean age of 45 years and are twice as common in women as in men. Depending on the size of the cyst, patients may present with complaints of abdominal pain, fever, and emesis. A midabdominal mass may be palpable upon examination of the abdomen. The diagnosis can usually be made preoperatively with ultrasonography or CT. Enucleation of the cyst at laparotomy is curative and can usually be accomplished because the mesenteric blood vessels and the intestinal wall are usually not adherent to the cyst wall. Internal drainage of the cyst into the

peritoneal cavity has also been successfully employed in the management of very large cysts. Aspiration alone has a very high rate of cyst recurrence. In those instances in which the cyst is not completely excised, the contents of the cyst and the internal architecture of the cyst wall must be carefully inspected and the cyst wall examined histologically to ensure a non-neoplastic etiology.

Acute Mesenteric Lymphadenitis

Acute mesenteric lymphadenitis is a syndrome of acute right lower quadrant abdominal pain associated with mesenteric lymph node enlargement and a normal appendix. Generally, the diagnosis is made upon exploration of the abdomen of a patient suspected of having acute appendicitis at which time a normal appendix and enlarged mesenteric lymph nodes are discovered. This syndrome occurs most commonly in children and young adults and occurs with equal frequency in males and females.

Numerous causative agents have been implicated in the pathobiology of acute mesenteric lymphadenitis, including viral, bacterial, parasitic, and fungal infections. *Yersinia enterocolitica* in particular has been associated with this syndrome in children. Culture and histologic examination of the enlarged lymph nodes, stool culture, and antibody titers have been used to identify causative agents but are not routinely employed in the management of these patients.

The symptom complex associated with acute mesenteric lymphadenitis is similar to that of acute appendicitis and includes the acute onset of periumbilical pain, which shifts to the right lower quadrant over time. Physical examination demonstrates right lower quadrant tenderness with abdominal wall muscular rigidity and rebound tenderness. Nausea, vomiting, and anorexia may also be present but are not dominant symptoms. Generally, the patient's temperature and white blood cell count are normal or only slightly elevated.

The diagnosis is made at the time of operation for presumed acute appendicitis, at which time a normal-appearing appendix is found with enlarged mesenteric lymph nodes. Excision of an enlarged lymph node with culture and nodal histology may provide information regarding the etiology but is not routinely employed.

Mesenteric Panniculitis

Mesenteric panniculitis is a rare inflammatory disease of the mesentery characterized by fat necrosis, acute and chronic inflammation, and fibrosis. It is postulated that these three pathologic features represent different stages of the same disease. Grossly, this condition is characterized by marked thickening of the mesentery of the small intestine with irregular areas of discoloration suggesting fat necrosis. There may also be multiple discrete nodules on the mesentery, or the disease may appear as a single matted mass. The process most often involves the root of the small bowel mesentery and frequently encompasses the mesenteric vessels. In advanced cases, mesenteric venous and lymphatic obstruction may be present. The mesocolon may also be affected but less frequently than the small bowel mesentery.

Mesenteric panniculitis is twice as common in males as females and occurs most commonly in the fifth decade of life. Most patients are asymptomatic, and the diagnosis is discovered incidentally upon imaging for an unrelated condition. Of those patients with symptoms, abdominal pain or symptoms of intestinal obstruction with nausea, vomiting, and abdominal distention are most common. An abdominal mass is palpable in more than half of patients. Laboratory studies are usually normal, except that the erythrocyte sedimentation rate and C-reactive protein levels may be elevated.

The differential diagnosis of mesenteric panniculitis includes a heterogenous group of conditions that alter the density of the mesenteric fat, including a variety of inflammatory and neoplastic causes. Differentiation of mesenteric panniculitis from peritoneal carcinomatosis, carcinoid tumor, and mesenteric and retroperitoneal sarcomas is particularly important. Following is a list of the CT characteristics of mesenteric panniculitis, which have been well described[34]:

1. A fatty mass arising from the base of mesentery, which has well-delineated margins separating it from normal mesentery, a feature described as a *tumoral pseudocapsule*
2. The presence of normal adipose tissue surrounding mesenteric vessels, termed *fat ring sign*
3. The presence of normal mesenteric vessels coursing through the fatty mass without evidence of vascular involvement or deviation
4. An intra-abdominal mass that displaces adjacent bowel loops without invading them

Laparotomy or laparoscopy with biopsy of the involved mesentery remains necessary for definitive diagnosis.

Most patients with mesenteric panniculitis experience spontaneous resolution of their symptoms. Of those without improvement, corticosteroids and a variety of other anti-inflammatory and immunosuppressive agents have been reported to be successful in improving the symptoms and radiographic findings. Operative management is indicated only in those cases in which there is confusion regarding the diagnosis and for treatment of intestinal obstruction.

Intra-abdominal (Internal) Hernias

Internal Hernias Due to Developmental Defects

There are three general mechanisms by which developmental abnormalities cause the formation of internal hernias:

1. Abnormal retroperitoneal fixation of the mesentery resulting in anomalous positioning of the intestine (e.g., mesocolic or paraduodenal hernias)
2. Abnormally large internal foramina or fossae (e.g., foramen of Winslow and supravesical hernias)
3. Incomplete mesenteric surfaces with the presence of an abnormal opening through which the intestine herniates (e.g., mesenteric hernias)

The anatomic and radiographic features of both acquired and congenital internal hernias are the subject of an excellent review by Martin and colleagues.[35]

Mesocolic (or Paraduodenal) Hernias

Mesocolic hernias are unusual congenital hernias in which the small intestine herniates behind the mesocolon. They result from abnormal rotation of the midgut and have been categorized as either right or left. A right mesocolic hernia occurs when the prearterial limb of the midgut loop fails to rotate around the superior mesenteric artery. This results in the majority of the small intestine remaining to the right of the superior mesenteric artery. Normal counterclockwise rotation of the cecum and proximal colon into the right side of the abdomen and its fixation to the posterolateral peritoneum cause the small intestine to become trapped behind the mesentery of the right side of the colon. The ileocolic, right colic, and middle colic vessels lie within the anterior wall of the sac, and the superior mesenteric artery courses along the medial border of the neck of the hernia (Fig. 43-12A). It is postulated that left mesocolic hernias occur as a consequence of in utero herniation of the small intestine between the inferior mesenteric vein and the posterior parietal attachments of the descending mesocolon to the retroperitoneum. The inferior mesenteric artery and vein are integral components of the hernia sac (see Fig. 43-12B). About 75% of mesocolic hernias occur on the left side.

Patients with paraduodenal hernias most commonly present with symptoms of acute or chronic small bowel obstruction. Barium radiographs will demonstrate displacement of the small intestine to the left or the right side of the abdomen. CT with IV contrast may demonstrate displacement of the mesenteric vessels and evidence of intestinal obstruction, if present.

The operative management of patients with a right mesocolic hernia involves incision of the lateral peritoneal reflections along the right colon with reflection of the right colon and cecum to the left. The entire gut then assumes a position simulating that of nonrotation of both the prearterial and postarterial segments of the midgut. Opening the neck of the hernia will injure the superior mesenteric vessels and fail to free the herniated bowel (see Fig. 43-12C).

The operative management of patients with a left mesocolic hernia consists of incision of the peritoneal attachments and adhesions along the right side of the inferior mesenteric vein with reduction of the herniated small intestine from beneath the inferior mesenteric vein. The vein is then allowed to return to its normal position on the left side of the base of the mesentery of the small intestine. The neck of the hernia may be closed by suturing the peritoneum adjacent to the vein to the retroperitoneum (see Fig. 43-12D).

Mesenteric Hernias

Mesenteric hernias occur when the intestine herniates through an abnormal orifice in the mesentery of the small intestine or colon. The most common location for these hernias is near the ileocolic junction, although defects in the sigmoid mesocolon have also been described. Patients present with intestinal obstruction resulting from compression of the loops of bowel at the neck of the hernia or by torsion of the herniated segment. Management of

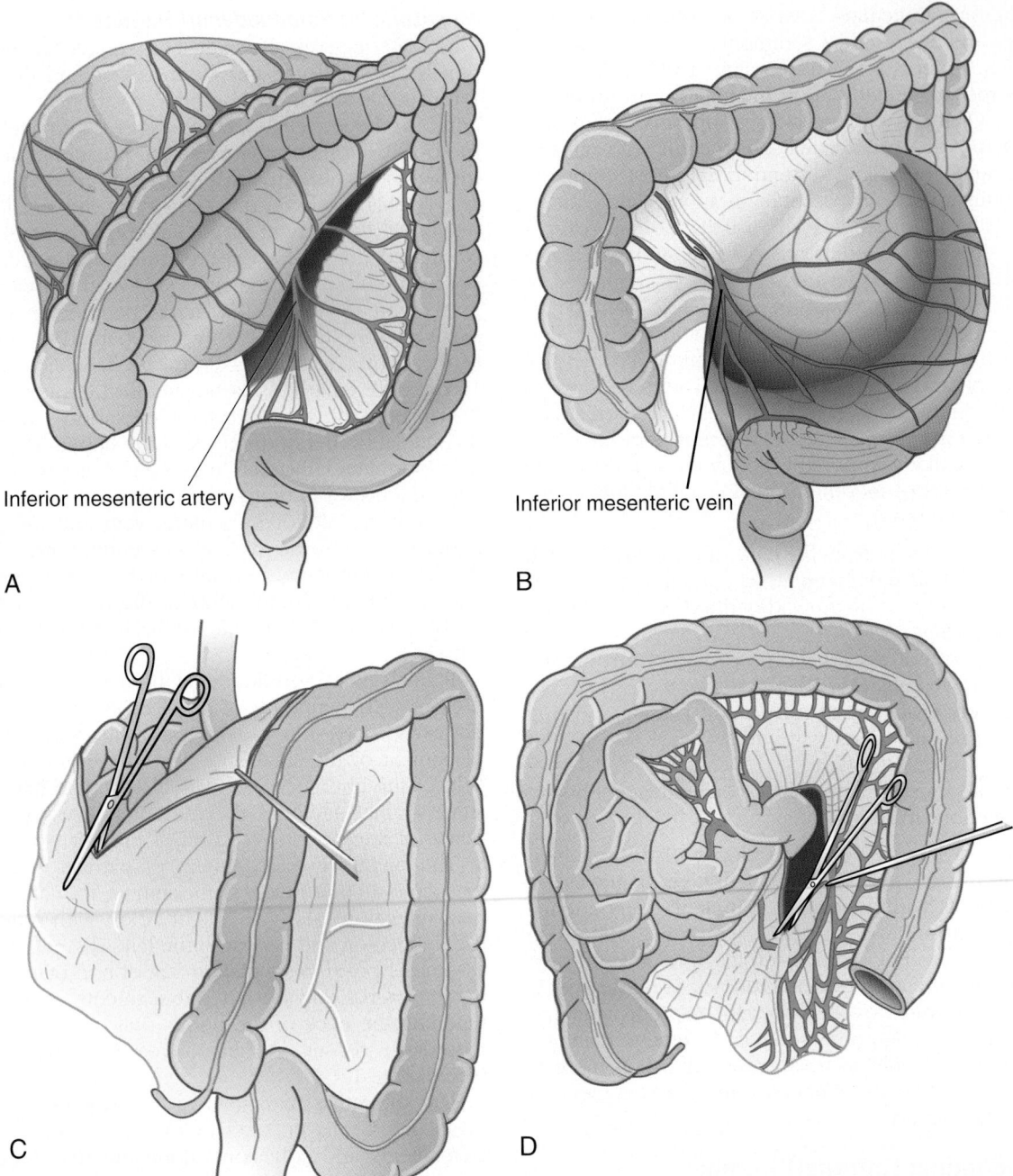

Inferior mesenteric artery

Inferior mesenteric vein

A

B

C

D

Figure 43-12 A, Right mesocolic (paraduodenal) hernia. Note that the anterior wall of a right mesocolic hernia is the ascending mesocolon. The hernia orifice lies to the right of the midline, and the superior mesenteric artery and ileocolic artery course along the anterior border of the hernia neck. **B,** Left mesocolic (paraduodenal) hernia. The hernia orifice is to the left of the midline, and the herniated intestine lies behind the anterior wall of the descending mesocolon. **C,** A right mesocolic hernia is repaired by division of the lateral peritoneal attachments of the ascending colon, reflecting it toward the left side of the abdomen. The small and large intestine then assumes a position simulating that of nonrotation of both the prearterial and postarterial segments of the midgut. Opening the neck of the hernia will injure the superior mesenteric vessels and fail to free the herniated bowel. **D,** A left mesocolic hernia is reduced by incising the hernia sac along an avascular plane immediately to the right of the inferior mesenteric vessels. **A** and **B,** From Brigham RA, d'Avis JC: Paraduodenal hernia. In Nyhus LM, Condon RE [eds]: Hernia, 3rd ed. Philadelphia, JB Lippincott, 1989, pp 484 and 485. **C** and **D,** From Brigham R, Fallon WF, Saunders JR, et al: Paraduodenal hernia: Diagnosis and surgical management. Surgery 96:498, 1984.)

these patients involves reduction of the hernia and closure of the mesenteric defect.

Acquired Internal Hernias

Acquired internal hernias result from the creation of abnormal mesenteric defects after operative procedures or trauma. Most commonly, these result from inadequate closure (or dehiscence of) mesenteric defects created during the performance of gastrojejunostomy, colostomy, ileostomy or bowel resection. The creation of a small space allows the herniation of the small intestine through the mesenteric rent and the development of intestinal obstruction. Internal hernias, including strangulated hernias, have most recently been noted after the performance of operations for morbid obesity, especially Roux-en-Y gastric bypass.[36,37] The treatment of these patients is operative reduction of the hernia and closure of the peritoneal defect.

Malignancies of the Mesentery

Similar to the peritoneum and omentum, the most common neoplasm involving the mesentery is metastatic disease from an intra-abdominal adenocarcinoma. This may result from the direct invasion of the primary tumor (or its lymphatic metastases) into the mesentery or from the transperitoneal spread of the malignancy into the mesentery. Distortion and fixation of the mesentery by the tumor itself or by the resultant desmoplastic reaction, as in carcinoid tumors of the gastrointestinal tract, may cause intestinal obstruction. The most common primary malignancy of the mesentery is a desmoid tumor.

Mesenteric Desmoid

Mesenteric desmoid accounts for less than 10% of sporadic desmoid tumors; however, it is a particularly common tumor in patients with FAP. In this group of patients, 70% of the desmoid tumors are intra-abdominal, and one half to three fourths of these involve the mesentery.[3,4] The association between desmoid tumor and FAP is particularly strong in that subset of patients with Gardner's syndrome. Patients with FAP and family history of desmoid tumors have a 25% chance of developing a desmoid tumor.[3]

Although mesenteric desmoid tumors tend to be aggressive, there is considerable variability in their growth rate during the course of the disease. In fact, the biology of intra-abdominal desmoid may be characterized by initial rapid growth followed by stability, or even regression.[38] Mesenteric desmoid, by virtue of its relationship to vital structures and its ability to infiltrate adjacent organs, may however cause significant complications requiring operative management, including intestinal obstruction, ischemia and perforation, hydronephrosis, and even aortic rupture. Despite these complications, the overall 10-year survival rate for patients with intra-abdominal desmoids has been as high as 60% to 70%.[4,38]

The recurrence rate after attempted resection has been reported between 60% and 85%.[4] Given the high likelihood of recurrence and prolonged survival, even in the

setting of advanced disease, some authors have suggested that a trial of watchful waiting along with minimally toxic agents such as sulindac and antiestrogen therapy may be the best strategy, particularly in patients with minimal symptoms.[38] In this nascent era of target-specific biologic therapy, clinical response to imatinib by patients with heavily treated desmoid tumor has been reported. Imatinib mesylate, specifically designed to inhibit the Bcr-Abl tyrosine kinase rendered constitutive by the Philadelphia chromosome translocation in chronic myeloid leukemia (CML), also inhibits the tyrosine kinase receptor for platelet-derived growth factor (PDGF) and c-kit. The observation that patients with desmoid tumors have partial tumor response and arrest of disease progression while on oral imatinib offers an alternative to surgical resection of desmoid tumors arising in the mesentery.[39]

RETROPERITONEUM

Anatomy

The retroperitoneal space lies between the peritoneum and the posterior parietal wall of the abdominal cavity and extends from the diaphragm to the pelvic floor. This space contains the contiguous lumbar and iliac fossae. The lumbar fossa extends from the 12th thoracic vertebra and lateral lumbocostal arch superiorly to the base of the sacrum, iliac crest, and iliolumbar ligament inferiorly. The floor of the space is formed by the fascia overlying the quadratus lumborum and psoas major muscles. This space contains varying amounts of fatty areolar tissue as well as the adrenal glands, kidneys, ascending and descending colon and duodenum. It is also traversed by the ureter, renal vessels, gonadal vessels, inferior vena cava, and aorta. The iliac fossa is contiguous with the lumbar fossa superiorly, the lateral and anterior preperitoneal spaces of the abdominal wall, and the pelvis inferiorly. The iliacus muscle with its investing fascia is the floor of the iliac fossa. This fossa contains the iliac vessels, ureter, genitofemoral nerve, gonadal vessels, and iliac lymph nodes.

Retroperitoneal Operative Approaches

The aorta, vena cava, iliac vessels, kidneys, and adrenal glands may be approached operatively through the retroperitoneal space. Specific operative procedures performed through the retroperitoneum include extirpative procedures such as adrenalectomy and nephrectomy as well as aortic aneurysmorrhaphy and renal transplantation. The advantages to this approach over a transabdominal approach follow:

1. Less postoperative ileus facilitating a more rapid resumption of a diet
2. No intra-abdominal adhesions, thus decreasing the likelihood of subsequent small bowel obstruction
3. Less intraoperative evaporative fluid losses with less dramatic intravascular fluid shifts
4. Fewer respiratory complications, such as atelectasis and pneumonia

Retroperitoneal Abscesses

Retroperitoneal abscesses may be classified as primary if the infection results from hematogenous spread or secondary if it is related to an infection in an adjacent organ. The conditions associated with the development of retroperitoneal abscesses are shown in Table 43-3, and the anatomic relationship of retroperitoneal abscesses to surrounding structures is shown in Figure 43-13. Infections originating from the kidney and gastrointestinal tract most commonly underlie the development of retroperitoneal abscesses. Renal causes include infections related to renal lithiasis or previous urologic operative procedures. Gas-

trointestinal causes include appendicitis, diverticulitis, pancreatitis, and Crohn's disease. In one series from an urban center, tuberculosis of the spine was a common cause of retroperitoneal abscesses, with *Mycobacterium tuberculosis* being the second most common bacterial isolate, after *E. coli*.[40]

The bacteriology of retroperitoneal abscesses is related to the etiology. Infections originating from the kidney are often monomicrobial, involving gram-negative rods such as *Proteus mirabilis* and *E. coli*. Abscesses associated with diseases of the gastrointestinal tract involve *E. coli*, *Enterobacter* species, enterococci, and anaerobic species such as *Bacteroides*. These infections are multimicrobial, involving species such as gram-negative bacilli, enterococci, and anaerobic species. Infections from hematogenous spread are usually monomicrobial and related to staphylococcal species. Tuberculosis of the spine is an important cause of retroperitoneal abscesses in immunocompromised individuals and those immigrating from underdeveloped countries.

The most common symptoms of retroperitoneal abscesses include abdominal or flank pain (60%-75%), fever and chills (30%-90%), malaise (10%-22%), and weight loss (12%).[41,42] Patients with psoas abscesses may have referred pain to the hip, groin, or knee. The duration of symptoms is usually longer than 1 week. Patients with retroperitoneal abscesses often have concurrent, chronic illnesses such as renal lithiasis, diabetes mellitus, human immunodeficiency virus (HIV) infection, or malignancies. CT demonstrates a low-density mass within the retroperitoneum with surrounding inflammation. Gas may be present in as many as one third of these lesions.[40] CT provides important information regarding the location of the abscess as well as its relationship to contiguous organs, hence likely sources of the infection.

Table 43-3 **Etiology and Relative Frequency of Retroperitoneal Abscesses**

ETIOLOGY	FREQUENCY (%)
Renal diseases	47
Gastrointestinal diseases, including diverticulitis, appendicitis, and Crohn's disease	16
Hematogenous spread from remote infections	11
Abscesses complicating operative procedures	8
Bone infections, including tuberculosis of the spine	7
Trauma	4.5
Malignancies	4
Miscellaneous causes	3

These data were compiled from three retrospective reviews[40-42] of 134 patients treated between 1971 and 2001.

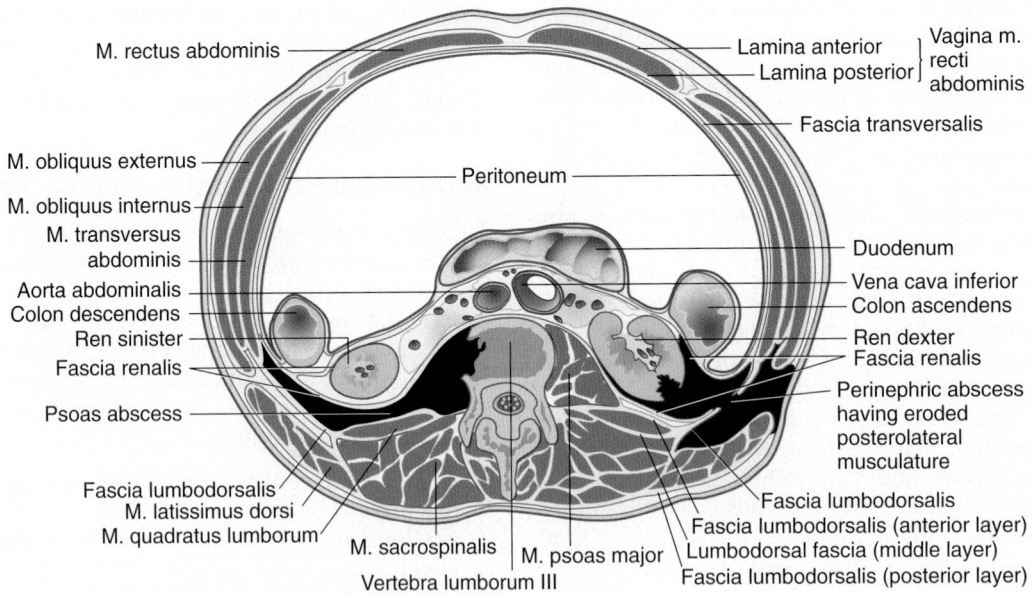

Figure 43-13 The anatomic relationships of retroperitoneal abscesses to surrounding structures. A psoas abscess is shown *on the left* and a perinephric abscess *on the right*. (From McVay C: Anson and McVay's Surgical Anatomy, 6th ed. Philadelphia, WB Saunders, 1984, p 735.)

Treatment of retroperitoneal abscesses includes appropriate antibiotics and adequate drainage. Many reports have demonstrated the efficacy of CT-guided drainage in managing this aspect of the treatment.[40,42] In one study, 86% of abscesses resolved with this approach.[42] Operative drainage through a retroperitoneal approach is indicated for those lesions not amenable to percutaneous drainage or those lesions that fail percutaneous drainage. The mortality rate for patients with retroperitoneal abscesses is related, in large part, to the presence of significant medical comorbidities. In one study in which 72% of patients had significant concurrent medical problems, the overall mortality rate was 26%, and the major complication rate was 50%.[41] In another recent study, in which many fewer patients had diabetes or other systemic illnesses, the mortality rate was only 1.6%.[42]

Retroperitoneal Hematomas

Retroperitoneal hematomas most commonly occur after blunt or penetrating injuries, in the setting of abdominal aortic or visceral artery aneurysms, or after acute or chronic anticoagulation or fibrinolytic therapy. The diagnosis and management of retroperitoneal hematomas occurring in the setting of trauma or aneurysmal rupture are considered in detail in Chapters 20, 65, and 67. Bleeding into the retroperitoneum also may complicate anticoagulant therapy, including low-molecular-weight heparin, for medical conditions such as atrial fibrillation or deep venous thrombosis. Retroperitoneal hematomas have also been described in patients undergoing fibrinolytic therapy for peripheral or coronary arterial thrombosis as well as in patients with bleeding diatheses such as hemophilia.

Patients present with abdominal or flank pain, which may radiate into the groin, labia, or scrotum. Clinical evidence of acute blood loss may be present depending on the volume of blood lost and the rapidity in which the patient bled. A palpable abdominal mass may be present as well as physical evidence of ileus. The complete blood count may provide evidence of subacute or chronic blood loss or platelet deficiency. The prothrombin and partial thromboplastin time may demonstrate a coagulopathy. Microscopic hematuria is a common finding on urinalysis. CT establishes the diagnosis by demonstrating a high-density mass in the retroperitoneum with surrounding stranding in the retroperitoneal tissue planes. These findings are readily distinguishable from the low-density mass characteristic of retroperitoneal abscesses.

Patients who develop retroperitoneal hematomas as a result of anticoagulation are best managed by the restoration of circulating blood volume and correction of the underlying coagulopathy. In rare circumstances, arteriography with embolization of a bleeding artery or operative exploration is required to stop the bleeding.

Retroperitoneal Fibrosis

Retroperitoneal fibrosis is an uncommon inflammatory condition characterized by the proliferation of fibrous tissue in the retroperitoneum. Seventy percent of cases are idiopathic (termed *Ormand disease*), whereas 30% are associated with various drugs (most notably, ergot alkaloids or dopaminergic agonists), infections, trauma, retroperitoneal hemorrhage or retroperitoneal operations, radiation therapy, or primary or metastatic neoplasms. Many of the idiopathic cases are associated with inflammatory abdominal aortic aneurysms or vasculitis syndromes. The fibrosis is usually confined to the central and paravertebral spaces between the renal arteries and sacrum and tends to encase the aorta, inferior vena cava, and ureters. The process usually begins at the level of the aortic bifurcation and spreads cephalad. In 15% of instances, the fibrotic process extends outside of the retroperitoneum to also involve the peripancreatic and periduodenal spaces, the pelvis, and the mediastinum.

Patients present with a vague constellation of symptoms, including abdominal or flank pain, weight loss, malaise, and hypertension. Scrotal or leg edema caused by lymphatic obstruction may also be present. Laboratory tests often provide evidence of renal insufficiency and anemia. Other laboratory abnormalities include an elevated erythrocyte sedimentation rate and an elevated C-reactive protein level.

The diagnosis is based on the patients' history and IV urography demonstrating hydronephrosis and hydroureter associated with delayed excretion and medial deviation of the ureters. Most commonly, the disease is bilateral, although unilateral cases do occur. CT without IV contrast will show a fibrous plaque that is usually isodense or slightly hyperdense compared with surrounding muscle. MRI of early benign retroperitoneal fibrosis may show areas of high signal intensity on T2-weighted images as a result of the abundant fluid content and hypercellularity associated with the acute inflammation. In the mature and quiescent stage of benign retroperitoneal fibrosis, the low signal intensity on both T1- and T2-weighted images is similar to that of psoas muscle. Malignant retroperitoneal fibrosis has signal intensities similar to early benign disease, that is, early enhancement with contrast.

Malignant retroperitoneal fibrosis may result from direct spread of malignant cells entrapping the ureter or from multiple metastases causing a severe desmoplastic reaction in the retroperitoneum. Hence, differentiating malignant from benign fibrosis is important and requires multiple biopsies of the retroperitoneal fibrotic tissue. Katz and colleagues[43] have reported good success with Tru-Cut needle biopsies under CT guidance. Primary, idiopathic retroperitoneal fibrosis is treated with ureteral stenting and immunosuppression including methylprednisolone, azathioprine, or penicillamine. Others have reported success with tamoxifen.[44] Most secondary cases of retroperitoneal fibrosis are treated with midline transperitoneal ureterolysis that includes wrapping the ureter with an omental flap or lateral retroperitoneal ureteral transposition. In one report of 14 patients undergoing ureterolysis with an omental flap, 12 had relief of ureteral obstruction on follow-up IV urograms.[43]

Retroperitoneal Malignancies

Malignancies in the retroperitoneum may result from the following:

1. Extracapsular growth of a primary neoplasm of a retroperitoneal organ such as the kidney, adrenal, colon, or pancreas
2. Development of a primary germ cell neoplasm from embryonic rest cells
3. Development of a primary malignancy of the retroperitoneal lymphatic system, for example, lymphoma
4. Metastases from a remote primary malignancy into a retroperitoneal lymph node, for example, testicular cancer
5. Development of a malignancy of the soft tissue of the retroperitoneum, for example, sarcomas and desmoid tumors

The most common primary malignancy of the retroperitoneum is a sarcoma.

Retroperitoneal Sarcoma

About 15% of all soft tissue sarcomas occur in the retroperitoneum, and about 8300 new cases of retroperitoneal sarcomas present in the United States each year.[45,46] Patients with von Recklinghausen's disease and Li-Fraumeni syndrome have an increased incidence of sarcoma. Furthermore, patients with mutations of the *p53* and *RB-1* genes also appear to have a predilection for the development of sarcoma, suggesting that these genes may play an important regulatory role in the malignant transformation to sarcoma.

Most patients with retroperitoneal sarcomas present with an asymptomatic abdominal mass, often after the primary tumor has reached a considerable size. Abdominal pain is present in half of patients, and less common symptoms include gastrointestinal hemorrhage, early satiety, nausea and vomiting, weight loss, and lower extremity swelling. Symptoms related to nerve compression by the tumor, such as lower extremity paresthesia and paresis, have also been associated with retroperitoneal sarcoma. CT and MRI provide important information regarding size and precise location of the primary tumor and its relationship to major vascular structures as well as the presence or absence of metastatic disease. Preoperative imaging studies provide important clues to the diagnosis; hence, CT-guided core biopsy is usually reserved for lesions significantly likely to be lymphoma or germ cell tumor. A CT scan of a large retrohepatic sarcoma is shown in Figure 43-14.

The goal of sarcoma treatment is complete en bloc resection of the tumor and any involved adjacent organs. Lymph node metastases by sarcoma are rare (<5%); therefore, radical lymphadenectomy is not indicated unless there is gross evidence of lymph node involvement at the time of resection. The prognostic factors in retroperitoneal sarcoma include the size of the tumor and the histologic grade. Rates of resectability of the primary retroperitoneal sarcoma vary widely, based on the extent of disease at presentation, the surgeon's experience, and the institution's referral pattern. Local recurrence after complete resection of retroperitoneal sarcoma is common, occurring in 40% to 80% of cases.[47,48] Although there is no difference in the rate of local recurrence when comparing high-grade and low-grade sarcomas, the median

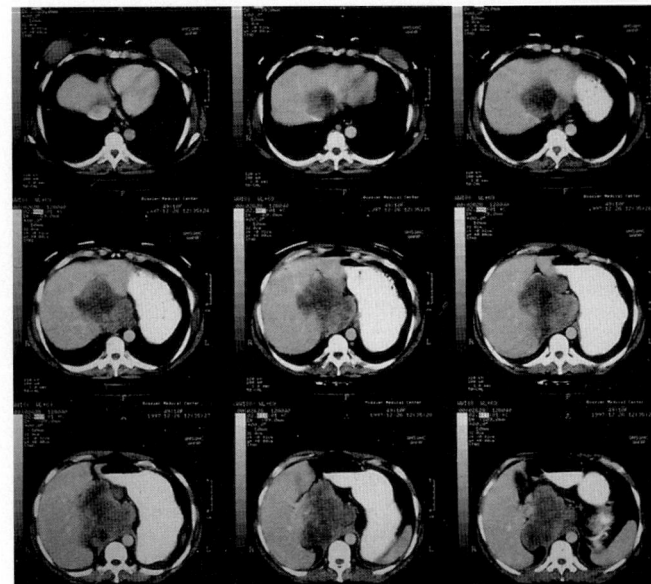

A

B

Figure 43-14 A, CT of the upper abdomen of a patient with a large sarcoma originating from the upper retroperitoneum. **B,** Intraoperative photograph.

time to recurrence is much shorter in high-grade than in low-grade sarcoma (15 months versus 42 months).[49] Additionally, patients with high-grade sarcoma also have a higher risk for systemic disease and death than patients with low-grade sarcoma.[47,48,50]

In patients with recurrent disease, complete resection of recurrent tumor is beneficial. In a report by Lewis and colleagues at the Memorial Sloan-Kettering Cancer Center,[47] of the 61 patients with recurrent sarcoma, 35 underwent complete resection. This group of patients had a significantly higher survival rate than those undergoing incomplete resection (60% versus 18% 5-year disease-specific survival). Unlike extremity sarcoma, the role for external-beam irradiation for local control after surgical resection is limited by the low tolerance for radiation injury of the surrounding normal tissue. External-beam radiation therapy and combined external-beam irradiation and intraoperative brachytherapy have been used for local control of these malignancies. Unfortunately, the potential benefits of radiation therapy after complete resection have been offset by the early and late radiation toxicity.

As with radiation therapy, most of the literature on the use of chemotherapy has been on extremity sarcoma. Specific retrospective studies on the efficacy of postoperative chemotherapy for retroperitoneal sarcoma have not shown significant benefits.[48] Limited experience with preoperative chemotherapy and radiation therapy for sarcoma has also been disappointing. As such, adjuvant therapy (chemotherapy and radiation therapy) in retroperitoneal sarcoma is offered in the context of a clinical trial. It may also play a role in the palliation of symptomatic inoperable disease.

Selected References

Guarner C, Runyon BA: Spontaneous bacterial peritonitis: Pathogenesis, diagnosis and management. Gastroenterologist 3:311-328, 1995.

> This is an outstanding review of the causes, diagnosis, and management of patients with spontaneous bacterial peritonitis.

Martin LC, Merkle EM, Thompson WM: Review of internal hernias: Radiographic and clinical findings. AJR Am J Roentgenol 186:703-717, 2006.

> This is a thorough and well-illustrated review of the types of congenital and acquired internal hernias.

Runyon BA, Montano AA, Akrividadis EA, et al: The serum-ascites albumin gradient is superior to the exudates-transudate concept in the differential diagnosis of ascites. Ann Intern Med 117:215-220, 1992.

> This well-written paper describes and defends the use of serum-ascites albumin gradient in the elucidation of the pathophysiology of ascites formation.

Thorek P: Anatomy in Surgery, 2nd ed. Philadelphia, JB Lippincott, 1962.
McVay C: Anson and McVay's Surgical Anatomy, 6th ed. Philadelphia, WB Saunders, 1984.

> Thorek's Anatomy in Surgery and Anson and McVay's Surgical Anatomy are classic texts of anatomy, beautifully illustrated and written from a surgeon's perspective.

Willwerth BM, Zollinger RM, Izant RJ: Congenital mesocolic (paraduodenal) hernia: Embryologic basis of repair. Am J Surg 128:358-361, 1974.

> This is a classic description of right and left mesocolic hernias. The authors suggest an embryologic basis for the occurrence of these hernias as well as a clear description of their management.

References

1. Cherry WB, Mueller PS: Rectus sheath hematoma: Review of 126 cases at a single institution. Medicine (Baltimore) 85:105-110, 2006.
2. Biermann JS: Desmoid tumors. Curr Treat Options Oncol 1:262-266, 2000.
3. Gurbuz AK, Giardiello FM, Petersen GM, et al: Desmoid tumours in familial adenomatous polyposis. Gut 35:377-381, 1994.
4. Kulaylat MN, Karakousis CP, Keaney CM, et al: Desmoid tumour: A pleomorphic lesion. Eur J Surg Oncol 25:487-497, 1999.
5. Gronchi A, Casali PG, Mariani L, et al: Quality of surgery and outcome in extra-abdominal aggressive fibromatosis: A series of patients surgically treated at a single institution. J Clin Oncol 21:1390-1397, 2003.
6. Nuyttens JJ, Rust PF, Thomas CR Jr, et al: Surgery versus radiation therapy for patients with aggressive fibromatosis or desmoid tumors: A comparative review of 22 articles. Cancer 88:1517-1523, 2000.
7. Klein WA, Miller HH, Anderson M, et al: The use of indomethacin, sulindac, and tamoxifen for the treatment of desmoid tumors associated with familial polyposis. Cancer 60:2863-2868, 1987.
8. Runyon BA: Paracentesis of ascitic fluid: A safe procedure. Arch Intern Med 146:2259-2261, 1986.
9. Sandhu BS, Sanyal AJ: Management of ascites in cirrhosis. Clin Liver Dis 9:715-732, viii, 2005.
10. Fattovich G, Giustina G, Degos F, et al: Morbidity and mortality in compensated cirrhosis type C: A retrospective follow-up study of 384 patients. Gastroenterology 112:463-472, 1997.
11. Rosner MH, Gupta R, Ellison D, et al: Management of cirrhotic ascites: Physiological basis of diuretic action. Eur J Intern Med 17:8-19, 2006.
12. Cattau EL Jr, Benjamin SB, Knuff TE, et al: The accuracy of the physical examination in the diagnosis of suspected ascites. JAMA 247:1164-1166, 1982.
13. Runyon BA, Montano AA, Akrividadis EA, et al: The serum-ascites albumin gradient is superior to the exudate-transudate concept in the differential diagnosis of ascites. Ann Intern Med 117:215-220, 1992.
14. Gines P, Cardenas A, Arroyo V, et al: Management of cirrhosis and ascites. N Engl J Med 350:1646-1654, 2004.
15. Trotter J, Pieramici E, Everson GT: Chronic albumin infusions to achieve diuresis in patients with ascites who are not candidates for transjugular intrahepatic portosystemic shunt (TIPS). Dig Dis Sci 50:1356-1360, 2005.
16. Baniel J, Foster RS, Rowland RG, et al: Management of chylous ascites after retroperitoneal lymph node dissection for testicular cancer. J Urol 150:1422-1424, 1993.
17. Huang Q, Jiang ZW, Jiang J, et al: Chylous ascites: Treated with total parenteral nutrition and somatostatin. World J Gastroenterol 10:2588-2591, 2004.
18. Almakdisi T, Massoud S, Makdisi G: Lymphomas and chylous ascites: Review of the literature. Oncologist 10:632-635, 2005.
19. Guarner C, Runyon BA: Spontaneous bacterial peritonitis: Pathogenesis, diagnosis, and management. Gastroenterologist 3:311-328, 1995.
20. Runyon BA: Early events in spontaneous bacterial peritonitis. Gut 53:782-784, 2004.
21. Gomez F, Ruiz P, Schreiber AD: Impaired function of macrophage Fc gamma receptors and bacterial infection in alcoholic cirrhosis. N Engl J Med 331:1122-1128, 1994.
22. Such J, Guarner C, Enriquez J, et al: Low C3 in cirrhotic ascites predisposes to spontaneous bacterial peritonitis. J Hepatol 6:80-84, 1988.
23. Runyon BA: Patients with deficient ascitic fluid opsonic activity are predisposed to spontaneous bacterial peritonitis. Hepatology 8:632-635, 1988.
24. Sort P, Navasa M, Arroyo V, et al: Effect of intravenous albumin on renal impairment and mortality in patients with cirrhosis and spontaneous bacterial peritonitis. N Engl J Med 341:403-409, 1999.

25. Fernandez J, Navasa M, Garcia-Pagan JC, et al: Effect of intravenous albumin on systemic and hepatic hemodynamics and vasoactive neurohormonal systems in patients with cirrhosis and spontaneous bacterial peritonitis. J Hepatol 41:384-390, 2004.

26. Sanai FM, Bzeizi KI: Systematic review. Tuberculous peritonitis: Presenting features, diagnostic strategies and treatment. Aliment Pharmacol Ther 22:685-700, 2005.

27. Shakil AO, Korula J, Kanel GC, et al: Diagnostic features of tuberculous peritonitis in the absence and presence of chronic liver disease: A case control study. Am J Med 100:179-185, 1996.

28. Kavanagh D, Prescott GJ, Mactier RA: Peritoneal dialysis–associated peritonitis in Scotland (1999-2002). Nephrol Dial Transplant 19:2584-2591, 2004.

29. Loggie BW, Fleming RA, McQuellon RP, et al: Prospective trial for the treatment of malignant peritoneal mesothelioma. Am Surg 67:999-1003, 2001.

30. Eltabbakh GH, Piver MS, Hempling RE, et al: Clinical picture, response to therapy, and survival of women with diffuse malignant peritoneal mesothelioma. J Surg Oncol 70:6-12, 1999.

31. Park BJ, Alexander HR, Libutti SK, et al: Treatment of primary peritoneal mesothelioma by continuous hyperthermic peritoneal perfusion (CHPP). Ann Surg Oncol 6:582-590, 1999.

32. Jivan S, Bahal V: Pseudomyxoma peritonei. Postgrad Med J 78:170-172, 2002.

33. Sugarbaker PH, Shmookler B, Ronnett BM, et al: Pseudomyxoma peritonei. Br J Surg 86:842, 1999.

34. Sabate JM, Torrubia S, Maideu J, et al: Sclerosing mesenteritis: Imaging findings in 17 patients. AJR Am J Roentgenol 172:625-629, 1999.

35. Martin LC, Merkle EM, Thompson WM: Review of internal hernias: Radiographic and clinical findings. AJR Am J Roentgenol 186:703-717, 2006.

36. Cho M, Carrodeguas L, Pinto D, et al: Diagnosis and management of partial small bowel obstruction after laparoscopic antecolic antegastric Roux-en-Y gastric bypass for morbid obesity. J Am Coll Surg 202:262-268, 2006.

37. Garza E Jr, Kuhn J, Arnold D, et al: Internal hernias after laparoscopic Roux-en-Y gastric bypass. Am J Surg 188:796-800, 2004.

38. Smith AJ, Lewis JJ, Merchant NB, et al: Surgical management of intra-abdominal desmoid tumours. Br J Surg 87:608-613, 2000.

39. Heinrich MC, McArthur GA, Demetri GD, et al: Clinical and molecular studies of the effect of imatinib on advanced aggressive fibromatosis (desmoid tumor). J Clin Oncol 24:1195-1203, 2006.

40. Paley M, Sidhu PS, Evans RA, et al: Retroperitoneal collections: Aetiology and radiological implications. Clin Radiol 52:290-294, 1997.

41. Crepps JT, Welch JP, Orlando R 3rd: Management and outcome of retroperitoneal abscesses. Ann Surg 205:276-281, 1987.

42. Manjon CC, Sanchez AT, Lara JD, et al: Retroperitoneal abscesses. Scand J Nephrol 37:139-144, 2003.

43. Katz R, Golijanin D, Pode D, et al: Primary and postoperative retroperitoneal fibrosis: Experience with 18 cases. Urology 60:780-783, 2002.

44. Owens LV, Cance WG, Huth JF: Retroperitoneal fibrosis treated with tamoxifen. Am Surg 61:842-844, 1995.

45. Feig BW: Retroperitoneal sarcomas. Surg Oncol Clin N Am 12:369-377, 2003.

46. Jemal A, Murray T, Samuels A, et al: Cancer statistics, 2003. CA Cancer J Clin 53:5-26, 2003.

47. Lewis JJ, Leung D, Woodruff JM, et al: Retroperitoneal soft-tissue sarcoma: Analysis of 500 patients treated and followed at a single institution. Ann Surg 228:355-365, 1998.

48. Singer S, Corson JM, Demetri GD, et al: Prognostic factors predictive of survival for truncal and retroperitoneal soft-tissue sarcoma. Ann Surg 221:185-195, 1995.

49. Jaques DP, Coit DG, Hajdu SI, et al: Management of primary and recurrent soft-tissue sarcoma of the retroperitoneum. Ann Surg 212:51-59, 1990.

50. Hassan I, Park SZ, Donohue JH, et al: Operative management of primary retroperitoneal sarcomas: A reappraisal of an institutional experience. Ann Surg 239:244-250, 2004.

CHAPTER 44

Hernias

Mark A. Malangoni, MD   and   Michael J. Rosen, MD

Inguinal Hernias
Femoral Hernias
Special Problems
Ventral Hernias
Unusual Hernias

More than 600,000 hernias are repaired annually in the United States, making hernia repair one of the most common operations performed by general surgeons. Despite the frequency of this procedure, no surgeon has ideal results, and complications such as postoperative pain, nerve injury, infection, and recurrence continue to challenge surgeons.

Hernia is derived from the Latin word for rupture. A hernia is defined as an abnormal protrusion of an organ or tissue through a defect in its surrounding walls. Although a hernia can occur at various sites of the body, these defects most commonly involve the abdominal wall, particularly the inguinal region. Abdominal wall hernias occur only at sites where the aponeurosis and fascia are not covered by striated muscle (Box 44-1). These sites most commonly include the inguinal, femoral, and umbilical areas, the linea alba, the lower portion of the semilunar line, and sites of prior incisions (Fig. 44-1). The so-called neck or orifice of a hernia is located at the innermost musculoaponeurotic layer, whereas the hernia sac is lined by peritoneum and protrudes from the neck. There is no consistent relationship between the area of a hernia defect and the size of a hernia sac.

A hernia is *reducible* when its contents can be replaced within the surrounding musculature, and it is *irreducible* or *incarcerated* when it cannot be reduced. A *strangulated* hernia has compromised blood supply to its contents, which is a serious and potentially fatal complication. Strangulation occurs more often in large hernias that have small orifices. In this situation, the small neck of the hernia obstructs arterial blood flow, venous drainage, or both to the contents of the hernia sac. Adhesions between the contents of the hernia and the peritoneal lining of the sac can provide a tethering point that entraps the hernia contents and predisposes to intestinal obstruction and strangulation. A more unusual type of strangulation is a Richter's hernia. In Richter's hernia, a small portion of the antimesenteric wall of the intestine is trapped within the hernia, and strangulation can occur without the presence of intestinal obstruction.

An *external* hernia protrudes through all layers of the abdominal wall, whereas an *internal* hernia is a protrusion of intestine through a defect within the peritoneal cavity. An *interparietal* hernia occurs when the hernia sac is contained within a musculoaponeurotic layer of the abdominal wall. In broad terms, most abdominal wall hernias can be separated into inguinal and ventral hernias. This chapter focuses on the specific aspects of each of these conditions individually.

INGUINAL HERNIAS

Inguinal hernias are classified as either *direct or indirect*. The sac of an indirect inguinal hernia passes from the internal inguinal ring obliquely toward the external inguinal ring and ultimately into the scrotum. In contrast, the sac of a direct inguinal hernia protrudes outward and forward and is medial to the internal inguinal ring and inferior epigastric vessels. Although it sometimes can be difficult to distinguish between an indirect and a direct inguinal hernia, this distinction is of little importance because the operative repair of these types of hernias is similar. A pantaloon-type hernia occurs when there is an indirect and direct hernia component.

Incidence

Hernias are a common problem; however, their true incidence is unknown. It is estimated that 5% of the population will develop an abdominal wall hernia, but the prevalence may be even higher. About 75% of all

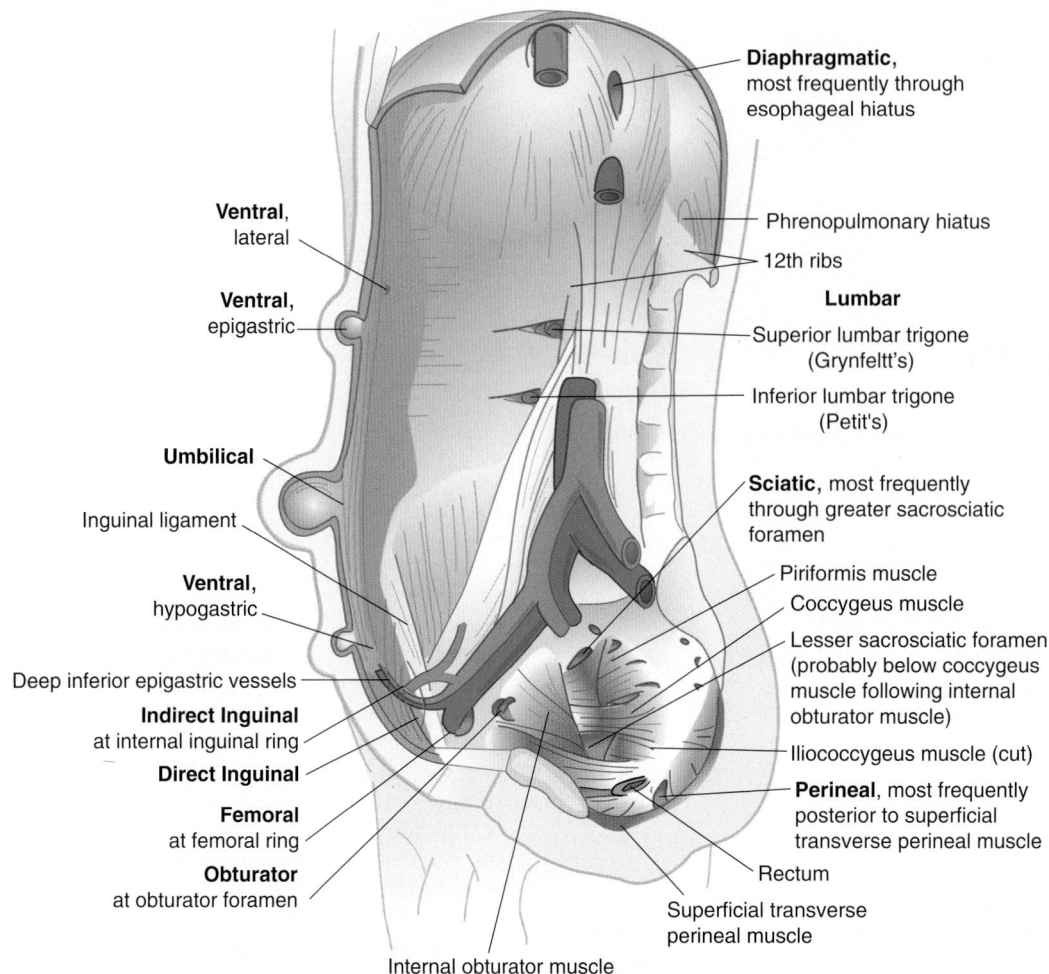

Figure 44-1 Types of abdominal wall hernias. (From Dorland's Illustrated Medical Dictionary, 26th ed, Philadelphia, WB Saunders, 1985, plate XXI.)

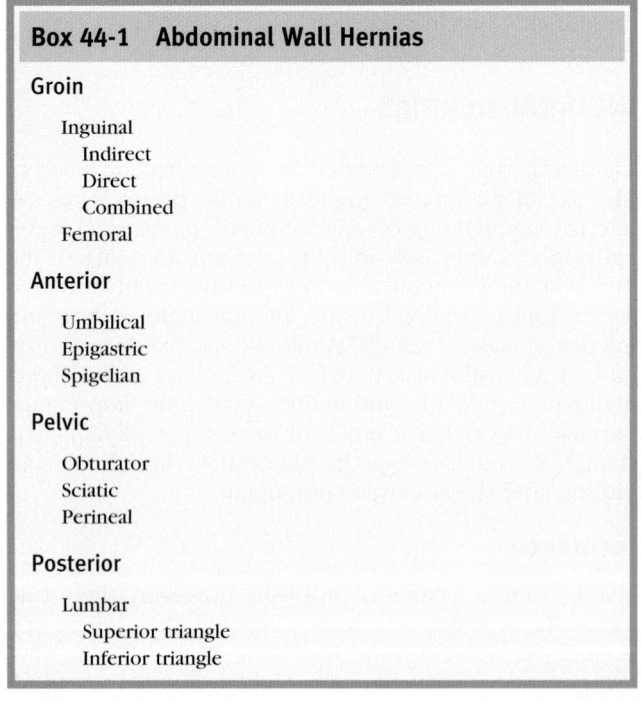

Box 44-1 Abdominal Wall Hernias

Groin

Inguinal
  Indirect
  Direct
  Combined
Femoral

Anterior

Umbilical
Epigastric
Spigelian

Pelvic

Obturator
Sciatic
Perineal

Posterior

Lumbar
  Superior triangle
  Inferior triangle

hernias occur in the inguinal region. Two thirds of these are indirect, and the remainder are direct inguinal hernias.

Men are 25 times more likely to have a groin hernia than are women. An indirect inguinal hernia is the most common hernia, regardless of gender. In men, indirect hernias predominate over direct hernias at a ratio of 2:1. Direct hernias are very uncommon in women. The female-to-male ratio in femoral and umbilical hernias, however, is about 10:1 and 2:1, respectively. Although femoral hernias occur more frequently in women than in men, inguinal hernias remain the most common hernia in women. Femoral hernias are rare in men. Ten percent of women and 50% of men who have a femoral hernia either have or will develop an inguinal hernia.

Both indirect inguinal and femoral hernias occur more commonly on the right side. This is attributed to a delay in atrophy of the processus vaginalis after the normal slower descent of the right testis to the scrotum during fetal development. The predominance of right-sided femoral hernias is thought to be due to the tamponading effect of the sigmoid colon on the left femoral canal.

The prevalence of hernias increases with age, particularly for inguinal, umbilical, and femoral hernias. The

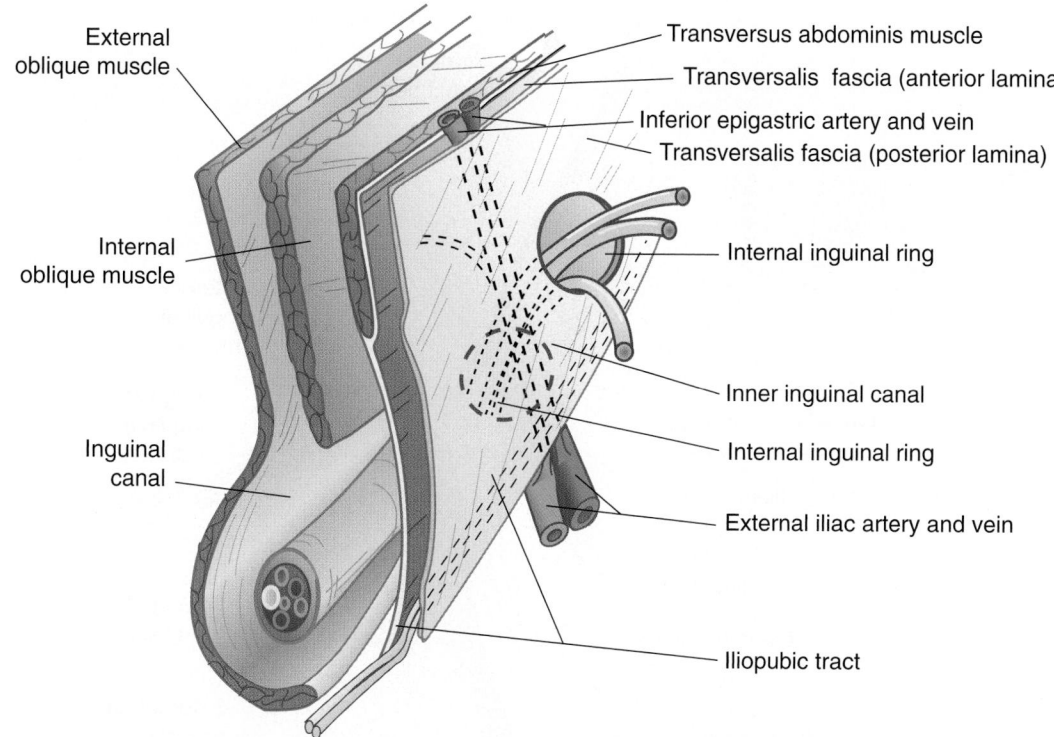

Figure 44-2 Nyhus's classic parasagittal diagram of the right midinguinal region illustrating the muscular aponeurotic layers separated into anterior and posterior walls. The posterior laminae of the transversalis fascia have been added, with the inferior epigastric vessels coursing through the abdominal wall medially to the inner inguinal canal. (From Read RC: The transversalis and preperitoneal fasciae: A re-evaluation. In Nyhus LM, Condon RE [eds]: Hernia, 4th ed. Philadelphia, JB Lippincott, 1995, pp 57-63.)

likelihood of strangulation and need for hospitalization also increase with aging. Strangulation, the most common serious complication of a hernia, occurs in only 1% to 3% of groin hernias and is more common at the extremes of life. Most strangulated hernias are indirect inguinal hernias; however, femoral hernias have the highest rate of strangulation (15%-20%) of all hernias, and for this reason, it is recommended that all femoral hernias be repaired at the time of discovery.

Anatomy

Anatomy of the Groin

The surgeon must have a comprehensive understanding of the anatomy of the groin to properly select and utilize various options for hernia repair. In addition, the relationships of muscles, aponeuroses, fascia, nerves, blood vessels, and spermatic cord structures in the inguinal region must be mastered to obtain the lowest incidence of recurrence and to avoid complications. These anatomic considerations must be understood from both the anterior and posterior approaches because both approaches are useful in different situations (Figs. 44-2 and 44-3).

From anterior to posterior, the groin anatomy includes the skin and subcutaneous tissues, below which are the superficial circumflex iliac, superficial epigastric, and external pudendal arteries and accompanying veins. These vessels arise from and drain to the proximal femoral artery and vein, respectively, and are directed superiorly. If encountered during operation, these vessels can be retracted or even divided when necessary.

External Oblique Muscle and Aponeurosis

The external oblique muscle fibers are directed inferiorly and medially and lie deep to the subcutaneous tissues. The aponeurosis of the external oblique muscle is formed by a superficial and deep layer. This aponeurosis, along with the bilaminar aponeuroses of the internal oblique and transversus abdominis, forms the anterior rectus sheath and, finally, the linea alba by linear decussation. The external oblique aponeurosis serves as the superficial boundary of the inguinal canal. The inguinal ligament (Poupart's ligament) is the inferior edge of the external oblique aponeurosis and extends from the anterior superior iliac spine to the pubic tubercle, turning posteriorly to form a shelving edge. The lacunar ligament is formed by the insertion of the inguinal ligament to the pubis. The lacunar ligament forms the medial border of the femoral space. The external (superficial) inguinal ring is an ovoid opening of the external oblique aponeurosis that is positioned superior and slightly lateral to the pubic tubercle. The spermatic cord exits the inguinal canal through the external inguinal ring.

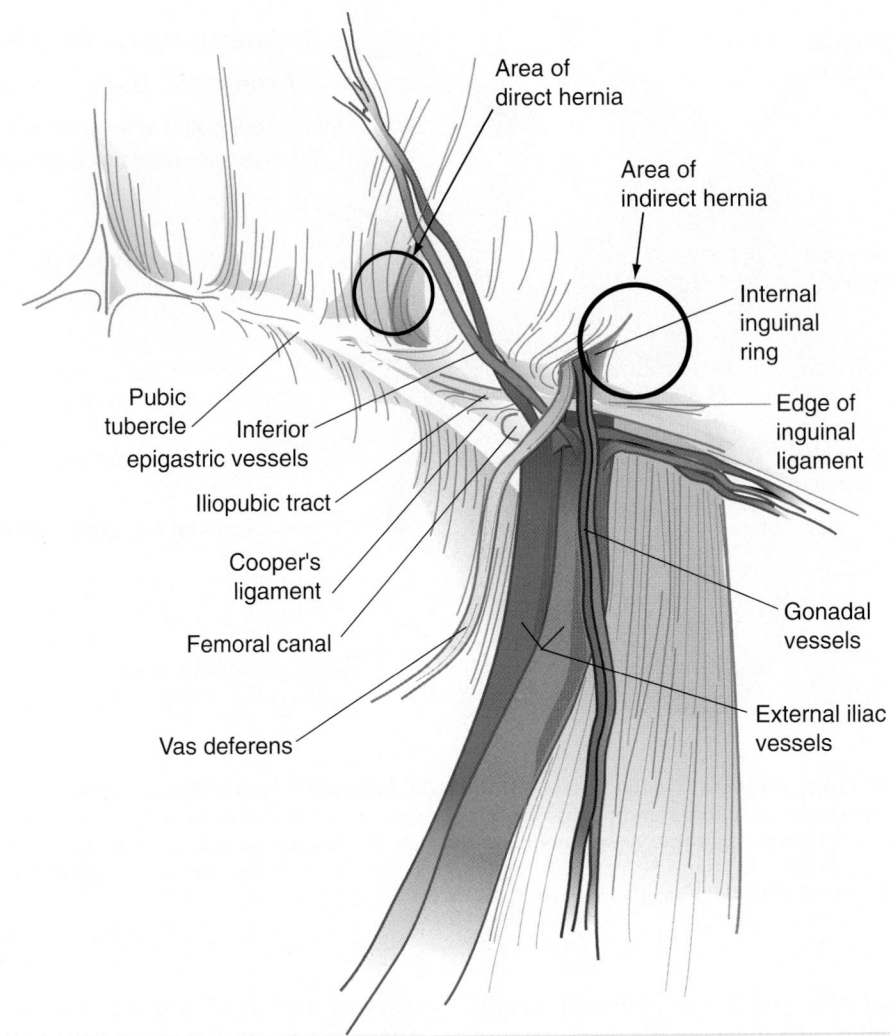

Area of
direct hernia

Area of
indirect hernia

Internal
inguinal
ring

Edge of
inguinal
ligament

Pubic
tubercle
Inferior
epigastric vessels

Iliopubic tract

Cooper's
ligament

Femoral canal

Gonadal
vessels

External iliac
vessels

Vas deferens

Figure 44-3 Anatomy of the important preperitoneal structures in the right inguinal space. (From Talamini MA, Are C: Laparoscopic hernia repair. In Zuidema GD, Yeo CJ [eds]: Shackelford's Surgery of the Alimentary Tract, 5th ed. Philadelphia, WB Saunders, 2002, vol 5, p 140.)

Internal Oblique Muscle and Aponeurosis

The internal oblique muscle fibers are directed superiorly and laterally in the upper abdomen; however, they run in a transverse direction in the inguinal region. The internal oblique muscle serves as the cephalad (or superior) border of the inguinal canal. The medial aspect of the internal oblique aponeurosis fuses with fibers from the transversus abdominis aponeurosis to form a conjoined tendon. This structure actually is present in only 5% to 10% of patients and is most evident at the insertion of these muscles on the pubic tubercle. The cremasteric muscle fibers arise from the internal oblique and encompass the spermatic cord. These muscle fibers are essential to the cremasteric reflex but have little relevance to hernia repairs.

Transversus Abdominis Muscle and Aponeurosis and Transversalis Fascia

The transversus abdominis muscle layer is oriented transversely throughout most of its area; in the inguinal region,

these fibers course in a slightly oblique downward direction. The strength and continuity of this muscle and aponeurosis are important for the prevention of inguinal hernia.

The aponeurosis of the transversus abdominis covers both anterior and posterior surfaces. The lower margin of the transversus abdominis arches along with the internal oblique muscle over the internal inguinal ring to form the *transversus abdominis aponeurotic arch*. The transversalis fascia is the connective tissue layer that underlies the abdominal wall musculature. The transversalis fascia, sometimes referred to as the *endoabdominal fascia,* is a component of the inguinal floor. It tends to be more dense in this area but still remains relatively thin.

The iliopubic tract is a continuation of the transverse abdominis aponeurosis and fascia at the upper border of the femoral sheath. The iliopubic tract also forms the inferior crus of the deep inguinal ring. The superior crus of the deep ring is formed by the transversus abdominis aponeurotic arch. The iliopubic tract is located posterior to the inguinal ligament, and it crosses over the femoral vessels and inserts on the anterior superior iliac spine and inner lip of the wing of the ilium.

The iliopubic tract is an extremely important structure in the repair of hernias from both the anterior and posterior approaches. It comprises the inferior margin for most anterior repairs. The portion of the iliopubic tract lateral to the internal inguinal ring serves as the inferior border below which staples or tacks are not placed during a laparoscopic inguinal hernia repair because the femoral, lateral femoral cutaneous, and genitofemoral nerves are located inferior to the iliopubic tract. Although it cannot always be visualized during posterior repairs, if the tacking device cannot be palpated on the anterior abdominal wall, one must assume it is below the iliopubic tract.

Cooper's Ligament

Cooper's ligament is formed by the periosteum and fascia along the superior ramus of the pubis. This structure is posterior to the iliopubic tract and forms the posterior border of the femoral canal. In about 75% of patients, there will be a vessel that crosses the lateral border of Cooper's ligament and is a direct communication from the obturator and iliac vessels. This is also known as the *corona mortis*. In laparoscopic repairs, if this is injured, troublesome bleeding can result.

Inguinal Canal

The inguinal canal is about 4 cm in length and is located 2 to 4 cm cephalad to the inguinal ligament. The canal extends between the internal (deep) inguinal and external (superficial) inguinal rings. The inguinal canal contains the spermatic cord and the round ligament of the uterus.

The spermatic cord is composed of cremasteric muscle fibers, the testicular artery and accompanying veins, the genital branch of the genitofemoral nerve, the vas deferens, the cremasteric vessels, the lymphatics, and the processus vaginalis. The cremaster muscle arises from the lowermost fibers of the internal oblique muscle and encompasses the spermatic cord in the inguinal canal. The cremasteric vessels are branches of the inferior epigastric vessels and pass through the posterior wall of the inguinal canal through their own foramen. These vessels supply the cremaster muscle and can be divided to expose the floor of the inguinal canal during hernia repair without damaging the testis.

The inguinal canal is bounded superficially by the external oblique aponeurosis. The internal oblique and transversus abdominis musculoaponeurosis form the cephalad wall of the inguinal canal. The inferior wall of the inguinal canal is formed by the inguinal ligament and lacunar ligament. The posterior wall or floor of the inguinal canal is formed by the transversalis fascia and the aponeurosis of the transversus abdominis muscle.

Hesselbach's triangle refers to the margins of the floor of the inguinal canal. The inferior epigastric vessels serve as its superolateral border, the rectus sheath as medial border, and the inguinal ligament as the inferior border. Direct hernias occur within Hesselbach's triangle, whereas indirect inguinal hernias arise lateral to the triangle. It is

not uncommon, however, for medium and large indirect inguinal hernias to involve the floor of the inguinal canal as they enlarge.

The iliohypogastric and ilioinguinal nerves and the genital branch of the genitofemoral nerve are the important nerves in the groin area (Fig. 44-4). The iliohypogastric and ilioinguinal nerves provide sensation to the skin of the groin, the base of the penis, and the ipsilateral upper medial thigh. The iliohypogastric and ilioinguinal nerves lie beneath the internal oblique muscle to a point just medially and superior to the anterior superior iliac spine, where they penetrate the internal oblique muscle and lie beneath the external oblique aponeurosis. The main trunk of the iliohypogastric nerve runs on the anterior surface of the internal oblique muscle and aponeurosis medial and superior to the internal ring. The iliohypogastric nerve may provide an inguinal branch that joins the ilioinguinal nerve. The ilioinguinal nerve runs anterior to the spermatic cord in the inguinal canal and branches at the superficial inguinal ring. The genital branch of the genitofemoral nerve innervates the cremaster muscle and the skin on the lateral side of the scrotum and labia. This nerve lies on the iliopubic tract and accompanies the cremaster vessels to form a neurovascular bundle.

Preperitoneal Space

The preperitoneal space contains adipose tissue, lymphatics, blood vessels, and nerves. The nerves of the preperitoneal space of specific concern to the surgeon include the lateral femoral cutaneous nerve and the genitofemoral nerve. The lateral femoral cutaneous nerve originates as a root of L2 and L3 and is occasionally a direct branch of the femoral nerve. This nerve courses along the anterior surface of the iliac muscle beneath the iliac fascia and passes either under or through the lateral attachment of the inguinal ligament at the anterior superior iliac spine. This nerve runs beneath or occasionally through the iliopubic tract lateral to the internal inguinal ring.

The genitofemoral nerve usually arises from the L2 or the L1 and L2 nerve roots. It divides into genital and femoral branches on the anterior surface of the psoas muscle. The genital branch enters the inguinal canal through the deep ring, whereas the femoral branch enters the femoral sheath lateral to the artery.

The inferior epigastric artery and vein are branches of the external iliac vessels and are important landmarks for laparoscopic hernia repair. These vessels course medial to the internal inguinal ring and eventually lie beneath the rectus abdominis muscle immediately beneath the transversalis fascia. The inferior epigastric vessels serve to define the types of inguinal hernia. Indirect inguinal hernias occur lateral to the inferior epigastric vessels, whereas direct hernias occur medial to these vessels.

The vas deferens courses through the preperitoneal space from caudad to cephalad and medial to lateral to join the spermatic cord at the deep inguinal ring.

Femoral Canal

The boundaries of the femoral canal are the iliopubic tract anteriorly, Cooper's ligament posteriorly, and the

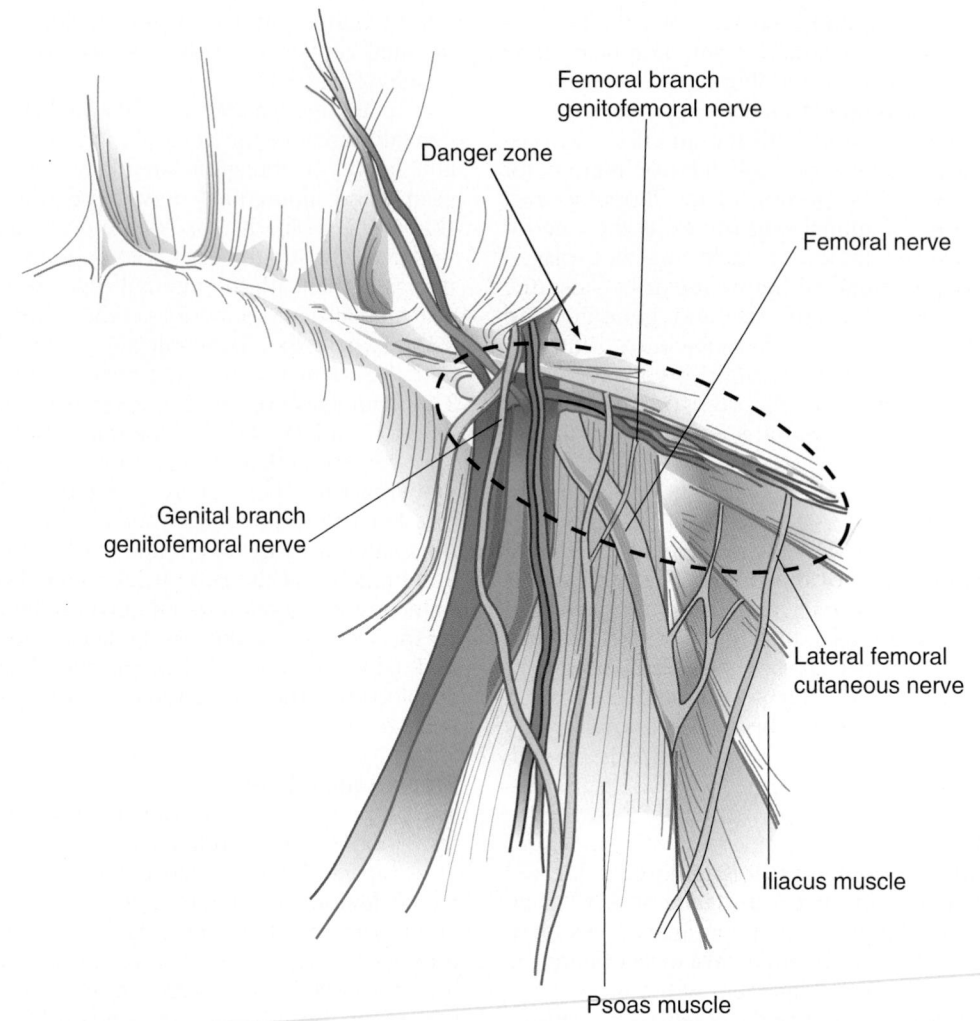

Femoral branch
genitofemoral nerve

Danger zone

Femoral nerve

Genital branch
genitofemoral nerve

Lateral femoral
cutaneous nerve

Iliacus muscle

Psoas muscle

Figure 44-4 Important nerves and their relationship to inguinal structures (right side is illustrated). (From Talamini MA, Are C: Laparoscopic hernia repair. In Zuidema GD, Yeo CJ [eds]: Shackelford's Surgery of the Alimentary Tract, 5th ed. Philadelphia, WB Saunders, 2002, vol 5, p 140.)

femoral vein laterally. The pubic tubercle forms the apex of the femoral canal triangle. A femoral hernia occurs through this space and is medial to the femoral vessels.

Diagnosis

A bulge in the inguinal region remains the main diagnostic finding in most groin hernias. There may be associated pain or vague discomfort in the region, but groin hernias are usually not extremely painful unless incarceration or strangulation has occurred. In the absence of physical findings, alternative causes for pain need to be entertained. Occasionally, patients may experience paresthesias related to compression or irritation of the inguinal nerves by the hernia. Masses other than hernias can occur in the groin region. Physical examination alone often differentiates between a groin hernia and these masses (Box 44-2).

The inguinal region is examined with the patient in both supine and standing positions. The examiner

Box 44-2   Differential Diagnosis of Groin Masses
Inguinal hernia
Hydrocele
Inguinal adenitis
Varicocele
Ectopic testis
Lipoma
Hematoma
Sebaceous cyst
Hidradenitis of inguinal apocrine glands
Psoas abscess
Lymphoma
Metastatic neoplasm
Epididymitis
Testicular torsion
Femoral hernia
Femoral adenitis
Femoral artery aneurysm or pseudoaneurysm

visually inspects and palpates the inguinal region, observing for asymmetry, bulges, or a mass. Having the patient cough or perform a Valsalva maneuver can facilitate identification of a hernia. The examiner places a fingertip over the inguinal canal and repeats the examination. Finally, a fingertip is placed into the inguinal canal by invaginating the scrotum to detect a small hernia. A bulge moving lateral to medial in the inguinal canal suggests an indirect hernia. If a bulge progresses from deep to superficial through the inguinal floor, a direct hernia is suspected. This distinction is not critical because repair is approached the same way regardless of the type of hernia. A bulge identified below the inguinal ligament is consistent with a femoral hernia.

A bulge of the groin described by the patient that is not demonstrated on examination presents a dilemma. Having the patient stand or ambulate for a period of time may allow the undiagnosed hernial mass to become visible or palpable. If a hernia is strongly suspected but undetectable, repeat examination at another time may be helpful.

Ultrasonography also can aid in the diagnosis. There is a high degree of sensitivity and specificity for ultrasound in the detection of occult direct, indirect, and femoral hernias.[1] Other imaging modalities are less useful. Computed tomography (CT) of the abdomen and pelvis may be useful for the diagnosis of obscure and unusual hernias as well as atypical groin masses.[2] Occasionally, laparoscopy can be both diagnostic and therapeutic for particularly challenging cases.

Classification

Numerous classification systems for groin hernias exist. One simple and widely used system is the Nyhus classification (Box 44-3). Although their purpose is to promote a common language and understanding for physician communication and to allow appropriate comparisons of therapeutic options, these classifications are incomplete and contentious. Most surgeons continue to describe

---

Box 44-3 Nyhus Classification of Groin Hernia

Type I: Indirect inguinal hernia—internal inguinal ring normal (e.g., pediatric hernia)

  Type II: Indirect inguinal hernia—internal inguinal ring dilated but posterior inguinal wall intact; inferior deep epigastric vessels not displaced

  Type III: Posterior wall defect

    A. Direct inguinal hernia
    B. Indirect inguinal hernia—internal inguinal ring dilated, medially encroaching on or destroying the transversalis fascia of Hesselbach's triangle (e.g., massive scrotal, sliding, or pantaloon hernia)
    C. Femoral hernia

  Type IV: Recurrent hernia

    A. Direct
    B. Indirect
    C. Femoral
    D. Combined

---

hernias by their type, location, and the volume of the hernia sac.

Nonoperative Management

Most surgeons recommend operation on discovery of a symptomatic inguinal hernia because the natural history of a groin hernia is that of progressive enlargement and weakening, with the potential for incarceration and strangulation. However, in patients with minimal symptoms, the clinician is often faced with balancing the risk for hernia-related complications such as hernia incarceration and bowel strangulation with the potential for complications in both the short and long term. Fitzgibbons and colleagues recently reported the first prospective randomized trial of a watchful waiting strategy for patients with asymptomatic or minimally symptomatic inguinal hernias.[3] These investigators randomized more than 700 men to either a watchful waiting or open tension-free hernia repair. The risk for hernia incarceration in the watchful waiting group was extremely low at 1.8 per thousand patient-years, or 0.03% of study participants. Almost one fourth of the patients assigned to watchful waiting crossed over to the surgical group, most commonly for pain related to the hernia that limited activity. Despite the seemingly high crossover rate, those patients who had later operation did not have increased surgical site infections, longer operative times, or higher recurrence rates than those who were initially assigned to early repair. This study provides conclusive evidence that a strategy of watchful waiting is safe for elderly patients with asymptomatic or minimally symptomatic inguinal hernias, and that even though almost 25% of patients eventually undergo repair, when they do, the operative risks and complication rates are no different than those of patients undergoing prophylactic repair.

Patients electing nonoperative management can occasionally have symptomatic improvements with the use of a truss. This approach is more commonly used in Europe. Correct measurement and fitting are important. Hernia control has been reported in about 30% of patients. Complications associated with the use of a truss include testicular atrophy, ilioinguinal or femoral neuritis, and hernia incarceration. It is generally agreed that nonoperative management is not used for femoral hernias because of the high incidence of associated complications, particularly strangulation.

Operative Repair

Anterior Repairs

Anterior repairs are the most common operative approach for inguinal hernias. Tension-free repairs are now standard, and there are a variety of different types. Older tissue types of repair are rarely indicated except for cases with simultaneous contamination or concomitant bowel resections when placement of a mesh prosthesis may be contraindicated.

There are some technical aspects of operation common to all anterior repairs. Open hernia repair is begun by making a transversely oriented linear or slightly curvilinear incision 2 to 3 cm above and parallel to the inguinal ligament. Dissection is continued through the subcutaneous tissues and Scarpa's fascia. The external oblique fascia and external inguinal ring are identified. The external oblique fascia is incised through the superficial inguinal ring to expose the inguinal canal. The ilioinguinal and iliohypogastric nerves are identified and mobilized to avoid transection and entrapment. The spermatic cord is mobilized at the pubic tubercle by a combination of blunt and sharp dissection. Improper mobilization of the spermatic cord too lateral to the pubic tubercle can cause confusion in the identification of tissue planes and essential structures and may result in disruption of the floor of the inguinal canal.

The cremasteric muscle of the mobilized spermatic cord is separated parallel to its fibers from the underlying cord structures. The cremasteric artery and vein, which join the cremaster muscle near the inguinal ring, are usually cauterized or ligated and divided. When an indirect hernia is present, the hernia sac is located deep to the cremaster muscle and anterior and superior to the spermatic cord structures. Incising the cremaster muscle in a longitudinal direction and dividing it circumferentially near the internal inguinal ring help expose the indirect hernia sac. The hernia sac is carefully dissected from adjacent cord structures and dissected to the level of the internal inguinal ring. The sac is opened and examined for visceral contents if it is large; however, this step is unnecessary in small hernias. The sac can be mobilized and placed within the preperitoneal space, or the neck of the sac can be ligated at the level of the internal ring, and any excess sac excised. If a large hernia sac is present, it can be divided using the electrocautery to facilitate ligation. It is not necessary to excise the distal portion of the sac. If the sac is broad based, it may be easier to displace it into the peritoneal cavity rather than to ligate it. Direct hernia sacs protrude through the floor of the inguinal canal and can be reduced below the transversalis fascia before repair. A lipoma of the cord represents retroperitoneal fat that has herniated through the deep inguinal ring and needs to be suture ligated and removed.

A sliding hernia presents a special challenge in handling the hernia sac. With a sliding hernia, a portion of the sac is composed of visceral peritoneum covering part of a retroperitoneal organ, usually the colon or bladder. In this situation, the grossly redundant portion of the sac (if present) is excised and the peritoneum reclosed. The organ and sac then can be reduced below the transversalis fascia, similar to a direct hernia.

Tissue Repairs

Although tissue repairs have largely been abandoned because of unacceptably high recurrence rates, they remain useful in certain situations. In strangulated hernias where bowel resection is necessary, mesh prostheses are contraindicated, and a tissue repair is necessary. Available options for tissue repair include iliopubic tract, Shouldice, Bassini, and McVay repairs.

The iliopubic tract repair approximates the transversus abdominis aponeurotic arch to the iliopubic tract with the use of interrupted sutures (Fig. 44-5). The repair begins at the pubic tubercle and extends laterally past the internal inguinal ring. This repair was initially described using a relaxing incision (see later); however, many surgeons who use this repair do not perform a relaxing incision.

The Shouldice repair emphasizes a multilayer imbricated repair of the posterior wall of the inguinal canal with a continuous running suture technique. After completion of the dissection, the posterior wall of the inguinal canal is reconstructed by superimposing running suture lines progressing from deep to more superficial layers. The initial suture line secures the transversus abdominis aponeurotic arch to the iliopubic tract. Next, the internal oblique and transversus abdominis muscles and aponeuroses are sutured to the inguinal ligament. The Shouldice repair is associated with a very low recurrence rate and a high degree of patient satisfaction in highly selected patients.

The Bassini repair is performed by suturing the transversus abdominis and internal oblique musculoaponeurotic arches or conjoined tendon (when present) to the inguinal ligament. This once popular technique is the basic approach to nonanatomic hernia repairs and was the most popular type of repair done before the advent of tension-free repairs.

Cooper's ligament, or the McVay repair, has traditionally been popular for the correction of direct inguinal hernias, large indirect hernias, recurrent hernias, and femoral hernias. Interrupted, nonabsorbable sutures are used to approximate the edge of the transversus abdominis aponeurosis to Cooper's ligament. When the medial aspect of the femoral canal is reached, a transition suture is placed to incorporate Cooper's ligament and the iliopubic tract. Lateral to this transition stitch, the transversus abdominis aponeurosis is secured to the iliopubic tract. An important principle of this repair is the need for a relaxing incision. The relaxing incision is made by reflecting the external oblique aponeurosis cephalad and medial to expose the anterior rectus sheath. An incision is then made in a curvilinear direction beginning 1 cm above the pubic tubercle throughout the extent of the anterior sheath to near its lateral border. This relieves tension on suture line and results in decreased postoperative pain and hernia recurrence. The fascial defect is covered by the body of the rectus muscle, which prevents herniation at the relaxing incision site. The McVay repair is particularly suited for strangulated femoral hernias because it provides obliteration of the femoral space without the use of mesh.

Tension-Free Inguinal Hernia Repair

The tension-free repair has become the dominant method of inguinal hernia repair (Fig. 44-6). Recognizing that tension in a repair is the principal cause of recurrence, current practices in hernia management employ a synthetic mesh prosthesis to bridge the defect, a concept first popularized by Lichtenstein. There are several options for placement of mesh during anterior inguinal herniorrhaphy, including the Lichtenstein approach, the plug-and-patch technique, or the sandwich technique with both an anterior and preperitoneal piece of mesh.

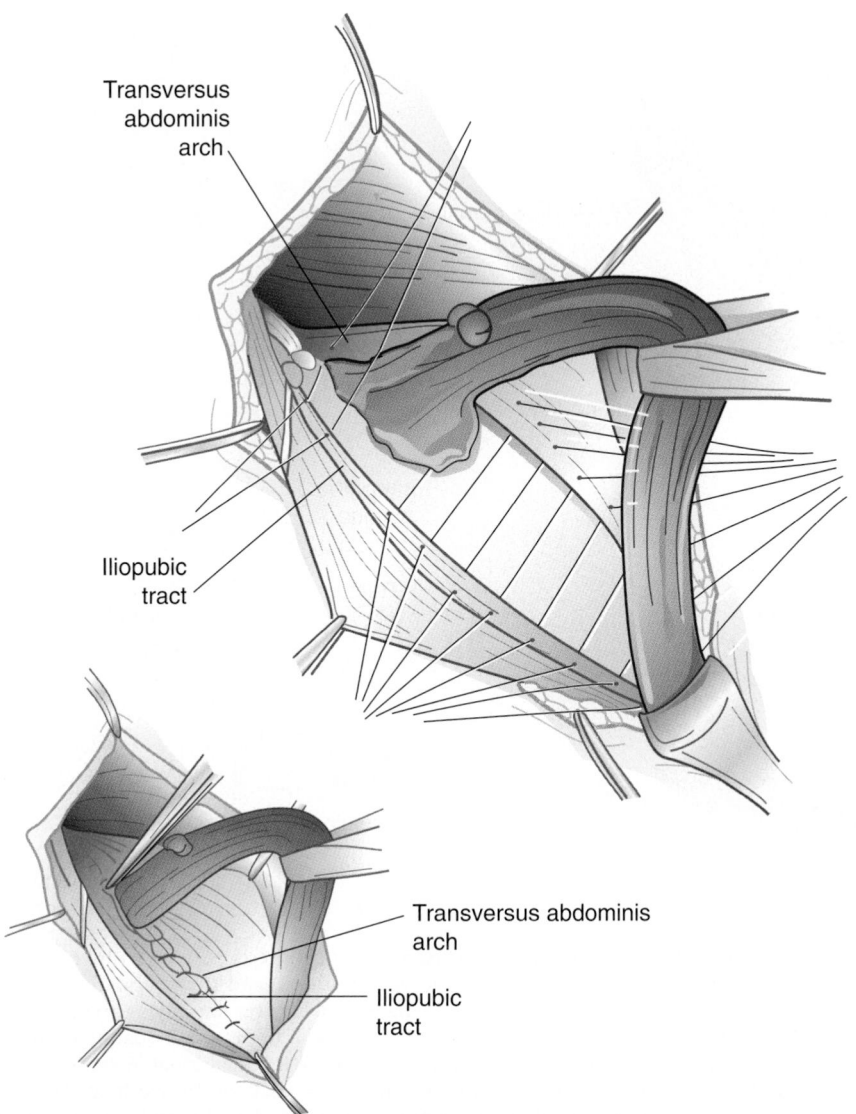

Transversus
abdominis
arch

Iliopubic
tract

Transversus abdominis
arch

Iliopubic
tract

Figure 44-5 Iliopubic tract repair. *Top,* Sutures lateral to the cord complete reconstruction of the deep inguinal ring. These sutures encompass the transversus abdominis arch above and the cremaster origin and iliopubic tract below. *Bottom,* The complete repair is ready for wound closure. The reconstruction of the deep ring should be snug but also loose enough to admit the tip of a hemostat. (From Condon RE: Anterior iliopubic tract repair. In Nyhus LM, Condon RE [eds]: Hernia, 2nd ed. Philadelphia, JB Lippincott, 1974, p 204.)

In the Lichtenstein repair, a piece of prosthetic nonabsorbable mesh is fashioned to fit the canal. A slit is cut into the distal, lateral edge of the mesh to accommodate the spermatic cord. There are various preformed, commercially available prostheses available for use. Monofilament, nonabsorbable suture is used in a continuous fashion beginning at the pubic tubercle and running a length of suture in both directions toward the superior aspect above the internal inguinal ring to the level of the tails of the mesh. The mesh is sutured to the aponeurotic tissue overlying the pubic bone medially, continuing superiorly along the transversus abdominis or conjoined tendon. The inferolateral edge of the mesh is sutured to the iliopubic tract or the shelving edge of the inguinal (Poupart's) ligament to a point lateral to the internal

inguinal ring. At this point, the tails created by the slit are sutured together around the spermatic cord, snugly forming a new internal inguinal ring. The ilioinguinal nerve and genital branch of the genitofemoral nerve are placed with the cord structures and are passed through this newly fashioned internal inguinal ring.

The tension-free mesh repair has been modified from the original Lichtenstein repair. Gilbert reported using a cone-shaped plug of polypropylene mesh that, when inserted into the internal inguinal ring, would deploy like an upside-down umbrella and occlude the hernia. This plug is sewn to the surrounding tissues and held in place by an additional overlying mesh patch. This patch may not need to be secured by sutures; however, to do so requires dissection to create a sufficient space between

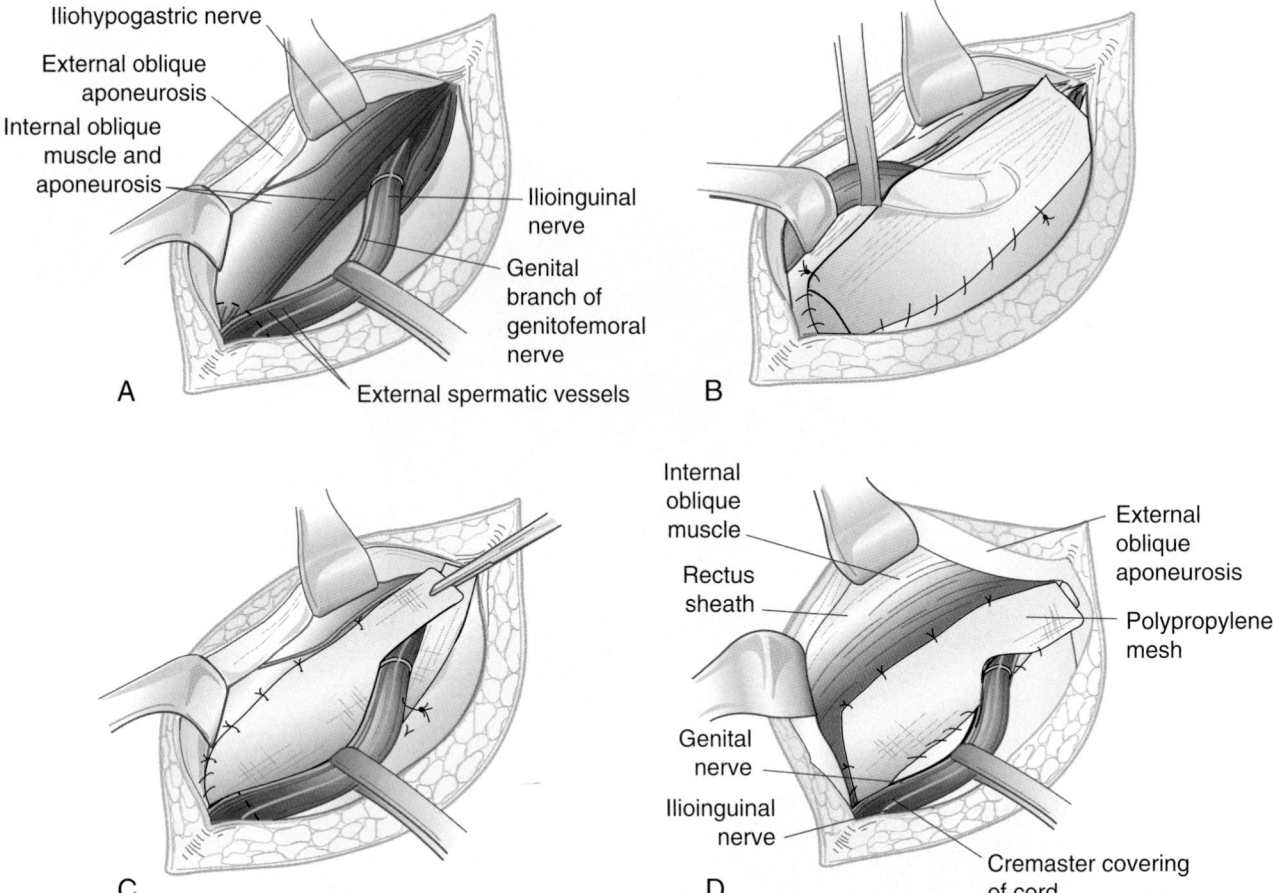

Figure 44-6 The Lichtenstein tension-free hernia repair. **A,** This procedure is performed by careful dissection of the inguinal canal. High ligation of an indirect hernia sac is performed, and the spermatic cord structures are retracted inferiorly. The external oblique aponeurosis is separated from the underlying internal oblique muscle high enough to accommodate a 6- to 8-cm wide mesh patch. Overlap of the internal oblique muscle edge by 2 to 3 cm is necessary. A sheet of polypropylene mesh is fashioned to fit the inguinal canal. A slit is made in the lateral aspect of the mesh, and the spermatic cord is placed between the two tails of the mesh. **B,** The spermatic cord is retracted in the cephalad direction. The medial aspect of the mesh overlaps the pubic bone by approximately 2 cm. The mesh is secured to the aponeurotic tissue overlying the pubic tubercle using a running suture of nonabsorbable monofilament material. The suture is continued laterally by suturing the inferior edge of the mesh to the shelving edge of the inguinal ligament to a point just lateral to the internal inguinal ring. **C,** A second monofilament suture is placed at the level of the pubic tubercle and continued laterally by suturing the mesh to the internal oblique aponeurosis or muscle approximately 2 cm from the aponeurotic edge. **D,** The lower edges of the two tails are sutured to the shelving edge of the inguinal ligament to create a new internal ring made of mesh. The spermatic cord structures are placed within the inguinal canal overlying the mesh. The external oblique aponeurosis is closed over the spermatic cord. (Reproduced from Arregui ME, Nagan RD [eds]: Inguinal Hernia: Advances or Controversies? Oxford, England, Radcliffe Medical, 1994.)

the external and internal oblique for the patch to lie flat over the inguinal canal. This so-called plug-and-patch repair, an extension of Lichtenstein's original mesh repair, has become the most commonly performed primary anterior inguinal hernia repair. Although this repair can be done without suture fixation by some experienced surgeons, many secure both plug and patch with several monofilament nonabsorbable sutures, especially for very weak inguinal floors or large defects.

The sandwich technique involves a bilayered device with three polypropylene components. An underlay circular patch provides a posterior repair similar to the laparoscopic approach, a connector functions similar to a plug, and an onlay patch covers the posterior inguinal floor. This repair has been deemed the *Prolene Hernia System* (PHS). The use of interrupted fixating sutures is not mandatory, but most surgeons place three or four fixation sutures in this repair.

Another option for a tension-free mesh repair involves a preperitoneal approach using a self-expanding polypropylene patch.[4] A pocket is created in the preperitoneal space by blunt dissection, and then a preformed mesh patch is inserted into the hernia defect that expands to cover the direct, indirect, and femoral spaces. The patch

Table 44-1 Prospective Randomized Trials Comparing Various Open Tension-Free Inguinal Hernia Approaches

STUDY	YEAR	PATIENTS	COMPLICATIONS (%)	MEAN FOLLOW-UP (mo)	RECURRENCE (%)
Nienhuijs et al[7]	2005	PHS 111	14	15	1
		Plug 113	9		3.5
		Lichtenstein 110	10		2.7
Vironen et al[8]	2006	PHS 150	26	12	0
		Lichtenstein 150	28		0.6
Kingsnorth et al[6]	2002	PHS 103	N/A	12	0
		Lichtenstein 103	N/A		2
Kingsnorth et al[5]	2000	Lichtenstein 68	9	1.5	0
		Plug 73	0		0
Total		PHS 364	33	10	0.25
		Lichtenstein 431	12		1.3
		Plug 186	4.5		1.8

PHS, Prolene Hernia System.

lies parallel to the inguinal ligament. It can remain without suture fixation, or a tacking suture can be placed.

Results of Anterior Tension-Free Inguinal Hernia Repair

Several recent prospective randomized trials have compared various anterior mesh inguinal hernia repairs. A compilation of these studies can be found in Table 44-1.[5-8] With nearly 1000 patients randomized to these different approaches, recurrence rates were minimal (0%-3.5%) with short-term follow-up (average <1 year). Depending on how complications were defined, reported rates ranged from 4.5% to 33%. Despite the randomized nature of these trials, caution must be used when interpreting the results. First, most of these patients were highly selected, and most trials excluded recurrent hernias, obese individuals, and large inguinal hernias. Second, the duration of follow-up is too short to identify all potential recurrences. Additionally, some follow-up results were completed by telephone interviews and not by physical exam. Regardless, these trials demonstrate that, in experienced hands, all three approaches for anterior tension-free hernia repair result in acceptable recurrence rates with minimal morbidity in appropriately selected patients.

Preperitoneal Repair

The open preperitoneal approach is useful for the repair of recurrent inguinal hernias, sliding hernias, strangulated hernias, and femoral hernias. A transverse skin incision is made 2 cm above the internal inguinal ring and is directed to the medial border of the rectus sheath. The muscles of the anterior abdominal wall are incised transversely, and the preperitoneal space is identified. If further exposure is needed, the anterior rectus sheath can be incised and the rectus muscle retracted medially. The preperitoneal tissues are retracted cephalad to visualize the posterior inguinal wall and the site of herniation. The inferior epigastric artery and veins are generally beneath the mid portion of the posterior rectus sheath and usually do not need to be divided. The posterior approach avoids mobilization of the spermatic cord and injury to the

sensory nerves of the inguinal canal, which is particularly important for hernias previously repaired through an anterior approach. If the peritoneum is incised, it is sutured closed to avoid evisceration of intraperitoneal contents into the operative field. The transversalis fascia and transversus abdominis aponeurosis are identified and sutured to the iliopubic tract. Femoral hernias repaired by this approach require closure of the femoral canal by securing the repair to Cooper's ligament. A mesh prosthesis is frequently used to reinforce the closure of the femoral canal, particularly with large hernias.

Laparoscopic Management

The application of minimally invasive surgical techniques to inguinal hernia repair has added to the ongoing debate about the best inguinal hernia repair. Laparoscopic inguinal hernia repair is another method of tension-free mesh repair, based on a preperitoneal approach. The laparoscopic approach provides the mechanical advantage of placing a large piece of mesh behind the defect covering the myopectineal orifice and using the natural forces of the abdominal wall to anchor the mesh in place. Proponents tout quicker recovery, less pain, better visualization of anatomy, utility in fixing all inguinal hernia defects, and decreased surgical site infections. Critics emphasize longer operative times, technical challenges, and increased cost. Although controversy exists about the utility of laparoscopic repair of primary unilateral inguinal hernias, most agree that this approach has advantages for patients with bilateral or recurrent hernias.[9] Adopting practice guidelines for the performance of laparoscopic hernia repairs may help control costs.

When considering the laparoscopic approach for repair of inguinal hernias, the surgeon has several options. Initially, laparoscopic repairs involved placing a large piece of mesh in an intraperitoneal position, similar to a laparoscopic ventral hernia repair. This approach has largely been abandoned secondary to high recurrence rates and the drawbacks of intraperitoneal mesh. The remaining two techniques include a totally extraperitoneal (TEP) and a transabdominal preperitoneal (TAPP) approach. The main difference between these two techniques is the sequence of gaining access to the preperitoneal space. In the TEP approach, the dissection begins in the preperitoneal space using a balloon dissector. In the TAPP repair, the preperitoneal space is accessed after initially entering the peritoneal cavity. Each approach has its merits. Using the TEP approach, the preperitoneal dissection is quicker, and the potential risk for intraperitoneal visceral damage is minimized. However, the use of dissection balloons is costly, the working space is more limited, and it may not be possible to create a working space if the patient has had a prior preperitoneal operation. Additionally, if a large tear in the peritoneal flap is created during a TEP approach, the potential working space can become obliterated, necessitating conversion to a transabdominal approach. For these reasons, knowledge of a transabdominal technique is essential when performing laparoscopic inguinal hernia repairs. The transabdominal approach allows immediate identification of the groin anatomy before extensive dissection and disruption of natural tissue planes. The larger working space of the peritoneal cavity can make early experience with the laparoscopic approach safer and easier.

There are no absolute contraindications to laparoscopic inguinal hernia repair other than the inability to tolerate general anesthesia. Patients who have had extensive prior lower abdominal surgery can require significant adhesiolysis and may be best approached anteriorly. In particular, patients who have had a radical retropubic prostatectomy with the preperitoneal space previously dissected can make accurate safe dissection challenging.

In the TEP approach, an infraumbilical incision is used. The anterior rectus sheath is incised, the ipsilateral rectus abdominis muscle is retracted laterally, and blunt dissection is used to create a space beneath the rectus. A dissecting balloon is inserted deep to the posterior rectus sheath, advanced to the pubic symphysis, and inflated under direct laparoscopic vision (Fig. 44-7). After it is opened, the space is insufflated, and additional trocars are placed. A 30-degree laparoscope provides the best visualization of the inguinal region (see Fig. 44-3). The inferior epigastric vessels are identified along the lower portion of the rectus muscle and retracted anteriorly. Cooper's ligament must be cleared from the pubic symphysis medially to the level of the external iliac vein. The iliopubic tract is also identified. Care must be taken to avoid injury to the femoral branch of the genitofemoral nerve and the lateral femoral cutaneous nerve, which are located lateral to and below the iliopubic tract (see Fig. 44-4). Lateral dissection is carried out to the anterior superior iliac spine. Finally, the spermatic cord is skeletonized.

In the TAPP approach, an infraumbilical incision is used to gain access to the peritoneal cavity directly. Two 5-mm ports are placed lateral to the inferior epigastric vessels at the level of the umbilicus. A peritoneal flap is created high on the anterior abdominal wall extending from the median umbilical fold to the anterior superior iliac spine. The remainder of the operation proceeds similar to a TEP procedure.

A direct hernia sac and associated preperitoneal fat is gently reduced by traction if it has not already been reduced by balloon expansion of the peritoneal space. A small indirect hernia sac is mobilized from the cord structures and reduced into the peritoneal cavity. A large sac may be difficult to reduce. In this case, the sac is divided with cautery near the internal inguinal ring, leaving the distal sac in situ. The proximal peritoneal sac is closed with a loop ligature to prevent pneumoperitoneum from occurring. After all hernias are reduced, a 12×14 cm piece of polypropylene mesh is inserted through a trocar and unfolded. It covers the direct, indirect, and femoral spaces and rests over the cord structures. It is imperative that the peritoneum is dissected at least 4 cm off the cord structures to prevent the peritoneum from encroaching beneath the mesh, which can lead to recurrence. The mesh is carefully secured with a tacking stapler to Cooper's ligament from the pubic tubercle to the external iliac vein, anteriorly to the posterior rectus musculature and transversus abdominis aponeurotic arch at least 2 cm above the hernia defect, and laterally to the iliopubic tract. The mesh extends beyond the pubic symphysis and below the spermatic cord and peritoneum (Fig. 44-8). The mesh is not fixed in this area, and tacks are not placed inferior to the iliopubic tract beyond the external iliac artery. Staples placed in this area may injure the femoral branch of the genitofemoral nerve or the lateral femoral cutaneous nerve. Staples are also avoided in the so-called triangle of doom bounded by the ductus deferens medially and the spermatic vessels laterally to avoid injury to the external iliac vessels and femoral nerve. As long as one can palpate the tip of the tacking device, these structures are avoided.

Results of Laparoscopic Inguinal Hernia Repair

Several randomized controlled trials have directly compared various laparoscopic inguinal hernia repairs to a multitude of open techniques. One of the most significant limitations of these series is the inclusion of multiple laparoscopic and open approaches. Additionally, some series compare the laparoscopic approach to open anatomic repairs that have largely been abandoned by most surgeons.[10] In Table 44-2, several recent prospective randomized trials evaluating laparoscopic versus open tension-free inguinal hernia repairs are presented.[11-13]

An extensive systematic review of randomized controlled trials was recently published by the European Union Hernia Trialists Collaboration.[14] These authors reported a meta-analysis in 2002 analyzing data from 4165 patients in 25 trials. Based on the available data, the laparoscopic repair resulted in a more rapid return to normal activity and decreased persistent postoperative pain. The recurrence rate for the laparoscopic repair was lower compared with open nonmesh repairs; however, open and laparoscopic mesh repairs had similar recurrence rates. A recently published prospective trial sponsored by the Veterans Administration randomized 1983 patients to receive either an open Lichtenstein repair or a laparoscopic repair, of which 90% were TEP repairs.[13] Most surgeons in this study had minimal experience with the laparoscopic approach; only 25 prior repairs were

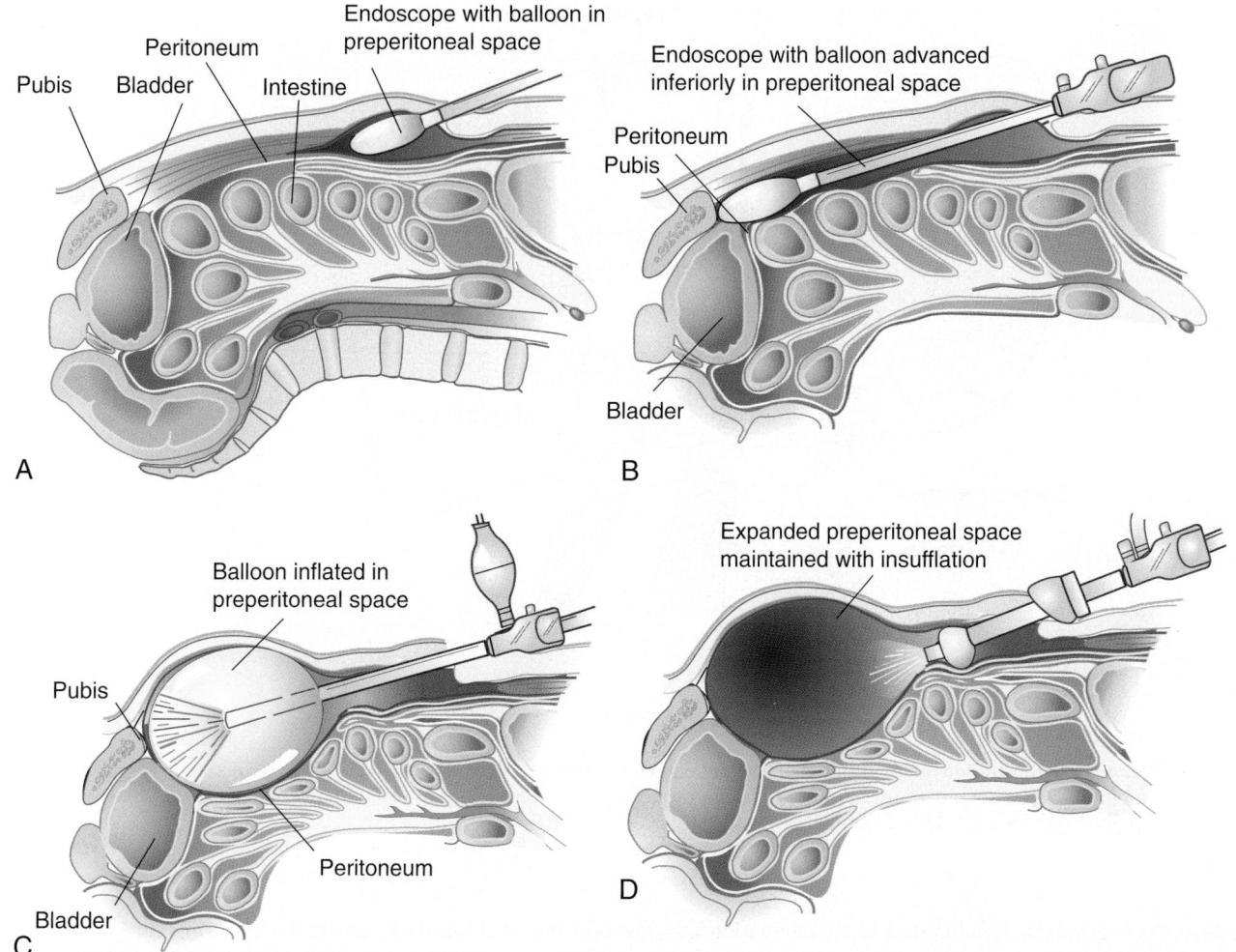

Figure 44-7 The total extraperitoneal (TEP) laparoscopic hernia repair. **A,** The TEP approach for laparoscopic hernia repair is demonstrated. Access to the posterior rectus sheath is gained in the periumbilical region. A balloon dissector is placed on the anterior surface of the posterior rectus sheath. **B,** The balloon dissector is advanced to the posterior surface of the pubis in the preperitoneal space. **C,** The balloon is inflated, thereby creating an optical cavity. **D,** The optical cavity is insufflated by carbon dioxide, and the posterior surface of the inguinal floor is dissected. (From Shadduck PP, Schwartz LB, Eubanks WS: Laparoscopic inguinal herniorrhaphy. In Pappas TN, Schwartz LB, Eubanks WE [eds]: Atlas of Laparoscopic Surgery. Philadelphia, Current Medicine, 1996. Copyright 1996 by Current Medicine. Reproduced by permission of the publisher.)

necessary to be eligible to enroll patients, which is consistent with the seemingly high conversion rate of 5%. Despite these factors, these investigators found a two-fold higher incidence of recurrence after laparoscopic repair (10%) than open repair (5%). This difference in recurrence remained for primary hernias (10% laparoscopic versus 4% open); however, recurrent hernias repaired by the laparoscopic approach tended to have fewer re-recurrences (10% versus 14%). In another publication from this same group, it was noted that surgeon inexperience with laparoscopy and surgeon age of more than 45 years were both predictors of recurrence after laparoscopic repair.[15] What can be concluded from this trial? This trial demonstrates that the laparoscopic repair of inguinal hernias has a definite learning curve in order to achieve an acceptably low recurrence rate. However, the dilemma of obtaining adequate technical proficiency to use this technique remains challenging.

FEMORAL HERNIAS

A femoral hernia occurs through the femoral canal that is bounded superiorly by the iliopubic tract, inferiorly by Cooper's ligament, laterally by the femoral vein, and medially by the junction of the iliopubic tract and Cooper's ligament (lacunar ligament). A femoral hernia produces a mass or bulge below the inguinal ligament. On occasion, some femoral hernias will present over the inguinal canal. In this situation, the femoral hernia sac still exits inferior to the inguinal ligament through the femoral canal but ascends in a cephalad direction.

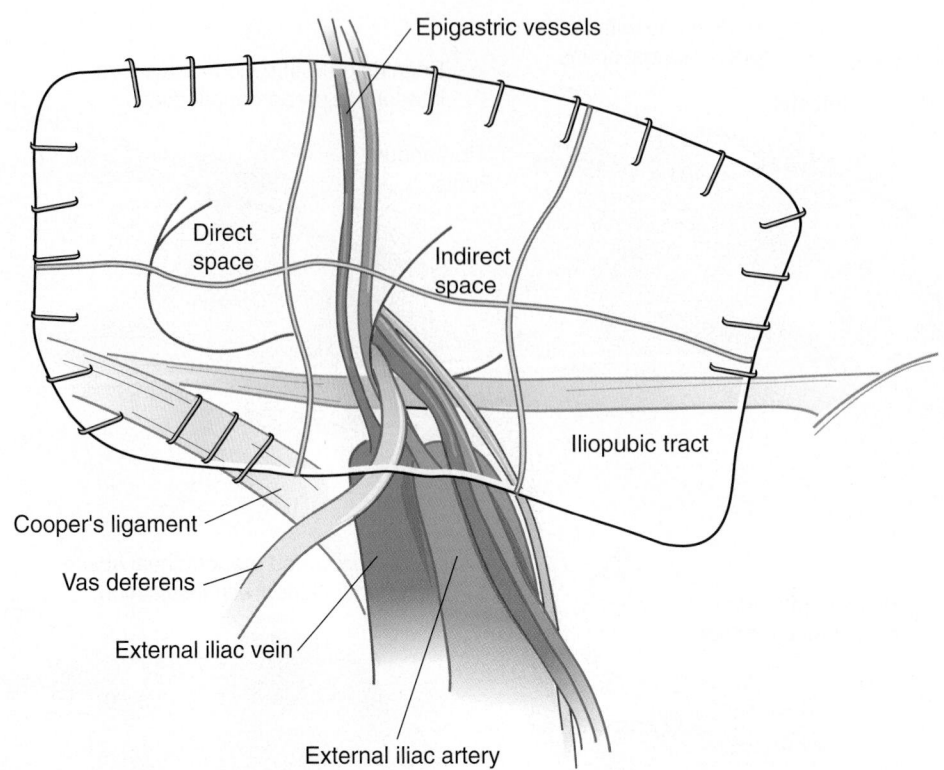

Epigastric vessels

Direct space

Indirect space

Iliopubic tract

Cooper's ligament

Vas deferens

External iliac vein

External iliac artery

Figure 44-8 Illustration of prosthetic mesh placement for the total extraperitoneal (TEP) hernia repair. (From Corbitt J: Laparoscopic transabdominal transperitoneal patch hernia repair. In Ballantyne GH [ed]: Atlas of Laparoscopic Surgery. Philadelphia, WB Saunders, 2000, p 511.)

Table 44-2 Prospective Randomized Trials Comparing Laparoscopic Inguinal Hernia Repair With Open Tension-Free Repairs

STUDY	YEAR	APPROACH (N)	COMPLICATIONS (%)	MEAN FOLLOW-UP (mo)	RECURRENCE (%)
Bringman et al[11]	2003	TEP 92	9.8	20	2.2
		Plug 104	15.4		1.9
		Lichtenstein 103	20.4		0
Lal et al[12]	2003	TEP 25	12	13	0
		Lichtenstein 25	4		0
Neumayer et al[13]	2004	TEP (90%)/TAPP (10%) 989	39	24	10
		Lichtenstein 994	33		5

TAPP, transabdominal preperitoneal; TEP, totally extraperitoneal.

A femoral hernia can be repaired using the standard Cooper's ligament repair, a preperitoneal approach, or a laparoscopic approach. The essential elements of femoral hernia repair include dissection and reduction of the hernia sac and obliteration of the defect in the femoral canal, either by approximation of the iliopubic tract to Cooper's ligament or by placement of prosthetic mesh to obliterate the defect. The incidence of strangulation in femoral hernias is high; therefore, all femoral hernias should be repaired, and incarcerated femoral hernias have the hernia sac contents examined for viability. In cases of compromised bowel, the Cooper's ligament approach is the preferred technique because mesh is contraindicated. When the incarcerated contents of a femoral hernia cannot be reduced, dividing the lacunar ligament can be helpful.

SPECIAL PROBLEMS

Sliding Hernia

A sliding hernia occurs when an internal organ comprises a portion of the wall of the hernia sac. The most common viscus involved is the colon or urinary bladder. Most sliding hernias are a variant of indirect inguinal hernias,

Table 44-3 Complications After Open and Laparoscopic Inguinal Hernia Repair

COMPLICATION	OPEN REPAIR (N = 994) (%)	LAPAROSCOPIC REPAIR (N = 989) (%)
Intraoperative complications	1.9	4.8
Postoperative complications	19.4	24.6
Urinary retention	2.2	2.8
Urinary tract infection	0.4	1.0
Orchitis	1.1	1.4
Surgical site infection	1.4	1.0
Neuralgia, pain	3.6	4.2
Life-threatening complications	0.1	1.1
Long-term complications	17.4	18.0
Seroma	3.0	9.0
Orchitis	2.2	1.9
Infection	0.6	0.4
Chronic pain	14.3	9.8
Recurrence	4.9	10.1

From Neumayer L, Giobbie-Hurder A, Jonassen O, et al: Open mesh versus laparoscopic mesh repair of inguinal hernias. N Engl J Med 350:1819-1827, 2004.

although femoral and direct sliding hernias can occur. The primary danger associated with a sliding hernia is the failure to recognize the visceral component of the hernia sac before injury to the bowel or bladder. The sliding hernia contents are reduced into the peritoneal cavity, and any excess hernia sac is ligated and divided. After reduction of the hernia, one of the aforementioned techniques can be used for repair of the inguinal hernia.

Recurrent Hernia

The repair of recurrent inguinal hernias is challenging, and results are associated with a higher incidence of secondary recurrence. Recurrent hernias almost always require placement of prosthetic mesh for successful repair. Recurrences after anterior hernia repair using mesh are best managed by either a laparoscopic or open posterior approach with placement of a second prosthesis.

Strangulated Hernia

Repair of a suspected strangulated hernia is most easily done using a preperitoneal approach. With this exposure, the hernia sac contents can be directly visualized and their viability assessed through a single incision. The constricting ring is identified and can be incised to reduce the entrapped viscus with minimal danger to the surrounding organs, blood vessels, and nerves. If it is necessary to resect strangulated intestine, the peritoneum can be opened and resection done without the need for a second incision.

Bilateral Hernias

The approach to repair of bilateral inguinal hernias is based on the extent of the hernia defect. Simultaneous repair of bilateral hernias has traditionally been associated with a recurrence rate approximately twice that of unilateral repair. The use of a giant prosthetic reinforcement of the visceral sac (Stoppa repair)[16] or the laparoscopic repair is appropriate for simultaneous repair of bilateral inguinal hernias, although bilateral anterior repair through separate incisions can be used.

Complications

There are a myriad of complications related to open and laparoscopic inguinal hernia repair (Table 44-3). Some are general complications that are related to underlying diseases and the effects of anesthesia. These will vary by patient population and risk. In addition, there are technical complications that are directly related to the repair. Technical complications are affected by the experience of the surgeon and are more frequent after repair of recurrent hernias. There is increased scarring and disturbed anatomy with hernia recurrence that can result in an inability to identify important structures at operation. This is the principal reason that we recommend using a different approach for recurrent hernias.

Although the overall complication rate from hernia repair has been estimated to be about 10%, many of these complications are transient and can be addressed easily. More serious complications from a large experience are listed in Table 44-3.

Surgical Site Infection

The risk for surgical site (wound) infection is estimated to be 1% to 2% after open inguinal hernia repair and less with laparoscopic repairs. These are clean operations, and the risk for infection is primarily influenced by associated patient diseases. Most would agree that there is no need to use routine antimicrobial prophylaxis for hernia repair.[17] Patients who have significant underlying disease, as reflected by an American Society of Anesthesiology (ASA) score of more than 3, receive perioperative antimicrobial prophylaxis with cefazolin, 1 to 2 g, given intravenously 30 to 60 minutes before the incision. Either clindamycin, 600 mg intravenously, or erythromycin, 250 mg intravenously, can be used for patients allergic to penicillin. Only a single dose of antibiotic is necessary. The placement of prosthetic mesh does not increase the risk for infection and does not affect the need for prophylaxis. The risk for infection can be decreased by using proper operative technique, preoperative antiseptic skin preparation, and appropriate hair removal. There is an increased risk for infection for patients who have had prior hernia incision infections, chronic skin infections, or an infection at a distant site. These infections are treated before elective operation.

Nerve Injuries

Nerve injuries are an infrequent and under-recognized complication of inguinal hernia repair. Injury can occur from traction, electrocautery, transection, and entrapment. The use of prosthetic mesh can result in dysesthesias that are usually temporary. The nerves most commonly affected during open hernia repair are the ilioinguinal, genital branch of the genitofemoral, and iliohypogastric. During laparoscopic repair, the lateral femoral cutaneous and genitofemoral nerves are most often affected.[18] Rarely, the main trunk of the femoral nerve can be injured during either open or laparoscopic inguinal hernia repair.

Transient neuralgias can occur and are usually self-limited and resolve within a few weeks after operation. Persistent neuralgias usually result in pain and hyperesthesia in the area of distribution. Symptoms are often reproduced by palpation over the point of entrapment. Transection of a sensory nerve usually results in an area of numbness corresponding to the distribution of the involved nerve.

With more recent attention to patient outcomes, chronic groin pain after open inguinal hernia repair has replaced recurrence as the primary complication after open inguinal hernia repair. Several large series with systematic follow-up have reported pain rates ranging from 29% to 76%.[7,19] Strategies of routine nerve division in open surgery have not been associated with a reduction in chronic pain in mesh-based anterior repairs.[20] In contrast, routine ilioinguinal nerve division is associated with significantly more sensory disturbances. By operating in a remote area to the commonly injured nerves and judicious appropriately placed tacks, chronic groin pain intuitively is less in laparoscopic repairs. Laparoscopic series and randomized controlled trials comparing laparoscopic and open repairs have reported significantly lower rates of chronic post-operative inguinal pain.

Various approaches to management of residual neuralgia have been described. These include analgesics, local anesthetic nerve blocks, transcutaneous electrical stimulation, and various medications. Patients presenting with nerve entrapment syndromes are usually best treated by repeat exploration with neurectomy. Mesh removal is usually needed as well. Laparoscopic nerve injuries are minimized by not placing any tacks or staples below the lateral portion of the iliopubic tract. If nerve entrapment occurs, patients undergo reoperation to remove the offending tack or staple.

Ischemic Orchitis

Ischemic orchitis occurs from thrombosis of the small veins of the pampiniform plexus within the spermatic cord. This results in venous congestion of the testis, which becomes swollen and tender 2 to 5 days after operation. The process continues for an additional 6 to 12 weeks and usually results in testicular atrophy. Orchiectomy is rarely necessary.

The incidence of ischemic orchitis can be minimized by avoiding unnecessary dissection within the spermatic cord. The incidence can increase with dissection of the distal portion of a large hernia sac and among patients who have anterior operations for hernia recurrence or for spermatic cord pathology. In these situations, the use of a posterior approach is preferred.

Injury to the Vas Deferens and Viscera

Injury to the vas deferens and the intra-abdominal viscera is unusual. Most of these injuries occur in patients with sliding inguinal hernias when there is failure to recognize the presence of intra-abdominal viscera in the hernia sac. With large hernias, the vas deferens can be displaced in an enlarged inguinal ring before its entry into the spermatic cord. In this situation, the vas deferens is identified and protected.

Hernia Recurrence

Hernia recurrence rates are variable but can be as low as 1% to 3% over a 10-year period of follow-up. Most hernias recur within the first 2 years after repair. In general, recurrences are lowest with tension-free repairs and higher with anatomic repairs.[10,21-25]

Hernia recurrences are usually due to technical factors, such as excessive tension on the repair, missed hernias, failure to include an adequate musculoaponeurotic margin in the repair, and improper mesh size and placement.[26] Recurrence also can result from failure to close a patulous internal inguinal ring, the size of which is always assessed at the conclusion of the primary operation. Other factors that can cause hernia recurrence are chronically elevated intra-abdominal pressure, a chronic cough, deep incisional infections, and poor collagen formation in the wound. Recurrences are more common among patients with direct hernias and usually involve the floor of the inguinal canal near the pubic tubercle, where suture line tension is greatest. The use of a relaxing incision when there is excessive tension at the time of primary hernia repair is helpful to reduce recurrence.

Most recurrent hernias require use of prosthetic mesh for successful repair.[27-30] Choosing a different approach (usually posterior) avoids dissection through scar tissue, improves visualization of the defect and reduction of the hernia, and decreases the incidence of complications, particularly ischemic orchitis and injury to the ilioinguinal nerve. Recurrences after initial prosthetic mesh repairs can be due to displaced prostheses or the use of a prosthetic of inadequate size. Recurrences are best managed by placing a second prosthesis through a different approach.

The Shouldice repair has been demonstrated to have a recurrence rate of less than 2%, which is the lowest rate of recurrence among repairs that do not use a tension-free approach.[31] A recent meta-analysis of 58 reports comparing synthetic mesh techniques to nonmesh repairs demonstrated a nearly 60% reduction in recurrence with the use of mesh.[14] This same report concluded that there was no difference in the rate of hernia recurrence between laparoscopic and open approaches that used mesh.

Recurrence is more common after repair of recurrent hernias and is directly related to the number of previous attempts at repair. Large population-based studies report a re-recurrence rate of 4% to 5% overall.[27] Tension-free and mesh-based repairs have the lowest rates of reoperation after recurrence and provide a reduction in recurrence of about 60% compared with more traditional repairs.[28,30]

Quality of Life

The major quality indicators that have been assessed for hernia repair are postoperative pain and return to work. Tension-free and laparoscopic mesh-based approaches have been demonstrated to be less painful than nonmesh repairs. Laparoscopic repairs have the least amount of postoperative pain and have been shown to provide a marginal advantage in reducing time off work.[9]

VENTRAL HERNIAS

A ventral hernia is defined by a protrusion through the anterior abdominal wall fascia. These defects can be categorized as spontaneous or acquired or by their location on the abdominal wall. Epigastric hernias occur from the xyphoid process to the umbilicus, umbilical hernias occur at the umbilicus, and hypogastric hernias are rare spontaneous hernias that occur below the umbilicus in the midline. Acquired hernias typically occur after surgical incisions and are therefore termed *incisional hernias.* Although not a true hernia, diastasis recti can present as a midline bulge. In this condition, the linea alba is stretched, resulting in bulging at the medial margins of the rectus muscles. Abdominal wall diastasis can occur at other sites besides the midline. There is no fascial ring or hernia sac, and unless significantly symptomatic, surgical correction is avoided.

Incidence

Based on national operative statistics, incisional hernias account for 15% to 20% of all abdominal wall hernias; umbilical and epigastric hernias constitute 10% of hernias. Incisional hernias are twice as common in women as in men. As a result of the almost 4 million laparotomies performed annually in the United States and the 2% to 30% incidence of incisional hernia, almost 150,000 ventral hernia repairs are performed each year.[32] Several technical and patient-related factors have been linked to the occurrence of incisional hernias. There is no conclusive evidence that demonstrates that the type of suture or

technique of incisional closure at the primary operation affects hernia formation.[33] Patient-related factors linked to ventral hernia formation include obesity, older age, male gender, sleep apnea, emphysema, and prostatism. It has been proposed that the same factors associated with destruction of the collagen in the lung result in poor wound healing with increased hernia formation. Wound infection has been linked to hernia formation.

Anatomy

The anatomy of the anterior abdominal wall is straightforward and considerably easier to grasp than the anatomy of the inguinal area. The lateral musculature is composed of three layers, with the fascicles of each directed obliquely at different angles to create a strong envelope for the abdominal contents. Each of these muscles forms an aponeurosis that inserts into the linea alba, a midline structure joining both sides of the abdominal wall. The external oblique is the most superficial muscle of the lateral abdominal wall. Deep to the external oblique lies the internal oblique muscle. The fibers of the external oblique course in an inferomedial direction (as hands in pockets), whereas those of the internal oblique muscle run deep to and opposite to the external oblique. The deepest muscular layer of the abdominal wall is the transversus abdominis muscle. Its fibers course in a horizontal direction. These three lateral muscles give rise to aponeurotic layers lateral to the rectus, which contribute to the anterior and posterior layers of the rectus sheath.

The medial extension of the external oblique aponeurosis forms the anterior layer of the rectus sheath. At the midline, the two anterior rectus sheaths form the tendinous linea alba. On either side of the linea alba are the rectus abdominis muscles, the fibers of which are directed longitudinally and run the length of the anterior abdominal wall. Below each rectus muscle lies the posterior layer of the rectus sheath, which also contributes to the linea alba.

Another important anatomic structure of the anterior abdominal wall is the arcuate line, which is located 3 to 6 cm below the umbilicus. The arcuate line delineates the point below which the posterior rectus sheath is absent. Above the arcuate line, the aponeurosis of the internal oblique muscle contributes to both the anterior and posterior rectus sheaths and the aponeurosis of the transversus abdominis muscle passes posterior to the rectus muscle to form the posterior rectus sheath. Below the arcuate line, the internal oblique and transversus abdominis aponeuroses pass completely anterior to the rectus muscle (Fig. 44-9). The rectus abdominis muscles are nearly fused below the arcuate line with the transversalis fascia directly behind them.

Diagnosis

The evaluation of abdominal wall hernias requires diligent physical examination. As with the inguinal region, the anterior abdominal wall is evaluated with the patient in both standing and supine positions, and a Valsalva maneuver is also useful to demonstrate the site and size of a hernia. Imaging modalities may play a greater role

Section above arcuate line

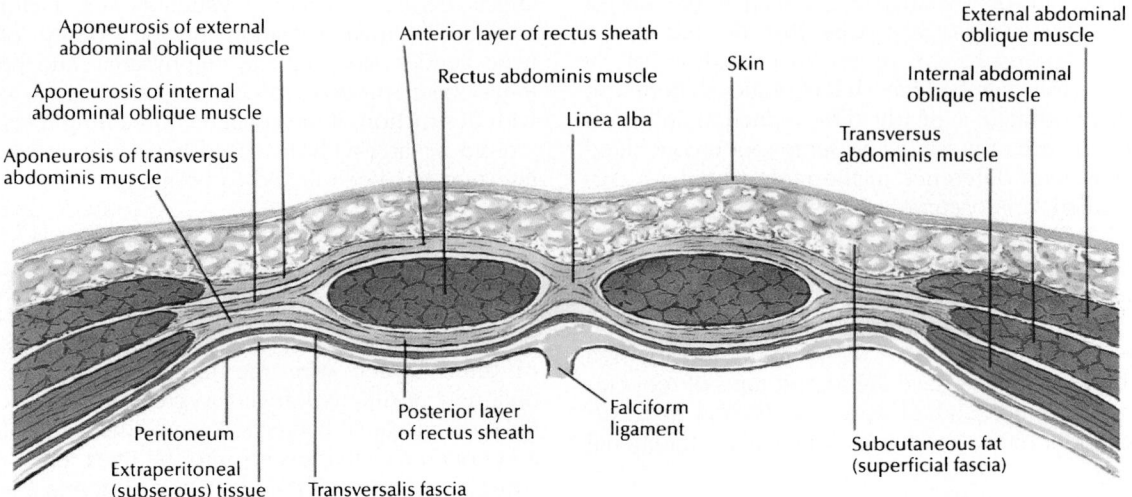

Aponeurosis of internal abdominal oblique muscle splits to form anterior and posterior layers of rectus sheath.
Aponeurosis of external abdominal oblique muscle joins anterior layer of sheath; aponeurosis of transversus abdominis
muscle joins posterior layer. Anterior and posterior layers of rectus sheath unite medially to form linea alba

Section below arcuate line

Aponeurosis of internal abdominal oblique muscle does not split at this level but passes completely anterior
to rectus abdominis muscle and is fused there with both aponeurosis of external abdominal oblique muscle
and that of transversus abdominis muscle. Thus posterior wall of rectus sheath is absent below arcuate line
and rectus abdominis muscle lies on transversalis fascia

Figure 44-9 Cross sections of the rectus abdominis muscle and aponeurosis above and below the arcuate line. (From Netter FT: Atlas of Human Anatomy. Summit, NJ, Ciba-Geigy, 1989, plate 235.)

in diagnosis of more unusual hernias of the abdominal wall.

Classification

Umbilical Hernia

The umbilicus is formed by the umbilical ring of the linea alba. Intra-abdominally, the round ligament (ligamentum teres) and the paraumbilical veins join into the umbilicus superiorly, and the median umbilical ligament (obliterated urachus) enters inferiorly. Umbilical hernias in infants are congenital and are quite common. They close spontaneously in most cases by the age of 2 years. Those that persist after the age of 5 years are frequently repaired surgically, although complications related to these hernias in children are unusual. There is a strong predisposition toward the development of these hernias in individuals of African descent. In the United States, the incidence of umbilical hernia is eight times higher in African Americans than in white infants.

Umbilical hernias in adults are largely acquired. These hernias are more common in women and in patients with conditions that result in increased intra-abdominal pressure, such as pregnancy, obesity, ascites, or abdominal distention. Umbilical hernia is more common among individuals who have only a single midline aponeurotic decussation compared with the normal decussation of fibers from all three lateral abdominal muscles. Strangulation is unusual in most patients; however, strangulation or rupture can occur in chronic ascitic conditions. Small asymptomatic umbilical hernias barely detectable on examination need not be repaired. Adults who have symptoms, a large hernia, incarceration, thinning of the overlying skin, or uncontrollable ascites should have hernia repair. Spontaneous rupture of umbilical hernias in patients with ascites can result in peritonitis and death.

Classically, repair was done using the vest-over-pants repair proposed by Mayo, which employs imbrication of superior and inferior fascial edges. Because of increased tension on the repair and recurrence rates of almost 30% with long-term follow-up, however, the Mayo repair is rarely performed today. Instead, small defects are closed primarily after separation of the sac from the overlying umbilicus and the surrounding fascia. Defects greater than 3 cm are closed using prosthetic mesh.[34] There are multiple techniques to place this mesh and no prospective data have conclusively found clear advantages of one technique over another. Options for mesh implantation include bridging the defect, placing a preperitoneal underlay of mesh reinforced with suture repair, or placing it laparoscopically. The laparoscopic technique requires general anesthesia and probably is reserved for large defects or recurrent umbilical hernias.[25] There is no universal consensus on the most appropriate method of umbilical hernia repair.

Epigastric Hernia

About 3% to 5% of the population has epigastric hernias.[35] Epigastric hernias are two to three times more common in men. These hernias are located between the xiphoid process and umbilicus and are usually within 5 to 6 cm of the umbilicus. Like umbilical hernias, epigastric hernias are more common in individuals with a single aponeurotic decussation. The defects are small and often produce pain out of proportion to their size owing to incarceration of preperitoneal fat. They are multiple in up to 20% of patients, and about 80% are just off the midline.[35] Repair usually consists of excision of the incarcerated preperitoneal tissue and simple closure of the fascial defect similar to umbilical hernias. Small defects can be repaired under local anesthesia. Uncommonly, these defects can be sizable and contain omentum or other intra-abdominal viscera and may require mesh repairs. Epigastric hernias are better repaired because the defect is small and fat that has herniated from within the peritoneal cavity is difficult to reduce.

Incisional Hernia

Of all hernias encountered, incisional hernias can be the most frustrating and difficult to treat. Incisional hernias occur as a result of excessive tension and inadequate healing of a previous incision, which is often associated with surgical site infection. These hernias enlarge over time, leading to pain, bowel obstruction, incarceration, and strangulation. Obesity, advanced age, malnutrition, ascites, pregnancy, and conditions that increase intra-abdominal pressure are factors that predispose to the development of an incisional hernia. Obesity can cause an incisional hernia to occur, owing to increased tension on the abdominal wall provided by the excessive bulk of a thick pannus and large omental mass. Chronic pulmonary disease and diabetes mellitus have also been recognized as risk factors for the development of incisional hernia. Medications such as corticosteroids and chemotherapeutic agents and surgical site infection can contribute to poor wound healing and increase the risk for developing an incisional hernia.

Large hernias can result in loss of abdominal domain, which occurs when the abdominal contents no longer reside in the abdominal cavity. These large abdominal wall defects also can result from the inability to close the abdomen primarily because of bowel edema, abdominal packing, peritonitis, and repeat laparotomy. With loss of domain, the natural rigidity of the abdominal wall becomes compromised, and the abdominal musculature is often retracted. Respiratory dysfunction can occur because these large ventral defects cause paradoxical respiratory abdominal motion. Loss of abdominal domain also can result in bowel edema, stasis of the splanchnic venous system, urinary retention, and constipation. Return of displaced viscera to the abdominal cavity during repair may lead to increased abdominal pressure, abdominal compartment syndrome, and acute respiratory failure.

Operative Repair

Primary repair of incisional hernias can be done when the defect is small (≤2 cm in diameter) and there is viable surrounding tissue. Larger defects (>2-3 cm in diameter) have a high recurrence rate if closed primarily and are repaired with a prosthesis.[36] Recurrence rates vary between 10% and 50% and are typically reduced by more than half with the use of prosthetic mesh.[37] Prosthetic material may be placed as an onlay patch to buttress a tissue repair, interposed between the fascial defect, sandwiched between tissue planes, or put in an intraperitoneal position. Depending on its location, several important properties of the mesh must be considered.

A variety of synthetic mesh products are available. Desirable characteristics of a synthetic mesh include being chemically inert, resistant to mechanical stress while maintaining compliance, sterilizable, noncarcinogenic, inciting minimal inflammatory reaction, and hypoallergenic. The ideal mesh has yet to be defined. Polypropylene mesh has been used extensively and allows for ingrowth of native fibroblasts and incorporation into the surrounding fascia. It is semirigid, somewhat flexible, and porous. Placing polypropylene mesh in an intraperitoneal position directly apposed to the bowel is avoided because of unacceptable rates of enterocutaneous fistula formation.[38] When placing mesh in an intraperitoneal position, several options are available. Polypropylene mesh can be used as long as omentum can be interposed between the mesh and hollow viscera. Another choice is to use expanded polytetrafluoroethylene (ePTFE). This product differs from other synthetic meshes in that it is flexible and smooth. Fibroblast proliferation occurs through the pores, but PTFE is impermeable to fluid. Unlike polypropylene, PTFE is not incorporated into the native tissue. Encapsulation occurs slowly, and infection can occur during the encapsulation process. When infected, PTFE almost always must be removed. Composite mesh is a newer product that combines attributes of both polypropylene and PTFE by layering the two substances on top of one another. The PTFE surface serves as a protective interface against the bowel, and the polypropylene side faces superficially to be incorporated into the native fascial tissue. Other dual-sided meshes have placed various collagen-based antiadhesive barriers on one side of either polypropylene or polyester products. The newest development in prostheses for ventral hernia repair is nonsynthetic or natural tissue mesh. These mesh products are largely composed of acellular collagen that is harvested from either porcine intestinal submucosa or dermis, or they are made from human-derived acellular tissue matrix from cadaveric dermis. These biosynthetic meshes are expensive alternatives to other mesh products and are currently used primarily when there is active infection or significant contamination, settings in which permanent mesh products are contraindicated. There are no data comparing the effectiveness of these natural tissue alternatives to synthetic mesh repairs.

With general agreement that all but the smallest incisional hernias are repaired with mesh, the surgeon has a variety of techniques for placing the mesh. The onlay technique involves primary closure of the fascia defect and placement of a polypropylene mesh over the anterior fascia. The major advantage of this approach is that the mesh is placed outside the abdominal cavity avoiding direct interaction with the abdominal viscera. However, disadvantages include that it requires a large subcutaneous dissection, increasing the likelihood of seroma formation; the superficial location of the mesh places it in jeopardy of contamination if the incision becomes infected; and the repair is usually under tension. Prospective analysis of this technique is not available, but a retrospective review reports recurrence rates of 28%.[39]

It is highly desirable to have the mesh placed beneath the fascia. With a wide overlap of mesh and fascia, the natural forces of the abdominal cavity act to hold the mesh in place. This can be accomplished using several techniques. With the use of available dual-type mesh, after reopening the prior incision, the mesh can be placed in an intraperitoneal position at least 2 cm beyond the fascial margin and secured with interrupted mattress sutures. This technique requires raising subcutaneous flaps and may be in direct contact with the mesh and abdominal contents. Alternatively, a piece of polypropylene mesh can be placed with an extensive fascial underlay within either the retrorectus or preperitoneal space, as popularized by Rives and Stoppa.[16,40] In this technique, a large piece of mesh is placed in the retromuscular space on top of either the posterior rectus sheath or peritoneum. This space must be dissected laterally on both sides of the linea alba to a distance of 8 to 10 cm beyond the defect. The prosthetic mesh extends 5 to 6 cm beyond the superior and inferior borders of the defect. It does not need to be sutured because it is held in place by intra-abdominal pressure (Pascal's principle), allowing eventual incorporation into the surrounding tissues. The mesh can be secured laterally with several sutures. This approach avoids contact between the mesh and the abdominal viscera and has been shown in long-term studies to have a respectable recurrence rate of 14% in large incisional hernias.[16]

The laparoscopic approach for ventral hernia repair relies on the same principles as the retrorectus repair; however, the mesh is placed within the peritoneal cavity. The use of laparoscopic ventral hernia repair has been increasing, particularly for large defects. Trocars are placed lateral to the hernia defect. In general, scope placement and trocar location are not consistent and depend on the size and location of the hernia. The hernia contents are reduced, and adhesions are lysed. The surface area of the defect is measured, and a piece of mesh is fashioned with at least 4 cm of overlap around the defect. The mesh is rolled, placed into the abdomen, and deployed. It is secured to the anterior abdominal wall with preplaced mattress sutures that are passed through separate incisions, and tacking staples are placed between these sutures to secure the mesh 4 cm beyond the defect. The advantages of this approach are quicker recovery time and less postoperative pain. Incisional complications are less with the laparoscopic approach because large incisions and subcutaneous undermining are avoided.

Massive ventral hernias can present a particular challenge. Originally, methods to gradually stretch the abdominal wall were used to allow for restoration of abdominal domain and closure. This was accomplished by insufflation of air into the abdominal cavity to create a progressive pneumoperitoneum. Repeated administrations of increasing volumes of air over 1 to 3 weeks allowed the muscles of the abdominal wall to become lax enough for primary closure of the defect. We have not found this technique to be successful in most cases. Instead we perform a staged resection of ePTFE dual mesh for these patients with loss of abdominal domain and lateral retraction of the abdominal wall musculature. The initial stage involves reduction of the hernia and placement of a large sheet of ePTFE dual mesh secured to the fascial edges with a running suture. Subsequent stages involve serial elliptical excision of the mesh until the fascia can be approximated in the midline without tension. Finally, the mesh is excised, and the fascia is reapproximated with component separation and an alloderm onlay patch if necessary.

Another recent development for the repair of complex or large ventral defects is the components separation technique (Fig. 44-10). This involves separating the lateral

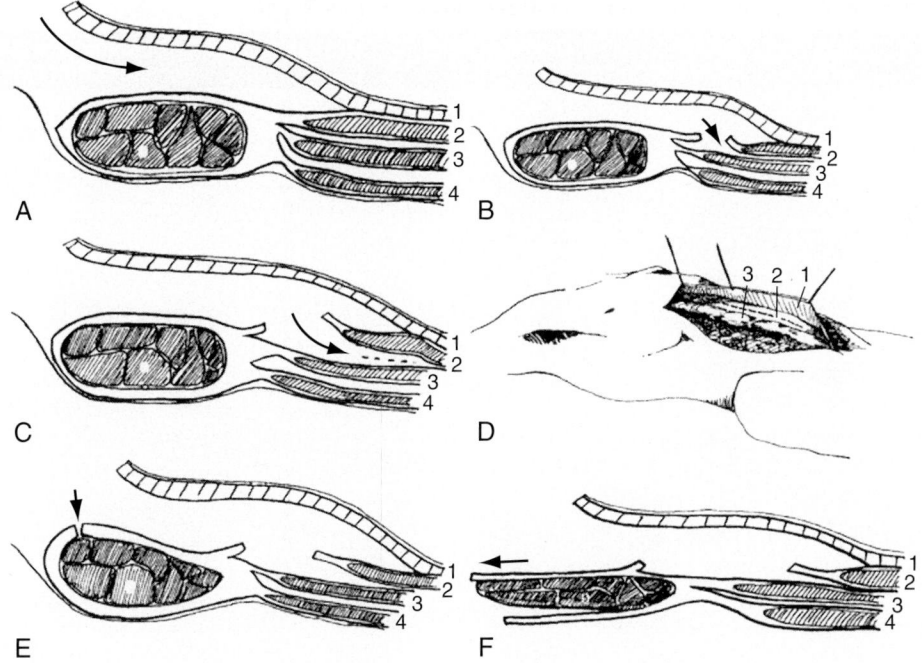

Figure 44-10 Components separation technique. **A,** The skin and subcutaneous fat are dissected free from the anterior sheath of the rectus abdominis muscle and the aponeurosis of the external abdominal oblique muscle. **B,** The external abdominal oblique is incised 1 to 2 cm lateral to the rectus abdominis muscle. **C,** The external abdominal oblique is separated from the internal abdominal oblique. **D,** The dissection is carried to the posterior axillary line. **E,** Additional length can be achieved by incising the posterior rectus sheath above the arcuate line. **F,** Care must be taken to avoid damaging the nerves and blood supply that enter the rectus abdominis posteriorly. (deVries Reilingh TS, van Goor H, Rosman C, et al: Components separation technique for the repair of large abdominal wall hernias. J Am Coll Surg 196:32-37, 2003.)

muscular layers of the abdominal wall to allow their advancement. Primary fascial closure at the midline is often possible, eliminating the need for mesh insertion. This procedure is performed by raising large subcutaneous flaps above the external oblique fascia. These flaps are carried laterally past the linea semilunaris. This dissection itself can provide some advancement of the abdominal wall. Large perforating subcutaneous vessels are carefully preserved to prevent ischemic necrosis of the skin flaps. A relaxing incision is made on the lateral external oblique aponeurosis from the costal margin to the pubis. The external oblique is then bluntly separated in the avascular plane away from the internal oblique, allowing its advancement. Further relaxing incisions can be performed on the aponeurotic layers of the internal oblique, transversus abdominis, or posterior rectus sheath. These techniques, when applied to both sides of the abdominal wall, can yield up to 20 cm of mobilization. Although this technique often allows tension-free closure of these large defects, recurrence rates of up to 30% have been documented without the use of prosthetic reinforcement in large hernias. It is important that patients understand that a lateral bulge is not uncommon after releasing the external oblique aponeurosis. Because of these factors, we typically reinforce this repair with a biologic prosthetic onlay. This technique is very useful in patients who have had damage-control laparotomies performed or in other situations in which large hernia defects exist.[41]

Results of Incisional Hernia Repairs

Only two prospective randomized trials have compared laparoscopic and open ventral hernia repairs.[42,43] Although both of these studies are small, with fewer than 100 patients in both studies combined, the results tend to favor a laparoscopic approach. The incidences of postoperative complications and recurrence were less in hernias repaired laparoscopically. Several retrospective reports demonstrate similar advantages for a laparoscopic approach. Based on the comparative trials listed in Table 44-4, laparoscopic incisional hernia repair results in fewer postoperative complications, a lower infection rate, and decreased hernia recurrence.[42-48] Until an appropriately powered prospective randomized trial is performed, the ideal approach will largely be based on surgeon expertise and preference.

UNUSUAL HERNIAS

Spigelian Hernia

A spigelian hernia occurs through the spigelian fascia, which is composed of the aponeurotic layer between the

Table 44-4 **Comparison of Studies of Laparoscopic and Open Ventral Hernia Repair**

STUDY	YEAR	NO. OF PATIENTS	COMPLICATIONS (%)	MESH INFECTION (%)	SURGICAL SITE INFECTION (%)	RECURRENCE (%)
McGreevy et al[45]	2003	Lap.: 65	8	3	0	—
		Open: 71	21	0	10	—
Raftopoulos et al[46]	2003	Lap.: 50	28	2	2	2
		Open: 22	45	0	5	18
Wright et al[48]	2002	Lap.: 90	17	1	1	1
		Open: 90	34	1	7	4
Robbins et al[47]	2001	Lap.: 18	—	6	6	—
		Open: 31		13	0	—
DeMaria et al[43]	2000	Lap.: 21	62	5	5	5
		Open: 18	72	11	22	0
Chari et al[44]	2000	Lap.: 14	14	0	—	—
		Open: 14	14	7	—	—
Carbajo et al[42]	1999	Lap.: 30	67	0	0	3
		Open: 30	20	10	17	6
Total		Lap.: 288	39	2.8	2.8	2.8
		Open: 276	41	6	12	7

rectus muscle medially and the semilunar line laterally. Nearly all spigelian hernias occur at or below the arcuate line. The absence of posterior rectus fascia may contribute to an inherent weakness in this area. These hernias are often interparietal, with the hernia sac dissecting posterior to the external oblique aponeurosis. Most spigelian hernias are small (1-2 cm in diameter) and develop during the fourth to seventh decades of life. Patients often present with localized pain in the area without a bulge because the hernia lies beneath the intact external oblique aponeurosis. Ultrasound or CT of the abdomen can be useful to establish the diagnosis.

A spigelian hernia is repaired because of the risk for incarceration associated with its relatively narrow neck. The hernia site is marked before operation. A transverse incision is made over the defect and carried through the external oblique aponeurosis. The hernia sac is opened and dissected free of the neck of the hernia and either excised or inverted. The defect is closed transversely by simple suture repair of the transversus abdominis and internal oblique muscles, followed by closure of the external oblique aponeurosis. Larger defects are repaired using a mesh prosthesis. Recurrence is uncommon.

Obturator Hernia

The obturator canal is formed by the union of the pubic bone and ischium. This canal is covered by a membrane pierced by the obturator nerve and vessels. Weakening of the obturator membrane may result in enlargement of the canal and formation of a hernia sac, which can lead to intestinal incarceration and strangulation. The patient can present with evidence of compression of the obturator nerve, which causes pain in the medial aspect of the thigh (Howship-Romberg sign). Nearly one half of patients

with obturator hernia present with complete or partial bowel obstruction. An abdominal CT can establish the diagnosis if necessary.

A posterior approach, either open or laparoscopic, is preferred. This approach provides direct access to the hernia. Patients with compromised bowel should have a preperitoneal open repair. After reduction of the hernia sac and contents, any preperitoneal fat within the obturator canal is reduced. The obturator nerve can be manipulated gently with a blunt nerve hook to facilitate reduction of the fat pad. The obturator foramen is repaired with sutures or a small piece of prosthetic mesh, with care to avoid injury to the obturator nerve and vessels.

Lumbar Hernia

Lumbar hernias can be either congenital or acquired and occur in the lumbar region of the posterior abdominal wall. Hernias through the superior lumbar triangle (Grynfeltt's triangle) are more common. The superior lumbar triangle is bounded by the 12th rib, paraspinal muscles, and internal oblique muscle. Less common are hernias through the inferior lumbar triangle (Petit's triangle), which is bounded by the iliac crest, latissimus dorsi muscle, and external oblique muscle. Weakness of the lumbodorsal fascia through either of these areas results in progressive protrusion of extraperitoneal fat and a hernia sac. Lumbar hernias are not prone to incarceration.

Satisfactory suture repair is difficult because of the immobile bony margins of these defects. Repair is best done by placement of prosthetic mesh, which can be sutured to the margins of the hernia. There is usually sufficient fascia over the bone to anchor the mesh.

Interparietal Hernia

Interparietal hernias are rare and occur when the hernia sac lies between layers of the abdominal wall. Interparietal hernias most frequently occur in previous incisions. Spigelian hernias are nearly always interparietal.

The correct preoperative diagnosis of interparietal hernia can be difficult. Many patients with complicated interparietal hernias present with intestinal obstruction. Abdominal CT can assist in the diagnosis. Large interparietal hernias usually require placement of prosthetic mesh for closure. When this cannot be done, the separation of components technique may be useful to provide natural tissues to obliterate the defect.

Sciatic Hernia

The greater sciatic foramen can be a site of hernia formation. These hernias are extremely unusual and difficult to diagnose and frequently are asymptomatic until intestinal obstruction occurs. The most common symptom is the presence of an uncomfortable or slowly enlarging mass in the gluteal or intragluteal area. Sciatic nerve pain can occur, but sciatic hernia is a rare cause of sciatic neuralgia.

A transperitoneal approach is preferred if bowel obstruction or strangulation is suspected. Hernia contents can usually be reduced with gentle traction. Prosthetic mesh repair is usually preferred. A transgluteal approach can be used if the diagnosis is certain and the hernia is reducible. With the patient prone, an incision is made from the posterior edge of the greater trochanter across the hernia mass. The gluteus maximus muscle is opened, and the sac is visualized. Either the muscle edges of the defect are reapproximated with interrupted sutures, or the defect is obliterated with mesh.

Perineal Hernia

Perineal hernias are caused by congenital or acquired defects and are very uncommon. These hernias also may occur after abdominoperineal resection or perineal prostatectomy. The hernia sac protrudes through the pelvic diaphragm. Primary perineal hernias are rare, occur most commonly in older, multiparous women, and can be quite large. Symptoms are usually related to protrusion of a mass through the defect that is worsened by sitting or standing. A bulge is frequently detected on bimanual rectal-vaginal examination.

Perineal hernias are generally repaired through a transabdominal approach or combined transabdominal and perineal approaches. After the sac contents are reduced, small defects may be closed with nonabsorbable suture, whereas large defects are repaired with prosthetic mesh.

Complications

Mesh Infection

Mesh infections are serious complications that can be very difficult to treat. If ePTFE becomes infected, it requires removal with the resultant morbidity of another defect that often must be closed under tension leading to inevitable recurrence. In open ventral hernia repair, incisional and mesh infections are not infrequent. Using the laparoscopic technique and placing a large piece of mesh without undermining large subcutaneous tissue flaps wound complications is accomplished rarely. In a series of almost 1000 patients who had laparoscopic ventral hernia repair, mesh infections occurred in less than 1% of cases.[49] Perhaps the greatest advantage of the laparoscopic approach for repairing ventral hernias is this reduction in infectious complications.

Seromas

Seroma formation can occur after laparoscopic and open ventral hernia repair. In open ventral hernia repair, drains are often placed in an attempt to obliterate the dead space caused by the hernia and tissue dissection. These drains can cause mesh contamination, and seromas can form after drain removal. With laparoscopic repair, the hernia sac is not resected, and a seroma cavity will result. Most of these seromas will resolve over time as the mesh becomes incorporated on the hernia sac. Preoperative discussions with the patient detailing the expectations of a temporary seroma are imperative before laparoscopic ventral hernia repair. We reserve aspiration for symptomatic or persistent seromas after 6 to 8 weeks.

Enterotomy

Intestinal injury during adhesiolysis can be catastrophic. Management of an enterotomy during a hernia repair is controversial and depends on the segment of intestine injured (small versus large bowel) and amount of spillage. Options include aborting the hernia repair, using a primary tissue or biologic tissue repair, or performing a delayed repair using prosthetic mesh in 3 to 4 days. When there is gross contamination, the use of prosthetic mesh is contraindicated.

Selected References

Anson BJ, McVay CB: Inguinal hernia: The anatomy of the region. Surg Gynecol Obstet 66:186, 1938.

Condon RE: Surgical anatomy of the transversus abdominis and transversalis fascia. Ann Surg 173:1, 1971.

Nyhus LM: An anatomic reappraisal of the posterior inguinal wall, with special consideration of the iliopubic tract and its relation to groin hernias. Surg Clin North Am 44:1305, 1960.

These three references are classic descriptions of the anatomy of the groin. All are well illustrated.

Anthony T, Bergen PC, Kim LT, et al: Factors affecting recurrence following incisional herniorrhaphy. World J Surg 24:95-100, 2000.

Excellent report comparing primary and mesh repairs for incisional hernia in a Veterans Administration hospital.

EU Hernia Trialists Collaboration: Repair of groin hernia with synthetic mesh. Meta-analysis of randomized controlled trials. Ann Surg 235:322-332, 2002.

Excellent meta-analysis of tension-free repairs compared with other methods. It demonstrates a 60% reduction in recurrence among mesh repairs.

Gilbert AI: Sutureless repair of inguinal hernia. Am J Surg 163:331, 1992.

> This report describes the "plug and patch" tension-free inguinal hernia repair.

Lichtenstein IL, Shulman AG, Amid PK, et al: The tension-free hernioplasty. Am J Surg 157:188, 1989.

> This article reports excellent results of a large number of tension-free hernia repairs.

Lowham AS, Filipi CJ, Fitzgibbons RJ Jr: Mechanisms of hernia recurrence after preperitoneal mesh repair: Traditional and laparoscopic. Ann Surg 225:422-431, 1997.

> This article outlines the important causes for inguinal hernia recurrence. These principles also apply to other hernias.

Stoppa RE: The treatment of complicated groin and incisional hernias. World J Surg 13:545, 1989.

> Reference describing the giant prosthetic reinforcement of the visceral sac (Stoppa) repair and its indications.

References

1. Bradley M, Morgan D, Pentlow B, et al: The groin hernia: An ultrasound diagnosis? Ann R Coll Surg Engl 85:178-180, 2003.
2. Della Santa V, Groebli Y: [Diagnosis of non-hernia groin masses]. Ann Chir 125:179-183, 2000.
3. Fitzgibbons RJ, Jr., Giobbie-Hurder A, Gibbs JO, et al: Watchful waiting vs repair of inguinal hernia in minimally symptomatic men: A randomized clinical trial. JAMA 295:285-292, 2006.
4. Kugel RD: Minimally invasive, nonlaparoscopic, preperitoneal, and sutureless, inguinal herniorrhaphy. Am J Surg 178:298-302, 1999.
5. Kingsnorth AN, Porter CS, Bennett DH, et al: Lichtenstein patch or Perfix plug-and-patch in inguinal hernia: A prospective double-blind randomized controlled trial of short-term outcome. Surgery 127:276-283, 2000.
6. Kingsnorth AN, Wright D, Porter CS, et al: Prolene Hernia System compared with Lichtenstein patch: A randomised double blind study of short-term and medium-term outcomes in primary inguinal hernia repair. Hernia 6:113-119, 2002.
7. Nienhuijs SW, van Oort I, Keemers-Gels ME, et al: Randomized trial comparing the Prolene Hernia System, mesh plug repair and Lichtenstein method for open inguinal hernia repair. Br J Surg 92:33-38, 2005.
8. Vironen J, Nieminen J, Eklund A, et al: Randomized clinical trial of Lichtenstein patch or Prolene Hernia System for inguinal hernia repair. Br J Surg 93:33-39, 2006.
9. Voyles CR, Hamilton BJ, Johnson WD, et al: Meta-analysis of laparoscopic inguinal hernia trials favors open hernia repair with preperitoneal mesh prosthesis. Am J Surg 184:6-10, 2002.
10. Liem MS, van Duyn EB, van der Graaf Y, et al: Recurrences after conventional anterior and laparoscopic inguinal hernia repair: a randomized comparison. Ann Surg 237:136-141, 2003.
11. Bringman S, Ramel S, Heikkinen TJ, et al: Tension-free inguinal hernia repair: TEP versus mesh-plug versus Lichtenstein. A prospective randomized controlled trial. Ann Surg 237:142-147, 2003.
12. Lal P, Kajla RK, Chander J, et al: Randomized controlled study of laparoscopic total extraperitoneal versus open Lichtenstein inguinal hernia repair. Surg Endosc 17:850-856, 2003.
13. Neumayer L, Giobbie-Harder A, Jonasson O, et al: Open mesh versus laparoscopic mesh repair of inguinal hernia. N Engl J Med 350:1819-1827, 2004.
14. Repair of groin hernia with synthetic mesh: Meta-analysis of randomized controlled trials. Ann Surg 235:322-332, 2002.
15. Neumayer LA, Gawande AA, Wang J, et al: Proficiency of surgeons in inguinal hernia repair: Effect of experience and age. Ann Surg 242:344-348; discussion, 348-352, 2005.
16. Stoppa RE: The treatment of complicated groin and incisional hernias. World J Surg 13:545-554, 1989.
17. Taylor EW, Byrne DJ, Leaper DJ, et al: Antibiotic prophylaxis and open groin hernia repair. World J Surg 21:811-814; discussion, 814-815, 1997.
18. Grant AM, Scott NW, O'Dwyer PJ: Five-year follow-up of a randomized trial to assess pain and numbness after laparoscopic or open repair of groin hernia. Br J Surg 91:1570-1574, 2004.
19. Nienhuijs SW, Boelens OB, Strobbe LJ: Pain after anterior mesh hernia repair. J Am Coll Surg 200:885-889, 2005.
20. Picchio M, Palimento D, Attanasio U, et al: Randomized controlled trial of preservation or elective division of ilioinguinal nerve on open inguinal hernia repair with polypropylene mesh. Arch Surg 139:755-758; discussion 759, 2004.
21. Johansson B, Hallerback B, Glise H, et al: Laparoscopic mesh versus open preperitoneal mesh versus conventional technique for inguinal hernia repair: A randomized multicenter trial (SCUR Hernia Repair Study). Ann Surg 230:225-231, 1999.
22. Juul P, Christensen K: Randomized clinical trial of laparoscopic versus open inguinal hernia repair. Br J Surg 86:316-319, 1999.
23. Lichtenstein IL, Shulman AG, Amid PK, et al: The tension-free hernioplasty. Am J Surg 157:188-193, 1989.
24. Swanstrom LL: Laparoscopic hernia repairs: The importance of cost as an outcome measurement at the century's end. Surg Clin North Am 80:1341-1351, 2000.
25. Wright BE, Beckerman J, Cohen M, et al: Is laparoscopic umbilical hernia repair with mesh a reasonable alternative to conventional repair? Am J Surg 184:505-508; discussion, 508-509, 2002.
26. Lowham AS, Filipi CJ, Fitzgibbons RJ Jr, et al: Mechanisms of hernia recurrence after preperitoneal mesh repair: Traditional and laparoscopic. Ann Surg 225:422-431, 1997.
27. Haapaniemi S, Gunnarsson U, Nordin P, et al: Reoperation after recurrent groin hernia repair. Ann Surg 234:122-126, 2001.
28. Janu PG, Sellers KD, Mangiante EC: Recurrent inguinal hernia: Preferred operative approach. Am Surg 64:569-573; discussion, 573-564, 1998.
29. Nyhus LM, Pollak R, Bombeck CT, et al: The preperitoneal approach and prosthetic buttress repair for recurrent hernia: The evolution of a technique. Ann Surg 208:733-737, 1988.
30. Shulman AG, Amid PK, Lichtenstein IL: The 'plug' repair of 1402 recurrent inguinal hernias: 20-year experience. Arch Surg 125:265-267, 1990.
31. Simons MP, Kleijnen J, van Geldere D, et al: Role of the Shouldice technique in inguinal hernia repair: A systematic review of controlled trials and a meta-analysis. Br J Surg 83:734-738, 1996.
32. Read RC, Yoder G: Recent trends in the management of incisional herniation. Arch Surg 124:485-488, 1989.

33. Rucinski J, Margolis M, Panagopoulos G, et al: Closure of the abdominal midline fascia: Meta-analysis delineates the optimal technique. Am Surg 67:421-426, 2001.
34. Arroyo A, Garcia P, Perez F, et al: Randomized clinical trial comparing suture and mesh repair of umbilical hernia in adults. Br J Surg 88:1321-1323, 2001.
35. Muschaweck U: Umbilical and epigastric hernia repair. Surg Clin North Am 83:1207-1221, 2003.
36. Luijendijk RW, Hop WC, van den Tol MP, et al: A comparison of suture repair with mesh repair for incisional hernia. N Engl J Med 343:392-398, 2000.
37. Anthony T, Bergen PC, Kim LT, et al: Factors affecting recurrence following incisional herniorrhaphy. World J Surg 24:95-100; discussion, 101, 2000.
38. Leber GE, Garb JL, Alexander AI, et al: Long-term complications associated with prosthetic repair of incisional hernias. Arch Surg 133:378-382, 1998.
39. de Vries Reilingh TS, van Geldere D, Langenhorst B, et al: Repair of large midline incisional hernias with polypropylene mesh: Comparison of three operative techniques. Hernia 8:56-59, 2004.
40. Rives J, Pire JC, Flament JB, et al: [Treatment of large eventrations. New therapeutic indications apropos of 322 cases]. Chirurgie 111:215-225, 1985.
41. Ewart CJ, Lankford AB, Gamboa MG: Successful closure of abdominal wall hernias using the components separation technique. Ann Plast Surg 50:269-273; discussion, 273-264, 2003.
42. Carbajo MA, Martin del Olmo JC, Blanco JI, et al: Laparoscopic treatment vs open surgery in the solution of major incisional and abdominal wall hernias with mesh. Surg Endosc 13:250-252, 1999.
43. DeMaria EJ, Moss JM, Sugerman HJ: Laparoscopic intraperitoneal polytetrafluoroethylene (PTFE) prosthetic patch repair of ventral hernia: Prospective comparison to open prefascial polypropylene mesh repair. Surg Endosc 14:326-329, 2000.
44. Chari R, Chari V, Eisenstat M, et al: A case controlled study of laparoscopic incisional hernia repair. Surg Endosc 14:117-119, 2000.
45. McGreevy JM, Goodney PP, Birkmeyer CM, et al: A prospective study comparing the complication rates between laparoscopic and open ventral hernia repairs. Surg Endosc 17:1778-1780, 2003.
46. Raftopoulos I, Vanuno D, Khorsand J, et al: Comparison of open and laparoscopic prosthetic repair of large ventral hernias. J Soc Laparoendosc Surg 7:227-232, 2003.
47. Robbins SB, Pofahl WE, Gonzalez RP: Laparoscopic ventral hernia repair reduces wound complications. Am Surg 67:896-900, 2001.
48. Wright BE, Niskanen BD, Peterson DJ, et al: Laparoscopic ventral hernia repair: Are there comparative advantages over traditional methods of repair? Am Surg 68:291-295; discussion, 295-296, 2002.
49. Heniford BT, Park A, Ramshaw BJ, et al: Laparoscopic repair of ventral hernias: Nine years' experience with 850 consecutive hernias. Ann Surg 238:391-399; discussion, 399-400, 2003.

Acute Abdomen

Russell G. Postier, MD   and   Ronald A. Squires, MD

DEFINITION

The term *acute abdomen* refers to signs and symptoms of abdominal pain and tenderness, a clinical presentation that often requires emergency surgical therapy. This challenging clinical scenario requires a thorough and expeditious workup to determine the need for operative intervention and to initiate appropriate therapy. Many diseases, some of which are not surgical or intraabdominal, can produce acute abdominal pain and tenderness. Therefore, every attempt is made to make a correct diagnosis so that the chosen therapy, often a laparoscopy or laparotomy, is appropriate.

The diagnoses associated with an acute abdomen vary according to age and gender.[1,2] Appendicitis is more common in the young, whereas biliary disease, bowel obstruction, intestinal ischemia and infarction, and diverticulitis are more common in elderly patients. Chapter 71 deals specifically with abdominal pain in children. Most of these diagnoses result from infection, obstruction, ischemia, or perforation.

Nonsurgical causes of an acute abdomen can be divided into three categories: endocrine and metabolic, hematologic, and toxins or drugs[3] (Table 45-1). Endocrine and metabolic causes include uremia, diabetic crisis, addisonian crisis, acute intermittent porphyria, acute hyperlipoproteinemia, and hereditary Mediterranean fever. Hematologic disorders are sickle cell crisis, acute leukemia, and other blood dyscrasias. Toxins and drugs causing an acute abdomen include lead and other heavy metal poisoning, narcotic withdrawal, and black widow spider poisoning. It is important to keep these possibilities in mind when evaluating a patient with acute abdominal pain.

Because of the potential surgical nature of the acute abdomen, an expeditious workup is necessary (Table 45-2). The workup proceeds in the usual order of history, physical examination, laboratory, and imaging studies. Although imaging studies have increased the accuracy with which the correct diagnosis can be made, the most important part of the evaluation remains a thorough history and careful physical examination. Laboratory and imaging studies, although usually needed, are directed by the findings on history and physical examination.

ANATOMY AND PHYSIOLOGY

Abdominal pain is conveniently divided into visceral or parietal components. Visceral pain tends to be vague and poorly localized to the epigastrium, periumbilical region, or hypogastrium, depending on its origin from the primitive foregut, midgut, or hindgut (Fig. 45-1). It is usually the result of distention of a hollow viscus. Parietal pain corresponds to the segmental nerve roots innervating the peritoneum and tends to be sharper and better localized. Referred pain is pain perceived at a site distant from the source of stimulus. For example, irritation of the diaphragm may produce pain in the shoulder. Common referred pain sites and their accompanying sources are listed in Table 45-3. Determining whether the pain is

Table 45-1 Nonsurgical Causes of Acute Abdomen

Endocrine and Metabolic Causes
Uremia
Diabetic crisis
Addisonian crisis
Acute intermittent porphyria
Hereditary Mediterranean fever

Hematologic Causes
Sickle cell crisis
Acute leukemia
Other blood dyscrasias

Toxins and Drugs
Lead poisoning
Other heavy metal poisoning
Narcotic withdrawal
Black widow spider poisoning

Table 45-2 Surgical Acute Abdominal Conditions

Hemorrhage
Solid organ trauma
Leaking or ruptured arterial aneurysm
Ruptured ectopic pregnancy
Bleeding gastrointestinal diverticulum
Arteriovenous malformation of gastrointestinal tract
Intestinal ulceration
Aortoduodenal fistula after aortic vascular graft
Hemorrhagic pancreatitis
Mallory-Weiss syndrome
Spontaneous rupture of spleen

Infection
Appendicitis
Cholecystitis
Meckel's diverticulitis
Hepatic abscess
Diverticular abscess
Psoas abscess

Perforation
Perforated gastrointestinal ulcer
Perforated gastrointestinal cancer
Boerhaave's syndrome
Perforated diverticulum

Obstruction
Adhesion related small or large bowel obstruction
Sigmoid volvulus
Cecal volvulus
Incarcerated hernias
Inflammatory bowel disease
Gastrointestinal malignancy
Intussusception

Ischemia
Buerger's disease
Mesenteric thrombosis or embolism
Ovarian torsion
Ischemic colitis
Testicular torsion
Strangulated hernias

visceral, parietal, or referred is important and can usually be done with a careful history.

Introduction of bacteria or irritating chemicals into the peritoneal cavity can cause an outpouring of fluid from the peritoneal membrane. The peritoneum responds to inflammation by increased blood flow, increased permeability, and the formation of a fibrinous exudate on its surface. The bowel also develops local or generalized paralysis. The fibrinous surface and decreased intestinal movement cause adherence between the bowel and omentum or abdominal wall and help to localize inflammation. As a result, an abscess may produce sharply localized pain with normal bowel sounds and gastrointestinal function, whereas a diffuse process, such as a perforated duodenal ulcer, produces generalized abdominal pain with a quiet abdomen. Peritonitis may affect the entire abdominal cavity or a portion of the visceral or parietal peritoneum.

Peritonitis is peritoneal inflammation from any cause. It is usually recognized on physical examination by severe tenderness to palpation, with or without rebound tenderness, and guarding. Peritonitis is usually secondary to an inflammatory insult, most often gram-negative infections with enteric organisms or anaerobes. It can result from noninfectious inflammation, a common example being pancreatitis. Primary peritonitis occurs more commonly in children and is most often due to *Pneumococcus* or hemolytic *Streptococcus* species infection.[4] Adults with end-stage renal disease on peritoneal dialysis can develop infections of their peritoneal fluid, with the most common organisms being gram-positive cocci.[5] Adults with ascites and cirrhosis can develop primary peritonitis, and in these cases, the organisms are usually *Escherichia coli* and *Klebsiella* species.

HISTORY

A detailed and organized history is essential to formulating an accurate differential diagnosis and subsequent treatment regimen. Modern advances in imaging cannot and will never replace the need for a skilled clinician's bedside examination. The history must focus not only on the investigation of the pain complaints but also on past problems and associated symptoms. Questions must be open-ended whenever possible and structured to disclose the onset, character, location, duration, radiation, and chronology of the pain experienced. It is tempting to ask questions such as, "is the pain sharp" or "does eating make it worse?" This specific yes or no style can speed up the history taking by not allowing the patient to narrate, but it stands to miss vital details and potentially skew the responses. A much better questioning style would be "how does the pain feel to you" or "does anything make the pain better or worse?" Often, additional information can be gained by observing how the patient describes the pain that is experienced. Identifying the pain with one finger often indicates pain that is much more localized and typical of parietal innervation or peritoneal inflammation, as compared with illustrating the area of discomfort with the palm of the hand, which

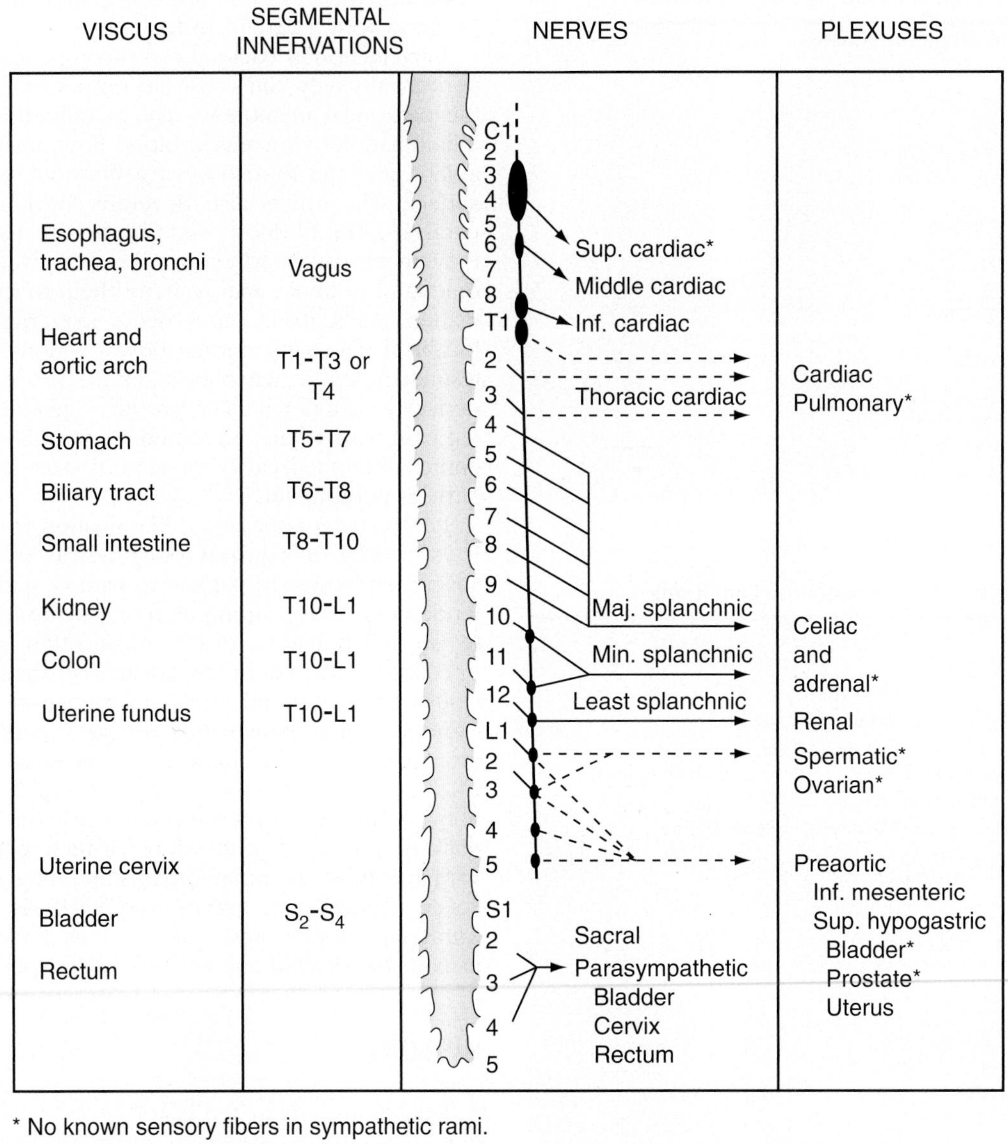

VISCUS	SEGMENTAL INNERVATIONS	NERVES	PLEXUSES
Esophagus, trachea, bronchi	Vagus	Sup. cardiac* / Middle cardiac / Inf. cardiac	
Heart and aortic arch	T1–T3 or T4	Thoracic cardiac	Cardiac Pulmonary*
Stomach	T5–T7		
Biliary tract	T6–T8		
Small intestine	T8–T10		
Kidney	T10–L1	Maj. splanchnic	Celiac and adrenal*
Colon	T10–L1	Min. splanchnic	
Uterine fundus	T10–L1	Least splanchnic	Renal Spermatic* Ovarian*
Uterine cervix			Preaortic Inf. mesenteric Sup. hypogastric Bladder* Prostate* Uterus
Bladder	S_2–S_4	Sacral Parasympathetic Bladder Cervix Rectum	
Rectum			

* No known sensory fibers in sympathetic rami.

Figure 45-1 **Sensory innervation of the viscera.** (From White JC, Sweet WH: Pain and the neurosurgeon. Springfield, IL, Charles C Thomas, 1969, p 526.)

Table 45-3 Locations of Referred Pain and Its Causes

Right Shoulder
Liver
Gallbladder
Right hemidiaphragm

Left Shoulder
Heart
Tail of pancreas
Spleen
Left hemidiaphragm

Scrotum and Testicles
Ureter

is more typical of the visceral discomfort of bowel or solid organ disease.

The intensity and severity of the pain are related to the underlying tissue damage. Sudden onset of excruciating pain suggests conditions such as intestinal perforation or arterial embolization with ischemia, although other conditions, such as biliary colic, can present suddenly as well. Pain that develops and worsens over several hours is typical of conditions of progressive inflammation or infection such as cholecystitis, colitis, or bowel obstruction. The history of progressive worsening, in contrast to intermittent episodes of pain, can help to differentiate infectious processes that worsen with time, as opposed to the spasmodic, colicky pain associated with bowel obstruction, biliary colic from cystic duct obstruction, or genitourinary obstruction (Figs. 45-2 to 45-4). Equally

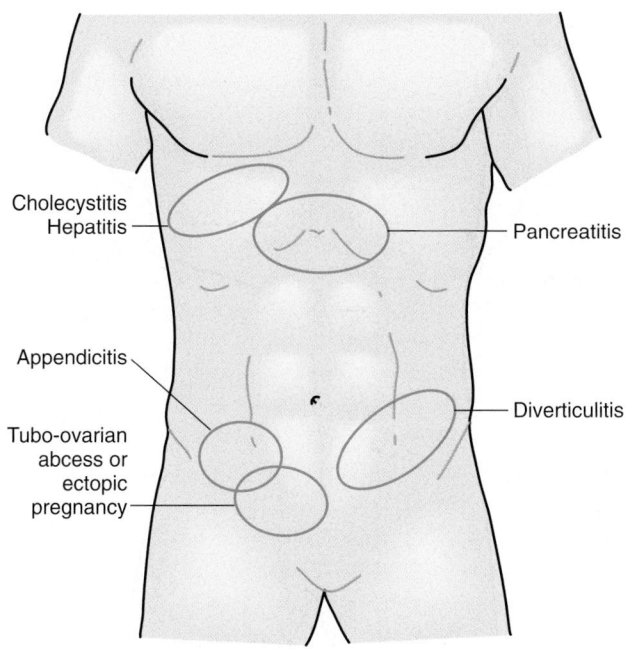

Figure 45-2 Character of pain: gradual, progressive pain.

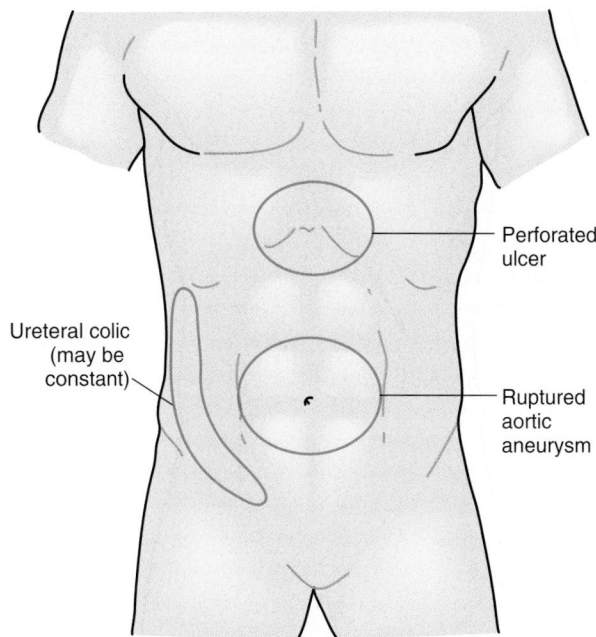

Figure 45-4 Character of pain: sudden, severe pain.

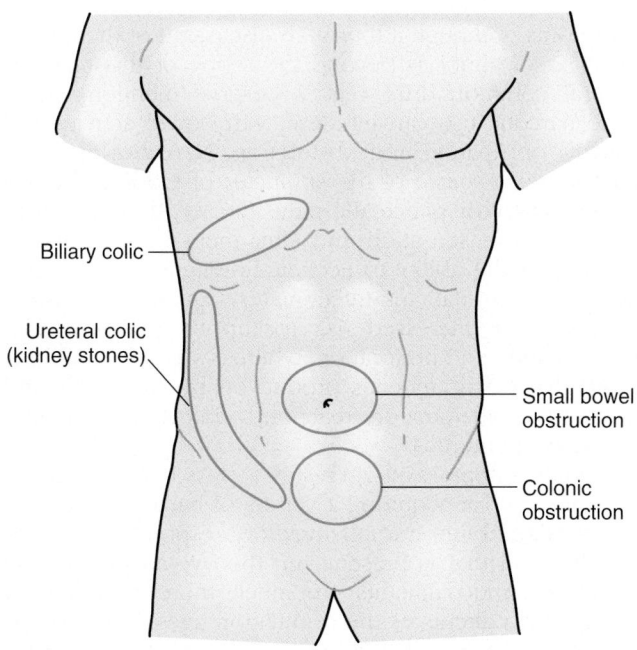

Figure 45-3 Character of pain: colicky, crampy, intermittent pain.

important as the character of the pain are its location and radiation. Tissue injury or inflammation can trigger both visceral and somatic pain. Solid organ visceral pain in the abdomen is generalized in the quadrant of the involved organ, such as liver pain across the right upper quadrant of the abdomen. Small bowel pain is perceived as poorly localized periumbilical pain, whereas colon pain is centered between the umbilicus and the pubic symphysis. As inflammation expands to involve the peritoneal

surface, parietal nerve fibers from the spine allow for focal and intense sensation. This combination of innervation is responsible for the classic diffuse periumbilical pain of early appendicitis, which later shifts to become an intense focal pain in the right lower abdomen at McBurney's point. If the clinician focuses on the character of the current pain and does not thoroughly investigate its onset and progression, he or she will miss these strong historical clues (Figs. 45-5 and 45-6). Pain may also extend well beyond the diseased site. The liver shares some of its innervation with the diaphragm and may create referred pain to the right shoulder from the C3 to C5 nerve roots. Genitourinary pain is another source of pain that commonly has a radiating pattern. Symptoms are primarily in the flank region, originating from the splanchnic nerves of T11 to L1, but pain often radiates to the scrotum or labia through the hypogastric plexus of S2-S4.

Activities that exacerbate or relieve the pain are also important. Eating often worsens the pain of bowel obstruction, biliary colic, pancreatitis, diverticulitis, or bowel perforation. Food can provide relief from the pain of nonperforated peptic ulcer disease or gastritis. Clinicians often recognize that they are evaluating peritonitis during the history. Patients with peritoneal inflammation avoid any activity that stretches or jostles the abdomen. They describe worsening of the pain with any sudden body movement and will realize that there is less pain if their knees are flexed. The car ride to the hospital can be agonizing, with the patient feeling every bump along the way.

Associated symptoms can be important clues to the diagnosis. Nausea, vomiting, constipation, diarrhea, pruritus, melena, hematochezia, or hematuria can all be helpful symptoms if present and recognized. Vomiting

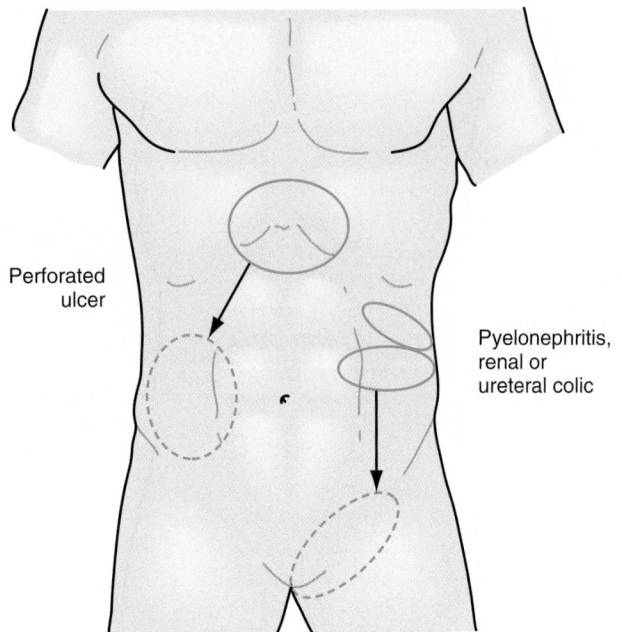

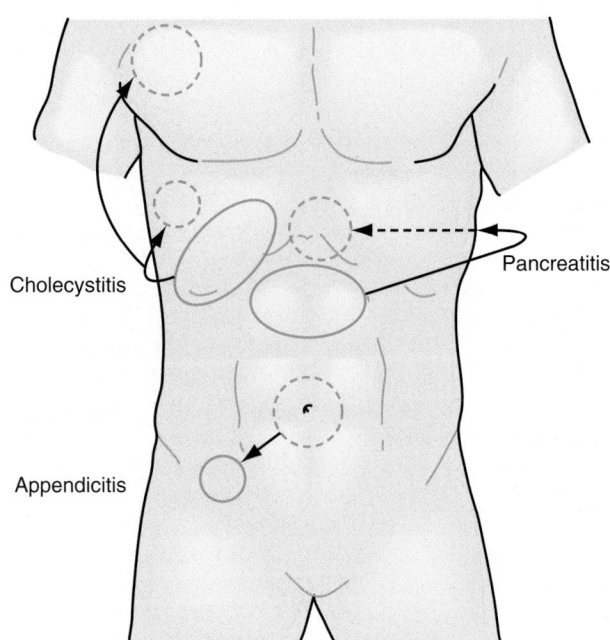

Figure 45-5 Referred pain. *Solid circles* are primary or most intense sites of pain.

Figure 45-6 Referred pain. *Solid circles* are primary or most intense sites of pain.

may result from severe abdominal pain of any etiology or from mechanical bowel obstruction or ileus. Vomiting is more likely to precede the onset of significant abdominal pain in many medical conditions, whereas the pain of an acute *surgical* abdomen presents first and stimulates vomiting through medullary efferent fibers that are triggered by the visceral afferent pain fibers. Constipation or obstipation can be a result of either mechanical obstruction or decreased peristalsis. It may represent the primary problem and require laxatives and prokinetic agents, or merely be a symptom of an underlying condition. A careful history includes whether the patient is continuing to pass any gas or stool from the rectum. A complete obstruction is more likely to be associated with subsequent bowel ischemia or perforation due to the massive distention that can occur. Diarrhea is associated with several medical causes of acute abdomen, including infectious enteritis, inflammatory bowel disease, and parasitic contamination. Bloody diarrhea can be seen in these conditions as well as in colonic ischemia.

The past medical history can potentially be more helpful than any other single part of the patient's evaluation. Previous illnesses or diagnoses can greatly increase or decrease the likelihood of certain conditions that would otherwise not be highly considered. Patients may, for example, report that the current pain is very similar to the kidney stone passage they experienced a decade prior. On the other hand, a prior history of appendectomy, pelvic inflammatory disease, or cholecystectomy can significantly shape the differential diagnosis. During the abdominal examination, all scars on the abdomen must be accounted for by the medical history obtained.

A history of medications and a gynecologic history of female patients are very important. Medications can both create acute abdominal conditions or mask their symptoms. Although a thorough discussion of the impact of all medications is beyond the scope of this chapter, several common drug classes deserve mention. High-dose narcotic use can interfere with bowel activity and lead to obstipation and obstruction. Narcotics also can contribute to spasm of the sphincter of Oddi and exacerbate biliary or pancreatic pain. Clearly, they also may suppress pain sensation and alter mental status, which can impair the ability to accurately diagnose the condition. Nonsteroidal anti-inflammatory agents are associated with an increased risk for upper gastrointestinal inflammation and perforation, whereas steroids can block protective gastric mucous production by chief cells and reduce the inflammatory reaction to infection, including advanced peritonitis.

Immunosuppressant agents as a class both increase a patient's risk for acquiring a variety of bacterial and viral illnesses and blunt the inflammatory response, diminishing the pain that is present and the overall physiologic response. Anticoagulants are much more prevalent in emergency patients as the population ages. These drugs may be the cause of gastrointestinal bleeds, retroperitoneal hemorrhages, or rectus sheath hematomas. They also can complicate the preoperative preparation of the patient and can cause substantial morbidity if their use goes unrecognized. Finally, recreational drugs can play a role in patients with an acute abdomen. Chronic alcoholism is strongly associated with coagulopathy and portal hypertension from liver impairment. Cocaine and methamphetamine can create an intense vasospastic reaction, which can create life-threatening hypertension as well as cardiac or intestinal ischemia.

The gynecologic health, and specifically the menstrual history, is crucial in evaluation of lower abdominal pain in young women. The likelihood of ectopic pregnancy, pelvic inflammatory disease, mittelschmerz, or severe endometriosis is heavily influenced by the details of the gynecologic history.

Little has changed in the technique or goals of history taking since Dr. Zachary Cope first published his classic paper on the diagnosis of acute abdominal pain in 1921.[6] An exception is the application of computers to the so-called art of history taking, which has been extensively studied in Europe.[7-11] Data were collected by physicians on detailed standardized forms during history and physical examination and entered into computers programmed with a medical database of diseases and their associated signs and symptoms. The computer-generated diagnosis based on mathematical probabilities was as much as 20% more accurate than the diagnosis determined by physicians left to their own methods. Statistically significant improvement was identified in timely laparotomy, shortened hospital stays, and reduced need for surgery and hospitalization.[7] It is interesting and important to note, however, that statistically significant improvement in accuracy and efficiency has been realized without computer assistance when similar standardized forms are used for data collection. This has also been observed in the settings of trauma and critical care.

PHYSICAL EXAMINATION

An organized and thoughtful physical examination is critical to the development of an accurate differential diagnosis and the subsequent treatment algorithm. Despite newer technologies, including high-resolution computed tomography (CT) scanning, ultrasound, and magnetic resonance imaging (MRI), the physical examination remains a key part of a patient's evaluation and must not be minimized. A skilled clinician will be able to develop a narrow and accurate differential diagnosis in most patients at the conclusion of the history and physical examination. Laboratory and imaging studies can then be used to further confirm the suspicions, reorder the proposed differential diagnosis, or less commonly, suggest unusual possibilities not yet considered.

The physical examination always begins with a general inspection of the patient, followed by inspection of the abdomen itself. Patients with peritoneal irritation experience worsened pain with any activity that moves or stretches the peritoneum. These patients typically lie very still in the bed during the evaluation and often maintain flexion of their knees and hips to reduce tension on the anterior abdominal wall. Disease states that cause pain without peritoneal irritation, such as ischemic bowel and ureteral and biliary colic, typically cause patients to continually shift and fidget in bed while trying to find a position that lessens their discomfort (Fig. 45-7). Other important clues, such as pallor, cyanosis, and diaphoresis, may be observed during the general inspection as well.

Abdominal inspection addresses the contour of the abdomen, including whether it appears distended or scaphoid or whether a localized mass effect is observed. Special attention is paid to all scars present, and if surgical in nature, scars need to correlate with the past surgical

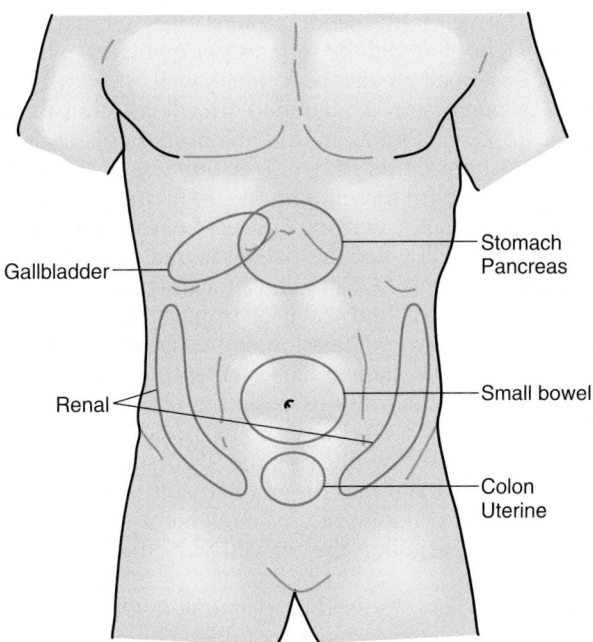

Figure 45-7 Common locations for visceral pain.

history provided. Fascial hernias may be suspected and can be confirmed during palpation of the abdominal wall. Evidence of erythema or edema of skin may suggest cellulitis of the abdominal wall, whereas ecchymosis is sometimes observed with deeper necrotizing infections of the fascia or abdominal structures such as the pancreas.

Auscultation can provide useful information about the gastrointestinal tract and the vascular system. Bowel sounds are typically evaluated for their quantity and quality. A quiet abdomen suggests an ileus, whereas hyperactive bowel sounds are found in enteritis and early ischemic intestine. The pitch and pattern of the sounds are also considered. Mechanical bowel obstruction is characterized by high-pitched "tinkling" sounds that tend to come in rushes and are associated with pain. Far-away, "echoing" sounds are often present when significant luminal distention exists. Bruits heard within the abdomen reflect turbulent blood flow within the vascular system. These are most frequently encountered in the setting of high-grade arterial stenoses of 70% to 95% but can also be heard if an arteriovenous fistula is present. The clinician can also subtly test for the location and degree of pain during the auscultatory exam by varying the position and amount of pressure applied with the stethoscope. These data can then be compared with the findings during palpation and evaluated for consistency. Even though few patients intentionally try to deceive their physician, some may exaggerate their pain complaints so as not to be disregarded or taken lightly.

Percussion is used to assess for gaseous distention of the bowel, free intra-abdominal air, degree of ascites, or presence of peritoneal inflammation. Hyperresonance, commonly referred to as *tympany to percussion,* is characteristic of underlying gas-filled loops of bowel. In the setting of bowel obstruction or ileus, this tympany is heard throughout all but the right upper quadrant, where the liver lies beneath the abdominal wall. If localized dullness to percussion is identified anywhere other than the right upper quadrant, an abdominal mass displacing the bowel is considered. When liver dullness is lost and resonance is uniform throughout, free intra-abdominal air is suspected. This air rises and collects beneath the anterior abdominal wall when the patient is in a supine position. Ascites is detected by looking for fluctuance of the abdominal cavity. A fluid wave or ripple can be generated by a quick, firm compression of the lateral abdomen. The resulting wave then travels across the abdominal wall. Movement of adipose tissue in the obese abdomen can be mistaken for a fluid wave. False-positive examinations can be avoided by pressing the ulnar surface of the examiner's open palm into the midline soft tissue of the abdominal wall to minimize any movement of the fatty tissue while generating the wave with the opposite hand.

Peritonitis is also assessed by percussion. Older, traditional writings teach a technique of deep compression of the abdominal wall followed by abrupt release. This practice is excruciating in the setting of peritoneal inflammation and can create significant discomfort even in its absence. More sensitive and reliable methods can and should be used. Firmly tapping the iliac crest, the flank, or the heel of an extended leg will jar the abdominal viscera and elicit characteristic pain when peritonitis is present.

The final major step in the abdominal examination is palpation. Palpation typically provides more information than any other single component of the abdominal exam. In addition to revealing the severity and exact location of the abdominal pain, palpation can further confirm the presence of peritonitis as well as identify organomegaly or an abnormal mass lesion. Palpation always begins gently and away from the reported area of pain. If considerable pain is induced at the outset of palpation, the patient is likely to voluntarily guard and continue to do so, limiting the information obtained. Involuntary guarding, or abdominal wall muscle spasm, is a sign of peritonitis and must be distinguished from voluntary guarding. To accomplish this, the examiner applies consistent pressure to the abdominal wall away from the point of maximal pain while asking the patient to take a slow, deep breath. In the setting of voluntary guarding, the abdominal muscles will relax during the act of inspiration, whereas if involuntary, they remain spastic and tense.

Pain, when focal, suggests an early or well-localized disease process, whereas diffuse pain upon palpation is present with extensive inflammation or late presentations. If pain is diffuse, careful investigation is carried out to determine where the pain is greatest. Even in the setting of extreme contamination from perforated peptic ulcers or colonic diverticula, the site of maximal tenderness often points to the underlying source.

Numerous unique physical findings have come to be associated with specific disease conditions and are well described as examination signs (Table 45-4). Murphy's sign of acute cholecystitis results when inspiration during palpation of the right upper quadrant results in sudden worsening of pain due to descent of the liver and gallbladder toward the examiners hand. Several signs help to localize the site of underlying peritonitis, including the obturator sign, the psoas sign, and Rovsing's sign. Others, such as Fothergill's sign and Carnett's sign, help distinguish intra-abdominal disease from that of the abdominal wall.

Digital rectal examination needs to be performed in all patients with acute abdominal pain, checking for the presence of a mass, pelvic pain, or intraluminal blood. A pelvic examination is included in all women when evaluating pain located below the umbilicus. Gynecologic and adnexal processes are best characterized by a thorough speculum and bimanual evaluation.

LABORATORY STUDIES

A number of laboratory studies are considered routine in the evaluation of a patient with an acute abdomen (Table 45-5). They help to confirm that inflammation or an infection is present and also aid in the elimination of some of the most common nonsurgical conditions. A complete blood count with differential is valuable because most patients with an acute abdomen have either a leukocytosis or bandemia. Measurement of serum electrolytes, blood urea nitrogen, and creatinine assists in evaluating the effect of such factors as vomiting or third-space fluid losses. In addition, it may suggest an endocrine or metabolic diagnosis as the cause of the patient's problem. Serum amylase and lipase determinations may suggest pancreatitis as the cause of the abdominal pain but can also be elevated in other disorders such as small bowel infarction or duodenal ulcer perforation. Normal serum amylase and lipase levels do not exclude pancreatitis as a possible diagnosis because of the effects of chronic inflammation on enzyme production and timing factors. Liver function tests, including total and direct bilirubin, serum aminotransferase, and alkaline phosphatase, are helpful in evaluating potential biliary tract causes of acute abdominal pain. Lactate levels and arterial blood gas determinations can be helpful in diagnosing intestinal ischemia or infarction. Urine testing such as urinalysis is helpful in the diagnosis of bacterial cystitis, pyelonephritis, and certain endocrine abnormalities, such as diabetes or renal parenchymal disease. Urine culture, although it can confirm a suspected urinary tract infection and direct antibiotic therapy, is not available in time to be helpful in the evaluation of an acute abdomen. Urinary measurements of human chorionic gonadotropin can either suggest pregnancy as a confounding factor in the patient's presentation or aid in decision making regarding therapy. The fetus of a pregnant patient with an acute abdomen is best protected by providing the best care to the mother, including an operation if indicated.[12] Stool testing for occult blood can be helpful in the evaluation of these patients but is nonspecific. Stool for ova and parasite evaluation, as well as culture and toxin assay for

Table 45-4 Abdominal Examination Signs

SIGN	DESCRIPTION	DIAGNOSIS/CONDITION
Aaron sign	Pain or pressure in epigastrium or anterior chest with persistent firm pressure applied to McBurney's point	Acute appendicitis
Bassler sign	Sharp pain created by compressing appendix between abdominal wall and iliacus	Chronic appendicitis
Blumberg's sign	Transient abdominal wall rebound tenderness	Peritoneal inflammation
Carnett's sign	Loss of abdominal tenderness when abdominal wall muscles are contracted	Intra-abdominal source of abdominal pain
Chandelier sign	Extreme lower abdominal and pelvic pain with movement of cervix	Pelvic inflammatory disease
Charcot's sign	Intermittent right upper abdominal pain, jaundice, and fever	Choledocholithiasis
Claybrook sign	Accentuation of breath and cardiac sounds through abdominal wall	Ruptured abdominal viscus
Courvoisier's sign	Palpable gallbladder in presence of painless jaundice	Periampullary tumor
Cruveilhier sign	Varicose veins at umbilicus (caput medusae)	Portal hypertension
Cullen's sign	Periumbilical bruising	Hemoperitoneum
Danforth sign	Shoulder pain on inspiration	Hemoperitoneum
Fothergill's sign	Abdominal wall mass that does not cross midline and remains palpable when rectus contracted	Rectus muscle hematomas
Grey Turner's sign	Local areas of discoloration around umbilicus and flanks	Acute hemorrhagic pancreatitis
Iliopsoas sign	Elevation and extension of leg against resistance creates pain	Appendicitis with retrocecal abscess
Kehr's sign	Left shoulder pain when supine and pressure placed on left upper abdomen	Hemoperitoneum (especially from splenic origin)
Mannkopf's sign	Increased pulse when painful abdomen palpated	Absent if malingering
Murphy's sign	Pain caused by inspiration while applying pressure to right upper abdomen	Acute cholecystitis
Obturator sign	Flexion and external rotation of right thigh while supine creates hypogastric pain	Pelvic abscess or inflammatory mass in pelvis
Ransohoff sign	Yellow discoloration of umbilical region	Ruptured common bile duct
Rovsing's sign	Pain at McBurney's point when compressing the left lower abdomen	Acute appendicitis
Ten Horn sign	Pain caused by gentle traction of right testicle	Acute appendicitis

Table 45-5 Helpful Laboratory Studies in the Acute Abdomen

Hemoglobin
White blood cell count with differential
Electrolytes, blood urea nitrogen, creatinine
Urinalysis
Urine human chorionic gonadotropin
Amylase, lipase
Total and direct bilirubin
Alkaline phosphatase
Serum aminotransferase
Serum lactate levels
Stool for ova and parasites
Clostridium difficile culture and toxin assay

Clostridium difficile, can be helpful if diarrhea is a component of the patient's presentation.

IMAGING STUDIES

Improvements in imaging techniques, especially multidetector CT, have revolutionized the diagnosis of the acute abdomen. The most difficult diagnostic dilemmas of the past, appendicitis in young women and ischemic bowel in elderly patients, can now be diagnosed with much greater certainty and speed[13-15] (Figs. 45-8 and 45-9). This has resulted in more rapid operative correction of the problem with less morbidity and mortality. Despite its usefulness, CT is not the only imaging technique available and is also not the first step in imaging for most patients. In addition, none of the imaging techniques take the place of a careful history and physical examination.

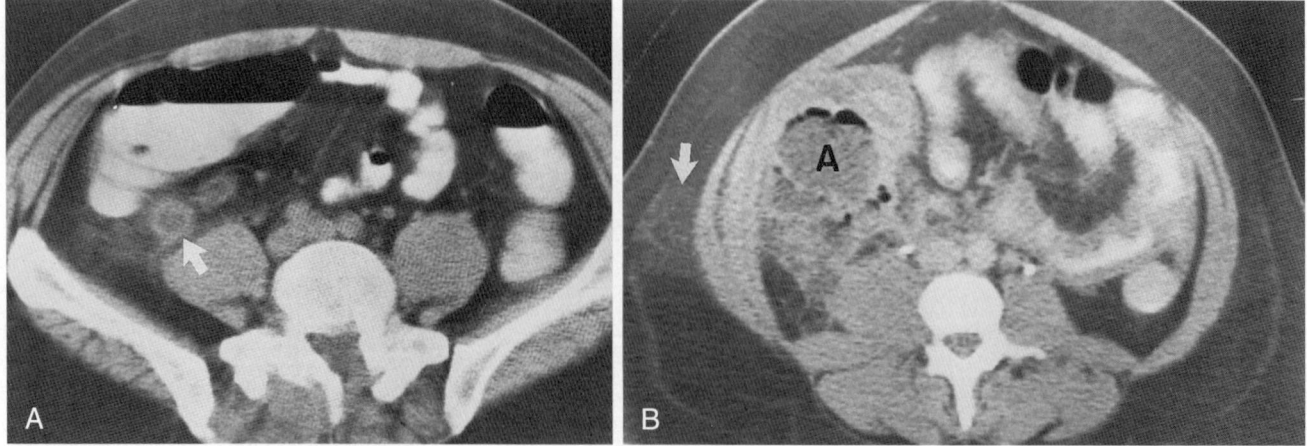

Figure 45-8 Appendicitis. **A,** CT scan of uncomplicated appendicitis. A thick-walled, distended, retrocecal appendix (*arrow*) is seen with inflammatory change in the surrounding fat. **B,** CT scan of complicated appendicitis. A retrocecal appendiceal abscess (A) with an associated phlegmon posteriorly found in a 3-week postpartum, obese woman. Inflammatory change extends through the flank musculature into the subcutaneous fat (*arrow*).

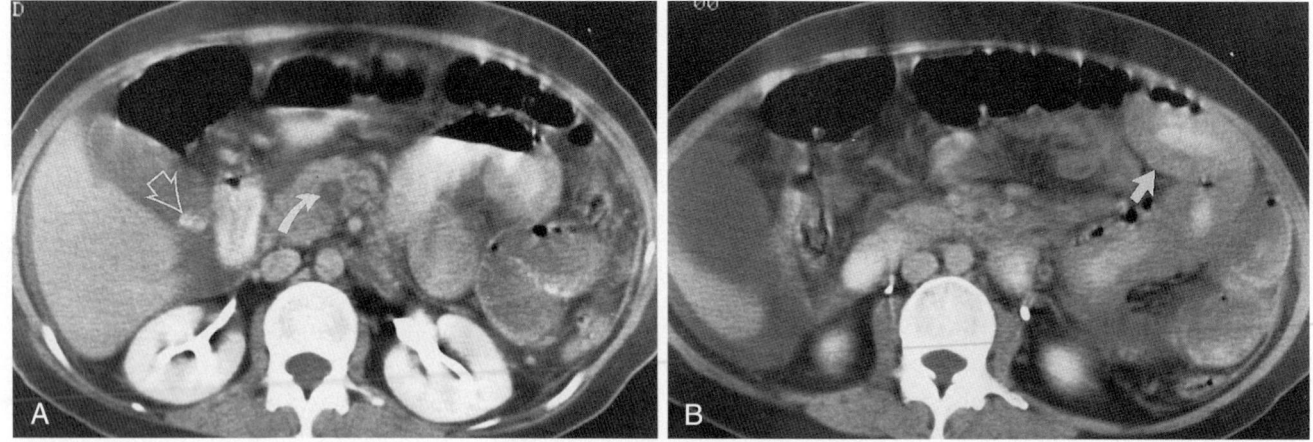

Figure 45-9 Small bowel infarction associated with mesenteric venous thrombosis. **A,** Note the low-density thrombosed superior mesenteric vein (*solid arrow*) and incidental gallstones (*open arrow*). **B,** Thickening of proximal small bowel wall (*arrow*) coincided with several feet of infarcting small bowel at time of operation.

Plain radiographs continue to play a role in imaging of patients with acute abdominal pain. Upright chest radiographs can detect as little as 1 mL of air injected into the peritoneal cavity. Lateral decubitus abdominal radiographs can also detect pneumoperitoneum effectively in patients who cannot stand. As little as 5 to 10 mL of gas may be detected with this technique.[16] These studies are particularly helpful in patients suspected of having a perforated duodenal ulcer because about 75% of these patients have a large enough pneumoperitoneum to be visible (Fig. 45-10). This obviates the need for further evaluation in most patients, allowing for laparotomy with little delay.

Plain films also show abnormal calcifications. About 5% of appendicoliths, 10% of gallstones, and 90% of renal stones contain sufficient amounts of calcium to be radiopaque. Pancreatic calcifications seen in many patients with chronic pancreatitis are visible on plain films, as are the calcifications in abdominal aortic aneurysms, visceral

artery aneurysm, and atherosclerosis in visceral vessels.

Upright and supine abdominal radiographs are very helpful in identifying gastric outlet obstruction and obstruction of the proximal, mid, or distal small bowel. They can also aid in determining whether a small bowel obstruction is complete or partial by the presence or absence of gas in the colon. Colonic gas can be differentiated from small intestinal gas by the presence of haustral markings owing to the taenia coli present in the colonic wall. Obstructed colon appears as distended bowel with haustral markings (Fig. 45-11). Associated distention of small bowel may also be present, especially if the ileocecal valve is incompetent. Plain films can also suggest volvulus of either the cecum or sigmoid colon. Cecal volvulus is identified by a distended loop of colon in a comma shape, with the concavity facing inferiorly and to the right. Sigmoid volvulus characteristically has the appearance of a bent inner tube, with its apex in the right upper quadrant (Fig. 45-12).

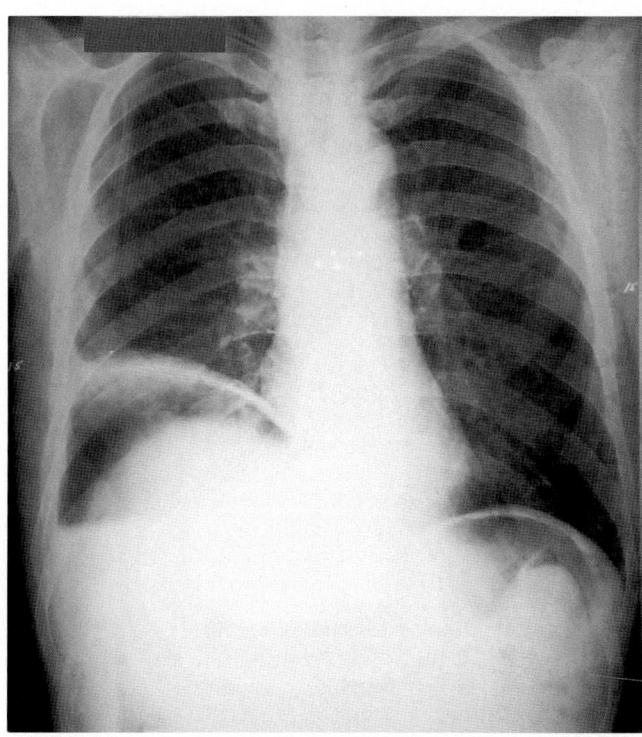

Figure 45-10 Upright chest radiograph depicting moderate-sized pneumoperitoneum consistent with perforation of abdominal viscus.

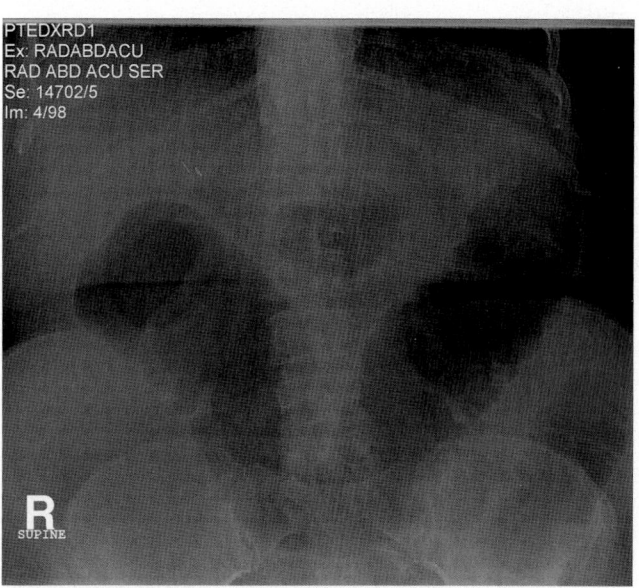

Figure 45-11 Upright abdominal x-ray in a patient with an obstructing sigmoid adenocarcinoma. Note the haustral markings on the dilated transverse colon that distinguished this from small intestine.

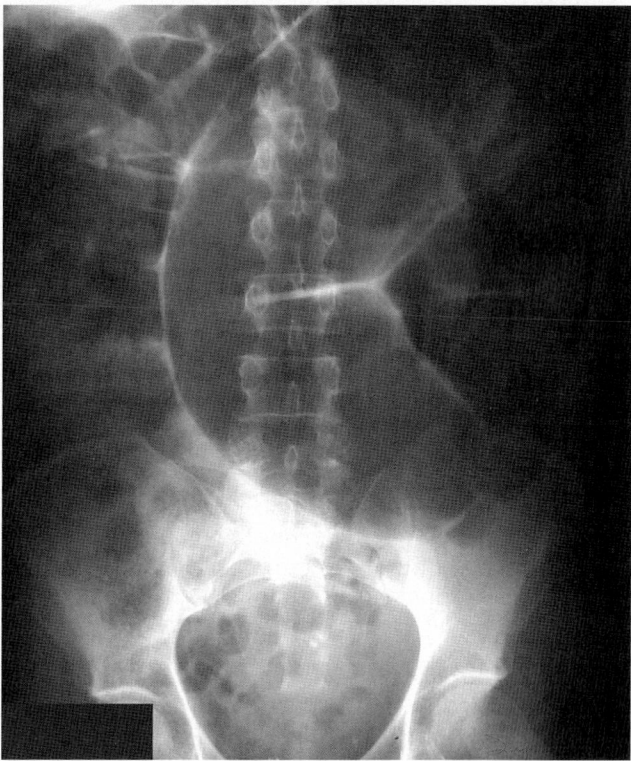

Figure 45-12 Upright abdominal x-ray in a patient with a sigmoid colon volvulus. Note the characteristic appearance of a "bent inner tube" with its apex in the right upper quadrant.

Abdominal ultrasonography is extremely accurate in detecting gallstones and in assessing gallbladder wall thickness and the presence of fluid around the gallbladder.[17,18] It is also good at determining the diameter of the extrahepatic and intrahepatic bile ducts. Its usefulness in detecting common bile duct stones is limited. Abdominal and transvaginal ultrasonography can aid in the detection of abnormalities of the ovaries, adnexa, and uterus. Ultrasound can also detect intraperitoneal fluid. The presence of abnormal amounts of intestinal air in most patients with an acute abdomen limits the ability of ultrasonography to evaluate the pancreas or other abdominal organs. There are important limits to the value of ultrasonography in the diagnosis of diseases that present as an acute abdomen. Ultrasound images are more difficult for most surgeons to interpret than are plain radiographs and CT images. Many hospitals have radiologic technologists available at all times to perform CT, but this is often not the case with ultrasonography. Because CT has become more widely available and less likely to be hindered by abdominal air, it is becoming the secondary imaging modality of choice in the patient with an acute abdomen, following plain abdominal radiographs.

A number of studies have demonstrated the accuracy and utility of CT of the abdomen and pelvis in the evaluation of acute abdominal pain.[13-15] Many of the most common causes of acute abdomen are readily identified by CT scanning, as are their complications. A notable example is appendicitis. Plain films and even barium enemas add little to the diagnosis of appendicitis,

however, a well-performed CT scan using oral, rectal, and intravenous (IV) contrast is highly accurate in this disease. CT is also excellent in differentiating mechanical small bowel obstruction from paralytic ileus and can usually identify the transition point in mechanical

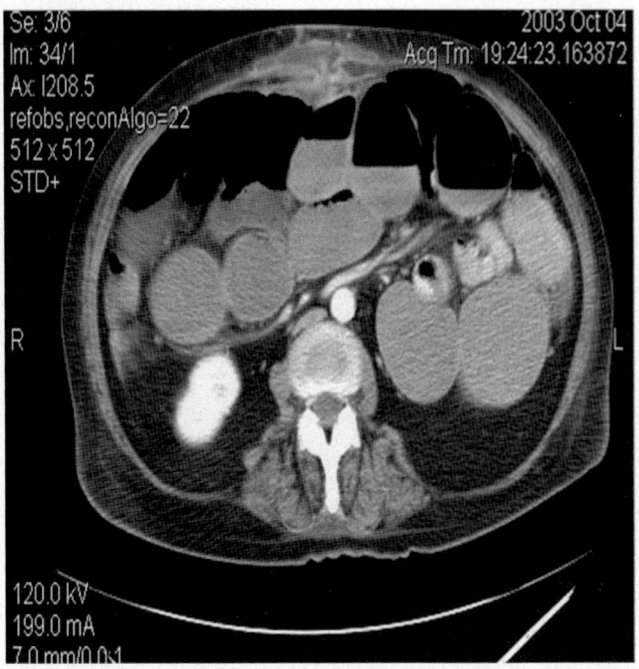

Figure 45-13 CT scan of a patient with a partial small bowel obstruction. Note the presence of dilated small bowel and decompressed small bowel. The decompressed bowel contains air, indicating a partial obstruction.

Table 45-6   **Findings Associated With Surgical Disease in the Setting of Acute Abdominal Pain**

Physical Exam and Laboratory Findings
Abdominal compartment pressure >30 mm Hg
Worsening distention after gastric decompression
Involuntary guarding or rebound tenderness
Gastrointestinal hemorrhage requiring >4 units of blood without stabilization
Unexplained systemic sepsis
Signs of hypoperfusion (acidosis, pain out of proportion to exam findings, rising liver function tests)

Radiographic Findings
Massive dilation of intestine
Progressive dilation of stationary loop of intestine (sentinel loop)
Pneumoperitoneum
Extravasation of contrast from bowel lumen
Vascular occlusion on angiography
Fat stranding or thickened bowel wall with systemic sepsis

Diagnostic Peritoneal Lavage (1000 mL)
Greater than 250 white blood cells per milliliter
Greater than 300,000 red blood cells per milliliter
Bilirubin level higher than plasma level (bile leak)
Particulate matter (stool)
Creatinine level higher than plasma level (urine leak)

obstruction (Fig. 45-13). Some of the most difficult diagnostic dilemmas, including acute intestinal ischemia, can often be identified by this method.

DIAGNOSTIC LAPAROSCOPY

A number of studies have confirmed the utility of diagnostic laparoscopy in patients with acute abdominal pain.[19-21] The purported advantages include a high sensitivity and specificity, the ability to treat a number of the conditions causing an acute abdomen laparoscopically, decreased morbidity and mortality, decreased length of stay, and decreased overall hospital costs. It may be particularly helpful in the critically ill intensive care patient, especially if a laparotomy can be avoided.[22] With advances in equipment and increased availability, this technique is being used with greater frequency in these patients.

DIFFERENTIAL DIAGNOSIS

The differential diagnosis of acute abdominal pain is extensive. Conditions range from the mild and self-limited to the rapidly progressive and fatal. All patients must therefore be seen and evaluated immediately upon presentation and reassessed at frequent intervals for changes in condition. Although many acute abdomen diagnoses require surgical intervention for resolution, it is important to keep in mind that many causes of acute abdominal pain are medical in etiology[23] (see Table 45-1). Develop-

ment of the differential diagnosis begins during the history and is further clarified during the physical examination. Refinements are then made with the assistance of laboratory analysis and imaging studies so that typically, one or two diagnoses rise above the rest. To be successful, this process requires a comprehensive knowledge of the medical and surgical conditions that create acute abdominal pain in order to allow individual disease features to be matched to patient demographics, symptoms, and signs.

Certain physical examination, laboratory, and radiographic findings are highly correlated with surgical disease. At times, some patients will be too unstable to undergo comprehensive evaluations that require transportation to other departments such as radiology. In this setting, peritoneal lavage can provide information suggesting pathology requiring surgical intervention. The lavage can be performed under local anesthesia at the patient's bedside. A small incision is made in the midline adjacent to the umbilicus, and dissection is carried down to the peritoneal cavity. A small catheter or IV tubing is inserted, and 1000 mL of saline is infused. A sample of fluid is then allowed to siphon back out into the empty saline bag and is analyzed for cellular or biochemical anomalies (Table 45-6). This technique can provide sensitive evidence of hemorrhage or infection as well as some types of solid or hollow organ injury.

Patients having emergency or life-threatening surgical disease are taken for immediate laparotomy, whereas urgent diagnoses allow time for stabilization, hydration, and preoperative preparation as needed. The remaining acute abdomen patients are grouped as those with surgical conditions that sometimes require surgery, those with medical diseases, and those who as yet remain unclear. Hospitalized patients who do not go urgently to the operating room must be reassessed frequently and preferably by the same examiner in order to recognize potentially serious changes in condition that alter the diagnosis or suggest development of complications.

Although the goal of every surgeon is to make the correct diagnosis preoperatively and have planned the best possible surgical procedure before entering the operating suite, it must be emphasized that a clear diagnosis cannot be developed in every patient. Surgeons must always be willing to accept uncertainty and commit to abdominal exploration when examination findings warrant. Laboratory and imaging studies, although helpful, must never replace the bedside clinical judgment of an experienced surgeon. Patients are far more likely to be seriously or fatally harmed by delaying surgical treatment in order to perform confirmatory tests than by misdiagnoses discovered at operation. Laparoscopy has proved to be a valuable tool when the diagnosis is unclear. The presence of surgical disease can be confirmed in all but the most hostile abdominal environments, and as a surgeon's experience grows, he or she is able to treat more and more conditions laparoscopically. Even when conversion to open technique is required, laparoscopic evaluation facilitates more accurate positioning of the laparotomy incision, thereby reducing its length.

PREPARATION FOR EMERGENCY OPERATION

Patients with an acute abdomen vary greatly in their overall state of health at the time the decision to operate is made. Regardless of the patient's severity of illness, all patients require some degree of preoperative preparation. IV access is obtained and any fluid or electrolyte abnormalities corrected. Nearly all patients will require antibiotic infusions. The bacteria common in acute abdominal emergencies are gram-negative enteric organisms and anaerobes. Infusion of antibiotics to cover these organisms is started after a presumptive diagnosis is made. Patients with generalized paralytic ileus, as manifested by absent or hypoactive bowel sounds, benefit from a nasogastric tube to decrease the likelihood of vomiting and aspiration. Foley catheter bladder drainage to assess urine output, a measure of adequacy of fluid resuscitation, is indicated in most patients. Preoperative urine output of 0.5 mL/kg/hour, along a with systolic blood pressure of at least 100 mm Hg and a pulse rate of 100 beats/minute or less, is indicative of adequate intravascular volume. A common electrolyte abnormality requiring correction is hypokalemia. If significant potassium repletion is necessary, a central venous line is required. The ability to give potassium through a peripheral line is limited by the development of phlebitis. Preoperative acidosis may respond to fluid repletion and IV bicarbonate infusion. Acidosis due to intestinal ischemia or infarction may be refractory to preoperative therapy. Significant anemia is uncommon, and preoperative blood transfusions are usually unnecessary. However, most patients should have blood typed and crossmatched and available at operation. There is an inherent uncertainty in the operation that will be required in these patients, and having crossmatched blood available avoids transfusion delay if unexpected intraoperative events occur. The need for preoperative stabilization of patients must be weighed against the increased morbidity and mortality associated with a delay in the treatment of some of the surgical diseases that present as an acute abdomen. The underlying nature of the disease process, such as infarcted bowel, may require surgical correction before stabilization of the patient's vital signs and restoration of acid-base balance can occur. Deciding when the maximum benefit of preoperative therapy in these patients has been achieved requires good surgical judgment.

ATYPICAL PATIENTS

Pregnancy

Acute abdominal pain presenting in the pregnant patient creates several unique diagnostic and therapeutic challenges. Special emphasis must be placed on the possibility of gynecologic and surgical diseases when acute abdominal pain develops during pregnancy owing to their frequency and morbidity if left unrecognized. Laparoscopy has had a major impact on the diagnosis and treatment of the gravid female with acute abdominal pain and is now routinely employed for many clinical situations. Short-term follow-up has suggested equal or superior safety with the laparoscopic approach, yet large series of long-term safety data are not currently available.[24-27] The greatest threat facing the pregnant patient with acute abdominal pain is the potential for delayed diagnosis. Delays in receiving surgical treatment have proved far more morbid than the operations themselves.[12,27,28] Delays occur for several reasons. Many times, symptoms are attributed to the underlying pregnancy, including abdominal pains, nausea, vomiting, and anorexia. Pregnancy can also alter the presentation of some disease processes and make the physical examination more challenging because of the enlarged uterus in the pelvis. The appendix rises out of the pelvis to within a few centimeters of the right anterolateral costal margin late in the third trimester[29] (Fig. 45-14). Laboratory studies, such as white blood cell counts and other chemistries, are also altered in pregnancy, making recognition of disease more difficult. In addition, physicians may hesitate to perform typical imaging studies such as plain abdominal films or CT scans because of concern about radiation exposure to the developing fetus. The lack of radiologic information can take a physician out of his or her diagnostic routine and cause the physician to place extra emphasis on other modalities, such as vital signs and laboratory studies, which can confuse or underestimate the existing condition. Finally, physicians naturally tend to be more conservative when treating pregnant patients. Surgery, especially within the pelvis, is associated with increased risk for spontaneous abortion in the

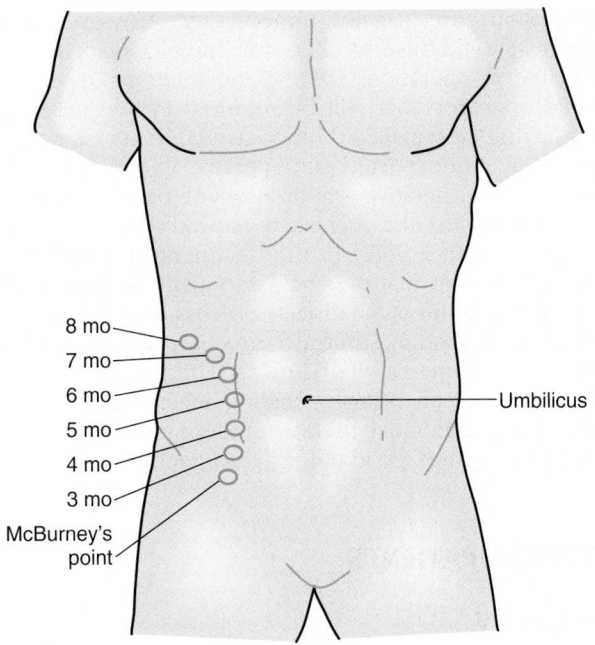

8 mo
7 mo
6 mo
5 mo
4 mo
3 mo
McBurney's point

Umbilicus

Figure 45-14 Location of maternal normal appendix during fetal gestation.

first trimester and progressively increasing risk for preterm labor in the second and third trimesters. The overall risk attributed to surgery and anesthesia is estimated at 4% to 6%, but some authors have reported incidences as high as 38%.[12,27,30,31] Perioperative risk is minimized by maintaining physiologic O_2 and CO_2 levels during surgery, avoiding episodes of hypotension, and performing minimal manipulation of the uterus.

Appendicitis is the most common nonobstetric disease requiring surgery, occurring in 1 of 1500 pregnancies.[26,32] Its symptoms typically consist of right lateral abdominal pain, nausea, and anorexia. Fever is uncommon unless perforated with abdominal sepsis. Symptoms are sometimes attributed to the underlying pregnancy, and a high index of suspicion must be maintained. Laboratory studies can also be misleading. Leukocytosis as high as 16,000 cells/mm³ is common in pregnancy, and labor can increase the count to 21,000 cells/mm³. Many authors have suggested that a neutrophil shift of more than 80% is suspicious for an acute inflammatory process, such as appendicitis, yet others have observed that only 75% of patients with proven appendicitis had a shift, whereas as many as 50% of patients with a shift and pain were found to have a normal appendix.[12,27,33] Ultrasound has been relied on as the first imaging tool in many centers. Graded compression ultrasound has been shown to have a sensitivity of 86% in the nonpregnant patient.[26] In a case series of 42 pregnant women with suspected appendicitis, graded compression ultrasound was found to be 100% sensitive, 96% specific, and 98% accurate.[34] Three women were excluded from the analysis because of a technically inadequate exam owing to advanced gestational age (>35 weeks). Helical CT scanning has been

established as a valuable tool for evaluation of the non-pregnant patient and shows promise as a second-line study in pregnancy. Compared to traditional CT scans, helical CT can provide a much faster study, with radiation exposures of about 300 cGy to the fetus.[26] MRI is also beginning to play a role. MRI is capable of demonstrating the normal appendix and can also recognize an enlarged appendix, periappendiceal fluid, and inflammation.[35] There is currently no large series documenting the success of MRI diagnosis of appendicitis; however, a recent study documented successful evaluation of 10 of 12 pregnant women.[36]

The added difficulties in evaluating the pregnant patient with right lower quadrant abdominal pain have resulted in a significantly higher negative appendectomy rate as compared with nonpregnant peers. False-positive diagnoses leading to negative appendectomies occur in 15% to 35% of pregnant women presenting with lower abdominal pain.[27] Although this diagnostic error rate would be unacceptable in a typical young healthy female, it is widely accepted owing to the fetal mortality suffered when appendicitis progresses to perforation before surgery. Perioperative fetal loss associated with appendectomy for early appendicitis is 3% to 5%; this rate climbs to more than 20% in the setting of perforation.[37]

The second and third most common surgical diseases seen in pregnancy are biliary tract disorders and bowel obstructions. Surgery for biliary disease occurs in 1 to 6 per 10,000 pregnancies.[38] Symptoms of pain, nausea, and anorexia are the same as in nonpregnant patients. Even though the elevated estrogen levels are generally more lithogenic, the incidence of disease is similar to that in nongravid women.[26] With few exceptions, the evaluation and treatment during pregnancy are similar to those in all patients with biliary disease. Ultrasound is the diagnostic test of choice. Alkaline phosphatase is elevated secondary to elevated estrogen, and normal values must be adjusted. Nuclear scans of the biliary tract pose minimal risk to the fetus, but a Foley catheter is placed so that isotope cleared by the kidneys does not collect adjacent to the uterus.

Most surgeons try to treat simple biliary colic with conservative management in the first and third trimesters and plan elective laparoscopic cholecystectomy for the second trimester or the postpartum period to minimize fetal risk. Gallstone pancreatitis and acute cholecystitis need to be managed more carefully. Gallstone pancreatitis has been associated with fetal loss rates as high as 60%.[39] If a woman does not respond quickly to conservative treatment with hydration, bowel rest, analgesia, and judicious use of antibiotics, surgical treatment is performed.

Bowel obstructions are much less common, occurring in about 1 or 2 per 4000 deliveries, and the underlying cause is adhesions in two thirds of cases. Volvulus is the second most common cause, occurring in 25% of cases, compared with only 4% of the nonpregnant population.[26] Signs and symptoms are typical but must not be attributed to morning sickness. Colicky abdominal pain with rapid abdominal distention keys the clinician to the diagnosis. Three periods during gestation are associated with an increased risk for obstruction and correlate with rapid changes in uterine size.[27] The first is from 16 to 20 weeks' gestation, when the uterus grows beyond the pelvis. The second is from 32 to 36 weeks, when the fetal head descends, and the third is in the early post-partum period. The evaluation is the same as for any patient, and there can be no hesitation to obtain abdominal x-rays if the situation warrants. As with other acute inflammatory processes in the abdomen, the maternal and fetal morbidity is most affected by delayed definitive treatment.

Acute Abdomen in the Critically Ill

The critically ill patient with a potential acute abdomen is a difficult challenge for intensivists and surgeons alike. Many of the underlying diseases and treatments encountered in the intensive care unit can predispose to acute abdominal disease. At the same time, unrecognized abdominal illness can be responsible for patients lingering in a critical state. Critically ill patients are often unable to appreciate symptoms to the same degree as healthy peers because of nutritional or immune compromise, narcotic analgesia, or antibiotic use. Many of these patients have an altered mental status or are intubated and cannot provide detailed information to their providers.

Cardiopulmonary bypass (CPB) has been associated with several acute abdominal illnesses. Mesenteric ischemia, paralytic ileus, Ogilvie's syndrome, stress peptic ulceration, acute acalculous cholecystitis, and acute pancreatitis have all been linked to the low-flow state of CPB, and their incidence appears tied to the length of the cardiac procedure.[40,41] Vasoactive medications and ventilator support have also been linked to hypoperfusion and similar abdominal processes.

When an acute abdominal complication occurs in an intensive care patient, it has a dramatic effect on outcome. Gajic studied 77 patients who experienced abdominal catastrophe while recovering in the medical intensive care unit.[42] Acute abdominal diagnoses included peptic ulcer, ischemic bowel, cholecystitis, bowel obstruction, and bowel inflammation. The APACHE III score on admission predicted an overall mortality rate of 31% in this group, yet they experienced an actual mortality rate of 63%. The development of a secondary acute abdominal illness doubled their observed mortality. Despite many of these patients having factors that could delay diagnosis, including antibiotics, analgesics, altered mental states, and intubations, 84% were still recognized as having abdominal pain, 95% as having abdominal tenderness, 73% as having abdominal distention, and 33% as having free intra-abdominal air. Intensivists must maintain a high index of suspicion for the development of intra-abdominal disease and consult with surgeons early to maximize recovery potential. Surgeons must then work to exclude the possibility of abdominal disease using all of the methods described in this chapter as well as bedside ultrasound, paracentesis, or minilaparoscopy so that early surgical intervention can be appropriately undertaken.

Immunocompromised Patients With Acute Abdomen

Immunocompromised patients have variable presentations with acute abdominal diseases. The variability is highly correlated to the degree of immunosuppression. There is no reliable test for determining the degree of immunosuppression experienced by a given patient, so estimates are made by associations with certain disease states or medications. Mild to moderate compromise is experienced by elderly, malnourished, and diabetic patients; transplant recipients on routine maintenance therapy; cancer patients; renal failure patients; and HIV patients with CD4 counts higher than 200 cells/mm³. Although patients in this group have the same types of illnesses and infections as their immunocompetent peers, they still can present in an atypical fashion. Abdominal pain and systemic signs and symptoms are often tied to the development of inflammation. These patients may not be able to mount a full inflammatory response and therefore may experience less abdominal pain, delayed development of fever, and a blunted leukocytosis.

Severely compromised patients would typically include transplant recipients having received high-dose therapy for rejection during the past 2 months; cancer patients on chemotherapy, especially with neutropenia; and HIV patients with CD4 counts of less than 200 cells/mm³. These patients present very late in their course, often with little or no pain, no fever, and vague constitutional symptoms, followed by an overwhelming systemic collapse. In addition, these patients may suffer from atypical infections, including peritoneal tuberculosis, fungal infections including aspergillosis and endemic mycoses, or a variety of viruses including cytomegalovirus and Epstein-Barr virus. When an abdominal infection does occur, it is less likely to be walled off as a localized infection because of the lack of inflammatory reaction. All severely immunocompromised patients require prompt and thorough evaluation for any persistent abdominal complaints. All patients requiring hospitalization receive a surgical consult to aid in timely diagnosis and treatment. High-resolution CT scanning can be of great benefit in these patients, but a low threshold for laparoscopy or laparotomy needs to be maintained in those with equivocal diagnostic tests and persistent symptoms that remain unexplained.

Acute Abdomen in the Morbidly Obese

Morbid obesity creates numerous challenges to the accurate diagnosis of acute abdominal processes. Many authors describe alterations in the signs and symptoms of peritonitis in the morbidly obese.[43-45] Findings of overt peritonitis are often late and usually ominous, leading to sepsis, organ failure, and death.[43] Abdominal sepsis is a much more subtle diagnosis in this population and may only be associated with symptoms such as malaise, shoulder pain, hiccups, or shortness of breath.[44] Exam findings can also be difficult to interpret. Severe abdominal pain is not common, and less specific findings, such as tachycardia, tachypnea, pleural effusion, or fever, may be the

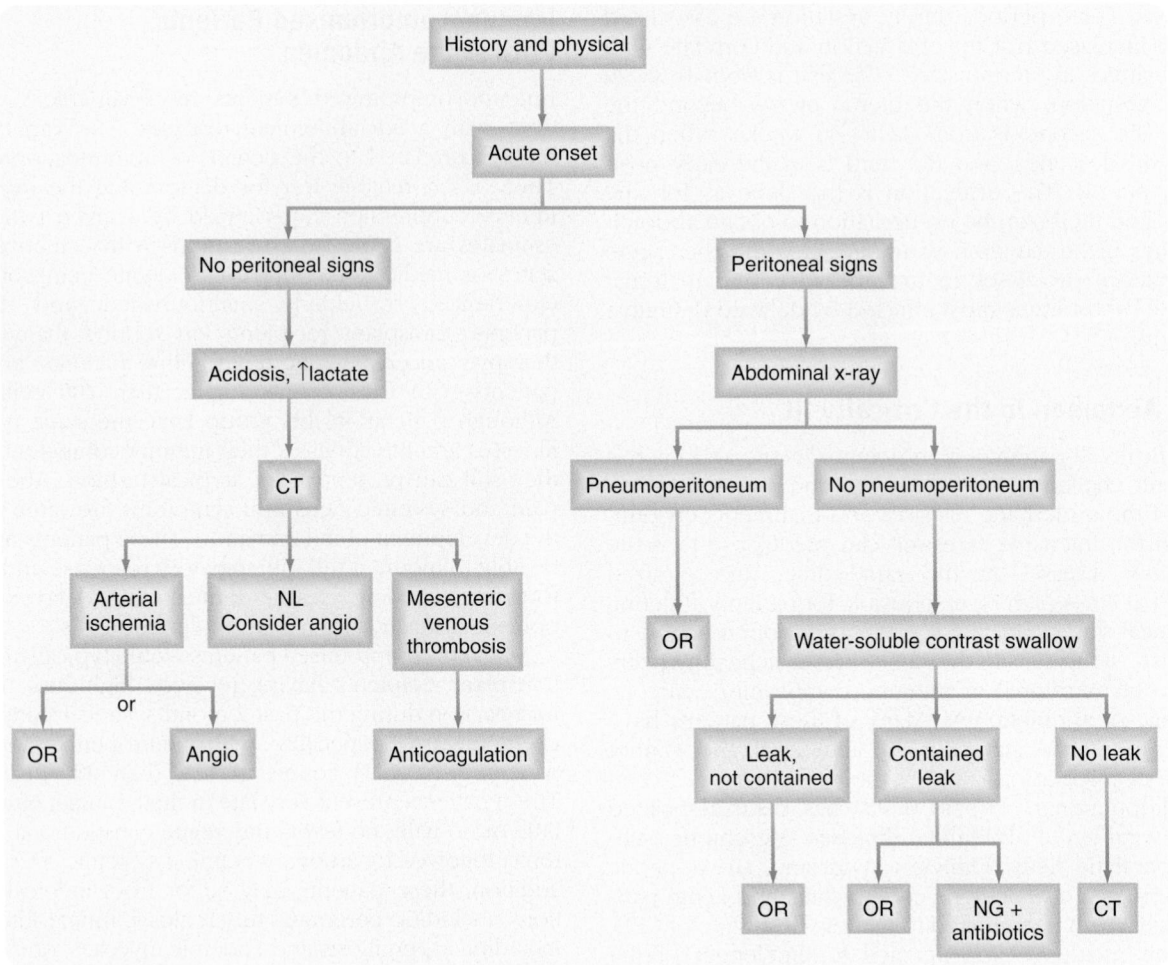

Figure 45-15 Algorithm for the treatment of acute-onset severe, generalized abdominal pain. CT, computed tomography; NG, nasogastric tube; NL, normal study; OR, operation.

primary observation.[45] Appreciation of distention or intra-abdominal mass is also very difficult because of the size and thickness of the abdominal wall.

Abdominal imaging is also adversely affected by obesity. Plain abdominal radiographs can require multiple images to view the entire abdomen, and clarity is reduced. CT and MRI scanning may be impossible to perform as a patient's girth or weight exceeds the size of the scanning aperture or the weight limit of the mechanized bed. In these settings, a high index of suspicion and low threshold for surgical exploration must be maintained. Laparoscopy is a valuable tool in these patients. Specially designed trocars and hand-assist ports for the morbidly obese abdominal wall are now readily available and greatly facilitate minimally invasive exploration of the abdomen.

TREATMENT ALGORITHMS FOR ACUTE ABDOMEN

Algorithms can aid in the diagnosis of the patient with an acute abdomen. As stated earlier, computer-assisted diagnosis has been shown to be more accurate than clinical judgment alone in a number of acute abdominal disease states. Algorithms are the basis for computer diagnosis and can be useful in making clinical decisions. The algorithms presented in Figures 45-15 to 45-20 are helpful in acute abdomen patients and can allow for both a focused workup and expeditious therapy.

SUMMARY

Evaluation and management of the patient with acute abdominal pain remains a challenging part of a surgeon's practice. Although advances in imaging techniques, use of algorithms, and computer assistance have improved the diagnostic accuracy for the conditions causing the acute abdomen, a careful history and physical examination remain the most important part of the evaluation. Even with these tools at hand, the surgeon must often make the decision to perform a laparoscopy or laparotomy with a good deal of uncertainty as to the expected findings. Increased morbidity and mortality associated with a delay in the treatment of many of the surgical

Text continued on p 1197

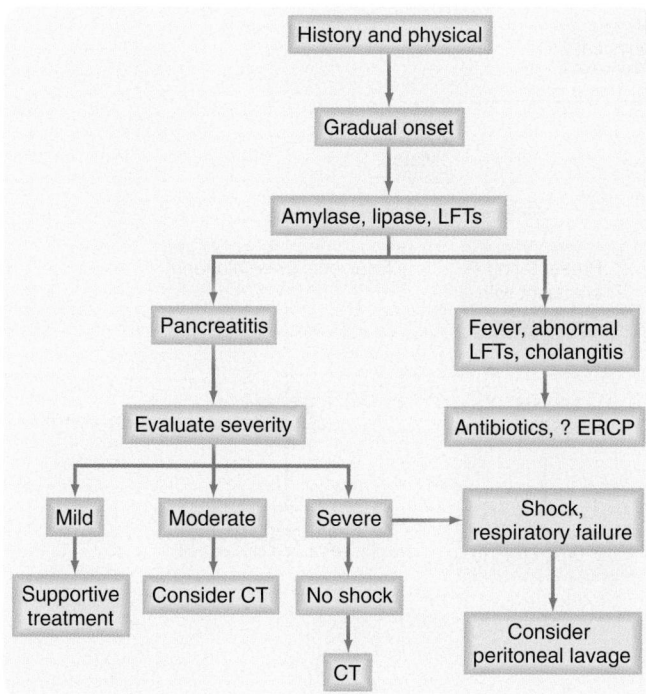

Figure 45-16 Algorithm for the treatment of gradual-onset severe, generalized abdominal pain. CT, computed tomography; ERCP, endoscopic retrograde cholangiopancreatography; LFTs, liver function tests.

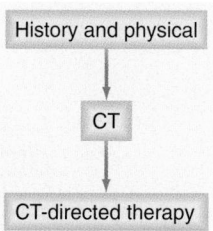

Figure 45-18 Algorithm for the treatment of left upper quadrant abdominal pain. CT, computed tomography.

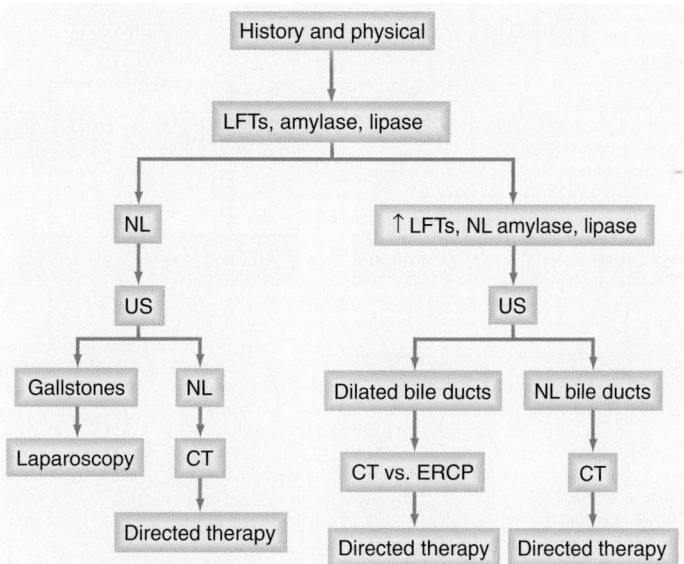

Figure 45-17 Algorithm for the treatment of right upper quadrant abdominal pain. CT, computed tomography; ERCP, endoscopic retrograde cholangiopancreatography; LFTs, liver function tests; NL, normal study; US, ultrasound.

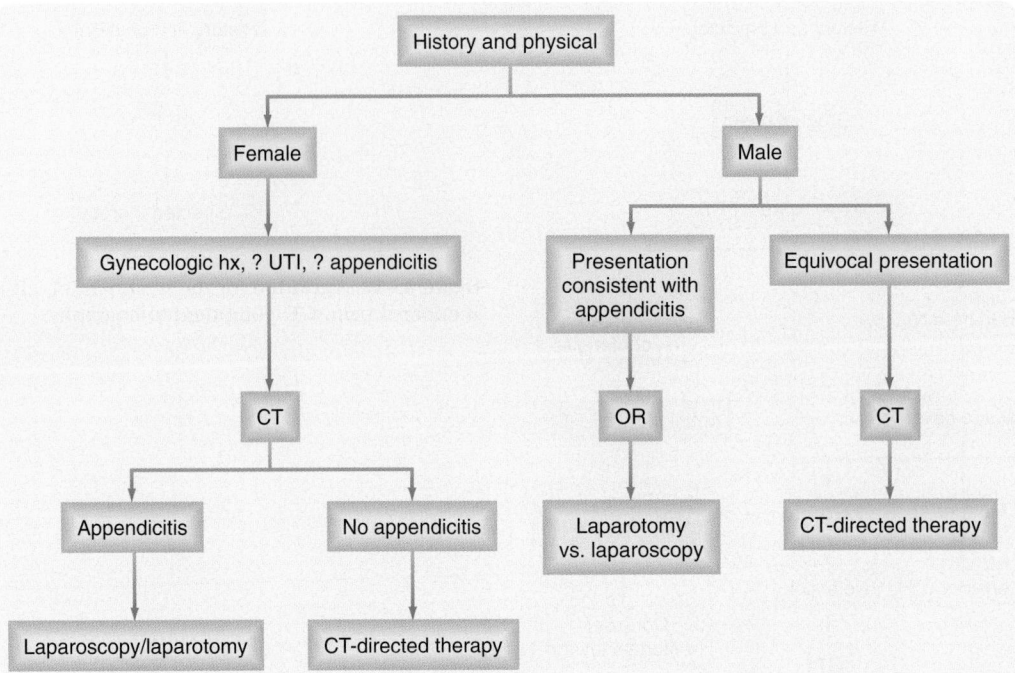

Figure 45-19 Algorithm for the treatment of right lower quadrant abdominal pain. CT, computed tomography; hx, history; OR, operation; UTI, urinary tract infection.

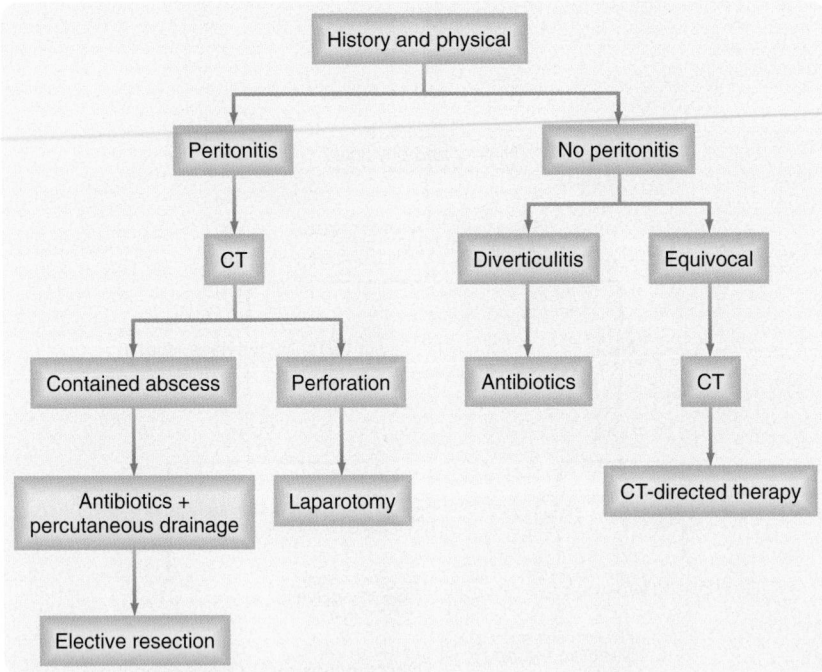

Figure 45-20 Algorithm for the treatment of left lower quadrant abdominal pain. CT, computed tomography.

causes of the acute abdomen argue for an aggressive and expeditious surgical approach.

Selected References

Ahmad TA, Shelbaya E, Razek SA, et al: Experience of laparoscopic management in 100 patients with acute abdomen. Hepatogastroenterology 48:733-736, 2001.

> A description of the usefulness of laparoscopy in a large series of patients with acute abdomen. A good review of this important diagnostic and therapeutic tool.

Cademartiri F, Raaijmaker RHJM, Kuiper JW, et al: Multi-detector row CT angiography in patients with abdominal angina. Radiographics 24:969-984, 2004.

> A good review of the CT characteristics of acute mesenteric ischemia. This outlines the radiographic findings that have greatly assisted in the diagnosis of this otherwise difficult condition.

Graff LG, Robinson D: Abdominal pain and emergency department evaluation. Emerg Med Clin North Am 19:123-136, 2001.

> Good review of the spectrum of patients presenting with acute abdominal pain.

Macari M, Balthazar EJ: The acute right lower quadrant: CT evaluation. Radiol Clin North Am 41:1117-1136, 2003.

> A modern discussion of the role of CT in the evaluation of patients with right lower quadrant abdominal pain.

Silen W: Cope's Early Diagnosis of the Acute Abdomen, 21st ed. New York, Oxford University Press, 2005.

> This is a classic monograph stressing the importance of history and physical examination in the diagnosis of the acute abdomen. The presentation of nearly all diseases presenting as an acute abdomen are presented. A must read for the surgical resident.

Steinheber FU: Medical conditions mimicking the acute surgical abdomen. Med Clin North Am 57:1559-1567, 1973.

> This classic article nicely reviews the various medical conditions that can present as an acute abdomen. It is well written and remains pertinent to the evaluation of these patients.

References

1. Brewer BJ, Golden GT, Hitch DC, et al: Abdominal pain: An analysis of 1,000 consecutive cases in a University Hospital emergency room. Am J Surg 131:219-223, 1976.
2. Graff LGT, Robinson D: Abdominal pain and emergency department evaluation. Emerg Med Clin North Am 19:123-136, 2001.
3. Steinheber FU: Medical conditions mimicking the acute surgical abdomen. Med Clin North Am 57:1559-1567, 1973.
4. Gilbert JA, Kamath PS: Spontaneous bacterial peritonitis: An update. Mayo Clin Proc 70:365-370, 1995.
5. Nathens AB, Rotstein OD, Marshall JC: Tertiary peritonitis: Clinical features of a complex nosocomial infection. World J Surg 22:158-163, 1998.
6. Silen W: Cope's Early Diagnosis of the Acute Abdomen, 21st ed. New York, Oxford University Press, 2005.
7. Paterson-Brown S, Vipond MN: Modern aids to clinical decision-making in the acute abdomen. Br J Surg 77:13-18, 1990.
8. de Dombal FT: Computers, diagnoses and patients with acute abdominal pain. Arch Emerg Med 9:267-270, 1992.
9. Adams ID, Chan M, Clifford PC, et al: Computer aided diagnosis of acute abdominal pain: A multicentre study. Br Med J (Clin Res Ed) 293:800-804, 1986.
10. Wellwood J, Johannessen S, Spiegelhalter DJ: How does computer-aided diagnosis improve the management of acute abdominal pain? Ann R Coll Surg Engl 74:40-46, 1992.
11. McAdam WA, Brock BM, Armitage T, et al: Twelve years' experience of computer-aided diagnosis in a district general hospital. Ann R Coll Surg Engl 72:140-146, 1990.
12. Kort B, Katz VL, Watson WJ: The effect of nonobstetric operation during pregnancy. Surg Gynecol Obstet 177:371-376, 1993.
13. Macari M, Balthazar EJ: The acute right lower quadrant: CT evaluation. Radiol Clin North Am 41:1117-1136, 2003.
14. Cademartiri F, Raaijmakers RH, Kuiper JW, et al: Multi-detector row CT angiography in patients with abdominal angina. Radiographics 24:969-984, 2004.
15. Lee R, Tung HK, Tung PH, et al: CT in acute mesenteric ischaemia. Clin Radiol 58:279-287, 2003.
16. Miller RE, Nelson SW: The roentgenologic demonstration of tiny amounts of free intraperitoneal gas: Experimental and clinical studies. AJR Am J Roentgenol 112:574-585, 1971.
17. Bortoff GA, Chen MY, Ott DJ, et al: Gallbladder stones: Imaging and intervention. Radiographics 20:751-766, 2000.
18. Hanbidge AE, Buckler PM, O'Malley ME, et al: From the RSNA refresher courses: Imaging evaluation for acute pain in the right upper quadrant. Radiographics 24:1117-1135, 2004.
19. Ahmad TA, Shelbaya E, Razek SA, et al: Experience of laparoscopic management in 100 patients with acute abdomen. Hepatogastroenterology 48:733-736, 2001.
20. Perri SG, Altilia F, Pietrangeli F, et al: [Laparoscopy in abdominal emergencies. Indications and limitations]. Chir Ital 54:165-178, 2002.
21. Riemann JF: Diagnostic laparoscopy. Endoscopy 35:43-47, 2003.
22. Pecoraro AP, Cacchione RN, Sayad P, et al: The routine use of diagnostic laparoscopy in the intensive care unit. Surg Endosc 15:638-641, 2001.
23. Hickey MS, Kiernan GJ, Weaver KE: Evaluation of abdominal pain. Emerg Med Clin North Am 7:437-452, 1989.
24. Lachman E, Schienfeld A, Voss E, et al: Pregnancy and laparoscopic surgery. J Am Assoc Gynecol Laparosc 6:347-351, 1999.
25. Fatum M, Rojansky N: Laparoscopic surgery during pregnancy. Obstet Gynecol Surv 56:50-59, 2001.
26. Sharp HT: The acute abdomen during pregnancy. Clin Obstet Gynecol 45:405-413, 2002.
27. Tarraza HM, Moore RD: Gynecologic causes of the acute abdomen and the acute abdomen in pregnancy. Surg Clin North Am 77:1371-1394, 1997.
28. Fallon WF Jr, Newman JS, Fallon GL, et al: The surgical management of intra-abdominal inflammatory conditions during pregnancy. Surg Clin North Am 75:15-31, 1995.
29. Baer J, Reis R, Arens R: Appendicitis in pregnancy with changes in position and axis of the normal appendix in pregnancy. JAMA 52:1359-1364, 1932.
30. Hunt MG, Martin JN Jr, Martin RW, et al: Perinatal aspects of abdominal surgery for nonobstetric disease. Am J Perinatol 6:412-417, 1989.
31. Kammerer WS: Nonobstetric surgery in pregnancy. Med Clin North Am 71:551-560, 1987.
32. Mazze RI, Kallen B: Appendectomy during pregnancy: A Swedish registry study of 778 cases. Obstet Gynecol 77:835-840, 1991.

33. Tamir IL, Bongard FS, Klein SR: Acute appendicitis in the pregnant patient. Am J Surg 160:571-575; discussion 575-576, 1990.

34. Lim HK, Bae SH, Seo GS: Diagnosis of acute appendicitis in pregnant women: Value of sonography. AJR Am J Roentgenol 159:539-542, 1992.

35. Brown MA, Birchard KR, Semelka RC: Magnetic resonance evaluation of pregnant patients with acute abdominal pain. Semin Ultrasound CT MR 26:206-211, 2005.

36. Cobben LP, Groot I, Haans L, et al: MRI for clinically suspected appendicitis during pregnancy. AJR Am J Roentgenol 183:671-675, 2004.

37. Mahmoodian S: Appendicitis complicating pregnancy. South Med J 85:19-24, 1992.

38. Lanzafame RJ: Laparoscopic cholecystectomy during pregnancy. Surgery 118:627-631; discussion 631-633, 1995.

39. Printen KJ, Ott RA: Cholecystectomy during pregnancy. Am Surg 44:432-434, 1978.

40. Tsiotos GG, Mullany CJ, Zietlow S, et al: Abdominal complications following cardiac surgery. Am J Surg 167:553-557, 1994.

41. Welling RE, Rath R, Albers JE, et al: Gastrointestinal complications after cardiac surgery. Arch Surg 121:1178-1180, 1986.

42. Gajic O, Urrutia LE, Sewani H, et al: Acute abdomen in the medical intensive care unit. Crit Care Med 30:1187-1190, 2002.

43. Mehran A, Liberman M, Rosenthal R, et al: Ruptured appendicitis after laparoscopic Roux-en-Y gastric bypass: Pitfalls in diagnosing a surgical abdomen in the morbidly obese. Obes Surg 13:938-940, 2003.

44. Byrne TK: Complications of surgery for obesity. Surg Clin North Am 81:1181-1193, vii-viii, 2001.

45. Hamilton EC, Sims TL, Hamilton TT, et al: Clinical predictors of leak after laparoscopic Roux-en-Y gastric bypass for morbid obesity. Surg Endosc 17:679-684, 2003.

CHAPTER 46

Acute Gastrointestinal Hemorrhage

Ali Tavakkolizadeh, MD   Joel E. Goldberg, MD   and   Stanley W. Ashley, MD

Approach to the Patient With Acute Gastrointestinal
Hemorrhage
Acute Upper Gastrointestinal Hemorrhage
Acute Lower Gastrointestinal Hemorrhage
Acute Gastrointestinal Hemorrhage From an Obscure
Source
Summary

Acute gastrointestinal (GI) hemorrhage is a common clinical problem with diverse manifestations. Such bleeding may range from trivial to massive and can originate from virtually any region of the GI tract, including the pancreas, liver, and biliary tree. Although no demographic group is spared, the annual incidence of about 170 cases per 100,000 adults increases steadily with advancing age, and the disease is slightly more common in men than women.[1] Furthermore, GI hemorrhage accounts for 1% to 2% of acute admissions, resulting in more than 300,000 annual hospitalizations in the United States.[2] It is also a common complication in patients hospitalized for other illness, especially surgical patients. Although the total economic burden of GI hemorrhage has not been formally assessed, annual estimates suggest that diverticular bleeding alone costs in excess of 1.3 billion dollars.[3]

Management of these patients is frequently multidisciplinary, involving emergency medicine, gastroenterology, intensive care, surgery, and interventional radiology. The importance of early surgical consultation in the care of these patients cannot be overemphasized.[4] In addition to aiding in the resuscitation of the unstable patient, in some settings the surgical endoscopist establishes the diagnosis and initiates therapy. Even when the gastroenterologist assumes this role, the early collaboration of the surgeon permits the establishment of goals and limits for initial

nonoperative therapy. Ultimately 5% to 10% of patients hospitalized for bleeding require operative intervention, and prompt surgical consultation permits more time for preoperative preparation and evaluation as well as patient and family education should urgent surgery become necessary.[1]

Most patients with an acute GI hemorrhage stop bleeding spontaneously. This allows time for a more elective evaluation. However, in almost 15% of cases, major bleeding persists, requiring emergent resuscitation, evaluation, and treatment.[5] Improvements in the management of these patients, primarily by early endoscopy and directed therapy, has significantly reduced the length of hospitalization. Despite this, the mortality rate remains greater than 5% and is significantly higher in those patients initially hospitalized for other reasons. This discrepancy between therapeutic advances and outcomes is probably related to the aging of the population with an increase in its comorbidities. Currently, the patient requiring operative intervention is both older and sicker than in the past.

Hemorrhage can originate from any region of the GI tract and is typically classified based on the location relative to the ligament of Treitz. Upper GI hemorrhage (proximal to the ligament of Treitz) accounts for more than 80% of acute bleeding.[1] Peptic ulcer disease (PUD) and variceal hemorrhage are the most common etiologies. Most lower GI bleeding originates from the colon, with diverticula and angiodysplasias accounting for the majority of cases. In less than 5% of patients, the small intestine is responsible.[1] *Obscure bleeding* is defined as hemorrhage that persists or recurs after negative endoscopy. Occult bleeding is not apparent to the patient until presentation with symptoms related to the anemia. Determination of the site of bleeding is important for directing diagnostic interventions with minimal delay. However, attempts to localize the source never precede appropriate resuscitative measures.

APPROACH TO THE PATIENT WITH ACUTE GASTROINTESTINAL HEMORRHAGE

In patients with GI bleeding, several fundamental principles of initial evaluation and management must be followed. A well-defined and logical approach to the patient with GI hemorrhage is outlined in Figure 46-1. On presentation, a rapid initial assessment permits a determination of the urgency of the situation. Resuscitation is initiated with stabilization of the patient's hemodynamic status and the establishment of a means for monitoring ongoing blood loss. A careful history and physical examination provides clues to the etiology and source of the bleeding and identifies any complicating conditions or medications. Specific investigation then proceeds to refine the diagnosis. Therapeutic measures are then initiated, and bleeding is controlled and recurrent hemorrhage prevented.

Initial Assessment

Adequacy of the patient's airway and breathing takes first priority. After this is assured, the patient's hemodynamic status becomes the dominant concern and forms the basis for further management. The presentation of GI bleeding is variable, ranging from hemoccult-positive stool on rectal exam to exsanguinating hemorrhage. Initial evaluation focuses on rapid assessment of the magnitude of both the preexisting deficits and ongoing hemorrhage. Continuous reassessment of the patient's circulatory status determines the aggressiveness of subsequent evaluation and intervention. The history of the bleeding, both its magnitude and frequency, also provides some guidance.

The severity of the hemorrhage can be generally determined based on simple clinical parameters. Obtundation, agitation, and hypotension (systolic blood pressure <90 mm Hg in the supine position), associated with cool, clammy extremities, are consistent with hemorrhagic shock and suggest a loss of more than 40% of the patient's blood volume. A resting heart rate of more than 100 beats/minute with a decreased pulse pressure implies a 20% to 40% volume loss. In patients without shock, postural changes are elicited by allowing the patient to sit up with the legs dangling for 5 minutes. A fall in blood pressure of more than 10 mm Hg or an elevation of the pulse of more than 20 beats/minute again reflects at least a 20% blood loss. Patients with lesser degrees of bleeding may have no detectable alterations in their hemodynamic status.

The hematocrit is not a useful parameter for assessing the degree of hemorrhage in the acute setting because the proportion of red blood cells (RBCs) and plasma initially lost is constant. The hematocrit does not fall until plasma is redistributed into the intravascular space and resuscitation with crystalloid solution is begun. Likewise, the absence of tachycardia may be misleading; some patients with severe blood loss may actually have bradycardia secondary to vagal slowing of the heart. Hemodynamic signs are less reliable in the elderly and patients taking β-blocker medications.

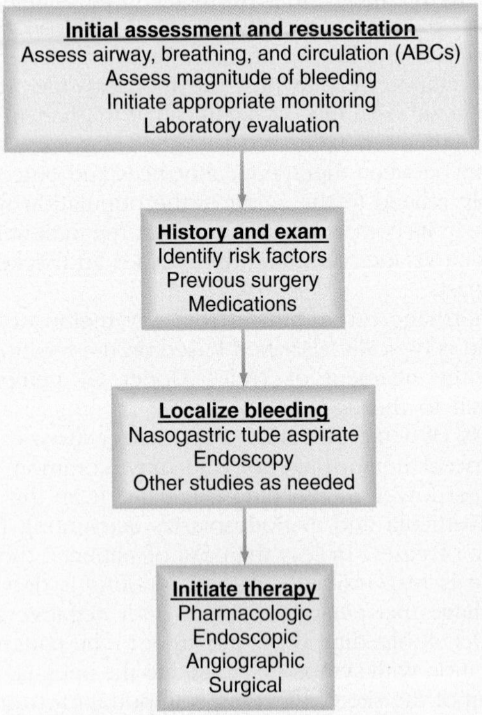

Risk Stratification

Not all patients with GI bleeding require hospital admission or emergent evaluation. For example, the patient with a small amount of rectal bleeding that has ceased can generally be evaluated on an outpatient basis. Clearly, in many patients, the decision making is less straightforward. Others require admission and observation but may be further evaluated with endoscopy on a more elective basis. Several prognostic factors, shown in Box 46-1, have been associated with adverse outcomes, including the need for emergent operation and death.[6] These factors

---

Initial assessment and resuscitation
Assess airway, breathing, and circulation (ABCs)
Assess magnitude of bleeding
Initiate appropriate monitoring
Laboratory evaluation

↓

History and exam
Identify risk factors
Previous surgery
Medications

↓

Localize bleeding
Nasogastric tube aspirate
Endoscopy
Other studies as needed

↓

Initiate therapy
Pharmacologic
Endoscopic
Angiographic
Surgical

Figure 46-1 General approach to the patient with acute GI hemorrhage.

Box 46-1   Risk Factors for Morbidity and Mortality in Acute Gastrointestinal Hemorrhage

Age >60 yr
Comorbid disease
  Renal failure
  Liver disease
  Respiratory insufficiency
  Cardiac disease
Magnitude of the hemorrhage
  Systolic blood pressure <100 mm Hg on presentation
  Transfusion requirement
Persistent or recurrent hemorrhage
Onset of hemorrhage during hospitalization
Need for surgery

are considered during the initial assessment and resuscitation of patients with GI hemorrhage. For instance, patients older than 60 years of age have higher mortality rates than their younger counterparts and are evaluated more cautiously. This increased morbidity may be a reflection of concomitant disease. The deleterious effects of cardiac, renal, pulmonary, and hepatic comorbidity all are considered when evaluating patients with GI bleeding. For example, one study estimated that bleeding patients with significant renal disease have a mortality rate of nearly 30%; this increases to 65% in the presence of acute renal failure.[7] Other factors, including the magnitude of the initial hemorrhage, persistence or recurrence of the bleeding, and the onset of bleeding during hospitalization for another illness, also contribute to increased morbidity and mortality.

Considerable recent effort has been devoted to the development of risk scoring tools to facilitate patient triage. These scoring systems have been used to predict the risk for rebleeding and mortality, to evaluate the need for intensive care unit (ICU) admission, and to determine the need for urgent endoscopy. For example, the BLEED classification schema uses five criteria[8]: ongoing bleeding; a systolic blood pressure of less than 100 mm Hg; a prothrombin time of greater than 1.2 times control; altered mental status; and an unstable comorbid disease process that would require ICU admission. If any one of these criteria is present, the model predicts an about three-fold increase in the risk for either recurrent hemorrhage, the need for surgical intervention, or death. Such scoring systems have been almost exclusively used in research studies and are significantly more accurate when endoscopic findings are included. Until these schema have been prospectively validated for everyday clinical practice, they are only applied in the context of clinical judgment.

Resuscitation

The more severe the bleeding, the more aggressive the resuscitation. In fact, the single leading cause of morbidity and mortality in these patients is multiorgan failure related to inadequate initial or subsequent resuscitation. Intubation and ventilation are initiated early if there is any question of respiratory compromise. In patients with evidence of hemodynamic instability and those in whom ongoing bleeding is suspected, two large-bore intravenous lines are placed, preferably in the antecubital fossae. Unstable patients receive a 2 L bolus of crystalloid solution, usually lactated Ringer's, which most closely approximates the electrolyte composition of whole blood. The response to the fluid resuscitation is noted. Blood is sent immediately for type and crossmatch, hematocrit, platelet count, coagulation profile, routine chemistries, and liver function tests. A Foley catheter also is inserted for assessment of end-organ perfusion. In elderly patients and those with significant cardiac, pulmonary, or renal disease, placement of a central venous or pulmonary artery catheter is considered for closer monitoring. The oxygen-carrying capacity of the blood can be maximized by administering supplemental oxygen. Frequently, these

patients benefit from early admission to and management in the ICU.

The decision to transfuse blood depends on the response to the fluid challenge, the age of the patient, whether concomitant cardiopulmonary disease is present, and whether the bleeding continues. The initial effects of crystalloid infusion and the patient's ongoing hemodynamic parameters are the primary criteria. Once again, this process requires clinical judgment. For example, a young, healthy patient with an estimated blood loss of 25% who responds to the fluid challenge with a normalization of hemodynamics may not need any blood products, whereas an elderly patient with a significant cardiac history and the same blood loss probably requires transfusion. Although the hematocrit may require 12 to 24 hours to fully equilibrate, it is commonly employed as one index of the need for blood replacement. In general, the hematocrit is maintained above 30% in elderly patients and above 20% in young, otherwise healthy patients. Likewise, the propensity of the suspected lesion to continue bleeding or to rebleed must play a role in this decision. For example, esophageal varices are very likely to continue to bleed, and transfusion might be considered earlier than in a patient with a Mallory-Weiss tear, which has a low rebleeding rate. In general, packed RBCs are the preferred form of transfusion, although whole blood, preferably warmed, may be employed in circumstances of massive blood loss.

History and Physical Examination

After the severity of the bleeding is assessed and resuscitation initiated, attention is directed to the history and physical examination. The history helps to make a preliminary assessment of the site and cause of bleeding and of significant medical conditions that may determine or alter the course of management.

Obviously, the characteristics of the bleeding provide important clues. The time of onset, volume, and frequency are important in estimating blood loss. Hematemesis, melena, and hematochezia are the most common manifestations of acute hemorrhage. Hematemesis is the vomiting of blood and is usually caused by bleeding from the upper GI tract, although rarely bleeding from the nose or pharynx can be responsible. It may be bright red or older and therefore take on the appearance of coffee grounds. Melena, the passage of black, tarry, and foul-smelling stool, generally suggests bleeding from the upper GI tract. Although the melanotic appearance typically results from both the gastric acid, which converts hemoglobin to hematin, and the actions of digestive enzymes and luminal bacteria in the small intestine, blood loss from the distal small bowel or right colon may have this appearance, particularly if transit is slow. Melena must not be confused with the greenish character of the stool in patients taking iron supplements. These can be distinguished by performing a guaiac test, which tests negative in those on iron supplementation. Hematochezia refers to bright red blood from the rectum that may or may not be mixed with stool. Although this typically reflects a distal colonic source, if the magnitude is

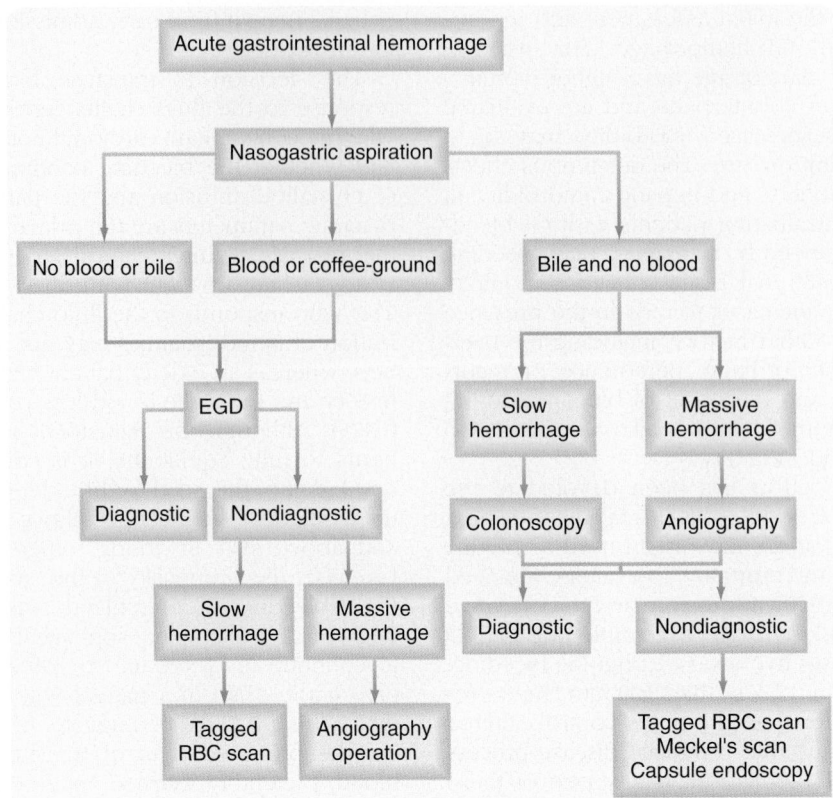

Figure 46-2 Algorithm for the diagnosis of acute GI hemorrhage. EGD, esophagogastroduodenoscopy; RBC, red blood cell.

significant, even upper GI hemorrhage may produce hematochezia.

The medical history may provide clues to the diagnosis. Chronic blood loss may lead to non-GI end-organ symptoms such as syncope, angina, and even myocardial infarction. Antecedent vomiting may suggest a Mallory-Weiss tear, whereas weight loss raises the specter of malignancy. Even demographic data may prove useful: elderly patients bleed from lesions such as angiodysplasias, diverticula, ischemic colitis, and cancer, whereas younger patients bleed from peptic ulcers, varices, and Meckel's diverticulum. A history of GI disease, bleeding, or operation immediately begins to focus the differential diagnosis. Antecedent epigastric distress may point to a peptic ulcer, whereas previous aortic surgery suggests the possibility of an aortoenteric fistula. A history of liver disease prompts a consideration of variceal bleeding. Medication use may also be revealing. A history of ingestion of salicylates, nonsteroidal anti-inflammatory drugs (NSAIDs), or selective serotonin-reuptake inhibitors (SSRIs) is common, particularly in elderly patients.[9] These medications are associated with GI mucosal erosions seen typically in the upper GI tract, but occasionally they can occur in the small bowel and colon. GI bleeding in the setting of anticoagulation therapy, either warfarin or low-molecular-weight heparin, is still most commonly the result of GI pathology and is not ascribed to the anticoagulation alone.[10]

Physical examination may also be revealing. Bleeding from the oropharynx and nose can occasionally simulate symptoms of a more distal source and must always be examined. Abdominal examination is only occasionally helpful, but it is important to exclude masses, splenomegaly, and adenopathy. Epigastric tenderness is suggestive, but not diagnostic, of gastritis or peptic ulceration. The stigmata of liver disease, including jaundice, ascites, palmar erythema, and caput medusae, may suggest bleeding related to varices, although these patients commonly bleed from other sources as well. Occasionally the physical exam may reveal clues to more obscure diagnoses such as the telangiectasias of Osler-Weber-Rendu disease or the pigmented lesions of the oral mucosa in Peutz-Jeghers syndrome. A rectal exam and anoscopy are performed to exclude a low-lying rectal cancer or bleeding from hemorrhoids.

Localization

Subsequent management of the patient with acute GI hemorrhage depends on localization of the site of the bleeding. An algorithm for the diagnosis of acute GI hemorrhage is shown in Figure 46-2.

Although melena is usually the result of bleeding from the upper GI tract, it can be the result of bleeding from the small bowel or colon. Likewise, hematochezia is sometimes the consequence of brisk upper GI bleeding.

The first step in distinguishing these possibilities is the insertion of a nasogastric (NG) tube and examination of the aspirate. Although hematemesis is usually diagnostic of an upper GI bleed, the tube is still useful to assess the rate of ongoing bleeding and to remove blood from the stomach to permit endoscopy. If the aspirate is positive, this effectively localizes the lesion. The presence of red blood or coffee-ground appearance suggests an upper source. Testing for occult blood is rarely necessary. The return of bile from a gastric aspirate suggests that the duodenum has been sampled. Although a bilious nonbloody gastric aspirate generally excludes the upper GI tract, these findings can occasionally be misleading. One study found that only 6 of 10 yellow-green NG aspirates tested positive for bile.[11] Likewise, almost 20% of patients with a clear aspirate are still bleeding from an upper GI source.[2] In patients with melena or even hematochezia from an upper lesion, the NG aspirate may be negative in the presence of significant duodenal bleeding and a competent pylorus preventing duodenogastric reflux. These considerations suggest that, although the findings of the NG aspirate can be helpful, virtually all patients with significant bleeding need to undergo upper endoscopy.

Esophagogastroduodenoscopy (EGD) under these circumstances is highly accurate in both identifying an upper GI lesion and, if negative, directing attention to a lower GI source. To maximize efficacy, EGD is performed within 24 hours even in stable patients.[12] Early EGD with directed therapy has been shown to reduce resource utilization and transfusion requirements and to shorten hospital stay. Accuracy may be limited by either active bleeding or abnormal anatomy as a result of previous surgery. Occasionally patients may have multiple lesions, and if there is no active bleeding, specificity is reduced. For example, patients with varices frequently have mucosal erosions that may have been the original source. Clinicians need to be aware that EGD in the urgent or emergent setting is associated with a significant increase in the incidence of complications, including aspiration, respiratory depression, and GI perforation, when compared with elective procedures. Airway protection is critical and may require endotracheal intubation if it has not been performed previously. Volume resuscitation must not be interrupted by the examination.

As shown in Figure 46-2, subsequent evaluation depends on the results of the EGD and the magnitude of the bleeding. Angiography or even surgery may prove necessary for massive hemorrhage, from either the upper or lower GI tract. For slow or intermittent bleeding from the lower GI tract, colonoscopy is now the initial diagnostic maneuver of choice. When this is nondiagnostic, the tagged RBC scan is usually employed. For obscure bleeding, usually from the small bowel, capsule endoscopy is becoming the appropriate study. These diagnostic procedures are discussed in greater detail later.

Therapy

Depending on the source of the bleeding, a variety of therapeutic options are available. These include pharma-

cologic, endoscopic, angiographic, and surgical modalities. Pharmacologic, endoscopic, and surgical therapies are, for the most part, site specific and are discussed further in appropriate sections later. Angiographic techniques are somewhat more generic and include selective angiography with either infusion of a vasoconstrictor, typically vasopressin, or embolization. Embolic agents include temporary materials such as gelatin sponge (e.g., Gelfoam) and autologous clot or permanent devices such as coils. There are few data comparing the efficacy of these techniques.

For most patients, bleeding has ceased, and therapeutic options are applied to prevent recurrence. The risk for recurrent bleeding, and therefore the need for preventive intervention, depends on the characteristics of the lesion, the magnitude of the initial hemorrhage, and the specific patient. For example, although the risk for recurrent diverticular hemorrhage is relatively low, elective colonic resection may still be appropriate in a patient with significant coronary disease who has already suffered a major hemorrhage.

For the about 15% of patients who continue to bleed, therapy is more urgent. In patients with hemodynamic instability, an appropriate goal is to institute therapy within 2 hours of presentation. This depends on the development of institution-specific protocols for the multidisciplinary management of these patients.[2] The availability of an endoscopist trained in techniques of hemostasis and of an appropriate support staff is critical. Likewise, angiographic expertise must be immediately accessible. Despite the variety of relatively new modalities for nonoperative control of bleeding, the early involvement of the surgical team remains essential.

Traditional series have demonstrated that the morbidity and mortality of operation for GI bleeding increase significantly in patients who have lost more than 6 units of blood. This increase is particularly marked in elderly patients and those with major comorbid conditions, suggesting that intervention in these patients needs to be earlier than in young, healthy patients who might otherwise be better operative candidates. Although improvements in supportive care and directed therapy, particularly endoscopic, may have moderated this approach to a degree, surgical therapy must always be a serious consideration in the context of blood loss of this magnitude.

ACUTE UPPER GASTROINTESTINAL HEMORRHAGE

Upper GI bleeding refers to bleeding that arises from the GI tract proximal to the ligament of Treitz and accounts for nearly 80% of significant GI hemorrhage. The causes of upper GI bleeding are best categorized as either nonvariceal or bleeding related to portal hypertension (Table 46-1). The nonvariceal causes account for about 80% of such bleeding, with PUD being the most common.[1] In the remaining 20% of patients, most of whom have cirrhosis, portal hypertension can lead to the develop-

Table 46-1 Common Causes of Upper Gastrointestinal Hemorrhage

NONVARICEAL BLEEDING	(80%)	PORTAL HYPERTENSIVE BLEEDING	(20%)
Peptic ulcer disease	30-50%	Gastroesophageal varices	>90%
Mallory-Weiss tears	15-20%	Hypertensive portal gastropathy	<5%
Gastritis or duodenitis	10-15%	Isolated gastric varices	Rare
Esophagitis	5-10%		
Arteriovenous malformations	5%		
Tumors	2%		
Other	5%		

Adapted from Ferguson CB, Mitchell RM: Nonvariceal upper gastrointestinal bleeding: Standard and new treatment. Gastroenterol Clin North Am 34:607-621, 2005.

ment of gastroesophageal varices, isolated gastric varices, or hypertensive portal gastropathy, any of which can be the source of an acute upper GI bleed. Although patients with cirrhosis are at high risk for developing variceal bleeding, even in these patients, nonvariceal sources account for most of the episodes of GI hemorrhage.[2] However, because of the greater morbidity and mortality of variceal bleeding, patients with cirrhosis is generally assumed to have variceal bleeding and appropriate therapy initiated, until an emergent EGD has demonstrated another cause.

The foundation of diagnosis and management of patients with an upper GI bleed is an EGD. Multiple studies have demonstrated that early EGD (within 24 hours) results in reductions in blood transfusion requirements, a decrease in the need for surgery, and a shorter length of hospital stay. Endoscopic identification of the source of bleeding also permits an estimate of the risk for subsequent or persistent hemorrhage as well as facilitating operative planning, should that prove necessary. In general, 20% to 35% of patients undergoing EGD will require a therapeutic endoscopic intervention, and 5% to 10% will eventually require surgery.[12]

Although the best tool for localization of the bleeding source is an EGD, in 1% to 2% of patients with upper GI hemorrhage, the source cannot be identified because of excessive blood impairing visualization of the mucosal surface.[13] Aggressive lavage of the stomach with room temperature normal saline solution before the procedure can be helpful. Recent evidence has suggested that a single bolus injection of intravenous erythromycin, which stimulates gastric emptying, can significantly improve visualization.[14] If identification of the source is still not possible, angiography may be appropriate in the reasonably stable patient, although operative intervention must be seriously considered if the blood loss is extreme or the patient hemodynamically unstable. Tagged RBC scan is seldom necessary with a confirmed upper GI bleed, and contrast studies are usually contraindicated because they will interfere with subsequent maneuvers.

Specific Causes of Upper Gastrointestinal Hemorrhage

Nonvariceal Bleeding

Peptic Ulcer Disease

PUD still represents the most frequent cause of upper GI hemorrhage, accounting for about 40% of all cases.[2] About 10% to 15% of patients with PUD develop bleeding at some point in the course of their disease. Bleeding is the most frequent indication for operation and the principal cause of death. PUD is discussed in more detail in Chapter 44; this discussion focuses only on bleeding from ulcer disease.

The epidemiology of peptic ulcer has continued to change. The incidence of uncomplicated PUD has declined dramatically. This recent change has been attributed to better medical therapy, including proton pump inhibitors (PPIs) and regimens for eradication of *Helicobacter pylori*. Although the need for operation for perforated PUD has declined as well, surgical intervention for bleeding PUD has remained relatively stable.[15] In fact, some population-based studies have documented an increase in PUD bleeding requiring hospital admission in elderly patients.[16] Today, when surgery for upper GI hemorrhage is undertaken, such operations are typically confined to the eldest and often the sickest patient.

Bleeding develops as a consequence of acid-peptic erosion of the mucosal surface. Although chronic blood loss is common with any ulcer, significant bleeding typically results when there is involvement of an artery, either of the submucosa or, with penetration of the ulcer, an even larger vessel. Although duodenal ulcers are more common than gastric ulcers, gastric ulcers bleed more commonly; as a result, in most series, the relative proportions are nearly equal. The most significant hemorrhage occurs when duodenal or gastric ulcers penetrate into branches of the gastroduodenal artery or left gastric artery, respectively.

Management Figure 46-3 outlines an approach to management. Strategies depend on the appearance of the lesion at endoscopy. Endoscopic therapy is instituted if

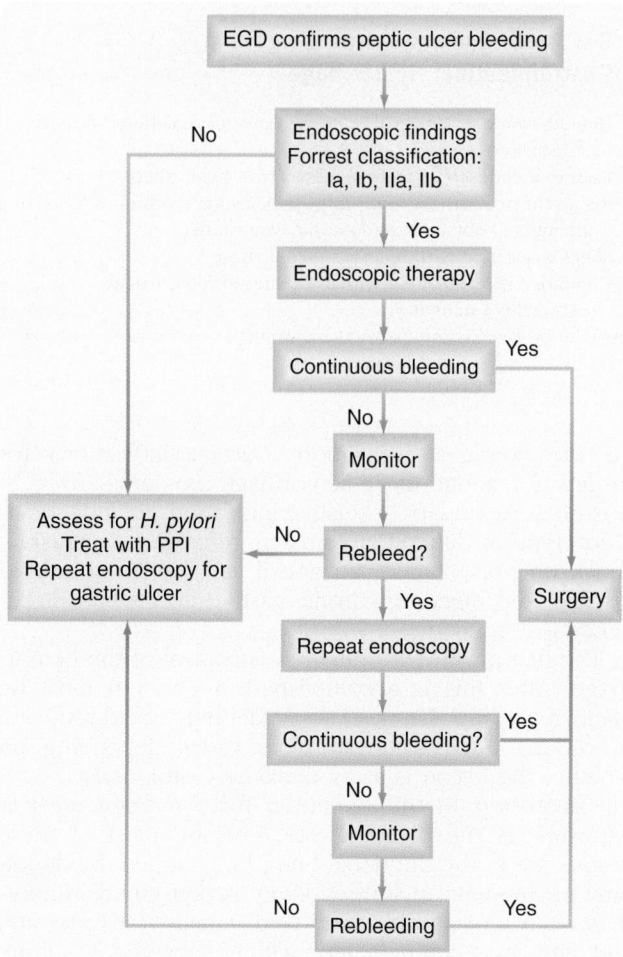

Figure 46-3 Algorithm for the diagnosis and management of nonvariceal upper GI bleeding. EGD, esophagogastroduodenoscopy; PPI, proton pump inhibitor.

Table 46-2 Forrest Classification of Endoscopic Findings and Rebleeding Risks in Peptic Ulcer Disease

CLASSIFICATION	REBLEEDING RISK
Grade Ia: Active, pulsatile bleeding	High
Grade Ib: Active, nonpulsatile bleeding	High
Grade IIa: Nonbleeding visible vessel	High
Grade IIb: Adherent clot	Intermediate
Grade IIc: Ulcer with black spot	Low
Grade III: Clean, nonbleeding ulcer bed	Low

ing ulcer test positive for *H. pylori*.[19] This has generated some controversy as to the importance of *H. pylori* treatment in patients with a bleeding peptic ulcer. However, several studies and a large meta-analysis have shown that *H. pylori* treatment and eradication, in patients who test positive for the infection, results in decreased rebleeding.[20] Importantly, after the *H. pylori* has been eradicated, there is no need for long-term acid suppression, and there is no increased risk for further bleeding with this approach.[21] In patients who are taking ulcerogenic medications, such as NSAIDs or SSRIs, and who present with a bleeding GI lesion, these medications are stopped, and the patient is started on a nonulcerogenic alternative. Recent evidence has, however, questioned the enhanced GI safety of COX-2 inhibitors.

Endoscopic Management After the bleeding ulcer has been identified, effective local therapy can be delivered endoscopically to control the hemorrhage. The available endoscopic options include epinephrine injection, heater probes and coagulation, and the application of hemoclips. Epinephrine injection (1:10,000) to all four quadrants of the lesion is very successful in controlling the hemorrhage. It has been shown that large-volume injection (>13 mL) is associated with better hemostasis, suggesting that the endoscopic injection works in part by compressing the bleeding vessel and inducing tamponade.[23] Epinephrine injection alone is associated with a high rebleeding rate, and therefore the standard practice is to provide combination therapy. This usually means the addition of thermal therapy to the injection. The sources of thermal energy can be heater probes, monopolar or bipolar electrocoagulation, laser, or argon plasma coagulator. The most commonly used therapies are electrocoagulation for bleeding ulcers and argon plasma coagulator for superficial lesions. A combination of injection with thermal therapy achieves hemostasis in 90% of bleeding PUD cases. The role of hemoclips is less clear, and several studies have reported mixed results. Hemoclips (Fig. 46-4), which can be difficult to apply, may be particularly effective when dealing with a spurting vessel because they provide immediate control of hemorrhage.

Rebleeding of an ulcer is associated with a significant increase in mortality, and careful observation of patients at high risk for rebleeding using criteria previously described is important. In those that rebled, the role of

bleeding is active or, when bleeding has already stopped, if there is a significant risk for rebleeding. The ability to predict the risk for rebleeding permits prophylactic therapy, closer monitoring, and earlier detection of hemorrhage in high-risk patients. The Forrest classification was developed in an attempt to assess this risk based on endoscopic findings, and to stratify the patients into low-, intermediate-, and high-risk groups[17] (Table 46-2). Endoscopic therapy is recommended in cases of active bleeding as well as a visible vessel (Forrest I to IIa). In cases of an adherent clot (Forrest IIb), the clot is removed and the underlying lesion evaluated. Ulcers with a clean base or a black spot, secondary to hematin deposition, are generally not treated endoscopically.

Medical Management In cases of an acute peptic ulcer bleed, PPIs have been shown to reduce the risk for rebleeding and the need for surgical intervention. Therefore, patients with a suspected or confirmed bleeding ulcer are started on a PPI.[18] Unlike perforated ulcers, which are commonly associated with *H. pylori* infection, the association between *H. pylori* infection and bleeding is less strong. Only 60% to 70% of patients with a bleed-

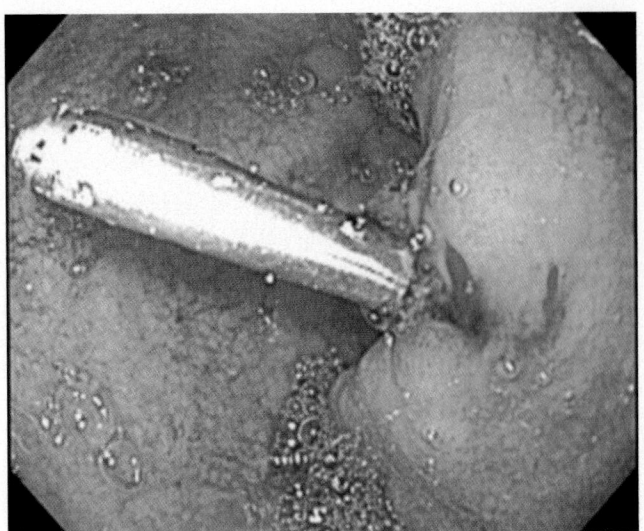

Figure 46-4 Hemoclip that has been applied to a bleeding duodenal ulcer. (Courtesy of Linda S. Lee, MD, Brigham and Women's Hospital.)

a second attempt at endoscopic control has been controversial but recently validated. For example, one recent study demonstrated that a second attempt at endoscopic hemostasis is successful in 75% of patients.[24] Although this will fail in 25% of patients who will then require emergent surgery, there does not appear to be any increase in morbidity or mortality with such management policy. Therefore, most clinicians would now encourage a second attempt at endoscopic control before surgical intervention.

Surgical Management Despite significant advances in endoscopic therapy, about 10% of patients with bleeding ulcers still require surgical intervention for effective hemostasis. Identifying patients who are likely to fail endoscopic therapy is difficult, however, and timing of surgery is controversial. To assist in this decision-making process, several clinical and endoscopic parameters have been employed to identify patients at high risk for failed endoscopic therapy. These include shock and a low hemoglobin level at presentation. At the time of endoscopy, although the Forrest classification is the most important indicator of rebleeding risk, the location and size of the ulcer also have significance. Ulcers greater than 2 cm, posterior duodenal ulcers, and gastric ulcers have a significantly higher risk for rebleeding.[25,26] Patients with these ulcer characteristics require closer monitoring and possibly earlier surgical intervention. Clearly, clinical judgment and local expertise must play a critical role in this decision.

Indications for surgery have traditionally been based on the blood transfusion requirements. Increased blood transfusions have been clearly associated with increased mortality. Although a less definitive criterion than it was in the past, most surgeons still consider an ongoing blood transfusion requirement in excess of 6 units an indication for surgical intervention, particularly in elderly patients, although an 8- to 10-unit loss may be more acceptable

for the younger population. Current indications for surgery for peptic ulcer hemorrhage are summarized in Box 46-2. Secondary or relative indications include a rare blood type or difficult crossmatch, refusal of transfusion, shock on presentation, advanced age, severe comorbid disease, and bleeding chronic gastric ulcer when malignancy is a concern.

The first priority at operation is control of the hemorrhage. After this is accomplished, a decision must be made regarding the need for a definitive acid-reducing procedure. Each of these steps varies depending on whether the lesion is a duodenal or gastric ulcer.

The first step in the operation for *duodenal ulcer* is exposure of the bleeding site. Because most of these lesions are in the duodenal bulb, longitudinal duodenotomy or duodenal pyloromyotomy is performed. Hemorrhage can typically be controlled initially with pressure and then direct suture ligation with nonabsorbable suture. When ulcers are positioned anteriorly, typically four-quadrant suture ligation suffices. A posterior ulcer eroding into the pancreaticoduodenal or gastroduodenal artery may require suture ligature of the vessel proximal and distal to the ulcer.

After the bleeding has been addressed, a definitive acid-reducing operation is considered. With the identification of the role of *H. pylori* infection in the pathogenesis of duodenal ulcers, the utility of such a procedure has recently been questioned based on the argument that simple closure and subsequent treatment for *H. pylori* is sufficient to prevent recurrence. In contrast to perforated ulcer, for which there is convincing evidence to support such an approach, current data do not exist for bleeding duodenal ulcers. Although this controversy will continue to evolve, at the present time an acid-reducing procedure still appears appropriate in most patients.

Historically, the choice between various operative procedures has been based on the hemodynamic condition of the patient and whether there is a long-standing history of refractory ulcer disease. The different operations for PUD are discussed in greater detail in Chapter 47. Because the pylorus has often been opened in a longitudinal fashion to control the bleeding, closure as a pyloroplasty combined with truncal vagotomy is the most frequently used operation for bleeding duodenal ulcer. There is some evidence to suggest that parietal cell vagotomy may represent a better therapy for a bleeding duodenal ulcer in the stable patient, although some of this benefit may be abrogated if the pylorus has been divided. Surgeon experience with this procedure may be the determining factor. In a patient who has a known history of refractory duodenal ulcer disease or who has failed more conservative surgery, antrectomy with truncal vagotomy may be more appropriate. However, this procedure is more complex and is rarely undertaken in a hemodynamically unstable patient.

For bleeding *gastric ulcers,* similar to bleeding duodenal ulcers, control of bleeding is the immediate priority. This may require gastrotomy and suture ligation, which, if no other procedure is performed, is associated with about a 30% risk for rebleeding.[27] In addition, because of the approximate 10% incidence of malignancy, gastric ulcer resection is generally indicated. Simple excision alone is associated with rebleeding in as many as 20% of patients, so that distal gastrectomy is generally preferred, although excision combined with vagotomy and pyloroplasty may be considered in the high-risk patient. Bleeding ulcers of the proximal stomach near the gastroesophageal junction are more difficult to manage. Proximal or near-total gastrectomy is associated with a particularly high morbidity in the setting of acute hemorrhage. Options include distal gastrectomy combined with resection of a tongue of proximal stomach to include the ulcer; or vagotomy and pyloroplasty combined with either wedge resection or simple oversewing of the ulcer.

Mallory-Weiss Tears

Mallory-Weiss tears are mucosal and submucosal tears that occur near the gastroesophageal junction. Classically, these lesions develop in alcoholic patients after a period of intense retching and vomiting after binge drinking, but they can occur in any patient who has a history of repeated emesis. The mechanism, proposed by Mallory and Weiss in 1929, is forceful contraction of the abdominal wall against an unrelaxed cardia, resulting in mucosal laceration of the proximal cardia as a result of the increase in intragastric pressure.

Mallory-Weiss tears account for 5% to 10% of cases of upper GI bleeding.[2] They are usually diagnosed based on history. Endoscopy is frequently employed to confirm the diagnosis. To avoid missing the lesion, it is important to perform a retroflexion maneuver and view the area just below the gastroesophageal junction. Most tears occur along the lesser curvature. Supportive therapy is often all that is necessary because 90% of bleeding episodes are self-limited, and the mucosa often heals within 72 hours.

In rare cases of severe ongoing bleeding, local endoscopic therapy with injection or electrocoagulation may be effective. Angiographic embolization, usually with absorbable material such as gelatin sponge, has been successfully employed in cases of failed endoscopic therapy. If these maneuvers fail, high gastrotomy and suturing of the mucosal tear is indicated. It is important to rule out the diagnosis of variceal bleeding in cases of failed endoscopic therapy by a thorough examination of

the gastroesophageal junction. Recurrent bleeding from a Mallory-Weiss tear is uncommon.

Stress Gastritis

Stress-related gastritis is characterized by the appearance of multiple superficial erosions of the entire stomach, most commonly in the body. It is thought to result from the combination of acid and pepsin injury in the context of ischemia from hypoperfusion states, although NSAIDs produce a very similar appearance. In the 1960s and 1970s, it was a commonly encountered lesion in critically ill patients, with significant morbidity and mortality from bleeding. These lesions are different from the solitary ulcerations, related to acid hypersecretion, that occur in patients with severe head injury (Cushing's ulcers). When stress ulceration is associated with major burns, these lesions are referred to as Curling's ulcers. In contrast to NSAID-associated lesions, significant hemorrhage from stress ulceration was a common phenomenon.

Today, with improvements in the management of shock and sepsis, as well as widespread use of acid-suppressive therapy, significant bleeding from such lesions is rarely encountered. The overuse of acid-suppressive therapy in this setting, however, has resulted in considerable cost and perhaps some risk to patients, with an increased incidence of nosocomial pneumonia secondary to gastric colonization. These issues have generated interest in the identification of specific subgroups that are at high risk for stress gastritis to permit a more selective approach to prophylactic therapy. The Canadian Critical Care Trial group prospectively reviewed more than 2200 patients admitted to the ICU and demonstrated an incidence of clinically significant bleeding in only 0.1% of patients considered at low risk for bleeding from stress-related gastritis.[28] Factors increasing the risk for hemorrhage from stress gastritis included ventilator dependence for greater than 48 hours and coagulopathy. For patients with these risk factors, clinically significant bleeding from stress-related gastritis occurred in 3.4%. Patients with these risk factors are given prophylactic therapy with antacids, histamine-2 (H_2)-receptor antagonists, PPIs, or sucralfate (Carafate). The primary prophylactic measure remains aggressive and appropriate resuscitation.

In patients who develop significant bleeding, acid-suppressive therapy is often successful in controlling the hemorrhage. In rare cases when this fails, consideration is given to administration of octreotide or vasopressin selectively through the left gastric artery, endoscopic therapy, or even angiographic embolization. Historically, these cases were more commonly seen and dealt with surgically. The surgical choices included vagotomy and pyloroplasty, with oversewing of the hemorrhage, or near-total gastrectomy. These procedures were associated with mortality rates as high as 60%. Fortunately, with enhanced awareness and better prophylaxis, surgery is rarely indicated in these patients.

Esophagitis

The esophagus is infrequently the source of significant hemorrhage. When it does occur, it is most commonly

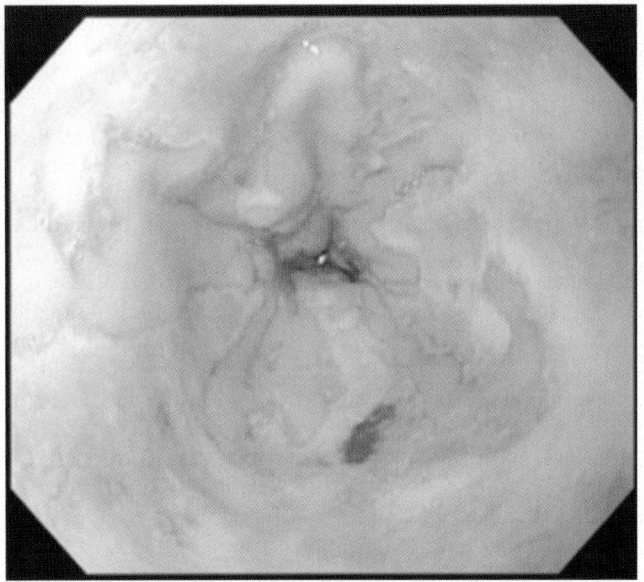

Figure 46-5 Bleeding esophageal ulcer secondary to herpes esophagitis. (Courtesy of Scott A. Hande, MD, Brigham and Women's Hospital.)

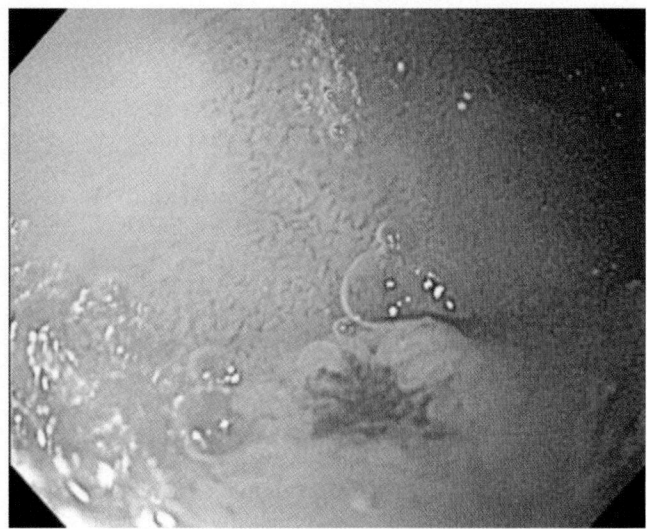

Figure 46-6 Bleeding Dieulafoy's lesion of the stomach. (Courtesy of Linda S. Lee, MD, Brigham and Women's Hospital.)

the result of esophagitis. Esophageal inflammation secondary to repeated exposure of the esophageal mucosa to the acidic gastric secretions in gastroesophageal reflux disease (GERD) leads to an inflammatory response, which can result in chronic blood loss. Ulceration may accompany this process, but the superficial mucosal ulcerations generally do not bleed acutely, but rather present as anemia or guaiac-positive stools. A variety of infectious agents may also cause esophagitis, particularly in the immunocompromised host (Fig. 46-5). With infection, hemorrhage can occasionally be massive. Other causes of esophageal bleeding include medications, Crohn's disease, and radiation.

Treatment typically includes acid-suppressive therapy. Endoscopic control of the hemorrhage, usually with electrocoagulation or heater probe, is often successful. In patients with an infectious etiology, targeted therapy is appropriate. Operation is seldom necessary.

Dieulafoy's Lesion

Dieulafoy's lesions are vascular malformations found primarily along the lesser curve of the stomach within 6 cm of the gastroesophageal junction, although they can occur elsewhere in the GI tract (Fig. 46-6). They represent rupture of unusually large vessels (1-3 mm) that are found in the gastric submucosa. Erosion of the gastric mucosa overlying these vessels leads to hemorrhage. The mucosal defect is usually small (2-5 mm) and may be difficult to identify. Given the large size of the underlying artery, bleeding from a Dieulafoy's lesion can be massive.

Initial attempts at endoscopic control are often successful. Application of thermal or sclerosant therapy is effective in 80% to 100% of cases. In cases that fail endoscopic therapy, angiographic coil embolization can be successful. If these approaches fail, surgical intervention may be necessary; owing to difficulties in visualization

and palpation of these lesions, prior endoscopic tattooing can facilitate the procedure. A gastrotomy is performed, and attempts are made at identifying the bleeding source. The lesion can then be oversewn. In cases in which the bleeding point is not identified, a partial gastrectomy may be necessary.

Gastric Antral Vascular Ectasia

Also known as "watermelon stomach," gastric antral vascular ectasia (GAVE) is characterized by a collection of dilated venules appearing as linear red streaks converging on the antrum in longitudinal fashion, giving it the appearance of a watermelon. Acute severe hemorrhage is rare in GAVE, and most patients present with persistent, iron deficiency anemia from continued occult blood loss. Endoscopic therapy is indicated for persistent, transfusion-dependent bleeding and has been reportedly successful in up to 90% of patients. The preferred endoscopic therapy is argon plasma coagulation (Fig. 46-7). Those failing endoscopic therapy are considered for antrectomy.

Malignancy

Malignancies of the upper GI tract are usually associated with chronic anemia or hemoccult-positive stool rather than episodes of significant hemorrhage. On occasion, malignancies present as ulcerative lesions that bleed persistently. This is perhaps most characteristic of the GI stromal tumor (GIST), although it may occur with a variety of other lesions, including leiomyomas and lymphomas. Although endoscopic therapy is often successful in controlling hemorrhage, the rebleeding rate is high; therefore, when a malignancy is diagnosed, surgical resection is indicated. The extent of resection is dependent on the specific lesion and on whether the resection is believed to be curative or palliative. Palliative resections for control of bleeding usually entail wedge resections. Standard cancer operations are indicated when

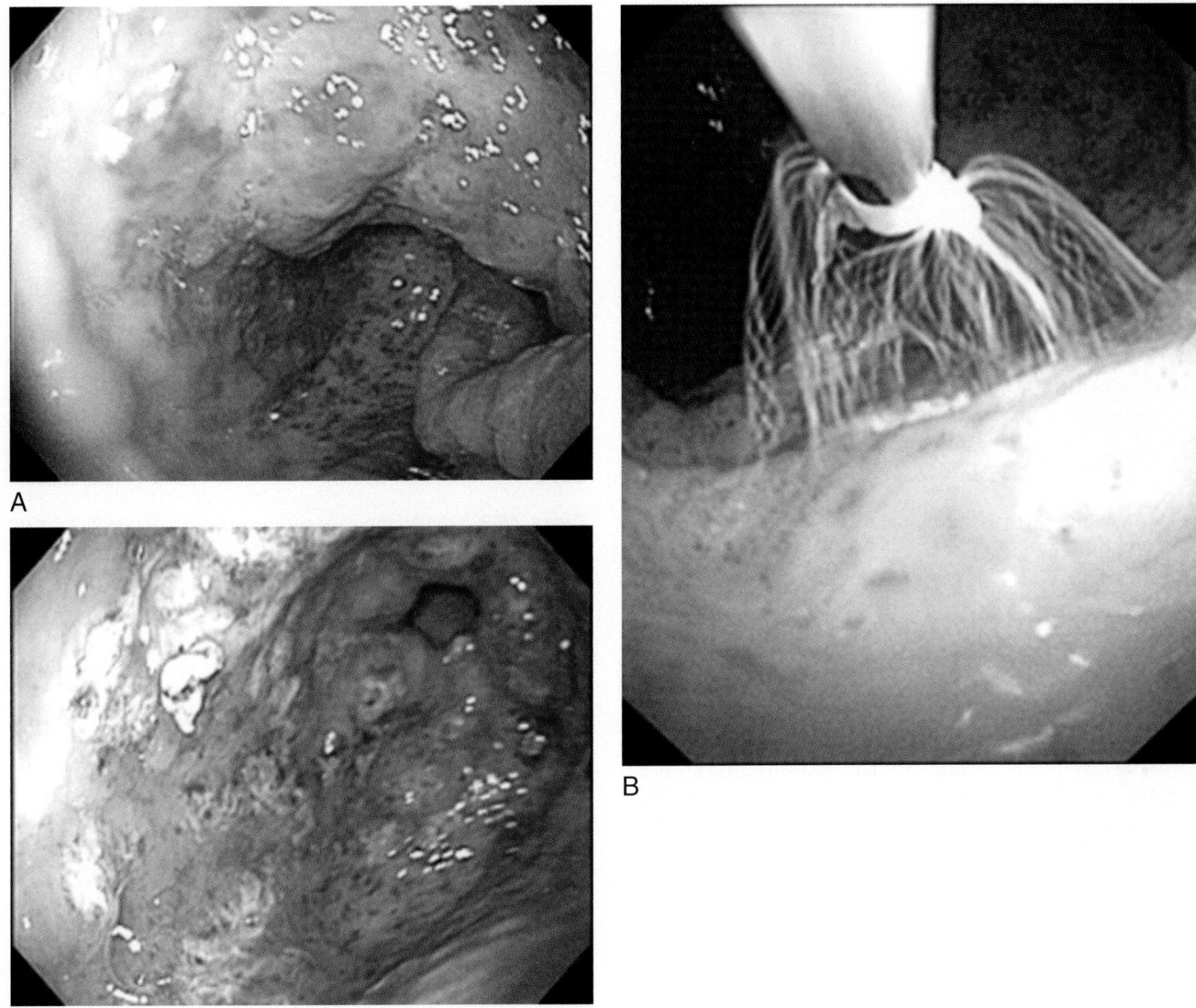

Figure 46-7 A, Gastric antral vascular ectasia (GAVE) can be seen in the gastric antrum, giving the stomach a watermelon appearance. **B,** Argon plasma coagulation therapy of a GAVE. **C,** Posttherapy appearance of the GAVE. (Courtesy of David L. Carr-Locke, MD, Brigham and Women's Hospital.)

possible, although this may depend on the hemodynamic stability of the patient.

Aortoenteric Fistula

Primary aortoduodenal fistulas are rare lesions developing in up to 1% of aortic graft cases. They typically develop in the setting of a previous abdominal aortic aneurysm repair, although they may occur as a result of an inflammatory or infectious aortitis. Although the interval between surgery and hemorrhage can be days to years, the median interval is about 3 years. The sequence is thought to involve development of a pseudoaneurysm at the proximal anastomotic suture line in the setting of an infection, with subsequent fistulization into the overlying duodenum.

Aortoenteric fistula is considered in all patients with GI hemorrhage with a known abdominal aortic aneurysm or a previous prosthetic aneurysm repair. Hemorrhage in this situation is often massive and fatal unless immediate surgical intervention is undertaken. Typically, patients with bleeding from an aortoenteric fistula will present first with a "sentinel bleed." This is a self-limited episode that heralds the subsequent massive, and often fatal, hemorrhage. This prompts urgent EGD because diagnosis at this stage can be lifesaving. Any evidence of bleeding in the distal duodenum (3rd or 4th portion) is considered diagnostic. Computed tomographic (CT) scan with intravenous contrast will demonstrate air around the graft (suggestive of an infection), possible pseudoaneurysm, and rarely the presence of intravenous contrast in the duodenal lumen.

Therapy includes ligation of the aorta proximal to the graft, removal of the infected prosthesis, and extra-anatomic bypass. The defect in the duodenum is often

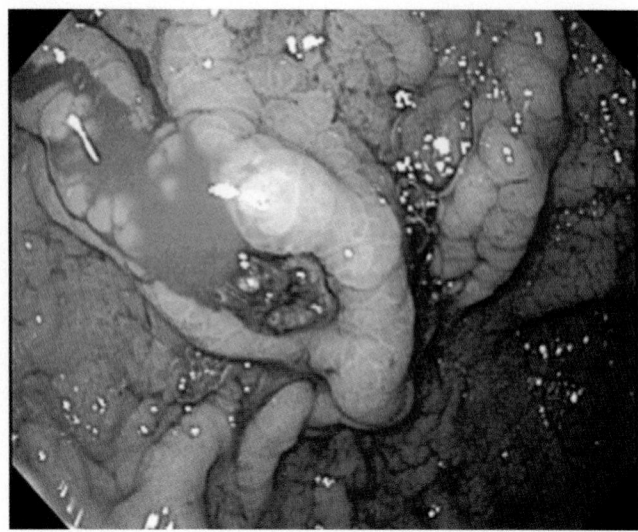

Figure 46-8 Bleeding from a percutaneous endoscopic gastrostomy site. (Courtesy of David L. Carr-Locke, MD, Brigham and Women's Hospital.)

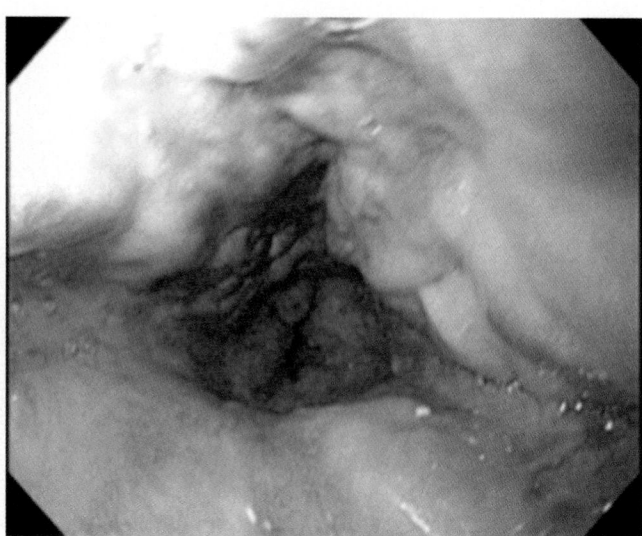

Figure 46-9 Nonbleeding esophageal varices secondary to cirrhosis. (Courtesy of David L. Carr-Locke, MD, Brigham and Women's Hospital.)

small and can be repaired primarily. This is a complex and often morbid procedure.

Hemobilia

Hemobilia is often a difficult diagnosis to make. It is typically associated with trauma, recent instrumentation of the biliary tree, or hepatic neoplasms. This unusual cause of GI bleeding is suspected in anyone who presents with hemorrhage, right upper quadrant pain, and jaundice. Unfortunately, this triad is seen in less than half of patients, and a high index of suspicion is required. Endoscopy can be helpful by demonstrating blood at the ampulla. Angiography is the diagnostic procedure of choice. If diagnosis is confirmed, angiographic embolization is the preferred treatment.

Hemosuccus Pancreaticus

Another rare cause of upper GI bleeding is bleeding from the pancreatic duct, or hemosuccus pancreaticus. This is typically caused by erosion of a pancreatic pseudocyst into the splenic artery. It presents with abdominal pain and hematochezia. As with hemobilia, it is a difficult diagnosis to make and requires a high index of suspicion in patients with abdominal pain, blood loss, and a past history of pancreatitis. Angiography is diagnostic and permits embolization, which is often therapeutic. In cases that are amenable to a distal pancreatectomy, this procedure often results in cure.

Iatrogenic Bleeding

Upper GI bleeding may follow therapeutic or diagnostic procedures. As described, hemobilia may be iatrogenic in nature, particularly after percutaneous transhepatic procedures. Another common cause of iatrogenic bleeding is endoscopic sphincterotomy. This can occur in up to 2% of cases. It is often mild and self-limited. Late hemorrhage usually occurs within the first 48 hours and

may require injection of the area with epinephrine. Surgical intervention is rarely required.

Percutaneous endoscopic gastrostomy (PEG) placement is an increasingly common procedure. Bleeding rates of up to 3% have been reported. Although most of these cases reflect bleeding from the incision site, some are due to bleeding from the gastric mucosa (Fig. 46-8). This can often be controlled endoscopically.

Upper GI bleeding can also be seen in patients who have recently undergone upper GI surgery. Any of the lesions previously mentioned could be responsible for postoperative hemorrhage, and these possibilities are considered. In cases in which a resection and anastomosis have been performed, the source of the bleeding may be the suture or the staple line. In cases in which bleeding is persistent and an intervention is needed, endoscopists are often concerned by the potential for suture or staple line disruption. However, it is safe to perform a diagnostic or even therapeutic EGD, providing that minimal insufflation is used and the procedure is performed with care.[29]

Bleeding Related to Portal Hypertension

Upper GI bleeding is a serious complication of portal hypertension, most often in the setting of cirrhosis. Cirrhosis and portal hypertension are covered in more detail in Chapter 53; only bleeding related to portal hypertension is discussed here.

Hemorrhage related to portal hypertension is most commonly the result of bleeding from varices. These dilated submucosal veins develop in response to the portal hypertension, providing a collateral pathway for decompression of the portal system into the systemic venous circulation. Although they are most common in the distal esophagus, they also may develop in the stomach and the hemorrhoidal plexus of the rectum. They can reach sizes of 1 to 2 cm, and as they enlarge, the overlying mucosa becomes increasingly tenuous and excoriated with bleeding occurring with minimal trauma. Portal hypertensive gastropathy, diffuse dilation of the mucosal and submucosal venous plexus of the stomach associated with overlying gastritis, is an incompletely understood entity. Endoscopically, the stomach acquires a snakeskin-like appearance with cherry-red spots. This entity uncommonly produces major hemorrhage.

Gastroesophageal varices (Fig. 46-9) develop in about 30% of patients with cirrhosis and portal hypertension, and 30% in this group develop variceal bleeding. Compared with nonvariceal bleeding, variceal hemorrhage is associated with an increased risk for rebleeding, need for transfusions, increased hospital stay, and mortality. Hemorrhage is frequently massive, accompanied by hematemesis and hemodynamic instability. The hepatic functional reserve, estimated by Child's criteria described in Chapter 53, correlates very closely with outcomes in these patients. Despite improvements in the medical management of these patients, the 6-week mortality rate after the first hemorrhage is about 20%.[30]

Management

As with other causes of GI bleeding, adequate resuscitation is imperative (Fig. 46-10). Fluid resuscitation in patients with cirrhosis is a delicate balance. These patients frequently have hyperaldosteronism associated with fluid retention and ascites. Animal studies have demonstrated that a rapid correction of fluid deficits and blood pressure increases the risk for further bleeding from varices.[31] Central venous pressure monitoring is indicated in most of these patients, and early admission to an ICU setting

is considered. A low threshold for intubation is appropriate. Defects in coagulation are common and need to be aggressively corrected. A significant percentage of patients with variceal bleeding have underlying sepsis, which may be associated with an aggravation in portal hypertension and lead to variceal bleeding. It has been demonstrated that, in those patients with variceal bleeding, a 7-day course of a quinolone, such as ofloxacin, lowers the risk of rebleeding by about 50%.[32] Based on these data, it has been recommended that patients with variceal bleeding be given an empiric course of a broad spectrum antibiotic for 7 days, and this therapy is initiated upon admission.

Medical Management In patients with cirrhosis, pharmacologic therapy to reduce portal hypertension is considered even while preparing for emergent EGD. Vasopressin produces splanchnic vasoconstriction and has been shown to significantly reduce bleeding when compared with placebo. Unfortunately, this agent results in significant cardiac vasoconstriction, with resulting myocardial ischemia. Although vasopressin has been combined with nitroglycerin in clinical practice, somatostatin or its synthetic analogue, octreotide, is now the vasoactive agent of choice.[33] Somatostatin, a natural peptide (with a very short half-life) that induces splanchnic vasoconstriction without cardiac side effects, has been used worldwide. Although studies have demonstrated its efficacy in controlling variceal bleeding, this agent has not been readily available in the United States, and in its place, octreotide, a longer-acting somatostatin analogue, has become the usual agent. Continuous intravenous infusion of these

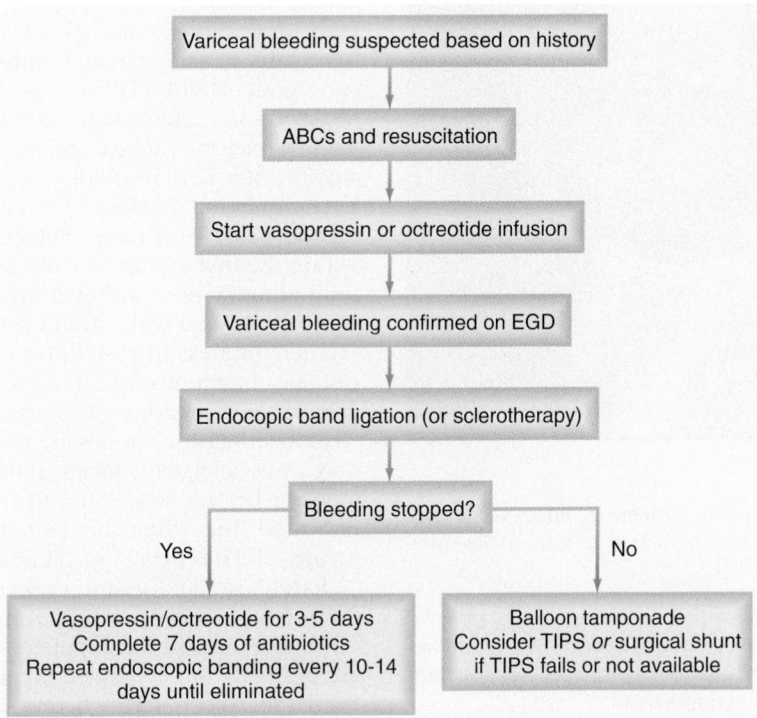

Figure 46-10 Algorithm for diagnosis and management of GI hemorrhage related to portal hypertension. EGD, esophagogastroduodenoscopy; TIPS, transjugular intrahepatic portosystemic shunt.

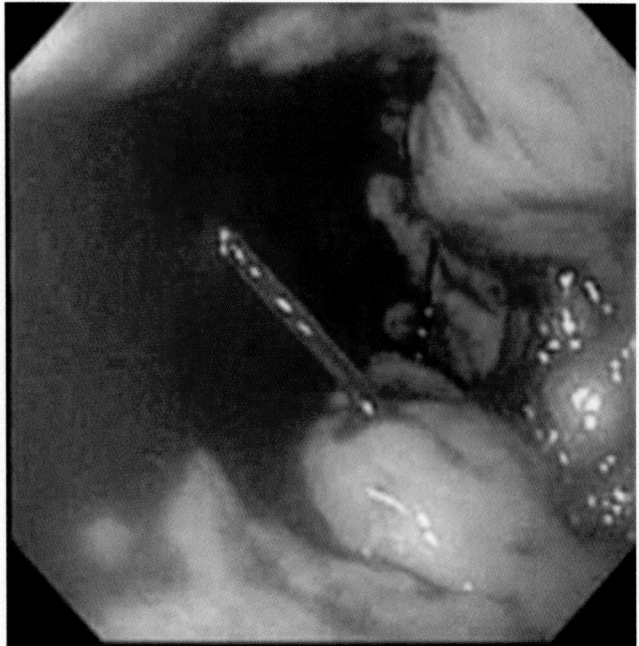

A

B

Figure 46-11 A, Actively bleeding varices. **B,** Effective control after variceal banding. (Courtesy of David L. Carr-Locke, MD, Brigham and Women's Hospital.)

agents results in temporary control of bleeding and allows time for resuscitation and to perform the appropriate diagnostic and therapeutic maneuvers.

Endoscopic Management Early EGD is critical to evaluate the source of bleeding because more than half of bleeding is caused by nonvariceal sources, including peptic

ulcer, gastritis, and Mallory-Weiss tears. Subsequent management is based on the endoscopic findings. If bleeding esophageal varices are identified, both sclerotherapy and variceal banding have been shown to control hemorrhage effectively. Although sclerotherapy, which may use a variety of agents, is an easier procedure to perform, it is also associated with perforation, mediastinitis, and stricture. Banding appears to have a lower complication rate and, when expertise is available, is the therapy of choice[34] (Fig. 46-11). These endoscopic approaches, sometimes with as many as three treatments over 24 hours, control the hemorrhage in up to 90% of patients with esophageal varices. Unfortunately, gastric varices are not effectively managed by endoscopic techniques.

Other Management In cases in which pharmacologic or endoscopic therapies fail to control the hemorrhage, balloon tamponade can be successful in temporizing the hemorrhage. The Sengstaken-Blakemore tube consists of a gastric tube with esophageal and gastric balloons. The gastric balloon is inflated, and tension is applied to the gastroesophageal junction. If this does not control the hemorrhage, the esophageal balloon is inflated as well, compressing the venous plexus between them. The Minnesota tube includes a proximal esophageal lumen for aspirating swallowed secretions. These tubes are associated with a high rate of complications related to both aspiration and inappropriate placement with esophageal perforation. Hemorrhage recurs on deflation in up to 50% of patients. Currently, balloon tamponade is reserved for patients with massive hemorrhage to permit more definitive therapies.

In cases of severe variceal bleeding that cannot be controlled endoscopically, emergent portal decompression is indicated. This is required in about 10% of patients with variceal bleeding.[30] This is most commonly achieved by means of percutaneous transjugular intrahepatic portosystemic shunt (TIPS). The TIPS procedure can be lifesaving in patients who are hemodynamically unstable from refractory variceal bleeding and is associated with significantly less morbidity and mortality than surgical decompression. Studies have shown that TIPS can control bleeding in 95% of cases. Rebleeding occurs in up to 20% within the first month, usually related to occlusion. Long-term patency rates are even lower although many cases can be salvaged with careful surveillance and percutaneous techniques. In cases in which TIPS is not available or fails, emergent surgical intervention is indicated. Emergent surgical options are discussed in Chapter 55.

Isolated gastric varices are managed in much the same way as esophageal varices, although endoscopic therapy tends to be less successful. Pharmacotherapy is primarily indicated, but when this fails, portal decompression by means of TIPS or a surgical shunt is recommended.

Rarely, isolated gastric varices occur after splenic vein thrombosis. This is most commonly seen in the setting of pancreatitis. In these patients, central portal pressures are normal, but left-sided hypertension, decompressed from the spleen through the short gastric vessels, produces the varices. Although the risk for variceal bleeding was thought to be high in this group and splenectomy was routinely recommended, recent data suggest that the

Table 46-3 Differential Diagnosis of Lower Gastrointestinal Hemorrhage

COLONIC BLEEDING (95%)	%	SMALL BOWEL BLEEDING (5%)
Diverticular disease	30-40	Angiodysplasias
Ischemia	5-10	Erosions or ulcers (potassium, NSAIDs)
Anorectal disease	5-15	Crohn's disease
Neoplasia	5-10	Radiation
Infectious colitis	3-8	Meckel's diverticulum
Postpolypectomy	3-7	Neoplasia
Inflammatory bowel disease	3-4	Aortoenteric fistula
Angiodysplasia	3	
Radiation colitis/proctitis	1-3	
Other	1-5	
Unknown	10-25	

Adapted from Strate LL: Lower gastrointestinal bleeding: Epidemiology and diagnosis. Gastroenterol Clin North Am 34:643-664, 2005.

incidence of variceal bleeding is in fact low (4%; mean follow-up, 34 months), and splenectomy is not routinely undertaken.[35]

Unlike variceal hemorrhage, bleeding from portal hypertensive gastropathy is not amenable to endoscopic treatment because of the diffuse nature of the mucosal abnormalities. The underlying pathology involves elevated portal venous pressures; therefore, pharmacologic therapies aimed at reducing portal venous pressure are indicated. If pharmacologic therapy fails to control acute bleeding, TIPS is considered.

Prevention of Rebleeding

After the initial bleeding has been controlled, prevention of recurrent hemorrhage needs to be a priority. When no further therapy is undertaken, about 70% of patients have another hemorrhagic event within 2 months. The risk for rebleeding is highest in the initial few hours to days following a first episode. Medical therapy to prevent recurrence includes a nonselective β-blocker, such as nadolol, and an antiulcer agent, such as a PPI or carafate. These are combined with endoscopic band ligation repeated every 10 to 14 days until all varices have been eradicated.

Although this aggressive approach results in a significant lowering of the rebleeding rate to less than 20%, it requires intensive medical follow-up and supervision.[36] In patients who are medically noncompliant or unable to tolerate such therapy, portal decompression is considered. The choice between TIPS and operative decompression in the stable patient depends on the residual liver function. In general, patients who have reduced liver capacity and are on the liver transplantation list are considered for TIPS. This procedure provides a temporizing measure and avoids postoperative scarring of the porta hepatis, which could complicate the transplantation. Unfortunately, TIPS is associated with hepatic encephalopathy in about 25% of patients and with shunt complications, such as thrombosis, in up to 30% after 1

year. In those with good liver function who do not qualify for transplantation, surgical decompression is preferred. This provides a more endurable long-term decompression, with a lower rate of hepatic encephalopathy. In those with good hepatic reserve, these advantages are thought to counterbalance the increased operative morbidity and mortality. The preferred elective shunt is a selective distal splenorenal shunt.

ACUTE LOWER GASTROINTESTINAL HEMORRHAGE

When compared with upper GI hemorrhage, lower GI bleeding is a much less common reason for hospitalization; in fact, it is about one fifth as common as bleeding from a location proximal to the ligament of Treitz.[37] In more than 95% of patients with lower GI bleeding, the source of hemorrhage is the colon. The small intestine is only occasionally responsible for lower GI bleeding, and because these lesions are not typically diagnosed with the combination of upper and lower endoscopy, they are considered in the section on obscure causes of GI bleeding. In general, the incidence of lower GI bleeding increases with age, and the etiology is often age related (Table 46-3). Specifically, vascular lesions and diverticular disease affect all age groups but have an increasing incidence in middle-aged and elderly patients. In children, intussusception is most commonly responsible, whereas Meckel's diverticulum must be considered in young adults. The clinical presentation of lower GI bleeding ranges from severe hemorrhage with diverticular disease or vascular lesions to a minor inconvenience secondary to an anal fissure or hemorrhoids.[37]

Diagnosis

Lower GI bleeding typically presents with hematochezia, which can range from bright-red blood to old clots. If the bleeding is slower or from a more proximal source,

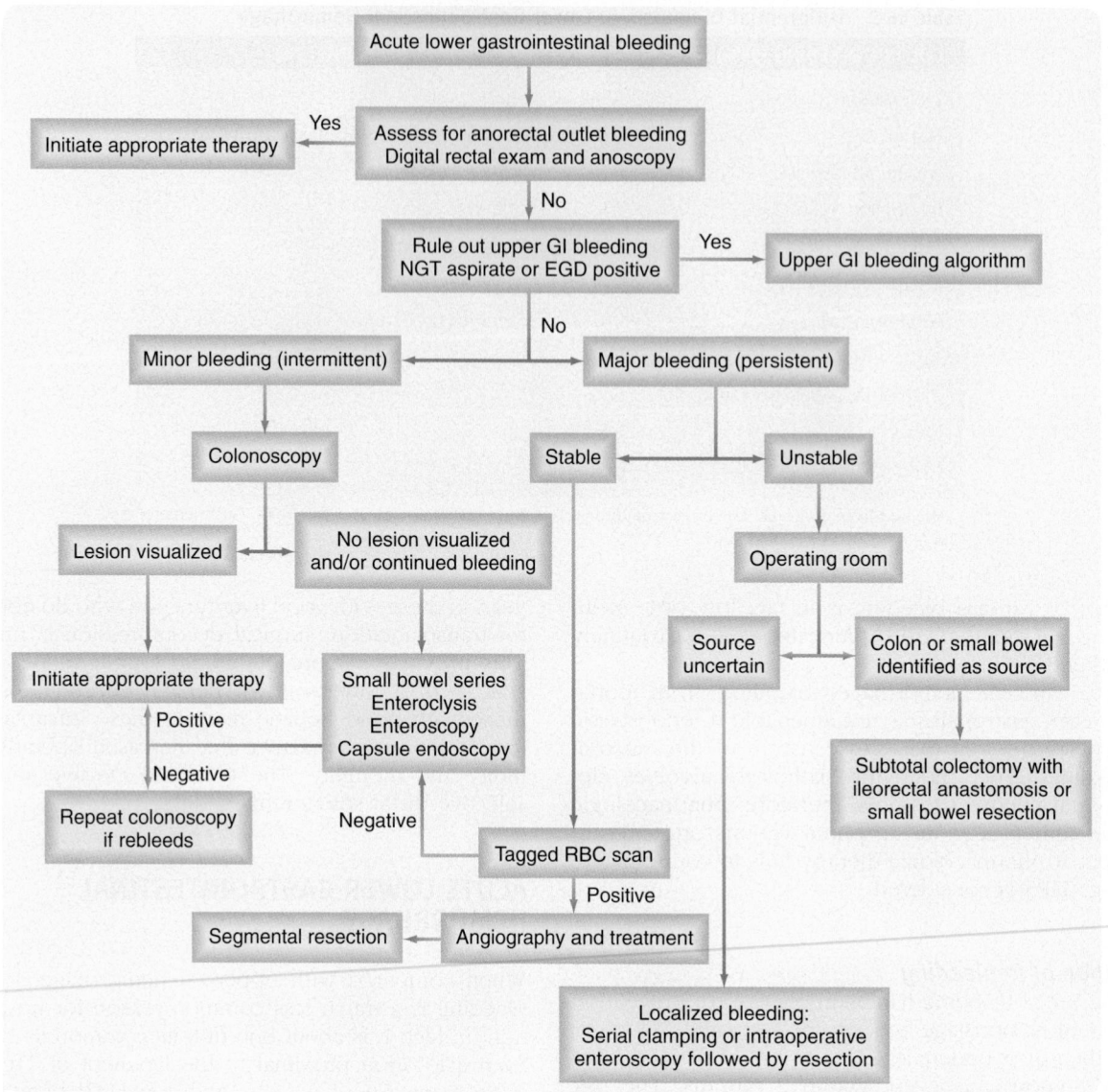

Figure 46-12 Algorithm for diagnosis and management of lower GI hemorrhage. EGD, esophagogastroduodenoscopy; NGT, nasogastric tube; RBC, red blood cell.

lower GI bleeding often presents as melena. Hemorrhage from the lower GI tract tends to be less severe and more intermittent, and it more commonly ceases spontaneously than upper GI bleeding. When compared with EGD for upper GI bleeding, the diagnostic modalities for lower GI bleeding are not as sensitive or specific in making an accurate diagnosis. Diagnostic evaluation is further complicated by the observation that, in up to 40% of patients with lower GI bleeding, more than one potential source of hemorrhage is identified. If more than one source is identified, it is critical to confirm the responsible lesion before initiating aggressive therapy. This approach may occasionally require a period of observation with several episodes of bleeding before a definitive diagnosis can be made. In fact, in up to 25% of patients with lower GI hemorrhage, the bleeding source is never accurately identified.

An algorithm for the evaluation of lower GI hemorrhage is shown in Figure 46-12. After resuscitation has been initiated, the first step in the workup is to rule out anorectal bleeding with a digital rectal exam and anoscopy or sigmoidoscopy. With significant bleeding, it is also important to eliminate an upper GI source. An NG aspirate that contains bile and no blood effectively rules out upper tract bleeding in most patients. However, when emergent surgery for life-threatening hemorrhage is being contemplated, preoperative or intraoperative EGD is usually appropriate. This is particularly relevant if blind subtotal colectomy for massive hemorrhage is being considered.

Subsequent evaluation depends on the magnitude of the hemorrhage. With major or persistent bleeding, the workup progresses depending on the patient's hemodynamic stability. The truly unstable patient who continues to bleed and requires ongoing aggressive resuscitation belongs in the operating room for expeditious diagnosis and surgical intervention. When hemorrhage is intermediate, resuscitation and hemodynamic stability permit a more directed evaluation and therapeutic intervention. Colonoscopy is the mainstay of diagnosis because it allows both visualization of the pathology and therapeutic intervention in colonic, rectal, and distal ileal sources of bleeding. The usual adjuncts to colonoscopy include tagged RBC scan and angiography. If these modalities are not diagnostic, the source of the hemorrhage is considered obscure (these lesions and their evaluation are considered in the final section).

Colonoscopy

Colonoscopy is most appropriate in the setting of minimal to moderate bleeding; major hemorrhage interferes significantly with visualization, and the diagnostic yield is low. In addition, in the unstable patient, sedation and manipulation may be associated with additional complications and can interfere with resuscitation. Although the blood is cathartic, gentle preparation with polyethylene glycol, either orally or through an NG tube, can improve visualization. Findings may include an actively bleeding site, clot adherent to a focus of mucosa or a diverticular orifice, or blood localized to a specific colonic segment, although this can be misleading because of retrograde peristalsis in the colon. Polyps, cancers, and inflammatory causes can frequently be seen. Unfortunately, angiodysplasias are often very difficult to visualize, particularly in the unstable patient with mesenteric vascular constriction. Diverticula are identified in most patients, whether they are the source of the hemorrhage or not. Despite these limitations, recent studies report that colonoscopy is successful in identifying the bleeding source in up to 95% of patients. Most of the bleeding is secondary to angiodysplasias or diverticula.[38]

Radionuclide Scanning

Radionuclide scanning with technetium-99m (^{99m}Tc)-labeled RBCs is the most sensitive but least accurate method for localization of GI bleeding. With this technique, the patient's own RBCs are labeled and reinjected. The labeled blood is extravasated into the GI tract lumen, creating a focus that can be detected scintigraphically. Initially, images are collected frequently and then at 4 hour intervals for up to 24 hours. The tagged RBC scan can detect bleeding as slow as 0.1 mL/min and is reported to be more than 90% sensitive[37] (Fig. 46-13). Unfortunately, the spatial resolution is lacking, and blood may move retrograde in the colon or distally in the small bowel. Reported accuracy of localization is in the range of only 40% to 60%, and it is particularly inaccurate in distinguishing right- from left-sided colonic bleeding. The RBC scan is not usually employed as a definitive study before surgery but instead as a guide to the utility of angiography; if the RBC scan is negative or only positive after several hours, angiography is unlikely to be revealing. Such an approach avoids the significant morbidity of the angiogram.

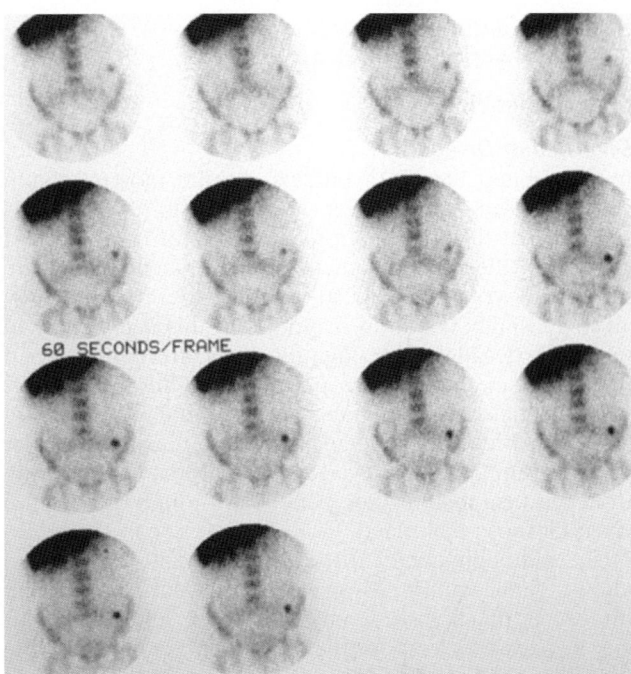

Figure 46-13 A positive red blood cell scan localizing the bleeding to the left lower quadrant. (Courtesy of Richard A. Baum, MD, Brigham and Women's Hospital.)

Mesenteric Angiography

Selective angiography, using either the superior or inferior mesenteric arteries, can detect hemorrhage in the range of 0.5 to 1.0 mL/min and is generally only employed in the diagnosis of ongoing hemorrhage. It can be particularly useful in identifying the vascular patterns of angiodysplasias. It may also be used for localizing actively bleeding diverticula. In addition, it has therapeutic capability. Catheter-directed vasopressin infusion can provide temporary control of bleeding, permitting hemodynamic stabilization, although as many as 50% of patients experience rebleeding when the medication is discontinued. It can also be employed for embolization. Although the more limited collateral circulation of the colon has made angiography less appealing than in the upper GI tract, recent series have suggested that these techniques can be applied safely in most patients. Typically, such therapy is reserved for patients whose underlying condition precludes surgical therapy. Unfortunately, angiography is associated with a significant risk for complications, including hematomas, arterial thrombosis, contrast reactions, and acute renal failure.

Treatment

Therapeutic approaches for lower GI bleeding are clearly dependent on the lesion identified. The criteria for operation are similar to those with upper GI hemorrhage, shown in Box 46-2, although there is a stronger tendency to delay surgery until the site is clearly localized.

Specific Causes of Lower Gastrointestinal Bleeding

Colonic Bleeding

Diverticular Disease

In the United States, diverticula are the most common cause of significant lower GI bleeding. Some series suggest that diverticula are responsible for up to 55% of cases.[37] In the past, diverticula were thought to be rare in patients younger than 40 years of age, but it is now an increasingly common diagnosis in this age group. In the ninth decade of life, diverticulosis affects more than two thirds of the Western population. Only 3% to 15% of individuals with diverticulosis experience episodes of bleeding. Bleeding generally occurs at the neck of the diverticulum and is believed to be secondary to bleeding from the vasa recti as they penetrate through the submucosa. Of those that bleed, more than 75% stop spontaneously, although about 10% rebleed within 1 year and almost 50% within 10 years.[37] Although diverticular disease is much more common on the left side, right-sided disease is responsible for more than half of the episodes of bleeding.

The best method of diagnosis and treatment is colonoscopy, although success is sometimes limited by the large amount of hemorrhage. If the bleeding diverticulum can be identified, epinephrine injection may control the bleeding. Electrocautery can also be used, and most recently, endoscopic clips have been successfully applied to control the hemorrhage. If bleeding ceases with these maneuvers or spontaneously, expectant management may be appropriate, although this requires clinical judgment based on the magnitude of the hemorrhage and the patient's comorbid conditions, particularly cardiac disease.

If none of these maneuvers is successful or if hemorrhage recurs, angiography with embolization can be considered, although the perceived risk for ischemic complications limits the use of this procedure. Usually, under these circumstances, colonic resection is indicated. Certainty of the bleeding site is critical. Blind hemicolectomy is associated with rebleeding in more than half of patients, and operation based on tagged RBC scan localization alone can result in recurrent hemorrhage in up to one third of patients.[39] Subtotal colectomy does not eliminate the risk for recurrent hemorrhage and, when compared with segmental resection, is accompanied by a significant increase in the morbidity, particularly diarrhea in elderly patients, in whom the remaining rectum may never effectively adapt. The mortality rate of emergent subtotal colectomy for bleeding is as high as 30%.[39,40]

Angiodysplasia

In some reports, hemorrhage secondary to angiodysplasia accounts for up to 40% of lower GI bleeding; however, most recent reports place the incidence much lower than that.[37] Angiodysplasias of the intestine, also referred to as *arteriovenous malformations* (AVMs), are distinct from hemangiomas and true congenital AVMs. They are thought to be acquired degenerative lesions secondary to progressive dilation of normal blood vessels within the submucosa of the intestine. Angiodysplasias are distributed equally between the sexes and are almost uniformly found in patients older than 50 years of age. These lesions are notably associated with aortic stenosis and renal failure, especially in elderly patients. The hemorrhage tends to arise from the right side of the colon, with the cecum being the most common location, although angiodysplasias can occur anywhere in the colorectum and small bowel. Most patients present with chronic bleeding; in up to 15% of patients, hemorrhage may be massive. Bleeding stops spontaneously in most cases, but about half of patients experience rebleeding within 5 years. These lesions can be diagnosed by either colonoscopy or angiography. Angiodysplasia appears as red stellate lesions with a surrounding rim of pale mucosa and can be treated with sclerotherapy or electrocautery. Angiography demonstrates dilated, slowly emptying veins and sometimes early venous filling. If these lesions are discovered incidentally, no further therapy is indicated. In acutely bleeding patients, angiodysplasias have been successfully treated with intra-arterial vasopressin, selective gel foam embolization, endoscopic electrocoagulation, or injection with sclerosing agents. If these measures fail or bleeding recurs and the lesion has been localized, segmental resection, most commonly right colectomy, is effective.

Neoplasia

Colorectal carcinoma is an uncommon cause of significant lower GI hemorrhage but is probably the most important one to rule out because about 150,000 individuals are diagnosed each year with this cancer in the United States. The bleeding is usually painless, intermittent, and slow in nature. Frequently, it is associated with iron deficiency anemia. Polyps can also bleed, but more commonly, the bleeding occurs after a polypectomy. Although bleeding in the pediatric population is discussed in Chapter 71, juvenile polyps are the second most common cause of bleeding in patients younger than 20 years of age. Occasionally other colonic neoplasms, most notably GISTs, can be associated with massive hemorrhage. The best diagnostic tool is colonoscopy. If the bleeding is attributable to a polyp, it can be treated with endoscopic therapy.

Anorectal Disease

The major causes of anorectal bleeding are internal hemorrhoids, anal fissures, and colorectal neoplasia. Although hemorrhoids are by far the most common of these entities, they account for only 5% to 10% of all acute lower GI bleeding. In general, anorectal hemorrhage is not massive and presents as bright-red blood per rectum that is seen in the toilet bowl and on the toilet paper. Most hemorrhoidal bleeding arises from internal hemorrhoids, which are painless and often accompanied by prolapsing tissue that reduces spontaneously or has to be manually reduced by the patient (Fig. 46-14). Anal fissure, on the other hand, produces painful bleeding after a bowel movement; bleeding is only occasionally the main symptom in these patients (Fig. 46-15).

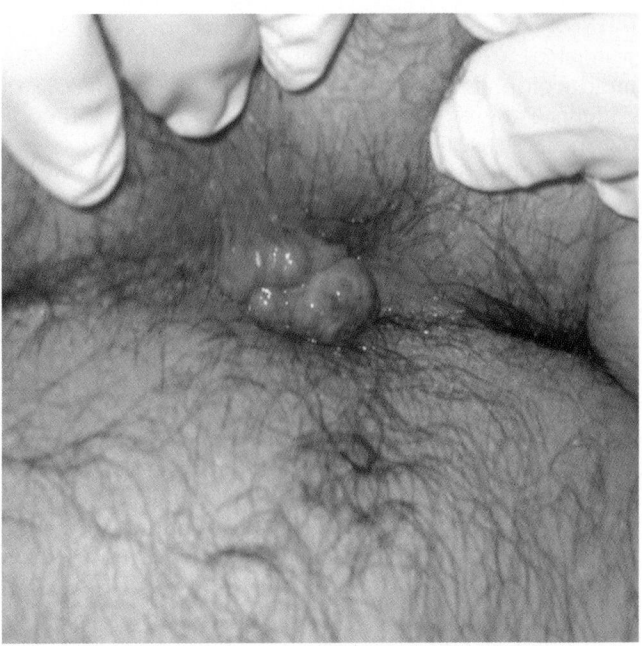

Figure 46-14 Bleeding and prolapsed hemorrhoids.

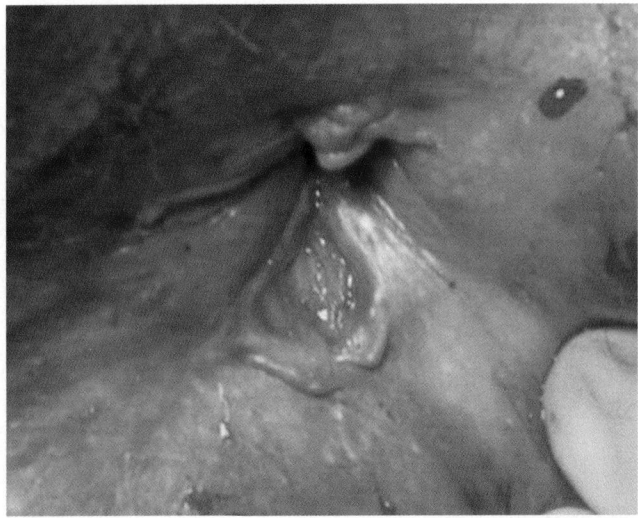

Figure 46-15 Anal fissure that can be a source of lower GI bleeding.

Because anorectal disease is common, a careful investigation to rule out all other sources of bleeding, especially malignancy, is imperative before lower GI bleeding is attributed to anorectal pathology. Anal fissures can be treated medically with stool-bulking agents (e.g., Metamucil), increased water intake, stool softeners, and topical nitroglycerin ointment or diltiazem to relieve sphincter spasm and promote healing. Internal hemorrhoids are treated with bulking agents, increased dietary fiber, and adequate hydration. A variety of office-based interventions, including rubber band ligation, injectable sclerosing agents, and infrared coagulation, have also been employed. If these measures fail, surgical hemorrhoidectomy may be needed. Most anorectal bleeding is self-limited and responds to dietary and local measures.

Colitis

Inflammation of the colon is caused by a multitude of disease processes, including inflammatory bowel disease (Crohn's disease, ulcerative colitis, and indeterminate colitis), infectious colitis (O157:H7 *Escherichia coli,* cytomegalovirus [CMV], *Salmonella, Shigella,* and *Campylobacter* species, and *Clostridium difficile*), radiation proctitis after treatment for pelvic malignancies, and ischemia.

Ulcerative colitis is much more likely than Crohn's disease to present with GI bleeding. Ulcerative colitis is a mucosal disease that starts distally in the rectum and progresses proximally to occasionally involve the entire colon. Patients can present with up to 20 bloody bowel movements per day. These episodes are accompanied by abdominal cramping, tenesmus, and occasionally abdominal pain. The diagnosis is confirmed by a careful history and flexible lower endoscopy with biopsy. Medical therapy with steroids, 5-aminosalicylic acid (ASA) compounds, immunomodulatory agents, and supportive care

are the mainstays of treatment. Surgical therapy is rarely indicated in the acute setting unless the patient develops a toxic megacolon or hemorrhage that is refractory to medical management.

In contrast, Crohn's disease typically is associated with guaiac-positive diarrhea and mucus-filled bowel movements but not with bright-red blood. Crohn's disease can affect the entire GI tract. It is characterized by skip lesions, transmural thickening of the bowel wall, and granuloma formation. The diagnosis is established with endoscopy and contrast studies. Medical management consists of steroids, antibiotics, immunomodulators, and 5-ASA compounds. Because Crohn's disease is a relapsing and remitting disease, surgical therapy is used as a last resort. Massive colonic hemorrhage complicates ulcerative colitis in up to 15% of affected patients, whereas it only occurs in 1% of those with Crohn's colitis.[41]

Infectious colitis can cause bloody diarrhea. The diagnosis is usually established from the history and stool culture. *C. difficile* and CMV colitis deserve special attention. *C. difficile* colitis usually presents with explosive, foul-smelling diarrhea in a patient with prior antibiotic use or hospitalization. Bloody bowel movements are not common but can be present, especially in severe cases in which there is associated mucosal sloughing. In North America, there has been an upsurge in the frequency and severity of *C. difficile*–associated colitis during the past decade. Treatment consists of stopping antibiotics, supportive care, and oral or intravenous metronidazole or oral vancomycin. CMV colitis is suspected in any immunocompromised patient who presents with bloody diarrhea. Endoscopy with biopsy confirms the diagnosis, and the treatment is intravenous ganciclovir.

Radiation proctitis has become much more common in the past several decades as the use of radiation to treat rectal cancer, prostate cancer, and gynecologic malignancies has increased. Patients present with bright-red blood

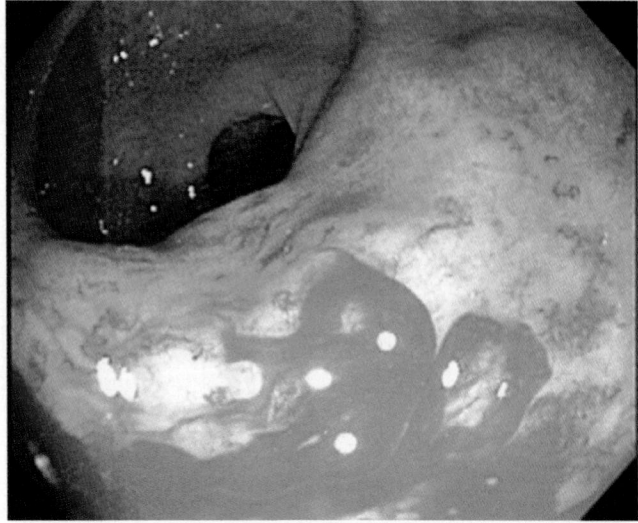

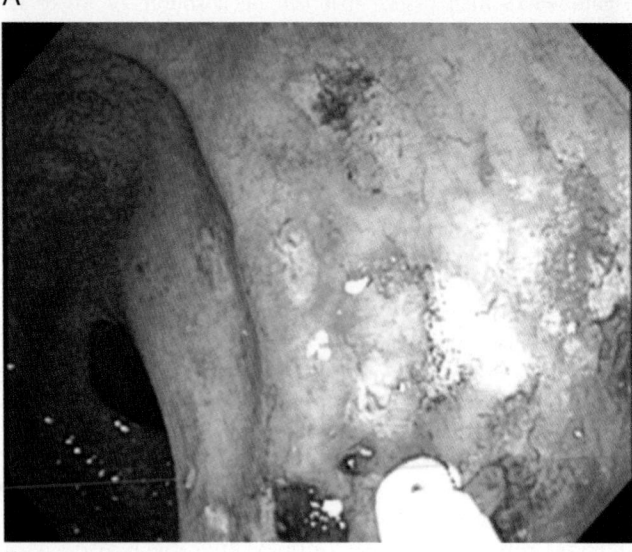

Figure 46-16 A, Rectal bleeding secondary to radiation damage. **B,** Effective control after application of argon plasma coagulation treatment. (Courtesy of David L. Carr-Locke, MD, Brigham and Women's Hospital.)

per rectum, diarrhea, tenesmus, and crampy pelvic pain. Flexible endoscopy reveals the characteristic bleeding telangiectasias (Fig. 46-16). Treatment consists of antidiarrheals, hydrocortisone enemas, and endoscopic argon plasma coagulator. In cases of persistent bleeding, ablation with 4% formalin solution usually works well.[42]

Mesenteric Ischemia
Mesenteric ischemia can be secondary to either acute or chronic arterial or venous insufficiency. Predisposing factors include preexisting cardiovascular disease (atrial fibrillation, congestive heart failure, and acute myocardial infarction), recent abdominal vascular surgery, hypercoagulable states, medications (vasopressors and digoxin), and vasculitis. Acute colonic ischemia is the most common

form of mesenteric ischemia. It tends to occur in the watershed areas of the splenic flexure and the rectosigmoid colon, but can be right-sided in up to 40% of patients. Patients present with abdominal pain and bloody diarrhea. CT scanning often shows a thickened bowel wall. The diagnosis is generally confirmed with flexible endoscopy, which reveals edema, hemorrhage, and a demarcation between the normal and abnormal mucosa. Treatment focuses on supportive care consisting of bowel rest, intravenous antibiotics, cardiovascular support, and correction of the low-flow state. In 85% of cases, the ischemia is self-limited and resolves without incident, although some patients develop a colonic stricture. In the other 15% of cases, surgery is indicated because of progressive ischemia and gangrene. Marked leukocytosis, fever, increased fluid requirement, tachycardia, acidosis, and peritonitis all indicate a failure of the ischemia to resolve and the need for surgical intervention. During the surgery, resection of the ischemic intestine and creation of an end ostomy is indicated.[43]

ACUTE GASTROINTESTINAL HEMORRHAGE FROM AN OBSCURE SOURCE

Obscure GI hemorrhage is defined as bleeding that persists or recurs after an initial negative evaluation with both EGD and colonoscopy. Obscure bleeding can be further subdivided into obscure-occult or obscure-overt bleeding. Obscure-occult bleeding is characterized by iron deficiency anemia or guaiac-positive stools without visible bleeding. If initial upper and lower endoscopy fail to identify a source for obscure-occult bleeding and the patient has no systemic signs of disease, a CT scan is usually performed to rule out a small bowel neoplasm. When this is negative, these patients are often treated with iron therapy and more than 80% resolve their symptoms in less than 2 years.[44] Obscure-overt bleeding is characterized by recurrent or persistent visible bleeding.[45]

Obscure bleeding can be frustrating for both the patient and the clinician. This is particularly true for obscure-overt bleeding, which cannot be localized despite aggressive diagnostic measures. One study from a tertiary referral center reported that the typical patient with obscure-overt bleeding had suffered intermittent episodes of hemorrhage for 26 months, had undergone up to 20 diagnostic tests, and had received an average of 20 units of blood before the etiology was identified.[46] Fortunately, obscure-overt bleeding is responsible for only about 1% of all GI bleeding. The differential diagnosis of obscure-overt bleeding is long and varied (Table 46-4) and includes a variety of small bowel lesions not described here.

Diagnosis

Repeat Endoscopy
The cause of obscure-overt bleeding is often a common lesion that is missed on initial evaluation. Repeat upper and lower endoscopy is a valuable tool in identifying

Table 46-4 **Differential Diagnosis of Obscure Gastrointestinal Bleeding**

UPPER GI	SMALL BOWEL	COLON
Angiodysplasia	Crohn's disease	Colitis
Peptic ulcer disease	Meckel's diverticulum	Ulcerative colitis
Aortoenteric fistula	Lymphoma	Crohn's colitis
Neoplasia	Radiation enteritis	Ischemic colitis
HIV-related causes	Ischemia	Radiation colitis
Dieulafoy's lesion	HIV-related causes	Infections colitis
Lymphoma	Bacterial infection	Solitary rectal ulcer
Sarcoidosis	Metastatic disease	Amyloidosis
Hemobilia	Angiodysplasia	Lymphoma
Hemosuccus pancreaticus		Endometriosis
GAVE		Angiodysplasia
Metastatic cancer		Neoplasia
		HIV-related causes
		Hemorrhoids

GAVE, gastric antral vascular ectasia; HIV, human immunodeficiency virus.
Adapted and modified from McFadden DW: Occult and obscure sources of gastrointestinal bleeding. In Cameron JL (ed): Current Surgical Therapy, 8th ed. Philadelphia, Mosby, 2004, pp 117-121.

missed lesions because up to 35% of patients have the bleeding source identified on second-look endoscopy. Most cases of obscure GI hemorrhage, however, are from a source distal to the ligament of Treitz. When repeat endoscopy fails to identify an obscure-overt bleeding source, investigation of the small bowel is warranted. This proceeds in an orderly fashion, depending on the degree of bleeding and the patient's hemodynamic status.

Conventional Imaging

The next step is probably a tagged RBC scan, although its utility in this setting has not been established, and as discussed previously, it may be misleading. Angiography may be more useful but usually requires significant ongoing hemorrhage. Provocative testing, which involves administering anticoagulants, fibrinolytics, or vasodilators to increase hemorrhage during angiography, has been employed in small series with favorable results; reluctance to induce uncontrolled hemorrhage has limited its use. Small bowel enteroclysis, which uses a tube to infuse barium, methylcellulose, and air directly into the small bowel, provides better imaging than simple small bowel follow-through. Because the yield has been reported to be very low, and the test is poorly tolerated, it is now rarely used. It can identify gross lesions such as small bowel tumors, inflammatory conditions such as Crohn's disease, and small bowel ulcerations. The limitation of small bowel radiography is that it cannot visualize angiodysplasias, the main cause of obscure small bowel hemorrhage.

In younger patients, usually less than 30 years of age, part of the initial evaluation is a Meckel's diverticulum scan. Meckel's diverticulum with ectopic acid-secreting

mucosa can ulcerate the small bowel and produce bleeding. The Meckel's scan is performed by administration of ^{99m}Tc-pertechnetate, which is taken up by the ectopic gastric mucosa in the diverticulum and localized with scintigraphy.

Small Bowel Endoscopy

The hemodynamically stable patient undergoes small bowel enteroscopy. Usually performed with a pediatric colonoscope, this is referred to as *push endoscopy*. It can reach about 50 to 70 cm past the ligament of Treitz in most cases and permits endoscopic management of some lesions. Overall, push enteroscopy is successful in 40% of patients. Sonde *pull endoscopy* uses an enteroscope that passes passively into the very distal small bowel. A balloon on the end of the scope permits normal small bowel peristalsis to carry the scope into the ileum; the mucosa is visualized as the scope is removed. This technique is cumbersome, does not permit intervention, and has largely been abandoned with the advent of capsule endoscopy.

Video Capsule Endoscopy

Capsule endoscopy uses a small capsule with a video camera that is swallowed and acquires video images as it passes through the GI tract. This modality permits visualization of the entire GI tract, but offers no interventional capability. It is also very time consuming because someone has to watch the video to identify the bleeding source, and then a means to deal with the pathology has to be developed. Despite this, capsule endoscopy is an excellent tool in the patient who is hemodynamically stable but continues to bleed. This technique has reported success rates as high as 90% in identifying small bowel pathology.[47] It is usually well tolerated, although it is contraindicated in patients with obstruction or a motility disorder.

Intraoperative Endoscopy

Intraoperative enteroscopy is reserved for patients who have transfusion-dependent obscure-overt bleeding in whom an exhaustive search has failed to identify a bleeding source. This typically uses a pediatric colonoscope introduced through the mouth or through an enterotomy in the small bowel made by the surgeon. In the latter technique, a sterile colonoscope is passed onto the field and is introduced into the small bowel and passed bidirectionally, with the surgeon assisting to pass the bowel over the scope. Any suspicious areas are marked for possible resection or are treated endoscopically. Because laparotomy has already been accomplished, it is usually preferable to resect the suspect areas.

Treatment

Obscure GI hemorrhage requires a careful approach to diagnosis and management. Specific causes and their management are listed later. Up to 25% of cases of obscure lower GI hemorrhage remain without a diagnosis, and 33% to 50% of patients experience rebleeding within 3 to 5 years.[45] Management strategies generally depend on the identification of a lesion. Iron replacement combined with intermittent transfusion is occasionally necessary although this approach is far from appealing.

Specific Causes of Small Bowel Bleeding

Angiodysplasias

Angiodysplasias are the most common cause of small intestinal bleeding, accounting for 40% of cases in elderly patients and 10% in younger patients. Most small intestinal vascular ectasias appear to occur in the jejunum, followed by the ileum and then the duodenum. The usual diagnostic tools are generally unsuccessful in identifying these lesions. Angiography is rarely positive. Rather, most small bowel vascular lesions require enteroscopy or capsule endoscopy for identification. In cases of severe hemorrhage requiring emergent operative intervention, intraoperative endoscopy may be helpful. Endoscope-directed segmental small bowel resection is the treatment of choice. Occasionally these lesions are diffuse; this may occur in hereditary hemorrhagic telangiectasia (Osler-Weber-Rendu disease), acute renal failure, or von Willebrand's disease. In this situation, there has been limited experience with estrogen and progesterone treatment but some studies suggest that these agents may be of benefit.

Neoplasia

Small bowel tumors are not very common but can be sources of occult or overt GI bleeding. Bleeding typically results from erosion of the mucosa overlying the tumor. GISTs have the greatest propensity for bleeding. Small bowel tumors are typically diagnosed by small bowel contrast series or spiral CT scan. Treatment involves surgical resection.

Crohn's Disease

Patients with Crohn's disease may also present with small bowel bleeding in association with terminal ileitis. Bleeding is not generally significant, nor is it usually the only presenting symptom. Diagnosis is established by small bowel contrast series, and initial treatment is medical.

Meckel's Diverticulum

Meckel's diverticulum is a true diverticulum in that it contains all layers of the small bowel wall. It is a congenital remnant of the omphalomesenteric duct, occurring in about 2% of the general population. Often, heterotopic tissue is present at the base of the diverticulum. Bleeding from Meckel's diverticulum is usually from an ulcerative lesion on the ileal wall opposite the diverticulum, caused by acid production by ectopic gastric mucosa. If nuclear medicine imaging is negative and bleeding is relatively brisk, angiography may be helpful in the diagnosis. Surgical management usually requires a segmental resection incorporating the opposing ileal mucosa, which is typically the site of bleeding.

Diverticula

Unlike Meckel's diverticulum, small intestinal diverticula are false diverticula that do not involve all layers of the bowel. Bleeding from small bowel diverticula can present a diagnostic challenge. Capsule endoscopy or small intestinal contrast studies can make the diagnosis of diverticula, and in the absence of other sources of bleeding, it may be assumed that the diverticula are the source of bleeding. In cases of profuse bleeding, angiography or intraoperative endoscopy may be used to identify the bleeding source.

SUMMARY

Despite significant recent advances, acute GI hemorrhage remains a major clinical problem. Prompt resuscitation is the first priority while evaluation of the magnitude and source of the bleeding is initiated simultaneously. These maneuvers establish whether the bleeding is from the upper or lower GI tract and assess the risk for ongoing or recurrent hemorrhage, determining the urgency of the subsequent evaluation. Endoscopy plays an increasing role in the diagnosis and management of bleeding from both the upper and lower GI tracts. In most cases, upper GI and colonic sources can be promptly identified and managed. Obscure GI bleeding, often from a small intestinal source, remains more difficult to localize, although recent refinements in capsule endoscopy represents a significant advance. The surgeon continues to play a critical role in this management strategy.

Selected References

Barkun A, Bardou M, Marshall JK: Consensus recommendations for managing patients with nonvariceal upper gastrointestinal bleeding. Ann Intern Med 139:843-849, 2003.

This summary of the recommendations from a recent consensus conference on upper GI bleeding reflects the most up-to-date clinical data on the benefits of early endoscopic diagnosis and therapy. Recent efforts to develop tools for risk stratification are summarized.

Gralnek IM: Obscure-overt gastrointestinal bleeding. Gastroenterology 128:1424-1430, 2005.

A recent concise discussion of the diagnostic approach to obscure bleeding, including the roles of small bowel fiberoptic and capsule endoscopy.

Jensen DM, Machicado GA, Jutabah R, et al: Urgent colonoscopy for the diagnosis and treatment of severe diverticular hemorrhage. N Engl J Med 342:78-82, 2000.

This well-designed clinical study demonstrates the efficacy of urgent colonoscopy and therapy in the management of lower GI hemorrhage. Although this remains controversial, this study is perhaps the most definitive.

Rockey DC (ed): Gastrointestinal bleeding. Gastroenterol Clin North Am 34:581-752, 2005.

A very current monograph covering all aspects of GI hemorrhage.

Strate LL: Lower GI bleeding: Epidemiology and diagnosis. Gastroenterol Clin North Am 34:643-664, 2005.

A clear, concise recent review on the epidemiology of lower GI hemorrhage.

References

1. Peura DA, Lanza FL, Gostout CJ, et al: The American College of Gastroenterology Bleeding Registry: Preliminary findings. Am J Gastroenterol 92:924-928, 1997.
2. Rockey DC: Gastrointestinal bleeding. Gastroenterol Clin North Am 34:581-588, 2005.
3. Strate LL, Saltzman JR, Ookubo R, et al: Validation of a clinical prediction rule for severe acute lower intestinal bleeding. Am J Gastroenterol 100:1821-1827, 2005.
4. Barkun A, Bardou M, Marshall JK: Consensus recommendations for managing patients with nonvariceal upper gastrointestinal bleeding. Ann Intern Med 139:843-857, 2003.
5. Dulai GS, Gralnek IM, Oei TT, et al: Utilization of health care resources for low-risk patients with acute, nonvariceal upper GI hemorrhage: an historical cohort study. Gastrointest Endosc 55:321-327, 2002.
6. Das A, Wong RC: Prediction of outcome of acute GI hemorrhage: A review of risk scores and predictive models. Gastrointest Endosc 60:85-93, 2004.
7. Lieberman D: Gastrointestinal bleeding: initial management. Gastroenterol Clin North Am 22:723-736, 1993.
8. Kollef MH, O'Brien JD, Zuckerman GR, Shannon W: BLEED: A classification tool to predict outcomes in patients with acute upper and lower gastrointestinal hemorrhage. Crit Care Med 25:1125-1132, 1997.
9. Tata LJ, Fortun PJ, Hubbard RB, et al: Does concurrent prescription of selective serotonin reuptake inhibitors and non-steroidal anti-inflammatory drugs substantially increase the risk of upper gastrointestinal bleeding? Aliment Pharmacol Ther 22:175-181, 2005.
10. Rubin TA, Murdoch M, Nelson DB: Acute GI bleeding in the setting of supratherapeutic international normalized ratio in patients taking warfarin: Endoscopic diagnosis, clinical management, and outcomes. Gastrointest Endosc 58:369-373, 2003.
11. Cuellar RE, Gavaler JS, Alexander JA, et al: Gastrointestinal tract hemorrhage: The value of a nasogastric aspirate. Arch Intern Med 150:1381-1384, 1990.
12. Cooper GS, Chak A, Way LE, et al: Early endoscopy in upper gastrointestinal hemorrhage: Associations with recurrent bleeding, surgery, and length of hospital stay. Gastrointest Endosc 49:145-152, 1999.
13. Cheng CL, Lee CS, Liu NJ, et al: Overlooked lesions at emergency endoscopy for acute nonvariceal upper gastrointestinal bleeding. Endoscopy 34:527-530, 2002.
14. Frossard JL, Spahr L, Queneau PE, et al: Erythromycin intravenous bolus infusion in acute upper gastrointestinal bleeding: A randomized, controlled, double-blind trial. Gastroenterology 123:17-23, 2002.
15. Lassen A, Hallas J, Schaffalitzky de Muckadell OB: Complicated and uncomplicated peptic ulcers in a Danish county 1993-2002: A population-based cohort study. Am J Gastroenterol 101:945-953, 2006.
16. Higham J, Kang JY, Majeed A: Recent trends in admissions and mortality due to peptic ulcer in England: Increasing frequency of haemorrhage among older subjects. Gut 50:460-464, 2002.
17. Heldwein W, Schreiner J, Pedrazzoli J, et al: Is the Forrest classification a useful tool for planning endoscopic therapy of bleeding peptic ulcers? Endoscopy 21:258-262, 1989.
18. Khuroo MS, Khuroo MS, Farahat KL, et al: Treatment with proton pump inhibitors in acute non-variceal upper gastrointestinal bleeding: A meta-analysis. J Gastroenterol Hepatol 20:11-25, 2005.
19. Schilling D, Demel A, Nusse T, et al: *Helicobacter pylori* infection does not affect the early rebleeding rate in patients with peptic ulcer bleeding after successful endoscopic hemostasis: A prospective single-center trial. Endoscopy 35:393-396, 2003.
20. Gisbert JP, Khorrami S, Carballo F, et al: *H. pylori* eradication therapy vs. antisecretory non-eradication therapy (with or without long-term maintenance antisecretory therapy) for the prevention of recurrent bleeding from peptic ulcer. Cochrane Database Syst Rev 4:CD004062, 2003.
21. Liu CC, Lee CL, Chan CC, et al: Maintenance treatment is not necessary after *Helicobacter pylori* eradication and healing of bleeding peptic ulcer: A 5-year prospective, randomized, controlled study. Arch Intern Med 163:2020-2024, 2003.
22. Hippisley-Cox J, Coupland C, Logan R: Risk of adverse gastrointestinal outcomes in patients taking cyclo-oxygenase-2 inhibitors or conventional non-steroidal anti-inflammatory drugs: Population based nested case-control analysis. BMJ 331:1310-1316, 2005.
23. Lin HJ, Hsieh YH, Tseng GY, et al: A prospective, randomized trial of large- versus small-volume endoscopic injection of epinephrine for peptic ulcer bleeding. Gastrointest Endosc 55:615-619, 2002.
24. Lau JY, Sung JJ, Lam YH, et al: Endoscopic retreatment compared with surgery in patients with recurrent bleeding after initial endoscopic control of bleeding ulcers. N Engl J Med 340:751-756, 1999.
25. Guglielmi A, Ruzzenente A, Sandri M, et al: Risk assessment and prediction of rebleeding in bleeding gastroduodenal ulcer. Endoscopy 34:778-786, 2002.
26. Chung IK, Kim EJ, Lee MS, et al: Endoscopic factors predisposing to rebleeding following endoscopic hemostasis in bleeding peptic ulcers. Endoscopy 33:969-975, 2001.
27. Bass B, Wolpert S: Management of the complications of peptic ulcer disease. Problems Gen Surg 14:54-68, 1997.

28. Cook DJ, Fuller HD, Guyatt GH, et al: Risk factors for gastrointestinal bleeding in critically ill patients. Canadian Critical Care Trials Group. N Engl J Med 330:377-381, 1994.

29. Stiegmann GV: Endoscopic approaches to upper gastrointestinal bleeding. Am Surg 72:111-115, 2006.

30. Chalasani N, Kahi C, Francois F, et al: Improved patient survival after acute variceal bleeding: A multicenter, cohort study. Am J Gastroenterol 98:653-659, 2003.

31. Castaneda B, Morales J, Lionetti R, et al: Effects of blood volume restitution following a portal hypertensive-related bleeding in anesthetized cirrhotic rats. Hepatology 33:821-825, 2001.

32. Hou MC, Lin HC, Liu TT, et al: Antibiotic prophylaxis after endoscopic therapy prevents rebleeding in acute variceal hemorrhage: a randomized trial. Hepatology 39:746-753, 2004.

33. Corley DA, Cello JP, Adkisson W, et al: Octreotide for acute esophageal variceal bleeding: A meta-analysis. Gastroenterology 120:946-954, 2001.

34. Avgerinos A, Armonis A, Manolakopoulos S, et al: Endoscopic sclerotherapy versus variceal ligation in the long-term management of patients with cirrhosis after variceal bleeding: A prospective randomized study. J Hepatol 26:1034-1041, 1997.

35. Heider TR, Azeem S, Galanko JA, et al: The natural history of pancreatitis-induced splenic vein thrombosis. Ann Surg 239:876-880, 2004.

36. de la Pena J, Brullet E, Sanchez-Hernandez E, et al: Variceal ligation plus nadolol compared with ligation for prophylaxis of variceal rebleeding: a multicenter trial. Hepatology 41:572-578, 2005.

37. Strate LL: Lower GI bleeding: Epidemiology and diagnosis. Gastroenterol Clin North Am 34:643-664, 2005.

38. Jensen DM, Machicado GA, Jutabha R, et al: Urgent colonoscopy for the diagnosis and treatment of severe diverticular hemorrhage. N Engl J Med 342:78-82, 2000.

39. Bender JS, Wiencek RG, Bouwman DL: Morbidity and mortality following total abdominal colectomy for massive lower gastrointestinal bleeding. Am Surg 57:536-540, 1991.

40. Setya V, Singer JA, Minken SL: Subtotal colectomy as a last resort for unrelenting, unlocalized, lower gastrointestinal hemorrhage: Experience with 12 cases. Am Surg 58:295-299, 1992.

41. Pardi DS, Loftus EV, Jr., Tremaine WJ, et al: Acute major gastrointestinal hemorrhage in inflammatory bowel disease. Gastrointest Endosc 49:153-157, 1999.

42. Saclarides TJ, King DG, Franklin JL, et al: Formalin instillation for refractory radiation-induced hemorrhagic proctitis: Report of 16 patients. Dis Colon Rectum 39:196-199, 1996.

43. Walker AM, Bohn RL, Cali C, et al: Risk factors for colon ischemia. Am J Gastroenterol 99:1333-1337, 2004.

44. Rockey DC, Cello JP: Evaluation of the gastrointestinal tract in patients with iron-deficiency anemia. N Engl J Med 329:1691-1695, 1993.

45. Gralnek IM: Obscure-overt gastrointestinal bleeding. Gastroenterology 128:1424-1430, 2005.

46. Szold A, Katz LB, Lewis BS: Surgical approach to occult gastrointestinal bleeding. Am J Surg 163:90-92, 1992.

47. Pennazio M, Santucci R, Rondonotti E, et al: Outcome of patients with obscure gastrointestinal bleeding after capsule endoscopy: Report of 100 consecutive cases. Gastroenterology 126:643-653, 2004.

CHAPTER 47

Stomach

David W. Mercer, MD   Emily K. Robinson, MD

Anatomy
Physiology
Peptic Ulcer Disease
Stress Gastritis
Gastric Neoplasia
Other Gastric Lesions

ANATOMY

Gross Anatomy

Divisions

Wallace P. Ritchie, Jr. called the stomach an *elegant organ,* once thought to be the seat of the soul, always handy to bring to the dinner table, and a recognized source of ecstasy and grief. It originates as a dilation in the tubular embryonic foregut during the fifth week of gestation. By the seventh week, it descends, rotates, and further dilates with a disproportionate elongation of the greater curvature into its normal anatomic shape and position. Following birth, it is the most proximal abdominal organ of the alimentary tract (Fig. 47-1). The most proximal region of the stomach is called the *cardia* and attaches to the esophagus. Immediately proximal to the cardia is a physiologically competent lower esophageal sphincter. Distally, the pylorus connects the distal stomach (antrum) to the proximal duodenum. Although the stomach is fixed at the gastroesophageal (GE) junction and the pylorus, its large mid portion is mobile. The fundus represents the superior-most part of the stomach and is floppy and distensible. It is bounded superiorly by the diaphragm and laterally by the spleen. The body of the stomach represents the largest portion and is also referred to as the *corpus.* The body also contains most of the parietal cells and is bounded on the right by the relatively straight lesser curvature and on the left by the longer greater curvature. At the angularis incisura, the lesser curvature abruptly angles to the right. It is at this point that the body of the stomach ends and the antrum begins. Another important anatomic angle (angle of His) is that which the fundus forms with the left margin of the esophagus.

Most of the stomach resides within the left upper quadrant of the abdomen. The left lateral segment of the liver usually covers a large portion of the stomach anteriorly. The diaphragm, chest, and abdominal wall bound the remainder of the stomach. Inferiorly, the stomach is attached to the transverse colon, spleen, caudate lobe of the liver, diaphragmatic crura, and retroperitoneal nerves and vessels. Superiorly, the GE junction is found about 2 to 3 cm below the diaphragmatic esophageal hiatus in the horizontal plane of the seventh chondrosternal articulation, a plane only slightly cephalad to that containing the pylorus. The gastrosplenic ligament attaches the proximal greater curvature to the spleen.

Blood Supply

As shown in Figure 47-2, most of the blood supply to the stomach is from the celiac artery. There are four main arteries: the left and right gastric arteries along the lesser curvature and the left and right gastroepiploic arteries along the greater curvature. In addition, a substantial quantity of blood may be supplied to the proximal stomach by the inferior phrenic arteries and by the short gastric arteries from the spleen. The largest artery to the stomach is the left gastric artery, and it is not uncommon (15%-20%) for an aberrant left hepatic artery to originate from it. Consequently, proximal ligation of the left gastric artery may result in acute left-sided hepatic ischemia because the aberrant left hepatic artery occasionally represents the only arterial flow to the left hepatic lobe. The right gastric artery arises from the hepatic artery (or the gastroduodenal artery). The left gastroepiploic artery originates from the splenic artery, and the right gastroepiploic originates from the gastroduodenal artery. The extensive anastomotic connection between these major vessels assures that, in most cases, the stomach will survive if three out of four arteries are ligated, provided that the arcades along the greater and lesser curvatures are not disturbed. In general, the veins of the stomach parallel the arteries. The left gastric (coronary) and right gastric veins usually drain into the portal vein. The right

gastroepiploic vein drains into the superior mesenteric vein, and the left gastroepiploic vein drains into the splenic vein.

Lymphatic Drainage

Generally, the lymphatic drainage of the stomach parallels the vasculature and essentially drains into four zones of lymph nodes, as depicted in Figure 47-3. The superior gastric group drains lymph from the upper lesser curvature into the left gastric and paracardial nodes. The suprapyloric group of nodes drains the antral segment on the lesser curvature of the stomach into the right suprapancreatic nodes. The pancreaticolienal group of nodes drains lymph high on the greater curvature into the left gastroepiploic and splenic nodes. The inferior gastric and subpyloric group of nodes drains lymph along the right gastroepiploic vascular pedicle. All four zones of lymph nodes drain into the celiac group and into the thoracic duct. Although the aforementioned lymph nodes drain different areas of the stomach, it remains widely recognized that gastric cancers may metastasize to any of the four nodal groups regardless of the cancer location. In addition, the extensive submucosal plexus of lymphatics accounts for the fact that there is frequently

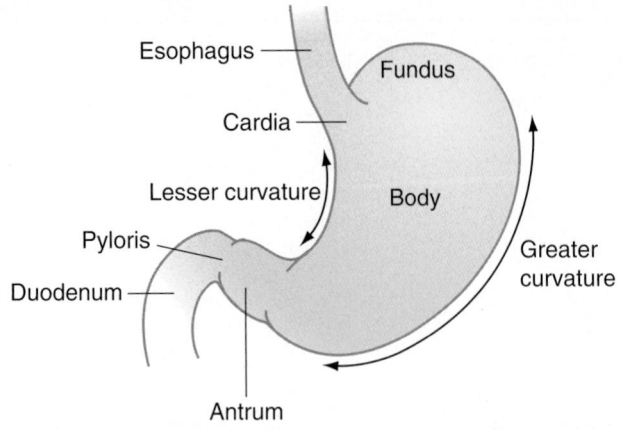

Figure 47-1 Divisions of the stomach. (From Zuidema G: Shackelford's Surgery of the Alimentary Tract, 4th ed. Philadelphia, WB Saunders, 1995.)

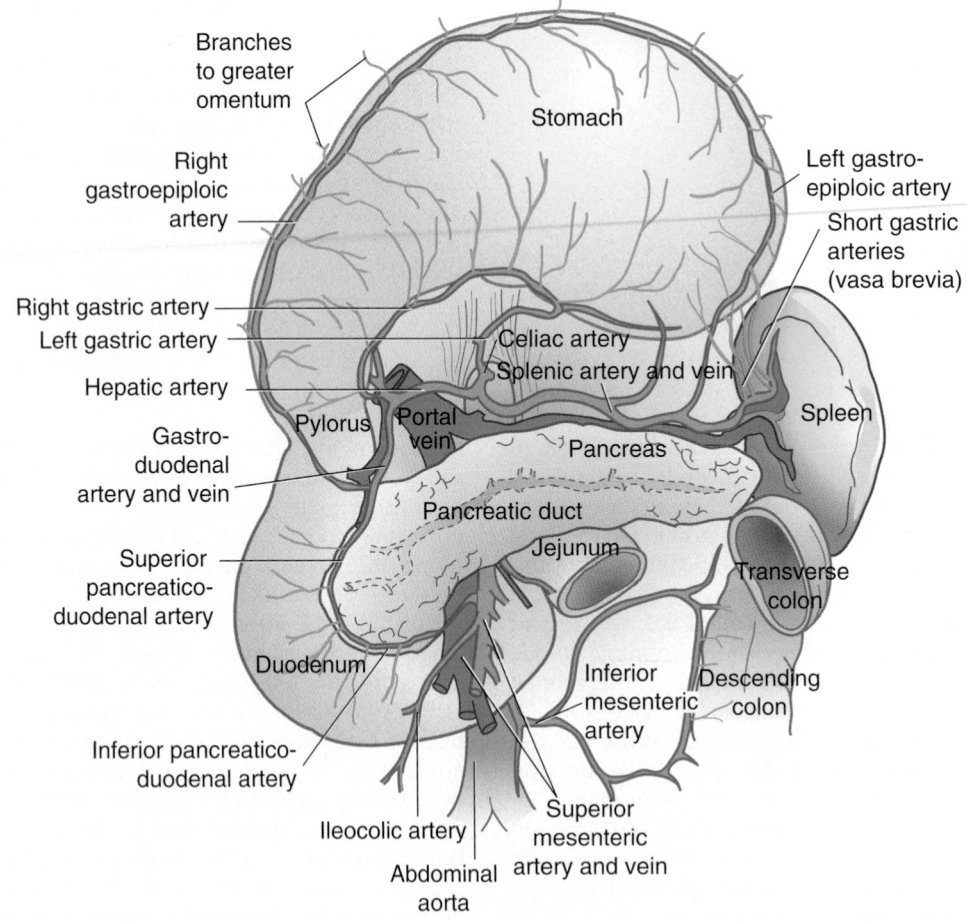

Figure 47-2 Blood supply to the stomach and duodenum with anatomic relationships to the spleen and pancreas. The stomach is reflected cephalad. (From Zuidema G: Shackelford's Surgery of the Alimentary Tract, 4th ed. Philadelphia, WB Saunders, 1995.)

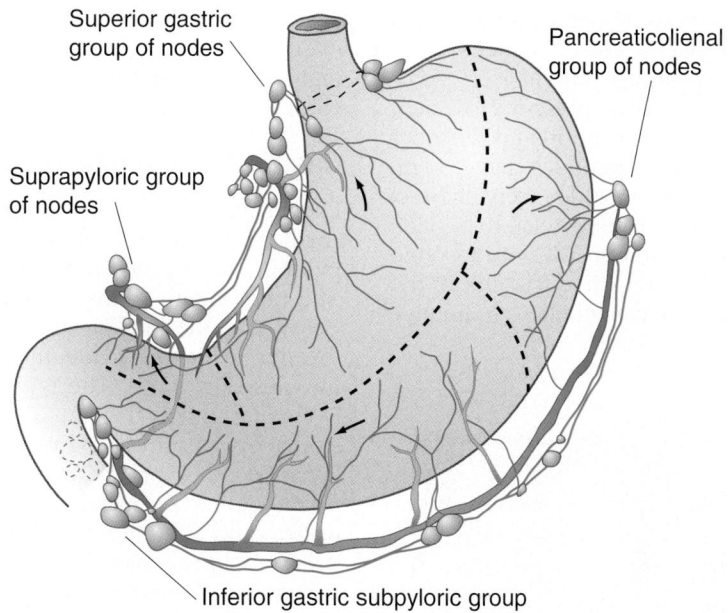

Superior gastric
group of nodes

Pancreaticolienal
group of nodes

Suprapyloric group
of nodes

Inferior gastric subpyloric group

Figure 47-3 Lymphatic drainage of the stomach. (From Moody F, McGreevy J, Miller T: Stomach. In Schwartz SI, Shires GT [eds]: Principles of Surgery, 5th ed. New York, McGraw-Hill, 1989.)

microscopic evidence of malignant cells several centimeters from the resection margin of gross disease.

Innervation

As shown in Figure 47-4, the extrinsic innervation of the stomach is both parasympathetic through the vagus and sympathetic through the celiac plexus. The vagus nerve originates in the vagal nucleus in the floor of the fourth ventricle and traverses the neck in the carotid sheath to enter the mediastinum, where it divides into several branches around the esophagus. These branches coalesce above the esophageal hiatus to form the left and right vagus nerves. However, it is not uncommon to find more than two vagal trunks at the distal esophagus. At the GE junction, the left vagus is anterior, and the right vagus is posterior (LARP mnemonic).

As shown in Figure 47-4, the left vagus gives off the hepatic branch to the liver and then continues along the lesser curvature as the anterior nerve of Latarjet. Although not shown, the so-called criminal nerve of Grassi is the first branch of the right or posterior vagus nerve and is recognized as a potential etiology of recurrent ulcers when left undivided. The right nerve also gives a branch off to the celiac plexus and then continues posteriorly along the lesser curvature. As depicted, a truncal vagotomy is performed above the celiac and hepatic branches of the vagi, whereas a selective vagotomy is performed below. A highly selective vagotomy is performed by dividing the crow's feet to the proximal stomach while preserving the innervation of the antral and pyloric parts of the stomach. Most (>90%) of the vagal fibers are afferent, carrying stimuli from the gut to the brain. Efferent vagal fibers originate in the dorsal nucleus of the medulla and synapse with neurons in the myenteric and submucosal plexuses. These neurons utilize acetylcholine as their neurotransmitter and influence gastric motor func-

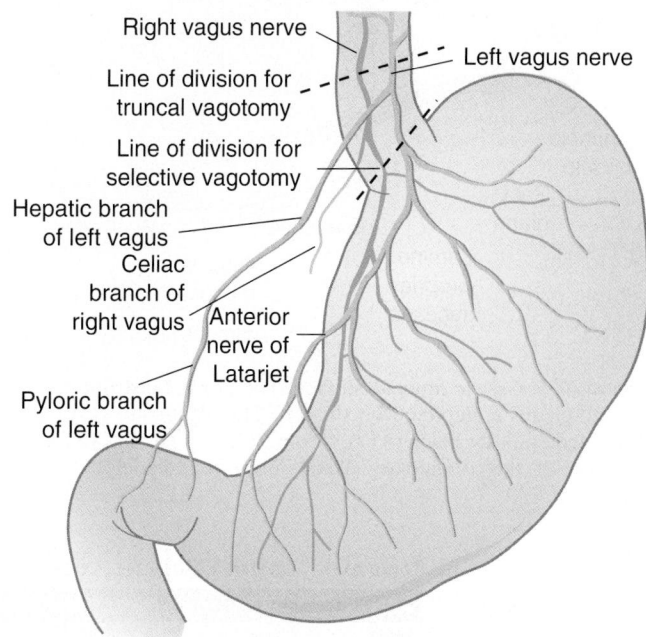

Right vagus nerve

Left vagus nerve

Line of division for
truncal vagotomy

Line of division for
selective vagotomy

Hepatic branch
of left vagus

Celiac
branch of
right vagus

Anterior
nerve of
Latarjet

Pyloric branch
of left vagus

Figure 47-4 Vagal innervation of the stomach. The line of division for truncal vagotomy is shown and is above the hepatic and celiac branches of the left and right vagus nerves, respectively. The line of division for selective vagotomy is shown and occurs below the hepatic and celiac branches. (From Mercer D, Liu T: Open truncal vagotomy. In Operative Techniques in General Surgery 5:8-85, 2003.)

tion and gastric secretion. In contrast, the sympathetic nerve supply comes from T5 to T10, traveling in the splanchnic nerve to the celiac ganglion. Postganglionic fibers then travel with the arterial system to innervate the stomach.

The intrinsic or enteric nervous system of the stomach consists of neurons in Auerbach's and Meissner's autonomic plexuses. In these locations, cholinergic, serotoninergic, and peptidergic neurons are present. However, the function of these neurons remains poorly understood. Nevertheless, a number of neuropeptides have been localized to these neurons and include acetylcholine, serotonin, substance P, calcitonin gene–related peptide (CGRP), bombesin, cholecystokinin (CCK), and somatostatin. Consequently, it is oversimplified to think of the stomach as only containing parasympathetic (cholinergic

input) and sympathetic (adrenergic input) supply. Moreover, the parasympathetic nervous system contains adrenergic neurons, and the sympathetic system also contains cholinergic neurons.

Gastric Morphology

Except for the exact lesser and greater curvatures and a small posterior area at the proximal cardia and distal pyloric antrum, the stomach is covered by peritoneum. The peritoneum forms the outer serosa of the stomach. Below it is the thicker muscularis propria, or muscularis externa, which is made up of three layers of smooth muscles (Fig. 47-5). The middle layer of smooth muscle is circular and is the only complete muscle layer of the stomach wall. At the pylorus, this middle circular muscle layer becomes progressively thicker and functions as a true anatomic sphincter. The outer muscle layer is longitudinal and continuous with the outer layer of longitudinal esophageal smooth muscle. Within the layers of the muscularis externa is a rich plexus of autonomic nerves and ganglia called *Auerbach's myenteric plexus.* The submucosa lies between the muscularis externa and mucosae and is a collagen-rich layer of connective tissue that is the strongest layer of the gastric wall. In addition, it contains the rich anastomotic network of blood vessels and lymphatics and contains Meissner's plexus of autonomic nerves. The mucosa consists of surface epithelium, lamina propria, and muscularis mucosae. The latter is on the luminal side of the submucosa and is probably responsible for the rugae that greatly increase epithelial surface area. It also marks the microscopic boundary for invasive and noninvasive gastric carcinoma. The lamina propria represents a small connective tissue layer and contains capillaries, vessels, lymphatics, and nerves necessary to support the surface epithelium.

Gastric Glandular Organization

Gastric mucosa consists of columnar glandular epithelia. The functions of the glands and the cells lining the glands vary according to the region of the stomach in which they are found (Table 47-1). The endocrine cells such as

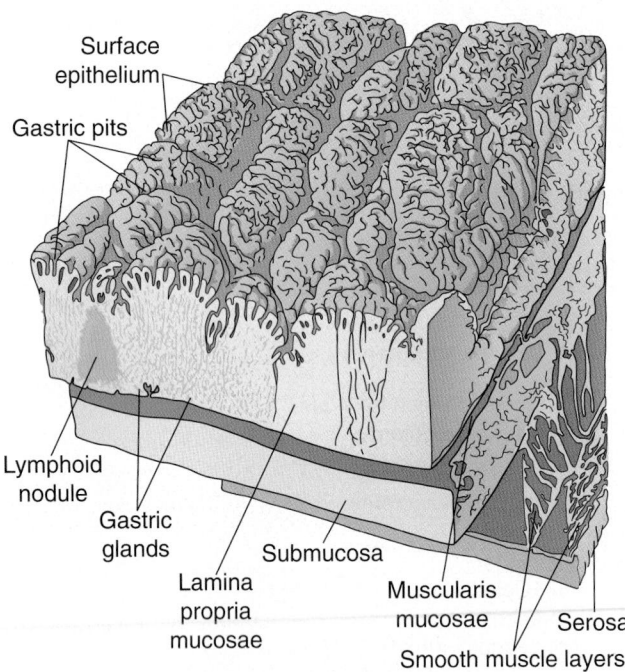

Figure 47-5 Gastric mucosa surface. The normal distribution of gastric glands is depicted on the left. The glands are gray, and the gastric pits are black (×17). (From Zuidema G: Shackelford's Surgery of the Alimentary Tract, 4th ed. Philadelphia, WB Saunders, 1995.)

Table 47-1 Gastric Cell Types, Location, and Function

CELLS	LOCATION	FUNCTION
Parietal	Body	Secretion of acid and intrinsic factor
Mucus	Body, antrum	Mucus
Chief	Body	Pepsin
Surface epithelial	Diffuse	Mucus, bicarbonate, prostaglandins (?)
Enterochromaffin-like	Body	Histamine
G	Antrum	Gastrin
D	Body, antrum	Somatostatin
Gastric mucosal interneurons	Body, antrum	Gastrin-releasing peptide
Enteric neurons	Diffuse	Calcitonin gene–related peptide, others
Endocrine	Body	Ghrelin

the gastrin (G) cells or somatostatin (D) cells can be either open or closed. Open-type endocrine cells have their microvilli on the apical membranes, which allows direct contact with gastric contents. The microvilli likely possess chemical and pH sensors, which signal the cell to secrete their pre-stored peptides. In contrast, closed-type endocrine cells do not have microvilli in contact with the gastric lumen. In the antrum, there are G cells and D cells that are of the open-type variety. In contrast, the D cells located in the fundus or body of the stomach are of the closed-type variety and are in direct contact with the acid-secreting parietal cells. In the cardia, the mucosa is arranged in branched glands that primarily secrete mucus, and the pits are short. In the fundus and body, the glands are more tubular and the pits longer. In the antrum, the glands are more branched. The luminal ends of the gastric glands and pits are lined with mucus-secreting surface epithelial cells, which extend down into the necks of the glands for variable distances. In the cardia, the glands are predominantly mucus secreting. In the body, the glands are lined from the neck to the base mostly with parietal and chief cells (Fig. 47-6). There are a few parietal cells in the fundus and proximal antrum, but none in the cardia or prepyloric antrum. Biopsy specimens taken from the stomach have demonstrated that parietal cells account for 13% of epithelial cells, whereas chief cells account for 44%; mucus cells account for 40%; and endocrine cells account for 3%.

PHYSIOLOGY

General Considerations

The principal function of the stomach is to prepare ingested food for digestion and absorption as it is propulsed into and through the small intestine. The initial period of digestion requires that solid components of a meal be stored for several hours while they undergo a reduction in size and breakdown into their basic metabolic constituents.

Receptive relaxation of the proximal stomach enables the stomach to function as a storage organ. Receptive relaxation refers to the process whereby the proximal portion of the stomach relaxes in anticipation of food intake. This relaxation enables liquids to pass easily from the stomach along the lesser curvature, whereas the solid food settles along the greater curvature of the fundus. In contrast to liquids, emptying of solid food is facilitated by the antrum, which pumps solid food components into and through the pylorus. The antrum and pylorus function in a coordinated fashion, allowing entry of food components into the duodenum and also returning material to the proximal stomach until it is appropriate for delivery into the duodenum.

In addition to storing food, the stomach participates in digestion of a meal. For example, starches undergo enzymatic breakdown through the activity of salivary amylase, although the pH within the center of the gastric bolus needs to be greater than pH 5. Peptic digestion metabolizes a meal into fats, proteins, and carbohydrates

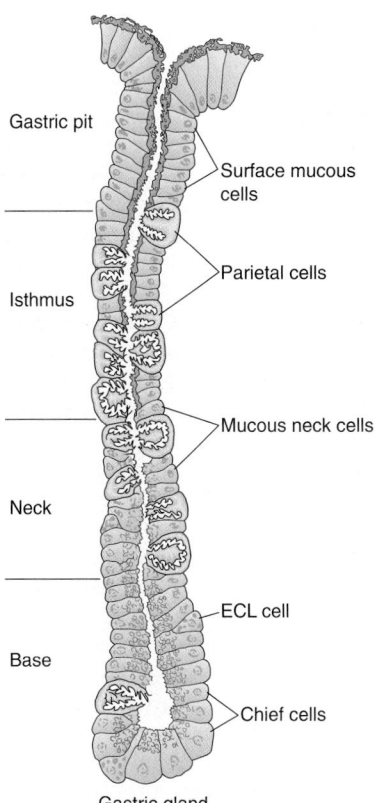

Figure 47-6 Cells residing within a gastric gland. ECL, enterochromaffin-like. (From Zuidema G: Shackelford's Surgery of the Alimentary Tract, 4th ed. Philadelphia, WB Saunders, 1995.)

by breaking down cell walls. Although the duodenum and proximal small intestine are primarily responsible for digestion of a meal, the stomach clearly facilitates this process.

Regulation of Gastric Function

Gastric function is under both neural and hormonal control, and both systems interact to provide additional regulation. Hormonal mediators of gastric function are usually peptides or amines that interact with their target cells in one of three ways: endocrine, paracrine, or neurocrine. Endocrine cells release peptides from their basolateral membranes into the bloodstream where they circulate, arrive at target cells, and exert their hormonal effects. In contrast, paracrine cells release their peptides locally, arriving at target cells by diffusion across the interstitial space. Finally, neurocrine mediators are released from nerve endings, diffuse across to the synapsed target cell, and bind to a receptor. It is noteworthy that some peptides such as somatostatin can act as either endocrine or paracrine mediators of gastric function, depending on the circumstances. Moreover, the precise state of any target cell is dependent on the relative balance of endocrine, paracrine, and neurocrine signals converging on it.

Gastric Peptides

Gastrin

Synthesis and Action

Gastrin is produced by G cells located in the gastric antrum (see Table 47-1). It is synthesized as a pre-propeptide and undergoes post-translational processing to produce biologic reactive gastrin peptides. Several molecular forms of gastrin exist. G-34 (big gastrin), G-17 (little gastrin), and G-14 (mini gastrin) have been identified. However, 90% of antral gastrin is released as the 17–amino acid peptide, although G-34 predominates in the circulation because its metabolic half-life is longer than that of G-17. The pentapeptide sequence contained at the carboxyl terminus of gastrin is the biologically active component and is identical to that found on another gut peptide, CCK. CCK and gastrin differ by tyrosine sulfation sites. The release of gastrin is stimulated by food components contained within a meal, especially protein digestion products. Luminal acid inhibits the release of gastrin. Somatostatin (see later) has paracrine actions on antral G cells and acts to inhibit gastrin release. In the antral location, somatostatin and gastrin release are functionally linked, and an inverse reciprocal relationship exists between these two peptides.[1] Moreover, somatostatin exerts a tonic inhibitory effect on gastrin release and likely mediates the inhibitory effects of luminal acid on gastrin release.

Gastrin is the major hormonal regulator of the gastric phase of acid secretion following a meal. Although parietal cells possess receptors to gastrin and exogenous gastrin elicits gastric acid secretion, it is likely that histamine, released from enterochromaffin-like (ECL) cells, is the principle mediator of this action. Evidence supporting this concept is the finding that gastrin-stimulated gastric acid secretion is significantly blunted after administration of histamine-2 (H_2)-receptor antagonists. Both exogenous gastrin and endogenous gastrin have been shown to prevent gastric injury from luminal irritants, suggesting that gastrin also plays a role in the intrinsic gastric mucosal defense system.[2] Gastrin also has considerable trophic effects on the parietal cells and the gastric ECL cells. In fact, prolonged hypergastrinemia from any cause leads to mucosal hyperplasia as well as an increase in the number of ECL cells and, under some circumstances, is associated with the development of gastric carcinoid tumors.[3]

Hypergastrinemia

Hypergastrinemia can result from a variety of causes. Disease states associated with hypergastrinemia are separated into those that are ulcerogenic (excess acid secretion) and those that are nonulcerogenic (normal or low acid secretion). Table 47-2 lists common causes of chronic hypergastrinemia. Hypergastrinemia that results from administration of antisecretory agents is an appropriate response caused by loss of feedback inhibition of gastrin release by luminal acid. Lack of acid causes a reduction in somatostatin release, which in turn causes increased release of gastrin from antral G cells. Hypergastrinemia

Table 47-2 Causes of Hypergastrinemia

ULCEROGENIC CAUSES	NONULCEROGENIC CAUSES
Antral G-cell hyperplasia or hyperfunction	Antisecretory agents (PPIs)
Retained excluded antrum	Atrophic gastritis
Zollinger-Ellison syndrome	Pernicious anemia
Gastric outlet obstruction	Acid-reducing procedure (vagotomy)
Short-gut syndrome	*Helicobacter pylori* infection Chronic renal failure

can also occur in the setting of pernicious anemia or uremia, or following surgical procedures such as vagotomy or retained gastric antrum after gastrectomy. In contrast, gastrin levels increase inappropriately in patients with gastrinoma (Zollinger-Ellison syndrome [ZES]). These gastrin-secreting tumors are not located in the antrum and secrete gastrin autonomously.

Somatostatin

Synthesis and Action

Somatostatin is produced by D cells and exists endogenously as either the 14– or 28–amino acid peptide. The predominant molecular form in the stomach is somatostatin-14. It is produced by diffuse neuroendocrine cells located in both the fundus and the antrum. In these locations, D cell cytoplasmic extensions have direct contact with the parietal cells and the G cells, where it presumably exerts its actions through paracrine effects on acid secretion and gastrin release.[4] Somatostatin is able to directly inhibit parietal cell acid secretion but can also indirectly inhibit acid secretion through inhibition of gastrin release and down-regulation of histamine release from ECL cells. The principal stimulus for somatostatin release is antral acidification, whereas acetylcholine from vagal fibers inhibits its release.

Effects of Helicobacter pylori on Somatostatin

Basal and stimulated gastrin concentrations are significantly increased in patients infected with *Helicobacter pylori*. It has been proposed that *H. pylori* causes a decrease in antral D cells with a resultant decrease in somatostatin levels. The reduction in somatostatin causes disinhibition of antral G cells, leading to increased gastrin release.[4] Interestingly, eradication of *H. pylori* restores the antral D-cell population, causing an increase in antral somatostatin with a resultant decrease in gastrin levels.[4] These data suggest that infection with *H. pylori* decreases antral D cells and somatostatin levels to cause an increase in gastrin release, which in turn leads to an increase in gastric acid secretion. However, although *H. pylori*–infected patients with duodenal ulcer disease usually have enhanced acid secretion, there are a number of *H. pylori*–positive healthy volunteers with no peptic ulcer disease (PUD) who have little or no increase in acid secretion when compared with *H. pylori*–negative volunteers. Nevertheless, cure of the infection in patients with duodenal ulcer has been demonstrated by some investigators to diminish acid secretion.[4]

Gastrin-Releasing Peptide

Bombesin was discovered in 1970 in an extract prepared from skin of the amphibian *Bombina bombina*. Its mammalian counterpart is gastrin-releasing peptide (GRP). GRP staining by immunoreactivity is particularly prominent in nerves ending in the acid-secreting and the gastrin-secreting portions of the stomach and is found in the circular muscular layer. In the antral mucosa, GRP stimulates gastrin and somatostatin release by binding to receptors located on the G and D cells, respectively. It is rapidly cleared from the circulation by a neutral endopeptidase and has a half-life of about 1.4 minutes. Peripheral administration of exogenous GRP stimulates gastric acid secretion, whereas central administration in the ventricles inhibits acid secretion. The inhibitory pathway activated is not mediated by a humoral factor, is unaffected by vagotomy, and appears to involve the sympathetic nervous system.

Histamine

Histamine plays a prominent role in parietal cell stimulation. Administration of H_2-receptor antagonists almost completely abolishes gastric acid secretion in response to both gastrin and acetylcholine. These data suggest that histamine may be a necessary intermediary of gastrin- and acetylcholine-stimulated acid secretion. Histamine is stored in the acidic granules of ECL cells as well as in resident mast cells. Its release is stimulated by gastrin, acetylcholine, and epinephrine following receptor-ligand interactions on ECL cells. In contrast, somatostatin inhibits gastrin-stimulated histamine release through interactions with somatostatin receptors located on the ECL cell. Thus, the ECL cell plays an essential role in parietal cell activation that possesses both stimulatory and inhibitory feedback pathways that modulate the release of histamine and therefore acid secretion.

Ghrelin

Ghrelin is a 28–amino acid peptide predominantly produced by endocrine cells of the oxyntic mucosa of the stomach, with substantially lower amounts derived from the bowel, pancreas, and other organs. Removal of the acid-producing part of the stomach decreases circulating ghrelin by 80%. Ghrelin appears to be under endocrine and metabolic control, has a diurnal rhythm, likely plays a major role in the neuroendocrine and metabolic response to changes in nutritional status, and may be a major anabolic hormone. Ghrelin displays a strong growth hormone–releasing action that is mediated by the activation of growth hormone secretagogue receptor type 1a. Human studies have shown a dose-dependent stimulation of growth hormone release with exogenous administration of ghrelin. Although the most significant response to ghrelin is growth hormone release, exogenous administration also causes increases in prolactin, adrenocorticotropin hormone, cortisol, and aldosterone. Recent studies have additionally reported that ghrelin influences

the insulin-signaling system, implicating ghrelin in glucose homeostasis. Exogenous ghrelin reduces insulin secretion and has powerful effects on islet cells, suggesting that endogenous ghrelin may contribute to the physiologic control of insulin and glucagon release.

In human volunteers, ghrelin administration enhances appetite and increases food intake. Interestingly, in patients who have undergone a gastric bypass, ghrelin levels are 77% lower than matched obese controls, a finding not seen after other forms of antiobesity surgery. Although the mechanism responsible for suppression of ghrelin levels after gastric bypass is unknown, these data suggest that ghrelin may be responsive to the normal flow of nutrients across the stomach. Other studies have suggested that ghrelin leads to a switch toward glycolysis and away from fatty acid oxidation, which would favor fat deposition. It appears that ghrelin is up-regulated in times of negative energy balance and down-regulated in times of positive energy balance, although the precise role of ghrelin in energy metabolism remains unclear. Ghrelin may come to have a role in the treatment and prevention of obesity.

Gastric Acid Secretion

Gastric acid secretion by the parietal cell is regulated by three local stimuli: acetylcholine, gastrin, and histamine. These three stimuli account for basal and stimulated gastric acid secretion. Acetylcholine is the principal neurotransmitter modulating acid secretion and is released from the vagus and parasympathetic ganglion cells. Vagal fibers innervate not only parietal cells but also G cells and ECL cells to modulate release of their peptides. Gastrin has hormonal effects on the parietal cell and stimulates histamine release. Histamine has paracrine-like effects on the parietal cell and, as shown in Figure 47-7, plays a central role in the regulation of acid secretion by the parietal cell after its release from ECL cells. As depicted, somatostatin exerts inhibitory actions on gastric acid secretion. Release of somatostatin from antral D cells is stimulated in the presence of intraluminal acid to a pH of 3 or less. After its release, somatostatin inhibits gastrin release through paracrine effects and also modifies histamine release from ECL cells. In some patients with PUD, this negative feedback response is defective. Consequently, the precise state of acid secretion by the parietal cell is dependent on the overall influence of the positive and negative stimuli.

Basal Acid Secretion

In the absence of food, the secretory status of the parietal cell varies among species. In humans, there is always a basal level of acid secretion that is roughly 10% of maximal acid output. Basal acid secretion also exhibits a circadian variation, with nighttime acid secretion greater than daytime. Under basal conditions, 1 to 5 mmol/hour of hydrochloric acid is secreted, and this is reduced by 75% to 90% after vagotomy or administration of atropine. These findings suggest that acetylcholine plays a significant role in basal gastric acid secretion. However, H_2-receptor blockade diminishes the magnitude of acid

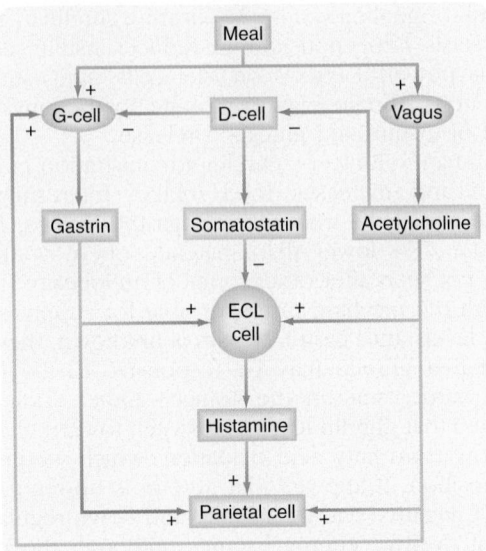

Figure 47-7 The central role of the enterochromaffin-like (ECL) cell in regulation of acid secretion by the parietal cell is shown. As demonstrated, ingestion of a meal stimulates vagal fibers to release acetylcholine (cephalic phase). Binding of acetylcholine to M_3 receptors located on the ECL cell, parietal cell, and G cell results in the release of histamine, hydrochloric acid, and gastrin, respectively. Binding of acetylcholine to M_3 receptors on D cells results in the inhibition of somatostatin release. Following a meal, G cells are also stimulated to release gastrin, which interacts with receptors located on ECL cells and parietal cells to cause the release of histamine and hydrochloric acid (gastric phase). Release of somatostatin from D cells decreases histamine release and gastrin release from ECL cells and G cells, respectively. In addition, somatostatin inhibits parietal cell acid secretion (not shown). The principal stimulus for activation of D cells is antral luminal acidification (not shown). (From Zuidema G: Shackelford's Surgery of the Alimentary Tract, 4th ed. Philadelphia, WB Saunders, 1995.)

secretion by 90%, suggesting that histamine also plays an important intermediary role in this process. Thus, it appears likely that basal acid secretion is due to a combination of cholinergic and histaminergic input.

Stimulated Acid Secretion

Cephalic Phase
Ingestion of food is the physiologic stimulus for acid secretion. Three phases of the acid secretory response to a meal have been described: cephalic, gastric, and intestinal. These three phases are interrelated and occur concurrently not consecutively.

The cephalic phase originates with the sight, smell, thought, or taste of food, which stimulates neural centers in the cortex and hypothalamus. Although the exact mechanisms by which senses stimulate acid secretion remain to be fully elucidated, it is hypothesized that several sites are stimulated in the brain. These higher centers transmit signals to the stomach by the vagus nerves, which release acetylcholine that, in turn, activates muscarinic receptors located on target cells. Acetylcho-

line directly increases acid secretion by the parietal cell and can both inhibit and stimulate gastrin release, the net effect being a slight increase in gastrin levels. Although the intensity of the acid secretory response in the cephalic phase surpasses that of the other phases, it accounts for only 20% to 30% of the total volume of gastric acid produced in response to a meal in humans because of the short duration of the cephalic phase.

Gastric Phase
The gastric phase of acid secretion begins when food enters the gastric lumen. Digestion products of ingested food interact with microvilli of antral G cells to stimulate gastrin release. Food also stimulates acid secretion by causing mechanical distention of the stomach. Gastric distention activates stretch receptors in the stomach to elicit the long vagovagal reflex arc. It is abolished by proximal gastric vagotomy and is, at least in part, independent of changes in serum gastrin levels. However, antral distention also causes gastrin release in humans, and this reflex has been called the *pyloro-oxyntic reflex.* In humans, mechanical distention of the stomach accounts for about 30% to 40% of the maximal acid secretory response to a peptone meal, with the remainder due to gastrin release. The entire gastric phase accounts for most (60%-70%) of meal-stimulated acid output because it lasts until the stomach is empty.

Intestinal Phase
The intestinal phase of gastric secretion remains poorly understood but appears to be initiated by entry of chyme into the small intestine. It occurs after gastric emptying and lasts as long as partially digested food components remain within the proximal small bowel. It accounts for only 10% of the acid secretory response to a meal and does not appear to be mediated by serum gastrin levels. It is hypothesized that a distinct acid stimulatory peptide hormone (entero-oxyntin) that is released from small bowel mucosa may mediate the intestinal phase of acid secretion.

Cellular Basis of Acid Secretion
Gastrin Receptors
Gastrin initiates its biologic actions by activation of surface membrane receptors. These receptors are members of the classical G protein–coupled 7-transmembrane-spanning receptor family and are classified as either type A or type B CCK receptors. The gastrin or CCK-B receptor has high affinity for both gastrin and CCK, whereas the type A CCK receptors have affinity for sulfated CCK analogues and a low affinity for gastrin.[2] Binding of gastrin with the CCK-B receptor has been coupled to elevated intracellular calcium levels.

Muscarinic Receptors
Acetylcholine exerts its effect on the parietal cell through interactions with the M_3 subtype of the muscarinic receptor family. This receptor is also coupled to increased levels of intracellular calcium.

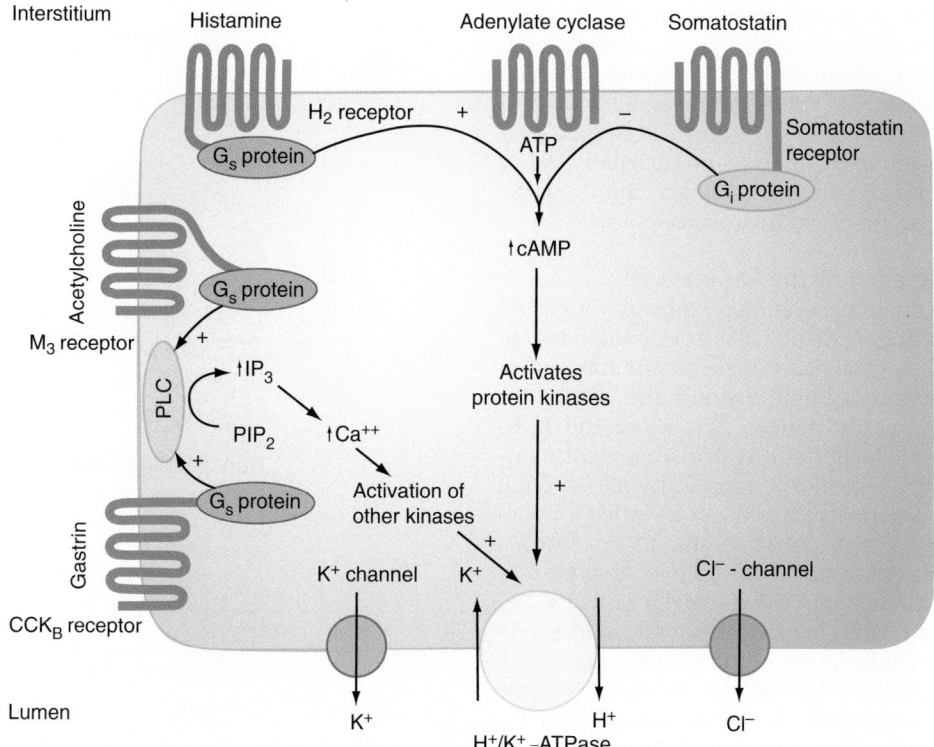

Figure 47-8 Intracellular signaling events within parietal cell are depicted. As shown, histamine binds to H_2 receptors, stimulating adenylate cyclase through a G protein–linked mechanism. Adenylate cyclase activation causes an increase in intracellular cyclic AMP levels, which in turn activates protein kinases. Activated protein kinases stimulate a phosphorylation cascade with a resultant increase in levels of phosphoproteins that activate the proton pump. Activation of the proton pump leads to extrusion of cytosolic hydrogen in exchange for extracytoplasmic potassium. In addition, chloride is secreted through a chloride channel located on the luminal side of the membrane. Gastrin binds to type B cholecystokinin receptors and acetylcholine binds to M_3 receptors. Following the interaction of gastrin or acetylcholine with their receptors, phospholipase C is stimulated through a G protein–linked mechanism to convert membrane-bound phospholipids into inositol triphosphate (IP_3). IP_3 stimulates the release of calcium from intracellular calcium stores, leading to an increase in intracellular calcium that in turn activates protein kinases, which activate the H/K-ATPase. ATP, adenosine triphosphate; ATPase, adenosine triphosphatase; cAMP, cyclic adenosine monophosphate; G_s protein, stimulatory guanine nucleotide protein; G_i, inhibitory guanine nucleotide protein; PLC, phospholipase C; PIP_2, phosphatidylinositol 4,5 diphosphate. (From Zuidema G: Shackelford's Surgery of the Alimentary Tract, 4th ed. Philadelphia, WB Saunders, 1995.)

Histamine Receptors

Histamine receptors are also of the family of G protein–coupled 7-transmembrane-spanning receptors. On the parietal cell, the H_2 subtype binds histamine to cause activation of adenylate cyclase, which increases intracellular cyclic adenosine monophosphate (AMP) levels.

Somatostatin Receptors

Somatostatin receptors are also 7-transmembrane-spanning receptors, and there are at least five different types. Binding of somatostatin with its receptors is coupled to one or more inhibitory guanine nucleotide–binding proteins. The different somatostatin receptors also appear to have divergent pharmacologic effects because one somatostatin receptor may associate with an inhibitory G protein, whereas another may not. Parietal cell somatostatin receptors appear to be a single subunit of glycoproteins having a molecular weight of 99 kd with equal affinity for somatostatin-14 and somatostatin-28. Somatostatin can inhibit parietal cell secretion through

both G protein–dependent and G protein–independent mechanisms. However, the ability of somatostatin to exert its inhibitory actions on cellular function is primarily thought to be mediated through inhibition of adenylate cyclase with a resultant reduction in cyclic AMP levels.

Second Messengers

The two second messengers principally involved in stimulation of acid secretion by parietal cells are intracellular cyclic AMP and calcium. Synthesis of these two messengers in turn activates a variety of protein kinases and phosphorylation cascades. Although these protein kinases become activated and phosphorylate a variety of parietal cell proteins, little is known about the precise phosphorylation pathways that result in activation of the proton pump that is ultimately responsible for acid secretion. Nevertheless, the intracellular events following ligand binding to receptors on the parietal cell are demonstrated in Figure 47-8. As depicted, histamine causes an increase in intracellular cyclic AMP, which activates protein kinases to initiate a cascade of phosphorylation events that culminate in activation of the H/K-ATPase. In contrast, acetylcholine and gastrin stimulate phospholipase C, which converts membrane-bound phospholipids into inositol triphosphate (IP_3) to mobilize calcium from intracellular stores. Increased intracellular calcium activates other protein kinases that likewise ultimately activate the H/K-ATPase to initiate secretion of hydrochloric acid.

Activation and Secretion by the Parietal Cell

The H/K-ATPase is the final common pathway for gastric acid secretion by the parietal cell. It is composed of two subunits, an α-catalytic (100-kd) subunit and a glycoprotein-β (60-kd) subunit. During the resting or nonsecreting state, gastric parietal cells store the H/K-ATPase within intracellular tubulovesicular elements. Cellular relocation of the proton pump subunits through cytoskeletal rearrangements must occur in order for acid secretion to increase in response to stimulatory factors. The subsequent insertion and heterodimer assembly of the H/K-ATPase subunits into the microvilli of the secretory canaliculus causes an increase in gastric acid secretion. A KCl efflux pathway must exist to supply potassium to the extracytoplasmic side of the pump. Cytosolic hydrogen is secreted by the H/K-ATPase in exchange for extracytoplasmic potassium (see Fig. 47-8), which is an electroneutral exchange and therefore does not contribute to the transmembrane potential difference across the parietal cell. Secretion of chloride is accomplished through a chloride channel moving chloride from the parietal cell cytoplasm to the gastric lumen. The secretion or exchange of hydrogen for potassium, however, does require energy in the form of adenosine triphosphate (ATP) because hydrogen is being secreted against a gradient of more than a million-fold. Because of this large energy requirement, the parietal cell also has the largest mitochondrial content of any mammalian cell, with a mitochondrial compartment representing 34% of its cell volume. In response to a secretagogue, the parietal cell undergoes a conformational change, and a several-fold increase in the canalicular surface area occurs (Fig. 47-9). In contrast to stimulated acid secretion, cessation of acid secretion requires endocytosis of the H/K-ATPase with regeneration of cytoplasmic tubulovesicles containing the subunits, and this occurs through a tyrosine-based signal. The tyrosine-containing sequence is located on the cytoplasmic tail of the β subunit and is highly homologous to the motif responsible for internalization of the transferrin receptor.

More than 1 billion parietal cells are found within the normal human stomach and are responsible for secreting about 20 millimoles of hydrochloric acid per hour in response to a protein meal. Each individual parietal cell secretes 3.3 billion hydrogen ions per second, and there is a linear relationship between maximal acid output and parietal cell number. However, gastric acid secretory rates may be altered in patients with upper gastrointestinal (GI) diseases. For example, gastric acid is often increased in patients with duodenal ulcer or gastrinoma, whereas it is decreased in patients with pernicious anemia, gastric atrophy, gastric ulcer, or gastric cancer. The lower secretory rates observed in gastric ulcer patients are typically for proximal gastric ulcers, whereas distal, antral, or prepyloric ulcers are associated with acid secretory rates similar to those obtained in duodenal ulcer patients.

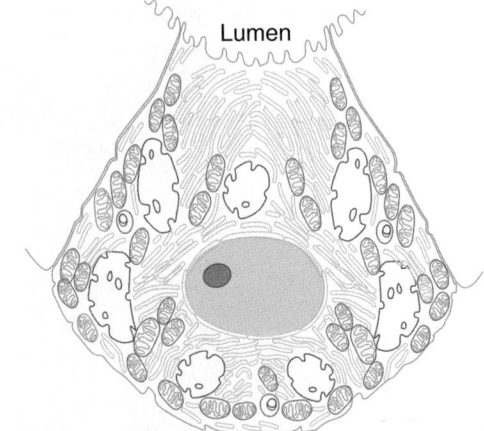

Nonsecreting parietal cell

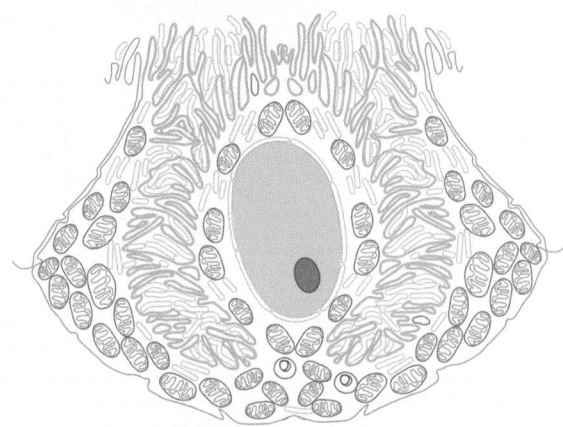

Acid-secreting parietal cell

Figure 47-9 Diagrammatic representation of resting and stimulated parietal cell. Note the morphologic transformation between the nonsecreting parietal cell and the stimulated parietal cell with increases in secretory canalicular membrane surface area. (From Mulholland MW: Anatomy and physiology. In Greenfield LJ, Mulholland MW [eds]: Surgery: Scientific Principles and Practice. Philadelphia, JB Lippincott, 1993.)

Pharmacologic Regulation of Gastric Acid Secretion

Site-specific receptor antagonists for histamine, gastrin, and acetylcholine inhibit gastric acid secretion by competitive inhibition of the receptor. The best known site-specific antagonists are the group collectively known as the H_2-receptor antagonists. The most potent of the H_2-receptor antagonists is famotidine, followed by ranitidine, nizatidine, and cimetidine. The half-life for famotidine is 3 hours and is about 1.5 hours for the others. All undergo hepatic metabolism, are excreted by the kidney, and do not differ much in bioavailability. The newest class of antisecretory agents, the substituted benzimidazoles, of which omeprazole is a prime example, inhibits acid secretion more completely because these agents irreversibly inhibit the proton pump. These proton pump inhibitors are weak acids with a pKa of 4 and therefore become selectively localized in the secretory canaliculus of the parietal cell, which is the only structure in the body with a pH of less than 4. After oral administration, these agents are absorbed into the bloodstream as prodrugs and then selectively concentrate in the secretory canaliculus. At low pH, they become ionized and activated with formation of an active sulfur group. Because the proton pump is located on the luminal surface, the transmembrane pump proteins are also exposed to acid or low pH. The cysteine residues on the α subunit form a covalent disulfate bond with activated benzimidazoles, which irreversibly inhibits the proton pump. Because of the covalent nature of this bond, these proton pump inhibitors have more prolonged inhibition of gastric acid secretion than H_2 blockers. In order for recovery of acid secretion to occur, new protein pumps need to be synthesized. As a result, these agents have a longer duration of action than their plasma half-life, with intragastric pH being maintained higher than 3 for 18 hours or more.

One notable side effect of the proton pump inhibitors is that an elevation of serum gastrin levels occurs, an effect also found in response to the other antisecretory agents. However, 24-hour plasma gastrin levels are greater after proton pump inhibitors than with H_2-receptor antagonists, and this effect is accompanied by hyperplasia of G cells and ECL cells when these agents are administered chronically. For example, chronic administration of omeprazole was found to cause ECL hyperplasia that could progress to carcinoid tumors in rats.[4] These tumors were more common in females than in males and occurred only when the rats were at the end of their natural life span. This sequence of events, however, was not specific for omeprazole and was reproduced by other agents that caused prolonged inhibition of acid secretion and resultant hypergastrinemia. Note that the effects on gastric acidity are reversed after discontinuation of these agents, and gastric acidity returns to normal levels.

Functions of Gastric Acid

Gastric acid plays a critical role in digestion of a meal. It is required to convert pepsinogen (see later) into pepsin, which is necessary for hydrolysis of proteins into polypeptides. Gastric acid also elicits the release of secretin from the duodenum, which results in pancreatic bicarbonate secretion. In addition, gastric acid functions to limit colonization of the upper GI tract with bacteria. Colonization of the stomach and duodenum is known to occur in patients with achlorhydria or in patients receiving antisecretory agents. Interestingly, there is evidence for causation between gastric colonization and the subsequent development of nosocomial pneumonias in the intensive care unit.[5] Gastric luminal alkalinization attenuates the natural bactericidal effect of gastric acid, creating an environment conducive to bacterial overgrowth. It is noteworthy that the pathogens involved in nosocomial pneumonia, the principal infection of patients with multiple organ dysfunction syndrome in the intensive care

unit, are frequently found in gastric aspirates and appear to temporally colonize the stomach before the development of clinical pneumonia.[5] However, some studies challenge the importance of increased gastric colonization with bacterial pathogens on subsequent nosocomial pneumonia development.

Gastric Analysis

There are numerous ways to assess acid secretion in the stomach. Aspiration of gastric contents through a nasogastric tube is probably the most accurate. The study requires complete emptying of gastric contents followed by instillation and recovery of 50 mL of saline. The stomach is then aspirated every 5 minutes for 1 hour and the aspirates pooled in 15-minute aliquots. At the end of 1 hour, the stomach is stimulated to secrete acid by intravenous (IV) administration of a secretogogue such as histamine (2 μg/kg) or pentagastrin (6 μg/kg). Aspiration of the stomach continues with four 15-minute collections obtained over a 1-hour period. The volume of collections is measured, and each aliquot is titrated to determine the amount of hydrogen ions present. The rate of secretion is expressed as the number of milliequivalents produced per hour during the basal or unstimulated state and during maximal and peak acid output. Maximal acid output (MAO) is obtained by averaging the output of the two final 15-minute periods. Peak acid output is the highest rate of secretion obtained during a 15-minute period following secretogogue stimulation. Basal acid output (BAO) is generally about 2 to 3 mEq/hour, and MAO is in the range of 10 to 15 mEq/hour.

Other Gastric Secretory Products

Gastric Juice

Gastric juice is the result of secretion by the parietal cells, chief cells, and mucus cells, in addition to swallowed saliva and duodenal refluxate. The electrolyte composition of parietal and nonparietal gastric secretion varies with the rate of gastric secretion. Parietal cells secrete an electrolyte solution that is isotonic with plasma and contains 160 mmol/L. The pH of this solution is 0.8. The lowest intraluminal pH commonly measured in the stomach is 2, owing to dilution of the parietal cell secretion by other gastric secretions, which also contain sodium, potassium, and bicarbonate.

Intrinsic Factor

Intrinsic factor is a 60,000-dalton mucoprotein secreted by the parietal cell that is essential for the absorption of vitamin B_{12} in the terminal ileum. It is secreted in amounts that far exceed those necessary for vitamin B_{12} absorption. In general, its secretion parallels that of gastric acid secretion, yet the secretory response is not necessarily linked to acid secretion. For example, proton pump inhibitors do not block intrinsic factor secretion in humans, nor do they alter absorption of labeled vitamin B_{12}. Intrinsic factor deficiency can develop in the setting of pernicious anemia or in patients undergoing total gastrectomy, and both groups of patients require vitamin B_{12} supplementation.

Pepsinogen

Pepsinogens are proteolytic proenzymes with a molecular weight of 42,500 that are secreted by the glands of the gastroduodenal mucosa. Two types of pepsinogens are secreted. Group 1 pepsinogens are secreted by chief cells and by mucus neck cells located in the glands of the acid-secreting portion of the stomach. Group 2 pepsinogens are produced by surface epithelial cells throughout the acid-secreting portion of the stomach as well as the antrum and the proximal duodenum. Consequently, group 1 pepsinogens are secreted by the same glands that secrete acid, whereas group 2 pepsinogens are secreted by acid-secreting and by gastrin-secreting mucosa. In the presence of acid, both forms of pepsinogen are converted to pepsin by removal of a short amino-terminal peptide. Pepsins become inactivated at a pH of greater that 5, although group 2 pepsinogens are active over a wider range of pH values than the group 1 pepsinogens. As a result, group 2 pepsinogens may be involved in peptic digestion in the setting of increased gastric pH, which commonly occurs in the setting of stress or in patients with gastric ulcer.

Mucus and Bicarbonate

Mucus and bicarbonate combine to neutralize gastric acid at the gastric mucosal surface. They are secreted by the surface mucus cells and by mucus neck cells located in the acid-secreting and antral portions of the stomach. Mucus is a viscoelastic gel that contains about 85% water and 15% glycoproteins. It provides a mechanical barrier to injury by contributing to the unstirred layer of water found at the luminal surface of the gastric mucosa. It also provides an impediment to ion movement from the lumen to the apical cell membrane and is relatively impermeable to pepsins. Mucus is in a constant state of flux because it is secreted continuously by mucosal cells on one hand and solubilized by luminal pepsin on the other. Mucus production is stimulated by vagal stimulation, cholinergic agonists, prostaglandins, and some bacterial toxins. In contrast, anticholinergic drugs and nonsteroidal anti-inflammatory drugs (NSAIDs) inhibit its secretion. *H. pylori,* on the other hand, secretes various proteases and lipases that break down mucin and impair the protective function of the mucus layer.

In the acid-secreting portion of the stomach, bicarbonate secretion is an active process, whereas in the antrum, both active and passive secretion of bicarbonate occurs. The magnitude of bicarbonate secretion, however, is considerably less than acid secretion. Yet, although the luminal pH is 2, the pH observed at the surface epithelial cell is usually 7. The pH gradient found at the epithelial surface is due to the aforementioned unstirred layer of water contained within the mucus gel and to the continuous secretion of bicarbonate by the surface epithelial cells. In fact, gastric cell surface pH remains greater than 5 until the luminal pH is less than 1.4. However, the luminal pH in duodenal ulcer patients is frequently less than 1.4, so the cell surface is exposed to lower pH in these patients. This reduction in pH may reflect a reduction in gastric bicarbonate secretion, as well as decreased duodenal bicarbonate secretion, and may explain why some duodenal ulcer patients have a higher relapse rate after treatment.

Motility

Gastric motility is regulated by extrinsic and intrinsic neural mechanisms as well as by myogenic control. The extrinsic neural controls are mediated through parasympathetic (vagus) and sympathetic pathways, whereas the intrinsic controls involve the enteric nervous system already discussed in the Anatomy section. In contrast, myogenic control resides within the excitatory membranes of the gastric smooth muscle cells. When the cell membrane potential exceeds its threshold potential, an action potential is generated and results in muscle contraction. There is a gradient in resting potential from −48 mV in the gastric pacemaker cells of Cajal, located in the proximal stomach, to a resting potential of −75 mV in the pylorus. This change in resting potential may in part be responsible for the reduced rate of contractions observed in the distal stomach when compared with the proximal stomach.

Fasting Gastric Motility

The electrical basis of gastric motility begins with the depolarization of pacemaker cells located in the mid body of the stomach along the greater curvature. Once initiated, slow waves travel at 3 cycles per minute in a circumferential and antegrade fashion toward the pylorus. In addition to these slow waves, gastric smooth muscle cells are capable of producing action potentials, which are associated with larger changes in membrane potential than slow waves. In comparison to slow waves, which are not associated with gastric contractions, action potentials are associated with actual muscle contractions. During fasting, the stomach goes through a cyclical pattern of electrical activity composed of slow waves and electrical spikes, which has been termed the *myoelectric migrating complex* (MMC). Each cycle of the MMC lasts 90 to 120 minutes and is made up of four phases of electrical activity. Phase I of the MMC is the quiescent phase, during which slow waves are present without action potentials, therefore resulting in an increase in gastric tone but no gastric contraction. In phase II of the MMC, the motor spikes are associated with slow waves and occasional gastric contractions. During phase III, motor spike activity is associated with each slow wave, resulting in forceful gastric contractions every 15 to 20 seconds. The net effect of phase III MMC activity is clearance of large indigestible food substances contained within the stomach. Phase IV activity is characterized as a brief period of recovery before the next MMC cycle. The net effects of the MMC are frequent clearance of gastric contents during periods of fasting. The exact regulatory mechanisms of MMC activities are unknown, but these activities remain intact after vagal denervation.

Postprandial Gastric Motility

Ingestion of a meal results in a decrease in the resting tone of the proximal stomach and fundus, referred to as *receptive relaxation* and *gastric accommodation.* Because these reflexes are mediated by the vagus nerves, interruption of vagal innervation to the proximal stomach, such as by truncal vagotomy or proximal gastric vagotomy, can eliminate these reflexes, with resultant early satiety and rapid emptying of ingested liquids. In addition to its storage function, the stomach is responsible for the mixing and grinding of ingested solid food particles. This activity involves repetitive forceful contractions of the mid and antral portions of the stomach, causing food particles to be propelled against a closed pylorus, with subsequent retropulsion of solids and liquids. The net effect is a thorough mixing of solids and liquids and sequential shearing of solid food particles to smaller than 1 mm.

The emptying of gastric contents is under the influence of well-coordinated neural and hormonal mediators. Systemic factors, such as anxiety, fear, depression, and exercise, can affect the rate of gastric motility and emptying. Additionally, the chemical and mechanical properties and the temperature of the intraluminal contents can influence the rate of gastric emptying. In general, liquids empty more rapidly than solids, and carbohydrates empty more readily than fats. Increases in the concentration or acidity of liquid meals causes a delay in gastric emptying. In addition, hot and cold liquids tend to empty at a slower rate than ambient temperature fluids. These responses to luminal stimuli are regulated by the enteric nervous system. Osmoreceptors and pH-sensitive receptors in the proximal small bowel have also been shown to be involved in the activation of feedback inhibition of gastric emptying. Inhibitory peptides proposed to be active in this setting include CCK, glucagon, vasoactive intestinal peptide, and gastric inhibitory polypeptide.

Abnormal Gastric Motility

Symptoms of abnormal gastric motility are nausea, fullness, early satiety, abdominal pain, and discomfort. Although mechanical obstruction can and should be ruled out with upper endoscopy or radiographic contrast studies, objective evaluation of a patient with a suspected motility disorder can be accomplished with gamma scintigraphy, real-time ultrasound, and magnetic resonance imaging (MRI). Gastric motility disorders that are most commonly encountered in clinical practice are gastric dysmotility following vagotomy, delayed gastric emptying associated with diabetes mellitus, and gastric motility dysfunction related to *H. pylori* infection. Vagotomy results in loss of receptive relaxation and gastric accommodation in response to meal ingestion with resultant early satiety, postprandial bloating, accelerated emptying of liquids, and a delay in emptying of solids. Clinical manifestations of diabetic gastropathy, which can occur in insulin-dependent or insulin-independent patients, closely resemble the clinical picture of postvagotomy gastroparesis. Furthermore, structural changes have been identified in the vagus nerve of patients with diabetes, suggesting that a diabetic autonomic neuropathy may be responsible. However, the metabolic effects of diabetes have also been implicated. Specifically, hyperglycemia has been shown to cause a decrease in contractility of

the gastric antrum, an increase in pyloric contractility, and a suppression of phase III activity of the MMC. Suppression of phase III MMC activity is thought to be responsible for the accumulation of gastric bezoars seen in some diabetic patients. In contrast, hyperinsulinemia, which is often associated with non–insulin-dependent diabetes, may play a role in the gastroparesis seen in non–insulin-dependent diabetes because it also leads to suppression of phase III MMC activity.[6]

H. pylori–infected patients with nonulcer dyspepsia have also been demonstrated to have impaired gastric emptying that is accompanied by a reduction in gastric compliance.[7] In rats, lipopolysaccharide derived from *H. pylori* causes a reduction in gastric emptying of a liquid meal for up to 12 hours by an unknown mechanism. Regardless of the etiology of gastroparesis, treatment consists of prokinetic agents, such as metoclopramide and erythromycin, that have been shown to have some benefit, although the evidence is more compelling in diabetes.

Gastric-Emptying Studies

There are a number of ways to assess gastric emptying. The saline load test is perhaps the simplest and is accomplished by instilling a known volume of saline into the stomach and aspirating the amount remaining at a certain time. For example, some recommend instillation of 750 mL and then aspirating at 30 minutes. If the return is less than 200 mL, this indicates normal gastric function. In contrast, gastric dysfunction is usually present if there is greater than 400 mL of saline present at the end of 30 minutes. Alternatively, fluoroscopic procedures can also provide information on gastric emptying and may reveal mechanical causes that could contribute to a delay, such as gastric outlet obstruction. However, the computerized radionucleotide scans are more commonly used to assess gastric emptying. This can be done with radiolabeled liquids or with a radiolabeled solid meal. After a mechanical obstruction has been ruled out, gastric emptying studies using these radionucleotide scans can be particularly helpful in patients with gastric atony from associated illness such as diabetes or in postgastrectomy patients.

Gastric Barrier Function

Gastric barrier function depends on a number of physiologic and anatomic factors. These include but are not limited to cell membranes, tight junctions, cell renewal processes, mucus secretion, alkaline secretion, and arterial pH. Blood flow also plays a role in gastric mucosal defense by providing nutrients and delivering oxygen to ensure that those intracellular processes that underlie mucosal resistance to injury can proceed unabated. Decreased gastric mucosal blood flow has minimal effects on lesion production until it approaches 50% of normal. When blood flow is reduced by more than 75%, marked mucosal injury results, and this is exacerbated in the presence of luminal acid. After damage does occur, injured surface epithelial cells are replaced rapidly by migration of surface mucus cells located along the basement membranes. This process is referred to as *restitution* or *reconstitution*. It occurs within minutes and does not require cell division.

Exposure of the stomach to noxious agents causes a reduction in the potential difference across the gastric mucosa. In normal gastric mucosa, the potential difference across the mucosa is -30 to -50 mV and results from the active transport of chloride into the lumen and sodium into the blood whose gradients are maintained by the activity of the Na/K-ATPase. Damage disrupts the tight junctions between mucosal cells, causing the epithelium to become leaky to ions (i.e., Na^+ and Cl^-) and a resultant loss of the high transepithelial electrical resistance normally found in gastric mucosa. In addition, damaging agents like NSAIDs or aspirin possess carboxyl groups that are nonionized at low intragastric pH because they are weak acids. Consequently, they readily enter the cell membranes of gastric mucosal cells because they are now lipid soluble, whereas they will not penetrate the cell membranes at neutral pH because they are ionized. Upon entry into the neutral pH environment found within the cytosol, they become reionized, will not exit the cell membrane, and are toxic to the mucosal cells.

Peptic ulcers are caused by increased aggressive factors, decreased defense factors, or both.[8] This in turn leads to mucosal damage and subsequent ulceration. Protective (or defensive) factors include mucosal bicarbonate secretion, mucus production, blood flow, growth factors, cell renewal, and endogenous prostaglandins. Damaging (or aggressive) factors include hydrochloric acid secretion, pepsins, ethanol ingestion, smoking, duodenal reflux of bile, ischemia, NSAIDs, hypoxia, and most notably *H. pylori*.

PEPTIC ULCER DISEASE

Epidemiology

PUD remains one of the most prevalent and costly GI diseases. The annual incidence of active ulcer (gastric ulcer and duodenal ulcer) in the United States is about 1.8%, or roughly 500,000 thousand new cases per year. In addition, there are about 4 million ulcer recurrences yearly.[9] During the past couple of decades, elective admissions have decreased dramatically while admissions for complications related to ulcer disease have shown little change. It is estimated that 3 to 4 million patients are seen by a physician each year for diagnosis and treatment of PUD and that an additional 3 to 4 million patients are self-medicating. Moreover, it is estimated that more than 130,000 operations for PUD are performed yearly and that about 9000 patients die from complications of their PUD yearly. Interestingly, hospitalization rates have decreased for duodenal ulcer but have remained stable for gastric ulcer.[9] Although the decreasing hospitalization rate for duodenal ulcer may represent a true decrease in incidence, it is more likely a change in hospitalization patterns, with a lower rate of elective hospitalizations. In contrast, gastric ulcer is also more likely to occur in elderly patients, and admissions for bleeding gastric ulcers have increased during the past several years.[9] The

increase in gastric ulcer complicated by hemorrhage is also associated with an increase in NSAID ingestion. It is noteworthy that PUD in the United States has decreased in males and increased in females.[9] Although the reason for the decrease in males is unknown, it may reflect the decrease in smoking among males during the past 2 decades. It is speculated that the increase in females with PUD is in part due to an increase in smoking and an increase in NSAID ingestion.

H. pylori may represent the most drastic change in our understanding of PUD and has led many experts to conclude that PUD is, in reality, an infectious disease. Interestingly, human gastric bacteria were first discovered in the early 1900s. In the 1920s, urease was erroneously thought to be produced by humans and to be protective. In the 1950s, these previously observed bacteria were dismissed as contaminants. However, in the 1970s, gastric bacteria were rediscovered and found to be associated with inflammation. Twelve years later, the first successful culture of the organism was accomplished by Marshall and Warren, who named it *Campylobacter pyloridis*. Then, in 1987, it was reported that eradication of the organism reduced duodenal ulcer recurrence. After reclassification of the organism to *H. pylori* in 1989, the National Institutes of Health (NIH) convened a consensus panel that issued guidelines for management of ulcer disease, taking *H. pylori* into account. Consequently, any treatment plan for PUD, both medical and surgical, requires that *H. pylori* be taken into account. The association between *H. pylori* and PUD is discussed in more detail under Pathophysiology.

Pathogenesis

Helicobacter pylori Infection

It is now believed that 90% of duodenal ulcers and roughly 75% of gastric ulcers are associated with *H. pylori* infection. When this organism is eradicated as part of ulcer treatment, ulcer recurrence is extremely rare. Warren and Marshall were the first to identify and isolate the organism and note its close relationship with the inflammatory gastritis that occurred in the stomach. The organism is a spiral or helical gram-negative rod with 4 to 6 flagella and resides in gastric-type epithelium within or beneath the mucus layer, which protects it from both acid and antibiotics. Its shape and flagella aid its movement through the mucus layer, and it produces a variety of enzymes that help it adapt to a hostile environment. Most notably, it is one of the most potent producers of urease of any bacteria yet described. This enzyme is capable of splitting urea into ammonia and bicarbonate, creating an alkaline microenvironment in the setting of an acidic gastric milieu, which facilitates establishing a diagnosis of this organism by various laboratory tests. The organism is microaerophilic, and the optimal temperature for isolation is 35°C to 37°C, with growth occurring after 2 to 5 days. Interestingly, *H. pylori* can only live in gastric epithelium because only gastric epithelium expresses specific adherence receptors in vivo that can be recognized by the organism. Thus, it can also be found in heterotopic gastric mucosa in proximal esophagus and Barrett's esophagus, in gastric metaplasia in the duodenum and Meckel's diverticulum, and in heterotopic gastric mucosa in the rectum.

The mechanisms responsible for *H. pylori*–induced GI injury remain to be fully elucidated, but three potential mechanisms have been proposed:

1. Production of toxic products to cause local tissue injury
2. Induction of a local mucosal immune response
3. Increased gastrin levels with a resultant increase in acid secretion

Some of the locally produced toxic mediators include breakdown products from urease activity (i.e., ammonia), cytotoxins, a mucinase that degrades mucus and glycoproteins, phospholipases that damage epithelial cells and mucus cells, and platelet-activating factor, which is know to cause mucosal injury and thrombosis in the microcirculation. In contrast, *H. pylori*–induced mucosal immune responses may also contribute to GI injury. *H. pylori* is known to cause a local inflammatory reaction in the gastric mucosa and to produce chemotactic factors that attract neutrophils and monocytes. Activated monocytes and neutrophils, in turn, produce a number of proinflammatory cytokines and reactive oxygen metabolites.

In patients with *H. pylori* infection, basal and stimulated gastrin levels are significantly increased, presumably secondary to a reduction in antral D cells caused by infection with *H. pylori*. However, the association of acid secretion with *H. pylori* is not as straightforward. Although *H. pylori*–positive healthy volunteers had a small increase or no increase in acid secretion as compared with *H. pylori*–negative volunteers, *H. pylori*–infected patients with duodenal ulcers did have a marked increase in acid secretion.[10]

Peptic ulcers are also strongly associated with antral gastritis. A multitude of studies done before the *H. pylori* era demonstrated that almost all peptic ulcer patients had histologic evidence of antral gastritis. It was later found that the only patients with gastric ulcers and no gastritis were those ingesting aspirin. It is now recognized that most cases of histologic gastritis are due to *H. pylori* infection. Even 25% of the patients with an NSAID-associated ulcer have evidence of a histologic antral gastritis, as opposed to 95% of those with non–NSAID-associated ulcers. In most cases, the infection tends to be confined initially to the antrum and results in antral inflammation. Other evidence supporting a causal role for *H. pylori* in histologic gastritis comes from two separate volunteer physicians who ingested inocula of *H. pylori* after first confirming normal gross and microscopic gastric mucosa. Both men developed gastric *H. pylori* infection. Acute inflammation was observed histologically on days 5 and 10. By 2 weeks, it had been replaced by chronic inflammation with evidence of a mononuclear cell infiltration. These two reports provide documentation that *H. pylori* can cause histologic gastritis. Furthermore, eradication of *H. pylori* improves gastric histology. However, histologic gastritis does not necessarily equate with symptoms of dyspepsia.

H. pylori represents a chronic infection found worldwide. After a person is infected, usually in childhood, it is probably for life because spontaneous remission is rare. There tends to be an inverse relationship between infection and socioeconomic status. The reasons for this remain poorly understood but may be due to factors such as sanitary conditions, familial clustering, and crowding. In fact, one study documented familial clustering of *H. pylori* infection, demonstrating that *H. pylori* in one household member is associated with a greater chance of infection in other members.[11] In this study, other family members of a child with *H. pylori* infection had exceptionally high rates of seropositivity—more than 75% had evidence of infection. In another study, *H. pylori* infection was most common in the lowest socioeconomic class (85%), intermediate in the middle class (52%), and lowest in the highest class (11%). Data such as these, combined with the evidence of familial clustering of *H. pylori* infection, provide strong evidence that the infection is transmitted by a person-to-person route and that the infection is commonly acquired early in life.[12]

Developing countries have a higher rate of *H. pylori* infection, and this is especially true in children. Multiple studies have demonstrated what appears to be a steady, linear increase in acquisition of *H. pylori* infection with age, especially in the United States and Northern European nations. *H. pylori* prevalence also varies with racial and ethnic groups, which is true even in the United States. Whites tend to have the lowest rates of infection, whereas in a study from Houston, African American rates of infection at each age about doubled those of whites. This difference in prevalence among different racial and ethnic groups is probably related to lower socioeconomic status and to poorer living conditions during childhood in the nonwhite subjects.

H. pylori infection is associated with a number of common upper GI disorders. In the United States, normal blood donors have an overall prevalence of about 20% to 55%, with variations by age and ethnicity of the population. *H. pylori* infection is virtually always present in the setting of active chronic gastritis and is present in most duodenal (>90%) and gastric (60%-90%) ulcer patients. Noninfected gastric ulcer patients tend to be NSAID users. There is a less strong association with nonulcer dyspepsia that is probably in the range of about 50%. In addition, most gastric cancer patients show evidence of past *H. pylori* infection. However, although the association is strong, no causal relationship has been proved. There is also a strong association between mucosa-associated lymphoid tissue (MALT) lymphoma and *H. pylori* infection. Interestingly, regression of these lymphomas has been demonstrated after eradication of the organism; therefore, *H. pylori* eradication is attempted before chemotherapy.

Limited data are available to estimate the lifetime risk for developing an ulcer in patients with *H. pylori* infection. However, in a serologic study from Australia with a mean period of evaluation of 18 years, 15% of *H. pylori*–positive subjects developed verified duodenal ulcer, as compared with 3% of seronegative individuals. Another study evaluated patients after 10 years in

Scandinavia. This study was related to the presence or absence of histologic gastritis at the time of their initial assessments. Because *H. pylori* causes most cases of histologic gastritis, this observation was used as a marker for *H. pylori* infection. In this study, 11% of the patients with histologic gastritis developed PUD over a 10-year period, compared with only 1% of those without gastritis. Another factor implicating a causative role for *H. pylori* and ulcer formation is that eradication of *H. pylori* dramatically reduces ulcer recurrence. Numerous prospective trials now document that patients with *H. pylori* infection and non-NSAID ulcer disease who have documented eradication of the organism virtually never (<2%) develop recurrent ulcers. Patients who do develop recurrent ulcers are usually NSAID users.

Nonsteroidal Anti-inflammatory Drugs

After *H. pylori* infection, ingestion of NSAIDs is the most common cause of PUD. As previously mentioned, hospitalizations for bleeding upper GI lesions are increasing along with increased NSAID use. Most of the increased NSAID use has occurred in women older than 50 years, which is also the group with the increase in bleeding gastric ulcers. The increased risk for bleeding has been documented in placebo-controlled trials with chronic aspirin use for prevention of recurrent heart attack or stroke. Furthermore, the increased risk for bleeding and ulcerations is proportional to the daily dosage of NSAID. In addition, the risk for complications increases with age older than 60, patients having a prior GI event, or concurrent use of steroids or anticoagulants.[13] Consequently, the ingestion of NSAIDs remains an important factor in ulcer pathogenesis, especially in relationship to the development of complications and death.[14] The role of NSAIDs in PUD becomes even more meaningful if one considers the fact that roughly 3 million people in the United States take daily NSAIDs, and about 1 in 10 patients taking daily NSAIDs have an acute ulcer. In addition, 2% to 4% of NSAID users have GI complications each year, and more than 3000 deaths and 25,000 hospitalizations per year are attributable to NSAID-induced GI complications. Moreover, when compared with the

general population, NSAID users have a 2- to 10-fold increased risk for GI complications.

NSAID ingestion not only causes acute gastroduodenal injury but also is associated with chronic gastroduodenal injury.[14] This risk for mucosal injury or ulceration is roughly proportional to the anti-inflammatory effect associated with each NSAID.[14] The acute gastroduodenal lesions typically appear within 1 to 2 weeks of ingestion of the NSAIDs and range from mucosal hyperemia to superficial gastric erosions. In contrast, chronic injury typically occurs after 1 month and may be seen in the stomach as erosions or as ulcerations in the gastric antrum or in the duodenum. In comparison to *H. pylori* ulcers, which are more frequently found in the duodenum, NSAID-induced ulcers are more frequently found in the stomach. *H. pylori* ulcers are also nearly always associated with chronic active gastritis, whereas gastritis is not frequently found with an NSAID-induced ulcer, occurring about 25% of the time. In addition, when NSAID use is discontinued, the ulcers usually do not recur, whereas with *H. pylori*–related ulcers, there is a 50% to 80% recurrence rate in 1 year unless the organism is eradicated.

Acid

There is a linear relationship between MAO and parietal cell number. However, gastric acid secretory rates are altered in patients with upper GI diseases. Basal acid secretion is normally in the 1- to 8-mmol/hour rate, and the response to pentagastrin ranges from 6 to 40 mmol/hour. In diseases such as pernicious anemia, gastric atrophy, and gastric cancer, both basal and pentagastrin-stimulated acid output is decreased. In contrast, gastric secretory rates are increased in patients with duodenal ulcer and gastrinoma. In fact, an adequate level of acid secretion is a prerequisite for duodenal ulcers, and their presence is rare in patients who have a maximal acid output of less than 12 to 15 mmol/hour. For type I and type IV gastric ulcers (see Gastric Ulcer Pathophysiology, later), which are not associated with excessive acid secretion, acid acts as an important cofactor, exacerbating the underlying ulcer damage and attenuating the ability of the stomach to heal. For patients with type II or type III gastric ulcers, gastric acid hypersecretion does seem to be more common, and consequently they behave more like duodenal ulcers. However, ulcers may also be caused by nonacid disorders such as Crohn's disease, pancreatic rests, syphilis, *Candida* species infection, or malignant diseases.

Duodenal Ulcer Pathophysiology

Duodenal ulcer is a disease of multiple etiologies. The only relatively absolute requirements are acid and pepsin secretion in combination with either infection with *H. pylori* or ingestion of NSAIDs. Many secretory abnormalities are found in patients with duodenal ulcer disease, and clearly not every patient has the same secretory abnormalities (Table 47-3). The more common secretory abnormalities relate to decreased bicarbonate secretion, increased nocturnal acid secretion, increased duodenal acid load, and increased daytime acid secretion. Although there is a strong correlation between parietal cell number

Table 47-3 Frequency of Secretory Abnormalities in Duodenal Ulcer Patients

Decreased duodenal bicarbonate secretion: 70%
Increased nocturnal acid secretion: 70%
Increased duodenal acid load: 65%
Increased daytime acid secretion: 50%
Increased pentagastrin-stimulated maximal acid output: 40%
Increased sensitivity to gastrin: 35%
Increased basal gastrin: 35%
Increased gastric emptying: 30%
Decreased pH inhibition of gastrin release: 25%
Increased postprandial gastrin release: 25%

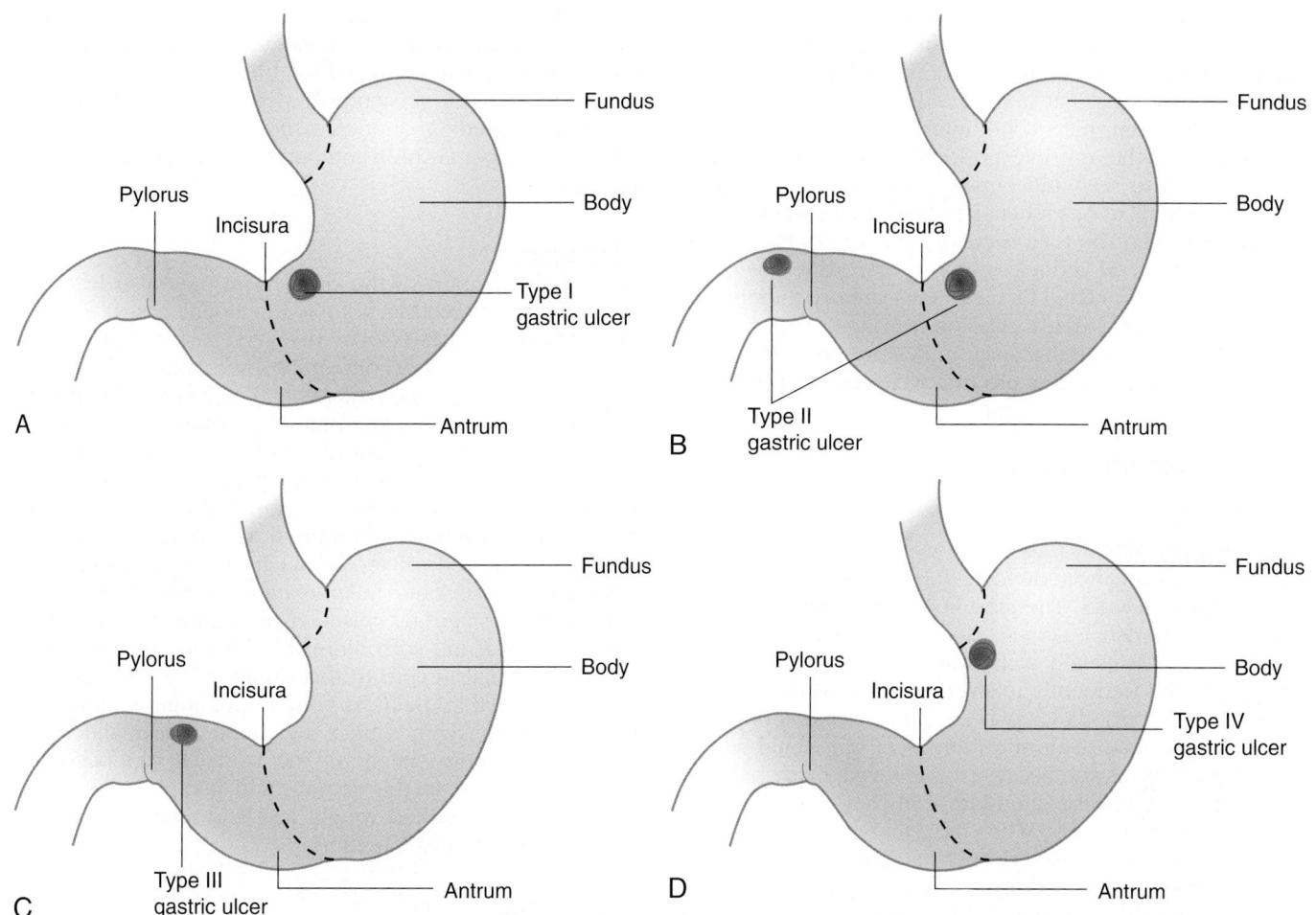

Figure 47-10 A, Location of type I gastric ulcer. **B,** Location of type II gastric ulcer. **C,** Location of type III gastric ulcer. **D,** Location of type IV gastric ulcer. (From Kauffman G Jr, Conter R: Stress ulcer and gastric ulcer. In Greenfield LJ, Mulholland MW [eds]: Surgery: Scientific Principles and Practice. Philadelphia, JB Lippincott, 1993.)

and MAO, only patients with duodenal ulcers have an increase in mean parietal cell number, whereas gastric ulcer patients do not. However, about 70% of patients with duodenal ulcers have MAOs that fall within the normal range. Because the overlap between duodenal ulcer patients and normal subjects is so great, acid secretory testing is of little value in establishing a diagnosis of duodenal ulcer.

Gastric Ulcer Pathophysiology

Gastric ulcers can occur anywhere in the stomach, although they usually present on the lesser curvature near the incisura, as shown in Figure 47-10. About 60% of ulcers are located in this location and are classified as type I gastric ulcers. These ulcers generally are not associated with excessive acid secretion and may in fact have low to normal acid output. Most occur within 1.5 cm of the histologic transition zone between the fundic and antral mucosa and are not associated with duodenal, pyloric, or prepyloric mucosal abnormalities. In contrast, type II gastric ulcers (~15%) are located in the body of the stomach in combina-

tion with a duodenal ulcer. These types of ulcers usually are associated with excess acid secretion. Type III gastric ulcers are prepyloric ulcers and account for about 20% of the lesions. These ulcers also behave like duodenal ulcers and are associated with hypersecretion of gastric acid. Type IV gastric ulcers occur high on the lesser curvature near the gastroesophageal junction. The incidence of type IV gastric ulcers is less than 10%, and they are not associated with excessive acid secretion. Finally, some ulcers may appear on the greater curvature of the stomach, but the incidence is less than 5%.

Gastric ulcers rarely develop before the age of 40 years, and the peak incidence occurs between the ages of 55 and 65 years. They are more likely to occur in lower than higher social economic classes and are slightly more common in the nonwhite than the white population. The exact pathogenesis of a benign gastric ulcer remains unknown. Some conditions that may predispose to gastric ulceration are age older than 40, sex (female-to-male ratio of 2:1), ingestion of barrier-breaking drugs such as aspirin or NSAIDs, abnormalities in acid and pepsin secretion, gastric stasis through delayed gastric emptying, coexisting duodenal ulcer, duodenal gastric reflux of bile, gastritis, and infection with *H. pylori*. Some clinical conditions that may predispose to gastric ulceration include chronic alcohol intake, smoking, long-term corticosteroid therapy, infection, and intra-arterial therapy. With regard to acid and pepsin secretion, the presence of acid appears to be essential to the production of gastric ulcer; however, the total secretory output appears to be less important. Nevertheless, it is noteworthy that rapid healing follows antacid therapy, antisecretory therapy, or vagotomy, even when the lesion-bearing portion of the stomach is left intact because, in the presence of gastric mucosal damage, acid is ulcerogenic even when present in normal or less than normal amounts.

Clinical Manifestations

Duodenal Ulcer

Abdominal Pain

Patients suffering from duodenal ulcer disease can present in a variety of ways. The most common symptom associated with duodenal ulcer disease is midepigastric abdominal pain that is usually well localized. The pain is usually tolerable and frequently relieved by food. Moreover, the pain may be episodic, may be seasonal in the spring and fall, or may relapse during periods of emotional stress. For these reasons and because it is relieved, many patients do not seek medical attention until they have had the disease for many years. When the pain becomes constant, this suggests that there is deeper penetration of the ulcer, and referral of pain to the back is usually a sign of penetration into the pancreas. Diffuse peritoneal irritation is usually a sign of free perforation.

Perforation

About 5% of the time, a penetrating ulcer will penetrate through the duodenum into the free peritoneal cavity and elicit a chemical peritonitis. The patient can typically recall the exact time of onset of abdominal pain that is frequently accompanied by fever, tachycardia, dehydration, and ileus. Abdominal examination reveals exquisite tenderness, rigidity, and rebound. A hallmark of free perforation is the demonstration of free air underneath the diaphragm on an upright chest radiograph. This complication of duodenal ulcer disease represents a surgical emergency. After the diagnosis is made, operation is performed in an expeditious fashion following appropriate fluid resuscitation.

Bleeding

The most common cause of death in patients with PUD is bleeding in those who have major medical problems or are older than 65 years.[15] Because the duodenum has an abundant blood supply and the gastroduodenal artery lies directly posterior to the duodenal bulb, GI bleeding from a duodenal ulcer is fairly common. Most cases of massive upper GI hemorrhage are in fact secondary to a bleeding duodenal ulcer following penetration of that ulcer into the gastroduodenal artery. Fortunately, most of the ulcers are superficial or are located on portions of the duodenum that are not adjacent to the gastroduodenal artery or its branches. Consequently, most duodenal ulcers present with only minor bleeding episodes that are detected by the presence of melanotic or guaiac-positive stool. Bleeding duodenal ulcers account for about 25% of all upper GI bleeding patients who present to the hospital.

Obstruction

Acute inflammation of the duodenum may also lead to mechanical obstruction with a functional gastric outlet obstruction manifested by delayed gastric emptying, anorexia, or nausea accompanied by vomiting. In cases of prolonged vomiting, patients may become dehydrated and develop a hypochloremic hypokalemic metabolic alkalosis secondary to loss of gastric juice rich in hydrogen, chloride, and potassium ions. In this setting, fluid resuscitation requires replacement of the chloride and potassium deficiencies in addition to nasogastric suction for relief of the obstructed stomach. In addition to acute inflammation, chronic inflammation of the duodenum may lead to recurrent episodes of healing followed by repair and scarring with ultimately fibrosis, and stenosis of the duodenal lumen. In this situation, the obstruction is accompanied by painless vomiting of large volumes of gastric contents with similar metabolic abnormalities as seen in the acute situation. The stomach can become massively dilated in this setting, and it rapidly loses its muscular tone. Marked weight loss and malnutrition are also common in this situation.

Gastric Ulcer

Gastric ulcer represents a clinical challenge in that it is often impossible to differentiate between gastric carcinoma and benign ulcer. Like duodenal ulcers, gastric ulcers are also characterized by recurrent episodes of quiescence and relapse. They also cause pain, bleeding, and obstruction and can perforate. On occasion, benign ulcers have also been found to result in spontaneous gastrocolic fistulas. Surgical intervention is required in 8% to 20% of those patients developing complications from their gastric ulcer disease. Hemorrhage occurs about 35% to 40% of the time at some point during the course of gastric ulceration. Usually, patients who develop significant bleeding from their gastric ulcers are older, are less likely to stop bleeding, and have higher morbidity and mortality rates than patients bleeding from duodenal ulcer. Hemorrhage is most frequently observed in patients with type II and III gastric ulcers, and patients with type IV gastric ulcers may also present with life-threatening hemorrhage. The most frequent complication of gastric ulceration, however, is perforation. Most perforations occur along the anterior aspect of the lesser curvature. In general, older patients have increased rates of perforations, and larger ulcers are associated with more morbidity and higher mortality rates. Similar to duodenal ulcer, gastric outlet obstruction can also occur in patients with type II or III gastric ulcer. However, one must carefully differentiate between benign obstruction and obstruction secondary to antral carcinoma.

Zollinger-Ellison Syndrome

ZES is a clinical triad consisting of gastric acid hypersecretion, severe PUD, and non-β islet cell tumors of the pancreas. The tumors are known to produce gastrin and are referred to as *gastrinomas.* These tumors are usually localized to the head of the pancreas, duodenal wall, or regional lymph nodes. About one half of these gastric tumors are multiple, and two thirds are malignant. About one fourth are associated with multiple endocrine neoplasia syndrome (MEN 1). Pathophysiologic features of ZES that distinguish it from duodenal ulcer are present and are all explained either by the actions of gastrin to stimulate gastric acid secretion and mucosal growth or by association with production of other hormones in the MEN 1 syndrome.

Hypergastrinemia associated with ZES accounts for most, if not all, of the clinical symptoms experienced by patients. Abdominal pain and PUD are the hallmarks of the syndrome and typically occur in more than 80% of patients. About one half of patients also exhibit diarrhea secondary to increased gastric acid secretion. Weight loss and steatorrhea also occur secondary to decreased duodenal and jejunal pH and inactivation of lipase. Esophagitis from gastroesophageal reflux is also common. Endoscopy frequently demonstrates prominent gastric rugal folds, reflecting the trophic effect of hypergastrinemia on the gastric fundus in addition to evidence of PUD. Gastrinoma and ZES are always considered and ruled out in patients who have recurrent or intractable PUD despite eradication of *H. pylori* and appropriate antisecretory therapy; multiple or atypically located ulcers; PUD associated with significant diarrhea; PUD associated with symptoms of MEN 1 such as hyperparathyroidism or occurring in a kindred of MEN 1 patients; large gastric rugae on endoscopy; or in those patients with other pancreatic endocrine tumors. Similarly, patients undergoing elective surgical intervention for PUD have the possibility of gastrinoma included in their preoperative evaluation.

Provocative tests are usually not required to establish the diagnosis of ZES because fasting and stimulated plasma gastrin levels are usually elevated. Most patients with gastrinoma have elevated fasting serum gastrin levels (>200 pg/mL), and values greater than 1000 pg/mL may be diagnostic. However, hypergastrinemia may be present in other disease states. Basal acid output of greater than 15 mEq/h (or >5 mEq/h in those with previous antiulcer surgery) supports the diagnosis. The secretin test is the most sensitive and specific provocative test for gastrinoma and aids in the differentiation between gastrinomas and other causes of ulcerogenic hypergastrinemia (see Table 47-2). IV administration of secretin (2 U/kg) is given and serum gastrin samples are measured before and after secretin administration at 5-minute intervals for 30 minutes. An increase in serum gastrin of greater than 200 pg/mL above basal levels is specific for gastrinoma versus other causes of hypergastrinemia, which do not demonstrate this response.

After diagnosis of gastrinoma, acid suppression therapy is initiated, preferably with a proton pump inhibitor. Medical management is indicated preoperatively and in patients with metastatic or unresectable gastrinoma. Localization of the gastrinoma is performed before operative intervention occurs. Noninvasive methods include computed tomography (CT) scanning, MRI, endoscopic ultrasound, and ^{111}In-octreotide scintigraphy (somatostatin receptor imaging). Invasive modalities may be used if noninvasive methods fail to localize the tumor. These include selective visceral angiography, percutaneous transhepatic portal venous sampling for gastrin, and the selective arterial secretin stimulation test. In patients with resectable gastrinomas, surgical resection is performed that includes tumor resection from the duodenum, pancreas, and regional lymph nodes. Total gastrectomy is rarely indicated and is reserved for patients who are noncompliant with acid suppression therapy or when the tumor cannot be localized.

Diagnosis

History and physical examination are probably of limited value in distinguishing between gastric and duodenal ulceration. Routine laboratory studies include a complete blood count, liver chemistries, serum creatinine, and calcium levels. A serum gastrin level should also be obtained in patients with ulcers that are refractory to medical therapy or require surgery. An upright chest radiograph is usually performed when ruling out perforation. The two principal means of diagnosing peptic ulcers are upper GI radiography and fiberoptic endoscopy. Contrast radiography is less expensive, and most (90%) can be diagnosed accurately. However, about 5% of ulcers that appear radiographically benign are malignant. *H. pylori* testing (see below) should also be done in all patients with suspected PUD.

H. pylori Testing

Diagnostic tests for *H. pylori* are divided between tests that do or do not require a sample of gastric mucosa. The noninvasive tests available are serology and the carbon-labeled urea breath test. The invasive tests available are the rapid urease test, histology, and culture. Noninvasive tests do not require endoscopy, whereas invasive tests do.

Serology

Because *H. pylori* infection elicits a local as well as a systemic immunoglobulin G (IgG)-mediated immune response, serology can be used to diagnose *H. pylori.* There are a variety of enzyme-linked immunosorbent assay (ELISA) laboratory-based tests available as well as some rapid office-based immunoassays. Serology is the diagnostic test of choice when endoscopy is not indicated and has about 90% sensitivity and specificity associated with it. Serology testing, however, is not without its limitations because antibody titers can remain high for a year or more, and consequently, this test cannot be used to assess eradication after therapy.

Urea Breath Test

Another noninvasive test used for diagnosing *H. pylori* is the carbon-labeled urea breath test. This test is based on the ability of *H. pylori* to hydrolyze urea. Its sensitivity and specificity are both greater than 95%. The test is performed by having the patient ingest a carbon isotope–labeled urea using either ^{14}C or ^{13}C. If ^{13}C is used, mass spectrometry is required, whereas it is not required for ^{14}C, but ^{14}C is associated with a low level of radiation exposure. After ingestion of the carbon isotope, urea will be metabolized to ammonia and labeled bicarbonate if *H. pylori* infection is present. The labeled bicarbonate is excreted in the breath as labeled carbon dioxide, which is then quantified. The urea breath test is less expensive than endoscopy and samples the entire stomach. False-negative results can occur if the test is done too soon after treatment, so it is usually best to test 4 weeks after therapy is finished. The urea breath test is the method of choice to document eradication.

Rapid Urease Assay

The method of choice to diagnosis *H. pylori* if endoscopy is employed is the rapid urease test. This is another test based on the ability of *H. pylori* to hydrolyze urea. The enzyme urease catalyzes degradation of urea to ammonia and bicarbonate, creating an alkaline environment that can be detected by a pH indicator. Consequently, endoscopy is performed and gastric mucosal tissue biopsied. Mucosal biopsy samples are placed into a liquid or solid medium containing urea and a pH indicator. Sensitivity is about 90% and specificity 98%, and the results are available within hours.

Histology

Endoscopy can also be performed with biopsy samples of gastric mucosa followed by histologic visualization of *H. pylori*. *H. pylori* is identified by its appearance and colonization sites with routine hematoxylin and eosin stains or with special stains such as silver, Giemsa, or Genta, for improved visibility. Sensitivity is about 95% and specificity 99%. This test is widely available and affords the clinician the ability to assess the severity of gastritis as well as to confirm the presence or absence of the organism.

Culture

Culturing of gastric mucosa obtained at endoscopy can also be performed to diagnosis *H. pylori*. The sensitivity is about 80% and specificity 100%. However, it requires laboratory expertise, it is not widely available, it is relatively expensive, and diagnosis requires up to 3 to 5 days until a diagnosis is made. Nevertheless, it does provide the opportunity to perform antibiotic sensitivity testing on isolates should the need arise.

H. pylori *Testing Summary*

In summary, it is not necessary to perform endoscopy to diagnose *H. pylori*. Serology is the test of choice for initial diagnosis when endoscopy is not required. If, however, endoscopy is to be performed, the rapid urease assay and histology are both excellent options, but the cost advantage lies with the rapid urease assay. After treatment, the urea breath test is the method of choice but again should not be performed until 4 weeks after therapy

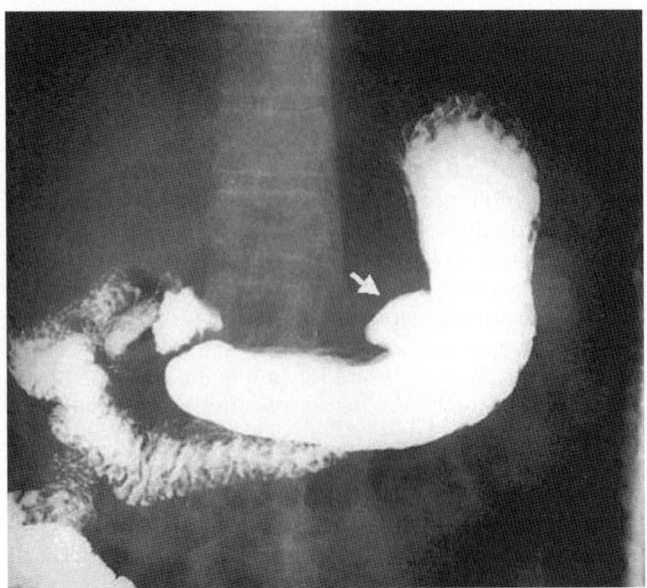

Figure 47-11 There is a large benign-appearing gastric ulcer protruding medially from the lesser curvature of the stomach (*arrow*) just above the gastric incisura. (Courtesy of Agnes Guthrie, MD, Department of Radiology, University of Texas Medical School, Houston.)

ends. If the breath test is unavailable, endoscopy may be performed in selected patients such as those with bleeding ulcers or other complications of their PUD.

Upper Gastrointestinal Radiography

Diagnosis of peptic ulcer by upper GI radiography requires the demonstration of barium within the ulcer crater, which is usually round or oval, and may or may not be surrounded by edema. This study is useful to determine the location and the depth of penetration of the ulcer as well as the extent of deformation from chronic fibrosis. A characteristic barium radiograph of a peptic ulcer is demonstrated in Figure 47-11. The ability to detect ulcers on radiography does require the technical skills and abilities of the radiologist but is also dependent on the size and location of the ulcer. With single-contrast radiographic techniques, as many as 50% of duodenal ulcers may be missed, whereas with double-contrast studies, 80% to 90% of ulcer craters can be detected. The location of a gastric ulcer is of little predictive value in establishing malignancy as benign, and malignant ulcers can occur anywhere in the stomach. However, the size of the gastric ulcer may have some predictive value in that larger lesions are more likely to be malignant than smaller ones. In addition, the finding of an ulcer with an associated mass; interrupted, fused, or nodular mucosal folds approaching the margin of the crater; or an ulcer with irregular filling defects in the ulcer crater is suggestive of a malignancy.

Fiberoptic Endoscopy

Endoscopy is the most reliable method of diagnosing a gastric ulcer. When multiple biopsies and brushings for cytology are performed, the probability of diagnosing a malignancy is in excess of 90%. In general, benign ulcers have smoother, more regular, rounded edges with a flat, smooth ulcer base. Malignancy is more often associated with a mass that may protrude into the lumen or have folds surrounding the ulcer crater that are nodular, clubbed, fused, or stop short of the ulcer margin. Again, multiple biopsy specimens are necessary for any of these ulcers because ruling out a malignancy is mandatory. Clinical symptoms or signs that may prompt early endoscopic evaluation include major weight loss, symptoms of gastric outlet obstruction, a palpable abdominal mass, guaiac-positive stool, or blood loss anemia. In addition to providing diagnostic abilities, endoscopy provides the ability to sample tissue for *H. pylori* testing and may also be used for therapeutic purposes in the setting of GI bleeding (see Approach to the Patient Bleeding From Peptic Ulcer Disease) or in the therapy of obstruction (see later).

Treatment

Medical Management

Drugs may heal ulcers by a variety of mechanisms. Some of the mechanisms by which medications may be used include eradication of *H. pylori* infection, neutralization or inhibition of acid secretion, or other mechanisms. Lifestyle modifications are also in order. Cigarette smoking has clearly been shown to retard ulcer healing and should be avoided. Discontinuation of aspirin or NSAIDs should also be undertaken if possible. Because coffee strongly stimulates acid secretion, and because alcohol may damage the mucosa, their ingestion should be moderate at most.

Antacids

Antacids are the oldest form of therapy for PUD. Antacids reduce gastric acidity by reacting with hydrochloric acid, forming a salt and water to inhibit peptic activity by raising pH. Antacids differ greatly in their buffering ability, absorption, taste, and side effects. They are most effective when ingested 1 hour after a meal. If taken on an empty stomach, the antacids are emptied rapidly and have only a transient buffering effect. However, if taken after meals, they are retained in the stomach and exert their buffering action for longer periods of time. The minimum dose of antacids required to produce optimal healing rates represents only a few tablets or liquid doses of antacids per day, usually in doses of 200 to 1000 mmol/day. This dosage level produces minimal side effects and results in about 80% ulcer healing at 1 month. The mechanism for ulcer healing at lower doses is not clear because gastric acidity is only neutralized for brief periods. Magnesium antacids tend to be the best buffers but can cause significant diarrhea by a cathartic action. In contrast, aluminum acids precipitate with phosphorous and can occasionally result in hypophosphatemia and sometimes constipation. Consequently, although antacids may heal duodenal ulcers with an efficacy comparable to that observed with H$_2$-receptor antagonists, many patients have found large, frequent doses to be unacceptable.

H$_2$-Receptor Antagonists

The H$_2$-receptor antagonists are structurally similar to histamine. Variations in the ring structure and the side chains cause differences in potency and side effects. The currently available H$_2$-receptor antagonists differ in their potency but only modestly in half-life and bioavailability. All undergo hepatic metabolism and are excreted by the kidney. Famotidine is probably the most potent, and cimetidine is the least potent. Continuous IV infusion of H$_2$-receptor antagonists has been shown to produce more uniform acid inhibition than intermittent administration. The fluctuating effects of intermittently administered H$_2$-receptor antagonists are probably caused by the relatively short half-life of these agents, which ranges from 1.5 to 3 hours. Many randomized controlled trials indicate that all H$_2$-receptor antagonists result in duodenal ulcer healing rates from 70% to 80% after 4 weeks and from 80% to 90% after 8 weeks of therapy. Split-dose, evening, and nighttime therapy are all effective, but again, continuous IV infusion produces the most uniform acid inhibition.

Proton Pump Inhibitors

The most potent antisecretory agents are the substituted benzimidazoles, also known as the proton pump inhibitors. These agents covalently bond to the catalytic (α) subunit of the proton pump and negate all types of acid secretion from all types of secretogogues. Not surprisingly, proton pump inhibitors provide more complete inhibition of acid secretion than the H$_2$-receptor antagonists. Inhibition of acid secretion is also more prolonged than with H$_2$-receptor antagonism because of the irreversible inhibition of the enzyme caused by the covalent bond to the proton pump. Both H$_2$-receptor antagonists and proton pump inhibitors are effective at night, but proton pump inhibitors are more effective during the day. Proton pump inhibitors also produce more rapid healing of ulcers than standard H$_2$-receptor antagonists. In fact, data from eight trials revealed that a 20-mg dose of omeprazole had a 14% advantage at 2 weeks and a 9% advantage at 4 weeks when compared with a 300-mg dose of cimetidine. Proton pump inhibitors have a healing rate of 85% at 4 weeks and 96% at 8 weeks. It is also worth mentioning that proton pump inhibitors require an acidic environment within the gastric lumen in order to become activated and bind to the proton pump at the secretory canaliculus. Thus, utilization of antacids or H$_2$-receptor antagonists in combination with proton pump inhibitors could have deleterious effects by promoting an alkaline environment and thereby preventing activation of the proton pump inhibitor. Consequently, antacids and H$_2$-receptor antagonists should not be used in combination with proton pump inhibitors.

Sucralfate

Sucralfate is structurally related to heparin but does not have any anticoagulant effects. It has been shown to be quite effective in the treatment of ulcer disease, although its exact mechanism of action is not entirely understood. It is an aluminum salt of sulfated sucrose that disassociates under the acidic conditions in the stomach. It is speculated that the sucrose polymerizes and binds to protein in the ulcer crater to produce a kind of protective coating that can last for up to 6 hours. It has also been suggested that it may bind and concentrate endogenous basic fibroblast growth factor, which appears to be important in mucosal healing. Duodenal ulcer healing after 4 to 6 weeks of treatment with sucralfate (1 g four times daily) is superior to placebo and comparable to H$_2$-receptor antagonists such as cimetidine. Similar healing rates have been reported with twice daily dosing (2 g twice daily 30 minutes before breakfast and at bedtime).

Treatment of H. pylori Infection
The clinician has three major goals when faced with a patient with ulcer disease:

1. Symptoms need to be relieved
2. The ulcer needs to be healed
3. Recurrence must be prevented

Antisecretory agents with acid suppression have traditionally achieved the first two goals. With NSAID-related ulcers, discontinuation of NSAIDs achieves the third goal. However, in the setting of non-NSAID ulcers, which are usually secondary to *H. pylori*, eradication of *H. pylori* can also almost completely prevent recurrence of ulcers. For duodenal ulcers, the recurrence rate after successful healing is roughly 72% if no additional therapy is employed. If H$_2$-receptor antagonists are used as maintenance therapy, patients still have a 25% recurrence rate. However, if *H. pylori* is eradicated, only 2% of the patients have an ulcer recurrence. Various triple regimens for *H. pylori* eradication have emerged. Most of these employ a proton pump inhibitor in combination with antibiotics such as metronidazole, clarithromycin, or amoxicillin. These regimens are usually 2 weeks in duration, have the advantage of not containing bismuth, and are only given twice a day. Some of these triple regimens are currently available in a packet such as Helidac. Eradication rates for these new triple regimens are about 90% (still not 100%). For failures, or in patients with high metronidazole resistance, quadruple therapy with bismuth added to the triple regimen is recommended. In February 1994, the NIH convened a consensus conference on *H. pylori* in PUD. At this conference, the following recommendations were made (Table 47-4). All patients with gastric or duodenal ulcers who were infected with *H. pylori*, regardless of whether a first presentation or recurrence, should be treated. *H. pylori*–infected ulcer patients receiving maintenance treatment or with a history of complicated or refractory disease should also be treated. The NIH added that there was no reason to consider routine detection or treatment in the absence of ulcers and concluded that NSAID use should not alter treatment. The NSAID should be discontinued if possible, but if *H. pylori* is present, *H. pylori* should be treated. However, because proton pump inhibitors have been shown to be more effective than H$_2$-receptor antagonists in patients taking NSAIDs, they should be used. If patients cannot discontinue the NSAIDs, then cotherapy with an antise-

Table 47-4 NIH Consensus Panel Recommendations for *Helicobacter pylori* Treatment

Patients with active peptic ulcer disease who are *H. pylori* positive
  Use of nonsteroidal anti-inflammatory drugs should not alter treatment.
  Document eradication in those with complications.

Ulcer patients in remission who are *H. pylori* positive, including patients on maintenance H$_2$-receptor antagonist therapy

H. pylori–positive patients with mucosa-associated lymphoid tissue (MALT) lymphoma

Controversial issues in *H. pylori*–positive patients
  First-degree relatives of gastric cancer patients
  Immigrants from countries with high prevalence of gastric cancer
  Individuals with gastric cancer precursor lesions (intestinal metaplasia)
  Non–ulcer dyspepsia patients who insist on eradication (benefit vs. risk)
  Patients on long-term antisecretory therapy for reflux disease

cretory agent or misoprostol, a prostaglandin analogue, might be of benefit. This same strategy should be employed for those patients taking NSAIDs and at risk for complications (i.e., age >60 years, prior GI event, concurrent use of steroids or anticoagulants). For patients with complications such as bleeding or perforation, documentation of eradication was also considered imperative. Again, this is most easily performed with a urea breath test. Although not recommended by the NIH, *H. pylori*–positive patients with MALT lymphoma should also be treated. In nonulcer dyspepsia, the infected patient who insists upon eradication of *H. pylori* needs to be advised of the benefits or lack of benefits *H. pylori* eradication might have because it is unlikely that eradication will improve symptoms, and it is possible that it will contribute to the emergence of antibiotic resistance. It is also important to remember that the success of therapy for *H. pylori* depends on the correct use of the regimens. One cannot substitute ampicillin for amoxicillin, and one cannot substitute doxycycline for tetracycline. Appropriate dosages need to be used, the recommended frequency of administration adhered to, and the duration of drug therapy enforced.

Approach to the Patient Bleeding From Peptic Ulcer Disease
About 80% of upper GI bleeds are self-limited. The overall mortality rate of 8% to 10% for those who continue to bleed or in whom bleeding recurs has not changed dramatically during the past several decades despite an older and probably sicker patient population. The initial step in management of patients with acute upper GI hemorrhage is adequate initial and ongoing resuscitation. After resuscitation, endoscopy is performed to assess the cause and severity of the bleed, which will dictate the required intensity of therapy and predict the risks for further bleeding and death. Several factors are associated with continued

or recurrent bleeding and increase the risk for mortality. Most studies have demonstrated that mortality increases with age, such as the American Society for Gastrointestinal Endoscopy (ASGE) study, which found a mortality rate of 8.7% in patients 60 years old or younger and of 13.4% in those older than 60 years.[16] The severity of the initial bleed is also an adverse prognostic factor. This includes the presence of shock, a high transfusion requirement, or bright-red blood in the nasogastric tube or in the stool. Interestingly, recurrent bleeding increased the mortality rate from 8% to 30% in one study and from 7% to 44% in another. The onset of bleeding in a hospital was also associated with a higher mortality rate (33%) compared with those who bled outside of the hospital or before admission (7%). In the ASGE study, eight disease categories were looked at to assess their contribution to the mortality rate in patients with upper GI bleeding. These disease states included cardiac, central nervous system, GI, hepatic, neoplastic, pulmonary, renal, and stress. In the absence of any concomitant disease, the mortality rate was 2.5%. However, if there were three concomitant diseases, the mortality rate rose to 14.6%. With six concomitant diseases, the mortality rate rose to 66.7%. Stigmata of recent hemorrhage from peptic ulcers also predict an adverse prognostic sign. These stigmata included a visible vessel on endoscopy, oozing of bright-red blood, and fresh or old blood clot at the base of the ulcer. When a visible vessel was seen, it was associated with a 50% rebleeding rate, whereas other signs were associated with a lower rebleeding rate of about 8%. In the ASGE study, pumping or oozing lesions had a significantly greater mortality rate (16%) and need for surgery (24%) when compared with those with clot or no blood (mortality 6.7%, surgery 11%). In addition, patients undergoing emergency surgery had a 30% mortality rate, compared with 10% for those undergoing elective surgery. Mortality also rises with increased severity of bleeding, which correlates with transfusion requirement. If no units are transfused, the mortality rate is about 2%; for 1 to 3 units, about 5%; for 4 to 6 units, about 12%; for 7 to 9 units, about 15%; and when more than 10 units are used, the mortality rate rises to about 35%. A pumping or oozing lesion in the ASGE study was associated with a transfusion requirement greater than 5 units (37.6%), which was significantly different when compared with patients who had a clot or no blood on the lesion. In the latter group, only 20% required more than 5 units of blood. Pumping lesions were seen in only 5.5% of the cases in the ASGE study, as compared with the 24.2% frequency of oozing lesions. The risk for rebleeding in a patient with no active bleeding and overlying clot varies from 8% to 30%. The visible vessel is regarded as the one sign of recent hemorrhage that is associated with the highest incidence of rebleeding. In patients with a visible vessel, rebleeding has occurred in 56% of patients in one study, compared with 8% of those with oozing and 0% of those with no signs of recent hemorrhage. Mortality was also limited to those patients with visible vessels.

Endoscopy remains the investigation of choice for patients with upper GI bleeding from PUD. As previously mentioned, endoscopy provides the opportunity not only for diagnosis but also for therapy. Hemostatic methods currently employed include thermotherapy (heater probe, multipolar or bipolar electrocoagulation) as well as injection of ethanol or epinephrine solutions. When the bleeding is controlled, long-term medical therapy includes antisecretory agents, usually in the form of a proton pump inhibitor, plus testing for *H. pylori* with treatment if positive. If *H. pylori* is present, documentation of eradication should be performed after therapy. If the bleeding continues or recurs, surgery may be indicated; this is discussed later in the sections Bleeding Duodenal Ulcers and Bleeding Gastric Ulcers.

Surgical Procedures for Peptic Ulcer and Its Complications

Despite advances in medical therapy to inhibit acid secretion and to eradicate *H. pylori,* surgery remains important in managing these patients. It is noteworthy that during the past 2 decades, there has been an increase in emergency operations performed for complications of peptic ulcers while the number of operations for elective indications has decreased markedly. Moreover, there is a high recurrence rate for peptic ulcerations after discontinuation of medical therapy. Thus, there is a renewed interest in operative management of patients suffering from PUD. Although the indications for surgery have not changed dramatically during the past several decades, the type of operation performed has changed in the *H. pylori* era.[17]

The four classic indications for surgery on peptic ulcers are intractability, hemorrhage, perforation, and obstruction. Elective surgery for intractability is becoming more rare as medical therapy becomes more effective. The recognition of *H. pylori* and its eradication suggest that the intractability indication for surgery may apply only to patients in whom the organism cannot be eradicated or who cannot be taken off NSAIDs. In contrast to uncomplicated ulcers, the incidence of ulcers with complications requiring surgery does not appear to have diminished, and therefore familiarity with the various methods for treating bleeding, perforation, and obstruction is essential.

One goal of ulcer surgery is to prevent gastric acid secretion. Subtotal gastrectomy was considered optimal management for duodenal and gastric ulcers until Dragstedt's description of vagotomy and its impact on ulcer healing and recurrence. As described later, there are three levels of vagotomy that can be performed, and these are shown in Figure 47-4. Vagotomy decreases peak acid output by about 50%, whereas vagotomy plus antrectomy, which removes the gastrin-secreting portion of the stomach, decreases peak acid output by about 85%.

Truncal Vagotomy

As shown in Figure 47-4, truncal vagotomy is performed by division of the left and right vagus nerves above the hepatic and celiac branches just above the GE junction. Truncal vagotomy is probably the most common operation performed for duodenal ulcer disease. Most surgeons employ some form of drainage procedure in association with truncal vagotomy. The classic truncal vagotomy, in combination with a Heineke-Mikulicz pyloroplasty, is

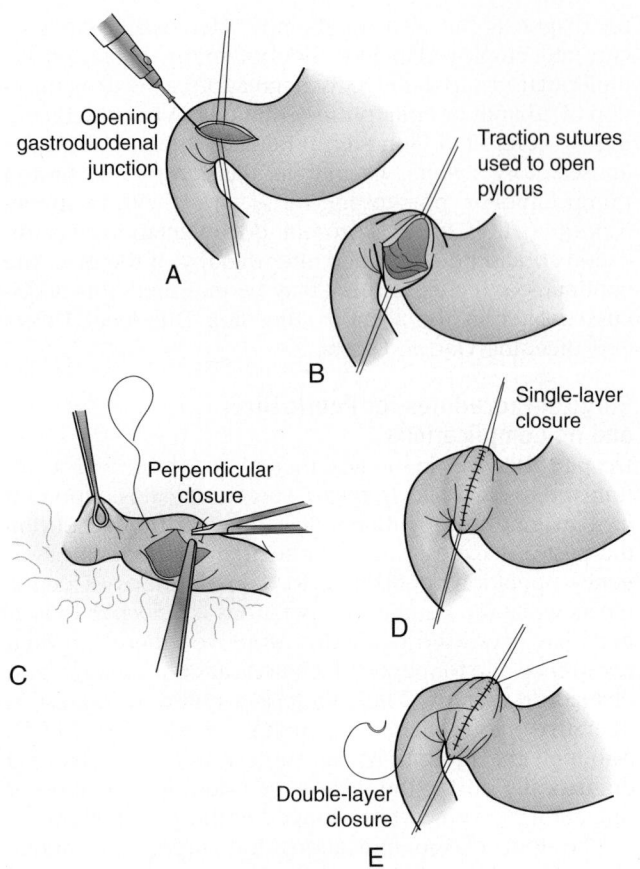

Figure 47-12 A to **E**, Heineke-Mikulicz pyloroplasty. (From Soreide JA, Soreide A: Pyloroplasty. Oper Tech Gen Surg 5:65-72, 2003.)

shown in Figure 47-12. When the duodenal bulb is scarred, a Finney pyloroplasty or Jaboulay gastroduodenostomy may be a useful alternative. In general, there is little difference in the side effects associated with the type of drainage procedure performed, although bile reflux may be more common after gastroenterostomy, and diarrhea is more common after pyloroplasty. The incidence of dumping is about the same for both. From a technical standpoint, truncal vagotomy and pyloroplasty represent an uncomplicated procedure that can be performed quickly, making it especially attractive for patients who are hemodynamically unstable from bleeding ulcers.

Highly Selective Vagotomy (Parietal Cell Vagotomy)

The highly selective vagotomy is also called the *parietal cell vagotomy* or the *proximal gastric vagotomy*. This procedure was developed after recognition that truncal vagotomy, in combination with a drainage procedure or gastric resection, adversely affected the pyloral antral pump function. This procedure divides only the vagus nerves supplying the acid-producing portion of the stomach within the corpus and fundus. This procedure preserves the vagal innervation of the gastric antrum so that there is no need for routine drainage procedures. Consequently, the incidence of postoperative complications is less. In general, the nerves of Latarjet are identified anteriorly and posteriorly, and the crow's feet innervating the fundus and body of the stomach are divided. These nerves are divided up until a point about 7 cm proximal to the pylorus or the area in the vicinity of the gastric antrum. Superiorly, division of these nerves is carried to a point at least 5 cm proximal to the gastroesophageal junction on the esophagus that is shown in Figure 47-13. Ideally, two or three branches to the antrum

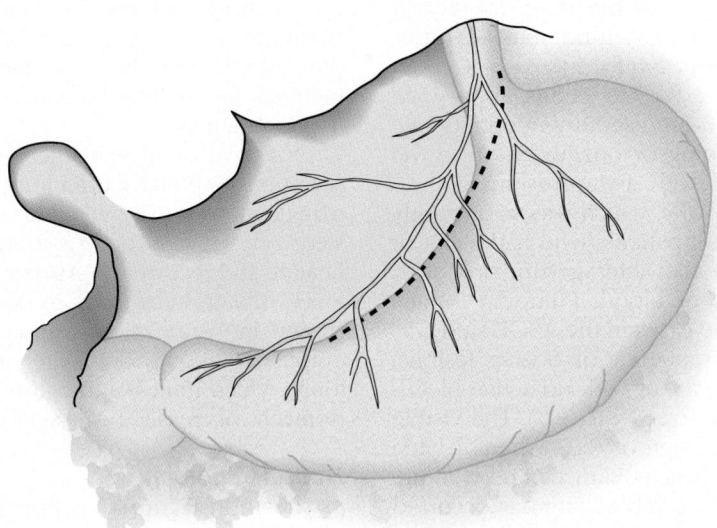

Figure 47-13 Anterior view of the stomach and the anterior nerve of Latarjet. The *dotted line* represents the line of dissection for parietal cell or highly selective vagotomy. Note that the last major branches of the nerve are left intact and that the dissection begins 7 cm from the pylorus. At the gastroesophageal junction, the dissection is well away from the origin of the hepatic branches of the left vagus. (From Kelly KA, Teotia SS: Proximal gastric vagotomy. In Baker RJ, Fischer JE [eds]: Mastery of Surgery. Philadelphia, Lippincott Williams & Wilkins, 2001.)

and pylorus should be preserved. The criminal nerve of Grassi represents a very proximal branch of the posterior trunk of the vagus, and great attention needs to be taken to avoid missing this branch in the division process because it is frequently cited as a predisposition for ulcer recurrence if left intact.

The recurrence rates after highly selective vagotomy are variable and depend on the skill of the operator and the duration of follow-up. Lengthy longitudinal follow-up is necessary to evaluate the results of this procedure because of the consistently reported rise in recurrent ulceration with time. Recurrence rates of 10% to 15% are reported for this procedure when performed by skilled surgeons. These compare very favorably or are even slightly higher than those reported after truncal vagotomy in combination with pyloroplasty. However, truncal vagotomy with pyloroplasty is more commonly associated with postvagotomy dumping syndrome and postvagotomy diarrhea. The moderate ulcer recurrence rate with highly selective vagotomy is considered acceptable by many surgeons because recurrences in this scenario are usually responsive to medical therapy with proton pump inhibitors. Interestingly, when the results of this procedure are broken down by the preoperative ulcer site, there appear to be strong data suggesting that prepyloric ulcers are more likely to be associated with recurrence than duodenal ulcers, for unclear reasons. As a result, parietal cell vagotomy is not the procedure of choice for prepyloric ulcers.

Truncal Vagotomy and Antrectomy

The most common indications for antrectomy or distal gastrectomy are gastric ulcer and large benign gastric tumors. Relative contraindications include cirrhosis, extensive scarring of the proximal duodenum that leaves a difficult or tenuous duodenal closure, and previous operations on the proximal duodenum, such as choledochoduodenostomy. When done in combination with truncal vagotomy, it is far more effective at reducing acid secretion and recurrence than either truncal vagotomy in combination with a drainage procedure or highly selective vagotomy. In fact, the recurrence rate for ulceration after truncal vagotomy and antrectomy is about 0% to 2%, and this procedure probably represents the gold standard with regard to recurrence rates. However, this low recurrence rate needs to be balanced against postgastrectomy and postvagotomy syndromes (see later) that rarely occur after highly selective vagotomy but appear in 20% of patients undergoing antrectomy.

Distal gastrectomy or antrectomy requires reconstruction of GI continuity that can be accomplished by either a gastroduodenostomy (Billroth I procedure; Fig. 47-14) or gastrojejunostomy (Billroth II procedure) using one of several modifications (Fig. 47-15). For benign diseases, gastroduodenostomy is usually favored because it avoids the problem of retained antrum syndrome, duodenal stump leak, and afferent loop obstruction associated with gastrojejunostomy after resection. If the duodenum is significantly scarred, gastroduodenostomy may be technically more difficult, necessitating gastrojejunostomy. If a gastrojejunostomy is performed, the loop of jejunum

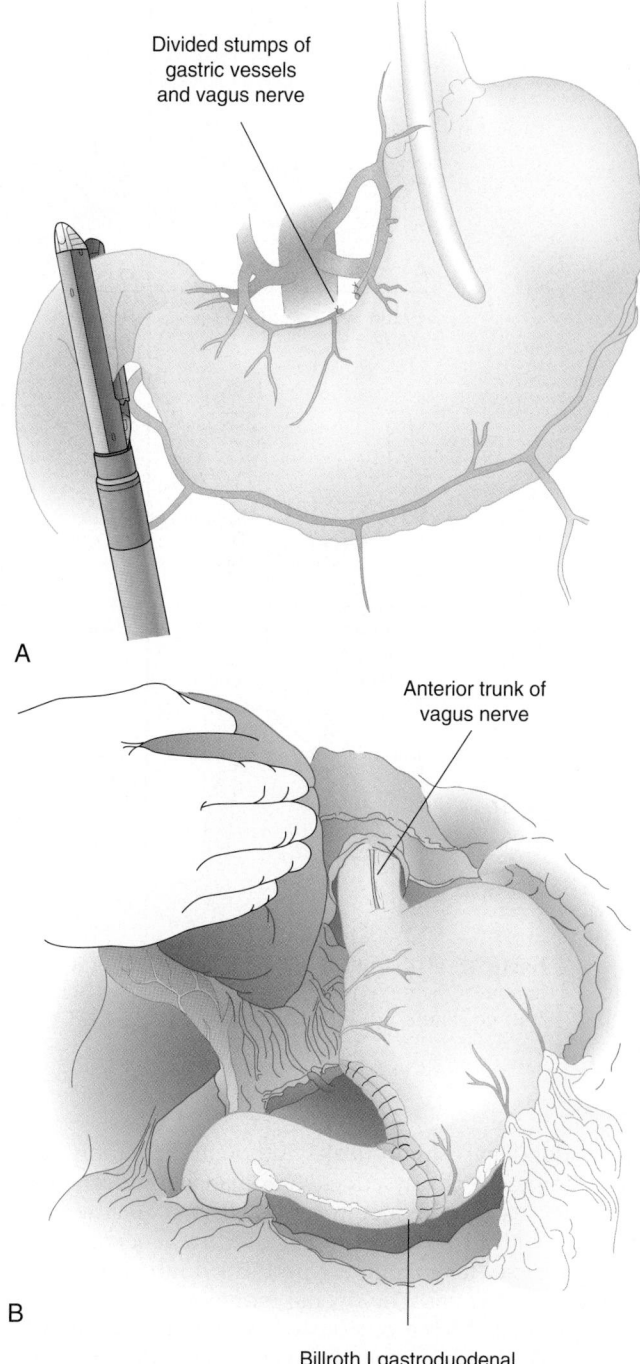

Figure 47-14 Hemigastrectomy with Billroth I (gastroduodenal) anastomosis. (From Dempsey D, Pathak A: Antrectomy. Oper Tech Gen Surg 5:86-100, 2003.)

chosen for anastomosis is usually brought through the transverse mesocolon in a retrocolic fashion rather than in front of the transverse colon in an antecolic fashion. The retrocolic anastomosis minimizes the length of the afferent limb and decreases the likelihood of twisting or kinking that could potentially lead to afferent loop obstruction and predispose to the devastating complication

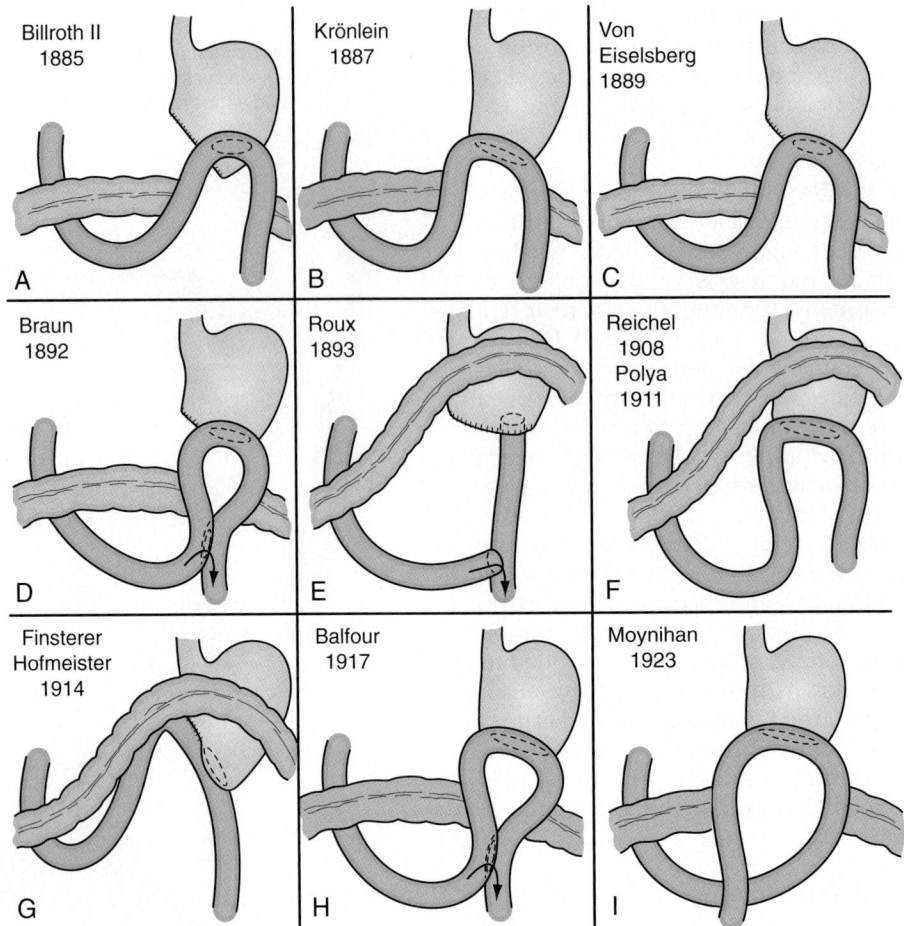

Figure 47-15 Billroth II operation and some of its modifications. (From Soybel DI, Zinner MJ: Stomach and duodenum: Operative procedures. In Zinner MJ, Schwartz SI, Ellis H [eds]: Maingot's Abdominal Operations, vol I, 10th ed. Stamford, CT, Appleton & Lange, 1997.)

of a duodenal stump leak. Although vagotomy and antrectomy are clearly effective at managing ulcerations, they are used infrequently today in the treatment of patients with PUD, as described later. In general, operations of lesser magnitude are performed more frequently in the *H. pylori* era. The overall mortality rate for antrectomy is about 2% but obviously is higher in patients with comorbid conditions such as insulin-dependent diabetes or immunosuppression. About 20% of patients develop some form of postgastrectomy or postvagotomy complications, and these are described later.

Subtotal Gastrectomy

Subtotal gastrectomy is rarely performed today for treatment of patients with PUD. It is usually reserved for patients with underlying malignancies or patients who have developed recurrent ulcerations after truncal vagotomy and antrectomy. The latter scenario assumes that medical therapy has been unable to heal the recurrent ulcer and that ZES has been ruled out. After subtotal gastrectomy, restoration of GI continuity can be accomplished with either a Billroth II anastomosis or via a Roux-en-Y gastrojejunostomy.

Laparoscopic Procedures

Not surprisingly, since the advent of laparoscopic cholecystectomy, many surgeons have applied minimally invasive surgical approaches to gastric surgery. Both parietal cell vagotomy and posterior truncal vagotomy with anterior seromyotomy (Taylor procedure) can be accomplished laparoscopically and represent effective antiulcer operations. However, long-term results are still unavailable to compare with those of the openly performed procedures. Dumping syndrome and postvagotomy diarrhea are similar in incidence to that observed after open highly selective vagotomy. Major concerns regarding this operation relate primarily to its efficacy and prevention of recurrent ulcers. Because incomplete innervation predisposes patients to recurrent ulcerations after highly selective vagotomy, anterior seromyotomy might place patients at risk for recurrence because of failure to completely denervate the parietal cell mass. Laparoscopic approaches can also be used for repair of simple perforations and offer clear advantages to the formal laparotomy required in open procedures.

Surgical Indications

Surgical intervention is required in 8% to 20% of patients developing complications from their PUD. Surgical therapy serves several purposes. It salvages patients from life-threatening complications associated with perforation, hemorrhage, and gastric outlet obstruction. It provides cure for the disease in the form of protection from recurrence, and it rules out the potential for malignancy in the case of gastric ulcerations. The indications for surgery are intractable abdominal pain, bleeding, perforation, and obstruction. For all patients with ulcers being considered for elective surgery, antisecretory agents should probably be discontinued for about 72 hours before operation in order to allow gastric acidity to return to normal values, which minimizes bacterial overgrowth and the extent of contamination. The recommended operations for patients suffering from complications related to their PUD are shown in Table 47-5, and the rationale is described later. In patients undergoing surgery for PUD, it is recommended that all have *H. pylori* testing and, if positive, treatment and documentation of eradication. NSAIDs should be discontinued. Minimally invasive surgery can be applied to most of the procedures, and the technical aspects are summarized by Dubois.[18] The reader is reminded that much of the surgical literature is retrospective and predates modern medical therapy, NSAID use, and *H. pylori*. However, an excellent review of the clinical trials relevant to the surgical management of PUD is provided by Harbison and Dempsey.[19]

Intractable Duodenal Ulcer

Intractability is loosely defined as failure of an ulcer to heal after an initial trial of 8 to 12 weeks of therapy or if patients relapse after therapy has been discontinued. This is unusual for duodenal ulcer disease in the *H. pylori* era; however, it still exists for benign gastric ulcers in which malignancy needs to be ruled out. For any intractable ulcer, adequate duration of therapy, *H. pylori* eradication, and elimination of NSAID use must be confirmed. A serum gastrin level should also be obtained in patients with ulcers refractory to medical therapy to rule out gastrinoma. Although rarely seen today, intractable duodenal ulcer should be treated by parietal cell vagotomy. Although this can be performed openly, many prefer a laparoscopic approach. The laparoscopic technology currently available allows performance of parietal cell vagotomy in exactly the same way it is performed openly and probably provides better visualization. Proximal gastric vagotomy is associated with a morbidity rate of less than 1% and a mortality rate of less than 0.5%. Unfortunately, the recurrence rate is roughly 5% to 25%. Some surgeons prefer a Taylor procedure in which the posterior truncal vagotomy is performed laparoscopically and then an endoscopic GI stapler is used to perform a seromyotomy across the anterior portion of the stomach to divide all the vagal fibers coursing through the seromuscular layer.

Table 47-5 Surgical Treatment Recommendations for Complications Related to Peptic Ulcer Disease

Duodenal Ulcer
Intractable: parietal cell vagotomy
Bleeding: truncal vagotomy with pyloroplasty and oversewing of bleeding vessel
Perforation: patch closure with treatment of *H. pylori* with or without parietal cell vagotomy (see text)
Obstruction: rule out malignancy and parietal cell vagotomy with gastrojejunostomy

Gastric Ulcer
Intractable
- Type I: distal gastrectomy with Billroth I
- Type II or III: distal gastrectomy with truncal vagotomy
Bleeding
- Type I: distal gastrectomy with Billroth I
- Type II or III: distal gastrectomy with truncal vagotomy
Perforated
- Type I, stable: distal gastrectomy with Billroth I
- Type I, unstable: biopsy, patch, and treatment for *H. pylori*
- Type II or III: patch closure with treatment of *H. pylori*
Obstruction: rule out malignancy and antrectomy with vagotomy
Type IV: depends on ulcer size, distance from the gastroesophageal junction, and degree of surrounding inflammation (see text)
Giant gastric ulcers: distal gastrectomy, with vagotomy reserved for type II and III gastric ulcers

Though some are concerned about dividing vagal innervation to the celiac ganglion and to the rest of the viscera, there is considerable evidence that preserving vagal innervation of the celiac axis and small bowel does little to reduce the side effects of vagotomy. Thus, the Taylor procedure appears to be equivalent to parietal cell vagotomy, and the side effects are not any greater. It has also been suggested that anterior lesser curve seromyotomy and posterior truncal vagotomy result in acid suppression that is similar in magnitude to that achieved after highly selective vagotomy or truncal vagotomy with drainage. Gastric emptying following the Taylor procedure is also similar to that of highly selective vagotomy (increased emptying of liquids and normal emptying of solids), and dumping and diarrhea are less than that observed after truncal vagotomy and drainage.

Intractable Gastric Ulcer

Type I Gastric Ulcer

For type I gastric ulcers, malignancy remains a major concern, and excision of the ulcer is necessary. Consequently, distal gastrectomy (40%-50%) is recommended with a Billroth I anastomosis. Vagotomy is not necessary, although 15% of type I gastric ulcers may be type II, in which case a truncal vagotomy should be added. The morbidity rate associated with a distal gastrectomy without vagotomy and Billroth I reconstruction is about 3% to 5% for elective treatment of type I gastric ulcers. Mortality rates range from 1% to 2%, and mortality is associated with a recurrence rate of less than 5%. It is important to remember, however, that the presentation of a nonhealing gastric ulcer in the *H. pylori* era should raise serious concerns about the presence of underlying malignancy. If malignancy is encountered, a subtotal gastrectomy with a Billroth II gastrojejunostomy or Roux-en-Y gastrojejunostomy should be performed. Vagotomy usually is not necessary for the type I gastric ulcer because it is not dependent on gastric acid. Although technically more difficult, a parietal cell vagotomy with wedge excision of the ulcer could also be performed. Because intractable PUD is so uncommon, it is again important to ensure that adequate time has elapsed and appropriate therapy has been administered to allow healing of the ulcer to occur. This includes confirmation that *H. pylori* has been eradicated and that NSAIDs have been eliminated as a potential cause. Most patients with a type I gastric ulcer should, in fact, heal following appropriate medical therapy as described earlier in the Medical Management section.

Type II or Type III Gastric Ulcers

Assuming that the ulcer has had adequate time to heal and that *H. pylori* has been eradicated, a distal gastrectomy in combination with truncal vagotomy should be performed. Several studies have demonstrated that patients undergoing highly selective vagotomy for type II or III gastric ulcers have a poorer outcome than those undergoing resection. However, there are still some who advocate performing a laparoscopic parietal cell vagotomy and reserve resection for those who develop ulcer recurrence. Management of type IV gastric ulcers is discussed separately, later.

Bleeding Duodenal Ulcers

Endoscopic management of PUD complicated by bleeding is successful in more than 75% of patients. Rebleeding occurs in 10% to 30% of cases, and almost all fatal rebleeding occurs within the first 24 hours. The available evidence suggests that rebleeding can also be handled endoscopically, although in patients who are elderly or have hypotension, large ulcers (>2 cm), or comorbidities, we advocate surgery.[20] As a result of aggressive endoscopic management, the patients who come to surgery are usually sicker, more elderly, and more likely to have complications. For patients with bleeding duodenal ulcers requiring surgery, we recommend oversewing the ulcer with a U stitch along with truncal vagotomy and pyloroplasty. Because most of these patients are elderly, have bled a significant amount, and have some degree of hypotension, the more time-consuming parietal cell vagotomy is usually not performed. Although not proved successful, there are some who advocate opening the duodenum, ligating the gastroduodenal vessel, closing the duodenum, and then eradicating *H. pylori*. The clear exception to this would be if the patient had received therapy in the past for *H. pylori* and failed or if the patient was known to be *H. pylori*–negative. In this situation, an acid-reducing procedure with some type of vagotomy is clearly indicated. Most surgeons would not perform any form of gastrectomy for a bleeding duodenal ulcer.

It is also important to remember that in those patients receiving endoscopic management of their bleeding ulcer, treatment with endoscopy needs to be as prompt and aggressive as possible, and the patient needs to be watched closely for signs of rebleeding. Furthermore, assuming that the gastroenterologist or surgical endoscopist can stop the bleeding and is confident that it can be managed by endoscopy, the patient still needs to be treated with a proton pump inhibitor and undergo therapy for *H. pylori* after testing.

Bleeding Gastric Ulcers

For bleeding type I gastric ulcers, a distal gastrectomy with Billroth I anastomosis is recommended. Some have advocated adding vagotomy for patients who continue to take NSAIDs, although the data on this are unclear. Alternatively, if patients need to stay on NSAIDs, they should be given misoprostol, a prostaglandin analogue, because it has been found to have a 40% reduction in serious GI complications in those patients who have to stay on NSAIDs.[21] For type II and III bleeding gastric ulcers, distal gastrectomy, in combination with vagotomy, is indicated.

Perforated Duodenal Ulcers

Simple omental patch closure, patch closure with parietal cell vagotomy, or patch closure with truncal vagotomy and drainage are options for patients with perforated duodenal ulcer. Simple patching of the perforation is recommended in patients in poor medical condition, hemodynamically unstable patients, and patients with exudative peritonitis (>24 hours of contamination) followed by treatment of *H. pylori*.[22] If the patient is known to be *H. pylori*–negative, presents with a chronic history, requires NSAID use, or is thought to be at risk for noncompliance with therapy, we recommend adding parietal cell vagotomy. Patch closure of the duodenum can be performed either laparoscopically or openly. In some cases, patients present with a sealed perforation. In one study from Hong Kong, these patients were treated prospectively and successfully with nonoperative management.[23] The successfully managed patients were hemodynamically stable and without signs of toxicity. Unfortunately, the patients who failed were the ones in whom it would be most desirable to use nonoperative management (i.e., the elderly and the very ill). In this situation, upper GI radiography needs to demonstrate that the ulcer is indeed sealed. Nonoperative therapy in this situation would also include treatment for *H. pylori* and acid suppression. For all perforated duodenal ulcer patients who are *H. pylori*–positive, documentation of *H. pylori* eradication with a urea breath test is mandatory, and it is paramount that the patients are compliant with their medications to treat *H. pylori* regardless of whether they are managed surgically or nonoperatively.

Perforated Gastric Ulcer

For perforated type I gastric ulcers that occur in stable patients, distal gastrectomy with Billroth I anastomosis is recommended. In unstable patients, simple patching of the gastric ulcer with biopsy and treatment for *H. pylori*, if positive, is recommended. However, even if the biopsy is negative, the risk for malignancy still needs to be ruled out; therefore, documentation of healing is required with repeat endoscopy and biopsy, if unhealed. Adding vagotomy for perforated type I gastric ulcers is unlikely to be of any value. Because they behave like duodenal ulcers, type II and III gastric ulcers can be simply treated with patch closure with or without truncal vagotomy and pyloroplasty, depending on the medical condition, hemodynamic status, and extent of peritonitis, followed by treatment for *H. pylori*. Again, this assumes that patients are *H. pylori*–positive.

Gastric Outlet Obstruction

Gastric outlet obstruction is the least common indication for surgery. It is more common with duodenal and type III gastric ulcers and requires that malignancy be ruled out. Obstruction is an unusual presentation for type I gastric ulcers, and its presence should suggest an occult malignancy. All patients with gastric outlet obstruction require preoperative nasogastric decompression for several days, correction of fluid and electrolyte imbalances, antisecretory therapy, and endoscopy with biopsies before surgical intervention. The first principle is to categorize the patient as either acutely or chronically obstructed. If the patient is acutely obstructed, the patient should be treated nonoperatively with nasogastric decompression, IV fluid, nutritional support as needed, and acid-suppressive therapy. *H. pylori* should be tested for and treated. For chronic obstruction from a benign duodenal ulcer, we recommend parietal cell vagotomy with a gastrojejunostomy followed by treatment of *H. pylori*. Endoscopic balloon dilation has also been tried in this situation, although those who benefit from this procedure are likely those with acute gastric outlet obstruction and not those with chronic gastric outlet obstruction. The physiologic argument for doing the parietal cell vagotomy with a gastrojejunostomy, as opposed to truncal vagotomy, is that it maintains innervation to the chronically obstructed antrum. As a result, the patient may have fewer chronic emptying problems than if a truncal vagotomy was performed. For obstructing type II or III gastric ulcers, we recommend gastrectomy with vagotomy followed by treatment for *H. pylori*.

Type IV Gastric Ulcers

The type IV gastric ulcer presents a difficult management problem.[24] The surgical treatment depends on the ulcer size, the distance from the GE junction, and the degree of surrounding inflammation. Whenever possible, the ulcer should be excised. The most aggressive approach is to perform a gastrectomy that includes a small portion of the esophageal wall and ulcer followed by a Roux-en-Y esophogogastrojejunostomy to restore intestinal continuity. For type IV gastric ulcers that are located 2 to 5 cm from the gastroesophageal junction, a distal gastrectomy with a vertical extension of the resection to include the lesser curvature with the ulcer can be performed (i.e., Pauchet procedure) (Fig. 47-16). After resection, bowel continuity is restored with an end-to-end gastroduodenostomy. The Csendes procedure may be useful in stable patients or the Kelling-Madlener operation in unstable ones. Some have even advocated leaving the ulcer in

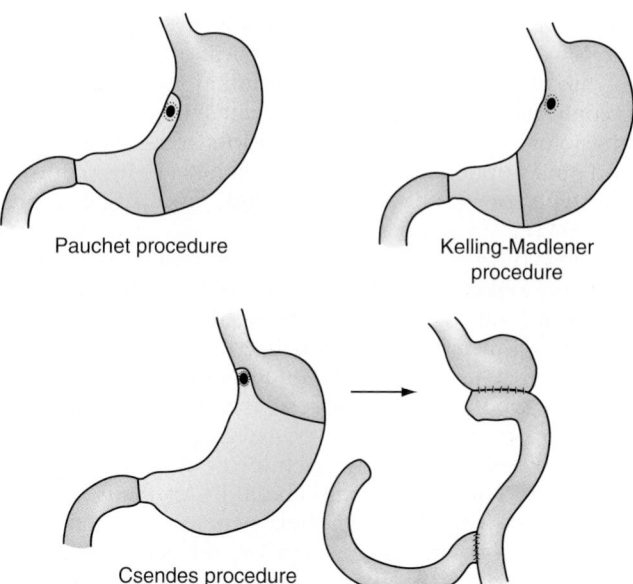

Figure 47-16 Operations for high-lying ulcers near the gastroesophageal junction (type IV). (Adapted from Seymour NE: Operations for peptic ulcer and their complications. In Feldman M, Scharschmidt BF, Sleisenger MH [eds]: Gastrointestinal and Liver Disease, 6th ed. Philadelphia, WB Saunders, 1998.)

place or locally excising it in conjunction with truncal vagotomy and pyloroplasty.

Giant Gastric Ulcers

Giant gastric ulcers are defined as ulcers with a diameter of 2 cm or greater. They are usually found on the lesser curvature and have a higher incidence of malignancy (10%) than smaller ones. It is not uncommon for these ulcers to penetrate into contiguous structures such as the spleen, pancreas, liver, or transverse colon and be falsely diagnosed as an unresectable malignancy, despite normal biopsy results. The incidence of malignancy probably ranges from 6% to 30% and increases with the size of the ulcer. Giant gastric ulcers have a high likelihood of developing complications (i.e., perforation, bleeding). Medical therapy heals 80% of these ulcers, although repeat endoscopy is indicated in 6 to 8 weeks. For complications or failure to heal, the operation of choice is gastrectomy including the ulcer bed, with vagotomy reserved for type II and III gastric ulcers. In the high-risk patient with significant underlying comorbid conditions, a local excision combined with vagotomy and pyloroplasty may be considered; otherwise, resection has the highest chance for successful outcome.

Postgastrectomy Syndromes

Postoperative Complications for Peptic Ulcer Disease

The overall mortality rate for vagotomy and pyloroplasty or a vagotomy with antrectomy is about 1% or less, whereas for highly selective vagotomy, it is about 0.05%. Postoperative complications include bleeding, infection, and delayed gastric emptying, which can occur in roughly 5% of patients after vagotomy and pyloroplasty or vagotomy and antrectomy. Highly selective vagotomy has the lowest rate of associated complications, which occur in only about 1% of patients. In addition to these early complications, gastric surgery results in a number of physiologic derangements due to loss of reservoir function, interruption of the pyloric sphincter mechanism, the type of gastric reconstruction, and vagal nerve transection.

These disorders are collectively referred to as *postgastrectomy syndromes*. Although the physiologic derangements account for most symptoms, there are also some psychological elements associated with the disease process that remain poorly understood. About 25% of patients who undergo surgery for PUD subsequently develop some degree of postgastrectomy syndrome, although this frequency is much lower in highly selective vagotomy. Fortunately, only about 1% of them become permanently disabled from their symptoms. When these postgastrectomy symptoms develop, it has become more apparent that every attempt should be made to avoid reoperation because many of these patients lack a clearly definable mechanical or physiologic defect and many of the problems persist despite reoperation. If reoperation is attempted, it should not be performed until an adequate trial of conservative therapy has been administered for an adequate period of time.

Postgastrectomy Syndromes Secondary to Gastric Resection

Dumping Syndrome

Dumping syndrome refers to a symptom complex that occurs following ingestion of a meal when a portion of the stomach has been removed or the normal pyloric sphincter mechanism has become disrupted. Dumping syndrome exists in either a late or an early form, with the early form occurring more frequently.

Early Dumping

The early form of dumping syndrome usually occurs within 20 to 30 minutes after ingestion of a meal and is accompanied by both GI and cardiovascular symptoms. The GI symptoms include nausea and vomiting, a sense of epigastric fullness, eructations, cramping abdominal pain, and often explosive diarrhea. The cardiovascular symptoms include palpitations, tachycardia, diaphoresis, fainting, dizziness, flushing, and occasionally blurred vision. The symptoms characteristically occur while the patient is seated at the table eating or shortly after eating. This symptom complex can develop after any operation on the stomach but is more common after partial gastrectomy with the Billroth II reconstruction, in which as many as 50% to 60% of patients may develop this complication, especially if more that two thirds of the stomach has been removed. It is far less commonly observed following the Billroth I gastrectomy or after vagotomy and drainage procedures. Usually, the GI symptoms are more common, and only rarely does the full-blown symptom complex occur with the cardiovascular and vasomotor aberrations noted previously.

Although the exact sequence of events responsible for this syndrome remains to be fully defined, it is generally agreed that it occurs because of the rapid passage of food of high osmolarity from the stomach into the small intestine. This occurs because gastrectomy or interruption of the pyloric sphincteric mechanism prevents the stomach from preparing its contents and delivering them to the proximal bowel in the form of small particles in isotonic solution. The resultant hypertonic food bolus passes into the small intestine, which induces a rapid shift of extracellular fluid into the intestinal lumen to achieve isotonicity. After this shift of extracellular fluid, luminal distention occurs and induces the autonomic responses listed previously.

The symptoms associated with early dumping syndrome appear to be secondary to the release of several humoral agents, such as serotonin, bradykinin-like substances, neurotensin, and enteroglucagon. Usually, the symptoms of dumping are sufficiently obvious that the diagnosis can be made on this basis alone; however, if there is doubt, gastric emptying scans can be obtained that demonstrate rapid gastric emptying. Alternatively, a provocative test can also be done in the form of a 200-mL meal of 50% glucose solution and water. Patients with early dumping syndrome have their symptoms elicited after ingestion of this glucose solution.

Most patients subjected to gastric surgery complain of some dumping-like symptoms after surgery. Most, however, experience spontaneous relief and require no specific therapy. In those situations in which symptoms are prolonged, dietary measures are usually sufficient. These dietary measures include avoiding foods containing large amounts of sugar, frequent feeding of small meals rich in protein and fat, and separating liquids from solids during a meal. In the past, serotonin antagonists were given to these patients with marginal benefit. Recently, however, the long-acting somatostatin analogue octreotide acetate (Sandostatin) has been shown to be highly effective in preventing the development of symptoms, both vasomotor and GI. This synthetic analogue has been shown to inhibit the hormonal responses associated with this syndrome and to completely abolish the associated diarrhea. This peptide not only inhibits gastric emptying but also induces a fasting or interdigestive small bowel motility pattern in patients with dumping syndrome such that intestinal transit of the ingested meal is prolonged. The side effects associated with administration of this synthetic peptide are relatively benign; however, the agent is somewhat expensive.

In the fewer than 1% of patients who fail to respond to the conservative measures mentioned earlier, operative intervention may become necessary. The physiologic rationale behind surgery is to improve the gastric reservoir function, decrease rapid gastric emptying, or ideally accomplish both goals. Although a variety of surgical procedures have been used to manage early dumping, the use of isoperistaltic or antiperistaltic jejunal segments has had the greatest success in dealing with this problem in most centers. This procedure is done using a 10- to 20-cm loop of jejunum and interposing it between the stomach and small intestine in an isoperistaltic fashion.

This loop dilates over time and, therefore, promotes the reservoir function. In the antiperistaltic approach, a jejunal segment 10 cm in length is used, and the jejunum is twisted on its mesentery so that its distal end is anastomosed to the stomach and its proximal end to the small intestine. This reversal in peristalsis permits the loop to act as a substitute pylorus and delay the rate of gastric emptying. Another technique is the creation of a long-limb Roux-en-Y anastomosis to delay gastric emptying. Whether this approach is superior to the use of isoperistaltic or antiperistaltic jejunal segments has yet to be determined.

Late Dumping

The syndrome of late dumping appears 2 to 3 hours after a meal and is far less common than early dumping. The basic defect in this order is also rapid gastric emptying; however, it is related specifically to carbohydrates being delivered rapidly into the proximal intestine. When carbohydrates are delivered to the small intestine, they are quickly absorbed, resulting in hyperglycemia, which triggers the release of large amounts of insulin to control the rising blood sugar. This results in an actual overshooting such that a profound hypoglycemia occurs in response to the insulin. This activates the adrenal gland to release catecholamines, which results in diaphoresis, tremulousness, light-headedness, tachycardia, and confusion. The symptom complex is indistinguishable from insulin shock.

These patients should be advised to ingest frequent small meals and to reduce their carbohydrate intake. Some patients have found benefit with pectin either alone or in combination with acarbose, an α-glucoside hydrolase inhibitor that delays carbohydrate absorption through impairment of intraluminal starch and sucrose digestion. If conservative measures fail, the use of an antiperistaltic loop of jejunum between the residual gastric pouch and intestine has been shown to effectively manage this problem. The antiperistaltic limb accomplishes a delay in gastric emptying and also results in flattening of the glucose tolerance curve to alleviate the hypoglycemic symptomatology.

Metabolic Disturbances

A number of metabolic consequences arise after gastric procedures but are more common and serious after partial gastrectomy than after vagotomy. The incidence after gastrectomy is also much greater if a Billroth II as opposed to a Billroth I procedure is used for reconstruction. As for dumping, the severity of these disturbances is directly related to the extent of gastric resection.

The most common metabolic defect appearing after gastrectomy is anemia. Two types have been identified, and one is related to deficiency in iron and the other to an impairment in vitamin B_{12} metabolism. Iron deficiency anemia is more common than vitamin B_{12} deficiency anemia. More than 30% of patients undergoing gastrectomy suffer from iron deficiency anemia. The exact cause remains to be fully understood but appears to be related to a combination of decreased iron intake, impaired iron absorption, and chronic subliminal blood loss secondary to the hyperemic, friable gastric mucosa primarily involving the margins of the stoma where the stomach connects to the small intestine. In general, the addition of iron supplements to the patient's diet corrects this metabolic problem.

Megaloblastic anemia can also occur after gastrectomy, especially when more than 50% of the stomach is removed such as occurs during subtotal gastrectomy. Megaloblastic anemia from vitamin B_{12} deficiency only rarely develops after partial gastrectomy. Vitamin B_{12} deficiency occurs secondary to poor absorption of the substance owing to lack of intrinsic factor secretion in the gastric juice. If a patient develops a macrocytic anemia, serum vitamin B_{12} levels should be obtained. If the vitamin B_{12} level is abnormal, the patient should be treated with intramuscular injections of cyanocobalamin every 3 to 4 months indefinitely because its administration orally is not a reliable route. The other cause of macrocytic anemia is a folate deficiency, which is rare after gastric resection but may coexist with either an iron or vitamin B_{12} deficiency. Folate deficiency can usually be corrected by dietary supplementation.

Another common metabolic disturbance after gastric resections is impaired absorption of fat. On occasion, steatorrhea may be seen after a Billroth II gastrectomy and may occur as a result of inadequate mixing of bile salts and pancreatic lipase with ingested fat because of the duodenal bypass. If this occurs, a deficiency in uptake of fat-soluble vitamins may also occur. In the setting of steatorrhea, pancreatic replacement enzymes are often effective in decreasing fat loss.

Both osteoporosis and osteomalacia have also been observed after gastric resection and appear to be caused by deficiencies in calcium. If fat absorption is also present, the calcium malabsorption is further aggravated because fatty acids bind calcium. The incidence of this problem also increases with the extent of gastric resection and is usually associated with a Billroth II gastrectomy. Development of bone disease generally occurs about 4 to 5 years after surgery. Treatment of this disorder usually requires calcium supplements (1-2 g/day) in conjunction with vitamin D (500-5000 units daily).

Postgastrectomy Syndromes Related to Gastric Reconstruction

A number of disorders can develop after gastric resection as a result of the technique used to reestablish GI continuity. Patients undergoing Billroth II gastrectomy are more likely to encounter these problems than those undergoing other types of reconstruction. The afferent loop and retained antrum syndromes occur only in patients with this type of gastrectomy.

Afferent Loop Syndrome

Afferent loop syndrome occurs as a result of partial obstruction of the afferent limb that is unable then to empty its contents. As shown in Figure 47-17, afferent loop syndrome can occur from a variety of causes. It can arise secondary to kinking and angulation of the afferent limb, internal herniation behind the efferent limb, stenosis of the gastrojejunal anastomosis, a redundant twisting

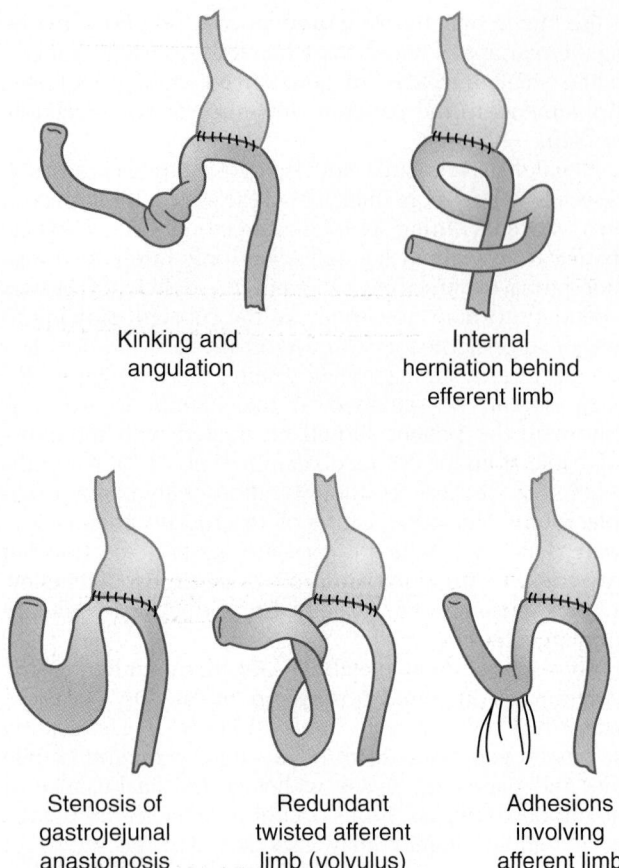

Kinking and
angulation

Internal
herniation behind
efferent limb

Stenosis of
gastrojejunal
anastomosis

Redundant
twisted afferent
limb (volvulus)

Adhesions
involving
afferent limb

Figure 47-17 Causes of afferent loop syndrome.

of the afferent limb with a resultant volvulus, or adhesions involving the afferent limb. The syndrome usually occurs when the afferent limb is greater than 30 to 40 cm in length and has been anastomosed to the gastric remnant in an antecolic fashion. Although acute afferent loop syndrome can occur, it is usually found chronically.

After obstruction of the afferent limb, there is an accumulation of pancreatic and hepatobiliary secretion within the limb, resulting in its distention. Pancreatic and hepatobiliary secretion occur in response to ingestion of food in the gastric remnant or passage of food into the efferent loop. Accumulation of these secretions results in distention, which causes epigastric discomfort and cramping. In the setting of partial obstruction, the intraluminal pressure increases to forcefully empty its contents into the stomach, resulting in bilious vomiting that is often projectile but offers immediate relief of symptoms. There is no food contained within the vomitus because the ingested meal has already passed into the efferent limb. In the setting of complete obstruction, necrosis and perforation of the loop can occur as the obstruction is a closed loop because the duodenum proximally has already been closed during the Billroth II gastrectomy. In this situation, constant abdominal pain is noted and may be more pronounced in the right upper quadrant with radiation into the interscapular area. Like any

complete bowel obstruction, this is a surgical emergency and requires immediate attention. In most patients with afferent loop syndrome, the obstruction is only partial. Whether or not a patient seeks medical attention is dependent on the degree of afferent loop obstruction present. If the obstruction has been present for a long period of time, it can also be aggravated by the development of the blind loop syndrome. In this situation, bacterial overgrowth occurs in the static loop, and the bacteria bind with vitamin B_{12} and deconjugated bile acids. This results in a systemic deficiency of vitamin B_{12} with the development of megaloblastic anemia.

The acute form of afferent loop obstruction, which is rare, may occur within a few days after operation or may develop quite unexpectedly years after the Billroth II gastrectomy. In both circumstances, it is caused by the acute blockage of the afferent limb such as that seen with volvulus or herniation of the afferent loop posterior to the efferent limb. If the resulting obstruction is of the closed-loop type, it requires immediate operative intervention. A palpable abdominal mass may be present in about one third of patients, although the associated pain and tenderness are usually severe enough to indicate the necessity of urgent operative intervention.

In contrast to the diagnosis of acute afferent obstruction, diagnosing chronic afferent loop obstruction may be more problematic. Although symptoms may suggest this diagnosis, it is sometimes difficult to establish the diagnosis. On occasion, the dilated afferent loop may be seen on plain films of the abdomen, or a contrast barium study of the stomach may delineate the presence of an obstructed loop. Failure to visualize the afferent limb on upper endoscopy is also suggestive of the diagnosis. Radionuclide studies imaging the hepatobiliary tree have also been used with some success in diagnosing this syndrome. Normally, the radionuclide should pass into the stomach or distal small bowel after being excreted into the afferent limb. If there is failure to do so, the possibility of an afferent loop obstruction should be considered. The medical usefulness of radionuclide studies remains to be determined.

For both forms of afferent loop syndrome, acute and chronic, operation is indicated because it is a mechanical problem, not a functional problem. A long afferent limb is usually the underlying problem, and treatment therefore involves the elimination of this loop. Some have advocated converting the Billroth II construction into a Billroth I anastomosis, whereas others have advocated an enteroenterostomy below the stoma, which is technically easier. Creation of a Roux-en-Y can also be done, but a concomitant vagotomy should also be performed to prevent marginal ulceration from the diversion of duodenal contents from the gastroenteric stoma.

Efferent Loop Obstruction
Obstruction of the efferent limb is usually quite rare. The most common cause of efferent loop obstruction is herniation of the limb behind the anastomosis in a right-to-left fashion. This can occur with both antecolic and retrocolic gastrojejunostomies. The preference for herniation in the right-to-left direction is probably a result of

the fact that gastrojejunostomies lie to the left of the main mass of the small intestine, making it mechanically easier for herniation to occur from right to left. With this type of herniation, obstruction of the efferent limb is usually all that occurs; however, it may also compress the mesentery of the afferent limb, compromising its blood supply or obstructing the afferent limb as well. Efferent loop obstruction may occur anytime after surgery; however, more than 50% of cases do so within the first postoperative month. Establishing a diagnosis is difficult. Initial complaints may include left upper quadrant abdominal pain that is colicky in nature, bilious vomiting, and abdominal distention. The diagnosis is usually established by a contrast barium study of the stomach with failure of barium to enter the efferent limb. Operative intervention is almost always necessary and consists of reducing the retroanastomotic hernia and closing the retroanastomotic space to prevent recurrence of this condition.

Alkaline Reflux Gastritis

After gastrectomy, reflux of bile is fairly common. In a small percentage of patients, this reflux is associated with severe epigastric abdominal pain accompanied by bilious vomiting and weight loss. It is usually not relieved by food or antacids. The vomiting may occur at any time during the day or night and can even awaken patients from sleep. Although the diagnosis can be made by taking a careful history, HIDA scans are usually diagnostic, demonstrating biliary secretion into the stomach and even into the esophagus in severe cases. Upper endoscopy can also be performed with multiple biopsy samples taken away from the stoma, and the gastric fluid can be analyzed for bile acid concentrations. On endoscopy, the mucosa is frequently friable and beefy-red, and superficial mucosal ulcerations may be apparent on microscopy. Iron deficiency anemia and weight loss are also common.

Most patients suffering from alkaline reflux gastritis have had gastric resection performed with a Billroth II anastomosis. Symptomatology may occur at any time after the operation. Although bile reflux appears to be the inciting event, a number of issues remain unanswered with respect to the role of bile in its pathogenesis. For example, many patients have reflux of bile into the stomach following gastrectomy without any symptoms. Moreover, there is no clear correlation between the volume of bile or its composition and the subsequent development of alkaline reflux gastritis. Although it is clear the syndrome does exist, caution needs to be exercised to be sure that it is not overdiagnosed. After a diagnosis is made, therapy is directed at relief of symptoms. Unfortunately, most of the medical therapies that have been tried to treat alkaline reflux gastritis have not shown any consistent benefit. Thus, for those patients with intractable symptoms, surgery is recommended. The surgical procedure of choice usually means converting the Billroth II anastomosis into a Roux-en-Y gastrojejunostomy in which the Roux limb has been lengthened to 41 to 46 cm.

Retained Antrum Syndrome

Because the antral mucosa may extend past the pyloric muscle for a distance of 0.5 cm, the syndrome of retained gastric antrum may occur after partial gastrectomy even if the resection is carried beyond the pyloric sphincter. A Billroth II anastomosis can therefore result in the development of a retained antrum syndrome if residual antrum is left in the duodenal stump. In this situation, the retained antrum is continually bathed in alkaline pH from the duodenal, pancreatic, and biliary secretions that, in turn, stimulate the release of large amounts of gastrin with a resultant increase in acid secretion. This highly ulcerogenic circumstance is responsible for about 9% of recurrent ulcers after previous surgery for PUD and is associated with an incidence of recurrent ulceration as high as 80%. It can be eliminated if biopsy confirmation of duodenal mucosa is obtained after resection of the proximal duodenum at the time of the Billroth II gastrectomy.

In patients who develop a recurrent ulcer after previous gastrectomy for ulcer disease in which a Billroth II anastomosis was performed, a technetium scan may prove helpful in diagnosing retained antrum. In patients with a retained antrum, this scan demonstrates a hot spot that is adjacent to the area where normal uptake of technetium by the gastric mucosa of the remaining stomach occurs. If a retained antrum is diagnosed, H_2-receptor blockade or proton pump inhibitors may prove helpful in controlling acid hypersecretion. If this is ineffective, either conversion of the Billroth II to a Billroth I reconstruction or excision of the retained antral tissue in the duodenal stump is indicated.

Postvagotomy Syndromes

Postvagotomy Diarrhea

About 30% or more of patients suffer from diarrhea after gastric surgery. For most patients, it is not severe and usually disappears within the first 3 to 4 months. For some patients, the diarrhea is part of the dumping syndrome previously described. However, vagotomy is also associated with alterations in stool frequency. Truncal vagotomy has been reported to result in increased frequency of daily bowel movements in 30% to 70% of patients. In some, the diarrhea may occur 2 to 3 times weekly or manifest itself once or twice a month. In others, it may be more explosive and result in soiled clothing. Most patients with postvagotomy diarrhea have their symptoms resolve over time. In those patients whose symptoms fail to resolve, cholestyramine, an anionic exchange resin that absorbs bile salts rendering them unabsorbable and inactive, can significantly diminish the severity of diarrhea. However, because postvagotomy diarrhea is usually self-limited, treatment should be symptomatic. Treatment with cholestyramine should show signs of improvement within 1 to 4 weeks of initiation of treatment. Four grams of cholestyramine with meals three times daily followed by an adjustment to a maintenance dosage should decrease bowel movements to once or twice a day. Only in rare cases is operative therapy necessary for postvagotomy diarrhea. When diarrhea has remained incapacitating for at least 1 year after initial gastric surgery, the diarrhea fails to respond to cholestyramine therapy, and other causes have been ruled out, surgery is indicated. This should involve no more than 1% of all patients undergoing vagotomy. The operative procedure of choice is to interpose a 10-cm segment of reverse jejunum 70 to 100 cm from the ligament of Treitz. This has led to sustained relief of diarrhea in most patients subjected to this operation.

Postvagotomy Gastric Atony

After vagotomy, gastric emptying is delayed. This is true for both truncal and selective vagotomies but not in the case of highly selective or parietal cell vagotomy. With selective or truncal vagotomy, patients lose antral pump function and therefore have a reduction in their ability to empty solids. In contrast, emptying of liquids is accelerated because of loss of receptive relaxation in the proximal stomach, which regulates liquid emptying. Although most patients undergoing vagotomy and a drainage procedure manage to adequately empty their stomach, some patients have persistent gastric stasis that results in retention of food within the stomach for several hours. This may be accompanied by a feeling of fullness and occasionally abdominal pain. In still rarer cases, it may be associated with a functional gastric outlet obstruction. The diagnosis of gastroparesis is confirmed on scintigraphic assessment of gastric emptying. However, other causes of delayed gastric emptying, such as diabetes mellitus, electrolyte imbalance, drug toxicity, and neuromuscular disorders, must also be excluded. In addition, a mechanical cause of gastric outlet obstruction, such as postoperative adhesions, afferent or efferent loop obstruction, and internal herniations, must be ruled out. Endoscopic examination of the stomach also needs to be performed to rule out any anastomotic obstructions. In those patients with a functional gastric outlet obstruction and documented gastroparesis, pharmacotherapy is usually employed. The agents most commonly used are prokinetic agents such as metoclopramide and erythromycin. Metoclopramide exerts it prokinetic effects by acting as a dopamine antagonist and has cholinergic-enhancing effects as a result of facilitation of acetylcholine release from enteric cholinergic neurons. In contrast, erythromycin markedly accelerates gastric emptying by binding to motilin receptors on GI smooth muscle cells, where it acts as a motilin agonist. One of these two agents usually is sufficient to enhance gastric tone and improve gastric emptying.

Incomplete Vagal Transection

When performing vagotomy, it is important to denervate the acid-secreting portion of the stomach. If not performed properly, it predisposes the patient to the possible development of recurrent ulcer formation. The type of vagotomy performed influences the likelihood of this problem. In highly selective vagotomy, incomplete vagotomy is rarely a problem because of the meticulous dissection required during this procedure. In contrast, truncal vagotomy may be associated with incomplete transection because of the variability in size of the two trunks and

their anatomic position. Either vagus nerve may be incompletely transected during truncal vagotomy, although the right vagus nerve is more frequently transected inadequately than the left. In contrast to the left vagus nerve, which usually hugs the anterior esophageal surface, the right vagus nerve is frequently buried in the periesophageal tissue, potentially leading to incomplete transection. Histologic confirmation of vagal transection decreases the incidence of incomplete vagotomy.

STRESS GASTRITIS

Stress gastritis has been referred to as *stress ulcerations, stress erosive gastritis,* and *hemorrhagic gastritis.* These lesions may lead to life-threatening gastric bleeding and by definition occur after physical trauma, shock, sepsis, hemorrhage, or respiratory failure. They are characterized by multiple, superficial (nonulcerating) erosions that begin in the proximal or acid-secreting portion of the stomach and progress distally. They may also occur in the setting of central nervous system disease such as that seen with Cushing's ulcer or as a result of thermal burn injury involving more than 30% of the body surface area (Curling's ulcer).

Stress gastritis lesions typically change with time. They may be detected within hours after injury and are considered early if they appear within the first 24 hours. These early lesions are typically multiple and shallow, with discrete areas of erythema along with focal hemorrhage or an adherent clot. If the lesion erodes into the submucosa, which contains the blood supply, frank bleeding may result. On microscopy, these lesions appear as wedged-shaped mucosal hemorrhages with coagulation necrosis of the superficial mucosal cells. They are almost always seen in the fundus of the stomach and only rarely in the distal stomach. Acute stress gastritis can be classified as late if there is a tissue reaction or organization around a clot, or if an inflammatory exudate is present. This picture may be seen by microscopy 24 to 72 hours after injury. Late lesions appear identical to regenerating mucosa around a healing gastric ulcer. Both types of lesions can be seen endoscopically.

Pathophysiology

Although the precise mechanisms responsible for the development of stress gastritis remain to be fully elucidated, current evidence suggests a multifactorial etiology. These stress-induced gastric lesions appear to require the presence of acid. Other factors that may predispose to the development of these lesions include impaired mucosal defense mechanisms against luminal acid such as a reduction in blood flow, a reduction in mucus, a reduction in bicarbonate secretion by mucosal cells, or a reduction in endogenous prostaglandins. All these factors render the stomach more susceptible to damage from luminal acid with the resultant hemorrhagic gastritis. Stress is considered present when hypoxia, sepsis, or organ failure occurs. When stress is present, mucosal ischemia is thought to be the main factor responsible for the breakdown of these normal defense mechanisms. In this setting, luminal acid is then able to damage the compromised mucosa. There is little evidence to suggest that increased gastric acid secretion occurs in this situation. However, the presence of luminal acid appears to be a prerequisite for this form of gastritis to evolve. Moreover, complete neutralization of luminal acid or antisecretory therapy precludes the development of experimental stress gastritis.

The frequency of life-threatening hemorrhage from stress gastritis appears to be diminishing and may be related to improvements in our ability to manage critically ill patients. Consequently, there are few well-designed, prospective, randomized trials to identify risk factors for patients at risk for developing this disease process. With the studies that have been performed with a limited number of patients, other risk factors or predisposing clinical conditions have been identified. These include the presence of adult respiratory syndrome, multiple trauma, major burn over 35% of body surface area, oliguric renal failure, large transfusion requirements, hepatic dysfunction, hypotension, prolonged surgical procedures, and sepsis from any source. A direct correlation has also been identified between acute upper GI hemorrhage and the severity of the underlying critical illness.

Most studies probably underestimate the true incidence of stress gastritis unless endoscopy is performed because at least one study has shown that gastric erosions are present in almost every patient with a life-threatening injury. The major predisposing condition appears to be sepsis. Major thermal burns also significantly increase the risk for development of stress gastritis. In severely burned patients, one study demonstrated that gastric erosions are present in 93% of these patients on endoscopy and that the occurrence of severe acute upper GI hemorrhage was about 25% to 50%.

Presentation and Diagnosis

More than 50% of patients develop their stress gastritis within 1 to 2 days after a traumatic event. The only clinical sign may be painless upper GI bleeding that may be delayed at onset. The bleeding is usually slow and intermittent and may be detected by only a few flecks of blood in the nasogastric tube or an unexplained drop in the hemoglobin. On occasion, there may be profound upper GI hemorrhage that is accompanied by hypotension and hematemesis. The stool is frequently guaiac-positive, although melena and hematochezia are rare. Endoscopy is required to confirm the diagnosis and to differentiate stress gastritis from other sources of GI hemorrhage.

Therapy

Any patient with upper GI bleeding requires prompt and definitive fluid resuscitation with correction of any coagulation or platelet abnormalities. If blood is required, it should be administered without delay, and if there are specific clotting abnormalities or platelet deficiencies,

fresh frozen plasma and platelets should likewise be administered. In patients being treated for sepsis, broad-spectrum antibiotics, in conjunction with source control of the infection, need to be undertaken. Treatment of the underlying sepsis plays a major role in treating the underlying gastric erosions. Saline lavage of the stomach through a nasogastric tube will help to remove any pooled blood and to prevent gastric distention, which stimulates gastrin release. Nasogastric decompression also removes noxious substances such as bile and pancreatic juice that could potentially further compromise the stomach. More than 80% of patients who present with upper GI hemorrhage stop bleeding using this approach. When the nasogastric tube aspirate is clear, indicating that bleeding has ceased, intraluminal gastric pH should be maintained at greater than 5.0 with antisecretory agents. Usually this involves the utilization of proton pump inhibitors or, alternatively, H_2-receptor antagonists with or without combination antacid therapy. There is little evidence to suggest that endoscopy with electrocautery or heater probe coagulation has any benefit in the therapy of bleeding from acute stress gastritis. However, some studies suggest that acute bleeding can be effectively controlled by selective infusion of vasopressin into the splanchnic circulation through the left gastric artery. Vasopressin is administered by continuous infusion through the catheter at a rate of 0.2 to 0.4 IU/min for a maximum of 48 to 72 hours. If the patient has underlying cardiac or liver disease, vasopressin should not be used. Although vasopressin may decrease blood loss, it has not been shown to result in improved survival. Other angiographic techniques that can be employed include embolization of the left gastric artery if bleeding is identified on angiography. However, the extensive plexus of submucosal arterial vessels within the stomach makes this approach less appealing and not as successful.

Bleeding that recurs or persists requiring more than 6 units of blood (3000 mL) is an indication for operation. Because most of the lesions are in the proximal stomach or fundus, a long anterior gastrotomy should be made in this area. The gastric lumen is cleared of blood and the mucosal surface inspected for bleeding points. All bleeding areas are oversewn with figure-of-eight stitches taken deep within the gastric wall. Most of the superficial erosions are not actively bleeding and therefore do not require ligature unless a blood vessel is seen at it base. The operation is completed by closing the anterior gastrotomy and then performing a truncal vagotomy and pyloroplasty to reduce acid secretion. The incidence of rebleeding is less than 5% if bleeding points are carefully looked for and secured. Less commonly, a partial gastrectomy, in combination with vagotomy, is performed. Rarely, and only in patients with life-threatening hemorrhage refractory to other forms of therapy, should total gastrectomy be performed

Prophylaxis

Because of the high mortality rate in patients with acute stress gastritis who develop massive upper GI hemorrhage, high-risk patients should be treated prophylactically. Because mucosal ischemia may alter a number of mucosal defense mechanisms that enable the stomach to withstand luminal irritants and protect itself from injury, every effort should be made to correct any perfusion deficits from shock.

Sepsis needs to be controlled with antibiotics and source control; ventilatory support needs to be optimized in addition to correcting any systemic acid-base abnormalities or electrolyte abnormalities; and patients require adequate nutrition preferably through the enteral route, which is associated with fewer infectious complications. In addition to optimizing patient care, several medical therapies are available for prophylaxis, and most are aimed at neutralizing or preventing acid secretion.

The patients at risk for stress gastritis in the intensive care setting appear to be patients with respiratory failure and underlying coagulopathy.[25] For patients who do not have coagulopathy or require mechanical ventilation for less than 48 hours, one study suggested that prophylaxis for stress gastritis was unnecessary.[25]

Antacids can be administered as prophylaxis for stress gastritis and have an efficacy of 96%. This usually requires hourly administration of antacids (30-60 mL) by nasogastric tube to maintain the intraluminal gastric pH above 3.5. If the pH can be maintained above 5.0, more than 99.9% of acid will be neutralized, and pepsin will be inactive. Interestingly, in a review of data collected from 16 prospective trials (2133 patients), 3.7% of patients given antacids had evidence of blood loss, compared with 17.4% given cimetidine for prophylaxis against stress gastritis and 27.3% for those given placebo. Thus, there appears to be no significant advantage of H_2 blockers over antacids. In fact, most studies have demonstrated that it is easier to maintain a pH greater than 5 with antacids than with standard intermittent doses of H_2-receptor antagonist. However, recent data suggest that continuous infusions of the H_2-receptor antagonists provide more consistent maintenance of intraluminal gastric pH than do standard intermittent infusions.

Whether continuous infusion of H_2-receptor antagonists has a better clinical outcome or improves drug safety has yet to be determined. Nevertheless, H_2-receptor antagonists have about a 97% efficacy when used as medical prophylaxis for stress gastritis.

Sucralfate has also been used for prophylaxis against stress gastritis and, like antacids and H_2-receptor antagonists, is extremely efficacious, in the 90% to 97% range. Sucralfate, 1 g every 6 hours, appears to be just as effective as antacids or cimetidine. This form of prophylaxis has the added effect of allowing the stomach to maintain its normal pH and thus prevent bacterial overgrowth. This latter effect may be beneficial because several studies have suggested that gastric luminal alkalinization predisposes the stomach to bacterial overgrowth and subsequent nosocomial pneumonia. Exogenous prostaglandins have also been used as stress gastritis prophylaxis agents, although their efficacy appears to be much less than that of the other agents.

GASTRIC NEOPLASIA

Benign Tumors

Gastric Polyps

Gastric polyps are usually an incidental finding on endoscopy, detected in 2% to 3% of gastroscopic evaluations. Fundic gland polyps constitute 47% of all gastric polyps and have no malignant potential. Typically, they present as multiple 2- to 3-mm sessile lesions in the body and fundus, most commonly in healthy gastric mucosa. Most cases are sporadic, but gastric polyps can occur in 53% of patients with familial adenomatous polyposis or Gardner's syndrome. Although the polyps themselves are non-neoplastic, retrospective studies have reported colorectal neoplasms in up to 60% of patients with gastric fundic gland polyps.[26]

Hyperplastic polyps are among the most frequently observed polyps and compose 28% to 75% of all gastric polyps. The lesions are typically less than 1.5 cm in size and arise in a setting of chronic atrophic gastritis 40% to 75% of the time. Most commonly, the chronic atrophic gastritis is secondary to *H. pylori* infection, the treatment of which may result in polyp regression. Although the hyperplastic polyp itself is non-neoplastic, dysplastic changes may occasionally develop in the polyp. Frank adenocarcinoma is detected in 2% of hyperplastic polyps. When detected, endoscopic polypectomy is indicated for histologic examination.

Adenomatous polyps have a distinct risk for malignancy. They account for 10% of all gastric polyps and most commonly are antral, sessile, solitary, and eroded. The adenomas can present as tubular, tubulovillous, or villous. Gastric adenocarcinoma may be found in 21% of cases, with increased risk with larger size and villous histology. Polyps more than 4 cm in diameter may harbor carcinoma 40% of the time. Focal carcinomas were found in 6% of flat tubular adenomas and 33% of villous and tubulovillous adenomas. Additionally, the presence of gastric adenomas is a marker for increased risk for developing adenocarcinoma in another part of the stomach. Coincident carcinomas have been reported in 8% to 59% of cases.[27] Endoscopic polypectomy is sufficient treatment if the entire polyp is removed and there is no invasive cancer in the specimen. Operative excision is recommended for sessile lesions larger than 2 cm, polyps found to have areas of invasive tumor, or polyps that are symptomatic secondary to pain or bleeding. Because of the increased risk for coincident gastric carcinoma, these patients should be followed closely by serial endoscopies.

Ectopic Pancreas

Ectopic pancreatic tissue arises during embryonal development during the fusion of the dorsal and ventral pancreatic buds. The ectopic pancreatic tissue is implanted in the bowel wall and carried to its final location. The incidence of ectopic pancreatic tissue is 1% to 2% in autopsy series, with 70% of cases occurring in the stomach, duodenum, and jejunum. Most patients with gastric ectopic pancreatic tissue are asymptomatic, whereas others present with symptoms similar to those of PUD. The most common presenting symptoms are abdominal pain (45%), epigastric discomfort (12%), nausea and vomiting (10%), and bleeding (8%). The mass can be visualized on upper GI endoscopy; however, tissue diagnosis can be difficult because of the submucosal location of the rests. Endoscopic ultrasonography can be a useful adjunct for diagnosis as well as for guided biopsy. Pancreatic rests that cause symptoms are treated by surgical excision.

Malignant Tumors

Adenocarcinoma

Epidemiology

Gastric carcinoma was the most common cancer worldwide in the 1980s and is now surpassed only by lung cancer as the leading cause of cancer deaths. There is substantial geographic variation in the incidence of gastric carcinoma internationally, with higher rates in Japan and some parts of South America and lower rates in Western Europe and the United States.

Gastric cancer is the 14th most common cancer in the United States, the incidence of which has been decreasing over the past 70 years. About 22,000 patients are diagnosed with gastric cancer each year, of whom 11,500 will die. Gastric cancer in the United States is twice as common in men as it is in women, and the incidence is higher among U.S. black men than white men.[28] The incidence also increases with age, peaking in the seventh decade. Studies of migrant populations from areas of high incidence to areas of low incidence suggest that environmental exposure as well as other cultural or genetic factors influence the predisposition to gastric cancer. The risk for gastric cancer in individuals who migrated from the highest risk areas in Japan persisted even when they adopted a Western diet. However, offspring who adopted a Western-style diet had a markedly decreased risk. There has been a noticeable shift in the site of gastric cancer from the distal stomach to the more proximal stomach over the past several decades. The incidence of adenocarcinoma of the gastric cardia has increased steadily, whereas the incidence of cancer in other anatomic subsites has decreased. The increase was most noticeable for white men and is possibly linked to a history of smoking or heavy alcohol use.

Risk Factors

Most epidemiologic studies investigating the role of diet in relation to the development of gastric cancer associate diets low in animal protein and fat, high in complex carbohydrates, high in salted meats and fish, and with high levels of nitrates or *H. pylori* in drinking water with an increased risk for gastric cancer. It appears that the long-term ingestion of nitrates in dried, smoked, and salted food contributes to this increased risk. Nitrates are converted to carcinogenic nitrites by bacteria. Such bacteria may be introduced through consumption of partially decayed foods, a practice that is more common in the lower social economic strata worldwide. Conversely, the consumption of raw vegetables, citrus fruits, and high-

Table 47-6 Factors Associated With Increased Risk for Developing Stomach Cancer

| **Nutritional** |
| Low fat or protein consumption |
| Salted meat or fish |
| High nitrate consumption |
| High complex-carbohydrate consumption |
| **Environmental** |
| Poor food preparation (smoked, salted) |
| Lack of refrigeration |
| Poor drinking water (well water) |
| Smoking |
| **Social** |
| Low social class |
| **Medical** |
| Prior gastric surgery |
| *Helicobacter pylori* infection |
| Gastric atrophy and gastritis |
| Adenomatous polyps |
| Male gender |

fiber breads is associated with a lower risk for gastric cancer. The ascorbic acid and β-carotene found in fruits and vegetables act as antioxidants, whereas ascorbic acid can also prevent the conversion of nitrates to nitrites (Table 47-6).

Other factors associated with an increased risk for gastric cancer include low socioeconomic status (except in Japan), cigarette smoking, male gender, and *H. pylori* infection. The presence of IgG antibodies to *H. pylori* in a given population correlates with the local incidence and mortality rates of gastric cancer. Different strains of this organism elicit different levels of antibody response. For example, infection with the *cagA* strain elicits more mucosal inflammation than *cagA*-negative strains and also confers a greater risk for developing gastric cancer.[29] Interestingly, host genetic factors also tend to play a role by which individuals with *H. pylori* infection will eventually develop gastric cancer. Interleukin-1 gene cluster polymorphisms, which enhance the production of interleukin-1β, are associated with an increased risk for hypochlorhydria induced by *H. pylori* and thus gastric cancer.[30] Therefore, the familial clustering of *H. pylori* infection associated with inherited genetic polymorphisms linked to hypochlorhydria may explain the increase in cancer risk in individuals with a family history of gastric cancer.

Balfour first reported a correlation between prior gastric surgery for benign disease and the subsequent development of gastric cancer in 1922. Subsequent meta-analyses support the conclusion that there is an increased risk for gastric remnant cancer in patients with prior partial gastrectomy. However, the risk is only observed after a latency of 15 years and is increased in patients operated on for gastric but not duodenal ulcers. The incidence of malignancy ranges from 2% to 6% in gastric remnants, and a variety of causative factors have been proposed to include alkaline duodenal gastric reflux as well as increased *N*-nitroso compounds secondary to bacterial overgrowth. The development of atrophic gastritis along with gastritis cystica profunda can be associated with dysplasia in 5% of patients, for which surveillance endoscopy is indicated.

Patients with pernicious anemia are also at increased risk for developing gastric cancer. Pernicious anemia is an autoimmune gastritis of the oxyntic mucosa and increases the risk for gastric cancer, as do other types of chronic inflammation. Achlorhydria is the defining feature of this condition because the autoimmune reaction destroys chief and parietal cells. The mucosa becomes very atrophic and develops antral and intestinal metaplasia. The relative risk for a patient with pernicious anemia developing gastric cancer is about 2.1 to 5.6.

The presence of gastric polyps can increase a patient's risk for gastric cancer. Hyperplastic polyps, the most common histologic type, are benign. However, their presence is associated with an increased risk for gastric cancer because they form in stomachs with established gastritis, a known risk factor for carcinoma.

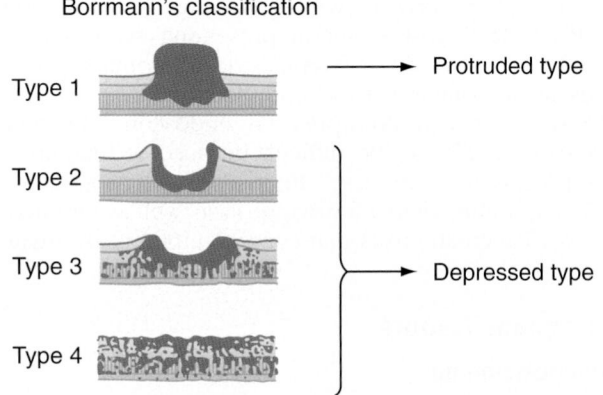

Figure 47-18 Borrmann's pathologic classification of gastric cancer based on gross appearance. (From Iriyama K, Asakawa T, Koike H, et al: Is extensive lymphadenectomy necessary for surgical treatment of intramucosal carcinoma of the stomach? Arch Surg 124:309, 1989. Copyright 1989, American Medical Association.)

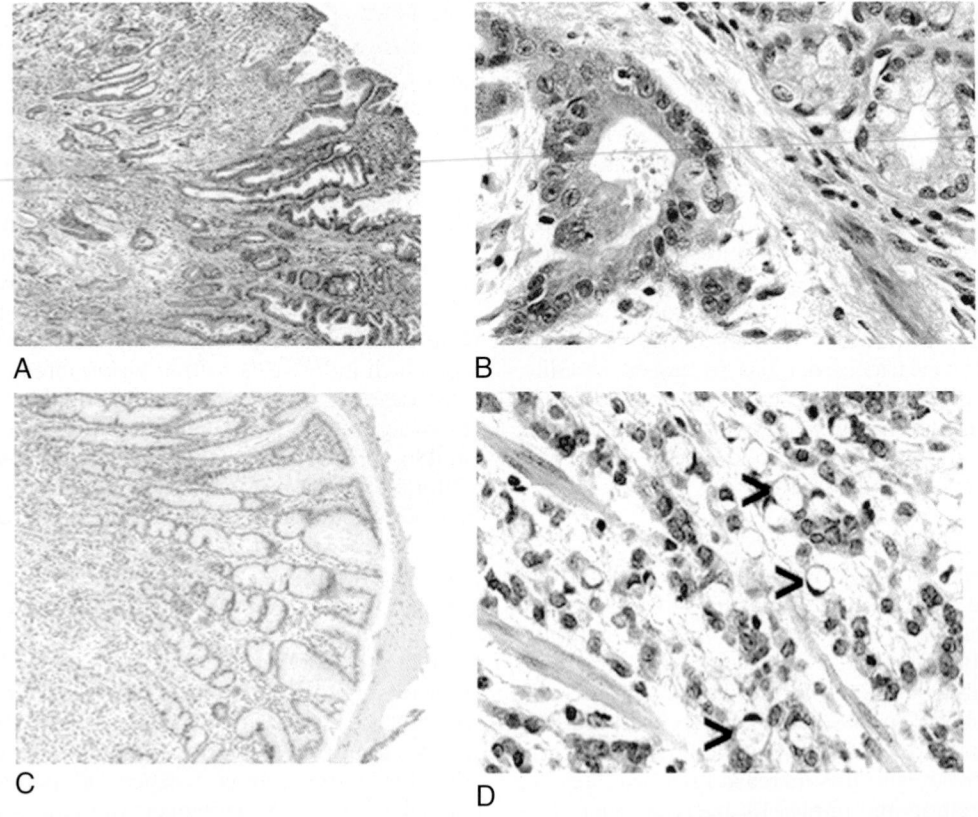

Figure 47-19 Photomicrographs of gastric adenocarcinoma. **A,** Gastric adenocarcinoma intestinal type (H&E, ×25). **B,** Gastric adenocarcinoma intestinal type (H&E, ×400). **C,** Gastric adenocarcinoma diffuse type (H&E, ×25). **D,** Gastric adenocarcinoma diffuse type (H&E, ×400). *Arrows* on signet ring cells. (Courtesy of Dr. Marylee Kott, Department of Pathology, University of Texas Health Science Center, Houston.)

Adenomatous polyps carry a distinct risk for the development of malignancy in the polyp. Mucosal atypia is frequent, and progression from dysplasia to carcinoma in situ has been observed. The risk for the development of carcinoma is about 10% to 20% and increases with increasing size of the polyp. Endoscopic removal is indicated for pedunculated lesions and is sufficient if the polyp is completely removed and there are no foci of invasive cancer on histologic examination. If the polyp is larger than 2 cm, is sessile, or has a proven focus of invasive carcinoma, operative excision is warranted.

Recently, several genetic alterations have been identified that are associated with gastric adenocarcinoma. These changes can be classified as the activation of oncogenes, the inactivation of tumor suppressor genes, the reduction of cellular adhesion, the reactivation of telomerase, and the presence of microsatellite instability. The c-*met* proto-oncogene is the receptor for the hepatocyte growth factor and is frequently overexpressed in gastric cancer, as are the k-*sam* and c-*erbB2* oncogenes. The inactivation of the tumor suppressor genes *p53* and *p16* has been reported in both diffuse and intestinal-type cancers, whereas adenomatous polyposis coli (*APC*) gene mutations tend to be more frequent in intestinal-type gastric cancers. Additionally, a reduction or loss in the cell adhesion molecule E-cadherin can be found in about 50% of diffuse-type gastric cancers.[31] Microsatellite instability can be found in about 20% to 30% of intestinal-type gastric cancer. Microsatellites are lengths of DNA in which a short (one to five nucleotides) motif is repeated several times. Microsatellite instability reflects a gain or loss of repeat units in a germline microsatellite allele, indicating the clonal expansion that is typical of a neoplasm.

Pathology

Ninety-five percent of all malignant gastric neoplasms are adenocarcinomas. Other histologic types include squamous cell carcinoma, adenoacanthoma, carcinoid tumors, GI stromal tumors, and lymphoma. Numerous pathologic classification schemes of gastric cancer have been proposed. The Borrmann classification system was developed in 1926 and remains useful today for the description of endoscopic findings. The Borrmann system divides gastric carcinoma into five types depending on the lesion's macroscopic appearance. Borrmann type 1 represents polypoid or fungating lesions; type 2, ulcerating lesions surrounded by elevated borders; type 3, ulcerating lesions with infiltration into the gastric wall; type 4, diffusely infiltrating lesions; and type 5, lesions that do not fit into any of the other categories (Fig. 47-18). *Linitis plastica* is the term to describe type 4 carcinoma when it involves the entire stomach. The original histologic classification system was developed by Borders in 1942. Borders classified gastric carcinomas according to the degree of cellular differentiation, independent of morphology, and ranged from 1 (well differentiated) to 4 (anaplastic). Many other classification systems have been proposed; however, the most useful and widely used system remains the one proposed by Lauren in 1965. The Lauren system separates gastric adenocarcinoma into intestinal or diffuse types based on histology (Fig. 47-19).

This schema characterizes two varieties of gastric adenocarcinoma that manifest different pathology, epidemiology, pathogenesis, and prognosis (Table 47-7). The intestinal variant typically arises in the setting of a recognizable precancerous condition such as gastric atrophy or intestinal metaplasia. Men are more commonly affected than women, and the incidence of the intestinal-type gastric adenocarcinoma increases with age. The intestinal variety is well differentiated with a tendency to form glands. Metastatic spread is generally hematogenous to distant organs.

The intestinal type is also the dominant histology in areas in which gastric cancer is epidemic, suggesting an environmental etiology. Correa and colleagues proposed a model for the pathogenesis of the intestinal type that is based on progression from gastritis to carcinoma over the course of several decades (Fig. 47-20). An intermediate step in Correa's model of gastric cancer development is intestinal metaplasia. Intestinal metaplasia is defined by the replacement of the gastric mucosa with epithelium that resembles small bowel mucosa. This replacement is effected by gastric stem cells, which are diverted from gastric cell–specific pathways into the pathway of the small intestine secondary to persistent irritation of the gastric mucosa, most commonly from *H. pylori* infection. Intestinal metaplasia can be subclassified into complete type I and the incomplete types II and III. The types differ based on the patterns of mucin core protein (MUC) expression as well as cell type composition. Type I is characterized by the presence of absorptive cells, Paneth cells, and goblet cells secreting sialomucins, whereas the incomplete types are characterized by the presence of columnar and goblet cells secreting sialomucins, sulfomucins, or both. The risk for progression from intestinal metaplasia to gastric cancer is higher in the type III metaplasia than in type I.[32] A wide range of molecular alterations in intestinal metaplasia have been described and may affect the transformation into gastric cancer. These include overexpression of cyclooxygenase-2 and cyclin D2, *p53* mutations, microsatellite instability, decreased

Table 47-7 Lauren Classification System

INTESTINAL	DIFFUSE
Environmental	Familial
Gastric atrophy, intestinal metaplasia	Blood type A
Men>women	Women>men
Increasing incidence with age	Younger age group
Gland formation	Poorly differentiated, signet ring cells
Hematogenous spread	Transmural/lymphatic spread
Microsatellite instability *APC* gene mutations	Decreased E-cadherin
p53, p16 inactivation	*p53, p16* inactivation

APC, adenomatous polyposis coli.

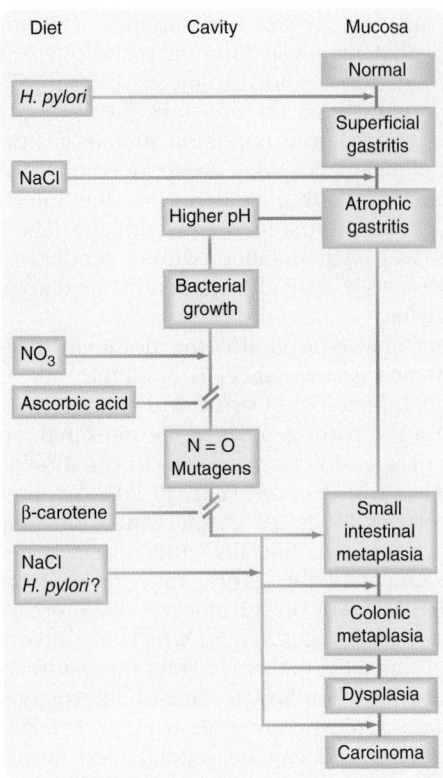

Figure 47-20 Correa model of the pathogenesis of human gastric adenocarcinoma. (From Correa P: Human gastric carcinogenesis: A multistep and multifactoral process. First Cancer Society Award Lecture on Cancer Epidemiology and Prevention. Cancer Res 52:6735, 1992.)

p27 expression, and alterations in transcription factors like CDX1 and CDX2.[33] It is clear that intestinal metaplasia is a risk factor for the development of gastric carcinoma; however, not every patient with intestinal metaplasia develops invasive cancer.

The recent description of a metaplastic cell lineage expressing the intestinal mucosal trefoil peptide, spasmolytic polypeptide, in the gastric remnant of patients with dysplasia has led to the concept that spasmolytic polypeptide–expressing metaplasia (SPEM) may be a precursor to gastric adenocarcinoma. SPEM is associated with chronic *H. pylori* fundic gastritis and is expressed in gastric mucosa adjacent to gastric adenocarcinomas.[34] Additionally, the identification of SPEM in the setting of gastritis has been associated with the subsequent development of gastric carcinoma.[35] Although studies evaluating the prevention of gastric adenocarcinoma by *H. pylori* eradication have been inconclusive, better risk stratification is needed to demonstrate effectiveness. Further elucidation of the molecular alterations associated with SPEM may facilitate the development of alternative chemopreventive strategies.

The diffuse form of gastric adenocarcinoma is poorly differentiated, lacks gland formation, and is composed of signet ring cells. The diffuse variant consists of tiny clusters of small uniform cells, tends to spread submucosally,

has less inflammatory infiltration, and metastasizes early. The route of spread is generally by transmural extension and through lymphatic invasion. The diffuse form does not generally arise in the setting of prior gastritis, is more common in women, and affects a slightly younger age group. The diffuse form also has an association with blood type A and familial occurrences, suggesting a genetic etiology. Intraperitoneal metastases are frequent, and in general, the prognosis is less favorable for patients with diffuse-subtype histology.

In 1990, the World Health Organization (WHO) recommended another classification system for gastric cancers that is based on morphologic features. In the WHO system, gastric cancer is divided into five main categories: adenocarcinoma, adenosquamous cell carcinoma, squamous cell carcinoma, undifferentiated carcinoma, and unclassified carcinoma. Adenocarcinomas are further subdivided into four types according to their growth pattern: papillary, tubular, mucinous, and signet ring. Each type is further subdivided by degree of differentiation. Although widely used, the WHO classification system offers little in terms of patient management, and there are a significant number of gastric cancers that do not fit into their categories. There is little evidence that any of the above classification systems can add to the prognostic information provided by the American Joint Cancer Commission (AJCC) tumor node metastases (TNM) staging system (Table 47-8).

Clinical Presentation

Gastric adenocarcinoma lacks specific symptoms early in the course of the disease. Patients often ignore early vague epigastric discomfort and indigestion, which are often mistaken for gastritis, leading to symptomatic treatment for 6 to 12 months before diagnostic studies are ordered. The epigastric pain is similar to pain caused by benign ulcers and similarly may mimic angina. Typically, however, the pain is constant, nonradiating, and unrelieved by food ingestion. More advanced disease may present with weight loss, anorexia, fatigue, or vomiting. Symptoms often reflect the site of origin of the tumor. Proximal tumors involving the gastroesophageal junction often present with dysphagia, whereas distal antral tumors may present as gastric outlet obstruction. Diffuse mural involvement by tumor, as occurs in linitis plastica, leads to decreased distensibility of the stomach and complaints of early satiety. Clinically significant GI bleeding is rare, but as many as 15% of patients may develop hematemesis, and 40% of patients are anemic. Very large tumors may erode through the stomach and into the transverse colon, presenting as large bowel obstruction.

Physical signs develop late in the course of the disease and are most commonly associated with locally advanced or metastatic disease. Patients may present with a palpable abdominal mass, a palpable supraclavicular (Virchow's) or periumbilical (Sister Mary Joseph's) lymph node, peritoneal metastasis palpable by rectal examination (Blummer's shelf), or a palpable ovarian mass (Krukenberg's tumor). As the disease progresses, patients may develop hepatomegaly secondary to metastasis, jaundice, ascites, and cachexia.

Table 47-8 TNM Classification of Carcinoma of the Stomach

CATEGORY	CRITERIA
Primary Tumor (T)	
TX	Primary tumor cannot be assessed
T0	No evidence of primary tumor
Tis	Carcinoma in situ: intraepithelial tumor without invasion of the lamina propria
T1	Tumor invades lamina propria or submucosa
T2	Tumor invades muscularis propria or subserosa
T2a	Tumor invades muscularis propria
T2b	Tumor invades subserosa
T3	Tumor penetrates serosa (visceral peritoneum) without invasion of adjacent structures
T4	Tumor invades adjacent structures
Regional Lymph Nodes (N)	
NX	Regional lymph node(s) cannot be assessed
N0	No regional lymph node metastasis
N1	Metastasis in 1 to 6 regional lymph nodes
N2	Metastasis in 7 to 15 regional lymph nodes
N3	Metastasis in more than 15 regional lymph nodes
Distant Metastasis (M)	
MX	Distant metastasis cannot be assessed
M0	No distant metastasis
M1	Distant metastasis

Stage Grouping

Stage	T	N	M
Stage 0	Tis	N0	M0
Stage 1A	T1	N0	M0
Stage IB	T1	N1	M0
	T2a/b	N0	M0
Stage II	T1	N2	M0
	T2a/b	N1	M0
	T3	N0	M0
Stage IIIA	T2a/b	N2	M0
	T3	N1	M0
	T4	N0	M0
Stage IIIB	T3	N2	M0
Stage IV	T4	N1-3	M0
	T1-3	N3	M0
	Any T	Any N	M1

From AJCC Cancer Staging Manual, 6th ed. New York, Springer-Verlag, 2001.

Preoperative Evaluation

When gastric cancer is suspected based on history and physical examination, flexible upper endoscopy is the diagnostic modality of choice. Although double-contrast barium upper GI radiography is cost-effective with 90% diagnostic accuracy, the inability to distinguish benign from malignant gastric ulcers makes endoscopy preferable. During endoscopy, multiple biopsy samples (seven or more) should be obtained around the ulcer crater to facilitate histologic diagnosis. Biopsy of the ulcer crater itself may reveal only necrotic debris. When multiple biopsy specimens are taken, the diagnostic accuracy of the procedure approaches 98%. The addition of direct brush cytology to multiple biopsy specimens may increase the diagnostic accuracy of the study. Additionally, the size, location, and morphology of the tumor should be noted and other mucosal abnormalities carefully evaluated. In select patients with advanced disease, esophagogastroduodenoscopy provides a means for palliation through the use of laser ablation, dilation, or tumor stenting. Although not included in the National Comprehensive Cancer Network guidelines for the evaluation of gastric adenocarcinoma, some centers are using endoscopic ultrasonography (EUS) to assist in the staging of this disease. EUS can gauge the extent of gastric wall invasion as well as evaluate local nodal status. However, EUS cannot reliably distinguish tumor from fibrosis; therefore, it is not a good modality for evaluating response to therapy. Overall, staging accuracy with EUS is about 75%. Correct assignment of tumor stage by EUS is poor for AJCC T2 lesions (38%) but better for T1 (80%) and T3 (90%) lesions. Overall accuracy of nodal staging is 77%.[36] Although the accuracy of nodal staging can be improved by fine-needle aspiration biopsy, the application of this technique is limited by technical challenges. Because of the previously described limitations, the use of EUS in the evaluation of gastric cancer is largely confined to regional referral centers.

When the diagnosis of gastric cancer is confirmed, further studies should include a complete blood count, serum chemistries to include liver function tests, coagulation studies, chest x-ray, and CT scan of the abdomen. In women, a pelvic CT scan or ultrasound is also recommended. CT of the chest may be needed for proximal gastric cancers. CT can readily detect the presence of visceral metastatic disease as well as malignant ascites. The major limitations of CT are in the evaluation of early gastric primaries and in the detection of small (<5 mm) metastases in the liver or on peritoneal surfaces. The reported accuracy for CT staging of lymph node metastasis ranges from 25% to 86%.[37]

Because of the inaccuracy of CT and other modalities for the detection of macrometastases smaller than 5 mm on the peritoneal surface or liver, laparoscopy is recommended as the next step in the evaluation of patients with locoregional disease. Laparoscopy can detect metastatic disease in 23% to 37% of patients judged to be eligible for potentially curative resection by current-generation CT scanning. Sarela and associates[38] further defined the indications for staging laparoscopy by evaluating preoperatively available factors that predict M1 disease. In their institutional review, occult metastatic disease was found at laparoscopy only in patients in whom lymphadenopathy was detected by high-quality spiral CT and in patients whose tumors were located either at the gastroesophageal junction or diffusely throughout the stomach.

To determine the natural history of patients with laparoscopically detected M1 disease treated without primary resection, a retrospective review was performed.[39] In this single institutional review of 97 patients with M1 disease detected at laparoscopy and treated with chemotherapy and no resection, half of patients required no palliative intervention, and only 12% ultimately required

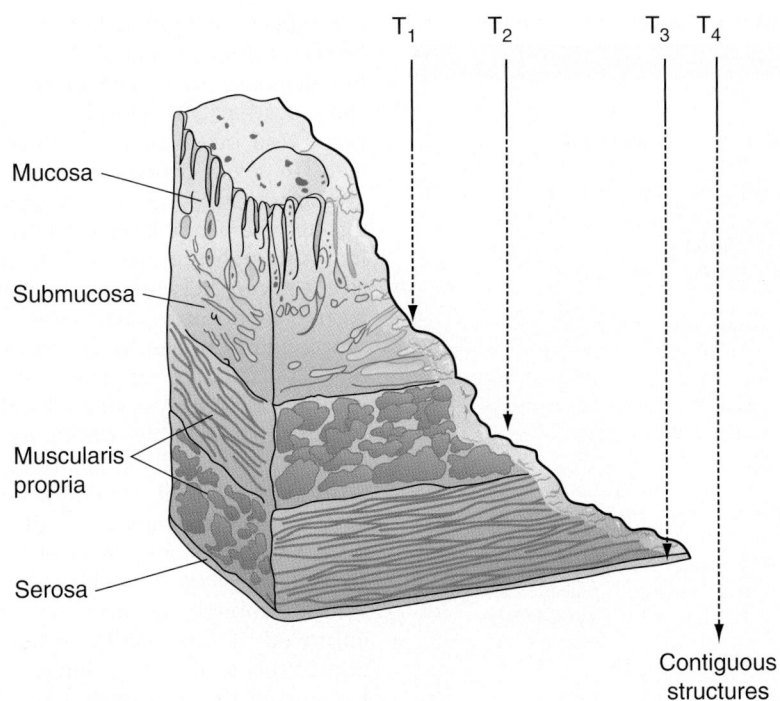

T₁ T₂ T₃ T₄

Mucosa

Submucosa

Muscularis
propria

Serosa

Contiguous
structures

Figure 47-21 T stage as defined by depth of penetration into the gastric wall. (From Alexander HR, Kelsen DG, Tepper JC: Cancer of the stomach. In De Vita VT, Hellman S, Rosenberg SA [eds]: Cancer: Principles and Practice of Oncology, 5th ed. Philadelphia, Lippincott-Raven, 1997.)

laparotomy. Procedures for gastric or GE junction obstruction were required in 33%, whereas 33% of patients required a blood transfusion. The median survival time of 10 months and estimated 1-year survival rate of 39% with a procedural-related mortality rate of 1% compare favorably to other series of gastric resection with M1 disease, in which median survival was reported to be 8 to 12 months, with a 1-year survival rate of 28% to 50% and a perioperative mortality rate of 2% to 19%. Laparoscopy may therefore improve palliation by avoiding a nontherapeutic laparotomy in patients presumed to have localized gastric cancer. The addition of laparoscopic ultrasonography may increase the sensitivity of laparoscopic staging in gastric cancer as it has in other abdominal malignancies. However, given the limitations of the available data and the operator-dependent nature of the technique, further investigation is required to define the role of ultrasound in the staging of gastric cancer.

Cytologic analysis of peritoneal fluid or of fluid obtained by peritoneal lavage may reveal the presence of free intraperitoneal gastric cancer cells, identifying patients with otherwise occult carcinomatosis. Patients with positive findings on peritoneal cytology have a poor prognosis, similar to that of patients with macroscopic stage IV disease. However, false-positive results can be obtained, and not all studies confirm the prognostic significance of positive findings. More sensitive methods of detecting free intraperitoneal gastric cancer cells, such as immunostaining and reverse-transcriptase polymerase chain reaction for carcinoembryonic antigen (CEA) messenger RNA, are under investigation.

Staging

Many staging systems have been proposed for gastric adenocarcinoma. A basic understanding of the older systems is necessary to understand the literature. The pathologic staging system currently in use worldwide is the AJCC TNM staging system. TNM stands for tumor, nodes, and metastasis and is based on depth of primary tumor invasion through the gastric wall (Fig. 47-21), the number of involved lymph nodes, and the presence or absence of distant metastasis. The TNM system can adequately stratify patients into distinct groups with different risks for tumor-related death. A major revision occurred in the AJCC staging system for gastric cancer in 1997 when nodal status stratification was changed from location of nodes to number of positive nodes. In the current staging system, a minimum of 15 nodes must be evaluated for accurate staging. Nodal staging is then determined by the number of positive nodes, with pN1 reflecting 1 to 6 positive nodes, pN2 designating 7 to 15 positive nodes, and pN3 more than 15 positive nodes. Some data suggest location of the primary (cardia compared with distal tumors) may independently predict survival. However, the current AJCC staging system does not reflect the poorer prognosis for proximal gastric tumors noted in some studies.

The term *R status* was first described by Hermanek in 1994 and is used to describe the tumor status after resection. R0 describes a microscopically margin-negative resection, in which no gross or microscopic tumor remains in the tumor bed. R1 indicates removal of all macroscopic disease, but microscopic margins are positive for tumor.

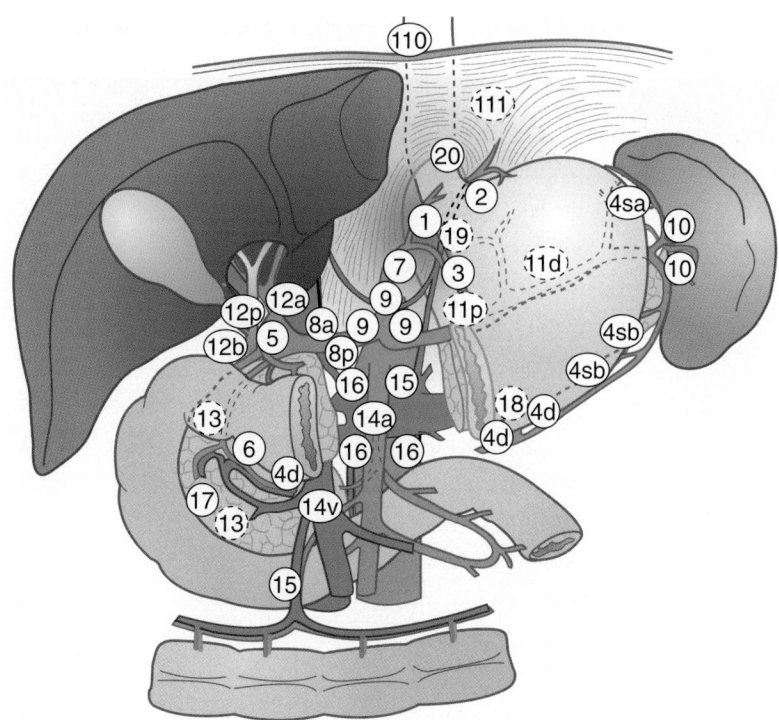

Figure 47-22 Lymph node station numbers as defined by the Japanese Gastric Cancer Association. (From Japanese Gastric Cancer Association: Japanese Classification of Gastric Carcinoma, 2nd English ed. Gastric Cancer 1:10-24, 1998.)

R2 indicates gross residual disease. Because the extent of resection can influence survival, some authors include this R designation to complement the TNM system. Long-term survival can be expected only after an R0 resection; therefore, a significant effort should be made to avoid R1 or R2 resections.

Knowledge of the older staging systems and the Japanese system is crucial to the understanding of the debate regarding lymphadenectomies for gastric cancer. In the previous edition of Union Internationale Contre le Cancer (UICC) TNM system, N categories were defined by the location of lymph node metastases relative to the primary. In 1982, UICC and AJCC agreed to define pN1 as 3 cm or less from the primary and pN2 as greater than 3 cm from the primary or nodal metastases along named blood vessels. The Japanese Classification for Gastric Carcinoma (JCGC) staging system was designed to describe the anatomic locations of nodes removed during gastrectomy. Sixteen distinct anatomic locations of lymph nodes are described (Fig. 47-22), with the recommendation for nodal basin dissection dependent on the location of the primary. The lymph node stations or echelons are numbered and then further classified into groups of echelons that correspond to the location of the primary and reflect the likelihood of harboring metastases (Table 47-9). The presence of metastasis to each lymph node group then determines the N classification. For example, metastases to any of the group 1 lymph nodes in the absence of disease in more distant lymph node groups is classified as N1.

Surgical Treatment

The optimal surgical management of gastric cancer must be tailored to the extent and location of disease. In the absence of distant metastatic spread, aggressive surgical resection of the gastric tumor is justified. The extent of gastric resection is determined by the need to obtain a resection margin free of microscopic disease. Because gastric tumors are characterized by extensive intramural spread, a line of resection at least 6 cm from the tumor mass is necessary to ensure a low rate of anastomotic recurrence. The appropriate surgical procedure should be determined by the location of the tumor and the known pattern of spread.

Tumors of the cardia and proximal stomach account for 35% to 50% of all gastric adenocarcinomas. In general, proximal tumors are more advanced at presentation than more distant tumors, so curative resections are rare. For proximal lesions, either total gastrectomy or proximal gastric resection is necessary to remove the tumor (Fig. 47-23).

Although there is no evidence that one operation is better than the other for tumor removal, there is abundant evidence that proximal gastric resection results in higher morbidity and mortality than total gastrectomy. In a series by Buhl, patients with a proximal gastric resection had higher incidences of dumping, heartburn, and reduced appetite than patients treated with distal or total gastrectomy.[40] In the Norwegian Stomach Cancer Trial, the morbidity and mortality rates after proximal gastric resections

Table 47-9 Grouping of Regional Lymph Nodes (Groups 1-3) by Location of Primary Tumor According to the Japanese Classification of Gastric Carcinoma

LYMPH NODE STATION (NO.)	DESCRIPTION	LOCATION OF PRIMARY TUMOR IN STOMACH		
		Upper Third	Middle Third	Lower Third
1	Right paracardial	1	1	2
2	Left paracardial	1	3	M
3	Lesser curvature	1	1	1
4sa	Short gastric	1	3	M
4sb	Left gastroepiploic	1	1	3
4d	Right gastroepiploic	2	1	1
5	Suprapyloric	3	1	1
6	Infrapyloric	3	1	1
7	Left gastric artery	2	2	2
8a	Anterior comm. hepatic	2	2	2
8p	Posterior comm. hepatic	3	3	3
9	Celiac artery	2	2	2
10	Splenic hilum	2	3	M
11p	Proximal splenic	2	2	2
11d	Distal splenic	2	3	M
12a	Left hepatoduodenal	3	2	2
12b,p	Posterior hepatoduodenal	3	3	3
13	Retropancreatic	M	3	3
14v	Superior mesenteric vein	M	3	2
14a	Superior mesenteric artery	M	M	M
15	Middle colic	M	M	M
16al	Aortic hiatus	3	M	M
16a2,b1	Para-aortic, middle	M	3	3
16b2	Para-aortic, caudal	M	M	M

M, lymph nodes regarded as distant metastasis.

were 52% and 16%, respectively, compared with 38% and 8% for total gastrectomy. Thus, total gastrectomy should be considered the procedure of choice for proximal gastric lesions. Distal tumors account for about 35% of all gastric cancers. Because recent studies have indicated no difference in 5-year survival between patients undergoing potentially curative subtotal versus total gastrectomy, subtotal gastrectomy is appropriate for patients in whom a negative margin resection can be performed. Studies of patients with recurrent gastric cancer have noted the median proximal margin of resection in patients with a recurrence to be 3.5 cm versus 6.5 cm in patients who did not develop a recurrence. Thus, a luminal margin of 5 to 6 cm is recommended with frozen-section analysis when a subtotal gastric resection is performed for adenocarcinoma.

The role of extended lymphadenectomy in the surgical treatment of gastric cancer remains controversial. Extended lymph node dissections for the treatment of gastric cancer have best been described by the Japanese, and subsequently the JCGC D categories are used to define the extent of lymphatic dissection performed. In the JCGC system, lymph node basins are numbered and subsequently grouped according to the location of the primary. The groupings, according to primary site, are as listed in Table 47-9. A D1 resection refers to the removal of group 1 lymph nodes, D2 to dissection of group 1 and 2, and D3 resection to a D2 resection plus removal of para-aortic lymph nodes. To effect complete removal of station 10 (parasplenic) and station 11 (parapancreatic), Japanese surgeons perform splenectomy and partial pancreatectomy during D2 resections for primaries whose drainage includes these echelons (see Table 47-9). Because of the increased morbidity in the patients receiving these adjunctive resections, Western surgeons do not typically resect the spleen or pancreas unless involved by direct extension from a T4 tumor.

Splenectomy is no longer advocated as a routine adjunctive procedure to gastrectomy for cancer. The purpose of splenectomy in gastric cancer, aside from managing direct tumor extension, is for removal of lymph nodes at the splenic hilus (station 10) as a part of an

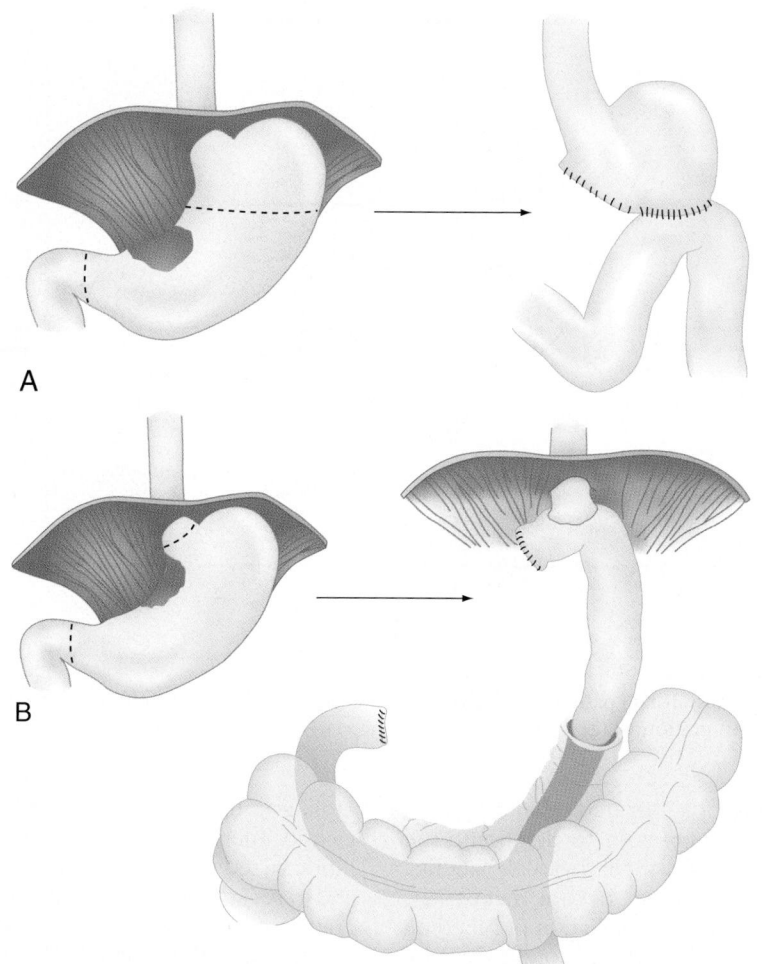

Figure 47-23 A, Subtotal gastrectomy with a Billroth II anastomosis. **B,** Total gastrectomy with a Roux-en-Y anastomosis.

extended lymph node resection (D2) for proximal gastric cancer. However, multivariate analysis in the Dutch trial comparing D1 and D2 resections for gastric cancer indicated that splenectomy carried a major risk for hospital death (hazard ratio, 2.16) and overall complications (hazard ratio, 2.13).[41] It is clear that any extended resection is accompanied by an increase in morbidity and mortality without an improvement in survival. Thus, local organ resection, especially of the spleen, pancreas, or transverse colon, should be performed only when needed to accomplish an R0 resection.

Extended D2 lymph node dissections are routinely performed in Japan and have been demonstrated in studies performed in that country to provide a survival benefit over more limited D1 dissections. The first evidence of a survival benefit for an extended dissection was in 1981 by Kodama and colleagues,[42] who reported a 39% 5-year survival rate after a D2 dissection compared to 18% for D1. Multiple other Japanese studies have confirmed these findings. However, randomized controlled trials in the West of D2 versus D1 dissections for gastric cancer have failed to demonstrate a survival benefit for the extended dissections. The British trial

reported an elevated postoperative morbidity (28% for D1 and 46% for D2) and mortality (6.5% for D1 and 13% for D2) in the D2 arm without any difference in 5-year survival (35% for D1 and 32% for D2).[43] Similarly, the Dutch trial also observed increased morbidity (25% for D1 and 43% for D2) and mortality (6.5% for D1 and 13% for D2) with no survival benefit associated with the extended resection.[44] Extended lymph node dissections for gastric cancer remain an investigational treatment option and should be performed at specialized centers in the context of a clinical trial. Per National Comprehensive Cancer Network (NCCN) guidelines, in the United States, a minimum of a D1 resection is recommended with excision of at least 15 lymph nodes for evaluation.

Palliative Treatment

Because 20% to 30% of gastric cancer patients present with stage IV disease, clinicians must be familiar with different methods of palliative treatment. The goal of palliative treatment is the relief of symptoms with minimal morbidity. Surgical palliation of advanced gastric cancer may include resection or bypass alone or in conjunction

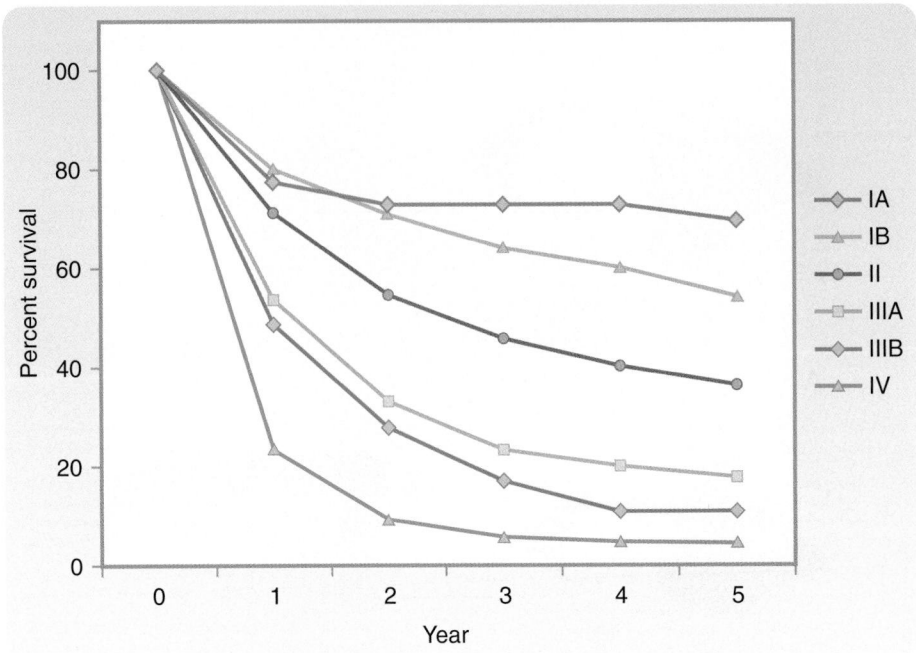

Figure 47-24 Survival rates for all patients with gastric carcinoma stratified by combined American Joint Committee on Cancer (AJCC), 5th edition, stage.

with percutaneous, endoscopic, or radiotherapy techniques. Complete staging is necessary to determine the appropriate method of palliation for individual patients. In the presence of peritoneal disease, hepatic metastases, diffuse nodal metastases, or ascites, palliation of bleeding or proximal gastric obstruction would preferably be obtained nonoperatively. Nonoperative therapies include laser recannulization and endoscopic dilation with or without stent placement. Patients who undergo stent placement for gastric outlet obstruction are frequently able to tolerate solid foods and may not require additional interventions.

Adjuvant Therapy

In a review of the National Cancer Database, Hundahl and colleagues[45] reported that only 29% of patients undergoing gastrectomy for gastric adenocarcinoma received some type of adjuvant treatment, whereas 71% were treated by surgery alone. These practice trends reflected the lack of convincing data to support the use of chemotherapy or radiation therapy in the management of gastric adenocarcinoma. However, many investigators believe the standard of care has changed on the basis of the Southwest Cancer Oncology Group trial (INT-00116). This trial evaluated two cycles of 5-fluorouracil and leucovorin with subsequent concurrent chemoradiotherapy, using the same chemotherapeutic agents, as adjuncts following an R0 resection of gastric adenocarcinoma. The median survival time for the surgery-only arm was 27 months, compared with 36 months ($P = .005$) for the chemoradiotherapy group. The 3-year survival rates were 41% in the surgery-only group, compared with 50% in the chemoradiation therapy group ($P = .005$).[46] These data would support the addition of postoperative chemo-

radiation to the treatment of patients with resectable gastric adenocarcinoma. More recently, a British MRC randomized trial (MAGIC) demonstrated improved overall and disease-free survival in patients treated with preoperative or postoperative chemotherapy (epirubicin, cisplatin, and 5-fluorouracil. The 5-year overall survival rate was 23% in the control arm, compared with 39% ($P = .009$) in those patients who received chemotherapy.[47]

Neoadjuvant chemotherapy is currently under investigation and has yielded some promising results. A few studies have demonstrated acceptable toxicities, with an increased number of patients completing all planned therapy and undergoing R0 resections compared with historic controls. Currently, NCCN guidelines recommend adjuvant chemoradiation with a 5-fluorouracil–based regimen following complete surgical resection for patients with T3, T4, or node-positive cancers. Additionally, patients with microscopically positive resection margins should also have adjuvant therapy.

Outcomes

Overall 5-year survival rates after the diagnosis of gastric cancer are 10% to 21%. Stage-stratified 5-year survival for all patients and those undergoing surgical excision is depicted in Figures 47-24 and 47-25. Patients who undergo a potentially curative resection have a better prognosis, with a 5-year survival rate of 24% to 57%.

Recurrence rates after gastrectomy remain high, ranging from 40% to 80% depending on the series. Most recurrences occur within the first 3 years. The locoregional failure rate ranges from 38% to 45%, whereas peritoneal dissemination as a component of failure occurs in 54% of patients in several series. Isolated distant metastases are uncommon because most patients with distant failure

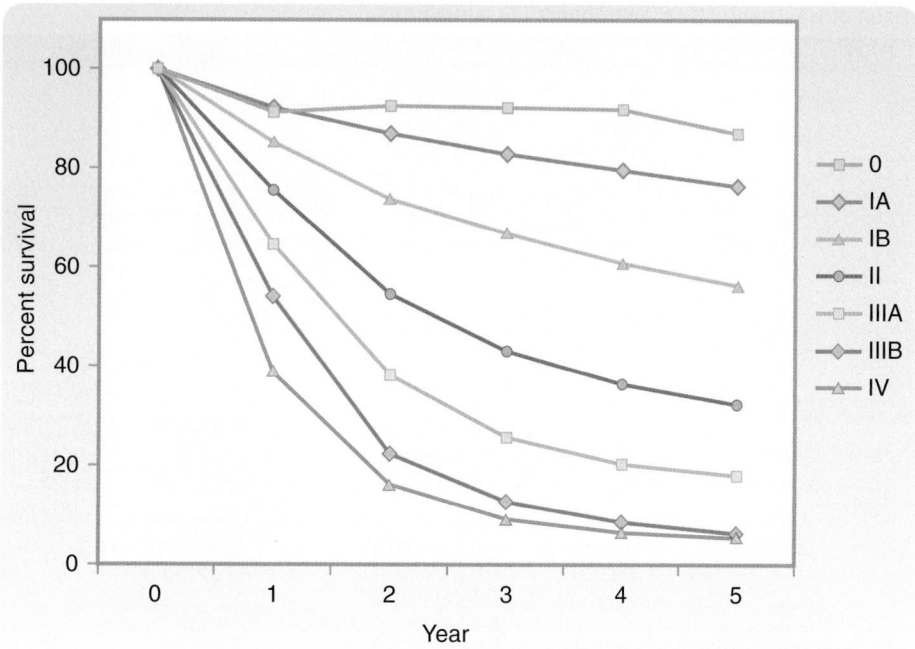

Figure 47-25 Survival rates for gastric cancer patients undergoing gastrectomy as stratified by combined American Joint Committee on Cancer (AJCC), 5th edition, stage.

have locoregional recurrence as well. The most common sites of locoregional recurrence are the gastric remnant at the anastomosis, in the gastric bed, and in the regional nodes. Hematogenous spread occurs to the liver, lung, and bone.

Surveillance

All patients should be followed systematically. Because most recurrences occur within the first 3 years, surveillance examinations are more frequent in the first several years. Follow-up should include a complete history and physical examination every 4 months for 1 year, then every 6 months for 2 years, and then annually thereafter. Laboratory examinations, including complete blood counts and liver function tests, should be obtained as clinically indicated. Many clinicians obtain chest x-rays as well as CT scans of the abdomen and pelvis routinely, whereas others obtain studies only when clinically suspicious of a recurrence. Yearly endoscopy should be considered in patients who have undergone a subtotal gastrectomy.

Gastric Lymphoma

Epidemiology

The stomach is the most common site of lymphomas in the GI system. However, primary gastric lymphoma is still relatively uncommon, accounting for less than 15% of gastric malignancies and 2% of lymphomas. Patients often present with vague symptoms, namely epigastric pain, early satiety, and fatigue. Constitutional B symptoms are very rare. Although overt bleeding is uncommon, more than half of patients present with anemia. Lymphomas occur in older patients, with the peak incidence in the

sixth and seventh decades, and are more common in men (male-to-female ratio of 2:1). Gastric lymphomas, like carcinomas, most commonly occur in the gastric antrum but can arise from any part of the stomach. Patients are considered to have gastric lymphoma if the stomach is the exclusive or predominant site of disease.

Pathology

In the management of gastric lymphomas, as in the management of nodal lymphomas, it is important to determine not only the stage of disease but also the subtype of lymphoma. There are multiple classification systems for lymphomas (Table 47-10). The most common gastric lymphoma is diffuse large B-cell lymphoma (55%), followed by extranodal marginal cell lymphoma (MALT) (40%), Burkitt's lymphoma (3%), and mantle cell and follicular lymphomas (each <1%).

Diffuse large B-cell lymphomas most commonly are primary lesions; however, they may also occur from progression of less aggressive lymphomas such as chronic lymphocytic leukemia/small lymphocytic lymphoma (CLL/SLL), follicular lymphoma, or MALT lymphoma. Immunodeficiencies and *H. pylori* infection are risk factors for the development of primary diffuse large B-cell lymphoma.

In 1983, Isaacson and Wright noted that the histology of primary low-grade gastric B-cell lymphoma resembled that of MALT.[48] Subsequently, the MALT lymphoma concept was extended to include other extranodal low-grade B-cell lymphomas of the salivary gland, lung, and thyroid. These organs lack native lymphoid tissue; the lymphomas at these sites arise from the MALT acquired as a result of chronic inflammation. MALT lymphomas

Table 47-10 Comparison of Gastrointestinal Lymphoma Classifications

WHO CLASSIFICATION	REAL	WORKING	LUKES-COLLINS	KLEL	RAPPAPORT
Extranodal marginal zone lymphoma (MALT lymphoma)	—	Small cleaved cell type	Small cleaved cell type	Immunocytoma	Well-differentiated lymphocytic
Follicular lymphoma	Follicular center lymphoma	Small cleaved cell type	Small cleaved cell type	Centroblastic/centrocytic, follicular and diffuse	Nodular, poorly differentiated lymphocytic
Mantle cell lymphoma	—	—	—	Centrocytic	Intermediately or poorly differentiated lymphocytic, diffuse or nodular
Diffuse large B-cell lymphoma	Diffuse large B-cell lymphoma	Large cleaved follicular center cell	Large cleaved follicular center cell	Centroblastic, B-immunoblastic	Diffuse mixed lymphocytic and histiocytic
Burkitt's lymphoma	Burkitt's lymphoma	Small noncleaved follicular center cell	Small noncleaved follicular center cell	Burkitt's lymphoma with intracytoplasmic immunoglobulin	Undifferentiated lymphoma, Burkitt's type

MALT, mucosa-associated lymphoid tissue; WHO, World Health Organization.

were recently reclassified as *extranodal marginal zone lymphomas of MALT-type*. Gastric MALT lymphoma is most commonly preceded by *H. pylori*–associated gastritis. Evidence of *H. pylori* infection can be found in almost every instance of gastric MALT lymphoma. Epidemiologic studies have also linked *H. pylori* infection with gastric lymphomas. Genetically, MALT lymphoma is characterized by the translocations t(1;14)(p22;q32) and t(11;18)(q21;q21), both of which result in impaired responsiveness to apoptotic signaling and increased nuclear factor κB activity. Recent evidence suggests that the t(11;18)(q21;q21) and Bcl-10 nuclear expression may predict for nonresponsiveness to treatment by *H. pylori* eradication and lymphoma regression.

Burkitt's lymphomas of the stomach are associated with Epstein-Barr virus infections as they are in other sites. Burkitt's lymphoma is very aggressive and tends to affect a younger population than other types of gastric lymphomas. Burkitt's is most commonly found in the cardia or body of the stomach as opposed to the antrum.

Evaluation

Endoscopy generally reveals nonspecific gastritis or gastric ulcerations, with mass lesions being unusual. Occasionally a submucosal growth pattern will render endoscopic biopsies nondiagnostic. Endoscopic ultrasound is useful to determine the depth of gastric wall invasion, specifically to identify patients at risk for perforation secondary to full-thickness involvement of the gastric wall. Evidence of distant disease should be sought through upper airway examination, bone marrow biopsy, and CT of the chest and abdomen to detect lymphadenopathy. Any enlarged lymph nodes should undergo biopsy. *H. pylori* testing should be performed by histology and, if negative, confirmed by serology.

Staging

The best staging system remains controversial. When possible, the TNM staging system should be used (using the criteria proposed for gastric carcinoma). Several other staging systems for primary gastric non-Hodgkin's lymphoma are available (Table 47-11).

Treatment

Most centers employ a multimodality treatment program for patients with gastric lymphoma. The role of resection in gastric lymphoma remains controversial, and many patients are now being treated with chemoradiation therapy alone. The risk for perforation in patients treated with chemotherapy has been overstated in the past and approaches 5%. The most common chemotherapeutic combination is CHOP (cyclophosphamide, doxorubicin, vincristine, and prednisone). A prospective, nonrandomized study evaluating patients with early-stage (stage IE, IIE) disease demonstrated similar disease-free 5-year survival rates in patients treated with surgery, chemotherapy, and radiation therapy versus chemotherapy and radiation therapy alone (82% versus 84.4%; NS).[49] Radiation therapy is limited in usefulness for larger tumors, with local control rates dropping from 100% for tumors 3 cm or smaller to 60% to 70% for tumors larger than 6 cm.[50] Late complications of radiation therapy, such as stricture, enteritis, and secondary tumor formation, can be significant. The overall risk for severe radiation complications after treatment to 30 Gy for GI tumors can approach 30% at 10 years. Thus, treatment should be individualized, with careful consideration given to treating a younger patient with high-dose GI radiation.

Patients who present with late-stage disease are not amenable to surgical cure and should be referred for chemotherapy. The diagnosis of lymphoma discovered

Table 47-11 Staging Systems for Primary Gastrointestinal Non-Hodgkin's Lymphoma

ANN ARBOR*	RAO ET AL†	MUSSHOFF‡	DESCRIPTION	RELATIVE INCIDENCE (%)
IE	IE	IE	Tumor confined to gastrointestinal tract	26
IIE	IIE	IIE	Tumor with spread to regional lymph nodes	26
IIE	IIIE	IIE	Tumor with nodal involvement beyond regional lymph nodes (para-aortic, iliac)	17
IIIE–IV	IVE	IIIE–IV	Tumor with spread to other intra-abdominal organs (liver, spleen) or beyond abdomen (chest, bone marrow)	31

*Carbone PP, Kaplan HS, Musshoff K, et al: Report of the Committee on Hodgkin's Disease Staging Classification. Cancer Res 31:1860-1861, 1971.
†Rao AR, Kagan AR, Kagan AR, et al: Management of gastrointestinal lymphoma. Am J Clin Oncol 7:213-219, 1984.
‡Musshoff K: [Clinical staging classification of non-Hodgkin's lymphomas (author's trans, German)]. Strahlentherapie 153:218-221, 1977.
From Bozzetti F, Audisio RA, Giardini R, Gennari L: Role of surgery in patients with primary non-Hodgkin's lymphoma of the stomach: An old problem revisited. Br J Surg 80:1102, 1993.

unexpectedly at operation can be confirmed by frozen section. Additionally, fresh tissue should be sent for fluorescence-activated cell sorting, immunohistochemistry, and genetic analysis. Consideration should be given to performing a bone marrow aspiration at the time of surgery. If isolated stage IE or IIE lymphoma is encountered, surgical removal of all gross disease is ideal. Patients with disseminated lymphoma cannot be cured surgically, and the operation should focus on obtaining enough tissue for diagnosis and the repair of perforations.

Recent evidence suggests that early-stage MALT lymphomas as well as some cases of very limited diffuse large B-cell lymphoma may be effectively treated by *H. pylori* eradication alone. Successful eradication resulted in remission in more than 75% of cases. However, careful follow-up is necessary, with repeat endoscopy in 2 months to document clearance of the infection as well as biannual endoscopy for 3 years to document regression. Some patients continue to demonstrate the lymphoma clone after *H. pylori* eradication, suggesting the lymphoma became dormant rather than disappearing.

The presence of transmural tumor extension, nodal involvement, transformation into a large cell phenotype, t(11;18), or nuclear *BCL-10* expression all predict failure after *H. pylori* eradication alone. Additionally, a small subset of MALT lymphoma patients are *H. pylori*–negative. In these patients, consideration should be given to surgical resection, radiation, and chemotherapy. The 5-year disease-free survival rate with multimodality treatment is greater than 95% in stage IE and 75% in stage IIE disease.

Gastric Sarcomas

Epidemiology

Gastric sarcomas arise from mesenchymal components of the gastric wall and constitute about 3% of all gastric malignancies. Gastrointestinal stromal tumors (GISTs) are the most common mesenchymal tumor of the GI tract and are most frequently located in the stomach (60%-70%). Patients usually present after the fourth decade, with the mean age of 60 years at diagnosis.

Pathology

Initially thought to arise from smooth muscle cells, GISTs were previously classified as leiomyomas or leiomyosarcomas. Histologically, they appear to arise from the muscularis propria and most likely originate from the cells of Cajal, autonomic nerve–related GI pacemaker cells that regulate intestinal motility. GISTs are defined as cellular, spindle cell, or occasionally pleomorphic mesenchymal tumors located in the GI tract and express the Kit (CD117, stem cell factor receptor) protein. Kit is a transmembrane tyrosine kinase receptor, the ligand for which is stem cell factor. The Kit protein is detected by immunohistochemistry and can reliably distinguish GISTs from true smooth muscle neoplasms. Most GISTs (70%-80%) also are positive for CD34, a hematopoietic progenitor cell antigen. Recently, a new activating mutation has been detected in GI stromal tumors. A subset of GISTs lack c-*kit* mutations and have intragenic activation mutations in a related tyrosine kinase receptor, platelet-derived growth factor-α.

Staging

No current staging system exists for GISTs; however, several factors have been identified that correlate with clinical behavior. Tumors that show low mitotic frequency (5 or fewer mitoses per 50 high-power fields [HPF]) usually have a benign behavior. Tumors with mitotic counts of more than 5 per 50 HPF are considered malignant, whereas tumors with more than 50 mitoses per 50 HPF are classified as high-grade malignant. Malignancy is also associated with tumors greater than 5 cm in size, cellular atypia, necrosis, or local invasion. c-*kit* mutations occur predominantly in malignant GISTs and are an unfavorable prognostic marker. Most c-*kit* mutations occur in exon 11 and result in activation of c-*kit*. More than 80% of gastric GISTs are classified as benign according to the previous criteria. However, many histologically malignant-appearing lesions never metastasize, whereas rarely, benign-appearing lesions do. Benign gastric GISTs occur more frequently than malignant ones (3:1 versus 5:1). Because GISTs with low mitotic counts and malignant behavior are generally larger, this has led to the designation of *uncertain malignant potential* for a significant number of GISTs.

Clinical Manifestations and Evaluation

The most common presentations of gastric GISTs are GI bleeding and pain or dyspepsia. Endoscopy may be the first diagnostic test if patients present with bleeding; however, as the neoplasm grows intramurally, the true extent of the tumor can best be assessed with CT. Double-contrast upper GI series may show a smooth-edged filling defect. Endoscopic biopsy is diagnostic in about half of cases. Percutaneous or endoscopic biopsy should only be performed if the results would obviate the need for surgery.

Treatment

The goal of surgery is a margin-negative resection to include en bloc resection of adjacent organs if involved by direct extension. If at the time of surgical resection the histology is uncertain, a frozen section should be performed because the diagnosis of adenocarcinoma or lymphoma would change the surgical management. Rupture of the tumor should be avoided to prevent inoculation of the peritoneal cavity with tumor cells. Because lymph node metastases are rare (<10%), there is no known added benefit of extended lymphadenectomy. Most recurrences occur in the first 2 years, presenting as local disease frequently associated with liver metastases. Other common patterns of failure include peritoneal recurrences. Salvage surgery to resect recurrent disease has not been demonstrated to improve survival. The overall 5-year survival rate for gastric GISTs is 48% (19%-56%), with survival rates after complete surgical resection ranging from 32% to 63%. Indices that independently predict recurrence include mitotic rate of more than 15 mitoses per 30 HPF, mixed cytomorphology (spindle cell and epithelioid), presence of deletion/insertion c-*kit* exon 11 mutations, and male sex.

Until recently, there was no good adjuvant therapy for GISTs. Radiation therapy has not been proved effective in the management of GISTs, and only 5% of tumors respond to doxorubicin-based cytotoxic chemotherapy. Imatinib mesylate (formerly ST1517, now Gleevec [Novartis]) is a competitive inhibitor of certain tyrosine kinases, including the kinases associated with the transmembrane receptor Kit and platelet-derived growth factor receptors. Initial studies showed very encouraging results, with 54% of patients exhibiting at least a partial response.[51] Imatinib mesylate is approved for use in CD117-positive unresectable and metastatic GISTs. Further studies are ongoing; patients with a diagnosis of GIST should be considered for enrollment in one of the many active clinical trials.

OTHER GASTRIC LESIONS

Hypertrophic Gastritis (Ménétrier's Disease)

Ménétrier's disease (hypoproteinemic hypertrophic gastropathy) is a rare, acquired, premalignant disease characterized by massive gastric folds in the fundus and corpus of the stomach, giving the mucosa a cobblestone or cerebriform appearance. Histologic examination reveals foveolar hyperplasia (expansion of surface mucous cells) with absent parietal cells. The condition is associated with protein loss from the stomach, excessive mucus production, and hypochlorhydria or achlorhydria. The cause of Ménétrier's disease is unknown, but it has been associated with cytomegalovirus infection in children and *H. pylori* infection in adults. Additionally, increased transforming growth factor-α has been noted in the gastric mucosa of patients with the disease. Patients often present with epigastric pain, vomiting, weight loss, anorexia, and peripheral edema. Typical gastric mucosal changes can be detected by radiographic or endoscopic examination. Biopsy should be performed to rule out gastric carcinoma or lymphoma. Twenty-four-hour pH monitoring reveals hypochlorhydria or achlorhydria, and a chromium-labeled albumin test reveals increased GI protein loss. Medical treatment has yielded inconsistent results; however, some benefit has been shown through the use of anticholinergic drugs, acid suppression, octreotide, and *H. pylori* eradication. Total gastrectomy should be performed in patients who continue to have massive protein loss despite optimal medical therapy or if dysplasia or carcinoma develops.

Mallory-Weiss Tear

Mallory-Weiss tears are related to forceful vomiting, retching, coughing, or straining that results in disruption of the gastric mucosa high on the lesser curve at the gastroesophageal junction. They account for 15% of acute upper GI hemorrhages and are rarely associated with massive bleeding. The overall mortality rate for the lesion is 3% to 4%, with the greatest risk for massive hemorrhage in alcoholic patients with preexisting portal hypertension. Most patients with active bleeding can be managed by endoscopic methods such as multipolar electric coagulation, epinephrine injection, endoscopic band ligation, or endoscopic hemoclipping. Angiographic intra-arterial infusion of vasopressin or transcatheter embolization may be of use in very selective high-risk cases. The need for operative intervention is rare. If surgery is required, the lesion at the gastroesophageal junction is approached through an anterior gastrotomy and the bleeding site oversewn with several deep 2-0 silk ligatures to reapproximate the gastric mucosa in an anatomic fashion.

Dieulafoy's Gastric Lesion

Dieulafoy's lesions account for 0.3% to 7% of nonvariceal upper GI hemorrhages. Bleeding from a gastric Dieulafoy's lesion is caused by an abnormally large (1-3 mm), tortuous artery coursing through the submucosa. Erosion of the superficial mucosa overlying the artery occurs secondary to the pulsations of the large submucosal vessel. The artery is then exposed to the gastric contents, and further erosion and bleeding occurs. Generally, the mucosal defect is 2 to 5 mm in size and is surrounded by normal-appearing gastric mucosa. The lesions generally occur 6 to 10 cm from the gastroesophageal junction generally in the fundus near the cardia. In one series, 67% were located high in the body of the stomach, with

25% in the gastric fundus. Dieulafoy's lesions are more common in men (2:1), with the peak incidence in the fifth decade. Most patients present with hematemesis. The classic presentation of a patient with a Dieulafoy's lesion is sudden onset of massive, painless, recurrent hematemesis with hypotension. Detection and identification of the Dieulafoy's lesion can be difficult. Esophagogastroduodenoscopy is the diagnostic modality of choice, correctly identifying the lesion in 80% of patients. Because of the intermittent nature of the bleeding, repeated endoscopies may be needed to correctly identify the lesion. If the lesion can be identified endoscopically, attempts should be made to stop the bleeding using endoscopic modalities such as multipolar electrocoagulation, heater probe, noncontact laser photocoagulation, injection sclerotherapy, band ligation, or endoscopic hemoclipping. Angiography can be useful in cases in which endoscopy could not definitely identify the source. Angiographic findings may include a tortuous, ectatic artery in the distribution of the left gastric artery with accompanied contrast extravasation in the setting of acute bleeding. Gelfoam embolization has been reported to successfully control bleeding in patients with Dieulafoy's lesion, though the reported experience is limited.

Surgery was once the only therapy for Dieulafoy's lesion and is now reserved for patients in whom other modalities have failed. The surgical management consists of gastric wedge resection to include the offending vessel. The difficulty at the time of surgery is locating the lesion unless it is actively bleeding. The surgical procedure can be greatly facilitated by asking the endoscopist to tattoo the stomach when the lesion is identified. The traditional surgical approach has been through laparotomy with wide gastrotomy to identify the lesion with subsequent wide wedge resection. The lesion can also be approached laparoscopically, combined with intraoperative endoscopy. A wedge resection is performed with a linear stapling device using endoscopic transillumination to determine the resection margin.

Gastric Varices

Gastric varices are broadly classified by Sarin into two types, gastroesophageal varices and isolated gastric varices. Isolated gastric varices are subclassified into type 1, varices located in the fundus of the stomach; and type 2, isolated ectopic varices located anywhere in the stomach.

Gastric varices can develop secondary to portal hypertension, in conjunction with esophageal varices, or secondary to sinistral hypertension from splenic vein thrombosis. In generalized portal hypertension, the increased portal pressure is transmitted by the left gastric vein to esophageal varices and by the short and posterior gastric veins to the fundic plexus and cardia veins. Isolated gastric varices tend to occur secondary to splenic vein thrombosis. Splenic blood flows retrograde through the short and posterior gastric veins into the varices, then hepatopetally through the coronary vein into the portal vein. Left-to-right retrograde flow through the gastroepi-

ploic vein to the superior mesenteric vein can explain the development of ectopic varices in the stomach.

The incidence of bleeding from gastric varices has been reported between 3% and 30%, but in most series, it is less than 10%. However, the incidence of bleeding can be as high as 78% in patients with splenic vein thrombosis and fundic varices. There are limited data on risk factors associated with hemorrhage in patients with gastric varices, although increasing size of the varices or worse Child's status increases the risk for bleeding.

Gastric varices in the setting of splenic vein thrombosis are readily treated by splenectomy. Patients with bleeding gastric varices should have an abdominal ultrasound to document splenic vein thrombosis before surgical intervention because gastric varices are most often associated with generalized portal hypertension.

Gastric varices in the setting of portal hypertension should be managed like esophageal varices. The patient should be volume resuscitated with attention paid to correction of abnormal coagulation profiles. Temporary tamponade can be attempted with a Sengstaken-Blakemore tube. Endoscopy serves as a diagnostic as well as a therapeutic tool. Successful eradication of the esophageal varices through banding or sclerotherapy often results in obliteration of the gastric varices. As gastric varices arise in the submucosa, a common complication associated with gastric variceal sclerotherapy is ulceration. A major problem with gastric varices is rebleeding, 50% of which is secondary to ulcers. Endoscopic variceal band ligation can achieve hemostasis in about 89% of patients; however, concerns about gastric perforations with this technique have tempered its use. Transjugular intrahepatic portosystemic shunting (TIPS) can be effective in controlling gastric variceal hemorrhage, with rebleeding rates of about 30%. A gastrorenal shunt between gastric varices and the left renal vein is present in 85% of patients with gastric varices. This spontaneous shunt decompresses the portal system and lessens the efficacy of TIPS. A balloon catheter can be inserted into the gastrorenal shunt through the left renal vein and the shunt occluded by inflating the balloon. A sclerosant (ethanolamine oleate) is then injected and left to remain until clots have formed in the varices. Balloon-occluded retrograde transvenous obliteration has been reported to have a high success rate (100%), with a low recurrence rate (0%-5%). The major complication of this procedure is aggravation of esophageal varices secondary to a rise in portal pressure as a consequence of occluding the gastrorenal shunt. Additionally, ethanolamine oleate can cause hemolysis (treated by haptoglobin administration) with subsequent renal damage.

Gastric Volvulus

Gastric volvulus is an uncommon condition. Torsion occurs along the stomach's longitudinal axis (organoaxial) in about two thirds of cases and along the vertical axis (mesenteroaxial) in one third of cases (Fig. 47-26). Most commonly, organoaxial gastric volvulus occurs acutely and is associated with a diaphragmatic defect, whereas mesenteroaxial volvulus is partial (<180 degrees),

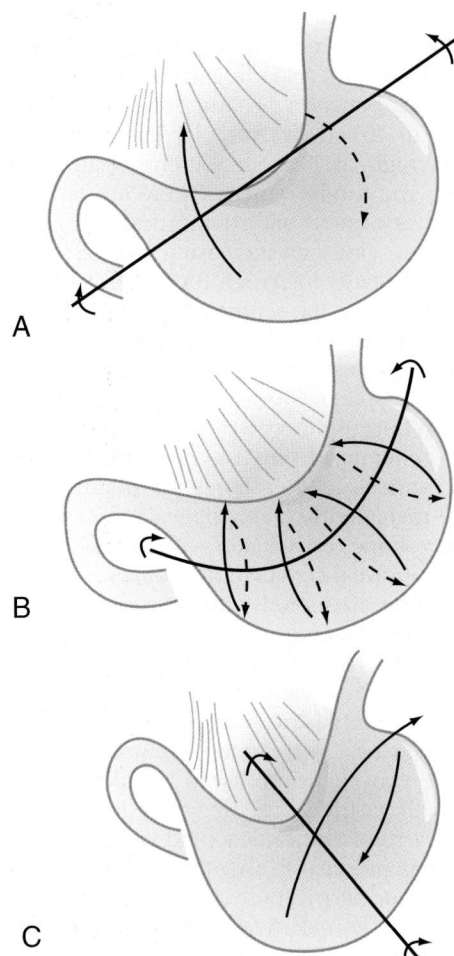

Figure 47-26 Torsion of the stomach along the longitudinal axis (organoaxial) (**A** and **B**) and along the vertical axis (mesoaxial) (**C**). (From Dalgaard JG: Volvulus of the stomach. Acta Chir Scand 103:131, 1952.)

recurrent, and not associated with a diaphragmatic defect. In adults, the diaphragmatic defects are most commonly traumatic or paraesophageal hernias, whereas in children, congenital defects such as the foramen of Bochdalek or eventration are involved. The major symptoms at presentation are abdominal pain that is acute in onset, distention, vomiting, and upper GI hemorrhage. The sudden onset of constant and severe upper abdominal pain, recurrent retching with production of little vomitus, and the inability to pass a nasogastric tube constitute Borchardt's triad. Plain films of the abdomen reveal a gas-filled viscus in the chest or upper abdomen. The diagnosis can be confirmed by barium contrast study or upper GI endoscopy. Acute volvulus is a surgical emergency. Through a transabdominal approach, the stomach is reduced and uncoiled. The diaphragmatic defect is repaired with consideration given to a fundoplication in the setting of a paraesophageal hernia. In the unusual case in which strangulation has occurred (5%-28%), the compromised segment of stomach is resected. Spontaneous volvulus, without an associated diaphragmatic defect, is treated by detorsion and fixation of the stomach by gastropexy or tube gastrostomy.

Bezoars

Bezoars are collections of nondigestible materials, usually of vegetable origin (phytobezoar) but also of hair (trichobezoar). Phytobezoars are most commonly found in patients who have undergone surgery of the stomach and have impaired gastric emptying. Diabetics with autonomic neuropathy are also at risk. The symptoms of gastric bezoars include early satiety, nausea, pain, vomiting, and weight loss. A large mass may be palpable on physical exam and the diagnosis confirmed by a barium examination or endoscopy. Dan and coworkers in 1959 were the first to suggest enzymatic therapy to attempt dissolution of the bezoar. Papain, found in Adolph's Meat Tenderizer (AMT), is given in a dose of one teaspoon in 150 to 300 mL water several times daily. The sodium concentration in AMT is high, so hypernatremia may result if large quantities are administered. Alternative enzymes such as cellulase have been used with some success. Generally, enzymatic débridement is followed by aggressive Ewald tube lavage or endoscopic fragmentation. Failure of these therapies would necessitate surgical removal.

Trichobezoars are concretions of hair, generally found in long-haired girls or women who often deny eating their own hair (trichophagy). Symptoms include pain from gastric ulceration and fullness from gastric outlet obstruction with occasional gastric perforation and small bowel obstruction. Trichobezoars tend to form a cast of the stomach, with strands of hair having been observed as far distally as the transverse colon. Small trichobezoars may respond to endoscopic fragmentation, vigorous lavage, or enzymatic therapy. However, these techniques are of limited usefulness, and larger trichobezoars require surgical removal. The small bowel should be examined to be certain additional bezoars are not present. The trichophagy requires psychiatric care because recurrent bezoar formation is common.

Annotated References

Bonenkamp JJ, Hermans J, Sasako M, van de Velde CJ: Extended lymph-node dissection for gastric cancer. Dutch Gastric Cancer Group. N Engl J Med 340:908-914, 1999.

> Prospective randomized trial in 80 Dutch hospitals comparing D1 with D2 lymph-node dissection for gastric cancer in terms of morbidity. The results in Dutch patients do not support the routine use of D2 lymph-node dissection in patients with gastric cancer.

Cook DJ, Fuller HD, Guyatt GH, et al: Risk factors for gastrointestinal bleeding in critically ill patients. Canadian Critical Care Trials Group. N Engl J Med 330:377-381, 1994.

> A prospective multicenter cohort study evaluating the potential risk factors for stress ulceration in patients admitted to intensive care units and the occurrence of clinically important gastrointestinal bleeding (defined as overt bleeding in association with hemodynamic compromise or the need for blood transfusion). Few critically ill patients had clinically important gastrointestinal bleeding, and therefore prophylaxis against stress ulcers can be safely withheld from critically ill patients unless they have coagulopathy or require mechanical ventilation.

Cuschieri A, Weeden S, Fielding J, et al: Patient survival after D1 and D2 resections for gastric cancer: Long-term results of the MRC randomized surgical trial. Surgical Co-operative Group. Br J Cancer 79:1522-1530, 1999.

> In this prospective trial D1 resection (removal of regional perigastric nodes) was compared with D2 resection (extended lymphadenectomy to include level 1 and 2 regional nodes). In a multivariate analysis, clinical stages II and III, old age, male sex and removal of spleen and pancreas were independently associated with poor survival. These findings indicate that the classical Japanese D2 resection offers no survival advantage over D1 surgery. However, the possibility that D2 resection without pancreatico-splenectomy may be better than standard D1 resection cannot be dismissed by the results of this trial.

Demetri GD, von Mehren M, Blanke CD, et al: Efficacy and safety of imatinib mesylate in advanced gastrointestinal stromal tumors. N Engl J Med 347:472-480, 2002.

> Prospective, open label, randomized, multicenter trial to evaluate the activity of imatinib in patients with advanced gastrointestinal stromal tumor. Imatinib induced a sustained objective response in more than half of patients with an advanced unresectable or metastatic gastrointestinal stromal tumor.

Driks MR, Craven DE, Celli BR, et al: Nosocomial pneumonia in intubated patients given sucralfate as compared with antacids or histamine type 2 blockers: The role of gastric colonization. N Engl J Med 317:1376-1382, 1987.

> A prospective randomized trial evaluating the rate of nosocomial pneumonia among 130 patients given mechanical ventilation in an intensive care unit who were receiving as prophylaxis for stress ulcer either sucralfate (n = 61), which does not raise gastric pH, or conventional treatment with antacids, histamine type 2 (H_2) blockers, or both (n = 69). The rate of pneumonia was twice as high in the antacid-H_2 group as in the sucralfate group (95% confidence interval, 0.89 to 4.58; P = .11). In patients receiving mechanical ventilation, the use of a prophylactic agent against stress-ulcer bleeding that preserves the natural gastric acid barrier against bacterial overgrowth may be preferable to antacids and H_2 blockers.

Dubois F. New surgical strategy for gastroduodenal ulcer: laparoscopic approach. World J Surgery 24:270-6, 2000.

> Summary of application of minimally invasive surgery in surgical treatment of PUD.

Fries JF, Miller SR, Spitz PW, et al: Toward an epidemiology of gastropathy associated with nonsteroidal antiinflammatory drug use. Gastroenterology 96:647-55, 1989.

> The thesis of this paper is that gastropathy associated with nonsteroidal anti-inflammatory drugs (NSAIDs) is the most frequent and, in aggregate, the most severe drug side effect in the United States. Patients on NSAIDs had a hazard ratio for gastrointestinal (GI) hospitalization that was 6.45 times that of patients not on NSAIDs. The syndrome of NSAID-associated gastropathy can be estimated to account for at least 2600 deaths and 20,000 hospitalizations each year in patients with rheumatoid arthritis alone.

Harbison SP, Dempsey DT: Peptic Ulcer Disease: Current Problems in Surgery 42:335-454, 2005.

> Excellent review of the clinical trials relevant to the surgical management of PUD.

Hundahl SA, Phillips JL, Menck HR, et al: The National Cancer Data Base Report on poor survival of U.S. gastric carcinoma patients treated with gastrectomy: Fifth Edition American Joint Committee on Cancer staging, proximal disease, and the "different disease" hypothesis. Cancer 88:921-932, 2000.

> A review of the management of gastric cancer patients in the United States diagnosed during the years 1985-1996 and treated with gastrectomy. Based on a review of the National Cancer Data Base (NCDB) reports.

Koch P, del Valle F, Berdel WE, et al: Primary gastrointestinal non-Hodgkin's lymphoma: II. Combined surgical and conservative or conservative management only in localized gastric lymphoma—results of the prospective German Multicenter Study GIT NHL 01/92. J Clin Oncol 19:3874-3883, 2001.

> Prospective non-randomized multi-center trial of patients with primary gastrointestinal non-Hodgkin's lymphomas undergoing combined surgical and conservative treatment (CSCT) versus conservative treatment (CT) alone for primary gastric lymphoma (PGL) in localized stages. The study showed no survival benefit through the addition of surgery. Although the study was not randomized, a stomach-conserving approach may be favored.

Koniaris LG, Drugas G, Katzman PJ, Salloum R: Management of gastrointestinal lymphoma. J Am Coll Surg 197:127-141, 2003.

> Excellent review of gastrointestinal lymphomas and their management.

Macdonald JS, Smalley SR, Benedetti J, et al: Chemoradiotherapy after surgery compared with surgery alone for adenocarcinoma of the stomach or gastroesophageal junction. N Engl J Med 345:725-730, 2001.

> First study to show adjuvant chemoradiotherapy to be of benefit in patients with gastric adenocarcinoma. Postoperative chemoradiotherapy should be considered for all patients at high risk for recurrence of adenocarcinoma of the stomach or gastroesophageal junction who have undergone curative resection.

Ng EK, Lam YH, Sung JJ, et al: Eradication of *Helicobacter pylori* prevents recurrence of ulcer after simple closure of duodenal ulcer perforation: Randomized controlled trial. Ann Surg 231:153-158, 2000.

> A randomized trial to determine whether eradication of *Helicobacter pylori* could reduce the risk of ulcer recurrence after simple closure of perforated duodenal ulcer. The data suggest that eradication of *H. pylori* prevents ulcer recurrence in patients with *H. pylori*-associated perforated duodenal ulcers. Immediate acid-reduction surgery in the presence of generalized peritonitis is unnecessary.

References

1. Saffouri B, Weir GC, Bitar KN, et al: Gastrin and somatostatin secretion by perfused rat stomach: Functional linkage of antral peptides. Am J Physiol 238:G495-501, 1980.
2. Mercer DW, Cross JM, Smith GS, et al: Protective action of gastrin-17 against alcohol-induced gastric injury in the rat: Role in mucosal defense. Am J Physiol 273:G365-373, 1997.
3. Carney JA, Go VL, Fairbanks VF, et al: The syndrome of gastric argyrophil carcinoid tumors and nonantral gastric atrophy. Ann Intern Med 99:761-766, 1983.
4. Queiroz DM, Mendes EN, Rocha GA, et al: Effect of *Helicobacter pylori* eradication on antral gastrin- and somatostatin-immunoreactive cell density and gastrin and somatostatin concentrations. Scand J Gastroenterol 28:858-864, 1993.
5. Driks MR, Craven DE, Celli BR, et al: Nosocomial pneumonia in intubated patients given sucralfate as compared with antacids or histamine type 2 blockers. The role of gastric colonization. N Engl J Med 317:1376-1382, 1987.

6. Abrahamsson H: Gastrointestinal motility disorders in patients with diabetes mellitus. J Intern Med 237:403-409, 1995.

7. Saslow SB, Thumshirn M, Camilleri M, et al: Influence of *H. pylori* infection on gastric motor and sensory function in asymptomatic volunteers. Dig Dis Sci 43:258-264, 1998.

8. Soll AH: Pathogenesis of peptic ulcer and implications for therapy. N Engl J Med 322:909-916, 1990.

9. Kurata JH: Ulcer epidemiology: An overview and proposed research framework. Gastroenterology 96:569-580, 1989.

10. Peterson WL, Barnett CC, Evans DJ Jr, et al: Acid secretion and serum gastrin in normal subjects and patients with duodenal ulcer: the role of *Helicobacter pylori*. Am J Gastroenterol 88:2038-2043, 1993.

11. Drumm B, Perez-Perez GI, Blaser MJ, et al: Intrafamilial clustering of *Helicobacter pylori* infection. N Engl J Med 322:359-363, 1990.

12. Dooley CP, Cohen H, Fitzgibbons PL, et al: Prevalence of *Helicobacter pylori* infection and histologic gastritis in asymptomatic persons. N Engl J Med 321:1562-1566, 1989.

13. Laine L: Approaches to nonsteroidal anti-inflammatory drug use in the high-risk patient. Gastroenterology 120:594-606, 2001.

14. Fries JF, Miller SR, Spitz PW, et al: Toward an epidemiology of gastropathy associated with nonsteroidal antiinflammatory drug use. Gastroenterology 96:647-655, 1989.

15. Kurata JH, Elashoff JD, Haile BM, et al: A reappraisal of time trends in ulcer disease: Factors related to changes in ulcer hospitalization and mortality rates. Am J Public Health 73:1066-1072, 1983.

16. Silverstein FE, Gilbert DA, Tedesco FJ, et al: The national ASGE survey on upper gastrointestinal bleeding. I. Study design and baseline data. Gastrointest Endosc 27:73-79, 1981.

17. Stabile BE: Redefining the role of surgery for perforated duodenal ulcer in the *Helicobacter pylori* era. Ann Surg 231:159-160, 2000.

18. Dubois F: New surgical strategy for gastroduodenal ulcer: Laparoscopic approach. World J Surg 24:270-276, 2000.

19. Harbison SP, Dempsey DT: Peptic ulcer disease. Curr Probl Surg 42:346-454, 2005.

20. Laine Il, Peterson WL. Bleeding peptic ulcer. N Engl J Med 331:717-727, 1994.

21. Silverstein FE, Graham DY, Senior JR, et al: Misoprostol reduces serious gastrointestinal complications in patients with rheumatoid arthritis receiving nonsteroidal anti-inflammatory drugs: A randomized, double-blind, placebo-controlled trial. Ann Intern Med 123:241-249, 1995.

22. Ng EK, Lam YH, Sung JJ, et al: Eradication of *Helicobacter pylori* prevents recurrence of ulcer after simple closure of duodenal ulcer perforation: Randomized controlled trial. Ann Surg 231:153-158, 2000.

23. Crofts TJ, Park KG, Steele RJ, et al: A randomized trial of nonoperative treatment for perforated peptic ulcer. N Engl J Med 320:970-973, 1989.

24. Aoki T: Current status of and problems in the treatment of gastric and duodenal ulcer disease: Introduction. World J Surg 24:249-327, 2000.

25. Cook DJ, Fuller HD, Guyatt GH, et al: Risk factors for gastrointestinal bleeding in critically ill patients. Canadian Critical Care Trials Group. N Engl J Med 330:377-381, 1994.

26. Eidt S, Stolte M: Gastric glandular cysts—investigations into their genesis and relationship to colorectal epithelial tumors. Z Gastroenterol 27:212-217, 1989.

27. Oberhuber G, Stolte M: Gastric polyps: An update of their pathology and biological significance. Virchows Arch 437:581-590, 2000.

28. Smith RA, Cokkinides V, Eyre HJ: American Cancer Society guidelines for the early detection of cancer, 2006. CA Cancer J Clin 56:11-25; quiz, 49-50, 2006.

29. Israel DA, Peek RM: Pathogenesis of *Helicobacter pylori*–induced gastric inflammation. Aliment Pharmacol Ther 15:1271-1290, 2001.

30. Figueiredo C, Machado JC, Pharoah P, et al: *Helicobacter pylori* and interleukin 1 genotyping: An opportunity to identify high-risk individuals for gastric carcinoma. J Natl Cancer Inst 94:1680-1687, 2002.

31. Becker KF, Atkinson MJ, Reich U, et al: E-cadherin gene mutations provide clues to diffuse type gastric carcinomas. Cancer Res 54:3845-3852, 1994.

32. Leung WK, Sung JJ: Review article: Intestinal metaplasia and gastric carcinogenesis. Aliment Pharmacol Ther 16:1209-1216, 2002.

33. Leedham SJ, Schier S, Thliveris AT, et al: From gene mutations to tumours: Stem cells in gastrointestinal carcinogenesis. Cell Prolif 38:387-405, 2005.

34. Yamaguchi H, Goldenring JR, Kaminishi M, Lee JR: Identification of spasmolytic polypeptide expressing metaplasia (SPEM) in remnant gastric cancer and surveillance postgastrectomy biopsies. Dig Dis Sci 47:573-578, 2002.

35. Halldorsdottir AM, Sigurdardottrir M, Jonasson JG, et al: Spasmolytic polypeptide–expressing metaplasia (SPEM) associated with gastric cancer in Iceland. Dig Dis Sci 48:431-441, 2003.

36. Willis S, Truong S, Gribnitz S, et al: Endoscopic ultrasonography in the preoperative staging of gastric cancer: Accuracy and impact on surgical therapy. Surg Endosc 14:951-954, 2000.

37. Mani NB, Suri S, Gupta S, et al: Two-phase dynamic contrast-enhanced computed tomography with water-filling method for staging of gastric carcinoma. Clin Imaging 25:38-43, 2001.

38. Sarela AI, Miner TJ, Karpeh MS, et al: Clinical outcomes with laparoscopic stage M1, unresected gastric adenocarcinoma. Ann Surg 243:189-195, 2006.

39. Sarela AI, Lefkowitz R, Brennan MF, et al: Selection of patients with gastric adenocarcinoma for laparoscopic staging. Am J Surg 191:134-138, 2006.

40. Buhl K, Schlag P, Herfarth C: Quality of life and functional results following different types of resection for gastric carcinoma. Eur J Surg Oncol 16:404-409, 1990.

41. Bonenkamp JJ, Hermans J, Sasako M, et al: Extended lymph-node dissection for gastric cancer. Dutch Gastric Cancer Group. N Engl J Med 340:908-914, 1999.

42. Kodama Y, Sugimachi K, Soejima K, et al: Evaluation of extensive lymph node dissection for carcinoma of the stomach. World J Surg 5:241-248, 1981.

43. Cuschieri A, Weeden S, Fielding J, et al: Patient survival after D1 and D2 resections for gastric cancer: Long-term results of the MRC randomized surgical trial. Surgical Cooperative Group. Br J Cancer 79:1522-1530, 1999.

44. Hartgrink HH, van de Velde CJ, Putter H, et al: Extended lymph node dissection for gastric cancer: Who may benefit? Final results of the randomized Dutch gastric cancer group trial. J Clin Oncol 22:2069-2077, 2004.

45. Hundahl SA, Phillips JL, Menck HR. The National Cancer Data Base Report on poor survival of U.S. gastric carcinoma patients treated with gastrectomy: Fifth Edition American Joint Committee on Cancer staging, proximal disease, and the "different disease" hypothesis. Cancer 88:921-32, 2000.

46. Macdonald JS, Smalley SR, Benedetti J, et al: Chemoradiotherapy after surgery compared with surgery alone for adenocarcinoma of the stomach or gastroesophageal junction. N Engl J Med 345:725-730, 2001.

47. Cunningham D, Allum WH, Stenning SP, et al: Perioperative chemotherapy versus surgery alone for resectable gastroesophageal cancer. N Engl J Med 355:11-20, 2006.

48. Isaacson P, Wright DH: Malignant lymphoma of mucosa-associated lymphoid tissue. A distinctive type of B-cell lymphoma. Cancer 52:1410-1416, 1983.

49. Koch P, del Valle F, Berdel WE, et al: Primary gastrointestinal non-Hodgkin's lymphoma. II. Combined surgical and conservative or conservative management only in localized gastric lymphoma—results of the prospective German Multicenter Study GIT NHL 01/92. J Clin Oncol 19:3874-3883, 2001.

50. Koniaris LG, Drugas G, Katzman PJ, et al: Management of gastrointestinal lymphoma. J Am Coll Surg 197:127-141, 2003.

51. Demetri GD, von Mehren M, Blanke CD, et al: Efficacy and safety of imatinib mesylate in advanced gastrointestinal stromal tumors. N Engl J Med 347:472-480, 2002.

Small Intestine

B. Mark Evers, MD

The small intestine is a marvel of complexity and efficiency. The primary role of the small intestine is the digestion and absorption of dietary components after they leave the stomach. This process depends on a multitude of structural, physiologic, endocrine, and chemical factors. Exocrine secretions from the liver and pancreas enable complete digestion of the foodstuffs. The enlarged surface area of the small intestinal mucosa then absorbs these nutrients. In addition to its role in digestion and absorption, the small bowel is the largest endocrine organ in the body and is one of the most important organs of immune function. Given its essential role and complexity, it is amazing that diseases of the small bowel are not more frequent. In this chapter, the normal anatomy and physiology of the small intestine are described, as well as disease processes involving the small bowel, which include obstruction, inflammatory diseases, neoplasms, diverticular disease, and various miscellaneous problems.

EMBRYOLOGY

The primitive gut is formed during the fourth week of fetal human gestation.[1] The endodermal layer gives rise to the epithelial lining of the digestive tract, and the splanchnic mesoderm surrounding the endoderm gives rise to the muscular connective tissue and all of the other layers of the intestine. Except for the duodenum, which is a primitive foregut structure, the small intestine is derived from the midgut. During the fifth week of fetal development, when the intestinal length is rapidly increasing, herniation of the midgut occurs through the umbilicus (Fig. 48-1). This midgut loop has both a cranial and caudal limb, with the cranial limb developing into the distal duodenum, jejunum, and proximal ilium and the caudal limb becoming the distal ilium and proximal two thirds of the transverse colon. The juncture of the cranial and caudal limbs is where the vitelline duct joins to the yolk sac. This duct structure normally becomes obliterated before birth; however, it can persist as a Meckel diverticulum in about 2% of the population. This midgut herniation persists until about 10 weeks of fetal gestation, when the intestine returns to the abdominal cavity. After completing a 270-degree rotation from its initial starting point, the proximal jejunum reenters the abdomen and occupies the left side of the abdomen with subsequent loops lying more to the right. The cecum enters last and is located temporarily in the right upper quadrant; however, with time, it descends to its normal position in the right lower quadrant. Congenital anomalies of gut malrotation and fixation can occur during this process.

The primitive small bowel is lined by a sheet of cuboidal cells until about the ninth week of gestation, when villi begin to form in the proximal intestine and then proceed in a caudal fashion until the entire small bowel and even the colon, for a period of time, are lined by these finger-like projections. Crypt formation begins in

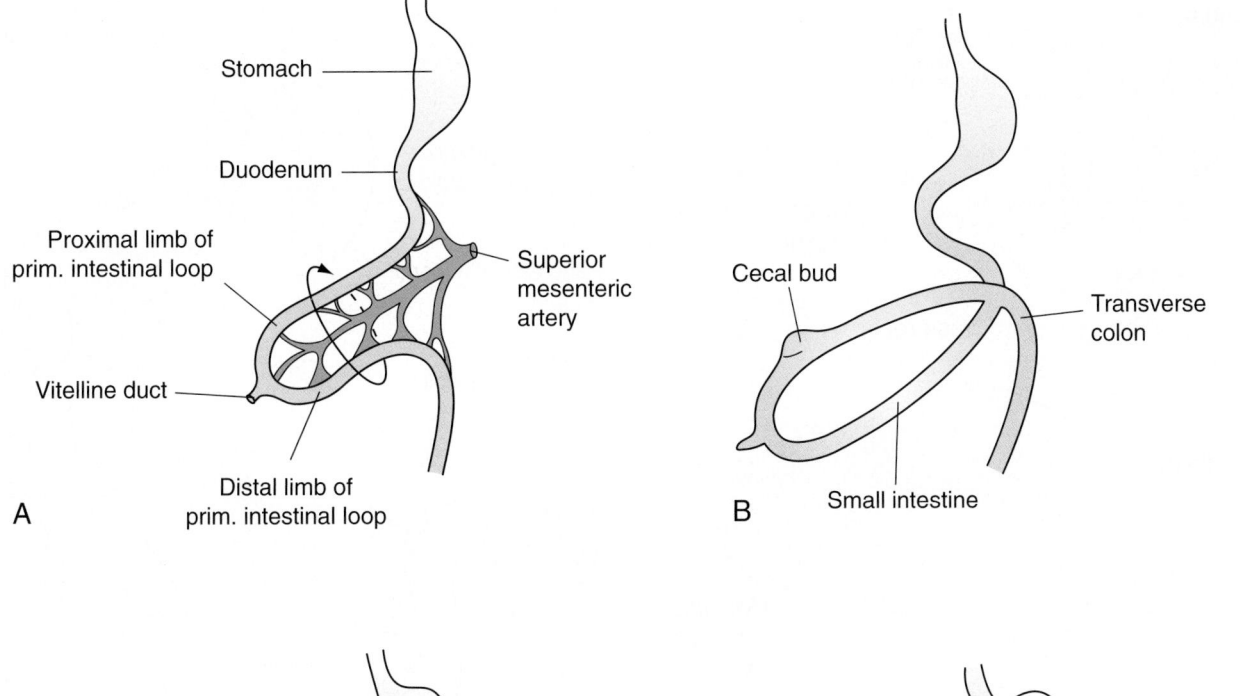

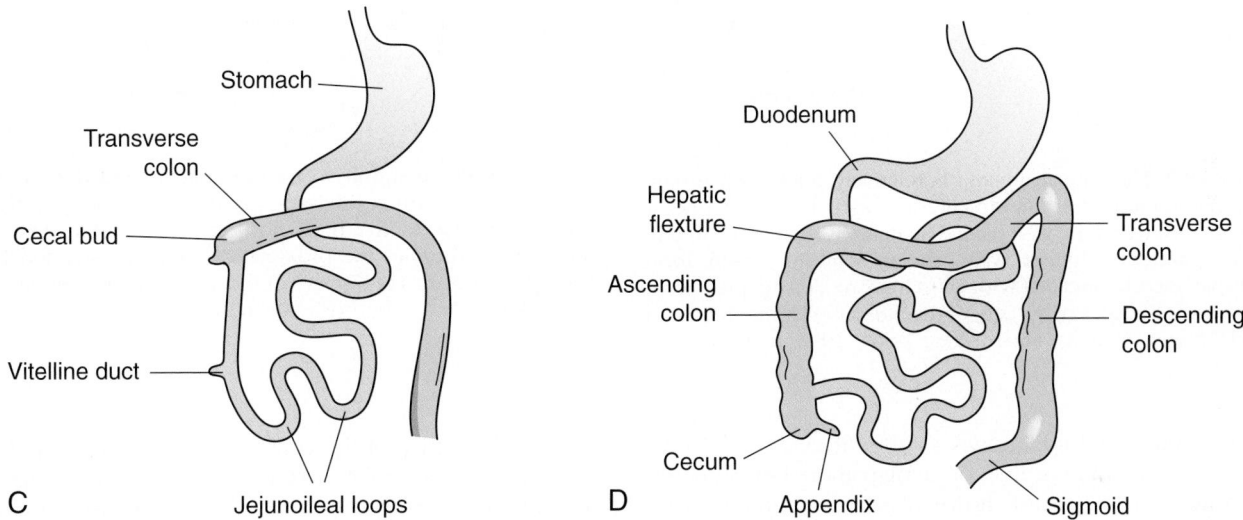

Figure 48-1 Rotation of the intestine. **A,** The intestine after a 90-degree rotation around the axis of the superior mesenteric artery, the proximal loop on the right, and the distal loop on the left. **B,** The intestinal loop after a further 180-degree rotation. The transverse colon passes in front of the duodenum. **C,** Position of the intestinal loops after reentry into the abdominal cavity. Note the elongation of the small intestine, with formation of the small intestine loops. **D,** Final position of the intestines after descent of the cecum into the right iliac fossa. (From Podolsky DK, Babyatshy MW: Growth and development of the gastrointestinal tract. In Yamada T [ed]: Textbook of Gastroenterology, Vol. 2. Philadelphia, JB Lippincott, 1995, Chap 23, with permission. Adapted from Sadler TW [ed]: Langman's Medical Embryology, 5th ed. Baltimore, Williams & Wilkins, 1985.).

the 10th to 12th weeks of gestation. The crypt layer of the small bowel is the site of continual cell renewal and proliferation. As the cells ascend the crypt-villus axis, proliferation ceases, and cells differentiate into one of the four main cell types: *absorptive enterocytes,* which compose about 95% of the intestinal cell population; *goblet cells; Paneth cells;* and *enteroendocrine cells.* Cells are eventually extruded into the intestinal lumen. Amazingly, this entire process of complete renewal of the intestinal lining occurs in less than 1 week in humans.

ANATOMY

Gross Anatomy

General Description

The entire small intestine, which extends from the pylorus to the cecum, measures 270 to 290 cm, with duodenal length estimated at about 20 cm, jejunal length at 100 to 110 cm, and ileal length at 150 to 160 cm. The jejunum begins at the duodenojejunal angle, which is supported

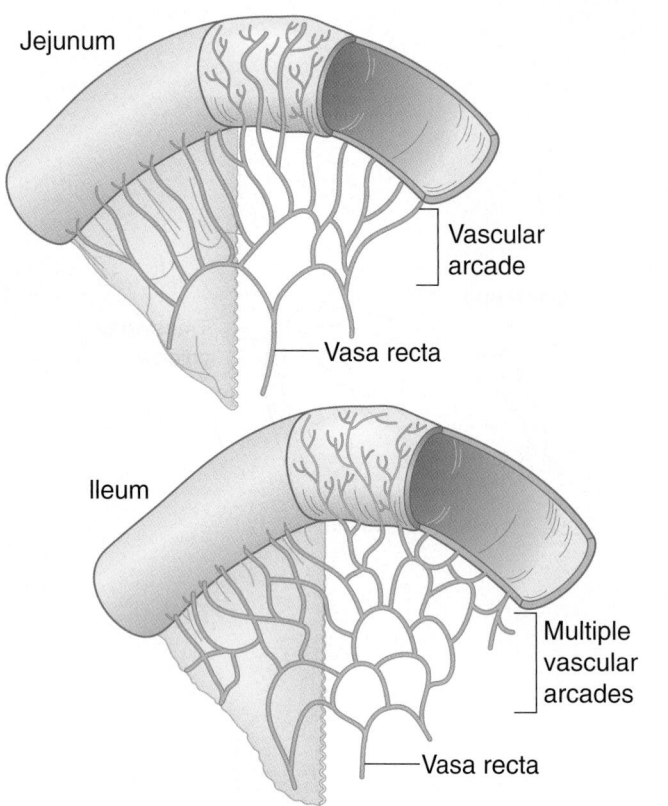

Figure 48-2 The jejunal mucosa is relatively thick with prominent plicae circulares; the mesenteric vessels form only one or two arcades with long vasa recta. The ileum is smaller in circumference and has thinner walls; the mesenteric vessels form multiple vascular arcades with short vasa recta. (Adapted from Thompson JC: Atlas of Surgery of the Stomach, Duodenum, and Small Bowel. St Louis, Mosby–Year Book, 1992, p 263.)

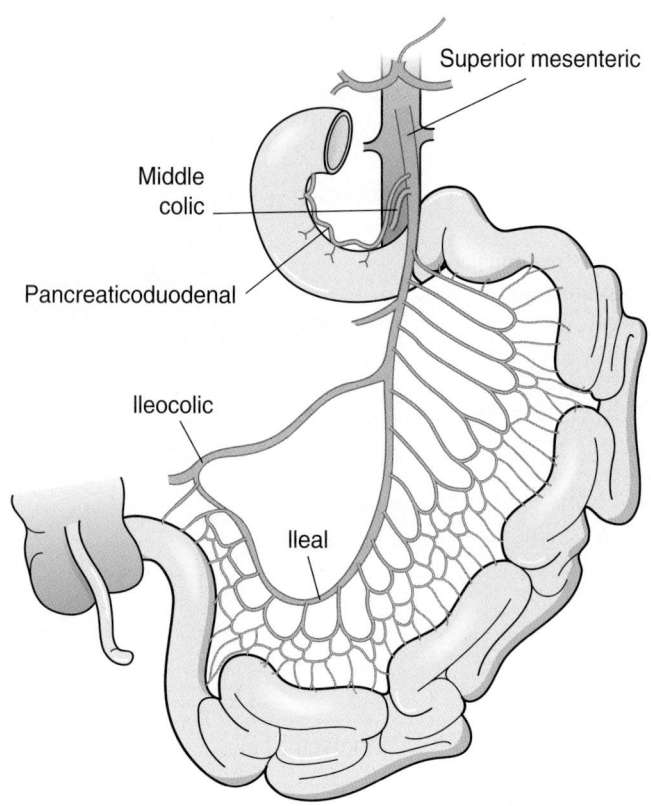

Figure 48-3 Blood supply to the jejunoileum and distal duodenum is entirely from the superior mesenteric artery, which courses anterior to the third portion of the duodenum. The celiac artery supplies the proximal duodenum. (Adapted from Thompson JC: Atlas of Surgery of the Stomach, Duodenum, and Small Bowel. St Louis, Mosby–Year Book, 1992, p 265.)

by a peritoneal fold known as the *ligament of Treitz.* There is no obvious line of demarcation between the jejunum and the ileum; however, the jejunum is commonly considered to make up the proximal two fifths of the small intestine, and the ileum makes up the remaining three fifths. The jejunum has a somewhat larger circumference, is thicker than the ileum, and can be identified at surgery by examining mesenteric vessels (Fig. 48-2). In the jejunum, only one or two arcades send out long, straight vasa recta to the mesenteric border, whereas the blood supply to the ileum may have four or five separate arcades with shorter vasa recta. The mucosa of the small bowel is characterized by transverse folds (*plicae circulares*), which are prominent in the distal duodenum and jejunum.

Neurovascular-Lymphatic Supply

The small intestine is served by rich vascular, neural, and lymphatic supplies, all traversing through the mesentery. The base of the mesentery attaches to the posterior abdominal wall to the left of the second lumbar vertebra and passes obliquely to the right and inferiorly to the right sacroiliac joint. The blood supply of the small bowel, except for the proximal duodenum that is sup-

plied by branches of the celiac axis, comes entirely from the superior mesenteric artery (Fig. 48-3). The superior mesenteric artery courses anterior to the uncinate process of the pancreas and the third portion of the duodenum, where it divides to supply the pancreas, distal duodenum, entire small intestine, and ascending and transverse colon. There is an abundant collateral blood supply to the small bowel provided by vascular arcades coursing in the mesentery. Venous drainage of the small bowel parallels the arterial supply, with blood draining into the superior mesenteric vein, which joins the splenic vein behind the neck of the pancreas to form the portal vein.

The innervation of the small bowel is provided by both parasympathetic and sympathetic divisions of the autonomic nervous system, which in turn provide the efferent nerves to the small intestine. Parasympathetic fibers are derived from the vagus, and they traverse the celiac ganglion and affect secretion, motility, and probably all phases of bowel activity. Vagal afferent fibers are present but apparently do not carry pain impulses. The sympathetic fibers come from three sets of splanchnic nerves and have their ganglion cells usually in a plexus around the base of the superior mesenteric artery. Motor

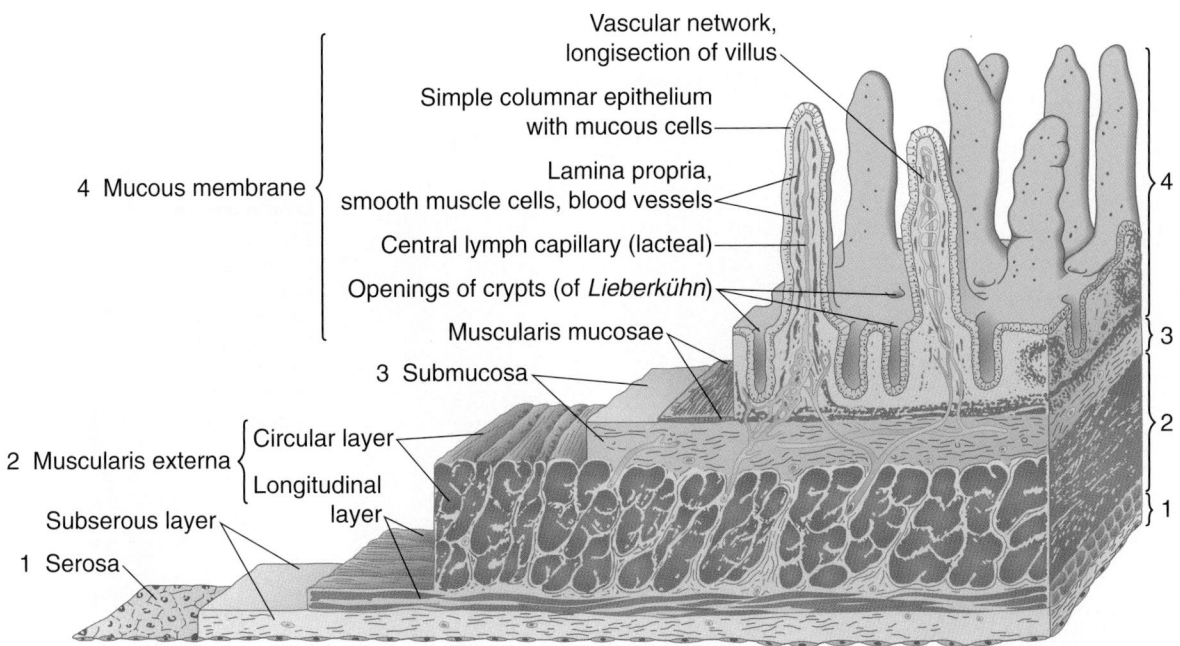

Figure 48-4 Layers of the small intestine. A large surface is provided by villi for the absorption of required nutriments. The solitary lymph follicles in the lamina propria of the mucous membrane are not labeled. In the stroma of both sectioned villi are shown the central chyle (lacteal) vessels or the villous capillaries. (From Sobotta J, Figge FHJ, Hild WJ: Atlas of Human Anatomy. New York, Hafner, 1974.)

impulses affect blood vessel motility and probably gut secretion and motility. Pain from the intestine is mediated through general visceral afferent fibers in the sympathetic system.

The lymphatics of the small intestine are noted in major deposits of lymphatic tissue, particularly in the Peyer patches of the distal small bowel. Lymphatic drainage proceeds from the mucosa through the wall of the bowel to a set of nodes adjacent to the bowel in the mesentery. Drainage continues to a group of regional nodes adjacent to the mesenteric arterial arcades and then to a group at the base of the superior mesentery vessels. From there, lymph flows into the cisterna chyli and then up the thoracic ducts to ultimately empty into the venous system located in the neck. The lymphatic drainage of the small intestine constitutes a major route for transport of absorbed lipid into the circulation and likewise plays a major role in immune defense and also in the spread of cells arising from cancers of the gut.

Microscopic Anatomy

The small bowel wall consists of four layers: serosa, muscularis propria, submucosa, and mucosa (Fig. 48-4).

The *serosa* is the outermost layer of the small intestine and consists of visceral peritoneum, a single layer of flattened mesoepithelial cells that encircles the jejunoileum, and the anterior surface of the duodenum.

The *muscularis* propria consists of two muscle layers, a thin outer longitudinal layer, and a thicker inner circular layer of smooth muscle. Ganglion cells from the myenteric (Auerbach) plexus are interposed between the

muscle layers and send neural fibers into both layers, thus providing electrical continuity between the smooth muscle cells and permitting conduction through the muscle layer.

The *submucosa* consists of a layer of fibroelastic connective tissue containing blood vessels and nerves. It is the strongest component of the intestinal wall and therefore must be included in anastomotic sutures. It contains elaborate networks of lymphatics, arterioles, and venules and an extensive plexus of nerve fibers and ganglion cells (Meissner plexus). The nerves from the mucosa and submucosa muscle layers are interconnected by small nerve fibers, and cross connections between adrenergic and cholinergic elements have been described.

The *mucosa* can be divided into three layers: muscularis mucosae, lamina propria, and epithelial layer (Fig. 48-5). The *muscularis mucosae* is a thin layer of muscle that separates the mucosa from the submucosa. The *lamina propria* is a connective tissue layer between the epithelial cells and the muscularis mucosae that contains a variety of cells, including plasma cells, lymphocytes, mast cells, eosinophils, macrophages, fibroblasts, smooth muscle cells, and noncellular connective tissue. The lamina propria, the base on which the epithelial cells lie, serves a protective role in the intestine to combat microorganisms that penetrate the overlying epithelium, secondary to a rich supply of immune cells. Plasma cells actively synthesize immunoglobulins and other immune cells in the lamina propria and release various mediators (e.g., cytokines, arachidonic acid metabolites, and histamines) that can modulate various cellular functions of the overlying epithelium. The *epithelial layer* is a continual

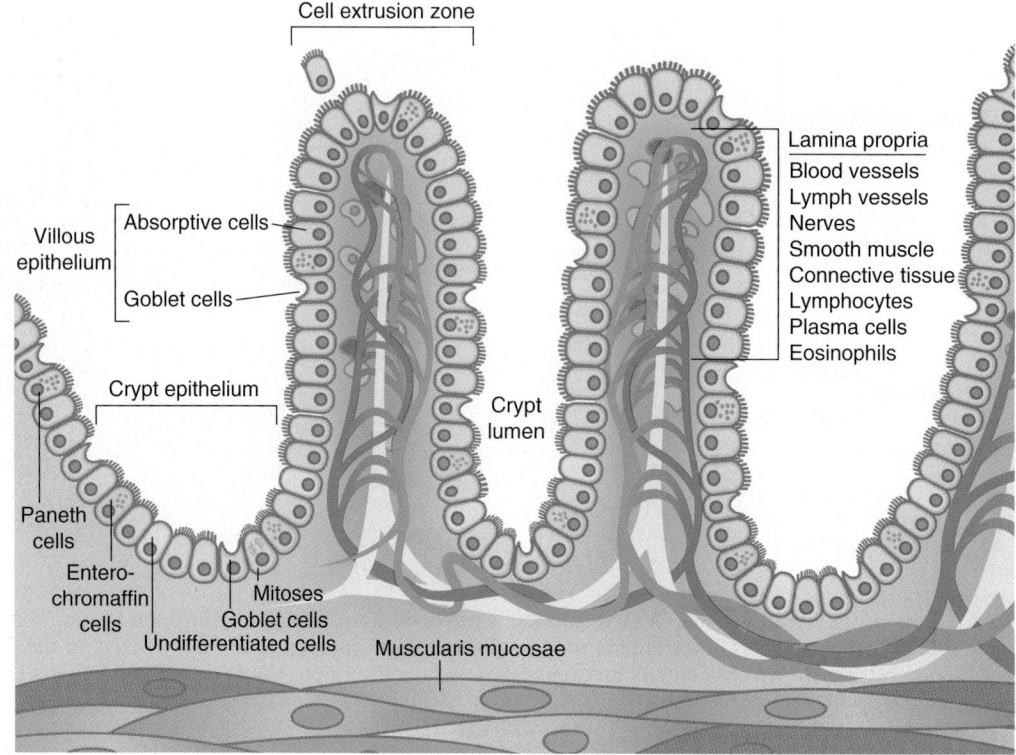

Figure 48-5 Schematic diagram of the histologic organization of the small intestinal mucosa. (Adapted from Keljo DJ, Gariepy CE: Anatomy, histology, embryology, and developmental anomalies of the small and large intestine. In Feldman M, Scharschmidt BF, Sleisenger MH [eds]: Sleisenger & Fordtran's Gastrointestinal and Liver Disease: Pathology/Diagnosis/Management. Philadelphia, WB Saunders, 2002, p 1646.)

sheet of epithelial cells covering the villi and lining the crypts. The main functions of the crypt epithelium are cell renewal and exocrine, endocrine, water, and ion secretion; the main functions of the villus epithelium are digestion and absorption. Four main cell types are contained in the mucosal layer:

1. Goblet cells, which secrete mucus
2. Paneth cells, which secrete lysozyme, tumor necrosis factor (TNF), and the cryptidins, which are homologues of leukocyte defensins and thought to be related to the host mucosal defense system
3. Absorptive enterocytes
4. Enteroendocrine cells, of which there are more than 10 distinct populations that produce the gastrointestinal hormones

Microscopically, the mucosa is designed for maximal absorptive surface area with villi protruding into the lumen. Villi are tallest in the distal duodenum and proximal jejunum and shortest in the distal ileum. Absorptive enterocytes represent the main cell type in the mucosa and are responsible for digestion and absorption. Their luminal surface is covered by microvilli that rest on a terminal web. The microvilli increase the absorptive capacity by 30-fold. To further increase absorption, the microvilli are covered by a fuzzy coat of glycoprotein, the *glycocalyx.*

PHYSIOLOGY

Digestion and Absorption

The complex process of digestion and eventual absorption of nutrients, water, electrolytes, and minerals is the main role of the small intestine. Liters of water and hundreds of grams of food are delivered to the small intestine daily; and, with remarkable efficiency, nearly all food is absorbed, except for indigestible cellulose. The stomach initiates the process of digestion with the breakdown of solids to particles 1 mm or smaller, which are then delivered to the duodenum, where pancreatic enzymes, bile, and brush border enzymes continue the process of digestion and eventual absorption through the small intestinal wall.[2] The small bowel is primarily responsible for absorption of the dietary components (carbohydrates, proteins, and fats), as well as ions, vitamins, and water.

Carbohydrates

An adult consuming a normal Western diet will ingest 300 to 350 g of carbohydrates a day, with about 50% consumed as starch, 30% as sucrose, 6% as lactose, and the remainder as maltose, trehalose, glucose, fructose, sorbitol, cellulose, and pectins.[2] Dietary starch is a polysaccharide consisting of long chains of glucose molecules (Fig. 48-6). Amylose makes up about 20% of starch in the diet and is broken down at the α-1,4 bonds by salivary (i.e., ptyalin) and pancreatic amylases that convert amylose to maltotriose and maltose. Amylopectin, making up about 80% of dietary starch, has branching points every 25 molecules along the straight glucose chains; the α-1,6 glucose linkages in amylopectin produce the end products of amylase digestion: maltose, maltotriose, and the residual branch saccharides, the dextrins. In general, the starches are almost totally converted into maltose and other small glucose polymers before they have passed beyond the duodenum or upper jejunum. The remainder of carbohydrate digestion occurs as a result of brush border enzymes of the luminal surface.

The brush border of the small intestine contains the enzymes lactase, maltase, sucrase-isomaltase, and trehalase, which split the disaccharides, as well as other small glucose polymers, into their constituent monosaccharides (Table 48-1). Lactase hydrolyzes lactose into glucose and galactose. Maltase hydrolyzes maltose to produce glucose monomers. Sucrase-isomaltase is a complex of two subunits; sucrase hydrolyzes sucrose to yield glucose and fructose, and isomaltase hydrolyzes the α-1,6 bonds in α-limit dextrins to yield glucose. Glucose represents more than 80% of the final products of carbohydrate

digestion, with galactose and fructose usually representing no more than 10% of the products of carbohydrate digestion.

The carbohydrates are absorbed in the form of monosaccharides. Transport of the released hexoses (glucose, galactose, and fructose) is carried by specific mechanisms involving active transport. The major routes of absorption are by three membrane carrier systems: sodium glucose transporter 1 (SGLT-1), glucose transporter 5 (GLUT-5), and glucose transporter 2 (GLUT-2)[2] (Fig. 48-7). Glucose and galactose are absorbed by a carrier-mediated active transport mechanism, which involves the cotransport of Na^+ (SGLT-1 transporter). As Na^+ diffuses into the inside of the cell, it pulls the glucose or galactose along with it, thus providing the energy for transport of the monosaccharide. The exit of glucose from the cytosol into the intracellular space is predominantly due to a Na^+-independent carrier (GLUT-2 transporter) located at the basolateral membrane. Fructose, the other significant monosaccharide, is absorbed from the intestinal lumen through a process of facilitated diffusion. The carrier involved for fructose absorption is GLUT-5, which is located in the apical membrane of the enterocyte. This transport process does not depend on Na^+ or energy. Fructose exits the basolateral membrane by another facilitated diffusion process involving the GLUT-2 transporter.

Protein

Protein digestion is initiated in the stomach, where gastric acid denatures proteins.[2] Digestion is continued in the small intestine, where the protein comes in contact with pancreatic proteases. Pancreatic trypsinogen is secreted in the intestine by the pancreas in an inactive form but becomes activated by the enzyme enterokinase, a brush border enzyme in the duodenum. Activated trypsin then activates the other pancreatic proteolytic enzyme precursors. The endopeptidases, which include trypsin, chymotrypsin, and elastase, act on peptide bonds at the interior of the protein molecule, producing peptides that are substrates for the exopeptidases (carboxypeptidases), which serially remove a single amino acid from the carboxyl end of the peptide (Table 48-2). This results in

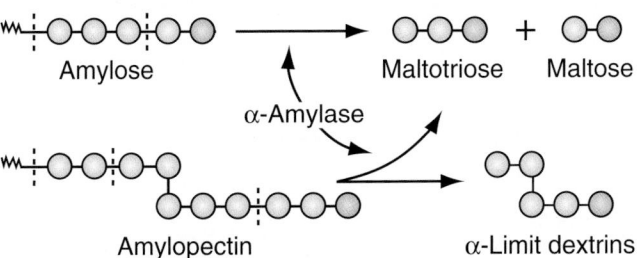

Figure 48-6 Action of pancreatic α-amylase on linear (amylose) and branched (amylopectin) forms of starch to produce the breakdown products maltotriose, maltose, and dextrins. (Adapted from Alpers DH: Digestion and absorption of carbohydrates and proteins. In Johnson LR, Alpers DH, Christensen J, et al [eds]: Physiology of the Gastrointestinal Tract, 3rd ed, Vol. 2. New York, Raven, 1994, p 1727.)

Table 48-1 Characteristics of Brush Border Membrane Carbohydrases

ENZYME	SUBSTRATE	PRODUCTS
Lactase	Lactose	Glucose Galactose
Maltase (glucoamylase)	α-1,4-linked oligosaccharides up to nine residues	Glucose
Sucrase-isomaltase (sucrose-α-dextrinase)		
Sucrase	Sucrose	Glucose Fructose
Isomaltase	α-Limit dextrin	Glucose
Both enzymes	α-Limit dextrin α-1,4-link at nonreducing end	Glucose
Trehalase	Trehalose	Glucose

From Marsh MN, Riley SA: Digestion and absorption of nutrients and vitamins. In Feldman M, Sleisenger MH, Scharschmidt BF (eds): Sleisenger and Fordtran's Gastrointestinal and Liver Disease: Pathophysiology/Diagnosis/Management, Vol 2. Philadelphia, WB Saunders, 1998, p 1480.

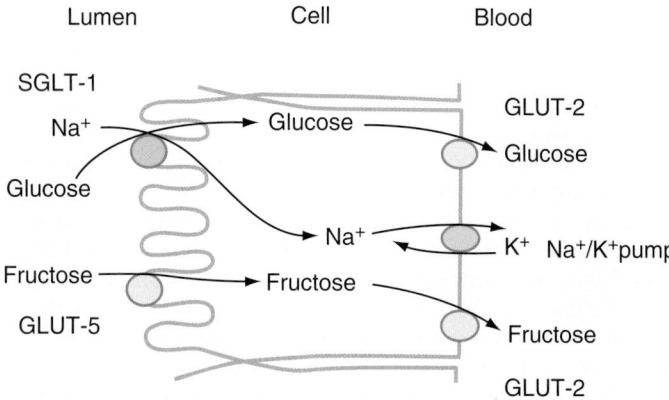

Lumen   Cell   Blood

Figure 48-7 Model for glucose, galactose, and fructose transport across the intestinal epithelium. Glucose and galactose are transported into the enterocyte across the brush border membrane by the Na^+/glucose cotransporter (SGLT-1) and then transported out across the basolateral membrane down their concentration gradients by GLUT-2. The low intracellular Na^+ driving uphill sugar transport across the brush border is maintained by the Na^+/K^+ pump on the basolateral membrane. Glucose and galactose therefore stimulate Na^+ absorption across the epithelium. Fructose is transported across the cell down the concentration gradient across the brush border and basolateral membranes. GLUT-5 is the brush border fructose transporter, whereas GLUT-2 handles fructose transport across the basolateral membrane. (From Wright EM, Hirayama BA, Loo DDF, et al: Intestinal sugar transport. In Johnson LR, Alpers DH, Christensen J, et al [eds]: Physiology of the Gastrointestinal Tract, 3rd ed. New York, Raven Press, 1994, p 1752.)

Table 48-2 Principal Pancreatic Proteases

ENZYME	PRIMARY ACTION
Endopeptidases	Hydrolyze interior peptide bonds of polypeptides and proteins
Trypsin	Attacks peptide bonds involving basic amino acids; yields products with basic amino acids at carboxyl-terminal end
Chymotrypsin	Attacks peptide bonds involving aromatic amino acids, leucine, glutamine, and methionine; yields peptide products with these amino acids at carboxyl-terminal end
Elastase	Attacks peptide bonds involving neutral aliphatic amino acids; yields products with neutral amino acids at carboxyl-terminal end
Exopeptidases	Hydrolyze external peptide bonds of polypeptides and protein
Carboxypeptidase A	Attacks peptides with aromatic and neutral aliphatic amino acids at carboxyl-terminal end
Carboxypeptidase B	Attacks peptides with basic amino acids at carboxyl-terminal end

From Castro GA: Digestion and absorption. In Johnson LR (ed): Gastrointestinal Physiology. St Louis, CV Mosby, 1991, pp 108-130.

splitting the complex proteins into dipeptides, tripeptides, and some larger proteins, which are absorbed from the intestinal lumen by an Na^+-mediated active transport mechanism and digested further by enzymes in the brush border and in the cytoplasm of the enterocytes (Fig. 48-8). These peptidase enzymes include amino peptidases and several dipeptidases, which split the remaining larger polypeptides into tripeptides and dipeptides and some amino acids. The amino acids, dipeptides, and tripeptides are easily transported through the microvilli into the epithelial cells, where, in the cytosol, additional peptidases hydrolyze the dipeptides and tripeptides into single amino acids, which then pass through the epithelial cell membrane into the portal venous system. In normal humans, digestion and absorption of protein are usually 80% to 90% completed in the jejunum.

Fats

Emulsification of Fats

Most adults in North America consume 60 to 100 g/day of fat. Triglycerides, the most abundant fats, are composed of a glycerol nucleus and three fatty acids; small quantities of phospholipids, cholesterol, and cholesterol esters also are found in the normal diet. Essentially all fat digestion occurs in the small intestine, where the first step is the breakdown of fat globules into smaller sizes to facilitate further breakdown by water-soluble digestive

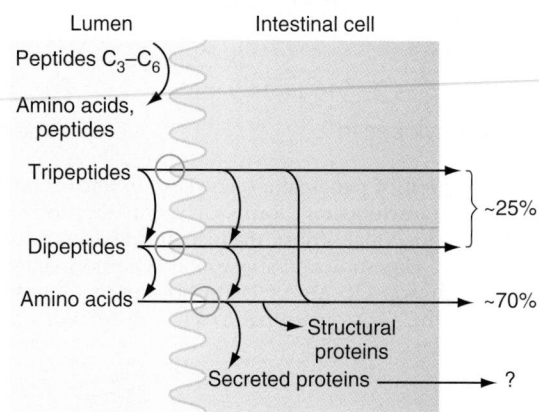

Lumen   Intestinal cell

Figure 48-8 Digestion and absorption of proteins. (Adapted from Alpers DH: Digestion and absorption of carbohydrates and proteins. In Johnson LR, Alpers DH, Christensen J, et al [eds]: Physiology of the Gastrointestinal Tract, 3rd ed, Vol 2. New York, Raven Press, 1994, p 1733.)

enzymes, a process called *emulsification.*[2] This process is facilitated by bile from the liver, which contains bile salts and the phospholipid lecithin. The polar parts of the bile salts and lecithin molecules are soluble in water, whereas the remaining portions are soluble in fat. Therefore, the fat-soluble portions dissolve in the surface layer of the fat globules, and the polar portions, projecting outward, are soluble in the surrounding aqueous fluids. This arrangement renders the fat globules more accessible to fragmentation by agitation in the small intestine. Therefore, a major function of bile salts, and especially lecithin in the bile, is to allow the fat globules to be readily fragmented by agitation in the intestinal lumen. With the increase in surface area of the fat globules resulting from the action of the bile salts and lecithin, the fats can now be readily attacked by pancreatic lipase, the most crucial enzyme in the digestion of triglycerides, which splits triglycerides into free fatty acids and 2-monoglycerides.

Micelle Formation

Fat digestion is further accelerated by bile salts, which, secondary to their amphipathic nature, can form micelles. Micelles are small spherical globules composed of 20 to 40 molecules of bile salts with a sterol nucleus that is highly fat soluble and a hydrophilic polar group that projects outward. The mixed micelles thus formed are arrayed so that the insoluble lipid is surrounded by the bile salts oriented with their hydrophilic ends facing outward. Therefore, as quickly as the monoglycerides and free fatty acids are formed from lipolysis, they become dissolved in the central hydrophobic portion of the micelles, which then act to carry these products of fat hydrolysis to the brush borders of the epithelial cells, where absorption occurs.

Intracellular Processing

The monoglycerides and free fatty acids, which are dissolved in the central lipid portion of the bile acid micelles, are absorbed through the brush border owing to their highly lipid-soluble nature and simply diffuse into the interior of the cell.[2] After disaggregation of the micelle, bile salts remain within the intestinal lumen to enter into the formation of new micelles and act to carry more monoglycerides and fatty acids to the epithelial cells. The released fatty acids and monoglycerides in the cell re-form into new triglycerides. This re-formation of a triglyceride occurs in the cell through the interactions of intracellular enzymes that are associated with the endoplasmic reticulum.

The major pathway for resynthesis involves synthesis of triglycerides from 2-monoglycerides and coenzyme A (CoA)-activated fatty acids. Microsomal acyl-CoA lipase is necessary to synthesize acyl-CoA from the fatty acid before esterification. These reconstituted triglycerides then combine with cholesterol, phospholipids, and apoproteins to form chylomicrons that consist of an inner core containing triglycerides and a membranous outer core of phospholipids and apoproteins. The chylomicrons pass from the epithelial cells into the lacteals, where they pass through the lymphatics into the venous system. From 80% to 90% of all fat absorbed from the gut is absorbed in this manner and transported to the blood by way of the thoracic lymph in the form of chylomicrons. Small quantities of short- to medium-chain fatty acids may be absorbed directly into the portal blood rather than being converted into triglycerides and absorbed into the lymphatics. These shorter-chain fatty acids are more water soluble, which allows for the direct diffusion into the bloodstream.

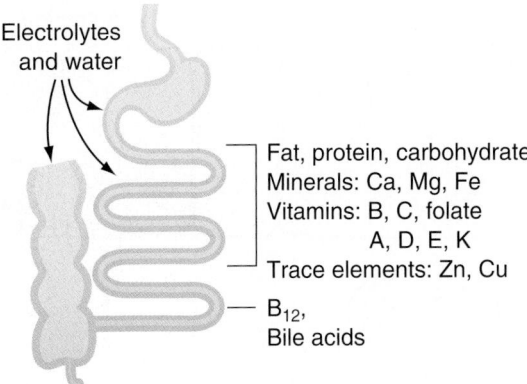

Figure 48-9 Absorption of water and electrolytes in the small bowel and colon. (Adapted from Westergaard H: Short bowel syndrome. In Feldman M, Scharschmidt BF, Sleisenger MH [eds]: Gastrointestinal and Liver Disease: Pathophysiology, Diagnosis, Management. Philadelphia, WB Saunders, 1998, p 1549.)

Enterohepatic Circulation

The proximal intestine absorbs most of the dietary fat. Although the unconjugated bile acids are absorbed into the jejunum by passive diffusion, the conjugated bile acids that form micelles are absorbed in the ileum by active transport and are reabsorbed from the distal ileum. The bile acids then pass through the portal venous system to the liver for secretion as bile. The total bile salt pool in humans is 2 to 3 g, and it recirculates about six times every 24 hours (the enterohepatic circulation of bile salts).[2] Almost all of the bile salts are absorbed, with only about 0.5 g lost in the stool every day; this is replaced by resynthesis from cholesterol.

Water, Electrolytes, and Vitamins

Eight to 10 L of water per day enters the small intestine. Much of this is absorbed, with only about 500 mL or less leaving the ileum and entering the colon[2] (Fig. 48-9). Water may be absorbed by the process of simple diffusion. In addition, water may be drawn in and out of the cell through a process of osmotic pressure, resulting from active transport of sodium, glucose, or amino acids into cells.

Electrolytes can be absorbed in the small bowel by active transport or by coupling to organic solute.[2] Na^+ is absorbed by active transport through the basolateral membranes. Cl^- is absorbed in the upper part of the small intestine by a process of passive diffusion. Large quantities of HCO_3^- must be reabsorbed, and this is accomplished in an indirect fashion. As the Na^+ is absorbed, H^+ is secreted into the lumen of the intestine. It then combines with HCO_3^- to form carbonic acid, which then dissociates to form water and carbon dioxide. The water remains in the chyme, but the carbon dioxide is readily absorbed in the blood and subsequently expired. Calcium is absorbed, particularly in the proximal intestine (duodenum and jejunum), by a process of active transport; absorption appears to be facilitated by an acid environment and is enhanced by vitamin D and parathyroid hormone. Iron is absorbed as either a heme or nonheme

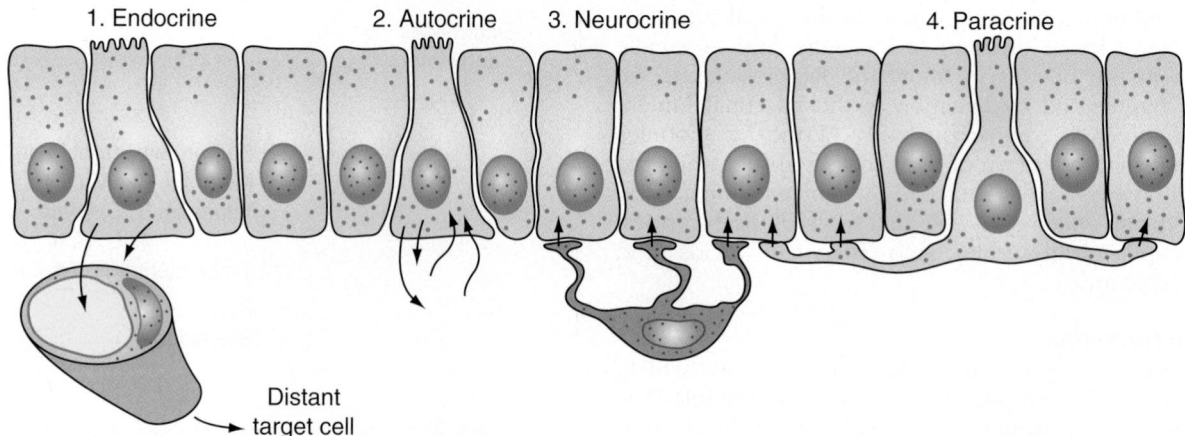

Figure 48-10 Actions of intestinal hormones may be via endocrine, autocrine, neurocrine, or paracrine effects. (Adapted from Miller LJ: Gastrointestinal hormones and receptors. In Yamada T, Alpers DH, Laine L, et al [eds]: Textbook of Gastroenterology, 3rd ed, Vol 1. Philadelphia, Lippincott Williams & Wilkins, 1999, p 37.)

component in the duodenum by an active process. Iron then is either deposited within the cell as ferritin or transferred to the plasma bound to transferrin. The total absorption of iron is dependent on body stores of iron and the rate of erythropoiesis; any increase in erythropoiesis increases iron absorption. Potassium, magnesium, phosphate, and other ions also can be actively absorbed throughout the mucosa.

Vitamins are either fat soluble (e.g., A, D, E, and K) or water soluble (e.g., ascorbic acid [vitamin C], biotin, nicotinic acid, folic acid, riboflavin, thiamine, pyridoxine [vitamin B_6], and cobalamin [vitamin B_{12}]).[2] The fat-soluble vitamins are carried in mixed micelles and transported in chylomicrons of lymph to the thoracic duct and into the venous system. The absorption of water-soluble vitamins appears to be more complex than originally thought. Vitamin C is absorbed by an active transport process that incorporates a sodium-coupled mechanism as well as a specific carrier system. Vitamin B_6 appears to be rapidly absorbed by simple diffusion into the proximal intestine. Thiamine (vitamin B_1) is rapidly absorbed in the jejunum by an active process similar to the sodium-coupled transport system for vitamin C. Riboflavin (vitamin B_2) is absorbed in the upper intestine by facilitated transport. The absorption of vitamin B_{12} occurs primarily in the terminal ileum. Vitamin B_{12} is derived from cobalamin, which is freed in the duodenum by pancreatic proteases. The cobalamin binds to intrinsic factor, which is secreted by the stomach, and is protected from proteolytic digestion. Specific receptors in the terminal ileum take up the cobalamin–intrinsic factor complex, probably by translocation. In the ileal enterocyte, free vitamin B_{12} is bound to an ileal pool of transcobalamin II, which transports it into the portal circulation.

MOTILITY

Food particles are propelled through the small bowel by a complex series of muscular contractions.[2] Peristalsis consists of intestinal contractions passing aborally at a rate of 1 to 2 cm/second. The major function of peristalsis is the movement of intestinal chyme through the intestine. Motility patterns in the small bowel vary greatly between the fed and fasted states. Pacesetter potentials, which are thought to originate in the duodenum, initiate a series of contractions in the fed state that propel food through the small bowel.

During the interdigestive (fasting) period between meals, the bowel is regularly swept by cyclical contractions that move aborally along the intestine every 75 to 90 minutes. These contractions are initiated by the migrating myoelectric complex (MMC), which is under the control of both neural and humoral pathways. Extrinsic nerves to the small bowel are vagal and sympathetic. The vagal fibers have two functionally different effects: one is cholinergic and excitatory, and the other is peptidergic and probably inhibitory. Sympathetic activity inhibits motor function, whereas parasympathetic activity stimulates it. Although intestinal hormones are known to affect small intestinal motility, the one peptide that has been clearly shown to function in this regard is motilin, which is found at its peak plasma level during phase III (intense bursts of myoelectrical activities resulting in regular, high-amplitude contractions) of MMCs.

ENDOCRINE FUNCTION

Gastrointestinal Hormones

The gastrointestinal hormones are distributed along the length of the small bowel in a spatial-specific pattern. In fact, the small bowel is the largest endocrine organ in the body.[3] Although often classified as hormones, these agents do not always function in a truly endocrine fashion (i.e., discharged into the bloodstream, where an action is produced at some distant site) (Fig. 48-10). Sometimes, these peptides are discharged and act locally in a paracrine or an autocrine manner. In addition, these peptides may serve as neurotransmitters (e.g., vasoactive intestinal peptide). The gastrointestinal hormones play a major role

Table 48-3 Gastrointestinal Hormones

HORMONE	LOCATION	MAJOR STIMULANTS OF PEPTIDE SECRETION	PRIMARY EFFECTS
Gastrin	Antrum, duodenum (G cells)	Peptides, amino acids, antral distention, vagal and adrenergic stimulation, gastrin-releasing peptide (bombesin)	Stimulates gastric acid and pepsinogen secretion Stimulates gastric mucosal growth
Cholecystokinin	Duodenum, jejunum (I cells)	Fats, peptides, amino acids	Stimulates pancreatic enzyme secretion Stimulates gallbladder contraction Relaxes sphincter of Oddi Inhibits gastric emptying
Secretin	Duodenum, jejunum (S cells)	Fatty acids, luminal acidity, bile salts	Stimulates release of water and bicarbonate from pancreatic ductal cells Stimulates flow and alkalinity of bile Inhibits gastric acid secretion and motility and inhibits gastrin release
Somatostatin	Pancreatic islets (D cells), antrum, duodenum	Gut: fat, protein, acid, other hormones (e.g., gastrin, cholecystokinin) Pancreas: glucose, amino acids, cholecystokinin	Universal "off" switch: Inhibits release of gastrointestinal hormones Inhibits gastric acid secretion Inhibits small bowel water and electrolyte secretion Inhibits secretion of pancreatic hormones
Gastrin-releasing peptide (mammalian equivalent of bombesin)	Small bowel	Vagal stimulation	Universal "on" switch: Stimulates release of all gastrointestinal hormones (except secretin) Stimulates gastrointestinal secretion and motility Stimulates gastric acid secretion and release of antral gastrin Stimulates growth of intestinal mucosa and pancreas
Gastric inhibitory polypeptide	Duodenum, jejunum (K cells)	Glucose, fat, protein adrenergic stimulation	Inhibits gastric acid and pepsin secretion Stimulates pancreatic insulin release in response to hyperglycemia
Motilin	Duodenum, jejunum	Gastric distention, fat	Stimulates upper gastrointestinal tract motility May initiate the migrating motor complex
Vasoactive intestinal peptide	Neurons throughout the gastrointestinal tract	Vagal stimulation	Primarily functions as a neuropeptide Potent vasodilator Stimulates pancreatic and intestinal secretion Inhibits gastric acid secretion
Neurotensin	Small bowel (N cells)	Fat	Stimulates growth of small and large bowel mucosa
Enteroglucagon	Small bowel (L cells)	Glucose, fat	Glucagon-like peptide-1: Stimulates insulin release Inhibits pancreatic glucagon release Glucagon-like peptide 2: Potent enterotrophic factor
Peptide YY	Distal small bowel, colon	Fatty acids, cholecystokinin	Inhibits gastric and pancreatic secretion Inhibits gallbladder contraction

in pancreaticobiliary and intestinal secretion and motility. In addition, certain gastrointestinal hormones exert a trophic effect on both normal and neoplastic intestinal mucosa and pancreas.[4] The location, major stimulants of release, and primary effects of the more important gastrointestinal hormones are summarized in Table 48-3. In addition, the diagnostic and therapeutic uses of gastrointestinal hormones are listed in Table 48-4. (For a more in-depth discussion of the structure, molecular biology,

physiologic functions, and uses of these hormones, the reader is referred to references 5 and 6.)

Receptors

The gastrointestinal hormones interact with their cell surface receptors to initiate a cascade of signaling events that eventually culminate in their physiologic effects. These hormones primarily signal through G protein–

Table 48-4 Diagnostic and Therapeutic Uses of Gastrointestinal Hormones

HORMONE	DIAGNOSTIC/THERAPEUTIC USES
Gastrin	Pentagastrin (gastrin analogue) used to measure maximal gastric acid secretion
Cholecystokinin	Biliary imaging of gallbladder contraction
Secretin	Provocative test for gastrinoma Measurement of maximal pancreatic secretion
Glucagon	Suppresses bowel motility for endocrine spasm Relieves sphincter of Oddi spasm Provocative test for insulin, catecholamine, and growth hormone release
Somatostatin analogues	Treatment of carcinoid diarrhea and flushing Decrease secretion from pancreatic and intestinal fistulas Ameliorate symptoms associated with hormone-overproducing endocrine tumors Treatment of esophageal variceal bleeding

coupled receptors that traverse the plasma membrane seven times and represent the largest group of receptors found in the body. The heterotrimeric G proteins, which are composed of α, β, and γ subunits, are the molecular switches for signal transduction. Agonist binding to the seven-transmembrane domain receptor is thought to cause a conformational change in the receptor that allows it to interact with the G proteins. Intracellular second messengers that can then be activated include cyclic adenosine monophosphate, Ca^{2+}, cyclic guanosine monophosphate, and inositol phosphate.

In addition to the gastrointestinal hormones, a number of other peptides and growth factors are located in the gastrointestinal mucosa, including epidermal growth factor, transforming growth factor-α and -β, insulin-like growth factor, fibroblast growth factor, and platelet-derived growth factor. These peptides play a role in cell growth and differentiation and act through tyrosine kinase receptors, which have a single membrane-spanning domain.

A third class of surface receptors, the ion channel–linked receptors, are found most commonly in cells of neuronal lineage and usually bind specific neurotransmitters. Examples include receptors for excitatory (acetylcholine and serotonin) and inhibitory (γ-aminobutyric acid, glycine) neurotransmitters. These receptors undergo a conformational change on binding of the mediator, which allows passage of ions across the cell membrane and results in changes in voltage potential.

IMMUNE FUNCTION

During the course of a normal day, we ingest a number of bacteria, parasites, and viruses. The large surface area of the small bowel mucosa represents a potential major portal of entry for these pathogens; the small intestine serves as a major immunologic barrier in addition to its important role in digestion and endocrine function. As a result of constant antigenic exposure, the intestine possesses abundant lymphoid cells (i.e., B and T lymphocytes) and myeloid cells (macrophages, neutrophils, eosinophils, and mast cells). To deal with the constant barrage of potential toxins and antigens, the gut has evolved into a highly organized and efficient mechanism for antigen processing, humoral immunity, and cellular immunity. The gut-associated lymphoid tissue is localized in three areas: Peyer patches, lamina propria lymphoid cells, and intraepithelial lymphocytes.

The Peyer patches are unencapsulated lymphoid nodules that constitute an afferent limb of the gut-associated lymphoid tissue that recognizes antigens through the specialized sampling mechanism of the microfold (M) cells contained within the follicle-associated epithelium (Fig. 48-11). Antigens that gain access to the Peyer patches activate and prime B and T cells in that site. The M cells cover the lymphoid follicles in the gastrointestinal tract and provide a site for the selective sampling of intraluminal antigens. Activated lymphocytes from intestinal lymphoid follicles then leave the intestinal tract and migrate into afferent lymphatics that drain into mesenteric lymph nodes. Furthermore, these cells migrate into the lamina propria. The B lymphocytes become surface immunoglobulin (IgA)-bearing lymphoblasts, which serve a critically important role in mucosal immunity.

B lymphocytes and plasma cells, T lymphocytes, macrophages, dendritic cells, eosinophils, and mast cells are scattered throughout the connective tissue of the lamina propria. About 60% of the lymphoid cells are T cells. These T lymphocytes are a heterogeneous group of cells and can differentiate into one of several types of T-effector cells. Cytotoxic T-effector cells directly damage the target cells. T-helper cells are effector cells that help mediate induction of other T cells or the induction of B cells to produce humoral antibodies. T-suppressor cells perform just the opposite function. About 40% of the lymphoid cells in the lamina propria are B cells, which are primarily derived from precursors in Peyer patches. These B cells and their progeny, plasma cells, are predominantly focused on IgA synthesis and, to a lesser extent, on IgM, IgG, and IgE synthesis.

The intraepithelial lymphocytes are located in the space between the epithelial cells that line the mucosal surface and lie close to the basement membrane. It is suspected that most of the intraepithelial lymphocytes are T cells. On activation, the intraepithelial lymphocytes may acquire cytolytic functions that can contribute to epithelial cell death through apoptosis. These cells may be important in the immunosurveillance against abnormal epithelial cells.

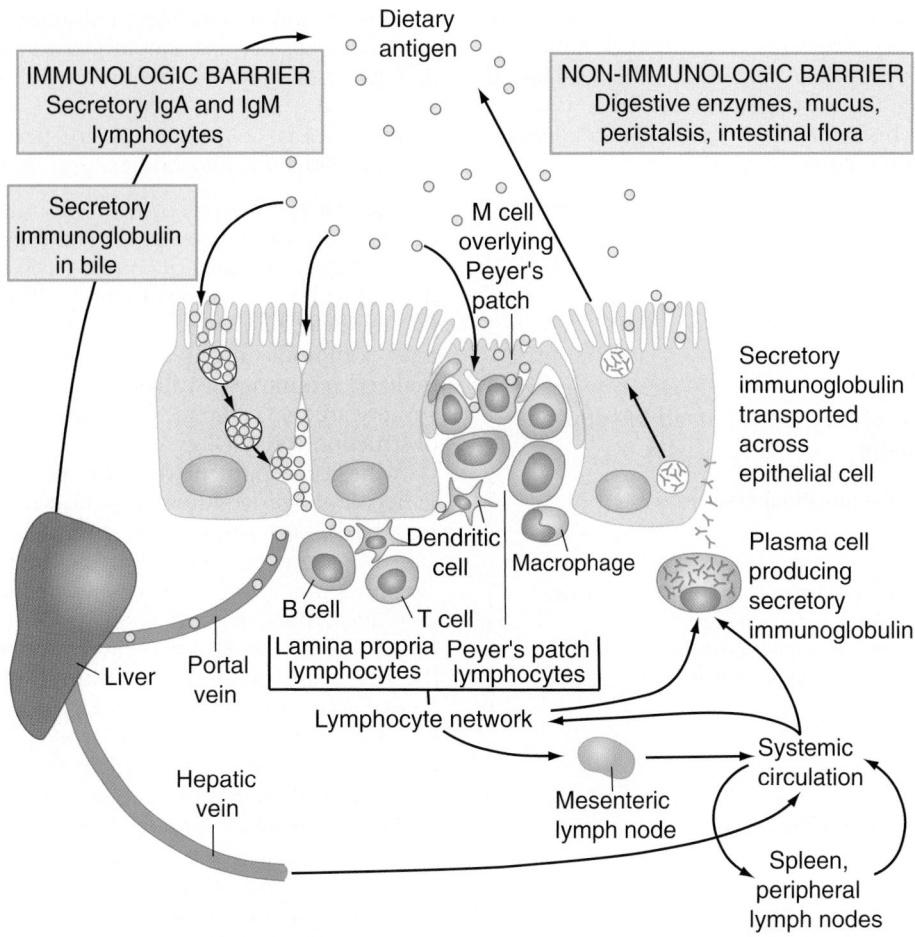

Figure 48-11 The mucosal barrier of the gut. Antigens contact specialized microfold (M) cells overlying Peyer's patches, which then process and present the antigen to the immune system. When B lymphocytes are stimulated by antigenic material, the cells develop into antibody-forming cells that secrete various types of immunoglobulins (Igs), the most important of which is IgA. (Adapted from Duerr RH, Shanahan F: Food allergy. In Targan SR, Shanahan F [eds]: Immunology and Immunopathology of the Liver and Gastrointestinal Tract. New York, Igaku-Shoin, 1990, p 510.)

As already stated, one of the major protective immune mechanisms for the intestinal tract is the synthesis and secretion of IgA. The intestine contains more than 70% of the IgA-producing cells in the body. IgA is produced by plasma cells in the lamina propria and is secreted into the intestine, where it can bind antigens at the mucosal surface. The IgA antibody traverses the epithelial cell to the lumen by means of a protein carrier (the secretory component) that not only transports the IgA but also protects it against the intracellular lysosomes. IgA does not activate complement and does not enhance cell-mediated opsonization or destruction of infectious organisms or antigens, which sharply contrasts to the role of other immunoglobulins. Secretory IgA inhibits the adherence of bacteria to epithelial cells and prevents their colonization and multiplication. In addition, secretory IgA neutralizes bacterial toxins and viral activity and blocks the absorption of antigens from the gut.

OBSTRUCTION

The description of patients presenting with small bowel obstruction dates back to the 3rd or 4th century, when Praxagoras created an enterocutaneous fistula to relieve a bowel obstruction. Despite this success with operative therapy, the nonoperative management of these patients with attempted reduction of hernias, laxatives, ingestion of heavy metals (e.g., lead or mercury), and leeches to remove toxic agents from the blood was the rule until the late 1800s, when antisepsis and aseptic surgical techniques made operative intervention safer and more acceptable. A better understanding of the pathophysiology of bowel obstruction and the use of isotonic fluid resuscitation, intestinal tube decompression, and antibiotics have greatly reduced the mortality rate for patients with mechanical bowel obstruction.[7] However, patients with a bowel obstruction still represent some of the most difficult and vexing problems that surgeons face with regard to the correct diagnosis, the optimal timing of therapy, and the appropriate treatment. Ultimate clinical decisions regarding the management of these patients dictates a thorough history and workup and a heightened awareness of potential complications.

Etiology

The causes of a small bowel obstruction can be divided into three categories (Box 48-1):

Box 48-1 Causes of Mechanical Small Intestinal Obstruction in Adults

Lesions Extrinsic to the Intestinal Wall

Adhesions (usually postoperative)
Hernia
   External (e.g., inguinal, femoral, umbilical, or ventral hernias)
   Internal (e.g., congenital defects such as paraduodenal,
      foramen of Winslow, and diaphragmatic hernias or
      postoperative secondary to mesenteric defects)
Neoplastic
   Carcinomatosis
   Extraintestinal neoplasms
Intra-abdominal abscess

Lesions Intrinsic to the Intestinal Wall

Congenital

Malrotation
Duplications/cysts

Inflammatory

Crohn's disease
Infections
   Tuberculosis
   Actinomycosis
   Diverticulitis

Neoplastic

Primary neoplasms
Metastatic neoplasms

Traumatic

Hematoma
Ischemic stricture

Miscellaneous

Intussusception
Endometriosis
Radiation enteropathy/stricture

Intraluminal/Obturator Obstruction

Gallstone
Enterolith
Bezoar
Foreign body

Adapted from Tito WA, Sarr MG: Intestinal obstruction. In Zuidema GD (ed): Surgery of the Alimentary Tract. Philadelphia, WB Saunders, 1996, pp 375-416.

---

1. Obstruction arising from extraluminal causes such as adhesions, hernias, carcinomas, and abscesses
2. Obstruction intrinsic to the bowel wall (e.g., primary tumors)
3. Intraluminal obturator obstruction (e.g., gallstones, enteroliths, foreign bodies, and bezoars)

The cause of small bowel obstruction has changed dramatically during the past century.[8] At the turn of the 20th century, hernias accounted for more than half of mechanical intestinal obstructions. With the routine elective repair of hernias, this cause has dropped to the third most common cause of small bowel obstruction in industrialized countries. Adhesions secondary to previous surgery are by far the most common cause of small bowel obstruction today (Fig. 48-12).

Adhesions, particularly after pelvic operations (e.g., gynecologic procedures, appendectomy, and colorectal resection), are responsible for more than 60% of all causes of bowel obstruction in the United States. This preponderance of lower abdominal procedures to produce adhesions that result in obstruction is thought to be due to the fact that the bowel is more mobile in the pelvis and more tethered in the upper abdomen.

Malignant tumors account for about 20% of the cases of small bowel obstruction. Most of these tumors are metastatic lesions that obstruct the intestine secondary to peritoneal implants that have spread from an intra-abdominal primary tumor such as ovarian, pancreatic, gastric, or colonic. Less often, malignant cells from distant sites, such as breast, lung, and melanoma, may metastasize hematogenously and account for peritoneal implants and result in an obstruction. Large intra-abdominal tumors may also cause small bowel obstruction through extrinsic compression of the bowel lumen. Primary colonic cancers (particularly those arising from the cecum and ascending colon) may present as a small bowel obstruction. Primary small bowel tumors can cause obstruction but are exceedingly rare.

Hernias are the third leading cause of intestinal obstruction and account for about 10% of all cases. Most commonly, these represent ventral or inguinal hernias. Internal hernias, usually related to prior abdominal surgery, can also result in small bowel obstruction. Less common hernias can also produce obstruction, such as femoral, obturator, lumbar, and sciatic hernias.

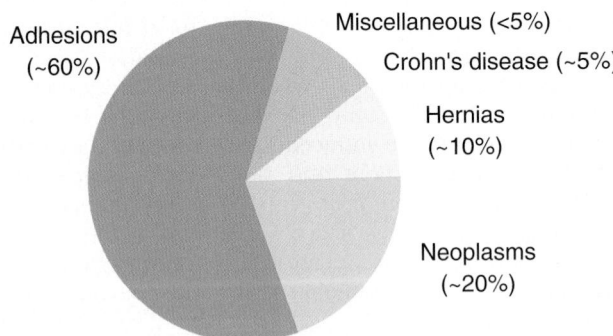

Figure 48-12 Common causes of small bowel obstruction in industrialized countries.

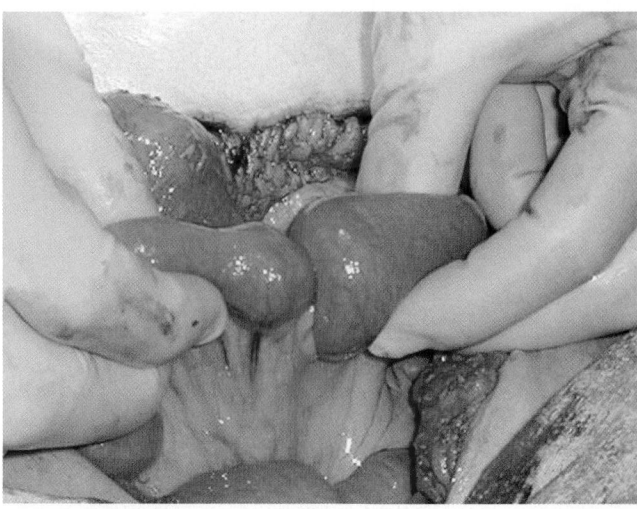

Figure 48-13 Jejunojejunal intussusception in an adult patient. (Courtesy of Steven Williams, MD, Nampa, Idaho.)

Crohn's disease is the fourth leading cause of small bowel obstruction and accounts for about 5% of all cases. Obstruction can result from acute inflammation and edema, which may resolve with conservative management. In patients with long-standing Crohn's disease, strictures can develop that may require resection and reanastomosis or strictureplasty.

An important cause of small bowel obstruction that is not routinely considered is obstruction associated with an intra-abdominal abscess, commonly from a ruptured appendix, diverticulum, or dehiscence of an intestinal anastomosis. The obstruction may occur as a result of a local ileus in the small bowel adjacent to the abscess. In addition, the small bowel can form a portion of the wall of the abscess cavity and become obstructed by kinking of the bowel at this point.

Miscellaneous causes of bowel obstruction account for 2% to 3% of all cases but should be considered in the differential diagnosis. These include intussusception of the bowel, which in the adult is usually secondary to a pathologic lead point such as a polyp or tumor (Fig. 48-13); gallstones, which can enter the intestinal lumen by a cholecystenteric fistula and cause obstruction; enteroliths originating from jejunal diverticula; foreign bodies; and phytobezoars.

Pathophysiology

Early in the course of an obstruction, intestinal motility and contractile activity increase in an effort to propel luminal contents past the obstructing point. The increase in peristalsis that occurs early in the course of bowel obstruction is present both above and below the point of obstruction, thus accounting for the finding of diarrhea that may accompany partial or even complete small bowel obstruction in the early period. Later in the course of obstruction, the intestine becomes fatigued and dilates, with contractions becoming less frequent and less intense.

As the bowel dilates, water and electrolytes accumulate both intraluminally and in the bowel wall itself. This massive third-space fluid loss accounts for the dehydration and hypovolemia. The metabolic effects of fluid loss depend on the site and duration of the obstruction. With a proximal obstruction, dehydration may be accompanied by hypochloremia, hypokalemia, and metabolic alkalosis associated with increased vomiting. Distal obstruction of the small bowel may result in large quantities of intestinal fluid into the bowel; however, abnormalities in serum electrolytes are usually less dramatic. Oliguria, azotemia, and hemoconcentration can accompany the dehydration. Hypotension and shock can ensue. Other consequences of bowel obstruction include increased intra-abdominal pressure, decreased venous return, and elevation of the diaphragm, compromising ventilation. These factors can serve to further potentiate the effects of hypovolemia.

As the intraluminal pressure increases in the bowel, a decrease in mucosal blood flow can occur. These alterations are particularly noted in patients with a closed-loop obstruction in which greater intraluminal pressures are attained. A closed-loop obstruction, produced commonly by a twist of the bowel, can progress to arterial occlusion and ischemia if left untreated and may potentially lead to bowel perforation and peritonitis.

In the absence of intestinal obstruction, the jejunum and proximal ileum of the human are virtually sterile. With obstruction, however, the flora of the small intestine changes dramatically, in both the type of organism (most commonly *Escherichia coli, Streptococcus faecalis,* and *Klebsiella* species) and the quantity, with organisms reaching concentrations of 10^9 to 10^{10}/mL. Studies have shown an increase in the number of indigenous bacteria translocating to mesenteric lymph nodes and even systemic organs. However, the overall importance of this bacterial translocation on the clinical course has not been entirely defined.

Clinical Manifestations and Diagnosis

A thorough history and physical examination are critical to establishing the diagnosis and treatment of the patient with an intestinal obstruction. In most patients, a meticulous history and physical examination complemented by plain abdominal radiographs are all that is required to establish the diagnosis and to devise a treatment plan. More sophisticated radiographic studies may be necessary in certain patients in whom the diagnosis and cause are uncertain. However, a computed tomography (CT) scan of the abdomen should not be the starting point in the workup of a patient with intestinal obstruction.

History

The cardinal symptoms of intestinal obstruction include colicky abdominal pain, nausea, vomiting, abdominal distention, and a failure to pass flatus and feces (i.e., obstipation). These symptoms may vary with the site and duration of obstruction. The typical crampy abdominal pain associated with intestinal obstruction occurs in paroxysms at 4- to 5-minute intervals and occurs less

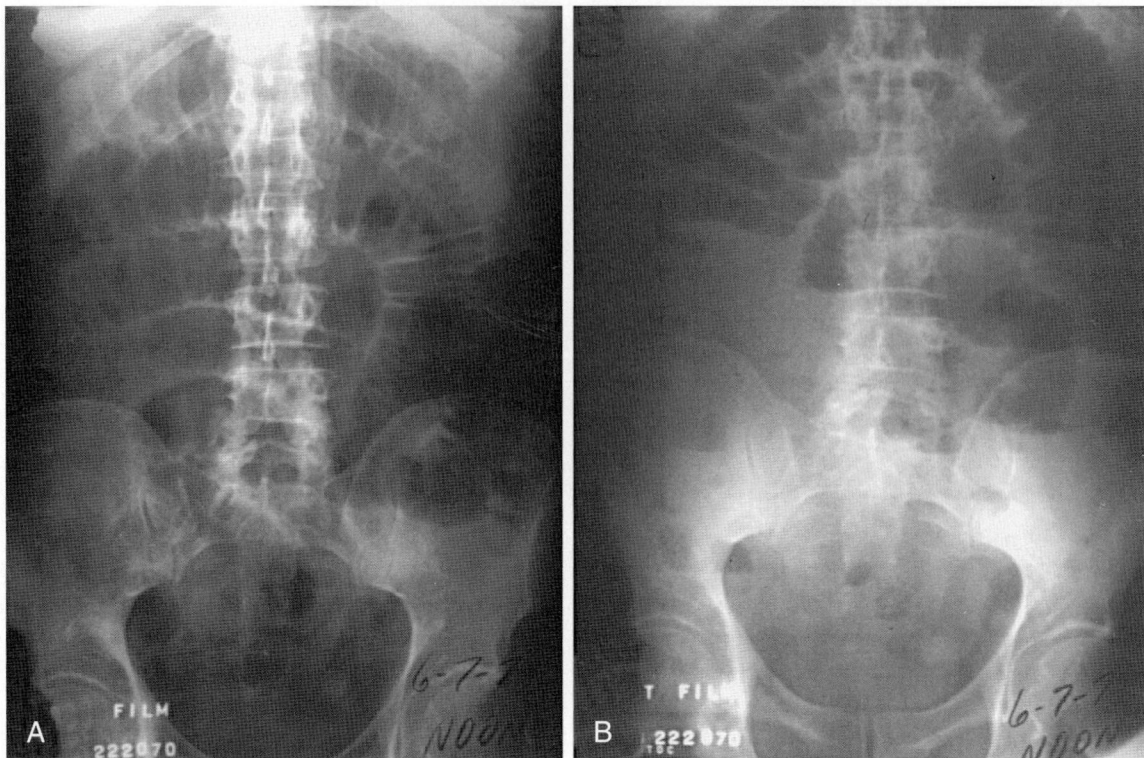

Figure 48-14 Plain abdominal radiographs of a patient with a complete small bowel obstruction. **A,** Supine film shows dilated loops of small bowel in an orderly arrangement, without evidence of colonic gas. **B,** Upright film shows multiple, short air-fluid levels arranged in a stepwise pattern. (Courtesy of Melvyn H. Schreiber, MD, The University of Texas Medical Branch.)

frequently with distal obstruction. Nausea and vomiting are more common with a higher obstruction and may be the only symptoms in patients with gastric outlet or high intestinal obstruction. An obstruction located distally is associated with less emesis, and the initial and most prominent symptom is the cramping abdominal pain. Abdominal distention occurs as the obstruction progresses, and the proximal intestine becomes increasingly dilated. Obstipation is a later development, and it must be reiterated that patients, particularly in the early stages of bowel obstruction, may relate a history of diarrhea that is secondary to increased peristalsis. Therefore, the important point to remember is that a complete bowel obstruction cannot be ruled out based on a history of loose bowel movements. The character of the vomitus is also important to obtain in the history. As the obstruction becomes more complete with bacterial overgrowth, the vomitus becomes more feculent, indicating a late and established intestinal obstruction.

Physical Examination
The patient with intestinal obstruction may present with tachycardia and hypotension, demonstrating the severe dehydration that is present. Fever suggests the possibility of strangulation. Abdominal examination demonstrates a distended abdomen, with the amount of distention somewhat dependent on the level of obstruction. Previous surgical scars should be noted. Early in the course of bowel obstruction, peristaltic waves can be observed,

particularly in thin patients, and auscultation of the abdomen may demonstrate hyperactive bowel sounds with audible rushes associated with vigorous peristalsis (i.e., borborygmi). Late in the obstructive course, minimal or no bowel sounds are noted. Mild abdominal tenderness may be present with or without a palpable mass; however, localized tenderness, rebound, and guarding suggest peritonitis and the likelihood of strangulation. A careful examination must be performed to rule out incarcerated hernias in the groin, the femoral triangle, and the obturator foramen. A rectal examination should be performed to assess for intraluminal masses and to examine the stool for occult blood, which may be an indication of malignancy, intussusception, or infarction.

Radiologic and Laboratory Examinations
The diagnosis of intestinal obstruction is often immediately evident after a thorough history and physical examination. Therefore, plain radiographs usually confirm the clinical suspicion and define more accurately the site of obstruction. The accuracy of diagnosis of the small intestinal obstruction on plain abdominal radiographs is estimated to be about 60%, with an equivocal or a nonspecific diagnosis obtained in the remainder of cases. Characteristic findings on supine radiographs are dilated loops of small intestine without evidence of colonic distention. Upright radiographs demonstrate multiple air-fluid levels, which often layer in a stepwise pattern (Fig. 48-14). Plain abdominal films may also demonstrate the cause of the

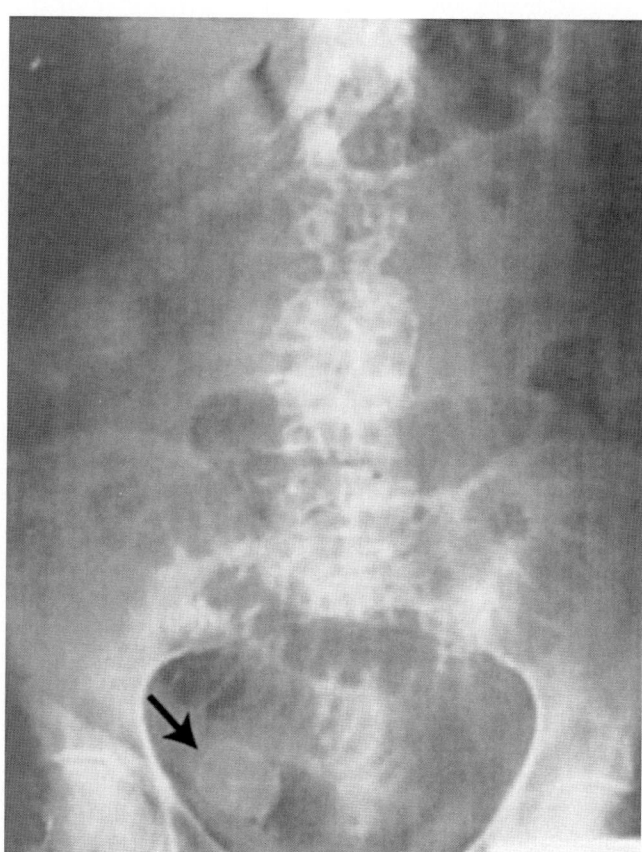

Figure 48-15 Plain abdominal film shows complete bowel obstruction caused by a large radiopaque gallstone *(arrow)* obstructing the distal ileum.

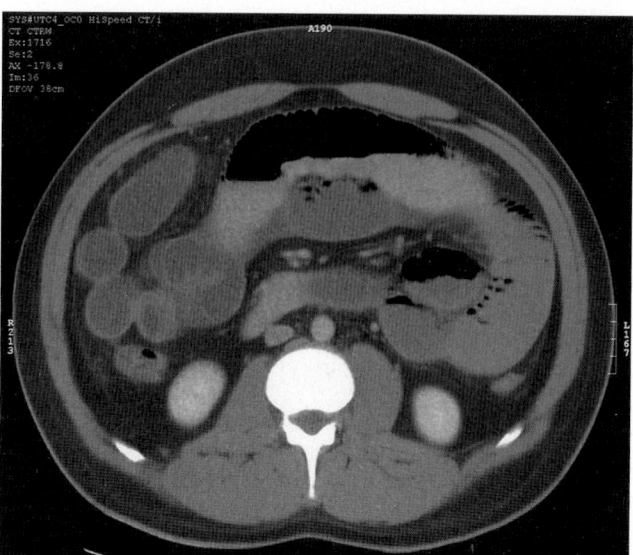

Figure 48-16 CT scan through the mid abdomen shows dilated small bowel loops filled with fluid and decompressed ascending and descending colon. These are typical CT findings in small bowel obstruction. (Courtesy of Eric Walser, MD, The University of Texas Medical Branch.)

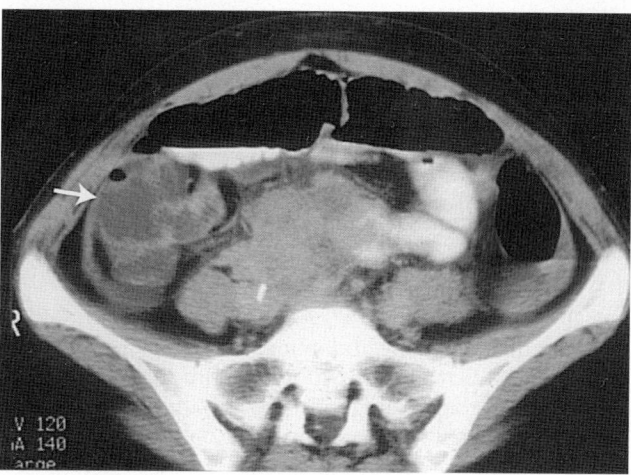

Figure 48-17 CT scan of the abdomen of a patient with a mechanical bowel obstruction secondary to an abscess in the right lower quadrant *(arrow)*. Multiple dilated and fluid-filled loops of small bowel are noted. (Courtesy of Melvyn H. Schreiber, MD, The University of Texas Medical Branch.)

obstruction (e.g., foreign bodies or gallstones) (Fig. 48-15). In uncertain cases or when one is unable to differentiate partial from complete obstruction, further diagnostic evaluations may be required.

In the more complex patient in whom the diagnosis is not readily apparent, CT has proved to be beneficial (Fig. 48-16). CT is particularly sensitive for diagnosing complete or high-grade obstruction of the small bowel and for determining the location and cause of obstruction. The CT examination is less sensitive, however, in patients with partial small bowel obstruction.[9] In addition, CT is helpful if an extrinsic cause of bowel obstruction (e.g., abdominal tumors, inflammatory disease, or abscess) is suggested (Fig. 48-17). CT has also been described as useful in determining bowel strangulation. Unfortunately, CT findings associated with strangulation are those of irreversible ischemia and necrosis.

Barium studies have been a useful adjunct in certain patients with a presumed obstruction. In particular, enteroclysis, which involves the oral insertion of a tube into the duodenum to instill air and barium directly into the small intestine and to follow the movement fluoroscopically, has been helpful in the assessment of obstruction.[10,11] Enteroclysis has been advocated as the definitive study in patients in whom the diagnosis of low-grade, intermittent small bowel obstruction is clinically uncertain. In addition, barium studies can precisely demonstrate the level of the obstruction as well as the cause of the obstruction in certain instances (Fig. 48-18). The main disadvantages of enteroclysis are the need for nasoenteric intubation, the slow transit of contrast material in patients with a fluid-filled hypotonic small bowel, and the enhanced expertise required by the radiologist to perform this procedure.

Ultrasound has been reported to be useful in pregnant patients because radiation exposure is a concern. Magnetic resonance imaging (MRI) has been described in patients with obstruction; however, it appears to be no better diagnostically than CT.

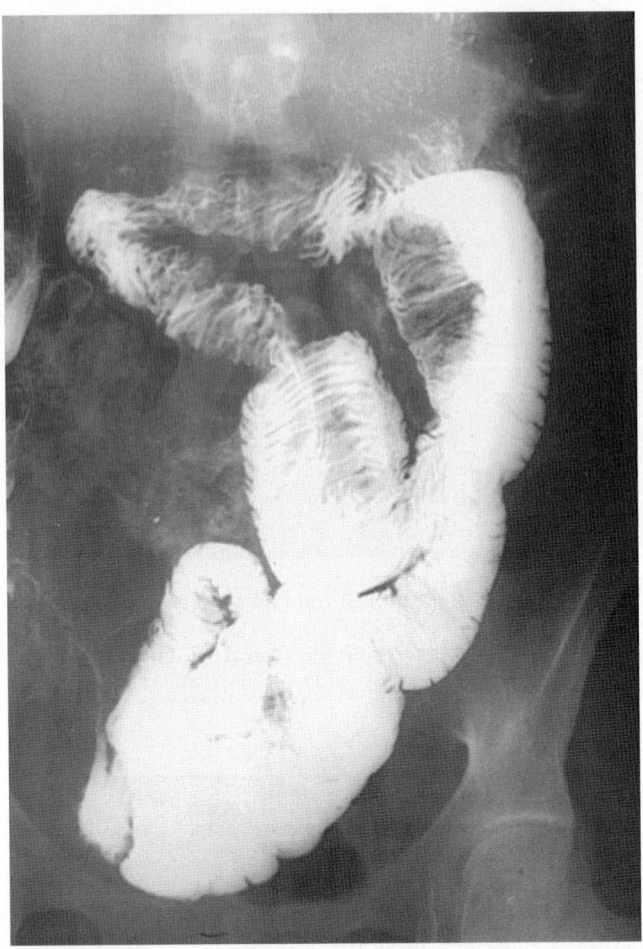

Figure 48-18 Barium study demonstrates jejunojejunal intussusception. (Courtesy of Melvyn H. Schreiber, MD, The University of Texas Medical Branch.)

To summarize, plain abdominal radiographs are usually diagnostic of bowel obstruction in more than 60% of the cases, but further evaluation (possibly by CT or barium radiography) may be necessary in 20% to 30% of cases. CT examination is particularly useful in patients with a history of abdominal malignancy, in postsurgical patients, and in patients who have no history of abdominal surgery and present with symptoms of bowel obstruction. Barium studies are recommended in patients with a history of recurring obstruction or low-grade mechanical obstruction to precisely define the obstructed segment and degree of obstruction.

Laboratory examinations are not helpful in the actual diagnosis of patients with small bowel obstruction but are extremely important in assessing the degree of dehydration. Patients with a bowel obstruction should routinely have laboratory measurements of serum sodium, chloride, potassium, bicarbonate, and creatinine. The serial determination of serum electrolytes should be performed to assess the adequacy of fluid resuscitation. Dehydration may result in hemoconcentration, as noted by an elevated hematocrit. This value should be monitored because fluid resuscitation results in a decrease in the hematocrit, and some patients (e.g., those with intes-

tinal malignancies) may require blood transfusions before surgery. In addition, the white blood cell count should be assessed. Leukocytosis may be found in patients with strangulation; however, an elevated white blood cell count does not necessarily denote strangulation. Conversely, the absence of leukocytosis does not eliminate strangulation as a possibility.

Simple Versus Strangulating Obstruction

Most patients with small bowel obstruction are classified as having simple obstructions that involve mechanical blockage of the flow of luminal contents without compromised viability of the intestinal wall. In contrast, strangulation obstruction, which usually involves a closed-loop obstruction in which the vascular supply to a segment of intestine is compromised, can lead to intestinal infarction. Strangulation obstruction is associated with an increased morbidity and mortality risk, and therefore recognition of early strangulation is important. In differentiating from simple intestinal obstruction, classic signs of strangulation have been described and include tachycardia, fever, leukocytosis, and a constant, noncramping abdominal pain. However, a number of studies have convincingly shown that no clinical parameters or laboratory measurements can accurately detect or exclude the presence of strangulation in all cases.[12]

CT examination is useful only in detecting the late stages of irreversible ischemia (e.g., pneumatosis intestinalis, portal venous gas). Various serum determinations, including lactate dehydrogenase, amylase, alkaline phosphatase, and ammonia levels, have been assessed with no real benefit. Initial reports have described some limited success in discriminating strangulation by measuring serum D-lactate, creatine phosphokinase isoenzyme (particularly the BB isoenzyme), or intestinal fatty acid–binding protein; however, these are only investigational and cannot be widely applied to patients with obstruction. Finally, noninvasive determinations of mesenteric ischemia have been described using a superconducting quantum interference device (SQUID) magnetometer to noninvasively detect mesenteric ischemia. Intestinal ischemia is associated with changes in the basic electrical rhythm of the small intestine. This technique remains investigational and is not in widespread clinical use.

To reiterate, it is important to remember that bowel ischemia and strangulation cannot be reliably diagnosed or excluded preoperatively in all cases by any known clinical parameter, combination of parameters, or current laboratory and radiographic examinations.

Treatment

Fluid Resuscitation and Antibiotics

Patients with intestinal obstruction are usually dehydrated and depleted of sodium, chloride, and potassium, requiring aggressive intravenous (IV) replacement with an isotonic saline solution such as lactated Ringer's. Urine output should be monitored by the placement of a Foley catheter. After the patient has formed adequate urine, potassium chloride should be added to the infusion if needed. Serial electrolyte measurements, as well as hematocrit and white blood cell count, are performed to assess the adequacy of fluid repletion. Because of large fluid requirements, patients, particularly the elderly, may require central venous assessment and, in some cases, the placement of a Swan-Ganz catheter. Broad-spectrum antibiotics are given prophylactically by some surgeons based on the reported findings of bacterial translocation occurring even in simple mechanical obstructions. In addition, antibiotics are administered as a prophylaxis for possible resection or inadvertent enterotomy at surgery.

Tube Decompression

In addition to IV fluid resuscitation, another important adjunct to the supportive care of patients with intestinal obstruction is nasogastric suction. Nasogastric suction with a Levin tube empties the stomach, reducing the hazard of pulmonary aspiration of vomitus and minimizing further intestinal distention from preoperatively swallowed air. The use of long intestinal tubes (e.g., Cantor or Baker tubes) has been advocated by some groups. However, prospective randomized trials demonstrated no significant differences with regard to the decompression achieved, the success of nonoperative treatment, or the morbidity rate after surgical intervention compared with the use of nasogastric tubes. Furthermore, the use of these long tubes has been associated with a significantly longer hospital stay, duration of postoperative ileus, and postoperative complications in some series. Therefore, it appears that long intestinal tubes offer no benefit in the preoperative setting over nasogastric tubes.

Patients with a partial intestinal obstruction may be treated conservatively with resuscitation and tube decompression alone. Resolution of symptoms and discharge without the need for surgery have been reported in 60% to 85% of patients with a partial obstruction.[8] Enteroclysis can assist in determining the degree of obstruction, with higher-grade partial obstructions requiring earlier operative intervention. Although an initial trial of nonoperative management of most patients with partial small bowel obstruction is warranted, it should be emphasized that clinical deterioration of the patient or increasing small bowel distention on abdominal radiographs during tube decompression warrants prompt operative intervention. The decision to continue to treat a patient nonoperatively with a presumed bowel obstruction is based on clinical judgment and requires constant vigilance to ensure that the clinical course has not changed.

Operative Management

In general, the patient with a complete small bowel obstruction requires operative intervention. A nonoperative approach to selected patients with complete small intestinal obstruction has been proposed by some, who argue that prolonged intubation is safe in these patients provided that no fever, tachycardia, tenderness, or leukocytosis is noted. Nevertheless, one must realize that nonoperative management of these patients is undertaken at a calculated risk of overlooking an underlying strangulation obstruction and delaying the treatment of intestinal strangulation until after the injury becomes irreversible. Retrospective studies report that a 12- to 24-hour delay of surgery in these patients is safe but that the incidence of strangulation and other complications increases significantly after this time period.

The nature of the problem dictates the approach to management of the obstructed patient. Patients with intestinal obstruction secondary to an adhesive band may be treated with lysis of adhesions. Great care should be used in the gentle handling of the bowel to reduce serosal trauma and avoid unnecessary dissection and inadvertent enterotomies. Incarcerated hernias can be managed by manual reduction of the herniated segment of bowel and closure of the defect.

The treatment of patients with an obstruction and a history of malignant tumors can be particularly challenging. In the terminal patient with widespread metastasis, nonoperative management, if successful, is usually the best course; however, only a small percentage of cases of complete obstruction can be successfully managed nonoperatively. In this case, a simple bypass of the obstructing lesion, by whatever means, may offer the best option rather than a long and complicated operation that may entail bowel resection.

An obstruction secondary to Crohn's disease will often resolve with conservative management if the obstruction is acute. If a chronic fibrotic stricture is the cause of the obstruction, then a bowel resection or strictureplasty may be required.

Patients with an intra-abdominal abscess can present in a manner indistinguishable from those with mechanical bowel obstruction. CT is particularly useful in diagnosing the cause of the obstruction in these patients; drainage of the abscess percutaneously may be sufficient to relieve the obstruction.

Radiation enteropathy, as a complication of radiation therapy for pelvic malignancies, may cause bowel obstruction. Most cases can be treated nonoperatively with tube decompression and possibly corticosteroids, particularly during the acute setting. In the chronic setting, nonoperative management is rarely effective and will require laparotomy with possible resection of the irradiated bowel or bypass of the affected area.

At the time of exploration, it can sometimes be difficult to evaluate bowel viability after the release of a strangulation. If intestinal viability is questionable, the bowel segment should be completely released and placed in a warm, saline-moistened sponge for 15 to 20 minutes and then reexamined. If normal color has returned and peristalsis is evident, it is safe to retain the bowel. A prospective controlled trial comparing clinical judgment with the use of a Doppler probe or the administration of fluorescein for the intraoperative discrimination of viability found that the Doppler flow probe added little to the conventional clinical judgment of the surgeon. In difficult borderline cases, fluorescein fluorescence may supplement clinical judgment. Another approach to the assessment of bowel viability is the so-called second look laparotomy 18 to 24 hours after the initial procedure. This decision should be made at the time of the initial operation. A second-look laparotomy is clearly indicated in a patient whose condition deteriorates after the initial operation.

Some groups have evaluated the efficacy of laparoscopic management of acute small bowel obstruction. The laparoscopic treatment of small bowel obstruction appears to be effective and leads to a shorter hospital stay in a highly selected group of patients.[13,14] Patients fitting the criteria for consideration of laparoscopic management include those with the following symptoms:

1. Mild abdominal distention allowing adequate visualization
2. Proximal obstruction
3. Partial obstruction
4. Anticipated single-band obstruction

In particular, laparoscopic treatment was of greatest benefit in patients who had undergone less than three previous operations, were seen early after the onset of symptoms, and were thought to have adhesive bands as the cause. Currently, patients who have advanced, complete, or distal small bowel obstructions are not candidates for laparoscopic treatment. Unfortunately, most patients with obstruction are in this group. Similarly, patients with matted adhesions or carcinomatosis or those who remain distended after nasogastric intubation should be managed with conventional laparotomy. Therefore, the future role of laparoscopic procedures in the treatment of these patients remains to be defined.

Management of Specific Problems

Recurrent Intestinal Obstruction

All surgeons can readily (and most often painfully) remember the complicated patient with multiple previous abdominal operations and a "frozen" abdomen who presents with yet another bowel obstruction. An initial nonoperative trial is usually desirable and often safe. In those patients who do not respond conservatively, reoperation is required. This can often be a long and arduous procedure with great care taken to prevent enterotomies. In these difficult patients, various surgical procedures and pharmacologic agents have been tried in an effort to prevent recurrent adhesions and obstruction.

External plication procedures have been described in which the small intestine or its mesentery is sutured in large, gently curving loops.[15] Common complications have included the development of fistulas, gross leakage, peritonitis, and death. For this reason, and because of the low overall success rate, these procedures have largely been abandoned. Several series have reported moderate success with internal fixation or stenting procedures using a long intestinal tube inserted through the nose, a gastrostomy, or even a jejunostomy and left in place for 2 weeks or longer.[16] Complications associated with these tubes include prolonged drainage of bowel contents from the tube insertion site, intussusception, and difficult removal of the tube, which may require surgical reexploration.

Pharmacologic agents, including corticosteroids and other anti-inflammatory agents, cytotoxic drugs, and antihistamines, have been used with limited success. The use of anticoagulants, such as heparin, dextran solutions, dicumarol, and sodium citrate, has modified the extent of adhesion formation, but their side effects far outweigh their efficacy. Intraperitoneal instillation of various proteinases (e.g., trypsin, papain, and pepsin), which cause enzymatic digestion of the extracellular protein matrix, has been unsuccessful. Hyaluronidase has been of questionable value, and conflicting results have been obtained with fibrinolytic agents such as streptokinase, urokinase, and fibrinolytic snake venoms. In a prospective, multicenter trial, Becker and colleagues[17] reported that the use of a hyaluronate-based, bioresorbable membrane reduced the incidence and severity of postoperative adhesion formation. Another study by Vrijland and associates[18] found that placement of this membrane reduced the severity, but not the incidence, of postoperative adhesion in patients undergoing a Hartmann procedure. Longer term, randomized studies will be required to completely determine the efficacy of this material to prevent adhesions and ultimately prevent bowel obstructions. This could represent a significant advance if the long-term incidence of obstruction is likewise shown to be reduced.

To date, the most effective means of limiting the number of adhesions is a good surgical technique, which includes the gentle handling of the bowel to reduce serosal trauma, avoidance of unnecessary dissection, exclusion of foreign material from the peritoneal cavity (the use of absorbable suture material when possible, the avoidance of excessive use of gauze sponges, and the removal of starch from gloves), adequate irrigation and removal of infectious and ischemic debris, and preservation and use of the omentum around the site of surgery or in the denuded pelvis.

Acute Postoperative Obstruction

Small bowel obstruction that occurs in the immediate postoperative period presents a challenge in both the diagnosis and treatment.[19] Diagnosis is often difficult because the primary symptoms of abdominal pain and nausea or emesis may be attributed to a postoperative ileus. Electrolyte deficiencies, particularly hypokalemia, can be a cause of ileus and should be corrected. Plain abdominal films are usually not helpful in distinguishing an ileus from obstruction. CT may be useful in this regard and, in particular, enteroclysis studies may be quite helpful in determining whether an obstruction exists and, if so, the level of the obstruction. Conservative management should be attempted for a partial obstruction. Complete obstruction requires reoperation and correction of the underlying problem.

Ileus

An ileus is defined as intestinal distention and the slowing or absence of passage of luminal contents without a demonstrable mechanical obstruction. An ileus can result from a number of causes, including drug induced, metabolic, neurogenic, and infectious (Box 48-2).

Pharmacologic agents that can produce an ileus include anticholinergic drugs, autonomic blockers, antihistamines, and various psychotropic agents, such as haloperidol and tricyclic antidepressants. One of the more common causes of drug-induced ileus in the operative patient is the use of opiates, such as morphine or meperidine. Metabolic causes of ileus are common and include hypokalemia, hyponatremia, and hypomagnesemia. Other metabolic causes include uremia, diabetic coma, and hypoparathyroidism. Neurogenic causes of an ileus include postoperative ileus, which occurs after abdominal operations. Spinal injury, retroperitoneal irritation, and orthopedic procedures on the spine or pelvis can result in an ileus. Finally, a number of infectious causes can result in an ileus; common infectious causes include pneumonia, peritonitis, and generalized sepsis from a nonabdominal source.

Patients often present in a manner similar to those with a mechanical small bowel obstruction. Abdominal distention, usually without the colicky abdominal pain, is the typical and most notable finding. Nausea and vomiting may occur but may also be absent. Patients with an ileus may continue to pass flatus and diarrhea, and this may help distinguish these patients from those with a mechanical small bowel obstruction.

Radiologic studies may help to distinguish ileus from small bowel obstruction. Plain abdominal radiographs may reveal distended small bowel as well as large bowel loops. In cases that are difficult to differentiate from obstruction, barium studies may be beneficial.

The treatment of an ileus is entirely supportive with nasogastric decompression and IV fluids. The most effective treatment to correct the underlying condition may be aggressive treatment of the sepsis, correction of any metabolic or electrolyte abnormalities, and discontinuation of medications that may produce an ileus. Pharmacologic agents have been used but for the most part have been ineffective. Drugs that block sympathetic input (e.g., guanethidine) or stimulate parasympathetic activity (e.g., bethanechol or neostigmine) have been tried. In addition, hormonal manipulation, using cholecystokinin or motilin, has been evaluated, but the results have been inconsistent. IV erythromycin has been ineffective, and cisapride, although apparently beneficial in stimulating gastric motility, does not appear to alter intestinal ileus.

INFLAMMATORY DISEASES

Crohn's Disease

Crohn's disease is a chronic, transmural inflammatory disease of the gastrointestinal tract of unknown cause. Crohn's disease can involve any part of the alimentary tract from the mouth to the anus but most commonly affects the small intestine and colon. The most common clinical manifestations are abdominal pain, diarrhea, and weight loss. Crohn's disease can be complicated by intestinal obstruction or localized perforation with fistula formation. Both medical and surgical treatments are palliative; however, operative therapy can provide effective symptomatic relief for those patients with complications from Crohn's disease and produces a reasonable long-term benefit.

History

The first documented case of Crohn's disease was described by Morgagni in 1761. In 1913, the Scottish surgeon Dalziel described nine cases of intestinal inflammatory disease. However, it is the landmark paper by Crohn, Ginzburg, and Oppenheimer in 1932 that provided, in eloquent detail, the pathologic and clinical findings of this inflammatory disease in young adults.[20] This classic paper crystallized the description of this inflammatory condition. Although many different (and sometimes misleading) terms have been used to describe this disease process, *Crohn's disease* has been universally accepted as its name.

Incidence and Epidemiology

Crohn's disease is the most common primary surgical disease of the small bowel, with an annual incidence of 3 to 7 cases per 100,000 of the general population; the incidence is highest in North America and Northern Europe.[21] Crohn's disease primarily attacks young adults in the second and third decades of life. However, a bimodal distribution is apparent with a second, smaller peak occurring in the sixth decade of life. Crohn's disease is more common in urban dwellers, and although earlier reports suggested a somewhat higher female predominance, the two genders are affected equally. The risk for developing Crohn's disease is about two times higher in smokers than in nonsmokers. Several studies have indicated an increased incidence of Crohn's disease in women using oral contraceptives; however, more recent studies have shown no differences. Although Crohn's disease is uncommon in African blacks, blacks in the United States have rates similar to whites. Certain ethnic groups, particularly Jews, have a greater incidence of Crohn's disease than do age- and gender-matched control subjects. There is a strong familial association, with the risk for developing Crohn's disease increased about 30-fold in siblings and 14- to 15-fold for all first-degree relatives. Other analyses supporting a genetic role for Crohn's disease show a concordance rate of 67% in monozygotic twins.

Etiology

The cause of Crohn's disease remains unknown. A number of potential causes have been proposed, with the most likely possibilities being infectious, immunologic, and genetic.[21,22] Other possibilities that have met with various levels of enthusiasm include environmental and dietary factors, smoking, and psychosocial factors. Although these latter factors may contribute to the overall disease process, it is unlikely that they represent the primary etiologic mechanism for Crohn's disease.

Infectious Agents

Although a number of infectious agents have been proposed as potential causes of Crohn's disease, the two that have received the most attention are mycobacterial infections, particularly *Mycobacterium paratuberculosis,* and the measles virus. The existence of atypical mycobacteria as a cause for Crohn's disease was proposed by Dalziel in 1913. Subsequent studies using polymerase chain reaction (PCR) techniques have confirmed the presence of mycobacteria in intestinal samples of patients with Crohn's disease. Transplantation of tissue from patients with Crohn's disease has resulted in ileitis, but antimicrobial therapy directed against mycobacteria has not been effective in ameliorating the disease process.

Immunologic Factors

Immunologic abnormalities that have been demonstrated in patients with Crohn's disease have included humoral as well as cell-mediated immune reactions directed against intestinal cells, suggesting an autoimmune phenomenon. Attention has focused on the role of cytokines, such as interleukin (IL)-1, IL-2, IL-8, and TNF-α, as contributing factors in the intestinal inflammatory response. The role of the immune response remains controversial in Crohn's disease and may represent an effect of the disease process rather than an actual cause.

Genetic Factors

Genetic factors play an important role in the pathogenesis of Crohn's disease because the single strongest risk factor for developing disease is having a relative with Crohn's disease. European and American studies reported the presence of a locus on chromosome 16q (called the *IBD1* locus).[23,24] Independent investigative groups identified the *IBD1* locus as the *CARD15/NOD2* gene, a member of the CED4/APAF1 superfamily of apoptosis regulatory proteins, which mediates the innate immune response to microbial pathogens, leading to NF-κB activation.[23] Individuals with allelic variants of *CARD15/NOD2* have a 40-fold relative risk for Crohn's disease compared with the general population; the *IBD1* locus appears to be relatively specific for Crohn's disease and not ulcerative colitis. Other inflammatory bowel disease genomic regions include *IBD2* on chromosome 12q (observed more in ulcerative colitis) and *IBD3,* containing the major histocompatibility complex region located on chromosome 6p. Putative *IBD* loci have been identified on chromosomes 5q, 19p, 7q, and 3p.

Even with strong evidence for a genetic link to Crohn's disease, it is worth reiterating that there is a substantially less than 100% concordance rate between monozygotic twins, suggesting that simple mendelian inheritance cannot account for the pattern of occurrence. Therefore, it is likely that multiple causes (e.g., environmental factors) contribute to the etiology and pathogenesis of this disease.

Pathology

The most common sites of occurrence of Crohn's disease are the small intestine and colon. The involvement of both large and small intestine has been noted in about 55% of patients. Thirty percent of patients present with small bowel disease alone, and in 15%, the disease appears limited to the large intestine. The disease process is discontinuous and segmental. In patients with colonic disease, rectal sparing is characteristic of Crohn's disease and helps to distinguish it from ulcerative colitis. Perirectal and perianal involvement occurs in about one third of patients with Crohn's disease, particularly those with colonic involvement. Crohn's disease can also involve the mouth, esophagus, stomach, duodenum, and appendix. Involvement of these sites can accompany disease in the small or large intestine, but in only rare cases have these locations been the only apparent sites of involvement.

Gross Pathologic Features

At exploration, thickened grayish-pink or dull purple-red loops of bowel are noted, with areas of thick gray-white exudate or fibrosis of the serosa. Areas of diseased bowel separated by areas of grossly appearing normal bowel called *skip areas* are commonly encountered. A striking finding of Crohn's disease is extensive fat wrapping caused by the circumferential growth of the mesenteric fat around the bowel wall (Fig. 48-19). As the disease progresses, the bowel wall becomes increasingly thickened, firm, rubbery, and virtually incompressible. The uninvolved proximal bowel may be dilated secondary to obstruction of the diseased segment. Involved segments often are adherent to adjacent intestinal loops or other viscera, with internal fistulas common in these areas. The mesentery of the involved segment is usually thickened, with enlarged lymph nodes often noted.

On opening the bowel, the earliest gross pathologic lesion is a superficial aphthous ulcer noted in the mucosa. As the disease progresses, the ulceration becomes pronounced, and complete transmural inflammation results. The ulcers are characteristically linear and may coalesce to produce transverse sinuses with islands of normal mucosa in between, thus giving the characteristic cobblestone appearance.

Microscopic Features

Mucosal and submucosal edema may be noted microscopically before any gross changes. A chronic inflammatory infiltrate appears in the mucosa and submucosa and extends transmurally. This inflammatory reaction is characterized by extensive edema, hyperemia, lymphangiectasia, an intense infiltration of mononuclear cells, and lymphoid hyperplasia. Characteristic histologic lesions of Crohn's disease are noncaseating granulomas with Langerhans' giant cells. Granulomas appear later in the course

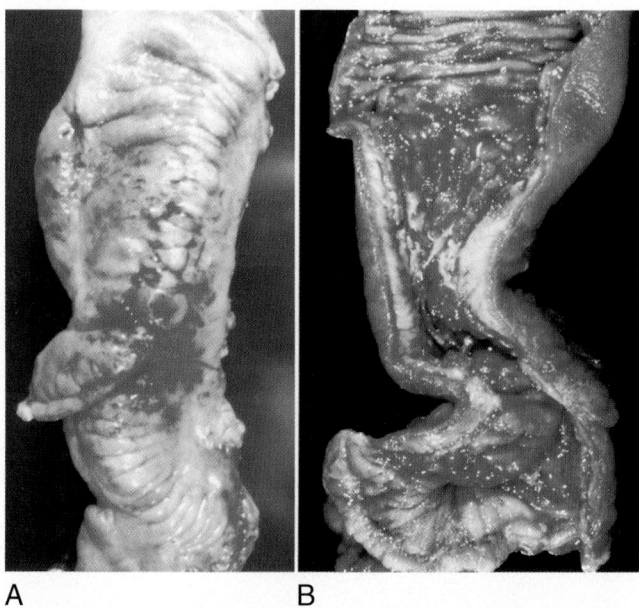

A   **B**

Figure 48-19 Gross pathologic features of Crohn's disease. **A,** Serosal surface demonstrates extensive "fat wrapping" and inflammation. **B,** Resected specimen demonstrates marked fibrosis of the intestinal wall, stricture, and segmental mucosal inflammation. (Courtesy of Mary R. Schwartz, MD, Baylor College of Medicine.)

and are found in the wall of the bowel or in regional lymph nodes in 60% to 70% of patients (Fig. 48-20).

Clinical Manifestations

Crohn's disease can occur at any age, but the typical patient is a young adult in the second or third decade of life. The onset of disease is often insidious, with a slow and protracted course. Characteristically, there are symptomatic periods of abdominal pain and diarrhea interspersed with asymptomatic periods of varying lengths. With time, the symptomatic periods gradually become more frequent, more severe, and longer lasting. The most common symptom is intermittent and colicky abdominal pain, most commonly noted in the lower abdomen. The pain, however, may be more severe and localized and may mimic the signs and symptoms of acute appendicitis. Diarrhea is the next most frequent symptom and is present, at least intermittently, in about 85% of patients. In contrast to ulcerative colitis, patients with Crohn's disease typically have fewer bowel movements, and the stools rarely contain mucus, pus, or blood. Systemic nonspecific symptoms include a low-grade fever (present in about one third of the patients), weight loss, loss of strength, and malaise.

The main intestinal complications of Crohn's disease include obstruction and perforation. Obstruction occurs as a result of chronic fibrosing lesions, which eventually narrow the lumen of the bowel, producing partial or near-complete obstruction. Free perforations into the peritoneal cavity leading to a generalized peritonitis can occur in patients with Crohn's disease, but this presentation is rare. More commonly, fistulas occur between the

sites of perforation and adjacent organs, such as loops of small and large intestine, the urinary bladder, the vagina, the stomach, and sometimes the skin, usually at the site of a previous laparotomy. Localized abscesses can occur near the sites of perforation. Patients with Crohn's colitis may develop toxic megacolon and present with a marked colonic dilation, abdominal tenderness, fever, and leukocytosis.

Long-standing Crohn's disease predisposes to cancer of both the small intestine and colon.[25] The relative risk for adenocarcinoma of the small bowel in Crohn's disease is at least 100-fold greater than in matched control subjects. These carcinomas typically arise at sites of chronic disease and more commonly occur in the ileum. Most are not detected until the advanced stages, and prognosis is poor. Although this relative risk for small bowel cancer in Crohn's disease is quite high, the absolute risk is still small. Of greater concern is the development of colorectal cancer in patients with colonic involvement and a long duration of disease. Although the cancer risk is lower in Crohn's disease than in patients with extensive ulcerative colitis, recent evidence indicates that with the same duration and anatomic extent of disease, the risk for cancer in Crohn's disease of the colon is at least as great as that in ulcerative colitis. Dysplasia is the putative precursor lesion for Crohn's-associated cancer. Although the dysplasia-carcinoma sequence has not been as extensively studied in Crohn's disease compared with ulcerative colitis, patients with long-standing Crohn's disease should have an equally aggressive colonoscopic surveillance regimen as patients with extensive ulcerative colitis. Extraintestinal cancer, such as squamous cell carcinoma of the vulva and anal canal and Hodgkin's and non-Hodgkin's lymphomas, may be more frequent in patients with Crohn's disease.

Perianal disease (fissure, fistula, stricture, or abscess) is common and occurs in 25% of patients with Crohn's disease limited to the small intestine, 41% of patients with ileocolitis, and 48% of patients with colonic involvement alone. Perianal disease may be the sole presenting feature in 5% of patients and may precede the onset of intestinal disease by months or even years. Crohn's disease should be suspected in any patient with multiple, chronic perianal fistulas.

Extraintestinal manifestations of Crohn's disease may be present in 30% of patients (Box 48-3). The most common symptoms are skin lesions, which include erythema nodosum and pyoderma gangrenosum, arthritis and arthralgias, uveitis and iritis, hepatitis and pericholangitis, and aphthous stomatitis. In addition, amyloidosis, pancreatitis, and nephrotic syndrome may occur in these patients. These symptoms may precede, accompany, or appear independent of the underlying bowel disease.

Diagnosis

A diagnosis of Crohn's disease should be considered in patients with chronic, recurring episodes of abdominal pain, diarrhea, and weight loss. Typically, the diagnostic modalities most commonly used include barium contrast studies and endoscopy.[26] Barium radiographic studies of the small bowel reveal a number of characteristic

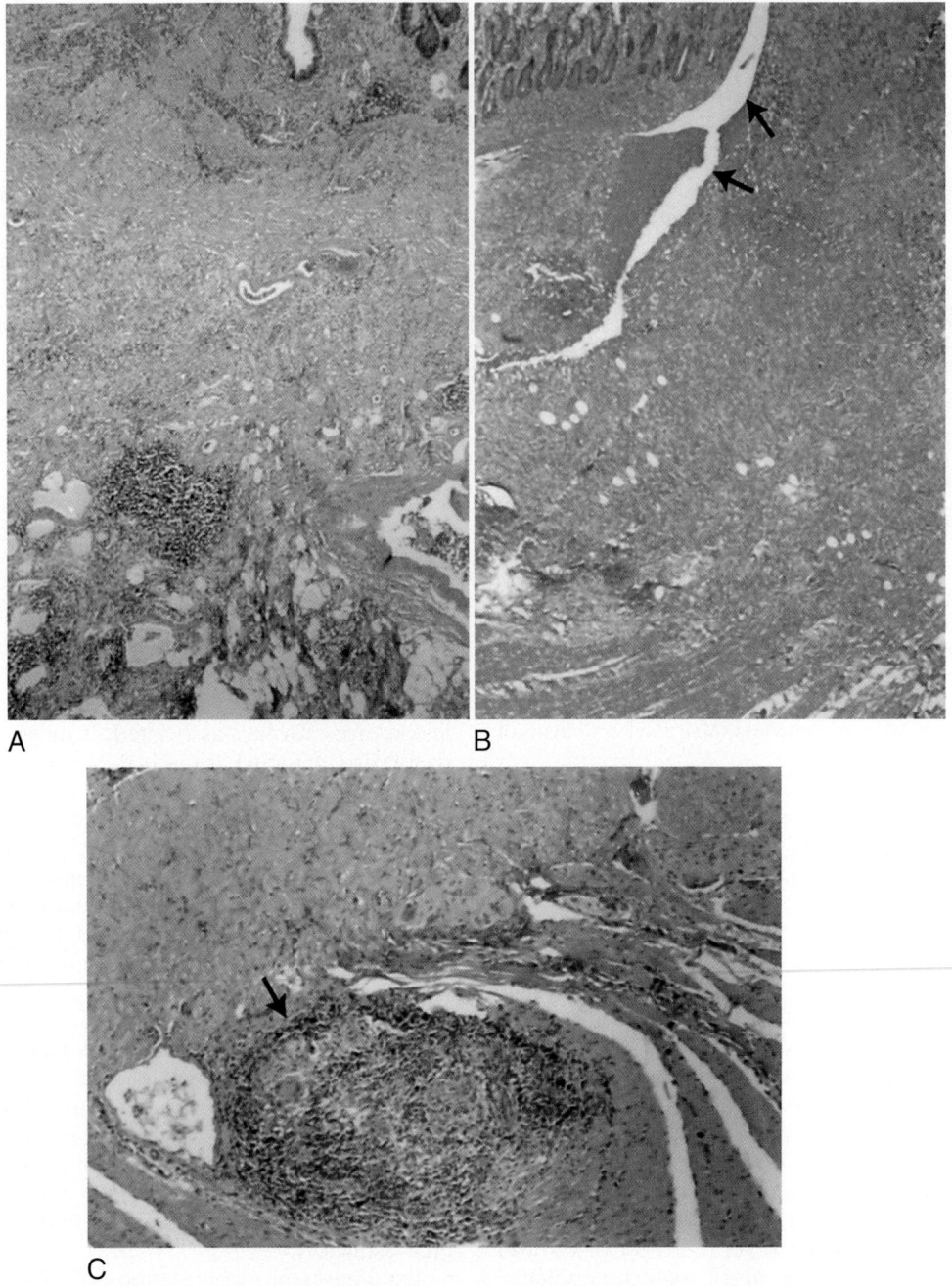

Figure 48-20 Microscopic features of Crohn's disease. **A,** Transmural inflammation. **B,** Fissure ulcer *(arrows)*. **C,** Noncaseating granuloma located in the muscular layer of the small bowel *(arrow)*. (Courtesy of Mary R. Schwartz, MD, Baylor College of Medicine.)

findings, including a cobblestone appearance of the mucosa composed of linear ulcers, transverse sinuses, and clefts. Long lengths of narrowed terminal ileum (Kantor string sign) may be present in long-standing disease (Fig. 48-21). Segmental and irregular patterns of bowel involvement may be noted. Fistulas between adjacent bowel loops and organs may be apparent (Fig. 48-22).

CT may be useful in demonstrating the marked transmural thickening, and it can also greatly aid in diagnosing extramural complications of Crohn's disease (Fig. 48-23).

Ultrasonography has limited value in the evaluation of patients with Crohn's disease, but it is useful in the assessment of undiagnosed right lower quadrant pain. When the colon is involved, sigmoidoscopy or colonoscopy may reveal characteristic aphthous ulcers with granularity and a normal-appearing surrounding mucosa. With more progressive and severe disease, the ulcerations involve more and more of the bowel lumen and may be difficult to distinguish from ulcerative colitis. However, the presence of discrete ulcers and cobbleston-

Box 48-3 Extraintestinal Manifestations of Crohn's Disease

Skin

Erythema multiforme
Erythema nodosum
Pyoderma gangrenosum

Eyes

Iritis
Uveitis
Conjunctivitis

Joints

Peripheral arthritis
Ankylosing spondylitis

Blood

Anemia
Thrombocytosis
Phlebothrombosis
Arterial thrombosis

Liver

Nonspecific triaditis
Sclerosing cholangitis

Kidney

Nephrotic syndrome
Amyloidosis

Pancreas

Pancreatitis

General

Amyloidosis

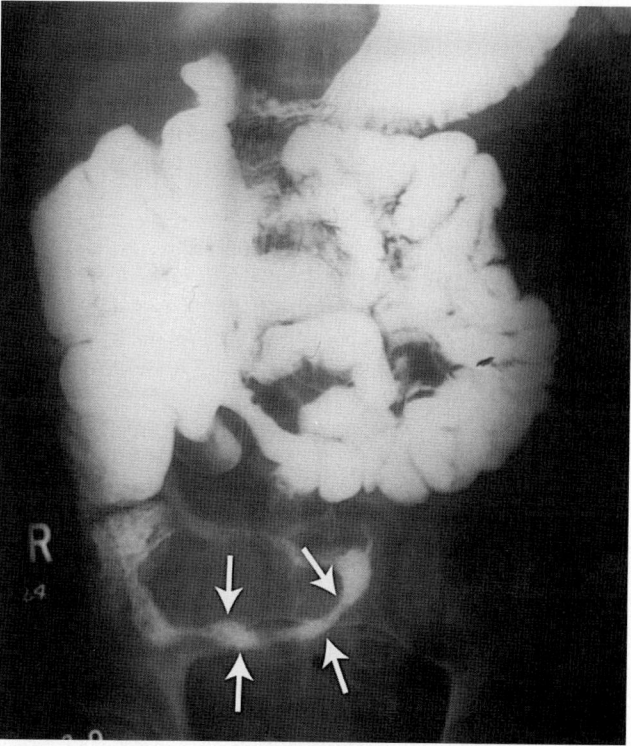

Figure 48-21 Small bowel series in a patient with Crohn's disease demonstrates a narrowed distal ileum *(arrows)* secondary to chronic inflammation and fibrosis. (Courtesy of Melvyn H. Schreiber, MD, The University of Texas Medical Branch.)

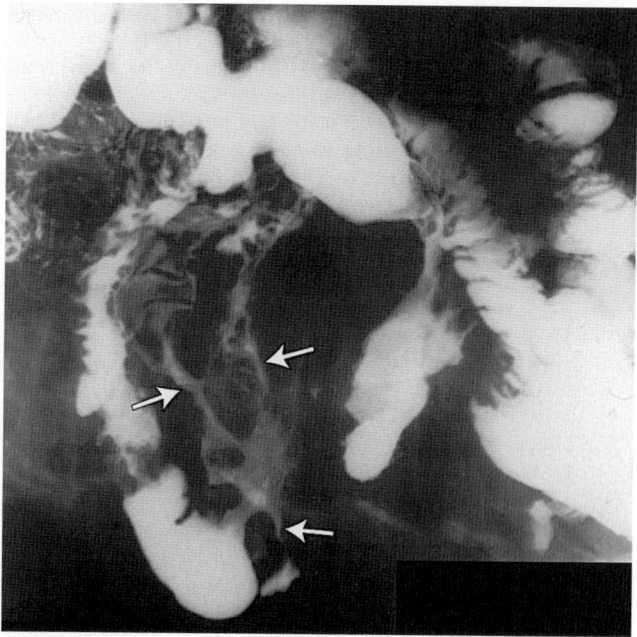

Figure 48-22 Crohn's disease with multiple short fistulous tracts communicating between the distal loops of ileum and the proximal colon *(arrows)*. (Courtesy of Melvyn H. Schreiber, MD, The University of Texas Medical Branch; adapted from Evers BM, Townsend CM Jr, Thompson JC: Small intestine. In Schwartz SI [ed]: Principles of Surgery, 7th ed. New York, McGraw-Hill, 1999, p 1233, with permission of The McGraw-Hill Companies.)

ing, as well as the discontinuous segments of involved bowel, favors a diagnosis of Crohn's disease. Intubation of the ileocecal valve during colonoscopy allows examination and biopsy of the terminal ileum. Serologic markers may also be useful in the diagnosis of Crohn's disease. In particular, perinuclear antineutrophil cytoplasmic antibody (pANCA) and anti-*Saccharomyces cerevisiae* (ASCA) are two autoantibodies associated with inflammatory bowel disease. A large cohort study reported a specificity of 92% for Crohn's disease in patients who were ASCA positive/pANCA negative and of 98% for ulcerative colitis in patients who were ASCA negative/pANCA positive.

The differential diagnosis of Crohn's disease includes both specific and nonspecific causes of intestinal inflammation. Bacterial inflammation, such as that caused by *Salmonella* and *Shigella;* intestinal tuberculosis; and protozoan infections, such as amebiasis, may present as an ileitis. In the immunocompromised host, rare infections, particularly mycobacterial and cytomegaloviral, have become more common and may cause ileitis. Acute distal ileitis may be a manifestation of early Crohn's disease, but it also may be unrelated, such as when it is caused by a bacteriologic agent (e.g., *Campylobacter* or *Yersinia*). Patients usually present in a similar fashion to those presenting with acute appendicitis with a sudden onset of right lower quadrant pain, nausea, vomiting, and fever. These entities normally resolve spontaneously; and when noted during surgery, no biopsy or resection should be performed.

In most instances, Crohn's disease of the colon can be readily distinguished from ulcerative colitis; however, in 5% to 10% of patients, the delineation between Crohn's and ulcerative colitis may be difficult, if not impossible, to make (Table 48-5). Ulcerative colitis nearly always involves the rectum most severely, with lessening inflam-

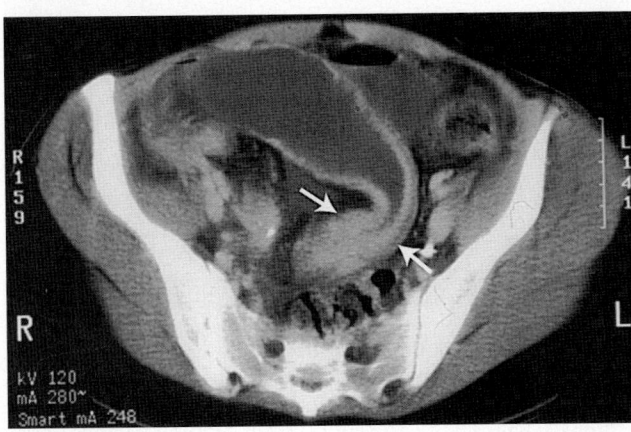

Figure 48-23 CT scan of a patient with Crohn's disease demonstrates marked thickening of the bowel *(arrows)* with a high-grade partial small bowel obstruction and dilated proximal intestine. (Courtesy of Melvyn H. Schreiber, MD, The University of Texas Medical Branch; adapted from Evers BM, Townsend CM Jr, Thompson JC: Small intestine. In Schwartz SI [ed]: Principles of Surgery, 7th ed. New York, McGraw-Hill, 1999, p 1233, with permission of The McGraw-Hill Companies.)

mation from the rectum to the ileocolic area. In contrast, Crohn's disease may be worse on the right side of the colon than on the left side, and sometimes the rectum is spared. Ulcerative colitis also demonstrates continuous involvement from rectum to proximal segments, whereas Crohn's disease is segmental. Although ulcerative colitis involves the mucosa of the large intestine, it does not extend deep into the wall of the bowel, as does Crohn's disease. Bleeding is a more common symptom in ulcerative colitis. Perianal involvement and rectovaginal fistulas are unusual in ulcerative colitis but are more common in Crohn's disease. Other endoscopic features of Crohn's disease are skip lesions, asymmetrical involvement of bowel, and the cobblestone appearance that results from ulcerations interspersed with islands of edematous mucosa.

Management

Medical Therapy

There is no cure for Crohn's disease, so both medical and surgical therapy is mainly palliative and directed toward relieving acute exacerbations or complications of the disease.[27,28] Drugs that have demonstrated efficacy in the induction and maintenance of remission include aminosalicylates (e.g., sulfasalazine, mesalamine), corticosteroids, immunosuppressive agents (e.g., azathioprine, 6-mercaptopurine, and methotrexate), antibiotics, and infliximab (an anti-TNF-α antibody). Other innovative therapies based on selective molecular targets are currently being analyzed.

Aminosalicylate Sulfasalazine (Azulfidine), an aminosalicylate, is the most commonly prescribed drug for Crohn's disease. The active moiety of sulfasalazine is 5-aminosalicylic acid. Sulfasalazine is taken orally and has been shown in randomized, controlled trials to be efficacious in patients with Crohn's disease. A clear benefit is noted in patients with colitis and ileocolitis, whereas the

Table 48-5 Diagnosis of Crohn's Colitis Versus Ulcerative Colitis

	CROHN'S COLITIS	ULCERATIVE COLITIS
Symptoms and Signs		
Diarrhea	Common	Common
Rectal bleeding	Less common	Almost always
Abdominal pain (cramps)	Moderate to severe	Mild to moderate
Palpable mass	At times	No (unless large cancer)
Anal complaints	Frequent (>50%)	Infrequent (<20%)
Radiologic Findings		
Ileal disease	Common	Rare (backwash ileitis)
Nodularity, fuzziness	No	Yes
Distribution	Skip areas	Rectum extending upward and continuously
Ulcers	Linear, cobblestone, fissures	Collar-button
Toxic dilation	Rare	Uncommon
Proctoscopic Findings		
Anal fissure, fistula, abscess	Common	Rare
Rectal sparing	Common (50%)	Rare (5%)
Granular mucosa	No	Yes
Ulceration	Linear, deep, scattered	Superficial, universal

effectiveness of sulfasalazine alone in the treatment of Crohn's disease limited to the small bowel is controversial. In contrast to its use in ulcerative colitis, sulfasalazine has not been conclusively proved to maintain remission in Crohn's disease or to prevent recurrence after surgery. Newer sulfasalazine-like drugs (e.g., mesalamine) that provide for a slow release of 5-aminosalicylic acid during their passage through the small bowel and the colon are being evaluated. Clinical trials have demonstrated efficacy of mesalamine at a dosage of 4 g/day without an increase in side effects. Studies are being conducted to evaluate even higher dosages. Mesalamine is considered first-line therapy for Crohn's disease.

Corticosteroids Corticosteroids, particularly prednisone, have been beneficial in the induction of remission in active Crohn's disease. However, they are ineffective in maintaining remission in Crohn's disease. Newer corticosteroids have been evaluated, of which budesonide has been found to be the most promising. In one study, high-dose budesonide was more effective than placebo in achieving remission in patients with active Crohn's disease. Although the combination of sulfasalazine and corticosteroids may be used to maintain patients for short periods after resolution of an acute inflammatory exacerbation, the long-term use of these compounds, either alone or in combination, has not been shown to be of benefit in preventing recurrence of disease. Given a relatively good response to mesalamine and its relative safety, budesonide may be considered an alternative to mesalamine as first-line therapy for patients with active Crohn's disease.

Antibiotics Certain antibiotics have also been found to be effective in the primary therapy of Crohn's disease.[29] The antibiotic used most is metronidazole, which has been shown in some studies to result in significant improvement in disease activity. Other antibiotics that have been used with varying success include ciprofloxacin, tetracycline, ampicillin, and clindamycin. The mechanism of action of antibiotics in Crohn's disease is unclear, and side effects of these antibiotics preclude their long-term use. Therefore, antibiotics may play an adjunctive role in the treatment of Crohn's disease and, in selected patients, may be useful in treating perianal disease, enterocutaneous fistulas, or active colonic disease.

Immunosuppressive Agents The immunosuppressive agents azathioprine and 6-mercaptopurine are effective in the treatment of Crohn's disease. Despite the potential toxicity, these drugs have proved to be relatively safe in these patients, with the most common side effects including pancreatitis, hepatitis, fever, and rash. The most disconcerting implications of these immunosuppressants are bone marrow suppression and the potential for malignancy. Other immunosuppressive agents that have been used with some effectiveness include methotrexate, cyclosporine, and tacrolimus (FK-506). Tacrolimus inhibits the production of IL-2 by T-helper cells and, in a recent randomized multicenter trial, was found to be effective for fistula improvement, but not fistula remission, in patients with perianal Crohn's disease.[30]

Anticytokine and Cytokine Therapies Perhaps the most promising therapy to emerge in recent years is the introduction of immunomodulatory treatments using cytokines and anticytokines.[27] Monoclonal antibodies to TNF-α have shown promise, with clinical trials demonstrating a rapid control of active Crohn's disease, tissue healing, and potential remission. A randomized controlled trial demonstrated that infliximab, a chimeric monoclonal antibody to TNF-α, is both efficacious and safe in the treatment of moderate-to-severe Crohn's disease and resulted in fistula closure in 46% of patients compared with only 13% of patients receiving placebo.[31] Although highly effective in certain Crohn's patients with fistulas, not every patient responds to infliximab. Also, there is an increased risk for tuberculosis reactivation, invasive fungal and other opportunistic infections, demyelinating central nervous system lesions, activation of latent multiple sclerosis, and exacerbating congestive heart disease.[32] Promising results have also been obtained using the anti-inflammatory cytokine IL-10. A multicenter randomized trial found that IL-10 demonstrated significant improvement in the clinical status in 46% of patients with Crohn's disease compared with 19% of placebo control subjects.

Novel Therapies Other therapeutic agents under investigation include IL-1 receptor antagonists, anti-IL-12, anti–IL-18, and anti–interferon-γ antibodies, anti–adhesion molecule antibodies, and growth factors. Compounds are also being evaluated that block certain signaling pathways (e.g., NF-κB, MAP kinases, and PPARγ); in limited studies, some of these compounds have shown clinical improvements.[33] A recent trial has also been reported using natalizumab, a recombinant humanized monoclonal antibody against α$_4$-integrin, with efficacy in reducing signs and symptoms of Crohn's disease that was at least similar to that of infliximab.

Nutritional Therapy

Nutritional therapy in patients with Crohn's disease has been used with varying success. The use of chemically defined elemental diets has been shown in some studies to reduce disease activity, particularly in patients with disease localized to the small bowel.[34] Liquid polymeric diets may be as effective as elemental feedings and are more acceptable to patients. With few exceptions, standard elemental diets have not been effective in the maintenance of remission in Crohn's disease. Total parenteral nutrition (TPN) has also been shown to be of use in patients with active Crohn's disease; however, complication rates exceed those for enteral nutrition. Although the primary role of nutritional therapy is questionable in patients with inflammatory bowel disease, there is definitely a secondary role for nutritional supplementation to replenish depleted nutrient stores, allowing intestinal protein synthesis and healing, and for preparing patients for operation.

Surgical Treatment

Although medical management is indicated during acute exacerbations of disease, most patients with chronic Crohn's disease require surgery some time during the course of their illness. In patients with more than 20 years of disease, the cumulative probability of surgery was 78%. The indications for operation are limited to complications that include intestinal obstruction, intestinal perforation with fistula formation or abscess, free perforation, gastrointestinal bleeding, urologic complications, cancer, and perianal disease.[35] Children with Crohn's disease and resulting systemic symptoms, such as growth retardation, may benefit from resection. The extraintestinal complications of Crohn's disease, although not primary indications for operation, often subside after resection of involved bowel, with the exception of ankylosing spondylitis and hepatic complications.

Operative therapy in patients with Crohn's disease should be specifically directed to the complication, and only the segment of bowel involved in the complicating process should be resected. Even if adjacent areas of bowel are clearly diseased, they should be ignored. Early in the history of the surgical therapy of Crohn's disease, surgeons tended to perform wider resections with the hope of cure or significant remission. However, repeated wide resections resulted in no greater remissions or cure and led to the short bowel syndrome, which is a devastating surgical complication. Frozen sections to determine microscopic disease are unreliable and are not recommended. *Therefore, operative treatment of a complication should be limited to that segment of bowel involved with the complication, and no attempt should be made to resect more bowel even though grossly evident disease may be apparent.*

The role of laparoscopic surgery for patients with Crohn's disease has been gaining acceptance as an alternative surgical approach. In appropriately selected patients, for example, those with localized abscesses, simple intra-abdominal fistulas, perianastomotic recurrent disease and disease limited to the distal ileum where ileocecectomy is indicated, this technique appears feasible and safe. Randomized clinical trials are required to assess the potential future role of laparoscopic surgery in the management of patients with Crohn's disease.

Management of Specific Problems

Acute Ileitis

Patients can present with acute abdominal pain localized to the right lower quadrant and signs and symptoms consistent with a diagnosis of acute appendicitis. At exploration, the appendix is found to be normal, but the terminal ileum is edematous and beefy red, with a thickened mesentery and enlarged lymph nodes. This condition, known as *acute ileitis,* is a self-limited disease. Acute ileitis may be a manifestation of early Crohn's disease but is most often unrelated. Bacteriologic agents such as *Campylobacter* or *Yersinia* may result in acute ileitis. Intestinal resection should not be performed. Although in the past the management of the appendix was controversial, it is clear now that in the absence of acute inflammatory involvement of the appendix or the cecum, appendectomy should be performed. This eliminates the appendix as a source of abdominal pain in the future.

Obstruction

Intestinal obstruction is the most common indication for surgical therapy in patients with Crohn's disease. Obstruc-

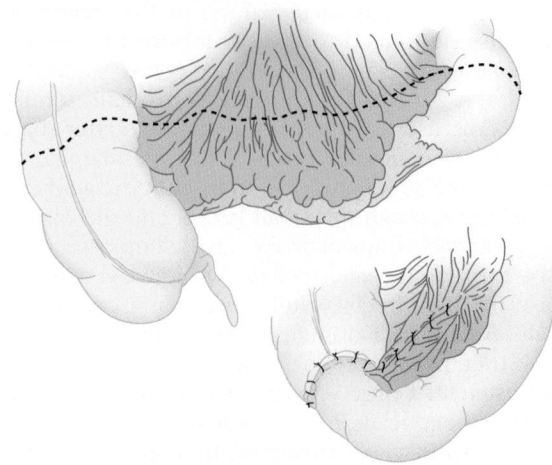

Figure 48-24 Resection of the ileum, ileocecal valve, cecum, and ascending colon for Crohn's disease of the ileum. Intestinal continuity is restored by end-to-end anastomosis.

tion in these patients is often partial, and nonoperative management is indicated initially. Operative intervention is required in instances of complete obstruction and in patients with partial obstruction whose condition does not resolve with nonoperative management. The treatment of choice of intestinal obstruction in patients with Crohn's disease is segmental resection of the involved segment with primary reanastomosis. This may involve segmental resection and primary anastomosis of a short segment of ileum if this is the site of the complication. More commonly, the cecum is involved contiguously with the terminal ileum, in which case resection of the involved terminal ileum and colon is required and the ileum is anastomosed to the ascending or transverse colon (Fig. 48-24).

In selected patients with obstruction caused by strictures (either single or multiple), one option is to perform a strictureplasty that effectively widens the lumen but avoids intestinal resection. Strictureplasty is performed by making a longitudinal incision through the narrowed area of the intestine followed by closure in a transverse fashion in a manner similar to a Heineke-Mikulicz pyloroplasty (Fig. 48-25A). For longer diseased segments (>10 cm), the strictureplasty can be performed similar to a Finney pyloroplasty (see Fig. 48-25B) or a side-to-side isoperistaltic strictureplasty. Strictureplasty has the most application in those patients in whom multiple short areas of narrowing are present over long segments of intestine, in those patients who have already had several previous resections of the small intestine, and when the areas of narrowing are due to fibrous obstruction rather than acute inflammation. This procedure preserves intestine and is associated with complication and recurrence rates comparable to resection and reanastomosis.

In the past, bypass procedures were commonly used. Currently, bypass with exclusion is used only in elderly, poor-risk patients; patients who have had several prior resections and cannot afford to lose any more bowel; and patients in whom resection would necessitate entering an abscess or endangering normal structures.

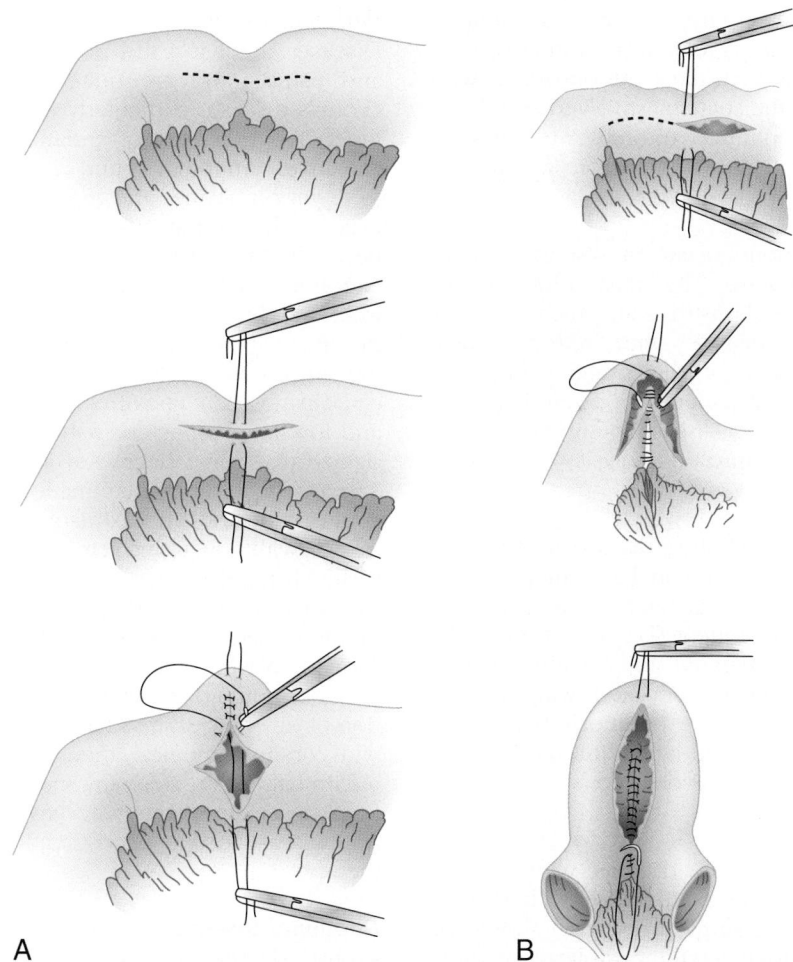

A   B

Figure 48-25 A, Technique of short strictureplasty in the manner of a Heineke-Mikulicz pyloroplasty. **B,** For longer diseased segments, strictureplasty may be performed in a manner similar to Finney pyloroplasty. (Adapted with permission from Alexander-Williams J, Haynes IG: Up-to-date management of small-bowel Crohn's disease. In Advances in Surgery. St Louis, Mosby, 1987, pp 245-264.)

Fistula

Fistulas in patients with Crohn's disease are relatively common and are usually to adjacent small bowel, colon, or other surrounding viscera (e.g., bladder). The presence of a radiographically demonstrable enteroenteric fistula without any signs of sepsis or other complications is not in itself an indication for surgery. However, many of these patients will require eventual resection as the disease progresses and the patients have progressively worsening abdominal pain. Enterocutaneous fistulas may develop but are rarely spontaneous and are more likely to follow resection or drainage of intra-abdominal abscesses. Ideally, enterocutaneous fistulas should be managed by excising the fistula tract along with the diseased segment of intestine and performing a primary reanastomosis. If the fistula forms between two or more adjacent loops of diseased bowel, the involved segments should be excised. Alternatively, if the fistula involves an adjacent normal organ, such as the bladder or colon, only the segment of the diseased small bowel and fistulous tract should be resected, and the defect in the normal

organ should simply be closed. Most patients with ileosigmoid fistulas do not require resection of the sigmoid because the disease is usually confined to the small bowel. However, if the segment of sigmoid is also found to have Crohn's disease, it should be resected along with the segment of diseased small bowel.

Free Perforation

Perforation into the free peritoneal cavity occurs occasionally but is not common in patients with Crohn's disease. When this occurs, the segment of involved bowel should be resected and, in the presence of minimal contamination, a primary anastomosis should be performed. If generalized peritonitis is present, a safer option may be to perform enterostomies until the intra-abdominal sepsis is controlled and then return for restoration of intestinal continuity.

Gastrointestinal Bleeding

Although anemia from chronic blood loss is common in patients with Crohn's disease, life-threatening gastrointestinal hemorrhage is rare. The incidence of hemorrhage is more common in patients with Crohn's disease involving the colon rather than the small bowel. As with the other complications, the segment involved should be resected and intestinal continuity restored. Arteriography may be useful to localize the bleeding before surgery.

Urologic Complications

Genitourinary complications occur in 4% to 35% of patients with Crohn's disease. The most common urologic complication is ureteral obstruction, which is usually secondary to ileocolic disease with retroperitoneal abscess. Surgical treatment of the primary intestinal disease is adequate in most patients. In a few instances of long-standing inflammatory disease, periureteric fibrosis may be present and require ureterolysis.

Cancer

Patients with long-standing Crohn's disease of the small bowel and, in particular, the colon have an increased incidence of cancer. The management of these patients is the same as that of any patient (i.e., resection of the cancer with appropriate margins and regional lymph nodes). Patients with cancer associated with Crohn's disease commonly have a worse prognosis than those who do not have Crohn's, based largely on the fact that the diagnosis in these patients is delayed.

Colorectal Disease

The same principle applies to patients with Crohn's disease limited to the colon as to those with disease to the small bowel; that is, surgical resection should be limited to the segment producing the complications. Indications for surgery include a lack of response to medical management or complications of Crohn's colitis, which include obstruction, hemorrhage, perforation, and toxic megacolon. Depending on the diseased segments, operations commonly include segmental colectomy with colocolonic anastomosis, subtotal colectomy with ileoproctostomy, and in patients with extensive perianal and rectal disease, total proctocolectomy with Brooke ileostomy. Patients with toxic megacolon should undergo colectomy, closure of the proximal rectum, and end ileostomy.

A particularly troubling problem after proctocolectomy in patients with Crohn's disease is delayed healing of the perineal wound. Several series have reported that 25% to 60% of perineal wounds are open 6 months after surgery. Persistent nonhealing wounds require excision with secondary closure. Large cavities or sinuses may be filled using well-vascularized pedicles of muscle (gracilis, semimembranosus, rectus abdominis) or omentum or by using an inferior gluteal myocutaneous graft.

Although controversial, continence-preserving operations, such as ileoanal pouch anastomoses or continent ileostomies (Kock pouch) that have been used in patients with ulcerative colitis, are not recommended for patients with Crohn's colitis because of the high rate of recurrence of Crohn's disease in the pouch, fistulas to the anastomosis, and peripouch abscesses.

Perianal Disease

Diseases involving the perianal region include fissures and fistulas and are quite common in patients with Crohn's disease, particularly those with colonic involvement. The treatment of perianal disease should be conservative. Antibiotics and immunosuppressive agents (e.g., azathioprine and 6-mercaptopurine) have been used with varying success. Encouraging reports have been obtained using the TNF-α antibody infliximab and tacrolimus. Wide excision of abscesses or fistulas is not indicated, but more conservative interventions, including the liberal placement of drainage catheters and noncutting setons, are preferable. Definitive fistulotomy is indicated in most patients with superficial, low trans-sphincteric, and low intersphincteric fistulas, although one must recognize that some degree of anal stenosis may occur as a result of chronic inflammation. High trans-sphincteric, suprasphincteric, and extrasphincteric fistulas are usually treated with noncutting setons. Fissures usually are lateral, relatively painless, large, and indolent and usually respond to conservative management. Abscesses should be drained, but large excisions of tissue should not be performed. Advancement flap closure of perineal fistulas may be required in certain instances. Selective construction of diverting stomas has good results when combined with optimal medical therapy to induce remission of inflammation. Proctectomy may be infrequently required in a subset of patients who have persistent and unremitting disease despite conservative medical and surgical therapy.

Duodenal Disease

Crohn's disease of the duodenum occurs in 2% to 4% of patients with Crohn's disease. Operative intervention is uncommon. The primary indication for surgery in these patients is duodenal obstruction that does not respond to medical therapy. The use of gastrojejunostomy to bypass the disease rather than duodenal resection is the procedure of choice. Strictureplasties have been performed with success in selected patients.

Prognosis

Operations directed at Crohn's disease are not curative. They provide patients with often significant symptomatic relief. High rates of recurrence are reported in most series.[36] It is important, however, to note how recurrence is defined in these studies. Endoscopic evidence of recurrence is detected in about 70% of patients within 1 year of surgery and in 85% by 3 years. Most of these recurrences are asymptomatic. If defined exclusively by the need for reoperation, however, recurrence rates are only 25% to 30% at 5 years and 40% to 50% at 20 years. To put this in perspective, after a first resection for Crohn's disease, about 45% of patients will ultimately require a second operation, of whom only 25% will require a third operation. Overall, nearly 90% of people undergoing operation for Crohn's disease will never require more than one additional operation. Despite the risk for recurrence, many patients who have had surgery for Crohn's disease wish that they had had their operation sooner.

Performed for proper indications, surgery almost invariably rehabilitates those disabled by Crohn's disease. The overwhelming majority of such patients report relief of symptoms after surgery, restoration of a feeling of well-being and the ability to eat normally, and a reduction in the need for medical therapy.

Standardized mortality rates in patients with Crohn's disease are increased in those patients whose disease began before the age of 20 and in those who have had disease present for longer than 13 years. Long-term survival studies have suggested that patients with Crohn's disease have a death rate that is about two to three times higher than that in the general population. Gastrointestinal cancer remains the leading cause of disease-related death in patients with Crohn's disease; other causes of disease-related deaths include sepsis, thromboembolic complications, and electrolyte disorders.

Typhoid Enteritis

Typhoid fever remains a significant problem in developing countries, most commonly in areas with contaminated water supplies and inadequate waste disposal. Children and young adults are most often affected. Improvements in sanitation have decreased the incidence of typhoid fever in industrialized countries; however, about 500 cases per year are still reported in the United States.

Typhoid enteritis is an acute systemic infection of several weeks' duration caused primarily by *Salmonella typhosa*. The pathologic events of typhoid fever are initiated in the intestinal tract after oral ingestion of the typhoid bacillus. These organisms penetrate the small bowel mucosa, making their way rapidly to the lymphatics and then systemically. Hyperplasia of the reticuloendothelial system, including lymph nodes, liver, and spleen, is characteristic of typhoid fever. Peyer patches in the small bowel become hyperplastic and may subsequently ulcerate with complications of hemorrhage or perforation.

The diagnosis of typhoid fever is confirmed by isolating the organism from blood (positive in 90% of the patients during the first week of the illness), bone marrow, and stool cultures. In addition, the finding of high titers of agglutinins against the O and H antigens is strongly suggestive of typhoid fever. Assays for the diagnosis of *S. typhosa* using PCR have been developed but are still experimental.

Treatment of typhoid fever and uncomplicated typhoid enteritis is accomplished by antibiotic administration. Chloramphenicol, ampicillin, amoxicillin, and trimethoprim-sulfamethoxazole have all been used as therapy with good results. In addition, short courses of third-generation cephalosporins have been used successfully to treat typhoid fever.

Complications requiring potential surgical intervention include hemorrhage and perforation. The incidence of hemorrhage was reported to be as high as 20% in some series, but with the availability of antibiotic treatment, this figure has decreased. When hemorrhage occurs, transfusion is indicated and usually suffices. Rarely, laparotomy must be performed for uncontrollable, life-threatening hemorrhage. Intestinal perforation through an ulcerated Peyer patch occurs in about 2% of cases. Typically, it is a single perforation in the terminal ileum, and simple closure of the perforation is the treatment of choice. With multiple perforations, which occur in about one fourth of the patients, resection with primary anastomosis or exteriorization of the intestinal loops may be required.

Enteritis in the Immunocompromised Host

The AIDS epidemic, as well as the widespread use of immunosuppressive agents after organ transplantation, has resulted in a number of rare and exotic pathogens infecting the gastrointestinal tract. Almost all patients with AIDS have gastrointestinal symptoms during their illness, the most common of which is diarrhea. However, the surgeon may be asked to evaluate the immunocompromised patient with abdominal pain, an obvious acute abdomen, or gastrointestinal bleeding; a number of protozoal, bacterial, viral, and fungal organisms may be responsible.

Protozoa

Protozoa (e.g., *Cryptosporidium, Isospora,* and *Microsporidium*) are the most frequent class of pathogens causing diarrhea in patients with AIDS. The small bowel is the most common site of infection. Diagnosis is established most often by acid-fast stain of the stool or duodenal secretions. Symptoms are most commonly related to diarrhea, which may be at times intractable. Current treatment regimens have not been entirely effective.

Bacteria

Infections by enteric bacteria are more frequent and more virulent in HIV-infected individuals than in healthy hosts. *Salmonella, Shigella,* and *Campylobacter* are associated with higher rates of both bacteremia and antibiotic resistance in the immunocompromised patient. The diagnosis of *Shigella* or *Salmonella* may be established by stool cultures. The diagnosis of *Campylobacter,* however, may be more difficult, with stool cultures often negative. These enteric infections manifest clinically with high fever, abdominal pain, and diarrhea that may be bloody. Abdominal pain may mimic an acute abdomen. Bacteremia should be treated by administration of parenteral antibiotics; ciprofloxacin is an attractive choice if the organisms are multiply resistant.

Diarrhea caused by *Clostridium difficile* is more common among patients with AIDS owing to the increased antibiotic use in this population compared with healthy hosts. Diagnosis is by standard assays of stool for *C. difficile* enterotoxin. Treatment with metronidazole or vancomycin is usually effective.

Mycobacteria

Mycobacterial infection is a frequent cause of intestinal disease in immunocompromised hosts. This can be

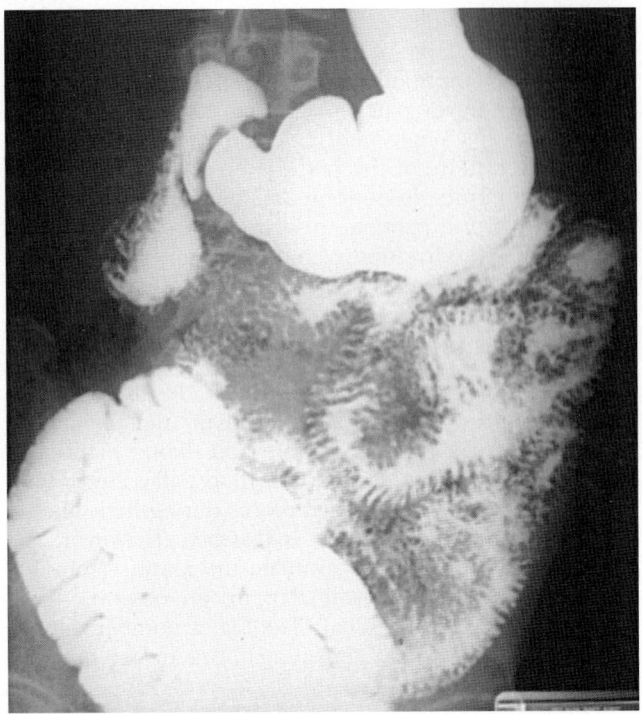

Figure 48-26 Barium radiograph of a patient with AIDS shows thickened intestinal folds consistent with enteritis secondary to atypical mycobacterium. (Courtesy of Melvyn H. Schreiber, MD, The University of Texas Medical Branch.)

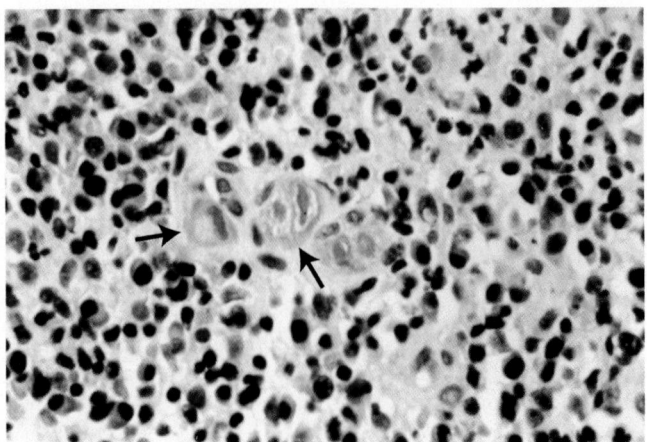

Figure 48-27 Microscopic section of small bowel in a patient with AIDS who has cytomegalovirus enteritis. Multiple large cells with both intranuclear and intracytoplasmic inclusions typical of cytomegalovirus are demonstrated *(arrows)*. (Courtesy of Mary R. Schwartz, MD, Baylor College of Medicine.)

secondary to either *Mycobacterium tuberculosis* or *Mycobacterium avium* complex (MAC), which is an atypical mycobacterium related to the type that causes cervical adenitis (scrofula). The usual route of infection is by swallowed organisms that directly penetrate the intestinal mucosa. The luminal gastrointestinal tract is involved by MAC, with massive thickening of the proximal small intestine often noted (Fig. 48-26). Clinically, patients with MAC present with diarrhea, fever, anorexia, and progressive wasting.

The most frequent site of intestinal involvement of *M. tuberculosis* is the distal ileum and cecum, with 85% to 90% of patients demonstrating disease at this site. The gross appearance can be ulcerative, hypertrophic, or ulcerohypertrophic. The bowel wall appears thickened, and often an inflammatory mass surrounds the ileocecal region. Acute inflammation is apparent, as well as strictures and even fistula formation. The serosal surface is normally covered with multiple tubercles, and mesenteric lymph nodes are frequently enlarged and thickened; on sectioning, caseous necrosis is noted. The mucosa is hyperemic, edematous, and, in some cases, ulcerated. Histologically, the distinguishing lesion is a granuloma, with caseating granulomas found most commonly in the lymph nodes. Most patients complain of chronic abdominal pain, which may be nonspecific, weight loss, fever, and diarrhea.

The diagnosis of mycobacterial infection is made by identification of the organism in tissue, either by direct visualization with an acid-fast stain, by culture of the excised tissue, or by PCR techniques. Radiographic examinations usually reveal a thickened mucosa with distorted mucosal folds and ulcerations. CT may be useful and shows a thickening of the ileocecal valve and cecum.

The treatment of *M. tuberculosis* is similar in the immunocompromised or nonimmunocompromised host. The organism is usually responsive to multidrug, antimicrobial therapy. The therapy for MAC infection is evolving; drugs that have been successfully used in vivo and in vitro include amikacin, ciprofloxacin, cycloserine, and ethionamide. Clarithromycin has also been successfully used in combination with other agents. Surgical intervention may be required for intestinal tuberculosis, particularly *M. tuberculosis*. Obstruction and fistula formation are the leading indications for surgery; however, with modern treatment, most fistulas now respond to medical management. Regarding ulcerative complications, surgery may be necessary when free perforation, perforation with abscess, or massive hemorrhage occurs. The treatment is usually resection with anastomosis.

Viruses

Cytomegalovirus (CMV) is the most common viral cause of diarrhea in immunocompromised patients. Clinical manifestations include intermittent diarrhea accompanied by fever, weight loss, and abdominal pain. The manifestations of enteric CMV infection result from mucosal ischemic ulcerations, which account for the high rate of perforations noted with CMV. As a result of the diffuse, ulcerating involvement of the intestine, patients may present with abdominal pain, peritonitis, or hematochezia. Diagnosis of CMV is made by demonstrating viral inclusions. The most characteristic form is an intranuclear inclusion, which is often surrounded by a halo, producing a so-called owl's-eye appearance. There may also be cytoplasmic inclusions (Fig. 48-27). Cultures for CMV are usually positive when inclusion bodies are present, but these cultures are less sensitive and specific than histopathologic identification. Once diagnosed, the treatment for CMV is usually affected by ganciclovir. An alternative to ganciclovir is foscarnet, a pyrophosphate analogue that inhibits viral replication. Other, less common viral infections have been reported and include adenovirus, rotavirus, and novel enteric viruses such as astrovirus and picornavirus.

Fungi

Fungal infections of the intestinal tract have been recognized in patients with AIDS. Gastrointestinal histoplasmosis occurs in the setting of systemic infection, often in association with pulmonary and hepatic disease. Diagnosis is made by fungal smear and culture of infected tissue or blood. The infection is most commonly treated by the administration of amphotericin B. Coccidioidomycosis of the intestinal tract is rare and, like histoplasmosis, occurs in the context of systemic infection.

NEOPLASMS

General Considerations

Small bowel neoplasms are exceedingly rare despite the fact that the small bowel constitutes about 80% of the total length of the gastrointestinal tract and makes up more than 90% of the mucosal surface area.[37] Only 5% of all gastrointestinal neoplasms and only 1% to 2% of all malignant tumors of the gastrointestinal tract occur in the small bowel. More than 5000 new cases of primary small intestinal cancer occur yearly in the United States (equally distributed between men and women), with more than 1000 estimated cancer deaths. The reasons for this decreased incidence in cancer despite the rapidly proliferating mucosa are entirely speculative but may include such factors as the rapid transit of luminal contents; the high turnover rate of small bowel epithelial cells, which may minimize carcinogenic exposure; the alkalinity of small intestinal contents; the high level of IgA in the intestinal wall; and the low bacterial count of small intestinal luminal contents.

The mean age at onset is about 59 years; the mean age of the presentation is 62 years for benign tumors and about 57 years for malignant lesions. Similar to other cancers, there appears to be a geographic distribution, with the highest cancer rates found among the Maori of New Zealand and ethnic Hawaiians. The incidence of small bowel cancer is particularly low in India, Romania, and other parts of Eastern Europe. Although as previously stated, the incidence of small bowel cancer is exceedingly small, there appears to be a disturbing trend of increased rates since the mid 1980s, possibly reflecting the spread of AIDS and the increase in neoplasms, such as lymphomas, that occur in the immunocompromised host.

The incidence of small bowel neoplasia varies considerably, with benign lesions identified more often in autopsy series. In contrast, malignant neoplasms account for 75% of symptomatic lesions that lead to surgery. This reflects the fact that most benign neoplasms are asymptomatic and therefore are not found unless as an incidental finding. Leiomyomas and adenomas are the most frequent of the benign tumors. Benign lesions appear to be more common in the distal small bowel, but these numbers may be somewhat misleading, owing to the relatively short length of the duodenum. In fact, per unit area, duodenal tumors are most frequent. Depending on the series, either adenocarcinoma or carcinoid tumor is the most common malignant neoplasm. Adenocarcinomas are more numerous in the proximal small bowel, whereas the other malignant lesions are more common in the distal intestine. Patients with Crohn's disease and familial adenomatous polyposis are at a higher risk for small bowel neoplasms than the general population. Although the molecular genetics of small bowel neoplasms have not been entirely characterized, similar to colorectal cancers, mutations of the K-*ras* gene are commonly found. Allelic losses, particularly involving tumor suppressor genes at chromosome locations 5q (the *APC* gene), 17q (the *p53* gene), and 18q (the *DCC* [Deleted in Colon Cancer] and *DPC4* [*SMAD4*] genes), have been noted in some small bowel cancers.

Numerous risk factors and associated conditions have been described with relation to neoplasia of the small bowel. These include patients with familial adenomatous polyposis, hereditary nonpolyposis colorectal cancer (HNPCC), Peutz-Jeghers syndrome, Crohn's disease, gluten-sensitive enteropathy (i.e., celiac sprue), and biliary diversion (e.g., previous cholecystectomy). Controversial factors that may contribute to small bowel cancers include smoking, heavy alcohol consumption (>80 g/day of ethanol), and consumption of red meat or salt-cured foods.

Diagnosis

Owing to the insidious nature of many of the small bowel neoplasms, a high index of suspicion must be present for these neoplasms to be diagnosed. In most series, a correct preoperative diagnosis is made in only 20% to 50% of symptomatic patients. An upper gastrointestinal tract series with small intestinal follow-through yields an accurate diagnosis in 50% to 70% of patients with malignant neoplasms of the small intestine (Fig. 48-28). CT enteroclysis appears to be an even more sensitive technique, with a diagnostic accuracy of about 90%.[11]

Flexible endoscopy may be useful, particularly in diagnosing duodenal lesions, and often the colonoscope can be advanced into the terminal ileum for visualization and biopsy of ileal neoplasms. Push enteroscopy has not been used routinely to evaluate lesions in the small bowel because this test may take up to 8 hours to perform and may not visualize the entire small bowel. The use of swallowed radiotelemetry capsules (e.g., capsule endoscopy) that transmit images of the bowel wall may be of diagnostic value as this technique becomes more widely available.[38]

Plain films may confirm the presence of an obstruction; however, for the most part, they are useless in making a diagnosis of small bowel neoplasms. Angiography is of value in diagnosing and localizing tumors of vascular origin. CT of the abdomen can prove particularly

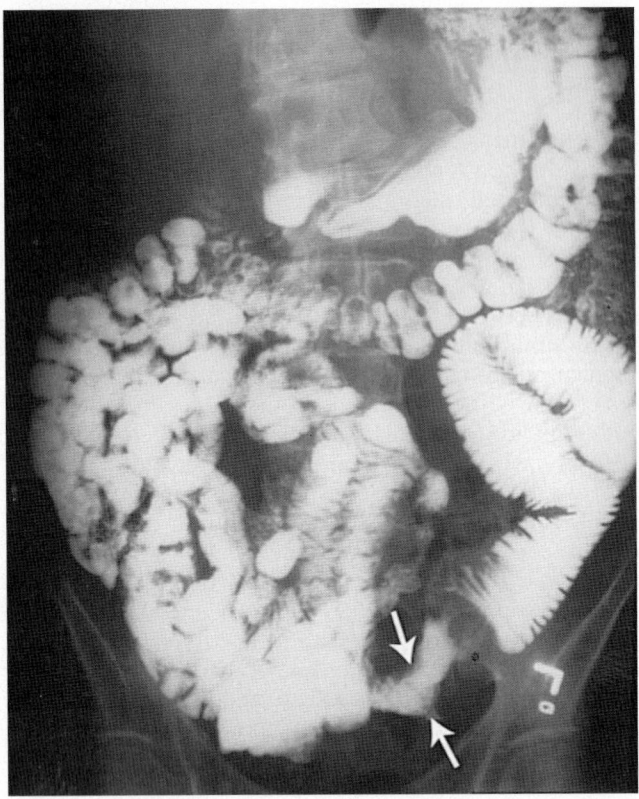

Figure 48-28 Barium radiograph demonstrates a typical "apple-core" lesion *(arrows)* caused by adenocarcinoma of the small bowel, producing a partial obstruction with dilated proximal bowel. (Courtesy of Melvyn H. Schreiber, MD, The University of Texas Medical Branch.)

useful in detecting extraluminal tumors such as gastrointestinal stromal tumors (GISTs) and can provide helpful information regarding staging of malignant cancers (Fig. 48-29). Ultrasonography has not proved to be effective in making the preoperative diagnosis of small bowel neoplasm. Despite the sophisticated imaging and diagnostic modalities, diagnosis of a small bowel tumor is often achieved only at the time of surgical exploration, performed either as an elective procedure or as an emergency procedure.

Benign Neoplasms

The most common benign neoplasms include benign GISTs, adenomas, and lipomas. Adenomas are the most common benign tumors reported in autopsy series, but GISTs are the most common benign small bowel lesions that produce symptoms.

Clinical Manifestations

Symptoms associated with small bowel neoplasms are often vague and nonspecific and may include dyspepsia, anorexia, malaise, and dull abdominal pain (often intermittent and colicky). These symptoms may be present for months or years before surgery. Most patients with benign neoplasms remain asymptomatic, and the neoplasms are only discovered at autopsy or as incidental findings at laparotomy or upper gastrointestinal radiologic studies. Of the remainder, pain, most often related to obstruction, is the most frequent complaint. Most frequently, obstruction is the result of intussusception, and benign small tumors are the most common cause of this condition in adults. Hemorrhage is the next most common

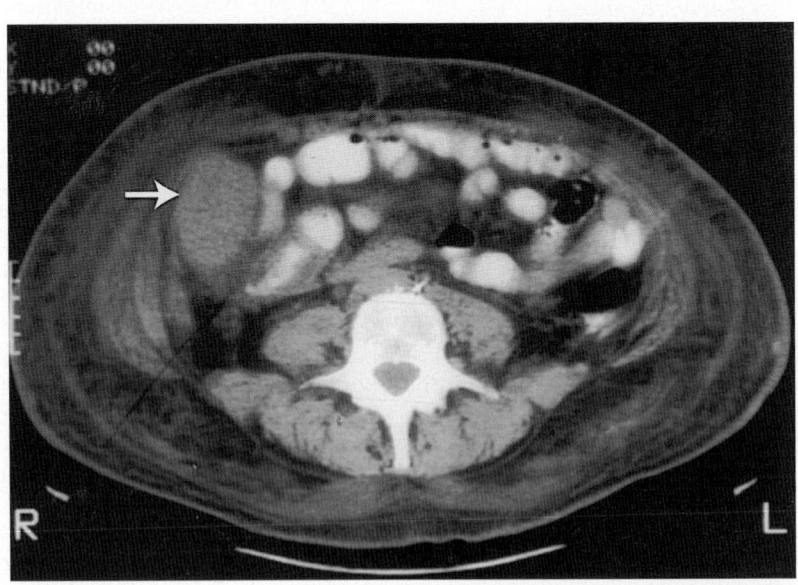

Figure 48-29 CT scan of abdomen demonstrates a small bowel neoplasm *(arrow)*. (Courtesy of Melvyn H. Schreiber, MD, The University of Texas Medical Branch.)

symptom. Bleeding is usually occult; hematochezia or hematemesis may occur, although life-threatening hemorrhage is uncommon.

Treatment

Surgical treatment of benign tumors is nearly always indicated because of the risk for subsequent complications and because the diagnosis of benign disease cannot be made without microscopic evaluation. The complications of benign neoplasms that most often require treatment include bleeding and obstruction. Segmental resection and primary anastomosis are most commonly used except for very small lesions, which may be excised by enterotomy. The entire small bowel should be searched for other lesions because they are often multiple.

Pathology

Leiomyomas, benign tumors of smooth muscle origin, are the most common symptomatic benign neoplasms of the small bowel. In recent years, as the origin of these tumors has become more clear, pathologists have shifted from designations such as leiomyoma or leiomyosarcoma to the term *stromal tumors* (i.e., GISTs).[39] Currently, these tumors are thought to arise from the interstitial cell of Cajal, an intestinal pacemaker cell of mesodermal descent. These tumors are made up of spindle (70%) and epithelioid (30%) cells, and benign GISTs are three to four times more common than malignant GISTs. Most (>90%) GISTs express CD117, the *c-kit* proto-oncogene protein that is a transmembrane receptor for the stem cell growth factor, and 70% to 80% express CD34, the human progenitor cell antigen; less frequently, these tumors stain positive for actin and desmin.[40] The incidence is equal in men and in women, and they are most frequently diagnosed in the fifth decade of life. Grossly, they are firm, gray-white lesions with a whorled appearance noted on cut surface; microscopic examination demonstrates well-differentiated smooth muscle cells. These tumors may grow intramurally and cause obstruction. Alternatively, the tumors demonstrate intramural and extramural growth, sometimes achieving considerable size and eventually outgrowing their blood supply and resulting in bleeding manifestations, which is the most common indication for surgery in patients with benign stromal tumors. Surgical resection is necessary for appropriate treatment. Mitotic counts higher than 2 per 50 high-power fields imply an increased risk for local recurrence.

Adenomas account for about 15% of all benign small bowel tumors and are of three primary types: true adenomas, villous adenomas, and Brunner gland adenomas. Twenty percent of adenomas are found in the duodenum, 30% are found in the jejunum, and 50% are found in the ileum. Most of these lesions are asymptomatic, with most occurring singly and found incidentally at autopsy. The most common presenting symptoms are bleeding and obstruction. Villous adenomas of the small bowel are rare but do occur, are most commonly found in the duodenum, and may be associated with the familial polyposis syndrome. These lesions have a propensity for malignant degeneration and may be of relatively large size (>5 cm) in diameter. They are usually noted secondary to abdomi-

nal pain or bleeding; obstruction may also occur. The malignant potential of these lesions is reportedly between 35% and 55%. The treatment of choice is segmental resection, although, in the duodenum, polypectomy may be performed if the tumor is histologically benign. Invasive changes necessitate more extensive resection, such as a pancreaticoduodenectomy. Brunner gland adenomas represent benign hyperplastic lesions arising from the Brunner glands of the proximal duodenum. These adenomas may produce symptoms mimicking those of peptic ulcer disease. Diagnosis can usually be accomplished by endoscopy and biopsy, and symptomatic lesions in an accessible region should be resected by simple excision. There is no malignant potential for Brunner gland adenomas, and a radical resection should not be used.

Lipomas, which are also included in the category of stromal tumors, are most common in the ileum and present as single intramural lesions located in the submucosa. They occur most commonly in the sixth and seventh decades of life and are more frequent in men. Less than one third of these tumors are symptomatic; and of these, the most common manifestations are obstruction and bleeding from superficial ulcerations. The treatment of choice for symptomatic lesions is excision. Lipomas do not have malignant potential, and, therefore, when found incidentally, they should be removed only if the resection is simple.

Hamartomas of the small bowel occur as part of the Peutz-Jeghers syndrome, an inherited syndrome of mucocutaneous melanotic pigmentation and gastrointestinal polyps. The pattern of inheritance is simple mendelian dominant with a high degree of penetrance. The classic pigmented lesions are small, 1- to 2-mm, brown or black spots located in the circumoral region of the face, buccal mucosa, forearms, palms, soles, digits, and perianal area. The entire jejunum and ileum are the most frequent portions of the gastrointestinal tract involved with these hamartomas; however, 50% of patients may also have rectal and colonic lesions, and 25% of patients have gastric lesions. The most common symptom is recurrent colicky abdominal pain, usually as a result of intermittent intussusception. Lower abdominal pain associated with a palpable mass has been reported to occur in one third of patients. Hemorrhage as a result of autoamputation of the polyps occurs less frequently and is most commonly manifested by anemia. Acute life-threatening hemorrhage is uncommon but may occur. Although once considered a purely benign disease, adenomatous changes have been reported in 3% to 6% of hamartomas. Extracolonic cancers are common, occurring in 50% to 90% of patients (small intestine, stomach, pancreas, ovary, lung, uterus, and breast). The small intestine represents the most frequent site for cancer, with a relative risk of 520 compared with the general population. The treatment of complications of Peutz-Jeghers syndrome is directed mainly at the complication of obstruction or persistent bleeding. Resection should be limited to the segment of bowel that is producing complications and most often involves a limited resection. Because of the widespread nature of intestinal involvement, cure is not possible, and extensive resections are not indicated.

Hemangiomas are developmental malformations consisting of submucosal proliferation of blood vessels. They can occur at any level of the gastrointestinal tract, and the jejunum is the most commonly affected small bowel segment. Hemangiomas account for 3% to 4% of all benign tumors of the small bowel and are multiple in 60% of patients. Hemangiomas of the small bowel may occur as part of an inherited disorder known as Osler-Weber-Rendu disease. In addition to the small bowel, hemangiomas may also be present in the lung, liver, and mucous membranes. Patients with Turner's syndrome are likely also to have cavernous hemangiomas of the intestine. The most common symptom of small bowel hemangiomas is intestinal bleeding. Angiography and ^{99m}Tc–red blood cell scanning are the most useful diagnostic studies. If a hemangioma is localized preoperatively, resection of the involved segment of intestine is warranted. If not identified, intraoperative transillumination and palpation can be helpful.

Malignant Neoplasms

The most common malignant neoplasms of the small bowel in the approximate order of frequency are adenocarcinomas, carcinoid tumors, malignant GISTs, and lymphomas. Because of differences in clinical presentation, diagnosis, and treatment, carcinoid tumors are considered separately.

Clinical Manifestations

In contrast to benign lesions, malignant neoplasms almost always produce symptoms, the most common of which include pain and weight loss. Obstruction develops in 15% to 35% of patients and, in contrast to the intussusception produced by benign lesions, is usually the result of tumor infiltration and adhesions. Diarrhea with tenesmus and passage of large amounts of mucus may occur. Adenocarcinomas may produce the typical constricting apple-core lesions similar to those observed in the colon. Gastrointestinal bleeding, manifested by anemia and guaiac-positive stools or occasionally by melena or hematochezia, occurs to varying degrees with malignant lesions and is more common with leiomyosarcomas. A palpable mass may be felt in 10% to 20% of patients, and perforations develop in about 10%, usually secondary to lymphomas and sarcomas.

Pathology

Adenocarcinomas constitute about 50% of the malignant tumors of the small bowel in most reported series. The peak incidence is in the seventh decade of life, and most series show a slight male predominance. Most of these tumors are located in the duodenum and proximal jejunum (Fig. 48-30). Those arising in association with Crohn's disease tend to occur at a somewhat younger age, and more than 70% arise in the ileum. Tumors of the duodenum tend to present somewhat earlier than those occurring in the most distal intestine, with symptoms of jaundice and chronic bleeding. Adenocarcinomas of the jejunum and ileum usually produce symptoms that may be more nonspecific and include vague abdominal

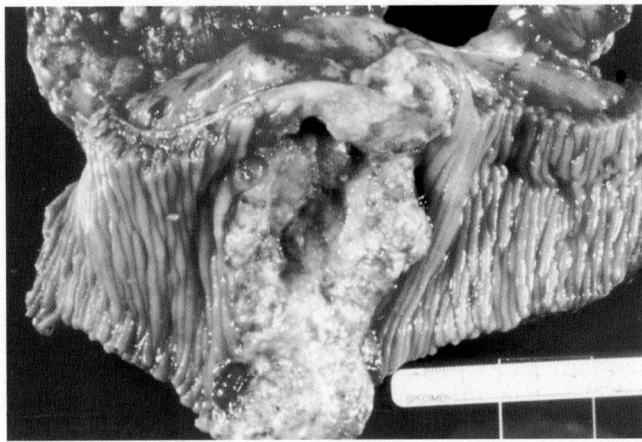

Figure 48-30 **Large circumferential mucinous adenocarcinoma of the jejunum.** (Courtesy of Mary R. Schwartz, MD, Baylor College of Medicine.)

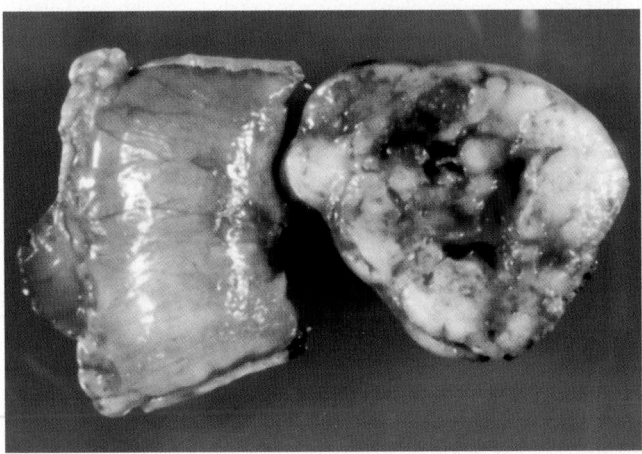

Figure 48-31 **Small bowel leiomyosarcoma (malignant gastrointestinal stromal tumor) with hemorrhagic necrosis.** (Courtesy of Mary R. Schwartz, MD, Baylor College of Medicine.)

pain and weight loss. Intestinal obstruction and chronic bleeding can also occur. Perforation is uncommon. As with adenocarcinomas in other organs, survival of patients with small bowel adenocarcinomas is related to the stage of disease at the time of diagnosis. Unfortunately, diagnosis is often delayed, and the disease is advanced at the time of surgery, secondary to a number of factors (e.g., the vagueness of symptoms, absence of physical findings, and lack of clinical suspicion owing to the rarity of these lesions).

Malignant GISTs, which arise from mesenchymal tissue, constitute about 20% of malignant neoplasms of the small bowel (Fig. 48-31). These tumors are more common in the jejunum and ileum, typically are diagnosed in the fifth and sixth decades of life, and occur with a somewhat more male preponderance. Malignant GISTs are greater than 5 cm at the time of diagnosis in 80% of patients. GISTs mostly arise from the muscularis propria and generally grow extramurally. Most common indications for surgery include bleeding and obstruction,

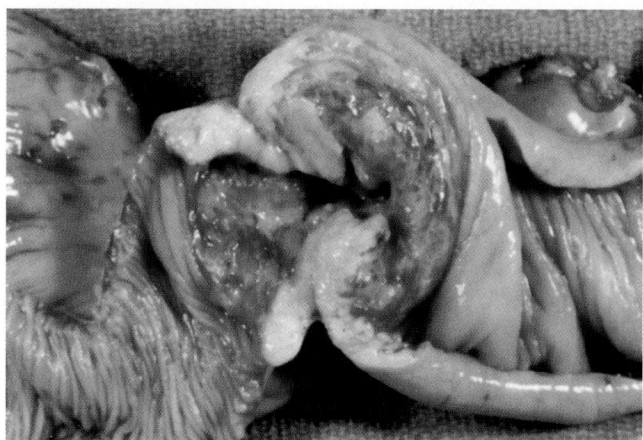

Figure 48-32 Gross photograph of primary lymphoma of the ileum shows replacement of all layers of the bowel wall with tumor. (Courtesy of Mary R. Schwartz, MD, Baylor College of Medicine.)

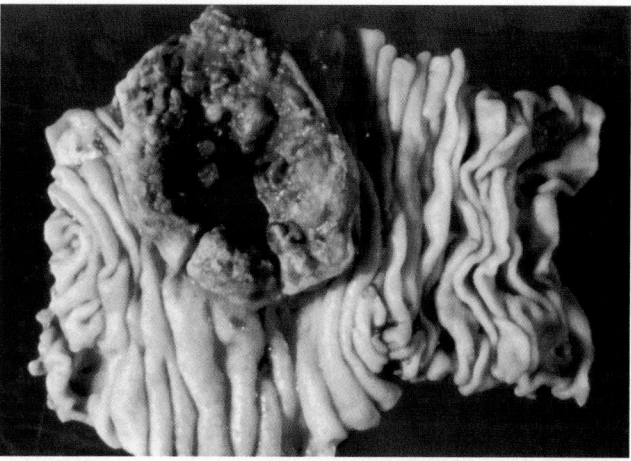

Figure 48-33 Small bowel lymphoma presents as perforation and peritonitis. (Courtesy of Mary R. Schwartz, MD, Baylor College of Medicine.)

although free perforation may occur as a result of hemorrhagic necrosis in large tumor masses. Typically, GISTs tend to invade locally and spread by direct extension into adjacent tissues and hematogenously to the liver, lungs, and bone; lymphatic metastases are unusual. The most useful indicators of survival and the risk for metastasis include the size of the tumor at presentation, the mitotic index, and evidence of tumor invasion into the lamina propria.

Malignant lymphomas involve the small bowel primarily or as a manifestation of systemic disease. Primary gastrointestinal lymphomas, of which about one third occur in the small bowel, account for 5% of all lymphomas.[41] Lymphomas constitute 7% to 25% of small bowel malignant tumors in the adult; in children younger than age 10 years, they are the most common intestinal neoplasm. Lymphomas are most commonly found in the ileum, where there is the greatest concentration of gut-associated lymphoid tissue. Increased risk for developing primary small bowel lymphomas has been reported in patients with celiac disease and immunodeficiency states (e.g., AIDS). Grossly, small intestine lymphomas are usually large, with most larger than 5 cm; they may extend beneath the mucosa (Fig. 48-32). Microscopically, there is often diffuse infiltration of the intestinal wall. Symptoms of small bowel lymphoma include pain, weight loss, nausea, vomiting, and change in bowel habits. Perforation may occur in up to 25% of the patients (Fig. 48-33). Fever is uncommon and suggests systemic involvement.

Treatment

The treatment of adenocarcinomas and lymphomas of the small bowel is wide resection including regional lymph nodes (Fig. 48-34). This may require pancreatico-duodenectomy (Whipple operation) for duodenal lesions. Often, surgical resection for cure is not possible. Therefore, palliative resection should be performed to prevent further complications of bleeding, obstruction, and perforation. If this is not possible, bypass of the involved

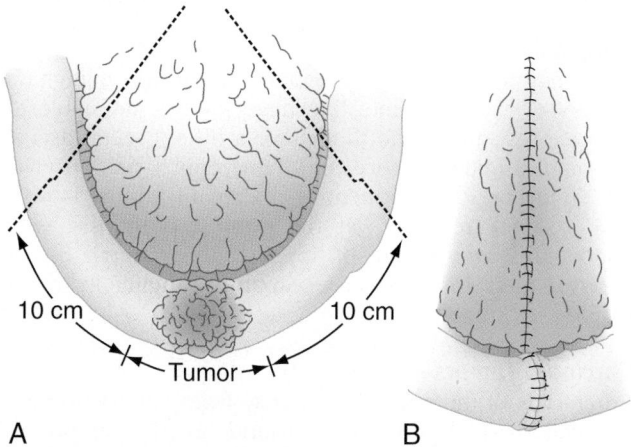

Figure 48-34 Surgical management of carcinoma of the small bowel. **A,** Malignant tumors should be resected with a wide margin of normal bowel and a wedge of mesentery to remove the immediate draining lymph nodes. **B,** End-to-end anastomosis of the small bowel and repair of the mesentery. (Adapted from Thompson JC: Atlas of Surgery of the Stomach, Duodenum, and Small Bowel. St Louis, Mosby–Year Book, 1992, p 299.)

segment may provide relief of symptoms. For GISTs, segmental bowel resection is required; wide margins and extensive lymph node dissection are not necessary. Resection of organ segments that have been invaded with tumor and of hepatic metastases appears to confer an improvement in survival.

Adjuvant radiation and chemotherapy have little role in the treatment of patients with adenocarcinomas of the small bowel. Radiotherapy and chemotherapy, combined with surgical excision, provide the best survival rates for patients with lymphomas. The adjuvant treatment of GISTs may be favorably impacted by recent reports demonstrating an effect on GIST tumor progression using the tyrosine kinase inhibitor imatinib mesylate (Gleevec; formerly referred to as STI571), which blocks the unregulated mutant c-*kit* (CD117) tyrosine kinase.[42] Imatinib also

Table 48-6   Secretory Products of Carcinoid Tumors

AMINES	TACHYKININS	PEPTIDES	OTHER
5-HT	Kallikrein	Pancreatic polypeptide (40%)	Prostaglandins
5-HIAA (88%)	Substance P (32%)	Chromogranins (100%)	
5-HTP	Neuropeptide K (67%)	Neurotensin (19%)	
Histamine		HCGα (28%)	
Dopamine		HCGβ	
		Motilin (14%)	

HCG, human chorionic gonadotropin; 5-HIAA, 5-hydroxyindoleacetic acid; 5-HT, 5-hydroxytryptamine; 5-HTP, 5-hydroxytryptophan.
Values in parentheses represent percentage frequency.

inhibits the Bcr-Abl and platelet-derived growth factor (PDGF) receptor tyrosine kinases. Mutations in c-*kit* are thought to represent the primary cause of the proliferative capacity and malignant potential of GIST. Clinical trials are underway using imatinib for metastatic and primary GIST, and the results appear encouraging.

Prognosis

Only half of the patients operated on for malignant tumors of the small intestine have lesions amenable to curative resection. One third have a distant metastasis at the time of initial surgery, and the overall 5-year survival rate after surgical treatment of malignant tumors is only 25%. Adenocarcinoma has the poorest prognosis, with an overall survival rate of 15% to 20%. Overall 5-year survival rates for GISTs are variable, ranging from 7% to 56%.

Carcinoid Tumors

Carcinoids of the small bowel arise from enterochromaffin cells (Kulchitsky cells) found in the crypts of Lieberkühn.[43] These cells are also known as *argentaffin cells* because of their staining by silver compounds. These tumors were first described by Lubarsch in 1888; in 1907, Oberndorfer coined the term *Karzinoide* to indicate the carcinoma-like appearance and the presumed lack of malignant potential. Carcinoid tumors have been reported in a number of organs, including most commonly the lungs, bronchi, and gastrointestinal tract. Most patients with small bowel carcinoids are in the fifth decade of life.

Carcinoids may be classified by the embryologic site of origin and secretory product. Carcinoid tumors may be derived from the foregut (respiratory tract, thymus), midgut (jejunum, ileum and right colon, stomach, and proximal duodenum), and hindgut (distal colon and rectum). Foregut carcinoids characteristically produce low levels of serotonin (5-hydroxytryptamine) but may secrete 5-hydroxytryptophan or adrenocorticotropic hormone. Midgut carcinoids are characterized by having high serotonin production. Hindgut carcinoids rarely produce serotonin but may produce other hormones, such as somatostatin and peptide YY. The gastrointestinal tract is the most common site for carcinoid tumors. After the appendix, the small intestine is the second most frequently affected site in the gastrointestinal tract. In the small intestine, carcinoids almost always occur within the last 2 feet of the ileum. Carcinoid tumors have a variable malignant potential and are composed of multipotential cells with the ability to secrete numerous humoral agents, the most prominent of which are serotonin and substance P (Table 48-6). In addition to these substances, carcinoid tumors have been found to secrete corticotropin, histamine, dopamine, neurotensin, prostaglandins, kinins, gastrin, somatostatin, pancreatic polypeptide, calcitonin, and neuron-specific enolase.

The primary importance of carcinoid tumors is the malignant potential of the tumors themselves. Although the carcinoid syndrome, which is characterized by episodic attacks of cutaneous flushing, bronchospasm, diarrhea, and vasomotor collapse, can occur and is quite dramatic in its most florid form, it occurs in only a small percentage of patients with malignant carcinoids.

Pathology

Carcinoid tumors may arise in organs derived from the foregut, midgut, and hindgut. Seventy to 80% of carcinoids are asymptomatic and found incidentally at the time of surgery. In the gastrointestinal tract, more than 90% of carcinoids are found in three sites: the appendix (45%), the ileum (28%), and the rectum (16%) (Table 48-7). The malignant potential (ability to metastasize) is related to location, size, depth of invasion, and growth pattern. Only about 3% of appendiceal carcinoids metastasize, but about 35% of ileal carcinoids are associated with metastasis. Most (~75%) gastrointestinal carcinoids are less than 1 cm in diameter, and about 2% of these are associated with metastasis. In contrast, carcinoid tumors 1 to 2 cm in diameter and larger than 2 cm are associated with metastasis in 50% and 80% to 90% of cases, respectively.

Grossly, these tumors are small, firm submucosal nodules that are usually yellow on cut surface (Fig. 48-35). They tend to grow very slowly, but after invasion of the serosa, there often is an intense desmoplastic reaction producing mesenteric fibrosis, intestinal kinking, and intermittent obstruction. Small bowel carcinoids are multicentric in 20% to 30% of patients. This tendency to multicentricity exceeds that of any other malignant neoplasm of the gastrointestinal tract. Another unusual observation is the frequent coexistence of a second primary malignant neoplasm of a different histologic type. This

Table 48-7 **Distribution of Gastrointestinal Carcinoids: Incidence of Metastases and of Carcinoid Syndrome**

SITE	CASES	AVERAGE METASTASIS (%)	CASES OF CARCINOID SYNDROME
Esophagus	1		0
Stomach	93 (2%)	23	8
Duodenum	135 (4%)	20	4
Jejunoileum	1032 (28%)	34	91
Meckel's diverticulum	42 (1%)	19	3
Appendix	1686 (45%)	2	6
Colon	91 (2%)	60	5
Rectum	592 (16%)	18	1
Ovary	34	6	17
Biliary tract	10	30	0
Pancreas	2		1
Total	3718		136

Adapted from Cheek RC, Wilson H: Carcinoid tumors. Curr Probl Surg (November):4-31, 1970.

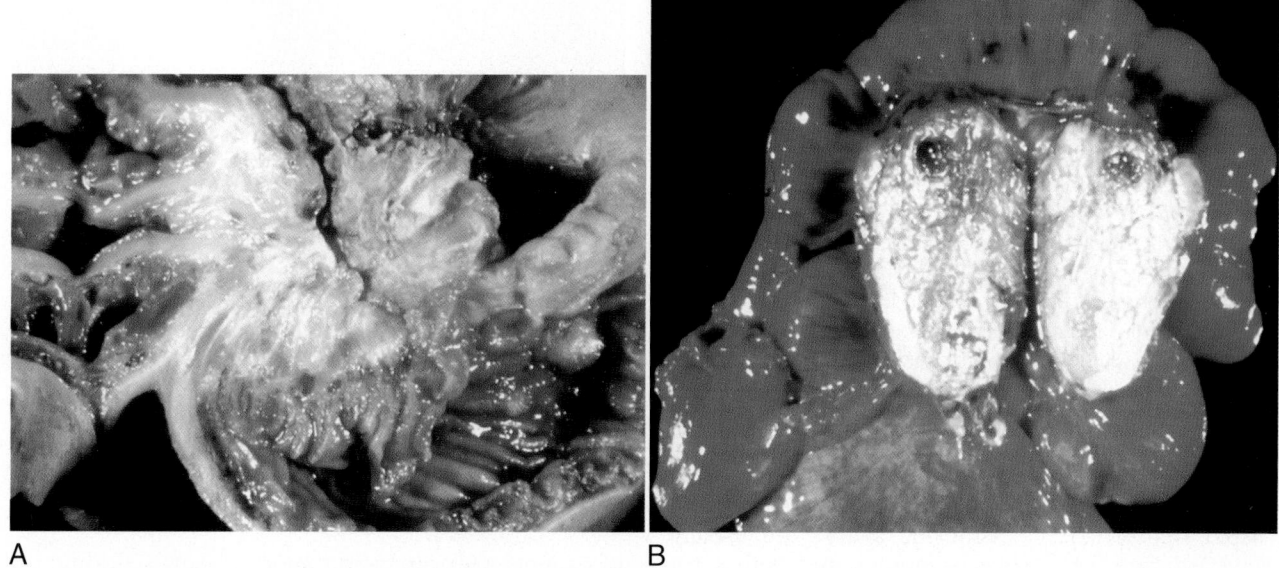

Figure 48-35 Gross pathologic characteristics of carcinoid tumor. **A,** Carcinoid tumor of the distal ileum demonstrates the intense desmoplastic reaction and fibrosis of the bowel wall. **B,** Mesenteric metastases from a carcinoid tumor of the small bowel. (Adapted from Evers BM, Townsend CM Jr, Thompson JC: Small intestine. In Schwartz SI [ed]: Principles of Surgery, 7th ed. New York, McGraw-Hill, 1999, p 1245, with permission of The McGraw-Hill Companies.)

usually is a synchronous adenocarcinoma (most commonly in the large intestine) that can occur in 10% to 20% of patients with carcinoid tumors. Carcinoid tumors are associated with multiple endocrine neoplasia type 1 in about 10% of cases.

Clinical Manifestations

Carcinoid Tumors In the absence of carcinoid syndrome, symptoms of patients with carcinoid tumors of the small bowel are similar to those of patients with small bowel tumors of other histologic types. The most common symptoms include abdominal pain, which is variably

associated with partial or complete small intestinal obstruction. Obstructive symptoms are often caused by intussusception but may occur secondary to a local desmoplastic reaction, apparently produced by humoral agents elaborated by the tumor. Diarrhea and weight loss may also occur. The diarrhea is a result of a partial bowel obstruction rather than a secretory diarrhea that is noted in patients with the malignant carcinoid syndrome.

Malignant Carcinoid Syndrome The malignant carcinoid syndrome is a relatively rare disease, occurring in fewer than 10% of patients with carcinoid tumors. The syndrome is most commonly associated with carcinoid tumors of the gastrointestinal tract, particularly from the small bowel, but carcinoids in other locations, such as the bronchus, pancreas, ovary, and testes, have also been described in association with the syndrome. The classic description of the carcinoid syndrome typically includes vasomotor, cardiac, and gastrointestinal manifestations. A number of humoral factors are produced by carcinoid tumors, but those considered to contribute to the carcinoid syndrome include serotonin, 5-hydroxytryptophan (a precursor of serotonin synthesis), histamine, dopamine, kallikrein, substance P, prostaglandin, and neuropeptide K. Most patients who exhibit malignant carcinoid syndrome have massive hepatic replacement by metastatic disease. However, tumors that bypass the liver, specifically ovarian and retroperitoneal carcinoids, may produce the syndrome in the absence of liver metastasis.

Common symptoms and signs include cutaneous flushing (80%); diarrhea (76%); hepatomegaly (71%); cardiac lesions, most commonly right heart valvular disease (41%-70%); and asthma (25%). Cutaneous flushing in the carcinoid syndrome may be of four varieties: *diffuse erythematous,* which is short lived and normally affects the face, neck, and upper chest; *violaceous,* which is similar to diffuse erythematous flush except that the attacks may be longer and patients may develop a permanent cyanotic flush with watery eyes and injected conjunctivae; *prolonged flushes,* which may last up to 2 to 3 days and involve the entire body and be associated with profuse lacrimation, hypotension, and facial edema; and a *bright-red patchy flushing,* which is typically seen with gastric carcinoids. The diarrhea associated with carcinoid syndrome is episodic (usually occurring after meals), watery, and often explosive. Increased circulating serotonin levels are thought to be the cause of the diarrhea because the serotonin antagonist methysergide effectively controls the symptom. Cardiac lesions of carcinoid tumors mainly involve the right side of the heart and are usually limited to the tricuspid and pulmonary valves. The three most common cardiac lesions are pulmonary stenosis (90%), tricuspid insufficiency (47%), and tricuspid stenosis (42%). Asthmatic attacks are usually observed during the flushing symptom, and both serotonin and bradykinin have been implicated in this symptom. Malabsorption and pellagra (dementia, dermatitis, and diarrhea) are occasionally present and are thought to be caused by excessive diversion of dietary tryptophan.

Diagnosis

The elevation of various humoral factors forms the basis for diagnostic tests in patients with carcinoid tumors and the carcinoid syndrome. Carcinoid tumors produce serotonin, which is then metabolized in the liver and the lung to the pharmacologically inactive 5-hydroxyindoleacetic acid. Elevated urinary levels of 5-hydroxyindoleacetic acid measured over 24 hours with high-performance liquid chromatography are highly specific. A potentially useful marker of neuroendocrine tumors is plasma concentrations of chromogranin A, a protein made in the secretory granules, which is elevated in more than 80%

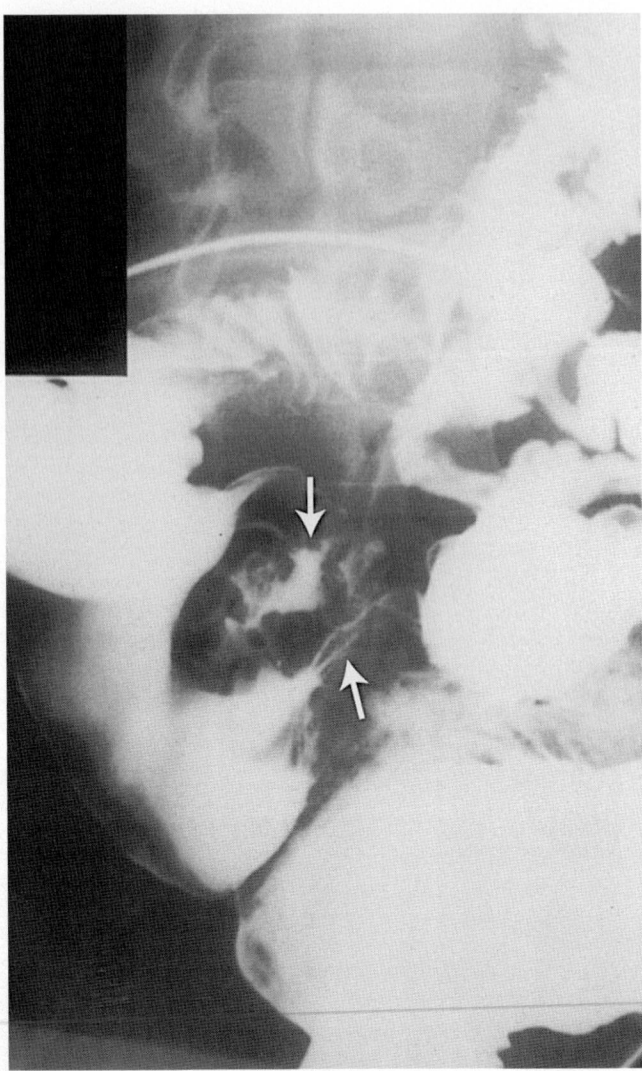

Figure 48-36 Barium radiograph of a carcinoid tumor of the terminal ileum demonstrates fibrosis with multiple filling defects and high-grade partial obstruction *(arrows).* (Courtesy of Melvyn H. Schreiber, MD, The University of Texas Medical Branch.)

of patients with carcinoid tumors. Plasma serotonin, substance P, neurotensin, neurokinin A, and neuropeptide K can be measured, but these peptides may not be elevated in all patients. Provocative tests using pentagastrin, calcium, or epinephrine may be used to reproduce the symptoms of carcinoid tumors. The administration of pentagastrin is the safest and most reliable and the most frequently used; however, with the accuracy of current diagnostic tests, there are relatively few indications today for provocative tests.

Carcinoid tumors of the small intestine are rarely diagnosed preoperatively. Barium radiographic studies of the small bowel may exhibit multiple filling defects as a result of kinking and fibrosis of the bowel (Fig. 48-36). There are a number of imaging techniques used to diagnose the extent and spread of carcinoid tumors. Angiography and high-resolution ultrasonography can provide information on mesenteric involvement as well as hepatic involvement. Angiography may show an abnormal arrangement of mesenteric arteries and narrowing of branches associated with poor accumulation of contrast medium and poor venous drainage of the tumor area. In addition, encasement and pseudoaneurysm formation, typical of a malignant process in the mesentery, may be noted. CT is useful in detecting hepatic and lymph node metastases and the extent of bowel wall and mesenteric involvement. A novel imaging study that takes advantage of the fact that many of these tumors possess somatostatin receptors is somatostatin receptor scintigraphy using ^{111}In-labeled pentetreotide. This scintigraphic localization study has shown encouraging results, with a higher reported sensitivity than conventional imaging techniques, such as CT, in delineating and localizing carcinoid tumors.

Treatment

The treatment of patients with small bowel carcinoid tumors is based on tumor size and site and presence or absence of metastatic disease.[43] For primary tumors of less than 1 cm in diameter without evidence of regional lymph node metastasis, a segmental intestinal resection is adequate. For patients with lesions larger than 1 cm, with multiple tumors or with regional lymph node metastasis, regardless of the size of the primary tumor, wide excision of bowel and mesentery is required. Lesions of the terminal ileum are best treated by right hemicolectomy. Small duodenal tumors can be excised locally; however, more extensive lesions may require pancreaticoduodenectomy. In addition to treatment of the primary tumor, it is important that the abdomen be thoroughly explored for multicentric lesions.

Caution should be exerted in the anesthetic management of patients with carcinoid tumors because anesthesia may precipitate a carcinoid crisis characterized by hypotension, bronchospasm, flushing, and tachycardia predisposing to arrhythmias. The treatment of carcinoid crisis is IV octreotide given as a bolus of 50 to 100 μg, which may be continued as an infusion at 50 μg/hour. In addition, IV antihistamine and hydrocortisone may be of some benefit.

In patients with carcinoid tumors and widespread metastatic disease, surgery is still indicated. In contrast to metastases from other tumors, there is a definite role for surgical debulking, which, in many series, provides beneficial symptomatic relief. This may involve hepatic resection by either wedge resection or formal hepatic lobectomy. In the case of widespread multiple hepatic metastases, hepatic artery ligation or percutaneous embolization has produced good results. Others have reported regression of tumors when hepatic artery occlusion was combined with chemotherapy, concluding that combined modality therapy should be further evaluated. The role of liver transplantation in the treatment of metastatic carcinoid tumors is unclear, and the number of patients in whom this has been attempted has been small. A 5-year survival rate of 69% has been reported among highly selected patients who underwent liver transplantation for metastatic carcinoid tumors.

Medical therapy for patients with malignant carcinoid syndrome is primarily directed toward the relief of symptoms caused by the excess production of humoral factors.[43] Various long-acting analogues of somatostatin, such as octreotide (Sandostatin), relieve symptoms (diarrhea and flushing) of the carcinoid syndrome in most patients. In addition to the relief of symptoms using octreotide, tumor regression has been reported in some patients. There is no doubt of the important role of somatostatin analogues in the control of symptoms; however, their potential role in tumor inhibition has not been resolved. Results using newer somatostatin analogues with a slow-release formulation (e.g., Sandostatin LAR) in patients with carcinoid tumors are pending. Interferon-α has also been shown to provide symptomatic relief in patients with carcinoid syndrome. A clinical trial that evaluated the use of interferon-α in more than 100 patients with carcinoid syndrome identified decreases in urinary 5-hydroxyindoleacetic acid in 42% of patients and tumor regression in 15%. However, the increased incidence of side effects (e.g., fever, fatigue, anorexia, and weight loss) precludes the widespread use of this drug.

Serotonin receptor antagonists have been used with limited success. Methysergide is no longer used owing to the incidence of retroperitoneal fibrosis. Ketanserin and cyproheptadine have been shown to provide some control of symptoms, and other antagonists, such as ondansetron, may be even more effective.

Cytotoxic chemotherapy has had only limited success. The role of chemotherapy is confined predominantly to patients with metastatic disease who are symptomatic and unresponsive to other therapies. The most frequent combination used is streptozotocin and 5-fluorouracil or cyclophosphamide, which may result in some tumor regression in up to one third of the patients. The duration of response, however, is short lived. The use of cisplatin and etoposide has shown some promise only in patients with well-differentiated carcinoids. Results using dacarbazine (DTIC) are conflicting.

In summary, the treatment of carcinoid tumors requires a multidisciplinary approach, and combined modalities may be the best option, including surgical debulking, hepatic artery embolization or chemoembolization, and medical therapy. In addition, newer therapies are being developed that may be useful in the future.[43] The expression of neuroendocrine peptide receptors on carcinoid tumors and their avid uptake of ^{111}In-octreotide and ^{123}I-labeled metaiodobenzylguanidine (MIBG) for scintigraphic scanning have led to the development of novel receptor-targeted therapy. In a small series of carcinoid tumors, this therapy resulted in decreased size and reduced 5-hydroxyindoleacetic acid output with repeated high-dose ^{111}In-octreotide. Studies with ^{131}I-MIBG therapy have shown up to a 60% response in patients. Most recently, ^{90}Y-labeled octreotide has been reported to be of therapeutic benefit in a limited group of patients; controlled trials are planned for the future.

Prognosis

Carcinoid tumors have the best prognosis of all small bowel tumors, whether the disease is localized or metastatic. Resection of a carcinoid tumor localized to its primary site approaches a 100% survival rate. Five-year survival rates are about 65% among patients with regional disease and 25% to 35% among those with distant metastasis. When widespread metastatic disease precludes cure, extensive resection for palliation is indicated. In fact, long-term palliation often can be obtained because these tumors are relatively slow growing. A number of factors have been evaluated in an attempt to identify patients with carcinoid tumors who have a poor prognosis. Probably the most useful factor identified is an elevated level of chromogranin A, which was found to be an independent predictor of an adverse prognosis.

Metastatic Neoplasms

Metastatic tumors involving the small bowel are much more common than primary neoplasms. The most common metastases to the small intestine are those arising from other intra-abdominal organs, including the uterine cervix, ovaries, kidneys, stomach, colon, and pancreas. Small intestinal involvement is by either direct extension or implantation of tumor cells. Metastases from extra-abdominal tumors are rare but may be found in patients with adenocarcinoma of the breast and carcinoma of the lung. Cutaneous melanoma is the most common extra-abdominal source to involve the small intestine, with involvement of the small intestine noted in more than half of patients dying from malignant melanoma (Fig. 48-37). Common symptoms include anorexia, weight loss, anemia, bleeding, and partial bowel obstruction. Treatment is palliative resection to relieve symptoms or, occasionally, bypass if the metastatic tumor is extensive and not amenable to resection.

DIVERTICULAR DISEASE

Diverticular disease of the small intestine is relatively common. It may present as either true or false diverticula. A true diverticulum contains all layers of the intestinal wall and is usually congenital. False diverticula consist of mucosa and submucosa protruding through a defect in the muscle coat and are usually acquired defects. Small bowel diverticula may occur in any portion of the small intestine. Duodenal diverticula are the most common acquired diverticula of the small bowel, and Meckel's diverticulum is the most common true congenital diverticulum of the small bowel.

Duodenal Diverticula

Incidence and Etiology

First described by Chomel, a French pathologist, in 1710, diverticula of the duodenum are relatively common, representing the second most common site for diverticulum formation after the colon. The incidence of duodenal diverticula is varied depending on the age of the patient and the method of diagnosis. Upper gastrointestinal radiographic studies identify duodenal diverticula in 1% to 5% of all studies, whereas some autopsy series report the incidence as being as high as 15% to 20%. Duodenal diverticula occur twice as often in women as in men and

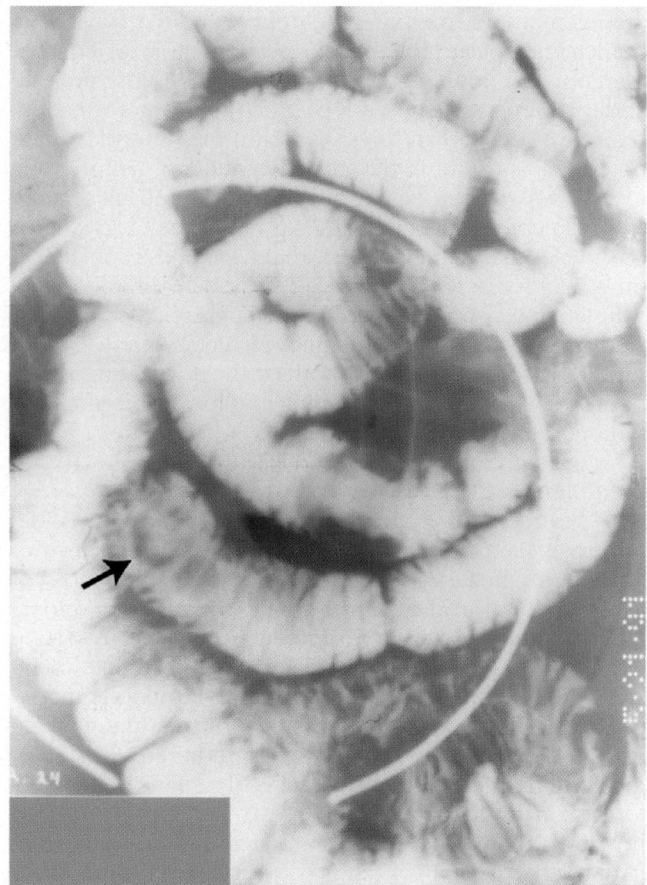

A

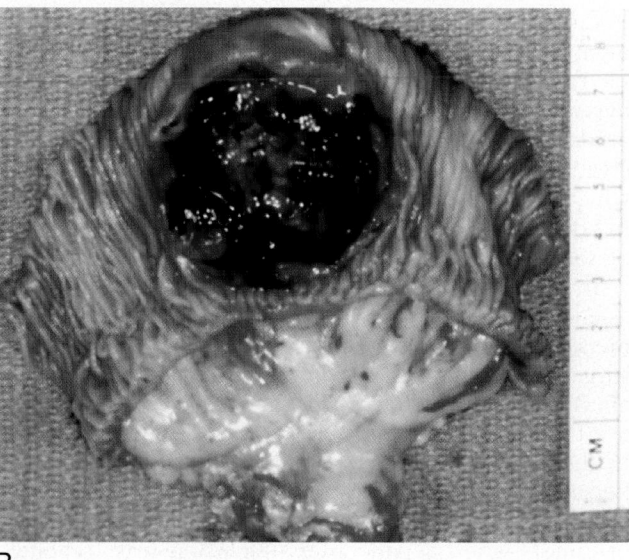

B

Figure 48-37 A, Barium radiograph shows "target lesions" consistent with metastatic melanoma of the small bowel *(arrow).* **B,** Gross specimen demonstrating metastatic melanoma to the small bowel. (**A,** Courtesy of Melvyn H. Schreiber, MD, The University of Texas Medical Branch. **B,** Courtesy of Mary R. Schwartz, MD, Baylor College of Medicine.)

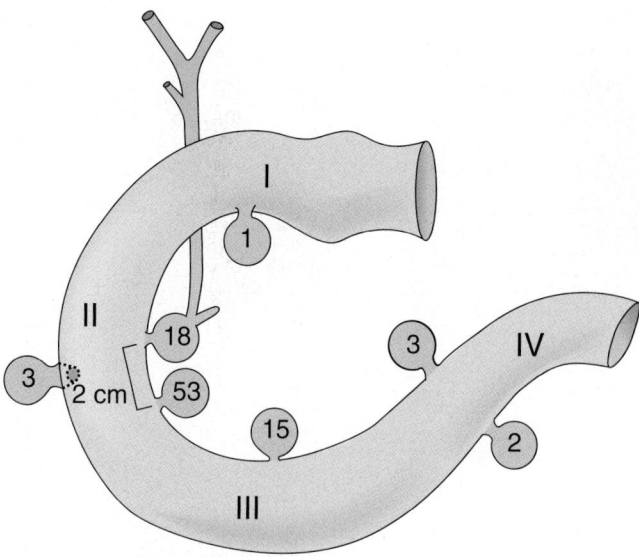

Figure 48-38 Distribution of 95 duodenal diverticula within the four portions of the duodenum. (From Eggert A, Teichmann W, Wittmann DH: The pathologic implication of duodenal diverticula. Surg Gynecol Obstet 154:62-64, 1982, with permission.)

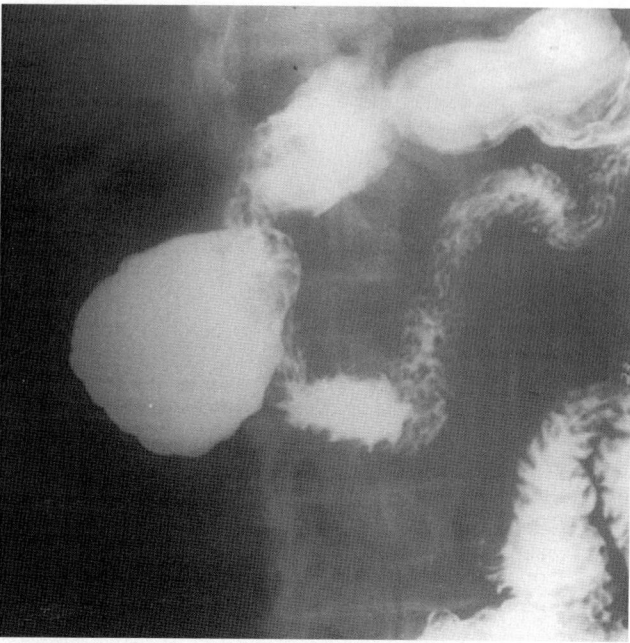

Figure 48-39 Large diverticulum arises from the second portion of the duodenum. (Courtesy of Melvyn H. Schreiber, MD, The University of Texas Medical Branch.)

are rare in patients younger than age 40 years. They have been classified as congenital or acquired, true or false, and intraluminal or extraluminal. Two thirds to three fourths of duodenal diverticula are found in the periampullary region (within a 2-cm radius of the ampulla) and project from the medial wall of the duodenum (Fig. 48-38).

Clinical Manifestations

The important thing to remember is that the overwhelming majority of duodenal diverticula are asymptomatic and are usually noted incidentally by an upper gastrointestinal series for an unrelated problem (Fig. 48-39). Diagnosis may also be obtained by upper gastrointestinal endoscopy or suggested by plain abdominal films showing an atypical gas bubble; CT can identify large diverticula. Less than 5% of duodenal diverticula will require surgery because of a complication of the diverticulum itself. Major complications of duodenal diverticula include obstruction of the biliary or pancreatic ducts that may contribute to cholangitis and pancreatitis, respectively; hemorrhage; perforation; and rarely, blind loop syndrome.

Only those diverticula associated with the ampulla of Vater are significantly related to complications of cholangitis and pancreatitis. In these patients, the ampulla most often enters the duodenum at the superior margin of the diverticulum rather than through the diverticulum itself. The mechanism proposed for the increased incidence of complications of the biliary tract is the location of the perivaterian diverticula that may produce mechanical distortion of the common bile duct as it enters the duodenum, resulting in partial obstruction and stasis. Hemorrhage can be caused by inflammation, leading to erosion of a branch of the superior mesenteric artery. Perforation of

duodenal diverticula has been described but is rare. Finally, stasis of intestinal contents within a distended diverticulum can result in bacterial overgrowth, malabsorption, steatorrhea, and megaloblastic anemia (i.e., blind loop syndrome). Symptoms related to duodenal diverticula in the absence of any other demonstrable disease usually are nonspecific epigastric complaints that can be treated conservatively and may actually prove to be the result of another problem not related to the diverticulum itself.

Treatment

As stated previously, most duodenal diverticula are asymptomatic and benign; when they are found incidentally, they should be left alone. Several operative procedures have been described for the treatment of the symptomatic duodenal diverticulum. The most common and most effective treatment is diverticulectomy, which is most easily accomplished by performing a wide Kocher maneuver that exposes the duodenum. The diverticulum is then excised, and the duodenum is closed in a transverse or longitudinal fashion, whichever produces the least amount of luminal obstruction. Because of the close proximity of the ampulla, careful identification of the ampulla is essential to prevent injury to the common bile duct and the pancreatic duct. For diverticula that are embedded deep within the head of the pancreas, a duodenotomy is performed with invagination of the diverticulum into the lumen, which is then excised, and the wall is closed (Fig. 48-40A to C). Alternative methods that have been described for duodenal diverticula associated with the ampulla of Vater include an extended sphincteroplasty through the common wall of the ampulla in the diverticulum (see Fig. 48-40D to F).

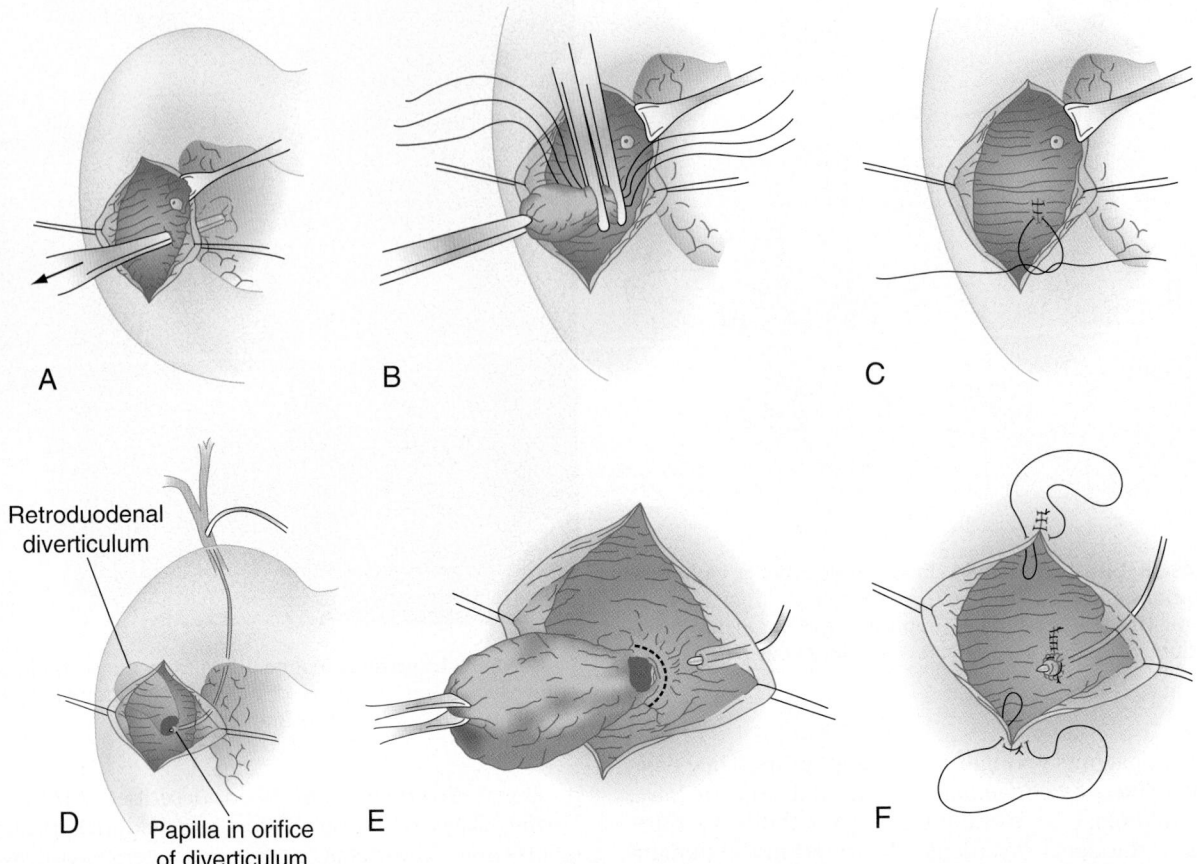

A

B

C

Retroduodenal
diverticulum

D   Papilla in orifice
of diverticulum

E

F

Figure 48-40 **A** to **C,** Treatment of a diverticulum protruding into the head of the pancreas. The duodenum is opened vertically. A clamp is used to invert the diverticulum into the lumen, where it is excised and the posterior wall defect is closed. **D** to **F,** Management of the unusual duodenal diverticula that arise in the periampullary location. A tube stent should be placed into the common bile duct and passed distally into the duodenum to facilitate identification and later dissection of the sphincter of Oddi. The diverticulum is inverted into the lumen of the duodenum. The round opening in the wall of the base of the diverticulum is the site at which the ampullary structures were freed by a circumferential incision. The *heavy broken line* in **E** shows the line of division of the base of the diverticulum, which is accomplished by free-hand dissection. After the diverticulum has been removed, the stent and enveloping papilla are protruded into the defect left by the division of the base of the diverticulum. The mucosa and muscle wall of the papilla are then sewn circumferentially to the wall of the duodenum. (Adapted from Thompson JC: Atlas of Surgery of the Stomach, Duodenum and Small Bowel. St Louis, Mosby–Year Book, 1992, pp 209-213.)

The treatment of a perforated diverticulum may require procedures similar to those described in patients with massive trauma-related defects of the duodenal wall. The perforated diverticulum should be excised and the duodenum closed with a serosal patch from the jejunal loop. If the surrounding inflammation is severe, it may be necessary to divert the enteric flow away from the site of the perforation with a gastrojejunostomy or duodenojejunostomy. Interruption of duodenal continuity proximal to the perforated diverticulum may be accomplished with a row of staples. Great care should be taken if the perforation is adjacent to the papilla of Vater. Intraluminal duodenal diverticula have been described but are highly uncommon and, if symptomatic, can be completely excised if they arise at a site distant from the ampulla. However, if a symptomatic intraluminal diverticulum is encountered associated with the ampulla of Vater, sub-

total resection of the diverticulum should be carried out to protect the entry of the biliary-pancreatic ducts.

Jejunal and Ileal Diverticula

Incidence and Etiology

Diverticula of the small bowel are much less common than duodenal diverticula, with an incidence ranging from 0.1% to 1.4% noted in autopsy series and 0.1% to 1.5% noted in upper gastrointestinal studies. Jejunal diverticula are more common and are larger than those in the ileum. These are false diverticula, occurring mainly in an older age group (after the sixth decade of life). These diverticula are multiple, usually protrude from the mesenteric border of the bowel, and may be overlooked at surgery because they are embedded within the small bowel mesentery (Fig. 48-41). The cause of jejunoileal

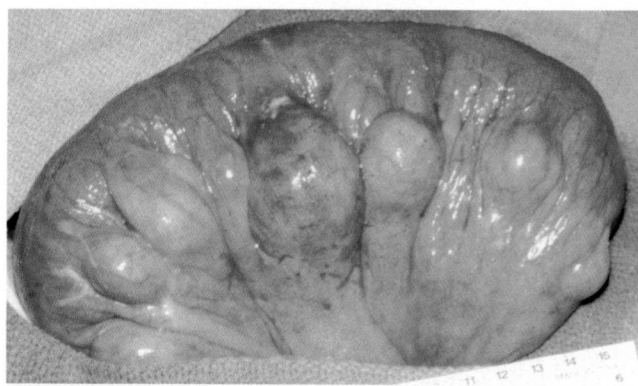

Figure 48-41 Multiple large jejunal diverticula located in the mesentery in an elderly patient presenting with obstruction secondary to an enterolith. (Adapted from Evers BM, Townsend CM Jr, Thompson JC: Small intestine. In Schwartz SI [ed]: Principles of Surgery, 7th ed. New York, McGraw-Hill, 1999, p 1248, with permission of The McGraw-Hill Companies.)

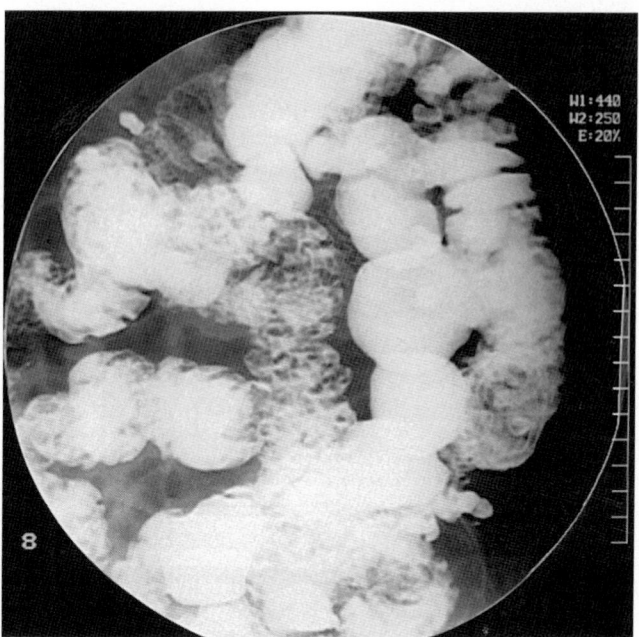

Figure 48-42 Multiple jejunal diverticula demonstrated by a barium contrast upper gastrointestinal study. (Courtesy of Melvyn H. Schreiber, MD, The University of Texas Medical Branch.)

diverticulosis is thought to be a motor dysfunction of the smooth muscle or the myenteric plexus, resulting in disordered contractions of the small bowel, generating increased intraluminal pressure, and resulting in herniation of the mucosa and submucosa through the weakest portion of the bowel (i.e., the mesenteric side).

Clinical Manifestations
Jejunoileal diverticula are usually found incidentally at laparotomy or during the performance of an upper gastrointestinal study (Fig. 48-42); the great majority remain asymptomatic. Acute complications such as intestinal obstruction, hemorrhage, or perforation can occur but are rare. Chronic symptomatology includes vague chronic abdominal pain, malabsorption, functional pseudo-obstruction, and chronic low-grade gastrointestinal hemorrhage. Acute complications are diverticulitis, with or without abscess or perforation; gastrointestinal hemorrhage; and intestinal obstruction. Stasis of intestinal flow with bacterial overgrowth (i.e., blind loop syndrome), owing to the jejunal dyskinesia, may lead to deconjugation of bowel salts and uptake of vitamin B_{12} by the bacterial flora, resulting in steatorrhea and megaloblastic anemia, with or without neuropathy.

Treatment
For incidentally noted, asymptomatic jejunoileal diverticula, no treatment is required. Treatment of complications of obstruction, bleeding, and perforation is usually by intestinal resection and end-to-end anastomosis. Patients presenting with malabsorption secondary to the blind loop syndrome and bacterial overgrowth within the diverticulum can usually be given antibiotics. Obstruction may be caused by enteroliths that form in a jejunal diverticulum and are subsequently dislodged and obstruct the distal intestine. This condition may be treated by enterotomy and removal of the enterolith, or sometimes the enterolith can be milked distally into the cecum. When the enterolith causes obstruction at the level of the diver-

ticulum, bowel resection is necessary. When a perforation of a jejunoileal diverticulum is encountered, resection with reanastomosis is required because lesser procedures such as simple closure, excision, and invagination are associated with greater mortality and morbidity rates. In extreme cases, such as diffuse peritonitis, enterostomies may be required if judgment dictates that reanastomosis may be risky.

Meckel's Diverticulum
Incidence and Etiology
Meckel's diverticulum is the most commonly encountered congenital anomaly of the small intestine, occurring in about 2% of the population. It was reported initially in 1598 by Hildanus and then described in detail by Johann Meckel in 1809. Meckel's diverticulum is located on the antimesenteric border of the ileum 45 to 60 cm proximal to the ileocecal valve and results from incomplete closure of the omphalomesenteric, or vitelline, duct. An equal incidence is found among men and women. Meckel's diverticulum may exist in different forms, ranging from a small bump that may be easily missed to a long projection that communicates with the umbilicus by a persistent fibrous cord (Fig. 48-43) or, much less commonly, a patent fistula. The usual manifestation is a relatively wide-mouth diverticulum measuring about 5 cm in length, with a diameter of up to 2 cm (Fig. 48-44). Cells lining the vitelline duct are pluripotent; therefore, it is not uncommon to find heterotopic tissue within the Meckel diverticulum, the most common of which is gastric mucosa (present in 50% of all Meckel's diverticula). Pancreatic mucosa is encountered in about 5% of diverticula;

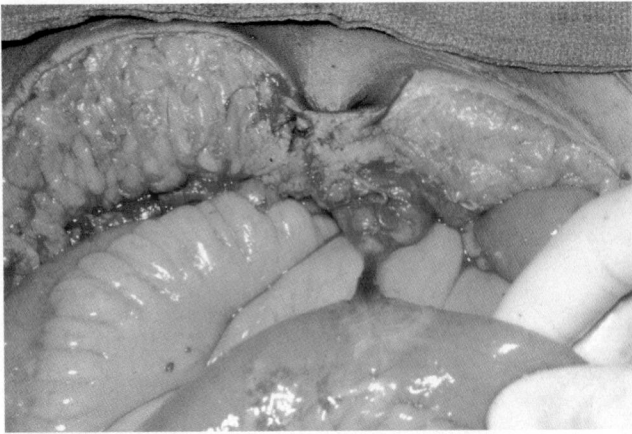

Figure 48-43 Omphalomesenteric remnant persisting as a fibrous cord from the ileum to the umbilicus.

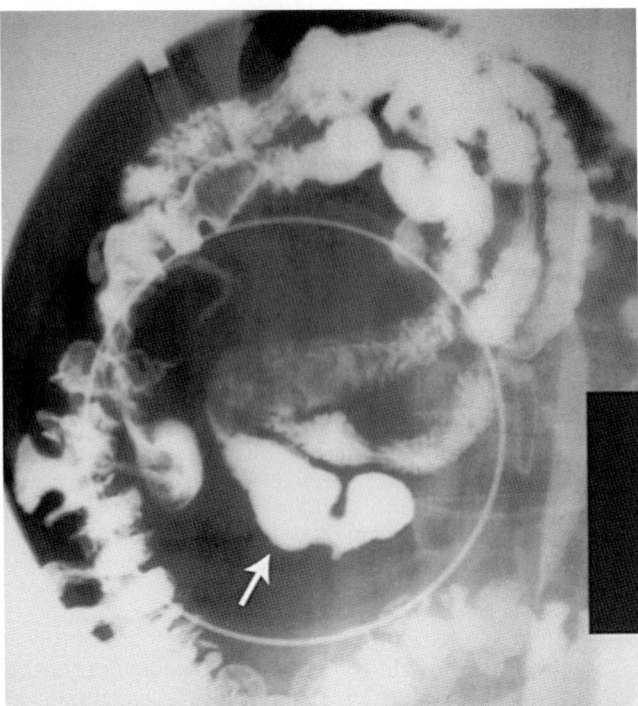

Figure 48-45 Barium radiograph demonstrates an asymptomatic Meckel's diverticulum *(arrow).* (Courtesy of Melvyn H. Schreiber, MD, The University of Texas Medical Branch.)

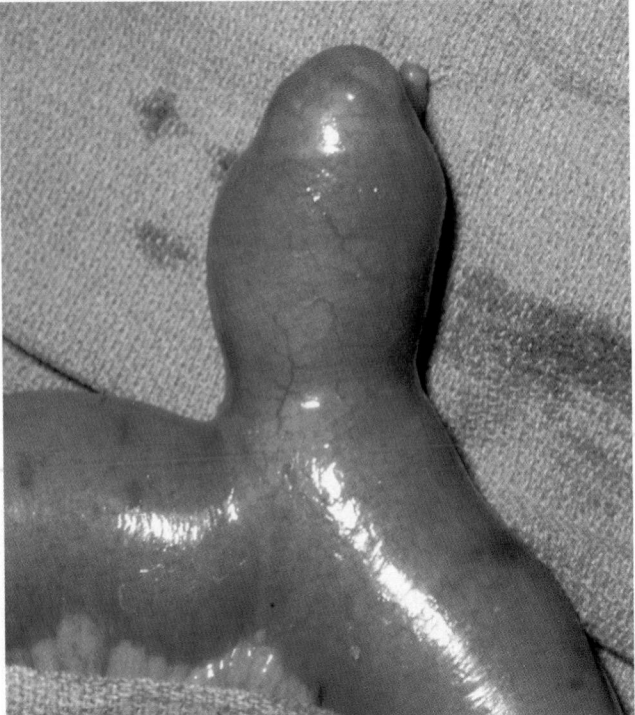

Figure 48-44 Common presentation of a Meckel diverticulum projecting from the antimesenteric border of the ileum.

less commonly, these diverticula may harbor colonic mucosa.

Clinical Manifestations

Most Meckel's diverticula are entirely benign and are incidentally discovered during autopsy, laparotomy, or barium studies (Fig. 48-45). The most common clinical presentation of Meckel's diverticulum is gastrointestinal bleeding, which occurs in 25% to 50% of patients who present with complications; hemorrhage is the most common symptomatic presentation in children aged 2 years or younger. This complication may present as acute massive hemorrhage, as anemia secondary to chronic bleeding, or as a self-limiting recurrent episodic event. The usual source of the bleeding is a chronic acid-induced ulcer in the ileum adjacent to a Meckel's diverticulum that contains gastric mucosa.

Another common presenting symptom of Meckel's diverticulum is intestinal obstruction, which may occur as a result of a volvulus of the small bowel around a diverticulum associated with a fibrotic band attached to the abdominal wall, intussusception, or, rarely, incarceration of the diverticulum in an inguinal hernia (Littre's hernia). Volvulus is usually an acute event and, if allowed to progress, may result in strangulation of the involved bowel. In intussusception, a broad-based diverticulum invaginates and then is carried forward by peristalsis. This may be ileoileal or ileocolic and present as acute obstruction associated with an urge to defecate, early vomiting, and, occasionally, the passage of the classic currant-jelly stool. A palpable mass may be present. Although reduction of an intussusception secondary to Meckel's diverticulum can sometimes be performed by barium enema, the patient should still undergo resection of the diverticulum to negate subsequent recurrence of the condition.

Diverticulitis accounts for 10% to 20% of symptomatic presentations. This complication is more common in adult patients. Meckel's diverticulitis, which is clinically indistinguishable from appendicitis, should be considered in the differential diagnosis of a patient with right lower quadrant pain. Progression of the diverticulitis may lead to perforation and peritonitis. It is important to remember that when the appendix is found to be normal during exploration for suspected appendicitis, the distal

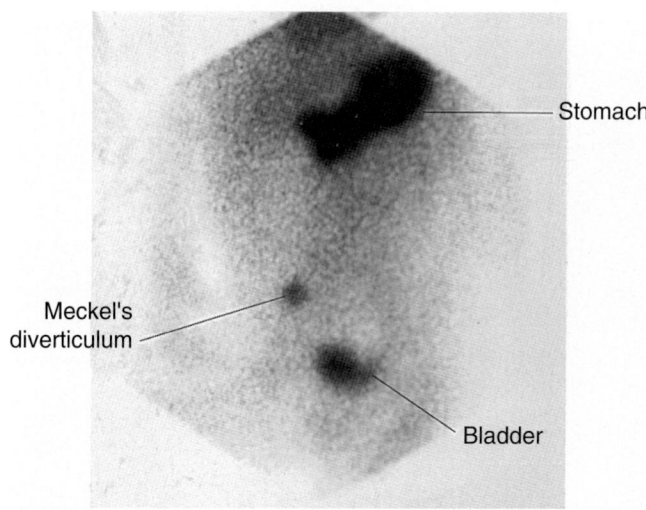

Figure 48-46 ⁹⁹ᵐTc-pertechnetate scintigraphy in a child demonstrates a Meckel's diverticulum clearly differentiated from the stomach and bladder. (Courtesy of Melvyn H. Schreiber, MD, The University of Texas Medical Branch.)

ileum should be inspected for the presence of an inflamed Meckel's diverticulum. Finally, much rarer complications of Meckel's diverticula include neoplasms, with the most common benign tumors reported as leiomyomas, angiomas, and lipomas. Malignant neoplasms include adenocarcinomas, which commonly originate from the gastric mucosa, sarcoma, and carcinoid tumor.

Diagnostic Studies

The diagnosis of Meckel's diverticulum may be difficult. Plain abdominal radiographs, CT, and ultrasonography are rarely helpful. In children, the single most accurate diagnostic test for Meckel's diverticula is scintigraphy with sodium ⁹⁹ᵐTc-pertechnetate. The ⁹⁹ᵐTc-pertechnetate is preferentially taken up by the mucus-secreting cells of gastric mucosa and ectopic gastric tissue in the diverticulum (Fig. 48-46). The diagnostic sensitivity of this scan has been reported as high as 85%, with a specificity of 95% and an accuracy of 90% in the pediatric age group.

In adults, however, ⁹⁹ᵐTc-pertechnetate scanning is less accurate because of the reduced prevalence of ectopic gastric mucosa within the diverticulum. The sensitivity and specificity can be improved by the use of pharmacologic agents such as pentagastrin and glucagon or histamine-2 (H_2)-receptor antagonists (e.g., cimetidine). Pentagastrin indirectly increases the metabolism of mucus-producing cells, whereas glucagon inhibits peristaltic dilution and washout of intraluminal radionuclide. Cimetidine may be used to increase the sensitivity of scintigraphy by decreasing the peptic secretion, but not the radionuclide uptake, and retarding the release of pertechnetate from the diverticular lumen, thus resulting in higher radionuclide concentrations in the wall of the diverticulum. In adult patients, when nuclear medicine findings are normal, barium studies should be performed. In patients with acute hemorrhage, angiography is sometimes useful.

Treatment

The treatment of a symptomatic Meckel's diverticulum should be prompt surgical intervention with resection of the diverticulum or resection of the segment of ileum bearing the diverticulum. Segmental intestinal resection is required for treatment of patients with bleeding because the bleeding site usually is in the ileum adjacent to the diverticulum. Resection of the diverticulum for nonbleeding Meckel's diverticula can be performed using either a hand-sewn technique or stapling across the base of the diverticulum in a diagonal or transverse line so as to minimize the risk for subsequent stenosis. Reports have demonstrated the feasibility and safety of laparoscopic diverticulectomy. Long-term outcomes with this procedure, however, are lacking.

Although the treatment of complicated Meckel's diverticulum is straightforward, controversy still exists regarding the optimal treatment of Meckel's diverticulum noted as an incidental finding. It is generally recommended that asymptomatic diverticula found in children during laparotomy be resected. The treatment of Meckel's diverticula encountered in the adult patient, however, remains controversial. In a landmark paper by Soltero and Bill,[44] which formed the basis of the surgical management of asymptomatic Meckel's diverticula in adults for a number of years, the likelihood of a Meckel's diverticulum becoming symptomatic in the adult patient was estimated as 2% or less; morbidity rates from incidental removal, which were reported to be as high as 12% in some studies, far exceeded the potential for prevention of disease. This study was criticized, however, because it was not a population-based analysis. An epidemiologic population-based study by Cullen and associates[45] challenged the practice of ignoring an incidentally found Meckel's diverticulum. A 6.4% rate of development of complications from the Meckel's diverticulum was calculated to occur over a lifetime. This incidence of complications does not appear to peak during childhood as originally thought. Therefore, the recommendation from this study was that an incidentally found Meckel's diverticulum should be removed at any age up to 80 years as long as no additional conditions (e.g., peritonitis) made removal hazardous. The rates of short- and long-term postoperative complications from prophylactic removal were low (~2%), and death was related to the primary operation or the general health of the patient and not to the diverticulectomy. Therefore, this study, as well as other recent studies, suggests that the issue of prophylactic diverticulectomy in adults should be reevaluated and that, in selected asymptomatic patients, diverticulectomy may be beneficial and safer than originally reported.

MISCELLANEOUS PROBLEMS

Small Bowel Ulcerations

Ulcerations of the small bowel are relatively uncommon and may be attributed to Crohn's disease, typhoid fever, tuberculosis, lymphoma, and ulcers associated with gastrinoma (Table 48-8). Drug-induced ulcerations can occur

Table 48-8 Causes of Small Intestine Ulceration

Infections	Tuberculosis, syphilis, cytomegalovirus, typhoid, parasites, *Strongyloides* hyperinfection, *Campylobacter, Yersinia*
Inflammatory	Crohn's disease, systemic lupus erythematosus, celiac disease, ulcerative enteritis
Ischemia	Mesenteric insufficiency
Idiopathic	Primary ulcer, Behçet's syndrome
Drug induced	Potassium, indomethacin, phenylbutazone, salicylates, antimetabolites
Radiation	Therapeutic, accidental
Vascular	Vasculitis, giant cell arteritis, amyloidosis (ischemic lesion), angiocentric lymphoma
Metabolic	Uremia
Hyperacidity	Zollinger-Ellison syndrome, Meckel's diverticulum, stomal ulceration
Neoplastic	Lymphoma, adenocarcinoma, melanoma
Toxic	Acute jejunitis (β-toxin–producing *Clostridium perfringens*), arsenic
Mucosal lesions	Lymphocytic enterocolitis

Adapted from Rai R, Bayless TM: Isolated and diffuse ulcers of the small intestine. In Feldman M, Scharschmidt BF, Sleisenger MH (eds): Gastrointestinal and Liver Disease: Pathophysiology/Diagnosis/Management. Philadelphia, WB Saunders, 1998, pp 1771-1778.

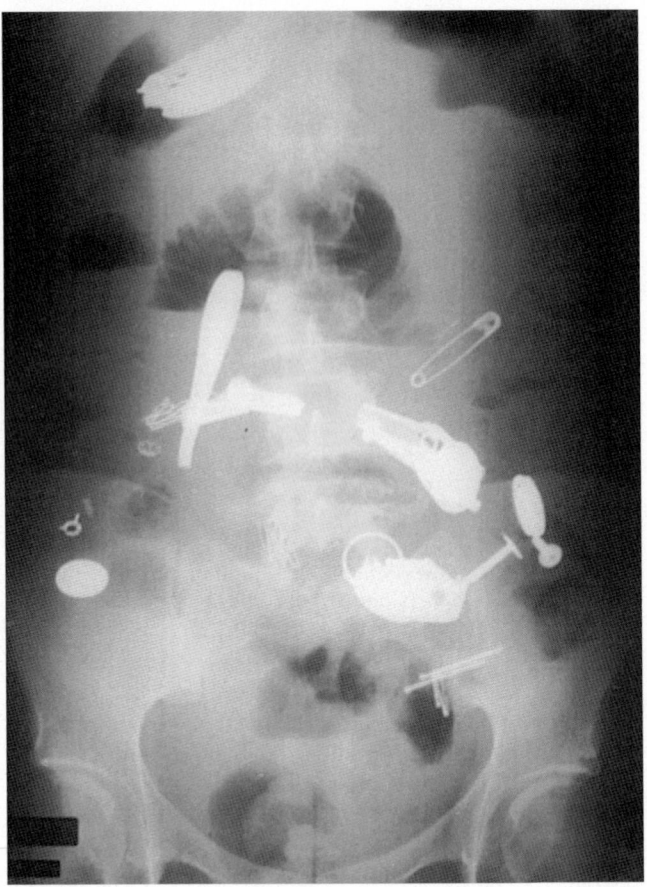

Figure 48-47 Plain abdominal film demonstrates a number of ingested foreign bodies in a patient presenting with a small bowel obstruction. (Courtesy of Melvyn H. Schreiber, MD, The University of Texas Medical Branch.)

and have been, in the past, attributed to enteric-coated potassium chloride tablets and corticosteroids. In addition, ulcerations of the small intestine in which no causative agent can be identified have been described. Reports suggest that small bowel complications from nonsteroidal anti-inflammatory drugs (NSAIDs) may be more common than originally considered. NSAID-induced ulcers occur more commonly in the ileum, with single or multiple ulcerations noted. Complications necessitating operative intervention include bleeding, perforation, and obstruction. In addition to ulcerations, NSAIDs are known to induce an enteropathy characterized by increased intestinal permeability leading to protein loss and hypoalbuminemia, malabsorption, and anemia. Treatment of complications from small bowel ulcerations is segmental resection and intestinal reanastomosis.

Ingested Foreign Bodies

Ingested foreign bodies, which can lead to subsequent perforation or obstruction of the gastrointestinal tract, are swallowed, usually accidentally, by children or adults. These include glass and metal fragments, pins, needles, toothpicks, fish bones, coins, whistles, toys, and broken razor blades, among others (Fig. 48-47). Intentional ingestion of foreign bodies is sometimes seen in the incarcer-

ated and the mentally deranged. For most patients, treatment is observation, which allows the safe passage of these objects through the intestinal tract. If the object is radiopaque, progress can be followed by serial abdominal films. Cathartic agents are contraindicated. Sharp, pointed objects such as needles, razor blades, or fish bones may penetrate the bowel wall. If abdominal pain, tenderness, fever, or leukocytosis occurs, immediate laparotomy and surgical removal of the offending object are indicated. Laparotomy is also required for intestinal obstruction.

Small Bowel Fistulas

Enterocutaneous fistulas are most commonly iatrogenic, usually the result of a surgical misadventure (e.g., anastomotic leakage, injury of the bowel or blood supply, laceration of the bowel by wire mesh, or retention suture).[46] In addition, fistulas may result from erosion by suction catheters, adjacent abscesses, or trauma. Contributing factors in some patients may include previous radiation therapy, intestinal obstruction, inflammatory bowel disease, mesenteric vascular disease, or intra-abdominal sepsis. Less than 2% of enterocutaneous fistulas occur spontaneously, and they are usually the result of Crohn's disease.

Recognition of enterocutaneous fistulas is usually not difficult. The typical clinical presentation is that of a febrile, postoperative patient with an erythematous wound. When a few skin sutures are removed, a purulent or bloody discharge is noted; leakage of enteric contents then occurs, sometimes immediately, but often within 1 or 2 days. If the diagnosis is in doubt, confirmation can be obtained by oral administration of a nonabsorbable marker, such as charcoal or Congo red, or by injection of water-soluble contrast medium into the fistula. This is the most common presentation of a small bowel fistula in which the process is more or less walled off in the immediate area of damage to the small bowel. Less commonly, small bowel fistulas may present as generalized peritonitis.

Enterocutaneous fistulas are classified according to their location and volume of daily output. These factors dictate both treatment and morbidity and mortality rates. In general, the more proximal the fistula in the intestine, the more serious the problem, with greater fluid and electrolyte loss. The drainage has a greater digestive capacity, and the distal segment is not available for absorption of nutrients. High-output fistulas are those that discharge 500 mL or more per 24 hours. Factors that prevent the spontaneous closure of fistulas are shown in Box 48-4.

Radiographic investigation of the fistula by injection of water-soluble contrast material through the fistula tract should be carried out early to delineate the presence and extent of any abscess cavities; to obtain information about the length of the tract, the extent of bowel wall disruption, and the location of the fistula; and to determine whether a distal obstruction is present. CT is helpful in determining whether underlying collections of fluid or pus are present. Often, these collections can be drained percutaneously.

The major complications associated with small bowel fistulas include sepsis, fluid and electrolyte depletion, necrosis of the skin at the site of external drainage, and malnutrition. Mortality rates for patients with enterocutaneous fistulas remain high, with some series reporting a 15% to 20% mortality rate.

Box 48-4   Factors Preventing Spontaneous Fistula Closure

High output (>500 mL/24 hr)
Severe disruption of intestinal continuity (>50% of bowel circumference)
Active inflammatory bowel disease of bowel segment
Cancer
Radiation enteritis
Distal obstruction
Undrained abscess cavity
Foreign body in the fistula tract
Fistula tract <2.5 cm long
Epithelialization of fistula tract

Treatment

Successful management of patients with intestinal fistulas requires establishment of controlled drainage, usually using a sump suction apparatus; management of sepsis; prevention of fluid and electrolyte depletion; protection of the skin; and provision of adequate nutrition.[46] The control of fistula output is most easily accomplished by intubation of the fistula tract with a drain. Protection of the skin around the fistulous opening is important to prevent excoriation and destruction of the skin. This is most easily accomplished by using Stomahesive appliances with applications of zinc oxide, aluminum paste ointment, or karaya powder. The suction catheter can be brought out through the end of the Stomahesive bag, which is cut to just fit the fistulous opening. This will allow for collection and accurate measurement of the output. The use of TPN has been an important advance in the management of patients with enterocutaneous fistulas and significantly prevents the problems of malnutrition.

The volume depletion that occurs from a proximal small bowel fistula may present a formidable problem. Agents that inhibit gut motility, such as codeine or diphenoxylate, are generally not helpful. The long-acting somatostatin analogue octreotide has been used in patients with enterocutaneous fistulas, with a successful decrease in the volume of output. Some series have reported that octreotide significantly improved the rate of fistula closure, whereas other studies have failed to document this increased closure rate. However, there is no doubt that octreotide greatly ameliorates the problems associated with a massive volume loss and allows better control of the fistula tract.

When sepsis has been controlled and nutritional therapy has been instituted, a course of conservative management should be followed. Some have advocated conservative management for up to 3 months to allow for spontaneous closure. However, others have shown that, after sepsis was controlled, more than 90% of small intestinal fistulas that closed did so within 1 month. Fewer than 10% of the fistulas closed after 2 months, and none closed spontaneously after 3 months. Therefore, a reasonable management plan would be to follow a conservative course for 4 to 6 weeks, at which time, if closure has not been obtained, surgical management should be considered. This period of conservative management not only allows those fistulas to heal spontaneously but also allows for optimization of nutritional status and control of the wound and fistula sites. Also, a reasonable delay permits the peritoneal reaction and inflammation to subside, thus making a second operation easier and safer.

Surgery is most easily accomplished by entering the previous abdominal wound, with great care taken to avoid further damage to adherent bowel. The preferred operation is fistula tract excision and segmental resection of the involved segment of intestine and reanastomosis. Simple closure of the fistula after removing the fistula tract almost always results in a recurrence of the fistula. If an unexpected abscess is encountered or if the bowel wall is rigid and distended over a long distance, thus making primary anastomosis unsafe, exteriorization of both ends of the intestine should be accomplished. Various bypass procedures have also been described as part of a staged approach in which exclusion of the segment containing the fistula is accomplished in the first reoperation and then another operation is required for resection of the involved segment and the fistula tract. Although this may be necessary in extreme circumstances, this is certainly not the preferred surgical management.

In summary, enterocutaneous fistulas occur most commonly as a result of a previous operative procedure. Once identified, radiologic studies must be performed to define the precise location as well as other factors, such as a surrounding abscess cavity or disruption of the bowel wall. This is most directly accomplished by a fistulogram, although CT may also be helpful in certain patients. The key elements to treating an enterocutaneous fistula include the control of sepsis, fluid and electrolyte depletion, skin necrosis, and malnutrition. Most of these fistulas heal spontaneously within 4 to 6 weeks of conservative management. If closure is not accomplished after this time, surgery is indicated.

Pneumatosis Intestinalis

Pneumatosis intestinalis is an uncommon condition presenting as multiple gas-filled cysts of the gastrointestinal tract. The cysts may be located in the subserosa, submucosa, and, rarely, muscularis layer and vary in size from microscopic to several centimeters in diameter. They can occur anywhere along the gastrointestinal tract, from the esophagus to the rectum; however, they are most common in the jejunum, followed by the ileocecal region and the colon. Extraintestinal structures such as mesentery, peritoneum, and the falciform ligament may also be involved. There is an equal incidence among males and females, and this condition most commonly occurs in the fourth to seventh decades of life. Pneumatosis in neonates is usually associated with necrotizing enterocolitis. The cause of pneumatosis intestinalis has not been completely delineated. A number of theories have been proposed, of which the mechanical, mucosal damage, bacterial, and pulmonary theories appear to be the most promising.

Most cases of pneumatosis intestinalis are associated with chronic obstructive pulmonary disease or the immunocompromised state (e.g., AIDS; after transplantation; in association with leukemia, lymphoma, vasculitis, or collagen vascular disease; and in those patients taking chemotherapy or corticosteroids).[47] Other associated conditions include inflammatory, obstructive, or infectious conditions of the intestine; iatrogenic conditions such as endoscopy and jejunostomy placement; ischemia; and extraintestinal diseases such as diabetes. Pneumatosis not associated with other lesions is referred to as *primary pneumatosis.*

Grossly, the cysts resemble cystic lymphangiomas or hydatid cysts. On histologic section, the involved portion has a honeycomb appearance. The cysts are thin walled and break easily. Spontaneous rupture gives rise to pneumoperitoneum. Symptoms are nonspecific, and in pneu-

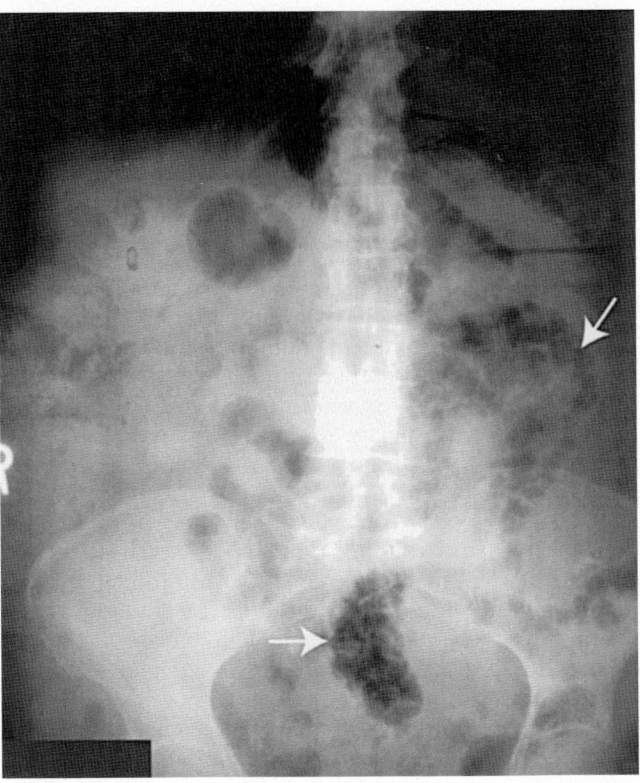

Figure 48-48 Plain abdominal film demonstrates pneumatosis intestinalis *(arrows).* (Courtesy of Melvyn H. Schreiber, MD, The University of Texas Medical Branch.)

matosis associated with other disorders, the symptoms may be those of the associated disease. Symptoms in primary pneumatosis intestinalis, when present, include most commonly diarrhea, abdominal pain, abdominal distention, nausea, vomiting, weight loss, and mucus in stools. Hematochezia and constipation have also been described. Complications associated with pneumatosis intestinalis occur in about 3% of cases and include volvulus, intestinal obstruction, hemorrhage, and intestinal perforation. Most commonly, pneumoperitoneum occurs in these patients, usually in association with small bowel rather than large bowel pneumatosis. Peritonitis is unusual. In fact, pneumatosis intestinalis represents one of the few cases of sterile pneumoperitoneum and should be considered in the patient with free abdominal air but no evidence of peritonitis.

The diagnosis is usually made radiographically by plain abdominal or barium studies. On plain films, pneumatosis intestinalis appears as radiolucent areas within the bowel wall, which must be differentiated from luminal intestinal gas (Fig. 48-48). The radiolucency may be linear or curvilinear or appear as grapelike clusters or tiny bubbles. Alternatively, barium contrast or CT studies can be used to confirm the diagnosis. Visualization of intestinal cysts has also been described by ultrasound.

No treatment is necessary unless one of the very rare complications supervenes, such as rectal bleeding, cyst-induced volvulus, or tension pneumoperitoneum. Prognosis in most patients is that of the underlying disease.

The important point is to recognize that pneumatosis intestinalis is a benign cause of pneumoperitoneum. Treatment should be directed at the underlying cause of the pneumatosis, and surgical intervention should be predicated on the clinical course of the patient.

Blind Loop Syndrome

Blind loop syndrome is a rare condition manifested by diarrhea, steatorrhea, megaloblastic anemia, weight loss, abdominal pain, and deficiencies of the fat-soluble vitamins (A, D, E, and K), as well as neurologic disorders. The underlying cause of this syndrome is bacterial overgrowth in stagnant areas of the small bowel produced by stricture, stenosis, fistulas, or diverticula (e.g., jejunoileal or Meckel's diverticulum). Under normal circumstances, the upper gastrointestinal tract contains fewer than 10^5 bacteria/mL, mostly gram-positive aerobes and facultative anaerobes. However, with stasis, the number of bacteria increases with excessive proliferation of aerobic and anaerobic bacteria (bacteroides, anaerobic lactobacilli, coliforms, and enterococci are likely to be present in varying numbers). The bacteria compete for vitamin B_{12}, producing systemic deficiency of vitamin B_{12} and megaloblastic anemia.

The syndrome can be confirmed by a series of laboratory investigations. Bacterial overgrowth can be diagnosed with cultures obtained through an intestinal tube or by indirect tests such as the ^{14}C-xylose or ^{14}C-cholylglycine breath tests. Excessive bacterial use of ^{14}C substrate leads to an increase in $^{14}CO_2$. After bacterial overgrowth and steatorrhea are confirmed, a Schilling test (^{57}Co-labeled vitamin B_{12} absorption) may be performed, which should reveal a pattern of urinary excretion of vitamin B_{12} resembling that of pernicious anemia (a urinary loss of 0%-6% of vitamin B_{12} compared with the normal of 7%-25%). In patients with blind loop syndrome, vitamin B_{12} excretion is not altered by the addition of intrinsic factor, but a course of a broad-spectrum antibiotic (e.g., tetracycline) should return vitamin B_{12} absorption to normal.

Treatment of patients with blind loop syndrome includes parenteral vitamin B_{12} therapy and a broad-spectrum antibiotic, most commonly tetracycline or amoxicillin-clavulanate potassium (Augmentin). An alternative choice is the combination of a cephalosporin (e.g., cephalexin [Keflex]) and metronidazole. If these agents are not effective, chloramphenicol may be used. For most patients, a single course of therapy (7-10 days) is sufficient, and the patient may remain symptom-free for months. Prokinetic agents have been used without real success. Surgical correction of the condition producing stagnation and blind loop syndrome produces a permanent cure and is indicated in those patients who require multiple rounds of antibiotics or are on continuous therapy.

Radiation Enteritis

Radiation therapy is commonly used as adjuvant therapy for various abdominal and pelvic cancers. In addition to tumor cells, however, other rapidly dividing cells in

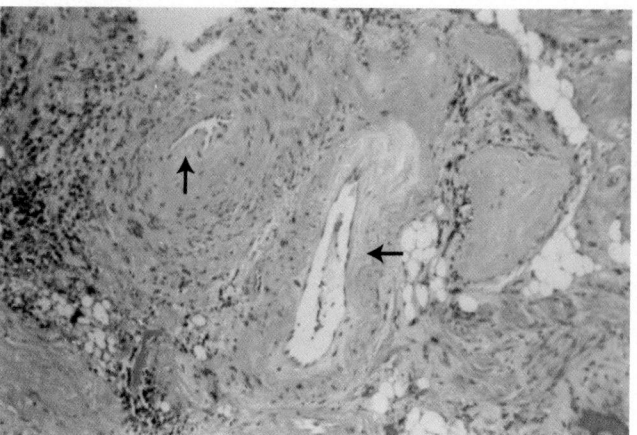

Figure 48-49 Photomicrograph of the ileum of a patient with ulceration and stricture secondary to radiation enteritis. Note the obliterative arteritis, thickened arterial walls, and submucosal fibrosis *(arrows)*, which are characteristic findings of chronic radiation injury. (Courtesy of Mary R. Schwartz, MD, Baylor College of Medicine.)

normal tissues may be affected by radiation. Surrounding normal tissue such as the small intestinal epithelium may sustain severe, acute, and chronic deleterious effects. The amount of radiation appears to correlate with the probability of developing radiation enteritis. Serious late complications are unusual if the total radiation dosage is less than 4000 cGy; morbidity risk increases with dosages exceeding 5000 cGy. Other factors, including previous abdominal operations, preexisting vascular disease, hypertension, diabetes, and adjuvant treatment with certain chemotherapeutic agents such as 5-fluorouracil, doxorubicin, dactinomycin, and methotrexate, contribute to the development of enteritis after radiation treatments. A previous history of laparotomy increases the risk for enteritis, presumably owing to adhesions that fix portions of the small bowel into the irradiated field. Radiation damage tends to be acute and self-limiting, with symptoms consisting mainly of diarrhea, abdominal pain, and malabsorption. The late effects of radiation injury are the result of damage to the small submucosal blood vessels with a progressive obliterative arteritis and submucosal fibrosis, resulting eventually in thrombosis and vascular insufficiency[48] (Fig. 48-49). This injury may produce necrosis and perforation of the involved intestine, but more commonly, it leads to stricture formation with symptoms of obstruction or small bowel fistulas.

Radiation enteritis may be minimized by adjusting ports and dosages of radiation to deliver optimal treatment specifically to the tumor and not to surrounding tissues. Placement of radiopaque markers, such as titanium clips, at the time of the original operation facilitates better targeting of the radiation treatment. Methods designed to exclude the small bowel from the irradiated field include reperitonealization, omental transposition, and placement of absorbable mesh slings.

Numerous pharmacologic interventions have also been described to reduce the side effects of radiation enteritis. Sucralfate has been shown to be of value in preventing the diarrhea associated with abdominal radiation. Superoxide dismutase, a free radical scavenger, has been used successfully to reduce complications. Other compounds that have been evaluated include glutathione, antioxidants (e.g., vitamin A, vitamin E, β-carotene), and histamine antagonists. The most effective radioprotectant agent appears to be amifostine (WR-2721), a sulfhydryl compound that is converted intracellularly to an active metabolite, WR-1065, which in turn binds to free radicals and protects the cell from radiation injury. Other agents that may prove useful in the prevention of the acute symptoms of acute radiation enteritis include glutamine-enriched enteral formulas and the hormones bombesin, growth hormone, glucagon-like peptide 2, and insulin-like growth factor I, which have demonstrated effectiveness in experimental studies in preventing or reducing symptoms associated with radiation enteritis.

The treatment of acute radiation enteritis is directed at controlling symptoms. Antispasmodics and analgesics may alleviate abdominal pain and cramping, and diarrhea usually responds to opiates or other antidiarrheal agents. The use of corticosteroids for acute radiation enteritis is of uncertain value. Dietary manipulation, including oral elemental diets, has also been advocated to ameliorate the acute effects of radiation enteritis; however, results are conflicting.

Operative intervention may be required in a subgroup of patients with the chronic effects of radiation enteritis. This subgroup of patients represents only a small percentage (2%-3%) of the total number of patients who have received abdominal or pelvic irradiation. Indications for operation include obstruction, fistula formation, perforation, and bleeding, with obstruction being the most common presentation. Operative procedures include a bypass or resection with reanastomosis. Advocates for bypass procedures contend that this procedure is safer and controls the symptoms better than resection. Advocates of resection contend that the high morbidity and mortality rates previously reported with resection and reanastomosis reflect inadequate resection and anastomosis of diseased intestine. In patients presenting with obstruction, extensive lysis of adhesions should be avoided. Obstruction due to rigid, fixed intestinal loops in the pelvis is best bypassed. If resection and reanastomosis are planned, at least one end of the anastomosis should be from intestine outside the irradiated field. An incidence as high as 50% of anastomotic breakdown has been reported after resection and anastomosis involving diseased segments of bowel, owing to the poor healing qualities of the irradiated tissue. Macroscopic findings may not be accurate in evaluating the full extent of radiation damage. Frozen sections and laser Doppler flowmetry have been used to assist resection and anastomosis. However, reports of the clinical usefulness of these techniques are conflicting. Perforation of the intestine should be treated with resection and anastomosis. When reanastomosis is thought to be unsafe, the ends should be exteriorized.

Radiation enteritis can be a relentless disease process. Almost half of patients who survive their first laparotomy for radiation bowel injury require further surgery for ongoing bowel damage. Up to 25% of these patients die of radiation enteritis and complications from its management.

Short Bowel Syndrome

The short bowel syndrome results from a total small bowel length that is inadequate to support nutrition. Seventy-five percent of cases of short bowel syndrome occur from massive intestinal resection.[49] In the adult, mesenteric occlusion, midgut volvulus, and traumatic disruption of the superior mesenteric vessels are the most frequent causes. Multiple sequential resections, most commonly associated with recurrent Crohn's disease, account for 25% of patients. In neonates, the most common cause of short bowel syndrome is bowel resection secondary to necrotizing enterocolitis. The clinical hallmarks of short bowel syndrome include diarrhea, fluid and electrolyte deficiency, and malnutrition. Other complications include an increased incidence of gallstones due to disruption of the enterohepatic circulation and of nephrolithiasis from hyperoxaluria. Specific nutrient deficiencies must be prevented, and levels must be monitored closely; these nutrients include iron, magnesium, zinc, copper, and vitamins. The likelihood that a patient with short bowel syndrome will be permanently dependent on TPN is thought to be primarily influenced by the length, location, and health of the remaining intestine. In patients with short bowel syndrome, postabsorptive levels of plasma citrulline, a nonprotein amino acid produced by intestinal mucosa, may provide an indicator to differentiate transient from permanent intestinal failure.

The bowel has a remarkable capacity to adapt after small bowel resection; in many instances, this process of intestinal adaptation, called *adaptive hyperplasia,* effectively prevents severe complications resulting from the markedly decreased surface area that is available for absorption and digestion. However, any adaptive mechanism can be overwhelmed, and adaptation can be inadequate if too much small bowel is lost. Although there is considerable individual variation, resection of up to 70% of the small bowel usually can be tolerated if the terminal ileum and ileocecal valve are preserved. Length alone, however, is not the only determining factor of complications related to small bowel resection. For example, if the distal two thirds of the ileum, including the ileocecal valve, is resected, significant abnormalities of absorption of bile salts and vitamin B_{12} may occur, resulting in diarrhea and anemia, although only 25% of the total length of the small bowel has been removed. Proximal bowel resection is tolerated much better than distal resection because the ileum can adapt and increase its absorptive capacity more efficiently than the jejunum.

Treatment

The most important aspect to remember about short bowel syndrome is prevention. In patients with Crohn's disease, resections limited to the particular complication should be performed. In addition, during surgery for problems related to intestinal ischemia, the smallest possible resection should be performed, and, if necessary, second-look operations should be carried out to allow the ischemic bowel to demarcate, thus potentially preventing unnecessary extensive resection of the bowel.

After massive small bowel resection, the treatment course may be divided into early and late phases. In its early phase, treatment is primarily directed at the control of diarrhea, replacement of fluid and electrolytes, and prompt institution of TPN.[50] Volume losses may exceed 5 L/day, and vigorous monitoring of intake and output with adequate replacement must be carried out. Diarrhea in this early phase can be caused by a multitude of sources. For example, hypergastrinemia and gastric hypersecretion occur after massive small bowel resection and greatly contribute to diarrhea after a massive small bowel resection. Acid hypersecretion can be managed by H_2-receptor antagonists or proton pump blockers, such as omeprazole. Diarrhea may also be caused by ileal resection, resulting in disruption of the enterohepatic circulation and excessive amounts of bile salts entering the colon. Cholestyramine may be beneficial when diarrhea is related to the cathartic effects of unabsorbed bile salts in the colon. In addition, the judicious use of agents that inhibit gut motility (e.g., codeine and diphenoxylate) may be helpful. The long-acting somatostatin analogue octreotide also appears to reduce the amount of diarrhea during the early phase of short bowel syndrome. Some studies suggest that octreotide may inhibit gut adaptation; other studies, however, have not confirmed this deleterious effect of octreotide.

As soon as the patient has recovered from the acute phase, enteral nutrition should begin so that intestinal adaptation may be started early and proceed successfully.[51] The most common types of enteral diets are elemental (Vivonex, Flexical) and polymeric (Isocal, Ensure). Controversy exists regarding the optimal diet for these patients. Initially, a high-carbohydrate, high-protein diet is appropriate to maximize absorption. Milk products should be avoided, and diet should be begun at iso-osmolar concentrations and with small amounts. As the gut adapts, the osmolality, volume, and caloric content can be increased. The provision of nutrients in their simplest forms is an important part of the treatment. Simple sugars, dipeptides, and tripeptides are rapidly absorbed from the intestinal tract. Reduction in dietary fat has long been considered to be important in the treatment of patients with short bowel syndrome. Supplementation of the diet with 100 g or more of fat, however, should be carried out, often requiring the use of medium-chain triglycerides, which are absorbed in the proximal bowel. Vitamins, especially fat-soluble vitamins, as well as calcium, magnesium, and zinc supplementation, should be provided. The roles of hormones administered systemically and glutamine administered enterally are being evaluated. The hormones neurotensin, bombesin, and glucagon-like peptide 2 (GLP-2) have demonstrated marked mucosal growth in various experimental studies and have been shown to prevent the gut atrophy associated with TPN in experimental studies; combination

therapy appears more efficacious than single-agent administration. In addition, limited clinical studies using GLP-2 show improved intestinal absorption and nutritional status in patients with short bowel syndrome.[52]

Two other hormones not derived from the gut that have been evaluated extensively in various experimental and limited clinical trials include growth hormone and insulin-like growth factor I.[53] In an uncontrolled clinical trial, Byrne and colleagues used a combination of growth hormone, glutamine, and a modified diet and demonstrated a reduction in or elimination of TPN requirements in some refractory patients with severe short bowel syndrome and TPN dependence.[54] However, in a double-blind, placebo-controlled randomized study, Scolapio and associates demonstrated only modest improvements in electrolyte absorption but no improvements in small bowel morphology, stool losses, or macronutrient absorption using the combination of glutamine and growth hormone.[55] In contrast, a study by Seguy and colleagues suggested that a 3-week course of low-dose growth hormone significantly improved intestinal absorption in TPN-dependent patients.[56] Given the conflicting results in these studies, the potential efficacy of this treatment in TPN-dependent patients remains to be defined. The combination of various trophic hormones with glutamine and a modified diet may prove more efficacious in this difficult group of patients.

A number of surgical strategies have been attempted in patients who are chronically TPN dependent with limited success; these include procedures to delay intestinal transit time, methods to increase absorptive area, and small bowel transplantation.[57] Methods to delay intestinal transit time include the construction of various valves and sphincters, with inconsistent results reported. Antiperistaltic segments of small intestine have been constructed to slow the transit, thus allowing additional contact time for nutrient and fluid absorption. Moderate successes have been described with this technique. Other procedures, including colonic interposition, recirculating loops of small bowel, and retrograde electrical pacing, have been tried but were found to be unsuccessful in humans and were largely abandoned. Surgical procedures to increase absorptive area include the intestinal tapering and lengthening procedure originally described by Bianchi.[57] This procedure improves intestinal function by correcting the dilation and ineffective peristalsis of the remaining intestine, as well as by doubling the intestinal length while preserving the mucosal surface area. Although beneficial in selected patients, potential complications can include necrosis of divided segments and anastomotic leaks.

Intestinal transplantation has improved with the introduction of the new immunosuppressive agent tacrolimus (FK506).[58] Intestinal transplantation procedures have included primarily isolated small intestinal grafts and combined liver–small intestinal grafts with a few more extensive cluster grafts in a large series reported from the International Intestinal Transplant Registry. Under tacrolimus treatment, 1-year graft and patient survival rates were 65% and 83%, respectively, for isolated bowel transplantation and 65% and 68% for liver–small bowel trans-

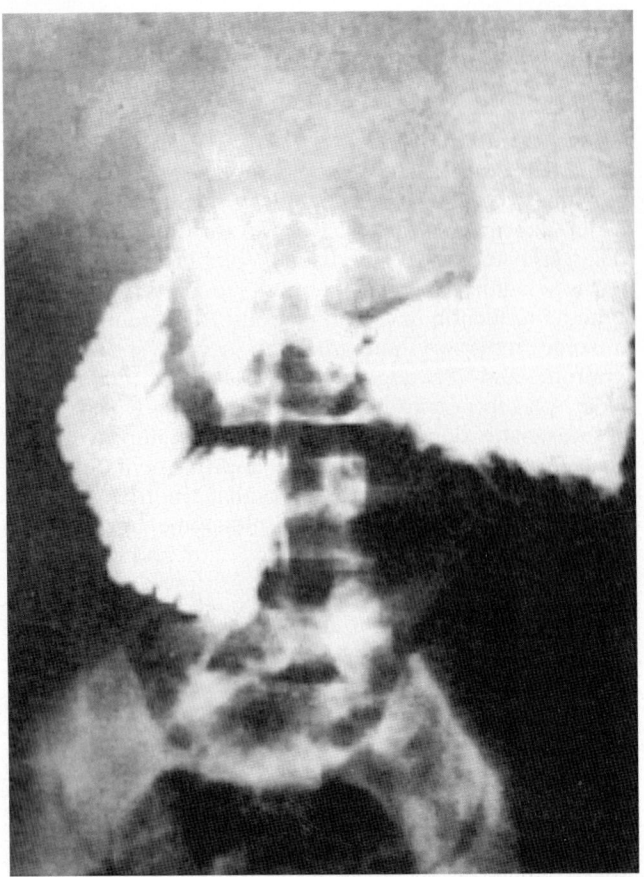

Figure 48-50 Barium radiograph demonstrates obstruction of the third portion of the duodenum secondary to superior mesenteric artery compression as a consequence of burn injury. (Adapted from Reckler JM, Bruck HM, Munster AM, et al: Superior mesenteric artery syndrome as a consequence of burn injury. J Trauma 12:979-985, 1972.)

plantation. Seventy-eight of the 86 survivors in this series had stopped TPN and were receiving oral nutrition. The largest experience in the United States has been at the University of Pittsburgh, where the reported patient survival rate has been 72% at 1 year, 53% at 2 years, and 42% at 3 years. Currently, liver–small intestine transplantation has a survival rate similar to that of kidney and heart transplantation. The challenges of small bowel transplantation continue to be the need for better immunosuppression and earlier detection of rejection. An alternative to intestinal transplantation is mucosal stem cell transplantation, which involves transplanting enterocytes onto a biomatrix and achieving regeneration of intestinal mucosa. This procedure is, at best, preliminary but has shown some promise in experimental studies.

Vascular Compression of the Duodenum

Vascular compression of the duodenum, also known as *superior mesenteric artery syndrome* or *Wilkie's syndrome,* is a rare condition characterized by compression of the third portion of the duodenum by the superior

mesenteric artery as it passes over this portion of the duodenum. Symptoms include profound nausea and vomiting, abdominal distention, weight loss, and postprandial epigastric pain, which varies from intermittent to constant depending on the severity of the duodenal obstruction. Weight loss usually occurs before the onset of symptoms and contributes to the syndrome.

This syndrome is most commonly seen in young asthenic individuals, with women being more commonly affected than men. Predisposing factors for vascular compression of the duodenum, aside from weight loss, include supine immobilization, scoliosis, and the placement of a body cast (sometimes called the *cast syndrome*). An association between vascular compression of the duodenum and peptic ulcer has been observed. Vascular compression of the duodenum has been reported in association with anorexia nervosa and after proctocolectomy and J-pouch anal anastomosis, resection of an arteriovenous malformation of the cervical cord, abdominal aortic aneurysm repair, and orthopedic procedures, usually spinal surgery. One report in the literature describes a family with a preponderance of vascular compression of the duodenum.

Diagnosis of this condition is made by barium upper gastrointestinal series (Fig. 48-50) or hypotonic duodenography, which demonstrates abrupt or near-total cessation of flow of barium from the duodenum to the jejunum. CT has been useful in certain instances. Treatment of this syndrome varies. Conservative measures are tried initially and have been increasingly successful as definitive treatment. The operative treatment of choice for vascular compression of the duodenum is duodenojejunostomy.

Selected References

Becker JM, Dayton MT, Fazio VW, et al: Prevention of postoperative abdominal adhesions by a sodium hyaluronate-based bioresorbable membrane: A prospective, randomized, double-blind multicenter study. J Am Coll Surg 183:297-306, 1996.

Prospective study showing decreased adhesions with a hyaluronate-based membrane. This is the first randomized clinical study to suggest a decrease in adhesion formation using these membranes.

Bianchi A: From the cradle to enteral autonomy: The role of autologous gastrointestinal reconstruction. Gastroenterology 130:S138-146, 2006.

Concise review of the role for bowel lengthening procedures as one operative strategy for the treatment of short gut syndrome. This review is written by one of the innovators of these techniques.

Crohn BB, Ginzburg L, Oppenheimer GD: Regional ileitis: A pathologic and clinical entity. JAMA 99:1323-1329, 1932.

This landmark paper succinctly crystallizes the clinical course, differential diagnosis, and pathologic findings of regional ileitis in young adults. Although other terms have been applied to this disease process, based on the descriptions in this classic paper, Crohn's disease has been universally accepted as the name.

Cullen JJ, Kelly KA, Moir CR, et al: Surgical management of Meckel's diverticulum: An epidemiologic, population-based study. Ann Surg 220:564-569, 1994.

This study, which was a carefully performed, epidemiologic, population-based analysis, challenges the prior dogma of selective resection of incidentally discovered Meckel's diverticula in the adult patient.

DeCosse JJ, Rhodes RS, Wentz WB, et al: The natural history and management of radiation-induced injury of the gastrointestinal tract. Ann Surg 170:369-384, 1969.

This report, presented at the annual meeting of the American Surgical Association in 1969, is a landmark article that clearly delineates the clinical features, complications, and management of patients with radiation enteritis.

Hayanga AJ, Bass-Wilkins K, Bulkley GB: Current management of small-bowel obstruction. Adv Surg 39:1-33, 2005.

This recent review nicely summarizes the current modalities for diagnosis and treatment of small bowel obstruction.

Korzenik JR, Podolsky DK: Evolving knowledge and therapy of inflammatory bowel disease. Nat Rev Drug Discov 5:197-209, 2006.

Succinct recent review which provides an up-to-date synopsis of current and emerging treatment for IBD.

Sarr MG, Bulkley GB, Zuidema GD: Preoperative recognition of intestinal strangulation obstruction: Prospective evaluation of diagnostic capability. Am J Surg 145:176-182, 1983.

Important study which clearly shows that no diagnostic test or study can accurately predict strangulation of the intestine. All surgical trainees should read this.

Thomas RP, Hellmich MR, Townsend CM Jr, Evers BM: Role of gastrointestinal hormones in the proliferation of normal and neoplastic tissues. Endocr Rev 24:571-599, 2003.

This review summarizes the effects of various gastrointestinal hormones on the growth of normal tissues and gastrointestinal cancers; possible treatment options are discussed.

Woodside KJ, Townsend CM, Jr., Evers BM: Current management of gastrointestinal carcinoid tumors. J Gastrointest Surg 8:742-756, 2004.

Thorough overview of gastrointestinal carcinoid tumors and the current treatment strategies.

References

1. Moore KL, Persaud TVN: The digestive system. In Moore KL, Persaud TVN (eds): The Developing Human: Clinically Oriented Embryology, 7th ed. Philadelphia, Elsevier, 2003, pp 255-286.
2. Chung DH, Evers BM: The digestive system. In O'Leary J (ed): The Physiologic Basis of Surgery, 3rd ed. Philadelphia, Lippincott Williams & Wilkins, 2002, pp 457-490.
3. Englander EW, Greeley JGH: Postpyloric gastrointestinal peptides. In Johnson LR (ed): Physiology of the Gastrointestinal Tract, 4th ed. San Diego: Elsevier, 2005, pp 121-160.
4. Thomas RP, Hellmich MR, Townsend CM Jr, et al: Role of gastrointestinal hormones in the proliferation of normal and neoplastic tissues. Endocr Rev 24:571-599, 2003.
5. Dockray GJ: Gastrointestinal hormones: Gastrin, cholecystokinin, somatostatin, and ghrelin. In Johnson LR (ed): Physiology of the Gastrointestinal Tract, 4th ed. San Diego, Elsevier, 2005, pp 91-120.
6. Gariepy CE, Dickinson CJ: Translation and posttranslation processing of gastrointestinal peptides. In Johnson LR (ed): Physiology of the Gastrointestinal Tract, 4th ed. San Diego, Elsevier, 2005, pp 31-62.
7. Wangensteen OH: Historical aspects of the management of acute intestinal obstruction. Surgery 65:363-383, 1969.
8. Hayanga AJ, Bass-Wilkins K, Bulkley GB: Current management of small-bowel obstruction. Adv Surg 39:1-33, 2005.
9. Mak SY, Roach SC, Sukumar SA: Small bowel obstruction: Computed tomography features and pitfalls. Curr Probl Diagn Radiol 35:65-74, 2006.
10. Maglinte DD, Heitkamp DE, Howard TJ, et al: Current concepts in imaging of small bowel obstruction. Radiol Clin North Am 41:263-283, 2003.
11. Schmidt S, Felley C, Meuwly JY, et al: CT enteroclysis: Technique and clinical applications. Eur Radiol 16:648-660, 2006.
12. Sarr MG, Bulkley GB, Zuidema GD: Preoperative recognition of intestinal strangulation obstruction: Prospective evaluation of diagnostic capability. Am J Surg 145:176-182, 1983.
13. Nagle A, Ujiki M, Denham W, et al: Laparoscopic adhesiolysis for small bowel obstruction. Am J Surg 187:464-470, 2004.
14. Szomstein S, Lo Menzo E, Simpfendorfer C, et al: Laparoscopic lysis of adhesions. World J Surg 30:535-540, 2006.
15. Childs WA, Phillips RB: Experience with intestinal plication and a proposed modification. Ann Surg 152:258-265, 1960.
16. Sprouse LR 2nd, Arnold CI, Thow GB, et al: Twelve-year experience with the Thow long intestinal tube: A means of preventing postoperative bowel obstruction. Am Surg 67:357-360, 2001.
17. Becker JM, Dayton MT, Fazio VW, et al: Prevention of postoperative abdominal adhesions by a sodium hyaluronate-based bioresorbable membrane: A prospective, randomized, double-blind multicenter study. J Am Coll Surg 183:297-306, 1996.
18. Vrijland WW, Tseng LN, Eijkman HJ, et al: Fewer intraperitoneal adhesions with use of hyaluronic acid-carboxymethylcellulose membrane: a randomized clinical trial. Ann Surg 235:193-199, 2002.
19. Sajja SB, Schein M: Early postoperative small bowel obstruction. Br J Surg 91:683-691, 2004.
20. Crohn BB, Ginzburg L, Oppenheimer GD: Regional ileitis: A pathologic and clinical entity. JAMA 99:1323-1329, 1932.
21. Sartor RB: Mechanisms of disease: Pathogenesis of Crohn's disease and ulcerative colitis. Nat Clin Pract Gastroenterol Hepatol 3:390-407, 2006.
22. Hanauer SB: Inflammatory bowel disease: epidemiology, pathogenesis, and therapeutic opportunities. Inflamm Bowel Dis 12(Suppl 1):S3-9, 2006.
23. Gaya DR, Russell RK, Nimmo ER, et al: New genes in inflammatory bowel disease: Lessons for complex diseases? Lancet 367:1271-1284, 2006.
24. Ahmed FE: Role of genes, the environment and their interactions in the etiology of inflammatory bowel diseases. Expert Rev Mol Diagn 6:345-363, 2006.
25. Jess T, Gamborg M, Matzen P, et al: Increased risk of intestinal cancer in Crohn's disease: A meta-analysis of population-based cohort studies. Am J Gastroenterol 100:2724-2729, 2005.
26. Stange EF, Travis SP, Vermeire S, et al: European evidence based consensus on the diagnosis and management of Crohn's disease: Definitions and diagnosis. Gut 55(Suppl 1):i1-15, 2006.

27. Van Assche G, Vermeire S, Rutgeerts P: Emerging biological treatments in inflammatory bowel diseases. Dig Dis 24:131-136, 2006.

28. Domenech E: Inflammatory bowel disease: Current therapeutic options. Digestion 73(Suppl 1):67-76, 2006.

29. Gionchetti P, Rizzello F, Lammers KM, et al: Antibiotics and probiotics in treatment of inflammatory bowel disease. World J Gastroenterol 12:3306-3313, 2006.

30. Sandborn WJ: What's new: Innovative concepts in inflammatory bowel disease. Colorectal Dis 8(Suppl 1):3-9, 2006.

31. Hommes DW, Oldenburg B, van Bodegraven AA, et al: Guidelines for treatment with infliximab for Crohn's disease. Neth J Med 64:219-229, 2006.

32. Bratcher JM, Korelitz BI: Toxicity of infliximab in the course of treatment of Crohn's disease. Expert Opin Drug Saf 5:9-16, 2006.

33. Korzenik JR, Podolsky DK: Evolving knowledge and therapy of inflammatory bowel disease. Nat Rev Drug Discov 5:197-209, 2006.

34. O'Sullivan M, O'Morain C: Nutrition in inflammatory bowel disease. Best Pract Res Clin Gastroenterol 20:561-573, 2006.

35. Hancock L, Windsor AC, Mortensen NJ: Inflammatory bowel disease: The view of the surgeon. Colorectal Dis 8(Suppl 1):10-14, 2006.

36. Rutgeerts P: Strategies in the prevention of post-operative recurrence in Crohn's disease. Best Pract Res Clin Gastroenterol 17:63-73, 2003.

37. Blanchard DK, Budde JM, Hatch GF 3rd, et al: Tumors of the small intestine. World J Surg 24:421-429, 2000.

38. Eliakim AR: Video capsule endoscopy of the small bowel (PillCam SB). Curr Opin Gastroenterol 22:124-127, 2006.

39. Berman J, O'Leary TJ: Gastrointestinal stromal tumor workshop. Hum Pathol 32:578-582, 2001.

40. DeMatteo RP: The GIST of targeted cancer therapy: A tumor (gastrointestinal stromal tumor), a mutated gene (c-kit), and a molecular inhibitor (STI571). Ann Surg Oncol 9:831-839, 2002.

41. Jackson LN, Evers BM: Gastrointestinal lymphomas. In Yeo CJ (ed): Shackelford's Surgery of the Alimentary Tract, 6th ed. Philadelphia: Elsevier, 2007, pp 1199-1212.

42. van Oosterom AT, Judson I, Verweij J, et al: Safety and efficacy of imatinib (STI571) in metastatic gastrointestinal stromal tumours: A phase I study. Lancet 358:1421-1423, 2001.

43. Woodside KJ, Townsend CM Jr, Evers BM: Current management of gastrointestinal carcinoid tumors. J Gastrointest Surg 8:742-756, 2004.

44. Soltero MJ, Bill AH: The natural history of Meckel's diverticulum and its relation to incidental removal: A study of 202 cases of diseased Meckel's diverticulum found in King County, Washington, over a fifteen year period. Am J Surg 132:168-173, 1976.

45. Cullen JJ, Kelly KA, Moir CR, et al: Surgical management of Meckel's diverticulum: An epidemiologic, population-based study. Ann Surg 220:564-569, 1994.

46. Evenson AR, Fischer JE: Current management of enterocutaneous fistula. J Gastrointest Surg 10:455-464, 2006.

47. Braumann C, Menenakos C, Jacobi CA: Pneumatosis intestinalis: A pitfall for surgeons? Scand J Surg 94:47-50, 2005.

48. DeCosse JJ, Rhodes RS, Wentz WB, et al: The natural history and management of radiation-induced injury of the gastrointestinal tract. Ann Surg 170:369-384, 1969.

49. Buchman AL: Etiology and initial management of short bowel syndrome. Gastroenterology 130:S5-S15, 2006.

50. Matarese LE, Steiger E: Dietary and medical management of short bowel syndrome in adult patients. J Clin Gastroenterol 40:S85-93, 2006.

51. Tappenden KA: Mechanisms of enteral nutrient-enhanced intestinal adaptation. Gastroenterology 130:S93-99, 2006.

52. Jeppesen PB: Glucagon-like peptide-2: Update of the recent clinical trials. Gastroenterology 130:S127-131, 2006.

53. Scolapio JS: Short bowel syndrome: Recent clinical outcomes with growth hormone. Gastroenterology 130:S122-126, 2006.

54. Byrne, TA, Morrissey TB, Nattakom TV, et al: Growth hormone, glutamine, and a modified diet enhance nutrient absorption in patients with severe short bowel syndrome. JPEN 19:296-302, 1995.

55. Scolapio JS, Camilleri M, Fleming CR, et al: Effect of growth hormone, glutamine, and diet on adaptation in short bowel patients: A randomized, controlled study. Gastroenterology 113:1074-1081, 1997.

56. Seguy D, Vahedi K, Kapel N, et al: Low-dose growth hormone in adult home parenteral nutrition–dependent short bowel patients: A positive study. Gastroenterology 124:293-302, 2003.

57. Bianchi A: From the cradle to enteral autonomy: The role of autologous gastrointestinal reconstruction. Gastroenterology 130:S138-146, 2006.

58. Abu-Elmagd KM: Intestinal transplantation for short bowel syndrome and gastrointestinal failure: Current consensus, rewarding outcomes, and practical guidelines. Gastroenterology 130:S132-137, 2006.

CHAPTER 49

The Appendix

John Maa, MD   and   Kimberly S. Kirkwood, MD

Embryology and Anatomy
Appendicitis
Neoplasms

About 8% of people in Western countries have appendicitis at some time during their life, with a peak incidence between 10 and 30 years of age.[1] Acute appendicitis is the most common general surgical emergency, and early surgical intervention improves outcomes. The diagnosis of appendicitis can be elusive, and a high index of suspicion is important in preventing serious complications from this disease.

EMBRYOLOGY AND ANATOMY

The appendix, ileum, and ascending colon are all derived from the midgut. The appendix first appears at the 8th week of gestation as an outpouching of the cecum and gradually rotates to a more medial location as the gut rotates and the cecum becomes fixed in the right lower quadrant.

The appendiceal artery, a branch of the ileocolic artery, supplies the appendix. Histologic examination of the appendix indicates that goblet cells, which produce mucus, are scattered throughout the mucosa. The submucosa contains lymphoid follicles, leading to speculation that the appendix might have an important, as yet undefined, immune function early in development. The lymphatics drain into the anterior ileocolic lymph nodes. In adults, the appendix has no known function.

The length of the appendix varies from 2 to 20 cm, and the average length is 9 cm in adults. The base of the appendix is located at the convergence of the taeniae along the inferior aspect of the cecum, and this anatomic relationship facilitates identification of the appendix at operation. The tip of the appendix may lie in a variety of locations. The most common location is retrocecal but within the peritoneal cavity. It is pelvic in 30% and retroperitoneal in 7% of the population.[2] The varying location of the tip of the appendix likely explains the myriad of symptoms that are attributable to the inflamed appendix.

APPENDICITIS

Historical Perspective

In 1886, Reginald Fitz of Boston correctly identified the appendix as the primary cause of right lower quadrant inflammation. He coined the term *appendicitis* and recommended early surgical treatment of the disease. Richard Hall reported the first survival of a patient after removal of a perforated appendix, which launched focused attention on the surgical treatment of acute appendicitis. In 1889, Chester McBurney described characteristic migratory pain as well as localization of the pain along an oblique line from the anterior superior iliac spine to the umbilicus. McBurney described a right lower quadrant muscle-splitting incision for removal of the appendix in 1894. The mortality rate from appendicitis improved with the widespread use of broad-spectrum antibiotics in the 1940s. Recent advances have included improved preoperative diagnostic studies, interventional radiologic procedures to drain established periappendiceal abscesses, and the use of laparoscopy to confirm the diagnosis and exclude other causes of abdominal pain. Laparoscopic appendectomy was first reported by the gynecologist Kurt Semm in 1982 but has only gained widespread acceptance in recent years.

Pathophysiology

Obstruction of the lumen is believed to be the major cause of acute appendicitis.[2] This may be due to inspissated stool (fecalith or appendicolith), lymphoid hyperplasia, vegetable matter or seeds, parasites, or a neoplasm. The lumen of the appendix is small in relation to its length, and this configuration may predispose to closed-loop obstruction. Obstruction of the appendiceal lumen contributes to bacterial overgrowth, and continued secretion of mucus leads to intraluminal distention and increased wall pressure. Luminal distention produces the visceral pain sensation experienced by the patient as periumbilical pain. Subsequent impairment of lymphatic and venous drainage leads to mucosal ischemia. These findings in combination promote a localized inflammatory process that may progress to gangrene and perforation. Inflammation of the adjacent peritoneum gives rise to localized pain in the right lower quadrant. Although there is considerable variability, perforation typically occurs after at least 48 hours from the onset of symptoms and is accompanied by an abscess cavity walled-off by the small intestine and omentum. Rarely, free perforation of the appendix into the peritoneal cavity occurs that may be accompanied by peritonitis and septic shock and can be complicated by the subsequent formation of multiple intraperitoneal abscesses.

Bacteriology

The flora in the normal appendix is very similar to that in the colon, with a variety of facultative aerobic and anaerobic bacteria. The polymicrobial nature of perforated appendicitis is well established. *Escherichia coli, Streptococcus viridans,* and *Bacteroides* and *Pseudomonas* species are frequently isolated, and many other organisms may be cultured (Table 49-1). Among patients with acute nonperforated appendicitis, cultures of peritoneal fluid are frequently negative and are of limited use. Among patients with perforated appendicitis, peritoneal fluid cultures are more likely to be positive, revealing colonic bacteria with predictable sensitivities.[3] Because it is rare that the findings alter the selection or duration of antibiotic use, some authors have challenged the traditional practice of obtaining cultures.[3,4]

Diagnosis

History

Appendicitis needs to be considered in the differential diagnosis of nearly every patient with acute abdominal pain. Early diagnosis remains the most important clinical goal in patients with suspected appendicitis and can be made primarily on the basis of the history and physical exam in most cases. The typical presentation begins with periumbilical pain (due to activation of visceral afferent neurons) followed by anorexia and nausea. The pain then localizes to the right lower quadrant as the inflammatory process progresses to involve the parietal peritoneum overlying the appendix. This classic pattern of migratory pain is the most reliable symptom of acute appendicitis.[5] A bout of vomiting may occur, in contrast to the repeated bouts of vomiting that typically accompany viral gastroenteritis or small bowel obstruction. Fever ensues, followed by the development of leukocytosis. These clinical features may vary. For example, not all patients become anorexic. Consequently, the feeling of hunger in an adult patient with suspected appendicitis should not necessarily deter one from surgical intervention. Occasional patients have urinary symptoms or microscopic hematuria, perhaps owing to inflammation of periappendiceal tissues adjacent to the ureter or bladder, and this may be misleading. Although most patients with appendicitis develop an adynamic ileus and absent bowel movements on the day of presentation, occasional patients may have diarrhea. Others may present with small bowel obstruction related to contiguous regional inflammation. Therefore, appendicitis needs to be considered as a possible cause of small bowel obstruction, especially among patients without prior abdominal surgery.

Physical Examination

Patients with acute appendicitis typically look ill and are lying still in bed. Low-grade fever is common (~38°C). Examination of the abdomen usually reveals diminished bowel sounds and focal tenderness with voluntary guarding. The exact location of the tenderness is directly over the appendix, which is most commonly at McBurney's point (located one third of the distance along a line drawn from the anterior superior iliac spine to the umbilicus). The normal appendix is mobile, so it may become inflamed at any point on a 360-degree circle around the base of the cecum. Thus, the site of maximal pain and tenderness can vary. Peritoneal irritation can be elicited on physical examination by the findings of voluntary and involuntary guarding, percussion, or rebound tenderness. Any movement, including coughing (*Dunphy's sign*), may cause increased pain. Other findings may include pain in the right lower quadrant during palpation of the left lower quadrant (*Rovsing's sign*), pain on internal rota-

Table 49-1   Bacteria Commonly Isolated in Perforated Appendicitis

ANAEROBIC	PATIENTS (%)
Bacteroides fragilis	80
Bacteroides thetaiotaomicron	61
Bilophila wadsworthia	55
Peptostreptococcus species	46
AEROBIC	
Escherichia coli	77
Streptococcus viridans	43
Group D streptococcus	27
Pseudomonas aeruginosa	18

Adapted from Bennion RS, Thompson JE: Appendicitis. In Fry DE (ed): Surgical Infections. Boston, Little, Brown, 1995, pp 241-250.

tion of the hip (*obturator sign,* suggesting a pelvic appendix), and pain on extension of the right hip (*iliopsoas sign,* typical of a retrocecal appendix).

Rectal and pelvic examinations are most likely to be negative. However, if the appendix is located within the pelvis, tenderness on abdominal examination may be minimal, whereas anterior tenderness may be elicited during rectal examination as the pelvic peritoneum is manipulated. Pelvic examination with cervical motion may also produce tenderness in this setting.

If the appendix perforates, abdominal pain becomes intense and more diffuse, and abdominal muscular spasm increases, producing rigidity. The heart rate rises, with an elevation of temperature above 39°C. The patient may appear ill and require a brief period of fluid resuscitation and antibiotics before the induction of anesthesia. Occasionally, pain may improve somewhat after rupture of the appendix, although a true pain-free interval is uncommon.

Laboratory Studies

The white blood cell count is elevated with more than 75% neutrophils in most patients. A completely normal leukocyte count and differential is found in about 10% of patients with acute appendicitis. A high white blood cell count (>20,000/mL) suggests complicated appendicitis with either gangrene or perforation. A urinalysis can also be helpful in excluding pyelonephritis or nephrolithiasis. Minimal pyuria, frequently seen in elderly women, does not exclude appendicitis from the differential diagnosis because the ureter may be irritated adjacent to the inflamed appendix. Although microscopic hematuria is common in appendicitis, gross hematuria is uncommon and may indicate the presence of a kidney stone. Other blood tests are generally not helpful and are not indicated in the patient with suspected appendicitis.

Radiography

Although they are commonly obtained, the indiscriminate use of *plain abdominal radiographs* in the evaluation of patients with acute abdominal pain is unwarranted. In one study of 104 patients with acute onset of right lower quadrant pain, interpretation of plain x-rays changed the management of only 6 patients (6%), and in one case contributed to an unnecessary laparotomy.[6] A calcified appendicolith is visible on plain films in only 10% to 15% of patients with acute appendicitis; however, its presence strongly supports the diagnosis in a patient with abdominal pain. Plain abdominal films may be useful for the detection of ureteral calculi, small bowel obstruction, or perforated ulcer, but such conditions are rarely confused with appendicitis. Failure of the appendix to fill during a *barium enema* has been associated with appendicitis, but this finding lacks both sensitivity and specificity because up to 20% of normal appendices do not fill.

Among patients with abdominal pain, *ultrasonography* has a sensitivity of about 85% and a specificity of more than 90% for the diagnosis of acute appendicitis. Sonographic findings consistent with acute appendicitis include an appendix of 7 mm or more in anteroposterior diameter, a thick-walled, noncompressible luminal structure

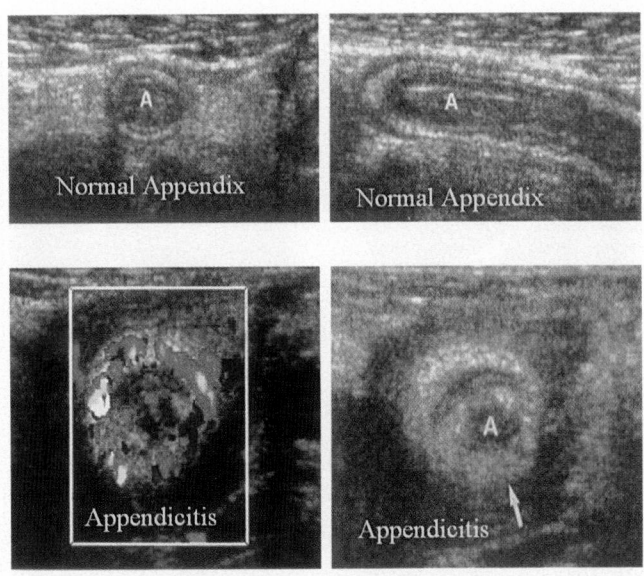

Figure 49-1 Ultrasound of a normal appendix (**top**) illustrating the thin wall in both coronal (*left*) and longitudinal (*right*) planes. In appendicitis, there is distention and wall thickening (**bottom,** *right*), and blood flow is increased, leading to the so-called ring-of-fire appearance. A, appendix.

seen in cross section referred to as a *target lesion,* or the presence of an appendicolith (Fig. 49-1). In more advanced cases, periappendiceal fluid or a mass may be found. Ultrasonography has the advantages of being a noninvasive modality requiring no patient preparation that also avoids exposure to ionizing radiation. For these reasons, it is commonly used in children and in pregnant patients with equivocal clinical findings suggestive of acute appendicitis. Disadvantages of ultrasonography include operator-dependent accuracy and difficulty interpreting the images by those other than the operator. Because performance of the study may require hands-on participation by the radiologist, ultrasonography may not be readily available at night or on weekends. *Pelvic ultrasound* can be especially useful in excluding pelvic pathology, such as tubo-ovarian abscess or ovarian torsion, that may mimic acute appendicitis.

Computed tomography (CT) is commonly used in the evaluation of adult patients with suspected acute appendicitis. Improved imaging techniques, including the use of 5-mm sections, have resulted in increased accuracy of CT scanning,[7] which has a sensitivity of about 90% and a specificity of 80% to 90% for the diagnosis of acute appendicitis among patients with abdominal pain. Controversy remains as to the importance of intravenous, oral gastrointestinal, and rectal contrast in improving diagnostic accuracy. In general, CT findings of appendicitis increase with the severity of the disease. Classic findings include a distended appendix greater than 7 mm in diameter and circumferential wall thickening, which may give the appearance of a halo or target (Fig. 49-2). As inflammation progresses, one may see periappendiceal fat stranding, edema, peritoneal fluid, phlegmon, or a periappendiceal abscess. CT detects appendicoliths in about

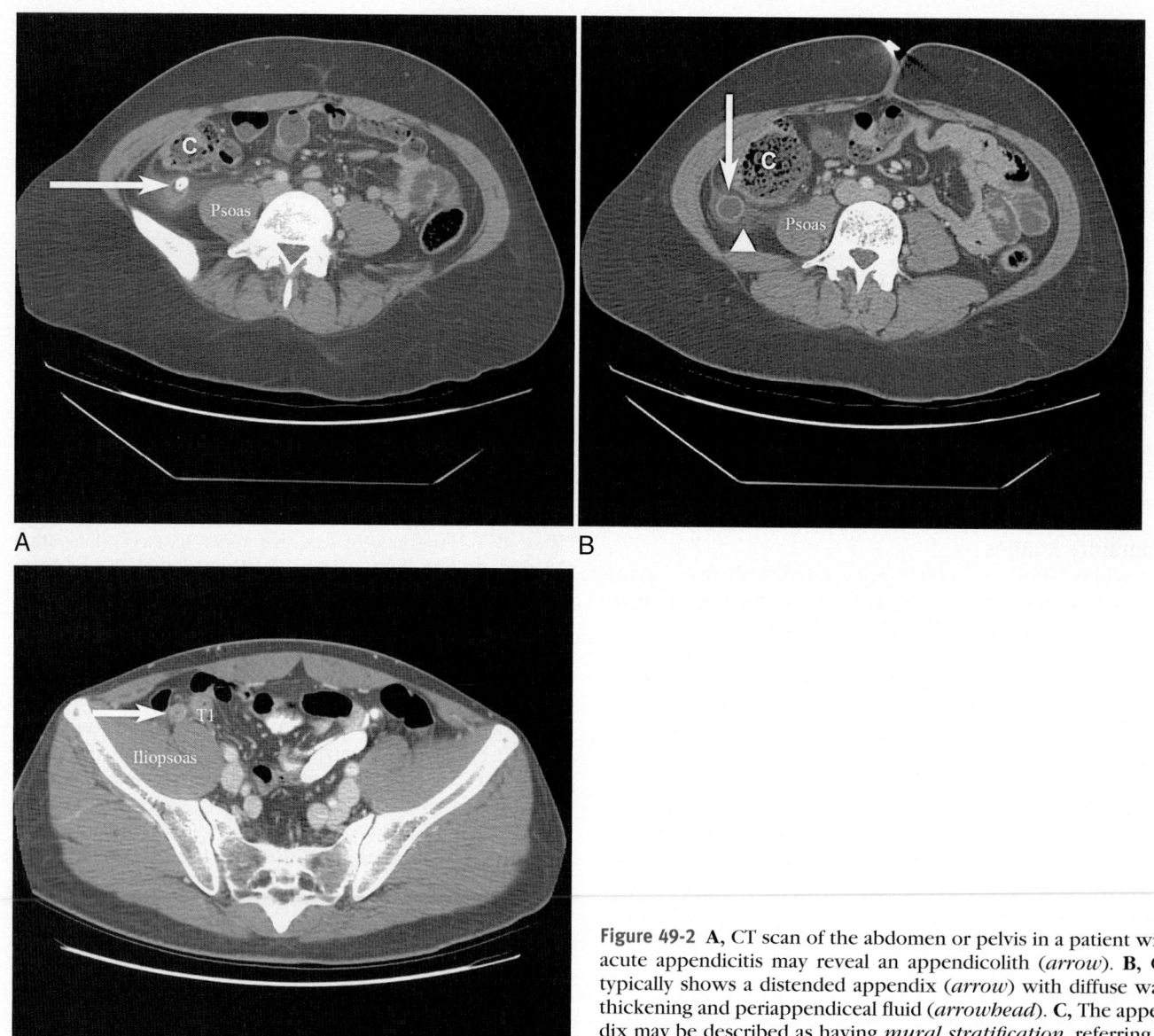

A

B

C

Figure 49-2 A, CT scan of the abdomen or pelvis in a patient with acute appendicitis may reveal an appendicolith (*arrow*). **B,** CT typically shows a distended appendix (*arrow*) with diffuse wall-thickening and periappendiceal fluid (*arrowhead*). **C,** The appendix may be described as having *mural stratification,* referring to the layers of enhancement and edema within the wall *(arrow),* and this may also be referred to as a *target sign.* C, cecum; TI, terminal ileum.

50% of patients with appendicitis and also in a small percentage of people without appendicitis. Among patients with abdominal pain, the positive predictive value of the finding of an appendicolith on CT remains high at about 75%.

Should CT be used *routinely* in the diagnostic evaluation of patients with suspected appendicitis? In our opinion, no. In the setting of typical right lower quadrant pain and tenderness with signs of inflammation in a young patient, a CT scan is unnecessary, wastes valuable time, and exposes the patient to the risks for allergic contrast reaction, nephropathy, aspiration pneumonitis, and ionizing radiation. The latter carries increased risk in children in whom the rate of radiation-induced cancer has been estimated at 0.18% following an abdominal CT scan.[8] Moreover, a negative study may be misleading,

particularly early in the inflammatory process. CT has proved most valuable among older patients in whom the differential diagnosis is lengthy, the clinical findings may be confusing, and appendectomy carries increased risk.[9,10] Among patients with atypical symptoms, CT scan may reduce the negative appendectomy rate (i.e., the fraction of pathologically normal appendices that are removed). Selective use of CT scans seems most appropriate, and as always, the study needs to be obtained only in settings in which it has a significant potential to alter management.

The morbidity of perforated appendicitis far exceeds that of a negative appendectomy. Thus, the strategy has been to set a low enough threshold for removal of the appendix so as to minimize the cases of missed appendicitis. With increased use of CT scans, the frequency of negative explorations has declined in recent years without an accompanying rise in the number of perforations. A recent analysis of more than 75,000 patients in 1999 to 2000 revealed a negative appendectomy rate of 6% in men and 13.4% in women.[9]

Diagnostic Laparoscopy

Although most patients with appendicitis will be accurately diagnosed based on history, physical exam, laboratory studies, and if necessary, imaging techniques, there are a small number in whom the diagnosis remains elusive. For these patients, diagnostic laparoscopy can provide both a direct examination of the appendix and a survey of the abdominal cavity for other possible causes of pain. We use this technique primarily for women of childbearing age in whom preoperative pelvic ultrasound or CT scan fails to provide a diagnosis. Concerns about the possible adverse effects of a missed perforation and peritonitis on future fertility sometimes prompt earlier intervention in this patient population.

Differential Diagnoses

The differential diagnosis of appendicitis can include almost all causes of abdominal pain, as described in the classic treatise "Cope's Early Diagnosis of the Acute Abdomen."[11] A useful rule is never to place appendicitis lower than second in the differential diagnosis of acute abdominal pain in a previously healthy person. The diagnosis of appendicitis is particularly difficult in the very young and in the elderly. It is in these groups that diagnosis is most often delayed and perforation occurs most frequently. Imaging studies are strongly considered here. Because of increasing concerns about radiation-induced cancers among children,[8] ultrasonography is the preferred initial imaging modality in this group. Ultrasonography was shown to change the disposition of 59% of children with abdominal pain that had already been evaluated by the surgical team.[12] For older patients, CT has the advantages of detection of the broader array of conditions, such as diverticulitis and malignancy, found in the differential diagnosis.

In *infants*, nonfocal findings such as lethargy, irritability, and anorexia may be present in the early stages, with vomiting, fever, and pain apparent as the disease progresses. Ultrasound is useful in the evaluation of appendicitis and other acute abdominal emergencies, such as pyloric stenosis, in infants.

In *preschool-aged children*, the differential diagnosis includes intussusception, Meckel's diverticulitis, and acute gastroenteritis. Intussusception may be distinguished by the colicky nature of the pain, with intervening pain-free periods, and the absence of peritonitis. Meckel's diverticulitis is relatively uncommon, but its presentation is similar to that of appendicitis with the exception that the pain and tenderness typically localize in the periumbilical region. Gastroenteritis can be difficult to distinguish from acute appendicitis in any age group. Typically, diarrhea and vomiting occur early and persistently in gastroenteritis, and focal abdominal tenderness and peritoneal signs are uncommon. However, it is advisable to discuss with parents of a child suspected of having gastroenteritis the importance of re-evaluation within 12 to 24 hours if the child develops worsening abdominal pain, or other signs of clinical deterioration, because misdiagnosed appendicitis remains high on the list of considerations.

In *school-aged children*, gastroenteritis often presents with abdominal pain and diarrhea without fever or leukocytosis. The most common mimicker of appendicitis in this population is mesenteric lymphadenitis, which may be caused by a wide variety of enteric infections.[13] Ultrasonography may be helpful in identifying enlarged lymph nodes in the region of the ileal mesentery in conjunction with thickening of the ileal wall and a normal appendix, in which case appendectomy may be avoided. It is important to bear in mind that enlarged mesenteric lymph nodes may also be the result of acute appendicitis. Inflammatory bowel disease is also considered in children, particularly if there is a history of recurrent episodes of abdominal pain. Constipation and functional pain are common in this age group. Although constipation may be associated with relatively severe pain, there are no peritoneal signs, fever, or leukocytosis, and the diagnosis is supported by a recent history of hard stools. Functional pain is usually somewhat milder, recurrent, and self-limited.

In *adults*, it is important to consider other regional inflammatory conditions, such as pyelonephritis, colitis, and diverticulitis. The pain and tenderness of pyelonephritis are typically located in the flank and are accompanied by high fever and white blood cell count as well as pyuria. Colitis is often accompanied by diarrhea, and the location of the pain typically outlines the trajectory of the colon. In Crohn's colitis, diarrhea is uncommon, but there is often a pattern of recurrent symptoms. The onset of right-sided diverticulitis is typically insidious, worsening over a period of days, and involves a larger area of the right lower abdomen than does appendicitis. CT scan is helpful in identifying the inflamed diverticula and enhancement of cecal wall thickening that accompanies this diagnosis.

The differential diagnosis for appendicitis among *women* in their childbearing years is broad and accounts for the higher incidence of false-positive diagnoses in this group. Pelvic pathology that may mimic acute appendicitis includes pelvic inflammatory disease (PID), tubo-ovarian abscess, ruptured ovarian cyst or ovarian torsion, and ectopic pregnancy, among others.[14] These conditions are typically distinguished from acute appendicitis by the absence of gastrointestinal symptoms. *Pelvic ultrasound* is especially helpful in these patients because of its high sensitivity and specificity for the diagnosis of pelvic pathology. If a normal appendix is also seen, appendicitis is unlikely.

Appendicitis is the most common nonobstetric surgical disease of the abdomen during *pregnancy*. Diagnosis may be difficult because symptoms of nausea, vomiting, and anorexia, as well as elevated white blood cell count, are common during pregnancy. Moreover, the location of tenderness varies with gestation. After the 5th month of gestation, the appendix is shifted superiorly above the iliac crest, and the appendiceal tip is rotated medially

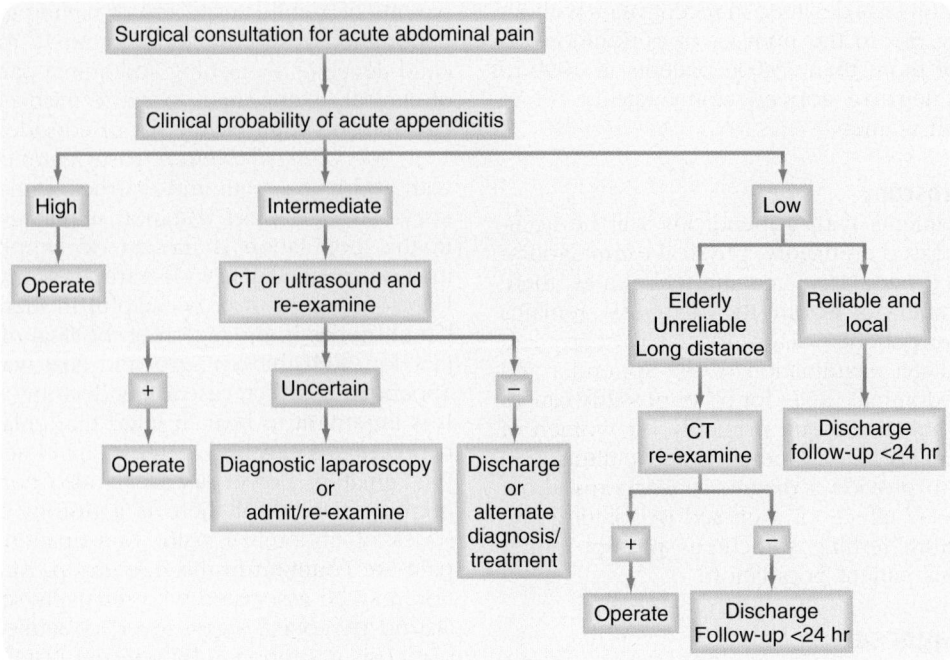

Figure 49-3 Algorithm for the evaluation and management of patients with possible acute appendicitis based on surgical assessment of clinical probability of the diagnosis.

into the right upper quadrant by the gravid uterus. Ultrasound is helpful both in establishing the diagnosis and the location of the inflamed appendix. In cases in which ultrasound has been equivocal, magnetic resonance imaging (MRI) has been used successfully, thereby avoiding ionizing radiation exposure to the developing fetus. The main challenge is to recognize the possibility of appendicitis in pregnant patients and intervene promptly because peritonitis significantly increases the rate of fetal loss (2.6%-10.9% in one meta-analysis).[15] Laparoscopic appendectomy has been performed through the second trimester of pregnancy, although data are lacking comparing the safety of this approach to the open procedure.

Appendicitis in the *elderly* can be difficult to diagnose because many patients delay in seeking care and present atypically. Fever is uncommon, the white blood cell count may be normal, and many older patients with appendicitis do not experience right lower quadrant pain. About one half of older patients are incorrectly diagnosed at the time of admission, and these patients have a much higher rate of perforation at the time of surgery because of delays in operative intervention.[10] More than 50% of older patients have perforated appendicitis, compared with less than 20% for younger patients. Diverticulitis and bowel obstruction are common misdiagnoses in this patient population, and the differential diagnosis also includes malignancies of the gastrointestinal tract and reproductive system, perforated ulcers, and cholecystitis, among others. CT has become an invaluable tool in the evaluation of abdominal pain among older patients, and its use has shortened preoperative hospital delays.[10]

Diagnostic Algorithm

Patients in whom the diagnosis of appendicitis is being considered should have a surgical evaluation (Fig. 49-3). Early involvement of the surgical team in the diagnostic evaluation of these patients may improve diagnostic accuracy and help to avoid expensive and unnecessary diagnostic studies.[16] Experienced clinicians accurately diagnose appendicitis based on a combination of history, physical exam, and laboratory studies about 80% of the time. We stratify patients based on their clinical findings starting with the extremes, which are easier to identify. Patients with a *high* probability of uncomplicated appendicitis undergo surgery. Patients suspected of having an appendiceal abscess undergo further imaging, typically ultrasonography for children or CT for adults. The next step in the evaluation of patients in whom the likelihood of appendicitis is believed to be *low* is determined by the probability and severity of alternate diagnoses under consideration. Many of these patients will be discharged with a planned follow-up visit or phone call the next day. Most older patients with abdominal pain undergo CT before discharge because of the high prevalence of surgical pathology in this patient population. The remaining patients are believed to have an *intermediate* probability of having appendicitis. Children and pregnant women in this category typically undergo abdominal ultrasonography. Women in their childbearing years may undergo pelvic ultrasonography or CT scan depending on the index of suspicion of pelvic pathology. Among patients that would otherwise be admitted to the hospital for observation, CT may reduce hospital costs by reducing length of stay. Following the completion of imaging

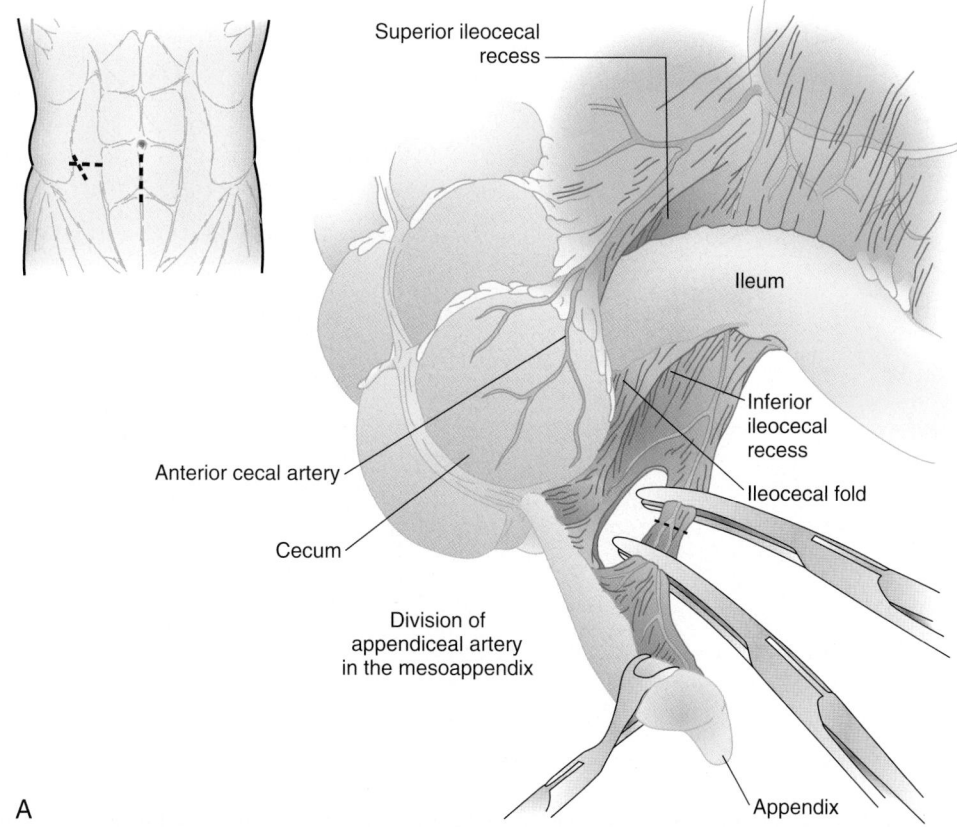

Superior ileocecal recess

Ileum

Inferior ileocecal recess

Ileocecal fold

Anterior cecal artery

Cecum

Division of appendiceal artery in the mesoappendix

Appendix

A

Figure 49-4 A, *Left,* Location of possible incisions for an open appendectomy. *Right,* Division of the mesoappendix.

Continued

studies, the patient is re-examined to determine whether pain and tenderness have localized to the right lower quadrant. If the diagnosis remains uncertain at this point, patients either undergo diagnostic laparoscopy, especially in fertile women, are admitted for observation and re-examination, or are discharged with follow-up the next day.

Treatment

Most patients with acute appendicitis are managed by prompt surgical removal of the appendix. A brief period of resuscitation is usually sufficient to ensure the safe induction of general anesthesia. Preoperative antibiotics cover aerobic and anaerobic colonic flora. For patients with nonperforated appendicitis, a single preoperative dose of antibiotics reduces postoperative wound infections and intra-abdominal abscess formation.[17] Postoperative oral antibiotics do not further reduce the incidence of infectious complications in these patients.[18] For patients with perforated or gangrenous appendicitis, we continue postoperative intravenous antibiotics until the patient is afebrile.[19,20]

Several prospective randomized studies have compared laparoscopic and open appendectomy, and the overall differences in outcomes remain small. The percentage of appendectomies performed laparoscopically

continues to increase.[21] Obese patients had less pain and shorter hospital stays after laparoscopic versus open appendectomy.[22] Patients with perforated appendicitis had lower rates of wound infections following laparoscopic removal of the appendix.[23,24] Patients treated laparoscopically had improved quality-of-life scores 2 weeks after surgery[25] and lower readmission rates.[21] As compared with open appendectomy, the laparoscopic approach involves higher operating room costs, but these have been counterbalanced in some series by shorter lengths of stay.[21] For patients in whom the diagnosis remains uncertain after the preoperative evaluation, diagnostic laparoscopy is useful because it allows the surgeon to examine the remainder of the abdomen, including the pelvis, for abnormalities. Our practice is to perform appendectomies laparoscopically in fertile women, obese patients, and cases of diagnostic uncertainty; otherwise, the approach is determined by patient or surgeon preference.

Open appendectomy is usually easily performed through a transverse right lower quadrant incision (Davis-Rockey) or an oblique incision (McArthur-McBurney) (Fig. 49-4, inset). In cases with a large phlegmon or diagnostic uncertainty, a subumbilical midline incision may be used. For uncomplicated cases we prefer a transverse, muscle-splitting incision lateral to the rectus abdominis muscle over McBurney's point. Local anes-

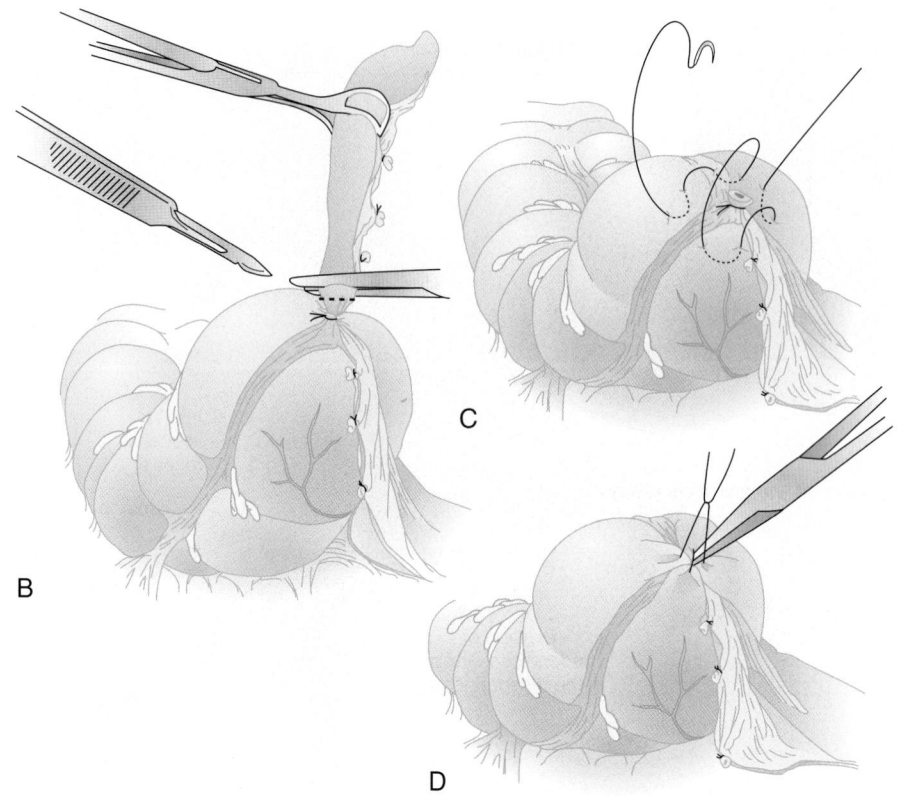

Figure 49-4, cont'd B, Ligation of the base and division of the appendix. **C,** Placement of purse-string suture or **Z** stitch. **D,** Inversion of the appendiceal stump. (From Ortega JM, Ricardo AE: Surgery of the appendix and colon. In Moody FG [ed]: Atlas of Ambulatory Surgery. Philadelphia, WB Saunders, 1999.)

thetic, administered before the incision, reduces post-operative pain.[26] After the peritoneum is entered, the inflamed appendix is identified by its firm consistency and delivered into the field. Particular attention is paid to gentle handling of the inflamed tissues to minimize the risk for rupture during the procedure. In difficult cases, enlarging the incision and working down the trajectory of the taeniae on the cecum will often facilitate localization and delivery of the appendix. The meso-appendix is divided between clamps and ties (see Fig. 49-4A). The base of the appendix is skeletonized at its junction with the cecum. A heavy absorbable tie is placed around the base of the appendix, and the specimen is clamped and divided (see Fig. 49-4B). An absorbable purse-string suture or Z stitch is placed into the cecal wall (see Fig. 49-4C), and the appendiceal stump is inverted into a fold in the wall of the cecum (see Fig. 49-4D). Simple ligation and inversion probably have equivalent outcomes. If the base of the appendix and adjacent cecum are extensively indurated, an ileocecal resection is performed. The wound is closed primarily in most cases because the wound infection rate is less than 5%.

Laparoscopic appendectomy offers the advantage of diagnostic laparoscopy combined with the potential for shorter recovery and incisions that are less conspicuous. If a CT scan was obtained preoperatively, it needs to be reviewed by the surgeon for useful information regarding the position of the appendix relative to the cecum. After injection of local anesthetic, we place a 10-mm port into the umbilicus, followed by a 5-mm port in the suprapubic midline region and a 5-mm port midway between the first 2 ports and to the left of the rectus abdominis muscle (Fig. 49-5, inset). The 5-mm, 30-degree scope is moved to the central port with the surgeon and assistant both on the patient's left. With the patient in Trendelenburg's position and rotated left-side down, we gently sweep the terminal ileum medially and follow the taeniae of the cecum caudad to locate the appendix, which is then elevated. The mesoappendix is divided using a 5-mm harmonic scalpel or Liga-Sure, or between clips, depending on the thickness of this tissue (see Fig. 49-5A). We typically encircle the appendix with two heavy absorbable Endoloops cinched down at the base of the appendix and then place a third Endoloop about 1 cm distally and divide the appendix (see Fig. 49-5B and C). In cases in which the base is indurated and friable, we use a 30-mm endoscopic stapler to divide the appendix. For most cases, however, the considerable added cost of the stapler is unwarranted. Any spillage of fluid is promptly aspirated, and similarly any identified appendicoliths are removed to prevent postoperative abscess formation. The appendix is placed into a specimen bag and removed with the port through the umbilical wound (see Fig. 49-5D). Fascia at the 10-mm trocar site is closed, and all wounds are closed primarily.

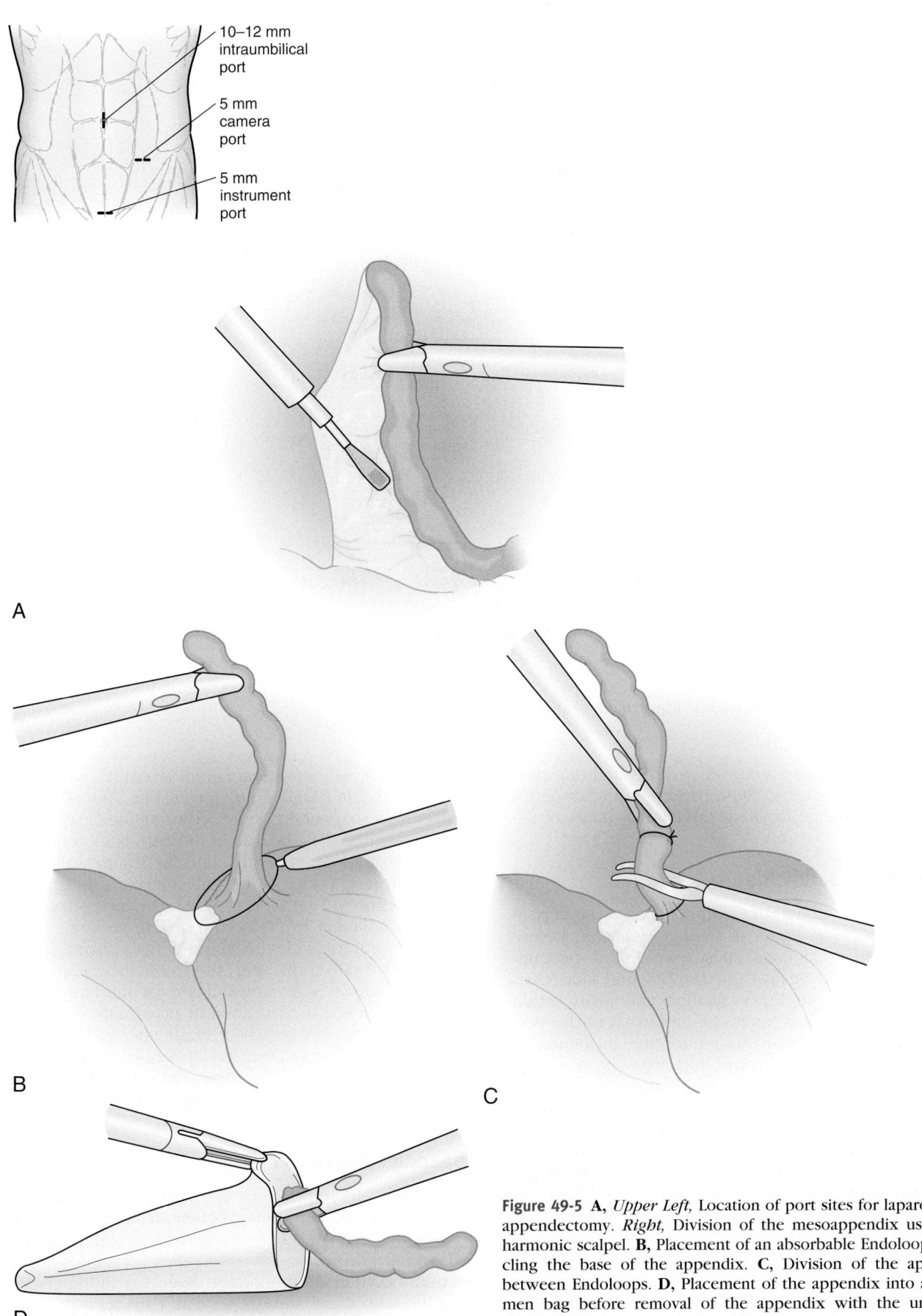

Figure 49-5 A, *Upper Left,* Location of port sites for laparoscopic appendectomy. *Right,* Division of the mesoappendix using the harmonic scalpel. **B,** Placement of an absorbable Endoloop encircling the base of the appendix. **C,** Division of the appendix between Endoloops. **D,** Placement of the appendix into a specimen bag before removal of the appendix with the umbilical port.

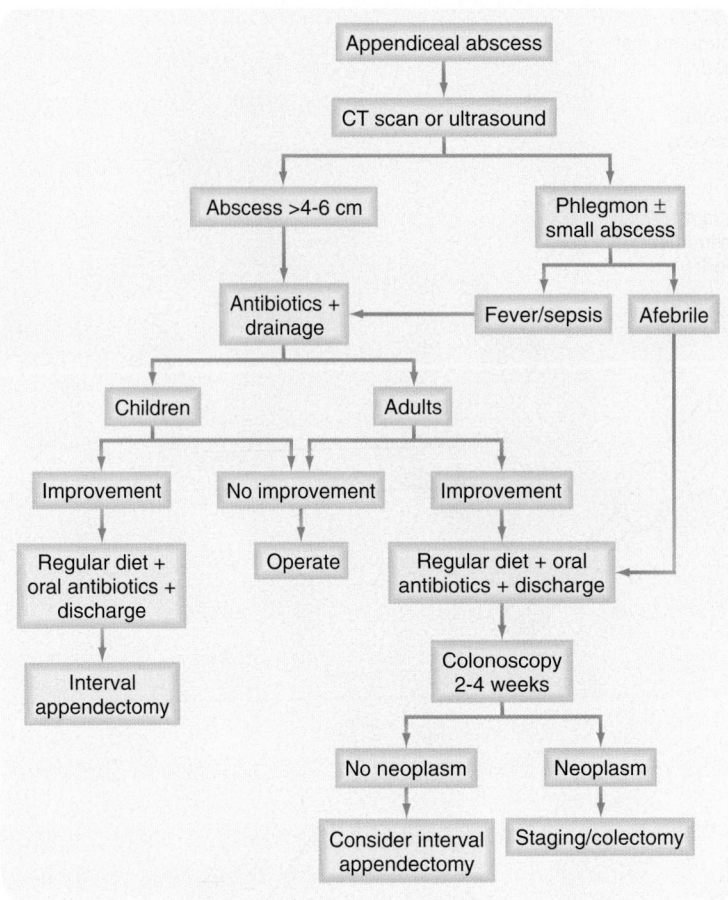

Figure 49-6 Algorithm for the management of appendiceal abscess.

Patients are offered an unrestricted diet and oral pain medication after surgery. Most patients with nonperforated appendicitis are discharged within 24 hours of the procedure.

Perforated Appendicitis

Patients with perforation of the appendix may be very ill and require several hours of fluid resuscitation before safe induction of general anesthesia. Broad-spectrum antibiotics directed against gut aerobes and anaerobes are initiated early in the evaluation and resuscitation phase. In children, a laparoscopic approach to the perforated appendix appears to reduce the incidence of postoperative wound infections and ileus and is associated with shorter hospital stays and lower costs.[27] Recent studies in adults suggest that patients successfully treated laparoscopically realize similar benefits, albeit with a higher risk for conversion to an open procedure than for patients with simple appendicitis.[28,29] We usually begin with a diagnostic laparoscopy and use a rolled gauze to gently sweep adherent loops of small bowel away from the cecum, thereby exposing the appendix. Depending on the ease of completing that task, a decision is made whether or not to convert to an open appendectomy. Any pus encountered during the dissection is aspirated and sent for Gram stain and culture. Oozing from the

severely inflamed retroperitoneum is easily controlled with argon beam coagulation, if available. The inflamed, indurated mesoappendix is divided using the LigaSure or harmonic scalpel. The taeniae of the cecum are followed onto the base of the appendix, and the stump is divided either between Endoloops or with a stapler, depending on the integrity of the tissues. When the mesoappendix is densely adherent to the cecum or retroperitoneum, it may be helpful to divide the stump of the appendix with the stapler before dividing the mesoappendix. The abdomen and pelvis are irrigated and the fluid aspirated. We leave a closed-suction drain in place only if a well-defined residual abscess cavity exists after reflection of the small bowel away from the appendiceal bed. Antibiotics may be altered, if necessary, based on the culture results and are continued until the patient is afebrile postoperatively.

Appendiceal Abscess

Patients who present late in the course of appendicitis with a mass and fever may benefit from a period of nonoperative management, which reduces complications and overall hospital stay[30,31] (Fig. 49-6). Imaging studies are useful both in confirming the diagnosis and in evaluating the size of any abscess present. Patients with large abscesses, greater than 4 to 6 cm in size, and especially those patients with abscess and high fever, benefit from abscess drainage. This may be accomplished via the transrectal or transvaginal route using ultrasound guidance if the abscess is suitably located,[32] or by a percutaneous image-guided approach. Those patients with smaller abscesses or phlegmon and who are not sick may be successfully managed initially with antibiotics alone. Patients who continue to have fever and leukocytosis after several days of nonoperative treatment are likely to require appendectomy during the same hospitalization, whereas those who improve promptly may be considered for interval appendectomy.[33]

After nonoperative treatment of suspected late appendicitis, adults undergo *colonoscopy* or barium enema because colon cancer is detected in about 5% of cases.[34] The risk for *recurrent appendicitis* is about 15% to 25% after nonoperative treatment and warrants consideration of *interval appendectomy*. We typically perform this procedure laparoscopically about 6 weeks after the initial bout of appendicitis. Interval appendectomy is associated with low morbidity and a short hospital stay. The procedure is routinely performed in children. The decision about whether to proceed with interval appendectomy for adult patients includes factors such as patient age, comorbid conditions, and prior abdominal surgery.

Chronic or Recurrent Appendicitis

A small number of patients report episodic bouts of right lower abdominal pain in the absence of an acute febrile illness. Some are found to have appendicoliths on CT[35] or sonographic evidence of an enlarged appendiceal diameter[36]; most of these will have both surgical and pathologic evidence of chronic inflammation of the appendix and relief of symptoms after appendectomy. These findings support the notion that appendicitis represents a spectrum of inflammatory changes that may, in rare cases, wax and wane.

The dilemma is more difficult when the report of pain is not accompanied by other clinical or radiographic findings. These patients fall into the category of those with chronic abdominal pain, and pathologically confirmed appendiceal inflammation is rarely found in these patients. We have sought evidence of appendiceal pathology before appendectomy for chronic pain using ultrasound, CT, or both, in combination with colonoscopy to exclude other causes of pain.

Normal-Appearing Appendix

If a normal-appearing appendix is identified at the time of surgery, should it be removed? This question has been raised again after the introduction of the laparoscopic approach; consensus is lacking on this point. Although it is difficult to know how many patients benefit from this practice, removal of the appendix adds little morbidity to the procedure. In some cases, pathologic abnormalities that were not apparent on visual inspection are identified.[37-39] Our practice is to remove the appendix and perform a thorough search for other causes of the patient's symptoms. We specifically examine the small intestine for Meckel's diverticulum and Crohn's disease, the mesentery

for lymphadenopathy, and the pelvis for abscesses, ovarian torsion, and hernias.

Appendicitis in Elderly Patients

Older patients with appendicitis are more likely to delay seeking treatment, present with atypical findings, and have a higher rate of perforation at the time of presentation (see Differential Diagnoses, earlier). CT is widely used in older patients both to establish the diagnosis of appendicitis and to exclude neoplasms, diverticulitis, and other confounding conditions. Perforation and abscess formation are relatively common operative findings among older patients with appendicitis.[40] Elderly people have an increased incidence of cardiovascular, renal, and pulmonary complications after appendectomy. Analysis of a large administrative database showed that the laparoscopic approach was associated with a shorter hospitalization and a higher probability of discharge to home (rather than a skilled nursing facility) than open appendectomy for older patients with both perforated and nonperforated appendicitis.[41] Following risk adjustment among groups, the benefits of laparoscopic appendectomy appear to be more pronounced for older patients than for their younger counterparts.[42]

Treatment Algorithm

Our approach to the treatment of appendicitis is summarized in Figure 49-7. Patients are considered to have so-called simple appendicitis if the duration of symptoms is less than 48 hours or imaging studies show the absence of a large abscess or phlegmon. These patients typically undergo appendectomy. For patients with an atypical or long history and those who present during the recovery phase, imaging studies are obtained. CT is typically selected for nonpregnant adults and ultrasound for pregnant women and children. Occasionally, these patients are found to have radiographic features of simple appendicitis and undergo appendectomy. More commonly, a phlegmon is found. An associated large abscess (>4-6 cm) is drained either percutaneously, if it is located in the iliac fossa, or transrectally, if it is in the lower pelvis. Patients who are systemically ill are treated with antibiotics and bowel rest and re-evaluated. If they do not improve, we perform an open appendectomy. Similarly, sick patients with a phlegmon or a small abscess are treated with antibiotics and bowel rest and re-evaluated for signs of improvement as described earlier. Some patients present during the recovery phase from the acute illness and may be managed as outpatients. Adults who are managed nonoperatively during their initial presentation undergo colonoscopy 2 to 4 weeks after their acute illness to exclude colitis or neoplasms. We typically remove the appendix in these patients 6 to 8 weeks after the initial presentation. The procedure is performed laparoscopically as an outpatient.

Outcomes

The mortality rate after appendectomy is less than 1%. The morbidity of perforated appendicitis is higher than

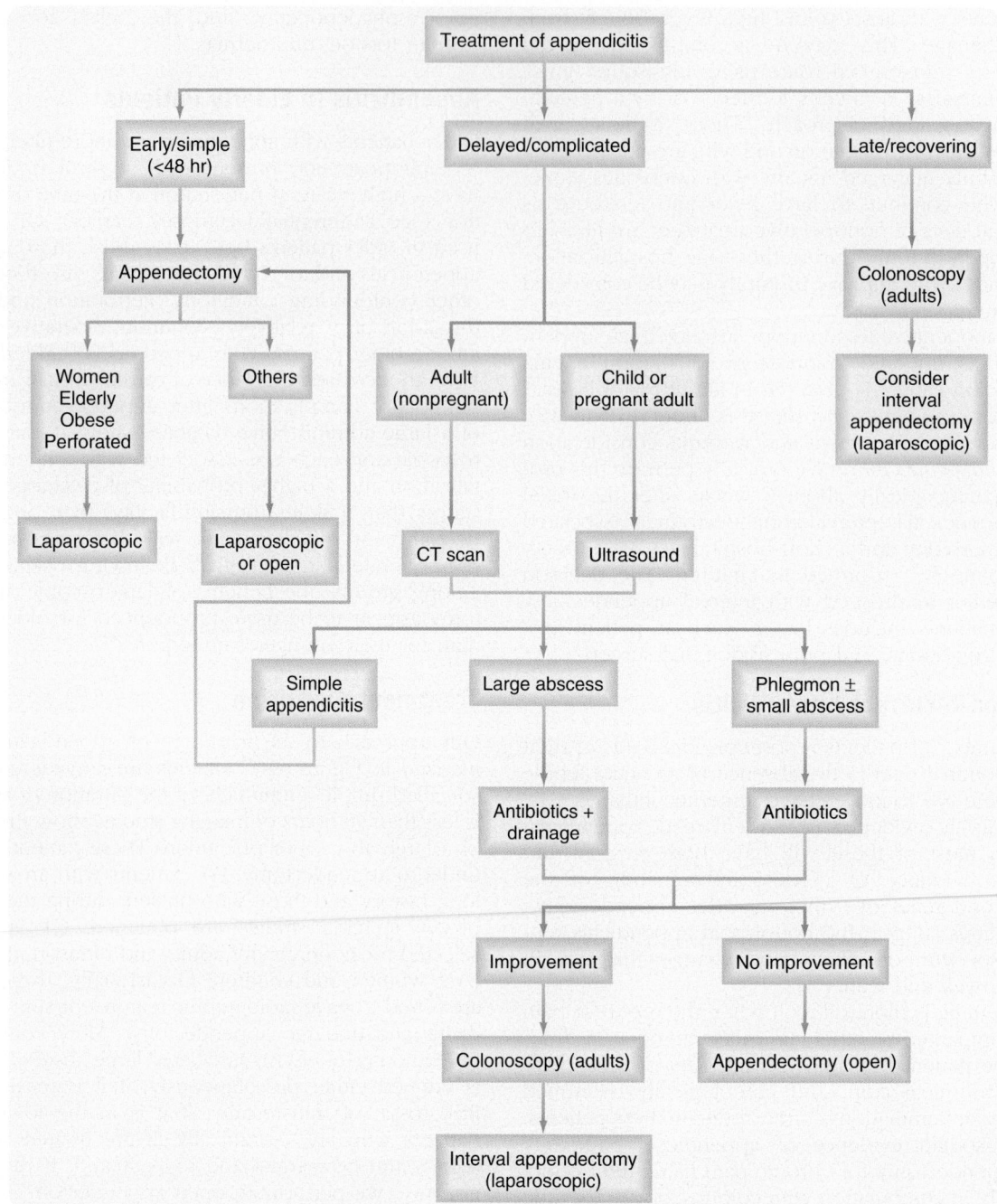

Figure 49-7 Algorithm summarizing the treatment of acute appendicitis.

that of nonperforated cases and is related to increased rates of wound infection, intra-abdominal abscess formation, increased hospital stay, and delayed return to full activity.

Surgical site infections are the most common complications seen after appendectomy. About 5% of patients with uncomplicated appendicitis develop wound infections after open appendectomy. Laparoscopic appendectomy is associated with a lower incidence of wound infections; this difference is magnified among groups of patients with perforated appendicitis (14% versus 26%).[43] Patients with a fever and leukocytosis and a normal-

appearing wound after appendectomy undergo CT or ultrasonography to exclude an intra-abdominal abscess. Similarly, if pus emanates from a fascial opening during wound inspection, an imaging study is obtained to identify any undrained intra-abdominal fluid collections. In this situation, we place a percutaneous drain into the collection to divert the infected material away from the fascia and facilitate wound healing. For pelvic abscesses that are located in proximity to the rectum or vagina, we prefer ultrasound-guided transrectal or transvaginal drainage, thereby avoiding the discomfort of a percutaneous perineal drain.[32]

Small bowel obstruction occurs in less than 1% of patients after appendectomy for uncomplicated appendicitis and in 3% of patients with perforated appendicitis who are followed for 30 years.[44] About one half of these patients present with bowel obstruction during the first year.

The risk for *infertility* following appendectomy in childhood appears to be small.[45] A history of either simple or perforated appendicitis was sought in a large cohort of infertile patients and compared with the frequency of appendicitis in pregnant women; no significant differences were found.[46]

There are rare reports of appendicocutaneous or appendicovesical *fistulas* after appendectomy, typically for perforated appendicitis. Fistulas to the skin generally close after any local infection is treated. Fistulas to the bladder have been successfully diagnosed and treated laparoscopically in recent years.

NEOPLASMS

Primary tumors of the appendix are rare. They are usually diagnosed after pathologic inspection of the appendix removed for suspected appendicitis. Although it was previously believed that carcinoid tumors were the most common appendiceal neoplasms, analysis of the Surveillance, Epidemiology, and End Results (SEER) database indicates that mucinous tumors of the appendix are more common.[9]

Appendiceal *carcinoids* are neuroendocrine tumors that are usually of the enterochromaffin cell type. They frequently contain sustentacular cells that express S-100.[47] Although they are classified as malignancies, most appendiceal carcinoids exhibit benign behavior patterns. These tumors tend to occur in patients in their 40s, and most are localized to the appendix at the time of presentation.[9] For lesions smaller than 1 cm that are located in the tip of the appendix, appendectomy is curative nearly 100% of the time.[9] Appendiceal carcinoids that are larger than 1 to 2 cm, involve the base of the appendix, or invade the mesoappendix, may exhibit a more aggressive biologic behavior and warrant consideration of right hemicolectomy. A large population-based study showed that goblet cell histology was associated with a particularly poor prognosis among carcinoids.[48] As with other neuroendocrine tumors, patients with appendiceal carcinoids may present with second primary tumors, especially of the gastrointestinal and genitourinary tracts, and this likelihood was recently estimated at 18.2%.[49] Thus, these patients undergo colonoscopy and other screening procedures, as appropriate, based on the age of the patient and additional risk factors.

Noncarcinoid tumors of the appendix are rare tumors that typically present as appendicitis in an older patient. The duration of symptoms is usually longer. A mild anemia may be present[50]; however, the diagnosis is not usually made preoperatively. The mucinous adenocarcinoma cell type is most common and has a better prognosis after resection than does the colon or signet-ring cell type, with 5-year survival rates approaching 50%.[9]

Some patients with mucinous tumors present with a distended appendix containing mucus, called a *mucocele*. Right hemicolectomy is recommended for noncarcinoid cancers larger than 1 cm.

A *mucocele* of the appendix is the result of obstruction of the appendiceal orifice with distention of the appendix caused by intraluminal accumulation of mucoid material. The mucosa of the appendix may contain benign epithelium associated with a retention cyst, mucosal hyperplasia, or low-grade atypia noted in low-grade appendiceal mucinous neoplasms. However, the epithelium may also exhibit malignant changes as with mucinous adenocarcinoma.[51] Intact mucoceles smaller than 2 cm are nearly always benign.[52] A *retention cyst* results from chronic obstruction of the proximal lumen, usually by fibrous tissue, which leads to a simple mucocele that is lined by flattened cuboidal epithelium and is cured by appendectomy. Larger mucoceles are more likely to be neoplastic. Every effort is made to keep the mucocele intact during extraction, including placing the specimen in a bag or converting a laparoscopic procedure to open if necessary.[52] The mesoappendix is removed with the appendix to determine lymph node status, but a right hemicolectomy is not indicated unless there is invasion of the base of the appendix by tumor.[53]

Mucoceles that have ruptured are more likely to be associated with spread of epithelial cells in mucoid fluid throughout the peritoneal cavity, so-called pseudomyxoma peritonei, or mucinous carcinomatosis of appendiceal origin. The appendix is the most common source of mucoid fluid collections in the abdomen. Patients may present with appendicitis or in a less acute fashion with increased abdominal girth, an ovarian mass or an inguinal hernia (in men) due to intraperitoneal accumulation of mucoid material. Preoperative imaging studies may reveal enlargement of the ovaries due to entrapment of mucinous tumor cells within ovarian tissue, or focal mucinous fluid collections in the pelvis, left paracolic gutter, subhepatic space, splenic hilum, and omentum. Appendiceal mucinous neoplasms have several unique characteristics of which the surgeon needs to be aware. Although nearly all patients have peritoneal dissemination of tumor cells at the time of diagnosis, most of these neoplasms are noninvasive.[53] Nodal and liver metastases are uncommon, whereas locoregional recurrence of mucinous tumors, which ultimately impair small bowel function, is typical. The bulk of the peritoneal tumor is an important prognostic factor independent of histologic grade.[51] An aggressive surgical approach involving extensive removal of the peritoneum and perioperative intraperitoneal chemotherapy may improve survival for these patients, especially if performed early in the course of this disease before tumor cells become trapped in scar tissue surrounding the viscera.[53]

Selected References

Guller U, Hervey S, Purves H, et al: Laparoscopic versus open appendectomy: Outcomes comparison based on a large administrative database. Ann Surg 239(1), 43-52, 2004.

Based on a representative large U.S. nationwide database, this was the first investigation that showed that laparoscopic appendectomy has significant advantages over the open approach with respect to length of hospital stay, rate of routine discharge, and postoperative in-hospital morbidity. The advantages of laparoscopy for the specific subset of elderly patients were addressed in this publication as well as in a second article from this group published in Surgery 2004;135:479-488.

Mazuski JE, Sawyer RG, Nathens AB, et al: The Surgical Infection Society guidelines on antimicrobial therapy for intra-abdominal infections: Evidence for the recommendations. Surg Infect (Larchmt) 3(3), 175-233, 2002.

A comprehensive review of various antibiotics and their uses for various abdominal infectious processes is presented, based on the consensus of the Surgical Infection Society. The charts that summarize appropriate agents and recommended durations of therapy are particularly useful.

McGory ML, Maggard MA, Kang H, et al: Malignancies of the appendix: Beyond case series reports. Dis Colon Rectum 48(12), 2264-2271, 2005.

Based on a review of the SEER database from 1973 to 2001, this study is one of the few population-based analyses of appendiceal carcinomas. It contains important epidemiologic information about the relative incidence of carcinoid and noncarcinoid appendiceal tumors. Surgical treatment recommendations are also discussed.

Prystowsky JB, Pugh CM, Nagle AP: Current problems in surgery: Appendicitis. Curr Probl Surg 42(10), 688-742, 2005.

An eloquent and very readable review of the subject, this article offers a particularly thoughtful discussion of the pathophysiology of acute appendiceal inflammation.

Silen W: Cope's Early Diagnosis of the Acute Abdomen, 20th ed. New York, Oxford University Press, 2000.

This short treatise provides a masterful account of the nuances of the clinical presentations among patients with acute abdominal inflammatory processes.

References

1. Addiss DG, Shaffer N, Fowler BS, et al: The epidemiology of appendicitis and appendectomy in the United States. Am J Epidemiol 132:910-925, 1990.
2. Prystowsky JB, Pugh CM, Nagle AP: Current problems in surgery: Appendicitis. Curr Probl Surg 42:688-742, 2005.
3. Gladman MA, Knowles CH, Gladman LJ, et al: Intra-operative culture in appendicitis: Traditional practice challenged. Ann R Coll Surg Engl 86:196-201, 2004.
4. Soffer D, Zait S, Klausner J, et al: Peritoneal cultures and antibiotic treatment in patients with perforated appendicitis. Eur J Surg 167:214-216, 2001.
5. Lee SL, Ho HS: Acute appendicitis: Is there a difference between children and adults? Am Surg 72:409-413, 2006.
6. Boleslawski E, Panis Y, Benoist S, et al: Plain abdominal radiography as a routine procedure for acute abdominal pain of the right lower quadrant: Prospective evaluation. World J Surg 23:262-264, 1999.
7. Weltman DI, Yu J, Krumenacker J Jr, et al: Diagnosis of acute appendicitis: Comparison of 5- and 10-mm CT sections in the same patient. Radiology 216:172-177, 2000.
8. Brenner D, Elliston C, Hall E, et al: Estimated risks of radiation-induced fatal cancer from pediatric CT. AJR Am J Roentgenol 176:289-296, 2001.
9. McGory ML, Maggard MA, Kang H, et al: Malignancies of the appendix: Beyond case series reports. Dis Colon Rectum 48:2264-2271, 2005.
10. Storm-Dickerson TL, Horattas MC: What have we learned over the past 20 years about appendicitis in the elderly? Am J Surg 185:198-201, 2003.
11. Silen W: 20. New York: Oxford University Press, 2000.
12. Kaiser S, Jorulf H, Soderman E, et al: Impact of radiologic imaging on the surgical decision-making process in suspected appendicitis in children. Acad Radiol 11:971-979, 2004.
13. Macari M, Hines J, Balthazar E, et al: Mesenteric adenitis: CT diagnosis of primary versus secondary causes, incidence, and clinical significance in pediatric and adult patients. AJR Am J Roentgenol 178:853-858, 2002.
14. Bau A, Atri M: Acute female pelvic pain: Ultrasound evaluation. Semin Ultrasound CT MR 21:78-93, 2000.
15. Cohen-Kerem R, Railton C, Oren D, et al: Pregnancy outcome following non-obstetric surgical intervention. Am J Surg 190:467-473, 2005.
16. Kosloske AM, Love CL, Rohrer JE, et al: The diagnosis of appendicitis in children: Outcomes of a strategy based on pediatric surgical evaluation. Pediatrics 113:29-34, 2004.
17. Andersen BR, Kallehave FL, Andersen HK: Antibiotics versus placebo for prevention of postoperative infection after appendicectomy. Cochrane Database Syst Rev CD001439, 2005.
18. Taylor E, Berjis A, Bosch T, et al: The efficacy of postoperative oral antibiotics in appendicitis: A randomized prospective double-blinded study. Am Surg 70:858-862, 2004.
19. Mazuski JE, Sawyer RG, Nathens AB, et al: The Surgical Infection Society guidelines on antimicrobial therapy for intra-abdominal infections: Evidence for the recommendations. Surg Infect (Larchmt) 3:175-233, 2002.
20. Taylor E, Dev V, Shah D, et al: Complicated appendicitis: Is there a minimum intravenous antibiotic requirement? A prospective randomized trial. Am Surg 66:887-890, 2000.
21. Nguyen NT, Zainabadi K, Mavandadi S, et al: Trends in utilization and outcomes of laparoscopic versus open appendectomy. Am J Surg 188:813-820, 2004.
22. Enochsson L, Hellberg A, Rudberg C, et al: Laparoscopic vs open appendectomy in overweight patients. Surg Endosc 15:387-392, 2001.
23. Bendeck SE, Nino-Murcia M, Berry GJ, et al: Imaging for suspected appendicitis: Negative appendectomy and perforation rates. Radiology 225:131-136, 2002.
24. Towfigh S, Chen F, Mason R, et al: Laparoscopic appendectomy significantly reduces length of stay for perforated appendicitis. Surg Endosc 20:495-499, 2006.
25. Katkhouda N, Mason RJ, Towfigh S, et al: Laparoscopic versus open appendectomy: A prospective randomized double-blind study. Ann Surg 242:439-448; discussion 448-450, 2005.
26. Lohsiriwat V, Lert-akyamanee N, Rushatamukayanunt W: Efficacy of pre-incisional bupivacaine infiltration on postoperative pain relief after appendectomy: Prospective double-blind randomized trial. World J Surg 28:947-950, 2004.
27. Aziz O, Athanasiou T, Tekkis PP, et al: Laparoscopic versus open appendectomy in children: A meta-analysis. Ann Surg 243:17-27, 2006.
28. Ball CG, Kortbeek JB, Kirkpatrick AW, et al: Laparoscopic appendectomy for complicated appendicitis: An evaluation of postoperative factors. Surg Endosc 18:969-973, 2004.
29. Bresciani C, Perez RO, Habr-Gama A, et al: Laparoscopic versus standard appendectomy outcomes and cost compari-

sons in the private sector. J Gastrointest Surg 9:1174-1180; discussion 1180-1171, 2005.

30. Brown CV, Abrishami M, Muller M, et al: Appendiceal abscess: Immediate operation or percutaneous drainage? Am Surg 69:829-832, 2003.

31. Vane DW, Fernandez N: Role of interval appendectomy in the management of complicated appendicitis in children. World J Surg 30:51-54, 2006.

32. Sudakoff GS, Lundeen SJ, Otterson MF: Transrectal and transvaginal sonographic intervention of infected pelvic fluid collections: A complete approach. Ultrasound Q 21:175-185, 2005.

33. Nadler EP, Reblock KK, Vaughan KG, et al: Predictors of outcome for children with perforated appendicitis initially treated with non-operative management. Surg Infect (Larchmt) 5:349-356, 2004.

34. Lai HW, Loong CC, Chiu JH, et al: Interval appendectomy after conservative treatment of an appendiceal mass. World J Surg 30:352-357, 2006.

35. Giuliano V, Giuliano C, Pinto F, et al: Chronic appendicitis "syndrome" manifested by an appendicolith and thickened appendix presenting as chronic right lower abdominal pain in adults. Emerg Radiol 12:96-98, 2006.

36. Cobben LP, de Van Otterloo AM, Puylaert JB: Spontaneously resolving appendicitis: Frequency and natural history in 60 patients. Radiology 215:349-352, 2000.

37. Chiarugi M, Buccianti P, Decanini L, et al: "What you see is not what you get." A plea to remove a 'normal' appendix during diagnostic laparoscopy. Acta Chir Belg 101:243-245, 2001.

38. Greason KL, Rappold JF, Liberman MA: Incidental laparoscopic appendectomy for acute right lower quadrant abdominal pain. Its time has come. Surg Endosc 12:223-225, 1998.

39. Teh SH, O'Ceallaigh S, McKeon JG, et al: Should an appendix that looks 'normal' be removed at diagnostic laparoscopy for acute right iliac fossa pain? Eur J Surg 166:388-389, 2000.

40. Hui TT, Major KM, Avital I, et al: Outcome of elderly patients with appendicitis: Effect of computed tomography and laparoscopy. Arch Surg 137:995-998; discussion 999-1000, 2002.

41. Harrell AG, Lincourt AE, Novitsky YW, et al: Advantages of laparoscopic appendectomy in the elderly. Am Surg 72:474-480, 2006.

42. Guller U, Hervey S, Purves H, et al: Laparoscopic versus open appendectomy: Outcomes comparison based on a large administrative database. Ann Surg 239:43-52, 2004.

43. So JB, Chiong EC, Chiong E, et al: Laparoscopic appendectomy for perforated appendicitis. World J Surg 26:1485-1488, 2002.

44. Andersson RE: Small bowel obstruction after appendicectomy. Br J Surg 88:1387-1391, 2001.

45. Andersson R, Lambe M, Bergstrom R: Fertility patterns after appendicectomy: Historical cohort study. BMJ 318:963-967, 1999.

46. Urbach DR, Marrett LD, Kung R, et al: Association of perforation of the appendix with female tubal infertility. Am J Epidemiol 153:566-571, 2001.

47. Carr NJ, Sobin LH: Neuroendocrine tumors of the appendix. Semin Diagn Pathol 21:108-119, 2004.

48. McCusker ME, Cote TR, Clegg LX, et al: Primary malignant neoplasms of the appendix: A population-based study from the surveillance, epidemiology and end-results program, 1973-1998. Cancer 94:3307-3312, 2002.

49. Modlin IM, Lye KD, Kidd M: A 5-decade analysis of 13,715 carcinoid tumors. Cancer 97:934-959, 2003.

50. Todd RD, Sarosi GA, Nwariaku F, et al: Incidence and predictors of appendiceal tumors in elderly males presenting with signs and symptoms of acute appendicitis. Am J Surg 188:500-504, 2004.

51. Misdraji J, Yantiss RK, Graeme-Cook FM, et al: Appendiceal mucinous neoplasms: A clinicopathologic analysis of 107 cases. Am J Surg Pathol 27:1089-1103, 2003.

52. Dhage-Ivatury S, Sugarbaker PH: Update on the surgical approach to mucocele of the appendix. J Am Coll Surg 202:680-684, 2006.

53. Sugarbaker PH: New standard of care for appendiceal epithelial neoplasms and pseudomyxoma peritonei syndrome? Lancet Oncol 7:69-76, 2006.

Colon and Rectum

Robert D. Fry, MD   Najjia Mahmoud, MD   David J. Maron, MD   Howard M. Ross, MD
and   John Rombeau, MD

EMBRYOLOGY OF THE COLON AND RECTUM

No comprehensive discussion of colorectal anatomy is complete without a thorough understanding of the genesis of the gastrointestinal tract. Knowledge of the developmental anatomy of the foregut, midgut, and hindgut establishes a context in which to consider mature structural and functional anatomic relationships.

The endodermal roof of the yolk sac gives rise to the primitive gut tube. At the beginning of the third week of development, the gut tube is divided into three regions: the *midgut*, which opens ventrally, positioned between the *foregut* in the headfold and the *hindgut* in the tailfold. Development progresses through these stages: physiologic herniation, return to the abdomen, and fixation. The acquisition of length and formation of dedicated blood and lymphatic supplies takes place during this time (Fig. 50-1).

Foregut-derived structures end at the second portion of the duodenum and rely on the celiac artery for blood supply. The midgut, extending from the duodenal ampulla to the distal transverse colon, is based on the superior mesenteric artery. The distal one third of the transverse colon, descending colon, and rectum evolve from the hindgut fold and are supplied by the inferior mesenteric artery. Venous and lymphatic channels mirror their arterial counterparts and follow the same embryologic divisions. At the dentate line, endoderm-derived tissues fuse with the ectoderm-derived *proctodeum,* or ingrowth from the anal pit.

Distal rectal development is complex. The cloaca is a specialized area of the primitive distal rectum composed of both endoderm- and ectoderm-derived tissues. This area is incorporated into the anal transition zone, which surrounds the dentate line in the adult. The cloaca exists in a continuum with the hindgut, but at about the sixth week, it begins to divide and differentiate into anterior urogenital and posterior anal and sphincter elements. Simultaneously, the urogenital and gastrointestinal tracts are separated by caudal migration of the urogenital septum. During the 10th week of development, the external anal sphincter is formed from the posterior cloaca as the descent of the urogenital septum becomes complete. The internal anal sphincter is formed by the 12th week from enlarged circular muscle layers of the rectum.

ANATOMY OF THE COLON, RECTUM, AND PELVIC FLOOR

The colon and rectum constitute a tube of variable diameter about 150 cm in length. The terminal ileum empties into the cecum through a thickened, nipple-shaped invagination, the ileocecal valve. The cecum is a capacious sac-like segment of the proximal colon with an

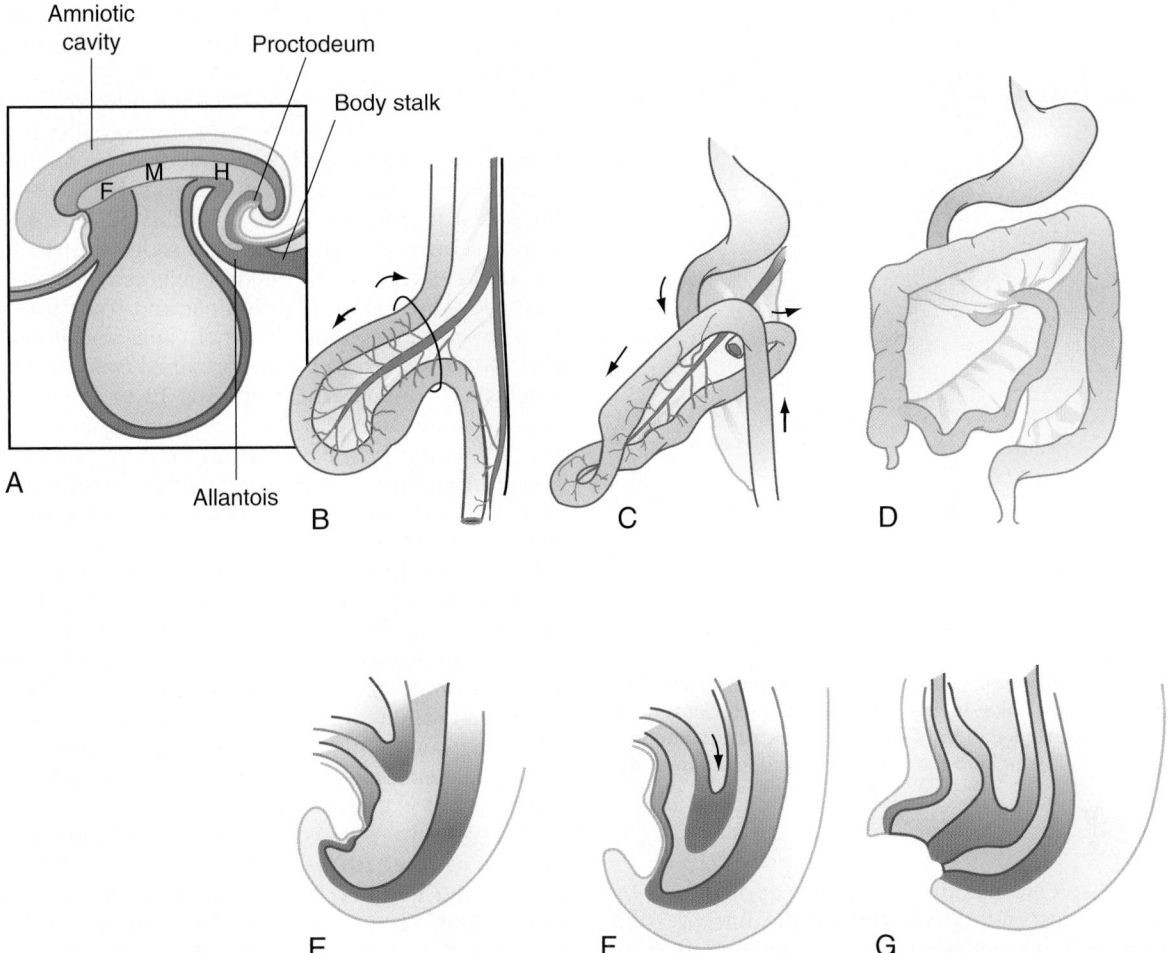

Figure 50-1 A, At the third week of development, the primitive tube can be divided into three regions: the foregut in the head fold, the hindgut with its ventral allantoic outgrowth in the smaller tail fold, and the midgut between these two portions. Stages of development of the midgut: physiologic herniation (**B**), return to the abdomen (**C**), and fixation (**D**). At the sixth week, the urogenital septum migrates caudally (**E**) and separates the intestinal and urogenital tracts (**F, G**). (From Corman ML [ed]: Colon and Rectal Surgery, 4th ed. Philadelphia, Lippincott-Raven, 1998, p 2.)

average diameter of 7.5 cm and length of 10 cm. Although it is distensible, acute dilation of the cecum to a diameter of greater than 12 cm, an event that can be measured by a plain abdominal radiograph, can result in ischemic necrosis and perforation of the bowel wall. Surgical intervention may be required when this degree of cecal distention is caused by obstruction or pseudo-obstruction (Fig. 50-2).

The appendix extends from the cecum about 3 cm below the ileocecal valve as a blind-ending elongated tube 8 to 10 cm in length. The proximal appendix is fairly constant in location, whereas the end can be located in a wide variety of positions relative to the cecum and terminal ileum. Most commonly, it is retrocecal (65%), followed by pelvic (31%), subcecal (2.3%), preileal (1.0%), and retroileal (0.4%). Clinically, the appendix is found at the convergence of the taeniae coli. Another clinical aid useful in detecting the location of the appendix through a small abdominal incision is the identification of the fold of Treves, the only antimesenteric epiploic appendage

normally found on the small intestine, marking the junction of the ileum and cecum.

The ascending colon, about 15 cm in length, runs upward toward the liver on the right side; like the descending colon, the posterior surface is fixed against the retroperitoneum, whereas the lateral and anterior surfaces are true intraperitoneal structures. The *white line of Toldt* represents the fusion of the mesentery with the posterior peritoneum. This subtle peritoneal landmark serves the surgeon as a guide for mobilizing the colon and mesentery from the retroperitoneum.

The transverse colon is about 45 cm in length. Hanging between fixed positions at the hepatic and splenic flexures, it is completely invested in visceral peritoneum. The nephrocolic ligament secures the hepatic flexure and directly overlies the right kidney, duodenum, and porta hepatis. The phrenocolic ligament lies ventral to the spleen and fixes the splenic flexure in the left upper quadrant. The angle of the splenic flexure is higher, more acute, and more deeply situated than that of the hepatic

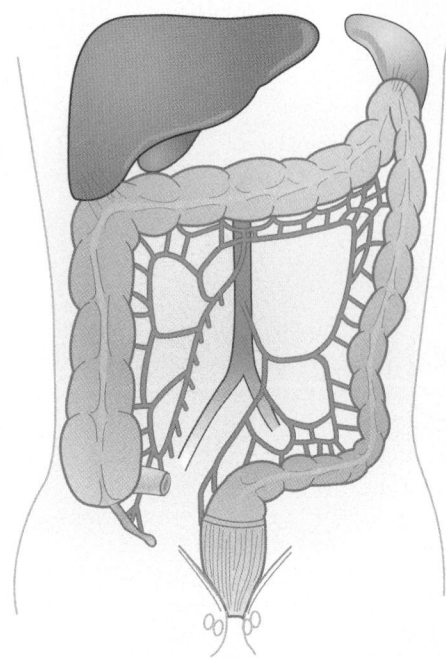

Figure 50-2 Anatomy of the colon and rectum: coronal view. The diameter of the right colon is larger than the diameter of the left side. Note the higher location of the splenic flexure compared with the hepatic flexure, and the extraperitoneal location of the rectum.

flexure. The splenic flexure is typically approached by dissecting the descending colon along the line of Toldt from below and then entering the lesser sac by reflecting the omentum from the transverse colon. This maneuver allows mobilization of the flexure to be achieved with minimal traction required for exposure. Attached to the superior aspect of the transverse colon is the greater omentum, a fused double layer of visceral and parietal peritoneum (four total layers) that contains variable amounts of stored fat. Clinically, it is quite useful in preventing adhesions between surgical abdominal wounds and underlying bowel and is often used to cover intraperitoneal contents as incisions are closed. The omentum can be mobilized and placed between the rectum and vagina after repair of a high rectovaginal fistula, or used to fill the pelvic and perineal space left after excision of the rectum. The living tissue of the greater omentum makes a good patch in difficult situations, such as treatment of a perforated duodenum, when closure of inflamed and friable tissues is impossible or ill-advised.

The descending colon lies ventral to the left kidney and extends downward from the splenic flexure for about 25 cm. It is smaller in diameter than the ascending colon. At the level of the pelvic brim, there is a transition between the relatively thin-walled, fixed, descending colon and the thicker, mobile sigmoid colon. The sigmoid colon varies in length from 15 to 50 cm (average, 38 cm) and is very mobile. It is a small-diameter, muscular tube on a long, floppy mesentery that often forms an omega loop in the pelvis. The mesosigmoid is frequently attached to the left pelvic sidewall, producing a small recess in

the mesentery known as the *intersigmoid fossa*. This mesenteric fold is a surgical landmark for the underlying left ureter.

The rectum, along with the sigmoid colon, serves as a fecal reservoir. There is some controversy in the definition of the proximal and distal extent of the rectum. Some consider the rectosigmoid junction to be at the level of the sacral promontory; others, at the point at which the taeniae converge. Anatomists consider the dentate line the distal extent of the rectum, whereas surgeons typically view this union of columnar and squamous epithelium as existing within the anal canal and consider the end of the rectum to be the proximal border of the anal sphincter complex. The rectum is 12 to 15 cm in length and lacks taeniae coli or appendices epiploicae. It occupies the curve of the sacrum in the true pelvis, and the posterior surface is almost completely extraperitoneal in that it is adherent to presacral soft tissues and thus is outside of the peritoneal cavity. The anterior surface of the proximal third of the rectum is covered by visceral peritoneum. The peritoneal reflection is 7 to 9 cm from the anal verge in men and 5 to 7.5 cm in women. This anterior peritonealized space is called the *pouch of Douglas* or the *pelvic cul-de-sac* and may serve as the site of so-called drop metastases from visceral tumors. These peritoneal metastases can form a mass in the cul-de-sac (called *Bloomer's shelf*) that can be detected by a digital rectal examination.

The rectum possesses three involutions or curves known as the *valves of Houston*. The middle valve folds to the left, and the proximal and distal valves fold to the right. These valves are more properly called *folds* because they have no specific function as impediments to flow. They are lost after full surgical mobilization of the rectum, a maneuver that may provide about 5 cm of additional length to the rectum, greatly facilitating the surgeon's ability to fashion an anastomosis deep in the pelvis.

The posterior aspect of the rectum is invested with a thick, closely applied mesorectum. A thin layer of investing fascia (fascia propria) coats the mesorectum and represents a distinct layer from the presacral fascia against which it lies. During proctectomy for rectal cancer, mobilization and dissection of the rectum proceed between the presacral fascia and the fascia propria. Total mesorectal excision is a well-described oncologic maneuver that makes good use of the tissue planes investing the rectum to achieve a relatively bloodless rectal and mesorectal dissection. The lymphatics are contained within the mesorectum, and total mesorectal excision adheres to the basic surgical oncologic principle of removal of the cancer in continuity with its blood and lymphatic supply. Resection of the rectum using this technique and based on a thorough understanding of anatomy has been shown to markedly reduce the incidence of subsequent local recurrence of rectal cancer.

Pararectal Fascia

The endopelvic fascia is a thick layer of parietal peritoneum that lines the walls and floor of the pelvis. The

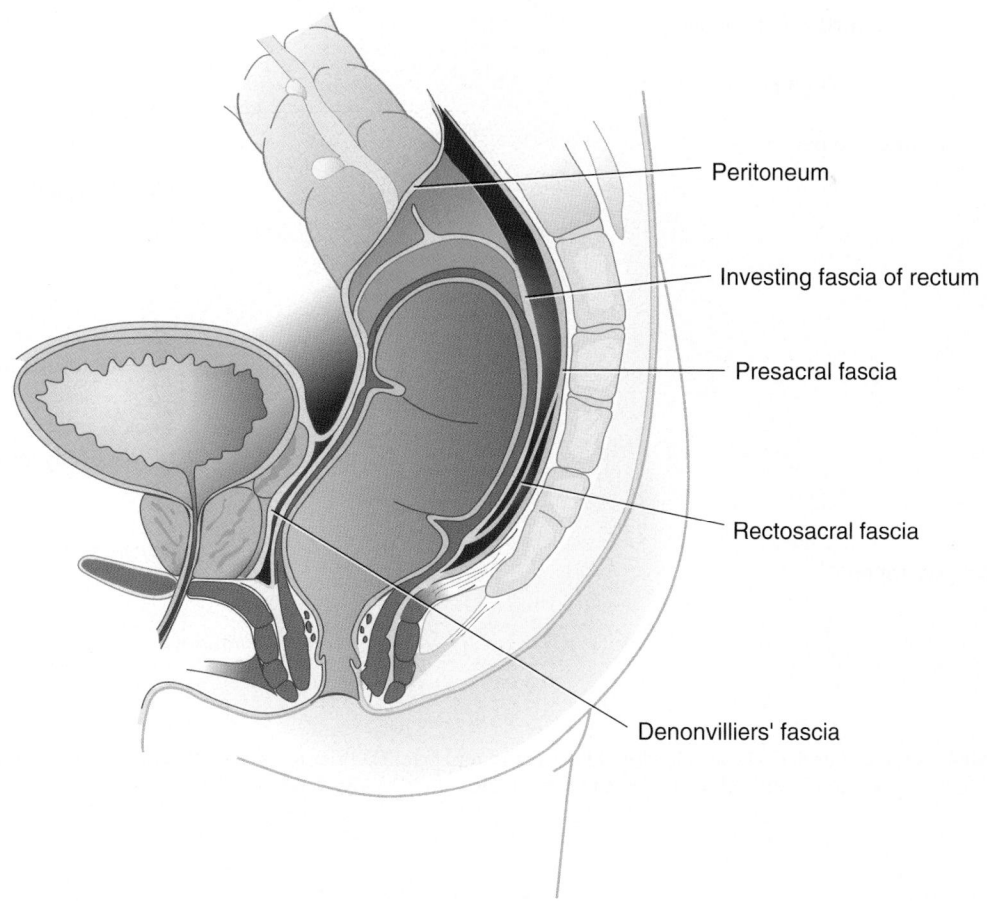

Figure 50-3 **Endopelvic fascia.** (From Gordon PH, Nivatvongs S [eds]: Principles and Practice of Surgery for the Colon, Rectum and Anus, 2nd ed. St Louis, Quality Medical Publishing, 1999, p 10).

portion that is closely applied to the periosteum of the anterior sacrum is the presacral fascia. The fascia propria of the rectum is a thin condensation of the endopelvic fascia that forms an envelope around the mesorectum and continues distally to help form the lateral rectal stalks. The lateral rectal stalks or ligaments are actually anterolateral structures containing the middle rectal artery. The stalks reside in close proximity to the mixed autonomic nerves (containing both sympathetic and parasympathetic nerves), and division of these structures close to the pelvic sidewall may result in injury to these nerves, resulting in impotence and bladder dysfunction (Fig. 50-3).

The rectosacral fascia, or Waldeyer's fascia, is a thick condensation of endopelvic fascia connecting the presacral fascia to the fascia propria at the level of S4 and extends to the anorectal ring. Waldeyer's fascia is an important surgical landmark, and its division during dissection from an abdominal approach provides entry to the deep retrorectal pelvis. Dissection between the fascia propria and the presacral fascia follows the principles of surgical oncology and minimizes the risk for vascular or neural injuries. Disruption of the presacral fascia may lead to injury of the basivertebral venous plexus, resulting in massive hemorrhage. Disrupting the fascia propria

during an operation for rectal cancer may significantly increase the incidence of subsequent recurrence of cancer in the pelvis if mesorectum is then left behind.

Pelvic Floor

The muscles of the pelvic floor, like those of the anal sphincter mechanism, arise from the primitive cloaca. The pelvic floor, or diaphragm, consists of the pubococcygeus, iliococcygeus, and puborectalis, a group of muscles that together form the levator ani. The pelvic diaphragm resides between the sacrum, obturator fascia, ischial spines, and pubis. It forms a strong floor that supports the pelvic organs and, together with the external anal sphincter, regulates defecation. The levator hiatus is an opening between the decussating fibers of the pubococcygeus that allows egress of the anal canal, urethra, and dorsal vein in men and the anal canal, urethra, and vagina in women. The puborectalis is a strong U-shaped sling of striated muscle coursing around the rectum just above the level of the anal sphincters. Relaxation of the puborectalis straightens the anorectal angle and permits descent of feces; contraction produces the opposite effect. The puborectalis is in a state of continual contraction, a factor vital to the maintenance of continence.

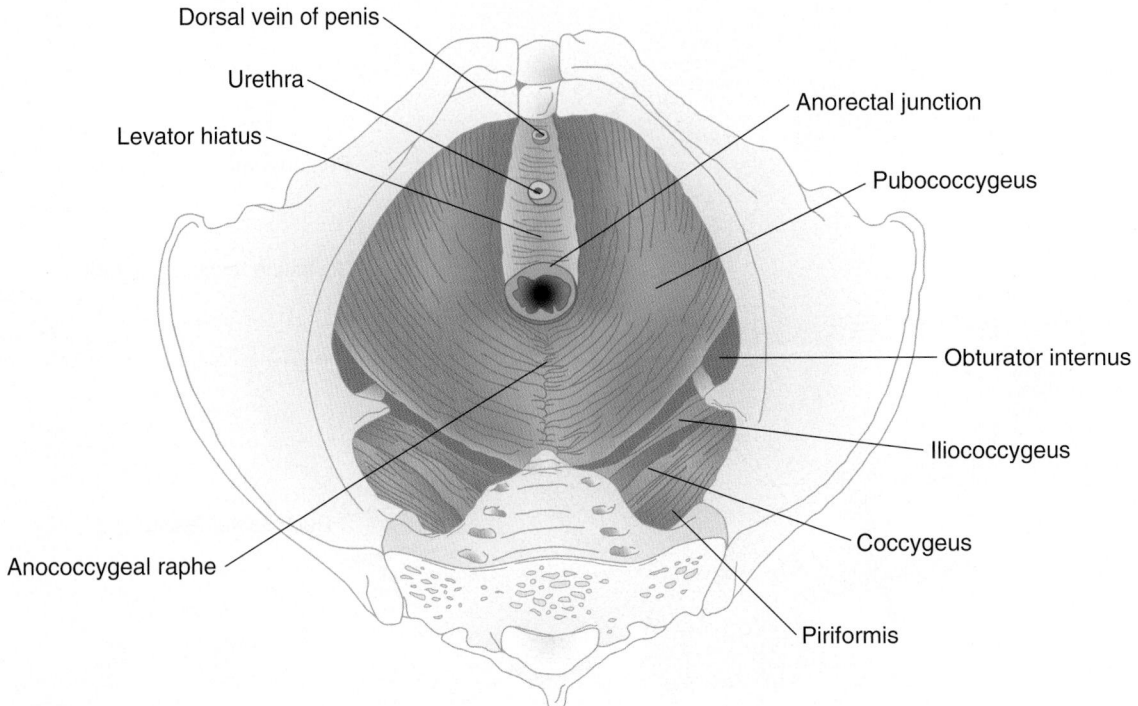

Figure 50-4 Levator muscles. (From Gordon PH, Nivatvongs S [eds]: Principles and Practice of Surgery for the Colon, Rectum and Anus, 2nd ed. St Louis, Quality Medical Publishing, 1999, p 18.)

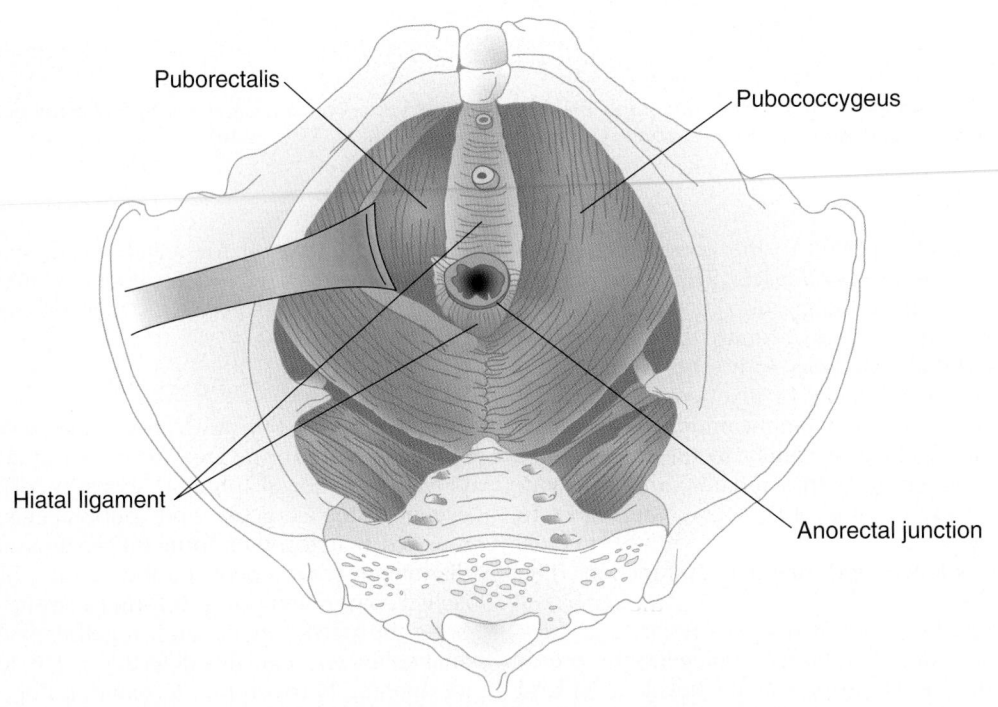

Figure 50-5 Hiatal ligament. (From Gordon PH, Nivatvongs S [eds]: Principles and Practice of Surgery for the Colon, Rectum and Anus, 2nd ed. St Louis, Quality Medical Publishing, 1999, p 18.)

Puborectalis dysfunction is an important cause of defecation disorders. The pubococcygeus and iliococcygeus most likely participate in continence by applying lateral pressure to narrow the levator hiatus (Figs. 50-4 and 50-5).

Arterial Supply and Venous and Lymphatic Drainage

Knowledge of the embryologic development of the intestinal tract provides an excellent foundation for

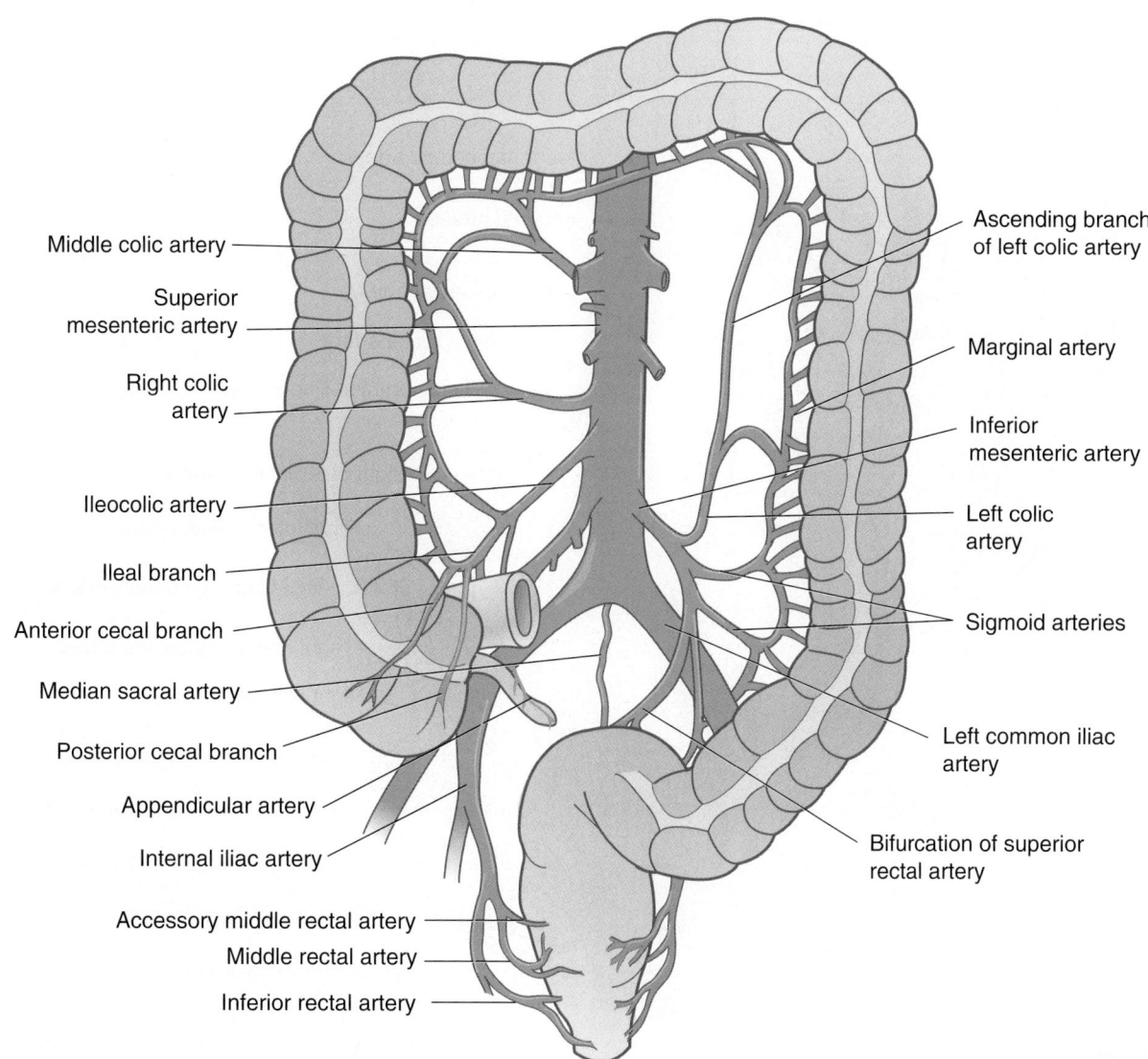

Figure 50-6 Arterial supply of the colon. (From Gordon PH, Nivatvongs S [eds]: Principles and Practice of Surgery for the Colon, Rectum and Anus, 2nd ed. St Louis, Quality Medical Publishing, 1999, p 23.)

understanding the anatomic blood supply. The foregut is supplied by the celiac artery, the midgut by the superior mesenteric artery (SMA), and the hindgut by the inferior mesenteric artery (IMA) (Figs. 50-6 and 50-7). Anatomic redundancy confers survival advantages, and in the intestinal tract, this feature is provided by extensive communication between the major arteries and the collateral blood supply (Fig. 50-8). The territory of the SMA ends at the distal portion of the transverse colon, and that of the IMA begins in the region of the splenic flexure. A large collateral vessel, the marginal artery, connects these two circulations and forms a continuous arcade along the mesenteric border of the colon. Vasa recta from this artery branch off at short intervals and directly supply the bowel wall (Fig. 50-9). The SMA supplies the entire small bowel, giving off 12 to 20 jejunal and ileal branches to the left and up to three main colonic branches to the right. The ileocolic artery is the most constant of these branches and supplies the terminal ileum, cecum, and appendix.

The right colic artery is absent in 2% to 18% of specimens; when present, it may arise directly from the SMA, or as a branch of the ileocolic or middle colic artery. It supplies the ascending colon and hepatic flexure and communicates with the middle colic artery through collateral marginal artery arcades. The middle colic artery is a proximal branch of the SMA. It generally divides into a right and a left branch, which supply the proximal and distal transverse colon, respectively. Anatomic variations of the middle colic artery include complete absence in 4% to 20% and presence of an accessory middle colic artery in 10% of specimens. The left branch of the middle colic artery may supply territory also supplied by the left colic artery through the collateral channel of the marginal artery. This collateral circulation in the area of the splenic flexure is the most inconsistent of the entire colon and has been referred to as a *watershed area,* vulnerable to ischemia in the presence of hypotension. In some studies, up to 50% of specimens lack clearly identified arteries in

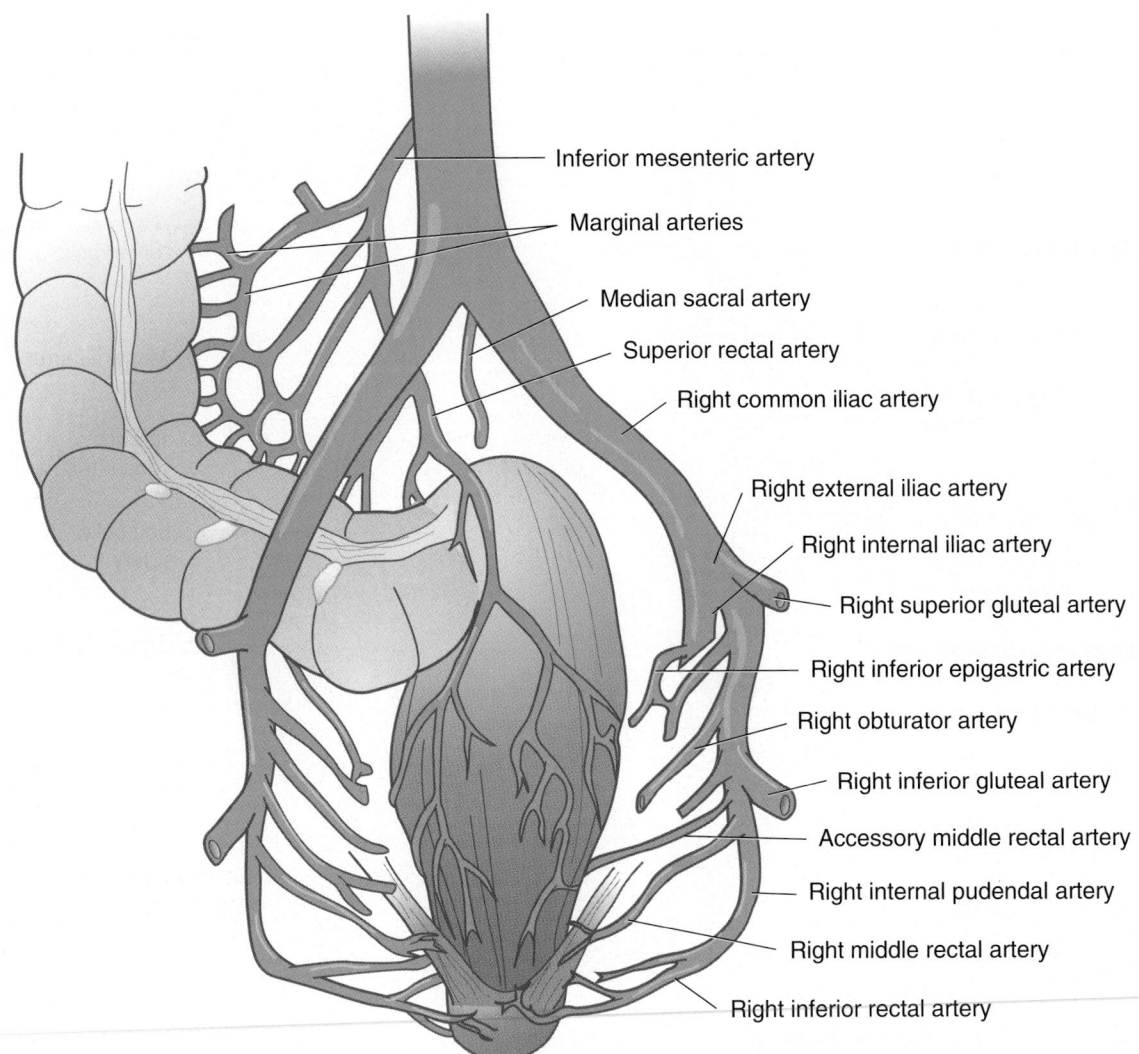

Inferior mesenteric artery

Marginal arteries

Median sacral artery

Superior rectal artery

Right common iliac artery

Right external iliac artery

Right internal iliac artery

Right superior gluteal artery

Right inferior epigastric artery

Right obturator artery

Right inferior gluteal artery

Accessory middle rectal artery

Right internal pudendal artery

Right middle rectal artery

Right inferior rectal artery

Figure 50-7 Arterial supply of the rectum. (From Gordon PH, Nivatvongs S [eds]: Principles and Practice of Surgery for the Colon, Rectum and Anus, 2nd ed. St Louis, Quality Medical Publishing, 1999, p 24.)

a small segment of colon at the confluence of the blood supplies of the midgut and hindgut. These individuals rely on adjacent vasa recta in this area for arterial supply to the bowel wall. In practice, surgeons avoid making anastomoses in the region of the splenic flexure for fear that the blood supply will not be sufficient to permit healing of the anastomosis, a situation that could lead to anastomotic leak and sepsis.

The IMA originates from the aorta at the level of L2 to L3, about 3 cm above the aortic bifurcation. The left colic artery is the most proximal branch, supplying the distal transverse colon, splenic flexure, and descending colon. Two to six sigmoid branches collateralize with the left colic artery and form arcades that supply the sigmoid colon and contribute to the marginal artery.

The arc of Riolan is a collateral artery first described by Jean Riolan (1580-1657) that directly connects the proximal SMA with the proximal IMA and may serve as a vital conduit when one or the other of these arteries is occluded. It is also known as the *meandering mesenteric artery* and is highly variable in size. Flow can be either forward (IMA stenosis) or retrograde (SMA stenosis), depending on the site of obstruction. Such obstruction results in increased size and tortuosity of this meandering artery that may be detected by arteriography; the presence of a large arc of Riolan thus suggests occlusion of one of the major mesenteric arteries (Fig. 50-10).

The IMA terminates in the superior rectal (superior hemorrhoidal) artery, which courses behind the rectum in the mesorectum, branching and then entering the rectal submucosa. Here, the capillaries form a submucosal plexus in the distal rectum at the level of the anal columns. The anal canal also receives arterial blood from the middle rectal (hemorrhoidal) and inferior rectal (hemorrhoidal) arteries. The middle rectal artery is a branch of the internal iliac artery. It is variable in size and enters the rectum anterolaterally, passing alongside and slightly anterior to the lateral rectal stalks. It has been reported to be absent in 40% to 80% of specimens studied. The inferior rectal artery is a branch of the pudendal artery,

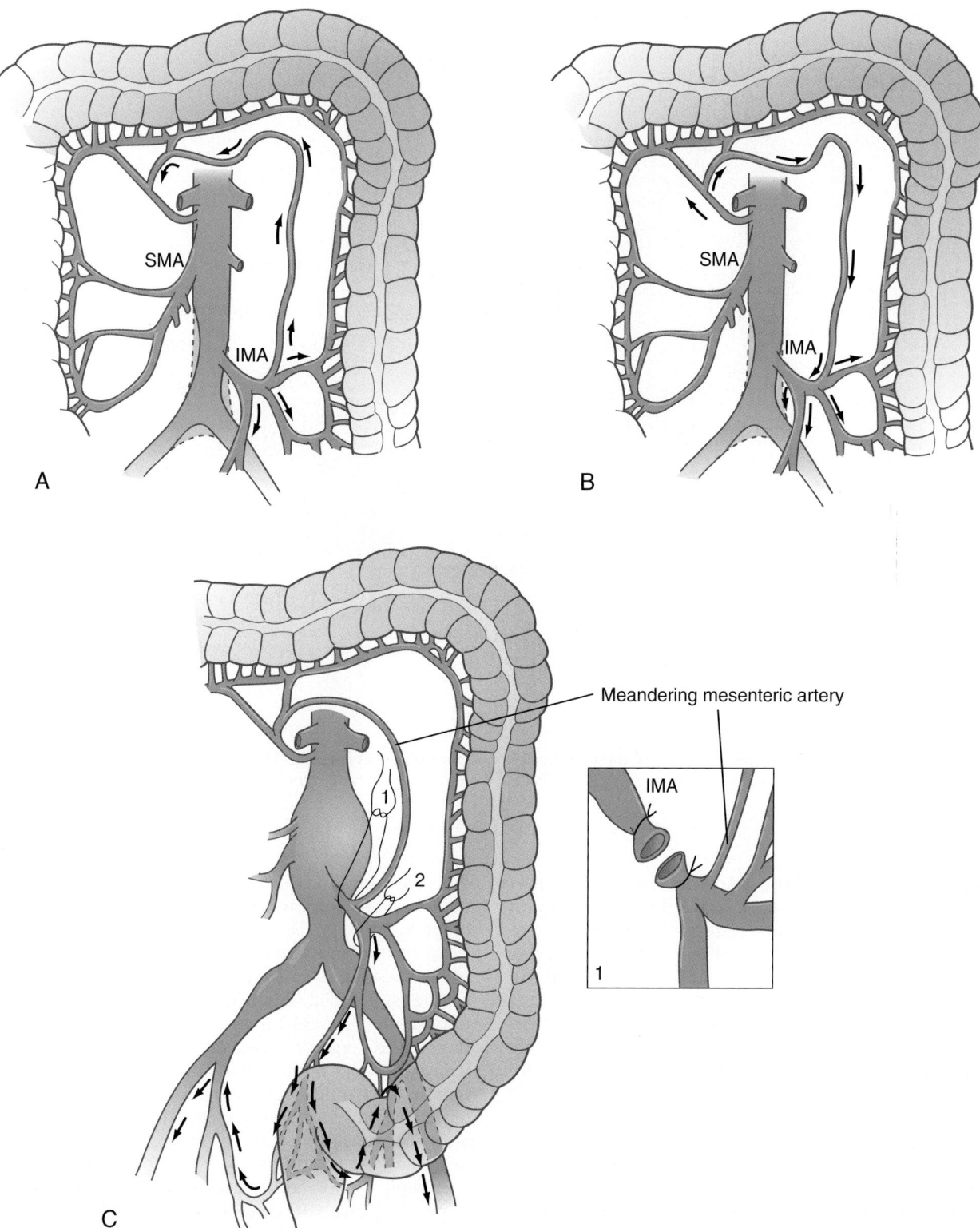

SMA

IMA

A

SMA

IMA

B

Meandering mesenteric artery

IMA

1

C

Figure 50-8 Pathologic anatomy and occlusion of the superior mesenteric artery (SMA) and the inferior mesenteric artery (IMA). **A,** Occlusion of SMA. **B,** Occlusion of IMA. **C,** Location for ligating IMA: **1,** correct location of ligation (see *inset*); **2,** incorrect location of ligation. (From Gordon PH, Nivatvongs S [eds]: Principles and Practice of Surgery for the Colon, Rectum and Anus, 2nd ed. St Louis, Quality Medical Publishing, 1999, p 28.)

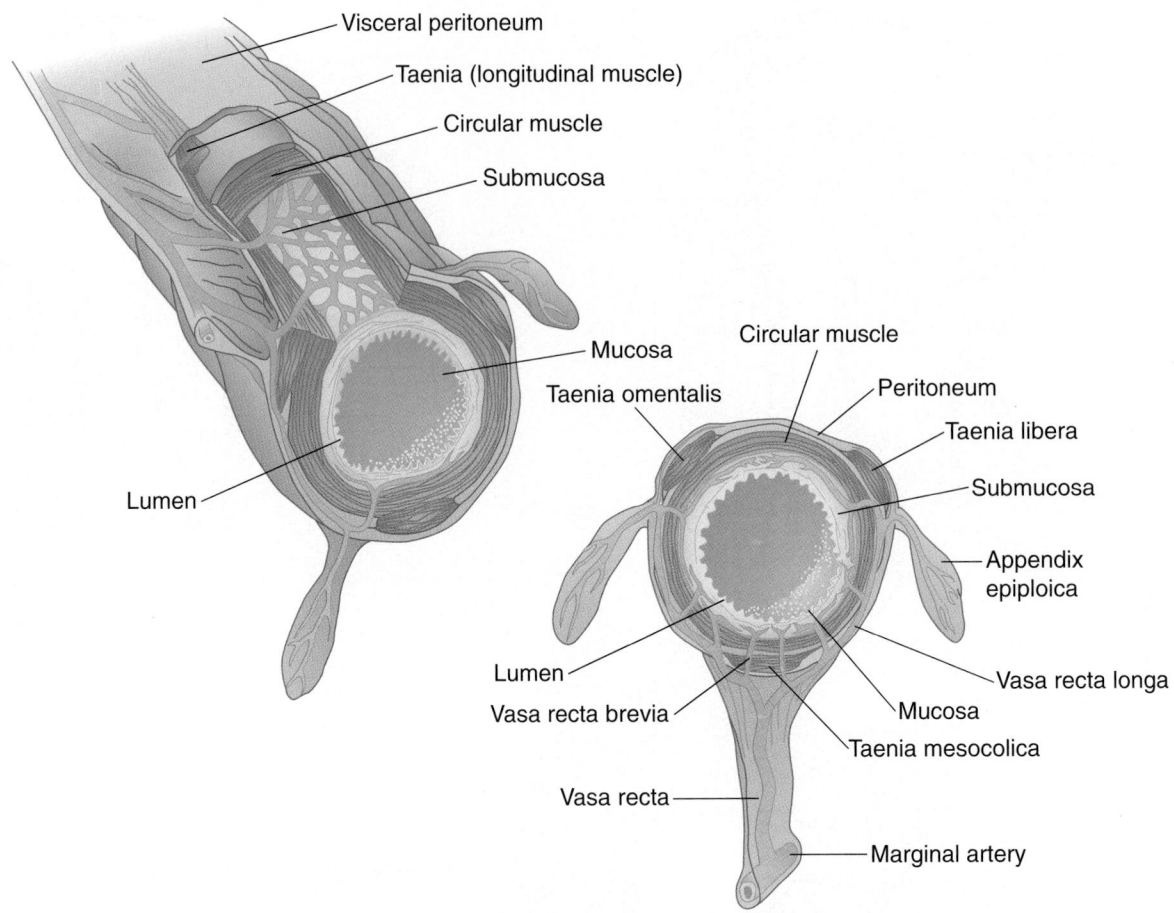

Figure 50-9 Cross-sectional anatomy of the colon, with vasa brevia and vasa recta. (From Gordon PH, Nivatvongs S [eds]: Principles and Practice of Surgery for the Colon, Rectum and Anus, 2nd ed. St Louis, Quality Medical Publishing, 1999, p 26.)

which itself is a more distal branch of the internal iliac. From the obturator canal, it traverses the obturator fascia, ischiorectal fossa, and external anal sphincter to reach the anal canal. This vessel is encountered during the perineal dissection of an abdominoperineal resection.

The venous drainage of the colon and rectum mirrors the arterial blood supply. Venous drainage from the right and proximal transverse colon empties into the superior mesenteric vein, which coalesces with the splenic vein to become the portal vein. The distal transverse colon, descending colon, sigmoid, and most of the rectum drain into the inferior mesenteric vein, which empties into the splenic vein to the left of the aorta. The anal canal is drained by the middle and inferior rectal veins into the internal iliac vein and subsequently the inferior vena cava. The bidirectional venous drainage of the anal canal accounts for differences in patterns of metastasis from tumors arising in this region (Fig. 50-11).

Lymphatic drainage also follows the arterial anatomy. The wall of the large bowel is supplied with a rich network of lymphatic capillaries that drain to extramural channels paralleling the arterial supply. Lymphatics from

the colon and proximal two thirds of the rectum ultimately drain into the para-aortic nodal chain, which empties into the cisterna chyli. Lymphatics draining the distal rectum and anal canal may drain either to the para-aortic nodes or laterally, through the internal iliac system, to the superficial inguinal nodal basin. Although the dentate line roughly marks the level where lymphatic drainage diverges, classic studies by Block and Enquist using dye injection demonstrated that spread through lymphatic channels occurs to adjacent pelvic organs, such as the vagina and broad ligament, when injections are administered as high as 10 cm proximal to the dentate line (Figs. 50-12 and 50-13).

Lymph nodes are commonly grouped into levels depending on their location. Epicolic nodes are located along the bowel wall and in the epiploicae. Nodes adjacent to the marginal artery are paracolic. Intermediate nodes are located along the main branches of the large blood vessels; primary nodes are located on the superior or inferior mesenteric artery. Lymph node invasion by metastatic cancer is an important prognostic factor for patients with colorectal cancer. Accurate pathologic assessment of lymph nodes is essential for accurate

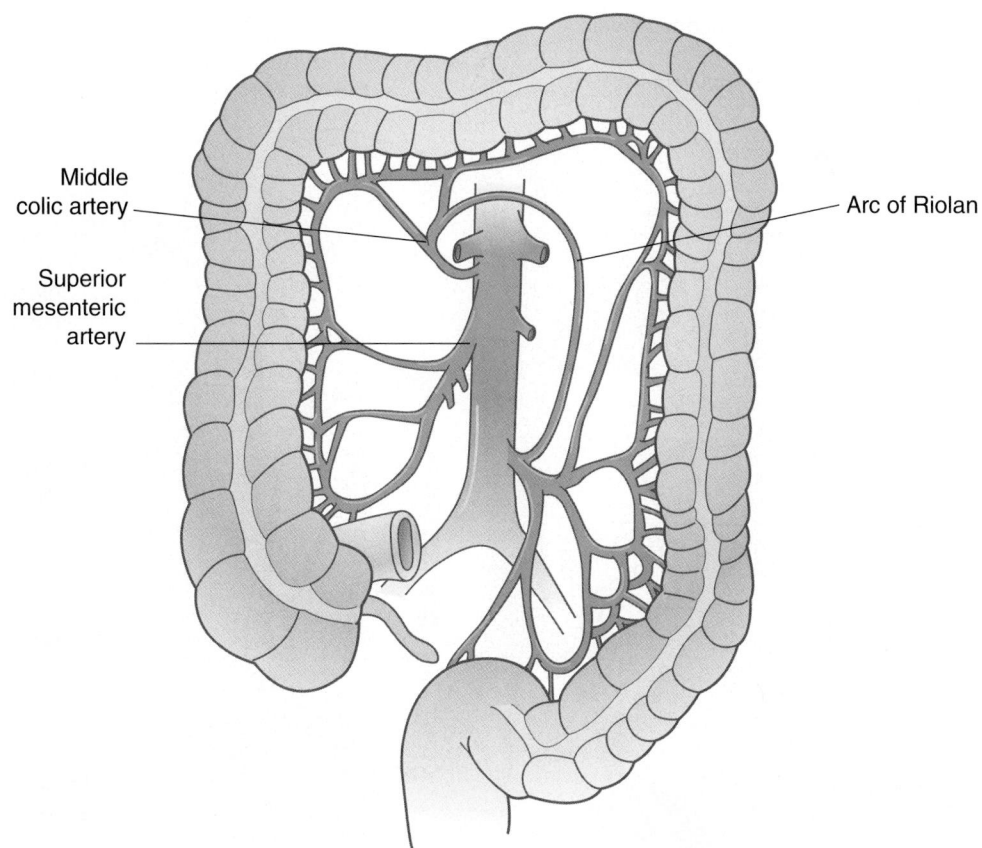

Middle colic artery

Superior mesenteric artery

Arc of Riolan

Figure 50-10 Arc of Riolan. (From Gordon PH, Nivatvongs S [eds]: Principles and Practice of Surgery for the Colon, Rectum and Anus, 2nd ed. St Louis, Quality Medical Publishing, 1999, p 27.)

staging, which serves as a determinant for treatment of patients with colorectal cancer.

Nerves

Preganglionic sympathetic nerves from T6 to T12 synapse in preaortic ganglia. Postsympathetic fibers then course along blood vessels to reach the right and transverse colon. The right and transverse colon parasympathetic supply comes from the right vagus nerve. Parasympathetic fibers follow branches of the superior mesenteric artery to synapse in the wall of the bowel. The left colon and rectum receive sympathetic supply from the preganglionic lumbar splanchnics of L1 to L3. These synapse in the preaortic plexus located above the aortic bifurcation, and the postganglionic elements follow the branches of the IMA and superior rectal artery to the left colon, sigmoid, and rectum. The lower rectum, pelvic floor, and anal canal receive postganglionic sympathetics from the pelvic plexus. The pelvic plexus is adherent to the pelvic sidewalls and is adjacent to the lateral stalks. It receives sympathetic branches from the presacral plexus, which condense at the sacral promontory into the left and right hypogastric nerves. These sympathetic nerves, which descend into the pelvis dorsal to the superior rectal artery, are responsible for delivery of semen to the posterior prostatic urethra. Failure to preserve at least one

of the hypogastric nerves during rectal dissection results in ejaculatory dysfunction in males.

The pelvic parasympathetic nerves, or nervi erigenti, arise from S2 to S4. Preganglionic parasympathetic nerves merge with postganglionic sympathetics after the latter emerge from the sacral foramina. These nerve fibers, through the pelvic plexus, surround and innervate the prostate, urethra, seminal vesicles, urinary bladder, and muscles of the pelvic floor. Rectal dissection may disrupt the pelvic plexus and its subdivisions, resulting in neurogenic bladder and sexual dysfunction. Rates of bladder and erectile dysfunction after rectal surgery are as high as 45%. Degree and type of dysfunction are affected by the level of the neurologic injury. A high inferior mesenteric artery ligation severing the hypogastric nerves near the sacral promontory results in sympathetic dysfunction characterized by retrograde ejaculation and bladder dysfunction. Injury to the mixed parasympathetic and sympathetic periprostatic plexus results in impotence and atonic bladder.

PHYSIOLOGY OF THE COLON

In a broad sense, the function of the colon is the recycling of nutrients, whereas the function of the rectum is

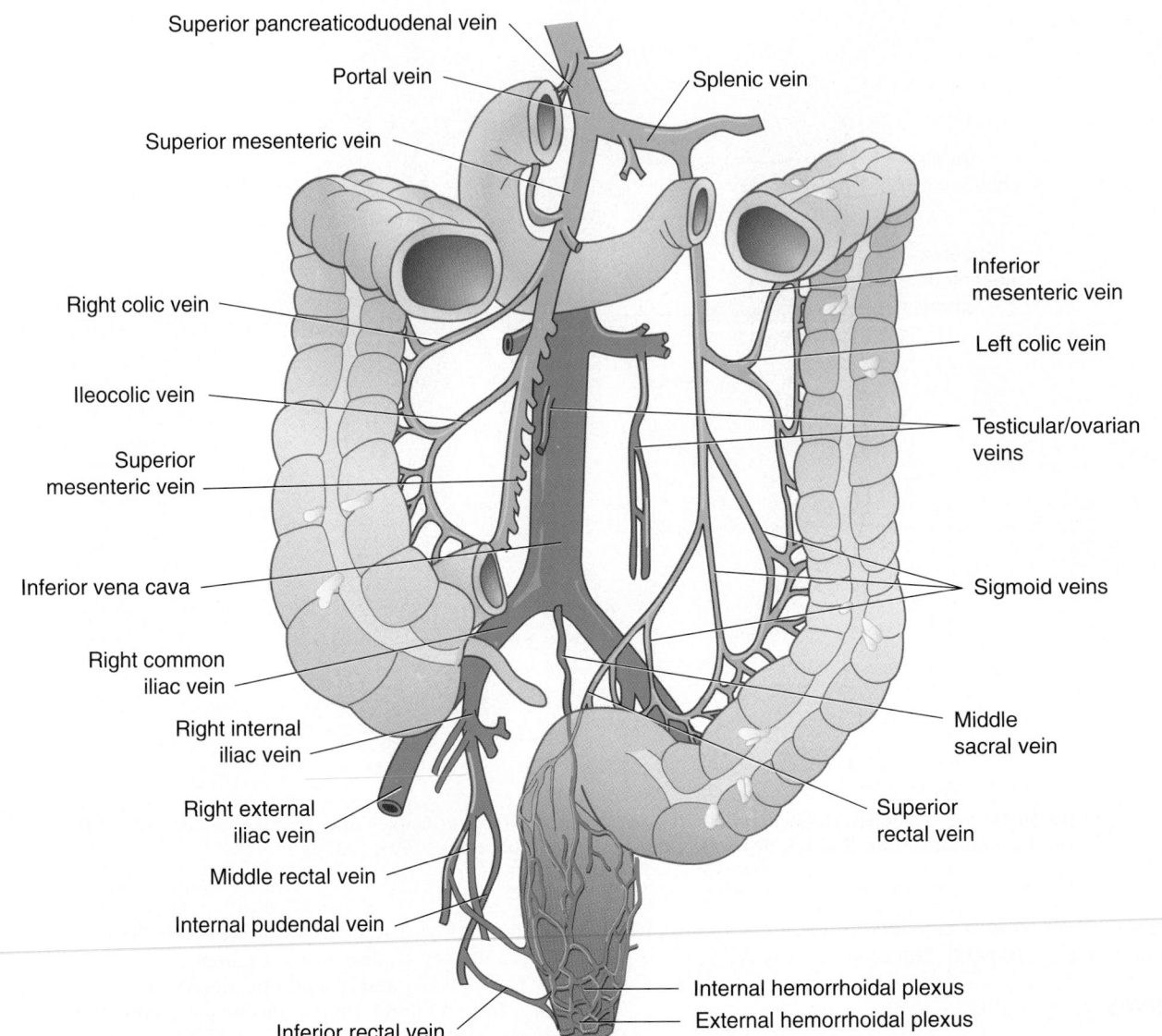

Figure 50-11 Venous drainage of the colon and rectum. (From Gordon PH, Nivatvongs S [eds]: Principles and Practice of Surgery for the Colon, Rectum and Anus, 2nd ed. St Louis, Quality Medical Publishing, 1999, p 30.)

the elimination of stool. The recycling of nutrients depends on the metabolic activity of the colonic flora, on colonic motility, and on mucosal absorption and secretion. Stool elimination involves dehydration of colonic contents and defecation.

Recycling of Nutrients

During the digestive process, ingested nutrients are diluted within the intestinal lumen by biliopancreatic and gastrointestinal (GI) secretions. The small intestine absorbs most ingested nutrients as well as some of the fluid and bile salts secreted into the lumen. However, the ileal effluent is still rich in water, electrolytes, and nutrients that resist digestion. The colon has the functions to recover these substances and to avoid unnecessary losses of fluids, electrolytes, nitrogen, and energy. To accom-

plish this, the colon depends highly on its bacterial flora.

Colonic Flora

The colonic microbiota plays an important role in several areas of human physiology. This complex congregate of microorganisms confers great metabolic potential on the colon, primarily through its degradative abilities. Many hundreds of different types of bacteria, varying widely in physiology and biochemistry, exist in the various microhabitats of the colon: the lumen, the mucin layer, and the mucosal surface. Cultures from colonoscopic biopsies reveal aerobic counts (aerobes and facultative organisms) ranging from 2.4×10^3 to 1.3×10^6 colony-forming units (cfu)/sample biopsy (5.6 mg) and total anaerobic counts 10 to 10^2 times higher at 1.4×10^5 to 10^7 cfu/sample.

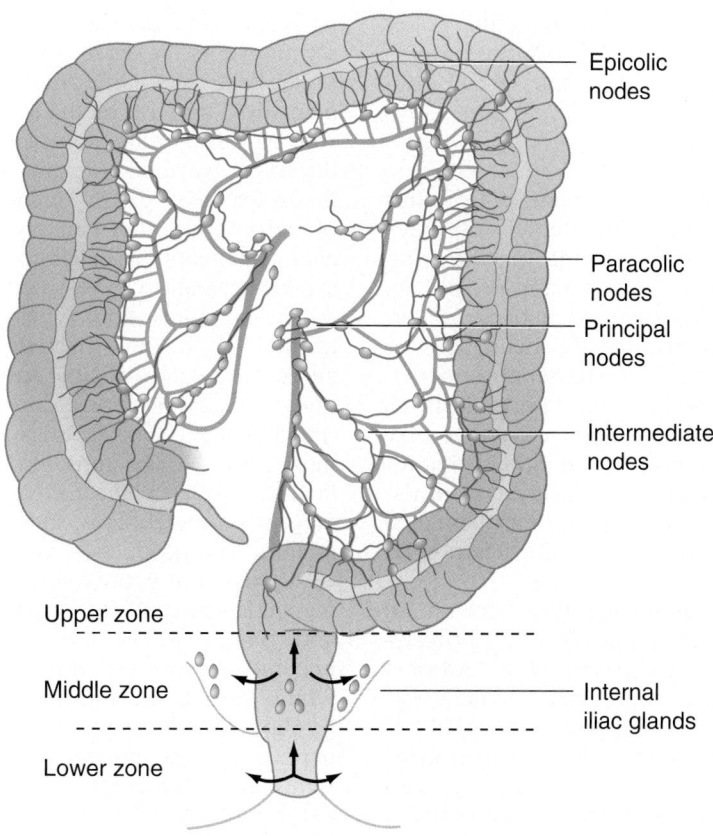

Figure 50-12 Lymphatic drainage of the colon. (From Corman ML [ed]: Colon and Rectal Surgery, 4th ed. Philadelphia, Lippincott-Raven, 1998, p 21.)

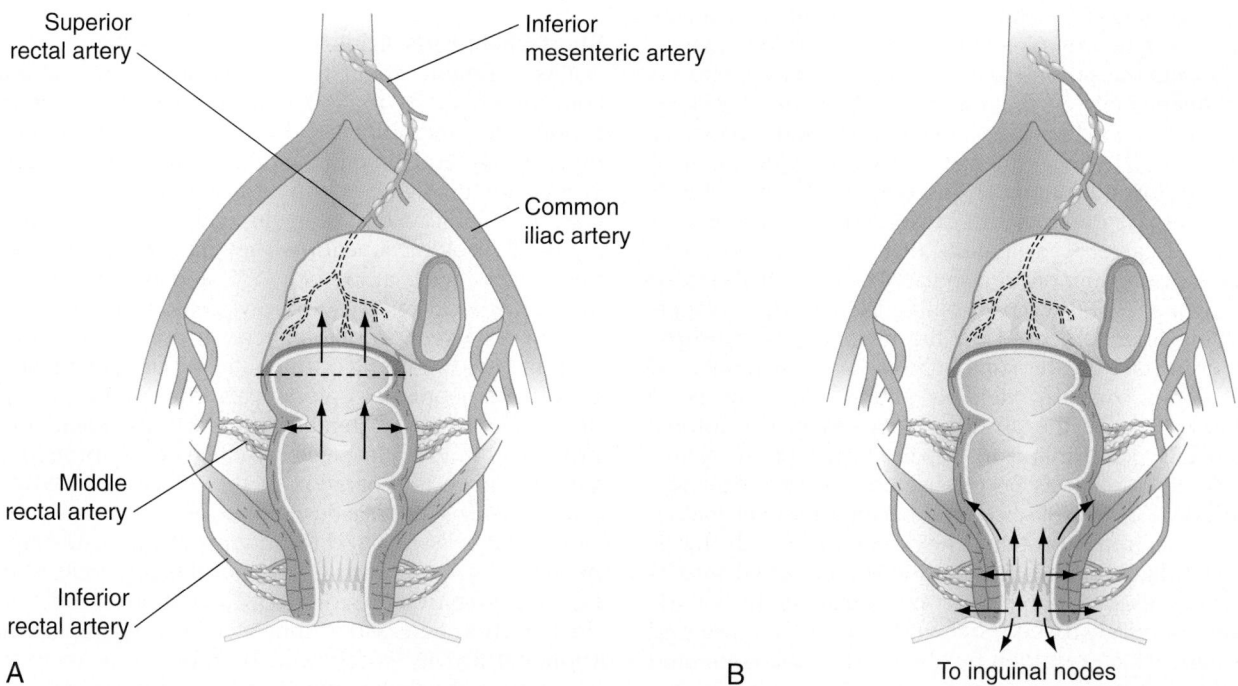

Figure 50-13 Lymphatic drainage of the rectum (**A**) and anal canal (**B**). (From Gordon PH, Nivatvongs S [eds]: Principles and Practice of Surgery for the Colon, Rectum and Anus, 2nd ed. St Louis, Quality Medical Publishing, 1999, p 32.)

Bacteroides species predominate throughout the colon (range, 8.6×10^4 to 1.4×10^7 cfu/sample), composing 66% of total counts from proximal colon and 68.5% from rectum.

Fermentation

Both microbiota and host obtain clear benefits from this association. Although the host provides energy substrates from diet and desquamated cellular debris, together with a relatively stable environment for bacteria to proliferate, bacteria supply the host with *butyrate*, a bacterial fermentation product that has become the main fuel for colonic epithelial cells. Furthermore, bacterial fermentation products are also absorbed and used systemically as a source of energy. One patient population that may benefit from colonic absorption of energy is that of patients with short bowel syndrome. Preservation of the colon in these patients can provide as much as 0.8 megajoule (MJ) per day and reduce carbohydrate excretion by fivefold.

The main sources of energy for intestinal bacteria are complex carbohydrates: starches and nonstarch polysaccharides (NSPs), also known as *dietary fiber*. Carbohydrate metabolism is of great importance in the colon because generically, and in terms of absolute numbers, most cultivable microorganisms are saccharolytic. However, the most complex carbohydrates are degraded in a multistep process by a consortium of bacteria rather than by one specific bacterial species. Although NSPs are the main substrate for bacterial fermentation in the colon, not all types of NSPs are equally fermented. *Lignin* is a noncarbohydrate component of plants that is not fermented by human colonic flora and attracts water, thus producing bulk. *Celluloses*, which are primarily found in leafy vegetables, are only partially fermented, whereas *fruit pectins* are completely fermented by colonic bacteria. Colonic transit time and bulking of stool depend on the fermentability of the various NSPs ingested. Poorly fermented NSPs increase luminal bulk and accelerate transit time. Highly fermentable NSPs provide minimal bulk and slow transit time. Consequently, the type of NSP has an impact on both the cause and the treatment of colonic diseases. Constipation, diverticulosis, and colon cancer are uncommon in populations with a high intake of roughage (i.e., water-insoluble NSPs). Thus, water-insoluble fibers are used for the treatment of constipation. Conversely, water-soluble NSPs are easily fermented by colonic bacteria, yielding short-chain fatty acids (SCFAs). Because the absence of SCFAs in the colonic lumen has been linked to impaired absorption, water-soluble NSPs, such as pectin, are used to treat diarrhea.

In addition to NSPs, colonic bacteria ferment malabsorbed starch and protein. The fraction of starch that is not well digested and absorbed in the upper GI tract is known as resistant starch (RS). In this manner, the caloric content of malabsorbed starch and proteins is transferred to SCFAs, which can then be absorbed by the colon and thereby recovered as a calorie supply. It is estimated that about 10% of the daily energy expenditure of a normal subject is obtained from the absorption of SCFAs by the colon.

In subjects fed a diet high in RS, breath hydrogen and serum SCFAs are increased compared with subjects fed a diet low in RS. Other gases produced by bacterial fermentation are CO_2, methane (CH_4), and nitrogen (N_2), as well as odoriferous sulfur-containing gases. Gases produced by bacterial fermentation compose about 74% of flatus. Excessive gas production from a high consumption of fermentable fiber can produce a feeling of bloating, although bloating is usually more a sign of irritable bowel syndrome than of excessive fiber fermentation.[1]

The amounts and types of fermentation products formed by colonic bacteria depend on the relative amounts of each available substrate, their chemical structures and compositions, and the fermentation strategies (biochemical characteristics and catabolite regulatory mechanisms) of bacteria. Protein fermentation, or putrefaction, results in the formation of a number of potentially toxic metabolites, including phenols, indoles, and amines. The production of these substances is inhibited or repressed in many intestinal microorganisms by a fermentable source of carbohydrate. Because of the anatomy and physiology of the colon, putrefactive processes become quantitatively more important in the distal colon, where carbohydrate is more limiting. The more distal location of colon cancer is probably due to the greater exposure to carcinogens formed by protein putrefaction. Although carbohydrates and proteins entering the colon can be salvaged by bacteria and recycled to the benefit of the host, bacterial metabolism of malabsorbed lipids can be harmful to the host. It has been proposed that lipidic bacterial metabolites can act as detergents in the colon, leading to mucosal injury and reactive hyperproliferation, which in turn can promote tumor development.[2]

Short-Chain Fatty Acids

SCFAs constitute about two thirds of the colonic anion concentration (70 to 130 mmol/L), mainly as acetate, propionate, and butyrate. Besides their action on gut morphology and function, SCFAs influence GI motility. SCFAs are involved in the so-called ileocolonic brake (i.e., the inhibition of gastric emptying by nutrients reaching the ileocolonic junction). They may involve hormonal messengers, such as peptide YY, and neural pathways, as well as local reflexes and myogenic responses.

Butyrate exerts trophic effects on normal colonocytes both in vitro and in vivo. In contrast, butyrate arrests the growth of neoplastic colonocytes and inhibits the preneoplastic hyperproliferation induced by some tumor promoters in vitro. Its selective effects on G-protein activation explain this paradox of the effects of butyrate in normal versus neoplastic colonocytes.[3] Human colonic carcinoma cells exposed to butyrate accumulate simultaneously in G_0 to G_1 and G_2 to M of the cell cycle. During this transition from G_0 to G_1 to G_2 to M arrest, mitochondrial electron transport is enhanced. This change in mitochondrial activity is followed by changes in membrane potential and cellular growth arrest. Butyrate also regulates the expression of molecules involved in colonocyte adhesion. Butyrate-stimulated differentiation inhibits cell proliferation across collagen I, collagen IV, and laminin and decreases β_1-, β_1-, and α_2-integrin subunit surface expression.

Urea Recycling

For many years, urea was thought to be the end product of nitrogen metabolism in humans. This is true in the sense that humans, and mammals in general, do not produce urease. However, colonic bacteria are rich in urease. When urea is labeled with a tracer (radioisotope or heavy isotope) and injected intravenously, 10% of the urea nitrogen is not recovered in urine but rather is incorporated into body protein. Bacteria firmly adherent to the colonic epithelium mediate this process of urea recycling, which produces urease. A low-protein and high-fiber diet such as that of the Papua New Guinea highlanders further increases urea recycling. These individuals ingest only 10 mg of protein per kilogram per day and have normal health with normal muscle mass and serum proteins. Adaptation to this low-protein diet has made the colon very efficient in recycling nitrogen to the point that it may even absorb some essential amino acids (lysine). Urea recycling has been exploited as a therapy for renal failure by excluding nonessential amino acids from the diet to promote maximal urea recycling and diminish the need for dialysis. The one pathologic condition in which urea recycling is not beneficial is liver failure. When the liver cannot reuse the urea nitrogen absorbed by the colon, ammonia crosses the blood-brain barrier and produces false neurotransmitters, which result in hepatic coma.

Absorption

The total absorptive area of the colon is estimated at about 900 cm^2. Between 1000 and 1500 mL of fluid is poured into the cecum by the daily ileal effluent. The total volume of water in stool is only 100 to 150 mL/day. This 10-fold reduction in water across the colon represents the most efficient site of absorption in the GI tract per surface area. The net absorption of sodium is even higher: Although the ileal effluent contains 200 mEq/L of sodium, stool contains only 25 to 50 mEq/L. One major difference between sodium and water absorption in the colon is that although water is absorbed passively, sodium requires active transport. Sodium is transported against chemical and electrical gradients at the expense of energy consumption.

The colonic epithelium can use various fuels; however, *n*-butyrate is oxidized in preference to glutamine, glucose, or ketone bodies. Because mammalian cells do not produce *n*-butyrate, the colonic epithelium relies on luminal bacteria to produce it through the fermentation of dietary fiber. The lack of *n*-butyrate, such as that resulting from the inhibition of fermentation by broad-spectrum antibiotics, leads to less sodium and water absorption and, thus, diarrhea. Conversely, the perfusion of the colonic lumen with *n*-butyrate stimulates sodium and water absorption. *n*-Butyrate, acetate, and propionate are SCFAs produced through bacterial fermentation; these constitute the main anions in stool. Other physiologic effects of SCFAs on the colon include stimulation of

blood flow, mucosal cell renewal, and regulation of intraluminal pH for homeostasis of the bacterial flora.

In addition to recovering sodium and water, the colonic mucosa absorbs bile acids. The colon absorbs bile acids that escape absorption by the terminal ileum, thus making the colon part of the enterohepatic circulation. Bile acids are passively transported across the colonic epithelium by nonionic diffusion. When the colonic absorptive capacity is exceeded, colonic bacteria deconjugate bile acids. Deconjugated bile acids can then interfere with sodium and water absorption, leading to secretory, or choleretic, diarrhea. Choleretic diarrhea is seen early after right hemicolectomy as a transient phenomenon and more permanently after extensive ileal resection.

Secretion

The physiologic role of colon secretion is demonstrated in patients with chronic renal failure. Uremic patients can remain normokalemic while ingesting a normal amount of potassium before requiring dialysis. This phenomenon is associated with a compensatory increase in colonic secretion and fecal excretion of potassium. This effect is blocked by spironolactone, which illustrates the effect of aldosterone on colonic potassium secretion. Potassium secretion requires both Na^+, K^+ ATPase and Na^+, K^+ 2Cl cotransport on the basolateral membrane and an apical potassium channel.

Many forms of colitis are associated with increased potassium secretion, such as inflammatory bowel disease (IBD), cholera, and shigellosis. In addition, some forms of colitis impair colonic absorption or produce secretion of chloride; examples are collagenous and microscopic colitis and congenital chloridorrhea. Chloride is secreted by colonic epithelium at a basal rate, which is increased in pathologic conditions such as cystic fibrosis and secretory diarrhea. Secretion of chloride also requires the coupling of Na^+, K^+ ATPase and Na^+, K^+ 2Cl cotransport to exit passively through the apical membrane. Calcium and cyclic adenosine monophosphate both stimulate chloride secretion, whereas bicarbonate and SCFAs inhibit chloride secretion.

Colonic secretion of H^+ and bicarbonate is coupled to the absorption of Na^+ and Cl, respectively. It is through these exchangers that the colon is linked to systemic acid-base metabolism. The supply of H^+ and bicarbonate for these exchangers is maintained by the hydration of CO_2 catalyzed by colonic carbonic anhydrase. Changes in systemic pH induce changes in the activity of carbonic anhydrase eliciting elimination of H^+ or bicarbonate as needed to bring systemic pH back to normal.

Motility

Fermentation in the colon is made possible by its distinctive morphology. The colon can be divided into three anatomic segments: the right colon, the left colon, and the rectum. The right colon is the fermentation chamber of the human GI tract, with the cecum being the colonic segment where bacteria are most metabolically active. The left colon is a site of storage and dehydration of stool. Colonic transit rate is a determinant of stool SCFA concentration, including butyrate, and of distal colonic pH. This may explain the interrelations among colonic cancer, dietary fiber intake, stool elimination, and stool pH.[4] Transit through the colon is controlled by the autonomic nervous system. Parasympathetic nervous fibers supply the colon through the vagi and the pelvic nerves. Nerve fibers reaching the colon arrange themselves in several plexuses: the subserosal, myenteric (Auerbach), submucosal (Meissner), and mucosal plexuses. The neurons of the myenteric plexus concentrate along the taeniae but are sparse between them, where the longitudinal muscle layer is thin. Sympathetic nerve fibers originate in the superior and inferior mesenteric ganglia and reach the colon by way of perivascular plexuses.

The motility pattern is different in the three anatomic segments. In the right colon, antiperistaltic, or retropulsive, waves generate retrograde flow of colonic contents back to the cecum. In the left colon, contents are propelled caudad by tonic contractions, separating them into a series of globular masses. A third type of contraction, called *mass peristalsis,* is interspersed with the propulsive and retropulsive contractions and occurs at varying intervals, more frequently after meals. Each mass peristaltic contraction is able to advance a column of colonic contents through one third of the colonic length.

The colon responds to the ingestion of a meal with an increase in the number of migrating and nonmigrating long spike bursts of potentials peaking at 15 minutes after the meal.[5] This increase in electrical activity is followed by an increase in colonic tone. The increased postprandial contractility is greater in the sigmoid than in the transverse colon. The effects of a meal on colonic motility are commonly called the *gastrocolic reflex.*

Formation of Stool

The frequency of defecation is just as variable among individuals as is their perception of abnormal stool frequency. An individual who passes more than three loose stools per day is considered as having diarrhea, whereas fewer than three weekly stools is considered constipation. Any frequency within that range is considered normal, although many individuals will still seek medical attention for what they perceive as either diarrhea or constipation. Many factors influence colonic transit rate. Colonic transit is longer in women than in men and longer in premenopausal women than postmenopausal women. Conversely, colonic transit is shortened in smokers. In normal subjects, supplementation with NSPs does not shorten colonic transit time, although it does increase fecal weight. In patients with idiopathic constipation, however, NSPs, in the form of psyllium seeds, shorten colonic transit and increase stool weight.[6]

Defecation

Normal defecation requires adequate colonic transit time, stool consistency, and fecal continence. Fecal continence implies deferment of stool elimination; discrimination among gas, liquid, and solid stool; and selective elimination of gas without stool. There is some controversy regarding the actual role of the rectum under resting conditions. Some propose that the rectum is simply a conduit, which under resting conditions should be empty. If stool arrives at the rectum, the anorectal inhibitory reflex is triggered, forcing the subject to hold defecation by voluntary contraction of the external sphincter. However, any surgeon who performs routine rigid proctosigmoidoscopies in the office is well aware that a patient can have a rectum full of stool without any awareness. This leads to the opposing view, which regards the rectum as a reservoir. Just as stool triggers the anorectal inhibitory reflex, it also triggers a rectocolic reflex. This reflex allows continuous filling of the rectum with fecal material until the colon is emptied.

The mechanisms involved in fecal continence are not fully understood. A certain reservoir capacity is needed to achieve fecal continence. A stiff, nondistensible rectum such as in radiation proctitis may produce incontinence even when the sphincter muscles are competent. Some of the internal and external sphincter muscle fibers are necessary for adequate continence, although many patients have part of the sphincter severed during a fistulotomy and are still continent. Probably, the only factor certainly needed for fecal continence is innervation of the sphincter. Not only the motor nerve fibers, which produce contraction of the sphincter fibers, but also all of the sensory innervation are important to adequately empty the rectum.

BOWEL PREPARATION BEFORE SURGERY

Purging the feces and reducing the concentration of colonic intraluminal bacteria before operations on the colon have long been basic tenets of surgery. The normal, or autochthonous, microbial organisms in the colon compose up to 90% of the dry weight of feces, reaching concentrations up to 10^9 organism/mL of feces. The anaerobic *Bacteroides* is the most common colonic microbe, whereas *Escherichia coli* is the most common aerobe. *Pseudomonas, Enterococcus, Proteus, Klebsiella,* and *Streptococcus* species are also present in large numbers.

The process of preparing the colon for an elective operation has traditionally involved two factors: purging the fecal contents (mechanical preparation) and administration of antibiotics effective against colonic bacteria. Tradition has held that an unprepared colon (i.e., one that contains intraluminal feces) poses an unacceptably high rate of failure of the anastomosis to heal. However, recent experience with primary repair of colonic injuries by trauma surgeons, along with reports from European surgeons describing elective operations conducted safely without the use of preoperative purging, have caused reconsideration concerning the true value of purging the colon before colonic surgery. Because the colonocytes receive nutrition from intraluminal free fatty acids produced by fermentation from colonic bacteria, there are concerns that purging may actually be detrimental to the healing of a colonic anastomosis. However, in the United States at the present time, the colon is generally cleansed in preparation for colonic operations. Effective cleansing is mandatory for adequate colonoscopy or contrast enema.

Although the use of preoperative parenteral antibiotics is well accepted and validated, the related issue of preoperative oral antibiotic use is controversial. A multiplicity of bowel preparation regimens and antibiotic combinations are in current use. A clear superiority of one above another is not present; however, for some patients, certain bowel preparations may have adverse physiologic consequences. Knowledge of the history of bowel preparation practices, current controversies, and data is useful.

Mechanical bowel cleansing methods are used for both colonoscopy and elective surgery. Complete bowel obstruction and free perforation are absolute contraindications to bowel preparation. For colonoscopy, properties of various preparations are judged by safety, patient tolerance, and efficacy or preparation quality. In the past, 4 to 5 days of clear liquids along with laxatives such as senna, castor oil, and bisacodyl; whole bowel nasogastric irrigation; mannitol irrigation; and repeated enemas were among the regimens used. Patient tolerance of these methods is poor, associated with dehydration, electrolyte abnormalities, and severe abdominal cramping, and are generally not well tolerated by elderly or infirm patients.

In the 1980s, polyethylene glycol solution (PEG), a nonabsorbed sodium sulfate–based liquid, was developed as an oral mechanical bowel preparation. Patients are required to drink at least 2 to 4 liters of the solution along with additional fluids. Abdominal cramping, nausea, and vomiting are common side effects of the preparation, and prophylactic antiemetics are often routinely administered. Sodium phosphate solution (Fleet's Phosphosoda) was developed in response to patient dissatisfaction with the large fluid volume required for PEG preparation and has been found in most trials to be a more tolerable preparation with higher rates of patient satisfaction and compliance. The smaller volume (45 mL taken twice) seems to be the main benefit because the side effects are similar. Sodium phosphate pills (Visicol) were recently introduced as an alternative to liquids. The regimen consists of ingesting a total of 40 pills, with 3 pills taken every 15 minutes with 8 oz of fluid. Sodium phosphate, whether in liquid or pill form, has been linked more frequently than PEG to rare, but serious, electrolyte imbalances. In patients with impaired renal function, hyperphosphatemia, hypernatremia, hypokalemia, and hypocalcemia can occur. For this reason, PEG is the recommended bowel preparation in patients with renal insufficiency, cirrhosis, ascites, or congestive heart failure. Investigation comparing efficacy of mechanical bowel preparation has focused on comparisons between PEG and sodium phosphate solutions.

Cohen and colleagues demonstrated a 90% "excellent" or "good" bowel preparation with sodium phosphate versus 70% with 4 L PEG.[7] Frommer found that sodium phosphate results in a cleaner bowel than PEG with no difference in infectious complications.[8] On the other hand, Poon and colleagues found that there was no difference in bowel cleanliness when the volume of PEG was reduced to 2 liters and compared with 90 mL of sodium phosphate, and that the reduced volume enhanced patient compliance.[9] A Canadian study found the use of sodium phosphate to be associated with increased patient compliance and an eight-fold cost reduction when compared with PEG.[10] Ultimately, patient comfort and economic factors may determine mechanical bowel preparation practices if efficacy is similar.

For patients undergoing colonoscopy, the quality of the bowel preparation is essential for obtaining an accurate exam. For segmental resections, however, the necessity of mechanical bowel preparation has come under scrutiny. A study comparing infectious complications in mechanically prepared bowel (PEG solution) versus unprepared bowel in patients undergoing segmental resection failed to reveal differences in any type of infectious complication.[11] Both groups received parenteral antibiotics. Zmora and associates looked at left-sided anastomoses only and found that there was no significant difference between overall infection rates in unprepared (13.2%) versus prepared bowel (12.5%).[12] The wound infection rates in this study did not significantly differ either, at 6.6% in the prepared group and 10% in the unprepared group. Although studies of this type have been relatively small and significantly underpowered, they point to the future possibility of avoiding the discomfort of bowel preparation and the small attendant risk for electrolyte irregularities and dehydration.

Antibiotic use in colorectal surgery is a well-established practice that reduces infectious complications. Elective colorectal cases are classified as clean-contaminated and, as such, benefit from routine single-dose administration of parenteral antibiotics 30 minutes before incision. There is evidence to show that when operative times are prolonged, additional doses at 4-hour intervals reduce wound infection. When the operation is completed, postoperative administration of antibiotics for a clean-contaminated case such as a routine segmental resection does not further reduce infectious complications and may promote *Clostridium difficile* colitis, *Candida* infection, and the emergence of bacterial antibiotic resistance. Polk and Lopez-Mayer showed a reduction in postoperative infection rates from 30% to 8% with the routine use of preoperative parenteral antibiotics.[13] Gomez-Alonzo and colleagues repeated these results, showing a drop from 39% to 9%.[14] Antibiotics active against both aerobes and anaerobes are ideal: second- or third-generation cephalosporins alone, or combination of a fluoroquinolone plus metronidazole or clindamycin is typical. The use of additional oral antibiotics to theoretically further reduce the bacterial load is widely accepted, but not as well validated. In a survey of colon and rectal surgeons, 87% indicated that both oral and parenteral antibiotic usage is part of their routine preparation for elective colon operations.[15] A preparation often used consists of erythromycin base (1 g) and neomycin (1 g) given in three preoperative doses the day before surgery. However, this regimen is associated with a high incidence of nausea and abdominal cramps, and some surgeons prefer to prescribe oral ciprofloxacin or metronidazole.

In studies comparing oral and parenteral antibiotics, a decrease in wound infection rate from 36% to 6.5% was seen with intravenous administration, whereas others comparing a combination of oral plus parenteral antibiotics, versus oral alone, found that the addition of intravenous antibiotics reduced infectious complications by half (22% to 11%). It is notable that there have been no prospective randomized trials examining this issue and that most retrospective reviews are poorly powered. Although it is clear that preoperative parenteral antibiotics reduce wound infection rates, oral antibiotics do not clearly benefit the patient either by reducing wound infection or by decreasing intra-abdominal abscess or leaks. The rate of intra-abdominal abscess is more dependent on technical factors affecting anastomotic integrity than on antibiotic prophylaxis.

DIVERTICULAR DISEASE

A diverticulum is an abnormal sac or pouch protruding from the wall of a hollow organ, which is, for the purposes of this discussion, the colon. A *true diverticulum* is composed of all layers of the intestinal wall, whereas a *false diverticulum,* or *pseudodiverticulum,* lacks a portion of the normal bowel wall. The diverticula that commonly occur in the human colon are protrusions of mucosa through the muscular layers of the intestine. Because these mucosal herniations are devoid of the normal muscular layers, they are pseudodiverticula (Fig. 50-14).

Diverticulosis and *diverticular disease* are terms used to indicate the presence of colonic diverticula. Diverticulosis is a common condition of Western society and seems to be an unfortunate product of the Industrial Revolution. It is interesting that there seem to be no specimens of colonic diverticulosis in anatomic or medical museums in Europe that were archived before the Industrial Revolution. The process of roller-milling wheat flour was introduced in Europe about a quarter of a century earlier than the appearance of diverticulosis, which was initially observed in the first decade of the 20th century. It has been postulated that the decreased consumption of unprocessed cereals and the increased consumption of sugar and meat by the general population are factors largely responsible for the appearance of diverticulosis. During the past 75 years, the amount of fiber consumed by individuals in North America and Western Europe has decreased, whereas the prevalence of diverticulosis has increased significantly. The formation of diverticula is also related to aging. Diverticula are rare in individuals younger than 30 years, but at least two thirds of Americans will have developed colonic diverticula by the age of 80 years.

Further evidence that a diet low in fiber and high in carbohydrates and meat contributes to the incidence of diverticulosis is the observation that diverticulosis is rare in sub-Saharan African blacks who consume a high-fiber diet; however, blacks in Johannesburg who consume a low-fiber diet have the same incidence of diverticulosis as South African whites.

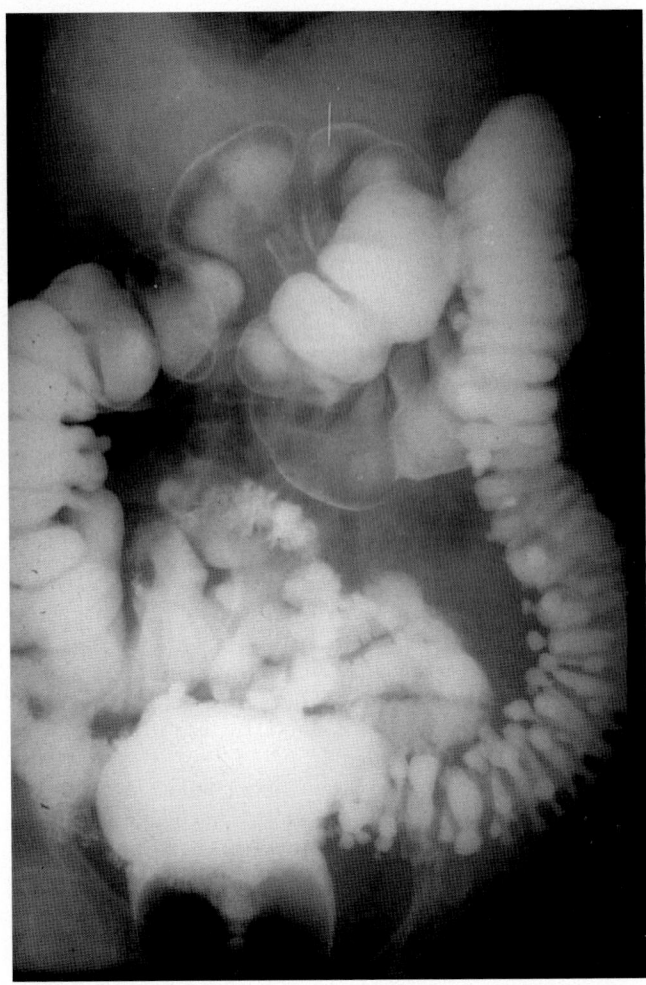

Figure 50-14 Barium enema with extensive sigmoid diverticulosis.

Pathogenesis

Diverticula are actually herniations of mucosa through the colon at sites of penetration of the muscular wall by arterioles. These sites are on the mesenteric side of the antimesenteric taeniae. In some cases, the arteriole penetrating the wall can be displaced over the dome of the diverticulum. This close relationship between the artery and diverticulum is responsible for the massive hemorrhage that occasionally can complicate diverticulosis (Fig. 50-15).

There is often a striking hypertrophy of the muscular layers of the colonic wall associated with diverticulosis. This thickening of the colonic wall, most commonly affecting the sigmoid colon, may precede the appearance of diverticula. Diverticula most commonly affect the sigmoid colon and are confined to the sigmoid in about half of patients with diverticulosis. The next most common area involved is the descending colon (~40% of affected individuals), and the entire colon has diverticula in 5% to 10% of patients with diverticulosis. Even in patients with diverticula involving the entire colon, the muscular thickening characteristic of the disease is usually confined to the sigmoid (Fig. 50-16).

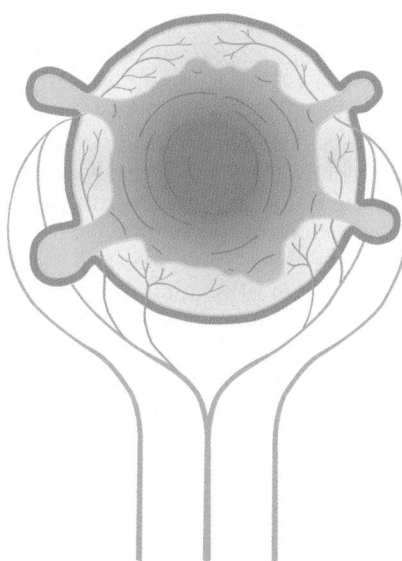

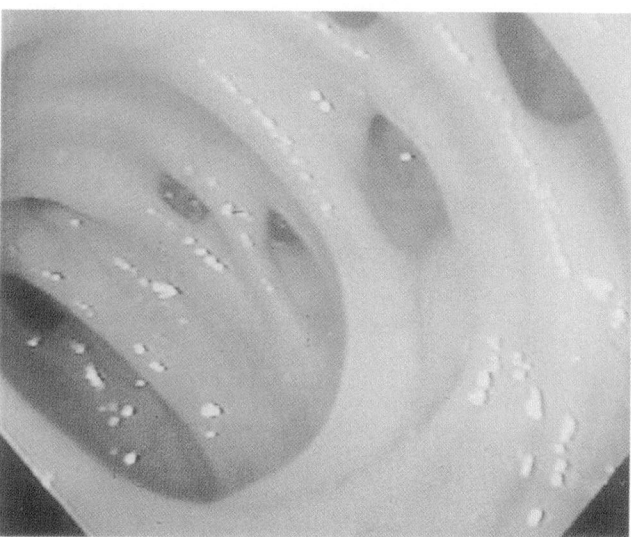

Figure 50-16 Colonoscopic view of diverticula.

Figure 50-15 Pathogenesis of diverticular disease. Diverticula are herniations of the mucosa through the points of entry of blood vessels across the muscular wall. Because the diverticula are formed only by the mucosa rather than by the entire wall of the intestine, they are called *false diverticula*. Note that the diverticula form only between the mesenteric taenia and each of the two lateral taeniae. Because there are no perforating vessels, diverticula do not form on the antimesenteric side of the colon.

The sigmoid colon, the most common site of diverticula formation, is also the segment of colon with the smallest luminal diameter. If the colonic lumen contains a large volume of fiber, the contractile pressure required to propel the feces forward is low. In such circumstances, the colonic pressure in the sigmoid is only slightly above atmospheric pressure. However, with the decreased amount of fiber provided by today's typical dietary regimens, there is decreased colonic luminal content requiring generation of increased colonic pressures to propel the feces forward. Colonic pressures as high as 90 mm Hg can be generated by contraction of the narrow sigmoid colon. These high intraluminal pressures are thought to be responsible for the herniations of mucosa through the anatomically weak points in the colonic wall.

Diverticulitis

Diverticulitis is the result of a perforation of a colonic diverticulum. The term is somewhat of a misnomer because the disease is actually an extraluminal pericolic infection caused by the extravasation of feces through the perforated diverticulum. *Peridiverticulitis* would actually be the term to more appropriately describe the infectious process. Recognition that the infection is actually caused by a perforation of the colon, an event that is often controlled by the body's natural defenses, provides a basis for understanding the signs and symptoms of the disease as well as the rationale for determining appropriate diagnostic tests and treatment.

The sigmoid colon is the segment of large bowel with the highest incidence of diverticula, and it is by far the

most frequent site for involvement with diverticulitis. Patients with diverticulitis usually complain of left lower quadrant abdominal, pain which my radiate to the suprapubic area, left groin, or back. Alteration in bowel habit is a very common complaint, and fever, chills, and urinary urgency are common. This is an infectious, inflammatory process, and rectal bleeding is not usually associated with an attack of diverticulitis.

The physical findings are dependent on the site of perforation, the amount of contamination, and the presence or absence of secondary infection of adjacent organs. The most common physical finding is tenderness of the left lower abdomen. There may be voluntary guarding of the left abdominal musculature, and a tender mass in the left lower abdomen is suggestive of a phlegmon or abscess. Abdominal wall distention may be detected if there is associated ileus or small bowel obstruction secondary to the inflammatory process. A rectal or vaginal examination may reveal a tender fluctuant mass typical of a pelvic abscess.

Sigmoid diverticulitis should be distinguished from cancer of the rectosigmoid, although it is seldom necessary to establish the distinction on an emergency basis. However, the surgical approach to diverticulitis is significantly different than that required for a perforated sigmoid cancer, and if urgent operation is indicated, an effort should be made to exclude the diagnosis of cancer. A limited sigmoidoscopic examination may at times be helpful in such circumstances. However, air should not be insufflated through the endoscope because of distention of the colon and the possibility that increased colonic pressure could force more bacteria through the perforation into the peritoneal cavity. The sigmoidoscope can seldom be advanced beyond 12 cm in a patient with diverticulitis, and the exam is usually only useful to exclude a cancer of the rectum as a cause of the symptoms.

The diagnosis of diverticulitis can often be presumed with a fair degree of reliability by a careful history and

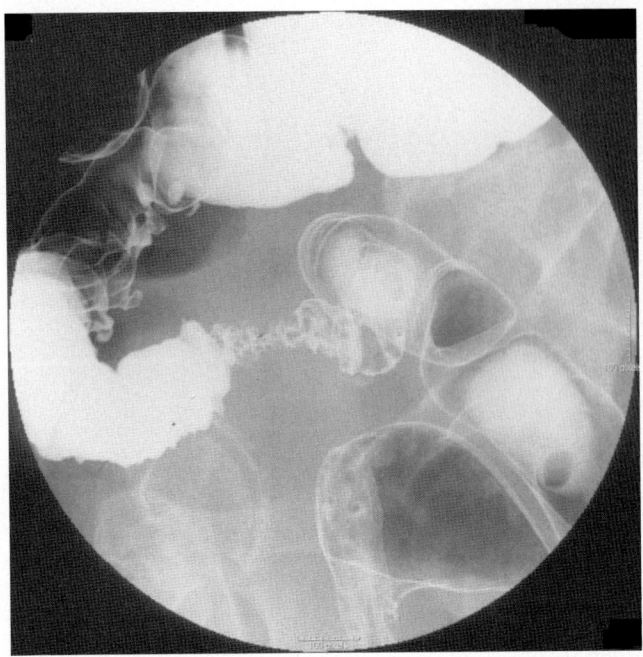

Figure 50-17 Barium enema in a patient with a previous attack of diverticulitis. Note stricture in sigmoid colon. Colonoscopy was necessary to exclude cancer.

physical examination, and it is reasonable to begin treatment with antibiotics on this evidence alone. However, if the diagnosis is in doubt, four diagnostic tests can be considered: computed tomography (CT) of the abdomen, magnetic resonance imaging (MRI), abdominal ultrasound, and water-soluble contrast enema. CT and MRI provide essentially the same information and advantages. There has been more experience with CT, and this is considered by most surgeons to be the preferred test to confirm the suspected diagnosis of diverticulitis. It reliably reveals the location of the infection, the extent of the inflammatory process, the presence and location of an abscess, and the sympathetic involvement of other organs, with secondary complications such as ureteral obstruction or a fistula to the bladder. In addition, an abscess detected by CT may often be drained by a percutaneous approach with the aid of CT guidance.

Ultrasound of the abdomen offers many of the advantages of CT, including the possibility of percutaneous drainage of an abscess with ultrasound guidance. The selection among CT, MRI, and ultrasound examinations varies considerably among institutions, but all three techniques have been shown to be useful in establishing the diagnosis of diverticulitis, especially when an abscess has complicated the disease.

The use of a contrast enema in the evaluation of a patient suspected of having diverticulitis has diminished considerably because of the advantages offered by the noninvasive tests described previously. An enema carries the risk for increasing the colonic pressure and causing further extravasation of feces through the perforated diverticulum. Some studies have shown an advantage of the contrast enema in distinguishing acute diverticulitis

from perforated cancer, but many surgeons believe the risk associated with a contrast enema outweighs the potential gain. If a contrast enema is used, the contrast should be water soluble. Water-soluble contrast enemas do not carry the risk for barium-fecal peritonitis, but there is still a considerable risk for extravasation of contrast material from the colon that may aggravate the infection and spread the extent of the peritonitis.

Diverticulitis obviously presents in a variety of ways with a broad spectrum of severity, from a single episode of mild self-limited disease, to repeated episodes that respond to antibiotics, to fulminant complicated disease characterized by life-threatening sepsis. Hinchey and associates[16] described a practical classification system that provides some organization of the broad clinical spectrum of the disease:

- Stage I: pericolic or mesenteric abscess
- Stage II: walled-off pelvic abscess
- Stage III: generalized purulent peritonitis
- Stage IV: generalized fecal peritonitis

Appropriate treatment obviously must be individualized based on the severity of the disease.

Uncomplicated Diverticulitis

Uncomplicated diverticulitis (disease not associated with free intraperitoneal perforation, fistula formation, or obstruction) can often be treated with antibiotics on an outpatient basis. If the patient has significant pain characteristic of localized peritonitis, hospitalization and intravenous antibiotics are indicated. The use of morphine should be avoided because of the increased intracolonic pressure associated with that drug; meperidine has been reported to decrease intraluminal pressure and is a more appropriate analgesic.

Patients with uncomplicated diverticulitis usually respond promptly to antibiotic treatment, with marked improvement in symptoms within 48 hours. After the symptoms have subsided for at least 3 weeks, investigative studies should be conducted to establish the presence of diverticula and to exclude cancer, which can mimic diverticulitis. The preferred test is a colonoscopic examination, which can directly visualize the colonic lumen even in the presence of numerous diverticula. A barium enema can demonstrate the extent of the diverticular disease, but a sigmoid cancer may be hidden by the numerous contrast-filled diverticula of the sigmoid colon, a fact that considerably diminishes the value of the contrast enema in the evaluation of the patient with diverticulosis (Fig. 50-17).

A first attack of uncomplicated diverticulitis that responds to antibiotic therapy is generally treated nonoperatively, with the introduction of a high-fiber diet. A recent population-based study demonstrated that only a small percentage (5.5%) of patients who recovered from an initial episode of uncomplicated diverticulitis required subsequent emergency colectomy or colostomy.[17] The chances of a second attack of diverticulitis are relatively low, less than 25%. The management of patients younger than 45 years affected by an attack of uncomplicated diverticulitis is somewhat controversial. Many surgeons have recommended an elective sigmoidectomy following recovery in young patients because the natural history of diverticulitis in the young is not well understood, and there may be a high risk for recurrence of the disease over the expected long life span. However, Vignati and colleagues studied 40 patients younger than 50 years who were hospitalized with diverticulitis and followed for up to 9 years.[18] Two thirds of these patients did not require surgery during the follow-up period. These results are similar to the expectations for patients older than 50 years, and the authors concluded that younger patients should be treated in the same manner as patients whose first attack of diverticulitis occurs after the age of 50 years.

If a patient suffers recurrent attacks of diverticulitis, surgical treatment should be considered. It has generally been recommended that sigmoidectomy be offered after two uncomplicated attacks of diverticulitis to prevent a future complicated episode that would require emergency operation or a colostomy. However, recent studies have thrown some doubt on this concept. It appears that the need for a colostomy to be fashioned is highest with the first attack of diverticulitis, and the recommendation that sigmoidectomy be offered after two attacks on the basis of avoiding a colostomy in the future has to be reconsidered in light of recent evidence. Chapman and associates found that patients with more than two episodes of diverticulitis are not at increased risk for poor outcomes if they should subsequently develop complicated diverticulitis, and that morbidity and mortality were not significantly different between patients with multiple episodes of diverticulitis compared with those suffering only one or two prior attacks.[19] Salem and colleagues determined that performing colectomy after the fourth episode of diverticulitis, rather than after the second episode, in patients older than 50 years resulted in 0.5% fewer deaths, 0.7% fewer colostomies, and a reduction in cost per patient.[20] The recommendation for sigmoidectomy because of recurrent attacks of diverticulitis obviously needs to consider the patient's overall health and lifestyle, frequency of the attacks, and debility associated with each attack.

Diverticulitis in the immunocompromised host represents a special challenge for the surgeon. Selective sigmoidectomy after a single attack of diverticulitis should be considered in such patients because of their diminished ability to combat an infectious insult. There is some suggestion that medical therapy is less effective in these patients, resulting in an increased incidence of emergent surgery. Unfortunately, mortality rates after surgery are higher than those in patients whose immune system is not compromised.

A growing trend in elective surgery for diverticular disease has been the utilization of a laparoscopic approach. Most studies reveal a hospital length of stay 2 to 3 days shorter for patients undergoing sigmoidectomy by a laparoscopic approach when compared with patients receiving a standard midline incision. A hand-assisted laparoscopic has been advocated by some surgeons, who believe this technique facilitates the division of fused tissue planes and the blunt disruption of fistula tracts.

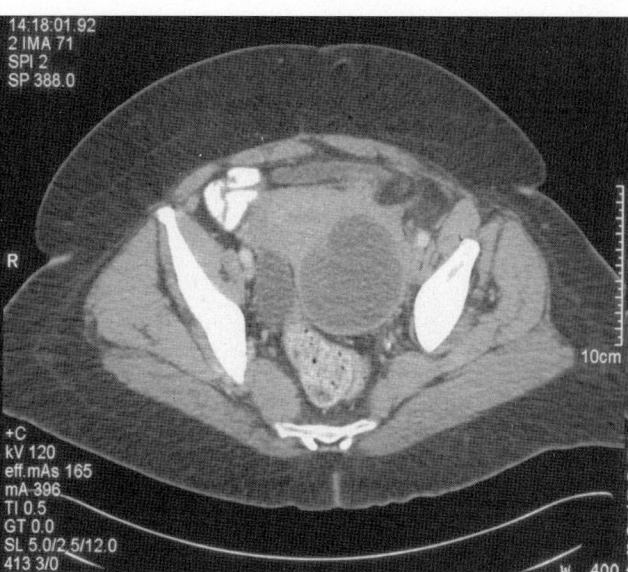

Figure 50-18 Computed tomography scan of pelvis showing diverticulitis with abscess.

Complicated Diverticulitis

Abscess

As discussed earlier, an abscess complicating diverticulitis is usually confined to the pelvis. Typically, patients with pelvic abscesses caused by diverticulitis have significant pain, fever, and leukocytosis. The abdominal, pelvic, or rectal examination may detect a tender, fluctuant mass, and a CT scan, MRI, or ultrasound will confirm the diagnosis and location of the abscess. Unless the abscess is small (<2 cm in diameter), it should be drained, and the preferred method of drainage is a percutaneous route guided by CT or ultrasound. Occasionally, a pelvic abscess can be drained into the rectum through a transanal approach. These methods of drainage are highly preferable to a transabdominal approach by laparotomy, which risks spreading the contents of the abscess throughout the peritoneal cavity (Fig. 50-18).

Adequate drainage of the abscess, accompanied by administration of intravenous antibiotics, usually results in a rapid clinical improvement. Although a fistula may result from the sigmoid colon to the insertion site of the percutaneous catheter that provided drainage, this can be easily handled at the time of elective surgery when the intense intra-abdominal infection has subsided.

Elective surgery should be offered after the patient has completely recovered from the infection, usually about 6 weeks after drainage of the abscess. At that time, it is usually feasible to excise the diseased sigmoid colon and fashion an anastomosis between the descending colon and rectum, thus avoiding a colostomy. It is essential to remove all the colon that is abnormally thickened and to incorporate rectum that is not inflamed or thickened into the distal component of the anastomosis. A major cause of recurrent diverticulitis after sigmoidectomy is failure to completely remove the entire abnormally thickened bowel that is associated with this disease. If the distal

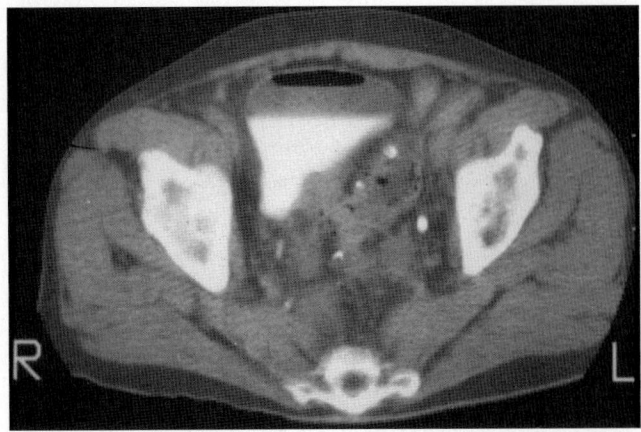

Figure 50-19 Computed tomography scan of pelvis. The patient has diverticulitis, and air in the bladder indicates a fistula between the sigmoid and the bladder.

sigmoid colon is not resected, the rate of recurrent diverticulitis is unnecessarily elevated. Benn and coworkers found the rate of recurrent diverticulitis to be 12% if the distal sigmoid was not resected, compared with 6% if the anastomosis was to the top of the rectum.[21] It is seldom necessary to mobilize the rectum further than 2 cm below the sacral promontory to obtain normal bowel for a satisfactory anastomosis. Although diverticula may be present throughout the colon, it is not necessary to excise the entire colon in such circumstances; only the colon that is thickened and brittle (usually the entire sigmoid) needs to be resected.

Fistula

A fistula between the sigmoid colon and the skin (which may result from percutaneous drainage of an abscess), bladder, vagina, or small bowel is a relatively frequent complication of diverticulitis. Such a fistula commonly forms when an abscess is either drained or necrotizes into an adjacent organ or onto the skin. The source of the infection (the perforated diverticulum) continues to supply the fistula, and cure will not be achieved until the source is eradicated by excising the diseased sigmoid colon. Diverticulitis is a more common cause of a fistula between the colon and bladder than is Crohn's disease or cancer. Sigmoid-vesical fistulas are more common in men than women because the uterus prevents the sigmoid from adhering to the bladder in women. Women with sigmoid fistulas have usually had a prior hysterectomy.

Symptoms of a sigmoid-vesical fistula include pneumaturia (passage of air from the urethra classically noted at the end of micturition), fecaluria, and recurring urinary tract infections. The fistula may cause significant urosepsis in men, with prostatic hypertrophy causing a relative obstruction of the distal urinary tract. The most reliable test to confirm the suspicion of a fistula between the intestine and the bladder is a CT scan, which may demonstrate air in the bladder (Fig. 50-19). A barium enema will fail to reveal a fistula half of the time, and an intravenous pyelogram is even less accurate. Cystoscopy usually reveals cystitis and bullous edema at the site of

the fistula, but the test is helpful to exclude cancer (colon or bladder) as the cause of the fistula.

Initial treatment of any fistula caused by diverticulitis is to control the infection and reduce the associated inflammation. A fistula arising from the colon is rarely a cause for emergency surgery; in fact, the patient's condition is often improved when the abscess fistulizes and drains. Antibiotics should be administered to reduce the adjacent cellulitis, and diagnostic steps should be taken to confirm the cause of the fistula before a definitive operation is undertaken. A colonoscopy should be done to examine the sigmoid mucosa and exclude colon cancer (or Crohn's disease) as the cause of the fistula. Every effort should be made to rule out cancer because the operation for a sigmoid-vesical fistula secondary to sigmoid cancer requires en bloc excision of the involved organs, a more extensive operation than is required to interrupt the nonmalignant fistula and excise the diseased (but benign) sigmoid colon.

Fistulas caused by diverticulitis can usually be treated by a one-stage operation, taking down the fistula and excising the sigmoid colon, then fashioning an anastomosis between the descending colon and the rectum. The secondary organs involved (usually the bladder) will heal once the source of the infection, the sigmoid colon, is removed. The bladder defect is usually so small that no closure is necessary, and healing will occur if the bladder is drained with a Foley catheter or suprapubic cystostomy for 7 days after the operation. Larger bladder openings may require suture closure with absorbable (chromic) sutures combined with drainage. If there is significant inflammation in the abdomen and pelvis, despite a so-called cooling-off period, the use of ureteral stents placed preoperatively can facilitate identification of the ureters and minimize inadvertent ureteral injury. A technique of early identification of the ureter and proximal-to-distal dissection of the sigmoid colon facilitates the resection when a phlegmon caused by diverticulitis obliterates the normal anatomy.

Generalized Peritonitis

Generalized peritonitis resulting from diverticulitis can have two causes: (1) a diverticulum perforates into the peritoneal cavity, and the perforation is not sealed by the body's normal defenses, or (2) an abscess that is initially localized expands and suddenly bursts into the unprotected peritoneal cavity. In the former instance, the peritoneal cavity is contaminated with feces; in the latter, contamination is from pus containing enteric bacteria. In either situation, the result is an overwhelming infection that requires immediate operative intervention. Fortunately, both of these circumstances are relatively rare.

Patients with generalized peritonitis caused by a perforated diverticulum exhibit diffuse abdominal tenderness, with voluntary and involuntary guarding over the entire abdomen. Abdominal radiographs or CT scans may reveal intraperitoneal free air, but the absence of extraintestinal air does not exclude the diagnosis. Signs of generalized sepsis include an elevated white blood count, fever, tachycardia, and hypotension. Immediate celiotomy is mandatory to identify and excise the segment of colon containing the perforation. Under such circumstances, it is not safe to restore intestinal continuity because of the high likelihood that an intestinal anastomosis will not heal when fashioned in such a hostile infectious environment. The proper operation in this situation is to resect the diseased sigmoid colon, construct a colostomy using noninflamed descending colon, and suture the divided end of the rectum closed. This procedure is called *Hartmann's operation,* after Henri Hartmann, the French surgeon who described this technique in 1921. Hartmann's operation, although initially described for the treatment of cancer, is the most common technique for emergency operations required for control of infection secondary to diverticulitis.

Eliminating the source of infection by excising the perforated sigmoid colon, establishing diversion of the feces with a colostomy, and controlling the peritoneal infection by irrigating the peritoneal cavity and administering intravenous antibiotics, along with appropriate generalized and nutritional support, should result in resolution of the infection. When the patient has recovered completely from the illness, usually after a period of at least 10 weeks, taking down the colostomy and fashioning an anastomosis between the descending colon and the rectum will restore intestinal continuity.

Obstruction

Intestinal obstruction associated with diverticular disease occurs in two circumstances. The first is relatively unusual and is caused by narrowing of the sigmoid due to the muscular hypertrophy of the bowel wall. This type of stricture rarely causes antegrade mechanical obstruction, but it occasionally presents a diagnostic problem if a contrast study reveals a sigmoid stricture in an area containing numerous diverticula. It may be impossible for the radiologist to exclude a cancer as a cause of the stricture. In such cases, the stenosis may prevent the passage of a colonoscope for adequate evaluation, and sigmoidectomy may be the only remedy if cancer cannot be ruled out.

The more common type of intestinal obstruction is small bowel obstruction associated with the infectious and inflammatory aspect of diverticulitis. The small bowel may become adherent to the phlegmon or abscess, with obstruction caused by the infectious process. In such circumstances, the appropriate treatment is to pass a nasogastric tube to relieve the upper intestinal secretions while addressing the obstruction by treating the infection with antibiotics and percutaneous drainage of the abscess.

COLONIC VOLVULUS

Volvulus describes the condition in which the bowel becomes twisted on its mesenteric axis, a situation that results in partial or complete obstruction of the bowel lumen and a variable degree of impairment of its blood supply. The condition most commonly affects the colon. Although colonic volvulus is relatively rare in the United States, ranking behind cancer and diverticulitis, it is responsible for about 5% of cases of large bowel obstruction. However, in Russia, volvulus accounts for about half of all causes of colonic obstruction, and it is a common cause of colonic obstruction in Iran, India, and some parts of Africa.

Any portion of the large bowel can torse if that segment is attached to a long and floppy mesentery that is fixed to the retroperitoneum by a narrow base of origin. However, the mesenteric anatomy is such that volvulus is most common in the sigmoid colon, with less frequent occurrences involving the right colon and terminal ileum (usually referred to as *cecal volvulus*), the cecum alone (the condition permitted by a highly mobile cecum, called a *cecal bascule,* that is mobile in a caudad to cephalad direction), and most rarely, the transverse colon.

Sigmoid volvulus accounts for two thirds to three fourths of all cases of colonic volvulus. The condition is permitted by an elongated segment of bowel accompanied by a lengthy mesentery with a very narrow parietal attachment, a situation that allows the two ends of the mobile segment to come close together and twist around the narrow mesenteric base. Associated factors include chronic constipation and aging, with the average age of presentation being in the seventh to eighth decade of life. There is an increased incidence of the condition in institutionalized patients afflicted with neuropsychiatric conditions and treated with psychotropic drugs. These medications may predispose to volvulus by affecting intestinal motility. The increased incidence of volvulus in Third World countries has been attributed to a diet high in fiber and vegetables.

Sigmoid volvulus may present as acute or subacute intestinal obstruction with signs and symptoms indistinguishable from those caused by cancer of the distal colon. There is usually a sudden onset of severe abdominal pain, vomiting, and obstipation. The abdomen is usually markedly distended and tympanitic, with the distention often more dramatic than would be associated with other causes of obstruction. There is always the possibility that the condition can be associated with ischemia caused either by mural ischemia associated with the increased tension of the distended bowel wall or by arterial occlusion caused by torsion of the mesenteric arterial supply; therefore, severe abdominal pain, rebound tenderness, and tachycardia are ominous signs.

There may be a history of previous episodes of acute volvulus that spontaneously resolved, and in such circumstances, marked abdominal distention may occur with minimal tenderness.

The radiographic findings are often dramatic and enable prompt diagnosis and treatment (Fig. 50-20). They usually reveal a markedly dilated sigmoid colon with the appearance of a bent inner tube with its apex in the right upper quadrant. An air-fluid level may be seen in the dilated loop of colon, and gas is usually absent from the rectum. CT reveals a characteristic mesenteric whorl, although the diagnosis can usually be established on the

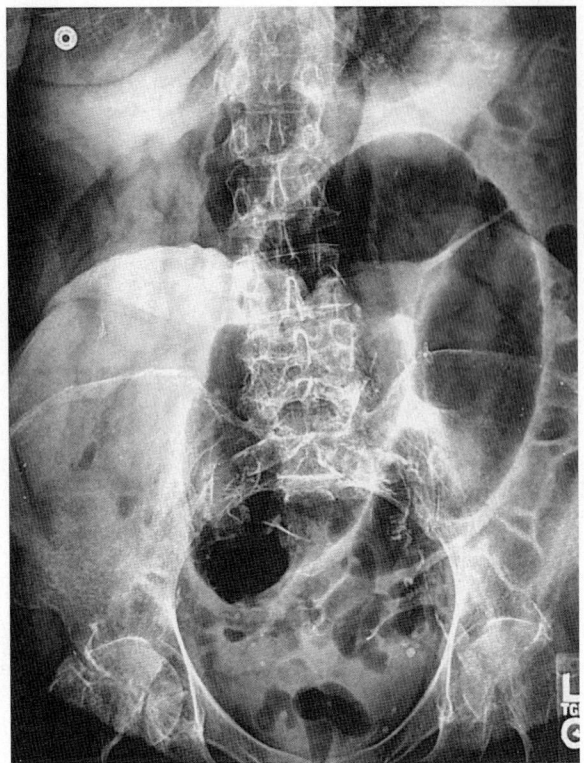

Figure 50-20 Plain film of sigmoid volvulus. Note appearance of "bent inner tube."

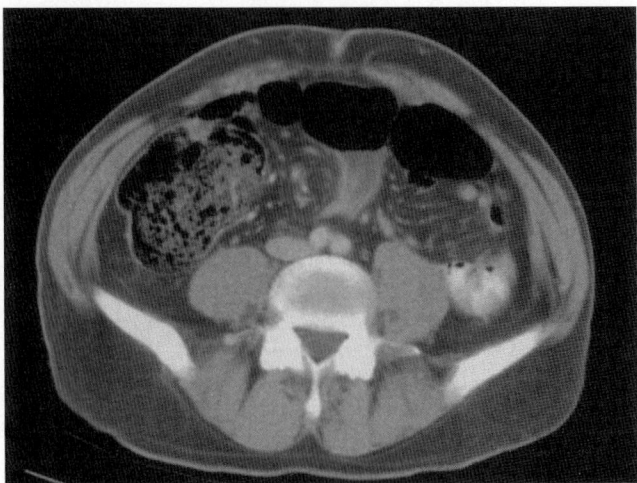

Figure 50-21 Computed tomography scan of abdomen in patient with sigmoid volvulus. Note characteristic whorl in mesentery.

basis of the clinical presentation and the plain film of the abdomen (Fig. 50-21). A contrast enema typically demonstrates the point of obstruction with the pathognomonic "bird's beak" deformity revealing the twist that obstructs the sigmoid lumen (Fig. 50-22).

Treatment of the sigmoid volvulus begins with appropriate resuscitation and in most cases involves nonoperative decompression. Decompression relieves the acute problem and allows resection as an elective procedure, which can be accomplished with reduced morbidity and mortality. Patients with signs of colonic necrosis are not eligible for nonoperative decompression.

Decompression can occur by placement of a rectal tube through a proctoscope or the use of a colonoscope. Often, a soft rectal tube can be inserted under direct vision through the twist of the volvulus while the patient is in the emergency room. Decompression results in a sudden gush of gas and fluid, with a decrease in the abdominal distention. The reduction should be confirmed with an abdominal radiograph. The rectal tube should be taped to the thigh and left in place for 1 or 2 days to allow continued decompression and to prevent immediate recurrence of the volvulus. The bowel can then be cleansed with cathartics and a complete colonoscopic examination performed. If a rectal tube cannot be passed as described, detorsion of the volvulus with the colonoscope should be attempted. If detorsion of the volvulus cannot be accomplished with either a rectal tube or colonoscope, laparotomy with resection of the sigmoid colon (Hartmann's operation) is required.

Even if detorsion of the sigmoid is successful, elective sigmoid resection is indicated in most cases because of the extremely high recurrence rate (approaching 50%). The operation can be conducted through a small left lower quadrant incision or by a laparoscopic approach. Because the elongated colon and mesentery require virtually no mobilization, resection with primary anastomosis is easily accomplished. Colonoscopy should be performed before elective resection to exclude an associated neoplasm.

Although the term *cecal volvulus* is ingrained in the literature, true volvulus of the cecum probably never occurs. There is a well-recognized condition in which the cecum folds in a cephalad direction anteriorly over a fixed ascending colon. Although gangrene may develop, this is exceedingly rare because there is not major vessel obstruction. This so-called cecal bascule commonly causes intermittent bouts of abdominal pain because the mobile cecum permits intermittent episodes of isolated cecal obstruction that are spontaneously relieved as the cecum falls back into its normal position.

The condition commonly referred to as cecal volvulus is actually a cecocolic volvulus and consists of an axial rotation of the terminal ileum, cecum, and ascending colon with concomitant twisting of the associated mesentery. This is a relatively rare condition, accounting for less than 2% of all cases of adult intestinal obstruction and about one fourth of all cases of colonic volvulus in the United States. Cecocolic volvulus is possible because of a lack of fixation of the cecum to the retroperitoneum. Studies on cadavers have shown that between 11% and 22% of people have a right colon that is sufficiently mobile to allow a volvulus to occur. Factors that have been implicated in causing a cecal volvulus include previous surgery, pregnancy, malrotation, and obstructing lesions of the left colon. Cecocolic volvulus is somewhat more common in women, whereas sigmoid volvulus occurs with equal frequency in both sexes. Cecocolic volvulus affects a younger age group (most common in the late 50s) than sigmoid volvulus.

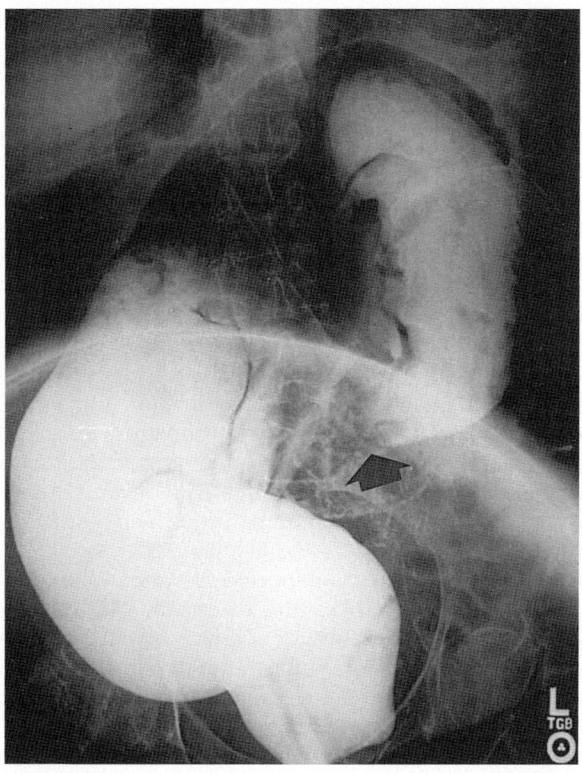

Figure 50-22 Barium enema of sigmoid volvulus. Contrast and air fill rectum and distal sigmoid colon. The contrast stops abruptly at the point of torsion.

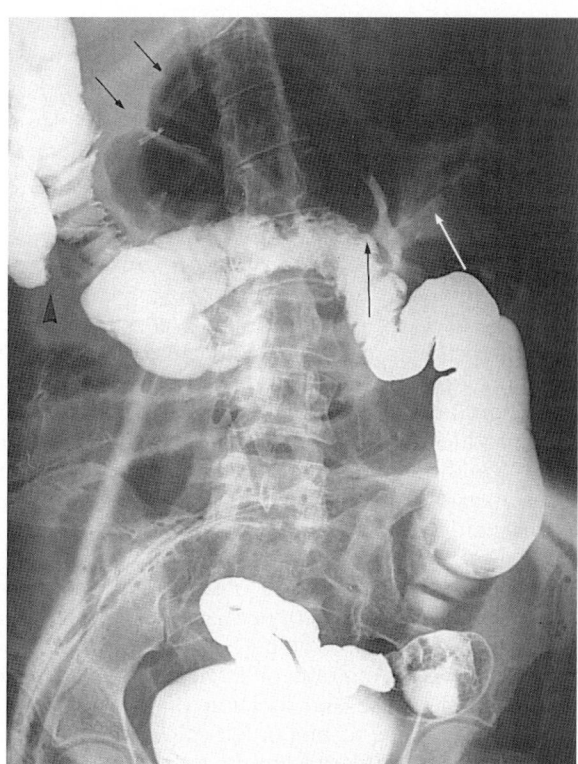

Figure 50-23 Barium enema in a patient with cecal volvulus. The contrast stops abruptly at the proximal end of the hepatic flexure (*arrowhead*). The dilated, air-filled cecum crosses the midline of the abdomen toward the left upper quadrant (*arrows*). (Courtesy of Dina F. Caroline, MD, PhD, Temple University Hospital.)

The typical presentation of patients with cecocolic volvulus is the sudden onset of abdominal pain and distention. In the early phases of a cecocolic volvulus, the pain is mild or moderate in intensity. If the condition is not relieved and ischemia occurs, the pain increases significantly. Physical examination may reveal asymmetric distention of the abdomen, with a tympanitic mass palpable in either the left upper quadrant or midabdomen. Plain radiographs of the abdomen reveal a dilated cecum that is usually displaced to the left side of the abdomen. The distended cecum usually assumes a gas-filled comma shape, the concavity of which faces inferiorly and to the right. Occasionally the distended cecum appears as a circular shape with a narrow, triangular density pointing superiorly and to the right. Haustral markings in the distended loop indicate that the dilated bowel is colon. The torsion results in obstruction of the small bowel, and the radiographic pattern of dilated small intestine can cause diagnostic difficulty.

Although there have been reports of detorsion of cecocolic volvulus with a colonoscope, most cases require operation to correct the volvulus and prevent ischemia. If ischemia has already occurred, immediate operation is obviously required. Contrast enema is helpful to confirm the diagnosis and to exclude a carcinoma of the distal bowel as a precipitating cause of the volvulus (Fig. 50-23).

Right colectomy is the procedure of choice. Primary anastomosis is usually preferred unless the volvulus has resulted in frankly gangrenous bowel, in which case resec-

tion of the gangrenous bowel with ileostomy is a safer approach. There have been many reports of correcting cecocolic volvulus with cecopexy, which should avoid the complication associated with an anastomosis. However, the operation to provide fixation of the cecum is extensive and entails elevating and attaching a flap of peritoneum over the surface of the cecum and ascending colon. The recurrence rates are high with cecopexy, and right colectomy remains the procedure of choice for most surgeons.

Volvulus of the transverse colon is extremely rare and tends to be associated with other abnormalities such as congenital bands, distal obstructing lesions, and pregnancy. Clinical features are indistinguishable from other causes of large bowel obstruction. Radiologic examination is not particularly useful because many cases are misdiagnosed as sigmoid volvulus. A contrast study may show a bird's beak deformity indicating a volvulus. In such cases, colonoscopic reduction may result in detorsion and relief of obstruction. Elective resection should follow to prevent recurrence.

LARGE BOWEL OBSTRUCTION AND PSEUDO-OBSTRUCTION

Large bowel obstruction can be classified as dynamic (mechanical) or adynamic (pseudo-obstruction). Mechanical obstruction is characterized by blockage of the large bowel (luminal, mural, or extramural), resulting in increased intestinal contractility as a physiologic response to relieve the obstruction. Pseudo-obstruction is characterized by the absence of intestinal contractility, often associated with decreased or absent motility of the small bowel and stomach.

Colorectal cancer is the single most common cause of large intestinal obstruction in the United States, whereas colonic volvulus is the more common cause in Russia, Eastern Europe, and Africa. About 2% to 5% of patients with colorectal cancer in the United States present with complete obstruction. Intraluminal causes of colorectal obstruction include fecal impaction, inspissated barium, and foreign bodies. Intramural causes, in addition to carcinoma, include inflammation (diverticulitis, Crohn's disease, lymphogranuloma venereum, tuberculosis, and schistosomiasis), Hirschsprung's disease (aganglionosis), ischemia, radiation, intussusception, and anastomotic stricture. Extraluminal causes include adhesions (the most common cause of small bowel obstruction, but rarely a cause of colonic obstruction), hernias, tumors in adjacent organs, abscesses, and volvulus.

The signs and symptoms of large bowel obstruction depend on the cause and location of the obstruction. Cancers arising in the rectum or left colon are more likely to obstruct than those arising in the more capacious proximal colon. Regardless of the cause of the blockage, the clinical manifestations of large bowel obstruction include the failure to pass stool and flatus associated with increasing abdominal distention and cramping abdominal pain.

The colon becomes distended as gas (about two thirds is swallowed air, the remainder includes the products of bacterial fermentation), stool, and liquid accumulate proximal to the site of blockage. If the obstruction is the result of a segment of colon trapped by a hernia or by a volvulus, the blood supply can become compromised, or strangulated; initially, the venous return is blocked, causing localized swelling that can, in turn, occlude the arterial supply with resultant ischemia that, if uncorrected, can progress to necrosis, or gangrene. Initially, the strangulation involves only the entrapped, or incarcerated, segment of bowel, but the colon proximal to that segment becomes progressively dilated because of the obstruction.

Another route to vascular compromise of the obstructed colon occurs if the bowel proximal to the point of obstruction distends to the extent that the intramural pressure within the intestinal wall exceeds the capillary pressure, depriving the bowel of adequate oxygenation. This route to ischemic necrosis can occur with both mechanical obstruction and pseudo-obstruction.

A *closed-loop obstruction* occurs when both the proximal and distal parts of the bowel are occluded. A strangulated hernia or volvulus almost always leads to this condition. The more common form of closed-loop obstruction, however, is seen when a cancer occludes the lumen of the colon in the presence of a competent ileocecal valve. In this situation, increasing colonic distention causes the pressure in the cecum to become so

high that the vessels in the bowel wall are occluded, and necrosis and perforation can occur.

The treatment of large bowel obstruction obviously depends on the cause of the obstruction, and specific treatments are covered in the discussion of those entities. However, some principles of diagnosis and treatment can be generalized. The obstruction needs to be relieved with some expediency before compromise of the blood supply results in ischemia and gangrene. The diagnosis should be established to guide appropriate treatment. History and physical examination provide important clues. The abdomen should be palpated for masses, the groins inspected for hernias, and a digital rectal examination performed to exclude rectal cancer. Plain films of the abdomen provide considerable information concerning the location of the obstruction and in some situations may be diagnostic of a volvulus. A CT scan may be helpful in revealing an inflammatory process such as an abscess associated with diverticulitis. If a volvulus or distal sigmoid cancer is suspected, a water-soluble contrast enema may establish the diagnosis. The treatment options vary considerably, depending on the diagnosis, and it is very helpful to establish the diagnosis before an operation to properly guide therapy. If the cause of the obstruction is a cancer of the distal or mid rectum, the preferred treatment is to relieve the obstruction by a loop colostomy, subsequently treat the cancer with neoadjuvant chemoradiation, with the plan to resect the primary lesion at a later time. On the other hand, if the obstructing cancer is in the sigmoid colon, the surgical options include Hartmann's operation (sigmoidectomy with descending colostomy and closure of the rectal stump), sigmoidectomy with primary colorectal anastomosis (with or without intraoperative colonic lavage), or abdominal colectomy with ileorectal anastomosis.

Right-sided colonic obstruction, whether by cancer or the result of volvulus, is generally treated by resection and primary anastomosis of the ileum and transverse colon.

Pseudo-obstruction of the colon (also called *Ogilvie's syndrome,* after its description by Sir Heneage Ogilvie in 1948) describes the condition of distention of the colon, with signs and symptoms of colonic obstruction, in the absence of an actual physical cause of the obstruction. Ogilvie described two patients with clinical features of colonic obstruction despite a normal barium enema. Both patients underwent laparotomy for the condition; neither had mechanical obstruction, but both had unsuspected malignant disease involving the area of the celiac axis and semilunar ganglion. The cause of the dilation was attributed to the malignant infiltration of the sympathetic ganglia. Subsequently there have been numerous descriptions of cases of colonic distention in the absence of mechanical obstruction and without malignant involvement of the visceral autonomic nerves. Very few cases of pseudo-obstruction have malignant infiltration of the autonomic nerves as the cause; in fact, the exact pathogenesis of the syndrome remains unknown, and it has been associated with a heterogeneous group of conditions.

Primary pseudo-obstruction is a motility disorder that is either a familial visceral myopathy (hollow visceral myopathy syndrome) or a diffuse motility disorder involving the autonomic innervation of the intestinal wall. The latter may be modified by a disturbance of intestinal hormones or may be principally due to disordered autonomic innervation.

Secondary pseudo-obstruction is more common and has been associated with neuroleptic medications, opiates, severe metabolic illness, myxedema, diabetes mellitus, uremia, hyperparathyroidism, lupus, scleroderma, Parkinson's disease, and traumatic retroperitoneal hematomas. One mechanism thought to play a role in the pathogenesis is sympathetic overactivity overriding the parasympathetic system. Indirect support for this theory has been derived from the success in treating the syndrome with neostigmine, a parasympathomimetic agent. Further support comes from reports of immediate resolution of the syndrome after administration of an epidural anesthetic that provides sympathetic blockade.

Pseudo-obstruction may present in acute or chronic forms. The acute variety most commonly affects patients with chronic renal, respiratory, cerebral, or cardiovascular disease. It usually involves only the colon, whereas the chronic form affects other parts of the gastrointestinal tract, usually presents as bouts of subacute and partial intestinal obstruction, and tends to recur periodically.

Acute colonic pseudo-obstruction should be suspected when a medically ill patient suddenly develops abdominal distention. The abdomen is tympanitic, usually nontender, and bowel sounds are usually present. Plain abdominal radiographs reveal a distended colon, with the right and transverse segments tending to be most dramatically affected. The radiologic appearance is one of large bowel obstruction.

The most useful investigation is a water-soluble contrast enema, which should be performed in all patients in whom the diagnosis is suspected, provided their condition is stable enough to warrant the procedure. The contrast enema can reliably differentiate between mechanical obstruction and pseudo-obstruction, a differentiation that is essential to guide appropriate therapy.

Colonoscopy is the alternative diagnostic investigation for pseudo-obstruction and has the attractive advantage that it can be used for treatment. However, at the present time, the water-soluble contrast enema is generally the preferred initial test.

When the diagnosis of acute pseudo-obstruction is suspected, treatment should accompany the diagnostic evaluation. Initial treatment includes nasogastric decompression, replacement of extracellular fluid deficits, and correction of electrolyte abnormalities. All medications that inhibit bowel motility, such as opiates, should be discontinued. Patient response is monitored by serial abdominal examinations and radiographs. Most patients improve with this regimen. Until the mid-1990s, the treatment usually used when the colonic distention failed to resolve with supportive measures was colonoscopic decompression. Although this approach was generally successful, it required skilled personnel and equipment and carried the risk for colonic perforation from both instrument trauma and insufflation. In addition, the procedure often had to be repeated because of recurrence of the colonic distention.

At the present time, the trend has been to treat this condition with neostigmine, a parasympathomimetic agent. It is obviously imperative that mechanical obstruction be excluded (either by water-soluble contrast enema or colonoscopy) before the administration of neostigmine because the subsequent high pressures generated in the colon against a distal obstruction could cause colonic perforation.

Neostigmine enhances parasympathetic activity by competing with acetylcholine for acetylcholinesterase binding sites. In the treatment of colonic pseudo-obstruction, 2.5 mg of neostigmine is given intravenously over 3 minutes. The resolution of the condition is indicated within less than 10 minutes of administration of the drug, by the passage of stool and flatus by the patient. The recurrence rates following the administration of neostigmine appear to be far lower than those associated with colonoscopic decompression, with satisfactory decompression being achieved in about 90% of patients after a single administration of the medication.[22]

A significant side effect of neostigmine is bradycardia, and all patients must be monitored by telemetry during administration of the drug. Atropine must be immediately available, and patients with significant cardiac disease are not candidates for this treatment.

INFLAMMATORY BOWEL DISEASE

Inflammatory bowel disease (IBD) is a term generally used to denote two diseases of unknown etiology with similar general characteristics: *ulcerative colitis* and *Crohn's disease*. The distinction between the two entities can usually be established based on clinical and pathologic criteria, including history and physical examination, radiologic and endoscopic studies, gross appearance, and histology. However, in about 10% to 15% of patients with inflammatory disease confined to the colon, a clear distinction cannot be made, and the disease is labeled *indeterminate colitis*. The medical and surgical management of ulcerative colitis and Crohn's disease often differ significantly, so each entity is discussed separately here. A comparison of the characteristics of ulcerative colitis and Crohn's disease is presented in Table 50-1.

Ulcerative Colitis

Epidemiology and Etiology

Ulcerative colitis occurs more commonly in developed countries and is relatively unusual in Asia, Africa, and South America. There appears to be a seasonal variation in the activity of the disease, with onset as well as relapse occurring statistically more often between August and January. The incidence of the disease has remained relatively stable during the past 20 years, with new cases reported as 4 to 6 cases per 100,000 white adults per year

Table 50-1 Comparisons of Ulcerative Colitis and Crohn's Colitis

	ULCERATIVE COLITIS	CROHN'S COLITIS
Gross Appearance		
Thickened wall	0	4+
Thickened mesentery	0	3+
Serosal "fat wrapping"	0	4+
Segmental disease	0	4+
Microscopic Appearance		
Transmural	0	4+
Lymphoid aggregates	0	4+
Granulomas	0	3+
Clinical Features		
Bleeding per rectum	3+	1+
Diarrhea	3+	3+
Obstructive symptoms	1+	3+
Anal/perianal disease	Rare	4+
Risk for cancer	2+	3+
Small bowel disease	0	4+
Colonoscopic Features		
Distribution	Continuous	Discontinuous
Rectal disease	4+	1+
Friability	4+	1+
Aphthous ulcers	0	4+
Deep longitudinal ulcers	0	4+
Cobblestoning	0	4+
Pseudopolyps	2+	2+
Operative Treatment		
Total proctocolectomy	Curative	Combined disease: colon + rectum
Segmental resection	Rare	Absence of anorectal disease
Ileal pouch	Preferred by most patients	Contraindicated
Complications		
Postoperative recurrence	0	4+
Fistulas	Rare	4+
Sclerosing cholangitis	1+	Rare
Cholelithiasis	0	2+
Nephrolithiasis	0	2+

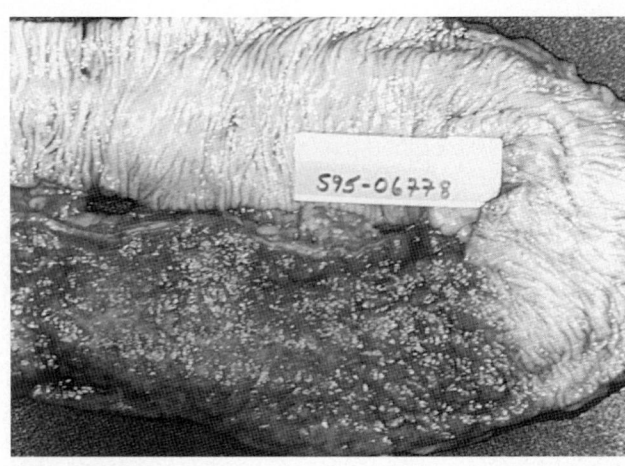

Figure 50-24 Ulcerative colitis, macroscopic appearance of left-sided colitis. The left side of the colon displays continuous disease manifested as erythema and granularity of the mucosal surface, whereas the right colon appears normal.

included inadequate fiber intake, chemical food additives, refined sugars, and cow's milk. However, none of these have been demonstrated to play a definitive role. Infectious agents, including *C. difficile* and *Campylobacter jejuni,* have been implicated as playing a causative role in the pathogenesis, but such a role has not been confirmed.

Smoking appears to confer a protective effect against the development of ulcerative colitis, as well as providing a therapeutic influence; nicotine has been reported to induce remission in some cases. This is in contrast to Crohn's disease, which is more common in smokers and appears to be aggravated by the habit. Both ulcerative colitis and Crohn's disease are more common among women who use oral contraceptives compared with those who do not. Patients who have had an appendectomy appear to be at increased risk for developing ulcerative colitis.[23]

A family history of IBD is a significant risk factor. Several studies have demonstrated the existence of family aggregates with ulcerative colitis and a high degree of concordance in monozygotic twins. The genetic predisposition for ulcerative colitis is not inherited in a classic mendelian pattern, suggesting the influence of environmental factors on an individual's susceptibility. Two genetic abnormalities found to be associated with ulcerative colitis are variations in DNA repair genes and class II major histocompatibility complex genes. Patients with ulcerative colitis display specific alleles of group HLA and DR2 (HLA-DRB1), with an association between certain alleles and expression of the disease. The DR1501 allele is associated with a more benign course, whereas the DR1502 allele is associated with a more virulent form of the disease.

Another theory of the etiology of IBD concerns an altered immunologic response to both external and host antigens. Although anticolon antibodies have been identified in both blood and tissue of patients with IBD, there is little evidence that these play a pathogenic role. Other

with a prevalence between 40 and 100 cases per 100,000. All ages are susceptible, but it more commonly affects patients younger than 30 years. A small secondary peak in the incidence occurs in the sixth decade. Both sexes are equally affected, but the condition is more common in Caucasians, Jews, and persons of northern European ancestry.

Although the cause of ulcerative colitis is unknown, its prevalence in industrialized countries and the increased incidence among individuals who migrate from low-risk to high-risk areas suggest an environmental influence. Speculation on the influence of dietary factors has

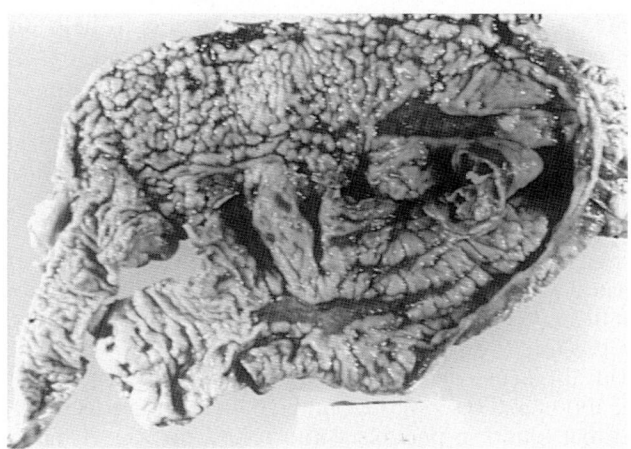

Figure 50-25 Ulcerative colitis, macroscopic appearance of pancolitis. Because the entire colon is involved with inflammatory changes, this specimen represents a case of universal colitis or pancolitis. The distal colon shows a large longitudinal ulcer with heaped-up adjacent mucosa. In the midportion of the colon, the mucosa is relatively flat and featureless. In the right side of the colon, there are multiple projections, or pseudopolyps, creating a cobblestone appearance. The ileocecal valve is edematous and irregular, whereas the terminal ileum is spared. (Courtesy of M. Markowitz Haber, MD, Hahnemann University Hospital.)

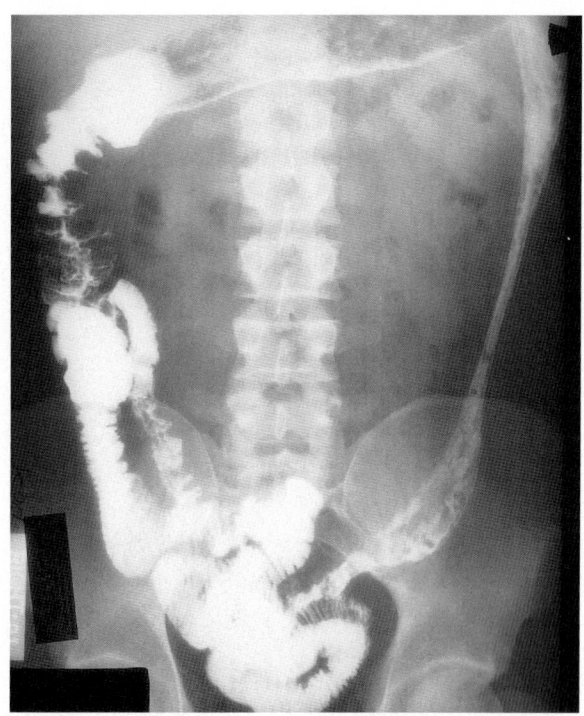

Figure 50-26 Stricture in chronic ulcerative colitis. Colonoscopy revealed chronic inflammation, but no dysplasia or cancer.

studies have shown that defective cell-mediated immunity, leukocyte chemotactic impairment, and abnormalities of antigen-specific helper and suppressor T cells may be involved in the pathogenesis.

Pathologic Features

Gross Appearance

Ulcerative colitis is a disease in which the major pathologic process involves the mucosa and submucosa of the colon, with sparing of the muscularis. Despite the disease's name, ulceration of the mucosa is not invariably present. In fact, the typical gross appearance of ulcerative colitis is hyperemic mucosa. Friable and granular mucosa is common in more severe cases, and ulceration may not be readily evident, especially early in the course of the disease. However, ulceration may appear and vary widely, from small superficial erosions to patchy ulceration of the full thickness of the mucosa (Fig. 50-24). The rectum is invariably involved with the inflammatory process. In fact, rectal involvement (proctitis) is the *sine qua non* of the disease, and the diagnosis should be seriously questioned if the rectal mucosa is not affected. The mucosal inflammation extends in a continuous fashion for a variable distance into the more proximal colon. Pseudopolyps, or inflammatory polyps, represent regeneration of inflamed mucosa and are composed of a variable mixture of non-neoplastic colonic mucosa and inflamed lamina propria (Fig. 50-25).

As implied earlier, a diagnostic characteristic of ulcerative colitis is continuous, uninterrupted inflammation of the colonic mucosa beginning in the distal rectum and extending proximally to a variable distance. This is in contrast to Crohn's disease, in which normal segments of colon (skipped areas) may be interspersed between distinct segments of colonic inflammation. The entire colon, including the cecum and appendix, may be involved in ulcerative colitis. In contrast to Crohn's disease, ulcerative colitis does not involve the terminal ileum except in cases of backwash ileitis, when the ileal mucosa may appear inflamed in the presence of extensive proximal colonic involvement. However, in such cases, contrast studies usually reveal the inflamed ileum to be dilated, in contrast to the frequently narrowed and contracted ileum characteristic of Crohn's disease.

Colonic strictures can occur in 5% to 12% of patients with chronic ulcerative colitis. Although such strictures are most often benign and caused by hypertrophy of the muscularis, cancer must be excluded as the cause of any colonic stricture occurring in the setting of ulcerative colitis. Three important features are suggestive of malignant strictures:

1. Appearance later in the course of ulcerative colitis (60% after 20 years versus 0% before 10 years)
2. Location proximal to the splenic flexure (86% malignant)
3. Large bowel obstruction caused by the stricture (Fig. 50-26)

Histologic Appearance

The typical microscopic finding in ulcerative colitis is inflammation of the mucosa and submucosa. The most characteristic lesion is the crypt abscess, in which collections of neutrophils fill and expand the lumina of individual crypts of Lieberkühn (Fig. 50-27). Crypt abscesses,

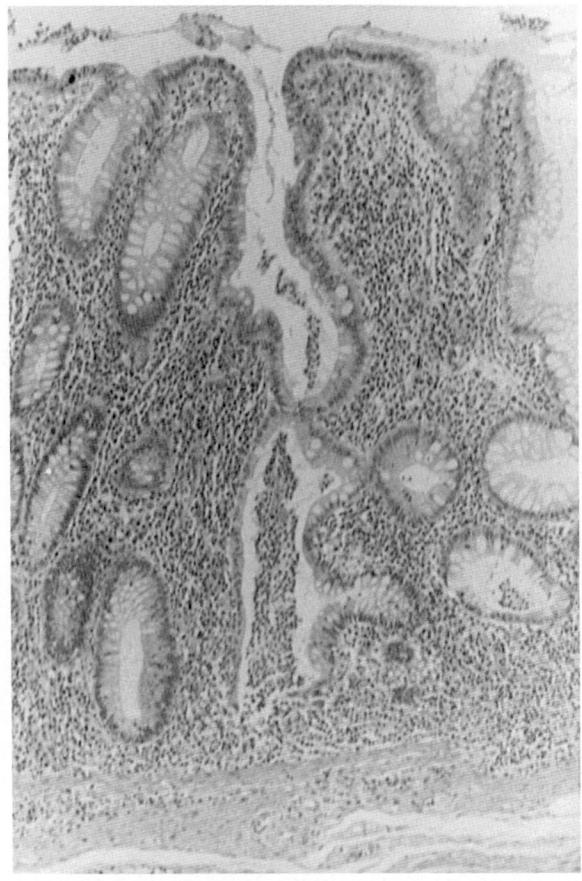

Figure 50-27 Active ulcerative colitis. The glands are irregular with branching, and focally, the long axis of the gland is horizontal rather than perpendicular. A central crypt abscess is present. There are increased numbers of chronic inflammatory cells throughout the lamina propria.

however, are not specific for ulcerative colitis and can be seen in Crohn's disease and infectious colitis. Hematochezia often results from the marked vascular congestion. Crypt branching may be seen in chronic ulcerative colitis and is an important characteristic. The number of goblet cells in the crypts is diminished, as is mucus production.

It has been stressed that the inflammatory process in ulcerative colitis spares the muscular coats of the colon, a characteristic that differentiates the entity from Crohn's disease (the latter is characterized by transmural inflammation, or involvement of all layers of the intestinal wall). However, in rare cases of severe inflammation characteristic of toxic megacolon in patients with ulcerative colitis, all layers of the colon may be involved, and perforation may occur if treatment is delayed. However, the inflammatory process in such circumstances is atypical and may be related to factors such as prolonged colonic distention with vascular compromise.

Numerous studies have demonstrated that antineutrophil cytoplasmic antibodies (ANCAs) with a perinuclear staining pattern (pANCA) are seen in up to 86% of patients with mucosal ulcerative colitis. The presence of

pANCA has been used as a diagnostic test to help differentiate ulcerative colitis from Crohn's disease.

Clinical Presentation

Ulcerative colitis and colonic Crohn's disease often have similar clinical presentations. Both may present with diarrhea and the passage of mucus. Patients with ulcerative colitis tend to have more urgency than those with Crohn's disease, likely because ulcerative colitis is invariable associated with distal proctitis. Rectal bleeding is also common in ulcerative colitis; although it may be present in patients with Crohn's disease, it is typically not as severe. Patients with the acute onset of ulcerative colitis often complain of abdominal discomfort, but the pain is seldom as severe as that found in patients with Crohn's disease. A tender abdominal mass is suggestive of a phlegmon or abscess more commonly associated with Crohn's.

Perianal disease is an uncommon finding in patients with ulcerative disease, whereas it may be the only presenting symptom of Crohn's disease. It is an interesting and seemingly paradoxical fact that rectal involvement is present in virtually 100% of patients with ulcerative colitis, whereas anal involvement is very rare. In contrast, patients with Crohn's disease may have normal rectal mucosa (so-called rectal sparing), although anal disease (fissures, fistulas, abscesses) is common.

Extraintestinal Manifestations

Extraintestinal manifestations of ulcerative colitis include arthritis, ankylosing spondylitis, erythema nodosum, pyoderma gangrenosum, and primary sclerosing cholangitis. Arthritis, particularly of the knees, ankles, hips, and shoulders, occurs in about 20% of patients, typically in association with increased activity of the intestinal disease. Ankylosing spondylitis occurs in 3% to 5% of patients and is most prevalent in patients who are HLA-B27 positive or have a family history of ankylosing spondylitis. Erythema nodosum arises in 10% to 15% of patients with ulcerative colitis and often occurs in conjunction with peripheral arthropathy. Pyoderma gangrenosum typically presents on the pretibial region as an erythematous plaque that progresses into an ulcerated, painful wound. Most patients who develop this condition have underlying active inflammatory bowel disease. Arthritis, ankylosing spondylitis, erythema nodosum, and pyoderma gangrenosum typically improve or completely resolve after colectomy.

Primary sclerosing cholangitis (PSC) occurs in 5% to 8% of patients with ulcerative colitis. Most patients with inflammatory bowel disease who develop PSC are younger than 40 years of age, and the majority are men. Genetics likely play a role because patients with ulcerative colitis who have the HLA-B8 or HLA-DR3 haplotype are 10 times more likely to develop PSC. Patients with PSC and ulcerative colitis typically have a more quiescent disease course; however, the risk for colon cancer in these patients is up to five times greater than in patients with ulcerative colitis alone. These tumors are more likely to arise proximal to the splenic flexure. Primary sclerosing cholangitis may be asymptomatic and diagnosed only by abnormal laboratory studies, or it may present with symptoms of obstructive jaundice and abdominal pain. The disease is progressive and ultimately fatal unless liver transplantation is undertaken. Colectomy has no effect on the course of PSC.

Diagnosis

Endoscopic examination of the colon and rectum is essential in the diagnosis of inflammatory bowel disease. In the acute phase of the disease, proctosigmoidoscopy is often sufficient because the rectum is invariably inflamed in patients with ulcerative colitis. Complete colonoscopy offers little additional information in the acute setting and increases the risk for colonic perforation. The presence of diffuse, confluent, symmetric disease from the dentate line proximally is consistent with ulcerative colitis, and the mucosal appearance can vary from loss of the normal vessel pattern secondary to edema in the early stages of the disease to frank ulceration in the more advanced disease. If the inflammation extends beyond the level of the sigmoidoscope, a full colonoscopy should be obtained after the disease is under control.

Conditions other than ulcerative colitis can present with similar symptoms of diarrhea and bleeding, and it is important to identify these conditions because their treatments may be considerably different. Crohn's disease has features similar to ulcerative colitis; however, the rectum is spared in 40% of patients with Crohn's colitis, even in the presence of perianal disease. An upper gastrointestinal radiograph with a small bowel follow-through should be obtained to rule out the possibility of small bowel involvement, a finding that would suggest Crohn's disease. Collagenous colitis is a condition that generally occurs in women older than 50 years. It typically presents with profuse watery diarrhea and is characterized histologically by marked thickening of the colonic subepithelial basement membrane. On endoscopic evaluation, the mucosa appears normal in most patients, and the diagnosis is made by endoscopic biopsy. Treatment of collagenous colitis is typically medical.

In addition to multiple mucosal biopsy specimens from serial sites, stool samples should be sent to the laboratory to look for bacteria and ova and parasites. Infectious conditions that mimic ulcerative colitis include colitis caused by *C. difficile, Entamoeba histolytica, C. jejuni,* and *Salmonella enteritidis.*

Risk for Carcinoma

One of the most serious sequelae of mucosal ulcerative colitis is the development of colorectal carcinoma. The most important risk factors include prolonged duration of the disease, pancolonic disease, continuously active disease, and severity of the inflammation. The cumulative risk for cancer increases with the duration of the disease, reaching 25% at 25 years, 35% at 30 years, 45% at 35 years, and 65% at 40 years.[24] Patients with disease confined to the left side of the colon have a lower risk for developing carcinoma than patients with disease involving the entire colon. Carcinomas arising in ulcerative colitis tend to be poorly differentiated and highly aggressive tumors. As briefly discussed previously, a colonic

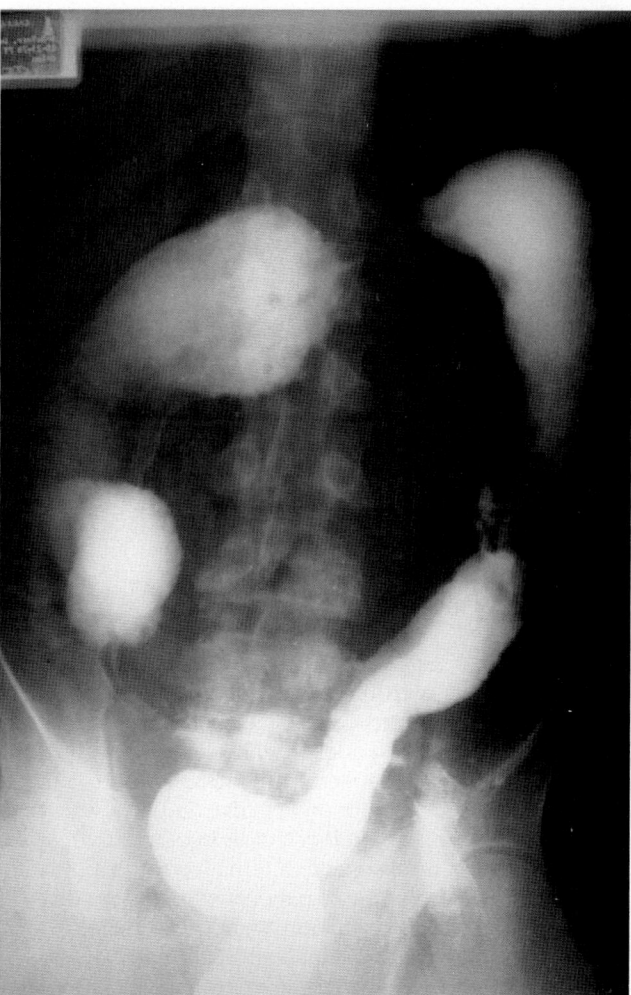

Figure 50-28 Barium enema demonstrating stricture in transverse colon of patient with ulcerative colitis of 15 years' duration.

stricture in a patient with ulcerative colitis must be presumed carcinoma until proved otherwise. If malignancy cannot be ruled out by endoscopy, the presence of a stricture is an indication for operative intervention (Figs. 50-28 to 50-30).

There is considerable debate regarding the optimal method of surveillance colonoscopy in patients with ulcerative colitis. The American Cancer Society guidelines recommend surveillance colonoscopy every 1 to 2 years beginning 8 years after the onset of pancolitis and 12 to 15 years after the onset of left-sided colitis. This strategy is based on the premise that a dysplastic lesion can be detected endoscopically before invasive carcinoma has developed (Fig. 50-31). Traditionally, 10 random biopsy specimens have been recommended; however, several studies have recently suggested that at least 30 specimens be obtained.

The risk for cancer varies with the degree of dysplasia, with carcinoma found in 10% of colons displaying low-grade dysplasia, in 30% to 40% with high-grade dysplasia, and in more than 50% of colons with dysplasia associated

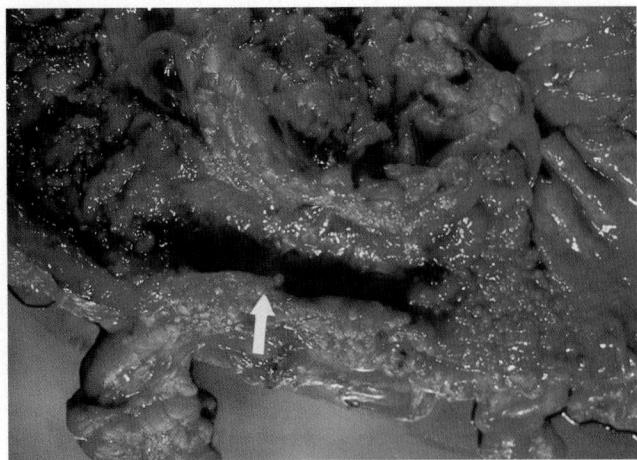

Figure 50-29 Resected colon from patient in Figure 50-28, revealing the stricture (*arrow*) to be invasive cancer. The patient had liver metastases.

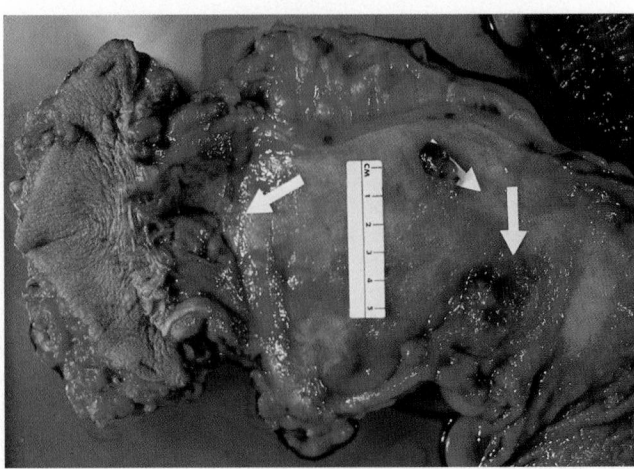

Figure 50-30 Resected rectum from patient in Figure 50-28, showing invasive cancers in rectum (*arrows*).

with a lesion or mass (DALM). Neoplastic lesions of the colon of patients with ulcerative colitis can develop in a DALM lesion or in a coincidental adenoma, and about 25% of carcinomas in patients with ulcerative colitis are not associated with dysplasia elsewhere in the colon.[25]

A meta-analysis of 10 prospective studies was performed to determine whether colonoscopic surveillance of dysplasia was a reasonable alternative to prophylactic colectomy.[26] Less than 3% of patients who had no dysplasia during the initial evaluation went on to develop evidence of dysplasia. In patients with high-grade dysplasia, however, 32% were found to have invasive carcinoma at the time of colectomy. These tumors tended to be of earlier stages when compared with tumors in patients in whom the diagnosis of cancer was made before colectomy. Other studies have shown no benefit to colonoscopic surveillance. Patients therefore need to be counseled about the potential for dysplasia so that they can rationally take part in their management. When high-grade dysplasia is found and has been confirmed by a second independent pathologist, proctocolectomy should be recommended. This is also true for patients who have DALM. If low-grade dysplasia is confirmed, strong consideration should also be given to proctocolectomy.

Flow cytometry of colonoscopic biopsies may also be useful in detecting dysplasia. Several studies have demonstrated a strong correlation between DNA aneuploidy and polyploidy and the presence of dysplasia. Although the presence of these abnormalities should not serve as an indication for colectomy, they may indicate a need for more frequent colonoscopic surveillance.

Medical Therapy

There are multiple medications available for use in the treatment of ulcerative colitis. These medications can be grouped into three broad categories: aminosalicylates, corticosteroids, and immunomodulatory drugs.

The most common therapy in the treatment of mild to moderate ulcerative colitis involves aminosalicylates. Sul-

fasalazine is composed of a molecule of 5-aminosalicylic acid (5-ASA) linked by a diazo bond to sulfapyridine. 5-ASA is released in the colon when bacterial azo reductases cleave the diazo bond; its actions involve blocking the cyclooxygenase and lipoxygenase pathways of arachidonic acid metabolism and scavenging free radicals in the colonic mucosa. Its usefulness is limited by toxicity, most of which is attributed to the sulfapyridine portion of the drug. Newer 5-ASA medications, including Asacol and Pentasa, have been developed that do not contain sulfapyridine, thereby minimizing side effects. Salicylates can be used in the treatment of active disease at higher doses and also play a role in maintaining remission at lower doses.

Corticosteroids are highly effective in the treatment of active ulcerative colitis and can be administered orally, intravenously, or topically through enemas. Steroids act to block phospholipase A_2, thereby decreasing prostaglandins and leukotrienes. Side effects of steroid therapy, including hypertension, diabetes mellitus, osteoporosis, and increased susceptibility to infection, preclude long-term therapy with these medications. Hydrocortisone enemas delivered two or three times per day are often very effective in the treatment of disease limited to the rectum and left side of the colon; these have the benefit of less absorption and therefore fewer systemic side effects. Newer steroid analogues have been developed that act locally in the colon and are then inactivated during first pass in the liver. Budesonide, a water-soluble analogue of hydrocortisone, has recently been shown to be as effective as prednisolone with far fewer side effects, including much less adrenal suppression.

Immunomodulatory medications are often used in the long-term management of patients with ulcerative colitis. 6-Mercaptopurine (6-MP), a purine analogue, and its precursor azathioprine, act by causing chromosome breaks and inhibiting the proliferation of rapidly dividing cells such as lymphocytes (T cells more than B cells). Azathioprine and 6-MP are useful in inducing remission

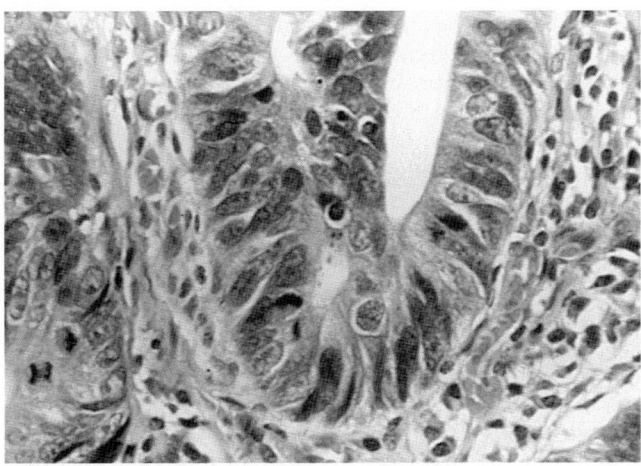

Figure 50-31 High-grade colonic dysplasia in ulcerative colitis. Nuclei are large, pleomorphic, hyperchromatic, and crowded. Cells have a high nucleus-to-cytoplasm ratio. Mitotic figures are easily identified. Note that the tubular lumen is irregular with a row of cells seen centrally, suggesting a transition to intramucosal carcinoma. (Courtesy of M. Markowitz Haber, MD, Hahnemann University Hospital.)

in patients who are refractory to 5-ASA, and their use allows steroids to be tapered or minimized in more than half of patients. Side effects of these medications include reversible bone marrow suppression and pancreatitis, and measurement of 6-MP metabolites has been proposed as a method to guide dosing to help avoid toxicity. Cyclosporine is an immunosuppressant used frequently in solid organ transplantation that inhibits interleukin-2 (IL-2) gene transcription, thereby reducing the activation of lymphocytes. Cyclosporine has serious potential side effects, including nephrotoxicity, hepatotoxicity, seizures, and lymphoproliferative disorders, and is typically reserved for use in acute severe ulcerative colitis and refractory Crohn's disease.

Indications for Surgery

Indications for the surgical management of mucosal ulcerative colitis include fulminant colitis with toxic megacolon, massive bleeding, intractable disease, and dysplasia or carcinoma (Box 50-1). Malnutrition and growth retardation may necessitate resection in pediatric and adolescent patients.

Fulminant Colitis and Toxic Megacolon

Patients with fulminant colitis typically present with high fever, severe abdominal pain, tenderness, tachycardia, and leukocytosis. These patients require hospitalization with intravenous hydration, nasogastric decompression, high-dose intravenous steroids if the patient is steroid dependent, and broad-spectrum antibiotics. Intravenous hyperalimentation may be useful depending on the patient's nutritional status and length of illness before the fulminant episode. Patients should be closely monitored with serial abdominal exams and leukocyte counts. Deterioration or lack of improvement within 24 to 48 hours of the initiation of medical treatment warrants an urgent

---

Box 50-1   Ulcerative Colitis—Indications for Surgery

Intractability
Dysplasia-carcinoma
Massive colonic bleeding
Toxic megacolon

---

procedure because the mortality rate is increased four-fold in patients with colonic perforation.

Toxic megacolon is a serious, life-threatening condition that can occur in patients with ulcerative colitis, Crohn's colitis, and infectious colitides such as pseudomembranous colitis, in which the bacterial infiltration of the walls of the colon creates a dilation of the colon that progresses to the point of imminent perforation. This decompensation results in a necrotic, thin-walled bowel in which pneumatosis can often be seen radiographically. Although some patients with toxic megacolon have been successfully treated medically, a high rate of recurrence with subsequent urgent operation has been reported. Aggressive preoperative stabilization is required, using volume resuscitation with crystalloid solutions to prevent dehydration secondary to third-space fluid losses, stress-dose steroids for patients previously on steroid therapy, and broad-spectrum antibiotics.

Although restorative proctocolectomy with ileal pouch–anal anastomosis (IPAA) as a single-staged procedure has been reported for toxic megacolon, proctectomy and anastomosis are generally ill advised in the acutely ill patient with an unprepared bowel. Total proctocolectomy in the urgent setting carries a prohibitively high mortality rate, and the leak rate from a primary anastomosis is unacceptably high. Whereas the goal in elective surgery is to remove all the colonic or dysplastic mucosa, the aim in emergent surgery is to rescue the patient from a life-threatening situation. A total abdominal colectomy with ileostomy and preservation of the rectum is therefore the preferred operation for this condition. This procedure can be expeditiously performed with relatively low morbidity and mortality, and it serves the main purpose of removing the diseased colon and avoiding a difficult and morbid pelvic dissection.

Preserving the rectum leaves the option of fashioning an ileorectal anastomosis in the future (Fig. 50-32). This is particularly important in patients in whom the diagnosis is unclear and a subsequent ileoanal pouch might be contraindicated (e.g., in Crohn's disease). Some controversy exists regarding management of the distal segment of bowel. The remaining rectum or rectosigmoid can be delivered as a mucous fistula placed subcutaneously, or closed as a Hartmann's pouch. Each management strategy has its proponents, but no randomized prospective trial has been performed to date that has shown superiority of any of these options.

The so-called blow-hole procedure was advocated in the past for treatment of patients with severe toxic megacolon in whom the distended colonic wall was so thin and fragile that any handling during the conduct of an

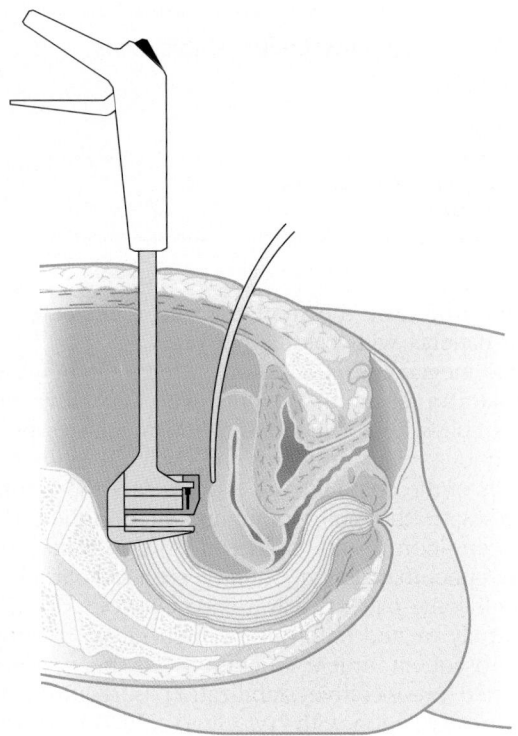

Figure 50-32 Closure of rectal stump after resection of abdominal colon.

operation would risk perforation of the colon with massive peritoneal contamination. Currently, it is distinctly unusual that operative intervention is delayed to such a degree, but the operation may be advantageous in such dire circumstances. The technique consists of performing a skin-level (blow-hole) transverse colostomy (and sometimes the left colon is decompressed with a simultaneous, second sigmoid skin level colostomy). Fashioning a loop ileostomy is an essential component of this operation. The operation was often rewarded with dramatic improvement in the patient's condition. After recovery from the acute illness (usually over a period of several months), the patient could then be treated with restorative proctocolectomy with IPAA, or total procto-colectomy, depending on the circumstances.

Massive Bleeding

Massive hemorrhage from ulcerative colitis is an uncommon event, occurring in less than 5% of patients requiring operation. Patients obviously require resuscitation and stabilization before surgery, with replenishment of extracellular volume and transfusions as needed. Subtotal colectomy is the procedure of choice and will usually suffice. However, if bleeding continues from the remaining rectal mucosa, emergency proctectomy may be required.

Intractability

Colitis with debilitating symptoms refractory to medical therapy is the most common indication for operative therapy. Patients with intractable disease have persistent symptoms such as crampy abdominal pain, frequent

bowel movements, stool urgency, and anemia, which may result in deterioration of the patient's social and professional relationships. It has been demonstrated that patients' quality of life after surgery for ulcerative colitis is improved, regardless of the procedure performed. Complications of long-term steroid therapy, such as diabetes mellitus, avascular necrosis of the femoral head, cataracts, psychiatric problems, osteoporosis, and weight gain, are a frequent indication for surgical resection, even though the patient's symptoms may be controlled while on steroids. Elective surgery should also be considered in patients with significant extracolonic manifestations refractory to nonoperative measures.

Dysplasia or Carcinoma

The finding of dysplastic changes in the colon or carcinoma is an indication for surgical intervention as discussed previously. The presence of cancer may influence the procedure selected or the sequence of staged procedures. It does not exclude the possibility of performing an ileoanal pouch, but the location and stage of the cancer must be taken into consideration.

Operations

Elective surgical options for ulcerative colitis include total proctocolectomy with ileostomy, restorative proctocolectomy with IPAA, and total proctocolectomy with a continent ileal reservoir (Kock pouch). Segmental colectomy for ulcerative colitis (in contrast to Crohn's disease) has been shown to be an inadequate procedure for controlling disease. For example, in the case of colitis confined to the left side, a proctosigmoidectomy with end descending colostomy or coloanal anastomosis invariably results in the recurrence of disease within the remaining colon within a short time and is contraindicated.

In the past, abdominal colectomy with ileorectal anastomosis has been advocated for patients with ulcerative colitis and rectal sparing. However, such patients are exceedingly rare. The inflammatory process typical of ulcerative colitis virtually always involves the rectum, and an anastomosis of the ileum to the inflamed rectum invariably results in intractable diarrhea. Patients with true rectal sparing and left colitis most likely have Crohn's disease. In that situation, a segmental colectomy or subtotal colectomy with rectal anastomosis is an appropriate procedure.

Total Proctocolectomy With End Ileostomy

Total proctocolectomy has the advantage of removing all diseased mucosa, thereby preventing further inflammation or the potential for progression to dysplasia or carcinoma. The major disadvantage of this procedure is the need for a permanent ileostomy. In addition, despite improvements in bowel preparation, antibiotics, and surgical technique, total proctocolectomy still has a fairly high morbidity rate. Most of the morbidity is related to perineal wound healing, adhesions, the ileostomy, and complications of pelvic dissection. Perineal wound problems may be reduced if an intersphincteric proctectomy is performed. This approach involves a dissection between the internal and external sphincters, preserving the external sphincter and levator ani for a more secure perineal wound closure.

Total proctocolectomy with end ileostomy was one of the earliest operations performed for ulcerative colitis, and despite advances in sphincter-saving procedures, continues to have a role. Elderly patients, those with poor sphincter function, and patients with carcinomas in the distal rectum may be candidates for this procedure. All patients should be marked for an ileostomy preoperatively in the sitting and standing positions. The preferred site of the stoma is within the body of the rectus abdominis muscle at the summit of the infraumbilical fat mound on the right side, away from bony prominences, the umbilicus, and the midline incision.

Total Proctocolectomy With Continent Ileostomy

The continent ileostomy was introduced by Kock in 1969 and became popular in the 1970s because it offered control of evacuations for patients with an ileostomy. A single-chambered reservoir is fashioned by suturing several limbs of ileum together after the antimesenteric border has been divided. The outflow tract is intussuscepted into the reservoir to create a valve that provides obstruction to the pouch contents (continence). As the pouch distends, pressure over the valve causes it close and retain stool, permitting patients to wear a simple bandage over a skin-level stoma. Between two and four times per day, the patient introduces a tube through the valve to evacuate the pouch.

The major problem with the Kock pouch is the high complication rate necessitating reoperation in up to half of patients. The most common problem is a slipped valve, which occurs when the intussuscepted limb everts, and the "continent" nipple is lost. This leads to either the inability of the pouch to remain continent or the inability to intubate the pouch, leading to spontaneous emptying of the pouch as it overflows. Revision of the nipple valve corrects this problem. Other complications include inflammation of the ileal pouch mucosa ("pouchitis") in 15% to 30% of cases, fistula formation (10%), and stoma stricture (10%).

Since the introduction of restorative proctocolectomy and IPAA, the popularity of the continent ileostomy has declined, and it is seldom used. High complication and reoperation rates have dampened enthusiasm among surgeons for the technique. Although ulcerative colitis patients in whom IPAA is contraindicated may be candidates, realistically, only a very few centers presently offer the operation. Currently, the most common surgery related to continent ileostomies is revisional surgery. The Kock procedure should not be performed in obese patients, debilitated patients, or any patient with physical or mental handicap that would prohibit safe catheterization of the reservoir. The procedure is contraindicated in patients with Crohn's disease because of the high incidence of recurrence of Crohn's causing failure of the pouch.

Total Proctocolectomy With Ileal Pouch–Anal Anastomosis

Restorative proctocolectomy with IPAA has become the most common definitive operation for the surgical treat-

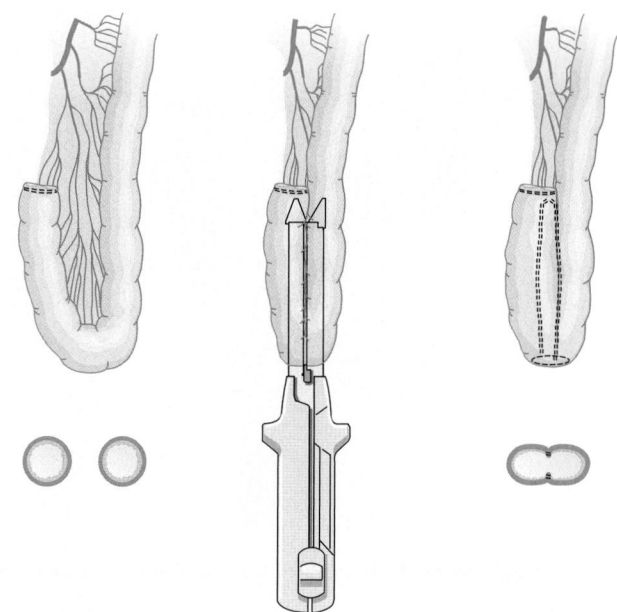

Figure 50-33 Creation of an ileal J pouch using a cutting linear stapler. For replacement of the rectum, a reservoir is created from the distal ileum. The stapler joins two limbs of intestine with staples while dividing the intervening wall. The diameter of the pouch so created is twice as large as the original diameter of the ileum.

ment of ulcerative colitis. The procedure involves a near-total proctocolectomy with preservation of the anal sphincter complex. A single-chambered pouch is fashioned from the distal 30 cm of the ileum (Fig. 50-33) and sutured to the anus using a double-stapled technique (Fig. 50-34). Alternatively, a hand-sewn anastomosis may be fashioned between the pouch and the anus after stripping the distal rectal mucosa from the internal anal sphincter (mucosectomy) (Fig. 50-35).

Some controversy exists concerning the advantages of performing a mucosectomy, especially as a routine component of the procedure. The double-stapling technique may leave a small remnant of rectal mucosa at the anastomosis, which, in theory, is at risk for the development of dysplasia and cancer. Large retrospective long-term analyses of outcomes of this technique have failed to bear this out. Mucosectomy has, however, been complicated by cancer arising at the anastomosis and extraluminally in the pelvis, evidently from islands of glands that remained after the mucosa was incompletely removed. Although cancer is exceedingly rare, the mucosectomy technique may conceal retained rectal mucosa in more than 20% of patients. The double-stapling technique permits surveillance and biopsy of the remaining mucosa. Avoiding the mucosectomy preserves the anal transition zone, which contains nerve endings involved in differentiating liquid and solid stool from gas, and is thus thought to provide superior postoperative continence.

Controversy also exists regarding temporary fecal diversion. The pouch and anastomosis were traditionally

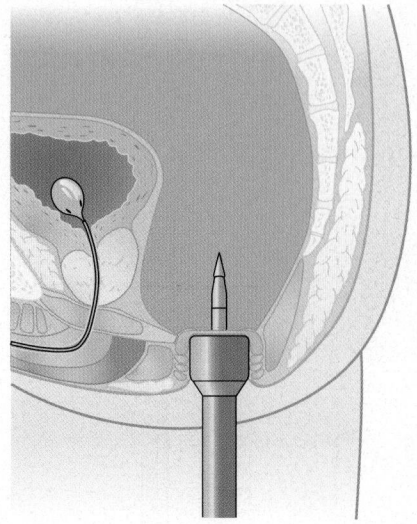
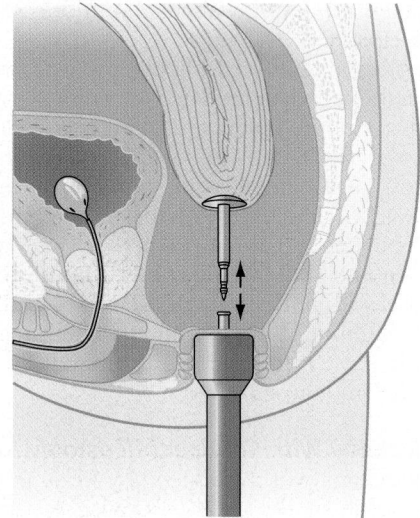

Figure 50-34 Fashioning of stapled ileal pouch–anal anastomosis.

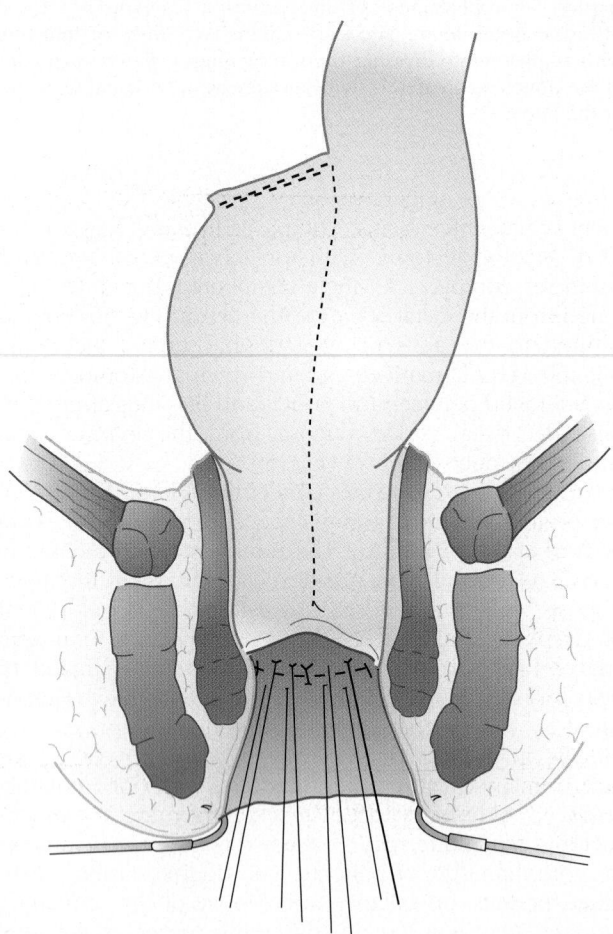

Figure 50-35 Hand-sewn ileal pouch–anal anastomosis following anorectal mucosectomy.

protected with a diverting loop ileostomy; however, there are some proponents of the single-stage procedure without diversion. This approach has the advantage of a single operation that avoids the complications that accompany an ileostomy. Disadvantages, however, include an increased risk for pelvic sepsis caused, usually, by anastomotic leak of a pouch suture line or the anal anastomosis. Most surgeons routinely perform a two-stage operation in high-risk patients, particularly those patients taking steroids preoperatively.

Patients who undergo total proctocolectomy and IPAA typically have between five and seven bowel movements in a 24-hour period. Function continues to improve with time, with numerous studies demonstrating a decrease in the number of daily bowel movements during the ensuing 3 to 24 months after reestablishment of continuity.

Restorative proctocolectomy and IPAA are associated with both early and late complications. A common complication is small bowel obstruction, occurring in up to 27% of patients. Bowel obstruction after IPAA tends to be severe and requires surgery in almost half of cases. Another significant complication is pelvic sepsis. Anastomotic and pouch suture line leaks are devastating complications that can lead to pelvic abscess and seriously threaten the integrity and functionality of the pouch. Treatment of pelvic sepsis secondary to pouch leaks usually requires a diverting ileostomy and drainage of any abscesses. Delayed ileostomy closure after resolution of IPAA complications has no deleterious functional effects. A pouch-vaginal fistula is a specific form of pelvic sepsis that is difficult to manage and occurs in up to 7% of women. Persistence of the fistula after surgical closure (and often temporary diversion) usually signifies underlying Crohn's disease and may result in the loss of the pouch in a significant number of patients.

Inflammation of the mucosa of the ileal pouch, or *pouchitis,* occurs in 7% to 33% of patients with ulcerative colitis treated by IPAA. Pouchitis typically presents with

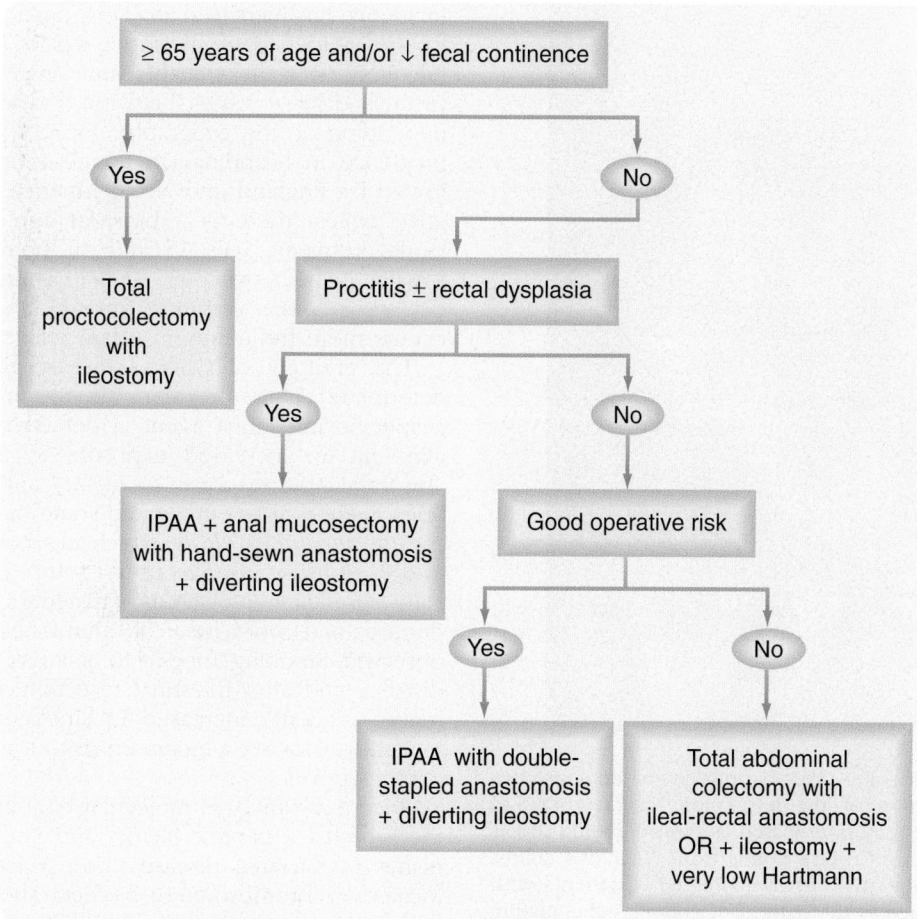

Figure 50-36 Elective operations for ulcerative colitis. IPAA, ileal pouch–anal anastomosis.

increased stool frequency, fever, bleeding, cramps, and dehydration. The cause is unknown but may be related to bacterial overgrowth, mucosal ischemia, or other local factors. Episodes usually respond to rehydration and oral antibiotics (usually metronidazole or ciprofloxacin). Probiotics have recently been reported to provide dramatic resolution in some cases of pouchitis resistant to antibiotic therapy. The diagnosis of Crohn's disease must also be entertained in patients with significant pouchitis that does not respond to medical treatment.

In some cases, the preoperative distinction between Crohn's disease and ulcerative colitis can be difficult, and the pathologist may label the disease "indeterminate colitis." Patients with Crohn's disease are not candidates for IPAA, because of the very high incidence of recurrent inflammation in the pouch that can cause abscesses, fistulas, and loss of the reservoir. Patients with indeterminate colitis who undergo restorative proctocolectomy and IPAA who do not develop Crohn's disease have results that are more encouraging, and patients with indeterminate colitis are generally considered candidates for IPAA if they understand that they are at increased risk for pouch complications related to underlying Crohn's disease.

Summary of Elective Operations

A suggested algorithm for elective operations for patients with intractable mucosal ulcerative colitis is presented in Figure 50-36. Elderly patients or those with fecal incontinence should undergo a total proctocolectomy with an end ileostomy. Younger patients with no evidence of rectal dysplasia should undergo restorative proctocolectomy and IPAA with a double-stapled anastomosis and diverting loop ileostomy. Patients with confirmed rectal dysplasia should be treated with mucosectomy and a hand-sewn IPAA. Patients with significant debility who are poor operative candidates should undergo a total abdominal colectomy with a very low Hartmann closure and an end ileostomy.

Postoperative Care

Postoperative care after restorative proctocolectomy with IPAA is similar to other major colorectal procedures. Nasogastric tubes are usually removed at the completion of the procedure, and liquid diets are offered to patients in the early recovery period. Diet is advanced with return of bowel function as evidenced by ileostomy function. If a pelvic drain is used, it is typically removed after 48 to

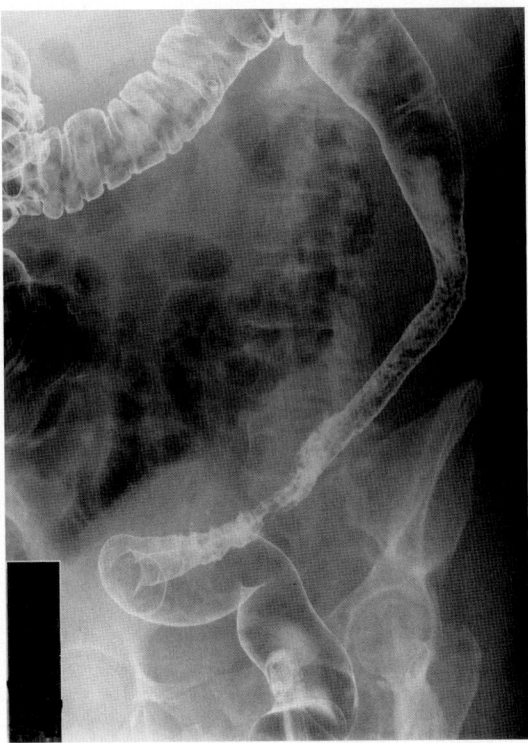

Figure 50-37 Crohn's colitis. This barium enema demonstrates segmental inflammation of the left colon, characteristic of Crohn's disease. The rectum is spared, a clinical finding that is useful in distinguishing Crohn's colitis from ulcerative colitis. The rectal mucosa is virtually always affected in patients with ulcerative colitis, whereas the pattern of colonic inflammation is variable in Crohn's colitis.

72 hours. Bladder catheters are typically left in place for 3 to 4 days depending on the difficulty of pelvic dissection. A water-soluble contrast enema is performed about 10 weeks postoperatively to ensure an intact IPAA. If the enema shows a leak, the contrast examination is repeated in 6 weeks; close to 95% of anastomotic leaks heal in the absence of pelvic sepsis. If the radiograph shows no leak, the diverting ileostomy is closed.

Crohn's Colitis

Originally described as *regional ileitis,* Crohn's disease is a nonspecific inflammatory bowel disease that may affect any segment of the gastrointestinal tract. Fifteen percent of patients with Crohn's have disease limited to the colon. The inflammatory process may affect the entire colon and mimic ulcerative colitis, or it may affect only segments of the colon (Fig. 50-37). This section discusses Crohn's colitis; additional discussions of Crohn's disease are found elsewhere in this text.

Epidemiology and Etiology

A rapid increase in the incidence of Crohn's disease occurred between 1965 and 1980, and since then, the incidence has increased at a slow pace. This is in contrast to the incidence of ulcerative colitis, which has been relatively constant over the same time. The incidence of Crohn's disease varies between 1 and 10 per 100,000 depending on the geographic location, with the highest incidence in Scandinavian countries and Scotland, followed by England and North America. Similar to ulcerative colitis, there is a bimodal age distribution with peaks between ages 15 and 30 years and a second, smaller peak between 55 and 80 years of age. Crohn's disease is more common among Jewish patients and occurs more frequently in urban residents.

The etiology of Crohn's disease has not yet been determined. Three prevalent theories include response to a specific infectious agent, a defective mucosal barrier allowing an increased exposure to antigens, and an abnormal host response to dietary antigens. One infectious agent that has generated some interest is *Mycobacterium paratuberculosis,* which has been isolated in up to 65% of tissue samples from Crohn's patients. A statistically significant association between the onset of Crohn's disease and prior use of antibiotics has also been observed. Smoking appears to be a risk factor for Crohn's disease, and after intestinal resection, the risk of recurrence is greatly increased in smokers. Several studies have also shown an increased risk in patients taking oral contraceptives.

Recent advances in molecular biology have intensified the search for genetic factors and pathogenetic mechanisms in Crohn's disease. The *NOD2/CARD15* gene, located on chromosome 16, has been shown to be involved in the activation of nuclear factor kappa-B (NF-κB), a transcription factor that plays a significant role in Crohn's disease. Specific genotypes may also determine susceptibility, location, and behavior of Crohn's disease.[27]

Pathologic Features

Gross Appearance

Crohn's disease is a transmural, predominantly submucosal inflammation characterized by a thickened colonic wall. The affected mucosa observed by endoscopy is often described as having a cobblestone appearance. In severe disease, the bowel wall may be entirely encased by creeping fat of the mesentery, and strictures may develop in the small and large intestine. The mucosa may demonstrate long, deep linear ulcers that appear like "railroad tracks" or "bear claws" (Fig. 50-38). Normal mucosa may intervene between areas of inflammation, causing "skip areas" characteristic of the disease.

Histologic Appearance

Crohn's disease is characterized microscopically by transmural inflammation, submucosal edema, lymphoid aggregation, and ultimately fibrosis. The pathognomonic histologic feature of Crohn's disease is the noncaseating granuloma, a localized, well-formed aggregate of epithelioid histocytes surrounded by lymphocytes and giant cells (Fig. 50-39). Granulomas are found in 50% of specimens resected in Crohn's disease; however, the number identified by colonoscopic biopsy is far smaller.

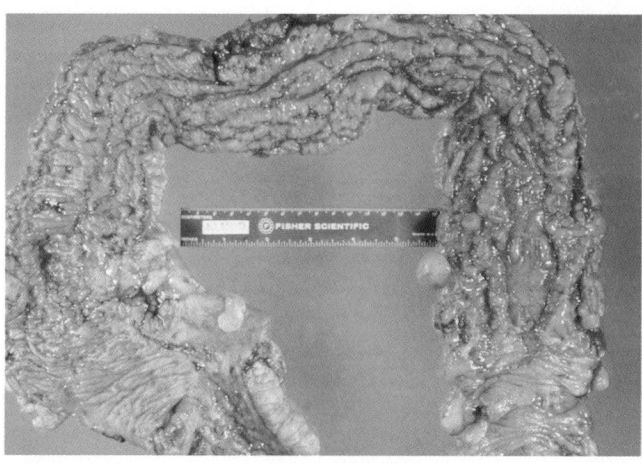

Figure 50-38 Crohn's colitis. Linear ulceration of the mucosa, giving appearance of a railroad track or bear claw ulcers.

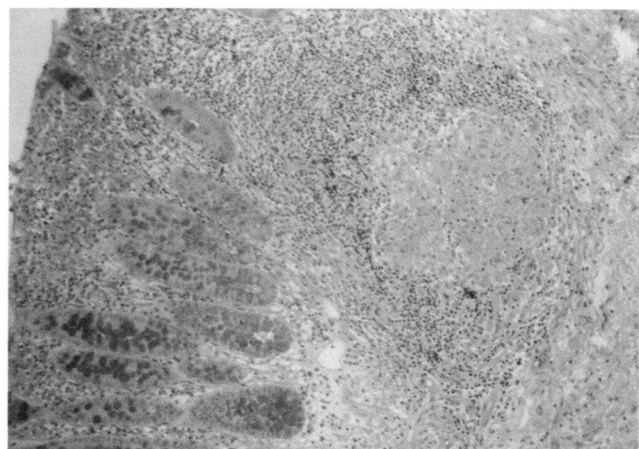

Figure 50-39 Crohn's colitis with noncaseating granuloma.

Clinical Presentation

Patients with Crohn's disease may present with a wide spectrum of severity, from subtle symptoms to overwhelming fulminant disease. The characteristic triad of symptoms—abdominal pain, diarrhea, and weight loss—mimic viral gastroenteritis or irritable bowel syndrome. Other symptoms may include anorexia, fever, and recurrent oral aphthous ulcers. Patients with a family history of Crohn's disease tend to present with more extensive disease. In contrast to ulcerative colitis, in which the rectum is invariably involved, only half of patients with Crohn's colitis have rectal disease. Two thirds of patients with Crohn's colitis have involvement of the entire colon.

Anal disease, including anal fistulas, fissures, strictures, edematous skin tags, and erosion of the anoderm, occurs in up to 30% of patients with Crohn's disease of the terminal ileum and in more than 50% of patients with colonic disease. Anal disease in a patient with colitis suggests a diagnosis of Crohn's disease because primary anal disease is unusual in patients with ulcerative colitis.

Diagnosis

The differential diagnosis of Crohn's colitis includes ulcerative colitis and various infectious agents. As with patients with ulcerative colitis, stool should be sent for culture and examined for ova and parasites. The diagnosis of Crohn's colitis is made by a combination of clinical, endoscopic, and radiologic features. Barium enema may not demonstrate any abnormalities in mild and early disease; colonoscopy is the more sensitive diagnostic modality. The disease is often patchy in distribution; however, some patients may have granular and friable mucosa in a continuous pattern involving the entire colon and rectum. Edema of the mucosa and aphthous ulcers are present in early Crohn's disease, with deep linear ulcers present in more severe disease and strictures more prevalent in chronic disease. It is at times difficult to distinguish Crohn's disease from ulcerative colitis, particularly if the rectum is involved. Biopsy samples should be obtained. However, unless a granuloma is identified,

distinguishing between the two diseases may still be difficult.

An air-contrast enema may provide useful information in making the diagnosis and determining the extent of the disease. Characteristic radiologic findings in Crohn's colitis are skip lesions, contour defects, longitudinal and transverse ulcers, a cobblestone-like mucosal pattern, strictures, thickening of the haustral margin, and irregular nodular defects. A small bowel series or enteroclysis should be performed in all patients with suspected Crohn's disease or ulcerative colitis. Involvement of the small intestine strongly favors the diagnosis of Crohn's disease (Fig. 50-40). CT may demonstrate thickening of the colon, adenopathy, or intra-abdominal abscess.

Medical Therapy

The medical treatment of Crohn's disease is similar to that of ulcerative colitis and includes aminosalicylates, steroids, and immunomodulatory medications (6-MP, azathioprine, and cyclosporine). One immunomodulatory drug that deserves mention in the treatment of Crohn's disease is infliximab, a monoclonal anti–tumor necrosis factor-α (anti–TNF-α) antibody designed to block the TNF-α receptor in an effort to decrease inflammation. Infliximab is given as an intravenous infusion to treat Crohn's disease in steroid-dependent or intractable patients and has also been shown to be of use in patients with chronic draining fistulas. Although initial response rates have been favorable, it is yet unclear whether long-term administration is effective, and higher rates of lymphoma have been reported in patients treated with infliximab.

Indications for Surgery

The indications for surgery in patients with Crohn's colitis are presented in Box 50-2. Operative treatment in Crohn's disease is intended to relieve symptoms when medical management has failed, correct complications, and prevent the development of cancer. It must be remembered that Crohn's disease is a pan-gastrointestinal

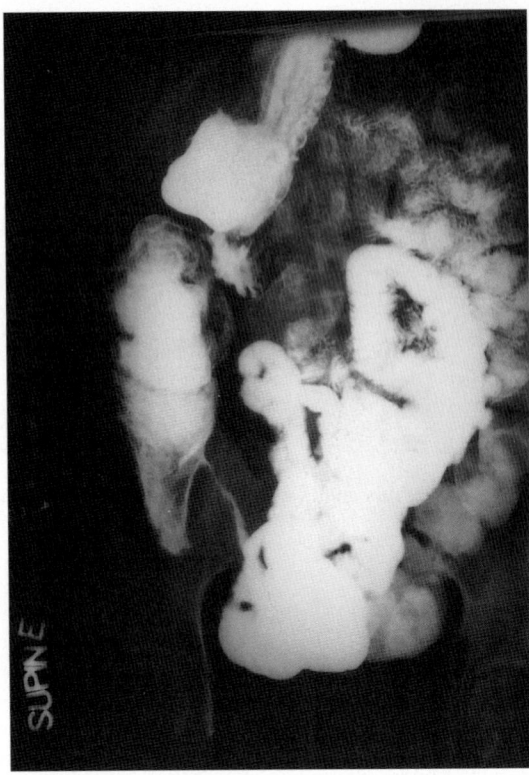

Figure 50-40 Small bowel contrast study demonstrating "string sign" caused by inflammation and narrowing of the terminal ileum.

Box 50-2 Crohn's Colitis—Indications for Surgery

Intractability
Intestinal obstruction
Intra-abdominal abscess
Fistulas
Fulminant colitis
Toxic megacolon
Massive bleeding
Cancer
Growth retardation

---

disease, and therefore surgical intervention may not cure the patient.

Intractability

Patients who fail to respond to optimal medical therapy for Crohn's disease and remain debilitated are often referred for surgical consultation. As with ulcerative colitis, this represents the most common indication for operative treatment for Crohn's disease.

Intestinal Obstruction

Intestinal obstruction in Crohn's disease may be caused by active inflammation, a fibrotic stricture from chronic disease, or an abscess or phlegmon causing a mass effect. Adhesions from previous abdominal operations must also be considered. Obstruction typically involves the small intestine, although large bowel obstruction from strictures

may occur. Initial treatment includes bowel rest, nasogastric decompression, intravenous fluids, and anti-inflammatory medications, usually steroids. Obstruction caused by a strictured anastomosis may be treated by endoscopic balloon dilation.

Intra-abdominal Abscess

An intra-abdominal abscess in Crohn's disease is the result of intestinal perforation caused by transmural inflammation. An abscess is usually diagnosed by CT scan and can often be managed nonoperatively with CT-guided percutaneous drainage and antibiotics. If percutaneous drainage is not feasible or the patient does not respond to this therapy, laparotomy, drainage of the abscess, and resection of the involved bowel are indicated.

Fistulas

Fistulas may develop between the intestine and any other intra-abdominal organ, including the bladder, bowel, uterus, vagina, and stomach. Up to 35% of patients with Crohn's disease develop such fistulas, most of which involve the small intestine. Asymptomatic enteroenteric or enterocolic fistulas may not require operative therapy. A common fistula associated with Crohn's disease is an ileosigmoid fistula. This usually is caused by ileal disease with secondary involvement of the sigmoid. Symptomatic patients should undergo resection of the terminal ileum. When the inflammation in the sigmoid colon is minimal, the sigmoid defect can be primarily closed. Extensive inflammation in the sigmoid, however, requires resection of the sigmoid colon as well. Colovesical and colovaginal fistulas require resection of the diseased bowel and closure of the bladder or vagina with interposition of omentum between the bowel and the contiguous organ.

Enterocutaneous fistulas in Crohn's disease may develop spontaneously (typically with ileal disease) or as the result of an early postoperative anastomotic breakdown. Patients are initially treated with bowel rest and drainage of any intra-abdominal abscess. Parenteral nutrition and medical treatment of the disease may result in spontaneous closure of the fistula; however, operative treatment is often necessary.

Fulminant Colitis and Toxic Megacolon

Patients with Crohn's disease may present with fulminant colitis in a fashion similar to patients with ulcerative colitis presenting with toxic megacolon. Fulminant colitis typically presents with high fever, severe abdominal pain, tenderness, tachycardia, and leukocytosis. Patients should be monitored in an intensive care unit and given intravenous fluids, bowel rest, antibiotics, and steroids. If there is evidence of clinical deterioration, or if there is no significant improvement within a short period, subtotal colectomy with an end ileostomy is indicated. Patients with toxic megacolon due to Crohn's disease undergo surgical treatment similar to those with toxic megacolon due to ulcerative colitis. Because the pathologic process in Crohn's disease involves inflammation of the entire bowel wall, the colonic dilation characteristic of toxic megacolon may not

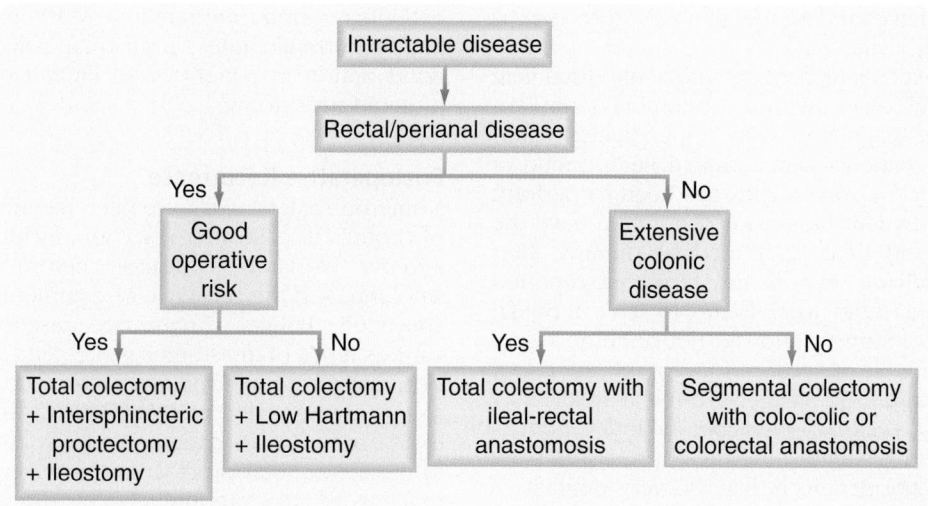

Figure 50-41 Elective operations for Crohn's colitis.

occur in patients with Crohn's disease, but the toxicity of the colitis may be no less severe.

Massive Bleeding

Massive bleeding, although less common in Crohn's disease than in ulcerative colitis, can occur in up to 13% of patients in some series. The terminal ileum represents the most common site of bleeding. If the disease involves the colon and spares the ileum, and the bleeding does not respond to medical therapy, flexible sigmoidoscopy or proctoscopy should be performed to rule out a rectal source. Appropriate operative treatment in the rare instances of colonic bleeding for Crohn's colitis is abdominal colectomy and ileostomy or ileorectal anastomosis if the rectum is not inflamed.

Cancer

The risk for development of carcinoma of the colon is not as high as the risk in long-standing, chronic ulcerative colitis, but it is present; therefore, patients with chronic, active disease require periodic colonoscopic surveillance and biopsy. The presence of high-grade dysplasia is an indication for colectomy. Patients who have undergone intestinal bypass for Crohn's disease have an increased risk for developing carcinoma; therefore, a bypassed segment of Crohn's disease should be resected if possible.

Extracolonic Manifestations

Extraintestinal manifestations of Crohn's disease are similar to those associated with ulcerative colitis. With the exception of primary sclerosing cholangitis, cirrhosis, and ankylosing spondylitis, most extracolonic manifestations of Crohn's disease improve after resection of the diseased bowel.

Growth Retardation

Young patients with Crohn's disease and ulcerative colitis may be have impaired growth and mental development.

Growth failure is often the result of prolonged inadequate caloric intake; therefore, nutritional support is an important component of care in these patients. Resection of severely diseased segments of bowel before puberty may help to eliminate growth retardation and premature closure of bone epiphyses.

Operations

Because surgical intervention is not curative, medical therapy is the mainstay of treatment of Crohn's disease. Recurrence rates after surgery are high, and the risk continues with the passage of time. Therefore, an important principle in the surgical treatment of Crohn's disease is to resect only enough intestine to improve symptoms or correct complications. Intestine should be resected with the aim of obtaining margins free of disease by gross inspection. Frozen sections of the margins of resection are unnecessary because positive microscopic margins are not predictive of postoperative recurrence. Resection of grossly normal-appearing intestine may eventually lead to a short bowel syndrome, with insufficient absorptive surface to maintain nutrition. A suggested algorithm for elective operations for patients with intractable Crohn's disease is presented in Figure 50-41.

Ileocecal Resection

Ileocecal resection is indicated in patients with severe disease of the terminal ileum resulting in obstruction or perforation. It typically involves resection of about 6 to 12 inches of the terminal ileum and cecum, with an anastomosis created between the ileum and ascending colon. The terminal ileum is transected 2 cm proximal to the grossly apparent Crohn's disease. The technique of feeling a sharp mesenteric-bowel margin correlates well with the intraluminal disease and prevents removing additional uninvolved small intestine. In most series, the recurrence rate of Crohn's disease requiring re-resection in patients who have undergone ileocolic resection is roughly 50% in 10 years.

Occasionally, patients presenting with acute distal ileal disease (fever, right lower quadrant abdominal pain, leukocytosis) are misdiagnosed with appendicitis. Traditional therapy for patients with terminal ileitis found at the time of surgery for appendicitis has been to perform an appendectomy when the cecum is normal, leave the ileum in place, and treat with medical therapy after surgery. A contradictory experience, however, reported that 92% of patients who were found to have terminal ileitis at the time of surgery and did not undergo resection required ileocolic resection for complications of Crohn's disease within 12 years.[28] Terminal ileitis may also be caused by *Yersinia enterocolitica* and *Campylobacter* species, and distinguishing these processes from Crohn's disease intraoperatively may be very difficult.

Total Proctocolectomy With End Ileostomy

Total proctocolectomy with end ileostomy involves removing all of the abdominal colon, rectum, and anus and is indicated in patients with Crohn's disease involving the entire colon and rectum or when fecal incontinence is too severe to warrant preserving the rectum. Disadvantages of this procedure include delayed healing of the perineal wound and problems with malabsorption. Intersphincteric proctectomy decreases the incidence of perineal wound complications. Rapid small bowel transit and malabsorption of nutrients may occur more frequently after this procedure in patients with Crohn's disease as compared with patients with ulcerative colitis because variable amounts of terminal ileum may be involved in the disease process.

Total Abdominal Colectomy With Ileorectal Anastomosis or End Ileostomy

Total abdominal colectomy with ileorectal anastomosis is indicated in patients with Crohn's colitis with sparing of the rectum and anus and offers the best functional results in patients who wish to maintain intestinal continuity. After this procedure, patients may expect to have between four and six bowel movements per day. The major disadvantage of the operation is the high likelihood of recurrence requiring completion proctectomy and ileostomy. Numerous studies have shown that roughly 50% of patients require proctectomy within 10 years. Patients who are poor operative candidates may best be served with a total abdominal colectomy and proximal proctectomy with low Hartmann's closure and end ileostomy.

Segmental Colon Resection

Between 10% and 20% of patients with Crohn's colitis have disease limited to a segment of colon. Segmental colon resection may therefore be an option in patients with limited colonic disease associated with stricture or obstruction. It is contraindicated in patients with severe rectal or anal disease. As with total abdominal colectomy and ileorectal anastomosis, the major disadvantage of segmental colon resection is the high rate of recurrence requiring subsequent operations. Within 5 years, recurrence rates range between 30% and 50%, with 60% of patients requiring reoperation by 10 years. Despite these high recurrence rates, segmental colectomy may be a good option in patients with limited disease who wish to avoid an ostomy.

Postoperative Recurrence

Numerous risk factors have been identified for recurrence of Crohn's disease after resection, including duration and severity of Crohn's disease before initial resection, smoking, and the presence of granulomas in the resected specimen. Longer disease-free resection margins and various types of anastomoses (i.e., end-to-side or side-to-side) have not been shown to affect recurrence rates. The reoperative rate for patients with Crohn's disease is 4% to 5% per year. In patients with Crohn's disease limited to the colon, total proctocolectomy has the lowest recurrence, with rates varying between 10% and 25%, depending on the length of follow-up.

Maintaining remission of Crohn's disease after resection remains an area of active investigation. Options include treatment with 5-ASA compounds, antibiotics, and the thiopurines azathioprine and 6-MP. A meta-analysis demonstrated an 18% reduction in postoperative recurrence in patients treated with 4 g/day of 5-ASA.[29] Metronidazole given for 3 months after surgery also has been shown to decrease recurrence; however, the side effects of long-term treatment with this medication preclude its routine use. In comparison with 5-ASA, azathioprine has been shown to have equal reduction in postoperative recurrence, with an increased benefit in patients who had undergone at least one previous resection.[30] Prophylaxis is typically begun within 2 weeks after surgery.

INFECTIOUS COLITIS

Various forms of infectious enteritis are brought to the attention of the surgeon because they may present as an acute abdomen, masquerade as Crohn's disease or ulcerative colitis, result from standard treatment for a surgical procedure (prophylactic antibiotics for intestinal operations), or progress to the point that surgical treatment is required. The initial evaluation of a patient with diarrhea suspected of having inflammatory bowel disease should include stool samples to be evaluated for *C. jejuni*, *Y. enterocolitica*, *Salmonella typhi*, and *C. difficile*.

C. jejuni is a leading cause of infectious colitis worldwide and has become one of the major causes of infectious diarrhea in the United States. *C. jejuni* is a curved, microaerophilic, gram-positive rod. Symptoms and findings of *Campylobacter* enteritis are similar to other nonspecific IBDs and include bloody diarrhea, abdominal pain, fever, nausea, and vomiting. Toxic megacolon resulting from *C. jejuni* is rare but has been reported. Endoscopic evaluation usually shows an edematous, inflamed mucosa, and histologic examination is usually nonspecific; dark-field microscopy may identify the organism. Treatment of *Campylobacter* enteritis is with ciprofloxacin.

Y. enterocolitica also can cause enteric infection, most commonly in infants, young children, and young adults. It typically occurs in the ileocecal region, thereby mimicking appendicitis as well as Crohn's disease. Patients infected with *Yersinia* typically present with bloody diarrhea and abdominal pain. Diagnosis is made by isolation of the bacteria from the stool. Radiographically, the terminal ileum may demonstrate a coarse, irregular, nodular mucosal pattern with ulcerations; however, because the disease is confined to the mucosa and submucosa, the characteristic string sign seen in Crohn's disease is absent. *Yersinia* enteritis will often resolve with supportive care alone; however, in more severe cases, patients should be treated with aminoglycosides or trimethoprim-sulfamethoxazole.

S. typhi causes an infectious enterocolitis in 16 million people worldwide annually and is the cause of typhoid fever. Invasion of the mucosa and submucosa of the small bowel and colon leads to an inflammatory reaction and release of an endotoxin from the bacterial cell. Severe septicemia may also occur if the organism enters the bloodstream. Toxic megacolon and intestinal perforation have been reported with *S. typhi* infection, and on rare occasions, patients may develop massive lower gastrointestinal bleeding. Gangrenous cholecystitis has also been reported with typhoid fever. Diagnosis is based on culture of the organism from the stool or blood. Medical management includes treatment with fluoroquinolones or third-generation cephalosporins. Surgical intervention is warranted in cases of peritonitis secondary to perforation and generally requires resection of the affected bowel or diversion.

C. difficile is a gram-positive, spore-forming anaerobic microorganism that is related to the bacteria that cause tetanus and botulism. The organism has two forms: an active, infectious form that is difficult to culture and cannot survive in the environment for prolonged periods, and an inactive spore that can survive for long periods and can be often be found in hospitals, operating rooms, nursing homes, and extended care facilities. The spores can enter the intestinal tract and transform into the active form of the organism. Usually the growth of the active organism is suppressed by the normal (autochthonous) bacteria of the colon, but antibiotics that suppress the colonic flora permit overgrowth of *C. difficile,* which releases toxins that cause diarrhea.

C. difficile produces two toxins (A and B), both of which are important in the pathogenesis of pseudomembranous colitis. Toxin A, the toxin that directly leads to the development of colitis, is released by the bacterium and binds to a colonocyte glycoprotein receptor. This leads to the destruction of the colonocyte and the release of inflammatory mediators. Toxin A is also a chemoattractant for neutrophils and activates macrophages and mast cells, resulting in further inflammation and systemic symptoms of sepsis. Toxin B is also a potent cytotoxin and has the potential to cause colitis even in strains of *C. difficile* that do not produce toxin A.

C. difficile colitis typically begins within 4 to 9 days after the initiation of antibiotics, although 25% of patients may not become symptomatic until up to 10 weeks after a course of antibiotics. Clinically, it may present as diarrhea, self-limited colitis, pseudomembranous colitis, toxin megacolon, or fulminant colitis. Diarrhea is often accompanied by crampy abdominal pain and anorexia, and patients may also have fever, leukocytosis, and electrolyte abnormalities.

Laboratory diagnosis can be made by demonstrating the toxins in the stool with an enzyme-linked immunosorbent assay (ELISA). These tests can be performed within hours; however, their accuracy is not 100%. Therefore, a negative test does not rule out the disease. The test of choice to confirm the suspected diagnosis is the stool cytotoxin test, which has a high sensitivity (94%-100%) and specificity (99%). A stool sample is filtered and added to cultured fibroblasts. A cytopathic effect that is neutralized by specific antiserum confirms the diagnosis. The test is expensive and requires overnight incubation and a tissue culture facility. If the diagnosis remains unclear, proctoscopy or flexible sigmoidoscopy may reveal inflamed mucosa covered by yellowish plaquelike membranes, or *pseudomembranes*. These pseudomembranes are composed of a mixture of inflammatory cells, fibrin, and bacterial and cellular components; they are seen in roughly 25% of patients with mild disease and 87% of patients with fulminant colitis.

Treatment should be tailored to the severity of the disease. For mild cases (patients without fever, abdominal pain, or leukocytosis), cessation of all antibiotics may be the only treatment necessary. Patients with more severe diarrhea or toxic symptoms should be treated by discontinuing the causative antibiotics and administering antibiotics directed against *C. difficile.* Vancomycin (oral) or metronidazole (oral or intravenous) are equally effective against the organism, and improvement is usually seen within 3 days of initiating therapy. Treatment is usually continued for 10 days, but relapse occurs in about 25% of cases after cessation of treatment. Recurrence is treated with a repeated course of vancomycin or metronidazole.

Severe cases of *C. difficile* colitis may progress to a fulminant disease and toxic megacolon. In such circumstances, abdominal colectomy with ileostomy is indicated. Unfortunately, the mortality rate associated with *C. difficile* colitis of such severity that colectomy is required is greater than 50%.

There have been reports of outbreaks of especially severe *C. difficile* colitis that are associated with a higher mortality rate than expected with the usual strains. This strain has a defective gene, *TxcD,* which is associated with extremely high toxin production by the bacteria. The currently used diagnostic tests do not distinguish this strain from the usual strain, but it responds to treatment with metronidazole or vancomycin.

COLONIC ISCHEMIA

Colonic ischemia (CI) is the most common form of intestinal ischemia. Most attacks are transient and resolve spontaneously; thus, the entity is often misdiagnosed or unrecognized. Although the etiology of many cases of CI is obscure, aortic surgery, arteriosclerotic disease, and conditions causing transient hypotension have been implicated. Other factors associated with the disease include the use of oral contraceptives, cocaine abuse, hereditary coagulopathies, long-distance running, and certain bacterial pathogens, including cytomegalovirus (CMV) and *E. coli O157:H7*.[31]

As described previously, the colon is supplied with arterial blood from the superior and inferior mesenteric arteries. There are collateral channels that may develop between these major mesenteric arteries; it is not unusual for the marginal artery or the arc of Riolan to provide collateral circulation adequate to sustain the left colon if the inferior mesenteric artery has been gradually occluded by atherosclerosis. Indeed, the IMA is frequently occluded in conditions requiring aortic surgery, and in such circumstances, transection of the IMA does not require reimplantation. However, in this situation, the left colon is dependent on collateral blood supply, and transient hypotension at the time of the vascular procedure or immediately after surgery may result in ischemic injury to the vulnerable colonic mucosa.

The spectrum of CI includes transient ischemia, chronic ischemia, and gangrene. The disease is usually segmental in nature. If the ischemia is limited to the most vulnerable layer of the intestine, the mucosa, the disease may be transient, and recovery may be complete. More significant ischemia involving the muscularis may result in scarring and a chronic stricture. Ischemia affecting the full thickness of the bowel wall may result in gangrene with perforation and fecal peritonitis.

The signs and symptoms of colonic ischemia include abdominal pain, hematochezia, and fever. These symptoms vary considerably depending on the severity of the ischemia and the length as well as the thickness of the colon that is affected. Ischemia limited to a small segment of mucosa may cause cramping abdominal pain and passage of a small amount of blood; more significant mucosal ischemia may result in more severe abdominal pain and tenderness over the affected segment of colon, bacterial translocation, fever, leukocytosis, and acidosis; compromise of blood supply to the full thickness of the colonic wall will result in severe abdominal pain, fever, leukocytosis, acidosis, and signs of peritonitis.

Rapid and accurate diagnosis permits institution of supportive measures or withdrawal of offending medications (i.e., oral contraceptives) that may halt the progression of the disease and prevent mucosal ischemia from progressing to transmural gangrene. Early diagnosis is obviously facilitated by a high suspicion for colonic ischemia in the setting of mild to moderate abdominal pain, fever, and bloody diarrhea.

Radiologic investigation of CI usually begins with a plain film of the abdomen. The resulting picture is often nonspecific, but findings suggestive of colonic ischemia include an ileus, an isolated segment of distended colon, or, more specifically, *thumbprinting*—a sign caused by intestinal wall edema or submucosal hemorrhage. Free intraperitoneal air can result from gangrene causing intestinal perforation.

The use of barium enema for the diagnosis of acute colonic ischemia has become obsolete. The risk for perforation and barium peritonitis in this circumstance is unacceptable. Water-soluble contrast studies also carry a risk for perforation of the compromised intestine and should be avoided in the acute setting. However, contrast enemas are useful and acceptable for the detection and evaluation of a stricture that may have developed because of ischemia.

Flexible sigmoidoscopy provides the advantage of direct visualization of the colonic mucosa. Bacterial or viral cultures may be obtained, and biopsies may be taken. Unfortunately, biopsies of the mucosa in this setting are typically nonspecific and uninformative. The segment of large bowel most prone to ischemia is the sigmoid. Cases of isolated ischemic proctitis have been reported but are rare. All segments of the colon may be involved, but rarely is it necessary to visualize the colon beyond the level of the splenic flexure to establish the diagnosis. The finding of hemorrhagic, dusky mucosa is typical. Patches of inflammation may be interspersed with healthy-appearing mucosa. The major disadvantage of endoscopic diagnosis of CI is the inability to distinguish between mucosal and transmural gangrene.

CT with intravenous contrast is useful in such circumstances. This modality also may permit visualization of the arterial supply to the entire intestine. Arteriography is not indicated unless it is believed that acute mesenteric ischemia involves the small intestine. Arteriography does not change the management or outcome of clinically apparent colonic ischemia.

Treatment of CI depends on the presentation and severity of signs and symptoms (Fig. 50-42). Hospital admission, intravenous fluids, bowel rest, and general supportive measures until the patient is pain-free usually are adequate treatment for mucosal ischemia. Because loss of integrity of the mucosa may result in bacterial translocation, broad-spectrum antibiotics are generally advocated for the treatment of CI. Level 1 evidence for antibiotic treatment in humans is nonexistent, but antibiotics are associated with increased survival in rat models of CI.

There is a recognized risk for CI after abdominal aortic operations, and the diagnosis must be considered when abdominal pain, fever, leukocytosis, or acidosis occurs after this type of operation. Flexible sigmoidoscopy is indicated to establish the diagnosis. Monitoring of the patient includes serial abdominal examinations and frequent recording of vital signs, urine output, blood pH, and white blood cell count. Supportive measures are provided as described earlier. If transmural gangrene is suspected, immediate operation is indicated.

Although surgical intervention for CI is relatively uncommon, when it is indicated, the procedure of choice is partial or total colectomy with or without an end stoma (Box 50-3). Unlike mesenteric ischemia involving the small bowel, revascularization procedures to establish blood flow to the colon are not indicated. Indications for operation in CI are fairly straightforward. Colonic perforation is a clear indication for laparotomy and resection of

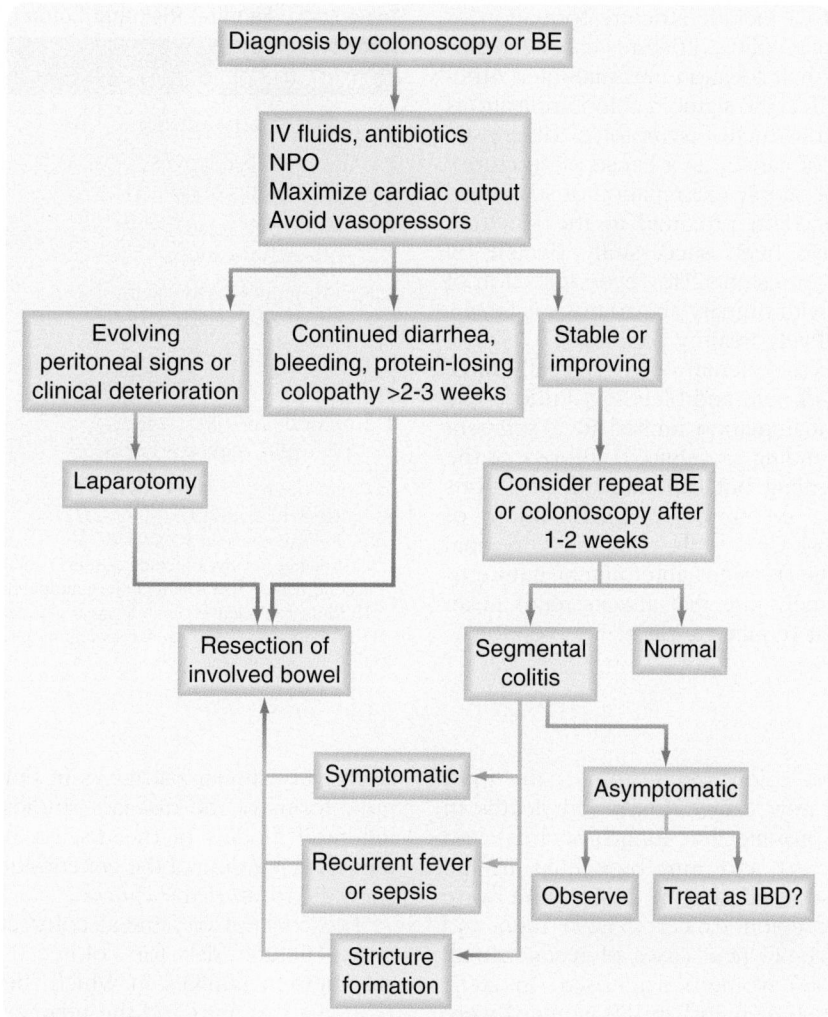

Figure 50-42 Management of colonic ischemia. BE, barium enema; IV, intravenous; NPO, nil per os; IBD, inflammatory bowel disease.

Box 50-3   Colonic Ischemia—Indications for Surgery

Acute Indications

Peritoneal signs
Massive bleeding
Universal fulminant colitis with or without toxic megacolon

Subacute Indications

Failure of an acute segmental ischemic colitis to respond within 2 to 3 weeks, with continued symptoms or a protein-losing colopathy
Apparent healing but with recurrent bouts of sepsis

Chronic Indications

Symptomatic colon stricture
Symptomatic segmental ischemic colitis

---

the ischemic segment with end ileostomy or colostomy. Total colonic ischemia is rare, but cases have been reported to mimic fulminant colitis or toxic megacolon. Such cases require treatment by total colectomy and end ileostomy. Although quite rare, massive bleeding in the setting of acute ischemic colitis is a serious and life-threatening occurrence. Subtotal colectomy with an end ileostomy is usually indicated in this situation unless the specifically involved segment of colon can be accurately identified and resected.[32]

Indications for surgery in subacute situations are uncommon. However, patients who remain symptomatic, with pain, bleeding, diarrhea or recurrent bouts of sepsis for 2 to 3 weeks after presentation with no improvement may require operation. Whether to fashion an anastomosis in this setting is unclear. The nature of this disease and the potential for serious septic complications argues for creation of a stoma.

Chronic sequelae of CI include stricture formation as well as chronic segmental colitis. Strictures can be symptomatic depending on their location and diameter. Strictures most commonly affect the sigmoid colon. Indications for treatment include obstructive symptoms, diagnostic uncertainty (suspicion of cancer as a cause of stricture), and impediment to endoscopic examination of suspected colonic lesions in the colon proximal to the stricture. Ischemic strictures have been successfully dilated by endoscopic techniques and stents. However, resection of the strictured segment with primary anastomosis is generally advocated for relatively healthy patients.

Patients with chronic segmental colitis typically have intermittent symptoms of pain and bleeding. Endoscopic examination reveals inflammation limited to a segment of colon (usually descending or sigmoid). Biopsy of the friable tissue is unrevealing but can rule out infectious etiologies. Frequently, colonoscopic examination of patients after a bout of CI reveals completely normal mucosa, testifying to the transient, intermittent nature of the attacks. It is extremely rare that attacks recur in an intermittent fashion that requires surgical intervention.

NEOPLASIA

Adenocarcinoma of the colon and rectum is the third most common site of new cancer cases and deaths in both men (following prostate and lung/bronchus) and women (following breast and lung/bronchus) in the United States. It is estimated that in 2007, there were 112,340 new cases of colon cancer (55,290 men and 57,050 women) and 41,420 new cases of rectal cancer (23,840 men and 17,580 women) diagnosed. In 2007, 52,180 Americans (26,000 men and 26,180 women) were predicted to die of colorectal cancer. The lifetime risk for developing colorectal cancer in the United States is 5.79% (1 in 17) for men and 5.37% (1 in 19) for women. The risk for developing invasive colorectal cancer increases with age, with more than 90% of new cases being diagnosed in patients older than 50 years. The overall incidence of colorectal cancer decreased at a rate of 2.1% per year from 1998 to 2003, and the death rate decreased 2.8% annually over the period from 2001 to 2003.[33]

Colorectal cancer occurs in hereditary, sporadic, or familial forms. Hereditary forms of colorectal cancer have been extensively described and are characterized by family history, young age at onset, and the presence of other specific tumors and defects. Familial adenomatous polyposis (FAP) and hereditary nonpolyposis colorectal cancer (HNPCC) have been the subject of many recent investigations that have provided significant insights into the pathogenesis of colorectal cancer.

Sporadic colorectal cancer occurs in the absence of family history, generally affects an older population (60-80 years of age), and usually presents as an isolated colon or rectal lesion. Genetic mutations associated with the cancer are limited to the tumor itself, unlike hereditary disease, in which the specific mutation is present in all cells of the affected individual. Nevertheless, the genetics of colorectal cancer initiation and progression proceed

Table 50-2 Familial Risk and Colon Cancer

FAMILIAL SETTING	APPROXIMATE LIFETIME RISK OF COLON CANCER
General U.S. population	6%
1 first-degree relative* with colon cancer	2- to 3-fold increased
2 first-degree relatives* with colon cancer	3- to 4-fold increased
First-degree relative* with colon cancer diagnosed ≤50 yr	3- to 4-fold increased
1 second- or third-degree relative‡ with colon cancer	1.5-fold increased
2 second- or third-degree relatives‡ with colon cancer	2- to 3-fold increased
1 first-degree relative* with adenomatous polyp	2-fold increased

*First-degree relatives include parents, siblings, and children.
†Second-degree relatives include grandparents, aunts, and uncles.
‡Third-degree relatives include great-grandparents and cousins.
From Burt RW: Colon cancer screening. Gastroenterology 119:837-853, 2000, with permission.

along very similar pathways in both hereditary and sporadic forms of the disease. Studies of the relatively rare inherited models of the disease have greatly enhanced the understanding of the genetics of the far more common sporadic form of the cancer.

The concept of familial colorectal cancer is relatively new. Lifetime risk for colorectal cancer increases for members in families in which the index case is young (<50 years of age) and the relative is close (first degree). The risk increases as the number of family members with colorectal cancer rises (Table 50-2). An individual who is a first-degree relative of a patient diagnosed with colorectal cancer before the age of 50 years is twice as likely as the general population to develop the cancer. This more subtle form of inheritance is currently the subject of much investigation. Genetic polymorphisms, gene modifiers, and defects in tyrosine kinases have all been implicated in various forms of familial colorectal cancer.

Colorectal Cancer Genetics

The field of colorectal cancer genetics was revolutionized in 1988 by the description of the genetic changes involved in the progression of a benign adenomatous polyp to invasive carcinoma.[34] Since then, there has been an explosion of additional information about the molecular and genetic pathways resulting in colorectal cancer. Tumor suppressor genes, DNA mismatch repair genes, and proto-oncogenes all contribute to colorectal neoplasia, both in the sporadic and inherited forms. The Fearon-Vogelstein adenoma-carcinoma multistep model of colorectal neoplasia represents one of the best-known models of carcinogenesis (Fig. 50-43). This sequence of tumor progression involves damage to proto-oncogenes

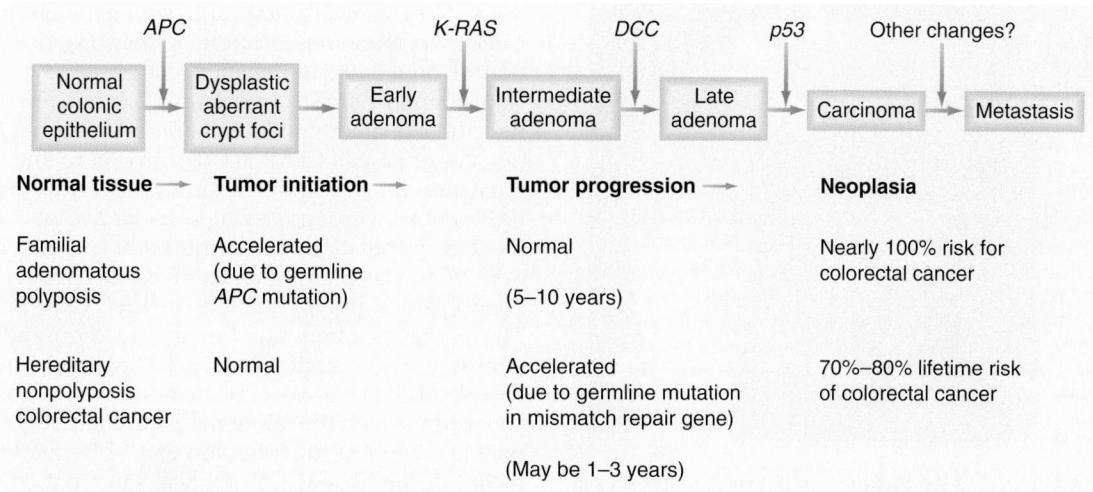

Figure 50-43 The adenoma-carcinoma sequence in sporadic and hereditary colorectal cancer. (From Ivanovich JL, Read TE, Ciske DJ, et al: Am J Med 107:68-77, 1999.)

Table 50-3 Gene Mutations that Cause Colon Cancer

MUTATION TYPE	GENES INVOLVED	TYPE OF DISEASE CAUSED
Germline	*APC*	Familial adenomatous polyposis
	MMR	HNPCC (Lynch syndrome)
Somatic	Oncogenes: *myc ras src erbB2*	Sporadic disease
	Tumor suppressor genes: *TP53 DCC APC*	
	MMR genes: *bMSH2 bMLH1 bPMS1 bPMS2 bMSH6 bMSH3*	
Genetic polymorphism	*APC*	Familial colon cancer in Ashkenazi Jewish persons

DCC, deleted in colorectal carcinoma; HNPCC, hereditary nonpolyposis colorectal cancer; MMR, mismatch repair.

and tumor suppressor genes. The multistep carcinogenesis model can serve as a template to illustrate how certain early mutations produce accumulated defects resulting in neoplasia. The specific contributing mutations in genes such as *APC* have been intensely studied. It is important to view this model and others as progressive and in flux while interconnected cell cycle control pathways and new functions for well-known genes are becoming recognized (Table 50-3).

Specific Mutations

Tumor Suppressor Genes

Tumor suppressor genes produce proteins that inhibit tumor formation by regulating mitotic activity and providing inhibitory cell cycle control. Tumor formation occurs when these inhibitory controls are deregulated by mutation. Point mutations, loss of heterozygosity (LOH), frameshift mutations, and promoter hypermethylation are all

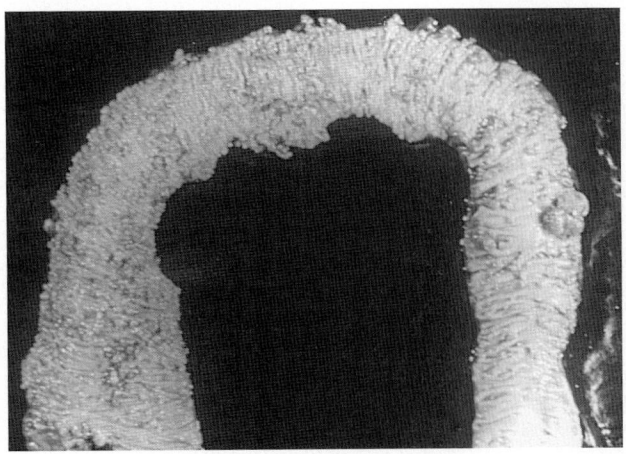

Figure 50-44 Familial adenomatous polyposis, macroscopic appearance. The colon has been opened longitudinally, exposing the mucosa. Thousands of small polyps are seen throughout the colon (note the large one on the left side). (Courtesy of M. Markowitz Haber, MD, Hahnemann University Hospital.)

types of genetic changes that can cause failure of a tumor suppressor gene. These genes are often referred to as *gatekeeper genes* because they provide cell cycle inhibition and regulatory control at specific checkpoints in cell division. The failure of regulation of normal cellular function by tumor suppressor genes is appropriately described by the term *loss of function.* Both alleles of the gene must be nonfunctional to initiate tumor formation.

The adenomatous polyposis coli (*APC*) gene is a tumor suppressor gene located on chromosome 5q21. Its product is 2843 amino acids in length and forms a cytoplasmic complex with GSK-3β (a serine-threonine kinase), β-catenin, and axin. β-Catenin, a multifunctional protein, is a structural component of the epithelial cell adherens junctions and the actin cytoskeleton; it also binds in the cytoplasm to Tcf/LEF and is then transported into the nucleus, where it activates transcription of genes like *c-myc* and others that regulate cellular growth and proliferation. *APC* therefore participates in cell cycle control by regulating the intracytoplasmic pool of β-catenin.

The Wnt signaling proteins are closely associated with the *APC*-β-catenin pathway. *APC* also influences cell cycle proliferation by regulating Wnt expression. Wnt gene products are extracellular signaling molecules that help regulate tissue development throughout the organism. The Wnt signaling proteins are closely associated with the *APC*-β-catenin pathway. Under normal conditions, reduced intracytoplasmic β-catenin levels inhibit Wnt expression. When *APC* is mutated however, β-catenin levels rise, and Wnt is activated. Overexpression of Wnt leads to activation of Wnt target genes such as cyclin D1 and *Myc,* which drive cell proliferation and tumor formation.[35]

The earliest mutations in the adenoma-carcinoma sequence occur in the *APC* gene. The earliest phenotypic change present is known as *aberrant crypt formation,* and the most consistent genetic aberrations within these cells are abnormally short proteins known as *APC* trunca-

tions. Most clinically relevant derangements in *APC* are truncation mutations created by inappropriate transcription of premature termination codons.

A germline *APC* truncation mutation is responsible for the autosomal dominant–inherited disease, FAP. Thirty percent of cases of FAP are de novo germline mutations, thus presenting without a family history of the disease. FAP is rare, with an estimated incidence of 1 in 8000 of the U.S. population, occurring without gender predilection. It is classically characterized by greater than 100 adenomatous polyps present in the colon and rectum. These polyps often number in the thousands and are almost always manifest by the late second or early third decade of life (Fig. 50-44). Because some of these polyps proceed through the adenoma-carcinoma sequence, most patients with FAP die of colon cancer by the fifth decade of life in the absence of surgical intervention. FAP is of great interest to those studying sporadic colorectal cancer because *APC* truncation mutations similar to those found in APC patients occur in 85% of sporadic colorectal cancers.

Most *APC* truncation mutations occur in the *mutational cluster region* of the gene, an area responsible for β-catenin binding. However, genotype-phenotype correlations exist with mutations in other regions of the gene. For example, mutations close to the 5' end of the gene produce a short truncated protein that causes the syndrome known as *attenuated FAP* or (AFAP). These patients usually have far less than the hundreds of polyps usually associated with FAP, and the disease has a tendency to spare the rectum.

Classic FAP is characterized by truncation mutations occurring in the gene from codon 1250 to codon 1464. Mutations occurring further along the gene toward the 3' end are quite rare and most likely result in either a much attenuated phenotype or no detectable abnormality (Fig. 50-45).

The variability of the FAP phenotype is also demonstrated by the presence or absence of extraintestinal manifestations of disease. In the past, the term *Gardener's syndrome* was used to describe the coexpression of profuse colonic adenomatous polyps along with osteomas of the mandible and skull, desmoid tumors of the mesentery, and periampullary neoplasms.

Many other associated disorders have been subsequently described, including thyroid papillary tumors, medulloblastomas, hypertrophic gastric fundic polyps, and congenital hypertrophy of the retinal pigmented epithelium of the iris (CHRPE). The expression of extraintestinal manifestations of FAP is dependent on mutation location, with most of these signs seen only when the truncation occurs in a very small area of the mutational cluster region.

Another *APC* mutation implicated in about 25% of colorectal cancers afflicting Ashkenazi Jewish descendants is the I1307 point mutation caused by substitution of a lysine for isoleucine at codon 1307. This was initially believed to be a genetic polymorphism—a substitution that does not affect the protein structure. However, it is now recognized as probably the most important cause of familial colorectal cancer in this population.

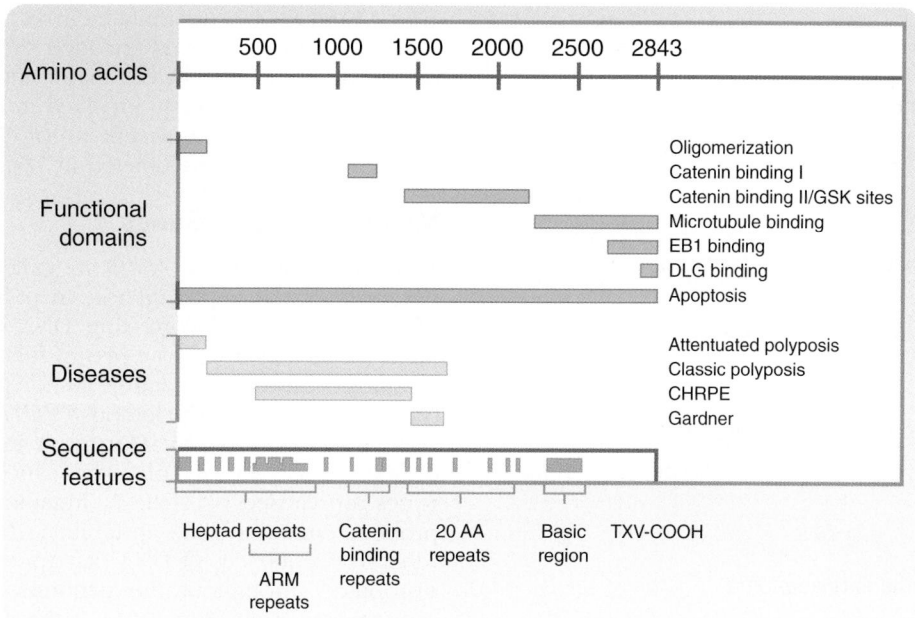

Figure 50-45 Functional and pathogenic properties of *APC*. APC is a protein heterodimer 2843 amino acids in length. The figure depicts the functional domains of APC schematically as *blue* bars where regional mutations result in loss of protein binding as described in the column on the right side of the figure. Mutations in these regions result in truncations that may affect cellular structure and cell signaling such as the inability to bind catenins and interference with microtubule binding. Cellular processes such as apoptosis are affected by mutations occurring at many sites along the gene. Some mutational affects are unknown, such as those preventing EB1 and DLG binding (proteins with unclear functions). Diseases are similarly represented by *tan bars*. Mutations within the regions depicted result in the disease phenotypes described in the right column, including attenuated polyposis, classic polyposis, congenital hypertrophy of the retinal pigmented epithelium (CHRPE), and Gardner's syndrome (extraintestinal manifestations of familial adenomatous polyposis [FAP]). (From Kinzler KW, Vogelstein B: Lessons from hereditary colorectal cancer. Cell 87:159-170, 1996.)

MYH Mutations and *MYH*-associated Polyposis

Recently, a number of families were characterized with a phenotype resembling that of FAP or AFAP, but without a discoverable *APC* gene defect. In 2002, a report of a Welsh family ("family N") with apparent recessive inheritance of multiple colorectal polyps and a cancer was published. Upon analysis of tumor *APC,* frequent somatic mutations were found characterized by G : C to T : A substitutions typically caused by oxidative DNA damage. The authors found that those family members affected had two distinct mutations in the *MYH* gene, a gene responsible for base excision-repair and used to repair oxidative DNA damage. From several subsequent surveys of kindreds with familial colorectal cancer or polyp inheritance patterns, it has become clear that multiple *MYH* mutations exist, and may coexist in the same patient.[36] The mutation has been characterized in Northern European, Indian, and Pakistani populations, appears to affect the production of polyps and tumors by promoting *APC* defects, and is called *MYH-associated polyposis* (MAP). Although the proportion of colorectal cancers attributable to germline *MYH* mutations is unknown, all patients with biallelic *MYH* mutations are at increased risk for colorectal cancer. Greater numbers of polyps (100-1000), and even extracolonic manifestations such as duodenal adenomas, are associated with the presence of more than one germline *MYH* mutation in a single patient.[36]

It is evident that the MAP phenotype is highly variable and that clinical management, for now, should follow guidelines previously established for FAP and AFAP. Surgery in carriers who have polyps is either IPAA or ileorectal anastomosis, depending on the status of the rectum. Colonoscopic and duodenal surveillance every 1 or 2 years for those with biallelic mutations is warranted given the uncertainty of the natural history of the disease.

It remains unclear whether heterozygotes are at increased risk for colorectal cancer; all offspring of those with the disease can be reasonably assured that they are heterozygotes unless they too have multiple polyps (an extremely unlikely event). However, it is certain that patients with MAP need to be distinguished from those with FAP or AFAP because it implies increased risk in siblings rather than offspring. For those with biallelic mutations, spouses can also be tested in the unlikely event that both spouses possess a recessive *MYH* allele.[37]

The most frequently mutated tumor suppressor gene in human neoplasia is *p53* (*TP53*), located on chromosome 17p. Mutations in *p53* are present in 75% of colorectal cancers and occur rather late in the adenoma-carcinoma sequence. Under normal conditions, *p53* acts by inducing apoptosis in response to cellular damage, or by causing G_1 cell-cycle arrest, allowing DNA repair mechanisms to occur. One of the features of mutated *p53* is that it is

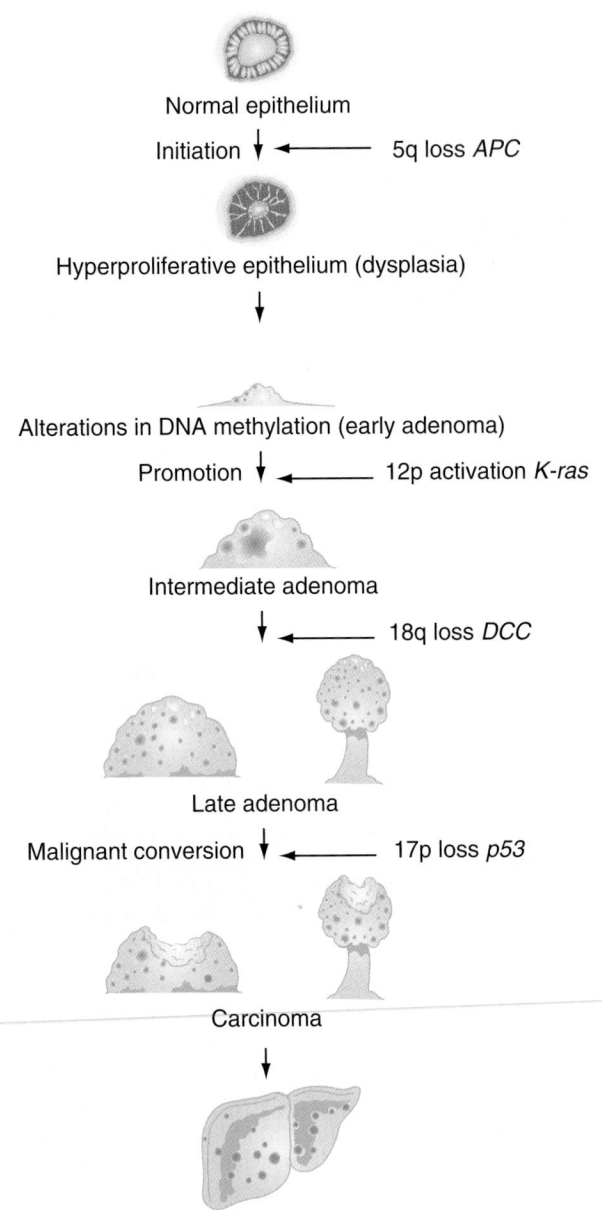

Normal epithelium

Initiation ↓ ◄——— 5q loss *APC*

Hyperproliferative epithelium (dysplasia)

↓

Alterations in DNA methylation (early adenoma)

Promotion ↓ ◄——— 12p activation *K-ras*

Intermediate adenoma

↓ ◄——— 18q loss *DCC*

Late adenoma

Malignant conversion ↓ ◄——— 17p loss *p53*

Carcinoma

↓

Metastasis

Figure 50-46 **Model of colorectal carcinogenesis.** (Modified from Corman ML [ed]: Colon and Rectal Surgery, 4th ed. Philadelphia, Lippincott-Raven, 1998, p 593, after Fearon ER, Vogelstein B: A genetic model of colorectal cancer tumorigenesis. Cell 61:759, 1990. With permission.)

unable to activate the *BAX* gene to induce apoptosis. For its role in regulating apoptosis, *p53* is known as the *guardian of the genome.* The minority of colon cancer patients who have intact *p53* in their tumors may possess a survival advantage. Several recent studies have indicated that prognostic significance may be related to tumor *p53* status.[38]

A number of genes on chromosome 18q are implicated in colorectal cancer, including *SMAD2, SMAD4,* and *DCC.* SMAD proteins are involved in the transforming growth factor-β (TGF-β) signal transduction pathway.

SMAD2 and *SMAD4* are mutated in 5% to 10% of sporadic colorectal cancer. *DCC* is encoded by a large gene and is involved in cell-cell or cell-matrix interactions. It is not clear how *DCC* is directly involved in colorectal neoplasia. *DPC4* is a gene adjacent to *DCC* and may be the tumor suppressor gene deleted in 18q mutations.

Mismatch Repair Genes

Mismatch repair genes (*MMR*) are called *caretaker* genes because of their important role in policing the integrity of the genome and correcting DNA replication errors. *MMR* genes that undergo a loss of function contribute to carcinogenesis by accelerating tumor progression. Mutations in *MMR* genes (including *hMLH1, hMSH2, hMSH3, hPMS1, hPMS2,* and *hMSH6*) result in the HNPCC syndrome. About 3% of colorectal cancers in the United States are caused by HNPCC. Mutations in *MMR* genes produce microsatellite instability. Microsatellites are repetitive sequences of DNA that appear to be randomly distributed throughout the genome. Stability of these sequences is a good measure of the general integrity of the genome. *MMR* gene mutations result in errors in S phase when DNA is newly synthesized and copied. Microsatellite instability exists in 10% to 15% of sporadic tumors and in 95% of tumors in patients with HNPCC. Even so, only 50% of patients diagnosed with HNPCC have readily identifiable *MMR* mutations.

Oncogenes

Proto-oncogenes are genes that produce proteins that promote cellular growth and proliferation. Mutations in proto-oncogenes typically produce a gain of function and can be caused by mutation in only one of the two alleles. After mutation, the gene is called an *oncogene.* Overexpression of these growth-oriented genes contributes to the uncontrolled proliferation of cells associated with cancer. The products of oncogenes can be divided into categories. For example, growth factors (TGF-β, epidermal growth factor, insulin-like growth factor); growth factor receptors (*erbB2*), signal transducers (*src, abl, ras*); and nuclear proto-oncogenes and transcription factors (*myc*) are all oncogene products that appear to have a role in the development of colorectal neoplasia. The *ras* proto-oncogene is located on chromosome 12, and mutations are believed to occur early in the adenoma-carcinoma sequence. Mutated *ras* has been found to be present in aberrant crypt foci as well as adenomatous polyps. Activated *ras* leads to constitutive activity of the protein, which stimulates cellular growth. Fifty percent of sporadic colon cancers possess *ras* mutations, and current trials of farnesyl transferase inhibitors, which block a step in *ras* post-translational modification, may hold therapeutic promise.[35]

Adenoma-Carcinoma Sequence

The adenoma-carcinoma sequence is now recognized as the process through which most colorectal carcinomas develop. Clinical and epidemiologic observations have long been cited to support the hypothesis that colorectal carcinomas evolve through a progression of benign

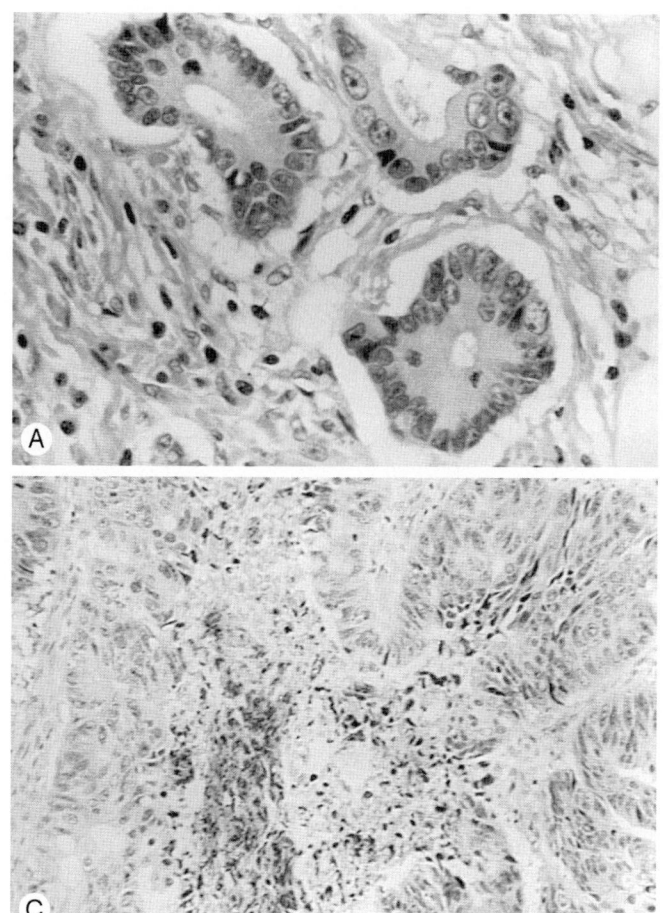

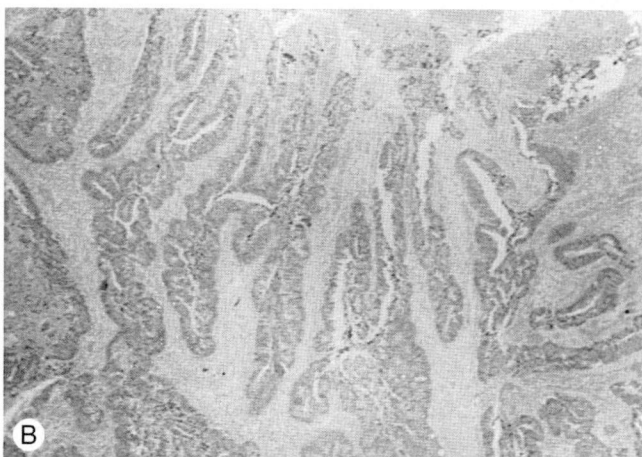

Figure 50-47 Colon carcinoma, microscopic appearance. **A,** Neoplastic glands present within desmoplastic stroma. **B,** Neoplastic glands in region of ulcerated surface. **C,** Neoplastic glands with extensive central necrosis present within desmoplastic stroma. (Courtesy of M. Markowitz Haber, MD, Hahnemann University Hospital.)

polyps to invasive carcinoma, and the elucidation of the genetic pathways to cancer described earlier has confirmed the validity of this hypothesis. However, before the molecular genesis of colorectal cancer was appreciated, there was considerable controversy about whether colorectal cancer arose de novo or evolved from a polyp that was initially a benign precursor. Although there have been a few documented instances of tiny colonic cancers arising de novo from normal mucosa, these instances are rare, and the validity of the adenoma-carcinoma sequence is now accepted by virtually all authorities. The historical observations that lead to the hypothesis are of interest because of the therapeutic implications implicit in an understanding of the adenoma-carcinoma sequence. Observations that provided support for the hypothesis include the following:

- Larger adenomas are found to harbor cancers more often than smaller ones, and the larger the polyp, the higher the risk for cancer. Although the cellular characteristics of the polyp are important, with villous adenomas carrying a higher risk than tubular adenomas, the size of either polyp is also important. The risk for cancer in a tubular adenoma smaller than 1 cm in diameter is less than 5%, whereas the risk for cancer in a tubular adenoma larger than 2 cm is 35%. A villous

adenoma larger than 2 cm in size carries a 50% chance of containing a cancer.
- Residual benign adenomatous tissue is found in most invasive colorectal cancers, suggesting progression of the cancer from the remaining benign cells to the predominant malignant ones.
- Benign polyps have been observed to develop into cancers. There have been reports of the direct observation of benign polyps that were not removed progressing over time into malignancies.
- Colonic adenomas occur more frequently in patients who have colorectal cancer. Nearly one third of all patients with colorectal cancer will also have a benign colorectal polyp.
- Patients who develop adenomas have an increased lifetime risk for developing colorectal cancer.
- Removal of polyps decreases the incidence of cancer. Patients with small adenomas have a 2.3 times increased risk for cancer after the polyp is removed, compared with an 8-fold increased incidence of colorectal cancer in patients with polyps who do not undergo polypectomy.
- Populations with a high risk for colorectal cancer also have a high prevalence of colorectal polyps.
- Patients with FAP will develop colorectal cancer virtually 100% of the time in the absence of surgical inter-

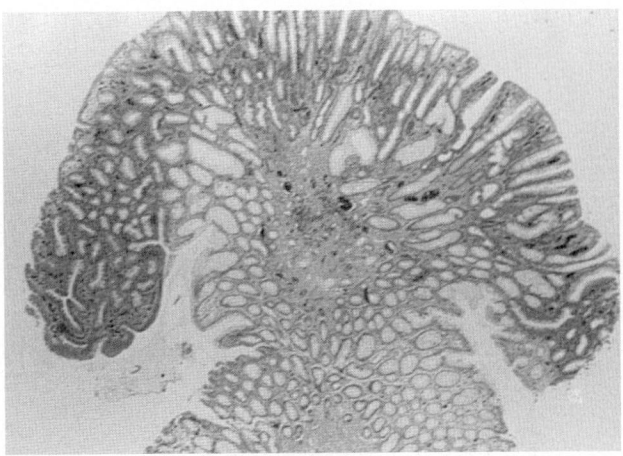

Figure 50-48 Pedunculated adenomatous polyp, microscopic appearance at low-power magnification. The head of the polyp is lined with dysplastic epithelium, whereas the stalk is lined with nondysplastic epithelium. (Courtesy of M. Markowitz Haber, MD, Hahnemann University Hospital.)

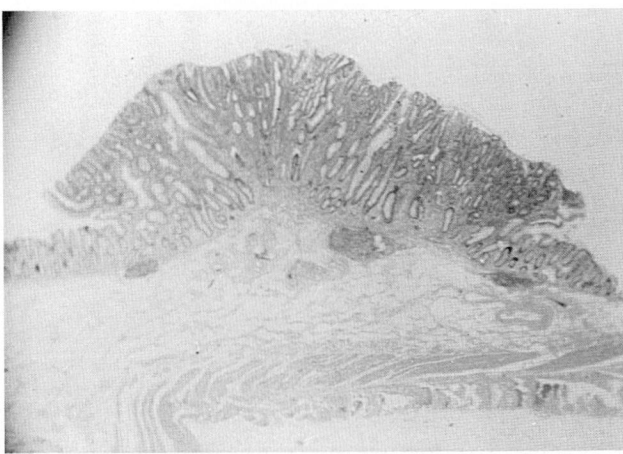

Figure 50-49 Sessile adenomatous polyp, microscopic appearance at low-power magnification. This small tubular adenoma is called *sessile* because of its broad base, the preservation of the muscularis mucosae underneath, and the absence of a stalk. (Courtesy of M. Markowitz Haber, MD, Hahnemann University Hospital.)

vention. The adenomas that characterize this syndrome are histologically the same as sporadic adenomas.

- The peak incidence for the discovery of benign colorectal polyps is 50 years of age. The peak incidence for the development of colorectal cancer is 60 years of age. This suggests a 10-year time span for the progression of an adenomatous polyp to a cancer. It has been estimated that a polyp larger than 1 cm has a cancer risk of 2.5% in 5 years, 8% in 10 years, and 24% in 20 years.

These observations and the studies by molecular biologists document that colonic mucosa progresses through stages to the eventual development of an invasive cancer. Colonic epithelial cells lose the normal progression to maturity and cell death and begin proliferating in a more and more uncontrolled manner. With this uncontrolled proliferation, the cells accumulate on the surface of the bowel lumen as a polyp. With more proliferation and increasing cellular disorganization, the cells extend though the muscularis mucosae to become invasive carcinoma. Even at this advanced stage, the process of colorectal carcinogenesis generally follows an orderly sequence of invasion of the muscularis mucosae, pericolic tissue, lymph nodes, and finally, distant metastasis (Figs. 50-46 and 50-47).

Colorectal Polyps

A colorectal polyp is any mass projecting into the lumen of the bowel above the surface of the intestinal epithelium. Polyps arising from the intestinal mucosa are generally classified by their gross appearance as pedunculated (with a stalk) (Fig. 50-48) or sessile (flat, without a stalk) (Fig. 50-49). They are further classified by their histologic

appearance as tubular adenoma (with branched tubular glands), villous adenoma (with long finger-like projections of the surface epithelium) (Fig. 50-50), or tubulovillous adenoma (with elements of both cellular patterns). The most common benign polyp is the tubular adenoma, constituting about 65% to 80% of all polyps removed. About 10% to 25% of polyps are tubulovillous, and 5% to 10% are villous adenomas. Tubular adenomas are most often pedunculated; villous adenomas are more commonly sessile. The degree of cellular atypia is variable across the span of polyps, but there is generally less atypia in tubular adenomas, and severe atypia or dysplasia (precancerous cellular change) is found more often in villous adenomas. The incidence of invasive carcinoma being found in a polyp is dependent on the size and histologic type of the polyp. As mentioned previously, there is less than a 5% incidence of carcinoma in an adenomatous polyp less than 1 cm in size, whereas there is a 50% chance that a villous adenoma greater than 2 cm in size will contain a cancer.

The treatment of an adenomatous or villous polyp is removal, usually by colonoscopy. The presence of any polypoid lesion is an indication for a complete colonoscopy and polypectomy, if feasible. Polyps on a stalk are often removed by a snare passed through the colonoscope, whereas sessile (flat) polyps present technical problems with this technique because of danger of perforation associated with the snare technique. Although it may be feasible to elevate the sessile polyp from the underlying muscularis with saline injection, permitting subsequent endoscopic excision, sessile lesions often require segmental colectomy for complete removal (Fig. 50-51).

As described earlier, adenomatous polyps should be considered precursors of cancer, and when cancer arises in a polyp, careful consideration needs to be given to

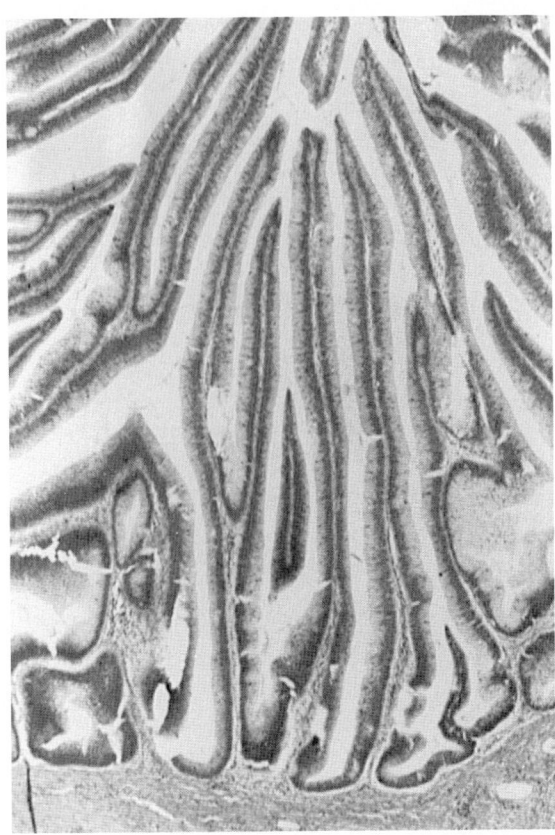

Figure 50-50 Villous adenoma. This photomicrograph reveals the finger-like projections that give the appearance of villi. (Courtesy of M. Markowitz Haber, MD, Hahnemann University Hospital.)

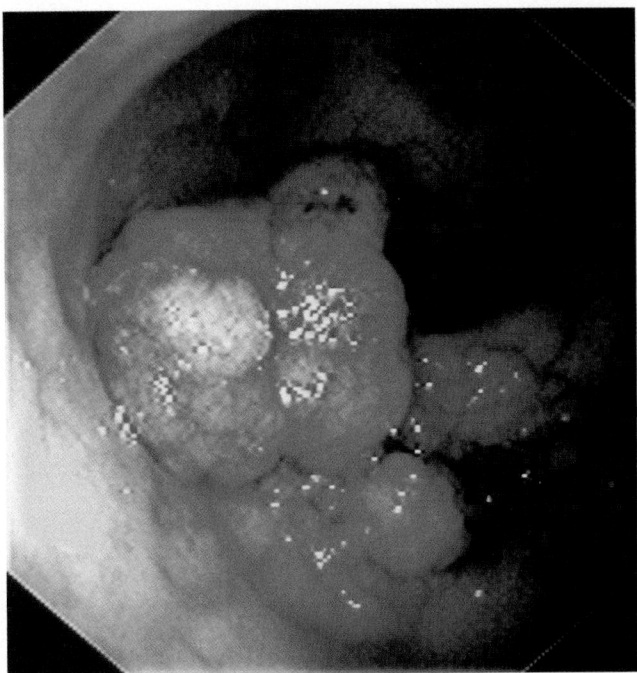

Figure 50-51 Colonoscopic view of sessile polyp. This polyp proved to be a carcinoma after it was removed by segmental resection.

ensure the adequacy of treatment. *Invasive carcinoma* describes the situation in which malignant cells have extended through the muscularis mucosae of the polyp, whether it is a lesion on a stalk or a sessile lesion. Carcinoma confined to the muscularis mucosae does not metastasize, and the cellular abnormalities should be described as atypia. Complete excision of this type of polyp is adequate treatment.

If invasive carcinoma penetrates the muscularis mucosae, consideration of the risk for lymph node metastasis and local recurrence is required to determine whether a more extensive resection is required. Haggitt and colleagues[39] proposed a classification for polyps containing cancer according to the depth of invasion as follows (Fig. 50-52):

- Level 0: Carcinoma does not invade the muscularis mucosae (carcinoma-in-situ or intramucosal carcinoma).
- Level 1: Carcinoma invades through the muscularis mucosae into the submucosa but is limited to the head of the polyp.
- Level 2: Carcinoma invades the level of the neck of the polyp (junction between the head and the stalk).
- Level 3: Carcinoma invades any part of the stalk.
- Level 4: Carcinoma invades into the submucosa of the bowel wall below the stalk of the polyp but above the muscularis propria.

By definition, all sessile polyps with invasive carcinoma are level 4 by Haggitt's criteria.

If a polyp contains a histologically poorly differentiated invasive carcinoma, or if there are cancer cells observed in the lymphovascular spaces, there is a greater than 10% chance of metastases, and these lesions should be treated aggressively.

A pedunculated polyp with invasion to levels 1, 2, and 3 has a low risk for lymph node metastasis or local recurrence, and complete excision of the polyp is adequate if the poor prognostic factors mentioned earlier are not present. A sessile polyp containing invasive cancer has at least a 10% chance of metastasis to regional lymph nodes, but if the lesion is well or moderately differentiated, there is no lymphovascular invasion noted, and the lesion can be completely excised, the depth of invasion by the cancer may provide useful prognostic information. There is a high risk for lymph node and distant metastasis associated with sessile cancers in the rectum, and these lesions should be treated aggressively.

Hyperplastic polyps are the most common colonic polyps, but they are usually quite small and composed of cells showing dysmaturation and hyperplasia. The small diminutive polyps have been regarded as benign in nature with no neoplastic potential. The histologic appearance of these polyps is serrated (saw-toothed) (Fig. 50-53). Ninety percent of these polyps are less than 3 mm in size, and these diminutive lesions are generally considered to have no malignant potential. However, adenomatous changes can be found in hyperplastic polyps, and for this reason, the polyps should be excised for histologic examination. Recently, these serrated adenomas have been observed to be associated with

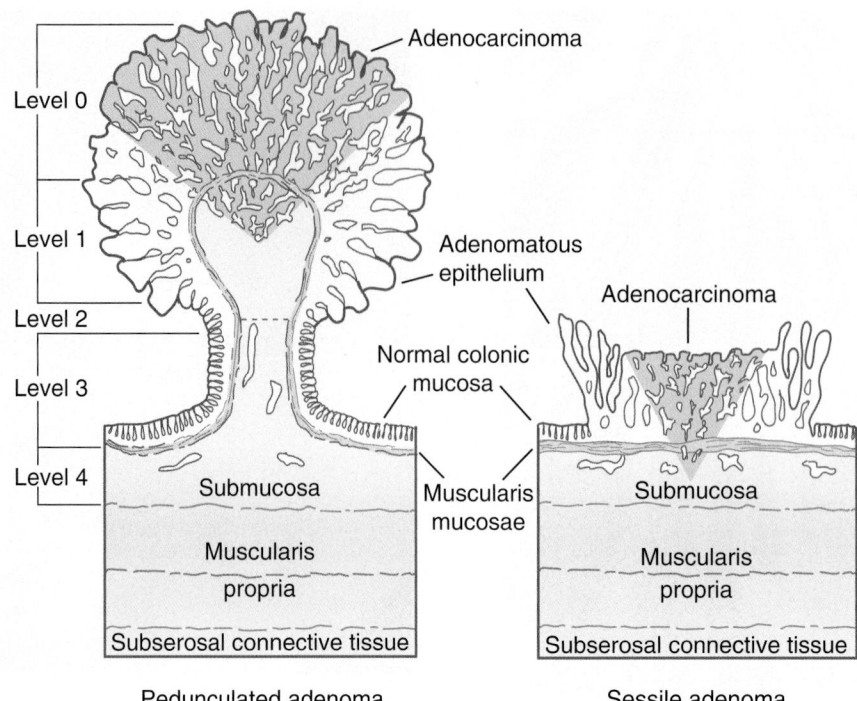

Figure 50-52 Anatomic landmarks of pedunculated and sessile adenomas. (From Haggitt RC, Glotzbach RE, Soffer EE, et al: Prognostic factors in colorectal carcinoma arising in adenomas: Implications for lesions removed by endoscopic polypectomy. Gastroenterology 89:328-336, 1985.)

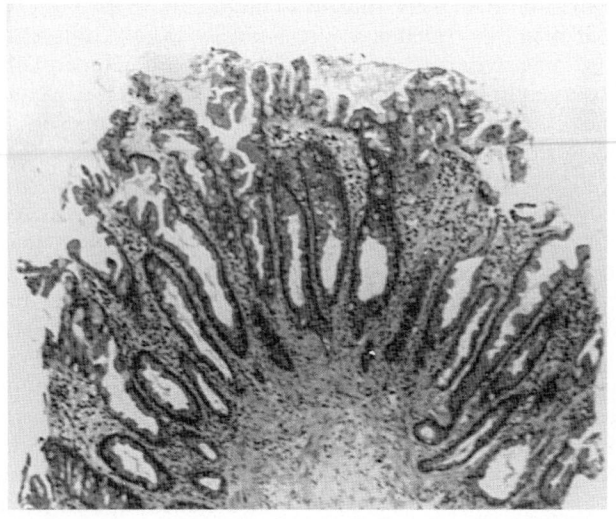

Figure 50-53 Hyperplastic polyp. Elongated tubular glands are lined by epithelium with abundant pink cytoplasm and a tufted appearance, seen predominantly at the surface and at the luminal portion of the gland. This gives the glands a serrated, or saw-toothed, appearance. (Courtesy of M. Markowitz Haber, MD, Hahnemann University Hospital.)

development of cancers that predominate in the right side of the colon, more frequently in elderly women and smokers. These serrated adenomas appear to be associated with the microsatellite instability characteristic of defects in DNA repair mechanisms.[40]

Hereditary Cancer Syndromes

Peutz-Jeghers syndrome is an autosomal dominant syndrome characterized by the combination of hamartomatous polyps of the intestinal tract and hyperpigmentation of the buccal mucosa, lips, and digits (Table 50-4). Germline defects in the tumor suppressor serine/threonine kinase 11 (*STK11*) gene are implicated in this rare autosomal dominant–inherited disease. Although the syndrome was first described by Hutchinson in 1896, later separate descriptions by Peutz and then Jeghers in the 1940s brought recognition to the condition. The syndrome is associated with an increased (2%-10%) risk for cancer of the intestinal tract, with cancers reported throughout the intestinal tract, from the stomach to the rectum. There is also an increased risk for extraintestinal malignancies, including cancer of the breast, ovary, cervix, fallopian tubes, thyroid, lung, gallbladder, bile ducts, pancreas, and testicles.

The polyps may cause bleeding or intestinal obstruction (from intussusception). If surgery is required for these symptoms, an attempt should be made to remove as many polyps as possible with the aid of intraoperative endoscopy and polypectomy. Any polyp that is larger than 1.5 cm should be removed if possible. It is reasonable to survey the colon endoscopically every 2 years, and patients should be screened periodically for malignancies of the breast, cervix, ovary, testicle, stomach, and pancreas.

Juvenile polyps are benign polyps composed of cystic dilations of glandular structures within the fibroblastic stroma of the lamina propria. They are relatively uncommon, yet may cause bleeding or intussusception. For these reasons, the polyps should be treated by endoscopic removal.

Multiple polyposis coli is an autosomal dominant syndrome with high penetrance that carries an increased risk for both gastrointestinal and extraintestinal cancer. The syndrome is usually discovered because of GI bleeding, intussusception, or hypoalbuminemia associated with protein loss through the intestine. The juvenile polyps in this syndrome are predominately hamartomas, but the hamartomas may contain adenomatous elements, and adenomatous polyps also are common. There is an increased cancer risk in afflicted individuals, with a malignant potential of at least 10% in patients with multiple juvenile polyps. Mutations in the tumor suppressor gene *SMAD4* are believed to cause up to 50% of reported cases.

In patients with relatively few juvenile polyps, endoscopic polypectomy should be done. However, patients with numerous polyps should be treated with abdominal colectomy, ileorectal anastomosis, and frequent endoscopic surveillance of the rectum. If the diffuse form of polyposis involves the rectal mucosa, consideration should be given to restorative proctocolectomy with IPAA.

FAP is the prototypical hereditary polyposis syndrome. The discovery of the gene responsible for the transmission of the disease, the *APC* gene, located on chromosome 5q21, lagged behind the first descriptions of cases of FAP by an entire century. In 1863, Virchow reported a 15-year-old boy with multiple colonic polyps. In 1882, Cripps described the occurrence of numerous colonic polyps in multiple family members. In 1927, Cockayne demonstrated that FAP was genetically transmitted in an autosomal dominant fashion. Dukes was the first to establish some form of a familial tumor registry, which he reported with Lockhart-Mummery in 1930. Throughout the 20th century, many reports described various extraintestinal manifestations associated with FAP. In 1986, Lemuel Herrera demonstrated that the underlying genetic abnormality was a mutation in the *APC* gene.

The common expression of the syndrome is the invariable presence of multiple colonic polyps, the frequent occurrence of gastric, duodenal, and periampullary polyps, and the occasional association of extraintestinal manifestations, including epidermoid cysts, desmoid tumors in the abdomen, osteomas, and brain tumors. Gastric and duodenal polyps occur in about half of affected individuals. Most of the gastric polyps represent fundic gland hyperplasia, rather than adenomatous polyps, and have limited malignant potential. However, duodenal polyps are adenomatous in nature and should be considered premalignant. Patients with FAP have an increased risk for ampullary cancer. Adenomatous polyps and cancer have also been found in the jejunum and ileum of patients with FAP. Rare extraintestinal malignancies in FAP patients include cancers of the extrahepatic bile ducts, gallbladder, pancreas, adrenals, thyroid, and liver. An interesting marker for FAP is CHRPE, which can be detected by indirect ophthalmoscopy in about 75% of affected individuals.

The gene is expressed in 100% of patients with the mutation. Autosomal dominance results in expression in 50% of offspring. There is a negative family history in 10% to 20% of affected individuals, who apparently acquire the syndrome as the result of a spontaneous mutation. All patients with the defective gene will develop cancer of the colon if left untreated. The average age of discovery of a new patient with FAP is 29 years. The average age of a patient who is newly discovered to have colorectal cancer related to FAP is 39 years. Eponymous polyposis syndromes now recognized to belong to the general disorder of FAP include Gardner's syndrome (colonic polyps, epidermal inclusion cysts, osteomas) and Turcot's syndrome (colonic polyps and brain tumors).

Osteomas usually present as visible and palpable prominences in the skull, mandible, and tibia of individuals with FAP. They are virtually always benign. Radiographs of the maxilla and mandible may reveal bone cysts, supernumerary and impacted molars, or congenitally absent teeth. Desmoid tumors can present in the retroperitoneum and abdominal wall of affected patients, usually after surgery. These tumors seldom metastasize but are often locally invasive, and direct invasion of the mesenteric vessels, ureters, or walls of the small intestine can result in death.

Surgical treatment of patients with FAP is directed at removal of all affected colonic and rectal mucosa. Restorative proctocolectomy with IPAA has become the most commonly recommended operation. The procedure is usually accompanied by a distal rectal mucosectomy to ensure that all premalignant colonic mucosa is removed, and the IPAA is fashioned between the ileal pouch and the dentate line of the anal canal. Patients who undergo this procedure for FAP have a better functional result than patients similarly treated for ulcerative colitis, in that the incidence of inflammation in the ileal pouch (pouchitis) is much lower in patients with FAP than in patients with ulcerative colitis.

An alternative approach, total abdominal colectomy with ileorectal anastomosis, was used extensively before the development of the technique of IPAA and has certain advantages. If an FAP patient has relatively few polyps in the rectum, consideration may be given to this option. The abdominal colon is resected and an anastomosis fashioned between the ileum and rectum. It is technically a simpler operation to perform, and the pelvic dissection is avoided. This eliminates the potential complication of injury to the autonomic nerves that could result in impotence. In addition, there is theoretically less risk for anastomotic leak from the relatively simple ileorectal anastomosis fashioned in the peritoneal cavity, compared with the long suture (or staple) lines required to form the ileal pouch and then fashion the anastomosis between the ileal pouch and the anus.

An additional argument in favor if abdominal colectomy and ileorectal anastomosis is the observation that sulindac and celecoxib have been observed to cause the regression of adenomatous polyps in some patients with FAP.[41] The disadvantages are that the rectum remains at high risk for the formation of new precancerous polyps,

Text continued on p 1404

Table 50-4 Hereditary Cancer Syndromes

	HEREDITARY NONPOLYPOSIS COLON CANCER	HEREDITARY ADENOMATOUS POLYPOSIS SYNDROMES		HEREDITARY HAMARTOMATOUS POLYPOSIS SYNDROMES			
		Familial Adenomatous Polyposis/Gardner's Syndrome	Turcot's Syndrome	Cowden's Disease	Familial Juvenile Polyposis	Peutz-Jeghers Syndrome	Ruvalcaba-Myhre-Smith Syndrome (Bannayan-Zonana Syndrome)
GI Features	Small number of colorectal polyps	Hundreds to thousands of colorectal polyps; duodenal adenomas and gastric polyps, usually fundic gland	Colorectal polyps, which may be few or resemble classic familial adenomatous polyposis	Polyps most commonly of colon and stomach	Juvenile polyps mostly in the colon but throughout GI tract Defined by ≥ 10 juvenile polyps	Small number of polyps throughout GI tract but most common in small intestine	Hamartomatous GI polyps, usually lipomas, hemangiomas, or lymphangiomas
Other Clinical Features	Muir-Torre variant: sebaceous adenomas, keratoacanthomas, sebaceous epitheliomas, and basal cell epitheliomas	Osteomas, desmoid tumors, epidermoid cysts, and congenital hypertrophy of retinal epithelium	Brain tumors, including cerebellar medulloblastoma and glioblastomas	Mucocutaneous lesions, thyroid adenomas and goiter, fibroadenomas and fibrocystic disease of the breast, uterine leiomyomas, and macrocephaly	Congenital abnormalities in at least 20%, including malrotation, hydrocephalus, cardiac lesions, Meckel's diverticulum, and mesenteric lymphangioma	Pigmented lesions of skin; benign and malignant genital tumors	Dysmorphic facial features, macrocephaly, seizures, intellectual impairment, and pigmented macules of shaft and glans of penis
Malignancy Risk	70%-80% lifetime risk for colorectal cancer; 30%-60% lifetime risk for endometrial cancer; ↑ risk for ovarian cancer, gastric carcinoma, transitional cell carcinoma of the ureters and renal pelvis, small bowel cancer, and sebaceous carcinoma	Colorectal cancer risk approaches 100%; ↑ risk for periampullary malignancy, thyroid carcinoma, central nervous system tumors, and hepatoblastoma	Colorectal carcinoma and brain tumors	10% risk for thyroid cancer and up to 50% risk for adenocarcinoma of breast in affected women	9% to 25% risk for colorectal cancer; ↑ risk for gastric, duodenal, and pancreatic cancer	↑ Risk for GI malignancy and pancreatic cancer and adenoma malignum of cervix; unknown risk for breast cancer	Malignant GI tumors identified but lifetime risk for malignancy unknown

Screening Recommendations						
Colonoscopy at age 20-25 yr; repeat every 1-3 yr Transvaginal ultrasound or endometrial aspirate at age 20-25 yr; repeat annually (expert opinion only)	Flexible proctosigmoidoscopy at age 10-12 yr; repeat every 1-2 yr until age 35; after age 35 repeat every 3 yr Upper GI endoscopy every 1-3 yr starting when polyps first identified	Same as for familial adenomatous polyposis Also consider imaging of the brain	Annual physical exam with special attention to thyroid Mammography at age 30 or 5 yr before earliest breast cancer case in the family Routine colon cancer surveillance (expert opinion only)	Screening by age 12 yr if symptoms have not yet arisen Colonoscopy with multiple random biopsies every several years (expert opinion only)	Upper GI endoscopy, small bowel radiography, and colonoscopy every 2 yr; pancreatic ultrasound and hemoglobin levels annually; gynecologic examination, cervical smear, and pelvic ultrasound annually; clinical breast exam and mammography at age 25 yr; clinical testicular exam and testicular ultrasound in males with feminizing features (expert opinion only)	No known published recommendations

Genetic Basis

AD *MLH1* (chromosome 3p) *MSH2* (chromosome 2p) *MSH6/GTMP* (chromosome 2p) *PMS1* (chromosome 2q) *PMS2* (chromosome 7q)	AD *APC* (chromosome 5q)	AD *APC* mutations identified predominantly in families with cerebellar medulloblastoma *MLH1, PMS2* mutations identified in families with predominance of glioblastomas	AD *PTEN* (chromosome 10q)	AD inheritance in some families Subset of families with mutation in *SMAD4 (DRC4)* (chromosome 10q)	AD *STK11* (chromosome 19p)	AD *PTEN* (chromosome 10q) in some families

Genetic Testing

Clinical testing of *MLH1* and *MSH2* genes available	Clinical testing of *APC* gene available	Clinical testing of *APC* and *MLH1* genes available	Research testing of *PTEN* gene available	Families being collected for research studies only	Research testing of *STK11* gene available	Research testing of *PTEN* gene available

AD, autosomal dominant; GI, gastrointestinal; ↑, increased.

a proctoscopic examination is required every 6 months to detect and destroy any new polyps, and there is a definite increased risk for cancer arising in the rectum with the passage of time.

It has been suggested that genetic testing may help make a decision between restorative proctocolectomy with IPAA and abdominal colectomy with ileorectal anastomosis. It has been observed that the risk for rectal cancer is almost three times higher in FAP patients with a mutation after codon 1250 than in patients with mutations before this codon. This fact may influence the decision to offer abdominal colectomy with ileorectal anastomosis to patients whose mutation occurs proximal to codon 1250 if proctoscopic examination should reveal no or few polyps in the rectum.

Patients who choose to be treated by abdominal colectomy with ileorectal anastomosis should realize that the risk for developing rectal cancer is real and has been shown to be 4%, 5.6%, 7.9%, and 25% at 5, 10, 15, and 20 years after the operation, respectively.[42] Even though sulindac and celecoxib can produce partial regression of polyps, semiannual surveillance of the rectal mucosa is required, and about one third of patients treated by abdominal colectomy and ileorectal anastomosis develop florid polyposis of the rectum that will require proctectomy (and either ileostomy or IPAA) within 20 years.

As discussed earlier, polyps of the stomach and duodenum are not uncommon in patients with FAP. The gastric polyps are usually hyperplastic and do not require surgical removal. However, the duodenal and ampullary polyps are usually neoplastic and require attention. A reasonable surveillance program is for upper gastrointestinal surveillance every 2 years after the age of 30 years and endoscopic polypectomy, if possible, to remove all large adenomas from the duodenum. If numerous polyps are identified, the endoscopy obviously should be repeated with greater frequency. If an ampullary cancer is discovered at an early stage, pancreatoduodenectomy (Whipple procedure) is indicated.

The abdominal desmoid tumor can be an especially vexing and difficult extraintestinal manifestation of FAP. After surgical procedures, dense fibrous tissue forms in the mesentery of the small intestine or within the abdominal wall in some patients with FAP. If the mesentery is involved, the intestine can be tethered or invaded directly by the tumor. The locally invasive tumor can also encroach on the vascular supply to the intestine. Small desmoid tumors confined to the abdominal wall are appropriately treated by resection, but the surgical treatment of mesenteric desmoids is dangerous and generally futile. There have been sporadic reports of regression of desmoid tumors after treatment with sulindac, tamoxifen, low-dose methotrexate, radiation, and various types of chemotherapy. The initial treatment is usually with sulindac or tamoxifen.[43]

The ability to identify the genetic mutation in most patients with FAP (although the mutation may not be identified in as many as 20% of patients with a well-documented, transmissible FAP syndrome) permits a method of screening family members at risk for inheriting the mutation. It is imperative that the *APC* mutation is clearly identified in the DNA of a family member known to have the disease. The DNA of other family members can then be directly analyzed, requiring only a venipuncture. If the analysis demonstrates non inheritance of a mutated *APC* gene, the individual can avoid yearly endoscopic screening and should require only occasional colonoscopy.

HNPCC is the most frequently occurring hereditary colorectal cancer syndrome in the United States and Western Europe. It accounts for about 3% of all cases of colorectal cancer and for about 15% of such cancers in patients with a family history of colorectal cancer. Dr. Alder S. Warthin, chairman of pathology at the University of Michigan, initially recognized this hereditary syndrome in 1985. Dr. Warthin's seamstress prophesied that she would die of cancer because of her strong family history of endometrial, gastric, and colon cancer. Dr. Warthin's investigations of her family's medical records revealed a pattern of autosomal dominant transmission of the cancer risk. This family (Family G) has been further studied and characterized by Dr. Henry Lynch, who described the prominent features of the syndrome, including onset of cancer at a relative young age (mean, 44 years), proximal distribution (70% of cancers located in the right colon), predominance of mucinous or poorly differentiated (signet cell) adenocarcinoma, increased number of synchronous and metachronous cancers, and, despite all these poor prognostic indicators, a relatively good outcome after surgery. Two hereditary syndromes were initially described. Lynch I syndrome is characterized by cancer of the proximal colon occurring at a relatively young age, whereas Lynch II syndrome is characterized by families at risk for both colorectal cancer and extracolonic cancers, including cancers of endometrial, ovarian, gastric, small intestinal, pancreatic, and ureteral and renal pelvic origin.

Before the genetic mechanisms underlying the Lynch syndromes were understood, the syndromes were defined by the Amsterdam Criteria, which required three criteria for the diagnosis:

1. Colorectal cancer in three family members (first-degree relatives)
2. Involvement of at least two generations
3. At least one affected individual being younger than 50 years at the time of diagnosis

These requirements were recognized as being too restrictive, and the modified Amsterdam Criteria expanded the cancers to be included to not only colorectal but also endometrial, ovarian, gastric, pancreatic, small intestinal, ureteral, and renal pelvic cancers. Further liberalization for identifying patients with HNPCC occurred with the introduction of the Bethesda criteria (Box 50-4).

Molecular biologists have demonstrated that the increased cancer risk in these syndromes is due to malfunction of the DNA repair mechanism. Specific genes that have been shown to be responsible for the syndrome include *hMSH2* (located on chromosome 2p21), *hMLH1* (3p21), *hMSH6* (2p16-21), and *hPMS2* (7p21). A mutation in *hMSH2* has been shown to be responsible for the cancer prevalence in Cancer Family G. Mutations in *hMSH2* or *hMLH1* account for more than 90% of identifiable mutations in patients with HNPCC. The initially reported difference in types of cancers occurring in Lynch I and II syndromes cannot be accounted for by mutations in specific mismatch repair genes. The cancer family syndrome involving *hMSH6* is characterized by an increased incidence of endometrial carcinoma.

Box 50-4   Clinical Criteria for Hereditary Nonpolyposis Colorectal Cancer (HNPCC)

Amsterdam Criteria

At least three relatives with colon cancer and all of the following:
   One affected person is a first-degree relative of the other two affected persons
   Two successive generations affected
   At least one case of colon cancer diagnosed before age 50 years
   Familial adenomatous polyposis excluded

Modified Amsterdam Criteria

Same as the Amsterdam criteria, except that cancer must be associated with HNPCC (colon, endometrium, small bowel, ureter, renal pelvis) instead of specifically colon cancer

Bethesda Criteria

The Amsterdam criteria or one of the following:
   Two cases of HNPCC-associated cancer in one patient, including synchronous or metachronous cancer
   Colon cancer and a first-degree relative with HNPCC-associated cancer and/or colonic adenoma (one case of cancer diagnosed before age 45 years and adenoma diagnosed before age 40 years)
   Colon or endometrial cancer diagnosed before age 45 years
   Right-sided colon cancer that has an undifferentiated pattern (solid-cribriform) or signet-cell histopathologic characteristics diagnosed before age 45 years
   Adenomas diagnosed before age 40 years

HNPCC, hereditary nonpolyposis colorectal cancer.

The mainstay of the diagnosis of HNPCC is a detailed family history. Still, it should be remembered that as many as 20% of newly discovered cases of HNPCC are caused by spontaneous germline mutations, so a family history may not accurately reflect the genetic nature of the syndrome. Colorectal cancer, or an HNPCC-related cancer, arising in a person younger than 50 years should raise the suspicion of this syndrome. Genetic counseling and genetic testing can be offered. If the individual proves to have HNPCC by identification of a mutation in one of the known mismatch repair genes, then other family members can be tested after obtaining genetic counseling. However, failure to identify a causative mismatch repair gene mutation in a patient with a suggestive history does not exclude the diagnosis of HNPCC. In as many as 50% of patients with a family history that clearly demonstrates HNPCC-type transmission of cancer susceptibility, DNA testing will fail to identify the causative gene.

The management of patients with HNPCC is somewhat controversial, but the need for close surveillance in patients known to carry the mutation is obvious. It is usually recommended that a program of surveillance colonoscopy should begin at the age of 20 years. Colonoscopy is repeated every 2 years until the age of 35 years, and then annually thereafter. In women, periodic vacuum curettage is begun at age 25 years, as are pelvic ultrasound and CA-125 levels. Annual tests for occult blood in the urine should also be obtained because of the risk for ureteral and renal pelvic cancer (Table 50-5).

It has been shown that annual colonoscopy and removal of polyps when found will decrease the incidence of colon cancer in patients with HNPCC. However, there have been well-documented cases of invasive colon cancers occurring 1 year after a negative colonoscopy. It is obvious that the slow evolution from benign polyp to invasive cancer is not a feature of the pathogenesis in HNPCC patients, and this phenomenon of accelerated

---

Table 50-5   Screening Recommendations for FAP and HNPCC

LIFETIME CANCER RISK		SCREENING RECOMMENDATIONS
Familial Adenomatous Polyposis (FAP)		
Colorectal cancer	100%	Colonoscopy annually, beginning age 10-12 yr
Duodenal or periampullary cancer	5%-10%	Upper GI endoscopy every 1-3 yr, beginning age 20-25 yr
Pancreatic cancer	2%	Possible periodic abdominal ultrasound
Thyroid cancer	2%	Annual thyroid examination
Gastric cancer	<1%	Upper GI endoscopy as for duodenal and periampullary
Central nervous system cancer	<1%	Annual physical examination
Hereditary Nonpolyposis Colorectal Cancer (HNPCC)		
Colorectal cancer	80%	Colonoscopy, every 2 yr beginning age 20 yr, annually after age 40 yr or 10 years younger than earliest case in family
Endometrial cancer	40%-60%	Pelvic exam, transvaginal ultrasound, endometrial aspirate every 1-2 yr, beginning age 25-35 yr
Upper urinary tract cancer	4%-10%	Ultrasound and urinalysis every 1-2 yr; start at age 30-35 yr
Gallbladder and biliary cancer	2%-18%	No recommendation
Central nervous system cancer	<5%	No recommendation
Small bowel cancer	<5%	No recommendation

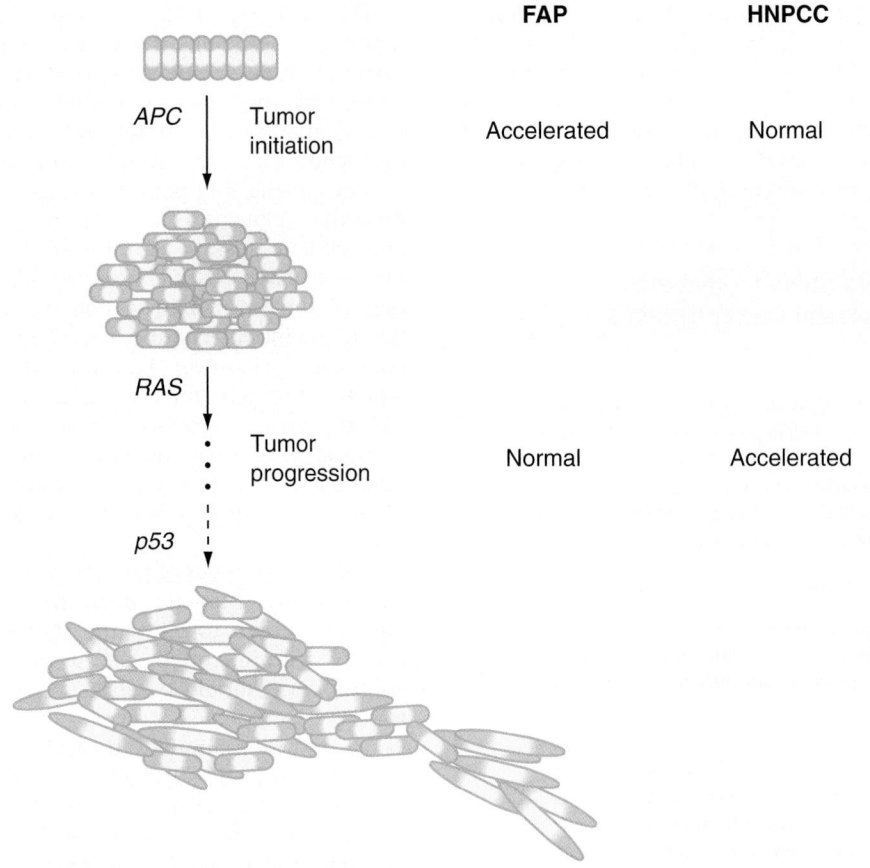

	FAP	HNPCC
APC — Tumor initiation	Accelerated	Normal
RAS / *p53* — Tumor progression	Normal	Accelerated

Figure 50-54 Comparison of the development of cancer in familial adenomatous polyposis (FAP) and hereditary nonpolyposis colorectal cancer (HNPCC) patients. (From Kinzler KW, Vogelstein B: Lessons from hereditary colorectal cancer. Cell 87:159-170, 1966.)

carcinogenesis mandates frequent (annual) colonoscopic examinations. Even with annual colonoscopic examinations, there is a documented risk for colon cancer, but when a cancer arises while the patient is under a vigorous surveillance program, the cancer stage is usually favorable (Fig. 50-54).

When colon cancer is detected in a patient with HNPCC, an abdominal colectomy and ileorectal anastomosis is the procedure of choice. If the patient is a woman with no further plans for childbearing, prophylactic total abdominal hysterectomy and bilateral salpingo-oophorectomy are recommended. The rectum remains at risk for development of cancer, and annual proctoscopic examinations are mandatory after abdominal colectomy. Other forms of cancer associated with HNPCC are treated according to the same criteria as in nonhereditary cases. The role of prophylactic colectomy for patients with HNPCC has been considered in some instances, but this concept has not received universal acceptance. It is an interesting but well-documented fact that the prognosis is better for cancer patients with HNPCC than for non-HNPCC patients with cancer of the same stage.

Sporadic Colon Cancer

It is important to recognize the increased risk for cancer in patients with hereditary cancer syndromes, but by far the most common form of colorectal cancer is sporadic in nature, without an associated strong family history.

Although the cause and pathogenesis of adenocarcinoma are similar throughout the large bowel, significant differences in the use of diagnostic and therapeutic modalities separate colonic from rectal cancers. This distinction is largely due to the confinement of the rectum by the bony pelvis. The limited mobility of the rectum allows MRI to generate better images and increases its sensitivity. In addition, the proximity of the rectum to the anus permits easy access of ultrasound probes for more accurate assessment of the extent of penetration of the bowel wall and the involvement of adjacent lymph nodes. The limited accessibility of the rectum, the proximity to the anal sphincter, and the close association with the autonomic nerves supplying the bladder and genitalia require special and unique consideration when planning treatment for cancer of the rectum. Therefore, colon and rectal adenocarcinomas are discussed separately.

The signs and symptoms of colon cancer are varied, nonspecific, and somewhat dependent on the location of the tumor in the colon as well as the extent of constriction of the lumen caused by the cancer. During the past several decades, the incidence of cancer in the right colon has increased in comparison to cancer arising in the left colon and rectum. This is an important consideration, in that at least half of all colon cancers are located proximal to the area that can be visualized by the flexible sigmoidoscope. Colorectal cancers can bleed, causing red blood to appear in the stool (hematochezia). Bleeding from right-sided colon tumors can cause dark, tarry stools (melena). Often, the bleeding is asymptomatic and detected only by anemia discovered by a routine hemoglobin determination. Iron deficiency anemia in any male or nonmenstruating female should lead to a search for a source of bleeding from the gastrointestinal tract. Bleeding is often associated with colon cancer, but in about one third of patients with a proven colon cancer, the hemoglobin is normal and the stool tests negative for occult blood.

Cancers located in the left colon are often constrictive in nature. Patients with left-sided colon cancers may notice a change in bowel habit, most often reported as increasing constipation. Sigmoid cancers can mimic diverticulitis, presenting with pain, fever, and obstructive symptoms. At least 20% of patients with sigmoid cancer also have diverticular disease, making the correct diagnosis difficult at times. Sigmoid cancers can also cause colovesical or colovaginal fistulas. Such fistulas are more commonly caused by diverticulitis, but it is imperative that the correct diagnosis be established because treatment of colon cancer is substantially different than treatment of diverticulitis.

Cancers in the right colon more often present with melena, fatigue associated with anemia, or, if the tumor is advanced, abdominal pain. Although obstructive symptoms are more commonly associated with cancers of the left colon, any advanced colorectal cancer can cause a change in bowel habits and intestinal obstruction (Figs. 50-55 and 50-56).

Colonoscopy is the gold standard for establishing the diagnosis of colon cancer. It permits biopsy of the tumor to verify the diagnosis while allowing inspection of the entire colon to exclude metachronous polyps or cancers (the incidence of a synchronous cancer is about 3%). Colonoscopy is generally performed even after a cancer is detected by barium enema to obtain a biopsy and to detect (and remove) small polyps that may be missed by the contrast study (Fig. 50-57).

In patients with tumors causing complete obstruction, the diagnosis is most properly established by resection of the tumor without the benefit of preoperative colonoscopy. A water-soluble contrast enema is often useful in such circumstances to establish the anatomic level of the obstruction. Primary anastomosis between the proximal colon and the colon distal to the tumor has been avoided in the past in the presence of obstruction because of a high risk for anastomotic leak associated with such an approach. Thus, such patients were usually treated by

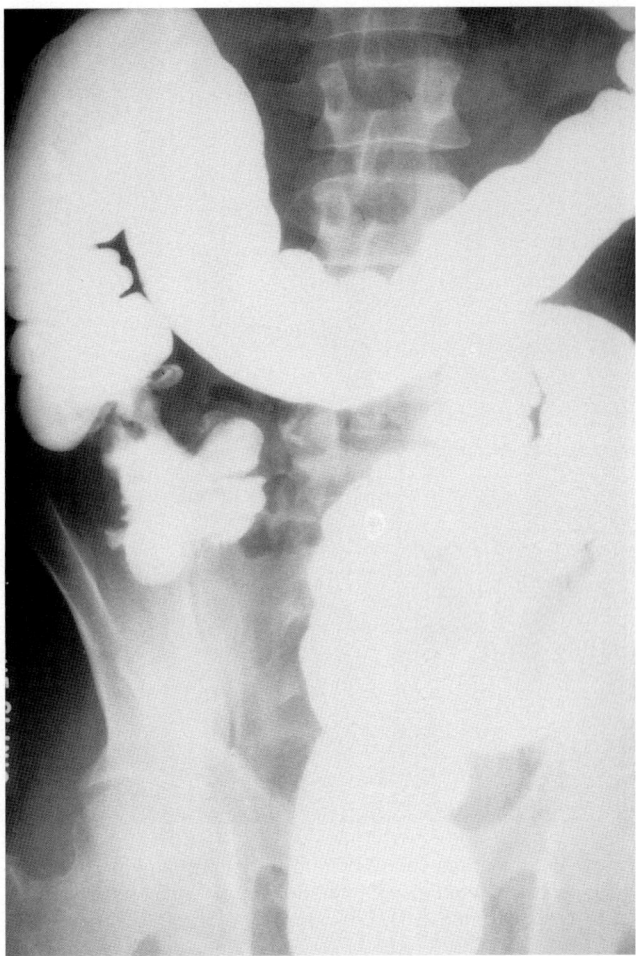

Figure 50-55 Barium enema demonstrating "apple core" or "napkin ring" lesion, caused by a constricting carcinoma.

resection of the segment of colon containing the obstructing cancer, suture closure of the distal sigmoid or rectum, and constructing a colostomy (Hartmann's operation). Intestinal continuity could be reestablished later, after the colon had been cleansed with purgatives, by taking down the colostomy and fashioning a colorectal anastomosis.

Alternatives to this approach have been to resect the segment of left colon containing the cancer and then cleanse the remaining colon with saline lavage by inserting a catheter through the appendix or ileum into the cecum and irrigating the contents from the colon. A primary anastomosis between the prepared colon and the rectum can then be fashioned without the need for a temporary colostomy. A third approach occasionally used for obstructing cancers of the sigmoid colon is to resect the tumor and the entire colon proximal to the tumor and fashion an anastomosis between the ileum and the distal sigmoid colon (subtotal colectomy and ileosigmoid anastomosis). This approach has the advantage of avoiding a temporary colostomy and eliminating the need to search for synchronous lesions in the colon proximal to the cancer. However, patients treated by this approach may have more frequent bowel movements.

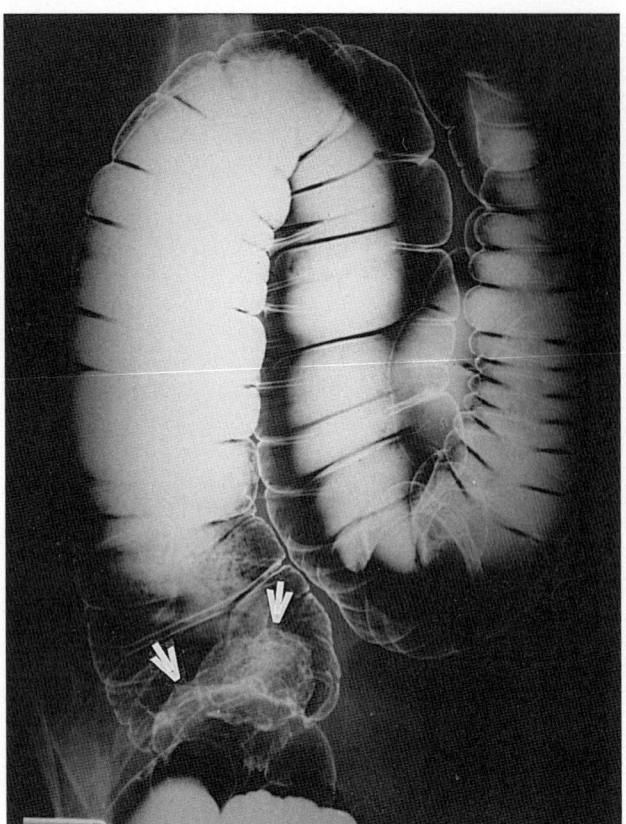

Figure 50-56 Barium enema demonstrating a polypoid carcinoma arising in the cecum of a 35-year-old woman (*arrows*). (Courtesy of Dina F. Caroline, MD, PhD, Temple University Hospital.)

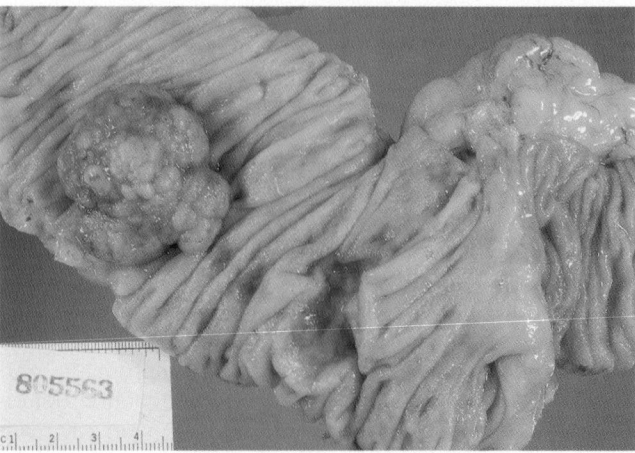

Figure 50-57 Resected right colon containing large benign sessile polyp adjacent to an ulcerated carcinoma.

More recently, endoscopic techniques have been developed that permit the placement of a stent introduced with the aid of a colonoscope that traverses the obstructed tumor and expands, recreating a lumen, relieving the obstruction, and permitting a bowel prep and elective operation with primary colorectal anastomosis.[44]

The approaches discussed previously concern obstruction of the left colon. Complete obstruction of the right colon or cecum by cancer occurs less frequently. These patients present with signs and symptoms of a small bowel obstruction. If an obstruction of the proximal colon is suspected, a water-soluble contrast study is useful to verify the diagnosis and evaluate the distal colon for the presence of a synchronous lesion. Obstructing cancer of the proximal colon is treated by right colectomy with primary anastomosis between the ileum and the transverse colon.

Patients with tumors that are not obstructing should undergo a thorough evaluation for metastatic disease. This includes a thorough physical examination, chest x-ray, liver function tests, and carcinoembryonic antigen (CEA) level. Most surgeons now obtain a CT or MRI to more thoroughly inspect the liver for metastases and to search for other intra-abdominal pathology.

The presence of hepatic metastatic disease does not preclude the surgical excision of the primary tumor.

Unless the hepatic metastatic disease is extensive, excising the primary cancer can provide excellent palliation. Bleeding and obstruction caused by the tumor can be avoided, and if the metastatic disease in the liver is resectable, the patient may yet be cured.

The objective of surgery for colon adenocarcinoma is the removal of the primary cancer with adequate margins, regional lymphadenectomy, and restoration of the continuity of the gastrointestinal tract by anastomosis. The extent of resection is determined by the location of the cancer, its blood supply and draining lymphatic system, and the presence or absence of direct extension into adjacent organs. It is important to resect the lymphatics (which parallel the arterial supply) to the greatest extent possible in order to render the abdomen free of lymphatic metastases if possible. Should hepatic metastases subsequently be detected, they may still be resected for cure in some instances if the abdominal disease has been completed eradicated.

To restore the continuity of the gastrointestinal tract, an anastomosis is fashioned with either sutures or staples, joining the ends of the intestine (small or large). It is important that both segments of the intestine used for the anastomosis have excellent blood supply and that there be no tension on the anastomosis. For lesions involving the cecum, ascending colon, and hepatic flexure, a right hemicolectomy is the procedure of choice. This involves removal of the bowel from 4 to 6 cm proximal to the ileocecal valve to the portion of the transverse colon supplied by the right branch of the middle colic artery (Fig. 50-58). An anastomosis is fashioned between the terminal ileum and the transverse colon. An extended right hemicolectomy is the procedure of choice for most transverse colon lesions and involves division of the right and middle colic arteries at their origin, with removal of the right and transverse colon supplied by these vessels. The anastomosis is fashioned between the terminal ileum and the proximal left colon. A left hemicolectomy (i.e., resection from the splenic flexure to the rectosigmoid junction) is the procedure of choice for tumors of the descending colon, whereas a sigmoidectomy is appropriate for tumors of the sigmoid colon. Most surgeons prefer to avoid incorporating the proximal sigmoid colon into an anastomosis because of the often tenuous blood supply from the inferior mesenteric artery and the frequent involvement of the sigmoid with diverticular disease.

Abdominal colectomy (sometimes called *subtotal colectomy or total colectomy*) entails removal of the entire colon from the ileum to the rectum, with continuity restored by an ileorectal anastomosis. Because of loss of the absorptive and storage capacity of the colon, this procedure causes an increase in stool frequency. Patients younger than 60 years generally tolerate this well, with gradual adaptation of the small bowel mucosa, increased water absorption, and an acceptable stool frequency of one to three movements daily. In older individuals, however, abdominal colectomy may result in significant chronic diarrhea. Abdominal colectomy is indicated for patients with multiple primary tumors, for individuals with HNPCC, and occasionally for patients with completely obstructing sigmoid cancers.

The chances that the patient has been cured by an operation performed to remove a colorectal cancer is dependent on several factors, including technical aspects of the operation, such as the complete removal of all tumor, certain biologic properties of the cancer that are poorly understood, and the stage of the disease.

Staging may be defined as the process by which objective data are assembled to try to define the state of progression of the disease. Separate items of data are summated to provide a designated stage for an individual patient's disease, from which inferences may be drawn regarding the relative likelihood of residual disease and hence the chance of cure without further treatment and the advisability of considering further treatment. The ideal staging system would provide one ultimately important and simple item of information: Has the operation cured the patient, or will he or she die unless further intervention prevents it? Thus, there would be just two categories: the cured and those destined to die of their disease. Unfortunately, no system extant even remotely approaches that goal. Still, every attempt should be made to accurately assess the extent of the disease to provide guidance for prognosis and the need for further treatment.

At the present time, the stage of the tumor is assessed by indicating the depth of penetration of the tumor into the bowel wall (T stage), the extent of lymph node involvement (N stage), and the presence or absence of distant metastases (M stage). For most of the past half century, the standard staging system was based on a system developed and modified by Cuthbert Dukes, a pathologist at St. Mark's Hospital in London. The classification was developed for rectal cancer, but it was generally also used to describe the stage of colon cancer. The Dukes classification is simple to remember and is still frequently used. Dukes' stage A cancer is confined to the bowel wall. Stage B cancer penetrates the bowel wall, and stage C cancer indicates lymph node metastases. Kirklin and colleagues, from the Mayo Clinic, established a distinction between tumors that partially penetrated the

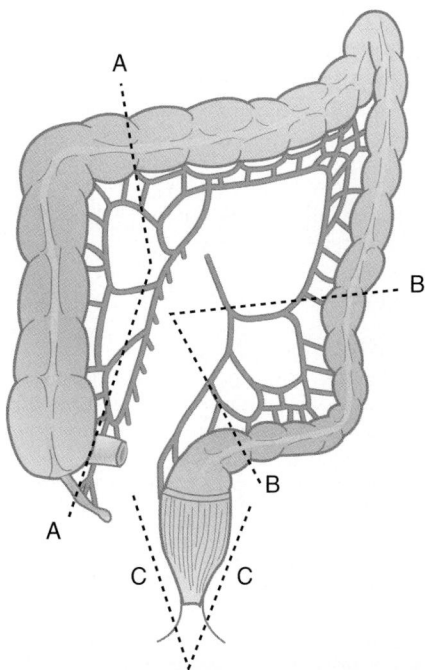

Figure 50-58 Operative procedures for right-sided colon cancer, sigmoid diverticulitis, and low-lying rectal cancer. A right hemicolectomy (A) involves resection of a few centimeters of terminal ileum and colon up to the division of the middle colic vessels into right and left. A sigmoidectomy (B) consists of removing the colon between the partially retroperitoneal descending colon and the rectum. An abdominoperineal resection of the rectum (C) is performed in a combined approach through the abdomen and through the perineum for the resection of the entire rectum and anus.

muscularis propria (B1) and those that fully penetrated this layer (B2). Astler and Coller further separated the tumors that had invaded lymph nodes but did not penetrate the entire bowel wall (C1) from tumors that invaded lymph nodes and did penetrate the entire wall (C2). Turnbull and associates from the Cleveland Clinic added stage D for tumors with distant metastasis. All these modifications in various combinations are still in use and are often called *modified Dukes classification.*

The classification in use by most hospitals in the United States was developed by the American Joint Committee on Cancer (AJCC) and was approved by the International Union Against Cancer (UICC).[45] This classification, known as the TNM (tumor, node, metastasis) system, combines clinical information obtained preoperatively with data obtained during surgery and after histologic examination of the specimen. There have been some modifications in the system since its introduction in 1987. The surgeon is now encouraged to score the completeness of the resection as follows: R0 for complete tumor resection with all margins negative; R1 for incomplete tumor resection with microscopic involvement of a margin, and R2 for incomplete tumor resection with gross residual tumor not resected (Table 50-6).

There are four possible stages of colorectal cancer within the AJCC system. In stage I, there is no lymph node metastasis, and the tumor is either T1 or T2 (up to

Table 50-6   AJCC TNM Staging System for Colorectal Cancer

Primary Tumor (T)

TX	Primary tumor cannot be assessed
T0	No evidence of primary tumor
Tis	Carcinoma in situ: intraepithelial or invasion of lamina propria*
T1	Tumor invades submucosa
T2	Tumor invades muscularis propria
T3	Tumor invades through the muscularis propria into the subserosa, or into nonperitonealized pericolic or perirectal tissues
T4	Tumor directly invades other organs or structures and/or perforates visceral peritoneum[†]

Regional Lymph Nodes (N)[‡]

NX	Regional lymph nodes cannot be assessed
N0	No regional lymph node metastasis
N1	Metastasis in 1 to 3 regional lymph nodes
N2	Metastasis in 4 or more regional lymph nodes

Distant Metastasis (M)

MX	Distant metastasis cannot be assessed
M0	No distant metastasis
M1	Distant metastasis

Stage Grouping

STAGE	T	N	M	DUKES[§]	MAC[§]
0	Tis	N0	M0		
I	T1	N0	M0	A	A
	T2	N0	M0	A	B1
IIA	T3	N0	M0	B	B2
IIB	T4	N0	M0	B	B3
IIIA	T1-T2	N1	M0	C	C1
IIIB	T3-T4	N1	M0	C	C2/C3
IIIC	Any T	N2	M0	C	C1/C2/C3
IV	Any T	Any N	M1		D

Histologic Grade (G)

GX	Grade cannot be assessed
G1	Well differentiated
G2	Moderately differentiated
G3	Poorly differentiated
G4	Undifferentiated

*Tis includes cancer cells confined within the glandular basement membrane (intraepithelial) or lamina propria (intramucosal) with no extension through the muscularis mucosae into the submucosa.

[†]Direct invasion in T4 includes invasion of other segments of the colorectum by way of the serosa: for example, invasion of the sigmoid colon by a carcinoma of the cecum. Tumor that is adherent to other organs or structures macroscopically is classified T4. However, if no tumor is present in the adhesion microscopically, the classification should be pT3. The V and L substaging should be used to identify the presence or absence of vascular or lymphatic invasion.

[‡]A tumor nodule in the pericolorectal adipose tissue of a primary carcinoma without histologic evidence of residual lymph node in the nodule is classified in the pN category as a regional lymph node metastasis if the nodule has the form and smooth contour of a lymph node. If the nodule has an irregular contour, it should be classified in the T category and also coded as V1 (microscopic venous invasion) or as V2 (if it was grossly evident), because there is a strong likelihood that it represents venous invasion.

[§]Dukes B is a composite of better (T3N0M0) and worse (T4N0M0) prognostic groups, as is Dukes C (Any TN1M0 and Any TN2M0). MAC is the modified Astler-Coller classification.

Note: The y prefix is to be used for those cancers that are classified after pretreatment, whereas the r prefix is to be used for those cancers that have recurred. Used with permission of the American Joint Committee on Cancer (AJCC), Chicago, Illinois. The original and primary source for this information is the *AJCC Cancer Staging Manual, Sixth Edition* (2002) published by Springer-Verlag New York. (For more information, visit www.cancerstaging.net.) Any citation or quotation of this material must be credited to the AJCC as its primary source. The inclusion of this information herein does not authorize any reuse or further distribution without the expressed, written permission of Springer-Verlag New York, Inc., on behalf of the AJCC. © 2002 National Comprehensive Cancer Network, Inc. All rights reserved.

muscularis propria). Patients who undergo appropriate resection of T stage 1 colon cancer have a 5-year survival rate of about 90%. Stage II is now subdivided into IIA (if the primary tumor is T3) and IIB (for T4 lesions), with no lymph node metastasis. The 5-year survival rate for patients with stage II colon cancer treated by appropriate surgical resection is about 75%. Stage III cancer is characterized by lymph node metastasis and is now subdivided into IIIA (T1-T2, N1, M0), IIIB (T3-T4, N1, M0), and IIIC (any T, N2, M0). In the latest version of the staging system (2003), smooth metastatic nodules in the pericolic or perirectal fat are considered lymph node metastasis and should be included in N staging. Irregularly contoured metastatic nodules in the peritumoral fat are considered vascular invasion. The survival for stage III cancer treated by surgery alone has been about 50%. Distant metastatic disease (stage IV) carries a poor prognosis, with a 5-year survival rate of less than 5%.

Further treatment and follow-up of patients treated by segmental colectomy for colon cancer is directed by the stage of the disease. About 85% of recurrences are detected within 2 years of the time of resection, so follow-up strategy should be especially intensive during that period.

A reasonable strategy to follow patients with stage I colon cancer is a colonoscopic examination 1 year after the operation, to inspect the anastomosis but also to detect any new or missed polyps. The colonoscopy should be repeated annually if any polyps are detected and removed, until an examination reveals the absence of polyps. Then a colonoscopy should be offered every 5 years unless a strong family history or other genetic risk factor is present, in which case more frequent endoscopic examinations are obviously indicated. A CEA level should be obtained every 3 months during the first 2 years, even if the preoperative CEA was normal. A rising CEA level requires further tests to search for metastatic disease, including a CT scan (or MRI) of the abdomen and chest, and possible positron emission tomography (PET) scan. The goal of close follow-up testing is to detect early recurrence that is amenable to treatment. Isolated hepatic or pulmonary metastases are amenable to resection, with a 5-year survival rate of 20%. Multiple or unresectable metastases may respond to modern chemotherapeutic agents.

Postoperative treatment of patients with stage II colon cancer is somewhat controversial. To date, no large randomized trial has shown a benefit from adjuvant chemotherapy for this rather heterogeneous group of patients. An attempt to stratify the patients may identify a subset that would benefit from chemotherapy. The 5-year survival rate of patients with stage IIA disease is 85%, compared with 72% for stage IIB disease, which is actually worse than for those patients with node-positive stage IIIA disease. The American Society of Clinical Oncology (ASCO) currently suggests a course of 5-flurouracil (5-FU)-based adjuvant chemotherapy for stage II patients with at least one poor prognostic indicator including insufficient lymph node sampling (<12 nodes resected with the specimen), T4 lesions, poorly differentiated histology, or bowel perforation. Whether oxaliplatin-based regimens should be used in stage II disease in addition to 5-FU/leucovorin is controversial, but current practice in most areas appears to favor the addition of oxaliplatin in early-stage disease. Further follow-up of stage II patients includes a CEA level every 3 months for 2 years, then every 6 months for a total of 5 years, and yearly CT scans of the abdomen and chest for at least the first 3 years.

Patients with stage III disease clearly benefit from adjuvant chemotherapy. The addition of oxaliplatin to the 5-FU/leucovorin regimen (FOLFOX) has resulted in an improvement of disease-free survival rates at 3 years to 78% (compared with 73% with 5-FU/leucovorin alone). Irinotecan (Camptosar) has been investigated as an addition to 5-FU–based therapy in the adjuvant setting, based on its benefit against metastatic disease. Unfortunately, irinotecan has not demonstrated efficacy in the adjuvant setting and is not currently used for the treatment of stage III patients.

The method of delivery of the chemotherapeutic agents is evolving. Continuous-infusion 5-FU is now generally considered to be superior to bolus infusions, with less toxicity. Recently, an oral fluoropyrimidine, capecitabine (Xeloda), has been shown to be at least equivalent to intravenous 5-FU and may have superior efficacy.

The treatment of stage IV patients depends on the location and extent of the metastases. Isolated hepatic or pulmonary lesions may be amenable to resection. Chemotherapy is indicated, with exciting new agents complementing the 5-FU regimens that remain the keystone of therapy. The newest agents that have been shown to be effective for metastatic disease and are now being studied in the adjuvant setting are the monoclonal antibodies bevacizumab (Avastin) and cetuximab (Erbitux). Cetuximab binds to and inhibits the epidermal growth factor receptor, which is overexpressed in 60% to 80% of colorectal cancers and is associated with a shorter survival time. This agent has shown clinical efficacy in patients with metastatic colorectal cancer, both as monotherapy and in combination with irinotecan and FOLFOX. Bevacizumab, a vascular endothelial growth factor inhibitor, has also improved survival when added to regimens that include irinotecan, 5-FU/leucovorin, or oxaliplatin. Both of these drugs, coupled with FOLFOX chemotherapy, are being studied in the adjuvant setting.

Rectal Cancer

Cancers arising in the distal 15 cm of the large bowel share many of the genetic, biologic, and morphologic characteristics of colon cancers. However, the unique anatomy of the rectum, with its retroperitoneal location in the narrow pelvis and proximity to the urogenital organs, autonomic nerves, and anal sphincters, makes surgical access relatively difficult. In addition, precise dissection in appropriate anatomic planes is essential because dissection medial to the endopelvic fascia investing the mesorectum may doom the patient to local recurrence of the disease, and dissection laterally to the avascular anatomic space risks injury to the mixed autonomic nerves, causing impotence in men and bladder dysfunction in both sexes.

Furthermore, the biologic properties of the rectum, combined with its anatomic distance from the small intestine afforded by its retroperitoneal pelvic location, provides an opportunity for treatment by radiation therapy that is not feasible for colon tumors. The large bowel can tolerate properly delivered radiation doses up to 6000 cGy, whereas such levels of radiation targeted at colon tumors would include small bowel in the treatment field. The small bowel cannot withstand radiation doses of this level without complications of radiation enteritis, including stricture, hemorrhage, and perforation.

The treatment of rectal cancer has changed significantly during the past 20 years, and there is considerable controversy today concerning the precise role of surgery, radiation therapy, and chemotherapy, and the ideal timing of each modality with relation to the others. Although information from clinical trials has provided data supporting the multimodality treatment of rectal cancer, the criteria for patient selection remains controversial. However, some generalities can be made at the present time:

- Radiation therapy offers significant benefit to many patients with rectal cancer, and preoperative radiation is superior to postoperative radiation. Until recently, preoperative radiation (combined with chemotherapy) has generally been reserved for locally advanced distal rectal cancers (within 10 cm of the anal verge, stage II or higher), but a recent analysis based on a cooperative 7-year trial of the National Research Council (NRC) of the United Kingdom and the National Cancer Institute of Canada (NCIC) has shown that short-term preoperative radiation (25 Gy over 5 days) results in a significant reduction in the local recurrence rate and improved disease-free survival for all stages of rectal cancer.[46]
- Chemotherapy that has shown efficacy in the adjuvant setting in the treatment of colon cancer is also beneficial in the adjuvant setting for patients with rectal cancer. The combination of neoadjuvant (preoperative) radiation (usually 4500-5040 cGy) with infusional 5-FU/leucovorin (and more recently with the addition of oxaliplatin) often results in dramatic reduction in tumor size (down-staging), and may result in apparent complete eradication of the tumor in up to 25% of cases.
- Neoadjuvant chemoradiation may increase the ability of the surgeon to preserve continence by down-staging the cancer, in some instances shrinking the size of the tumor to permit the achievement of a cancer-free margin at the distal extent of the resection, when a clear margin that would permit an anastomosis in the anal canal could not be achieved without such shrinkage.
- The best course of neoadjuvant treatment has not yet been determined. In Europe, the short course of radiation (25 Gy), followed by extirpative surgery (either low anterior resection or abdominal perineal resection), is the most common approach. In the United States, stage II or higher rectal cancers are more commonly treated with preoperative chemoradiation consisting of 4500 to 5040 cGy of radiation in conjunction with infusional 5-FU-based chemotherapy. The radiation is delivered over a period of 5 to 6 weeks, and surgery (low anterior resection or abdominal perineal resection) is done 6 to 10 weeks after the completion of the radiation therapy. A diverting stoma (either ileostomy or transverse colostomy) is usually fashioned (with irradiated rectum) to protect the anastomosis,

and the stoma is then closed 10 weeks later, when studies show satisfactory healing of the anastomosis. In Europe, a diverting stoma is not usually done, and the anastomotic leak rates appear quite low.
- Neoadjuvant therapy is not a substitute for a properly performed surgical procedure. As discussed later, dissection in the proper plane is essential to achieve adequate margins and remove the rectal lymphatics that may harbor metastases. A total mesorectal resection is appropriate for cancer of the mid and distal rectum, but the mesorectum can be divided below a cancer of the proximal rectum (>10 cm above the anus) to allow preservation of the distal rectum for the anastomosis. If a total mesorectal excision is performed and the anal sphincters are preserved, the anastomosis to establish continence will need to join the colon to the anus.

The most common symptom of rectal cancer is hematochezia. Unfortunately, this is often attributed to hemorrhoids, and the correct diagnosis is consequently delayed until the cancer has reached an advanced stage. Other symptoms include mucus discharge, tenesmus, and change in bowel habit.

The differential diagnosis of rectal cancer include ulcerative colitis, Crohn's proctocolitis, radiation proctitis, and procidentia. Occasionally, so-called hidden rectal prolapse or internal intussusception of the sigmoid into the rectum can produce a solitary rectal ulcer that mimics an ulcerating cancer. It is thought that the chronic trauma from the recurrent intussusception results in ulceration of the rectal mucosa. Instead of a solitary rectal ulcer, this mucosal trauma from intussusception can sometimes produce the entity of *colitis cystica profunda,* a polypoid lesion that is characterized by the presence of benign columnar epithelium and mucous cysts residing deep to the muscularis mucosae. This histologic pattern can be confused with invasive adenocarcinoma, and it is obviously important to recognize this completely benign entity.

The preoperative assessment of patients with rectal cancer is similar to that described for patients with colon cancer, with some significant differences: the requirement for precise characterization of the cancer with respect to proximity to the anal sphincters, and the extent of invasion as determined by depth of penetration into the bowel wall and spread to adjacent lymph nodes. A complete colonoscopic examination should be done to exclude synchronous tumors in the colon, but the precise location of the rectal tumor is best determined by examination with a rigid proctosigmoidoscope. Rigid proctosigmoidoscopy should be done even if the tumor has been diagnosed with a colonoscopic examination because the flexible scope may not accurately measure the exact distance from the tumor to the anal sphincter. The depth of penetration can be estimated by digital rectal exam (superficially invasive tumors are mobile, whereas the lesions become tethered and fixed with increasing depth of penetration), and endorectal ultrasound (EUS) or MRI with endorectal coil can provide fairly accurate assessment of the extent of invasion of the bowel wall (Fig. 50-59).

Tumors located in the distal 3 to 5 cm of the rectum present the greatest challenge for the surgeon. Thorough and adequate assessment of tumors in this location is mandatory to select the proper treatment. If the tumor is confined to the submucosa (uT1, N0), excision by a transanal approach is an attractive option. In such circumstances, the incidence of lymphatic metastases is less than 8%, a factor that should be considered when contemplating the mortality and morbidity that would be associated with an abdominal perineal resection in a frail or elderly patient. Cancers in this location that invade or penetrate the muscular wall of the rectum have a high incidence of local recurrence after transanal excision (>20%), and consideration should be given to treatment that is more aggressive than local excision. The preferred course of treatment requires consideration of many factors, including the patient's overall health and preferences. However, consideration should be given to more aggressive treatment for a T2 rectal cancer: either chemoradiation or formal surgical excision (proctectomy with total mesorectal excision).

After the location and stage of the cancer are determined, various options need to be considered for the optimal treatment of the rectal cancer. Other important considerations include the presence or absence of comorbid conditions and the patient's body habitus (an obese male with a narrow pelvis presents technical difficulties different than in a thin woman with a wide pelvis). The appropriate operation should be tailored to eradicate the tumor while preserving function to the fullest extent possible. The following procedures all are useful in certain circumstances.

Local Excision

Local excision of a rectal cancer is an excellent operation for a small cancer in the distal rectum that has not penetrated into the muscularis. This is accomplished through a transanal approach, and usually involves excision of the full thickness of the rectal wall underlying the tumor. Local excisions do not allow complete removal of lymph nodes in the mesorectum, and therefore operative staging is limited. The operation is indicated for mobile tumors that are less than 4 cm in diameter, that involve less than 40% of the rectal wall circumference, and that are located within 6 cm of the anal verge. These tumors should be stage T1 (limited to the submucosa) or T2 (limited to the muscularis propria), well or moderately differentiated histologically, and with no vascular or lymphatic invasion. There should be no evidence of nodal disease on preoperative ultrasound or MRI. Adherence to these principles results in acceptable local recurrence rates compared with treatment by abdominal perineal resection. Local excision is also used for palliation of more advanced cancer in patients with severe comorbid disease, in whom extensive surgery carries a high risk for morbidity or mortality. Various technical approaches have been described to achieve transanal local excision, including use of a special proctoscope equipped with a magnifying camera (transanal endoscopic microsurgery), but all approaches require the complete excision of the cancer with adequate margins of normal tissue. Although many

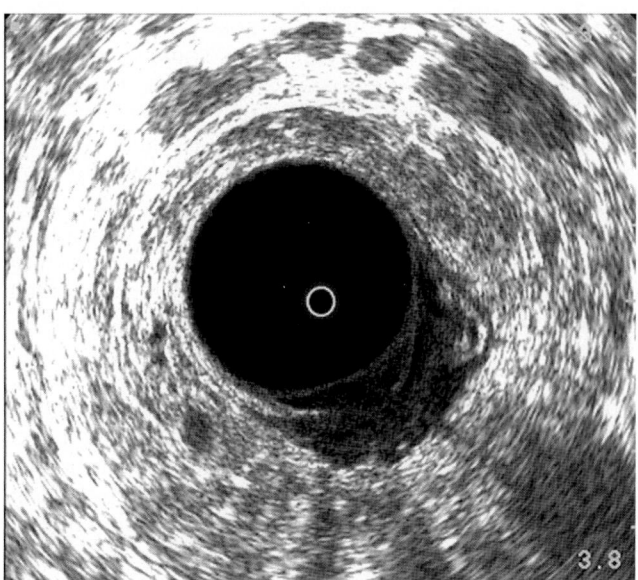

Figure 50-59 Endorectal ultrasound of patient with T3, N1 rectal cancer. The cancer penetrates through all layers of the rectal wall, and an enlarged lymph node is clearly visible.

surgeons suture the rectal defect closed after the local excision, this is not mandatory because the operative site is below the peritoneal reflection. Unfortunately, as experience has accumulated with this approach, it has become clear that close follow-up is mandatory, in that about 8% of T1 lesions recur, and the recurrence rate for T2 lesions has been shown in some series to exceed 20%.[47] As discussed previously, most clinicians feel that local excision is not adequate treatment for a T2 rectal cancer, and further treatment is required, either adjuvant radiation plus chemotherapy or radical excision (either low anterior resection or abdominal perineal resection).

Transanal Endoscopic Microsurgery

Transanal endoscopic microsurgery (TEM) is an approach for local excision of favorable rectal tumors (T1 cancers and sessile polyps) through a device designed to provide access to the mid and proximal rectum. The endosurgical device is a large (4 cm in diameter) proctoscope through which four functions (carbon dioxide insufflation, water irrigation, suction, and monitoring of intrarectal pressure) are simultaneously regulated. The TEM scope itself is closed and sealed, so that the rectum distends when carbon dioxide is insufflated into the system. This distention facilitates visualization that is afforded by binocular lenses attached to the system.

The scope is inserted through the anus and positioned in a fashion to provide the optimum visualization and access to the tumor. Positioning of the scope is critical for success of the operation, and the patient must be placed in the proper position on the operating table to permit the scope to be adequately secured in a stable position. Long operating instruments are then inserted through ports in the system and used to excise the tumor under direct vision. The advantages of the technique include excellent exposure to tumors in a difficult area of access. However, the technique is somewhat difficult to perfect, the equipment is expensive, and the number of lesions amenable to this approach is relatively small. The complications associated with the technique are the same as for standard transanal local excision: bleeding, urinary retention, perforation into the peritoneal cavity, and fecal soilage. The dilation of the anal sphincters by the large scope may be associated with subsequent fecal incontinence, but this appears to be a transient problem in most circumstances.

Fulguration

The technique of fulguration, which eradicates the cancer by using an electrocautery device that destroys the tumor by creating a full-thickness eschar at the tumor site, requires extension of the eschar into the perirectal fat, thus destroying both the tumor and the rectal wall. The procedure can be used only for lesions below the peritoneal reflection. Complications associated with this approach are postoperative fever and significant bleeding that can occur as late as 10 days after the operation. Obviously, this technique cannot provide a specimen to assess the pathologic stage because the tumor and margins are disintegrated by fulguration. The procedure is reserved for patients with a prohibitive operative risk and limited life expectancy, and it has largely been replaced by transanal excision, which provides the advantage of examination and more adequate staging of the specimen.

Abdominal Perineal Resection

The complete excision of the rectum and anus, by concomitant dissection through the abdomen and perineum, with suture closure of the perineum and creation of a permanent colostomy was first described by Ernest Miles and is thus sometimes referred to as the *Miles procedure.* The rectum and sigmoid colon are mobilized through an abdominal incision. The pelvic dissection, done through the abdominal incision, mobilizes the mesorectum in continuity with the tumor-bearing rectum. The pelvic dissection is carried to the level of the levator ani muscles. The perineal portion of the operation excises the anus, the anal sphincters, and the distal rectum. The operation may be accomplished sequentially or simultaneously using an abdominal surgeon and surgeon in the perineal field. An abdominal perineal resection is indicated when the tumor involves the anal sphincters, when the tumor is too close to the sphincters to obtain adequate margins, or in patients in whom sphincter-preserving surgery is not possible because of unfavorable body habitus or poor preoperative sphincter control.

Low Anterior Resection

Resection of the rectum through an abdominal approach offers the advantage of completely removing the portion of bowel containing the cancer and the mesorectum, which contains the lymphatic channels that drain the tumor bed. The term *anterior resection* (an abbreviation for the more correct term, *anterior proctosigmoidectomy with colorectal anastomosis*) indicates resection of the proximal rectum or rectosigmoid, above the peritoneal reflection. The term *low anterior resection* indicates that the operation entails resection of the rectum below the peritoneal reflection through an abdominal approach. The sigmoid colon is almost always included with the resected specimen because diverticulosis often involves the sigmoid, and the blood supply to the sigmoid is often not adequate to sustain an anastomosis if the inferior mesenteric artery is transected. For cancers involving the lower half of the rectum, the entire mesorectum (which contains the lymph channels draining the tumor bed) should be excised in continuity with the rectum. This technique, *total mesorectal excision,* produces the complete resection of an intact package of the rectum and its adjacent mesorectum, enveloped within the visceral pelvic fascia with uninvolved circumferential margins. The use of the technique of total mesorectal excision has resulted in a significant increase in 5-year survival rates (50% to 75%), a decrease in local recurrence rate (30% to 5%), and a decrease in the incidence of impotence and bladder dysfunction (85% to <15%).

Intestinal continuity is reestablished by fashioning an anastomosis between the descending colon and the rectum, a feat that has been greatly facilitated by the introduction of the circular stapling device. After the colorectal anastomosis has been completed, it should be inspected with a proctoscope inserted through the anus. If there is concern about the integrity of the anastomosis, or if the patient has received high-dose preoperative chemoradiation, a temporary proximal colostomy should be made to permit complete healing of the anastomosis. The colostomy can be closed in about 10 weeks if proctoscopy and contrast studies verify the integrity of the anastomosis.

An end-to-end anastomosis between the descending colon and the distal rectum or anus may result in significant alteration of bowel habits attributed to the loss of the normal rectal capacity (Fig. 50-60). Patients treated with this operation often experience frequent small bowel movements (low anterior resection syndrome or clustering). This problem has been addressed by fashioning a colonic J pouch as the proximal component of the anastomosis (Fig. 50-61). As experience has accumulated with this approach, it appears that improvement in bowel function is significant for cancers located in the distal rectum, but if the anastomosis is created above 9 cm from the anal verge, there is little benefit of a J pouch compared with an end-to-end anastomosis. The limbs of the J pouch should be relatively short (6 cm) because patients with larger J pouches have a significant incidence of difficulty with evacuation.

In obese patients and in patients with a narrow pelvis, it may not be technically feasible to fashion a J pouch as the proximal component of the low pelvic anastomosis because the bulk of the pouch simply will not fit into the narrow pelvis. In such circumstances, a reservoir can be devised with a coloplasty. This technique provides a rectal reservoir by making an 8- to 10-cm colotomy 4 to 6 cm from the divided end of the colon. The colotomy is closed transversely to provide increased rectal space and capacitance (Figs. 50-62 and 50-63).[48]

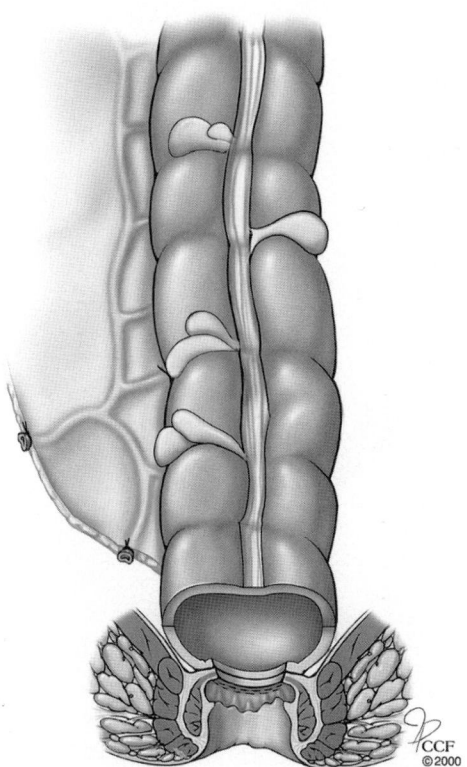

Figure 50-60 Anastomosis between descending colon and anus, following complete resection of the rectum. The absence of the rectum often results in frequent, small bowel movements, a phenomenon known as "clustering" or "low anterior resection syndrome." (Copyright © Cleveland Clinic Foundation, 2000.)

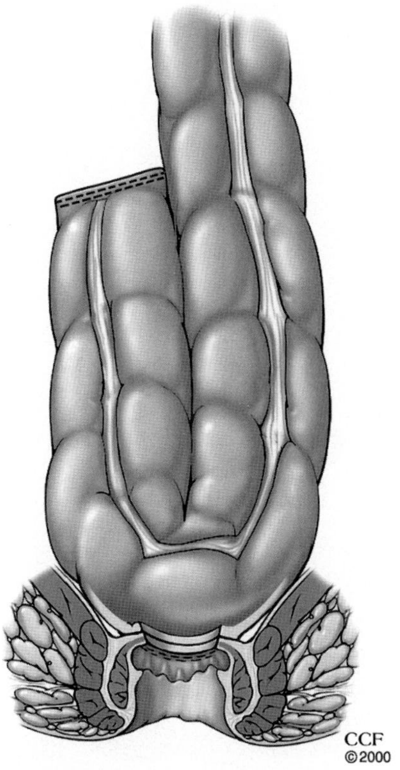

Figure 50-61 J pouch fashioned from descending colon to form proximal portion of coloanal anastomosis. This increases the "capacitance" to decrease the frequency of bowel movements. (Copyright © Cleveland Clinic Foundation, 2000.)

Sphincter-Sparing Abdominal Perineal Resection With Coloanal Anastomosis

Abdominal perineal resection is at times required because a cancer in the distal rectum cannot be resected with adequate margins while preserving the anal sphincter. However, the use of preoperative radiation and chemotherapy has been shown, in some instances, to shrink the tumor to an extent that acceptable margins can be achieved. If the anal sphincters do not need to be sacrificed to achieve adequate margins based on oncologic principles, a permanent stoma may be avoided with a sphincter-sparing abdominal perineal resection with an anastomosis between the colon and the anal canal. This operation has particular application for young patients with rectal tumors who have a favorable body habitus and good preoperative sphincter function. The operation can be conducted in a variety of ways, but all methods involve mobilizing the sigmoid colon and pelvic rectum through an abdominal approach, dissecting the rectal mucosa from the anal sphincters at the level of the dentate line, and completing the resection of the most distal rectum through the anal approach. An anastomosis is then fashioned between the descending colon and the anus, often using a J pouch or coloplasty procedure described previously for the low colorectal anastomosis. The anastomosis is made with sutures placed through a transanal approach by the surgeon in the perineal field.

Colorectal Cancer Prevention and Screening

Cancer prevention can be divided into a discussion of primary and secondary prevention.

Primary prevention is the identification of environmental factors responsible for cancer, and then modification of those factors to reduce risk. Examples of this strategy include dietary modification, avoidance of environmental hazards, and chemoprevention.

Secondary prevention involves finding a precursor lesion or cancer at a stage when metastasis and death can be prevented.

Cancer screening is the cornerstone of secondary prevention. Colorectal cancer is a preventable disease. An understanding of defined risk factors and screening options is essential for every health care practitioner. Our understanding of the natural history of colorectal cancer, precancerous conditions, patient risk factors, and the efficacy of screening options is currently in flux. Even so, obtaining a basic facility with the current evidence should be the goal.

Colorectal cancer is an ideal candidate for screening strategies for the following reasons:

1. It is a common and serious problem.
2. Precursor lesions exist.
3. It is slow growing.
4. Testing is available.

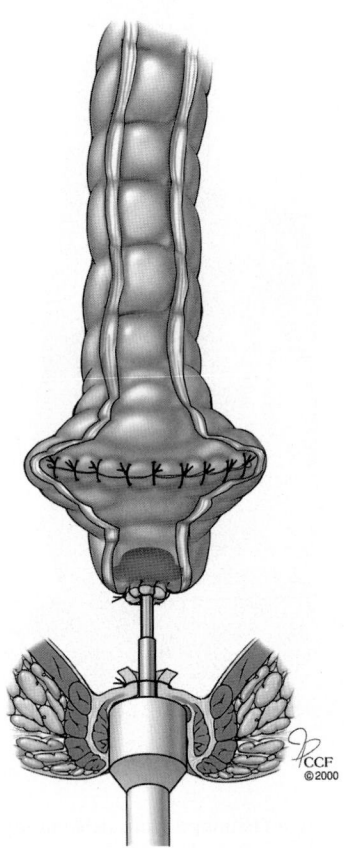

Figure 50-62 A coloplasty is performed by making an 8- to 10-cm colotomy 4 to 6 cm from the cut end of the colon. The longitudinal colotomy is made between the taeniae on the antimesenteric side. It is closed transversely with absorbable sutures. An end-to-end stapled anastomosis then joins the colon to the distal rectum or anus. (Copyright © Cleveland Clinic Foundation, 2000.)

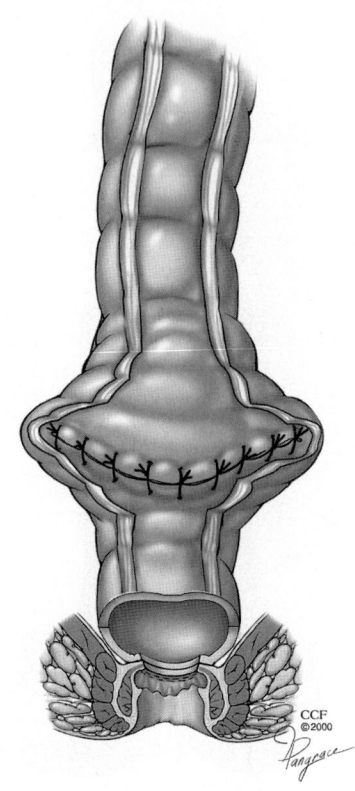

Figure 50-63 The completed stapled coloplasty with anastomosis. (Copyright © Cleveland Clinic Foundation, 2000.)

In 1993, the National Polyp Study Workgroup published a landmark study documenting a 76% to 90% reduction in colorectal cancer incidence compared with reference populations when adenomatous colon polyps are removed endoscopically. A year before this, both Selby and Newcomb independently showed a 60% to 70% rectal cancer mortality reduction following sigmoidoscopy and polypectomy. Clearly, intervention results in mortality reduction.

Far more controversial is the choice of screening method. This area of prevention is rapidly changing, and updated recommendations occur frequently. Patients are risk-stratified with frequency and method of screening dictated by category (see Table 50-5). By far, most patients (70%) are of average risk; these patients have no personal or family history of colorectal cancer or polyps, and no predisposing conditions such as ulcerative colitis or Crohn's disease.

The most difficult risk category to define is the moderate-risk group. The American College of Gastroenterologists stratified these patients into two groups.[49] Patients with one first-degree relative with colorectal cancer diagnosed after age 60 years are twice as likely as an average-risk individual to develop colorectal cancer themselves. Furthermore, their risk for colorectal cancer at age 40 years is the same as the general population's risk at age 50 years. Therefore, these individuals are considered at moderately increased risk—screening recommendations are the same as for average-risk patients but should begin at age 40 years. Patients with a strong family history of colorectal cancer include those with multiple first-degree relatives with colorectal cancer, or a single first-degree relative with cancer diagnosed before 60 years of age. Overall risk for developing cancer for this cohort is three to four times the average. Patients at high risk for developing colorectal cancer are those with a hereditary cancer syndrome such as FAP or HNPCC or with either ulcerative or Crohn's colitis.

Perhaps the most frequently used, and least well understood, screening tool is fecal occult blood testing (FOBT). It has the advantage of being inexpensive, easy-to-use, and interpretable by primary care physicians. In randomized studies, use of FOBT alone annually with three consecutive stools produced a colorectal cancer-specific mortality reduction rate of 33%. Unfortunately, the false-negative rate using FOBT alone is unacceptably high. Only 30% to 50% of cancers were detectable in most series. A recent study conducted by the Veterans Administration Study Group documented that only 24% of colorectal cancers produced a positive result.[50] Only 7.0% of patients with polyps produced positive FOBT (compared with 6.4% of polyp-free patients). In short, FOBT alone is not an adequate test for either polyps or colorectal cancer in any risk group.

For average-risk individuals, combining FOBT with flexible sigmoidoscopy at 5-year intervals is deemed acceptable as a screening option. In 2001, the Veterans Administration Cooperative Study Group published the results of a large study (2885 patients) comparing FOBT and flexible sigmoidoscopy with colonoscopy.[51] All patients underwent FOBT followed by full colonoscopy. The flexible sigmoidoscopy portion of the exam was carefully documented. Although sigmoidoscopy alone identified 70.3% of all cancers, the combination of FOBT and flexible sigmoidoscopy failed to detect 24% of proximal cancers. Flexible sigmoidoscopy is a valuable tool that can be done in an office-based setting by general practitioners without a full bowel preparation. However, poor preparation, patient discomfort, and variable technique may limit the accuracy of the exam. Polyps detected by flexible sigmoidoscopy should prompt full colonoscopic exam. Flexible sigmoidoscopy alone or with FOBT is not an adequate exam for those in either the strong family history or high-risk group.

Double-contrast barium enema (DCBE) was once the diagnostic mainstay for lower gastrointestinal disease. The advent of flexible fiberoptics has largely supplanted its use. Even so, it has retained a place in the screening armamentarium for the average-risk patient. In 2000, the National Polyp Study Work Group compared DCBE and colonoscopy in a prospective double-blinded trial in patients with a history of polyps.[52] All 862 study subjects underwent both types of exam. Colonoscopists were blinded to the results of the antecedent barium enema. Forty-five percent of colonoscopies revealed adenomatous polyps, compared with only 26% of DCBEs. The rate of detection on DCBE is significantly influenced by size. Only 48% of polyps 1.0 cm or greater in size were detected on DCBE.

Colonoscopy is considered the screening gold standard. It is the test of choice for patients with greater-than-average risk and has the advantage of providing a way to intervene in the natural history of colorectal cancer by facilitating endoscopic polypectomy. However, it has several disadvantages. It is the most morbid screening method. Colonic perforation (1 per 2000-1 per 2500 exams), as well as significant bleeding (<1% of exams), can occur. Colonoscopy requires a full bowel preparation accompanied by fasting, sedation, and a skilled endoscopist. Finally, colonoscopy is the most expensive screening test available. Even considering these limitations, the use of colonoscopy has become commonplace. It is the screening test recommended for average-risk individuals; indeed, it may be the most cost-effective test if administered once every 10 years as recommended. For those with greater-than-average risk, colonoscopy is mandatory both for initial screening and for follow-up. Several good studies have endeavored to establish reliable accuracy

statistics for colonoscopy. Studies pairing back-to-back colonoscopies have demonstrated a 15% polyp miss rate.[53] In the National Polyp Study Work Group trial, colonoscopic examination revealed a 20% overall polyp miss rate. Clearly, the gold standard could be improved upon, particularly for polyps smaller than 1.0 cm.

PELVIC FLOOR DISORDERS AND CONSTIPATION

Disorders of the pelvic floor can be classified as primarily colorectal, urologic, or gynecologic. Often, problems requiring the attention of multiple specialists present in a synchronous fashion, a condition known as *complex prolapse*. Rectal prolapse (procidentia), enterocele, rectocele, and functional disorders of the muscles of the pelvic floor (anismus, levator spasm) are among the pelvic floor disorders that surgeons treat. A *functional disorder* is defined by the concurrent presence of normal anatomy and abnormal function. Surgeons are often consulted concerning functional disorders of the large bowel or pelvic floor. These problems do not usually require operative intervention; in fact, the surgical literature is replete with examples of failed operations to correct these problems. However, the signs and symptoms of these disorders mimic surgical diseases and require proper recognition and treatment. Although chronic constipation is often considered an example of a functional problem, surgery is a consideration in a select number of patients who fail medical management. The surgical evaluation and management of these disorders is discussed in this section.

Testing and Evaluation
Anorectal Physiology Laboratory
Anorectal physiology testing refers to the systematic evaluation of anal canal resting and squeeze pressures, anal reflexes, pudendal nerve conduction velocities, and electromyogram (EMG) muscle fiber recruitment. Measurement of anal canal pressures (manometry) involves the use of water-filled balloons attached to catheters and transducers placed in the anal canal. The measurement of resting and squeeze pressures at various points in the anal canal reflects the strength, tone, and function of the internal and external sphincter. Normal resting and squeeze values are 40 to 80 mm Hg. Resting pressure reflects the function of the internal sphincter, whereas squeeze pressure measures external sphincter (voluntary muscle) contributions. Measurement of anal canal pressures is useful in the evaluation of conditions ranging from incontinence to obstructive defecation. *EMG recruitment* refers to the motor unit potential of the puborectalis muscle and is compared for rest, squeeze, and push (simulated defecation). An increase in the recruitment of fibers during straining is pathognomonic for the syndrome of paradoxic puborectalis, or inappropriate puborectalis contraction. Pudendal nerve terminal motor latency (PNTML) times are measured with a special transducer attached to a glovelike apparatus designed to be worn on the finger and hand. A digital rectal exam is

required with application of the finger electrode to the right and left levator ani complex. Values between 1.8 and 2.2 msec are normal. Prolonged values are seen in traumatic injuries of the vagina or anal canal (obstetric in etiology), sacral nerve root damage, or in chronic diseases such as diabetes.

Defecography

Defecography is an extremely useful modality for determining the precise nature of various pelvic floor abnormalities. Barium paste is placed in both the vagina and the rectum after the patient ingests water-soluble contrast to opacify the small bowel. As the patient evacuates the rectal barium paste, abnormalities occurring during the act of defecation can be recorded with fluoroscopic videotaping. A vast amount of both functional and anatomic information can be gathered from this test. The presence of multiple anatomic abnormalities such as rectocele, enterocele, and vaginal vault prolapse can be efficiently evaluated. Functional problems such as paradoxical puborectalis syndrome have very characteristic defecography patterns and can be evaluated in this way. Many contributing anatomic problems can be readily identified.

Rectal Prolapse (Procidentia)

Etiology and Symptoms

Most information regarding how patients develop rectal prolapse is based on observation of the clinical characteristics of those suffering from the problem. The condition was documented in the Hippocratic Corpus, and since then, descriptions of both etiologies and rectifying procedures have been numerous. However, two competing theories of rectal prolapse did evolve. Alexis Moschcowitz proposed in 1912 that a rectal prolapse was caused by a sliding herniation of the pouch of Douglas through the pelvic floor fascia into the anterior aspect of the rectum. His theory was based on the fact that the pelvic floor of prolapse patients is mobile and unsupported and the observation that other adjacent structures can occasionally be seen alongside the rectal component of the prolapse. With the advent of defecography in 1968, however, Broden and Snellman were able to show convincingly that procidentia is basically a full-thickness rectal intussusception starting about 3 inches above the dentate line and extending beyond the anal verge. Both explanations take into consideration the weakness of the pelvic floor in rectal prolapse cases, the concept of herniation, and the observation that there are abnormal anatomic features that characterize this condition.

Women aged 50 years and older are six times as likely as men to present with rectal prolapse. The peak age of incidence is the seventh decade in women, whereas the relatively few men afflicted with the syndrome may develop prolapse at the age of 40 years or less. One striking characteristic of young male patients is their tendency to have psychiatric disorders, and many are institutionalized. Young male patients with procidentia also tend to take constipating medications and report significant symptoms related to bowel function.

Anatomy and Pathophysiology of Prolapse

Patients with prolapse are frequently found to have specific anatomic characteristics. Diastasis of the levator ani, an abnormally deep cul-de-sac, a redundant sigmoid colon, a patulous anal sphincter, and loss of the rectal sacral attachments are commonly described.

Large case reviews aimed at elucidating other predisposing factors support several observations. Chronic or lifelong constipation with a component of straining is present in more than 50% of patients. Fifteen percent experience diarrhea. Contrary to the common assumption that rectal prolapse is a consequence of multiparity, 35% of patients with rectal prolapse are nulliparous. Once a prolapse is apparent, fecal incontinence becomes a predominant symptomatic feature, occurring in 50% to 75% of cases. Proximal bilateral pudendal neuropathy is present in incontinent prolapse patients and is responsible for denervation atrophy of the external sphincter musculature. This finding is absent in normal controls. It is speculated that pudendal nerve damage is responsible for pelvic floor and anal sphincter weakening and may be the underlying cause of a spectrum of pelvic floor disorders. Pudendal nerve damage can result from direct trauma (obstetric injury), chronic diseases such as diabetes, and neoplastic processes causing sacral nerve root damage.

Symptoms of prolapse progress as the prolapse develops. Often, the prolapse initially comes down with defecation or straining, only to spontaneously reduce afterward. Patients describe a mass or large lump that they may have to push back in after defecation (Fig. 50-64). The presenting complaint may be the concurrent

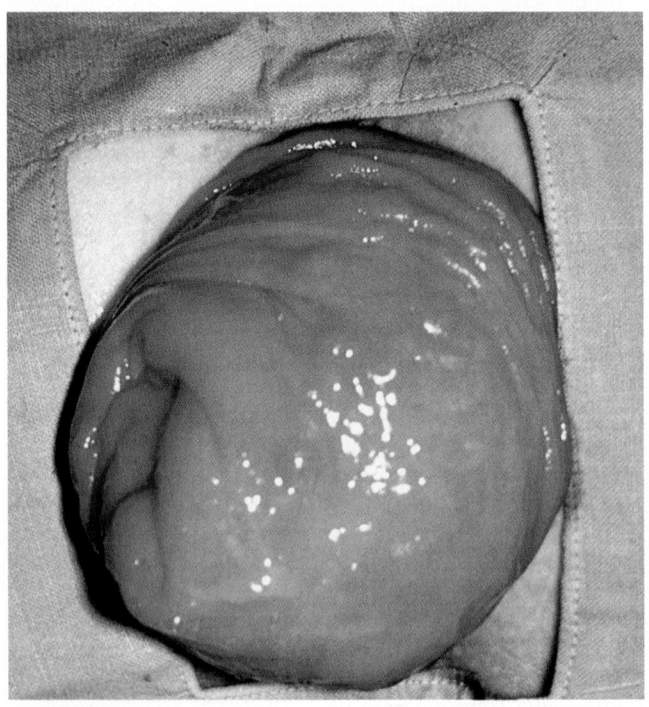

Figure 50-64 Procidentia, or rectal prolapse. The entire rectum has protruded through the anal canal.

fecal incontinence that results from the prolapse, or a sensation of chronic moisture and mucous drainage in the perineal area. Minimal or spontaneously reducible prolapses may progress to chronically prolapsed rectum requiring digital reduction. Chronically prolapsed rectal mucosa may become thickened or ulcerated and cause significant bleeding. Occasionally, the presentation of rectal prolapse can be dramatic when the prolapsed segment becomes incarcerated below the level of the anal sphincter. Emergent operative therapy is indicated in this situation.

Differential Diagnosis and Investigation

A common pitfall in the diagnosis of rectal prolapse is the potential for confusion with prolapsed incarcerated internal hemorrhoids. These conditions may be distinguished by close inspection of the direction of the prolapsed tissue folds. In the case of rectal prolapse, the folds are always concentric, whereas hemorrhoidal tissue develops radial invaginations defining the hemorrhoidal cushions. Prolapsed, incarcerated hemorrhoids produce extreme pain and can be accompanied by fever and urinary retention. Unless incarcerated, rectal prolapse is easily reducible and painless.

Before operative intervention, a careful history, physical examination, and colonoscopy should be performed. Thirty-five percent of patients with rectal prolapse complain of urinary incontinence, and another 15% have a significant vaginal vault prolapse. These symptoms will require evaluation and potential multidisciplinary surgical intervention.

If the diagnosis is suspected from the history, but not detected on physical exam, confirmation can be obtained by asking the patient to produce the prolapse by straining while on a toilet. Inspection of the perineum with the patient in the sitting or squatting position is helpful for this purpose. In the event that the prolapse is still elusive, defecography, a technique described in the section Testing and Evaluation, may reveal the problem.

Although uncommon, a neoplasm may form the lead point for a rectal intussusception. For this reason, and because this age group has the highest incidence of colorectal neoplasia, colonoscopy or barium enema should precede an operation. A significant finding on colonoscopic inspection may change the operative approach.

Anal manometry and pudendal nerve terminal motor latencies can be ordered preoperatively to further evaluate symptoms of incontinence. However, rarely do these test results change the operative strategy. A finding of increased nerve conduction periods (nerve damage) may have postoperative prognostic significance for continence, although more studies are required to confirm this. Those patients with evidence of nerve damage may have a higher rate of incontinence after surgical correction of the prolapse. Decreased anal squeeze or resting pressures are expected with this condition and may predate the actual development of the prolapse. Routine manometric studies for obvious prolapse are usually not done.

Operative Repair

The number of procedures described in the literature both historically and in recent times is breathtaking. More than 50 types of repair have been documented—most of historical interest only. Approaches have generally included anal encirclement, mucosal resection, perineal proctosigmoidectomy, anterior resection with or without rectopexy, rectopexy alone, and a host of procedures involving the use of synthetic mesh affixed to the presacral fascia. The apparent enthusiasm and ingenuity of surgeons in their quest to define the ideal prolapse operation only serves to highlight its elusiveness. Two predominant approaches, abdominal and perineal, are considered in the operative repair of rectal prolapse. The surgical approach is dictated by the comorbidities of the patient, the surgeon's preference and experience, and the patient's age. It is generally believed that the perineal approach results in less perioperative morbidity and pain and a reduced length of hospital stay. These advantages have, until recently, been considered to be offset by a higher recurrence rate. Recent data are unclear on this point, however, and a properly executed perineal operation may yield the same good long-term results as abdominal procedures. This point will be clarified by ongoing long-term studies. The advent of laparoscopic options may also provide advantages, but for now, recurrence data are scant.

The Ripstein repair has many advocates and involves placement of a prosthetic mesh around the mobilized rectum with attachment of the mesh to the presacral fascia below the sacral promontory. Recurrence rates for this procedure range from 2.3% to 5%. The bowel is mechanically prepared for this procedure with a polyethylene glycol or sodium phosphate solution. The procedure involves mobilizing the rectum on both sides posteriorly down to the coccyx. Ripstein described division of the upper portion of the lateral rectal ligaments, but others advocate leaving them wholly intact because the rates of postoperative constipation are fully 50% greater in patients with divided lateral stalks. After mobilization of the rectum, a 5-cm band of rectangular mesh is placed around its anterior aspect at the level of the peritoneal reflection, and both sides of the mesh are sutured with nonabsorbable suture to the presacral fascia, about 1 cm from the midline. Sutures are used to secure the mesh to the rectum anteriorly, and the rectum is pulled upward and posteriorly. Various materials have been recommended to secure the rectum, including autologous fascia lata, synthetic nonabsorbable products such as Marlex (Davol, Inc. subsidiary of C. R. Bard, Inc. Cranston, RI), Teflon (E. I. duPont de Nemours & Co., Wilmington, DE), and absorbable prosthetics such as polyglycolic acid. The recurrence rates for all these materials are less than 10%, although follow-up times and evaluation criteria between studies have varied, and strict comparisons cannot be made. Complications include large bowel obstruction, erosion of the mesh through the bowel, ureteric injury or fibrosis, small bowel obstruction, rectovaginal fistula, and fecal impaction. Postoperative morbidity rates are 20%, but most of these complications are minor. Although mesh rectopexy results in significant

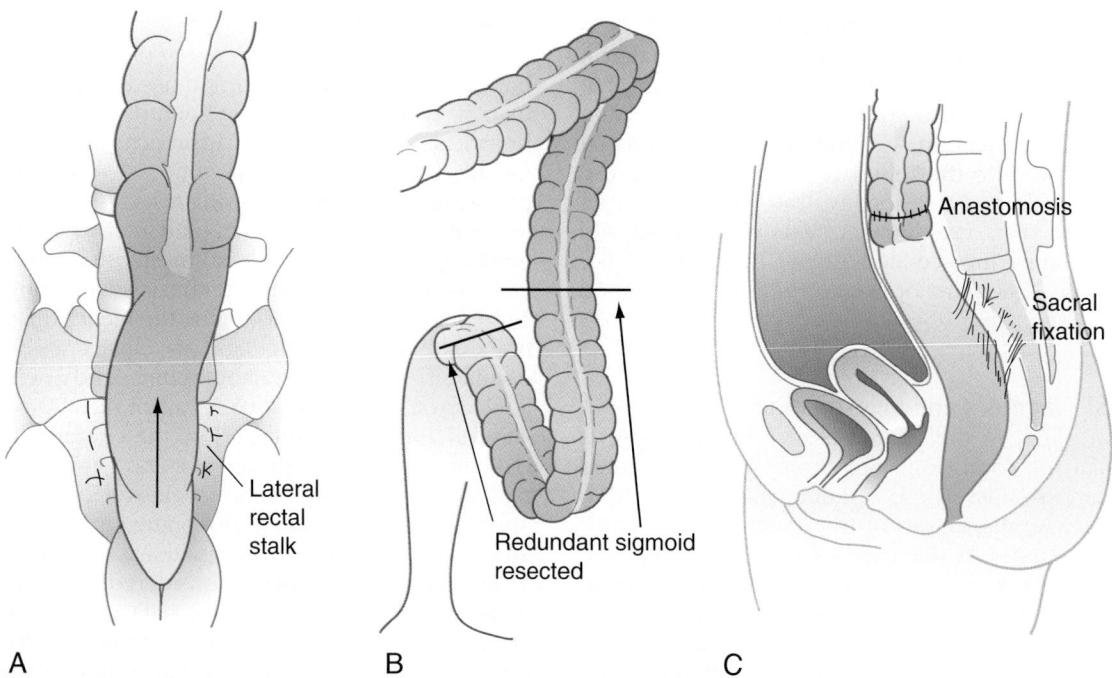

Figure 50-65 Anterior resection with rectopexy, or the Frykman-Goldberg procedure, for rectal prolapse. **A,** After full mobilization by sharp dissection, the tissues lateral to the rectal wall are swept away laterally. **B,** Resection of the redundant sigmoid colon. **C,** Anastomosis is completed, and rectopexy sutures are placed. (From Gordon PL, Nivatvongs S [eds]: Principles and Practice of Surgery for the Colon, Rectum, and Anus, 2nd ed. St Louis, Quality Medical Publishing, 1999.)

improvement in fecal incontinence (50%), no rectal prolapse operation should be advocated as a procedure to restore continence; and patients, especially those with prolapse for more than 2 years, should be warned of the possibility that incontinence could persist.

A significant complication of this operation is the incidence of new-onset or worsened constipation. Fifteen percent of patients experience constipation for the first time after Ripstein rectopexy, and at least 50% of those who are constipated preoperatively are made worse. Although some of these difficulties are attributed to complications of the procedure such as mesh stricture, obstruction at the level of the repair, or rectal dysfunction following lateral stalk division, a subset of patients will be found to have slow-transit constipation characterizing a global motility disorder. Some authors advocate routine preoperative transit studies to select these patients out, but usually a good bowel habit history will suffice. The etiology of any severe, unremitting postoperative defecation or obstruction problem should be investigated with a barium enema and perhaps with a small bowel study. Strictures, obstructions, adhesions, and fistulas may be identified by the radiograph.

Fiber, fluids, and stool softeners are useful in the management of functional constipation following rectal prolapse repairs of any type. Occasionally, mild laxatives such as milk of magnesia, magnesium citrate, or polyethylene glycol–based therapies may be necessary for short periods. Newer treatments for constipation involve oral administration of 5-HT$_4$ receptor agonists (tegaserod

maleate) and may prove invaluable in the short-term treatment of this problem.

The Wells procedure is an alternative mesh technique that reduces the incidence of rectal obstruction by eliminating the anterior placement of the mesh. The mesh is affixed to the posterior aspect of the rectal fascia propria and then to the presacral fascia as previously described. The Ivalon (polyvinyl alcohol) sponge is a method that at one point was popular among European surgeons, but has since fallen out of favor. The sponge is placed posteriorly in the deep pelvis in a manner similar to the Wells technique. In fact, Wells initially described this procedure. Although postoperative recurrence rate results have been as good as those involving synthetic nonabsorbable mesh, and reported evacuation disorders have been low, a disturbing feature of the Ivalon sponge is a high rate of pelvic abscess necessitating sponge removal. Although polyvinyl alcohol is a sarcoma-producing carcinogen in rats, this effect has not been demonstrated in humans.

Resection rectopexy is a technique first described by Frykman and Goldberg in 1969 and popularized in the United States in the past 30 years (Fig. 50-65). Lack of artificial mesh, ease of operation, and reduction of redundant sigmoid colon are the principle attractions of the procedure. Recurrence rates are low, ranging from 2% to 5%, and major complication rates range from 0% to 20% and relate either to obstruction or anastomotic leak. Basically, the sigmoid colon and rectum are mobilized to the level of the levators. The lateral ligaments are divided, elevated from the deep pelvis, and sutured to the presacral fascia. The mesentery of the sigmoid colon is then divided, with preservation of the inferior mesenteric artery, and a tension-free anastomosis is created. A revised version of this procedure involves preservation of the lateral stalks and unilateral fastening of the rectal mesentery to the sacrum at the level of the sacral promontory. Sigmoid resection is a unique and controversial feature of this procedure. It appears to reduce constipation by 50% in those who complain preoperatively of this symptom in some studies. Others have argued that sigmoidectomy is an inadequate operation for a chronic motility problem that affects the entire bowel and that those patients should be formally evaluated preoperatively and subtotal colectomy recommended if colonic inertia is detected. Interestingly, in patients who complain of incontinence before surgery, this symptom consistently improves in about 35%, even with the sigmoid resection. A variant of this procedure involves forgoing the sigmoid resection in those who report no history of constipation and whose predominant complaint is fecal incontinence.

Perineal proctosigmoidectomy was first introduced by Mikulicz in 1899 and remained the favored treatment for prolapse in Europe for many years. Miles advocated this procedure in the United Kingdom, and it was promoted in the United States by Altemeier at the University of Cincinnati. As the abdominal approaches gained favor, principally because of the reduced recurrence rates, the perineal approach was increasingly reserved only for those with the highest operative risk. However, renewed interest in the technique has accompanied recent studies showing reduced recurrence rates, and a number of surgeons feel that strong consideration should be given to this technique when repairing prolapse in young men who have an increased risk for autonomic nerve injury resulting in impotence.

The Altemeier procedure combines a perineal proctosigmoidectomy with an anterior levatoroplasty (Fig. 50-66). The latter procedure is performed to correct the levator diastasis commonly associated with this condition. Theoretically, restoration of fecal continence is enhanced by this additional maneuver. As always, the large bowel is mechanically cleansed. The patient is placed in the prone jackknife position, and a Foley catheter is placed. The rectal mucosa is serially grasped with Babcock or Allis clamps until a full-thickness prolapse is demonstrated. A full-thickness circumferential incision is made 1.5 cm proximal to the dentate line. The low peritoneal reflection can usually be incised anteriorly and the peritoneal cavity entered. The mesentery of the rectum and sigmoid colon is sequentially clamped and tied until no redundant bowel remains. The colon is transected at this point, and an anastomosis is fashioned between the colon and the anal canal with either sutures or staples.

Patients undergoing perineal proctosigmoidectomy are general older and with significantly more comorbidities than those who are considered for abdominal repair. Complication rates are less than 10%, and recurrence rates have been reported as high as 16%, although, as mentioned, recent series demonstrate significantly lower recurrence rates. Complications include bleeding from the staple or suture line, pelvic abscess, and rarely dehiscence of the suture line, with perineal evisceration. Lack of an abdominal incision, reduced pain, and reduced length of hospitalization make this procedure an attractive option.

Anal encirclement is one of the oldest surgical techniques for rectal prolapse described. Thiersch described silver wire anal encirclement in 1891. Since then, it has been tried with a wide variety of materials, including stainless steel wire, nonabsorbable mesh, small Silastic bands, nylon suture, and polypropylene. This technique is reserved by most surgeons for patients of the highest surgical risk because it can be done under local anesthesia. With the patient in the prone jackknife or lithotomy position, the anal area is sterilely prepped and draped. Two small lateral incisions are made, and the wire or suture is introduced with a curved needle into one and brought out the other. This is repeated, and a knot is tied and buried laterally. The orifice should be snug but should easily admit an index finger. Anal encirclement does not correct the fecal incontinence associated with prolapse, and the recurrence rate is high (>30%). In addition, although the mortality rate is 0%, the morbidity rate is high. Erosion of the wire into the sphincter, anovaginal fistula formation, rectal prolapse incarceration, fecal impaction, and infection can occur. Reoperative rates of 7% to 59% are reported in the literature. The safety of current anesthetic techniques and the low morbidity and relative functional success of perineal proctectomy have made anal encirclement, for the most part, a procedure of the past.

Internal Prolapse and Solitary Rectal Ulcer Syndrome

Two areas of controversy related to rectal prolapse involve the treatment of solitary rectal ulcer syndrome (SRUS) and internal intussusception of the rectal mucosa. Although identified as an ulcer, the gross pathology of SRUS can range from a typical crater-like ulcer with a fibrinous central depression to a polypoid lesion. It is always located on the anterior aspect of the rectum 4 to 12 cm from the anal verge and is thought to correspond to the location of the puborectalis "sling." It is frequently, although not exclusively, associated with internal intussusception or full-thickness rectal prolapse. Patients are typically young and female, however, with an average age of 25 years and a history of straining and difficult evacuation.

The rectal ulcer is usually found on proctoscopy or flexible sigmoidoscopy and commonly presents with rectal bleeding in the setting of straining or constipation. The etiology of SRUS remains somewhat unclear, but speculation centers on chronic ischemia. The fold with the ulcer is thought to form the lead point of an intussusception into the anal canal. Chronic, repeated straining or prolapse of this lead point produces ischemia, tissue breakdown, and ulceration. Possible digital self-disimpaction may also be a contributing factor. Histology reveals a thick layer of fibrosis obliterating the lamina

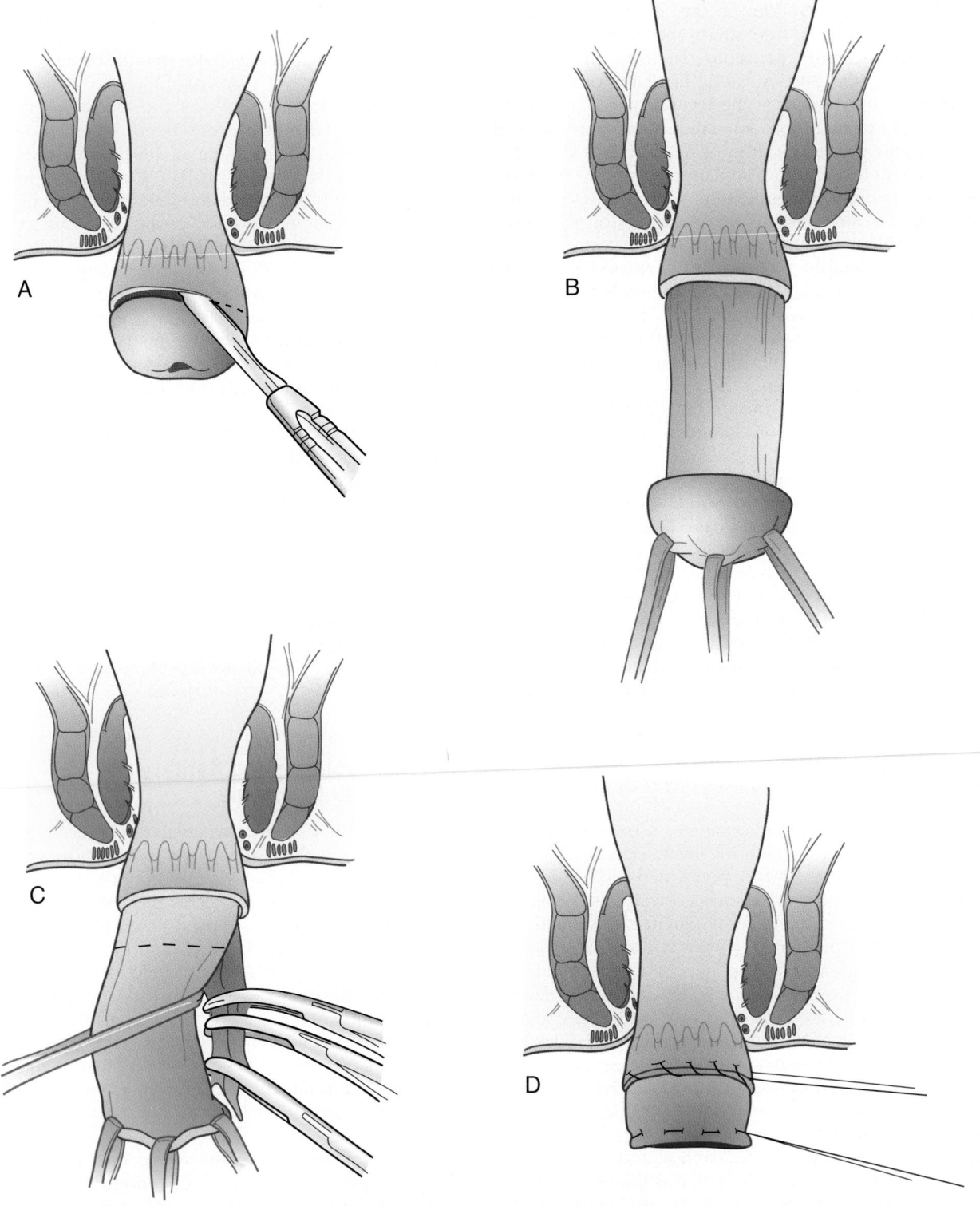

Figure 50-66 Altemeier perineal rectosigmoidectomy. **A,** Circumferential incision of rectum proximal to dentate line. **B,** Delivery of redundant rectum and sigmoid colon. **C,** Ligation of blood supply to rectum. **D,** Placement of purse-string suture on proximal bowels and excision of redundant colon and rectum. Whip stitch placed on rectal stump.

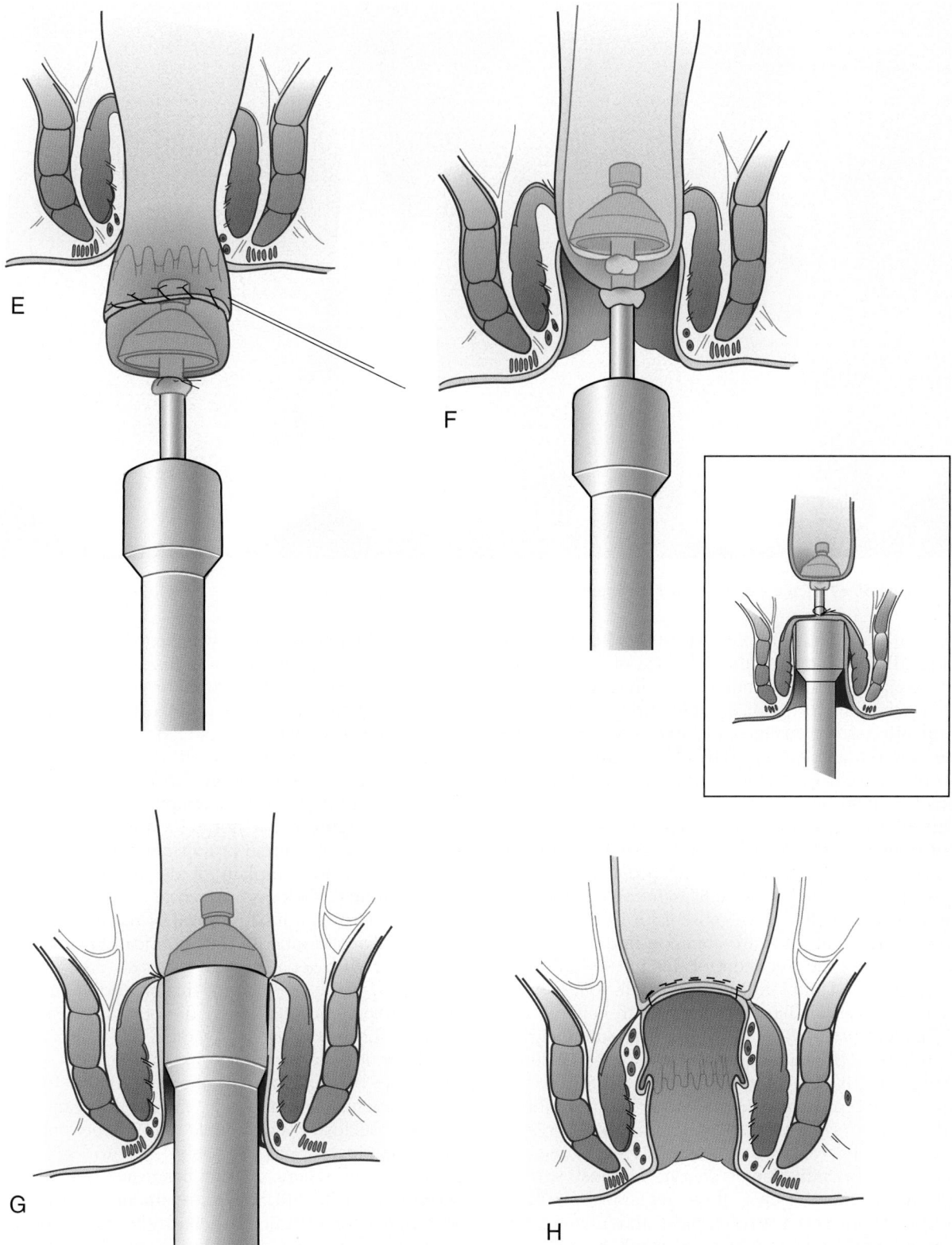

Figure 50-66, cont'd **E**, Proximal purse-string suture secured around central shaft. **F**, Proximal bowel advanced through anus and distal purse-string tied. **G**, Approximation of anvil to cartridge and activation of stapler. **H**, Completed anastomosis. (From Gordon PL, Nivatvongs S [eds]: Principles and Practice of Surgery for the Colon, Rectum, and Anus, 2nd ed. St Louis: Quality Medical Publishing, 1999.)

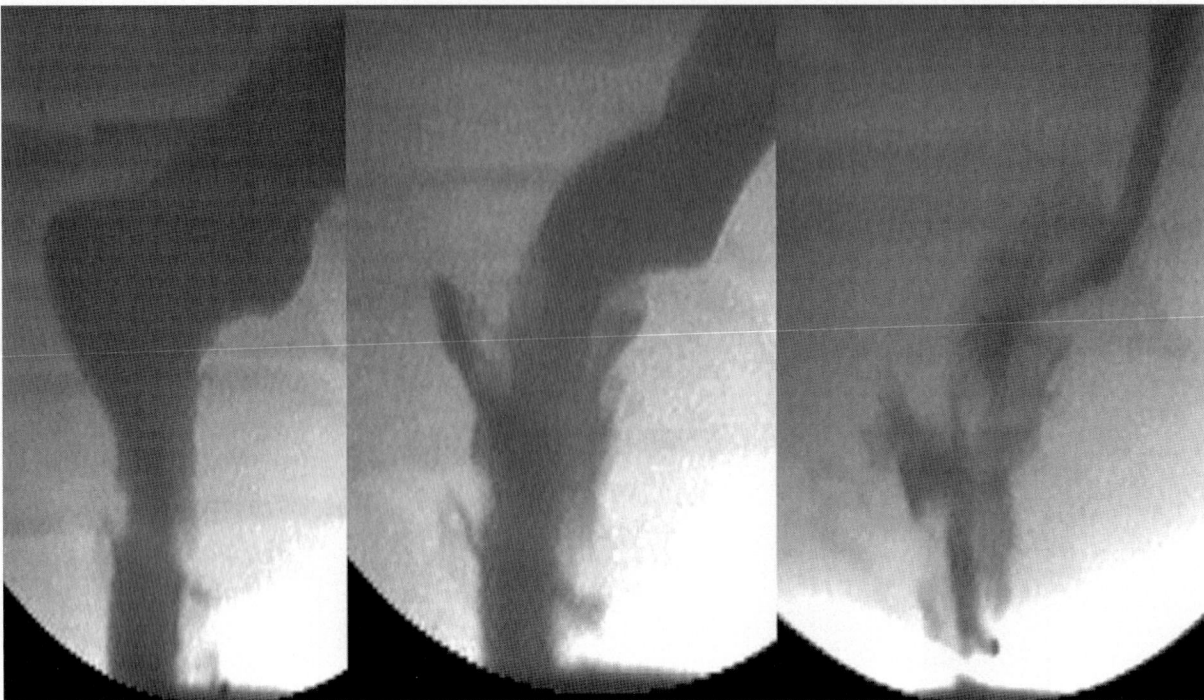

Figure 50-67 Defecography showing progression of internal intussusception.

propria and a central fibrinous exudate. Other common pathologic findings include the presence of mucus-filled glands misplaced in the submucosa and lined with normal colonic epithelium (i.e., colitis cystica profunda). Differentiating SRUS from malignancy, infection, or Crohn's disease is important, but not difficult. The anterior location in the context of classic symptoms and pathologic findings is conclusive.

Diagnostic evaluation by defecography is the radiologic procedure of choice and usually reveals the underlying disorder. Full-thickness rectal prolapse, internal prolapse, paradoxical puborectalis syndrome (failure of relaxation of the pelvic floor musculature on straining) and thickened rectal folds are common findings.

Data regarding the treatment of this unusual disorder are retrospective, and studies are small, but several common observations have been made. In general, one third of patients with SRUS also suffer from full-thickness rectal prolapse. Abdominal prolapse repairs have resulted in a cure rate of 80% in patients with SRUS and full-thickness rectal prolapse. In the same study, patients treated with the same procedure for mucosal prolapse and SRUS faired far worse—only 25% of patients responded to operative intervention. In most studies, dietary management, pelvic floor retraining (biofeedback), and short-term use of topical anti-inflammatory medications containing mesalamine result in remission for those with either internal prolapse or pelvic muscle dysfunction. Prompt diagnosis of the underlying problem and appropriate treatment can be difficult but are the keys to cure. Local excision usually results in a larger, nonhealing wound and has no role in management. Rarely, symptoms of severe bleeding, pain, and spasm may require a temporary diverting sigmoid colostomy.[54]

Internal intussusception was first described in the late 1960s when defecography was first developed and came into widespread use. The condition is also called *internal* or *hidden prolapse* and is confined to the rectal mucosa and submucosa, which separates from the muscularis mucosae layer and slides down the anal canal (Fig. 50-67). Internal intussusception can be identified in a significant proportion of the asymptomatic population and appears to represent a normal variant. However, there are advocates of internal prolapse repair when it is found in patients who complain of dysfunctional defecation. The transanal Delorme mucosal resection procedure involves circumferential removal of redundant anal canal and distal rectal mucosa and imbrication of the muscularis layer with serial vertical sutures. Although satisfactory results were reported for this procedure in the 1990s, recent experience has been discouraging, and enthusiasm for the procedure has waned.

Abdominal repairs such as the Ripstein procedure have also been advocated as an alternative for symptomatic patients. Unfortunately, the results of these studies are not conclusive. Of patients who underwent repair by an abdominal approach, only 24% to 38% reported improvement, whereas a significant number experienced worsening. Like SRUS, the treatment of patients with incomplete or obstructed defecation should be initially evaluated with defecography. Data do not currently support operative intervention for these disorders when internal intussusception alone is present.[55]

Rectocele

A rectocele is an abnormal sac-like projection of the anterior rectum that extends from the distal rectum to the

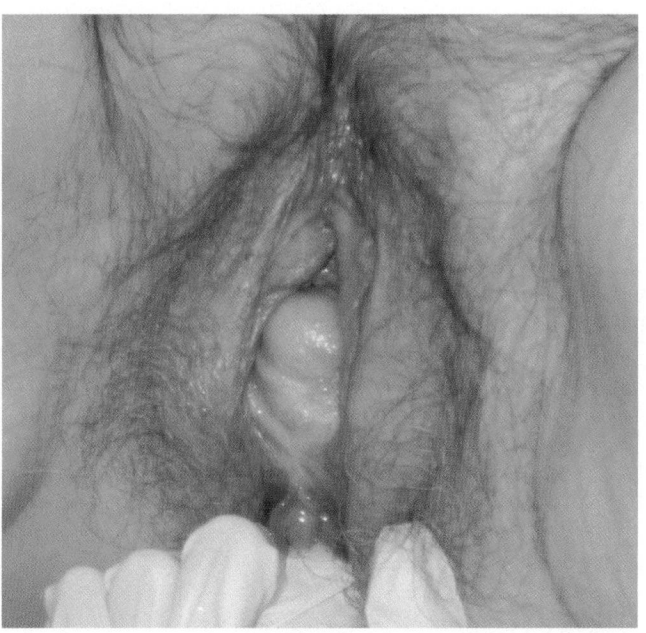

Figure 50-68 Digital anorectal examination demonstrating anterior rectocele protruding from the vaginal introitus.

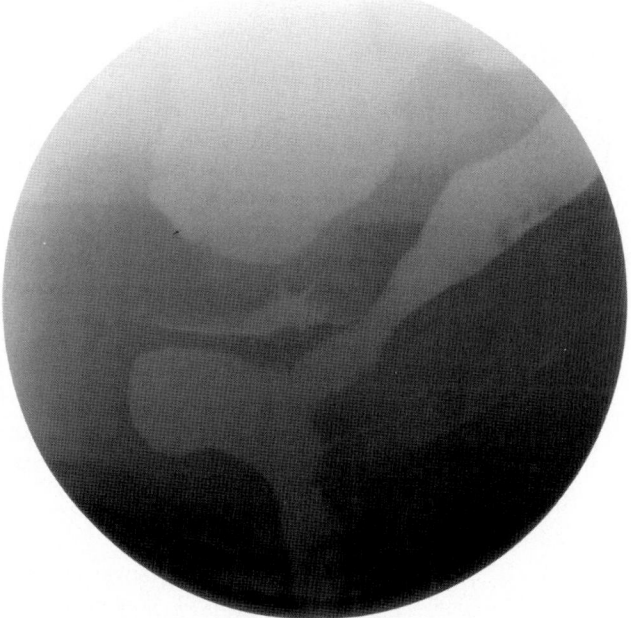

Figure 50-69 Triple-contrast radiograph demonstrates large anterior rectocele. Contrast material is also in the vagina and small intestine.

distal anal canal. It usually begins just above the sphincter complex (Figs. 50-68 and 50-69). The etiology of rectoceles is multifactorial. Stretching of the endopelvic fascia from antecedent pelvic floor injury, followed by chronic increased intra-abdominal pressure, causes an anterior full-thickness herniation of the rectum into the vagina. Rectal pressures are higher than those in the vagina; therefore, pressure tends to push the rectum anteriorly and stretch and shift the rectovaginal septum as well. The major symptom of rectocele is *stool trapping,* a form of obstructed defecation. Women commonly describe requiring vaginal pressure to reduce the bulge, effectively stenting the anterior rectum and enabling defecation.

Criteria for operative intervention include symptomatic stool trapping requiring digital evacuation or vaginal support and large protruding rectoceles that push vaginal mucosa beyond the introitus producing dryness, ulceration, and discomfort. Although small rectoceles are common, it is rare that a rectocele smaller than 2 cm is symptomatic.

There are two major operative approaches to rectoceles: transanal and transvaginal. Although the transvaginal approach has been criticized by surgeons because the repair is done on the low-pressure side of the rectovaginal septum, it does have certain distinct advantages. The bowel is fully prepped, and the patient is placed in the lithotomy position. After the submucosal injection of lidocaine with 1% epinephrine, a swath of vagina is excised starting at the vaginal introitus and carried to the apex of the vagina. The size of this segment is determined by the depth of the rectocele. The goal is to excise a full-thickness segment of vagina, dissect out and reduce an enterocele if one is found in the rectovaginal septum, and then obliterate the deep cul-de-sac by suturing the

cut edges of vagina closed and allowing the space to contract by fibrosis.

Alternatively, several approaches for the transanal correction of rectocele have been described. This technique is probably best described by Sullivan, who expects 80% of patients to have good to excellent results. An incision is made longitudinally in the rectum over the bulge above the sphincters. The incision's length varies with the size of the rectocele. The underlying vagina is exposed and imbricated to obliterate the sac, and the rectum is separately imbricated and closed over that with absorbable sutures. Unfortunately, direct comparisons in the literature between these techniques are absent. However, the largely unsubstantiated argument is made by surgeons that a repair based in the high pressure, or rectal side, of the bulge may reduce recurrence. No matter the technique, patient selection and follow-up are crucial. In one study, only 54% of patients who underwent rectocele repair obtained relief from their symptoms of obstructive defecation. Paradoxical puborectalis syndrome was not ruled out and was responsible for continued problems. Postoperative biofeedback therapy is appropriate in these cases. Defecography evaluation is helpful to distinguish these problems before surgery.

Constipation

Constipation is a symptom, and it is often used by patients to describe different problems. It occurs frequently in older populations; in one survey, 50% of women and 30% of men older than 65 years were affected. Although functional constipation appears to occur most often in elderly patients, a small subset of patients present at a young age with severe unremitting symptoms. These

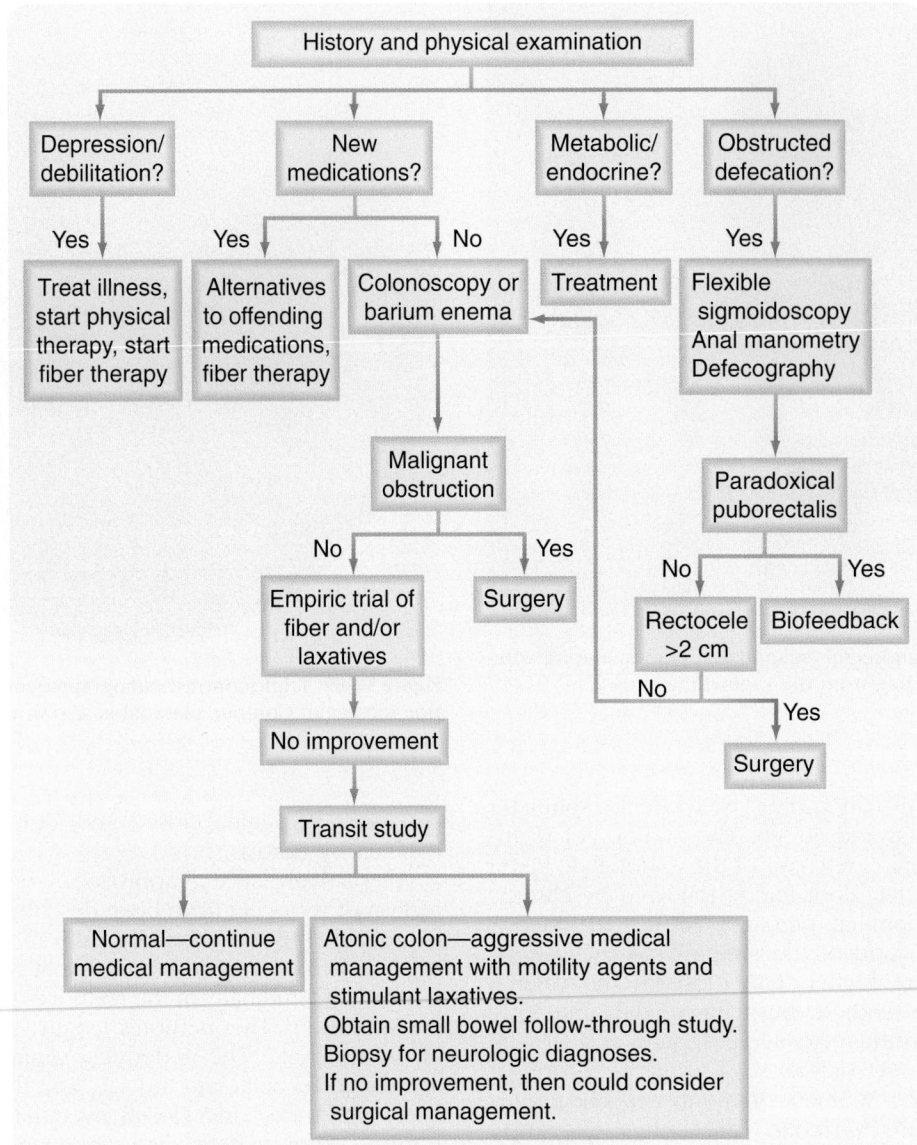

Figure 50-70 Algorithm for management of patients with constipation.

patients are evaluated differently and are discussed in detail later. Although most individuals describe constipation in terms of reduced stool frequency, up to 25% use the term to indicate straining, excessive pushing, or a feeling of incomplete defecation. Normal stool frequencies range from three times per week to three times per day. The causes of constipation are numerous, but the evaluation of constipation is relatively straightforward, and the indications for surgery are few (Fig. 50-70). The initial evaluation of constipation should elicit information regarding acuteness of symptoms, stool frequency, changes in stool form, presence or absence of blood in the stool, new medications, and any newly diagnosed illnesses. The physical exam should always include a rectal exam and proctoscopy. New-onset constipation can be divided into categories for further diagnostic consideration. These categories are depression or debilita-

tion, new medications, endocrine conditions such as hypothyroidism, and obstructed defecation. For the purposes of this chapter, we will focus on surgically correctable causes, while recognizing that, by far, most constipation is chronic and functional and is rectified simply by the addition of fluid and fiber to the diet.

A patient whose symptoms include straining and incomplete defecation with a normal stool frequency should be evaluated for obstructive defecation. The best way to obtain the most information is through physical exam and defecography. Symptomatic rectoceles are those that fail to empty completely on defecogram. Associated anatomic abnormalities (e.g., vaginal vault prolapse and enterocele) can be concurrently corrected. Anal manometry with EMG recruitment is an invaluable investigatory tool for the patient with normal anatomy and suspected paradoxical puborectalis syndrome. Biofeedback therapy is indicated in these cases. Occasionally, both surgically correctable rectocele and functional defecatory disorders coexist. In this situation, biofeedback is usually initiated, and then rectocele repair is done subsequently.

The primary concern for the physician evaluating new-onset constipation is to rule out large bowel malignancy. A patient who presents with complaints of an acute change in bowel habits should be evaluated by colonoscopy in the absence of obvious etiologies such as narcotic usage. Suspect medications should be immediately stopped, and re-evaluation should take place shortly thereafter. No improvement or a guaiac-positive stool should lead to colonoscopic exam. Barium enema is acceptable as well, but flexible sigmoidoscopy, even combined with stool guaiac testing, fails to detect 25% of right-sided malignancies.[50] A normal colonoscopic examination is reassuring and should lead to trials of dietary therapy. Fluid intake should be increased to 2 L/day at minimum, and fiber therapy should be instituted. Caffeinated beverages should be avoided. There are many other laxative-based strategies for the short-term treatment of functional constipation. Long-term failure to respond to these strategies necessitates further investigation.

Transit Studies

Measurement of colonic transit time is a valuable aid in the establishment of a diagnosis of slow-transit constipation or colonic inertia. Although many different techniques exist to assess colonic transit times, two main goals of testing are to establish whole gut and segmental transit values. A common and simple test has been devised by Martelli to do both. The patient is asked to refrain from the use of laxatives or constipating medications such as iron supplements for three to four days before the test. The patient ingests a capsule containing 20 radiopaque markers, and an abdominal x-ray is obtained on each subsequent day for a total of 7 days or until the markers are expelled. The capsules are quantified in three areas of the colon: right, left, and rectosigmoid. Normal subjects expel 80% of markers within 5 days after ingestion. Slow-transit constipation is diagnosed in patients who fail to meet these criteria.

Slow-Transit Constipation (Colonic Inertia)

It has been estimated that 2% of the population suffers from chronic, unremitting functional constipation. Most patients are female, with a mean age of less than 30 years. Most of these individuals will report that they were constipated as children and that the constipation worsened during adolescence and early adulthood. Bowel movement frequency is widely variable and ranges from once or twice a week to once every 2 to 3 weeks. Abdominal pain, bloating, and nausea accompany the constipation and make these patients miserable. Frequent use of over-the-counter laxatives and enemas characterize this group, and concurrent psychiatric conditions such as depression are common. Although malignancy in this group is exceedingly rare, it should be ruled out. A barium enema is a useful initial exam; not only does it screen for large

obvious lesions, but the morphology of the colon and the presence of dilation can also be evaluated. A transit study is the next diagnostic step. Biopsies are usually not indicated unless a strong suspicion of neuropathic constipation is harbored. A loss of the argyrophil plexus with a marked increase in Schwann cells indicating extrinsic damage to the myenteric plexus may be found. This damage is thought to result from chronic laxative abuse. A delay in gastric emptying and small bowel follow-through has been noted in some patients, implying a global motility problem. This motility problem may be responsible for the mixed surgical outcomes reported.

An aggressive bowel regimen is always the first course of action after diagnosis of slow-transit constipation. A combination of laxatives, fiber, and polyethylene glycol–based solutions can be helpful. A new class of laxative approved for short-term use is 5-HT$_4$ receptor agonists. These may prove beneficial and merit investigation.

Surgery for idiopathic colonic inertia is controversial. The most commonly described procedure is subtotal colectomy with ileorectal anastomosis. Traditionally, only patients with symptoms in the setting of megacolon or megarectum were considered for operative intervention. More and more patients with a normal-caliber colon and severe refractory constipation have been referred for surgery. The costs and inconvenience associated with medical therapy for severe chronic constipation are not inconsiderable. Intuitively, surgery may seem like an attractive option. However, the data concerning lasting cure are unclear. In most series that include more than 20 patients and have longer than 2-year follow-up, results range from 33% to 94% success rates (regular defecation without the use of laxatives). The wide range of results is concerning. It has been noted that often the symptoms of nausea, bloating, and abdominal pain can persist and can be accompanied by incapacitating diarrhea. In effect, many patients trade one symptom complex for another. There have been a few small prospective studies exercising strict selection criteria for surgery that includes normal defecography results and diffuse delay on transit study. These patients appear to fair best in follow-up, enjoying a 94% success rate as defined by good or excellent patient satisfaction scores.[56] Subtotal colectomy with ileorectal anastomosis is an option for patients with normal-caliber colonic inertia, but it should not be advocated as a perfect solution. Careful selection criteria applied to motivated, psychologically well-adjusted individuals results in the best long-term surgical results.

Slow-Transit Constipation (Colonic Inertia) With Megacolon

A small but important subset of constipation is neurologic in origin. In contrast to colonic inertia with a normal colon, as a group, 50% of these patients are male. Surgical intervention is usually indicated in these cases because medical therapy eventually fails. Among these entities, Chagas' disease, adult Hirschsprung's disease, and neuronal intestinal dysplasia will be considered. Commonly, all these etiologies present with slow-transit constipation in the presence of a dilated colon. A dilated rectum is a variable finding and is typically absent in Hirschsprung's disease.

Hirschsprung's disease is occasionally diagnosed in adulthood. These patients are typically young men in their 20s with lifelong evacuation complaints. Commonly, in these cases, a short, distal segment of rectum is involved. The remainder of the colon is dilated from chronic distal partial obstruction. Stool is characteristically absent from the distal rectum, similar to the physical finding in children. Barium enema characteristically demonstrates a narrow distal rectum with proximal dilated colon. Anal manometric findings reveal an absent recto-anal inhibitory reflex (RAIR) indicating that the rectum has lost its neurologically mediated ability to relax in response to the presence of a fecal load. Histologic diagnosis is made on biopsy of the distal rectal mucosa at least 3 cm above the dentate line to avoid the normal aganglionic segment in this area. Suction mucosal and superficial punch biopsies are both diagnostic and can be done in the office setting. Acetylcholinesterase staining of the submucosa and lamina propria reveals an increased number of large brown-stained nerve fibers and is considered 99% accurate in establishing the diagnosis. A discussion of surgical interventions for this problem is found in the chapter on pediatric surgery.

Megacolon is the most common complication of intestinal trypanosomiasis. The organism involved is *Trypanosoma cruzi,* a parasite endemic to South America. Nerve damage resulting from trypanosomiasis causes megacolon and megarectum. Fecal impaction and sigmoid volvulus are the most common complications. Subtotal colectomy for this problem results in a residual dyskinetic rectum, therefore, pull-through procedures with excision of the colon and rectum and creation of an ileal reservoir (ileal J pouch or Park's pouch) are preferable.

Neuronal intestinal dysplasia describes two distinct congenital defects of the intestinal mural ganglia. Type A is seen predominantly in children and consists of hypoplasia of the sympathetic innervation. Type B is present in both children and adults and is characterized by dysplasia of the submucosal plexus resulting in weak forward propulsion of stool. Histologically, hyperplasia and giant ganglia with 7 to 10 nerve cells are present. Acetylcholinesterase staining shows a dense plexus of parasympathetic fibers with increased activity. Laxative therapy in these individuals is usually a short-term strategy, and most patients fail treatment. Surgical resection with ileorectal anastomosis is the treatment of choice.

LAPAROSCOPIC COLON RESECTION

The first laparoscopic colon resections were performed in 1991. The experience gained by surgeons performing laparoscopic cholecystectomy provided the impetus to develop the laparoscopic colon resection. Patients undergoing laparoscopic cholecystectomy had smaller incisions, less postoperative pain, shorter hospital stays, and earlier return to work. These benefits were achieved while preserving the time-honored technical aspects of removal of the gallbladder. The goals of laparoscopic colectomy are similar to those of laparoscopic cholecys-

tectomy. The technical requirements and principles of colonic resection cannot be compromised in an effort to avoid the detriment of a standard midline incision. Earlier return to physical activity must be reliably provided. In nearly all studies investigating the implementation of laparoscopic colon resection for various diseases, patients have been discharged 2 to 3 days earlier than patients treated by open colon resection. Laparoscopic colectomy has not been associated with an increased incidence of complications. Data suggest that pulmonary and immune system function is better maintained after laparoscopic operation. Body image satisfaction subsequent to the diminished incision size is well documented. The benefits of laparoscopic colon resection have been found in all age groups, including elderly patients.

The accelerated return of bowel function has facilitated earlier discharge from the hospital. The propulsive movement of intestinal content in the nonfed surgical patient is dependent on the migrating motor complex. The migrating motor complex is inhibited by bowel handling, opiate intake, and catecholamine (stress hormone) levels. It is hypothesized that laparoscopic colon resection provides earlier return of bowel function because there is less handling of the bowel, and the benefit of the smaller incision includes decreased catecholamine release and decreased narcotic requirement.

Virtually all colon and rectal diseases amenable to surgical treatment are amenable to treatment by a laparoscopic approach. Ileocecectomy for Crohn's disease; right, left, and low anterior colon resection for colon polyps and cancer; ileostomy and colostomy creation and closure; sigmoid resection for diverticulitis; and proctocolectomy with ileoanal J pouch formation for ulcerative colitis are all performed regularly at centers with colon and rectal surgeons who have advanced laparoscopic training. The indications for surgery are the same, whether the approach is through a standard incision or by laparoscopic technique. The laparoscopic surgeon essentially performs a proven operation by a technique that reduces the length of the abdominal incision.

There are various nuances of the techniques used by laparoscopic surgeons. Laparoscopic techniques of colon resection invariably involve laparoscopic mobilization of the diseased colonic segments. The postoperative recovery benefit of laparoscopic colon resection is not altered if hand-assisted techniques are employed or if bowel division and anastomosis are performed intracorporeally or extracorporeally.

In the first decade after the development of laparoscopic colectomy, there was a concern that laparoscopic colon resection for cancer might not achieve cure rates established by standard oncologic operations. These concerns seemed especially pertinent given a report from Europe in 1994 of a high rate of port site cancer recurrence. As experience has accumulated, port site recurrence appears equivalent to recurrence of cancer in the incision of patients treated by conventional operation.

If the operation is conducted correctly, proximal and distal resection margins and lymph node harvest are the same, whether a laparoscopic or conventional incision

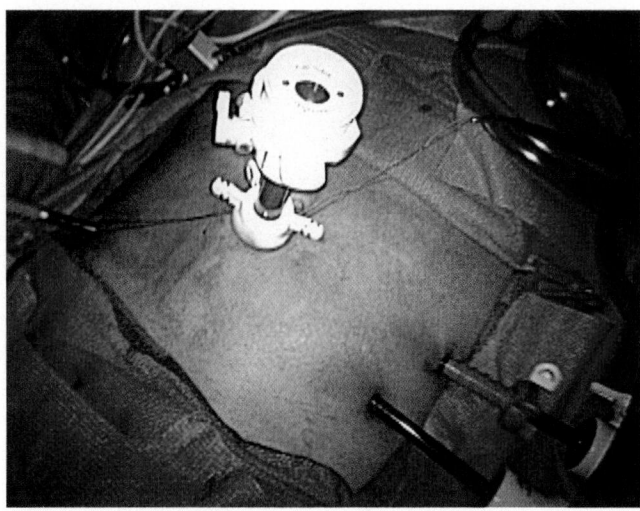

Figure 50-71 Standard port placement.

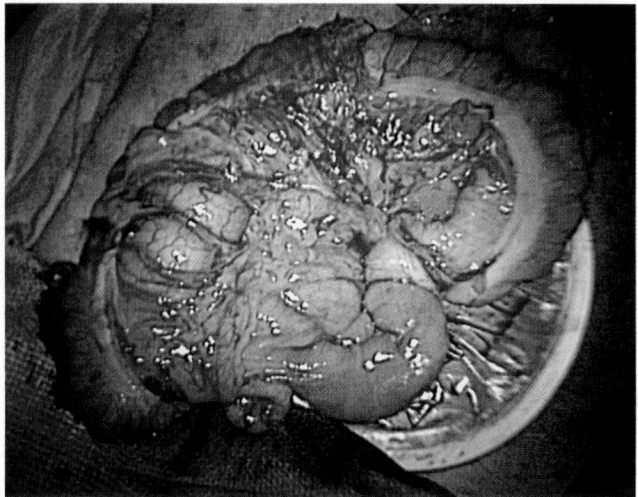

Figure 50-72 This illustrates the right colon, mobilized and delivered through a small midline wound. The right colon is being resected to excise an endoscopically unresectable polyp discovered at colonoscopy. It is valuable to note the ink tattoo that marked the location of the polyp.

approach is used. A landmark multi-institutional prospective randomized trial of patients undergoing curative colon cancer resection was reported in 2004.[57] This study demonstrated noninferiority of laparoscopic colectomy when compared with operation conducted through a conventional midline incision. In the hands of experienced surgeons, laparoscopic colectomy was proved not only safe but also equally efficacious with regard to survival. The study also demonstrated decreased pain medicine requirement and shorter hospital stay of patients in the laparoscopic group.

Surgeons who participated in this trial had an experience of at least 20 prior laparoscopic colon resections and had to submit a video documenting the technical procedure. In an effort to have these results recreated by surgeons throughout the world, surgical societies have suggested that surgeons should have performed at least 20 laparoscopic colon resections for benign disease before the performance of a laparoscopic cancer resection.

Laparoscopic Colon Resection— Technical Notes and Highlights

Equipment

The performance of a laparoscopic colon resection requires instruments that will allow gentle handling of small and large bowel. We use 5-mm atraumatic Babcock graspers. A vessel sealant device permits the efficient division of vascularized structures within the abdomen. Although not commonly required, we have ready access to endoscopic loop ligature devices should vascular pedicles bleed after division.

Positioning and Port Placement

Although there are many reported optimal patient and port positions, individual preferences determine practice. Some important constants exist. Foremost is the development and utilization of a standardized setup and operative routine. Efficiencies develop that are of benefit to the entire operative team if each operation is not performed as if it is the surgeon's first. In general, all ports should be separated by 4 fingerbreadths. Visualization is optimized by the placement of the camera port as far as possible from a hand-assist device. Utilization of a split-leg patient position allows the surgeon to stand between the patient's legs and enhances the ability to reach all quadrants of the abdomen.

Conversion

At times, regardless of surgeon experience, the safe completion of an operation requires the need to make a larger incision. Many reasons for conversion exist, including adhesions from prior surgery, bleeding, obesity, inability to identify key structures (like the ureter), and failure to move an operation to completion. We consider conversion not to be a technical shortcoming, but rather a necessary step to ensure an appropriate operation. Patients whose operations were converted from laparoscopic to open have not experienced adverse short- or long-term outcomes. Our advice is to convert early in an operation to minimize operating time. Part of the learning curve in laparoscopic colectomy is earlier recognition of the need to convert a laparoscopic operation.

Right Colon Resection

Our technique utilizes four ports, with a camera port created through an infraumbilical 10-mm incision. Two 5-mm ports are placed in the left lower quadrant. The first is 2 to 3 fingerbreadths superior and medial to the anterior superior iliac spine. The next is 4 fingerbreadths superior to this. Mobilization begins at the terminal ileum and proceeds to the hepatic flexure. The omentum is then taken off the transverse colon. The hepatic flexure attachments are divided with a tissue sealant device. Once mobilized, we generally create a window around the ileocolic pedicle toward its origin and divide the pedicle intracorporeally. A 3- to 5-cm inferior extension

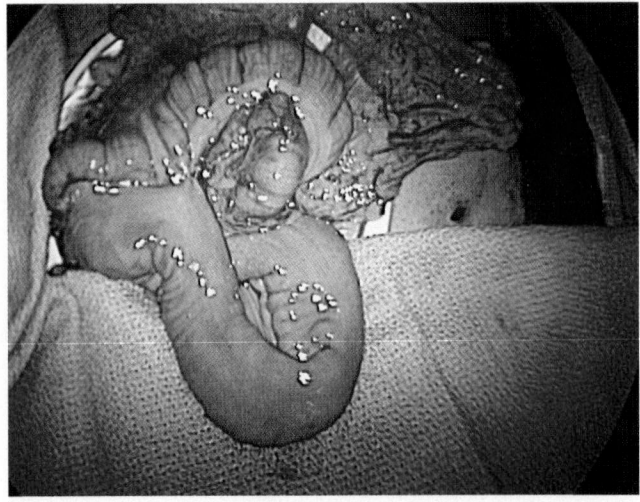

Figure 50-73 This represents a completed right colon resection with ileotransverse colon anastomosis. The exteriorized anastomosis is ready to be returned to the abdomen.

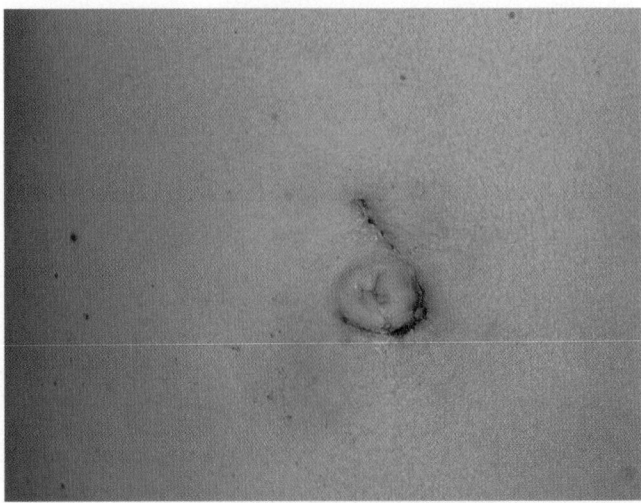

Figure 50-74 This represents the immediate postoperative cosmetic result after total abdominal colectomy.

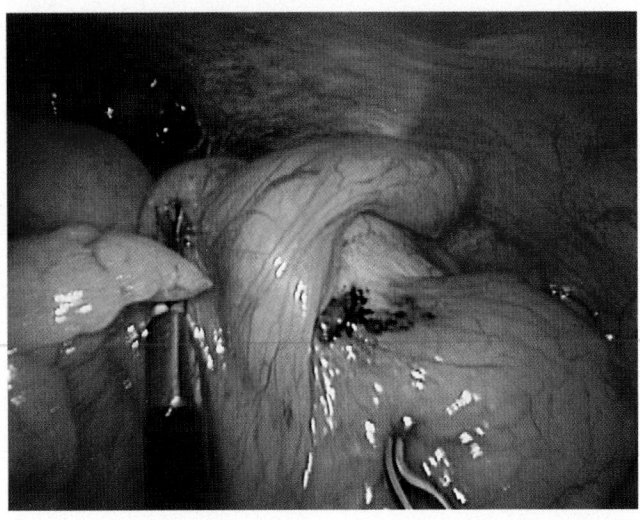

A

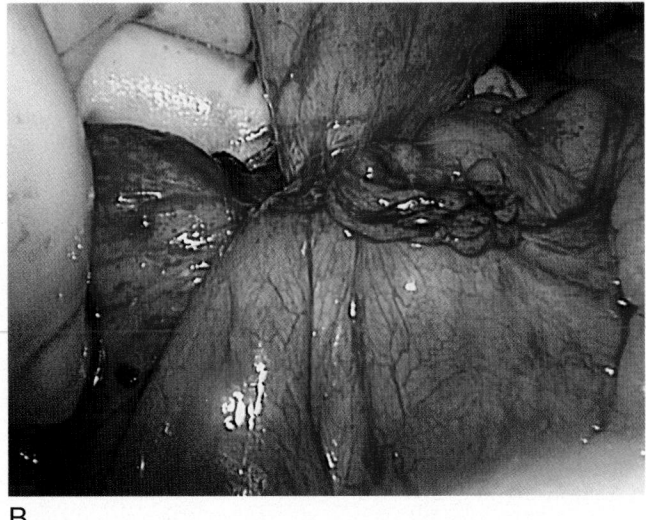

B

Figure 50-75 A, The laparoscopic identification of a colonic "tattoo." The ink on the colon wall corresponds to the endoluminal location of a polyp. **B,** Hand-assisted division of a colovesical fistula.

of the camera insertion site is created and a wound protector placed in the wound. The terminal ileum, right colon, hepatic flexure, and transverse colon are delivered into the wound. Bowel division and stapled anastomosis are performed extracorporeally in standard fashion. The anastomosis is returned to the abdomen.

Figure 50-71 illustrates standard port placement. Figure 50-72 illustrates the mobilized right colon resected to excise an endoscopically unresectable polyp discovered at colonoscopy. It is valuable to note the ink tattoo that marked the location of the polyp. Figure 50-73 represents ileocecal Crohn's disease, mobilized then delivered through a 4-cm wound. Figure 50-74 represents a typical postoperative cosmetic result of a laparoscopic right colon resection.

Hand-Assisted Laparoscopic Colon Resection

Even if a surgeon has the skills and desire to completely mobilize the colon and divide all vasculature intracorporeally, the specimen must be removed. Surgeons and device manufacturers have taken advantage of the need to make an incision of a few centimeters for specimen extraction. Hand-assist devices allow surgeons to place a single hand into a patient's abdomen through this wound while not losing pneumoperitoneum. Such techniques return the sense of touch to the surgeon, facilitating such maneuvers as finger fracture of a diverticular phlegmon off the pelvic sidewall, division of a colovesical fistula, and speeding of the division of vascular structures. Hand-assist devices lower the threshold for surgeons to attempt laparoscopic techniques. Figure 50-75 illustrates the division of a colovesical fistula that formed in response to diverticulitis. Recovery benefits are similar whether hand-assisted laparoscopic techniques are employed or "pure" laparoscopic surgery is performed.

Clearly, many approaches to colectomy exist. Many surgeons perform a medial-to-lateral approach when the vascular pedicle is divided early in the operation. We believe it is important for surgeons to be facile with all mobilization techniques.

Selected References

Gordon PL, Nivatvongs S (eds): Principles and Practice of Surgery for the Colon, Rectum, and Anus, 2nd ed. St Louis: Quality Medical Publishing, Inc, 1999.

This text provides excellent anatomic illustrations and detailed descriptions of diverticular disease and common colorectal disorders.

Corman ML (ed): Colon and Rectal Surgery, 5th ed. Philadelphia: Lippincott Williams & Wilkins, 2004.

Describes colorectal operative procedures in detail with excellent illustrations.

Pemberton JH, Swash M, Henry MM (eds): The Pelvic Floor: Its Function and Disorders. Philadelphia, WB Saunders, 2002.

Excellent in-depth discussion of pelvic floor disorders and colonic motility disorders.

Zinzler KW, Vogelstein B: Lessons from hereditary colorectal Cancer. Cell 87:159-170, 1996.

Excellent and thorough description of the genetics of colorectal cancer.

References

1. Levitt MD, Furne J, Olsson S: The relation of passage of gas and abdominal bloating to colonic gas production. Ann Intern Med 124:422-424, 1996.
2. Vonk RJ, Kalivianakis M, Minich DM, et al: The metabolic importance of unabsorbed dietary lipids in the colon. Scand J Gastroenterol Suppl 222:65-67, 1997.
3. Velazquez OC, Lederer HM, Rombeau JL: Butyrate and the colonocyte: Implications for neoplasia. Dig Dis Sci 41:727-739, 1996.
4. Lewis SJ, Heaton KW: Increasing butyrate concentration in the distal colon by accelerating intestinal transit. Gut 41:245-251, 1997.
5. Medeiros JA, Pontes FA, Mesquita OA: Is colonic electrical activity a similar phenomena to small-bowel electrical activity? Dis Colon Rectum 40:93-99, 1997.
6. Ashraf W, Park F, Lof J, et al: Effects of psyllium therapy on stool characteristics, colon transit and anorectal function in chronic idiopathic constipation. Aliment Pharmacol Ther 9:639-647, 1995.
7. Cohen SM, Wexner SD, Binderow SR, et al: Prospective, randomized, endoscopic-blinded trial comparing precolonoscopy bowel cleansing methods. Dis Colon Rectum 37:689-696, 1994.
8. Frommer D: Cleansing ability and tolerance of three bowel preparations for colonoscopy. Dis Colon Rectum 40:100-104, 1997.
9. Poon CM, Lee DW, Mak SK, et al: Two liters of polyethylene glycol-electrolyte lavage solution versus sodium phosphate as bowel cleansing regimen for colonoscopy: A prospective randomized controlled trial. Endoscopy 34:560-563, 2002.
10. Vanner SJ, MacDonald PH, Paterson WG, et al: A randomized prospective trial comparing oral sodium phosphate with standard polyethylene glycol-based lavage solution (Golytely) in the preparation of patients for colonoscopy. Am J Gastroenterol 85:422-427, 1990.
11. Miettinen RP, Laitinen ST, Makela JT, et al: Bowel preparation with oral polyethylene glycol electrolyte solution vs. no preparation in elective open colorectal surgery: Prospective, randomized study. Dis Colon Rectum 43:669-675; discussion 675-667, 2000.
12. Zmora O, Pikarsky AJ, Wexner SD: Bowel preparation for colorectal surgery. Dis Colon Rectum 44:1537-1549, 2001.
13. Polk HC Jr, Lopez-Mayer JF: Postoperative wound infection: A prospective study of determinant factors and prevention. Surgery 66:97-103, 1969.
14. Gomez-Alonso A, Lozano F, Perez A, et al: Systemic prophylaxis with gentamicin-metronidazole in appendicectomy and colorectal surgery: A prospective controlled clinical study. Int Surg 69:17-20, 1984.
15. Solla JA, Rothenberger DA: Preoperative bowel preparation: A survey of colon and rectal surgeons. Dis Colon Rectum 33:154-159, 1990.
16. Hinchey EJ, Schaal PG, Richards GK: Treatment of perforated diverticular disease of the colon. Adv Surg 12:85-109, 1978.
17. Anaya DA, Flum DR: Risk of emergency colectomy and colostomy in patients with diverticular disease. Arch Surg 140:681-685, 2005.
18. Vignati PV, Welch JP, Cohen JL: Long-term management of diverticulitis in young patients. Dis Colon Rectum 38:627-629, 1995.
19. Chapman JR, Dozois EJ, Wolff BG, et al: Diverticulitis: A progressive disease? Do multiple recurrences predict less favorable outcomes? Ann Surg 243:876-883, 2006.
20. Salem L, Veenstra DL, Sullivan SD, et al: The timing of elective colectomy in diverticulitis: A decision analysis. J Am Coll Surg 199:904-912, 2004.
21. Benn PL, Wolff BG, Ilstrup DM: Level of anastomosis and recurrent colonic diverticulitis. Am J Surg 151:269-271, 1986.
22. Trevisani GT, Hyman NH, Church JM: Neostigmine: Safe and effective treatment for acute colonic pseudo-obstruction. Dis Colon Rectum 43:599-603, 2000.
23. Koutroubakis IE, Vlachonikolis IG, Kouroumalis EA: Role of appendicitis and appendectomy in the pathogenesis of ulcerative colitis: A critical review. Inflamm Bowel Dis 8:277-286, 2002.
24. Ohman U: Colorectal carcinoma in patients with ulcerative colitis. Am J Surg 144:344-349, 1982.
25. Mayer R, Wong WD, Rothenberger DA, et al: Colorectal cancer in inflammatory bowel disease: A continuing problem. Dis Colon Rectum 42:343-347, 1999.
26. Bernstein CN, Shanahan F, Weinstein WM: Are we telling patients the truth about surveillance colonoscopy in ulcerative colitis? Lancet 343:71-74, 1994.
27. Ahmad T, Armuzzi A, Bunce M, et al: The molecular classification of the clinical manifestations of Crohn's disease. Gastroenterology 122:854-866, 2002.
28. Weston LA, Roberts PL, Schoetz DJ Jr, et al: Ileocolic resection for acute presentation of Crohn's disease of the ileum. Dis Colon Rectum 39:841-846, 1996.
29. Camma C, Viscido A, Latella G: Mesalamine in the prevention of clinical and endoscopic post-operative recurrence of Crohn's disease: A meta-analysis. Dig Liver Dis 34:A86, 2002.

30. Ardizzone S, Maconi G, Sampietro GM, et al: Azathioprine and mesalamine for prevention of relapse after conservative surgery for Crohn's disease. Gastroenterology 127:730-740, 2004.

31. American Gastroenterological Association Medical Position Statement: Guidelines on intestinal ischemia. Gastroenterology 118:951-953, 2000.

32. Brandt LJ, Boley SJ: AGA technical review on intestinal ischemia. American Gastrointestinal Association. Gastroenterology 118:954-968, 2000.

33. Jemal A, Siegel R, Ward E, et al: Cancer statistics, 2007. CA Cancer J Clin 57:43-66, 2007.

34. Vogelstein B, Fearon ER, Hamilton SR, et al: Genetic alterations during colorectal-tumor development. N Engl J Med 319:525-532, 1988.

35. Neibergs HL, Hein DW, Spratt JS: Genetic profiling of colon cancer. J Surg Oncol 80:204-213, 2002.

36. Sieber OM, Lipton L, Crabtree M, et al: Multiple colorectal adenomas, classic adenomatous polyposis, and germ-line mutations in MYH. N Engl J Med 348:791-799, 2003.

37. Sampson JR, Jones S, Dolwani S, et al: MutYH (MYH) and colorectal cancer. Biochem Soc Trans 33:679-683, 2005.

38. Calvert PM, Frucht H: The genetics of colorectal cancer. Ann Intern Med 137:603-612, 2002.

39. Haggitt RC, Glotzbach RE, Soffer EE, et al: Prognostic factors in colorectal carcinomas arising in adenomas: Implications for lesions removed by endoscopic polypectomy. Gastroenterology 89:328-336, 1985.

40. Jass JR, Young J, Leggett BA: Evolution of colorectal cancer: Change of pace and change of direction. J Gastroenterol Hepatol 17:17-26, 2002.

41. Steinbach G, Lynch PM, Phillips RK, et al: The effect of celecoxib, a cyclooxygenase-2 inhibitor, in familial adenomatous polyposis. N Engl J Med 342:1946-1952, 2000.

42. Heiskanen I, Jarvinen HJ: Fate of the rectal stump after colectomy and ileorectal anastomosis for familial adenomatous polyposis. Int J Colorectal Dis 12:9-13, 1997.

43. Soravia C, Berk T, McLeod RS, et al: Desmoid disease in patients with familial adenomatous polyposis. Dis Colon Rectum 43:363-369, 2000.

44. Dauphine CE, Tan P, Beart RW Jr, et al: Placement of self-expanding metal stents for acute malignant large-bowel obstruction: A collective review. Ann Surg Oncol 9:574-579, 2002.

45. Greene FL, Page, DL, Fleming ID, et al: AJCC Cancer Staging Manual, 6th ed. New York, Springer-Verlag, 2002.

46. Quirke P, Sebag-Montefiore D, Steele R, et al: Local recurrence after rectal cancer resection is strongly related to the plane of surgical dissection and is further reduced by preoperative short course radiotherapy: Preliminary results of the Medical Research Council (MRC) CR07 trial [abstract]. J Clin Oncol 24(149S):3512, 2006.

47. Steele GD Jr, Herndon JE, Bleday R, et al: Sphincter-sparing treatment for distal rectal adenocarcinoma. Ann Surg Oncol 6:433-441, 1999.

48. Mantyh CR, Hull TL, Fazio VW: Coloplasty in low colorectal anastomosis: Manometric and functional comparison with straight and colonic J-pouch anastomosis. Dis Colon Rectum 44:37-42, 2001.

49. Rex DK, Johnson DA, Lieberman DA, et al: Colorectal cancer prevention 2000: Screening recommendations of the American College of Gastroenterology. Am J Gastroenterol 95:868-877, 2000.

50. Lieberman DA, Weiss DG: One-time screening for colorectal cancer with combined fecal occult-blood testing and examination of the distal colon. N Engl J Med 345:555-560, 2001.

51. Lieberman DA, Weiss DG, Bond JH, et al: Use of colonoscopy to screen asymptomatic adults for colorectal cancer. Veterans Affairs Cooperative Study Group 380. N Engl J Med 343:162-168, 2000.

52. Winawer SJ, Stewart ET, Zauber AG, et al: A comparison of colonoscopy and double-contrast barium enema for surveillance after polypectomy. National Polyp Study Work Group. N Engl J Med 342:1766-1772, 2000.

53. Hixson LJ, Fennerty MB, Sampliner RE, et al: Prospective study of the frequency and size distribution of polyps missed by colonoscopy. J Natl Cancer Inst 82:1769-1772, 1990.

54. Lawler LP, Fleshman JW: Solitary rectal ulcer, rectocele, hemorrhoids and pelvic pain. In Pemberton JH, Swash M, Henry MM (eds): The Pelvic Floor: Its Function and Disorders. Philadelphia, WB Saunders, 2002, pp 358-384.

55. Fleshman JW, Kodner IJ, Fry RD: Internal intussusception of the rectum: a changing perspective. Neth J Surg 41:145-148, 1989.

56. Wexner SD, Daniel N, Jagelman DG: Colectomy for constipation: Physiologic investigation is the key to success. Dis Colon Rectum 34:851-856, 1991.

57. The Clinical Outcomes of Surgical Therapy Study Group: A comparison of laparoscopically assisted and open colectomy for colon cancer. N Engl J Med 350:2050-2059, 2004.

CHAPTER 51

Anus

Heidi Nelson, MD   and   Robert R. Cima, MD

Disorders of the Anal Canal
Pelvic Floor Disorders
Common Benign Anal Disorders
Less Common Benign Anal Disorders
Neoplastic Disorders

DISORDERS OF THE ANAL CANAL

The anal canal can be the site of rare lesions. Most conditions arising in this area, however, are common and benign but may be incapacitating and interfere with the daily quality of life of patients. Moreover, these disorders are often misdiagnosed or maltreated, leading at times to disastrous consequences. A better knowledge of the functional anatomy of this portion of the gastrointestinal tract, as well as recent changes in our understanding of its physiology and that of the pelvic floor, should facilitate diagnosis and management of these ailments and result in more favorable outcomes.

Anatomy

The anal canal, which extends for a distance of about 4 cm from the anorectal ring to the hairy skin of the anal verge, is the most distal portion of the alimentary canal. Its lining, as well as its musculature, has important features that, together with the pelvic floor structures, contribute significantly to the regulation of defecation and continence. Its borders include the coccyx posteriorly, the ischiorectal fossa and its contents bilaterally, and the perineal body and vagina in women and the urethra in men anteriorly.

Anal Canal Lining

The epithelium that lines the anal canal differs at various levels. The characteristically serrated dentate (or pectinate) line made up of anal valves anatomically demarcates the cephalad, pleated mucosa from the caudad, smooth anoderm mucosa. The proximal mucosa is corrugated into a series of 12 to 14 columns of Morgagni with corresponding crypts between each fold. Opening into these crypts are a variable number of anal glands, which traverse the submucosa to enter the internal sphincter to terminate in the intersphincteric plane. Thus, infection of these cryptoglandular structures may result in fistulas that can be expected to communicate with the dentate line area.

The mucosa of the upper anal canal, like that of the rectum, is pinkish and is lined by columnar epithelium, whereas the mucosa distal to the dentate line is paler and lined by squamous epithelium devoid of hair and glands. The change between the two types of epithelium, however, is not abrupt, and the mucosa of the so-called transitional zone, which lies immediately proximal to the dentate line, consists of layers of cuboidal cells interspersed with tongues of columnar epithelium, which is purplish in color. Differences between the rectal columnar mucosal lining and anal squamous lining have several important clinical implications. For example, diseases affecting the rectal mucosa, such as ulcerative colitis, can extend within the transitional zone area but not distal to the dentate.[1] Cancers proximal to the dentate are typically adenocarcinomas, and those distal are squamous or cloacogenic. At the anal verge, the lining acquires the characteristics of normal skin with its apocrine glands, and this is where infectious complications of the apocrine glands, hidradenitis suppurativa, present. Further, this differentiation also demarcates differences in sensory perception, which influences the surgical approaches to

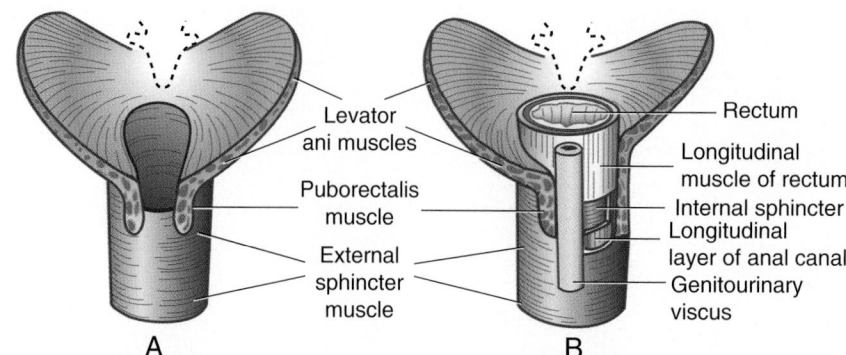

Figure 51-1 The anal canal mechanism comprises two components, visceral and somatic, each of which is tubular. The visceral tube is enclosed by a skeletal muscle tube by means of which continence is maintained. **A,** Diagrammatic representation of the skeletal muscle component. **B,** Composite arrangement after insertion of a simple visceral component. (From Parks AG, Gordon PH, Hardcastle JD: A classification of fistula-in-ano. Br J Surg 63:1-12, 1976.)

anorectal conditions. For example, internal hemorrhoids can be treated with rubber band ligation without the need for local anesthesia. Excision of external hemorrhoids requires the application of local anesthesia to the sensitive perianal skin.

Anal Canal Musculature

The anal canal musculature with its sphincteric apparatus is the terminal muscular channel of the gastrointestinal tract and can be conceptualized as two tubular structures overlying each other. The inner component is the continuation of the smooth circular layer of the rectum forming the thickened and rounded internal sphincter that ends 1.5 cm below the dentate line slightly cephalad to the external sphincter (intersphincteric groove). The outer component is a continuous sheet of striated muscle constituting the pelvic floor, which comprises the levator ani muscle, the puborectalis muscle, and the external sphincter (Fig. 51-1). The latter is elliptical and engulfs the anal canal and the internal sphincter, beyond which it terminates in a subcutaneous portion. The other two portions, namely the superficial and deep divisions, constitute a single muscular unit, which is continuous superiorly with the puborectalis and levator ani muscles. The external sphincter, bulbospongiosus, and transverse perineal muscles meet together centrally on the perineum to constitute the perineal body. The funnel-shaped configuration of the paired levator ani muscles form the major part of the pelvic floor, and their fibers decussate medially with the contralateral side to fuse with the perineal body around the prostate or vagina.

The internal sphincter, which is innervated by the autonomic nervous system, is independent of voluntary control, whereas the external sphincter, which is supplied by the inferior rectal branch of the internal pudendal nerve and the perineal branch of the fourth sacral nerve, is under voluntary control.

Physiology

The physiology of the anal canal and pelvic floor is complex, but the advent of more sophisticated means to evaluate its functions, such as manometry, defecography, evacuability testing, and electromyography, has improved our understanding of it. The principal function of the anal canal is the regulation of defecation and maintenance of continence. The ability to control defecation depends on the coordinated functions of the sensory and muscular activities of the anus; the compliance, tone, and evacuability of the rectum; the muscular activities of the pelvic floor; and the consistency, volume, and timing of the colonic fecal movements. Perturbations of any of the critical functions can result in fecal incontinence (Table 51-1).

The anal canal, which has a mean length of 4 cm, lengthens with squeezing of the external sphincter and shortens with straining.[2] Resting pressure, or tone, which depends largely on the internal sphincter, averages 90 cm H_2O and is lower in women and older patients than in men and younger patients. This high-pressure zone increases resistance to the passage of stool. Squeeze pressure, generated by contraction of the external anal sphincter and puborectalis muscle, more than doubles intra-anal canal resting pressure. This maximal increase lasts but for a minute at the most, and consequently, squeeze pressure serves only to prevent leakage on presentation of the rectal content to the proximal anal canal at inappropriate times. The principal mechanism that provides continence is the pressure differential between the rectum (6 cm H_2O) and the anal canal (90 cm H_2O).[3] The anorectal angle is produced by the anterior pull of the puborectalis muscle as it encircles the rectum at the anorectal ring and contributes to fecal continence. This angle may act as a flap valve[4] or have a sphincter-like function.[5] Maneuvers that sharpen this angle augment continence, whereas those that straighten it favor defecation.

Anorectal sensation allows discrimination of the character of the enteric content (gas, liquids, or solids) and detection of the need to pass that content through sensory receptors located either in the rectal muscular wall or in the pelvic floor musculature. The fact that such sensations persist after proctectomy and ileoanal anastomosis[6] suggests that the receptors are situated in the pelvic floor.

Table 51-1   **Common Causes of Fecal Incontinence**

CATEGORY	MECHANISM	COMMON CAUSES
Functional	Fecal impaction; dilated internal anal sphincter	Pelvic floor dyssynergia (difficulty relaxing sphincter when defecating), drug side effect, idiopathic, spinal cord injury
	Diarrhea; rapid transit and/or large volume	Irritable bowel syndrome; infectious and metabolic causes of diarrhea
	Cognitive/psychological; social indifference	Dementia, psychosis, willful soiling
Sphincter weakness	Sphincter muscle injury	Obstetric trauma, motor vehicle crash, foreign body trauma
	Pudendal nerve injury	Obstetric trauma, diabetic peripheral neuropathy, multiple sclerosis, idiopathic
	Central nervous system injury	Spina bifida, traumatic spinal cord injury, cerebrovascular accident, multiple sclerosis
Sensory loss	Afferent nerve injury: unable to detect rectal filling	Diabetic neuropathy, spinal cord injury, multiple sclerosis

Adapted from Whitehead WE, Wald A, Norton NJ: Treatment options for fecal incontinence. Dis Colon Rectum 44:134, 2001.

For the enteric content to reach the anal canal for discrimination, the internal sphincter must relax while the rectum distends and contracts (rectal anal inhibitory reflex). This reflex involves inhibitory neurons of the myenteric plexus, which innervates the internal sphincter, and intramural nerves and neurotransmitters. Transient relaxation of the internal anal sphincter brings the rectal content into contact with the sensory mucosa of the proximal anal canal so that it can be recognized. Other factors important to continence include rectal compliance, tone, and capacity; rectal filling and emptying; and stool volume and consistency.

Diagnostic Evaluation of the Anus

Systematic evaluation of anorectal disorders includes a careful history and physical examination of the anal canal area before elaborate laboratory testing.

History

Important symptoms include bleeding, pain, discharge (mucoid, purulent, or fecal), and change in bowel habits. It is also paramount to know about associated illnesses, medications, family history, bleeding tendency, and exposure through travel or sexual contacts.

Bleeding is a common presenting symptom of both benign and malignant conditions of the anus and large bowel. Details regarding the type of bleeding can help differentiate between anorectal and large bowel disorders. Inquiry into the type of bleeding should include whether the blood is dark or bright red or associated with clots, whether it is mixed with the stool or separate, and whether it drips into the toilet bowl or only appears on the toilet paper. Blood that drips, is separate from stools, and is bright red is most commonly seen with bleeding internal hemorrhoids. Blood on toilet tissue may be associated with minor hemorrhoidal disease but also with anal fissure. Clots or melena indicate colonic or more proximal bleeding, respectively. Although a careful bleeding history may suggest a specific etiology, consideration must always be given to proximal bowel evaluation to exclude the possibility of more serious conditions, such as cancer. This is particularly important when examination cannot confirm a bleeding source; when patients are at increased risk for cancer by age or family history; and when bleeding does not resolve promptly after treatment of the presumed source. When there is doubt, evaluate the proximal bowel.

Anorectal pain occurring during or immediately after stooling that is described as severe is usually associated with anal fissure. Pain that may or may not be related to stooling and is throbbing in nature most often is seen with an abscess or poorly draining fistula. Pain totally unrelated to stooling is likely to be associated with proctalgia fugax or levator ani syndrome, a condition characterized by painful episodes of short duration (<20-30 minutes) occurring often at night and relieved by walking, warm baths, or other maneuvers. To ascertain change in bowel habits, it is necessary to establish by careful inquiry the previous pattern of bowel habit. Indeed, constipation may mean different conditions to different patients, and it is important to know whether the condition is of recent onset or chronic to determine the course of investigation.

Physical Examination

The left lateral position, with the buttocks projecting slightly beyond the edge of the table, and the prone jackknife position are both suitable for evaluation of anal conditions. Inspection with good lighting should precede any other type of examination. Skin tags, excoriations, scars, and any changes in color or appearance of perianal skin are easily recognized. A patulous anus may indicate incontinence and possibly prolapse. Inspection while straining may help determine the presence of hemorrhoidal or rectal prolapse in multiparous women, and a protruding anus may be an indication of descending perineum syndrome. A careful and systematic digital examination with a well-lubricated index finger gradually inserted into the anal canal helps the examiner to appreciate any mass, induration, or stricturing as well as to

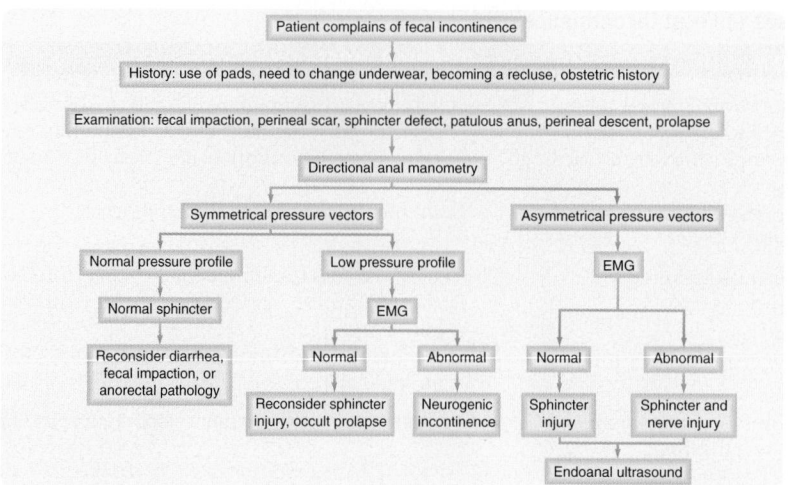

Figure 51-2 Investigation of fecal incontinence. EMG, electromyogram. (From Sagar PM, Pemberton JH: Anorectal and pelvic floor function: Relevance to continence, incontinence, and constipation. Gastroenterol Clin North Am 25:173, 1996.)

assess the resting tone and strength of the squeeze pressure of the anal sphincter. In men, the prostate should be palpated; in women, the posterior vaginal wall should be pushed forward to detect rectocele.

After the preliminary evaluation has been completed, proctosigmoidoscopy after enema preparation enables satisfactory visualization of the anorectum. Early signs of mucosal inflammation include the loss of the vascular pattern with erythema, granularity, friability, and even ulcerations. Gross lesions, such as polyps or carcinoma, should be readily identifiable. Any suspicious area or mass should be sampled for biopsy, with the patient's permission, so that a precise histopathologic diagnosis can be established. On withdrawing the scope, the anorectal area can be assessed for mucosal prolapse, hemorrhoids, fissure, polyps, and so forth. The anoscope can also be used for the same purpose; it optimizes the evaluation of lesions confined to the anus.

Other investigations may include barium enema, flexible sigmoidoscopy or colonoscopy, and stool examination, especially if infectious diarrhea or sexually transmitted disease (STD) is suspected. Special studies, such as manometry, defecography, and electromyography, may help in the assessment of anorectal incontinence, constipation, or any other pelvic floor disorders. More recently, ultrasonography and magnetic resonance imaging (MRI) have shown promise in the evaluation of anorectal suppurative processes. The indications and usefulness of these tests are discussed later under the specific disorders.

PELVIC FLOOR DISORDERS

Incontinence

Clinical Evaluation

Voluntary control of defecation is obviously desirable; fecal incontinence is often a disabling condition. Deter-

mining the extent and nature of the problem should start by distinguishing true incontinence (i.e., complete loss of solid stools) from minor incontinence (i.e., occasional staining from seepage or urgency). Seepage of mucus from prolapsing hemorrhoids or from a large secretory villous polyp, urgency from colitis or proctitis, and overflow incontinence from fecal impaction may be confused with true incontinence. After true incontinence is established, the severity of the disability should be assessed by seeking information on control of flatus, liquid and solid stool, and effect on lifestyle and activities[7] (Fig. 51-2). Fecal incontinence may be multifactorial; hence, details regarding possible causes and associated gastrointestinal disorders should be sought in the patient's history (see Table 51-1).

Defects in the sphincter may be the result of trauma from previous surgical procedures for hemorrhoids, fissures, or fistulas; forceful dilation of the anal canal; impalement injury; or obstetric injuries either directly because of a tear or breakdown of episiotomy repair or indirectly from stretching of the pudendal nerve during labor, which may develop decades later. Other possible causes include radiation damage, primary anal diseases, aging, and neurogenic processes. When associated with other neurologic findings or risk factors, more extensive neurologic evaluations should be performed. Associated gastrointestinal disorders, such as diarrhea, can aggravate disorders of continence.[8] Physical examination should confirm a weak resting tone and squeeze pressure or a patulous anus and the presence of scars, defects, deformities, or keyhole abnormalities. Examination can also exclude the presence of prolapse, hemorrhoids, or other contributory or associated anorectal abnormalities. Endoscopy excludes the diagnoses of proctitis, fecal impaction, rectal polyps, and colitis cystica profunda.

Additional testing can be restricted to a few tests depending on the extent of findings at examination.[8,9] Anal manometry confirms the extent of impairment of the internal and external sphincters by the resting and

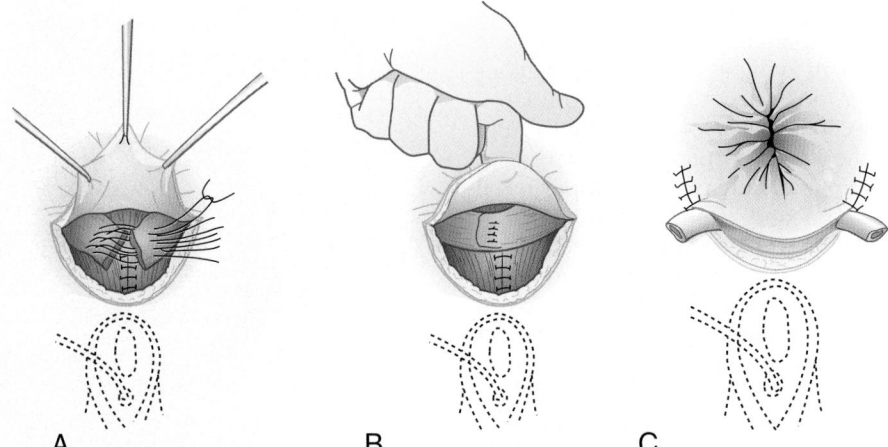

Figure 51-3 Overlapping sphincteroplasty. **A,** A curvilinear incision is made midway between the anus and the introitus, limited in its posterolateral extent to avoid pudendal nerve injury. The external sphincter ends are dissected, the scar excised when extensive, and the muscle ends reapproximated using overlapping suture technique. The levator ani muscles are also reapproximated. **B,** Tightness is judged by digital rectal examination. **C,** The wound edges are closed over drains, at times using a Y configuration to lengthen the perineal body. (By permission of Mayo Foundation.)

squeeze pressures, respectively. Manometry can also identify asymmetry, suggesting anatomic defects amenable to repair. Endoanal ultrasound has been recommended to detect occult defects and, in some centers with expertise, is considered more accurate than clinical or conventional methods of evaluation. Finally, electromyography of the pelvic floor can be used to differentiate between anatomic and neurogenic sources of incontinence, and pudendal nerve terminal motor latency testing can predict the likelihood of successful repair.[8,9]

Medical Management

Treatment may be nonoperative, including medications to slow transit or increase stool consistency or diet and sphincter exercises, but in general, results from these approaches have been disappointing, except for cases of mild incontinence.[8] Biofeedback training for strengthening of the anal musculature and improvement of anorectal sensation has been widely applied, particularly in cases of generalized weakness in which repairable anatomic defects are not identified. Variable rates of success have been reported, with typically 75% experiencing at least modest reduction in incontinence frequency and 50% accomplishing complete continence.[8] Biofeedback can also be used before or after surgical repair to optimize results. Another nonsurgical approach is to maximize evacuation regularity; this can be accomplished with the assistance of suppositories or daily tap-water enemas.[8] Accidental eliminations are minimized if the rectum is empty between evacuations.

Surgical Repair

An expanding number of surgical options are available for correction of fecal incontinence, including everything from direct sphincter repair to artificial sphincter implantation and colostomy diversion. For discrete anatomic defects, the most common surgical approach is the direct overlapping sphincteroplasty, in which the separated muscular ends are dissected, reapproximated, and sutured[10] (Fig. 51-3). Fecal diversion is not typically required for these repairs unless there are extenuating circumstances. The overlapping sphincteroplasty is associated with low rates of morbidity and mortality and reasonable rates of success with good to excellent results achieved in 55% to 68% of patients,[8] but direct repair of anterior sphincter defects from obstetric injuries can be expected to restore fecal continence in 59% of patients. For nonanatomic defects, postanal repair has been advocated by some authorities as a useful surgical option. Because rates of continence from the postanal repair are reported as low as 35% in specialty-focused centers, it has a rather limited role in the overall management of incontinence.[11]

Anal encirclement, such as with a Thiersch wire or other prosthetic material, is discouraged as a definitive strategy and has largely been replaced by the use of implantable artificial sphincters or the application of neoanal muscular sphincters, or the application of sacral nerve stimulation.[12] Early results from these approaches are encouraging. On rare occasions, a patient may be so disabled from incontinence and refractory to medical and surgical therapies that an end colostomy may be acceptable.

Prolapse of the Rectum

Pathogenesis and Clinical Presentation

Prolapse of the rectum, or procidentia, is an uncommon problem of obscure etiology characterized by full-thickness eversion of the rectal wall through the anus. The exact cause is unclear, but the disorder tends to predominate in women, in those who strain excessively, and in those with chronic mental disorders. Pregnancy and delivery cannot be important because the condition can occur in men and in nulliparous women. Studies would strongly support the concept that rectal prolapse is the result of intussusception or infolding of the rectum or rectosigmoid.[13] As the intussusception progresses caudally, the intussusceptum gradually pulls the upper rectal wall away from its sacral and lateral moorings. With continued straining, the bowel continues to roll inside out until initially the mucocutaneous junction and eventually the rectal wall evert completely. This progressive phenomenon may explain why some patients have occult or hidden prolapse and why the sigmoid mesentery may elongate, the cul-de-sac may deepen, and the pelvic floor musculature may increasingly weaken. Such findings have been implicated as causative, but it is more likely that they are the result of the prolonged process of gradual prolapsing of the rectum.

The symptoms of early prolapse may be vague, including discomfort or a sensation of incomplete evacuation during defecation. A long history of constipation and excessive straining is common. When prolapse is complete, protrusion of the rectum is noted as a mass during and after defecation. In patients with occult prolapse, a feeling of pressure and a sensation of incomplete evacuation may be the only symptoms.

Preoperative Evaluation

The preoperative assessment of the patient should focus on establishing the extent of the prolapse; the patient's overall health status; the presence of associated bowel conditions, such as constipation; and complications, such as incontinence. All these factors influence the operative strategy. At history, nearly half of patients[14] have constipation, and most have fecal incontinence.[15-17] By observing the patient while straining on the commode, the presence and extent of the prolapse can be verified. Complete prolapse demonstrates full-thickness rectal protrusion with concentric rings (Fig. 51-4). Frail elderly patients and those with high-risk comorbid conditions or limited life expectancy are ideally suited for perineal procedures. Young patients, particularly those with constipation or evidence of defecating disorders, are best served with resection and fixation, using open or laparoscopic approaches.

Complete lower gastrointestinal tract evaluations are performed as indicated. On endoscopy, redness of the anterior rectal mucosa or a solitary rectal ulcer 6 to 8 cm anteriorly may be present. A number of additional tests can be ordered but have limited value and are not typically required. Manometry documents the presence of sphincter damage but does not predict recovery. An abnormal pudendal nerve terminal motor latency predicts a high risk for postoperative anal incontinence but rarely influences the management.[15] Defecography can demonstrate the extent of prolapse and transit studies the extent of constipation. Because a patient with significant prolongation in transit time may respond better to a more extensive colonic resection, this may be indicated in select patients with constipation.

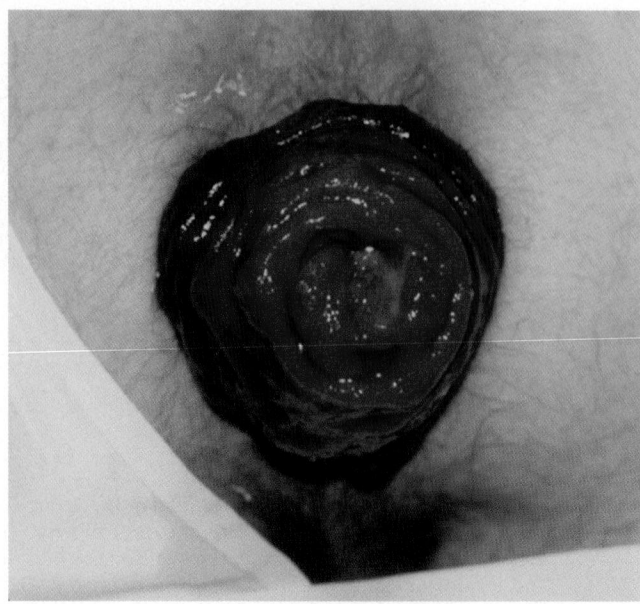

Figure 51-4 Complete rectal prolapse. The everted rectal wall appears as a tubular mass made up of several concentric mucosal folds. (By permission of Mayo Foundation.)

Surgical Correction

Two general approaches are used to achieve surgical correction of rectal prolapse: the perineal approach, which includes the Delorme and the Altemeier procedures, and the abdominal approach, which includes but is not limited to anterior resection with or without rectopexy and mesh fixation. The perineal approach is less taxing on the patient and yet has a higher recurrence rate; thus, it is ideally suited for patients with high operative risk and a limited life expectancy. An abdominal approach is preferred for young healthy patients because they can tolerate the procedure with low risk and are less likely to suffer a recurrence requiring reoperation.

Perineal Procedures

The Delorme procedure is essentially a mucosal proctectomy and muscularis plicating procedure (Fig. 51-5). It is ideally applied to patients with up to 3 to 4 cm of prolapse, even though the mucosal tube resected can extend up to 15 cm. Even in frail, elderly patients, the Delorme procedure is associated with low rates of mortality and major morbidity, about 1% and 14%, respectively.[17] Incontinence improves in as many as 69% of patients.[17] Prolapse recurrence is not uncommon and is likely underestimated because this procedure is performed in patients with limited life expectancies and therefore short follow-up.

The Altemeier procedure is similar to the Delorme, but rather than a mucosal resection, a full-thickness rectal resection is performed starting 1 or 2 cm above the dentate. The bowel and attendant mesentery are resected. Because the pelvic cavity is entered, injury to small bowel must be avoided. A full-thickness anastomosis is accomplished after the full extent of resection is completed. For

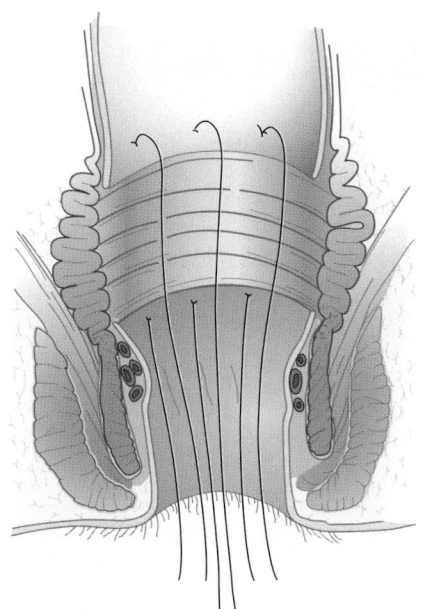

Figure 51-5 Schematic representation of Delorme repair of complete rectal prolapse. Mucosal proctectomy is followed by muscular plication, anastomosing the proximal extent of the mucosal resection site to the distal mucosa, just proximal to the dentate. (By permission of Mayo Foundation.)

patients with incontinence, a levatorplasty may be added to the resection. Results are similar to those described for the Delorme procedure.[16]

Abdominal Procedures

The abdominal options include bowel resection and rectopexy with or without mesh, performed either alone or together. Complete mobilization of the rectum is required for the abdominal procedures; debate exists about whether the lateral stalks should be preserved.[18] Preservation of the stalks is thought to yield better functional results but a greater risk for recurrence.[14] Although the entire rectum is mobilized to the level of the levatores, if resection and anastomosis are being performed, they should be performed high rather than low in the rectum, essentially an anterior resection. This minimizes the risk for anastomotic complications. Rectopexy is performed by securing the rectum to the presacral tissues. Resection with rectopexy is associated with low recurrence rates (0%-9%)[14,15] and can be performed safely, with morbidity and mortality rates commensurate with any large bowel resection. Constipation improves in up to half of patients and incontinence in most patients.[14]

Rectopexy alone with mesh fixation is a well-described procedure, preferred by some centers. The risks for resection and anastomosis are avoided, and recurrence rates are generally low. Complications can result, however, from the presence of a foreign body, and symptoms of constipation are often aggravated. The abdominal procedures can be performed through standard laparotomy or using laparoscopic techniques. Results suggest that postoperative recovery is typically faster after laparoscopic

resection with rectopexy. Furthermore, rates of morbidities, mortality, recurrence, and functional improvement are the same with laparoscopic and open techniques.[19]

Incontinence and Biofeedback

Because incontinence resulting from chronic stretching may or may not cause permanent pudendal nerve damage, many patients note improvement in continence after prolapse repair. The role of biofeedback for treating persistent postoperative incontinence or for preventing recurrent prolapse in patients with obvious pelvic floor dysfunction and a tendency toward excessive straining is not well established. That it can be beneficial to some patients and that it is noninvasive encourage its use in select patients.

Rectocele

Clinical Evaluation

Patients with a rectocele present with a bulge or prolapse of the anterior rectal wall into the vagina. Symptoms attributable to a rectocele include the presentation of a vaginal bulge, inability to completely evacuate during defecation, and in most cases the necessity to digitally evacuate through the vagina or through the rectum or perineum. The etiology of rectoceles remains unclear and is probably multifactorial because it is associated with a constellation of a number of pelvic floor disorders, including constipation, paradoxical muscular contraction, and neuropathies or anatomic disorders from childbirth.[20] Rectocele may coexist with other defecation disorders such as slow-transit constipation or pelvic floor dysfunction, including pelvic organ prolapse, in which factors such as age, parity, obesity, constipation, pelvic surgery, and a number of pulmonary and medical conditions may play a role.[20] Associated disorders must be addressed to achieve resolution of all symptoms. A careful physical examination will reveal the size of the defect where the rectum prolapse extends to the vagina.

Defecography, which can demonstrate dynamic information on the process of rectal emptying, is the only test that is specifically diagnostic for a rectocele.[20] It is probably the most useful test for understanding the relevance of the rectocele in the defecation process even though there is no exact correlation between any single test finding and the results from surgery.[20] Further colorectal evaluations and tests can be ordered as appropriate for other symptoms or coexisting disorders.

Treatment

The optimization of bowel function through proper diet, fiber supplements, and good bowel habits is always appropriate as complementary therapy. Medical therapies, specifically biofeedback, have met with limited success, providing only partial relief in most patients but major relief in only a minority of patients.[21]

Surgical Treatment

Patients with rectoceles should be considered for surgical correction if the rectocele is greater than 2 cm and the patient has to perform digitally assisted defecation.[22]

Table 51-2   Internal Hemorrhoids: Grading and Management

GRADE	SYMPTOMS AND SIGNS	MANAGEMENT
First degree	Bleeding; no prolapse	Dietary modifications*
Second degree	Prolapse with spontaneous reduction Bleeding, seepage	Rubber band ligation Coagulation Dietary modifications
Third degree	Prolapse requiring digital reduction Bleeding, seepage	Surgical hemorrhoidectomy Rubber band ligation Dietary modifications
Fourth degree	Prolapsed, cannot be reduced Strangulated	Surgical hemorrhoidectomy Urgent hemorrhoidectomy Dietary modifications

*Dietary modifications include increasing consumption of fiber, bran, or psyllium and water. Dietary modifications are always appropriate for the management of hemorrhoids, if not for acute care then for chronic management, and for prevention of recurrence after banding and/or surgery.

Although gynecologic surgeons often perform a transvaginal repair, the defect between the vagina and the rectum can be corrected using a transperineal approach (with or without mesh and including a levatorplasty) or using a transanal repair, with an anal mucosa flap and a plication technique without mesh.[22] The repair should extend 7 to 10 cm above the anal canal. Symptomatic improvement can be anticipated in 73% to 79% of properly selected patients.[22] Best results can be expected in patients who have a small rectocele, require digital-assisted evacuation, are without evidence of anismus, and are repaired using a transperineal approach.[22,23]

COMMON BENIGN ANAL DISORDERS

Hemorrhoids

Clinical Presentation and Diagnostic Evaluations
Within the normal anal canal exist specialized, highly vascularized "cushions" forming discrete masses of thick submucosa containing blood vessels, smooth muscle, and elastic and connective tissue.[24] They are located in the left lateral, right anterior, and right posterior quadrants of the canal to aid in anal continence. The term *hemorrhoids* should be restricted to clinical situations in which these "cushions" are abnormal and cause symptoms. The cause of hemorrhoids remains unknown. They may be no more than the downward sliding of anal cushions associated with gravity, straining, and irregular bowel habits. Hemorrhoids can be considered external or internal; the diagnosis is based on the history, physical examination, and endoscopy. External hemorrhoids are covered with anoderm and are distal to the dentate line; they may swell, causing discomfort and difficult hygiene, but cause severe pain only if actually thrombosed. Internal hemorrhoids cause painless, bright red bleeding or prolapse associated with defecation. Internal hemorrhoids are classified according to the extent of prolapse, which influences treatment options (Table 51-2). The patient

may report dripping or even squirting of blood in the toilet bowl. Chronic occult bleeding leading to anemia is rare, and other causes of anemia must be excluded. Prolapse below the dentate line area can occur, especially with straining, and may lead to mucus and fecal leakage and pruritus. Pain is not usually associated with uncomplicated hemorrhoids but more often with fissure, abscess, or external hemorrhoidal thrombosis.

The physical examination should include inspection during straining, preferably on a commode; digital rectal examination; and anoscopy (Fig. 51-6). Digital examination enables assessment of internal and external hemorrhoidal disease and anal canal tone and exclusion of other lesions, especially low rectal or anal canal neoplasms. Because virtually all anorectal symptoms are ascribed to "hemorrhoids" by patients, it is essential that other anorectal pathologies be considered and excluded. Anoscopy is the definitive examination, but a flexible proctosigmoidoscopy should always be added to exclude proximal inflammation or neoplasia. Colonoscopy or barium enema should be added if the hemorrhoidal disease is unimpressive, the history is somewhat uncharacteristic, or the patient is older than 40 years or has risk factors for colon cancer, such as a family history. Depending on degree of disease, treatment falls into two main categories: nonsurgical and hemorrhoidectomy.

Nonoperative Management
In many patients, hemorrhoidal symptoms can be ameliorated or relieved by simple measures, such as better local hygiene, avoidance of excessive straining, and better dietary habits supplemented by medication to keep stools soft, formed, and regular (see Table 51-2). A wide array of fiber supplements are now available over the counter. Symptoms of bleeding but not prolapse can be significantly reduced over a period of 30 to 45 days with the use of fiber supplements. Over-the-counter suppositories and anal salves, although popular, have never been tested for efficacy. Even though all patients should be

counseled on dietary and fiber recommendations, patients with prolapse and internal plus external hemorrhoids benefit from additional interventions.

In the absence of symptomatic external hemorrhoids, second- and some third-degree internal hemorrhoids can be treated with office procedures that produce mucosal fixation. Although sclerotherapy, infrared coagulation, heater probe, and bipolar electrocoagulation all have been described, the simplest, most effective, and most widely applied office procedure is rubber band ligation. Rubber band ligation can be performed in the office without sedation through an anoscope using a ligator (Fig. 51-7). Preferably, only one site should be banded each time. Because severe perineal sepsis and even deaths have been reported after rubber band ligation, patients should be instructed to return to the emergency department if delayed or undue pain, inability to void, or a fever develops.[25] With one or more applications, symptoms are alleviated in 79% of patients.[26] Because of the risk for bleeding and sepsis, it is preferable that patients are not taking antiplatelet or blood-thinning medications and that subacute bacterial endocarditis prophylaxis is administered to patients at risk. Rubber band ligation should be avoided in immunodeficient patients.

Surgical Treatment

Hemorrhoidectomy is the best means of curing hemorrhoidal disease and should be considered whenever patients fail to respond satisfactorily to repeated attempts at conservative measures; hemorrhoids are severely prolapsed and require manual reduction; hemorrhoids are complicated by strangulation or associated pathology, such as ulceration, fissure, fistula; or hemorrhoids are associated with symptomatic external hemorrhoids or large anal tags. The choice of anesthesia should be individualized based on the patient's preference, build, and medical status. In most instances, local or regional anesthesia with mild sedation can be used effectively. For

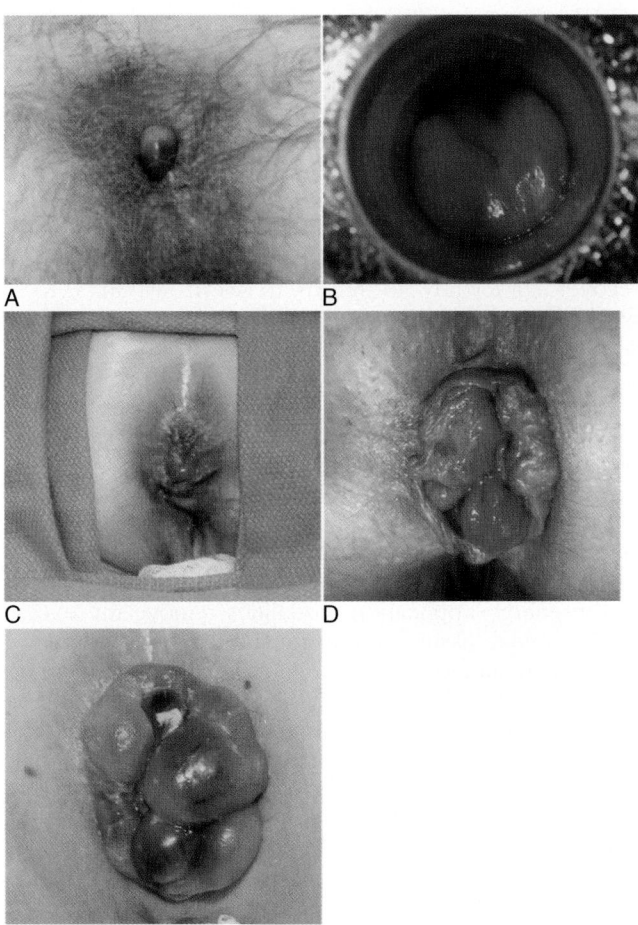

Figure 51-6 Hemorrhoids. **A,** Thrombosed external. **B,** First-degree internal viewed through anoscope. **C,** Second-degree internal prolapsed, reduced spontaneously. **D,** Third-degree internal prolapsed, requiring manual reduction. **E,** Fourth-degree strangulated internal and thrombosed external. (By permission of Mayo Foundation.)

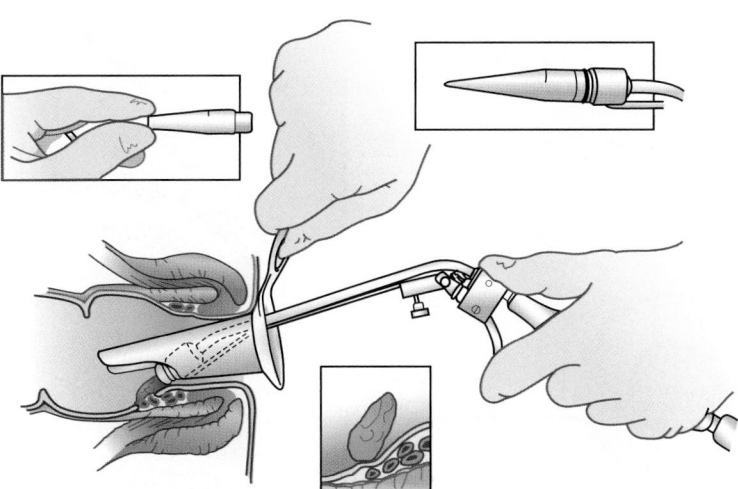

Figure 51-7 The band is advanced onto the end of the ligator instrument using a conical attachment (*insets*). The hemorrhoid is identified at a level proximal to the dentate; this area is tested for sensation before banding. Occluding the suction port of the ligator instrument draws the hemorrhoid into the open end of the ligator, at which time the instrument is fired. The banded hemorrhoid typically sloughs in a week's time. (By permission of Mayo Foundation.)

simple thrombosed external hemorrhoids, excision in the office is best performed early in the course of the disease, during the period of maximum pain (Fig. 51-8). To remove complex internal or external hemorrhoids, an open or closed hemorrhoidectomy can be performed as an outpatient procedure.

Closed hemorrhoidectomy provides simultaneous excision of internal and external hemorrhoids (Fig. 51-9).

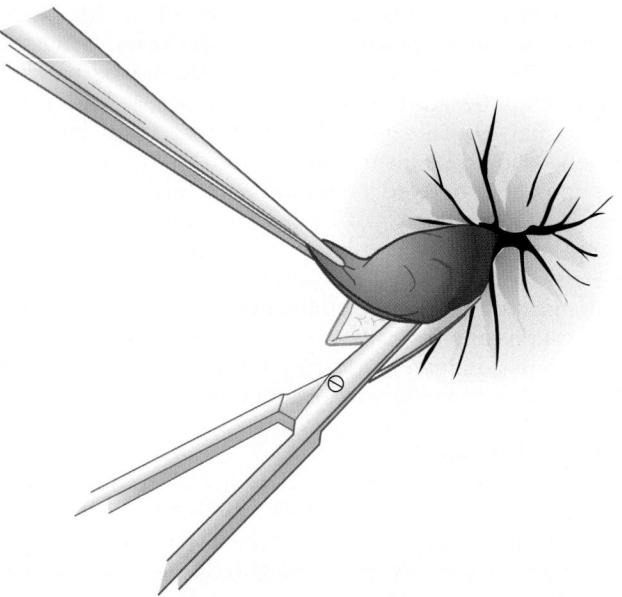

Figure 51-8 Excision of thrombosed external hemorrhoid. The area is infiltrated with local anesthetic, and the thrombosed hemorrhoid is excised sharply. The wound is left open. (By permission of Mayo Foundation.)

Preoperative and intraoperative assessment determines the number and location of hemorrhoids requiring excision; typically, three bundles are identified in the right anterior, right posterior, and left lateral positions. The use of a large operative scope retractor, such as the Fansler, ensures that sufficient anoderm is preserved to avoid the long-term complication of anal stenosis. Postoperative complications include fecal impaction, infection, urinary retention, and rarely arterial bleeding. Patients typically recover sufficiently to return to work within 1 to 2 weeks.[27] As an alternative to the closed technique, the surgical wounds can be left open to reduce postoperative pain, but at the expense of longer healing times.

Newer technology and techniques have been applied to the operative treatment of hemorrhoids with the promise of less postoperative pain. The two main categories of newer treatments involve either the application of ultrasonic or controlled electrical energy such as the Harmonic Scalpel and Liga-Sure, respectively, or a new operative approach to hemorrhoidal tissue excision. Both of the energy application modalities remove the excess hemorrhoidal tissue and coagulate or seal the blood vessels simultaneously with minimal lateral thermal injury to nearby tissue. It is thought that the reduction in trauma to the surrounding anal canal mucosa and the underlying anal sphincter will decrease postoperative edema and pain. A number of small single institutional reports have evaluated both of these new technologies compared to traditional excisional hemorrhoidectomy.[28] These studies all demonstrated decreased postoperative pain and analgesic use in the Harmonic Scalpel or Liga-Sure groups compared with traditional techniques with similar short-term success rates.

Another operative technique developed to treat circumferential prolapsed and bleeding hemorrhoids was

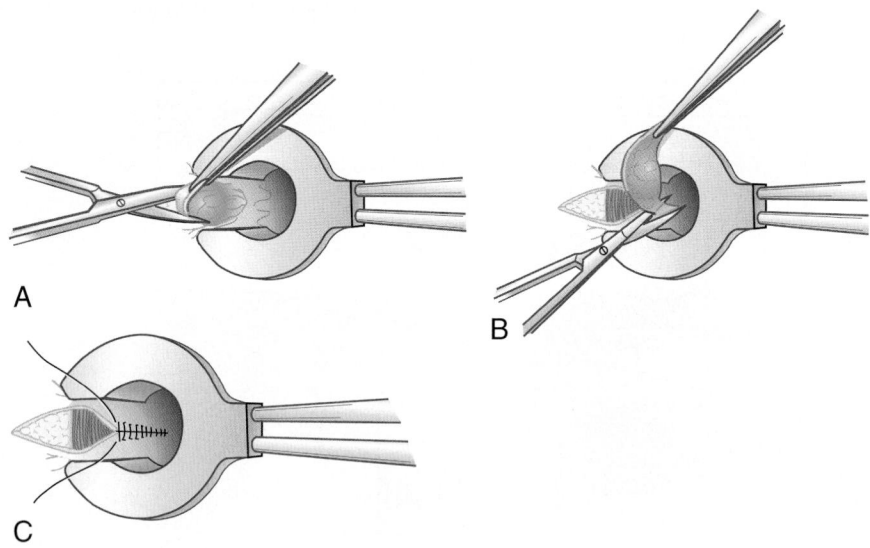

Figure 51-9 Closed hemorrhoidectomy. **A,** Hemorrhoidal tissues are sharply excised starting just beyond the external component and working proximally, finishing with resection of the internal component. **B,** The sphincter muscles are preserved by dissecting only the tissues superficial to them. **C,** The pedicle is transfixed and the defect closed with a running absorbable suture. (By permission of Mayo Foundation.)

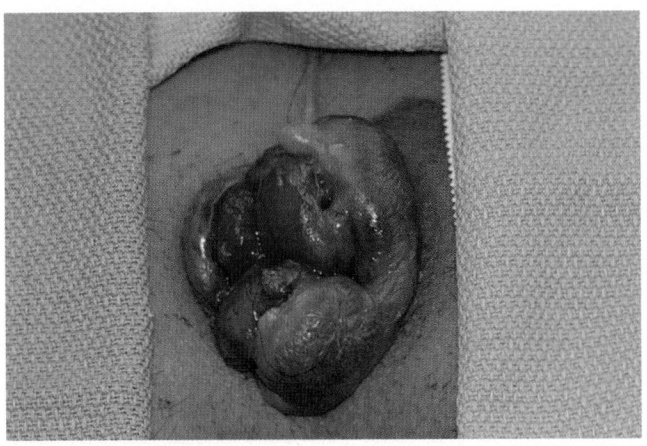

A

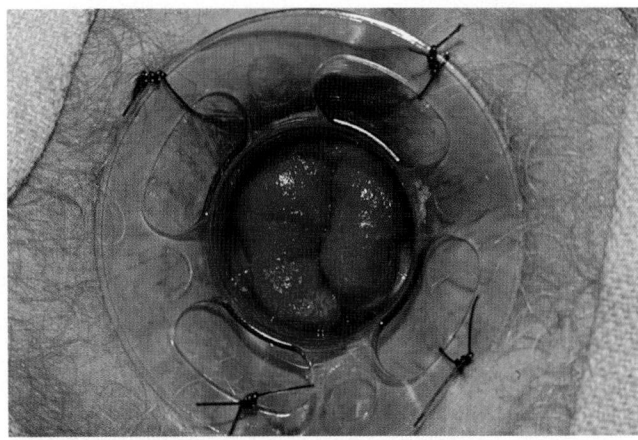

B

Figure 51-10 A, Grade 4 hemorrhoid before reduction. **B,** Placement of stapling device obturator.

first described by Longo.[29] Longo's technique, commonly referred to as the *stapled hemorrhoidectomy* or *stapled hemorrhoidopexy,* excises a circumferential portion of the lower rectal and upper anal canal mucosa and submucosa and performs a reanastomosis with a circular stapling device. As a result, the prolapsed anal cushions are retracted into their normal anatomic positions within the anal canal. In addition, the terminal branches of the inferior hemorrhoidal artery are disrupted, and blood flow into the cushions is thereby decreased. The primary physiologic appeal of this operation is that it leaves the richly innervated anal canal tissue and perianal skin intact, thus reducing the pain usually associated with excisional hemorrhoidectomy. Initially, stapled hemorrhoidopexy was performed with a large standard end-to-end anastomosis (EEA) stapler. Recently, however, a dedicated stapling device specifically designed for this operation was introduced into clinical practice. The stapled hemorrhoidopexy consists of five steps:

1. Reduce the prolapsed tissue.
2. Gently dilate the anal canal to allow it to accept the instrument.
3. Place a purse-string suture (Fig. 51-10).
4. Place and fire the stapler (Fig. 51-11).
5. Control any bleeding from the staple line.

By far the most important technical consideration is proper placement of the purse-string suture. The suture should be at least 3 to 4 cm above the dentate line; if it is too low, a portion of the dentate line may be excised, which could lead to a severe prolonged pain syndrome or to persistent fecal urgency. In addition, the purse-string suture must be placed so as to incorporate all of the redundant tissue circumferentially; failure to do so may lead to incomplete excision and predispose to recurrent prolapse. Finally, extreme care must be exercised in placing the purse-string suture in women so that the vagina is not entrapped anteriorly.

Several randomized, controlled trials comparing stapled hemorrhoidopexy with conventional excisional hemorrhoidectomy have been performed.[30-33] The stapled hemorrhoidopexy was associated with significantly less

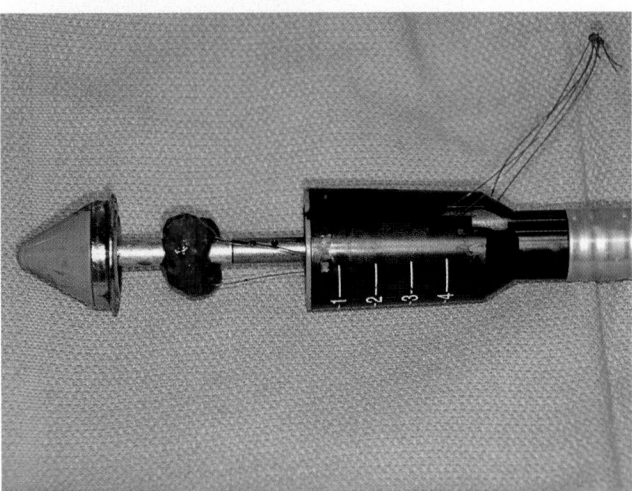

Figure 51-11 Stapling device with circumferential excision of anal canal and hemorrhoid mucosa.

postoperative pain overall, less pain with the first bowel movement, and earlier resumption of normal activities. In none of the trials was there any significant difference between the two procedures with regard to impairment of continence, which was an initial concern in view of the size of the stapler. In 2003, long-term follow-up of patients in one of the original stapled hemorrhoidopexy trials was reported.[34] At a minimum follow-up of 33 months, there were no significant differences between the two procedures with respect to quality of life, symptoms, or functional outcomes. Although stapled hemorrhoidopexy appears simple, it has been associated with a number of serious complications, including anastomotic dehiscence necessitating colostomy, rectal perforation, severe pelvic infection, and acute rectal obstruction and therefore training before use is strongly recommended.

Anal Fissures

Clinical Presentation and Diagnostic Evaluations

An anal fissure is a linear ulcer of the lower half of the anal canal, usually located in the posterior commissure

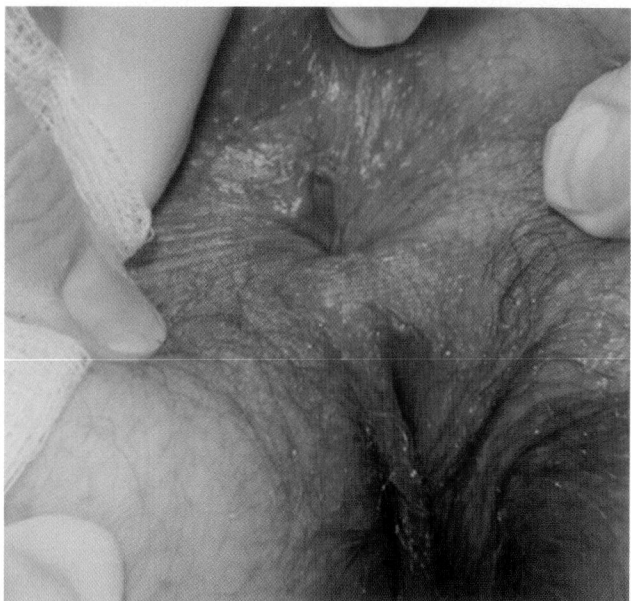

Figure 51-12 Posterior anal fissure. (By permission of Mayo Foundation.)

in the midline (Fig. 51-12). Often misnamed as *rectal fissures,* in fact, these lesions truly involve just the anal tissues and are typically best seen by visually inspecting the anal verge with gentle separation of the gluteal cleft. Location may vary, and an anterior midline fissure is seen more often in women, although most fissures in women and men reside in the posterior midline. Characteristic associated findings include a sentinel pile or tag externally and an enlarged anal papilla internally. Fissures away from these two locations should raise the possibility of associated diseases, especially Crohn's disease, hidradenitis suppurativa, or STDs. Because it involves the highly sensitive squamous epithelium, fissure in ano is often a painful condition. With defecation, the ulcer is stretched, causing pain and mild bleeding.

The diagnosis is secured by the typical history of pain and bleeding with defecation, especially if associated with prior constipation and confirmed by inspection after gently parting the posterior anus. Digital as well as proctoscopic examination may trigger severe pain, interfering with the ability to visualize the ulcer. An endoscopic examination should be performed, but it can be delayed 4 to 6 weeks, until the pain is resolved with medical management or until surgery is performed for those cases refractory to medical therapy.

Pathogenesis

The exact cause of anal fissures is unknown, but many factors appear likely, such as the passage of large, hard stools, which may be the initiating factor; inappropriate diet; previous anal surgery; childbirth; and laxative abuse. Numerous authors have documented higher than normal resting anal canal pressures and reduced anal blood flow in the posterior midline.[35] It is therefore believed that anal fissures are the result of anal sphincter hypertonia and

subsequent mucosal ischemia. New information regarding the pathogenesis of anal fissures has led to the introduction of several new medical approaches, including the application of nitric oxide donors (e.g., nitroglycerin), calcium-channel blockers (e.g., diltiazem and nifedipine), and botulinum injections, all of which allow for internal sphincter relaxation.

Medical Management

Medical therapies for anal fissures are gaining in popularity, particularly for acute fissures, that is, those presenting within 3 to 6 weeks of symptom onset. The traditional first-line therapy for acute fissures is treatment with warm sitz baths and bran or bulking agents, with rates of fissure healing reported as 87%.[36] Hydrocortisone and lidocaine have been advocated as local topical therapies for acute fissures; however, prospective, randomized evaluations show no benefit over sitz baths and bran.[36] Because improving the dietary and bowel evacuation habits of patients is a good long-term strategy for reducing colon, rectal, and anal problems in general and for reducing the risk for fissures specifically, counseling on proper diet and institution of commercial bulking agents (e.g., psyllium seeds) are always indicated.

Patients with chronic fissures should be started on the acute fissure regimen but are typically also started on other therapies simultaneously, including nitroglycerin or isosorbide dinitrate, theoretically producing "reversible chemical sphincterotomy." For nitroglycerin, the limiting side effects are headaches and tachyphylaxis, which can be reduced by instructing the patient to rest lying down while applying the ointment. The topical application of diltiazem (2%) produces fewer side effects and similar efficacy as nitroglycerin.[37] Fissure healing can be anticipated in about 70% of patients with chronic fissures using nitroglycerin or diltiazem.[37]

The concept of reversible chemical sphincterotomy has also been applied to the technique of internal sphincter injection of botulinum toxin (Botox), a technique that transiently produces striated muscle denervation leading to muscle paralysis and relaxation.[38] It has been recommended as a nonsurgical treatment of fissures, with a low risk for complications. In the treatment of chronic anal fissure, such relaxation of the internal anal sphincter is thought to promote increased blood flow to the affected perianal skin, allowing the fissure to heal. The literature documents a variable success rate, but 60% to 80% has been achieved.[39,40] A Cochrane review of the literature on nonsurgical therapies for anal fissure, however, demonstrated no convincing evidence that botulinum injections were any more effective than placebo.[41] The most common side effect associated with botulinum toxin injections is temporary incontinence to flatus in up to 10% of patients with rarely any events of temporary fecal incontinence. Unfortunately, there is no standardized fashion reported in the administration of botulinum toxin regarding the appropriate dose, site of injection, or number or timing of injections that may contribute to the variable success that is reported. However, in patients who have not responded to standard dietary measures and medical therapy, such as topical nitroglycerin or

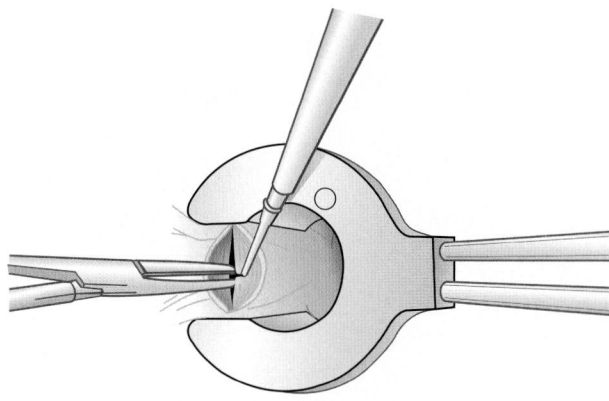

Figure 51-13 Partial lateral internal sphincterotomy, closed technique. With an operating scope in place, a small transverse incision is made along the intersphincteric groove. The mucosa is elevated, and the underlying internal sphincter is elevated and divided to release the tight band. (By permission of Mayo Foundation.)

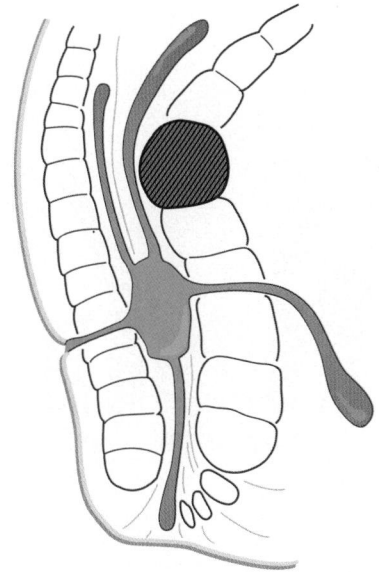

Figure 51-14 The various modes of spread from the primary locus in the intersphincteric zone of the midanal canal. The puborectalis muscle has been *crosshatched* for easy recognition. (From Parks AG, Gordon PH, Hardcastle JD: A classification of fistula-in-ano. Br J Surg 63:4, 1976.)

calcium channel blockers, and who are at high risk for complications from surgery or wish to avoid surgery, botulinum injection may be a reasonable alternative treatment.

Surgical Treatment

Patients with chronic fissures who fail medical therapy either for persistent or recurrent disease and those who develop complications can benefit from surgical therapy. The anal stretch procedure (the Lord procedure) is no longer favored, and the most commonly performed procedure is the partial lateral internal sphincterotomy. An alternate surgical approach is the anorectal advancement flap. The flap procedure is particularly attractive for patients with low anal pressures, that is, those who have failed previous sphincterotomy despite a postoperative lowering of anal pressure, and for those with severe anal stenosis. The management of fissures in the setting of Crohn's disease is discussed in the section on perianal Crohn's disease.

Partial lateral internal sphincterotomy can be performed using the closed or open (Fig. 51-13) technique, depending on surgeon preference, training, and experience. Although open sphincterotomy is more appealing from a training standpoint because the internal sphincter can be directly visualized and the extent of transection more readily quantitated, results from the literature do not support better healing rates for the open technique and generally describe a greater frequency of complications. In the past, fissure excision was described as part of the sphincterotomy procedure; it is now accepted that fissure excision is not necessary for achieving complete fissure healing. When open and closed sphincterotomy are considered together, large series confirm high success rates, with rates of fissure nonhealing and recurrence as low as 0% to 10%.[42] Early and late complications can occur after lateral internal sphincterotomy, including urinary retention, bleeding, and abscess or fistula formation as well as seepage and, rarely, incontinence.[42]

Anorectal Suppuration

Although anorectal suppuration may have several causes, by far the most common is a nonspecific infection of cryptoglandular origin. Other causes are rare, except for Crohn's disease and hidradenitis suppurativa. The pathogenesis of abscesses and fistulas is usually the same, with the abscess representing the acute phase and the fistula the chronic sequela.

Abscess

Infection originates in the intersphincteric plane, most likely in one of the anal glands. This may result in a simple intersphincteric abscess, or it may extend vertically either upward or downward (Fig. 51-14), horizontally (Fig. 51-15), or circumferentially (Fig. 51-16), resulting in a number of clinical presentations.

Clinical Presentation: Types of Abscesses

An intersphincteric abscess is limited to the primary site of origin and may be asymptomatic or result in severe, throbbing pain that resembles the pain of a fissure. Pain persisting after adequate treatment of a coexisting fissure should raise suspicion of an underlying, unrecognized intersphincteric abscess. A perianal abscess results from the vertical downward spread of the intersphincteric infection to the anal margin and presents as a tender swelling, which can be misinterpreted as a thrombosed external hemorrhoid.

If the infection spreads vertically upward, an intermuscular abscess within the rectal wall or a supralevator abscess may develop, depending on which side of the longitudinal muscle the infection has tracked. These

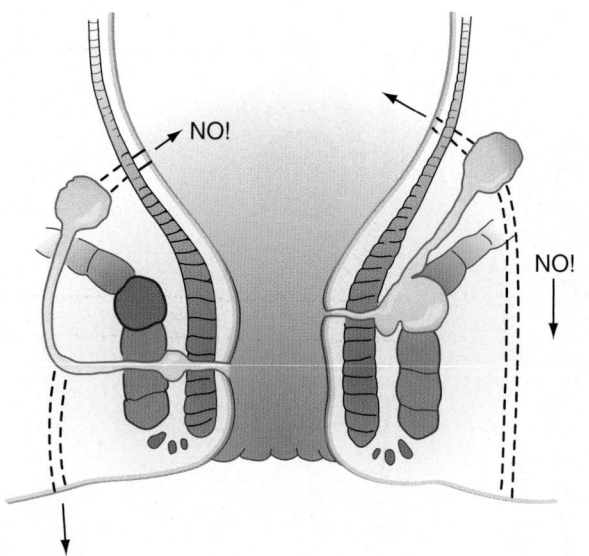

Figure 51-15 Diagram demonstrates the two ways in which an acute pararectal abscess can form. It is essential that drainage be carried out in a way appropriate to the type. If incorrectly performed, a different extrasphincteric or suprasphincteric fistula may ensue. (From Parks AG, Gordon PH, Hardcastle JD: A classification of fistula-in-ano. Br J Surg 63:10, 1976.)

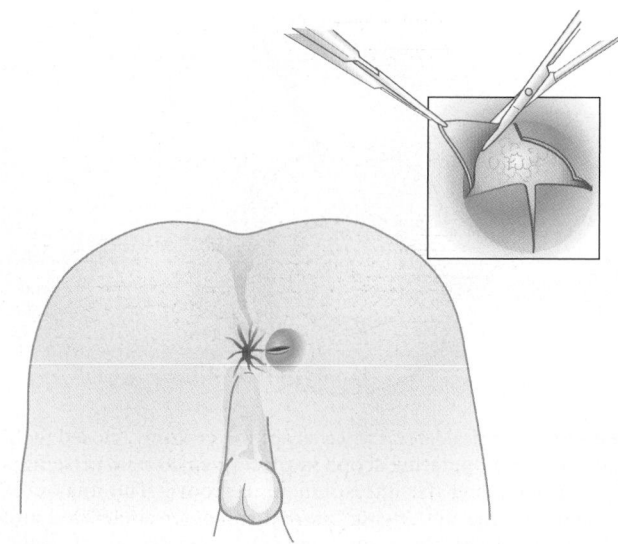

Figure 51-17 Incision and drainage of an anorectal abscess. A cruciate incision is made and the wound probed for loculations. The wound edges are kept open to facilitate proper drainage by excising the corners of the cruciate (*inset*) and packing the cavity. (By permission of Mayo Foundation.)

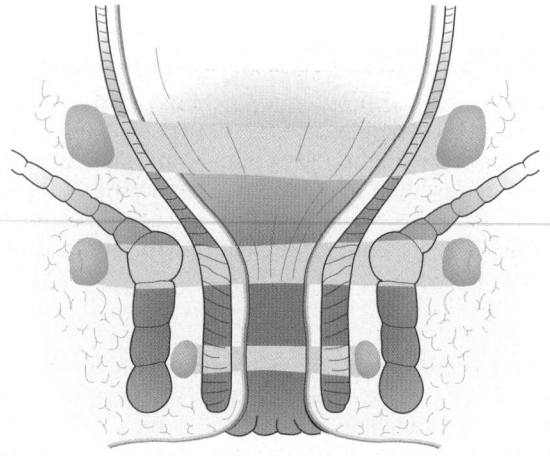

Figure 51-16 Diagram illustrates the three planes in which circumferential spread, or "horseshoeing," can occur. (From Parks AG, Gordon PH, Hardcastle JD: A classification of fistula-in-ano. Br J Surg 63:11, 1976.)

abscesses are difficult to diagnose because the patient may complain of vague discomfort, external manifestations are absent, and the presence of rectal induration and swelling may be clearly established only with the aid of an examination under anesthesia.

Horizontal spread of infection may track across the internal sphincter into the anal canal or in the opposite direction across the external sphincter into the ischiorectal fossa to form an ischiorectal abscess. The abscess may be large, especially if neglected or treated only with antibiotics and allowed to expand to the roof of the fossa or even through it into the supralevator space after tra-

versing the levator ani muscle and downward to the perianal skin. The patient may complain of pain and fever before an erythematous mass is detectable. Ultimately, an obvious red, fluctuant mass is visible. The infectious process may spread circumferentially from one side to the other of the intersphincteric space, the supralevator space, or the ischiorectal fossa, producing the complex, horseshoe abscess.

Treatment

Abscesses should be drained when diagnosed. Simple and superficial abscesses can most often be drained under local anesthesia in the office setting in patients who are otherwise healthy. Patients who manifest systemic symptoms; those who are immunocompromised for any reason, including acquired immunodeficiency syndrome (AIDS), diabetes, cancer therapies, or chronic medical immunosuppression; and those with complex, complicated abscesses are best treated in a hospital setting.

An intersphincteric abscess is drained by dividing the internal sphincter at the level of the abscess. For a perianal abscess, a simple skin incision is all that is necessary (Fig. 51-17). Both an intermuscular abscess and a supralevator abscess, so long as it is not an ischiorectal abscess extension, need to be drained into the lower rectum and upper anal canal. An ischiorectal abscess requires immediate, wide local drainage through an appropriate cruciform incision through the skin and subcutaneous tissue overlying the infected space. At times, these abscesses are sufficiently deep that needle localization of the purulent material may be required to guide the surgeon for optimizing the skin incision site. The cavity should be gently digitalized to break down loculations. Neglected

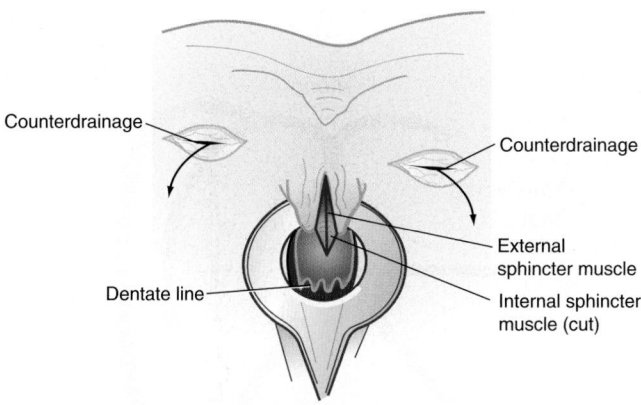

Figure 51-18 Modification of Hanley's technique for incision and drainage of a horseshoe abscess. (From Gordon PH: Anorectal abscesses and fistula-in-ano. In Gordon PH, Nivatvongs S [eds]: Principles and Practice of Surgery for the Colon, Rectum, and Anus, 2nd ed. St. Louis, Quality Medical, 1992, p 232.)

Table 51-3 Classification of Anorectal Fistulas

Intersphincteric (the most common): The fistula track is confined to the intersphincteric plane.

Trans-sphincteric: The fistula connects the intersphincteric plane with the ischiorectal fossa by perforating the external sphincter.

Suprasphincteric: Similar to trans-sphincteric, but the track loops over the external sphincter and perforates the levator ani.

Extrasphincteric: The track passes from the rectum to perineal skin, completely external to the sphincteric complex.

Adapted from classification by Parks AG, Gordon PH, Hardcastle JD: A classification of fistula-in-ano. Br J Surg 63:1, 1976.

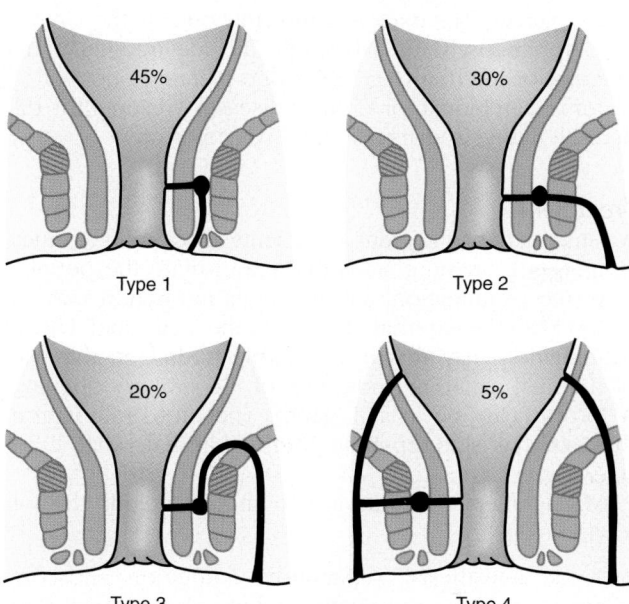

Figure 51-19 The four main anatomic types of fistulas. The external sphincter mass is regarded as the keystone, and the prefixes trans, supra, and extra refer to it. The puborectalis muscle has been *crosshatched* for easy recognition. Type 1, intersphincteric; type 2, trans-sphincteric; type 3, suprasphincteric; type 4, extrasphincteric. (From Parks AG, Gordon PH, Hardcastle JD: A classification of fistula-in-ano. Br J Surg 63:5, 1976.)

abscesses can lead to devastating, necrotizing infections of the perineum that can spread and become lethal. Failure of response to local treatment or recurrent abscesses may suggest inadequate drainage with residual pus, the presence of a fistula, or immunoincompetence. Under these circumstances, antibiotics may be useful, together with examination under anesthesia after preliminary evaluation by computed tomography (CT) of the pelvis and perineum. For horseshoe abscess, the deep postanal space should be drained through a posterior midline incision extending from the subcutaneous portion of the external sphincter over the abscess to the tip of the coccyx, separating the superficial external sphincter and thus unroofing the postanal space and its ischioanal extension (Fig. 51-18). Para-anal incisions can be made and setons placed to drain the anterior extensions of a horseshoe abscess.

Fistula in Ano

Anorectal sepsis can be complicated by a fistula in ano in about 25% of patients during the acute phase of sepsis or within 6 months thereafter.[43] Most fistulas derive from sepsis originating in the anal canal glands at the dentate line. The path of a fistula is determined by the local anatomy; most commonly, they track in the fascial or fatty planes, especially the intersphincteric space between the internal and the external sphincter into the ischiorectal fascia. In such instances, the track passes directly to the perineal skin. In some cases, circumferential spread may also occur in the ischiorectal fossa, with the track passing from one fossa to the contralateral one through the posterior rectum, a fistula known as the horseshoe fistula. Fistulas usually fall under four main anatomic categories as described by Parks and colleagues in 1976[44] (Table 51-3 and Fig. 51-19).

Clinical Presentation: Types of Fistulas

Intersphincteric fistulas are the most common anal fistulas, and in most cases, the infection passes directly down-

ward to the anal margin. However, there are some variants of this type of fistula that are less common and more complex to treat. For instance, the track may travel upward in the rectal wall (higher track), with or without a perineal opening. Rarely, an intersphincteric fistula originates in the pelvis from the colon.[44] In trans-sphincteric fistulas, the track traverses the external sphincter to travel through the ischiorectal fossa and end at the perineal skin. If it passes through the muscle at a low level, it is uncomplicated and readily treatable; if, however, it penetrates the upper portion of the sphincter (high blind track), it constitutes a more difficult therapeutic dilemma.

Indeed, it may be felt digitally through the wall of the rectum and may lead the surgeon to create an artificial connection with the rectum by forceful probing, a situation that can be difficult to correct. Suprasphincteric fistulas are rare, difficult to treat, and may be hazardous if dealt with by inexperienced surgeons.

The track may first travel upward in the intersphincteric plane before taking a lateral direction over the top of the puborectalis and finally downward through the ischiorectal fossa to the perineal skin. Because its trajectory is above all muscles of importance to continence, division of all external muscles results in incontinence. Moreover, the fistula may have an additional extension into the pelvis that runs parallel to the rectum (high blind track). In this instance, an indurated area can be palpated through the rectal wall. Finally, extrasphincteric fistula is rare, and its treatment is also hazardous. It travels from the perineal skin to the rectal wall above the levator ani that it pierces. The track is completely outside the sphincteric apparatus. Causes typically include trauma, either external or internal (e.g., fish bone piercing one wall of rectum), carcinoma, or Crohn's disease. Treatment is difficult, lengthy, and usually involves colostomy.

Treatment

A fistula may first present as an acute abscess or, at times, simply as a draining sinus that may irritate the perineal skin. On examination, subcutaneous induration may be traced from the external opening to the anal canal. Digital examination may reveal a palpable nodule in the wall of the anal canal, an indication of the primary opening. A probe can be eased gently (not forcefully) from the external skin opening to the internal, anal canal opening.

Management of fistula in ano should include the following steps:

1. Under anesthesia, palpation for induration, anoscopy for inspection, and gentle probing along the dentate for internal openings allows accurate definition of the abnormal anatomy. The Goodsall rule (Fig. 51-20) is useful for anticipating the anatomy of simple fistulas. If the internal opening cannot be identified by direct probing, it should be identified by probing the external opening or by injecting a mixture of methylene blue and peroxide into the track using a pediatric feeding tube (Fig. 51-21A).
2. Drainage of primary intersphincteric infection in all types of fistulas, as well as the primary track across the external sphincter and secondary tracks within the anorectal fossa, is key. For superficial fistulas involving small quantities of sphincter muscle, primary fistulotomy is simple and definitive. For anterior fistulas in women and fistulas involving greater than one fourth to one half the bulk of sphincter muscles, seton placement should be preferred over primary fistulotomy (see Fig. 51-21 B to D).
3. Close follow-up and careful nursing of the wound by a physician-nurse team involve sitz baths and wound dressing to ensure healing from the depth of the wound to the surface. A seton of monofilament nylon

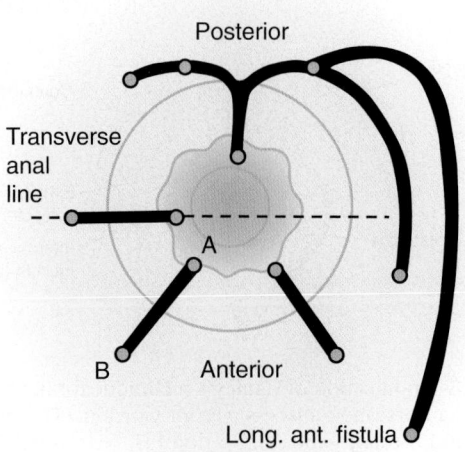

Figure 51-20 The Goodsall rule. The usual relationship of primary and secondary fistula orifices is diagrammed. The internal (primary orifice) is marked A. The rule predicts that if a line is drawn transversely across the anus, an external opening (B) anterior to this line will lead to a straight radial tract, whereas an external opening that lies posterior to the line will lead to a curved tract and an internal opening in the posterior commissure. The long anterior fistula is an exception to the rule. (From Schrock TR: Benign and malignant disease of the anorectum. In Fromm O [ed]: Gastrointestinal Surgery. New York, Churchill Livingstone, 1985, p 612.)

tied loosely around the fistulous track may be used to drain the trans-sphincteric track traveling above the anal valves for a suprasphincteric fistula. The seton may be removed 2 to 3 months later, at which time the track may heal spontaneously. If not, the track may be divided because fibrosis may cause minimal separation of the cut ends. For more straightforward trans-sphincteric fistulas, a cutting seton can be placed at surgery and tightened in the office. This divides the track gradually over a few weeks and minimizes the sphincter defect and the risk for significant fecal incontinence.

In rare circumstances with complex, deep, or recurrent fistulas, newer alternatives to fistulotomy are preferred to avoid the complication of fecal incontinence. Currently, there are two therapies that use biologic material to promote the closure of fistulas without division of any sphincter muscle: injection of fibrin glue into the fistula track and insertion of a porcine small intestinal submucosa (SIS) plug. Both products are thought to promote healing of the track by providing a naturally derived extracellular matrix to act as scaffolding, allowing ingrowth of host tissue for incorporation and remodeling. Fibrin glue is a multicomponent system with the primary agents being human pooled plasma fibrinogen and thrombin. Once prepared, the fibrin glue components are injected into the anal fistula track. Over a matter of minutes, the glue hardens and fills the entire track. Initially, successful fistula closure rates of nearly 70% were

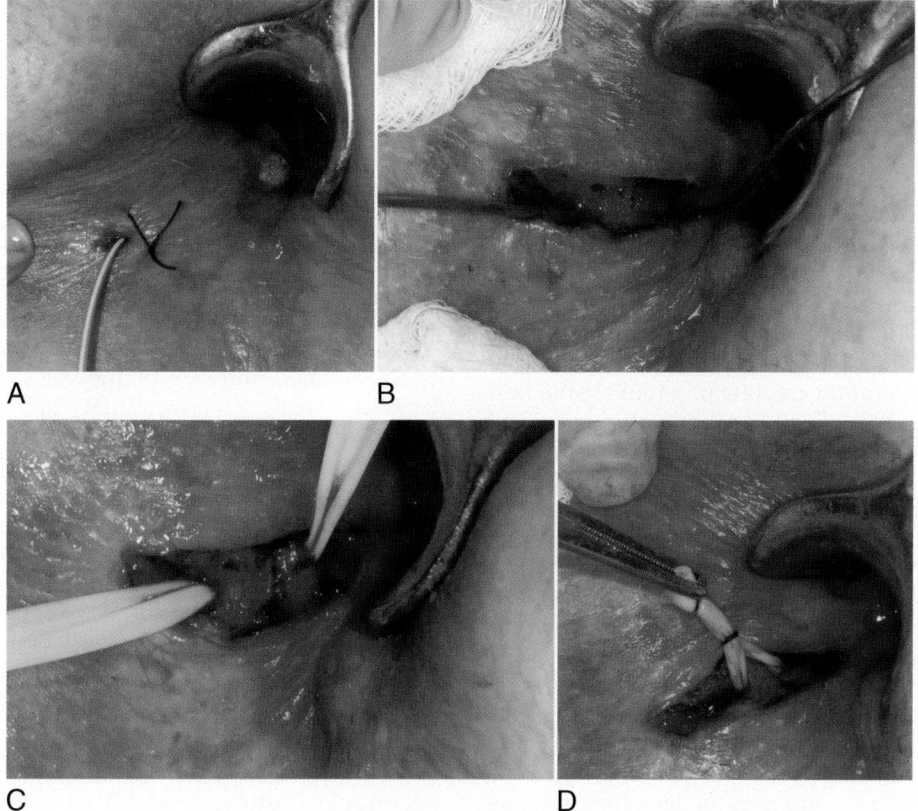

Figure 51-21 Seton placement. **A,** If the primary opening cannot be identified by gentle probing along the dentate line, methylene blue plus peroxide injections may better delineate the internal fistula source. **B,** A probe is passed from the primary to the secondary openings, and the skin is incised to reveal the tract and interposed sphincter muscle. **C,** An elastic cutting seton can be placed when generous muscle requires division. **D,** The seton is tightened in the operating room and again once or twice in the office to allow for fibrosis and gradual sphincter transection. (By permission of Mayo Foundation.)

reported.[45] More recently, a comprehensive review of the literature reported that fibrin glue injection resulted in a broad range of successful fistula closure from 14% to 60%.[39] This review included a randomized control trial of fibrin glue compared to standard treatment of fistulas which demonstrated no difference in closure rate or patient satisfaction with the procedure.[45] The only real difference was that fibrin glue patients returned to work earlier than the conventionally treated patients.

Based on this premise of providing scaffolding for tissue in-growth, a new biologically based product has recently become available, SurgiSis Anal Fistula Plug. This cone-shaped product is made of a porcine SIS. It is physically inserted into the fistula and then secured to the internal and external opening of the anal fistula with absorbable suture. Over time, tissue from the fistula wall will grow into the SIS plug and replace the matrix of the plug with new viable tissue that obliterates the fistula track. There has only been one recently published report of the use of an SIS plug in the treatment of benign anal fistulas.[46] In this small series, patients were treated either with fibrin glue or an SIS plug. The 3-month fistula closure was 60% in the fibrin glue and 87% in the SIS plug group. Although the success rate of fistula closure for both of these products is variable or relatively

unknown because of their recent clinical introduction, the benefit is that there is no permanent injury to the anal sphincter mechanism and, therefore, no risk for incontinence related to the treatment. If either modality fails to close the fistula, the patient has not been harmed.

Difficult and persistent high fistulas can be treated by sliding flap advancement made of mucosa, submucosa, and circular muscle to cover the internal opening. The Goodsall rule (see Fig. 51-20) is of little help in defining the anatomy of complex and recurrent fistulas. Diagnostic tests such as pelvic MRI and endorectal ultrasound and treatment by a specialist may be helpful here.

Pilonidal Disease

Pilonidal infections and chronic pilonidal sinuses typically occur in the midline of the sacrococcygeal skin of young men. Although the exact pathogenesis of pilonidal disease remains elusive and controversial, hair seems to play a central role in the process of infection and in the perpetuation of granulation tissue in sinuses. This is consistent with the clinical observation that pilonidal patients are often hirsute and that pilonidal disease rarely occurs in populations with less body hair.[47] It is uncommon for pilonidal disease to be confused with clinical disorders such as anal fistulas, skin disorders, underlying malignancies, or true sacrococcygeal sinuses.

Acute Management

Patients presenting acutely with new-onset disease may have a painful fluctuant abscess or a draining infected sinus. Both can be managed with simple office therapies, with more definitive procedures reserved for patients who suffer from a recurrence. Abscess can be drained in the office or emergency department using local anesthesia. Typically, the fluctuance extends to either side of the midline cleft, and incision and drainage down to the subcutaneous tissues off the midline provides for the best drainage and fastest healing. For both abscesses and sinuses, hair should be removed from the wound, and local skin should be shaved weekly to prevent the reintroduction of hair. Laser depilation can also be used to accomplish long-lasting, but temporary, hair removal. Ideally, these patients should be seen weekly in the office for wound care until there is complete healing. Most do not require further care; those who do can be treated as described in the following section.

Operative Management

For those patients who have recurring infections, more definitive operative management is warranted. Numerous procedures have been described in the literature, ranging from simple incision and drainage to complex plastic flaps for cleft obliteration.[47]

Incision and curettage are advocated by some as the simplest approach to pilonidal disease. After a probe is placed in the sinus, an incision is made over the probe, incising the overlying pits followed by curetting the granulation tissue.[47] Daily care with dry dressings and weekly office visits are required for postoperative management. Wound healing typically requires 4 to 7 weeks, and recurrence rates vary from 1% to 20%.[47] A more common approach is the simple excision without closure. The entire pilonidal cyst is removed and the wound left to heal by secondary intention, typically requiring 8 to 21 weeks. Recurrence rates are low with this technique, at 2% to 3%.[47] It is appealing to consider excision with immediate closure of the wound because wound healing takes only 2 to 7 weeks; however, recurrences are more likely to occur at rates of 11% to 29%.[47] A technique that is intermediate to the excision with or without closure is that of marsupialization, where the wound edges are approximated to the fibrous base of the pilonidal cyst. Reducing the size of the wound reduces the healing times to less than 5 weeks and keeps recurrence rates low at between 1% and 4%.[47]

Most other procedures described for pilonidal disease focus on off-midline procedures such as the Bascom[48] or a plastic flap reconstruction like the Limberg[49] or Karydakis.[47] The Bascom procedure involves the excision of the midline pits coupled with a lateral incision for off-midline drainage of the underlying abscess.[48] With minimal postoperative care, these wounds heal in 4 weeks, and recurrence rates are as low as 10%.[48] The rhomboid excision and Limberg flap are one example of

a flap technique for complete removal of the site of disease and subsequent primary tissue closure.[49] The disadvantage of the flap techniques include the complexity of the procedures; the necessity for inpatient hospitalization, typically less than a week; and the fact that recurrences can still occur in 5% of cases.[49]

LESS COMMON BENIGN ANAL DISORDERS

Rectovaginal Fistula

A rectovaginal fistula is a communication between the epithelial-lined surfaces of the rectum and the vagina. Patients usually complain that they pass gas, mucus, blood, or stool through the vagina. Rectovaginal fistulas may be congenital or acquired through trauma, inflammatory bowel disease, irradiation, neoplasia, infection, or other rare causes. For those fistulas associated with a history of trauma, anal manometry and endoanal ultrasound can determine the severity of underlying sphincter defect and help guide surgical therapies. Rectovaginal fistulas are classified as high or low depending on whether they can be corrected transabdominally or transperineally, respectively.

Surgical Repair

Rectovaginal fistulas need not be corrected immediately, and delay depends on the underlying disease, the size of the fistula, the presence of active inflammation, and the severity of the symptoms. Some fistulas may close spontaneously, whereas others, like those associated with inflammatory bowel disease, may heal with medical therapy alone. High rectovaginal fistulas require a transabdominal approach, whereas low rectovaginal fistulas can be approached transvaginally, transrectally, transperineally, trans-sphincterically, or transanally.

The most common surgical approaches to the low-lying fistula (typically a true anovaginal fistula) are the endorectal advancement flap, sphincteroplasty, and transperineal procedures.[50] An endorectal advancement flap consists of a flap raised of rectal mucosa and underlying internal sphincter that is advanced to cover the primary fistula's opening in the rectum or anus after the fistula's opening has been excised and the underlying muscle reapproximated. The flap is best suited for the first attempt at repair or in patients without evidence of an underlying sphincter defect and is accordingly associated with a healing rate of 50%. The transperineal repair completely excises the fistula tract and accomplishes a primary reapproximation of the internal, external, and levator muscles in discrete layers. Success rates are as high as 85% to 100% in patients with associated sphincter defects who have already failed other approaches.[50]

For high rectovaginal fistulas, a transabdominal approach is necessary. Whether a portion or the entire rectum is sacrificed depends on the nature and extent of the underlying disease. This approach involves mobilization of the rectovaginal septum, division of the fistula, and a layer closure of the rectal and vaginal defects. In some cases, no rectal resection is necessary, and a live pedicle of tissue may be interposed between the two anastomotic structures to supplement the repair. When rectal tissues are involved by severe irradiation changes, inflammatory bowel disease, or neoplasia, rectal excision is required. Whenever possible, the sphincter apparatus can be preserved using either a low anterior resection or coloanal anastomosis.[50] Whether the outcome of such procedures is favorable or not depends on the underlying disease, selection of patients, and experience and expertise of the surgeon.

In the setting of Crohn's disease, the low anovaginal fistula represents a unique challenge. Primary repair avoids the need for a permanent stoma and can be accomplished in up to 68% of patients using a variety of horizontal, linear, and sleeve advancement flaps.

Condyloma Acuminatum

Condyloma acuminatum is a perineal wart disease caused by the human papillomavirus (HPV); some types are transmitted through sexual contact. Certain types, such as HPV-6 and HPV-11, are found in benign warts, whereas others, such as HPV-16 and HPV-18, are more aggressive and more commonly associated with dysplasia and malignancies. Its incidence has increased considerably since the mid-1960s, and it is the most common STD seen by colorectal surgeons, with a million new cases seen yearly. Most patients with anal condylomata have a history of anal-receptive intercourse, and the occurrence of anal HPV infection is strongly related to human immunodeficiency virus (HIV)-associated immunosuppression.

Clinical Presentation

The usual symptoms include pruritus ani, bleeding, pain, discharge, and wetness. Examination reveals pinkish-white warts of varying sizes that may coalesce to form a mass, often foul smelling (Fig. 51-22). Anoscopy may reveal extension in the anal canal. A giant form of the disease has been observed rarely (Buschke-Löwenstein disease). Such lesions can invade, fistulize, and be associated with verrucous carcinoma and squamous cell carcinomas. The diagnosis is based on direct inspection of the perineum and genital organs; anoscopy and proctosigmoidoscopy must be performed because the disease extends intra-anally and a small percentage of patients have only intra-anal disease. The diagnosis is confirmed histologically. Anal warts must be differentiated from condylomata molluscum contagiosum, secondary syphilis, and enlarged anal papillae.

Treatment

Many treatments have been proposed and used, but none offers complete resolution of the disease process. Podophyllin, which is cytotoxic to condylomata but irritating to normal skin, must be applied to the warts. Its use should be limited to minimal disease and extra-anal warts and not repeated because of local complications and potential systemic toxicity. It requires no anesthesia and is inexpensive, but the results are often disappointing. Dichloroacetic acid (bichloracetic acid) can be used to destroy both perianal and intra-anal warts, and it is less

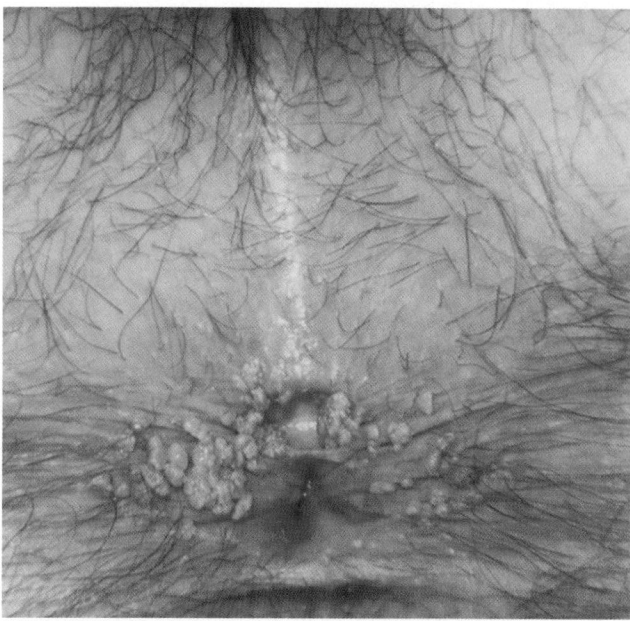

Figure 51-22 Perianal condyloma acuminatum. (By permission of Mayo Foundation.)

irritating than podophyllin. The recurrence rate with both agents is much higher than with surgical excision. Intramuscular or intralesional interferon-beta is somewhat effective but may be complicated by systemic symptoms and an influenza-like syndrome.

Electrocauterization with a needle tip is effective and used extensively, often in combination with excision. Local, regional, or general anesthesia is necessary. Carbon dioxide laser can also be effective but is more expensive and offers no added benefits. With either technique, vapors should be aspirated. Excision with small scissors is preferred because it is precise, provides a tissue diagnosis, minimizes destruction of intervening skin, and can be used on larger lesions (Fig. 51-23). General or regional anesthesia is necessary.

None of the therapeutic options is completely satisfactory; they all are associated with a significant chance of recurrence. Combination of treatments may be valuable. Because recurrence is frequent, close follow-up of patients is recommended.

Sexually Transmitted Diseases and Acquired Immunodeficiency Syndrome

STDs, formerly referred to as venereal diseases, are exceeded in frequency only by the common cold and influenza. Multiple partners and anal-receptive intercourse increases the risk for STD transmission.[51] STDs can be bacterial, viral, or parasitic in origin (Table 51-4), and a variety of sexual practices may favor their development.

Clinical Presentation

Patients with bacterial STDs may have no symptoms or may have symptoms of pruritus, bloody or mucopurulent

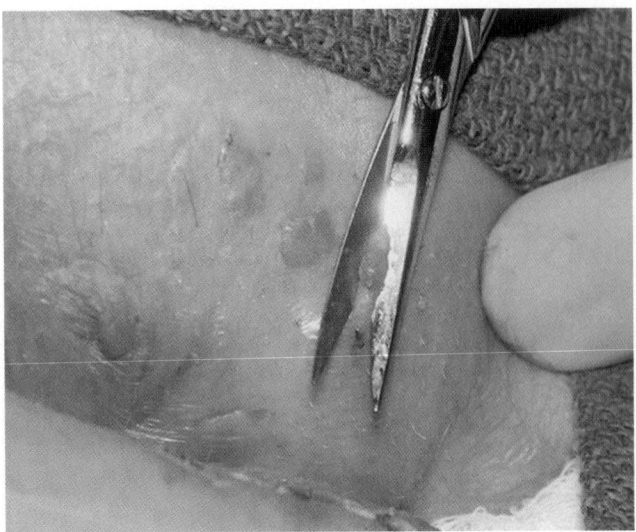

Figure 51-23 Sharp excision of perianal condyloma is facilitated by the raising of the lesion by the injection of a local anesthetic agent. (By permission of Mayo Foundation.)

Table 51-4 Organisms That Cause Sexually Transmitted Diseases

Bacterial
Neisseria gonorrhoeae
Treponema pallidum
Haemophilus ducreyi
Chlamydia species
Shigella flexneri
Campylobacter species
Viral
Herpes simplex
Human papillomavirus
Molluscum contagiosum
Parasitic
Entamoeba histolytica
Giardia lamblia
Cryptococcus species
Isospora belli

rectal discharge, tenesmus, perineal or rectal pain, diarrhea, and fever. Depending on the etiologic agent, proctoscopy may reveal proctitis, discharge (mucopurulent in gonorrhea or *Campylobacter* species infection, bloody in chlamydial infection), anal ulcerations, and abscesses. The diagnosis is based on the clinical signs and physical examination, including endoscopy and cultures of stool or discharge specimens. Treatment is based on the causative agent.

Patients with viral STDs may complain of anorectal pain, discharge, bleeding, and pruritus. In molluscum contagiosum, the patient has painless dermal lesions that are flattened, round, and umbilicated. Endoscopy may reveal vesicles, ulcers, and diffuse friability as in herpes or anal warts in condylomata. The diagnosis is based on cultures, scrapings, or excisional biopsy. Herpes is best treated with acyclovir, whereas the other viral lesions are treated by destruction or excision.[51]

Patients with parasitic STDs have more systemic symptoms, such as fever, abdominal cramping, and bloody diarrhea. Ulcerations due to *Entamoeba histolytica* are typically hourglass shaped, whereas they are more diffuse when caused by *Giardia lamblia*. Diagnosis is based on biopsy specimens or scrapings and specific stains. *E. histolytica* and *G. lamblia* are treated with metronidazole, and *Isospora belli* is managed with cotrimoxazole.

Acquired Immunodeficiency Syndrome

Anorectal pathology is common in patients who are HIV positive, affecting about one third of patients at some point in their disease.[52] Anorectal pain, the presence of a mass, and bleeding per rectum are the most frequent presenting complaints.[52] In a consecutive series of 260 HIV-positive patients, the most frequently occurring diseases were condylomata (42%), fistulas (34%), and fissures (32%).[52] For benign noninfectious disorders, fissures and ulcers are the most common presenting problem.

This is uniquely different from HIV-negative patients, in whom the primary presenting diagnoses are hemorrhoids and skin tags.[53] In seeing patients with HIV, it is important to distinguish between anal fissures that are amenable to medical therapy or lateral internal sphincterotomy and anal ulcers that respond best to operative evaluation, biopsy, viral culture, débridement, and topical antiviral therapy.[53] Herpes, cytomegalovirus, and *Chlamydia* species are the most typical infectious agents.[52]

Neoplastic disorders in HIV-positive patients include condyloma, anal intraepithelial neoplasia, epidermoid carcinoma, and Kaposi sarcoma, the incidence of each of these being higher in HIV-positive than HIV-negative patients.[52-54] Although therapies for anal condyloma are no different based on HIV status, the recurrence rates appear to be higher for HIV-positive than HIV-negative patients. For the management of in situ and invasive squamous cell carcinoma, it appears that the CD4 count and concomitant treatment with antiretroviral therapy are keys to success with local excision and radiation plus chemotherapy, respectively.

Best-practice strategies for anorectal conditions complicating HIV are likely to evolve as we acquire more effective therapies to treat HIV-infected patients.

Hidradenitis Suppurativa

Hidradenitis suppurativa is a chronic inflammatory process affecting the apocrine glands of the perianal region characterized by abscesses and sinus formation. Although recent dermatologic investigations call into question the site of origin of hidradenitis, implicating occluding spongiform infundibulofolliculitis, a follicular disease, hidradenitis has traditionally been considered the result of keratotic debris plugging the apocrine gland. The plugging event is followed by bacterial proliferation, suppurative infection, gland rupture, and spread of inflammation to surrounding subcutaneous tissues. Numerous tracks and pits develop, and the tissues become

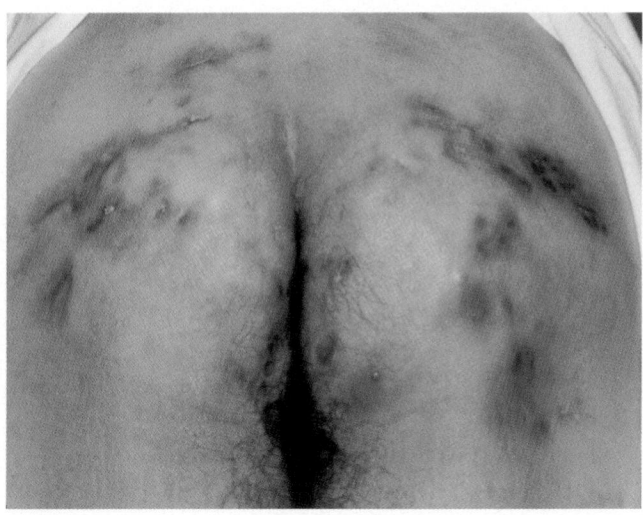

Figure 51-24 Hidradenitis suppurativa. (By permission of Mayo Foundation.)

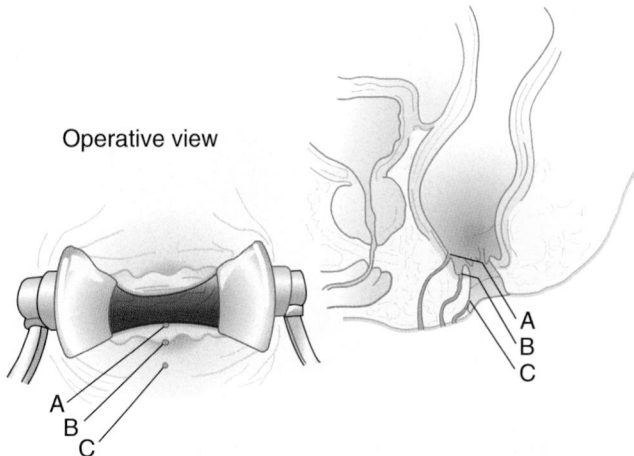

Operative view

Figure 51-25 Relationship of fistulous tracks in Crohn's disease, above dentate line (A); cryptoglandular abscess/fistula disease at dentate line (B); and hidradenitis suppurativa, distal to dentate line (C). (From Culp CE: Chronic hidradenitis suppurativa of the anal canal: A surgical skin disease. Dis Colon Rectum 26:669-676, 1983.)

fibrotic and thickened from the persistent inflammatory response. A number of factors have been implicated in the development and perpetuation of hidradenitis, including the use of depilatories, close shaving, poor personal hygiene, tight-fitting and synthetic clothing, and antiperspirants. The most common bacterial organisms identified include *Streptococcus milleri* and *Staphylococcus aureus, Staphylococcus epidermidis,* and *Staphylococcus hominis.*[55]

Clinical Presentation

Clinically, patients may complain of burning, itching, and hyperhidrosis. Affected patients frequently have seborrheic skin and sometimes have involvement of other areas where apocrine sweat glands are present, such as the axillae and the mammary, inguinal, and genital regions. The affected areas have a purplish appearance with drainage of watery pus. In advanced cases, numerous fistulous tracks are readily identified, and the appearance is classic (Fig. 51-24). When the condition presents early and there are limited fistulous tracks around the anal and perianal tissues, hidradenitis must be differentiated from other types of fistulas, such as those arising from Crohn's disease or infected crypts. Fistulas from hidradenitis arise distal to the dentate in the anal skin, allowing their differentiation from cryptoglandular fistulas, which communicate with the dentate line, and Crohn's disease, which may track to the anorectum proximal to the dentate line[56] (Fig. 51-25). Hidradenitis is more common in women and blacks; however, perianal hidradenitis is more common in men.

Treatment

Perianal hidradenitis can present in one of several states from early acute to late chronic and severe forms and can present alone or with associated complications, such as severe anal fibrosis and incontinence, or even co-presentation with squamous malignancies.[55] To exclude the possibility of coexisting cancer, biopsies should be performed with liberal indications. For early, limited

disease, emphasis should be placed on incision and drainage of infections and prevention of recurrences. The role of oral antibiotic treatment, typically erythromycin, is not established but often recommended. Although not proved, frequent cleansing and warm-water soaking, avoidance of tight-fitting and synthetic clothing, and avoidance of local chemical irritants may help prevent further disease or may reduce the severity of active disease.

When hidradenitis sinus tracks are well established but relatively superficial, they can be unroofed, or laid open.[56] Because these tracks are lined by epithelium, the floor of the track can be preserved; this facilitates rapid healing and minimizes scarring. For more extensive and deeper disease, wide excision may be required. Although wide excision is thought to be more effective for advanced cases, it is associated with recurrence rates of about 50%, when both same-site and new-site disease are considered. In cases of aggressive wide excision, large wounds can be managed primarily, with delayed healing, flaps, or skin grafts. Wound closure can be tailored to the specific conditions of each patient. Skin grafting offers the advantage of early wound coverage with a reduction in pain and time to complete healing but requires compliance with delicate postoperative wound care. Healing by secondary intention requires less delicate wound care but takes 2 to 3 months for complete healing to be accomplished.[55]

Crohn's Disease of the Anorectum

Clinical Presentation

Anal manifestations of Crohn's disease can be most devastating because of their painful nature and their threat to the patient's continence,[57] and they occur in nearly 20% of patients with Crohn's disease. Patients may suffer from fissures, fistulas, and abscesses. Symptoms and signs of anal Crohn's disease may include pain, swelling, bleed-

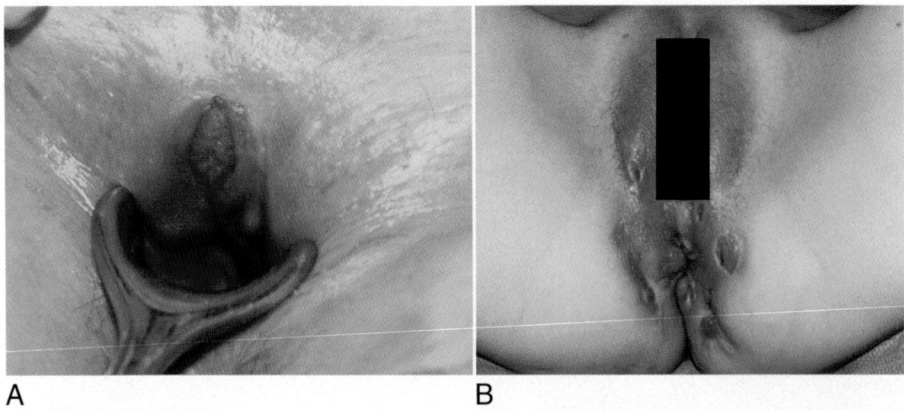

Figure 51-26 Perineal Crohn's disease. **A,** Characteristic of Crohn's fissures are the shaggy edges, deep ulceration, and granulation tissue. **B,** Uncontrolled perianal Crohn's with multiple fistulas can present as a "watering pot" perineum. (By permission of Mayo Foundation.)

ing, soilage or frank incontinence, and fever. Pain may be due to skin excoriation and maceration, hemorrhoids, fissures, or abscess and fistula disease[57] (Fig. 51-26). Edematous, purplish tags are characteristic of the disease. Bleeding may be from distal proctitis, fissures, hemorrhoids, or granulating fistulas. Soilage may result from prolapsing rectal mucosa, seepage of liquid stool, drainage from abscess, or poor continence. Poor continence may result from sphincter damage caused by the disease or aggressive surgery, anoperineal fistulas, rectovaginal fistulas, or loss of rectal compliance.[57]

Evaluation and Treatment

Anorectal examination should include inspection, digital examination, anoscopy, and proctosigmoidoscopy. If the examination cannot be performed satisfactorily because of pain, the patient should be evaluated under anesthesia. The remainder of the gastrointestinal tract should also be assessed. Although conservatism is paramount in importance, patients should not be undertreated if treatment is indicated. Surgery is usually warranted for pain resulting from a poorly draining or undrained abscess. Fissures caused by Crohn's disease are often multiple and located off the midline; they usually respond to conservative measures, such as sitz baths, stool softeners, and oral analgesics. Occasionally, excision of skin tags surrounding deep ulcers to favor better drainage and gentle stretch may be sufficient. Sphincterotomy and fissurectomy should be avoided when perianal Crohn's disease is present. Metronidazole and immunosuppressive drugs, such as steroids, 6-mercaptopurine, azathioprine (Imuran), and cyclosporine, have produced mixed results in the medical treatment of Crohn's perianal disease.[57] However, the introduction of the anti–tumor necrosis factor antibody, infliximab, for the medical management of Crohn's disease has significantly altered the treatment of Crohn's and specifically perianal disease.[58]

Fistulas represent a special challenge in Crohn's disease[59] (Fig. 51-27). In a number of trials, infliximab has been very successful in the treatment of fistulizing perianal Crohn's disease with closure rates between 25% and 67%.[60] The most successful strategy is a staged approach to perianal disease. Control of local sepsis is an essential first step. Abscesses need to be drained and fistula tracts require chronic drainage with noncutting setons. Once the perianal sepsis is controlled, infliximab treatment is initiated. After two to three infliximab infusions, the setons are removed to permit closure of the fistulas. If the fistulas do not close and the local sepsis has resolved, definitive surgical therapy may be undertaken. Using this staged approach in a small series of patients, van der Hagen and colleagues reported a 100% fistula closure rate at a median follow-up of 19 months.[61] A number of definitive surgical options for Crohn's perianal fistulas have been proposed. For very superficial fistulas, unroofing the track is highly successful, although healing may be prolonged. The use of local mucosal or skin advancement flaps to close fistula openings have met with variable success. Most studies report a 60% to 75% long-term closure rate.[62] Other treatment options include the use of biologic material such as fibrin glue or tissue plugs. Although these products have been used in small series so their true efficacy cannot be reported, their ease of use and low morbidity make them an attractive therapeutic option. Unfortunately, in some patients, a proctectomy may ultimately be required. The dissection should be done in the intersphincteric plane to favor better perineal healing and help reduce the risk for sexual dysfunction.

It is now increasingly recognized that patients with Crohn's disease can also present with common anorectal conditions such as fissures, abscesses, and fistulas. In the absence of evidence of rectal or perianal Crohn's, these conditions may be best treated using standard approaches. Although caution is advised against aggressive approaches when treating a Crohn's patient with anorectal problems, undertreatment of symptomatic conditions is also discouraged.

NEOPLASTIC DISORDERS

Neoplasms of the anal area are rare and represent a wide spectrum of benign and malignant tumors. Benign lesions

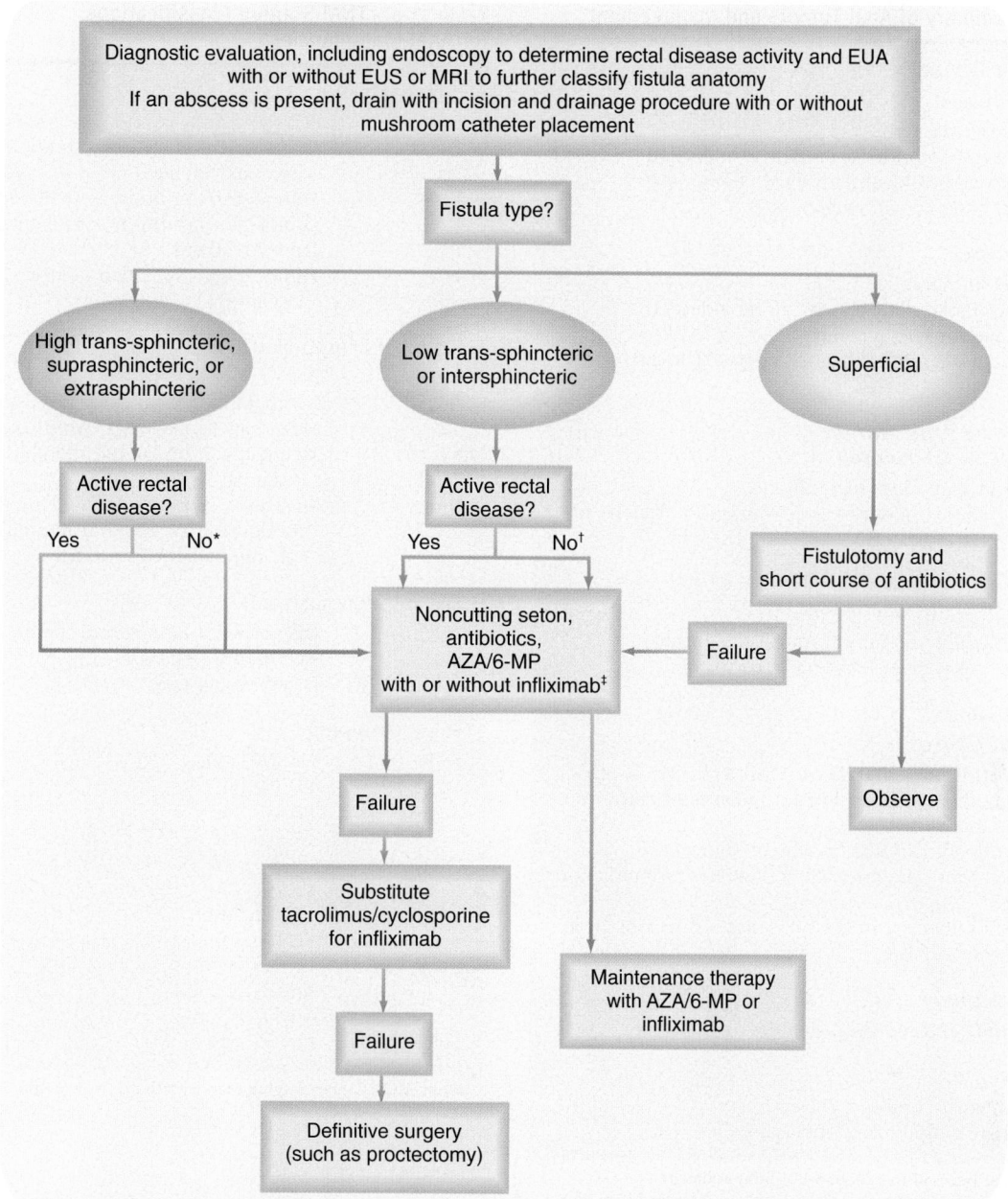

Figure 51-27 Treatment algorithm for perianal Crohn's disease. If the fistula is simple, endorectal advancement flap (*) or fistulotomy (†) can be considered. Use of infliximab should be favored if the fistula is complex, recurrent, or associated with active rectal inflammation (‡). 6-MP, 6-mercaptopurine; AZA, azathioprine; EUA, examination under anesthesia; EUS, endoscopic ultrasonography; MRI, magnetic resonance imaging. (From Schwartz DA, Pemberton JH, Sandborn WJ: Diagnosis and treatment of perianal fistulas in Crohn disease. Ann Intern Med 135:906-918, 2001.)

may range from innocuous in situ Bowen's disease to clinically aggressive verrucous lesions; malignant lesions range from favorable early-stage squamous cell cancers of the anal margin to anal canal adenocarcinoma and melanoma.[63] In all instances, it is essential for clinicians to consider tumor location with reference to clear landmarks, such as anal verge, dentate line, and anorectal ring. For a number of reasons, the anatomy of the anus should be differentiated into two parts: the anal margin and the anal canal. Although it is not always possible to

determine readily the exact anatomic origin of a large, bulky anal tumor, distinguishing between margin and canal tumors is directly relevant to the management of these tumors. For example, as described in more detail later, a squamous cell tumor of the margin is treated with excision, similar to any skin cancer, yet squamous cell cancer of the canal is treated with radiation plus chemotherapy[64] (Table 51-5).

Historically, two different lines of differentiation between the anal margin and canal have been described:

Table 51-5 Summary of Anal Tumors and Management

Anal Margin Tumors

Bowen's Disease

Accurate lesion mapping
Wide local excision with flap repair as indicated
Exclude presence of locally invasive component or
  associated gynecologic malignancy

Paget's Disease

Accurate lesion mapping
Wide local excision with flap repair as indicated
Exclude underlying malignancy
APR and chemotherapy/radiation therapy if invasive
  adenocarcinoma present

*Basal Cell and Anal Margin
Squamous Cell Carcinoma*

Local excision with clear margins
Radiation or chemotherapy in poor-prognosis lesions or
  recurrence as indicated

Verrucous Carcinoma

Wide local excision; APR if extensive
Combined-modality therapy if transformation to
  squamous cell cancer has occurred

Anal Canal Tumors

Epidermoid Cancer

Local excision if favorable T1
Combined-modality, external-beam radiation therapy plus
  5-FU plus mitomycin
APR if incontinent or local treatment failure or
  recurrence after combined chemotherapy and radiation
  therapy
Triple-modality therapy in bulky T3 and T4 lesions (role
  of APR controversial)

Adenocarcinoma

APR with 5-FU and radiation therapy as indicated

Melanoma

APR if potentially curable
Local excision if established metastases

APR, abdominal perineal resection; 5-FU, 5-fluorouracil.
Adapted from McMurrick PJ, Nelson H, Goldberg RM, Haddock MG:
Cancer of the anal canal. In Torosian MH (ed): Integrated Cancer
Management. New York, Marcel Dekker, 1999, p 200.

Table 51-6 TNM Staging Classifications
for Anal Malignancies

Primary Tumor (T)

Tx	Primary tumor cannot be assessed
T0	No evidence of primary tumor
Tis	Carcinoma in situ
T1	Tumor <2.0 cm in greatest dimension
T2	Tumor >2.0 cm but not >5.0 cm
T3	Tumor >5.0 cm
T4	Tumor of any size that invades adjacent organ(s)

Regional Lymph Nodes (N)

Nx	Regional lymph nodes cannot be assessed
N0	No regional lymph node metastasis
N1	Metastasis in perirectal lymph node(s)
N2	Metastasis in unilateral internal iliac and/or inguinal lymph node(s)
N3	Metastasis in perirectal and inguinal lymph nodes and/or bilateral internal iliac and/or inguinal lymph nodes

Distant Metastasis (M)

Mx	Distant metastasis cannot be assessed
M0	No distant metastasis
M1	Distant metastasis

Stage Grouping

Stage 0	Tis, N0, M0
Stage I	T1, N0, M0
Stage II	T2, N0, M0
	T3, N0, M0
Stage IIIA	T1, N1, M0
	T2, N1, M0
	T3, N1, M0
	T4, N0, M0
Stage IIIB	T4, N1, M0
	Any T, N2, M0
	Any T, N3, M0
Stage IV	Any T, any N, M1

From AJCC Cancer Staging Manual, 6th ed. New York, Springer-Verlag,
2002.

number of staging classifications have been described,
the most widely applied is the TNM (Table 51-6).

Clinical Evaluations

Preoperative assessment should include a complete
history and physical examination. The nature and duration of local anal symptoms, such as a mass, bleeding,
and pruritus, and distant manifestations, such as weight
loss, should be documented. The perianal area should
be closely inspected for skin alterations. Digital examination helps establish tumor location, tumor mobility or
fixity, and the integrity of the sphincter mechanism.
Anoscopy or rigid proctosigmoidoscopy can verify the
size and location of the tumor in relationship to the
dentate line, anal verge, or anorectal ring. Examining for
organomegaly and groin adenopathy, as well as performing CT, chest radiography, and assessments of localizing

the surgical canal and the anatomic canal. For the anatomic canal, the dentate line separates canal from margin,
based on differences in histology and lymphatic drainage.
Proximal or cephalad to the dentate, the epithelium is
transitional then columnar, and the lymphatics typically
drain toward the superior hemorrhoidal to the inferior
hemorrhoidal vessels. Distal or caudad to the dentate, the
epithelium is squamous, and the lymphatic drainage is
more typically toward the inguinal lymphatics. For the
surgical canal, the anal verge separates canal from margin.
From a practical standpoint, the surgical canal is easy to
apply, predicts the behavior of anal tumors, and is incorporated into the TNM staging classification. Although a

symptoms, is important when evaluating a malignant lesion.

Anal Margin Tumors

Bowen's Disease and Anal Intraepithelial Neoplasia

The condition of anal squamous cell carcinoma in situ (Bowen's disease) was originally described by John T. Bowen in 1912 and redescribed as anal intraepithelial neoplasia (AIN) in 1985.[65] The exact relationship between the two conditions has yet to be clarified; the histologies are the same and the clinical distinctions are challenging because the conditions are rare. From a historical perspective, Bowen's disease was described before the clinical recognition of HPV and before the outbreak of HIV; thus, the contribution of viral infections to the original Bowen's disease is not established.

Patients with perianal Bowen's disease typically present with no symptoms or with minor complaints, such as burning or pruritus. Skin changes are variable (Fig. 51-28) and can show erythematous changes, thickening and fissuring, or brown-red plaques or even nodules. Such subtle physical findings can be difficult to differentiate from psoriasis, eczema, leukoplakia, and monilial infections. The description of AIN considers both perianal and anal canal disease. It may be completely asymptomatic and detected during surgery for other conditions such as hemorrhoids, or as part of a screening program for high-risk individuals. Less important than the distinction of Bowen's and AIN are the points regarding diagnostic and therapeutic strategies that should be considered once the histology is confirmed.

A proper medical history, including a sexual history, should ascertain risks for exposure to or the known presence of HIV and HPV. Subtyping HPV will identify patients at high risk for cancer, including types 16, 18, 31, 33, 35, 39, 45, 51, and 52 and at low risk, 6, 11, 42, 43, and 44.[66] Patients positive for HPV should be evaluated for other genital sites of viral damage and be considered for treatment with topical imidazoquinolones for perianal disease and in the future with antiviral vaccines.[67] HIV patients should be treated and those with active disease followed closely. At least one long-term series of patients with immunosuppression showed a heightened risk for the subsequent development of invasive anal squamous cell carcinoma during follow-up.[68]

In addition to diagnosing and treating underlying viral conditions, the neoplastic disease itself needs to be properly diagnosed with mapping, and treated according to the extent and location of the disease. In situ lesions that are unifocal and visible can be managed with mapping and excision to achieve negative margins. The resulting defects are often of sufficient size to require wound closure with other than primary approximation; V-Y advancement flaps work well for most defects (Fig. 51-29). Multifocal disease can be mapped at multiple levels and in four quadrants. Perianal multifocal disease can be treated with imiquimod or 80% trichloroacetic acid. Multifocal anal canal disease is typically ablated. All cases are closely monitored for recurrence and for invasive disease. Five percent of Bowen's disease pre-

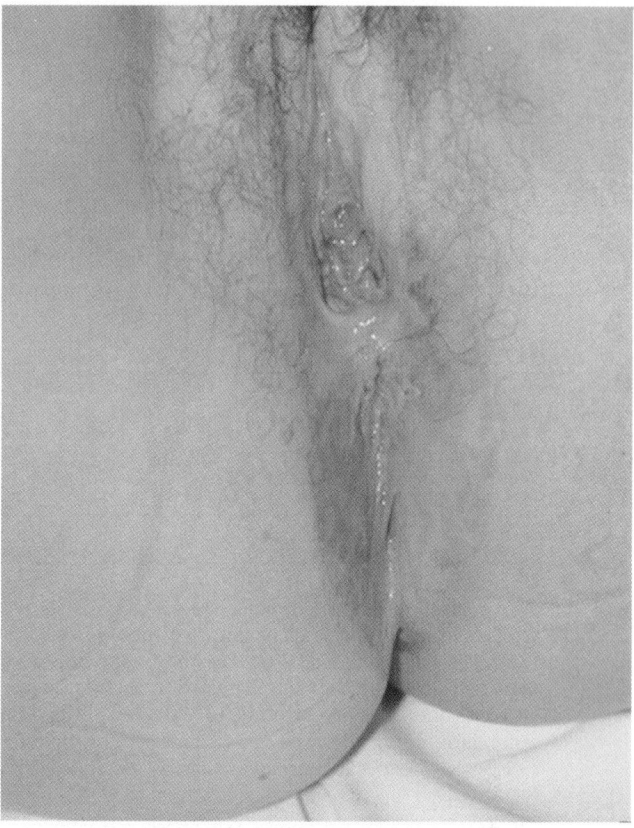

Figure 51-28 Bowen's disease. (By permission of Mayo Foundation.)

sents with invasive disease[63] and is treated as in the section Epidermoid Carcinoma, later.

Paget's Disease

Extramammary Paget's disease of the anus is a rare intraepithelial adenocarcinoma. The presence of intraepithelial adenocarcinoma in an area of squamous epithelium has led to speculation about the origin of Paget's cells. A number of concepts have been proposed, including the possibility that they are derived from pluripotent epidermal stem cells, arise from apocrine or sweat glands, or are metastatic from underlying adenocarcinomas. Unlike Bowen's disease, Paget's disease is more common in older patients, is associated with an underlying carcinoma in 50% to 86% of patients, and has a poor prognosis.[63] The typical appearance of Paget's disease is that of well-demarcated eczematoid plaque with whitish gray ulcerations or papillary lesions[63] (Fig. 51-30). As is true for Bowen's disease, Paget's disease can have a variable and at times a subtle appearance and can be confused with other dermatologic conditions, such as hyperkeratosis, eczema, or lichen sclerosus et atrophicus. Histology demonstrates the presence of periodic acid–Schiff positive Paget cells, confirming the diagnosis.

Treatment is based on the local extent of the disease and on the presence or absence of underlying malignancies. More limited Paget's disease can be widely excised and the defect closed primarily or with V-Y advancement flaps. Biopsies of the proximal anal canal and distal anal

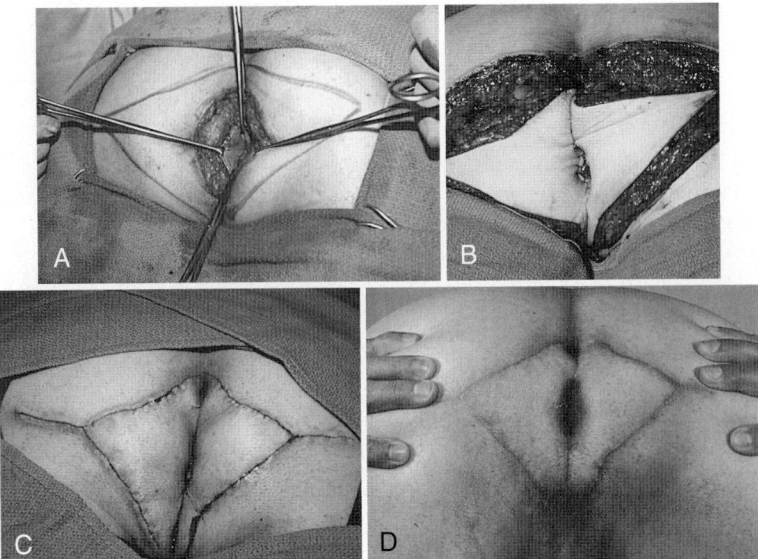

Figure 51-29 V-Y advancement flap for perianal Bowen's disease. **A,** Circumferential excision is performed with wide margins, histologically negative for Bowen's disease. The residual defect will be closed by advancing surrounding V-shaped islands of skin and underlying tissue. The Allis clamps expose the anal canal. **B,** The V-shaped flaps are advanced and anastomosed to the residual anal canal at the dentate line. **C,** Closure of the flap wounds converts the V-shaped wounds to Y-shaped suture lines. **D,** Six months after surgery, the perianal scars are soft, compliant, and without stenosis. The patient has normal sphincter tone and a good functional outcome. (From Nelson H, Dozois RR: Anal neoplasms. Perspect Colon Rectal Surg 7:22, 1994.)

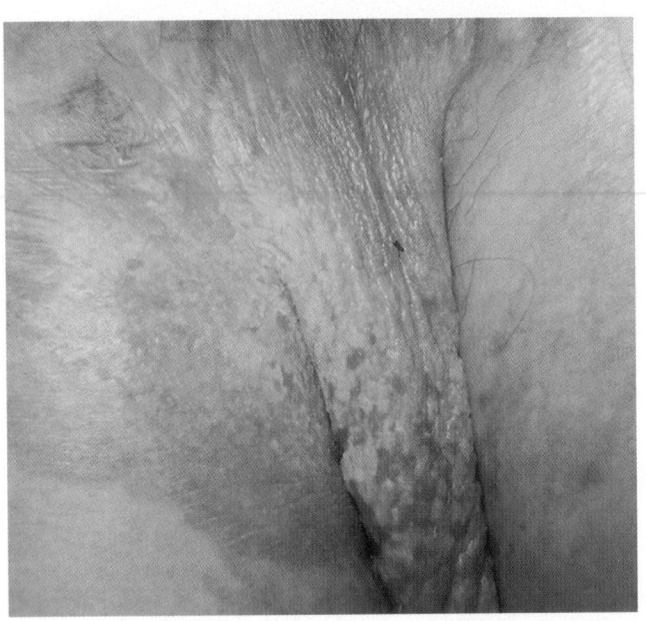

Figure 51-30. Paget's disease. (By permission of Mayo Foundation.)

skin margins can help map the extent of resection.[63] An alternative to wide excision for patients without invasive cancer and who are poor operative candidates is a course of topical retinoic acid (0.025%). Topical application is performed to the affected area until it generates discomfort; then it is applied every other day. Close observation is advised and biopsies for symptoms recommended.[69] Patients with underlying rectal adenocarcinoma should

undergo abdominal perineal resection (APR), whereas those with epidermoid anal canal cancer can be treated with combined radiation and chemotherapy.[70] For patients with an invasive component, treated with radical therapy, the 5-year crude survival rate is only 54%.[71] After surgery, patients should be monitored closely for recurrence.

Basal Cell Carcinoma

Basal cell carcinoma is a rare type of anal canal tumor. Macroscopically, these lesions have the same pearly borders with central depression that other basal cell cancers of the skin have (Fig. 51-31). On occasion, it may be difficult to differentiate a cloacogenic (or basaloid) carcinoma arising in the transitional zone from a basal cell cancer arising in the anal skin. The distinction is crucial because of the dramatic behavioral difference and is based on location as well as histologic features.[63] Most often, these tumors can be treated adequately by wide local excision, reserving APR for extensive lesions.[63] Because nearly one third of patients experience recurrence, close follow-up is indicated.

Squamous Cell Carcinoma

Although the oncologic behavior of squamous cell carcinoma resembles that of skin tumors elsewhere, the location of these lesions results in site-specific symptoms, such as a mass, chronic pruritus, bleeding, pain, and associated fistulas and condylomata.[63] Wide local excision is recommended for early anal margin squamous cell carcinoma with excellent results. Recurrences may be managed by re-excision or by APR, especially if locally advanced. Lymphadenectomy is indicated for those rare

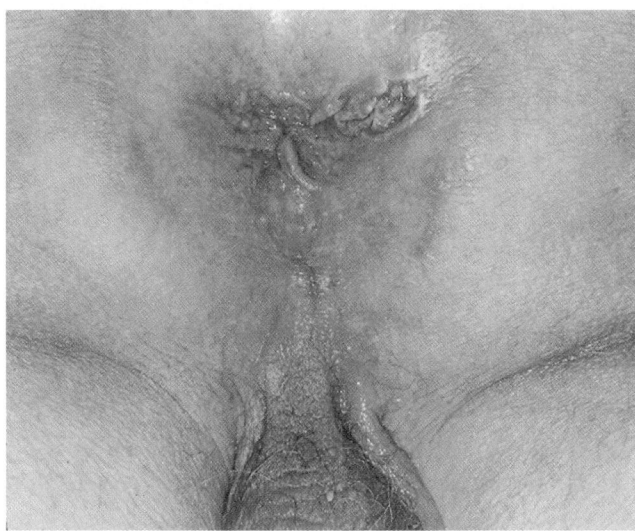

Figure 51-31 Basal cell carcinoma of anal margin. (By permission of Mayo Foundation.)

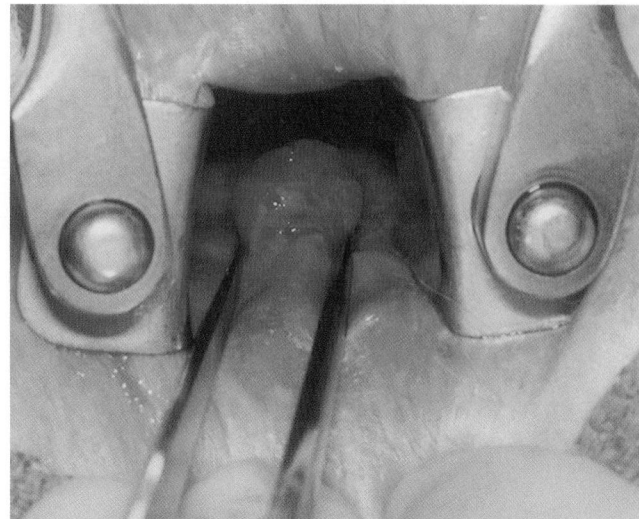

Figure 51-32 Squamous cell carcinoma of anal canal. (By permission of Mayo Foundation.)

patients (<10%) presenting with evidence of regional lymph node metastases.

Verrucous Carcinoma

Verrucous carcinoma, also referred to as *giant condyloma acuminatum* or *Buschke-Löwenstein tumor,* is poorly defined and best considered as intermediate lesions between condyloma acuminatum and invasive squamous cell carcinomas based on their common HPV etiology.[63] The large, wartlike lesions are soft and slow growing. They may fistulize, become infected, and undergo malignant transformation.[63] Radical wide local excision or APR is recommended. A poor prognosis can be expected for tumors progressing to invasive squamous cell carcinoma, although some may respond favorably to combined irradiation and chemotherapy.

Anal Canal Neoplasms

Epidermoid Carcinoma

Tumors arising in the anal canal or in the transitional zone that have a squamous, basaloid, cloacogenic, or mucoepidermoid epithelium share a similar behavior in clinical presentation, response to treatment, and prognosis[63] and are considered collectively. They typically present as a mass, sometimes with bleeding and pruritus (Fig. 51-32). At the time of diagnosis, nearly one fourth of these are superficial or in situ; half are less than 3 cm in size, and the other half are larger.[63] About 71% have deep tumor penetration; 25% are node positive, and 6% present with distant metastases.

In the past, treatment modalities have included either surgery alone or radiation therapy alone. Patients with tumors confined to epithelial or subepithelial tissue have been treated by local excision and patients with more advanced lesions by APR. The introduction of multimodality therapy combining irradiation and chemotherapy promised to preserve continence, avoid colostomy, and

offer similar survival advantage. In keeping with this concept, local excision alone remains an option for superficial, early-stage lesions, which have been associated with variable survivorship (61%-87%; 100% in at least one study) if the lesion was smaller than 2 cm. Although some small superficial lesions can be treated with local excision, most patients are best treated with combined chemotherapy and irradiation.

Combined-modality therapy has evolved as the preferred alternative to radical surgery because, in theory, surgical mortality and morbidity are largely avoided, intestinal continuity is preserved, and survival compares favorably with that after surgery. Nigro and colleagues[70] were the first to promote radiation therapy plus chemotherapy as definitive treatment for epidermoid anal canal malignancies. The current Nigro protocol includes external-beam radiation therapy to the pelvic tumor and pelvic and inguinal nodes, to a total dose of 3000 cGy starting on day 1 using 15 fractions (200 cGy/day).[70] Systemic chemotherapy includes 5-fluorouracil (5-FU), 1000 mg/m^2 for 24 hours as continuous infusion for 4 days, commencing on day 1 and again on day 28 (two cycles total). Mitomycin C is delivered as an intravenous bolus at 15 mg/m^2 starting on day 1 only. Many institutions have modified the pelvic radiation doses, approximating the doses typically delivered in rectal cancer. Although some reports have described comparable results using radiation therapy alone, current studies support the continued use of 5-FU and mitomycin C.[72] Although radiation plus chemotherapy has largely replaced the need for APR in anal canal cancers, there remain subsets of patients in whom APR may be considered appropriate as either single-modality or combined-modality therapy. Such groups would include patients who are already in need of a stoma for fecal incontinence, those for whom chemotherapy or radiation therapy is contraindicated, and those whose disease fails to resolve completely after radiation therapy plus chemotherapy.

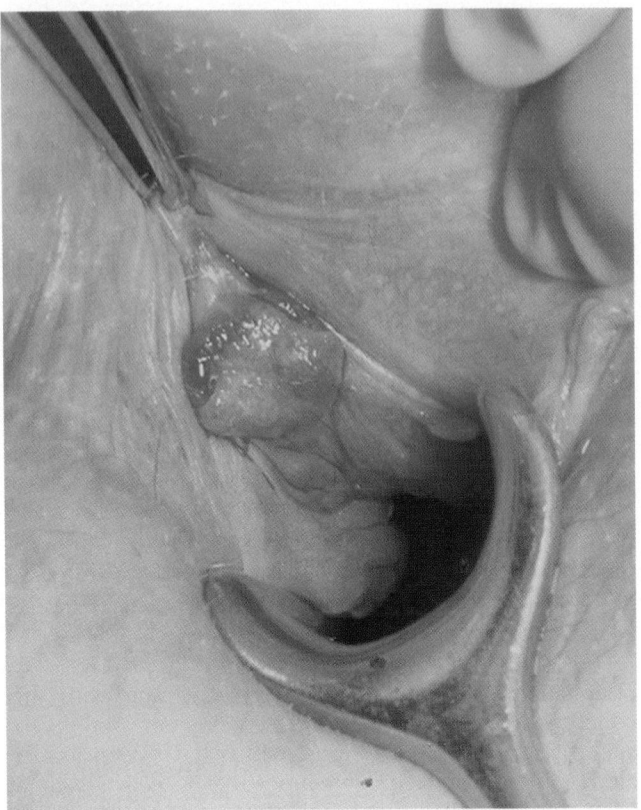

Figure 51-33 Anal canal amelanotic melanoma. (By permission of Mayo Foundation.)

Despite high success rates with combination radiation and chemotherapy, some cases of locally advanced disease reoccur or fail to completely respond in the locoregional tumor bed. Whether patients with recurrent or persistent disease are treated with surgery or further radiation and chemotherapy hinges on their willingness and ability to undergo surgery. The standard treatment of surgical candidates is APR. Between 50% and 57% of patients treated with salvage APR can expect a 5-year cure.[73,74] In contrast, only 27% of patients treated with salvage radiation and concurrent cisplatin-based chemotherapy can expect to be cured.[73]

Melanoma

Melanoma involving the anal canal can produce a mass, pain, or bleeding and is not infrequently amelanotic (Fig. 51-33). Overall, the outlook for patients with such tumors is poor, with a 5-year survival rate hovering around 10% to, at most, 26%.[75] The survivorship, however, depends on the stage of the disease. In general, survival is poor whether the surgery is conservative or radical. APR appears reasonable for advanced lesions if complete resection and palliation are to be achieved. Recent results of local excision and APR seem comparable. Some centers describe better survival for APR, and others show no difference; it remains a controversial subject.[75,76] Prophylactic inguinal node dissection offers no benefit.

Adenocarcinoma

True adenocarcinomas of the anal canal are extremely rare. They originate from anal ducts and are often extramucosal in location. Because of their rarity, their diagnosis is frequently delayed. Like melanoma, the tumor is occasionally found incidentally during hemorrhoidectomy. Whether the tumor is locally excised or widely removed by APR, the prognosis is poor.[63] Because it is conceivable that some adenocarcinomas arise in the rectum but appear as anal adenocarcinomas, it is appealing to give benefit of the doubt and treat these cases as a primary rectal cancer with trimodality therapy, that is, surgery plus irradiation plus chemotherapy. This not only provides appropriate therapy for a misdiagnosed rectal primary but also may improve results for primary anal adenocarcinomas, which are otherwise associated with universally fatal outcomes.

Other Tumors

Connective tissue sarcomas, such as leiomyosarcoma, rhabdomyosarcoma, and myoblastoma, are rare in the anal canal. Lymphoma of the anus is unusual. Carcinoid tumors can occasionally originate from anal canal endocrine cells, and APR may be required, especially for those exceeding 2 cm in size.

Selected References

Abbasakoor F, Boulos PB: Anal intraepithelial neoplasia. Br J Surg 92:277-290, 2005.

A comprehensive review of evolving diagnostic and treatment issues pertinent to anal intraepithelial neoplasia.

Billingham RP, Isler JT, Kimmins MH, et al: The diagnosis and management of common anorectal disorders. Curr Probl Surg 41:586-645, 2004.

An in-depth review of current diagnostic and therapeutic approaches to common conditions of the anus and distal rectum.

Hulme-Moir M, Bartolo DC: Hemorrhoids. Gastroenterol Clin North Am 30:183-197, 2001.

This article provides a well-referenced, comprehensive review of the classification, etiology, anatomy, diagnosis, and treatment of hemorrhoids.

McMurrick PJ, Nelson H, Goldberg RM, Haddock MG: Cancer of the anal canal. In Torosian MH (ed): Integrated Cancer Management. New York, Marcel Dekker, 1999, pp 195-205.

The multidisciplinary authorship of this publication uniquely offers an in-depth description of current practices in the management of anal cancer.

Nelson R: Operative procedures for fissure in ano. Cochrane Database Syst Rev Apr 18 (2):CD002199, 2005.

An evidence-based review of best data on five different surgical approaches to chronic anal fissure.

Nicholls RJ, Dozois RR (eds): Surgery of the Colon and Rectum. New York, Churchill Livingstone, 1997.

This well-illustrated compendium of commonly performed colorectal and anal procedures is clearly written and comprehensive.

Parks AG, Gordon PH, Hardcastle JD: A classification of fistula-in-ano. Br J Surg 63:1-12, 1976.

> A classic description of anorectal suppurative disease, this article includes the acute phase (abscesses) and chronic phase (fistulas). The anatomic descriptions, data, and classification schema are still relevant today.

Ryan DP, Compton CC, Mayer RJ: Carcinoma of the anal canal. N Engl J Med 342:792-800, 2000.

> A comprehensive review of the epidemiologic association, primary therapies, and expected outcomes for patients with carcinoma of the anal canal.

Whitehead WE, Wald A, Norton NJ: Treatment options for fecal incontinence. Dis Colon Rectum 44:131-144, 2001.

> This article represents a summary review of a Consensus Conference on Treatment Options in Fecal Incontinence.

References

1. Ambroze WL, Pemberton JH, Dozois RR, et al: Does retaining the anal transition zone (ATZ) fail to extirpate chronic ulcerative colitis (CUC) after ileal-pouch anal anastomosis (IPAA)? Dis Colon Rectum 34:P20, 1991.
2. Kerremans R: Morphological and Physiological Aspects of Anal Continence and Defecation. Brussels, Arscia, Ultgavon, 1969.
3. Ferrara A, Pemberton JH, Levin KE, et al: Relationship between anal canal tone and rectal motor activity. Dis Colon Rectum 36:337-342, 1993.
4. Parks AG: Royal Society of Medicine, Section of Proctology; Meeting 27, November 1974. President's Address. Anorectal incontinence. Proc R Soc Med 68:681-690, 1975.
5. Bartolo DCC, Roe AM, Locke-Edmunds JC, et al: Flap-valve theory of anorectal continence. Br J Surg 73:1012-1014, 1986.
6. Beart RW Jr, Dozois RR, Wolff BG, et al: Mechanisms of rectal continence: Lessons from the ileoanal procedure. Am J Surg 149:31-34, 1985.
7. Sagar PM, Pemberton JH: Anorectal and pelvic floor function: Relevance of continence, incontinence, and constipation. Gastroenterol Clin North Am 25:163-182, 1996.
8. Whitehead WE, Wald A, Norton NJ: Treatment options for fecal incontinence. Dis Colon Rectum 44:131-144, 2001.
9. Rudolph W, Galandiuk S: A practical guide to the diagnosis and management of fecal incontinence. Mayo Clin Proc 77:271-275, 2002.
10. Gordon PH: Anal incontinence. In Gordon PH, Nivatvongs S (eds): Principles and Practice of Surgery for the Colon, Rectum, and Anus. St Louis, Quality Medical, 1992, pp 337-359.
11. Matsuoka H, Mavrantonis C, Wexner SD, et al: Postanal repair for fecal incontinence: Is it worthwhile? Dis Colon Rectum 43:1561-1567, 2000.
12. Malouf AJ, Vaizey CJ, Nicholls RJ, et al: Permanent sacral nerve stimulation for fecal incontinence. Ann Surg 232:143-148, 2000.
13. Theuerkauf FJ Jr, Beahrs OH, Hill JR: Rectal prolapse: Causation and surgical treatment. Ann Surg 171:819-835, 1970.
14. Huber FT, Stein H, Siewert JR: Functional results after treatment of rectal prolapse with rectopexy and sigmoid resection. World J Surg 19:138-143, 1995.
15. Birnbaum EH, Stamm L, Rafferty JF, et al: Pudendal nerve terminal motor latency influences surgical outcome in treatment of rectal prolapse. Dis Colon Rectum 39:1215-1221, 1996.
16. Kimmins MH, Evetts BK, Isler J, et al: The Altemeier repair: Outpatient treatment of rectal prolapse. Dis Colon Rectum 44:565-570, 2001.
17. Lechaux JP, Lechaux D, Perez M: Results of Delorme's procedure for rectal prolapse: Advantages of a modified technique. Dis Colon Rectum 38:301-307, 1995.
18. Bachoo P, Brazzelli M, Grant A: Surgery for complete rectal prolapse in adults. Cochrane Database Syst Rev, Issue 4, 2002.
19. Stevenson ARL, Stitz RW, Lumley JW: Laparoscopic-assisted resection-rectopexy for rectal prolapse: Early and medium follow-up. Dis Colon Rectum 41:46-54, 1998.
20. Goh JT, Tjandra JJ, Carey MP: How could management of rectoceles be optimized? ANZ J Surg 72:896-901, 2002.
21. Mimura T, Roy AJ, Storrie JB, et al: Treatment of impaired defecation associated with rectocele by behavioral retraining (biofeedback). Dis Colon Rectum 43:1267-1272, 2000.
22. Van Laarhoven CJ, Kamm MA, Bartram CI, et al: Relationship between anatomic and symptomatic long-term results after rectocele repair for impaired defecation. Dis Colon Rectum 42:204-211, 1999.
23. Tjandra JJ, Ooi BS, Tang CL, et al: Transanal repair of rectocele corrects obstructed defecation if it is not associated with anismus. Dis Colon Rectum 42:1544-1550, 1999.
24. Hulme-Moir M, Bartolo DC: Hemorrhoids. Gastroenterol Clin North Am 30:183-197, 2001.
25. Shemesh EI, Kodner IJ, Fry RD, et al: Severe complication of rubber band ligation of internal hemorrhoids. Dis Colon Rectum 30:199-200, 1987.
26. Bayer I, Myslovaty B, Picovsky BM: Rubber band ligation of hemorrhoids: Convenient and economic treatment. J Clin Gastroenterol 23:50-52, 1996.
27. Gencosmanoglu R, Sad O, Koc D, et al: Hemorrhoidectomy: Open or closed technique? A prospective, randomized clinical trial. Dis Colon Rectum 45:70-75, 2002.
28. Khan S, Pawlak SE, Eggenberger JC, et al: Surgical treatment of hemorrhoids: Prospective, randomized trial comparing closed excisional hemorrhoidectomy and the Harmonic Scalpel technique of excisional hemorrhoidectomy. Dis Colon Rectum 44:845-849, 2001.
29. Longo A: Treatment of haemorrhoids disease by reduction of mucosa and haemorrhoidal prolapse with a circular-suturing device: A new procedure. Proceedings of the Sixth World Congress of Endoscopic Surgery, Rome, Italy, 1998, p 777.
30. Ho YH, Cheong WK, Tsang C, et al. Stapled hemorrhoidectomy: Cost and effectiveness. Randomized, controlled trial including incontinence scoring, anorectal manometry, and endoanal ultrasound assessments at up to three months. Dis Colon Rectum 43:1666, 2000.
31. Cheetham MJ, Mortensen NJ, Nystrom PO, et al: Persistent pain and faecal urgency after stapled haemorrhoidectomy. Lancet 356:730, 2000.
32. Ganio E, Altomare DF, Gabrielli F, et al: Prospective randomized multicentre trial comparing stapled with open haemorrhoidectomy. Br J Surg 88:669, 2001.
33. Palimento D, Picchoi M, Attasasio U, et al: Stapled and open hemorrhoidectomy: Randomized controlled trial of early results. World J Surg 27:203, 2003.
34. Smyth EF, Baker RP, Wilken BJ, et al: Stapled versus excision haemorrhoidectomy: Long-term follow up of a randomised controlled trial. Lancet 361:1437, 2003.
35. Lund JN, Binch C, McGrath J, et al: Topographical distribution of blood supply to the anal canal. Br J Surg 86:496-498, 1999.

36. Jensen SL: Treatment of first episodes of acute anal fissure: Prospective randomised study of lignocaine ointment versus hydrocortisone ointment or warm sitz baths plus bran. BMJ 292:1167-1169, 1986.

37. Kocher HM, Steward M, Leather AJ, et al: Randomized clinical trial assessing the side effects of glyceryl trinitrate and diltiazem hydrochloride in the treatment of chronic anal fissure. Br J Surg 89:413-417, 2002.

38. Minguez M, Herreros B, Espi A, et al: Long-term follow-up (42 months) of chronic anal fissure after healing with botulinum toxin. Gastroenterology 123:112-117, 2002.

39. Whiteford MH, Kilkenny J III, Hyman N, et al: The Standards Practice Task Force and the American Society of Colon and Rectal Surgeons. Practice parameters for the treatment of perianal abscess and fistula-in-ano. Dis Colon Rectum 48:1337-1372, 2005.

40. Brisinad G, Maria G, Bentivoglio AR, et al: A comparison of injections of botulinum toxin and topical nitroglycerin ointment for the treatment of chronic anal fissure. N Engl J Med 341:65-69, 1999.

41. Mentes BB, Irkorucu O, Akin M, et al: Comparison of botulinum toxin injection and lateral internal sphincterotomy for the treatment of chronic anal fissure. Dis Colon Rectum 46:232-237, 2003.

42. Madoff RD, Fleshman JW: AGA technical review on the diagnosis and care of patients with anal fissure. Gastroenterology 124:235-245, 2003.

43. Henrichsen S, Christiansen J: Incidence of fistula-in-ano complicating anorectal sepsis: A prospective study. Br J Surg 73:371-372, 1986.

44. Parks AG, Gordon PH, Hardcastle JD: A classification of fistula-in-ano. Br J Surg 63:1-12, 1976.

45. Lindsey I, Smilgin-Humphreys MM, Cunningham C, et al: A randomized, controlled trial of fibrin glue versus conventional treatment for anal fistula. Dis Colon Rectum 45:1608-1615, 2002.

46. Johnson EK, Gau JU, Armstrong DN: Efficacy of anal fistula plug vs fibrin glue in closure of anorectal fistulas. Dis Colon Rectum 49:1-6, 2006.

47. da Silva JH: Pilonidal cyst: Cause and treatment. Dis Colon Rectum 43:1146-1156, 2000.

48. Senapati A, Cripps NP, Thompson MR: Bascom's operation in the day-surgical management of symptomatic pilonidal sinus. Br J Surg 87:1067-1070, 2000.

49. Urhan MK, Kucukel F, Topgul K, et al: Rhomboid excision and Limberg flap for managing pilonidal sinus: Results of 102 cases. Dis Colon Rectum 45:656-659, 2002.

50. Saclarides TJ: Rectovaginal fistula. Surg Clin North Am 82:1261-1272, 2002.

51. El-Attar SM, Evans DV: Anal warts, sexually transmitted diseases, and anorectal conditions associated with human immunodeficiency virus. Prim Care 26:81-100, 1999.

52. Barrett WL, Callahan TD, Orkin BA: Perianal manifestations of human immunodeficiency virus infection: Experience with 260 patients. Dis Colon Rectum 41:606-612, 1998.

53. Nadal SR, Manzione CR, Galvao VM, et al: Perianal diseases in HIV-positive patients compared with a seronegative population. Dis Colon Rectum 42:649-654, 1999.

54. Place RJ, Gregorcyk SG, Huber PJ, et al: Outcome analysis of HIV-positive patients with anal squamous cell carcinoma. Dis Colon Rectum 44:506-512, 2001.

55. Mitchell KM, Beck DE: Hidradenitis suppurativa. Surg Clin North Am 82:1187-1197, 2002.

56. Culp CE: Chronic hidradenitis suppurativa of the anal canal: A surgical skin disease. Dis Colon Rectum 26:669-676, 1983.

57. Abcarian H: Perianal Crohn's disease. Semin Colon Rectal Surg 5:210, 1994.

58. Poupardin C, Lemann M, Gendre J, et al: Efficacy of infliximab in Crohn's disease. Results of a retrospective multicenter study with a 15-month follow-up. Gastroenterol Clin Biol 30:247-252, 2006.

59. Schwartz DA, Pemberton JH, Sandborn WJ: Diagnosis and treatment of perianal fistulas in Crohn disease. Ann Intern Med 135:906-918, 2001.

60. Poritz L: How should complex perianal Crohn's disease be treated in the Remicade era? J Gastrointest Surg 10(5):633-634, 2006.

61. van der Hagen S, Baeten C, Soeters P, et al: Anti-TNF-alpha (Infliximab) used as induction treatment in case of active proctitis in a multistep strategy followed by definitive surgery of complex anal fistulas in Crohn's disease: A preliminary report. Dis Colon Rectum 48:758-767, 2005.

62. Singh B, Mortensen N, Jewell D, George B: Perianal Crohn's disease. Br J Surg 91:801-814, 2004.

63. Nelson H, Dozois RR: Anal neoplasms. Perspect Colon Rectal Surg 7:16, 1994.

64. McMurrick PJ, Nelson H, Goldberg RM, et al: Cancer of the anal canal. In Torosian MH (ed): Integrated Cancer Management. New York, Marcel Dekker, 1999, pp 195-205.

65. McCance DJ, Clarkson PK, Dyson JL, et al: Human papillomavirus types 6 and 16 in multifocal intraepithelial neoplasias of the female lower genital tract. Br J Obstet Gynaecol 92:1093-1100, 1985.

66. Chang GJ, Berry JM, Jay N, et al: Surgical treatment of high-grade anal squamous intraepithelial lesions. Dis Colon Rectum 45:453-458, 2002.

67. Stanley M. Genital human papillomavirus infections: Current and prospective therapies. J Natl Cancer Inst Monogr 31:117-124, 2003.

68. Scholefeld JH, Castle MT, Watson NFS: Malignant transformation of high-grade anal intraepithelial neoplasia. Br J Surg 92:1133-1136, 2005.

69. McCarter DM, Quan SHQ, Busam K, et al: Long-term outcome of perianal Paget's disease. Dis Colon Rectum 46:612-616, 2003.

70. Nigro ND, Vaitkevicius VK, Considine B Jr: Dynamic management of squamous cell cancer of the anal canal. Invest New Drugs 7:83-89, 1989.

71. Jensen SL, Sjolin KE, Shokouh-Amiri MH, et al: Paget's disease of the anal margin. Br J Surg 75:1089-1092, 1988.

72. UKCCCR Anal Cancer Trial Working Party: UK Coordinating Committee on Cancer Research: Epidermoid anal cancer: Results from the UKCCCR randomised trial of radiotherapy alone versus radiotherapy, 5-fluorouracil, and mitomycin. Lancet 348:1049-1054, 1996.

73. Longo WE, Vernava AM, Wade TP, et al: Recurrent squamous cell carcinoma of the anal canal: Predictors of initial treatment failure and results of salvage therapy. Ann Surg 220; 40-49, 1994.

74. Pocard M, Tiret E, Nugent K, et al: Results of salvage abdominoperineal resection for anal cancer after radiotherapy. Dis Colon Rectum 41:1148-1493, 1998.

75. Brady MS, Kavolius JP, Quan SH: Anorectal melanoma: A 64-year experience at Memorial Sloan-Kettering Cancer Center. Dis Colon Rectum 38:146-151, 1995.

76. Bullard KM, Tuttle TM, Rothenberger DA, et al: Surgical therapy for anorectal melanoma. J Am Coll Surg 196:206-211, 2003.

CHAPTER 52

The Liver

Michael D'Angelica, MD   and   Yuman Fong, MD

Historical Perspective
Anatomy and Physiology
Infectious Diseases
Neoplasms
Hemobilia
Viral Hepatitis and the Surgeon

HISTORICAL PERSPECTIVE

The surface anatomy of the liver was described as early as 2000 years before Christ by the ancient Babylonians. Even Hippocrates understood and described the seriousness of liver injury. Francis Glisson, in 1654, was the first physician to accurately describe the essential anatomy of the blood vessels of the liver. The beginnings of liver surgery are accurately described as rudimentary excisions of eviscerated liver from penetrating trauma. The first documented case of a partial hepatectomy is usually credited to Berta in 1716, who amputated a portion of protruding liver in a patient with a self-inflicted stab wound.[1,2]

In the late 1800s, while the first gastrectomies and cholecystectomies were being performed in Europe, surgery on the liver was regarded as dangerous, if not impossible. J. W. Elliot, in his report on liver surgery for trauma in 1897, said that the liver was so "friable, so full of gaping vessels and so evidently incapable of being sutured that it had always seemed impossible to successfully manage large wounds of its substance." European surgeons began to experiment with techniques of elective liver surgery on animals in the late 1800s. The credit for the first elective liver resection is a matter of debate, and

many surgeons have been given credit, but it certainly occurred during this time period.[1]

The early 1900s saw some small, but significant advances in liver surgery. Techniques for suturing major hepatic vessels and the use of cautery for small vessels were applied and reported on. The most significant advance of that time was probably that of J. Hogarth Pringle, who in 1908 described digital compression of the hilar vessels to control hepatic bleeding from traumatic injuries. The modern era of hepatic surgery was ushered in by the development of a better understanding of liver anatomy and formal anatomic liver resection. Credit for the first anatomic liver resection is usually given to Lortat-Jacob, who performed a right hepatectomy in 1952 in France. Pack from New York and Quattelbaum from Georgia performed a similar operation within the next year and were unlikely to have had any knowledge of Lortat-Jacob's report. Descriptions of the segmental nature of liver anatomy by Couinaud and Woodsmith and Goldburne in 1957 opened the door even further to the modern era of liver surgery.[1,2]

Despite these improvements, hepatic surgery was plagued by tremendous operative morbidity and mortality from the 1950s into the 1980s. Operative mortality rates in excess of 20% were common and usually related to massive hemorrhage.[1] Many surgeons were reluctant to perform hepatic surgery because of these results, and understandably many physicians were reluctant to refer patients for hepatectomy. Nonetheless, with the courage of patients, their families, and persistent surgeons, safe hepatic surgery has been realized. A complete list is not possible here, but courageous hepatic surgeons such as Blumgart, Bismuth, Longmire, Fortner, Schwartz, Starzl, and Ton deserve mention. Advances in anesthesia, intensive care, and antibiotics have also contributed tremendously to the safety of major hepatic surgery. Total hepatectomy with liver transplantation and live donor

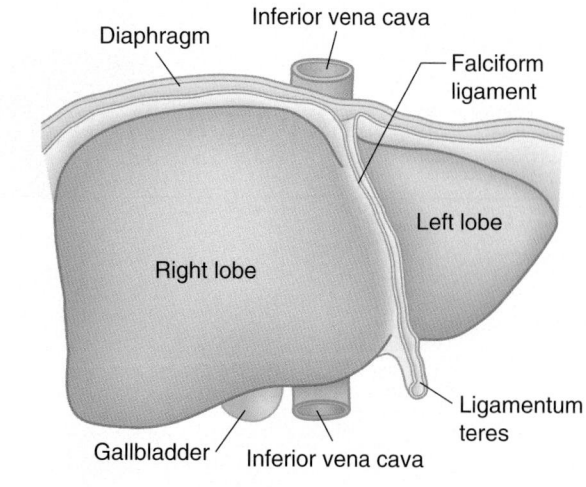

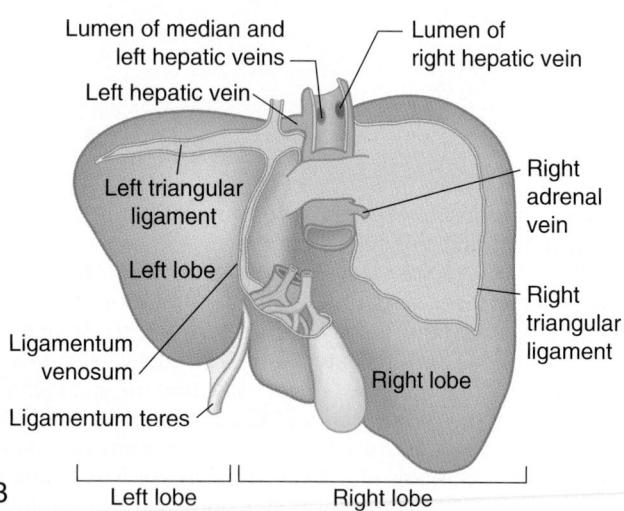

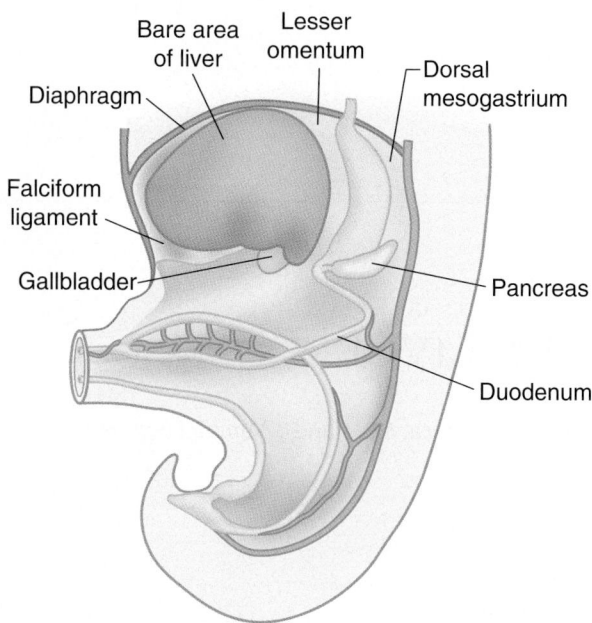

Figure 52-2 An approximately 36-day-old embryo is shown. The extensions of the septum transversum can be seen developing as the liver protrudes into the abdominal cavity, stretching out and forming the lesser omentum and the falciform ligament. The liver is completely invested in visceral peritoneum except for a portion next to the diaphragm known as the *bare area.* (From Sadler TW: Langman's Medical Embryology, 5th ed. Baltimore, William & Wilkins, 1985.)

Figure 52-1 A, Historically, the liver was divided into right and left lobes by the external marking of the falciform ligament. On the inferior surface of the falciform ligament, the ligamentum teres can be seen entering the umbilical fissure. **B,** The posterior and inferior surface of the liver is shown. The liver embraces the inferior vena cava (IVC) posteriorly in a groove. The lumens of the three major hepatic veins and the right adrenal vein can be seen directly entering the IVC. The bare area, bounded by the right and left triangular ligaments, is illustrated. To the left of the IVC is the caudate lobe, which is bounded on its left side by a fissure containing the ligamentum venosum. The lesser omentum terminates along the edge of the ligamentum venosum; thus, the caudate lobe lies within the lesser sac, and the rest of the liver lies in the supracolic compartment. A layer of fibrous tissue can be seen bridging the right lobe to the caudate lobe posterior to the IVC, encircling the IVC. This ligament of tissue must be divided on the right side when mobilizing the right liver off of the IVC. (From Blumgart LH, Hann LE: Surgical and radiologic anatomy of the liver and biliary tract. In Blumgart LH, Fong Y [eds]: Surgery of the Liver and Biliary Tract. London, WB Saunders, 2000, pp 3-34.)

partial hepatectomy for transplantation are now performed routinely in specialized transplantation centers. Partial hepatectomy for a large number of indications is now performed throughout the world in specialized centers with mortality rates of 5% or less. In fact, partial hepatectomy performed on normal livers is now consistently performed with mortality rates of 1% to 2%.[1-3]

Safe hepatic surgery and its liberal use in the management of a wide variety of diseases is now reality. The future, however, demands improvement and further innovation. Minimally invasive approaches to liver surgery have been developed and used in significant numbers, but the indications for this technique are still unclear. Thermal ablative techniques to treat hepatic tumors have exploded in popularity, but their indications remain undefined. Lastly, techniques to further improve the safety of liver resection, such as portal vein embolization to induce preoperative hypertrophy of the future liver remnant, have been developed and used, but also lack definition of optimal indications.

ANATOMY AND PHYSIOLOGY

Gross Anatomy

A precise knowledge of the anatomy of the liver is an absolute prerequisite to performing surgery on the liver or biliary tree. With the development of hepatic surgery during the past few decades, a greater appreciation for the complex anatomy beyond the misleading minimal external markings has been realized. The days of using the falciform ligament as the only marker of a left and

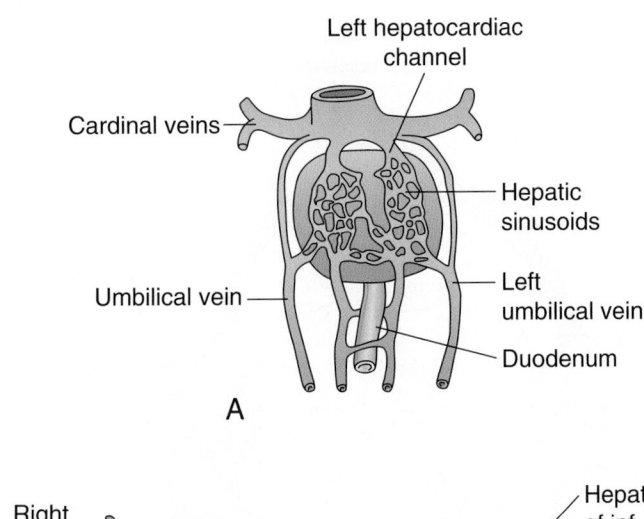

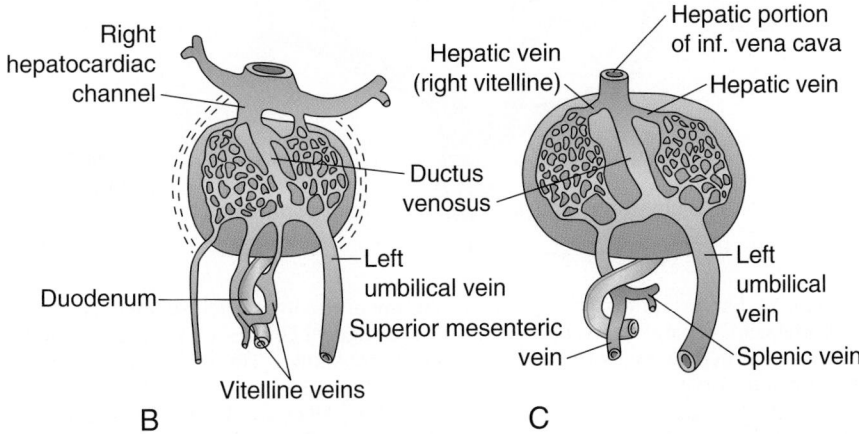

Figure 52-3 A, Umbilical and vitelline vein development of a 5-week-old embryo. The hepatic sinusoids have developed, and although there are channels that bypass these sinusoids, the vitelline and umbilical veins are beginning to drain into them. **B,** In the 2nd month, the vitelline veins drain directly into the hepatic sinusoids. The ductus venosus has formed and accepts oxygenated blood from the left umbilical vein, bypasses the hepatic sinusoids, and directly enters the hepatocardiac channel. **C,** By the 3rd month, the vitelline veins have formed into the portal system (splenic, superior mesenteric, and portal vein). The right umbilical vein has disappeared, and the left umbilical vein (future ligamentum teres) drains into the sinus venosus, bypassing the hepatic sinusoids. Note the development of the inferior vena cava and the hepatic veins. (From Sadler TW: Langman's Medical Embryology, 5th ed. Baltimore, William & Wilkins, 1985.)

right side of the liver are over, and the anatomic contributions of Couinaud (see later) and the description of the segmental nature of the liver need to be embraced and studied by students of hepatic surgery.

General Description and Topography

The liver is a solid gastrointestinal organ whose mass (1200-1600 g) largely occupies the right upper quadrant of the abdomen. The costal margin coincides with the lower margin and the superior surface is draped over by the diaphragm. Most of the right liver and most of the left liver is covered by the thoracic cage. The liver extends superiorly to the height of the fifth rib on the right and the sixth rib on the left. The posterior surface straddles the inferior vena cava (IVC). A wedge of liver extends to the left half of the abdomen across the epigastrium to lie above the anterior surface of the stomach and under the central and left diaphragm. The superior surface of the liver is convex and is molded to the diaphragm, whereas the inferior surface is mildly concave and extends to a sharp anterior border.

The liver is invested in the peritoneum except for the gallbladder bed, the porta hepatis, and posteriorly on either side of the IVC in two wedge-shaped areas (called the *bare area* of the liver to the right of the IVC). The peritoneal duplications on the liver surface are referred to as *ligaments*. The diaphragmatic peritoneal duplications are referred to as the *coronary ligament*, whose lateral margins on either side are the right and left triangular ligaments. From the center of the coronary ligament emerges the falciform ligament, which extends anteriorly as a thin membrane connecting the liver surface to the diaphragm, abdominal wall, and umbilicus. The ligamentum teres (the obliterated umbilical vein) runs along the inferior edge of the falciform ligament from the umbilicus to the umbilical fissure. The umbilical fissure is on the inferior surface of the left liver and contains the left portal triad. The falciform ligament, the most obvious surface

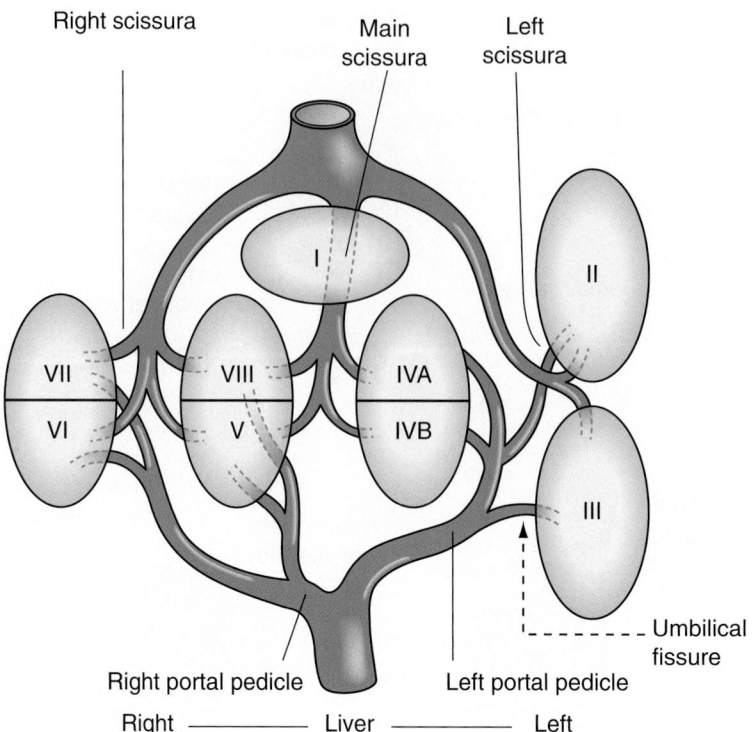

Right scissura   Main scissura   Left scissura

Figure 52-4 A schematic demonstrating the segmental anatomy of the liver. Each segment receives its own portal pedicle (triad of portal vein, hepatic artery, and bile duct). The eight segments are illustrated, and the four sectors, divided by the three main hepatic veins running in scissurae, are shown. The umbilical fissure (not a scissura) is shown to contain the left portal pedicle. (From Blumgart LH, Hann LE: Surgical and radiologic anatomy of the liver and biliary tract. In Blumgart LH, Fong Y [eds]: Surgery of the Liver and Biliary Tract. London, WB Saunders, 2000, pp 3-34.)

marking of the liver, historically was used to mark the division of the right and left lobes of the liver in early descriptions of hepatic anatomy. However, this description is inaccurate and of minimal utility to the hepatobiliary surgeon (see later for detailed segmental anatomy). On the posterior surface of the left liver, running from the left portal vein in the porta hepatis toward the left hepatic vein and the IVC, is the ligamentum venosum (obliterated sinus venosus), which also runs in a fissure (Fig. 52-1). Hepatic arterial and portal venous blood flow enter the liver at the hilum and branch throughout the liver as a single unit that also includes the bile ducts (portal triad). These portal triads are invested in a peritoneal sheath that invaginates at the hepatic hilum. Venous drainage is through hepatic veins that empty directly into the IVC.[4]

Normal Development and Embryology

The liver primordium is formed in the third week of gestation as an outgrowth of endodermal epithelium (known as the *hepatic diverticulum,* or *liver bud*). The connection between the hepatic diverticulum and the future duodenum narrows to form the bile duct, and an outpouching of the bile duct forms into the gallbladder and cystic duct. Hepatic cells develop cords and intermingle with the vitelline and umbilical veins to form hepatic sinusoids. Simultaneously, hematopoietic cells, Kupffer cells, and connective tissue form from the meso-

derm of the septum transversum. The mesoderm of the septum transversum connects the liver to the ventral abdominal wall and to the foregut. As the liver protrudes into the abdominal cavity, these structures are stretched into thin membranes, ultimately forming the falciform ligament and the lesser omentum, respectively. The mesoderm on the surface of the developing liver differentiates into visceral peritoneum except superiorly, where contact between the liver and mesoderm (future diaphragm) is maintained, forming a bare area devoid of visceral peritoneum (Fig. 52-2).

The primitive liver plays a central role in fetal circulation. The vitelline veins carry blood from the yolk sac to the sinus venosus and ultimately form a network of veins around the foregut (future duodenum) that drain into the developing hepatic sinusoids. These vitelline veins eventually fuse to form the portal, superior mesenteric, and splenic veins. The sinus venosus, which empties into the fetal heart, ultimately becomes the hepatocardiac channel and then the hepatic veins and posthepatic IVC. The umbilical veins, which are paired early on, carry oxygenated blood to the fetus. Initially, the umbilical veins drain into the sinus venosus, but at 5 weeks, they begin to drain into the hepatic sinusoids. The right umbilical vein ultimately disappears, and the left umbilical vein later drains directly into the hepatocardiac channel, bypassing the hepatic sinusoids through the ductus venosus. In the adult liver, the remnant of the left umbilical vein becomes the ligamentum teres, which runs

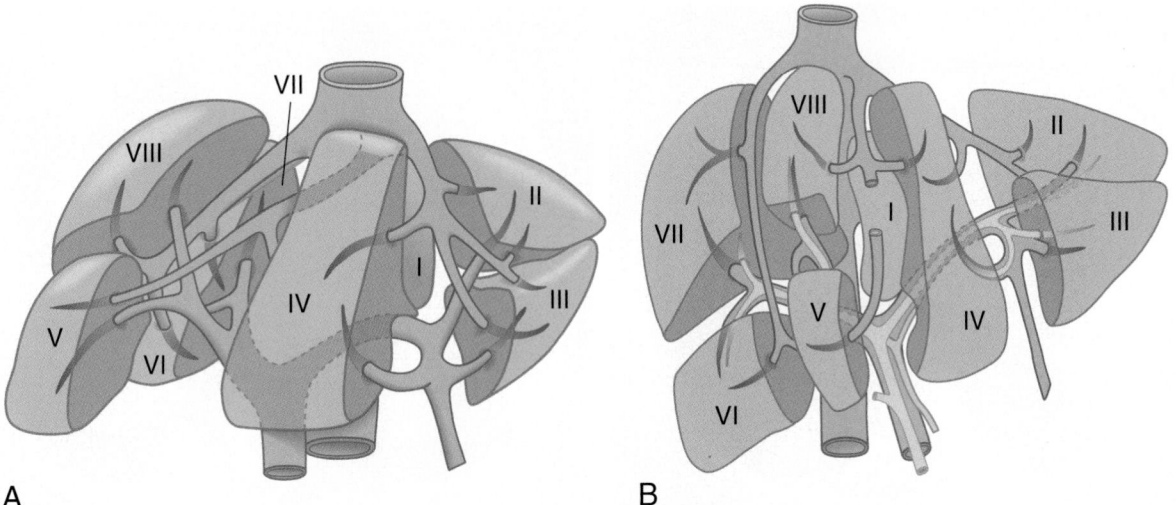

A   B

Figure 52-5 Segmental anatomy of the liver as seen at laparotomy in the anatomic position **(A)** and in the ex vivo position **(B).** (From Blumgart LH, Hann LE: Surgical and radiologic anatomy of the liver and biliary tract. In Blumgart LH, Fong Y [eds]: Surgery of the Liver and Biliary Tract. London, WB Saunders, 2000, pp 3-34.)

in the falciform ligament into the umbilical fissure and the remnant of the ductus venosus becomes the ligamentum venosus at the termination of the lesser omentum under the left liver (Fig. 52-3).

The fetal liver plays an important role in hematopoiesis. In the 10th week of gestation, the liver is 10% of the body weight, which is due to developing hepatic sinusoids and active hematopoiesis. During the last 2 months of intrauterine life, hepatic hematopoiesis decreases, and the weight of the liver is decreased to 5% of body weight. By the 12th week of gestation, bile forms in hepatic cells, along with the simultaneous development of the gall-bladder and bile duct, allowing drainage of bile into the foregut.[5]

Functional Anatomy

Historically, the liver was divided into left and right lobes by the obvious external landmark of the falciform ligament. Not only was this description oversimplified, but it was also anatomically incorrect in relationship to the blood supply to the liver. Later, more accurate descriptions of the lobar anatomy of the liver were developed. The liver was divided into right and left lobes determined by portal and hepatic vein branches. Briefly, a plane without any surface markings running from the gall-bladder to the left side of the IVC (known as the *portal fissure,* or *Cantlie's line*) divided the liver into right and left lobes. The right lobe was further divided into anterior and posterior segments. The left lobe was divided into a medial segment (also known as the *quadrate lobe*) that lies to the right of the falciform ligament and umbilical fissure and a lateral segment lying to the left. This system, although anatomically more correct, is only sufficient for mobilization of the liver and simple hepatic procedures. It does not describe the more intricate and functional segmental anatomy that is essential to understand before pursuing complex hepatobiliary surgery.[1]

The functional anatomy (Figs. 52-4 and 52-5) of the liver is composed of eight segments, each of which is supplied by a single portal triad (also called a *pedicle*)

composed of a portal vein, hepatic artery, and bile duct. These segments are further organized into four sectors that are separated by scissurae containing the three main hepatic veins. The four sectors are even further organized into the right and left liver (the phrase *right and left liver* is preferable to *right and left lobe* because there is no external mark that allows the identification of the right and left liver). This system was originally described in 1957 by Woodsmith and Goldburne as well as Couinaud and defines hepatic anatomy as it is most relevant to surgery of the liver.[4] The functional anatomy is more often seen as cross-sectional imaging, and Figure 52-6 shows the anatomy in this context.

The main scissura contains the middle hepatic vein, which runs in an anteroposterior direction from the gall-bladder fossa to the left side of the vena cava and divides the liver into right and left hemi-livers. The line of the main scissura is also known as *Cantlie's line.* The right liver is divided into an anterior (segments V and VIII) and posterior (segments VI and VII) sector by the right scissura, which contains the right hepatic vein. The right portal pedicle, composed of the right hepatic artery, portal vein, and bile duct, splits into right anterior and posterior pedicles that supply the segments of the anterior and posterior sectors.

The left liver has a visible fissure along its inferior surface called the *umbilical fissure.* The ligamentum teres (containing the remnant of the umbilical vein) runs into this fissure. The falciform ligament is contiguous with the umbilical fissure and ligamentum teres. The umbilical fissure is *not* a scissura, does not contain a hepatic vein, and in fact, contains the left portal pedicle (triad containing the left portal vein, hepatic artery, and bile duct), which runs in this fissure, branching to feed the left liver. The left scissura runs posterior to the ligamentum teres and contains the left hepatic vein. The left liver is split into an anterior (segments III and IV) and posterior (segment II—the only sector composed of a single segment) sector by the left scissura.

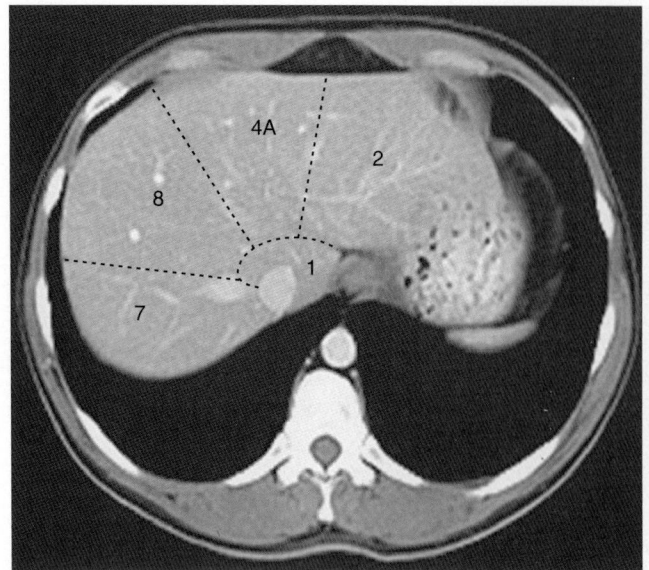

A

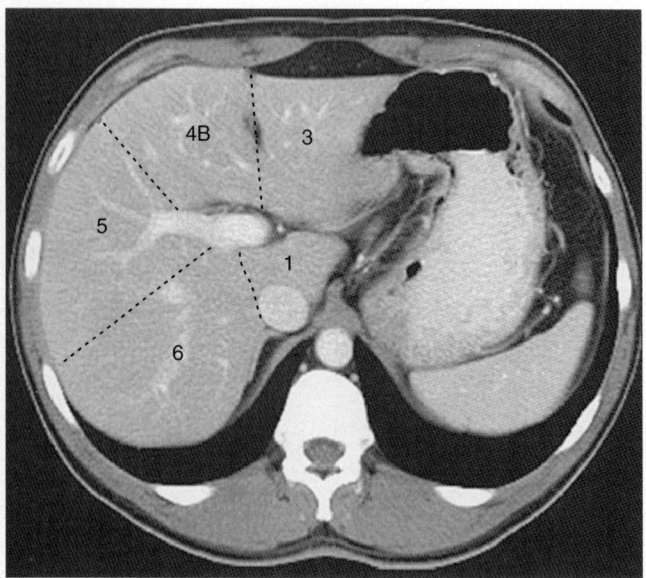

B

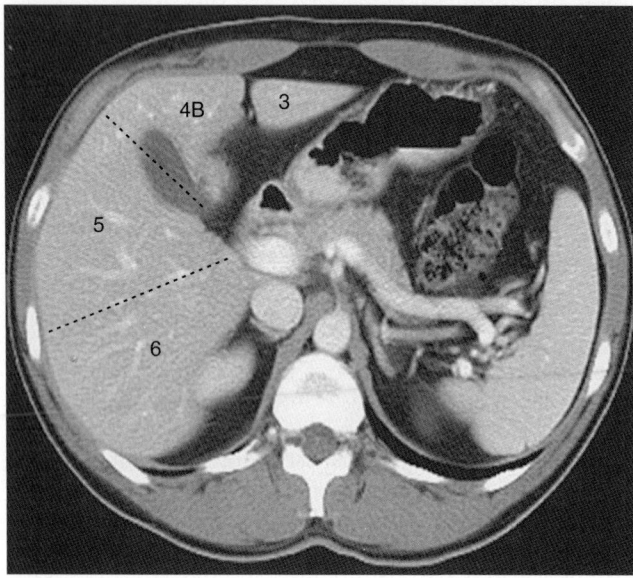

C

Figure 52-6 Segmental anatomy of the liver is demonstrated at three levels on contrast-enhanced CT images. **A,** At the level of the hepatic veins, segment I is seen posteriorly embracing the vena cava. Segment II is separated from segment IVA by the left hepatic vein. Segment IVA is separated from segment VIII by the middle hepatic vein, and segment VIII is separated from segment VII by the right hepatic vein. **B,** At the level of the portal vein bifurcation, segment III is visible as it hangs inferiorly in its anatomic position and is separated from segment IVB by the umbilical fissure. Note that segment II is not visible at this level. Terminal branches of the middle hepatic vein separate segment IVB from segment V, and terminal branches of the right hepatic vein separate segment V from segment VI. Note that segments IVA, VIII, and VII are not visible at this level. Segment I is seen posterior to the portal vein and embracing the vena cava. **C,** Below the portal bifurcation, one can see the inferior tips of segments III and IVB. The terminal branches of the middle hepatic vein and the gallbladder mark the separation of segment IVB from segment V. Segments V and VI are separated by the distal branches of the right hepatic vein. Note how the right liver hangs well inferior to the left liver.

At the hilum of the liver, the right portal triad has a short extrahepatic course of about 1 to 1.5 cm before entering the substance of the liver and branching into anterior and posterior sectoral branches. The left portal triad, however, has a long extrahepatic course of up to 3 or 4 cm and runs transversely along the base of segment IV in a peritoneal sheath that is the upper end of the lesser omentum. The left portal triad, as it runs along the base of segment IV, is separated from the liver substance by connective tissue known as the hilar plate (Fig. 52-7). The continuation of the left portal triad runs anteriorly and caudally in the umbilical fissure and gives branches to segments II and III and recurrent branches to segment IV.

The caudate lobe (segment I) is the dorsal portion of the liver and embraces the IVC on its posterior surface and lies posterior to the left portal triad inferiorly and the left and middle hepatic veins superiorly. The main bulk of the caudate lobe is to the left of the IVC, but inferiorly, it traverses between the IVC and left portal triad, where it fuses to the right liver (segments VI and VII). This part of the caudate lobe is known as the right portion or the caudate process. The left portion of the caudate lobe lies in the lesser omental bursa and is covered anteriorly by the gastrohepatic ligament (lesser omentum) that separates it from segments II and III anteriorly. The gastrohepatic ligament attaches to the ligamentum venosum (sinus venosus remnant) along the left side of the left portal triad (Fig. 52-8).

The vascular inflow and biliary drainage to the caudate lobe comes from both the right and left systems. The right side of the caudate (the caudate process) largely derives its portal venous supply from the right portal vein or the bifurcation of the main portal vein, whereas the

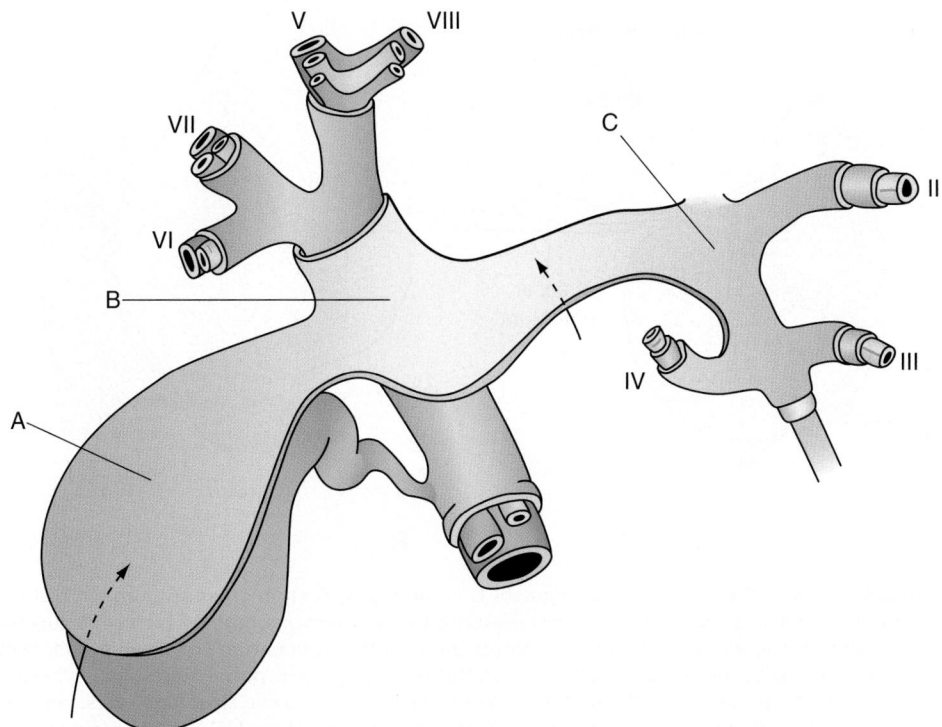

Figure 52-7 The plate system is illustrated. A, The cystic plate between the gallbladder and the liver. B, The hilar plate at the biliary confluence at the base of segment IV. C, The umbilical plate above the umbilical portion of the portal vein. The *arrows* show the plane of dissection of the cystic plate for cholecystectomy and the hilar plate for exposure of the hepatic duct confluence and the main left hepatic duct. (From Blumgart LH, Hann LE: Surgical and radiologic anatomy of the liver and biliary tract. In Blumgart LH, Fong Y [eds]: Surgery of the Liver and Biliary Tract. London, WB Saunders, 2000, pp 3-34.)

left portion of the caudate derives its portal venous inflow from the left main portal vein. The arterial supply and the biliary drainage of the right portion are generally through the right posterior sectoral system and the left portion through the left main vessels. The hepatic venous drainage of the caudate is unique in that multiple small veins drain posteriorly directly into the IVC.

The posterior edge of the left side of the caudate terminates into a fibrous component that attaches to the crura of the diaphragm and also runs posteriorly, wrapping behind the IVC and attaching to segment VII of the right liver. Up to 50% of the time, this fibrous component is composed either partially or completely of liver parenchyma, and thus liver tissue may completely encircle the IVC. This important structure is known as the *IVC ligament* and is important when mobilizing the right liver or the caudate lobe off of the vena cava.

Anomalous development of the liver is uncommonly encountered. Complete absence of the left liver has been reported. A tongue of tissue extending inferiorly off of the right liver has been described (Riedel's lobe). Rare cases of supradiaphragmatic liver in the absence of a hernia sac have been noted.[4]

Portal Vein

The portal vein provides about 75% of hepatic blood flow, and although it is postcapillary and largely deoxy-genated, its large-volume flow rate provides 50% to 70% of the liver's oxygenation. The lack of valves in the portal venous system provides a system that can accommodate high flow at low pressure because of the low resistance and allows measurement of portal venous pressure anywhere along the system.

The portal vein forms behind the neck of the pancreas at the confluence of the superior mesenteric vein and the splenic vein at the height of the second lumbar vertebra. The length of the main portal vein ranges from 5.5 to 8 cm, and its diameter is usually about 1 cm. Cephalad to its formation behind the neck of the pancreas, the portal vein runs behind the first portion of the duodenum and into the hepatoduodenal ligament, where it runs along the right border of the lesser omentum, usually posterior to the bile duct and hepatic artery.

The portal vein divides into main right and left branches at the hilum of the liver. The left branch of the portal vein runs transversely along the base of segment IV and into the umbilical fissure, where it gives off branches to segments II and III and feedback branches to segment IV. The left portal vein also gives off posterior branches to the left side of the caudate lobe. The right portal vein has a short extrahepatic course and usually enters the substance of the liver, where it splits into anterior and posterior sectoral branches. These sectoral branches can occasionally be seen extrahepatically and can come off

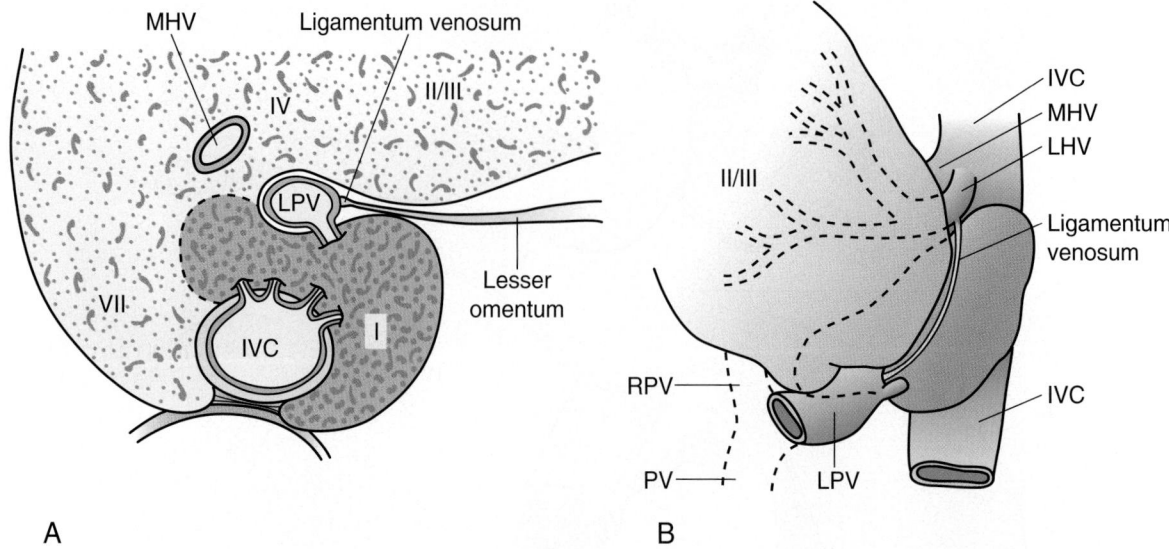

Figure 52-8 The anatomy of the caudate lobe (segment I) is shown. **A,** Seen in cross section, most of the caudate is to the left of the inferior vena cava (IVC) and lies posterior to the lesser omentum, which separates the caudate from segments II and III. The termination of the lesser omentum at the ligamentum venosum is demonstrated. The caudate traverses to the right, insinuating itself between the IVC and the left portal vein (LPV), where it attaches to the right liver. Note the proximity of the middle hepatic vein (MHV) to these structures. **B,** Segments II and III have been rotated to the patient's right, exposing the left side of the caudate. LHV, left hepatic vein; PV, portal vein. (From Blumgart LH, Hann LE: Surgical and radiologic anatomy of the liver and biliary tract. In Blumgart LH, Fong Y [eds]: Surgery of the Liver and Biliary Tract. London, WB Saunders, 2000, pp 3-34.)

the main portal vein before its bifurcation. There is usually a small branch off the right portal vein or at the bifurcation that comes off posteriorly to supply the caudate process[4] (Fig. 52-9).

There are a number of connections between the portal venous system and the systemic venous system. Under conditions of high portal venous pressure, these portosystemic connections may enlarge secondary to collateral flow. This concept is reviewed in more detail in Chapter 53, but the most significant portosystemic collateral locations are listed:

1. Submucosal veins of the proximal stomach and distal esophagus, which receive portal flow from the short gastric veins and the left gastric vein and can result in varices with the potential for intestinal hemorrhage
2. Umbilical and abdominal wall veins, which recanalize from flow through the umbilical vein in the ligamentum teres, resulting in caput medusae
3. Superior hemorrhoidal plexus, which receives portal flow from inferior mesenteric vein tributaries and yields large hemorrhoids
4. Other retroperitoneal communications yielding collaterals that can make abdominal surgery hazardous

The anatomy of the portal vein and its branches is relatively constant and has much less variation than the ductal and hepatic arterial system. The portal vein is rarely found anterior to the neck of the pancreas and the duodenum. Entrance of the portal vein directly into the vena cava has also been described. Rarely, a pulmonary vein may enter the portal vein. Lastly, there may be a congenital absence of the left branch of the portal vein.

In this situation, the right branch courses through the right liver and curves around peripherally to supply the left liver.[4]

Hepatic Artery

The hepatic artery, representing high-flow oxygenated systemic arterial flow, provides about 25% of the hepatic blood flow and 30% to 50% of its oxygenation. A number of smaller perihepatic arteries derived from the inferior phrenic and the gastroduodenal arteries also supply the liver. These vessels are important sources of collateral blood flow in the event of occlusion of the main hepatic arterial inflow. In the case of ligation of the right or left hepatic artery, intrahepatic collaterals almost immediately provide for nutrient blood flow.

The common description of the arterial supply to the liver and biliary tree is present only about 60% of the time (Fig. 52-10). The celiac trunk originates directly off the aorta just below the aortic diaphragmatic hiatus and gives off three branches: the splenic artery, the left gastric artery, and the common hepatic artery. The common hepatic artery passes forward and to the right along the superior border of the pancreas and runs along the right side of the lesser omentum, where it ascends toward the hepatic hilum lying anterior to the portal vein and to the left of the bile duct. At the point that the common hepatic artery begins to head superiorly toward the hepatic hilum, it gives off the gastroduodenal artery, followed by the supraduodenal artery and then the right gastric artery. The common hepatic artery beyond the takeoff of the gastroduodenal artery is called the *proper hepatic artery* and divides into right and left branches at the hilum. The left hepatic artery heads vertically toward the umbilical fissure to supply segments I, II, and III. The left hepatic artery usually gives off a middle hepatic artery branch that heads toward the right side of the umbilical fissure and supplies segment IV. The right hepatic artery usually runs posterior to the common hepatic bile duct and enters Calot's triangle (bordered by the cystic duct, common hepatic duct, and the liver edge), where it gives off the cystic artery to supply the gallbladder and then continues into the substance of the right liver.

Unlike portal vein anatomy, hepatic arterial anatomy is extraordinarily variable (Fig. 52-11). An accessory vessel is described as an aberrant origin of a branch that is in addition to the normal branching pattern. A replaced vessel is described as an aberrant origin of a branch that substitutes for the lack of the normal branch. Most often, the hepatic artery originates off of the celiac trunk, but different branches of the entire hepatic arterial system can originate off of the superior mesenteric artery (SMA). The right and left hepatic arteries can also arise separately off of the celiac axis. Replaced or accessory right hepatic arteries come off the SMA and are present about 10% to 20% of the time.

Hepatic vessels replaced to the SMA run behind the head of the pancreas, posterior to the portal vein in the portacaval space. The right hepatic artery, in its usual branching pattern, can also course anterior to the common hepatic duct. A replaced or accessory left hepatic artery is present about 7% to 18% of the time, originating from the left gastric artery and coursing within the lesser omentum heading toward the umbilical fissure. Other important variations include the origin of the gastroduodenal artery, which has been found to originate from the right hepatic artery and is occasionally duplicated. The anatomy of the cystic artery is also quite variable, and knowledge of these variations is of particular importance in the performance of cholecystectomy (Fig. 52-12). An accessory cystic artery can originate from the proper hepatic artery or the gastroduodenal artery, where it runs anterior to the bile duct. A single cystic artery can originate anywhere off of the proper hepatic artery or the gastroduodenal artery, or directly from the celiac axis. These variant cystic arteries can run anterior to the bile duct and are not necessarily present in the triangle of Calot. All these variations in hepatic arterial anatomy are of obvious importance during hepatic resection, hepatic arterial pump placement, cholecystectomy, and hepatic interventional radiologic procedures.[4]

Hepatic Veins

The three major hepatic veins drain from the superior and posterior surface of the liver directly into the IVC (see Figs. 52-4, 52-5, and 52-6). The right hepatic vein runs in the right scissura (between the anterior and posterior sectors of the right liver) and drains most of the right liver after a short (1-cm) extrahepatic course into the right side of the IVC. The left and middle hepatic veins usually join intrahepatically and enter the left side of the IVC as a single vessel, although they may drain separately. The left hepatic vein runs in the left scissura

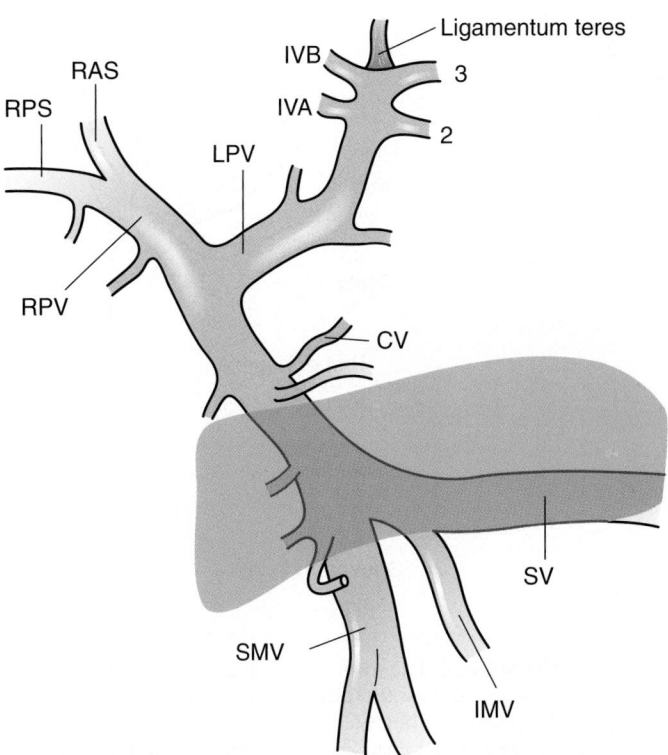

Figure 52-9 The anatomy of the portal vein is demonstrated. The superior mesenteric vein (SMV) joins the splenic vein (SV) posterior to the neck of the pancreas (*shaded*) to form the portal vein. Note the entrance of the inferior mesenteric vein (IMV) into the splenic vein—the most common anatomic arrangement. In its course superiorly in the edge of the lesser omentum posterior to the common bile duct and hepatic artery, the portal vein receives venous effluent from the coronary vein (CV). At the hepatic hilum, the portal vein bifurcates into a larger right portal vein and a smaller left portal vein. The left portal vein runs transversely at the base of segment IV and enters the umbilical fissure to supply the segments of the left liver. Just before the umbilical fissure, the left portal vein (LPV) usually gives off a sizable branch to the caudate lobe. The right portal vein (RPV) enters the substance of the liver and splits into a right anterior sectoral (RAS) and right posterior sectoral (RPS) branch. It also gives off a posterior branch to the right side of the caudate lobe/caudate process. (From Blumgart LH, Hann LE: Surgical and radiologic anatomy of the liver and biliary tract. In Blumgart LH, Fong Y [eds]: Surgery of the Liver and Biliary Tract. London, WB Saunders, 2000, pp 3-34.)

(between segments II and III) and drains segments II and III, and the middle hepatic vein runs in the portal scissura (between segment IV and the anterior sector of the right liver) draining segment IV and some of the anterior sector of the right liver. The umbilical vein is an additional vein that runs under the falciform ligament, between the left and middle veins, and usually empties into the left hepatic vein. Multiple small venous branches from the right posterior sector and the caudate lobe drain posteriorly directly into the IVC. A substantial inferior accessory right hepatic vein is commonly encountered. There is often a venous tributary from the caudate that drains superiorly into the left hepatic vein.[4]

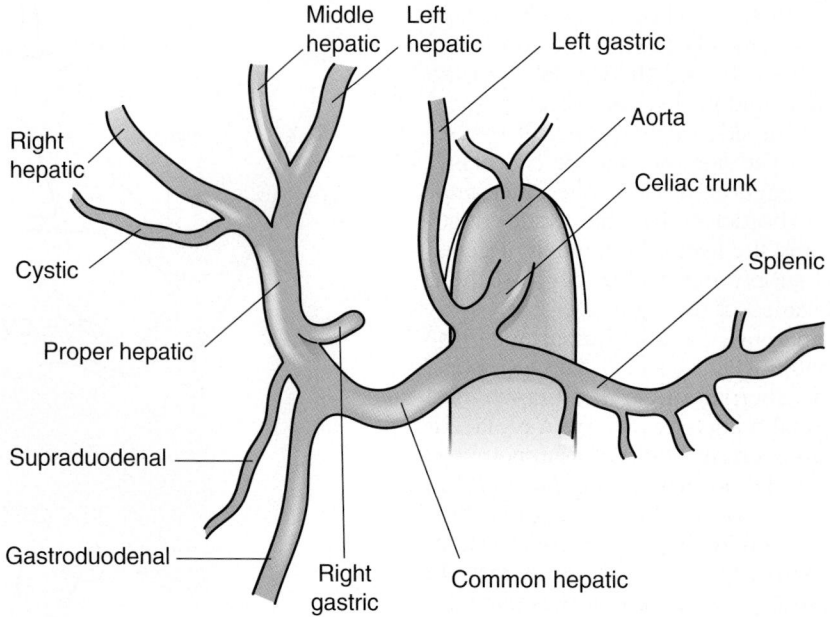

Figure 52-10 The most common anatomy of the celiac axis and hepatic arterial system is demonstrated. The celiac axis, just below the diaphragmatic hiatus, trifurcates into the splenic, left gastric, and common hepatic arteries. The common hepatic artery heads to the right and turns superiorly toward the hilum. At the point of this turn, the gastroduodenal artery is given off, and the proper hepatic artery is formed. The common hepatic artery gives off right and left hepatic arteries in the hilum. Note the middle hepatic artery off of the proximal left hepatic artery, which goes on to supply segment IV. The cystic artery most commonly comes off the right hepatic artery within the triangle of Calot. (From Blumgart LH, Hann LE: Surgical and radiologic anatomy of the liver and biliary tract. In Blumgart LH, Fong Y [eds]: Surgery of the Liver and Biliary Tract. London, WB Saunders, 2000, pp 3-34.)

Biliary System

The intrahepatic bile ducts are terminal branches of the main right and left hepatic ductal branches that invaginate Glisson's capsule at the hilum along with corresponding portal vein and hepatic artery branches, forming the peritoneal covered portal triads. Along these intrahepatic portal pedicles, the bile duct branches are usually superior to the portal vein, whereas the hepatic artery branches run inferiorly. The left hepatic bile duct drains segments II, III, and IV, which constitute the left liver. The intrahepatic ductal branches of the left liver join to form the main left duct at the base of the umbilical fissure, where the left hepatic duct courses transversely across the base of segment IV to join the right hepatic duct at the hilum. In its transverse portion, the left hepatic duct drains 1 to 3 small branches from segment IV. The right hepatic duct drains the right liver and is formed by the joining of the anterior sectoral duct (draining segments V and VIII) and the posterior sectoral duct (draining segments VI and VII). The posterior sectoral duct runs in a horizontal and posterior direction, whereas the anterior sectoral duct runs vertically. The main right hepatic duct bifurcates just above the right portal vein. The short right hepatic duct meets the longer left hepatic duct, forming the confluence anterior to the right portal vein, constituting the common hepatic duct. The caudate lobe (segment I) has its own biliary drainage, which is usually through both right and left systems, although in up to 15% of cases, drainage is through the left system only, and in 5%, it is through the right system only.[4]

The common hepatic duct drains inferiorly, and below the takeoff of the cystic duct is referred to as the *common bile duct*. The common bile or hepatic duct runs along the right side of the hepatoduodenal ligament (free edge of the lesser omentum) to the right of the hepatic artery and anterior to the portal vein. The common bile duct continues inferiorly (usually ~10-15 cm in length and 6 mm in diameter) behind the first portion of the duodenum and into the head of the pancreas in an inferior and slightly rightward direction. The intrapancreatic distal common bile duct then joins with the main pancreatic duct (of Wirsung), with or without a common channel, and enters the second portion of the duodenum through the major papilla of Vater. At the choledochoduodenal junction, a complex muscular complex known as the *sphincter of Oddi* regulates bile flow and prevents reflux of duodenal contents into the biliary tree. There are three major parts to this sphincter: the sphincter choledochus, which is a circular muscle that serves to regulate bile flow and the filling of the gallbladder; the pancreatic sphincter, present to variable degrees, which surrounds the intraduodenal pancreatic duct; and the sphincter ampullae, made up of longitudinal muscle, which serves to prevent duodenal reflux.[4]

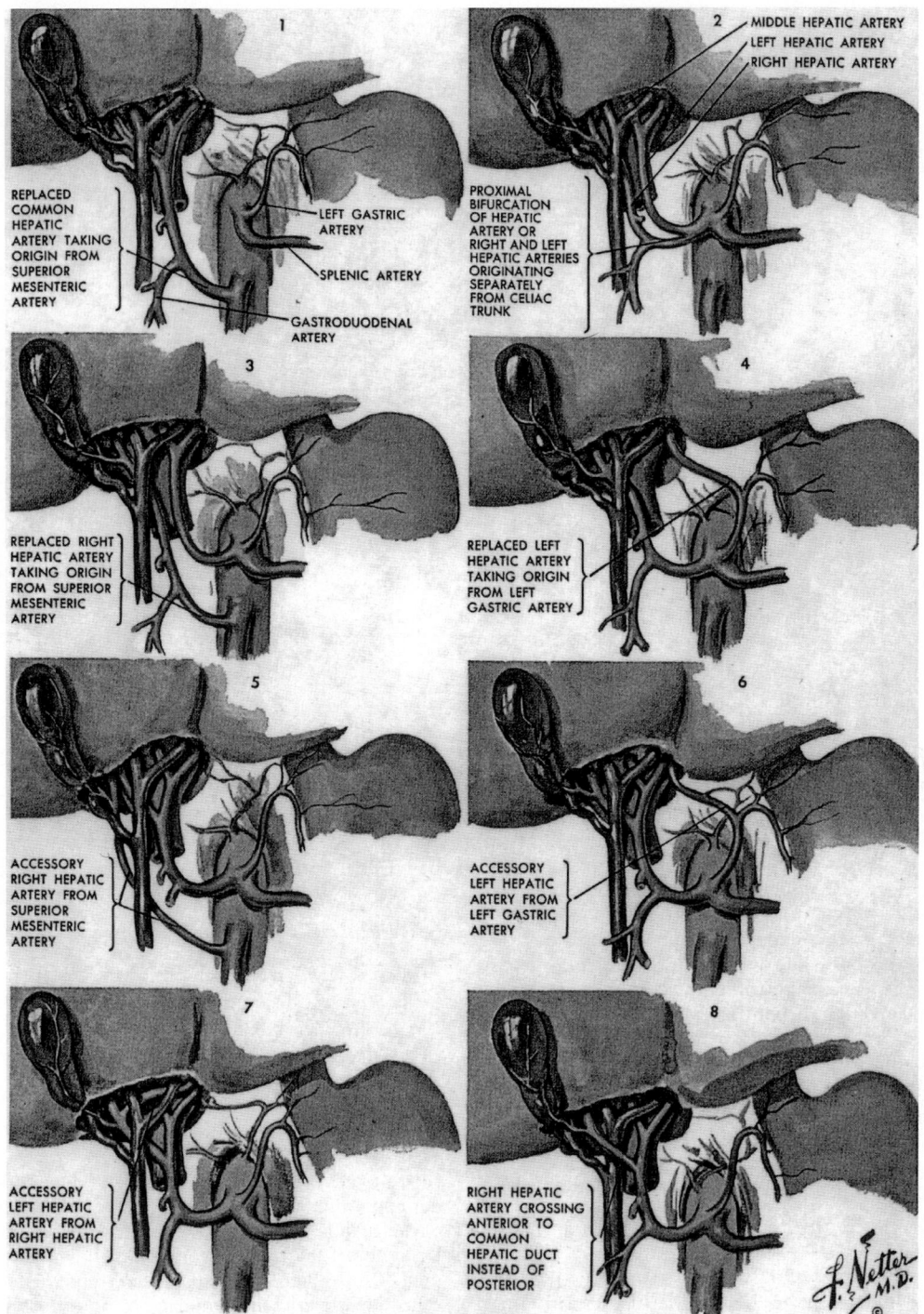

Figure 52-11 The variable anatomy of the hepatic artery is demonstrated. The common hepatic artery can originate off of the superior mesenteric artery instead of the celiac axis. A replaced or accessory right hepatic artery comes off the superior mesenteric artery and runs posterior to the head of the pancreas, to the right of the portal vein and behind the common bile duct into the hilum. A replaced or accessory left hepatic artery originates off of the left gastric artery and runs through the lesser omentum into the umbilical fissure. (From Netter FH: Liver, biliary tract and pancreas. In Netter FH: The Netter Collection of Medical Illustrations. Teterboro, NJ, ICON Learning Systems, 2001.)

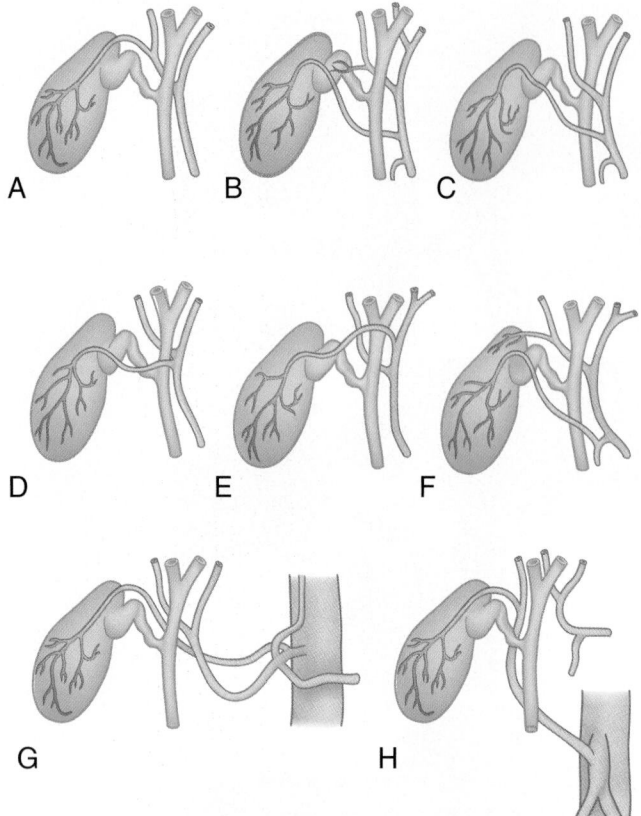

Figure 52-12 Variations in the anatomy of the cystic artery are demonstrated. **A,** Most common anatomy. **B,** Double cystic artery—one off the proper hepatic artery. **C,** Origin off the proper hepatic artery and coursing anterior to the bile duct. **D,** Originating off of the right hepatic artery and coursing anterior to the bile duct. **E,** Originating from the left hepatic artery and coursing anterior to the bile duct. **F,** Originating off the gastroduodenal artery. **G,** Originating off of the celiac axis. **H,** Originating from a replaced right hepatic artery. (From Blumgart LH, Hann LE: Surgical and radiologic anatomy of the liver and biliary tract. In Blumgart LH, Fong Y [eds]: Surgery of the Liver and Biliary Tract. London, WB Saunders, 2000, pp 3-34.)

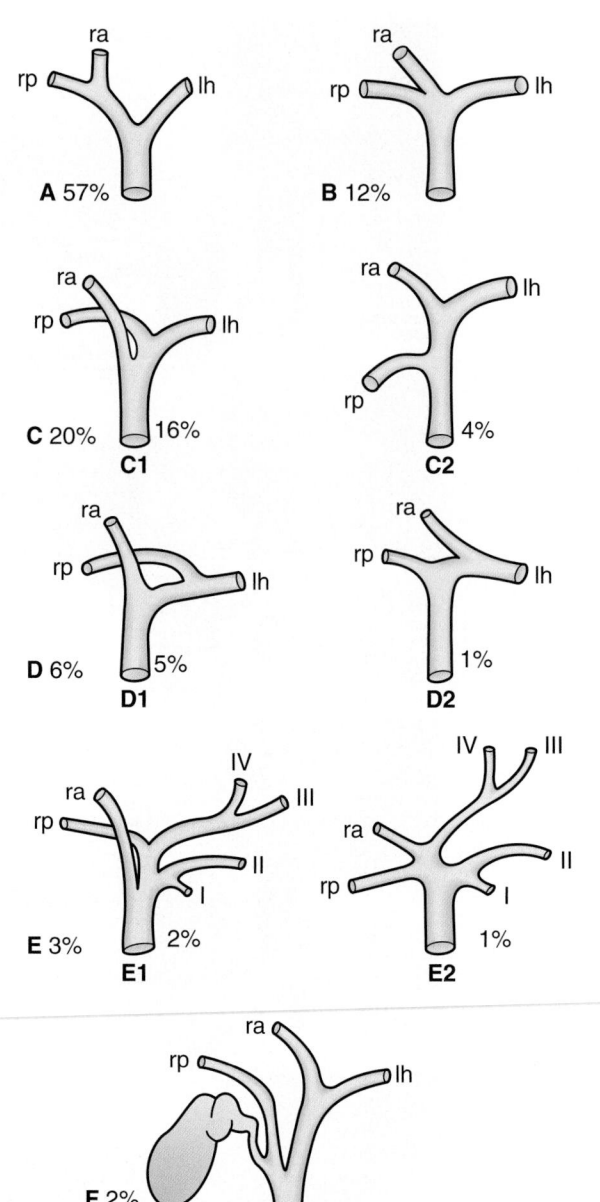

Figure 52-13 Variations of the hepatic duct confluence. **A,** Most common anatomy. **B,** Trifurcation at the confluence. **C,** Either of the right sectoral ducts drains into the common hepatic duct. **D,** Either of the right sectoral ducts drains into the left hepatic duct. **E,** Absence of a hepatic duct confluence. **F,** Absence of right hepatic duct and drainage of right posterior sectoral duct (rp) into the cystic duct. ra, right anterior sectoral duct; lh, left hepatic duct. (From Blumgart LH, Hann LE: Surgical and radiologic anatomy of the liver and biliary tract. In Blumgart LH, Fong Y [eds]: Surgery of the Liver and Biliary Tract. London, WB Saunders, 2000, pp 3-34.)

The gallbladder is a biliary reservoir that lies against the inferior surface of segments IV and V of the liver, usually making an impression against it. A peritoneal layer covers most of the gallbladder except for the portion adherent to the liver. Where the gallbladder is adherent to the liver, there is a layer of fibroconnective tissue known as the *cystic plate*, which is an extension of the hilar plate (see Fig. 52-7). Variable in size, but usually about 10 cm long and 3 to 5 cm wide, the gallbladder is composed of a fundus, body, infundibulum, and neck that ultimately empties into the cystic duct. The fundus usually projects just slightly beyond the liver edge anteriorly and when folded on itself is described as a *Phrygian cap*. Continuing toward the bile duct, the body of the gallbladder is usually in close proximity to the second portion of the duodenum and the transverse colon. The infundibulum (or Hartmann's pouch) hangs forward

along the free edge of the lesser omentum and can fold in front of the cystic duct. The portion of gallbladder between the infundibulum and the cystic duct is the neck of the gallbladder. The cystic duct is variable in its length, its course, and its insertion into the main biliary tree. The

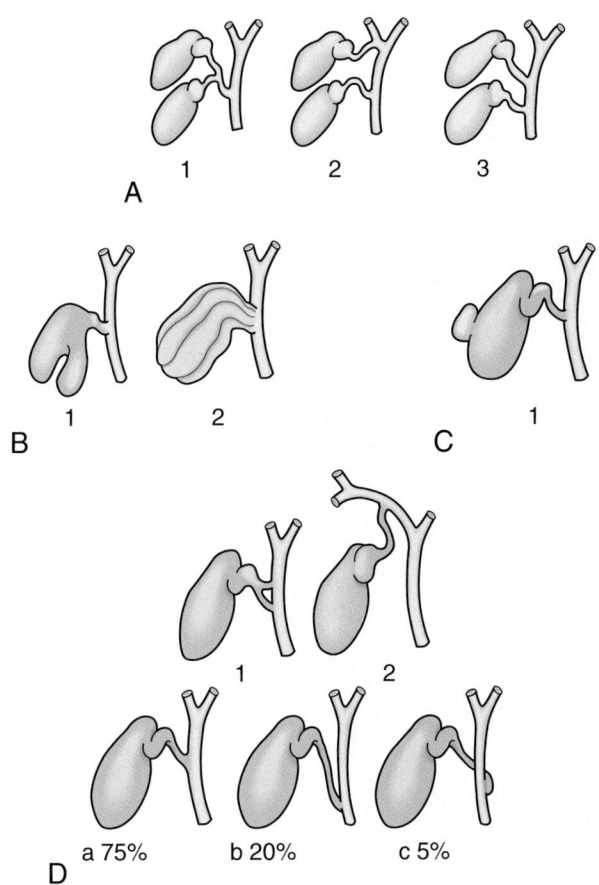

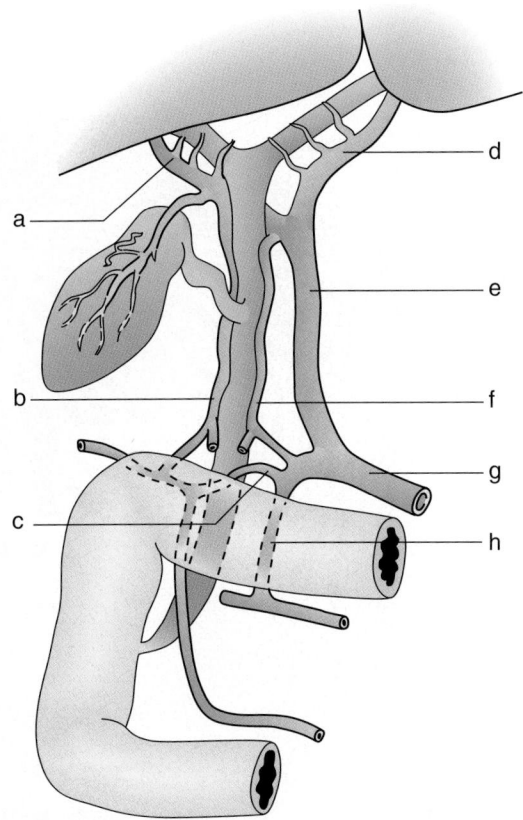

Figure 52-14 Variations in the anatomy of the gallbladder and cystic duct. **A,** Bilobar gallbladder. **B,** Septations of the gall-bladder. **C,** Diverticulum of the gallbladder. **D,** Variations in cystic duct anatomy. **The three types of union of the cystic duct and common hepatic duct are illustrated.** (From Blumgart LH, Hann LE: Surgical and radiologic anatomy of the liver and biliary tract. In Blumgart LH, Fong Y [eds]: Surgery of the Liver and Biliary Tract. London, WB Saunders, 2000, pp 3-34.)

Figure 52-15 The blood supply to the common bile duct and common hepatic duct is illustrated. a, Right hepatic artery; b, 9:00 artery; c, retroduodenal artery; d, left hepatic artery; e, proper hepatic artery; f, 3:00 artery; g, common hepatic artery; h, gastroduodenal artery. (From Blumgart LH, Hann LE: Surgical and radiologic anatomy of the liver and biliary tract. In Blumgart LH, Fong Y [eds]: Surgery of the Liver and Biliary Tract. London, WB Saunders, 2000, pp 3-34.)

first portion of the cystic duct is usually tortuous and contains mucosal duplications, referred to as the *fold of Heister,* that regulate the filling and emptying of the gallbladder. Most commonly, the cystic duct joins the hepatic duct to form the common bile duct.[4]

Knowledge of the multiple and frequent variations in the anatomy of the biliary tree is absolutely essential to perform hepatobiliary procedures. Anomalies of the hepatic ductal confluence are common, with the normal anatomy described previously present about two thirds of the time. The most common anomalies of the biliary confluence involve variations in the insertion of the right sectoral ducts (more commonly, the posterior sectoral duct). The confluence can be a trifurcation of the right anterior sectoral, right posterior sectoral, and left hepatic ducts. Either of the right sectoral ducts can drain into the left hepatic duct, the common hepatic duct, the cystic duct, or rarely the gallbladder (Fig. 52-13). Anomalies of the gallbladder itself are rare. Agenesis of the gallbladder,

bilobar gallbladder with two ducts or a single duct, and septations and congenital diverticulum of the gallbladder have all been described. Anomalies of the position of the gallbladder are more common and include an intrahepatic position or rarely presence on the left side of the liver. The gallbladder can also have a long mesentery, which can predispose to torsion. The position and entry of the cystic duct into the main ductal system is variable. Double cystic ducts draining a unilocular gallbladder and drainage into hepatic duct branches have been reported. Usually, the cystic duct joins the common hepatic duct at an angle, but it can run parallel and enter it more distally. In the latter situation, the cystic duct can be fused to the hepatic duct along its parallel course by connective tissue. The cystic duct can also run a spiral course anteriorly or posteriorly and enter the left side of the hepatic duct. Lastly, the cystic duct can be very short or even absent[4] (Fig. 52-14).

The supraduodenal and infrahilar bile duct are predominantly supplied by two axial vessels that run in a

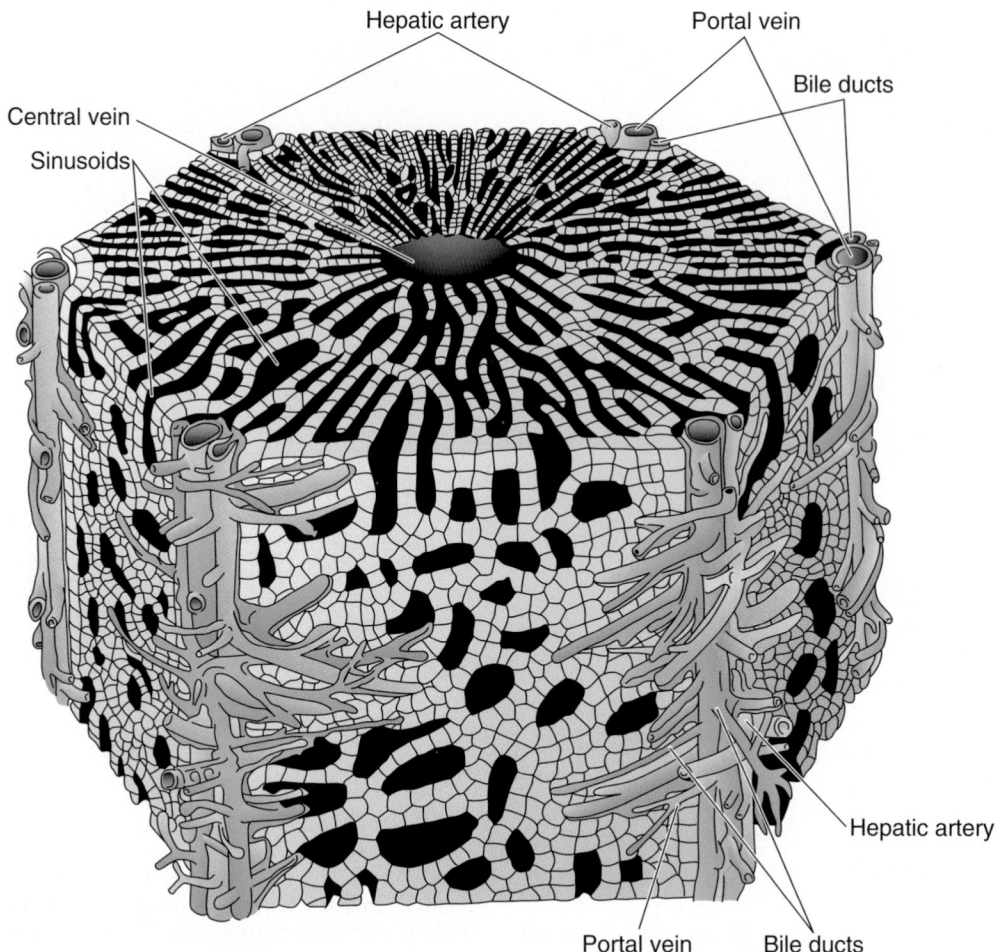

Figure 52-16 Schematic illustration of a hepatic lobule seen as a three-dimensional polyhedral unit. The terminal portal triads (hepatic artery, portal vein, and bile duct) are at each corner and give off branches along the sides of the lobule. Hepatocytes are in single-cell sheets with sinusoids on either end aligned radially toward a central hepatic venule. (From Ross MH, Reith EJ, Romrell LJ: The liver. In Ross RH, Reith EJ, Romrell LJ: Histology: A Text and Atlas. Baltimore, Williams & Wilkins, 1989, pp 471-478.)

3- and 9-o'clock position. These vessels are derived from the superior pancreaticoduodenal, right hepatic, cystic, gastroduodenal, and retroduodenal arteries. It has been estimated that only 2% of the arterial supply to this portion of the bile duct is segmental and arises directly off of the proper hepatic artery. The bile duct and its bifurcation in the hilum derive their arterial supply from a rich network of multiple small branches from surrounding vessels. Similarly, the retropancreatic bile duct derives its arterial supply from the retroduodenal artery, which provides a rich network of multiple small branches[4] (Fig. 52-15). Venous drainage of the bile duct parallels the arterial supply and drains into the portal venous system. The venous drainage of the gallbladder empties into the veins that drain the bile duct and does not flow directly to the portal vein.

Nerves
The innervation of the liver and biliary tract is by sympathetic fibers originating from T7 through T10 and parasympathetic fibers from both vagal nerves. The sympathetic fibers pass through celiac ganglia before giving off postganglionic fibers to the liver and bile ducts. The right-sided celiac ganglia and right vagal nerve form an anterior hepatic plexus of nerves that runs along the hepatic artery. The left-sided celiac ganglia and left vagal nerve form a posterior hepatic plexus that runs posterior to the bile duct and portal vein. The hepatic arteries are supplied by sympathetic fibers, and the gallbladder and extrahepatic bile ducts receive innervation from both sympathetic and parasympathetic fibers. The clinical significance of these nerves is still not well understood. Pain elicited from acute distention of the liver (and thus the liver capsule) is referred to the right shoulder because of innervation of the capsule from the phrenic nerve.

Lymphatics
Most lymph node drainage from the liver is to the hepatoduodenal ligament. Lymphatic drainage usually continues along the hepatic artery to the celiac lymph nodes

and from there to the cisterna chyli. Lymphatic drainage can also follow the hepatic veins to lymph nodes in the area of the suprahepatic inferior vena cava and through the diaphragmatic hiatus. The lymphatic drainage of the gallbladder and most of the extrahepatic biliary tract is generally into the lymph nodes of the hepatoduodenal ligament. This drainage can also follow along the hepatic artery to the celiac lymph nodes, but can also run to lymph nodes behind the head of the pancreas or in the inter-aortocaval groove.

Microscopic Anatomy

The Functional Unit of the Liver

The organization of hepatic parenchyma into microscopic functional units has been described in a number of ways and referred to as an *acinus* or a *lobule* (Fig. 52-16). This was originally described by Rappaport and was modified by Matsumoto and Kawakami.[6] A lobule is made up of a central terminal hepatic venule surrounded by four to six terminal portal triads forming a polygonal unit. This unit is lined on its periphery (between each terminal portal triad) by terminal portal triad branches. In between the terminal portal triads and the central hepatic venule, hepatocytes are arranged in plates, one cell thick, surrounded on each side by endothelium-lined and blood-filled sinusoids. Blood flows from the terminal portal triad through the sinusoids into the terminal hepatic venule. Bile is formed in the hepatocytes and emptied into terminal canaliculi that form on the lateral walls of the intercellular hepatocyte, ultimately coalescing into bile ducts and flowing toward the portal triads. This functional hepatic unit provides a structural basis for the many metabolic and secretory functions of the liver.

Between the terminal portal triad and the central hepatic venule, there are three zones that differ in their enzymatic makeup and exposure to nutrients and oxygenated blood. Although there is debate as to the shape of these zones and their relationship to the basic lobular unit, in general, zones 1 through 3 fan out from the terminal portal triad toward the central hepatic venule. Zone 1, the periportal zone, is exposed to an environment rich in nutrients and oxygen. Zones 2 (intermediate zone) and 3 (perivenular zone) are exposed to environments less rich in oxygen and nutrients. The cells of the different zones differ enzymatically and respond differently to toxin exposure as well as hypoxia. This anatomic arrangement also explains the phenomenon of centrilobular necrosis from hypotension because zone 3 is the most susceptible to decreases in oxygen delivery.[7]

Hepatic Microcirculation

Terminal portal vessels directly supply sinusoids, providing a constant but minimal flow into this low-volume system. The terminal hepatic arterial branches both empty into the sinusoids and provide a plexus of vessels around the terminal small bile ducts, supplying nutrients. Arterial branches provide a pulsatile, low-volume flow that enhances flow in the sinusoids. Arterial and portal vein flow vary inversely in the sinusoids and can be compensatory. Local control of blood flow in the sinusoids likely depends on arteriolar sphincters as well as on contraction of the sinusoidal lining by endothelial and stellate cells. Blood flow through sinusoids empties directly into terminal hepatic venules at the center of a functional lobule.[8]

The endothelium-lined sinusoids of the hepatic lobule provide the functional unit of the liver where afferent blood flow is exposed to functional hepatic parenchyma before being drained into hepatic venules (Fig. 52-17). The hepatic sinusoids are 7 to 15 μm wide but can increase in size 10-fold, yielding a low-resistance and low-pressure (generally 2-3 mm Hg) system. The sinusoidal endothelial cells account for 15% to 20% of the total number of hepatic cells. Sinusoidal endothelial cells are separated from hepatocytes by the space of Disse, which is an extravascular fluid compartment into which hepatocytes project microvilli. Key aspects of these endothelial cells are that they lack intercellular junctions, have no basement membrane, and contain multiple and large fenestrations. This arrangement provides for the maximal contact of hepatocyte membranes, an extravascular fluid compartment (space of Disse), and blood in the sinusoidal space. Thus, this system permits free bidirectional movement of solutes (high- and low-molecular-weight substances) into and out of hepatocytes, providing tremendous filtration potential. The fenestrations of the endothelial cells restrict movement of molecules between the sinusoids and hepatocytes and vary in response to exogenous as well as endogenous mediators.[7,8]

Other cell types are found along the sinusoidal lining. Kupffer cells, derived from the macrophage-monocyte system, are irregular stellate-shaped cells that also line the sinusoids, insinuating between endothelial cells. Kupffer cells are phagocytic, can migrate along sinusoids to areas of injury, and play a major role in the trapping of foreign substances and initiating an inflammatory response. Major histocompatibility complex II antigens are expressed on Kupffer cells but do not confer efficient antigen presentation compared with macrophages elsewhere in the body. Other lymphoid cells also exist in hepatic parenchyma, such as natural killer cells and CD4 and CD8 T cells that provide the liver with innate immunity. Hepatic stellate cells (also known as *Ito cells* or *lipocytes*) are cells high in lipid content (accounting for their phenotypic identification) found in the space of Disse. They have dendritic processes that contact hepatocyte microvilli and also wrap around endothelial cells. The major function of these stellate cells appears to be vitamin A storage and synthesis of extracellular collagen. In acute and chronic hepatic inflammatory states, these cells are activated to a myofibroblast-like state that is associated with morphologic changes, cellular contractility, decreases in intracellular vitamin A, and production of extracellular collagen. Stellate cells appear to play a central role in the development and progression of hepatic fibrosis and are the target for the development of antifibrosis drugs.

The Hepatocyte

Hepatocytes are complex and multifunctional cells that make up 60% of the cellular mass and 80% of the cyto-

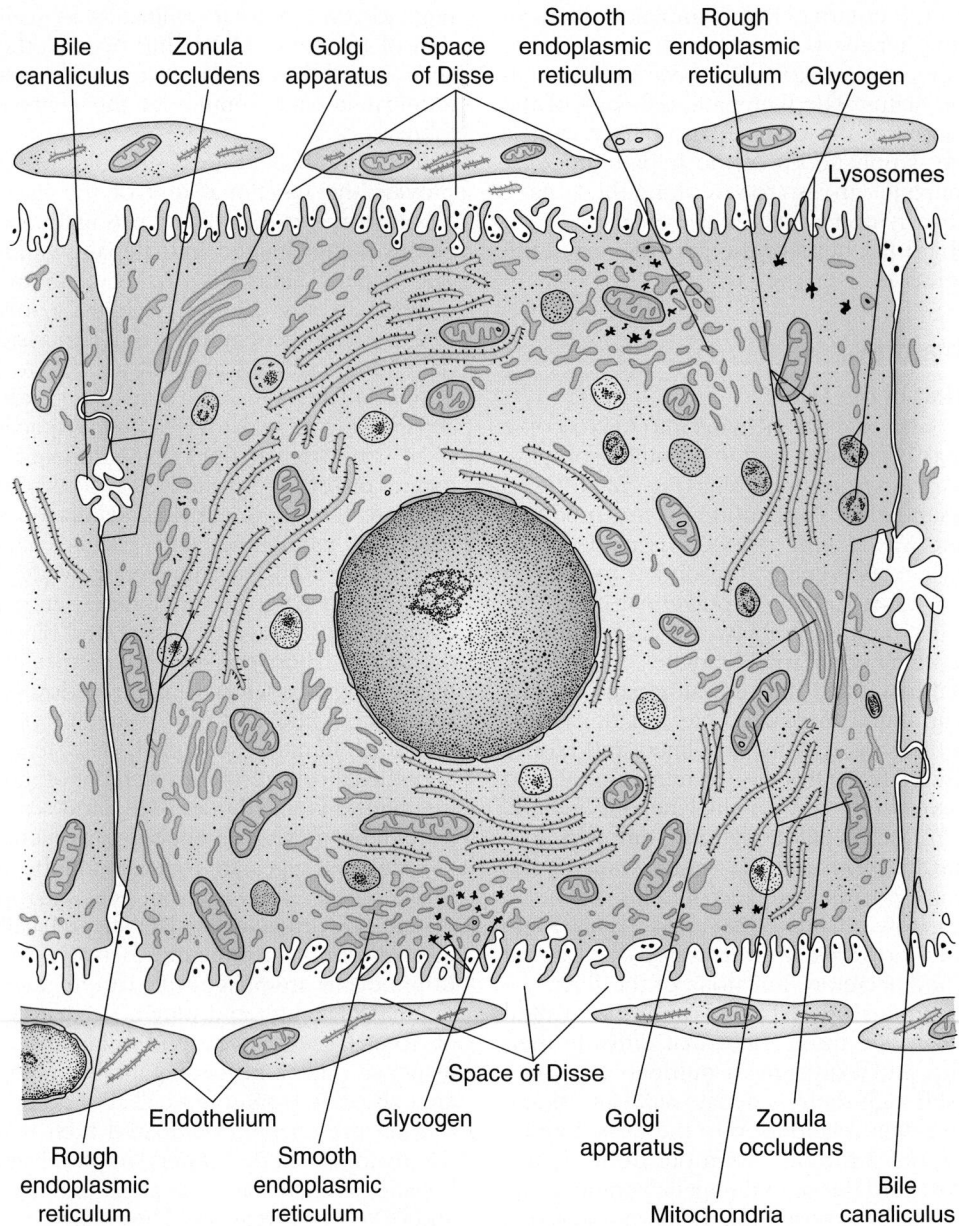

Figure 52-17 Illustration of a hepatocyte. Intracellular organelles are depicted. The endothelial-lined sinusoids on two sides of the cell are seen. In between the microvilli of the plasma membrane of the hepatocyte and the sinusoids, the extracellular fluid space of Disse is demonstrated. Along the lateral intercellular plasma membrane, bile canaliculi are formed by the apposing cells where microvilli extend into the canaliculus. Envisioning the cell in three dimensions, the bile canaliculi form a ring around each hepatocyte. (From Ross MH, Reith EJ, Romrell LJ: The liver. In Ross RH, Reith EJ, Romrell LJ: Histology: A Text and Atlas. Baltimore, Williams & Wilkins, 1989, pp 471-478.)

plasmic mass of the liver (see Fig. 52-17). Morphologically, the hepatocyte is polyhedral, with a central spherical nucleus. As mentioned earlier, hepatocytes are arranged in single-cell-layer plates that are lined on either side by blood-filled sinusoids. Every hepatocyte has contact with adjacent hepatocytes, the biliary space (bile canaliculus), and the sinusoidal space, allowing its broad range of functions. Among the many essential functions performed

by the hepatocyte are uptake, storage, and release of nutrients; synthesis of multiple plasma proteins, glucose, fatty acids, and lipids; production and secretion of bile (and thus digestion of dietary fats); and degradation and detoxification of toxins.

The plasma membrane of the hepatocyte is organized into three specific domains. The sinusoidal membrane is exposed to the space of Disse and has multiple microvilli that provide a surface specialized in the active transport of substances between the blood and hepatocyte. The lateral domain exists between neighboring hepatocytes and contains gap junctions that provide for intercellular communication. The canalicular membrane is a tube containing microvilli formed by two apposing hepatocytes. These bile canaliculi are sealed by zonulae occludentes (tight junctions), which prevent escape of bile. The bile canaliculi form a ring around the hepatocyte and drain into small bile ducts known as *canals of Herring* that ultimately empty into a bile duct at a portal triad. The canalicular membrane contains adenosine triphosphate (ATP)-dependent active transport systems that enable solutes to be secreted into the canalicular membrane against large concentration gradients.[7]

The hepatocyte is one of the most diverse and metabolically active cells in the body, which is reflected in its abundance of organelles. There are 1000 mitochondria per hepatocyte, occupying 20% of the cell volume. Mitochondria generate energy (ATP) through oxidative phosphorylation and provide the energy for the metabolic demands of the hepatocyte. The hepatocyte mitochondria are also essential for fatty acid oxidation. An extensive system of interconnected membrane complexes made up of smooth and rough endoplasmic reticulum and the Golgi complex comprise the hepatocyte microsomal fraction. These complexes have a diverse range of functions, including synthesis of secretory and structural proteins, metabolism of lipids and glucose, production and metabolism of cholesterol, glycosylation of secretory proteins, bile formation and secretion, and drug metabolism. Lysosomes are intracellular single-membrane vesicles that contain a number of enzymes and that both store and degrade exogenous and endogenous substances.[6,7] The monoclonal antibody HepPar-1 (hepatocyte paraffin-1) identifies a unique antigen on hepatocyte mitochondria and is widely used to identify hepatocytes or hepatocellular neoplasms.

Function

The unique anatomic arrangement of the liver described previously provides a remarkable landscape upon which the multiple central and critical functions of this organ can be carried out. The liver is the center of metabolic homeostasis and serves as the regulatory site for energy metabolism by coordinating the uptake, processing, and distribution of nutrients and their subsequent energy products. The liver also synthesizes a large number of proteins, enzymes, and vitamins that participate in a tremendously broad range of bodily functions. Lastly, the liver detoxifies and eliminates many exogenous and endogenous substances, serving as the major filter of the human body. The sections that follow summarize this broad range of functions.

Energy

The liver is the critical intermediary between dietary sources of energy and the extrahepatic tissues that require this energy. The critical and central nature of the liver in regulating the body's energy metabolism is evidenced by the fact that despite accounting for only 4% of body weight, the liver consumes about 28% of total body blood flow and 20% of the total oxygen consumed by the body. The liver also expends about 20% of the total kilocalories used by the whole body.

The liver receives dietary byproducts through the portal circulation and sorts them, metabolizes them, and distributes them to the systemic circulation. The liver also plays a major role in regulating systemic sources of energy, such as fatty acids and glycerol from adipose tissues, and lactate, pyruvate, and certain amino acids from skeletal muscle. The two major sources of energy that the liver releases into the extrahepatic circulation are glucose and acetoacetate. Glucose is derived from glycogenolysis of stored glycogen and from gluconeogenesis from lactate, pyruvate, glycerol, propionate, and alanine. Acetoacetate is derived from the oxidation of fatty acids. Storage lipids, such as triacylglycerols and phospholipids, are synthesized and stored as lipoproteins by the liver as well. These can be circulated in the systemic circulation to the peripheral tissues. These complex and essential functions are regulated by hormones, the overall nutritional state of the organism, and the requirements of obligate glucose-requiring tissues.[9]

Functional Heterogeneity

To add to the metabolic complexity of the liver, hepatocytes vary in their function depending on their location within the functional lobule. This functional heterogeneity of hepatocytes is anatomically related to their location within the three zones of the lobule and is specifically related to the distance from the incoming portal triad. For example, cells located in the periportal zone (zone 1) are exposed to a high concentration of substrate, and uptake of oxygen and solutes is greater. A critically important function of hepatocytes, however, is their ability to change their metabolic functionality and be recruited to perform specific functions under varying physiologic conditions regardless of anatomic location. The sinusoids are also variable in form and function. Sinusoids in the periportal zone are narrower and more tortuous, facilitating increased uptake of substrate by the hepatocyte in this area. In contrast, sinusoids in zone 3 (perivenous) have larger fenestrations, allowing uptake of larger molecules.

Enzymatic makeup, plasma membrane proteins, and ultrastructure are also heterogenous among the hepatocyte population. This cellular protein variability can also be distinguished based on the hepatocyte location within the lobule. Glucose uptake and release, bile formation, and synthesis of albumin and fibrinogen take place in the periportal zone, whereas glucose catabolism, xenobiotic metabolism, and synthesis of α_1-antitrypsin and α-fetoprotein (AFP) occur in the perivenous zone. Another example of enzymatic heterogeneity according to lobular zones is the location of the urea cycle enzymes in zone 3 adjacent to the terminal hepatic vein. The functional hepatocyte heterogeneity and its anatomic relationship to the lobular unit account for patterns of damage from metabolic or physiologic insults to the liver.[8]

Table 52-1 **Solute Concentrations of Hepatic Bile**

SOLUTE	CONCENTRATION
Na^+	132-165 mEq/L
K^+	4.2-5.6 mEq/L
Ca^{2+}	1.2-4.8 mEq/L
Mg^{2+}	1.4-3.0 mEq/L
Cl^-	96-126 mEq/L
HCO_3^-	17-55 mEq/L
Bile acids	3-45 mM
Phospholipid	25-810 mg/dL
Cholesterol	60-320 mg/dL
Protein	300-3000 mg/L

Blood Flow

The blood supply to the liver is dual and comes from the portal vein and the hepatic artery. The portal vein provides about 75% of the blood flow to the liver, which is oxygen poor but rich in nutrients. The hepatic artery provides the other 25% of the blood flow and is oxygen rich, representing systemic arterial flow. The large flow rate of the portal vein is still able to provide 50% to 70% of the afferent oxygenation to the liver. Overall, hepatic blood flow represents about one fourth of the cardiac output, demonstrating its central role in whole body metabolism. Hepatic blood flow is decreased during exercise and increased after ingestion of food (carbohydrates have the most profound effect on hepatic blood flow). Hepatic arterial pressure is representative of systemic arterial pressure. Portal pressures are generally 6 to 10 mm Hg, and sinusoidal pressure is usually 2 to 4 mm Hg.

Hepatic blood flow is regulated by a variety of factors. Differences in afferent and efferent vessel pressures, as well as muscular sphincters located at the inlet and outlet of the sinusoids, play a major role. Muscular sphincter tone is regulated by the autonomic nervous system, circulating hormones, bile salts, and metabolites. Specific endogenous factors known to affect hepatic blood flow include glucagon, histamine, bradykinin, prostaglandins, nitric oxide, and many gut hormones, such as gastrin, secretin, and cholecystokinin. The sinusoids themselves, primarily through contraction and expansion of their endothelial cells, Kupffer cells, and stellate cells, are also primary regulators of hepatic blood flow.[8]

A one-way reciprocal relationship between hepatic artery and portal vein flow has been demonstrated. Increases in hepatic arterial flow accompany decreases in portal vein flow, but the opposite does not occur. Hepatic arterial compensation, however, cannot provide complete compensation to support hepatic parenchyma in the case of total portal vein occlusion, which is likely the cause of ipsilateral atrophy in the case of a portal vein branch occlusion. Experimental evidence suggests that the buildup of adenosine in the liver plays an important role in this hepatic arterial compensatory response.

Bile Formation

Bile production and secretion is one of the major functions of the liver. The physiologic role of bile is twofold: first to dispose of certain substances secreted into bile and second to provide enteric bile salts to aid in the digestion of fats. Bile is a substance containing organic and inorganic solutes that is produced by an active process of secretion and subsequent concentration of these solutes. The concentration of inorganic solutes in bile in the main biliary tree resembles that of plasma (Table 52-1). In the case of bile loss (e.g., from an external biliary fistula), the high concentrations of protein and electrolytes must be considered when replacing the losses. The osmolality of bile is about 300 mOsm/kg and is accounted for by the inorganic solutes. The major organic solutes in bile are bile acids, bile pigments, cholesterol, and phospholipids.

The contents of bile are generally absorbed from the bloodstream through sinusoids into the hepatocyte through the sinusoidal membrane. Bile is initially secreted by hepatocytes into the canaliculi through specialized microvilli-containing lateral membranes of the hepatocytes that form the canaliculi. Tight junctions along the canalicular membranes prevent leakage of bile in the normal state, but also provide a route for paracellular secretion of solutes and water into bile. The canaliculi ultimately coalesce into larger bile ductules containing biliary epithelium, which then form the intrahepatic and extrahepatic biliary tree. Thus, the liver, in part, serves as an epithelial structure that moves solutes from blood to bile and provides a route of secretion of bile into the intestines.

About 1500 mL of bile is secreted daily, 80% of which is secreted by hepatocytes into canaliculi. Canalicular bile flow is largely due to water flow in response to active solute transport. Bile acids are transported from the sinusoidal blood into the hepatocyte by ATP-requiring active transport. Intracellular transport to the canalicular membrane is through bile acid–binding proteins that are transported by a vesicular system derived from the Golgi apparatus. The bile acids are then actively pumped into the canaliculus through an ATP-requiring active transport system. It is well recognized that bile flow has a linear association with bile acid secretion, known as *bile acid–dependent flow*. Because bile acids are micellar in bile and do not provide osmotic potential, it is likely that flow related to bile acid secretion is secondary to ions that accompany the bile acids (counter-ions). Bile flow can also occur in the near absence of bile acid secretion and is know as *bile acid–independent flow*. Experimental evidence suggests that bile acid–independent flow is at least partially the result of biliary glutathione secretion.

After bile has passed from the canaliculi to the biliary ductules and main bile ducts, bile undergoes further reabsorption and secretion. The epithelial cells of the biliary lining actively reabsorb and secrete water and electrolytes. Secretion is generally through a chloride channel that is activated by secretin (its most powerful activator) and its subsequent activation of cyclic adenosine monophosphate (cAMP) production. There is generally a net secretion of water and electrolytes (accounting for the other 20% of biliary secretion), and in particular, bile becomes highly enriched in bicarbonate ions. Many organic substances, such as glutathione, are degraded in the biliary tree. It is important to note that many drugs can be secreted into the biliary tree in a highly concentrated form (e.g., ceftriaxone). The gallbladder acts as the reservoir of the biliary tree, whose function is to store bile in the fasting state. The gallbladder reabsorbs water, concentrating stored bile, and secretes mucin. Contraction of the gallbladder is mediated hormonally (largely through cholecystokinin) in response to a meal, with the simultaneous relaxation of the sphincter of Oddi and release of bile into the duodenum.[10]

Enterohepatic Circulation

Bile salts are primarily produced in the liver and secreted to be used in the biliary tree and the intestine. The primary bile salts cholic acid and chenodeoxycholic acid are produced in the liver from cholesterol and subsequently conjugated with glycine or taurine within the hepatocyte. Once secreted in the gut, the primary bile acids are modified by intestinal bacteria, forming secondary bile acids deoxycholic acid and lithocholic acid. Bile acids are reabsorbed passively in the jejunum and actively in the ileum into the portal venous system, where up to 90% of the bile acids are extracted by hepatocytes. Only a small fraction spills over into the systemic circulation because of efficient hepatic extraction, accounting for low levels of plasma bile acids. After hepatic extraction, bile acids are recirculated into canaliculi and back into the biliary tree, completing the circuit. A small amount of intestinal bile acids are not absorbed by the portal system and are excreted in the stool. Thus, the active secretion of bile salts from hepatocyte to bile and from ileal enterocytes to the portal vein is the engine behind the enterohepatic circulation.

The enterohepatic circulation is more than a unique physiologic mechanism of reusing physiologically valuable bile acids. This circulation of bile constitutes the major mechanism of eliminating excess cholesterol by consuming cholesterol in the production of bile salts as well as accumulating cholesterol in mixed micelles formed by organic biliary solutes with eventual fecal loss. Bile salts also play a critical role in the absorption of dietary fats, fat-soluble vitamins, and lipophilic drugs. Water movement from hepatocytes into bile and water absorption through the small bowel are also regulated by bile salts. Thus, the enterohepatic circulation is central to a number of solubilization, transport, and regulatory functions.[11]

Bilirubin Metabolism

Bilirubin is the result of heme breakdown. An early phase of heme breakdown, accounting for 20% of bilirubin, is from hemoproteins (heme-containing enzymes) and occurs within 3 days of labeling with radioactive heme. A late phase of heme breakdown, accounting for 80% of bilirubin, is from senescent red blood cells and occurs in about 110 days (life span of a red blood cell) after administering labeled radioactive heme. Heme is initially broken down into a green biliverdin by heme oxygenase, which is then broken down into the orange bilirubin by biliverdin reductase.

Circulating bilirubin is bound to albumin, which protects many organs from the potentially toxic effects of this compound. The bilirubin-albumin complex enters hepatic sinusoidal blood, where it enters the space of Disse through the large sinusoidal fenestrations. The bilirubin-albumin complex is disassociated in this space. Free bilirubin is then internalized into the hepatocyte, where it is conjugated to glucuronic acid. Conjugated bilirubin is then secreted in an energy-dependent fashion into canalicular bile against a large concentration gradient. Bilirubin is then secreted with bile into the gastrointestinal tract. Within the gastrointestinal tract, bilirubin is deconjugated by intestinal bacteria to a group of compounds known as *urobilinogens*. These urobilinogens are further oxidized and reabsorbed into the enterohepatic circulation and secreted into bile. A small percentage of the reabsorbed urobilinogens are excreted into urine. It is these oxidized urobilinogens that account for the colored compounds that contribute to the yellow color of urine and the brown color of stool.

Bilirubin has long been known to be a toxic compound and is the agent responsible for neonatal encephalopathy and cochlear damage secondary to severe unconjugated hyperbilirubinemia (kernicterus). The binding of serum bilirubin to albumin protects the tissues from exposure to bilirubin, but binding sites can be overwhelmed by increasing amounts of bilirubin or displaced by other binding agents, such as many drugs. The mechanism of bilirubin toxicity appears to be related to a number of its effects. Free bilirubin can uncouple oxidative phosphorylation, inhibit ATPase, reduce glucose metabolism, and inhibit a broad spectrum of protein kinase activity.

Portosystemic shunts, such as those seen with cirrhosis and portal hypertension, decrease the first-pass hepatic clearance of bilirubin, resulting in a mildly increased serum unconjugated hyperbilirubinemia. A number of disorders can result in a serum unconjugated hyperbilirubinemia, such as the aforementioned neonatal hyperbilirubinemia, increased bilirubin load (hemolytic syndromes), and inherited enzymatic deficiencies such as Crigler-Najjar syndrome and Gilbert syndrome. Disorders presenting with serum conjugated hyperbilirubinemia include cholestasis syndromes, Dubin-Johnson syndrome, and Rotor's syndrome.[12]

Carbohydrate Metabolism

The liver is the center of carbohydrate metabolism because it is the major regulator of storage and distribution of glucose to the peripheral tissues and in particular to the glucose-dependent tissues such as the brain and erythrocytes. Both liver and muscle are capable of storing glucose in the form of glycogen, but only the liver is able to break down glycogen to provide glucose for systemic circulation. Broken down muscular glycogen can only be used within muscle and is therefore not a source of systemically circulated glucose.[13]

In the fed state, carbohydrate absorbed through the intestines (mostly glucose) is circulated systemically. Carbohydrate reaching the liver is rapidly converted to its storage form glycogen (up to 65 g of glycogen per kilogram of liver tissue). Excess carbohydrate is mostly converted to fatty acids and stored in adipose tissue. In the postabsorptive state (between meals, nonfasting), there is no further systemic glucose coming directly from the gut, and the liver becomes the primary source of circulating glucose by the breakdown of glycogen. This is crucial for the brain and erythrocytes, which rely on glucose for their metabolism. Most other tissues in the postabsorptive state begin to rely on fatty acids derived from adipose tissue as their primary fuel. Highly active muscle may deplete its own glycogen and depend on liver-derived glucose for substrate in the postabsorptive state. After 48 hours of fasting, hepatic glycogen is depleted, and the liver shifts from glycogen breakdown to gluconeogenesis. The substrate for hepatic gluconeogenesis is mostly from amino acids (mainly alanine) derived from muscle breakdown, but it also comes from glycerol derived from adipose breakdown. During a prolonged fast, fatty acids from adipose breakdown are β-oxidized in the liver, releasing ketone bodies, which then become the primary fuel of the brain.[13]

Transition in and out of these various metabolic states and regulation of carbohydrate metabolism are mostly from glucose concentration in sinusoidal blood and hormonal (insulin, catecholamines, and glucagon) influence. In the fasting state, during anaerobic metabolism, lactate, largely from muscle, is produced. The liver uses this lactate and, by conversion to pyruvate and entrance into gluconeogenic pathways, produces glucose. This cycle is known as the *Cori cycle*.[13]

Derangements of carbohydrate metabolism are common in liver disease. Cirrhotic patients often demonstrate abnormal glucose tolerance. The mechanism of this is not completely clear but is probably related to an associated insulin resistance. This phenomenon is not due to shunting of glucose-containing blood away from the liver. Hypoglycemia is a distinctly uncommon entity in chronic liver disease owing to the remarkable resilience of the liver and its metabolic function. Only with massive hepatocyte loss in fulminant hepatic failure does gluconeogenesis fail and hypoglycemia ensue.[13]

Lipid Metabolism

Fatty acids are synthesized in the liver during states of glucose excess when the liver's ability to store glycogen has been exceeded. Adipocytes have a limited ability to synthesize fatty acids, and therefore, the liver is the predominant source of synthesized fatty acids, although they are largely stored in adipose tissue. During lipolysis, free fatty acids are transported to the liver, where their metabolism takes place. Fatty acids in the liver undergo either esterification with glycerol to form triglycerides for storage or transportation or oxidation-yielding energy in the form of ATP and ketone bodies. In general, this process is regulated by the nutritional state; starvation favors oxidation, and the fed state favors esterification.[13]

There is a constant cycling of fatty acids between the liver and adipose tissue that is under a delicate balance. This balance can easily be offset, resulting in fatty infiltration of the liver. A few factors influence this balance. Hepatic uptake of fatty acids is a function of plasma concentrations. Although there is no limit in the liver's ability to esterify fatty acids, its ability to dispose of or breakdown fatty acids is limited. The liver is also limited in its ability to secrete triglycerides in the form of lipoproteins. Therefore, conditions of increased circulating fatty acids can easily override the liver's ability to handle them, resulting in fatty accumulation in the liver, known as *steatosis,* or its advanced counterpart, *steatohepatitis.* A number of conditions have been associated with hepatic steatosis, such as diabetes, steroid use, starvation, obesity, and extensive cytotoxic chemotherapy. Fatty liver associated with alcohol intake is multifactorial and related to increased lipolysis, reduced oxygenation, and augmented esterification of hepatic fatty acids, and it may also be related to relative starvation in the chronic alcoholic patient.[13]

Protein Metabolism

The liver is also a central site for the metabolism of proteins and is involved in protein synthesis, catabolism of proteins into energy or storage forms, and managing excess amino acids and nitrogen waste. Ingested protein is broken down into amino acids and circulated throughout the body, where it is used as the building blocks for proteins, enzymes, hormones, and nucleotides. Excess amino acids not used in peripheral tissues are generally handled by the liver, where they are oxidized for energy (providing 50% of the liver's energy needs) or converted into glucose, ketone bodies, or fats. When amino acids are catabolized for energy production throughout the body, ammonia, glutamine, glutamate, and aspartate are produced. These products are largely dealt with in the liver, where the waste nitrogen is converted to urea by the urea cycle. The urea is generally excreted in the urine. The liver, therefore, is central and critical to whole body's nitrogen balance as well as amino acid metabolism.[14]

Although the liver can catabolize most amino acids, yielding energy or other storable energy forms such as glucose or fats, a notable exception are the branched-chain amino acids. Branched-chain amino acids cannot be catabolized in the liver and are mostly dealt with by muscle. It has been postulated that this is something of a so-called safety net that helps to spare the liver some of the demands of protein and amino acid metabolism.[14]

The liver also is the main site of synthesis for many proteins that are involved in such wide-ranging and critical functions as coagulation, transport, iron binding, and protease inhibition. Examples of these proteins are α_1-antitrypsin, ceruloplasmin, and iron-storage and iron-binding proteins. Albumin is made exclusively in the liver and is the predominant serum-binding protein. Hepatic insufficiency or specific genetic abnormalities can result in altered amounts and function of these proteins, with wide-ranging pathologic effects.

The liver is also responsible for the so-called acute phase response, a protein synthetic response by the liver to trauma or infection. The purpose of the response is to restrict organ damage, maintain vital hepatic function, and control defense mechanisms. The response is incited by proinflammatory cytokines such as interleukin-1 (IL-1), IL-6, and tumor necrosis factor (TNF), which induce acute phase protein gene expression in the liver. Some of the well-known hepatic acute phase proteins are α_1-, α_2-, and β-globulin, C-reactive protein, and serum amyloid A. An equally important part of this response is its termination. Anti-inflammatory cytokines such as IL-1 receptor antagonist, IL-4, and IL-10 appear to play an important role. The acute phase response is usually over in 24 to 48 hours, but in the context of ongoing injury, it can be prolonged.

Vitamin Metabolism

Along with the intestine, the liver is responsible for the metabolism of the fat-soluble vitamins A, D, E, and K. These vitamins are obtained exogenously and absorbed in the intestine. Their adequate intestinal absorption is critically dependent on adequate fatty acid micellization, which requires bile acids. Vitamin A is from the retinoid family and is involved in normal vision, embryonic development, and adult gene regulation. Storage of vitamin A is solely in the liver and is thought to be in the stellate cells (Ito cells). Overingestion of vitamin A can result in hepatic toxicity. Vitamin D is involved in calcium and phosphorus homeostasis, and one of its activation steps (25-hydroxylation) occurs in the liver. Vitamin E is a potent antioxidant and protects membranes from lipid peroxidation and free radical formation. Vitamin K is a critical cofactor in the post-translational γ-carboxylation of the hepatically synthesized coagulation factors II, VII, IX, and X and proteins C and S (so-called vitamin K–dependent factors), which is essential to their activity. Cholestasis syndromes result in inadequate absorption of these vitamins secondary to poor micellization in the intestine. The associated vitamin deficiency syndromes such as metabolic bone disease (D), neurologic disorders (E), and coagulopathy (K) can subsequently occur.

The liver is also involved in the uptake, storage, and metabolism of a variety of water-soluble vitamins. These vitamins include thiamin, riboflavin, B_6, B_{12}, folate, biotin, and pantothenic acid. The liver is responsible for converting some of these water-soluble vitamins to active coenzymes, transforming some to storage metabolites; others are involved in the enterohepatic circulation (e.g., vitamin B_{12}).

Coagulation

The liver is responsible for synthesizing almost all of the identified coagulation factors as well as many of the fibrinolytic system components and several plasma regulatory proteins of coagulation and fibrinolysis. As mentioned previously, the liver is critical in the absorption of vitamin K, synthesizes the vitamin K–dependent coagulation factors, and contains the enzyme that activates these factors. Additionally, the reticuloendothelial system of the liver clears activated clotting factors, activated complexes

of the coagulation and fibrinolytic systems, and the end products of fibrin degradation. Diseases of the liver are also often associated with thrombocytopenia, qualitative abnormalities of platelets, vitamin K deficiency, impaired modulation of vitamin K–dependent coagulation factors, and disseminated intravascular coagulation. It is no surprise, therefore, that liver disease is firmly associated with coagulation disorders that are often challenging to deal with.

Warfarin, one of the most commonly dispensed anticoagulants, acts in the liver by blocking vitamin K–dependent activation of factors II, VII, IX, and X. Factor VII has the shortest half-life of the coagulation factors, and its deficiency is manifested clinically as abnormalities of the measured prothrombin time. Patients with hepatic synthetic dysfunction similarly have abnormal prothrombin times.

Metabolism of Drugs and Toxins (Xenobiotics)

The human body is exposed to an inordinate amount of foreign chemicals in a lifetime, posing a challenge to our bodies to be able to detoxify and eliminate these potentially harmful substances. Many of these chemicals are not incorporated into cellular metabolism and are referred to as *xenobiotics*. The liver plays a central role in handling these chemicals through an enormously complex and numerous set of enzymes and reaction pathways that are increasingly recognized as newer chemicals are discovered.

Hepatic-based reactions to xenobiotics are broadly classified into phase I and II reactions. Phase I reactions, through oxidation, reduction, and hydrolysis, increase the polarity and thus water solubility of compounds. This, in turn, allows for easier excretion. It is important to realize that phase I reactions do not necessarily detoxify chemicals and may in fact create toxic metabolites. An example of phase I reactions is the cytochrome P-450 system. Phase II reactions generally act to create a less toxic or less active byproduct. This is generally accomplished through transferase reactions in which a compound is usually coupled to a conjugate, rendering the xenobiotic less dangerous.[15]

Regeneration

The liver possesses the unique quality of adjusting its volume to the needs of the body. This is observed clinically in its regeneration after partial hepatectomy or after toxic injury. It is additionally seen in liver transplant recipients in that liver size mismatches adjust to the new host. This quality is highly conserved evolutionarily because of the critical functions of the liver and the fact that the liver is the first line of exposure to ingested toxic agents.

Liver regeneration is a hyperplastic response of all cell types of the liver in which ultimately the microscopic anatomy of the functional liver is maintained. Much of the information we have about the regenerative response of the liver is based on experimental evidence in rodents. Normally quiescent hepatocytes rapidly reenter the cell cycle after partial hepatectomy. Maximal hepatocyte DNA synthesis occurs 24 to 36 hours after partial hepatectomy, and maximal DNA synthesis of the other cell types occurs 48 to 72 hours later. Most of the increase in hepatic mass in rodents is seen by 3 days after partial hepatectomy and is usually nearly complete in 7 days.[16]

In the late 1960s, it was recognized that circulating factors were responsible, in part, for the regenerative response, and during the past 35 years, a large amount of research has gone into the humoral and genetic control of hepatic regeneration. The major circulating factors that have been identified (largely from rodent studies) are hepatocyte growth factor, epidermal growth factor, transforming growth factors, insulin, glucagon, and the cytokines TNF, IL-1, and IL-6. These factors, when infused into a normal host, do not result in hepatic growth, indicating that hepatocytes must be primed in some way before responding to these growth factors. Remarkable progress in the understanding of liver regeneration has been made as a result of improved genetic and molecular biologic techniques. Hundreds of genes involved at all stages of regeneration have been identified by complementary DNA (cDNA) array techniques. Additionally, numerous cytokine-dependent and growth factor–independent pathways have been further defined. A complete description is beyond the scope of this chapter, and many questions still remain.[16]

Future Developments

The study of the liver and its physiology continues to be a remarkable and exciting field. As the fields of molecular biology and genetic manipulation have exploded, so has the field of hepatology. Given the lack of alternative options to transplantation for patients with end-stage liver failure, tissue engineering and attempts to provide exogenous hepatic functional support continue to be researched. Liver repopulation with transplanted cells (hepatocytes or liver stem cells) may provide future options for patients with liver failure as well.

Although the identification of specific and reliable markers for hepatic stem cells has been elusive, the concept of stem cells and bone marrow–derived precursor cells and their potential utility in hepatic repopulation has slowly become accepted and is an exciting area of research. Ongoing genetic comparisons of normal and diseased liver using cDNA array technology will provide clues into the genetic regulation of liver diseases. Great strides have been made in the effectiveness of gene therapy, and many groups continue to study liver-directed gene therapy strategies to treat acquired and inherited disorders. Ongoing molecular biology studies are researching hepatic cell cycle regulation with implications for regeneration and hepatocarcinogenesis. Research into the pathogenesis of hepatic fibrosis and, perhaps more exciting, reversing this process are ongoing and likely to result in significant advances over the next few decades.

Assessment of Liver Function

A wide variety of tests are available to evaluate hepatic diseases. Screening for hepatic disease, assessing hepatic function, diagnosing specific disorders, and prognosticating are critical in the management of hepatic pathology.

For the surgeon, assessment of hepatic function and estimating the ability of a hepatic remnant to be sufficient after liver resection are also of obvious importance. Unfortunately, most measures of hepatic disease are gross and lack sensitivity, specificity, and accuracy. We have divided these tests into the following categories: routine screening tests, specific diagnostic tests, and quantitative tests of hepatic function.

Screening blood tests are often used to simply ask the question, Is there pathology in the hepatobiliary system? Standard liver function tests (LFTs) are generally not tests of function and are not always specific to hepatic pathology. Nonetheless, they are valuable as a general screening tool that can provide the basic tools to recognize the presence of hepatic disease and give clues about the etiology of that disease. Total bilirubin, direct bilirubin (conjugated), and indirect bilirubin (unconjugated) levels can be affected by a number of processes related to the metabolism of bilirubin. Unconjugated hyperbilirubinemia can be a reflection of increased bilirubin production (e.g., hemolysis), drug effects, inherited enzymatic disorders, and the physiologic jaundice of the newborn. Conjugated hyperbilirubinemia is generally a result of cholestasis or mechanical biliary obstruction but can also be seen in some inherited disorders and hepatocellular disease.

The transaminases alanine aminotransferase (ALT) and aspartate aminotransferase (AST) are the most common serum markers of hepatocellular necrosis, with subsequent leak of these intracellular enzymes into the circulation. AST is found in a variety of other organs (heart, muscle, and kidney), but ALT is liver specific. The level of elevation of these enzymes has never been shown to be of prognostic value. Alkaline phosphatase (ALP) is expressed in liver, bile ducts, bone, intestine, placenta, kidney, and leukocytes. Isoenzyme determinations can sometimes be helpful in distinguishing the source of an elevated ALP. Elevations of ALP in hepatobiliary diseases are generally secondary to cholestasis or biliary obstruction and are caused by increased production of the enzyme. ALP can also be elevated in malignant disease of the liver. γ-Glutamyltranspeptidase (GGT) is an enzyme in many organs aside from the liver (kidney, seminal vesicle, spleen, pancreas, heart, and brain) and can be elevated in diseases affecting any of these. It is induced by alcohol intake and is elevated in biliary obstruction. It is also a nonspecific marker of liver disease but can be helpful in determining whether an elevated alkaline phosphatase is from hepatic pathology. 5′-Nucleotidase is also found in a wide variety of organs beside the liver, but increased levels are fairly specific to hepatic pathology. Like GGT, it can be helpful in determining whether an elevated ALP is secondary to hepatic pathology.

Albumin is synthesized exclusively in the liver and can be used as a general measure of hepatic synthetic function. Because chronic malnutrition and acute injury or inflammation can decrease albumin synthesis, these factors must be taken into account when evaluating a low serum albumin level. Because of the remarkable protein synthetic capacity of the liver, hypoalbuminemia as a marker of liver disease lacks sensitivity, and tremendous decreases in hepatic function are required to be reflected in albumin levels. In general, it is most helpful in chronic liver disease. Clotting factors are largely synthesized in the liver, and abnormalities of clotting can be a marker of diminished hepatic synthetic function. Measures of specific clotting factors such as factors V and VII have been used to evaluate hepatic function in the transplant population. The prothrombin time is the best test to measure the effects of hepatic disease on clotting and is usually a marker of advanced chronic liver disease. Hepatic pathology can also affect clotting through intravascular coagulation and vitamin K malabsorption.[11,17]

After screening tests, along with clinical findings, have suggested liver disease, specific tests can be used to help elucidate the etiology and guide treatment if necessary. Hepatitis serologies are important to determine the presence of viral hepatitis. Autoimmune antibodies are used to diagnose primary biliary cirrhosis (antimitochondrial), primary sclerosing cholangitis (antineutrophil), and autoimmune hepatitis. α_1-Antitrypsin and ceruloplasmin levels assist in the diagnosis of α_1-antitrypsin deficiency and Wilson's disease, respectively. Tumor markers such as AFP and carcinoembryonic antigen (CEA) can be helpful in the diagnosis and management of primary and metastatic tumors of the liver.

The LFTs discussed previously, in general, are gross and nonspecific and contain little, if any, prognostic value. Many attempts have been made to formulate dynamic and quantitative tests of hepatic function based on the liver's ability to clear various exogenously administered substances. Despite many years of research, it still remains unclear whether these tests of hepatic function are any better than scoring systems derived from simple blood tests and clinical observations.

The aminopyrine breath test is based on the clearance, by the hepatic P-450 system, of radiolabeled aminopyrine. A breath test measuring radiolabeled CO_2 as a breakdown product of aminopyrine is performed after administration at a specified time. The results largely depend on the functional hepatic mass, which is generally not depleted until end-stage liver disease. There are varying results of studies comparing the aminopyrine breath test to standard LFTs and scoring systems. Its main value appears to be prognosis in chronic liver disease, but it is clearly not an effective test to detect subclinical hepatic dysfunction. Substances such as antipyrine and caffeine can evaluate liver function in a similar way with similar results. The lidocaine clearance test yields similar information to the aminopyrine test because it is based on its clearance by the hepatic P-450 test. Lidocaine clearance is dependent on blood flow and a complex distribution process, but measurement of one of its metabolites, monoethylglycinexylidide (MEGX), has greatly simplified the test. This test has been shown to have some prognostic value in the transplant population. The galactose elimination test is based on the liver's role in phosphorylating galactose and converting it to glucose. The rate at which galactose is eliminated from the bloodstream can be a measure of hepatic function. Problems related to this test are that the enzymes involved are genetically heterogeneous, and considerable extrahepatic metabo-

Table 52-2 Child-Pugh Classification

FACTOR	NO. OF POINTS		
	1	2	3
Bilirubin (mg/dL)	<2	2-3	>3
Albumin (g/dL)	>3.5	2.8-3.5	<2.8
Protime (increased seconds)	1-3	4-6	>6
Ascites	None	Slight	Moderate
Encephalopathy	None	Minimal	Advanced

Grade A, 5-6 points; grade B, 7-9 points; grade C, 10-15 points.

lism occurs. Additionally, multiple blood draws are necessary making the test cumbersome. The value of this test has also largely been in assessing prognosis in chronic liver disease rather than in screening. Indocyanine green is a dye removed by the liver through a carrier-mediated process and excreted into bile. This dye is rapidly cleared from the bloodstream and is not metabolized. This is the only test that has been shown to have some prognostic ability in cirrhotic patients undergoing liver resection, although this is not universally demonstrated in studies, nor is it universally accepted.[11,17]

Lastly, a large number of scoring systems based on clinical observation and standard blood tests have been proposed. The most commonly used system is Pugh's modification of the Child score (Table 52-2). Although all these systems are less than perfect and not universally accepted, the Child-Pugh score is commonly used in cirrhotic patients who require liver surgery. Mortality and survival rates after hepatectomy have been shown to correlate with this score but are not always related to liver failure. Child's B and C patients generally have high perioperative mortality after any partial hepatectomy, whereas Child's A patients can generally withstand a major hepatectomy. The presence of portal hypertension has been shown to predict poor outcome after partial hepatectomy. The presence of portal hypertension in cirrhotic patients is usually manifested as thrombocytopenia, splenomegaly, and the presence of intra-abdominal varices on imaging. The best evidence for portal hypertension is a hepatic vein wedge pressure of more than 10 mm Hg, which has been shown to correlate strongly with postoperative liver failure.[11,17]

INFECTIOUS DISEASES

Pyogenic Abscess

Epidemiology
Oschsner and DeBakey, in their classic paper on pyogenic liver abscess in 1938, described 47 cases and reviewed the world literature.[18] This was the largest experience of the time and the first serious attempt to study this disease. At that time, pyogenic liver abscess was largely a disease of people in their 20s and 30s and mostly the result of acute appendicitis. With the marked change in medical care during the past 60 years—notably

Table 52-3 Percentage of Pyogenic Abscesses Attributable to Specific Cause

YEARS	NO. OF PATIENTS	PORTAL VEIN	HEPATIC ARTERY	BILIARY TREE	DIRECT EXTENSION	TRAUMA	CRYPTOGENIC
1927-1938 1 study*	622	42	—	—	17	4	20
1945-1982 8 studies	521	17	9	38	10	4	16
1970-1999 8 studies	1264	5	3	38	1	2	43

*1927-1938 is the Ochsner/DeBakey classic study that reviewed 575 previously reported cases and 47 new cases.

effective antibiotics, prompt effective treatments for acute inflammatory disorders, and an aging population—the spectrum of this disease has changed. Pyogenic liver abscess is now mostly seen in patients 50 to 60 years old and is more often related to biliary tract disease or is cryptogenic.

The incidence of pyogenic liver abscess has remained similar over 60 years. Ochsner and Debakey reported an incidence of 8 per 100,000 hospital admissions in 1938,[1] whereas in 1975, Pitt and Zuidema reported 13 per 100,000 hospital admissions. Two large autopsy studies, one from 1901 and one from 1960, reported similar incidences of pyogenic liver abscess: 0.45% and 0.59%, respectively.[3] More recent studies from the 1980s and 1990s have suggested small but significant increases in the incidence of pyogenic liver abscess (as high as 22 per 100,000 hospital admissions).[19,20] This may reflect better, more available, and more frequently used high-quality imaging techniques. Hospital admission practices surely affect these statistics as well. A recent population-based study from North America calculated an annual incidence of 2.3 cases per 100,000 population. There are no significant gender, ethnic, or geographic differences in disease frequency, and the male-to-female ratio is about 1.5:1. Comorbid conditions associated with pyogenic abscess are prior diabetes and a history of malignancy.[20]

Pathogenesis

The liver is probably exposed to portal venous bacterial loads on a regular basis and clears this bacterial load without problems in the usual circumstance. The development of a hepatic abscess occurs when the inoculum of bacteria, regardless of the route of exposure, exceeds the liver's ability to clear it. This results in tissue invasion, neutrophil infiltration, and the formation of an organized abscess. The potential routes of hepatic exposure to bacteria follow:

1. Biliary tree
2. Portal vein
3. Hepatic artery
4. Direct extension of a nearby focus of infection
5. Trauma

The relative contribution of these routes to the formation of hepatic abscess is summarized in Table 52-3.[21]

Along with cryptogenic infections, infections from the biliary tree are presently the most common identifiable

cause of hepatic abscess. Biliary obstruction results in bile stasis with the potential for subsequent bacterial colonization, infection, and ascension into the liver. This process is known as ascending suppurative cholangitis. The nature of biliary obstruction is mostly related to stone disease or malignancy. In Asia, intrahepatic stones and cholangitis (recurrent pyogenic cholangitis—see later) are a common cause, whereas in the Western world, malignant obstruction is becoming a more predominant factor. Other factors associated with increased risk include Caroli's disease, biliary *Ascaris* species infection, and biliary tract surgery. The common link between all causes of hepatic abscess from the biliary tree is obstruction and bacteria in the biliary tree. Previous biliary-enteric anastomosis has also been associated with hepatic abscess formation, likely due to unimpeded exposure of the biliary tree to enteric organisms.[19-21]

The portal venous system drains the gastrointestinal tract, and therefore, any infectious disorder of the gastrointestinal tract can result in an ascending portal vein infection (pyelophlebitis) with exposure of the liver to large amounts of bacteria. Historically, untreated appendicitis was considered the most common cause of hepatic abscess, but with the advent of antibiotics and the development of prompt and effective treatment of acute abdominal infections, portal venous infections of the liver have become less common. The most common causes of pyelophlebitis are diverticulitis, appendicitis, pancreatitis, inflammatory bowel disease, pelvic inflammatory disease, perforated viscus, or omphalitis in the newborn. Hepatic abscess has also been associated with colorectal malignancy.[21]

Any systemic infection (endocarditis, pneumonia, osteomyelitis) can result in bacteremia and infection of the liver through the hepatic artery. Multiple microabscess formation is a relatively common finding at autopsy in patients dying of sepsis, but these patients are generally not included in analyses of pyogenic liver abscess. Hepatic abscess from systemic infections may also reflect an altered immune response, such as in patients with malignancy, acquired immunodeficiency syndrome, or disorders of granulocyte function. Children with chronic granulomatous disease are particularly susceptible.

Hepatic abscess can be the result of direct extension of an infective process. Common examples of this include suppurative cholecystitis, subphrenic abscess, perinephric abscess, and even perforation of the intestine directly into the liver.

Penetrating and blunt trauma can result in an intrahepatic hematoma or an area of necrotic liver, which can subsequently develop into an abscess. Bacteria may have been introduced from the trauma, or the affected area may be seeded from systemic bacteremia. Hepatic abscesses associated with trauma can present in a delayed fashion, up to weeks after the injury. Other mechanisms of iatrogenic hepatic necrosis, such as hepatic artery embolization or, more recently, thermal ablative procedures, can be complicated by abscess. This is an uncommon complication of these procedures but is seen more often when there has been a previous biliary-enteric anastomosis.

Commonly, no cause for a hepatic abscess is found. Cryptogenic abscesses predominate in many series and are more common in recent case series.[20,21] Possible explanations for cryptogenic hepatic abscess are undiagnosed abdominal pathology, resolved infective process at the time of presentation, and host factors such as diabetes or malignancy rendering the liver more susceptible to transient hepatic artery or portal vein bacteremias. In patients with cryptogenic hepatic abscess who have had computed tomography (CT) and ultrasonography, it has been argued that a diligent search for a cause should ensue. In series evaluating colonoscopy and endoscopic retrograde cholangiopancreatography (ERCP) in patients with cryptogenic abscess, the yield has been low and often is only fruitful in patients with some objective finding that might have suggested a subclinical abnormality (e.g., mildly elevated bilirubin). In general, these patients undergo a thorough history, physical examination, and laboratory workup in search of abnormalities in the intestinal tract or biliary tree. Further invasive procedures are based on clinical suspicions raised by this workup.

Pathology and Microbiology

Most hepatic abscesses involve the right lobe of the liver, accounting for three fourths of cases. The explanation for this is not known, but preferential laminar blood flow to the right side has been postulated. The left lobe is involved about 20% of the time, and the caudate lobe is uncommonly involved (5%). Bilobar involvement with multiple abscesses is uncommon. About half of hepatic abscesses are solitary. The size of hepatic abscesses can vary from less than a millimeter to several centimeters in diameter and can be multiloculated or a single cavity. At abdominal exploration, hepatic abscesses appear tan and are fluctuant to palpation, although deeper abscesses may not be visible and can be difficult to feel. Surrounding inflammation can cause adhesion to local structures.

Studies on the microbiology of hepatic abscesses have been variable for a number of reasons. In early series, sterile abscesses were commonly reported but probably reflected inadequate culture techniques, whereas in modern series, few abscesses are sampled before the administration of antibiotics. Additionally, the heterogeneity of the routes of infection makes the microbiology variable. Abscesses from pyelophlebitis or cholangitis tend to be polymicrobial, with a high preponderance of gram-negative rods. Systemic infections, on the other hand, usually cause infection with a single organism.[21]

Although the rate of sterility reported by Ochsner's review in 1938 was about 50%, series in the 1990s report sterile abscesses in about 10% to 20% of cases. Many hepatic abscesses are polymicrobial in nature and account for about 40% of cases. Some authors suggest that solitary abscesses are more likely to be polymicrobial.[19,21] Anaerobic organisms are involved about 40% to 60% of the time. The most common organisms cultured are *Escherichia coli* and *Klebsiella pneumoniae*. Other common organisms encountered are *Staphylococcus aureus, Enterococcus* species, *Streptococcus viridans,* and *Bacteroides* species. *Klebsiella* is frequently associated with gas-forming abscesses. Enterococci and viridans streptococci are generally found in polymicrobial abscesses, whereas staphylococcal infections are typically single organism. Uncommonly encountered organisms (<10% of cultures) include *Pseudomonas, Proteus, Enterobacter, Citrobacter, Serratia,* β-hemolytic streptococci, microaerophilic streptococci, *Fusobacterium, Clostridium,* and other rare anaerobes. Blood cultures are positive in about 50% to 60% of cases.[21] Of note, highly resistant organisms in patients with indwelling biliary catheters, multiple episodes of cholangitis, and repeated use of antibiotics are being encountered as the use of these catheters becomes more common. Fungal and mycobacterial hepatic abscesses are rare and are almost always associated with immunosuppression, usually from chemotherapy.

Clinical Features

The classic description of the presenting symptoms of hepatic abscess are fever, jaundice, and right upper quadrant pain and tenderness. Unfortunately, this presentation is present only 10% of the time. Fever, chills, and abdominal pain are the most common presenting symptoms, but there is a broad array of nonspecific symptoms that can be found[19-21] (Table 52-4). A recent study from Taiwan of 133 patients found fever in 96% of patients, chills in 80%, abdominal pain in 53%, and jaundice in 20%. Many of the symptoms, such as malaise and vomiting, are constitutional in nature. Involvement of the diaphragm may result in symptoms of cough or dyspnea. Rarely, patients present with peritonitis secondary to rupture. Cases of rupture into the pleural space or pericardium have been reported but are distinctly uncommon. The duration of presenting symptoms is variable, ranging from an acute illness to a chronic presentation lasting months. It has been suggested that acute presentation is associated with identifiable abdominal pathology, whereas a chronic presentation is often associated with a cryptogenic abscess. A rare complication specific to *Klebsiella* hepatic abscesses is endogenous endophthalmitis, occurring in about 3% of cases. This serious complication is more common in diabetic patients. Early diagnosis and treatment represent the best chance to preserve visual function.

On physical exam, fever and right upper quadrant tenderness are the most common findings, tenderness being present about 40% to 70% of the time. Jaundice is found about 25% of the time and is often secondary to underlying biliary disease. Chest findings are often found

Table 52-4 **Percentage of Pyogenic Abscesses With Noted Symptoms**

YEARS	NO. OF PATIENTS	FEVER, CHILLS	NIGHT SWEATS	MALAISE	ANOREXIA, WEIGHT LOSS	NAUSEA, VOMITING	DIARRHEA	ABDOMINAL PAIN	CHEST PAIN	COUGH
1927-1938 1 study*	333	94	—	—	—	33	—	92	—	—
1945-1982 8 studies	494	88	8	58	62	40	17	66	14	13
1970-1995 10 studies	1314	72	9	25	33	30	14	59	16	16

*1927-1938 is the Ochsner/DeBakey classic study that reviewed 286 previously reported cases and 47 new cases.

and are present in about one fourth of cases. Hepatomegaly is also commonly noted and present about half of the time. Ascites, splenomegaly, and severe sepsis are uncommon signs.

Nonspecific abnormalities of blood tests are common in pyogenic abscesses. Leukocytosis is present in 70% to 90% of patients, and anemia is commonly encountered. Abnormalities of LFTs are generally present. ALP is mildly elevated in 80% of cases, whereas total bilirubin is elevated 20% to 50% of the time. Transaminases are mildly elevated about 60% of the time. Severe abnormalities of LFTs are almost always associated with underlying biliary disease. Hypoalbuminemia and mild elevations of the prothrombin time can be present and reflect a degree of chronicity. None of these blood tests specifically helps to diagnose a hepatic abscess, but they can suggest a liver abnormality that often leads to imaging studies.

The most essential element to making the diagnosis of hepatic abscess is radiographic imaging. Chest x-rays are abnormal about 50% of the time, and findings generally reflect subdiaphragmatic pathology such as an elevated right hemidiaphragm, right pleural effusion, or atelectasis. Occasionally, these can be left-sided findings in the case of an abscess involving the left liver. Plain abdominal x-rays, in rare cases, can be helpful. They can show air-fluid levels or portal venous gas (Fig. 52-18).

Ultrasound and CT are the mainstays in diagnostic modalities for hepatic abscess. Ultrasound usually demonstrates a round or oval area that is less echogenic than the liver and can reliably distinguish solid from cystic lesions. The limitations of ultrasound are in its relative inability to visualize lesions high up in the dome of the liver and the fact that it is a user-dependent modality. The sensitivity of ultrasound in diagnosing hepatic abscess is 80% to 95%. CT demonstrates findings similar to ultrasound, and lesions are of lower attenuation than surrounding hepatic parenchyma. High-quality CT can demonstrate very small abscesses and can more easily pick up multiple small abscesses. The abscess wall usually shows an intense enhancement on contrast-enhanced CT. The sensitivity of CT in diagnosing hepatic abscess is 95% to 100%. Both CT and ultrasound are useful in diagnosing other intra-abdominal pathology, such as biliary disease (ultrasound) or inflammatory disorders like appendicitis or diverticulitis (CT).[19-21] Magnetic resonance imaging

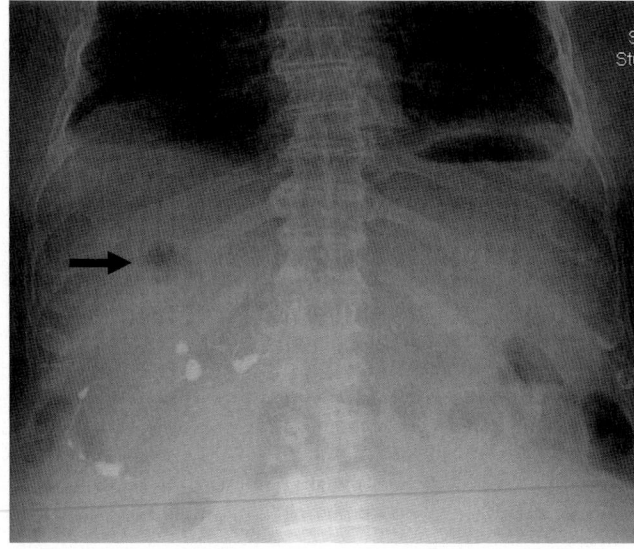

Figure 52-18 Plain abdominal x-ray demonstrating an abnormal collection of air in the right upper quadrant consistent with a pyogenic hepatic abscess (*black arrow*).

(MRI) can be very helpful in distinguishing the etiology of many hepatic masses but does not appear to have any distinct advantage over CT in diagnosing hepatic abscess.

Differential Diagnosis

Differentiating pyogenic abscess from other cystic infective diseases of the liver, such as amebic abscess or echinococcal cyst, is important because of differences in treatment. Pyogenic abscess (as discussed later) is largely treated by antibiotics and drainage. Amebic abscess is largely treated by antibiotics, and echinococcal cysts often require surgical management. Fortunately, echinococcal cysts can usually be diagnosed by history and characteristic radiologic findings (see later). The presentations of amebic and pyogenic abscess, however, are more similar, with some notable exceptions that are critical in distinguishing the two (Table 52-5). Amebic abscesses generally occur in young Hispanic males in North America, whereas pyogenic abscess tends to occur

Table 52-5 Features of Amebic Versus Pyogenic Liver Abscess

CLINICAL FEATURES	AMEBIC ABSCESS	PYOGENIC ABSCESS
Age (yr)	20-40	>50
Male-to-female ratio	≥10:1	1.5:1
Solitary vs. multiple	Solitary 80%*	Solitary 50%
Location	Usually right liver	Usually right liver
Travel in endemic area	Yes	No
Diabetes	Uncommon (~2%)	More common (~27%)
Alcohol use	Common	Common
Jaundice	Uncommon	Common
Elevated bilirubin	Uncommon	Common
Elevated alkaline phosphatase	Common	Common
Positive blood culture	No	Common
Positive amebic serology	Yes	No

*In acute amebic abscess, 50% are solitary.

in patients 50 to 60 years of age with no predominant gender or race. Fever is common in both, but chills and symptoms of a severe acute bacteremia are more common in pyogenic abscess. Serologic tests for *Entamoeba histolytica* antibodies are nearly always positive in patients with amebic abscesses but are uncommon in those with pyogenic abscess. A recent study comparing 471 patients with amebic abscess to 106 patients with pyogenic abscess found age over 50 years, pulmonary findings on physical exam, multiple abscesses, and low amebic serology titers to be independently predictive of pyogenic abscess.[22] Occasionally, differentiating the two is not possible, and diagnostic aspiration or a trial of antiamebic antibiotics may be necessary. Unfortunately, aspiration is only diagnostic in amebic abscess about 10% to 20% of the time.[23]

Treatment

Before the availability of antibiotics and the routine use of drainage procedures, untreated hepatic pyogenic abscess was almost uniformly fatal. It was not until the classic review by Ochsner and DeBakey in 1938 that routine surgical drainage was employed and dramatic reductions in mortality were noted. Open surgical drainage of pyogenic abscesses was the sole treatment (with the addition of antibiotics eventually) for hepatic abscess until the 1980s. Since the 1980s, less invasive percutaneous drainage techniques, along with the use of intravenous (IV) antibiotics, have been employed. Laparotomy is generally reserved for failures of percutaneous drainage.

When the diagnosis of pyogenic hepatic abscess is suspected, broad-spectrum IV antibiotics are started immediately to control ongoing bacteremia and its associated complications. Blood cultures and cultures of the abscess from aspiration are sent for aerobic and anaerobic cultures. In immunosuppressed patients, mycobacterial

and fungal cultures of the aspirate need to be considered. Patients who are at risk for amebic infections have amebic serologies drawn. Until cultures have specifically identified the offending organism, broad-spectrum antibiotics covering gram-negatives, gram-positives, and anaerobes are used. Combinations such as ampicillin, an aminoglycoside, and metronidazole or a third-generation cephalosporin with metronidazole are appropriate. The optimal duration of antibiotic treatment is not well defined and must be individualized depending on the success of the drainage procedure. Antibiotics are certainly continued while there is evidence of ongoing infection, such as fever, chills, or leukocytosis. Beyond this, it is unclear how long to continue antibiotics, but recommendations usually are for 2 or more weeks.

Percutaneous drainage procedures for pyogenic hepatic abscesses were first reported in 1953 but did not gain widespread acceptance until the 1980s with the development of high-quality imaging and expertise in interventional radiologic techniques.[24] During the past 20 years, percutaneous catheter drainage has become the treatment of choice for most patients (Fig. 52-19). Success rates range from 69% to 90%.[19-21,24] The obvious advantages are the simplicity of treatment (usually employed at the time of radiologic diagnosis) and avoidance of general anesthesia and a laparotomy. Relative contraindications to percutaneous catheter drainage include the presence of ascites, coagulopathy, or proximity to vital structures. Percutaneous drainage of multiple abscesses is usually met with a higher failure rate, but reports demonstrate a high enough success rate that percutaneous approaches need to be made first, reserving surgery for percutaneous failures. A recent retrospective study comparing surgical with percutaneous drainage for large (>5 cm) abscesses showed a better success rate with surgical drainage. Despite this, two thirds of the percutaneous treatments were successful, and the overall morbidity and mortality rates were similar. There has never been a randomized

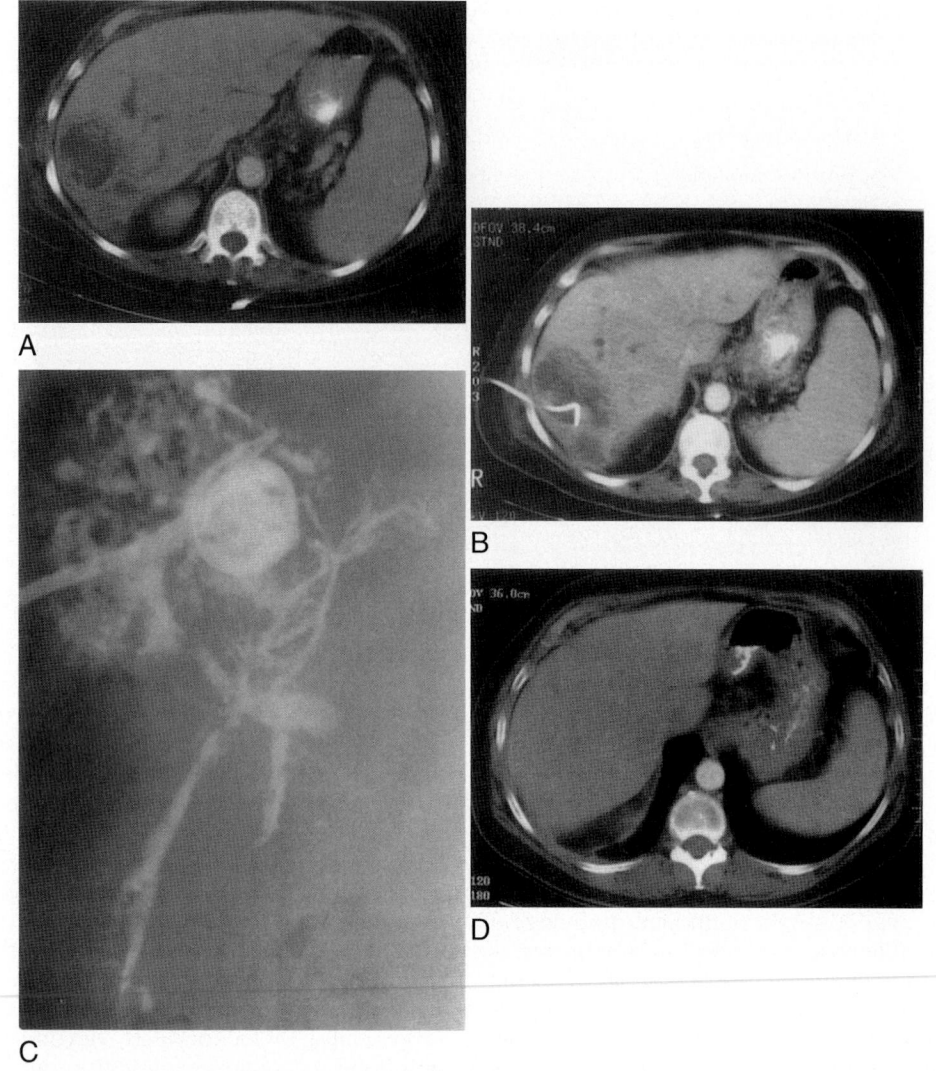

C

Figure 52-19 A, CT scan demonstrating multiloculated hepatic abscess in the right liver. **B,** CT scan at the time of percutaneous drainage. **C,** Contrast study through the drainage catheter demonstrating typical irregular loculated-type appearance as well as communication with the biliary tree. **D,** Follow-up CT scan 3 months after treatment demonstrating complete resolution of abscess. (From Brown KT, Getrajdman GI: Interventional radiologic techniques in the liver and biliary tract. In Blumgart LH, Fong Y [eds]: Surgery of the Liver and Biliary Tract. London, WB Saunders, 2000, pp 575-594).

prospective comparison between percutaneous and surgical therapy for hepatic abscess, but case series suggest that for most cases, there are similar success rates and mortality rates. Modern series attempting to compare these two techniques retrospectively must be read with caution because most patients treated surgically have failed other, less invasive techniques. In general, surgery is reserved for patients who require surgical treatment of the primary pathology (e.g., appendicitis) or for those who have failed percutaneous techniques. Note that laparoscopic drainage procedures have been reported with some success and can be considered a reasonable option to pursue in selected cases.

Percutaneous aspiration without the placement of a drain has been investigated by a number of groups. Success rates are generally 60% to 90% and are somewhat similar to those for percutaneous catheter drainage.[19,24] Usually, however, more than one aspiration is required, and one fourth of patients require three or more aspirations. One randomized trial has evaluated percutaneous aspiration versus percutaneous catheter drainage. Success rates were 60% in the aspiration group and 100% in the catheter group, but all but one patient in the aspiration group had a single aspiration. Another recent randomized trial compared aspiration alone to catheter drainage. Sixty-four randomized patients were analyzed, and there were similar outcomes in terms of treatment success rate, hospital stay, antibiotic duration, and mortality. In the aspiration-only group, 40% required two aspirations, and 20% required three aspirations.[24] In general, catheter drainage remains the treatment of choice, although a trial of a single aspiration is reasonable to consider.

Some investigators have reported success with antibiotics alone. Most of these patients, however, have had a diagnostic aspiration and thus at least a partial drainage. Additionally, other series have reported that antibiotic treatment without drainage carries a prohibitively high mortality rate (59%-100%).[19] In patients who are not surgical candidates or who absolutely refuse any invasive procedure, an attempt at antibiotic treatment is reasonable; however, this is not recommended in all other situations.

Liver resection is occasionally required for hepatic abscess. This may be required for an infected hepatic malignancy, hepatolithiasis, or intrahepatic biliary stricture. If hepatic destruction from infection is severe, some patients may benefit from resection.

Outcome

Mortality from pyogenic hepatic abscess has dramatically improved during the past 60 years. Before the routine use of surgical drainage, pyogenic abscess was uniformly fatal. With the routine use of surgical drainage and the use of IV antibiotics, mortality was reduced to about 50%, a figure that stayed relatively constant from 1945 until the early 1980s. Since the 1980s, mortality has been reported from 10% to 20%, and series from the 1990s now routinely demonstrate a mortality rate of less than 10%.[19,21,24] A number of studies have analyzed factors predictive of a poor outcome in patients with hepatic pyogenic abscess. The presence of malignancy, factors associated with malignancy (jaundice, markedly elevated LFTs), or signs of sepsis appear to be a consistent marker of poor prognosis. Signs of chronic disease, such as hypoalbuminemia, also are often associated with a poor outcome. Lastly, signs of severe infection, such as marked leukocytosis, Acute Physiology and Chronic Health Evaluation (APACHE) II scores, abscess rupture, bacteremia, and shock, are also associated with mortality.[19,21]

Amebic Abscess

Epidemiology

Amebiasis is largely a disease of tropical and developing countries but is also a significant problem in developed countries because of immigration and travel between countries. *E. histolytica* is endemic in Mexico, India, Africa, and parts of Central and South America. In 1995, the World Health Organization estimated that 40 to 50 million people suffer from amebic colitis or amebic liver abscess worldwide, resulting in 40,000 to 100,000 deaths each year.[23] Before this, estimates of amebiasis were unreliable because *E. histolytica* (the pathogenic form) was not differentiated from *Entamoeba dispar* (the nonpathogenic form). Male homosexuals with diarrhea, previously thought to harbor *E. histolytica,* have been found in fact to be infected with *E. dispar,* which requires no treatment. Epidemiologic studies specifically addressing *E. histolytica* infections estimate that as many as 55% of a population in endemic regions are infected, although less than half are symptomatic.[25]

In contrast to pyogenic hepatic abscesses, patients with amebic liver abscesses tend to be Hispanic males, aged 20 to 40 years, with a history of travel to (or origination from) an endemic area. Poverty and cramped living conditions are associated with higher rates of infection. A male preponderance of greater than 10:1 has been reported in almost all studies. For unclear reasons, menstruating women have a low incidence of invasive amebiasis, and pregnancy appears to abrogate this resistance. Heavy alcohol consumption is commonly reported and may render the liver more susceptible to amebic infection. Patients with impaired host immunity also appear to be at higher risk for infection and have higher mortality rates. Patients with amebic liver abscess without a history of travel to an endemic area often have an associated immunosuppression, such as human immunodeficiency virus (HIV) infection, malnutrition, chronic infection, or chronic steroid use.[23,25]

Pathogenesis

E. histolytica is a protozoan and exists as a trophozoite or as a cyst. All other species in the genus *Entamoeba* are considered nonpathogenic, and not all strains of *E. histolytica* are considered virulent. Ingestion of *E. histolytica* cysts through a fecal-oral route is the cause of amebiasis. Humans are the principal host, and the main source of infection is human contact with a cyst-passing carrier. Contaminated water and vegetables are also a route of human infection. Once ingested, the cysts are not degraded in the stomach and pass to the intestines where the trophozoite is released and passed on to the colon. In the colon, the trophozoite can invade mucosa, resulting in disease.

It is believed that the trophozoites reach the liver through the portal venous system. There is no evidence for trophozoites passing through lymphatics. As implied by its name, *E. histolytica* trophozoites have the capacity to lyse tissues through a complex set of events, including cell adherence, cell activation, and subsequent release of multiple enzymes resulting in necrosis. The major mechanism is probably enzymatic cellular hydrolysis. Amebic liver abscesses are thus formed by progressing, localized hepatic necrosis resulting in a cavity containing acellular proteinaceous debris surrounded by a rim of invasive amebic trophozoites. Early development of an amebic liver abscess is associated with an accumulation of polymorphonuclear leukocytes, which are then lysed by the trophozoites.[23,25]

Antiamebic antibodies develop rapidly in patients with invasive disease or amebic hepatic abscess. Secretory immunoglobulin A (IgA) antibodies have been shown in vitro to inhibit adherence to colonic epithelium; however, the development of these antibodies does not halt the progression of disease. Interestingly, children who lack antiamebic IgG have innate resistance to invasive infection, suggesting an alternative immune-mediated response. There is now evidence that a cell-mediated T-helper response is probably the major mechanism of resistance.[25]

Table 52-6 Signs, Symptoms, and Laboratory Findings in Amebic Liver Abscess in a Recent Extensive Literature Review

	AVERAGE	RANGE	NO. OF CASES REVIEWED
Symptoms and Signs			
Abdominal pain (%)	92	73-100	1701
Fever (%)	90	72-100	2192
Abdominal tenderness (%)	78	40-100	1424
Hepatomegaly (%)	62	20-100	1539
Anorexia (%)	47	28-89	499
Weight loss (%)	39	11-83	871
Diarrhea (%)	23	12-40	1426
Jaundice (%)	22	5-50	1630
Laboratory Tests			
Stool cysts/ trophozoites (%)	12	4-30	4908
Amebae in cyst aspirate (%)	42	30-76	1402
Hemoglobin (g/dL)	12.1	10.2-12.8	229
Alk. phosphatase (% >120 U/L)	76	65-91	589
Total bilirubin (g/dL)	1.4	0.8-2.4	509
Albumin (g/dL)	2.8	2.3-3.4	404
AST (× upper limit normal)	1.7	1.0-2.5	459

Pathology

Hepatic amebic abscess is essentially the result of lique-faction necrosis of the liver, producing a cavity full of blood and liquefied liver tissue. The appearance of this fluid is typically described as *anchovy sauce,* and the fluid is odorless unless secondary bacterial infection has taken place. The progressive hepatic necrosis continues until Glisson's capsule is reached because the capsule is resistant to hydrolysis by the amebae and thus amebic abscesses tend to abut the liver capsule. Because of the resistance of Glisson's capsule, the cavity is typically crisscrossed by portal triads protected by this peritoneal sheath. Early on, the formed cavity is ill defined, with no real fibrous response around the edges, but a chronic abscess can ultimately develop a fibrous capsule and may even calcify. Like pyogenic abscesses, amebic abscesses tend to occur mainly in the right liver.[25]

Clinical Features

About 80% of patients with amebic liver abscess present with symptoms lasting from a few days to 4 weeks. Most recent reports find the duration of symptoms typically to be less than 10 days. The presenting clinical signs and symptoms are summarized in Table 52-6.[23,25] The typical clinical picture is a patient 20 to 40 years of age who has recently traveled to an endemic area, with fever, chills, anorexia, right upper quadrant pain and tenderness, and hepatomegaly. The abdominal pain is typically constant, dull, and localized to the right upper quadrant. Although some studies report higher numbers, about one fourth of

patients have diarrhea despite an obligatory colonic infection. Synchronous hepatic abscess is found in one third of patients with active amebic colitis. Jaundice, as a result of a large abscess compressing the biliary tree, is not as rare as was once thought, with an average of 22% of patients presenting with this feature worldwide. Weight loss and myalgias may occur when symptoms have been present for weeks. Pleuritic or shoulder pain can occur if there is irritation of the diaphragm. Symptoms and tenderness may be epigastric or left sided if the abscess is located in the left liver. Rupture into the peritoneum with peritonitis occurs infrequently and more often with left-sided abscesses. Rare cases of rupture into the pleural space, pericardium, and other intra-abdominal organs have been reported.[25]

Laboratory abnormalities are common in amebic abscess. Patients typically have a mild to moderate leukocytosis without eosinophilia. Anemia is common. Mild abnormalities of LFTs, including albumin, prothrombin time, ALP, AST, and bilirubin levels, are typical. The most common LFT abnormality is an elevated prothrombin time.[23,25] Because more than 70% of patients with amebic liver abscess do not have detectable amebae in their stool, the most useful laboratory evaluation is the measurement of circulating antiamebic antibodies, which are present in 90% to 95% of patients. A number of serologic tests have been devised over the years. An indirect hemagglutinin test was used extensively in the past and has a sensitivity of 90%. This test has largely been replaced by enzyme immunoassays (EIAs), which are simple, rapidly performed, and inexpensive. The EIA has a reported sensitivity of 99% and specificity greater than 90% in patients with hepatic abscess. Unfortunately, the presence of antibodies may reflect old infection, and interpretation can be difficult in endemic areas. Ongoing studies are focusing on identifying specific *E. histolytic* antigens in an attempt to identify acute infection.[23]

Patients presenting acutely (symptoms for <10 days) versus those with a chronic presentation (symptoms for >2 weeks) differ clinically. Acute presentations are typically more dramatic with high fevers, chills, and significant abdominal tenderness. In the acute presentation, half of patients present with multiple lesions, whereas with the chronic presentation, greater than 80% of patients have single right-sided lesion. A more complicated course tends to ensue in the acute presentation, but response to therapy is similar in both groups.

Radiologic studies are a critical element in the diagnosis of amebic liver abscess. Plain chest radiographs are abnormal in about half of cases, usually demonstrating elevated right diaphragm, pleural effusion, or atelectasis.[25] Abdominal ultrasound has a reported accuracy of about 90% when combined with a typical history and clinical presentation. Typical findings on abdominal ultrasound are a rounded lesion abutting the liver capsule (see earlier) without significant rim echoes interpreted as an abscess wall. The contents of the cavity are usually hypoechoic and nonhomogeneous (Fig. 52-20). These findings on ultrasound are found in 40% to 70% of cases. Abdominal CT scan is probably more sensitive than ultrasound and is helpful in differentiating amebic from pyogenic abscess, with rim enhancement noted in the latter (Fig. 52-21). CT can also be helpful in identifying simple cysts and necrotic tumors. MRI of the liver has no distinct advantages over CT or ultrasound in typical cases but may be helpful in differentiating atypical lesions. Nuclear medicine studies such as gallium scanning or technetium-99m liver scans can be helpful in differentiating pyogenic from amebic abscesses because the latter typically do not contain leukocytes and therefore do not light up on these scans.[23,25]

When the previously outlined workup is still not definitive and diagnostic uncertainty persists, two options are considered. A therapeutic trial of antiamebic drugs in which rapid improvement occurs in most cases of amebic abscess can be helpful. In situations in which amebic serology is inconclusive and therapeutic trial of antibiotics is either deemed inappropriate or has failed to improve symptoms, consideration is given to diagnostic aspiration. A pyogenic abscess would have bacteria and leukocytes, whereas an amebic abscess would contain the typical anchovy sauce appearance. Cultures of amebic abscess are usually negative and do not contain leukocytes. In cases in which neoplasm or hydatid disease is given serious consideration, aspiration should not be performed.

Differential Diagnosis

The differential diagnosis of an amebic liver abscess can be broad and include such diseases as viral hepatitis, echinococcal disease, cholangitis, cholecystitis, or even other inflammatory abdominal disorders such as appendicitis. Malignant lesions of the liver can also have similar presentations in atypical situations. Occasionally, primary pulmonary disorders must be considered. In the main, the most important distinction to be made is between pyogenic and amebic abscess. The essential elements of this distinction are summarized in Table 52-5 and in the section on Pyogenic Abscess.[23]

Management

The mainstay of treatment for amebic abscesses is metronidazole (750 mg orally three times per day for 10 days), which is curative in more than 90% of patients. Clinical improvement is usually seen within 3 days. Other nitroimidazoles (secnidazole, tinidazole) are also as effective and are commonly used outside of the United States. If response to metronidazole is poor or the drug is not tolerated, other agents can be used. Emetine hydrochloride is effective against invasive amebiasis (particularly in the liver) but requires intramuscular injections and has serious cardiac side effects. A more attractive option is chloroquine, but this is a less effective agent. After treatment of the liver abscess, it is recommended that luminal agents such as iodoquinol, paromomycin, and diloxanide furoate are administered to treat the carrier state.[23]

Therapeutic needle aspiration of amebic abscesses has been proposed. Small randomized trials comparing metronidazole with or without aspiration have shown minor benefits with aspiration, but no major improvement to justify routine aspiration. In general, aspiration is recommended for diagnostic uncertainty (see earlier), failure to respond to metronidazole therapy in 3 to 5 days, or in

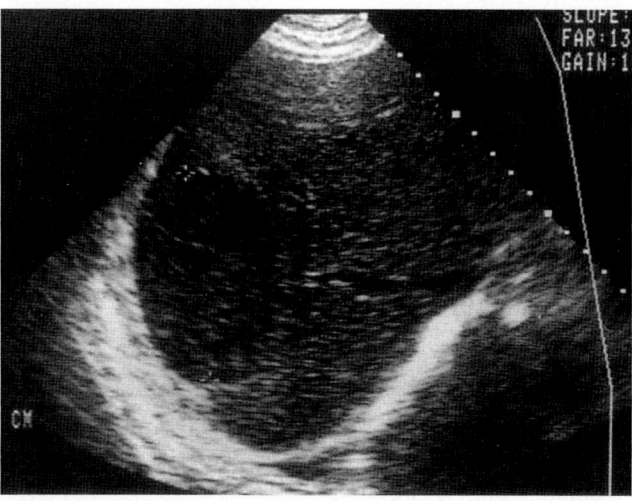

Figure 52-20 Typical ultrasound of an amebic hepatic abscess. Note the peripheral location, rounded shape with poor rim, and internal echoes. (From Thomas PG, Ravindra KV: Amebiasis and biliary infection. In Blumgart LH, Fong Y [eds]: Surgery of the Liver and Biliary Tract. London, WB Saunders, 2000, pp 1147-1166.)

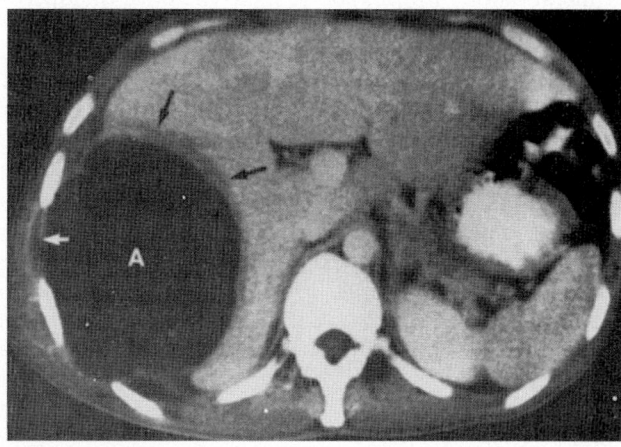

Figure 52-21 CT scan of amebic abscess. The lesion is peripherally located and round. Rim is nonenhancing but shows peripheral edema (*black arrows*). Note the extension into the intercostal space (*white arrow*).

abscesses felt to be at high risk for rupture. Abscesses larger than 5 cm in diameter and in the left liver are thought to be a higher risk for rupture, and aspiration needs to be considered.[23,26]

Outcome

Although amebic liver abscess usually responds rapidly to treatment, there are uncommon complications that the practitioner must be aware of. The most frequent complication of amebic abscess is rupture into the peritoneum, pleural cavity, or pericardium.[23] Size of the abscess appears to be the most important risk factor for rupture, and the overall incidence of rupture ranges from 3% to

17%. Most peritoneal ruptures tend to be contained by the diaphragm, abdominal wall or omentum, but rupture can fistulize into a hollow viscus. A peritoneal rupture usually presents as abdominal pain, peritonitis, and either a mass or generalized distention. Laparotomy was advocated in the past for this complication, but now many cases are managed successfully with percutaneous drainage. Laparotomy is indicated in cases of doubtful diagnosis, hollow viscus perforation, fistulization resulting in hemorrhage or sepsis, and failure of conservative therapy. Rupture into the pleural space usually results in a large and rapidly accumulated effusion that collapses the involved lung. Treatment consists of thoracentesis, but if secondary bacterial infection ensues, more aggressive surgical approaches may be necessary. Rupture can occur into the bronchi and is usually self-limited with postural drainage and bronchodilators. Rarely, a left-sided abscess may rupture into the pericardium and can present as an asymptomatic pericardial effusion or even tamponade.[26] This must be treated with aspiration. Other complications include compression of the biliary tree or inferior vena cava from a very large abscess and development of a brain abscess.

The mortality rate for all patients with amebic liver abscess is about 5% and does not appear to be affected by the addition of aspiration to metronidazole therapy or chronicity of symptoms. When an abscess ruptures, the mortality rate is reported to be from 6% to as high as 50%. Factors independently associated with poor outcome are elevated serum bilirubin (>3.5 mg/dL), encephalopathy, hypoalbuminemia (<2.0 g/dL), multiple abscess cavities, abscess volume greater than 500 mL, anemia, and diabetes.[23] Although clinical improvement after adequate treatment with antiamebic agents is the rule, radiologic resolution of the abscess cavity is usually delayed. The average time to radiologic resolution is 3 to 9 months and can take as long as years in some patients. Studies have shown that more than 90% of the visible lesions disappear radiologically, but a small percentage of patients are left with a clinically irrelevant residual lesion.[26]

Hydatid Cyst

Hydatid disease, or echinococcosis, is a zoonosis that occurs primarily in sheep-grazing areas of the world, but is common worldwide because the dog is a definitive host. Echinococcosis is endemic in Mediterranean countries, the Middle East, the Far East, South America, Australia, New Zealand, and East Africa. Humans contract the disease from dogs, and there is no human-to-human transmission.[27,28]

There are three species of *Echinococcus* that cause hydatid disease. *Echinococcus granulosus* is the most common, whereas *E. multilocularis* and *E. oligartus* account for a small number of cases. Dogs are the definitive host of *E. granulosus,* in which the adult tapeworm is attached to the villi of the ileum. Eggs are passed (up to thousands of ova daily) and deposited with the dog's feces. Sheep are the usual intermediate host, but humans

are an accidental intermediate host. Humans are an end stage to the parasite. In the human duodenum, the parasitic embryo releases an oncosphere containing hooklets that penetrate the mucosa, allowing access to the bloodstream. In the blood, the oncosphere reaches the liver (most commonly) or lungs, where the parasite develops its larval stage known as the *hydatid cyst.*[27,28]

Three weeks after infection, a visible hydatid cyst develops and then slowly grows in a spherical manner. A pericyst, a fibrous capsule derived from host tissues, develops around the hydatid cyst. The cyst wall itself has two layers: an outer gelatinous membrane (ectocyst) and an inner germinal membrane (endocyst). Brood capsules are small intracystic cellular masses in which future worm heads develop into scoleces. In a definitive host, the scoleces would develop into an adult tapeworm, but in the intermediate host, they can only differentiate into a new hydatid cyst. Freed brood capsules and scoleces are found in the hydatid fluid and form the so-called hydatid sand. Daughter cysts are true replicas of the mother cyst. Hydatid cysts can die with degeneration of the membranes, development of cystic vacuoles, and calcification of the wall. Calcification of a hydatid cyst, however, does not always imply that the cyst is dead.[27,28]

Hydatid cysts are diagnosed in equal numbers of men and women at an average age of about 45 years. About three fourths of hydatid cysts are located in the right liver and are singular. The clinical presentation of a hydatid cyst is largely asymptomatic until complications occur. The most common presenting symptoms are abdominal pain, dyspepsia, and vomiting. The most frequent sign is hepatomegaly. Jaundice and fever are each present in about 8% of patients.[27,28] Bacterial superinfection of a hydatid cyst can occur and present like a pyogenic abscess. Rupture of the cyst into the biliary tree or bronchial tree, or free rupture into the peritoneal, pleural, or pericardial cavities, can occur. Free ruptures can result in disseminated echinococcosis and a potentially fatal anaphylactic reaction. In cases of diagnostic uncertainty, a battery of serologic tests are available to evaluate antibody response, but all are plagued by low sensitivity and specificity.[27,28]

Ultrasound is most commonly used worldwide for the diagnosis of echinococcosis because of its availability, affordability, and accuracy. A number of findings on ultrasound can be diagnostic and depend on the stage of the cyst at the time of the exam. A simple hydatid cyst is well circumscribed with budding signs on the cyst membrane and may contain free-floating hyperechogenic hydatid sand. A rosette appearance is seen when daughter cysts are present. The cyst can be filled with an amorphous mass, which can be diagnostically misleading. Calcifications in the wall of the cyst are highly suggestive of hydatid disease and can be helpful in the diagnosis (Fig. 52-22). Similar findings are seen on CT or MRI. These cross-sectional imaging studies can also evaluate extrahepatic disease and demonstrate detailed hepatic anatomic relationships to the cyst. In patients with suspected biliary involvement, ERCP or percutaneous transhepatic cholangiography (PTC) may be necessary.

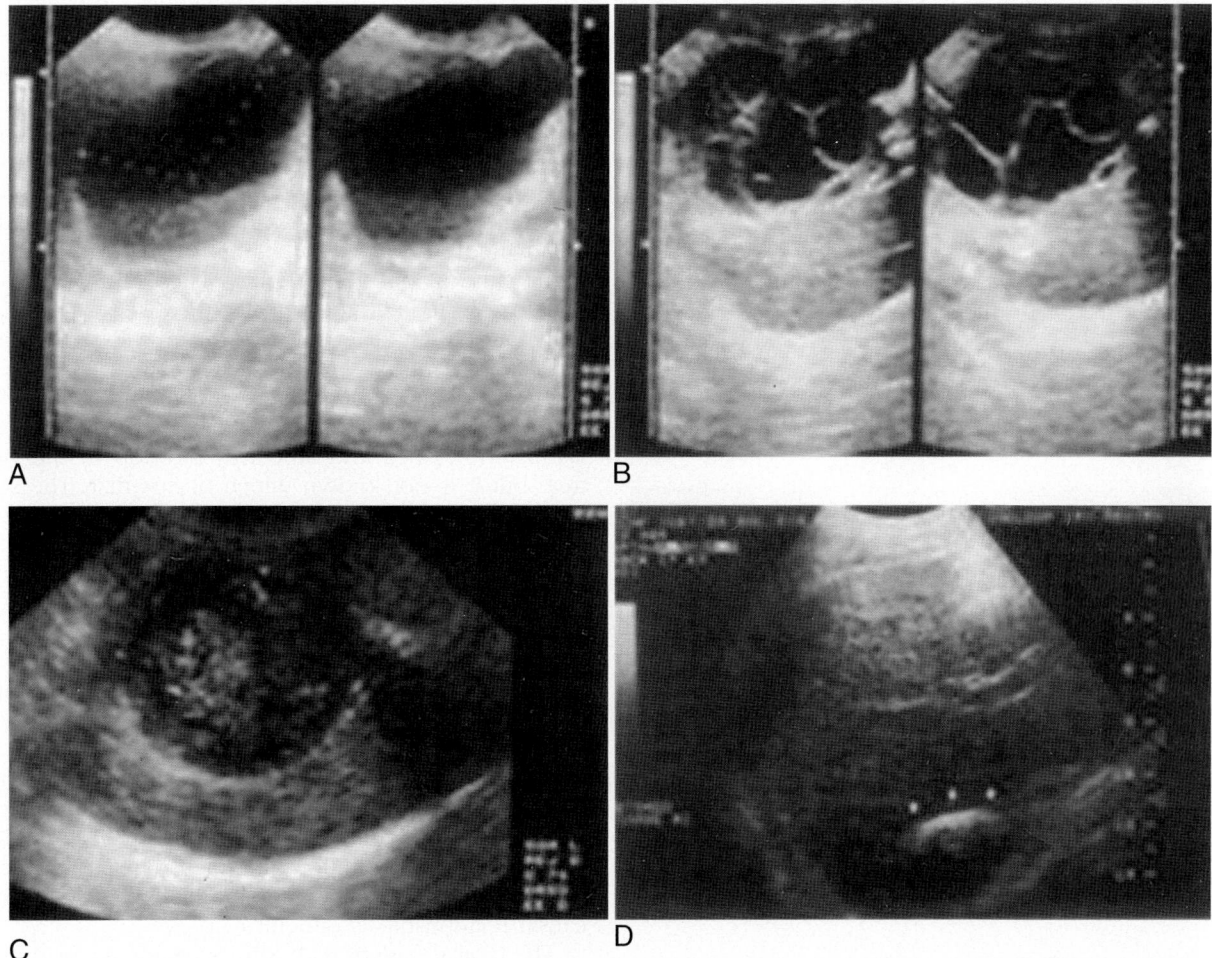

Figure 52-22 Ultrasound demonstrating typical characteristics of hydatid cyst at varying stages. **A,** Simple hydatid cyst with "hydatid sand." **B,** "Daughter and granddaughter" cysts and typical rosette appearance. **C,** Hydatid cyst filled with amorphous mass giving a solid or semisolid appearance. **D,** Calcified cyst with "eggshell" appearance. (From Thomas PG, Ravindra KV: Amebiasis and biliary infection. In Blumgart LH, Fong Y [eds]: Surgery of the Liver and Biliary Tract. London, WB Saunders, 2000, pp 1147-1166.)

The treatment of hepatic hydatid cysts is primarily surgical. In general, most cysts are treated, but in elderly patients with small, asymptomatic, densely calcified cysts, conservative management is appropriate. In preparation for an operation, preoperative steroids have been recommended but are not universally used. The anesthesiologist has epinephrine and steroids available for the potential of an anaphylactic reaction. A number of operations have been used, but in general, the abdomen is completely explored, the liver mobilized, and the cyst exposed. Packing off of the abdomen is important because rupture can result in anaphylaxis and diffuse seeding. Usually, the cyst is then aspirated through a closed-suction system and flushed with a scolicidal agent such as hypertonic saline. The cyst is then unroofed, which can then be followed by a number of possibilities, including excision (or pericystectomy), marsupialization procedures, leaving the cyst open, drainage of the cyst, omentoplasty, or partial hepatectomy to encompass the

cyst. Total pericystectomy or formal partial hepatectomy can also be performed without entering the cyst[28] (Fig. 52-23). Radical (resection) and conservative (drainage and evacuation) surgical approaches appear to be equally effective at controlling disease, although a prospective comparison has never been done.[29] When bile duct communication is diagnosed at operation or preoperatively, it must be meticulously sought out. Simple suture repair is often sufficient, but major biliary repairs, approaches through the common bile duct, or postoperative ERCP may be necessary.[28,29] Laparoscopic techniques for drainage and unroofing of cysts have been reported in a number of series with encouraging results. Recurrence rates after surgical treatment range from 1% to 20% but are generally 5% or less in experienced centers.[29]

In the past, percutaneous aspiration of hydatid cysts was contraindicated because of the risk for rupture and uncontrolled spillage. In recent years, however, a number of authors have reported percutaneous aspiration and

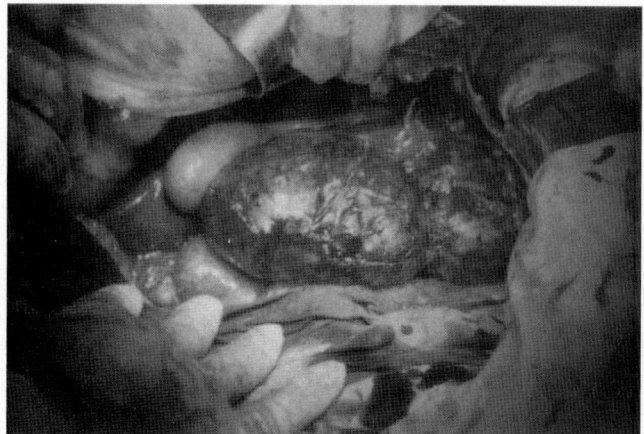

A

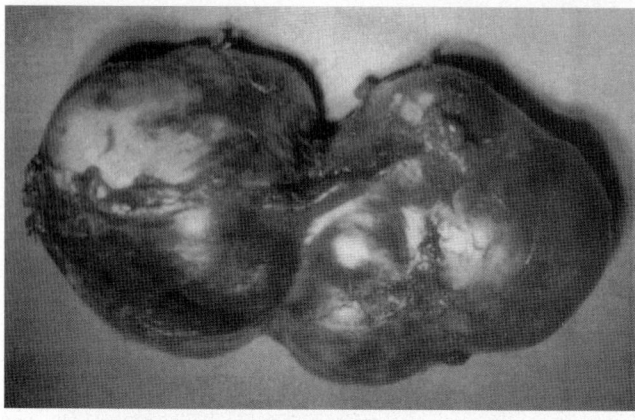

B

Figure 52-23 **A** and **B,** Peripheral hydatid cyst of the left liver and intact specimen after pericystectomy. Note that the entire pericyst has been removed. (From Milicevic MN: Hydatid disease. In Blumgart LH, Fong Y [eds]: Surgery of the Liver and Biliary Tract. London, WB Saunders, 2000, pp 1167-1204.)

injection of scolicidal agents with high success rates in highly selected patients. This technique is known as PAIR (puncture, aspiration, injection, and reaspiration) and has become more accepted in some institutions. Two randomized trials, one comparing PAIR to surgery (N=50) and one comparing PAIR to medical therapy, have shown similar success rates. These trials are small and have significant methodologic problems, limiting the ability to draw firm conclusions.[30] Although surgery remains the treatment of choice, further prospective trials are clearly indicated to address this interesting and potentially useful technique. Chemotherapy for echinococcosis with albendazole or mebendazole is effective at shrinking cysts in many patients with *E. granulosus,* but cyst disappearance occurs in fewer than 50% of patients. Preoperative treatment may decrease the risk for spillage and is a reasonable and safe practice.[29] Chemotherapy without definitive resection or drainage is only considered for widely disseminated disease or patients with poor surgical risk.

Recurrent Pyogenic Cholangitis

Recurrent pyogenic cholangitis (RPC) is a syndrome of repeated attacks of cholangitis secondary to biliary stones and strictures that involve the extrahepatic and intrahepatic ducts. The condition has many names but is often referred to as *Oriental cholangiohepatitis* or *hepatolithiasis.* The disease is almost exclusively found in Asians and Asian medical centers but is also seen in Asian immigrants throughout the world. Males and females are equally affected and, historically, the disease strikes at an early age (20-40 years) in patients from lower socioeconomic classes.

The etiology of RPC is unknown but is related to recurrent infection of biliary radicals with gut bacteria. Ultimately, stones and strictures develop in the biliary tree, but it is not known which occurs first. The stones are bilirubinate stones, and in some patients, no stones are found, and only biliary sludge is demonstrated. An association between RPC and *Clonorchis sinensis* and *Ascaris lumbricoides* infection has been noted, but a true causal relationship has never been proved.

Strictures can be found anywhere in the biliary tree but more commonly involve the intrahepatic main hepatic ducts and most often involve the left hepatic duct. The gallbladder is only involved in about 20% of cases. Cirrhosis and liver failure are only seen in long-standing disease, usually after multiple operations. Other complications include choledochoduodenal fistula and acute pancreatitis from common bile duct stones. An increased incidence of cholangiocarcinoma has been noted, but a causal relationship is difficult to prove.

The typical patient with RPC is young, Asian, and of a lower socioeconomic background who presents with repeated bouts of cholangitis. The symptoms and presentation are those of cholangitis: fever, right upper quadrant abdominal pain, and jaundice. Biliary obstruction is usually incomplete; therefore, marked jaundice and pruritus are not common. There is usually leukocytosis and abnormal LFTs consistent with biliary obstruction. Evaluation of the anatomic distribution of disease is critical to formulating a sound therapeutic plan. A combination of ultrasound, CT, and direct cholangiography is often necessary to evaluate these patients. Direct cholangiography performed endoscopically or transhepatically is considered an important study complementing the cross-sectional imaging. Magnetic resonance cholangiopancreatography (MRCP) can combine cross-sectional imaging and cholangiography in one noninvasive test and may ultimately replace direct cholangiography.

In an acute presentation, most patients improve with conservative management, allowing time for radiologic studies and planning of a definitive operation, which is the treatment of choice. If intervention is necessary during the acute phase, it must focus on adequate decompression of the biliary tree through open common bile duct exploration or endoscopic papillotomy or stenting.[31] Although nonoperative approaches such as percutaneous transhepatic cholangioscopic lithotomy (PTCSL) have been developed, surgery remains the treatment of choice. PTCSL is generally used in poor-risk surgical patients and

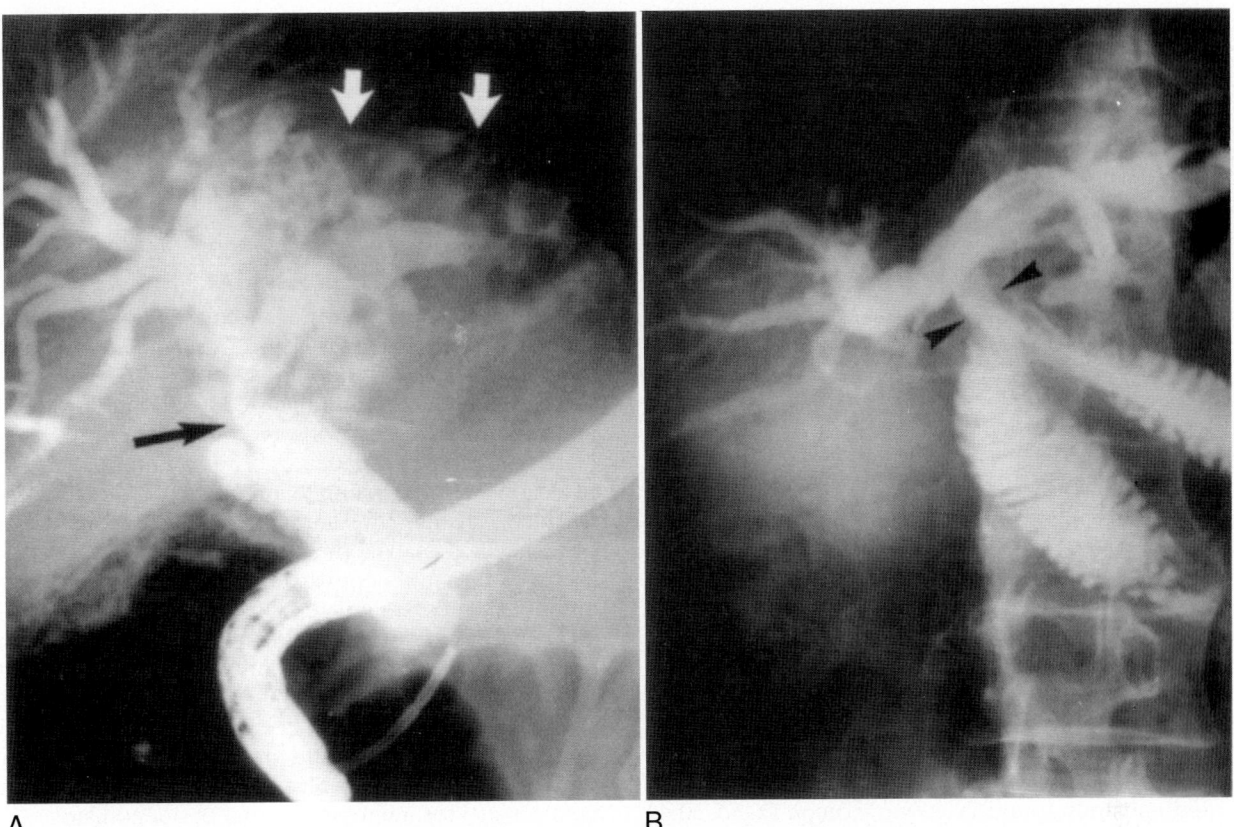

Figure 52-24 A, Cholangiogram of a patient with recurrent pyogenic cholangitis and a common hepatic duct stricture (*black arrow*). There are numerous stones inside dilated left ducts (*white arrows*). **B,** A hepaticojejunostomy to the segment III duct (*arrowheads*) has been performed, and a flexible choledochoscope is shown passing through the anastomosis into the peripheral left ducts. All stones have been cleared. (From Fan ST, Wong J: Recurrent pyogenic cholangitis. In Blumgart LH, Fong Y [eds]: Surgery of the Liver and Biliary Tract. London, WB Saunders, 2000, pp 1205-1225.)

in those who have failed surgical treatment. Stone clearance rates are high (>80%) and necessary for a successful long-term outcome. Unfortunately, stone recurrence is common and mostly related to the presence of biliary strictures.[32]

The goal of operative approaches is to clear the biliary tree of stones and to bypass, resect, or dilate strictures. Many cases only require exploration of the common bile duct with or without hepaticojejunostomy. In complicated cases, providing permanent access to the biliary tree for interventional radiologic procedures by extending the end of the Roux-en-Y loop hepaticojejunostomy to the skin or subcutaneous space has been a successful approach (Fig. 52-24). Other potentially necessary procedures include strictureplasty or partial hepatectomy. Partial hepatectomy is advocated for patients with intrahepatic strictures, hepatic atrophy, liver abscess, or suspicion of cholangiocarcinoma.[31,32]

In large series from Asia, where surgery and hepatectomy are liberally applied, surgical mortality rates are 1%, and with aggressive treatment, there is an almost 100% stone clearance rate. Long-term outcome is excellent, with a less than 5% stone recurrence rate. Long-term survival is mostly related to the presence of cholangio-

carcinoma, which is found in about 10% of cases. Particularly complicated cases can have a higher rate of recurrent symptoms.[31,32]

NEOPLASMS

Solid Benign Neoplasms

It is estimated that benign focal liver masses are present in about 10% to 20% of the population in developed countries. With the increasing use of rapidly improving radiologic exams, these entities are being encountered more frequently. Familiarity with the clinical characteristics, natural history, imaging characteristics, and indications for surgery in these tumors is essential. Many benign lesions can be adequately characterized by modern imaging studies such as CT, ultrasound, and MRI, but in unclear cases, serum tumor markers (AFP, CEA) and a search for a primary tumor (in the case of suspected metastases) is carried out. Ultimately, a resection might be necessary to make a definitive diagnosis. Laparoscopic techniques for assessment, biopsy, and resection have become an important diagnostic technique as well.[33]

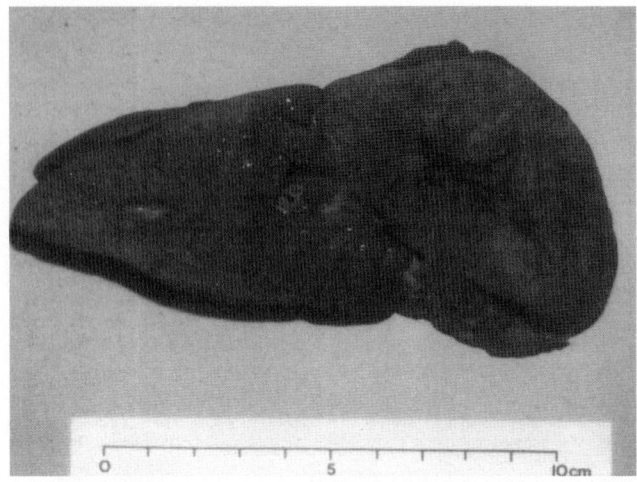

Figure 52-25 Cross section of resected focal nodular hyperplasia. Note the well-defined central scar. (From Hugh TJ, Poston GJ: Benign liver tumors and masses. In Blumgart LH, Fong Y [eds]: Surgery of the Liver and Biliary Tract. London, WB Saunders, 2000, pp 1397-1422.)

Liver Cell Adenoma

Liver cell adenoma (LCA) is a relatively rare benign proliferation of hepatocytes in the context of a normal liver. It is predominantly found in young women (aged 20-40 years) and is often associated with steroid hormone use such as oral contraceptive pills (OCPs).[33] The female-to-male ratio is approximately 11:1. LCAs are usually singular, but multiple lesions have been reported in 12% to 30% of cases. The presence of 10 or more adenomas is termed *adenomatosis*. Interestingly, cases with multiple adenomas are not associated with OCP use and do not have as dramatic a female preponderance. Histologically, LCAs are composed of cords of benign hepatocytes containing increased glycogen and fat. Bile ductules are not seen, and the normal architecture of the liver is not present in these lesions. Hemorrhage and necrosis are commonly seen.[34] Molecular studies have recently identified genetic signatures associated with a higher risk for malignant transformation.

Patients with LCA present with symptoms about 50% to 75% of the time. Upper abdominal pain is common and may be related to hemorrhage into the tumor or local compressive symptoms. Physical exam is usually unrevealing, and tumor markers are normal. Dramatic presentations with free intraperitoneal rupture and bleeding can occur. CT usually demonstrates a well-circumscribed heterogenous mass that shows early enhancement during the arterial phase. MRI scans of LCA have specific imaging characteristics, including a well-demarcated heterogenous mass containing fat or hemorrhage. Although in the past, imaging studies lacked the accuracy to diagnose LCA, modern-day imaging techniques can accurately identify most of these tumors.[35] Ultimately, however, resection may be necessary to secure a diagnosis in difficult cases.

The two major risks of LCA are rupture (with potentially life-threatening intraperitoneal hemorrhage) and malignant transformation. Quantifying the risk for rupture is difficult, but it has been estimated to be as high as 30% to 50% and may be related to size. Although there are numerous reports of transformation of LCA into hepatocellular carcinoma, the true risk for transformation is probably low.[33]

Patients who present with acute hemorrhage need emergent attention. If possible, hepatic artery embolization is a helpful and usually effective temporizing maneuver. Once stabilized and appropriately resuscitated, a laparotomy and resection of the mass is required. Symptomatic masses, likewise, are resected. Patients with asymptomatic LCA who take OCPs can be watched for regression after stopping the OCPs, although progression and rupture have been observed in this setting. Behavior of LCA during pregnancy has been unpredictable, and resection before a planned pregnancy is usually recommended. Overall, the surgeon must compare the risks of expectant management with serial imaging studies and AFP measurements against those of resection. Most authorities recommend resection because of a very low mortality in experienced hands and the previously mentioned risks of observation. Margin status is not important in these resections, and limited resections can be performed. The management of adenomatosis is controversial, but large lesions should probably be resected because of the risk for rupture. Occasionally, liver transplantation is necessary for aggressive forms of adenomatosis.[33]

Focal Nodular Hyperplasia

Focal nodular hyperplasia (FNH) is the second most common benign tumor of the liver and is predominantly discovered in young women. FNH is usually a small (<5 cm) nodular mass arising in a normal liver that involves the right and left liver equally. The mass is characterized by a central fibrous scar with radiating septa, although no central scar is seen in about 15% of cases (Fig. 52-25). Microscopically, FNH contains cords of benign-appearing hepatocytes divided by multiple fibrous septa originating from a central scar. Typical hepatic vascularity is not seen, but atypical biliary epithelium is found scattered throughout the lesion. The central scar often contains a large artery that branches out into multiple smaller arteries in a spoke-wheel pattern.[33]

The etiology of FNH is not known, but the most common theory is that FNH is related to a developmental vascular malformation. Female hormones and OCPs have been implicated in the development and growth of FNH, but the association is weak and difficult to prove. Occasional cases of resolution of symptoms after stopping OCPs have been reported. In recent years, nonclassic forms of FNH have been described. Telangiectatic FNH with or without atypia and mixed hyperplastic and adenomatous FNH account for about 20% of cases, occur more frequently in men, and are more difficult to characterize radiologically.[3]

In most patients, FNH presents as an incidental finding at laparotomy or more commonly on imaging studies. If symptoms are noted, they are most often vague abdominal pain, but a variety of nonspecific symptoms have been described. It is often difficult to ascribe these reported symptoms to the presence of FNH, and therefore, other possible causes must be sought.[5] Physical examination is usually unrevealing, and mild abnormalities of LFTs may be found. Serum AFP levels are normal.

With advances in hepatobiliary imaging, most cases of FNH can be diagnosed radiologically with reasonable certainty. Contrast-enhanced CT and MRI have become accurate methods of diagnosing FNH. These scans usually demonstrate a homogeneous mass with a central scar that rapidly enhances during the arterial phase of contrast administration. When no central scar is seen, however, radiologic diagnosis is difficult, and differentiating from liver cell adenoma or a malignant mass (especially fibrolamellar hepatocellular carcinoma) can sometimes be impossible.[35] Occasionally, histologic confirmation is necessary, and resection is recommended for definitive diagnosis. Fine-needle aspiration for the diagnosis of FNH has been recommended but is often unrevealing.[33]

The natural history of FNH is not fully understood, but in general, FNH is a benign and indolent tumor. Asymptomatic patients mostly remain so over long periods of time. Rupture, bleeding, and infarction are exceedingly rare, and malignant degeneration of FNH has never been reported. The treatment of FNH, therefore, depends on diagnostic certainty and symptoms. Asymptomatic patients with typical radiologic features do not require treatment. If diagnostic uncertainty exists, resection may be necessary for histologic confirmation. Symptomatic patients are thoroughly investigated to look for other pathology to explain the symptoms. Careful observation of symptomatic FNH with serial imaging is reasonable because symptoms may resolve in a significant number of cases. Patients with persistent symptomatic FNH or an enlarging mass need to be considered for resection. Because FNH is a benign diagnosis, resection must be performed with minimal morbidity and mortality.[33]

Hemangioma

Hemangioma is the most common benign tumor of the liver. It occurs in women more commonly than men (3:1 ratio) and at a mean age of about 45 years. Small capillary hemangiomas are of no clinical significance, whereas the larger cavernous hemangiomas more often come to the attention of the liver surgeon (Fig. 52-26). Cavernous hemangiomas have been associated with FNH and are also theorized to be congenital vascular malformations. Enlargement of hemangiomas are by ectasia rather than neoplasia. They are usually single and less than 5 cm in diameter, and they occur equally in the right and left liver. Lesions greater than 5 cm are arbitrarily called *giant hemangiomas*. Involution or thrombosis of hemangiomas can result in dense fibrotic masses that may be difficult to differentiate from malignancy. Microscopically, they are endothelium-lined, blood-filled spaces that are separated by thin, fibrous septa.[33]

Most commonly, hemangiomas are asymptomatic and incidentally found on imaging studies. Large compressive masses may cause vague upper abdominal symptoms.

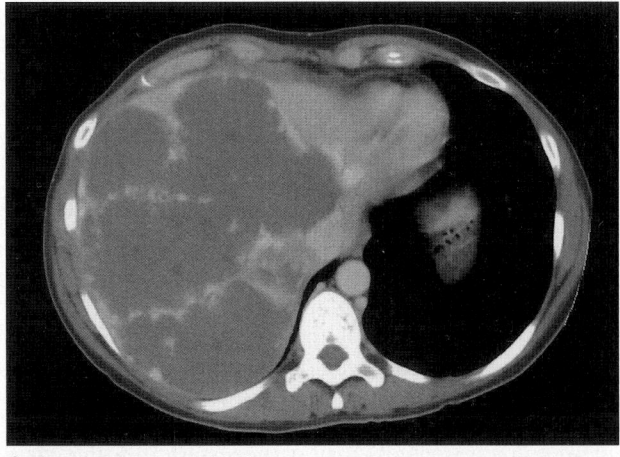

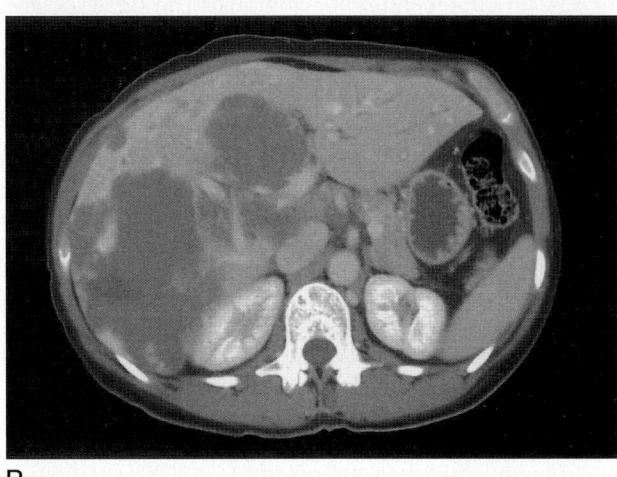

Figure 52-26 A and **B,** CT scans of a large cavernous hemangioma showing displacement of left and middle hepatic veins and abutment of the left portal vein. The mass was symptomatic and required an extended right hepatectomy to remove.

Symptoms ascribed to a liver hemangioma, however, mandate a search for other pathology because in about half of cases, an alternative cause of symptoms will be found. Rapid expansion or acute thrombosis can, on occasion, cause symptoms. Spontaneous rupture of liver hemangiomas is exceedingly rare. An associated syndrome of thrombocytopenia and consumptive coagulopathy known as *Kasabach-Merritt syndrome* is rare but well described.[33]

LFTs and tumor markers are usually normal in liver hemangiomas. Radiologic investigation can reliably make the diagnosis in most cases. CT and MRI are usually sufficient if a typical peripheral nodular enhancement pattern is seen. Labeled red blood cell scans are an accurate test but are rarely necessary if high-quality CT and MRI are available.[35] Percutaneous biopsy of a suspected hemangioma is potentially dangerous and inaccurate and is therefore not recommended.

The natural history of liver hemangioma is generally benign, and it appears that most of these tumors remain stable over long periods of time with a low risk for rupture or hemorrhage. Growth and development of symptoms do occur, however, occasionally requiring resection. There has never been a report of malignant degeneration of a liver hemangioma. An asymptomatic patient with a secure diagnosis can therefore be simply observed. Symptomatic patients undergo a thorough evaluation, looking for alternative explanations for the symptoms, but are candidates for resection if no other cause is found. Rupture, change in size, and development of the Kasabach-Merritt syndrome are indications for resection. In rare cases of diagnostic uncertainty, resection may be necessary to make a definitive diagnosis. Resection of liver hemangiomas should be performed with minimal morbidity and mortality. The preferred approach to resection is enucleation with inflow control, but anatomic resections may be necessary in some cases. Surgery on large central hemangiomas can be associated with significant morbidity.[33]

Liver hemangiomas in children account for about 12% of all childhood hepatic tumors. They are usually multifocal and can involve other organs. Large hemangiomas in children can result in congestive heart failure secondary to arteriovenous shunting. Untreated symptomatic childhood hemangiomas are associated with a 70% mortality rate, but small capillary hemangiomas almost all resolve. Symptomatic childhood hemangiomas may be treated medically for congestive heart failure, with therapeutic embolization. Radiation and chemotherapeutic agents have been used, but experience is limited. Resection may be necessary for symptomatic lesions or for rupture.[36]

Other Benign Tumors

Most benign solid liver tumors are LCA, FNH, or hemangiomas. An array of other benign hepatic tumors exists, but these are rare and can be difficult to differentiate from malignancy. Macroregenerative nodules (previously known as *adenomatous hyperplasia*) are single or multiple, well-circumscribed, bile-stained, bulging surface nodules that occur primarily in cirrhotic patients and result from the hyperplastic response to chronic liver injury. These lesions have malignant potential and can be very difficult to distinguish from hepatocellular carcinoma. Nodular regenerative hyperplasia (NRH) is a benign, diffuse, micronodular (usually <2 cm) process that is associated with lymphoproliferative disorders, collagen vascular diseases, and the use of steroids or chemotherapy. NRH has no malignant potential and is not associated with cirrhosis. Biopsy may be necessary to distinguish these focal nodules from malignancy.

Mesenchymal hamartomas (MHs) are rare solitary tumors of childhood that account for 5% of pediatric liver tumors. These are usually large cystic masses found in the right liver that present as progressive painless abdominal distention. Resection of MH may be necessary in the case of large lesions causing a mass effect. Fatty tumors of the liver are rarely encountered but can usually be distinguished by typical characteristics on CT or MRI. Fatty tumors of the liver include primary lipoma, myelolipoma (also containing hematopoietic tissue), angiolipoma (also containing blood vessels), and angiomyolipoma (also containing smooth muscle). Focal fatty change in

the liver can be confused with a neoplastic process and is becoming more common with improved imaging and the increasing incidence of hepatic steatosis. Benign fibrous tumors of the liver exist and can become large and symptomatic, requiring resection. Inflammatory pseudotumor of the liver is a localized mass of inflammatory cells that can mimic a neoplasm. The etiology of these inflammatory lesions is not known but may be related to thrombosed vessels or old abscesses. Other, extremely rare benign hepatic tumors include leiomyomas, myxomas, schwannomas, lymphangiomas, and teratomas.[36]

Intrahepatic biliary cystadenomas or bile duct adenomas are rare but can cause biliary symptoms. Biliary hamartoma and biliary hyperplasia are often seen as small white surface lesions that can mimic small metastatic tumors at abdominal exploration. Adrenal and pancreatic rests have also been found in the liver.

Primary Solid Malignant Neoplasms

Hepatocellular Carcinoma

Epidemiology

Hepatocellular carcinoma (HCC) is the most common primary malignancy of the liver and one of the most common malignancies worldwide, accounting for more than 1 million deaths annually. The geographic distribution of HCC is clearly related to the incidence of hepatitis B virus (HBV) infection. The highest incidence of disease (>10-20 per 100,000) is found in Southeast Asia and tropical Africa, and the lowest incidence (1-3 per 100,000) is found in Australia, North America, and Europe. In high incidence areas, rates are variable. For example, Taiwan has an incidence of 150 per 100,000, whereas Singapore has an incidence of 28 per 100,000. Epidemiologic evidence strongly suggests that HCC is largely related to environmental factors, with incidence in immigrants eventually taking on that of the local population after several generations. An exception to this observation is that whites living in high prevalence areas tend to have a low incidence of HCC. This is likely related to the continuation of the lifestyle and environment of their home country. It is probable that the variation in incidence rates among immigrants is related to HBV carrier rates. Recent publications have noted a significant rise in the incidence of HCC in the United States and other Western countries during the past 30 years. The explanation of this rising incidence is not understood, but emergence of hepatitis C virus (HCV) infection and immigration patterns have been suggested.[37,38]

HCC is two to eight times more common in males than in females in low and high incidence areas. Although sex hormones may play a minor role in the development of HCC, the higher incidence in males is probably related to higher rates of associated risk factors such as HBV infection, cirrhosis, smoking, alcohol abuse, and higher hepatic DNA synthesis in cirrhosis. In general, the incidence of HCC increases with age, but a tendency to develop HCC earlier in high incidence areas has been noted. For example, in Mozambique, 50% of patients with HCC are younger than 30 years of age. This may be related to the differing age at infection and natural histories of HBV and HCV infections.[37,38]

Etiology

A large number of associations between hepatic viral infections, environmental exposures, alcohol use, smoking, genetic metabolic diseases, cirrhosis, OCPs, and the development of HCC have been recognized. Overall, 75% to 80% of HCC cases are related to HBV (50%-55%) or HCV (25%-30%) infection. What is also clear from research is that the development of HCC is a complex and multistep process that involves any number of these risk factors.

Many years of research have documented a clear association between persistent HBV infection and the development of HCC. Studies estimate relative risks of 5 to 100 for the development of HCC in HBV-infected individuals compared with noninfected individuals. Other evidence includes the following observations: geographic areas high in HBV infection have high rates of HCC; HBV infection precedes the development of HCC; the sequence of HBV infection to cirrhosis to HCC is well documented; and the HBV genome is found in the HCC genome. HBV has no known oncogenes, but insertional mutagenesis into hepatocytes may be a contributing factor to the development of HCC. Another proposed mechanism is related to cirrhosis and chronic hepatic inflammation, which is present in 60% to 90% of patients with HBV infection and HCC. Cirrhosis, however, is not a prerequisite for the development of HBV-related HCC. It is important to note that the risk for HCC is not simply related to HBV exposure but requires chronic infection (i.e., chronically positive hepatitis B surface antigen). There is a higher risk for persistent infection (carrier state) when the infection is acquired at birth or during early childhood. Familial clustering of HCC is probably related to early vertical transmission of the virus and establishment of the chronic carrier state.

HCV has recently been discovered to be a major cause of chronic liver disease in Japan, Europe, and the United States, where there is a relatively low rate of HBV infection. Antibodies to HCV are found in 76% of patients with HCC in Japan and Europe and in 36% of patients in the United States. HBV and HCV infection are both independent risk factors for the development of HCC but probably act synergistically when an individual is infected with both viruses. Although the natural history of HCV infection is not completely understood, it appears to be one of chronic infection with a benign early course but with ultimate development of cirrhosis and HCC. Studies on the rates of progression to cirrhosis estimate a median time of 30 years, but differing progression rates yield a range of less than 20 years to more than 50 years. Factors associated with a more rapid progression include male gender, chronic alcohol use, and older age at infection. HCV is an RNA virus that does not integrate into the host genome, and therefore, the pathogenesis of HCV-related HCC may be more related to chronic inflammation and cirrhosis rather than direct carcinogenesis.[37,38]

The true relationship of cirrhosis and HCC is difficult to ascertain, and suggestions of causation remain speculative. Cirrhosis is not required for the development of HCC, and HCC is not an inevitable result of cirrhosis. The relationship of cirrhosis and HCC is further complicated by the fact that they share common associations. Furthermore, some associations (e.g., HBV infection, hemochromatosis) are associated with higher risk for HCC, whereas others (e.g., alcohol, primary biliary cirrhosis) are associated with a lower risk for HCC. Research has demonstrated that cirrhotic livers with higher DNA replication rates are associated with the development of HCC.

Chronic alcohol abuse has been associated with an increased risk for HCC, and there may be a synergistic effect with HBV and HCV infection. Alcohol causes cirrhosis but has never been shown to be directly carcinogenic to hepatocytes and likely acts as a cocarcinogen. Cigarette smoking has been linked to the development of HCC, but the evidence is not consistent, and the contributing risk independent of viral hepatitis is likely small. Aflatoxin, produced by *Aspergillus* species, is a powerful hepatotoxin. With chronic exposure, aflatoxin acts as a carcinogen and increases the risk for HCC. The offending fungi grow on grains, peanuts, and food products in tropical and subtropical regions, and intake of contaminated foods results in aflatoxin exposure. Levels of aflatoxin in implicated foods are regulated in the United States. A variety of chemicals have been implicated as carcinogens related to HCC and include nitrites, hydrocarbons, solvents, pesticides, and vinyl chloride. Thorotrast (colloidal thorium dioxide) is an angiographic medium that was used in the 1930s that emits high levels of long-lasting radiation and has been associated with hepatic fibrosis, angiosarcoma, cholangiosarcoma, and HCC. Associations with inherited metabolic liver diseases, such as hereditary hemochromatosis, α_1-antitrypsin deficiency, and Wilson's disease, have also been implicated as risk factors for HCC. Associations with hormonal manipulations, such as the use of OCPs and anabolic steroids, have been suggested but are weak and are probably specifically better linked to adenoma and well-differentiated HCC. Current research is focusing on relationships of HCC with diabetes, obesity, and nonalcoholic fatty liver disease.[38]

Clinical Presentation

Most commonly, patients presenting with HCC are men 50 to 60 years of age who complain of right upper quadrant abdominal pain and weight loss and have a palpable mass. In countries endemic for HBV, presentation at a young age is common and probably related to childhood infection. Unfortunately, in unscreened populations, HCC tends to present at a late stage because of the lack of symptoms in early stages. Presentation at this advanced stage is often with a vague right upper quadrant abdominal pain that sometimes radiates to the right shoulder. Nonspecific symptoms of advanced malignancy such as anorexia, nausea, lethargy, and weight loss are common. Another common presentation of HCC is hepatic decompensation in a patient with known mild cirrhosis or even in patients without previously recognized cirrhosis.

On rare occasions, HCC can present as a rupture with the sudden onset of abdominal pain followed by hypo-

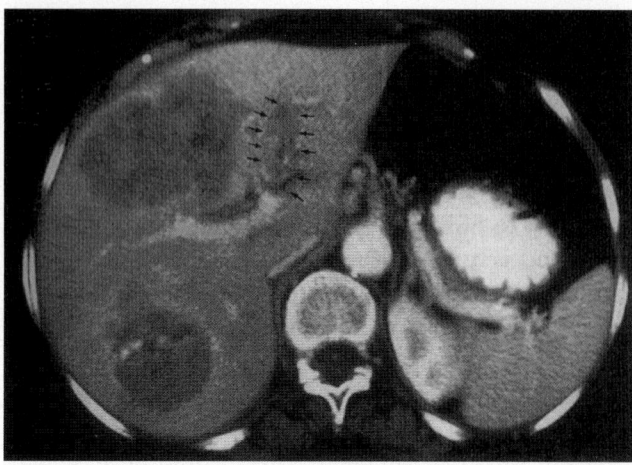

Figure 52-27 Contrast-enhanced CT scan demonstrating multifocal hepatocellular carcinoma. The left portal vein is invaded and expanded by tumor. (From Roddie ME, Adam A: Computed tomography of the liver and biliary tree. In Blumgart LH, Fong Y [eds]: Surgery of the Liver and Biliary Tract. London, WB Saunders, 2000, pp 309-340.)

volemic shock secondary to intraperitoneal bleeding. Other rare presentations include hepatic vein occlusion (Budd-Chiari syndrome), obstructive jaundice, hemobilia, or fever of unknown origin. Less than 1% of cases of HCC present with a paraneoplastic syndrome, most commonly hypercalcemia, hypoglycemia, and erythrocytosis. Small, incidentally noted tumors are becoming a more common presentation because of the knowledge of specific risk factors, screening programs for diagnosed HBV or HCV infection, and the increasing use of high-quality abdominal imaging.[37,38]

Diagnosis

Radiologic investigation is a critical part of the diagnosis of HCC. In the past, liver radioisotope scans and angiography were common methods of diagnosis, but ultrasound, CT, and MRI have replaced these studies. Ultrasound plays a significant role in screening and early detection of HCC, but definitive diagnosis and treatment planning rely on CT and MRI. Contrast-enhanced CT and MRI protocols aimed at diagnosing HCC take advantage of the hypervascularity of these tumors, and arterial phase images are critical to adequately assess the extent of disease. CT and MRI also evaluate the extent of disease in terms of peritoneal metastases, nodal metastases, and extent of vascular and biliary involvement. Detection of bland or tumor thrombus in the portal venous system is also very important and can be done with any of the above modalities[35,37] (Fig. 52-27).

AFP measurements can be very helpful in the diagnosis of HCC. An AFP level greater than 20 ng/mL is noted in about three fourths of documented cases of HCC. False-positive elevations of serum AFP can be seen in inflammatory disorders of the liver, such as chronic active viral hepatitis. Specificity and positive predictive values of AFP improve with higher cutoff levels (e.g., 400 ng/mL), but at the cost of sensitivity. With the improvements

in imaging technology and the ability to detect smaller tumors, AFP is largely used as an adjunctive test in patients with liver masses. In fact, a hypervascular mass consistent with HCC combined with an AFP higher than 400 ng/mL is diagnostic. AFP levels are particularly useful in monitoring treated patients for recurrence after normalization of levels.[37]

Percutaneous needle biopsies of liver lesions suspected of being HCC are only necessary in patients who are being considered for nonoperative therapies. Patients with appropriate risk factors and suggestive radiology (with or without an elevated AFP) who are candidates for potentially curative surgical therapy do not require preoperative biopsy. Percutaneous fine-needle aspiration of HCC does run a small risk of tumor cell spillage (estimated to be ~1%) and rupture or bleeding (especially in cirrhotic livers and subcapsular tumors).

After the diagnosis of HCC has been made, the patient must be staged in order to develop an appropriate treatment plan. Most patients with HCC have two diseases, and survival is as much related to the tumor as it is to cirrhosis. Staging, therefore, includes an extent of disease workup as well as an extent of cirrhosis workup.

In assessing the extent of disease, the common sites of metastases must be considered. HCC largely metastasizes to the lung, bone, and peritoneum, and the preoperative history focuses on symptoms referable to these areas. Extent of disease in the liver, including macrovascular invasion and the presence of multiple liver masses, must also be considered. Cross-sectional abdominal imaging, including arterial-phase images (discussed earlier), yields information on extent of disease in the liver as well as on peritoneal disease. A preoperative chest x-ray is mandatory and is followed with CT if any abnormalities are present. Routine bone scans are not performed unless there are suggestive symptoms or signs.

Assessment of liver function is absolutely critical in considering treatment options for a patient with HCC. Liver resection is considered the treatment of choice for HCC, and the risk for postoperative liver failure and death must be considered. This risk is related to the degree of cirrhosis, the amount of liver resected (functional liver reserve), and the regenerative response. Other successful treatments are available for HCC, such as ablative techniques, embolization techniques, and liver transplantation, and therefore, a complete assessment of tumor and liver function must ensue. A number of assessments of liver function are available and are described in an earlier section. Generally, they are divided into a clinical assessment and functional tests. Many clinical assessment schemes are described (see earlier), but most commonly, Child's status (as modified by Pugh) is used. Child's C patients are not candidates for resectional therapy, whereas Child's A patients can usually tolerate some extent of liver resection. Many consider Child's B patients candidates for operation, but they are generally borderline, and therapy must be individualized. Outside of scoring systems, it has been recently demonstrated that significant portal hypertension regardless of biochemical assessments is highly predictive of postoperative liver failure and death. Portal hypertension can be assessed directly through hepatic vein wedge pressures but is usually obvious on high-quality imaging in the form of splenomegaly, cirrhotic-appearing liver, and varices. Blood work usually demonstrates marked cytopenias, typically thrombocytopenia. Functional tests of liver function are well described (see earlier) but are not routinely used in most Western centers because the results of studies evaluating predictive value have been mixed.

Staging laparoscopy has recently been employed as a staging tool in HCC and spares about one in five patients a nontherapeutic laparotomy. Laparoscopy yields additional information about extent of disease in the liver, extrahepatic disease, and cirrhosis. The yield of laparoscopy is dictated by the extent of disease and is only selectively employed. The presence of clinically apparent cirrhosis, radiologic evidence of vascular invasion, or bilobar tumors increased the yield to 30%, whereas without these factors, the yield is 5%.

A number of staging systems for HCC exist, but none has ever been shown to be particularly superior, and they probably depend on the specific population being staged and the etiology of HCC in that particular population. The TNM staging system is not routinely used for HCC; it does not accurately predict survival because it does not take liver function into account. The Okuda staging system is an older but simple and effective system that takes into account liver function and tumor-related factors. It adds up a single point for the presence of tumor involving more than 50% of the liver, presence of ascites, albumin less than 3 g/dL, and bilirubin more than 3 mg/dL and reliably distinguishes patients with a prohibitively poor prognosis from those with potential for long-term survival. The most well-validated staging system is the Cancer of the Liver Italian Program (CLIP), which was rigorously developed and has been prospectively validated (Table 52-7). An example of a scoring system that is probably population specific is the Chinese University Prognostic Index (CUPI), which takes into account TNM stage, symptoms, ascites, and AFP, bilirubin, and alkaline phosphatase levels and appears to largely apply to HBV-related HCC in China.[37]

Pathology

Histologically, HCC is graded as well, moderately, or poorly differentiated. The grade of HCC, however, has never been shown to accurately predict outcome. Grossly, the growth patterns of HCC have been classified in a number of ways. The most useful scheme divides HCC into three distinct growth patterns that have a distinct relationship to outcome. This type of HCC is connected to the liver by a small vascular stalk and is easily resected without sacrifice of a significant amount of non-neoplastic liver tissue. The hanging type of HCC can grow to substantial size without involving much normal liver tissue. The pushing type of HCC is well demarcated and often contains a fibrous capsule. It is characterized by growth that displaces vascular structures rather than invading them. The pushing type of HCC is usually resectable. The last type is called the *infiltrative type* of HCC and tends to invade vascular structures even at a

Table 52-7 The Cancer of the Liver Italian Group Score (CLIP)*

CLINICAL PARAMETERS	CUTOFF VALUES	POINTS
Child-Pugh stage	A	0
	B	1
	C	2
Tumor morphology	Uninodular, <50% extension	0
	Multinodular, <50% extension	1
	Massive or extension >50%	2
AFP (ng/dL)	<400	0
	>400	1
Portal vein thrombosis	No	0
	Yes	1

*Score ranges from 0 to 6; scores of 4 to 6 are generally considered advanced disease, whereas scores of 0 to 3 have the potential for long-term survival.

AFP, α-fetoprotein.

small size. Resecting the infiltrative type is often possible, but positive histologic margins are common. Small tumors less than 5 cm in size usually do not fall into any of these groups and are often discussed as a separate entity. Lastly, HCC can present in a multifocal manner. Most HCCs probably start as a single tumor, but ultimately multiple satellite lesions can develop secondary to portal vein invasion and metastases. Multifocal tumors throughout the liver probably represent the end stage of HCC with multiple metastases and multiple primary tumors.[34]

Treatment

There are a large number of treatment options for patients with HCC, reflecting the heterogeneity of this disease as well as the lack of a proven superior treatment except for complete resection (Table 52-8). Deciding on a treatment regimen for any one patient must take into consideration the stage of malignancy, the condition of the patient, the condition of the liver, and the experience of the treating physicians.

Complete excision of HCC either by partial hepatectomy or by total hepatectomy and transplantation is the treatment of choice when possible because it has the highest chance of long-term survival. In general, however, only 10% to 20% of patients are considered to have resectable disease. Historically, mortality rates for partial hepatectomy ranged from 1% to 20%, but if performed in healthy patients without advanced cirrhosis, most modern series have a mortality rate less than 5%. Advances in surgical technique have allowed the development of limited segmental resections when appropriate, which preserves functional liver and improves early postoperative recovery. Selection of the appropriate patient for resection is critical and must take into account the condition of the liver as well as the extent of disease. Patients with Child's B or C cirrhosis or portal hypertension do

Table 52-8 **Treatment Options for Hepatocellular Carcinoma**

Surgical
Resection
Orthotopic liver transplantation

Ablative
EtOH injection
Acetic acid injection
Thermal ablation (cryotherapy, radiofrequency ablation, microwave)

Transarterial
Embolization
Chemoembolization
Radiotherapy

Combination Transarterial and Ablative

External-beam Radiation Therapy

Systemic
Chemotherapy
Hormonal
Immunotherapy

not tolerate resection. The volume of the future liver remnant (FLR) is also an important consideration and is associated with postoperative complications and mortality. Preoperative portal vein embolization is an effective strategy to increase the volume and function of the FLR and is used liberally in patients with Childs A cirrhosis being considered for a major resection with a small FLR. The overall postresection survival rates for HCC are 58% to 100% at 1 year, 28% to 88% at 3 years, 11% to 75% at 5 years, and 19% to 26% at 10 years. These results obviously depend on the stage of the tumor as well as the degree of cirrhosis in particular series, but give a sense of the possibilities. A variety of prognostic factors predictive of survival after resection have been identified, but none are universally agreed on. The most commonly cited negative prognostic factors are tumor size, cirrhosis, infiltrative growth pattern, vascular invasion, intrahepatic metastases, multifocal tumors, lymph node metastases, margin less than 1 cm, and lack of a capsule. The best outcomes are found in patients with single small tumors, but size alone does not contraindicate resection. Multifocal tumors and major vascular invasion are generally associated with a poor outcome, but some groups advocate resection in highly selected patients.[37,39,40]

Theoretically, liver transplantation is the ideal treatment for HCC because it addresses both the liver dysfunction and the HCC. The limitations of transplantation are the need for chronic immunosuppression as well as the lack of organ donors. There is a growing interest in the use of partial hepatectomy from live donors, which addresses the latter point but remains a somewhat controversial approach. Early series of transplantation for

HCC had high recurrence rates and relatively poor long-term survival. This has largely been attributed to the fact that most of these patients were being transplanted for advanced disease. Refinements in patient selection, namely, patients with single tumors less than 5 cm or multiple tumors no more than three in number and 3 cm in size have resulted in improved outcomes. Long-term survival rates in recent years with more stringent selection criteria have ranged from 50% to 85%. Recent studies have begun to expand the indications for liver transplantation without a major effect on long-term survival but likely with an increase in overall recurrence rates. Comparing results of resection to transplantation is difficult, and the two are viewed as complementary rather than competitive. Patients with advanced cirrhosis (Child's B and C) and early-stage HCC are considered for transplantation, whereas those with Child's A cirrhosis have similar results with transplantation and resection and should probably undergo resection.[40]

A number of nonsurgical local ablative therapies are available for the treatment of small tumors. Percutaneous ethanol injection (PEI) is a useful technique for ablating small tumors. The tumor is killed by a combination of cellular dehydration, coagulative necrosis, and vascular thrombosis. Most tumors less than 2 cm in size can be ablated with a single application of PEI, but larger tumors may require multiple injections. Long-term survival after PEI for tumors less than 5 cm has been reported to range from 24% to 40%, but no randomized trials have compared PEI to resection. Percutaneous injection of acetic acid is a technique similar to PEI but has stronger necrotizing abilities, making it more useful in septated tumors.[41]

Thermal ablative techniques that freeze or heat tumors to destroy them have become very popular in recent years. Cryotherapy uses a specialized cryoprobe to freeze and thaw tumor and surrounding liver tissue with resulting necrosis. Cryotherapy is usually performed at laparotomy or laparoscopically but has recently been performed with percutaneous techniques. One advantage is that the ice ball formed is easily monitored with ultrasound. Disadvantages include a heat-sink effect, limiting the utility of freezing near major blood vessels and a relatively high complication rate of 8% to 41%. Reported 2-year survival rates for cryoablation of HCC range from 30% to 60%, but no studies comparative to resection exist. Radiofrequency ablation (RFA) uses high-frequency alternating current to create heat around an inserted probe, resulting in temperatures greater than 60°C and immediate cell death. Although initially limited to smaller tumors, improvements in technology have created RFA probes reportedly able to ablate tumors as large as 7 cm. Nonetheless, the efficacy of RFA for HCCs larger than 3 to 5 cm is limited. RFA is also limited by the protective effect of blood vessels and does not ablate well in these areas. RFA can easily be performed percutaneously with low complication rates, and optimal guidance systems are being developed. Recent trials have suggested that RFA is superior to PEI for limited HCC for local tumor control but not survival. No long-term data for RFA of HCC exist.[41]

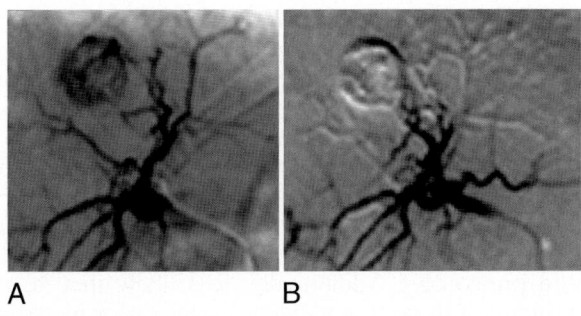

A   **B**

Figure 52-28 Angiogram demonstrating hypervascular hepatocellular carcinoma before **(A)** and after **(B)** embolization.

Table 52-9 Comparison of Standard Hepatocellular Carcinoma (HCC) and Fibrolamellar Hepatocellular Carcinoma (FHCC)

CHARACTERISTIC	HCC	FHCC
Male-to-female ratio	2:1-8:1	1:1
Median age (yr)	55	25
Tumor	Invasive	Well circumscribed
Resectability	<25%	50%-75%
Cirrhosis	90%	5%
α-fetoprotein positive	80%	5%
Hepatitis B positive	65%	5%

Transarterial therapy for HCC is based on the fact that most of the tumor's blood supply is from the hepatic artery. Hepatic arterial infusion (HAI) chemotherapy using 5-fluorouracil (5-FU)-based compounds, cisplatin, and doxorubicin has been studied in limited numbers. Response rates of 25% to 60% have been reported, but the requirement of a laparotomy to place the pump and associated hepatic toxicity limits the applicability of this approach to highly selected patients.[17] Percutaneous transarterial embolization can induce ischemic necrosis in HCC, resulting in response rates as high as 50% (Fig. 52-28). Attempts to improve the efficacy of arterial embolization have included adding chemotherapeutic agents (chemoembolization) to the embolization particles and oils such as lipiodol that are selectively taken up by HCC. Randomized trials have not shown chemoembolization to be superior to embolization alone. Seven randomized trials have compared embolization or chemoembolization with conservative management. Two of these trials and a meta-analysis have confirmed an overall survival advantage to embolization strategies. The selection of appropriate candidates for embolization is important, and treatment is generally limited to patients with preserved liver function and asymptomatic multinodular tumors without vascular invasion. Poor selection will result in a higher incidence of treatment-induced liver failure, offsetting the potential benefits.

External-beam radiation therapy (EBRT) has a limited role in the treatment of HCC, although occasional dramatic responses are seen. EBRT is limited by damage to normal liver parenchyma and to surrounding organs, but newer methods of conformal radiotherapy and breath-gated techniques are improving the utility of this treatment modality. Intra-arterial injections of iodine-131 with lipiodol or yttrium-90 in glass microspheres have been used to deliver localized radiation to HCC with reports of dramatic response rates. Transarterial radiotherapy is potentially promising for HCC as primary therapy or as adjuvant therapy.

Systemic chemotherapy with a variety of agents has been ineffective for the treatment of HCC and has a minimal role in the treatment of HCC. Response rates are generally less than 20% and of short duration. Systemic immunotherapy and hormonal therapy have been used in small numbers of patients with HCC with some early promising results, but to date have not demonstrated superiority to standard regimens.

With the bewildering number of available treatment strategies for HCC, it is no surprise that combinations of therapies and adjuvant or neoadjuvant strategies in conjunction with resection have been attempted. Two randomized trials have demonstrated a survival benefit to specific adjuvant strategies after resection of HCC. The first is the use of the retinoid polyprenoic acid, and the second is transarterial iodine-131 lipiodol treatment. Further studies and larger trials are awaited to confirm these promising strategies.

Distinct Variants of HCC

Fibrolamellar HCC (FHCC) is a variant of HCC with remarkably different clinical features that are summarized in Table 52-9. This tumor generally occurs in younger patients without a history of cirrhosis. The tumor is usually well demarcated and encapsulated and may have a central fibrotic area. The central scar can make distinguishing this tumor from FNH difficult. Histologically, FHCC is composed of large polygonal tumor cells embedded in a fibrous stroma forming lamellar structures (Fig. 52-29). FHCC does not produce AFP, but is associated with elevated neurotensin levels. In general, FHCC has a better prognosis than HCC. This is likely related to high resectability rates, lack of chronic liver disease, and a more indolent course. Long-term survival can be expected in about 50% to 75% of patients after complete resection, but recurrence is common and occurs in at least 80% of patients. The presence of lymph node metastases predicts a worse outcome. Resection of lymph node metastases and recurrent disease has been advocated because of a lack of alternative therapy and the possibility of long-term survival.[37]

Rarely, HCC can present as a mixed hepatocellular-cholangiocellular tumor, with cellular differentiation of both types present. Whether this is two separate tumors growing into each other or mixed differentiation of the same tumor is not known. These mixed tumors tend to take on a worse prognosis than standard HCC. A clear cell variant of HCC exists where the cells contain a clear cytoplasm. These tumors can resemble renal cell neo-

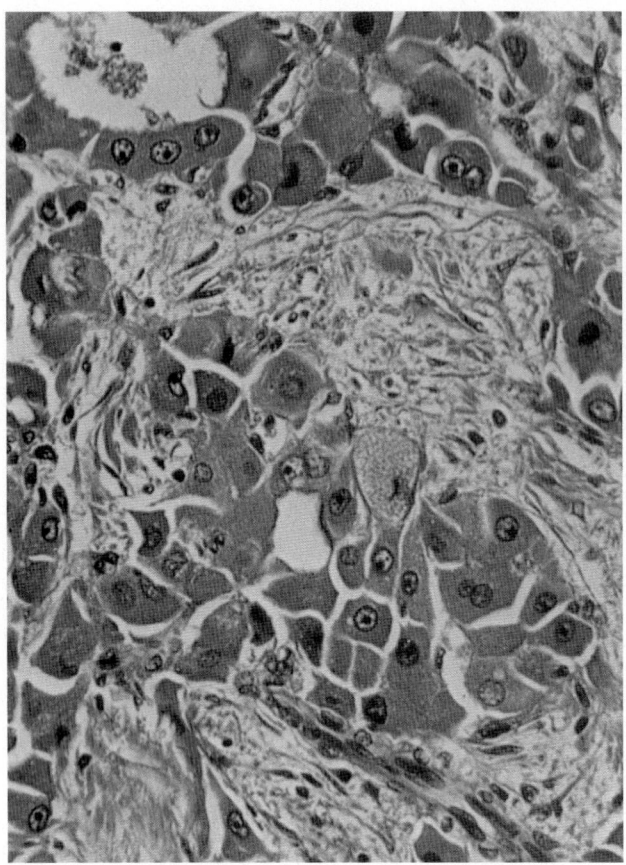

Figure 52-29 Fibrolamellar hepatocellular carcinoma. Abundant collagen is evident interconnecting clusters of cells. The cells are often in single-layer sheets. An acinus is present in the left upper field.

plasms. The clear cell variant may have a better prognosis than standard HCC, but this is a subject of debate. A pleomorphic or giant cell variant of HCC has been reported. Cells in this type are multinucleated, pleomorphic, and large and likely originate from primary hepatic cells. Some HCCs show evidence of sarcomatoid differentiation and are referred to as a *sarcomatoid variant* or *carcinosarcoma*. These tumors tend not to produce AFP and have a higher incidence of metastases at presentation.[34,37]

Childhood HCC is a distinct entity that comprises almost one fourth of pediatric liver tumors, but rarely occurs in infancy. Viral hepatitis is associated with childhood HCC in Asia, but less so in the United States. Inherited metabolic liver diseases (discussed earlier) are often associated with childhood HCC. As in adult HCC, complete resection is the only potentially curative treatment. There is a high incidence of multifocality, vascular invasion, and extrahepatic metastases resulting in relatively poor long-term survival rates of 10% to 20%.[36]

Intrahepatic Cholangiocarcinoma

Cholangiocarcinoma is an uncommon neoplasm with an incidence of 1 to 2 per 100,000 in the United States and can develop anywhere along the biliary tree from the ampulla of Vater to the peripheral intrahepatic bile ducts.

Most (40%-60%) of these tumors involve the biliary confluence (Klatskin's tumor), but about 10% emanate from intrahepatic ducts, presenting as a liver mass. Intrahepatic cholangiocarcinoma (IHC) is the second most common primary hepatic neoplasm and has also been referred to as *peripheral cholangiocarcinoma* or *cholangiolar carcinoma*. Studies on the incidence and natural history of IHC have been confused by the fact that many series include mixed hepatocellular-cholangiocarcinoma (discussed previously). Additionally, it is likely that, in the past, many of these tumors were mistaken for metastatic adenocarcinoma because biopsy is unable to differentiate the two. Historically, the most common risk factors for the development of cholangiocarcinoma (all types) were primary sclerosing cholangitis, choledochal cyst disease, and recurrent pyogenic cholangitis. Recent epidemiologic evidence has now linked IHC to HCV infection, HIV infection, cirrhosis, and diabetes. Recent increases in the diagnosis of IHC in the United States are likely related to better recognition of the disease and perhaps the rise in HCV infections in the 1960s and 1970s.

The clinical presentation of IHC is similar to HCC. The most common symptoms are right upper abdominal pain and weight loss. Jaundice occurs in about one fourth of patients. In recent years, patients are more often presenting with incidentally found liver masses on cross-sectional imaging. Unlike HCC, the AFP level will be normal, although CEA levels can be elevated in some cases. Most often, a search for a primary tumor with endoscopy and imaging of the chest will ensue and will not yield any information. If a biopsy has been performed, it is often read as adenocarcinoma. On CT and MRI, IHC is seen as a focal hepatic mass that may be associated with peripheral biliary dilation. The mass typically has peripheral or central enhancement on contrast-enhanced scans. Intrahepatic metastases, lymph node metastases, and growth along the biliary tree are commonly encountered.

Complete resection is the treatment of choice for IHC. Resectability rates generally range from 60% to 90%, and long-term survival in unresected patients is rare. If completely resected, 3-year survival rates range from 16% to 61%, and 5-year survival rates range from 24% to 44%. Factors associated with a poor outcome include intrahepatic metastases, lymph node metastases, vascular invasion, and positive margins. There is little known about the utility of radiation and chemotherapy for IHC due to the rarity of the disease, and their use is not routine. Chemotherapy is largely considered ineffective for IHC, but improvements in chemotherapy for other gastrointestinal tumors will hopefully translate into improved outcomes. Regional hepatic artery chemotherapy is under study and may be a promising approach.[42]

Other Primary Malignant Neoplasms

Hepatoblastoma is the most common primary hepatic tumor of childhood. There are about 50 to 70 new cases per year in the United States. Rare cases of adult hepatoblastoma have been reported, but overall, the median age of presentation is 18 months, and almost all cases occur before the age of 3 years. Recently, hepatoblastoma has been associated with the familial polyposis syndrome. There are a number of histologic subtypes, but in general, the tumor is derived from fetal or embryonic hepatocytes, and there are often mesenchymal elements present. Most often, this tumor presents as an asymptomatic mass. Mild anemia and thrombocytosis are commonly found at presentation. Serum AFP levels are elevated in 85% to 90% of patients and can serve as a useful marker for therapeutic response. Most studies support the use of chemotherapy followed by resection, and survival appears to be dependent on complete resection. Chemotherapy can serve to downstage tumors, facilitating resection. In patients without metastatic disease or the anaplastic variant, long-term survival rates of 60% to 70% can be expected with complete resection. Interestingly, 50% of patients with pulmonary metastases can be cured with resection of the hepatic tumor and chemotherapy or resection of the pulmonary metastases.[34,36]

A variety of sarcomas can rarely present as primary liver tumors but must always be considered metastatic lesions until proven otherwise. Angiosarcoma is probably the best described primary hepatic sarcoma because of its well-known association with vinyl chloride or Thorotrast exposure. Angiosarcoma typically presents as multiple hepatic masses and can present in childhood. Long-term survival is uncommon with primary hepatic angiosarcoma. A variety of other sarcomas, including leiomyosarcoma, malignant fibrous histiocytoma, embryonic sarcoma, and primary hepatic rhabdoid tumor, have been described but are rare. The latter two lesions are typically seen in children.

Non-Hodgkin's lymphoma can present primarily in the liver with or without extrahepatic disease. Primary hepatic lymphoma is treated like lymphoma elsewhere in the body if the diagnosis can be made before a liver resection. Primary hepatic neuroendocrine tumors or carcinoid tumors have been described but are probably extremely rare. Distinguishing the rare primary hepatic neuroendocrine tumor from a metastatic lesion can be difficult because the extrahepatic primary tumor can be radiologically occult for many years, and the liver is the most common site of metastases. Malignant germ cell tumors of the liver, including teratomas, choriocarcinomas, and yolk sac tumors, are very rare and are principally described in children. Epithelioid hemangioendothelioma of the liver is a rare malignant vascular tumor that presents with multiple bilateral hepatic masses. Extrahepatic metastases occur in about one fourth of patients, and clinical behavior is unpredictable. Most patients ultimately die of liver failure, but cases of successful transplantation have been reported.

Metastatic Tumors

The most common malignant tumors of the liver are metastatic lesions. The liver is a common site of metastases from gastrointestinal tumors presumably because of dissemination through the portal venous system. The most relevant metastatic tumor of the liver to the surgeon is colorectal cancer because of the well-documented potential for long-term survival after complete resection.

However, a large number of other tumors commonly metastasize to the liver. Included among these are cancers of the upper gastrointestinal system (stomach, pancreas, biliary), genitourinary system (renal, prostate), neuroendocrine system, breast, skin (melanoma), soft tissue (retroperitoneal sarcoma), and gynecologic system (ovarian, endometrial, cervix). The large majority of metastatic liver tumors occur with extrahepatic disease, have unresectable liver disease, or are not curable with resection, limiting the role of the surgeon to highly selected cases. It is worth re-emphasizing that metastatic adenocarcinoma of the liver from an unknown primary tumor is often in fact a primary intrahepatic cholangiocarcinoma, and this diagnosis must always be kept in mind.

Traditionally, when a cancer had spread to a distant site, it was considered a systemic disease in which locoregional therapies (i.e., surgery) were not effective. Some metastatic tumors to the liver and, in particular, metastatic colorectal cancer to the liver have been shown to be an exception to this rule. More than 30 years of clinical research has documented that metastatic colorectal cancer isolated in the liver can be resected with the potential for long-term survival and cure.[43] Advances in systemic and regional chemotherapy have also broadened the number of patients eligible for surgical therapy and probably have improved long-term survival after resection. Patient selection is by far the most important aspect of surgical therapy for metastatic disease in the liver, and clinical follow-up of resected patients has identified those most and least likely to benefit. Although long-term survival is common and occurs in up to 50% of patients in modern series, recurrence and chronic multimodal therapy are common, occurring in most patients. Therefore, realistic expectations and honest patient education are an important aspect of treatment. Tumors other than colorectal cancer presenting as isolated or limited hepatic metastases can also be resected for potential long-term survival, but data on these other tumors are sparse and less compelling than those on colorectal cancer.

Colorectal

There are more than 50,000 cases of colorectal liver metastases a year in the United States. Most of these cases are associated with widespread disease or unresectable hepatic disease, and it is estimated that about 5% to 10% of these patients are candidates for a potentially curative liver resection. With improved response rates to modern chemotherapy and advances in hepatic surgery, however, more patients are now candidates for hepatectomy than in the past. In the distant past, patients with hepatic colorectal metastases generally presented with symptoms and signs of advanced malignancy, such as pain, ascites, jaundice, weight loss, and a palpable mass. In fact, presentation with such symptoms is a poor prognostic sign, and few of these patients are candidates for therapy outside of chemotherapy or supportive care. This has led most practitioners to carefully follow patients with resected primary colorectal cancer who are potential candidates for aggressive therapy with serial physical exams, cross-sectional imaging studies, LFTs, and CEA levels. Although not supported by randomized trials, clinical observation has been that patients carefully followed with the above tests are the ones often found to have resectable disease and the greatest potential for long-term survival. Some patients are found to have synchronous metastatic disease at the time of diagnosis of the primary colorectal cancer on preoperative imaging or at laparotomy.[43]

CEA is normally only secreted in utero but is secreted by most colorectal cancers. Although an elevated CEA is not specific for recurrent colorectal cancer, a rising CEA on serial exams and a new solid mass on imaging studies are diagnostic of metastatic disease. Mild elevations in LFTs are common in metastatic colorectal cancer to the liver but are not effective as a screening tool. The most common elevated tests are ALP, GGT, and lactate dehydrogenase (LDH).[25] Imaging of hepatic metastases is generally adequate with good-quality CT. Most practitioners use thin-cut (5 mm), high-resolution, dynamic, contrast-enhanced helical scanning techniques. Timing with IV contrast corresponds to the portal venous phase to maximize hepatic parenchymal enhancement, which enhances the disparity between parenchyma and tumor. Contrast-enhanced MRI can be useful to characterize hepatic lesions of uncertain significance (see earlier).

After a patient who presents with a hepatic colorectal metastasis is considered a candidate for surgical therapy, a complete extent-of-disease workup must be performed. Colonoscopy is performed if it has been more than 1 year since the last exam to rule out local recurrence or metachronous lesions. Complete abdominal and pelvic cross-sectional imaging must also be performed. A chest CT is often performed but is of low yield, and a chest x-ray is sufficient. Many studies have evaluated the added benefit of PET scans to detect occult extrahepatic disease. About 25% of patients have a change in management based on PET scan findings, but this is highly variable depending on the quality of cross-sectional imaging and patient selection (Fig. 52-30). Staging laparoscopy before definitive laparotomy identifies about half of all unresectable patients. Overall, 10% of patients are spared a nontherapeutic laparotomy, and the yield of laparoscopy correlates with the number of poor prognostic factors present and can be used selectively.

No prospective trial comparing surgery to no treatment or chemotherapy has ever been done (or is likely to ever be done). Therefore, the rationale for liver resection comes from retrospective comparisons of these treatment strategies. The surgeon must understand the natural history of colorectal liver metastases left untreated or treated with systemic chemotherapy in order to appropriately interpret survival data associated with hepatectomy. Before the 1980s, most hepatic metastases were left untreated. Two key studies retrospectively identified patients with isolated single hepatic metastases or multiple but resectable tumors who received no therapy. One study documented a 10% 3-year survival and the other a 2% 5-year survival for patients with limited and potentially resectable disease. It was clear from these studies that long-term survival is extremely rare without treatment and also that survival is closely related to the extent of disease. In the past, 5-FU–based systemic chemother-

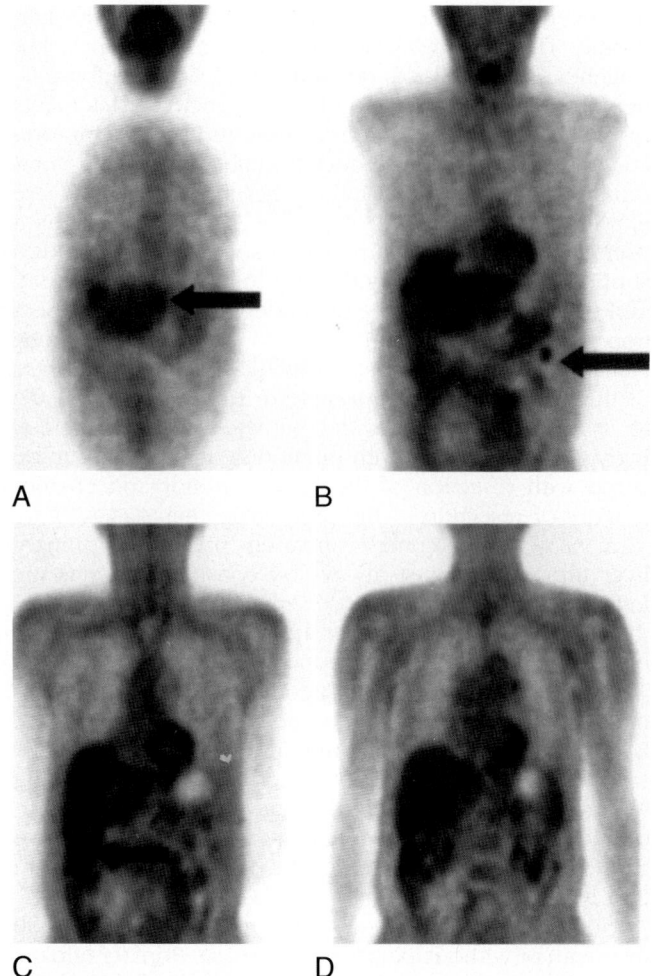

Figure 52-30 Positron emission tomography scan in a patient diagnosed with colorectal cancer synchronously metastatic to the liver after resection of the colonic tumor. The scan demonstrates hypermetabolic activity throughout the liver but also shows two areas in the left upper quadrant consistent with an omental lesion as well as an anastomotic recurrence. A recent CT scan demonstrated liver disease only. (From Akhurst T, Larson SM: The role of nuclear medicine in the diagnosis and management of hepatobiliary diseases. In Blumgart LH, Fong Y [eds]: Surgery of the Liver and Biliary Tract. London, WB Saunders, 2000, pp 271-308.)

apy was ineffective as a sole therapy for hepatic colorectal metastases, with median survival times of about 12 months and response rates of 20% to 30%. Tremendous advances in systemic chemotherapy for metastatic colorectal cancer have recently been achieved. Combination chemotherapy, including 5-FU with irinotecan or oxaliplatin, combined with targeted antiangiogenic antibodies such as bevacizumab (anti–vascular endothelial growth factor antibody), have now resulted in response rates higher than 50% and median survival times of 20 months and longer for patients with advanced disease.[44] Although response rates and survival have improved, durable complete response and 5-year survival is extremely rare with the use of chemotherapy alone.

Table 52-10 Results of Hepatic Resection for Hepatic Colorectal Metastases in Selected Series With Greater Than 100 Patients

AUTHOR	NO. OF PATIENTS	OPERATIVE MORTALITY RATE (%)	1-YEAR SURVIVAL RATE (%)	5-YEAR SURVIVAL RATE (%)	10-YEAR SURVIVAL RATE (%)	MEDIAN SURVIVAL (mo)
Adson, 1984	141	2	82	25	—	24
Hughes, 1986	607	—	—	33	—	—
Schlag, 1990	122	4	85	30	—	32
Doci, 1991	100	5	—	30	—	28
Gayowski, 1994	204	0	91	32	—	33
Scheele, 1995	469	4	83	33	20	40
Fong, 1995	577	4	85	35	—	40
Jenkins, 1997	131	4	81	25	—	33
Rees, 1997	150	1	94	37	—	—
Jamison, 1997	280	4	84	27	20	33
Fong, 1999	1001	3	89	37	22	42
Minagawa, 2000	235	0	—	35	26	37
Scheele, 2000	597	—	—	36	—	35
Choti, 2002	226	1	—	40*	26	46
Abdalla, 2004	190	—	—	58	—	NR

*The 5-year survival rate in the patients operated on in the most modern time period in this study was 58%.
NR, not reached.

The sporadic partial hepatectomy performed for metastatic colorectal cancer before the 1980s was appropriately viewed with great skepticism. The high morbidity and mortality for liver surgery at that time and the questionable rationale of resecting blood-borne metastases were the major issues. During the past 25 years, however, large series have demonstrated that liver surgery can now be practiced with acceptable safety and that patients with isolated and resectable hepatic metastases have the potential for long-term survival. Five-year survival rates range from 25% to 58%, and there is a clear trend toward longer survival in the more modern series (Table 52-10). Perioperative mortality in experienced centers is consistently less than 5% and in many modern series is less than 2%. Almost all series demonstrate that nearly half of patients undergoing a liver resection for metastatic colorectal cancer will survive 3 years, and 1 in 5 patients will survive 10 years. Despite the low operative mortality, it must be stated that liver surgery is still associated with significant morbidity rates of 30% to 50%. Complications are most commonly bleeding, bile leak, abscess, and other generalized cardiorespiratory complications. With improvements in chemotherapy, a higher proportion of patients undergoing hepatectomy have been treated preoperatively, and recent studies have shown preoperative chemotherapy to be associated with hepatic toxicity and higher rates of postoperative liver failure.[43,45]

From these large series, we have learned a lot about prognostic factors and which patients are most likely to benefit from a liver resection for hepatic colorectal metas-tases. Although not all studies agree, a list of poor prognostic factors exists and includes extrahepatic metastases, involved lymph nodes with the primary colorectal tumor, synchronous presentation (or shorter disease-free interval), larger number of tumors, bilobar involvement, CEA elevation greater than 200 ng/mL, size of largest hepatic tumor over 5 cm, and involved histologic margins.[43] In a series of 1001 liver resections from Memorial Sloan-Kettering Cancer Center (MSKCC), a multivariate analysis identified five preoperative factors as the most influential on outcome. These included size greater than 5 cm, disease-free interval less than 1 year, more than 1 tumor, lymph node–positive primary, and a CEA greater than 200 ng/mL. Utilizing these five factors, we have developed a risk score predictive of recurrence after liver resection[45] (Table 52-11).

Traditionally, the presence of extrahepatic disease, four or more hepatic metastases, close margins, and the inability to resect all disease in the liver have been considered contraindications to hepatectomy. The only one of these historic contraindications that holds true today is the inability to resect all disease. Recent publications have shown that hepatectomy for four or more metastases is associated with an approximate 5-year survival rate of 33% despite a recurrence rate of at least 80%. Although the width of the closest margin has been shown to be associated with outcome, it is often confounded by its relationship to an overall poor prognostic tumor (i.e., multiple synchronous tumors). However, close or involved margins do not appear to preclude the possibility of long-

Table 52-11   **Clinical Risk Score and Survival in 1001 Patients Undergoing Liver Resection for Metastatic Colorectal Cancer***

SCORE	1-YEAR SURVIVAL RATE (%)	3-YEAR SURVIVAL RATE (%)	5-YEAR SURVIVAL RATE (%)	MEDIAN SURVIVAL (mo)
0	93	72	60	74
1	91	66	44	51
2	89	60	40	47
3	86	42	20	33
4	70	38	25	20
5	71	27	14	22

*Each of the following 5 risk factors equals one point: node-positive–primary, disease-free interval less than 12 months, greater than 1 tumor, size greater than 5 cm, carcinoembryonic antigen level greater than 200 ng/mL. Score is total number of points in an individual patient.

term survival. Nonetheless, attempts at wide margins greater than 1 cm are appropriate when possible. Resection of extrahepatic metastases that present simultaneously with liver metastases has recently been shown to be associated with long-term survival in highly selected cases. The sites that appear to be associated with the best outcomes in this situation are limited lung metastases, locoregional recurrences of the primary tumor, and portal lymph nodes. Patient selection is critical for this aggressive approach and generally requires preoperative chemotherapy to exclude progression and consideration of the overall bulk of disease.

Although long-term survival after liver resection for hepatic colorectal metastases is clearly possible, recurrence of disease is common. Overall, about two thirds of cases recur, but in high-risk situations (i.e., four or more tumors, extrahepatic disease), recurrence rates are generally 80% or higher. About half of the recurrences are isolated to the liver, and a small number of these patients (~5% of all patients undergoing liver resection) are candidates for a second liver resection. These highly selected patients who undergo a second liver resection with complete removal of all disease can expect further 5-year survival rates of 30% to 40%. Limited and isolated lung recurrences can also be resected with the potential for further long-term survival. Furthermore, multiple lines of effective chemotherapy are now available and are associated with prolongation of survival. Because of the potential for further effective therapeutic interventions after liver resection, patients eligible for such treatment are followed with serial CEA and imaging studies to detect recurrences at an early and potentially treatable phase.

Adjuvant systemic chemotherapy after liver resection for metastatic colorectal cancer is often given, but is not supported by prospective trials. A number of retrospective comparisons have been performed, but no prospective trials support the routine use of adjuvant postoperative systemic chemotherapy. However, with the improved efficacy of systemic chemotherapy and the known benefit of adjuvant therapy for lymph node–positive primary colon cancer, it is likely to be effective as an adjuvant to hepatectomy. In practice, systemic chemotherapy is frequently used after liver resection and likely contributes to the improving overall long-term survival. Neoadjuvant chemotherapy for resectable metastases is also a common strategy to treat occult systemic disease and can also

be helpful in selecting patients for resection because patients who progress while on chemotherapy have a poor outcome after hepatectomy. A convincing argument for adjuvant therapy with the use of HAI chemotherapy can be made. The rationale for adjuvant hepatic artery chemotherapy is based on the fact that liver metastases derive most of their blood supply from the hepatic artery, and regional infusion of chemotherapeutic agents such as fluorodeoxyuridine (FUDR) have hepatic extraction rates of 90%, providing high local concentrations with minimal systemic toxicity. Furthermore, about half of all recurrences after hepatectomy involve the liver, and therefore, controlling the liver is likely to affect long-term outcome. There is clearly a higher response rate for liver tumors with HAI therapy compared with systemic therapy. A trial from MSKCC comparing HAI therapy with systemic chemotherapy to systemic chemotherapy alone demonstrated significantly lower recurrence rates (9% and 36%, respectively) and a survival advantage at 2 years (86% versus 72%, respectively).[46] Other trials have shown HAI therapy with FUDR to be more effective than hepatectomy alone, with significantly improved disease-free survival.

For patients with unresectable disease, preoperative chemotherapy has been shown to convert some patients to complete resection. A critical observation in these patients is that outcome after complete resection appears to be as good as for patients whose disease is resectable at initial presentation. Strategies to extend the limits of liver resection have used parenchyma-preserving segmental resections, two-stage operations, and thermal ablative techniques such as cryoablation or RFA. Thus, multiple bilobar tumors can be extirpated by a combination of resection and ablation with preservation of sufficient hepatic parenchyma. In our series of patients with extensive hepatic disease treated with a combination of resection and ablation, the 3-year survival rate was 47%.

In summary, the treatment of hepatic colorectal metastases is evolving at a rapid pace, and improvements in hepatic surgery and chemotherapy have greatly improved prospects for patients. Chemotherapy has improved, but long-term survival with this modality alone is extremely rare. Combinations of chemotherapy and complete resection of hepatic metastases are associated with long-term survival in up to 50% of patients in modern series. Long-term survival also appears to be possible in patients undergoing resection of extensive hepatic metastases and limited extrahepatic disease. Complete resection of hepatic metastases appears to be a critically important treatment modality that is necessary for long-term survival.

Neuroendocrine

Liver metastases from neuroendocrine tumors are common but vary according to the primary tumor type. Examples of primary tumors that commonly metastasize to the liver are gastrinomas, glucagonomas, somatostatinomas, and nonfunctional neuroendocrine tumors. Insulinomas and carcinoid tumors metastasize to the liver less commonly. There are two issues to consider when planning therapy for metastatic neuroendocrine tumors. First, these are slow-growing, indolent tumors, with which long-term survival is common even in the absence of treatment. Thus, assessing the effects of any treatment is difficult. Second, these tumors often secrete functional neuropeptides that can create debilitating syndromes of hormonal excess. Thus, the goal of treatment is more focused on quality of life rather than prolongation of life.

A number of effective nonsurgical therapies exist for neuroendocrine liver metastases. Long-acting somatostatin analogues are useful for alleviating hormonal symptoms and may have a cytostatic role as well. Liver tumors can also be treated by hepatic arterial embolization or thermoablative approaches. Combinations of these therapies can be very effective in cytoreducing tumor loads and alleviating symptoms of hormonal excess.

Liver resection can play a role in patients whose tumor can be completely encompassed. Because these tumors are indolent, any therapy must be delivered with minimal morbidity, and this has been the case in experienced hepatobiliary units. Five-year survival rates ranging from 50% to 75% can be expected if a complete resection is accomplished. Retrospective comparisons have suggested that this survival is better than that in untreated patients, but selection bias accounts for at least some of this difference. Because of the rarity of this diagnosis, no prospective data exist. The other role surgery plays is in those patients who have failed medical therapy and have recalcitrant symptoms of hormonal excess. If preoperative staging suggests that at least 90% of tumor can be removed without prohibitive operative risk, surgical cytoreduction is reasonable. Symptom improvement can be expected in most patients if adequate cytoreduction is achieved. Formal resections with wide margins are not necessary for neuroendocrine tumors, and techniques such as enucleations or wedge resections are good options.[47] Thermoablative approaches, such as cryoablation or RFA, are also attractive alternatives in this type of cytoreductive surgery. Recently, laparoscopic RFA has been used, although long-term follow-up data are not available.

Noncolorectal, Non-neuroendocrine

A number of other tumors can present as isolated liver metastases, but these are uncommon situations, and therefore, data for these situations are sparse. A long list of primary tumors that can present like this exists and includes breast, lung, melanoma, soft tissue sarcoma, Wilms', ocular melanoma, upper gastrointestinal (gastric, pancreas, esophagus, gallbladder), adrenocortical, urologic (bladder, renal cell, prostate, testicular), and gynecologic (uterine, cervix, ovarian). General principles that must be considered when dealing with these tumors as isolated liver metastases are similar to those of metastatic colorectal cancer. Prognosis tends to be dismal if there is extrahepatic disease, multiple tumors, large tumors, or a short disease-free interval, and patients need to be carefully selected for surgery based on these factors.

Although rare reports of long-term survival after resection of isolated liver metastases from upper gastrointestinal tumor exist, in general, these patients have a dismal prognosis, and liver resection is not recommended. In most series, liver resection for genitourinary tumors has the best prognosis and in well-selected patients liver resection is considered. Breast, melanoma, and sarcoma patients rarely present with isolated liver metastases, and in the situation of a long disease-free interval or long-term stability on chemotherapy, liver resection is considered. In general, liver resection for metastatic noncolorectal, non-neuroendocrine tumors has to be considered cytoreductive and is only used in the most favorable situation, as described previously. Liver resection can also be an effective therapy for symptomatic tumors in patients who have a reasonable life expectancy and no other effective therapy.

Cystic Neoplasms

Simple Cyst

Simple cysts of the liver contain serous fluid, do not communicate with the biliary tree, and do not have septations. They are generally spherical or ovoid and can be as large as 20 cm. Large cysts can compress normal liver, inducing regional atrophy and sometimes compensatory hypertrophy. In 50% of cases, the cysts are singular. Histologically, a single layer of cuboidal or columnar cells that have no atypia line these cysts. Simple cysts are generally regarded as congenital malformations.

Simple cysts are a relatively common finding in adults and in the main are asymptomatic incidental radiologic findings. Occasionally, a large cyst will cause symptoms. Although CT demonstrates anatomic relationships, ultrasound is a helpful test to confirm a single thin-walled simple cyst. Hydatid disease, cystadenoma, and metastatic neuroendocrine tumors are the most important differential diagnoses to consider. A thick or nodular wall raises the suspicion of a cystadenoma but can represent hemorrhage. The most common complication is intracystic bleeding, but overall, complications are rare. Treatment of simple hepatic cysts is only indicated if they are symptomatic or if there is diagnostic uncertainty. Because most cysts are asymptomatic, a thorough evaluation of the etiology of the symptoms must be carried out before attributing them to the cyst. Nonsurgical treatment consists of aspiration and injection of a sclerosing agent. Few studies have documented long-term follow-up of sclerotherapy for hepatic cysts. Surgical therapy is achieved by fenestration or unroofing of the portion of the cyst that is extrahepatic. This can be performed at laparotomy with good long-term results or through laparoscopic approaches. The latter approach is favored, but long-term efficacy is not well documented.[48]

Cystadenoma and Cystadenocarcinoma

Cystadenoma of the liver is a rare neoplasm that usually presents as a large cystic mass (usually 10-20 cm). The cyst has a globular external surface with multiple protruding cysts and locules of various sizes. The fluid contained in these cysts is usually mucinous. Microscopically, atypical cuboidal or columnar cells resting on a basement membrane line the cysts. The epithelium often forms polypoid or papillary projections.

Cystadenoma of the liver mainly affects women older than 40 years. Although many cystadenomas are asymptomatic, symptoms can include abdominal pain, anorexia, nausea, and abdominal distention. The diagnosis is usually suspected by a combination of cross-sectional imaging (CT or MRI) and ultrasound. Ultrasound usually demonstrates a cystic structure with varying wall thickness, nodularity, septations, and fluid-filled locules. Importantly, contrast-enhanced CT demonstrates enhancement of the cyst wall and septa. Hydatid disease must always be considered in the differential diagnosis. Cystadenoma tends to grow slowly but can eventually progress to its malignant counterpart cystadenocarcinoma. Cystadenocarcinoma is an extremely rare malignancy with little documentation of its natural history and outcome after resection. Malignant degeneration is typically suggested on imaging with large projections and a markedly thickened wall. The treatment of cystadenoma or cystadenocarcinoma is complete excision and can be done with an enucleation if there is no evidence of invasive malignancy. Leaving any disease behind risks recurrence and the development of cystadenocarcinoma.[48]

Polycystic Liver Disease

Liver cysts are commonly seen in patients with the autosomal dominant–inherited adult polycystic kidney disease. Histologically, the cysts are similar to simple cysts (see earlier), the main difference between the two entities being the number of cysts. When liver cysts are present in patients with adult polycystic kidney disease, they are always multiple. Additionally, there are usually numerous microscopic hepatic cysts as well as the grossly visible macrocysts. Despite the large number of liver cysts, hepatic parenchyma and function are usually preserved. Liver cysts are always preceded by kidney cysts, and the prevalence of liver cysts in adult polycystic kidney disease increases with age. Before the age of 20 years, the prevalence of liver cysts is 0%, whereas it is 80% after the age of 60 years.

Liver cysts in patients with adult polycystic kidney disease are generally asymptomatic, but in a few patients, large, numerous cysts may cause abdominal pain and distention. LFTs are almost always normal. Rare complications can occur and include infection or intracystic bleeding. Ultrasound and CT show multiple simple cysts throughout the liver and kidneys. Treatment of polycystic

liver disease is reserved for severe symptoms related to large cysts and complications. Treatment is by percutaneous aspiration with or without sclerotherapy, fenestration (by laparotomy or laparoscopy), hepatic resection, or orthotopic liver transplantation. Liver transplantation is only used with progressive disease after fenestration or resection with liver or renal dysfunction. In the context of renal failure, a combined kidney and liver transplantation may be appropriate.[48]

Bile Duct Cysts

Bile duct cysts or choledochal cysts are congenital dilations of the biliary tree that are usually diagnosed in childhood but can present in adulthood. Because of the risk for malignancy and recurrent cholangitis, treatment is excision with reestablishment of bilioenteric continuity. Most bile duct cysts involve the extrahepatic biliary tree, but in type IV cysts, there is involvement of the extrahepatic bile duct and intrahepatic ducts, whereas Caroli's disease (type V) is characterized by multiple intrahepatic cysts. Thus, bile duct cysts must be considered in the differential diagnosis of a patient with multiple hepatic cystic lesions. The intrahepatic lesion of type IV bile duct cysts and Caroli's disease is multifocal dilation of the segmental bile ducts that are separated by portions of normal-caliber bile ducts. About half the cases of Caroli's disease are associated with congenital hepatic fibrosis, and the cysts are diffusely located throughout the liver. In the other half of cases, the dilations may be confined to a part of the liver, usually the left liver. Recurrent bacterial cholangitis usually dominates the clinical course of these diseases, and death usually ensues within 5 to 10 years without adequate treatment. When intrahepatic bile duct cysts are localized, hepatic resection with or without biliary reconstruction is the treatment of choice. Treatment of diffuse hepatic involvement is poor, and probably the only effective treatment is transplantation in complicated cases.[48]

Principles of Hepatic Resection

Although liver resections were performed in the late 1800s, it wasn't until 1952 that Lortat-Jacob was given credit for the first true anatomic right hepatectomy. This event ushered in the modern era of hepatic surgery, but early series were plagued by high morbidity and mortality rates, which were largely related to massive intraoperative blood loss. Series from the 1970s and 1980s often reported mortality rates in excess of 10% and were often as high as 20%, especially for major resections. This high mortality limited the use of liver resection, and there was reluctance to refer patients for such operations. During the past 2 decades, a number of advances have improved perioperative outcome dramatically for major hepatic surgery. The understanding that the majority of blood loss during a liver resection comes from the hepatic veins prompted surgeons to do these operations with a low central venous pressure (CVP). We perform partial hepatectomy with a central line in place, the patient positioned in mild Trendelenburg's position, with fluid restriction and venodilators if necessary to maintain a

CVP below 5. The other major advance has been an improved understanding of the segmental anatomy of the liver, making intrahepatic dissection safer and more precise. There are numerous techniques to transect liver tissue and many methods to coagulate and control vessels, but the most important concept is that dividing liver tissue is a dissection requiring complete understanding of the vascular anatomy within the liver.[1,2]

In experienced centers, the perioperative mortality rate is routinely 5% or less and depends on a number of factors. The three most critical factors related to perioperative morbidity are blood loss, the amount of normal liver resected, and the condition of the liver (e.g., cirrhosis). The performance of a partial hepatectomy must be performed with these factors in mind to minimize morbidity. In a recent review of more than 1800 liver resections over a 10-year period from MSKCC, the operative mortality rate was 3.1%. The median blood loss was 600 mL, and two thirds of the patients did not require a red blood cell transfusion. Overall, postoperative morbidity was 45%, but the median hospital stay was 8 days. Morbidity was mostly related to blood loss and the extent of resection. Minor resections were associated with a mortality rate of 1%. Most complications and deaths were seen in patients with complex biliary tumors, cirrhosis and HCC, and extensive resections.[3] Improving outcomes after partial hepatectomy continue, and experienced hepatobiliary centers report mortality rates that approach 1% to 2%, with fewer and fewer patients requiring perioperative blood transfusions. As a result of the increasing safety of hepatic surgery, liver resection has become the treatment of choice for a long list of malignant and benign hepatic conditions.

Bile leaks are a problem in cases requiring complex biliary reconstruction but also occur in about 10% to 20% of hepatectomies without biliary reconstruction. Careful ligation of biliary radicals is of obvious importance in minimizing this complication. Because of the regenerative capacity of the liver, resections of up to 80% of normal noncirrhotic livers can be performed with functional compensation within a few weeks. Many resections encompass tumors as well as normal liver, and the concepts of functional liver parenchyma and future liver remnant volume are important because there is often compensatory hypertrophy of normal liver when tumors occupy a significant amount of the liver volume. The risk

for hepatic dysfunction is minimal if the reduction of functional liver parenchyma is less than 50% but begins to increase when this number approaches 20% or 25%. Patients with cirrhosis have much higher rates of postoperative liver dysfunction because of impaired regenerative capacity as well as impaired primary liver function. Liver failure, extrahepatic multiorgan failure, and death are serious hazards to performing major liver resections in cirrhotic patients. In general, patients with Child's B or C cirrhosis or portal hypertension do not tolerate liver resections, and patient selection is therefore critical. Ascites and infectious complications are also common problems after major liver resection. One strategy to minimize postoperative liver dysfunction and morbidity after major hepatectomy is to percutaneously embolize the portal vein on the side of the liver to be resected. In about 4 weeks, this induces atrophy of the liver parenchyma to be resected and hypertrophy of the future liver remnant, increasing the relative volume of the future liver remnant. One prospective trial has shown this to be a beneficial strategy in cirrhotic patients.

Techniques of liver resection differ according to the disease being treated. In benign hepatic diseases requiring resection, the indications for operation are usually symptoms or infection. Removal of normal liver is kept to a minimum in these cases, and techniques such as enucleation are appropriate, although major resections are occasionally necessary. For malignant disease, a margin of normal tissue is important, and formal anatomic resections yield the best results. Techniques such as wedge resections often result in higher rates of margin involvement and disease recurrence and must be used carefully and sparingly.

Detailed knowledge of liver anatomy is essential to the practice of safe hepatic surgery and is reviewed in an earlier section. Unfortunately, descriptions of liver anatomy and of common liver resections have yielded a huge number of names that can be confusing to the student. A recent consensus conference conducted in Brisbane with the assistance of the American Hepato-Pancreato-Biliary Association (AHPBA) has published new guidelines for this terminology (Table 52-12; Fig. 52-31). In general, the term *lobectomy* is not preferred because there are no external markings on the liver denoting a lobe. When in doubt, always revert back to the numerical segments of the liver if there is any

Table 52-12 Nomenclature for Most Common Major Anatomic Hepatic Resections*

SEGMENTS	COUINAUD, 1957	GOLDSMITH AND WOODBURNE, 1957	BRISBANE, 2000
V-VIII (Fig. 52-31A)	Right hepatectomy	Right hepatic lobectomy	Right hemi-hepatectomy
IV-VIII[†] (Fig. 52-31C)	Right lobectomy	Extended right hepatic lobectomy	Right trisectionectomy
II-IV (Fig. 52-31B)	Left hepatectomy	Left hepatic lobectomy	Left hemi-hepatectomy
II, III (Fig. 52-31D)	Left lobectomy	Left lateral segmentectomy	Left lateral sectionectomy
II, III, IV, V, VIII[†] (Fig. 52-31E)	Extended left hepatectomy	Extended left lobectomy	Left trisectionectomy

*The original terminology is based on the anatomic descriptions of Couinaud and of Goldsmith and Woodburne. The Brisbane 2000 terminology from an American Hepato-Pancreatico-Biliary Association (AHPBA) consensus conference is also listed.
[†]Another common name for these operations is *right* or *left trisegmentectomy*.

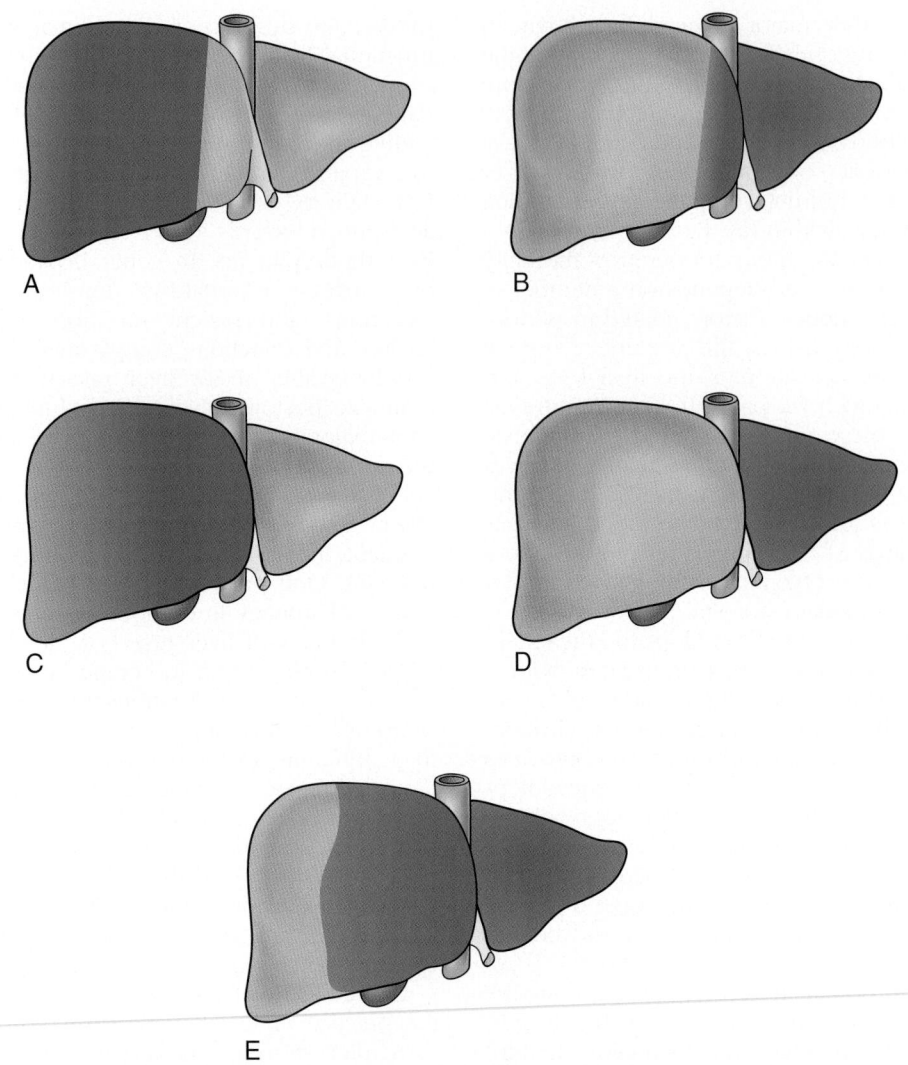

Figure 52-31 The commonly performed major hepatic resections are indicated by the *shaded areas*. **A,** Right hepatectomy, right hepatic lobectomy, or right hemi-hepatectomy (segments V-VIII). **B,** Left hepatectomy, left hepatic lobectomy, or left hemi-hepatectomy (segments II-IV). **C,** Right lobectomy, extended right hepatic lobectomy, or right trisectionectomy (trisegmentectomy) (segments IV-VIII). **D,** Left lobectomy, left lateral segmentectomy, or left lateral sectionectomy (segments II-III). **E,** Extended left hepatectomy, extended left lobectomy, or left trisectionectomy (trisegmentectomy) (segments II, III, IV, V, VIII). See Table 52-12. (From Blumgart LH, Jarnagin W, Fong Y: Liver resection for benign disease and for liver and biliary tumors. In Blumgart LH, Fong Y [eds]: Surgery of the Liver and Biliary Tract. London, WB Saunders, 2000, pp 1639-1714.)

confusion about the description of a liver resection. Recall that the right liver is comprised of segments V through VIII, and *right hepatectomy* and *right hemi-hepatectomy* are appropriate terms for resection of these segments. Segments II through IV compose the left liver, and *left hepatectomy* and *left hemi-hepatectomy* are appropriate terms for resection of these segments. A right hepatectomy can be extended farther to the left to include segment IV, and a left hepatectomy can be extended farther to the right to include segments V and VIII. Terms such as *extended right/left hepatectomy, right/left trisectionectomy,* and *trisegmentectomy,* are appropriate to describe these resections (see Table 52-12; see Fig. 52-31). Resection of segments II and III is a commonly per-

formed sublobar resection and is often referred to as a *left lateral segmentectomy* and *left lateral sectionectomy.* Other common sublobar resections, such as that of the right posterior sector (segments VI and VII) or the right anterior sector (segments V and VII), are referred to as *right posterior sectorectomy/sectionectomy* and *right anterior sectorectomy/sectionectomy,* respectively. Single-segment or bisegmental resections can always be simply referred to by a numerical description of the segments to be resected.

A detailed discussion of the techniques of liver resection is beyond the scope of this chapter and requires specialty training. General principles, however, need to be mentioned. A liver resection must consider the disease to be treated and the goals of the operation, whether a margin-negative resection of a malignancy or the removal of benign tissue to alleviate symptoms. The most basic steps can be distilled down to inflow (portal vein, hepatic artery, bile duct) control, outflow (hepatic veins) control, and parenchymal transection with preservation of a liver remnant of adequate size with intact inflow, biliary drainage, and venous outflow. The most common approach to an anatomic resection, in the most common order, is mobilization of the liver to be resected, dissection of inflow and outflow structures, division of the inflow, division of the outflow, and parenchymal transection.

Mobilization of the liver involves division of the right or left triangular ligaments, freeing up the liver from the diaphragm. Often, the liver must be mobilized completely off of the vena cava (which it straddles), and this requires careful dissection and division of multiple retrohepatic caval venous branches. For major resections, the hepatic vein of the resected portion of liver is often encircled before the resection. There are a variety of techniques to dissect, control, and divide inflow vessels. Classic inflow control is obtained by a dissection of the liver hilum with control of the portal vein and hepatic artery to the hemi-liver to be resected. These can be suture-ligated or can be divided with vascular staplers. Unless tumor proximity mandates, we advocate dividing the bile duct within the liver substance to absolutely minimize contralateral biliary injuries related to anatomic anomalies. Inflow control can also be obtained by dissection of the intrahepatic inflow pedicle to the anatomic section of liver to be resected. Recall that the inflow structures invaginate peritoneum at the hepatic hilus and run intrahepatically as an invested pedicle of the three inflow structures. The inflow pedicle can be encircled by making flanking hepatotomies or by splitting parenchyma down to the pedicle of interest. The pedicle can usually be divided with a vascular stapler, but suture ligation is sometimes necessary. Classically, the hepatic vein is divided in its extrahepatic position and can also usually be done with a vascular stapler. The hepatic vein can also be divided within the substance of the liver during parenchymal transection. There are numerous methods of parenchymal transection, ranging from complex ultrasonic irrigators to radiofrequency energy coagulators to a simple clamp crushing technique. All of these, in experienced hands, can be used effectively to minimize blood loss, and it is important to develop a specific technique that you are comfortable with. Ultimately, parenchymal transection is about dissecting intrahepatic anatomy, controlling vascular and biliary structures, minimizing blood loss, and avoiding injury to the future liver remnant.[49]

HEMOBILIA

A case of lethal hemobilia secondary to penetrating abdominal trauma was first described by Glisson in 1654. It was not until 1948 that Sandblom coined the term *hemobilia* in his seminal paper on the subject. Hemobilia is defined as bleeding into the biliary tree from an abnormal communication between a blood vessel and bile duct. It is a rare condition that is often difficult to distinguish from common causes of gastrointestinal bleeding. The most common causes of hemobilia in modern times are iatrogenic trauma, accidental trauma, gallstones, tumors, inflammatory disorders, and vascular disorders. Major hemobilia is relatively uncommon, whereas minor inconsequential hemobilia is a common consequence of gallstone disease or interventional hepatic procedures.[50-53]

Etiology

In recent years, the most common cause of hemobilia has become iatrogenic trauma to the liver and biliary tree. Before the 1980s, the ratio of hemobilia attributed to accidental trauma compared with iatrogenic trauma was 2:1. Recent reviews put iatrogenic trauma as the cause of hemobilia in 40% to 60% of cases. Percutaneous liver biopsy results in hemobilia in less than 1% of cases, but percutaneous transhepatic biliary drainage (PTBD) procedures yield an incidence of 2% to 10%. Likewise, surgical exploration of the biliary tree can result in hemobilia from direct injury or arterial pseudoaneurysm. A number of cases of hemobilia following cholecystectomy have been reported in recent years. Hemobilia secondary to accidental trauma is more common with blunt than penetrating abdominal trauma and occurs with a reported incidence of 0.2% to 3%. Risk factors for the development of hemobilia following accidental trauma are central hepatic rupture with a cavity, the use of packs, and inadequate drainage. The gallbladder can be a source of bleeding from trauma, gallstones, or acalculous cholecystitis. Primary vascular pathology such as aneurysm, angiodysplasia, and hemangiomas are rare causes of hemobilia. Malignant tumors of the liver, biliary tree, gallbladder, and pancreas; parasitic infection; hepatic abscess; and cholangitis are uncommon causes of hemobilia.[50-52]

Presentation

Portal venous bleeding into the biliary tree is rare, minor, and self-limited unless the portal pressure is elevated. Arterial hemobilia, the most common source, can be dramatic, however. Clinical sequelae of hemobilia are related to blood loss and the formation of potentially occlusive blood clots in the biliary tree. The classic triad of symptoms and signs of hemobilia are upper abdominal pain, upper gastrointestinal hemorrhage, and jaundice. In a recent review, all three were present in 22% of patients. Minor hemobilia generally runs an uneventful asymptomatic clinical course. The symptoms and signs of major hemobilia are melena (90% of cases), hematemesis (60% of cases), biliary colic (70% of cases), and jaundice (60% of cases). Upper gastrointestinal bleeding seen in conjunction with biliary symptoms must always raise the suspicion of hemobilia. One interesting aspect of hemobilia is the tendency for delayed presentations (up to weeks) and recurrent brisk but limited bleeding over months and even years. Blood clots in the biliary tree can masquerade as stones if hemobilia goes unrecognized. These clots can cause cholangitis, pancreatitis, and cholecystitis.[50,52]

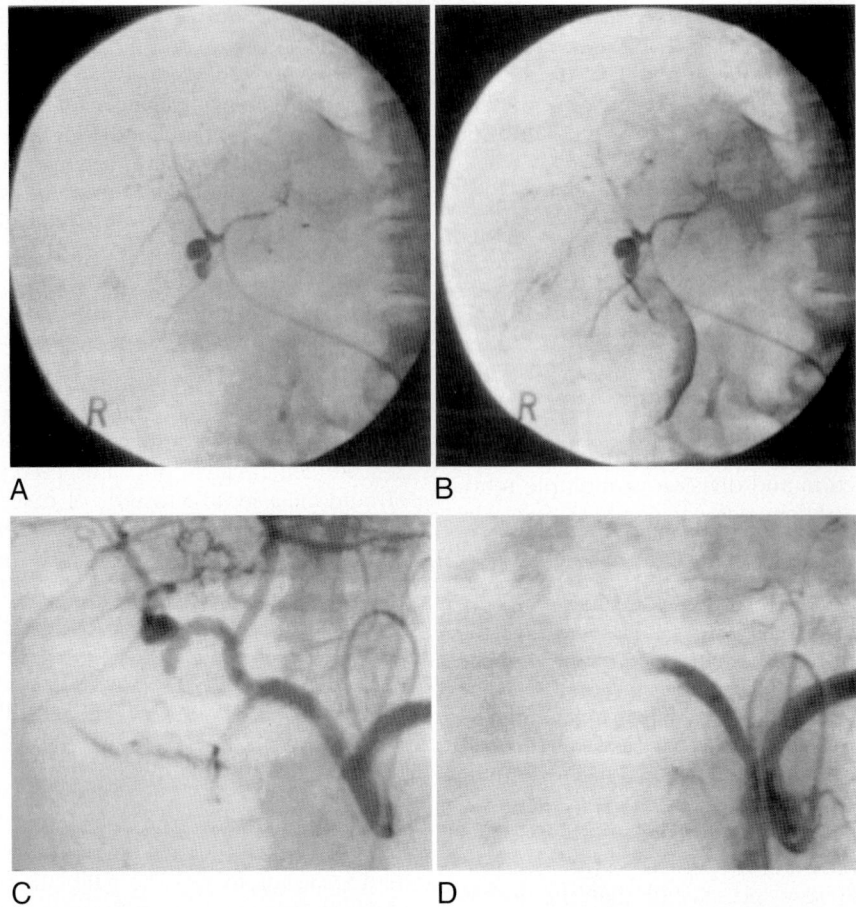

Figure 52-32 Classic findings of hemobilia are demonstrated. After a complicated cholecystectomy, an iatrogenic pseudoaneurysm developed and ruptured into the biliary tree. Exsanguinating hemobilia ensued. The diagnosis was made by endoscopy and then treated by arterial embolization. **A,** Arteriogram demonstrating a pseudoaneurysm of the hepatic artery at the hilum. **B,** A few seconds later, the contrast is seen flowing down the hepatic duct with evidence of clot in the biliary tree. **C** and **D,** The same aneurysm before and after successful embolization. (From Sandblom JP: Hemobilia and bilhemia. In Blumgart LH, Fong Y [eds]: Surgery of the Liver and Biliary Tract. London, WB Saunders, 2000, pp 1319-1342.)

Diagnostic Workup

When hemobilia is suspected, the first evaluation is upper gastrointestinal endoscopy, which rules out other sources of hemorrhage and may visualize bleeding from the ampulla of Vater. Upper endoscopy is only diagnostic of hemobilia in about 10% of cases, however. If upper endoscopy is diagnostic and conservative management is planned, no further studies are necessary. Ultrasound or CT may be helpful in demonstrating intrahepatic tumor or hematoma. Evidence of active bleeding into the biliary tree may be seen on contrast-enhanced CT in the form of pooling contrast, intraluminal clots, or biliary dilation. CT may also show risk factors associated with hemobilia, such as cavitating central lesions and aneurysms. Arterial angiography is now recognized as the test of choice when significant hemobilia is suspected and will reveal the source of bleeding in about 90% of cases. Cholangiography demonstrates blood clots in the biliary tree, which may appear as stringy defects or smaller spherical defects. The latter may be difficult to distinguish from stones.

Treatment and Outcome

The treatment of hemobilia must be focused on stopping bleeding and relieving biliary obstruction. Most cases of minor hemobilia can be managed conservatively with correction of coagulopathy, adequate biliary drainage (only if necessary), and close observation. In a recent review of 171 reported cases from 1996 to 1999, 43% of cases were successfully managed conservatively. The first line of therapy for major hemobilia is transarterial embolization (TAE), and success rates of 80% to 100% are reported. Angiography with TAE is indicated for major hemobilia requiring blood transfusion[51] (Fig. 52-32).

Surgery is indicated when conservative therapy and TAE have failed. It is important to note that surgical treatment of hemobilia is rarely necessary, and that even in cases in which a laparotomy may be mandated for other reasons, TAE is still the therapy of choice for hemobilia because of lower morbidity. Surgical approaches generally involve ligation of bleeding vessels, excision of aneurysm, or nonselective ligation of a main hepatic artery.

Hepatic resection may be necessary for failed arterial ligation or for cases of severe trauma or tumor. Hemorrhage from the gallbladder or hemorrhagic cholecystitis mandate cholecystectomy. There are isolated reports of successful management of hemobilia with endoscopic coagulation, somatostatin, and vasopressin. The management of hemobilia following PTBD usually consists of removal of the catheter or replacement with larger catheters but may require TAE.[51]

At the time of Sandblom's report from 1972, the mortality rate for hemobilia was at least 25%.[52] A report from 1987 noted a mortality rate of 12%. In a review of cases from 1996 through 1999, only four deaths were reported.[51] There has clearly been a reduction in mortality from hemobilia, which is probably related to two factors. First, the incidence of minor self-limited hemobilia has increased secondary to the rising number of percutaneous hepatic procedures. Second, improvements in selective angiography and TAE have greatly improved the treatment of major hemobilia.

Bilhemia

Bilhemia is an extremely rare condition in which bile flows into the bloodstream either through the hepatic veins or portal vein branches. This flow occurs in the context of high intrabiliary pressure, exceeding that of the venous system. The cause can be gallstones eroding into the portal vein or accidental or iatrogenic trauma. The condition can be fatal secondary to embolization of large amounts of bile into the lungs. Most often, however, bile flow is low, and the fistula spontaneously closes. The clinical presentation is that of rapidly increasing jaundice, marked direct hyperbilirubinemia without elevation of hepatocellular enzymes and septicemia. The best test to make this diagnosis is endoscopic retrograde cholangiopancreatography. Treatment is directed at lowering intrabiliary pressures either through stents or sphincterotomy.[50]

VIRAL HEPATITIS AND THE SURGEON

Epidemics of jaundice were noted in ancient civilizations and recorded by Hippocrates. During World War II, these epidemics were called *catarrhal jaundice,* and more than 28,000 cases were documented at that time. Epidemiologic studies in the 1940s documented the difference between blood-borne hepatitis (hepatitis B) and enteric hepatitis (hepatitis A). The most important discovery was that of the Australia antigen by Blumberg and associates in 1965. This antigen proved to be the hepatitis B surface antigen (HBsAg) and provided a means of differentiating the two types of hepatitis and characterizing the epidemiology of this disease. This discovery also ultimately led to the development of hepatitis B vaccines based on this antigen with obvious and profound effects worldwide. Further research ultimately led to the discovery of the delta virus (hepatitis D) and hepatitis C (explaining cases of non-A, non-B hepatitis). Hepatitis E has been found to be a unique enteral form of infectious hepatitis, and

hepatitis G virus was recently discovered and is being defined.[53-55]

Viral hepatitis is a major health problem and is the most common cause of liver disease worldwide. Although fulminant acute hepatitis is uncommon, more than 5 million people suffer with chronic hepatitis. It is estimated that more than 15,000 patients die each year of viral hepatitis in the United States. Viral hepatitis is not a surgical disease but has important consequences for surgeons and surgical patients. For any surgeon performing hepatic surgery, the functional state of the liver is extremely important, and patients with chronic viral hepatitis require special attention before any surgical intervention. Additionally, chronic viral hepatitis is a common cause of hepatocellular carcinoma. Lastly, the risk for transmission from patient to surgeon and visa versa is an issue with which all surgeons need to be familiar.

Definition

Viral hepatitis is an infection of the liver by one of six known viruses that have diverse genetic compositions and structures. Hepatitis viruses A, C, D, E, and G have RNA genomes, whereas HBV has a DNA genome that replicates through RNA intermediates. Hepatitis A virus (HAV) and hepatitis E virus (HEV) are both responsible for forms of epidemic hepatitis and are transmitted by a fecal-oral route. HBV is the only one with the potential to integrate into host genomes, although this is not required for replication. HCV virus replicates in the cytoplasm of hepatocytes and has complex mechanisms of evading host immunity through hypervariable areas in its genome. The hepatitis D virus (HDV) requires the presence of HBV infection for replication and infectivity and can alter the clinical course of HBV infection. The hepatitis G virus (HGV) has been recently discovered and has similarities to HCV, but has no definitive association with clinical hepatitis.[53-55]

Diagnosis

Table 52-13 summarizes the serologic tests and their implications for HAV, HBV, and HCV. The diagnosis of HAV infection relies on the determination of antibodies to HAV. Both IgM and IgG antibodies are present early in the infection, but only IgG persists long-term. HAV antigens and tests for HAV RNA have been developed but are generally restricted to research laboratories.[53]

HBV infection has been characterized by a number of antigens and antibodies (Fig. 52-33). HBsAg is the hallmark of the diagnosis of HBV infection and appears in the serum from 1 to 10 weeks after infection. HBsAg usually disappears in 4 to 6 months, but persistence in the serum implies chronic infection. Anti-HBs antibodies usually appear during a window period after the disappearance of HBsAg and mark recovery after HBV infection. Anti-HBs antibodies are also induced by the HBV vaccine. The hepatitis core antigen (HBcAg) is an intracellular antigen that is not detectable in serum. Anti-HBc antibodies, however, are detectable early after infection and persist after recovery and in chronic infections.

Table 52-13 **Serologic Evaluation of the Most Common Viral Hepatitides**

VIRUS	ANTIGEN NAME	INTERPRETATION	ANTIBODY NAME	INTERPRETATION
Hepatitis A (HAV)	HAV antigen	Acute infection	Anti-HAV IgM	Acute infection
			Anti-HAV IgG	Immunity
Hepatitis B (HBV)	HBsAg	Acute or chronic infection	Anti-HBs	Immunity
	HBeAg	HBV replication, infectivity	Anti-HBc	All phases of infection
			Anti-HBe	Late convalescence
Hepatitis C (HCV)	None	—	Anti-HCV	Late convalescence or chronic infection

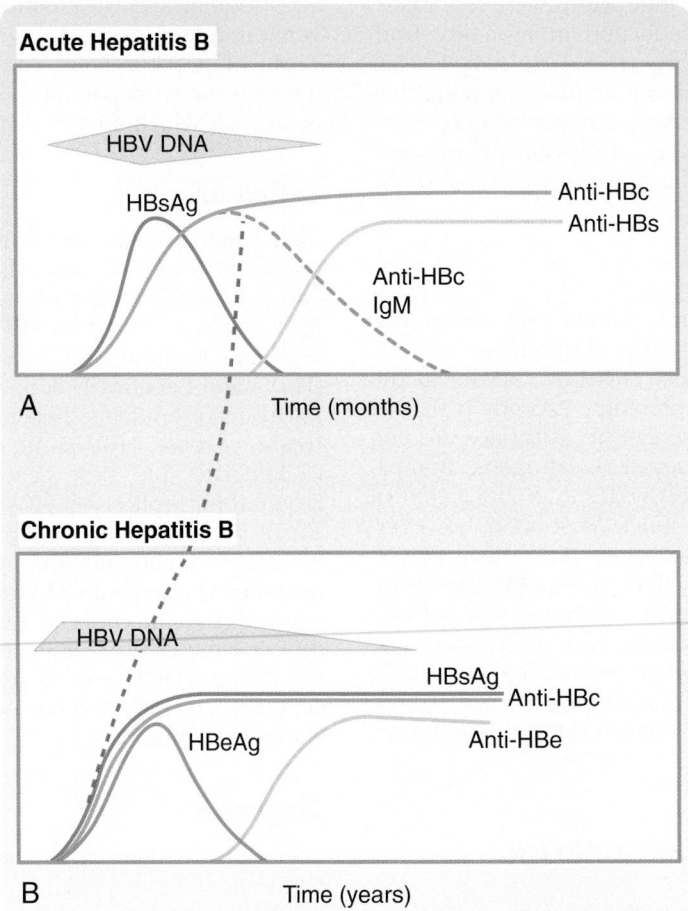

Figure 52-33 Serologic markers in acute hepatitis B virus (HBV) infection **(A)** and chronic HBV infection **(B).** (From Doo EC, Lian TJ: The hepatitis viruses. In Schiff ER, Sorrell MF, Maddrey WC [eds]: Schiff's Diseases of the Liver. Philadelphia, Lippincott-Raven, 1999, pp 725-744.)

Hepatitis B e antigen (HBeAg) is a secretory protein that is a marker of HBV replication and infectivity. It is usually present early and may persist for years in chronic infection, but it usually disappears within months in the absence of chronic infection. Seroconversion to anti-HBe antibodies is usually associated with the resolution of infection; however, recent studies have shown that many patients who have seroconverted often have measurable HBV DNA, albeit at low levels. Quantification of HBV DNA in the serum has now become the most accurate way of assessing HBV activity. Recent evidence has shown that many patients thought to have resolved acute HBV may have persistent viral infection and may be at risk for ongoing hepatitis or reactivation.[54]

The diagnosis of HCV infection relies on detection of antibodies to multiple HCV antigens. The most recent immunoassays are highly specific and sensitive. No specific HCV antigen tests exist, but a variety of quantitative and qualitative tests for HCV RNA exist. These tests of HCV RNA have become very important in confirming the diagnosis in unclear cases as well as in assessing responses to therapy.[55]

HDV co-infection of HBV-infected patients is best diagnosed by detection of HDV RNA, which can be measured in serum. The HDV antigen can be detected in liver specimens. HEV infection can be diagnosed by measurement of antibodies in serum or by detection of the virus or its components in feces, serum, or liver.[54]

Epidemiology and Transmission

The incidence of HAV has fallen dramatically since the introduction of effective vaccines, but vaccination is not routine in all countries. HAV is common in Third World countries, with seropositivity rates approaching 100% in some populations. Infection occurs in childhood and is facilitated by poor hygiene and sanitation. Infection rates are much lower in developed countries. In the United States, about 10% of children and 35% of adults have been infected with HAV. Despite vaccination availability, 6000 cases were reported in the United States in 2004, likely representing an estimated 60,000 cases nationwide. The primary route of HAV infection is the fecal-oral route. Ingestion of contaminated water or food, as well as person-to-person contact, accounts for most cases. Parenteral transmission is possible, but uncommon. Sexual transmission has been documented in homosexual men.[53]

HBV is a major worldwide health problem. There are more than 300 million carriers and 250,000 associated deaths annually. The prevalence of HBV infection has considerable geographic variation. Low prevalence areas, such as the United States and Western Europe, have carrier rates of 0.1% to 2%, and transmission is generally through sexual contact or IV drug abuse. Carrier rates in intermediate prevalence areas such as Japan and Singapore range from 3% to 5%. In high prevalence areas such as Southeast Asia and sub-Saharan Africa, carrier rates range from 10% to 20%. Transmission in high prevalence areas is largely perinatal and horizontal during childhood.[54]

Transfusion-associated HBV was common in the 1960s, and the risk has been estimated to be as high as 50% at that time. Current screening programs and limitation of blood donation to voluntary donors has decreased the risk for acquiring HBV from a blood transfusion to less than 1 in 100,000. Percutaneous transmission through the use of any contaminated needle is a major route of HBV infection and is common in IV drug abusers. Sexual transmission is common in low prevalence countries and is estimated to account for about 30% of cases in the United States. There is a particularly high incidence in male homosexuals and heterosexuals with multiple sexual partners. Perinatal HBV infection accounts for less than 10% of cases in the United States but is common in endemic areas, with rates of transmission of 90% in some areas. Horizontal transmission among children is common and is probably related to minor breaks in skin and mucous membranes. HBV is the most commonly transmitted virus among health care personnel, and transmission is usually patient to patient or patient to worker. Rare cases of physician-to-patient transmission have been reported. Needle-stick risk has been related to HBeAg positivity.

HCV is the most common cause of chronic liver disease in the United States, with an estimated prevalence of 1.8% accounting for 3.9 million infected people. New infection typically occurs at young age (20-39 years), and the most common risk factor is IV drug abuse. Health care workers have higher carrier rates than the general public. Transmission among health care workers is usually related to needle-stick incidents, and the risk for transmission is higher than that of HIV and HBV. In the past, blood transfusion was the major cause of HCV infection, accounting for at least 85% of cases. Currently, less than 2% of acute infections are due to transfusions, and the risk associated with transfusion is estimated to be between 0.001% and 0.0001%. Although HCV has never been documented in semen, it is estimated that about 20% of HCV infections are due to sexual transmission. Risk for sexual transmission appears to be related to number of partners and the presence of other sexually transmitted diseases. Monogamous sexual partners of HCV-infected people occasionally test positive for HCV in the absence of other risk factors, but this appears to be distinctly rare. Perinatal transmission has been documented but is rare. No identifiable risk factors are found in 30% to 40% of HCV cases.[55]

HDV infection occurs worldwide, with a variable distribution that parallels HBV infection. About 5% of HBsAg-positive patients also harbor HDV infection. Transmission of HDV is parenteral and can only occur in patients previously infected with HBV.[54]

HEV is endemic in Southeast and Central Asia and occurs with low frequency in other areas of the world. HEV outbreaks are usually large, affecting hundreds to thousands of people at once, and often follow large rains and flooding. There are particularly high attack and mortality rates in pregnant women. Transmission is by a fecal-oral route and is usually related to contaminated drinking water or food. Person-to-person and vertical transmissions are rare.[53]

Pathogenesis and Clinical Characteristics

The pathogenesis of hepatic injury from these viral infections is not completely understood. For all the viruses discussed in this section, the hepatic inflammation appears to be due to either direct cytotoxicity or to immune-related phenomena. Combinations of these two mechanisms probably underlie the etiology of hepatitic damage.

Humans are the only host for HAV, and no reservoir of infection has been identified. After oral intake, HAV can survive the acidic gastric pH, but the mechanism of hepatic uptake is not known. HAV infection results in acute inflammation of the liver and has no associated chronic sequelae. The most recent data suggest that hepatocyte damage is most likely an immunopathologic response rather than direct hepatotoxicity. Most children younger than 2 years with HAV infection are asymptomatic, whereas after the age of 5 years, 80% of patients develop symptoms. A fulminant hepatitis develops in 1% to 5% of cases, and the mortality rate is generally less than 1%.[53]

About 70% of patients with acute HBV infection have subclinical or anicteric hepatitis; the other 30% have icteric hepatitis. The incubation period for HBV ranges from 1 to 4 months. A prodromal serum sickness–like syndrome may develop, followed by a multitude of constitutional symptoms such as malaise, anorexia, and nausea. The constitutional symptoms last about 10 days and are then followed by jaundice in 30% of patients. Clinical symptoms usually disappear within 3 months. Fulminant hepatic failure develops in 0.1% to 0.5% of cases. Nearly 80% of patients with fulminant HBV-related hepatitis die unless liver transplantation is performed.[54]

Risk for chronic HBV infection is related to immunocompetence and age. Immunocompetent adults have a risk of less than 5%, whereas 30% of children and 90% of infants develop chronic disease. Most cases of chronic HBV infection are asymptomatic, but some patients may experience exacerbations of symptoms. Laboratory tests may be entirely normal in HBV carriers, or mild elevations of ALT and AST may be the only findings. Progression to cirrhosis is marked by hepatic synthetic dysfunction and often cytopenia related to hypersplenism. Extrahepatic manifestations of HBV infection due to circulating immune complexes occur in about 10% to 20% of patients and include polyarteritis nodosa, glomerulonephritis, essential mixed cryoglobulinemia, and papular acrodermatitis. The sequelae of chronic HBV infection range from nothing to cirrhosis to hepatocellular carcinoma to hepatic failure or to death. It has been noted that patients thought to have previously cleared their infections can experience a reactivation, especially during a period of immunosuppression. Although in nonendemic areas, the long-term risk appears to be low, in endemic areas, chronic HBV infection is a significant cause of morbidity and mortality.[54]

Acute HCV infection generally presents with mild elevation of hepatocellular enzymes, and 80% of cases occur between 5 and 12 weeks after infection. Symptoms occur in less than 30% of patients and are usually so mild and nonspecific that they do not affect daily life. Jaundice occurs in less than 20% of patients, and fulminant hepatic failure due to HCV is extremely uncommon. Chronic HCV infection develops in about two thirds of patients, whereas the other one third appear to clear the infection. Most cases of chronic HCV infection are asymptomatic without evidence of overt liver disease and only present with mildly elevated hepatocellular enzymes. Despite this quiet clinical course, patients with chronic HCV infection are at risk for developing cirrhosis and hepatocellular carcinoma. Estimates put the risk of cirrhosis at 2% to 20% at a 20- to 30-year interval. The risk for developing HCC from that point has been estimated at 1% to 4% per year. Progression of liver damage can be quite variable, and several factors appear to affect the rate of progression. Factors associated with a more rapid progression include male gender, older age at infection, immunosuppression (e.g., HIV infection), coinfection with HBV, moderate alcohol intake, and obesity. A variety of extrahepatic manifestations, such as autoimmune disorders

and lymphoma, can occur with HCV infection and are likely related to circulating immune complexes.[55]

The clinical presentation of HDV infection is related to a complex relationship between the degree of both HBV and HDV infection. Simultaneous coinfection with high expression of HBV and HDV results in higher rates of acute fulminant hepatitis, and superinfection in a previous HBV carrier generally results in more rapidly progressive chronic liver damage. Some milder forms of acute HDV infection, however, are associated with decreased expression of HDV and repression of HBV infection.[54]

HEV has a different histologic picture than the other viral hepatitides in that a cholestatic type of hepatitis is seen in more than half of patients. HEV is introduced orally, and it is not known how the virus travels to the liver. The incubation period of HEV ranges from 2 to 9 weeks. The most common form of illness is acute icteric hepatis, and most series report jaundice in more than 90% of cases. Asymptomatic forms of the disease occur and are probably more common than the icteric form, but the actual frequency is unknown. The disease is usually self-limited, but fulminant hepatic failure can occur in a small percentage of patients. Overall, the mortality rate is probably significantly less than 1%. Pregnant women tend to have a more severe clinical course, and mortality rates range from 5% to 25%.[53]

Prevention

HAV prophylaxis has largely relied on sanitary measures and administration of serum immunoglobulin. Recent development of safe and effective HAV vaccines, however, has made the use of pre-exposure immunoglobulin unnecessary. Serum immunoglobulin is still the therapy of choice for postexposure prophylaxis and may be safely given along with active immunization. In the United States, the Centers for Disease Control and Prevention have recently recommended universal vaccination of children based on the safety and efficacy of the vaccine in high-risk populations. Public health policies are working on vaccination schemes to eradicate HAV in high-risk populations throughout the world, but cost-benefit analyses have not supported universal vaccination in all countries. Likewise, HEV prophylaxis has focused on sanitary measures, particularly strategies aimed at drinking water. Immunoglobulin has not been successful in pre-exposure or postexposure prevention of HEV infection, but anti-HEV antibodies appear to be effective in attenuating the clinical syndrome. Vaccines for HEV infection have been developed and are currently being evaluated in clinical trials.[53]

Remarkable advances have been made in the prevention of HBV infection. In the past, prevention of HBV infection was limited to passive immunization with immunoglobulin containing high titers of antibody to HBsAg. Currently, immunoglobulin immunization is only used in postexposure prophylaxis. HBsAg-containing vaccines have been developed with good safety and efficacy profiles. These vaccines are used primarily for pre-exposure prophylaxis but can also be used in a postexposure setting along with immunoglobulin. HBV vaccination is recommended for high-risk groups such as health care workers. There are also schemes for HBV vaccination to prevent perinatal transmission, and currently all children who are 11 or 12 years old need to be vaccinated if not done previously. HBV DNA-based vaccines have recently been developed, and a combined HBV and HAV vaccine has recently been approved. Although no vaccine is available for HDV, effective HBV prevention prevents HDV infection.[54]

The only effective preventive strategy for HCV infection relies on public health principles aimed at the major risk factors for transmission. Conventionally prepared anti-HCV immunoglobulin has been evaluated in a number of trials and was never demonstrated to prevent transfusion-related non-A, non-B hepatitis. Screening of blood donors has rendered this issue irrelevant today. Unfortunately, because of a variety of obstacles, a successful HCV vaccine has not been produced.[55]

Treatment

Treatment for HAV or HEV infection is supportive in nature and is generally aimed at correcting dehydration and providing adequate caloric intake. Although fatigue may mandate significant periods of rest, hospitalization is not usually necessary except in cases of fulminant liver failure.

The treatment of HBV infection is largely aimed at patients with chronic active disease. The two licensed therapies are interferon-α (IFN-α) and the nucleoside analogue lamivudine. IFN-α is an immunomodulatory agent with some antiviral properties that can induce a virologic response in 35% to 40% of patients. However, long-term benefit with IFN-α therapy has not been proved. Many nucleoside analogues for the treatment of HBV have been developed and probably work through inhibition of DNA synthesis. They have similar viral response rates to IFN-α, are inexpensive, are given orally, and have few side effects. On the other hand, nucleoside analogues often require long-term therapy (>1 year), and the development of resistant HBV mutants has been documented. Randomized trials have shown oral lamivudine to be effective at decreasing the risk for cirrhosis progression and HCC. Newer antiviral agents are in development and are likely to improve outcomes.[54]

During the past 15 years, tremendous advances in the treatment of HCV infection have occurred. A benefit for IFN-α in the treatment of non-A, non-B hepatitis was originally demonstrated in 1986 before the discovery of HCV. With current IFN-α treatment regimens, *complete viral response* (defined as sustained loss of serum viral RNA) occurs in 12% to 20% of patients. The addition of ribavirin to IFN-α has resulted in response rates of 35% to 45%. In the most recent trials, treatment with pegylated IFN-α and ribavirin for 48 weeks resulted in viral clearance in 55% of patients. The specific genotype appears to be predictive of response, with some types resulting in response rates of 80% and others of 45%. Relapse is possible but usually occurs with monotherapy and short-

ened courses of therapy. Because therapy with IFN-α has significant side effects, controversies such as indications for treatment and optimal doses and duration of treatment are still being evaluated.[55]

Selected References

Blumgart LH, Fong Y: Surgical options in the treatment of hepatic metastasis from colorectal cancer. Curr Probl Surg 32:333-421, 1995.

Although published in 1995, this complete review of the subject clearly outlines the rationale for liver resection of hepatic colorectal metastases and remains relevant to the practicing hepatobiliary surgeon today.

Blumgart LH, Hann LE: Surgical and radiologic anatomy of the liver and biliary tract. In Blumgart LH, Fong Y (eds): Surgery of the Liver and Biliary Tract. London, WB Saunders, 2000, pp 3-34.

A comprehensive and clinically oriented review of hepatobiliary anatomy. The text is specifically oriented toward surgery of the liver and biliary tree.

Fong Y, Fortner J, Sun RL, et al: Clinical score for predicting recurrence after hepatic resection for metastatic colorectal cancer: Analysis of 1001 consecutive cases. Ann Surg 230:309-318, 1999.

The largest single-institution series of liver resection for metastatic colorectal cancer. A very useful prognostic scoring system is presented.

Foster JH, Berman MM: Solid Liver Tumors. Philadelphia, WB Saunders, 1977.

A classic and comprehensive monograph that contains a complete history of liver surgery.

Green MHA, Duell RM, Johnson CD, et al: Haemobilia. Br J Surg 88:773-786, 2001.

A recent comprehensive and concise review of the subject.

Jarnagin WR, Gonen M, Fong Y, et al: Improvement in perioperative outcome after hepatic resection: Analysis of 1,803 consecutive cases over the past decade. Ann Surg 236:397-406; discussion 406-407, 2002.

One of the largest series of hepatic resections that documents the remarkable improvement in perioperative outcomes.

Johannsen EC, Sifri CD, Madoff LC: Infections of the liver: Pyogenic liver abscess. Infect Dis Clin N Am 14:547-563, 2000.

An excellent and modern review of all aspects of pyogenic liver abscess.

Lau WY: Primary hepatocellular carcinoma. In Blumgart LH, Fong Y (eds): Surgery of the Liver and Biliary Tract. London, WB Saunders, 2000, pp 1423-1450.

Comprehensive review of the subject from an innovative researcher in the field.

Ochsner A, DeBakey M, Murray S: Pyogenic abscess of the liver. Am J Surg 40:292-319, 1938.

A classic landmark study on pyogenic abscesses of the liver. This was the first serious attempt to study hepatic abscesses and ushered in the modern era of treatment.

Saxena R, Zucker SD, Crawford JM: Anatomy and physiology of the liver. In Zakim D, Boyer TD (eds): Hepatology: A Textbook of Liver Disease. Philadelphia, WB Saunders, 2003, pp 3-30.

An excellent overview of the microscopic anatomy of the liver and basic hepatic physiology from a comprehensive hepatology textbook.

References

1. Foster JH, Berman MM: Solid Liver Tumors. Philadelphia: WB Saunders, 1977.
2. Fortner JG, Blumgart LH: A historic perspective of liver surgery for tumors at the end of the millennium. J Am Coll Surg 193:210-222, 2001.
3. Jarnagin WR, Gonen M, Fong Y, et al: Improvement in perioperative outcome after hepatic resection: Analysis of 1,803 consecutive cases over the past decade. Ann Surg 236:397-406; discussion 406-407, 2002.
4. Blumgart LH, Hann LE: Surgical and radiologic anatomy of the liver and biliary tract. In Blumgart LH, Fong Y (eds): Surgery of the Liver and Biliary Tract. London, WB Saunders, 2000, pp 3-34.
5. Sadler TW: Langman's Medical Embryology, 5th ed. Baltimore, William & Wilkins, 1985.
6. Rappaport AM, Wanless IR: Physioanatomic considerations. In Schiff L, Schiff ER (eds): Diseases of the Liver. Philadelphia, JB Lippincott, 1993.
7. Saxena R, Zucker SD, Crawford JM: Anatomy and physiology of the liver. In Zakim D, Boyer TD (eds): Hepatology: A Textbook of Liver Disease. Philadelphia, WB Saunders, 2003, pp 3-30.
8. McCuskey RS, Reilly FD: Hepatic microvasculature: Dynamic structure and its regulation. Semin Liver Dis 13:1, 1993.
9. Seifert S, England S: Energy metabolism. In Arias IM (ed): The Liver: Biology and Pathobiology. New York, Raven Press, 1994.
10. Muller M, Jansen PLM: Mechanisms of bile secretion. In Zakim D, Boyer TD (eds): Hepatology: A Textbook of Liver Disease. Philadelphia, WB Saunders, 2003, pp 271-290.
11. Zimmermann H, Reichen J: Assessment of liver function in the surgical patient. In Blumgart LH, Fong Y (eds): Surgery of the Liver and Biliary Tract. London, WB Saunders, 2000, pp 35-64.
12. Chowdhury JR, Chowdhury NR, Jansen PLM: Bilirubin metabolism and its disorders. In Zakim D, Boyer TD (eds): Hepatology: A Textbook of Liver Disease. Philadelphia, WB Saunders, 2003, pp 233-270.
13. Zakim D: Metabolism of glucose and fatty acids by the liver. In Zakim D, Boyer TD (eds): Hepatology: A Textbook of Liver Disease. Philadelphia, WB Saunders, 2003, pp 49-80.
14. Cooper AJL: Amino acid metabolism and synthesis of urea. In Zakim D, Boyer TD (eds): Hepatology: A Textbook of Liver Disease. Philadelphia, WB Saunders, 2003, pp 81-126.
15. Vessey DA: Hepatic metabolism of xenobiotics in humans. In Zakim D, Boyer TD (eds): Hepatology: A Textbook of Liver Disease. Philadelphia, WB Saunders, 2003, pp 185-232.
16. Taub R: Liver regeneration: from myth to mechanism. Nat Rev Mol Cell Biol 5:836-847, 2004.
17. Schneider PD: Preoperative assessment of liver function. Surg Clin North Am 84:355-373, 2004.
18. Ochsner A, DeBakey M, Murray S: Pyogenic abscess of the liver. Am J Surg 40:292-319, 1938.
19. Pope IM, Poston GJ: Pyogenic liver abscess. In Blumgart LH, Fong Y (eds): Surgery of the Liver and Biliary Tract. London, WB Saunders, 2000, pp 1135-1145.
20. Kaplan GG, Gregson DB, Laupland KB: Population-based study of the epidemiology of and the risk factors for pyogenic liver abscess. Clin Gastroenterol Hepatol 2:1032-1038, 2004.
21. Johannsen EC, Sifri CD, Madoff LC: Infections of the liver: Pyogenic liver abscess. Infect Dis Clin N Am 14:547-563, 2000.
22. Lodhi S, Sarwari AR, Muzammil M, et al: Features distinguishing amoebic from pyogenic liver abscess: A review of 577 adult cases. Trop Med Int Health 9:718, 2004.
23. Hughes MA, Petri WA: Infections of the liver: Amebic liver abscess. Infect Dis Clin N Am 14:565-582, 2000.
24. Yu SCH, Ho SSM, Lau WY, et al: Treatment of pyogenic liver abscess: Prospective randomized comparison of catheter drainage and needle aspiration. Hepatology 39:932-938, 2004.
25. Wells C, Arguedas M: Amebic liver abscess. South Med J 97:673, 2004.
26. Blessmann J, Khoa ND, Van An L, et al: Ultrasound patterns and frequency of focal liver lesions after successful treatment of amebic liver abscess. Trop Med Int Health 11:504-508, 2006.
27. Dziri C: Hydatid disease: Continuing serious public health problem. Introduction. World J Surg 25:1-3, 2001.
28. McManus DP, Zhang W, Li J, et al: Echinococcosis. Lancet 362:1295-304, 2003.
29. Dziri C, Haouet K, Fingerhut A: Treatment of hydatid cyst of the liver: Where is the evidence? World J Surg 28:731-736, 2004.
30. Moghaddam N, Abrishami A, Malekzadeh R: Percutaneous needle aspiration, injection and reaspiration with or without benzimidazole coverage for uncomplicated hepatic hydatid cysts. Cochrane Database Syst Rev 2:CD003623, 2006.
31. Chen D, Poon R, Liu CL, et al: Immediate and long-term outcomes of hepatectomy for hepatolithiasis. Surgery 135:386-393, 2004.
32. Chen C, Huang M, Yang J, et al: Reappraisal of percutaneous transhepatic cholangioscopic lithotomy for primary hepatolithiasis. Surg Endosc 19:505-509, 2005.
33. Gibbs JF, Litwin AM, Kahlenbert MS: Contemporary management of benign liver tumors. Surg Clin N Am 84:463-480, 2004.
34. Zimmerman A: Tumors of the liver—pathologic aspects. In Blumgart LH, Fong Y (eds): Surgery of the Liver and Biliary Tract. London, WB Saunders, 2000, pp 1343-1396.
35. Fulcher AS, Sterling RK: Hepatic neoplasms: Computed tomography and magnetic resonance imaging features. J Clin Gastroenterol 34:463-471, 2002.
36. LaQuaglia MP: Liver tumors in children. In Blumgart LH, Fong Y (eds): Surgery of the Liver and Biliary Tract. London, WB Saunders, 2000, pp 1397-1422.
37. Lau WY: Primary hepatocellular carcinoma. In Blumgart LH, Fong Y (eds): Surgery of the Liver and Biliary Tract. London, WB Saunders, 2000, pp 1423-1450.
38. Bosch FX, Ribes J, Cleries R, et al: Epidemiology of hepatocellular carcinoma. Clin Liver Dis 9:191-211, 2005.
39. Ribero D, Abdalla EK, Thomas MB, et al: Liver resection in the treatment of hepatocellular carcinoma. Expert Rev Anticancer Ther 6:567-579, 2006.
40. Sutcliffe R, Maguire D, Portmann B, et al: Selection of patients with hepatocellular carcinoma for liver transplantation. Br J Surg 92:11-18, 2006.
41. Lencioni R, Crocetti L: A critical appraisal of the literature on local ablative therapies for hepatocellular carcinoma. Clin Liver Dis 9:301-314, 2005.

42. Weber SM, Jarnagin WR, Klimstra D, et al: Intrahepatic cholangiocarcinoma: Resectability, recurrence pattern, and outcomes. J Am Coll Surg 193:384-391, 2001.

43. Blumgart LH, Fong Y: Surgical options in the treatment of hepatic metastasis from colorectal cancer. Curr Probl Surg 32:333-421, 1995.

44. Kelly H, Goldberg RM: Systemic therapy for metastatic colorectal cancer: Current options, current evidence. J Clin Oncol 23:4553-4560, 2005.

45. Fong Y, Fortner J, Sun RL, et al: Clinical score for predicting recurrence after hepatic resection for metastatic colorectal cancer: Analysis of 1001 consecutive cases. Ann Surg 230:309-318, 1999.

46. Kemeny N, Huang Y, Cohen AM, et al: Hepatic arterial infusion of chemotherapy after resection of hepatic metastases from colorectal cancer. N Engl J Med 341:2039-2048, 1999.

47. Sarmiento JM, Heywood G, Rubin J, et al: Surgical treatment of neuroendocrine metastases to the liver: Plea for resection to increase survival. J Am Coll Surg 197:29-37, 2003.

48. Farges O, Menu Y, Benhamou JP: Non-parasitic cystic diseases of the liver and intrahepatic biliary tree. In Blumgart LH, Fong Y (eds): Surgery of the Liver and Biliary Tract. London, WB Saunders, 2000, pp 1245-1260.

49. Blumgart LH, Jarnagin W, Fong Y: Liver resection for benign disease and for liver and biliary tumors. In Blumgart LH, Fong Y (eds): Surgery of the Liver and Biliary Tract. London, WB Saunders, 2000, pp 1639-1714.

50. Sandblom JP: Hemobilia and bilhemia. In Blumgart LH, Fong Y (eds): Surgery of the Liver and Biliary Tract. London, WB Saunders, 2000, pp 1319-1342.

51. Green MHA, Duell RM, Johnson CD, et al: Haemobilia. Br J Surg 88:773-786, 2001.

52. Sandblom P: Hemobilia (Biliary Tract Hemorrhage): History, Pathology, Diagnosis, Treatment. Springfield: Charles C. Thomas, 1972.

53. Koff RS: Hepatitis A and E. In Zakim D, Boyer TD (eds): Hepatology: A Textbook of Liver Disease. Philadelphia, WB Saunders, 2003, pp 939-959.

54. Nair S, Perrillo RP: Hepatitis B and D. In Zakim D, Boyer TD (eds): Hepatology: A Textbook of Liver Disease. Philadelphia, WB Saunders, 2003, pp 959-1016.

55. Hoffnagle JH, Heller T: Hepatitis C. In Zakim D, Boyer TD (eds): Hepatology: A Textbook of Liver Disease. Philadelphia, WB Saunders, 2003, pp 1017-1062.

Surgical Complications of Cirrhosis and Portal Hypertension

Layton F. Rikkers, MD

Historical Review

Anatomy, Physiology, and Pathophysiology of Portal Hypertension

Evaluation of the Patient With Cirrhosis

Variceal Hemorrhage

Ascites and the Hepatorenal Syndrome

Encephalopathy

HISTORICAL REVIEW

Cirrhosis was first described in a 4th-century BC hippocratic aphorism: In cases of jaundice it is a bad sign when the liver becomes hard.[1] Although the deleterious effect of alcohol on the liver was appreciated by Galen and his contemporaries in the 2nd century AD, alcoholic liver disease as an entity was first recognized by Baillie and other English writers after the "gin plague" in the 18th century. Shortly thereafter, Laënnec introduced the term *cirrhosis,* which was derived from the Greek word *kirrhos,* meaning "orange-yellow." Nineteenth-century European and English pathologists, including Carswell and Rokitansky, described the gross and histopathologic characteristics of the disease. Although alcoholic cirrhosis was thought to be due to toxins other than alcohol or to malnutrition during much of the 20th century, recent investigations have established alcohol as a hepatotoxin.

Cirrhosis is the end result of a variety of mechanisms causing hepatocellular injury, including toxins (alcohol), viruses (hepatitis B and hepatitis C), prolonged cholestasis (extrahepatic and intrahepatic), autoimmunity (lupoid hepatitis), and metabolic disorders (hemochromatosis, Wilson's disease, α_1-antitrypsin deficiency). Although the mechanisms are diverse, the pathologic response is uniform: hepatocellular necrosis followed by fibrosis and nodular regeneration. Each of these elements may exist alone (necrosis, uncomplicated hepatitis; fibrosis, congenital hepatic fibrosis; nodular regeneration, partial nodular transformation), but all three are required for the development of cirrhosis. Cirrhosis is always a diffuse process and may be classified either morphologically or by etiology. Alcoholic cirrhosis, which is usually micronodular, and posthepatitic cirrhosis, which is generally macronodular, are the two most common varieties in the United States. Because the pathologic responses to various mechanisms of hepatocellular injury are so similar, occasionally the cause cannot be ascertained (cryptogenic cirrhosis).

Cirrhosis causes two major phenomena: hepatocellular failure and portal hypertension. Even after the noxious agent is removed (e.g., abstinence from alcohol), the disease may progress. Although the mechanism is not clear, both ischemia, secondary to extensive fibrosis and intrahepatic and extrahepatic shunts, and autoimmune factors may play roles. The altered hepatic architecture and perisinusoidal fibrosis cause increased hepatic vascular resistance, resulting in portal hypertension and its associated complications of variceal hemorrhage, encephalopathy, ascites, and hypersplenism.

Autopsy studies suggest an incidence of cirrhosis of between 3.5% and 5%. Only 10% to 15% of heavy drinkers develop alcoholic cirrhosis. Because of the large number of alcoholic people in the United States, as well as a significant percentage of patients with nonalcoholic causes of chronic liver disease, cirrhosis presently ranks as the sixth leading cause of death between the ages of 35 and 54 years. Hepatic failure and variceal hemorrhage are the first and second most common causes of death, respectively, in patients with cirrhosis.

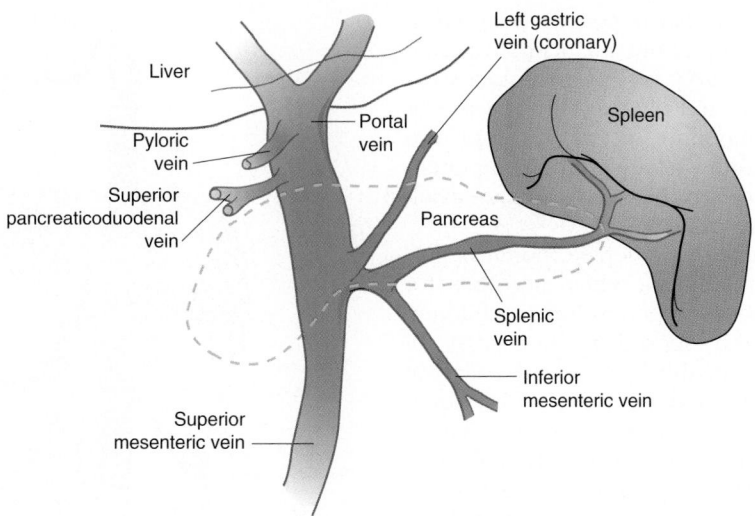

Figure 53-1 The extrahepatic portal venous circulation. (From Rikkers LF: Portal hypertension. In Goldsmith H [ed]: Practice of Surgery. Philadelphia, Harper & Row, 1981, pp 1-37.)

Historically, the treatment of cirrhosis has been the treatment of the complications of portal hypertension. Medical treatment of cirrhosis with antifibrogenesis drugs, such as colchicine, has been ineffective. In contrast, since 1980, the surgical management of chronic liver disease with hepatic transplantation has been highly successful, with long-term survival rates generally above 70%. A major challenge to the physician or surgeon managing patients with cirrhosis is to determine when definitive treatment (transplantation) rather than palliative treatment (e.g., interventions to prevent recurrent variceal hemorrhage) should be applied.

ANATOMY, PHYSIOLOGY, AND PATHOPHYSIOLOGY OF PORTAL HYPERTENSION

The liver is a unique organ in that it has a dual blood supply: portal venous and hepatic arterial. The portal vein is formed from the confluence of the superior mesenteric and splenic veins behind the neck of the pancreas and is 6 to 8 cm in length (Fig. 53-1). The left gastric, or coronary, vein drains the distal esophagus and lesser curvature of the stomach, generally entering the portal vein near its origin. The splenic vein lies beneath the pancreas and is usually joined by the inferior mesenteric vein just before its confluence with the superior mesenteric vein.

The hepatic artery, one of three major branches of the celiac axis, lies medial to the common bile duct and portal vein in the hepatoduodenal ligament. Common variations include origins of the right and left hepatic arteries from the superior mesenteric artery and the left gastric artery, respectively, both of which occur in nearly 20% of the population.

Hepatic blood flow averages 1500 mL/minute, which represents about 25% of the cardiac output. The portal vein contributes two thirds of the total hepatic blood flow, whereas hepatic arterial perfusion accounts for more than half of the liver's oxygen supply. The volume of portal venous flow is indirectly regulated by vasoconstriction and vasodilation of the splanchnic arterial bed. In contrast, hepatic arterioles respond to circulating catecholamines and sympathetic nervous stimulation; thus, hepatic arterial flow is directly regulated. Even intense vasoconstrictive influences, however, can be overcome by a hepatic arterial autoregulatory or *buffer* response, which maintains total hepatic blood flow as near to normal as possible when portal perfusion is decreased in patients with shock or either disease-induced or surgically created portosystemic shunts.[2]

Many splanchnic hormones are important regulators of hepatic metabolism. Insulin is particularly important because it is a hepatotropic hormone and is essential for maintenance of liver structure and function. Thus, even if the quantity of hepatic blood flow is maintained in the normal range by hepatic arterial compensation for decreased portal flow, hepatic physiology may be impaired.

Because increased portal venous resistance is usually the initiator of portal hypertension, classifications of this disorder are generally based on the site of elevated resistance. In addition to the increased passive resistance secondary to fibrosis and regenerative nodules, a component of the increased hepatic vascular resistance is due to active vasoconstriction caused by norepinephrine, endothelin, and other humoral vasoconstrictors. However, increased portal venous inflow secondary to a hyperdynamic systemic circulation and splanchnic hyperemia is a major contributor to the maintenance of portal hypertension as portosystemic collaterals develop. The cause of the elevated cardiac output and splanchnic hyperemia is not known, but splanchnic hormones, such as glucagon, and decreased sensitivity of the splanchnic vasculature to catecholamines probably play a role.[3] Increased production of nitrous oxide and prostacyclin by vascular endothelium is also an important factor.[3] An improved understanding of the pathophysiology of portal hypertension has therapeutic implications because drugs are available that can alter these responses.

The most common cause of prehepatic portal hypertension is portal vein thrombosis, which accounts for about half of cases of portal hypertension in children. When the portal vein is thrombosed in the absence of liver disease, hepatopetal (to the liver) portal collateral vessels develop to restore portal perfusion. This combination is termed *cavernomatous transformation of the portal vein*. Isolated splenic vein thrombosis (left-sided portal hypertension) is usually secondary to pancreatic inflammation or neoplasm. The result is gastrosplenic venous hypertension, with superior mesenteric and portal venous pressures remaining normal. The left gastroepiploic vein becomes a major collateral vessel, and gastric, rather than esophageal, varices develop. This variant of portal hypertension is important to recognize because it is easily reversed by splenectomy alone.

The site of increased resistance in intrahepatic portal hypertension may be at the presinusoidal, sinusoidal, or postsinusoidal level. Frequently, more than one level is involved. The most common cause of intrahepatic, presinusoidal hypertension is schistosomiasis. In addition, many causes of nonalcoholic cirrhosis also result in presinusoidal portal hypertension, especially early in their course. Alcoholic cirrhosis, the most common cause of portal hypertension in the United States, usually causes increased resistance to portal flow at the sinusoidal (secondary to deposition of collagen in the Disse space) and postsinusoidal (secondary to regenerating nodules distorting small hepatic veins) levels. Other postsinusoidal causes of portal hypertension are rare and include Budd-Chiari syndrome (hepatic vein thrombosis), constrictive pericarditis, and heart failure. Rarely, increased portal venous flow alone, secondary either to massive splenomegaly (idiopathic portal hypertension) or a splanchnic arteriovenous fistula, causes portal hypertension.

Portal hypertension is defined by a portal pressure above 5 mm Hg. Somewhat higher pressures (8-10 mm Hg) are required to stimulate portosystemic collateralization. Collateral vessels usually develop where the portal and systemic venous circulations are in close proximity (Fig. 53-2). The collateral network through the coronary and short gastric veins to the azygos vein is the most important one clinically because it results in formation of esophagogastric varices; however, other sites include a recanalized umbilical vein from the left portal vein to the epigastric venous system (caput medusae), retroperitoneal collateral vessels, and the hemorrhoidal venous plexus. In addition to extrahepatic collateral vessels, a significant fraction of portal venous flow passes through both anatomic and physiologic (capillarization of hepatic sinusoids) intrahepatic shunts. As hepatic portal perfusion decreases, hepatic arterial flow generally increases (buffer response).[2]

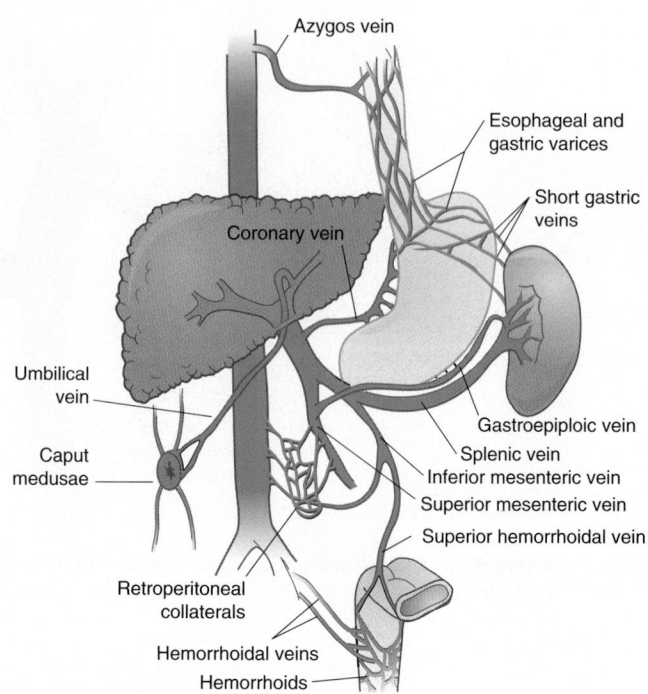

Figure 53-2 Portosystemic collateral pathways develop where the portal venous and systemic venous systems are in close apposition. (From Rikkers LF: Portal hypertension. In Miller TA [ed]: Physiologic Basis of Modern Surgical Care. St. Louis, CV Mosby, 1988, pp 417-428.)

EVALUATION OF THE PATIENT WITH CIRRHOSIS

Key aspects of the assessment of a patient with suspected chronic liver disease or one of the complications of portal hypertension are the following:

1. Diagnosis of the underlying liver disease
2. Estimation of functional hepatic reserve
3. Definition of portal venous anatomy and hepatic hemodynamic evaluation
4. Identification of the site of upper gastrointestinal hemorrhage, if present

These diagnostic categories take on varying levels of importance depending on the clinical situation. For example, estimation of functional hepatic reserve is useful in determining the risk associated with therapeutic intervention and whether definitive (hepatic transplantation) or palliative (e.g., endoscopic variceal ligation or shunt procedure) treatment is indicated. Knowledge of portal anatomy and physiology guides the surgeon in selecting an appropriate operation for control of variceal bleeding. Precise identification of the site of bleeding is essential because hemorrhage secondary to portal hypertension may be from esophageal varices, gastric varices, ectopic varices, portal hypertensive gastropathy (PHG), or portal colopathy, and because a significant fraction of patients with portal hypertension bleed from other lesions.

History and Physical Examination

In a patient with nonspecific constitutional complaints such as weight loss, malaise, and weakness, a past history of chronic alcoholism, hepatitis, complicated biliary disease, or exposure to hepatotoxins leads one to include cirrhosis in the differential diagnosis. Subtle clues to the presence of underlying chronic liver disease on physical examination are spider angiomas, palmar erythema, testicular atrophy, and gynecomastia. A palpable spleen in association with these signs suggests portal hypertension. Confirmatory evidence of cirrhosis is provided by signs of hepatic functional decompensation or advanced portal hypertension, such as jaundice, ascites, palpation of a firm irregular liver edge, dilated abdominal wall veins, and impairment of mental status or the presence of asterixis (liver flap).

Laboratory Tests

Cirrhosis is often accompanied by anemia, leukopenia, and thrombocytopenia. Anemia may result from bleeding, nutritional deficiencies, hemolysis, or bone marrow depression secondary to alcoholism. Although many patients with portal hypertension have some degree of hypersplenism, it is unusual to find a platelet count of less than 50,000 per mm³ or a white blood cell count of less than 2000 per mm³. The degree of thrombocytopenia has been found to be a quite accurate predictor of the presence of esophageal varices.[4] In addition to thrombocytopenia, coagulation may be impaired by a prolonged prothrombin time because many of the coagulation factors are synthesized by the liver and by primary fibrinolysis, which is present in many patients with chronic liver disease.

A chemistry profile is helpful in both the diagnosis and assessment of severity of cirrhosis. Hypoalbuminemia and a prolonged International Normalized Ratio (INR) are usually reliable indices of chronic rather than acute liver disease. Elevation of the hepatocellular enzymes aspartate aminotransferase and alanine aminotransferase to more than three times their normal level is indicative of significant, ongoing hepatocellular necrosis, which is often present in patients with alcoholic hepatitis and chronic active hepatitis resulting from a variety of causes. Increased disease activity may be an important risk factor in patients who undergo surgery. A ratio of alanine aminotransferase to aspartate aminotransferase of greater than 2 is highly suggestive of alcohol as the cause of liver disease. Although mild elevations of the enzymes alkaline phosphatase and γ-glutamyl transpeptidase are nonspecific, marked increases in these enzymes are indicative of either intrahepatic or extrahepatic cholestasis (primary or secondary biliary cirrhosis). In the absence of prior blood transfusions, a total bilirubin level of greater than 3 mg per 100 mL is indicative of severe hepatic decompensation and a high operative risk status.

Hepatitis serology is obtained in most patients with cirrhosis. A significant fraction of patients with hepatitis B and hepatitis C develop cirrhosis, whereas hepatitis A generally causes only acute liver disease. One of the most common internal malignancies worldwide is hepatocellular carcinoma, which is frequently secondary to hepatitis B or hepatitis C infection. This malignancy, however, frequently develops in patients with other causes of cirrhosis and occasionally in patients without chronic liver disease. Unexpected hepatic functional deterioration in a patient with cirrhosis is often a result of the development of hepatocellular carcinoma, which can be diagnosed in about 60% of patients by an elevated α-fetoprotein level. All newly diagnosed cirrhotic patients are screened for hepatocellular carcinoma by determination of α-fetoprotein level and by obtaining a computed tomography (CT) scan of the liver.

Common serum electrolyte abnormalities in cirrhosis are hyponatremia, hypokalemia, and metabolic alkalosis. These metabolic disorders are secondary to hyperaldosteronism, diarrhea, and recurrent emesis, which frequently accompany cirrhosis. Deleterious consequences of metabolic alkalosis are shift of the oxyhemoglobin dissociation curve to the left, which impairs tissue oxygen delivery, and conversion of ammonium chloride to ammonia, which facilitates transport of this purported cerebral toxin across the blood-brain barrier.

Liver Biopsy

Percutaneous liver biopsy is a useful technique for establishing the cause of cirrhosis and for assessing activity of the liver disease. Percutaneous liver biopsy is not done when either coagulopathy or moderate ascites is present. In these situations, liver tissue can be obtained by means of a transjugular venous approach or laparoscopy. Laparoscopic biopsy reduces the false-negative rate for diagnosing cirrhosis as compared with the blind biopsy techniques.

Measurement of Hepatic Functional Reserve

The time-honored method of assessing hepatic functional reserve is Child's classification or one of its modifications. The most commonly used scheme is the Child-Pugh classification (Table 53-1), which includes two clinical vari-

Table 53-1   Child-Pugh Criteria for Hepatic Functional Reserve

Clinical and laboratory measurement	PATIENT SCORE FOR INCREASING ABNORMALITY		
	1	**2**	**3**
Encephalopathy (grade)	None	1 or 2	3 or 4
Ascites	None	Mild	Moderate
Bilirubin (mg/dL)	1-2	2.1-3	≥3.1
Albumin (g/dL)	≥3.5	2.8-3.4	≤2.7
Prothrombin time (increase, s)	1-4	4.1-6	≥6.1

Grade A, 5-6; grade B, 7-9; grade C, 10-15

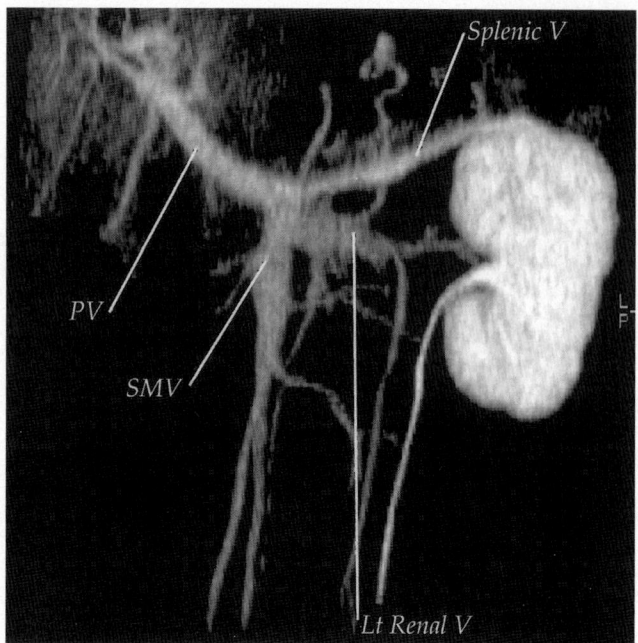

Figure 53-3 A three-dimensional reconstruction of a computed tomography angiogram. The portal vein (PV), superior mesenteric vein (SMV), splenic vein, and left renal vein are clearly demonstrated. The ready availability of these scans has decreased the need for more invasive techniques such as visceral angiography.

ables in addition to three biochemical indices.[5] Although not a direct measure of hepatic functional reserve, no other test has surpassed it with respect to predicting operative outcome or assessing long-term prognosis in the unoperated patient. The serum bilirubin level is interpreted in the context of recent blood transfusions, which may transiently elevate it but are not indicative of further impairment of hepatic functional reserve. In most clinical series, operative mortality rates for Child-Pugh class A, B, and C patients are in the range of 0% to 5%, 10% to 15%, and greater than 25%, respectively. The Model for End-Stage Liver Disease (MELD) scale that consists of serum bilirubin and creatinine levels, INR, and etiology of liver disease has recently been found to be as predictive of mortality as the Child-Pugh score.[6]

True quantitative measures of hepatocellular function, such as galactose elimination capacity, aminopyrine breath test, indocyanine green clearance, and hepatic clearance of amino acids, are not available in most institutions. These tests, however, may be valuable indicators of limited hepatic reserve in some patients with nearly normal conventional liver function tests. Now that hepatic transplantation has become a realistic option for many patients with cirrhosis, accurate quantitation of hepatocellular function to determine which patients are transplantation candidates has become even more important.

Hepatic Hemodynamic Assessment

In patients with alcoholic cirrhosis and many varieties of nonalcoholic cirrhosis, portal pressure can be indirectly estimated by measurement of hepatic venous wedge pressure (HVWP). Because HVWP is normal in patients with presinusoidal portal hypertension, portal pressure in these patients can be measured only directly by transhepatic or umbilical venous cannulation of the portal venous system or by percutaneous puncture of the spleen.

The portal pressure is expressed as the portal pressure gradient, which is the difference between the portal pressure and the inferior vena cava pressure. It is an important measurement because a gradient in excess of 10 mm Hg is necessary for varices to form, and a pressure higher than 12 mm Hg is required for varices to bleed.

Because splanchnic venous thrombosis may be the cause of portal hypertension or develop as a result of cirrhosis, portal venous anatomy needs to be defined before performing a portosystemic shunt operation. Although selective visceral angiography has been the most frequently used method for visualization of the portal venous system and for qualitative estimation of hepatic portal perfusion, this relatively invasive approach is presently being replaced in many institutions by less invasive methods such as CT angiography, Doppler ultrasonography, and magnetic resonance imaging. CT angiograms can delineate the location, size, and patency status of all veins (e.g., splenic vein and left renal vein) to be used in creation of a portosystemic shunt[7] (Fig. 53-3). Magnetic resonance imaging has also been successfully utilized to visualize the portal venous circulation. This technique is particularly appropriate for patients with an allergy to radiopaque contrast.

Doppler ultrasonography is a noninvasive technique for assessment of portal venous patency, direction of portal flow, and shunt patency status.[8] Because of its noninvasiveness, Doppler ultrasonography has become a standard for the evaluation of most patients with chronic liver disease because direction of portal flow and its velocity can be diagnostic of associated portal hypertension. Ultrasound is also useful for assessing liver size, spleen size, and the presence of liver masses. It can also detect ascites in its earliest stages (≥100 mL). Doppler ultrasound is less accurate in assessing superior mesenteric and splenic vein anatomy and flow characteristics. Likewise, Doppler ultrasonography usually accurately assesses patency status of surgically constructed shunts unless there is overlying bowel gas. Doppler ultrasound has also been used to evaluate patency and narrowing of a transjugular intrahepatic portosystemic shunt (TIPS), but it is less accurate than direct cannulation through a systemic venous approach.

Diagnosis of Bleeding

In the absence of hematemesis, a nasogastric tube is inserted to determine whether bleeding is from the upper gastrointestinal tract. The key procedure for diagnosing the site of upper gastrointestinal hemorrhage in a patient with portal hypertension is endoscopy. Before endoscopy, the patient needs to be hemodynamically stabilized and the stomach evacuated of blood clots with a large-bore lavage tube.

Upper gastrointestinal tract bleeding in patients with portal hypertension is caused by the portal hypertension in about 90% of instances. The remaining 10% of patients bleed from Mallory-Weiss tears, gastric ulcers, and duodenal ulcers, all of which are more common in patients with alcoholic cirrhosis than in the general population. Portal hypertensive bleeding is most commonly from esophagogastric varices (esophageal varices, 80%; gastric varices, 20%). Gastric varices most commonly occur in association with esophageal varices, but they occasionally occur alone. Isolated gastric varices raise the suspicion of splenic vein thrombosis. Hemorrhage from gastric fundal varices can be especially severe and is associated with a higher likelihood of recurrent bleeding and mortality than bleeding from esophageal varices. The endoscopic diagnosis of variceal hemorrhage can be established by observing a bleeding varix (~25% of patients) or by observation of moderate- to large-sized varices and no other lesions in a patient who has recently experienced a major upper gastrointestinal tract hemorrhage (loss of >2 units of blood).

The only nonvariceal causes of portal hypertensive bleeding are PHG and, much less commonly, portal colopathy.[9] The frequency of PHG is unknown, but it is probably more common after eradication of varices by endoscopic sclerotherapy or banding. PHG mainly involves the fundus and body of the stomach and, when mild, has an endoscopic appearance of a white reticular network with enclosed erythematous areas. The more severe form of PHG includes granular mucosa and cherry-red spots, both of which indicate a higher risk for bleeding.[9] PHG is associated with increased gastric mucosal perfusion and reflects a hyperemic rather than a congestive pathophysiologic change. Because varices and PHG often coexist, it may be difficult to determine which lesion is responsible for any given episode of bleeding. Occasionally, massive bleeding in a patient with cirrhosis makes an endoscopic diagnosis initially impossible, in which case endoscopy is repeated after bleeding is controlled. Gastric varices may be difficult to recognize endoscopically even in nonbleeding patients. Endoscopic ultrasound is a more sensitive diagnostic test than endoscopy alone for detection of gastric varices.

VARICEAL HEMORRHAGE

Bleeding from esophagogastric varices is the single most life-threatening complication of portal hypertension, responsible for about one third of all deaths in patients with cirrhosis. About one half of the deaths are due to uncontrolled bleeding. The risk for death from bleeding is mainly related to the underlying hepatic functional reserve. Patients with extrahepatic portal venous obstruction and normal hepatic function rarely die from bleeding varices, whereas those with decompensated cirrhosis (Child-Pugh class C) may face a mortality rate in excess of 50%. The greatest risk for rebleeding from varices is within the first few days after the onset of hemorrhage; the risk declines rapidly between then and 6 weeks after

hemorrhage onset, when it returns to the prehemorrhage risk level.[10]

Pathogenesis

Varices in the distal esophagus and proximal stomach are a component of the collateral network that diverts high-pressure portal venous flow through the left and right gastric veins and the short gastric veins to the azygous system. Less commonly, varices develop at other sites in the gastrointestinal tract but are less prone to rupture in those locations. Esophagogastric varices do not bleed until portal pressure exceeds 12 mm Hg, and then they bleed in only one third to one half of patients.[5] The pathogenesis of variceal rupture is incompletely understood but is most likely multifactorial.

The pathophysiology of variceal rupture is based on Laplace's law.[11] Although it has been observed that variceal size, magnitude of portal pressure, and thickness of the epithelium overlying the varix all significantly separate bleeders from nonbleeders, the overlap between groups is large when any one of these variables is considered independently. Laplace's law states that variceal wall tension is directly related to transmural pressure and varix radius and inversely related to variceal wall thickness, thus combining all three of these variables. Because all of these parameters cannot be measured clinically, there are inherent inaccuracies in predicting which patients with varices may bleed. The three key variables that are predictive of variceal bleeding are Child-Pugh class, variceal size, and the presence and severity of red wale markings (indicative of epithelial thickness).[12] The capacity to predict variceal bleeding is especially important when considering prophylactic therapy (treatment of varices that have not previously bled).

Treatment

Therapy for portal hypertension and variceal bleeding has evolved during the past 100 years. The many treatment modalities available suggest that no single therapy is entirely satisfactory for all patients or for all clinical situations. Sequential therapies are often necessary. Nonoperative treatments are generally preferred for acutely bleeding patients because they are often high operative risks because of decompensated hepatic function. Therapies that are effective (a low rebleeding rate) and minimally alter hepatic physiology are optimal for long-term prevention of recurrent bleeding. Only treatments associated with minimal morbidity and mortality can be considered for prophylaxis because many patients will be treated unnecessarily (only one third to one half of patients with varices eventually bleed).

History of Treatment for Portal Hypertension

Table 53-2 presents a chronology of the treatment of portal hypertension, which began with the description of the Eck fistula (end-to-side portacaval shunt) in 1877.[1] Eck's main concerns were to determine whether survival was possible after complete portal flow diversion and to develop a treatment for ascites. Probably the most important contribution to this field was made by Pavlov's group

Table 53-2 History of Treatment of Portal Hypertension

INVESTIGATORS	CONTRIBUTION
Eck, 1877	Portacaval shunt (dog)
Pavlov, 1893	Encephalopathy (dog)
Vidal, 1903	Clinical portacaval shunt (ascites)
Westphal, 1930	Balloon tamponade
Crafoord and Frenckner, 1939	Endoscopic sclerotherapy
Blakemore et al, 1945	Clinical portacaval and splenorenal shunts (bleeding)
Sengstaken and Blakemore, 1950	Balloon tamponade
Kehne, 1956	Vasopressin
Warren et al, 1967	Distal splenorenal shunt
Starzl, 1967	First successful liver transplantation
Inokuchi, 1968	Left gastric–vena caval shunt
Rosch, 1969	Transjugular intrahepatic portosystemic shunt (TIPS) in animals
Johnston and Rodgers, 1973	Reintroduction of endoscopic sclerotherapy
Sugiura and Futagawa, 1973	Extensive esophagogastric devascularization
Calne, 1980	Cyclosporine for transplantation
Lebrec, 1981	Propranolol for bleeding
Colapinto, 1983	TIPS in humans

Data from Chen TS, Chen PS: Understanding the Liver. Westport, CT, Greenwood Press, 1984.

in 1893.[13] These investigators perfected the technique of portacaval shunting and, after carefully observing 20 surviving dogs, described in detail the syndrome of "meat intoxication" or portosystemic encephalopathy, which they believed was due to intestinally absorbed cerebral toxins bypassing their site of metabolism in the liver. They also found from autopsy studies that dogs with encephalopathy had patent portacaval shunts and atrophic livers, whereas animals with normal cerebral function and preserved hepatic structure had thrombosed shunts and maintenance of hepatic portal perfusion through collateral vessels.

The modern era of treatment of variceal hemorrhage can be dated from the mid 1940s, when the portacaval and conventional splenorenal shunts were introduced into clinical practice. Although balloon tamponade and endoscopic sclerosis of varices were initially described in the 1930s, these were found to be only temporizing measures. During the ensuing 20 years, several varieties of nonselective shunts (complete portal decompression and portal flow diversion) were described, and the por-

tacaval shunt was evaluated in randomized, controlled trials. Motivated by the discouraging results of these trials, the concept of selective variceal decompression (distal splenorenal shunt) was introduced in 1967. An initial wave of enthusiasm for the distal splenorenal shunt (partial portal flow diversion) was followed by several randomized trials, which produced inconsistent results. A resurgence in interest of endoscopic sclerotherapy occurred in the 1970s, initially in Europe and South Africa and then in the United States.

Although pharmacotherapy with vasopressin was first used for acute hemorrhage in 1956, drug treatment for long-term prevention of initial or recurrent hemorrhage is a phenomenon of the 1980s. Improved immunosuppression (cyclosporine) and surgical techniques have led to the widespread application of hepatic transplantation for patients with end-stage liver disease. Finally, a nonoperative means of portal decompression (TIPS), first described in animals in 1969, has more recently been applied to the problem of variceal bleeding and, along with endoscopic therapy, is presently the most widely used intervention for this complication of portal hypertension.

Treatment of the Acute Bleeding Episode

Because many patients with acute variceal bleeding have decompensated hepatic function secondary to either recent alcoholism or hypotension, they are at high risk for emergency surgical intervention. In addition, these patients often have other complications of chronic liver disease, such as encephalopathy, ascites, coagulopathy, and malnutrition. Therefore, emergency treatment should be nonoperative whenever possible. Endoscopic treatment (sclerosis or ligation), which has become the mainstay of nonoperative treatment of acute hemorrhage in most centers, controls bleeding in more than 85% of patients, allowing an interval of medical management for improvement of hepatic function, resolution of ascites and encephalopathy, and enhancement of nutrition before definitive treatment for prevention of recurrent bleeding. Pharmacotherapy can be initiated in any hospital, and some trials suggest that it is just as effective as endoscopic treatment. Balloon tamponade, which is infrequently used, can be lifesaving in patients with exsanguinating hemorrhage and when the other nonoperative methods are not successful. TIPS has replaced operative shunts for managing acute variceal bleeding when pharmacotherapy and endoscopic treatment fail to control bleeding. Emergency surgical intervention in most centers is reserved for selected patients who are not TIPS candidates.

Resuscitation and Diagnosis

The highest priority in emergency management is restoration of circulating blood volume, which needs to be accomplished before upper gastrointestinal endoscopy. Although initial resuscitation is usually with isotonic crystalloid solutions, a minimum of 6 units of blood are typed and crossmatched for most patients with variceal bleeding. Volume status is assessed by central venous pressure measurements, urinary output, and a Swan-Ganz pulmonary artery catheter if necessary. If the prothrombin time is prolonged more than 3 seconds, fresh frozen plasma is a component of the resuscitation volume. Although moderate hypersplenism is a common accompaniment of portal hypertension, platelet transfusions are necessary only when the platelet count is less than 50,000 per mm^3.

Endoscopy to determine the cause of bleeding is performed as soon as the patient is stabilized. If a bleeding esophageal varix is observed or suspected because of an overlying clot, sclerotherapy or variceal ligation is performed during the initial endoscopy if the expertise is available. Endoscopic sclerotherapy is also effective for acutely bleeding PHG. Endoscopic variceal ligation and injection with cyanoacrylate (not available for use in the United States) have been shown to be efficacious for bleeding gastric varices.[14]

Because infections are common in patients with bleeding varices, prophylactic antibiotics are initiated. They have been shown to decrease the infection rate by more than 50%, decrease rebleeding, and improve survival.[15]

Randomized trials have shown that somatostatin and its longer-acting analogue octreotide are as efficacious as endoscopic treatment for control of acute variceal bleeding.[16] These splanchnic vasoconstrictors are associated with fewer adverse side effects than vasopressin, the mainstay for acute pharmacotherapy in the past. Because of their ease of administration and effectiveness, these newer drugs may return pharmacotherapy to a more central role in the treatment of acute portal hypertensive bleeding, especially when endoscopic treatment is unlikely to be effective (failed chronic endoscopic therapy, gastric varices, and PHG). Somatostatin is administered as a 250-μg intravenous (IV) bolus, followed by a continuous infusion of 250 μg/hour for 2 to 4 days. Octreotide is given as an IV bolus of 50 μg followed by an infusion of 25 to 50 μg/hour for a similar length of time. Because of the minimal adverse effects and ease of administration, octreotide is now commonly used as an adjunct to endoscopic therapy. The combination of octreotide and endoscopic therapy is more effective in controlling bleeding than octreotide alone and is the preferred treatment for most patients.[17] If vasopressin is used, it needs to be given as an initial bolus of 20 units over 20 minutes followed by an infusion of 0.2 to 0.4 units/minute. Because of the adverse systemic effects of vasopressin, nitroglycerine is simultaneously infused at an initial rate of 40 μg/minute and then titrated to achieve blood pressure control.

Balloon Tamponade

The major advantages of variceal tamponade with the Sengstaken-Blakemore tube are immediate cessation of bleeding in more than 85% of patients and widespread availability of this device, including small community hospitals (Fig. 53-4). Significant disadvantages of balloon tamponade are frequent recurrent hemorrhage in up to 50% of patients after balloon deflation, considerable discomfort for the patient, and a high incidence of serious

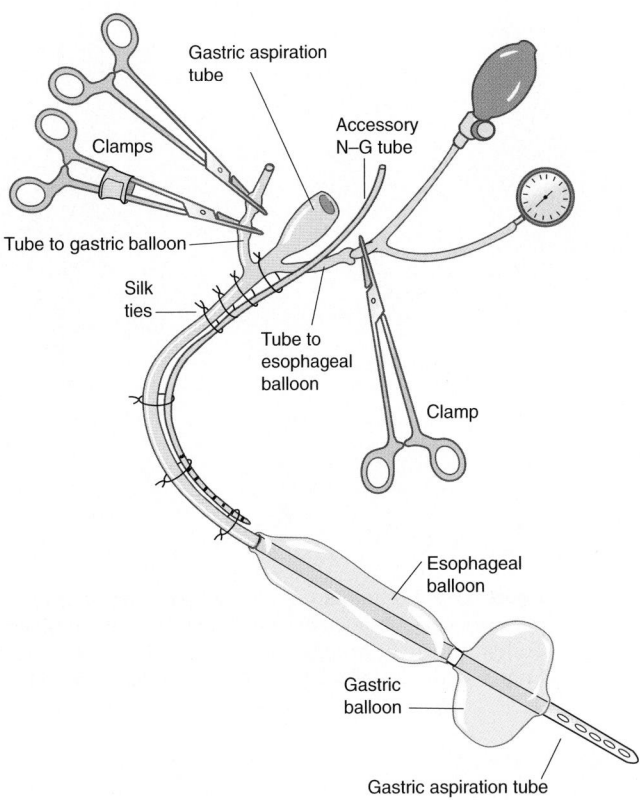

Figure 53-4 The modified Sengstaken-Blakemore tube. Note the accessory nasogastric (N-G) tube for suctioning of secretions above the esophageal balloon and the two clamps, one secured with tape, to prevent inadvertent decompression of the gastric balloon. (From Rikkers LF: Portal hypertension. In Goldsmith H [ed]: Practice of Surgery. Philadelphia, Harper & Row, 1981, pp 1-37.)

complications when the device is used by inexperienced personnel. The potentially lethal complications of esophageal perforation secondary to intraesophageal inflation of the gastric balloon, ischemic necrosis of the esophagus secondary to overinflation of the esophageal balloon, and aspiration can be avoided by using balloon tamponade only in an intensive care unit and adhering to a strict protocol. Patients in whom balloon tamponade is used have their airway controlled by endotracheal intubation. Controlled trials have demonstrated that balloon tamponade is as effective as pharmacotherapy and endoscopic therapy in controlling acute variceal bleeding.

Because of the effectiveness of endoscopic treatment and pharmacotherapy for acute variceal bleeding, balloon tamponade is infrequently required. It may be lifesaving, however, when exsanguinating hemorrhage prevents acute endoscopic treatment and in patients in whom sclerotherapy has failed and who do not respond to pharmacotherapy. Because balloon deflation is followed by a high rebleeding rate, definitive treatment, such as endoscopic therapy, TIPS, or operation, is planned for most patients in whom the Sengstaken-Blakemore tube is used.

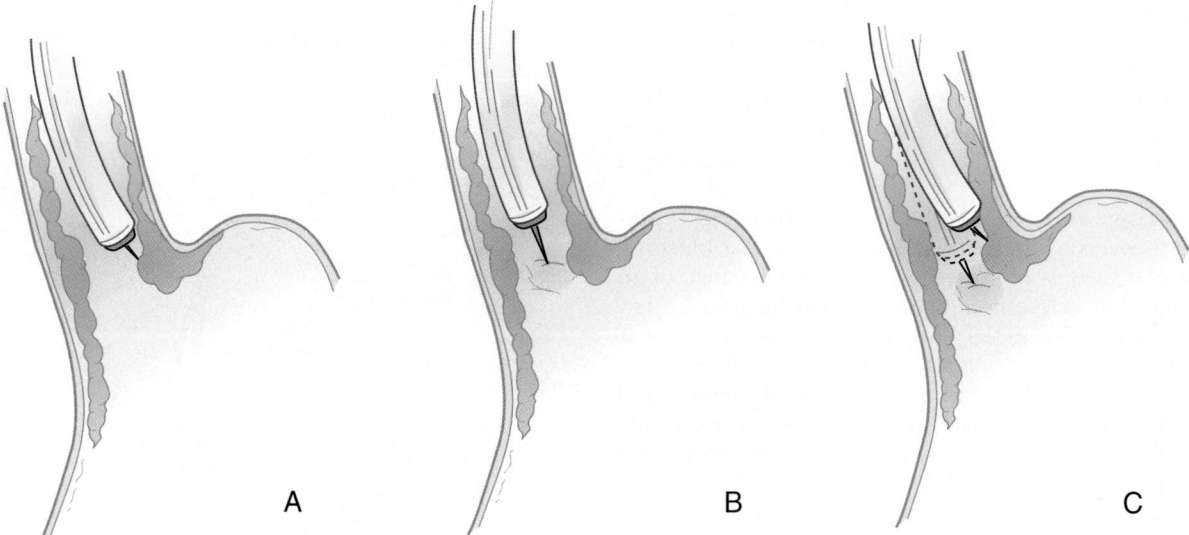

Figure 53-5 Techniques of endoscopic sclerotherapy. A flexible endoscope is used for intravariceal injection (**A**), paravariceal (submucosal) injection (**B**), and combined paravariceal and intravariceal injection (**C**). (Modified from Terblanche J, Burroughs AK, Hobbs EF: Controversies in the management of bleeding esophageal varices. N Engl J Med 320:1393-1398, 1989. Copyright 1989 Massachusetts Medical Society. All rights reserved.)

Endoscopic Treatment

Endoscopic treatment (variceal sclerosis or ligation) is the most commonly used therapy for both management of the acute bleeding episode and prevention of recurrent hemorrhage. In the acute setting, sclerotherapy and band ligation have been shown to be equally efficacious. Ligation is associated with fewer complications, but it is more difficult to do in the acutely bleeding patient. Both techniques require a skilled endoscopist and stop the bleeding in 80% to 90% of patients.[18]

Both intravariceal and paravariceal techniques of sclerosant injection are used, and often these two techniques are purposefully or inadvertently combined (Fig. 53-5). The most commonly used sclerosants in the United States are sodium morrhuate and sodium tetradecyl sulfate.

When experienced personnel are available, the initial sclerotherapy injections can often be done during the endoscopy, at which diagnosis of variceal bleeding is made. Each varix is usually injected with 1 to 2 mL of sclerosant just above the esophagogastric junction and 5 cm proximal to it. Alternatively, each varix can be ligated with a rubber band, as shown in Figure 53-6. A subsequent treatment session is planned for 4 to 6 days later. Additional endoscopic treatments depend on the effectiveness of the initial treatments in controlling bleeding and on whether endoscopic therapy has been selected as definitive treatment for that patient.

Minor complications of sclerotherapy, including retrosternal chest pain, esophageal ulceration, and fever, occur commonly. More serious complications, which account for the 1% to 3% mortality rate of this procedure, are esophageal perforation, worsening of variceal hemorrhage, and aspiration pneumonitis. Failure of endoscopic

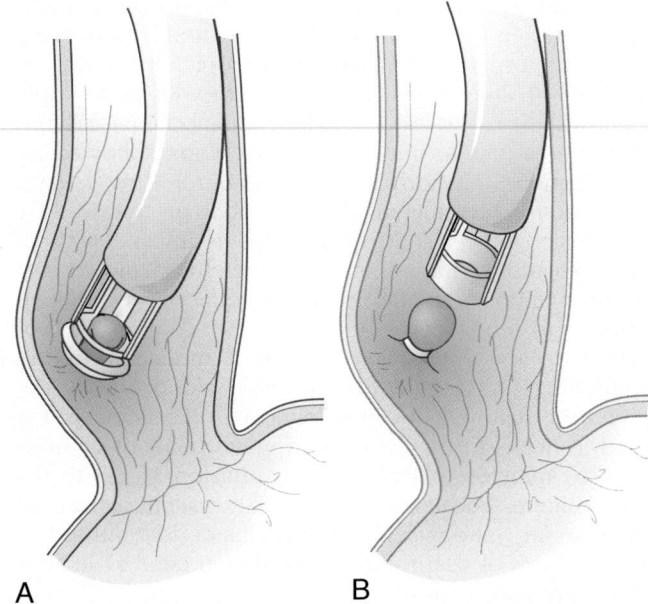

Figure 53-6 Endoscopic ligation of esophageal varices. **A,** The varix is drawn into the ligator by suction. **B,** An O-ring is applied. (From Turcotte JG, Roger SE, Eckhauser FE: Portal hypertension. In Greenfield LJ, Mulholland MW, Oldham KT [eds]: Surgery: Scientific Principles and Practice. Philadelphia, JB Lippincott, 1993, p 899.)

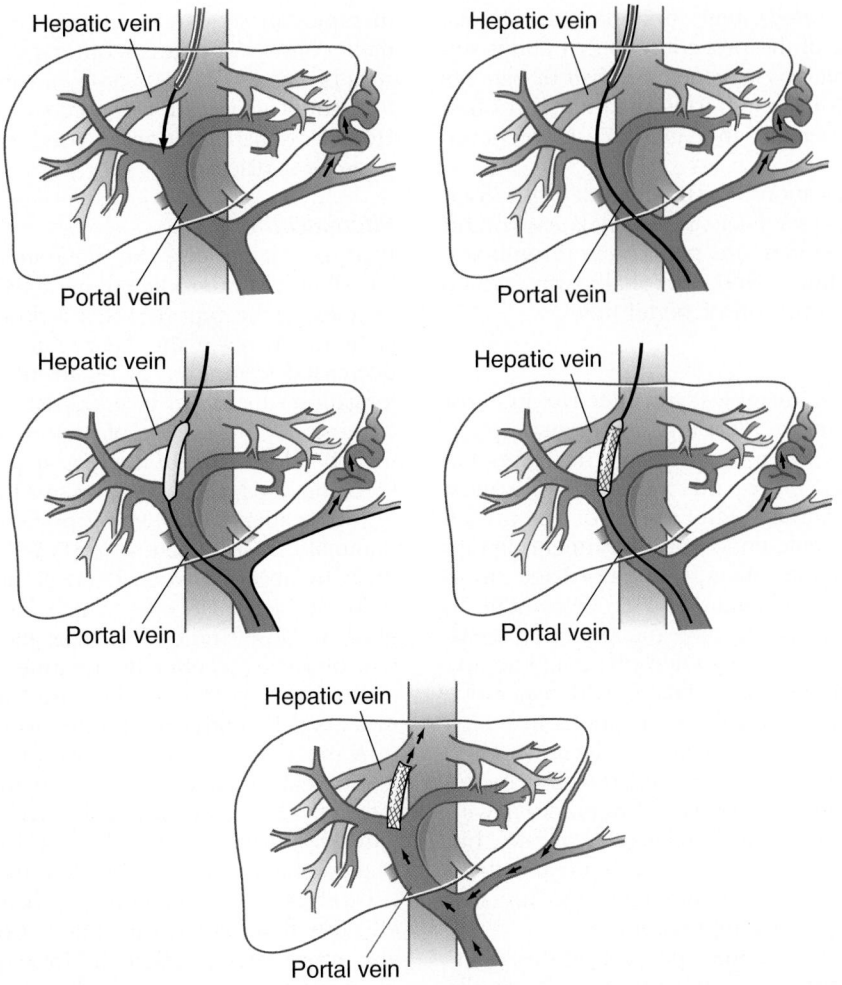

Figure 53-7 Transjugular intrahepatic portosystemic shunt. A needle is advanced from a hepatic vein to a major portal vein branch *(top left)* and a guidewire is placed *(top right)*. A hepatic parenchymal tract is created by balloon dilation *(middle left)*, and an expandable metal stent is placed *(middle right)*, thereby creating the shunt *(bottom)*. (From Zemel G, Katzen BT, Becker GJ, et al: Percutaneous transjugular portosystemic shunt. JAMA 266:390, 1991. Copyright 1991, American Medical Association.)

treatment is declared when two sessions fail to control hemorrhage. Unless urgent surgery is performed in such patients, the mortality rate exceeds 60%.

Transjugular Intrahepatic Portosystemic Shunt

TIPS is a technique that accomplishes portal decompression without an operation. Because of the complexity of the procedure, an experienced interventional radiologist is required. Access is gained to a major intrahepatic portal venous branch by puncture through a hepatic vein. A parenchymal tract between hepatic and portal veins is then created with a balloon catheter, and a 10-mm expandable metal stent is inserted, thereby creating the shunt (Fig. 53-7).

In large series, the success rate of TIPS has been more than 95%, but experience with this technique is limited in acutely bleeding patients, who generally make up only a small fraction of patients receiving TIPS. At the present time, TIPS is not recommended as initial therapy for acute

variceal hemorrhage but is used only after less invasive treatments, such as endoscopic therapy and pharmacotherapy, have failed to control bleeding. TIPS is effective in stopping bleeding in this setting.[19] Mortality is related to the status of hepatic function.

One clear indication for TIPS is as a short-term bridge to liver transplantation for patients in whom endoscopic treatment has failed. In addition to controlling bleeding, advantages in this situation are that the lower portal pressure may make the transplantation operation easier and that the shunt is removed when the recipient liver is excised. Patients with advanced hepatic functional decompensation (Child's class C), even those who are not transplantation candidates, are better served by TIPS than by an emergency operation when less invasive approaches fail to control bleeding.

Hemodynamic studies suggest that TIPS is a nonselective shunt, and several investigations have demonstrated a similar frequency of encephalopathy after TIPS as has been previously reported after nonselective shunts. Another disadvantage of the procedure is that shunt stenosis or occlusion develops in as many as half of patients within 1 year of TIPS insertion. This situation can often be remedied by repeated angiographic intervention, however.

Absolute contraindications to TIPS include right-sided heart failure and polycystic liver disease. Relative contraindications to the procedure are portal vein thrombosis, hypervascular liver tumors, and encephalopathy, which can be worsened by diversion of portal flow.

Emergency Surgery

Although nonoperative therapies are effective in most patients with acute variceal bleeding, emergency operation is promptly done when less invasive measures fail to control hemorrhage or are not indicated. The most common situations requiring either urgent or emergency surgery are failure of acute endoscopic treatment, failure of long-term endoscopic therapy, hemorrhage from gastric varices or PHG, and failure of TIPS placement. In most institutions, TIPS has become the preferred treatment for acute variceal bleeding when pharmacotherapy and endoscopic treatment have failed, with operative procedures being reserved for those situations in which TIPS is not indicated or not available. Selection of the appropriate emergency operation is guided mainly by the experience of the surgeon. Esophageal transection with a stapling device is rapid and relatively simple, but rebleeding rates after this procedure are high, and there is little evidence that operative mortality rates are less than after surgical portal decompression.

A commonly performed shunt operation in the emergency setting is the portacaval shunt because it rapidly and effectively decompresses the portal venous circulation. Impressive results have been achieved by Orloff,[20] but not by others, when the emergency portacaval shunt is used as routine therapy for acute variceal bleeding. In patients who are not actively bleeding at the time of surgery and in those in whom bleeding is temporarily controlled by pharmacotherapy or balloon tamponade, a more complex operation, such as the distal splenorenal shunt, may be appropriate. The major disadvantage of emergency surgery is that operative mortality rates exceed 25% in most reported series. Early postoperative mortality is usually related to the status of hepatic functional reserve rather than to the type of emergency operation selected.

Prevention of Recurrent Hemorrhage

After a patient has bled from varices, the likelihood of a repeat episode exceeds 70%. Because most patients with variceal hemorrhage have chronic liver disease, the challenge of long-term management is both prevention of recurrent bleeding and maintenance of satisfactory hepatic function. Options available for definitive treatment include pharmacotherapy, chronic endoscopic treatment, TIPS, three hemodynamic types of shunt operations (nonselective, selective, and partial), a variety of nonshunt procedures, and hepatic transplantation. The most effective treatment regimen usually uses two or more of these

therapies in sequence. In most institutions, initial treatment consists of pharmacotherapy or endoscopic therapy with portal decompression by means of TIPS or an operative shunt reserved for failures of first-line treatment. Hepatic transplantation is used for patients with end-stage liver disease.

Pharmacotherapy

Pharmacotherapy for the prevention of recurrent variceal bleeding was introduced in 1984 by Lebrec and colleagues,[21] who reported that a dose of propranolol sufficient to decrease the heart rate by 25% resulted in a decreased frequency of recurrent hemorrhage and prolongation of survival in good-risk patients with alcoholic cirrhosis. The objective of pharmacotherapy is to reduce the HVWP below 12 mm Hg, a level at which variceal bleeding does not occur. Invasive hemodynamic monitoring of patients taking propranolol has demonstrated minimal or no reduction of HVWP in many patients and no correlation between decrease in portal pressure and reduction in pulse rate, which has been the parameter used in most studies to assess therapeutic effect. Thus, two obstacles to effective treatment with drugs are variability of response to the drug and lack of an easily measured hemodynamic index to monitor therapy.

A meta-analysis of controlled trials of nonselective β-adrenergic blockade has shown that this treatment significantly decreases the likelihood of recurrent hemorrhage and demonstrates a trend toward decreased mortality.[22] The combination of a β-blocker and a long-acting nitrate (isosorbide 5-mononitrate) has been shown to be more effective than variceal ligation.[23] Combination therapy is also more effective than β-blockade alone.[24] Long-term pharmacotherapy is used only in compliant patients who are observed closely by their physicians. Although an attractive approach because of its noninvasiveness, pharmacotherapy, like endoscopic therapy, is associated with a high incidence of rebleeding.

Endoscopic Therapy

Since the late 1970s, chronic endoscopic therapy has become the most common treatment for prevention of recurrent variceal hemorrhage. The increasing popularity of endoscopic treatment can be attributed to several factors:

1. Several gastroenterologists and surgeons have expressed disenchantment with shunt surgery.
2. Endoscopic therapy is less invasive than surgery.
3. There are no adverse hemodynamic effects of endoscopic therapy.
4. Endoscopic treatment can be administered by gastroenterologists to whom most patients are initially referred.
5. Several controlled trials have confirmed its therapeutic efficacy.

The objective of chronic endoscopic therapy is to eradicate esophageal varices (see Figs. 53-5 and 53-6). Although the timing of repeat sessions varies from series to series, variceal eradication is usually successful in about two thirds of patients. After eradication is achieved, diagnostic endoscopy is performed at 6-month to 1-year intervals because varices do recur and can bleed. Some investigators have noted an increased frequency of bleeding from gastric varices and PHG after eradication of esophageal varices.

Several controlled trials and a meta-analysis comparing endoscopic sclerotherapy to variceal ligation have shown a significant advantage to the latter technique.[25] Complications are less frequent after variceal ligation, and fewer treatment sessions are required to eradicate varices (see Fig. 53-6). Additionally, rebleeding and mortality rates appear to be lower after variceal ligation. The combination of variceal ligation and pharmacotherapy with nonselective β-blockade is more effective than variceal ligation alone.[26]

Several controlled trials comparing chronic endoscopic therapy to conventional medical management have been completed.[27] Although fewer patients receiving endoscopic treatment than medical treatment experienced rebleeding in all of the investigations, recurrent bleeding still occurred in about half of endoscopic therapy patients. Rebleeding is most frequent during the initial year, and the rebleeding rate decreases by about 15% per year thereafter. Although a single episode of recurrent hemorrhage does not signify failure of therapy, uncontrolled hemorrhage, multiple major episodes of rebleeding, and hemorrhage from gastric varices and PHG all require that endoscopic therapy be abandoned and another treatment modality substituted. Endoscopic treatment failure secondary to rebleeding occurs in as many as one third of patients. Thus, chronic endoscopic therapy is a rational initial treatment for many patients who bleed from esophageal varices, but subsequent treatment with TIPS, a shunt procedure, a nonshunt operation, or hepatic transplantation is anticipated for a significant percentage of patients. Because of its relatively high failure rate, a course of chronic endoscopic therapy is not undertaken for noncompliant patients and those living a long distance from advanced medical care.

Transjugular Intrahepatic Portosystemic Shunt

TIPS is being increasingly used as a definitive treatment for patients who bleed from portal hypertension (see Fig. 53-7). A major limitation of TIPS, however, is a high incidence (up to 50%) of shunt stenosis or shunt thrombosis within the first year. Shunt stenosis, which is usually secondary to neointimal hyperplasia, is more common than thrombosis and can often be resolved by balloon dilation of the TIPS or, in some cases, by placement of a second shunt. Total shunt occlusion occurs in 10% to 15% of patients. Both shunt stenosis and shunt thrombosis are often followed by recurrent portal hypertensive bleeding. TIPS stenosis and occlusion may become less frequent as TIPS technology improves (e.g., covered stents).

Angiographic and Doppler ultrasound studies suggest that TIPS, when it effectively decompresses varices, is a nonselective shunt and completely diverts portal flow. Clinical evidence of the nonselectivity of TIPS is its effectiveness in resolving medically intractable ascites

and a fairly high frequency of post-TIPS encephalopathy (~30%).[28]

TIPS has been compared to chronic endoscopic therapy in 11 randomized controlled trials.[28] Fewer patients rebled after TIPS (19%) than after endoscopic treatment (47%), but encephalopathy was significantly more common in TIPS patients (34%). TIPS dysfunction developed in 50% of patients. The major advantage of TIPS is that it is nonoperative. Because of this, it would appear to be the ideal therapy when only short-term portal decompression is required. Thus, liver transplantation candidates who fail endoscopic or pharmacotherapy are well suited for TIPS followed by transplantation when a donor organ becomes available. The patient is protected from bleeding in the interim, and the transplantation procedure may also be facilitated by the lower portal pressure. Another group of patients in whom TIPS may be advantageous includes those with advanced hepatic functional decompensation who are unlikely to survive long enough for the TIPS to malfunction. Because it functions as a side-to-side portosystemic shunt, TIPS is also effective in the treatment of medically intractable ascites.

Portosystemic Shunts

Portosystemic shunts are clearly the most effective means of preventing recurrent hemorrhage in patients with portal hypertension. These procedures are effective because they all, to some degree, decompress the portal venous system by shunting portal flow into the low-pressure systemic venous system. Diversion of portal blood, however, which contains hepatotropic hormones, nutrients, and cerebral toxins, is also responsible for the adverse consequences of shunt operations, namely portosystemic encephalopathy and accelerated hepatic failure. Depending on whether they completely decompress, compartmentalize, or partially decompress the portal venous circulation, portosystemic shunts can be classified as nonselective, selective, or partial. In addition to variceal decompression, the goal of selective and partial portosystemic shunts is preservation of hepatic portal perfusion, thereby preventing or minimizing the adverse consequences of these procedures.

Nonselective Shunts Commonly used varieties of nonselective shunts, all of which completely divert portal flow, include the end-to-side portacaval shunt (Eck fistula), the side-to-side portacaval shunt, large-diameter interposition shunts, and the conventional splenorenal shunt (Fig. 53-8). The end-to-side portacaval shunt is the prototype of nonselective shunts and is the only shunt procedure that has been compared to conventional medical management in randomized, controlled trials.[27] Figure 53-9 combines survival data from the four controlled investigations of the therapeutic portacaval shunt (performed in patients with prior variceal hemorrhage). The most common causes of death in medically treated and shunted patients were rebleeding and accelerated hepatic failure, respectively. Although no survival advantage could be demonstrated for shunt patients, all of these studies had a crossover bias in favor of medically treated patients, several of whom received a shunt when they developed

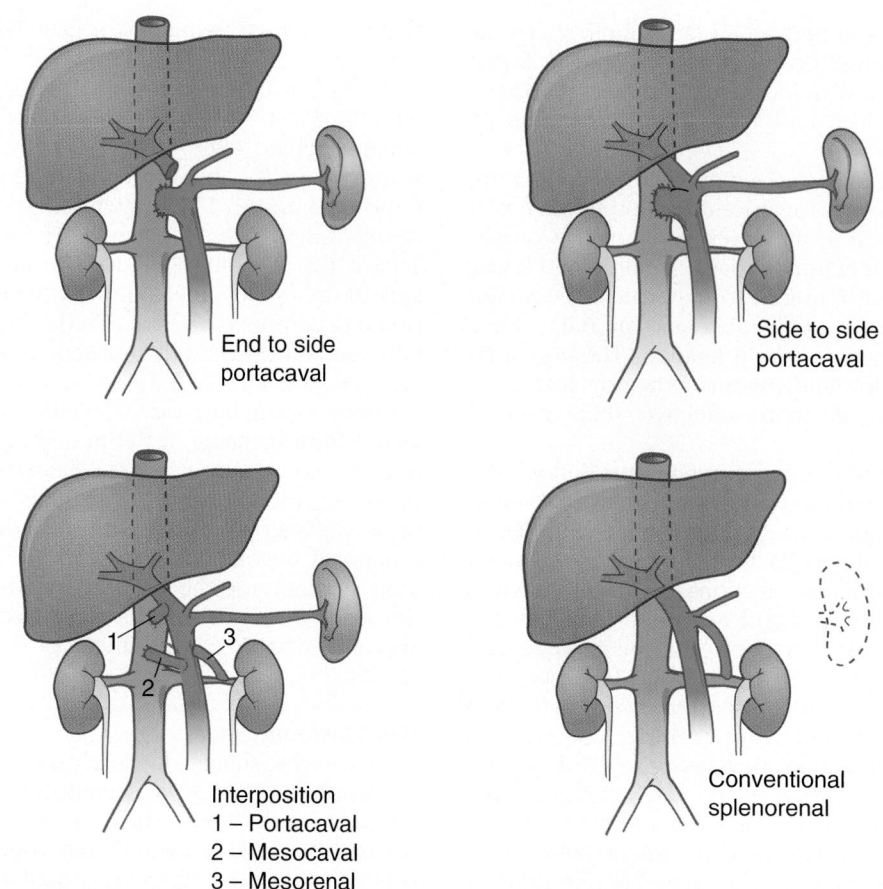

End to side
portacaval

Side to side
portacaval

Interposition
1 – Portacaval
2 – Mesocaval
3 – Mesorenal

Conventional
splenorenal

Figure 53-8 Nonselective shunts completely divert portal blood flow away from the liver. (From Rikkers LF: Portal hypertension. In Moody FG [ed]: Surgical Treatment of Digestive Disease. Chicago, Year Book Medical, 1986, pp 409-424.)

intractable recurrent variceal hemorrhage. In addition, nearly all of the trial patients had alcoholic cirrhosis; therefore, these results do not necessarily apply to other causes of portal hypertension. Other important findings of these randomized trials include reliable control of bleeding in shunted patients, variceal rebleeding in more than 70% of medically treated patients, and spontaneous, often severe, encephalopathy in 20% to 40% of shunted patients.

All of the other nonselective shunts in Figure 53-8 maintain continuity of the portal vein, thereby connecting the portal and systemic venous systems in a side-to-side fashion. Therefore, these procedures decompress both the splanchnic venous circulation and the intrahepatic sinusoidal network. Because the liver and intestines are both important contributors to ascites formation, side-to-side portosystemic shunts are the most effective shunt procedures for relieving ascites as well as preventing recurrent variceal bleeding. Because they completely divert portal flow like the end-to-side portacaval shunt, however, side-to-side shunts also accelerate hepatic failure and lead to frequent postshunt encephalopathy.

Synthetic grafts or autogenous vein may be interposed between the portal and systemic venous circulations at a variety of locations (see Fig. 53-8). A major disadvantage

of prosthetic interposition shunts is a high graft thrombosis rate that approaches 35% during the late postoperative interval. This problem can be avoided by using autogenous vein (internal jugular vein) rather than a prosthetic graft. On the other hand, advantages of these shunts are that they are relatively easy to construct; the hepatic hilum is avoided, thereby making subsequent liver transplantation less complicated; and they can be easily occluded if intractable postshunt encephalopathy develops.

The conventional splenorenal shunt consists of anastomosis of the proximal splenic vein to the renal vein. Splenectomy is also done. Because the smaller proximal rather than the larger distal end of the splenic vein is used, shunt thrombosis is more common after this procedure than after the distal splenorenal shunt. Although early series noted that postshunt encephalopathy was less common after the conventional splenorenal shunt than after the portacaval shunt, subsequent analyses have suggested that this low frequency of encephalopathy was probably a result of restoration of hepatic portal perfusion after shunt thrombosis developed in many patients. A conventional splenorenal shunt that is of sufficient caliber to remain patent gradually dilates and eventually causes complete portal decompression and portal flow

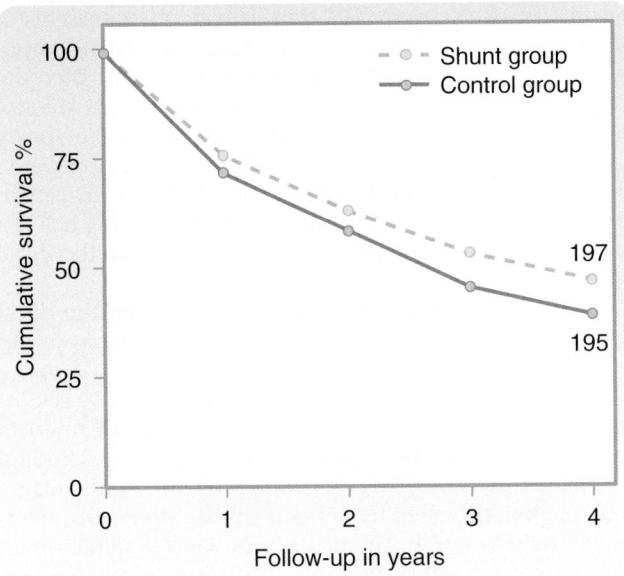

Figure 53-9 Cumulative survival data from four controlled trials of the portacaval shunt versus conventional medical management. (From Boyer TD: Portal hypertension and its complications: Bleeding esophageal varices, ascites, and spontaneous bacterial peritonitis. In Zakim D, Boyer TD [eds]: Hepatology: A Textbook of Liver Disease. Philadelphia, WB Saunders, 1982, pp 464-499.)

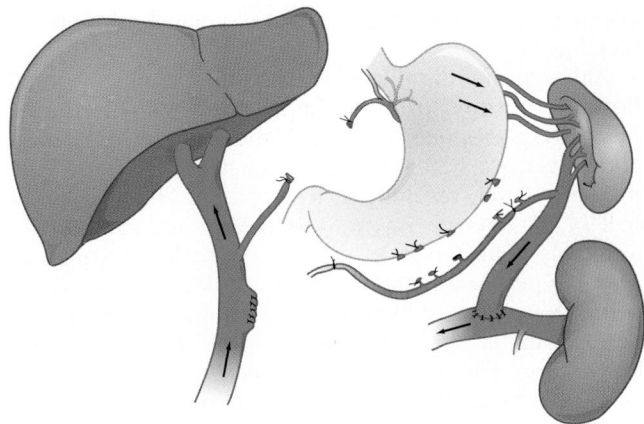

Figure 53-10 The distal splenorenal shunt provides selective variceal decompression through the short gastric veins, spleen, and splenic vein to the left renal vein. Hepatic portal perfusion is maintained by interrupting the umbilical vein, coronary vein, gastroepiploic vein, and any other prominent collaterals. (From Salam AA: Distal splenorenal shunts: Hemodynamics of total versus selective shunting. In Baker RJ, Fischer JE [eds]: Mastery of Surgery. 4th ed. Philadelphia, Lippincott Williams & Wilkins, 2001, pp 1357-1366.)

diversion. A purported advantage of the procedure is that hypersplenism is eliminated by splenectomy. The thrombocytopenia and leukopenia that accompany portal hypertension, however, are rarely of clinical significance, making splenectomy an unnecessary procedure in most patients.

In summary, nonselective shunts effectively decompress varices. Because of complete portal flow diversion, however, they are complicated by frequent postoperative encephalopathy and accelerated hepatic failure. Side-to-side nonselective shunts effectively relieve ascites and prevent variceal hemorrhage. Presently, nonselective shunts are only rarely indicated. TIPS (also a nonselective shunt) is the preferred therapy for most situations in which nonselective shunts were previously utilized (e.g., patients with both variceal bleeding and medically intractable ascites). Generally, a nonselective shunt is constructed only when a TIPS cannot be done or fails.

Selective Shunts The hemodynamic and clinical shortcomings of nonselective shunts stimulated development of the concept of selective variceal decompression. In 1967, Warren and colleagues introduced the distal splenorenal shunt; and in the following year, Inokuchi and associates[29] reported their initial results with the left gastric–vena caval shunt. The latter procedure consists of interposition of a vein graft between the left gastric (coronary) vein and the inferior vena cava and, thus, directly and selectively decompresses esophagogastric varices. Only a minority of patients with portal hypertension, however, have appropriate anatomy for this operation; experience with it has been limited to Japan, and no controlled trials have been conducted.

The distal splenorenal shunt consists of anastomosis of the distal end of the splenic vein to the left renal vein and interruption of all collateral vessels, such as the coronary and gastroepiploic veins, connecting the superior mesenteric and gastrosplenic components of the splanchnic venous circulation (Fig. 53-10). This results in separation of the portal venous circulation into a decompressed gastrosplenic venous circuit and a high-pressure superior mesenteric venous system that continues to perfuse the liver. Although the procedure is technically demanding, it can be mastered by most well-trained surgeons who are knowledgeable in the principles of vascular surgery.

Not all patients are candidates for the distal splenorenal shunt. Because sinusoidal and mesenteric hypertension is maintained and important lymphatic pathways are transected during dissection of the left renal vein, the distal splenorenal shunt tends to aggravate rather than relieve ascites. Thus, patients with medically intractable ascites do not undergo this procedure. However, the larger population of patients who develop transient ascites after resuscitation from a variceal hemorrhage are candidates for a selective shunt. Another contraindication to a distal splenorenal shunt is prior splenectomy. A splenic vein diameter of less than 7 mm is a relative contraindication to the procedure because the incidence of shunt thrombosis is high when using a small-diameter vein.

Although selective variceal decompression is a sound physiologic concept, the distal splenorenal shunt remains controversial after an extensive clinical experience spanning almost 40 years.[30,31] The key questions regarding this procedure are, How effective is it in preserving hepatic portal perfusion? Is it superior to nonselective shunts with respect to duration or quality of survival? Is it more effective than TIPS for long-term control of variceal bleeding?

Although the distal splenorenal shunt results in portal flow preservation in more than 85% of patients during the early postoperative interval, the high-pressure mesenteric venous system gradually collateralizes to the low-pressure shunt, resulting in loss of portal flow in about half of patients by 1 year. The degree and duration of portal flow preservation depend on both the cause of portal hypertension and the technical details of the operation (extent to which mesenteric and gastrosplenic venous circulations are separated). Henderson and coworkers[32] have shown that portal flow is maintained in most patients with nonalcoholic cirrhosis and noncirrhotic portal hypertension (e.g., portal vein thrombosis). In contrast, portal flow rapidly collateralizes to the shunt in patients with alcoholic cirrhosis.

Modification of the distal splenorenal shunt by purposeful or inadvertent omission of coronary vein ligation results in early loss of portal flow. Even when all major collateral vessels are interrupted, portal flow may be gradually diverted through a pancreatic collateral network (pancreatic siphon). This pathway can be discouraged by dissecting the full length of the splenic vein from the pancreas (splenopancreatic disconnection), which results in better preservation of hepatic portal perfusion, especially in patients with alcoholic cirrhosis. However, this extension of the procedure makes it technically more challenging, which may be a significant disadvantage in an era when fewer shunts are being done because of increased use of endoscopic therapy, TIPS, and hepatic transplantation.

Six of the seven controlled comparisons of the distal splenorenal shunt to nonselective shunts have included predominantly alcoholic cirrhotic patients.[27,31] None of these trials has demonstrated an advantage to either procedure with respect to long-term survival. Three of the studies have found a lower frequency of encephalopathy after the distal splenorenal shunt, whereas the other trials have shown no difference in the incidence of this postoperative complication. In contrast to survival, encephalopathy is a subjective end point that was assessed with a variety of methods in the different trials. Another important end point in comparing treatments for variceal hemorrhage is the effectiveness with which recurrent bleeding is prevented. In nearly all uncontrolled and controlled series of the distal splenorenal shunt, this procedure has been equivalent to nonselective shunts in preventing recurrent hemorrhage. Mainly because of these inconsistent results of the controlled trials, there is no consensus as to which shunting procedure is superior in patients with alcoholic cirrhosis. Because the quality of life (encephalopathy rate) was significantly better in the distal splenorenal shunt group in three of the trials, however, there appears to be an advantage to selective variceal decompression even in this population.[33]

Considerably fewer data are available regarding selective shunting in nonalcoholic cirrhosis and in noncirrhotic portal hypertension. Because hepatic portal perfusion after the distal splenorenal shunt is better preserved in these disease categories, one might expect improved results. A single controlled trial in patients with schistosomiasis (presinusoidal portal hypertension) demonstrated a lower frequency of encephalopathy after the distal splenorenal shunt than after a conventional splenorenal shunt (nonselective).[34] The large Emory University series of the distal splenorenal shunt has demonstrated better survival in patients with nonalcoholic cirrhosis than in those with alcoholic cirrhosis.[30] However, this has not been a consistent finding in all centers in which the distal splenorenal shunt is performed.

Several controlled trials have also compared the distal splenorenal shunt with chronic endoscopic therapy.[35] In these investigations, recurrent hemorrhage was more effectively prevented by selective shunting than by sclerotherapy, but hepatic portal perfusion was maintained in a significantly higher fraction of patients undergoing sclerotherapy. Despite this hemodynamic advantage, encephalopathy rates have been similar after both therapies. The two North American trials were dissimilar with respect to the effect of these treatments on long-term survival. Sclerotherapy with surgical rescue for the one third of sclerotherapy failures resulted in significantly better survival than selective shunt alone in one study.[36] In this investigation, 85% of sclerotherapy failures could be salvaged by surgery.

In contrast, a similar investigation conducted in a sparsely populated area (Intermountain West and Plains) showed superior survival after the distal splenorenal shunt.[37] Only 31% of sclerotherapy failures could be salvaged by surgery in this trial. The survival results of these two studies suggest that endoscopic therapy is a rational, initial treatment for patients who bleed from varices if sclerotherapy failure is recognized and such patients promptly undergo surgery or TIPS. However, patients living in remote areas are less likely to be salvaged by shunt surgery when endoscopic treatment fails, and a selective shunt may be preferable initial treatment for such patients.

In a nonrandomized comparison to TIPS, the distal splenorenal shunt had lower rates of recurrent bleeding, encephalopathy, and shunt thrombosis.[38] Ascites was less prevalent after TIPS. A multicenter randomized trial comparing TIPS and the distal splenorenal shunt for the elective treatment of variceal bleeding in good-risk cirrhotic patients showed generally equivalent results for these two procedures.[39] Rebleeding rates were not significantly different between the distal splenorenal shunt (6%) and TIPS (11%), but this represents the lowest reported rate of rebleeding following TIPS, likely secondary to the meticulous surveillance of TIPS patency by duplex ultrasound and angiography. Frequent reintervention in TIPS patients (82% compared with 11% for distal splenorenal shunt patients) was necessary to achieve these results. In this trial, postshunt encephalopathy and survival were similar after the two procedures.

Partial Shunts The objectives of partial and selective shunts are the same:

1. Effective decompression of varices
2. Preservation of hepatic portal perfusion
3. Maintenance of some residual portal hypertension

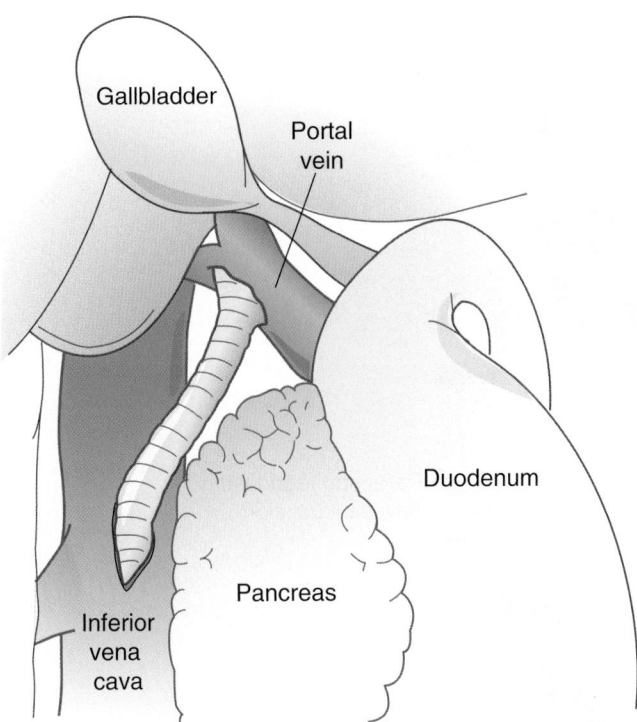

Initial attempts at partial shunting consisted of small-diameter vein-to-vein anastomoses, but these generally either thrombosed or dilated with time, thereby becoming nonselective shunts.

More recently, a small-diameter interposition portacaval shunt using a polytetrafluoroethylene graft, combined with ligation of the coronary vein and other collateral vessels, has been described (Fig. 53-11). When the prosthetic graft is 10 mm or less in diameter, hepatic portal perfusion is preserved in most patients, at least during the early postoperative interval.[40] Early experience with this small-diameter prosthetic shunt is that fewer than 15% of shunts have thrombosed, and most of these have been successfully opened by interventional radiologic techniques. A prospective randomized trial of partial (8 mm in diameter) and nonselective (16 mm in diameter) interposition portacaval shunts has shown a lower frequency of encephalopathy after the partial shunt but similar survival after both types of shunts.[41] The number of patients included in this investigation was small, however, and further trials need to be done to confirm this finding. In another controlled trial, the small-diameter interposition shunt was discovered to have a lower overall failure rate than TIPS.[42]

Nonshunt Operations

The objectives of these procedures are either ablation of varices or, more commonly, extensive interruption of collateral vessels connecting the high-pressure portal venous system with the varices. One exception is splenectomy, which is effective in left-sided portal hypertension caused by splenic vein thrombosis.

The simplest nonshunt operation is transection and reanastomosis of the distal esophagus with a stapling device. This operation, which has generally been used in the emergency setting, is frequently followed by recurrent hemorrhage. The most effective nonshunt operation is extensive esophagogastric devascularization combined with esophageal transection and splenectomy (Fig. 53-12). The Sugiura procedure preserves the coronary and paraesophageal veins to maintain a portosystemic collateral pathway and thus discourage re-formation of varices. In Japan, the results with this operation have been excellent, with rebleeding rates of less than 10%.[43] Extensive devascularization procedures, however, have generally been less successful in North American patients with alcoholic cirrhosis. Long-term follow-up in American series has revealed rebleeding rates of 35% to 55%, which are similar to the endoscopic therapy experience.[44] In many centers, esophagogastric devascularization procedures are mainly used for unshuntable patients with diffuse splanchnic venous thrombosis and for patients with distal splenorenal shunt thrombosis.

Hepatic Transplantation

Liver transplantation is not a treatment for variceal bleeding per se, but rather needs to be considered for all patients who present with end-stage hepatic failure whether or not it is accompanied by bleeding. Transplantation in patients who have bled secondary to portal hypertension is the only therapy that addresses the underlying liver disease in addition to providing reliable portal decompression. Because of economic factors and a limited supply of donor organs, liver transplantation is not available to all patients. Additionally, transplantation is not indicated for some of the more common causes of variceal bleeding, such as schistosomiasis (normal liver function) and active alcoholism (noncompliance).

There is accumulating evidence that variceal bleeders with well-compensated hepatic functional reserve (Child's class A and B+) are better served by nontransplantation strategies initially.[45,46] The first-line treatment for such patients is pharmacologic and endoscopic therapy, with portal decompression by means of an operative shunt or TIPS reserved for those who fail first-line therapy and for circumstances in which pharmacologic or endoscopic treatment would be risky (e.g., patients with gastric varices and those geographically separated from tertiary medical care).

Patients with variceal bleeding who are transplantation candidates include nonalcoholic cirrhotic patients and abstinent alcoholic cirrhotic patients with either limited hepatic functional reserve (Child's class B and C) or a poor quality of life secondary to their disease (e.g., encephalopathy, fatigue, or bone pain). In these patients, the acute hemorrhage is treated with endoscopic therapy and pharmacotherapy and the patient's transplantation candidacy immediately activated. If endoscopic treatment

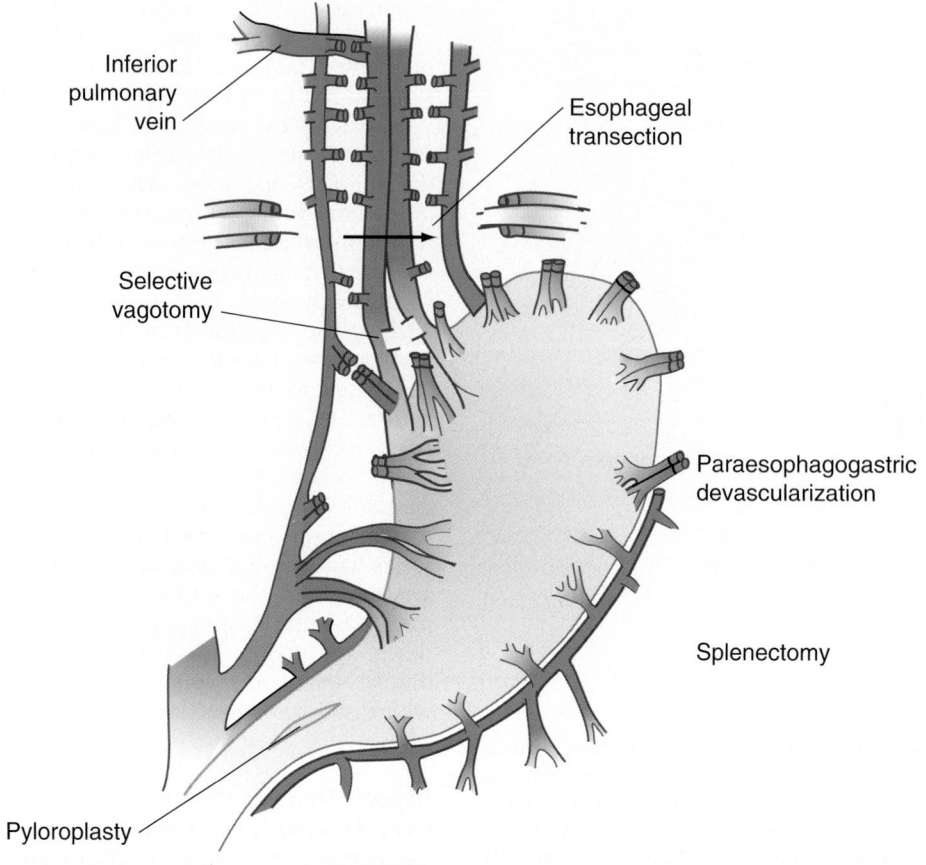

Inferior
pulmonary
vein

Esophageal
transection

Selective
vagotomy

Paraesophagogastric
devascularization

Splenectomy

Pyloroplasty

Figure 53-12 The Sugiura procedure combines esophageal transection, extensive esophagogastric devascularization, and splenectomy. The paraesophageal collateral vessels are preserved to discourage re-formation of varices. (Modified from Sugiura M, Futagawa S: Further evaluation of the Sugiura procedure in the treatment of esophageal varices. Arch Surg 112:1317, 1977. Copyright 1977, American Medical Association.)

and pharmocotherapy are ineffective, a TIPS is inserted as a short-term bridge to transplantation.

If a nontransplantation procedure (e.g., operative shunt or TIPS) is performed initially, these patients are carefully assessed at 6-month to 1-year intervals and hepatic transplantation considered when other complications of cirrhosis develop or hepatic functional decompensation is evident either clinically or by careful assessment with quantitative tests of liver function.

Overall Treatment Plan

An algorithm for definitive management of variceal hemorrhage is shown in Figure 53-13. Patients are first grouped according to their transplantation candidacy. This decision is based on multiple factors: etiology of portal hypertension, abstinence for alcoholic cirrhotic patients, the presence or absence of other diseases, and physiologic rather than chronologic age. Transplantation candidates with either decompensated hepatic function or a poor quality of life secondary to their liver disease undergo transplantation as soon as possible. Most future transplantation and nontransplantation candidates undergo initial endoscopic treatment, pharmacotherapy,

or both unless they bleed from gastric varices or PHG or live in remote geographic locations and have limited access to emergency tertiary care. Patients who live in remote locations and those who fail endoscopic and drug therapy receive a selective shunt or TIPS. A recent controlled trial has shown that if careful surveillance of TIPS patency and frequent TIPS reinterventions are done, these procedures are equally efficacious. Until improvements in TIPS technology (e.g., covered stents) are fully realized, the distal splenorenal shunt is likely to remain a more durable long-term solution and a reasonable alternative for TIPS failure.[47] However, TIPS is much more commonly done, and few surgeons who are experienced in shunt surgery remain. Therefore, it is likely that operative shunts will play an even lesser role in the management of variceal bleeding in the future than they do presently. Patients with medically intractable ascites in addition to variceal bleeding are best treated with TIPS when less invasive measures fail to control bleeding. If the TIPS eventually fails, an open side-to-side type shunt can then be constructed if the patient has reasonable hepatic function and is not a transplantation candidate. TIPS is clearly indicated for patients with endoscopic treatment failure who may require transplantation in the

DEFINITIVE THERAPY

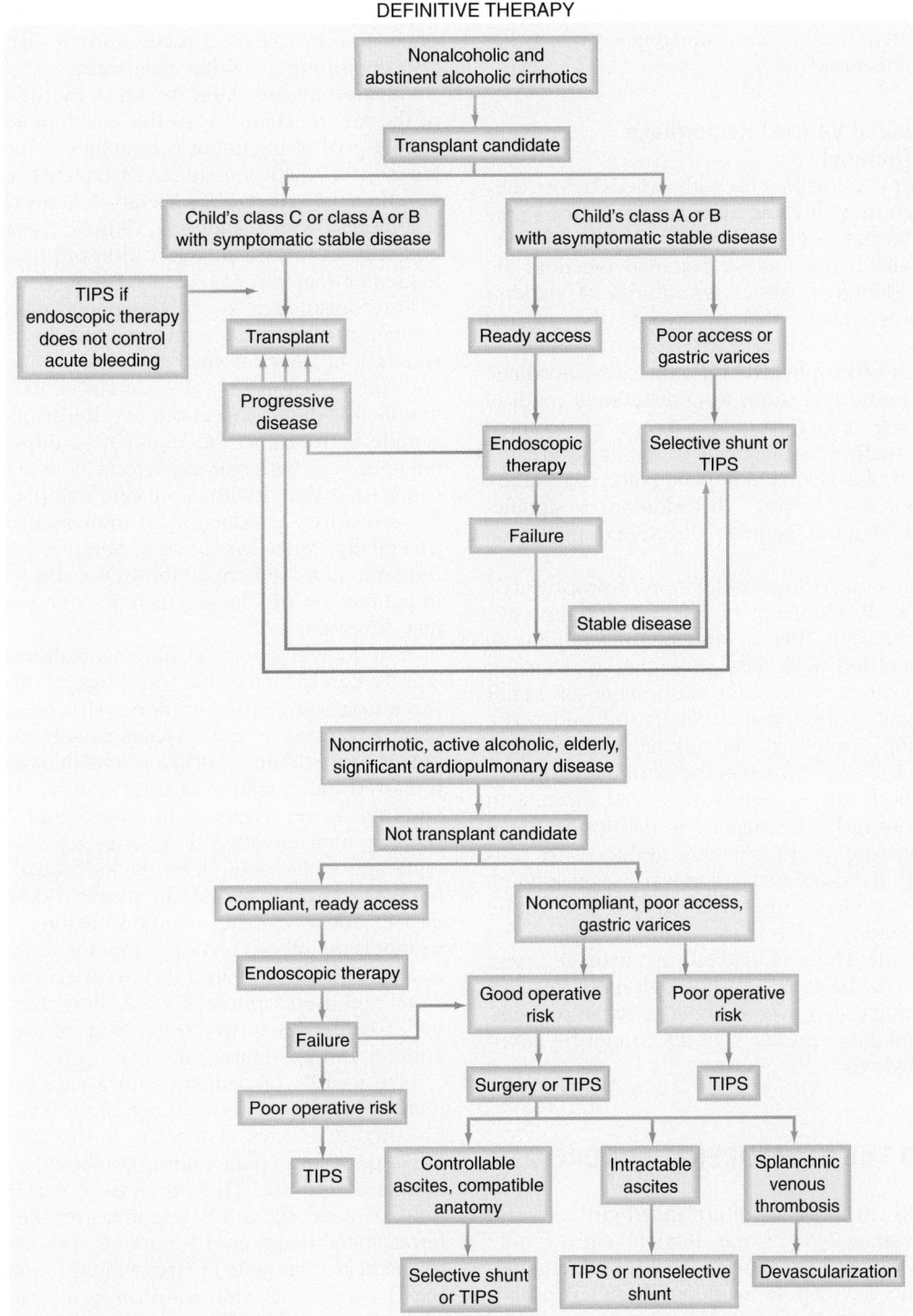

Figure 53-13 Algorithm for definitive therapy of variceal hemorrhage (see text). TIPS, transjugular intrahepatic portosystemic shunt. (Modified from Rikkers LF: Portal hypertension. In Levine BA, Copeland E, Howard R, et al [eds]: Current Practice of Surgery, Vol. 3. New York, Churchill Livingstone, 1995.)

near future and for nontransplantation candidates with advanced hepatic functional deterioration. Future transplantation candidates are carefully monitored so that they undergo transplantation at the appropriate time before they become poor operative risks.

The treatment algorithm for variceal bleeding has changed considerably since the 1970s, during which time endoscopic therapy, liver transplantation, and TIPS have become available to these patients. Nontransplantation operations are now necessary less frequently, the survival results are better because high operative risk patients are managed by other means, and emergency surgery has nearly been eliminated.[48]

Prevention of Initial Variceal Hemorrhage (Prophylactic Therapy)

The rationale for treating patients with varices before they bleed is the high mortality rate associated with the initial hemorrhage. Because only one third of patients with varices eventually bleed, unless potential bleeders are more reliably identified, about two thirds of patients undergoing prophylactic therapy would be treated unnecessarily.

The first trials of prophylaxis for variceal hemorrhage compared the portacaval shunt to conventional medical therapy. In these investigations, survival of shunted patients was actually less than that of medically treated patients because of accelerated hepatic failure secondary to complete portal diversion.[27] In addition, a significant fraction of shunted patients developed postshunt encephalopathy.

The major impetus for reconsideration of prophylactic therapy was the development of relatively noninvasive treatments (endoscopic therapy and pharmacotherapy), which are associated with less morbidity than major operative procedures, and the development of better methods to identify varices that are likely to bleed.[12] The gold standard for prophylactic therapy has become nonselective β-blockade.[12,27] This therapy is offered to most patients with moderate or large varices and those with small varices with red color signs. The risk for an initial variceal hemorrhage is significantly reduced by this approach, and in some trials, survival is prolonged. However, many patients may not tolerate β-blockade because of adverse side effects such as hypotension and sexual dysfunction. These individuals are managed with endoscopic variceal ligation that, although more invasive than pharmacotherapy, is even more effective in preventing an initial bleeding episode.[12,49] TIPS cannot be advocated for prophylaxis.[50]

ASCITES AND THE HEPATORENAL SYNDROME

Ascites is usually an indicator of advanced cirrhosis and is associated with a 2- to 5-year survival rate of only 50%.[51] Patients with ascites refractory to medical management, those who develop spontaneous bacterial peritonitis, and those who evolve to the hepatorenal syndrome have a particularly poor prognosis.

Portal hypertensive ascites is initiated by altered hepatic and splanchnic hemodynamics, which cause transudation of fluid into the interstitial space. When the rate of interstitial fluid formation exceeds the lymph drainage capacity, ascites accumulates. This pathophysiologic process results in an intravascular volume deficit, which initiates compensatory mechanisms such as aldosterone secretion, to restore plasma volume. Both the liver and intestines are important sites of ascites formation, and clinically significant ascites is rare in patients with extra-hepatic portal hypertension. The hypoalbuminemia that often accompanies advanced chronic liver disease may also contribute to ascites formation.

Because avid sodium retention by the kidneys is one of the key mechanisms in the development of ascites, a central goal of treatment is to achieve a negative sodium balance. A small percentage of patients with ascites can be effectively treated by dietary salt restriction and bed rest alone. More commonly, diuretic therapy is required and will resolve this complication of portal hypertension in greater than 90% of patients. Because secondary hyperaldosteronism is a key pathogenetic mechanism in the formation of ascites, a rational first-line diuretic is spironolactone. A combination of salt restriction (2 g/day) and spironolactone in a dose of 100 to 400 mg/day results in effective diuresis in about two thirds of patients. Furosemide is added to the regimen in those patients who fail to diurese with spironolactone alone. Diuretic therapy can be associated with significant complications because it can lead to a reduction in intravascular volume and, potentially, renal dysfunction. Serum electrolytes, blood urea nitrogen, and creatinine values are followed closely in patients on diuretics, which are discontinued if azotemia develops.

As a general guideline, patients with new-onset ascites that is barely detectable on physical examination are placed on salt restriction alone. However, patients with more advanced or tense ascites usually require the combination of sodium restriction and diuretic therapy. The preferred initial spironolactone dose is 100 mg per day, and this can be advanced to a maximum dose of 400 mg per day until effective diuresis is achieved. If treatment with spironolactone alone is ineffective or results in hyperkalemia, furosemide in an initial dose of 40 mg per day is added to the regimen. During diuresis, body weight is monitored carefully and not allowed to decrease at a rate of more than 1 lb/day in patients with ascites alone and no peripheral edema. More aggressive diuresis will usually result in contraction of the intravascular volume and azotemia.

Five to 10% of patients with ascites are refractory to medical treatment and require more invasive measures. The two mainstays of therapy in this group of patients are large-volume paracentesis combined with IV albumin administration and TIPS. Because it can be done in the outpatient setting and is less invasive, the generally preferred initial treatment for patients with ascites refractory to medical treatment is large-volume paracentesis combined with IV albumin infusion in a dose of 6 to 8 g/L of ascites removed.[51] After large-volume paracentesis, ascites is less likely to recur in patients treated with spironolactone than in those not on a diuretic. TIPS is more effective in preventing ascites reaccumulation than large-volume paracentesis, but survival is similar after the two procedures.[52] As in patients treated with TIPS for variceal bleeding, major disadvantages of this therapy are a fairly high rate of encephalopathy and eventual TIPS dysfunction in most patients. TIPS is used in patients who require frequent paracentesis for management of their ascites and in those who are intolerant of large-volume paracentesis.

Although initially effective in most patients, a surgically placed peritoneovenous shunt is seldom used in the management of medically refractory ascites because of its associated complications such as occlusion, infection, and disseminated intravascular coagulation. Additionally, controlled trials have shown that this relatively simple operation, which can be done under local anesthesia, is no more effective than medical management in prolonging patient survival. A surgically constructed side-to-side portosystemic shunt, like TIPS, is also effective in relieving ascites. However, because of the associated morbidity and mortality, these operations are infrequently done and are used only in ascitic patients who have bled from esophagogastric varices and in whom TIPS is either not indicated or has failed.

Cirrhotic patients with ascites who develop fever, abdominal tenderness, or worsening hepatic or renal function undergo a diagnostic paracentesis to rule out spontaneous bacterial peritonitis. This complication of ascites is associated with a mortality rate of about 25% per episode. The diagnosis is made with an ascitic fluid polymorphonuclear count of greater than 250 per mm^3 or a positive ascites culture. The most common organisms causing spontaneous bacterial peritonitis are aerobic gram-negative organisms, which likely come from the bowel by bacterial translocation. Before culture results are available, antibiotic therapy is initiated when spontaneous bacterial peritonitis is suspected. A 5- to 10-day course of either cefotaxime or a combination of amoxicillin and clavulanic acid have been shown to be effective treatment.[53] Because spontaneous bacterial peritonitis recurs in more than 70% of patients, prophylactic therapy with oral norfloxacin is initiated as soon as IV therapy is completed and continued until ascites is resolved.

Another life-threatening complication of portal hypertension is the hepatorenal syndrome that develops almost exclusively in patients with tense ascites and declining hepatic function. When renal failure is rapidly progressive, the prognosis is poor, with a median survival of about 2 weeks. In other patients, renal failure develops more gradually, and the prognosis is somewhat better. The only reliable treatment for the hepatorenal syndrome is liver transplantation. Because the renal failure is functional rather than structural, after hepatic function is improved and portal hypertension is relieved, the kidneys recover. A few small series have suggested that renal function may improve in patients with the hepatorenal syndrome after insertion of a TIPS. However, in this setting, TIPS is regarded as a bridge to liver transplantation in the near future.

ENCEPHALOPATHY

Portosystemic encephalopathy is a psychoneurologic syndrome that may have a variety of manifestations, including alterations in the level of consciousness, intellectual deterioration, personality changes, and neurologic findings such as the flapping tremor asterixis. Although the pathogenesis of these alterations is unclear, they occur in patients with either significant hepatocellular dysfunction or portosystemic shunting. The shunts may be congenital, spontaneously form secondary to portal hypertension, or surgically or radiologically (TIPS) constructed. The most common setting for the development of encephalopathy is in patients with cirrhosis who undergo a procedural shunt. Nonselective shunts, such as the operative portacaval shunt and TIPS, are frequently followed by encephalopathy (20%-40% of patients), whereas this complication is less common in patients who receive a selective shunt, such as the distal splenorenal shunt.

Most theories of the pathogenesis of encephalopathy are based on circulating cerebral toxins that are intestinally absorbed and bypass the liver by means of shunts or fail to be inactivated by the liver's decreased metabolic capacity. Purported cerebral toxins include ammonia, mercaptans, and γ-aminobutyric acid. The false neurotransmitter hypothesis, based on the high ratio of aromatic to branched-chain amino acids present in the blood of patients with chronic liver disease, has also been proposed to explain the psychoneurologic disturbances observed. Almost certainly the syndrome is multifactorial with the bulk of evidence supporting ammonia as the main cerebral toxin. However, the severity of encephalopathy does not correlate well with blood ammonia levels.

Encephalopathy develops spontaneously in less than 10% of patients, and this form of the syndrome is almost entirely confined to those patients who undergo a procedural shunt. More commonly, one or more of the following precipitating factors induce the syndrome: gastrointestinal hemorrhage, excessive diuresis, azotemia, constipation, sedatives, infection, and excess dietary protein. In fact, when encephalopathy develops in a patient with cirrhosis who is otherwise stable, gastrointestinal bleeding or a subtle infection is suspected. Most of the precipitating factors cause an increase in blood ammonia.

Key to the management of encephalopathy is identifying and then eliminating whatever precipitating factors are responsible. Dietary protein is restricted, infections are treated, all sedatives are discontinued, and intestinal catharsis is accomplished.

Most episodes of encephalopathy are acute and develop over a period of hours to days. Such episodes may first present with subtle personality changes and sleep disturbances. As encephalopathy progresses, disorientation, slurred speech, confusion, and eventually coma may develop. The characteristic flapping tremor asterixis is commonly present and represents an inability to actively maintain posture or position. Neither asterixis nor the psychoneurologic manifestations of this syndrome are specific to portosystemic encephalopathy and may also be present in other types of metabolic dysfunction such as renal failure. Nearly all cases of acute encephalopathy are induced by one or more precipitating factors that need to be identified and eliminated. Chronic encephalopathy is considerably less common than acute encephalopathy and generally occurs in patients with either a surgical nonselective portosystemic shunt or TIPS.

Pharmacologic treatment of encephalopathy is indicated for patients with chronic, intermittent symptoms and for those with persistent, acute psychoneurologic disturbances despite elimination of precipitating factors. The only drugs with proven effectiveness are neomycin, a poorly absorbed antibiotic that suppresses urease-containing bacteria, and lactulose, a nonabsorbable disaccharide that acidifies colonic contents and also has a cathartic effect. A likely mechanism of action of both of these drugs is a decrease in the amount of intestinal ammonia and inhibition of its absorption. Acute episodes of encephalopathy can be treated equally effectively with neomycin and lactulose. Neomycin is administered orally in a dose of 1.5 g every 6 hours. In the acute setting, lactulose is given in a dose of 30 g every 1 or 2 hours until a cathartic effect is noted. The patient is then maintained with 20 to 30 g of lactulose 2 to 4 times a day or as needed to result in two soft bowel movements daily. Comatose patients can be treated with lactulose enemas. Lactulose is the mainstay of therapy for chronic encephalopathy because long-term use of neomycin may cause nephrotoxicity or ototoxicity in some patients. Protein restriction is also a component of the therapeutic regimen. The comatose patient is treated initially exclusively with glucose supplements as IV fluids. As encephalopathy lessens, 0.5 to 1.2 g/kg/day of amino acids or proteins are provided. When an oral diet is resumed, it initially consists of 40 to 60 g/day of protein, which can then be gradually increased to a maintenance level of 60 to 80 g/day.

Unproven therapies for encephalopathy include the enteral or parenteral administration of branched-chain amino acids and the drug flumazenil, a selective antagonist of benzodiazepine receptors. Neither of these treatments has been clearly established in randomized controlled trials.

Interventional procedures or surgery have improved cerebral function in some patients with encephalopathy by interrupting a surgically constructed portosystemic shunt or TIPS. Likewise, in isolated cases, occlusion of a major portosystemic collateral, such as the coronary vein, has reversed encephalopathy after the selective distal splenorenal shunt. Although both total colectomy and colonic exclusion have resolved encephalopathy in some patients, the high morbidity and mortality rates after these operations in patients with decompensated hepatic disease have prevented their widespread use.

Selected References

D'Amico G, Pagliaro L, Bosch J: The treatment of portal hypertension: A meta-analytic review. Hepatology 22:332-354, 1995.

Since the 1960s, countless controlled trials comparing the various treatments for variceal bleeding have been conducted throughout the world. These authors have painstakingly tabulated the results of all these trials and applied meta-analysis when appropriate.

Garcia-Tsao G: Current management of the complications of cirrhosis and portal hypertension: Variceal hemorrhage, ascites, and spontaneous bacterial peritonitis. Gastroenterology 120:726-748, 2001.

This is a superb review of the pathophysiology, diagnosis, and treatment of the major life-threatening complications of portal hypertension.

Henderson JM, Barnes DS, Geisinger MA: Portal hypertension. Curr Probl Surg 35:379-452, 1998.

This is a superb and complete monograph on the pathophysiology, diagnosis, and treatment of complications of portal hypertension. The expertise of the authors represents the disciplines of surgery, gastroenterology, and interventional radiology.

Henderson JM, Boyer TD, Kutner MH, et al: Distal splenorenal shunt versus transjugular intrahepatic portal systemic shunt for variceal bleeding: A randomized trial. Gastroenterology 130:1643-51, 2006.

This is a multi-institutional randomized controlled trial assessing the relative effectiveness of distal splenorenal shunt and TIPS for the long-term control of variceal bleeding in child's class A and B cirrhotic patients. These two treatments were found to be equivalent except for the necessity of multiple re-interventions in the TIPS patients.

Rikkers LF: The changing spectrum of treatment for variceal bleeding. Ann Surg 228:536-546, 1998.

A series of 263 consecutive patients undergoing a variety of operations for variceal bleeding from 1978 to 1996 is presented. Four eras, separated by the times when endoscopic treatment, liver transplantation, and TIPS were introduced, are analyzed. The author concludes that these innovations have decreased the need for and improved the results of portal hypertension surgery, which is still indicated for selected patients.

Sandhu BS, Sanyal AJ: Management of ascites in cirrhosis. Clin Liver Dis 9:715-732, 2005.

This is an excellent, comprehensive, and practical review of the treatment of ascites in patients with cirrhosis.

Wright AS, Rikkers LF: Current management of portal hypertension. J Gastrointest Surg 9:992-1005, 2005.

This is a quite concise and fairly comprehensive review of the management of patients with variceal bleeding. Treatment of the acutely bleeding patient as well as prevention of rebleeding are discussed in detail. An up-to-date list of references is included.

References

1. Chen TS, Chen PS: Understanding the Liver: A History. Westport, CT, Greenwood, 1984.
2. Biernat J, Pawlik WW, Sendor R, et al: Role of afferent nerves and sensory peptides in the mediation of hepatic artery buffer response. J Physiol Pharmacol 56:133-145, 2005.
3. Laleman W, Van Landeghem L, Wilmer A, et al: Portal hypertension: From pathophysiology to clinical practice. Liver Int 25:1079-1090, 2005.
4. Bressler B, Pinto R, El Ashry D, et al: Which patients with primary biliary cirrhosis or primary sclerosing cholangitis should undergo endoscopic screening for oesophageal varices detection? Gut 54:407-410, 2005.
5. Pugh RN, Murray-Lyon IM, Dawson JL, et al: Transection of the oesophagus for bleeding oesophageal varices. Br J Surg 60:646-649, 1973.
6. Kamath PS, Wiesner RH, Malinchoc M, et al: A model to predict survival in patients with end-stage liver disease. Hepatology 33:464-470, 2001.
7. Sheth S, Horton KM, Fishman EK: Vascular sequelae of cirrhosis: Evaluation with dual-phase helical CT. Abdom Imaging 27:720-727, 2002.

8. Li FH, Hao J, Xia JG, et al: Hemodynamic analysis of esophageal varices in patients with liver cirrhosis using color Doppler ultrasound. World J Gastroenterol 11:4510-4515, 2005.
9. Rondonotti E, Villa F, Signorelli C, et al: Portal hypertensive enteropathy. Gastrointest Endosc Clin N Am 16:277-286, 2006.
10. Smith JL, Graham DY: Variceal hemorrhage: A critical evaluation of survival analysis. Gastroenterology 82:968-973, 1982.
11. Garcia-Tsao: Portal hypertension. Curr Opin Gastroenterol 22:254-262, 2006.
12. deFranchis R: Evolving consensus in portal hypertension: Report of the Baveno IV consensus workshop on methodology of diagnosis and therapy in portal hypertension. J Hepatol 43:167-176, 2005.
13. Hahn M, Massen O, Nenki M, et al: De ecksche fistel zwischen der unteren hohlvene und der pfortaden und folgen fur den organismus. Arch Exp Pathol Pharmakol 32:162, 1893.
14. Tan PC, Hou MC, Lin HC, et al: A randomized trial of endoscopic treatment of acute gastric variceal hemorrhage: N-butyl-2-cyanoacrylate injection versus band ligation. Hepatology 43:690-697, 2006.
15. Bernard B, Nguyen KE, Opolon P, et al: Antibiotic prophylaxis (ABP) for the prevention of bacterial infections in cirrhotic patients with gastrointestinal bleeding (GB): A meta-analysis. Hepatology 29:1655-1661, 1999.
16. Escorsell A, Bordas JM, Ruiz del Arbol L, et al: Randomized controlled trial of sclerotherapy versus somatostatin infusion in the prevention of early rebleeding following acute variceal hemorrhage in patients with cirrhosis. J Hepatol 29:779-788, 1998.
17. Villanueva C, Ortiz J, Sabat M, et al: Somatostatin alone or combined with emergency sclerotherapy in the treatment of acute esophageal variceal bleeding: a prospective randomized trial. Hepatology 30:384-389, 1999.
18. De Franchis R, Primignani M: Endoscopic treatments for portal hypertension. Semin Liver Dis 19:439-455, 1999.
19. Vangeli M, Patch D, Burroughs AK: Salvage TIPS for uncontrolled variceal bleeding. J Hepatol 37:703-704, 2003.
20. Orloff MJ, Orloff MS, Orloff SL, et al: Three decades of experience with emergency portacaval shunt for acutely bleeding esophageal varices in 400 unselected patients with cirrhosis of the liver. J Am Coll Surg 180:257-272, 1995.
21. Lebrec D, Poynard T, Bernuau J, et al: A randomized controlled study of propranolol for prevention of recurrent gastrointestinal bleeding in patients with cirrhosis: A final report. Hepatology 4:355-358, 1984.
22. Bernard B, Lebrec D, Mathurin P, et al: Beta-adrenergic antagonists in the prevention of gastrointestinal rebleeding in patients with cirrhosis: a meta-analysis. Hepatology 25:63-70, 1997.
23. Villanueva C, Miñana J, Ortiz J, et al: Endoscopic ligation compared with combined treatment with nadolol and isosorbide mononitrate to prevent recurrent variceal bleeding. N Engl J Med 345:647-655, 2001.
24. Gournay J, Masliah C, Martin T, et al: Isosorbide mononitrate and propranolol compared with propranolol alone for the prevention of variceal rebleeding. Hepatology 31:1239-1245, 2000.
25. Laine L, Cook D: Endoscopic ligation compared with sclerotherapy for treatment of esophageal variceal bleeding: A meta-analysis. Ann Intern Med 123:280-287, 1995.
26. de la Pena J, Brullet E, Sanchez-Hernandez E, et al: Variceal ligation plus nadolol compared with ligation for prophy-laxis of variceal rebleeding: A multicenter trial. Hepatology 41:572-578, 2005.
27. D'Amico G, Pagliaro L, Bosch J: The treatment of portal hypertension: A meta-analytic review. Hepatology 22:332-354, 1995.
28. Papatheodoridis GV, Goulis J, Leandro G, et al: Transjugular intrahepatic portasystemic shunt compared with endoscopic treatment for prevention of variceal rebleeding: A meta-analysis. Hepatology 30:612-622, 1999.
29. Inokuchi K, Beppu K, Koyanagi N, et al: Fifteen years' experience with left gastric–venous caval shunt for esophageal varices. World J Surg 8:716-721, 1984.
30. Henderson JM: Role of distal splenorenal shunt for long-term management of variceal bleeding [review]. World J Surg 18:205-210, 1994.
31. Jin GL, Rikkers LF: Selective variceal decompression: Current status [review]. HPB Surg 5:1-15, 1991.
32. Henderson JM, Millikan WJJ, Wright-Bacon L, et al: Hemodynamic differences between alcoholic and nonalcoholic cirrhotics following distal splenorenal shunt: Effect on survival? Ann Surg 198:325-334, 1983.
33. Rikkers LF: Is the distal splenorenal shunt better? Hepatology 8:1705-1707, 1988.
34. da Silva LC, Strauss E, Gayotto LC, et al: A randomized trial for the study of the elective surgical treatment of portal hypertension in mansonic schistosomiasis. Ann Surg 204:148-153, 1986.
35. Spina GP, Henderson JM, Rikkers LF, et al: Distal splenorenal shunt versus endoscopic sclerotherapy in the prevention of variceal rebleeding: A meta-analysis of 4 randomized clinical trials. J Hepatol 16:338-345, 1992.
36. Henderson JM, Kutner MH, Millikan WJJ, et al: Endoscopic variceal sclerosis compared with distal splenorenal shunt to prevent recurrent variceal bleeding in cirrhosis: A prospective, randomized trial. Ann Intern Med 112:262-269, 1990.
37. Rikkers LF, Jin G, Burnett DA, et al: Shunt surgery versus endoscopic sclerotherapy for variceal hemorrhage: Late results of a randomized trial. Am J Surg 165:27-32, 1993.
38. Khaitiyar JS, Luthra SK, Prasad N, et al: Transjugular intrahepatic portosystemic shunt versus distal splenorenal shunt: A comparative study. Hepatogastroenterology 47:492-497, 2000.
39. Henderson JM, Boyer TD, Kutner MH, et al: Distal splenorenal shunt versus transjugular intrahepatic portal systemic shunt for variceal bleeding: A randomized trial. Gastroenterology 130:1643-1651, 2006.
40. Collins JC, Rypins EB, Sarfeh IJ: Narrow-diameter portacaval shunts for management of variceal bleeding [review]. World J Surg 18:211-215, 1994.
41. Sarfeh IJ, Rypins EB: Partial versus total portacaval shunt in alcoholic cirrhosis: Results of a prospective, randomized clinical trial. Ann Surg 219:353-361, 1994.
42. Rosemurgy AS, Serafini FM, Zweibel BR, et al: Transjugular intrahepatic portosystemic shunt vs. small-diameter prosthetic H-graft portacaval shunt: extended follow-up of an expanded randomized prospective trial. J Gastrointest Surg 4:589-597, 2000.
43. Idezuki Y, Kokudo N, Sanjo K, et al: Sugiura procedure for management of variceal bleeding in Japan. World J Surg 18:216-221, 1994.
44. Jin G, Rikkers LF: Transabdominal esophagogastric devascularization as treatment for variceal hemorrhage. Surgery 120:641-647, 1996.
45. Henderson JM: The role of portosystemic shunts for variceal bleeding in the liver transplantation era. Arch Surg 129:886, 1994.

46. Rikkers LF, Jin G, Langnas AN, et al: Shunt surgery during the era of liver transplantation. Ann Surg 226:51-57, 1997.

47. Elwood DR, Pomposelli JJ, Pomfret EA, et al: Distal spleno-renal shunt: Preferred treatment for recurrent variceal hemorrhage in the patient with well-compensated cirrhosis. Arch Surg 141:385-388, 2006.

48. Rikkers LF: The changing spectrum of treatment for variceal bleeding. Ann Surg 228:536-546, 1998.

49. Khuroo MS, Khuroo NS, Farahat KLC, et al: Meta-analysis: Endoscopic variceal ligation for primary prophylaxis of oesophageal variceal bleeding. Aliment Pharmacol Ther 21:347-361, 2005.

50. Boyer TD, Haskal ZJ: AASLD practice guideline: The role of transjugular intrahepatic portasystemic shunt in the management of portal hypertension. Hepatology 41:386-400, 2005.

51. Sandhu BS, Sanyal AJ: Management of ascites in cirrhosis. Clin Liver Dis 9:715-732, 2005.

52. D'Amico G, Luca A, Morabito A, et al: Uncovered transjugular intrahepatic portasystemic shunt for refractory ascites: A meta-analysis. Gastroenterology 129:1282-1293, 2005.

53. Ricart R, Soriano G, Novella M, et al: Amoxicillin-clavulanic acid versus cefotaxime in the therapy of bacterial infections in cirrhotic patients. J Hepatol 32:596-602, 2000.

CHAPTER 54

Biliary System

Ravi S. Chari, MD   and   Shimul A. Shah, MD

Anatomy

Physiology

General Considerations in Biliary Tract Pathophysiology

Benign Pathophysiologic Conditions

Malignant Biliary Disease

Although signs and symptoms of gallstones and extrahepatic biliary obstruction have been recognized for centuries, the surgical management of biliary tract disorders has evolved only recently. Advances in anesthesia, a better understanding of biliary anatomy and physiology, and improved surgical technique have allowed surgeons to manage both benign and malignant biliary disorders with increasing frequency and success in the past 10 years.

The first biliary tract operation is credited to John Stough Bobb of Indianapolis in 1867. He explored a 32-year-old woman with a large abdominal mass and discovered a massive gallbladder hydrops. Bobb made a cholecystotomy, removed the gallstones, and then sutured the gallbladder. In 1882, Carl Langenbuch of Berlin performed the first cholecystectomy for a patient with biliary colic. The patient survived the operation and was discharged from the hospital 8 weeks after surgery. The treatment of calculous gallbladder disease was revolutionized again, more than 100 years later, in 1986 when Mühe performed the first laparoscopic cholecystectomy.

Since the late 19th century, the operative management of extrahepatic biliary obstruction also evolved rapidly. The first biliary enteric anastomosis was performed by

Alexander von Winiwarter in Liège in 1880 on a patient with common bile duct obstruction due to choledocholithiasis who underwent a cholecystocolostomy. Monastryski performed the first palliative biliary bypass for malignant obstruction in 1887. Choledochotomy with stone extraction was first performed in 1889. However, the high mortality associated with this procedure led to the use of cholecystojejunostomy for biliary obstruction. This was popularized by Ludwig Courvoisier, who reported his first 10 cases in 1890 with an operative mortality rate of 20%. Choledochoduodenostomy was initially attempted for an impacted common duct stone by Oskar Sprengel in Germany in 1891 and then again following resection of a periampullary cancer in 1898 by William Stewart Halsted. The use of a Roux-en-Y jejunal limb to create a hepaticojejunostomy as commonly used today was first reported by Robert Dahl of Stockholm in 1909.

Advances in a variety of diagnostic and nonoperative modalities have been made in the 20th century and have further refined the management of patients with biliary tract disease. The diagnosis of gallstones was improved considerably by the development of oral cholecystography by Graham and Cole in 1924. In the 1950s, cholescintigraphy and endoscopic and transhepatic cholangiography were developed, permitting nonoperative imaging of the biliary tract. More recently, ultrasonography, computed tomography (CT), magnetic resonance imaging (MRI), and laparoscopy have vastly improved the ability to image the biliary tract. The detail of the liver and biliary tract outlined by CT and magnetic resonance cholangiopancreatography (MRCP) has enabled the surgeon to approach operative cases with a clear understanding of the anatomy and relationships of important structures in the porta hepatitis.

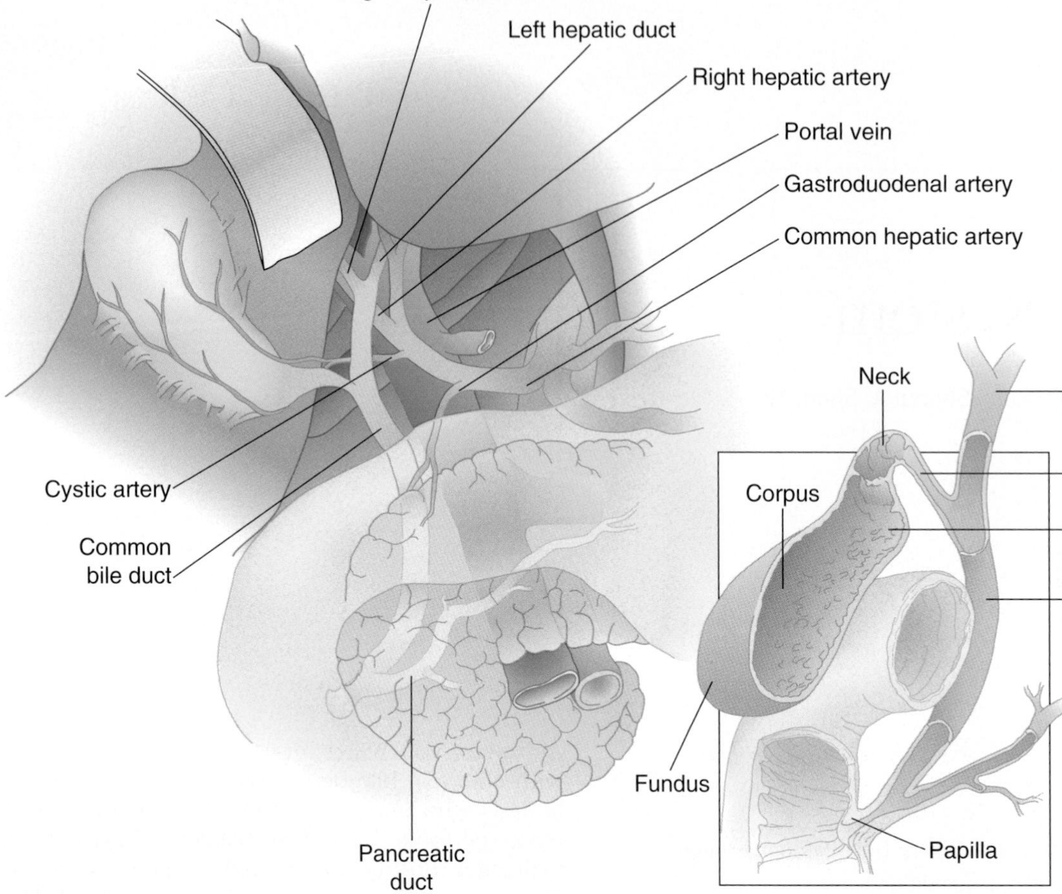

Right hepatic duct

Left hepatic duct

Right hepatic artery

Portal vein

Gastroduodenal artery

Common hepatic artery

Cystic artery

Common bile duct

Pancreatic duct

Neck

Corpus

Fundus

Common hepatic duct

Cystic duct

Hartmann's pouch

Common bile duct

Papilla

Figure 54-1 Anatomy of the biliary system and its relationship to surrounding structures.

ANATOMY

Extrahepatic Biliary Tract

The extrahepatic biliary tract consists of the bifurcation of the left and right hepatic ducts, the common hepatic duct, the common bile duct, and the cystic duct and gallbladder (Fig. 54-1). The left hepatic duct is formed by the ducts draining segments II, III, and IV of the liver, courses horizontally along the base of segment IV, and has an extrahepatic length of about 2 cm. The right hepatic duct is formed by the right posterior (segments IV and VII) and right anterior (segments V and VIII) hepatic ducts and has a shorter extrahepatic length. The hepatic duct bifurcation is usually extrahepatic and anterior to the portal vein bifurcation. The biliary confluence is separated from the posterior aspect of the caudate lobe (segment I) of the liver by the hilar plate, which consists of a fusion of connective tissue enclosing the biliary and vascular structures within the *Glisson capsule* (Fig. 54-2). The common hepatic duct lays anterolateral to the hepatic artery and portal vein in the hepatoduodenal ligament and joins the cystic duct to form the common bile duct. The common bile duct extends from the cystic duct–common hepatic duct junction inferiorly to the papilla of

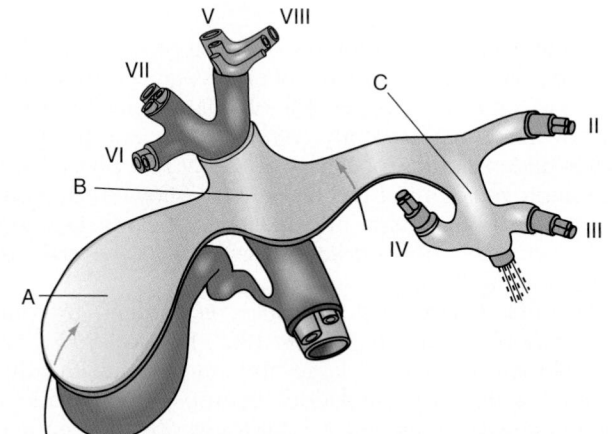

Figure 54-2 Anatomy of the hilar plate. Note the cystic plate (A) above the gallbladder, the hilar plate (B) above the biliary confluence, and the umbilical plate (C) above the umbilical portion of the portal vein. Large, curving arrows indicate plane of dissection of the cystic plate during cholecystectomy and of the hilar plate at the base of segment IV during approaches to the left hepatic duct. (From Blumgart LH, Hann LE: Surgical and radiological anatomy of the liver and biliary tract. In Blumgart LH, Fong Y [ed]: Surgery of the Liver and Biliary Tract. New York, WB Saunders, 2000, pp 13-14.)

Vater, where it empties into the duodenum. The common bile duct varies in length from 5 to 9 cm depending on its junction with the cystic duct and is divided into three segments: supraduodenal, retroduodenal, and intrapancreatic. The distal common bile duct and pancreatic duct may join outside the duodenal wall to form a long common channel, within the duodenal wall to form a short common channel, or they may enter the duodenum through two distinct ostia.

The gallbladder is a pear-shaped reservoir in continuity with the common hepatic and common bile ducts through the cystic duct. It is usually 7 to 10 cm in length, is 3 to 5 cm in diameter, and has a capacity of 30 to 60 mL. The gallbladder lies on the inferior surface of the liver partially enveloped in a layer of peritoneum. The gallbladder is anatomically divided into the fundus, body, infundibulum, and neck, which empties into the cystic duct. Both the gallbladder neck and the cystic duct contain spirally oriented mucosal folds known as the *valves of Heister*. The valves prevent the passage of gallstones and excessive distention or collapse of the cystic duct, despite variations in ductal pressure. The cystic duct varies in length from 1 to 5 cm and in diameter from 3 to 7 mm; it usually joins the common hepatic duct at an acute angle. Small veins and lymphatics course between the gallbladder fossa and the gallbladder wall, connecting the lymphatic and venous drainage of the liver and gallbladder. These connections are the cause of the direct inflammatory and carcinomatous spread from the gallbladder into the liver.

Anatomic variations in the cystic duct and hepatic ducts are common. Frequent variations in the hepatic ductal anatomy are shown in Figure 54-3. Drainage to the caudate lobe (segment I) is not shown but can arise directly from common bile duct, right hepatic duct, or left hepatic duct. Variations of the left hepatic duct are much less common than those of the right hepatic duct. The cystic duct usually enters the common bile duct at an acute angle, but may run parallel to the common hepatic duct for a variable distance before joining it, or may join the right hepatic duct or a segmental right hepatic duct. An accessory hepatic duct or cholecystohepatic duct (*duct of Luschka*) may also enter the gallbladder through the gallbladder fossa and, if encountered during a cholecystectomy, should be ligated to prevent a biliary fistula.

Anomalies of the gallbladder are much less frequent than variations in ductal anatomy. Agenesis of the gallbladder has been reported (~200 cases), and duplication of the gallbladder (two separate gallbladders, each with its own cystic duct) occurs in 1 of 4000 births.

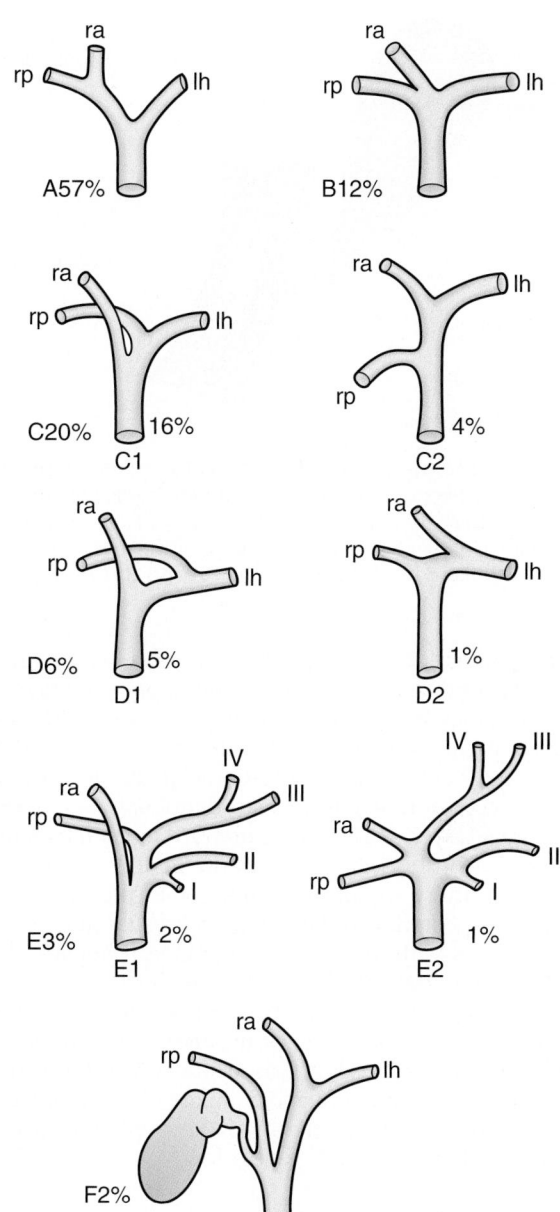

Figure 54-3 Variations in the confluence of the left and right hepatic ducts. **A,** Typical anatomy of the confluence. **B,** Trifurcation of left, right anterior, and right posterior hepatic ducts. **C,** Aberrant drainage of a right anterior (C1) or posterior (C2) sectoral hepatic duct into the common hepatic duct. **D-F,** Less common variations in hepatic ductal anatomy. (From Smadja C, Blumgart L: The biliary tract and the anatomy of biliary exposure. In Blumgart L [ed]: Surgery of the Liver and Biliary Tract. New York, Churchill Livingstone, 1994, pp 11-24.)

Vascular Anatomy

The blood supply to the extrahepatic biliary tree originates (1) distally from the gastroduodenal, retroduodenal, and posterosuperior pancreatoduodenal arteries and (2) proximally from the right hepatic and cystic arteries. These arteries supply the common bile and common hepatic ducts through branches running parallel to the duct in the 3- and 9-o'clock positions. The extrahepatic biliary tree is vulnerable to ischemic injury. To avoid disrupting the fragile inconstant blood supply to the duct, it is important not to strip the investing areolar tissue around it during dissection and isolation. Ischemia of the bile duct will not be readily evident at time of dissection but can result in biliary stricture or leak postoperatively.

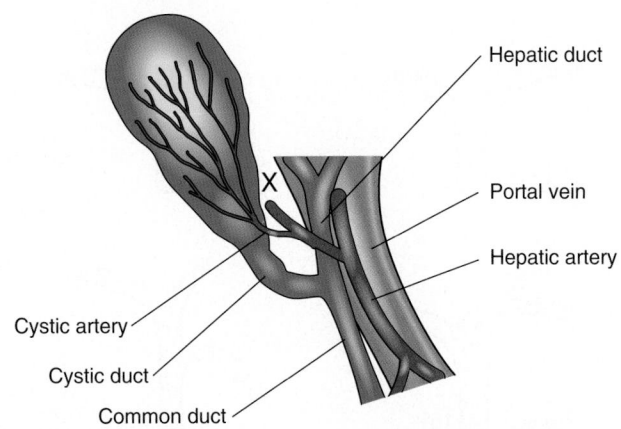

Figure 54-4 The triangle of Calot is bounded by the cystic duct, the common hepatic duct, and the inferior border of the liver. (From Gilchrist BF, Trunkey DD, Biliary Tract trauma. In Zuidema GD [ed]: Shackelford's surgery of the alimentary tract, 3rd ed. WB Saunders, Philadelphia, 1991, pp 257.)

The gallbladder is supplied by a single cystic artery, but in 12% of cases, a double cystic artery (anterior and posterior) may exist. The origin and course of the cystic artery is highly variable and is one of the most variable in the body. The cystic artery may originate from the left hepatic, common hepatic, gastroduodenal, or superior mesenteric arteries. The cystic artery divides into superficial and deep branches before entering the gallbladder. The cystic artery usually lies superior to the cystic duct and passes posterior to the common hepatic duct, but its course varies with its origin. The common hepatic duct, the liver, and the cystic duct define the boundaries of *Calot's triangle* (Fig. 54-4). Located within this triangle are important structures: the cystic artery, the right hepatic artery, and the cystic duct lymph node. The Calot node is the main route of lymphatic drainage of the gallbladder and is therefore commonly involved in inflammatory or neoplastic diseases of the gallbladder.

PHYSIOLOGY

Bile Ducts

The bile ducts, gallbladder, and sphincter of Oddi modify, store, and regulate the flow of bile. The liver produces 500 to 1000 mL of bile per day and excretes it into the bile canaliculi. During its passage through the bile ductules and hepatic duct, canalicular bile is modified by the absorption and secretion of electrolytes and water. The secretion of bile is responsive to neurogenic, humoral, and chemical stimuli. Vagal stimulation increases bile secretion, whereas splanchnic nerve stimulation results in decreased bile flow. The gastrointestinal hormone, secretin, stimulates bile flow primarily by increasing the active secretion of chloride-rich fluid by the bile ducts and ductules. Secretin release is stimulated by hydrochloric acid, proteins, and fatty acids in the duodenum. Bile ductular secretion is also stimulated by cholecystokinin (CCK), gastrin, and other hormones. The bile duct epi-

thelium is also capable of water and electrolyte absorption, which may be of primary importance in the storage of bile during fasting in patients who have previously undergone cholecystectomy.

Bile is composed of water, electrolytes, bile salts, proteins, lipids, and bile pigments. Sodium, potassium, calcium, and chlorine have the same concentration in bile as in plasma or extracellular fluid. The primary bile salts, cholate and chenodeoxycholate, are synthesized in the liver by cholesterol. They are conjugated there with taurine and glycine, and act within the bile as anions (bile acids) that are balanced by sodium. Bile salts are excreted into the bile by the hepatocyte and aid in the digestion and absorption of fats in the intestines. About 95% of the bile acid pool is reabsorbed and returned through the portal venous system to the liver, also known as the *enterohepatic circulation* (Fig. 54-5). The remaining 5% is excreted in the stool.

Cholesterol and phospholipids synthesized in the liver are the principal lipids found in bile. The synthesis of phospholipid and cholesterol by the liver is regulated in part by bile acids. The color of bile is due to the presence of the pigment bilirubin diglucuronide, which is the metabolic product from the breakdown of hemoglobin, and is present in bile in concentrations 100 times greater than plasma. Once in the intestine, bacteria convert it into urobilinogen, a small fraction of which is absorbed and secreted into the bile.

Gallbladder

The gallbladder concentrates and stores hepatic bile during the fasting state and delivers bile into the duodenum in response to a meal. Since the usual capacity of the gallbladder is only about 30 to 60 mL, the remarkable absorptive capacity of the gallbladder accounts for its ability to store much of the 600 mL of bile produced each day. The gallbladder mucosa has the greatest absorptive capacity per unit area of any structure in the body. Bile is usually concentrated 5- to 10-fold by the absorption of water and electrolytes leading to a marked change in bile composition.

Active NaCl transport by the gallbladder epithelium is the driving force for the concentration of bile. Water is passively absorbed in response to the osmotic force generated by solute absorption. The concentration of bile may affect the solubility of two important components of gallstones: calcium and cholesterol. Although the gallbladder mucosa absorbs calcium, this process is not nearly as efficient as for sodium or water, leading to greater relative increase in calcium concentration. As the gallbladder bile becomes concentrated, several changes occur in the capacity of bile to solubilize cholesterol. The solubility in the micellar fraction is increased, but the stability of phospholipid-cholesterol vesicles is greatly decreased. Because cholesterol crystal precipitation occurs preferentially by vesicular rather than micellar mechanisms, the net effect of concentrating bile is an increased tendency for cholesterol nucleation.

The gallbladder epithelial cell secretes at least two important products into the gallbladder lumen: glycopro-

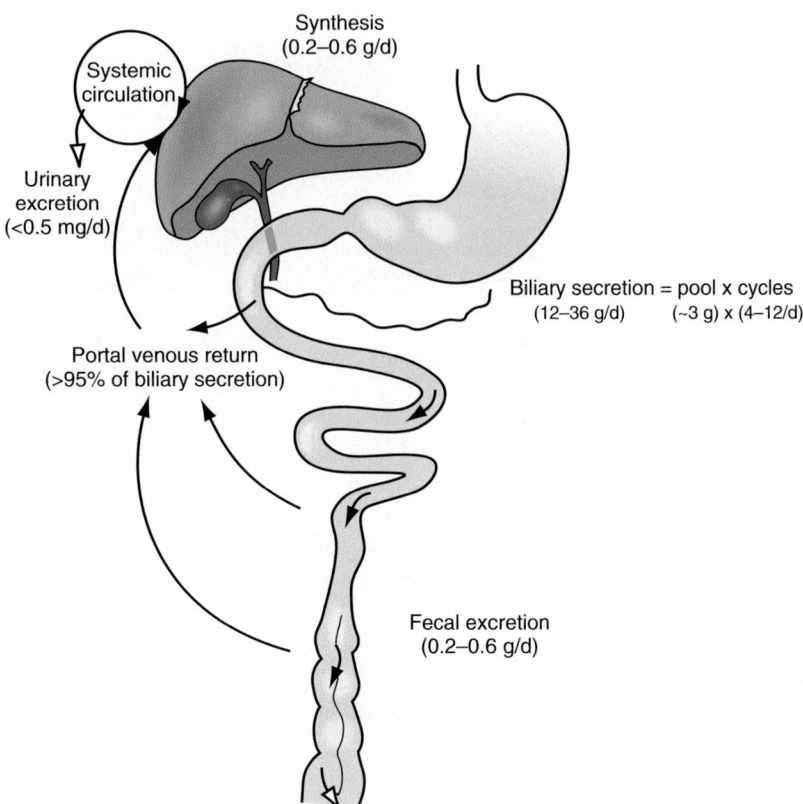

Figure 54-5 Enterohepatic circulation. (From Arias IM, Popper H, Jakoby WB, et al: The liver: Biology and pathobiology. Philadelphia: Raven Press, 1988, p 576.)

teins and hydrogen ions. Secretion of mucus glycoprotein occurs primarily from the glands of the gallbladder neck and cystic duct. The resultant mucin gel is believed to constitute an important part of the unstirred layer (diffusion-resistant barrier) that separates the gallbladder cell membrane from the luminal bile. This mucus barrier may be very important in protecting the gallbladder epithelium from the strong detergent effect of the highly concentrated bile salts found in the gallbladder. However, considerable evidence also suggests that mucin glycoproteins play a role as a pronucleating agent for cholesterol crystallization. The transport of hydrogen ions by the gallbladder epithelium leads to a decrease in gallbladder bile pH through a sodium-exchange mechanism. Acidification of bile promotes calcium solubility, thereby preventing its precipitation as calcium salts. The gallbladder's normal acidification process lowers the pH of entering hepatic bile from 7.5 to 7.8 down to 7.1 to 7.3.

The gallbladder fills from the continuous production of bile by the liver against the force of a contracted sphincter of Oddi. As the pressure within the common bile duct exceeds that within the gallbladder lumen, hepatic bile enters the gallbladder by retrograde flow through the cystic duct, wherein it is rapidly concentrated. Periods of filling are punctuated by brief episodes of partial emptying (~10%-15% of its volume) of concentrated gallbladder bile that are coordinated through the duodenum of phase III of the migrating myoelectric complex (MMC).

Following a meal, the gallbladder contracts in response to both a vagally mediated cephalic phase of activity and the release of CCK, the major regulator of gallbladder function. In the next 60 to 120 minutes, about 50% to 70% of gallbladder bile is steadily emptied into the intestinal tract. CCK is localized to the proximal small intestine, especially the duodenal epithelial cells, where its release is stimulated by intraluminal fat, amino acids, and gastric acid and inhibited by bile. In addition to stimulating gallbladder contractions, CCK also acts to functionally inhibit the normal phasic motor activity of the sphincter of Oddi. Gallbladder refilling then occurs gradually over the next 60 to 90 minutes.

Sphincter of Oddi

The sphincter of Oddi is a complex structure that is functionally independent from the duodenal musculature. It creates a high-pressure zone between the bile duct and the duodenum. The sphincter regulates the flow of bile and pancreatic juice into the duodenum, prevents the regurgitation of duodenal contents into the biliary tract, and also diverts bile into the gallbladder. The sphincter of Oddi also has very high-pressure phasic contractions, which play a role in preventing the regurgitation of duodenal contents into the biliary tract.

Both neural and hormonal factors influence the sphincter of Oddi. In response to CCK, both sphincter of Oddi pressure and phasic wave activity diminish. After a meal,

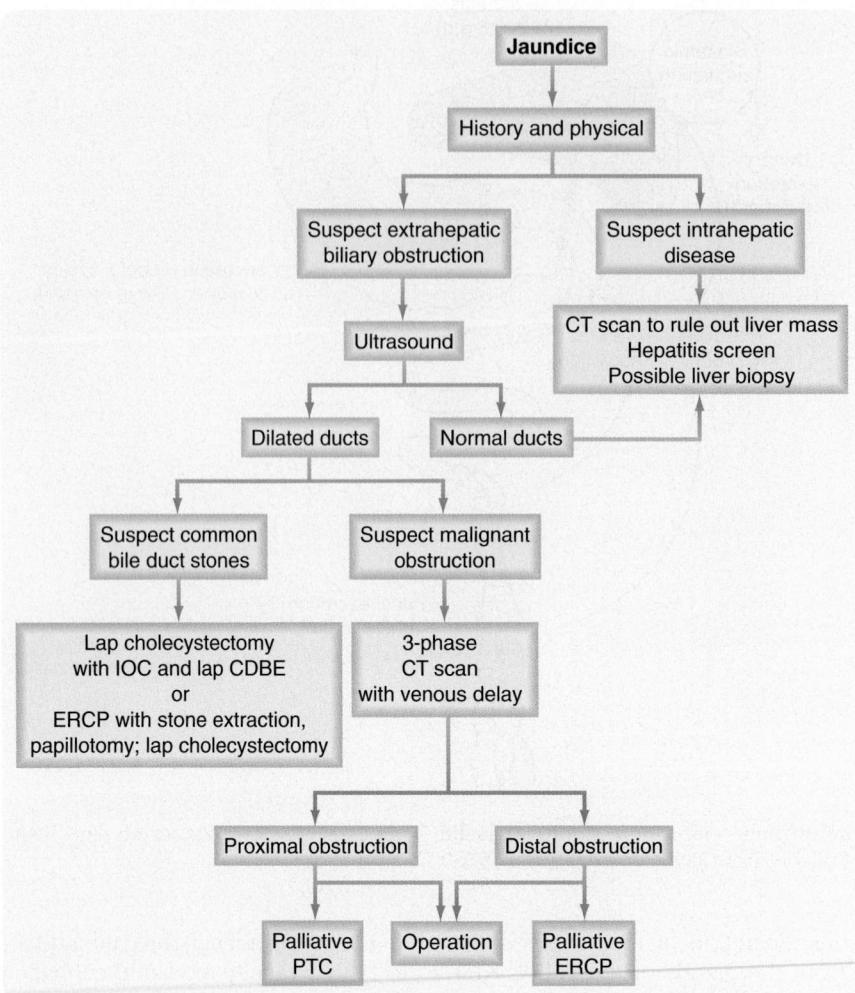

Figure 54-6 Diagnostic algorithm for patients presenting with jaundice. CBDE, common bile duct exploration; CT, computed tomography; ERCP, endoscopic retrograde cholangiopancreatography; IOC, intraoperative cholangiogram; lap, laparoscopic; PTC, percutaneous transhepatic cholangiography.

sphincter pressure relaxes in coordination with gallbladder contraction, thereby allowing the passive flow of bile into the duodenum. During fasting, high-pressure phasic contractions of the sphincter of Oddi persist through all phases of the MMC. Sphincter of Oddi activity appears to be coordinated with the partial gallbladder emptying and increases in the bile flow that occur during phase III of the MMC. This activity may be a preventive mechanism against the accumulation of biliary crystals during fasting.

GENERAL CONSIDERATIONS IN BILIARY TRACT PATHOPHYSIOLOGY

Symptoms

Symptoms attributable to biliary tract pathology are usually the result of obstruction, infection, or both. Obstruction can be extramural (e.g., pancreatic cancer), intramural (cholangiocarcinoma), or intraluminal (cho-

ledocholithiasis). Similar to infections in other parts of the body, biliary infections are usually due to three factors: a susceptible host, sufficient inoculum, and stasis. The most common symptoms related to biliary tract disease are abdominal pain, jaundice, fever, and nausea and vomiting.

Abdominal Pain

Gallstones and inflammation of the gallbladder are the most frequent causes of abdominal pain from biliary tract disease. Acute obstruction of the gallbladder by calculi results in *biliary colic,* a common misnomer because the pain is not colicky in the epigastrium or right upper quadrant. Biliary colic is a constant pain that builds in intensity, and can radiate to the back, interscapular region, or right shoulder. The pain is described as a bandlike tightness of the upper abdomen that may be associated with nausea and vomiting. This is due to a normal gallbladder contracting against a luminal obstruction, such as a gallstone impacted in the neck of the gallbladder, the cystic duct, or the common bile duct.

Table 54-1 Accuracy of Preferred Imaging Modalities for Different Biliary Tract Diagnoses Causing Right Upper Quadrant Pain

SUSPECTED DIAGNOSIS	IMAGING MODALITY	SENSITIVITY (%)	SPECIFICITY (%)
Cholelithiasis	Ultrasound	95	99
Acute calculous cholecystitis	Ultrasound	88	80
	HIDA	95	95
Acute acalculous cholecystitis	Ultrasound	36-93	17-89
	HIDA	70-80	90-100
Choledocholithiasis	ERCP	95	89
	MRC	95	98
	I/OP cholangiogram	78	97
	Lap ultrasound	80	99
Biliary dyskinesia	HIDA	94	80

ERCP, endoscopic retrograde cholangiopancreatography; HIDA, cholecystokinin hepatobiliary 2,6-dimethyl-iminodiacetic acid scan; I/OP, intraoperative; Lap, laparoscopic; MRC, magnetic resonance cholangiography.
From Trowbridge RL, Rutkowski NK, Shojania KG: Does this patient have acute cholecystitis? JAMA 289:80-86, 2003.

The pain is most commonly triggered by fatty foods, but it can also be initiated by other types of food or even occur spontaneously. An association with meals is present in only 50% of patients, and in these patients, the pain often develops more than 1 hour after eating.

The pain of biliary colic is distinct from that associated with acute cholecystitis. Although biliary colic can also be localized to the right upper quadrant, the pain of acute cholecystitis is exacerbated by touch, is somatic in nature, and is often associated with fever and leukocytosis. Irritation of the visceral and parietal peritoneum due to transmural inflammation from cholecystitis results in a positive *Murphy's sign*. This physical exam finding (in a patient abruptly arresting his or her inspiratory effort because of pain as the examiner palpates under the right costal margin) is indicative of acute cholecystitis.

Jaundice

When the serum concentration of bilirubin exceeds about 2.5 mg/dL, a yellowish discoloration of the sclera becomes evident (scleral icterus). Jaundice represents a similar discoloration of the skin, with serum bilirubin levels in excess of 5 mg/dL. The changes in color represent deposition of bile pigments in the affected tissues. The presence of conjugated bilirubin in the urine is one of the first changes noted by patients.

Workup and diagnosis of the jaundiced patient require an algorithm similar that in to Figure 54-6. Disorders resulting in jaundice can be divided into those causing "medical" jaundice, such as increased production, decreased hepatocyte transport or conjugation, or impaired excretion of bilirubin, and those causing "surgical" jaundice through impaired delivery of bilirubin into the intestine. Common causes of increased bilirubin production include the hemolytic anemias and acquired causes of hemolysis, including sepsis, burns, transfusion reactions, and medications. Impaired excretion of bilirubin leads to intrahepatic cholestasis and conjugated hyperbilirubinemia and can be due to conditions like viral or alcoholic hepatitis, cirrhosis, and drug-induced cholestasis.

Fever

Significant elevations in body temperature (≥38.0°C) represent a systemic manifestation of an initially localized inflammatory process. Bacterial contamination of the biliary system is a common feature of acute cholecystitis or choledocholithiasis with obstruction, and can be expected following percutaneous or endoscopic cholangiography. The combination of right upper quadrant abdominal pain, jaundice, and fever, known as *Charcot's triad,* signifies an active infection of the biliary system termed *acute cholangitis*. The addition of an altered mental status and hypotension to the above findings represents severe cholangitis and is termed *pentad of Reynolds*.

Laboratory Tests

Biliary colic, in the absence of gallbladder wall pathology or common bile duct obstruction, does not produce abnormal laboratory test values. On the other hand, obstructive choledocholithiasis is commonly associated with both liver dysfunction and acute cellular injury with resultant elevations in liver function tests. Hepatocellular injury results in increased levels of unconjugated or indirect reacting bilirubin due to an increase in bilirubin production or a decrease in hepatocyte uptake with conjugation. Conjugated or direct hyperbilirubinemia is due to defects in bilirubin excretion (intrahepatic cholestasis) or extrahepatic biliary obstruction. In addition to hyperbilirubinemia, an increased alkaline phosphatase level is virtually pathognomonic of bile duct obstruction. In patients with a high clinical suspicion of cholecystitis, but with associated elevations of bilirubin, alkaline phosphatase, and aminotransferase, cholangitis should be suspected. Serum transaminase (aspartate and alanine) levels can also be mildly elevated in biliary system disease, either because of direct injury of the liver adjacent to an inflamed gallbladder or from the effect of biliary sepsis on hepatocellular membrane integrity. Leukocytosis, composed primarily of neutrophils, is often present with acute cholecystitis or cholangitis, but is a nonspecific

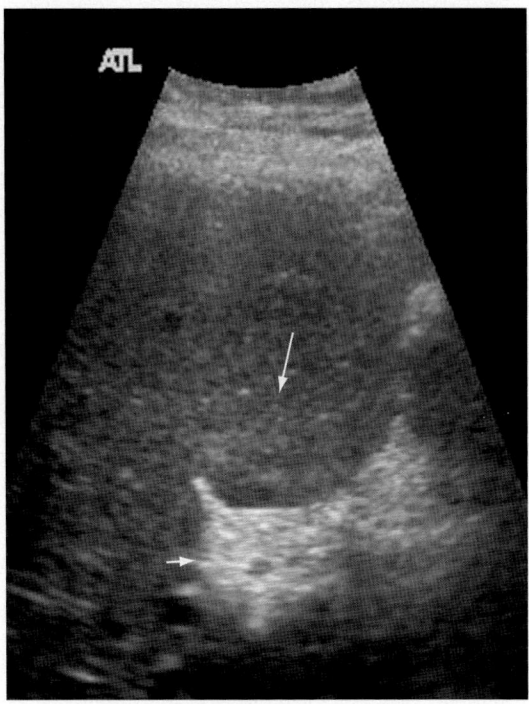

Figure 54-7 Ultrasound of liver identifying mass at hepatic duct bifurcation (*long arrow*), pressing on confluence of right and left hepatic ducts (*short arrow*).

finding that does not distinguish them from other infectious or inflammatory causes.

Studies

Plain Radiographs
Although frequently obtained during the initial evaluation of abdominal pain, plain radiographs of the abdomen in patients with complaints localized to the right upper quadrant are rarely helpful. Only about 15% of gallstones contain enough calcium to render them radiopaque and therefore visible on plain abdominal films. Plain films are important to exclude other potential diagnoses, such as perforated ulcer with free intraperitoneal air, bowel obstruction with dilated loops of bowel, or right lower lobe pneumonia on chest x-ray, that may mimic biliary tract disease.

Ultrasonography
Ultrasound of the abdomen is an extremely useful and accurate method for identifying gallstones and pathologic changes in the gallbladder consistent with acute cholecystitis. Abdominal ultrasound, if performed by an experienced operator, should be part of the routine evaluation of patients suspected of having gallstone disease, given the high specificity (>98%) and sensitivity (>95%) of this test for the diagnosis of cholelithiasis[1] (Table 54-1). In addition to identifying gallstones, ultrasound can also detail signs of cholecystitis such as thickening of the gallbladder wall, pericholecystic fluid, and impacted stone in the neck of the gallbladder. It is often the initial

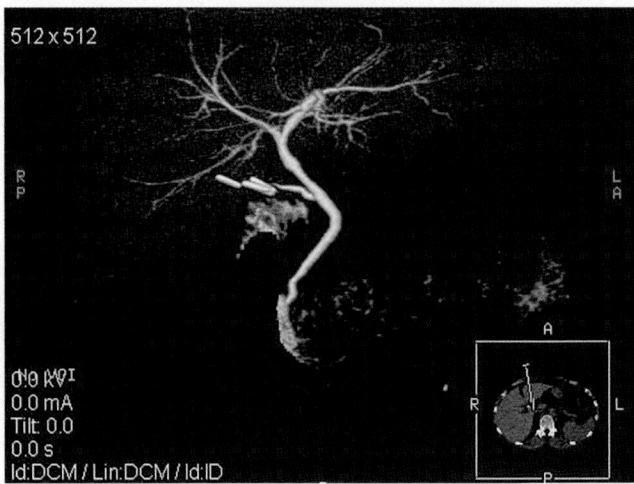

Figure 54-8 CT cholangiogram shows enhanced imaging of the biliary system comparable to MRC. Intrahepatic and extrahepatic biliary ducts are clearly seen in this patient for evaluation for living donor right hepatectomy.

screening test for patients with suspected extrahepatic biliary obstruction (Fig. 54-7). Dilation of the extrahepatic (>10 mm) or intrahepatic (>4 mm) bile ducts suggests biliary obstruction. Intraoperative ultrasound is now used frequently to further evaluate intrahepatic lesions, assess resectability, and determine involvement of vascular structures.[2]

Oral Cholecystography
Once considered the diagnostic test of choice for gallstones, oral cholecystography has been replaced by ultrasonography. It identifies filling defects in a visualized, opacified gallbladder after oral administration of a radiopaque compound that passes into the gallbladder. Oral cholecystography is of no value in patients with vomiting, biliary obstruction, jaundice, or hepatic failure.

Computed Tomography
Although abdominal CT scanning is probably the most informative single radiographic tool for examining intraabdominal pathology, its overall value for the diagnosis of biliary tract disease pales in comparison to ultrasonography. The disadvantage is largely because gallstones and bile appear nearly isodense on CT; that is, it is difficult to distinguish gallstones from bile, unless the stones are heavily calcified. CT identifies gallstones within the biliary tree and gallbladder with a sensitivity of only about 55% to 65%. Conversely, CT is more accurate at identifying the site and cause of extrahepatic biliary obstruction. Abdominal CT is a powerful tool for evaluating biliary tract disease when the differential diagnosis includes a question of hepatobiliary or pancreatic neoplasm, liver abscess, or hepatic parenchymal disease (e.g., biliary cirrhosis, organ atrophy). Use of CT cholangiogram provides improved definition of the biliary tract comparable to magnetic resonance cholangiography (MRC; Fig. 54-8). Angiograms have now essentially been replaced by triplephase liver CT angiogram.

Cholangiography

Cholangiography functionally involves the installation of contrast directly into the biliary tree and is the most accurate and sensitive method available to anatomically delineate the intrahepatic and extrahepatic biliary tree. It is most useful when the precise location or cause of biliary pathology needs to be ascertained. MRC is non-invasive and provides excellent anatomic detail. No contrast is administered because bile/water density is phase-contrasted. CT cholangiography requires the administration of intravenous (IV) contrast that is excreted in the biliary system. Neither of these is considered invasive. Both endoscopic retrograde cholangiopancreatography (ERCP) and percutaneous transhepatic cholangiography (PTC) are invasive procedures with a 2% to 5% risk of complications but offer the opportunity for a therapeutic intervention. ERCP is most useful in imaging patients with hepatobiliary malignancies and choledocholithiasis. It illustrates distal common bile duct or ampullary obstruction, can provide tissue samples for pathologic diagnosis, and can palliate patients with complete biliary obstruction using prosthetic stents. However, it gives no information regarding tumor size, local invasion, or distant spread, and is of limited use in staging.[2] Transhepatic cholangiography is the preferred technique in patients with proximal biliary obstruction or in patients in whom ERCP is not technically possible. Percutaneous transhepatic cholangiography can be followed by placement of transhepatic catheters, which can decompress the biliary system, function as anatomical landmarks during surgical reconstruction, or provide access for nonoperative dilation of strictures.

Scintigraphy

Biliary scintigraphy is useful to visualize the biliary tree, assess liver and gallbladder function, and diagnose several common disorders including cholecystitis. Although it is an excellent test to decide whether the common bile and cystic ducts are patent, biliary scintigraphy does not identify gallstones or give any detailed anatomic information. Nonvisualization of the gallbladder at 2 hours after injection is reliable evidence of cystic duct obstruction. Biliary scintigraphy followed by CCK administration is helpful for documenting biliary dyskinesia when gallbladder contraction accompanies biliary tract pain in patients without evidence of stones (CCK hepatobiliary 2,6-dimethyl-iminodiacetic acid [HIDA]). These agents are iminodiacetic acid (IDA)-based compounds and are processed in the liver and excreted (H originally stood for hydroxy, but today stands for hepatobiliary because other IDA derivatives, such as proisopropyl-IDA [PIPIDA], are more commonly used, but are still referred to as HIDA scans).

Laparoscopy

Advancement in laparoscopic skill has coincided with the increased use of laparoscopy for diagnosis and treatment of biliary tract disorders. It is most effective when used in conjunction with laparoscopic ultrasound in the staging and operative management of biliary malignancies. Intra-operative ultrasound is now used frequently to further evaluate intrahepatic lesions, assess resectability, and determine involvement of vascular structures.[2,3] Although the need for laparoscopy may have diminished as a result of advancements in radiologic techniques like CT, laparoscopy still best identifies micrometastases much beyond the discrimination of the CT scan; in addition, biopsy of micrometastases can be undertaken with the laparoscope.

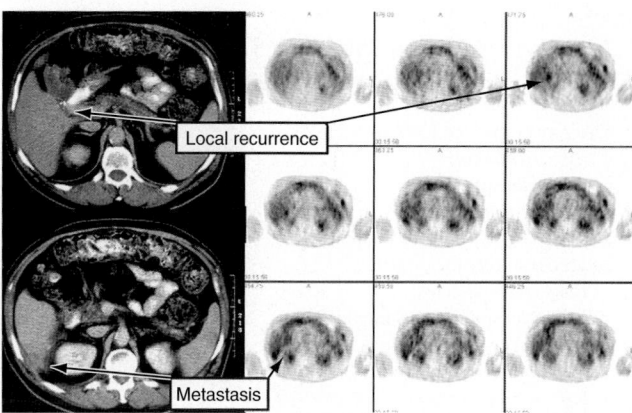

Figure 54-9 Fluorodeoxyglucose positron emission tomography (FDG-PET) imaging in a patient undergoing surveillance after treatment for cholangiocarcinoma. The FDG-PET images demonstrate FDG uptake corresponding to the hilum on the respective CT image, indicating local recurrence and metastatic spread.

FDG-PET Scanning

Fluorodeoxyglucose positron emission tomography (FDG-PET) is a whole-body technique that allows detection of unsuspected metastases that may lead to major changes in the surgical management of these patients. PET imaging with the fluorinated glucose analogue, [18]FDG, can be used to exploit the metabolic differences between benign and malignant cells for imaging purposes. Therefore, [18]FDG-PET imaging has become well established for differentiation of benign from malignant lesions, staging malignant lesions, detection of malignancy recurrence, and monitoring therapy for various malignancies (Fig. 54-9). Recent studies have shown that [18]FDG-PET is accurate in predicting the presence of nodular cholangiocarcinoma (mass >1 cm) and gallbladder carcinoma (sensitivity, 78%).[4] [18]FDG-PET is not useful for detection of carcinomatosis, and inflammatory changes related to biliary stents may cause interpretation difficulties.

Bacteriology

Bile in the gallbladder or bile ducts in the absence of gallstones or any other biliary tract disease is normally sterile. In the presence of gallstones or biliary obstruction, the prevalence of bactibilia increases. The percentage of positive gallbladder bile cultures among patients with symptomatic gallstones and chronic cholecystitis ranges from 11% to 30%. The prevalence of positive gallbladder bile cultures is higher in patients with acute cholecystitis than chronic cholecystitis (46% versus 22%) and increases further in the presence of common bile duct stones. Positive bile cultures are significantly more common in elderly (>60 years) patients with symptomatic gallstones than in younger patients (45% versus 16%).[5,6] Gram-negative aerobes are the organisms most frequently isolated from bile in patients with symptomatic gallstones, acute cholecystitis, or cholangitis (Box 54-1). *Escherichia coli* and *Klebsiella* species are the most common gram-negative bacteria isolated. However, *Pseudomonas* and *Enterobacter* species are being seen with increased frequency, particularly in patients with malignant biliary obstruction.[5] Other common isolates include the gram-positive aerobes, *Enterococcus* species, and *Streptococcus viridans*. Anaerobic bacteria, such as *Bacteroides* and *Clostridium* species, are infrequent but remain significant pathogens in biliary infections. *Candida* species are also being increasingly recognized as a significant biliary pathogen particularly in critically ill patients.

The source of bacteria in patients with biliary tract infections is controversial. Most theories favor an ascending route through the duodenum as the main source of biliary bacteria. The bacterial flora in the small intestine is similar to that detected in the biliary tract.

Antibiotic Selection
Antibiotics should be used prophylactically in most patients undergoing elective biliary tract surgery or other biliary tract manipulations such as ERCP or PTC. In low-risk patients undergoing laparoscopic cholecystectomy for biliary colic or chronic cholecystitis, there is no benefit of prophylactic antibiotics. In high-risk patients, such as elderly patients, patients with recent acute cholecystitis, and those with high risk for conversion to open cholecystectomy, a single dose of the first-generation cephalosporin, cefazolin, provides good coverage against the gram-negative aerobes commonly isolated from bile and skin flora.

Therapeutic antibiotics should be used in patients with acute cholecystitis and cholangitis and should cover gram-negative aerobes, gram-positive coverage, and anaerobes.

BENIGN PATHOPHYSIOLOGIC CONDITIONS
Calculous Biliary Disease
Epidemiology
Gallstones are among the most common gastrointestinal illness requiring hospitalization and frequently occur in young, otherwise healthy people with a prevalence of 11% to 36% in autopsy reports. Female sex, obesity, pregnancy, fatty foods, Crohn's disease, terminal ileal resection, gastric surgery, hereditary spherocytosis, sickle cell disease, and thalassemia are all associated with an increased risk for developing gallstones[7] (Box 54-2). Only first-degree relatives of patients with gallstones and *obesity* (defined as body mass index >30 kg/m²) have been identified as strong risk factors for development of symptomatic gallstone disease.[8]

Gallstone Pathogenesis
Gallstones represent an inability to maintain certain biliary solutes, primarily cholesterol and calcium salts, in a solubilized state. Gallstones are classified by their cholesterol content as either cholesterol or pigment stones. Pigment stones are further classified as either black or brown. Pure cholesterol gallstones are uncommon (10%), with most cholesterol stones containing calcium salts in their center, or nidus. In the United States, 70% to 80% of gallstones are cholesterol, and black pigment stones account for most of the remaining 20% to 30%.

Biliary sludge refers to a mixture of cholesterol crystals, calcium bilirubinate granules, and a mucin gel matrix. It is most commonly found in prolonged fasting states or with the use of parental nutrition. The finding of macromolecular complexes of mucin and bilirubin suggests that sludge may serve as the nidus for gallstone pathogenesis.

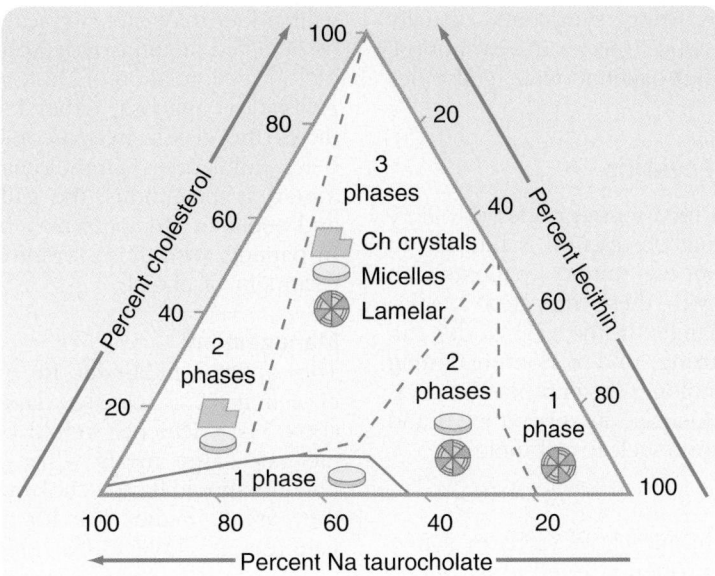

Figure 54-10 Triangular-phase diagram with axes plotted in percent cholesterol, lecithin (phospholipid), and the bile salt sodium taurocholate. Below the *solid line,* cholesterol is maintained in solution in micelles. Above the *solid line,* bile is supersaturated with cholesterol and precipitation of cholesterol crystals can occur. Ch, cholesterol. (From Donovan JM, Carey MC: Separation and quantitation of cholesterol "carriers" in bile. Hepatology 12:94S, 1990.)

Cholesterol Gallstones

The pathogenesis of cholesterol gallstones involves three stages:

1. Cholesterol supersaturation in bile
2. Crystal nucleation
3. Stone growth

Gallbladder mucosal and motor function plays a key role in gallstone formation. The key to maintaining cholesterol in solution is the formation of micelles, a bile salt–phospholipid-cholesterol complex, and cholesterol-phospholipid vesicles. In states of excess cholesterol production, these large vesicles may also exceed their capability to transport cholesterol, and crystal precipitation may occur. One third of biliary cholesterol is transported in micelles, but the cholesterol-phospholipid vesicles carry the majority of biliary cholesterol. By plotting the percentages of each component on triangular coordinates, the micellar zone in which cholesterol is completely soluble can be demonstrated (Fig. 54-10). In the area above the curve, bile is supersaturated with cholesterol, and precipitation of cholesterol crystals can occur.

Pigment Gallstones

Pigment stones contain less than 20% cholesterol and are dark owing to the presence of calcium bilirubinate. Otherwise, black and brown pigment stones have little in common and should be considered as separate entities. Black pigment stones are small and tarry, and are frequently associated with hemolytic conditions such as hereditary spherocytosis and sickle cell disease or cir-

rhosis. In hemolytic states, the bilirubin load and concentration of unconjugated bilirubin increases. Cirrhosis may lead to increased secretion of unconjugated bilirubin. These stones are usually not associated with infected bile and are located almost exclusively in the gallbladder. Black stones account for a high percentage of gallstones in Asian countries such as Japan compared with the Western hemisphere.

Brown pigment stones are soft and earthy in texture and are typically found in bile ducts, especially in Asian populations. Brown stones often contain more cholesterol and calcium palmitate and occur as primary common duct stones in Western patients with disorders of biliary motility and associated bacterial infection. Bacteria producing slime such as *E. coli* secrete β-glucuronidase that causes enzymatic hydrolysis of soluble conjugated bilirubin glucuronide to produce insoluble free bilirubin, which then precipitates with calcium.[9]

Natural History

Most patients remain asymptomatic from their gallstones. Although the mechanism is unclear, some patients develop symptomatic gallstones, with biliary colic caused by a stone obstructing the cystic duct. Additional complications related to gallstones include acute cholecystitis, choledocholithiasis with or without cholangitis, gallstone pancreatitis, gallstone ileus, and gallbladder carcinoma.

Gallstones are commonly found incidentally at laparotomy or on imaging either by ultrasonography or CT scan. Only 1% to 2% of asymptomatic individuals with gallstones develop serious symptoms or complications related to their gallstones per year; therefore, only about 1% require a cholecystectomy. Once symptomatic, patients tend to have recurring symptoms, usually repeated episodes of biliary colic.[10] Over a 20-year period, two thirds of asymptomatic patients with gallstones remain symptom-free.

Chronic Calculous Cholecystitis

Ongoing inflammation with recurrent episodes of biliary colic or pain from cystic duct obstruction is referred to as *chronic cholecystitis*. About two thirds of patients with gallstone disease present with these repeated attacks. Although the pathologic changes in the gallbladder can vary, repeated attacks, scarring, and a nonfunctioning gallbladder are the rule. Histologically, chronic cholecystitis is characterized by an increase in subepithelial and subserosal fibrosis and a mononuclear cell infiltrate.

Clinical Presentation

The primary symptom of chronic cholecystitis or symptomatic cholelithiasis is pain, often referred to as *biliary colic* (see earlier section, Abdominal Pain). The pain is constant and usually lasts 1 to 5 hours. The attacks usually last for more than 1 hour but subsides by 24 hours; if pain persists longer than 1 day, acute cholecystitis is likely the underlying etiology. The attacks are discrete and severe enough that patients can accurately recall and number them. Other symptoms such as nausea and vomiting often accompany each episode, and bloating and belching may also be present in 50% of cases. Fever and jaundice are rare with simple biliary colic. Patients without symptoms, about two thirds of patients with gallstones, develop symptoms infrequently and complications at an even lower rate. In most cases, treatment is not necessary in these asymptomatic patients. Patients with gallstones but an atypical presentation should have other causes of right upper quadrant pain ruled out such as peptic ulcer disease, pneumonia, renal calculi, liver disease, hernia, reflux, or angina.

The physical examination and liver function tests are usually completely normal in patients with chronic cholecystitis, particularly if they are pain-free. During an episode of biliary colic, mild right upper quadrant tenderness may also be present.

Diagnosis

The diagnosis of symptomatic gallstones or chronic calculous cholecystitis relies on the clinical presentation and evidence of gallstones on diagnostic imaging. The presence of symptoms, typically biliary colic, attributable to the gallbladder is necessary to consider any treatment for gallstones. An abdominal ultrasound is the standard diagnostic exam for gallstones (Fig. 54-11). Ultrasonography also provides important anatomic information for the surgeon—presence of polyps, common bile duct diameter, or any hepatic parenchymal abnormalities. Occasionally, patients with typical attacks of biliary pain have no evidence of stones on ultrasonography, or only sludge is present. If the patient has recurrent attacks of typical biliary colic and sludge is detected on two or more occasions, cholecystectomy is indicated. In addition to sludge and stones, cholesterolosis and adenomyomatosis of the

gallbladder may cause typical biliary symptoms and may be detected on ultrasonography. Cholesterolosis is caused by the accumulation of cholesterol in macrophages in the gallbladder mucosa, either locally or as polyps. It produces the classic macroscopic appearance of a "strawberry gallbladder." Granulomatous polyps develop in the lumen at the fundus; the gallbladder wall is thickened, and septa or strictures may be seen in the gallbladder. In patients with these symptoms, cholecystectomy is the treatment of choice.

Management

The optimal treatment for patients with symptomatic cholelithiasis is elective laparoscopic cholecystectomy (Box 54-3). Patients should be advised to avoid dietary fats and large meals while awaiting surgery. Diabetic patients should have a cholecystectomy promptly because they are at higher risk for acute cholecystitis or even gangrenous cholecystitis. Pregnant women with symp-

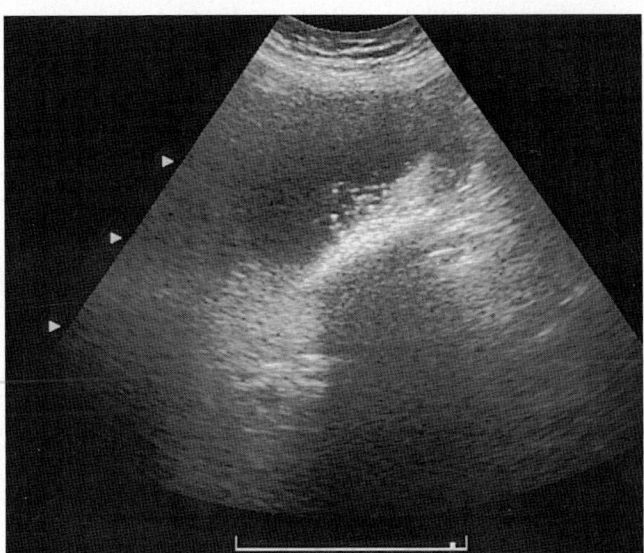

Figure 54-11 Gallbladder ultrasound in patient with biliary colic demonstrating multiple dependent echogenic foci with posterior acoustic shadowing consistent with gallstones.

Box 54-3   Indications for Cholecystectomy

Urgent*

Acute cholecystitis
Emphysematous cholecystitis
Empyema of the gallbladder
Perforation of the gallbladder
Previous choledocholithiasis with endoscopic duct clearance

Elective

Biliary dyskinesia
Chronic cholecystitis
Symptomatic cholelithiasis

*Within 24 to 72 hours.

tomatic gallstones who fail expectant management with dietary modification can safely undergo surgery during the second trimester. Cholecystectomy offers excellent long-term results for patients with symptomatic gallstones. About 90% of patients are rendered symptom-free after cholecystectomy. For patients with atypical symptoms or painless dyspepsia (fatty food intolerance, flatulence, belching, or bloating), the percentage of patients experiencing relief of symptoms falls.

Acute Calculous Cholecystitis

Pathophysiology

Acute cholecystitis is related to gallstones in 90% to 95% of cases. Obstruction of the cystic duct leading to biliary colic is the initial event in acute cholecystitis. If the cystic duct remains obstructed, the gallbladder distends, and the gallbladder wall then becomes inflamed and edematous. Initially, acute cholecystitis is an inflammatory process with a thickened and reddish wall with subserosal hemorrhage. The mucosa may show hyperemia and patchy areas of necrosis. In the most common scenario, the gallstone dislodges, and the inflammation will gradually resolve. In the most severe cases, this process can lead to ischemia and necrosis of the gallbladder wall (5%-10%). Acute gangrenous cholecystitis results in formation of an abscess or empyema within the gallbladder. When gas-forming organisms are part of the secondary bacterial infection, gas may be seen in the gallbladder lumen and in the wall of the gallbladder on imaging resulting in *emphysematous cholecystitis.*

Clinical Presentation

Right upper quadrant pain, similar in severity to but much longer in duration than pain from previous episodes of biliary colic, is the most common symptom of acute cholecystitis. Other common symptoms include fever, nausea, and vomiting. On physical exam, right upper quadrant tenderness and guarding are usually present inferior to the right costal margin, distinguishing the episode from simple biliary colic. When inflammation spreads to the peritoneum, patients develop more diffuse tenderness, guarding and rigidity. A mass, the gallbladder and adherent omentum, is occasionally palpable, and *Murphy's sign,* inspiratory arrest with deep palpation in the right upper quadrant, may also be present. A mild leukocytosis is usually present (12,000-14,000 cells/mm^3). In addition, mild elevations in serum bilirubin (>4 mg/dL), alkaline phosphatase, the transaminases, and amylase may be present. Severe jaundice is suggestive of common bile duct stones or obstruction of the bile ducts by severe pericholecystic inflammation secondary to impaction of a stone in the infundibulum of the gallbladder that mechanically obstructs the bile duct, known as *Mirizzi's syndrome.*

Diagnosis

Ultrasound is the most useful radiographic test for diagnosing acute cholecystitis, with sensitivity and specificity of 85% and 95%, respectively. It is sensitive for identifying the presence of gallstones. Ultrasound also shows the presence of thickening of the gallbladder wall (>4 mm), pericholecystic fluid, gallbladder distention, impacted stone, and a sonographic Murphy's sign (focal tenderness directly over the gallbladder).

Biliary radionuclide scanning is used less frequently today but may be helpful in atypical cases. No filling of the gallbladder with the radiotracer (^{99m}Tc-HIDA) after 4 hours indicates an obstructed cystic duct with a sensitivity and specificity for acute cholecystitis of 95%. A normal HIDA scan excludes acute cholecystitis. However, when the patient is fasting for more than 5 days, HIDA scan is much less helpful, with a 40% false-positive rate. CT scan, although performed frequently in patients with abdominal pain, may identify some of the findings mentioned previously, similar to ultrasonography, but is less sensitive than ultrasonography for acute cholecystitis.

Management

After the diagnosis of acute cholecystitis is made, IV fluids, antibiotics, and analgesia should be initiated. Antibiotics should cover gram-negative aerobes as well as anaerobes (see Box 54-1). More than half of patients with acute cholecystitis have positive cultures from the gallbladder bile. Because it is difficult to know who is secondarily infected, IV antibiotics are an appropriate part of the management.

Cholecystectomy is the definitive treatment for patients with acute cholecystitis. Early cholecystectomy performed within 2 to 3 days of presentation is preferred over interval or delayed cholecystectomy that is performed 6 to 10 weeks after initial medical therapy.[11,12] About 20% of patients fail initial medical therapy and require surgery during the initial admission or before the end of the planned cooling-off period.

Laparoscopic cholecystectomy is the preferred approach to patients with acute cholecystitis. Conversion to an open procedure should be made if the inflammation prevents adequate visualization of important structures. The conversion rate to an open cholecystectomy is higher (4%-35%) in the setting of acute cholecystitis than with chronic cholecystitis. Numerous studies have shown the morbidity rate, hospital stay, and time to return to work are lower in patients undergoing laparoscopic cholecystectomy than open cholecystectomy.[13-15] Early laparoscopic cholecystectomy, due to a reduced length of hospital stay and readmissions, is a more cost-effective approach than open cholecystectomy for acute cholecystitis.[16] Patients who are operated on early in the course of their illness (within 48 hours) are more likely to have their procedure completed laparoscopically (4% versus 23%) than patients with a longer duration of symptoms.[17] Additional factors predicting the need to convert to an open cholecystectomy include increased patient age, male gender, elevated American Society of Anesthesiologists class, obesity, and thickened gallbladder wall (>4 mm).

Acute cholecystitis may progress to empyema of the gallbladder, emphysematous cholecystitis, or perforation of the gallbladder despite antibiotic therapy. In each case, emergency cholecystectomy is indicated, if the patient can safely withstand an anesthetic. In most patients, cholecystectomy can be performed and is the best treatment of complicated acute cholecystitis. Occasionally, the inflammatory process obscures the structures in the triangle of Calot, precluding safe dissection and ligation of the cystic duct. In these patients, partial cholecystectomy, cauterization of the remaining gallbladder mucosa, and drainage avoid injury to the common bile duct. In patients considered too unstable to tolerate a laparotomy, percutaneous transhepatic cholecystostomy under local anesthesia can be performed to drain the gallbladder. This procedure leaves the gallbladder in place, which may be a source of ongoing sepsis. Drainage and IV antibiotics, followed by interval laparoscopic cholecystectomy, can then be performed after 3 to 4 months to allow the patient to recover and the acute inflammation to resolve.

Choledocholithiasis

Common bile duct stones are classified by their point of origin and are found in 6% to 12% of patients with stones in the gallbladder. Most common bile duct stones in Western countries form initially in the gallbladder and migrate through the cystic duct into the common bile duct. These stones are identified as secondary calculi to distinguish them from primary common bile duct stones, which form within the biliary tract. Common duct stones are also defined as *retained* if they are discovered within 2 years of cholecystectomy, or *recurrent* if they are detected more than 2 years after cholecystectomy. The secondary stones are usually of the brown pigment type. Identification of brown stones in the common bile duct should alert the surgeon to the high likelihood of recurrent stones and need for a biliary-enteric drainage procedure. The primary stones are associated with biliary stasis and infection and are more commonly seen in Asian populations. The causes of biliary stasis that lead to the development of primary stones include biliary stricture, papillary stenosis, tumors, or other (secondary) stones.

Presentation

Common bile duct stones may be silent and are often discovered incidentally. In these patients, biliary obstruction is transient, and laboratory tests may be normal. About 1% to 2% of patients with normal liver function tests managed with laparoscopic cholecystectomy without a routine cholangiogram for gallstones present with a retained stone after cholecystectomy.

Clinical features suspicious for biliary obstruction due to common bile duct stones include biliary colic, jaundice, lightening of the stools, and darkening of the urine. In addition, fever and chills may be present in patients with choledocholithiasis and cholangitis. Serum bilirubin (>3.0 mg/dL), serum aminotransferases, and alkaline phosphatase all are commonly elevated in patients with biliary obstruction but are neither sensitive nor specific for the presence of common duct stones. Of these, serum bilirubin has the highest positive predictive value (28%-

50%) for the presence of choledocholithiasis. However, laboratory values may be normal in as many as one third of patients with choledocholithiasis.

Diagnosis

Ultrasonography, commonly the first test, can document stones in the gallbladder and estimate the diameter of the common bile duct. A dilated bile duct (>8 mm in diameter) on ultrasonography in a patient with gallstones, jaundice and biliary pain is highly suggestive of choledocholithiasis. As stones in the distal bile duct slowly move down, bowel gas can preclude their visibility on ultrasound; echogenic shadows consistent with calculi in the common bile duct are visible in only 60% to 70% of patients with choledocholithiasis. Among patients with gallstones, the prevalence of choledocholithiasis is significantly higher in the setting of a dilated common bile duct (diameter >5 mm) than in patients with a nondilated duct (58% versus 1%).[18] MRC provides excellent anatomic detail, with sensitivity and specificity of 95% and 98%, respectively, for common bile duct stones, avoids the need for invasive ERCP in more than 50% of patients and can be used as a screening test for patients at low or moderate risk for having common duct stones before ERCP.

ERCP is the diagnostic and potentially therapeutic test of choice for patients with suspected common bile duct stones (Fig. 54-12). Cannulation of the ampulla of Vater and diagnostic cholangiography are achieved in more than 90% of cases. Minimal morbidity rates of less than 5% are now achieved in experienced hands and mainly consist of cholangitis and pancreatitis. Endoscopic ultrasound (EUS) can also be used to identify bile duct stones without cannulation of the ampulla and its associated risks, but it is less sensitive than ERCP.

Management

Endoscopic Cholangiography

The use of endoscopic cholangiography in patients with suspected common bile duct stones not only confirms the diagnosis but also provides ductal clearance of the stones and sphincterotomy before subsequent laparoscopic cholecystectomy. Endoscopic clearance of stones from the common bile duct can avoid the need for an open operation if expertise in laparoscopic common bile duct exploration is not available. Patients with worsening cholangitis, ampullary stone impaction, biliary pancreatitis, multiple comorbidities, and cirrhosis are considered good candidates for preoperative endoscopic therapy. When endoscopic evaluation is carried out routinely in all patients, 86% are normal. If clearance is not possible because of multiple stones, intrahepatic stones, impacted stones, difficulty with cannulation, duodenal diverticula, or biliary stricture, this information is known before surgery. Endoscopic sphincterotomy with stone extraction is well tolerated in most patients, with a 5% to 8% complication rate. Complete clearance of all common duct stones is achieved endoscopically in 71% to 75% of patients at the first procedure and in 84% to 95% of patients after multiple endoscopic procedures.[19]

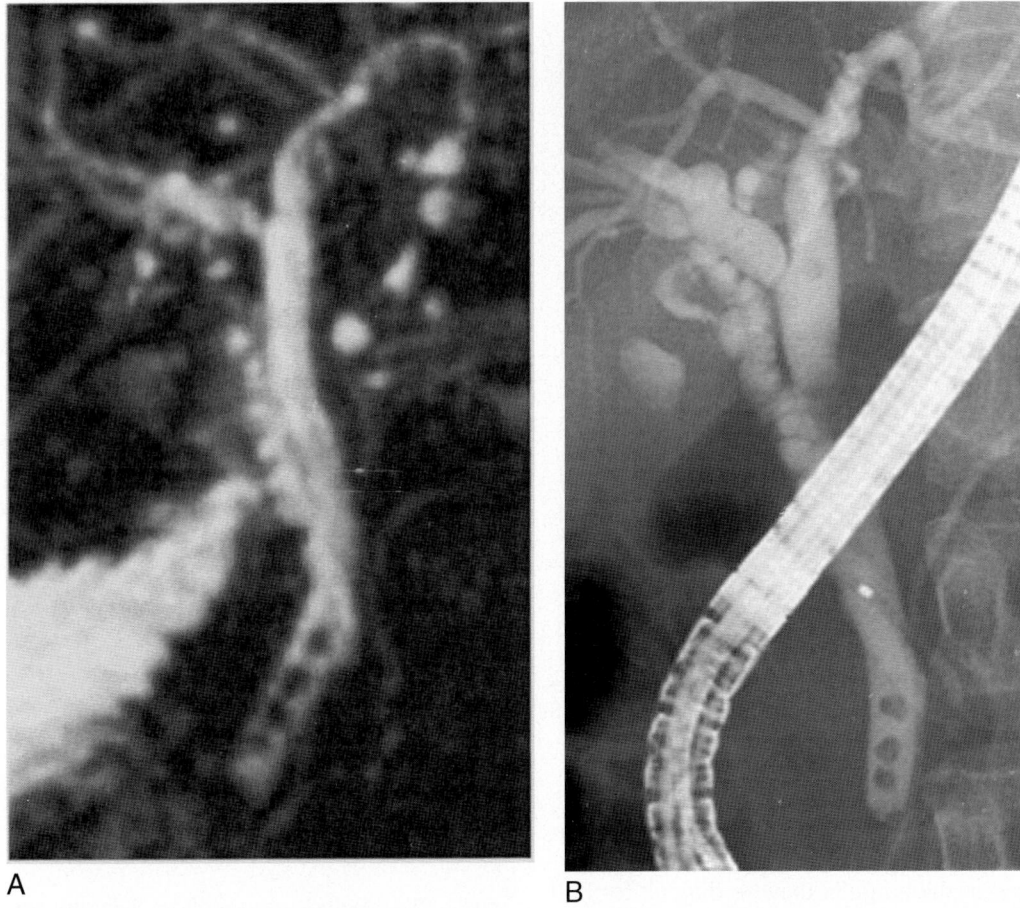

A   B

Figure 54-12 A, MRCP showing multiple, small stones in a nondilated common bile duct. **B,** Corresponding endoscopic retrograde cholangiopancreatography image. (From Moon JH, Cho YD, Cha SW, et al: The detection of bile duct stones in suspected biliary pancreatitis: Comparison of MRCP, ERCP, and intraductal US. Am J Gastroenterol 100:1051-1057, 2005.)

After endoscopic sphincterotomy and stone extraction, patients with gallstones still remain at high risk for developing future biliary complications. A significantly greater incidence of recurrent biliary symptoms is expected among patients managed with a wait-and-see approach versus laparoscopic cholecystectomy (47% versus 2%; $P > .0001$) after endoscopic stone extraction. Thirty-seven percent of patients managed expectantly later required cholecystectomy.[20] Therefore, prompt cholecystectomy after endoscopic clearance of the common bile duct should be performed during the hospital admission if the patient is fit for surgery. On the other hand, patients older than 70 years should have their ductal stones cleared endoscopically as their sole therapy; only about 15% become symptomatic from their gallbladder stones in their remaining lifetime, which can then be treated as symptoms arise.

Laparoscopic Common Bile Duct Exploration

An intraoperative cholangiogram at the time of cholecystectomy will also document the presence of common bile duct stones (Fig. 54-13). Laparoscopic common bile duct exploration through the cystic duct or with formal choledochotomy allows the stones to be retrieved during the

same procedure. If the expertise and instrumentation for laparoscopic common bile duct exploration are not available, a drain should be placed and left adjacent next to the cystic duct and an endoscopic cholangiogram performed the following day. An open common bile duct exploration should be performed if endoscopic intervention is not available or not feasible because of anatomic restrictions or expertise. If a choledochotomy is performed, a T tube is left in place. The purpose of the T tube is to provide access to the biliary system for postoperative radiologic stone extraction. The size of the tube is therefore of importance, in that tubes smaller than 16 French do not allow for postoperative radiologic instrumentation without dilation of the tract; a minimum of 4 to 6 weeks should pass for the tract to mature before instrumentation.

Open Common Bile Duct Exploration

With the increased use of endoscopic, percutaneous, and laparoscopic techniques, open common bile duct exploration is rarely performed today. It should be performed when a concomitant biliary drainage procedure is indicated. Open common bile duct exploration is associated with low operative mortality (1%-2%) and operative mor-

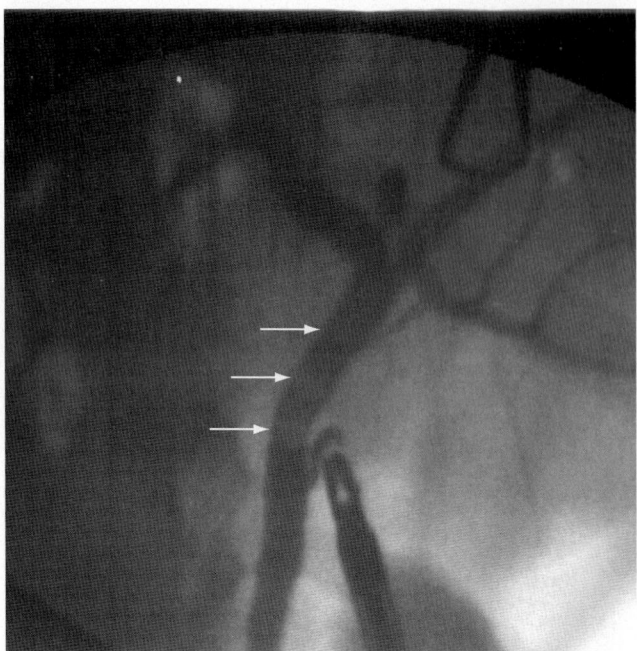

Figure 54-13 Intraoperative cholangiogram confirming the presence of common bile duct stones. Calculi are indicated with *arrows*. (Courtesy of Michael D. Holzman, MD.)

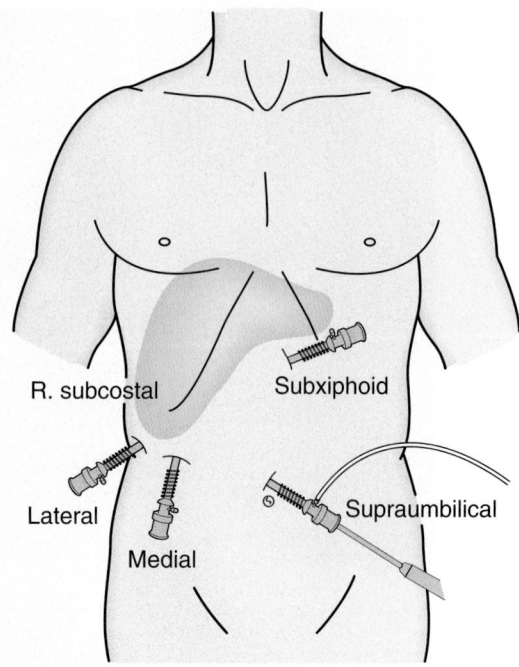

Figure 54-14 Trocar placement for laparoscopic cholecystectomy. The laparoscope is placed through a 10-mm port just above the umbilicus. Additional ports are placed in the epigastrium and subcostally in the midclavicular and near the anterior axillary lines. (From Cameron J: Atlas of Surgery, vol 2. Philadelphia, BC Decker, 1994.)

bidity (8%-16%). The rate of retained common bile stones using intraoperative choledochoscopy is less than 5%. Stones impacted in the ampulla may be difficult for both endoscopic ductal clearance and common bile duct exploration. In these cases, transduodenal sphincteroplasty and stone extraction should be performed; alternatively, if this is not successful, a choledochoduodenostomy or a Roux-en-Y choledochojejunostomy should be performed.

Gallstone Pancreatitis

Blockage of the pancreatic duct by an impacted stone or temporary obstruction by a stone passing through the ampulla may lead to pancreatitis by an unknown mechanism. An ultrasound in patients with acute pancreatitis of uncertain cause is critical to assess for gallstones and choledocholithiasis. An ERCP with sphincterotomy and stone extraction is the initial treatment and may relieve the pancreatitis. Once the pancreatitis has subsided, the gallbladder should be removed during the same admission. If the pancreatitis is self-limited, the stone has likely passed. For these patients, cholecystectomy and an intraoperative cholangiogram are indicated.

Biliary Dyskinesia

Patients who present with typical symptoms of biliary colic but have no evidence of gallstones on ultrasound exam should be investigated for biliary dyskinesia. Once other possible diagnoses have been excluded with CT scan, upper endoscopy, or ERCP, a CCK-Tc-HIDA scan should be performed to rule out biliary dyskinesia. CCK is infused IV after the gallbladder has been filled with

the ^{99m}Tc-labeled radionuclide. Twenty minutes after the administration of CCK, a gallbladder ejection fraction is determined. An ejection fraction less than 35% at 20 minutes is considered abnormal.

Patients with symptoms of biliary colic and an abnormal gallbladder ejection fraction should be managed with a laparoscopic cholecystectomy. Between 85% and 94% of patients with a low gallbladder ejection fraction and symptoms of biliary colic will be asymptomatic or improved by cholecystectomy. Commonly, there is histopathologic evidence of chronic cholecystitis.

Sphincter of Oddi Dysfunction

Pain similar to biliary colic with normal liver function tests and episodes of acute pancreatitis have been attributed to a poorly defined syndrome known as *dysfunction of the sphincter of Oddi*. The pathogenesis is unclear, but theories that have been postulated include gallstone migration inducing fibrosis of the sphincter, trauma, pancreatitis, and congenital anomalies. About 1% of patients undergoing cholecystectomy have sphincter of Oddi dysfunction. A dilated common bile duct (>12 mm diameter) or increase in common bile duct diameter in response to CCK is a typical ultrasound finding. Delayed emptying of contrast medium from the common bile duct after ERCP is also indicative of abnormal sphincter function. Ampullary manometry indicating an elevated basal sphincter pressure (>40 mm Hg) has been correlated with good results after treatment that consists of endoscopic or operative sphincterotomy.[21]

Surgery for Calculous Biliary Disease

Laparoscopic Cholecystectomy

Since the introduction of laparoscopic cholecystectomy, the number of cholecystectomies performed in the United States has increased from about 500,000 per year to 700,000 per year. Contraindications to laparoscopic cholecystectomy include coagulopathy, severe chronic obstructive pulmonary disease, end-stage liver disease, and congestive heart failure. Currently, the major contraindication to completing a laparoscopic cholecystectomy is inability to clearly identify all of the anatomic structures. The conversion rate for elective laparoscopic cholecystectomy should be around 5%, whereas the conversion rate in the setting of acute cholecystitis may be as high as 30%. Conversion to an open procedure is not a failure, and the possibility should be discussed with the patient preoperatively.

Patients undergoing laparoscopic cholecystectomy should be prepared and draped in a similar fashion to open cholecystectomy. The patient is supine on the operating table with the surgeon standing on the patient's left. The pneumoperitoneum is created with carbon dioxide gas, either with an open technique or by closed-needle technique. With the open technique, a small incision is made either above or below the umbilicus into the peritoneal cavity. A special blunt-tipped cannula (Hasson) with a gas-tight sleeve is inserted into the peritoneal cavity and anchored to the fascia. This technique is often used following previous abdominal surgery and should

avoid infrequent but life-threatening trocar injuries. In the closed technique, a special hollow insufflation needle (Veress) with a retractable cutting sheath is inserted into the peritoneal cavity through a periumbilical incision and used for insufflation. There is no difference in inadvertent bowel or tissue injury between the two techniques.

The laparoscope with the attached video camera is then inserted into the umbilical port and the abdomen inspected. The additional ports are inserted under direct vision (Fig. 54-14). The medial 5-mm cannula is used to grasp the gallbladder infundibulum (Fig. 54-15) and retract it laterally with the pull toward the right pelvis, to expose the triangle of Calot; it is important to widely expose the triangle of Calot with this direction of retraction to fully enable identification of possible aberrant biliary anatomy. This maneuver may require taking down the adhesions between the omentum or duodenum and the gallbladder. Most of the dissection can be performed using a dissector, hook, or scissors. The junction of the gallbladder and cystic duct is identified and dissection continued until the cystic artery and duct is clearly seen entering the gallbladder (Fig. 54-16). A helpful anatomic landmark is the cystic lymph node. Careful extended dissection of the base of the gallbladder off the liver bed is essential to define the duct and artery. The outdated infundibular technique of cystic duct dissection and identification does not fully expose the triangle of Calot and leads to misidentification and is a setup for bile duct injury. Partial dissection of the base of the gallbladder off the liver bed before dividing either the artery or cystic

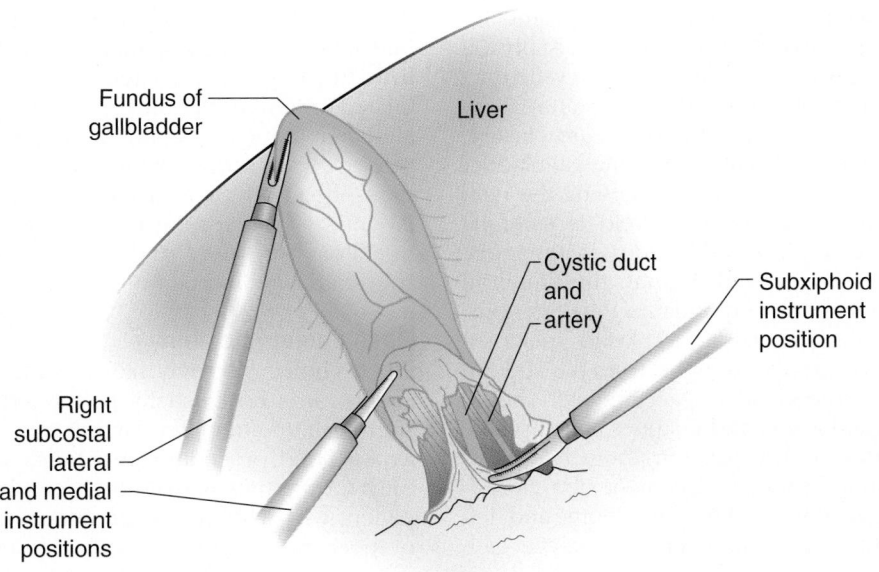

Figure 54-15 The gallbladder is retracted cephalad using the grasper on the gallbladder fundus and at the infundibulum, with the direction of pull toward the right pelvis. The peritoneum overlying the gallbladder infundibulum and neck and the cystic duct is divided bluntly, exposing the cystic duct. (From Cameron J: Atlas of Surgery, vol 2. Philadelphia, BC Becker, 1994.)

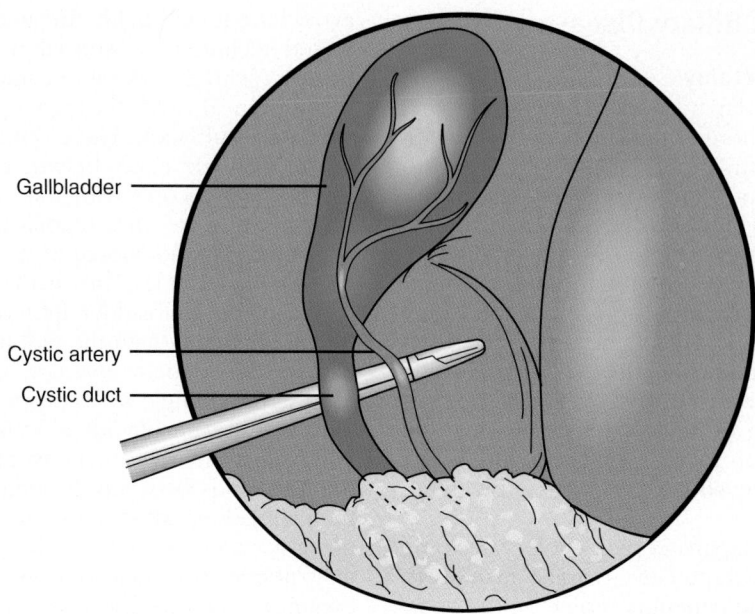

Gallbladder

Cystic artery
Cystic duct

Figure 54-16 View obtained after dissection within the triangle of Calot demonstrating the cystic duct and cystic artery clearly entering the gallbladder. At this point, it is safe to ligate and divide the cystic duct. Visualization of the common bile duct is not necessary. (From Strasberg SM, Hertl M, Soper NJ: An analysis of the problem of biliary injury during laparoscopic cholecystectomy. J Am Coll Surg 180:101-125, 1995.)

duct enables identification of all the anatomy and minimizes risk for bile duct injury.

The next step is ligation of the cystic artery. The artery is usually encountered running parallel to and behind the cystic duct. Clips are placed proximally and distally on the artery, which is then divided. If indicated, an intraoperative cholangiogram may now be performed by placing a hemoclip proximally on the cystic duct, incising the anterior surface of the duct, and passing a cholangiogram catheter into the cystic duct. Once the cholangiogram is completed, two clips are placed distally on the cystic duct, which is then divided. A large cystic duct may require placement of a pretied loop ligature or a standard suture tied laparoscopically for secure closure. Finally, the gallbladder is dissected out of the gallbladder fossa with electrocautery. Just before removing the gallbladder from the liver, the operative field is carefully searched for hemostasis. The gallbladder is then dissected off the liver and removed through the umbilical port. If the gallbladder is acutely inflamed, gangrenous, or entered during the dissection, a plastic specimen retrieval bag should be used for removal from the abdominal cavity. Any bile or blood that has accumulated should be irrigated and sucked away, and if stones were spilled, they should be retrieved. Any concern about bile accumulation or leak should prompt placement of a closed-suction drain through one of the 5-mm ports and left underneath the right lobe of the liver close to the gallbladder fossa.

Elective laparoscopic cholecystectomy can be safely performed as an outpatient procedure, and most centers in the United States have demonstrated a strong trend toward ambulatory cholecystectomy.[22] Among patients selected for outpatient management, 77% to 97% of patients can be successfully discharged without hospital admission.[23]

Intraoperative Cholangiogram or Ultrasound
Use of routine cholangiogram or ultrasound to identify so-called silent common bile duct stones is controversial. Routine intraoperative cholangiography will detect stones in about 7% of patients, outline the anatomy, and identify potential biliary injuries,[24] although it does not prevent them. A selective intraoperative cholangiogram should be performed when the patient has a history of abnormal liver function tests, a large duct and small stones, or a dilated common bile duct, or if preoperative endoscopic cholangiography was not performed in a patient with suspected choledocholithiasis (Box 54-4). Laparoscopic ultrasonography is as accurate as intraoperative cholangiography in detecting common bile duct stones but is operator dependent and requires expertise with ultrasound and interpretation of results.[25]

Open Cholecystectomy
Open cholecystectomy has become an uncommon procedure. It is now usually performed either as a conversion from an attempted laparoscopic cholecystectomy or as a second procedure in patients who require laparotomy for another reason. It should be performed in any patient who cannot tolerate pneumoperitoneum because of poor pulmonary or cardiac reserve (Box 54-5). An important consideration for open cholecystectomy is in patients in whom gallbladder cancer is suspected preoperatively.

From a technical standpoint, open cholecystectomy can be performed similarly to the laparoscopic approach. After the cystic artery and duct have been identified, the gallbladder is dissected from the liver bed, starting with the fundus. Alternatively, the retrograde technique can be used where the dissection is initiated with the fundus and the artery and duct identified, ligated, and divided as a final step. It is important to keep the dissection as close to the gallbladder as possible, to avoid dissection into the liver and subsequent bleeding. The dissection is carried proximally toward the cystic artery and the cystic duct, which are then ligated and divided.

Common Bile Duct Exploration

In patients with large and multiple stones or dilated ducts, and when endoscopic therapy fails, laparoscopic common bile duct exploration is indicated. If unsuccessful, conversion to open surgery is necessary, whereas postoperative ERCP should be used as the last resource. After intraoperative cholangiogram indicates the presence of choledocholithiasis, the surgeon is faced with many options. A wide array of techniques and tools are at a surgeon's disposal. The initial step is to determine the important factors regarding which modality of treatment will best serve the patient. Factors such as diameter and anatomy of the cystic and common bile ducts, number and size of CBD stones, clinical status of the patient, and most importantly, technical skill of the surgeon should all be considered.

Laparoscopic Approach

If the stones are small, use of saline irrigation through the cholangiogram catheter to flush the stones into the duodenum is all that is necessary. Relaxation of the sphincter of Oddi with glucagon may be helpful. If irrigation is unsuccessful, a balloon catheter may be passed through the cystic duct and down the common bile duct, where it is inflated and withdrawn to retrieve the stones. The next attempt should be made with a wire basket passed under fluoroscopic guidance to catch the stones. If needed, a flexible choledochoscope is inserted directly into the cystic duct (Fig. 54-17). The cystic duct may have to be dilated to allow its passage. Although most authors advocate first attempting a transcystic access, there are clear indications for a direct common bile duct exploration first. The most common scenarios are the presence of more than five common bile duct stones, stones larger than 9 mm, and common hepatic duct stones. Once in the common bile duct, the stones may be caught into

a wire basket under direct vision or pushed into the duodenum.

When the duct has been cleared, the cystic duct is ligated and cut and the cholecystectomy is completed. If the cystic duct cannot be dilated, a longitudinal choledochotomy should be made on the anterior wall. After adequate dissection, anterior choledochotomy can be used. A longitudinal incision is favored because of the pattern of terminal arterioles supplying the common bile duct. Postoperative biliary drainage with a T tube may then be necessary. Clearance of all common bile duct stones is achieved in 75% to 95% of cases with laparoscopic common bile duct exploration.[19] Many studies have shown similar efficacy of laparoscopic common bile duct exploration as endoscopic sphincterotomy and laparoscopic cholecystectomy, while demonstrating significant cost analysis in favor of common bile duct exploration at one setting.

Open Approach

With the increased use of endoscopic, percutaneous, and laparoscopic techniques to treat common bile duct stones, the open common bile duct exploration is rarely performed today. It is now commonly used as a last resort if the above therapies fail. The techniques and operative manipulations are similar to the laparoscopic approach. In patients with a nondilated bile duct (>4 mm), a transduodenal sphincterotomy should be performed and the duct explored through the sphincteroplasty. This avoids the need for a postoperative T tube and the potential for a late bile duct stricture. With the use of intraoperative choledochoscopy, the rate of retained common bile stones is less than 5%.

Drainage Procedures

If the stones cannot be cleared or when the duct is very dilated (>1.5 cm in diameter), a choledochal drainage procedure should be performed. Options for biliary drainage include a side-to-side choledochoduodenostomy or a choledochojejunostomy with a Roux-en-Y limb of jejunum. Surgeon preference dictates which approach is used. Use of the duodenum is preferred if the duodenum can be fully mobilized (Kocher maneuver) and there is minimal scarring. Any concerns about tension should prompt use of the jejunum either as an end-to-side or side-to-side configuration.

Transduodenal Sphincterotomy

In the current era, endoscopic sphincterotomy has replaced open transduodenal sphincterotomy. If an open procedure for common bile duct stones is being done in which the stones are impacted, recurrent, or multiple, the

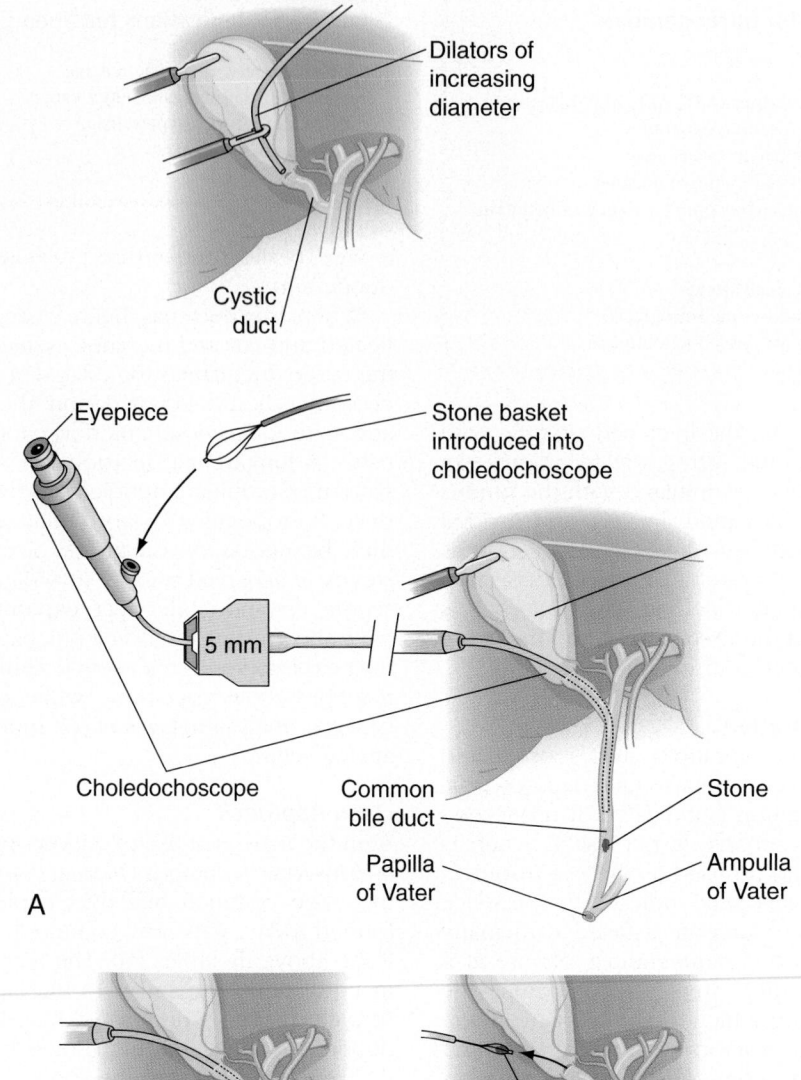

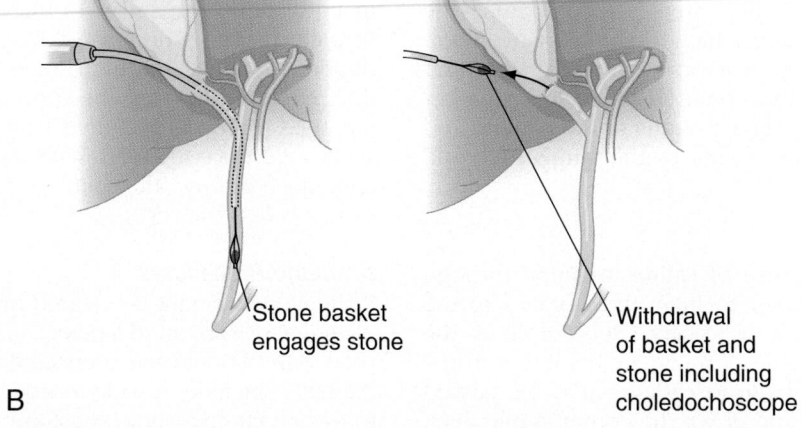

Figure 54-17 A, Laparoscopic common bile duct exploration. After dilation of the cystic duct, the flexible choledochoscope is inserted into the abdomen through the small trocar and maneuvered into the distal common bile duct. **B,** A stone basket is passed through the working channel of the choledochoscope and is used to snare a common duct stone. The stone basket and choledochoscope are withdrawn together. (From Curet M, Zucker K: Laparoscopic surgery of the biliary tract and liver. In Zuidema G [ed]: Shackelford's Surgery of the Alimentary Tract, 3rd ed. Philadelphia, WB Saunders, 1996, pp 257-278.)

transduodenal approach may be feasible. The duodenum is incised transversely. The sphincter then is incised at the 11-o'clock position to avoid injury to the pancreatic duct (Fig. 54-18). The impacted stones are removed, as are large stones, from the duct. There is no need to fully clear the duct of stones because they can now pass spontaneously through the cut sphincter.

Postcholecystectomy Syndromes

Because of the frequency of laparoscopic cholecystectomy being performed today, the surgeon should be aware of an entire spectrum of early problems inherent to this procedure. Identification and prompt treatment are critical for good outcomes (Fig. 54-19).

Bile Duct Injury and Ligation

Most benign strictures follow iatrogenic bile duct injury, most commonly during laparoscopic cholecystectomy. Most injuries are recognized intraoperatively or during the early postoperative period, and with appropriate management, the long-term results are acceptable. Long-term sequelae of unrecognized or inappropriately managed biliary strictures may lead to recurrent cholangitis, secondary biliary cirrhosis, and portal hypertension.

Pathogenesis

The incidence of biliary injuries rose sharply in the 1990s with the widespread use of laparoscopic cholecystectomy. Although the incidence of bile duct injuries during open cholecystectomy is only 0.1% to 0.2%, estimates of bile duct injuries and leaks after laparoscopic cholecystectomy are reported around 0.85% in several large studies.

A number of factors may be involved in the occurrence of bile duct injuries during laparoscopic cholecystectomy. These include acute or chronic inflammation, obesity, anatomic variations, and bleeding. Surgical technique with inadequate exposure and failure to identify structures before ligating or dividing them are the most common cause of significant biliary injury. The bile duct injury rate is increased in patients with complications of gallstones, including acute cholecystitis, pancreatitis, cholangitis, and obstructive jaundice. Surgeon training and experience were recognized as factors in early reports of laparoscopic bile duct injuries. As surgeon experience increases beyond 20 cases, the bile duct injury rate decreases. Recent reports have indicated that errors leading to laparoscopic bile duct injuries stem from misperception, not errors of skill, knowledge, or judgment. The primary cause of error in 97% of cases was a visual perceptual illusion, whereas only 3% of injuries were due to faults of technical skill.[26]

Aberrant biliary anatomy is often cited as a factor in biliary injuries. The bile duct may be narrow and can be mistaken for the cystic duct. The cystic duct may travel parallel to the common bile duct before joining it, misleading the surgeon to the wrong place. Also, the cystic duct may enter the right hepatic duct, and the right hepatic duct may run aberrantly, coursing through the

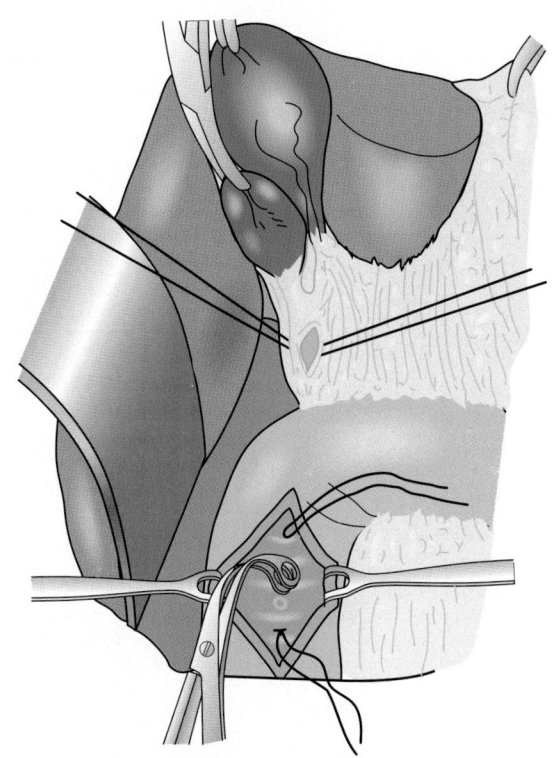

Figure 54-18 A transduodenal sphincterotomy can be used to remove distal bile duct stones that may be affected. An incision is made enlarging the papilla along the long axis of the duct, and the calculus is either expressed or removed using stone forceps. (From Zollinger RM Jr, Zollinger RM: Atlas of Surgical Operations, 7th ed. New York, McGraw Hill, 1993.)

triangle of Calot and entering the common hepatic duct. A number of other technical factors have been implicated in biliary injuries. The classic injury occurs when excessive cephalad retraction of the gallbladder may align the cystic duct with the common bile duct, allowing the latter to be mistaken for the cystic duct (Fig. 54-20). Careless use of electrocautery may lead to thermal injury. Dissection deep into the liver parenchyma may cause injury to intrahepatic ducts, and poor clip placement close to the hilar area or to structures not well visualized can result in a clip across the bile duct.

The routine use of intraoperative cholangiography to prevent bile duct injury is controversial.[24] It may limit the extent of injury, but does not seem to prevent it. However, if a bile duct injury is suspected during cholecystectomy, a cholangiogram must be obtained to identify the anatomy.

Presentation

Patients with bile duct injuries can present intraoperatively, in the early postoperative period, or months or years after the initial injury. About 25% of major ductal injuries are recognized intraoperatively because of bile leakage, an abnormal cholangiogram, or late recognition of the anatomy. The most common presentation of a complete occlusion of the common hepatic or bile duct

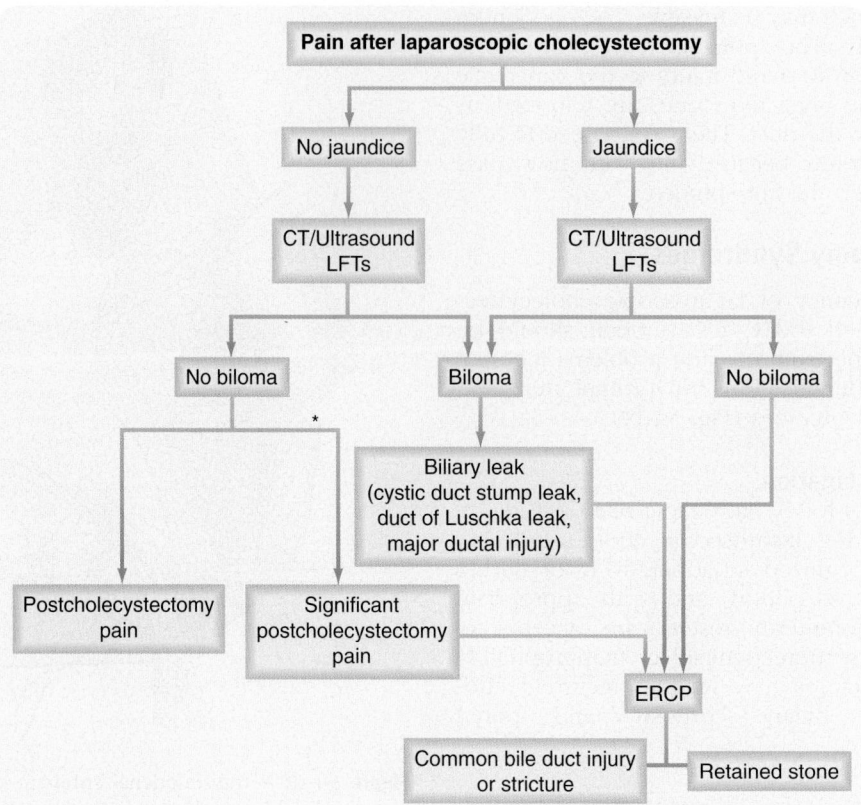

Figure 54-19 Workup and diagnostic algorithm of patients with right upper quadrant pain after laparoscopic cholecystectomy. CT, computed tomography; ERCP, endoscopic retrograde cholangiopancreatography; LFT, liver function test.
*Significant and persistent pain should by itself necessitate evaluation of the biliary system even if no biloma is found.

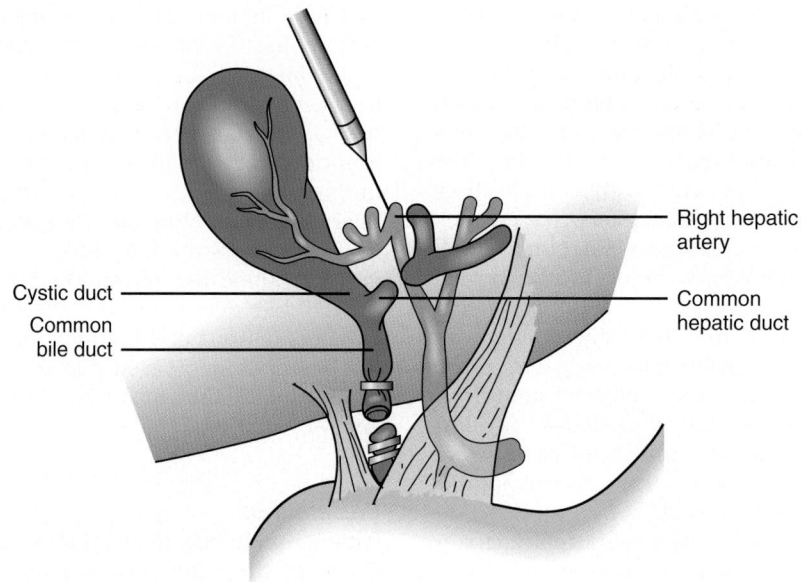

Figure 54-20 The classic laparoscopic cholecystectomy bile duct injury. The cystic duct and common bile duct are aligned by traction on the gallbladder. A segment of the common bile and hepatic ducts is resected. (From Branum G, Schmitt C, Baillie J, et al: Management of major biliary complications after laparoscopic cholecystectomy. Ann Surg 217:532-541, 1993.)

is jaundice with or without abdominal pain. Patients may also present months or years after prior surgery with cholangitis or cirrhosis secondary to a biliary tract injury.

Diagnosis and Management

The management of bile duct injury is dependent on the timing of diagnosis and extent and level of injury. Inappropriate management of biliary strictures may result in significant morbidity and mortality secondary to complications such as biliary cirrhosis or cholangitis. In a 12-year review of 130 patients with postoperative biliary strictures, the causes of mortality were all related to the presence of liver parenchymal disease with portal hypertension. Twenty-three of these patients had evidence of portal hypertension at the time of referral.[27]

Management of the Bile Duct Injury Recognized at the Time of Cholecystectomy Isolated, small, non–cautery-based partial lateral bile duct injury recognized at time of cholecystectomy can be managed with placement of a T tube. The T tube can be placed at the site of the injury if this is similar in size to a choledochotomy. However, if the biliary injury is more extensive, or if there is significant thermal damage owing to cautery-based trauma, or if the injury involves more than 50% of the circumference of the bile duct wall, an end-to-side choledochojejunostomy with a Roux-en-Y loop of jejunum should be performed. Similarly, major bile duct injuries, including transections of the common bile or common hepatic duct, can be repaired if recognized at the time of cholecystectomy. Isolated hepatic ducts smaller than 3 mm or those draining a single hepatic segment can be safely ligated. Ducts larger than 3 mm are more likely to drain several segments or an entire lobe and need to be reimplanted. It cannot be overstated that significant experience and judgment are critical to the decision to conduct a repair at the time of injury. If one is uncertain or underexperienced, and no colleague with sufficient expertise is immediately available, placing a drain followed by referral to an experienced center is the most appropriate course of action.

Management of the Bile Duct Injury Recognized After Cholecystectomy Most large series report the incidence of ductal injury after laparoscopic cholecystectomy to be 0.3% to 0.85%. Historically, after open cholecystectomy, 10% of patients presented within the first week, 70% within 6 months, and 80% within 1 year. In a recent study of 156 patients referred for management of biliary strictures resulting from bile duct injuries, 9.3% of injuries were recognized during laparoscopic versus 0% during open cholecystectomy.[28] In this series of 156 patients with postoperative biliary strictures, 49 patients (31.4%) presented with leaks, 42 (26.9%) presented with jaundice, and 50 (32.1%) presented with cholangitis.[28] In general, patients with a bile leak will present early, whereas patients with postoperative biliary strictures alone often present with jaundice or cholangitis months to years after the initial injury.

Diagnosis Abdominal imaging with ultrasonography or CT should be performed in patients with signs of abdominal pain or peritonitis, sepsis, or any other clinical sus-

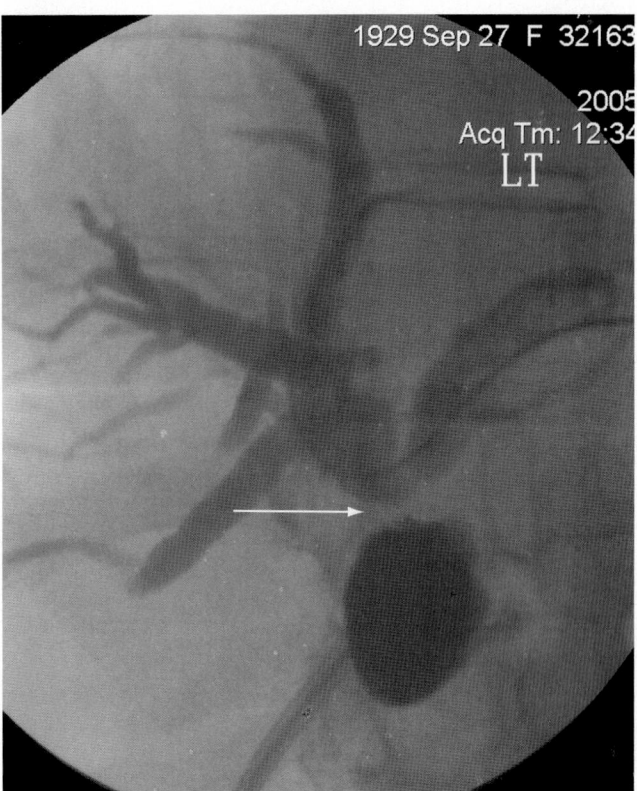

Figure 54-21 Transhepatic cholangiography confirming ligation of the common hepatic duct just distal to the bifurcation (*arrow*).

picion of biloma. Such patients must be stabilized with immediate parenteral antibiotics and image-guided percutaneous drainage of any fluid collections. Patients with signs and symptoms of cholangitis should undergo urgent cholangiogram with bile duct drainage. Cholangiography should be performed to establish the presence of ductal stricture, identify the level of the stricture, and identify the nature of the injury when necessary. In one study of 88 patients with bile duct injuries from laparoscopic cholecystectomy, attempts at repair were unsuccessful in 27 of 28 (96%) when preoperative cholangiograms were not performed, and 69% unsuccessful when data from cholangiograms were incomplete.[29] It is important that the method of cholangiography should provide detail of the intrahepatic ductal system and the bile duct confluence. Although PTC is the imaging method of choice for most postoperative biliary strictures, expertise with this is not available at all centers (Fig. 54-21). ERCP may be easier to obtain in a patient with a biliary stricture and cholangitis who requires urgent cholangiography and biliary decompression. However, this is only useful in patients with bile duct continuity. Cystic duct leaks or small tangential injuries can be treated with endoscopic stenting. In situations in which the biliary stricture is too tight to pass with ERCP, PTC may be performed for proximal biliary decompression.

CT arteriography should be considered in the preoperative evaluation of patients with benign biliary

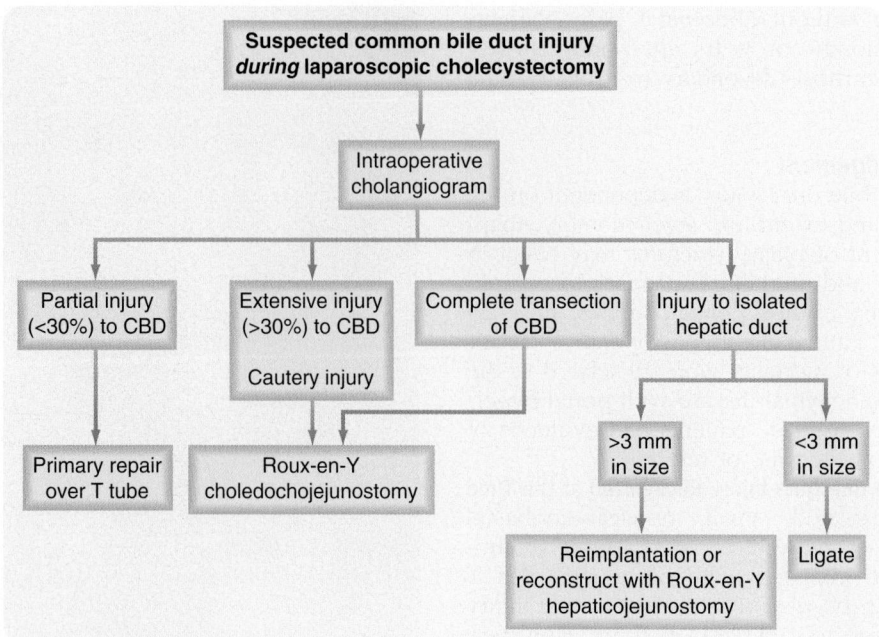

Figure 54-22 Suspected injury to the biliary tract during laparoscopic cholecystectomy and treatment.

strictures. Unrecognized injury to the hepatic artery or a portal vein branch occurs with a frequency of 12% to 47% concomitant with a bile duct injury. Certainly, if significant bleeding required urgent control at the time of the original operation, a vascular injury should be considered. However, the clinical consequences of hepatic artery injury are not fully known, but at least one study suggested that the presence of a right hepatic artery disruption should not affect the surgical repair of a bile duct injury.[30,31] In patients presenting with late strictures with evidence of liver dysfunction, a CT arteriogram should be performed to evaluate for evidence of portal hypertension.

Intraoperative Considerations

The management of postoperative biliary strictures following ductal injury depends on the degree of injury, the presence of stricture-induced complications, and the operative risk of the patient. After recognition of a bile duct injury or stricture, a multidisciplinary team consisting of experienced interventional radiologists, endoscopists, and surgeons, coordinated by an experienced hepatobiliary surgeon, should plan the following specific goals:

1. Control the infection (abscess or cholangitis)
2. Drain the biloma
3. Complete the cholangiography
4. Provide definitive therapy with controlled reconstruction or stenting (Fig. 54-22)

These goals do not mandate elaborate workup and delayed repair in all cases. Initial experience suggested that immediate repair of bile duct injury from cholecystectomy can give good results with low morbidity when performed properly; more recent data, however, suggest

that inexperience with the repairs leads to recurrent stricture, failure of the repair, and potentially secondary liver parenchymal damage from unrelieved obstruction.[32] Independent predictors of stricture recurrence after an initial operative repair include cholangitis before the initial repair, incomplete cholangiography, and primary repair within 3 weeks of the bile duct injury. When a bile duct injury is recognized at the time of cholecystectomy (or other operation), the surgeon should optimize all aspects of the patient's physiologic situation. If immediate repair is to be attempted, consultation with more experienced surgeons should be made. In those cases in which expertise is not available at the time of a recognized injury, or difficult circumstances preclude elaborate reconstructive attempts, external biliary drains will allow patient recovery and transfer to a center of excellence.

Successful repair of biliary strictures after appropriate preoperative management requires adherence to specific surgical principles:

1. Use of proximal bile duct with minimal inflammation
2. Creation of a tension-free anastomosis with the use of a Roux-en-Y jejunal limb
3. Direct mucosa-to-mucosa anastomosis

Historically, an end-to-end bile duct anastomosis was encouraged because it preserved the normal anatomy and theoretically reduced the possibility of cholangitis. However, multiple reports suggest that primary repair of the bile duct is associated with a 40% to 50% long-term failure rate. Direct operative biliary-enteric bypass is the gold standard procedure for the long-term treatment of biliary strictures. These procedures have low operative mortality and acceptable morbidity.

An adequate incision permitting full visualization is necessary for a good biliary-enteric anastomosis. A right subcostal incision extended to either the midline (hockey stick) or the left (chevron incision) is usually necessary. The liver should be completely freed from the diaphragm, and adhesions from previous operations should be taken down to facilitate creation of a Roux-en-Y jejunal limb if necessary (Fig. 54-23). The Hepp-Couinaud approach to bile duct reconstruction is the best option in most circumstances. This technique requires dissection of the hilar plate to expose the left hepatic duct and allow for a side-to-side anastomosis of the left hepatic duct to the Roux-en-Y jejunal limb. The use of a Roux-en-Y jejunal limb is favored over a direct choledochoduodenostomy or choledochojejunostomy because it also allows for the creation of an "access loop" of the proximal portion of the Roux-en-Y limb for future interventional radiologic access.

Interventional Radiologic and Endoscopic Techniques
Interventional radiologic techniques are useful in patients with bile duct injuries, leaks, or postoperative strictures. These techniques allow percutaneous drainage of abdominal fluid collections, preoperative identification of the ductal anatomy through percutaneous transhepatic cholangiography, and stricture dilation with or without placement of palliative stents for bile drainage in the patient whose overall physiologic status precludes a major operation. Percutaneous transhepatic dilation can be employed in patients with intrahepatic ductal disease and in patients in whom ERCP is not possible. It is often used as an adjunct to operative repair in order to assist with identification of the proximal biliary tree for reconstruction and for the dilation of anastomotic strictures.

The success rate of percutaneous transhepatic dilation is reported between 50% and 70%. Patients with anastomotic strictures (including biliary-enteric anastomotic strictures) have the highest success rates. A study of 89 patients treated for major bile duct injuries following laparoscopic cholecystectomy showed that by a mean follow-up of 27 months, percutaneous dilation yielded only a 64% success rate in ischemic strictures versus 92% at 33.4 months in patients with biliary-enteric anastomotic strictures.[33] In addition, although mortality following percutaneous dilation is low, complication rates are reported as high as 35%, and complications consist mainly of hemobilia, cholangitis, and bile leaks. These procedures often require multiple sessions of dilation to achieve long-term success rates.

When reported from large-volume centers, endoscopic and percutaneous methods of dilation have equivalent efficacy. Endoscopic dilation of benign extrahepatic biliary strictures is also a useful adjunctive option in patents with a dominant extrahepatic stricture causing clinical symptoms. In general, treatment of biliary strictures with this technique, as with interventional radiologic methods, requires multiple sessions of dilations, and nonischemic strictures (anastomotic strictures) respond best. Endoscopic dilation also has a low mortality rate, but it has a significant morbidity rate. The more common complications following endoscopic biliary interventions

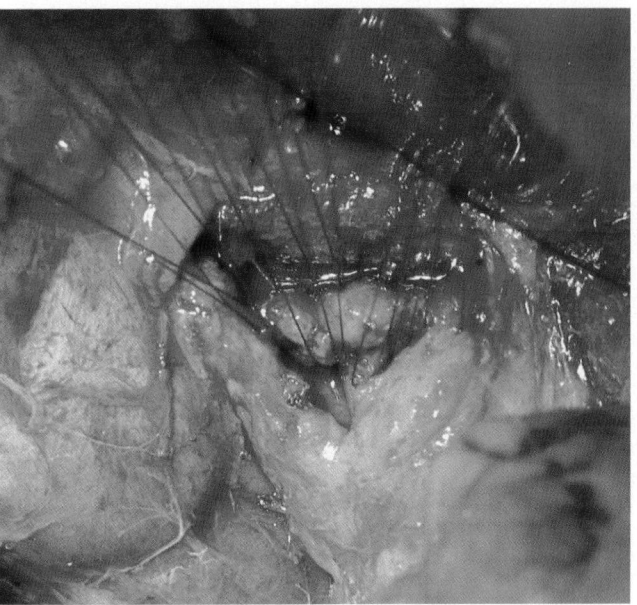

Figure 54-23 End-to-side biliary reconstruction with Roux-en-Y hepaticojejunostomy. Note than anterior row of PDS sutures is placed first to elevate anterior wall of bile duct and facilitate exposure.

include hemobilia, bile leak, pancreatitis, and cholangitis. In a study of 101 patients with benign biliary strictures, 66 patients were treated endoscopically, with a reported re-stricture rate of 18% at 3 months and a complication rate of 35%.[34] Although endoscopic and interventional radiologic procedures are not ideal long-term treatments for unresponsive biliary strictures, endoscopic stenting and drainage is a successful treatment option for cystic duct leak or small common bile duct leaks following laparoscopic cholecystectomy.

Careful long-term follow-up of patients with biliary strictures treated with percutaneous or endoscopic dilation methods is required because ischemic biliary strictures will not respond permanently to dilation. Early retreatment (through repeat dilation or biliary-enteric reconstruction) of postdilation recurrent strictures is essential to prevent secondary biliary cirrhosis. The risk for additive morbidity from the required repeat sessions and the risk for late stricture recurrence should be considered and discussed with patients when treatment options for benign biliary strictures are being considered.

Outcomes
Acceptable long-term results can be achieved in most patients undergoing operative repair of bile duct injuries. More than 90% of patients are free of jaundice and cholangitis after operative repair of a laparoscopic bile duct injury.[28] The best results are obtained when the injury is recognized during the cholecystectomy and repaired by an experienced biliary surgeon. Postoperative injuries identified in the presence of concomitant biliary leak should be repaired once the biliary leak has subsided and tissue planes are less inflamed, usually 6 weeks after initial laparoscopic cholecystectomy. Complications of

biliary reconstruction can be managed nonoperatively, and mortality rates have been less than 1%.[32] Common complications include recurrent cholangitis, external biliary fistula, bile leak, and hemobilia. Restenosis of a biliary-enteric anastomosis occurs in about 10% of patients, and may manifest up to 20 years later. About two thirds of recurrent strictures become symptomatic within 2 years after repair. The more proximal strictures are associated with a lower success rate than are distal ones. Percutaneous balloon dilation with stenting has a significantly lower success rate (64%) than operative repair. Although most patients are free of jaundice and cholangitis after operative repair of a bile duct injury, there appears to be a significant impact of the injury on the quality of life.[35]

Postcholecystectomy Pain

Abdominal pain or other symptoms originally attributed to the gallbladder may persist or recur months or years after cholecystectomy. Improvements in imaging have decreased the incidence of this pain, which was once reported to be as high as 20%. Patients presenting with right upper quadrant pain, jaundice, and chills shortly after cholecystectomy should be evaluated for retained stones or biliary leak. Other causes of abdominal pain in patients with normal liver function tests should also be investigated. Another possibility in a small number of patients with persistent pain following cholecystectomy is abnormalities in the sphincter of Oddi such as stenosing papillitis or sphincter dysfunction.

Retained Biliary Stones

Retained or recurrent stones following cholecystectomy present soon after (<4 weeks) surgery and are best treated endoscopically. If stones are found shortly after the cholecystectomy, they are classified as *retained;* those diagnosed months or years later are termed *recurrent.* Patients will present most commonly shortly after cholecystectomy with sharp, intense right upper quadrant pain and jaundice. Bilirubin and alkaline phosphatase elevation should prompt endoscopic clearance of biliary stones. Recurrent stones may be multiple and large. A generous endoscopic sphincterotomy will allow stone retrieval as well as spontaneous passage of retained and recurrent stones.

Biliary Leak

Leaks from the cystic duct stump or an unrecognized duct of Luschka may be problematic. The most common etiology for a cystic duct stump leak is an inflammation around the duct in the setting of acute cholecystitis, which dislodges placed clips. Bile leaks commonly present shortly after cholecystectomy (within 1 week) with right upper quadrant pain, fever, chills, and hyperbilirubinemia. Bile leak or bile peritonitis should be considered in any patient with persistent bloating or anorexia more than a few days after laparoscopic cholecystectomy. The port sites on the right side should be examined for bile staining. CT scan and ultrasound will confirm presence of a complex fluid collection in the right upper quadrant. Immediate operative intervention with wide drainage is only indicated if the patient is in septic shock. Attempts at early repair are dangerous and doomed for failure because of the inflammatory response incited by the bile leak. Percutaneous drainage of intra-abdominal fluid collections followed by an endoscopic biliary stenting resolves most leaks without need for operative intervention. If bile leaks fail to resolve after 6 weeks, further imaging with MRC and endoscopic imaging may be necessary to rule out a common bile duct injury. When the acute inflammation has resolved 6 to 8 weeks later, operative repair is performed.

Gallstone Ileus

Passage of a stone through a spontaneous biliary-enteric fistula leading to a mechanical bowel obstruction is known as *gallstone ileus.* Most (75%) of these fistulas develop between the gallbladder and duodenum, occur in elderly people, and account for 1% of all small bowel obstructions. Gallstone ileus may account for as many as 25% of cases of intestinal obstruction in patients older than 70 years who have no previous surgery or hernias on physical exam. Biliary-enteric fistulas usually follow an episode of acute cholecystitis with gangrene and perforation of the gallbladder wall into the adjacent viscus or from pressure necrosis from an impacted gallstone.

Presentation and Diagnosis

Nausea, vomiting, and abdominal pain, signs and symptoms of intestinal obstruction, are the common presentation of patients with gallstone ileus. A history of gallbladder-related symptoms is present in only half of the patients. The pain may be episodic and recurrent as the impacted stone temporarily obstructs the bowel lumen and then dislodges and moves distally, known as *tumbling obstruction.* Abdominal films will demonstrate evidence of an intestinal obstruction with pneumobilia or a calcified stone distant from the gallbladder (Fig. 54-24). The most common site of obstruction is the terminal ileum because of its narrow lumen.

Management

Relieving the obstruction by removing the gallstone through a proximal enterotomy is the initial management of gallstone ileus; the stone is "milked" proximally, and then removed from a healthy portion of bowel. Care should be given to examine the area of the impacted stone. If there has been ischemic compromise to that section of bowel, this portion should be resected to prevent postimpaction wall necrosis and leak. Thorough evaluation for other gallstones should be performed because 10% of patients will have recurrent obstruction. Takedown of the biliary-enteric fistula and cholecystectomy during the same procedure is warranted because recurrent cholecystitis and cholangitis are common. However, in patients with a significant inflammatory process in the right upper quadrant or who are unstable to withstand a prolonged operative procedure, the fistula can be addressed at a second laparotomy.

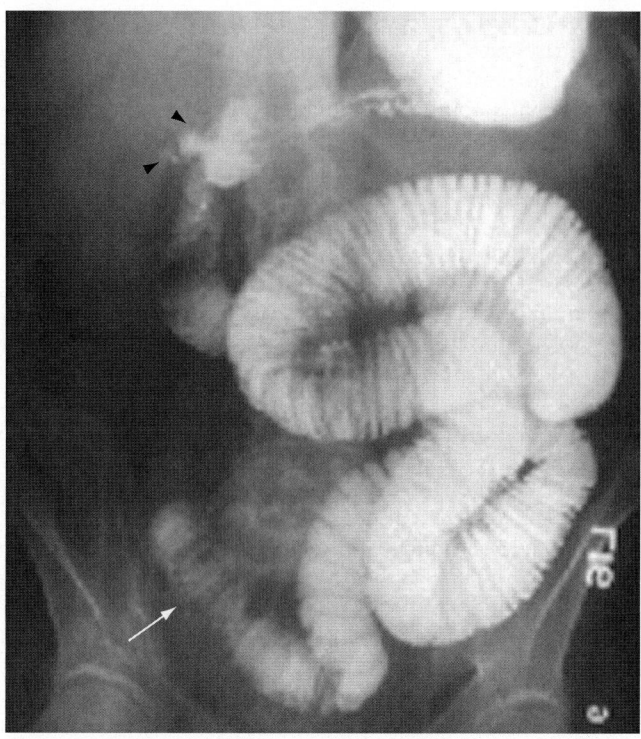

A

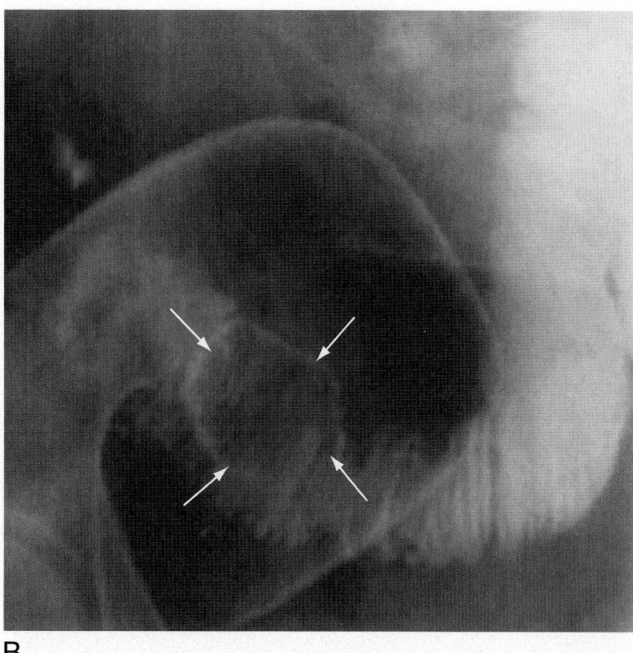

B

Figure 54-24 A posteroanterior radiograph obtained during a barium examination of the small bowel shows an irregular collection of barium in the right upper quadrant (**A,** *arrowheads*), representing partial filling of the cystic duct. Both jejunum and ileum are markedly dilated, with dilution of the barium in a pattern consistent with small bowel obstruction. There is abrupt termination of the barium column at the site of an oval intraluminal filling defect (**A,** *arrow*). A view of the end of the barium column shows luminal obstruction by a smooth intraluminal mass (**B,** *arrows*) with faint calcification of the peripheral rim. Exploratory laparotomy revealed a foreign body in the terminal ileum that was 4 cm by 4 cm and felt hard. (From Kaiser AM, Molmenti EP: Gallstone ileus. N Engl J Med 335:942, 1996.)

Recurrent Pyogenic Cholangitis

Cholangiohepatitis or intrahepatic stones are endemic in East Asia. It is uncommon in North America except in the Chinese population. It is more common in people with poor economic status and living standards. The infectious aspect of this disease is caused by bacterial contamination, usually biliary pathogens, and biliary parasites, such as *Clonorchis sinensis, Opisthorchis viverrini,* and *Ascaris lumbricoides.* Biliary sludge and dead bacterial cell bodies form brown pigment stones formed throughout the biliary tree, which cause partial obstruction. Biliary strictures and repeated episodes of cholangitis are the common clinical course and may lead to hepatic abscesses and cirrhosis. Patients are at risk for cholangiocarcinoma due to persistent biliary infection and irritation from stones and sludge.

Presentation

Patients with recurrent pyogenic cholangitis (RPC) commonly present with frequent episodes of pain, fever, and jaundice. MRC and PTC are the primary imaging modalities for monitoring of disease progression (Fig. 54-25). They are useful for identifying location and severity of stones and strictures and allow decompression of the biliary tree in a septic patient.

Management

Patients with RPC should be treated with a multidisciplinary approach including endoscopists, interventional radiologists, and surgeons because of the frequency and inaccessibility of strictures and stones. The long-term goal of therapy is to extract stones, remove debris, and relieve strictures. Because clearance of all stones at any one operation is difficult, Roux-en-Y hepaticojejunostomy with a subcutaneous afferent limb (Hudson loop) is a safe and effective way to provide access to the biliary tree for stone extractions.[36] Cholangiocarcinoma has been reported in 1% to 10% of patients with RPC; therefore, patients with adequate hepatic reserve and a dominant lobe with stones should undergo extended hepatectomy of the involved side, Roux-en-Y hepaticojejunostomy, and Hudson loop. This would remove the stones and reduce the future risk for cholangiocarcinoma. About 50% of patients require further percutaneous choledochoscopy or balloon dilation to clear any remaining stones or manage persistent strictures.

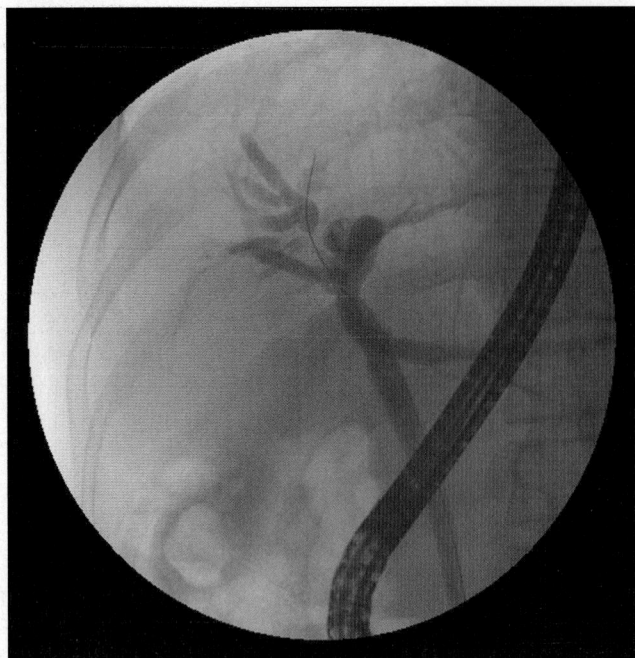

Figure 54-25 Endoscopic retrograde cholangiopancreatography of patient with recurrent pyogenic cholangitis. Note the presence of intrahepatic stone and stricturing of the bile ducts.

Noncalculous Biliary Disease

Acute Acalculous Cholecystitis

Acute inflammation of the gallbladder can occur without gallstones. Acute acalculous cholecystitis accounts for 5% to 10% of all patients with acute cholecystitis and is the diagnosis in about 1% to 2% of patients undergoing cholecystectomy. It has a more fulminant course than acute calculous cholecystitis and more commonly progresses to gangrene, empyema, or perforation. Acute acalculous cholecystitis occurs most frequently in elderly and critically ill patients after trauma, burns, long-term parenteral nutrition, and major operations such as abdominal aneurysm repair and cardiopulmonary bypass. Although the exact etiology is unclear, gallbladder stasis and ischemia have been implicated as causative factors. Stasis is common in critically ill patients not being fed enterally and may lead to colonization of the gallbladder with bacteria. Visceral ischemia is also common in patients with acute acalculous cholecystitis and may explain the high incidence of gallbladder gangrene.

The signs and symptoms of acute acalculous cholecystitis parallel acute calculous cholecystitis. Patients may also present with only unexplained fever, leukocytosis, and hyperamylasemia without right upper quadrant tenderness. If untreated, rapid progression to gangrene and perforation may occur.[37] Radiologic findings are also similar except for the absence of gallstones. Ultrasonography is the diagnostic test of choice, especially because it can be done at the bedside. Cholescintigraphy demonstrates absent gallbladder filling, but the false-positive rate may be as high as 40%.

Emergency cholecystectomy is the appropriate treatment for acute acalculous cholecystitis for patients who are stable enough to tolerate the anesthetic and procedure. Because of the high incidence of gangrene, perforation, and empyema, open cholecystectomy is often the preferred approach. Because most patients are critically ill, the morbidity rate of acute acalculous cholecystitis in recent series is 40%. If patients are unfit for surgery, percutaneous, ultrasound-guided, or CT-guided cholecystostomy is the treatment of choice. If the diagnosis is uncertain, percutaneous cholecystostomy can be both diagnostic and therapeutic. About 90% of patients will improve with percutaneous cholecystostomy.

Acute Cholangitis

Cholangitis is an ascending bacterial infection of the biliary ductal system with obstruction most commonly due to choledochal stones. Although cultures of the gallbladder and bile ducts are usually sterile, in the presence of common bile duct stones or other obstructing pathology, the incidence of positive bile cultures increases. The most common organisms present in the bile in patients with cholangitis include *E. coli*, *Klebsiella pneumoniae*, *Streptococcus faecalis*, and *Bacteroides fragilis*. Even in the presence of high bacteria counts, clinical cholangitis and bacteremia do not develop unless obstruction causes elevated intraductal pressures. Although stones are the most common cause of obstruction in cholangitis, other etiologies include benign and malignant strictures, anastomotic strictures, cholangiocarcinoma, and periampullary cancer.

Diagnosis

Cholangitis may be either self-limited or toxic with severe illness, including jaundice, fever, abdominal pain, mental status changes, and hypotension (Reynold's pentad). Fever and chills are the most common presentation and are due to cholangiovenous and cholangiolymphatic reflux. Normal biliary pressures range from 7 to 14 cm H_2O; in the presence of bactibilia and normal biliary pressures, hepatic vein blood and perihepatic lymph are sterile. However, with partial or complete biliary obstruction, intrabiliary pressures rise to 18 to 20 cm H_2O, and organisms rapidly appear in both the blood and lymph.

The most common causes of biliary obstruction are choledocholithiasis, benign strictures, biliary-enteric anastomotic strictures, and cholangiocarcinoma and periampullary cancer. Before 1980, choledocholithiasis was the cause of about 80% of the reported cases of cholangitis, but in recent years, malignant strictures have become a more frequent cause in tertiary referral centers. Leukocytosis, hyperbilirubinemia, and elevations of alkaline phosphatase and transaminases all are common in patients with cholangitis. Although ultrasound, CT, and MRI may be helpful in identifying the cause of obstruction, cholangiography is mandatory as a diagnostic and potentially therapeutic intervention. If ERCP is not available, PTC should be performed. Cholangiography will identify the level of and reason for obstruction, allow for culture and possible biopsy if a mass is present, and provide drainage of the bile ducts with stents, catheters, or dilation.

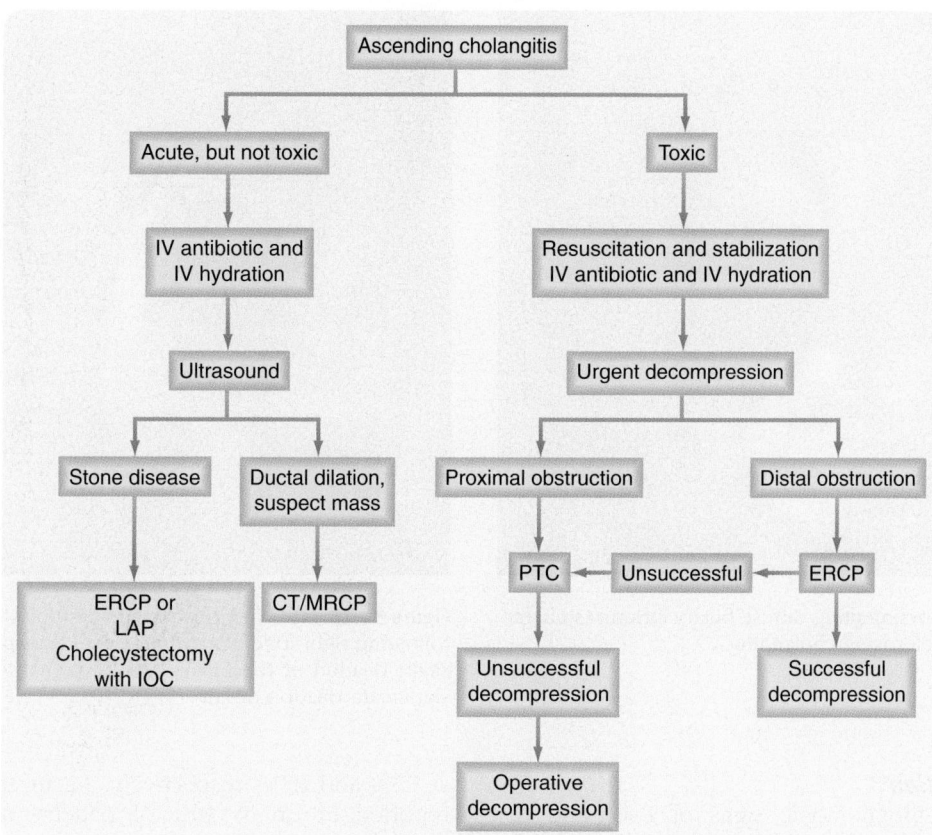

Figure 54-26 Diagnostic and therapeutic algorithm of patients with ascending cholangitis. CT, computed tomography; ERCP, endoscopic retrograde cholangiopancreatography; IOC, intraoperative cholangiogram; LAP, laparoscopic; MRCP; magnetic resonance cholangiopancreatography; PTC, percutaneous transhepatic cholangiography.

Management

IV antibiotics and aggressive hydration are the initial treatment in patients with acute cholangitis. Identifying severity of ascending cholangitis is crucial to the diagnostic and therapeutic management of the patient (Fig. 54-26). Patients in septic shock with toxic cholangitis may require intensive care unit monitoring and vasopressors to support blood pressure. Most patients will respond to these measures alone. However, in 15% of cases, urgent biliary decompression will be necessary. Biliary decompression may be performed endoscopically or by a percutaneous transhepatic route based on the level of the obstruction. Patients with a proximal hilar obstruction or a biliary-enteric anastomotic stricture should be drained transhepatically. Choledocholithiasis or suspected ampullary tumors are best accessed endoscopically. If ERCP or PTC is not possible, an emergent operation and decompression of the common bile duct with a T tube should be performed. Definitive operative therapy should be deferred until the cholangitis has been treated, the patient stabilized, and the diagnosis confirmed.

Overall, the mortality rate associated with an episode of gallstone cholangitis is about 2%, but is much higher in patients with toxic cholangitis (5%). Renal failure, hepatic abscess, and malignancy are all associated with higher morbidity and mortality. Hepatic abscess is frequently observed in patients with biliary pathology and should be considered in patients who do not respond to therapy.

Primary Sclerosing Cholangitis

Primary sclerosing cholangitis (PSC) is a cholestatic liver disease characterized by fibrotic strictures involving the intrahepatic and extrahepatic biliary tree in the absence of a known precipitating cause (Fig. 54-27). Some patients remain asymptomatic for years, whereas others rapidly progress to bile duct loss, cirrhosis, and liver failure. Genetic and immunologic factors appear to have a role in the pathogenesis of this disease. It is more common in certain HLA haplotypes such as B8/DR3.

The diseases with the strongest association with PSC are inflammatory bowel disease and primarily ulcerative colitis. The incidence of ulcerative colitis in patients with PSC ranges from 60% to 72%. Patients with PSC are at increased risk for developing cholangiocarcinoma. The risk for developing cholangiocarcinoma is 1% per year in patients with PSC. Between 10% and 15% of patients undergoing liver transplantation as treatment of PSC will have an unsuspected cholangiocarcinoma on explant analysis.

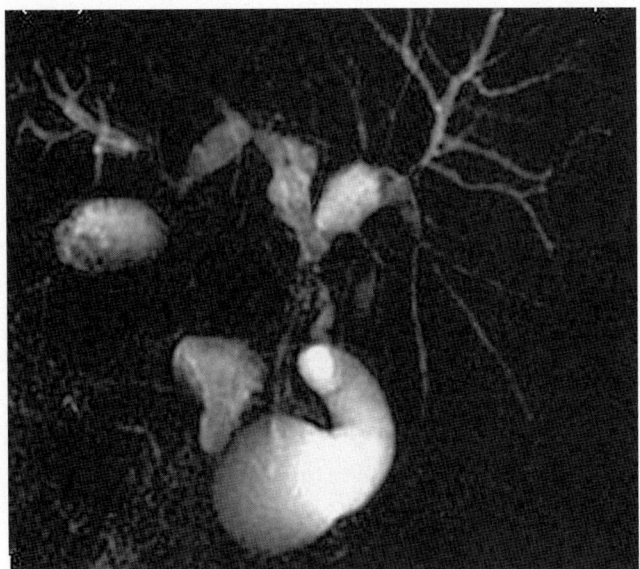

Figure 54-27 MRC documenting diffuse biliary strictures characteristic of primary sclerosing cholangitis.

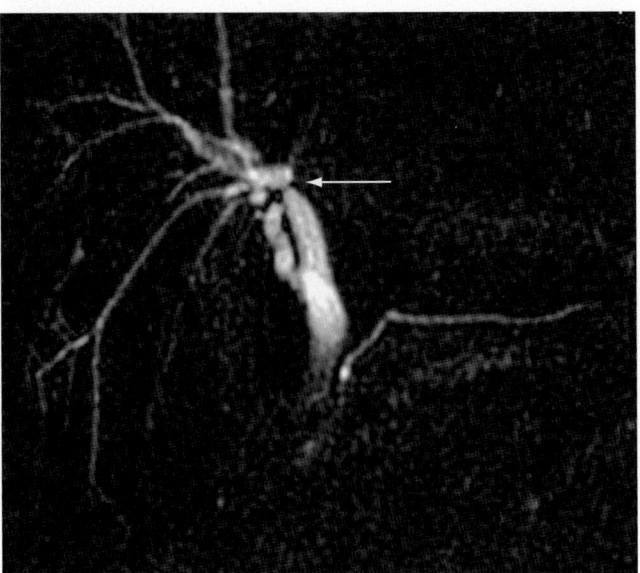

Figure 54-28 MRC demonstrating anastomotic stricture (*arrow*) following right lobe living donor liver transplantation. Note the slight dilation of the biliary tree proximal to the stricture and significant dilation distal.

Clinical Presentation

There are no pathognomonic signs of PSC, and the natural history is variable. Although patients can be asymptomatic for up to 15 years, prolonged disease ultimately leads to progressive hepatic failure. Mean age at presentation is 40 to 45 years, and most patients are male.[38] About 75% of patients are symptomatic at presentation with evidence of cholestatic liver disease such as jaundice, pruritus, and fatigue. Symptoms of bacterial cholangitis are uncommon. The condition is characterized by relapses and remissions, with quiescent periods. The median survival for patients with PSC from the time of diagnosis ranges from 10 to 12 years.

Diagnosis

Cholangiography confirms the diagnosis of PSC with evidence of diffuse multifocal strictures commonly found in both intrahepatic and extrahepatic bile ducts. Involvement of the extrahepatic ducts alone without intrahepatic duct involvement occurs in 5% to 10% of patients with PSC. Despite the presence of diffuse disease in most patients with PSC, the hepatic duct bifurcation is often the most severely strictured segment of the biliary tree. A liver biopsy to determine the degree of hepatic fibrosis or the presence of cirrhosis is also critical in selecting therapy.

Management

Primary sclerosing cholangitis is a progressive disease that eventually results in biliary cirrhosis. Patients with persistent biliary sepsis, biliary cirrhosis, and manifestations of end-stage liver disease (ascites, variceal bleeding) are best treated with liver transplantation. Five-year graft and patient survival after transplantation are excellent at 72% and 85%, respectively. Recurrent PSC has been reported in up to 10% of patients and may require retransplantation.

An important consideration in the management of PSC is the risk for superimposed cholangiocarcinoma, which occurs in 10% to 20% of cases.[39] Rapid onset of jaundice, pruritus, and weight loss may be clues to the diagnosis of cholangiocarcinoma but are not specific. Cancer antigen (CA) 19-9 may be helpful if levels are greater than 100 U/mL but is not predictive. Repeated brushings for cytology by endoscopic or percutaneous approaches should be employed to distinguish benign from malignant dominant strictures. Long-term survival in patients with a small incidental cholangiocarcinoma (<1 cm) is similar to that in patients without cancer. Historically, known cholangiocarcinoma in a patient with PSC has been a contraindication to liver transplantation, but data from the Mayo Clinic indicate that in carefully selected patients with extrahepatic cholangiocarcinoma who undergo neoadjuvant chemoradiation therapy, postoperative survival is similar to that in patients without cancer.[40]

Medical therapy for PSC has been disappointing. Ursodeoxycholate lowers serum bilirubin and transaminases but has not improved symptoms or delayed disease progression. Patients with recurrent biliary sepsis should be managed with antibiotics and surveillance if possible. Biliary strictures in patients with PSC have been dilated or stented using either the percutaneous or endoscopic route. These nonoperative procedures have produced short-term improvements in symptoms and serum bilirubin levels. Symptomatic patients with persistent jaundice with a dominant stricture may also be candidates for surgical therapy, but otherwise, the role of nontransplant

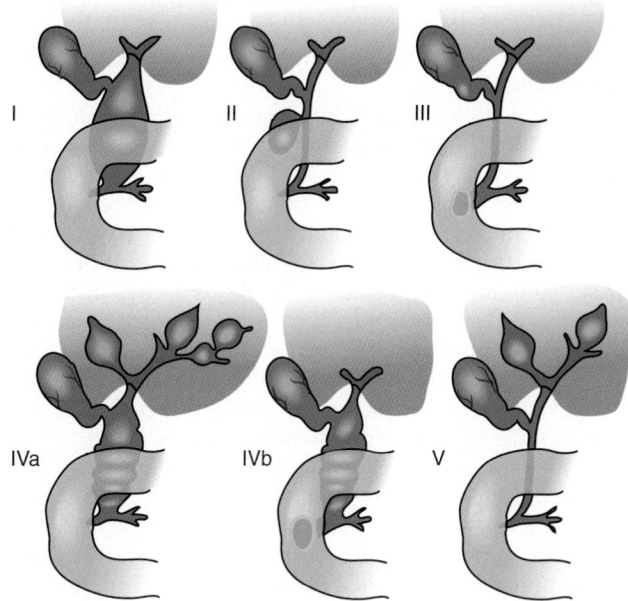

Figure 54-29 Todani modification of Alonso-Lej classification of choledochal cysts. (From Chijiiwa K, Koga A: Surgical management and long-term follow-up of patients with choledochal cysts. Am J Surg 165:238-242, 1993.)

surgery is limited. These patients are not common, however, because bilateral involvement is the usual presentation. Resection of the extrahepatic biliary tree with bilateral hepaticojejunostomies may have a role in patients without cirrhosis or significant fibrosis on biopsy, but timing, aggressiveness, and selection remain unclear. Limited data have shown that overall survival has been significantly longer in noncirrhotic patients treated with resection than in patients managed nonoperatively.[38] Liver transplantation has produced excellent results in patients with PSC and end-stage liver disease, with a 5-year actuarial patient survival rate of 72% and a 5-year graft survival rate of 72% reported.

Biliary Strictures

Benign bile duct strictures have numerous causes, including chronic pancreatitis, common bile duct stones, acute cholangitis, biliary obstruction due to cholecystolithiasis (Mirizzi's syndrome), PSC, RPC, post-transplantation strictures, and biliary-enteric anastomosis. Patients most commonly present with episodes of cholangitis or jaundice. Cholangiography provides diagnostic and therapeutic information regarding location, severity, and causes of biliary strictures. Percutaneous or endoscopic dilation and stent placement give good results in more than half of patients. Surgery with Roux-en-Y choledochojejunostomy or hepaticojejunostomy is the standard of care with excellent results in 80% to 90% of cases.[28]

Anastomotic biliary strictures after liver transplantation or biliary-enteric bypass can usually be managed nonoperatively (Fig. 54-28). Percutaneous transhepatic stents are required for patients with Roux-en-Y reconstruction because of difficulty accessing the papilla. This provides symptomatic relief but may not provide long-term success. Biliary strictures after duct-to-duct reconstruction are best treated with endoscopic stenting initially, and if unsuccessful, then Roux-en-Y biliary-enteric reconstruction.

Biliary Cysts

Cystic dilation of the biliary ducts, also known as a *choledochal cyst,* is an uncommon but serious condition that requires surgical treatment. Although choledochal cysts frequently present in infancy and childhood, the disease is more commonly diagnosed in adults. The incidence of choledochal cysts is only between 1 in 100,000 and 1 in 150,000 people in Western countries but is much more common in Japan. They occur three to eight times more commonly in women. This congenital disorder involves isolated or combined dilation of the extrahepatic or intrahepatic biliary tree.

Pathogenesis

The most commonly accepted theory is an anomalous pancreatic duct–biliary duct junction (APBDJ). A high common bile duct–pancreatic duct junction creates a long common channel. This results in reflux of pancreatic fluid into the distal common hepatic duct and results in mucosal injury, chronic inflammation, and weakening of the bile duct wall. This proposed mechanism is supported by elevated levels of amylase in choledochal cysts.

In 1977, Todani modified the Alonso-Lej classification (Box 54-6 and Fig. 54-29) and combined the extrahepatic and intrahepatic types into a classification that is currently used by most surgeons. Type I cysts are the most common and make up 50% of choledochal cysts.

Clinical Presentation

The classic clinical triad associated with choledochal cysts includes right upper quadrant pain, jaundice, and an abdominal mass. Only 10% of patients present with this triad. Adults have a slightly different presentation (abdominal pain and jaundice) than children because of a higher incidence of bile calculi or sludge and pancreatic-biliary ductal malformation.

Severe hepatobiliary complications may result from long-standing biliary cysts if left untreated. Portal hypertension may develop as a result of portal vein compression by the adjacent cyst or cirrhosis secondary to long-term biliary obstruction. Some patients may present with variceal hemorrhage as an initial manifestation. Very rarely, patients may present with bilious ascites and peritonitis as a result of rupture of a choledochal cyst, and pseudocysts may appear surrounding the common bile duct. Those patients also have a high incidence of developing sludge, cholelithiasis, or choledocholithiasis and have commonly had a prior cholecystectomy.

The incidence of carcinoma (bile duct, hepatic, or gallbladder in origin) in the choledochal cyst ranges from 2.5% to 26%, which is well above the rate of less than 1% for the general population. Many patients have biliary cancer at the time of initial presentation. Chronic inflammation caused by bile stagnation has been suggested as a possible mechanism for the development of cancer by causing metaplasia of the epithelium of the cystic wall.

Laboratory evaluation may demonstrate liver dysfunction in 60% of adult patients but is not specific. The diagnosis can be established with ultrasound or CT scan (Fig. 54-30A). Cholangiography is required to determine the type of choledochal cyst and plan operative treatment (see Fig. 54-30B). ERCP is more useful in defining the distal ductal anatomy and the presence of APBDJ, whereas PTC is useful in defining the proximal ductal anatomy and the presence of intrahepatic disease.

Management

The goals of management are to relieve symptoms and prevent long-term complications of biliary cysts such as cholangitis, portal hypertension, cirrhosis, and potential carcinoma. Cholecystectomy, resection of the extrahepatic biliary tract including the choledochal cyst, with Roux-en-Y hepaticojejunostomy is the appropriate treatment for type I and II choledochal cysts. The goal of cyst excision is to completely remove the lining mucosa of the bile duct cysts (Fig. 54-31), with oversewing of the distal duct. Simple enteric drainage (choledochocystojejunosotomy) of the bile duct cyst is associated with recurrent biliary stasis and infection[24] and does not prevent development of biliary malignancy. Todani and colleagues have reported a 10-year mean interval between internal drainage and detection of carcinoma.[41] Cholangiocarcinoma is uncommon in children with choledochal cysts, but the risk in adults may be as high as 30%. Resection of the extrahepatic cyst is also recommended for type IV cysts; if the intrahepatic cysts are confined to one side of the liver, hepatic resection of the involved liver is recommended. With long-standing Caroli's disease (Fig. 54-32), hepatic parenchymal damage may ensue from diffuse biliary dilation and periportal fibrosis and eventually result in cirrhosis and liver failure. Liver trans-

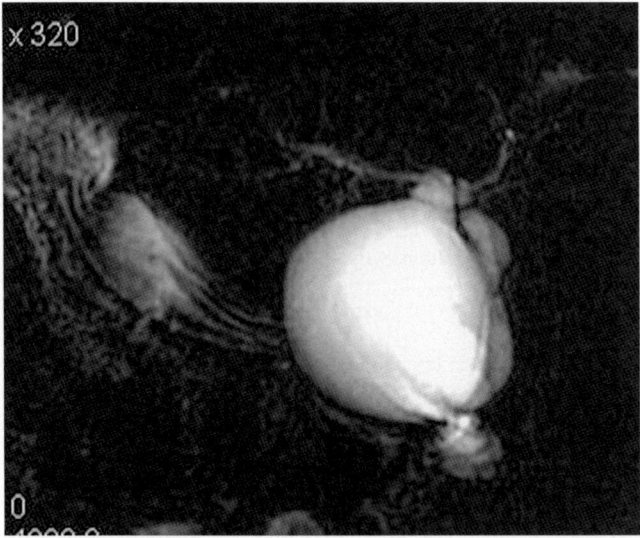

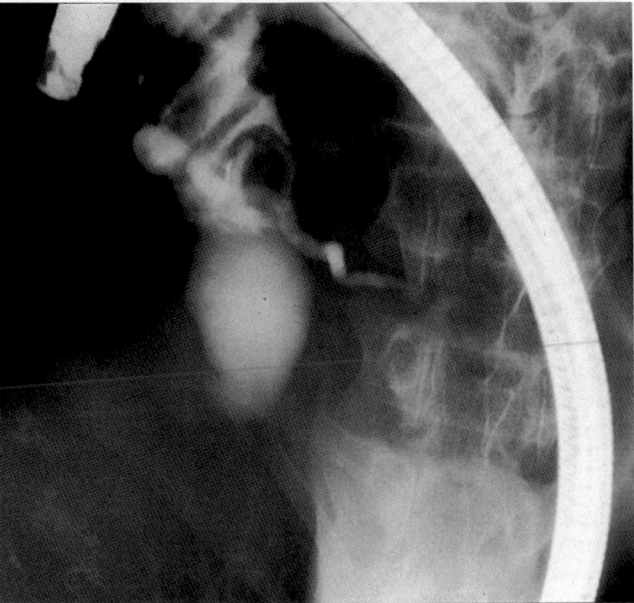

Figure 54-30 A, Computed tomography scan demonstrating type I choledochal cyst. **B,** Endoscopic retrograde cholangiopancreatography visualizing anatomy and relationship to nearby structures of choledochal cyst is important in operative planning. (From Shah SA, Alsoufi B, Callery MP: Bile duct cysts. Available online: http://www.unboundsurgery.com.)

plantation offers a potential cure without long-term complications of recurrences of Caroli's disease.

Polyploid Lesions of the Gallbladder

Benign masses classified as polyploid lesions of the gallbladder include benign pseudotumors, such as cholesterol polyps and adenomyomatosis, and adenomas, and appear in 3% to 7% of normal subjects undergoing abdominal ultrasound and in 2% to 12% of cholecystectomy specimens. Cholesterol polyps are the most common

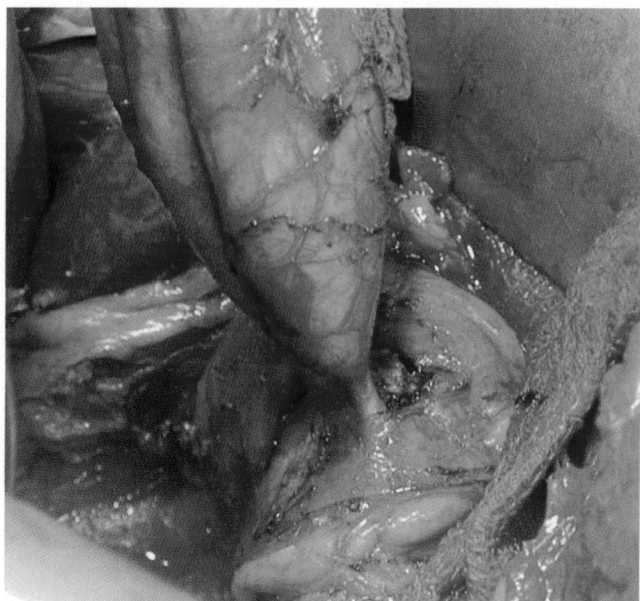

Figure 54-31 Operative photography demonstrating neck of biliary cyst during excision of a type I choledochal cyst.

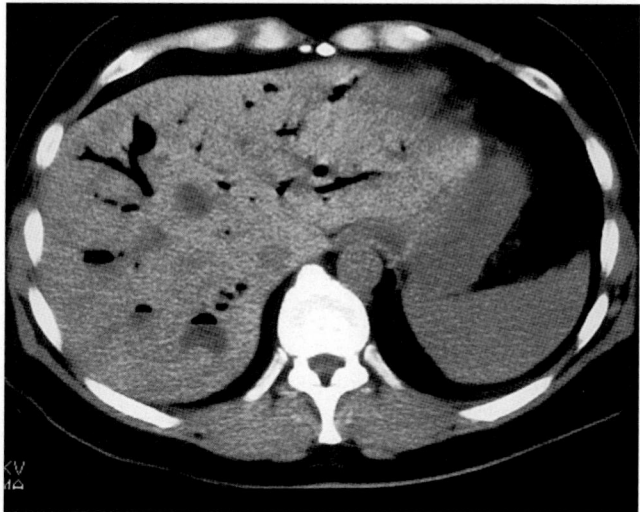

Figure 54-32 Computed tomography demonstrating Caroli's disease.

benign masses of the gallbladder and are usually smaller than 10 mm, have a characteristic echogenic pedunculated appearance on ultrasound, and are often multiple (30% of cases). Adenomyomatosis appears as a sessile polyp with characteristic microcysts on ultrasound and is often larger than 10 mm. Adenoma may be difficult to distinguish from adenocarcinoma of the gallbladder; the main differentiating feature is a lack of transmural invasion on ultrasound, which is sometimes difficult to accurately assess. Risk factors associated with malignancy are age older than 60 years, coexistence of gallstones, a documented increase in size, and size larger than 10 mm. All patients with symptomatic polyploid lesions of the

gallbladder should undergo laparoscopic cholecystectomy. Any patient with risk factors or a suspicion of in situ or frank adenocarcinoma should undergo open cholecystectomy. Lesions smaller than 10 mm that are asymptomatic and without ultrasound features of neoplasia may be safely observed with follow-up imaging.

Benign Biliary Masses

The most common benign tumor of the extrahepatic biliary tree is the papilloma or adenoma, which arises from the glandular epithelium lining the ducts. Most of these tumors are found in or close to the ampulla (47%). Jaundice is the presenting symptom in most patients but can also be accompanied by right upper quadrant pain. A benign adenomatous tumor should be included in the differential in all secondary operations performed for obstruction of the biliary system. It is a soft lesion, is difficult to palpate, and presents very little resistance to ductal probes. Treatment should consist of total resection of symptomatic lesions with some duct wall as well. High recurrence rates have been reported after simple curettage of the polyps. Lesions situated at the ampulla can usually be managed by transduodenal papillotomy or wide local excision.

Benign inflammatory tumors of the bile duct, known as *pseudotumors* and *benign fibrosing disease* can mimic biliary tract tumors. Their histology consists of only inflammatory cells and fibrosis. Pseudotumors appear to occur most frequently above the biliary bifurcation but are still usually extrahepatic. About 10% of resected cholangiocarcinomas are pseudotumors in origin.

MALIGNANT BILIARY DISEASE

Gallbladder Cancer

Cancer of the gallbladder is an aggressive malignancy that occurs predominantly in elderly people. Besides the exceptional cases detected incidentally at the time of cholecystectomy for gallstone disease, which are usually early stage, the prognosis for most patients is poor. Series from the Western hemisphere have reported 5-year survival rates of only 5% to 38%.[42-44] Unfortunately, many of these tumors are unresectable at presentation, and most must be managed nonoperatively. Recently, an aggressive surgical approach for patients with localized gallbladder cancer has produced encouraging results with an acceptable morbidity.

Incidence

Gallbladder cancer is the fifth most common gastrointestinal malignancy, with about 5000 new cases diagnosed annually in the United States. Cancer of the gallbladder is two to three times more common in women than men, in part because of the higher incidence of gallstones in women. More than 75% of patients with this malignancy are older than 65 years. The incidence of gallbladder cancer varies considerably with both ethnic background and geographic location. In the United States, gallbladder cancer is more common in Native Americans. Similarly,

Box 54-7   Risk Factors for Gallbladder Carcinoma

Gallstones
Porcelain gallbladder
Anomalous pancreatobiliary junction
Choledochal cysts
Adenomatous gallbladder polyps
Primary sclerosing cholangitis
Obesity
Salmonella typhi infection

Table 54-2   TNM Staging for Gallbladder Cancer

T1	Tumor invades lamina propria (T1a) or muscular (T1b) layer
T2	Tumor invades perimuscular connective tissue, no extension beyond the serosa or into the liver
T3	Tumor perforates the serosa (visceral peritoneum) and/or directly invades into liver and/or one other adjacent organ or structure such as the stomach, duodenum, colon, pancreas, omentum, or extrahepatic bile ducts
T4	Tumor invades main portal vein or hepatic artery or invades multiple extrahepatic organs and/or structures
N0	No lymph node metastases
N1	Regional lymph node metastases
M0	No distant metastases
M1	Distant metastases

Stage	Stage Grouping
IA	T1 N0 M0
IB	T2 N0 M0
IIA	T3 N0 M0
IIB	T1 N1 M0
	T2 N1 M0
	T3 N1 M0
III	T4 Any N M0
IV	Any T Any N M1

Adapted from Greene F, Page D, Fleming I, et al (eds): AJCC Cancer Staging Manual, 6th ed. New York, Springer-Verlag, 2002.

in Chile, the incidence of gallbladder cancer is particularly high.

Etiology

Several factors have been associated with an increased risk for developing gallbladder cancer (Box 54-7). Although not entirely clear, the pathogenesis is likely related to chronic inflammation. Among these factors, gallstones are the most common because of the high prevalence in the general population. The association between an APBDJ, a porcelain gallbladder, and other biliary disorders such as choledochal cysts and primary sclerosing cholangitis and gallbladder cancer has been recognized more recently.

A strong association has long been noted between gallbladder cancer and cholelithiasis, which is present in 75% to 90% of cases. The incidence of gallstones increases with age, and by age 75, about 35% of women and 20% of men in the United States have developed gallstones. The incidence of gallbladder cancer is about seven times more common in the presence of cholelithiasis and chronic cholecystitis than in people without gallstones. In addition, the risk for developing gallbladder cancer is higher in patients with symptomatic gallstones than in patients with asymptomatic gallstones. About 1% of all elective cholecystectomies performed for cholelithiasis harbor an occult gallbladder cancer.

Pathology and Staging

Ninety percent of cancers of the gallbladder are classified as adenocarcinoma. Squamous cell, oat cell, undifferentiated, and adenosquamous cancers and carcinoid tumors are much less frequent. Six percent of gallbladder adenocarcinomas demonstrate papillary features histopathologically; these tumors are commonly diagnosed while localized to the gallbladder and are also associated with an improved overall survival. At diagnosis, 25% of cancers are localized to the gallbladder wall, 35% have associated metastases to regional lymph nodes or extension into adjacent organs, and 40% have already metastasized to distant sites.

Lymphatic drainage from the gallbladder occurs in a predictable fashion and correlates with the pattern of lymph node metastases seen in gallbladder cancer. Hepatic involvement with gallbladder cancer can occur by direct invasion through the gallbladder bed, angiolymphatic portal tract invasion, or distant hematogenous spread. The current TNM classification of the American Joint Committee on Cancer (AJCC) is shown in Table 54-2. The appropriate management and overall prognosis are strongly dependent on tumor stage.

Clinical Presentation

Gallbladder cancer most often presents with right upper quadrant abdominal pain often mimicking cholecystitis and cholelithiasis. Weight loss, jaundice, and an abdominal mass are less common presenting symptoms. About 40% of patients present with symptoms of chronic cholecystitis, often with a recent change in the quality or frequency of the painful episodes. Another common presentation is similar to acute cholecystitis, with a short duration of pain associated with vomiting, fever, and tenderness. Signs and symptoms of malignant biliary obstruction with jaundice, weight loss, and right upper quadrant pain are also common. Patients can also present with symptoms of a nonbiliary malignancy with anorexia and weight loss in the absence of jaundice or, least commonly, with signs of gastrointestinal bleeding or obstruction. Gallbladder cancer is often misdiagnosed as chronic cholecystitis, pancreatic cancer, acute cholecystitis, choledocholithiasis, or gallbladder hydrops.

Diagnosis

Ultrasonography is often the first diagnostic modality used in the evaluation of patients with right upper quadrant abdominal pain. A heterogeneous mass replacing the gallbladder lumen and an irregular gallbladder wall are common sonographic features of gallbladder cancer. The sensitivity of ultrasound in the detection of gallbladder cancer ranges from 70% to 100%. CT scan usually demonstrates a mass replacing the gallbladder or extending into adjacent organs. Spiral CT also demonstrates the adjacent vascular anatomy. With newer magnetic resonance techniques, gallbladder cancers may be differentiated from the adjacent liver and biliary obstruction or encasement of the portal vein may also be easily visualized.

Cholangiography also may be helpful in diagnosing jaundiced patients with gallbladder cancer. The typical cholangiographic finding in gallbladder cancer is a long stricture of the common hepatic duct. Angiography, spiral CT, or MRI may identify encasement of the portal vein or hepatic artery. If radiographic studies suggest that the tumor is unresectable (liver or peritoneal metastases, portal vein encasement, or extensive hepatic invasion), a biopsy of the tumor is warranted and can be performed under ultrasound or CT guidance.

Management

The appropriate operative procedure for the patient with localized gallbladder cancer is determined by the pathologic stage. Patients with tumors confined to the gallbladder mucosa or submucosa (T1a) or confined to the gallbladder muscularis (T1b) are usually identified after cholecystectomy for gallstone disease and have an overall 5-year survival rate approaching 100% and 85%, respectively. Therefore, cholecystectomy is adequate therapy for patients with T1 tumors. Recurrent cancer at port sites and peritoneal carcinomatosis have been reported after laparoscopic cholecystectomy, even for patients with in situ disease; therefore, all port sites should be excised if a patient has had a previous laparoscopic cholecystectomy. Bile spillage occurs in 26% to 36% of laparoscopic cholecystectomies and appears to be even more common (50%) in cases of gallbladder cancer. Spillage is associated with poor survival even in early stage (T1 and T2) gallbladder cancer. Patients with preoperatively suspected gallbladder cancer should undergo open cholecystectomy to minimize the chance of bile spillage and tumor dissemination.

Cancer of the gallbladder with invasion beyond (stages II and III) the gallbladder muscularis is associated with an increased incidence of regional lymph node metastases and should be managed with an "extended cholecystectomy." This includes lymphadenectomy of the cystic duct, pericholedochal, portal, right celiac, and posterior pancreatoduodenal lymph nodes. Obtaining an R0 resection should be the goal of surgery and results in an improved survival compared with patients who have remaining microscopic or macroscopic disease.[42] Adequate clearance of the pericholedochal lymph nodes may be facilitated by resection of the common bile duct, but common duct resection is not always necessary; in those cases in which the cystic duct stump margin is positive for malignancy, common duct resection with Roux-en-Y reconstruction is mandatory. Extension into the hepatic

parenchyma is common, and extended cholecystectomy should incorporate at least a 2-cm margin beyond the palpable or sonographic extent of the tumor. For smaller tumors, this goal can be achieved with a wedge resection of the liver. For larger tumors, an anatomic liver resection (extended right hepatectomy) may be required to achieve a histologically negative margin. Staging laparoscopy should be performed in patients with gallbladder cancer, as a high proportion (50%-55%) of patients have hepatic or extrahepatic disease that is not detected by noninvasive staging modalities.

In most cases, therapy for gallbladder cancer is palliative. If a tissue diagnosis can be established in patients with an unresectable tumor, nonoperative palliation should be considered. Many of these patients have obstructive jaundice that can be managed with either an endoscopic or percutaneously placed biliary stent. Pain is another problem that should be treated aggressively to improve quality of life. Percutaneous celiac ganglion nerve block may reduce the need for narcotics.

The results of chemotherapy in the treatment of patients with gallbladder cancer have been quite poor. External-beam and intraoperative radiation therapy have both been used in the management of patients with gallbladder cancer. Unfortunately, no randomized data have demonstrated improved survival with either chemotherapy or radiation.

Survival

Survival in patients with gallbladder cancer is strongly influenced by the pathologic stage at presentation. Recent advances in surgical technique and aggressiveness of resection for gallbladder cancer have resulted in improved overall survival[42] (Fig. 54-33). Patients with cancer limited to the gallbladder mucosa and lamina propria (T1a) have an excellent prognosis. Invasion into the muscular wall (T1b) of the gallbladder increases the risk for recurrent cancer after curative resection. However, no difference

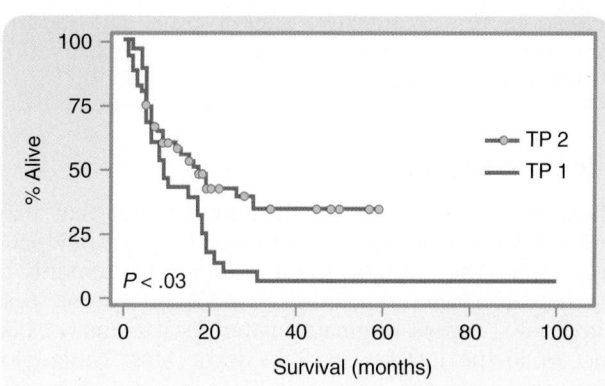

Figure 54-33 Improved survival due to an aggressive approach to gallbladder cancer comparing two time periods (TPs), 1990-1996 and 1996-2002 (*circles*) (*P* < .03). (From Dixon E, Vollmer CM, Sahajpal A, et al: An aggressive surgical approach leads to improved survival in patients with gallbladder cancer: A 12-year study at a North American Center. Ann Surg 241:385-394, 2005.)

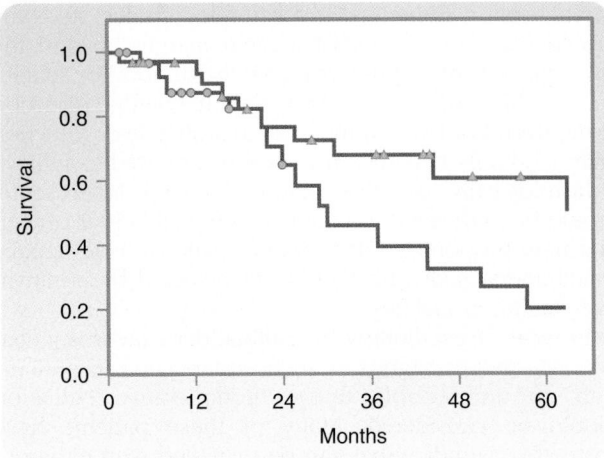

Figure 54-34 Survival following surgical resection for T2 gallbladder cancer. Patients undergoing radical resection (*triangles*) are compared with patients undergoing simple cholecystectomy (*circles*) (*P* > .05). (From Fong Y, Jarnigan W, Blumgart LH: Gallbladder cancer: Comparison of patients presenting initially for definitive operation with those presenting after prior non-curative intervention. Ann Surg 232:557-569, 2000.)

in 10-year survival has been demonstrated after simple cholecystectomy (100%) and extended cholecystectomy (75%) among patients with T1b gallbladder cancer. Invasion into the subserosa (T2) increases the risk for regional lymph node metastases to between 33% and 50%. Five-year survival in patients with T2 tumors is improved following extended cholecystectomy with lymphadenectomy and liver resection (59%-61%) compared with simple cholecystectomy (17%-19%)[43] (Fig. 54-34). Several groups have recently reported 5-year overall survival rates for resected patients with stages IIA and IIB gallbladder cancer of 28% to 63% and 19% to 25%, respectively. However, most patients with gallbladder cancer have advanced unresectable disease at the time of presentation. As a result, fewer than 15% of all patients with gallbladder cancer are alive after 5 years. The median survival for stage IV patients at the time of presentation is only 1 to 3 months.

Bile Duct Cancer

Cholangiocarcinoma is an uncommon tumor that may occur anywhere along the intrahepatic or extrahepatic biliary tree. These tumors are located most commonly at the hepatic duct bifurcation (60%-80% of cases). Less commonly, tumors originate in the distal common bile duct or in the intrahepatic bile ducts. Most cholangiocarcinomas present with jaundice, and the diagnosis of cholangiocarcinoma should be considered in every patient with obstructive jaundice. When possible, surgical resection does offer a chance for long-term disease-free survival. Many patients, however, will be candidates only for palliative bypass or operative or nonoperative intubation aimed to provide biliary drainage and prevent cholangitis and hepatic failure.

Incidence

The reported incidence of cholangiocarcinoma in the United States is 1 or 2 cases per 100,000 population. Incidence data from the American Cancer Society are difficult to interpret because intrahepatic bile duct cancers are included with primary liver cancers, whereas extrahepatic biliary cancers are in a separate category that includes gallbladder cancer. In the United States, an estimated 17,550 primary liver cancers will be diagnosed in 2005. Data from the National Cancer Institute Surveillance, Epidemiology, and End Results (SEER) program suggest that about 15% of these (2600 cases) will be intrahepatic cholangiocarcinomas. About 7000 cases of extrahepatic bile duct cancer are diagnosed annually in the United States, two thirds of which are gallbladder cancers. Thus, 2000 to 3000 cases per year are extrahepatic cholangiocarcinomas.

For unclear reasons, the incidence of intrahepatic cholangiocarcinoma has been rising over the past 2 decades in Europe and North America, Asia, Japan, and Australia, whereas rates of extrahepatic cholangiocarcinoma are declining internationally. The rising rates of intrahepatic cholangiocarcinoma have not been associated with an increase in the proportion of early-stage or smaller lesions. Furthermore, incidence rates do not appear to have reached a plateau.

Risk Factors

A number of diseases have been linked to cholangiocarcinoma, including primary sclerosing cholangitis, choledochal cysts, and hepatolithiasis. Characteristics common to these diseases include bile duct stones, biliary stasis, and infection. Bile duct cancers in patients with primary sclerosing cholangitis are most often extrahepatic, commonly occur near the hepatic duct bifurcation, and are difficult to differentiate from the multiple, benign strictures associated with this disease. As a general rule, the incidence of biliary tract cancers increases with age; the typical patient with cholangiocarcinoma is between 50 and 70 years of age. However, patients with PSC and those with choledochal cysts present nearly 2 decades earlier. In contrast to gallbladder cancer, for which female gender predominates, the incidence of cholangiocarcinoma is slightly higher in men. This probably reflects the higher incidence of PSC in men. Hepatolithiasis is also a definite risk factor for cholangiocarcinoma, which will develop in 5% to 10% of patients with intrahepatic stones. Hepatitis B and C are also now recognized as risk factors in the development of intrahepatic cholangiocarcinoma. At least two genetic disorders are associated with an increased risk for cholangiocarcinoma: the inherited "cancer family" syndrome termed *Lynch syndrome II,* and a rare inherited disorder called *multiple biliary papillomatosis;* the latter condition is characterized by multiple adenomatous polyps in the bile ducts, and repeated episodes of abdominal pain, jaundice, and acute cholangitis.

Prior biliary-enteric anastomosis may also increase the future risk for cholangiocarcinoma. Five percent of patients in a large Italian series developed cholangiocar-

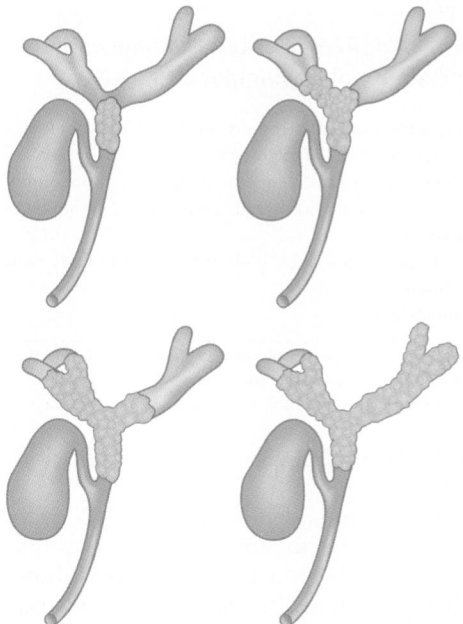

Figure 54-35 Bismuth classification of perihilar cholangiocarcinoma by anatomic extent. Type I tumors (*upper, left*) are confined to the common hepatic duct, and type II tumors (*upper, right*) involve the bifurcation without involvement of secondary intrahepatic ducts. Type IIIa and IIIb tumors (*lower, left*) extend into either the right or left secondary intrahepatic ducts, respectively. Type IV tumors (*lower, right*) involve the secondary intrahepatic ducts on both sides.

Table 54-3 Current American Joint Commission on Cancer TNM Staging System for Cholangiocarcinoma

Stage 0	Tis	N0	M0
Stage I	T1	N0	M0
Stage II	T2	N0	M0
Stage III	T1 or T2	N1 or N2	M0
Stage IVA	T3	Any N	M0
Stage IVB	Any T	Any N	M1

Tis, carcinoma *in situ;* T1, tumor invades the subepithelial connective tissue; T2, tumor invades perifibromuscular connective tissue; T3, tumor invades adjacent organs.

N0, no regional lymph node metastases; N1, metastasis to hepatoduodenal ligament lymph nodes; N2, metastasis to peripancreatic, periduodenal, periportal, celiac, and/or superior mesenteric artery lymph nodes.

M0, no distant metastasis; M1, distant metastasis.

Adapted from Greene F, Page D, Fleming I, et al (eds): AJCC Cancer Staging Manual, 6th ed. New York, Springer-Verlag, 2002.

cinoma between 11 and 18 years after a biliary-enteric anastomosis. The risk for bile duct cancer was higher after transduodenal sphincteroplasty and choledochoduodenostomy than after hepaticojejunostomy and was most strongly associated with recurrent episodes of cholangitis. Multiple other risk factors for cholangiocarcinoma have been identified, including liver flukes, Thorotrast, industrial chemicals, dietary nitrosamines, and exposure to dioxin.

Staging and Classification

Cholangiocarcinoma is best classified anatomically into three broad groups:

1. Intrahepatic
2. Perihilar
3. Distal

Intrahepatic tumors are treated like hepatocellular carcinoma with hepatectomy, when possible. The perihilar tumors make up the largest group and are managed with resection of the bile duct, preferably with hepatic resection. Distal tumors are managed in a fashion similar to other periampullary malignancies with pancreatoduodenectomy.

Cancers of the hepatic duct bifurcation have also been classified according to their anatomic location (Fig. 54-35). In this system, type I tumors are confined to the common hepatic duct, and type II tumors involve the bifurcation without involvement of secondary intrahe-

patic ducts. Types IIIa and IIIb tumors extend into either the right or left secondary intrahepatic ducts, respectively, and type IV tumors involve the secondary intrahepatic ducts on both sides.

Cholangiocarcinoma is also staged according to the tumor, node, metastasis (TNM) classification of the AJCC (Table 54-3). Using this system, stage IA tumors are limited to the bile duct, whereas stage IB tumors invade periductal tissues. Stage IIA tumors are locally advanced without lymph node metastases, and stage IIB tumors have regional lymph node metastases. Stage III tumors are locally advanced and unresectable, and stage IV tumors have distant metastases. Portal vein involvement and lobar atrophy have been reported as important prognostic factors for cholangiocarcinoma and may be incorporated in the classification in the future.[45]

Clinical Presentation

More than 90% of patients with perihilar or distal tumors present with jaundice. Patients with intrahepatic cholangiocarcinoma are rarely jaundiced until late in the course of the disease. Less common presenting clinical features include pruritus, fever, mild abdominal pain, fatigue, anorexia, and weight loss. Cholangitis is not a frequent presenting finding but most commonly develops after biliary manipulation. Except for jaundice, the physical examination is usually normal in patients with cholangiocarcinoma.

Diagnosis and Assessment of Resectability

At the time of presentation, most patients with perihilar and distal cholangiocarcinoma have a total serum bilirubin level greater than 10 mg/dL. Marked elevations in alkaline phosphatase are also routinely observed. Serum CA 19-9 may also be elevated in patients with cholangiocarcinoma, although levels may fall once biliary obstruction is relieved.

The radiologic evaluation of patients with cholangiocarcinoma should delineate the overall extent of the

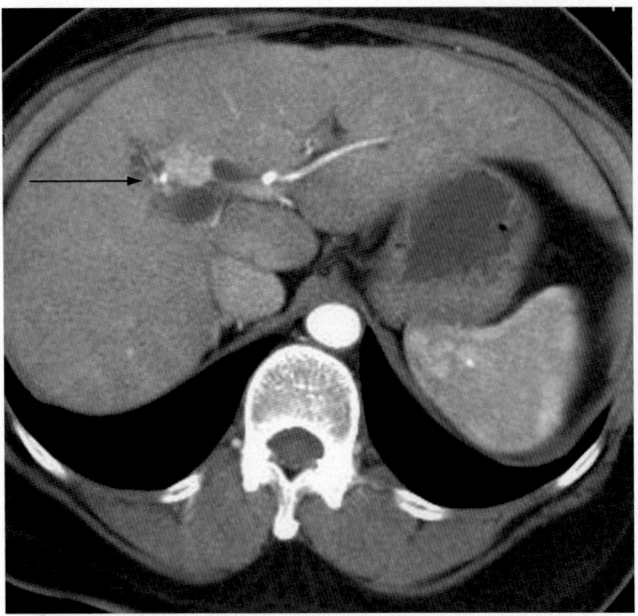

Figure 54-36 Computed tomography scan visualizes mass at hepatic duct bifurcation (*arrow*) resulting in bilateral biliary dilation and extensive perihilar malignancy.

tumor, including involvement of the bile ducts, liver, hilar vessels, and distant metastases. The initial radiographic studies consist of either abdominal ultrasound or CT scanning (Fig. 54-36). Intrahepatic cholangiocarcinomas are easily visualized on CT scans; however, perihilar and distal tumors are often difficult to visualize on ultrasound and standard CT scan. Cholangiocarcinoma can be enhanced by using delayed-phase CT acquisition (10 minutes after contrast injection). A hilar cholangiocarcinoma gives a picture of a dilated intrahepatic biliary tree and a normal or collapsed gallbladder and extrahepatic biliary tree. Distal tumors lead to dilation of the gallbladder and both the intrahepatic and extrahepatic biliary tree.

After documentation of bile duct dilation, biliary anatomy has been traditionally defined cholangiographically through either the percutaneous transhepatic or the endoscopic retrograde route. The most proximal extent of the tumor is the most important feature in determining resectability in patients with perihilar tumors, and the percutaneous route is favored in these patients because it defines the proximal extent of tumor involvement most reliably. PET will detect unsuspected distant or intrahepatic metastases in up to 30% of patients with cholangiocarcinoma. MRC offers good resolution of both the intrahepatic and extrahepatic biliary tree, but should be substituted with PTC or ERCP in patients that will require preoperative or palliative biliary drainage. Biliary drainage is necessary if the patient's bilirubin is more than 10 mg/dL, but it has been associated with an increased risk for cholangitis and longer postoperative hospital stay in patients with obstructive jaundice who then undergo resection.[46] Cholestasis, biliary cirrhosis, and liver dys-

Box 54-8 Radiologic Criteria to Suggest Unresectability of Cholangiocarcinoma

Bilateral hepatic duct involvement up to secondary radicals
Bilateral hepatic artery involvement
Encasement of the portal vein proximal to its bifurcation
Atrophy of one hepatic lobe with contralateral portal vein encasement
Atrophy of one hepatic lobe with contralateral biliary radical involvement
Distant metastasis

Adapted from Anderson CD, Pinson CW, Berlin J, Chari RS: Diagnosis and treatment of cholangiocarcinoma. Oncologist 9:43-57, 2004.

function develop rapidly in the face of unrelieved biliary obstruction.

Percutaneous fine-needle aspiration biopsy, brush and scrape biopsy, and cytologic examination of bile all have been used to establish a tissue diagnosis; however, the sensitivity in detecting a malignancy is low, and a benign result should be considered unreliable. Seven to 15% of patients with preoperative symptoms and imaging studies and intraoperative findings consistent with malignant biliary obstruction will ultimately have benign lesions on histologic analysis of resection specimens.

Management

Hepatic lobar atrophy and hepatic ductal extension predict the need for hepatectomy in order to achieve a margin-negative resection.[45,47] All available data must be used to distinguish resectability from unresectability (Fig. 54-37). Radiographic criteria that suggest unresectability of perihilar tumors include bilateral hepatic duct involvement up to secondary radicals, encasement or occlusion of the portal vein proximal to its bifurcation, atrophy of one liver lobe with encasement of the contralateral portal vein branch, involvement of bilateral hepatic arteries, or atrophy of one liver lobe with contralateral secondary biliary radical involvement (Box 54-8). Ipsilateral portal vein involvement and involvement of secondary biliary radicals do not preclude resection, nor does ipsilateral lobar atrophy.[48] Curative treatment of patients with cholangiocarcinoma is possible only with complete resection (R0).

Patients with unequivocal evidence of unresectable cholangiocarcinoma at initial evaluation are palliated nonoperatively. Nonoperative palliation can be achieved both endoscopically and percutaneously. Percutaneous biliary drainage has several advantages over endoscopic management in patients with perihilar cholangiocarcinoma, whereas endoscopic palliation is the preferred approach in patients with distal cholangiocarcinoma. More recently, metallic stents have been used to palliate patients with malignant biliary obstruction. These stents remain patent longer than plastic stents and require fewer subsequent manipulations.

Operative Approach

Surgical exploration should be undertaken in good-risk patients without evidence of metastatic or locally unre-

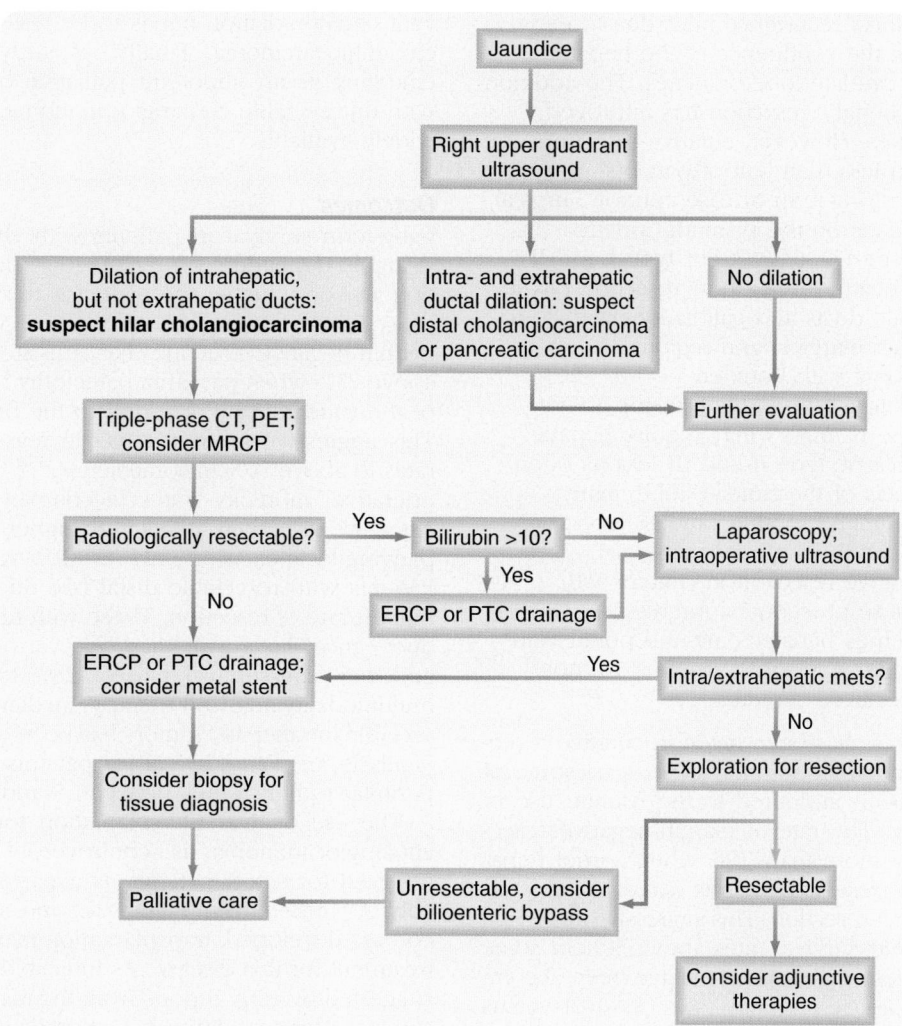

Figure 54-37 Flow chart depicting the workup and treatment of a patient with suspected hilar cholangiocarcinoma. CT, computed tomography; ERCP, endoscopic retrograde cholangiopancreatography; MRCP; magnetic resonance cholangiopancreatography; PTC, percutaneous transhepatic cholangiography. (From Anderson CD, Pinson CW, Berlin J, Chari RS: Diagnosis and treatment of cholangiocarcinoma. Oncologist 9:43-57, 2004.)

sectable disease; however, intraoperatively, more than half of these patients are found to have either peritoneal or hepatic metastases or, more likely, locally unresectable disease. Selective use of laparoscopy in patients with locally advanced but potentially resectable perihilar cholangiocarcinoma may avoid laparotomy in some patients with metastatic disease. In patients who are found to have extensive metastatic disease, the preoperatively placed biliary stents should be left in place. However, a cholecystectomy should be performed to avoid the risk of acute cholecystitis, which occurs in patients with long-term indwelling biliary stents. In patients with locally advanced unresectable perihilar tumors, several operative approaches are available for palliation, including a Roux-en-Y hepaticojejunostomy to segment III or V.

Distal cholangiocarcinoma—Distal lesions are usually treated with pancreaticoduodenectomy (Whipple's procedure). A pylorus-preserving operation is preferable and feasible in most patients, with 5-year survival rates averaging 15% to 25%, but can be as high as 54% in selected patients who undergo complete resection for node-negative disease. If resection is not possible owing to vascular encasement, cholecystectomy, Roux-en-Y hepaticojejunostomy proximal to the tumor, and a gastrojejunostomy to prevent gastric outlet obstruction should be performed.

Intrahepatic cholangiocarcinoma—Intrahepatic cholangiocarcinoma is treated by hepatic resection, and outcomes depend on disease stage (particularly the status of the lymph nodes) and the ability to achieve negative margins. There is a broad range of long-term outcomes in patients undergoing complete resection (3-year survival rates of 22%-66%).

Perihilar cholangiocarcinoma—For perihilar cholangiocarcinomas, bile duct resection alone leads to high local recurrence rates due to early involvement of the confluence of the hepatic ducts and the caudate lobe branches. The addition of a modified hepatic resection has improved resectability rates. However, curative resections are still possible in less than half of patients, and most do not achieve long-term disease control. Surgical treatment depends on the Bismuth-Corlette classification (see Fig. 54-35). For type I and II lesions, the procedure is en bloc resection of the extrahepatic bile ducts and gallbladder with 5- to 10-mm bile duct margins, and regional lymphadenectomy with Roux-en-Y hepaticojejunostomy. In addition to the above operations, type II tumors may require hepatic lobectomy. Because type II and III lesions often involve the ducts of the caudate lobe, many surgeons recommend routine caudate lobectomy. Type III and IV tumors are amenable to potentially curative resection in centers with expertise in these procedures. Aggressive techniques such as hepatectomy and portal vein resection to achieve negative margins are now routine in specialized centers.

Substantial progress has been made in curative resection for perihilar cholangiocarcinomas. At least some of this progress has been attributed to the routine use of partial hepatectomy. The rate of margin-negative resections is consistently more than 75% when partial hepatectomy (including resection of the caudate lobe) is added to the bile duct resection. This aggressive approach has resulted in 5-year survival rates above 50% in some series. However, these improvements have been accompanied by higher surgical mortality rates (8%-10% versus 2%-4%). The major prognostic factors are margin status and tumor stage. In addition to location, stage, and status of the resection margins, other factors influence outcome after resection.

Medical Therapy

Numerous reports have suggested that radiation therapy improves survival for patients with cholangiocarcinoma, especially when resection is impossible. External-beam radiotherapy has been delivered using a variety of innovative techniques, including intraoperative radiotherapy and brachytherapy with iridium-192 through percutaneous or endoscopic stents. However, no prospective, randomized trials have been reported, and a well-controlled, but not randomized, trial reported no benefit for postoperative adjuvant radiation. A survival benefit for postoperative radiation therapy may be limited to patients with local extension into the liver parenchyma and microscopic residual disease following resection. Chemotherapy has also not been shown to improve survival in patients with either resected or unresected cholangiocarcinoma. Given the potential radiosensitization effect of 5-fluorouracil or gemcitabine, the combination of radiation and chemotherapy may be more effective than either agent alone. As with gallbladder cancer, the role of adju-

vant chemoradiation needs to be tested in patients with cholangiocarcinoma. Finally, photodynamic therapy is emerging as an important palliative option for patients with unresectable cholangiocarcinoma, although it is not widely available.

Outcomes

Long-term survival in patients with cholangiocarcinoma is highly dependent on the stage of disease at presentation and on whether the patient is treated by a palliative procedure or complete tumor resection. The rate of margin-negative resections has consistently been reported above 75% when partial hepatectomy including resection of the caudate lobe is added to the biliary resection.[49,50] This aggressive approach has increased 5-year survival rates to above 50% in some series.[47,49] However, the perioperative mortality rates accompanying these more extensive resections are slightly higher than those accompanying local excision only (8%-10% versus 2%-4%).[49,51,52] Patients with resectable distal bile duct cancer have the highest rate of resection. Those with resectable distal bile duct cancer have a median survival of 32 to 38 months and a 5-year survival rate of 28% to 45%. Even with multimodality adjuvant therapy, median survival for unresectable intrahepatic tumors has been only 6 to 7 months. Similarly, median survival for patients with unresectable perihilar tumors varies between 5 and 8 months.

The use of liver transplantation for the treatment of cholangiocarcinoma is controversial and should be reserved for select patients as a part of research protocols. As more effective adjuvant and neoadjuvant protocols are developed, transplantation may be a more useful treatment for this disease. As indicated previously, this is suggested by early reports from the Mayo Clinic in which survival after neoadjuvant chemoradiation and liver transplantation was significantly improved over resection alone for stage I and II hilar cholangiocarcinoma.[40]

Metastatic and Other Tumors

Hepatocellular carcinoma and liver metastases can cause obstructive jaundice by direct extension into the perihilar bile ducts. Hepatocellular and metastatic colorectal carcinoma have also both been reported to "embolize" into the biliary tree. This rare phenomenon occurs when tumor cells are shed into the biliary tract and implant distally, leading to biliary obstruction when the tumor embolus increases in size. Hepatic cystadenomas and cystadenocarcinomas arise from the biliary epithelium, and these tumors or the mucin they produce may also cause bile duct obstruction.

Primary and secondary hepatic tumors can also produce biliary obstruction by metastasizing to hilar or pericholedochal lymph nodes. Hepatocellular carcinoma, colorectal carcinoma, and pancreatic carcinoma are the most common primary sites associated with biliary tract obstruction from lymph node metastases, although nodal metastases from a number of tumors including breast and ovarian cancer have been reported to cause bile duct obstruction. Lymphoma can also result in biliary obstruction and mimic either pancreatic cancer or perihilar cholangiocarcinoma. Although commonly extensive, lymphomas usually respond to chemotherapy, leading to resolution of the biliary obstruction.

Selected References

Anderson CD, Pinson CW, Berlin J, et al: Diagnosis and treatment of cholangiocarcinoma. Oncologist 9:43-57, 2004.

> Excellent review and summary of the modern treatment of cholangiocarcinoma.

Boerma D, Rauws EA, Keulemans YC, et al: Wait-and-see policy or laparoscopic cholecystectomy after endoscopic sphincterotomy for bile-duct stones: A randomised trial. Lancet 360:761-765, 2002.

> A randomized, prospective trial comparing observation versus laparoscopic cholecystectomy following endoscopic removal of stones. Recurrent biliary symptoms developed in 47% in the observation arm, and one third of these required cholecystectomy.

Cotton PB: Endoscopic management of bile duct stones (apples and oranges). Gut 25:587, 1984.

> This classic article describes problems and results of the endoscopic management of choledocholithiasis.

Dixon E, Vollmer CM Jr, Sahajpal A, et al: An aggressive surgical approach leads to improved survival in patients with gallbladder cancer: A 12-year study at a North American Center. Ann Surg 241:385-394, 2005.

> A review of the results in a single center over 12 years indicating that an aggressive approach to gallbladder cancer with extensive resection improves long-term survival.

Glenn F: Acute cholecystitis. Surg Gynecol Obstet 143:56, 1976.

> This is a classic review with more than 200 cases by the late master biliary tract surgeon. Serious risk factors and the increased mortality in elderly patients are stressed.

Nakeeb A, Comuzzie AG, Martin L, et al: Gallstones: Genetics versus environment. Ann Surg 235:842-849, 2002.

> An excellent study that examines the contribution of genetics to the pathogenesis of symptomatic gallstones.

Rea DJ, Heimbach JK, Rosen CB, et al: Liver transplantation with neoadjuvant chemoradiation is more effective than resection for hilar cholangiocarcinoma. Ann Surg 242:451-458, 2005.

> Pivotal paper in the renewed interest in liver transplantation in the management of cholangiocarcinoma.

Reisner RM: Gallstone ileus: A review of 1001 reported cases. Am Surg 60:441, 1994.

> An exhaustive review of all cases reported in the English language from 1953 to 1993. It covers all aspects of epidemiology, diagnosis, therapy, and complications.

Southern Surgeons Club: A prospective analysis of 1518 laparoscopic cholecystectomies. N Engl J Med 324:1073-1078, 1991.

> This classic paper is one of the first to identify and report outcomes following laparoscopic cholecystectomy.

Way LW, Stewart L, Gantert W, et al: Causes and prevention of laparoscopic bile duct injuries: Analysis of 252 cases from a human factors and cognitive psychology perspective. Ann Surg 237:460-469, 2003.

> Intriguing article examining the human factor in the causation of bile duct injury.

References

1. Trowbridge RL, Rutkowski NK, Shojania KG: Does this patient have acute cholecystitis? JAMA 289:80-86, 2003.
2. Potter MW, Shah SA, McEnaney P, et al: A critical appraisal of laparoscopic staging in hepatobiliary and pancreatic malignancy. Surg Oncol 9:103-110, 2000.
3. Weber SM, DeMatteo RP, Fong Y, et al: Staging laparoscopy in patients with extrahepatic biliary carcinoma: Analysis of 100 patients. Ann Surg 235:392-399, 2002.
4. Anderson CD, Rice MH, Pinson CW, et al: Fluorodeoxyglucose PET imaging in the evaluation of gallbladder carcinoma and cholangiocarcinoma. J Gastrointest Surg 8:90-97, 2004.
5. Thompson JE Jr, Pitt HA, Doty JE, et al: Broad spectrum penicillin as an adequate therapy for acute cholangitis. Surg Gynecol Obstet 171:275-282, 1990.
6. Thompson JE Jr, Bennion RS, Doty JE, et al: Predictive factors for bactibilia in acute cholecystitis. Arch Surg 125:261-264, 1990.
7. Bellows CF, Berger DH, Crass RA: Management of gallstones. Am Fam Physician 72:637-642, 2005.
8. Nakeeb A, Comuzzie AG, Martin L, et al: Gallstones: Genetics versus environment. Ann Surg 235:842-849, 2002.
9. Stewart L, Oesterle AL, Erdan I, et al: Pathogenesis of pigment gallstones in Western societies: The central role of bacteria. J Gastrointest Surg 6:891-903, 2002.
10. Glasgow RE, Cho M, Hutter MM, et al: The spectrum and cost of complicated gallstone disease in California. Arch Surg 135:1021-1025, 2000.
11. Lo CM, Liu CL, Fan ST, et al: Prospective randomized study of early versus delayed laparoscopic cholecystectomy for acute cholecystitis. Ann Surg 227:461-467, 1998.
12. Lai PB, Kwong KH, Leung KL, et al: Randomized trial of early versus delayed laparoscopic cholecystectomy for acute cholecystitis. Br J Surg 85:764-767, 1998.
13. Kiviluoto T, Siren J, Luukkonen P, et al: Randomised trial of laparoscopic versus open cholecystectomy for acute and gangrenous cholecystitis. Lancet 351:321-325, 1998.
14. Steiner CA, Bass EB, Talamini MA, et al: Surgical rates and operative mortality for open and laparoscopic cholecystectomy in Maryland. N Engl J Med 330:403-408, 1994.
15. Southern Surgeons Club: A prospective analysis of 1518 laparoscopic cholecystectomies. N Engl J Med 324:1073-1078, 1991.
16. Lau H, Lo CY, Patil NG, et al: Early versus delayed-interval laparoscopic cholecystectomy for acute cholecystitis: A metaanalysis. Surg Endosc 20:82-87, 2006.
17. Willsher PC, Sanabria JR, Gallinger S, et al: Early laparoscopic cholecystectomy for acute cholecystitis: A safe procedure. J Gastrointest Surg 3:50-53, 1999.
18. Liu TH, Consorti ET, Kawashima A, et al: Patient evaluation and management with selective use of magnetic resonance cholangiography and endoscopic retrograde cholangiopancreatography before laparoscopic cholecystectomy. Ann Surg 234:33-40, 2001.
19. Rhodes M, Sussman L, Cohen L, et al: Randomised trial of laparoscopic exploration of common bile duct versus

postoperative endoscopic retrograde cholangiography for common bile duct stones. Lancet 351:159-161, 1998.

20. Boerma D, Rauws EA, Keulemans YC, et al: Wait-and-see policy or laparoscopic cholecystectomy after endoscopic sphincterotomy for bile-duct stones: A randomised trial. Lancet 360:761-765, 2002.

21. Linder JD, Klapow JC, Linder SD, et al: Incomplete response to endoscopic sphincterotomy in patients with sphincter of Oddi dysfunction: Evidence for a chronic pain disorder. Am J Gastroenterol 98:1738-1743, 2003.

22. Lau H, Brooks DC: Transitions in laparoscopic cholecystectomy: The impact of ambulatory surgery. Surg Endosc 16:323-326, 2002.

23. Calland JF, Tanaka K, Foley E, et al: Outpatient laparoscopic cholecystectomy: Patient outcomes after implementation of a clinical pathway. Ann Surg 233:704-715, 2001.

24. Flum DR, Dellinger EP, Cheadle A, et al: Intraoperative cholangiography and risk of common bile duct injury during cholecystectomy. JAMA 289:1639-1644, 2003.

25. Halpin VJ, Dunnegan D, Soper NJ: Laparoscopic intracorporeal ultrasound versus fluoroscopic intraoperative cholangiography: After the learning curve. Surg Endosc 16:336-341, 2002.

26. Way LW, Stewart L, Gantert W, et al: Causes and prevention of laparoscopic bile duct injuries: Analysis of 252 cases from a human factors and cognitive psychology perspective. Ann Surg 237:460-469, 2003.

27. Chapman WC, Halevy A, Blumgart LH, et al: Postcholecystectomy bile duct strictures: Management and outcome in 130 patients. Arch Surg 130:597-602, 1995.

28. Lillemoe KD, Melton GB, Cameron JL, et al: Postoperative bile duct strictures: Management and outcome in the 1990s. Ann Surg 232:430-441, 2000.

29. Stewart L, Way LW: Bile duct injuries during laparoscopic cholecystectomy: Factors that influence the results of treatment. Arch Surg 130:1123-1128, 1995.

30. Stewart L, Robinson TN, Lee CM, et al: Right hepatic artery injury associated with laparoscopic bile duct injury: Incidence, mechanism, and consequences. J Gastrointest Surg 8:523-530, 2004.

31. Alves A, Farges O, Nicolet J, et al: Incidence and consequence of an hepatic artery injury in patients with postcholecystectomy bile duct strictures. Ann Surg 238:93-96, 2003.

32. Sicklick JK, Camp MS, Lillemoe KD, et al: Surgical management of bile duct injuries sustained during laparoscopic cholecystectomy: Perioperative results in 200 patients. Ann Surg 241:786-792, 2005.

33. Lillemoe KD, Martin SA, Cameron JL, et al: Major bile duct injuries during laparoscopic cholecystectomy: Follow-up after combined surgical and radiologic management. Ann Surg 225:459-468, 1997.

34. Davids PH, Tanka AK, Rauws EA, et al: Benign biliary strictures. Surgery or endoscopy? Ann Surg 217:237-243, 1993.

35. Melton GB, Lillemoe KD, Cameron JL, et al: Major bile duct injuries associated with laparoscopic cholecystectomy: Effect of surgical repair on quality of life. Ann Surg 235:888-895, 2002.

36. Cosenza CA, Durazo F, Stain SC, et al: Current management of recurrent pyogenic cholangitis. Am Surg 65:939-943, 1999.

37. Owen CC, Bilhartz LE: Gallbladder polyps, cholesterolosis, adenomyomatosis, and acute acalculous cholecystitis. Semin Gastrointest Dis 14:178-188, 2003.

38. Ahrendt SA, Pitt HA, Kalloo AN, et al: Primary sclerosing cholangitis: Resect, dilate, or transplant? Ann Surg 227:412-423, 1998.

39. Rosen CB, Nagorney DM, Wiesner RH, et al: Cholangiocarcinoma complicating primary sclerosing cholangitis. Ann Surg 213:21-25, 1991.

40. Rea DJ, Heimbach JK, Rosen CB, et al: Liver transplantation with neoadjuvant chemoradiation is more effective than resection for hilar cholangiocarcinoma. Ann Surg 242:451-458, 2005.

41. Todani T, Watanabe Y, Toki A, et al: Carcinoma related to choledochal cysts with internal drainage operations. Surg Gynecol Obstet 164:61-64, 1987.

42. Dixon E, Vollmer CM Jr, Sahajpal, A, et al: An aggressive surgical approach leads to improved survival in patients with gallbladder cancer: A 12-year study at a North American Center. Ann Surg 241:385-394, 2005.

43. Fong Y, Jarnagin W, Blumgart LH: Gallbladder cancer: Comparison of patients presenting initially for definitive operation with those presenting after prior noncurative intervention. Ann Surg 232:557-569, 2000.

44. Bartlett DL, Fong Y, Fortner JG, et al: Long-term results after resection for gallbladder cancer: Implications for staging and management. Ann Surg 224:639-646, 1996.

45. Jarnagin WR, Fong Y, DeMatteo RP, et al: Staging, resectability, and outcome in 225 patients with hilar cholangiocarcinoma. Ann Surg 234:507-517, 2001.

46. Figueras J, Llado L, Valls C, et al: Changing strategies in diagnosis and management of hilar cholangiocarcinoma. Liver Transpl 6:786-794, 2000.

47. Burke EC, Jarnagin WR, Hochwald SN, et al: Hilar cholangiocarcinoma: Patterns of spread, the importance of hepatic resection for curative operation, and a presurgical clinical staging system. Ann Surg 228:385-394, 1998.

48. Anderson CD, Pinson CW, Berlin J, et al: Diagnosis and treatment of cholangiocarcinoma. Oncologist 9:43-57, 2004.

49. Nakeeb A, Tran KQ, Black MJ, et al: Improved survival in resected biliary malignancies. Surgery 132:555-563, 2002.

50. Tsao JI, Nimura Y, Kamiya J, et al: Management of hilar cholangiocarcinoma: Comparison of an American and a Japanese experience. Ann Surg 232:166-174, 2000.

51. Nimura Y, Kamiya J, Kondo S, et al: Aggressive preoperative management and extended surgery for hilar cholangiocarcinoma: Nagoya experience. J Hepatobiliary Pancreat Surg 7:155-162, 2000.

52. Nagino M, Kamiya J, Arai T, et al: "Anatomic" right hepatic trisectionectomy (extended right hepatectomy) with caudate lobectomy for hilar cholangiocarcinoma. Ann Surg 243:28-32, 2006.

53. Todani T, Watanabe Y, Narusue M, et al: Congenital bile duct cysts: Classification, operative procedures, and review of thirty-seven cases including cancer arising from choledochal cyst. Am J Surg 134:263-269, 1977.

Exocrine Pancreas

Michael L. Steer, MD

The pancreas was first mentioned in the writings of Eristratos (310-250 BC) and given its name by Rufus of Ephesus (circa 100 AD). The name pancreas (Greek *pan,* all; *kreas,* flesh or meat) was used because the organ contains neither cartilage nor bone. Its main duct was described by Wirsung in 1642, whereas the enlargement of that duct at its junction with the common bile duct and its projection into the duodenum as a papilla were first described by Vater in 1720. Santorini, in 1734, described the accessory duct that bears his name.

ANATOMY

Location

The pancreas lies posterior to the stomach and lesser omentum in the retroperitoneum of the upper abdomen. It extends obliquely, rising slightly as it passes from the medial edge of the duodenal C loop to the hilum of the spleen. It lies anterior to the inferior vena cava, aorta, splenic vein, and left adrenal gland.

Regions

The pancreas is divided into four regions: the head and uncinate process, neck, body, and tail. The head lies within the duodenal C loop, and its uncinate process extends posteriorly and medially to lie behind the portal and superior mesenteric vein and superior mesenteric artery. The neck of the gland extends medially from the head to lie anterior to those vessels. The body extends laterally from the neck toward the spleen, whereas the tail extends into the splenic hilum.

Blood Supply and Lymph Nodes

Both the celiac trunk and the superior mesenteric artery provide the arterial supply to the pancreas. Variations are common, but for the most part, the body and tail are supplied by branches of the splenic artery, whereas the head and uncinate process receive their supply through arcades originating from the hepatic and gastroduodenal branch of the celiac artery and from the first branch of the superior mesenteric artery (Fig. 55-1A). Venous drainage is to the splenic, superior mesenteric, and portal veins (see Fig. 55-1B). The pancreas is drained by multiple lymph node groups. The major drainage of the pancreatic head and uncinate process is to the subpyloric, portal, mesenteric, mesocolic, and aortocaval nodes. The pancreatic body and tail, for the most part, are drained through nodes in the celiac, aortocaval, mesenteric, and mesocolic groups and through nodes in the splenic hilum.

Innervation

The pancreas is innervated by both sympathetic and parasympathetic components of the autonomic nervous system. The principal, and possibly only, pathway for pancreatic pain involves nociceptive fibers arising in the pancreas. They pass through the celiac ganglia to form

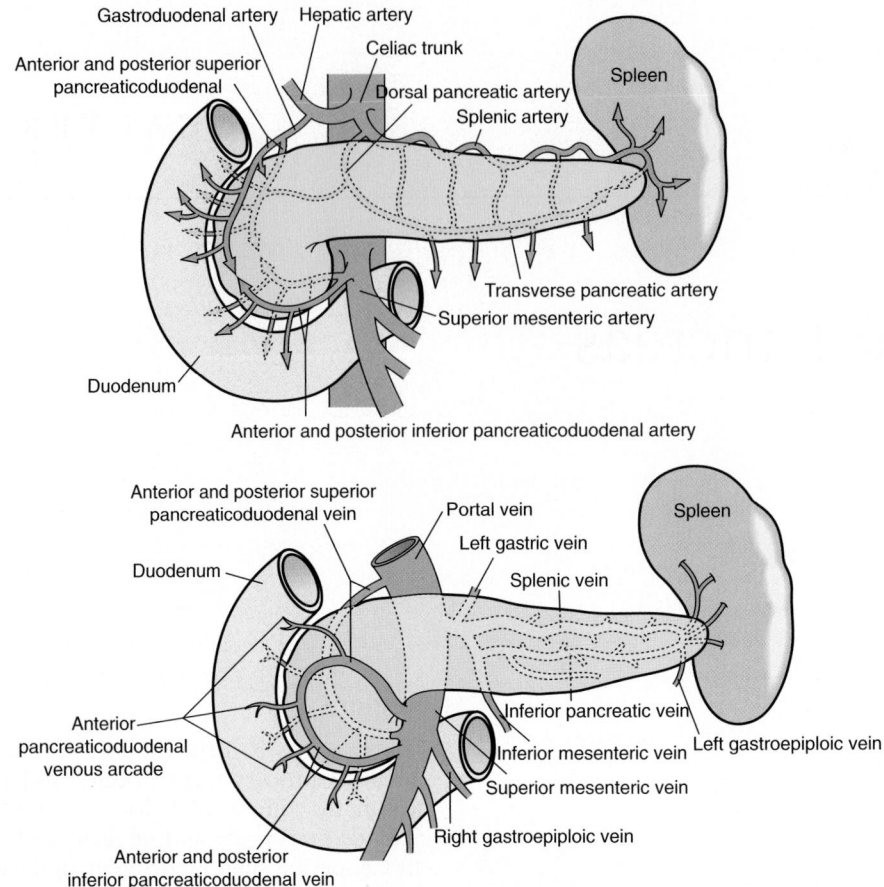

Figure 55-1 Arterial supply to the pancreas (*top*) and venous drainage of the pancreas (*bottom*). The pancreatic head is supplied by branches of the gastroduodenal and superior mesenteric arteries, whereas the body and tail are supplied by branches of the splenic artery. Venous drainage is to the splenic and superior mesenteric/portal veins. (From Skandalakis JE, Gray SW, Rowe JS Jr, et al: Anatomical complications of pancreatic surgery. Contemp Surg 15:17-50, 1979.)

the greater, lesser, and least splanchnic nerves that pass to cell bodies in the thoracic sympathetic chain. Efferent visceral motor supply to the pancreas is provided by both the sympathetic and parasympathetic systems. The latter involves preganglionic fibers arising from cell bodies in the vagal nuclei that travel through the posterior vagal trunk to the celiac plexus. Postganglionic fibers then innervate pancreatic islets, acini, ducts, and blood vessels. In general, the nerves of the pancreas travel with the blood vessels supplying the organ.

Ducts

The main pancreatic duct, or duct of Wirsung, arises in the tail of the pancreas and terminates at the papilla of Vater in the duodenum. It crosses the vertebral column between T12 and L2. Within the body and tail of the pancreas, the duct lies slightly cephalad to a line drawn midway between the superior and inferior edges. The duct is also more posterior than anterior. In adults, the duct within the head measures 3.1 to 4.8 mm in diameter and gradually tapers to measure 0.9 to 2.4 mm in the tail. With age, the duct diameter can increase. The duct of

Santorini (i.e., the minor, or accessory, pancreatic duct) is smaller than the main duct. It extends from the main duct to enter the duodenum at the lesser papilla. That papilla lies about 2 cm proximal and slightly anterior to the major papilla.

EMBRYOLOGY AND HISTOLOGY

Organogenesis

During the 4th week of gestation, two endodermal buds arise from the duodenum: the hepatic diverticulum, which is destined to form the liver, gallbladder, and bile ducts, and the dorsal pancreatic bud that forms the body and tail of the pancreas (Fig. 55-2). On the 32nd day of gestation, this hepatic diverticulum gives rise to a ventral pancreatic bud that eventually develops into the uncinate process and inferior part of the head of the pancreas. The dorsal pancreatic bud extends transversely across the abdomen, to lie anterior to the portal and mesenteric vessels. With time, as the duodenum rotates to form a C-loop configuration, the ventral pancreas and distal bile duct undergo

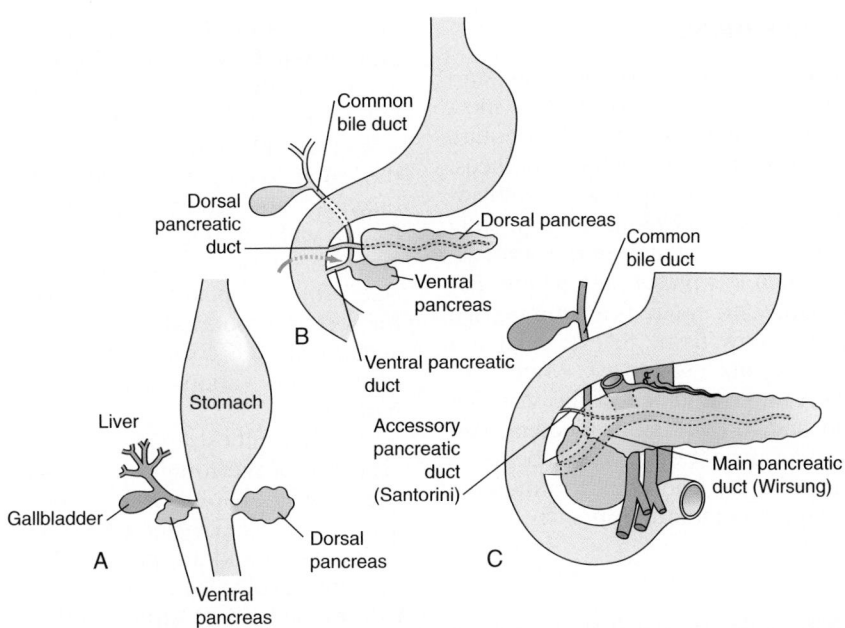

Figure 55-2 Organogenesis of the pancreas. **A,** Formation of dorsal and ventral pancreatic buds. **B,** Rotation of the ventral pancreas, distal bile duct, and major papilla. **C,** Fusion of the dorsal and ventral pancreata to form the adult pancreas. (From Skandalakis JE, Gray SW, Rowe JS Jr, et al: Anatomical complications of pancreatic surgery. Contemp Surg 15:17-50, 1979.)

clockwise rotation around the back of the duodenum to, finally, lie on the medial side of the duodenum, inferior and slightly posterior to the dorsal pancreas and posterior to the portal and mesenteric vessels. On the 37th day of gestation, the two pancreatic buds fuse, and in 90% of individuals, their duct systems also join.

Histology

The mature pancreas is an endocrine organ made up of the islets of Langerhans and an exocrine organ consisting of acinar and ductal cells. The acinar cells, so named because they are clustered like grapes on the stem of a vine, discharge their secretions into a centrally located acinar space that communicates with the main pancreatic duct. Most of the cells in the pancreas are acinar cells, and duct cells make up only 5% of pancreatic mass. Histologically, acinar cells have a high content of endoplasmic reticulum and an abundance of apically located eosinophilic zymogen granules. The cells lining the main pancreatic duct are tall columnar cells, and many contain mucin granules. With progression from the large ducts to the smaller intralobular and interlobular ducts, the lining cells become flatter, assuming a cuboidal configuration, and mucin granules are no longer seen. Centroacinar cells, located at the junction between ducts and acini, resemble acinar cells in size and shape but lack zymogen granules.

Cell Differentiation

The cells composing the pancreatic buds are homogeneous and indistinguishable from other endodermal cells of the primitive gut. These endodermal cells undergo stepwise differentiation, from an undifferentiated precursor into committed islet and exocrine cell precursors and then into either acinar cells or ductal cells. Some recently presented evidence has also suggested that transdifferentiation can occur, that is, that differentiated duct cells may give rise to islet or acinar cells.

CONGENITAL ANOMALIES

Pancreas Divisum

Failure of the dorsal and ventral pancreatic duct systems to join during embryogenesis (see Fig. 55-2) is referred to as *pancreas divisum*. It results in a pancreas with divided drainage because the dorsal pancreas drains, through the duct of Santorini, to empty at the lesser papilla, whereas the ventral pancreas, composed of the head and uncinate process, drains through Vater's papilla. Pancreas divisum has been noted in as many as 11% of autopsy cases. The significance of pancreas divisum remains controversial.[1] Some have suggested that it may contribute to the development of pancreatitis by establishing a condition of relative outflow obstruction because the major fraction of pancreatic exocrine secretion is obliged to exit through the relatively small orifice of the lesser papilla. On the other hand, the presence of pancreas divisum and the development of pancreatitis are, in most patients, not related to each other in a cause-and-effect manner, and the corollary of this may also be true; that is, attempts to widen the orifice of the dorsal duct at the lesser papilla in patients with pancreas divisum and pancreatitis are unlikely to be of benefit.

Ectopic and Accessory Pancreas

Pancreatic tissue at ectopic sites is not unusual, and most ectopic pancreatic tissue is functional. The most common sites are in the walls of the stomach, duodenum, or ileum; in Meckel's diverticulum; or at the umbilicus. Less common sites include the colon, appendix, gallbladder, omentum, and mesentery. Islet tissue is frequently present when ectopic pancreas is located in the stomach and duodenum but not when it is present elsewhere. For the most part, ectopic pancreatic tissue is a submucosal, irregular nodule of firm, yellow tissue that may have a central umbilication. Pancreatic secretions often exit through this umbilication into the lumen of the stomach or intestine. Ulceration and, on occasion, bleeding can be associated with these lesions. They may also be associated with obstruction or be the lead point for intussusception. Resection or bypass is indicated in such cases.

Annular Pancreas

Annular pancreas refers to the presence of a band of normal pancreatic tissue that partially or completely encircles the second portion of the duodenum and extends into the head of the pancreas. It usually contains a duct that joins the main pancreatic duct. The basis for annular pancreas is uncertain. It may result from failure of normal clockwise rotation of the ventral pancreas, or it may result from expansion of ectopic pancreatic tissue in the duodenal wall. It presents with varying degrees of duodenal obstruction that, in children, is often associated with other congenital anomalies. It may be totally asymptomatic or present later in life with obstructive symptoms if pancreatitis develops in the annular segment. Treatment usually involves bypass, through duodenojejunostomy, rather than resection.

Developmental Pancreatic Cysts

Solitary (congenital, duplication, or dermoid) cysts of the pancreas are rare. In contrast, multiple pancreatic cysts, lined with cuboidal epithelium, are more common. They are frequently associated with polycystic disease of the liver or kidney, and they can be seen in up to half of patients with von Hippel-Lindau disease. Pancreatic cysts only rarely become symptomatic, and in general, no treatment is indicated.

PHYSIOLOGY

About 2.5 liters of clear, colorless, bicarbonate-rich pancreatic juice, containing 6 to 20 g of protein, is secreted by the human pancreas each day. It plays a critical role in duodenal alkalinization and in food digestion.

Protein Secretion

With the possible exception of the lactating mammary gland, the exocrine pancreas synthesizes protein at a greater rate, per gram of tissue, than any other organ. More than 90% of that protein consists of digestive enzymes. Most of the digestive enzymes are synthesized and secreted by acinar cells as inactive proenzymes or zymogens that, in health, are activated only after they reach the duodenum where enterokinase activates trypsinogen and the trypsin catalyses the activation of the other zymogens. Some of the pancreatic digestive enzymes are synthesized and secreted in their active forms without the need for an activation step (e.g., amylase, lipase, ribonuclease). Acinar cells also synthesize proteins, including enzymes, that are not destined for secretion but, rather, are intended for use within the acinar cell itself. Examples of this latter group of proteins include the various structural proteins and lysosomal hydrolases.

Newly synthesized proteins are assembled within the cisternae of the rough endoplasmic reticulum and transported to the Golgi, where they are modified by glycosylation. Those destined for secretion pass through the Golgi stacks and are packaged within condensing vacuoles that evolve into zymogen granules as they migrate toward the luminal surface of the acinar cell. By a process involving membrane fusion and fission, the contents of the zymogen granules are then released into the acinar lumen.[2] Other proteins that are not destined for secretion are segregated away from the secretory pathway as they pass through the Golgi, and they are then targeted to their appropriate intracellular site.[3]

Secretion of protein from acinar cells is a regulated process. At rest, secretion occurs at a low or basal rate, but this rate can be markedly increased by secretory stimulation that, in the pancreas, is both hormonal and neural. Pancreatic acinar cells can express receptors for acetylcholine, cholecystokinin, secretin, and vasoactive intestinal peptide. Stimulation of secretion by either acetylcholine or cholecystokinin has been shown to involve activation of phospholipase C, generation of inositol triphosphate and diacyl glycerol, and a rise in intracellular ionized calcium levels that, by yet unidentified mechanisms, up-regulates the rate of secretory protein discharge at the apical cell membrane. In contrast, secretin and vasoactive intestinal peptide activate adenylate cyclase, increase cellular levels of cyclic adenosine monophosphate (AMP), and activate protein kinase A. This also leads to protein secretion at the apical pole. Recent studies indicate that human acinar cells may not possess receptors for cholecystokinin and that, in humans, cholecystokinin stimulation of secretion is mediated by intrapancreatic nerves that express cholecystokinin receptors.[4]

Electrolyte Secretion

Although stimulation of acinar cells results in the secretion of a small amount of serum-like fluid, most of the fluid and electrolytes secreted from the pancreas arise from duct cells[5] (Fig. 55-3). The earliest step in duct cell electrolyte secretion involves diffusion of circulating carbon dioxide into the duct cell, and that carbon dioxide is hydrated by carbonic anhydrase to yield carbonic acid. Subsequently, the carbonic acid dissociates into protons and bicarbonate ions. The protons diffuse out of the cell

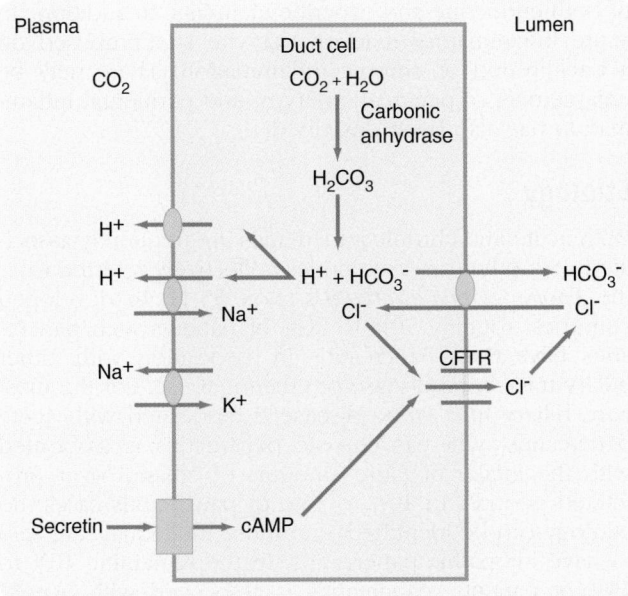

Figure 55-3 Secretion of bicarbonate-rich juice by duct cells. CO_2 diffuses into duct cells and is converted to H_2CO_3 by carbonic anhydrase. H_2CO_3 dissociates into HCO_3^- and H^+. The H^+ then exits at the basal side of the cell. Secretin stimulation increases cyclic adenosine monophosphate (cAMP), which accelerates apical chloride secretion through the cystic fibrosis transmembrane regulator (CFTR) chloride channel. The exchange of luminal Cl^- for cellular HCO_3^- results in net HCO_3^- secretion into the duct from the apex of the cell.

and are carried away in the circulation while the bicarbonate remains inside the cell. The fluid and electrolyte secretagogue secretin acts, through a cyclic AMP–mediated process, to stimulate chloride secretion, at the apical cell surface, through cystic fibrosis transmembrane regulator (chloride) channels. Then, through an apical chloride-bicarbonate exchanger, the actively secreted chloride is taken up again by the duct cell in exchange for bicarbonate. Taken together, the result of these events is the secretion of a bicarbonate-rich fluid into the duct and the discharge, into the circulation, of protons (see Fig. 55-3). In the absence of secretin stimulation, pancreatic juice has a more plasma-like composition because it is composed primarily of acinar cell secretions and there is little duct cell secretion of chloride to permit exchange with bicarbonate. With secretin stimulation, chloride secretion is increased, flow rates rise, and chloride-bicarbonate exchange results in juice that is rich in bicarbonate and poor in chloride.

Integrated Physiology

During the resting (interdigestive) phase of gastrointestinal function, pancreatic secretion is minimal and may be as low as 2% of that noted with maximal stimulation. The pancreatic response to a meal is a three-phase process that includes a cephalic phase, a gastric phase, and an intestinal phase. The cephalic phase, accounting for 10% to 15% of meal-stimulated pancreatic secretion, reflects the response to the sight, smell, or taste of food. It is believed to be almost exclusively mediated by peripherally released acetylcholine, which directly stimulates pancreatic secretion of enzymes and gastric secretion of acid. The acid indirectly stimulates pancreatic secretion of fluid and electrolytes by causing duodenal acidification and secretin release. The gastric phase of pancreatic secretion, accounting for 10% to 15% of meal-stimulated pancreatic secretion, reflects the response to gastric distention and the entry of food into the stomach. These events can cause release of gastrin and stimulate vagal afferents. By binding to cholecystokinin receptors, gastrin is itself a weak stimulant of pancreatic enzyme secretion. Vagal stimulation also increases enzyme secretion.

More important, however, gastrin and vagal stimulation cause gastric acid secretion, and this leads to duodenal acidification, release of secretin from the duodenum, and pancreatic secretion of fluid and electrolytes. The intestinal phase of pancreatic secretion reflects the response to food and gastric secretions entering the proximal intestine. Acidification of the duodenum and the presence of bile in the duodenum promote secretin release. In addition, in the duodenum and proximal small intestine, the presence of fat and protein, as well as their partial breakdown products, stimulates the release of cholecystokinin, and this cholecystokinin stimulates enzyme secretion from acinar cells. The intestinal phase of pancreatic secretion accounts for 70% to 75% of meal-stimulated pancreatic secretion.

Feedback Loop

Luminal proteins, referred to as *releasing factors,* have been described that can also stimulate cholecystokinin and secretin release. The most well characterized are the releasing factors for cholecystokinin.[6] Two forms are known, one apparently synthesized by duodenal cells (*cholecystokinin-releasing factor*) and the other secreted by the pancreas (*monitor peptide*). Both forms are subject to degradation by trypsin. Thus, with high-protein meals that quench intraduodenal tryptic activity, the releasing factor remains intact, cholecystokinin release is increased, and pancreatic secretion is stimulated.

In contrast, when food is absent from the duodenum, the proteolytic activity that remains unquenched within the lumen degrades the releasing factor and, as a result, cholecystokinin release and pancreatic secretion are reduced. Some have argued that this feedback loop may, at least in part, explain the pain of chronic pancreatitis because, with pancreatic insufficiency, intraluminal proteolytic activity would be low and cholecystokinin release would increase. Based on this concept, some have advocated administration of exogenous pancreatic enzymes as a treatment for the chronic pain of pancreatitis. Presumably, administration of exogenous enzymes to such patients would result in degradation of the releasing factor and reduce pancreatic stimulation. However, evidence supporting a physiologic role for these releasing factors comes almost exclusively from experiments using rodents, and the actual existence of a physiologic feedback loop in humans has not been established.

Box 55-1 Etiologies of Pancreatitis

Acute Pancreatitis

Abuse of ethanol
Biliary tract stones
Drugs
Endoscopic retrograde cholangiopancreatography
Hypercalcemia
Hyperlipidemia
Idiopathic
Infections
Ischemia
Parasites
Postoperative
Scorpion sting
Trauma

Chronic Pancreatitis

Autoimmune
Duct obstruction
Ethanol abuse
Hereditary
Hypercalcemia
Hyperlipidemia
Idiopathic

PANCREATITIS

Definition and Classification

Pancreatitis can be classified as either *acute* or *chronic* based on its clinical characteristics, pathologic changes, and natural history. Clinically, acute pancreatitis is usually characterized by the acute onset of symptoms in a previously healthy individual and the disappearance of those symptoms as the attack resolves. In contrast, patients with chronic pancreatitis may have had prior attacks or symptoms of either exocrine or endocrine insufficiency before the current attack, and their symptoms may persist even after resolution of the current attack. From a clinical standpoint, however, attacks of *either* acute or chronic pancreatitis can be characterized by the abrupt onset of symptoms that are often similar. Thus, without the test of time or a tissue sample, it may be difficult or impossible to determine whether a first attack is one of acute or chronic pancreatitis.

Pathology

The pathologic changes of acute pancreatitis include parenchymal and peripancreatic fat necrosis and an associated inflammatory reaction. The extent of these changes is directly related to the severity of an attack. In mild pancreatitis, changes frequently include interstitial edema and infiltration of inflammatory cells with relatively little necrosis, whereas in severe pancreatitis, extensive necrosis, thrombosis of intrapancreatic vessels, vascular disruption, and intraparenchymal hemorrhage can be seen. With infection, intrapancreatic or peripancreatic abscesses involving areas of necrosis can also develop. The major changes of chronic pancreatitis include fibrosis and loss

of both endocrine and exocrine elements. In addition, an acute inflammatory reaction may be superimposed on a background of chronic inflammation. There may be enlargement of pancreatic nerves, and perineural inflammation has also been described.

Etiology

Both acute and chronic pancreatitis are frequently associated with other disease entities collectively referred to as the *etiologies of pancreatitis* (Box 55-1). In developed countries, roughly 70% to 80% of patients with pancreatitis have their pancreatitis in association with either biliary tract stone disease or ethanol abuse. For the most part, biliary tract stone disease is associated with acute pancreatitis, whereas chronic pancreatitis is associated with the intake of large amounts of ethanol over protracted periods. In 10% to 15% of pancreatitis cases, no etiology can be identified, and those individuals are said to have idiopathic pancreatitis. In the remaining 10% to 15% of patients, pancreatitis is associated with one of many possible miscellaneous etiologies. In underdeveloped countries, particularly in Africa and Southeast Asia, pancreatitis is frequently termed either *tropical* or *nutritional*. Recent reports indicate that many patients with tropical pancreatitis have a form of hereditary pancreatitis caused by mutations of the genes that code for pancreatic secretory trypsin inhibitors. Affected individuals often complain of painful attacks, and they frequently develop pancreatic calcifications as well as diabetes. Ketoacidosis is uncommon.

Biliary Tract Stones

The onset of acute pancreatitis is frequently associated with the passage of biliary tract stones through the terminal biliopancreatic duct into the duodenum. Stones can be retrieved from the stools of roughly 90% of patients with stone-induced pancreatitis. There has been much speculation regarding the mechanisms by which such stones might cause pancreatitis. In 1901, Opie, a pathologist at Johns Hopkins University, noted a stone lodged in the terminal biliopancreatic duct of a patient who had died of severe pancreatitis. He suggested that the stone might have caused outflow obstruction from a *common biliopancreatic channel,* allowing bile to reflux into the pancreatic duct.[7] In a second publication based on observations made at another autopsy, Opie suggested that biliary pancreatitis could also occur when a stone, or the edema and inflammation caused by its passage, caused outflow obstruction of the pancreatic duct even in the absence of bile reflux. Although the bile reflux theory, often referred to as the *common channel theory,* was originally favored, subsequent studies have cast doubt on its validity, and most observers now believe that it is stone-induced pancreatic duct obstruction and ductal hypertension, rather than bile reflux, that triggers acute pancreatitis. Recent data derived from experiments using a model of pancreatitis induced in opossums also support the duct obstruction theory. Those experiments indicate that pancreatic duct obstruction, without bile duct obstruction or bile reflux, can cause pancreatitis and that the severity of pancreatitis is not worsened by bile reflux into the pancreatic duct.[8]

Abuse of Ethanol

The most frequent cause of morphologically defined chronic pancreatitis is ethanol abuse, but occasionally ethanol can also induce acute pancreatitis. There is no threshold rate of consumption below which ethanol consumption is not associated with an increased incidence of pancreatitis. The mean ethanol consumption among patients with ethanol-induced pancreatitis is 150 to 175 g/day. The mean duration of ethanol abuse for men is 18 ± 11 years and, for women, 11 ± 8 years. Ethanol-induced pancreatitis, like ethanol abuse itself, is more common in men than in women. Dietary factors, such as consumption of a high-protein diet with either high-fat or low-fat content, may contribute to the development of pancreatitis. Most observers currently believe that the chronic pancreatitis that follows prolonged ethanol abuse reflects repeated, but subclinical, episodes of acute pancreatic injury. These repeated episodes of pancreatic injury with necrosis eventually lead to the fibrosis that characterizes chronic pancreatitis.[9]

Many theories have been advanced to explain the mechanism by which ethanol might cause pancreatic injury. According to one theory, ethanol consumption causes hypertriglyceridemia and the generation of fatty acids as well as their ethyl ester metabolites that can injure the pancreas. Another theory suggests that ethanol ingestion causes intrapancreatic generation of oxygen-derived free radicals that can injure the pancreas. Others believe that ethanol acts directly on pancreatic acinar cells to cause injury or that it promotes secretion of pancreatic juice that is high in proteolytic enzyme content but low in enzyme inhibitor content. Theoretically, enzyme activation could occur under these conditions, and that activation could cause pancreatic injury. Secretion of an enzyme-rich fluid deficient in enzyme inhibitors could also lead to protein precipitation and the formation of intraductal plugs. Those plugs, by causing duct obstruction and ductal hypertension, could subsequently trigger pancreatic injury. Ethanol ingestion has also been reported to cause sphincter of Oddi spasm, and this could also contribute to ethanol-induced pancreatitis if it resulted in ductal hypertension. Each of these various theories has attractive features and its own proponents, but, at present, the actual mechanisms by which ethanol causes pancreatitis remain unclear.

Drugs

Exposure to certain drugs is, perhaps, the third most frequent cause of pancreatitis (Box 55-2), but the mechanisms by which those drugs cause pancreatitis is not known. Although many different drugs have been implicated, the strength of the data supporting a cause-and-effect relationship in pancreatitis varies considerably. Drugs associated with pancreatitis can be divided into the following three groups:

1. Those considered to be definite causes of pancreatitis because their use has been associated with the onset

---

Box 55-2 Drugs Associated With Pancreatitis

Definite Cause

5-Aminosalicylate
6-Mercaptopurine
Azathioprine
Cytosine arabinoside
Dideoxyinosine
Diuretics
Estrogens
Furosemide
Metronidazole
Pentamidine
Tetracycline
Thiazide
Trimethoprim-sulfamethoxazole
Valproic acid

Probable Cause

Acetaminophen
α-Methyl-DOPA
Isoniazid
L-Asparaginase
Phenformin
Procainamide
Sulindac

DOPA, dihydroxyphenylalanine

---

of pancreatitis and the disease has recurred when patients have been rechallenged with the drug
2. Those considered to be probable causes of pancreatitis because the incidence of disease is increased in individuals exposed to the drug
3. Those whose relationship to pancreatitis is just suspected because only anecdotal evidence has been presented to support such a relationship

In the past, there have been claims that steroids as well as histamine-2 (H_2) antagonists can cause pancreatitis, but there is little evidence to support those claims.

Obstruction

Even in the absence of biliary tract stones, pancreatic duct obstruction can cause pancreatitis. Thus, pancreatitis has been associated with duodenal lesions such as duodenal ulcers, duodenal Crohn's disease, and periampullary tumors. It can also be triggered by a periampullary diverticulum, particularly if that diverticulum is filled with debris or food particles. Pancreatitis can also be the result of a pancreatic duct stricture or disruption following blunt pancreatic trauma or duct obstruction caused by a pancreatic tumor. Most patients with obstruction-induced pancreatitis have chronic, rather than acute, pancreatitis. This type of chronic pancreatitis affects only the obstructed portion of the pancreas, and it can be cured by removing that part of the pancreas. Post-traumatic strictures, the result of blunt abdominal trauma, can cause pancreatitis. They usually occur where the pancreas passes over the vertebral column. Parasites such as *Ascaris* and *Clonorchis* species can also cause pancreatitis by obstructing the pancreatic duct. Pancreas divisum has also been described as a cause of obstructive pancreatitis. Presumably, that pancreatitis results from the relative obstruction that might occur at the lesser papilla when the major fraction of pancreatic secretion is forced to exit through that orifice. Most observers believe that pancreas divisum, which occurs in roughly 10% of individuals, is rarely the cause of pancreatitis.

Hereditary and Autoimmune Pancreatitis

There has been considerable recent interest in the few patients who develop pancreatitis on a hereditary basis. It is generally believed that spontaneous trypsinogen activation normally occurs to a slight degree within the pancreas but that, in health, the pancreas is protected from injury by the presence of trypsin inhibitors. In hereditary pancreatitis, genetic mutations are believed to cause this protective process to fail either because a trypsin that is resistant to inhibition is synthesized or because the trypsin inhibitors themselves are defective. In either case, the end result could be expected to be further intrapancreatic activation of trypsin and, possibly, other digestive enzymes, eventually leading to repeated episodes of pancreatitis. In hereditary pancreatitis, those attacks begin at a young age and lead to chronic changes, including fibrosis, calcifications, and loss of both exocrine and endocrine function. The incidence of pancreatic cancer is also markedly increased in patients with hereditary pancreatitis. Hereditary pancreatitis is an autosomal dominant disease with incomplete penetrance. Pancreatic cancer most frequently develops in those with a paternal pattern of inheritance.[10]

Pancreatitis can be the result of an autoimmune process, and, in those patients, it is frequently associated with other autoimmune diseases such as primary sclerosing cholangitis, Sjögren's syndrome, and primary biliary cirrhosis. Recently, a distinct form of autoimmune pancreatitis has been described in which there is a severe, sclerosing process characterized by intense lymphocyte and plasmacyte infiltration. It is frequently associated with bile as well as pancreatic duct strictures, pancreatic inflammation, and a pancreatic mass. Some refer to the disease as *lymphoplasmacytic autoimmune pancreatitis*. Most patients with this form of pancreatitis have elevated circulating immunoglobulin G (IgG) levels, and that elevation is mostly due to an elevation in the levels of IgG_4.[11] Perhaps the most important feature of this form of autoimmune pancreatitis is the fact that it frequently presents as an otherwise unexplained mass in the head of the pancreas and the sclerotic process can result in bile as well as pancreatic duct strictures (i.e., a so-called double-duct sign). Thus, it can easily be confused with pancreatic cancer. If correctly diagnosed, the mass as well as the strictures can completely resolve with steroid treatment.

Other Miscellaneous Causes of Pancreatitis

Pancreatitis can result from pancreatic trauma even without major duct disruption or stricture. In those cases, the inflammatory process is usually related to contusion or laceration of the gland and possibly disruption of small ducts. Pancreatitis can occur during the postoperative period in patients undergoing procedures on or near the pancreas or procedures associated with either hypoperfusion or atheroembolism (cardiopulmonary bypass, cardiac transplantation, renal transplantation). The injection of the pancreatic duct that occurs during endoscopic retrograde pancreatography or during sphincter of Oddi manometry can also cause pancreatitis. Both acute and chronic pancreatitis can be caused by metabolic abnormalities, especially those leading to hypercalcemia (i.e., hyperparathyroidism) and those leading to hyperlipidemia (type I, IV, or V hyperlipoproteinemias).

Hypercalcemia may result in pancreatitis by facilitating intrapancreatic digestive enzyme activation. Hyperlipidemia may lead to pancreatitis if the accompanying hyperchylomicronemia interferes with the pancreatic microcirculation or results in release of free fatty acids in the pancreatic microcirculation. Both hypercalcemia-induced pancreatitis and hyperlipidemia-induced pancreatitis can be prevented if the underlying metabolic abnormality is corrected by either parathyroidectomy or drug and dietary management of the hyperlipidemia. In places such as Trinidad, scorpion stings are a frequent cause of pancreatitis. Scorpion toxin contains a potent pancreatic secretagogue, and presumably, the excessive pancreatic stimulation that follows exposure to this toxin leads to pancreatic injury.

Idiopathic Pancreatitis

In most series, roughly 20% of patients have pancreatitis without an identifiable etiology. Some of those individuals have gallbladder sludge or microcrystals, and further attacks can be prevented by either cholecystectomy or biliary sphincterotomy. Other patients have been found to have sphincter of Oddi malfunction, sometimes associated with increased pressures in the pancreatic duct system, and they can be effectively treated by sphincterotomy with pancreatic septotomy. Therefore, these patients have forms of biliary pancreatitis rather than truly idiopathic pancreatitis. There remains, however, a significant group of patients with no identifiable cause for their pancreatitis. Recent studies by several independent groups have suggested that some of these patients may have subclinical mutations of the cystic fibrosis gene. In its most severe form, cystic fibrosis can cause pancreatic fibrosis and the loss of both exocrine and endocrine function as a result of the blockade of ducts with inspissated secretions. However, the patients with idiopathic pancreatitis related to cystic fibrosis have subclinical mutations of the cystic fibrosis transmembrane regulator gene. They do not have inspissated secretion, and their pancreatitis probably develops on another basis.

Pathophysiology of Acute and Chronic Pancreatitis

It is generally believed that acute pancreatitis is triggered by obstruction of the pancreatic duct and that the injury begins within pancreatic acinar cells. That injury is believed to include, and possibly be the result of, intra-acinar cell activation of digestive enzyme zymogens, including trypsinogen. Chronic pancreatitis is believed to reflect repeated episodes of subclinical acute pancreatitis with unrecognized pancreatic necrosis evolving into pancreatic fibrosis.

One of the central issues in our understanding of the cellular events leading to acute pancreatitis is how duct obstruction could result in intra-acinar cell enzyme activation. Perhaps one of the most widely accepted theories to explain this coupling is the so-called colocalization hypothesis.[12] This hypothesis is based on a number of studies that have used experimental models of pancreatitis induced in laboratory animals. In those studies, one of the earliest changes noted has been the colocalization of digestive enzyme zymogens such as trypsinogen with lysosomal hydrolases such as cathepsin B inside cytoplasmic vacuoles. Under these conditions, cathepsin B can activate trypsinogen, and trypsin can activate the other zymogens. According to the colocalization hypothesis, cathepsin B–mediated intra-acinar cell activation of the digestive enzymes leads to acinar cell injury and triggers an intrapancreatic inflammatory response. The intensity of that inflammatory response appears to regulate the severity of the pancreatitis and to couple pancreatitis to extrapancreatic events such as lung and renal injury.

Presentation of an Acute Attack

The clinical presentation, diagnosis, and management of an acute attack of pancreatitis are similar regardless of whether that attack is *acute* or *chronic* pancreatitis. In fact, many describe patients with chronic pancreatitis who present with acute symptoms as having *acute on chronic* pancreatitis. On the other hand, the long-term management of patients with acute and chronic pancreatitis may differ considerably. The former primarily involves elimination of the inciting cause, whereas for chronic pancreatitis, irreversible changes have usually occurred before diagnosis, and long-term management primarily involves treatment of pain and pancreatic exocrine and endocrine insufficiency. For these reasons, this discussion of clinical presentation focuses on issues relevant to an acute attack and does not make distinctions based on whether that is an attack of acute or chronic pancreatitis.

Symptoms

Abdominal pain, nausea, and vomiting are the dominant symptoms of pancreatitis. Typically, the pain is located in the epigastrium, but it may also involve both upper quadrants, the lower abdomen, or the lower chest. It may have a pleuritic component and be felt in one or both shoulders. Most patients describe the pain as being knifelike and radiating straight through to the mid-central back. It is usually abrupt in onset and slowly increases in magnitude to reach a maximal level. The pain is usually constant, although it may be somewhat relieved by leaning forward or lying on the side with the knees drawn upward. Patients with chronic pancreatitis frequently describe similar prior attacks that are often noted

to occur within 12 to 24 hours of ethanol consumption. The nausea and vomiting of pancreatitis usually persists even after the stomach has been emptied. The vomiting may lead to gastroesophageal tears (i.e., Mallory-Weiss syndrome) and upper gastrointestinal bleeding. Although vomiting and retching may be relieved by passage of a nasogastric tube, the pain usually persists even after gastric decompression. Some patients, especially those with postoperative pancreatitis who are already receiving analgesic medications, may not experience abdominal pain, and therefore, the diagnosis of pancreatitis may be particularly difficult.

Physical Findings

Pancreatitis patients are frequently noted to be rolling or moving around in search of a more comfortable position and, in this sense, they are unlike patients with a perforated viscus who often remain motionless because movement worsens their pain. Patients with severe pancreatitis usually appear ill and anxious. Hyperthermia is common and may be explained by the release of proinflammatory factors, including cytokines and chemokines, from the injured pancreas. Tachycardia, tachypnea, and hypotension caused by hypovolemia are common. Hypovolemia can also result in collapsed neck veins, dry skin, dry mucous membranes, and diminished subcutaneous elasticity. Because pleuritic and abdominal pain may make breathing difficult, breath sounds in the lower lung fields are usually diminished, and atelectasis may be present.

A pleural effusion can often be detected on either side, although it is more commonly found on the left. Patients with severe pancreatitis frequently develop an acute lung injury that can clinically present as the adult respiratory distress syndrome (ARDS). Occasionally, patients with pancreatitis have alterations in their mental status as a result of drug or ethanol exposure, hypotension, hypoxemia, or release of circulating toxic agents from the inflamed pancreas. Some degree of jaundice is common. In gallstone-induced acute pancreatitis, the jaundice may reflect distal bile duct obstruction, but jaundice can also occur in nonbiliary pancreatitis either as a result of duct obstruction caused by the inflamed pancreas or as a result of cholestasis induced by the severe illness itself. As a result of ileus, bowel sounds are usually diminished during an attack of pancreatitis, and the abdomen may become distended and tympanitic. Direct, percussion, and rebound abdominal tenderness, as well as both voluntary and involuntary guarding, are common. These findings may be localized to the epigastrium, or they may be diffusely present throughout the abdomen. An epigastric mass, reflecting the inflamed pancreas and surrounding tissues, may be felt in the upper abdomen or left upper quadrant. On rare occasions, flank ecchymoses (Grey Turner's sign) or periumbilical ecchymoses (Cullen's sign), which result from retroperitoneal hemorrhage, can be seen during severe pancreatitis. Occasionally, patients develop areas of tender subcutaneous induration and erythema that resemble erythema nodosum but that, in the case of pancreatitis, are caused by subcutaneous fat necrosis.

Diagnosis

Routine Blood Tests

Pancreatitis can induce a diffuse capillary leak syndrome that, when combined with vomiting, can result in significant fluid losses. The resulting hypovolemia can be marked. It usually leads to an increased hematocrit, hemoglobin, blood urea nitrogen, and creatinine. Serum albumin levels may be markedly depressed, particularly if fluid losses are corrected by administration of albumin-free crystalloid solutions. The serum electrolytes may be normal, but with significant vomiting, a hypochloremic metabolic alkalosis can develop. The white blood cell count is usually elevated with an associated left shift in the differential count. Blood glucose may be elevated either due to associated diabetes mellitus or as a result of increased glucagon and catecholamine release combined with diminished insulin release.

Hyperbilirubinemia is relatively common during the early stages of pancreatitis. It can be caused by either a biliary tract stone or by the inflamed (and possibly fibrotic) pancreas causing bile duct obstruction, and in this setting, cholangitis with positive blood cultures can be superimposed on the pancreatitis. On the other hand, the hyperbilirubinemia of pancreatitis can also reflect the nonobstructive cholestasis that often accompanies any severe illness. Hypertriglyceridemia is routinely noted in patients who have hyperlipidemia-induced pancreatitis. Hypertriglyceridemia can also be induced by exposure to ethanol, and therefore, the diagnosis of pancreatitis is always suspected when lactescent serum is found when evaluating an alcoholic patient with abdominal pain. Many patients with pancreatitis appear to have hypocalcemia, but for the most part, that hypocalcemia can be explained by the hypoalbuminemia that accompanies pancreatitis. Occasionally, however, patients with severe pancreatitis have a reduction in their free, ionized calcium that is not a reflection of hypoalbuminemia. This type of hypocalcemia is associated with a poor prognosis. Some of these patients manifest tetany and carpopedal spasm, making treatment with calcium mandatory. The mechanisms responsible for this type of pancreatitis-associated hypocalcemia are not clear. Most likely, it occurs because bone calcium stores do not respond to circulating parathormone. Patients with severe pancreatitis can also develop disseminated intravascular coagulation. In those cases, thrombocytopenia, elevated levels of fibrin degradation products, a decreased fibrinogen level, prolonged partial thromboplastin time, and a prolonged prothrombin time can be observed.

Amylase Measurement

Serum amylase activity is usually, but not always, elevated during pancreatitis, but the magnitude of that elevation does not parallel the severity of the attack. In fact, as many as 10% of patients with lethal pancreatitis may have near-normal or normal amylase levels. This could reflect the fact that pancreatitis-associated hyperamylasemia can be transient. Typically, amylase levels rise 2 to 12 hours after the onset of symptoms and then decline, so that 3 to 6 days after the onset of an attack, the serum amylase levels are usually normal. Elevations that persist beyond a week suggest either ongoing inflammation or the development of a complication such as pseudocyst, abscess, or pancreatic ascites. Urinary amylase levels remain elevated longer than serum amylase levels; thus, measurement of urinary amylase levels may be of diagnostic help in patients who present long after the onset of symptoms. Although amylase can enter the circulation from nonpancreatic sites, including the salivary glands, lung, prostate, and ovary, it is pancreatic amylase that accounts for the rise in circulating amylase activity during pancreatitis.

The mechanisms responsible for the hyperamylasemia of pancreatitis are not clear. Some have suggested that, during pancreatitis, amylase and other digestive enzymes may be secreted from the basolateral, as opposed to the apical, surface of acinar cells, and in this manner, they could gain access to the lymphatic and vascular system. On the other hand, some recent studies have indicated that cell-to-cell contacts are loosened during pancreatitis. This could allow enzymes in the duct to reach periacinar, lymphatic, and intravascular spaces.

The overall sensitivity and specificity of serum amylase determination in the diagnosis of pancreatitis depend on both the clinical presentation and the cutoff value chosen for the upper limit of normal. In some series, sensitivity and specificity values in the low-to-mid 90% range have been reported. Hyperamylasemia can be associated with acute cholecystitis, perforated viscus, bowel obstruction, and bowel infarction. These states can also be clinically confused with pancreatitis because they are also characterized by abdominal pain, nausea, vomiting, and abdominal tenderness. In most cases, patients with hyperamylasemia that is not due to pancreatitis have only mild elevations in the circulating amylase level (i.e., twofold to threefold elevations from the normal value), whereas those with pancreatitis usually have greater elevations. At one time, measurement of the clearance ratio between amylase and creatinine was advocated as a method by which pancreatitis-associated hyperamylasemia could be distinguished from non–pancreatitis-associated elevations of amylase activity. It was claimed that an elevated clearance rate was diagnostic of pancreatitis. Unfortunately, the so-called amylase-to-creatinine clearance ratio has not proved clinically useful because changes in this ratio are not specific to pancreatitis and elevated clearance ratios can be seen in other diseases.

Occasionally, serum amylase activity may be normal, even during the early stages of an attack. The basis for this phenomenon is not certain. In some cases, it may reflect overwhelming necrosis of the gland. Some patients with acute pancreatitis superimposed on advanced chronic pancreatitis do not develop hyperamylasemia because there is little residual and functional pancreatic exocrine tissue and, therefore, little pancreatic amylase to be released into the circulation. In some patients with hyperlipidemia-induced pancreatitis, hyperamylasemia may be masked by circulating amylase inhibitors. This is particularly true of patients with lactescent serum, in whom the circulating amylase activity may appear to be normal.

Macroamylasemia is a form of pancreatitis-independent hyperamylasemia that affects 0.5% of individuals. It occurs when amylase binds to an abnormal circulating albumin-like protein. Because of its large size, this protein prevents the normal clearance of amylase, and as a result, circulating levels of amylase rise. In some patients, episodes of abdominal pain can also occur, raising the suspicion that they have pancreatitis. In this situation, macroamylasemia can be distinguished from the hyperamylasemia of pancreatitis by simple measurement of urinary amylase activity. In the former, urinary amylase levels are very low.

Other Blood Tests

In addition to amylase, other enzymes and inflammatory mediators are released into the circulation during pancreatitis, and many have been the target of diagnostic or prognostic tests. Circulating lipase levels usually increase during pancreatitis. That increase usually parallels the rise in amylase activity, but the elevations of lipase activity may persist even after amylase activity has returned to normal. Thus, serum lipase measurement may be particularly helpful when patients are first seen several days after the onset of symptoms. Circulating levels of other pancreatic enzymes, including trypsinogen, phospholipase, elastase, and chymotrypsinogen, increase during pancreatitis, but measurement of these circulating enzymes is usually not performed because they add little to the information gained by the easier and more straightforward measurement of amylase activity. The activation peptides released during either trypsinogen, procarboxypeptidase, or prophospholipase activation are increased in the urine of patients with acute pancreatitis, and several studies have indicated that measurement of those activation peptides may aid in predicting the severity of an attack. Although methemalbumin levels sometimes rise during attacks of severe pancreatitis, and methemalbuminemia is indicative of a poor prognosis, methemalbumin levels are usually not measured. Circulating levels of several inflammatory mediators and acute phase reactants (e.g., interleukin [IL]-1, IL-6, tumor necrosis factor-α, and C-reactive protein) also increase during pancreatitis, and the magnitude of those increases can be used to predict the severity of an attack.

Imaging Studies

In general, the plain chest and abdominal radiographs are not particularly helpful in the diagnosis of pancreatitis, although they may be useful in patient management by revealing other causes for the patient's symptoms (e.g., pneumonia, perforated hollow viscus, mechanical bowel obstruction). In patients with pancreatitis, radiographs of the chest frequently reveal basal atelectasis and elevation of the diaphragm caused by splinting of respiration. Pleural effusions, most common on the left, can also be seen. Plain abdominal films usually show the gas pattern of a paralytic ileus, but occasionally, retroperitoneal gas bubbles indicating infection with gas-forming organisms can be seen. Pancreatic calcifications that are pathognomonic of chronic pancreatitis and are caused by the formation of calcified intraductal protein plugs may be seen on the routine abdominal films. Transcutaneous ultrasound may be useful in demonstrating the presence of gallbladder stones or dilated bile ducts, but ultrasound examination has limited value because of the presence of intestinal gas in the upper abdomen.

Computed tomography (CT) has been shown to be particularly helpful in the diagnosis and management of patients with pancreatitis. During the early stages of an attack, CT can image the upper abdomen and pancreas without being obscured by overlying or surrounding intestinal gas. When combined with bolus administration of intravenous (IV) contrast material, helical CT can detect the subtle changes of mild pancreatitis (i.e., pancreatic swelling and edema) as well as the changes of more severe pancreatitis (i.e., varying degrees of pancreatic necrosis and the presence of peripancreatic or intrapancreatic fluid collections). Both clinical and experimental studies have demonstrated the close parallel that exists between nonperfused pancreas seen on CT examination and necrosis seen on morphologic examination of the pancreas. At later times during the evolution of an attack, CT can be used to detect and follow pseudocysts and to permit fine-needle aspiration of areas suspected of harboring pancreatic infection. The timing of CT during an attack of pancreatitis is a matter of considerable controversy. One study, using an experimental model of pancreatitis in rodents, suggested that early CT with administration of IV contrast material could adversely affect the course of pancreatitis and worsen outcome,[13] but this conclusion has not been borne out by other studies,[14] and at present, it is generally believed that early performance of contrast-enhanced CT does not worsen pancreatitis. On the other hand, there may be little or no value in obtaining a CT scan in patients with obvious pancreatitis because early CT is unlikely to alter treatment. Early CT may be particularly helpful when the diagnosis of pancreatitis is in doubt. A normal pancreas imaged in a patient thought to have severe pancreatitis would prompt further diagnostic studies. Magnetic resonance imaging (MRI), which has the same sensitivity and specificity as CT in pancreatitis, has also been used in these patients. It provides information that is similar to that obtained by CT, but because of its ease of interpretation and ready availability, most clinicians prefer to use CT, rather than MRI, for the diagnosis and management of patients with pancreatitis.

Differential Diagnosis

The differential diagnosis of acute pancreatitis includes any process that can cause upper abdominal pain and tenderness, nausea, and vomiting (Box 55-3). Usually, but not always, the serum amylase or lipase levels are elevated in pancreatitis, but those enzymes can also be elevated in other conditions, including cholecystitis and cholangitis, perforated hollow viscus, bowel obstruction, and bowel infarction. In these patients, the CT does not suggest pancreatitis, and for the most part, enzyme elevations in these conditions are usually only twofold or threefold above normal. Occasionally, however, it may be difficult or even impossible to be certain that the patient actually has pancreatitis, and in these cases, a diagnostic exploratory laparotomy may be indicated.

Prognosis of an Acute Attack

The ultimate severity of an attack appears to be determined by events that occur within the first 24 to 48 hours. Most patients experience only a mild self-limited illness that can be expected to resolve with only supportive care, but about 10% of patients experience a severe attack. Severe attacks are more common in acute pancreatitis, but they can also occur when an acute attack is superimposed on chronic pancreatitis, that is, the so-called acute on chronic pancreatitis. Severe attacks are also more common in patients older than 60 years of age; those experiencing a first attack; those with postoperative pancreatitis; and those with methemalbuminemia, hypocalcemia, Grey Turner's sign, or Cullen's sign. The observation that the ultimate severity is determined by events that occur during the early stages of pancreatitis has prompted several groups of investigators to undertake studies designed to determine which clinical, chemical, or radiologic parameters might be used to identify those patients destined to experience a severe illness.

As a result, a number of prognostic schemes have been developed. Among the clinical scoring systems, the most widely used are those developed in New York by Ranson's group[15] (Table 55-1) and, in Glasgow, by Imrie's group.[16] Patients with fewer than three of the prognostic criteria can be expected to have a mild attack with little morbidity and a mortality rate of less than 1%. On the other hand, with the presence of more prognostic factors, increased morbidity and mortality can be expected, so that with three or four of Ranson's criteria, the mortality rate may reach 15%, and 50% of patients may need to be treated in an intensive care unit. Most patients with five or six signs will require intensive care, and with seven or eight of Ranson's signs, the mortality rate may reach 90%.

As an alternative to using clinical criteria, Balthazar and coworkers developed radiologic criteria for predicting a severe attack. In a prospective study employing contrast-enhanced CT examination,[17] they noted that the severity of an attack was related to the number of pancreatic fluid collections and the extent of pancreatic nonperfusion (i.e., necrosis) seen on CT examination. In addition to clinical and radiologic criteria, high levels of certain circulating factors can also be used to predict the evolution of a severe attack. Those factors include the following: C-reactive protein, phospholipase A_2, poly-

Table 55-1 Ranson's Prognostic Signs

ADMISSION	INITIAL 48 HOURS
Gallstone Pancreatitis	
Age > 70 yr	Hct fall >10
WBC >18,000/mm³	BUN elevation >2 mg/100 mL
Glucose > 220 mg/100 mL	Ca²⁺ <8 mg/100 mL
LDH >400 IU/L	Base deficit >5 mEq/L
AST >250 U/100 mL	Fluid sequestration >4 L
Nongallstone Pancreatitis	
Age >55 yr	Hct fall >10
WBC >16,000/mm³	BUN elevation >5 mg/100 mL
Glucose >200 mg/100 mL	Ca²⁺ <8 mg/100 mL
LDH >350 IU/L	PAO₂ <55 mm Hg
AST >250 U/100 mL	Base deficit >4 mEq/L
	Fluid sequestration >6 L

AST, aspartate transaminase; BUN, blood urea nitrogen; Ca²⁺, calcium; Hct, hematocrit; LDH, lactic dehydrogenase; PAO₂, arterial oxygen; WBC, white blood cell count.

Adapted from Ranson JHC, Rifkind KM, Roses DF, et al: Prognostic signs and the role of operative management in acute pancreatitis. Surg Gynecol Obstet 139:69-81, 1974; and Ranson JHC: Etiological and prognostic factors in human acute pancreatitis: A review. Am J Gastroenterol 77:633, 1982.

morphonuclear elastase, immunoreactive trypsin, IL-6, and pancreatitis-associated protein. High urinary levels of the activation peptides for trypsinogen, procarboxypeptidase, and prophospholipase also indicate a severe attack. The second version of the Acute Physiology and Chronic Health Evaluation (APACHE-II) scoring system has also been used to predict the severity of a pancreatitis attack. An APACHE-II score of 8 or more is generally indicative of a severe attack. The APACHE-II scoring system has the advantage of continually quantifying disease severity. Although the APACHE-II system can be used at the time of admission, recent studies have suggested that an admission score that worsens over the initial 48 hours of hospitalization despite aggressive treatment, or the score itself 48 hours after admission, may be particularly accurate in predicting the severity of the attack and a poor outcome.[18]

Although each of these scoring systems may predict the severity of an attack, there is also evidence that a good examination by an experienced clinician can accurately discriminate between mild and severe pancreatitis. Furthermore, none of the prognostic schemes are intended for use as a diagnostic tool in pancreatitis. Their ultimate value is in triaging patients to their appropriate care settings. In addition, they may be useful in clinical studies by permitting comparison of therapeutic outcomes for comparable patients stratified to different treatments.

Treatment of an Acute Attack

An acute attack of pancreatitis evolves in two, somewhat overlapping, phases. The initial phase, which lasts for 1 to 2 weeks, involves an acute inflammatory and autodigestive process that takes place within and around the pancreas. It may have systemic effects as well. In patients with severe pancreatitis, this initial phase of pancreatitis seamlessly evolves into a later phase that may last for weeks or months. This later phase of pancreatitis is primarily characterized by the development of local complications that are the result of necrosis, infection, and pancreatic duct rupture.

Initial Treatment

The initial management of patients with pancreatitis focuses on establishing the diagnosis, estimating its severity, addressing the major symptoms (i.e., pain, nausea, vomiting, and hypovolemia), and limiting its progression. Ideally, the diagnosis is established without exploratory surgery because exploration may increase the incidence of later pancreatic infection. On occasion, however, exploration may be required to establish the diagnosis with certainty, especially when the diagnosis is uncertain, and the patient has not responded favorably to aggressive nonoperative treatment. For the most part, patients with predicted severe pancreatitis are treated in an intensive care setting because it is in this group that fluid and respiratory management may be particularly challenging, and both morbidity and mortality are, essentially, confined to this group.

Management of Pain

The pain of pancreatitis may be severe and difficult to control. Most patients require narcotic medications. Meperidine and its analogues are probably preferable to morphine in this setting because morphine can induce spasm of the sphincter of Oddi, which could, at least theoretically, worsen biliary pancreatitis.

Fluid and Electrolyte Management

Aggressive fluid and electrolyte repletion is the most important element in the initial management of pancreatitis. Fluid losses can be enormous and can lead to marked hemoconcentration as well as hypovolemia. Inadequate fluid resuscitation during the early stages of pancreatitis can worsen the severity of an attack and lead to subsequent complications. The fluid depletion that occurs in pancreatitis results from the additive effects of losing fluid both externally and internally. The external fluid losses are caused by repeated episodes of vomiting and worsen by nausea that limits fluid intake. Repeated vomiting can result in a hypochloremic alkalosis. Internal fluid losses, which are usually even greater than the external losses, are caused by fluid sequestration into areas of inflammation (i.e., the peripancreatic retroperitoneum) and into the pulmonary parenchyma and soft tissues elsewhere in the body. These latter losses result from the diffuse capillary leak phenomenon that is triggered by proinflammatory factors released during pancreatitis. Total fluid losses may be so great that they lead to hypovolemia and hypoperfusion, and as a result, a metabolic acidosis can develop. Many of the patients with chronic pancreatitis are alcoholics who, even before the onset of pancreatitis, had hypoalbuminemia and hypomagnesemia. Those problems are exacerbated by the

losses of pancreatitis. The measured values for serum albumin may be even further depressed as fluid losses are treated with albumin-free crystalloid solutions. Although hypocalcemia is common particularly during a severe attack, the low total serum calcium is usually attributable to the low levels of circulating albumin, and no treatment is needed when ionized calcium is normal. Occasionally, however, ionized calcium levels may also be depressed, and tetany as well as carpopedal spasm can occur. Under those circumstances, aggressive calcium repletion is indicated.

During the first several days of a severe attack, circulating levels of many proinflammatory factors, including cytokines and chemokines, are elevated. This so-called cytokine storm, in many cases, triggers the systemic immune response syndrome, and as a result, the hemodynamic parameters of these patients may resemble those of sepsis associated with other disease states. Heart rate, cardiac output, and cardiac index usually rise, and total peripheral resistance falls. Hypoxemia can also occur as a result of the combined effects of increased intrapulmonary shunting and a pancreatitis-associated lung injury that closely resembles that seen in other forms of ARDS. Fluid management, although critical, may be particularly difficult when hypovolemia is combined with the respiratory failure of ARDS.

Treatment requires meticulous replacement of fluid and electrolyte losses. A fluid balance flow sheet is helpful, but parameters such as pulse rate, blood pressure, oxygen saturation, and urine output are notoriously unreliable for determining fluid needs in this setting. The hematocrit, however, can be quite useful because increased levels usually are accurate indicators of the magnitude of extracellular fluid loss. However, in a setting of blood loss or hemolysis, hematocrit measurements may lose their value in fluid management. Measurement of central filling pressures, using a Swan-Ganz or central venous pressure catheter, can be helpful in guiding fluid management, particularly when hypovolemia is combined with lung injury.

Role of Nasogastric Decompression

The nausea and vomiting of pancreatitis can result in significant fluid as well as electrolyte losses. Furthermore, retching can lead to gastroesophageal mucosal tears and result in upper gastrointestinal bleeding (i.e., the Mallory-Weiss syndrome). To increase patient comfort, nasogastric decompression may be needed, although the institution of nasogastric drainage has not been shown to alter the eventual outcome of an attack.

Role of Prophylactic Antibiotics

Several prospective and randomized trials have shown that prophylactic antibiotics can favorably affect the course of severe pancreatitis,[19-21] although a recent double-blind study detected no benefit with respect to the risk for developing infected pancreatic necrosis.[21] All the studies indicate that no benefit is observed when prophylactic antibiotics are given to patients with mild pancreatitis because patients with mild pancreatitis almost invariably recover quickly and without infectious complications. In patients with severe pancreatitis, benefit has been observed with regimens that included imipenem alone, imipenem with cilastatin, and cefuroxime. Selective gut decontamination with a combination of norfloxacin, colistin, and amphotericin has also been found to be beneficial, although that approach is labor intensive and not readily available. Although these recent studies argue strongly for administration of prophylactic antibiotics to patients with severe pancreatitis, there is an opposing view that is becoming increasingly widespread. According to that school of thought, administration of prophylactic antibiotics favors emergence of resistant organisms in the area of pancreatic injury. That may be particularly true for fungal strains such as *Candida*. Some have advocated adding antifungal agents such as fluconazole to the prophylactic antibiotic regimen, whereas others have argued that, because of the risk for infection with resistant organisms or fungi, antibiotics are not prophylactically used in the management of a severe attack.

Nutritional Support

Patients with severe pancreatitis may be unable to eat for prolonged periods and an alternative route for providing nutrition is required. Traditionally, these patients have been given parenteral nutrition administered through a central venous catheter. Widely differing opinions exist regarding the time that total parenteral nutrition should be started. Some advocate starting within the first day or two, whereas others delay starting total parenteral nutrition until the early phase of pancreatitis, characterized by extensive fluid shifts and high fluid requirements, has been completed. I favor the latter approach.

Several investigative groups have recently demonstrated that most patients with pancreatitis, including those with severe pancreatitis, can actually tolerate small amounts of enterally administered nutrients. They have shown that those nutrients can be tolerated if given either into the stomach (through a nasogastric tube) or into the small intestine (through a nasojejunal tube). Pancreatic infections are believed to occur because gut bacteria are translocated across the injured bowel wall adjacent to areas of pancreatic injury. Theoretically, enteral nutrition exerts a trophic effect on the injured bowel wall that could reduce this translocation and, thus, reduce the incidence of pancreatic infections. Studies evaluating this concept are currently underway,[22-24] but even in the absence of definitive results, I favor administration of trophic amounts of nutrients to patients with severe pancreatitis and begin that treatment within 72 hours of hospitalization.

Treatments of Limited or Unproven Value

Peritoneal dialysis, designed to eliminate the proinflammatory factors released into the abdomen during pancreatitis, might theoretically be expected to reduce the severity of pancreatitis. Indeed, early anecdotal studies did support the use of peritoneal dialysis in patients with severe pancreatitis, but a more recent, prospective, randomized multi-institutional study showed that peritoneal dialysis was of no benefit. Nasogastric decompression does not appear to alter the course or outcome of a pancreatitis attack, although it may provide for greater patient comfort during the early stages when nausea and vomiting are common. Other attempts to reduce gastrointestinal or pancreatic secretion (i.e., H_2 blockers, proton pump inhibitors, antacids, atropine, somatostatin, glucagon, calcitonin) have not been shown to be beneficial in the treatment of pancreatitis. Similarly, the use of antiinflammatory agents (i.e., steroids, prostaglandins, and indomethacin) has not been helpful, although recent experimental studies have suggested that specific inhibition of cyclooxygenase-2 might be beneficial.

Many attempts to treat pancreatitis with agents designed to inhibit activated proteolytic enzymes (e.g., aprotinin, gabexate mesylate) have failed to alter the course of pancreatitis unless their use is begun before the onset of the attack. Hypothermia, thoracic duct drainage, and plasmapheresis have been evaluated in experimental models of pancreatitis, but to date, there is little evidence that these modes of therapy are clinically useful. Many other approaches have also been tried (e.g., procainamide, isoproterenol, heparin, dextran, vasopressin). Although these forms of treatment have been supported by experimental animal studies, particularly when the treatment is begun before the onset of pancreatitis, human clinical trials have failed to show a beneficial effect on the course of patients with established pancreatitis, and at present, none of these treatments is commonly employed. Platelet-activating factor (PAF) is a proinflammatory factor that has been shown to promote worsening of experimental pancreatitis in animal models. Recently, several clinical trials have evaluated the effects of interfering with PAF action during severe clinical pancreatitis, but they have failed to show these anti-PAF agents beneficially alter the outcome of patients with severe pancreatitis. Therefore, anti-PAF agents are not currently used.

Treatment of Early Systemic Complications of Pancreatitis

The pathogenesis and management of the cardiovascular collapse, respiratory failure, renal failure, metabolic encephalopathy, gastrointestinal bleeding, and disseminated intravascular coagulation that complicate severe pancreatitis appear to be identical to those involved when these processes are superimposed on other disease states that are characterized by peritonitis and hypovolemia. Cardiovascular collapse is largely caused by hypovolemia, and its management requires aggressive fluid and electrolyte repletion. This may necessitate placement of a central venous or Swan-Ganz monitoring catheter. Changes in hematocrit, filling pressures, and cardiac output can be used to monitor the adequacy of treatment, but changes in blood pressure, pulse, and urine output do not accurately and reliably reflect the adequacy of fluid replacement.

The pulmonary manifestations of pancreatitis include atelectasis and acute lung injury. The latter appears to be similar to the acute lung injury caused by other systemic processes, including septic shock, ischemia and reperfusion, and massive blood transfusion. Management includes good pulmonary toilet combined with close monitoring of pulmonary function. For many patients, intubation and respiratory support may be required. Renal failure in pancreatitis is usually prerenal and is associated with a poor prognosis. In severe cases, dialysis, usually hemodialysis, may be required. Stress-induced gastroduodenal erosions account for most of the gastrointestinal bleeding in pancreatitis and prophylaxis with antacids, H_2-receptor antagonists, or proton pump inhibitors may be appropriate. Rarely, massive bleeding can result from injury to peripancreatic vascular structures, leading to hemorrhage into the retroperitoneum. The peripancreatic inflammatory process can also cause thrombosis of major gastrointestinal vessels and result in ischemic lesions involving the stomach, small intestine, or colon that can cause bleeding. Management of these complications of pancreatitis is similar to that involved when they occur in the absence of pancreatitis. Some patients with severe pancreatitis develop disseminated intravascular coagulation, but it rarely causes bleeding, and prophylactic heparinization is usually not indicated.

Role of Early Endoscopy and Stone Extraction

Patients with mild pancreatitis may ultimately require endoscopic duct clearance to prevent recurrent attacks, but they rarely benefit from early endoscopy because their pancreatitis generally resolves spontaneously within several days. On the other hand, the role of early endoscopic duct clearance in the initial management of patients with severe biliary pancreatitis is more controversial. Three randomized, controlled, prospective studies have differing results.[25-27] One study indicated that early stone clearance reduced the severity and mortality of biliary pancreatitis, whereas a second study indicated that early duct clearance reduced the incidence of infectious complications. The third study concluded that early endoscopy and duct clearance actually adversely affected the course of pancreatitis because it was associated with a high incidence of complications. At the present time, most experts would favor early (i.e., <48 hours after the onset of symptoms) endoscopic intervention in severe biliary pancreatitis, but further studies are needed.

Role and Timing of Cholecystectomy in Patients With Gallstone Pancreatitis

In general, patients with gallstone pancreatitis undergo some form of definitive treatment before discharge from the hospital, and that intervention takes place as soon as possible after resolution of their attack. Further delaying the intervention would increase the chances that additional stones might be passed and another attack of pancreatitis might be triggered. Intervening sooner, on the other hand, could introduce infection into the inflamed peripancreatic area or worsen the pancreatitis.

For purposes of therapeutic decision making, patients with gallstone pancreatitis can be divided into two groups: those who have or have had gallbladder-derived problems (cholecystitis or biliary colic) and those whose only problems are purely related to stones in the biliary ductal system (i.e., cholangitis and pancreatitis). Patients in the first group undergo cholecystectomy because that operation will prevent additional gallbladder attacks as well as eliminating the source of stones that might trigger another attack of pancreatitis. Patients in the second group, however, do not necessarily require cholecystectomy because their problem relates only to ductal stones. Theoretically, they could be treated simply by endoscopic stone clearance combined with endoscopic sphincterotomy, so that future stones are passed without becoming impacted in the ampulla and triggering either pancreatitis or cholangitis. Indeed, for poor surgical risk patients, the endoscopic approach is generally recommended. On the other hand, roughly 25% of patients treated in this manner will go on to develop gallbladder symptoms over the next 3 to 5 years.[28] Thus, good surgical risk patients are better managed by cholecystectomy.

Treatment of Later Complications

Definitions

In 1992, an international symposium was held to resolve the confusion that had arisen concerning the terminology used to describe the local complications of pancreatitis and the value of specific treatments for those complications.[29] The following definitions were agreed on at that conference:

1. *Acute Fluid Collections.* These occur during the early stages of severe pancreatitis in 30% to 50% of patients, they lack a wall of granulation or fibrous tissue, and more than half regress spontaneously. Most are peripancreatic, but some are intrapancreatic. Those that do not regress may evolve into pseudocysts or involve areas of necrosis.

2. *Pancreatic and Peripancreatic Necrosis.* These are areas of nonviable pancreatic or peripancreatic tissue that may be either sterile or infected. They typically include areas of fat necrosis, and the necrotic tissue has a puttylike or pastelike consistency. Some necrotic regions may evolve into pseudocysts, whereas others may be replaced by fibrous tissue.

3. *Pancreatic Pseudocyst.* These are collections of pancreatic juice, usually rich in digestive enzymes, that are enclosed by a nonepithelialized wall composed of fibrous and granulation tissue (Fig. 55-4). Pseudocysts can be intrapancreatic but are more commonly extrapancreatic and occupy the lesser peritoneal sac. Pseudocysts are usually round or oval in shape and are not present before 4 to 6 weeks after the onset of an attack. Before that time, the fluid collection lacks a defined wall and is usually either an acute fluid collection or a localized area of necrosis (see earlier). Pseudocysts may be colonized by microorganisms, but infection, as evidenced by the presence of pus, is less common. When pus is present, the infected pseudocyst is referred to as a *pancreatic abscess*. Leakage or rupture of a pseudocyst into the peritoneal cavity results in *pancreatic ascites*. A *pancreaticopleural fistula* results from erosion of a pseudocyst into the pleural space.

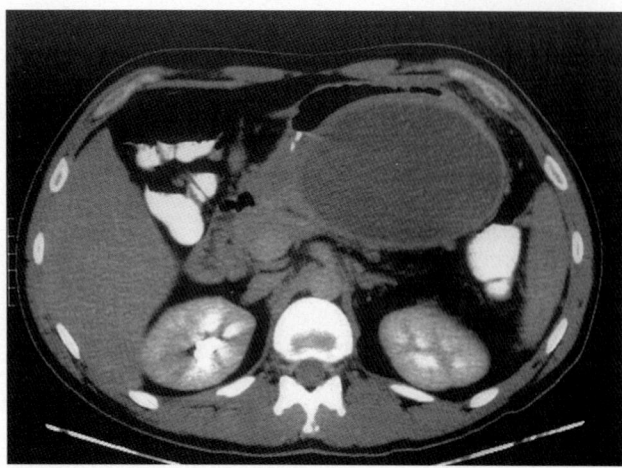

Figure 55-4 CT scan of pancreatic pseudocyst.

4. *Pancreatic Abscess and Infected Pancreatic Necrosis.* These are circumscribed intra-abdominal collections of pus, usually in proximity to the pancreas, which contain little or no necrotic tissue but arise as a consequence of pancreatitis. An infected pseudocyst is considered a pancreatic abscess. Pancreatic abscess and infected pancreatic necrosis represent the extremes of a spectrum that includes lesions with varying amounts of necrosis. Thus, in a pancreatic abscess, there is little necrosis, and the material has a liquid consistency, whereas in infected pancreatic necrosis, necrosis predominates, and the material is pastelike or puttylike.

Diagnosis

Contrast-enhanced CT is particularly valuable as a means of quantifying the extent of pancreatic necrosis (i.e., nonenhancement). The maturation of a pseudocyst can be followed by both contrast-enhanced CT and endoscopic ultrasound. Management of local pancreatitis complications is dependent on whether the lesion is sterile or infected (see later). Occasionally, infection can be diagnosed when plain abdominal films or CT scans reveal extraintestinal gas bubbles or air either within the area of inflammation or elsewhere in the retroperitoneum. When the clinical suspicion of infection is high, fine-needle aspiration of peripancreatic or intrapancreatic fluid for culture and Gram stain analysis may be particularly helpful.[30] The procedure is most frequently done with CT guidance, and it is safe when performed by experienced radiologists.

Management of Sterile and Infected Acute Fluid Collections

Sterile acute fluid collections usually resolve spontaneously, and no specific treatment is indicated. Attempts to drain acute fluid collections, either by using percutaneously placed drains or by intervening surgically, are discouraged as they are usually unnecessary, and furthermore, they are likely to lead to infection. Even without instrumentation, these fluid collections can become infected, but because they contain liquid pus with little or no necrotic tissue, they are amenable to transcutaneous catheter drainage along with antibiotic therapy. It is generally believed that aspirating fluid from any site near the pancreas yields information that is relevant to all the fluid collections and that sampling multiple sites is unnecessary.

Management of Sterile and Infected Necrosis

The role of surgical intervention in the management of patients with *sterile* pancreatic or peripancreatic necrosis has been the subject of considerable controversy.[31] Opinions range from those advocating aggressive débridement for patients with sterile necrosis who fail to rapidly improve on nonoperative treatment to those who claim that surgical intervention is virtually never indicated when the necrosis is sterile. Those taking the former position claim that removing the necrotic tissue (i.e., necrosectomy) reduces morbidity and speeds recovery, whereas those taking the latter position, including me, base their position on the fact that most people treated nonoperatively will eventually recover and some who undergo operation may actually be made worse by the operation.

There is, however, a general consensus that patients with *infected* necrosis require some form of intervention. Prospective studies have indicated that infection of areas of necrosis can occur at any time but that it usually occurs during the initial 3 to 4 weeks of an attack. Although some recent reports have indicated that highly selected patients might be adequately treated with antibiotics alone,[32] simple antibiotic therapy is generally considered to be inadequate because the necrotic tissue acts as a foreign body, making it impossible to sterilize the area with antibiotics alone. Combining antibiotic therapy with percutaneous catheter drainage may also not be adequate treatment because the pastelike necrotic tissue does not pass through the small-bore drainage catheters, and therefore, drainage is usually incomplete. Other methods of removing the necrotic tissue, either through a transpapillary endoscopic route or using minimally invasive surgical approaches with an operating nephroscope, have been tried, but experience with these techniques has been limited and essentially anecdotal. The conventional approach to managing infected necrosis involves laparotomy and surgical débridement of the infected, devitalized tissue. Repeated operations and débridement may be needed. The timing of the initial débridement appears to be closely related to the outcome; that is, those undergoing later operations do better and require fewer repeat operations than those undergoing early operation. Thus, in stable patients, delaying operative intervention may decrease the overall morbidity of an attack.

The goal of operation in patients with infected necrosis is to remove as much as possible of the infected, necrotic tissue and to provide drainage for the remaining viable exocrine tissue. Many different ways of achieving these goals have been described (Box 55-4), and although each has its advocates, none has been proved superior to the others. My practice is to perform repeat operations, each of which involves débridement and abdominal wall closure. At the time of the final débridement, drains and a feeding jejunostomy are placed. For the most part, the repeat laparotomies are performed every 2 to 3 days until no further débridement is possible or necessary.

Management of Pancreatic Pseudocysts

Most pseudocysts communicate with the pancreatic ductal system and contain a watery fluid that is rich in pancreatic digestive enzymes. Typically, patients with pseudocysts have persistent elevations of circulating pancreatic enzymes. Recent reports have shown that many pseudocysts eventually resolve without complications and that intervention is not mandatory in all cases unless the pseudocysts are symptomatic, enlarging, or associated with complications. The likelihood that a pseudocyst will resolve spontaneously, however, is dependent on its size. Large pseudocysts (i.e., >6 cm in diameter) are more likely to become symptomatic either because they are tender or because of their mass effect on adjacent organs. Those that compress the stomach or duodenum may cause gastric outlet obstruction with nausea and vomiting. Those that reduce the capacity of the stomach frequently cause early satiety, whereas those impinging on the bile duct can cause obstructive jaundice. Pancreatic pseudocysts that erode into a neighboring vessel can result in formation of a pseudoaneurysm with *hemosuccus pancreaticus* and upper gastrointestinal bleeding.

Symptomatic or enlarging pseudocysts can be treated by several methods. Those in the tail can be treated by excision (i.e., distal pancreatectomy), but excision in the setting of recent acute inflammation may be hazardous. Most patients who develop symptomatic pseudocysts are best managed by pseudocyst drainage. In poor surgical risk patients, percutaneous catheter drainage can be considered, but in my experience, that approach leads to considerable morbidity because of catheter-induced infection and the development of a prolonged external pancreatic fistula. Internal drainage can avoid these problems and seems preferable. Internal drainage can be accomplished either endoscopically (by transpapillary drainage, cystogastrostomy, or cystoduodenostomy) or surgically (by cystogastrostomy, cystoduodenostomy, or Roux-en-Y cystojejunostomy). The approach chosen depends primarily on the locally available expertise as well as the location of the pseudocyst, but endoscopic drainage may be preferable in poor surgical risk patients.

Pseudocysts that are directly adjacent to either the stomach or duodenum can be safely drained endoscopically if there are no intervening vessels. After endoscopic ultrasound and preliminary aspiration of the cyst fluid to confirm the diagnosis and exclude intervening vessels, endoscopic drainage is achieved by making an incision into the pseudocyst through the wall of the stomach or duodenum. To facilitate decompression, the opening is relatively large, and a pigtail catheter may be placed. Transpapillary drainage might be more appropriate for patients with pancreatic head pseudocysts whose CT and endoscopic ultrasound suggest that incising into the

---

> **Box 55-4   Management Options for Infected Pancreatic Necrosis**
>
> **Conventional Approach**
>
> Débridement with reoperation when clinically indicated or at planned intervals
> Débridement with open or closed packing and reoperation when clinically indicated or at planned intervals
> Débridement with continuous lavage
>
> **Unconventional Approach**
>
> Antibiotics alone
> Antibiotics with percutaneous drainage
> Antibiotics with endoscopic drainage
> Antibiotics with surgical drainage but not débridement
> Antibiotics with débridement through minimally invasive surgery

---

pseudocyst could be hazardous. At the time of endoscopic retrograde cholangiopancreatography (ERCP), a stent is passed into the pseudocyst through the papilla of Vater. Unfortunately, transpapillary drainage, particularly when incomplete, can allow bacteria to enter the pseudocyst and lead to development of an infected pseudocyst. Another transpapillary approach involves placing a stent across the duct defect rather than into the cyst through the defect. By excluding pancreatic juice from the pseudocyst, this bridging intraductal stent may permit the duct disruption to heal and the pseudocyst to resolve without drainage. Further experience with this technique will be needed before its ultimate use can be determined.

Surgical internal drainage of pseudocysts is usually accomplished by creating either a Roux-en-Y cystojejunostomy, a side-to-side cystogastrostomy, or a side-to-side cystoduodenostomy. The former is usually accomplished by directly anastomosing a defunctionalized Roux-en-Y limb of jejunum to the opened pseudocyst. Surgical cystogastrostomy (or cystoduodenostomy) has traditionally been accomplished by laparotomy and anterior gastrotomy (or lateral duodenotomy). A generous incision is then made through the posterior wall of the stomach (or medial wall of the duodenum) into the pseudocyst. Some surgeons now perform cystgastrostomy using a laparoscopic approach.

Management of Pancreatic Ascites and Pancreaticopleural Fistulas

Pancreatic ascites occurs when pancreatic juice gains entry into the peritoneal cavity either from a pancreatic duct disruption or from a leaking pseudocyst. The diagnosis can usually be made when high amylase levels are found in the ascitic fluid. The initial treatment usually is nonoperative and involves attempts to decrease pancreatic secretion by elimination of enteral feeding, institution of nasogastric drainage, and administration of the antisecretory hormone somatostatin. Repeat paracentesis may also be helpful. Roughly 50% to 60% of patients can be expected to respond to this treatment with resolution of pancreatic ascites within 2 to 3 weeks. Persistent or recurrent ascites can be treated either endoscopically or surgically. Endoscopic treatment involves endoscopic pancreatic sphincterotomy with or without placement of a transpapillary pancreatic duct stent. By reducing the resistance to drainage into the duodenum, and by bridging the site of duct disruption, this approach is designed to allow the site of leakage to seal. Surgical treatment of pancreatic ascites, usually preceded by performance of an ERCP to identify the site of duct disruption, involves either resection (for leaks in the pancreatic tail) or internal Roux-en-Y drainage (for leaks in the head and neck region). It seems most appropriate to attempt endoscopic treatment initially and to reserve surgical treatment for those patients who do not respond to endoscopic therapy.

The genesis of pancreaticopleural fistula is similar to that of pancreatic ascites, but in this case, the duct disruption is usually posterior, and the extravasated juice travels in a cephalad direction through the retroperitoneum to reach the thoracic cavity. Although the incidence of pancreaticopleural fistula is lower than that of pancreatic ascites, the management of both is similar.

Management of Pancreatitis-Induced False Aneurysms

Rarely, pancreatic pseudocysts or areas of pancreatic necrosis can erode into pancreatic or peripancreatic vascular structures. This results in the formation of a false aneurysm because the vessel communicates with the pseudocyst. That false aneurysm may either communicate with the ductal system or rupture into the free peritoneal cavity. The former leads to bleeding into the pancreatic duct (*hemosuccus pancreaticus*) and presents as transpapillary upper gastrointestinal bleeding. Rupture into the peritoneal cavity can lead to hemoperitoneum. Therapeutic angiographic embolization is most appropriate for the unstable patient, and this approach may also provide definitive treatment, particularly for those patients whose false aneurysm is in the pancreatic head. For those whose false aneurysm is in the tail of the pancreas, subsequent distal pancreatectomy, after the patient is stabilized, may provide more secure hemostasis.

Management of Pancreaticoenteric Fistulas

Pancreatic pseudocysts or areas of pancreatic necrosis can erode into the small intestine, duodenum, stomach, bile duct, or splenic flexure of the colon. Occasionally, this results in resolution of the pseudocyst, and no further treatment is needed. More often, however, such an event is accompanied by significant bleeding or signs of sepsis, and surgical intervention is usually required. Management of these fistulas is determined by the gastrointestinal organ involved.

Management of Pancreatitis-Induced Splenic Vein Thrombosis and Sinistral Varices

Because of the close proximity of the splenic vein to the pancreas, splenic vein thrombosis is not unusual in cases of severe pancreatitis. For the most part, it does not result in early symptoms, but it may eventually result in the

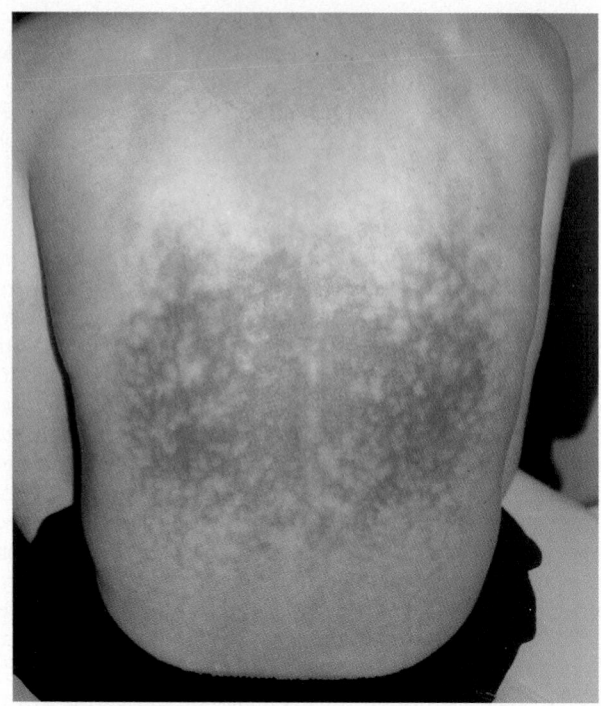

Figure 55-5 Erythema ab igne. Skin injury, characterized by keratinocyte injury and melanocyte activation, is induced by mild and repeated exposure to infrared sources. This patient with chronic pancreatitis repeatedly applied a heating pad to the painful area on his back.

formation of gastroesophageal varices. Splenectomy provides effective and definitive treatment when these sinistral varices bleed, but because bleeding occurs in fewer than 10% of these patients, prophylactic splenectomy is not generally performed.

CHRONIC PANCREATITIS

Pathology and Etiology of Chronic Pancreatitis

Chronic pancreatitis is characterized by irreversible changes, including pancreatic fibrosis and the loss of functional pancreatic exocrine or endocrine tissue. Most patients develop chronic pancreatitis as a result of prolonged ethanol abuse. It is generally believed that, in its earliest stages, chronic pancreatitis is an acute inflammatory process, and repeated episodes of subclinical acute pancreatic injury and necrosis lead to the fibrosis of chronic pancreatitis.

Diagnosis of Chronic Pancreatitis

There has been considerable confusion concerning the clinical distinction between chronic and acute pancreatitis. To a great extent, this confusion results from the fact that, from a clinical standpoint, attacks of chronic pancreatitis may be indistinguishable from those of acute pancreatitis. Fortunately, the initial management of acute

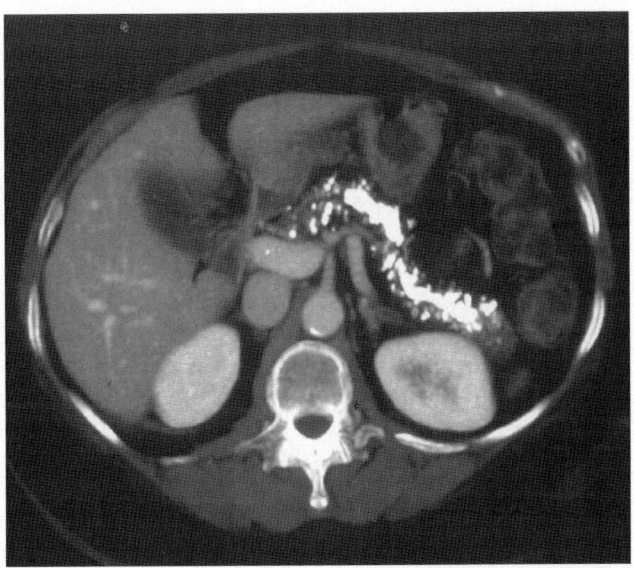

Figure 55-6 Pancreatic calcifications. CT scan showing multiple, calcified, intraductal stones in a patient with hereditary chronic pancreatitis.

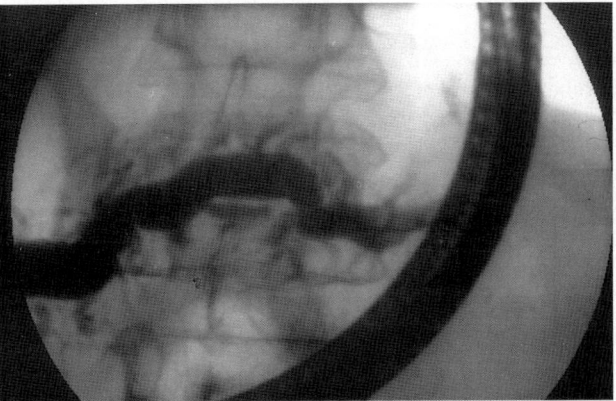

Figure 55-7 Endoscopic retrograde cholangiopancreatography in chronic pancreatitis. The pancreatic duct and its side branches are irregularly dilated.

or chronic pancreatitis attacks is identical, as is the management of complications such as infection, necrosis, and pseudocyst (see Treatment of an Acute Attack section, earlier). On the other hand, the two forms of pancreatitis have natural histories that differ considerably, and the long-term management of chronic pancreatitis presents challenges that are not inherent to the management of acute pancreatitis.

History

Patients with chronic pancreatitis may describe prior episodes of pancreatic-type abdominal pain, and 60% to 80% of patients have a long history of ethanol abuse. There may be a family history of pancreatitis suggestive of the presence of hereditary pancreatitis or a history of autoimmune diseases, including primary sclerosing cholangitis and Sjögren's syndrome, that raise suspicion of pancreatitis on an autoimmune basis. Diabetes mellitus or a history suggestive of malabsorption (i.e., steatorrhea) indicates that significant pancreatic endocrine or exocrine function has been lost, and this is most compatible with the diagnosis of chronic pancreatitis. Typically, patients with chronic pancreatitis have upper abdominal pain radiating to the back. It can be constant or episodic and triggered by drinking alcohol or eating. Repeated use of heating pads or hot water bottles to treat the chronic pain may result in skin lesions (erythema ab igne) that define the distribution of the pain (Fig. 55-5). Some patients experience no pain.

Imaging Studies

Radiographs or CT scans showing pancreatic calcifications are diagnostic of chronic pancreatitis (Fig. 55-6). Those calcifications reflect the deposition of calcium carbonate in the intraductal protein plugs that frequently, but not invariably, occur in chronic pancreatitis. Thus,

the absence of pancreatic calcifications does not rule out a diagnosis of chronic pancreatitis. Perhaps the most sensitive methods for diagnosing chronic pancreatitis are those that provide images of the pancreatic ductal system. ERCP, CT cholangiopancreatography, or magnetic resonance cholangiopancreatography may be particularly valuable in the diagnosis of chronic pancreatitis.

Chronic pancreatitis is characterized by irregularities of the pancreatic ducts, ductal strictures, and areas of duct dilation (Fig. 55-7). The major as well as the side-branch ducts may be involved. For unexplained reasons, some patients with chronic pancreatitis develop dilated main pancreatic ducts *(large duct disease),* whereas others retain ducts of normal or even smaller than normal caliber *(small duct disease).* Some patients with chronic pancreatitis can be shown to have major ducts that have the appearance of a "chain of lakes" or a "string of pearls" that is the result of segments of dilated duct separated by areas of ductal stricture. Transcutaneous and endoscopic ultrasound can also be used to diagnose chronic pancreatitis if duct dilation, calcifications, pseudocysts, or parenchymal fibrosis are seen. Ultrasound examination is more operator dependent and perhaps less sensitive than either CT or MRI.

Pancreatic Function Tests

The pancreas has considerable functional reserve, and more than 90% of exocrine function must be lost before steatorrhea develops. More subtle losses may be identified by performance of pancreatic function tests[33] that can be either noninvasive (so-called tubeless tests) or invasive (tube tests) (Box 55-5). Tubeless tests involve measuring the stool content of fat, measuring stool content of digestive enzymes, or orally administering a pancreatic digestive enzyme substrate and quantitating enzyme activity in the gut by measuring metabolic product in either the urine or exhaled gases. These tests, although nonintrusive, are notoriously insensitive, and therefore, normal results are not too helpful. The more invasive tube tests involve placement of a collecting tube in the duodenum and measuring pancreatic bicarbonate or

> **Box 55-5   Pancreatic Function Tests**
>
> **Tubeless Tests**
>
> *Fecal Tests*
>
> Fat stain
> 72-hour fat content
> Chymotrypsin, trypsin, elastase content
>
> *Indirect Tests*
>
> Bentiromide test
> Pancreolauryl test
> Breath tests
>
> **Tube Tests**
>
> Lundh test meal
> Secretin or cholecystokinin test

enzyme output after meal or hormone stimulation of the pancreas. These tests are more specific and sensitive than the tubeless tests, but they are still relatively insensitive, and they have a relatively high rate of false-negative results.

Natural History

Some patients with chronic pancreatitis have a painless disease that remains unrecognized until complications or loss of pancreatic function leads to the diagnosis. Most patients, however, have intermittent or constant pain that may limit lifestyle or mandate repeated hospitalizations. Ammann and Muellhaupt[34] have suggested that the painful pancreatitis experienced by many of these patients evolves into a painless disease as pancreatic function is lost, but the existence of this "burnout" phenomenon is highly controversial. More often, the disease remains painful, addicting doses of narcotics are required, and loss of function results in diabetes, steatorrhea, and profound weight loss.

Treatment of Pancreatic Malabsorption

The loss of pancreatic exocrine function in chronic pancreatitis affects the output of all pancreatic digestive enzymes, but it is mostly fat absorption that is abnormal, and it is the delivery of lipolytic enzyme activity to the small intestine that determines the success of treatment. In health, roughly 300,000 IU of lipase is secreted by the pancreas within 4 hours of ingesting a typical meal, but only 10% (30,000 IU) of secreted lipase is needed to allow for normal fat digestion and absorption. Theoretically, pancreatic malabsorption of fat is corrected by oral administration of exogenous lipase. Unfortunately, most orally administered lipase is inactivated as it traverses the acidic environment of the stomach, allowing only 8% to 15% of ingested lipase activity to reach the duodenum. Some of that lipase may be ineffective, either because of low duodenal pH (caused by inadequate pancreatic secretion of bicarbonate) or because the exogenously administered lipase arrives in the duodenum before or

after the ingested fat. The use of acid-inhibiting agents (e.g., proton pump inhibitors) and enterically coated microsphere delivery systems can partially compensate for these problems. Thus, treatment involves acid suppression, a low-fat diet, and lipase doses of 90 to 150,000 IU per meal, although control of steatorrhea is often incomplete even with this treatment.

Treatment of Pain in Chronic Pancreatitis

Medical Management

Complete abstinence from ethanol is advised for patients with alcohol-induced pancreatitis, but symptoms may persist even after complete abstinence. Attacks of hyperlipidemia-induced pancreatitis can be prevented by normalizing lipid levels with medication or dietary changes. Most patients with autoimmune pancreatitis are cured by administration of steroids. For most patients with painful chronic pancreatitis, intermittent or persistent pain remains a major issue, and analgesics of increasing potency are needed. Toskes[35] noted that some of their patients with painful chronic pancreatitis have diminished pain if pancreatic secretion is reduced either by oral administration of pancreatic enzymes or by administration of the inhibitory hormone somatostatin. However, the clinical results achieved using exogenous pancreatic enzymes to reduce the pain of chronic pancreatitis have been variable, and at this time, the role of enzyme administration for pain relief in these patients is highly controversial.

Endoscopic Management

The endoscopic treatment of chronic pancreatitis has not been tested by well-designed prospective, randomized trials; therefore, the ultimate value of these treatments remains to be established. Several endoscopic approaches have been described. Endoscopic pancreatic sphincterotomy has been reported to benefit some patients with elevated sphincter of Oddi pressures. Endoscopic minor pancreatic sphincterotomy has been used to treat patients with pancreatitis thought to be due to pancreas divisum. Pancreatic duct stones have also been removed or fragmented using an endoscopic approach with reported benefits. Finally, some patients with pancreatic duct strictures have been treated either by dilation of the stricture or by endoscopically placed stents that pass across the stricture, but the value of this treatment is unclear because the stents themselves can cause strictures.

Neuroablative Procedures

Pain from the pancreas is carried in sympathetic fibers that traverse the celiac ganglia, reach the sympathetic chain through the splanchnic nerves, and then ascend to the cortex. Celiac plexus nerve blocks performed either percutaneously or endoscopically have been employed to abolish this pain with inconsistent results. Recently, splanchnicectomy performed in the chest by a thoracoscopic approach has been used, with reports of transient improvement in 70% of patients and long-lasting pain control in 50%.[36] Experience with thoracoscopic splanchnicectomy has been only anecdotal, and randomized, prospective trials will be needed to determine its ultimate value.

Surgical Treatment of Chronic Pancreatitis

The two indications for surgical intervention are pain and concern about the possible presence of cancer. After the diagnosis of chronic pancreatitis has been established, surgical intervention is considered when (1) the pain is severe enough to limit the patient's lifestyle or reduce productivity, and (2) the pain persists despite complete abstinence from alcohol and administration of non-narcotic analgesics. Imaging studies are performed to define pancreatic and ductal anatomy because that will determine the surgical options. Finally, the risks and benefits of planned procedures must be clearly explained to the patient because, even with a technically successful operation, the pain may persist, and further deterioration in exocrine and endocrine function can still occur.

Drainage Procedures for Patients With Small Ducts

Patients with small (<4-6 mm) pancreatic ducts, but in whom pancreatitis is caused by obstruction at the ampullary level, may benefit from transduodenal sphincteroplasty of the common bile duct with division of the septum that lies between the pancreatic duct and bile duct (pancreatic septotomy). Sphincteroplasty of the lesser papilla might be appropriate for highly selected patients with pancreas divisum. On the other hand, most patients with chronic pancreatitis have multiple areas of duct stricture throughout the pancreas and are unlikely to benefit from these transduodenal procedures.

Drainage Procedures for Patients With Dilated Ducts

The ideal treatment for these patients involves creating an anastomotic connection between the dilated duct and the intestinal lumen. There is little agreement concerning the minimum duct size needed to perform these anastomoses. Ducts larger than 1 cm in diameter are, clearly, large enough, but many surgeons perform duct-to-intestine drainage procedures with ducts as small as 5 mm. Duct drainage operations were pioneered by Duval, who described a procedure that involved splenectomy, resection of the pancreatic tail, and then creation of an end-to-end anastomosis between the transected end of the pancreas and a Roux-en-Y limb of jejunum. This procedure often failed because the presence of multiple pancreatic duct strictures interfered with complete ductal decompression.

Puestow and Gillesby, in 1958, described an operation that involved longitudinally opening the entire duct and then invaginating the opened pancreas into a Roux-en-Y loop of jejunum. This allowed for more complete decompression but still required splenectomy. Later, Partington and Rochelle[37] modified the Puestow procedure by creating a side-to-side anastomosis between the opened duct and jejunum, thus eliminating the need for splenectomy (Fig. 55-8). In appropriately selected patients (i.e., those with large ducts and those with intraductal stones), longitudinal pancreaticojejunostomy, performed according to the Partington and Rochelle modification of the Puestow procedure, has been reported to result in

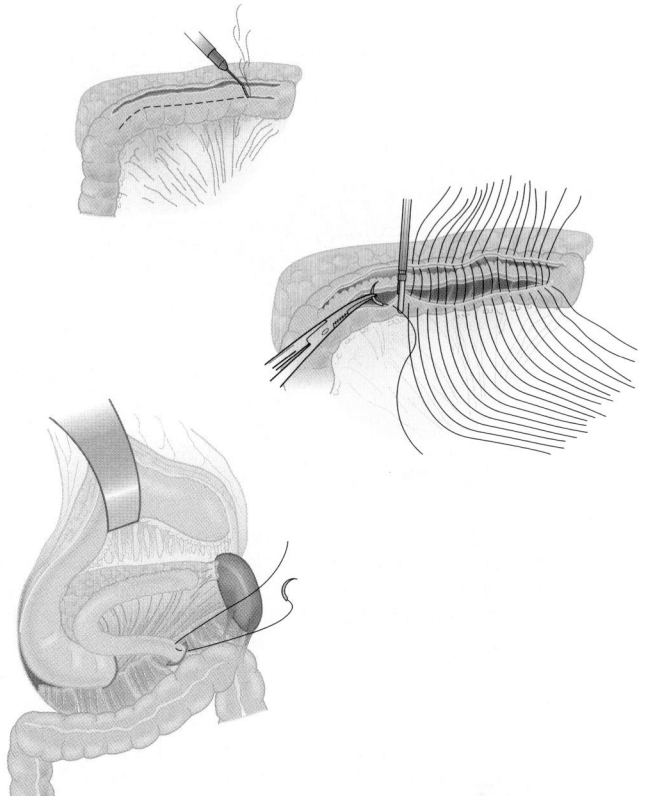

Figure 55-8 Partington and Rochelle modification of the Puestow procedure. The pancreatic duct is opened from the tail of the pancreas to the edge of the duodenum, and a side-to-side anastomosis is created joining a Roux-en-Y limb of jejunum to the opened pancreatic duct. (From Carey LC: Pancreatico-jejunostomy with cystoduodenostomy. In Malt RA [ed]: Surgical Techniques Illustrated. New York, WB Saunders, 1985, pp 396-405.)

immediate pain relief in more than 80% of patients and long-term pain relief in roughly 60% of patients. More recently, Ho and Frey[38] further modified the procedure by including removal of part of the pancreatic head, thereby marsupializing the duct as it dives deeply in the pancreas to reach the ampulla of Vater. This allows for an even more complete duct decompression and a longer longitudinal pancreaticojejunostomy. Both short- and long-term pain relief appear to be improved, and the procedure can be performed when the duct is only moderately dilated.

Resective Procedures

Painful chronic pancreatitis can be treated with resection of the body and tail of the pancreas (distal pancreatectomy), resection of the head and uncinate process of the pancreas (Whipple procedure), subtotal pancreatectomy that spares a rim of pancreas along the inner curve of the duodenum, or total pancreatectomy. Each of these procedures can either cause or worsen pancreatic exocrine and endocrine insufficiency, and in the case of total pancreatectomy, a brittle form of diabetes can occur. Most experts believe that it is the inflammatory process in the pancreatic head that controls both the severity of

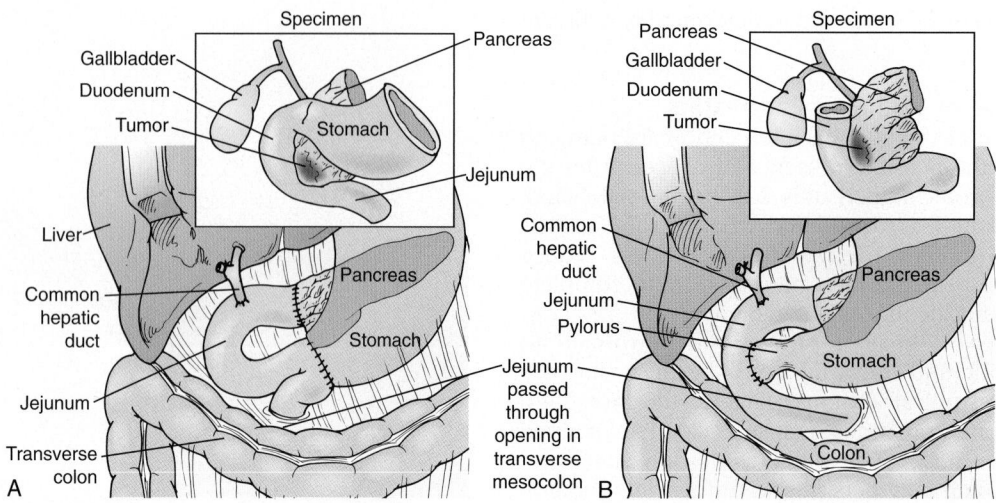

Figure 55-9 Standard and pylorus-preserving Whipple procedure. **A,** The standard Whipple involves resection of the gastric antrum, head of pancreas, distal bile duct, and entire duodenum with reconstruction as shown. **B,** The pylorus-preserving Whipple does not include resection of the distal stomach, pylorus, or proximal duodenum. (From Cameron, JL: Current status of the Whipple operation for periampullary carcinoma. Surg Rounds 77-87, 1988.)

symptoms and the further progression of the disease in the remainder of the gland. Perhaps because of this, resection of the pancreatic head has been shown to completely relieve the pain of chronic pancreatitis in 70% to 80% of patients. Resection of the pancreatic head can be accomplished by a standard pancreaticoduodenectomy (Whipple procedure) or by its pylorus-preserving modification (pylorus-preserving Whipple procedure)[39] (Fig. 55-9). Relief of symptoms by either procedure is comparable, but some claim that the quality of life and gastrointestinal function are better after the pylorus-preserving operation. Beger and colleagues have modified the Whipple procedure even further by coring out the head of the pancreas and preserving the duodenum and distal bile duct.[40] They claim that this duodenum-preserving pancreatic head resection yields results that are as good as or better than those achieved with the standard Whipple procedure.

Distal pancreatectomy is the ideal surgical procedure for patients whose chronic pancreatitis is confined to the pancreatic tail. This occurs in patients who develop a mid-duct stricture as a result of either necrotizing acute pancreatitis or trauma that injures the gland and duct as they cross the spine. Usually, distal pancreatectomy is combined with splenectomy for technical reasons, but in fact, the spleen can be preserved if its vascular supply is secure. Distal pancreatectomy is not performed for patients with diffuse, chronic pancreatitis that involves the entire gland, even if the pancreatic tail is the area most severely involved, because recurrence of pancreatitis in the head can be anticipated and further resection of the pancreas, in that case, would leave the patient without functioning pancreatic endocrine tissue.

The role of total or near-total pancreatectomy in the treatment of patients with chronic pancreatitis is not clear. These procedures may represent the only surgical option for patients who have failed drainage procedures or who have small ducts and have already undergone distal pancreatectomy. Some patients continue to experience severe pancreatic pain even after total pancreatectomy, and for this reason, the effects of total pancreatectomy on pain in chronic pancreatitis cannot be accurately predicted. On the other hand, it can be expected that patients undergoing total or near-total pancreatectomy will have brittle diabetes and severe steatorrhea. In combination with ongoing ethanol or drug abuse, the brittle diabetes and malnutrition may be unmanageable problems, and a high late mortality rate in these patients has been reported. In an attempt to avoid brittle diabetes in these patients, some surgeons have advocated harvesting and autotransplanting islets of Langerhans from the resected specimen.[41] Modest success at insulin independence has been achieved using this approach, but the ultimate role of islet reimplantation remains to be established. In the past, some surgeons have reimplanted the entire resected pancreas with mixed results, and the procedure is performed only rarely now.

BENIGN EXOCRINE TUMORS

Most benign pancreatic exocrine tumors are cystic, but not all cystic tumors are benign. Benign cystic tumors, which account for 10% to 15% of pancreatic tumors, are usually asymptomatic, but when symptoms develop, they are usually related to pressure or obstruction of an adjacent organ.

Serous Cystadenoma

Serous cystadenomas account for 20% to 40% of cystic pancreatic neoplasms. They are lined by a flattened

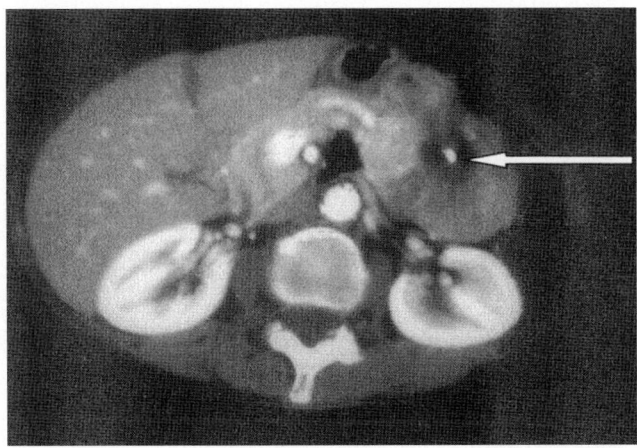

Figure 55-10 CT scan of serous (microcystic) cystadenoma. Note scar with central calcification *(arrow)*.

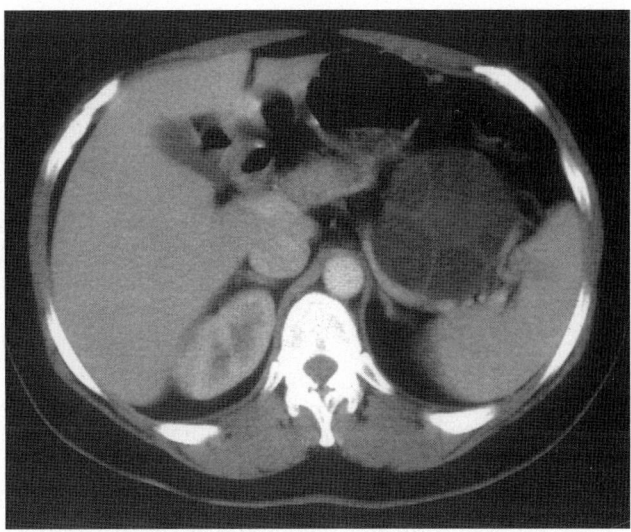

Figure 55-11 CT scan of mucinous (macrocystic) cystadenoma. Note multiple large cystic spaces. Microscopic examination revealed multiple areas of ovarian-like stroma.

epithelium with glycogen-rich cytoplasm that does not stain for mucins, and the finding of glycogen-rich cells on cytologic examination is diagnostic of a serous cystadenoma. Rare cases of malignant serous cystic lesions have been reported, but most are benign and have no malignant potential. Typically, they are large, spherical masses that contain a watery fluid and have a central, calcified stellate scar (Fig. 55-10). Oligocystic varieties, with large cystic spaces, can occur, but most are microcystic. They usually occur in the body or tail and are asymptomatic, but when located in the head, even benign serous cystadenomas can become symptomatic if they enlarge and compress adjacent structures. Resection is indicated when the diagnosis is in doubt or when they become symptomatic.

Mucinous Tumors

Mucinous tumors account for 20% to 40% of cystic tumors. Even if benign at the time of diagnosis, they are usually considered to have malignant potential. Two types have been described, but neither type usually communicates with the pancreatic duct. One form contains areas of ovarian-like stroma, is almost always found in women, and is almost always found in the pancreatic tail (Fig. 55-11). The more common type, however, lacks ovarian stroma and can be found anywhere in the pancreas. Some have argued that it may be a variant of intraductal papillary mucinous neoplasms (IPMNs; see later) that does not communicate with the duct.[42] It occurs equally in both sexes. For both types, imaging studies usually indicate that the lesion is composed of one or more very large cysts (i.e., macrocystic), although microcystic mucinous tumors can also occur. The cysts are lined by a columnar, mucin-producing, and sometimes papillary epithelium. Prolonged survival (i.e., >5 years) can be anticipated in more than 50% of patients if these tumors are resected before the development of invasive malignancy, but even after the development of malignant changes and invasion, long-term survival is still better than for ductal adenocarcinoma.

Intraductal Papillary Mucinous Tumor

IPMN, also known as *intraductal papillary mucinous tumor,* is another type of cystic pancreatic neoplasm. Although first described in Japan in the 1980s, it is now being recognized worldwide, and its incidence appears to be rapidly increasing. Both men and women are equally affected. IPMN can involve the major ducts *(main duct variety),* the smaller ducts *(branch duct variety),* or both types of ducts. It can be located in any or all parts of the pancreas, although involvement of the head appears to be its most common form. IPMN patients can experience pancreatitis when mucus, secreted by the tumor, transiently obstructs the orifice of the pancreatic duct. The diagnosis of IPMN can be made with near certainty if mucus is seen extruding through a large, fish-mouth-like papillary orifice at the time of endoscopy. The main or side-branch ducts involved with IPMN are usually lined by columnar mucin-producing cells that develop papillary projections. Other areas of the duct, although lined by normal epithelium, may be dilated as a result of prior obstructive episodes. IPMN is believed to follow an adenoma-carcinoma sequence, and it can be classified according to the Pan-IN classification scheme (Fig. 55-12) that categorizes tumors as having minimal or no dysplasia (PanIN-1), moderate dysplasia (PanIN-2), or severe dysplasia or carcinoma in situ (PanIN-3).[43] The natural history of tumors with only mild or no dysplasia is not known, but those with severe dysplasia or carcinoma in situ are likely to become locally invasive and metastasize if left unresected. Resection with, at worst, PanIN-1 changes at the margin, before development of invasive malignancy, is usually curative. This may mandate total pancreatectomy. When resection is performed after development of invasive malignancy, cure rates are relatively low.

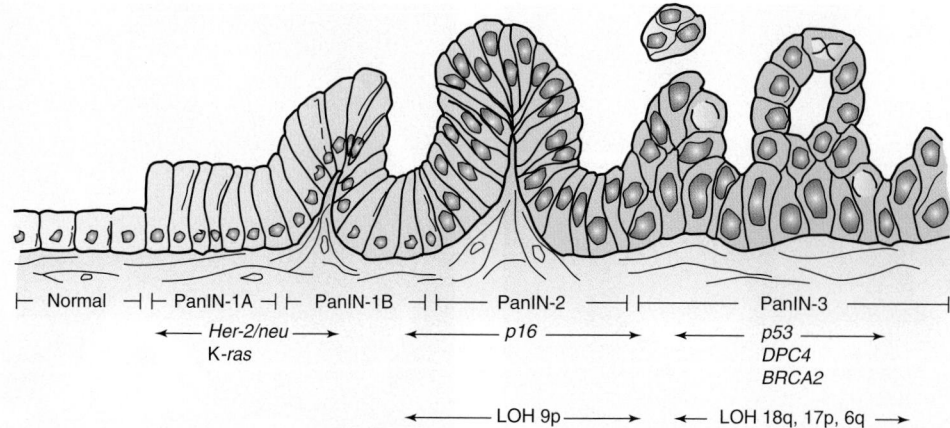

├─ Normal ─┤├─ PanIN-1A ─┤├─ PanIN-1B ─┤├─ PanIN-2 ─────┤├─ PanIN-3 ─────┤

◄─── *Her-2/neu* ───►   ◄─── *p16* ───►   ◄─── *p53* ───►
      K-ras   *DPC4*
                                                        BRCA2

◄─── LOH 9p ───►   ◄─── LOH 18q, 17p, 6q ───►

Figure 55-12 Progression model for pancreatic cancer. The progression from histologically normal ductal epithelium to low-grade pancreatic intraepithelial neoplasia (PanIN) to high-grade PanIN (left to right) is associated with the accumulation of specific genetic changes. Early changes include *Her-2*/neu and K-*ras* mutations; intermediate changes include *p16* mutations; and changes associated with either in situ or early invasive cancer include *p53*, *BRCA2,* and *DPC4* mutations. (From Wilentz RE, Iacobuzio-Donahoe CA, Argani P, et al: Loss of expression of DPC4 in pancreatic intraepithelial neoplasia: Evidence that DPC4 inactivation occurs late in neoplastic progression. Cancer Res 60:2002-2006, 2000.)

Management of Cystic Pancreatic Neoplasms

A recent history of pancreatitis, enzyme-rich fluid in the cyst, and communication between the cyst and the pancreatic duct suggests that the cystic lesion is a postpancreatitic (i.e., inflammatory) pseudocyst. Patients with asymptomatic pseudocysts can be left untreated. However, occasionally these features can also be associated with neoplastic cystic lesions; therefore, these patients must be closely followed. Serous cystadenomas, diagnosed by finding glycogen-rich cells on fine-needle aspiration biopsy, can also be followed without resection if they are not symptomatic.

The major challenge is distinguishing pseudocysts and serous cystadenomas from the other, malignant or potentially malignant, types of cystic pancreatic tumors. The finding of mucin in the cyst, mucin-secreting cells on biopsy, a high cyst fluid viscosity, or a high cyst fluid carcinoembryonic antigen (CEA) is suggestive, but not diagnostic, of a potentially malignant tumor.[44] Failure to observe these changes, however, does not exclude a malignant or potentially malignant mass. Because of these uncertainties, all neoplastic cysts are resected unless the diagnosis of a serous cystadenoma can be made with certainty. For those located in the pancreatic tail, a distal pancreatectomy is ideal, whereas cystic lesions in the pancreatic head present a greater decision-making challenge because resection would require pancreaticoduodenectomy. Cytologic examination of aspirated tissue, removed either transcutaneously or with endoscopic ultrasonographic guidance, may aid in the difficult management decision, but not infrequently, doubt persists, and in good surgical risk patients, pancreaticoduodenectomy is probably indicated.

Solid-Pseudopapillary Tumor of the Pancreas

Solid-pseudopapillary tumor, a relatively uncommon tumor, often occurs in young women and follows a benign course. Local resection is usually curative, although incomplete removal can result in local recurrence, and malignant varieties have been described. The tumors are usually large, round, and well-demarcated masses that can occur in any part of the pancreas. Histologically, the tumor is mostly solid and consists of monomorphous eosinophilic or clear cells that demonstrate a pseudopapillary architecture. In suitable operative candidates, solid-pseudopapillary tumors of the pancreas are resected.

MALIGNANT PANCREATIC TUMORS

Incidence and Epidemiology

Pancreatic cancer affects 25,000 to 30,000 people in the United States each year and is the fourth or fifth leading cause of cancer-related death in this country. It occurs more frequently in men than in women and is more common among blacks than whites. Roughly 80% of cases occur between 60 and 80 years of age, whereas less than 2% occur in people younger than 40 years. Other risk factors include a family history of pancreatic cancer or a history of either hereditary or chronic pancreatitis, cigarette smoking, and occupational exposure to carcinogens. The incidence of diabetes mellitus is increased in patients with pancreatic cancer, but the relationship of diabetes to pancreatic cancer is controversial. Some studies have indicated that diabetes is a risk factor for the development of pancreatic cancer, whereas others have argued that diabetes may be a manifestation of the cancer. Coffee drinking, which was once considered a risk factor, is no longer thought to play a role in the development of pancreatic cancer.

Pathology

Ductal adenocarcinoma and its variants account for 80% to 90% of all pancreatic neoplasms and for an even greater fraction of the malignant tumors. Roughly 70% of ductal cancers arise in the pancreatic head or uncinate process. Grossly, they appear as hard, irregular, gritty masses that are yellow-gray and are usually poorly demarcated. At the time of diagnosis, they are usually larger than 3 cm in diameter, and both nodal and distant metastases are also frequently present. Those originating in the body or tail of the pancreas are often larger and more likely to have spread before their presence is known. Microscopically, the degree of differentiation, mitotic index, and amount of mucus may vary considerably. They are frequently associated with an intense desmoplastic stromal reaction and fibrosis. A halo of chronic pancreatitis frequently surrounds the tumor, presumably caused by tumor-induced obstruction of neighboring ducts. Areas of vascular and lymphatic invasion within and around the tumor are commonly seen. In addition, perineural growth of the tumor is highly characteristic of this cancer and may account for the propensity of pancreatic cancer to extend into neighboring neural plexuses causing both upper abdominal and back pain.

Cancers such as mucinous noncystic carcinoma (colloid carcinoma), signet ring cell carcinoma, adenosquamous carcinoma, anaplastic carcinoma, giant cell carcinoma, and sarcomatoid carcinoma are considered to be variants of ductal adenocarcinoma that differ primarily in their degree of differentiation and their morphologic appearance. In addition to ductal adenocarcinoma, other cancers of the pancreas are known. Some of those cancers represent previously benign tumors that have undergone malignant change. For example, carcinoma in situ and invasive carcinoma can develop in areas of IPMN or within areas of mucinous cystic tumors. Other forms of pancreatic cancer include acinar cell carcinomas, which are most common in the 5th to 7th decades of life and most frequently present as large masses in the body or tail of the pancreas. Pancreatoblastoma is a rare form of pancreatic cancer that usually presents in young children. Nonepithelial cancers of all types, including leiomyosarcomas, liposarcomas, plasmacytomas, and lymphomas, can also develop within the pancreas, but these tumors are quite rare. Lymphomas of the pancreas, if diagnosed before resection, are usually best treated with chemoradiation.

Development and Molecular Biology

The following three types of genetic abnormalities have been observed in pancreatic cancers: activation of growth-promoting oncogenes, mutations that result in the inactivation of tumor suppressor genes, and excessive expression of growth factors or their receptors.[45] Almost all pancreatic cancers and most of the precursor lesions demonstrate codon 12 mutations of the K-*ras* oncogene. These and other mutations of K-*ras* are believed to be early events in pancreatic tumorigenesis. K-*ras* normally plays a key role in regulating many cellular events, including growth. Its activation is a guanosine triphosphate (GTP)-dependent event, terminated by GTP hydrolysis and dissociation of guanosine diphosphate (GDP). Oncogenic point mutations of K-*ras* interfere with that termination event, and as a result, K-*ras* becomes permanently activated, and a continuous growth signal is transmitted to the nucleus.

Mutation of the *p53* tumor suppressor gene is the most common genetic event in all human cancers, and it is observed in 75% of pancreatic cancers. The gene encodes a 53-kd nuclear phosphoprotein that plays an important role in regulating the cell cycle, DNA synthesis and repair, apoptosis, and cell differentiation. Although mutation of *p53* results in the loss of its function, *p53* mutations alone are not believed to be sufficient to cause malignant transformation. Mutations resulting in the functional loss of other tumor suppressor genes, including *p16, SMAD-4/DPC,* and *DCC,* are also commonly observed in pancreatic cancer. Other much less frequent tumor suppressor gene deletions that have been observed in pancreatic cancers result in the loss of the retinoblastoma gene and the adenomatous polyposis coli (*APC*) gene. DNA mismatch repair genes have also been reported to be mutated and functionally deleted in pancreatic cancers. These genes encode for enzymes that function to repair potentially pathologic DNA changes that occur during DNA replication.

Several growth factor systems are commonly upregulated in pancreatic cancer either by increased expression of their receptors or by increases in the relevant ligands. The most commonly observed changes involve the epidermal growth factor (EGF) receptor family that includes the EGF receptor (which responds to EGF and to transforming growth factor-α) and the HER2, HER3, and HER4 receptors. Overexpression of EGF receptors or its ligands is correlated with tumor invasiveness, enhanced potential for metastasis, and a poorer prognosis. Increased expression of HER2 is associated with a better differentiated phenotype. Other growth factor systems implicated in pancreatic cancer development include those for hepatocyte growth factor and for transforming growth factor-β.

It is now generally believed that pancreatic cancer evolves in a progressive, stepwise fashion, much like that observed for colon cancer. Precursor ductal lesions (see Fig. 55-12) have been identified, and the stepwise progression toward invasive cancer and metastasis has been related to the accumulated presence of multiple genetic abnormalities. K-*ras* mutations and *HER2*/neu overexpression are the earliest changes to occur. Alterations in *p16* are found primarily in PanIN-2 and PanIN-3. *DPC4, BRCA2,* and *p53* are inactivated during the later stages of cancer progression and are found almost exclusively in invasive lesions.

Table 55-2 **Signs and Symptoms of Pancreatic Cancer**

FREQUENT	INFREQUENT
Pancreatic Head Cancers	
Weight loss (92%)	Nausea (37%)
Pain (72%)	Weakness (35%)
Jaundice (82%)	Pruritus (24%)
Dark urine (63%)	Vomiting (37%)
Light stool (62%)	
Anorexia (64%)	
Pancreatic Body or Tail Cancers	
Weight loss (100%)	Jaundice (7%)
Pain (87%)	Dark urine (5%)
Weakness (43%)	Light stool (6%)
Nausea (45%)	Pruritus (4%)
Anorexia (33%)	
Vomiting (37%)	

Hereditary Pancreatic Cancer Syndromes

Pancreatic cancer has been observed to be increased in families with hereditary nonpolyposis colon cancer (HNPCC), those with familial breast cancer (associated with the *BRCA2* mutation), those with Peutz-Jeghers syndrome, those with ataxia-telangiectasia, and those with the familial atypical multiple mole melanoma (FAMMM) syndrome. Patients with hereditary pancreatitis are also at increased risk for developing pancreatic cancer. This is particularly true in those with a paternal pattern of inheritance who may have a 75% risk for developing pancreatic cancer.[46] Even in the absence of one of these familial cancer syndromes or hereditary pancreatitis, individuals with a family history of pancreatic cancer, especially those with two or more pancreatic cancer–affected first-degree relatives, have an increased risk for developing pancreatic cancer.

Symptoms and Signs

Pancreatic cancers are insidious tumors that can be present for long periods and grow extensively before they produce symptoms. The symptoms, once they develop, are determined by the location of the tumor in the pancreas (Table 55-2). Those in the head or uncinate process of the pancreas make their presence known by causing bile duct, duodenal, or pancreatic duct obstruction. Symptoms include unexplained episodes of pancreatitis, painless jaundice, nausea, vomiting, steatorrhea, and unexplained weight loss. With further spread beyond the pancreas, these patients may note upper abdominal or back pain when peripancreatic nerve plexuses are involved and ascites when peritoneal carcinomatosis or portal vein occlusion develops. Patients with tumors arising in the neck, body, or tail of the pancreas usually do not develop jaundice or gastric outlet obstruction. Their symptoms may be limited to unexplained weight loss and vague upper abdominal pain until the tumor has grown extensively and spread beyond the pancreas. New-onset diabetes mellitus is occasionally the first

symptom of an otherwise occult pancreatic cancer. Recent studies have suggested that this form of diabetes may be mediated by a factor released from the tumor that either inhibits insulin release from islets or induces peripheral insulin resistance. Unexplained migratory thrombophlebitis (Trousseau's syndrome) may be associated with pancreatic and other types of malignancy. It is probably a paraneoplastic phenomenon that results from a tumor-induced hypercoagulable state.

The physical findings in patients with pancreatic cancer are also dependent on the location, size, and extent of the tumor. Liver nodules indicative of metastases can sometimes be felt. Metastatic subumbilical ("Sister Mary Joseph node") and pelvic peritoneal ("Blumer's shelf") deposits, as well as left supraclavicular lymphadenopathy ("Virchow's node"), indicate the presence of distant metastases. Malignant ascites, caused by peritoneal carcinomatosis, may also be present. With portal, splenic, or superior mesenteric vein occlusion, mesenteric venous pressures may be increased, and collateral channels, including gastroesophageal varices and caput medusae, may develop. Distal common bile duct obstruction caused by the tumor often leads to bile duct and gallbladder distention. Thus, a palpable gallbladder in a patient with painless jaundice (i.e., Courvoisier's sign) suggests the presence of a periampullary neoplasm.

Blood Tests

Patients with pancreatic head lesions frequently have elevated bilirubin and alkaline phosphatase levels suggestive of obstructive jaundice. Other routine laboratory studies are usually normal. The two most widely used pancreatic cancer serum markers are the CEA and the Lewis blood group carbohydrate antigen CA 19-9. Both are frequently elevated in patients with advanced disease, but unfortunately, the circulating levels of these tumor markers are often normal in patients with early, potentially curable, tumors. Thus, using these tumor markers to screen patients with vague symptoms or those in high-risk groups has not been shown to be useful in detecting early disease. With a cutoff value of 37 U/mL, CA 19-9 has been reported to have a sensitivity of 86% and a specificity of 87%.[47] CA 19-9 can also be elevated in patients with cholangitis and jaundice not caused by pancreatic cancer. Extremely high levels of either CA 19-9 or CEA usually indicate unresectable or metastatic disease.

Imaging Studies

For most patients, the initial imaging study is a transcutaneous ultrasound examination. It may reveal a pancreatic mass and indicate whether that mass is solid or cystic. It can also aid in the diagnosis of jaundiced patients by revealing the presence of extrahepatic ductal dilation in the absence of demonstrable biliary tract stones. Transcutaneous ultrasound, regardless of its findings, is usually followed by helical contrast-enhanced CT, performed in conjunction with IV infusion of contrast material. Timed images are taken to permit visualization of the pancreas during the arterial phase, the parenchymal phase, and finally the venous phase of contrast perfusion. Pancreatic cancer usually appears as a hypodense mass with poorly demarcated edges. It may have a more hypodense center, indicating either central necrosis or cystic change, and the pancreatic duct to the left of the lesion may be dilated. When performed and interpreted by experienced radiologists, CT has a specificity for diagnosing pancreatic tumors of 95% or better. Its sensitivity depends on the size of the tumor, exceeding 95% for tumors larger than 2 cm in diameter. Much, if not all, of the information provided by CT can also be obtained with high-quality MRI. Although the sensitivity and specificity of MRI appear to equal those of CT, CT is currently more widely employed perhaps because it is cheaper, more user friendly, and more easily interpreted by clinicians. Positron emission tomography (PET) may be of value in diagnosing small pancreatic tumors that escape CT or MRI detection, but the sensitivity and specificity of PET scanning remain to be established.

ERCP may be particularly helpful in evaluating patients with obstructive jaundice without a detectable mass on CT or MRI. It can identify stones or other nonmalignant causes of obstructive jaundice, define the location of the bile duct obstruction, identify ampullary and periampullary lesions, and establish the diagnosis of IPMN if mucus is seen extruding through a fish-mouth papillary opening. The finding of superimposable bile duct and pancreatic duct strictures (i.e., the double-duct sign) on ERCP is highly suggestive of a pancreatic head cancer (Fig. 55-13), but benign processes, such as chronic pancreatitis or autoimmune pancreatitis, can also produce a double-duct sign. The role of ERCP in the management of patients with a mass on CT is more controversial. Many surgeons (including me) would argue that ERCP is not helpful because a malignant lesion cannot be entirely excluded by ERCP. Thus, resection is indicated, regardless of the ERCP findings.

Role of Biopsy

Biopsy to confirm the presence and identify the type of cancer is usually required before chemoradiation therapy of unresectable pancreatic tumors or neoadjuvant treatment of resectable tumors. Percutaneous biopsy, performed with either CT or ultrasound guidance, or transduodenal biopsy, performed with endoscopic ultrasound guidance, is routinely employed in these situations. Considerable controversy, however, surrounds the question of whether all patients with potentially resectable tumors should undergo preoperative biopsy. Biopsy might yield false-negative results, and at least theoretically, transcutaneous biopsy could promote intraperitoneal dissemination of the tumor. Performing the biopsy through a transduodenal approach would eliminate the concern of tumor dissemination, but even with this approach, a positive biopsy merely confirms the decision for resection, and a negative biopsy is inconclusive. For these reasons, most surgeons would not recommend routine preoperative biopsy for confirmation of the diagnosis in the management of patients with potentially resectable lesions. However, if this policy of not performing preoperative biopsy is followed, 5% to 10% of patients undergoing resection for suspected cancer will be found to have benign lesions.

Staging of Pancreatic Cancer

The American Joint Committee on Cancer (AJCC) staging system is widely used to stage pancreatic cancer (Table 55-3). This system uses the TNM classification to define the *t*umor extent, *n*odal metastases, and distant *m*etastases.[48] Tis, which denotes in situ cancer, corresponds to PanIN-3, that is, the most advanced of the ductal cancer precursor lesions (see Fig. 55-12). T1 and T2 cancers are confined to the pancreas and are either less than 2 cm or greater than 2 cm in diameter, respectively. T3 and T4 lesions extend beyond the pancreas. T3 lesions are con-

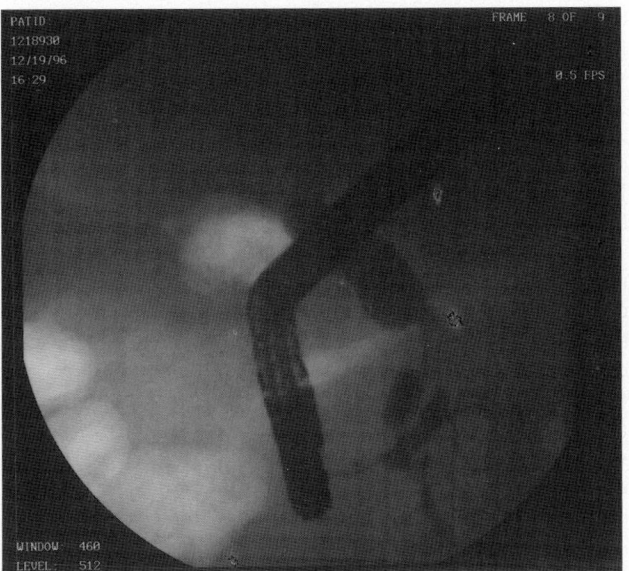

Figure 55-13 Endoscopic retrograde cholangiopancreatography showing double-duct sign. A stent traverses the bile duct stricture. Note closely adjacent bile and pancreatic duct strictures in patient with adenocarcinoma of the pancreatic head.

Table 55-3 American Joint Committee on Cancer: TNM System for Staging of Pancreatic Cancer

STAGE	T STATUS	N STATUS	M STATUS
Stage 0	Tis	N0	M0
Stage IA	T1	N0	M0
Stage IB	T2	N0	M0
Stage IIA	T3	N0	M0
Stage IIB	T1	N1	M0
	T2	N1	M0
	T3	N1	M0
Stage III	T4	Any N	M0
Stage IV	Any T	Any N	M1

Adapted from AJCC Cancer Staging Handbook, 6th ed. New York, Springer, 2002, pp 179-188.

sidered to be potentially resectable because they do not involve the celiac axis or superior mesenteric artery. They may involve the portal or superior mesenteric vein, and resection of the tumor may mandate venous resection and reconstruction. Long-term survival of patients undergoing major venous resection is poor, and it is not clear that those patients actually benefit from resection. T4 lesions are considered to be unresectable because they involve the critical peripancreatic arteries. N1 lesions have positive regional nodes, and M1 lesions have distant metastases, whereas N0 and M0 lesions lack both these features. Distant metastases are common, and they are most frequently located in the liver or lung or on the peritoneal surfaces of the abdomen.

Stage I and II cancers are amenable to resection. Poor prognostic signs include aneuploidy, large tumor size (T2), the presence of positive regional nodes (N1), and an incomplete resection at the pancreatic or retroperitoneal margin. The latter is most closely associated with poor survival. Stages III and IV cancers are considered to be unresectable, either because of distant metastases (stage IV) or because of major arterial involvement (stage III). Mean survival for patients with stage III tumors ranges from 8 to 12 months, whereas that for patients with stage IV tumors is only 3 to 6 months.

Preoperative staging of pancreatic cancers is usually accomplished using one or more of the standard imaging techniques, such as CT, MRI, or ultrasonography. High-resolution helical CT, with phased imaging for visualization of the pancreas and major peripancreatic vessels, is the most widely used method of evaluating tumor resectability. Circumferential encasement, invasion, or occlusion of the portal vein, superior mesenteric vein, or superior mesenteric artery is generally considered to be a sign of unresectability, although strictly speaking, resection is still technically possible if only the venous structures are involved. Partial encasement (i.e., involvement of 30% to 60% of the circumference of the vein) may result in distortion of the vein and the appearance of a teardrop-shaped rather than a round structure. In our experience, this is associated with a low resectability rate.[49]

Other CT changes suggestive of unresectability include extension beyond the pancreatic capsule and into the retroperitoneum, involvement of neural or nodal structures surrounding the origin of either the celiac axis or superior mesenteric artery, and extension of the tumor along the hepatoduodenal ligament. MRI provides information that is similar to that obtained by CT, but combining MRI with CT does not seem to provide additional information. There have been recent claims that endoscopic ultrasound may provide staging information that is superior to that obtained by either CT or MRI[50] because it permits better visualization of nodal structures and allows for determination of the depth of invasion for tumors involving the duodenal wall. Unfortunately, endoscopic ultrasound is operator dependent, and its applicability to preoperative staging is dependent on the locally available expertise. Theoretically, PET scanning might be useful in staging pancreatic cancers by permitting detection of small metastatic lesions that escape detection by standard cross-sectional imaging techniques, but the sensitivity and specificity of PET scans in this setting are not currently known.

Role of Laparoscopy in Staging

The role of staging laparoscopy in the management of pancreatic cancer is controversial. Proponents claim that 20% to 40% of patients believed to have stage I or II disease have unrecognized small metastases to peritoneal surfaces (e.g., diaphragm, liver) and that those metastases can be laparoscopically detected, thus preventing a needless laparotomy. Our own experience indicates that, with high-quality modern imaging techniques, few pancreatic head tumors are deemed unresectable at operation merely because they are found to have metastases that might have been found by laparoscopy. More commonly, unappreciated vascular involvement is the operative finding that prevents resection, and in those patients, benefit can still be provided by performance of bilioenteric, and possibly gastroenteric, bypass. The argument for preliminary laparoscopy would be more compelling in the case of patients with body or tail lesions because, with left-sided lesions, neither obstructive jaundice nor gastric outlet obstruction is likely to develop, and therefore, there is no role for surgical bypass in those patients. For these reasons, it is my practice to perform staging laparoscopy for potentially resectable body or tail lesions. For pancreatic head lesions that are deemed resectable by preoperative routine staging, laparoscopy is not advocated.

Resectional Surgery for Pancreatic Head and Uncinate Process Tumors

Tumors of the head, neck, and uncinate process of the pancreas account for about 70% of pancreatic tumors. They are generally resected by pancreaticoduodenectomy, with or without preservation of the pylorus and proximal duodenum (see Fig. 55-9). The two procedures yield similar survival rates and have similar morbidity. The pylorus-preserving operation is technically easier and faster, but it may be associated with a higher incidence of and more prolonged delayed gastric emptying. Both operations can be performed through a midline, bilateral subcostal, or right subcostal incision.

After a preliminary search for metastases or other reasons to abort resection, the retroperitoneal area behind the pancreatic head, the hepatoduodenal ligament, and the base of the transverse mesocolon must be carefully examined. The finding of involved peripancreatic nodes, even along the cephalad border of the pancreas near the portal vein, does not preclude resection, although it worsens prognosis. A tunnel (the so-called tunnel of love) needs to be developed behind the neck of the pancreas and anterior to the underlying visceral vessels before concluding that the lesion can be resected. After it is deemed resectable, irreversible steps can be taken. The gallbladder is usually removed, and the common bile duct is divided above the duodenum. The proximal gastrointestinal tract is divided at the level of the gastric antrum (standard Whipple) or first part of the duodenum (pylorus-preserving Whipple). The proximal jejunum is divided, and the neck of the pancreas is transected. Finally, the uncinate process of the pancreas is resected from the retroperitoneum along the lateral surface of the superior mesenteric artery, and the specimen is removed. Reconstruction can be accomplished in a variety of ways, but the most common involves a pancreaticojejunostomy (as an end-to-end or end-to-side), an end-to-side hepaticojejunostomy, and then an antecolic end-to-side gastrojejunostomy (standard Whipple) or duodenojejunostomy (pylorus-preserving Whipple) (see Fig. 55-9). Frequently, drains and a feeding jejunal tube are placed, the latter in anticipation of the delayed gastric emptying that frequently occurs, and the abdomen is closed.

Several reports, mostly from Japan, have suggested that extending the Whipple procedure to include an extensive retroperitoneal lymphadenectomy, and in some cases, total pancreatectomy, along with possible major venous resection, can result in increased long-term patient survival. This so-called extended radical pancreaticoduodenectomy is frequently followed by a prolonged delay in the return of gastrointestinal function and, on occasion, with incapacitating and persistent diarrhea. A recent prospective, randomized study in the United States has failed to show a survival benefit for this extended radical operation, and it is rarely performed in the United States.[51]

Complications of Pancreaticoduodenectomy

When performed by experienced surgeons in high-volume centers, the operative mortality rate of pancreaticoduodenectomy is 2% to 4%. Anastomotic leaks, intra-abdominal abscesses, and delayed gastric emptying account for most of the perioperative complications after pancreaticoduodenectomy. Leakage from the pancreatic anastomosis, resulting in a pancreatic fistula, occurs in 15% to 20% of patients. With adequate drainage, these fistulas usually heal within several weeks. Some pancreatic surgeons have claimed that administration of a somatostatin analogue to patients undergoing pancreaticoduodenectomy for cancer could reduce the incidence or duration of pancreatic fistula, but a recent randomized trial addressing this subject concluded that prophylactic administration of a somatostatin analogue in this setting is not beneficial. Biliary fistulas are much less common than pancreatic fistulas after pancreaticoduodenectomy, but they also usually heal if adequate drainage is achieved. Delayed gastric emptying occurs in 15% to 40% of patients and almost always resolves with time. Its occurrence is unpredictable, and it may persist for several weeks or even months. The basis for delayed gastric emptying after pancreaticoduodenectomy is not clear. Some have suggested that it is the result of removing the cells in the duodenum that secrete the promotility hormone motilin. Erythromycin, which has a structure that resembles motilin, acts as an agonist at motilin receptors and has been used to treat these patients. Success has been reported using this approach, but my experience with this use of erythromycin has been disappointing.

The endocrine pancreas has considerable functional reserve and, for that reason, most patients do not develop diabetes after resection of the pancreatic head. In fact, some patients with tumor-induced diabetes may have resolution of their diabetes after resection. In contrast, pancreatic malabsorption and steatorrhea are relatively common long-term problems. They may reflect exocrine secretory insufficiency, an obstruction at the pancreaticjejunal anastomosis, or poor postoperative mixing of secreted enzymes with food. Although distressing, postoperative malabsorption and steatorrhea are rarely incapacitating, but they require exogenously administered pancreatic enzymes.

Results of Pancreaticoduodenectomy for Pancreatic Cancer

Long-term survival, when the operation is performed for ductal adenocarcinoma, is unusual. Five-year survival rates of 15% to 20% have been reported from some centers, but rates of 10% to 15% are more common, and most of those patients who survive for 5 years succumb over the subsequent 5 years. A number of factors affect the survival rate. Perhaps the most influential is the presence or absence of tumor at the resection margin. Negative margins, in one study, were associated with a 26% 5-year survival rate, whereas positive margins were associated with an 8% 5-year survival rate. Extending the resection to a total pancreatectomy or to include more radical retroperitoneal lymph node resection does not appear to increase long-term survival. Other factors that affect long-term survival include tumor diameter, diploid or aneuploid DNA content, and lymph node status. The 5-year survival rate for node-positive patients, in one series, was reported to be 14%, whereas the 5-year survival rate for node-negative patients was 36%.

Resectional Surgery for Pancreatic Body and Tail Tumors

Most body and tail cancers have already metastasized to distant sites or extended locally to involve nodes, nerves, or major vessels by the time of diagnosis. Splenic vein involvement or occlusion is not uncommon and, by itself, is not a sign of nonresectability. On the other hand, involvement of the splenic and superior mesenteric vein confluence generally precludes resection. Resection involves a distal pancreatectomy either with or without concomitant splenectomy. Splenectomy is performed for malignant tumors, but splenic preservation is not contraindicated when benign tumors are being removed. After a thorough search for metastatic disease, the operation starts by dividing the gastrocolic omentum, short gastric vessels, and peritoneal reflections around the body and tail of the pancreas to elevate the spleen and pancreatic tail out of the retroperitoneum. The splenic artery and vein, in that order, are ligated, and the pancreas is transected to the right of the tumor, leaving an uninvolved margin. The resection margin can be either closed with a stapler or imbricated with sutures. Ideally, the transected duct is suture-ligated separately.

Complications of distal pancreatectomy include subphrenic abscess, which may occur in 5% to 10% of patients, and pancreatic duct leak, which has been reported to occur in up to 20% of patients. Both complications can usually be managed nonoperatively by percutaneous drainage, and reoperation is rarely required. Pancreatic duct leak usually results in the formation of a fluid collection that resembles a pseudocyst and that, following drainage, becomes a pancreaticocutaneous fistula. Some surgeons have advocated prophylactic administration of a somatostatin analogue to reduce the incidence or duration of pancreatic fistula after distal pancreatectomy, but there are no convincing data to support this practice. Somatostatin administration frequently reduces the output of these pancreatic fistulas, but it does not appear to alter the time of fistula closure.

Only 10% of cancers involving the tail or body of the pancreas are resectable at the time of diagnosis. The 5-year survival rate for patients who are deemed resectable (8%-14%) is somewhat lower than for patients with resectable cancer of the pancreatic head. Factors affecting long-term survival are similar to those for pancreatic head cancers.

Palliative Nonsurgical Treatment of Pancreatic Cancers

Establishing the diagnosis and relieving symptoms of jaundice, gastric outlet obstruction, and pain are the goals of palliative nonsurgical treatment. Tissue diagnosis can usually be made by CT- or ultrasound-guided percutaneous fine-needle aspiration of either the tumor or its metastases. Transduodenal fine-needle aspiration of the tumor with endoscopic ultrasound guidance and duct cytology obtained by brushings is an alternative method of establishing the diagnosis. Decompression of the obstructed biliary tract can be achieved using either an endoscopic or a percutaneous-transhepatic approach. The former has been shown, in randomized trials, to yield better results with fewer associated complications. At the time of ERCP, a transpapillary stent is placed across the obstructed segment of bile duct.

Either plastic or expandable metal stents can be used, but metal stents give more complete and more long-lasting relief of jaundice. Plastic stents can become obstructed by tumor or debris and, as a result, must be changed every 2 to 3 months. The percutaneous-transhepatic approach to duct decompression is usually reserved for patients in whom, for technical reasons, a stent cannot be placed endoscopically. Pancreatic tumors can extend into and obstruct the duodenum, leading to gastric outlet obstruction. This commonly occurs in the second portion of the duodenum in patients with pancreatic head cancers. Pancreatic body tumors can invade the third or fourth portion of the duodenum and also cause obstruction. Many of these patients can be palliated by endoscopic placement of expandable endoluminal metal stents into the duodenum.[52] For lesions that are not amenable to stents, surgical gastrojejunostomy may be required. Pain, which is a common symptom of pancreatic cancer, is usually caused by tumor invasion of the peripancreatic neural plexus. Most patients can be adequately treated with orally or transcutaneously administered analgesics. Narcotic medications may be required. When or if this fails, percutaneous CT-guided or endoscopic ultrasound-guided celiac plexus block may be helpful.

Palliative Surgical Management of Pancreatic Cancer

Most of the symptoms experienced by patients with unresectable pancreatic cancer can be relieved by nonsurgical means. Surgical palliation is, for the most part, employed for patients who are undergoing laparotomy for anticipated resectable disease and found to be unresectable at the time of surgery. In that situation, biliary tract decompression can be achieved by creating either a cholecystojejunostomy or a choledochojejunostomy. The former is most appropriate for patients with nondilated ducts in whom the cystic duct–common bile duct junction is far from the pancreatic tumor. Choledochojejunostomy, on the other hand, is performed when the tumor is close to or at the cystic duct–common bile duct junction and the bile duct is dilated. Either a loop or a Roux-en-Y segment of jejunum can be used with similar results.

Duodenal obstruction can be managed by creation of a side-to-side gastrojejunostomy in which an antecolic jejunal loop is anastomosed to the posterior wall of the gastric antrum. Duodenal obstruction, even in advanced pancreatic cancer, occurs in less than 25% of patients; therefore, considerable controversy surrounds whether a prophylactic gastrojejunostomy should be performed before the development of gastric outlet obstruction. The issue is further complicated by the fact that a gastrojejunostomy can cause delayed gastric emptying and result in symptoms identical to those experienced by patients with duodenal obstruction. It is my practice to perform gastrojejunostomy selectively (i.e., for patients whose tumor is locally advanced but without distant metastases [stage III lesions]) because these patients have an expected survival time of 8 to 12 months. I would not perform prophylactic gastrojejunostomy in patients with distant metastasis (stage IV lesions) because their expected survival time is only 3 to 6 months and they are less likely to develop duodenal obstruction before death. Palliation of pain can be achieved, intraoperatively, by injecting alcohol into the celiac plexus, and some surgeons routinely perform operative celiac plexus block at the time of surgical palliation. This is usually accomplished by injecting 15 to 20 mL of 50% ethanol into the celiac plexus on either side of the aorta, and in one randomized, prospective trial, this treatment has been reported to reduce postoperative pain and the need for postoperative analgesics in patients with unresectable pancreatic cancers. However, many patients with unresectable pancreatic cancer can be successfully managed with minimal or no narcotic analgesics, and when more severe pain occurs, results similar to those achieved by intraoperative chemical splanchnicectomy can be achieved using a percutaneous approach. For these reasons, many surgeons do not routinely perform intraoperative celiac plexus blocks.

Chemoradiation Therapy

Many different protocols for chemoradiation treatment of recurrent or unresectable pancreatic cancer have been described. The body of literature on this subject is quite large and beyond the scope of this review. For the most part, the best results have been achieved using radiation therapy combined with either 5-fluorouracil or gemcitabine. Patients undergoing resection may also benefit from adjuvant chemoradiation therapy. The frequently quoted Gastrointestinal Tumor Study Group (GITSG) report suggested that the combination of 5-fluorouracil with radiation therapy could increase the 2-year survival rate for patients with tumor-free resection margins from 18% to 43%.[53] This approach, although based on the experience with a very small group of patients, has been generally accepted and is widely employed.

Recently, the European Study Group for Pancreatic Cancer (ESPAC) has reported a different experience.[54] They conducted a large study evaluating adjuvant chemotherapy (5-fluorouracil), radiation therapy, both, or neither. A survival benefit was observed for those undergoing chemotherapy but not for those receiving either radiation therapy alone or combined chemoradiotherapy. Intraoperative radiation therapy, as adjuvant treatment, has been evaluated, but no benefit has been found. Neoadjuvant chemoradiation has also been used for patients believed to have resectable lesions, but good prospective, randomized studies have not been reported. Some have claimed that up to 15% of selected patients with locally advanced lesions deemed to be unresectable can be made resectable by aggressive administration of chemoradiation therapy. Although the specimens ultimately resected in these cases have frequently contained relatively little viable tumor, the long-term benefits achieved by resecting these advanced tumors are not known.

PANCREATIC AND PANCREATICODUODENAL TRAUMA

Three to 12% of patients with severe abdominal trauma have pancreatic injury. On average, these patients have 3.5 other organs injured, and isolated pancreatic injury is uncommon. Roughly two thirds of pancreatic injuries are the result of penetrating trauma, and the remaining one third are due to blunt trauma. Blunt abdominal trauma can cause damage that ranges from a mild contusion to a severe crushing injury. Classically, blunt injury is the result of midline upper abdominal trauma inflicted by objects as diverse as automobile seatbelts and bicycle handlebars. In these cases, the neck and body of the pancreas can be injured as they pass over the vertebral column. The mortality rate for pancreatic trauma is closely related to the nature of the injury. Thus, the mortality rate associated with blunt trauma is 17% to 19%; with stab wounds, it is 3% to 5%; with gunshot wounds, it is 15% to 22%; and with shotgun wounds, it is 46% to 56%.

Diagnosis

Serum amylase levels are elevated in most patients with significant pancreatic trauma, but they are also increased in up to 90% of severe abdominal trauma patients who do not have pancreatic injury. Thus, measurement of amylase at the time of hospital admission is not helpful in identifying those with pancreatic injury. On the other hand, a progressive rise in serum amylase activity is a more specific indicator of pancreatic injury. Contrast-enhanced CT, which is increasingly being used as a screening test in patients with major abdominal trauma, is the most useful noninvasive method of evaluating patients with suspected pancreatic injury, but even high-quality CT examinations may be either falsely negative or falsely positive. Changes suggestive of pancreatic injury include the presence of peripancreatic fluid collections, focal or diffuse enlargement of the gland, parenchymal disruption, and areas of diminished contrast perfusion. Frequently, serial CT examinations are needed because the changes indicative of pancreatic injury may not be present on examinations performed very soon after injury.

Ultimately, the management of pancreatic injuries depends on the presence of pancreatic duct disruption, major associated vascular injury, or significant injury to peripancreatic organs, especially the duodenum. Vascular and duodenal injury can be evaluated at the time of exploratory laparotomy, but the integrity of the pancreatic duct may be difficult to determine at the time of operation unless the pancreas is transected or pancreatic juice is seen to be extravasating from the region of the duct. In the absence of these findings, pancreatography is required to localize or exclude a duct injury. Intraoperative ductography can be performed either transduodenally after duodenotomy or, in a prograde fashion, from the cut end of the duct after resection of the pancreatic tail. Both these approaches are difficult and dangerous because, if the suture line fails, they can result in either a pancreatic or a duodenal fistula. Thus, if the patient is stable and duct injury is suspected, the surgeon needs to consider preoperative ERCP to determine whether the duct is intact. ERCP may have an even more important role in the evaluation of patients managed by delayed exploratory laparotomy after abdominal trauma because, in this setting, delineation of the site and extent of duct injury helps plan a definitive procedure.

Management

The Pancreas Organ Injury Scale,[55] developed by the American Association for the Surgery of Trauma, can be used to grade pancreatic injuries (Box 55-6). Management of pancreatic injuries is determined by the site and grade of that injury. Grade I injuries, which involve minor contusions or lacerations of the gland without duct injury, are treated expectantly. Drainage is usually not needed. On the other hand, grade II injuries, which involve major contusions or lacerations of the gland without duct injury, are traditionally treated by débridement, adequate hemostasis, and placement of sump drains.

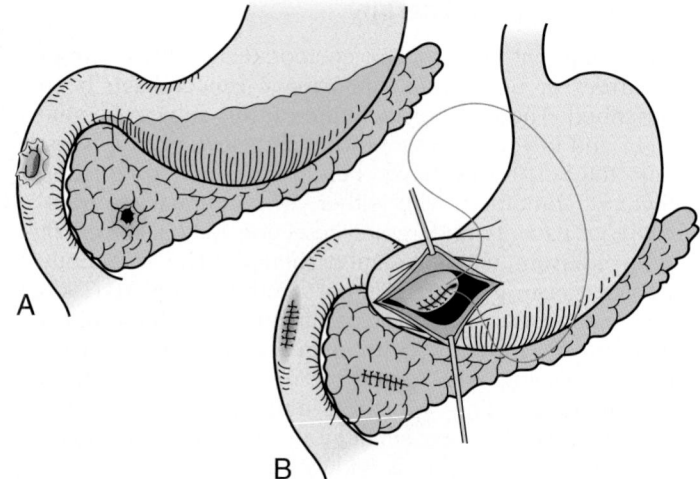

Figure 55-14 Pyloric exclusion with gastrojejunostomy. **A** and **B,** After repairing the duodenal injury, débriding the area of pancreatic injury, and achieving adequate hemostasis, a gastrotomy is performed, and the pylorus is closed with a slowly reabsorbable suture. A gastrojejunostomy is performed, and the area of injury is widely drained. (©1978 Baylor College of Medicine.)

Some surgeons advocate repairing the disrupted capsule and placing an omental patch into areas of devitalized parenchyma. Transection of the neck, body, or tail of the pancreas or parenchymal injury to those areas accompanied by duct injury is considered a grade III injury. The critical feature of these injuries is violation of the major pancreatic duct. Preoperative ERCP in stable patients may identify the presence and location of the duct injury in some patients, but because most patients are not stable enough to undergo preoperative ERCP, the status of the duct is uncertain at the time of operation. Occasionally, in such patients, the intraoperative finding of a transected gland, fat necrosis, or extravasation of clear fluid from the region of the duct establishes the presence of a duct injury. The classic treatment of grade III injuries involves resection of the pancreas to the left of the injury along with splenectomy. Because of the fear of overwhelming postsplenectomy sepsis, splenic conservation might be considered for children with grade III injuries. When the location of a grade III injury is to the right of the pancreatic neck, the surgeon needs to consider débriding the site of injury and conserving, rather than resecting, the uninjured body and tail by anastomosing it to a Roux-en-Y jejunal limb.

Grade IV and V injuries present the greatest surgical challenge because they involve the head of the pancreas and, in addition, usually involve the adjacent duodenum or papilla of Vater. Because of their location, grade IV and V injuries are also most likely to involve major adjacent vascular structures. The initial goal in managing these multiply injured patients is that of obtaining hemostasis, minimizing contamination by repairing torn bowel, and repairing associated injuries. In unstable patients and in those with major associated injuries, this damage control approach may be all that is done at the initial operation, and definitive repair may be postponed until the patient's condition has improved. On the other hand, some patients may require emergent pancreaticoduodenectomy as the initial procedure if they have uncontrollable hemorrhage from the head of the pancreas, injury

to adjacent major vessels that can only be controlled by removing the pancreatic head, or devitalization of the duodenal C loop and pancreatic head.

Short of radical resection, however, other options designed to divert gastric, pancreatic, and biliary secretions away from the duodenum need to be considered for the management of patients with grade IV and V injuries. These include duodenal diverticularization, pyloric exclusion or gastrojejunostomy, and triple-tube decompression. Duodenal diverticularization is accomplished by performing antrectomy and gastrojejunostomy to achieve gastric diversion, choledochostomy to divert bile if the ampulla is injured, tube duodenostomy for decompression of the duodenum, suture repair of any duodenal injuries, and extensive periduodenal and peripancreatic drainage. Pyloric exclusion with gastrojejunostomy (Fig. 55-14) is a simpler method of protecting the injured duodenum, and it does not permanently alter function.[56] Through a gastrotomy, the pylorus is closed with a purse-string suture, and an antecolic gastrojejunostomy is performed at the site of the gastrotomy. As with duodenal diverticularization, duodenal injuries are closed, and the area is extensively débrided. Use of a slowly absorbable suture for pyloric closure results in diversion of gastric secretions from the duodenum for about 2 to 3 weeks, but after 21 days (i.e., dissolution of the suture), more than 90% of patients are found to have a patent and functioning pylorus. Triple-tube decompression involves placement of a gastrostomy tube for drainage of the stomach, drainage of the duodenum through a tube passed retrogradely through a jejunostomy, and antegrade passage of a jejunostomy tube for provision of enteral nutrition. The rapidity and ease of this procedure make it an attractive choice, but subsequent dislodgment of the duodenal tube or inadequate diversion provided by the gastrostomy tube may limit its effectiveness.

Delayed Complications

The major delayed complications of severe pancreatic injuries involve the development of sterile or infected pseudocysts or other fluid collections and the ultimate development of a pancreatic duct stricture at a site of duct injury or transection. Classically, the duct stricture usually develops in the portion of the pancreas that overlies the spinal column. In many patients, the initial injury may go undetected, and even the trauma itself may be forgotten until the patient returns months or years later with recurrent episodes of obstructive chronic pancreatitis involving the pancreatic tail but sparing the pancreatic head. Management involves distal pancreatectomy.

Annotated References

Bradley EL III: A clinically based classification system for acute pancreatitis: Summary of the International Symposium on Acute Pancreatitis. Atlanta, GA, September 11-13, 1992. Arch Surg 128:586-590, 1993.

A conference summary article that outlines the definitions of terms currently used to describe the complications of pancreatitis.

Burch JM, Moore EE: Duodenal and pancreatic trauma. In Taylor MB, Gollan JL, Steer ML, Wolfe MM (eds): Gastrointestinal Emergencies. Baltimore, Williams & Wilkins, 1997, pp 995-1001.

A review of current surgical treatment for pancreatic and duodenal injuries.

Case RM: Pancreatic exocrine secretion mechanisms and control. In Beger HG, Warshaw AW, Buchler MW, et al (eds): The Pancreas. Oxford, Blackwell Science, 1998, pp 63-100.

An up-to-date summary of current concepts regarding the physiology of pancreatic exocrine secretion.

Chey WY, Chang TM: Neural hormonal regulation of exocrine pancreatic secretion. Pancreatology 1:320-335, 2001.

An up-to-date review of pancreatic exocrine physiology.

Hruban RH, Adsay NV, Albores-Saavedra J, et al: Pancreatic intraepithelial neoplasia: A new nomenclature and classification system for pancreatic duct lesions. Am J Surg Pathol 25:579-586, 2001.

A detailed description of criteria used to define ductal cancer precursor lesions in the pancreas.

Keith RG: Surgical management of chronic pancreatitis. World J Surg 27:1171-1274, 2003.

An issue of World Journal of Surgery that summarizes current surgical management of chronic pancreatitis and its complications.

Kloppel G, Kosmahl M: Cystic lesions and neoplasms of the pancreas: The features are becoming clearer. Pancreatology 1:648-655, 2001.

A review of cystic exocrine pancreatic lesions that focuses on their pathology and growth characteristics.

Opie EL: The etiology of acute hemorrhagic pancreatitis. Bull Johns Hopkins Hosp 12:182-192, 1901.

The classic paper by Opie that led to the common channel theory as an explanation for gallstone pancreatitis.

Skandalakis LJ, Rowe JS Jr, Gray SW, et al: Surgical embryology and anatomy of the pancreas. Surg Clin North Am 73:661-697, 1993.

A comprehensive overview of embryology and anatomy focused on issues relevant to pancreatic disease and pancreatic surgery.

Steer ML: The early intra-acinar cell events which occur during acute pancreatitis: The Frank Brooks Memorial Lecture. Pancreas 17:31-37, 1998.

A summary of recent experimental data defining the early events that occur within pancreatic acinar cells and that ultimately lead to pancreatitis.

Steer ML, Waxman I, Freedman S: Chronic pancreatitis. N Engl J Med 332:1482-1490, 1995.

A review of current concepts regarding the pathophysiology, diagnosis, and treatment of chronic pancreatitis.

Whipple AO, Parsons WB, Mullens CR: Treatment of carcinoma of the ampulla of Vater. Ann Surg 102:763-769, 1935.

The first successful two-stage radical pancreaticoduodenectomy for periampullary carcinoma.

Yeo CJ, Cameron JL, Lillemoe KD, et al: Pancreaticoduodenectomy with or without distal gastrectomy and extended retroperitoneal lymphadenectomy for periampullary adenocarcinoma. II. Randomized controlled trial evaluating survival, morbidity, and mortality. Ann Surg 236:355-368, 2002.

Randomized, prospective trial of conventional Whipple resection versus extended Whipple resection for pancreatic cancer showing no benefit of the more radical procedure.

References

1. Steer ML: Pancreas divisum and pancreatitis: Implications and rationale for treatment. In Beger HG, Buchler M, Ditschuneit H, Malfertheiner P (eds): Chronic Pancreatitis. New York, Springer-Verlag, 1990, pp 245-252.
2. Palade G: Intracellular aspects of the process of protein secretion. Science 189:347-358, 1975.
3. Kornfeld S: Trafficking of lysosomal enzymes in normal and disease states. J Clin Invest 77:1-6, 1986.
4. Owyang C, Logsdon CD: New insights into neurohumoral regulation of pancreatic secretion. Gastroenterology 127:957-964, 2004.
5. Case RM, Argent BE: Pancreatic duct cell secretion: Control and mechanisms of transport. In Go VLW, DiMagno EP, Gardner JD, et al (eds): The Pancreas: Biology, Pathobiology, and Disease, 2nd ed. New York, Raven Press, 1993, pp 301-350.
6. Case RM: Pancreatic exocrine secretion: Mechanisms and control. In Beger HG, Warshaw AW, Buchler MW, et al (eds): The Pancreas. Oxford, Blackwell Science, 1998, pp 63-100.
7. Opie EL: The etiology of acute hemorrhagic pancreatitis. Bull Johns Hopkins Hosp 12:182-192, 1901.
8. Lerch MM, Saluja AK, Runzi M, et al: Pancreatic duct obstruction triggers acute necrotizing pancreatitis in the opossum. Gastroenterology 104:853-861, 1993.

9. Kloppel G: Progression from acute to chronic pancreatitis: A pathologist's view. Surg Clin North Am 79:801-814, 1999.

10. Lowenfels AB, Maisonneuve P, Whitcomb DC: Risk factors for cancer in hereditary pancreatitis. International Hereditary Pancreatitis Study Group. Med Clin North Am 84:565-573, 2000.

11. Hamano H, Kawa S, Horiuchi A, et al: High serum IgG4 concentrations in patients with sclerosing pancreatitis. N Engl J Med 344:732-738, 2001.

12. Steer ML: The early intra-acinar cell events which occur during acute pancreatitis: The Frank Brooks Memorial Lecture. Pancreas 17:31-37, 1998.

13. Foitzik T, Bassi DG, Schmidt J, et al: Intravenous contrast medium accentuates the severity of acute necrotizing pancreatitis in the rat. Gastroenterology 106:207-214, 1994.

14. Kaiser AM, Grady T, Gerdes D, et al: Intravenous contrast medium does not increase the severity of acute necrotizing pancreatitis in the opossum. Dig Dis Sci 40:1547-1553, 1995.

15. Ranson JHC, Rifkind KM, Roses DF, et al: Prognostic signs and the role of operative management in acute pancreatitis. Surg Gynecol Obstet 139:69-81, 1974.

16. Imrie CW, Benjamin IS, Ferguson JC, et al: A single-centre double-blind trial of Trasylol therapy in primary acute pancreatitis. Br J Surg 65:337-341, 1978.

17. Balthazar EJ: Acute pancreatitis: Assessment of severity with clinical and CT evaluation. Radiology 223:603-613, 2002.

18. Khan AA, Parekh D, Young C, et al: Improved prediction of outcome in patients with severe acute pancreatitis by the APACHE II score at 48 hours after hospital admission compared with the APACHE II score at admission. Arch Surg 137:1136-1140, 2002.

19. UK guidelines for the management of acute pancreatitis. Working Party of the British Society of Gastroenterology, Association of Surgeons of Great Britain and Ireland, Pancreatic Society of Great Britain and Ireland, Association of Upper GI Surgeons of Great Britain and Ireland. Gut 54(Suppl 3):1-9, 2005.

20. Golub R, Siddiqi F, Pohl D: Role of antibiotics in acute pancreatitis: A meta-analysis. J Gastrointest Surg 2:496-503, 1998.

21. Isenmann R, Runzi M, Kron M, et al: Prophylactic antibiotic treatment in patients with predicted severe acute pancreatitis: A placebo-controlled, double-blind trial. Gastroenterology 126:997-1004, 2004.

22. Eatock FC, Chong P, Menezes N, et al: A randomized study of early nasogastric versus nasojejunal feeding in severe acute pancreatitis. Am J Gastroenterol 100:432-439, 2005.

23. Modena, JT, Cevasco LB, Basto CA, et al: Total enteral nutrition as prophylactic therapy for pancreatic necrosis infection in severe acute pancreatitis. Pancreatology 6:58-64, 2006.

24. Mark PE, Zaloga GP: Meta-analysis of parenteral nutrition versus enteral nutrition in patients with acute pancreatitis. BMJ 328:1407-1412, 2004.

25. Neoptolemos JP, Carr-Locke DL, London NJ, et al: Controlled trial of urgent endoscopic retrograde cholangiopancreatography and endoscopic sphincterotomy versus conservative treatment for acute pancreatitis due to gallstones. Lancet 2:979-983, 1988.

26. Folsch OR, Nitsche R, Ludtke R, et al: Early ERCP and papillotomy compared with conservative treatment for acute biliary pancreatitis. The German Study Group on Acute Biliary Pancreatitis. N Engl J Med 336:237-242, 1997.

27. Fan ST, Lai CS, Mok FPT, et al: Early treatment of acute biliary pancreatitis by endoscopic papillotomy. N Engl J Med 328:228-232, 1993.

28. Vazquez-Iglesias JL, Gonzalez-Conde B, Lopez-Roses L, et al: Endoscopic sphincterotomy for prevention of the recurrence of acute biliary pancreatitis in patients with gallbladder in situ: Long-term follow-up of 88 patients. Surg Endosc 18:1442-1446, 2004.

29. Bradley EL: A clinically based classification system for acute pancreatitis: Summary of the International Symposium on Acute Pancreatitis. Atlanta, GA, September 11-13, 1992. Arch Surg 128:586-590, 1993.

30. Gerzof SG, Banks PA, Robbins AH, et al: Early diagnosis of pancreatic infection by computed tomography–guided aspiration. Gastroenterology 93:1315-1320, 1987.

31. Vege SS, Baron TH: Management of pancreatic necrosis in severe acute pancreatitis. Clin Gastroenterol Hepatol 3:192-196, 2005.

32. Runzi M, Layer P: Nonsurgical management of acute pancreatitis: Use of antibiotics. Surg Clin North Am 79:759-765, 1999.

33. Chowdhury RS, Forsmark CE: Pancreatic function testing. Aliment Pharmacol Ther 17:733-750, 2003.

34. Ammann RW, Muellhaupt B: The natural history of pain in alcoholic chronic pancreatitis. Gastroenterology 116:1252-1257, 1999.

35. Toskes PP: Medical management of chronic pancreatitis. Scand J Gastroenterol Suppl 208:74-80, 1995.

36. Bradley EL: Nerve blocks and neuroablative surgery for chronic pancreatitis. World J Surg 27:1241-1248, 2003.

37. Partington PF, Rochelle EL: Modified Puestow procedure for retrograde drainage of pancreatic duct. Ann Surg 152:1037-1043, 1960.

38. Ho HS, Frey CF: The Frey procedure: Local resection of pancreatic head combined with lateral pancreaticojejunostomy. Arch Surg 136:1353-1358, 2001.

39. Traverso LW, Longmire WP: Preservation of the pylorus during pancreaticoduodenectomy. Surg Gynecol Obstet 146:959-962, 1978.

40. Beger HG, Schlosser W, Friess H, et al: Duodenum-preserving head resection in chronic pancreatitis changes the normal course of the disease: Single-center 26-year experience. Ann Surg 230:512-519, 1999.

41. Ahmad SA, Lowy AM, Wray CJ, et al: Factors associated with insulin and narcotic independence after islet autotransplantation in patients with severe chronic pancreatitis. J Am Coll Surg 201:680-687, 2005.

42. Tanaka M, Chari S, Adsay V, et al: International consensus guidelines for management of intraductal papillary mucinous neoplasms and mucinous cystic neoplasms of the pancreas. Pancreatology 6:17-32, 2006.

43. Hruban RH, Adsay V, Albores-Saavedra J, et al: Pancreatic intraepithelial neoplasia: A new nomenclature and classification system for pancreatic duct lesions. Am J Surg Pathol 25:579-586, 2001.

44. Brugge WR, Lewandrowski K, Lee-Lewandrowski E, et al: Diagnosis of pancreatic cystic neoplasms: A report of the cooperative pancreatic cyst study. Gastroenterology 126:1330-1336, 2004.

45. McCormick CSF, Lemoine NR: Molecular biological events in the development of pancreatic cancer. In Beger HG, Warshaw AL, Buchler MW, et al (eds): The Pancreas. Oxford, Blackwell Science, 1998, pp 907-921.

46. Lowenfels AB, Maisonneuve P, Whitcomb DC: Risk factors for cancer in hereditary pancreatitis. International Hereditary Pancreatitis Study Group. Med Clin North Am 84:565-573, 2000.

47. Safi F, Schlosser W, Falkenreck S, et al: Ca 19-9 serum course and prognosis of pancreatic cancer. Int J Pancreatol 20:155-162, 1996.

48. AJCC Cancer Staging Handbook, 6th ed. New York, Springer, 2002, pp 179-188.

49. Saldinger PF, Reilly M, Reynolds K, et al: Is CT angiography sufficient for prediction of resectability of periampullary neoplasms. J Gastrointest Surg 4:233-237, 2000.

50. Wiersema MJ: Accuracy of endoscopic ultrasound in diagnosing and staging pancreatic carcinoma. Pancreatology 1:625-632, 2001.

51. Yeo CJ, Cameron JL, Lillemoe KD, et al: Pancreaticoduodenectomy with or without distal gastrectomy and extended retroperitoneal lymphadenectomy for periampullary adenocarcinoma. II. Randomized controlled trial evaluating survival, morbidity, and mortality. Ann Surg 236:355-368, 2002.

52. Adler DG, Baron TH: Endoscopic palliation of malignant gastric outlet obstruction using self-expanding metal stents: Experience in 36 patients. Am J Gastroenterol 97:72-80, 2002.

53. Kalser NH, Ellenberg SS: Pancreatic cancer: Adjuvant combined radiation and chemotherapy following curative resection. Arch Surg 120:899-903, 1985.

54. Neoptolemos JP, Stocken DD, Friess H, et al: A randomized trial of chemoradiotherapy and chemotherapy after resection of pancreatic cancer. N Engl J Med 350:1200-1210, 2004.

55. Moore EE, Cogbill TH, Malangoni MA, et al: Organ injury scaling. II. Pancreas, duodenum, small bowel, colon, and rectum. J Trauma 30:1427-1429, 1990.

56. Burch JM, Moore EE: Duodenal and pancreatic trauma. In Taylor MB, Gollan JL, Steer ML, Wolfe MM (eds): Gastrointestinal Emergencies. Baltimore, Williams & Wilkins, 1997, pp 995-1001.

The Spleen

R. Daniel Beauchamp, MD   Michael D. Holzman, MD, MPH
Timothy C. Fabian, MD   and   Jordan A. Weinberg, MD

SPLENIC ANATOMY

The spleen develops from mesenchymal cells in the dorsal mesogastrium during the fifth week of gestation. The spleen is located in the posterior left upper quadrant of the abdomen. The convex smooth surface of the spleen faces superiorly, posteriorly, and to the left in relation to the abdominal surface of the diaphragm. The diaphragm separates the spleen from the pleura, the left lower lobe of the lung, and the adjacent 9th, 10th, and 11th ribs. The costodiaphragmatic recess of the pleura extends down as far as the inferior border of the normal-sized spleen. The normal size and weight vary somewhat; in adults, the approximate size of the spleen is 12 cm in length, 7 cm in width, and 3 to 4 cm in thickness. The average spleen weight in an adult is 150 g, with a range of 80 to 300 g.

The visceral relationships of the spleen are with the proximal greater curvature of the stomach, the tail of the pancreas, the left kidney, and the splenic flexure of the colon (Fig. 56-1). The parietal peritoneum adheres firmly to the splenic capsule, except at the splenic hilum. The peritoneum extends superiorly, laterally, and inferiorly, creating folds, which form the suspensory ligaments of the spleen. The splenophrenic and splenocolic ligaments are usually relatively avascular. The splenorenal ligament extends from the anterior left kidney to the hilum of the spleen as a two-layered fold in which the splenic vessels and the tail of the pancreas are invested. These two layers continue anteriorly and superiorly to the greater curvature of the stomach to form the two leaves of the gastrosplenic ligament through which the short gastric arteries and veins course.

A fibroelastic capsule commonly known as the splenic capsule invests the organ, and from it trabeculae pass into the parenchyma, branching to form a trabecular network that subdivides the organ into small compartments.

The splenic artery is a tortuous vessel that arises from the celiac trunk; it courses along the superior border of the pancreas (Fig. 56-2). The branches of the splenic artery include the numerous pancreatic branches, the short gastric arteries, the left gastroepiploic artery, and the terminal splenic branches. The splenic artery divides into several branches within the splenorenal ligament before entering the splenic hilum, where they branch again into these trabeculae as they enter the splenic pulp. Small arteriolar branches leave the trabeculae, and their adventitial coat becomes replaced by a sheath of lymphatic tissue that accompanies the vessels and their branches until they divide into capillaries. It is these lymphatic sheaths that make up the white pulp of the spleen and that are interspersed along the arteriolar vessels as lymphatic follicles. The interface between the white pulp and the red pulp is known as the *marginal zone*. As the arterioles lose their sheaths of lymphatic

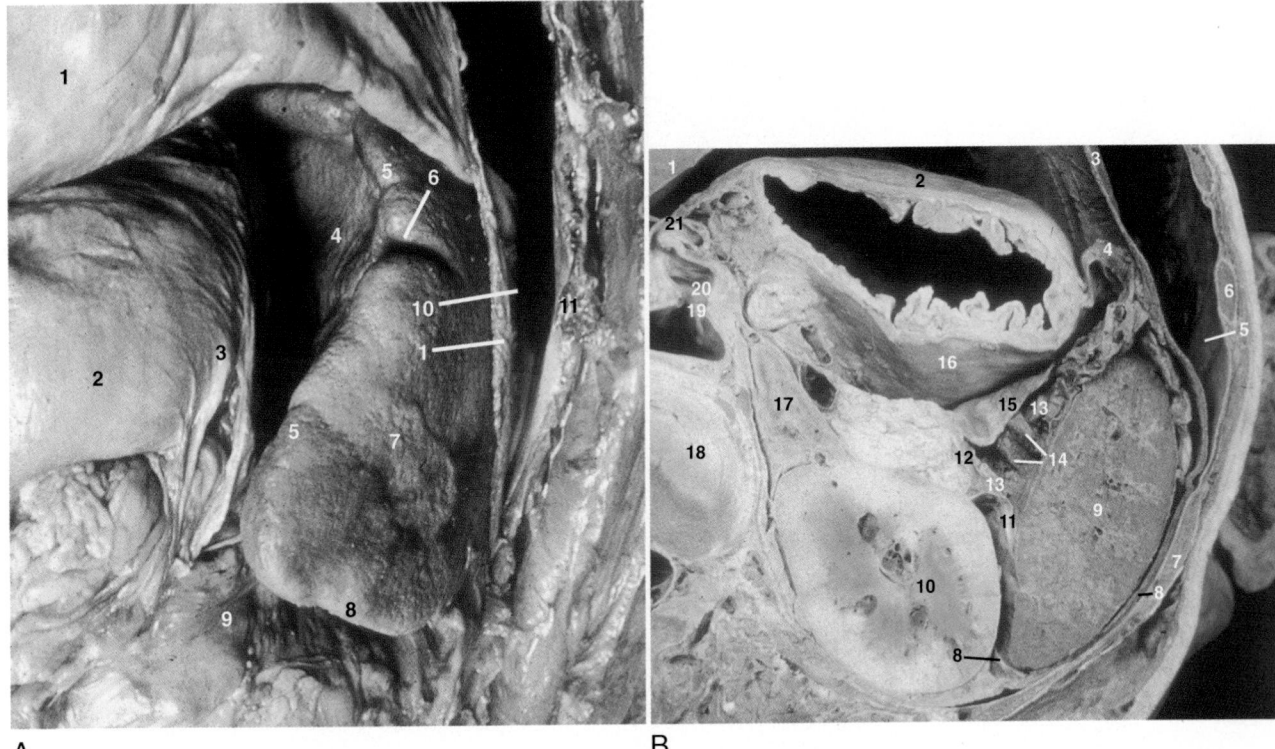

A

B

Figure 56-1 A, Spleen, from the front: (1) diaphragm, (2) stomach, (3) gastrosplenic ligament, (4) gastric impression, (5) superior border, (6) notch, (7) diaphragmatic surface, (8) inferior border, (9) left colic flexure, (10) costodiaphragmatic recess, (11) thoracic wall. The left upper abdominal and lower anterior thoracic walls have been removed and part of the diaphragm (1) turned upward to show the spleen in its normal position, lying adjacent to the stomach (2) and colon (9), with the lower part against the kidney (part B, 9 and 10). **B,** Spleen, in a transverse section of the left upper abdomen: (1) left lobe of liver, (2) stomach, (3) diaphragm, (4) gastrosplenic ligament, (5) costodiaphragmatic recess of pleura, (6) 9th rib, (7) 10th rib, (8) peritoneum of greater sac, (9) spleen, (10) left kidney, (11) posterior layer of lienorenal ligament, (12) tail of pancreas, (13) splenic artery, (14) splenic vein, (15) anterior layer of lienorenal ligament, (16) lesser sac, (17) left suprarenal gland, (18) intervertebral disk, (19) abdominal aorta, (20) celiac trunk, (21) left gastric artery. The section is at the level of the disk (18) between the 12th thoracic and 1st lumbar vertebrae and is viewed from below looking toward the thorax. The spleen (9) lies against the diaphragm (3) and left kidney (10) but separated from them by peritoneum of the greater sac (8). The peritoneum behind the stomach (2) forming part of the gastrosplenic (4) and ileorenal (15) ligaments belongs to the lesser sac (16). (From McMinn RMH, Hutchings RT, Pegington J, Abrahams PH: Color Atlas of Human Anatomy, 3rd ed. St Louis, Mosby-Year Book, 1993, pp 230-231.)

tissue, they traverse the marginal zone and enter the red pulp, which is composed of large branching, thin-walled blood vessels called *splenic sinuses* and *sinusoids,* and thin plates of cellular tissue composing the splenic cords.

The venous sinusoids empty into the veins of the red pulp, and these veins drain back along the trabecular veins that empty into at least five major tributaries, ultimately joining to form the splenic vein in the splenorenal ligament. The splenic vein runs inferior to the artery and posterior to the pancreatic tail and body. It receives several short tributaries from the pancreas. The splenic vein joins the superior mesenteric vein at a right angle behind the neck of the pancreas to form the portal vein. The inferior mesenteric vein often empties into the splenic vein; it may also empty into the superior mesenteric vein at or near the confluence of the splenic vein and superior mesenteric vein.

SPLENIC FUNCTION

The spleen has important hematopoietic functions during early fetal development, with both red and white blood cell production. By the fifth month of gestation, the bone marrow assumes the predominant role in hematopoiesis, and normally there is no significant hematopoietic function left in the spleen. Under certain pathologic conditions, however, such as myelodysplasia, the spleen can reacquire its hematopoietic function. Removal of the spleen does not usually result in anemia or leukopenia in an otherwise healthy person. Although the hematopoietic function is usually lost during fetal development, the spleen continues to function as a sophisticated filter because of the unique circulatory system and lymphoid organization, and it has blood cell monitoring and management functions as well as important immune functions throughout life.

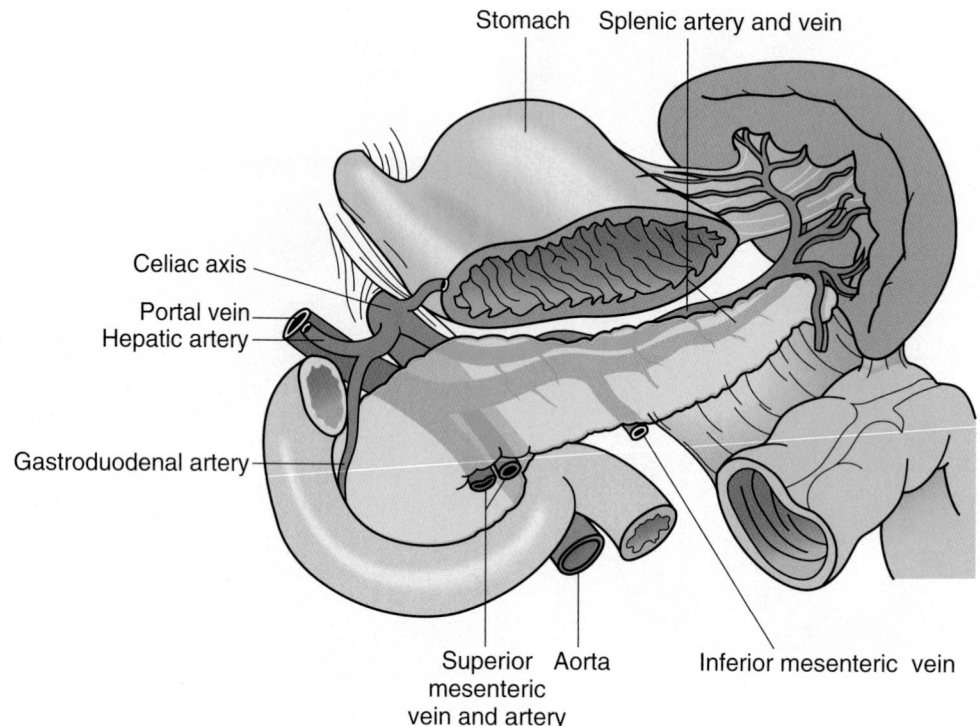

Figure 56-2 **The anatomic relationships of the splenic vasculature.** (From Economou SG, Economou TS: Atlas of Surgical Techniques. Philadelphia, WB Saunders, 1966, p 562.)

The functions of the spleen are closely linked to splenic structure and its unique circulatory system. The arteries flow through the white pulp (lymphoid tissues), after which part of the blood flow goes directly through endothelial cell–lined capillaries into the venous system ("closed" theory). Most of the blood flow, however, enters the macrophage-lined reticular meshwork, and the blood flows slowly back to the venous circulation through the venous sinuses ("open" theory). The formed blood elements must pass through slits in the lining of the venous sinuses; if they cannot pass, they are trapped in the spleen and ingested by splenic phagocytes (Fig. 56-3). Experimental animal studies have demonstrated that an intact splenic arterial system is necessary for optimal control of infection. Removal of the spleen results in loss of both the immunologic and filtering functions.

The most important function of the spleen is probably its mechanical filtration, which removes senescent erythrocytes and likely contributes to control of infection. The spleen is important in clearing circulating pathogens that reside within erythrocytes, for example, malarial parasites, or bacteria such as *Bartonella* species. Mechanical filtration by the spleen may also be important for removal of unopsonized, noningested bacteria from the circulation. It may be particularly important for clearing microorganisms for which the host has no specific antibody.

Splenic filtering function is important for maintaining normal erythrocyte morphology and function. Normal red blood cells are biconcave and deform relatively easily to facilitate both passage through the microvasculature and optimal oxygen and carbon dioxide exchange. The spleen is an important site for the processing of immature erythrocytes and for repair or destruction of deformed or aged erythrocytes. As immature red blood cells pass through the spleen, they may undergo several types of repair, including removal of nuclei and excessive cell membrane from immature cells to convert them from a spherical nucleated to a biconcave anucleated mature morphology. Erythrocytes may also undergo repair by having surface abnormalities such as pits or spurs removed. In the asplenic condition, there are several characteristic alterations in the morphologic appearance of the peripheral red blood cells, with the presence of target cells (immature cells), Howell-Jolly bodies (nuclear remnant), Heinz bodies (denatured hemoglobin), Pappenheimer bodies (iron granules), stippling, and spur cells. Aged red blood cells (120 days) that have lost enzymatic activity and membrane plasticity are trapped and destroyed in the spleen (Table 56-1).

The filtering function of the spleen is also an important factor in anemic conditions associated with abnormal red blood cell morphology. Abnormal erythrocytes that result from hereditary spherocytosis, sickle cell anemia, thalassemia, or pyruvate kinase deficiency are trapped by the splenic filtering mechanism, resulting in worsening anemia, symptomatic splenomegaly, and occasionally splenic infarction. In autoimmune hemolytic anemia, immunoglobulin G (IgG) bound to the cell membrane targets the red blood cells for splenic destruction by splenic macrophages. A similar IgG-dependent mechanism is involved in splenic platelet destruction in immune thrombocytopenic purpura (ITP).

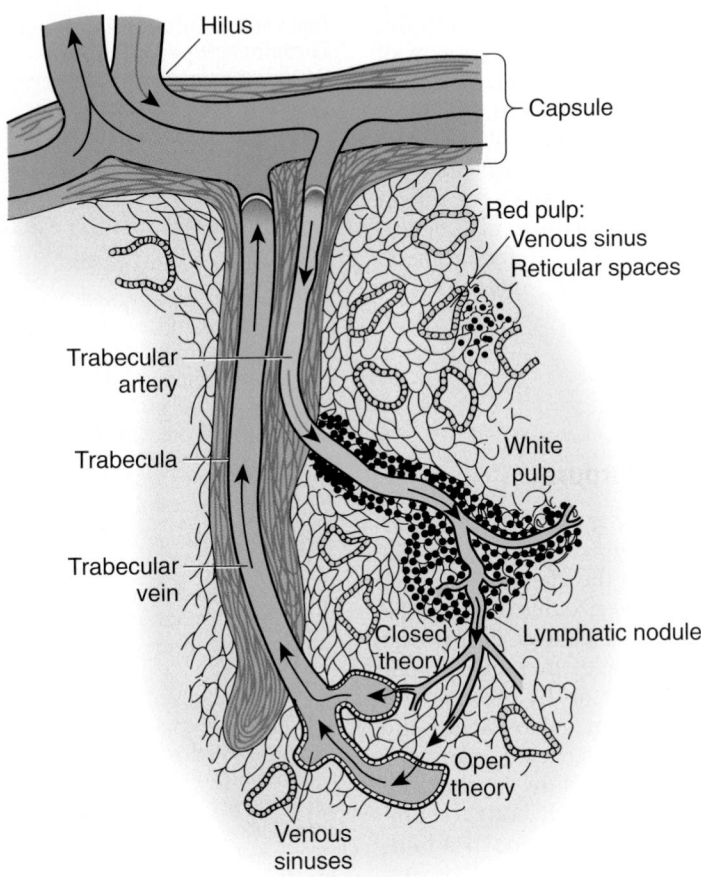

Figure 56-3 Structure of the sinusoidal spleen shows the open and closed blood flow routes. (From Bellanti JA: Immunology: Basic Processes. Philadelphia, WB Saunders, 1979.)

Table 56-1 Biologic Substances Removed by the Spleen

Normal Subjects
Red blood cell membrane
Red blood cell surface pits and craters
Howell-Jolly bodies
Heinz bodies
Pappenheimer bodies
Acanthocytes
Senescent red blood cells
Particulate antigen

Patients With Disease
Spherocytes (hereditary spherocytosis)
Sickle cells, hemoglobin C cells
Antibody-coated red blood cells
Antibody-coated platelets
Antibody-coated white blood cells

Modified from Eichner ER: Splenic function: Normal, too much and too little. Am J Med 66:311, 1979.

Another major function of the spleen is the maintenance of normal immune function and host defenses against certain types of infectious agents. It is well established that people lacking a spleen are at a significantly higher risk for overwhelming postsplenectomy infection (OPSI) with fulminant bacteremia, pneumonia, or meningitis, as compared with those with normal splenic function. Major pathogens in OPSI are organisms such as *Streptococcus pneumoniae,* in which polysaccharide capsules requiring both antibody and complement are important in host defense against these organisms. Asplenic subjects have defective activation of complement by the alternative pathway, leaving them more susceptible to infection.

Asplenic patients have a normal response to reimmunization to an antigen first encountered before splenectomy but do not have an optimal response to new antigen exposure, especially if the antigen is administered intravenously (IV). For organisms such as the encapsulated bacteria, much higher quantities of antibody are necessary for effective clearance. The spleen, with its specialized circulatory system and large supply of macrophages that are capable of ingestion of organisms not optimally opsonized with antibody, greatly enhances their clearance. Asplenic subjects have been found to have subnormal IgM levels, and their peripheral blood mononuclear cells exhibit a suppressed immunoglobulin response.

The spleen is a major site of production for the opsonins properdin and tuftsin, and removal of the spleen results in decreased serum levels of these factors.

Properdin can initiate the alternative pathway of complement activation to produce destruction of bacteria as well as foreign and abnormal cells. Tuftsin is a tetrapeptide that enhances the phagocytic activity of both polymorphonuclear leukocytes and mononuclear phagocytes. The spleen is the major site of cleavage of tuftsin from the heavy chain of IgG, and circulating levels of tuftsin are suppressed in asplenic subjects. Neutrophil function is decreased in asplenic patients, and the defect appears to result from the absence of a circulating mediator.

SPLENECTOMY FOR BENIGN HEMATOLOGIC CONDITIONS

Immune Thrombocytopenic Purpura

Immune thrombocytopenic purpura is also referred to as *idiopathic thrombocytopenic purpura*. A low platelet count, a normal bone marrow, and the absence of other causes of thrombocytopenia characterize this disease. ITP is principally a disorder of increased platelet destruction mediated by autoantibodies to platelet membrane antigens that results in platelet phagocytosis by the reticuloendothelial system. Bone marrow megakaryocytes are present in normal or sometimes increased numbers; however, there is relative marrow failure in that the marrow does not increase production sufficiently to compensate for platelet destruction in the spleen. In adults, ITP is more common in young women than men. Seventy-two percent of patients older than 10 years of age are women, and 70% of affected women are younger than 40 years of age. In children, ITP is manifested somewhat differently. It affects both sexes equally, and its onset is typically abrupt, with severe thrombocytopenia; however, spontaneous permanent remissions are the rule, occurring in about 80% of affected children. Children who develop the chronic thrombocytopenia are usually girls older than 10 years of age and present with a longer history of purpura.

Patients with ITP often present with a history of purpura, epistaxis, and gingival bleeding. Hematuria and gastrointestinal bleeding occur less commonly, and intracerebral hemorrhage is a rare but sometimes fatal event. The diagnosis of ITP requires exclusion of other causes of thrombocytopenia (Table 56-2). Apparent thrombocytopenia may be an artifactual report on a complete blood count because of in vitro platelet clumping or the presence of giant platelets. Mild thrombocytopenia may occur in 6% to 8% of otherwise normal pregnant women and in up to one fourth of women with preeclampsia. Several drugs are known to induce thrombocytopenia, including heparin, quinidine, quinine, and sulfonamides. Human immunodeficiency virus (HIV) infection and other viral infections may cause thrombocytopenia that may be mistaken for ITP. Other conditions that may be associated with thrombocytopenia include myelodysplasia, congenital thrombocytopenia, thrombotic thrombocytopenic purpura, chronic disseminated intravascular coagulation, autoimmune diseases such as systemic lupus erythematosus, and lymphoproliferative disorders such as chronic

Table 56-2 Differential Diagnosis of Immune Thrombocytopenic Purpura

Falsely Low Platelet Count
In vitro platelet clumping caused by ethylenediamine tetra-acetic acid (EDTA)-dependent or cold-dependent agglutinins
Giant platelets

Common Causes of Thrombocytopenia
Pregnancy (gestational thrombocytopenia, preeclampsia)
Drug-induced thrombocytopenia (common drugs include heparin, quinidine, quinine, and sulfonamides)
Viral infections, such as human immunodeficiency virus, rubella, infectious mononucleosis
Hypersplenism due to chronic liver disease

Other Causes of Thrombocytopenia That Have Been Mistaken for Immune Thrombocytopenic Purpura
Myelodysplasia
Congenital thrombocytopenias
Thrombotic thrombocytopenic purpura and hemolytic-uremic syndrome
Chronic disseminated intravascular coagulation

Thrombocytopenia Associated With Other Disorders
Autoimmune diseases, such as systemic lupus erythematosus
Lymphoproliferative disorders (chronic lymphocytic leukemia, non-Hodgkin's lymphoma)

From George JN, El-Harake MA, Raskob GE: Chronic idiopathic thrombocytopenic purpura. N Engl J Med 331:1207-1211, 1994.

lymphocytic leukemia (CLL) and non-Hodgkin's lymphoma (NHL).

Management of patients with ITP varies according to the severity of the thrombocytopenia.[1] Patients with asymptomatic disease and platelet counts above 50,000/mm³ may simply be followed with no specific treatment. Platelet counts above 50,000/mm³ are seldom associated with spontaneous clinically important bleeding, even with invasive procedures. Patients with platelet counts between 30,000 and 50,000/mm³ who do not have symptoms may also be observed without treatment; however, careful follow-up is essential in these patients because they are at risk for more severe thrombocytopenia. The initial medical treatment is with glucocorticoids, usually prednisone (1 mg/kg body weight per day). About two thirds of patients treated in this manner experience an increase in their platelet count to more than 50,000/mm³, usually within 1 week of treatment, although it sometimes requires up to 3 weeks. Up to 26% of patients may have a complete response with glucocorticoid therapy. Patients with platelet counts greater than 20,000/mm³ who are symptom-free, or who have only minor purpura, do not require hospitalization. Treatment of ITP is indicated in patients with platelet counts of less than 20,000 to 30,000/mm³ or for those with platelet counts of less than 50,000/mm³ and significant mucus membrane bleeding or risk factors for bleeding, such as hypertension, peptic ulcer disease, or a vigorous lifestyle.

Hospitalization is often required for patients with platelet counts of less than 20,000/mm³ who have significant mucous membrane bleeding and is necessary for all patients who experience severe life-threatening hemorrhage. Although platelet transfusions are necessary for controlling severe hemorrhage, they are seldom indicated in patients with ITP in the absence of severe hemorrhage. IV immunoglobulin is important in the management of acute bleeding and for preparing patients for operation or delivery in the case of pregnancy. The usual dose is 1 g/kg per day for 2 days. This dose increases the platelet count in most patients within 3 days. It also increases the efficacy of transfused platelets. Administration of IV immunoglobulin is also appropriate in patients with platelet counts of less than 20,000/mm³ who are being prepared for splenectomy.

Splenectomy was the first effective treatment described for ITP and was an established therapeutic modality long before glucocorticoid therapy was introduced in 1950.[1] About two thirds of patients achieve a complete response with normalization of platelet counts after splenectomy and require no further therapy. Splenectomy is indicated in patients with refractory severe symptomatic thrombocytopenia, patients requiring toxic doses of steroids to achieve remission, and patients with a relapse of thrombocytopenia after initial glucocorticoid treatment. Splenectomy is an appropriate consideration for patients who have had the diagnosis of ITP for 6 weeks and continue to have a platelet count of less than 10,000/mm³ whether or not bleeding symptoms are present. Splenectomy is also indicated for patients who have had the diagnosis of ITP for up to 3 months and have experienced a transient or incomplete response to primary therapy and have a platelet count of less than 30,000/mm³. Splenectomy is considered for women in the second trimester of pregnancy who have failed glucocorticoid and IV immunoglobulin therapy and have platelet counts of less than 10,000/mm³ or who have platelet counts of less than 30,000/mm³ and bleeding problems. Splenectomy is probably not indicated in nonbleeding patients who have had a diagnosis of ITP for 6 months, have platelet counts of greater than 50,000/mm³, and are not engaged in high-risk activities.

A systematic review of 436 published articles from 1966 to 2004[2] reported a complete response in 66% and complete or partial response in 88% of adult patients with a median follow-up of 29 months (range, 1-153 months). When series with adults and children were analyzed, 72% of ITP patients demonstrated a complete response to splenectomy. The frequency of complete responses was not different across the 58 years of patient accrual. Relapses occurred in a median of 15% of patients (range, 0%-51%) with a median follow-up of 33 months.

Multiple factors have been evaluated as predictors of successful splenectomy in the treatment of ITP. None of the 12 preoperative characteristics reported had consistently predicted response to splenectomy in this systematic review.[2] Of all analyzed variables in a multivariate model, age at the time of splenectomy was an independent variable that most often correlated with response. However, no specific age cutoff point is identified, and even though younger patients had more frequent responses, most of the older patients also responded to splenectomy. The principal site of platelet sequestration on preoperative indium-111 (¹¹¹In)-labeled platelet scintigraphy had previously been reported to be predictive of the efficacy of splenectomy. In a cumulative study of 564 patients with ITP, a predominant splenic sequestration site was associated with an 87% to 93% rate of good response after splenectomy. In comparison, in patients with hepatic sequestration, the response rate was significantly lower (7%-30%).[3] The long-term cure rates when predominantly splenic sequestration is present were not shown to be an independent predictor of success with splenotomy for ITP in nine other published studies. Previous response to glucocorticoids has been correlated with response in several case series, but in series with multivariate models, previous response to glucocorticoids was not an independent variable for predicting response.

Most patients who respond to splenectomy with increased platelet counts do so within the first 10 days after their operation. Durable platelet responses have been correlated with platelet counts greater than 150,000/mm³ by the third postoperative day or greater than 500,000/mm³ on the 10th postoperative day. The immediate response rates among series collected between 1980 and 1998 range from 71% to 95%, with relapse rates of 4% to 12%[4] (Tables 56-3 and 56-4).

For patients with chronic ITP who fail to achieve complete response after splenectomy, the options range from simple observation in patients with no bleeding symptoms and platelet counts of more than 30,000/mm³ to continued long-term prednisone therapy (Table 56-5). Single-agent treatment with azathioprine or cyclophosphamide may be considered, but response to these agents may require up to 4 months of treatment. Patients who fail to respond to splenectomy or have relapsing disease after an initial response must be investigated for the presence of accessory spleen. Accessory spleen may be found in as many as 10% of these patients. The presence of an accessory spleen may be suggested by the absence of asplenic red blood cell morphologic features and may also be identified by radionuclide imaging. Identification of an accessory spleen in a patient who remains severely thrombocytopenic and is otherwise fit for operation warrants surgical excision of the accessory spleen.

In a summary of splenectomy series for hematologic disease using either a laparoscopic or open approach, Katkhouda and colleagues[4] found that among 394 patients treated with laparoscopic splenectomy, 237 had ITP, and 15% had an accessory spleen (see Tables 56-3 and 56-4). From the combined series of patients treated for ITP, there was an immediate response rate to splenectomy of 85% and a relapse rate of 4%. These series spanned from 1994 through 1998. The same authors also summarized another six series of open splenectomy for hematologic disease spanning from 1980 to 1990 and totaling 749 patients, of which 508 patients underwent splenectomy for ITP. The incidence of accessory spleen in these combined series was 16%. For treatment of ITP, the immediate response rate was 81.3%, and the relapse rate was 12%.

Table 56-3 Hematologic Response After Laparoscopic Treatment of Immune Thrombocytopenia Purpura

STUDY	PATIENTS (N)	ITP (N)	AS (N [%])	IR (N [%])	RR (N [%])
Cadiere et al, 1994	17	8	2 (11.8)	NA	NA
Emmermann et al, 1995	27	20	2 (7.4)	19 (95.0)	0 at 14 mo
Poulin et al, 1995	22	22	6 (27.2)	NA	NA
Yee & Akpata, 1995	25	14	2 (8.0)	11 (76.0)	NA
Brunt et al, 1996	26	17	3 (11.5)	13 (76.0)	NA
Flowers et al, 1996[44]	43	22	4 (9.3)	18 (82.0)	0 at 21 mo
Gigot et al, 1996	18	16	7 (39.0)	NA	2 (12.5) at 14 mo
Smith et al, 1996	10	8	2 (20.0)	NA	0
Friedman et al, 1997	63	28	11 (17.5)	NA	NA
Park et al, 1997	22	8	2 (9.0)	NA	NA
Tsiotos & Schlinkert, 1997	18	18	1 (5.6)	17 (94.0)	0
Katkhouda et al, 1998[4]	103	67	17 (16.5)	56 (83.6)	4 (6.0) at 38 mo
Total	**394**	**237**	**59/394 (15.0)**	**134/158 (85.0)**	**6/151 (4.0)**

AS, total number of patients with accessory spleens; IR, immediate response in immune thrombocytopenic purpura (ITP); RR, relapse rate in ITP; NA, data not available.

From Katkhouda N, Hurwitz MB, Rivera RT, et al: Laparoscopic splenectomy: Outcome and efficacy in 103 consecutive patients. Ann Surg 228:568-578, 1998.

Table 56-4 Results in 749 Collected Cases of Open Splenectomy

STUDY	PATIENTS (N)	MORBIDITY (N [%])	MORTALITY (N [%])	ITP (N)	AS (N [%])	IR (N [%])	RR (N [%])
DiFino et al, 1980	37	9 (24.3)	0	37	2 (5.4)	27 (73.0)	9 (24.3)
Mintz et al, 1981	66	13 (14.1)	1 (1.4)	66	20 (28.2)	56 (84.8)	6 (9.0)
Musser et al, 1984[42]	306	118 (24.0)	18 (6.0)	65	58 (19.0)	50 (77.0)	NA
Jacobs et al, 1986	102	15 (14.7)	0	102	NA	95 (93.1)	11 (10.7)
Akwari et al, 1987	100	8 (8.0)	0	100	18 (18.0)	71 (71.0)	4 (4.0)
Julia et al, 1990	138	NA	NA	138	NA	114 (83.0)	23 (17.0)
Total	**749**	**163/611 (26.7)**	**19/611 (3.1)**	**508**	**98/611 (16.0)**	**413/508 (81.3)**	**53/443 (12.0)**

AS, total number of patients with accessory spleens; IR, immediate response in immune thrombocytopenic purpura (ITP); RR relapse rate in ITP; NA, data not available.

From Katkhouda N, Hurwitz MB, Rivera RT, et al: Laparoscopic splenectomy: Outcome and efficacy in 103 consecutive patients. Ann Surg 228:568-578, 1998.

About 10% to 20% of otherwise symptom-free patients infected with HIV develop ITP.[5] Splenectomy may be performed safely in this cohort of patients and produces sustained increases in platelet levels in more than 80%. Splenectomy does not increase the risk for progression to AIDS, and a recent cohort study suggested that the absence of a spleen during the asymptomatic phase of HIV infection may delay disease progression.[5]

Hereditary Spherocytosis

Hereditary spherocytosis is an autosomal dominant disease that results from a deficiency of spectrin, a red blood cell cytoskeletal protein. This protein defect causes a membrane abnormality in the red blood cells resulting in small, spherical, and rigid erythrocytes. These cells have increased osmotic fragility. These spherocytes are more susceptible to becoming trapped in the spleen and destroyed. The clinical features of this disease include anemia, occasionally with jaundice, and splenomegaly. The diagnosis is made by identification of spherocytes on the peripheral blood smear, an increased reticulocyte count, increased osmotic fragility, and a negative Coombs test.

Splenectomy decreases the rate of hemolysis and usually leads to resolution of the anemia. Splenectomy is usually performed in childhood shortly after diagnosis. Although splenectomy does not normalize the morphology of the red blood cells, it does reduce the trapping and premature destruction of them. It is generally recommended that the operation be delayed until after the fourth year of life to preserve immunologic function of the spleen in young children who are most at risk for OPSI. There is a high incidence of pigmented gallstones

Table 56-5 Treatment Options for Patients With Chronic Immune Thrombocytopenic Purpura
Unresponsive to Initial Glucocorticoid Therapy and Splenectomy

INTERVENTION	INDICATION	OUTCOME
Observation	No bleeding symptoms; platelet count of ≥30,000-50,000/mm³	Platelet count may remain stable, but the risk for more severe thrombocytopenia with serious bleeding is unknown
Prednisone	Symptomatic thrombocytopenia, with bleeding symptoms; platelet count of ≤30,000-50,000/mm³	Goal is a safe platelet count with a minimal dose, such as 10 mg every other day; steroid toxicity is the limiting factor
Azathioprine or cyclophosphamide	Symptomatic thrombocytopenia, with bleeding symptoms; platelet count of ≤30,000-50,000 mm³	Response may require 4 months of treatment; complete recovery may occur in 10%-40% of patients
Other regimens	Symptomatic thrombocytopenia, with bleeding symptoms; platelet count of ≤30,000-50,000 mm³	Some regimens promising in small, preliminary studies; in others, few patients recover completely
Resection of accessory spleen or spleens	Symptomatic thrombocytopenia in a patient who is a good candidate for surgery	Complete recoveries reported in a few patients; symptomatic improvement in some others
Observation (with glucocorticoid or intravenous immune globulin as needed to treat or prevent bleeding)	Unresponsive to treatment	Some patients require frequent supportive therapy; others have minimal symptoms despite severe thrombocytopenia; spontaneous remissions may occur

From George JN, El-Harake MA, Raskob GE: Chronic idiopathic thrombocytopenic purpura. N Engl J Med 331:1207-1211, 1994.

among patients with spherocytosis, similar to other hemolytic anemias, and ultrasound needs to be performed before splenectomy. If gallstones are present, it is appropriate to perform cholecystectomy at the time of the splenectomy.

Other anemias associated with erythrocyte structural abnormalities include hereditary elliptocytosis, hereditary pyropoikilocytosis, hereditary xerocytosis, and hereditary hydrocytosis. All these conditions result in abnormalities of the erythrocyte cellular membrane and increased red blood cell destruction. Splenectomy is indicated for the severe hemolytic anemia that commonly occurs in these conditions. An exception to this is the mild anemia that is usually of limited clinical significance in the condition of hereditary xerocytosis, in which splenectomy is not usually indicated.

Hemolytic Anemia Due to Erythrocyte Enzyme Deficiency

Glucose-6-phosphate dehydrogenase deficiency and pyruvate kinase deficiency are the two predominant hereditary conditions associated with hemolytic anemia. These deficiencies result in abnormal glucose use and metabolism, leading to increased hemolysis. Pyruvate kinase deficiency is an autosomal recessive condition in which there is decreased red blood cell deformability resulting in increased hemolysis. The spleen is the site of erythrocyte entrapment and destruction in patients with deficiency of pyruvate kinase. These patients often have splenomegaly, and splenectomy has been shown to decrease their transfusion requirements. For the previously mentioned reasons of preserving immunologic

function, splenectomy is usually delayed until after 4 years of age in patients with this condition.

Glucose-6-phosphate dehydrogenase deficiency is an X-linked hereditary condition that is most frequently seen in people of African, Middle Eastern, or Mediterranean ancestry. Hemolytic anemia occurs in most patients after exposure to certain drugs or chemicals. Splenectomy is rarely indicated in patients with glucose-6-phosphate dehydrogenase deficiency.

Hemoglobinopathies

Thalassemia and sickle cell disease are hereditary hemolytic anemias that result from abnormal hemoglobin molecules. This results in abnormal shape of the erythrocyte, which may be subject to splenic sequestration and destruction. Sickle cell anemia is the result of the homozygous inheritance of hemoglobin S. Hemoglobin S has a single amino acid substitution of a valine for a glutamic acid in the sixth position of the β-chain of hemoglobin A.

Sickling of erythrocytes may also occur in patients who coinherit hemoglobin S and other hemoglobin variants, such as hemoglobin C or sickle cell β-thalassemia. Sickle cell disease results in patients who are homozygous for hemoglobin S. About 0.5% of African Americans are homozygous for hemoglobin S, whereas about 8% are heterozygous for hemoglobin S. The heterozygotes have the sickle cell trait. Under conditions of reduced oxygen tension, hemoglobin S molecules crystallize within the cell, which results in an elongated, distorted cell with a crescent shape. These altered erythrocytes are rigid and incapable of deforming in microvasculature. This lack of deformation results in capillary occlusion and thrombosis, ultimately leading to microinfarction. This occurs with particular frequency in the spleen. The spleen is enlarged during the first decade of life in most patients with sickle cell disease, but progressive infarction caused by repeated attacks of vaso-occlusion results in autosplenectomy. The spleen in patients with sickle cell disease usually atrophies by adulthood, although splenomegaly may occasionally persist into adult life.

Thalassemias constitute a group of hemoglobin disorders that also result in hemolytic anemia. Thalassemias are inherited as autosomal dominant traits and occur as a result of a defect in hemoglobin synthesis. This results in variable degrees of hemolytic anemia. Splenic infarction, splenomegaly, and hypersplenism may be predominant features of either sickle cell disease or thalassemia.

Hypersplenism and acute splenic sequestration are life-threatening disorders in children with sickle cell anemia and thalassemia. In these conditions, there may be rapid splenic enlargement, resulting in severe pain and requiring multiple blood transfusions. In addition to acute splenic sequestration crisis, these patients may suffer from symptomatic massive splenomegaly causing discomfort and interfering with daily activities. Indications for splenectomy in patients with sickle cell disease include acute splenic sequestration crisis, hypersplenism, and splenic abscess. Children with sickle cell anemia often exhibit weight loss and poor growth; these conditions may be improved after splenectomy as the result of decreased whole-body, total protein turnover and decreased resting metabolic rate. Sickle cell disease–associated hypersplenism is characterized by anemia requiring transfusions as well as by leukopenia and thrombocytopenia. Splenectomy reduces the need for transfusions in these patients.

Splenic abscesses are not uncommon in patients with sickle cell anemia and are characterized by fever, abdominal pain, and a tender, enlarged spleen. Many patients with splenic abscess have leukocytosis. Thrombocytosis and Howell-Jolly bodies also occur in these patients, indicating functional asplenia. Common organisms involved in splenic abscess in patients with sickle cell anemia are *Salmonella* species, *Enterobacter* species, and other enteric organisms. In acute splenic sequestration crisis, the patients have severe anemia, splenomegaly, and an acute bone marrow response with erythrocytosis. They may exhibit a dramatic decrease in their hemoglobin levels along with abdominal pain and may undergo circulatory collapse. These patients need to be stabilized with hydration and transfusion and may require urgent splenectomy after stabilization.

SPLENECTOMY FOR MALIGNANCY

Lymphomas

Hodgkin's Disease

Hodgkin's disease is a malignant lymphoma that typically affects young adults in their 20s and 30s. Most patients have asymptomatic lymphadenopathy at the time of diagnosis, and most present with cervical node enlargement. A minority of patients, usually with more advanced disease, may present with constitutional symptoms such as night sweats, weight loss, and pruritus. Hodgkin's disease is histologically classified as lymphocyte-predominant, nodular-sclerosing, mixed-cellularity, or lymphocyte-depleted Hodgkin's disease.

The disease is pathologically staged according to the Ann Arbor classification. Stage I represents disease in a single lymphatic site, whereas stage II indicates the presence of disease in two or more lymphatic sites on the same side of the diaphragm. Stage III indicates the presence of lymphatic disease (includes splenic involvement) on both sides of the diaphragm. Stage IV disease is disseminated into extralymphatic sites such as liver, lung, or bone marrow. Subscript E indicates single or contiguous extralymphatic involvement in stages I to III, and subscript S represents splenic involvement. Patients with constitutional symptoms are classified as B (presence) or A (absence), for example, stage IIA or IIB.

Historically, staging laparotomy including splenectomy provided essential pathologic staging information that was necessary to select appropriate therapy for Hodgkin's disease. The purpose of staging laparotomy is to pathologically stage the presence and extent of disease below the diaphragm. In one of the larger reported series from 1985, 38.9% of 825 splenectomy specimens tested positive for involvement with Hodgkin's disease.[6] In half of the patients with splenic involvement, the spleen was the only site of intra-abdominal disease. The spleen was also involved in all of the 6.2% of patients with liver involvement. In this important series by Taylor and colleagues,[6] the clinical stage was changed in 43% of cases by laparotomy.

Advances in imaging techniques, with widespread availability of dynamic helical computed tomography (CT) scan and lymphangiography and increasing availability of fluorodeoxyglucose positron emission tomography imaging, have improved nonoperative staging of Hodgkin's disease. The improved nonoperative staging, along with the use of less toxic systemic chemotherapeutics for earlier stages of Hodgkin's disease, has led to a dramatic decrease in the numbers of patients requiring staging laparotomy. Patients at high risk for relapse, especially those with B symptoms and those with evidence of intra-abdominal involvement on one or more of the diagnostic imaging studies, require systemic chemotherapy and should not undergo a staging laparotomy. Staging laparotomy and splenectomy are appropriate for selected patients with an early clinical stage of disease (stage IA or IIA) in whom pathologic staging of the abdomen will significantly influence the therapeutic management. Early-stage Hodgkin's disease is often cured with radiation therapy alone.

When indicated, the staging laparotomy for Hodgkin's disease includes a thorough abdominal exploration, splenectomy with splenic hilar lymphadenectomy, bilateral wedge and core-needle liver biopsies, retroperitoneal lymphadenectomy, iliac crest bone marrow biopsy, and in premenopausal women, oophoropexy. The perioperative mortality rate for staging laparotomy should be less than 1%, and the risk of major complications has been less than 10%.[6]

Non-Hodgkin's Lymphomas

Splenomegaly or hypersplenism is a common occurrence during the course of NHL. Splenectomy is indicated for patients with NHL for treatment of massive splenomegaly when the bulk of the spleen contributes to abdominal pain, fullness, and early satiety. Splenectomy may also be effective in the treatment of patients who develop hypersplenism with associated anemia, thrombocytopenia, and neutropenia.

Splenectomy occasionally plays an important role in the diagnosis and staging of patients who present with isolated splenic disease. The most common primary splenic neoplasm is NHL. The spleen is involved in 50% to 80% of NHL patients, but fewer than 1% of patients present with splenomegaly without peripheral lymphadenopathy.[7] Disease that appears clinically confined to the spleen has been called *malignant lymphoma with prominent splenic involvement.* Most affected patients have low-grade NHL. There is frequent involvement of the splenic hilar lymph nodes, extrahilar nodes, bone marrow, and liver in these patients. About 75% exhibit clinical evidence of hypersplenism. In a series of 59 such patients reported by Morel and associates,[7] 40 underwent splenectomy, and 19 did not. Eighty-two percent of the cytopenic patients who underwent splenectomy had correction of their hematologic abnormalities postoperatively. For those patients with low-grade NHL who had spleen-predominant features, survival was significantly improved after splenectomy (median, 108 months) as compared with patients receiving similar treatment without splenectomy (median, 24 months).

Leukemia

Hairy Cell Leukemia

Hairy cell leukemia is a rare disease that represents about 2% of adult leukemias. Splenomegaly, pancytopenia, and neoplastic mononuclear cells in the peripheral blood and bone marrow characterize the disease. The "hairy" cells are usually B lymphocytes that have cell membrane ruffling, which appears as cytoplasmic projections under the light microscope. The patients are usually elderly men with palpable splenomegaly. About 10% of cases have an indolent course requiring no specific therapy, but most require therapy for cytopenias such as symptomatic anemia, infectious complications from neutropenia, or hemorrhage from thrombocytopenia. The pancytopenia results from the combined effects of hypersplenism and bone marrow replacement by leukemic cells. Therapy may also be required for massive splenomegaly. Patients with hairy cell leukemia have a twofold to threefold increased risk for diagnosis of a second primary malignancy at a median interval of 40 months after the diagnosis of hairy cell leukemia. Most of the second malignancies are solid tumors, and the types of tumors include prostate cancer, skin cancers, lung cancer, and gastrointestinal adenocarcinomas.

Splenectomy and interferon alfa-2 have been the standard treatment of hairy cell leukemia until recently; this approach is being replaced with systemic administration of purine analogues, such as 2-chlorodeoxyadenosine and deoxycoformycin, as initial treatment.[8] Splenectomy is still indicated for some patients with massive enlargement of the spleen or with evidence of hypersplenism that is refractory to medical therapy. Splenectomy provides a highly effective and sustained palliation of these problems, and most patients show definite hematologic improvement after the procedure. About 40% of patients experience normalization of their blood counts after splenectomy. The responses to splenectomy usually last for 10 or more years, and about half of patients will require no further therapy. Patients with diffusely involved bone marrow who do not have significant splenomegaly are far less likely to achieve a significant benefit from splenectomy. The current 4-year survival rate after diagnosis of hairy cell leukemia is about 80%, as compared with 60% for patients diagnosed in the 1970s.[9]

Chronic Lymphocytic Leukemia

CLL is a B-cell leukemia that is characterized by the progressive accumulation of relatively mature, but functionally incompetent, lymphocytes. CLL occurs more frequently in men and usually occurs after 50 years of age. Staging of CLL is according to the Rai staging system, which correlates well with prognosis. Stage 0 includes bone marrow and blood lymphocytosis only; stage I includes lymphocytosis and enlarged lymph nodes; stage II includes lymphocytosis and enlarged spleen, liver, or both; stage III includes lymphocytosis and anemia; and stage IV includes lymphocytosis with thrombocytopenia. Chlorambucil has long been the mainstay of medical therapy and was useful for the palliation of symptoms; however, there is increasing interest in using purine analogues, such as fludarabine, as first-line therapy, with some studies showing improved rates of remission.[9] Bone marrow transplantation has also become increasingly used in the treatment of CLL, and both allotransplantation and autotransplantation approaches are being investigated.

The role of splenectomy in the treatment of CLL continues to be for palliation of symptomatic splenomegaly and for treatment of cytopenia related to hypersplenism. Relief of bulk symptoms from splenomegaly is virtually always successful, whereas the hematologic response rates for correction of anemia and thrombocytopenia are between 60% and 70%.[10] Cusack and colleagues[10] reported a review of 77 consecutive patients with CLL (76% Rai stage III or IV) who underwent splenectomy at the University of Texas M. D. Anderson Cancer Center and who were compared with an age- and gender-matched cohort of CLL patients treated with fludarabine and no splenectomy. In this retrospective review, the patients with profound anemia and thrombocytopenia who underwent splenectomy had significantly better survival rates than the nonsplenectomy group.

Chronic Myelogenous Leukemia

Chronic myelogenous leukemia (CML) is a myeloproliferative disorder that results from neoplastic transformation of myeloid elements. CML was the first leukemic subset for which a chromosomal marker (the Philadelphia chromosome) was discovered. The Philadelphia chromosome is caused by a fusion of fragments of chromosomes 22 and 9 and results in the expression of the abnormal chimeric oncogenic protein p210bcr-abl. The disease is characterized by a progressive replacement of the normal diploid elements of the bone marrow with mature-appearing neoplastic myeloid cells.

CML may occur from childhood to old age. CML usually presents with an indolent or chronic phase that is asymptomatic. Progression to the accelerated phase is marked by the onset of symptoms such as fever, night sweats, and progressive splenomegaly; however, this phase may also be asymptomatic and detectable only from changes in the peripheral blood or bone marrow. The accelerated phase may give rise to the blastic phase, which is characterized by the previously listed symptoms as well as anemia, infectious complications, and bleeding. Splenomegaly with splenic sequestration of blood elements often contributes to these symptoms.

Treatment of CML is primarily medical and may include hydroxyurea, interferon alfa, and high-dose chemotherapy with bone marrow transplantation. Symptomatic splenomegaly and hypersplenism in patients with CML may be effectively palliated by splenectomy. Otherwise, the role of splenectomy in the treatment of CML has been controversial. Randomized studies of patients with CML have demonstrated no survival benefit when splenectomy is performed during the early chronic phase.[11] Splenectomy has also not resulted in a survival benefit when performed before allogeneic bone marrow transplantation. Thus, splenectomy before allogeneic bone marrow transplantation is recommended only for patients with significant splenomegaly.

Non-Hematologic Tumors of the Spleen

The spleen is a site of metastatic tumor in up to 7% of autopsies of cancer patients. The primary solid tumors that most frequently metastasize to the spleen are carcinomas of the breast, lung, and melanoma; however, virtually any primary malignancy may metastasize to the spleen.[12] Metastases to the spleen are often asymptomatic but may be associated with symptomatic splenomegaly or even spontaneous splenic rupture. Splenectomy may provide effective palliation in carefully selected symptomatic patients with splenic metastasis.

Vascular neoplasms are the most common primary splenic tumors that include both benign and malignant variants. Hemangiomas are usually incidental findings identified in spleens removed for other reasons. Angiosarcomas (or hemangiosarcomas) of the spleen have been associated with environmental exposure to thorium dioxide or monomeric vinyl chloride, but they most often occur spontaneously. Patients with these tumors may present with splenomegaly, hemolytic anemia, ascites, and pleural effusions or with spontaneous splenic rupture. These are highly aggressive tumors that have a poor prognosis. Lymphangiomas are usually benign endothelium-lined cysts that may become symptomatic by

causing splenomegaly. Lymphangiosarcoma within a cystic lymphangioma has been reported. Splenectomy is appropriate for diagnosis, treatment, or palliation of the conditions cited above.

SPLENECTOMY FOR MISCELLANEOUS BENIGN CONDITIONS

Splenic Cysts

Cystic lesions of the spleen have been recognized with increasing frequency since the advent of CT scanning and ultrasound imaging. Splenic cysts are classified as true cysts, which may be either nonparasitic or parasitic, and pseudocysts. Cystic-appearing tumors of the spleen include cystic lymphangiomas and cavernous hemangiomas, as discussed previously.[13] Primary true cysts of the spleen account for about 10% of all nonparasitic cysts of the spleen. Most nonparasitic cysts are pseudocysts and are secondary to trauma. The diagnosis of true splenic cysts is commonly made in the second and third decades of life. True cysts are characterized by a squamous epithelial lining, and many are considered congenital. These epithelial cells are often positive for CA 19-9 and carcinoembryonic antigen by immunohistochemistry, and patients with epidermoid cysts of the spleen may have elevated serum levels of one or both of these tumor-associated antigens.[13] Despite the presence of these tumor markers, these cysts are benign and apparently do not have malignant potential greater than any other native tissue.

Often, true splenic cysts are asymptomatic and found incidentally. When symptomatic, patients may complain of vague upper abdominal fullness and discomfort, early satiety, pleuritic chest pain, shortness of breath, left back or shoulder pain, or renal symptoms from compression of the left kidney. A palpable abdominal mass may be present. The presence of symptoms is often related to the size of the cysts, and cysts smaller than 8 cm are rarely symptomatic. Rarely, these cysts may present with acute symptoms related to rupture, hemorrhage, or infection. The diagnosis of splenic cysts is best made with CT imaging. Operative intervention is indicated for symptomatic cysts and for large cysts. Either total or partial splenectomy may provide successful treatment. The clear advantage of partial splenectomy is the preservation of splenic function. Preservation of at least 25% of the spleen appears sufficient to protect against pneumococcal pneumonia. Most recent reports describe successful experience with partial splenectomy, cyst wall resection, or partial decapsulation, which may be accomplished with either an open or laparoscopic approach.[13]

Most true splenic cysts are parasitic cysts in areas of endemic hydatid disease (*Echinococcus* species). Radiographic imaging may reveal cyst wall calcifications or daughter cysts. Although hydatid cysts are uncommon in North America, this diagnosis must always be excluded before the performance of invasive diagnostic or therapeutic procedures that may risk spillage of cyst contents. Serologic tests for *Echinococcus* species are often helpful in verifying the presence of parasites. As with hydatid cysts of the liver, spillage of cyst contents may precipitate an anaphylactic shock and risks intraperitoneal dissemination of infective scoleces. Splenectomy is the treatment of choice, and great care needs to be taken to avoid rupture of the cysts intraoperatively. The cysts may be sterilized by injection of a 3% sodium chloride solution, alcohol, or 0.5% silver nitrate, as has been recommended for hydatid cysts of the liver.

Pseudocysts account for 70% to 80% of all nonparasitic cysts of the spleen. A history of prior trauma can usually be elicited. Splenic pseudocysts are not epithelial lined. Radiographic imaging may demonstrate focal calcifications in up to half of cases. Most splenic pseudocysts are unilocular, and the cysts are smooth and thick-walled. Small asymptomatic splenic pseudocysts (<4 cm) do not require treatment and may undergo involution over time. When the pseudocysts are symptomatic, patients often present with left upper quadrant and referred left shoulder pain. Symptomatic pseudocysts are treated surgically. If the spleen can be safely and completely mobilized and partial splenectomy accomplished to include the cystic portion of the spleen, this technique offers effective therapy that preserves splenic function. Presented with less favorable conditions, the surgeon should not hesitate to perform total splenectomy. Successful percutaneous drainage has also been reported for splenic pseudocysts, although the success rate with this approach as compared with surgical intervention has not been determined. The 90% success rate of image-guided percutaneous drainage of unilocular splenic abscesses suggests that this may be a reasonable initial approach for the management of symptomatic splenic pseudocysts.[14]

Splenic Abscess

Splenic abscess is an uncommon and potentially fatal illness. The incidence in autopsy series approximates 0.7%.[15] The mortality rate for splenic abscess ranges from about 80% for multiple abscesses in immunocompromised patients to about 15% to 20% in previously healthy patients with solitary unilocular lesions. Predisposing illnesses include malignancies, polycythemia vera, endocarditis, previous trauma, hemoglobinopathy (e.g., sickle cell disease), urinary tract infection, IV drug abuse, and AIDS. About 70% of splenic abscesses result from hematogenous spread of the infecting organism from another location, as occurs with endocarditis, osteomyelitis, and IV drug abuse. Splenic abscess may also occur as the result of infection of a contiguous structure, such as the colon, kidney, or pancreas. Gram-positive cocci, such as *Staphylococcus, Streptococcus,* or *Enterococcus* species, and gram-negative enteric organisms are often the infectious agents. Splenic abscesses may also be caused by other fastidious organisms, including *Mycobacterium tuberculosis, Mycobacterium avium,* and *Actinomyces* species. Immunosuppressed patients may develop multiple fungal abscesses, typically from *Candida* species infection.

The clinical presentation of splenic abscess is often nonspecific and insidious, including abdominal pain, fever, peritonitis, and pleuritic chest pain. The abdominal pain is localized in the left upper quadrant less than half the time and is more often vague abdominal pain. Splenomegaly is present in a minority of patients. The diagnosis is made most accurately by CT; however, it may also be made with ultrasonography. Two thirds of splenic abscesses in adults are solitary, and the remaining one third are multiple. These ratios are reversed in children.[16]

The initial approach to treatment of splenic abscess depends on whether it is unilocular or multilocular. Unilocular abscesses are amenable to CT-guided drainage, and this approach, along with systemic antibiotic administration, has a success rate that is in excess of 75% and that may be as high as 90% when only patients with unilocular collections are considered.[17] Failure of a prompt clinical response to percutaneous drainage leads to splenectomy without delay. Multilocular abscesses are usually treated by splenectomy, with drainage of the left upper quadrant and antibiotic administration.

Wandering Spleen

Wandering spleen is a rare finding, accounting for only a fraction of a percent of all splenectomies. The spleen normally has peritoneal attachments (called *suspensory ligaments*) that fix the spleen in its usual anatomic position. Failure to form these attachments has been postulated to result from failure of the dorsal mesogastrium to fuse to the posterior abdominal wall during embryonic development. The result is an unusually long splenic pedicle. It has also been postulated that an acquired defect in splenic attachment may occur in multiparous women secondary to hormonal changes during pregnancy and associated abdominal laxity. Wandering spleen is most often diagnosed in children or in women between the ages of 20 and 40 years.

Most patients with wandering spleen are asymptomatic. Symptomatic patients often present with recurrent episodes of abdominal pain. This is likely related to tension on the vascular pedicle or intermittent torsion. Torsion of the splenic vessels may lead to venous congestion and splenomegaly. Severe and persistent pain is suggestive of splenic torsion and ischemia. On examination, a mobile abdominal mass may be present along with abdominal tenderness. The diagnosis may be most readily confirmed with a CT scan of the abdomen. The typical finding is the absence of a spleen in its normal position and the presence of a spleen in an ectopic location. IV contrast injection during the CT scan provides valuable information. Lack of contrast enhancement of the spleen suggests splenic torsion, as does a whorled appearance to the splenic pedicle. Lack of splenic perfusion on the CT scan may be helpful in guiding the operative decision for splenectomy versus splenopexy.[18]

SPLENIC TRAUMA

The most significant contemporary issue in managing splenic trauma is the role of nonoperative management. Advances in diagnostic techniques that have occurred since the early 1980s have led to alternative approaches to managing these injuries. In recent years, abdominal ultrasound and CT have permitted observation of the location and relative quantification of the amount of intra-abdominal hemorrhage, and CT has provided relatively good definition of the degree of anatomic splenic disruption. The main thrust of this section of the chapter is to trace those diagnostic developments in conjunction with the issues of clinical presentation and splenic anatomy in order to develop a logical platform for decision making.

General Considerations

Injury to the spleen is the most common indication for laparotomy after blunt mechanisms of injury. Motor vehicular crashes continue to be the major source of injury in industrialized nations. Other common mechanisms include motorcycle crashes, falls, pedestrian and vehicular incidents, bicycle crashes, and sports. Significant abdominal pain produced in the setting of nonvehicular blunt trauma is associated with a high incidence of significant intra-abdominal injury, with the spleen being the most commonly injured organ.

Directly surrounding the spleen are the left hemidiaphragm, splenic flexure of the colon, kidney, distal pancreas, and stomach (see Fig. 56-1). The relatively avascular ligaments described earlier in this chapter (splenophrenic, splenorenal, splenocolic, and gastrosplenic) secure the spleen in this left upper quadrant niche somewhat protected by the lower costal margins (see Fig. 56-1). Splenic injuries are produced by rapid deceleration, compression, energy transmission through the posterolateral chest wall over the spleen, or puncture from an adjacent rib fracture. Rapid deceleration results in the spleen continuing in a forward motion while being tethered at the point of attachment. Injuries produced by deceleration forces result in capsular avulsion along the various ligamentous attachments and linear or stellate fractures of varying depths. Because of its solid structural characteristics and density, energy transfer to the spleen is relatively efficient. Injuries caused by assaults or falls are usually a result of direct blows over the lower chest wall, with transmission of energy resulting in splenic lacerations and fractures.

The blood supply to the spleen is considerable. The spleen receives about 5% of the cardiac output. The blood supply is through the splenic artery and the short gastric vessels (see Fig. 56-2). The splenic arteries divide into several segmental vessels supplying the poles and midportion, and these arteries divide into second- and third-order vessels that course transversely within the spleen. Because of this extensive arterial supply, even superficial lacerations and capsular avulsions often yield substantial hemorrhage.

Diagnosis

The history and physical examination continue to be the basis from which splenic injury is diagnosed. Details concerning the mechanism of injury delineated in the previous section need to be sought. On physical examination, evidence of peritoneal irritation (tenderness, guarding, rebound) is sometimes apparent. Recently extravasated blood, however, is a fairly benign peritoneal irritant, and large amounts of blood may be contained in the free peritoneal cavity with minimal physical findings. In the era before diagnostic peritoneal lavage (DPL), physical examination was found to be accurate only 42% to 87% of the time. Perhaps more helpful than examination directed at the abdominal cavity is that focused in the left upper quadrant. Percussion tenderness or evidence of bruising and soft tissue contusion in the posterior left lower costal margin is usually present when direct blows have produced splenic injury. Complaints of left upper quadrant pain or of pain referred to the left shoulder (Kehr sign) are highly correlated with injury. At least one fourth of patients with left lower rib fractures have associated injury to the spleen.

Significant injury producing hemorrhage is indicated by the hemodynamic status of the patient. Hypotension or tachycardia should alert the clinician to the potential for splenic injury. At the initial trauma assessment, apparent injuries that may yield enough blood loss individually or in aggregate to produce physiologic changes in hemodynamics need to be noted. If blood loss from long bone or pelvic fractures or from external losses from lacerations cannot be attributed, an intra-abdominal source must be assumed, and the spleen is the most common source. Indeed, since the classic study by West and associates[19] of preventable deaths that directly contributed to the development of trauma systems in the United States, mortality from missed or delayed recognition of splenic hemorrhage has remained near the top of the list of causes of preventable death.

The diagnosis becomes more difficult in the presence of multiple injuries, which are both distracting to examination and confounding to interpretation of potential sources and volumes of blood loss. Furthermore, associated neurologic injury and substance abuse often add to the diagnostic difficulty. Closed head injury is associated in 30% to 40% of cases and compromises or eliminates the reliability of the physical examination. Spinal cord injury also eliminates reliance on abdominal examination. Substance abuse has been documented in about 40% of patients involved in motor vehicle crashes. Because of the unreliability of physical examination accounted for by these several concerns, more objective means of diagnosis have evolved.

Diagnostic Peritoneal Lavage

DPL was introduced by Root and colleagues in 1965.[20] That modality remained the standard diagnostic procedure for blunt abdominal trauma evaluations for the subsequent 20 years. Initially, results were interpreted from a grossly positive examination or from quantification of red and white blood cells in the large effluent. A positive DPL consisted of either 10 mL of gross blood aspirated with catheter insertion or a microscopically positive examination. For microscopic examination in adults, 1 L of crystalloid solution is instilled through a periumbilical catheter inserted by either open or closed technique. Assuming complete instillation of the liter, positive examinations consisted of a red blood cell count higher than 100,000/mm³ or a white blood cell count higher than 500/mm³ in the completely mixed effluent. The dilution factor that produces a red blood cell count of more than 100,000/mm³ accounts for about 30 to 40 mL of blood in the peritoneal cavity. A microscopically positive examination by white blood cell count criteria is indicative of peritoneal inflammation generally produced by hollow viscus injury.

After the introduction of DPL, multiple investigators demonstrated sensitivities approaching 99% and specificities in the range of 95% to 98%. Subsequent refinements included enzyme analysis of the effluent to enhance diagnostic accuracy of hollow viscus and pancreatic injury. An extraordinary amount of clinical research has been done on DPL-related issues. For several years, one could expect at least one presentation on DPL at any surgical meeting dealing with clinical trauma topics, and often multiple papers were presented.

Reliance on DPL as a standard screening procedure, however, came into scrutiny from two fronts. As CT began to be applied for trauma diagnostics, it was observed that small splenic injuries had occurred and that the patient remained hemodynamically stable. It was further noted that enough blood was present to have caused a positive lavage. Coincident with that development was the observation by surgeons that many of the positive DPL procedures led to laparotomies in which there was indeed a splenic injury, but often of a relatively trivial nature without active bleeding. Based on these parallel observations, the term *nontherapeutic laparotomy* began surfacing in the splenic injury literature, and it began to be appreciated that DPL was perhaps too sensitive.

Computed Tomography

Application of this technology for diagnosing abdominal injuries began in the early 1980s. Initial observations consisted of examinations done for other injuries at some interval after initial trauma evaluation (e.g., chest or pelvic CT). Injuries to the spleen and liver were noted incidentally and, although initially unrecognized, produced no sequelae. This led to questioning of both the routine reliance on DPL for screening and the necessity of operating on all splenic injuries. As opposed to DPL, CT permitted not only identification of intraperitoneal blood but also definition of individual organ injuries. This actually revolutionized the management of splenic injury. Heretofore, it was assumed that once injured, the spleen invariably continued bleeding. It was generally taught in surgical training programs that if the spleen was incidentally injured from retraction during elective celiotomy, splenectomy was required because of the high risk for continued or recurrent hemorrhage. The early incidental CT observations of damaged spleens in stable patients ushered in the era of nonoperative management.

The anatomic definition of injury provided objective criteria for classification of degrees of splenic injury. The American Association for the Surgery of Trauma developed a splenic injury grading scale through a consensus methodology[21] (Table 56-6). This scale has been useful

Table 56-6 American Association for the Surgery of Trauma Splenic Injury Scale (1994 Revision)

GRADE	TYPE	INJURY DESCRIPTION
I	Hematoma	Subcapsular, <10% surface area
	Laceration	Capsular tear, <1 cm parenchymal depth
II	Hematoma	Subcapsular, 10%-50% surface area; intraparenchymal, <5 cm in diameter
	Laceration	Capsular tear, 1-3 cm parenchymal depth, which does not involve a trabecular vessel
III	Hematoma	Subcapsular, >50% surface area or expanding; ruptured subcapsular or parenchymal hematoma Intraparenchymal hematoma >5 cm or expanding
	Laceration	>3 cm parenchymal depth or involving trabecular vessels
IV	Laceration	Laceration involving segmental or hilar vessels producing major devascularization (>25% of spleen)
V	Laceration	Completely shattered spleen
	Vascular	Hilar vascular injury which devascularizes spleen

Adapted from Moore EE, Cogbill TH, Jurkovich GJ, et al: Organ injury scaling: Spleen and liver (1994 revision). J Trauma 38:323, 1995.

for comparison of data among institutions. It has also provided a structure for a logical approach to management decisions. Advances in CT technology have continued to increase the value of evaluating intra-abdominal and retroperitoneal injury. The current generation of helical and spiral scanning technology is both rapid and high resolution. Previous technology required 15 to 20 minutes for complete examination, but current technology requires 1 to 2 minutes. The resolution permits more precise delineation of organ fracture and intraparenchymal vascular disruption. The newest generation of CT technology is multislice scanning. That approach allows for scanning of the torso in less than 10 seconds and, owing to a much higher number of accumulated images compared with standard helical technology, an even higher resolution is obtained. This technology is very promising to replace diagnostic angiography and may have profound importance in better defining solid organ injury and further minimizing failures of nonoperative management.

Ultrasound

During the 1990s, ultrasound was introduced and firmly established as an important diagnostic tool for evaluating blunt abdominal trauma. It was first used in Europe in the early 1980s.[22] A few years later, it was adopted by physicians in the United States. Its advantages include noninvasiveness, rapidity, and low cost. Ultrasound provides similar but somewhat more information than DPL.

The presence of free intraperitoneal fluid can be identified and semiquantitated. Acoustic windows are noted around solid interfaces. Those solid interfaces for trauma evaluation include the spleen, kidneys, liver, heart, and distended urinary bladder. The acronym FAST (focused abdominal sonogram for trauma) has been applied to this quick survey, which takes about 3 minutes to complete in experienced hands. Significant bowel distention, obesity, and subcutaneous emphysema compromise the examination. Initial concerns were with the sensitivity and reproducibility of FAST. There was also a question of whether this technology could be grasped easily enough to permit widespread application by surgeons, or whether the difficulty was such that only radiologists who had more extensive training could be relied on for accuracy.

Tso and colleagues[23] reported in 1992 on 163 stable patients evaluated by ultrasound before either DPL or CT and found a 91% sensitivity rate, with all cases of clinically significant hemoperitoneum being identified. A subsequent study by Bode and associates[24] involved 353 blunt abdominal trauma patients evaluated with ultrasound by a radiologist. These investigators reported a 93% specificity rate, 99% accuracy rate, and no nontherapeutic laparotomies. Rothlin and coworkers[25] reported a study of 290 patients in which ultrasound was performed by a surgeon. They found a 90% sensitivity rate and a 99% specificity rate for intra-abdominal injury. They also noted the ease of repeatability for follow-up of these patients. The reported data would suggest that with a structured training format, FAST can be expeditiously taught to practicing surgeons. The American College of Surgeons is vigorously involved in evaluating new technologies and is developing structured courses for teaching surgeons applications of ultrasound for evaluation of breast disease, intra-abdominal pathology, and trauma.

Ultrasound has emerged as a replacement for DPL. It appears to be as sensitive in detecting free intraperitoneal blood and is less invasive and quicker. The most important application is in evaluating the hemodynamically unstable patient with multiple injuries. A positive ultrasound would generally mandate expeditious exploratory laparotomy. The place for ultrasound use in the stable patient has been less clear. As nonoperative management has become so prominent, CT has become indispensable in defining the location and degree of organ injury. Ultrasound is not capable of accurately defining those anatomic characteristics. Technology is advancing rapidly, however, and it is likely that future generations of ultrasonography equipment will significantly improve resolution and anatomic definition. Furthermore, ultrasound may have a more positive impact on cost than is immediately apparent. As ultrasound has become more widely adopted and confidence in the modality has developed, it has become apparent that ultrasound can be applied for screening as an alternative to the more costly CT evaluation.

In a prospective study, Branney and associates[26] used ultrasound in the emergency department for screening stable patients. Their findings included a reduction in the number of CT examinations in patients with significant injury because those with negative examinations required no further studies. Sixty-five percent of the patients had no further studies, the number of admissions for observation decreased significantly, and no significant injuries were missed.

Issues Concerning Operation

Indications for Exploration

The clearest indication for urgent operation is hemodynamic instability. Unfortunately, this is not a binomial or discrete factor. The definition of stability is clearly associated with some degree of arbitrary assignment. This problem is underscored in the face of multiple organ system injury in which blood loss accumulates from external losses from lacerations and internal losses in fractures and soft tissues and thoracic and abdominal cavities. Optimal decisions become apparent in retrospect. Nonetheless, when in doubt, abdominal exploration is performed. The risks associated with nontherapeutic laparotomy are outweighed by the risks associated with shock secondary to prolonged intraperitoneal hemorrhage and the associated consequences of immunocompromise, multiple organ system dysfunction, and death.

Because there can be no standard criteria for hemodynamic instability, a general guideline is to operate for a systolic blood pressure below 90 mm Hg or a pulse of more than 120 beats/minute if there is not immediate response to 1 to 2 L of crystalloid resuscitation and when physical examination, ultrasound, or DPL indicates intra-abdominal blood loss. Indications for operation based on CT findings are delineated in a subsequent section of this chapter on nonoperative management.

Technical Issues

A midline incision is usually preferred for trauma exploration. This approach is expeditious and provides access to all areas of the abdominal cavity, including the retroperitoneum. A left subcostal approach may be preferred when laparotomy is directed by CT findings. The small bowel and lesser sac are easily evaluated from this incision. Extension to the right side provides outstanding exposure of the liver and access to the whole abdomen with the exception of the deepest portion of the pelvis. Both incisions are adequate, but the performance of a midline incision is quicker.

After rapid evacuation of free blood and clots to assess other sources of injury, including the liver and mesentery, the spleen is mobilized into the wound. Splenic mobilization is accomplished by the fundamental operative principle of traction and countertraction. In the case of splenic mobilization, traction and countertraction are based on the spleen and its suspensory ligaments. The operating surgeon applies dorsal and medial traction on the spleen with the hand splayed widely over the splenic surface to stretch and define clearly the splenorenal and splenophrenic ligaments. It appears that there is a natural tendency to place ventral traction on the spleen to "lift" it from the left upper quadrant, a maneuver that results in decapsulation over the posterior splenic surface and along the splenocolic ligament, producing iatrogenic trauma and increasing hemorrhage. After exposure of the splenorenal and splenophrenic ligaments, which is facilitated by the first assistant providing countertraction with tissue forceps, the ligaments can be divided under direct vision.

The incision begins at the phrenocolic ligament, continuing through the ligaments to the stomach in the vicinity of the highest short gastric vessels. Division occurs 1 to 2 cm from the spleen to avoid injury to both spleen and diaphragmatic muscle. Continued tension on the tissues allows gradual mobilization anterior to the spleen as deeper layers of filmy connective tissue planes are placed under tension and easily visualized and divided. The dissection progresses such that the left adrenal gland is visualized and left undisturbed in its posterior location. As this dissection progresses through these thin connective tissue planes, the posterior surface of the pancreas and the splenic vein densely adherent to the pancreas are visualized. The spleen–pancreas complex can be mobilized over the top of the aorta, taking care to avoid injury of the superior mesenteric artery. After this mobilization, the spleen and distal pancreas are delivered to the level of the subcutaneous tissue. Laparotomy pads are placed in the left upper quadrant to maintain the spleen in the wound. At this point, the degree of injury can be clearly evaluated and the decision for extirpation or repair made.

Splenectomy is usually indicated under the following circumstances:

1. Patient is unstable.
2. Other injuries require prompt attention.
3. Spleen is extensively injured with continuous bleeding.
4. Bleeding is associated with hilar injury.

There are both anterior (short gastric arteries) and posterior (splenic artery) blood supplies. After complete splenic mobilization, traction can be placed on the gastrosplenic ligament that places tension on and exposes the short gastric arteries. These are rapidly divided; with appropriate traction, the gastric wall is easily visualized, avoiding clamp injury. The spleen can then be grasped and elevated by the surgeon or assistant and the splenic artery identified at the superior border of the pancreas. The artery and vein are separately divided and ligated. Not infrequently, the tail of the pancreas extends right into the hilum, in which case it is generally more practical and safer to ligate the splenic vessels after they have divided in order to avoid the morbid complication of injury to the pancreatic tail. In the absence of pancreatic injury, drainage of the splenic fossa is not necessary.

As noted earlier in this chapter, thrombocytosis occurs in about half of postoperative patients in the initial weeks after splenectomy. The thrombocytosis may increase the risk for deep venous thrombosis. When the platelet count rises above 750,000/mm^3, many surgeons treat the patient with antiplatelet therapy, low-dose heparin, or low-molecular-weight heparin. Pimpl and colleagues[27] reviewed 37,000 autopsies over 20 years of adults who died after splenectomy and compared them with a deceased population of 403 who did not have splenectomy. These

investigators found higher incidence rates of lethal pneumonia, sepsis with multiple organ failure, purulent pyelonephritis, and pulmonary embolism in the splenectomy group. They concluded that splenectomy carries a considerable lifelong risk for severe infection and thromboembolism.

Splenorrhaphy

Attempts at splenic repair were initiated with appreciation of the entity of OPSI (see previous section). Additionally, it has been noted that splenic absence provides a relative dead space in the left upper quadrant, which often becomes occupied with blood clot or serum, creating a potential for subphrenic abscess. This occurrence is especially pronounced in the face of hollow viscus or pancreatic injuries. Those scenarios provide for bacterial colonization and culture media.

Splenorrhaphy techniques became widely applied in the late 1970s, reaching a peak in the mid 1980s. Their application has gradually decreased since that time in association with the rise of nonoperative management. Splenorrhaphy was applied to nearly half of splenic injuries at the height of its use. A general rule is that if more than one unit of blood is required for salvage, splenectomy is performed. Beyond that, the risks associated with transfusion generally outweigh the risks of OPSI. Four types of splenorrhaphy have been used:

1. Superficial hemostatic agents (cautery, oxidized cellulose, absorbable gelatin sponge, topical thrombin)
2. Suture repair
3. Absorbable mesh wrap
4. Resectional débridement

Superficial hemostatic approaches are useful for American Association for the Surgery of Trauma grade I and II injuries (see Table 56-6). They may also be adjunctive in higher grades of injury. The argon-beam coagulator has received some support, but there is no clinical evidence that it is superior to other approaches.

Suture repair of lacerations in grade II and III injuries has become common. When feasible, temporary occlusion of the splenic artery may reduce blood loss and facilitate repair. A problem with suture repair is the tendency for the sutures to tear the spleen further when tied. Pledgeted repairs reduce that occurrence. Many surgeons have used Teflon pledgets. The use of pledgets constructed of 2- to 3-cm absorbable gelatin sponge wrapped in oxidized cellulose and secured with suture ties to resemble a cigarette has been commonly applied (Fig. 56-4). These are placed along each edge of the laceration and secured with a running polypropylene suture. That approach has proved effective for both splenic and hepatic lacerations.

Mesh wrapping has been effectively used for grade III and some grade IV injuries. Investigators from Cook County Hospital provided some of the earliest data and description of this technique.[28] Disposable mesh, composed of either polyglycolic acid or polyglactin, has been used. If knitted mesh is used, a keyhole about 1 to 2 cm in diameter is cut in the middle of the mesh and is stretched, so that the spleen can be delivered through it,

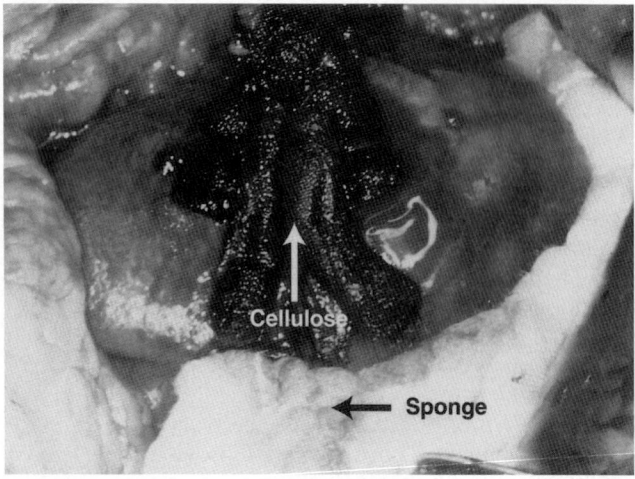

Figure 56-4 Pledgets constructed of gelatin sponge wrapped in oxidized cellulose are used to suture-repair a grade III splenic laceration.

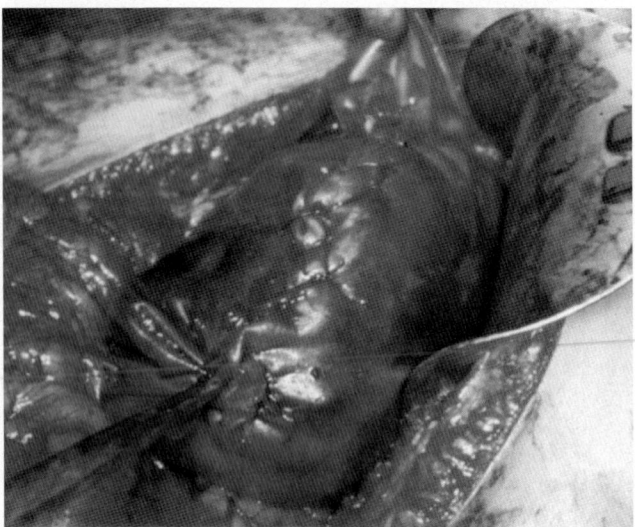

Figure 56-5 Splenorrhaphy of grade IV splenic laceration is accomplished by wrapping with woven polyglactin.

resulting in the keyhole around the splenic hilum. The edges of the mesh are then approximated with a running suture over the top, so that the spleen is effectively enclosed in a mesh sac. If woven mesh is used, it will not stretch; thus, the keyhole for surrounding the hilum is designed by dividing one side of a square piece of mesh to the center and constructing an appropriately sized circular hole. The mesh is tightened around the hilum by reapproximating the severed mesh. The mesh is secured over the top of the spleen as described previously (Fig. 56-5). This technique works surprisingly well, apparently through a tamponade effect.

Resectional débridement has been applied for major fractures, usually involving the upper or lower pole (grade II or IV). The raw surfaces are approximated. Pledgeted materials are of considerable benefit for reap-

proximating those edges. At least one third of the splenic mass is necessary to maintain immunocompetence.

As noted previously, in the past, splenic conservation through splenorrhaphy was applied to nearly half of all splenic injuries. That percentage decreased substantially in the 1990s and probably now accounts for no more than 10%. A high percentage of splenorrhaphy was accounted for by simple techniques for repair of grade I and II injuries. Most of those types of injury are now being managed nonoperatively. Most patients who currently undergo operation for splenic injury have active bleeding or destructive injuries requiring splenectomy. Heightened awareness of risk for transmission of viral disease, especially hepatitis, with blood transfusion has also dampened enthusiasm for splenic repair.

Nonoperative Management

The basis for nonoperative management can be traced to OPSI and incidental notation of splenic injury in the early years of CT scanning for trauma. Nonoperative management originated in pediatric surgery. For several years, general surgeons questioned the judgment of their pediatric surgical colleagues. With the passage of time, it has become clear that nonoperative management is logical. Nonoperative management in adults is somewhat more controversial but is gaining continuously wider acceptance as data accumulate.

Currently, 70% to 90% of children with splenic injury are successfully treated without operation, and 40% to 50% of adult patients with splenic injury are managed nonoperatively in large-volume trauma centers. The lower percentage of nonoperatively managed splenic injury in adults than in children has been a source of speculation. It has been suggested that anatomic differences between adults and children are responsible, including a more elastic, cartilaginous rib cage providing protection and more elastin in the spleen producing contraction and some degree of hemostasis in children. Powell and colleagues,[29] however, have produced data demonstrating that the differences in management of splenic injury between adults and children are most likely related to mechanisms of injury. Their analysis of 411 patients (293 adults and 118 children) found major differences in mechanism of injury in adults and children (P <.05), including the following: motor vehicle crash (67% in adults versus 24% in children), motorcycle crash (9% versus 1%), sports-related injury (2% versus 17%), falls (9% versus 25%), pedestrian and auto collision (4% versus 11%), and bicycle crash (1% versus 9%). Higher injury severity scores, lower Glasgow Coma Scale scores, and higher mortality rates indicated that adults were more severely injured.

A fundamental rule for consideration of nonoperative management is the requirement that the patient be hemodynamically stable. Additionally, institutional resources need to be such that the patient can be monitored in a critical care environment and that operating room facilities and personnel are available in the event of sudden bleeding that requires splenectomy. Most grade I and II injuries can be managed nonoperatively; these account

Table 56-7 Comparison of Results of Nonoperative Management of Blunt Splenic Injuries From Published Series

STUDY	Splenic Injuries (n)	CASES PLANNED Nonoperatively Managed (%)	Nonoperative Success (%)	Failure (%)
Shackford and Molin,[33] 1990	1866	13	69	31
Schurr et al,[36] 1995*	309	25	87	13
Smith et al,[34] 1996*	166	47	97	3
Morrell et al,[35] 1996	135	18	52	48
Davis et al,[30] 1998	524	61	94	6
Myers et al,[37] 1999	204	68	93	7
Cocanour et al,[32] 1999	368	57	86	14
Bee et al,[38] 2001	558	77	92	8

*Excluded grade IV and V injuries.

for about 60% to 70% of cases of nonoperative management.[30] Although CT scanning is the fundamental measure for selecting nonoperative management, it has shortcomings that must be taken into consideration. A report by Sutyak and coworkers[31] involving CT in 49 patients with splenic injury correlated surgical with CT findings. These investigators found that CT matched surgical grading in 10 patients, underestimated it in 18, and overestimated it in 6. They also reported that five injuries were missed by CT and that radiologists disagreed in their interpretations of 20% of scans. Note, however, that the CT scan used in this study was not the current state-of-the-art helical CT scan.

In early reports, most investigators expressed extreme caution regarding nonoperative management of grades III and IV, even with hemodynamic stability. As experience has accumulated, most feel comfortable with observing stable grade III injuries, and many have begun observing grade IV and V injuries.[30,32] Most of the early reports of nonoperative management in the 1980s were anecdotal, noting occasional successful management in highly selected cases. Since the 1990s, nonoperative management has become a more standardized approach. In a review in 1990, Shackford and Molin[33] reported on 1866 splenic injuries in which 13% were managed nonoperatively. Subsequently, Smith and colleagues[34] reported a 47% nonoperative management rate among 166 splenic injuries. These and most other reports have reserved nonoperative management for injury grades I through III.

Analysis of failure rates is important in evaluating criteria for selecting appropriate patients for nonoperative management. Although age greater than 55 years has been reported to be associated with high failure rates,[35] others have refuted that observation.[30,32] Nonoperative management failure rates from recent series are shown in Table 56-7.

An important finding that has been correlated with failed nonoperative management is the presence of a "vascular blush" on CT examination. Schurr and associates[36] reported on 309 blunt splenic injuries, of which 29% were managed nonoperatively. They noted a 13%

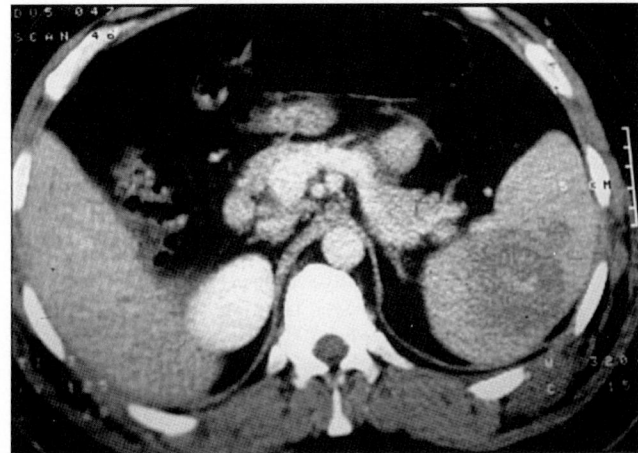

Figure 56-6 Computed tomography scan demonstrates "vascular blush" in an injured spleen.

failure rate; two thirds of the failures were associated with a vascular blush (Fig. 56-6). Those vascular blushes were proved to represent false aneurysms of intraparenchymal branches of the splenic artery (Fig. 56-7). The cause of failure from false aneurysms is gradual enlargement of the aneurysm, with rupture of the aneurysm and spleen. This pathophysiology most likely accounts for many of the instances of "delayed splenic rupture" noted from the past. Not all these pseudoaneurysms rupture, however. It appears likely that 30% to 40% spontaneously thrombose.[36] A subsequent study from the same institution by Davis and colleagues[30] dealt with 524 blunt splenic injuries during a 4.5-year period. In that report, a protocol was followed in which vascular blushes identified by CT were followed by angiography with embolization of the false aneurysm (Fig. 56-8). That approach yielded a failure rate of 5% for nonoperative management, a rate significantly lower ($P < .03$) than their prior experience.

Controversy exists concerning the need for follow-up CT evaluations. Some institutions have suggested that follow-up scans are unnecessary.[32,37] Davis and

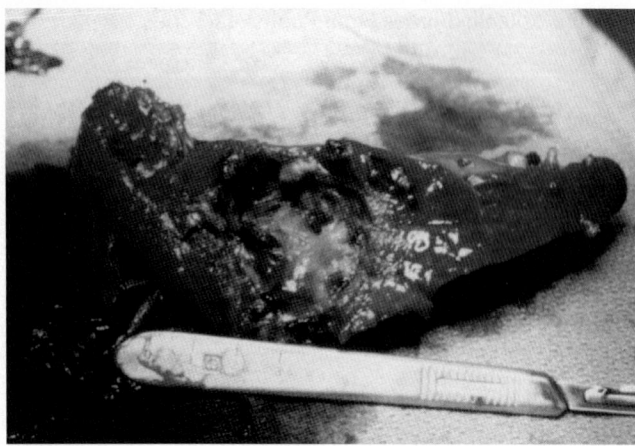

Figure 56-7 After splenectomy, the sectioned spleen demonstrated a false aneurysm, which corresponds to the vascular blush in Figure 56-6.

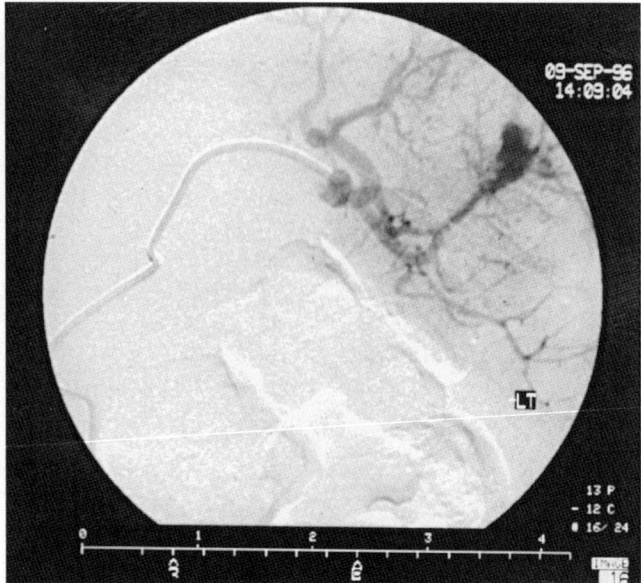

A

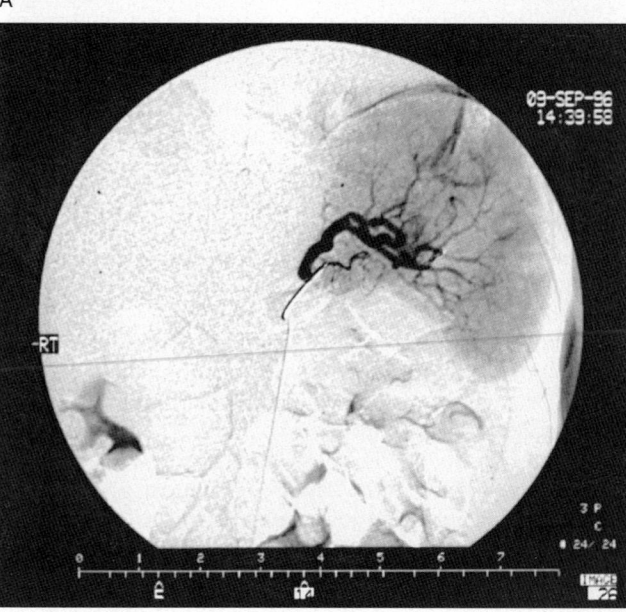

B

Figure 56-8 A and **B,** Angiographic embolization of a false aneurysm, which was demonstrated by helical computed tomography.

colleagues,[30] however, noted that 74% of vascular blushes were seen only in follow-up studies. Because a high rate of failure was noted with the finding, these investigators recommend follow-up scans within 2 to 3 days for all but the most trivial lesions. The reasons for absence of vascular blush on initial scans include missed by 1-cm cut protocol and lysis of initial clot.

The cause of other failures is less clear. Investigators have become more aggressive by including patients with higher injury grades (IV and V). Fifty-six of 106 grade IV and V injuries were nonoperatively managed with a failure rate of 18%.[30] This and subsequent reports have also correlated a higher failure rate with large amounts of free intraperitoneal blood on the admission CT scan (perisplenic and perihepatic and gutter and pelvis).[30,32,37] It seems intuitive that larger degrees of splenic injury as indicated by CT scan and by volume of intraperitoneal blood would be associated with higher failure rates.

In a recent report published by Bee and colleagues,[38] the published contraindications to nonoperative management (NOM) of blunt splenic injury were reviewed and compared with their experience with nonoperative failures. The published contraindications reviewed included age of 55 years or older, Glasgow Coma Scale score of 13 or less, admission blood pressure less than 100 mm Hg, major (grade III-V) injuries, and large amounts of hemoperitoneum. In their evaluation of 430 consecutive patients who were observed, the NOM failure rate was 8%. Multivariate analysis identified age of 55 or older and grades III to V as independent predictors of failure. They noted the highest failure rate (30%-40%) occurred in patients older than 55 years with major injury or moderate to large amounts of hemoperitoneum. They noted a mortality rate for successful NOM of 12%, compared with 9% for failed NOM, and thought that failed NOM was not significantly associated with adverse outcome. An ideal situation would be for 70% to 80% of cases to be manageable nonoperatively with a 1% to 2% failure rate. This may not be possible. Future clinical studies need to be designed to address these important issues of selection,

causes of failure, and use of adjunctive techniques, including embolization. We believe that advancing CT technology, which will better define the injuries, combined with clinical trials, will ultimately approach those numbers—high NOM rates coupled with very low failure rates.

No objective data are available related to recommendations for return to activity after splenic injury. For grade I and II injuries, 2 to 3 weeks is probably adequate healing time. For higher-grade injuries, 6 to 8 weeks is probably more appropriate, and many surgeons would obtain a CT scan at that time to evaluate degree of healing before return to excessive physical activity.

Table 56-8 Evidence-Based Classification of Medical Literature Adapted From Recommendations by the Agency for Health Care Policy and Research

Class I Evidence

Prospective, randomized controlled trials—the gold standard of clinical trials. Some may be poorly designed, have inadequate numbers, or suffer from other methodologic inadequacies and thus may not be clinically significant.

Class II Evidence

Clinical studies in which the data were collected prospectively and retrospective analyses that were based on clearly reliable data. These types of studies include observational studies, cohort studies, prevalence studies, and case-control studies.

Class III Evidence

Studies based on retrospectively collected data. Evidence used in this class includes clinical series, databases or registries, case reviews, case reports, and expert opinion.

Table 56-9 Categorization of Strengths of Recommendations Based on a Medical Literature Review of a Specified Topic* According to Methodologies Derived From the Agency for Health Care Policy and Research

Level 1

This recommendation is convincingly justifiable based on the available scientific information alone. It is usually based on class I data; however, strong class II evidence may form the basis for a level 1 recommendation, especially if the issue does not lend itself to testing in a randomized format. Conversely, weak or contradictory class I data may not be able to support a level 1 recommendation.

Level 2

This recommendation is reasonably justifiable by available scientific evidence and strongly supported by expert critical opinion. It is usually supported by class II data or a preponderance of class III evidence.

Level 3

This recommendation is supported by available data, but adequate scientific evidence is lacking. It is generally supported by class III data. This type of recommendation is useful for educational purposes and in guiding future studies.

*See Table 56-8.

Evidence-Based Medicine Evaluation

The use of evidence-based medicine (EBM) to address optimal management of clinical problems is gaining increased acceptance. One of the most important applications of EBM is to develop practice management guidelines. There are two basic methodologies. The first is through statistical methodology centered on meta-analysis. Rigorous meta-analytic techniques require randomized, controlled trials for analysis; however, there are relatively few randomized, controlled trials for addressing most questions in surgery. Therefore, a second methodology for EBM addresses questions through data classification and assessing confidence levels for recommendations. Extensive work on data classification has been done by the Canadian and U.S. Preventive Task Forces and by the Agency for Health Care Policy and Research of the United States Department of Health and Human Services.[39] A classification system based on that work is outlined in Table 56-8.

The Agency for Health Care Policy and Research has also developed a system of assessing confidence levels for recommendations based on that data classification system, which is presented in Table 56-9. Using those methodologies for data evaluation and assessment, the Eastern Association for the Surgery of Trauma (EAST) has published 11 patient management guidelines on their Internet website (*www.east.org*). One of those evidence-based guidelines addresses nonoperative management of splenic injury. To develop the guidelines for splenic injury, a study group consisting of seven surgeons identified 50 English-language clinical articles published between 1976 and 1996 addressing pertinent questions about blunt splenic injury management. The recommendations based on the classification and assessment of those published data are listed in Table 56-10. The EAST

evidence-based analysis demonstrates that there are neither class I data nor level I recommendations. Those findings make it clear that splenic injury management must be addressed by prospective, multi-institutional trials. A strong case for such trials can be made because splenic injury occurs at a high incidence and is associated with substantial cost and morbidity.

The intent of EBM-derived guidelines is that they be adopted at the local level into management schemes through clinical pathways and algorithms that consider resource availability and practice patterns. An algorithm developed from the EAST recommendations and their accompanying literature review is represented in Figure 56-9.

ELECTIVE LAPAROSCOPIC SPLENECTOMY

The technique of open splenectomy was described in detail in the previous section on splenic trauma. Many surgeons now prefer to use the laparoscopic approach for most elective splenectomies. The technique of laparoscopic splenectomy was first described in 1992.[40] In experienced hands, laparoscopic splenectomy can be performed as safely and effectively as open splenectomy, particularly for hematologic diseases in which the spleen size is normal or only slightly enlarged.[4] Early experiences with laparoscopic splenectomy have demonstrated many similarities to the early days of laparoscopic cholecystectomy. Operative time is longer for laparoscopic splenectomy, but the procedure offers the advantages of

Table 56-10 Eastern Association for the Surgery of Trauma*
Recommended Patient Management Guidelines
for the Nonoperative Management (NOM)
of Blunt Injuries to the Liver and the Spleen

Level I

There are insufficient data to suggest NOM as a level I
recommendation for the initial management of blunt
injuries to the liver and/or spleen in the
hemodynamically stable patient.

Level II

1. There are class II and mostly class III data to suggest
   that NOM of blunt hepatic and/or splenic injuries in a
   hemodynamically stable patient is reasonable.
2. Severity of hepatic or splenic injury (as suggested by
   computed tomography [CT] grade or degree of
   hemoperitoneum), neurologic status, and/or the
   presence of associated injuries are not
   contraindications to NOM.
3. Abdominal CT is the most reliable method to identify
   and assess the severity of the injury to the spleen or
   liver.

Level III

1. The clinical status of the patient should dictate the
   frequency of follow-up scans.
2. Initial CT of the abdomen should be performed with
   oral and intravenous contrast agents to facilitate the
   diagnosis of hollow viscus injuries.
3. Medical clearance to resume normal activity status
   should be based on evidence of healing.
4. Angiographic embolization is an adjunct in the NOM
   of the hemodynamically stable patient with hepatic
   and splenic injuries and evidence of ongoing
   bleeding.

*See their website at *www.east.org.*

more rapid postoperative recovery and shorter duration
of hospital stay, leading some to consider laparoscopic
splenectomy the standard of care for some hematologic
disorders requiring splenectomy.

Results of laparoscopic splenectomy for benign hematologic diseases, such as ITP, are compared with the
standard of open splenectomy, which is technically feasible in 100% of patients and is associated with a hospital
mortality rate of less than 1% and a morbidity rate of 10%
to 20%. In a retrospective literature review of 1358
patients who underwent open splenectomy, the rate of
wound-related complications was estimated to be 3%.
The mean postoperative hospital stay ranged from 7.5 to
11 days.[41,42] In patients with splenomegaly secondary to
malignant hematologic disorders, however, the operative
mortality rates are increased in the range of 0% to 18%,
and morbidity rates are increased in the range of 19% to
56%, respectively.[43]

In comparison, laparoscopic splenectomy can be completed in about 90% of properly selected patients. The
incidence of conversion to open splenectomy is between
0% and 20%. Most of the conversions are caused by
intraoperative bleeding, but lack of surgical experience, extensive adhesions,[44] large splenomegaly,[45] and
obesity[45,46] are also involved. A significant learning curve

is observed with laparoscopic splenectomy, and with
increasing experience, the conversion rate has been
reported to decrease dramatically.[44,46,47] Glasgow and
associates[47] reported a conversion rate of 36% during the
initial 11 laparoscopic splenectomies; during the subsequent operations, the conversion rate dropped to 0% to
5%.

In two reviews[3,4] of laparoscopic series that included
418 and 948 patients, respectively, the mean operative
time for laparoscopic splenectomy ranged from 88 to 261
minutes, with an open conversion rate ranging from
0% to 30% (Table 56-11). In a multivariate analysis by
Friedman and coworkers,[45] operative time was significantly related to patient age, hematologic diagnosis,
operative technique, and splenic weight. The perioperative morbidity rates averaged 8% and 12%, respectively
(range, 0%-30%), and the mortality rate was 0.7% (0%-
6%). Most deaths were attributable to the patient's underlying diseases or hematologic disorder. In the review by
Gigot and associates[3] of 984 patients, 119 had reported
complications. Bleeding was the most frequent perioperative complication and has been significantly linked to
the surgeon's learning curve.[44] The mean number of
patients requiring intraoperative or postoperative transfusions was 13%, ranging from 0% to 40%. Local complications, including wound-related complications (seroma,
hematoma, infection, evisceration, or incisional hernia),
occurred in 1.5%. Postoperative bleeding occurred in
1% of patients, and 73% of these cases required re-
exploration. Pancreatic complications (pancreatitis or
pancreatic fistula) occurred in 0.6% and subphrenic
abscess in 0.5%. General postoperative complications
occurred in 7.4%; most (3.2%) were pleuropulmonary.

Postoperative recovery after laparoscopic splenectomy
is surprisingly fast, as has previously been observed with
laparoscopic cholecystectomy. The length of stay ranged
from 1.8 to 6 days after laparoscopic splenectomy.[3,4] Most
patients are able to return to full activities within 1 week
if their underlying hematologic disorder allows. In Flowers'
study,[44] 9% of patients returned to work in 7 days, and all
patients with uncomplicated laparoscopic splenectomy
were fully recovered by 21 days regardless of profession.
Although a prospective, randomized comparison has not
been conducted, several retrospective case-control series
have compared the laparoscopic approach to an open
splenectomy (see Table 56-11). Although it is difficult to
extrapolate definitive data from these series because of
potential selection bias (patient age, diagnosis and indication, splenic weight, and major comorbid conditions), the
results are consistently in favor of the laparoscopic
approach. Each series has demonstrated an earlier resumption of diet, reduced postoperative analgesics, and
decreased postoperative hospital stay.

Despite the promising technical results of laparoscopic
splenectomy, the hematologic response and long-term
cure rates are the most important. Open splenectomy for
the treatment of ITP achieves a long-term cure rate of
65% to 90%. In clinical series of laparoscopic splenectomy, the mean follow-up is usually limited to 1 to 2
years. During this short follow-up, reports of 76% to 100%
success rates have been published. Similarly, Katkhouda

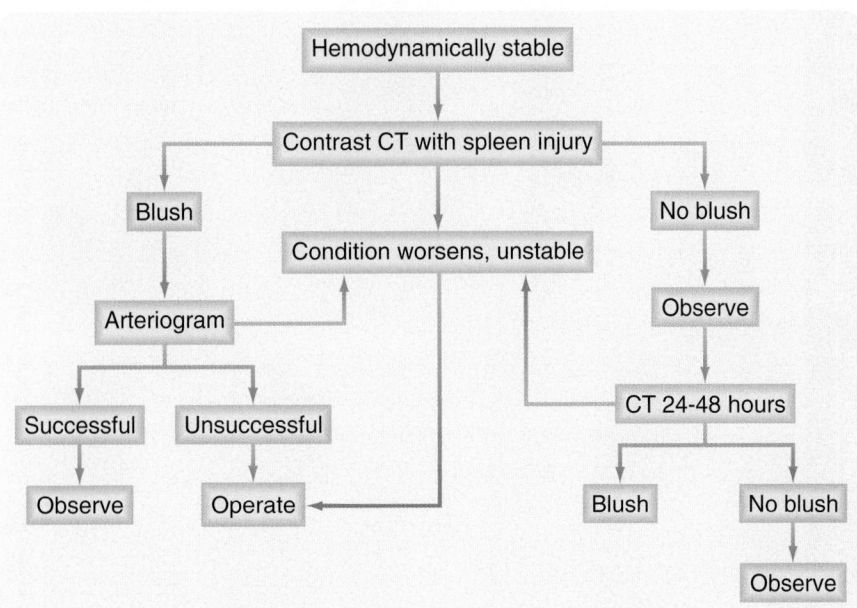

Figure 56-9 Algorithm for nonoperative management of splenic injuries in the hemodynamically stable patient. CT, computed tomography. (From Bee TK, Croce MA, Miller PR, et al: Failures of splenic nonoperative management: Is the glass half empty or half full? J Trauma 50:231, 2001.)

and associates[4] reported that the treatment of ITP appears to be at least as good after laparoscopic surgery as after the open technique in comparisons of separate series (see Tables 56-3 and 56-4). Gigot and colleagues[3] reported on 279 patients with ITP, and an absence of initial response or recurrent thrombocytopenia occurred in about 15% (Table 56-12).

The causes of recurrence in patients with ITP are multifactorial, but residual accessory spleens are well known to be one of the factors of recurrence. There have been several reported cases of recurrent thrombocytopenia secondary to retained accessory spleens (see Table 56-12). This issue of accessory spleens has been prominent in the discussion of the role of laparoscopic splenectomy. Autopsy studies have demonstrated that the incidence of accessory spleens in the normal population is about 10%. In clinical series, however, accessory spleens have been reported in 15% to 30% of patients. The incidence of accessory spleen in recently reviewed splenectomy series since 1980 is 15% to 16%.[4] The incidence probably correlates with the diligence of the search and is higher than commonly estimated because small accessory spleens are easily missed or mistaken for lymph nodes. Because accessory spleens are often easier felt than seen, it is likely that the incidence of missed splenunculi is higher at laparoscopic than open splenectomy. The reliability of laparoscopic exploration in dealing with the problem of accessory spleens is a key factor in establishing the long-term credibility of the laparoscopic approach.[3]

Although the indications for a laparoscopic splenectomy remain the same as for open splenectomy, some cases require caution in performing laparoscopically. Absolute contraindications to the laparoscopic approach include severe cardiopulmonary disease, cirrhosis, and

pregnancy. Variceal short gastric vessels compounded by the coagulopathy of liver disease present an unacceptable risk for operative hemorrhage and temper enthusiasm for the laparoscopic approach in patients with portal hypertension. Thrombocytopenia in pregnancy is frequently gestational. Surgery is reserved for the failure of medical management and associated with a fetal mortality rate of 31%. Although laparoscopic cholecystectomy has been shown to be safe in the second trimester of pregnancy, results of laparoscopic splenectomy in this rare patient population have not been reported.

Initially, splenomegaly was felt to be an absolute contraindication to the laparoscopic approach. Increasing experience and improvement of surgical devices have made this a relative contraindication. Splenic size and surgeon experience are the determining factors. Though technically feasible, laparoscopic splenectomy in the patient with splenomegaly can be a challenge. The introduction of hand-assisted laparoscopic surgery (HALS) has led some surgeons to approach these larger spleens with outcomes similar to the totally laparoscopic approach.[48]

The laparoscopic technique may be performed with the patient in the supine (or modified lithotomy) position or in the right lateral decubitus position. After induction of general anesthesia and endotracheal intubation, a nasogastric tube and a urinary catheter are inserted, and pneumatic compression stockings are applied. Appropriate patient positioning is of paramount importance to the successful completion of a laparoscopic splenectomy. With either the lateral or the supine approach, the patient is placed so that the kidney rest can be raised to maximize the space between the iliac crest and the costal margin. The patient is positioned so that the table may be flexed to create a wider working space. The patient is then placed in a reverse Trendelenburg position to

Table 56-11 Retrospective Case-Control Series Comparing Open and Laparoscopic Splenectomies in Adults

	YEE ET AL, 1995		RHODES ET AL, 1995		BRUNT ET AL, 1996		WATSON ET AL, 1997		DIAZ ET AL, 1997		FRIEDMAN ET AL, 1997		DELAITRE AND PITRE, 1997[46]		SMITH ET AL, 1996		GLASGOW ET AL, 1997[47]		ASHIZUME ET AL, 1996	
	OS	LS	OS	LS	OS	LS	OS	LS	OS	LS	OS	LS	OS	LS	OS	LS	OS	LS	OS	LS
Patients	25	25	11	24	20	26	47	13	15	15	74	63	28	28	10	10	28	52	41	10
Operative time (min)	156	198†	75	120	134	202†	84	88	116	196†	121	153	127	183*	131	261*	156	196†	249	100‡
Delay before regular diet (days)	4.3	2.1†	—	—	4.1	1.4‡	—	—	—	—	3.2	1.5*	—	—	4.4	1.9*	4.3	2	—	—
Blood loss (mL)	273	319	—	—	222	376	—	—	359	385	437	259	—	—	—	—	274	320	512	176*
Transfusion rate	12	16	—	—	15	10	13	0	—	—	27	3.5	36	29	20	40	18	27	—	—
Complications (%)	12	8	—	27	23	23	19	0	13	6.7	22	12	32	11	20	0	14	10	46	0
POHS	6.7	5.1*	7	3†	5.8	2.5‡	10	2‡	8.8	2.3†	6.7	3.5‡	8.6	5.1*	5.8	3*	6.7	4.8*	20	8.2
Total hospital costs USD×10³	13,433	9207	—	—	—	—	4224	2238	16,362	18,015	10,900	9700*	—	—	13,196	17,071	17,876	20,295	9264	6438†
Cure rate at FU in ITP (%)	76	81	—	—	75	75	83	92	75	80	—	—	86	93	—	81	81	74	63	80
Mean FU (mo)	—	—	—	—	6.5	6.5	60	14	20	29	13.5	19	—	—	—	—	—	—	—	—
AS detected (%)	24	8	—	—	5	5	6	15	23	12*	29	11	18	11	30	21	21	16	—	—
Return to full activity (days)	—	—	—	—	—	—	—	—	—	—	—	—	—	—	6 wk	—	—	1-2 wk	—	—

As, accessory spleen; FU, follow-up; ITP, immune thrombocytopenic purpura; LS, laparoscopic splenectomy; OS, open splenectomy; POHS, postoperative hospital stay; USD, U.S. dollars.

*P < .05.
†P < .001.
‡P = .0005.

From Gigot JF, Lengele B, Gianello P, et al: Present status of laparoscopic splenectomy for hematologic diseases: Certitudes and unresolved issues. Semin Laparosc Surg 5:159, 1998.

Table 56-12 Long-Term Hematologic Cure Rate After Laparoscopic Treatment of Immune Thrombocytopenic Purpura Patients

STUDY	PATIENTS (N)	MEAN FOLLOW-UP (mo [RANGE])	ABSENCE OF INITIAL RESPONSE AND/OR RECURRENT THROMBOCYTOPENIA	RESIDUAL ACCESSORY SPLEEN DETECTED
Emmermann et al, 1995	20	14 (1-28)	1	?
Yee et al, 1995	14	At discharge	4	1
Liew and Storey, 1995	6	?	1	1
Legrand et al, 1996	9	12 (1-26)	1	?
Parent et al, 1995	11	— (6-9)	1	?
Flowers et al,[44] 1996	22	21 (3-36)	4	?
Dexter et al, 1996	6	24 (17-33)	0	—
Zamir et al, 1996	15	— (2-36)	0	—
Katkhouda et al, 1996	20	20 (1-46)	0	—
Watson et al, 1997	13	14 (5-21)	1	1
Tsiotos and Schinkert, 1997	18	15 (0-30)	1	?
Lee and Kim, 1997	15	?	3	?
Glasgow et al,[47] 1997	16	?	4	1
Delaitre and Pitre,[46] 1997	26	— (3-48)	2	?
Decker et al, 1998	17	12.5 (1-28)	4	?
Trias et al, 1998	32	12 (-50)	9	3
Gigot, 1998*	19	45 (22-63)	6	3

*Unpublished data.

?, data not given despite treatment failures—not assessed; —, no treatment failures, therefore not assessed.

facilitate gravity retraction of the viscera away from the left upper quadrant.

In the supine approach, the surgeon stands to the left of the patient, and the first assistant and camera assistants stand to the right.[44] It is often easier for a right-handed surgeon to work from a position between the patient's legs, with the patient in a modified lithotomy position. The scrub nurse stands to the patient's left side near the foot of the table. Alternatively, the patient may be placed on a beanbag in a 60-degree right lateral decubitus position, with a right axillary roll. The left arm is supported by a splint. In this approach, the surgeon and the scrub nurse stand to the patient's right, and the assistants stand to the left. The spleen is suspended from its diaphragmatic attachments, and gravity retracts the stomach, transverse colon, and greater omentum, while placing the splenic hilum under tension. For both approaches, the video monitors are placed on each side of the table, at or above the level of the patient's shoulders.

Pneumoperitoneum is established to a pressure of 12 to 15 mm Hg, and three to five 2- to 12-mm diameter operating ports are used, with the camera port at the umbilicus or offset between the umbilicus and the left costal margin. The other port sites are arrayed in the positions depicted in Figure 56-10. The operation is begun with a thorough search of the abdominal cavity for the presence of accessory splenic tissue (Fig. 56-11). The stomach is retracted to the right to facilitate inspection of the gastrosplenic ligament. The splenocolic ligament, the greater omentum, and the phrenosplenic

ligament are then carefully inspected. The small and large bowel mesenteries, the pelvis, and the adnexal tissues are all inspected. The gastrosplenic ligament is opened and the area of the pancreatic tail inspected.

Our preference has been to use the lateral decubitus approach. The initial dissection is begun by mobilization of the splenic flexure of the colon. The splenocolic ligament is divided using sharp dissection. This mobilizes the inferior pole of the spleen and allows the spleen to be retracted cephalad. Great care is taken to avoid rupture of the splenic capsule during retraction.

The lateral peritoneal attachments of the spleen are then incised using either sharp dissection or ultrasonic shears. A 1-cm cuff of peritoneum is left along the lateral aspect of the spleen to be grasped if the spleen needs to be drawn medially. The lesser sac is entered along the medial border of the spleen. With the spleen elevated, the short gastric vessels and main vascular pedicle are visualized. The tail of the pancreas is also visualized and avoided at this point as it approaches the splenic hilum. The short gastric vessels are divided. This can be accomplished with several different modalities as long as the surgeon has familiarity with the device and its application. Currently available instrumentation for the control of splenic vessels include ultrasonic dissector, hemoclips, bipolar devices, Liga-Sure, or an endovascular stapling device. The use of hemoclips is minimized throughout the procedure and especially around the hilum because the clips may interfere with future applications of a stapling device. The stapler will not function if a clip is

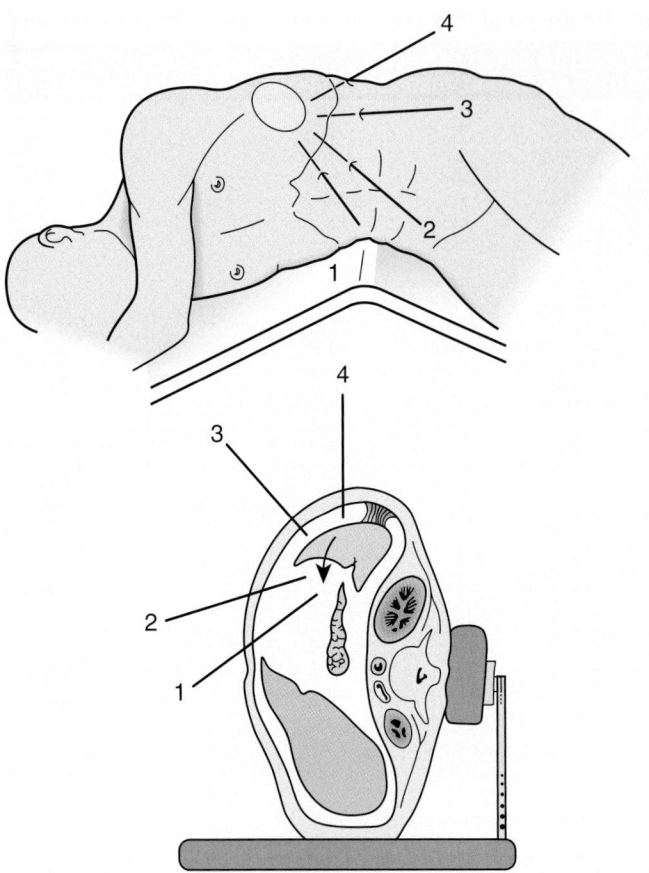

Figure 56-10 Strict lateral position of the patient for laparoscopic splenectomy. The table is angulated, giving forced lateral flexion of the patient to open the costophrenic space. Trocars are inserted along the left costal margin more posteriorly. The spleen is hanged by its peritoneal attachments. The numbered lines show the position of laparoscopic ports. (From Gigot JF, Lengele B, Gianello P, et al: Present status of laparoscopic splenectomy for hematologic diseases: Certitudes and unresolved issues. Semin Laparosc Surg 5:149, 1998.)

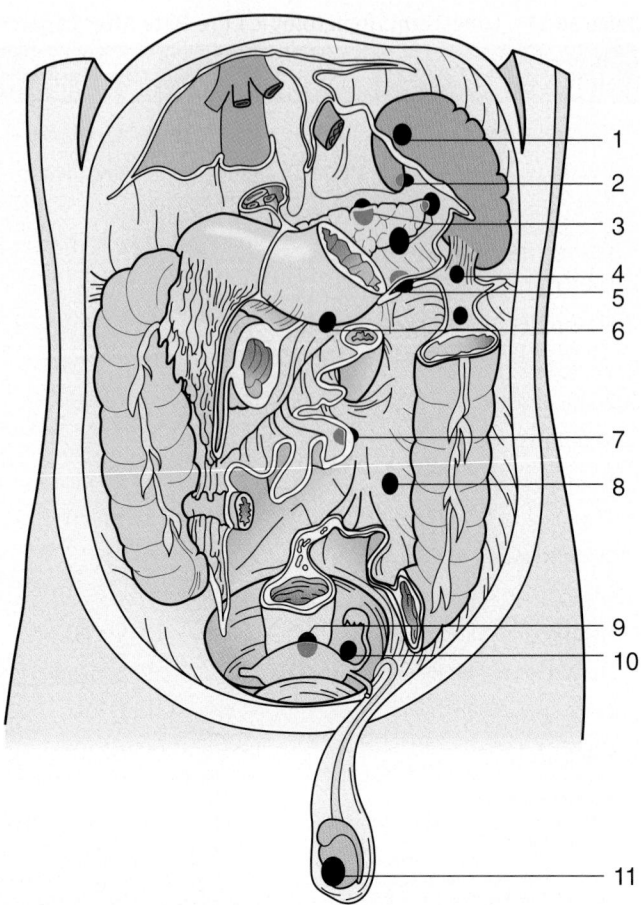

Figure 56-11 Usual location of accessory spleens: (1) gastrosplenic ligament, (2) splenic hilum, (3) tail of the pancreas, (4) splenocolic ligament, (5) left transverse mesocolon, (6) greater omentum along the greater curvature of the stomach, (7) mesentery, (8) left mesocolon, (9) left ovary, (10) Douglas pouch, (11) left testis. (From Gigot JF, Lengele B, Gianello P, et al: Present status of laparoscopic splenectomy for hematologic diseases: Certitudes and unresolved issues. Semin Laparosc Surg 5:156, 1998.)

caught within its jaws, and this can result in significant bleeding from hilar vessels.

After the short gastric vessels have been divided, the splenic pedicle may be carefully dissected from both the medial and lateral aspects (an advantage over the anterior approach). After the artery and vein are dissected, the vessels are divided by application of endoscopic vascular staplers or suture ligatures. In the more common distributed mode, there are multiple vascular branches that enter the spleen; these arise from the main vascular trunks about 2 to 3 cm from the hilum.[4] For this reason, we generally try to keep our dissection 2 cm from the splenic capsule. Several branches may still be encountered, however, and are controlled individually if necessary. A pedicle formed by the artery and vein that enters the hilum as a compact bundle is known as the *magistral mode*. In this circumstance, the pedicle is transected en bloc using a linear vascular stapler. The tail of the pancreas should be well visualized as the staplers are applied to avoid injury to this structure. The surgeon must be

acutely aware of the position of the tail of the pancreas during the hilar division. The pancreatic tail lies within 1 cm of the splenic hilum in 75% of patients and touches the splenic hilum in 30%.

After the hilar vessels have been controlled, the completely devascularized spleen is suspended by a small cuff of avascular superior-pole splenophrenic attachments. This is left in place to facilitate entrapment of the spleen into the retrieval bag. To remove the detached spleen, a puncture-resistant nylon extraction bag is introduced through one of the trocar sites, typically the left lateral site. The bag is opened within the abdominal cavity, and the spleen is placed into the bag. The drawstring is grasped, and the bag is closed, leaving only the superior pole attachments to be divided at this stage. The open end of the closed bag is brought outside the abdomen through the supraumbilical or epigastric trocar site. The spleen is then morcellated with ring forceps and with finger fracture, and is removed in fragments (Fig. 56-12).

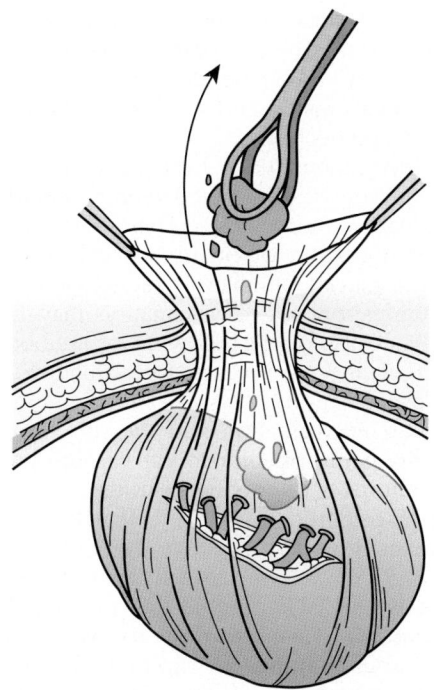

Figure 56-12 Extraction of the spleen within a heavy plastic bag. Instrumental morcellation of the organ with forceps. (From Gigot JF, Lengele B, Gianello P, et al: Present status of laparoscopic splenectomy for hematologic diseases: Certitudes and unresolved issues. Semin Laparosc Surg 5:154, 1998.)

In conditions requiring pathologic evaluation of an intact spleen, an incision adequate to enable removal of the bag containing the intact spleen is made. Care must be taken to avoid spillage of any fragments of spleen into either the abdominal cavity or the wound. The laparoscope is reinserted, and the splenic bed is assessed for hemostasis. At this point, drains may be placed if deemed necessary. The fascia of all trocar ports larger than 5 mm are closed.

LATE MORBIDITY AFTER SPLENECTOMY

Postsplenectomy thrombocytosis may be associated with both hemorrhagic and thromboembolic phenomena. This occurs particularly in patients with myeloproliferative disorders such as CML, agnogenic myeloid dysplasia, essential thrombocytosis, and polycythemia vera. Thrombosis of the mesenteric, portal, and renal veins may be life-threatening sequelae of postsplenectomy thrombocytosis. The lifelong risk for deep venous thrombosis and pulmonary embolism has not been well defined but may be significant. In review of 37,012 autopsies over a 20-year period, Pimpl and colleagues[27] identified 202 deceased adults who had a history of splenectomy and matched them with a cohort of 403 deceased patients who had not undergone splenectomy. Pulmonary embolism was the major or contributory cause of death more often in the splenectomy group (35.6%) than in the control group (9.7%).

OPSI is among the more devastating sequelae of asplenia and is the most common fatal late complication of splenectomy.[49] Hyposplenism in the neonatal period has been suggested to contribute to the poor outcomes from neonatal sepsis. The exact incidence of OPSI has been difficult to determine. The incidence of infection in postsplenectomy patients is likely to be underreported. In the autopsy series by Pimpl and colleagues,[27] lethal pneumonia was identified twice as often in autopsies of splenectomized patients than in controls (57.9% versus 24.1%), and lethal sepsis with multiple organ failure occurred in 6.9% of splenectomized versus 1.5% of autopsies on controls. One consistent observation is that the risk for OPSI is greater after splenectomy for malignancy or hematologic disease than for trauma. The risk also appears to be greater in young children (<4 years of age). The risk for fatal OPSI is estimated to be 1 per 300 to 350 patient-years follow-up for children, and 1 per 800 to 1000 patient-years follow-up for adults. The incidence of nonfatal infection and sepsis is likely to be significantly greater. A recent review of selected reported splenectomy series of 7872 total cases inclusive of both children and adults revealed 270 episodes of sepsis (3.5%), with 169 septic fatalities (2.1%).[50] Infection may occur at any time after splenectomy; in one recent series, most infections occurred more than 2 years after splenectomy, and 42% occurred more than 5 years after splenectomy.

OPSI typically begins with a prodromal phase characterized by fever and chills and nonspecific symptoms, including sore throat, malaise, myalgias, diarrhea, and vomiting. Patients may have had rigors for 1 to 2 days before seeking appropriate medical treatment. Pneumonia and meningitis may be present, but many cases have no identifiable focal site of infection and present with high-grade primary bacteremia. Progression of the illness is classically rapid, with the development of hypotension, disseminated intravascular coagulation, respiratory distress, coma, and death within hours of presentation. The mortality rate is between 50% and 70% for fully developed OPSI despite antibiotics and intensive care. Survivors often have a long and complicated hospital course with severe sequelae, such as peripheral gangrene requiring amputation, deafness from meningitis, mastoid osteomyelitis, bacterial endocarditis, and cardiac valvular destruction.

S. pneumoniae is the most frequently involved organism in OPSI and is estimated to be responsible for between 50% and 90% of cases. Other organisms involved in OPSI include *Haemophilus influenzae*, *Neisseria meningitidis*, *Streptococcus* species and other pneumococcal species, *Salmonella* species, and *Capnocytophaga canimorsus* (implicated in OPSI as a sequela of dog bites).

Prophylactic Treatment of Splenectomized Patients

Immunization
Many cases of delayed OPSI occurred in nonimmunized immunocompetent patients and before the current polyvalent pneumococcal vaccine (PPV23) that was

introduced in 1983, replacing the 14-valent vaccine licensed in 1977. PPV23 is composed of purified preparations of pneumococcal capsular polysaccharide antigens of 23 types of *S. pneumoniae* (25 μg each) that cause 88% of the bacteremic pneumococcal disease in the United States.

Currently, the standard of care for postsplenectomy patients includes immunization with polyvalent pneumococcal vaccine (PPV23), *H. influenzae* type b conjugate, and meningococcal polysaccharide vaccine within 2 weeks of splenectomy.[51] Despite this established standard, the literature reflects a diverse 11% to 75% postsplenectomy immunization rate. A recent report of 77 cases[52] of OPSI documented that only 31% of individuals had received pneumococcal vaccination before OPSI.

Most healthy adults show a twofold or greater rise in type-specific antibody within 2 to 3 weeks of vaccination. It has been clearly documented that after vaccination with PPV23, antibody levels decline after 5 to 10 years, and may fall to prevaccination levels. However, the relationship between antibody titer and protection from invasive disease is not certain. The ability to define the need for revaccination based on serology represents a clinical challenge. Even with vaccination, the development of a protective level of antibody against pneumococci is only about 50%. Currently available vaccines elicit a T-cell–independent response and do not produce a sustained increase in antibody titers. Subsequently, there is a lack of evidence that indicates a substantial increase in protection in most revaccinated persons.

Therefore, routine revaccination of immunocompetent persons who were previously vaccinated with PPV23 is not recommended by the Centers for Disease Control and Prevention (CDC). Revaccination is, however, recommended in high-risk individuals. Candidates for revaccination with PPV23 include the following[53]:

- Persons who received the 14-valent vaccine who are at highest risk for fatal pneumococcal infection (e.g., asplenic patients)
- Adults at highest risk who received the 23-valent vaccine 6 years prior
- Adults at highest risk who have shown a rapid decline in pneumococcal antibody levels (e.g., patients with nephrotic syndrome, those with renal failure, and transplant recipients)
- Children at highest risk (asplenia, nephritic syndrome, sickle cell anemia) who would be 10 years old at revaccination

Only one PPV23 revaccination dose is recommended for these high-risk persons, and it is administered 5 years after the initial dose. Rutherford and colleagues[54] examined the efficacy and safety of pneumococcal revaccination after splenectomy for trauma. Of 45 patients offered revaccination 2 or more years after primary vaccination, 24 patients demonstrated a lack of understanding of the postsplenectomy state, confirming poor patient understanding of postsplenectomy risk. After revaccination, 48% of patients demonstrated at least a twofold increase in at least one titer (serotype 6 and 23 pneumococcus). The CDC concluded that despite physician and patient education, pamphlets, and Medic Alert bracelets, patient retention regarding the risks of the postsplenectomy state was poor. They recommended that all splenectomy patients be revaccinated and re-educated between 2 and 6 years after splenectomy.

Similar recommendations have been made for other patients requiring surgical splenectomy, including those with hereditary spherocytosis. These recommendations include determination of pneumococcal antibody titers after immunization of every splenectomized patient because nonresponders to vaccination may be at high risk for OPSI. Subsequent follow-up of antibody titers is recommended at 3 to 5 years, to evaluate for possible need for revaccination.

Other than revaccination and the development of a more immunogenic pneumococcal vaccine preparation, additional efforts at improving host immunocompetence have been considered. Partial splenic salvage or splenic autotransplantation may improve the humoral immune response to PPV23.[55] The difficulty with splenic salvage techniques is the lack of objective functional immune testing in humans. This is also true for patients who have undergone angiographic embolization for cessation of splenic hemorrhage in trauma. No data are available regarding the risk of these patients for OPSI. Preclinical studies have examined the optimal site and amount of splenic tissue for autotransplantation. The most effective site of splenic autotransplantation was the omental pouch, and about 50% of the whole spleen would be necessary for prevention of pneumococcal sepsis. Although all efforts need to be made to preserve the spleen in trauma victims, the strategy of splenic autotransplantation seems to have limited applicability in humans at present.

Current information suggests that patient education regarding OPSI is poor. Educational interventions for trauma patients who required emergent splenectomy are necessary. Communication with and educational efforts for primary care providers who assume medical care for trauma victims is therefore extremely important regarding OPSI risk. Overwhelming postsplenectomy infection is preventable if appropriate precautions are taken.

Antibiotics

Penicillin prophylaxis is commonly practiced in children during the first few years after splenectomy, and some authorities have advocated this form of prophylaxis in adults, although data showing the efficacy of this treatment are lacking. OPSI has been reported in both adults and children taking prophylactic penicillin, despite penicillin-sensitive pneumococcal infection. Available data do not support the practice of long-term penicillin prophylaxis in asplenic adults. Another approach that appears rational is to provide the asplenic patient with a supply of oral antibiotics, such as amoxicillin, with instructions to begin taking the medication at the onset of rigor or a febrile illness if appropriate medical evaluation is not immediately available. Fever and rigor in an asplenic patient must prompt immediate aggressive empirical treatment with antibiotic coverage, even in the absence of culture data.

Selected References

Advisory Committee on Immunization Practices: Prevention of pneumococcal disease: Recommendations of the advisory committee on immunization practices (ACIP). MMWR Morb Mortal Wkly Rep 46:1-24, 1997.

This report of the Advisory Committee on Immunization Practices provides a summary of the epidemiology of pneumococcal infections as well as treatment and prophylaxis recommendations. Groups at high risk are discussed in detail, including patients who have undergone splenectomy.

Kojouri K, Vesely SK, Terrell DR, George JN: Splenectomy for adult patients with idiopathic thrombocytopenic purpura: A systematic review to assess long-term platelet count responses, prediction of response, and surgical complications. Blood 104:2623-2634, 2004.

This report comprehensively summarizes practice guideline recommendations for the treatment of idiopathic thrombocytopenic purpura (ITP). This review provides the evidence for the current treatment recommendations and the data for treatment outcomes for children and adults with ITP.

Gigot JF, Lengele B, Gianello P, et al: Present status of laparoscopic splenectomy for hematologic diseases: Certitudes and unresolved issues. Semin Laparosc Surg 5:147-167, 1998.

Gigot and colleagues nicely summarize the published experience on the role of laparoscopic splenectomy in the management of hematologic disorders. They provide useful technical tips for the practicing surgeon.

Katkhouda N, Hurwitz MB, Rivera RT, et al: Laparoscopic splenectomy: Outcome and efficacy in 103 consecutive patients. Ann Surg 228:568-578, 1998.

Katkhouda and colleagues show the safety and efficacy of laparoscopic splenectomy in a large series of patients. The discussion section of this article provides an extensive review of previously published series and provides helpful tables comparing the outcomes of open versus laparoscopic splenectomy.

References

1. George JN, Woolf SH, Raskob GE, et al: Idiopathic thrombocytopenic purpura: A practice guideline developed by explicit methods for the American Society of Hematology. Blood 88:3-40, 1996.
2. Kojouri K, Vesely SK, Terrell DR, et al: Splenectomy for adult patients with idiopathic thrombocytopenic purpura: A systematic review to assess long-term platelet count responses, prediction of response, and surgical complications. Blood 104:2623-2634, 2004.
3. Gigot JF, Jamar F, Ferrant A, et al: Inadequate detection of accessory spleens and splenosis with laparoscopic splenectomy: A shortcoming of the laparoscopic approach in hematologic diseases. Surg Endosc 12:101-106, 1998.
4. Katkhouda N, Hurwitz MB, Rivera RT, et al: Laparoscopic splenectomy: Outcome and efficacy in 103 consecutive patients. Ann Surg 228:568-578, 1998.
5. Tsoukas CM, Bernard NF, Abrahamowicz M, et al: Effect of splenectomy on slowing human immunodeficiency virus disease progression. Arch Surg 133:25-31, 1998.
6. Taylor MA, Kaplan HS, Nelsen TS: Staging laparotomy with splenectomy for Hodgkin's disease: The Stanford experience. World J Surg 9:449-460, 1985.
7. Morel P, Dupriez B, Gosselin B, et al: Role of early splenectomy in malignant lymphomas with prominent splenic involvement (primary lymphomas of the spleen): A study of 59 cases. Cancer 71:207-215, 1993.
8. Saven A, Burian C, Koziol JA, et al: Long-term follow-up of patients with hairy cell leukemia after cladribine treatment. Blood 92:1918-1926, 1998.
9. Montserrat E: Chronic lymphoproliferative disorders. Curr Opin Oncol 9:34-41, 1997.
10. Cusack JC, Jr., Seymour JF, Lerner S, et al: Role of splenectomy in chronic lymphocytic leukemia. J Am Coll Surg 185:237-243, 1997.
11. Results of a prospective randomized trial of early splenectomy in chronic myeloid leukemia. The Italian Cooperative Study Group on Chronic Myeloid Leukemia. Cancer 54:333-338, 1984.
12. Morgenstern L, Rosenberg J, Geller SA: Tumors of the spleen. World J Surg 9:468-476, 1985.
13. Sardi A, Ojeda HF, King D Jr: Laparoscopic resection of a benign true cyst of the spleen with the harmonic scalpel producing high levels of CA 19-9 and carcinoembryonic antigen. Am Surg 64:1149-1154, 1998.
14. Pachter HL, Hofstetter SR, Elkowitz A, et al: Traumatic cysts of the spleen: The role of cystectomy and splenic preservation: experience with seven consecutive patients. J Trauma 35:430-436, 1993.
15. Gadacz TR: Splenic abscess. World J Surg 9:410-415, 1985.
16. Faught WE, Gilbertson JJ, Nelson EW: Splenic abscess: Presentation, treatment options, and results. Am J Surg 158:612-614, 1989.
17. Gleich S, Wolin DA, Herbsman H: A review of percutaneous drainage in splenic abscess. Surg Gynecol Obstet 167:211-216, 1988.
18. Sayeed S, Koniaris LG, Kovach SJ, et al: Torsion of a wandering spleen. Surgery 132:535-536, 2002.
19. West JG, Trunkey DD, Lim RC: Systems of trauma care: A study of two counties. Arch Surg 114:455-460, 1979.
20. Root HD, Hauser CW, McKinley CR, et al: Diagnostic Peritoneal Lavage. Surgery 57:633-637, 1965.
21. Moore EE, Cogbill TH, Jurkovich GJ, et al: Organ injury scaling: Spleen and liver (1994 revision). J Trauma 38:323-324, 1995.
22. Halbfass HJ, Wimmer B, Hauenstein K, et al: [Ultrasonic diagnosis of blunt abdominal injuries]. Fortschr Med 99:1681-1685, 1981.
23. Tso P, Rodriguez A, Cooper C, et al: Sonography in blunt abdominal trauma: A preliminary progress report. J Trauma 33:39-43; discussion 43-34, 1992.
24. Bode PJ, Niezen RA, van Vugt AB, et al: Abdominal ultrasound as a reliable indicator for conclusive laparotomy in blunt abdominal trauma. J Trauma 34:27-31, 1993.
25. Rothlin MA, Naf R, Amgwerd M, et al: Ultrasound in blunt abdominal and thoracic trauma. J Trauma 34:488-495, 1993.
26. Branney SW, Moore EE, Cantrill SV, et al: Ultrasound-based key clinical pathway reduces the use of hospital resources for the evaluation of blunt abdominal trauma. J Trauma 42:1086-1090, 1997.
27. Pimpl W, Daput O, Kaindl H, et al: Incidence of septic and thromboembolic-related deaths after splenectomy in adults. Br J Surg 76:517-521, 1989.
28. Rogers FB, Baumgartner NE, Robin AP, et al: Absorbable mesh splenorrhaphy for severe splenic injuries: Functional studies in an animal model and an additional patient series. J Trauma 31:200-204, 1991.
29. Powell M, Courcoulas A, Gardner M, et al: Management of blunt splenic trauma: Significant differences between adults and children. Surgery 122:654-660, 1997.

30. Davis KA, Fabian TC, Croce MA, et al: Improved success in nonoperative management of blunt splenic injuries: Embolization of splenic artery pseudoaneurysms. J Trauma 44:1008-1013; discussion 1013-1005, 1998.

31. Sutyak JP, Chiu WC, D'Amelio LF, et al: Computed tomography is inaccurate in estimating the severity of adult splenic injury. J Trauma 39:514-518, 1995.

32. Cocanour CS, Moore FA, Arteaga BS: Age should not be a consideration for nonoperative management of blunt splenic injury. J Trauma 47:220(A), 1999.

33. Shackford SR, Molin M: Management of splenic injuries. Surg Clin North Am 70:595-620, 1990.

34. Smith JS Jr, Cooney RN, Mucha P Jr: Nonoperative management of the ruptured spleen: A revalidation of criteria. Surgery 120:745-750; discussion 750-741, 1996.

35. Morrell DG, Chang FC, Helmer SD: Changing trends in the management of splenic injury. Am J Surg 170:686-689; discussion 690, 1995.

36. Schurr MJ, Fabian TC, Gavant M, et al: Management of blunt splenic trauma: Computed tomographic contrast blush predicts failure of nonoperative management. J Trauma 39:507-512; discussion 512-503, 1995.

37. Myers LK, Tang B, Rosloniec EF, et al: Characterization of a peptide analog of a determinant of type II collagen that suppresses collagen-induced arthritis. J Immunol 161:3589-3595, 1998.

38. Bee TK, Croce MA, Miller PR, et al: Failures of splenic nonoperative management: Is the glass half empty or half full? J Trauma 50:230-236, 2001.

39. Agency for Health Care Policy and Research: Interim Manual for Clinical Practice Guideline Development. Rockville, MD: U.S. Department of Health and Human Services, Public Health Service, 1991.

40. Carroll BJ, Phillips EH, Semel CJ, et al: Laparoscopic splenectomy. Surg Endosc 6:183-185, 1992.

41. Chirletti P, Cardi M, Barillari P, et al: Surgical treatment of immune thrombocytopenic purpura. World J Surg 16:1001-1004; discussion 1004-1005, 1992.

42. Musser G, Lazar G, Hocking W, et al: Splenectomy for hematologic disease. The UCLA experience with 306 patients. Ann Surg 200:40-45, 1984.

43. Danforth DN Jr, Fraker DL: Splenectomy for the massively enlarged spleen. Am Surg 57:108-113, 1991.

44. Flowers JL, Lefor AT, Steers J, et al: Laparoscopic splenectomy in patients with hematologic diseases. Ann Surg 224:19-28, 1996.

45. Friedman RL, Fallas MJ, Carroll BJ, et al: Laparoscopic splenectomy for ITP: The gold standard. Surg Endosc 10:991-995, 1996.

46. Delaitre B, Pitre J: Laparoscopic splenectomy versus open splenectomy: A comparative study. Hepatogastroenterology 44:45-49, 1997.

47. Glasgow RE, Yee LF, Mulvihill SJ: Laparoscopic splenectomy: The emerging standard. Surg Endosc 11:108-112, 1997.

48. Romanelli JR, Kelly JJ, Litwin DE: Hand-assisted laparoscopic surgery in the United States: An overview. Semin Laparosc Surg 8:96-103, 2001.

49. Horowitz J, Smith JL, Weber TK: Postoperative complications after splenectomy for hematologic malignancies. Ann Surg 223, 290-296, 1996.

50. Hansen K, Singer DB: Asplenic-hyposplenic overwhelming sepsis: Postsplenectomy sepsis revisited. Pediatr Dev Pathol 4:105-121, 2001.

51. Shatz DV, Schinsky MF, Pais LB, et al: Immune responses of splenectomized trauma patients to the 23-valent pneumococcal polysaccharide vaccine at 1 versus 7 versus 14 days after splenectomy. J Trauma 44:760-765; discussion 765-766, 1998.

52. Waghorn DJ: Overwhelming infection in asplenic patients: Current best practice preventive measures are not being followed. J Clin Pathol 54:214-218, 2001.

53. Centers for Disease Control and Prevention; Atkinson W, Hamborsky J, McIntyre L, Worfe S (eds): Epidemiology and Prevention of Vaccine-Preventable Diseases, 10th ed. Washington, DC: Public Health Foundation, 2007.

54. Rutherford EJ, Livengood J, Higginbotham M, et al: Efficacy and safety of pneumococcal revaccination after splenectomy for trauma. J Trauma 39:448-452, 1995.

55. Leemans R, Harms G, Rijkers GT, et al: Spleen autotransplantation provides restoration of functional splenic lymphoid compartments and improves the humoral immune response to pneumococcal polysaccharide vaccine. Clin Exp Immunol 117:596-604, 1999.

CHEST

CHAPTER 57

Chest Wall and Pleura

David J. Sugarbaker, MD   and   Jeanne M. Lukanich, MD

Historical Perspectives
Chest Wall
Pleura

HISTORICAL PERSPECTIVES

Chest wall abscesses, tumors, and trauma were described as long ago as 2900 BC in the *Edwin Smith Surgical Papyrus*. Later, drainage of empyema and penetrating chest wall trauma and their sequelae were recorded.[1,2] However, the modern treatment of diseases of the chest wall and pleura would await several important medical developments and discoveries. The understanding of ventilatory physiology was of foremost importance. Forced respiration through the trachea was practiced for respiratory arrest such as drowning or morphine poisoning in the 19th century.

The first working iron lung was developed in 1876 by Wille for negative-pressure ventilation. Techniques for positive-pressure ventilation by tracheal intubation were described in the early 1900s but were not used clinically until much later in the century. Roentgen's discovery of the x-ray in 1895 was crucial for diagnosis because of limitations in clinical examination. During World War I, experience with open incision for empyema secondary to influenza led to physiologic studies by the Empyema Commission, which defined the problem of open pneumothorax and its consequences.[3] On the basis of these studies, closed aspiration or drainage of the pleural space, which prevented the introduction of air, was developed. During the next 50 years, surgery of the thorax became commonplace. The discovery and development of antibiotics during World War II, as well as advances in anesthesiology, greatly lessened the morbidity and mortality

of transpleural procedures and operations. Basic thoracic surgical techniques primarily focused on the treatment of pulmonary and pleural tuberculosis and suppurative diseases of the chest wall, pleura, and lung. Variations of these techniques are still widely employed today. Most recently, in the 1990s, the introduction of thoracoscopy into the specialty has altered the standard of practice in the treatment of diseases of the chest wall and pleura.

CHEST WALL

Anatomy

The thorax is a rigid, noncollapsible structural frame that houses and protects the thoracic organs and supports the upper extremities. Owing to specialized mechanics that allow for limited expansion, it provides for ventilation and phonation. The bony thorax consists of 12 paired ribs, multiple cartilages, and the sternum and clavicles arranged around the thoracic vertebrae. The ribs and sternum determine the size and shape of the thoracic cavity. The upper seven ribs (numbered 1-7) are true ribs because they articulate directly with the sternum by means of cartilages. The lower five ribs (numbered 8-12) are false ribs; they do not directly connect to the sternum anteriorly but, in most cases, connect with the costocartilage above them. Ribs 11 and 12 are floating ribs. They can be diminutive or large; they articulate only with the thoracic spine. Each rib is composed of a head, neck, and shaft. Each head has an upper facet, which articulates with the vertebral body above it, and a lower facet, which articulates with the corresponding thoracic vertebra to that rib, establishing the costovertebral joint. The neck of the rib has a tubercle with an articular facet; this articulates with the transverse process, creating the costotransverse joint and imparting strength to the posterior rib cage.

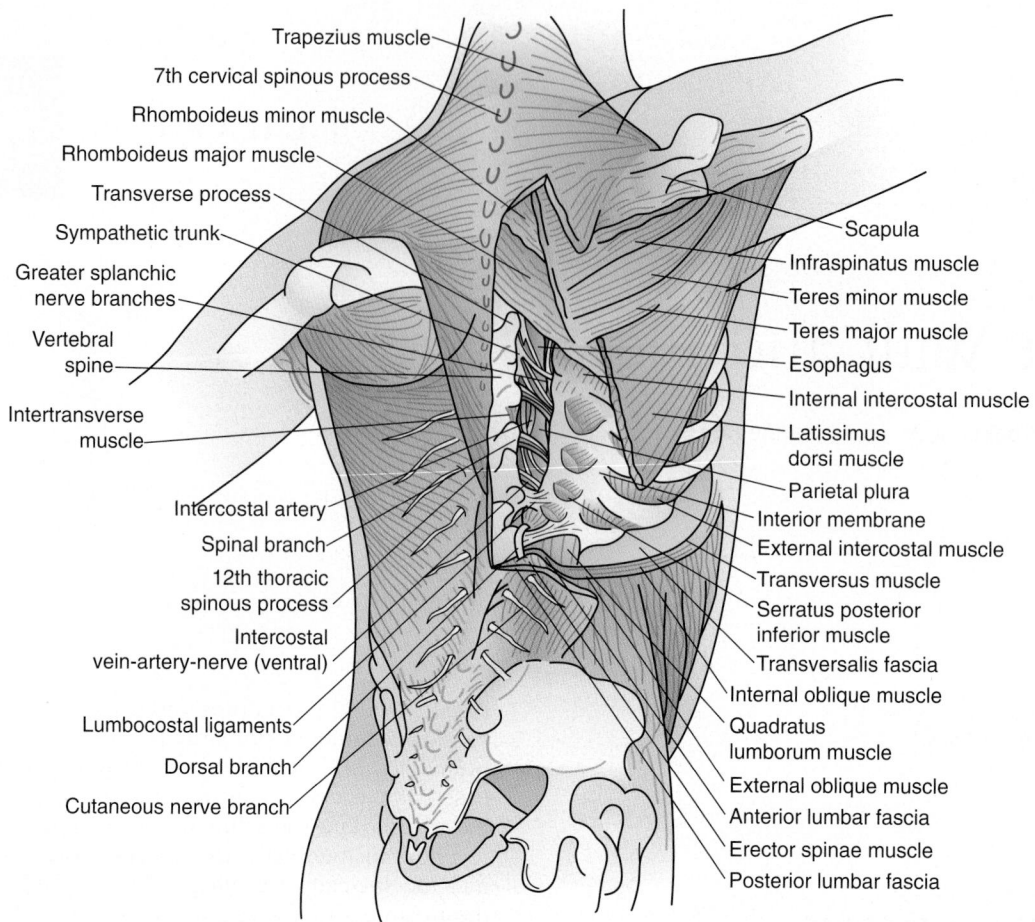

Trapezius muscle
7th cervical spinous process
Rhomboideus minor muscle
Rhomboideus major muscle
Transverse process
Sympathetic trunk
Greater splanchic nerve branches
Vertebral spine
Intertransverse muscle
Intercostal artery
Spinal branch
12th thoracic spinous process
Intercostal vein-artery-nerve (ventral)
Lumbocostal ligaments
Dorsal branch
Cutaneous nerve branch

Scapula
Infraspinatus muscle
Teres minor muscle
Teres major muscle
Esophagus
Internal intercostal muscle
Latissimus dorsi muscle
Parietal plura
Interior membrane
External intercostal muscle
Transversus muscle
Serratus posterior inferior muscle
Transversalis fascia
Internal oblique muscle
Quadratus lumborum muscle
External oblique muscle
Anterior lumbar fascia
Erector spinae muscle
Posterior lumbar fascia

Figure 57-1 **Musculature of the chest wall.** (From Ravitch MM, Steichen FM: Atlas of General Thoracic Surgery. Philadelphia, WB Saunders, 1988.)

The sternum is a flat bone, 15 to 20 cm in length, divided superiorly to inferiorly into the manubrium, body, and xiphoid. The manubrium articulates with the clavicles and first costal cartilage at its rostral aspect. The manubrium joins the body of the sternum at the angle of Louis, which corresponds to the anterior aspect of the junction of the second rib. The anterior cartilaginous attachments of the true ribs to the sternum, along with intercostal muscles and the hemidiaphragms, allow for movement of the ribs with respiration.

Beneath skin and subcutaneous tissue, the bony thorax is covered by three groups of muscles: the primary and secondary muscles for respiration and those attaching the upper extremity to the body. The primary muscles include the diaphragm and intercostal muscles. The intercostal muscles of the intercostal spaces include the external, internal, and transverse or innermost muscles. Eleven intercostal spaces, each associated numerically with the rib superior to it, contain the intercostal bundles (vein, artery, and nerve) that travel along the lower edge of each rib. All intercostal spaces are wider anteriorly, and each intercostal bundle falls away from the rib posteriorly to become more centrally located within each space.

The secondary muscles consist of the sternocleidomastoid, the serratus posterior, and the levatores costarum.

The third muscle group attaches the upper extremity to the body. The pectoralis major and minor muscles lie anteriorly and superficially. Posterior superficial musculature includes the trapezius and latissimus dorsi. Deep muscles include the serratus anterior and posterior, the levatores, and the major and minor rhomboids. These superficial and deep muscles help to hold the scapulae to the chest wall (Fig. 57-1). In respiratory distress, the deltoid, pectoralis, and latissimus dorsi muscles form a tertiary system for ventilatory assistance through fixation of the upper extremities.

Chest Wall Deformities

Infants and children present with a wide range of congenital chest wall deformities (Table 57-1). Although most of these young patients are asymptomatic, some defects can be life threatening and may be associated with other congenital malformations.

Depression Deformities (Pectus Excavatum)

Pectus excavatum (also called *funnel chest*) is the most common chest wall deformity, occurring in 1 of 400 children. Males are affected more frequently than females (4:1). Although a familial predisposition is not confirmed,

Table 57-1   Chest Wall Abnormalities

Depression deformities/pectus excavatum
Protrusion deformities/pectus carinatum
Poland's syndrome
Sternal defects
Cervical ectopia cordis
Thoracic ectopia cordis
Thoracoabdominal ectopia cordis
Bifid sternum

more than 30% of cases have a family history of chest wall anomalies. Pectus excavatum arises from imbalanced or excessive growth of the lower costal cartilages, causing posterior sternal depression. The depression can often be deeper on the right side than the left, causing a rotation of the sternum. Typically, the defect is diagnosed within the first year of life and worsens over time. A wide range of depression abnormalities is reported, varying from a mildly depressed sternum to sternal depression abutting the vertebral column with displacement of mediastinal organs, including the heart. About 20% of cases are associated with other musculoskeletal abnormalities such as scoliosis (15%) and Marfan syndrome, whereas congenital heart disease is seen in 1.5% of patients.

Most patients with pectus excavatum are asymptomatic at the time of presentation; however, some subjects report a decrease in respiratory reserve or pain along the costal cartilages with exercise. Occasionally, palpitations or murmurs are noted, particularly in the presence of mitral valve prolapse. Evaluation of baseline pulmonary function can be obtained with pulmonary function testing, exercise radiologic or physiologic studies, and ventilation-perfusion scans. Cardiovascular assessment can be performed using echocardiography or angiography. In severe cases, decreased stroke volume and cardiac output have been documented, along with a restrictive pattern (decreased maximal breathing capacity) on pulmonary function testing.

To assess the severity of this defect, a variety of methods have been used based on measurements obtained from chest radiography or chest computed tomography (CT). Most methods use the distance between the sternum and spine to create a ratio to compare the depth of the depression. Examples of these methods include a ratio of the sternovertebral distance divided by the anteroposterior diameter of the chest at the sternomanubrial joint or, alternatively, the depth of the chest wall defect and the maximal anteroposterior distance of the thorax.

The indications for operative intervention include cosmesis, psychosocial factors, and the presence of respiratory or cardiovascular insufficiency. Poor self-image is an important concern for many patients, particularly children and adolescents or young adults who are taunted by peers. Frequently, these individuals attempt to cover the defect with clothing and abstain from participating in activities that require their chests to be bare, such as swimming. Because of these concerns, early repair is supported, with best results reported between 2 and 8 years of age.[4]

Surgical repair of pectus excavatum has evolved from techniques developed by surgeons during the past 50 years. Five procedures are mentioned here. The first involves repositioning the sternum anteriorly by sternal osteotomy. The second is a modification of this procedure that involves supporting the repositioned sternum with a posterior strut (sternal strut). The third technique (sternal turnover) involves removing the sternum and repositioning it in a front-to-back rotated position before stabilization. The fourth technique for correction employs a Silastic mold that is implanted into the subcutaneous space to fill the defect without altering the thoracic cage.[5] The fifth technique is a minimally invasive procedure that avoids cartilage resection or sternal osteotomy, but utilizes an internal posterior sternal support. This technique has gained popularity during the past decade, but is less applicable in older patients and those with asymmetric deformities.

The most frequently used operative technique employs a small transverse inframammary or midline incision. Electrocautery is used to mobilize the soft tissue and to reflect the pectoralis muscles laterally and the rectus muscle inferiorly. After the involved costal cartilages are exposed, the deformed segments of cartilage are isolated subperichondrially for the length of the deformity and resected. The perichondrium is preserved to allow for growth of new cartilage over several months, creating a firm anterior chest wall. After the cartilages are removed, the pleura is mobilized away from the posterior surface of the sternum by blunt dissection. This maneuver allows the sternum to be completely freed from its "restrictive" attachments after the intercostal muscles laterally are divided. A transverse osteotomy is made through the sternomanubrial joint, permitting the sternum to be straightened. Fixation of the sternum in a slightly overcorrected position is essential to ensure good repair. A number of techniques for stabilizing the sternum have been used, including bioabsorbable struts, Marlex mesh, Dacron vascular grafts, and metallic wires and struts. At present, little evidence exists to support one technique over another. Drainage of the mediastinum is routinely performed postoperatively. Complications of surgical repair are rare and include wound infection and pneumothorax. Improvement of respiratory function and exercise capacity after repair has been reported. Early (1-year) cosmetic results are excellent (80%-90%) (Fig. 57-2), with recurrence varying from 5% to 15% with long-term follow-up.[6] A lengthy follow-up period is indicated in these patients, especially with regard to recurrence, because the rapid growth phase of puberty can alter dramatically the appearance of the chest wall.

Protrusion Deformities (Pectus Carinatum)

Pectus carinatum (also called *pigeon breast*) is a defect characterized by an anterior protrusion deformity of the sternum and costal cartilages. This condition affects males

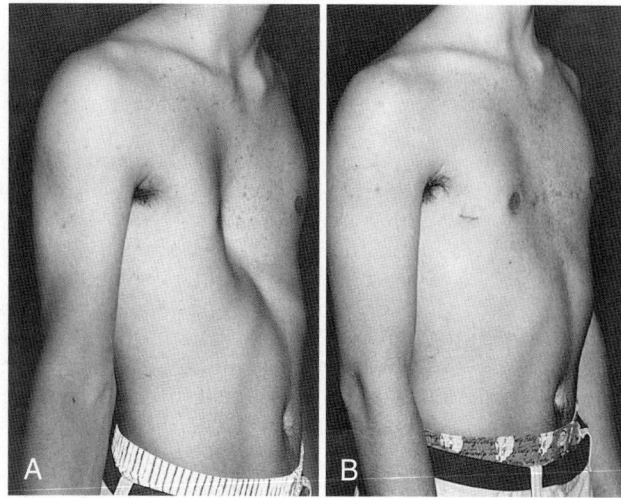

Figure 57-2 Patient with pectus excavatum. **A,** Preoperative. **B,** After repair. (From Shamberger RC, Hendren WH III: Congenital deformities of the chest wall and sternum. In Pearson FG, Cooper JD, et al [eds]: Thoracic Surgery, 2nd ed. Philadelphia, Churchill Livingstone, 2002, p 1352).

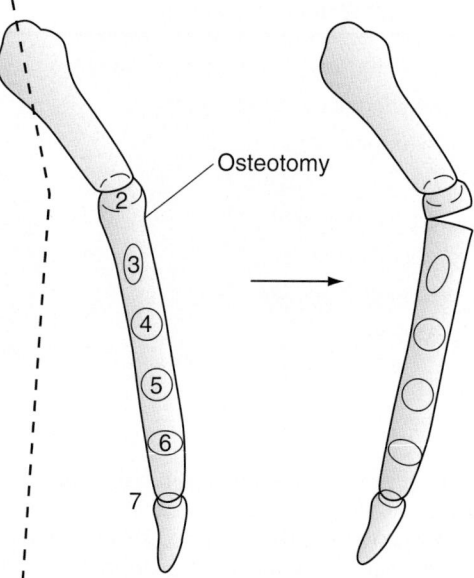

Figure 57-3 A single or double osteotomy after resection of the costal cartilages allows posterior displacement of the sternum to an orthotopic position in pectus carinatum. (From Shamberger RC: Congenital chest wall deformities. Curr Probl Surg 33:471, 1996.)

more than females (4:1) and presents less frequently than pectus excavatum by a ratio of about 1:5. The defect, which worsens as the child grows, typically is not appreciated until after the first decade of life. Similar to pectus excavatum, a familial predisposition (30%) and an association with scoliosis (15%) and congenital heart disease (20%) are reported.

Three types of defects have been described in pectus carinatum. The most frequent variant, an anterior displacement of the body of the sternum and symmetrical concavity of the costal cartilages, is termed *chondrogladiolar protrusion*. The second variety involves a lateral depression of the ribs on one or both sides of the sternum; Poland's syndrome frequently is associated with this type. The third and least common type, the pouter pigeon breast, consists of an upper or chondromanubrial prominence with protrusion of the manubrium and depression of the sternal body.

Symptoms are uncommon but may include exertional dyspnea or cardiac arrhythmias. Pulmonary function tests and echocardiography are useful for determining the extent of cardiopulmonary compromise. Frequently, distinguishing this defect from a neoplasm is a concern of the patient and family.

The initial repair of pectus carinatum involves mobilization of the skin and pectoralis muscle flaps through a transverse incision. The subsequent surgical correction is modified depending on the extent of the deformity. In patients with the chondrogladiolar or chondromanubrial deformity, the sternum can be straightened using an osteotomy (sometimes two) of the sternal table (Fig. 57-3). In the mixed deformity, the protrusion of the costal cartilages is corrected by using a subperichondrial resection of the involved costal cartilages. The oblique position of the sternum subsequently is fixed using a wedge-shaped osteotomy in the anterior sternal plate.

Shortening of the sternum may be required in all defect types. Complications arising from surgical intervention such as pneumothorax, wound infection, or dehiscence are rare. Excellent results commonly are obtained with few recurrences reported.

Poland's Syndrome

Poland's syndrome is a rare, nonfamilial disease of unknown cause that occurs in 1 per 30,000 births. The components of the syndrome include absence of the pectoralis major muscle, absence or hypoplasia of the pectoralis minor muscle, absence of costal cartilages, hypoplasia of breast and subcutaneous tissue (including the nipple complex), and a variety of hand anomalies. Occasionally, Poland's syndrome has been associated with Möbius' syndrome (facial palsy and abducens oculi palsy) or childhood leukemia.

Patients who present with absent ribs are considered candidates for surgical repair. Although a variety of surgical techniques have been described to correct this anomaly, an approach using a latissimus dorsi muscle flap with autologous rib grafts to reconstruct the chest wall commonly is used.[7]

Sternal Defects

During embryologic development, the body of the sternum arises from migrating cells (6th week) originating in the lateral plate mesoderm, which form two bands that fuse by the 10th week of gestation. The manubrium arises from primordia between the ventral ends of the clavicles. Abnormalities in the development of the sternum lead to four types of sternal clefts.

The upper sternal defects (cervical ectopia cordis) are associated with a broad defect that extends to the fourth costal cartilage in a U- or V-shaped appearance. Repair entails joining the sternal bands in the midline after performing oblique chondrotomies to provide protective coverage for the heart and great vessels. In severe cases, reconstruction of the defect with prosthetic material (e.g., Marlex mesh) is necessary to avoid excessive compression of the heart that would lead to bradycardia or hypotension. Complete clefts (thoracic ectopia cordis) are more extensive and frequently are associated with a crescentic anterior diaphragmatic defect and diastasis recti, which results in free communication between the peritoneum and pericardial cavities. Distal sternal clefts (thoracoabdominal ectopia cordis) are the most extensive defects and are associated with Cantrell's pentalogy. This group of anomalies is characterized by a distal cleft in the sternum, omphalocele, diaphragmatic cleft, pericardial defect, and congenital heart defect (ventricular septal defect, tetralogy of Fallot).[8] Bifid sternum is the least severe anomaly of the sternum and may be associated with facial hemangiomas.

Chest Wall Tumors

Chest wall tumors are rare neoplasms. They include tumors originating in the bone, cartilage, or soft tissue of the chest wall. Most bony chest wall tumors arise in the ribs (85%), with the remainder arising from the scapula, sternum, and clavicle.[9] These chest wall neoplasms commonly are classified as benign or malignant tumors of bone and soft tissue (Table 57-2). Malignant lesions are

further divided into primary or secondary (metastatic) tumors. Although metastatic disease to the ribs is the most common malignant chest wall tumor, primary bone tumors account for 7% to 8% of all chest wall malignancies.

The clinical presentation of chest wall tumors ranges from an asymptomatic lump to a painful and sometimes ulcerated mass. Pain usually indicates periosteal invasion and more commonly is associated with malignancy. The correct diagnosis of chest wall lesions relies on a thorough clinical evaluation (history and physical examination) and radiologic tests. In particular, chest radiography with rib tomograms and chest CT are helpful in delineating soft tissue or bony involvement. Magnetic resonance imaging (MRI) is useful in determining neural and vascular invasion. Bone scanning also may aid in the differential diagnosis to rule out the presence of satellite or metastatic disease.

The correct treatment of chest wall tumors requires pathologic confirmation to be obtained. Excisional rather than incisional biopsy, with a minimum of a 1- to 2-cm margin, is preferred. Incisional biopsy occasionally may be appropriate for a large tumor. Frequently, surgical resection is the treatment of choice and often requires a multidisciplinary team approach (e.g., plastic surgery, neurosurgery, orthopedic surgery, and thoracic surgery).

Bone

Benign

Fibrous dysplasia of bone accounts for more than 30% of benign chest wall tumors. Typically, these lesions present in the third or fourth decade of life, with equal frequency in men and women. They are slow growing and most commonly present as an asymptomatic mass in the lateral or posterior aspect of the rib. Pain may develop as the tumor enlarges and causes pressure symptoms or develops pathologic fractures. Albright's syndrome is suspected if these lesions are multiple and associated with precocious puberty and skin pigmentation. The diagnosis is assisted by the appearance of fusiform expansion in the posterior aspect of the rib with a characteristic "soap bubble" or "ground glass" appearance on chest radiography. Excision is indicated for symptom relief (pain) and to confirm the diagnosis.

Chondromas account for 15% to 20% of benign chest wall lesions. These lesions present in the second or third decade of life as asymptomatic, slowly growing tumors at the anterior costochondral junction. Males and females are affected equally. The tumors can arise in the medulla (enchondroma) or the periosteum (periosteal chondroma). On chest radiography, the neoplastic growth appears as a lytic lesion with sclerotic margins that may be difficult to distinguish from chondrosarcomas. As a result, wide excision of the lesion is necessary to rule out a malignant component.

Osteochondroma presents as a mass originating from the cortex of the rib. Symptoms depend on the direction of tumor growth. Inward-growing tumors are usually asymptomatic, whereas outward-growing tumors present

Table 57-2 Classification of Tumors of the Chest Wall

	BENIGN	MALIGNANT
Bone Tumors		
Bone	Osteoid osteoma	Osteosarcoma
	Aneurysmal bone cyst	Ewing's sarcoma
Cartilage	Enchondroma	Chondrosarcoma
	Osteochondroma	
Fibrous	Fibrous dysplasia	Malignant fibrous histiocytoma
Marrow	Eosinophilic granuloma	Plasmacytoma
Vascular	Hemangioma	Hemangiosarcoma
Soft Tissue		
Adipose	Lipoma and its variations	Liposarcoma
Muscle	Leiomyoma	Leiomyosarcoma
	Rhabdomyoma	Rhabdomyosarcoma
Neural	Neurofibroma	Neurofibrosarcoma
	Neurilemoma	Malignant schwannoma
		Askin's tumor (primitive neuroectodermal tumor)
Fibrous	Desmoid	Fibrosarcoma

Adapted from Faber LP, Somers J, Templeton AC: Chest wall tumors. Curr Probl Surg 32:663, 1995.

as a painless mass. Young males are most commonly affected. A characteristic finding on chest radiography is a pedunculated bony mass capped with viable cartilage. Familial osteochondromatosis is suspected if multiple lesions are noted. Complete excision is the treatment of choice; recurrences are rare.

Eosinophilic granuloma is a benign component of malignant fibrous histiocytosis, which primarily affects men. Patients present with skull and rib involvement that appears as expansile bone lesions on radiographic evaluation. Excisional biopsy is indicated for solitary lesions; radiotherapy is reserved for patients who present with multiple lesions.

Osteoid osteomas are rare tumors that arise in the bony cortex of the rib or vertebral arches. Young males most commonly are affected and present with sharp pain that is worse at night and is relieved by aspirin. A small radiolucent nidus encircled by a sclerotic margin is frequently seen on a chest radiograph. Indications for resection include cosmesis and relief of pain; resection of the entire rib is recommended.

Aneurysmal bone cysts commonly occur in the ribs and may arise as the result of chest wall trauma. The characteristic pattern of a blow-out lytic lesion frequently is seen on chest radiography. Complete excision is warranted for relief of pain.

Malignant

Chondrosarcoma is the most common malignant tumor of the chest wall, accounting for 20% of all bone tumors. These lesions arise in the third and fourth decades of life and may be associated with trauma to the chest or represent malignant degeneration of benign chondromas or osteochondromas. On chest radiography, a poorly defined tumor mass that is destroying cortical bone is observed. The anterior costochondral junctions of the sternum most frequently are involved. Resection with wide margins is the treatment of choice, with a 70% 5-year survival rate reported for complete excision.[10] Radiotherapy may be effective for control of local recurrences.

Osteosarcoma (osteogenic sarcoma) is a tumor that arises most frequently in the long bones of adolescents and young adults. In the chest, osteosarcomas account for 10% to 15% of malignant tumors. Typically, the tumor presents as a rapidly enlarging mass with a characteristic sunburst pattern on chest radiography. Because metastases are common at presentation, a complete radiographic evaluation of the lungs, liver, and bones is indicated. Five-year survival with complete excision and adjuvant chemotherapy approaches 60%.

Ewing's sarcoma is a bone tumor that arises most commonly in the pelvis, humerus, or femur of young males. It is the third most common malignant chest wall tumor (5%-10%). A mass that is intermittently painful is a common presentation in this disease. A characteristic onion peel appearance caused by periosteal elevation and bony remodeling is seen on the chest radiograph. Survival is about 50% at 5 years with multimodality therapy (chemotherapy, radiotherapy, and surgery).[11]

Solitary plasmacytoma is a rare tumor arising from plasma cells. Multiple myeloma is the same tumor arising

in more than one location. More than half of patients with an apparently solitary plasmacytoma of the bone develop multiple myeloma within 10 years. The tumor commonly presents as pain without a mass in older men. A diffuse, punched-out appearance of the bone caused by myelogenous deposits is seen on chest radiography. Systemic disease can be confirmed using serum protein electrophoresis, urinalysis (Bence Jones protein), and bone marrow aspiration. Incisional biopsy frequently is used to confirm the diagnosis, although a solitary plasmacytoma is resected completely. Radiotherapy is the primary mode of therapy, with a 5-year survival of 30% reported.[12]

Soft Tissue

Many benign tumors arise from the chest wall. These rare tumors are listed in Table 57-2 and are discussed in detail elsewhere in the text. Malignant degeneration rarely has been observed in some of these tumors, such as neurofibromas. Surgical excision is the preferred mode of therapy.

Soft tissue sarcomas are the most common malignant primary chest wall tumors. These lesions can arise anywhere in the thorax and usually are graded as low or high grade based on mitotic rate, cellular pleomorphism, and nuclear-to-cytoplasmic ratio. Incisional biopsy is performed to establish the diagnosis, and surgical excision with wide margins is used for definitive therapy. Of note, the pseudocapsule that surrounds the tumor and frequently contains microscopic disease is avoided during the resection to decrease the chance of local recurrence. Chemotherapy and radiotherapy are used frequently as adjuvant therapeutic modalities.

Metastatic

Metastatic neoplasms may involve the chest wall by direct extension, by progression of lymphatic disease, or by metastases from blood-borne deposits, with the latter being most common. Tumors that involve the chest wall by direct extension include breast and lung cancer. In breast cancer, locoregional recurrence involving the chest wall can occur in more than 10% of stage II lesions after mastectomy.[13] Recurrences are treated with resection and adjuvant radiotherapy and chemotherapy.

Chest wall invasion is reported in 5% of primary non–small cell lung cancer patients. Historically, these tumors have the best prognosis of all T3 lesions because they are readily amenable to resection. In 1985, a report by McCaughan and colleagues[14] noted that the actuarial 5-year survival rate for patients with chest wall invasion without lymph node involvement (T3, N0—stage IIB) was 56%, whereas patients with tumors with N1 or N2 nodal invasion had survival rates of 35% and 16%, respectively. In 1987, similar findings were reported by the Mayo Clinic. A 59% 5-year survival rate for patients with resected T3, N0 chest wall lesions was noted, compared with a 7% rate for patients with T3, N1-N2 disease. Therefore, nodal involvement is a strong prognostic determinant of survival. An evaluation of other prognostic factors from this series indicated that long-term survival was additionally affected by the extent of chest wall involvement and the ability to completely resect the tumor. For these reasons, the use of adjuvant radiotherapy for these patients has been investigated; however, a large trial has yet to confirm a survival advantage in this subset of patients with T3 tumors.

In 1924, Pancoast described posteroapical chest tumors characterized by arm pain, atrophy of hand muscles, bone destruction, and Horner's syndrome.[15] These tumors, which account for less than 5% of all non–small cell lung cancer, have been associated with a favorable survival, with a cumulative 5-year survival rate of more than 30%.[16] Controversy regarding the importance of nodal status in the survival of these patients exists; however, most series rarely report long-term survival with N2 disease.[17] For this reason, careful preoperative mediastinal lymph node staging is important to exclude inoperable N2 or N3 disease. Recently, efforts have focused on improving local control by using preoperative radiotherapy in conjunction with surgery. A preoperative radiotherapy dose of more than 50 Gy offers advantages, including a decrease in tumor size, thereby facilitating surgery, a reduction in number and dissemination of viable tumor cells, and a survival benefit. Most series report local control rates of 70% to 85% using this bimodality approach. Concurrent treatment with neoadjuvant chemotherapy and radiotherapy also is being used clinically.

Secondary chest wall metastases arise from sarcomas and breast, lung, kidney, and thyroid cancers. Surgical resection, formerly uncommon except for diagnosis, is gaining popularity because of its safety and efficacy (improvement in disease-free and overall survival) as reported in large series of patients undergoing one-step resection (with negative margins) and reconstruction. Lesions may be treated palliatively with radiotherapy.

Radiation-associated malignancies of the chest wall are uncommon. All varieties of malignant tumors have been reported in this setting. The latency period from radiation therapy to diagnosis ranges from 2 to more than 20 years. The primary treatment of these tumors is resection and reconstruction when possible. Outcomes after surgery appear to be similar (by type) for de novo and radiation-associated chest wall tumors.[18]

Reconstruction

Reconstruction of the chest wall requires an intricate knowledge of the anatomy of the chest defect and the availability of soft tissues and prosthetic materials to repair the defect. Defects in the anterior, superior, and lateral chest wall commonly are reconstructed if the defect is greater than 5 cm. Skeletal stabilization is obtained using a prosthetic mesh or patch or with methyl methacrylate. Posterior defects generally do not require reconstruction, particularly if they are adequately covered by the scapula in superior defects. Soft tissue reconstruction can be accomplished using a variety of techniques, such as myocutaneous flaps (latissimus dorsi, pectoralis major, rectus abdominis, trapezius, serratus anterior), omental transposition, tissue expansion, and microvascular composite tissue transfer. Frequently, the assistance

of other surgical specialties is beneficial in the reconstruction of complex defects.

Chest Wall Infections

Chest wall infections encompass those infections arising from skin, soft tissue, cartilage, and bony structures of the chest wall. Frequently, these infections occur after surgical intervention. Infections caused by tuberculosis or fungi are less common than those caused by bacteria but may be more difficult to eradicate. Management of chest wall infections ranges from antibiotic therapy to radical resection and débridement for more advanced or complicated infections.

Soft tissue infections commonly include superficial abrasions, carbuncles, or furuncles. Herpes zoster (shingles) also may present as painful lesions distributed along cutaneous nerve dermatomes and usually is self-limited, although antiherpes medications generally improve the time course and diminish the severity of symptoms. Life-threatening necrotizing (clostridial, streptococcal, or *Escherichia coli*) infections also may appear in diabetic or immunocompromised patients and require aggressive débridement with systemic antibiotic therapy.[19] Inflammatory breast carcinoma may mimic chest wall infection or breast abscess and requires a high index of suspicion to make the appropriate diagnosis. Although Mondor's disease frequently is misdiagnosed as a chest wall infection, it is actually a thrombophlebitis of the superficial veins of the breast and anterior chest wall. Ultrasound may be helpful in confirming this diagnosis.

Cartilage and bony structures occasionally may be the source of a chest wall infection. Costochondritis usually is self-limited, as in Tietze's syndrome. However, because the poor vascular supply of cartilage limits the exposure to systemic antibiotics, a small indolent infection may fester or progress and subsequently require radical débridement and reconstruction. Consideration needs to be given to early débridement in these situations. Bone infections arise primarily from surgical interventions such as median sternotomy. Although relatively uncommon today in the postantibiotic era, sternal wound infection occurs in 1% to 2% of operative cases. Thoracotomy infection is rare. Risk factors include trauma, chronic obstructive pulmonary disease, diabetes, prolonged mechanical ventilation, age, general debilitation, and division or use for revascularization of the internal thoracic arteries. Diagnosis can be confirmed with chest CT or gallium scan. Treatment of sternal osteomyelitis includes radical débridement, irrigation systems, systemic antibiotics, and muscle flap reconstruction. Occasionally, chest wall infections can arise from fungal infections, actinomycosis, or nocardiosis, and frequently lead to chest wall fistulas. Tuberculous chest wall infections are uncommon; however, the entity of lytic chest wall lesions arising from tuberculosis is becoming more common with the increased incidence of multidrug-resistant tuberculosis or mycobacterial organisms, more widespread use of immunosuppression, and the rising prevalence of HIV infection.

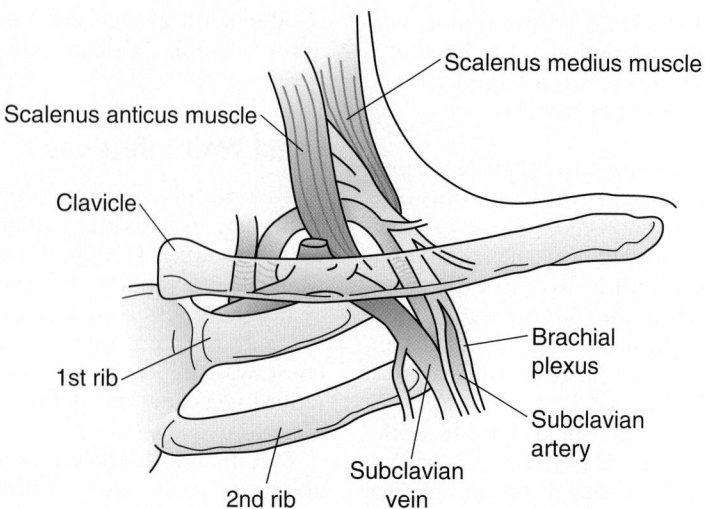

Figure 57-4 Relationship of the neurovascular bundle to the scalenus muscles, clavicle, and first rib. (From Urschel HC: Thoracic outlet syndromes. In Baue AE, Geha AS, Hammond GL, et al [eds]: Glenn's Thoracic and Cardio-vascular Surgery, 6th ed. Stamford, CT, Appleton & Lange, 1996, p 567. With permission of The McGraw-Hill Companies.)

Radiotherapy is an effective modality in the treatment of malignancies arising in the thorax such as Hodgkin's lymphoma, lung cancer, breast cancer, and other chest wall malignancies. It may be used to treat a tumor as first-line therapy, as adjuvant therapy, or for treatment of metastasis or local recurrences. Radiotherapy works by releasing free radicals and peroxidases into cells. These intermediaries cause destruction of rapidly dividing cells, such as neoplastic cells, by fracturing DNA molecules. These ionizing rays also cause a nonspecific injury and hence can damage surrounding normal tissue. Endothelial cells in blood vessels are particularly susceptible to injury, leading to arteritis and ischemic fibrosis. Therefore, poorly vascularized tissues such as bone and cartilage are very susceptible to radiation injury. A wide spectrum of injuries has been reported, ranging from erythema of the skin (radiodermatitis) to soft tissue ulceration with osteoradionecrosis and chondroradionecrosis. Although the severity of the injuries is dose dependent, standard doses of 45 to 50 Gy given over 4 to 6 weeks appear to limit complications. Prevention is the best treatment of radionecrosis. Currently, new techniques in administrating radiotherapy that increase the therapeutic effect while limiting toxicities are being explored. If radionecrosis develops in the chest wall, partial- or full-thickness resection with vascularized soft tissue flap reconstruction may be necessary if more conservative therapy fails.

Thoracic Outlet Syndrome

Thoracic outlet syndrome (TOS) refers to compression of the subclavian vessels and nerves of the brachial plexus in the region of the thoracic inlet. These neurovascular structures of the upper extremity may be compressed by a variety of anatomic structures, such as bone (cervical rib, long transverse process of C7, abnormal first rib,

osteoarthritis), muscles (scalenes), trauma (neck hematoma, bone dislocation), fibrous bands (congenital and acquired), or neoplasm. Symptoms most commonly develop secondary to neural compromise; however, vascular or neurovascular symptoms are reported. The patient population most commonly affected by TOS is middle-aged women. To understand the pathophysiology of TOS, knowledge of the relevant anatomy is essential.

At the apex of the thorax, the subclavian vessels and nerves of the brachial plexus traverse the cervicoaxillary canal en route to the upper extremity. The cervical portion of the canal is divided into two portions by the first rib. The first portion, the scalene triangle, is bound by the scalenus anticus anteriorly, scalenus medius posteriorly, and the first rib inferiorly. The clavicle and the first rib bind the second portion, the costoclavicular space[20] (Fig. 57-4). The route of neurovascular structures through these anatomic regions helps to explain the variable symptomatology that may be noted in patients with TOS.

The subclavian artery exits the chest behind the sternoclavicular joints and passes between the scalenus anticus and medius muscles. The trunks of the five spinal nerves (C5-C8, T1) accompany the artery after they exit their intervertebral foramina. The trunks become cords as the nerves run posterior to the pectoralis minor tendon. Distal to the pectoralis tendon, the cords subsequently divide into the major motor and sensory nerves of the upper extremity[21] (Fig. 57-5). The axillary vein passes posteriorly to the costocoracoid ligament and pectoralis minor tendons. The axillary vein becomes the subclavian vein as it passes anteriorly over the first rib. The subclavian vein joins the jugular venous system after passing between the scalenus anterior muscle and clavicle.

These subclavian vessels and the brachial plexus can be compressed at a variety of locations as they pass

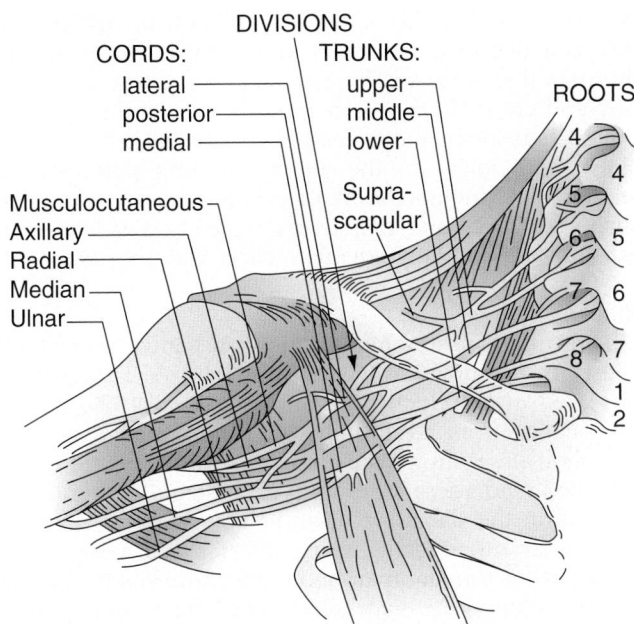

DIVISIONS

CORDS:
lateral
posterior
medial

TRUNKS:
upper
middle
lower

Supra-
scapular

ROOTS

Musculocutaneous
Axillary
Radial
Median
Ulnar

Figure 57-5 Detailed view of brachial plexus. (From Urschel HC, Razzuk M: Upper plexus thoracic outlet syndrome: Optimal therapy. Ann Thorac Surg 63:935-939, 1997. Reprinted with permission from the Society of Thoracic Surgeons.)

between the thoracic inlet and the upper extremity. From medial to lateral, these anatomic regions are as follows:

1. The interscalene triangle (artery and nerves)
2. The costoclavicular space (vein)
3. The subcoracoid area (artery, vein, nerves)

Diagnosis

The symptoms associated with TOS vary depending on the anatomic structure that is compressed. In more than 90% of cases, neurogenic manifestations are reported. Ulnar nerve (C8-T1) involvement is associated with motor weakness and atrophy of the hypothenar and interosseous muscles, as well as pain and paresthesia along the medial aspect of the arm and hand, the fifth finger, and the medial aspect of the fourth finger. Median nerve (C5-8, T1) involvement produces symptoms in the index and middle fingers, as well as in the flexor compartment of the forearm. Symptoms of subclavian artery compression include fatigue, weakness, coldness, ischemic pain, and paresthesia. Exercise or cold weather may precipitate or potentiate these symptoms. Thrombosis with distal embolization rarely can occur, producing vasomotor symptoms (Raynaud's phenomenon) in the hand or ischemic changes. Atypical chest pain (pseudoangina) also has been reported. Edema, venous distention, collateral formation, and cyanosis of the affected limb are manifestations of venous compression or occlusion. Patients with Paget-Schroetter syndrome present with effort-induced thrombosis of the axillary or subclavian vein secondary to unusual, repetitive, or excessive arm exertion or exercise.

Four provocative clinical maneuvers to evaluate a patient suspected of having TOS have been described. The loss or decrease of radial pulse or the reproduction of neurologic symptoms suggests a positive test.

1. *The Adson (Scalene) Test* causes narrowing of the space between the scalenus anticus and medius, resulting in compression of the subclavian artery and the brachial plexus. The patient is instructed to inspire maximally and hold his or her breath while the neck is fully extended and the head is turned toward the affected side. A decrease or loss of the ipsilateral radial pulse suggests compression.
2. *The Halsted (Costoclavicular) Test* is used to narrow the costoclavicular space between the first rib and the clavicle, thereby causing neurovascular compression. The patient is instructed to place his or her shoulders in a military position (drawn backward and downward). This maneuver causes changes in the radial pulse if compression of one or both subclavian arteries is present.
3. *The Wright (Hyperabduction) Test* causes the neurovascular structures to be compressed in the subcoracoid region by the pectoralis tendon, the head of the humerus, or the coracoid process. To perform the test, the patient's arm is hyperabducted 180 degrees. Compression is suspected with decrease or loss of the radial pulse.
4. *The Roos Test* is performed by having the patient abduct his or her arm 90 degrees with external rotation of the shoulder. Maintaining this body position, the modified Roos test is performed by opening and closing the hand rapidly for 3 minutes in an attempt to reproduce symptoms. Additionally, neurogenic compromise may be detected using provocative tests such as percussion of the nerve (Tinel's sign) or flexion of the elbow or wrist (Phalen's sign).

The radiologic evaluation of a patient suspected of having TOS includes chest and cervical spine radiography. Occasionally, these tests reveal bony abnormalities such as a cervical rib or bony degenerative changes. CT, MRI, or cervical myelograms are sometimes helpful to rule out narrowing of the intervertebral foramina or cervical disk pathology. Doppler studies or vascular imaging (angiogram/venogram) may be indicated if the extent of vascular impairment cannot be determined clinically or if an aneurysm or venous thrombosis is suspected.

Nerve conduction velocities can be very useful in differentiating the causes of neurologic symptoms reported by patients. Using electrodiagnostic testing, the velocity of action potential progression can be measured over proximal and distal segments of specific nerves, such as the median, ulnar, radial, and musculocutaneous nerves. By varying the points of stimulation along these nerves from the supraclavicular fossa to the wrist, the site of compression can be identified.

Management

After the diagnosis of TOS has been confirmed, the initial method of management is nonsurgical.[22] Improvements in postural sitting, standing, and sleeping positions are recommended first, along with behavior modification at work. Many patients also benefit from muscle stretching and strengthening exercises, as instructed by physiotherapists. With these measures and patient education, 50% to 90% of patients can be successfully treated.

Indications for surgical intervention include failure of conservative management, progression of sensory or motor symptoms, the presence of excessively prolonged ulnar or median nerve conduction velocities, narrowing or occlusion of the subclavian artery, and thrombosis of the axillary or subclavian vein. The initial operation for TOS includes complete removal of the first rib, with division of the scalenus anticus and medius. A first rib resection can be accomplished through a variety of approaches, including transaxillary, supraclavicular, infraclavicular, transthoracic, and posterior. A review by Urschel and Razzuk[21] of more than 2200 procedures suggested that the transaxillary approach alone is required to obtain satisfactory symptom relief from upper (median nerve) and lower plexus (ulnar nerve) compression. Brachial plexus injuries, vascular injuries, pleural effusion, winged scapula, and infection are complications that may arise secondary to first rib removal. Success rates with surgery approach 70% at 5 years. Results indicate better success rates (by 15%) in patients with non–work-related compared with work-related injuries contributing to their TOS. Recurrence of symptoms is documented in about 1% of patients.[21] Reoperation with removal of a persistent bony remnant or neurolysis of the brachial plexus then may be required.

Aneurysmal dilation of the subclavian artery requires close follow-up. Treatment using graft reconstruction occasionally is required for large aneurysms or thrombosis. Treatment of subclavian vein thrombosis is accomplished with thrombolytic and anticoagulant therapy and simultaneous surgical decompression.

Chest Wall Trauma

Trauma to the chest wall is common and can range from an isolated single rib fracture to flail chest. About 30% of patients presenting with significant trauma have a chest wall injury. Guidelines of the Advanced Trauma Life Support program (Airway, Breathing, Circulation, Disability, Exposure) always need to be followed in the preliminary assessment of these patients.[23] This organized approach helps to rule out injuries to the underlying viscera such as the lungs, heart, liver, and spleen, all of which frequently are associated with chest wall injury.

Chest radiography and chest CT scan often are obtained as part of the secondary survey in chest wall trauma. Chest radiographs frequently miss or underestimate extent and severity. Chest CT scan is a significantly more sensitive study for detection of osseous and pleural abnormalities and can readily distinguish chest wall from parenchymal injury, unlike chest radiography.

Soft Tissue

Blunt chest wall trauma commonly results in contusion with localized tissue swelling and hematoma formation. In severe cases, these injuries can progress to soft tissue infections or necrosis that require antibiotic therapy and

débridement. Initially, it often is difficult to distinguish between deep muscle injury and bony fractures, given the pain that is caused by these injuries. Chest radiography and chest CT can be helpful in making this distinction. When subcutaneous emphysema is palpable on the chest wall, injury to the airway or lung parenchyma leading to a pneumothorax or esophageal perforation is suspected. Circumferential burns to the chest wall require escharotomy to allow adequate chest wall expansion.

Ribs

Rib fractures are a common injury sustained after blunt chest wall trauma. A higher incidence of fractures is observed in the elderly owing to the loss of chest wall compliance from ossification of costal cartilage and to osteoporosis. Symptoms include pain on inspiration and localized tenderness. Chest and rib radiographs can help to confirm the diagnosis in an acute setting but cannot completely rule out this injury. From 3 to 6 weeks after injury, callus formation around the fracture site is evident on repeat films. The management of rib fractures depends on the number and location of the injuries. Upper thoracic rib fractures (T1-T4) are uncommon because of the relatively protected position of these ribs below the upper extremity girdle musculature. Fractures of the first two thoracic ribs usually are seen in high-velocity injuries and can be associated with aortic disruption (6%).[24] Similarly, fractures of the lower thoracic ribs (T11-T12) are uncommon because the ribs are short and less exposed. Frequently, fractures to ribs 11 and 12 are associated with injuries to underlying abdominal organs such as the spleen, liver, and diaphragm. Fractures to thoracic ribs 5 to 10 are most commonly reported. Injury to three or more ribs often requires hospitalization for analgesia and monitoring of respiratory status. Splinting from improperly controlled pain can lead to atelectasis, retained secretions, pneumonia, shunting, and hypoxia. This is a particular problem in the elderly population. Analgesia can be provided using oral, intravenous, or intramuscular opioid analgesics for mild-to-moderate injuries, or epidural analgesia or intercostal nerve blocks for more severe injuries. Delayed healing or chronic pain may be an issue for patients who present with fractures or dislocation of the costochondral junction.

Flail chest is a unique injury in which rib fractures lead to an unstable chest wall that results in a paradoxical motion during respiration. The injuries must occur along the same rib to produce the free-floating segment. This injury arises from blunt chest wall trauma such as direct impact from a steering wheel column. The diagnosis of flail chest is made on clinical examination. Pulmonary contusion is the most commonly associated injury. Maintenance of adequate ventilation is the goal of therapy. Stabilization of the chest wall has been attempted using weights and rib binders, as well as fixation devices such as pins and plates. Mechanical ventilation with positive-pressure ventilation also occasionally is used to treat injuries in the elderly or in those patients with underlying pulmonary disease. Some centers report a more rapid wean from mechanical ventilation with the use of internal fixation.[25]

Sternum

Although relatively uncommon, sternal injuries can occur secondary to blunt trauma of the anterior chest. Commonly, fracture of the sternomanubrial joint occurs and leads to severe localized pain. A step deformity may be palpable if fracture dislocation of the sternum has occurred. The diagnosis is made by clinical evaluation with the assistance of a lateral chest radiograph. Operative stabilization using internal fixation is indicated in isolated injuries to achieve analgesia or long-term cosmetic improvement. The main concern of sternal injuries is the potential for associated underlying injuries that can be life threatening, such as aortic disruption, cardiac contusion, cardiac arrhythmias, and pericardial effusion. Telemetry, serial electrocardiograms with cardiac enzymes, and echocardiography are used to rule out these injuries.

Clavicles and Scapulae

Clavicular fractures may be associated with injury to the brachial plexus or subclavian vessels that can lead to TOS with improper healing. The usual mechanism of injury is either a direct blow or shoulder-restraint injury. Scapular fracture is a high-velocity injury associated with injuries to the lung (contusion and pneumothorax) and ribs (fractures). Clavicular and scapular fractures generally are treated expectantly, except if joint function is impaired or pain is excessive.

Chest Wall Defects

A defect in the chest wall may create a direct communication between the pleural space and the exterior of the patient. If the wound is of sufficient size, an open pneumothorax develops. Clinical examination and chest radiography can confirm the diagnosis. Treatment involves closure of the defect with a dressing and chest tube drainage of the affected hemithorax. Occasionally, a flap-valve mechanism (sucking chest wound) is created by the soft tissue that surrounds the chest wall defect, resulting in lung collapse and paradoxical shifting of the mediastinum. The resulting tension pneumothorax is life threatening because of the diminished cardiac output that accompanies the mediastinal shift. Prompt needle decompression through the second intercostal space (midclavicular line) is required, followed by chest tube insertion to restore the mediastinum to midline. Very rarely, a problem of lung herniation through a chest wall defect that leads to strangulation has been observed. Lung herniation, which occasionally occurs after thoracic surgical procedures, is rarely clinically symptomatic.

PLEURA

Anatomy

The pleural cavity appears between the 4th and 7th gestational weeks and is lined by the splanchnopleurae and somatopleurae, which later form the visceral and parietal pleurae and account for anatomic differences in vascular, nervous, and lymphatic structure.[26] The pleural space is a potential cavity lining the chest wall and into which each lung protrudes. The visceral and parietal pleurae are smooth, serous membranes, continuous with each other at the lung hila and pulmonary ligaments. Humans have a divided pleural space or two individual pleural spaces, unlike some other mammals, because of the development of a complete mediastinum. Under normal circumstances, the pleural space contains only a small amount of pleural fluid.

The parietal pleura is divided into four areas.[26] The cervical pleura, or cupula, covers the apex of the hemithorax and extends above the level of the first rib to join stronger connective tissue known as the Sibson fascia. The costal pleura lines the inner surface of the sternum, ribs, and vertebrae and is attached to the chest wall by the endothoracic fascia, a layer of loose connective tissue. The mediastinal pleura covers the pericardium and other mediastinal structures. The diaphragmatic pleura lines the diaphragm, where it is tightly bound to the central tendon of the diaphragm. It forms the floor of the pleural cavity.

The visceral pleura covers both lungs and follows all fissures. The pleural spaces oppose one another anteriorly at the sternal angle but diverge to accommodate the heart. Under normal conditions, the parietal and visceral pleural membranes are separated by a thin layer of fluid, which functions as a lubricant and transmits the forces of breathing between lung and chest wall. This fluid is formed as an ultrafiltrate of plasma but contains molecules secreted by mesothelial cells of the pleura that have surfactant-like properties. The parietal pleura derives its arterial blood supply from systemic arteries, including the posterior intercostal, internal mammary, anterior mediastinal, and superior phrenic arteries. Its drainage is through venules and corresponding systemic veins. The dual blood supply of the visceral pleura is both systemic and pulmonary. Typically, pulmonary capillaries form a subpleural network for the visceral pleura. However, fibrosis and inflammation increase the contribution of radicular branches of the bronchial arteries to the visceral pleural arterial supply. Venous drainage is only by the low-pressure pulmonary veins. The lymphatic drainage of the parietal pleura is into regional lymph nodes, including intercostal, mediastinal, and phrenic nodes. Visceral pleural lymphatics form a subpleural plexus when they mesh with superficial lung lymphatics. This subpleural plexus subsequently drains into mediastinal lymph nodes. Parietal pleura is richly innervated by the intercostal nerves, except the mediastinal and central diaphragmatic parietal pleurae, which are innervated by the phrenic nerves. The visceral pleura is insensitive and is innervated by vagal branches and the sympathetic system.

Pleural Effusions

The movement of fluid across the pleural membranes is complicated but in general is governed by Starling's law of capillary exchange. This suggests that the flux of fluid is controlled by the balance of both oncotic and hydrostatic pressures within the pleural capillaries and pleural space. The net pressure difference moves fluid primarily

Table 57-3 Etiology of Transudative Effusions

Congestive heart failure
Cirrhosis
Nephrotic syndrome
Hypoalbuminemic conditions
Fluid retention/overload
Pulmonary embolism
Lobar collapse
Meigs' syndrome

Table 57-4 Etiology of Exudative Effusions

Malignant
Bronchogenic carcinoma
Metastatic carcinoma
Lymphoma
Mesothelioma
Pleural adenocarcinoma
Infectious
Bacterial/parapneumonic
Empyema
Tuberculosis
Fungal
Viral
Parasitic
Collagen-Vascular Disease Related
Rheumatoid arthritis
Wegener's granulomatosis
Systemic lupus erythematosus
Churg-Strauss syndrome
Abdominal/Gastrointestinal Disease Related
Esophageal perforation
Subphrenic abscess
Pancreatitis/pancreatic pseudocyst
Meigs' syndrome
Others
Chylothorax
Uremia
Sarcoidosis
After coronary artery bypass grafting
Postirradiation
Trauma
Dressler's syndrome
Pulmonary embolism with infarction
Asbestosis related

from the parietal pleura into the pleural space. From 5 to 10 L of fluid transgress the pleural space over a 24-hour period. However, the amount of fluid within the normal pleural space is quite small.[27] The balance of forces favors fluid reabsorption from the pleural cavity across the visceral pleura. Nevertheless, under physiologic conditions, most pleural fluid reabsorption is through lymphatics of the parietal pleura because protein that enters the pleural space cannot enter the relatively impermeable visceral pleural capillaries. The parietal pleura, with its lymphatics, has an enormous capacity for both protein and fluid removal. In addition, this pleural homeostasis is affected by other factors, including gravity, pleural fluid viscosity, pleural membrane thickness, and the distribution of lymphatic drainage sites throughout the parietal pleura.[26] Even a small imbalance of accumulation and absorption of pleural fluid will lead to the development of a pleural effusion. The mechanisms of this imbalance include the following:

1. Increased hydrostatic pressure
2. Increased negative intrapleural pressure
3. Increased capillary permeability
4. Decreased plasma oncotic pressure
5. Decreased or interrupted lymphatic drainage

About 300 mL of fluid is required for the development of costophrenic angle blunting seen on an upright chest radiograph. At least 500 mL of effusion is necessary for detection on clinical examination. Pleural effusions are classified as either transudates or exudates based on fluid protein and lactate dehydrogenase (LDH) concentrations. Transudative effusions occur as the result of a change in fluid balance in the pleural space. Exudative effusions suggest the disruption or integrity loss of pleura or lymphatics. An effusion is considered exudative if it meets any one of the following criteria[28]:

- Pleural fluid protein/serum protein greater than 0.5
- Pleural fluid LDH/serum LDH greater than 0.6
- Pleural fluid LDH 1.67 times normal serum

The etiology of pleural effusions is quite varied.[29] Some of the many causes are listed in Tables 57-3 and 57-4.

Benign

Many, but not all, benign pleural effusions are transudates. With chronicity, however, even initially transudative effusions may be exudative. Benign transudative effusions tend to be free flowing and layer dependently. Benign, noninfectious pleural effusions are drained completely by thoracentesis for diagnosis. Treatment of benign pleural effusions is directed toward treatment of the underlying disease, such as congestive heart failure or ascites.[29]

Recurrent benign pleural effusions are not uncommon and are treated aggressively. Repeat thoracenteses can be carried out. Medical management of the underlying cause must be maximized. Despite these efforts, some pleural effusions tend to recur and cause symptoms of dyspnea or chest pain or heaviness. Tube thoracostomy or thoracoscopic drainage with or without chemical pleurodesis then is warranted. Chest tube insertion is carried out in such a way (angled chest tube, low insertion site) that drainage is as complete as possible. Pleurodesis can be

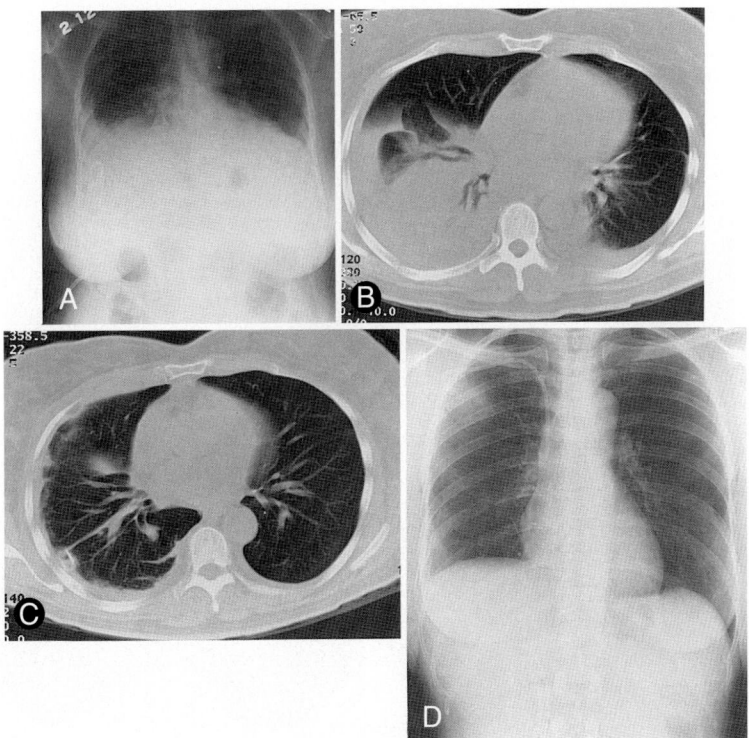

Figure 57-6 A, Chest radiograph demonstrates right pleural effusion after laparoscopic cholecystectomy. **B,** CT scan shows complicated (loculated) inflammatory effusion. **C,** CT scan from the postoperative period, after thoracoscopic débridement and decortication; note location of basilar chest tube. **D,** Follow-up chest radiograph after complete resolution.

carried out through the chest tube after chest tube outputs have decreased to less than 150 to 200 mL/day. Because tetracycline is no longer being manufactured for this purpose, alternatives are being used that are equally effective.[30] Doxycycline and minocycline can be instilled through the chest tube, as can sterile talc in slurry form. Typically, 300 mg of doxycycline or 2 to 5 g of talc in 100 to 200 mL of saline solution is instilled, and the chest tube is clamped at its exit site. The patient is turned at intervals for 1 hour to assist with distribution, and then the chest tube is replaced to suction drainage.

Thoracoscopic drainage of effusions with intraoperative chemical pleurodesis is currently widely used with excellent results.[31] Talc or doxycycline can be insufflated in its powdered form to cover all pleural surfaces. This procedure has the added advantage of being diagnostic in a pleural effusion whose cause is undiagnosed. The procedure does require general anesthesia with lung separation, and all patients may not be candidates (Fig. 57-6).

Thoracoscopy or thoracotomy with mechanical pleurodesis or pleurectomy is reserved for only the most recalcitrant effusions. A chronic pleural effusion may cause lung entrapment and not be amenable to procedures other than thoracotomy with decortication. Therefore, prompt attention to all benign pleural effusions is recommended.

Malignant

Malignancy is a common cause of pleural effusion. Most malignant pleural effusions are exudative. They are the second most common exudative effusive process. Metastatic breast and lung cancers are the most common malignancies that cause malignant effusions. Metastatic ovarian carcinoma is not uncommon. Lymphomas are an important cause of malignant effusion and account for 10% to 14% of all malignant pleural effusions.

Malignant pleural effusion is an effusion with positive cytopathology. Not all pleural effusions associated with malignancy are caused by direct or metastatic pleural involvement. Other mechanisms for their development (bronchial or lymphatic obstruction, hypoproteinemia, and sympathetic accumulation from infradiaphragmatic involvement) exist. Although repeated cytologic evaluation of a pleural effusion achieves high positive and negative predictive values, limitations are important. It is unreliable in establishing a diagnosis of lymphoma. Inflammation makes cytologic examination difficult and inaccurate. Malignant and reactive mesothelial cells have a similar appearance.

A malignant pleural effusion is best approached with a combination of treatment of the underlying disease (if available) and specific intervention of the effusion itself. Initial complete thoracentesis of a suspected malignant effusion is carried out for diagnostic (type of effusion,

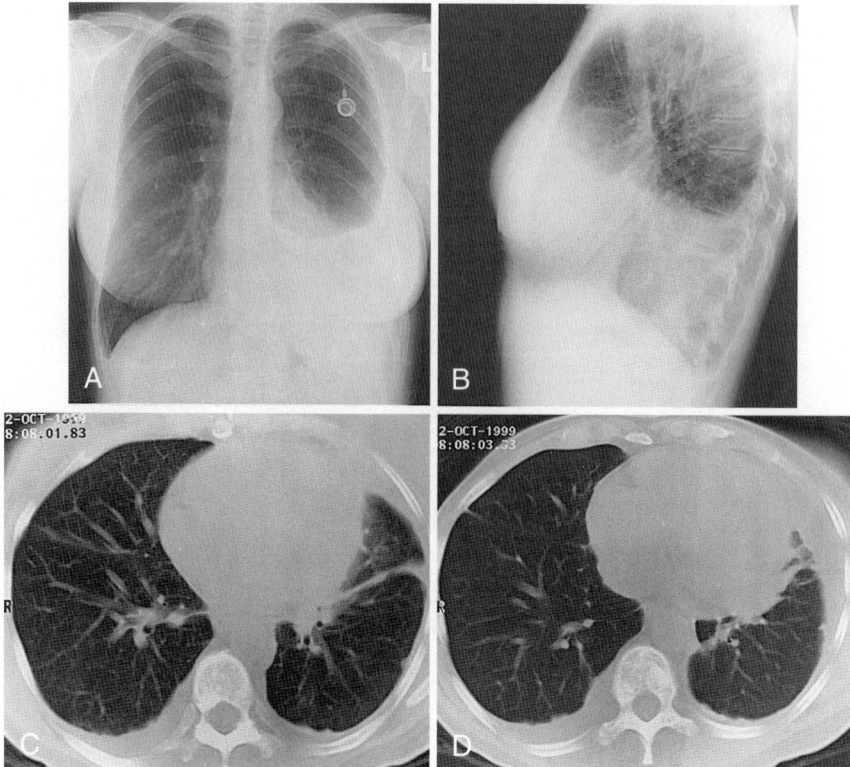

Figure 57-7 A and **B,** Posteroanterior and lateral chest radiographs demonstrate left malignant pleural effusion. **C** and **D,** CT scan cuts after video-assisted thoracic surgery drainage and talc pleurodesis.

expansibility of the lung) and therapeutic purposes. If the effusion reaccumulates, either repeat thoracentesis, chest tube insertion, or video-assisted thoracic surgery (VATS) drainage is indicated. Thoracentesis may be appropriate if the patient has minimal symptoms, has symptoms but is expected to have a prompt response to other therapy, is receiving chemotherapy and chest tube insertion is contraindicated (neutropenia), or is not a candidate for a more aggressive approach because of comorbid disease or stage of malignancy. A permanent pleural drainage catheter (Hickman, Groshong, PleurX) can facilitate repeated thoracenteses in both ambulatory and home-bound patients. Tube thoracostomy or VATS drainage of malignant effusions not only allows for continued emptying of the pleural space with visceral and parietal pleural apposition and possible adherence but also allows for chemical or mechanical pleurodesis. In addition to talc and doxycycline, bleomycin is an effective agent for chemical pleurodesis. VATS drainage has the added benefit of obtaining a definitive diagnostic biopsy if the pleural effusion is of an indeterminate cause (Fig. 57-7).

Yim and coworkers[32] reported their experience with thoracoscopic (VATS) management of malignant pleural effusions in 1996. Sixty-nine patients were treated without mortality or intraoperative complications; talc insufflation for prevention of recurrence was successful in 94%.

Local treatment of malignant effusions does not affect the systemic disease process but may provide significant symptomatic relief. Complications of these treatments include hemothorax, loculation of fluid, empyema, failure of pleurodesis with recurrence of effusion, and lung entrapment caused by inexpansile lung. Open surgical pleurectomy and pleurodesis is reserved for patients who fail other therapies and who have a reasonably long life expectancy.

Empyema

Empyema is a pyogenic or suppurative infection of the pleural space. Empyemas are the most common exudative type of pleural effusion. They may be classified into three categories based on the chronicity of the disease process.[33] The acute phase is characterized by pleural effusion of low viscosity and cell count. The transitional, exudative, or fibrinopurulent phase, which can begin after 48 hours, is characterized by an increase in white blood cells in the pleural effusion. The effusion is turbid, begins to loculate, and is associated with fibrin deposition on visceral and parietal pleurae and progressive lung entrapment. The organizing or chronic phase occurs after as little as 1 to 2 weeks and is associated with an ingrowth of capillaries and fibroblasts into the pleural rind and inexpansile lung.

An empyema may occur by direct contamination of the pleural space through wounds of the chest (trauma or surgery), by hematologic spread (bacteremia or sepsis), by direct extension from lung parenchymal infection

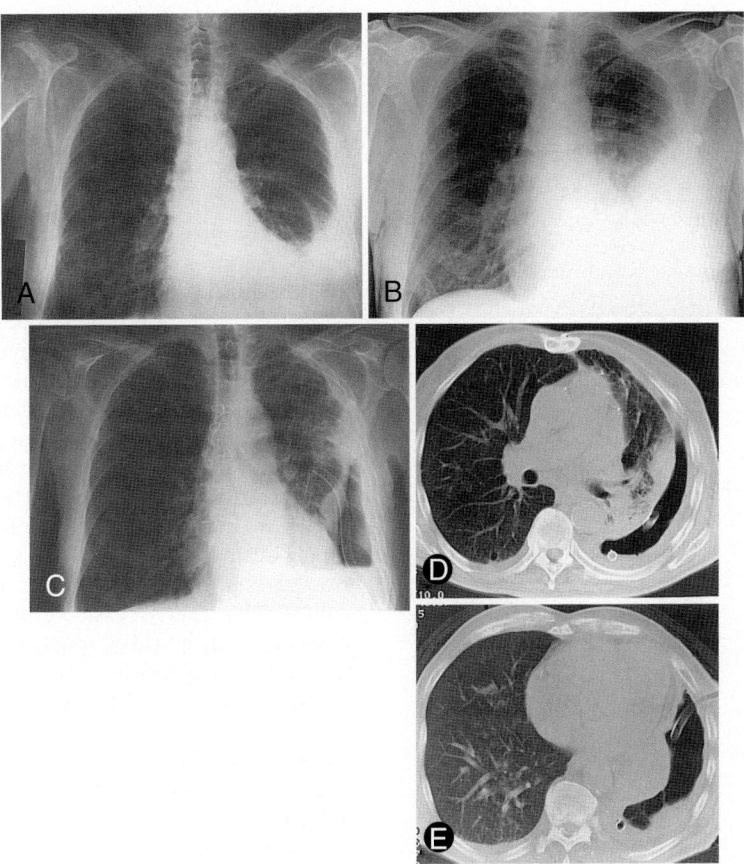

Figure 57-8 A, Chest radiograph shows left pleural effusion 1 year before treatment. **B,** Chest radiograph shows progression of left pleural process 2 months before treatment. **C,** Chest radiograph after left chest tube insertion for chronic empyema; note inexpansible left lung. **D** and **E,** CT scans show inexpansible left lung and basilar space with residual fluid.

(parapneumonic or postpneumonic), by rupture of an intrapulmonary abscess or infected cavity, or by extension from the mediastinum (esophageal perforation). Most often, empyemas are the result of a primary infectious process in the lung. Historically, these infections were commonly due to *Streptococcus* or *Pneumococcus pneumoniae;* today gram-negative and anaerobic organisms are common causes of empyema. Tuberculous empyema has had a recent resurgence.[29]

Most patients with acute or transitional phase empyema present with symptoms of their primary lung infection (cough, fever, sputum production), followed by symptoms of pleural effusion (chest pain and dyspnea) and systemic illness (anorexia, malaise, and sweats). Fever from empyema can be very high. Without intervention, a septic course will ensue. Chest radiography demonstrates a pleural effusion; chest CT may demonstrate a complicated effusion with loculations and a heterogeneous appearance to the effusion.

Treatment of empyema is dependent on its phase but involves the identification and systemic treatment (antibiotics) of the causative organism and complete drainage of the pleural space. In the acute and early fibrinopurulent phases, complete thoracentesis can be both diagnostic and therapeutic if the effusion is drained entirely. The

prior administration of antibiotics may lead to a sterile tap, but Gram stain (organisms), cell count (polymorphonuclear leukocytic predominance in bacterial empyema and lymphocytic predominance in tuberculous empyema), chemistries (protein, LDH, amylase, and glucose), and pH (<7.3) all can be useful in making the diagnosis.

Tube thoracostomy may be indicated for pleural drainage if thoracentesis fails or the empyema has progressed beyond its earliest stages. Chest tube insertion, however, can be ineffective if the empyema has become loculated or organized (Fig. 57-8). VATS empyema drainage with early pleural débridement has the added advantage of more complete pleural drainage by visualizing and breaking down loculations. Full lung expansion and the prevention of complications is the goal of the procedural intervention. Occasionally, radiologically guided catheter drainage can be a useful adjunct to these surgical procedures. Thoracotomy with débridement or formal decortication in later-stage empyema is reserved for treatment failures with persistent sepsis.

Management of parapneumonic effusion and empyema requires individualization of care owing to multiple factors that affect outcome. A patient's general health, existence of comorbidities, underlying pulmonary disease, and causative pathogen all dictate clinical outcome and

Table 57-5 Etiology of Chylothorax

Traumatic (Chest and Neck)
Blunt
Penetrating

Iatrogenic
Catheterization, particularly subclavian vein
Postsurgical
Excision of cervical/supraclavicular lymph nodes
Radical lymph node dissections of the neck
Radical lymph node dissections of the chest
Esophagectomy
Lobectomy or pneumonectomy
Mediastinal tumor resection
Thoracic aneurysm repair
Sympathectomy
Congenital cardiovascular surgery

Neoplasms
Lymphoma
Lung cancers
Esophageal cancers
Mediastinal malignancies
Metastatic carcinomas

Infectious
Tuberculous lymphadenosis
Mediastinitis
Ascending lymphangitis

Other
Lymphangioleiomyomatosis
Venous thrombosis

Congenital

have an impact on the relative risks and benefits of treatments. No algorithmic approach is applicable to all patients. Basic principles (established by Clagett and Geraci more than 40 years ago) that apply to all successful interventions include early detection of empyema, rapid and effective pleural drainage, and complete lung re-expansion. Effective treatments lead to decreased morbidity and mortality of empyema.[34]

Complications of empyema include empyema necessitatis (spontaneous decompression of pus through the chest wall), chronic empyema (with entrapped lung and pulmonary restrictive disease), osteomyelitis or chondritis of the ribs or vertebrae, pericarditis, mediastinitis, the development of a bronchopleural fistula, or disseminated infection of the central nervous system. Complications are best treated with prompt complete pleural drainage and débridement of infected tissues. Long-term (≥6 weeks) antibiotic therapy is required. Nutritional optimization plays an important role in treatment.

Chronic empyema is the result of failure to recognize or properly treat acute pneumonia or acute empyema, or failure (or incompleteness) of earlier intervention, and usually is associated with lung entrapment by a thick pleural peel or fibrothorax. This process can begin as early as 1 to 2 weeks and as late as 6 weeks after the

onset of the acute illness. Chronic empyema can mimic other systemic illnesses with symptoms of anorexia, weight loss, and lethargy. Debilitation is both a contributing factor to and an end result of this disease. Anemia is a common sign.

With chronic empyema, chest radiography demonstrates opacification of the affected hemithorax, particularly laterally and inferiorly, where thickened pleura abuts compressed lung. The interspaces are narrowed, and the hemithorax becomes contracted. CT of the chest is useful for defining the extent of pleural thickening and the exact location of the empyema cavity and to rule out other associated parenchymal disease.

The open surgical approaches for chronic empyema include variations of an open thoracostomy with rib resection or full thoracotomy with empyema evacuation and lung decortication.[33] The appropriate procedure depends on the patient's overall status and comorbidities. Open drainage involves removal of a portion of a rib or ribs at the most dependent portion of the empyema cavity. The pus is evacuated. This space can then be drained with a tube, packed with dressings (thoracic window), irrigated, or lined with a mobilized skin flap to prevent closure (Eloesser flap). Open drainage usually allows the cavity to constrict and eventually obliterate itself, although this can take many months. Delayed muscle flap closure of the space may be an option in selected patients.

Empyema evacuation and decortication is indicated for patients who are in otherwise good health and without significant underlying lung parenchymal disease. Resection of the thickened peel or cortex over the chest wall and lung permits expansion of chronically collapsed lung. Resolution of sepsis (early) and improvement in pulmonary function (late) are the expected results of this surgery. Often, extrapleural resection of the parietal pleura is necessary. Occasionally, pleuropneumonectomy is indicated in empyema with underlying destroyed lung (tuberculosis or bronchiectasis).

Chylothorax

Chylothorax is the accumulation of lymph within the pleural space. The incidence of chylothorax may be increasing because the number of thoracic surgical procedures and chest traumas continues to rise. Chylothorax characteristically is milky white fluid that contains a high concentration of emulsified fats (triglycerides, chylomicrons) and a lymphocytic predominance on cell count.[29] However, depending on the nutritional and dietary status of the patient, the effusion may be only slightly cloudy or even clear. Chylothorax occurs when the contents of the thoracic duct empty into the pleural space. In the nonsurgical setting, it is more common on the left side because of the anatomy of the thoracic duct. The underlying causes of chylothorax are numerous (Table 57-5).

Symptoms of chylothorax may mimic the effects of a pleural effusion (dyspnea, chest pain, fatigue), be attributable to underlying disease (infectious or neoplastic causes), or be the result of chronic metabolic (nutritional and immunologic) effects of a thoracic duct leak (loss of fat, protein, antibodies, and fat-soluble vitamins). Losses in fluid volume may be large (>3 L/day) and produce hemodynamic instability if not adequately replaced.

After diagnosis, management of a chylothorax consists initially of tube thoracostomy drainage (chest tube insertion) with complete lung re-expansion and supportive measures such as a low-fat or fat-free diet supplemented by medium-chain triglycerides and aggressive fluid, electrolyte, and nutritional replacement or correction. Often, these measures are enough to promote closure of the thoracic duct pleural fistula. If the chylothorax is caused by malignancy, primary treatment of the neoplasm may be necessary. Radiation therapy to the mediastinum has been useful in managing chylothorax secondary to lymphoma.

Conservative measures for the treatment of chylothorax generally are maintained for 1 to 2 weeks. If the chylous effusion has not responded to this management, surgical intervention is indicated.[33] The most common procedures are ligation of the thoracic duct or mass ligation of tissue at the diaphragmatic hiatus (generally through a right thoracotomy or right thoracoscopy) or direct closure of the duct injury. Instillation of olive oil or cream by nasogastric tube at the time of surgery can help to identify the duct and area of leakage. Rarely, pleurectomy and pleurodesis are useful adjuncts to these other surgical procedures for recalcitrant chylothorax. Most recently, minimally invasive techniques for thoracic duct obliteration through cisterna chyli cannulation or fenestration have been championed by interventional radiologists.

Pneumothorax

Pneumothorax is the accumulation of air within the pleural space. Pneumothoraces may be spontaneous or occur secondary to a traumatic, surgical, therapeutic, or disease-related event. A pneumothorax compresses lung tissue and reduces pulmonary compliance, ventilatory volumes, and diffusing capacity. These pathophysiologic consequences depend primarily on the size of the pneumothorax and condition of the underlying lung. If air enters the pleural space repeatedly (as with inspiration) and is unable to escape, positive pressure develops in the pleural space, causing compression or collapse of the entire lung, shifting of the mediastinum and heart away from the pneumothorax, and severe respiratory compromise with hemodynamic collapse. This situation is called a *tension pneumothorax* and requires immediate decompressive treatment. It may be the sequela of a pneumothorax from many causes.

Pneumothoraces may be classified as shown in Table 57-6. A primary spontaneous pneumothorax occurs without known cause or evidence of diffuse pulmonary disease or from subpleural blebs.[33] A secondary spontaneous pneumothorax occurs as the result of an underlying pulmonary process that predisposes to pneumothorax. Iatrogenic pneumothoraces are common and may be caused by thoracentesis, central venous catheterization, surgery, mechanical ventilation, or diagnostic lung biopsy.

Table 57-6 Classifications of Pneumothorax

Spontaneous
Primary
Secondary
   Chronic obstructive pulmonary disease (COPD)
   Bullous disease
   Cystic fibrosis
   Pneumocystis-related
   Congenital cysts
   Idiopathic pulmonary fibrosis (IPF)
   Pulmonary embolism
Catamenial
Neonatal

Traumatic
Penetrating
Blunt

Iatrogenic
Mechanical ventilation
Thoracentesis
Lung biopsy
Venous catheterization
Postsurgical

Other
Esophageal perforation

Patients with pneumothorax most commonly present with chest pain. It is often sharp and pleuritic and may lead to severe respiratory embarrassment or become dull and persistent. Dyspnea is the second most common symptom in patients with pneumothorax. Less common symptoms include nonproductive cough and orthopnea.

The diagnosis of primary spontaneous pneumothorax usually is established by history and physical examination and confirmed with chest radiography. Patients are often tall, thin men from 25 to 40 years of age. Physical findings may be normal if the pneumothorax is less than 25%. Characteristic physical findings include diminished chest excursion and hyperresonance on percussion of the affected side. Breath sounds are diminished to absent. Rarely, subcutaneous emphysema may be palpated or pneumomediastinum or pneumopericardium auscultated on cardiac examination.

A pneumothorax usually is seen on the standard posteroanterior chest radiograph with displacement of the visceral pleura from the parietal pleura by air in the pleural space. The area appears hyperlucent with absent pulmonary markings. An end-expiratory chest radiograph may appear to increase the size of the pneumothorax because of reduction in lung volume during forced expiration. Recognition of a pneumothorax may be difficult on portable supine or semirecumbent chest radiographs obtained in trauma or critically ill patients because of both the location of the least dependent pleural spaces (anterior, subdiaphragmatic) and associated radiographic findings. Patients with bullous disease also may have chest radiographs that are difficult to interpret; chest CT may be useful in these situations. The routine use of CT in patients with spontaneous primary pneumothorax is not warranted because the confirmation of apical blebs does not change treatment recommendations. The occurrence of apical blebs and bullae in these patients has been found to be greater than 85% in most recent surgical series.[35]

The treatment of a first-time spontaneous pneumothorax depends on the size of pneumothorax, associated symptoms, and pulmonary history. Smoking cessation is advocated for all smokers. Small pneumothoraces (<20%) that are stable may be monitored if the patient has few symptoms. Follow-up of a pneumothorax includes a chest radiograph to assess stability within 24 to 48 hours. An uncomplicated pneumothorax reabsorbs at a rate of about 1% per day. Indications for intervention include progressive pneumothorax, delayed pulmonary expansion, or development of symptoms.

Moderate (20%-40%) and large (>40%) pneumothoraces nearly always are associated with persistent symptoms that cause physical limitations and require intervention. Simple needle aspiration of a pneumothorax may relieve symptoms and can promote quicker lung re-expansion. It also may help to determine whether the initial fistula that caused the pneumothorax has sealed or if there is an ongoing air leak that requires chest tube insertion. This method is carried out using a standard thoracentesis kit and either an evacuated bottle or hand aspiration by a three-way stopcock and syringe. The needle generally is placed either anteriorly or laterally. The needle aspiration may be repeated, or a chest tube or needle catheter or thoracic vent drainage system may be inserted. It provides excellent management of iatrogenic pneumothoraces after central venous access or lung needle biopsy. This approach conservatively treats a sealed pneumothorax and identifies those with an active air leak for chest tube insertion.

Emergent needle decompression for tension pneumothorax is carried out on the affected side by placing an 18-gauge needle or angiocatheter into the hemithorax at the midclavicular line in the second anterior intercostal space. This emergency maneuver relieves the tension created within the thorax. It does not treat the pneumothorax; subsequent chest tube insertion is required.

Tube thoracostomy (chest tube insertion) and underwater seal drainage are the mainstays of treatment for spontaneous pneumothorax. Full re-expansion of the lung, even in the presence of a continuous leak, usually can be achieved with the application of suction to the thoracostomy drainage system. The classic location for chest tube insertion is the same as for emergency needle decompression because the tube can be inserted quickly and easily without the need for patient positioning. The preferred approach is through the fourth, fifth, or sixth intercostal space in the mid to anterior axillary line. This can be done under local anesthetic employing rib blocks or under intravenous procedural sedation. The chest tube needs to be directed upward to the apex of the hemithorax. Care must be taken to avoid the subcutaneous placement of a chest tube. Digital pleural dilation is recommended to confirm entrance into the chest cavity,

appreciate any adhesions, and allow passage of the chest tube without need for a stylet, which can cause damage to the lung or other intrathoracic structures.

Needle catheter and thoracic vent drainage systems may be employed for the treatment of a pneumothorax.[36] This system is comparable to a chest tube and drainage system, although the tube is of much smaller diameter and is inserted by means of the Seldinger technique or stylet. The end of the needle catheter drain is modified to be completely compatible with the many underwater seal drainage systems available. Many kits also include a unidirectional valve (Heimlich or Pneumostat, also available separately), which can be used in conjunction with either a catheter drain or conventional chest tube. The unidirectional valve and thoracic drain function as a one-way valve that lets air escape from the hemithorax, similar to an underwater seal. Patients may be discharged with these in place, to be removed at a later time after the leak has stopped.

Complications of chest tube insertion for pneumothorax are infrequent but include laceration of an intercostal vessel, laceration of the lung, intrapulmonary or extrathoracic placement of the chest tube, and infection. Re-expansion pulmonary edema is a rare complication that can be seen after treatment of a pneumothorax. It was first reported by Carlson and colleagues[37] in 1958 in this setting. Risk factors for this complication have not been consistently identified. Although re-expansion pulmonary edema is thought to be secondary to a sudden increase in capillary permeability, the exact mechanism of this increased permeability is unknown. Most cases have been reported after rapid lung re-expansion.

An air leak may be present for a variable amount of time after tube thoracostomy. Should the air leak persist for more than 72 hours or the lung not completely re-expand, surgical intervention is warranted. Primary spontaneous pneumothorax tends to recur with increasing frequency after each episode. The risk for first-time recurrence is about 25% to 30%. Surgery is recommended for a recurrence or the development of a contralateral pneumothorax. Surgical intervention for a first-time pneumothorax is recommended in situations that include bilateral simultaneous pneumothoraces, complete (100%) pneumothorax, pneumothorax associated with tension or borderline cardiopulmonary reserve, and in patients in high-risk professions or activities involving significant variations in atmospheric pressure, such as pilots and scuba divers. Surgery for complications of pneumothorax (empyema, hemothorax, or chronic pneumothorax) also is recommended in patients with first-time spontaneous pneumothorax.

Surgery for primary spontaneous pneumothorax has evolved over recent years from open thoracotomy (axillary or posterolateral) to a minimally invasive video-assisted technique (Fig. 57-9). The surgery carried out is identical, despite the differences in approach. Apical blebs are resected. The parietal pleura over the apex of the hemithorax can be removed (pleurectomy), abraded (mechanical pleurodesis), or treated with talc or tetracycline-like agents (chemical pleurodesis or poudrage). The

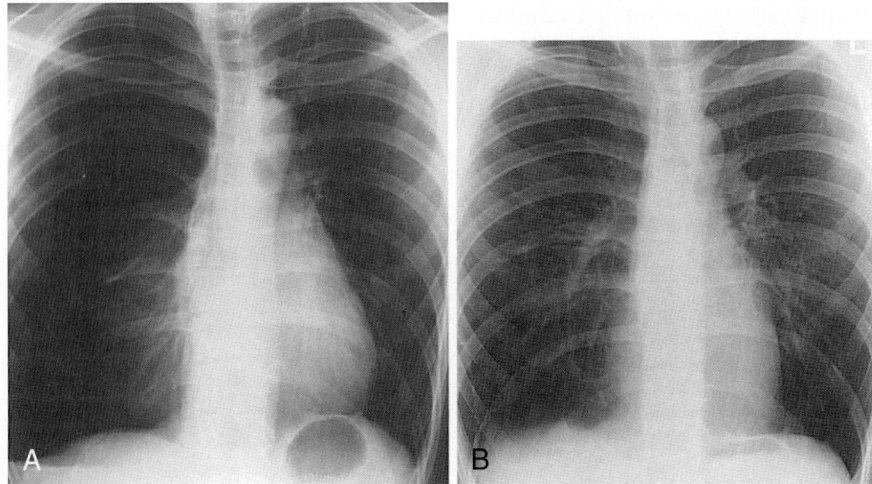

Figure 57-9 **A,** Chest radiograph demonstrates spontaneous right pneumothorax. Note left apical scarring from previous surgery for spontaneous left pneumothorax. **B,** Chest x-ray after thoracoscopic blebectomy and apical pleurectomy.

recurrence rate of these procedures, performed open or closed, is less than 5%. Naunheim and colleagues[38] reported their results on 113 consecutive patients treated with VATS blebectomy and pleurodesis in 1995. Their recurrence rate was 4%. More importantly, they found a reduced drainage time and complication rate and a shorter hospital stay with this approach. Patients also had a high acceptance rate of this procedure.

Treatment options for primary and secondary spontaneous pneumothorax are similar. However, patients with secondary pneumothorax generally are debilitated from a respiratory standpoint and may have other significant comorbid diseases. Treatment with tube thoracostomy alone has a high recurrence rate. Effective treatment must be individualized but needs to include chemical or surgical pleurodesis in combination with complete lung re-expansion and effective sealing of air leaks.

Mesothelioma

Mesothelioma is a rare neoplasm that arises from mesothelial cells lining the parietal and visceral pleura and can present in a localized or diffuse manner. The localized variant, the solitary fibrous tumor of the pleura, is a very uncommon benign neoplasm that usually presents as a well-defined, encapsulated tumor that is not associated with asbestos exposure. Historically, this was classified as a benign mesothelioma. Typically, the lesions are diagnosed as an asymptomatic mass on a chest radiograph. Complete surgical resection is the treatment of choice.

Diffuse malignant pleural mesothelioma presents as a locally aggressive tumor commonly associated with asbestos exposure (75%). A long latency period between asbestos exposure and the development of the disease has been reported.[39] Although smoking alone is not a reported risk factor, other factors such as radiation therapy

and various occupational exposures have been implicated. In the late 1990s, an association between simian virus 40 (SV 40) and mesothelioma was investigated.[40]

The clinical presentation of a patient with diffuse malignant pleural mesothelioma (MPM) is variable; therefore, a thorough clinical evaluation is essential. Dyspnea secondary to pleural effusion or encasement of the lung and chest pain from tumor infiltration into the chest wall and adjacent organs are the most commonly reported symptoms. Nonspecific symptoms such as weight loss, anorexia, night sweats, and weakness also are frequently noted. Physical signs vary depending on the stage of the neoplasm. Early in the disease, decreased breath sounds secondary to pleural effusion may be noted. In advanced stages of the disease, palpable tumor invading the chest wall and abdomen or nodal involvement may be identified.

Radiographic tests such as chest radiography, chest CT, and MRI play a major role in the evaluation of the patient with mesothelioma. Depending on the extent of disease, the chest radiographic findings may be quite variable. Typically, chest radiography demonstrates pleural thickening with or without pleural effusion. Chest CT and MRI are particularly effective in determining the presence of advanced disease, such as transdiaphragmatic involvement or mediastinal organ invasion.[41] Echocardiography also is helpful in ruling out pericardial invasion. In the future, positron emission tomography (PET) also may prove to be a useful tool in determining the extent of tumor invasion.

A number of techniques are used to confirm the diagnosis of MPM, including thoracocentesis of pleural effusion and pleural biopsy (open, VATS, and closed).[42] Open or VATS biopsy provides the best method to obtain a tumor sample sufficient to distinguish mesothelioma from other tumors such as adenocarcinoma and to determine the specific subtype of MPM. Frequently, immunohistochemistry techniques and electron microscopy performed by an experienced pathologist are required to confirm the diagnosis of MPM.[43]

Microscopically, malignant mesothelioma originates from mesothelial cells that line the pleural cavity. Three histologic subtypes of mesothelioma have been identified; these are epithelial, sarcomatous, and mixed histology. The histologic subtype has been shown to affect survival dramatically, with epithelial histology having a more favorable prognosis than the other two subtypes.[44,45]

Several staging systems for mesothelioma are used throughout the world. Although the Butchart tumor, node, metastasis (TNM) and Brigham staging systems are the most commonly used classifications, neither has been widely accepted.[44,46]

With supportive care, survival for mesothelioma ranges between 4 and 12 months. Attempts to improve survival have been made using a wide variety of therapeutic modalities. Treatment of this tumor using single-modality therapy such as radiotherapy, chemotherapy, or surgery has not demonstrated any improvement in survival.

Two surgical cytoreductive procedures, extrapleural pneumonectomy (EPP) or pleural pneumonectomy and pleurectomy/decortication, have been used in the treatment of MPM. In our experience, EPP is the more effective cytoreductive procedure because decorticating the tumor from the fissures and other recesses during pleurectomy can be difficult. The published results of pleurectomy/decortication in a multimodality setting indicate a median survival between 9 and 21 months and a mortality rate ranging from 1.5% to 5%.[47] Controversy surrounding the use of EPP is based on published trials that report high operative morbidity and mortality with no impact on patient survival when used as a single-modality therapy.[48] With advances in perioperative management and the development of multimodality approaches, long-term survival can, however, be obtained with EPP, with perioperative mortality rates of less than 3%.[44,47,49]

At the Brigham and Women's Hospital, a series of 183 patients who underwent trimodality therapy for MPM from 1980 to 1997 was reviewed in 1999.[44] The patients had undergone EPP followed by sequential chemotherapy (carboplatin/paclitaxel) and radiotherapy (55 Gy). Results from this series identified a favorable subgroup of patients who had epithelial histology, tumor-free resection margins, and negative extrapleural lymph nodes. This group of patients had a 46% 5-year survival and a median survival of 51 months. More recently, novel chemotherapeutic approaches have been advocated. Promising new agents are undergoing clinical trial for single modality and adjuvant therapy. Intraoperative intracavitary heated chemotherapy (cisplatin) administered at the time of either EPP or pleurectomy/decortication is being clinically utilized under protocol.[50,51]

Despite the overall improvement in survival with multimodality therapy, only 15% to 25% of patients are candidates for EPP. Thus, novel treatment strategies are being developed for this locally aggressive tumor using an intracavitary approach. These strategies include intracavitary chemotherapy, photodynamic therapy, immunotherapy, gene therapy, and vaccination therapy.

Selected References

Martin T, Fontana G, Olak J, et al: Use of pleural catheter for the management of simple pneumothorax. Chest 110:1169-1172, 1996.

> Retrospective review of 84 patients treated with a pleural catheter for iatrogenic or spontaneous pneumothorax demonstrates an 85% resolution rate with this therapy alone.

Naunheim KS, Mack MJ, Hazelrigg SR, et al: Safety and efficacy of video-assisted thoracic surgical techniques for the treatment of spontaneous pneumothorax. J Thorac Cardiovasc Surg 109:1198-1204, 1995.

> Review of 113 consecutive patients undergoing VATS treatment of spontaneous pneumothorax demonstrates low morbidity and recurrence rates. Univariate and multivariate analyses identify failure of bleb identification at surgery as the only significant independent predictor of recurrence.

Shamberger RC, Welch KJ: Surgical repair of pectus excavatum. J Pediatr Surg 23:615-622, 1988.

> Three-decade review of 704 patients with corrected pectus excavatum. Long-term follow-up documented major recurrence in 2% to 7% and identified total preservation of the perichondrial sheaths (resulting in full cartilage regeneration) as the key to a successful repair.

Sugarbaker DJ, Flores RM, Jaklitsch MT, et al: Resection margins, extrapleural nodal status, and cell type determine postoperative long-term survival in trimodality therapy of malignant pleural mesothelioma: Results in 183 patients. J Thorac Cardiovasc Surg 117:54-65, 1999.

> Review of 183 patients undergoing trimodality therapy for MPM demonstrated a 3.8% mortality rate and extended survival in patients with epithelial type, margin-negative, and extrapleural node-negative resection.

Webb WR, Ozmen V, Moulder PV, et al: Iodized talc pleurodesis for the treatment of pleural effusions. J Thorac Cardiovasc Surg 103:881-886, 1992.

> Prospective study of talc slurry pleurodesis in 34 patients demonstrating safety and efficacy for pleurodesis of benign or malignant pleural effusions.

Yim AP, Chung SS, Lee TW, et al: Thoracoscopic management of malignant pleural effusions. Chest 109:1234-1238, 1996.

> Single-institution experience of VATS management of malignant pleural effusions in 69 patients showing feasibility and safety.

References

1. Celsus: De Medicina. Spencer GW (trans). Cambridge, Harvard University Press, 1938.
2. Hippocrates: The Genuine Works of Hippocrates. Adams F (trans). New York, William Wood, 1929.
3. Graham EA, Bell RD: Open pneumothorax: Its relation to the treatment of acute empyema. Am J Med Sci 156:839, 1918.
4. Shamberger RC, Welch KJ: Chest wall deformities. In Ashcraft KW, Holder TM (eds): Pediatric Surgery, 2nd ed. Philadelphia, WB Saunders, 1993, p 146.
5. Crump HW: Pectus excavatum. Am Fam Physician 46:173-179, 1992.
6. Kowalewski J, Brocki M, Zolynski K: Long-term observation in 68 patients operated on for pectus excavatum: Surgical repair of funnel chest. Ann Thorac Surg 67:821-824, 1999.

7. Shamberger RC, Welch KJ, Upton J III: Surgical treatment of thoracic deformity in Poland's syndrome. J Pediatr Surg 24:760-766, 1989.

8. Cantrell JR, Haller JA, Ravitch MM: A syndrome of congenital defects involving the abdominal wall, sternum, diaphragm, pericardium, and heart. Surg Gynecol Obstet 107:1958.

9. Anderson BO, Burt ME: Chest wall neoplasms and their management. Ann Thorac Surg 58:1774-1781, 1994.

10. Burt M, Fulton M, Wessner-Dunlap S, et al: Primary bony and cartilaginous sarcomas of chest wall: Results of therapy. Ann Thorac Surg 54:226-232, 1992.

11. Miser JS, Kinsella TJ, Triche TJ, et al: Preliminary results of treatment of Ewing's sarcoma of bone in children and young adults: Six months of intensive combined modality therapy without maintenance. J Clin Oncol 6:484-490, 1988.

12. Faber LP, Somers J, Templeton AC: Chest wall tumors. Curr Probl Surg 32:661-747, 1995.

13. Pairolero PC, Arnold PG: Chest wall reconstruction. Ann Thorac Surg 32:325-326, 1981.

14. McCaughan BC, Martini N, Bains MS, et al: Chest wall invasion in carcinoma of the lung: Therapeutic and prognostic implications. J Thorac Cardiovasc Surg 89:836-841, 1985.

15. Pancoast H: Superior pulmonary sulcus tumor: Tumor characterized by pain, Horner's syndrome, destruction of bone and atrophy of hand muscles. JAMA 99:1391, 1932.

16. Paulson DL: Carcinomas in the superior pulmonary sulcus. J Thorac Cardiovasc Surg 70:1095-1104, 1975.

17. Taylor LQ, Williams AJ, Santiago SM: Survival in patients with superior pulmonary sulcus tumors. Respiration 59:27-29, 1992.

18. Mansour KA, Thourani, VH, Losken A, et al: Chest wall resections and reconstruction: A 25-year experience. Ann Thorac Surg 73:1720-1725; discussion 1725-1726, 2002.

19. Urschel JD, Takita H, Antkowiak JG: Necrotizing soft tissue infections of the chest wall. Ann Thorac Surg 64:276-279, 1997.

20. Urschel HC: Thoracic outlet syndromes. In Baue AE, Geha AS, Hammond GL, et al (eds): Glenn's Thoracic and Cardiovascular Surgery, 6th ed. Stamford, CT, Appleton & Lange, 1996, p 567.

21. Urschel HC Jr, Razzuk MA: Upper plexus thoracic outlet syndrome: Optimal therapy. Ann Thorac Surg 63:935-939, 1997.

22. Novak CB: Conservative management of thoracic outlet syndrome. Semin Thorac Cardiovasc Surg 8:201-207, 1996.

23. Feliciano DV: The diagnostic and therapeutic approach to chest trauma. Semin Thorac Cardiovasc Surg 4:156-162, 1992.

24. Poole GV: Fracture of the upper ribs and injury to the great vessels. Surg Gynecol Obstet 169:275-282, 1989.

25. Ahmed Z, Mohyuddin Z: Management of flail chest injury: Internal fixation versus endotracheal intubation and ventilation. J Thorac Cardiovasc Surg 110:1676-1680, 1995.

26. Lee KF, Olak J: Anatomy and physiology of the pleural space. Chest Surg Clin North Am 4:391-403, 1994.

27. Miserocchi G: Physiology and pathophysiology of pleural fluid turnover. Eur Respir J 10:219-225, 1997.

28. Light RW, Macgregor MI, Luchsinger PC, et al: Pleural effusions: The diagnostic separation of transudates and exudates. Ann Intern Med 77:507-513, 1972.

29. Hammar SP: The pathology of benign and malignant pleural disease. Chest Surg Clin N Am 4:405-430, 1994.

30. Robinson LA, Fleming WH, Galbraith TA: Intrapleural doxycycline control of malignant pleural effusions. Ann Thorac Surg 55:1115-1122, 1993.

31. Webb WR, Ozmen V, Moulder PV, et al: Iodized talc pleurodesis for the treatment of pleural effusions. J Thorac Cardiovasc Surg 103:881-886, 1992.

32. Yim AP, Chung SS, Lee TW, et al: Thoracoscopic management of malignant pleural effusions. Chest 109:1234-1238, 1996.

33. DeMeester TR, LaFontaine E: The pleura. In Sabiston DC Jr, Spencer FC (eds): Surgery of the Chest, 5th ed. Philadelphia, WB Saunders, 1990, p 444.

34. Vallieres E: Management of empyemas after lung resections. Chest Surg Clin N Am 12(3):571-585, 2002.

35. Schramel FM, Postmus PE, Vanderschueren RG: Current aspects of spontaneous pneumothorax. Eur Respir J 10:1372-1379, 1997.

36. Martin T, Fontana G, Olak J, et al: Use of pleural catheter for the management of simple pneumothorax. Chest 110:1169-1172, 1996.

37. Carlson RI, Classen KL, Gollan F, et al: Pulmonary edema following the rapid re-expansion of a totally collapsed lung due to a pneumothorax: A clinical and experimental study. Surg Forum 9:367, 1958.

38. Naunheim KS, Mack MJ, Hazelrigg SR, et al: Safety and efficacy of video-assisted thoracic surgical techniques for the treatment of spontaneous pneumothorax. J Thorac Cardiovasc Surg 109:1198-1204, 1995.

39. Price B: Analysis of current trends in United States mesothelioma incidence. Am J Epidemiol 145:211-218, 1997.

40. Pass HI, Donington JS, Wu P, et al: Human mesotheliomas contain the simian virus-40 regulatory region and large tumor antigen DNA sequences. J Thorac Cardiovasc Surg 116:854-859, 1998.

41. Patz EF Jr, Shaffer K, Piwnica-Worms DR, et al: Malignant pleural mesothelioma: Value of CT and MR imaging in predicting resectability. AJR Am J Roentgenol 159:961-966, 1992.

42. Sugarbaker DJ, Norberto JJ, Swanson SJ: Surgical staging and work-up of patients with diffuse malignant pleural mesothelioma. Semin Thorac Cardiovasc Surg 9:356-360, 1997.

43. Soosay GN, Griffiths M, Papadaki L, et al: The differential diagnosis of epithelial-type mesothelioma from adenocarcinoma and reactive mesothelial proliferation. J Pathol 163:299-305, 1991.

44. Sugarbaker DJ, Flores RM, Jaklitsch MT, et al: Resection margins, extrapleural nodal status, and cell type determine postoperative long-term survival in trimodality therapy of malignant pleural mesothelioma: Results in 183 patients. J Thorac Cardiovasc Surg 117:54-65, 1999.

45. Sugarbaker DJ, Garcia JP, Richards WG, et al: Extrapleural pneumonectomy in the multimodality therapy of malignant pleural mesothelioma: Results in 120 consecutive patients. Ann Surg 224:288-296, 1996.

46. Rusch VW: A proposed new international TNM staging system for malignant pleural mesothelioma. From the International Mesothelioma Interest Group. Chest 108:1122-1128, 1995.

47. Sugarbaker DJ, Norberto JJ, Swanson SJ: Extrapleural pneumonectomy in the setting of multimodality therapy for diffuse malignant pleural mesothelioma. Semin Thorac Cardiovasc Surg 9:373-382, 1997.

48. Rusch VW, Piantadosi S, Holmes EC: The role of extrapleural pneumonectomy in malignant pleural mesothelioma: A Lung Cancer Study Group trial. J Thorac Cardiovasc Surg 102:1-9, 1991.

49. Sugarbaker DJ, Strauss GM, Lynch TJ, et al: Node status has prognostic significance in the multimodality therapy of diffuse, malignant mesothelioma. J Clin Oncol 11:1172-1178, 1993.

50. Sugarbaker DJ, Richards W, Jaklitsch M, et al: Prevention, early detection and management of complications following 328 consecutive extrapleural pneumonectomies. Presented before the American Association for Thoracic Surgery, 83rd Annual Meeting, Boston, 2003.

51. Richards WG, Zellos L, Bueno R, et al: Phase I to II study of pleurectomy/decortication and intraoperative intracavitary hyperthermic cisplatin lavage for mesothelioma. J Clin Oncol 24(10):1561-1567, 2006.

CHAPTER 58

The Mediastinum

Thomas K. Varghese, Jr., MD   and   Christine L. Lau, MD

Anatomy
Primary Neoplasms
Primary Cysts

The mediastinum is the anatomic space that lies between the two pleural cavities and extends from the diaphragm to the thoracic inlet. Although it is the site of both localized disorders and systemic diseases, this chapter focuses on the primary tumors and cysts that characteristically present in the mediastinum. Other disease processes such as mediastinitis and mediastinal trauma can be found in chapters on heart, vascular system, and trauma.

ANATOMY

The mediastinum is defined by the following borders: the thoracic inlet superiorly, the diaphragm inferiorly, the sternum anteriorly, the vertebral column posteriorly, and the parietal pleura laterally. Although there are no definitive fascial or anatomic planes within the mediastinum, it is artificially subdivided into three compartments: the anterosuperior, middle, and posterior (Fig. 58-1). Contents of the anterosuperior compartment include the thymus gland, lymph nodes, and fat. The middle mediastinum or visceral compartment is defined as the space that contains the heart and pericardium, and contains the ascending and transverse aorta, brachiocephalic vessels, vena cavae, main pulmonary arteries and veins, phrenic and vagus nerves, trachea, bronchi, and lymph nodes. The posterior mediastinum is bounded anteriorly by the heart and trachea and extends posteriorly to the thoracic vertebral column and paravertebral gutters. It contains

the esophagus, descending aorta, azygos and hemiazygos veins, thoracic duct, sympathetic chain, and lymph nodes. Some elect to divide the mediastinum into four compartments: anterior, superior, middle, and posterior.

PRIMARY NEOPLASMS

Mediastinal tumors and cysts affect people of all ages, although they are more common in young and middle-aged adults. Most mediastinal masses are diagnosed in an asymptomatic patient on routine chest radiographs. Symptoms may occur as a result of local involvement of adjacent structures, tumor secretory factors, or immunologic factors. Benign lesions are more commonly asymptomatic, whereas malignant lesions generally produce clinical findings. The precise nature of a mediastinal lesion is dependent on histology. However, a tentative preoperative diagnosis can often be made by consideration of location of the tumor, age of the patient, presence or absence of local symptoms, and association of a specific systemic disease state.

With improvements in treatment modalities, the observation of a mediastinal mass, except in rare circumstances, cannot be justified. A classification of primary mediastinal tumors and cysts is shown in Table 58-1. The relative incidence of primary tumors in a combined series of 3805 patients is shown in Table 58-2. Although differences in the relative incidence of neoplasms and cysts exist in some series, the most common mediastinal masses are neurogenic tumors (23%), thymomas (21%), lymphomas (13%) and germ cell tumors (12%).

Mediastinal masses are most frequently located in the anterosuperior mediastinum (54%), with the posterior (26%) and middle mediastinum (20%) being less frequently involved.[1] Many of the mediastinal lesions occur in characteristic sites within the mediastinum. The masses

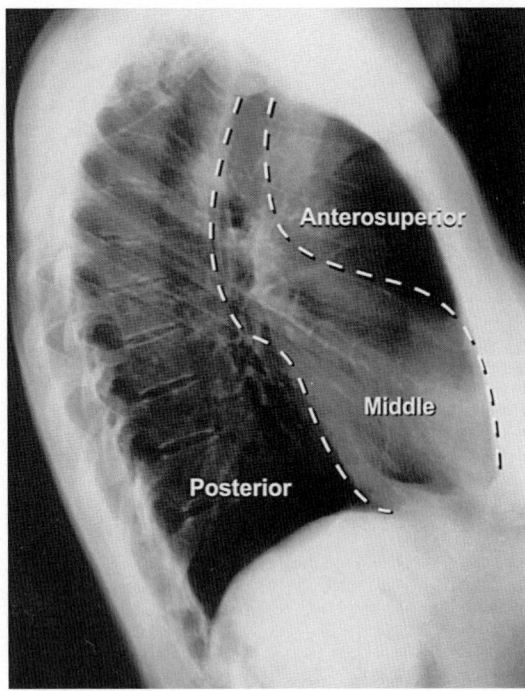

Figure 58-1 Lateral chest radiograph demonstrating the mediastinum divided into three anatomic subdivisions.

Table 58-1   Classification of Primary Mediastinal Tumors and Cysts

Neurogenic Tumors
Neurofibroma
Neurilemoma
Paraganglioma
Ganglioneuroma
Neuroblastoma
Chemodectoma
Neurosarcoma
Thymoma
Benign
Malignant
Lymphoma
Hodgkin's disease
Lymphoblastic lymphoma
Large cell lymphoma
Germ Cell Tumors
Teratodermoid
Benign
Malignant
Seminoma
Nonseminoma
Embryonal
Choriocarcinoma
Endodermal
Primary Carcinomas
Mesenchymal Tumors
Fibroma/fibrosarcoma
Lipoma/liposarcoma
Leiomyoma/leiomyosarcoma
Rhabdosarcoma
Xanthogranuloma
Myxoma
Mesothelioma
Hemangioma
Hemangioendothelioma
Hemangiopericytoma
Lymphangioma
Lymphangiomyoma
Lymphangiopericytoma
Endocrine Tumors
Intrathoracic thyroid
Parathyroid adenoma/carcinoma
Carcinoid
Cysts
Bronchogenic
Pericardial
Enteric
Thymic
Thoracic duct
Nonspecific
Giant Lymph Node Hyperplasia
Castleman's disease
Chondroma
Extramedullary Hematopoiesis

that occur most commonly in each of the three anatomic subdivisions are shown in Table 58-3. In addition, the location of the mass explains some of the typical symptoms related to a mediastinal mass because of compression or invasion of adjacent mediastinal structures. The common symptoms related to mechanical involvement with mediastinal structures are listed in Table 58-4.

Malignant neoplasms represent 42% of mediastinal masses in adults.[1] Lymphomas, thymomas, germ cell tumors, primary carcinomas, and neurogenic tumors are the most common. The relative frequency of mediastinal mass malignancy varies with the anatomic site in the mediastinum. Anterosuperior masses are most likely malignant (59%), relative to middle mediastinal masses (29%) and posterior mediastinal masses (16%). The relative percentage of lesions that are malignant also varies with age. Patients in the second through fourth decades of life have a greater proportion of malignant mediastinal masses. This period corresponds to the peak incidence of lymphomas and germ cell tumors. In contrast, in the first decade of life, a mediastinal mass is most likely benign (73%).

The incidence of mediastinal masses varies in infants, children, and adults. In a combined series of 712 children with mediastinal masses, neurogenic tumors (34%), primary cysts (16%), germ cell tumors (14%) and lymphomas (13%) were diagnosed most frequently.[2] The neurogenic tumors in children most commonly originate from sympathetic ganglion cells: gangliomas, ganglioneuroblastomas, and neuroblastomas. In contrast, neurilemomas and neurofibromas are the most common neurogenic tumors in adults. The childhood lymphomas are usually

Table 58-2 Primary Mediastinal Tumors and Cysts in 3805 Adult Patients

TYPE OF TUMOR	SABISTON AND SCOTT, 1952[35]	HERLITZKA AND GALE, 1958[36]	MORRISON, 1958[37]	LE ROUX, 1962[38]	HEIMBURGER AND BATTERSBY, 1965[39]	BOYD AND MIDELL, 1968[40]	BURKELL ET AL, 1969[41]	WYCHULIS ET AL, 1971[42]
Neurogenic tumor	20	35	101	30	21	11	13	212
Thymomas and thymic cysts	17	14	47	17	10	20	12	225
Lymphomas	11	12	33	0	9	20	12	107
Germ cell tumors	9	26	36	21	10	22	3	99
Enterogenous cysts (bronchogenic and enteric)	7	26	29	14	17	15	9	83
Pericardial cysts	2	17	13	20	4	6	4	72
Miscellaneous	23	29	30	3	7	2	4	118
Total	**89**	**159**	**289**	**105**	**78**	**96**	**57**	**916**

	FONTENELLE ET AL, 1971[43]	BENJAMIN ET AL, 1972[44]	RUBUSH ET AL, 1973[45]	OVRUM AND BIRKELAND, 1979[46]	NANDI ET AL, 1980[47]	PARISH ET AL, 1984[48]	DAVIS ET AL, 1987[1]	COHEN ET AL, 1991[49]
Neurogenic tumor	7	49	36	19	27	212	57	39
Thymomas and thymic cysts	18	34	51	10	18	206	67	45
Lymphomas	14	32	14	9	4	107	62	36
Germ cell tumors	3	27	14	5	7	99	42	23
Enterogenous cysts (bronchogenic and enteric)	2	12	8	0	0	83	50	36
Pericardial cysts	3	3	10	7	2	72	36	8
Miscellaneous	17	28	24	6	10	137	40	29
Total	**64**	**185**	**157**	**56**	**68**	**916**	**354**	**216**

	TOTAL FOR ALL SERIES	OVERALL INCIDENCE (%)
Neurogenic tumor	889	23
Thymomas and thymic cysts	811	21
Lymphomas	482	13
Germ cell tumors	446	12
Enterogenous cysts (bronchogenic and enteric)	391	10
Pericardial cysts	279	7
Miscellaneous	507	13
Total	**3805**	

of a non-Hodgkin's lymphoma variety. The germ cell tumors are most frequently benign teratomas. Pericardial cysts and thymomas are uncommon in children.

Clinical Features

The clinical presentation ranges from asymptomatic disease to symptoms related to mechanical effects of invasion or compression to systemic symptoms. Of patients with a mediastinal mass, 56% to 65% have symptoms at presentation. Patients with a benign lesion are more often symptom-free (54%) than are patients with a malignant neoplasm (15%). The most common features in a series of 400 patients were chest pain, fever, cough, and dyspnea (Table 58-5). Infants and children are more likely to present with symptoms or findings (78%) because of the relatively small space within the mediastinum.[2]

Symptoms related to compression or invasion of mediastinal structures, such as the superior vena caval syndrome, Horner's syndrome, hoarseness, and severe pain,

Table 58-3 **Differential Diagnosis of Mediastinal Tumors by Location**

Anterosuperior Mediastinum

95% of tumors in this compartment made up by the four "Ts":
Thymoma
Teratoma (germ cell tumors)
Thyroid goiter
"Terrible" lymphoma

Middle Mediastinum

Majority are cysts
Most common: congenital foregut cysts (20% of all mediastinal masses)
Bronchogenic cysts
Pericardial cysts
Most common tumor in middle mediastinum:
Lymphoma

Posterior Mediastinum

Neurogenic
Nerve sheath subtype
Benign
Malignant
Paraganglionic subtype
Benign
Malignant

Table 58-4 **Clinical Manifestations of Anatomic Compression or Invasion by Neoplasms of the Mediastinum**

Spinal cord compressive syndrome
Vena caval obstruction
Pericardial tamponade
Congestive heart failure
Dysrhythmias
Pulmonary stenosis
Tracheal compression
Esophageal compression
Vocal cord paralysis
Horner's syndrome
Phrenic nerve paralysis
Chylothorax
Chylopericardium
Pancoast's syndrome
Postobstructive pneumonitis

Table 58-5 **Presenting Symptoms in Patients With a Mediastinal Mass**

SYMPTOMS	PATIENTS (N=400)
Chest pain	30%
Fever, chills	20%
Dyspnea	16%
Cough	16%
Other Weight loss Superior vena cava syndrome Myasthenia gravis Fatigue Dysphagia Night sweats	<10%

Data from Davis RD, Oldham HN, Sabiston DC: Primary cysts and neoplasms of the mediastinum: Recent changes in clinical presentation, methods of diagnosis, management, and results. Ann Thorac Surg 44:229-237, 1987.

Table 58-6 **Systemic Syndromes Caused by Mediastinal Neoplasm Hormone Production**

SYNDROME	TUMOR
Hypertension	Pheochromocytoma, chemodectoma, ganglioneuroma, neuroblastoma
Hypoglycemia	Mesothelioma, teratoma, fibrosarcoma, neurosarcoma
Diarrhea	Ganglioneuroma, neuroblastoma, neurofibroma
Hypercalcemia	Parathyroid adenoma/carcinoma, Hodgkin's disease
Thyrotoxicosis	Thyroid adenoma/carcinoma
Gynecomastia	Nonseminomatous germ cell tumor

Examples of these syndromes include Cushing's syndrome, caused by ectopic production of adrenocorticotropic hormone, most frequently by neuroendocrine tumors; thyrotoxicosis, caused by a mediastinal goiter; hypertension and a hyperdynamic state, caused by pheochromocytoma; and hypercalcemia secondary to increased parathyroid hormone release from a mediastinal parathyroid adenoma.

In other syndromes, the pathophysiology is not as well understood (Table 58-7). Autoimmune mechanisms have been implicated in the association of myasthenia gravis and red blood cell aplasia with thymoma. In other cases, the pathophysiology is less defined: osteoarthropathy and neurogenic tumors; pain after ingestion of alcohol and the cyclic Pel-Ebstein fevers associated with Hodgkin's disease; and the opsoclonus-myoclonus syndrome and neuroblastoma.

Diagnosis

The goal of the diagnostic evaluation in a patient with a mediastinal mass is a precise histologic diagnosis so that

are more indicative of a malignant histologic diagnosis, although patients with a benign lesion, on occasion, present in this manner.

A number of primary mediastinal lesions produce hormones or antibodies that cause systemic symptoms, which may characterize a specific syndrome (Table 58-6).

Table 58-7   Systemic Syndromes Associated With Mediastinal Neoplasms

TUMOR	SYNDROME
Thymoma	Myasthenia gravis Red blood cell aplasia Aplastic anemia Hypogammaglobulinemia Progressive systemic sclerosis Hemolytic anemia Megaesophagus Dermatomyositis Systemic lupus erythematosus Myocarditis Collagen vascular disease
Lymphoma	Anemia, myasthenia gravis
Neurofibroma	Von Recklinghausen's disease
Carcinoid	Cushing's syndrome
Carcinoid, thymoma	Multiple endocrine adenomatosis
Thymoma, neurofibroma, neurilemoma, mesothelioma	Osteoarthropathy
Enteric cysts	Vertebral anomalies, peptic ulcer
Hodgkin's lymphoma	Alcohol-induced pain Pel-Ebstein fever
Neuroblastoma	Opsoclonus-myoclonus, erythrocyte abnormalities

optimal therapy can be performed. The preoperative evaluation of a patient with a mediastinal mass is intended to achieve the following:

1. Differentiate a primary mediastinal mass from masses of other causes that have a similar radiographic appearance
2. Recognize associated systemic manifestations that may affect the patient's perioperative course
3. Evaluate for possible compression by the mass of the tracheobronchial tree, pulmonary artery, or superior vena cava
4. Ascertain whether the mass extends into the spinal column
5. Determine whether the mass is a nonseminomatous germ cell tumor
6. Assess the likelihood of resectability
7. Identify significant factors of medical comorbidity and optimize overall medical condition

The initial diagnostic intervention needs to be a careful history and physical examination. The recognition of associated systemic syndromes with many neoplasms is necessary to avoid potentially serious intraoperative and postoperative complications. Although most systemic syndromes listed in Table 58-7 may be of little consequence regarding the planned surgical management, the association of myasthenia gravis, malignant hypertension,

hypogammaglobulinemia, hypercalcemia, and thyrotoxicosis with mediastinal neoplasms markedly affects appropriate management.

The posteroanterior and lateral chest radiographs provide important information concerning anatomic location and size of the tumor. Computed tomography (CT) with contrast medium enhancement is done routinely in patients with a mediastinal mass. CT allows for determination of location, size, shape, density and composition of the mass, calcification, edge characteristics, lymphadenopathy, and associated findings. In patients with a contraindication to the use of contrast dye and in those with surgical clips in the anatomic region of interest, magnetic resonance imaging (MRI) is used. Considerable information can be obtained regarding the relative invasiveness and malignant nature of the mediastinal mass with either CT or MRI. Tumor disruption of fat planes; irregularity of pleural, vascular, or pericardial margins by tumor; and infiltration into muscle or periosteum are useful for differentiating tumor compression from invasion. Resectability is better assessed than nonresectability using CT or MRI. MRI may be more useful than CT with certain posterior mediastinal masses in terms of evaluating foramen involvement in neurogenic tumors, and it has been shown to be superior to CT in diagnosing various cysts.[3] Additionally, MRI may provide information regarding the involvement of the tumor with major vascular or cardiac structures and may help detect whether the tumor is actually a vascular abnormality.

Echocardiography may be useful in the evaluation of mediastinal masses, especially tumors that occur in the middle mediastinum or in patients with tamponade or pulmonary stenosis. Echocardiography delineates the cystic nature of lesions, and it has been used to guide needle biopsy, especially with lesions adjacent to the chest wall. Although echocardiography is not as sensitive as MRI or CT, it is useful in determining the physiologic effect of tumor involvement of the pericardium, heart, or great vessels.

FDG (2-deoxy-2-[^{18}F] fluoro-D-glucose) positron emission tomography (PET) has played an increasing role in evaluation of mediastinal neoplasms, especially in determining the malignant potential of a mediastinal mass. One series reported the sensitivity and specificity of CT and PET in diagnosing tumor invasion and found PET to be superior (sensitivity, 90%; specificity, 92%; accuracy, 91%) to CT (sensitivity, 70%; specificity, 83%; accuracy, 77%). With thymic neoplasms, high FDG uptake was reflective of invasiveness and was seen in thymic carcinomas and invasive thymomas.[4] FDG-PET has a significantly higher sensitivity compared with gallium-67 (^{67}Ga) scintigraphy in pretherapy imaging of aggressive non-Hodgkin's lymphomas and Hodgkin's disease.[5]

Serologic evaluation is indicated in certain patients. Male patients in their second through fifth decades who have an anterosuperior mediastinal mass need to have α-fetoprotein and β-human chorionic gonadotropin (β-HCG) serologic studies obtained. A positive serology is indicative of a nonseminomatous germ cell tumor.

Patients with a mediastinal mass and a history of significant hypertension or hypermetabolism have urinary excretion of vanillylmandelic acid and catecholamines measured. This enables the initiation of appropriate perioperative adrenergic blockers in patients with hormonally active intrathoracic pheochromocytoma, paraganglioma, and neuroblastoma, limiting perioperative complications secondary to episodic catecholamine release. In these patients, nuclear scans using metaiodobenzylguanidine (MIBG) are useful in tumor location and in identifying sites of metastatic disease, particularly when located in the middle mediastinum.

Patients with contrast medium–enhancing lesions in the superior mediastinum who do not have symptoms are evaluated with an iodine-131 (^{131}I) scan. In a patient who does not have symptoms but has a positive scan indicative of a thyroid lesion and no identifiable active thyroid tissue elsewhere, careful observation without excision using serial CT scans to evaluate for growth is indicated.

Increased success has been reported in making a cytologic diagnosis preoperatively by using fine-needle biopsy techniques (18-22 gauge needle) with low morbidity and almost no mortality. CT, echocardiography, endoscopic ultrasound and endobronchial ultrasound, because of better localization of the mass and improved placement of the needle, have increased the sensitivity of the technique.[6,7] Although a cytologic diagnosis of benign or malignant differentiation between masses can be made in about 90% of patients, a precise histologic diagnosis is not always possible. Obtaining core biopsy specimens using cutting needles increases the accuracy of the precise histologic diagnosis and differentiation between benign and malignant lesions. Core biopsy techniques are particularly useful in the diagnosis of lymphomas, thymomas, and neural tumors. Recent advances in immunohistochemical and core biopsy techniques have allowed them to become more accurate for establishing the initial diagnosis of lymphoma, but it is probably better utilized for confirming recurrent disease.[8] Complications related to the procedure include pneumothorax in 20% to 25% of patients, with about 5% requiring tube thoracostomy; hemoptysis in 5% to 10%, with rare occurrences of significant hemorrhagic complications; and tumor seeding along the needle track, which is a theoretical but extremely rare complication. Needle biopsy techniques are particularly useful for evaluating patients in whom excisional therapy is not indicated but have limited yield in tumors with marked associated desmoplastic reaction, such as nodular sclerosing Hodgkin's lymphoma.

Poorly differentiated malignant tumors of the anterosuperior mediastinum, particularly thymomas, lymphomas, germ cell tumors, and primary carcinomas, can have remarkably similar cytologic and morphologic appearances. In addition to light microscopy using special staining techniques, immunostaining techniques and electron microscopy of multiple sections of the tumor may be necessary to establish an accurate diagnosis (Table 58-8).

When needle biopsy techniques are contraindicated or do not produce sufficient tissue for the histologic diagnosis, more invasive procedures are often required,

Table 58-8 Ultrastructural Characteristics of Mediastinal Tumors

TUMORS	ULTRASTRUCTURE
Carcinoid	Dense core granules, fewer monofilaments and desmosomes
Lymphoma	Absence of junctional attachments and epithelial features
Thymoma	Well-formed desmosome, bundles of tonofilaments
Germ cell	Prominent nucleoli, even chromatin, scant desmosomes, rare tonofilaments
Neuroblastoma	Neurosecretory granules, synaptic endings

such as mediastinoscopy, mediastinotomy, thoracoscopy, thoracotomy, or median sternotomy. Mediastinoscopy is a useful technique to evaluate and biopsy lesions of the middle mediastinum. This technique is often used to evaluate associated lymphadenopathy in this region. Biopsy of lesions in the anterosuperior mediastinum is best done using a limited anterior second or third interspace parasternal mediastinotomy or by thoracoscopy, which provides excellent exposure. Biopsies of posterior mediastinal masses may be approached thoracoscopically or through a limited posterolateral thoracotomy. A representative section of the tissue obtained is submitted for immediate frozen-section analysis to establish adequacy of the biopsy before closing. Importantly, the incision is not made in the portals for potential radiation therapy. Lesions that appear resectable are excised. Median sternotomy provides optimal exposure for lesions in the anterosuperior mediastinum. A transcervical approach using sternal elevators has been successfully used to resect tumors in the superior aspect of the anterosuperior mediastinum. Occasionally for extensive tumors of the anterosuperior mediastinum, a trans-sternal bilateral thoracotomy (clam shell) incision is indicated. Middle and posterior mediastinal masses are usually best excised through a posterolateral thoracotomy. Thoracoscopic and thoracoscopically assisted procedures are being used in diagnosing and treating a variety of mediastinal lesions in carefully selected patients.

Although most patients undergo surgical procedures safely, patients with large anterosuperior or middle mediastinal masses, particularly children, have an increased risk for severe cardiorespiratory complications during general anesthesia. Patients with posture-related dyspnea and superior vena caval syndrome are at increased risk, and attempts to obtain a histologic diagnosis are limited to needle biopsies or open procedures done with local anesthesia. If a general anesthesia is required and there is concern about airway obstruction, an awake fiberoptic intubation is performed, rigid bronchoscopy available, and, if at all possible, anesthesia provided with inhalational agents only; muscle paralysis needs to be avoided.

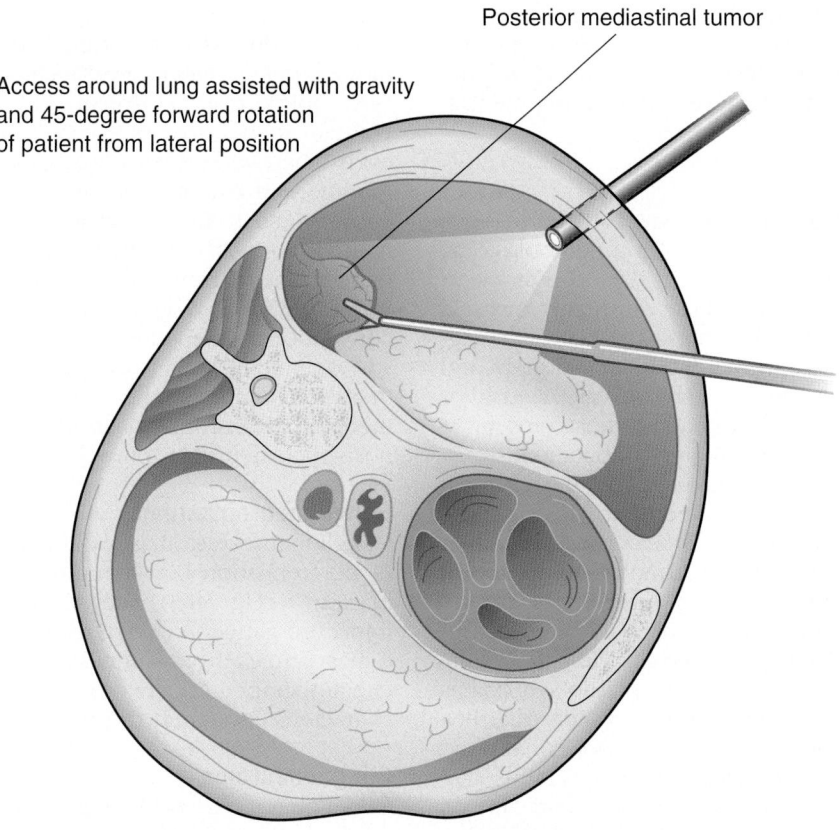

Posterior mediastinal tumor

Access around lung assisted with gravity
and 45-degree forward rotation
of patient from lateral position

Figure 58-2 The endoscopic dissector, scissors, and grasper can be introduced into the pleural cavity through the accessory intercostal space access sites to complete the tumor resection. The resected tumor can be put into a plastic bag and withdrawn through one of the access sites. The access site may have to be extended to allow tumor removal. Adequate hemostasis is essential. A chest tube (28 French) is inserted into the pleural cavity through the lowest access site for underwater sealed drainage. The other incisions are closed with sutures. (From Sabiston DC Jr: Atlas of Cardiothoracic Surgery. Philadelphia, WB Saunders, 1995, p 560.)

Neurogenic Tumors

Neurogenic tumors are the most common neoplasm, constituting 23% of all primary tumors and cysts. These tumors are usually located in the posterior mediastinum and originate from the sympathetic ganglia (ganglioma, ganglioneuroblastoma, and neuroblastoma), the intercostal nerves (neurofibroma, neurilemoma, and neurosarcoma), and the paraganglia cells (paraganglioma). Only rarely are neurogenic tumors located in the anterosuperior mediastinum. Although the peak incidence occurs in adults, neurogenic tumors make up a proportionally greater percentage of mediastinal masses in children (34%). Although most neurogenic tumors in adults are benign, a greater percentage of neurogenic tumors are malignant in children.

Many of these tumors are found on routine chest radiographs in patients who do not have symptoms. When present, symptoms are usually caused by mechanical factors, such as chest and back pain resulting from compression or invasion of intercostal nerve, bone, and chest wall; cough and dyspnea resulting from compression of the tracheobronchial tree; Pancoast's syndrome; and Horner's syndrome resulting from involvement of the

brachial and the cervical sympathetic chain. Symptoms may be systemic and related to production of neurohormonal agents.

Thoracoscopy has played an increasing role in both diagnosis and treatment of neurogenic tumors (Fig. 58-2). Benign neurogenic tumors are particularly amenable to thoracoscopic removal, and more rapid postoperative recovery is seen with thoracoscopic removal than with open excision. For malignant tumors, the standard of care remains thoracotomy.

About 10% of neurogenic tumors have extensions into the spinal column. These tumors are termed *dumbbell tumors* because of their characteristic shape resulting from the relatively large paraspinal and intraspinal portions connected by a narrow isthmus of tissue traversing the intervertebral foramen. Although 60% of patients with a dumbbell tumor have neurologic symptoms related to spinal cord compression, the significant proportion of patients without symptoms underscores the importance of evaluating all patients with a posterior mediastinal mass for possible intraspinal extension. MRI is preferred to evaluate the presence and extent of the intraspinal component. The recommended surgical approach to dumbbell tumors is a one-stage excision of the intraspinal component before resecting the thoracic component to minimize any spinal column hematoma. The incision used for the posterior laminectomy is extended into the appropriate interspace to allow resection of the mediastinal component.

Neuroblastoma

Neuroblastomas originate from the sympathetic nervous system. The most common location for a neuroblastoma is in the retroperitoneum; however, 10% to 20% occur primarily in the mediastinum. These are highly invasive neoplasms that have frequently metastasized before diagnosis. Biologically they can behave quite uniquely and have been known to spontaneously regress, mature, or proliferate aggressively. Unfortunately, most present at advanced stages and do not regress spontaneously or mature. Common sites of metastases are the regional lymph nodes, bone, brain, liver, and lung. Most of these tumors occur in children, and 75% occur in children younger than 4 years of age. The tumor is composed of small, round, immature cells organized in a rosette pattern. On ultrastructural examination, the presence of neurosecretory granules is characteristic. Patients usually have symptoms. A variety of paraneoplastic syndromes have been reported, including profuse watery diarrhea and abdominal pain related to vasoactive intestinal polypeptide production, the opsoclonus-polymyoclonus syndrome (an unexplained symptom complex characterized by cerebellar and truncal ataxia with rapid, darting eye movements [dancing eyes] that is possibly related to an autoimmune mechanism), and pheochromocytoma syndrome caused by catecholamine secretion. A 24-hour urine collection to measure catecholamines is obtained in children with a posterior mediastinal mass.

Neuroblastoma and ganglioneuroblastoma are staged as follows[8]:

Stage I: Well-circumscribed, noninvasive tumor; complete gross excision and residual microscopic disease; microscopically negative nodes

Stage IIA: Tumor invasion locally without extension across the midline; incomplete gross excision; microscopically negative nodes

Stage IIB: Tumor invasion locally without extension across the midline; complete or incomplete gross resection; positive nodes ipsilaterally but negative microscopically contralateral lymph nodes

Stage III: Unresectable tumor spread across the midline with node involvement (regional); or no extension across the midline with contralateral lymph nodes positive; or midline tumor with bilateral nodes positive

Stage IV: Tumor with metastasis (except as in stage IVS)

Stage IVS: Primary tumor localized, metastatic disease limited to liver, skin, and/or bone marrow in infants younger than 1 year of age

Therapy is determined by the stage of the disease: stage I, surgical excision; stage II, excision and radiation therapy; stages III and IV, multimodality therapy using surgical debulking, radiation therapy, and multiagent chemotherapy as well as a second-look exploration to resect residual disease when necessary. The usual chemotherapeutic agents used include cisplatin, vincristine, doxorubicin, cyclophosphamide, and etoposide. Children younger than 1 year of age have an excellent prognosis even when widespread disease is present. With increasing age and extent of involvement, however, the prognosis worsens. In the subset of patients with high-risk neuroblastomas, dose-intensive chemotherapy and autologous bone marrow transplantation resulted in improved event-free survival but not overall survival compared with conventional chemotherapy.[9] Treatment of patients with 13-*cis*-retinoic acid, a differentiating agent, after initial therapy also appeared to confer a benefit.[10] Interestingly, mediastinal neuroblastomas appear to have a better prognosis than neuroblastomas occurring elsewhere.

Ganglioneuroblastoma

Ganglioneuroblastomas exhibit an intermediate degree of differentiation between ganglioneuromas and neuroblastomas (Fig. 58-3). They are composed of mature and immature ganglion cells. Treatment of ganglioneuroblastomas ranges from surgical excision alone to various chemotherapeutic strategies depending on histologic characteristics, age at diagnosis, and stage of disease.

Ganglioneuroma

Ganglioneuromas are benign tumors originating from the sympathetic chain that are composed of ganglion cells and nerve fibers. These tumors typically present at an early age and are the most common neurogenic tumors occurring during childhood. The usual location is the paravertebral region. These tumors are well encapsulated and, when cross-sectioned, frequently exhibit areas of cystic degeneration. Surgical excision provides cure.

Neurilemoma, Neurofibroma, and Neurosarcoma

The most common neurogenic tumor is the neurilemoma or schwannoma (Fig. 58-4), which originates from perineural Schwann cells. They are benign, slow-growing neoplasms that frequently arise from a spinal nerve root, but can involve any thoracic nerve. These tumors are well circumscribed and have a defined capsule. They arise from the nerve sheath and extrinsically compress the nerve fibers. There are two morphologic patterns: Antoni type A, which has organized architecture with a cellular palisading pattern of growth; and Antoni type B, which has a loose reticular pattern of growth. The peak incidence of these tumors is in the third through fifth decades of life, with men and women being equally affected.

In contrast to neurilemomas, neurofibromas are poorly encapsulated and consist of randomly arranged spindle-shaped cells. These tumors originate as a proliferation of all the elements of the peripheral nerve. Although both neurilemomas and neurofibromas occur as a manifestation of neurofibromatosis (von Recklinghausen's disease), they must be differentiated from the two other common entities in the posterior mediastinum: meningioma and meningocele. Both neurilemomas and neurofibromas appear as spherical or lobulated paraspinous masses that

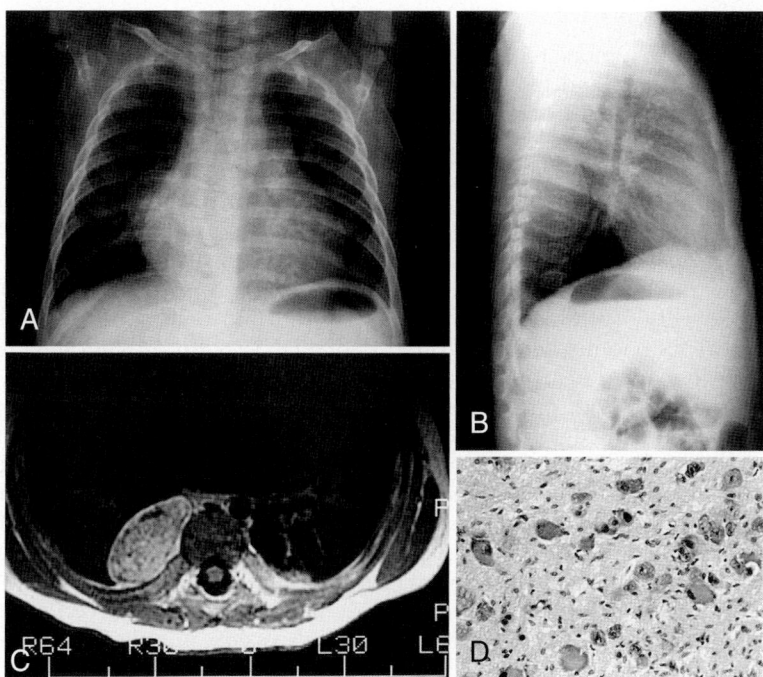

Figure 58-3 A and **B,** Chest radiographs of patient with ganglioneuroblastoma. **C,** MRI (cross-sectional) of tumor. **D,** Histopathologic examination of ganglioneuroblastoma shows mature component of tumor (H&E, ×250).

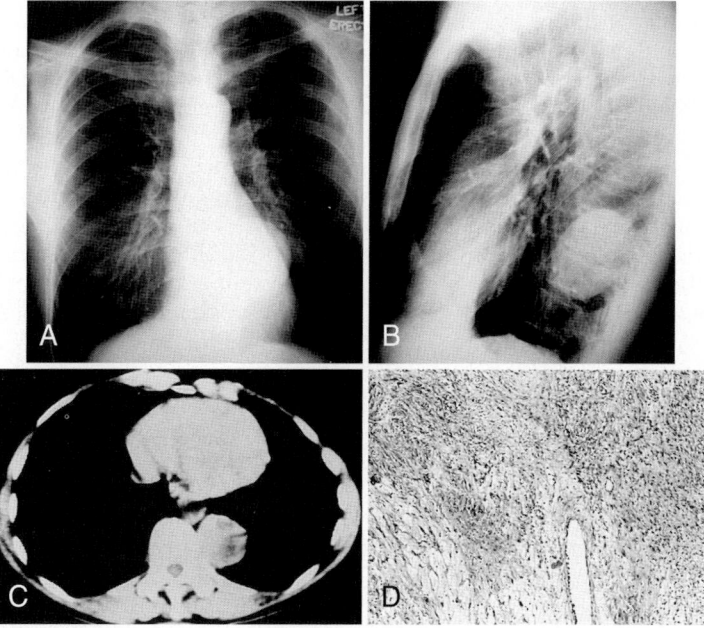

Figure 58-4 A and **B,** Chest radiographs of patient with a neurilemoma. **C,** CT scan of the tumor in the posterior mediastinum. **D,** Histopathologic examination of neurilemoma shows the highly cellular Antoni A areas and the less cellular Antoni B areas (H&E, ×68).

often span one to two posterior intercostal spaces, but can attain larger sizes. With both neurilemoma and neurofibroma, surgical excision results in cure.

Neurosarcomas originate by malignant degeneration of either neurilemomas or neurofibromas, in addition to developing de novo. These tumors usually occur in adults; however, patients with neurofibromatosis may develop neurosarcomas as children. These are rapidly growing tumors that frequently invade vital structures, preventing attempts at resection. Unless tumor excision is possible, the prognosis is extremely poor because of the unresponsiveness to adjuvant therapies.

Paraganglioma (Pheochromocytoma)

Mediastinal paragangliomas are rare tumors, representing less than 1% of all mediastinal tumors and less than 2% of all pheochromocytomas. Although most are found in the paravertebral sulcus, an increasing number of middle mediastinal paragangliomas occur in the branchial arch structures, coronary and aortopulmonary paraganglia, atria, and islands of tissue in the pericardium. The likelihood of functional activity of a paraganglioma is related to the site of origin: adrenal medulla, high likelihood; branchiomeric and intravagal, very low likelihood; and aortosympathetic and visceral autonomic, intermediate likelihood. Catecholamine production causes the classic constellation of symptoms associated with pheochromocytomas, including periodic or sustained hypertension, often accompanied by orthostatic hypotension, hypermetabolism manifested by weight loss, hyperhidrosis, palpitations, and headaches. Measurement of elevated levels of urinary catecholamines or their metabolites, the metanephrines and vanillylmandelic acid, usually establishes the diagnosis. Although adrenal pheochromocytomas often produce both epinephrine and norepinephrine, extra-adrenal paragangliomas rarely secrete epinephrine.

Tumor localization has improved remarkably through the use of CT and ^{131}I-MIBG scintigraphy, particularly when the tumors are hormonally active. Because of the high vascularity of these lesions, enhancement with contrast medium administration occurs during CT. Because of the accuracy of CT and MIBG scanning, rarely is selective venous angiography with serial sampling for catecholamine levels necessary for preoperative localization.

When appropriate, surgical resection is the optimal therapy. In patients with tumors involving the middle mediastinum, cardiopulmonary bypass may be necessary to enable resection. Preoperative embolization to reduce perioperative bleeding may be considered. Although half of tumors appear malignant morphologically, metastatic disease develops in only 3% of patients. In those with metastatic disease, α-methyltyramine, a tyrosine hydroxylase inhibitor that blocks the synthesis of catecholamines, is helpful in controlling symptoms.

About 10% of patients have multiple paragangliomas. They are more common in patients with multiple endocrine neoplasia syndromes, a family history of disease, and Carney's syndrome (pulmonary chondroma, gastric leiomyosarcoma, and extra-adrenal paraganglioma). In patients who have had excision of an adrenal pheochromocytoma and continue to have symptoms, a search for an extra-adrenal lesion is undertaken, with careful attention directed to the evaluation of the mediastinum.

Thymoma

Thymoma is the most common neoplasm of the anterosuperior mediastinum and the second most common mediastinal mass (21%). The peak incidence is in the third through fifth decades, but this tumor may occur throughout adulthood. Thymoma is rare in the first two decades of life. On a radiograph, it may appear as a small, well-circumscribed mass or as a bulky lobulated mass confluent with adjacent mediastinal structures (Fig. 58-5). Patients usually have symptoms at presentation, and symptoms may be related to local mass effects causing chest pain, dyspnea, hemoptysis, cough, and the superior vena caval syndrome. Thymomas, however, are frequently associated with systemic syndromes caused by immunologic mechanisms. Although the most common syndrome is myasthenia gravis, many other syndromes have been associated with thymomas, including red blood cell aplasia, pure white blood cell aplasia, aplastic anemia, Cushing's syndrome, hypogammaglobulinemia and hypergammaglobulinemia, dermatomyositis, systemic lupus erythematosus, progressive systemic sclerosis, hypercoagulopathy with thrombosis, rheumatoid arthritis, megaesophagus, and granulomatous myocarditis. These systemic syndromes often do not improve after successful control of the thymoma.

Most patients with myasthenia gravis do not have thymoma. The incidence is 10% to 42%, depending on the reporting medical center. Although red blood cell aplasia occurs in only 5% of patients with thymoma, 33% to 50% of adults with red blood cell aplasia have a thymoma. Because of the significant association between thymoma and these syndromes, an evaluation of the mediastinum with CT or MRI is recommended in all patients with myasthenia gravis and red blood cell aplasia.

Thymomas are epithelial neoplasms characterized by an admixture of epithelial cells and mature lymphocytes. They are histologically classified either by the predominance of epithelial or lymphocytic cells (lymphocytic, epithelial, mixed, and spindle) or by the morphologic resemblance to cortical or medullary epithelium.[11] Most thymomas are completely surrounded by a fibrous capsule. Unfortunately, a wide variance in the cellular composition is often present within the tumor and a consistent relationship is not present between the microscopic appearance and biologic behavior with regard to either tumor invasiveness or association with systemic syndromes.

Differentiation between benign and malignant disease is determined by the presence of gross invasion of adjacent structures, metastasis, or microscopic evidence of capsular invasion. Fifteen to 65 percent of thymomas are benign. The relative percentage is partially related to early surgical treatment of myasthenia gravis; when thymectomy is performed early in the course of myasthenia gravis, a greater percentage of thymomas are benign.

Whenever possible, the therapy for thymoma is surgical excision without removing or injuring vital structures. Even with well-encapsulated thymomas, extended thymectomy with eradication of all accessible mediastinal fatty areolar tissue is performed to ensure removal of all ectopic thymic tissue. In a series of 283 patients from the Mayo Clinic, 32% had locally invasive tumors, including 6% with metastases to the pleura and lungs.[12] Extended thymectomy has been shown to lower the number of tumor recurrences. The best operative exposure is obtained using a median sternotomy. Because many thy-

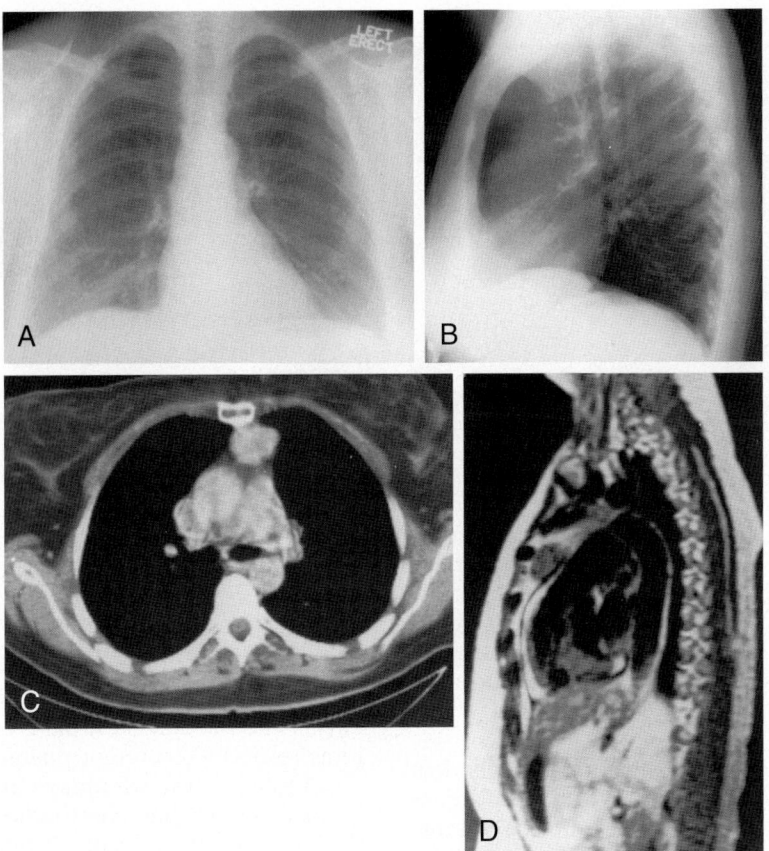

Figure 58-5 A and **B,** Chest radiographs of a patient with myasthenia gravis who had a benign thymoma. The tumor is poorly visualized, manifested only by an irregularity of the anterior cardiac border. **C,** CT scan clearly illustrates the tumor in the anterior mediastinum. **D,** Sagittal MRI of the mediastinum demonstrates a separation between the tumor and the pericardium. (**A-D** From Davis RD Jr, Oldham HN Jr, Sabiston DC Jr: The mediastinum. In Sabiston DC Jr, Spencer FC [eds]: Surgery of the Chest, 5th ed. Philadelphia, WB Saunders, 1990.)

momas are radiosensitive, the placement of surgical clips to outline the anatomic extent of disease aids in the determination of optimal radiation portals.

In 1939, Blalock and colleagues reported the beneficial effect of thymectomy in the treatment of myasthenia gravis.[13] For patients with myasthenia gravis without thymomas, extended transcervical thymectomy offers comparable results to trans-sternal procedures.[14] The perioperative management in patients with myasthenia gravis is extremely important to prevent complications. Anticholinesterase inhibitors are discontinued to decrease the amount of pulmonary secretions and prevent inadvertent cholinergic weakness. Plasmapheresis is used routinely within 72 hours of thymectomy. In most patients, plasmapheresis is effective in controlling generalized weakness. Also, careful attention to the maintenance of pulmonary function with chest physiotherapy, endotracheal suctioning, and bronchodilators is the mainstay of postoperative management. Although myasthenic patients with thymoma had a worse prognosis in past series, improvements in therapy for myasthenia gravis have allowed prognosis to be dependent on the stage of the disease rather than on the presence of myasthenia gravis.

Staging of thymoma is as follows[15]:

Stage I: Tumor is well encapsulated without evidence of gross or microscopic capsular invasion.
Stage II: Tumor exhibits pericapsular growth into adjacent fat or mediastinal pleura or microscopic invasion of the thymic capsule.
Stage III: Tumor invades adjacent organs.
Stage IVa: Intrathoracic metastatic spread occurs.
Stage IVb: Extrathoracic metastatic spread occurs (uncommon).

Complete surgical resection for stage I is sufficient treatment. The adjunctive use of radiation therapy for stage II and III disease is common practice. Tumors greater than 5 cm, locally invasive tumors, unresectable tumors, and metastatic tumors are treated following protocols that include chemotherapy,[16] followed by surgical exploration with the goal of complete resection and postoperative radiation therapy. The best results are seen with cisplatin-based regimens, with overall response rates of 70% to 100%.[16]

An aggressive surgical approach is recommended for invasive thymomas that includes radical resection and

Table 58-9   Classification of Germ Cell Tumors

Benign
Mature teratomas
Dermoid cysts

Malignant
Seminomas
Nonseminomatous germ cell tumors
   Immature teratoma
   Teratoma with malignant components
   Choriocarcinomas
   Embryonal cell carcinomas
   Endodermal cell (yolk sac) tumors
   Mixed germ cell tumors

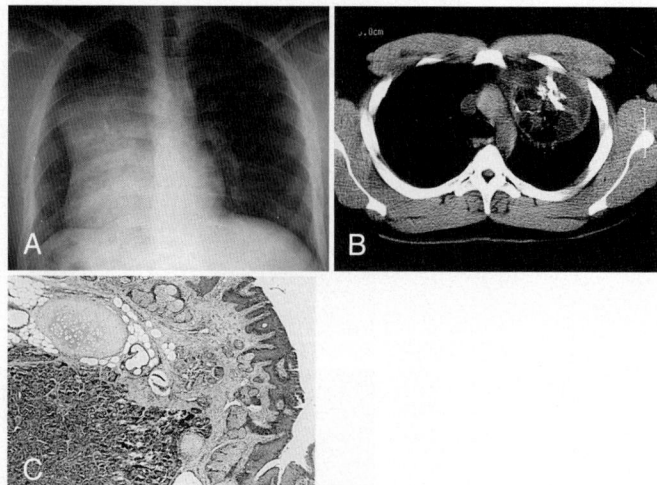

Figure 58-6 A, Chest radiograph of patient with teratoma. **B,** CT scan of tumor. **C,** Histopathologic examination of benign teratoma (H&E, ×52).

vascular reconstruction of the superior vena cava or its branches when invaded.[17] Using this aggressive approach to obtain complete resection, a significant difference in 5-year survival rates is seen in patients with stage III thymomas (94%) compared with those with incomplete resections (35%). Thymomas frequently show recurrence, and reoperation for recurrent disease has been recommended.[17]

The prognosis for patients with thymoma is dependent on clinical stage; 5- and 10-year survival rates are as follows: stage I, 90% to 96.2% and 66.7% to 86%; stage II, 70% to 96% and 55% to 75%; stage III, 50% to 69.6% and 21% to 58.3%; and stage IV, 50% to 100% and 0% to 40%.[18] Because thymomas have been reported to have late recurrences, cure rates need to be based on 10-year follow-up data.

Germ Cell Tumors

Germ cell tumors are benign and malignant neoplasms thought to originate from primordial germ cells that fail to complete the migration from the urogenital ridge and come to rest in the mediastinum. The anterosuperior mediastinum is the most common extragonadal primary site of these tumors. These tumors are classified as shown in Table 58-9. Although these lesions are identical histologically to germ cell tumors originating in the gonads, they are not considered to be metastatic from primary gonadal tumors. The current recommendations for evaluating the testes of a patient with mediastinal germ cell tumor are careful physical examination and ultrasonography. Biopsy is reserved for positive findings. Blind biopsy or orchiectomy is contraindicated.

Teratomatous Lesions

Teratomas are the most common mediastinal germ cell tumors. They are neoplasms composed of multiple tissue elements derived from the three primitive embryonic layers foreign to the area in which they occur. The peak incidence is in the second and third decades of life. There is no gender predisposition. These tumors are located most commonly in the anterosuperior mediastinum, although 3% to 8% are found in the posterior mediastinum. Symptoms, when present, are related to mechanical effects and include chest pain, cough, dyspnea, or symptoms related to recurrent pneumonitis.

Although germ cell tumors are rare, the diagnosis can be made on routine chest radiography by the identification of well-formed teeth. CT findings of a predominantly fatty mass with a denser dependent portion containing globular calcifications, bone, or teeth and a solid protuberance into a cystic cavity are considered specific. Despite occasional characteristic appearances using various imaging techniques, the diagnosis usually depends on microscopic examination.

The teratodermoid (dermoid) cyst is the simplest form. It is composed predominantly of derivatives of the epidermal layer, including dermal and epidermal glands, hair, and sebaceous material. Teratomas are histologically more complex (Fig. 58-6). The solid component of the tumor often contains well-differentiated elements of bone, cartilage, teeth, muscle, connective tissue, fibrous and lymphoid tissue, nerve, thymus, mucous and salivary glands, lung, liver, or pancreas. Malignant tumors are differentiated from benign tumors by the presence of primitive (embryonic) tissue or by the presence of malignant components. Immature teratomas contain combinations of mature epithelial and connective tissues with immature areas of mesenchymal and neuroectodermal tissues. Teratomas with malignant components are divided into categories based on the elements present.

Diagnosis and therapy rely on surgical excision. For those benign tumors of such large size or with involvement of adjacent mediastinal structures such that complete resection is impossible, partial resection has led to resolution of symptoms, frequently without relapse. For malignant teratomas, chemotherapy and radiation therapy, combined with surgical excision, are individualized for the type of malignant components contained in the tumors. The overall prognosis is poor for malignant tumors.

Malignant Nonteratomatous Germ Cell Tumors

Malignant germ cell tumors also occur predominantly in the anterosuperior mediastinum. Unlike benign teratomas, there is a marked male predominance. The peak incidence is in the third and fourth decades of life. Most cases are symptomatic, with chest pain, cough, dyspnea, and hemoptysis; the superior vena caval syndrome occurs commonly. The chest radiograph usually demonstrates a large anterior mediastinal mass that is often multilobular; frequently, there is evidence of intrathoracic spread of disease. CT and MRI are most helpful in defining the extent of involvement for the purpose of providing a means of following response to therapy and diagnosing relapses. These imaging modalities are also useful in determining impingement on vital structures that may contraindicate the use of general anesthesia. Serologic measurements of α-fetoprotein and β-HCG are useful for the following tasks: differentiating seminomas from nonseminomas, quantitatively assessing response to therapy in hormonally active tumors, and diagnosing relapse or failure of therapy before changes that can be observed in gross disease. Seminomas rarely produce β-HCG (<7%) and never produce α-fetoprotein; in contrast, more than 90% of nonseminomas secrete one or both of these hormones. This differentiation is important because of the marked radiosensitivity of seminomas and the relative radiosensitivity of nonseminomas.

Seminomas

Seminomas constitute 50% of malignant germ cell tumors and 2% to 4% of all mediastinal masses. Unlike other malignant germ cell tumors, seminomas usually remain intrathoracic with local extension to adjacent mediastinal and pulmonary structures. Although metastatic spread occurs first through lymphatics, hematogenous spread with extrathoracic involvement may develop late in the course of disease. Bone and lung are the most common sites of metastatic spread. Patients usually develop symptoms related to the mechanical effects of the tumor on adjacent structures. The superior vena caval syndrome occurs in 10% to 20% of patients. The histologic appearance of this tumor is characterized by large cells with round nuclei, scant cytoplasm, and abundant glycogen.

Therapy is determined by the stage of the disease. Occasionally, excision is possible without injury to vital structures and is recommended when possible. When complete resection is possible, the use of adjuvant therapy is unnecessary. Careful follow-up with serial CT examinations is required to diagnose recurrences. When excision is not possible, a biopsy sample of sufficient size to establish the diagnosis is obtained. Because these tumors are sensitive to irradiation and chemotherapy, cytoreductive resection before chemotherapy or radiation therapy is unnecessary and is contraindicated when vital structures are involved or when the procedure is technically difficult. Treatment varies somewhat based on extent of disease and usually consists of chemotherapy with or without secondary surgery or combination chemotherapy and radiation therapy. Radiation therapy alone is occasionally used for localized disease, but inferior results have been reported, and its sole use is discouraged.[19] Cisplatin-based chemotherapy is the treatment of choice; alternatively, carboplatin-based regimens can be used.

As discussed in the subsequent section on nonseminomatous mediastinal germ cell tumors, residual disease is surgically resected after chemotherapy. FDG-PET is of no apparent benefit in evaluation of postchemotherapy residual masses in patients with seminomas.[20] Recurrent disease is treated with salvage chemotherapy and selective consolidation. Excellent long-term survival rates have been seen with mediastinal seminoma, with a recent large multi-institutional series reporting an 88% 5-year survival rate.[21]

Nonseminomatous Tumors

Malignant nonseminomatous tumors include choriocarcinomas, embryonal cell carcinomas, immature teratomas, teratomas with malignant components, and endodermal cell (yolk sac) tumors, of which 40% are a mixture of tissue types. Malignant teratomas have already been discussed with other teratomatous lesions. The nonseminomas differ from seminomas in several aspects: they are more aggressive tumors that are frequently disseminated at the time of diagnosis; they are rarely radiosensitive; and more than 90% produce either β-HCG or α-fetoprotein. All patients with choriocarcinoma and some patients with embryonal cell tumors have elevated levels of β-HCG. α-Fetoprotein is most commonly elevated in patients with embryonal cell carcinomas and yolk sac tumors.

Like seminomas, most nonseminomatous neoplasms are symptomatic with chest pain, dyspnea, weight loss, cough, hemoptysis, fever, chills, and the superior vena caval syndrome. Children with these tumors may present with precocious puberty. Patients are predominantly men in their third or fourth decades. Chest radiographs usually reveal a large anterior mediastinal mass with frequent extension into lung parenchyma and adjacent mediastinal structures. In addition to superior vena caval obstruction, they may cause pulmonary stenosis and coarctation of the aorta. Characteristically, these tumors have extensive intrathoracic involvement and frequently have metastasized outside the thorax. Frequent sites of metastatic disease include brain, lung, liver, bone, and the lymphatic system, particularly the supraclavicular nodes. Chest wall involvement is common.

A number of chromosomal abnormalities are associated with an increased incidence of nonseminomatous germ cell tumors, including Klinefelter's syndrome, trisomy 8, and 5q deletion.[22] Additionally, mediastinal nonseminomas, but not testicular germ cell tumors, are associated with the development of rare hematologic malignancies, such as acute megakaryocytic leukemia, systemic mast cell disease, and malignant histiocytosis, as well as other hematologic abnormalities, including myelodysplastic syndrome and idiopathic thrombocytopenia refractory to treatment.

The local invasiveness of these tumors and their frequent metastasis usually preclude surgical resection of all disease at the time of diagnosis. Initially, operative intervention is necessary only to establish the histologic diagnosis in patients without elevations in serum α-fetoprotein or β-HCG.

Treatment of these nonseminomatous tumors currently is with cisplatin and etoposide-based regimens.[23] Serum markers α-fetoprotein and β-HCG are followed to assess response to treatment. If a complete serologic and radiologic response is achieved, patients are closely observed. If the disease progresses during therapy, salvage chemotherapy is initiated. If there is a serologic response but a radiographic abnormality remains, the patient is taken to the operating room and surgical removal of as much of the remaining tumor as possible is performed. The pathology of the resected postchemotherapy specimen appears to be the most significant predictor of survival.[24] The presence of residual disease after chemotherapy portends a poor prognosis and the need for additional chemotherapy. When tumor necrosis or a benign teratoma is found during surgical exploration after chemotherapy, an excellent or intermediate prognosis is conferred, respectively. Overall, 45% of patients with mediastinal nonseminomas are alive after 5 years.

Although salvage therapies have achieved cures in 20% to 50% of patients with relapsing or refractory testicular nonseminomatous tumors, salvage treatment protocols have been disappointing in those with mediastinal nonseminomatous tumors.[25] Residual tumor masses after salvage therapy are treated with secondary resection.

Lymphomas

Although the mediastinum is frequently involved in patients with lymphoma at some time during the course of their disease (40%-70%), it is infrequently the sole site of disease at the time of presentation. Hodgkin's and non-Hodgkin's lymphoma are distinct clinical entities with overlapping features. Although Hodgkin's represents only 25% to 30% of all lymphomas, 50% to 70% of patients with peripheral involvement and mediastinal disease have Hodgkin's, whereas 15% to 25% have non-Hodgkin's. Only 5% to 10% of patients with Hodgkin's and non-Hodgkin's lymphoma present solely with symptoms related to local mass effects, such as mediastinal involvement. Patients usually have symptoms; chest pain, cough, dyspnea, hoarseness, and superior vena caval syndrome are the most common clinical manifestations. Nonspecific systemic symptoms of fever and chills, weight loss, and anorexia are frequently noted and are important in the staging of patients with Hodgkin's lymphoma. Symptoms characteristic of Hodgkin's lymphoma include chest pain after consumption of alcohol and the cyclic fevers that were first described by Pel and Ebstein.

Characteristically, these tumors occur in the anterosuperior mediastinum or in the hilar region of the middle mediastinum. CT and MRI are useful in delineating the extent of disease, determining invasiveness into contiguous structures, differentiating the lesions from cardiovascular abnormalities, aiding the selection of radiation portals, following the response to therapy, and diagnosing relapse. Also, differentiation from thymomas and germ cell tumors, which usually are solitary masses, may be possible because lymphomas are usually composed

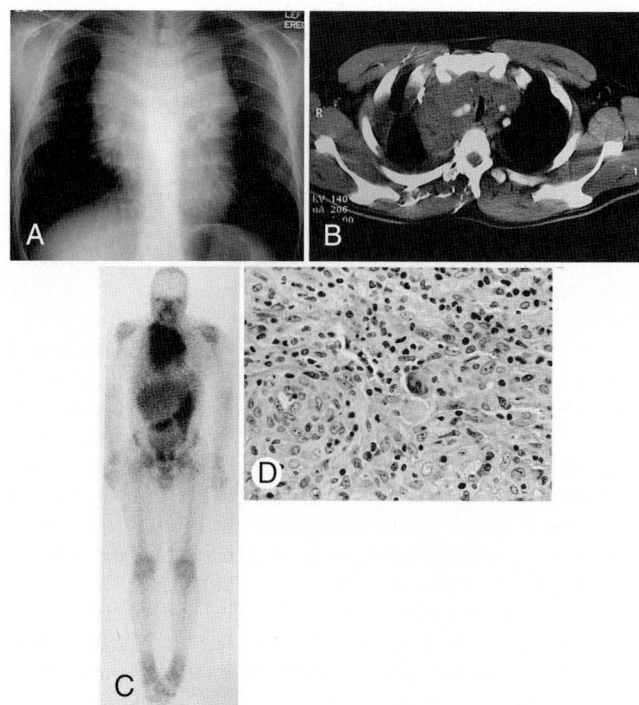

Figure 58-7 A, Chest radiograph of patient with Hodgkin's lymphoma. **B,** CT scan shows tracheal compression. **C,** Gallium scan of Hodgkin's lymphoma after 72 hours of uptake. **D,** Histopathologic examination of Hodgkin's lymphoma shows characteristic Reed-Sternberg cell (H&E, ×520).

of multiple nodules that appear as separate masses on CT.

Hodgkin's Lymphoma

Hodgkin's lymphoma is categorized histologically by the World Health Organization (WHO) classification, based on immunologic and molecular data first described in the Revised European-American Lymphoma classification (REAL concepts),[26] which divides these hematologic malignancies into two main groups: nodular lymphocyte predominant and classic Hodgkin's disease.[27]

Classic Hodgkin's disease is composed of nodular sclerosing, mixed cellularity, lymphocyte-rich classic disease, and lymphocyte-depleted types. The nodular sclerosing type is the most common type of Hodgkin's lymphoma (Fig. 58-7) seen in the mediastinum, occurring 55% to 75% of the time, followed by the lymphocyte-predominant type (40%). Nodular sclerosing lymphoma has a predilection for the thymus, whereas other variants tend to affect mediastinal lymph nodes and are not seen as commonly as an isolated mediastinal mass. The neoplastic cells in Hodgkin's disease are Reed-Sternberg cells or Reed-Sternberg variants, which are derived from germinal center B cells.

Treatment of Hodgkin's lymphoma is determined by the stage of disease and the prognostic factors related to the patient and the tumor. The Cotswold classification,[28] a modification of the Ann Arbor classification, is used for staging. Treatment is based on radiation therapy and chemotherapy. Surgical excision of all disease is rarely possible, and the surgeon's primary role is to provide sufficient tissue for diagnosis and to assist in pathologic staging. A needle biopsy is often unsuccessful because larger tissue samples are needed to make a histologic diagnosis, particularly with nodular sclerosing lesions. Thoracoscopy, mediastinoscopy, or mediastinotomy and, rarely, thoracotomy or median sternotomy may be necessary to obtain sufficient tissue. The role of staging laparotomy has been minimized, and its only current indication is for patients with clinically limited disease who opt for limited treatment.

Early- and intermediate-stage Hodgkin's disease is generally treated with combined chemotherapy and involved-field irradiation. Care needs to be taken that the heart does not receive more than 30 Gy of radiation. Early-stage disease with favorable prognostic factors was traditionally treated with radiation alone, but this treatment is currently not recommended because of high relapse rates. Patients with more advanced disease at presentation or with adverse prognostic factors are treated with extensive chemotherapy alone or with multimodality therapy. When bulky mediastinal disease is present, involved field or regional field irradiation is added.

Chemotherapeutic regimens used in Hodgkin's disease consist of various combinations, including MOPP (nitrogen mustard, vincristine [Oncovin], procarbazine, prednisone), ABVD (doxorubicin [Adriamycin], bleomycin, vinblastine, dacarbazine), MOPP plus ABVD, and other various combination regimens selected on an individual basis with attention to the toxicity of each regimen. Furthermore, dose-intensified chemotherapy has been introduced to treat advanced Hodgkin's disease. If cure is not achieved with conventional-dose chemotherapy, patients with Hodgkin's disease are considered candidates for high-dose chemotherapy with hematopoietic support.

Today most patients with Hodgkin's disease, whether localized or advanced, can be cured. Looking at all stages of Hodgkin's lymphoma with appropriate treatment, 5-year survival rates of about 90% can be achieved. Unfortunately, as the cure rate has improved over the past several decades, the long-term complications of treatment (secondary malignancies, coronary artery disease, and late pulmonary toxicity) have become more apparent. It has become increasingly possible to tailor specific treatments to individual risks of the patient, with patients with more favorable disease receiving less intensive and toxic therapy and more aggressive treatment protocols reserved for those with unfavorable disease.

Non-Hodgkin's Lymphoma

Non-Hodgkin's lymphoma, like Hodgkin's disease, is classified now by the WHO classification of lymphoid malignancies adopting the REAL concepts to define clinically relevant entities.[27] Mediastinal non-Hodgkin's lymphoma is usually of either lymphoblastic (60%) or large cell morphology (40%). Patients with non-Hodgkin's lymphoma usually have symptoms because of involvement of adjacent mediastinal structures. Superior vena caval syndrome is relatively common. Lymphoblastic lymphoma occurs predominantly in children, adolescents,

and young adults and represents 60% of cases of mediastinal non-Hodgkin's lymphoma. These tumors usually arise from the thymus, and patients often present with respiratory difficulties from a rapidly enlarging anterior mediastinal mass. This disease is two to four times more common in men and has an aggressive course with rapid dissemination to the central nervous system; bone marrow, which often progresses to a leukemic phase; gonads; and other visceral sites. Consensus now exists that lymphoblastic lymphoma and acute lymphoblastic leukemia represent different clinical presentations of the same biologic disease.[27] Differentiation of lymphoblastic lymphoma from acute lymphoblastic leukemia is arbitrary, determined by more than 25% bone marrow infiltration; higher degrees of bone marrow involvement are classified as acute lymphoblastic leukemia. Because lymphoblastic lymphoma infiltrates the thymus and is diffuse in appearance, it can be confused with a lymphocyte-predominant thymoma if not carefully studied.

Twenty percent of lymphoblastic lymphomas are from B-cell precursors; the remainder are from T-cell precursors and phenotypically express various stages of T-cell differentiation. High levels of terminal deoxynucleotidyl transferase activity are often present in lymphoblastic lymphoma. Histologically, these tumors are divided into convoluted, nonconvoluted, and large cell subtypes according to the appearance of the neoplastic cell nucleus. The convoluted type is present in 80% of cases, and the convoluted and nonconvoluted types preferentially involve the mediastinum.

Large cell non-Hodgkin's lymphomas of the mediastinum are a diverse group of lymphomas arising from both B-cell and T-cell lineage. These tumors are subdivided into primary mediastinal (thymic) large B-cell lymphoma and anaplastic large cell lymphoma of T-cell and null cell types. Additional variants of mediastinal large cell lymphomas have been identified: large cell lymphoma with marked tropism for germ centers and low-grade mucosa-associated lymphoma of the thymus.

Primary mediastinal B-cell lymphoma is by far the most common of the large cell lymphomas seen in the mediastinum. Studies have reported a slight female predominance and a young adult age at onset. Primary mediastinal B-cell lymphomas present with a rapidly growing mass located in the anterior mediastinum. These lymphomas likely originate from a native population of B cells located in the thymus. At diagnosis, these tumors are often limited to intrathoracic organs, but recurrence at extrathoracic sites, including the liver, kidneys, and central nervous system, is common.[29] Histologically, mediastinal large B-cell lymphoma tumors are often composed of large clear cells, which may appear compartmentalized by associated connective tissue (sclerosis). Because of this compartmentalization pattern, large cell lymphomas can be mistaken for seminomas, thymic undifferentiated carcinomas, or Hodgkin's lymphoma based on light microscopic appearance. Primary mediastinal B-cell lymphoma stains positive for CD20 and negative for CD3.[29]

The anaplastic large cell lymphoma of T-cell and null cell types was initially recognized by its expression of

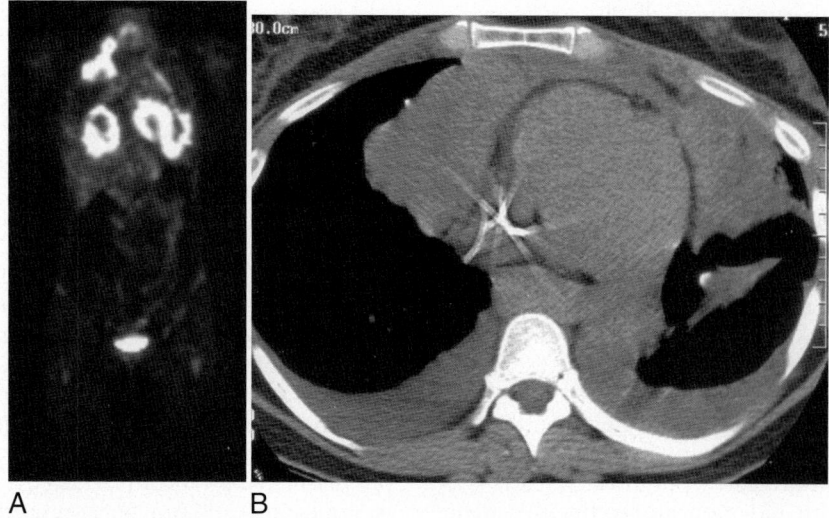

Figure 58-8 A, FDG positron emission tomography scan showing relapse of Hodgkin's disease evidenced by increased uptake in the mediastinum, along left chest wall, and in right neck. **B,** Chest CT scan of same patient as in **A.**

antigen for the Ki-1 (CD30) antibody. These tumors have only rarely been located primarily in the mediastinum; however, up to 75% of patients with these tumors have bulky mediastinal involvement in addition to their extrathoracic disease. Histologically, these tumors are composed of large cells and show marked nuclear pleomorphism.

Treatment of non-Hodgkin's lymphoma consists of aggressive anthracycline-containing chemotherapeutic regimens. After intensive chemotherapy, consolidation-involved field radiotherapy may be given.[30] In lymphoblastic lymphoma, central nervous system prophylaxis is given in conjunction with the standard chemotherapeutic regimen and consists of intrathecal chemotherapy, with or without cranial irradiation. Prophylactic treatment of the central nervous system is not needed in large cell lymphoma because of its infrequent involvement. Recently, the chimeric anti-CD20 monoclonal antibody rituximab, combined with standard chemotherapy, has shown promise in the initial treatment of diffuse large B-cell lymphoma. Poor response to initial doxorubicin-containing chemotherapy was a predictor of nonresponsiveness to subsequent chemotherapies. Bulky mediastinal disease at presentation and residual abnormality after initial chemotherapy were risk factors for relapse.[30] Patients in first response with poor prognostic factors, with refractory disease, or with recurrent lymphoma can be treated with high-dose chemotherapy and with either autologous bone marrow or peripheral stem cell transplantation. Anti-CD20 antibody may have a role in salvage therapy of patients with primary mediastinal B-cell lymphoma. With an aggressive approach, cure rates of 50% and greater have been achieved in patients with non-Hodgkin's lymphomas.

Residual Masses After Lymphoma Treatment

After treatment of lymphomas, residual abnormalities within the mediastinum are commonly noted radiograph-ically (64%-88%). Residual radiographic abnormalities are seen more commonly in patients with initial bulky mediastinal disease. Residual mediastinal abnormalities were not significantly associated with eventual disease relapse, except when treatment was with chemotherapy alone. CT cannot differentiate fibrosis or necrosis from residual tumor.

[67]Ga scintigraphy is a metabolic imaging technique and has proved valuable in the determination of neoplastic disease in residual mediastinal abnormalities after therapy. A negative ^{67}Ga scintigraphic scan has been predictive of absence of residual disease. In order to be useful after therapy, avidity of the lymphoma for ^{67}Ga needs to be confirmed before treatment.

The use of metabolic imaging with FDG-PET has shown promise as a noninvasive way to detect active mediastinal disease and predict relapse in patients with lymphoma (Fig. 58-8). Jerusalem and colleagues have shown that the use of FDG-PET can detect preclinical relapse of Hodgkin's disease, which may allow earlier treatment of patients with salvage chemotherapy when minimal disease is present.[31] More studies are required to determine whether earlier detection of relapse by FDG-PET will alter treatment management, be cost-effective, and improve survival. As in ^{67}Ga scintigraphy, rebound thymus hyperplasia can result in false-positive FDG-PET results.

Primary Carcinoma

Primary carcinomas of the mediastinum constitute between 3% and 11% of primary mediastinal masses in most series. The origin of these tumors is unknown. It is important to differentiate them from malignant thymomas, germ cell tumors, carcinoid tumors, lymphomas, mediastinal extension of bronchogenic carcinomas, and metastatic tumors, which may have a similar appearance by light microscopy. Metastatic disease in mediastinal lymph nodes is usually from bronchogenic or esophageal malignancies and rarely occurs with extrathoracic malignancies. The tumors most likely to metastasize to the mediastinum include those originating in the breast, head, neck, and genitourinary tract as well as melanomas. Primary carcinomas are usually of the large cell, undifferentiated morphology, although small cell and squamous cell tumors have been described. The use of electron microscopic examination of the tumor ultrastructure and immunostaining for surface antigens and cellular proteins better define the origin of some of these primary carcinomas and decrease the reported incidence.

These tumors occur with equal frequency in either sex. Most patients have symptoms from the local mass effects of the tumor. Extensive involvement within the thorax and often metastatic disease outside the thorax characterize this disease. Surgical excision is rarely possible. Unfortunately, the routine use of radiation therapy and chemotherapy has been unsuccessful in prolonging survival. Overall, the mean survival time is less than 1 year.

Endocrine Tumors

Thyroid Tumors

Although substernal extension of a cervical goiter is common, totally intrathoracic thyroid tumors are rare and make up only 1% of all mediastinal masses in the collected series. These tumors arise from heterotopic thyroid tissue, which occurs most commonly in the anterosuperior mediastinum but may also occur in the middle mediastinum between the trachea and esophagus as well as in the posterior mediastinum. Although there may be a demonstrable connection with the cervical gland (usually a fibrous connective tissue band), a true intrathoracic thyroid gland derives its blood supply from thoracic vessels.

The peak incidence is in the sixth and seventh decades. Women are more commonly affected. When these lesions occur in the anterosuperior or middle mediastinum, symptoms related to tracheal compression are often present, such as dyspnea, cough, wheezing, and stridor. When these tumors occur in the posterior mediastinum, esophageal compression manifested by dysphagia is common. Rarely, symptoms related to thyrotoxicosis may be the initiating factor for a patient to seek medical attention. On chest radiography, these lesions appear as sharply circumscribed, dense masses, occurring more frequently on the right. The administration of iodinated contrast material causes prolonged enhancement of thyroid tissue, and intrathoracic goiters are contrast medium–enhancing lesions when visualized by CT. When functioning thyroid tissue is present, the ^{131}I scan is usually diagnostic. Some of these neoplasms, however, are functionally inactive and are not identified by ^{131}I scanning.

Most of these tumors are adenomas, but carcinomas have been reported. If the lesion is identified as the sole functioning thyroid tissue and the patient does not have symptoms, surgical exploration and excision are not indicated. In these patients, frequent follow-up radiographic examinations are indicated to evaluate changes in the size and nature of the lesion. Otherwise, these lesions need to be resected because of their propensity to enlarge and compress adjacent structures. Because of the thoracic derivation of the blood supply, intrathoracic thyroid tumors are approached through the thorax, using either an anterolateral thoracotomy or a median sternotomy for anterior lesions or a posterolateral thoracotomy for posterior lesions. Substernal extensions of a cervical goiter can usually be excised using a cervical approach.

Parathyroid Tumors

Although parathyroid glands may occur in the mediastinum in 10% of patients, they are usually accessible through the cervical incision. Most often, these adenomas are found in the anterosuperior mediastinum (80%) embedded in or near the superior pole of the thymus. This anatomic relationship is the result of the common embryogenesis of the inferior parathyroid glands from the third branchial cleft. The superior parathyroid glands and the lateral lobes of the thyroid gland are derived from the fourth branchial pouch. Because they migrate with the lateral lobes of the thyroid gland to a paraesophageal position, parathyroid adenomas can also be found in the posterior mediastinum.

The clinical manifestations of a mediastinal parathyroid tumor are similar to those that occur with tumors of the cervical region; symptoms are related to the excess secretion of parathyroid hormone causing the hyperparathyroid syndrome. Preoperative attempts at anatomic localization are indicated. In patients whose preoperative studies have failed to locate the site of the responsible parathyroid gland, exploration of the mediastinum is often unsuccessful. Because of their small size, these neoplasms rarely cause symptoms related to mechanical effects and are not often visualized using conventional radiography. Using CT, MRI, thallium and technetium scanning, technetium-sestamibi scintigraphy, selective arteriography, and more recently FDG-PET, preoperative localization of these tumors can be made in greater than 80% of patients.[32] Venous angiography with selective sampling is useful for determining the size of the adenoma but is usually inadequate for defining the anatomic location.

Most frequently, the mediastinal adenoma may be excised after a negative exploration of the cervical region, through the existing cervical incision. Usually, the vascular supply to the adenoma extends from cervical blood vessels. In patients with persistent hyperparathyroidism, after cervical exploration if localization studies show residual parathyroid in the mediastinum, mediastinal exploration using a median sternotomy or thoracoscopy is indicated.

Parathyroid carcinomas have been reported and are usually hormonally active. Patients differ in clinical presentation in that they often have higher serum calcium levels and manifest more severe symptoms of hyperparathyroidism. When possible, surgical resection is the optimal therapy.

Unlike parathyroid adenomas and carcinomas, parathyroid cysts are usually not hormonally active. These cysts are defined by the presence of parathyroid cells identifiable within the cyst wall. Because these lesions are frequently larger than adenomas, symptoms related to local mass effects are more common, as is visualization on chest film. Surgical excision yields a cure.

Neuroendocrine Tumors

Mediastinal neuroendocrine tumors, previously known as carcinoid tumors, arise from cells of Kulchitsky located in the thymus. These tumors show a predilection for males in their 40s and 50s, are usually located in the anterosuperior mediastinum, and behave aggressively. Metastatic spread to mediastinal and cervical lymph nodes, liver, bone, skin, and lungs is present in at least 20% at presentation.[33] Fifty percent of thymic neuroendocrine tumors are hormonally active, often associated with Cushing's syndrome because of production of adrenocorticotropic hormone, less frequently associated with multiple endocrine neoplasia syndromes, and only rarely associated with carcinoid syndrome (0.6%).

In patients with hormonally inactive tumors, symptoms are related to local mass effects, leading to chest pain, dyspnea, cough, and the superior vena caval syndrome. Hormonally inactive neuroendocrine tumors tend to be larger and are frequently invasive locally.

The best chance for cure is surgical excision, but local invasion or metastatic spread often precludes complete excision. Adjuvant therapy is controversial, but irradiation should probably be added, particularly in patients with capsular invasion. Therapies that exploit the somatostatin receptors present on these tumors, such as radiolabeled octreotide, may hold promise.[33] Survival is significantly worse than with neuroendocrine tumors occurring elsewhere in the chest, and patients with tumors associated with an endocrinopathy have a particularly poor prognosis. Late recurrences are possible.

Mesenchymal Tumors

Mediastinal mesenchymal tumors originate from the connective tissue, striated and smooth muscle, fat, lymphatic tissue, and blood vessels present within the mediastinum, giving rise to a diverse group of neoplasms. Relative to other sites in the body, these tumors occur less commonly within the mediastinum. Mesenchymal tumors have been reported to occur in less than 10% of the primary masses in the various series. There is no apparent difference in incidence between genders. The soft tissue neoplasms include lipomas, liposarcomas, fibrosarcomas, fibromas, xanthogranulomas, leiomyomas, leiomyosarcomas, benign and malignant mesenchymomas, rhabdomyosarcomas, and mesotheliomas. These tumors have a similar histologic appearance and generally follow the same clinical course as the soft tissue tumors found elsewhere in the body. Fifty-five percent of these tumors are malignant. Surgical resection remains the primary therapy because poor results have been obtained using radiation therapy and chemotherapy.

Extramedullary Hematopoiesis

Extramedullary hematopoiesis occurs in all age groups, usually as a result of altered hematopoiesis. In the adult, this is typically a result of massive hemolysis, myelofibrosis, spherocytic anemia, or thalassemia. These lesions appear as bilateral, asymmetric paravertebral masses and enhance with contrast medium. Radionuclide imaging using technetium-99m (^{99m}Tc) sulfur colloid is a noninvasive method of diagnosing intrathoracic extramedullary hematopoiesis. Surgical resection is unnecessary unless there is invasion or compression of mediastinal structures. Radiation therapy can produce rapid shrinkage of these masses.

Giant Lymph Node Hyperplasia (Castleman's Disease)

Giant lymph node hyperplasia was initially described by Castleman.[34] Although the mediastinum was the site of disease in the initial report and in most patients, these tumors may develop wherever lymph nodes are present; the retroperitoneum and cervical, axillary, and pelvic regions are the most common nonmediastinal sites. Although these tumors are usually located in the anterosuperior mediastinum, they are also found in the posterior mediastinum and at the pericardiophrenic angle, where they may be confused with neurogenic tumors and pericardial cysts, respectively. Two distinct histologic entities exist: (1) hyaline vascular, characterized by small hyaline follicles and interfollicular capillary proliferation, and (2) plasma cell, characterized by large follicles with intervening sheets of plasma cells. Increasingly, it appears that there are different causes for the distinct histologic variants. The tumors most frequently appear as single, well-demarcated lesions. The hyaline vascular type represents 90% of Castleman's tumors, and these are most often discovered in patients without symptoms on a routine chest radiograph. Patients with the plasma cell type often exhibit systemic features, including fever, night sweats, anemia, and hypergammaglobulinemia. Surgical excision effects cure, although resection of the hyaline vascular type may be associated with significant hemorrhage because of extreme vascularity.

Castleman's disease may also be multicentric, characterized by generalized lymphadenopathy with morphologic features of giant lymph node hyperplasia. Patients most often have symptoms, including fever, chills, weight loss, and hepatosplenomegaly, and exhibit disordered immunity and autoimmune phenomena. Multicentric Castleman's disease has been associated with HIV infection and human herpesvirus 8. Unlike the benign clinical course of classic Castleman's disease, multicentric disease is a much more malignant disease, with death often occurring after infectious complications.

Chordoma

Chordomas are rare malignant tumors that may occur in the posterior mediastinum and originate from the primitive notochord. Men are affected twice as often as women, with the peak age of incidence in the fifth through seventh decades. Chest pain, cough, and dyspnea are the most common features. Spinal cord compression may follow extension into the spinal canal. Radical surgical excision is the only effective therapy. Despite resection, chordomas tend to recur at the surgical site, and most patients die of their disease.

PRIMARY CYSTS

Primary cysts of the mediastinum make up 18% of the mediastinal masses in the collected series. These cysts can be bronchogenic, pericardial, enteric, or thymic or may be of an unspecified nature. More than 75% of cases are asymptomatic, and these tumors rarely cause morbidity. Because of the proximity of vital structures within the mediastinum, however, with increasing size, even benign cysts may cause significant morbidity. In addition, these masses need to be differentiated from malignant tumors. Benign mediastinal cysts can be removed thoracoscopically.

Bronchogenic cysts are the most common primary cysts of the mediastinum, representing 50% to 60% of these cysts. They originate as sequestrations from the ventral foregut, the antecedent of the tracheobronchial tree. The bronchogenic cyst may lie within the lung parenchyma or the mediastinum. The cyst wall is composed of cartilage, mucous glands, smooth muscle, and fibrous tissue with a pathognomonic inner layer of ciliated respiratory epithelium. When bronchogenic cysts occur in the mediastinum, they are usually located proximal to the trachea or bronchi and may be just posterior to the carina. Rarely, a true communication between the cyst and the tracheobronchial tree exists, and an air-fluid level may be observed on chest radiograph.

Two thirds of bronchogenic cysts are asymptomatic. In infants, these cysts may cause severe respiratory compromise by compressing the trachea or the bronchus; compression of the bronchus may cause bronchial stenosis and recurrent pneumonitis. In children with recurrent pulmonary infections, CT may be useful in assessing the subcarinal space for possible bronchogenic cyst, an area that is poorly visualized using standard radiography. More often, bronchogenic cysts occur in older children and adults, in whom these cysts may cause symptoms of chest pain, dyspnea, cough, and stridor. Bronchogenic cysts appear as a smooth density at the level of the carina that may compress the esophagus on barium swallow. Differentiation from hilar structures may be difficult.

Surgical excision is recommended in all patients to provide definitive histologic diagnosis, alleviate symptoms, and prevent the development of associated complications. Malignant degeneration has been reported, as has the presence of a bronchial adenoma within the cysts.

Pericardial cysts are the second most frequently encountered cysts within the mediastinum. These cysts classically occur in the pericardiophrenic angles (Fig. 58-9), with 70% in the right pericardiophrenic angle, 22% in the left, and the remainder in other sites in the pericardium. Pericardial cysts may or may not have a communication with the pericardium. Numerous reports have

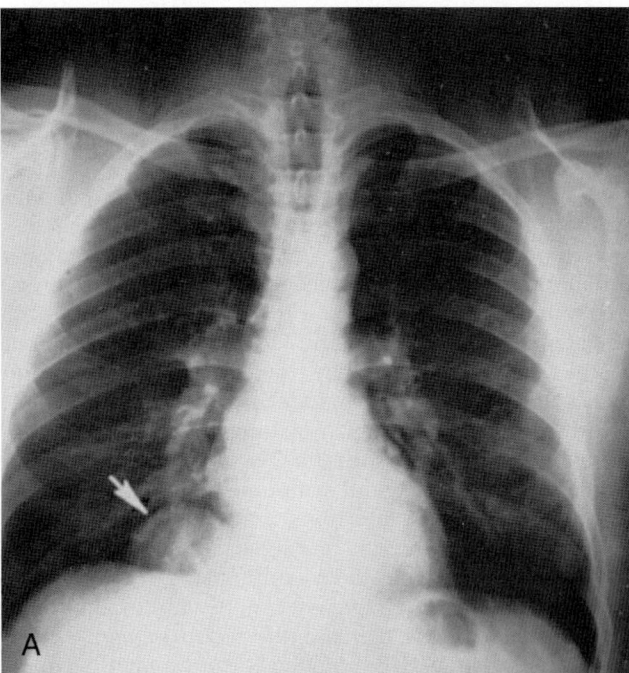

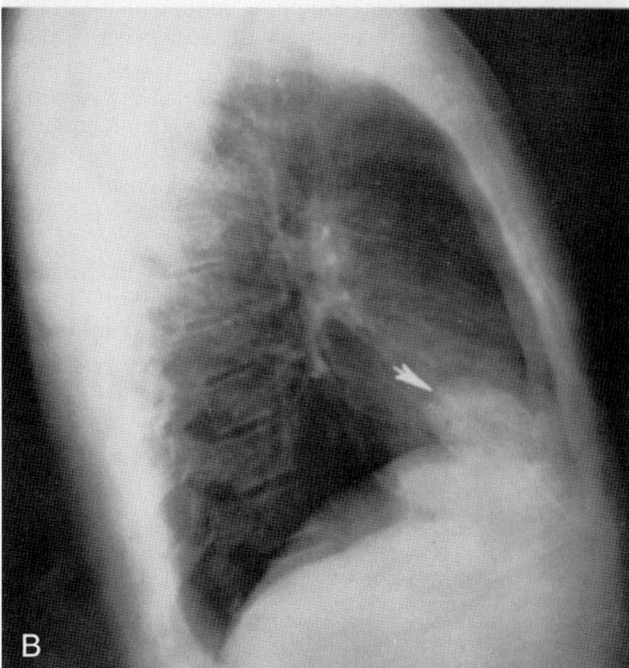

Figure 58-9 **A** and **B,** Chest radiographs show the typical location of a pericardial cyst in the right cardiophrenic angle. (From Sabiston DC Jr, Oldham HN Jr: The mediastinum. In Sabiston DC Jr, Spencer FC [eds]: Gibbon's Surgery of the Chest, 4th ed. Philadelphia, WB Saunders, 1983.)

described the characteristic CT appearance of pericardial cysts: pericardiophrenic location, near-water attenuation value, and smooth borders. Lesions demonstrating classic CT characteristics of pericardial cysts have been managed with needle aspiration and follow-up with serial CT rather than surgical excision. Surgical excision of pericardial cysts is indicated primarily for diagnosis and to differentiate these cysts from malignant lesions.

Enteric cysts (duplication cysts) arise from the posterior division of the primitive foregut, which develops into the upper division of the gastrointestinal tract. These cysts are found less frequently than bronchogenic or pericardial cysts and are most frequently located in the posterior mediastinum, usually adjacent to the esophagus. These lesions are composed of smooth muscle with an inner epithelial lining of esophageal, gastric, or intestinal mucosa. When gastric mucosa is present, peptic ulceration with perforation into the esophageal or bronchial lumina may occur, producing hemoptysis or hematemesis. Usually, enteric cysts have an attachment to the esophagus and may be embedded within the muscularis layer. Symptoms are usually related to compression of the esophagus, leading to obstruction that commonly presents as dysphagia. Compromise of the tracheobronchial tree with symptoms of cough, dyspnea, recurrent pulmonary infections, and chest pain also may result. Most enteric cysts are diagnosed in children, who are also more likely to have symptoms.

When enteric cysts are associated with anomalies of the vertebral column, they are referred to as *neuroenteric cysts*. Such cysts may be connected to the meninges, or, less frequently, a direct communication with the dural space may exist. In patients with neuroenteric cysts, preoperative evaluation for potential spinal cord involvement is mandatory. The vertebral anomalies associated with this syndrome include spina bifida, hemivertebrae, and a widened neural canal. Treatment is surgical excision, providing a definite histologic diagnosis as well as alleviating symptoms and preventing potential complications.

Nonspecific cysts include those lesions in which a specific epithelial or mesothelial lining cannot be identified. These lesions may originate in any of the aforementioned cysts by the destruction of the inner epithelial lining from an inflammatory or digestive process. Other causes include postinflammatory cysts and hemorrhagic cysts.

Selected References

Blalock A, Mason MF, Morgan HJ, et al: Myasthenia gravis and tumors of the thymic region. Ann Surg 110:544-561, 1939.

This landmark paper substantiates the use of thymectomy in the treatment of myasthenia gravis. In this paper, Blalock reports the successful removal of a 6 × 5 × 3-cm thymic tumor from a 19-year-old woman. Follow-up of this patient over a 3-year period demonstrated significant improvement in her symptoms of myasthenia.

Bokemeyer C, Nichols CR, Droz J-P, et al: Extragonadal germ cell tumors of the mediastinum and retroperitoneum: Results from an international analysis. J Clin Oncol 20:1864-1873, 2002.

This article characterizes the clinical and biologic features of extragonadal germ cell tumors. Based on currently available treatment strategies, it shows that, independent of primary tumor site, patients with pure seminomatous histology have an almost 90% long-term chance of cure. Unfortunately, only 45% of patients with mediastinal nonseminomas are alive at 5 years. Patients with nonseminomatous mediastinal primary tumors have a significantly inferior outcome compared with patients with nonseminomatous retroperitoneal primary tumors.

Davis RD, Oldham HN, Sabiston DC: Primary cysts and neoplasms of the mediastinum: Recent changes in clinical presentation, methods of diagnosis, management, and results. Ann Thorac Surg 44:229-237, 1987.

This study of 400 patients with mediastinal tumors is one of the largest in the literature. It emphasizes the major changes that have occurred in clinical presentation, diagnosis, and management of primary lesions of the mediastinum.

Masaoka A, Monden Y, Nakahara K, et al: Follow-up study of thymomas with special reference to their clinical stages. Cancer 48:2485-2492, 1981.

This article proposes the clinical staging system for thymomas that is most widely used today. This staging system allows for comparison between studies.

Shimosato Y, Mukai K: Atlas of Tumor Pathology, 3rd series, fascicle 21. Washington, DC, Armed Forces Institute of Pathology, 1997.

This comprehensive fascicle provides one of the best overall reviews available on tumors of the mediastinum, with special emphasis on thymic tumors.

Weihrauch MR, Re D, Scheidhauer K, et al: Thoracic positron emission tomography using ^{18}F-fluorodeoxyglucose for the evaluation of residual mediastinal Hodgkin disease. Blood 98:2930-2934, 2001.

This article shows the value of using FDG-PET to evaluate residual mediastinal masses after treatment of Hodgkin's disease. Hodgkin's disease patients with residual mediastinal masses with negative post-treatment FDG-PET are unlikely to relapse before 1 year. Positive post-treatment FDG-PET scans in patients with residual masses indicate a significantly higher risk for relapse and warrant further diagnostic procedures and closer follow-up.

References

1. Davis RD, Oldham HN, Sabiston DC: Primary cysts and neoplasms of the mediastinum: Recent changes in clinical presentation, methods of diagnosis, management, and results. Ann Thorac Surg 44:229-237, 1987.
2. Shields TW: Overview of primary mediastinal tumors and cysts. In Shields TW, LoCicero J, Ponn RB, Rusch VW (eds): General Thoracic Surgery, 6th ed. Philadelphia, Lippincott Williams & Wilkins, 2005, p 2491.
3. Nakata H, Egashira K, Watanabe H, et al: MRI of bronchogenic cysts. J Comput Assist Tomogr 17:267-270, 1993.
4. Kubota K, Yamada S, Kondo T, et al: PET imaging of primary mediastinal tumours. Br J Cancer 73:882-886, 1996.
5. Kostakoglu L, Leonard JP, Kuji I, et al: Comparison of fluorine-18 fluorodeoxyglucose positron emission tomography and Ga-67 scintigraphy in evaluation of lymphoma. Cancer 94:879-888, 2002.
6. Khoo K, Ho K, Nilsson B, et al: EUS-guided FNA immediately after unrevealing transbronchial needle aspiration in the evaluation of mediastinal lymphadenopathy: A prospective study. Gastrointest Endosc 63:215-220, 2006.
7. Panelli F, Erickson RA, Prasad VM: Evaluation of mediastinal masses by endoscopic ultrasound and endoscopic ultrasound-guided fine needle aspiration. Am J Gastroenterol 96:401-408, 2001.
8. Brodeur GM, Pritchard J, Berthold F, et al: Revisions of the international criteria for neuroblastoma diagnosis, staging, and response to treatment [comment]. J Clin Oncol 11:1466-1477, 1993.

9. Matthay KK: Intensification of therapy using hematopoietic stem-cell support for high-risk neuroblastoma. Pediatr Transplant 3:72-77, 1999.

10. Yanik GA, Levine JE, Matthay KK, et al: Pilot study of iodine-131-metaiodobenzylguanidine in combination with myeloablative chemotherapy and autologous stem-cell support for the treatment of neuroblastoma. J Clin Oncol 20:2142-2149, 2002.

11. Marino M, Müller-Hermelink HK: Thymoma and thymic carcinoma: Relation of thymoma epithelial cells to the cortical and medullary differentiation of thymus. Virchows Arch 407:119-149, 1985.

12. Morgenthaler TI, Brown LR, Colby TV, et al: Thymoma. Mayo Clin Proc 68:110-1123, 1993.

13. Blalock A, Mason MF, Morgan HJ, et al: Myasthenia gravis and tumors of the thymic region. Ann Surg 110:544-561, 1939.

14. Calhoun RF, Ritter JH, Guthrie TJ, et al: Results of transcervical thymectomy for myasthenia gravis in 100 consecutive patients. Ann Surg 230:555-559; discussion 559-561, 1999.

15. Wilkins EW, Grillo HC, Scannell G, et al: Role of staging in prognosis and management of thymoma. Ann Thorac Surg 51:888-892, 1991.

16. Loehrer PJ, Kim K, Chen M, et al: Phase II trial of cisplatin (P), Adriamycin (A), cyclophosphamide (C) plus radiotherapy in limited stage unresectable thymoma. Proc Am Soc Clin Oncol 14:433, 1995.

17. Yagi K, Hirata T, Fukuse T, et al: Surgical treatment for invasive thymoma, especially when the superior vena cava is invaded. Ann Thorac Surg 61:521-524, 1996.

18. Masaoka A, Monden Y, Nakahara K, et al: Follow-up study of thymomas with special reference to their clinical stages. Cancer 48:2485-2492, 1981.

19. Fizazi K, Culine S, Droz JP, et al: Initial management of primary mediastinal seminoma: Radiotherapy or cisplatin-based chemotherapy? Eur J Cancer 34:347-352, 1998.

20. Ganjoo KN, Chan RJ, Sharma M, et al: Positron emission tomography scans in the evaluation of postchemotherapy residual masses in patients with seminoma. J Clin Oncol 17:3457-3460, 1999.

21. Bokemeyer C, Droz JP, Horwich A, et al: Extragonadal seminoma: An international multicenter analysis of prognostic factors and long term treatment outcome. Cancer 91:1394-1401, 2001.

22. Nichols CR, Heerema NA, Palmer C, et al: Klinefelter's syndrome associated with mediastinal germ cell neoplasms. J Clin Oncol 5:1290-1294, 1987.

23. Ganjoo KN, Rieger KM, Kesler KA, et al: Results of modern therapy for patients with mediastinal nonseminomatous germ cell tumors. Cancer 88:1051-1056, 2000.

24. Kesler KA, Rieger KM, Ganjoo KN, et al: Primary mediastinal nonseminomatous germ cell tumors: The influence of postchemotherapy pathology on long-term survival after surgery. J Thorac Cardiovasc Surg 118:692-701, 1999.

25. Vuky J, Bains M, Bacik J, et al: Role of postchemotherapy adjunctive surgery in the management of patients with nonseminoma arising from the mediastinum. J Clin Oncol 19:682-688, 2001.

26. Harris NL, Jaffe ES, Stein H, et al: A revised European-American classification of lymphoid neoplasms: A proposal from The International Lymphoma Study Group. Blood 84:1361-1392, 1994.

27. Harris NL, Jaffe ES, Diebold J, et al: The World Health Organization classification of hematological malignancies report of the Clinical Advisory Committee Meeting, Airlie House, Virginia, November 1997. Mod Pathol 13:193-207, 2000.

28. Lister TA, Crowther D, Sutcliffe SB, et al: Report of a committee convened to discuss the evaluation and staging of patients with Hodgkin's disease: Cotswold Meeting. J Clin Oncol 7:1630, 1989.

29. van Besien K, Kelta M, Bahaguna P: Primary mediastinal B-cell lymphoma: A review of pathology and management. J Clin Oncol 19:1855-1864, 2001.

30. Lazzarino M, Orlandi E, Paulli M: Treatment outcome and prognostic factors for primary mediastinal (thymic) B-cell lymphoma: A multicenter study of 106 patients. J Clin Oncol 15:1646-1653, 1997.

31. Jerusalem G, Beguin Y, Fassotte MF, et al: Early detection of relapse by whole-body positron emission tomography in the follow-up of patients with Hodgkin's disease. Ann Oncol 14:123-130, 2003.

32. Hopkins CR, Reading CC: Thyroid and parathyroid imaging. Semin Ultrasound CT MR 16:279-295, 1995.

33. Chaer R, Massad MG, Evans A, et al: Primary neuroendocrine tumors of the thymus. Ann Thorac Surg 74:1733-1740, 2002.

34. Castleman B, Iverson L, Menendez VP: Localized mediastinal lymphoid hyperplasia resembling thymoma. Cancer 9:822-830, 1956.

35. Sabiston DC, Scott HW: Primary neoplasms and cysts of the mediastinum. Ann Surg 136:777-797, 1952.

36. Herlitzka AJ, Gale JW: Tumors and cysts of the mediastinum. Arch Surg 76:697-706, 1958.

37. Morrison IM: Tumors and cysts of the mediastinum. Thorax 13:294-307, 1958.

38. Le Roux BT: Cysts and tumors of the mediastinum. Surg Gynecol Obstet 115:695-703, 1962.

39. Heimburger IL, Battersby JS: Primary mediastinal tumors of childhood. J Thorac Cardiovasc Surg 50:92-103, 1965.

40. Boyd DP, Midell AI: Mediastinal cysts and tumors: An analysis of 96 cases. Surg Clin North Am 48:493-505, 1968.

41. Burkell CC, Cross JM, Kent HP, et al: Mass lesions of the mediastinum. Curr Prob Surg 2:57, 1969.

42. Wychulis AR, Payne WS, Clagett OT, et al: Surgical treatment of mediastinal tumors: A 40-year experience. J Thorac Cardiovasc Surg 62:379-392, 1971.

43. Fontenelle LJ, Armstrong RG, Stanford W, et al: The asymptomatic mediastinal mass. Arch Surg 102:98-102, 1971.

44. Benjamin SP, McCormack LJ, Effler DB, et al: Primary lymphatic tumors of the mediastinum. Cancer 30:708-712, 1972.

45. Rubush JL, Gardner IR, Boyd WC, et al: Mediastinal tumors: Review of 186 cases. J Thorac Cardiovasc Surg 65:216-222, 1973.

46. Ovrum E, Birkeland S: Mediastinal tumors and cysts: A review of 91 cases. Scand J Thorac Cardiovasc Surg 13:161-168, 1979.

47. Nandi P, Wong KC, Mok CK, et al: Primary mediastinal tumors: Review of 74 cases. J R Coll Surg Edinb 25:460-466, 1980.

48. Parish JM, Rosenow EC III, Muhm JR: Mediastinal masses: Clues to interpretation of radiologic studies. Postgrad Med 76:173-182, 1984.

49. Cohen AJ, Thompson L, Edwards FH, et al: Primary cysts and tumors of the mediastinum. Ann Thorac Surg 51:378-384, 1991.

Lung (Including Pulmonary Embolism and Thoracic Outlet Syndrome)

W. Roy Smythe, MD   Scott I. Reznik, MD   and   Joe B. Putnam, Jr., MD

ANATOMY

The development of the respiratory system begins at about 21 to 28 days' gestation as a ventral groove in the foregut. The bronchial tree is complete at about 16 weeks' gestation, and the lungs have subdivided into 15 to 26 divisions. The alveoli are lined by cuboidal cells to about the fourth month. These cells become flattened, and capillary buds develop at about 4 to 6 months. The true alveolar stage, with air sacs surrounded on all sides by capillaries, occurs from about 7 months' (26-28 weeks')

gestation to term. Alveolar proliferation continues to occur after birth. There are about 20 million alveoli at birth, which increase to about 300 million by age 10 years, with no more increase after that time. Eighty percent of the lung volume is air, 10% of the lung volume is blood, and about 10% of the lung volume is solid tissue.

The alveolar-capillary membrane typically consists of five layers: the alveolar epithelium, basement membrane, ground substance, basal membrane, and capillary endothelium. The pores of Kohn perforate and connect the alveoli, although it is unknown whether they can actually serve for collateral ventilation. Twenty-three generations of bronchi occur between the trachea and terminal alveoli. Alveoli make up about half of the entire lung volume. The ciliated tall columnar epithelium, as a single layer, lines the larger airways. These cells maintain a cuboidal shape in bronchioles and are flattened, thinned epithelial cells in alveoli. The interstitium is a narrow space between basement membrane of capillary endothelium and alveolar epithelium where gas exchange takes place in alveoli. The space is wider in submucosa, muscle, and cartilage in larger airways.

The alveoli are composed of type I and II cells in about equal number. However, type I cells constitute about 40% of the number of cells lining the alveoli but cover more than 90% of the alveolar lining and are for gas exchange. Type II alveolar cells are the granular pneumocytes, containing lipid inclusion bodies and manufacturing surfactant, a lipoprotein (dipalmitoyl-lecithin) that decreases surface tension. This substance maintains alveolar stability and fluid balance, preventing atelectasis and edema. Capillary endothelial cells have a nonspecific response to lung injury with edema, hyaline membrane formation, cellular infiltrates, and granuloma formation. Chronically, this process of lung injury is marked by diffuse fibrosis and honeycombing.

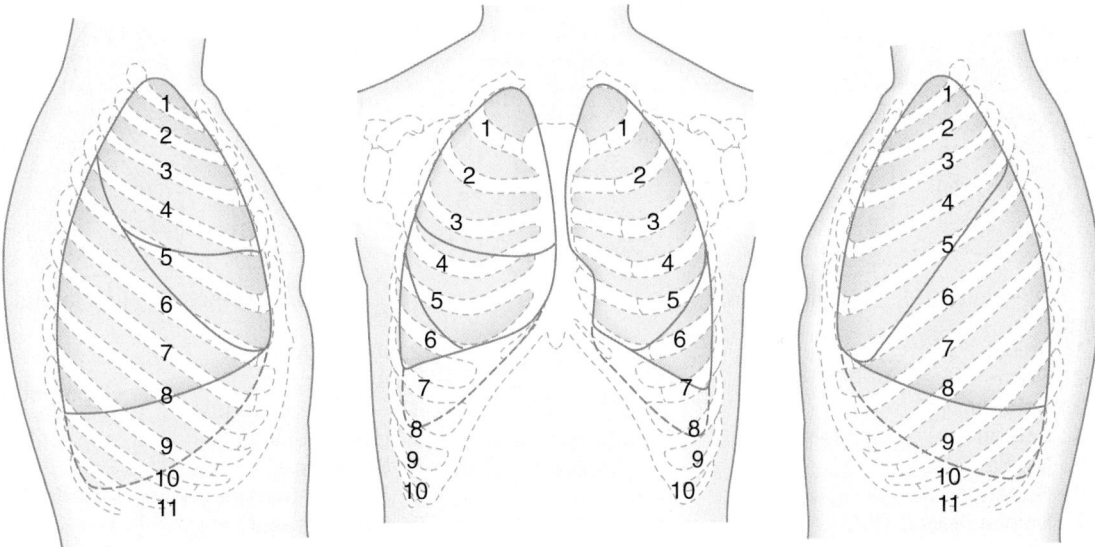

Figure 59-1 The relationships of the pleural reflections and the lobes of the lung to the ribs. The topographic anatomy and the relationship of the fissures of the lobes to ribs in inspiration and expiration are important in evaluation of the routine posteroanterior and lateral chest film.

The bony thorax consists of 12 ribs. The 11th and 12th ribs are so-called floating ribs and are not attached directly to the sternum. Ribs 1 to 5 are directly attached to the sternum by costal cartilages. The lower ribs (6-10) coalesce by way of the costal cartilages into the costal arch. The first rib is flat and travels from the first thoracic vertebra to the manubrium at the manubrium-clavicular junction. Through this relatively small area pass the great vessels, trachea, esophagus, and nerves. The remaining ribs gradually slope downward. The intercostal muscle layers assist with respiration and protect the thoracic structures. The extrinsic muscles of the chest, latissimus dorsi muscle, serratus anterior muscle, pectoralis major and minor muscles, and cervical muscles (sternocleidomastoid, scalene muscles) attach to the bony thorax, protect the chest wall itself, and may assist with ventilatory efforts in those with chronic obstructive pulmonary disease.

The right lung is composed of three lobes: the upper, middle, and lower. Two fissures separate these lobes. The major, or oblique, fissure separates the lower lobe from the upper and middle lobes. The minor or horizontal fissure separates the upper lobe from the middle lobe. The left lung has two lobes—the upper lobe and the lower lobe; the lingula is a portion of the left upper lobe and corresponds embryologically to the right middle lobe. A single oblique fissure separates the lobes (Fig. 59-1). The degree to which these fissures are anatomically complete, that is, completely separating adjacent lobes, is variable, but is of interest to the surgeon in regard to the approach that might be considered at the time of resection because an anatomically complete fissure facilitates easier hilar dissection.

The bronchopulmonary segments are divisions of each lobe that contain anatomically separate arterial, venous, and bronchial supply. There are 10 bronchopulmonary segments on the right and 8 bronchopulmonary segments on the left (Fig. 59-2).

The blood supply of the lung is twofold. Unoxygenated blood is pumped to the lung from the right ventricle by way of the pulmonary artery. After oxygenation in the lung, the blood is returned to the left atrium by way of the pulmonary veins. Blood supply to the bronchi is from the systemic circulation by bronchial arteries arising from the superior thoracic aorta or the aortic arch, either as discrete branches or in combination with the intercostal arteries. In most individuals, there are two left and one right main bronchial artery. In about one fourth of patients, the bronchial arteries arise as a common trunk.

Lymphatic vessels are present throughout the parenchyma and gradually coalesce toward the hilar areas of the lungs. Generally, lymphatic drainage from the lung affects the ipsilateral lymph nodes; however, flow of lymph from the left lower lobe may drain to the right mediastinal lymph nodes. Lymphatic drainage within the mediastinum moves cephalad. The pulmonary parenchyma does not contain a nerve supply; however, the parietal pleura has rich nerve endings. Generous local anesthesia is therefore necessary for chest tube insertion.

Anatomic variation in the lung is not uncommon, but rarely poses clinical difficulty if recognized. Pulmonary arterial branching variation is common, and more commonly affects the left upper lobe. An azygos lobe can be identified on about 0.5% of routine chest roentgenograms. Because of the position of the azygos vein within the substance of the right upper lobe, development continues around the azygos vein in an inferior-to-superior direction. The lung develops a double fold of visceral pleura associated with the azygos lobe that can be identified on chest x-ray as a so-called reverse comma sign.

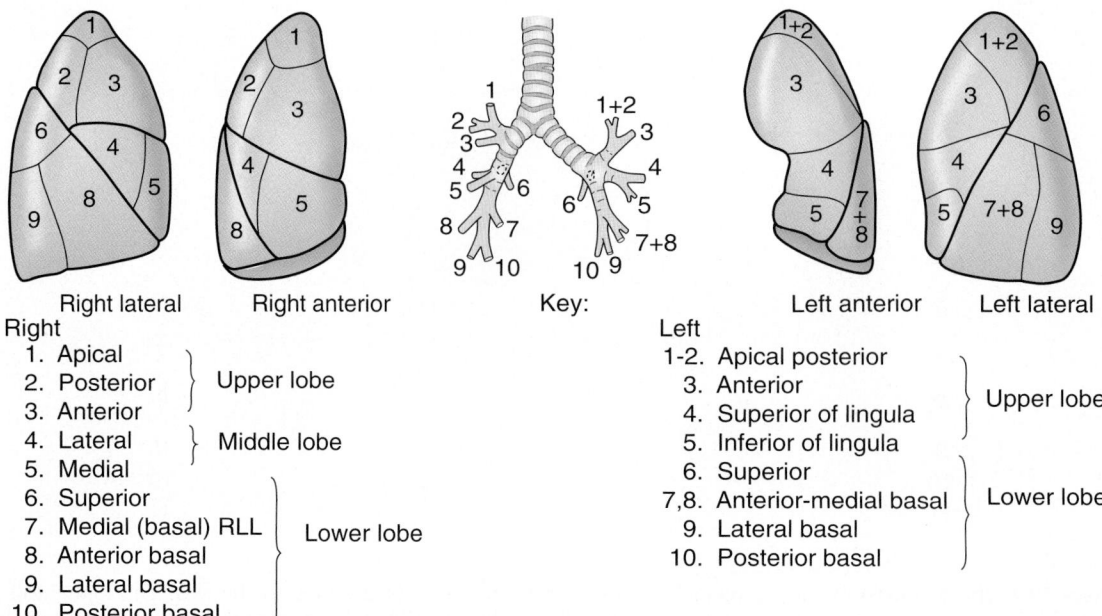

Figure 59-2 **Segments of the pulmonary lobes.** (Modified from Jackson CL, Huber JF: Correlated applied anatomy of the bronchial tree and lungs with a system of nomenclature. Dis Chest 9:319, 1943.)

Right
1. Apical   ⎱
2. Posterior ⎰ Upper lobe
3. Anterior
4. Lateral   ⎱ Middle lobe
5. Medial
6. Superior   ⎱
7. Medial (basal) RLL ⎰ Lower lobe
8. Anterior basal
9. Lateral basal
10. Posterior basal

Left
1-2. Apical posterior   ⎱
3. Anterior   ⎰ Upper lobe
4. Superior of lingula
5. Inferior of lingula
6. Superior   ⎱
7,8. Anterior-medial basal ⎰ Lower lobe
9. Lateral basal
10. Posterior basal

The azygos lobe is not a true anatomic lobe in that it does not have a separate segmental bronchus, although it may be involved by tuberculosis, cancer, or pulmonary metastasis, without involving the other portions of the lung. Other common variations include segmental lobar fissures, more commonly seen separating the superior segments from the lower right and left lobes proper, and the lateral segment of the lingula from the medial in the left upper lobe.

PULMONARY FUNCTION TESTS

Before pulmonary resection, patients are evaluated by a combination of pulmonary function tests, including spirometry (Fig. 59-3). Each of these tests measures a specific component of the patient's pulmonary function and, in some cases, measures the combined function of both the heart and the lungs. Spirometry measures the lung volumes and mechanical properties of lung elasticity, recoil, and compliance. Pulmonary function testing also evaluates gas exchange functions. Occasionally, this combined measurement of the cardiorespiratory axis serves as a more appropriate study to assess the patient's physiologic reserve.[1] Elevated P_{CO_2} is actually associated with increased surgical risk more significantly than hypoxia. A P_{CO_2} greater than 43 to 45 mm Hg suggests severe disease, with nearly a 50% functional loss of the lung, and may be associated in some cases with underlying pulmonary hypertension, which is another relative contraindication to surgical resection.

The predicted postoperative forced expiratory volume in 1 second (FEV_1) is the most commonly used predictor of postoperative pulmonary reserve. Typically, this is

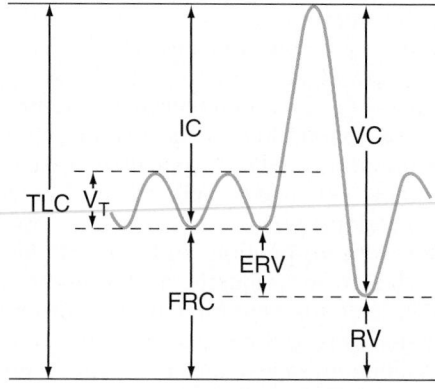

Figure 59-3 Spirometry. Subdivisions of lung volumes. ERV, expiratory reserve volume; FRC, functional residual capacity, that is, lung volume at end-expiration; IC, inspiratory capacity; RV, residual volume, that is, lung volume after forced expiration from FRC; TLC, total lung capacity; VC, vital capacity, that is, the maximal volume of gas inspired from RV; V_T, tidal volume.

greater than 0.8 liter. FEV_1 may be expressed as an actual value such as 0.9 liter per second or as a percentage, such as 68% of that predicted. The predicted value is based on height and weight in normal patients. In the past, it has been common to use the absolute value of the FEV_1 to guide decisions regarding resectability. However, this is dependent on the patient's size, and therefore less accurate than the percent predicted value that takes body habitus into account. Furthermore, it is the postoperative, and not necessarily the preoperative, predicted FEV_1 that is most important. Most patients with an FEV_1 in excess of 60% of predicted will tolerate an anatomic lobectomy, depending of course on other eval-

Section of Pulmonary Medicine
Pulmonary Function Report

Last Name: First Name:
Identification:
Age: 56 years   Room: Out-patient
Sex: male   Race: Caucasian
Height: 65 inches   Physician:
Weight: 177 lbs   Operator:
Date
Time

Spirometry		Pred	Pre BD	%Pred	Post BD	%Pred	%Chg
FVC	[l]	3.48	3.07	88	3.07	88	0
FEV$_1$	[l]	2.83	2.23	79	2.26	80	1
FEV$_1$/VC	[%]	80.81	72.26	89	69.78	86	−3
FEF 25–75	[l/s]	3.01	1.37	45	1.46	49	7
PEF	[l/s]	7.57	6.43	85	7.10	94	10
FIVC	[l]	3.48	3.09	89	3.24	93	5
FIV$_1$	[l]		3.09		3.24		5
FIV$_1$/FVC	[%]		100.00		100.00		0

Lung Volumes		Pred	Measured	%Pred
SVC	[l]	3.48	3.04	87
TLC	[l]	5.51	5.54	101
RV	[l]	1.96	2.49	127
RV/TLC	[%]	35.9	45.0	125
FRC-Box	[l]	2.24	3.01	134

Diffusion SB		Pred	Measured	%Pred
D$_{LCO}$ SB	[ml/min/mm Hg]	22.59	23.81	105
D$_{LCO}$ Hb Corr	[ml/min/mm Hg]	22.6	24.2	107
VA	[l]		5.27	
D$_{LCO}$/VA	[ml/min/mm Hg/l]	3.93	4.52	115
Hb	[g/100ml]		14.1	

Interpretation
Spirometry reveals an isolated reduction in mid-expiratory flows consistent with an obstructive small airways defect. Increased residual volume (RV) is consistent with air trapping. Following the inhalation of a bronchodilator, there is no improvement of the obstructive airway defect. The diffusing capacity is normal.

A

Figure 59-4 Pulmonary function report. **A,** The pulmonary function report provides complete spirometry data based on predicted values for height and weight. In this patient, the forced expiratory volume in 1 second (FEV$_1$) is 2.26 L after bronchodilators, which is 80% of predicted. The carbon monoxide diffusing capacity (D$_{LCO}$) is measured as 23.81 mL/min/mm Hg, which is 105% of predicted. FEF, forced expiratory flow; FIV$_1$, forced inspiratory volume in 1 second; FIVC, forced inspiratory vital capacity; FRC, functional reserve capacity; FVC, forced vital capacity; Hb, hemoglobin; PEF, peak expiratory flow; SB, single breath; SVC, slow vital capacity; TLC, total lung capacity; VA, alveolar volume; VC, vital capacity.

Continued

uable factors. If the FEV$_1$ is less than 60% of predicted, then further testing in an attempt to estimate postoperative FEV$_1$ could be considered. The quantitative xenon-133 ventilation-perfusion lung scan is used to evaluate lung function and to predict postoperative pulmonary function after pulmonary resection.

Tumors that compress the pulmonary artery may cause decreased perfusion to that lung. Tumors that impair ventilation by partial or complete obstruction of the bronchus have a corresponding reduction in ventilation values.

The surgeon can calculate or predict the postoperative FEV$_1$ by multiplying the preoperative value of the noninvolved lung by the percentage of xenon-133 activity within the noninvolved lung (Fig. 59-4). A postoperative FEV$_1$ of less than 30% predicted carries a high risk for oxygen, and even ventilator, dependence postoperatively, but a decision to deny surgical resection to this group of patients must be considered on an individual basis because some will do better than expected with careful selection at experienced centers.[2] Finally, it is

Patient Name:

Patient Number:

Date of Test:

REGIONAL PULMONARY FUNCTION STUDY (XENON-133)

Referring Physician: Patient's Age: 56 yrs Sex: Male   Height: 65 inches Weight: 177 lb

(Distribution of Volume, Ventilation and Perfusion expressed in %)

VOLUME, %

Right			Left
4	1	1	5
23	2	2	6
26	3	3	8
24	4	4	4
77			23

VENTILATION, %

Right			Left
3	1	1	4
23	2	2	4
29	3	3	6
29	4	4	2
84			16

PERFUSION, %

Right			Left
4	1	1	5
20	2	2	4
29	3	3	6
31	4	4	1
84			16

V̇/Q̇ INDICES

Right			Left
0.8	1	1	0.8
1.1	2	2	1.0
1.0	3	3	1.0
0.9	4	4	2.0

VENTILATORY CLEARANCE (T1/2 in seconds)

VENT GAS

Right			Left
17	1	1	99
11	2	2	99
11	3	3	99
9	4	4	26

PERFUSED GAS

Right			Left
19	1	1	218
16	2	2	21
20	3	3	16
12	4	4	20

INTERPRETATION:

There is severe, generalized hypoventilation and hypoperfusion throughout the left lung. Apical reduction in ventilation and perfusion is also noted on the right lung. The left lung contributes to approximately 16% of overall ventilation and 16% of overall perfusion.
Estimated post left pneumonectomy FEV_1 = 52 (1.5 L)
If indicated, resection of up to a left pneumonectomy should be functionally tolerated.

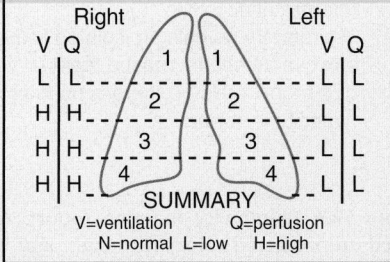

SUMMARY
V=ventilation   Q=perfusion
N=normal L=low H=high

Post BD FEV_1: 62% Pred   1.76 Liters

Involved lung: Left

B

Figure 59-4, cont'd B, The quantitative xenon ventilation-perfusion lung scan report provides the lung volume, the ventilation, and the perfusion to each lung. In this patient with a large hilar tumor, both ventilation and perfusion are reduced in the involved left lung compared with the uninvolved right lung. The predicted post–left pneumonectomy right lung function can be obtained by multiplying the right lung percent perfusion (84%) by the observed best FEV_1 (2.26 L). The resulting value, 1.9 L as a post–left pneumonectomy FEV_1, suggests that a left pneumonectomy would be functionally well tolerated.

important to understand that in the immediate postoperative period, primarily because of pain and other postoperative physiologic and emotional considerations, the objectively calculated postoperative predicted FEV_1 will likely not be realized.[3]

In a number of studies, the carbon monoxide diffusing capacity (DLCO) has been stressed as equally important to FEV_1 measurement in predicting postoperative compromise, and perhaps more important for long-term functional outcome.[4-6] DLCO can be measured by several methods, although the single-breath test is most commonly performed. The DLco measures the rate at which test molecules such as carbon monoxide move from the alveolar space to combine with hemoglobin in the red blood cells. The DLco is determined by calculating the difference between inspired and expired samples of gas. DLco levels less than 40% to 50% are associated with increased perioperative risk.[7]

The forced expiratory volume in 1 second to forced vital capacity ratio (FEV$_1$/FVC) describes the relationship between the FEV$_1$ and the total lung volume. In obstructive disease, the ratio is low (FEV$_1$ is low, and FVC is high); in restrictive disease, the ratio is about normal because both FEV$_1$ and FVC are reduced.

Maximal voluntary ventilation (MVV) describes the maximal movement of air into the lungs during a preset interval. MVV measures the effort, coordination, and compliance of the respiratory system. The test is typically conducted over a 12-second interval, and the results are expressed in liters per minute.

Flow-volume loops derived from spirometry describe the relationship between lung volume and airflow as the lung volume changes during a forced expiration and inspiration. The typical test consists of tidal breathing at rest, then maximal inspiratory effort to total lung capacity, then maximal expiratory effort to residual volume, concluding with maximal inspiratory effort to total lung capacity.

CARDIOPULMONARY EXERCISE TESTING

Cardiopulmonary exercise testing evaluates the cardiopulmonary axis, the ability of the respiratory system to take up oxygen in exchange for carbon dioxide, and the ability of the cardiovascular system to transport this oxygen to the tissues. The body's ability to accomplish this task at rest and when stressed with exercise can be measured by DLco, as described earlier, and $\dot{V}o_2$ max.

$\dot{V}o_2$ max can also be measured. Physiologic limits to the elevation in cardiac output depend on cardiac reserve and oxygen extraction. Typically, additional work is accompanied by an elevation in oxygen extraction. At some point, a plateau in the oxygen extraction is identified. Low of values $\dot{V}o_2$ max (<15 mL/min/kg) are associated with increased risk for surgical morbidity and mortality, and any value less than 10 mL/min/kg may be considered very high risk for resection if other parameters are not optimal.

Some thoracic surgeons have advocated stair climbing as a suitable measure of preoperative cardiopulmonary assessment.[8] If the patient can walk up one flight of stairs, a wedge resection generally is appropriate. If the patient can walk up two flights of stairs, a lobectomy is appropriate; and three flights of stairs, a pneumonectomy. The surgeon subjectively assesses breathlessness. This subjective evaluation is difficult to quantitate. In patients undergoing evaluation for lung volume reduction surgery or for lung transplantation, a 6-minute walk test is used for a measure of the cardiac and pulmonary reserve. Patients are told to walk as far and as fast as they can during this

time period. Distances of more than 1000 feet suggest an uncomplicated course. Although time-honored, in the current era, the use of more standardized techniques described in the foregoing sections would be recommended for the sake of patient and surgeon alike.

THORACIC INCISIONS

The choice of incision depends on the operation to be performed, the patient's underlying physiologic condition, and the anticipated benefits and limitations of the planned approach.

The posterolateral thoracotomy is the most frequent thoracic incision used. This incision may be used for operations on a single thorax, for pulmonary resection, esophageal surgery or resection, or resection of portions of the chest wall. The patient is placed in a lateral decubitus position with the side to be operated on placed up. An incision is made obliquely from a space between the spinous processes and the medial border of the scapula inferiorly to about 1 fingerbreadth below and in front of the tip of the scapula. The latissimus dorsi muscle may be divided; however, many surgeons prefer to spare this muscle and mobilize its lateral and inferior edge to facilitate additional exposure. The serratus anterior muscle is typically not divided but is simply mobilized along its lateral border. The chest is entered through the fifth intercostal space (the interspace just above the 6th rib) by dividing the intercostal muscles. The posterior portion of the sixth rib is often divided to facilitate exposure and to minimize the risk for breaking the rib. A thoracic epidural catheter is used to minimize postoperative pain.

The axillary thoracotomy may be created in two ways. A small transverse incision 3 to 4 cm underneath the axillary hairline (bordered posteriorly by the latissimus dorsi muscle and anteriorly by the pectoralis major muscle) is made. Another technique creates a vertical incision starting at the bottom of the axillary fat, just posterior to the pectoralis muscle, extending for 8 to 10 cm. Both these incisions provide access to the anteriorly placed hilum, but through the 4th, rather than the 5th, interspace considering the anteroinferior slope of the ribs. The serratus anterior muscle is mobilized by removing the slips from the ribs, and thus the subscapular space may be entered. Although it may not improve pain, there is increased shoulder girdle function in the immediate postoperative period. A similar posterior muscle-sparing incision for access through the 5th intercostal space may be performed by making a very small posterolateral incision overlying the respiratory triangle, and mobilizing the latissimus dorsi muscle posteriorly and the serratus anterior anteriorly.

The anterior or anterolateral thoracotomy is created by a curvilinear incision underneath the inferior border of the pectoralis major muscle at the inframammary fold. The incision extends from 2 to 3 cm medial to the sternum and then extends superiorly toward the anterior axillary line. The chest is then entered through the 4th or 5th intercostal space depending on the operation to be performed. The pectoralis major muscle may be mobilized to assist in obtaining the selected interspace. This approach is good for open lung biopsies in that all lobes of the lung can be reached with extremely easy access to the right middle lobe, or the lingular segment of the left upper lobe. However, the apex of the upper lobes may be difficult to reach. Supplemental techniques using video-assisted devices may be considered in addition to, or as an alternative to, open techniques.

A median sternotomy is performed using a vertical incision from the sternal notch to the xiphoid. A sternal saw is then used to divide the sternum in the midline. With gentle retraction, the sternum can be spread about 8 to 10 cm to allow access to both the right and left thorax. The pleura is opened in its anteromedial aspect, taking care to avoid the phrenic nerves. This approach is used for operations on the anterior mediastinum, for bilateral pulmonary metastasis resection, or when both lungs need to be explored or inspected for any reason. The sternum is usually closed with stainless steel wire.

The transverse sternotomy or "clamshell" incision is performed as an alternative to median sternotomy. This incision is larger and combines two anterior thoracotomy incisions with transverse division of the sternum at the fourth intercostal space. Both internal mammary arteries require ligation. The pectoralis major muscles of both sides generally need to be mobilized to access the appropriate (4th) interspace. This approach is ideal for accessing both the right and the left hilum, as well as providing additional exposure for large mediastinal tumors, bilateral hilar dissections, lung transplantation, or posterior-based metastases in both lungs. Care must be exercised in using this incision in those with compromised pulmonary function, however, because it often is more painful than a sternotomy.

Video-assisted thoracic surgery (VATS) or other minimally invasive techniques have been developed to treat some benign pulmonary conditions such as pneumothorax, to perform open lung biopsy, and to facilitate diagnosis and staging of thoracic malignancies. VATS continues to be used more commonly for treatment of thoracic malignancies. Although the use of minimally invasive techniques does minimize surgical trauma from the incisions, the individual surgeon must ensure that fundamentals of the operation are not compromised by such a limited approach, particularly in patients with known or suspected thoracic neoplasms. VATS is performed with the patient under general anesthesia with a double-lumen endotracheal tube, typically with the patient in a lateral decubitus position. A 1-cm incision is made over the central thorax, the muscles are gently spread, a trocar is inserted, and the thorax is entered. The thoracoscope is then introduced. One or more additional incisions are made to facilitate manipulation of the lung or other thoracic structures. The advantage of these techniques is the limited surgical trauma that occurs compared with conventional thoracotomy, and its attendant salutary effect on recovery, length of stay, and return to functional activity. It is now apparent that earliest stage (T1 N0 M0) tumors are safely amenable to this approach in experience hands.[9,10] However, the issues of complete nodal dissection and the theoretical increased risk for local recurrence for more advanced tumors following lung cancer resection by these methods have yet to be resolved definitively.

PERIOPERATIVE RISK

Certain comorbidities are associated with increased pulmonary risk, including smoking, poor overall health, increasing age, poorer pulmonary function or chronic obstructive pulmonary disease, asthma, and obesity. Optimization of medical care for these problems needs to be coordinated with planned pulmonary resection.[1]

Preoperative preparation begins with the first visit. If the patient is a smoker, he or she needs to be urged to stop immediately. Several studies have corroborated the importance of smoking cessation in prevention of serious postoperative pulmonary complications, and ideally, patients are smoke-free for a minimum of 2 weeks and preferably for 4 to 8 weeks before surgery.[11,12] Smoking cessation programs may be helpful for these patients, and all patients need to be offered pharmacologic assistance, such as bupropion hydrochloride and some form of nicotine supplementation, because this combination has demonstrated increased efficacy in smoking cessation efforts over counseling alone.[13,14]

Patients with chronic obstructive pulmonary disease (COPD) or asthma need to be medically optimized with bronchodilators for their pulmonary function before surgery. Obstructive pneumonia typically clears with antibiotic treatment of 7 to 10 days but may be more refractory if complete obstruction or early abscess formation is present. Occasionally, patients require intravenous (IV) antibiotics to clear infection before pulmonary resection. Steroids may be required in some patients but must be used with care in those scheduled for pneumonectomy in consideration of bronchial stump healing and the potential for bronchopleural fistula. Patients are taught to use incentive spirometry before surgery. The device is given to the patient for practice at home before surgery and is brought to the hospital for postoperative lung expansion. Patients are also educated about the rationale for their surgery and what to expect during their convalescence. Before surgery and during the perioperative period, deep venous thrombosis prophylaxis is provided by subcutaneous heparin or by sequential compression stockings. As well, perioperative antibiotics are used to minimize complications from infections.

Postoperative morbidity may also be minimized by adequate pain control with IV analgesics, usually patient-controlled analgesia (PCA), or by use of the thoracic epidural catheter. Some surgeons have successfully used intercostal nerve blocks after thoracotomy for postoperative pain relief. Pulmonary exercises to expand the lungs are performed by all patients after pulmonary resection. Incentive spirometry assists in expanding the lung and reducing the incidence of pulmonary morbidities. Postoperative positive airway pressure may be used effectively in some patients. Nasal bilevel positive airway pressure may delay or eliminate the need for intubation or reintubation after pulmonary resection. Mobilization is the key to avoidance of most perioperative complications. Patients are not sent to the intensive care unit routinely after lung resection unless there are comorbid indications because this will impede efforts to get the patient out of bed and ambulating. With adequate pain control, most patients are able to ambulate with assistance within 24 hours of surgery.

CONGENITAL LESIONS OF THE LUNG, TRACHEA, AND BRONCHI

Various congenital lung abnormalities can occur. Bilateral agenesis of the lungs is fatal. Unilateral agenesis may occur more frequently on the left (~70%) than on the right (~30%), with more than a 2:1 male-to-female ratio. Half of cases are isolated and compatible with life; however, half are associated with other abnormalities. The chest x-ray may demonstrate a small lucency on the involved side with a mediastinal shift. Isolated lobar agenesis is rare.

Hypoplasia of the lungs may occur as a result of interference with the development of the alveolar system during the last 2 months of gestation. This problem is seen in conjunction with lesions that compete with the lung for space in the pleural cavity. When this occurs, the number of branches in the airway decreases, as does the lining of the airways with cuboidal cells. Bochdalek's hernia is the most frequent cause of hypoplasia. Reversal of this condition in utero is being investigated.

Conditions associated with hypoplasia of the lungs include oligohydramnios, prune-belly syndrome (deficiency in the abdominal musculature, genitourinary abnormalities), scimitar syndrome (abnormal pulmonary vein draining into the inferior vena cava, demonstrated as a crescent along the right heart border on cardiac angiography), and dextrocardia. Isolated pulmonary hypoplasia is rare.

Hyaline membrane disease (or infant respiratory distress syndrome) is frequent in premature infants (24-28 weeks' gestation) and infants of diabetic mothers. At that gestation, the infants have an immature surfactant system. Hyaline membrane disease develops in the alveoli, causing congestion and a grossly deep-purple–appearing lung. Respiratory distress frequently ensues, requiring high concentrations of oxygen. The chest roentgenograms demonstrate a ground-glass appearance from the interstitial edema. As needs for oxygen and ventilator pressure increase to counteract this interstitial edema, pneumothorax frequently occurs. Ten to 30% of these infants do not survive.

Congenital cystic lesions generally occur secondary to separation of the pulmonary remnants from airway branchings. Diffuse cystic disease is a rare male-predominant (2:1) abnormality. This disease may usually involve one lobe or a portion of a lobe. Occasionally, the condition may be more generalized and consist of innumerable small cystic cavities lined with ciliated epithelium and containing clear mucus. The distribution within each of the lobes is about equal. Clinically, about one third of patients are without symptoms; one third have cough; and one third have infection or, rarely, hemoptysis. Treatment may be with antibiotics or, for more severe localized cases, with resection.

The differential diagnosis of cystic disease in the lung may be challenging. Various categories are considered. Cystic fibrosis is an autosomal recessive disorder that is found in white Americans. About 20% of patients with cystic fibrosis survive to the age of 30 years. Lung failure is the most frequent cause of death in most patients. Excessively thick mucus leads to inspissation, recurrent infections, bronchitis, and bronchiectasis. Pneumothorax secondary to air trapping is also found. Fibrosis and cystic changes on pathologic examinations are identified.

Tension cyst may be a complication of cystic disease. A rapid increase in the size of the cyst may cause mechanical ventilation problems as well as mediastinal shift. Resection, usually lobectomy, corrects this problem.

Pneumatoceles may develop as a result of childhood *Staphylococcus aureus* infection. They can be very large and may cause mechanical complications. These problems may resolve completely as the pneumonia resolves.

Congenital cystic adenomatoid malformations are closely related to a hamartoma without cartilage. Terminal bronchioles proliferate, yielding the "adenomatoid" malformation. The lung has the appearance of Swiss cheese and feels like a large rubbery mass. With air trapping and overdistention, respiratory distress may occur, which is optimally relieved by lobectomy.

Lobar emphysema frequently occurs as a congenital or infantile process. It rarely occurs after 6 months of age. Fifty percent of patients do not have an obvious cause. Twenty-five percent of patients have bronchial cartilage dysplasia, and 25% of cases are thought to be secondary to a variety of causes, such as bronchial atresia, mucosal valves, bronchostenosis, enlarged lymph nodes, and abnormal vessels. Bronchiolitis is probably the most common cause overall. The onset of rapidly progressive respiratory distress usually occurs from 4 to 5 days to several weeks after birth. Treatment is lobectomy.

Pulmonary sequestration occurs most commonly in the lower lobes (left lobe > right lobe) and within an area of embryonic lung tissue that has its blood supply from an anomalous systemic artery. This condition occurs secondary to an accessory lung bud caudal to the normal lung, but with a lack of absorption of primitive surrounding splanchnic vessels. During lung development, interlobar sequestration (75%) occurs early. Later, after the pleura forms, extralobar sequestration occurs (25%). The blood supply is from the systemic artery to the pulmonary vein (intralobar) or to the systemic veins (extralobar). Ninety-five percent of the systemic blood supply to the pulmonary sequestration comes from the thoracic aorta.

Kartagener's syndrome, an autosomal recessive condition, consists of sinusitis, bronchiectasis, and situs inversus. Dyskinetic cilia are a hallmark sign of this syndrome and affect both sperm and respiratory epithelium. Because of these dyskinetic cilia, bronchiectasis occurs in 20% to

25% of patients; however, with good medical supervision, these patients may live a full life span.

Congenital Abnormalities of the Trachea and Bronchi

Esophageal atresia with tracheoesophageal fistula is the most frequent abnormality of the trachea in infants. This topic is discussed under pediatric surgery.

Bronchial atresia is the second most frequent congenital pulmonary lesion after tracheoesophageal fistula. The lung tissue distal to the atresia expands and becomes emphysematous as a result of air entry through the pores of Kohn. With no exit for air or mucus because of this blind bronchial stump, emphysema from air trapping or development of a mucocele may occur. The chest roentgenograms may demonstrate hyperinflation of a lobe or a segment. The oval density may be identified between the hyperinflated lung and the hilum. The left upper lobe is the most frequently involved of all lobes within the lung. Diagnosis may be confirmed with bronchography or computed tomography (CT). The surgeon must rule out a mucus plug, adenoma, vascular compression, or sequestration.

Tracheal agenesis is a rare phenomenon and is fatal. The trachea is absent from the larynx to the carina, and bronchi communicate with the esophagus.

Tracheal stenosis is also rare and consists of generalized hypoplasia, a funnel-like trachea, and bronchial and segmental malformations. The right upper lobe bronchus may come from the trachea directly and may be associated with an aberrant left pulmonary artery (so-called pulmonary artery sling). Completely circular vascular rings are common. Repair is by incision of the trachea vertically and widening of the tracheal lumen.

Tracheomalacia can be identified by bronchoscopy. The surgeon will notice marked variation of the tracheal lumen with inspiration and expiration. The tracheal rings are ineffective in maintaining the lumen of the trachea, and with negative intrathoracic pressure, the trachea collapses. With the positive pressure exerted by exhalation, the trachea expands. Respiratory difficulty ensues from the intermittently collapsing trachea. Stent placement in adults or primary repair is required. This condition may have a congenital predisposition but is most often seen in adults with COPD.

Congenital Bronchopulmonary Malformations

Various congenital bronchopulmonary malformations include pulmonary sequestration, bronchogenic cysts, congenital lobar emphysema, and congenital cystic adenomatoid malformation. Lobectomy is commonly required, and this is one of the few current absolute indications for fetal surgical intervention when very large. Any thoracic cystic lesion that is enlarging on serial radiographs needs to be considered for resection. Asymptomatic cystic lesions may eventually produce compression of lung parenchyma, infection, or malignant degeneration.[15]

A bronchogenic cyst arises from a tracheal or bronchial diverticulum.[16] This diverticulum becomes completely separated from the trachea and is frequently found as an asymptomatic mass on routine chest roentgenograms. CT of the chest demonstrates this abnormality as a homogeneous-type mass, well circumscribed, and adjacent to the trachea (Fig. 59-5).

The bronchogenic cyst accounts for 10% of mediastinal masses in children and is located in the mid-mediastinum. The bronchogenic cyst arises from nests of cells that become isolated from the primitive lung bud. They are usually found in close association with the major bronchi or trachea but are not usually connected. The cyst may be adjacent to or involve the esophagus, or it may be located within the pulmonary substance. It is typically 2 to 10 cm, and the fluid is usually clear, although it may be cloudy. The wall of the cyst is of variable thickness and composed of fibrous tissue. This cyst wall may also have muscle-elastin cartilage in its composition. The inner lining usually consists of pseudostratified ciliated columnar epithelium. It may also have squamous or gastric mucosa, and it may or may not have a bronchial communication. Usually a bronchial or tracheal communication cannot be identified.

Clinically, the bronchogenic cyst occurs more frequently within the right mediastinum and is more common in men. Where there is no bronchial communication, the bronchogenic cyst typically is without symptoms, although tracheal compression, pain, and secondary infection may exist. The chest x-ray may identify a circle or ovoid density in proximity to a major air passage, or it may be noted simply as a mediastinal mass. With bronchial communication, the bronchogenic cyst is almost always symptomatic. Cough, fever, sputum production, or hemoptysis may occur. The chest roentgenograms may demonstrate an air-fluid level within a cystic structure within the mediastinum. The differential diagnosis may include lymphoma, teratoma, hamartoma, granuloma, and saccular aortic aneurysm (although these frequently have calcification).

Treatment consists of excision, even if the patient is asymptomatic, to confirm the diagnosis. Care is needed to protect the phrenic nerve, the superior vena cava, and the esophagus during the dissection because some fibrosis may be present from chronic inflammation. Typically, the bronchogenic cyst is simply enucleated from the mediastinum. If attached to a bronchus by a stalk, this stalk must be ligated. Actual open communication with the tracheobronchial tree is rare but has been noted. If a changing air-fluid level is noted, communication needs to be expected and evaluated by bronchoscopy to better plan the operative approach, especially in the subcarinal position.

Congenital Vascular Disorders

Congenital vascular disorders of the lungs may occur. In Swyer-James and Macleod's syndrome, there is idiopathic hyperlucent lung. This problem develops from chronic pulmonary infections such as bronchiectasis. As the consolidation persists, decreased pulmonary artery blood supply may cause an "autopneumonectomy" and a hyperlucent lung.

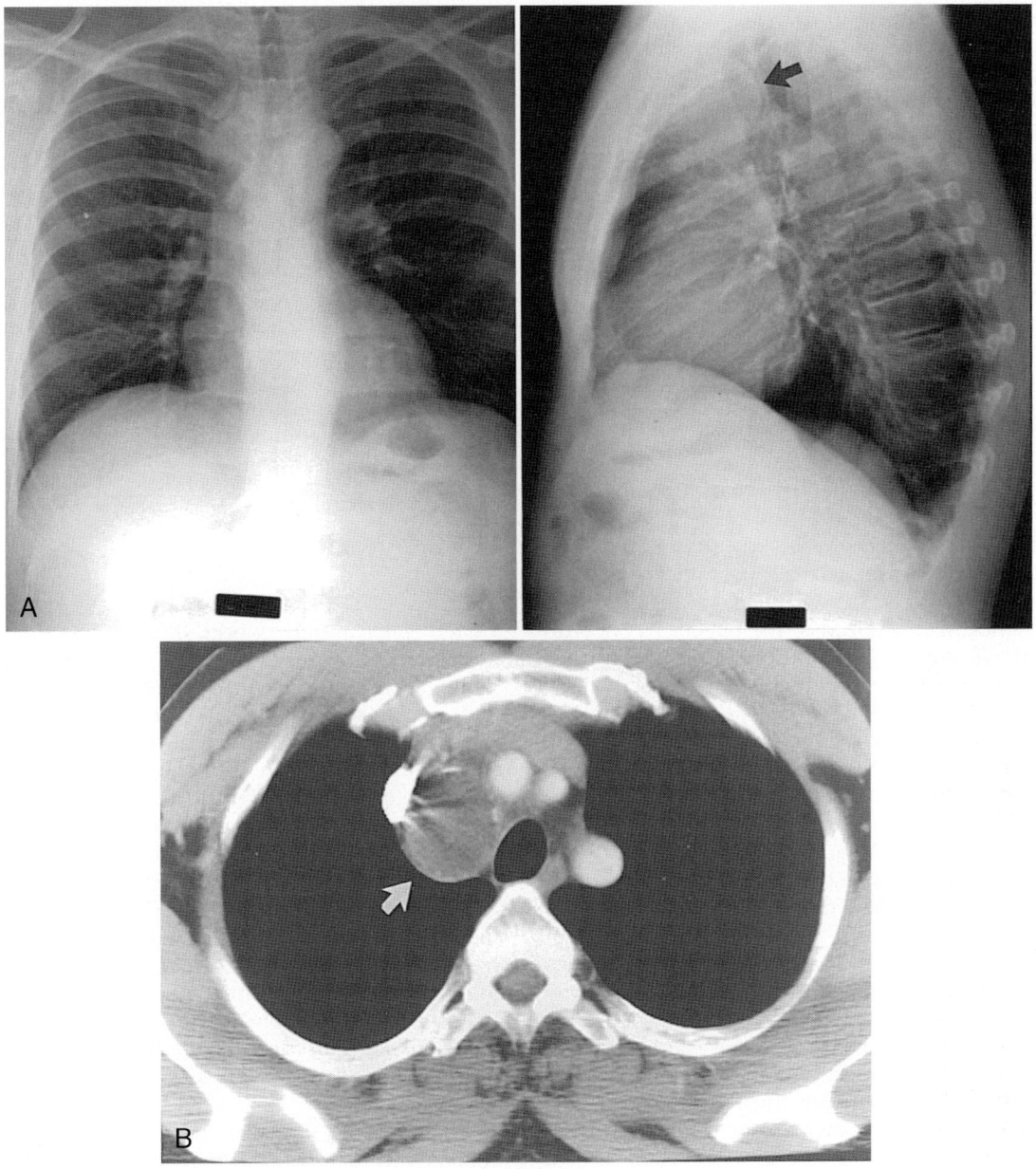

Figure 59-5 Two chest roentgenograms (**A**) and a CT scan (**B**) of the chest of a patient with a bronchogenic cyst (*arrow*).

Scimitar syndrome is associated with hypoplastic right lung with drainage of the pulmonary vein to the inferior vena cava. Usually, the anomaly is corrected using extracorporeal cardiopulmonary support. A patch from the pulmonary vein to the left atrium by way of an atrial septal defect corrects this problem.

Pulmonary arteriovenous malformations may exist as one or more pulmonary artery to pulmonary vein connections, bypassing the pulmonary capillary bed. This connection results in a right-to-left shunt. About one third of these patients have hereditary hemorrhagic telangiectasia (Osler-Weber-Rendu syndrome). About half the malformations are small (<1 cm) and tend to be multiple. As

well, half are greater than 1 cm and usually less than 5 cm, and tend to be subpleural. These lesions need to be considered in the differential diagnosis of any patient with hemoptysis that is unexplained on the basis of bronchoscopy or routine imaging. Either local resection or catheter embolization of these lesions can be curative.

Clinical features consist of small arterial venous malformations (shunting <25% of pulmonary blood flow). There is no true cyanosis; half of patients have no symptoms, and others may have exertional dyspnea and easy fatigability. Larger arterial venous malformations (which may shunt more than 25% of pulmonary blood flow) may present with cyanosis, dyspnea, and fatigability. The onset is frequently in adolescence or adulthood, and multiple lesions may be associated with congenital heart disease. With severe shunting, cyanosis, and clubbing, polycythemia (found in 20% overall) may occur. The differential diagnosis includes primary pulmonary hypertension, right-to-left cardiac shunts, or methemoglobinemia. Complications include pneumothorax, hemoptysis, cerebral thrombosis, or brain abscess. Cardiac output is not increased because resistance of the arterial venous malformation is equivalent to the pulmonary vascular resistance; therefore, no congestive heart failure or cardiac enlargement occurs. There is a continuous bruit present in about half of the patients with cyanosis. The chest x-ray may demonstrate a lobulated density frequently with larger lesions, but smaller lesions are rarely seen on plain film. For diagnosis, CT scan with contrast may be sufficient, although thin-cut magnetic resonance angiography is currently the gold standard, and some patients still require catheter angiography. The surgeon must consider resection of the arterial venous malformation if symptoms are present, the lesions are enlarging, or the lesion is large and sufficiently localized. If the patient has hereditary hemorrhagic telangiectasia, resection may be considered even if the lesions are of small size because solitary lesions will enlarge. The surgeon may consider lobectomy or wedge excision if adhesions are noted at the chest wall or diaphragm. Vascular control before excision is critical. Observation is recommended if lesions are small (<1-1.5 cm), without symptoms or hereditary hemorrhagic telangiectasia. Angiographic embolization can be helpful for multiple unresectable lesions and is more commonly being performed in lieu of surgery in selected cases at experienced centers.[17]

A pulmonary vascular sling consists of an anomalous or aberrant left pulmonary artery, which causes airway obstruction. Pulmonary vascular slings are commonly associated with other anomalies. In this particular anatomic variation, the aberrant left pulmonary artery arises from the right (main) pulmonary artery. The aberrant left pulmonary artery courses between the trachea and the esophagus to supply the left lung. More than 90% of patients have serious difficulty consisting of wheezing and stridor. Esophagoscopy will show the anomalous vessel anterior to the esophagus; bronchoscopy or bronchography will demonstrate the vessel posterior to the trachea. Surgical correction requires exploration of the left chest, division of the artery, and oversewing of the vessel as far as possible distal within the mediastinum. The reanastomosis to the main pulmonary artery is then performed.

Vascular rings make up 7% of all congenital heart problems. The most common vascular ring is double aortic arch, which occurs in 60% of all cases. The right, or posterior arch, is the larger and gives rise to the right carotid and right subclavian arteries. The ring wraps around both the trachea and the esophagus. A posterior indentation is noted in the esophagus on barium swallow. Simple division corrects the anomaly.

A right aortic arch with retroesophageal left subclavian artery and left ligamentum arteriosum occurs in about

25% to 30% of patients with vascular rings. Intracardiac defects occur with double aortic arch. Most of these infants require operation within the first weeks or months of life.

Most patients with vascular rings require only a careful history and barium swallow for diagnosis. Typically, one does not need bronchoscopy or esophagoscopy because it may be harmful; aortography adds little additional information. Repair is performed through the left chest. Division of the smaller arch, usually the left, is undertaken. The ligamentum is divided, and the trachea and the esophagus are freed from the surrounding tissues. When a retroesophageal right subclavian artery with left ligament occurs, the patient may complain of dysphagia. This clinical anomaly is often referred to as *dysphagia lusoria*. The differential diagnosis includes neuromotor diseases of the esophagus or stricture.

LUNG CANCER

Lung cancer is a significant public health problem in the United States and the world. In 2006, there were 174,470 new cases of cancer of the lung and bronchus estimated. Lung cancer is the most frequent cause of cancer death and accounts for 14% of all cancer diagnoses and 28% of all cancer deaths. Lung cancer is the most common cause of cancer death in women and the second most common cause of cancer death in men. The estimated deaths attributed to lung cancer in 2006 are about 162,460, exceeding the combined total deaths of breast, prostate, and colorectal cancer patients (Fig. 59-6). Lung cancer continues to be the leading cause of cancer death in both men and women. Although there are 70,000 more cases of prostate cancer than lung in men, the death rate for lung cancer is almost triple that of prostate cancer. Similarly for women, the incidence of breast cancer is three times greater than for lung, but there are almost twice as many lung cancer deaths than breast cancer deaths in this cohort.[18]

For men, the mortality rate for lung cancer declined significantly (decreasing 1.9%) in the period 1991 to 2003. However, since 1987, more women have died of lung cancer than breast cancer, which for almost 50 years was the major cause of death in women. The decreases in lung cancer incidence and the mortality rate in men probably reflect decreasing cigarette smoking over the previous 30 years. However, smoking cessation in women has lagged behind smoking cessation in men, and the incidence of lung cancer in women continues to climb, with an increase in mortality in this group of 2% from 1990 to 2003 (Figs. 59-7 and 59-8).

Among all groups studied, black men have both the highest incidence and the highest death rate from cancer of the lung and bronchus. Although the survival rates for lower-stage lung cancer have improved over time, the 5-year survival for all comers at all stages is only 15%. For localized disease, 5-year survival can approach 50% (stages I and II), for regional disease 20%, and for distant disease 2%. Unfortunately, only a small percentage (16%) are discovered when localized.[18]

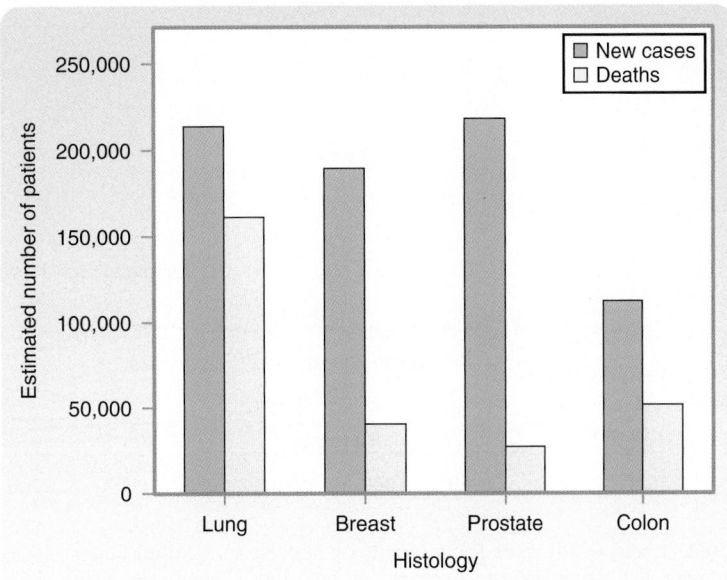

Figure 59-6 Estimated cancer statistics, United States 2007. New cases of cancer and cancer deaths for the four leading cancers in the United States are included. (From http://www.cancer.org/downloads/STT/CAFF2007 PWSecured.pdf. Reprinted by the permission of the American Cancer Society, Inc.)

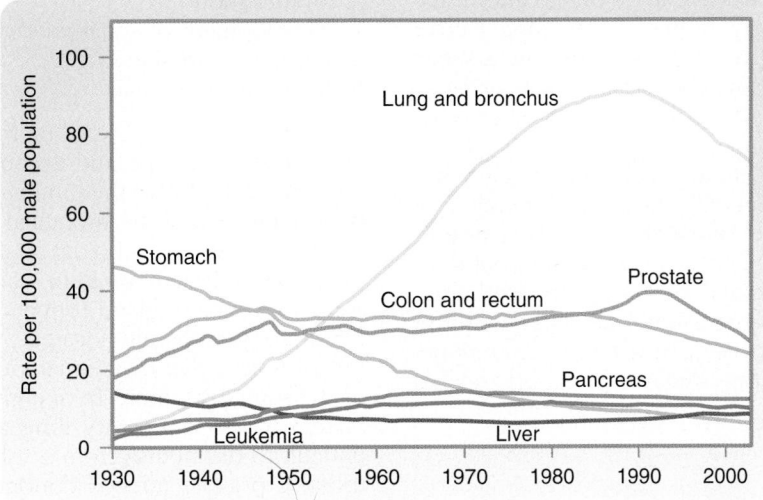

Figure 59-7 Age-adjusted cancer death rates for men, by site, in the United States (1930-2003) per 100,000, age-adjusted to the 2000 U.S. standard population. (From http://www.cancer.org/downloads/STT/Cancer_Statistics_ Combined_2007.ppt#6. Reprinted by permission of the American Cancer Society, Inc.)

Although local and systemic interventions may improve survival rates in these patients, accurate treatment depends on accurate and histologic staging before treatment and after resection. Anatomic resection of the involved lobe of the lung and mediastinal lymph node dissection provide optimal material for pathologic staging and optimal treatment (local control) for patients with stage I and II lung cancer. In advanced-stage (IIIA) patients, a multidisciplinary approach to the patient's treatment plan (with evaluation and recommendations by the surgeon, the medical oncologist, and the radiation oncologist before treatment) ensures an optimal treatment recommendation in a planned and structured manner. Earlier-stage patients (IB, IIA, and IIB) may eventually achieve

similar benefit. *In the future, knowledge of molecular changes that predispose to the development of lung cancer may provide strategies for chemoprevention or other treatments directed at genetic alterations in the cancer itself.* Many prospective protocols have been initiated through the efforts of oncologists throughout the world, in an attempt to better understand and evaluate various combinations of multidisciplinary treatments.

Etiology

Cigarette smoking is unequivocally the most important risk factor in the development of lung cancer. Smoking provides a 22-fold increased risk for lung cancer death

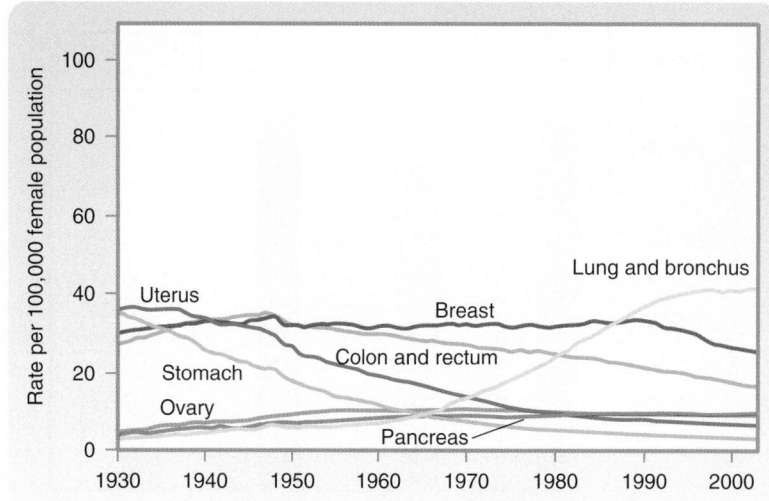

Figure 59-8 Age-adjusted cancer death rates for women, by site, in the United States (1930-2003) per 100,000, age-adjusted to the 2000 U.S. standard population. (From http://www.cancer.org/downloads/STT/Cancer_Statistics_Combined_2007.ppt#6 Reprinted by permission of the American Cancer Society, Inc.)

in men and a 12% increased risk in women. Other environmental factors that may predispose to lung cancer include industrial substances such as asbestos, arsenic, chromium, or nickel; organic chemicals, radon, or iatrogenic radiation exposure; air pollution; and other environmental (secondary) smoke in nonsmokers.

If cancers caused by cigarette smoking and heavy use of alcohol could be prevented, a significant number of lives would be saved. The American Cancer Society estimates that about 175,000 cancer deaths are attributed to tobacco use and an additional 19,000 cancer deaths per year are related to excessive alcohol use (frequently in combination with tobacco use). In the year 2000 alone, there were 4.8 million deaths estimated worldwide related to tobacco use.

Pathology

In general, there is a slight preponderance of lung cancer to develop in the right lung because the right lung has about 55% of the lung parenchyma, and there is a more favorable anatomic path for carcinogens to travel through the downwardly acutely angled right main-stem bronchus. As well, lung cancer more frequently occurs in the upper lobes than in lower lobes. The blood supply to these tumors, which arise from the bronchial epithelium, is from the bronchial arteries. A small percentage of patients may have a second focus or metastasis of lung cancer that increases the stage of the patient (see Staging of Lung Cancer). The progression of histologic changes in the lung that occurs from smoking is shown:

1. Proliferation of basal cells
2. Development of atypical nuclei with prominent nucleoli

3. Stratification
4. Development of squamous metaplasia
5. Carcinoma in situ
6. Invasive carcinoma

Adenocarcinoma (ACA) of the lung is the most frequent histologic type and accounts for about 45% of all lung cancers. ACA of the lung is derived from the mucus-producing cells of the bronchial epithelium. Microscopic features consist of cuboidal to columnar cells with adequate to abundant pink or vacuolated cytoplasm and some evidence of gland formation. Most of these tumors (75%) are peripherally located. ACA of the lung tends to metastasize earlier than squamous cell carcinoma (SCCA) of the lung, and more frequently to the central nervous system (CNS). A primary lung adenocarcinoma may be difficult to distinguish from a solitary metastasis of extrathoracic primary adenocarcinoma. When in doubt, one may treat for primary lung cancer with lobectomy and mediastinal lymph node dissection.

Bronchoalveolar carcinoma (BAC) of the lung is a subcategory of ACA but can be at times a more indolent disease. It has the best prognosis overall of any kind of lung cancer because it is highly differentiated and spreads along alveolar walls. BAC may present as a solitary nodule, multiple nodules, or diffuse parenchymal infiltrates. BAC may require resection to confirm the diagnosis. A solitary focus of bronchoalveolar carcinoma is treated in a manner similar to ACA. Multifocal disease is not amenable to surgical resection, and BAC is characteristically resistant to conventional chemotherapy.

SCCA of the lung occurs in about 30% of patients with lung cancer. About two thirds of these tumors are centrally located and tend to expand against the bronchus, causing extrinsic compression. These tumors are prone to undergo central necrosis and cavitation. SCCA tends to metastasize later than does ACA. Microscopically in SCCA, keratinization, stratification, and intercellular bridge formation are exhibited. SCCA may be more readily detected on sputum cytology than ACA.

A diagnosis of large cell undifferentiated carcinoma may be made in about 10% of all lung tumors. Specific cytologic features of SCCA or ACA are lacking. These tumors tend to occur peripherally and may metastasize relatively early. Microscopically, these tumors show anaplastic, pleomorphic cells with vesicular or hyperchromatic nuclei and abundant cytoplasm. Neuroendocrine histopathology in ACA can also portend a poorer prognosis and is somewhat more common in the large cell variant.

Small cell lung cancer represents about 20% of all lung cancers; about 80% are centrally located. The disease is characterized by an aggressive tendency to metastasize. It often spreads early to mediastinal lymph nodes and distant sites, especially bone marrow and brain. Small cell lung cancer appears to arise in cells derived from the embryologic neural crest. Microscopically, these cells appear as sheets or clusters of cells with dark nuclei and little cytoplasm. This oatlike appearance under the microscope provides the term *oat cell carcinoma* to this disease. Neurosecretory granules are evident on electron microscopy. This tumor is staged as *limited stage* (disease restricted to an ipsilateral hemithorax within a single radiation port) and *extensive stage* (obvious metastatic disease).

Most of these tumors are typically not treated by surgery because of extensive disease at presentation and their aggressive tendency to metastasize; chemotherapy and radiation are preferred, and prophylactic cranial irradiation needs to be discussed with the oncologist if the patient with limited- or extensive-stage disease responds well to first-line therapy. Complete responses may occur in about 30% of patients; however, the 5-year survival rate is only 5%. Relatively rare patients with very limited stage disease (mimicking stage I non–small cell lung cancer clinically) need to be considered for surgical resection, followed by more established systemic small cell therapy. Even in patients with clinically staged T1 N0 or T2 N0 tumors, mediastinoscopy precedes resection, and a positive mediastinoscopy would render the patient an inappropriate candidate for surgery.[19]

Lung Cancer Metastases

Lung cancer with metastases is characterized as stage IV (any T, any N, M1). Lung cancers most commonly metastasize to the pulmonary and mediastinal lymph nodes (lymphatic spread). Small cell carcinoma is the most aggressive tumor to metastasize to the lymph nodes. Typically, the pattern of spread is first to the hilar lymph nodes and then into the mediastinal (usually ipsilateral) lymph nodes. Tumors of the left lower lobe that metastasize to the mediastinal nodes involve the contralateral mediastinum in about 25% of patients.

Hematogenous spread of lung cancer is indiscriminate, and virtually all areas of the body are at risk. There is a particular predilection for non–small cell lung cancer to spread to the adrenal glands, lung, bone, and brain. ACA is more likely to metastasize to the CNS, but SCCA may as well. Bone metastases are usually osteolytic. Lung cancer is the second most common cause of bone metastasis after breast cancer. Metastases rarely occur distal to the elbow or distal to the knee.

It is important to remember that the biology of lymphatic and hematogenous metastasis is different and that a lack of mediastinal or hilar nodal involvement by no means precludes the ability of a non–small cell tumor to metastasize systemically. Patients with these "skip" metastases are not uncommon.

Detection of Lung Cancer

Patients with lung cancer typically are unfortunately most commonly first seen with symptoms and in advanced stage (stages III and IV). Because the pulmonary parenchyma does not contain nerve endings, many lung cancers grow to a large size before they cause local symptoms of hemoptysis, a change in sputum production, dyspnea, obstruction, or pain. With typical doubling times, a 3-cm tumor would have been present for well more than a year. Obstruction of a main-stem bronchus or lobar bronchus may impair mucus passage and cause postobstructive pneumonia, or a lesion irritating a bronchus or the pleural surface may lead to cough. Frequently, patients are seen by their local physician with clinical evidence of pneumonia of several days' onset. The pneumonia may be treated intermittently with antibiotics for a period of several weeks. If the clinical pneumonia does not clear, a chest x-ray is obtained, which frequently identifies the lung cancer. Earlier stages of lung cancer are occasionally found on a screening chest x-ray that is obtained when the patient goes to the physician for a routine physical examination or other nonthoracic-related problem.

Cytologic examination of sputum, chest x-ray, fiberoptic bronchoscopy, or fine-needle aspiration of the mass may further assist the clinician in making the diagnosis and establishing a more precise stage of the patient's lung cancer.

Screening of patients at high risk for lung cancer by sputum cytology or by chest x-ray does not provide a sensitive examination in the presence of small, resectable lung cancer. More recently, however, low-resolution CT of the chest has revealed small nodules undetectable on routine chest x-ray in some patients. Patients with benign nodules and patients identified with high likelihood of early-stage lung cancer were excluded. Some of these nodules have the potential to be lung cancer. Such early detection may improve subsequent survival rates; the improvement in survival during the past 20 years has been largely related to the ability to diagnose earlier-stage lesions. It is hoped that long-term survival rates will result from complete resection. A national trial evaluating the use of this modality in patients at higher risk for lung cancer development is ongoing at the time of publication of this text.

Staging of Lung Cancer

Patients with lung cancer may have specific treatment based on their physical characteristics and their anticipated survival outlook. These groupings have been described within the International System for Staging Lung Cancer. The system was adopted in 1986 and supported by the American Joint Committee on Cancer (AJCC) and the Union Internationale Contre Le Cancer (UICC). In 1997, the International System for Staging Lung Cancer was revised. This international staging system classified patients with lung cancer based on TNM characteristics (*T* corresponds to characteristics of the primary tumor, *N* to the regional and extrathoracic lymph nodes, and *M* to metastasis). Patients with similar survival outlooks were grouped together and their clinical characteristics examined.

Stage I disease is divided into stage IA and IB. Prior stage IIIA (T3 N0) patients had survival characteristics more like those of stage IIB. In 1997, these patients (T3 N0) were moved from stage IIIA to stage IIB to reflect this survival advantage.

The TNM definitions and stage groupings of the TNM subsets are listed in Boxes 59-1 and 59-2 and Table 59-1. Descriptions of T (tumor) and N (nodal) characteristics are given in Box 59-1. Stage grouping definitions are listed in Box 59-2 and Table 59-1. Representative descriptions of stages IA, IB, IIA, IIB, IIIA, and IIIB are shown in Figure 59-9. The lymph node map definitions are shown in Box 59-3. The regional lymph node classification schema is presented in Figure 59-10. This map presents a graphic representation of the mediastinal and pulmonary lymph nodes in relation to other thoracic structures for optimal dissection and correct anatomic labeling by the surgeon.

Lung cancer can be roughly grouped into three major categories:

1. *Stage I and II* tumors are completely contained within the lung and may be completely resected with surgery.
2. *Stage IV* disease includes metastatic disease and is not typically treated by surgery, except in those patients requiring surgical palliation.
3. *Resectable Stage IIIA and IIIB* tumors are locally advanced tumors with metastasis to the ipsilateral mediastinal (N2) lymph nodes (stage IIIA) or involving mediastinal structures (T4 N0 M0). These tumors, by their advanced nature, may be mechanically removed with surgery; however, surgery does not control the micrometastases that exist within the general area of the operation nor systemically.

Despite current surgical efforts, 5-year survival rates by stage are about 65% for stage I patients, 40% for stage II patients, 15% for stage III patients, and 5% for stage IV patients. Lung cancer staging allows physicians to group patients based on the extent of their disease and prospective survival, so that therapy can be applied in a systematic manner for which the patients will benefit. Staging also assists the physician in counseling the patient

Box 59-1 TNM Definitions

T—Primary Tumor

Tx Tumor proven by the presence of malignant cells in bronchopulmonary secretions but not visualized roentgenographically or bronchoscopically, or any tumor that cannot be assessed, as in a retreatment staging
T0 No evidence of primary tumor
Tis Carcinoma in situ
T1 A tumor that is 3 cm or less in greatest dimension, surrounded by lung or visceral pleura, and without evidence of invasion proximal to a lobar bronchus at bronchoscopy*
T2 A tumor more than 3 cm in greatest dimension, or a tumor of any size that either invades the visceral pleura or has associated atelectasis or obstructive pneumonitis extending to the hilar region. At bronchoscopy, the proximal extent of demonstrable tumor must be within a lobar bronchus or at least 2 cm distal to the carina. Any associated atelectasis or obstructive pneumonitis must involve less than an entire lung.
T3 A tumor of any size with direct extension into the chest wall (including superior sulcus tumors), diaphragm, or the mediastinal pleura or pericardium without involving the heart, great vessels, trachea, esophagus, or vertebral body, or a tumor in the main bronchus within 2 cm of the carina without involving the carina, or associated atelectasis or obstructive pneumonitis of entire lung
T4 A tumor of any size with invasion of the mediastinum or involving heart, great vessels, trachea, esophagus, vertebral body, or carina or presence of malignant pleural or pericardial effusion,† or with satellite tumor nodules within the ipsilateral, primary tumor lobe of the lung

N—Nodal Involvement

N0 No demonstrable metastasis to regional lymph nodes
N1 Metastasis to lymph nodes in the peribronchial or the ipsilateral hilar region, or both, including direct extension
N2 Metastasis to ipsilateral mediastinal lymph nodes and subcarinal lymph nodes
N3 Metastasis to contralateral mediastinal lymph nodes, contralateral hilar lymph nodes, or ipsilateral or contralateral scalene or supraclavicular lymph nodes

M—Distant Metastasis

M0 No (known) distant metastasis
M1 Distant metastasis present.‡ Specify site(s).

---

*The uncommon superficial tumor of any size with its invasive component limited to the bronchial wall, which may extend proximal to the main bronchus, is classified as T1.

†Most pleural effusions associated with lung cancer are due to tumor. There are, however, some patients in whom cytopathologic examination of pleural fluid (on more than one specimen) is negative for tumor and the fluid is nonbloody and is not an exudate. In such cases in which these elements and clinical judgment dictate that the effusion is not related to the tumor, the patients should be staged T1, T2, or T3, excluding effusion as a staging element.

‡Separate metastatic tumor nodules in ipsilateral nonprimary tumor lobes of the lung also are classified M1.

Data from Mountain CF: Revisions in the International System for Staging Lung Cancer. Chest 111:1710-1717, 1997; and Mountain CF, Dressler CM: Regional lymph node classification for lung cancer staging. Chest 111:1718-1723, 1997.

Table 59-1   TNM Subsets by Stage

Stages	
Stage 0	Carcinoma in situ
Stage 1A	T1 N0 M0
Stage 1B	T2 N0 M0
Stage IIA	T1 N1 M0
Stage IIB	T2 N1 M0
	T3 N0 M0
Stage IIIA	T3 N1 M0
	T1 N2 M0
	T2 N2 M0
	T3 N2 M0
Stage IIIB	T4 N0 M0
	T4 N1 M0
	T4 N2 M0
	T1 N3 M0
	T2 N3 M0
	T3 N3 M0
	T4 N3 M0
Stage IV	Any T, any N, M1

Simplified Mnemonic for TNM Subsets by Stage of Lung Cancer

	N0	N1	N2	N3
T1	IA	IIA	IIIA	IIIB
T2	IB	IIB	IIIA	IIIB
T3	IIB	IIIA	IIIA	IIIB
T4	IIIB	IIIB	IIIB	IIIB

Data from Mountain CF: Revisions in the International System for Staging Lung Cancer. Chest 111:1710-1717, 1997; and Mountain CF, Dressler CM: Regional lymph node classification for lung cancer staging. Chest 111:1718-1723, 1997.

and for the presence of cervical or supraclavicular lymph nodes. It is these lymph nodes in the cervical or supraclavicular areas that may provide, to the discerning physician, evidence of extrathoracic nodal metastasis (N3 disease). This extrathoracic nodal disease suggests treatment with nonsurgical means such as chemotherapy or radiation therapy.

Patients with lung cancer are usually 50 to 70 years of age; lung cancer is rarely seen in patients younger than 30 years old. Few patients are asymptomatic at the time of diagnosis. Most patients have bronchopulmonary symptoms such as cough (75%), dyspnea (60%), chest pain (50%), and hemoptysis (30%). Fever, wheezing, or stridor may also be present. Some patients have asymptomatic pulmonary nodules identified by screening chest x-ray obtained either for routine physical examination or for a related pulmonary problem.

Other symptoms may include hoarseness, superior vena cava syndrome, chest wall pain, Horner's syndrome, dysphagia, pleural effusion, or phrenic nerve paralysis. Nonspecific symptoms such as anorexia, malaise, fatigue, and weight loss may occur in up to 70% of patients, and patients with symptoms of any sort tend to have a poorer prognosis. Paraneoplastic syndromes are distant manifestations of lung cancer (not metastases) as revealed in

and the family as to potential therapy and prognosis. Figure 59-11 and Table 59-2 demonstrate the follow-up and survival based on the TNM subsets.

Preoperative Assessment of the Patient With Lung Cancer

The preoperative assessment includes the patient's history and physical examination with particular attention paid to the presence or absence of paraneoplastic syndromes

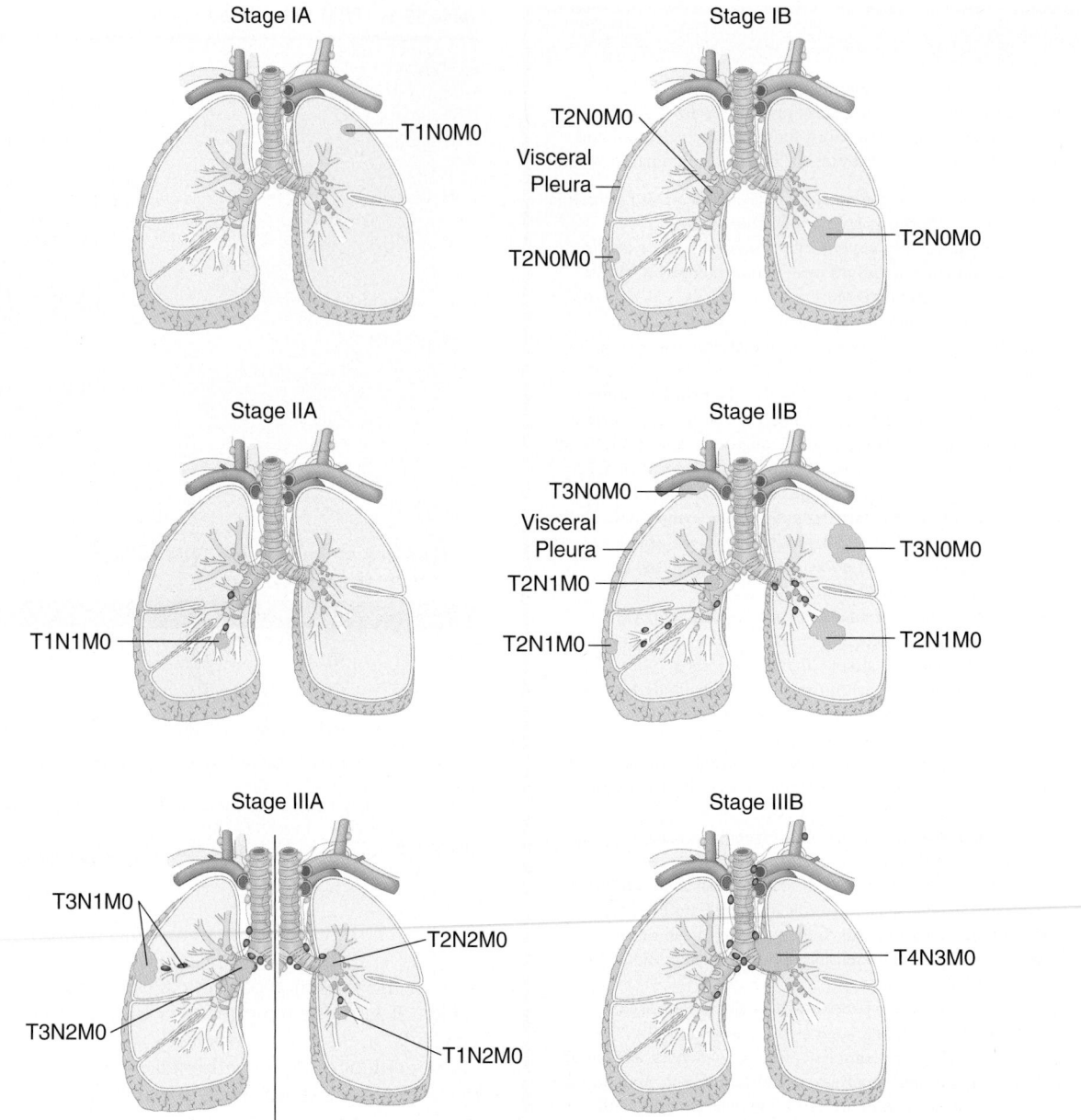

Figure 59-9 Stage groups based on TNM subsets. (From Mountain CF, Libshitz HI, Hermes KE: Lung Cancer: A Handbook for Staging, Imaging, and Lymph Node Classification. Houston, TX, Mountain, 1999, pp 1-71.)

extrathoracic nonmetastatic symptoms (Box 59-4). The lung cancer causes an effect on these extrathoracic sites by producing one or more biologic or biochemical substances. These various effects are grouped into paraneoplastic syndromes. Various criteria for nonresectability have been proposed and are listed in Box 59-5.

Radiographic Staging of Lung Cancer

The standard chest x-ray and CT scan of the chest and upper abdomen (to include the adrenals) are the most frequent diagnostic imaging studies performed in patients with lung cancer. The chest x-ray provides information

on the size, shape, density, and location of the tumor in relationship to the mediastinal structures. It is important that the CT scan be performed with IV contrast to delineate vascular structures. The chest x-ray is performed to evaluate the location of the mass, the presence or absence of thoracic lymphadenopathy, pleural effusion, pericardial effusion, pulmonary infiltrates, pneumonia, or consolidation. Changes in the contour of the mediastinum secondary to lymphadenopathy, and metastasis to ribs or other bone structure may be visualized. Clues to the histology may also be provided. Squamous carcinomas have a tendency to be large and central in location, adenocarcinoma tends to be more peripheral in its initial presenta-

Box 59-3   Lymph Node Map Definitions

N2 nodes—all N2 nodes lie within the mediastinal pleural envelope.

1. Highest mediastinal nodes: Nodes lying above a horizontal line at the upper rim of the brachiocephalic (left innominate) vein where it ascends to the left, crossing in front of the trachea at its midline.
2. Upper paratracheal nodes: Nodes lying above a horizontal line drawn tangential to the upper margin of the aortic arch and below the inferior boundary of number 1 nodes.
3. Prevascular and retrotracheal nodes: Pretracheal and retrotracheal nodes may be designated 3A and 3P. Midline nodes are considered to be ipsilateral.
4. Lower paratracheal nodes: The lower paratracheal nodes on the right lie to the right of the midline of the trachea between a horizontal line drawn tangential to the upper margin of the aortic arch and a line extending across the right main bronchus at the upper margin of the upper lobe bronchus and contained within the mediastinal pleural envelope; the lower paratracheal nodes on the left lie to the left of the midline of the trachea between a horizontal line drawn tangential to the upper margin of the aortic arch and a line extending across the left main bronchus at the level of the upper margin of the left upper lobe bronchus, medial to the ligamentum arteriosum and contained within the mediastinal pleural envelope.

Researchers may wish to designate the lower paratracheal nodes as number 4S (superior) and number 4I (inferior) subsets for study purposes; the number 4S nodes may be defined by a horizontal line extending across the trachea and drawn tangential to the cephalic border of the azygos vein; the number 4I nodes may be defined by the lower boundary of number 4S and the lower boundary of number 4, as described above.

Regional Lymph Node Classification

5. Subaortic (aortopulmonary window): Subaortic nodes are lateral to the ligamentum arteriosum or the aorta or left pulmonary artery and proximal to the first branch of the left pulmonary artery and lie within the mediastinal pleural envelope.
6. Para-aortic nodes (ascending aorta or phrenic): Nodes lying anterior and lateral to the ascending aorta and the aortic arch or the innominate artery, beneath a line tangential to the upper margin of the aortic arch.
7. Subcarinal nodes: Nodes lying caudad to the carina of the trachea, but not associated with the lower lobe bronchi or arteries within the lung.
8. Paraesophageal nodes (below carina): Nodes lying adjacent to the wall of the esophagus and to the right or left of the midline, excluding subcarinal nodes.
9. Pulmonary ligament nodes: Nodes lying within the pulmonary ligament, including those in the posterior wall and lower part of the inferior pulmonary vein.

N1 nodes—all N1 nodes lie distal to the mediastinal pleural reflection and within the visceral pleura.

10. Hilar nodes: The proximal lobar nodes, distal to the mediastinal pleural reflection and the nodes adjacent to the bronchus intermedius on the right; radiographically, the hilar shadow may be created by enlargement of both hilar and interlobar nodes.
11. Interlobar nodes: Nodes lying between the lobar bronchi.
12. Lobar nodes: Nodes adjacent to the distal lobar bronchi.
13. Segmental nodes: Nodes adjacent to segmental bronchi.
14. Subsegmental nodes: Nodes around the subsegmental bronchi.

Data from Mountain CF: Revisions in the International System for Staging Lung Cancer. Chest 111:1710-1717, 1997; and Mountain CF, Dressler CM: Regional lymph node classification for lung cancer staging. Chest 111:1718-1723, 1997.

---

tion, and a small cell carcinoma tends to have bulky mediastinal lymphadenopathy as well as large hilar and central tumors.

Specific attention needs to be paid to whether the mass has cavitation or not and its relationship to the thoracic structures and mediastinum, and whether it is limited or diffuse in appearance. Also sought is the presence or absence of segmental or lobar collapse or consolidation, hilar and mediastinal enlargement, or evidence of intrathoracic metastasis or extrapulmonary intrathoracic extension.

CT of the chest provides more detail than chest x-ray on the surface characteristics of the tumor, relationships of the tumor to the mediastinum and mediastinal structures, and metastasis to lung, bone, liver, and adrenals. Enlargement of the mediastinal lymph nodes can be identified if present. Although CT cannot accurately or consistently predict invasion, it can identify size and the density of mediastinal nodes. In a review article summarizing the accuracy of histologically confirmed CT evaluation of mediastinal lymph nodes using pooled data on 4793 patients, this modality was found to be 60% sensitive and 81% specific, with a positive predictive value of 53% and a negative predictive value of 82%.[20] Clearly, CT alone must be considered an imperfect tool for mediastinal staging.

A high-quality CT evaluation of the chest and upper abdomen to include the adrenals is mandatory because this is a frequent site of extrathoracic metastasis. This examination evaluates the presence or absence of enlarged (≥ 1 cm) mediastinal lymph nodes, and evaluates the liver, adrenals, and kidneys for metastasis. If mediastinal lymph nodes are enlarged (≥ 1 cm), invasive staging may be considered to define the extent of involvement of these lymph nodes with lung cancer metastases. The evaluation may consist of cervical mediastinoscopy, extended cervical mediastinoscopy, VATS, fine-needle aspiration by an extrathoracic or transesophageal route, or other staging modalities. The pathology of biopsied lymph nodes is reviewed before initiation of treatment. Other causes for enlarged lymph nodes include various infections and inflammatory processes.

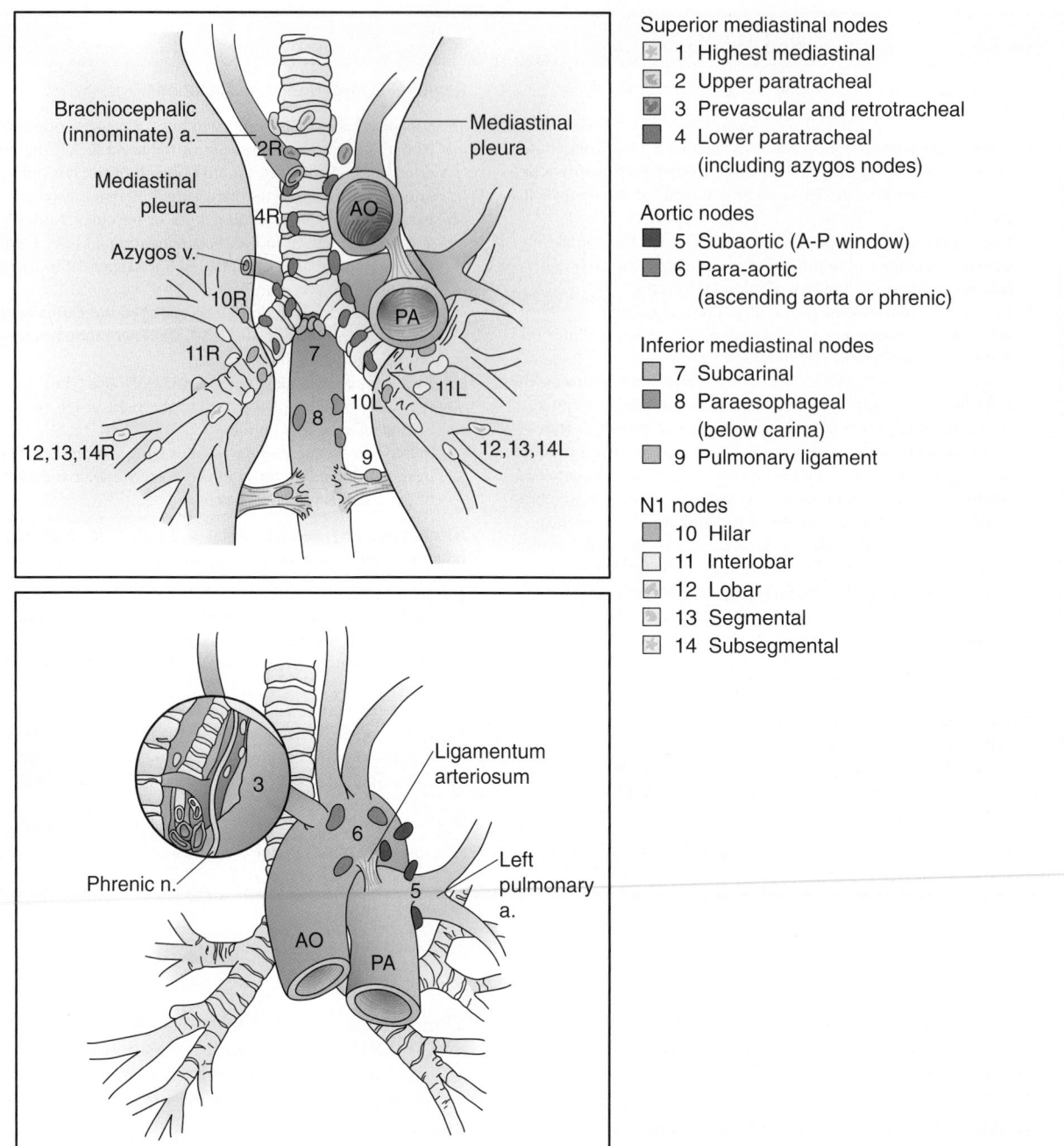

Superior mediastinal nodes
- ☒ 1 Highest mediastinal
- ☒ 2 Upper paratracheal
- ☒ 3 Prevascular and retrotracheal
- ☒ 4 Lower paratracheal
  (including azygos nodes)

Aortic nodes
- ☒ 5 Subaortic (A-P window)
- ☒ 6 Para-aortic
  (ascending aorta or phrenic)

Inferior mediastinal nodes
- ☒ 7 Subcarinal
- ☒ 8 Paraesophageal
  (below carina)
- ☒ 9 Pulmonary ligament

N1 nodes
- ☒ 10 Hilar
- ☒ 11 Interlobar
- ☒ 12 Lobar
- ☒ 13 Segmental
- ☒ 14 Subsegmental

Figure 59-10 Regional lymph node station location. AO, aorta; PA, pulmonary artery. (From Mountain CF, Libshitz HI, Hermes KE: Lung Cancer: A Handbook for Staging, Imaging, and Lymph Node Classification. Houston, TX, Mountain, 1999, pp 1-71.)

Positron emission tomography (PET) evaluation has been established as an important adjunct to mediastinoscopy for defining metastatic involvement of mediastinal nodes with lung cancer and other occult sites of metastases.[20,21] PET scanning is a method of determining the presence or absence of cancer based on the differential metabolism of cancer cells compared with normal tissues.[21-23] Cancer cells metabolize glucose more rapidly than normal cells. Using 18-fluorodeoxyglucose (18FDG) IV as a substrate, cancer cells take up the compound. With subsequent phosphorylation of this compound, FDG-phosphate with tracer is trapped within the cell and can be imaged with PET. PET-FDG scanning may be helpful in distinguishing between recurrent or persistent lung cancer and radiation fibrosis in patients having previous radiation therapy for their disease. The technique is not infallible; infectious and inflammatory conditions can image as avidly as neoplastic cells. The use of this modality, however, has increased the noninvasive accuracy of mediastinal lymph node staging and has more

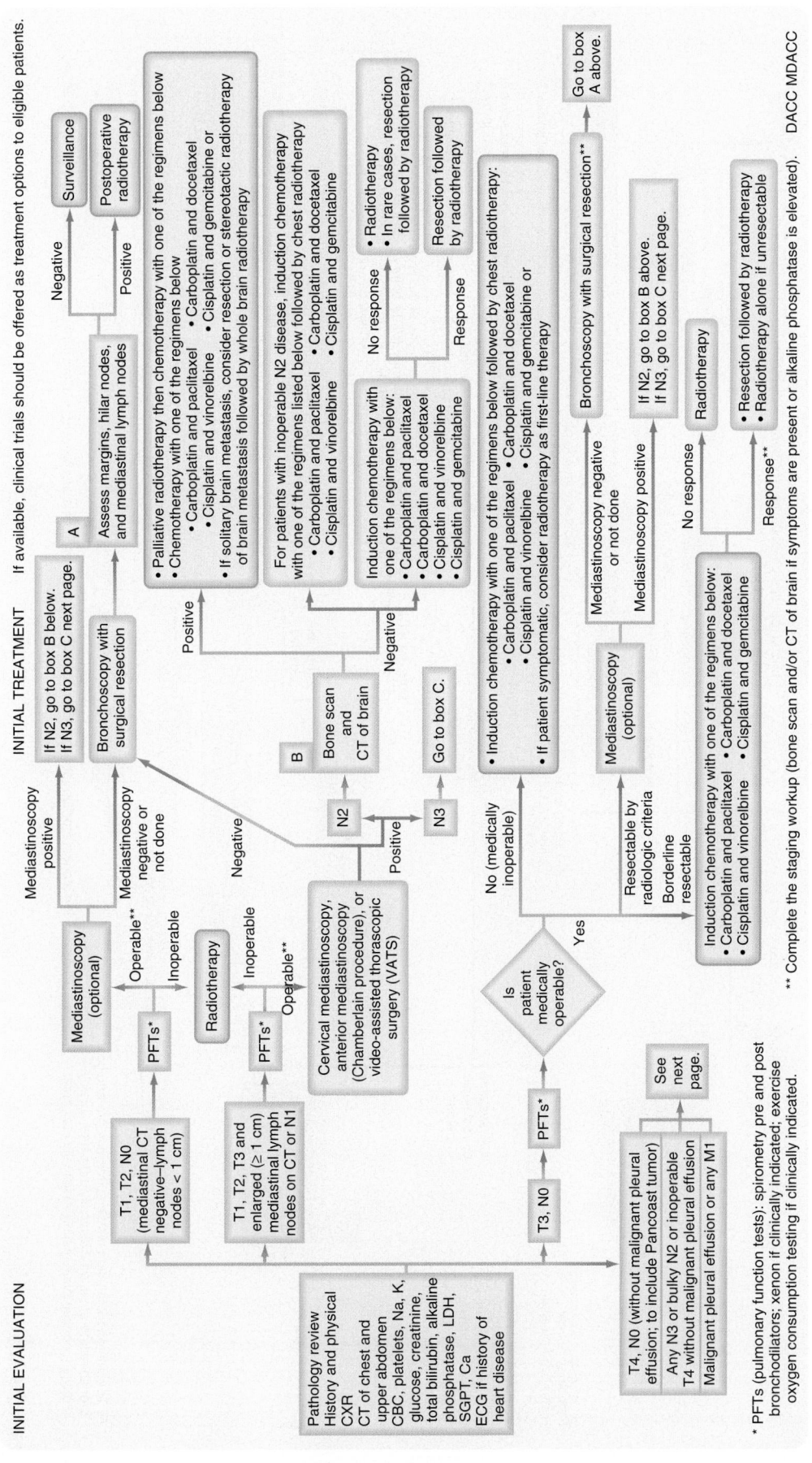

Figure 59-11 Postoperative guidelines for follow-up of patients with non-small cell lung cancer based on TNM grouping. (Copyright © The University of Texas M. D. Anderson Cancer Center, 1999.)

* PFTs (pulmonary function tests): spirometry pre and post bronchodilators; xenon if clinically indicated; exercise oxygen consumption testing if clinically indicated.

** Complete the staging workup (bone scan and/or CT of brain if symptoms are present or alkaline phosphatase is elevated.

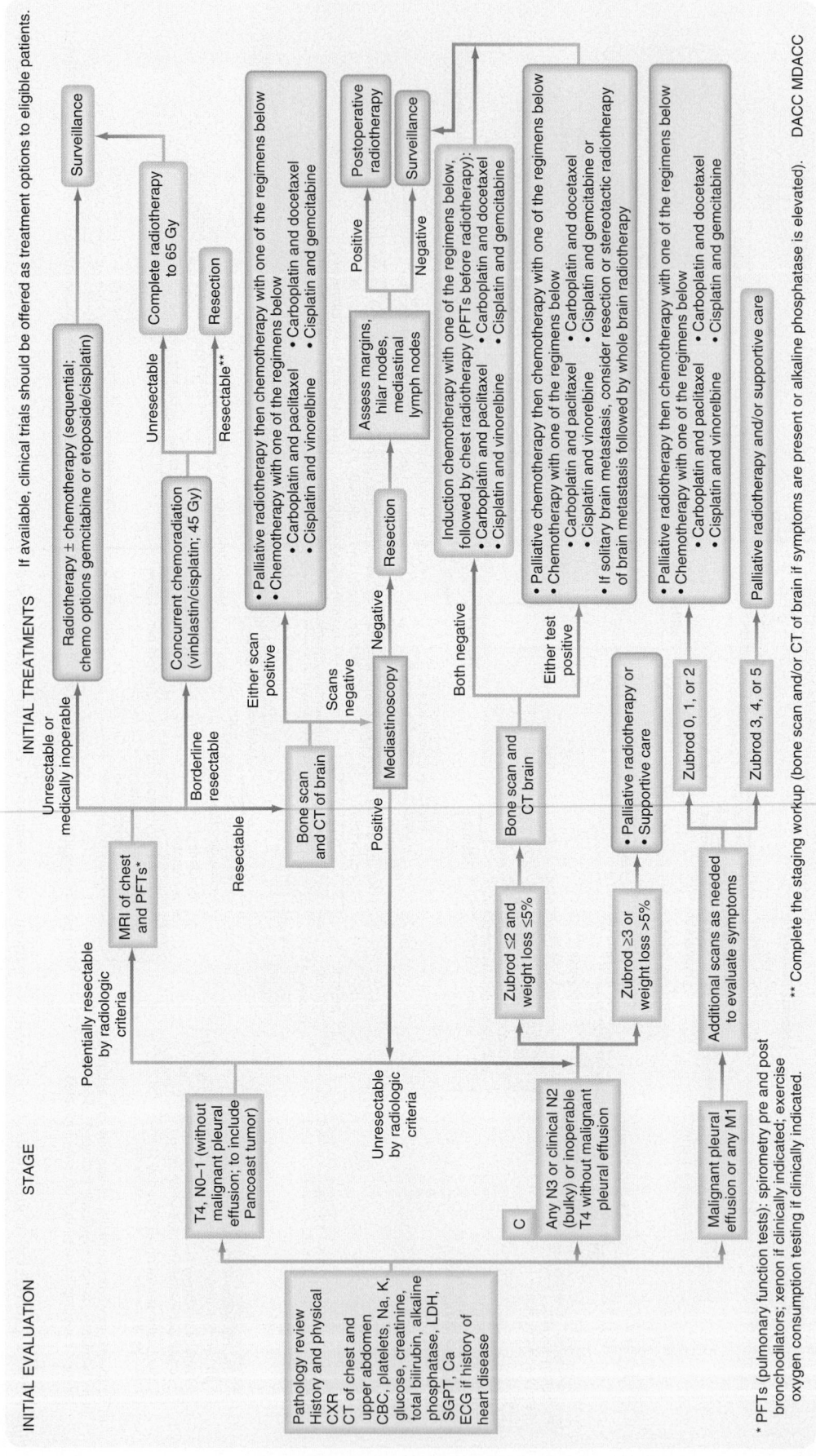

Figure 59-11, cont'd

Table 59-2 Postsurgical Survival Based on TNM Subsets From Mountain and Dressler and Naruke

| TNM SUBSET | MOUNTAIN, 1997 | | NARUKE, 1988 | |
	N	5-Yr Survival (%)	N	5-Yr Survival (%)
T1 N0 M0	511	67.0	245	75.5
T2 N0 M0	549	57.0	241	57.0
T1 N1 M0	76	55.0	66	52.5
T2 N1 M0	288	39.0	153	40.0
T3 N0 M0	87	38.0	106	33.3
T3 N1 M0	55	25.0	85	39.0
Any N2 M0	344	23.0	368	15.1

Data from Mountain CF: Revisions in the International System for Staging Lung Cancer. Chest 111:1710-1717, 1997; Mountain CF, Dressler CM: Regional lymph node classification for lung cancer staging. Chest 111:1718-1723, 1997; and Naruke T, Tomoyuki G, Tsuchiya R, Suemasa K: Prognosis and survival in resected lung carcinoma based on the new international staging system. J Thorac Cardiovasc Surg 96:440-447, 1988.

Box 59-4 Extrathoracic Nonmetastatic Symptoms (Paraneoplastic Syndromes)

General

Weight loss/cachexia
Fatigue
General malaise

Endocrine

Cushing's syndrome from adrenocorticotropic hormone secretion
Inappropriate antidiuretic hormone causing hyponatremia
Carcinoid syndrome
Hypercalcemia
Rarely, hypoglycemia or ectopic gonadotropins

Skeletal

Clubbing, 10% to 20%
Hypertrophic pulmonary osteoarthropathy (painful periosteal proliferation at the ends of long bones), 5%

Neuromuscular (about 15% and most common with small cell carcinoma)

Polymyositis
Myasthenia-like syndrome (Eaton-Lambert)
Peripheral neuropathy
Subacute cerebellar degeneration
Encephalopathy

Vascular thrombophlebitis

Box 59-5 Criteria for Nonresectability

Recurrent laryngeal nerve paralysis
Superior vena cava syndrome
Involvement of main pulmonary artery
Contralateral or supraclavicular node involvement
Ipsilateral mediastinal nodes if high (2R)
Malignant (or bloody) pleural effusion, which may cause dyspnea or pleuritic chest pain or may be asymptomatic
Malignant pericardial effusion
Phrenic nerve paralysis (relative contraindication)
Extrathoracic metastatic disease typically involving the brain, bone, adrenals, or liver
Involvement of trachea, heart, great vessel
Insufficient pulmonary reserve
Other signs that may suggest a more advanced tumor:
  Chest wall pain that may be described by the patient as dull, deep, and persistent
  Horner's syndrome from compression of the sympathetic nerve with unilateral ptosis, miosis, anhidrosis, and enophthalmos
  Phrenic nerve paralysis, with elevation of a hemidiaphragm from nerve paralysis
  Esophageal compression, yielding symptoms of dysphagia from extrinsic compression from enlarged subcarinal left nodes or direct invasion into the left main-stem and carina junction yielding a tracheoesophageal fistula

---

accurately predicted nodes that will require histologic sampling. Using pooled data from multiple studies, PET and CT combined have been shown to be more accurate for mediastinal staging than CT alone, with a positive predictive value of 78% and a high negative predictive value of 93%—a number that approaches invasive staging techniques.[20] In terms of metastatic disease, PET has been shown to demonstrate metastatic lesions not noted by CT and other conventional means in 10% to 20% of cases.[24]

Magnetic resonance imaging (MRI) is at times used to complement CT in evaluating the location of tumors within the chest. MRI has limited utility in the noninvasive staging of lung cancer patients. In the thorax, it may be used to further delineate vascular, bony spinal, or mediastinal involvement, and it is the most accurate means to evaluate brain metastases. When there is a question of invasion, the patient undergoes exploration. Frequently, these tumors may simply abut the structure without invasion. It has been recommended that MRI brain imaging be reserved for patients with stage I or II cancer with new symptoms only (vertigo, headache) and in all patients with stage III and IV cancer.[24]

Invasive Staging and Other Tests

Invasive staging such as bronchoscopy, mediastinoscopy, or fine-needle aspiration is usually considered after non-invasive staging evaluations. These staging procedures may be required for diagnosis to assist in the pretreatment planning for patients with a lung mass. Invasive staging of lung cancer is part of the clinical staging workup (cTNM) and typically includes bronchoscopy, mediastinoscopy, thoracoscopy, or other intrathoracic staging, as well as the complementary pathologic and histologic examinations that are done before definitive surgical resection. Surgical or pathologic staging (pTNM) provides the most accurate staging of the TNM status of the tumor. Invasive staging identifies patients with high likelihood of complete resection and those with metastases to mediastinal nodes for prospective clinical studies (protocols) or for definitive chemotherapy and radiation therapy.

Bronchoscopy is recommended before any planned pulmonary resection and can be performed with transbronchial biopsy to make a preoperative histologic diagnosis by the surgeon or a consultant. Regardless of previous procedures, the surgeon always performs a bronchoscopy before resection to independently assess the endobronchial anatomy, exclude secondary endobronchial primary tumors, and ensure that all known cancer will be encompassed by the planned pulmonary resection. For example, if the tumor is located in the right upper lobe orifice and involves a portion of the right main-stem bronchus or portion of the right bronchus intermedius, a sleeve lobectomy may be required to conserve the right middle and lower lobe, thereby avoiding a pneumonectomy.

Transbronchial biopsy may be performed with various gauges of needle through the flexible bronchoscope. This technique may be used in the biopsy of mediastinal nodes or other masses adjacent to the larger bronchi. As well, a transbronchial biopsy may obtain pulmonary parenchyma by forcing the flexible bronchoscope biopsy forceps through the terminal bronchioles into the lung parenchyma. Potential for hemorrhage and a pneumothorax exists. Use of fluorescence bronchoscopy after IV injection of hematoporphyrin derivatives localizes in situ and superficial tumors. These tumors fluoresce when illuminated with the light from a special laser. The overall sensitivity of transbronchial biopsy is about 76% and the specificity 96%. The average negative predictive value is 71%.[20]

Fine-needle aspiration by a transthoracic route may be about 95% accurate in patients with a poor operative risk. The negative predictive value of this procedure is similar to that of transbronchial biopsy, about 78%.[20]

Fine-needle aspiration is not always needed in the patient with good physiologic reserve who is otherwise an appropriate candidate for surgery (e.g., stages I and II) with a suggestive lesion on imaging studies, but an intraoperative biopsy must be performed before anatomic resection if possible. If the patient does have hard palpable lymph nodes in the cervical or supraclavicular area, fine-needle aspiration or biopsy may provide an accurate diagnosis of metastatic (N3) involvement. Otherwise, a superficial lymph node biopsy or a scalene node biopsy could be performed to obtain tissue for further evaluation. If this N3 lymph node is positive, the patient has stage IIIB cancer, and surgery is not recommended.

About 30% to 44% of newly diagnosed patients with non–small cell lung cancer have involvement of mediastinal lymph nodes. A mediastinoscopy or anterior mediastinotomy (Chamberlain procedure) or VATS is performed in all patients with enlarged (≥1 cm) lymph nodes based on the location of the enlarged lymph nodes, especially if PET is positive. This specific staging (pathologic staging) of mediastinal nodes is required before initiating surgical or medical management. Enlarged lymph nodes (≥1 cm) are more likely to be involved with metastases from lung cancer. Other causes of mediastinal lymphadenopathy include mediastinal inflammation, peripheral pulmonary obstruction, atelectasis, consolidation, bronchitis, pneumonitis, or pneumonia, or some patients may have normally enlarged lymph nodes. In one series of patients with N2-positive lymph nodes, the 5-year survival rate with enlarged lymph nodes on CT scan was 6.6%; with a negative scan, it was 13.5%.

Mediastinal lymph nodes larger than 1.5 cm are more likely to be associated with metastasis (>70%); however, normal-size lymph nodes (<1 cm) have a 7% to 15% chance of being involved. Some thoracic surgeons use CT to select patients for mediastinoscopy with enlarged lymph nodes (≥1 cm) because 90% of patients with a normal mediastinum have negative N2 lymph nodes after mediastinoscopy and pathologic examination. Some thoracic surgeons perform mediastinoscopy on every patient with lung cancer because small lymph nodes sometimes harbor metastasis (~11%); for example, reliance on radiologic staging may miss occult nodal metastases in 11% of patients with a radiographically "negative" mediastinum.

The advent of PET scan evaluation of the mediastinum has made the option of selective mediastinoscopy more appealing because its addition to CT increases the accuracy of noninvasive staging. Mediastinoscopy is recommended before the planned resection if the cancer is proximal, if pneumonectomy may be required, if the patient is at increased risk for the planned surgery or resection, if enlarged or PET-positive lymph nodes are noted on CT scan, or if neoadjuvant therapy is planned. Mediastinoscopy provides a means to assess the mediastinal lymph nodes by palpation and by biopsy for histologic diagnosis. Sensitivity for mediastinoscopy in this situation is 89%, and specificity is 100%. Anterior mediastinotomy or the Chamberlain procedure provides adequate assessment of the left-sided para-aortic and aortopulmonary window lymph nodes. VATS or VATS techniques may also be used to biopsy left hilar lymph nodes and to evaluate the intrathoracic manifestations of a cancer.

Mediastinoscopy can evaluate level 2R and 2L, 4R and 4L, and 7 nodal stations. Aortopulmonary window (level 5) or anterior mediastinum (level 6) can be evaluated using a left parasternal incision, the Chamberlain procedure, or extended mediastinoscopy anterior to the innominate artery. VATS techniques can evaluate enlarged level 5 or 6 lymph nodes and enlarged level 8 or 9 or low-level 7 lymphadenopathy. The extended mediastinoscopy technique is difficult and must only be attempted by those well-trained or experienced in the technique.

In the patient with a right upper lobe cancer, pathologically confirmed metastasis to region 5 (aortopulmonary window) or 6 (left anterior mediastinal) mediastinal lymph nodes (clinical stage IIIB) in the absence of extensive subcarinal adenopathy is extremely unlikely. However, region 4R lymphadenopathy may occur in 10% of patients with left lower lobe cancers. Left upper lobe cancers are unlikely to have 4R (right paratracheal) adenopathy in the absence of extensive subcarinal disease.

In certain patients, careful radiographic evaluation using both MRI and CT is necessary to plan treatment. For example, patients with local extension of lung cancer at the apex of the lung into the thoracic inlet may have characteristics of shoulder and arm pain, Horner's syndrome, and occasionally paresthesia in the ulnar nerve distribution of the hand (fourth and fifth fingers). Patients with all these characteristics may be classified as having Pancoast's syndrome. Pain comes from the C8 and T1 nerve roots. Sympathetic nerve involvement may result in Horner's syndrome (miosis, ptosis, anhidrosis, and enophthalmos). Typically, the first, second, and third ribs are involved and require resection, but the bony spine and intraforaminal spaces can also be involved. MRI is necessary, in addition to CT, to plan the surgical procedure.

Solitary Pulmonary Nodule

A solitary pulmonary nodule (SPN) is frequently a diagnostic and therapeutic dilemma.[25,26] An SPN may be defined as an asymptomatic lesion within the lung parenchyma that is smaller than 3 cm and is circumscribed. A lesion greater than 3 cm is considered a lung mass. Primary malignancy may be found in about 35% of SPNs and solitary metastatic lesions in another 23%. By age 50 years, 50% of SPNs harbor malignancy of some sort. In general, a patient with an SPN undergoes resection for definitive diagnosis and treatment; exceptions follow:

1. Patients who have a mass unchanged for longer than 2 years (documented on serial radiographic examinations)
2. Patients with benign patterns of calcification such as in hamartoma
3. Patients with masses clearly caused by an inflammatory process such as tuberculosis
4. Patients with prohibitive operative risk

If the mass represents active tuberculosis or another infectious process, the lesion may disappear after therapy. The only two consistent clinical predictors of benignity are calcification and stability of 2 years or more. Doubling time can be suggestive, with SPN having a doubling time of less than 1 month or more than 16 months, whereas non–small cell carcinoma usually doubles between 40 and 360 days. Morphology can be suggestive as well;

20% to 34% of spiculated lesions, compared with those that are well circumscribed, are malignant.

Fine-needle aspiration for diagnosis of a new SPN in a patient who is otherwise physiologically fit is often not needed or superfluous. It is only performed if the surgeon is trying to identify a reason not to operate (especially in high-risk patients) or if small cell carcinoma is expected. If the fine-needle aspiration is positive, resection of the nodule is recommended; nondiagnostic results cannot always be trusted, and surgery is recommended. The main problems with transthoracic biopsy of these lesions are the provision of a specific benign diagnosis and the fact that the sensitivity for a specific benign diagnosis was only about 12% to 15% in a number of studies.

MRI has little to no role in the evaluation of SPN; however, PET can be helpful. PET has been shown to have an accuracy of 94% in the diagnosis of benign nodules. PET is used if the appearance of the nodule is equivocal and the patient is a marginal surgical candidate.[26] Caveats include the fact that the spatial resolution of most PET units is greater than 5 cm only and that both bronchoalveolar carcinoma and carcinoid tumors can provide for false-negative scans.

Bronchoscopy for diagnostic purposes in the evaluation of SPN is reserved for experienced centers that are able to use a number of different imaging modalities to assist in approaching these more peripheral nodules, such as fluoroscopy, and on-site immediate pathology to allow for multiple attempts guided by tissue evaluation. The yield otherwise will be low.

A wedge resection may not always be possible, particularly if an SPN is located centrally within the lobe, but intermediate-depth lesions can be removed by carefully coring the lesion out with a needlepoint cautery. For an SPN in the absence of a cancer diagnosis that cannot be removed by wedge resection, a lobectomy is appropriate for diagnosis (and treatment) in the patient who is physiologically fit to undergo a lobectomy. If a cancer diagnosis is obtained, a mediastinal lymph node resection is performed. A pneumonectomy is not performed without a cancer diagnosis. I perform a mediastinal lymph node dissection, not sampling, to optimize pathologic staging of the mediastinal lymph nodes (Box 59-6).

Molecular Markers

Various molecular characteristics may be associated with a worse prognosis in patients with lung cancer.[28] DNA aneuploidy is associated with a poor survival rate. Oncogenes (K-*ras, myc, neu*) serve to regulate, in a positive sense, growth of tumors. K-*ras* mutation is the most frequent mutation, accounting for 90% of genetic mutations in ACA. This oncogene codes for a protein associated with signal transduction. Mutations in K-*ras* are associated with poor survival outlook. Overexpression of *HER2* oncogenes is associated with worse survival rate in patients with lung cancer. Tumor suppressor genes, such as *p53,* normally provide a negative influence on cell growth. If a tumor suppressor gene, such as *p53,* is

---

Box 59-6   Mediastinal Nodes to Be Dissected During Pulmonary Resection for Lung Cancer

The following mediastinal nodal stations should be inspected and dissected, and identified lymph nodes resected during a pulmonary resection for lung cancer.

Right Side (Level)

[2R]	If possible
4R	Paratracheal
7	Subcarinal
8R	Periesophageal
9R	Pulmonary ligament

Left Side (Level)

[2L]	If possible
[4L]	If possible
5	Aortopulmonary window
6	Anterior mediastinal, anterior to the ligamentum arteriosum
7	Subcarinal
8L	Periesophageal
9L	Pulmonary ligament

---

mutated, this negative influence is removed, and the tumor growth occurs unchecked.

Gene therapy trials to replace or modify this mutation are underway and have been shown to be safe when used in a clinical environment.[29] Mutations in the retinoblastoma (*RB*) gene are also associated with poor survival. If both *p53* and *RB* mutations are present, survival expectation is only 12 months, compared with 46 months in patients with normal expression of these proteins. A number of other molecular abnormalities have been identified for non–small cell lung cancer, including mutations of the *FHIT* gene, loss of heterozygosity and deletions on the short arm of chromosome 3, mutations in *EGFR*, and many others of diagnostic and prognostic significance. Several recent molecular expression profiling studies have been performed, and cell cycle, nucleotide metabolism, cell-cell adhesion, transcription, matrix protein, apoptosis, growth factor, and signal transduction genes have all been noted to be differentially expressed when compared with normal lung.[30,31] Using ratios of gene expression, investigators are beginning to determine more precise prognostic, treatment sensitivity, and diagnostic information for lung cancer.[32-35]

Treatment of Lung Cancer

Treatment options include surgery for localized disease, chemotherapy for metastatic disease, and radiation therapy for local control in patients whose condition is not amenable to surgery. Radiation therapy and chemotherapy together are better than chemotherapy or radiation therapy alone for primary treatment of advanced-stage lung cancer. Protocols evaluating chemotherapy, radiation, and surgery for advanced-stage lung cancer are ongoing.

Small cell lung cancer is frequently disseminated at diagnosis. Surgery is not the primary treatment for small cell carcinoma unless it mimics stage I non–small cell cancer at clinical staging presentation. Chemotherapy can provide patients with a survival advantage over no treatment. In patients with an SPN and no evidence of metastatic disease, resection (with wedge resection and frozen section) may reveal cancer. Lobectomy would be appropriate along with mediastinal lymph node dissection. If a wedge resection cannot be performed because of location in a patient with a suspicious nodule (spiculated, PET positive, greater than 1 cm), lobectomy for diagnosis would be appropriate in a physiologically fit individual.

The clinician treats non–small cell lung cancer based on the clinical stage at presentation. Survival depends on the cumulative mechanical and biologic effects of that treatment on the primary tumor and micrometastases. Despite the clinician's best efforts, survival expectations for advanced-stage lung cancer remain dismal for most patients. Even in earlier-stage cases (stages IB, IIA, and IIB), 5-year survival rates may only reach 55%, 50%, and 40%, respectively. In selected patients, combinations of surgery, chemotherapy, and radiation therapy may provide better survival results than a single modality alone. The choice of initial therapy (whether single modality or multimodality therapy) depends on the patient's clinical stage at presentation and the availability of prospective protocols. However, treatment options may vary, even among different subsets of patients within the same clinical stage. Pretreatment staging remains the critical step before initiating therapy.

Treatment of Early-Stage Lung Cancer: Stages IA, IB, IIA, IIB, and Early IIIA

Early-stage lung cancer (stages I and II) may successfully be treated with surgery alone; in most patients, this treatment yields long-term survival rates. Lobectomy is the procedure of choice for lung cancer confined to one lobe. Certain patients with lung cancer with chest wall involvement (T3 N0 M0) may be treated well with surgery alone as a local control modality. En bloc resection of the lung and involved chest wall with mediastinal lymphadenectomy results in about a 50% 5-year survival rate. In addition, T3 N0 M0 patients (with tumors <2 cm from the carina) have a 36% 5-year survival rate with surgical resection alone. Such improved survival rates based on the 1986 staging system have prompted the AJCC and UICC to propose the current (1997) staging system to account for such survival. This stage (T3 N0 M0) has been designated stage IIB.

Based on the favorable results of trials with advanced-stage disease, application of chemotherapy in earlier stages of lung cancer may improve survival expectations. Pisters and colleagues conducted a phase II trial to assess the feasibility (response, toxicity, resectability, and morbidity) of perioperative (a combination of neoadjuvant and adjuvant in selected patients) paclitaxel and carboplatin in patients with stages IB, IIA, IIB, and T3 N1 non–small cell lung cancer. All patients were N2 node-negative. Ninety-four patients were entered in the study, and all patients completed therapy. Major response (CR and PR) occurred in 50 patients (50 of 94, or 54%); 83 patients (90%) underwent exploration, and 75 (82%)

Table 59-3 Results of Randomized Trials for Advanced-Stage Lung Cancer

INVESTIGATORS	TREATMENT	PATIENTS (N)	RESECTION RATE	MEDIAN SURVIVAL (MO)	3-YR SURVIVAL
Rosell et al, 1994*	Surgery (+ radiation therapy)	30	90	8.0	0
	Chemosurgery (+ radiation therapy)	29	85	26.0	29
Roth et al, 1994†	Surgery	32	66	11.0	15
	Chemotherapy	28	61	64.0	56
Pass et al, 1992‡	Surgery	14	13	86	85
	Chemotherapy+surgery	15.6	28.7	23	50

*Rosell R, Gomez-Codina J, Camps C, et al: A randomized trial comparing preoperative chemotherapy plus surgery with surgery alone in patients with non–small-cell lung cancer. N Engl J Med 330:153-158, 1994.
†Roth JA, Fossella F, Komaki R, et al: A randomized trial comparing perioperative chemotherapy and surgery with surgery alone in resectable stage IIIA non–small-cell lung cancer. J Natl Cancer Inst 86:673-680, 1994.
‡Pass HI, Pogrebniak HW, Steinberg SM, et al: Randomized trial of neoadjuvant therapy for lung cancer: Interim analysis. Ann Thorac Surg 53:992-998, 1992.

underwent complete resection. Four pathologic complete responses were noted. The authors concluded that induction chemotherapy is feasible and has a high response rate in earlier stage patients.

Although promising, the results of this and other neoadjuvant treatment trials were supplanted by recent findings supporting the use of adjuvant chemotherapy in early-stage non–small cell lung cancer, and this is now considered the gold standard for multimodality therapy. As early as 1995, a meta-analysis was performed of adjuvant treatment studies in early-stage lung cancer that demonstrated a 13% reduction in the risk for death and an absolute benefit of chemotherapy of 5% at 5 years.

Although encouraging, these results were not statistically significant. Although several smaller trials continued to support the notion of adjuvant chemotherapy, the International Adjuvant Lung Trial (IALT) reported in 2004 was definitive. In this trial, 1867 patients with completely resected stage I to III non–small cell lung cancer were randomized, and the treatment group received one of four cisplatin-based adjuvant regimens. At the time of publication, the median follow-up was 56 months, and reproducible improvements in survival and disease-free survival were in the 5% range, both statistically significant.[36] A subsequent trial, examining the use of adjuvant vinorelbine and cisplatin versus observation in completely resected stage IB and II patients, demonstrated a clinically and statistically significant survival benefit at 5 years (69% in the treatment group, 54% control group).[37]

For stage IA lung cancer, anatomic resection (lobectomy), and mediastinal lymph node dissection alone is the preferred treatment. All patients staged IB-IIB are considered for adjuvant chemotherapy following resection.[38]

Treatment of Advanced-Stage Lung Cancer (Stages IIIA [N2], IIIB, IV)

Treatment decisions require accurate and complete staging as an integral component of pulmonary resection for lung cancer. For postoperative treatment decisions, mediastinal lymphadenectomy determines pathologic stage and provides information to the clinician as to

potential survival and the need for postresection therapy. For nodal stations to be identified and dissected during each lung cancer operation, see Box 59-6.

Most patients with histologically confirmed N2 disease have a biologically aggressive tumor with probable occult metastatic disease. Although pulmonary resection and mediastinal lymphadenectomy can provide some patients with improved survival rate and enhanced local control, most patients will not benefit from surgery as a sole modality for the treatment of pathologic stage IIIa non–small cell lung cancer. Neoadjuvant therapy (platinum based) before surgery for pathologic stage IIIA (N2) disease improves survival expectations over surgery alone (Table 59-3). A prospective trial for stage IIIA (N2) patients (RTOG 93-09) comparing neoadjuvant chemoradiotherapy and surgical resection with definitive chemotherapy and radiation therapy is ongoing.

Advanced-stage lung cancer, particularly with nodal spread, cannot typically be considered a disease effectively treated with a single modality (i.e., chemotherapy or radiation therapy). Surgery alone for stage IIIA (N2), IIIB, or IV lung cancer is infrequently performed because the risks of surgery usually exceed its benefits. The surgeon must balance the value of mechanical extirpation of the local disease (local disease control, pain relief, potential for improved survival) with the risks of a surgical procedure and potential improvement in survival length or quality of life. Typically, the risks exceed the benefits, and surgery is not considered; however, in some patients, surgery for advanced-stage lung cancer may receive benefit by local tumor control, palliation of symptoms, improved quality of life, and the potential for longer survival. Resection for isolated brain metastasis is warranted for improvement in quality of life and survival rate. The primary lung tumor can then be treated according to T and N stage.

Chemotherapy

Combination chemotherapy has been well tolerated and associated with a modest improvement in survival rate. Quality-of-life analysis of patients undergoing chemotherapy has demonstrated maintenance or improvement in quality of life.

Induction chemotherapy followed by radiation appears to improve survival rate in patients with locally advanced lung cancer as shown in prospective randomized studies. In these studies, cisplatin-based combination chemotherapy has been shown to improve survival expectation over and above that achieved with radiation alone.

Dillman and colleagues showed that patients given cisplatin at 100 mg/m² body surface area and vinblastine 5 mg/m² before radiation therapy (60 Gy over 6 weeks) were better off than patients who received the same radiation therapy but began it immediately and received no chemotherapy. This study was reviewed again in 1996. Dillman and colleagues provided data for 7 years of follow-up of induction chemotherapy before radiation therapy. The radiographic response was 56% for the chemotherapy and radiation therapy group and only 43% for the radiation therapy alone group ($P = .092$). Median survival rate was greater for the chemotherapy plus radiation therapy group at 13.7 months compared with the radiation alone group at 9.6 months ($P = .012$). The authors concluded that sequential chemotherapy plus radiation increased survival rate compared with radiation alone.

Le Chevalier and colleagues reported the results of a large prospective study evaluating radiation therapy (65 Gy) compared with radiation therapy and chemotherapy with cisplatin, vindesine, cyclophosphamide, and lomustine. The 2-year survival rates were 14% for radiation therapy alone and 21% for chemotherapy and radiation therapy ($P = .08$). Distant metastasis was significantly lower in the combined treatment group. Local control at 1 year was poor in both groups (17% for radiation therapy alone and 15% for combined therapy).

Sause and colleagues examined three treatment groups of locally advanced, surgically unresectable lung cancer patients:

1. Standard radiation therapy
2. Induction chemotherapy followed by standard radiation therapy
3. Twice-daily radiation therapy

They observed that chemotherapy plus radiation was superior to the other treatment arms (log rank $P = .03$). One-year survival and median survival rates were 46% and 11.4 months, respectively, for standard radiation therapy; 51% and 12.3 months for hyperfractionated radiation therapy; and 60% and 13.8 months for chemotherapy plus radiotherapy.

Concurrent chemotherapy and radiation therapy may provide better patient tolerance and improved survival rate compared with sequential chemotherapy and radiation therapy. A prospective multi-institutional trial is ongoing to evaluate chemotherapy, radiation, and surgery versus chemotherapy and radiation only to define the role of surgery in improving local control beyond that obtained with radiation alone.

Radiation Therapy

Like surgery, radiation therapy is a local control treatment modality. Prospective studies of preoperative radiation therapy alone in clinically resectable cases show that postoperative survival rates do not improve over surgery alone.

Postoperative radiation therapy may provide a local control advantage but no survival advantage in patients with complete resection of lung cancer. Postoperative radiation therapy has no significant survival benefit for patients without evidence of lymphatic metastasis. In a prospective randomized trial by the Lung Cancer Study Group (LCSG 773), local recurrence rates were reduced; however, survival rate was not improved. Radiation therapy can be effective palliative therapy in patients with symptomatic disease such as metastases to the bones or brain.

Complications of radiation therapy include esophagitis and fatigue. Radiation-induced myelitis of the spinal cord is devastating and can be minimized or eliminated by careful administration of the radiotherapy to avoid the spinal cord. Three-dimensional (conformal) radiotherapy and intensity-modulated radiation therapy may further concentrate dose to the treated area while minimizing radiation injury to surrounding tissues.

Lung Cancer Summary

The histologic (not radiologic) diagnosis of metastatic involvement of the enlarged (≥1 cm) mediastinal lymph nodes for lung cancer is the single most important piece of information to determine before treatment decisions are made. For lung cancer patients with negative mediastinal lymph nodes, anatomic pulmonary resection and intrathoracic mediastinal lymph node dissection are performed, and for those with AJCC stage IB and II, adjuvant chemotherapy is considered. For lung cancer patients with positive mediastinal lymph nodes, pulmonary resection is not performed alone, nor is it performed as the initial intervention in a combined treatment program. Rather, a combined program of chemotherapy and radiation therapy would provide these patients with the best chance of improved survival. Entry of these patients into prospective protocols is preferred.

PULMONARY METASTASES

Isolated pulmonary metastases represent a unique manifestation of systemic spread of a primary neoplasm. These patients, with metastases isolated only within the lungs, may have a biology more amenable to local or local and systemic treatment options than other patients with multiorgan metastases. Although primary tumors can be locally controlled with surgery or radiation, extraregional metastases are usually treated with systemic chemotherapy. Radiation therapy may be used to treat or palliate the local manifestations of metastatic disease, particularly when metastases occur within the bony skeleton and cause pain.

One of the first long-term survivors of any pulmonary metastasectomy was reported by Barney and Churchill after resection of a metastasis from a patient with renal cell carcinoma. Local control of the primary tumor was achieved, and the patient survived for 23 years after resection of the metastasis; the patient died of unrelated causes. Other authors have noted that certain clinical characteristics (prognostic indicators) may enable clinicians to identify patients with more favorable disease-free and overall survival expectations. Resection of solitary and multiple pulmonary metastases from sarcomas and various other primary neoplasms has been performed, with improved long-term survival rates in up to 40% of patients so treated.

Isolated pulmonary metastases, therefore, are not viewed as untreatable. Patients who have complete resection of all metastases have associated longer survival expectations than those whose metastases are unresectable. Long-term survival (>5 years) may be expected in about 20% to 30% of all patients with resectable pulmonary metastases (Box 59-7). Optimal (and more consistent) survival statistics await improvements in local control, systemic therapy, or regional drug delivery to the lungs.

Symptoms

Symptoms rarely occur from pulmonary metastases; therefore, diagnosis of metastases is routinely made on chest roentgenograms after primary tumor resection. Few (<5%) patients with metastases are first seen with symptoms of dyspnea, pain, cough, or hemoptysis. Rarely, pneumothorax from disruption of the peripheral pulmonary parenchyma develops in patients with peripheral sarcomatous metastases.

Diagnosis and Identification of Pulmonary Metastases

Routinely, clinicians may evaluate patients for pulmonary metastases based on screening chest roentgenograms. Although the specificity of chest x-rays exceeds 95% when nodules consistent with metastases are identified, their sensitivity (compared with CT of the chest) has prompted some clinicians to screen patients at high risk for recurrent metastases with CT chest scans. CT scans of the chest are sensitive and identify smaller nodules

earlier than conventional linear tomography, although these nodules may or may not be metastases.

MRI is not routinely helpful for the radiographic diagnosis of pulmonary metastases; rather, CT of the chest is preferred. MRI may assist the surgeon in planning the approach needed for resection of these complex intrathoracic neoplasms.

Benign granulomatous diseases may mimic metastases; however, in patients with a prior diagnosis of malignancy, these nodules are most likely metastases (>95%). Clinical stage I or II primary lung carcinoma may be indistinguishable from a solitary metastasis, particularly if the original tumor was SCCA or ACA. For these two histologies with solitary lesions, thoracotomy and lobectomy may be the procedure of choice. Mediastinal lymph node dissection would complete the staging. Fine-needle aspiration of thoracoscopic wedge excision may be helpful for diagnosis or staging of pulmonary changes in high-risk patients. In patients with lymphangitic spread of cancer, biopsy may be required to differentiate neoplasm from infection.

Surgical Treatment

Predictors for improved survival rate have been studied retrospectively for various tumor types. These predictors may allow the clinician to identify selected patients who will optimally benefit from pulmonary metastasectomy. These prognostic indicators are clinical, biologic, and molecular criteria, which describe the biologic interaction between the metastases and the patient and their association with prolonged survival. Pastorino and colleagues retrospectively reviewed more than 5000 patients with metastases treated with resection. Overall actuarial 5-year survival rate was 36%, 10-year survival rate was 26%, and 15-year survival rate was 22%. Cancer could generally be staged by the presence of favorable clinical indicators. These indicators included a disease-free interval of greater than 3 years, an SPN, and germ cell histology.

Surgical procedures for resection include single thoracotomy, staged bilateral thoracotomy, or median sternotomy. These procedures have almost no associated mortality rate and minimal morbidity. There are various advantages and disadvantages inherent to each incision. Patients with pulmonary metastases may also undergo multiple procedures for re-resection of metastases with prolonged survival expectations after complete resection.

Thoracoscopy may readily be used for diagnosis of metastatic disease; however, its use in treatment of metastatic disease is more controversial. In an elegant study, McCormack and colleagues conducted a prospective study of VATS resection for treatment of pulmonary metastases. Patients were screened with CT, followed by VATS, followed by open exploration. The authors found more nodules by thoracotomy and noted that VATS failed to identify all nodules. VATS is not the standard approach for resection in patients with pulmonary metastases. At present, VATS can be advocated only for diagnosis or staging of the extent of metastases. Follow-up on all patients is necessary at regular intervals because the likelihood of recurrence remains for a period of years.

Various prognostic indicators have been studied (Box 59-8). Regardless of histology, patients with pulmonary metastases isolated to the lungs that are *completely resected* have improved survival rates when compared with patients with unresectable metastases. Resectability consistently correlates with improved post-thoracotomy survival rates for patients with pulmonary metastases.

Surgery alone for treatment of pulmonary metastases will fail in a significant number of patients. Use of neoadjuvant or adjuvant therapy may allow for further prolonged survival or cure. Novel therapies such as identification of molecular events for therapy, gene transfer, or regional delivery of therapeutic agents to the lung by way of an isolated pulmonary system (isolated lung perfusion) may provide better and more directed therapy for patients with metastases. Cure in most patients represents a serendipitous occurrence in which the host biology, spread of tumor, response to chemotherapy, and surgical resection together render the patient disease-free.

MISCELLANEOUS LUNG TUMORS

Slow-growing lung tumors may arise from the epithelium, ducts, and glands of the bronchial tree and account for 1% to 2% of all lung neoplasms. Most are of low-grade malignant potential.

Carcinoid tumors (1% of lung neoplasms) arise from Kulchitsky (APUD) cells in bronchial epithelium. They have positive histologic reactions to silver staining and to chromogranin. Special stains and examination can identify neurosecretory granules by electron microscopy. These typical carcinoid tumors (least malignant) are the most indolent of the spectrum of pulmonary neuroendocrine tumors that include atypical carcinoid, large cell undifferentiated carcinoma, and small cell carcinoma (most malignant). Histologic findings include less than 2 to 10 mitoses per 10 high-power fields (HPFs).

Peripheral tumors are usually without symptoms, although central tumors may produce cough, hemoptysis, recurrent infection or pneumonia, bronchiectasis, lung abscess, pain, or wheezing. Symptoms may persist for many years without diagnosis, particularly if only an endobronchial component partially obstructs the airway. Stridor is often the presenting symptom of adenoid cystic tumors because these tumors are most often found in the trachea and main-stem bronchi. Carcinoid syndrome itself is not common and occurs with large tumors or extensive metastatic disease. The chest x-ray may reveal the tumor mass or the results of tracheobronchial traction, but about 25% are normal. CT may assist in localizing the tumor. Bronchoscopy is usually positive unless the nodule or mass is peripheral. Ninety-eight percent of adenoid cystic carcinomas can be identified with CT and bronchoscopy with biopsy. Seventy-five percent of carcinoids can be identified in this matter; and although they tend to bleed, biopsy can usually be performed safely.

Atypical carcinoid may have lymph node or vascular invasion with metastasis. The location is in the main-stem bronchi (20%), lobar bronchi (70%-75%), or peripheral bronchi (5%-10%). They rarely occur in the trachea. There is often some local invasion with involvement of peribronchial tissue. At bronchoscopy, most carcinoids are sessile, although a few are polypoid. The histology is that of small uniform cells with oval nuclei and interlacing cords of vascular connective tissue stroma. Mitoses are infrequent, but occasionally bizarre cells are noted. Atypical carcinoids are more pleomorphic and have more mitoses (>2-10 mitoses/HPF) than typical carcinoid. They have more prominent nucleoli but are more monotonous and have more cytoplasm than oat cell carcinoma. These tumors are more aggressive, with a 5-year survival rate of about 60%. These tumors tend to metastasize to the liver, bone, or adrenal. Electron microscopy can be used to identify neurosecretory granules.

Carcinoid syndrome is uncommon with lung carcinoids, although it might occur with very large or metastatic tumors. Carcinoid syndrome is related to the body's reaction to various vasoactive amines, such as serotonin, substance P, bradykinin, and histamine. Clinical manifestations include flushing, tachycardia, wheezing, and diarrhea. These tumors can produce other substances, such as adrenocorticotropic hormone, melanocyte-stimulating hormone, and antidiuretic hormone.

Surgical resection of typical carcinoid and atypical carcinoid is standard, with complete removal of the tumor and as much preservation of lung as possible. Lobectomy is the most common procedure; endoscopic removal is performed only for rare polypoid tumors if thoracotomy is contraindicated. Survival rate is typically 85% at 5 to

10 years. Patients with metastases tend to die of their disease. Large cell neuroendocrine tumors and small cell cancer are not typically treated with surgery and may be best treated with combinations of chemotherapy and radiation; survival of these patients is poor.

Adenoid cystic carcinoma is a slow-growing malignancy involving the trachea and main-stem bronchi that is similar to salivary gland tumors. Adenoid cystic carcinoma is more malignant than carcinoid tumors and has a slight female preponderance. The tumor typically involves the lower trachea, carina, and takeoff of the main-stem bronchi. One third of tumors may occur in the major bronchi; it is rarely peripheral. One third of patients have tumors that have metastasized at the time of treatment. These patients typically have involvement of the perineural lymphatics, regional nodes, or liver, bone, or kidneys. The tumor arises from ducts in the submucosa and spreads in that plane. Microscopic examination demonstrates cells with large nuclei and a small cytoplasm and surrounding cystic spaces (pseudoacinar type); the medullary type has a Swiss cheese appearance.

Treatment is wide en bloc resection with conservation of as much lung tissue as possible. Mediastinal lymph node dissection and frozen section control may be required to resect all the tumor. Radiation treatment alone may cure about one third of patients who are not amenable to surgical resection.

Mucoepidermoid carcinoma is rare in the bronchi, although the location is the same as carcinoid. This tumor may be of either high- or low-grade malignancy. Most are polypoid avascular submucosal masses that are gray to pink in color. Histologic examination reveals epidermoid cells with keratinization, mucin-producing cells lining cystic spaces, and intermediate cells in the cords. Treatment of these low-grade tumors is like that of carcinoid. The tumor is locally resected. High-grade tumors are treated like lung cancer with equivalent survival rates.

Benign tumors of the lung account for less than 1% of all lung neoplasms and arise from mesodermal origins (Box 59-9). Hamartomas are the most frequent benign lung tumor; hamartomas consist of normal tissue elements found in an abnormal location. Most commonly, hamartomas are manifested by overgrowth of cartilage. Hamartomas are typically identified at 40 to 60 years of age and have a 2:1 male-to-female predominance. They are usually peripheral. They grow slowly in the lung. The chest x-ray usually demonstrates a 2- to 3-cm mass that is sharply demarcated and frequently lobulated. It is usually not calcified, but the "popcorn" appearance on chest x-ray may provide the diagnosis of hamartoma. Cystic adenomatoid malformation may represent adenomatous hamartoma. The lesions usually occur in infants as cysts or immature elements in the lung.

Very low-grade malignancies include hemangiopericytoma and pulmonary blastoma that arises from embryonic lung tissue. Treatment is resection. Tumorlets are epithelial proliferative lesions that may resemble oat cell or carcinoid. These are typically incidental findings noted on examination of resected lung specimens. They rarely metastasize.

Box 59-9   Miscellaneous Lung Tumors

Hamartoma

Epithelial Origin Tumors

Papilloma: Single or multiple, squamous epithelium, occurs in childhood, probably viral, may require bronchial resection but frequently recur

Polyp: Inflammatory-squamous metaplasia on a stalk; bronchial resection may be needed; these do not usually recur

Mesodermal Origin Tumors

Fibroma: Most frequent mesodermal tumor
Chondroma
Lipoma
Leiomyoma: Intrabronchial or peripheral; conservative resection

Granular Cell Tumors

Rhabdomyoma
Neuroma
Hemangioma: Subglottic larynx or upper trachea of infants; radiation therapy
Lymphangioma: Similar to cystic hygroma—upper airway obstruction in neonates
Hemangioendothelioma: Newborn lungs, often progressive and lethal
Lymphangiomyomatosis: Rare, slowly progressive—death from pulmonary insufficiency; fine, multinodular lesions, loss of parenchyma and honeycombing; usually women in their reproductive years
Arteriovenous fistula: Congenital, right-to-left shunt; cyanosis, dyspnea on exertion, clubbing, brain abscess; associated with hereditary hemorrhagic telangiectasia of lower lobes

Inflammatory Tumors and Pseudotumors

Plasma cell granuloma
Pseudolymphoma
Xanthoma

Teratoma

Primary sarcomas of the lung occur rarely. They rarely break through the bronchial epithelium, and a cytologic evaluation by sputum is typically negative. The tumors are usually well circumscribed, asymptomatic, and solitary. Local invasion most frequently occurs, with blood-borne metastasis and lymphatic metastasis occuring less commonly. Resection, similar to lung carcinoma, is feasible in 50% to 60% of patients. Prognosis of patients with leiomyosarcoma is excellent, with about a 50% survival rate at 5 years; all others have poor survival expectations.

Lymphoma of the lung most commonly occurs as disseminated lymphoma involving the lung. The disseminated lymphoma occurs in 40% of patients with Hodgkin's disease and 7% in non-Hodgkin's disease. Primary lymphoma of the lung is rare. The diagnosis is usually made at surgery. A thorough evaluation for other primary sites of lymphoma is made if primary pulmonary lymphoma is suspected preoperatively.

TRACHEA

The trachea is about 11.8 cm long and ranges from 10 to 13 cm. There are 18 to 22 cartilaginous rings, and each ring is about 0.5 cm wide. The internal diameter in adults is 2.3 cm laterally and 1.8 cm anteroposteriorly. The larynx ends with the inferior edge of cricoid cartilage. The cricoid is the only complete cartilaginous ring in the trachea. The trachea begins about 1.5 cm below the vocal cords and is not rigidly fixed to surrounding tissues. Vertical movement is easily possible. The most rigid point of fixation is where the aortic arch forms a sling over the left main-stem bronchus. The innominate artery crosses over the anterior trachea in a left inferolateral to high right anterolateral direction. The azygos vein arches over the proximal right main-stem bronchus as it travels from posterior to anterior to empty into the superior vena cava. The esophagus is closely applied to the membranous trachea throughout its course. The esophagus is not a midline structure but more frequently lies just to the left of the midline of the trachea. The recurrent laryngeal nerves run in the tracheoesophageal groove on both the right and the left. Most commonly, the left recurrent laryngeal nerve lies close to the tracheoesophageal groove on the left and is a bit more laterally displaced on the right.

The trachea is up to 50% cervical with hyperextension in the young patient. The location of the carina is at the level of the angle of Louis anteriorly and the T4 vertebra posteriorly.

The blood supply to the trachea is lateral and segmental from the inferior thyroid, the internal thoracic, the supreme intercostal, and the bronchial arteries. One must never circumferentially dissect more than 1 to 2 cm of trachea that will remain in the patient, before or after reconstruction. The potential for tracheal necrosis is increased with circumferential dissection.

Stenosis of the trachea implies significant functional impairment. A normal, 2-cm trachea has a 100% peak expiratory flow rate. A 10-mm opening provides an 80% peak expiratory flow rate. At 5 to 6 mm, only a 30% expiratory flow rate is obtained.

Congenital lesions of the trachea may be lethal (e.g., tracheal atresia) or may provide significant functional impairment, depending on the extent of the stenosis. Stenosis may be generalized, funnel type, segmental (which is most common), or weblike. Treatment consists of dilation for resection of webs. For localized or segmental stenosis, resection and reanastomosis are performed. One needs to limit resection to one third or less of the trachea. A pericardial patch for a generalized or funnel-type stenosis may be required.

Vascular rings such as double aortic arch (right aortic arch with left ligamentum) may cause pulmonary insufficiency or dyspnea. The trachea is normal, and release of the ring provides relief of symptoms. This is in contrast to pulmonary artery sling, consisting of the left pulmonary artery coming from the right pulmonary artery traveling between the trachea and esophagus, which is identified by anterior indentation of the esophagus on barium swallow and by compression of the trachea.

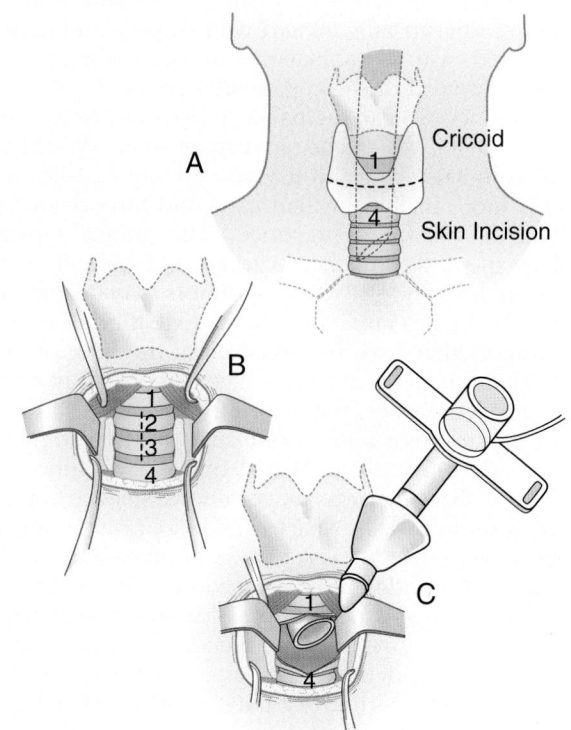

Figure 59-12 Technique of tracheostomy. **A,** An endotracheal airway is in place. With the patient's neck extended and centered in the midline, a short horizontal incision is made over the second or third tracheal ring after the level of the cricoid cartilage has been carefully palpated. The first and fourth tracheal cartilages are numbered. **B,** After horizontal division of the platysma, the strap muscles are separated in the midline, the cricoid is identified, and the thyroid isthmus usually is divided and sutured to allow easy access to the second and third tracheal rings. The second and third rings are incised vertically. Occasionally, an additional partial incision of the fourth ring is necessary. **C,** Smooth thyroid pole retractors are used to spread the opening in the trachea. The endotracheal tube is withdrawn to a point just above the incision. The tracheostomy tube is introduced with a small amount of water-soluble lubricant and with its large-volume cuff collapsed. The endotracheal airway is not removed until it is demonstrated that the tracheostomy tube is properly seated and permits suitable gas exchange. Closure is made with simple skin sutures. The flange of the tracheostomy tube is both sutured to the skin and tied with the usual tapes around the neck. On a rare occasion when an airway cannot be established from above, an emergency incision may be necessary over the cricothyroid membrane for rapid establishment of a temporary airway.

About half of patients have a separate tracheal stenotic problem (most commonly circumferential rings), and correction of the vascular sling alone would not correct the respiratory distress: the tracheal stenosis must also be treated. Congenital tracheomalacia, identified as a collapsible wall seen on bronchoscopy, may be related to chronic compression by the innominate artery and treated with aortopexy.

Tracheostomy is one of the most commonly performed operations. The technique is shown in Figure 59-12. For an elective procedure, the incision is made about 1 to 2 cm above the sternal notch. The strap muscles are separated in the midline to expose the trachea. Division of two tracheal cartilages (usually rings 2 and 3) is performed in a longitudinal (vertical) manner to insert the tracheostomy appliance. Occasionally, the thyroid isthmus must be divided. Rarely, a high innominate artery is encountered and must be protected.

Primary neoplasms of trachea include squamous cell carcinoma in about two thirds of patients and adenoid cystic carcinoma in other patients. Squamous cell carcinoma may be focal, diffuse, or multiple. The physical appearance may be exophytic or ulcerative. One third of these primary tracheal tumors have extensive local spread or metastases at initial presentation. Adenoid cystic carcinoma (previously called *cylindroma*) has a propensity for intramural and perineural spread. In adenoid cystic carcinoma, negative margins are important. Margin evaluation with frozen-section control is performed for stricture resection. Clinical features include dyspnea on exertion, wheezing, cough with or without hemoptysis, and recurrent pulmonary infections.

Secondary neoplasms of the trachea may include those related to laryngeal carcinomas with distal or inferior extension, recurrence of these laryngeal carcinomas at the tracheal stomal site, or other skip metastases. In patients with previous laryngectomy, anterior mediastinal tracheostomy may be required. Five centimeters of uninvolved trachea (i.e., negative margins at a minimum of 5 cm above the carina) is the minimal length of trachea that can remain to ensure optimal potential for recovery. To minimize innominate artery fistula, the trachea may be moved under the innominate artery. Cervical exenteration, with resection of tumor recurrence and portion of trachea, requires resection of the breastplate (manubrium, first rib, clavicles to the angle of Louis) before anterior mediastinal tracheostomy.

Involvement of the trachea because of local extension from bronchogenic carcinoma may contraindicate resection. Involvement of the trachea because of local extension of esophageal carcinoma may require palliative external-beam radiation or endoscopic palliation with laser, bronchoscopy, or esophagoscopy, or perhaps intraluminal brachytherapy. For thyroid carcinoma, resection of a short segment of trachea in continuity with thyroid may be performed with primary repair. However, resection is contraindicated for extensive anaplastic thyroid tumors because recurrence is rapid and risks often exceed anticipated benefits.

Infection and inflammation are uncommon causes of tracheal obstruction.

Tracheal Trauma

Penetrating injuries to the trachea are usually cervical; penetrating injuries that involve the mediastinal trachea are often lethal. Penetrating cervical injuries often involve the esophagus, and concurrent esophageal injury needs to be excluded by barium esophagogram or esophagoscopy. Neck exploration may be required.

Blunt trauma to the neck or trachea can produce lacerations, transections, or shattering injuries of both the cervical and mediastinal trachea.

Clinical features of a cervical injury are suggested by subcutaneous air in the neck, respiratory distress, and hemoptysis. Diagnosis is made by bronchoscopy.

Injury to the mediastinal trachea may be suggested by mediastinal or subcutaneous emphysema, pneumothorax of a lung that fails to expand after chest tube insertion, or a large air leak. Other clinical signs include respiratory distress and hemoptysis. Diagnosis is made by bronchoscopy. A chest tube may be inserted as initial management of a pneumothorax on screening trauma chest x-ray. If the lung does not completely inflate, a second chest tube may be inserted. If the pneumothorax or a continuous air leak persists, a bronchoscopy is recommended to exclude a mediastinal tracheal or bronchial injury. Anesthetic management with laryngeal mask airway may be helpful for initial examination for full visualization of the airway before endotracheal intubation.

Management of tracheal injuries includes control of airway, endotracheal intubation (using flexible bronchoscopy as a guide), or emergency tracheostomy. If emergency tracheostomy is considered, it is performed through the area of the tracheal tear (because this area is likely to be resected during the definitive reconstruction procedure). Cervical injuries may be treated conservatively. The endotracheal tube is placed distal to the lesion, and the cuff is kept inflated for about 2 days. This approach is indicated only if a small partial laceration is identified, there is little subcutaneous air, there is good apposition of lacerated tissue, and there are no other associated injuries. Cervical injury to trachea may also be treated with primary repair without tracheostomy. This approach is indicated with most knife wounds, many gunshot wounds, and occasional cases of blunt transections.

Primary repair of tracheal injury may be accomplished with tracheostomy, if the tracheostomy is performed distal to the repair. This approach is indicated for some blunt transections and some gunshot wounds. Alternatively, one may consider initial tracheostomy along with delayed repair. The tracheostomy may be best done through the damaged trachea. This approach is indicated for complex shattering injuries of the trachea, especially with significant laryngeal involvement.

For injuries to the mediastinal trachea, the surgical approach is thoracotomy through the right fourth intercostal space. Tracheostomy is rarely needed. Most patients have selective intubation of the left main-stem bronchus, double-lumen tube, or jet ventilation. Associated esophageal injuries are repaired primarily. Some tissue (e.g., the sternocleidomastoid or strap muscle) needs to be interposed between the two structures.

Postintubation injuries occur because of laryngeal or tracheal irritation from an indwelling endotracheal tube. This condition is usually reversible. Vocal cord fusion must occasionally be treated by division of the fissure. The cricoid is rarely injured but is difficult to repair. For patients with a tracheostomy stoma, postintubation injuries are common. Granulation tissue occurs, as does anterolateral stricture of the trachea. There are various predisposing factors, including too large a stoma, infection in the stoma, and excessive pressure from connecting systems. The cricoid may be damaged either by cricothyroidotomy or by too proximal a tracheostomy.

Low-pressure cuffs on the endotracheal tube have reduced cuff injuries. Pathogenesis is directly proportional to pressure necrosis. A wide spectrum of injury may occur, depending on depth of damage, including mucosal-tracheal stenosis, tracheomalacia, and full-thickness stricture. Clinical features of tracheal stenosis include dyspnea on exertion, stridor or wheezing (which is easily noted), and perhaps episodes of obstruction by small amounts of mucus.

Acquired tracheoesophageal fistula is the result of prolonged intubation with erosion posteriorly. Patients usually also have an indwelling nasogastric tube. The most common clinical appearance is that of a sudden appearance of copious secretions from the tracheobronchial tree or of methylene blue–colored tube feedings promptly appearing in the airway along with increasing difficulty ventilating the patient. Gastric distention may also occur.

The tracheoinnominate fistula may result from prolonged cuff erosion inferiorly and anteriorly in the trachea. Inappropriate low stoma may further increase the likelihood of a direct erosion of the trachea by the innominate artery. The tip of the endotracheal tube may predispose to erosions or granulomas within the trachea. Tracheoinnominate fistula may present with sudden exsanguinating hemorrhage. The patient usually has had one or more previous sentinel hemorrhages. Investigation of these sentinel hemorrhage episodes is imperative.

The principles of management of tracheal problems include a full evaluation of the larynx to ensure its integrity before tracheal repair. Direct or indirect endoscopy as well as fluoroscopy may be needed. A tracheal stenosis rarely demands a definitive procedure, either electively or emergently. However, emergency management of obstruction may include sedation, humidified air, or racemic epinephrine by nebulizer. In addition, dilation under general anesthesia may be helpful. The first choice of placement of the tracheostomy is through the stricture, then through the old tracheostomy site, then remote from the lesion. Exceptions include those stenoses immediately above the carina because they cannot readily be stented. Conservative measures can be supplemented on a chronic basis with a stent, especially if the patient is poor risk or has a partial-thickness lesion with potential for regression.

Contraindications to trachea repair include the following:

1. Inadequately treated laryngeal problem (which does not include single vocal cord paralysis)
2. Need for ventilatory support or permanent tracheostomy for patients with amyotrophic lateral sclerosis, myasthenia gravis, or quadriplegia
3. Use of high-dose steroids
4. Inflamed or recent tracheostomy

Poor pulmonary reserve is not a contraindication for repair in patients who have been weaned from the ventilator.

Various techniques may be considered for diagnosis of tracheal abnormalities. Plain films of the trachea and routine chest roentgenograms (posteroanterior, lateral, and oblique) are critical first steps. CT of the trachea is good for examining luminal compromise; however, it is less suitable than linear tomograms for longitudinal abnormalities. Fluoroscopy may be helpful for the diagnosis of tracheomalacia. A contrast tracheogram is not always necessary. If the patient has symptoms of dysphagia or if an esophageal cancer is suspected, a barium swallow is helpful to evaluate the extent of esophageal involvement.

Bronchoscopy is generally best deferred to the time of the proposed treatment. This approach avoids precipitating an acute episode of tracheal obstruction in an outpatient area. Exceptions to this rule may include highly complicated situations such as attempted previous repair or the need for urgent dilation. Both flexible and rigid bronchoscopes should be available, and the surgeon should be adept at their use.

The surgical management of tracheal problems may be complex. General inhalational anesthesia is used, and induction may take a long time if the stenosis is tight. If the stenosis is less than 5 to 6 mm, dilation may be required before passing the endotracheal tube. This may be performed with rigid bronchoscopy. If the stenosis is greater than 5 to 6 mm, the endotracheal tube may be positioned to a point above the stricture for induction. Stenoses that are subglottic must be dilated for intubation. The endotracheal tube often goes alongside tumors.

Surgical approaches to the trachea follow:

1. Purely cervical for the upper third
2. Cervicothoracic (with upper sternal split) (Fig. 59-13)
3. Cervical approach plus upper sternal split plus right fourth anterior thoracotomy to expose the entire trachea posteriorly and inferiorly (this approach is rarely used)

The right fourth posterolateral thoracotomy provides the best exposure of the lower trachea and carina (Fig. 59-14).

The cervical approach with or without an upper sternal split is usually used for tumors of the upper half of the trachea plus all benign tracheal stenoses (because these usually occur as a result of endotracheal tube placement). The posterolateral thoracotomy is used for tumors of the lower half of the trachea plus carinal reconstruction. Rigid bronchoscopy for diagnosis, biopsy, dilation, or treatment may be required if the tumor cannot be immediately resected (Fig. 59-15).

In general, the amount of trachea that can be resected is about 5 cm but varies from person to person. Various techniques can be used to achieve this resection without undue tension on the anastomosis. The anterior cervical approach plus mobilization of the trachea and neck flexion can allow for 4 to 5 cm of trachea resection. A suprahyoid release may achieve 1 cm of additional length, and mobilization of the right hilum, together with division of the pericardium around the right hilum, may achieve an additional 1.4 cm.

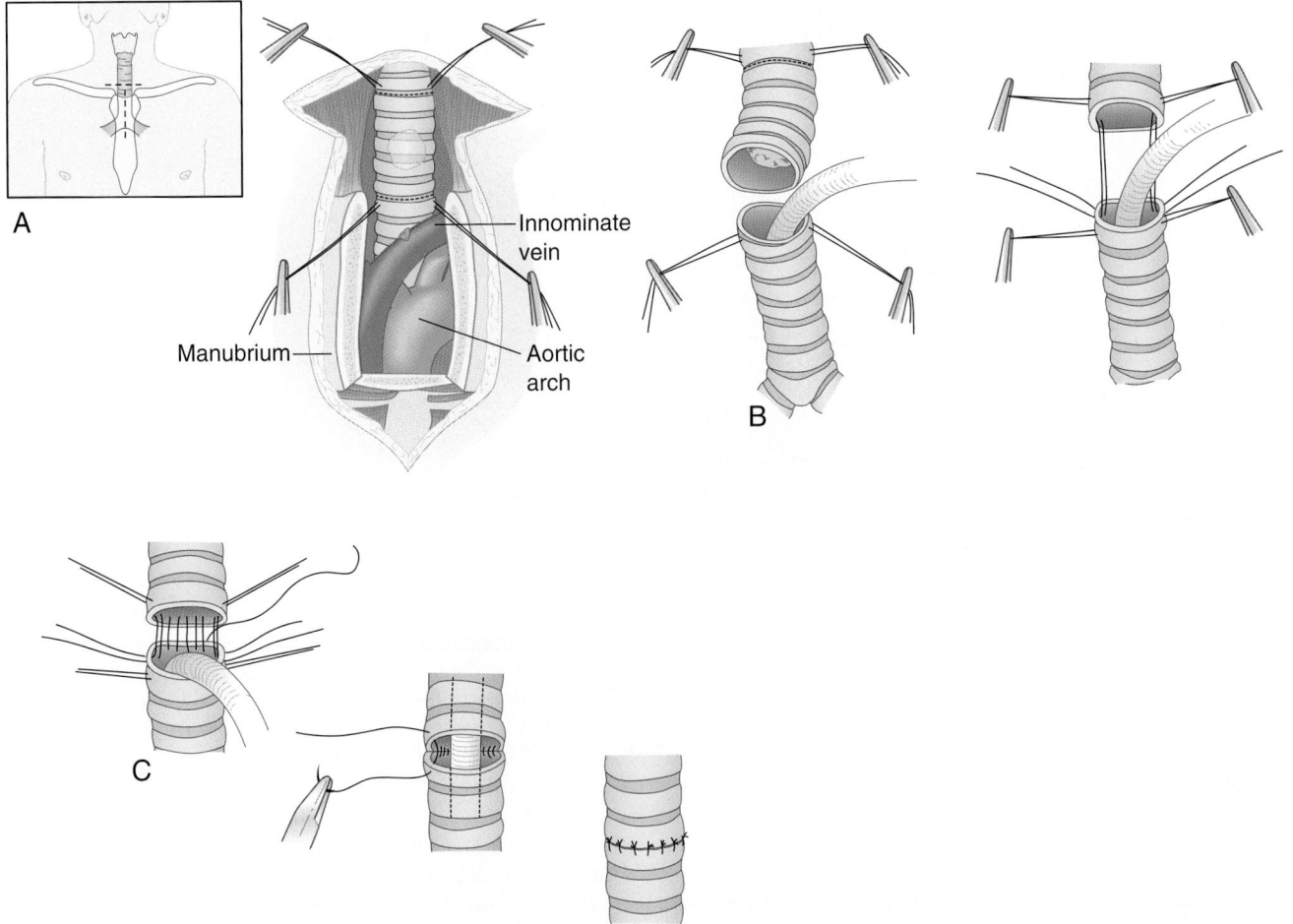

Figure 59-13 A, Exposure of the midtrachea through a cervical and partial sternal-splitting incision. The extent of the resection has been marked by sutures. **B,** After distal division, a sterile, armored endotracheal tube is placed. After proximal resection, two mattress sutures are placed in the edges of the cartilaginous rings. A simple, running suture completes the membranous anastomosis. **C,** At this point, the original endotracheal tube is positioned in the distal trachea so that the anastomosis can be completed with interrupted, simple sutures between cartilaginous rings.

The reconstruction of the upper trachea may be performed through a collar incision through an old tracheostomy site, which is convenient. Skin flaps are created superiorly to the thyroid prominence and inferiorly to the suprasternal notch. The sternal split is performed whenever indicated. The entire anterior length of the trachea is exposed, close to the tracheal wall. Limited circumferential dissection is performed around the trachea just below the lesion. Silk stay sutures are placed on either side below and later above the lesion. The trachea is transected just below the stricture or tumor. The endotracheal tube is placed across the operative field into the distal trachea. The diseased trachea is dissected superiorly and then transected above the lesion. Posterior mobilization and neck flexion are performed. Posterior sutures are placed with knots on the outside, and the patient is reintubated through the trachea. Anterior sutures are then placed and tied. No tracheostomy is performed. If ventilation is necessary, an endotracheal tube is used with the cuff away from the anastomosis.

A suprahyoid release as described by Montgomery achieves a little more than 1 cm of length by cutting the mylohyoid, the geniohyoid, and genioglossus muscles from the superior surface of the hyoid bone. The hyoid bone is transected on either side just medial to the digastric muscles. This technique probably yields less dysphagia or aspiration than the thyrohyoid release procedure.

Stenosis of the subglottic larynx or cricoid stenosis is a challenging technical procedure. The recurrent nerves innervate the larynx just superior to the posterolateral cricoid on each side. If the tracheal lesions only involve the anterior surface, the anterior cricoid can be removed and the distal trachea beveled to match the defect. This maneuver spares the recurrent laryngeal nerves. With circumferential involvement, it may be necessary to perform a laryngectomy. Otherwise, an attempt to preserve the larynx could be made. The anterior cricoid is removed with a rectangle of posterior cricoid. This leaves the posterolateral portions of the cricoid intact to protect the recurrent laryngeal nerves. The beveled trachea may

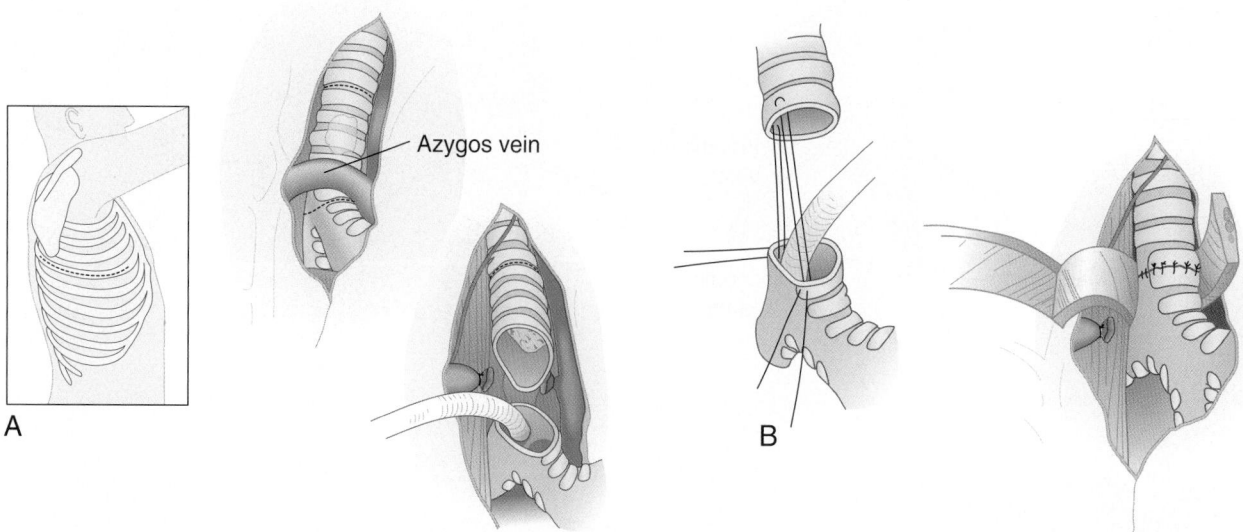

Azygos vein

A

B

Figure 59-14 A right serratus-sparing posterolateral thoracotomy is extended behind the scapula. Proximal and distal exposure shows a tracheal tumor near the bifurcation. **A,** After division of the azygos vein and the distal trachea, a sterile, armored endotracheal tube is placed into the left main-stem bronchus. After proximal resection, the interrupted mattress sutures are placed at the edges of the tracheal rings. **B,** After completion of the anastomosis (see Fig. 59-13), a vascularized intercostal muscle flap is placed around the anastomosis.

be brought up to this level along with a flap of membranous trachea posteriorly to match the posterior defect.

Reconstruction of the lower trachea is performed in the right fourth intercostal space. Intubation of the distal trachea or the left main stem is performed. Carinal reconstruction is usually performed for tumor and is the most feasible of alternative reconstructions chosen.

The technique of tracheostomy is best approached through cervical incision and a vertical incision through the second and third or the third and fourth tracheal rings. The tracheostomy cannot be placed too low because erosion of the innominate artery by the tracheostomy prosthesis may occur.

EMPHYSEMA

Emphysema is defined as dilation and destruction of the terminal air spaces. These air cavities may be defined as blebs—subpleural air space separated from the lung by a thin pleural covering with only minor alveolar communications—or bullae—larger than a bleb with some destruction of the underlying lung parenchyma. Microscopically, there are two important types of emphysema: centrilobular and panacinar. Centrilobular emphysema primarily involves the respiratory bronchioles; the distal alveoli may be normal. In severe cases, the distal alveoli may be damaged and incorporated into the central air space. Centrilobular emphysema is seen almost exclusively in smokers. It usually predominates in the upper lobes. Panacinar emphysema involves the entire distal lung unit, distorting and destroying alveoli and respira-

tory bronchioles alike; it can occur throughout the lung but may predominate in the lower lobes.[39]

Bullous emphysema either is congenital without general lung disease or a complication of COPD with more or less generalized lung disease. The challenge is to separate the disability related to the bullae from that caused by the chronic emphysema or chronic bronchitis. The DLCO is a good index of the state of severity of the generalized lung disease. On pulmonary angiography, bullae are cold and do not contain vessels. The bullae may compress normal lung with crowding of the relatively normal pulmonary vasculature. COPD may show abrupt narrowing and tapering of vessels. Surgical therapy includes resection of the bullae to leave functioning lung tissue.

Symptomatic patients with progressive dyspnea may undergo removal of the bullae with good results. The disease must be localized, with the air space occupying at least 40% to 50% of one hemithorax. The remaining "good" lung parenchyma is compressed by the bulla. Simple removal of the bulla alone is required. Lobectomy is seldom indicated because good lung tissue is removed, which is frequently needed for independent function by these patients with significant lung impairment. Operative mortality rate varies from 1.5% to 10%, depending on the patient's age and degree of emphysema. Pulmonary sepsis and prolonged air leaks are the most common nonfatal major complications. Proper treatment and preparation with pulmonary therapy before surgery, exercise programs, and thin strips of bovine pericardium or absorbable material to reinforce surgically stapled suture lines are helpful in preventing these complications.

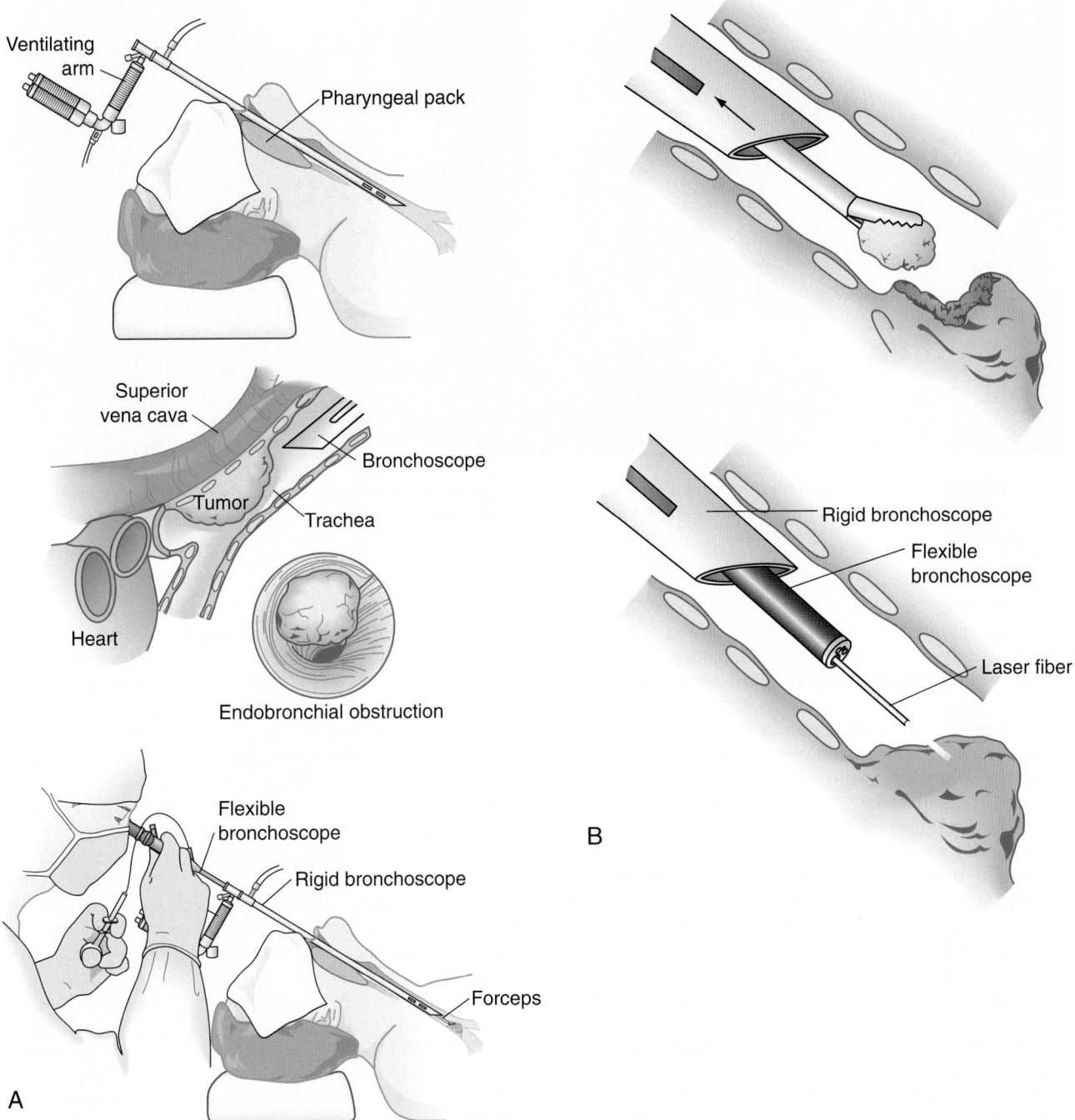

Figure 59-15 A, Proper technique for rigid bronchoscopy in a patient with a tracheal mass. *Top,* Pharyngeal packing is used to protect the esophagus. *Middle,* A nearly obstructing tumor is shown. *Bottom,* A flexible bronchoscope is placed into the rigid scope for the biopsy. This protects the airway. **B,** A technique for endoscopic resection of a tracheal mass with a rigid bronchoscope without (*top*) and with (*bottom*) use of the laser. (From Sugarbaker DJ, Mentzer SJ, Strauss G, Fried MP: Laser resection of endobronchial lesions: Use of the rigid and flexible bronchoscopes. Oper Tech Otolaryngol Head Neck Surg 3:93, 1992.)

Cysts are congenital air spaces lined by epithelium; pneumatoceles are an acquired postinflammatory air space with an epithelial lining. The cause is probably the result of biochemical alterations that permit alveolar wall destruction, often the result of staphylococcal pneumonia in children.

α_1-Antitrypsin deficiency is an autosomal recessive trait that affects 1% to 2% of all emphysema patients and commonly begins before the age of 40 years. Women are more likely than men to have this syndrome. Antitrypsin inhibits neutrophil elastase and other serine proteinases. This homeostatic function controls major proteolytic

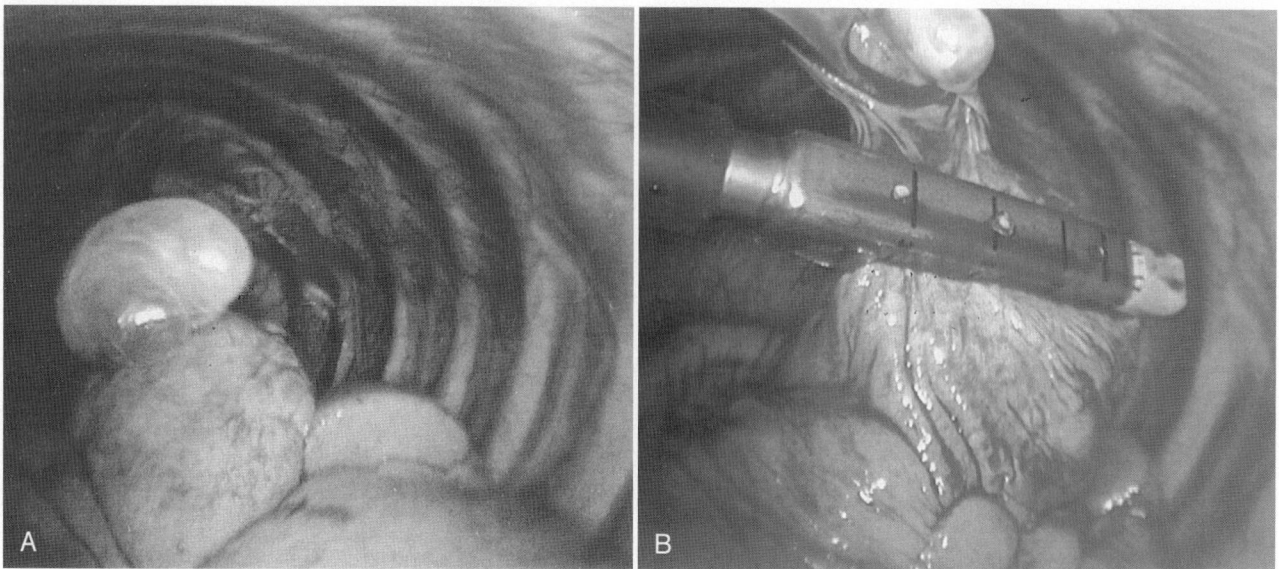

Figure 59-16 **A,** Thoracoscopic view of a typical apical bleb in a young patient who was first seen with spontaneous pneumothorax. **B,** Initial application of a linear stapler in excision of an apical bleb.

cascades. Absence of this serine proteinase inhibitor allows intrapulmonary elastase activity and neutrophil elastase activity (released from inflammatory cells) to act without control, thereby causing panacinar emphysema. Smoking significantly worsens α_1-antitrypsin deficiency and worsens this panacinar emphysema.

Indications for surgical intervention include a significantly large bulla (one third to one half of a hemithorax) with symptoms and only mild diffuse lung disease. The surgical treatment must be individualized because no criteria exist for predicting with certainty which patients will benefit from resection. Asymptomatic patients are generally observed, and infected bullae are resected. The mortality rate varies, and the patients experience variable improvement.

Pneumothorax may occur with emphysema. Conservative therapy often requires days to weeks of suction with chest tubes to obtain pleural symphysis. Resection of the bleb may be required (Fig. 59-16). If respiratory failure or pneumonia develops, tracheostomy will help in some patients, but makes it impossible for the patient to cough. Respiratory care and pulmonary hygiene are critical components of successful outcome.

Spontaneous pneumothoraces may also occur in patients without significant emphysema. The typical patient is a young adult or adolescent male between the ages of 15 and 30 years. These patients usually exhibit a tall thin body type. Smoking increases the risk by a factor of 20. Treatment options include observation, aspiration, tube thoracostomy, and operation. The classic indications for operation include recurrent pneumothorax either on the ipsilateral or contralateral side, failure of re-expansion of the lung, persistent air leak, tension pneumothorax, or hemopneumothorax. Other indications for operative intervention include a patient with a high-risk occupation such as a pilot or diver or someone with limited access

to medical care.[40] Many surgeons obtain a CT scan after re-expansion of the lung. If multiple blebs are identified, the patient is offered operation. The operative procedure includes resection of the bullous disease, an apical pleurectomy, and mechanical pleuroabrasion.

Treatment of emphysema is primarily medical, but there are surgical therapies. Although emphysema usually diffusely involves the lung, it may have a heterogenous distribution within the lung. These areas may be identified by CT and perfusion scan and subsequently resected. Often the disease predominates in the upper lobes and the superior segment of the lower lobes. Lung volume reduction surgery (LVRS) removes areas of greatest emphysematous involvement. The remaining lung tissue expands with improved elastic recoil, improved aeration and perfusion of the remaining lung, and improved chest wall mechanics. A recent prospective trial compared LVRS to best medical therapy. Patients with predominantly upper lobe emphysema and low exercise capacity had lower mortality with LVRS than medical therapy (RR = 0.47; P = .005). In patients with non–upper lobe emphysema and high exercise capacity, mortality was higher in the operative group (RR = 2.06, P = .02).[41] Endoscopic therapies have been developed, including airway bypass and one-way valves. These devices are still in the investigational stage.[42]

Lung transplantation is performed for COPD including α_1-antitrypsin deficiency. Pulmonary fibrosis, primary pulmonary hypertension, cystic fibrosis, and bronchiectasis are other indications for lung transplantation. The recipient is required to have a significant functional disability but be ambulatory. The recipient needs to be free of chronic and debilitating disease (e.g., no hepatic, renal, or cardiac disease), have no other effective therapy available, have a stable nutritional status, have good social and psychological support, and have several years of life potentially remaining outside of pulmonary disease. They need to have a life expectancy of less than 2 years because of pulmonary disease. The survival rates after lung transplantation are about 75% at 1 year, 60% at 2 years, and 50% at 5 years. The annual lung transplantation rate has begun to level off, and waiting times for lung transplants are currently about 18 months. As with any allograft, chronic immunosuppression is required. Combination immunosuppression regimens usually include cyclosporine or tacrolimus, azathioprine or mycophenolate mofetil, and glucocorticoids such as prednisone. Cytolytic therapy with antithymocyte globulin or OKT3 may be used for induction of immunosuppression or for rejection that fails to respond to steroid pulse therapy. Perioperative complications include ischemia-reperfusion injury, bronchial anastomotic dehiscence or stenosis, and vascular complications. The diagnosis and management of these complications can be challenging. Routine follow-up and screening for rejection are required. Transbronchial biopsy may be performed for diagnosis of acute rejection. Acute rejection usually occurs within 3 months of transplantation and manifests as dyspnea, chest x-ray with perihilar infiltrates, leukocytosis, and mild fever. FEV_1 is reduced. High-dose steroids may be used for treatment. Lung allografts appear more susceptible to chronic rejection than other commonly transplanted solid organs. Chronic lung rejection problems include bronchiolitis obliterans, which can be defined pathologically or by reduction in FEV_1 to less than 80% of the post-transplantation baseline.

Unilateral lung transplantation is more readily tolerated than bilateral lung transplantation; however, bilateral lung transplantation may have improved survival. The early mortality rate ranges from 8% to 21% as a result of infection or organ failure. Septic lung disease, such as cystic fibrosis or bronchiectasis, is an absolute indication for bilateral lung transplantation to prevent contamination of the allograft by the native lung. The 5-year survival rate approaches 60%.[43]

DIFFUSE LUNG DISEASE AND OPEN LUNG BIOPSY

The surgeon's role in diffuse lung disease is to obtain a diagnosis, typically by open lung biopsy. The patient has usually undergone several diagnostic bronchoscopies and often a transbronchial biopsy. The chest x-ray may demonstrate an alveolar pattern (fluffy with air bronchograms) or an interstitial pattern (ground-glass or granular appearance, indicating a diffuse increase in interstitial tissue) (Box 59-10).

Referrals for open lung biopsy fall into one of two categories. The first is an outpatient consult for a patient with increasing pulmonary symptoms. Often these patients are only mildly symptomatic. The biopsy may be necessary to confirm or rule out a specific diagnosis before embarking on aggressive medical therapy such as cyclophosphamide for Wegner's granulomatosis. The second category includes a critically ill patient, often

---

Box 59-10 Classification of Diffuse Lung Diseases

Infections (More Commonly Cause Focal Disease, Granuloma Formation)

Viruses—especially influenza, cytomegalovirus
Bacteria—tuberculosis, all kinds of regular bacteria, Rocky Mountain spotted fever
Fungi—all types can cause diffuse disease
Parasites—*Pneumocystis* species infection, toxoplasmosis, paragonimiasis, among others

Occupational Causes

Mineral dusts
Chemical fumes—NO_2 (silo filler's disease), Cl, NH_3, SO_2, CCl_4, Br, HF, HCl, HNO_3, kerosene, acetylene

Neoplastic Disease

Lymphangitic spread
Hematogenous metastases
Leukemia, lymphoma, bronchioloalveolar cell cancer

Congenital—Familial

Niemann-Pick, Gaucher's, neurofibromatosis, and tuberous fibrosis

Metabolic and Unknown

Liver disease, uremia, inflammatory bowel disease

Physical Agents

Radiation, O_2 toxicity, thermal injury, blast injury

Heart Failure and Multiple Pulmonary Emboli

Immunologic Causes

Hypersensitivity Pneumonia

Inhaled antigens
Farmer's lung (actinomycosis)
Bagassosis (sugar cane)
Malt workers (*Aspergillus* species)
Byssinosis (cotton)

Drug Reactions

Hydralazine, busulfan, nitrofurantoin (Macrodantin), hexamethonium, methysergide, bleomycin

Collagen Diseases

Scleroderma, rheumatoid, systemic lupus erythematosus, dermatomyositis, Wegener's granulomatosis, Goodpasture's syndrome

Other

Sarcoidosis
Histiocytosis
Idiopathic hemosiderosis
Pulmonary alveolar proteinosis
Diffuse interstitial fibrosis, idiopathic pulmonary fibrosis
Desquamative interstitial pneumonia
Eosinophilic pneumonia (*Note:* some are caused by drugs, actinomycosis, parasites)
Lymphangioleiomyomatosis

in the intensive care unit, requiring mechanical ventilation.

One of the most common conditions that triggers a referral for lung biopsy is sarcoidosis. Sarcoidosis affects the lungs in 90% of patients with this diagnosis, causing symptoms of dyspnea and dry cough. Foci of noncaseating epithelioid granulomas may be found in any part of the body. Ten to 20% of patients are asymptomatic, 20% to 40% are first seen with an acute form including fever and other significant symptoms, and 40% to 50% have insidious respiratory complaints without constitutional symptoms. Severe progressive pulmonary fibrosis may develop in 10% to 20% of patients. Bilateral hilar mediastinal lymph nodes are involved in 60% to 80% of patients. Although mediastinoscopy has a higher yield, bronchoscopic lung biopsy is often the first procedure of choice because bronchoscopy can be done without the need for a general anesthetic. Biopsy of these mediastinal lymph nodes may be required for diagnosis and often may be the only surgical procedure needed. If bronchoscopy and mediastinoscopy are nondiagnostic, then lung biopsy maybe indicated. Skin lesions such as erythema nodosum, plaques, squamous nodules, and maculopapular eruption occur in about 25% of patients, and eye involvement (uveitis) may occur in 25% of patients.

For diagnosis, clinical criteria and biopsy are needed. Bronchoscopy and transbronchial biopsy are good, and open lung biopsy is rarely needed. Steroids may be used for treatment.

An open lung biopsy is generally not necessary when the lung picture is typical of a previously known cause; however, open lung biopsy is generally necessary for those diseases for which the cause is not known.

Most lung biopsies can be performed using minimally invasive techniques. VATS lung biopsies can be performed using two or three ports. The patient must be able to tolerated single-lung ventilation and transport to the operating room. In patients who have undergone bronchoscopic biopsies, adequate time of up to 4 weeks must be allowed for the final culture results to be reported. Biopsies are sent for routine, fungal, and acid-fast bacillus culture. In immunocompromised patients, *Nocardia* cultures are considered. It is often helpful to sample more than one area of the lung. One method is to resect the radiographically worst-appearing region and the most normal-appearing area. The normal-appearing lung may exhibit early-stage disease and may aid the pathologist in making the diagnosis. Frozen section is only used to confirm that adequate samples of the pathologic process were obtained.

In the acute setting of a critically ill patient, an open lung biopsy is often not warranted for patients with diffuse lung disease or chronic ventilatory requirements. The value of open lung biopsy in this clinical setting is low and typically no better than best medical management in intensive care. An open lung biopsy is not performed unless the results will modify subsequent treatment such as the initiation of protocol-based treatment for experimental antibiotics. Often theses patients cannot tolerate single-lung ventilation or transfer to the operating room. In this small subset of patients, the

---

> **Box 59-11** **Causes of Adult Respiratory Distress Syndrome**
>
> Extrathoracic sepsis
> Blunt chest trauma
> Nonthoracic trauma
> Shock
> Burns
> Aspiration pneumonia
> Diffuse infectious pneumonia
> Nonbacterial pneumonia (viral, mycoplasma, legionnaires' disease, *Pneumocystis carinii*)
> Miscellaneous events
>   Smoke inhalation
>   Oxygen toxicity
>   Neurogenic pulmonary edema
>   Ingestion of toxic drugs
>   Acute hypersensitivity reactions

procedure can be performed in the intensive care unit through an anterolateral thoracotomy, and biopsy samples of the lingula or the right middle lobe can be obtained. These drastic measures are rarely indicated.

ACUTE RESPIRATORY DISTRESS SYNDROME

The acute, or adult, respiratory distress syndrome is a complex biologic and clinical process. This acute deterioration of pulmonary function occurs exclusive of pulmonary edema, pneumonia, or exacerbation of COPD. About 50,000 cases occur each year in the United States, with a mortality rate of 30% to 40%. Some causes of acute respiratory distress syndrome are listed in Box 59-11.

The initial clinical presentation of dyspnea, tachypnea, hypoxemia, and mild hypocapnia is nonspecific. A chest x-ray may show diffuse bilateral infiltrates secondary to increased interstitial fluid. Pathologically, vascular congestion occurs with alveolar collapse, edema, and inflammatory cell infiltration. The underlying mechanism is increased pulmonary capillary permeability with extravasation of intravascular fluid and protein into the interstitium and alveoli. The leukocyte is the most prominent mediator of this injury. Stimuli such as sepsis activate the complement pathway, causing recruitment of leukocytes to the site of the infection. The lung releases potent mediators such as oxygen free radicals, arachidonic acid metabolites, and proteases. If the underlying disease is not controlled, these changes progress to vascular thromboses and interstitial fibrosis and hyaline membrane deposition in the alveoli. This process causes hypoxemia, pulmonary hypertension, CO_2 retention, secondary infections, and eventually right heart failure, hypoxia, and death. Other criteria include impaired oxygenation with the PaO_2/FiO_2 ratio of less than 200 mm Hg. As well, pulmonary edema is present without cardiac failure, and a pulmonary capillary wedge pressure is less than 18 (noncardiac pulmonary edema).

The outcome of adult respiratory distress syndrome is related to the initial injury stimulus. Treatment is directed to improve oxygenation with optimal pulmonary hygiene, intubation, and pressure ventilation. Maintaining an inspired oxygen concentration as low as possible and positive end-expiratory pressure as low as possible to maintain adequate oxygenation and carbon dioxide exchange is helpful. Tidal volumes are kept lower than conventional protocols, such as 6 mL/kg.[44] Other strategies include permissive hypercapnia or changes in position. Prone or rotational therapy improves ventilation-perfusion matching by improving the distribution of perfusion.[45] A Swan-Ganz catheter maybe used to optimize hemodynamics, although randomized studies have not shown a survival benefit. Inotropes, corticosteroids, prostaglandin inhibitors, and oxygen free radical scavengers have been examined, yet, to date, they have failed to consistently improve pulmonary function or mortality rate for patients with adult respiratory distress syndrome.

HIGH-PRESSURE JET VENTILATION

High-pressure jet ventilation can be used during bronchoscopy, for carinal resection, and to improve oxygenation in patients with bronchopleural fistula or in the noncompliant lung in patients with respiratory failure. Complications include pneumothorax, hypotension at high driving pressures, blocked endotracheal tube from encrustation at the end of the tube, and a decrease in cardiac output, which may be prevented with inotropes. Its most frequent use is in managing respiratory failure in neonates.

BACTERIAL INFECTIONS

Bronchiectasis

Bronchiectasis is an infection of the bronchial wall and surrounding lung with sufficient severity to cause destruction and dilation of the air passages. This condition is decreasing in frequency and severity because of the use of antibiotics. There are numerous predisposing factors, including cystic fibrosis, α_1-antitrypsin deficiency, various immunodeficiency states, Kartagener's syndrome (sinusitis, bronchiectasis, situs inversus, and hypomotile cilia), and bronchial obstruction from foreign body, extrinsic lymph nodes that compress the bronchus, neoplasm, or mucus plug. The distribution is primarily in the basal segments of the lower lobes. Destructive changes and dilation of the bronchi accompany the infection.

With use of antibiotics, it has become rare to see an emaciated febrile patient coughing up large amounts of foul sputum accompanied by clubbing, cyanosis, and hemoptysis. Currently, frequent respiratory infections are typical, and sputum production is minimal except during exacerbations and acute infections. Mild hemoptysis may occur; massive hemoptysis is rare. Frequently, symptoms can be controlled with medical management such as chronic antibiotic therapy and postural drainage.

Evaluation begins with a history and physical exam and chest x-ray. The patient is specifically questioned about aspiration of a foreign body. The CT scan of the

chest has become the next step in the evaluation of a patient with suspected bronchiectasis. Bronchoscopy cannot differentiate bronchitis from bronchiectasis. Bronchoscopy can be performed to clear secretions and, when the diagnosis is suspected, to rule out cancer, foreign body, or stricture. Cultures may be obtained to facilitate antibiotic treatment. Bronchography is a method of diagnosis and may be required when surgery is being considered, although bronchography (Fig. 59-17A) has generally been replaced by CT. Dilation of the bronchi and no feathering of distal airways can be visualized. Medical treatment is optimized; this includes discontinuation of smoking and institution of postural drainage, bronchodilator medications, and oral antibiotics.

Surgical management may be performed if the disease is irreversible or if there is failure of medical therapy with recurrent pneumonia, hemoptysis affecting a normal lifestyle, or persistent sputum production greater than 1 to 2 ounces daily. The disease must be localized, and the patient needs to be physiologically suitable for resection. One segment of involvement with bronchiectasis is not enough to consider resection. Disease limited to but involving one lobe is best treated surgically. If bilateral bronchiectasis exists, medical management continues. Results of treatment are good in 80% to 90% of patients. Patients with severe bilateral bronchiectasis who have failed maximal medical management and are not candidates for resection may be candidates for lung transplantation.

Lung Abscess

The incidence of lung abscess is decreasing in frequency as a result of use of antibiotics.[46] A lung abscess may occur from an infection behind a blocked bronchus. The infection is usually anaerobic and may be associated with alcohol abuse, foreign body aspiration, a debilitated or elderly individual, or esophageal disease with aspiration. Lung abscess used to occur after tonsillectomy or tooth extraction, but this has become a rare event. Hematogenous spread from bacteremia may occur if congestive heart failure or debilitating disease is present, such as in elderly or very young patients, patients who use IV drugs, and patients taking steroids. These areas of infection are usually multiple and rarely require operative intervention. *Staphylococcus* bacteremia is frequently associated with lung abscess. Necrotizing pneumonia from *Klebsiella* species may rapidly destroy the involved lung with minimal surrounding reaction. The frequency of necrotizing pneumonia leading to lung abscess is decreasing with the use of antibiotics. Rupture of a lung abscess may yield empyema and pneumothorax. Lung abscess may also be superimposed on structural abnormalities, for example, a bronchogenic cyst, sequestration, bleb, or tuberculous or fungal cavities.

Lung abscesses secondary to aspiration are more commonly found on the right because of the less acute angle of the right main-stem bronchus. The abscess may occur in the lateral divisions of the anterior and posterior segments of the upper lobe, the axillary subsegment, or the superior segment of the lower lobe. Clinical features are

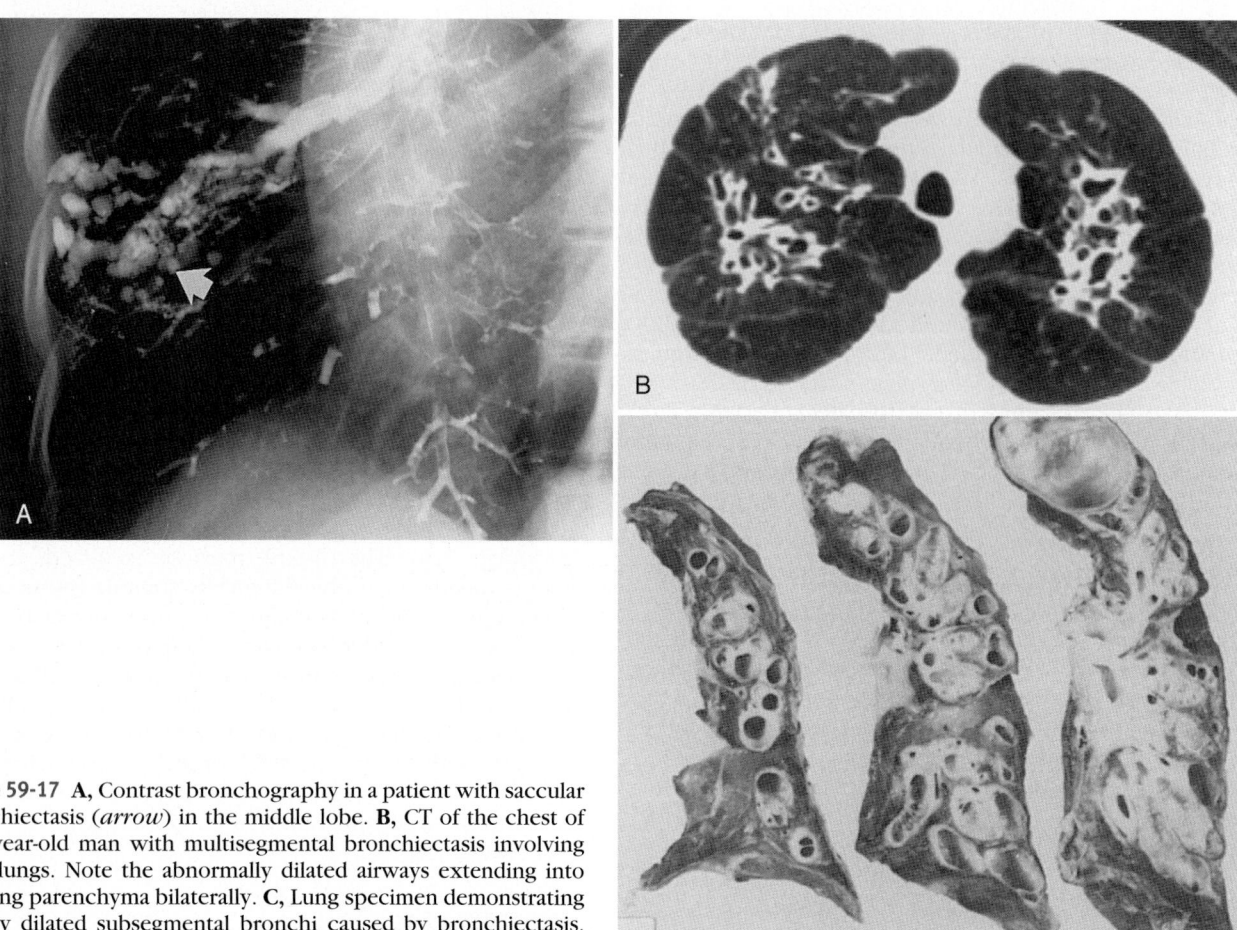

Figure 59-17 A, Contrast bronchography in a patient with saccular bronchiectasis (*arrow*) in the middle lobe. **B,** CT of the chest of a 30-year-old man with multisegmental bronchiectasis involving both lungs. Note the abnormally dilated airways extending into the lung parenchyma bilaterally. **C,** Lung specimen demonstrating grossly dilated subsegmental bronchi caused by bronchiectasis. (**C** from Bolman RM, Wolfe WG: Bronchiectasis and bronchopulmonary sequestration. Surg Clin North Am 60:867, 1980.)

similar to those of pneumonia, including fever, cough, leukocytosis, pleuritic pain, and sputum production. The chest x-ray and CT scan of the chest may demonstrate a rounded area of consolidation early and an air-fluid level on upright or decubitus chest x-ray later.

The differential diagnosis includes loculated empyema, which may be treated with drainage; epiphrenic diverticulum (in which the patient is not septic); or tuberculous or fungus cavity or a cavitary lung cancer (usually squamous cell carcinoma). Tubercular and fungus cavities do not retain fluid, so no air-fluid level is present; however, they may contain debris or a fungus ball. *Aspergillus* species infection may present in this manner (Fig. 59-18). Medical management is with antibiotics and pulmonary care (e.g., re-expansion). Bronchoscopy may be performed for diagnosis to rule out foreign body, stenosis, or cancer. Bronchoscopy may be used for treatment to assist in drainage of the cavity either directly or by way of transbronchial catheterization of the cavity. Most patients (85%-95%) respond to medical management with rapid decrease in fluid, collapse of the walls, and complete healing in 3 to 4 months. Patients with symptoms for longer than 3 months before treatment or cavities larger than 4 to 6 cm are less likely to respond.

Surgical therapy is indicated for persistent cavity (>2 cm and thick walled), failure to clear sepsis after 8 weeks of medical therapy, for hemoptysis (often small sentinel bleed before a massive bleed), and to exclude cancer. If a lung abscess ruptures into the pleural cavity, simple drainage may suffice, and the patient is managed for empyema or bronchopleural fistula. Lobectomy is typically required; the mortality rate is 1% to 5%. Occasionally, external drainage may be required in critically ill patients if pleural symphysis has occurred.

Other Bronchopulmonary Disorders

Bronchopulmonary disorders caused by inflammatory lymph node disease are usually caused by tuberculosis or histoplasmosis. Lobar atelectasis, hemoptysis, or broncholithiasis can occur. Bronchial compressive disease typically occurs most commonly in the middle lobe. More than 20% of cases are caused by cancer. This condition results in repeated infection in the same area of the lung, which usually responds to antibiotics. The differential diagnosis includes endobronchial tumors in adults and foreign body aspiration in children. Bronchoscopy is essential to rule out cancer and foreign body and to

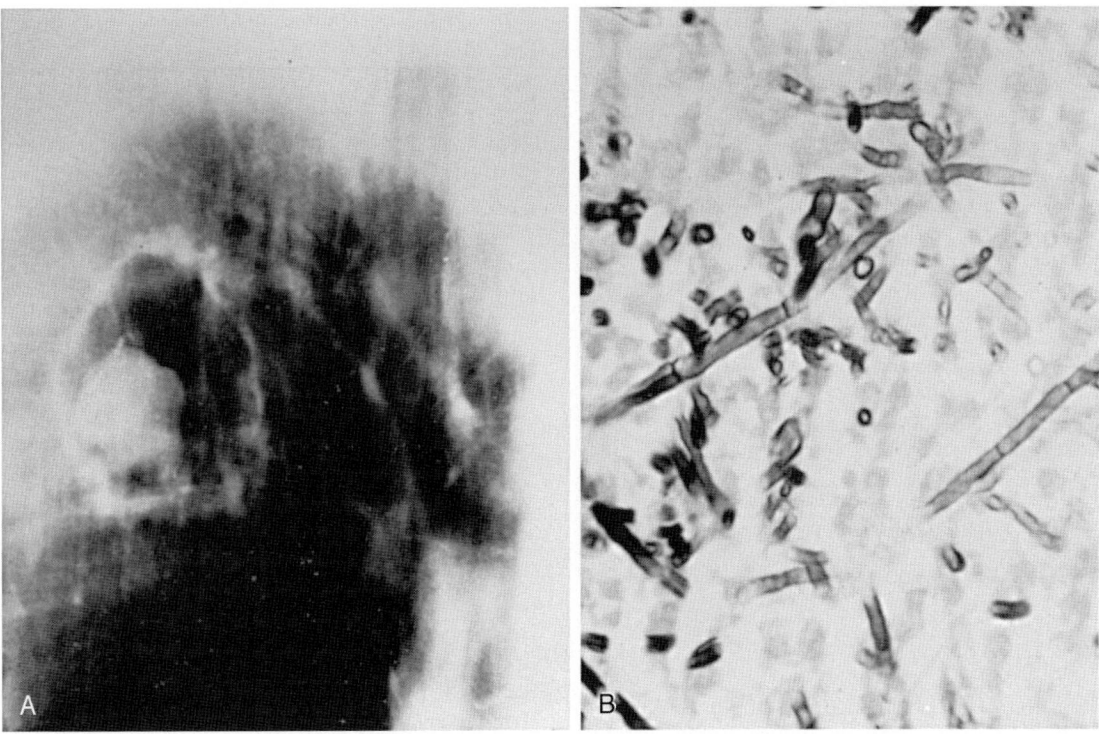

Figure 59-18 A, Linear tomogram of the lung demonstrates an aspergilloma ("fungus ball") within a large cavitary lesion within the lung parenchyma. The fungus ball is often unattached within the cavity and is located in the most gravity-dependent area of the cavity. It can alter its position as the patient changes position. **B,** The coarse, fragmented, septate mycelia of *Aspergillus fumigatus.* (**A** from Aslam PA, Larkin J, Eastridge CA, Hughes FA Jr: Endocavitary infusion through percutaneous endobronchial catheter. Chest 57:94, 1970. **B** from Takaro T: Thoracic mycotic infections. In Lewis' Practice of Surgery. New York, Hoeber Medical Division, Harper & Row, 1968.)

evaluate for stricture. Medical management is required to treat infection. Surgery is indicated to treat bronchostenosis, irreversible bronchiectasis, or severe recurrent infection.

Broncholithiasis is a calcified node tightly adherent to a bronchus. Innocent hemoptysis may occur even with a negative chest x-ray. Sudden bleeding caused by erosion of a small bronchial artery and mucosa by a spicule in the calcified node causes this hemoptysis. Bright red blood occurs, ranging from 5 to 500 mL, and usually stops with sedation and antitussive therapy. This type of hemoptysis is almost never massive (>600 mL in 24 hours). Bronchoscopy is possible during a bleeding episode to localize the site of the bleeding. Nasal or pharyngeal lesions need to be excluded.

Organizing pneumonia may replace lung parenchyma with scar tissue or persistent atelectasis or consolidation. Initially, an acute pneumonia develops, and then a persistent shadow. If the shadow or mass does not clear in 6 to 8 weeks, resection is performed to exclude carcinoma. The differential diagnosis includes pneumonia, congenital abnormality, and aneurysm of the aorta.

Mycobacterial Infections

Tuberculosis infects about 7% of patients exposed, and it develops in 5% to 10% of those patients infected. A primary infection develops. The exudative response progresses to caseous necrosis. Postprimary tuberculosis tends to occur in apical and posterior segments of the upper lobes and superior segments of the lower lobes. Healing occurs with fibrosis and contracture. Extensive caseation with cavitation may occur early. Coalescing areas of caseous necrosis may form cavities. There are frequently incomplete septations and lobulations. Septations supplied by bronchial arteries can cause hemoptysis if eroded and may be secondarily infected by other organisms.

Bronchoscopy may be required for patients not responding to medical management. Cancer should be excluded for a newly identified mass on chest x-ray even with a positive tuberculosis skin test and acid-fast bacillus–positive sputum. Medical management is with isonicotinic acid hydrazide (INH), rifampin, ethambutol, streptomycin, or pyrazinamide. The initial treatment for the disease is combination therapy (e.g., INH plus rifampin and pyrazinamide).

Surgical therapy may be considered when medical therapy fails and persistent tuberculosis-positive sputum remains, as well as when surgically correctable residua of tuberculosis may be of potential danger to the patient. This is not the same management as for atypical mycobacteria; many of these patients remain clinically well even with positive sputum. Some indications for surgery are listed in Box 59-12.

Box 59-12 Potential Indications for Surgery for Pulmonary Tuberculosis

Open positive cavity after 3 to 6 months of chemotherapy, especially if resistant mycobacteria

Persistent positive sputum with pathology (destroyed lung, atelectasis, bronchiectasis, bronchostenosis) amenable to resection

Negative sputum *but* destroyed lung, blocked cavity, tuberculoma—consider for resection

Localized infection with atypical mycobacteria

Tuberculous bronchiectasis of lower and middle lobes (usually occurs in upper lobes—good drainage; lower and middle lobes do not drain well)

Open negative cavities if thick walled, slow response, or unreliable patient

To exclude cancer

Recurrent or persistent hemoptysis: resection if greater than 600 mL of blood is lost in 24 hours or less

Pleural disease where indicated

Table 59-4 Extrapulmonary Manifestations of Fungal Infections

Actinomycosis	Cervicofacial, chest wall
Nocardiosis	Chest wall, central nervous system (CNS)
Histoplasmosis	Marrow, adrenal
Coccidioidomycosis	Bone (however, usually just lung)
Blastomycosis	Skin > genitourinary system
Cryptococcosis	CNS
Aspergillosis	CNS, blood vessels
Mucormycosis	Rhinocerebral, blood vessels

Surgical options include resection, which is the procedure of choice in most instances. Pleural adhesions and granulomas in peribronchial nodes and chronic inflammation make resection difficult. Preservation of lung tissue is a goal of the treatment. Surgical complications are doubled if the sputum is positive for *Mycobacterium tuberculosis* and decreased if remaining lung tissue is fully expanded. Infectious complications include empyema, bronchopleural fistula, and endobronchial spread of the disease and are associated with higher mortality rate. Tuberculosis infection of the pleural space without lung destruction is primarily treated medically.

Thoracoplasty or muscle flap interposition may be used to control the postresection empyema space. Collapse therapy, with thoracoplasty or plombage, is rarely, if ever, used to manage parenchymal disease alone. These techniques may be necessary in patients who fail medical management and who are not candidates for resection. Patients with extensive disease and positive sputum or chronic active endobronchial disease may also be considered. Plombage may be preferred over staged conventional thoracoplasty because it requires only one operation; there is no paradoxical chest motion and chest wall deformity. Cavernostomy, or external drainage of a tuberculous cavity with a chest tube or open drainage, may be used to control a large cavity with positive sputum or massive bleeding in a patient who is unable to tolerate resection or collapse therapy.

Fungal and Parasitic Infections

The surgical management of fungal infections includes diagnosis and management of complications of fungal disease. Frequently, cancer has to be excluded or other infectious or benign conditions confirmed. Medical management may be considered as initial treatment of fungal diseases in the lung and as part of the patient's overall management.

Immunocompromised patients suffer from *Aspergillus* species infection as the most frequent opportunistic infection, followed by *Candida* and *Nocardia* species and mucormycosis. Normal, or immunocompetent, patients may be affected by histoplasmosis, coccidioidomycosis, or blastomycosis. Both groups may be affected by actinomycosis and cryptococcosis. Although *Nocardia* and *Actinomyces* are bacteria, they are usually discussed with fungal infections. Diagnosis is most often made by sputum examination using potassium hydroxide preparations. Cultures are poor and may take some time for results to be obtained; Papanicolaou test cytology may be best. Silver methenamine stain is key to the evaluation. Extrapulmonary involvement of various fungal diseases is listed in Table 59-4. Most infections are self-limited and do not require treatment. IV or oral antifungal agents may be used for treatment of the diseases.

Histoplasmosis is the most common of all fungal infections in the United States and is most frequently a serious systemic fungal disease. *Histoplasma capsulatum* is endemic to the Mississippi and Ohio River valleys as well as portions of the southwestern United States. A high percentage of patients are affected, usually with a subclinical form of this disease. An inoculum (from the mycelial form found in soil, decaying materials, and bat or bird guano) can produce an acute pneumonic illness in immunocompetent hosts and usually resolves without specific treatment. The yeast form exists in macrophages or within the cytoplasm of the alveoli. Pathologic examination demonstrates granulomas (like tuberculosis) or caseating epithelioid granulomas. Calcified nodes in the lung, mediastinum, spleen, and liver may occur. The chest x-ray may demonstrate central or target calcification or concentric laminar calcification. Any form can have arthralgias or erythema nodosum or erythema multiforme. The localized form is usually an acute pneumonia, self-limited, and rarely severe. A solitary pulmonary nodule may be a residual finding of acute pneumonia and is resected unless proper calcification is identified. The lymphogenous reaction to *Histoplasma* causes mediastinal lymph node enlargement and may cause middle lobe syndrome, bronchiectasis, esophageal traction diverticulum, broncholithiasis with hemoptysis, tracheo-

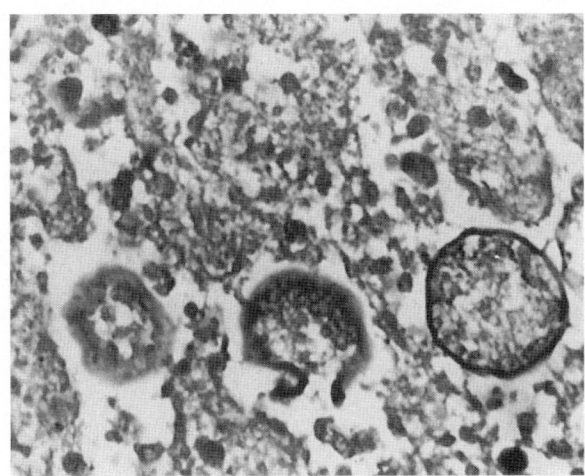

Figure 59-19 Microscopic section of a coccidioidal granuloma (×400) shows spherules packed with endospores. (From Scott S, Takaro T: Thoracic mycotic and actinomycotic infections. In Shields TW [ed]: General Thoracic Surgery, 4th ed. Baltimore, Williams & Wilkins, 1994.)

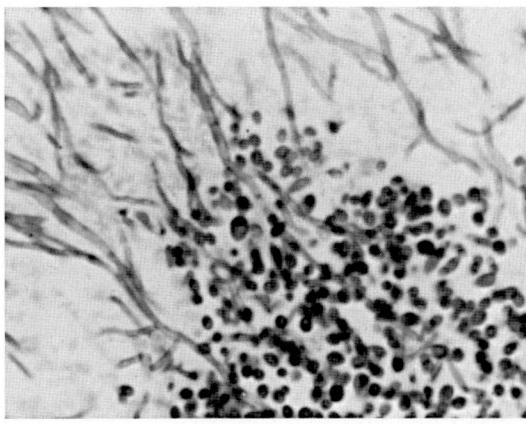

Figure 59-20 *Candida albicans* with both the mycelial and the yeast forms. (From Takaro T: Thoracic mycotic infections. In Lewis' Practice of Surgery. New York, Hoeber Medical Division, Harper & Row, 1968.)

esophageal fistula, constrictive pericarditis, or fibrosing mediastinitis with superior vena cava syndrome, or other problems relating to compression of mediastinal structures. In addition to the compressive symptoms, the lymphadenopathy caused by histoplasmosis may confound radiographic evaluation of the mediastinal lymph nodes in patients with lung cancer and may complicate lung resection.

Coccidioidomycosis is endemic to the Southwest and is localized in the soil. It is second only to histoplasmosis in frequency. Inhaling the organism results in a primary lung disease that is usually self-limited (Fig. 59-19). In endemic areas, coccidioidomycosis is a frequent cause of lung nodules, and resection may be required to rule out malignancy.

Treatment is often with amphotericin for patients who are severely ill, such as those who are immunocompromised and have positive sputum cultures. Other options include ketoconazole or itraconazole for non–life-threatening disease.

Surgery may be considered for treatment of cavitary disease or complications of cavitary disease. Amphotericin is used perioperatively. Indications for surgery include thick-walled or greater than 2-cm cavities, enlarging cavities, ruptured cavities, secondary bacterial infections, and severe recurrent hemoptysis.

Open lung biopsy may be required to make a diagnosis of cryptococcosis, which is widely disseminated in soil, dust, and pigeon guano. Pathologically, the organism appears as round, budding yeasts, with wide capsules and granulomas. It is the second most common lethal fungus after histoplasmosis. Lungs are frequently involved. The disease is usually mild. Meningitis is the most frequent cause of death. Any patient diagnosed with pulmonary cryptococcosis undergoes lumbar puncture to rule out CNS involvement. Surgery may be required for open lung biopsy for diagnosis or to exclude lung cancer.

Aspergillosis is an opportunistic infection, characterized by coarse fragmented septa and hyphae. There are three types of aspergillosis: aspergilloma, invasive pulmonary aspergillosis, and allergic bronchopulmonary aspergillosis. Aspergilloma is the most common form of aspergillosis. The fungus colonizes an existing lung cavity, commonly a tuberculosis cavity. The chest x-ray may demonstrate a crescent radiolucency next to a rounded mass. Cavities may form because of destruction of the underlying pulmonary parenchyma, and debris and hyphae may coalesce and form a fungus ball, which lies free in the cavity and can roll around on decubitus chest x-ray (see Fig. 59-18). Prophylactic resection is controversial, although some recommend resection if isolated disease is present in low-risk patients. Surgery is indicated for massive or recurrent hemoptysis or to rule out neoplasm. The procedure of choice is lobectomy. Invasive aspergillosis occurs in immunocompromised patients and presents with chest pain, cough, and hemoptysis. The treatment is primarily medical, although lung biopsy may be necessary for diagnosis. Allergic aspergillosis is diagnosed by bronchoscopy and represents the allergic reaction to chronic colonization with the fungus. It is usually treated medically. Rarely, resection is performed for localized bronchiectasis.

Mucormycosis is a rare, opportunistic, rapidly progressive infection; it occurs in immunocompromised patients, including those with diabetes. The appearance is that of a black mold; it has wide nonseptate branching hyphae. The infection causes blood vessels to thrombose and lung tissue to infarct. Clinically, the rhinocerebral form occurs much more frequently than the pulmonary form of consolidation and cavities. Medical management is with cessation of steroids and antineoplastic drugs, and initiation of amphotericin and control of diabetes are undertaken. The disease is often too advanced for effective treatment. Aggressive surgical and medical treatment may improve what is usually a grave prognosis.

Candida is a small, thin-walled budding yeast that occurs in immunocompromised patients (Fig. 59-20).

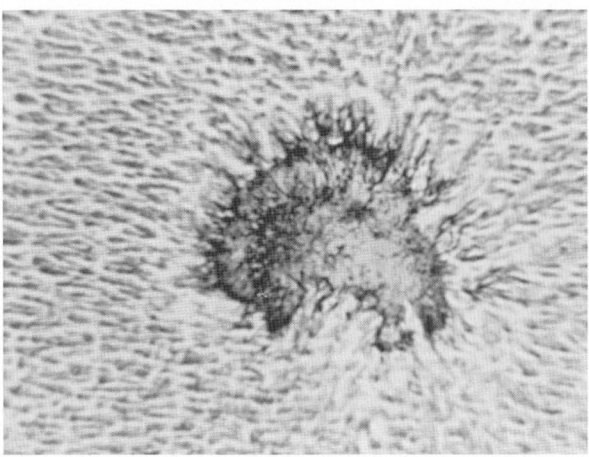

Figure 59-21 Actinomycotic granule shows branching filaments of a microscopic colony of *Actinomyces israelii*. (Gomori stain, ×250.)

Box 59-13   Causes of Hemoptysis

Lung cancer
Lung abscess
Cavitary aspergillosis
Tuberculosis
Bronchiectasis
Swan-Ganz catheterization
Cystic fibrosis
Broncholithiasis
Foreign body
Transbronchial lung biopsy

Lung involvement alone is rare. Surgery may be required to confirm the diagnosis.

Surgery may also be used to manage the sequelae and complications of parasitic infections. Infections with *Entamoeba histolytica* are usually confined to the right lower thorax and are related to extension from a liver abscess below the diaphragm by way of direct extension or lymphatics to the right thorax. Metronidazole (Flagyl) is usually effective, although Flagyl and tube drainage may be required for treatment of empyema. Open resection is infrequently required. Similarly, infection with *Echinococcus* species may occur. The hydatid cyst may rupture, flooding the lung or producing a severe hypersensitivity reaction. A lung abscess could occur with compression of the airway, great vessels, or esophagus. Surgery, if feasible, may include simple enucleation by way of cleavage of planes between the cyst and the normal tissue. Aspiration and hypertonic saline 10% may be performed before enucleation. Positive pressure on the lung needs to be maintained until the cyst is out to prevent contamination, soilage, or hypersensitivity reaction. Nonoperative therapy for small asymptomatic calcified cysts may be considered. Paragonimiasis is another common infection and common cause of hemoptysis in Asia.[47] In endemic areas, prevalence may reach 5%, and hemoptysis from paragonimiasis in one Asian population (16%) exceeded that from tuberculosis (3%).

Pneumocystis carinii is an opportunistic infection that is positive on silver methenamine stain. Bronchoalveolar lavage obtains the diagnosis in more than 90% of patients. However, lung biopsy may be required to confirm the diagnosis.

Actinomycosis is a bacterium that is not found free in nature. It produces a chronic anaerobic endogenous infection deep within a wound. "Sulfur granules" draining from infected sinuses are microcolonies (Fig. 59-21). The cervicofacial form is the most common. The thoracic form usually occurs as pulmonary parenchymal disease resembling cancer. The treatment is most commonly penicillin.

Surgery may occasionally be required for radical excision of chest wall disease and empyema.

Nocardiosis is caused by an aerobic bacterium widely disseminated in soil and domestic animals; it was formerly rare, although it is increasing in immunocompromised patients. Nocardiosis resembles actinomycosis in invading the chest wall and produces subcutaneous abscesses and sinuses draining sulfur granules. Surgery is performed to exclude cancer, to obtain a diagnosis, or to treat complications of the disease. Medical therapy may include sulfonamides.

MASSIVE HEMOPTYSIS

Massive hemoptysis may be defined as greater than 500 to 600 mL of blood loss from the lungs in 24 hours. However, the proximal airways may be occluded with as little as 150 mL of clotted blood; even lower volume hemoptysis may be life-threatening. The current mortality rate is about 13% and is related to drowning or suffocation rather than exsanguination. Causes of hemoptysis are listed in Box 59-13.

Diagnosis and treatment of massive hemoptysis typically include a chest x-ray and emergency bronchoscopy. Rigid bronchoscopy with an 8.5-mm or larger bronchoscope is needed. A 10-mm scope is preferred. Flexible bronchoscopy is usually inadequate for treatment of hemoptysis, but it may be considered for observation if active bleeding has stopped. Blood is typed and crossed and the interventional radiologist is notified if angiographic embolization is anticipated. Often, patients have been seen previously with slight hemoptysis and have undergone diagnostic evaluation consisting of a chest x-ray and CT of the chest. These studies may provide additional information to guide the surgeon in palliating hemoptysis. If the expertise is not available for emergent rigid bronchoscopy, the patient may be temporized by selective intubation of the contralateral main-stem bronchus under bronchoscopic guidance or by placing a double-lumen endotracheal tube to protect the contralateral lung parenchyma. A Fogarty balloon tip catheter or a bronchial blocking catheter may also be placed to occlude the bronchus from which the bleeding originates.

Box 59-14   Treatment Options for Massive Hemoptysis

Treatment of intrabronchial lesion by laser or topical epinephrine (transient effect only)
Definitive surgical resection (probably most applicable)
Expectant management (observation, cough suppression, rest)
Bronchoscopic lavage with iced saline
Fogarty catheter tamponade
Intracavitary instillation of antimicrobial medications for poor-risk patients with mycetomas
Cavernostomy with packing for patients too sick to undergo resection
Plombage (for active cavitary tuberculosis)
Bronchial arterial embolization by interventional radiology
Mass resection with large stapler *(last resort)*

Box 59-15   Potential Indications for Angiographic Catheterization

Cystic fibrosis
Bilateral chronic pulmonary disease and inability to localize a bleeding site
Nonresectable malignancy, primary or metastatic
Vital capacity of less than 40% of predicted value
Recurrent hemoptysis after surgery

Treatment options must be guided by the clinical situation and findings. Bronchoscopy under general anesthesia is performed and bleeding is controlled so as to prevent soiling the contralateral (uninvolved) lung. Conservative management may consist simply of bronchoscopy, clearing the airway of blood, cough suppression (with codeine), and rest (Box 59-14). The patient needs to be managed in a monitored or intensive care setting until stabilized.

Patients with hemoptysis from cystic fibrosis may do well with expectant treatment of hemoptysis, which may require tamponade using a balloon catheter. Patients with aspergilloma fungus balls are at high risk for fatal hemorrhage and are treated aggressively and undergo resection when possible. Broncholithiasis is another cause of hemoptysis. Broncholiths may form as a result of infection with *Histoplasmosis* or *Mycobacterium* species. Hemoptysis from broncholithiasis may require a bronchoplastic resection such as sleeve lobectomy after stabilization with bronchoscopic techniques.

Angiographic catheterization for massive hemoptysis may be considered in patients with hemoptysis and inability to localize a bleeding site. A relative contraindication to angiographic catheterization and embolization is the contribution of the bronchial arteries to the blood supply of the spinal cord or a common origin of the blood supply to the bronchi and the spinal cord. The risk for quadriplegia must be considered in light of the overall patient condition. Embolization is carried out with small particles of polyvinyl alcohol or other synthetic embolic material to occlude vessels at a peripheral level. Some reports show that bleeding is controlled in 70% of patients, but 50% rebleed. Embolization may be repeated. Angiographic catheterization indications are given in Box 59-15.

PULMONARY EMBOLISM

Pulmonary embolism is a spectrum of disease that ranges from the clinically insignificant pulmonary microembolus to a catastrophic instantaneously fatal massive pulmonary thrombus obstructing both pulmonary arteries.[48] Thrombi most commonly develop in the veins of the lower leg from stasis and a hypercoagulable state, and they propagate proximally to the deep veins of the leg and pelvis. As these clots become larger and as the veins become larger, the propensity for these clots to dislodge and embolize to the lungs increases. When this occurs, a chain reaction of events takes place: the pulmonary artery blood supply to those sections of the lung is occluded, vasoactive agents are released with elevation of pulmonary vascular resistance, a shunt develops as the pulmonary blood flow is redistributed, and pulmonary edema may occur. Alveolar dead space is increased, and gas exchange is impaired. Depending on the size of the thrombus or the patient's reaction to the embolic event, right ventricular work is increased. With increased afterload, right ventricular dysfunction or failure may occur. Right ventricular hypokinesis with a normal arterial blood pressure is a poor prognostic indicator. Paradoxical embolus from a patent foramen ovale may occur.

Pulmonary embolism may account for up to 3% of postoperative surgical deaths and has been found in 24% of 5477 patients in an autopsy series. Untreated pulmonary embolism has a 30% hospital mortality rate, whereas treated patients have a mortality rate estimated at about 2%. In the general population, the incidence of pulmonary embolus is estimated to be 1 in 1000 per year. Pulmonary embolism may occur in more than 250,000 patients annually in the United States with a mortality rate of 15% to 17%.

Risk factors for pulmonary embolus may include high body-mass index, malignancy, cigarette smoking, hypertension, and surgery. Activated protein C is an extremely potent anticoagulant. Resistance to activated protein C may be transmitted as an autosomal dominant trait in some patients with a propensity for venous thrombosis.[49] Routine laboratory tests in the past for a hypercoagulable state or pulmonary embolus included an assay of antithrombin III, protein C, and protein S; however, deficiencies in these proteins rarely occur.[48] Currently, recommended testing includes the following:

1. Factor V Leiden mutation (the most common hypercoagulable state)
2. Hyperhomocystinemia (readily treated with B vitamins)
3. Lupus anticoagulant (because intensive anticoagulation may be required)

Activated protein C is a potent endogenous anticoagulant. The genetic changes responsible for resistance to activated protein C are transmitted in an autosomal dominant manner. A point mutation occurs in the gene coding for coagulation factor V (which is responsible for activated protein C resistance). This is the factor V Leiden mutation, which makes activated factor V more difficult for activated protein C to cleave and inactivate. The risk for venous thrombosis in patients with this trait is increased twofold to fourfold. Plasma hyperhomocysteinemia is caused by deficiencies of folate and an inadequate supply of B vitamins (B_6 and B_{12}). Risk for deep vein thrombosis is increased two to three times in patients with hyperhomocysteinemia. When both hyperhomocysteinemia and factor V Leiden mutation are present, the risk for venous thrombosis is increased 10-fold. As well, patients with antiphospholipid antibodies or the lupus anticoagulant are associated with an increased risk for venous thrombosis. These patients may not have systemic lupus.

The clinical presentation of pulmonary embolus ranges from dyspnea, tachypnea, and chest pain to instant death. Chest pain, anxiety hypotension, hemoptysis, or cyanosis may occur. Physical examination may include signs of right ventricular dysfunction such as enlarged neck veins, and an accentuated second pulmonary sound on cardiac examination. About 40% of patients with pulmonary embolism have right ventricular dysfunction. The normal right ventricle with acute pulmonary embolism cannot tolerate a sustained mean pulmonary artery pressure of more than 40 mm Hg. These patients may be unresponsive to medical therapy, with persistent hypotension, hypoxia, and mean pulmonary artery pressure greater than 25 to 30 mm Hg despite anticoagulation and inotropes. Initial studies to be obtained include arterial blood gases, electrocardiogram (ECG), and chest x-rays.

The ECG may be normal but will usually exhibit an abnormality such as sinus tachycardia, an $S_1Q_3T_3$ pattern, right ventricular hypertrophy with strain, right bundle branch block, tachycardia, and T-wave inversion in the anterior chest leads (V_1-V_4).[50] Chest x-ray results are frequently normal. Westermark's sign (decreased pulmonary vascular markings peripherally) or Palla's sign (enlarged right descending pulmonary artery) may be present.

If the clinical likelihood is low, then a D-dimer enzyme-linked immunosorbent assay and ultrasound study of the lower extremities may be performed. The D-dimer is elevated in a number of conditions other than pulmonary embolism, including a recent major operation; however, a negative D-dimer assay suggests that the likelihood of pulmonary embolism is low. As well, hypoxia or hypercapnia is suggestive but not diagnostic of pulmonary embolism.

Other studies include ultrasound examination or impedance plethysmography of the lower extremities, ventilation-perfusion lung scan, echocardiography, high-resolution spiral CT of the chest, and pulmonary angiogram.

Ultrasound study of leg veins, even if negative, does not rule out pulmonary embolism. Helical CT using specific protocols has replaced ventilation-perfusion scans as the imaging modality of choice. CT scan is more widely available, especially at night, and can be performed more quickly than ventilation-perfusion scan. CT scan has the added benefit of imaging the entire chest, which may clarify the diagnosis, because the lung parenchyma, the pleural space, and the mediastinum are imaged. Some of the drawbacks to CT include need for IV contrast and high radiation dose. The sensitivity and specificity can range greatly and subsegmental thrombus can be missed. Furthermore, there is wide interobserver variability in interpreting the study.[51] Ventilation-perfusion lung scans are usually performed for any hemodynamically stable patient with suspicion of pulmonary embolism. If normal, the likelihood of pulmonary embolism is low. If decreased perfusion is matched by normal ventilation, a high probability of pulmonary embolism exists, and the patient receives treatment. Nondiagnostic results are difficult to interpret, and further studies may be required. The pulmonary arteriogram remains the gold standard for diagnosis. High-resolution helical CT of the chest with contrast may assist in defining the presence of thrombus in the proximal pulmonary arteries. The use of magnetic resonance pulmonary angiography is being studied.

The definitive study for pulmonary embolism is pulmonary arteriography, particularly for patients with cardiovascular collapse and hypotension, or when other studies are inconclusive. Lower extremity deep venous thrombosis itself may be an indication for treatment with anticoagulants.

Treatment of Pulmonary Embolus

Treatment of pulmonary embolus includes anticoagulation, oxygen, and analgesia. IV fluids, monitoring of central venous pressures, or use of inotropes may be required as dictated by the clinical situation. Heparin is the mainstay of treatment for pulmonary embolus. Heparin enhances antithrombin III activity to prevent propagation of the clot and to facilitate fibrinolysis. A bolus of heparin of 5000 to 10,000 units is given IV and followed by a continuous infusion of heparin (18 U/kg/hr; not to exceed 1600 U/hr). After therapeutic partial thromboplastin times have been achieved (ratio of activated partial thromboplastin time to the control ranges from 1.5-2.5), oral anticoagulation may be started with warfarin. Therapy for at least 3 to 5 days with heparin and warfarin sodium (Coumadin) is needed before adequate oral anticoagulation is achieved with the warfarin to discontinue the IV heparin. Warfarin is started at 5 mg/day to achieve an international normalized ratio (INR) of 2.0 to 3.0 (unfractionated heparin usually adds 0.5 to the INR). Routine anticoagulation monitoring is required. The duration of warfarin therapy is 3 months or longer.[52] Treatment greater than 6 months may carry increased risk. Low-molecular-weight heparins (LMWHs) are as safe and effective as unfractionated heparin. LMWHs have a longer half-life and more predictable dose response and are dosed by weight. Therapy with LMWHs does not usually require laboratory evaluation, and these drugs are administered subcutaneously. The level of anticoagulation can be measured with anti-Xa assays. LMWHs carry a lower risk for heparin-induced thrombocytopenia than unfractionated heparin. One significant disadvantage to LMWH therapy is the inability to completely reverse the anticoagulation with protamine. Fondaparinux is a synthetic anticoagulant with anti-Xa activity. It has been approved for use in the treatment of thromboembolic disease. It is administered subcutaneously and dosed based on weight once daily. It is not known to cause heparin-induced thrombocytopenia.[52]

Use of an inferior vena cava filter is considered in patients with pulmonary embolism when anticoagulation would carry increased risk (e.g., recent surgery, <24 hours postoperation, brain metastasis) or in patients with recurrent pulmonary emboli. The filter is placed below the renal veins at about the L3 vertebra level by way of the femoral or right jugular vein. The efficacy is 95%, and the risk for recurrent pulmonary embolism is 2% to 4%.

In patients with a serious hemodynamic and hypoxic response to pulmonary embolism (cardiogenic shock or hemodynamic instability) who do respond to resuscitation, heparin is initiated as standard therapy. In addition, thrombolytics (streptokinase or urokinase) may be given. Thrombolysis of clots occurs more quickly with thrombolytics than with heparin. Multivariate analysis suggests that thrombolysis and anticoagulation have better clinical outcomes than anticoagulation alone; however, the value of such treatment must be weighed against the risk for major hemorrhage. No prospective study has shown that the benefits of thrombolytic therapy in acute pulmonary embolism exceed the risks. Intracranial bleeding may occur in 3% of treated patients.[54] Other authors propose thrombolytic therapy in patients with right ventricular dysfunction.[55]

Further therapy may include catheter suction embolectomy for patients in whom thrombolytic therapy is ineffective. Venous (suction) or open (surgical) embolectomy may be performed to extract or obliterate the clot. IV pressors are frequently required. The open technique is infrequently performed and requires sternotomy (with consideration of femoral vein–to–femoral artery extracorporeal support before sternotomy) and bicaval cannulation, if possible, after sternotomy. The pulmonary artery is opened with a longitudinal incision, and gallstone forceps are used to extract proximal emboli, followed by use of Fogarty balloon catheters to extract emboli that are more distal.

Inferior vena cava interruption may be considered if all alternatives have been exhausted. Complications include chronic venous insufficiency of the lower extremities.

Chronic pulmonary embolism may develop with failure of the usual resolution of acute pulmonary emboli. Whereas most emboli will lyse, some become fibrotic and adhere to the pulmonary arterial wall. Symptoms of cor pulmonale, chronic dyspnea, right ventricular hypertrophy, and high right-sided pressures are all indications of chronic pulmonary embolism.

Indications for surgery follow:

1. Proximal pulmonary artery occlusion
2. Adequate collaterals with filling of distal pulmonary artery
3. High right-sided cardiac pressures and hypoxia
4. Minimally impaired lung function

The surgical approaches follow:

1. Unilateral thoracotomy without cardiopulmonary bypass
2. Standard cardiopulmonary bypass with proximal and distal control of pulmonary arteries
3. Cardiopulmonary bypass with total circulatory arrest (intermittent)

Incisions are patched with pericardium unless they are on the main pulmonary artery.

Prevention

Prevention of pulmonary embolism is considered in all patients having a major surgical procedure. All hospitalized patients must be evaluated and stratified for their risk for pulmonary embolism and the appropriate prophylaxis applied. Unfractionated heparin is most commonly used for perioperative prophylaxis and effectively reduces the rate of fatal pulmonary embolism. The dose is typically 5000 units three times daily and is continued until the patient is discharged and ambulatory. LMWHs are an alternative to unfractionated heparin because of their characteristics of improved bioavailability, improved absorption, once-daily injection, and reduced rates of heparin-induced thrombocytopenia. Mechanical compression devices to stimulate fibrinolysis (from stimulation of the venous endothelium) are effective in patients who are bed-bound; however, ambulatory patients are usually not compliant in their use within a general ward environment.

Pulmonary embolus, even in its treatable form, carries high morbidity and potential mortality risks. Patients with pulmonary embolism are given heparin, oral anticoagulants, or fractionated LMWH. Subsequent anticoagulation after discharge is required for periods up to 6 months. Patients with specific genetic characteristics are at increased risk for venous thrombolic events. Prevention of pulmonary embolism with some type of prophylaxis is initiated in all patients having major surgical procedures.

THORACIC OUTLET SYNDROME

Thoracic outlet syndrome may occur in 5% of the population in a mild form. Thoracic outlet syndrome may occur in three forms: neurogenic, venous, or arterial. The neurogenic form is by far the most common and the most difficult to diagnose and treat. Vascular compression may be documented; nerve compression and pain or paresthesias may require electromyelogram for diagnosis. The syndrome occurs more frequently in women than in men. The anatomy of thoracic outlet syndrome includes compression of the subclavian artery, the subclavian vein, or the brachial plexus, where it passes between the scalene muscles and over the first rib. Anomalous fibromuscular bands and cervical ribs may also compress the brachial plexus or subclavian vessels.

Clinical features of neurogenic thoracic outlet syndrome include intermittent symptoms of nerve compression in most patients, which include pain, paresthesias, and weakness. If the upper brachial plexus is involved, symptoms may be increased by turning or tilting the head. If the lower brachial plexus (C8-T1) is involved, pain may be noted in the supraclavicular fossa extending to the inner arm and involving the ring and small fingers. Venous thoracic outlet syndrome may be characterized by upper extremity edema, venous distention, or effort thrombosis, also known as *Paget-Schroetter syndrome*. Arterial compression may present with loss of radial pulse, upper extremity claudication, or thrombosis.

The diagnosis of neurogenic thoracic outlet syndrome is initially made clinically. A thorough history and physical exam, as well as a cervical spine x-ray series, can be performed to evaluate cervical spine disease. Maneuvers that may be performed in the clinic to help diagnose thoracic outlet syndrome include the Adson or scalene test, costoclavicular test, and arm claudication test. In the Adson test, the patient holds a deep breath, extends the neck maximally, and turns to face the affected side, while the clinician palpates the ipsilateral radial pulse. This test is positive if the pulse amplitude decreases or is abolished. The costoclavicular test is performed by having the patient pull the shoulders back and downward. Reproduction of neurologic symptoms or changes in the radial pulse are considered positive. Arm claudication may be elicited by positioning the patient with their shoulders down and back and the arms raised to 90 degrees with the elbows flexed. If exercise of the hands reproduces symptoms, the test is positive.

Neurogenic thoracic outlet syndrome needs to be confirmed with nerve conduction studies to localize the area of slowing of nerve conduction and to rule out other compression syndromes such as carpal tunnel syndrome. Electromyelogram or nerve conduction studies are helpful to rule out carpal tunnel syndrome. Patients with moderate to severe slowing of nerve conduction usually respond to nonoperative therapy.[39] Vascular thoracic outlet syndrome must be confirmed with objective studies. A venogram may be performed for significant venous symptoms. Noninvasive arterial studies may be helpful. Angiography may be performed if aneurysm, thrombus, or emboli are suspected.

Treatment is physical therapy for 2 to 12 months. Exercises to strengthen the shoulder girdle, neck stretching, hot and cold packs, and muscle relaxants are used. Repetitive mechanical and muscular trauma is avoided. Surgery is used as a last resort for severe pain, impaired motor function or atrophy, treatment failure, or need to improve quality of life. Patients who present with effort thrombosis undergo catheter-directed thrombolysis followed by surgical decompression of the thoracic outlet by first rib resection during the initial hospital admission.[56]

If surgery is required, transaxillary first rib resection allows complete resection with a good cosmetic result. Cervical ribs are also removed. The assistant must relax the arm and shoulders intermittently (every 5 minutes for at least 30 seconds). An anterior scalenectomy (total) may be performed through an anterior supraclavicular approach and is usually indicated for significant symptoms of upper plexus involvement. The results of surgical treatment are mixed, with 50% to 60% of patients having a good to excellent result, 20% to 30% having a fair or improved result, and 10% having no improvement. Recurrent symptoms may prompt surgical treatment in approximately one third of patients.[57] Recurrent thoracic outlet syndrome most often occurs in patients with neurogenic disease and may be caused by retained portions of the first rib or retained cervical rib. Recurrent thoracic outlet syndrome may be approached posteriorly. Before embarking on surgical treatment for recurrent symptoms, nerve conduction studies are repeated, and an extended trial of physical therapy is implemented.

References

1. Weisman IM: Cardiopulmonary exercise testing in the preoperative assessment for lung resection surgery: Semin Thorac Cardiovasc Surg 13:116-125, 2001.
2. Linden, PA, Bueno R, Colson YL, et al: Lung resection in patients with preoperative FEV1<35% predicted. Chest 127:1984-1990, 2005.
3. Varela G, Brunelli A, Rocco G, et al: Predicted versus observed FEV1 in the immediate postoperative period after pulmonary lobectomy. Eur J Cardiothoracic Surg 30:644-648, 2006.
4. Handy JR, Asaph JW, Skokan L, et al: What Happens to patients undergoing lung cancer surgery? Outcomes and quality of life before and after surgery. Chest 122:21-30, 2002.
5. Brunelli A, Refai MA, Salati M, et al: Carbon monoxide lung diffusion capacity improves risk stratification in patients without airflow limitation: Evidence for systematic measurement before lung resection. Eur J Cardiothoracic Surg 29:567-570, 2006.
6. Beckles MA, Spiro SG, Colice GL, Rudd RM: The physiologic evaluation of patients with lung cancer being considered for resectional surgery. Chest 123:105S-114S, 2003.
7. Wang J, Olak J, Ferguson MK: Diffusing capacity predicts operative mortality but not long-term survival after resection for lung cancer. J Thorac Cardiovasc Surg 117:581-586, 1999.
8. Brunelli A, Refai MA, Salati M, et al: Carbon monoxide lung diffusion capacity improves risk stratification in patients without airflow limitation: Evidence for systematic measurement before lung resection. Eur J Cardiothoracic Surg 29:567-570, 2006.
9. McKenna RJ, Houck W, Fuller CB: Video-assisted thoracic surgery lobectomy: Experience with 1,100 cases. Ann Thorac Surg 81:421-426, 2006.
10. Shigemura N, Akashi A, Nakagiri T, et al: Long-term outcomes after a variety of video-assisted thoracoscopic lobectomy approaches for clinical stage IA lung cancer: A multi-institutional study. J Thorac Cardiovasc Surg 132:507-512, 2006.

11. Barrera R, Shi W, Amar D, et al: Smoking and timing of cessation: Impact on pulmonary complications after thoracotomy. Chest 127:1977-1983, 2005.

12. Vaporciyan AA, Merriman KW, Ece F, et al: Incidence of major pulmonary morbidity after pneumonectomy: Association with timing of smoking cessation. Ann Thorac Surg 73:420-426, 2002.

13. The Tobacco Use and Dependence Clinical Practice Guideline Panel, Staff, and Consortium Representatives: A clinical practice guideline for treating tobacco use and dependence: A US public health service report. JAMA 283:3244-3254, 2000.

14. Cofta-Woerpel L, Wright KL, Wetter DW: Smoking cessation 1: Pharmacological treatments. Behav Med 32:47-56, 2006.

15. Evrard V, Ceulemans J, Coosemans W, et al: Congenital parenchymatous malformations of the lung. World J Surg 23:1123-1132, 1999.

16. McAdams HP, Kirejczyk WM, Rosado-de-Christenson ML, Matsumoto S: Bronchogenic cyst: Imaging features with clinical and histopathologic correlation. Radiology 217:441-446, 2000.

17. Ustunsoz B, Bozlar U, Kocaoglu M, et al: Mechanical coil embolization of pulmonary arteriovenous malformations. Diagn Interv Radiol 12:39-42, 2006.

18. U.S. Institutes of Health: Surveillance epidemiology and end results (SEER), 2006. Accessed October 17, 2006, at http://seer.cancer.gov/faststats/sites.

19. Simon GR, Wagner H: Small cell lung cancer. Chest 123:259S-269S, 2003.

20. Toloza EM: Noninvasive staging of non-small cell lung cancer: A review of the current evidence. Chest 123:137S-146S, 2003.

21. Boiselle PM, Patz EF Jr, Vining DJ, et al: Imaging of mediastinal lymph nodes: CT, MR, and FDG PET. Radiographics 18:1061-1069, 1998.

22. Coleman RE: PET in lung cancer: J Nucl Med 40:814-820, 1999.

23. Al Sugair A, Coleman RE: Applications of PET in lung cancer. Semin Nucl Med 28:303-319, 1998.

24. Silvestri GA, Margolis ML, Detterbeck F: The noninvasive staging of non-small cell lung cancer: The guidelines. Chest 123:147S-156S, 2003.

25. Gould MK, Lillington GA: Strategy and cost in investigating solitary pulmonary nodules. Thorax 53(Suppl 2):S32-S37, 1998.

26. Gambhir SS, Shepherd JE, Shah BD, et al: Analytical decision model for the cost-effective management of solitary pulmonary nodules. J Clin Oncol 16:2113-2125, 1998.

27. Tan BB, Flaherty KR, Kazerooni EA, Iannettoni MD: The solitary pulmonary nodule. Chest 123:89S-96S, 2003.

28. Fong KM, Sekido Y, Minna JD: Molecular pathogenesis of lung cancer. J Thorac Cardiovasc Surg 118:1136-1152, 1999.

29. Swisher SG, Roth JA, Nemunaitis J, et al: Adenovirus-mediated p53 gene transfer in advanced non-small-cell lung cancer. J Natl Cancer Inst 91:763-771, 1999.

30. Hofmann HS, Bartling B, Simm A, et al: Identification and classification of differentially expressed genes in non-small cell lung cancer by expression profiling on a global human 59.620-element oligonucleotide array. Oncol Rep 16:587-95, 2006.

31. McDoniels-Silver AL, Stone GD, Lubert RA, You M: Differential expression of critical cellular genes in human lung adenocarcinomas and squamous cell carcinomas in comparison to normal lung tissues. Neoplasia 4:141-50, 2002.

32. Raponi M, Zhang Y, Yu J, et al: Gene expression signatures for predicting prognosis of squamous cell and adenocarcinomas of the lung. Cancer Res 66:7466-7472, 2006.

33. D'Amico TA, Massey M, Herndon JE 2nd, et al: A biologic risk model for stage I lung cancer: Immunohistochemical analysis of 408 patients with the use of ten molecular markers. J Thorac Cardiovasc Surg 117:736-743, 1999.

34. Brooks KR, To K, Joshi MB, et al: Measurement of chemoresistance markers in patients with stage III non-small cell lung cancer: A novel approach for patient selection. Ann Thorac Surg 76:187-193, 2006.

35. Gordon GJ, Deters LA, Nitz MD, et al: Differential diagnosis of solitary lung nodules with gene expression ratios. J Thorac Cardiovasc Surg 132:621-627, 2006.

36. Arriagada R, Bergman B, Dunant A, et al, for the International Adjuvant Lung Cancer Trial Collaborative Group: Cisplatin-based adjuvant chemotherapy in patients with completely resected non-small-cell lung cancer. N Engl J Med 350:351-360, 2004.

37. Winton T, Livingston R, Johnson D, et al, for the National Cancer Institute of Canada Clinical Trials Group, National Cancer Institute of the United States Intergroup JBR, 10 Trial Investigators: Vinorelbine plus cisplatin vs. observation in resected non-small-cell lung cancer. N Engl J Med 352:2589-2597, 2005.

38. Smythe WR: Treatment of stage I non-small cell lung carcinoma. Chest 123:181S-187S, 2003.

39. Goldman L, Ausiello D: Cecil Textbook of Medicine. Philadelphia, WB Saunders, 2004.

40. Yang SC, Cameron DE: Current Therapy in Thoracic and Cardiovascular Surgery. Philadelphia, Mosby, 2004.

41. Fishman A, Martinez F, Naunheim K, et al: A randomized trial comparing lung-volume-reduction surgery with medical therapy for severe emphysema. N Engl J Med 348:2059-2073, 2003.

42. Venuta, F, Rendina EA, De Giacomo T, et al: Bronchoscopic procedures for emphysema treatment. Eur J Cardiothorac Surg 29:281-287, 2006.

43. Arcasoy SM, Kotloff RM: Lung transplantation. N Engl J Med 340:1081-1091, 1999.

44. Acute Respiratory Distress Syndrome Network: Ventilation with lower tidal volumes as compared with traditional tidal volumes for acute lung injury and the acute respiratory distress syndrome. N Engl J Med 342:1301-1308, 2000.

45. Mancebo J, Fernandez R, Blanch L, et al: A multicenter trial of prolonged prone ventilation in severe acute respiratory distress syndrome. Am J Respir Crit Care Med 173:1233-1239, 2006.

46. Hirshberg B, Sklair-Levi M, Nir-Paz R, et al: Factors predicting mortality of patients with lung abscess. Chest 115:746-750, 1999.

47. Blair D, Xu ZB, Agatsuma T: Paragonimiasis and the genus *Paragonimus*. Adv Parasitol 42:113-222, 1999.

48. Goldhaber SZ: Pulmonary embolism. N Engl J Med 339:93-104, 1998.

49. Cattaneo M, Franchi F, Zighetti ML, et al: Plasma levels of activated protein C in healthy subjects and patients with previous venous thromboembolism: Relationships with plasma homocysteine levels. Arterioscler Thromb Vasc Biol 18:1371-1375, 1998.

50. Kucher N, Goldhaber SZ: Management of massive pulmonary embolism. Circulation 112:E28-32, 2005.

51. Rahimtoola A, Bergin JD: Acute pulmonary embolism: An update on diagnosis and management. Curr Probl Cardiol 30:61-114, 2005.

52. Kearon C, Gent M, Hirsh J, et al: A comparison of three months of anticoagulation with extended anticoagulation

for a first episode of idiopathic venous thromboembolism [published erratum appears in N Engl J Med 22:34:298, 1999]. N Engl J Med 340:901-907, 1999.

53. Piazza G, Goldhaber SZ: Acute pulmonary embolism. II. Treatment and prophylaxis. Circulation 114: E42-47, 2006.

54. Elliott G: Thrombolytic therapy for venous thromboembolism. Curr Opin Hematol 6:304-308, 1999.

55. Goldhaber SZ: Thrombolytic therapy. Adv Intern Med 44:311-325, 1999.

56. Urschel HC Jr, Razzuk MA: Paget-Schroetter syndrome: What is the best management? Ann Thorac Surg 69:166-168, 2000.

57. Urschel HC Jr, Razzuk MA: Neurovascular compression in the thoracic outlet: Changing management over 50 years. Ann Surg 228:609-617, 1998.

CHAPTER 60

Congenital Heart Disease

Charles D. Fraser, Jr., MD   and   Kathleen E. Carberry, RN

HISTORY

The era of surgical treatment for congenital cardiac anomalies was initiated in November 1944 when Dr. Alfred Blalock and associates Vivien Thomas and Dr. Helen Taussig combined their unique talents and vision to treat a young child dying of cyanotic congenital heart disease.[1] This palliative operation involved the surgical creation of a systemic-to-pulmonary artery connection in the patient suffering from inadequate pulmonary blood flow; the procedure has since been recalled as "miraculous" and has carried the eponym, the *Blalock-Taussig shunt* (BT shunt) during the ensuing now more than half a century. The striking success of this simple concept and the reproducible nature of the operation in children suffering from otherwise fatal cardiac conditions emboldened subsequent surgical innovators to venture inside the congenitally malformed heart; initially asking a parent to serve as a biologic oxygenator using the technique of controlled cross-circulation and soon thereafter with the assistance of a mechanical, extracorporeal heart-lung

bypass pump.[2,3] With the aid of the ability to support the patient's circulation during intracardiac exploration, surgeons have sequentially attacked practically every described congenital cardiac anomaly. The prospect of meaningful survival for patients born with otherwise devastating congenital cardiac lesions is now expected in most, if not all, cases.

ADULTS WITH CONGENITAL HEART DISEASE

As a result of this success story, there is now a large and ever-growing population of adults with repaired or unrepaired congenital heart disease (CHD); estimates in the United States for 2005 place the number of adult patients surviving with repaired or palliated congenital cardiac lesions at more than 1 million persons.[4] This reality has been associated with new challenges in the ongoing medical maintenance of such patients, and particular focus on the care of patients with congenital cardiac lesions presenting for surgery for noncardiac illnesses. The evolving subspecialty of adult congenital heart disease, also known as grown-ups with congenital heart disease (GUCH), points to the unique needs of this population of patients.

TARGET AUDIENCE

This chapter is designed to provide medical students, general surgery residents, and practicing general surgeons a working tool to aid in their understanding of the features of anatomy and physiology in patients presenting for *general surgical procedures* in the setting of repaired or unrepaired congenital cardiac lesions. The large scope and breadth of the evolving field of congenital heart surgery precludes an exhaustive treatise on all

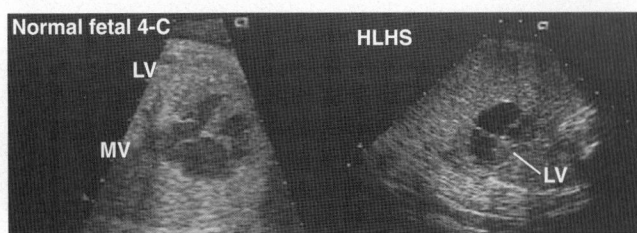

Figure 60-1 Normal fetal ultrasound (4-chamber) (*left*) and fetal ultrasound of a child with hypoplastic left heart syndrome (HLHS; *right*). LV, left ventricle; MV, mitral valve.

aspects of this specialty. Several excellent and thorough textbooks of congenital heart surgery will be referenced within this chapter, and the reader is encouraged to utilize these reference sources for additional, in-depth understanding of the lesions to be reviewed. Today's practicing general surgeon needs to be well versed in the basics of cardiac anatomy, physiology, and the specific derangements associated with the various known congenital cardiac lesions. Furthermore, there are few patients with complex congenital cardiac lesions that may be considered "cured" of their cardiac problem even after successful reconstructive surgery; it is imperative that the general surgeon who faces the need to perform a noncardiac operation on such a patient be familiar with the specific issues of ongoing concern in patients with congenital cardiac disease.

CURRENT PATHWAY FOR PRACTICING CONGENITAL HEART SURGERY

Before embarking on a review of the field, it is probably worthwhile to describe the setting in which patients with congenital heart disease seek and receive care in today's medical environment. With the development of sophisticated methods of fetal ultrasound, a large percentage of children requiring surgery for CHD are diagnosed during fetal life (Fig. 60-1). Although not yet confirmed as affecting overall survival rates, a fetal diagnosis of complex congenital heart disease is of inordinate help to the parents and medical management team. This is particularly important in the setting of lesions dependent on persistent patency of the ductus arteriosus for postnatal survival. In these individuals, survival after delivery is predicated on maintenance of ductal patency through the intravenous (IV) infusion of prostaglandin E_1 (PGE_1) initiated in the delivery suite often through an umbilical vein catheter.

An ever-growing number of congenital cardiac lesions are known to be associated with specific genetic mutations, many clearly inherited, some presumed sporadic. As such, a chromosomal analysis is frequently performed in individuals found to have major structural cardiac abnormalities; this analysis may be performed during fetal life through amniocentesis. The chromosomal evaluation is of benefit to the family when planning the risk of such an occurrence in future offspring. For the clini-

cian, knowledge of chromosomal abnormalities such as DiGeorge sequence, velocardiofacial syndrome, and Marfan syndrome in their patients, aids in the delivery of acute medical management.[5]

In general terms, the timing of surgery for various congenital cardiac conditions depends on the presenting symptomatology and the expectations for further associated complications. Children presenting with limited pulmonary blood flow or atretic pulmonary connections typically require surgery during the first few days of life and occasionally within hours of delivery. Lesions associated with excessive pulmonary blood flow result in early heart failure, which may manifest as poor feeding, tachypnea, or even respiratory failure. Such individuals are operated on during early infancy to ameliorate their symptoms and to prevent the development of pulmonary vascular disease.

The specialty of congenital heart surgery is now recognized as a subspecialty of cardiothoracic surgery. Congenital heart surgeons have been previously certified in cardiothoracic surgery by the American Board of Thoracic Surgery (ABTS) and have received additional fellowship training in the United States or abroad in congenital heart surgery. At present, no formal certification process exists for the specialty; however, the ABTS has recently recommended and approved a fellowship program format that will culminate in a qualifying examination and certificate.

Most pediatric cardiac surgery is performed in large, multispecialty children's hospitals in association with formal programs focused on the care of these complex patients. The management team includes pediatric cardiac anesthesiologists, perfusionists, and nursing staff. Focused pediatric cardiac intensive care units have been developed to optimize the patients' opportunity for recovery.[6]

Historically, pediatric cardiologists have provided the medical management of patients born with congenital heart disease. Pediatric cardiology is in a state of evolution as well. With the advances in catheter-based technology, lesions previously treated with surgery are now being addressed by interventional pediatric cardiologists. Examples include device closure of atrial and ventricular septal defects; occlusion of patent ductus arteriosus (PDA); and dilation and stenting of stenotic vessels in both the systemic and pulmonary circulation. For a more in-depth review of this specialty, the reader is referred to the excellent technical textbook recently written by Dr. Charles Mullins.[7]

The situation of care for adults with congenital heart disease is not as well organized as for children. This issue is of particular relevance to the general surgeon faced with operating on an adult patient with significant congenital heart disease. One overriding message needs to be clear to the general surgeon in this setting—*it must be assumed that in patients with previously repaired congenital cardiac lesions, even in the absence of overt cardiac symptomatology, the potential for significant perioperative cardiorespiratory derangement exists.* More simply stated, the presence of a surgical scar on the chest of a patient with known congenital heart disease does *not* suggest that the lesion has been cured. With this issue firmly in mind, the general surgeon may find it challenging to determine the best source for *qualified* consultation in such a patient. At present, most adult cardiologists are not adequately trained in congenital heart disease to be generally expected to provide competent consultation on adult patients with congenital heart disease.

On the other hand, pediatric cardiologists are not educated in adult medicine and cardiology—many feel very uncomfortable providing consultation on adult patients with congenital heart disease. As noted previously, the subspecialty of adult congenital heart disease is in a state of development, but at present, there are few practitioners who have been educated specifically to care for these patients.[8] These comments underscore the necessity of the practicing general surgeon to become familiar with the specific issues of concern for patients with congenital heart disease in order to ascertain that the patient's unique anatomic and physiologic issues have been evaluated properly. Adult patients with congenital heart disease who present for care in a center *without* a designated specialist qualified in the care of adults with congenital heart disease must be evaluated by a pediatric cardiologist in coordination with an adult cardiologist. Of equal importance, the anesthesiologists and intensivists caring for such a patient must have a working understanding of the complexities and nuances of the patient's cardiac condition.[9,10] The anesthetic management of patients with congenital heart disease undergoing general surgical procedures is complicated and can become disastrous if managed improperly.

ANATOMY, TERMINOLOGY, AND DIAGNOSIS

Anatomy and Terminology

One of the most intimidating aspects for the student of congenital heart disease is developing a level of comfort with the terminology used in describing specific lesions. To begin, a thorough and sound understanding of *normal* cardiac anatomy is mandatory. There are several excellent texts on this subject; in particular, the textbooks of cardiac anatomy edited by Benson Wilcox and Robert Anderson are especially concise and clear.[11] One issue of difficulty that challenges proper understanding of the patient's anatomy is the frequent use of abbreviations and eponyms for various congenital lesions (congenitally corrected transposition [ccTGA], ventricular inversion, and L-transposition all describe the same heart, but none provides a complete anatomic description). Unless otherwise clear to all parties involved in the care of these complicated patients, the anatomic description needs to be segmental and complete to avoid mistakes or misinterpretations of structure.

In describing congenital cardiac lesions, a segmental approach is used to determine the relationship of the various structural elements. The situs describes the relationship of sidedness; situs solitus (normal), situs inversus (reversed), or situs ambiguous (indeterminate). The cardiac elements described include (in sequence) the

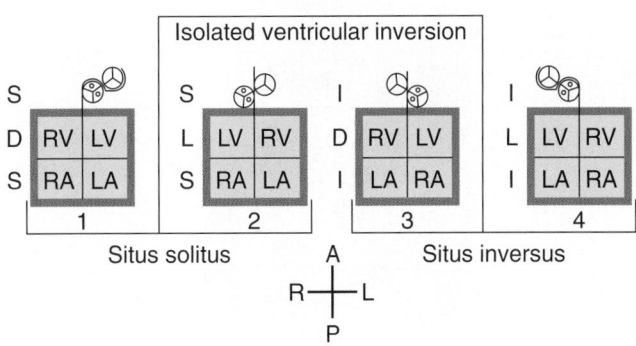

Figure 60-2 Model depicting cardiac morphology for "normal" hearts, that is, hearts with atrioventricular concordance and ventriculoarterial concordance using Van Praagh nomenclature. The vertical line above the box denotes position of the ventricular septum. (From Kirklin JW, Barratt Boyes BG: General considerations: Anatomy, dimensions, and terminology. In Cardiac Surgery, 2nd ed. New York, Churchill Livingstone, 1993.)

atria, the ventricles, and the great vessels. The relationship of the connections must be understood—connections are concordant (e.g., right atrium connecting to right ventricle) or discordant (e.g., right ventricle connecting to the aorta). The chamber sidedness must be clarified—a morphologic right atrium may be on the left side of the patient. The relationship and connections of the cardiac valves must then be assessed; connections may be normal, stenotic, atretic, or straddling. Of note to the general surgeon, abnormal sidedness of the cardiac structures is frequently associated with abnormal relationships of the thoracic and abdominal organs. A thorough assessment of the patient's anatomy is recommended before surgery.

There are two widely accepted and applied schools of cardiac morphologic description. The Van Praagh nomenclature uses abbreviations to sequentially describe the relationship of the atria, the ventricular looping, and the position of the aorta. The first letter describes the situs of the atrial chambers (and usually the abdominal organs); *S*—for situs solitus (normal), *I*—for situs inversus (reversed), or *A*—for situs ambiguous (indeterminate). The second letter describes the relationship of the embryologic looping of the ventricles; *D*—"dextro" looping or right-handed topology (normal) or *L*—for left-handed topology. The third and last letter describes the relationship of the aortic valve to the pulmonary valve; *D*—right sided and *L*—left sided (Fig. 60-2).

The Anderson nomenclature is more wordy and lengthy, but is perhaps a bit simpler to understand. The descriptions are again of the sequential relationship of the structures. Starting with the atria, the connections and relationships are sequentially described. Thus, the atrial sidedness is described, followed by the sequence of connections to the ventricles and then great vessels. Example: Atrial situs solitus (normal) with atrioventricular discordance (reversed) and ventriculoarterial discordance (reversed) describes the heart mentioned previously as

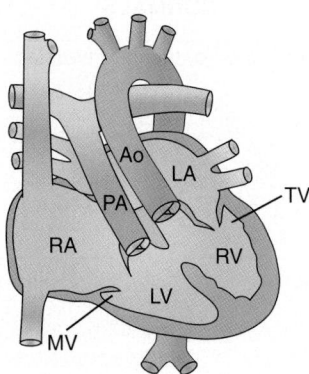

Figure 60-3 Congenitally corrected transposition of the great arteries. Atrial situs solitus (normal) with atrioventricular discordance and ventriculoarterial discordance using Anderson nomenclature. S, L, L by Van Praagh classification. Ao, aorta; LA, left atrium, LV, left ventricle; MV, mitral valve; RA, right atrium; RV, right ventricle; TV, tricuspid valve.

corrected transposition or S, L, L by the Van Praagh classification (Fig. 60-3).

Diagnosis

As with all aspects of surgery, there is a wide variety of highly sophisticated diagnostic tools available to examine cardiac structure and function. Despite the widespread availability and application of these tools, none has as of yet replaced or eliminated the necessity of a thorough history and physical examination. Most patients who have a history of congenital heart disease become very well informed about the specifics of their cardiac conditions, as do their parents. *A detailed review of the patient's past medical history is absolutely mandatory.* This includes securing, when possible, records from all previous diagnostic and procedural reports. It is disturbing how often an incorrect assumption is made about the patient's previous surgical history and anatomy, frequently in the setting where the patient's old operative report or clinical summary could easily clarify the misunderstanding.

Particularly in adults with congenital heart disease, there are specific points of medical history that must be elucidated. A history of palpitations, syncope, and neurologic deficit must be further investigated—the incidence of significant dysrhythmias in certain categories of adults with CHD is high and in many cases warrants further investigation including continuous monitoring (Holter) and electrophysiologic study.[12] A recent study of the adult patients undergoing congenital heart surgery at the Texas Children's Hospital during the past decade has demonstrated that *new-onset dysrhythmias* are the most frequently observed perioperative complication. Many of these are malignant dysrhythmias, such as ventricular tachycardia.[10]

Physical Examination

A complete physical examination in a patient with previously repaired congenital heart disease will often yield information critical to the proper planning of a general surgical procedure. Patients needs to be completely undressed and thoroughly examined. In many cyanotic patients, the color changes may be prominent, particularly in the nail beds and lips and mucous membranes. In other patients, cyanosis may be subtler, giving the patient a gray or even pale appearance. Previous surgical incisions need to be noted and reconciled with the known medical history. Thoracotomy incisions on either side may indicate a previous Blalock-Taussig shunt (using either the turned down, divided subclavian artery or with a prosthetic interposition graft, the so-called *modified* BT shunt). In patients with a left aortic arch, a left thoracotomy incision will be present if a previous coarctation repair has been carried out. Median sternotomy incisions or anterior thoracotomy incisions may indicate previous intra- or extracardiac surgery.

A complete vascular examination is often overlooked in patients with congenital heart disease. It is important to assess pulses and obtain blood pressure measurements in *all four extremities.* Patients who have existing or have previously had a BT shunt often have diminished or absent pulses in the upper extremity corresponding to the previous shunt. This may also be true in the left upper extremity in patients with previous coarctation repairs, especially if a subclavian flap angioplasty was performed (Waldhausen operation). Furthermore, a history of previous coarctation repair does not guarantee that the lower extremity pulses and blood pressures will be normal. Also, patients who have undergone previous cardiac catheterization may have chronically stenosed or occluded femoral vessels. All these issues may be of significance for monitoring and vascular access in a patient undergoing a general surgical procedure.

In a subsequent section, the Fontan procedure for single ventricle palliation will be reviewed. Briefly, this operation results in significant systemic venous hypertension (often in the range of 12 to 15 mm Hg). In patients with a Fontan circulation, physical examination may reveal hepatic congestion, ascites, pedal edema, venous varicosities, and jugular venous distention. In some individuals, macronodular hepatic cirrhosis may be suspected on the basis of a firm, fibrotic liver edge.[13]

Entire textbooks are dedicated to the physical examination of patients with cardiac disease and a thorough discussion of this issue, particularly the specifics of cardiac auscultation, is beyond the scope of this chapter. In general, however, the cardiac examination includes an assessment of the patient's rhythm, point of maximal impulse, and character of any auscultated murmurs. It must also be emphasized that the *absence* of a significant cardiac murmur does *not* rule out significant cardiac pathology.

Pulse Oximetry

Four-extremity pulse oximetry is an essential part of the clinical assessment of a patient with suspected congenital heart disease. In patients with ductal-dependent circulation to the lower body (severe aortic coarctation or aortic arch interruption), *differential cyanosis* may be presenting, indicating the ejection of desaturated systemic venous blood through the patent ductus to the descending aorta contrasted with fully saturated pulmonary venous blood ejected to the ascending aorta and, thereby, the upper extremities. Baseline (room air) saturations must be documented in all patients in whom an operative intervention is anticipated to establish the range of normal for a given patient.

Plain Radiography

Standard chest radiography with anteroposterior and lateral views is still an essential component of the assessment of a patient with congenital heart disease. Standard elements to be examined include a skeletal survey, assessment of the diaphragms and hepatic shadow, and location of the gastric bubble. The lung fields are assessed for pulmonary plethora (arterial or venous), air space disease, and presence of effusions. The cardiac silhouette may reveal much important information—cardiothoracic ratio indicative of cardiomegaly or pericardial effusion, presence of atrial enlargement, presence or absence of the pulmonary artery shadow, and arch sidedness (Fig. 60-4).

Electrocardiogram

The electrocardiogram (ECG) is of significant importance in assessing patients with congenital heart disease. The rate and rhythm must be noted, including the presence or absence of P-wave activity and axis. Many patients with congenital heart disease, especially those with complex conditions such as heterotaxy syndrome, may exhibit deranged or absent sinus node activity, giving rise to a predominant junctional rhythm, which may significantly compromise cardiac output. The QRS duration and axis yield important information concerning conduction delay and abnormal ventricular forces. For example, patients with atrioventricular canal defects are known to have left axis deviation. Furthermore, in patients undergoing repair of certain forms of congenital heart disease, there may be an early or late predisposition to malignant dysrhythmias. It is particularly important to elucidate a history of palpitations from a patient with repaired or unrepaired congenital heart disease—such a history may warrant further investigation with 24-hour continuous ECG monitoring (Holter).

Echocardiography

Noninvasive imaging is now well established as the primary diagnostic modality for structural cardiac disease. For most patients, excellent anatomic detail may be obtained using transthoracic imaging (two-dimensional). Standard images include subcostal, suprasternal, parasternal, and subxiphoid views and are oriented in both long and short axis directions. Furthermore, significant hemodynamic information may be inferred using echo Doppler blood flow velocities and interpreted using the modified Bernoulli formula (pressure gradient=$4V^2$, where V is echo velocity in m/sec). To properly assess the patient's cardiac lesion, segmental analysis of the cardiac structures, connections, and valves must be performed. A quantitative estimate of ejection fraction, shortening fraction, and valvular inflow velocity will aid in assessing

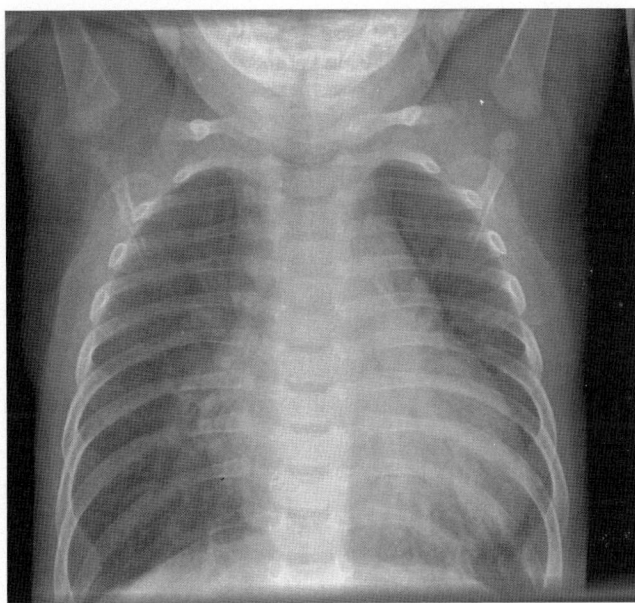

Figure 60-4 Cardiomegaly and increased pulmonary vascular markings in a patient with complete atrioventricular canal defect.

cardiac function. For most patients with congenital cardiac disease, adequate diagnostic information is attainable through echocardiography in the hands of a qualified pediatric cardiologist.

Magnetic Resonance Imaging and Computed Tomography

The fields of cardiac magnetic resonance imaging (MRI) and computed tomography (CT) are rapidly evolving as adjuncts to echocardiography for noninvasive structural and functional assessment of the heart. At present, MRI is being used with increasing frequency to provide anatomic detail in congenitally malformed hearts where echocardiographic detail is lacking or unattainable. This modality has proved particularly useful in imaging the extracardiac great vessels and systemic and pulmonary venous connections, and providing accurate estimates of cardiac function, especially right ventricular ejection fraction. CT may also be used for such imaging detail but does have the potential detrimental association with significant radiation exposure.

Cardiac Catheterization

Cardiac catheterization has long been considered the gold standard for diagnostic imaging of congenitally malformed hearts. With the current sophistication of echocardiography, this is no longer the case for most patients. Nonetheless, there are still circumstances in which diagnostic cardiac catheterization is necessary to obtain accurate anatomic detail. This may be the case in patients who for some reason have poor echo windows (although even this issue may be overcome using transesophageal echocardiography). More often, there are specifics of anatomic detail that neither echocardiography nor MRI

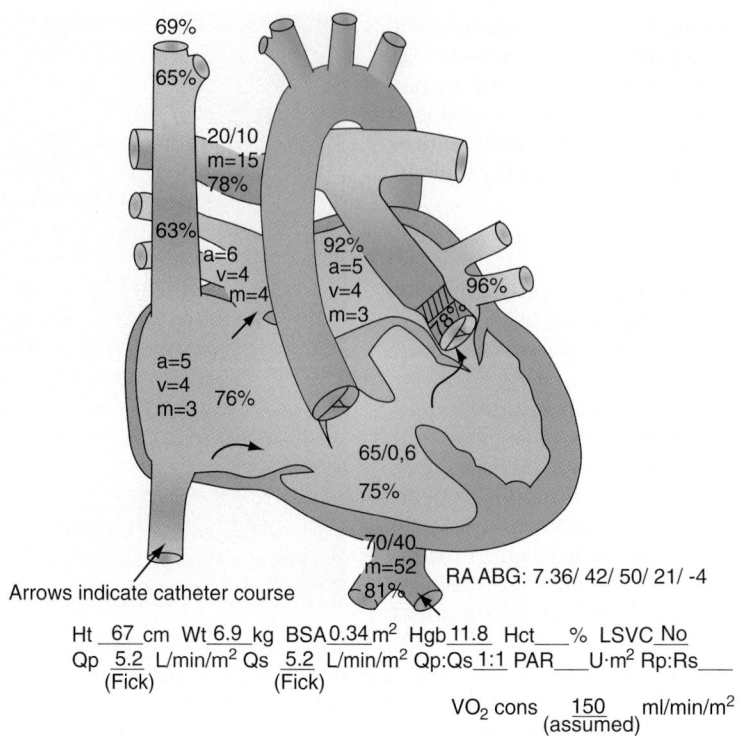

69%

65%

20/10
m=15
78%

63%
a=6
v=4
m=4

92%
a=5
v=4
m=3

96%

78%

a=5
v=4
m=3   76%

65/0,6

75%

70/40
m=52
81%   RA ABG: 7.36/ 42/ 50/ 21/ -4

Arrows indicate catheter course

Ht __67__ cm Wt __6.9__ kg BSA __0.34__ m² Hgb __11.8__ Hct___% LSVC __No__
Qp __5.2__ L/min/m² Qs __5.2__ L/min/m² Qp:Qs __1:1__ PAR___U·m² Rp:Rs___
    (Fick)   (Fick)

VO₂ cons __150__ ml/min/m²
          (assumed)

Figure 60-5 Hemodynamic information obtained following cardiac catheterization.

can delineate. Specific circumstances include branch pulmonary artery (or segmental) stenoses; origin and course of aortopulmonary collateral vessels; and fistulous connections and intracardiac communications (septal defects) not clarified by other imaging modalities.

More frequently, however, diagnostic cardiac catheterization is performed to obtain precise hemodynamic information needed to make an informed assessment of the consequences of the patient's cardiac lesions. Using oximetric measurements, pressure data, and thermodilution cardiac output determination, accurate assessment of the patient's hemodynamic profile is obtained. Measured or derived data include central venous pressure, atrial pressure, ventricular pressures (including end-diastolic pressure), shunt fraction (in the case of atrial or ventricular septal defects), pulmonary artery pressures, pulmonary capillary wedge pressure, systemic arterial pressure, and segmental oximetry of the various cardiac structures including systemic and pulmonary venous return (Fig. 60-5). Thus, critical information is obtained about the presence and degree of shunting, systemic and pulmonary vascular resistance, and cardiopulmonary function. It is without doubt that in certain clinical settings, these data are mandatory to a successful clinical management strategy. This may be particularly true in the adult patient with treated or untreated congenital cardiac disease requiring noncardiac surgery.

A thorough understanding of normal cardiorespiratory physiology is critical in interpreting data obtained at cardiac catheterization in the patient with congenital heart disease. Specifically, the normal pressure range,

pulse waveforms, and oxygen saturations for the various cardiac chambers must be compared against data obtained in a deranged circulation. The various cardiac chambers have normal pulse waveforms—in the atria there are characteristic waveforms—"a" wave corresponding to atrial contraction, "c" wave corresponding to atrioventricular valve closure, and "v" wave corresponding to atrial filling from venous return against the closed atrioventricular valve. Typical normal right atrial mean pressures range from 1 to 5 mm Hg, and left atrial pressures range from 2 to 10 mm Hg. Right ventricular pressure tracings in normal hearts demonstrate a more gradual upstroke when compared with the left ventricle. Filling or end-diastolic pressures range between 2 and 10 mm Hg in normal hearts. The normal right ventricular systolic pressure ranges from 15 to 30 mm Hg (and thus pulmonary artery systolic pressure) and the left ventricular systolic pressure ranges from 90 to 110 mm Hg.[7]

In normal hearts, there is a small, physiologically insignificant right-to-left shunt—this results from ventilation-perfusion mismatch in the lungs, and coronary venous return directly to the left ventricle (thebesian venous return). This physiologic shunt represents less than 5% of the cardiac output and in normal circumstances does not produce detectable systemic arterial desaturation. Thus, *significant systemic arterial desaturation represents a pathologic finding,* consistent with either pulmonary disease or intracardiac shunting or both. As noted previously, the origin and degree of intracardiac shunting may be assessed by echo study. In certain circumstances, however, cardiac catheterization is necessary to measure cardiac oximetry and to calculate shunt fraction and derive systemic and pulmonary vascular resistance. Using a derivation of the Fick principal, the ratio of pulmonary blood flow (Qp) to systemic blood flow (Qs) flow can be determined as follows[7]:

$$Qp/Qs = \text{SA } O_2 \text{ sat} - \text{MV } O_2 \text{ sat}/ \text{ PV } O_2 \text{ sat} - \text{PA } O_2 \text{ saturation}$$

where SA is systemic arterial, O_2 sat is oxygen saturation, MV is mixed venous, PV is pulmonary venous, and PA is pulmonary arterial.

Thus, in a patient with a mixed venous saturation of 60%, a pulmonary venous saturation of 100%, a systemic arterial saturation of 100% and a pulmonary arterial saturation of 80%, the $Qp/Qs = 100 - 60/100 - 80 = 40/20 = 2/1$.

Calculating vascular resistances may also be extremely important in determining operability in the patient with congenital heart disease. In many settings, a precise measure of vascular resistance is unnecessary based on the clinical evidence. For example, in the small child with a large ventricular septal defect seen on echocardiogram, the clinical findings of tachypnea, cardiomegaly, and failure to thrive confirm a large left-to-right shunt and thereby infers acceptable pulmonary vascular resistance. In less clear circumstances, however, a precise calculation may be very important in clinical decision making. The pulmonary vascular resistance may be calculated from cardiac catheterization data as follows[7]:

$$\text{Pulmonary vascular resistance (Rp)} = \text{mean pulmonary artery pressure (mm Hg)} - \text{mean left atrial pressure}$$
$$\text{(mm Hg)/pulmonary blood flow (Qp) (L/min/m}^2\text{)}$$

In general, patients with elevated Rp are further evaluated with pulmonary vasodilation—hyperventilation, hyperoxygenation, and inhaled nitric oxide—to determine whether the resistance is responsive. This information may be critical in patients who are otherwise marginal candidates.

Finally, it must be mentioned that cardiac catheterization is rapidly evolving as the primary *therapeutic* method for a number of important structural cardiac defects. In many children's hospitals, including Texas Children's Hospital, most catheterizations now performed are for interventional procedures rather than diagnostic. This may be particularly pertinent to the general surgeon faced with treating a patient with previous catheter-based correction of a cardiac defect. For example, the patient may have had an atrial or ventricular septal defect closed with an occluder device in the remote past. This information may have important ramifications for infectious exposure and vascular access.

PERIOPERATIVE CARE

Perioperative management of the patient with unrepaired or palliated congenital cardiac disease can be an extremely challenging proposition. Standard hemodynamic, respiratory, and pharmacologic manipulations that are appropriate for structurally normal hearts may be entirely inappropriate in settings of complex congenital heart disease. This is especially true in the operating room and

intensive care settings. General rules include a very thorough knowledge of the patient's intracardiac anatomy and expected physiology. It is certainly possible to make significant management errors based on incorrect physiologic expectations in the setting of incomplete understanding of the patient's anatomy. For example, in a patient with *unrepaired* tetralogy of Fallot (TOF) and associated significant right ventricular outflow tract obstruction, it is expected that the patient will exhibit some degree of systemic arterial desaturation. However, the patient with *repaired* tetralogy, with no residual intracardiac shunts, needs to be fully saturated. This is not an infrequent clinical scenario—a patient carrying a specific cardiac diagnosis, despite having undergone a successful correction, continues to be incorrectly presumed to have ongoing physiologic perturbation.

Anesthesia Pitfalls

Providing physiologic anesthetic management can be a very challenging proposition in patients with congenital cardiac disease, especially in situations including chronic single ventricle palliation, unrepaired congenital heart disease, chronic cyanosis, and situations of residual intracardiac pathology to name a few. It is an important general statement that standard anesthetic management paradigms may be completely inappropriate and potentially disastrous in the setting of complex congenital cardiac disease. A thorough understanding of the patient's anatomy is mandatory, along with knowledge of the potential for unexpected response to anesthetic agents and ventilator settings. The field of pediatric and congenital cardiac anesthesia has evolved relative to this specific clinical need, and the recent textbook by Andropoulos and colleagues is an excellent resource.[14]

Several points concerning anesthesia management merit discussion in this chapter. The first issue is vascular access for intraoperative and postoperative management. In patients with complex CHD, especially in those who have undergone previous complex surgical and catheterization procedures, obtaining appropriate vascular access may be very challenging. Typically, a large-bore, multilumen central venous line is necessary for appropriate resuscitation and monitoring of right-sided filling pressures. In some patients, the placement of a thermodilution pulmonary artery catheter (oximetric) must be considered because one cannot presume that right-sided filling pressures correlate well with left heart volume or functional status (e.g., in patients after the Fontan operation). Options for central access include percutaneous internal jugular or subclavian routes, with a secondary option of common femoral access to the inferior vena cava. Difficult access may occur in the setting of previous catheterization or venous reconstruction; this situation may be addressed with the aid of ultrasound-guided catheter placement, which has become a standard in many cardiac operating theaters. Arterial access for continuous blood pressure monitoring and blood gas sampling is important in many patients. Percutaneous radial arterial cannulation can be readily achieved in most patients; however, upper extremity blood pressure values may be factitiously altered by previous systemic-to-pulmonary artery shunts, previous aortic arch surgery (especially coarctation), and abnormalities of vascular origin (aberrant subclavian origin from the descending aorta).[9,14]

Ventilator management in the perioperative setting of congenital cardiac disease requires special understanding. In settings of large potential left-to-right shunts (e.g., unrepaired VSDs), hyperventilation and hyperoxygenation will promote excessive pulmonary blood flow and potentially diminish systemic cardiac output. Positive pressure ventilation, particularly positive end-expiratory pressure (PEEP), will negatively influence hemodynamics in many patients, especially in palliated single ventricle patients after the Fontan procedure.[9,14]

Finally, pharmacologic manipulation of the systemic and pulmonary vascular resistance and cardiac performance is an important adjunct in the perioperative management of patients with CHD. In general, a low-dose infusion of epinephrine (0.05 μg/kg/min) with the addition of a phosphodiesterase inhibitor is an effective pharmacologic cocktail to promote cardiac inotropic state, lower systemic and pulmonary vascular resistance, and limit tachycardia. Other agents frequently employed include dopamine, vasopressin, sodium nitroprusside, and nitroglycerin. Appropriate perioperative analgesia and sedation are also important aspects of the patient's management.[10]

LESION OVERVIEW

Defects Associated With Increased Pulmonary Blood Flow

Persistent Arterial Duct (Patent Ductus Arteriosus)

A persistent arterial duct or PDA is a frequently encountered congenital cardiac condition. The arterial duct is necessary during fetal life to shunt right ventricular blood away from the unventilated pulmonary vasculature (ductal flow is from pulmonary artery to aorta during fetal life). After the first breath at delivery of the neonate, ductal flow reverses and becomes left to right in most individuals. Over the first several hours or days of postnatal life, the PDA closes spontaneously, being completely closed in most people by 2 to 3 weeks of life.

In the absence of other congenital cardiac lesions (although a PDA may be present in association with other structural cardiac conditions and may in some patients be necessary for systemic or pulmonary blood flow), a PDA becomes pathologic related to its presence and the degree of left-to-right shunting. The amount of shunting produced relates to the size and geometry of the duct and the pulmonary vascular resistance. A PDA may be responsible for a large Qp:Qs and result in pulmonary overcirculation, left heart volume overload, and congestive heart failure (CHF). A large, unrestricted PDA will be associated with pulmonary hypertension; if left untreated, this situation will proceed to irreversible pulmonary vascular disease (Eisenmenger's syndrome) with the ultimate result of pulmonary and right heart failure (only treatable by pulmonary transplantation). Even with a small, pressure-restrictive PDA, there is an ongoing risk for pulmonary congestion and left heart volume overloading; endocarditis is an ever-present issue of concern for even small PDAs. As such, closure is recommended for all PDAs.

The gold standard of therapy for closure of PDA is surgery—usually accomplished through left thoracotomy using ductal division, ligation, or clipping (Fig. 60-6). This needs to be a low-risk procedure associated with minimal potential for persistence. Nonetheless, the invasive nature of this proven method has led to the development of alternative strategies for ductal occlusion. From a surgical perspective, many PDAs are amenable to thoracoscopic clipping through very small port incisions; robotic-assisted PDA occlusion has been performed in many patients with good result.[15] At present, however, most PDAs are occluded in the cardiac catheterization lab using a variety of occlusive devices. Even large defects in small babies have been successfully addressed. The long-term effects of the various devices remaining in the vascular tree are as of yet not fully understood; however, successful device closure appears to be an extremely effective and durable therapy.[16]

A PDA in an adult patient can be a challenging proposition. As noted earlier, a long-standing, large PDA may be associated with pulmonary vascular disease. Clearly, a right-to-left shunt in a PDA is cause for significant concern and warrants further investigation. In adults with PDAs, the arterial wall may calcify, making an attempt at ligation or division hazardous. In such patients, ductal occlusion may require resection of the adjacent descending aorta with either patch grafting or short-segment graft replacement (Dacron).

Aortopulmonary Septal Defect (Aortopulmonary Window)

An aortopulmonary septal defect is a communication between the ascending aorta and typically the main pulmonary artery. This is a rare defect, and it relates to the common embryologic origin of the arterial trunk and failure of complete separation into the aorta and pulmonary artery. Defects are classified by their location—type I is proximal, just above the aortic sinuses; type II—more distal on the ascending aorta and often involving the origin of the right pulmonary artery; type III—more distal and associated with separate origin of the right pulmonary artery from the aorta (Fig. 60-7). An aortopulmonary septal defect may occur in isolation or in association with other conditions, including interrupted aortic arch (IAA) and anomalous origin of a coronary artery. Defects are typically large and responsible for a large left-to-right shunt with systemic pulmonary artery pressures. Children with this problem typically present with CHF, failure to thrive, and frequent respiratory infections. Diagnosis may be made by echocardiography, MRI, or catheterization.

All aortopulmonary septal defects are surgically closed; this lesion is not amenable to catheter-based closure, and such an attempt is hazardous. A small defect may be ligated through a thoracotomy or median sternotomy approach, but this method is not recommended due

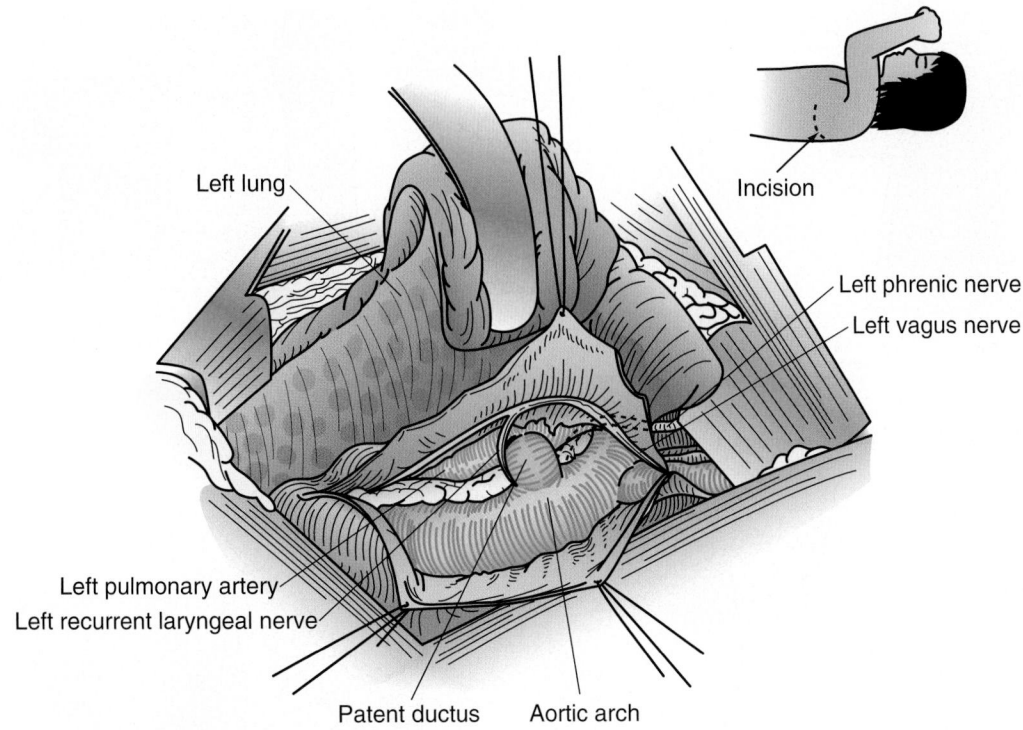

Figure 60-6 The anatomic relationships of a patent ductus arteriosus, exposed from a left thoracotomy. (From Castaneda AR, Jones RA, Mayer JE Jr, Hanley FL: Patent ductus arteriosus. In Cardiac Surgery of the Neonate and Infant. Philadelphia, WB Saunders, 1994.)

significant risk for rupture or incomplete closure. Surgical closure is accomplished with cardiopulmonary bypass support. Options for closure include complete division and separate patch repairs of the great vessel defects or a "sandwich" type of closure, using a patch to construct a common intervening wall; both methods are effective (Fig. 60-8).

Atrial Septal Defect

An isolated atrial septal defect (ASD) is one of the most common congenital cardiac lesions. The most frequently encountered ASD relates to a defect in the true interatrial wall as defined by the fossa ovalis. The defect develops as the result of incomplete closure of the embryologic patent foramen ovale; thus, the defect is a result of incomplete closure of the septum primum. Although the terminology can be confusing, these defects are typically termed *secundum atrial septal defects*. Defects present in a wide variety of configurations ranging from single small defects to multiple fenestrations to complete absence of the septum primum. The confines of the defect may extend from the inferior vena caval orifice up to the superior atrial wall adjacent to the aortic root (Fig. 60-9).

The primary pathophysiologic derangement in ASDs relates to a significant left-to-right shunt in the setting of normal pulmonary vascular resistance. It must be emphasized, however, that even in the setting of normal Rp, patients with ASDs are capable of transient right-to-left shunting, particularly during times of increased intrathoracic pressure. The effects of chronic, large left-to-right shunting (in some patients producing a Qp:Qs>3:1) include right heart volume overloading and enlargement. Most children are not overtly symptomatic but may exhibit some degree of exercise intolerance or frequent respiratory tract infection. Symptoms typically become more prevalent in adulthood and include dyspnea on exertion, palpitations, and ultimately evidence of right heart failure. Pulmonary vascular disease is not a typical finding in secundum ASDs, but one may demonstrate an ASD in patients with primary pulmonary hypertension.[17] A rare form of presentation relates to the potential of right-to-left shunting at the atrial level; the ever-present risk for paradoxical embolus and cerebrovascular accident must be considered in recommending ASD closure.

Most centers recommend ASD closure before school age. The standard therapy for ASDs for the past 50 years has been surgical closure using cardiopulmonary bypass support. The defect is closed using direct suture closure, autologous pericardium, or prosthetic patch material (Fig. 60-10). This is an effective method with low associated perioperative risk, including virtual absence of residual or recurrent defect in recent experience.[18] Minimally invasive techniques for ASD closure have also gained popularity.

The potential for closing defects using nonsurgical methods has led to the development of catheter-based therapies, which are now being widely applied to large numbers of patients worldwide for the treatment of ASD. The most commonly used device is the Amplatzer septal occluder (AGA Medical Corp, MN) device, which is a

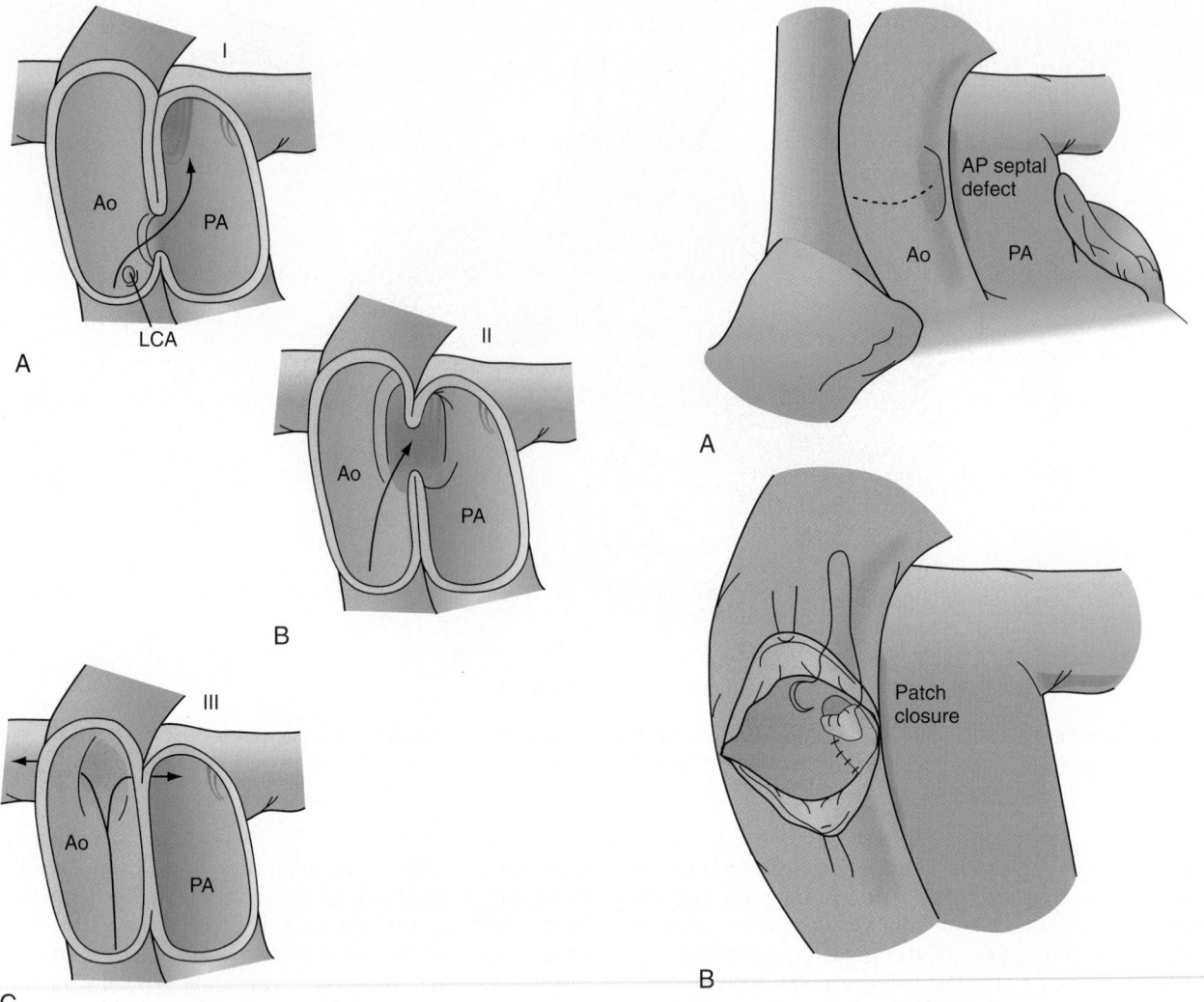

Figure 60-7 Native anatomy and classification of aortopulmonary septal defect. **A,** In type I, the communication is between the ascending aorta (Ao) and the main pulmonary artery (PA) on the posterior medial wall of the ascending aorta. The left main coronary artery (LCA) orifice may be close to the defect. **B,** In type II, the defect is more cephalad on the ascending aorta. **C,** In type III, the defect is more posterior and lateral in the aorta. The communication is with the right pulmonary artery, which may be completely separate from the main pulmonary artery. (Modified from Fraser CD: Aortopulmonary septal defects and patent ductus arteriosus. In Nichols DG, Ungerleider RM, et al [eds]: Critical Heart Disease in Infants and Children. Philadelphia, Mosby, 2006, pp 664-666.)

Figure 60-8 A, Surgical exposure of aortopulmonary (AP) septal defect includes a transverse incision in the ascending aorta (Ao). **B,** Aortopulmonary septal defect is closed by suturing a patch over the aortic side of the defect. PA, pulmonary artery. (Modified from Fraser CD: Aortopulmonary septal defects and patent ductus arteriosus. In Nichols DG, Ungerleider RM, Spevak PJ, et al [eds]: Critical Heart Disease in Infants and Children. Philadelphia, Mosby, 2006, pp 664-666.)

Nitinol metal mesh device, placed percutaneously and delivered with echo and fluoroscopic guidance. By report, more than 30,000 of these devices have been implanted to date, and reports indicate an acceptable procedure-related complication rate and successful closure rate. It is clear, however, that the long-term effects of having such a device in the mobile cardiac structures are not fully understood. Several recent reports have documented an alarming incidence of device erosion through the atrial wall and into the adjacent ascending aorta.[19-21] A recent case of late, severe endocarditis involving a previously placed Amplatzer ASD device highlights the need for ongoing observation of the long-term consequences of placing large prosthetic devices in the circulation.

Sinus venosus atrial septal defects occur as the result of the embryologic malalignment between either the superior or inferior vena cava. These defects are not associated with the ovale fossa. They are frequently associated with partial anomalous pulmonary venous return. A superior sinus venosus ASD occurs high in the atrium, near the orifice of the superior vena cava (SVC). This lesion is frequently associated with anomalous drainage of a portion of the right lung to the SVC. An inferior sinus venosus ASD is located low in the atrium, often extending into the inferior vena cava (IVC) orifice. This lesion

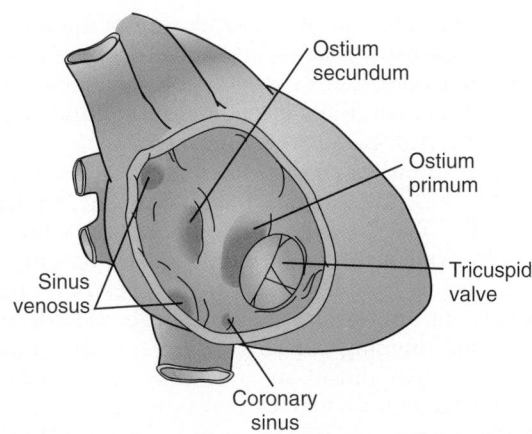

Figure 60-9 Types of atrial septal defects as viewed through the right atrium: ostium secundum, ostium primum, and sinus venosus. (Modified from Redmond JM, Lodge AJ: Atrial septal defects and ventricular septal defects. In Nichols DG, Ungerleider RM, Spevak PJ, et al [eds]: Critical Heart Disease in Infants and Children. Philadelphia, Mosby, 2006, p 580.)

is typically associated with anomalous pulmonary venous drainage of the entire right lung to the IVC (potentially intrahepatic); pulmonary sequestration and an abnormal systemic artery perfusing the right lower lobe (with origin from abdominal aorta) may also be present. In patients with total anomalous pulmonary venous return (TAPVR) to the IVC, the anomalous pulmonary vein may be readily obvious on plain chest radiograph and has been described as appearing like a saber (scimitar syndrome), first described by Sabiston and Neill.[22]

Surgery for sinus venosus ASDs is recommended for the same pathophysiologic reasons as secundum ASDs. The repair is not amenable to catheter techniques, and surgery is more complicated than for an isolated secundum ASD. Superior sinus venosus defects with partial anomalous pulmonary venous return (PAPVR) to the SVC may be treated with an intracardiac patch baffle, however, in the setting of high drainage of the anomalous pulmonary veins, an SVC translocation operation (Warden procedure) may be necessary.[23] Surgery for an inferior sinus venosus ASD with scimitar vein can be more complicated, potentially involving the need for a patch baffle within the intrahepatic inferior vena cava, which may require periods of hypothermic circulatory arrest.[24]

Ventricular Septal Defect

A ventricular septal defect (VSD) is a pathologic communication involving a defect in the interventricular septum. Defects are classified in terms of their location and surrounding structures. Patients may be entirely asymptomatic depending on the size and location of the VSD along with associated lesions and pulmonary vascular resistance. In the setting of otherwise normal cardiac morphology and appropriate pulmonary vascular resistance, the net shunt in patients with VSD is left to right—the Qp:Qs is dependent on the size of the defect and the pulmonary resistance. Large defects result in

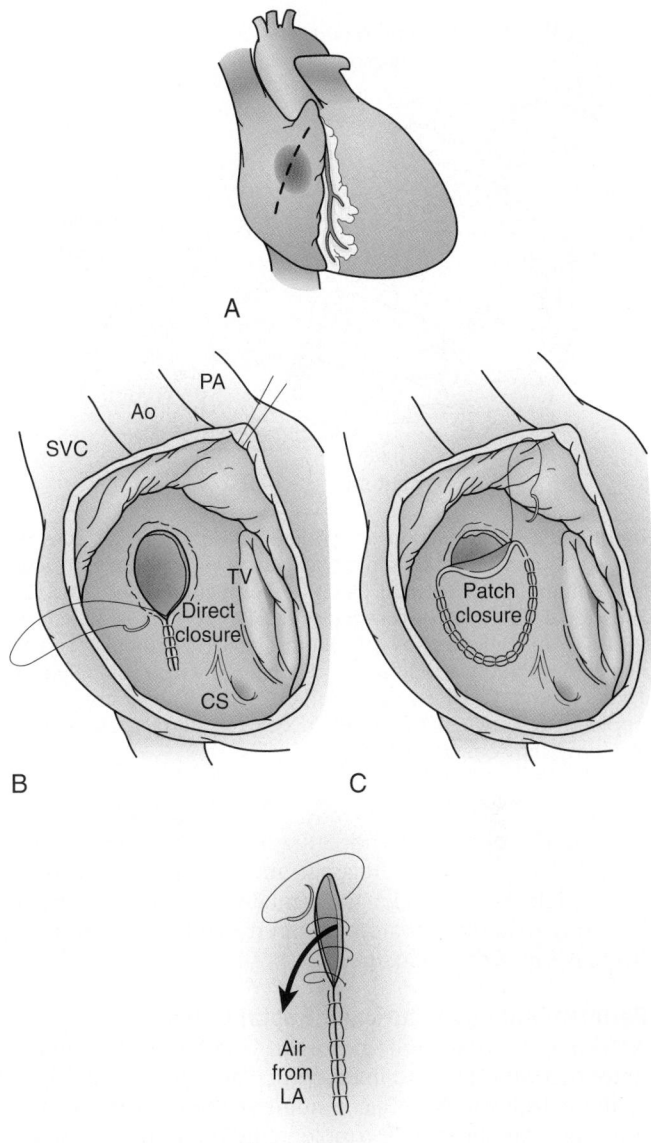

Figure 60-10 Surgical closure for atrial septal defect. **A,** Right atriotomy. **B,** Direct suture closure. Ao, aorta; CS, coronary sinus; PA, pulmonary artery; SVC, superior vena cava; TV, tricuspid valve. **C,** Patch closure. **D,** Deairing the left atrium (LA). (Modified from Redmond JM, Lodge AJ: Atrial septal defects and ventricular septal defects. In Nichols DG, Ungerleider RM, Spevak PJ, et al [eds]: Critical Heart Disease in Infants and Children. Philadelphia, Mosby, 2006, p 583.)

large shunts, high right ventricular and pulmonary artery pressures, and significant pulmonary overcirculation, CHF, and left heart volume overload. In such a setting, unrestrictive pulmonary blood flow exposes the patient to the risk for pulmonary vascular disease and Eisenmenger's syndrome.[25]

The ventricular septum can be best thought of in terms of the pathway of blood and the associated cardiac anatomy. Thus, the RV aspect of the septum has an inlet portion; midmuscular portion; apical, posterior, anterior,

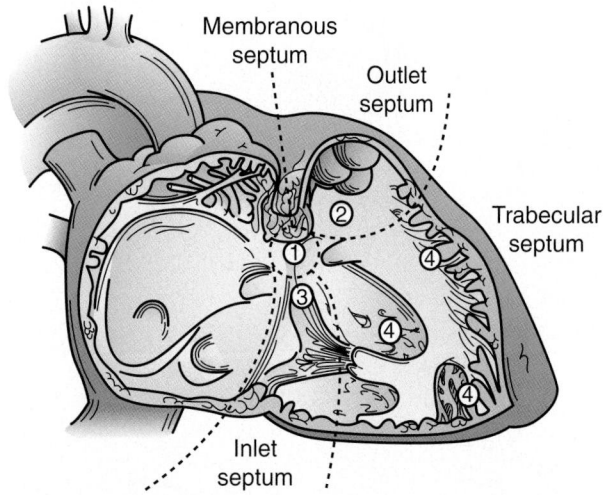

Figure 60-11 The location of various ventricular septal defects (VSDs) in the ventricular septum. (This is a view of the ventricular septum from the right side.) 1, Perimembranous VSD. 2, Subarterial VSD. 3, Atrioventricular canal-type VSD. 4, Muscular VSD. (From Tchervenkov CI, Shum-Tim D: Ventricular septal defect. In Baue AE, Geha AS, Hammond GL [eds]: Glenn's Thoracic and Cardiovascular Surgery, 6th ed. Stamford, CT, Appleton & Lange, 1996. Reproduced with permission of The McGraw-Hill Companies.)

and outlet portions; and subaortic component. This knowledge aids in the classification of VSDs. Furthermore, defects are understood relative to their embryologic origins and have varying propensities for spontaneous decrease in size or closure.

Perimembranous Ventricular Septal Defect

A *perimembranous* VSD occurs as a defect in the membranous portion of the interventricular septum—its associated margins include the annulus of the tricuspid valve, the muscular septum, and potentially the aortic annulus. The defects may be very large and have associated prolapse of either the noncoronary or right coronary aortic valve cusps. Perimembranous VSDs do exhibit a potential for spontaneous closure, particularly small defects presenting early in childhood.

Muscular Ventricular Septal Defect

Muscular VSDs occur in all aspects of the muscular interventricular septum. Margins of these defects are entirely muscle. The lesions may be isolated or involve multiple openings in the septum ("Swiss cheese septum"). Small defects have great potential for regression or spontaneous closure.

Subarterial (Supracristal or Outlet) Ventricular Septal Defect

Subarterial VSDs occur in association with the annulus of the aortic valve, pulmonary valve, or both. The defects are almost always associated with significant prolapse of the adjacent aortic valve cusp (usually right coronary cusp), which may lead to significant cusp distortion, aortic valve insufficiency, and even cusp perforation. The

only mechanism for spontaneous closure of these defects relates to the cusp prolapse and valve distortion, and is generally not complete or a favorable arrangement. All such defects are surgically closed because of the ongoing risk for aortic valve injury (Fig. 60-11).

The indications for surgery to close VSDs relate to the size of the VSD, the degree of shunting, and the associated lesions. Thus, small babies presenting with large VSDs, refractory heart failure, and large shunts undergo surgical closure of the defects in the newborn period irrespective of age or size. Other defects are addressed based on the ongoing concerns of left-to-right shunting, aortic valve cusp distortion, and risk for endocarditis. Asymptomatic patients with evidence of significant shunts and cardiomegaly are put forward for surgical therapy. Prophylactic closure of small defects in asymptomatic patients with normal cardiac size and function is advocated by some surgeons owing to the lifelong risk for endocarditis and comparative low risk for surgery.

Although catheter-based therapies for some VSDs have been achieved, particularly muscular defects, this mode of therapy is not yet widely applicable to most VSDs.[26] The complex relationship of many defects, including close association with the aortic valve and cardiac conduction tissue, makes the existing technology less than ideal.[27] At present, surgery remains the primary mode of therapy for VSD closure. Defects are approached with the aid of cardiopulmonary bypass support and may be closed with a variety of materials. including autologous pericardium (surgeon's preference), Dacron, polytetrafluoroethylene (PTFE), or homograft material. Surgical closure of VSDs are accomplished at low risk with high expectation of complete closure.[28] Challenging anatomic situations such as Swiss cheese septum or multiple apical muscular VSDs may be initially palliated by limiting pulmonary blood flow with a pulmonary artery band, and deferring corrective surgery to later in life.

Atrioventricular Septal Defect (Atrioventricular Canal Defect)

Atrioventricular septal defects (AVSDs) are a complex constellation of cardiac lesions involving deficiency of the atrial septum, ventricular septum, and atrioventricular valves. This lesion results from an embryologic maldevelopment involving the endocardial cushions—thus the term *endocardial cushion defect* is often applied. AVSDs may be *partial,* involving no ventricular level component; *intermediate* or *transitional,* involving a small, restrictive VSD; or *complete,* involving a large, nonrestrictive VSD. The atrioventricular valve tissue is always abnormal in AVSD, although there is great individual variability in terms of the severity of the valvular malformation and thereby valve function. Complete AVSDs are frequently seen in patients with trisomy 21,[29] but do occur in patients with normal chromosomes. The morphology of the septal defects in this condition is different than previously discussed. The ASD in this defect is termed a *primum* and is distinctly separate from the ovale fossa. There is displacement of the atrioventricular node and bundle of His to the inferior aspect of the primum defect and atrioven-

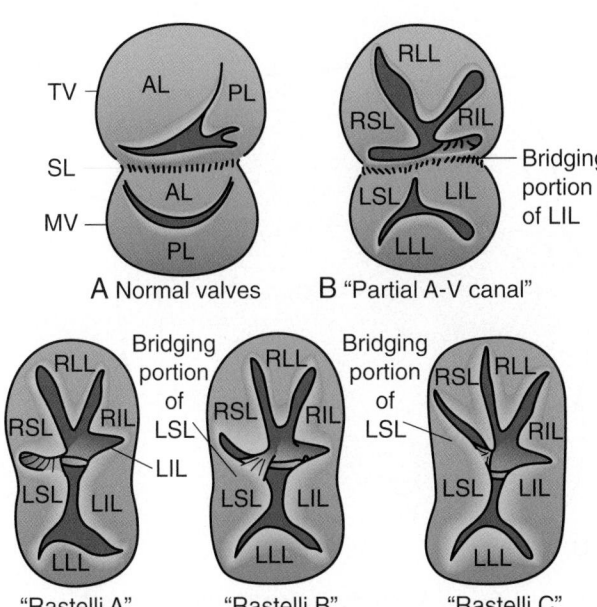

Figure 60-12 The Rastelli classification type A, B, or C. **A** to **C**, The difference in valve morphology in a normal, partial canal, and complete canal defect is illustrated. AL, anterior leaflet; A-V, atrioventricular; MV, mitral valve; PL, posterior leaflet; RIL, right inferior leaflet; RLL, right lateral leaflet; RSL, right superior leaflet; TV, tricuspid valve. (From Kirklin JW, Pacifico AD, Kirklin JK: The surgical treatment of atrioventricular canal defects. In Arciniegas E [ed]: Pediatric Cardiac Surgery. Chicago, Year Book Medical, 1985.)

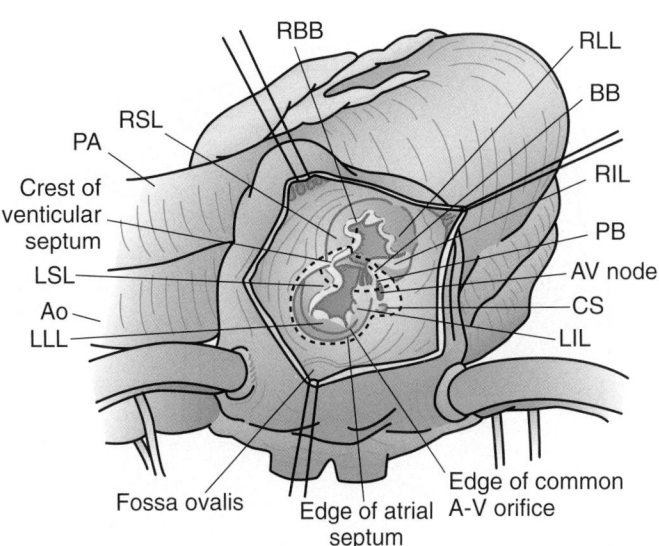

Figure 60-13 The position of the conducting system in complete atrioventricular canal defect (CAVC). The anatomic relationships and morphology of the common atrioventricular (A-V) valve are shown. The view is through a right atriotomy. Ao, aorta; BB, left bundle branch; CS, coronary sinus; LIL, left inferior leaflet; LLL, left lateral leaflet; LSL, left superior leaflet; PA, pulmonary artery; PB, penetrating bundle; RBB, right bundle branch; RIL, right inferior leaflet; RLL, right lateral leaflet; RSL, right superior leaflet. (From Bharati S, Lev M, Kirklin JW: Cardiac Surgery and the Conducting System. New York, Churchill Livingstone, 1983.)

tricular junction, a feature of critical importance during surgical repair. Patients with AVSD have an *inlet* VSD, which may extend into the subaortic region and have a component of septal malalignment. The chordal support of the atrioventricular valves has a variable relationship to the interventricular septum. The relationship of the chordal support and the superior bridging component of the left atrioventricular valve have been used to classify complete AVSD as described by Rastelli—type A with superior leaflet and chordal support committed to the left side of the ventricular septum; type B with straddling, shared chordal support; and type C with a "floating" left superior leaflet component and chordal support on the right side of the ventricular septum[30] (Fig. 60-12).

Patients with complete AVSD typically present in infancy with large left-to-right shunts, cardiomegaly, and CHF. In the absence of surgical treatment, patients exhibit severe failure to thrive, a susceptibility to severe respiratory infections, and potential for early development of pulmonary vascular disease. Surgical repair is recommended in infancy (usually before 6 months of life) but may be necessary in the newborn period in patients with refractory heart failure, especially in association with aortic arch anomalies. Patients with partial or intermediate defects may have their surgery deferred until later in childhood, depending on the degree of atrial level shunting and presence of atrioventricular valve regurgitation.

AVSD may also present in *unbalanced* forms with dominance of either the right- or left-sided components. In severely affected individuals, biventricular repair is not feasible, and patients are managed along a single ventricle pathway.[31] AVSD may also be found in association with TOF; this combination is associated with cyanosis, and repair is more challenging than for either condition considered in isolation.

Surgery is the primary mode of therapy for patients with AVSD. The goals of operation include complete closure of the atrial and ventricular septal defects and effective use of available atrioventricular valve tissue to achieve valve competence. As noted previously, the inferiorly displaced conduction tissue must be protected to avoid the complication of surgically induced atrioventricular block (Fig. 60-13). Patients are approached with the aid of cardiopulmonary bypass support. The atrial and ventricular septal components are closed either with a common patch (single-patch method) or separate patches (two-patch technique). This surgeon favors the two-patch method as superior in preserving atrioventricular valve tissue (Fig. 60-14). The critical component of the repair lies in the valve repair; typically after suspending the valve tissue to the reconstructed septum, the line of coaptation between the superior and inferior leaflet components (cleft) is closed; however, care must be exercised to avoid valvular stenosis.

Perioperative care is predicated on an accurate and hemodynamically favorable repair. Patients with long-standing pulmonary overcirculation may have potential

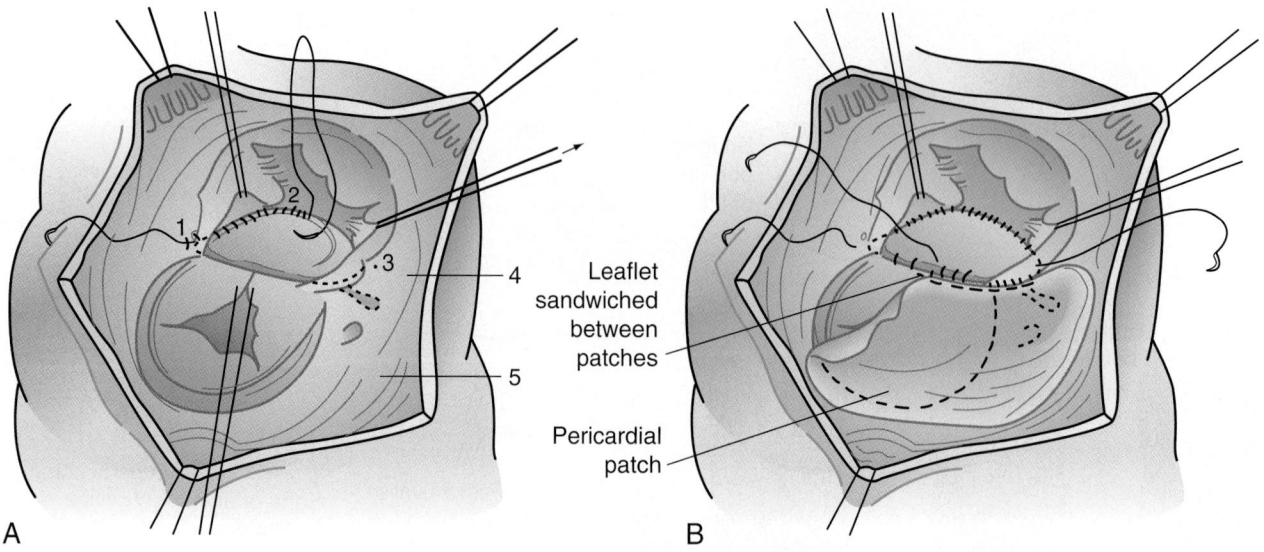

A

B

Leaflet
sandwiched
between
patches

Pericardial
patch

Figure 60-14 The two-patch closure of complete atrioventricular canal defect. A ventricular septal patch is placed first (**A**), and a separate patch is used to close the atrial septal defect (ASD) component. **B,** Note the position of the coronary sinus and conducting system relative to the ASD patch suture line, to avoid injury to the AV node. (From Kirklin JW, Barratt-Boyes BG: Cardiac Surgery. New York, Churchill Livingstone, 1986.)

for early perioperative pulmonary hypertensive crisis. This may require therapy including continuous sedation, hyperventilation, and, possibly, inhaled nitric oxide.[32]

The Adult Patient With AVSD

There are a number of patients with partial or transitional AVSD who survive well into adulthood without surgery. These patients have variable modes of presentation but may exhibit severe exercise intolerance, evidence of right heart dysfunction, some elevation of pulmonary vascular resistance, and possibly, atrial dysrhythmias, including atrial fibrillation. In such late presenting patients, cardiac catheterization is often recommended to rule out occult coronary artery lesions and to evaluate pulmonary vascular resistance. Nonetheless, in the absence of obvious surgical contraindication, surgery is recommended for adults with unrepaired AVSD to eliminate the chronic left-to-right shunt and repair the typically insufficient atrioventricular valves.

Other patients are now presenting well into adulthood with *previously repaired* AVSD. These patients may have a widely disparate constellation of findings, including atrial and ventricular dysrhythmias, valvular insufficiency or stenosis, and right heart dysfunction. In many individuals, secondary reparative surgery may become necessary. Furthermore, in the setting of a patient with remotely repaired AVSD requiring noncardiac surgery, it must be expected that there are potential ongoing hemodynamic concerns that will affect the perioperative course.

Persistent Arterial Trunk (Truncus Arteriosus)

Truncus arteriosus or persistent arterial trunk results from failure of separation of the embryonic arterial trunk and semilunar valves. It is almost always associated with a large, nonrestrictive VSD; it is typically perimembranous

and associated with varying degrees of truncal override of the interventricular septum, including 100% association of the trunk with the right ventricle. The condition is classified by the relationship of the origins of the pulmonary arteries; in type I truncus, there is a demonstrable common main pulmonary artery with subsequent origins of the branch pulmonary arteries; in type II truncus, the branch pulmonary arteries arise closely, but separately, from the trunk; and in type III, the branch pulmonary arteries are widely separated in origin on the ascending aorta (Fig. 60-15).

In distinction to aortopulmonary septal defect, patients with truncus have a single-outlet valve of highly variable morphology. The valve may have a very normal appearance with three well-formed and distinct cusps quite similar to a normal aortic valve. In other patients, the truncal valve may be severely malformed with multiple cusps, dysmorphic leaflets, and abnormal commissural relationships. The truncal valve morphology and function have significant bearing on patient symptoms and the difficulty of surgery. Patients with truncus frequently have coronary ostial abnormalities, including juxtacommissural origin and intramural course. There is an associated interruption of the aortic arch in as many as 25% of newborns presenting with truncus. Abnormalities of thymic genesis, T-cell function, and calcium homeostasis may be frequently seen in this group of patients in association with a chromosome 22 deletion (DiGeorge syndrome).[33]

Patients with truncus arteriosus present in the newborn period with unrestricted pulmonary blood flow and systemic pulmonary artery pressure. With the expected postnatal fall in pulmonary vascular resistance, massive pulmonary overcirculation, and CHF, patients may exhibit a wide pulse pressure due to diastolic runoff of blood into the pulmonary vasculature. This situation will be further exacerbated in the setting of significant truncal

Collett and Edwards

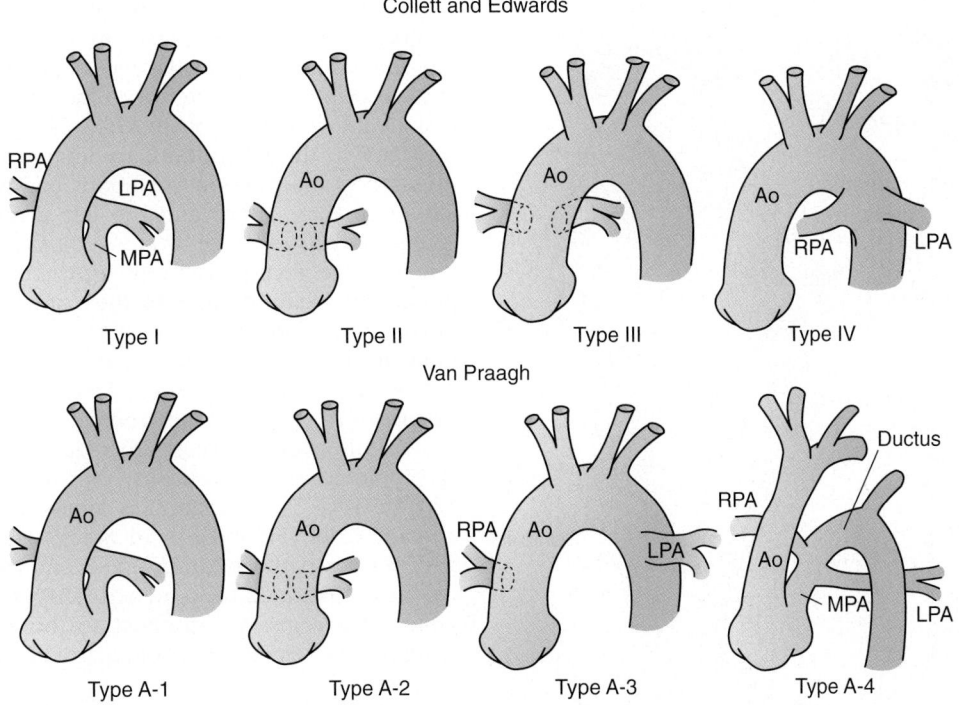

Van Praagh

Figure 60-15 Collett-Edwards and Van Praagh classification systems for persistent truncus arteriosus (see text for details). Ao, aorta; MPA, main pulmonary artery; LPA, left pulmonary artery; RPA, right pulmonary artery. (Modified from St. Louis, JD: Persistent truncus arteriosus. In Nichols DG, Ungerleider RM, Spevak PJ, et al [eds]: Critical Heart Disease in Infants and Children. Philadelphia, Mosby, 2006, p 690.)

valve insufficiency, resulting in poor systemic perfusion and cardiovascular collapse. Some infants can be initially managed with medical decongestive therapy (diuretics, angiotensin-converting enzyme inhibitors, and digoxin) and fortified nutritional support (through gastric intubation); however, this is a precarious arrangement. In the few individuals who successfully negotiate infancy, irreversible pulmonary vascular disease develops rapidly, and patients become inoperable. In other patients, refractory CHF results in poor weight gain, respiratory insufficiency, and susceptibility to infection. In many newborns with unrepaired truncus, the profound hemodynamic compromise places the patient at high risk for necrotizing enterocolitis (NEC). Patients with truncus and IAA have ductal-dependent systemic blood flow. They are therefore dependent on IV PGE₁ to maintain ductal patency until they undergo repair. Given these considerations, it is recommended that most patients presenting as newborns undergo repair in the first several weeks of life.

The surgical repair is performed on cardiopulmonary bypass support. Components of the repair include division of the common trunk and reconstruction of confluent central branch pulmonary arteries. The large ventricular septal defect is closed with a patch, typically performed through a right ventriculotomy. In patients with abnormal, insufficient truncal valves, a valve repair may be necessary. It is unusual to have to replace the truncal valve at the initial operation; most valves can be at least partially repaired to provide the patient an adequate aortic valve. Right ventricle–pulmonary artery con-

tinuity must then be established. Most surgeons prefer to interpose a valved conduit between the right ventriculotomy and pulmonary artery bifurcation (Fig. 60-16).

Conduit options are limited and include homograft (pulmonary artery or aorta, valved) or heterograft (bovine or porcine). Recent experience with a commercially available, glutaraldehyde-preserved bovine jugular vein valved-conduit (Contegra, Medtronic Inc., Minneapolis, MN) has been encouraging.[34] Successful truncus repair in infants using a direct, hooded anastomosis between the pulmonary artery bifurcation and the right ventriculotomy has also been reported.[35] Unfortunately, no available option offers the patient the lifetime solution of a connection capable of somatic growth along with a competent, durable pulmonary valve. As such, all infants undergoing successful truncus repair will be expected to require multiple subsequent cardiac surgeries as they outgrow their current right ventricle–pulmonary artery conduit. Recent experience with a percutaneously delivered, catheter-mounted pulmonary valve has been encouraging as an interim solution for such patients in an effort to limit the number of required cardiac reoperations.[36]

There are a growing number of adults surviving after childhood truncus repair. It is clear that all these patients require diligent longitudinal cardiology surveillance and that many will require reoperation. Issues of concern include late ventricular dysrhythmias (often related to surgical scarring from the previous right ventriculotomy), branch pulmonary artery stenosis, stenosis or insuffi-

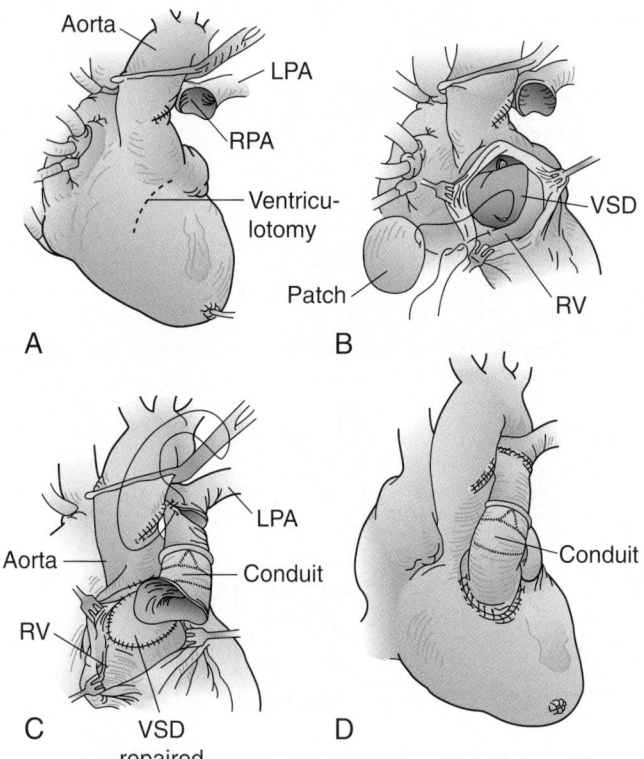

A

B

C

D

Figure 60-16 Surgical repair of truncus arteriosus. **A,** Origin of truncus arteriosus is excised and the truncal defect closed with direct suture. The incision is made high in the right ventricle (RV). LPA, left pulmonary artery; RPA, right pulmonary artery. **B,** Ventricular septal defect (VSD) is closed with a prosthetic patch. **C,** Placement of a valved conduit into the pulmonary arteries. **D,** Proximal end of conduit is anastomosed to the RV. (From Wallace RB: Truncus arteriosus. In Sabiston DC Jr, Spencer FC [eds]: Gibbons Surgery of the Chest, 3rd ed. Philadelphia, WB Saunders, 1976.)

ciency of the right ventricle–pulmonary artery conduit, truncal valve insufficiency, and right ventricular dysfunction.[37]

Abnormalities of Venous Drainage

Total Anomalous Pulmonary Venous Return

TAPVR results from embryonic failure of connection of the fetal pulmonary venous sinus to the left atrium. This fatal condition has a spectrum of clinical presentations and may be associated with additional complex structural cardiac disease, including single ventricle. In TAPVR, pulmonary venous return may take one of several pathways to return eventually to the right heart. Initial survival is predicated on an unobstructed pathway and an unrestricted atrial level communication such that sufficient intracardiac mixing affords the patient adequate systemic oxygenation. Patients with TAPVR are desaturated to varying degrees depending on the adequacy of the anomalous pathway, atrial mixing, and pulmonary function. The abnormal venous connection drains in several typical patterns.

In *supracardiac TAPVR*, the pulmonary veins drain to a vertical vein, which courses in a cephalad direction to join a systemic vein. In the most common variation, the vertical vein courses anterior to the left pulmonary artery to join the left innominate vein. This vein may course posterior to the left pulmonary artery, resulting in compression of the pulmonary venous pathway between the left pulmonary artery and the left main-stem bronchus (pulmonary artery "vise"). The vertical vein may also join the SVC or azygos vein. In *intracardiac TAPVR*, the pulmonary veins drain into the coronary sinus and, in most cases where the coronary sinus is intact, into the right atrium. This variant is rarely obstructed and may not be diagnosed until later in life in some patients. In *infracardiac TAPVR,* the vertical veins descend in a caudal direction, through the diaphragm to join the embryologic ductus venosus, then through the liver to join the IVC. This variation is almost always obstructed at some level (Fig. 60-17). In *mixed TAPVR,* the pulmonary venous pathway drains in several pathways to reach the heart. Frequently in mixed TAPVR, one or several pulmonary veins will connect to the SVC, with others draining either to an infracardiac or supracardiac connection.

Obstructed Total Anomalous Pulmonary Venous Return

Obstructed TAPVR is one of the few true surgical emergencies in congenital heart surgery and is diagnosed with transthoracic echo evaluation when the condition is suspected. This condition occurs when one of the previously mentioned drainage patterns is obstructed, resulting in severe pulmonary venous hypertension. Secondary effects include pulmonary edema, pulmonary artery hypertension, and profound hypoxemia. Interstitial pulmonary emphysema and frank pneumothorax may develop during efforts at vigorous ventilatory support in profoundly desaturated children. Patients with obstructed TAPVR may present within hours of birth in extremis and will not respond to resuscitative efforts. The only therapy useful in their management lies in the form of rapid surgical repair irrespective of the severity of the patient's preoperative status.

For other forms of TAPVR, elective surgical repair is recommended after the diagnosis is made. On occasion, the diagnosis is not made until later in childhood in patients with unobstructed vertical vein and widely patent atrial communication. These patients undergo elective repair to relieve the cyanosis, intracardiac mixing, and right heart volume overload.

Surgical repair of TAPVR requires cardiopulmonary bypass support and often periods of profound hypothermia and circulatory arrest are necessary. The principles of repair include identification of the pulmonary venous confluence and individual pulmonary veins. An anastomosis is constructed between the venous confluence and the left atrium using either a superolateral approach with the heart reflected to the patient's right or an incision directly through the interatrial septum and corresponding region of the posterior right atrial wall. The ASD and typically present PDA are closed as well (Fig. 60-18).

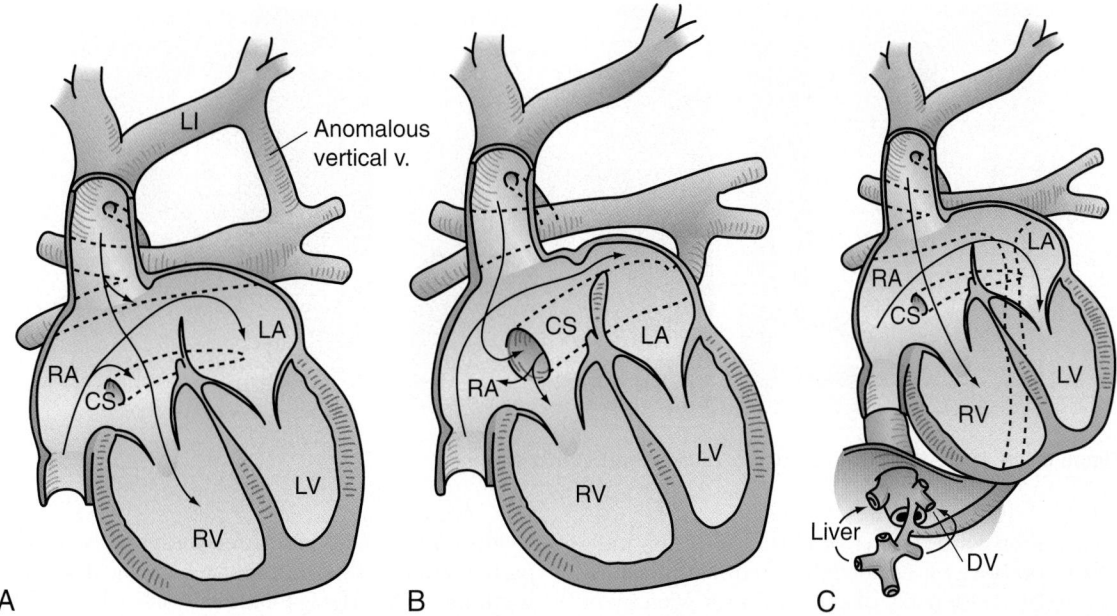

Figure 60-17 Types of total anomalous pulmonary venous connection (TAPVC). **A,** Supracardiac type with a vertical vein joining the left innominate (LI) vein. CS, coronary sinus; LA, left atrium; LV, left ventricle; RA, right atrium; RV, right ventricle. **B,** Intracardiac type with connection to the coronary sinus. **C,** Infracardiac type with drainage through the diaphragm through an inferior connecting vein. DV, ductus venosus. (From Hammon JW Jr, Bender HW Jr: Anomalous venous connections: Pulmonary and systemic. In Baue AE [ed]: Glenn's Thoracic and Cardiac Surgery, 5th ed. Norwalk, CT, Appleton & Lange, 1991. Reproduced with permission of the McGraw-Hill Companies.)

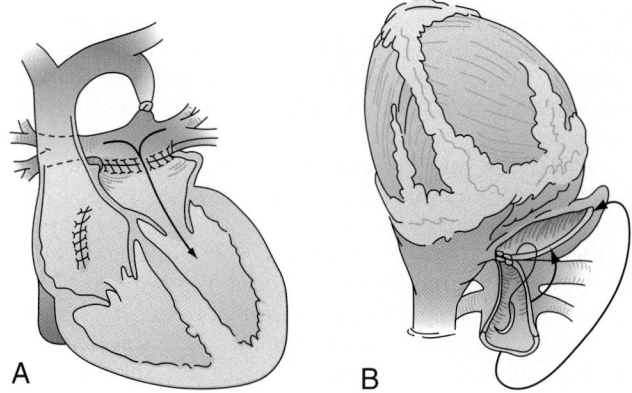

Figure 60-18 A, Repair of supracardiac total anomalous pulmonary venous connection (TAPVC) through a superior approach. **B,** Repair of infracardiac TAPVC. Elevating the apex of the heart to the right side exposes the left atrium and pulmonary confluence. Anastomosis is created as shown. (From Lupinetti FM, Kulik TJ, Beekman RH, et al: Correction of total anomalous pulmonary venous connection in infancy. J Thorac Cardiovasc Surg 106:880, 1993.)

Cor Triatriatum

Cor triatriatum is a rare condition in which the pulmonary veins enter a chamber posterior to the left atrium with a small connection to either right or left atrium. These patients exhibit evidence of pulmonary hypertension and variable desaturation. Surgical decompression is necessary to relieve the pulmonary venous obstruction and is

accomplished by resection of the membrane between the pulmonary venous chamber and left atrium.

A dreaded consequence of TAPVR occurs when there is a progressive, malignant sclerosing process involving the individual pulmonary veins. This process may be initiated by inaccurate surgery resulting in obstruction of the venous confluence and individual veins, or it may progress independent of surgical manipulation. The process may progress to intrapulmonary pulmonary venous stenoses. A technique to deal with the individual pulmonary venous stenoses has been developed that uses a pedicled flap of adjacent pericardium to augment the pulmonary venous orifices (sutureless technique), but this method is not applicable to all patients with pulmonary venous obstruction. Catheter-based dilation and stenting has been attempted in this setting but has been largely unsuccessful. In the most severe cases, the only meaningful surgical option is lung transplantation.

Anomalous Systemic Venous Drainage

Congenital abnormalities of systemic venous drainage may occur in isolation or in association with other significant structural cardiac defects. In the setting of an otherwise normal heart, the anomaly is frequently not of physiologic significance. The most common example of this is a persistent left SVC draining to the coronary sinus. In the absence of an intracardiac communication or unroofing of the coronary sinus, this is of anatomic significance only. In many cases, a persistent left SVC occurs with absence of a communicating innominate vein. This becomes important in situations of mechanical occlusion,

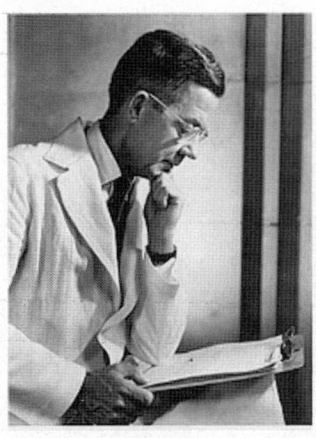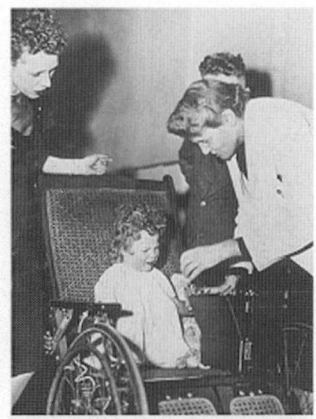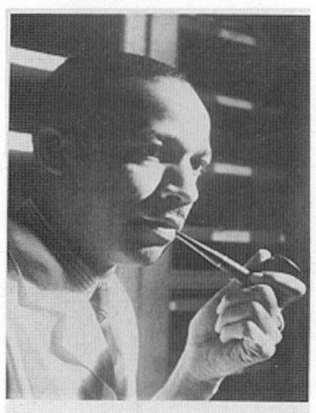

Figure 60-19 Drs. Alfred Blalock, Helen Taussig, and Vivien Thomas.

which may be seen with trauma or chronic venous intubation with thrombosis. It is not infrequent for a persistent left SVC to be incidentally discovered after placement of a left internal jugular central line, which is found to apparently track into the heart on plain chest radiography. A persistent left SVC becomes more significant in patients requiring intracardiac or extracardiac surgery. If the left SVC drains to an unroofed coronary sinus in a patient undergoing atrial septation, the patient will be profoundly desaturated after surgery. This situation requires either reconstruction of the coronary sinus or some other method to reroute the left SVC to the right atrium.

An interrupted IVC occurs most commonly in association with other structural cardiac disease. The IVC drainage in this setting is either to the azygos (azygos continuation) or hemiazygos vein and ultimately the SVC. In these patients, the hepatic veins drain into the atrium as a common confluence or as individual veins. The physiologic significance of interrupted IVC relates to the coexisting cardiac lesion and the necessity of appreciating the abnormality of systemic venous drainage in performing corrective surgery. In patients requiring noncardiac surgery or catheter intervention, the presence of an interrupted IVC is noted when an attempt is being made to pass a venous catheter from the groin into the heart.

Cyanotic Congenital Heart Disease

Tetralogy of Fallot
TOF is a common form of cyanotic congenital heart disease and is probably the most studied lesion in the era of surgical correction for congenital heart disease. Many believe that the Johns Hopkins Hospital was the birthplace of cardiac surgery; the first successful palliative operation for TOF was performed by Dr. Alfred Blalock with the able assistance of his laboratory technician in November of 1944.[1] Dr. Blalock was encouraged by the matriarch of pediatric cardiology, Dr. Helen Taussig (Fig. 60-19). Until very recently, some degree of controversy has surrounded the relative degree of contribution by these three individuals in bringing this historical event to

fruition. In actuality, all three individuals were significant participants in this momentous medical advance. While working at Vanderbilt Medical School, Dr. Blalock had charged his young and very capable laboratory technician, Vivien Thomas, with the development of a surgical model of pulmonary hypertension. Thomas and Blalock developed a method of anastomosing the left subclavian artery to the divided left pulmonary artery in a canine model. Specifically, Thomas worked out the technical details, including crafting the necessary surgical instruments, and mastered the operation. This work did not produce the desired effect; in fact, the canine pulmonary vascular resistance is almost infinitely low, and the animals did not develop a hypertensive pulmonary vasculature. Nonetheless, the technique was developed and published some 10 years in advance of the clinical application in 1944.

Dr. Blalock subsequently became the Chair of Surgery at Johns Hopkins. Dr. Taussig had, by that time, established a reputation as a meticulous diagnostician of complex congenital heart lesions. She had a large clinic of desperately ill children with disabling cyanosis—*blue babies*. At her suggestion (and probably her insistence), Dr. Blalock was convinced to attempt a surgical palliation for TOF by constructing in a human the subclavian to pulmonary artery anastomosis that had been perfected in the research laboratory (Fig. 60-20). Dr. Blalock performed the operation in conditions and with instruments that would be considered extremely crude by today's standards. Vivien Thomas stood immediately behind Dr. Blalock during that operation and many subsequent cases, providing instruction and encouragement. The clinical success was an earth-shattering event; literally hundreds of patients subsequently traveled to Johns Hopkins for surgical treatment, and the era of cardiac surgery was ushered in. These historical accounts are factual and are the result of personal interviews with many of the people in attendance at that event, including Dr. Vivien Thomas, Dr. H. Taussig, Dr. J. Alex Haller, and Dr. Denton Cooley.

The historical account of the development of the Blalock-Taussig shunt (BT shunt) has relevance to the practice of congenital heart surgery today. First, it is

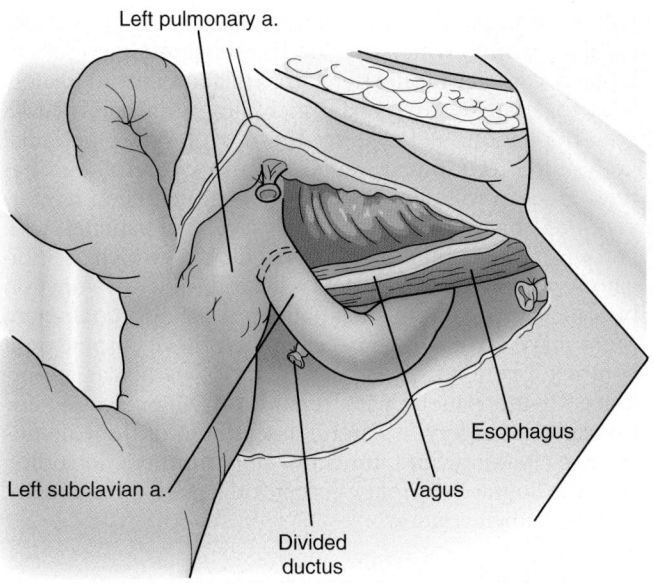

Figure 60-20 A Blalock-Taussig shunt.

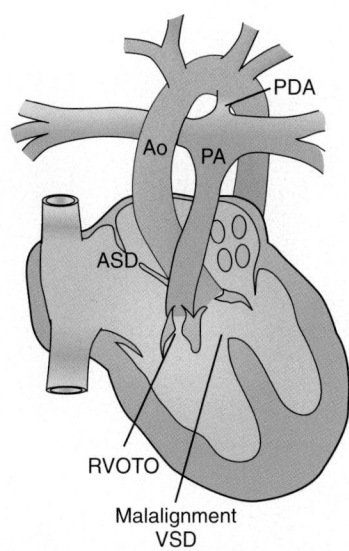

Figure 60-21 Anatomy of tetralogy of Fallot. A malalignment ventricular septal defect (VSD), aortic override, right ventricular outflow tract obstruction (RVOTO), and subsequent right ventricular hypertrophy. Ao, aorta; ASD, atrial septal defect; PA, pulmonary artery; PDA, patent ductus arteriosus. (Modified from Davis S: Tetralogy of Fallot with and without pulmonary atresia. In Nichols DG, Ungerleider RM, Spevak PJ, et al [eds]: Critical Heart Disease in Infants and Children. Philadelphia, Mosby, 2006, p 756.)

important that the facts surrounding this achievement are acknowledged. Second, this remarkably simple concept remains a frequently applied technique for children with inadequate pulmonary blood flow today. Finally, over the now more than 60 years of treatment of TOF, thousands of patients have been successfully treated, but most are *not* cured; many will require subsequent reoperative cardiac surgery even after complete repair.

The anatomic hallmark of TOF is anterior malalignment of the infundibular septum; this malalignment leaves a deficiency in the subaortic region—a *malalignment VSD,* which is usually perimembranous, large, and pressure nonrestrictive. The relative degree of malalignment influences the relationship of the aorta to the interventricular septum, producing varying degrees of *aortic override.* The deviated infundibular septum produces varying degrees of *right ventricular outflow tract obstruction.* The path of pulmonary blood flow may be impeded at multiple levels, including the infundibulum, the pulmonary valve and annulus, and the main and branch pulmonary arteries. Secondary *right ventricular hypertrophy* occurs relative to the degree and duration of the obstruction and is progressive, contributing to the propensity for the lesion to worsen over time (Fig. 60-21).

The pathophysiology of TOF relates to shunting of desaturated, systemic venous blood through the VSD to mix with the systemic cardiac output. The greater the degree of obstruction to pulmonary blood flow, the larger the right-to-left shunt and thereby the worse the desaturation. There are several modes of presentation. Newborns with TOF and severe right ventricular outflow tract obstruction (RVOTO) may present soon after birth with profound cyanosis; some will require PGE_1 to maintain ductal patency for adequate oxygenation. The other end of the spectrum occurs in children with little infundibular obstruction and normal pulmonary valve and branch pulmonary arteries. These patients may have net left-to-

right flow through the VSD, occasionally to the extent that they experience pulmonary overcirculation and CHF (so-called pink TOF). Most children present between these extremes; an initially mild to moderate degree of infundibular stenosis progresses over time to become severe with worsening desaturation. A TOF "spell" occurs when there is an acute change in cardiac inotropic state often in the setting of agitation and dehydration. The infundibular stenosis acutely worsens, and patients become profoundly desaturated; this may be an extremely serious event leading to brain damage or death. Acute treatment modalities include sedation, hydration, systemic afterload augmentation (α-adrenergic agonists), β-blockade to reduce the inotropic state, and even endotracheal intubation with supplemental inspired oxygen.

The natural history of untreated TOF is dismal, with most children succumbing to the ravages of progressive cyanosis before 10 years of age. Surgery remains the mainstay of therapy; medical and catheter-based therapy may be used to temporize; however, TOF is a surgical disease. The principles of surgical correction include patch closure of the VSD and relief of all levels of the right ventricular outflow tract obstruction (RVOTO) and pulmonary artery stenosis. The classic method of TOF repair uses a longitudinal incision through the RVOT, which provides an excellent transventricular view of the VSD, which is closed with a patch. The pulmonary artery, pulmonary valve, and annulus are incised if stenotic, and then the RVOT is patched. This method was used for many years but has the complicating feature of the long ventriculotomy with attendant right ventricular dysfunc-

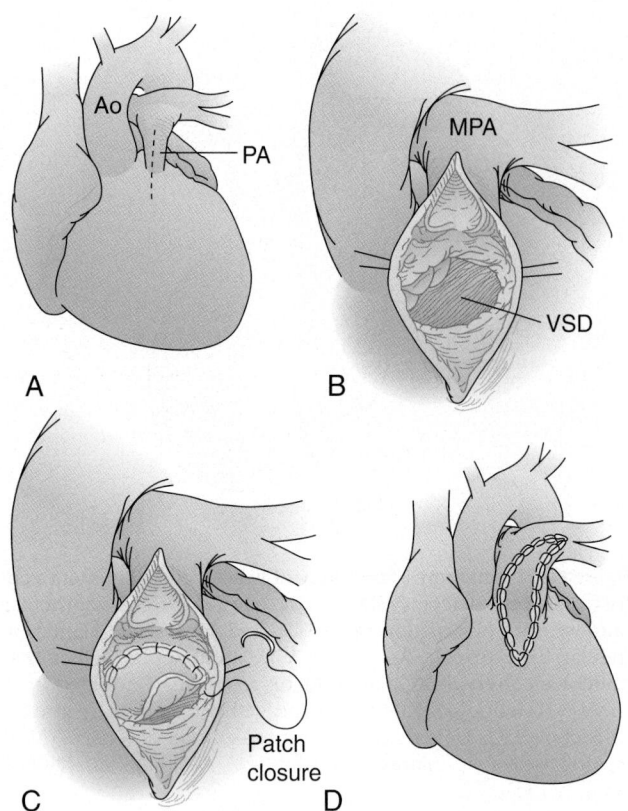

A

B

C

Patch closure

D

Figure 60-22 Complete repair of tetralogy of Fallot. **A,** Enlargement of the right ventricle–main pulmonary artery (MPA) connection with a transannular incision if necessary. Ao, aorta. **B,** Resection of muscle from the outflow tract and identification of edges of the ventricular septal defect (VSD). **C,** Patch closure of the VSD. **D,** Placement of a transmural patch if required.

patients with large right ventriculotomies develop endocardial scarring, which may be the substrate for ventricular tachycardia. Chronic right atrial dilation may ultimately lead to atrial dysrhythmias, including atrial tachycardia and fibrillation. Relative to these and other potential issues after TOF repair, patients require careful and lifelong medical follow-up. Many patients will need reintervention; this is frequently the case in patients with chronic, severe pulmonary insufficiency, which is indicated when right ventricle dilation and dysfunction become significant. In such patients, placing a competent pulmonary valve will be necessary to relieve chronic right ventricle overload. These issues are of particular importance to the patient with repaired TOF presenting for noncardiac surgery. A careful assessment of the patient's cardiac anatomy and function is performed, including echocardiography, Holter monitoring, and on occasion, cardiac catheterization.

Pulmonary Atresia and Intact Ventricular Septum

Pulmonary atresia with intact ventricular septum (PA/IVS) presents with profound desaturation and ductal-dependent pulmonary blood flow in the newborn period. The cardiac morphology in this condition varies widely. On the most severe end of the spectrum, patients have very small right ventricles, tiny tricuspid inlets, and often a *right ventricle–dependent coronary circulation*. In such cases, the right ventricle must remain hypertensive to provide flow to these segments of the coronary circulation. At the other end of the anatomic spectrum, patients have a relatively normal tricuspid valve and right ventricle. Most patients fall in between these extremes, with some degree of tricuspid valve and right ventricle underdevelopment.

Because patients are ductal dependent at birth, an assessment must be made as to whether the right heart will be capable of ultimately supporting a biventricular circulation. If the coronary circulation is truly right ventricle–dependent, decompressing the right ventricle will result in coronary insufficiency; in these situations, a palliative Blalock-Taussig shunt will be created in anticipation of promoting the patient down a single ventricle pathway. In other patients, the atretic pulmonary valve must be opened either with percutaneous balloon dilation or open surgical valvotomy. Over time, the hypertensive, often apparently underdeveloped right ventricle will improve in size and function and be capable of supporting all or a significant proportion of the cardiac output. At initial presentation, many patients have a large patent foramen ovale or ASD; in patients with a restrictive ASD and marginal right heart, an atrial septostomy (balloon) allows for atrial-level right-to-left shunting until the right ventricle improves. Ultimately, if the right ventricle is adequate, the ASD can be closed.

Pulmonary Atresia With Ventricular Septal Defect

Pulmonary atresia with ventricular septal defect (PA/VSD) is morphologically similar to TOF with the exception of an atretic pulmonary valve. Patients may have confluent, normal-sized pulmonary arteries perfused by a PDA. In

tion and often severe pulmonic insufficiency. An alternate method, the transatrial or transpulmonary approach, first proposed by Imai, has gained popularity during the past decade (Fig. 60-22). In this method, the VSD closure and RVOT resection are accomplished through a right atriotomy by way of the tricuspid valve. The main pulmonary artery and pulmonary annulus are only incised if stenotic, but there is no transmural infundibular incision. This method is technically more demanding than the classic method but may offer the patient improved long-term right ventricular function, as noted in recent large reported series.[38]

The long-term sequelae of TOF repair are continuing to unfold. It is clear that for most patients, successful childhood repair of TOF does not translate into a "cure." As patients age after TOF repair, a variety of long-term complications may develop. Patients with long RVOT incisions (transannular) will by necessity have severe pulmonary insufficiency and a noncontractile infundibulum. Over time, the effects of chronic right heart volume overload include right ventricle dilation and decreased function, often with progressive tricuspid insufficiency and elevated central venous pressure. Such patients may present with hepatomegaly, peripheral edema, and severe exercise intolerance. Dysrhythmias may frequently occur;

severe cases, the pulmonary arteries are discontinuous and the lungs are variably perfused by diminutive native branch pulmonary arteries and muscularized, collateral vessels originating from the descending aorta and brachiocephalic vessels. These major aortopulmonary collateral arteries (MAPCAs) have a propensity to develop severe stenoses as they are exposed to systemic arterial pressure. Many of these MAPCAs eventually occlude at an unpredictable rate during childhood. Because they may provide the only blood supply to some lung segments, patients will become progressively desaturated.

The goal of surgical therapy for PA/VSD is biventricular repair to achieve normal cardiac workload and systemic arterial saturations. In patients with confluent native pulmonary arteries of adequate caliber, the VSD is surgically closed and a valved conduit (homograft or heterograft) is interposed between the right ventricle and pulmonary bifurcation. In patients with PA/VSD and MAPCAs, the pulmonary arteries must be repaired by connecting the various lung segments into a common trunk through a process known as pulmonary artery unifocalization. Depending on the source and size of the MAPCAs and native pulmonary arteries, this may be a very challenging surgical procedure, but the goal is constructing a pulmonary tree as close to normal as possible, such that biventricular repair is feasible as previously described.

The long-term issues of repair of PA/VSD are not dissimilar to those concerns previously described for TOF. The addition of a right ventricle–pulmonary artery conduit guarantees the need for reoperation because no currently available conduit choice offers either the potential for somatic growth or an indefinitely durable valve.

Valvular Pulmonic Stenosis

Patients with isolated valvular pulmonary stenosis (PS) are almost always treated in infancy with a percutaneous balloon pulmonary valvotomy. The intermediate-term results of this treatment are good; however, all patients are left with significant pulmonary valve insufficiency and eventually require pulmonary valve replacement.

Conotruncal Anomalies

Transposition of the Great Arteries

Transposition of the great arteries (TGA) is a common cyanotic congenital cardiac lesion. In this section, discussion relates only to TGA in which there are two good ventricles identifiable as capable of independent function as the right and left ventricle. TGA is commonly referred to as D-TGA, in relationship to the typically normal "D" or dextro ventricular looping that occurs in association with the discordant ventriculoarterial connection and normal atrioventricular connection. TGA occurs in the setting of intact ventricular septum (TGA/IVS) or with associated VSD (TGA/VSD). In TGA/VSD, there may be associated aortic arch hypoplasia and coarctation. On the other extreme, there may be severe pulmonic and subpulmonic stenosis (left ventricular outflow tract obstruction [LVOTO]) or even pulmonary atresia (TGA/VSD with PA).

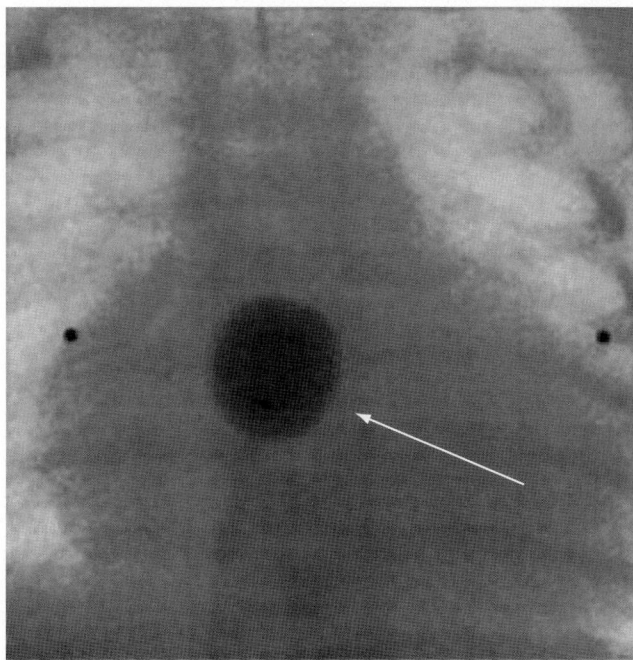

Figure 60-23 Angiogram during balloon atrial septostomy. The *arrow* points to the inflated balloon catheter at the atrial septum. The interventional cardiologist will forcefully pull the balloon across the patent foramen ovale to create an open, unobstructed secundum atrial septal defect.

Patients with TGA/IVS typically present in the early newborn period with profound cyanosis (associated with normal perinatal PDA closure). In the absence of a significant ASD, the cyanosis will be severe and progress to death if left untreated. Institution of IV PGE_1 is almost uniformly successful in reestablishing ductal patency that will improve the patient's arterial saturation by providing left-to-right shunting and improved pulmonary blood flow.

In most patients, a balloon atrial septostomy (BAS) is performed (percutaneous through either the umbilical vein or femoral vein) to allow atrial-level mixing (Fig. 60-23). This procedure is usually very effective in allowing sufficient atrial-level mixing so that the patient will be adequately saturated (70%-80%).

Following the procedure, the prostaglandin infusion can be discontinued. In TGA with significant VSD, there is often sufficient shunting at the level of the VSD to promote adequate systemic saturation; in fact, in patients with large VSDs, the predominant presenting symptom may be pulmonary *overcirculation* and CHF. Patients with TGA/PA clearly have ductal-dependent pulmonary blood flow. In patients with TGA/VSD and aortic arch hypoplasia or coarctation, PGE_1 may be necessary to maintain ductal patency and systemic perfusion. Echocardiography is the primary diagnostic modality for TGA.

The treatment of TGA has evolved significantly during the past 5 decades of surgical therapy for congenital cardiac disease. Initial success was achieved by surgical reconstruction to create a *physiologic* repair. The *atrial*

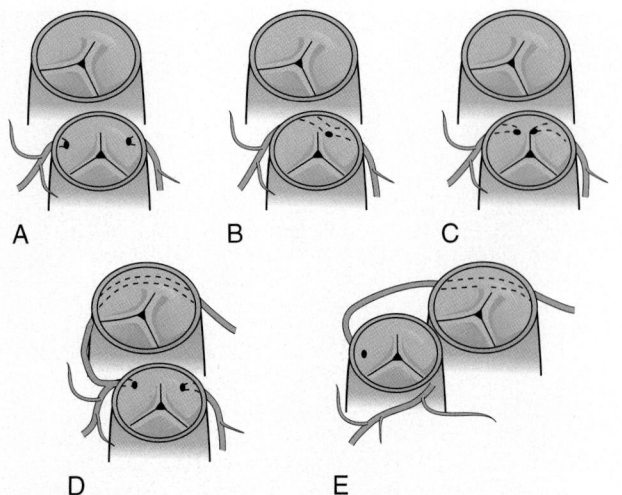

Figure 60-24 Five basic coronary artery configurations as described by Yacoub and Radley-Smith. (Modified from Mee R: The arterial switch operation. In Stark J, de Leval M [eds]: Surgery for Congenital Heart Defects, 2nd ed. Philadelphia, WB Saunders, 1994, p 484.)

switch operation involves a series of intra-atrial baffles using either a patch-channel (Mustard procedure)[39] or infolding of the native atrial wall and interatrial septum (Senning procedure).[40] Both operations achieve the same physiologic result: the systemic venous blood is redirected to the left ventricle (and thereby the pulmonary circulation) and the pulmonary venous blood to the right ventricle. After successful atrial switch, patients are fully saturated but are left with their morphologic right ventricle supporting the entire systemic cardiac output. Unfortunately, in many (perhaps ultimately all) patients undergoing the atrial switch procedure, the right ventricle becomes dysfunctional over time, which is manifested by dilation, decreased ejection fraction, tricuspid insufficiency, and dysrhythmias.[41] The observation of problems with the systemic right ventricle in patients after the atrial switch operation was the primary impetus behind the development and application of the arterial switch operation (ASO), which is now established as the surgical treatment of choice for patients with TGA. In the recent era, operative survival rates for the ASO are approaching 100%.[42,43]

The ASO provides both physiologic and *anatomic* correction of TGA by establishing ventriculoarterial concordance. The operation involves transection and translocation of the malposed great vessels. The technically challenging requirement of the ASO relates to the translocation of the coronary arteries to the pulmonary root (the neoaorta). As noted earlier, there are numerous possible branching patterns for the coronary arteries in TGA—some easily transferred in the ASO, others more challenging (including single coronary ostium and intramural course)[43] (Fig. 60-24). Nonetheless, precise surgical techniques have been described and successfully applied to all coronary branching patterns. Given this fact, and

the known benefit of aligning the morphologic left ventricle with the systemic circulation, the ASO is offered to all patients with TGA *irrespective* of coronary branching pattern. Thus, there is no need for precise anatomic definition before surgery; all patients will undergo the ASO.[44] In most patients undergoing the ASO, the pulmonary artery bifurcation is moved *anterior* to the reconstructed neoaorta to minimize the potential for pulmonary artery distortion and compression of the translocated coronary arteries—the maneuver of LeCompte (Fig. 60-25). Although there are interinstitutional biases in terms of nuances of treatment of TGA, the following surgical strategy is generally agreed on for this group of patients.

TGA/IVS

After BAS and weaning from PGE₁ if possible, newborns with TGA/IVS undergo semielective ASO in the first few days to weeks of life. Rarely, patients present with profound desaturation refractory to BAS and PGE₁; in this setting, an emergent ASO is indicated. In this surgeon's experience, this has been necessary in one patient during the past decade in an experience involving more than 200 newborn ASOs. For other patients, the ASO needs to be performed in a timely but nonemergent setting. Even in the presence of adequate systemic saturations, the patient's morphologic left ventricle is functioning in a low-pressure work environment (supporting the pulmonary circulation). Thus, left ventricle mass and function will *involute* rapidly in the first few weeks of life. By 6 weeks of life, the left ventricle may be incapable of supporting the normal systemic workload after the ASO. As such, the preferred timing for the operation is in the first 1 to 2 weeks of life.

TGA/VSD With or Without Arch Hypoplasia

There are several modes of presentation for patients with TGA/VSD. In patients with small, pressure-restrictive VSD, the presenting symptoms are similar to those of TGA/IVS. These patients require the ASO early in life, along with VSD closure before left ventricle involution. In patients with TGA and *nonrestrictive* VSD, there may be adequate mixing to allow reasonable systemic arterial saturation. In this setting, the left ventricle remains pressure-loaded and thereby does not involute; thus, the necessity of early promotion to the ASO is less time-compressed. Many newborns with TGA and large VSD are relatively asymptomatic soon after birth; they go on to develop CHF in the first 1 to 2 months of life as the normal fall in newborn pulmonary resistance occurs. This surgeon's preference in this group of patients is to follow closely for evidence of CHF and perform semielective ASO and VSD closure in the first 4 to 6 weeks of life. Some centers prefer to proceed with this surgery sooner; this appears to be a matter of surgeon preference and has not been shown to affect long-term outcome. In patients with TGA/VSD with arch hypoplasia or coarctation, early surgery is required. In this setting, the preferred treatment involves one-stage, complete correction including ASO, VSD closure, and aortic arch repair.

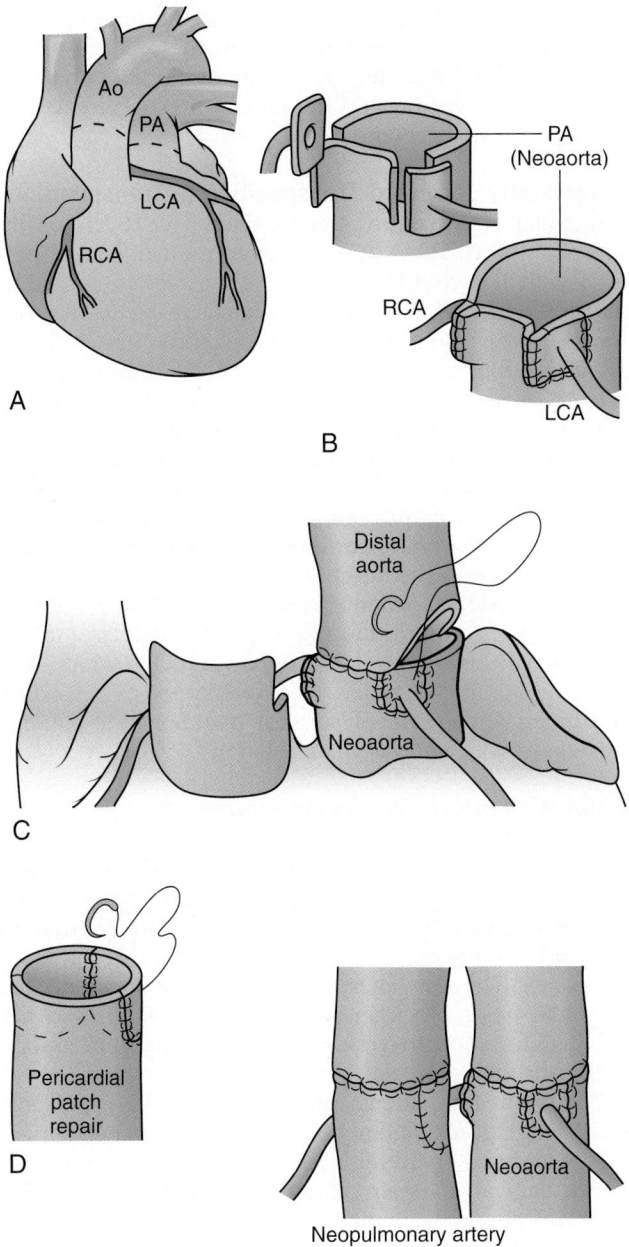

Figure 60-25 The arterial switch operation. **A,** The aorta (Ao) and pulmonary artery (PA) are transected above the sinuses of Valsalva. LCA, left coronary artery; RCA, right coronary artery. **B,** The coronaries are excised from the aorta and anastomosed to the pulmonary artery using a "trapdoor" technique. **C,** The distal aorta is brought behind the pulmonary artery (LeCompte maneuver) and anastomosed to the neoaorta. **D,** Separate pericardial patches are sutured to replace the excised coronary artery tissue from the aorta. **E,** Completed repair. (Modified from Karl TR, Kirshbom PM: Transposition of the great arteries and the arterial switch operation. In Nichols DG, Ungerleider RM, Spevak PJ, et al [eds]: Critical Heart Disease in Infants and Children. Philadelphia, Mosby, 2006, p 721.)

TGA/VSD With PS/LVOTO or PA

The issue of concern in this group of patients is the degree of left ventricular outflow tract obstruction (LVOTO). In patients with TGA/VSD and organic LVOTO with relatively normal pulmonary valve, the treatment strategy is as described previously with ASO, VSD closure, and LVOT resection. The situation becomes more complex in the setting of severe PS or pulmonary atresia. These patients may be ductal dependent as newborns (pulmonary atresia) and require either newborn complete correction or a palliative Blalock shunt in the newborn period followed by biventricular repair later in infancy (this surgeon's preference). The goal in these patients is to achieve biventricular repair to create an unobstructed connection between morphologic left ventricle and the systemic circulation. Several operations have been described and successfully utilized in this setting.

The *Rastelli procedure* involves an interventricular patch baffle, which commits the left ventricle to the aorta through the VSD. Typically, a right ventricle–pulmonary artery conduit is then placed to achieve pulmonary blood flow. Issues of concern include the potential for LVOT obstruction (at or below the level of the VSD) and the certain need for future right ventricle–pulmonary artery conduit revision. The *REV procedure* is designed to minimize the potential of LVOT obstruction and to utilize all possible native tissue-tissue connections to limit the potential need for future operation. This procedure involves resection of the muscular conus between aorta and pulmonary roots, interventricular baffle of the left ventricle to the aorta, and translocation of the native main pulmonary artery to the right ventricle (by a LeCompte maneuver) without the use of an intervening conduit. The final option involves *aortic root translocation,* which includes resection of the entire native aortic root and coronary origins, resection of the intervening muscular conus, and posterior translocation of the aortic root to the surgically enlarged pulmonary root to achieve a direct connection between the left ventricle and aorta. The VSD is then closed, and either a conduit is placed or a direct connection is created between the right ventricle and pulmonary arteries.

TGA in Adults

The long-term prognosis of adult patients who have undergone childhood repair of TGA is still incompletely understood; however, it is clear that all such patients require lifelong surveillance and have the potential of developing significant anatomic and functional cardiac problems. Patients who were treated with the atrial switch operation have a morphologic right ventricle supporting their systemic circulation, which will predictably fail in many patients. Although fully saturated, these patients may present later in life with signs and symptoms of CHF and dysrhythmia. For severely affected individuals, the only realistic option may ultimately be in the form of cardiac transplantation.

The long-term issues related to the ASO are less well understood, but issues of concern have been elucidated from several large series.[42,44] Despite technical advances in reconstructive methods, there is still a troubling incidence of postoperative supravalvular and branch pulmonic stenosis. The neoaortic root may dilate in some patients undergoing the ASO, leading to neoaortic insufficiency and coronary artery distortion. The fate of the surgically translocated coronary ostia is unclear; there is clearly a risk for late, sudden cardiac death related to unsuspected coronary insufficiency. As has been stated elsewhere in this chapter, for the adult patient undergoing noncardiac surgery after previous surgery for complex congenital cardiac disease including TGA, a high index of suspicion is warranted.

Double Outlet Right Ventricle

Double outlet right ventricle (DORV) occurs when both great vessels are anatomically committed to the RV. This may be in association with a subaortic VSD, a noncommitted (remote) VSD or a subpulmonary VSD (*Taussig-Bing anomaly*). As with other complex cardiac conditions, the goal of treatment relates to the presenting hemodynamic conditions and patient symptoms. The ultimate goal is to achieve a biventricular circulation when possible. Patients may present with severe cyanosis and require corrective or palliative therapy in the newborn period. Contrarily, they may present with unrestricted pulmonary blood flow and develop CHF. The challenging issue of constructing a biventricular repair relates to achieving unobstructed outlets from right and left ventricles. In patients with DORV with subaortic VSD and RVOT obstruction, reconstruction is similar to that for TOF. More remote VSDs may require enlargement with interventricular tunnel repair. For the Taussig-Bing anomaly, the relationship of the VSD to the pulmonary artery makes the ASO the procedure of choice. These patients often have RVOT obstruction and aortic arch

hypoplasia, which require attention at the time of complete correction. For rare individuals, the relationship of the great vessels and the complexity of the VSD preclude a biventricular repair, and the patient must be treated as a functional single ventricle.

Congenitally Corrected Transposition (L-Transposition)

Congenitally corrected transposition (ccTGA) or L-transposition (L-TGA) describes a constellation of conditions with the common feature of *atrioventricular and ventriculoarterial discordance*. This may be in association with VSD, pulmonic and subpulmonic stenosis, and displaced left atrioventricular valve ("ebsteinoid" left atrioventricular valve). In ccTGA, the morphologic mitral valve is right sided and associated with the morphologic left ventricle; the morphologic tricuspid valve is associated with the morphologic right ventricle. Patients with this condition are "physiologically corrected" in that, in the absence of ventricular-level shunting, they are fully saturated, hence the term *corrected* transposition. The age and mode of patient presentation in this condition depend on the contribution of associated defects and the function of the morphologic right ventricle (which acts as the systemic ventricle). Controversy exists regarding the timing and mode of surgical treatment for patients presenting with various manifestations of ccTGA.

ccTGA With Intact Ventricular Septum

Patients with ccTGA/IVS may be entirely asymptomatic throughout childhood and early adulthood. Frequently, the diagnosis is made incidentally. In other patients, the disease presents with symptoms of CHF in association with right ventricular dysfunction or left atrioventricular valve insufficiency. There is also a high incidence of complete heart block in patients with ccTGA, and the first manifestation may be this dysrhythmia with associated symptoms.

Treatment for patients presenting with CHF presents a challenging management scenario. For patients with ccTGA and preserved right ventricular function, left atrioventricular valve repair or replacement may be considered. Unfortunately, in many of these patients, the valvular insufficiency may be more a manifestation of declining systemic right ventricular function with septal shift and annular dilation rather than intrinsic valve pathology. In this setting, valve replacement will not correct the progression of right ventricular dysfunction. For patients with systemic right ventricular dysfunction, one option for treatment is through a complex reconstruction known as a *double switch* (Fig. 60-26). This procedure includes an atrial switch in combination with an arterial switch to align the morphologic left ventricle with the systemic circulation. In almost all patients with ccTGA/IVS and right ventricular dysfunction (and in the absence of structural LVOT obstruction), a period of left ventricle retraining will be required before the double-switch procedure. This relates to the fact that the left ventricle will have been functioning in the low-pressure pulmonary circulation and will be incapable of performing systemic work. Retraining or conditioning the left ventricle requires surgical creation of PS by the placement of a pulmonary

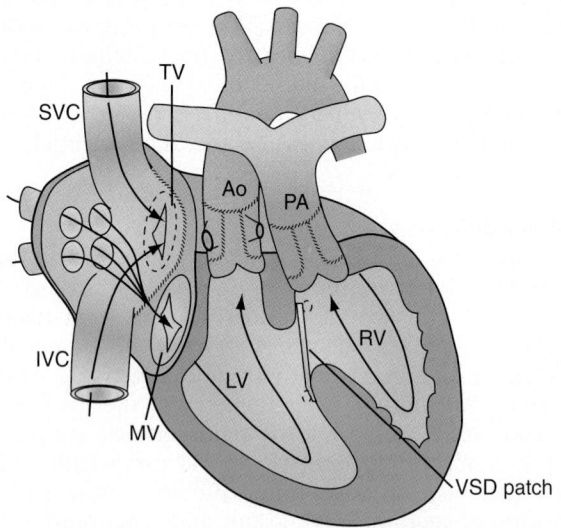

Figure 60-26 The double-switch operation (Senning and arterial switch). Ao, aorta; IVC, inferior vena cava; LV, left ventricle; MV, mitral valve; PA, pulmonary artery; SVC, superior vena cava; TV, tricuspid valve; VSD, ventricular septal defect. (Modified from Karl TR, Cochrane AD: Congenitally corrected transposition of the great arteries. In Mavroudis C, Backer CL [eds]: Pediatric Cardiac Surgery. Philadelphia, Mosby, 2003, p 488.)

artery band. Most surgeons agree that the left ventricle must work at or very near systemic blood pressure for many months (this surgeon favors a minimum of 6 months) before the double-switch operation. The double switch is a technically challenging operation with significant perioperative risk. Because of the small numbers of patients treated worldwide with this complicated surgical strategy, there are at present only limited data concerning the acute and midterm results.[45] An issue of concern centers on the long-term ability of the retrained left ventricle to function as the systemic ventricle. Nonetheless, patients with ccTGA and depressed right ventricular function have a poor prognosis otherwise, and as such, the complexity and risk of the double-switch process appear justified. The only other surgical option for these patients is cardiac transplantation.

ccTGA With VSD and Pulmonic Stenosis

Patients in this category are often well balanced and have mild cyanosis with minimal symptoms in childhood, whereas others with more severe PS or pulmonary atresia present early in life with symptomatic cyanosis. Treatment for the overtly cyanotic infant with ccTGA/PS is initially palliative in the form of a Blalock shunt. The ultimate goal for all patients is a biventricular circulation with normal arterial oxygen saturation. One option for such patients is to surgically close the VSD and place a conduit between the morphologic left ventricle and the pulmonary arteries to relieve the pulmonary obstruction. This classic repair benefits the patient by separating the systemic and pulmonary circulations and allowing normal oxygen tensions. The issue of concern in patients undergoing a classic repair is that the morphologic right ventricle must act independently as the systemic ventricle following repair. As noted previously, the ability of the right ventricle to support the systemic circulation may be of question over the long term in some patients. As such, an alternative strategy in these patients is to baffle the left ventricular outflow to the aorta through the VSD, then perform an atrial switch to reroute the systemic and pulmonary venous return and finally to place a conduit from the morphologic right ventricle to the pulmonary arteries. This option is a modification of the double-switch arrangement, affording the patient the benefit of a systemic left ventricle. Because the left ventricle has been working at systemic pressure before correction, a period of retraining is unnecessary.

Adult patients with ccTGA with or without previous surgery merit careful attention before any noncardiac operation. These patients may have a variety of complex ongoing cardiac issues including rhythm disturbance, ventricular dysfunction, and valvular insufficiency.

Left Ventricular Outflow Tract Obstruction

Left ventricular outflow tract obstruction (LVOTO) may present in isolation or in combination with other complex cardiac lesions. The physiologic consequences of severe LVOTO may be catastrophic, including diminished systemic cardiac output and tremendous left ventricular pressure overload. Newborns with severe LVOTO may

present in shock with diminished peripheral perfusion, cardiomegaly, and pulmonary congestion. There is a significant risk for NEC in these babies. In older patients, gradual onset of LVOTO may be initially asymptomatic, only to manifest over time as decreasing exercise tolerance and declining left ventricular function. Patients with severe LVOTO and cardiomegaly are at high risk for myocardial ischemia and sudden cardiac death. The resting ECG will often demonstrate left ventricular hypertrophy with strain pattern. If performed, an exercise stress test (EST) may demonstrate worrisome ST depression and ventricular dysrhythmias. Echocardiography is the primary diagnostic tool for patients with LVOTO. In rare cases, diagnostic cardiac catheterization may be considered to delineate the level of obstruction.

Valvular Aortic Stenosis

Congenital valvular aortic stenosis (AS) is a common cause of LVOTO. The degree of obstruction may range from mild in patients with a congenitally bicuspid aortic valve to severe in patients with critical AS with unidentifiable valve commissures and annular hypoplasia. Babies presenting with critical AS are often symptomatic early in the newborn period, presenting with shock and profoundly depressed ventricular function. In the current era, these patients are almost all taken to the cardiac catheterization laboratory for balloon aortic valvotomy. This procedure may be lifesaving in relieving the aortic stenosis and allowing for recovery of ventricular function. For most of the patients, however, the procedure is palliative with a significant incidence of recurrence of AS or development of significant aortic insufficiency (AI) following the procedure. In patients with AS refractory to balloon dilation, an open aortic valvotomy may be necessary (Fig. 60-27). Especially in small babies with adequate

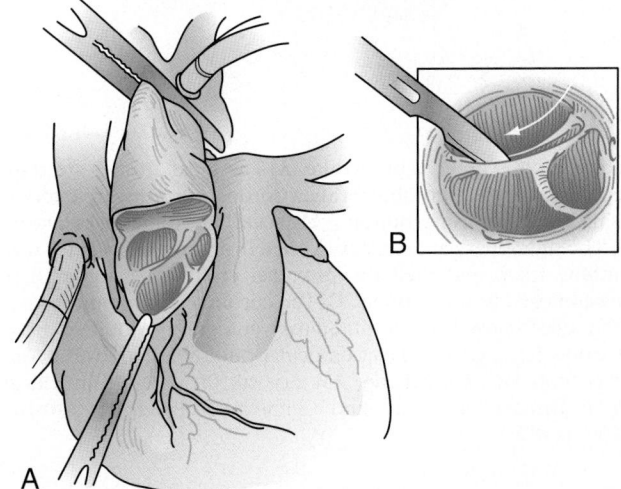

Figure 60-27 Close-up of the aortic valve demonstrates a surgical valvectomy. **A,** The valve is bicuspid with a prominent raphe in the anterior valve leaflet. **B,** The orifice is enlarged by incising the fused commissure between the two leaflets. (From Chang AC, Burke RP: Left ventricular outflow tract obstruction. In Chang AC, Hanley FL, Wernovsky G, Wessell DL [eds]: Pediatric Cardiac Intensive Care. Baltimore, Williams & Wilkins, 1998.)

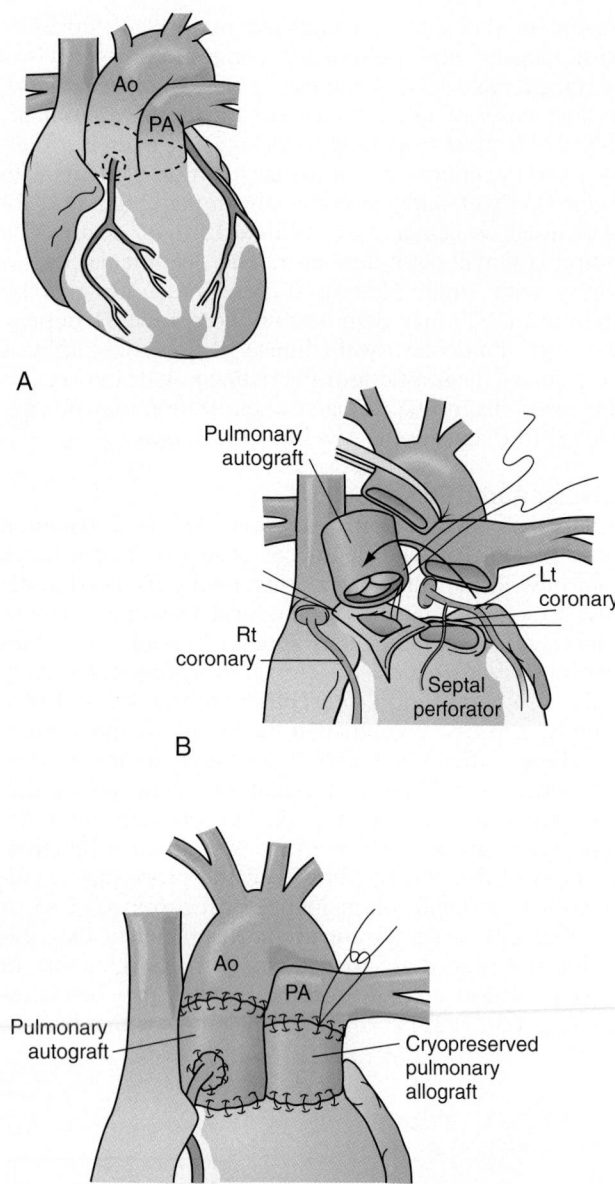

Figure 60-28 The Ross procedure. **A,** The great arteries are transected above the sinotubular ridge. Coronary arteries are excised using coronary artery buttons. Ao, aorta; PA, pulmonary artery. **B,** The pulmonary autograft is excised from the right ventricular outflow tract, and then the proximal end of the autograft is anastomosed to the annulus. **C,** The coronary artery buttons are then anastomosed to the pulmonary autograft. (Modified from St. Louis JD, Jaggers J: Left ventricular outflow tract obstruction. In Nichols DG, Ungerleider RM, Spevak PJ, et al [eds]: Critical Heart Disease in Infants and Children. Philadelphia, Mosby, 2006, p 615.)

annular dimension, a surgical valvotomy can be accomplished by an accurate incision down a rudimentary commissure or raphe to improve cusp mobility.

Recurrent AS after previous ballooning may be amenable to repeat dilation; however, when associated with significant AI, the patient will have to go to surgery.

Severe AI after previous balloon dilation is usually related to an avulsed cusp. In such instances, valve repair may be possible, but replacement may prove necessary. Recent published series have confirmed the utility of aortic valve repair procedures, which is a particularly attractive option for growing children.[46,47]

The decision to replace the aortic valve in growing children is clouded by the lack of an ideal aortic valve substitute, meaning a valve capable of life-long durability, appropriate somatic growth, easily implantable, and not requiring anticoagulation. Criteria for aortic valve replacement are beyond the scope of this chapter; however, severe valvular AS that is not amenable to catheter or open valvotomy is clearly an appropriate indication. Options for aortic valve replacement in children include mechanical prostheses, heterograft, homograft, and pulmonary autograft. A mechanical prosthesis may be considered in childhood; however, the valve size must be sufficient to afford adequate function as the patient grows. Most surgeons and cardiologists recommend therapeutic anticoagulation in children with mechanical valve prosthesis; this can be a challenging and potentially dangerous proposition in growing children and adolescents. As such, many surgeons believe the risk for such medical management outweighs the potential benefit of a theoretically durable valve.

Heterograft aortic valve prostheses historically have been associated with limited durability in children and, of course, are also not capable of somatic growth. The current era heterograft prostheses have not undergone sufficient use in children to provide useful data concerning improved durability. Human cadaver aortic valves (aortic homograft) have been used extensively in children and young adults. These valves are typically implanted as a complete aortic root replacement, which require coronary ostial implantation. Thus, the operation to place an aortic homograft is considerably more complex and with potentially higher risk. The positive features of aortic homograft include improved durability in comparison to heterograft and avoidance of anticoagulation. Nonetheless, these valves will eventually fail, necessitating a complicated reoperative aortic root replacement.

Pulmonary autograft aortic root replacement (Ross operation) involves translocation of the pulmonary valve to the aortic position with subsequent replacement of the pulmonary valve with either a homograft or heterograft valved conduit (Fig. 60-28). The theoretic advantages of the Ross procedure include the potential for somatic growth, avoidance of anticoagulation, and possibility of extended durability. Enthusiasm for this operation has been tempered by the recognition that the need for extension cardiac dissection to harvest the autograft, along with a more complex implantation, is associated with an increased operative risk. Furthermore, the unsupported pulmonary root may dilate in the presence of systemic arterial pressure, leading to progressive autograft aortic insufficiency. This observation has led to various modifications of the implantation technique to support the aortic annulus and even the sinus segment. Given these considerations and the certain need for reoperation to replace the right ventricular–pulmonary artery

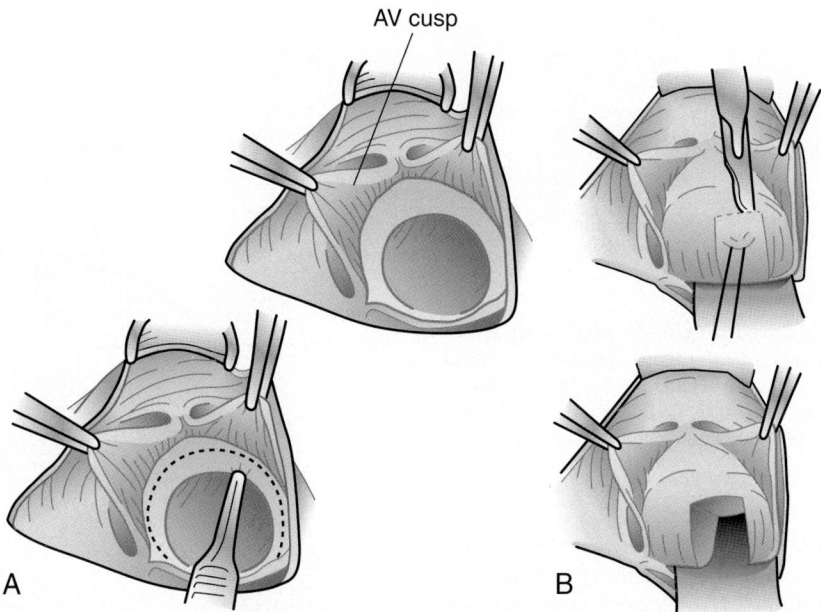

AV cusp

A   B

Figure 60-29 A, Excision of discrete subaortic stenosis. The aorta is opened obliquely, and the aortic valve leaflets are retracted to expose the subaortic membrane. The membrane is excised circumferentially along the *indicated line.* **B,** This is usually combined with a muscle resection. (From de Leval M: Surgery of the left ventricular outflow tract. In Stark J, de Leval M [eds]: Surgery for Congenital Heart Defects, 2nd ed. Philadelphia, WB Saunders, 1994.)

conduit, great caution must be exercised in the application of the Ross operation.

Fibromuscular Subaortic Stenosis
This condition is a progressive narrowing of the LVOT related to a dense fibrous membrane typically found in association with asymmetric protrusion of the interventricular septum into the outflow tract. The membrane is often concentric and becomes densely adherent to the septum and mitral valve. The membrane progresses toward and eventually onto the undersurface of the aortic valve cusps. This leads to progressive LVOTO as well as aortic valve cusp retraction and aortic insufficiency.

Echocardiography is the primary diagnostic tool in assessing the degree of obstruction and progression of subaortic stenosis. Unfortunately, echo is not accurate in assessing for subtle degrees of cusp extension. Cardiac catheterization is rarely needed to diagnose this condition; balloon dilation is of no use in treating the LVOTO.

Surgery is the mainstay of treatment for subaortic stenosis; however, there is disagreement concerning surgical indications. Most surgeons believe that new onset of any degree of aortic insufficiency in association with a subaortic membrane irrespective of the pressure gradient is an indication for surgery. In other patients, an escalating LVOT gradient, associated left ventricular hypertrophy, and the appropriate anatomic substrate are acceptable indications for operation.

Surgery for subaortic stenosis involves a transaortic resection of the subaortic membrane, including all attachments to the mitral valve, septum, and aortic valve cusps.

A septal myectomy is performed along with membrane resection in most patients (Fig. 60-29). Complications of the surgery include membrane recurrence, injury to the bundle of His, and iatrogenic VSD creation. Nonetheless, with careful operation, the risk for these complications is minimized.[48]

Tunnel Subaortic Stenosis
This is a more severe form of LVOTO that is often associated with aortic annular hypoplasia and valvular aortic stenosis. In severe cases, the LVOTO is not amenable to subaortic resection alone. In such cases, an aortic root enlarging procedure may be necessary to relieve the obstruction (aortoventriculoplasty or Konno procedure). This complex reconstruction typically is associated with the necessity of aortic valve replacement using one of the previously mentioned options. It is also of note that all degrees of LVOTO may be seen in association with multiple left heart obstructive lesions (Shone's syndrome[49]), which may require extensive reconstruction.[50]

Aortic Arch Anomalies
Aortic Coarctation
Coarctation of the aorta is one of the most frequently encountered congenital cardiac lesions. This condition has a wide range of presentations, from the severely symptomatic newborn with CHF and depressed ventricular function to the adult with proximal hypertension and minimal symptoms. Coarctation is classified relative to its association with the ligamentum arteriosus and aortic arch. An infantile or preductal aortic coarctation is seen in combination with a large PDA, which may have

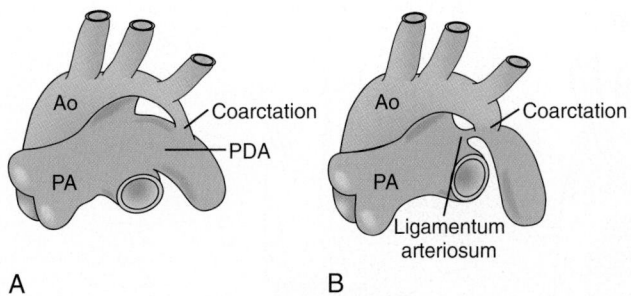

Figure 60-30 Coarctation of the aorta (Ao). PA, pulmonary artery; PDA, patent ductus arteriosus. **A,** Infantile or preductal coarctation. **B,** Adult coarctation. (From Backer CL, Mavroudis C: Coarctation of the aorta. In Mavroudis C, Backer CL [eds]: Pediatric Heart Surgery. Philadelphia, Mosby, 2003, p 252.)

predominantly right to left flow to the lower descending aorta. In this setting, the patient is ductal dependent for systemic blood flow until the coarctation is repaired, and a PGE₁ infusion must be maintained to prevent ductal closure. A periductal or juxtaductal coarctation occurs in the region of the ductal insertion and is distal to the aortic isthmus, which may be normal or hypoplastic (Fig. 60-30).

Aortic coarctation with or without aortic arch hypoplasia is frequently associated with intracardiac anomalies, including multiple left heart obstructive lesions (mitral stenosis, left ventricular hypoplasia or endocardial fibroelastosis, subaortic/aortic stenosis) known as Shone's syndrome.[49] Patients with large VSDs may present in infancy with severe aortic coarctation, with or without subaortic stenosis.

Aortic coarctation may be suspected on clinical examination by a significant upper-lower extremity blood pressure gradient and diminished or absent femoral and pedal pulses. In older patients with well-developed intercostal collateral arteries, a continuous murmur may be auscultated over the posterior thorax. Echocardiography is now the primary diagnostic modality for aortic coarctation. MRI and CT angiography may also be useful in some patients. In rare cases, cardiac catheterization is required to define the anatomy, but this modality is now more frequently used for treatment including balloon dilation with or without stenting.

Treatment strategies for aortic coarctation have evolved significantly since the first successful surgical treatment more than 60 years ago. Newborns presenting with severe aortic coarctation with or without associated ductal-dependent systemic blood flow are best treated by surgery. Initial enthusiasm regarding balloon dilation in these patients has diminished as it has become clear that there is a high incidence of recurrent coarctation after neonatal dilation.[51,52] Most congenital cardiac surgeons perform isolated coarctation repair through a left thoracotomy incision (3rd or 4th interspace) using resection of the coarctation and primary anastomosis. For patients with relative hypoplasia of the distal aortic arch, the anastomosis can be brought along the lesser curve of the aortic arch using an "extended" end-to-end method.

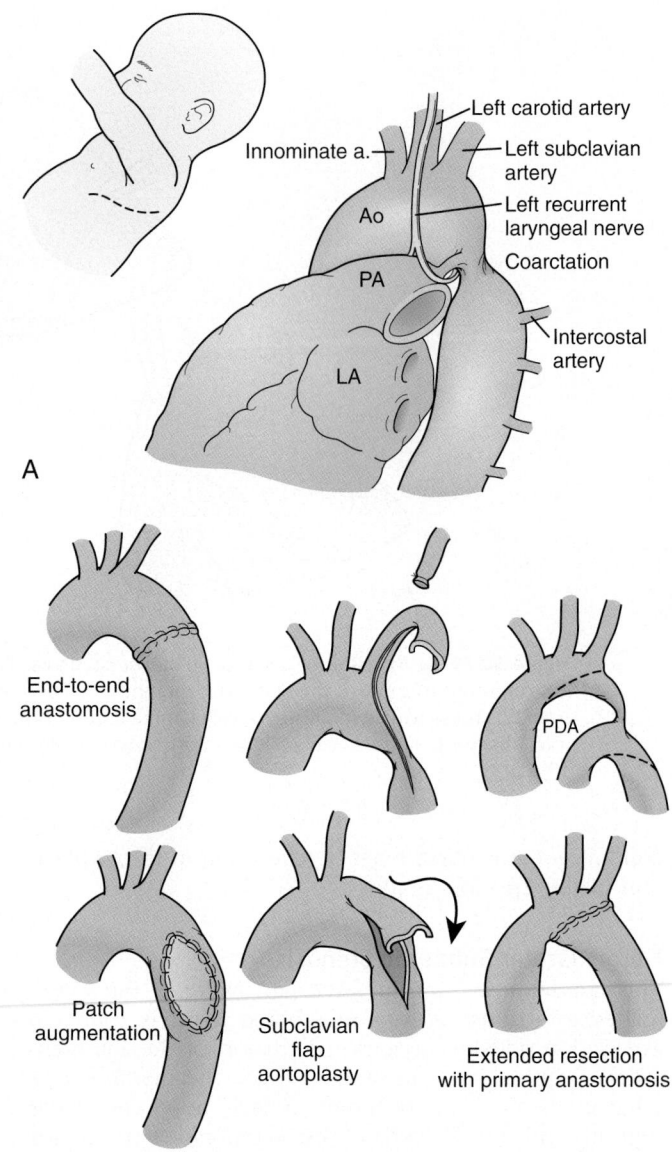

Figure 60-31 Surgical repair for aortic coarctation. **A,** Surgical incision and anatomic orientation. Ao, aorta; LA, left atrium; PA, pulmonary artery. **B,** Four different methods: end-to-end anastomosis; patch augmentation; subclavian flap aortoplasty; and extended resection with primary anastomosis. PDA, patent ductus arteriosus. (Modified from Hastings LA, Nichols DG: Coarctation of the aorta and interrupted aortic arch. In Nichols DG, Ungerleider RM, Spevak PJ, et al [eds]: Critical Heart Disease in Infants and Children. Philadelphia, Mosby, 2006, p 635.)

Other methods include subclavian artery flap aortoplasty (Waldhausen method) and prosthetic patch aortoplasty. The latter methods are today used less frequently than primary repair (Fig. 60-31). Catheter therapy as a primary treatment for aortic coarctation remains a controversial therapy in most surgeons' opinion. Although this methodology has been widely applied, its true comparability to surgery requires further prospective study. There are several issues of concern regarding angioplasty for coarctation. The balloon dilation results in transmural disruption of the aortic wall in many patients, and there is an acute and ongoing risk for aneurysm formation.[51,52] To limit this risk and minimize the potential of recurrence, off-label use of stents has occurred for treatment of coarctation. Obvious issues of concern include somatic growth and lifetime risk potential of a metal device in the descending aorta.

Another issue of controversy surrounds the concomitant treatment of coarctation and significant intracardiac pathology. Several series have now demonstrated superior outcomes for simultaneous therapy in selected groups of patients including neonates with large VSDs and coarctation with arch hypoplasia. This surgeon's approach to this circumstance has included one-stage complete repair of intracardiac defects along with aortic arch advancement through median sternotomy on cardiopulmonary bypass.[53]

Interrupted Aortic Arch

IAA results from lack of proper fusion and involution of the fetal aortic arches. This is a fatal condition without treatment, and IAA is frequently associated with serious intracardiac pathology. IAA is classified based on the level of the interruption: Type A is distal to the left subclavian artery; type B occurs between left subclavian and common carotid arteries; type C occurs proximal to the left subclavian artery (Fig. 60-32). There is a frequent finding of an aberrant right subclavian artery (retroesophageal) from the descending aorta. Survival for patients with IAA is initially predicated on ductal patency; thus, a PGE$_1$ infusion is required to stabilize the patients. Diagnosis is confirmed by echocardiography; other methods, including cardiac catheterization, are infrequently needed.

IAA requires surgical treatment in the newborn period, which typically involves simultaneous repair of intracardiac lesions (Fig. 60-33). Repair may be accomplished with the aid of an aortic arch augmentation patch, although Texas Children's Hospital has recently reported a series confirming that a primary tissue-tissue repair can be performed in most patients and minimizes the potential for recurrent aortic arch obstruction.[54]

SINGLE VENTRICLE

Single ventricle physiology is a frequently encountered form of congenital cardiac disease. Patients may present as newborns with inadequate pulmonary blood flow, excessive pulmonary blood flow, or balanced circulations. The single ventricle may be of right, left, or indeterminate morphology. Surgical treatment is required to provide adequate systemic oxygen delivery while protecting the pulmonary vasculature. The function of the single ventricle must be preserved to afford the patient the best possible long-term outcome.

The rapid evolution of successful palliation for patients with various forms of single ventricle during the past 30 years has led to a large and growing population of adults

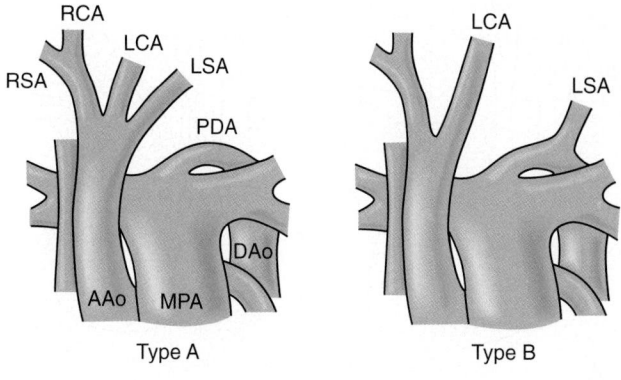

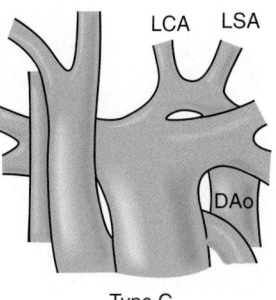

Figure 60-32 Classification of interrupted aortic arch. AAo, ascending aorta; DAo, descending aorta; LCA, left common carotid artery; LSA, left subclavian artery; MPA, main pulmonary artery; PDA, patent ductus arteriosus; RCA, right common carotid artery; RSA, right subclavian artery. (Modified from Monro JL: Interruption of aortic arch. In Stark J, de Laval M [eds]: Surgery for Congenital Heart Defects. Philadelphia, WB Saunders, 1994, p 299.)

with single ventricle. For most of these patients, lifelong cardiac attention is needed and the potential for subsequent cardiac reoperation is high. Patients in this category who present for noncardiac surgery may be especially difficult to manage.

An exhaustive discussion of the various forms of single ventricle is well beyond the scope of this chapter. As such, this discussion will be limited to common forms of single right and single left ventricle to provide examples of the surgical management strategies for single ventricle.

Tricuspid Atresia

Tricuspid atresia (TA) is the template single ventricle lesion for which most of our current palliative strategies were developed. Patients with TA have a single morphologic left ventricle and may have normally related or transposed great vessels (Fig. 60-34). They may present with excessive pulmonary blood flow and require pulmonary artery banding early in infancy to relieve pulmonary overcirculation and CHF. Contrarily, patients may have PS or pulmonary atresia and require creation of a Blalock shunt to provide adequate pulmonary blood flow and systemic oxygenation.

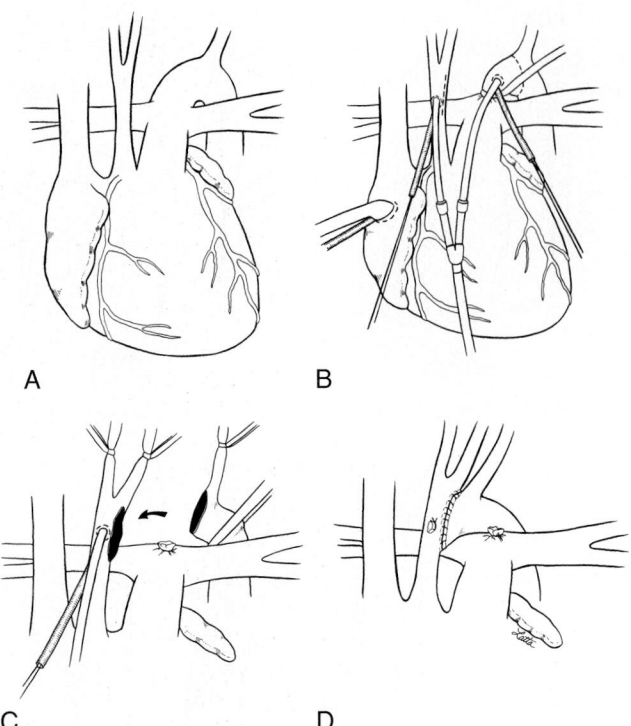

Figure 60-33 Type B interrupted aortic arch (**A**). Cannulation and site of incision for repair (**B**). The descending thoracic aorta is brought upward into the mediastinum (**C**) and then is anastomosed to the ascending aorta in an end-to-side fashion (**D**). (From Hirooka K, Fraser CD: One-stage neonatal repair of complex aortic arch obstruction or interruption. Tex Heart Inst J 24:317-321, 1997. Copyright 1997, Texas Heart Institute.)

As noted, the initial palliative goals in patients with TA include adequate systemic oxygenation, protection of ventricular function, and adequate pulmonary arterial growth. Patients with ductal-dependent pulmonary blood flow require a Blalock shunt in the newborn period. This surgeon's preference is to construct the shunt to the morphologic right pulmonary artery through a right thoracotomy. This allows shunt flow to be governed by the size of the subclavian artery. Furthermore, the right pulmonary artery is typically longer and runs in a more horizontal plane in comparison to the left pulmonary artery. This makes avoiding distortion of a lobar branch more facile. The goal of the shunt is to protect the pulmonary arteries, promote adequate pulmonary artery development, and support systemic arterial oxygenation for the first 4 to 6 months of life until the next planned stage of palliation (see Glenn and Fontan operations, later). The shunt is *not* designed for long-term use; thus, in most patients, a small interposition graft (expanded PTFE—3.0-4.0 mm) is selected. In the early era of single ventricle palliation, a variety of less well-controlled shunts were constructed, including classic Blalock (divided native subclavian artery to branch pulmonary artery), Pott's (side-to-side left pulmonary artery to descending aorta) and Waterston (side-to-side right pulmonary artery

to ascending aorta) (Fig. 60-35). These native tissue-tissue connections are capable of somatic growth but have the confounding risks for pulmonary overcirculation, pulmonary artery hypertension (potentially irreversible), and branch pulmonary artery distortion with hypoplasia. During the early stages of development of single ventricle palliation, many patients were treated with these poorly controlled shunts. As such, there are significant numbers of adult patients presenting with complications of these palliations, including chronic cardiac volume overload and decreased ventricular function, severe pulmonary artery distortion or isolation, pulmonary vascular disease, and profound cyanosis. These patients may present for surgery for noncardiac illness and are extremely difficult to manage.[55]

Hypoplastic Left Heart Syndrome

HLHS is the prototypical single right ventricle. Patients with this condition present with inadequate left heart structures ranging from mitral and aortic stenosis with left ventricular hypoplasia to almost complete absence of the left heart structures with aortic and mitral atresia (AA/MA). In the case of AA/MA, the ascending aorta is typically small (1-2 mm) and is perfused through *retrograde aortic arch flow* provided by the PDA. In HLHS, ductal closure results in rapid cardiovascular collapse with profound systemic hypoperfusion and hypoxia, followed quickly by death. Therefore, patients diagnosed in the antenatal period must be born in a facility qualified to immediately institute appropriate medical management, including the establishment of suitable vascular access (umbilical artery catheter) and institution of IV PGE_1 to maintain ductal patency. Patients undiagnosed at birth will typically have an early grace period of a few hours, but with the initiation of ductal closure, these children become critically ill and require aggressive resuscitation for survival. Without treatment, HLHS is a uniformly fatal condition. This fact is extremely poignant given that most children with HLHS are otherwise normal (Fig. 60-36).

After delivery, medical management is directed at maintaining ductal patency and balancing systemic and pulmonary blood flow. Balancing the circulations will become increasingly challenging with the normal decline in neonatal pulmonary vascular resistance (PVR) resulting in massive pulmonary overcirculation. As the overcirculation progresses, babies become tachypneic and may exhibit decreased systemic perfusion. NEC is a significant risk in these children, and many centers avoid enteral nutrition if there is any question of visceral malperfusion in an effort to minimize this potential. Other medical maneuvers include deliberate hypoventilation, low inspired oxygen concentration, and additional carbon dioxide to attempt to increase PVR and thereby limit pulmonary flow. These options are of limited utility in newborns with HLHS; over days to weeks, the children become progressively ill with pulmonary congestion and marginal systemic cardiac output. Patients fortunate enough to be maintained have the potential of develop-

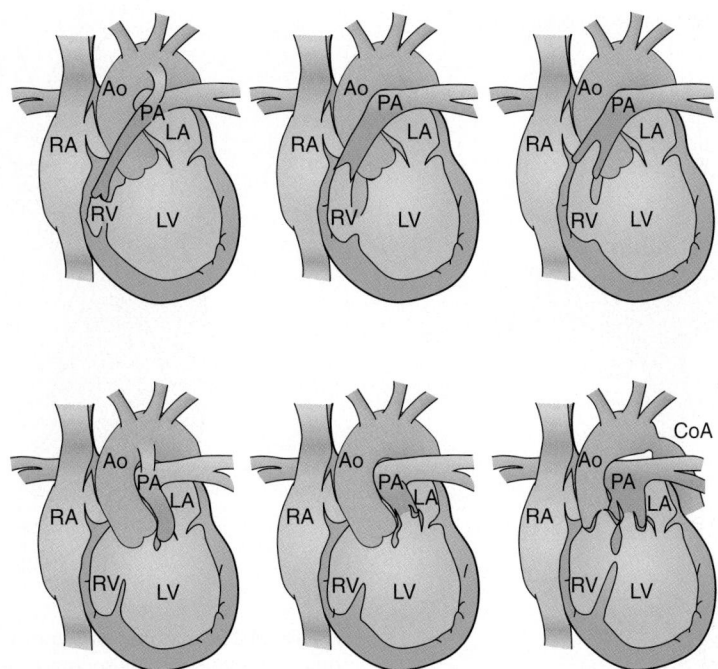

Figure 60-34 Anatomy of the various types of tricuspid atresia. *Top,* Normally related great vessels. *Bottom,* D-Transposition of the great vessels. Ao, aorta; CoA, coarctation of the aorta; LA, left atrium; LV, left ventricle; PA, pulmonary artery; RA, right atrium; RV, right ventricle. (Modified from Lok JM, Spevak PJ, Nichols DG: Tricuspid atresia. In Nichols DG, Ungerleider RM, Spevak PJ, et al [eds]: Critical Heart Disease in Infants and Children. Philadelphia, Mosby, 2006, pp 800-801.)

ing increased PVR as they age, and there is a known association with advanced age (>30 days) and increased operative mortality.

Surgery in the newborn period is the only realistic option for long-term survival in babies born with HLHS. In the current era, outcomes for surgical palliation of HLHS have come to be synonymous with the reputation of the treating center and surgeons. As with TA, patients with HLHS require a staged palliative approach. The first stage is, in all centers' experience, the most challenging and risk laden. The various first-stage options are described in the following sections.

Neonatal Cardiac Transplantation

Transplantation is a theoretically attractive option in babies with HLHS that replaces the malformed heart with a structurally normal one. Dr. Leonard Bailey has been an influential champion of this approach and was the first to report exciting results with transplantation in newborns with HLHS.[56] Furthermore, although there is an ever-present risk for rejection and infection in transplanted children, long-term, meaningful survival is possible and the quality of life of the recipients is quite good. Clearly, the option of cardiac transplantation is limited by the small numbers of suitable donor hearts and for most children with HLHS, waiting for a donor graft is unsuccessful. This has led most centers, including Texas Children's Hospital, to abandon cardiac transplantation as the primary mode of therapy for most neonates with HLHS.

Norwood Reconstruction

After initial work and success at Boston Children's Hospital, Dr. William Norwood and colleagues at the Children's Hospital of Philadelphia gained international attention for developing and implementing a reconstructive technique to palliate newborns with HLHS; this methodology now carries the widely used eponym of *Norwood's procedure.*[57] The Norwood procedure was gradually refined as experience accrued. The most common method involves surgical connection of the divided main pulmonary artery to the reconstructed aortic arch. In almost all children with HLHS, there is associated aortic arch hypoplasia with coarctation. As such, a critical feature of the operation is to reconstruct the aortic arch to provide unrestricted systemic blood flow. Most surgeons use some form of prosthetic material, commonly, pulmonary artery homograft patching. Some have reported accomplishing the arch reconstruction without the necessity of additional material.[58] After reconstructing the aortic arch, the divided main pulmonary artery is anastomosed to the arch and the small ascending aorta to create a neoaortic confluence providing systemic output from the right ventricle. The challenging feature of the reconstruction involves the accurate connection of this often miniscule ascending aorta to the confluence of the arch and main pulmonary artery stump. The opportunity for torsion and thereby coronary insufficiency is high; a recent multicenter report on outcomes for the Norwood procedure identified the diagnosis of aortic atresia as a risk factor for mortality.[59] The final element

CLASSIC RIGHT BLALOCK-TAUSSIG

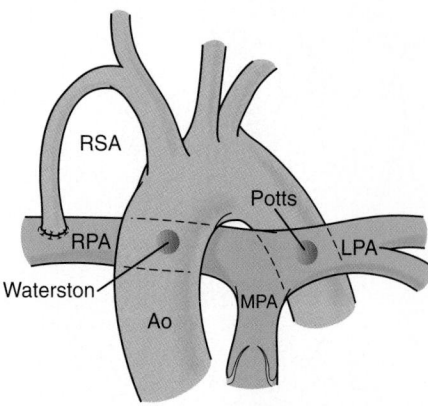

RIGHT MODIFIED BLALOCK-TAUSSIG

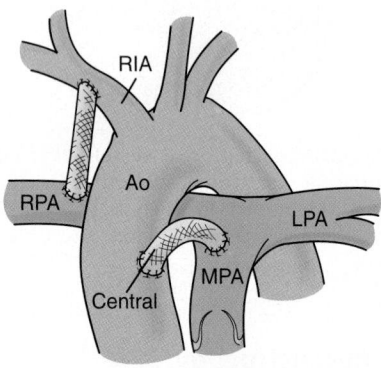

Figure 60-35 Various systemic-to-pulmonary artery shunts. Ao, aorta; MPA, main pulmonary artery; LPA, left pulmonary artery; RIA; right innominate artery; RPA, right pulmonary artery; RSA, right subclavian artery. (Modified from Marino BS, Wernovsky G, Greeley WJ: Single-ventricle lesions. In Nichols DG, Ungerleider RM, Spevak PJ, et al [eds]: Critical Heart Disease in Infants and Children. Philadelphia, Mosby, 2006, p 793.)

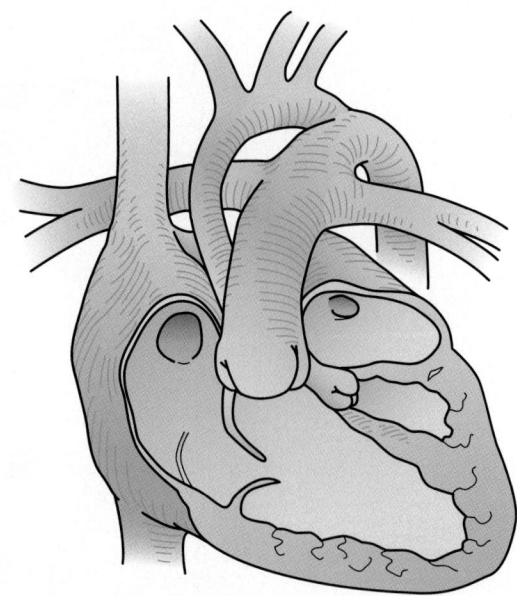

Figure 60-36 Anatomy of hypoplastic left heart syndrome. The tiny ascending aorta is seen arising from a markedly hypoplastic left ventricle. The ductus arteriosus is large, providing forward flow to the systemic circuit. The right ventricle is hypertrophied, and the pulmonary artery is enlarged. (From Wernovsky G, Bove EL: Single ventricle lesions. In Chang AC, Hanley FL, Wernovsky G, Wessell DL [eds]: Pediatric Cardiac Intensive Care. Baltimore, Williams & Wilkins, 1998.)

of the classic Norwood reconstruction is the creation of a controlled source of pulmonary blood flow in the form of a modified Blalock-Taussig shunt (Fig. 60-37).

Sano Modification of Norwood's Operation

Achieving survival after the Norwood operation is a challenging proposition, involving innumerable technical and medical details. At best, the patient after a Norwood procedure is fragile with a delicate balance between systemic and pulmonary blood flow. This fact and the observation of widely disparate outcomes for the procedure have led to a number of important advances in the treatment of these children. One issue relates to the difficulty of balancing the systemic to pulmonary artery shunt, which lowers diastolic blood pressure (and thereby coronary perfusion pressure) and volume loads the heart. Dr. Sunji Sano and colleagues from Okayama University in Japan were the first to report a series of babies under-

going a successful Norwood procedure, but with the modification of a *right ventricle to pulmonary artery conduit* rather than a Blalock shunt.[60] The theoretical advantage of this approach is the increase in diastolic pressure, creating a physiology more akin to a banded circulation rather than shunted. Early reports with this method have been encouraging, although patients do appear to become more rapidly desaturated as they age when compared with the shunted patients. The long-term effects of the right ventriculotomy on cardiac function are as of yet unknown.

Hybrid Procedure

The notion of a combined therapy between interventional cardiology and surgery for the first-stage palliation of HLHS has achieved significant attention in recent years. The idea is to minimize the risk of the first operation by banding the branch pulmonary arteries and delivering a stent into the ductus to maintain patency. This hybrid arrangement is designed to allow newborn survival such that a more complete reconstruction may be performed later in infancy in a larger child. There appears to be a significant learning curve with this approach as with any new procedure. Concerning features in addition to this include the effect of the banding on long-term pulmonary artery growth, the fact that cardiac perfusion is still retrograde through the aortic arch, and the risk profile of the more extensive reconstruction later in life. The true place for this mode of therapy is, at present, unclear, but it represents an important direction of

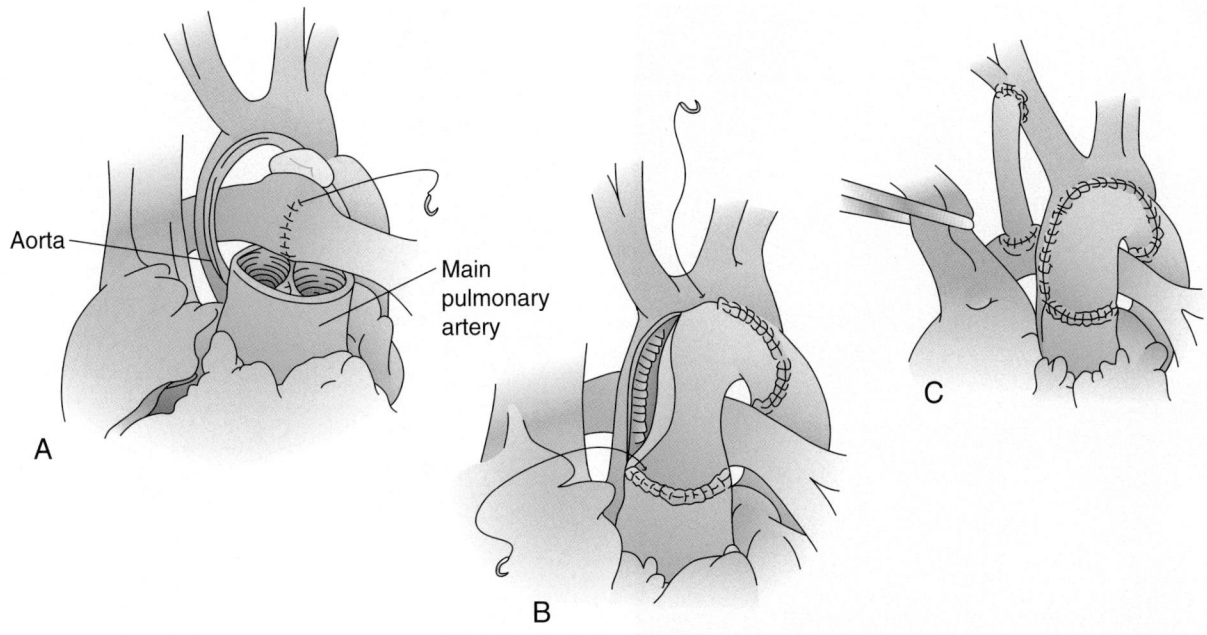

Figure 60-37 The Norwood procedure for first-stage palliation of hypoplastic left heart syndrome. **A,** The main pulmonary artery (MPA) is divided proximal to the bifurcation, the ductus arteriosus is ligated and divided, and the aortic arch is opened from the level of the transected MPA to a point distal to the ductal insertion in the descending aorta. **B,** A segment of homograft is cut to an appropriate size and shape. This is sutured into place, creating an unobstructed outflow from the right ventricle to the pulmonary artery and aorta. **C,** Polytetrafluoroethylene tube graft is placed from the innominate artery to the right pulmonary artery. The atrial septectomy is done while the patient is under circulatory arrest as well. (From Castaneda AR, Jonas RA, Mayer JE, Hanley FL: Hypoplastic left heart syndrome. In Cardiac Surgery of the Neonate and Infant. Philadelphia, WB Saunders, 1994.)

advancement to optimize the opportunity of survival for these children.[61]

Fontan Operation

The long-term goal of single ventricle palliation is to optimize ventricular function and promote systemic oxygen delivery. As noted earlier, patients with single ventricle who are either shunted or banded have ongoing concerns including systemic desaturation, continued intracardiac mixing, and chronic cardiac volume overload. The current strategy used to address these concerns utilizes direct connection between the branch pulmonary arteries and systemic venous return as initially proposed by Dr. Francis Fontan in the early 1970s. The Fontan operation is now the treatment of choice for children born with all varieties of single ventricle and, in suitable patients, provides acceptable long-term palliation. It must be recognized, however, that the Fontan circulation is not normal and, even in the best of circumstances, results in significant alteration in normal cardiorespiratory physiology.

The Fontan circulation is established by connecting the systemic venous return directly into isolated branch pulmonary arteries *without an intervening power source.* Thus, blood flow in the Fontan circuit is passive, being promoted only by the pressure differential between the systemic venous system and the pulmonary venous

atrium. As such, an impediment to flow in the systemic to pulmonary pathway will result in a poor Fontan outcome. Established criteria for creating an effective Fontan circulation include the ability to surgically connect the systemic venous return to the pulmonary arteries in an unobstructed manner, normal pulmonary artery architecture and resistance, normal pulmonary venous drainage and low left atrial pressure, absence of significant atrioventricular valve regurgitation, good ventricular function (and thereby, low ventricular end-diastolic pressure), an unobstructed systemic arterial outlet and good aortic valve function. Compromise of any of these elements may compromise the quality of the Fontan circulation.

The Fontan operation has undergone several technical modifications in the now more than 30 years of successful application to patients with single ventricle physiology. Many patients underwent an atriopulmonary connection in which the open right atrial appendage was directly anastomosed to the pulmonary artery bifurcation with surgical closure of the ASD. A large number of these patients are now presenting with extreme dilation of the right atrium with resulting sluggish flow, hepatic congestion, and atrial dysrhythmias (Fig. 60-38). Today, the most widely practiced modification of the Fontan operation is the *total cavopulmonary connection* (TCPC). First described by Professor Marc DeLeval, this operation involves connection of the divided SVC to the superior and inferior aspects of the right pulmonary artery (typi-

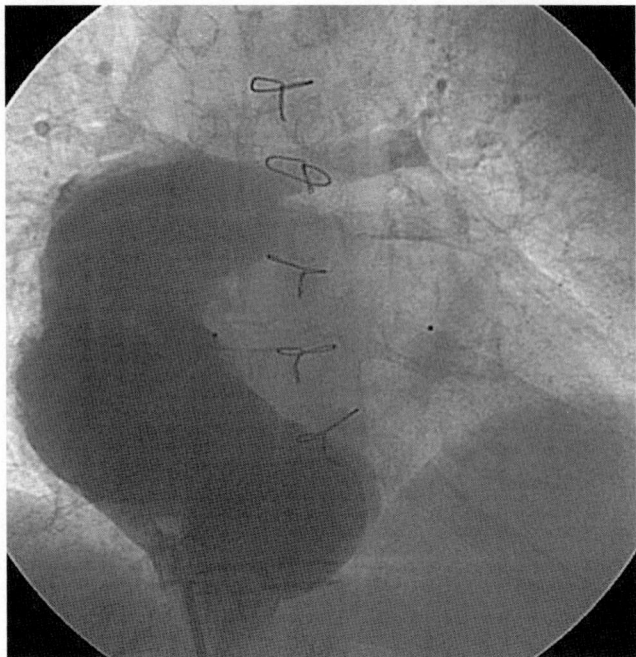

Figure 60-38 Angiogram of a dilated right atrium in a patient with an atriopulmonary Fontan connection.

cally somewhat offset) along with the creation of a channel to direct the IVC flow into the pulmonary arteries. The channel may be created using either a surgically created lateral tunnel in the right atrium (Fig. 60-39) or by interposing a conduit between the IVC and the pulmonary arteries (extracardiac Fontan) (Fig. 60-40).

The change from a volume-loaded circulation in shunted or banded single ventricle patients to a Fontan circulation results in acute volume unloading of the systemic ventricle. In the chronic overloaded heart, this acute change may be poorly tolerated with resultant diastolic dysfunction and decreased ventricular compliance. To deal with this problem, patients with single ventricle typically undergo an intervening stage of palliation in the form of a bidirectional, superior cavopulmonary anastomosis (Glenn shunt). The bidirectional Glenn shunt is constructed by anastomosing the cephalad end of the divided SVC to the superior aspect of the right pulmonary artery (Fig. 60-41). Other sources of pulmonary blood flow are typically eliminated, and thus, the heart is volume unloaded; however, systemic cardiac output is maintained because the IVC return is preserved. After the Glenn shunt, the patients are not fully saturated; typically patients run saturations of about 80%. Over time, the unloaded ventricle remodels, and the patient is promoted to reoperation and completion of the Fontan circulation.

Perioperative care of the Fontan patient can be challenging. The acute changes in cardiac volume loading may negatively affect cardiac output. Even in patients with "ideal" Fontan connections, the central venous pressure acutely rises to 12 to 15 mm Hg. Consequences of this increased venous pressure include pleural effusions, hepatic congestion, and ascites. In marginal Fontan can-

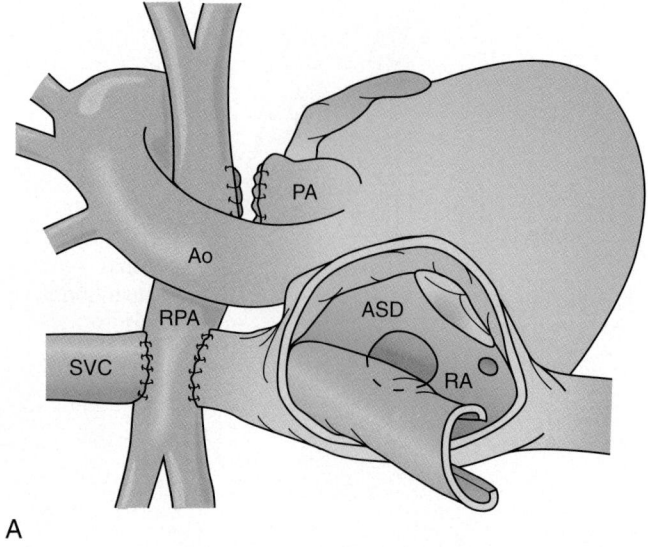

A

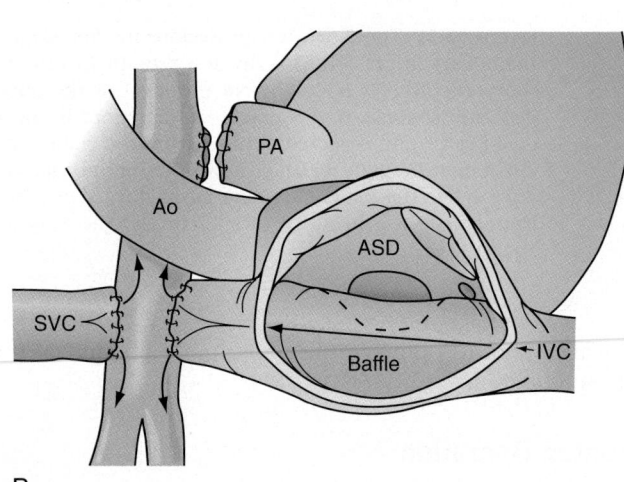

B

Figure 60-39 A and **B,** Lateral tunnel Fontan. Ao, aorta, ASD, atrial septal defect; IVC, inferior vena cava; RA, right atrium; RPA, right pulmonary artery; PA, pulmonary artery; SVC, superior vena cava. (Modified from Lok JM, Spevak PJ, Nichols DG: Tricuspid atresia. In Nichols DG, Ungerleider RM, Spevak PJ, et al [eds]: Critical Heart Disease in Infants and Children. Philadelphia, Mosby, 2006, p 813.)

didates, some surgeons routinely place an intentional "leak" or fenestration; the goal of such a fenestration is to preserve systemic ventricular volume loading and decrease systemic venous congestion at the expense of some degree of desaturation due to the right-to-left shunting. Any impediment to passive pulmonary blood flow will inhibit Fontan flow and result in right heart failure. Positive pressure ventilation, especially elevated levels of positive end-expiratory pressure, will impede pulmonary blood flow in the Fontan patient. Contrarily, early extubation and effective spontaneous ventilation will improve pulmonary blood flow in the Fontan patient.

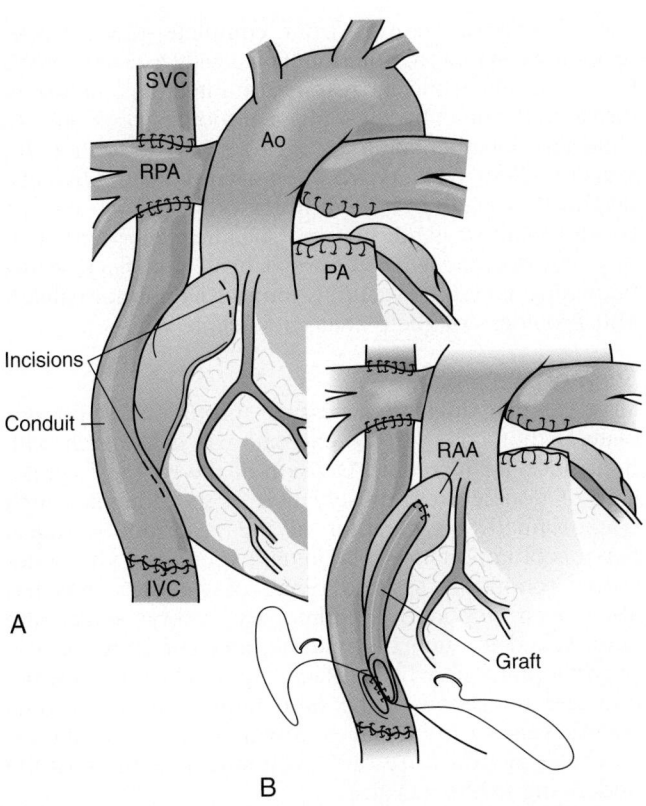

Figure 60-40 A, Extracardiac Fontan. Ao, aorta; IVC, inferior vena cava; PA, pulmonary artery; RPA, right pulmonary artery; SVC, superior vena cava. **B,** Creation of a fenestration in an extracardiac Fontan using a graft between the extracardiac conduit and the right atrial appendage (RAA). (Modified from Lok JM, Spevak PJ, Nichols DG: Tricuspid atresia. In Nichols DG, Ungerleider RM, Spevak PJ, et al [eds]: Critical Heart Disease in Infants and Children. Philadelphia, Mosby, 2006, p 814.)

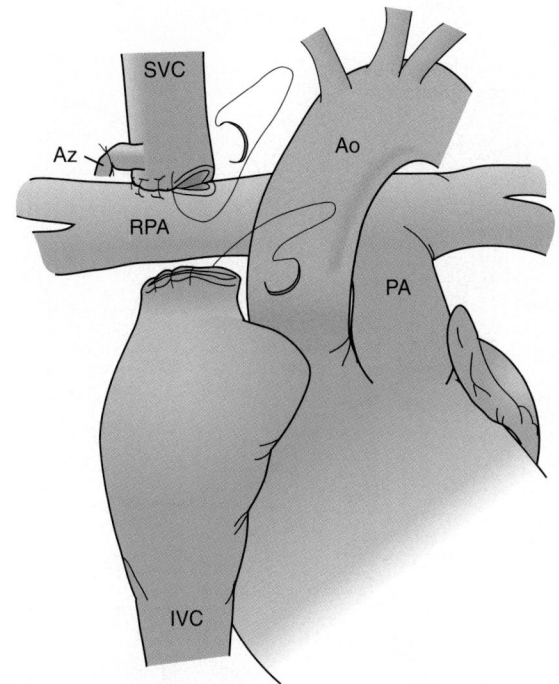

Figure 60-41 The bidirectional Glenn shunt. Ao, aorta; Az, azygos vein; IVC, inferior vena cava; PA, pulmonary artery; RPA, right pulmonary artery; SVC, superior vena cava. (Modified from Lok JM, Spevak PJ, Nichols DG: Tricuspid atresia. In Nichols DG, Ungerleider RM, Spevak PJ, et al [eds]: Critical Heart Disease in Infants and Children. Philadelphia, Mosby, 2006, p 809.)

The chronic complications of living with a Fontan circulation are still unfolding, but include chronic hepatic congestion and cirrhosis, protein-losing enteropathy, atrial dysrhythmias, and venous stasis disease.[62] Management of patients with failing Fontan circulations is especially challenging. These patients are at high risk for severe cardiac compromise while undergoing general anesthesia with positive-pressure ventilation or any procedure involving large fluid shifts, including abdominal surgery. Patients with chronic hepatic congestion may develop a coagulopathy related to a decrease in factor production.

MISCELLANEOUS ANOMALIES

Vascular Ring and Pulmonary Artery Sling

Vascular rings are abnormalities of the aortic arch and its branches, compressing the trachea, esophagus, or both. The ring may be either complete or partial. A pulmonary artery sling occurs when the left pulmonary artery arises from the right pulmonary artery, passing leftward between

the trachea and the esophagus. The trachea may be compressed, the cartilage may be soft, or there may be intrinsic stenosis of the trachea in the form of complete cartilage rings. Categorization of the defects is useful for description:

Complete vascular rings
- *Double arch:* Equal arches or left or right arch dominant (Fig. 60-42)
- *Right arch:* Left ligamentum arteriosus from anomalous left subclavian artery
- *Right arch:* Mirror image branching, with left ligamentum from descending aorta

Partial vascular rings
- *Left arch:* Aberrant right subclavian artery
- *Left arch:* Innominate artery compression

Pulmonary Artery Slings

The double aortic arch is the most common form of complete ring. Two arches arise from the ascending aorta, forming a true ring. The left arch is usually smaller. The right arch–left ligamentum complex is formed from persistence of the right fourth arch and regression of the left fourth arch. The anomalously arising left subclavian artery is often associated with a diverticulum at its base (Kommerell). In partial rings, the most common form is an aberrant right subclavian artery arising distal to the

ANTERIOR

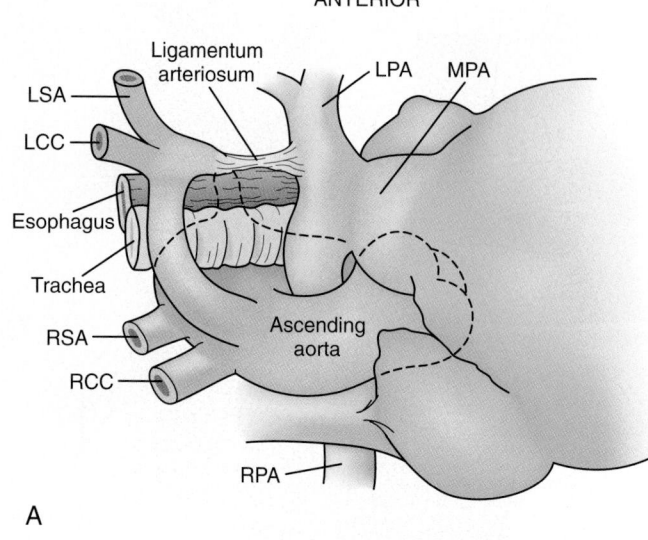

A

POSTERIOR

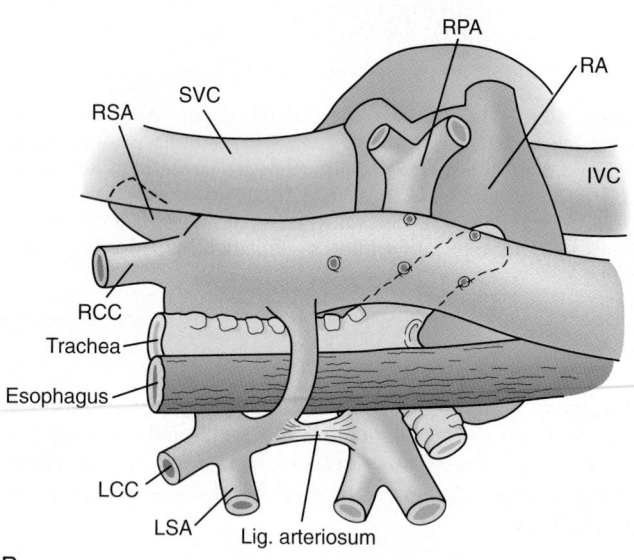

B

Figure 60-42 A and **B,** Double aortic arch. IVC, inferior vena cava; MPA, main pulmonary artery; LCC, left common carotid; LPA, left pulmonary artery; LSA, left subclavian artery; RA, right atrium; RCC, right common carotid; RSA, right subclavian artery; SVC, superior vena cava. (Modified from Jonas RA: Comprehensive Surgical Management of Congenital Heart Disease. New York, Oxford University Press, 2004, p 499.)

left subclavian artery with a left arch. The right subclavian artery passes behind the esophagus from left to right. Innominate artery compression arises from a more posterior and leftward origin of the innominate artery from a left arch, leading to anterior compression of the trachea.

Diagnosis and Indications for Intervention
Symptoms reflect the degree of tracheal and esophageal compression as well as the presence of coexistent tra-

cheomalacia or stenosis from complete rings. Upper respiratory symptoms predominate, with a characteristic brassy cough, recurrent respiratory infections, failure to thrive, and, sometimes, esophageal motility problems. In children, documentation of a ring is an indication for surgery. Older patients are often asymptomatic. Initially, diagnosis is made by a high index of suspicion, and the barium swallow is the first investigation. Echocardiography can document an abnormal head and neck vessel branching pattern, excluding intracardiac abnormalities. MRI provides complete anatomic detail.

Surgery
Most vascular rings are accessible through a left posteriolateral thoracotomy (the exception is a left arch with right-sided ligamentum). Division of the ring and, in the case of double arch, preservation of the dominant arch is performed. Preservation of the recurrent laryngeal nerve is of importance. The initial experience with endoscopic robotically assisted repair of vascular rings has also been reported.[15] Pulmonary artery slings are approached through the midline, and currently the use of cardiopulmonary bypass facilitates tracheal reconstruction and relocation of the right pulmonary artery (Fig. 60-43). Repair can be achieved with low risk. Symptoms may take months to resolve, with slow resolution of the underlying tracheomalacia.

Coronary Artery Anomalies

Anomalies occur as a result of anomalous origin, termination, courses, and aneurysm formation. Of these variables, only anomalous left coronary artery rising from the pulmonary artery (ALCAPA) and coronary artery fistulas are discussed. An ALCAPA is a rare lesion often lethal in early infancy. Untreated, the mortality rate approaches 90%.

Anomalous Left Coronary Artery Rising From the Pulmonary Artery

Anatomy and Pathophysiology
Developmentally, failure of the normal connection of the left coronary artery bud to the aorta results in an abnormal connection to the pulmonary artery. The abnormal origin can be situated in the main pulmonary artery or proximal branches. Associated abnormalities are rare but important to recognize because lowering of the pulmonary artery pressure by PDA ligation or closure of a VSD can be fatal if the ALCAPA is not noted. In utero, with equal pulmonary arterial and aortic pressures, satisfactory perfusion of the ALCAPA can occur. After birth, the pulmonary artery pressure falls, and left coronary artery perfusion decreases. Ischemia causes impaired ventricular function and myocardial infarcts and leads to left ventricular dilation. Papillary muscle dysfunction causes mitral regurgitation. Early coronary collateral development may prevent ongoing infarction.

Diagnosis and Indications for Intervention
ALCAPA is suspected in any infant with mitral regurgitation, ventricular dysfunction, or dilated cardiomyopathy.

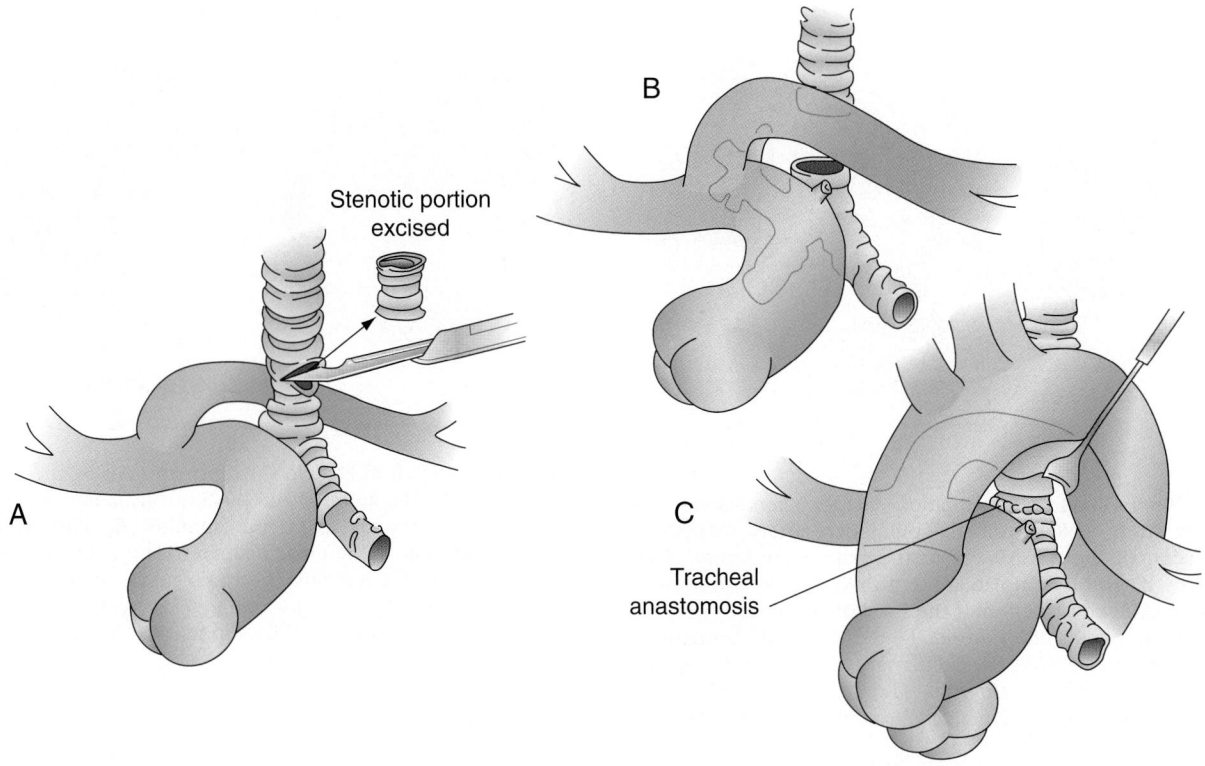

Figure 60-43 Method for the management of a pulmonary artery sling with associated tracheal stenosis, using cardiopulmonary bypass. **A,** Tracheal resection of the involved segment. **B,** Anterior translocation of the left pulmonary artery after transection of the trachea. **C,** Direct anastomosis of the trachea. (From Castaneda AR, Jonas RA, Mayer JE, Hanley FL: Vascular rings, slings, and tracheal anomalies. In Cardiac Surgery of the Neonate and Infant. Philadelphia, WB Saunders, 1994.)

Infants present with a low cardiac output and systemic heart failure. Feeding may also precipitate sudden death and angina in infants. Sudden death has been described in older children. ECG may reflect ischemic changes. The echocardiogram is usually diagnostic, but because this diagnosis is often confused with dilated cardiomyopathy, there is an argument in favor of catheterizing all patients with dilated cardiomyopathy in whom the coronary artery anatomy cannot be clearly defined on echocardiography. Secondary findings of dilated cardiac chambers and segmental wall motion abnormalities together with mitral regurgitation prompt a search for an ALCAPA. Diagnosis of an ALCAPA is an indication for intervention.

Surgery

A degree of ventricular dysfunction is usually present. Preoperative inotropic support and optimization of hemodynamics may be required before surgical intervention. Severe cardiomyopathy may rarely necessitate cardiac transplantation. Current experience indicates that creation of a dual coronary system is safe and reproducible and offers the best opportunity for recovery of function.[63] Operative considerations include optimal myocardial protection and prevention of left heart distention. Direct reimplantation of the ALCAPA into the ascending aorta is currently the procedure of choice (Fig. 60-44). Sometimes, limited mobility of the coronary artery will preclude reimplantation, and a surgically created

aorta–pulmonary artery–coronary artery tunnel is created: the Takeuchi procedure. Ligation of the ALCAPA is not recommended.

Postoperative management is directed toward maintaining adequate coronary perfusion and cardiac output. Mechanical support of the heart may be required temporarily. Mitral regurgitation usually improves, and valve replacement is rarely necessary. Current intervention has a low operative mortality. Risks for nonsurvival relate to preoperative ventricular dysfunction and cardiogenic shock. The Takeuchi repair is associated with tunnel complications such as obstruction, leak, aortic valve damage, and RVOTO in the long term.

Coronary Arteriovenous Fistula and Aneurysms

Isolated coronary artery fistula is more rare than ALCAPA. Drainage of coronary artery fistula is reported to terminate more commonly in the right side of the heart or pulmonary artery than in the left side of the heart. A shunt from the high-pressure coronary artery system into a low-pressure cardiac chamber may result in coronary steal and some degree of cardiac volume overload. Coronary artery aneurysms are associated with Kawasaki disease.

Diagnosis and Indications for Intervention

Presentation depends on the amount of functional compromise produced by the ischemia and volume overload.

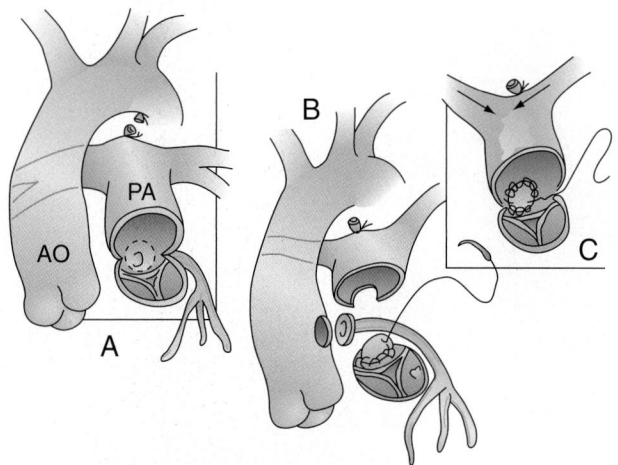

Figure 60-44 Direct reimplantation of the anomalous left coronary artery arising from the pulmonary artery (ALCAPA). **A,** Excision of the ALCAPA from the pulmonary artery (PA). AO, aorta. **B,** Aortic reimplantation of the coronary ostium into the aorta. **C,** Reconstruction of the PA with autologous pericardium. (From Vouhe PR, Tamisier D, Sidi D, et al: Anomalous left coronary artery from the pulmonary artery: Results of isolated aortic reimplantation. Ann Thorac Surg 54:621, 1992. Reprinted with permission from the Society of Thoracic Surgeons.)

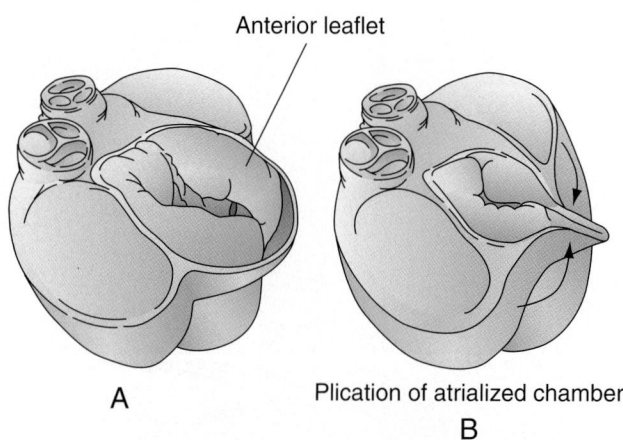

Figure 60-45 Repair of Ebstein's malformation using the Carpentier method. **A,** The anterior and posterior leaflets of the tricuspid valve are detached from the annulus. **B,** The atrium is plicated, reducing the annular diameter. The detached leaflets are reattached to the annulus. (From Ebstein's anomaly. In Castaneda AR, Jonas RA, Mayer JE, Hanley FL [eds]: Cardiac Surgery of the Neonate and Infant. Philadelphia, WB Saunders, 1994.)

Echocardiography may be able to delineate the anomaly, but coronary angiography is diagnostic. Details of coronary anatomy are essential for determining intervention. Interventional catheterization is useful for the obliteration of fistulas and terminal aneurysms.

Surgery

If the lesion is not amenable to transcatheter intervention, surgery is indicated. The options include suture ligation without bypass, cardiopulmonary bypass, and aneurysmectomy with closure of the fistula. Early and late mortality rates are low. Risk factors for death and ventricular dysfunction relate to coronary artery insufficiency and infarction after fistula ligation or aneurysmectomy.[64]

Ebstein's Anomaly of the Tricuspid Valve

Ebstein's anomaly of the tricuspid valve is a rare defect in which the tricuspid valve attachments are displaced into the right ventricle to varying degrees. Ebstein's anomaly includes a spectrum of abnormalities involving a degree of displacement of the tricuspid valve, variable right ventricular size, and variable pulmonary outflow obstruction. Associated abnormalities are an ASD, pulmonary atresia, and congenitally corrected transposition. The tricuspid valve's posterior and septal leaflets are variably displaced to the apex of the right ventricle. This results in an atrialized portion of the right ventricle. The anterior leaflet remains large and sail-like. The major hemodynamic issue is tricuspid incompetence with decreased pulmonary blood flow and, if an ASD is present, right-to-left shunting causing cyanosis. Long-standing tricuspid incompetence leads to volume overload of an abnormal right ventricle. Variable pulmonary outflow tract obstruction will limit effective pulmonary blood flow. If adequate pulmonary blood flow requires continued ductal patency, then the need for neonatal intervention is almost certain.

Diagnosis and Intervention

The more severe forms of Ebstein's anomaly present with cyanosis in infancy. Ill neonates tend to have a severe form of the disease, with a grossly inefficient right ventricle compounded by the high pulmonary resistance of the neonate or by pulmonary valve atresia. The mortality rate in this group is high. Older patients present in heart failure and may have cyanosis. Supraventricular dysrhythmias and the pre-excitation syndrome, Wolff-Parkinson-White, are associated with Ebstein's anomaly. Echocardiography is diagnostic. Critically ill neonates have poor survival rates, and surgery is indicated only after stabilization with PGE₁ and controlled ventilation. In the older patient, cyanosis and heart failure are indications to intervene, although recently, earlier intervention in the asymptomatic patient, before excessive right ventricular dilation, is being more actively pursued.

Surgery

In critically ill neonates, after stabilization, palliation with a systemic-to-pulmonary artery shunt may be required. The Starnes operation has allowed salvage in previously hopeless cases. This operation consists of patch closure of the tricuspid orifice, atrial septectomy, and a systemic-to-pulmonary artery shunt. In patients with less severe forms of this disease, tricuspid valve repair or replacement is also an option.[65,66] Surgical techniques for the treatment of Ebstein's anomaly are evolving, and outcomes are improving for this challenging group of patients[67] (Fig. 60-45).

Mitral Valve Anomalies

Most abnormalities of the mitral valve are associated with other complex lesions, for example, Shone's complex. More commonly, mitral disease in children is inflammatory in nature, that is, rheumatic disease or infective endocarditis. It may also be associated with collagen vascular disease and Marfan's syndrome.

Mitral Stenosis

Mitral stenosis is caused by obstruction at a supravalvular, valvular, or subvalvular level, singly or in combination. Supravalvular stenosis is due to a ring of fibrous tissue above the annulus of the mitral valve or attached to the proximal leaflets. Valvular stenosis involves the leaflets, with commissural fusion occurring with or without hypoplasia of the valve ring. Hypoplasia of the mitral valve is often associated with left ventricular hypoplasia. Frequently, the leaflets and subvalvular apparatus are dysplastic as well. Fusion of the leaflets can lead to an accessory orifice and produce mitral stenosis at a pure valvular level (so-called double-orifice mitral valve). Three types of subvalvular stenosis have been recognized: parachute mitral valve, hammock valve, and absence of one or both papillary muscles. Mitral regurgitation is a result of secondary annular dilation, congenital isolated clefts of the valve, and prolapse of the leaflets from abnormal chordae or papillary muscle insertion.

Echocardiography is diagnostic. Intervention includes balloon valvuloplasty, particularly for selected forms of rheumatic mitral stenosis, and surgical intervention. Intervention is timed to avoid irreversible sequelae related to either chronic volume overload or pulmonary hypertension. Surgical intervention in children is aimed at preserving the mitral valve. Valvuloplasty techniques have a valuable place in children. Prosthetic valves are the least desirable option. Bioprosthetic or tissue valves need to be avoided in children. Supra-annular placement of the prosthesis may be necessary. Repeat placement is ensured.

SUMMARY

This chapter provides a basic overview of the major congenital cardiac lesions and a framework of the diagnosis and treatment of these conditions. It must be emphasized that for most patients, the diagnosis of congenital heart disease, whether surgically treated or not, carries lifelong implications. For patients with congenital heart disease presenting for noncardiac surgery, a thorough understanding of the patient's unique anatomy and physiology is mandatory in deriving a rational management strategy. The reader is directed to several excellent textbooks of congenital heart disease for a more thorough review of each of the lesions reviewed in this chapter.

Selected References

Bailey LL, Nehlsen-Cannarella SL, Doroshow RW, et al: Cardiac allotransplantation in newborns as therapy for hypoplastic left heart syndrome. N Engl J Med 315(15):949-951, 1986.

This classic reference describes the first report of cardiac transplantation in newborns with HLHS. Although limited in its applicability because of limited donor organs, neonatal cardiac transplantation provided children born with HLHS a new option for survival.

Blalock A, Taussig HB: The surgical treatment of malformations of the heart in which there is pulmonary stenosis or pulmonary atresia. JAMA 128:189-202, 1945.

This landmark article describes the surgical procedure that commenced the era of elective cardiac surgery. Drs. Blalock and Taussig, and Vivian Thomas report the initial experience with palliative surgical treatment of patients with pulmonary stenosis or pulmonary atresia utilizing the Blalock-Taussig shunt.

Kirklin JW, Dushane JW, Patrick RT, et al: Intracardiac surgery with the aid of a mechanical pump-oxygenator system (gibbon type): Report of eight cases. Mayo Clin Proc 30:201-206, 1955.

This is a landmark article that demonstrated that open repairs of congenital cardiac defects utilizing mechanical pump-oxygenator systems could be performed with minimal risk to the patient.

Mustard W: Successful two-stage correction of transposition of the great vessels. Surgery 55:469-472, 1964.

This classic reference describes one of the initial surgical approaches to management of D-transposition of the great arteries (D-TGA). Although, the arterial switch operation is the surgical treatment of choice today for D-TGA, there are many adult congenital patients in the community who have been palliated with the Mustard operation. Understanding the operation and the resulting physiology is critical to general surgery management strategies for noncardiac operations.

Nichols DG, Ungerleider RM, Spevak PJ, et al (eds): Critical Heart Disease in Infants and Children, 2nd ed. Philadelphia, Mosby, 2006.

This textbook provides a comprehensive and current review of heart disease in infants and children. It contains numerous surgical drawings and diagnostic images to supplement the didactic material.

Norwood WI, Lang P, Casteneda AR, Campbell DN: Experience with operations for hypoplastic left heart syndrome. J Thorac Cardiovasc Surg 82:511-519, 1981.

In this landmark article, Norwood and others report the outcomes of a then new reconstructive surgical technique to palliate newborns with hypoplastic left heart syndrome. Until the Norwood operation, the only option for survival of patients with HLHS was cardiac transplantation. At most centers today, the Norwood operation is the primary mode of therapy for the majority of neonates with HLHS.

Senning A: Surgical correction of transposition of the great vessels. Surgery 45:966-980, 1959.

This classic reference describes the initial surgical approach to management of D-transposition of the great arteries (TGA). Although the arterial switch operation is the surgical treatment of choice today for D-TGA, there are many adult congenital patients in the community who have had the Senning operation. Understanding the operation and the resulting physiology is critical to general surgery management strategies for noncardiac operations.

Warden HE, Cohen M, Read RC, Lillehei CW: Controlled cross circulation for open intracardiac surgery: Physiologic studies and results of creation and closure of ventricular septal defects. J Thorac Surg 28:331-341; discussion 341-333, 1954.

This landmark article describes the technique of cross-circulation to facilitate cardiopulmonary bypass and intracardiac repair of congenital heart lesions. Lillehei and colleagues document the successful use of cross-circulation to correct defects such as ventricular septal defect.

Wilcox B, Cook A, Anderson R: Surgical Anatomy of the Heart, 3rd ed. Cambridge, UK: Cambridge University Press, 2004.

> This textbook provides an excellent reference manual for understanding the complex anatomy of the heart. It contains color photographs and diagrams. It is an invaluable resource to any student of cardiac surgery.

References

1. Blalock A, Taussig HB: The surgical treatment of malformations of the heart in which there is pulmonary stenosis or pulmonary atresia. JAMA 128:189-202, 1945.
2. Warden HE, Cohen M, Read RC, Lillehei CW: Controlled cross circulation for open intracardiac surgery: Physiologic studies and results of creation and closure of ventricular septal defects. J Thorac Surg 28:331-341; discussion 341-333, 1954.
3. Kirklin JW, Dushane JW, Patrick RT, et al: Intracardiac surgery with the aid of a mechanical pump-oxygenator system (gibbon type): Report of eight cases. Mayo Clin Proc 30:201-206, 1955.
4. Williams RG, Pearson GD, Barst RJ, et al: Report of the National Heart, Lung, and Blood Institute Working Group on research in adult congenital heart disease. J Am Coll Cardiol 47:701-707, 2006.
5. Towbin J: Genetics of Heart Disease. Pediatr Cardiol Today 2(8):1-8; 2004.
6. Moore J, Beekman III R, Case C, et al: Guidelines for Pediatric Cardiovascular Centers. Pediatrics 109:544-549, 2002.
7. Mullins C: Cardiac catheterization in congenital heart disease: Pediatric and adult. Malden, MA, Blackwell Futura, 2006.
8. Warnes CA: The adult with congenital heart disease: Born to be bad? J Am Coll Cardiol 46(1):1-8, 2005.
9. Galli KK, Myers LB, Nicolson SC: Anesthesia for adult patients with congenital heart disease undergoing noncardiac surgery. Int Anesthesiol Clin 39(4):43-71, 2001.
10. Mott AR, Fraser CD Jr, McKenzie ED, et al: Perioperative care of the adult with congenital heart disease in a free-standing tertiary pediatric facility. Pediatr Cardiol 23:624-630, 2002.
11. Wilcox B, Cook A, Anderson R: Surgical Anatomy of the Heart, 3rd ed. Cambridge, UK, Cambridge University Press, 2004.
12. Triedman JK: Arrhythmias in adults with congenital heart disease. Heart 87:383-389, 2002.
13. Ghaferi AA, Hutchins GM: Progression of liver pathology in patients undergoing the Fontan procedure: Chronic passive congestion, cardiac cirrhosis, hepatic adenoma, and hepatocellular carcinoma. J Thorac Cardiovasc Surg 129:1348-1352, 2005.
14. Andropoulos DB, Stayer SA, Russell IA: Anesthesia For Congenital Heart Disease, 1st ed. Malden, MA, Blackwell Futura, 2005.
15. Suematsu Y, Mora BN, Mihaljevic T, del Nido PJ: Totally endoscopic robotic-assisted repair of patent ductus arteriosus and vascular ring in children. Ann Thorac Surg 80:2309-2313, 2005.
16. Eerola A, Jokinen E, Boldt T, Pihkala J: The influence of percutaneous closure of patent ductus arteriosus on left ventricular size and function: A prospective study using two- and three-dimensional echocardiography and measurements of serum natriuretic peptides. J Am Coll Cardiol 47:1060-1066, 2006.
17. Sachweh JS, Daebritz SH, Hermanns B, et al: Hypertensive pulmonary vascular disease in adults with secundum or sinus venosus atrial septal defect. Ann Thorac Surg 81:207-213, 2006.
18. Hopkins RA, Bert AA, Buchholz B, et al: Surgical patch closure of atrial septal defects. Ann Thorac Surg 77:2144-2149; author reply 2149-2150, 2004.
19. Berdat PA, Chatterjee T, Pfammatter JP, et al: Surgical management of complications after transcatheter closure of an atrial septal defect or patent foramen ovale. J Thorac Cardiovasc Surg 120:1034-1039, 2000.
20. Amin Z, Hijazi ZM, Bass JL, et al: Erosion of Amplatzer septal occluder device after closure of secundum atrial septal defects: Review of registry of complications and recommendations to minimize future risk. Catheter Cardiovasc Interv 63:496-502, 2004.
21. Divekar A, Gaamangwe T, Shaikh N, et al: Cardiac perforation after device closure of atrial septal defects with the Amplatzer septal occluder. J Am Coll Cardiol 45:1213-1218, 2005.
22. Neill CA, Ferencz C, Sabiston DC, Sheldon H: The familial occurrence of hypoplastic right lung with systemic arterial supply and venous drainage "scimitar syndrome." Bull Johns Hopkins Hosp 107:1-21, 1960.
23. Dibardino DJ, McKenzie ED, Heinle, JS, et al: The Warden procedure for partially anomalous pulmonary venous connection to the superior vena caval vein. Cardiol Young 14(1):64-66, 2004.
24. Attenhofer Jost CH, Connolly HM, Danielson GK, et al: Sinus venosus atrial septal defect: Long-term postoperative outcome for 115 patients. Circulation 112:1953-1958, 2005.
25. Hopkins WE, Waggoner AD: Severe pulmonary hypertension without right ventricular failure: The unique hearts of patients with Eisenmenger syndrome. Am J Cardiol 89:34-38, 2002.
26. Diab KA, Hijazi ZM, Cao QL, Bacha EA: A truly hybrid approach to perventricular closure of multiple muscular ventricular septal defects. J Thorac Cardiovasc Surg 130:892-893, 2005.
27. McCarthy KP, Ching Leung PK, Ho SY: Perimembranous and muscular ventricular septal defects: Morphology revisited in the era of device closure. J Interv Cardiol 18:507-513, 2005.
28. Roos-Hesselink JW, Meijboom FJ, Spitaels SE, et al: Outcome of patients after surgical closure of ventricular septal defect at young age: Longitudinal follow-up of 22-34 years. Eur Heart J 25:1057-1062, 2004.
29. Formigari R, Di Donato RM, Gargiulo G, et al: Better surgical prognosis for patients with complete atrioventricular septal defect and Down's syndrome. Ann Thorac Surg 78:666-672; discussion 672, 2004.
30. Rastelli GC, Weidman WH, Kirklin JW: Surgical repair of the partial form of persistent common atrioventricular canal, with special reference to the problem of mitral valve incompetence. Circulation 31(Suppl 1):31-35, 1965.
31. De Oliveira NC, Sittiwangkul R, McCrindle BW, et al: Biventricular repair in children with atrioventricular septal defects and a small right ventricle: Anatomic and surgical considerations. J Thorac Cardiovasc Surg 130:250-257, 2005.
32. Journois D, Baufreton C, Mauriat P, et al: Effects of inhaled nitric oxide administration on early postoperative mortality in patients operated for correction of atrioventricular canal defects. Chest 128:3537-3544, 2005.
33. Khositseth A, Tocharoentanaphol C, Khowsathit P, Ruangdaraganon N: Chromosome 22q11 deletions in patients with conotruncal heart defects. Pediatr Cardiol 26:570-573, 2005.
34. Morales D, Braud, BE, Gunter KS, et al: Encouraging results for the Contegra conduit in the problematic right ventricle-

to-pulmonary artery connection. J Thorac Cardiovasc Surg 132:665-671, 2006.

35. Chen JM, Glickstein JS, Davies RR, et al: The effect of repair technique on postoperative right-sided obstruction in patients with truncus arteriosus. J Thorac Cardiovasc Surg 129:559-568, 2005.

36. Khambadkone S, Coats L, Taylor A, et al: Percutaneous pulmonary valve implantation in humans: results in 59 consecutive patients. Circulation 112:1189-1197, 2005.

37. Brown JW, Ruzmetov M, Okada Y, et al: Truncus arteriosus repair: Outcomes, risk factors, reoperation and management. Eur J Cardiothoracic Surg 20: 221-227, 2001.

38. Fraser CD, McKenzie ED, Cooley DA. Tetralogy of Fallot: Surgical management individualized to the patient. Ann Thorac Surg 71:1556-1561, 2001.

39. Mustard W: Successful two-stage correction of transposition of the great vessels. Surgery 55:469-472, 1964.

40. Senning A: Surgical correction of transposition of the great vessels. Surgery 45:966-980, 1959.

41. Dos L, Teruel L, Ferreira IJ, et al: Late outcome of Senning and Mustard procedures for correction of transposition of the great arteries. Heart 91:652-656, 2005.

42. Hutter PA, Kreb DL, Mantel SF, et al: Twenty-five years' experience with the arterial switch operation. J Thorac Cardiovasc Surg 124:790-797, 2002.

43. Yacoub MH, Radley-Smith: Anatomy of the coronary arteries in transposition of the great arteries and methods for their transfer in anatomical correction. Thorax 33(4):418-424, 1978.

44. DiBardino DJ, Allison AE, Vaughn WK, et al: Current expectations for newborns undergoing the arterial switch operation. Ann Surg 239:588-596, 2004.

45. Langley SM, Winlaw DS, Stumper O, et al: Midterm results after restoration of the morphologically left ventricle to the systemic circulation in patients with congenitally corrected transposition of the great arteries. J Thorac Cardiovasc Surg 125:1229-1241, 2003.

46. Tweddell JS, Pelech AN, Frommelt PC, et al: Complex aortic valve repair as a durable and effective alternative to valve replacement in children with aortic valve disease. J Thorac Cardiovasc Surg 129:551-558, 2005.

47. Fraser CD: Aortic valve repair. In Yang S, Cameron D (eds): Current Therapy in Thoracic and Cardiovascular Surgery. Philadelphia, Mosby, 2004.

48. Marasini M, Zannini L, Ussia GP, et al: Discrete subaortic stenosis: Incidence, morphology and surgical impact of associated subaortic anomalies. Ann Thorac Surg 75:1763-1768, 2003.

49. Shone JD, Sellers RD, Anderson RC, et al: The developmental complex of "parachute mitral valve," supravalvular ring of left atrium, subaortic stenosis, and coarctation of aorta. Am J Cardiol 11:714-725, 1963.

50. Brown JW, Ruzmetov M, Vijay P, et al: Operative results and outcomes in children with Shone's anomaly. Ann Thorac Surg 79:1358-1365, 2005.

51. Cowley CG, Orsmond GS, Feola P, et al: Long-term, randomized comparison of balloon angioplasty and surgery for native coarctation of the aorta in childhood. Circulation 111:3453-3456, 2005.

52. Fiore AC, Fischer LK, Schwartz T, et al: Comparison of angioplasty and surgery for neonatal aortic coarctation. Ann Thorac Surg 80:1659-1664; discussion 1664-1665, 2005.

53. Elgamal MA, McKenzie ED, Fraser CD Jr: Aortic arch advancement: The optimal one-stage approach for surgical management of neonatal coarctation with arch hypoplasia. Ann Thorac Surg 73:1267-1272; discussion 1272-1273, 2002.

54. Morales DSL, Scully PT, Braud, BE, et al: Interrupted aortic arch repair: Aortic arch advancement without a patch minimizes arch re-interventions. Ann Thoracic Surg (in press) 82:1577-1584, 2006.

55. Sittiwangkul R, Azakie A, Van Arsdell GS, et al: Outcomes of tricuspid atresia in the Fontan era. Ann Thorac Surg 77:889-894, 2004.

56. Bailey LL, Nehlsen-Cannarella SL, Doroshow RW, et al: Cardiac allotransplantation in newborns as therapy for hypoplastic left heart syndrome. N Engl J Med 315:949-951, 1986.

57. Norwood WI, Lang P, Castenada AR, Campbell DN: Experience with operations for hypoplastic left heart syndrome. J Thorac Cardiovasc Surg 82:511-519, 1981.

58. Fraser CD Jr, Mee RB: Modified Norwood procedure for hypoplastic left heart syndrome. Ann Thorac Surg 60(6 Suppl):546-549, 1995.

59. Ashburn DA, McCrindle BW, Tchervenkov CI, et al: Outcomes after the Norwood operation in neonates with critical aortic stenosis or aortic valve atresia. J Thorac Cardiovasc Surg 125:1070-1082, 2003.

60. Sano S, Ishino K, Kado H, et al: Outcome of right ventricle-to-pulmonary artery shunt in first-stage palliation of hypoplastic left heart syndrome: A multi-institutional study. Ann Thorac Surg 78:1951-1957; discussion 1957-1958, 2004.

61. Bacha EA, Daves S, Hardin J, et al: Single-ventricle palliation for high-risk neonates: The emergence of an alternative hybrid stage I strategy. J Thorac Cardiovasc Surg 131:163-171, 2006.

62. Jacobs ML, Pelletier G: Late complications associated with the Fontan circulation. Cardiol Young 16(Suppl 1):80-84, 2006.

63. Ando M, Mee RB, Duncan BW, et al: Creation of a dual-coronary system for anomalous origin of the left coronary artery from the pulmonary artery utilizing the trapdoor flap method. Eur J Cardiothorac Surg 22:576-581, 2002.

64. Kamiya H, Yasuda T, Nagamine H, et al: Surgical treatment of congenital coronary artery fistulas: 27 years' experience and a review of the literature. J Card Surg 17:173-177, 2002.

65. Carpentier A, Chauvaud S, Mace L, et al: A new reconstructive operation for Ebstein's anomaly of the tricuspid valve. J Thorac Cardiovasc Surg 96:92-101, 1988.

66. Starnes VA, Pitlick PT, Bernstein D, et al: Ebstein's anomaly appearing in the neonate: A new surgical approach. J Thorac Cardiovasc Surg 101:1082-1087, 1991.

67. Knott-Craig CJ, Overholt ED, Ward KE, et al: Repair of Ebstein's anomaly in the symptomatic neonate: An evolution of technique with 7-year follow-up. Ann Thorac Surg 73:1786-1792; discussion 1792-1793, 2002.

Acquired Heart Disease: Coronary Insufficiency

Victor A. Ferraris, MD, PhD   and   Robert M. Mentzer, Jr., MD

CORONARY ARTERY ANATOMY

The coronary arteries originate at the root of the aorta, behind the left and right cusps of the aortic valve. They provide the blood supply to the myocardium through the main epicardial conductance vessels and enter the myocardium by penetrating vessels called *resistance arteries*. These vessels then branch into a plexus of capillaries that are essentially contiguous with every myocyte (intercapillary distance at rest is 17 µm). The left main coronary artery (LMCA) rises from the left coronary sinus; it averages 2 cm in length, and varies from 1 to 4 cm. After coursing between the pulmonary artery and the left atrial appendage, it bifurcates into two major branches, the left anterior descending coronary artery (LAD) and the left circumflex coronary artery (LCA). In many instances, the vessel trifurcates; this occurs when the ramus medianus vessel originates between the anterior descending and the circumflex arteries. Occasionally, the LMCA is absent, and the LAD and LCA arise from common or separate ostia. Less commonly, a single coronary vessel arises from a common orifice and provides all cardiac blood flow (Fig. 61-1).

In general, the LAD supplies the anterior and left lateral portions of the left ventricle. The LAD proceeds distally behind the pulmonary trunk into the anterior intraventricular sulcus and provides a number of anterior perforating branches to the anterior interventricular septum. In most cases, the LAD wraps around the apex of the heart and forms an anastomosis with the posterior descending coronary artery (PDA), a branch of the right coronary artery (RCA). As the LAD follows the interventricular groove, it may give rise to one or more branches that course diagonally over the left anterior ventricular free wall. The first diagonal branch and the first septal perforator are usually the largest vessels arising from the LAD, and both the septals and the diagonals become smaller as the vessel progresses distally.

The LCA originates from the LMCA and follows a course posteriorly under the left atrial appendage and along the left atrioventricular (AV) groove. In most cases, the circumflex terminates as an obtuse marginal branch. It can, however, be the primary source of blood flow to the PDA. One to four obtuse marginal branches of varying size emerge from the main circumflex artery and course along the lateral and posterolateral aspects of the left ventricle. The branches that arise most distally are often referred to as *posterolateral branches* of the circumflex artery. These branches course parallel to the PDA, but provide no perforating branches into the intraventricular septum. In 10% of patients, the circumflex artery supplies the posterior descending and AV nodal arteries as it courses along the posterior intraventricular sulcus. This pattern of circulation defines a left dominant circulation (see Fig. 61-1).

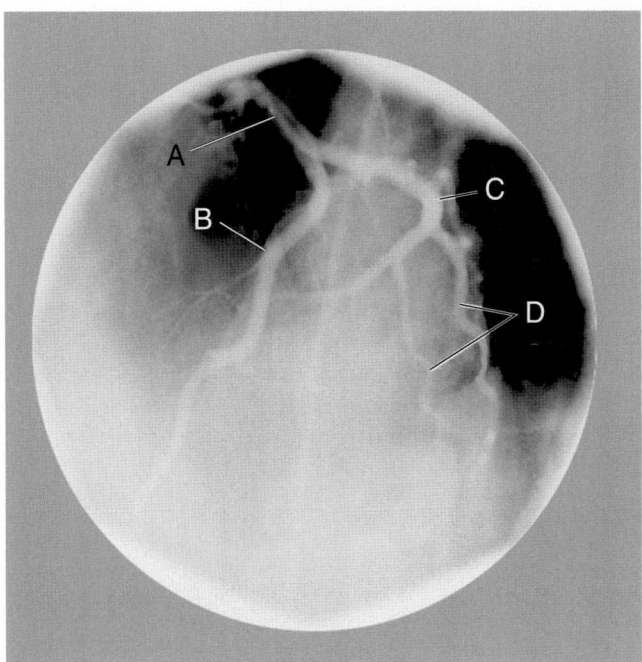

Figure 61-1 Left main coronary artery (A), left anterior descending coronary artery (B), left circumflex coronary artery (C), and obtuse marginal vessels (D). (Courtesy of David Booth, MD, Division of Cardiology, University of Kentucky, 2003.)

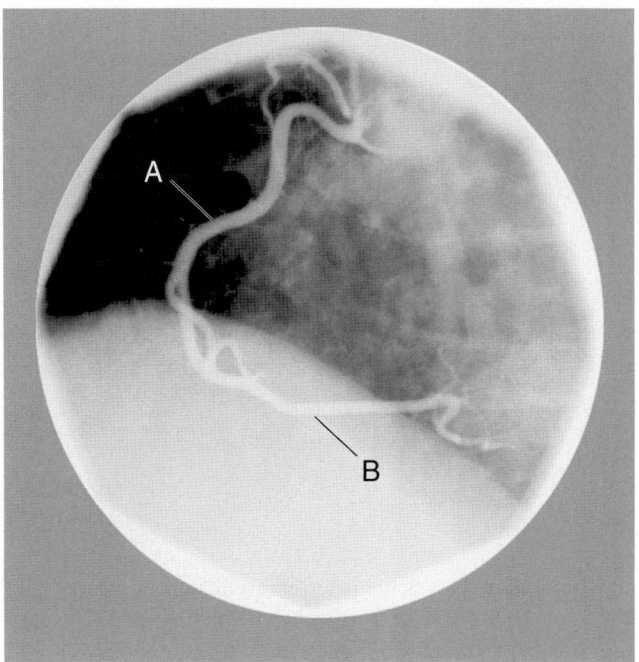

Figure 61-2 Right coronary artery (A) and posterior descending artery (B). (Courtesy of David Booth, MD, Division of Cardiology, University of Kentucky, 2003.)

The RCA supplies most of the right ventricle, as well as the posterior part of the left ventricle. The RCA emerges from its ostium in the right coronary sinus, passes deep in the right AV groove, and then proceeds to course over the anterior surface of the heart. At the superior end of the acute margin of the heart, the RCA turns posteriorly toward the crux and usually bifurcates into the PDA and the right posterolateral artery. The RCA also supplies multiple right ventricular branches (acute marginals) as well as branches to the AV node, although the latter may also arise from the left circumflex artery. In about 90% of patients, the RCA passes through the AV sulcus to the posterior interventricular sulcus and becomes the PDA. This pattern of circulation is referred to as a right dominant system. Occasionally, the PDA arises from both the RCA and the LCA and the circulation is considered to be codominant (Fig. 61-2). The sinoatrial node artery arises from the proximal RCA in 50% of patients, and many other small atrial branches arise from the RCA, but they are rarely of significance. Other prominent branches arising from the RCA include the acute marginal artery and anterior ventricular branches. Although the source of the PDA is often used clinically to define dominance of circulation in the heart, anatomists define it based on where the sinoatrial node artery arises. In 90% of patients, the RCA bifurcates into the posterior descending and the right posterolateral arteries. The AV node artery arises from the RCA in about 90% of patients.

The incidence of coronary artery anomalies is about 1%, and these congenital anomalies may or may not be clinically significant. Hemodynamically significant anomalies include coronary fistulas or origin of the coronary

artery from the pulmonary artery. Both may result in abnormal coronary perfusion. The most common congenital variation encountered during angiography is the origin of the circumflex artery from the RCA or the right coronary sinus, which occurs in about 0.5% of patients. Anomalous origin of the anterior descending artery from the right sinus of Valsalva or from the RCA is another common anomaly and is associated with tetralogy of Fallot.

A network of veins drains the coronary circulation, and the venous circulation can be divided into three systems: the coronary sinus and its tributaries, the anterior right ventricular veins, and the thebesian veins. Occlusive disease is uncommon in the venous system.

The coronary sinus predominantly drains the left ventricle and receives 85% of coronary venous blood. It lies within the posterior AV groove and empties into the right atrium. The anterior right ventricular veins travel across the right ventricular surface to the right AV groove, where they enter directly into the right atrium or form the small cardiac vein, which enters into the right atrium directly or joins the coronary sinus just proximal to its orifice. The thebesian veins are small venous tributaries that drain directly into the cardiac chambers and exit primarily into the right atrium and right ventricle.

NORMAL CORONARY ARTERY PHYSIOLOGY AND REGULATION OF BLOOD FLOW

Coronary Blood Flow

The coronary arteries deliver oxygen and other metabolic substrates to the myocardium and simultaneously remove

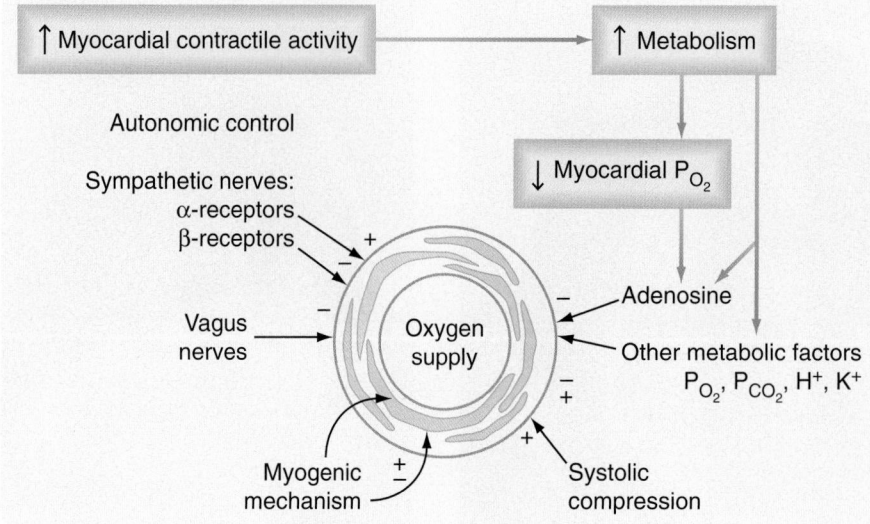

Figure 61-3 Schematic representation of factors that increase (+) or decrease (−) coronary vascular resistance. (From Berne RM, Levy MN [eds]: Physiology, 4th ed. St Louis, Mosby, 1998, p 483.)

carbon dioxide and metabolic degradation products through the process of transcapillary exchange. Relative to most other organ systems, the myocardium has a high rate of energy utilization. Normal coronary blood flow averages 225 mL/min or 0.7 to 0.9 mL/g of myocardium per minute and delivers 0.1 mL of oxygen per gram per minute to the myocardium. Under normal conditions, 75% of the delivered oxygen is extracted in the coronary capillary bed. The myocardium increases to 100% extraction during periods of stress.

Factors Influencing Coronary Vascular Resistance

In response to strenuous exercise, the healthy heart can increase myocardial blood flow fourfold to sevenfold. Increased blood flow occurs through a variety of means, including metabolic, physical, and neurohumoral regulatory mechanisms.

Metabolic

Local myocardial metabolism is the primary regulator of coronary blood flow, and blood flow is inversely related to vascular resistance (Fig. 61-3). There is a strong correlation between myocardial metabolic activity and the magnitude of coronary blood flow changes (Fig. 61-4). The mechanism by which increased myocardial metabolism promotes coronary blood flow has not yet been clearly elucidated. It is hypothesized that the decrease in oxygen supply to oxygen demand triggers release of a vasodilator substance from the myocardium, which in turn initiates relaxation of the coronary resistance vessels. This results in increased delivery of oxygen-rich blood. An example of this is the phenomenon of *reactive hyperemia*. When blood flow is transiently stopped by the occlusion of a vessel in the beating heart, blood flow immediately exceeds the normal baseline flow when the occlusion is removed. Blood flow returns to the baseline

level over a period of time proportional to the duration of the occlusion. Several metabolic factors are implicated as mediators of reactive hyperemia, including CO_2, decreased O_2 tension, hydrogen ions, lactate, potassium ions, and adenosine. Of these, adenosine is one of the leading candidates.

In the setting of ischemia or increased metabolic activity, adenosine, a potent vasodilator and degradation product of adenosine triphosphate (ATP), is produced, accumulates in the interstitial space, and relaxes the vascular smooth muscle. This results in vasomotor relaxation, coronary vasodilation, and increased blood flow. Although adenosine is a leading candidate, it may be only part of the process because adenosine receptor antagonists do not completely block reactive hyperemia. Another factor that may play an important role is nitric oxide (NO) that is produced from the endothelium. Nitric oxide is also called *endothelium-derived relaxing factor* (EDRF). In the absence of the endothelium, coronary arteries do not autoregulate, suggesting an endothelium-dependent mechanism for vasodilation and reactive hyperemia.

Physical Components of Vascular Resistance

Aortic pressure is a key factor responsible for myocardial perfusion. The coronary vasculature can compensate and maintain normal coronary perfusion pressures between systolic pressures of 60 and 180 mm Hg through the process of autoregulation. This is a process whereby baroreceptors promote local vasodilation or vasoconstriction through alterations in coronary diameter, so that coronary blood flow is maintained at a constant level. Extravascular compression of the coronaries during systole is another factor that plays an important role in the regulation of blood flow. During systole, the intracavitary pressures generated within the left ventricular wall exceed intracoronary pressure, and nutrient flow is

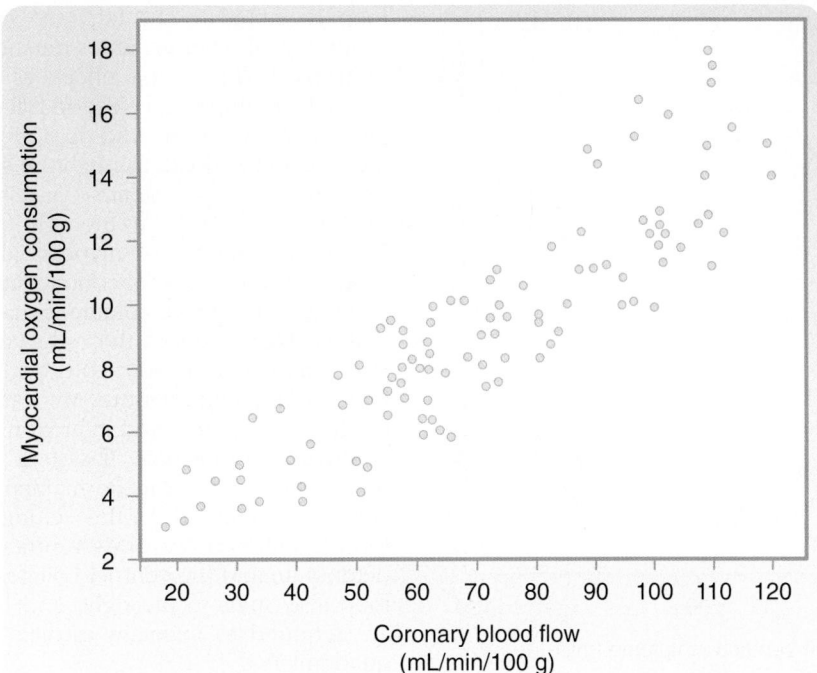

Figure 61-4 Relationship between myocardial oxygen consumption and coronary blood flow during a variety of interventions that increased or decreased myocardial metabolic rate. (From Berne RM, Levy MN [eds]: Physiology, 4th ed. St Louis, Mosby, 1998, p 482.)

impeded. This may result in the transient reversal in the direction of blood flow in the epicardial vessels during systole (see Fig. 61-3).

The heart rate also affects coronary artery blood flow. Tachycardia increases the proportion of the cardiac cycle in systole and results in the restriction of blood flow. In general, this is compensated by coronary vasodilation that occurs as a result of an increase in metabolic activity. Bradycardia prolongs diastole, and thus coronary flow and nutrient delivery is increased (see Fig. 61-3).

Neural and Neurohumoral

Stimulation of the cardiac sympathetic nerves indirectly increases coronary blood flow as a result of increased metabolic activity secondary to augmented myocardial contractility and tachycardia. Although α- and β-adrenergic receptors do exist in coronary vessels, the α-receptors are more prominent in the epicardial vessels, and the β-receptors are more prominent in the intramuscular vessels. Although both vasodilation and vasoconstriction can occur with activation of the receptors, these effects play a less important role than metabolic factors (see Fig. 61-3). Parasympathetic stimulation has only a slight vasodilatory effect on the coronary arteries and is not a significant contributor to the regulation of normal coronary blood flow.

MECHANICS OF PUMP FUNCTION

In the normal heart, an increase in intraventricular volume during diastole leads to an increase in the force of contraction. The association between end-diastolic volume and systolic pressure is known as the *Frank-Starling relationship* and is under the influences of hormonal and neuronal stimulation. For example, an increase in circulating catecholamines may result in more forceful contractions (inotropy), a rapid heartbeat (chronotropy), and more efficient relaxation (lusitropy). Ventricular performance is also determined, in part, by changes in preload and afterload. Preload varies as a result of changes in intravascular volume caused by alterations in systemic venous capacitance, pulmonary vascular capacitance, and ventricular compliance. *Preload* is a term that describes the intraventricular pressure immediately before contraction and is commonly referred to as the *filling pressure*. *Afterload* refers to the amount of pressure developed during ventricular systole that is required to eject blood against the pressure of the receiving vessel, aorta, or pulmonary artery. The greater the afterload is, the greater the energy requirements and consumption of oxygen. Afterload is the difference between the mean aortic pressure and central venous pressure divided by the cardiac output. The compliance of the ventricle is the change in volume per unit of pressure. The right ventricle is more compliant than the left ventricle and therefore may serve as a volume reservoir.

A graphic depiction of the relationship between ventricular pressure and volume during a single cardiac cycle facilitates an understanding of the mechanics of normal and abnormal ventricular contraction. This relationship is called a *pressure-volume loop,* and is shown for a normal heart in Figure 61-5. Diastolic filling begins at point A, and continues to point C. During the initial rapid filling from the atria, there is a slight fall in ventricular pressure

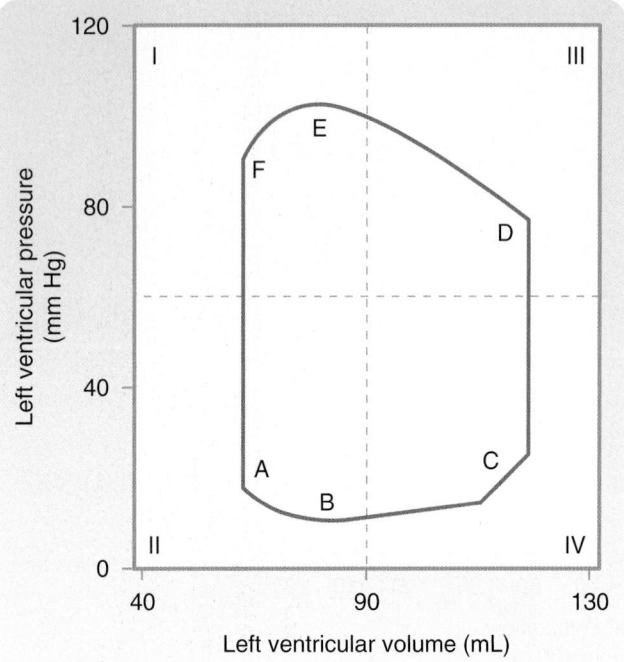

Figure 61-5 Pressure-volume loop during a single cardiac cycle. A variety of pathologic conditions bring about a shift in the pressure-volume loop to quadrants, here identified as quadrants I to V. A to C, diastolic filling; C to D, isovolumetric contraction; D to F, ventricular ejection; F to A, isovolumetric relaxation. (Courtesy of the Division of Cardiothoracic Surgery, University of Kentucky, 2003.)

associated with progressive ventricular relaxation. After active relaxation of the ventricle ceases (point B), the pressure slightly increases as a result of passive ventricular filling. Just before completion of filling (point C), an atrial contraction adds additional volume (the so-called atrial kick). During isovolumetric contraction, from point C to D, the ventricular pressure rapidly increases with no change in ventricular volume. When the pressure in the ventricle exceeds the pressure in the aorta, the aortic valve opens, point D, and the rapid phase of ejection begins. Between point D and E, ventricular pressure increases while ventricular volume declines. Between point E and F, both pressure and volume decline until ejection is complete and the aortic valve closes, point F. After the aortic valve is closed, a phase of isovolumetric relaxation occurs, point F to A, which is characterized by a rapid fall in pressure with no change in ventricular volume. When the ventricular pressure falls below the atrial pressure, the mitral valve opens, point A, and ventricular filling begins completing the cardiac cycle.

Pressure-volume loops are useful in understanding various physiologic and pathophysiologic conditions. The shape of the pressure-volume loop during systole is determined by the contractility of the heart and the afterload against which the ventricle is ejecting (represented by the line from point C through F in Fig. 61-5). In the setting of adrenergic stimulation, the pressure-volume

loop is shifted to the left (see Fig. 61-5, quadrant II). Assuming all other variables remain constant, the positive inotropic and lusitropic effects of adrenergic stimulation promote an improved ejection fraction (EF) that is associated with a lower end-diastolic filling pressure. An increase in afterload, as might be seen with hypertension or with aortic valve stenosis, is associated with a shift of the loop upward and to the right (see Fig. 61-5, quadrant III). In the setting of myocardial ischemia, there is a reduction in myocardial contractility and ventricular compliance. If the stroke volume is maintained, the pressure-volume loop shifts to the right (see Fig. 61-5, quadrant IV). This results in an acute decline in the EF and an increase in filling pressure. Myocardial fibrosis secondary to chronic ischemia and infarction can lead to decreased ventricular compliance. If systolic function is preserved, the stroke volume can be maintained if the filling pressures are increased. In this setting, the pressure-volume loop is shifted upward. As ventricular function begins to deteriorate and the ventricle dilates, the pressure-volume loop also shifts to the right, and higher filling pressures are required to maintain cardiac output (see Fig. 61-5, quadrant IV).

CORONARY ARTERY DISEASE

Pathogenesis

Coronary artery atherosclerosis is a progressive disease that begins early in life. Epicardial vessels are the most susceptible; intramyocardial arteries, the least. Initially, the internal elastic membrane undergoes rupture, degeneration, and regeneration. Deposition of mucopolysaccharides and proliferation of endothelial cells and fibroblasts follows initial intimal damage. Growth lesions appear in the form of small deposits of lipoid material visible beneath the intima. This ultimately progresses to plaque formation and obstruction of the arterial lumen. In the final stages of the disease, patients become symptomatic or die from a myocardial infarct as a result of marked narrowing of the vessel lumen or plaque rupture with coronary artery thrombosis.

Role of Inflammation

Although several mechanisms and many risk factors for disease development have been implicated, it appears that the primary causes of atherosclerotic CAD are endothelial injury induced by an inflammatory wall response and lipid deposition. There is evidence that an inflammatory response is involved in all stages of the disease, from early lipid deposition to plaque formation, plaque rupture, and coronary artery thrombosis. Early after initiation of an atherogenic diet in animals, endothelial cells begin to express selected adhesion molecules, such as the vascular cell adhesion molecule-1, that bind various classes of leukocytes, monocytes, and T-lymphocytes. After the leukocytes adhere to the endothelium, chemoattractant molecules promote transmigration and then penetrate the intima, where they participate in and perpetuate a local inflammatory response. The monocytes express

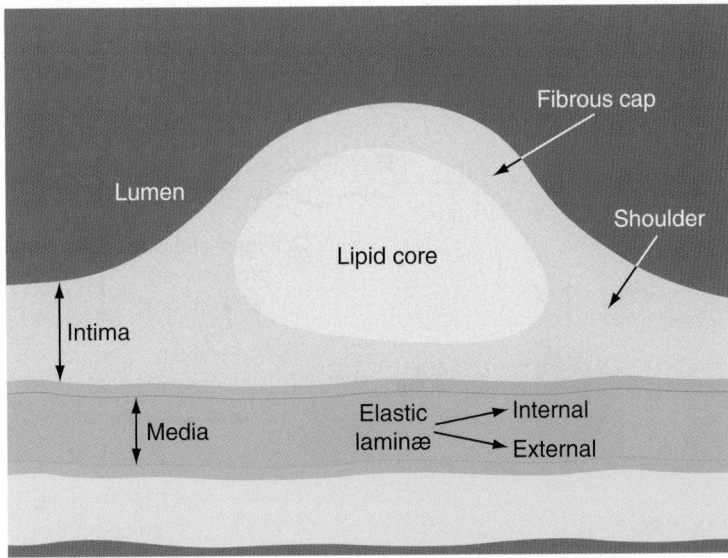

Figure 61-6 Anatomy of the atherosclerotic plaque. After the leukocytes have accumulated in the lesion, they often undergo death, sometimes by apoptosis, which can lead to a lipid core covered by a fibrous cap. (From Lipids Online, http://www.lipidsonline.org.)

scavenger receptors for modified lipoproteins, which allow them to ingest lipids. These modified lipids induce the expression of numerous adhesion molecules, chemokines, proinflammatory cytokines, and other mediators of inflammation in macrophages and vascular wall cells. The activated macrophages also release mitogens and chemoattractants, such as macrophage colony-stimulating factor and monocyte chemoattractant protein-1. These molecules promote and perpetuate ongoing mobilization of monocytes into the evolving plaque. Tissue signals likewise stimulate T cells to elaborate inflammatory cytokines, such as interferon-γ and tumor necrosis factor-β, which further stimulate the inflammatory process. Activated leukocytes also release fibrogenic mediators, which promote elaboration by local cells of a dense extracellular matrix. In addition to promoting the initiation of the atheroma, the inflammation precipitates the evolution of acute thrombotic complications. For instance, activated macrophages secrete proteolytic enzymes, which degrade the collagen that lends strength to the plaque's protective fibrous cap. This in turn renders the cap thin, weak, and prone to rupture.

Plaque Rupture

Several studies have shown that 70% to 80% of coronary thrombi occur where the fibrous cap of an atherosclerotic plaque has fissured or ruptured. Subsequent extension of the thrombus into the plaque with propagation of the thrombus downstream leads to an acute coronary event. According to the current paradigm, rupture of the fibrous cap leads to exposure of thrombogenic components of the plaque with subsequent activation of the platelets and coagulation pathways that result in thrombus formation and acute luminal compromise[2] (Figs. 61-6 and 61-7). Although the exact mechanism responsible for plaque

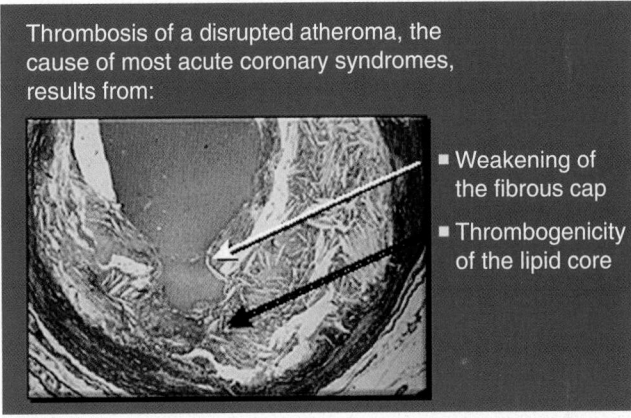

Thrombosis of a disrupted atheroma, the cause of most acute coronary syndromes, results from:

- Weakening of the fibrous cap
- Thrombogenicity of the lipid core

Figure 61-7 Thrombosis of a disrupted atheroma: weakening of the fibrous cap. Most coronary syndromes are caused by thrombosis of a disrupted atheroma, which can result from weakening of the fibrous cap and enhanced thrombogenicity of the lipid core. (Courtesy of Michael J. Davies, MD. From Lipids Online, http://www.lipidsonline.org.)

rupture is unknown, the five features of vulnerable or high-risk plaques that are prone to rupture are listed:

1. Large eccentric soft lipid core
2. Thin fibrous cap
3. Inflammation within the cap and adventitia
4. Increased plaque neovascularity
5. Evidence of outward or positive vessel remodeling

Thinner fibrous caps are at a higher risk for rupture. This is probably due to an imbalance between the synthesis and degradation of the extracellular matrix in the fibrous cap that results in an overall decrease in the collagen and

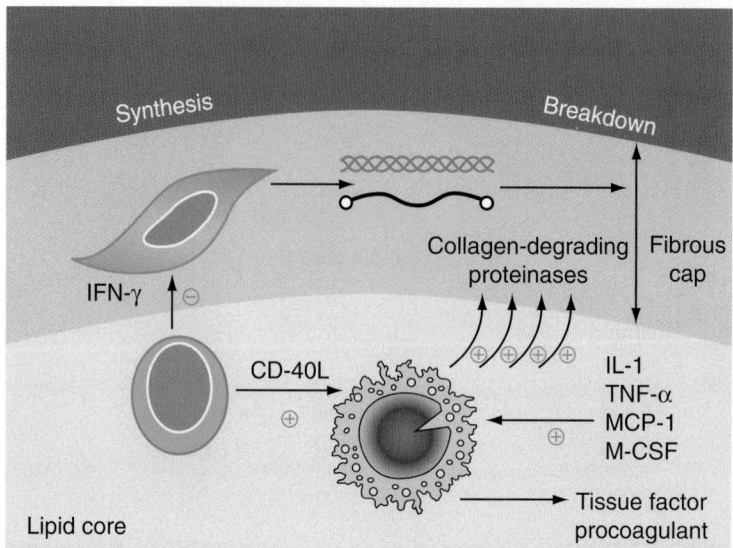

Figure 61-8 Matrix metabolism and integrity of the plaque's fibrous cap. This figure depicts the current understanding of the dynamics of the plaque's stability and thrombogenicity. The inflammatory cells can send molecular messages to the smooth muscle cells (interferon-γ [IFN-γ]) that inhibit the ability of this cell type to synthesize new collagen to strengthen the plaque's fibrous cap. In addition, the inflammatory cells can release proteolytic enzymes capable of degrading collagen and other structurally important constituents of the plaque's fibrous cap. Thus, when there is inflammation in the intima, the collagen responsible for the integrity of the plaque's fibrous cap is under double attack, subject to both decreased synthesis and increased degradation. This sets the stage for plaque disruption. The inflammatory cells also are responsible for signaling and producing increased quantities of tissue factor, a potent procoagulant deemed responsible for thrombosis of ruptured plaques. IL-1, interleukin-1; MCP-1, monocyte chemotactic protein-1; M-CSF, macrophage colony-stimulating factor. (From Libby P: Molecular bases of the acute coronary syndromes. Circulation 91:2844-2850, 1995. Source: Lipids Online-www.lipidsonline.org.)

matrix components (Fig. 61-8). Increased matrix breakdown may be due to matrix degradation as a result of metalloproteinase expressed by inflammatory cells within the plaque. Reduced production of extracellular matrix is likely to contribute as well. Although plaque rupture can lead to thrombosis and subsequent acute coronary syndrome (ACS), not all ruptures are symptomatic. The thrombotic response to plaque rupture is likely regulated by the thrombogenicity of the plaque's components. Tissue factor, secreted by activated macrophages and found in high concentrations within the lipid core of the plaque, is one of the most potent thrombogenic stimuli. Rupture of a vulnerable plaque may occur spontaneously or as a result of specific triggers, such as extreme physical activity, severe emotional distress, exposure to drugs, cold exposure, and acute infections. There are also circadian components to the onset of acute coronary syndromes.[1]

Lipid Metabolism

Epidemiologic evidence suggests that coronary artery atherosclerosis is closely linked to lipid metabolism, specifically cholesterol. Numerous studies have demonstrated that hydroxymethylglutaryl coenzyme-A reductase inhibitor (statin) therapy, aimed at lowering lipids, has resulted in a significant reduction in mortality. In one observational study of patients who received statin therapy and were known to have coronary artery disease (CAD),

statin treatment was associated with improved survival in all age groups.[2] There was a 30% adjusted risk reduction in mortality for those younger than 65 years, 44% for patients aged 65 to 79 years, and 50% for patients older than 79 years. The greatest survival benefit was derived in those patients with the highest quartile of high-sensitivity C-reactive protein (hs-CRP), a biomarker of inflammation and CAD.[3] Animal and human studies have demonstrated that statin therapy also modifies the lipid composition within plaques by lowering the amount of low-density lipoprotein (LDL) cholesterol and by stabilizing the plaque through a variety of mechanisms, including reduction in macrophage accumulation, collagen degradation, reduction in smooth muscle cell protease expression, and decrease in tissue factor expression. Thus, more aggressive statin use after coronary artery bypass grafting (CABG) may be indicated.

Fixed Coronary Obstructions

More than 90% of patients with symptomatic ischemic heart disease have advanced coronary atherosclerosis due to a fixed obstruction. Atherosclerotic plaques of the coronary arteries are either concentric (25%) or eccentric (75%). Eccentric lesions compromise only a portion of the lumen and, through vascular remodeling, the arterial lumen may remain patent until late in the disease process. The impact of an arterial stenosis on coronary blood flow can be appreciated in the context of Poiseuille's law. The volume of a homogeneous fluid passing per unit of time through a tube is directly proportional to the pressure difference between its ends and to the fourth power of its internal radius, and is inversely proportional to its length and to the viscosity of the fluid. Clinically, reductions in luminal diameter up to 60% have minimal impact on flow. When the cross-sectional area of the vessel has decreased by 75% or more, however, coronary blood flow is significantly compromised. Clinically, this often coincides with the onset of exertional angina. With a 90% reduction in luminal diameter, resistance is 256 times greater than a 60% stenosis, and coronary flow may be inadequate at rest.

ISCHEMIA AND MYOCARDIAL CELL INJURY

Myocardial ischemia can lead to reversible or irreversible injury. Ischemia of 15 to 20 minutes' duration is associated with postischemic myocardial dysfunction that lasts hours to days despite the restoration of normal coronary blood flow. This reversible injury is referred to as *myocardial stunning*. The mechanisms underlying stunning are complex but in general appear to be related to intracellular calcium overload and oxidative stress induced by reactive oxygen species (ROS) released at the time of reperfusion. Although intracellular calcium may return to normal levels early during reperfusion, transient increases can activate a variety of proteases, including protein kinase C (PKC), whose activation and subsequent action on contractile proteins can lead to myofibrillar injury. The incidence of myocardial stunning in patients after CABG surgery ranges from 20% to 80% depending on its definition and clinical manifestation. For example, as many as 75% of patients after CABG may be administered some form of inotropic support in the immediate postoperative period in order to maintain a satisfactory cardiac index, mixed venous saturation, blood pressure, and urinary output. In most patients, this is not associated with specific adverse outcomes. In the patient with severe preoperative myocardial dysfunction and limited cardiac reserve, however, myocardial stunning may result in a more profound reduction in cardiac output. These patients may require intensive inotropic support postoperatively and insertion of an intra-aortic balloon pump (IABP). In these patients, the mortality rate secondary to stunning may be as high as 10% to 15%.

Reversible contractile dysfunction that matches a reduction in resting coronary artery blood flow is termed *hibernating myocardium*. It is characterized by a balanced reduction in myocardial contractility and oxygen consumption and is typically found in patients with severe CAD who present with stable or unstable angina, myocardial infarction (MI), or congestive heart failure. By definition, it is reversible on restoration of normal coronary blood flow. Human tissue biopsies obtained from hibernating myocardium have shown a loss of myofibrils, glycogen accumulation, and interstitial fibrosis. Whether the contractile dysfunction in the hibernating myocardium is due to a reduction in coronary blood flow or a reduction in coronary reserve is unclear. It is also controversial whether chronic contractile dysfunction is caused by repetitive episodes of myocardial stunning, or is an adaptive mechanism to chronic myocardial ischemia. Characteristics that differentiate these two phenomena are summarized in Table 61-1.

MI represents cell death and necrosis. It is an irreversible injury that is associated with ischemia lasting more than 20 minutes. Because a gradient of ischemia may exist within the myocardium, not all cells are equally at risk for injury. Cells around the periphery of an ischemic zone and adjacent to the oxygen-rich blood in the ven-

Table 61-1   Characteristics of Reversible Postischemic Myocardial Dysfunction

STUNNING	HIBERNATION
Dysfunctional myocardium with normal or near-normal blood flow	Dysfunctional myocardium with reduced blood flow
Contractile abnormality reversible with time	Contractile abnormality reversible on reperfusion
Absence of irreversible damage	Absence of irreversible damage
Perfusion imaging (PET scan) normal or increased	Perfusion imaging (PET scan) increased
Contractile function decreased	Contractile function decreased
No metabolic deterioration during inotropic stimulation	Recruitment of inotropic reserve at the expense of metabolic recovery
Disruption of myofibrillar structure in canine model	Disruption of myofibrillar structure in canine model
Heart does not adapt to chronic underperfusion	Heart adapts to chronic underperfusion
Steady-state between perfusion and contraction not achieved	Steady-state between perfusion and contraction can be reached
Perfusion-contraction mismatching lasts from hours to days to months	Perfusion-contraction matching can be maintained for prolonged periods
Lack of evidence for dedifferentiation process in myocytes	Evidence for dedifferentiation process myocytes

PET, positron emission tomography.

tricular chamber may remain viable. In the absence of adequate collateral flow, sustained ischemia often results in a transmural infarction within 6 to 12 hours. Cell death leads to an inflammatory process that involves the migration of polymorphonuclear leukocytes into the ischemic area and removal of necrotic tissue by macrophages over days. This is followed by a fibroblastic response and neovascularization. Because the myocytes are incapable of regeneration, the infarcted tissue is ultimately replaced with noncontractile fibrous tissue.

Another cause of cardiomyocyte cell loss associated with ischemia is apoptosis, or programmed cell death. This phenomenon is a noninflammatory process that occurs as a result of reperfusion and may be associated with early and delayed cardiac muscle dysfunction. Some of the proposed mechanisms underlying apoptosis are the same mechanisms proposed for myocardial stunning, hibernation, and infarction, namely, generation of intracellular ROS or intracellular calcium overload. Apoptosis has been observed in humans with hibernating myocardium, acute myocardial infarction (AMI), and chronic heart failure. The characteristics of apoptotic death are morphologically and biochemically different from cell death secondary to cell necrosis. With necrosis, cell death is associated with swelling and rupture of the sarcolemmal, mitochondrial, and nuclear membranes and with nuclear chromatin clumping, and the dead cells are removed through an inflammatory process. In contrast, the apoptotic cell shrinks, the nucleus condenses and breaks into nucleosomes and DNA fragments, and the cells are phagocytized. There is some evidence that not all apoptotic cells are committed to cell death in the early stages of the process. Apoptosis represents one aspect of a continuum of ischemia. Its contribution to myocardial dysfunction after ischemia may be more relevant to the process of postischemic ventricular remodeling.

Finally, there is preclinical and circumstantial evidence in humans that an ischemic adaptive phenomenon exists in the human heart. This phenomenon is known as *ischemic preconditioning* (IPC). It is associated with a reduction in infarct size, apoptosis, and reperfusion-associated arrhythmias. IPC occurs when the heart is exposed to brief periods of sublethal ischemia before a period of prolonged ischemia. The underlying mechanism is unclear but most likely involves activation of cell surface receptors and intracellular transduction signaling pathways. Attempts to mimic the phenomenon pharmacologically could lead to the development of pharmacologic agents that are effective in increasing the heart's tolerance to ischemia.

CLINICAL MANIFESTATIONS AND DIAGNOSIS OF CORONARY ARTERY DISEASE

Clinical Presentation

One of the most typical manifestations of CAD is angina pectoris, a discomfort or sensation of heaviness, tightening, squeezing, or constricting in the chest. This discomfort is often retrosternal or left precordial and may radiate

from the chest. It is also characterized as discomfort in the jaw, shoulder, back, or arm. Patients often experience a disagreeable feeling similar to that of indigestion and may experience shortness of breath. Angina pectoris often presents while the patient is exercising, eating, or under emotional duress and usually subsides with rest. Patients with unstable angina typically have pain at rest or with minimal exertion that lasts more than 20 minutes. It is often severe in nature, new in onset (within 1 month), and occurs in a crescendo pattern. Angina is not, however, always present with myocardial ischemia. As many as 15% of patients with significant CAD do not present with angina. This silent ischemia occurs most frequently in patients with diabetes mellitus and is detected during electrocardiographic or echocardiographic monitoring during stress testing. In patients at risk for the disease, angina pectoris is graded according to a variety of classification systems, such as the New York Heart Association Functional Classification and the Canadian Cardiovascular Society Classification System (CCSCS). The latter is more specific for patients with angina pectoris. Using the CCSCS schema, class I patients are asymptomatic, class II patients experience slight limitation of ordinary activity, class III patients experience marked limitation of activity with ordinary physical activity, and class IV patients are unable to undertake any activity without discomfort. Classifications allow for the evaluation of the patient's condition followed over time and the assessment of therapeutic interventions.

In contrast to angina pectoris, MI often presents as crushing chest pain that may be associated with nausea, diaphoresis, anxiety, and dyspnea. Symptoms also include dizziness, fatigue, and vomiting. The pain or associated paresthesia often radiates to the neck and jaw and down the arm. Heart rate and blood pressure may be initially normal, but both increase in response to the duration and severity of pain. In as many as 40% of patients, the first manifestation of coronary artery disease is sudden death likely from malignant ventricular dysrhythmia caused by AMI. More than half of deaths from AMI occur in the prehospital setting. In-hospital fatalities account for 10% of all deaths from AMI, and an additional 10% of deaths occur in the first year after infarction.[4,5]

Physical Examination

It is possible for a patient to have extensive CAD with an unremarkable physical examination. Pertinent physical findings are more frequently associated with manifestations of atherosclerosis in general. The patient's mental status can vary from normal to anxious to confused. Eye examination may reveal a copper-wire sign, retinal hematoma or thrombosis secondary to vascular occlusive disease, and hypertension. The presence of neck bruits and thrills may reflect significant underlying carotid artery disease. Abnormal neck vein pulsations may be seen in patients with second- or third-degree heart block. The pulse may be weak or thready and suggest ectopic or premature ventricular beats. Often a precordial ectopic impulse may be palpated along the left lower sternal border, demarking enlargement of the left ventricle due to increased chamber compliance and bulging. A third heart sound can be noted with elevated left ventricular filling pressures. A fourth heart sound is commonly heard in patients with acute and chronic CAD, and heart murmurs may reflect ischemic papillary muscles and mitral valve insufficiency, aortic stenosis or insufficiency, and ventricular septal rupture. In patients with more advanced ischemic heart disease, auscultation of the chest may reveal rales, and examination of the abdomen may reveal hepatomegaly, right upper abdominal quadrant tenderness, ascites, and marked peripheral and presacral edema.

Laboratory Studies

Patients suspected of having CAD should undergo appropriate blood testing, including a lipid profile (cholesterol, triglycerides, LDL, high-density lipoprotein [HDL]) and perhaps an hs-CRP level. Elevated serum cholesterol is associated with an elevated risk for coronary heart disease (CHD). A 10% increase in serum cholesterol is associated with a 20% to 30% increase in heart disease. Clear benefits have been shown for dietary and drug regimens that lower serum cholesterol, and statins have been shown to reduce fatal and nonfatal CHD and slow the progression of bypass graft plaque progression.

There are also several markers of inflammation that are useful at predicting the development of CHD. These include hs-CRP, intercellular adhesion molecule-1, and cytokines such as interleukin-6 and tumor necrosis factor. The hs-CRP marker adds to the predictive value of total and HDL cholesterol in determining risk for future MI. Whether these markers can be used to better identify patients at risk and target therapeutic intervention remains to be determined.

Diagnostic Studies

Numerous methods and technologies are available to detect the presence of hemodynamically significant coronary artery stenoses and to assess cardiac function and myocardial viability. The information ultimately determines whether a patient should be treated medically or with percutaneous transluminal coronary angioplasty (PTCA), percutaneous coronary intervention (PCI), or CABG (Fig. 61-9). Many of these studies can be performed even if the patient is unable to exercise. The strengths and weaknesses of each method are shown in Box 61-1.

Chest Radiograph

The chest radiograph is helpful in identifying causes of chest discomfort or pain other than that due to CAD. With advanced CAD, there may be evidence of cardiomegaly, pulmonary edema, or pleural effusions, which are indicative of heart failure. Evidence of calcification in the coronary arteries, aortic or mitral valves, or aorta is also consistent with presumptive evidence of generalized atherosclerosis.

Electrocardiogram

A 12-lead resting electrocardiogram (ECG) should be obtained in patients suspected of having CAD and in those with episodes of chest discomfort or angina pectoris. The ECG is evaluated for evidence of left ventricular hypertrophy, ST-segment depression or elevation, ectopic beats, or Q waves. In addition, arrhythmias (atrial fibrillation or ventricular tachycardia) and conduction defects (left anterior fascicular block, right bundle branch block, left bundle branch block) are suggestive of CAD and MI. Persistent ST-segment elevation or an evolving Q wave is consistent with myocardial injury and ongoing ischemia. Fifty percent of patients will have normal ECG results despite the existence of significant CAD, and 50% of ECGs obtained during chest pain at rest will be normal. An exercise stress ECG is helpful in determining the extent of CAD and the prognosis. Exercise protocols, typically using a treadmill or bicycle, increase myocardial oxygen demand to elicit an ischemic threshold. A positive exercise ECG may show progressive flattening of the ST segment or ST-segment depression as exercise progresses. During the recovery phase, ST depression may persist, with down-sloping segments and T-wave inversion. Additional findings associated with an adverse prognosis and presence of multivessel occlusive disease include duration of symptom-limited exercise of less than 6 metabolic equivalents (METs), failure to increase systolic blood pressure to more than 120 mm Hg, or appearance of ventricular arrhythmias. For detection of CAD, the sensitivity and specificity of an exercise ECG approach 70% and 80%, respectively. The accuracy of exercise ECG testing is dependent on a patient achieving 85% to 90% of their age-predicted maximum exercise response (see Box 61-1).

Echocardiography

Surface and transesophageal echocardiography use reflected acoustic waves for cardiac imaging. Common indications for a resting echocardiogram include heart murmurs and suggested diagnoses such as aortic stenosis or insufficiency, hypertrophic cardiomyopathy, mitral valve stenosis or regurgitation, and congestive heart failure. Rest echocardiography can also reveal regional wall motion abnormalities, ventricular dilation, and wall thinning. The sensitivity and specificity of echocardiography can be enhanced with the administration of intravenous (IV) dobutamine in incremental doses, which is helpful in differentiating stunned, hibernating, and infarcted myocardium. A reduced inotropic response and evidence of new wall motion abnormalities are also indicative of myocardial ischemia (see Box 61-1).

Single-Photon Emission Computed Tomography

Exercise or pharmacologic stress thallium-201 (^{201}Tl) or technetium-99m (^{99m}Tc)-sestamibi single-photon emission computed tomography (SPECT) has a sensitivity for detecting CAD of 85% to 96%, and when gated with ECG, has a specificity of 90%. Compared with exercise ECG, both techniques are more accurate. They are particularly useful in patients with left ventricular hypertrophy or conduction abnormalities and in those unable to achieve 85% of their maximum predicted exercise response. In conjunction with ECG gating, ^{201}Tl SPECT imaging also provides useful data on regional wall thickening, global

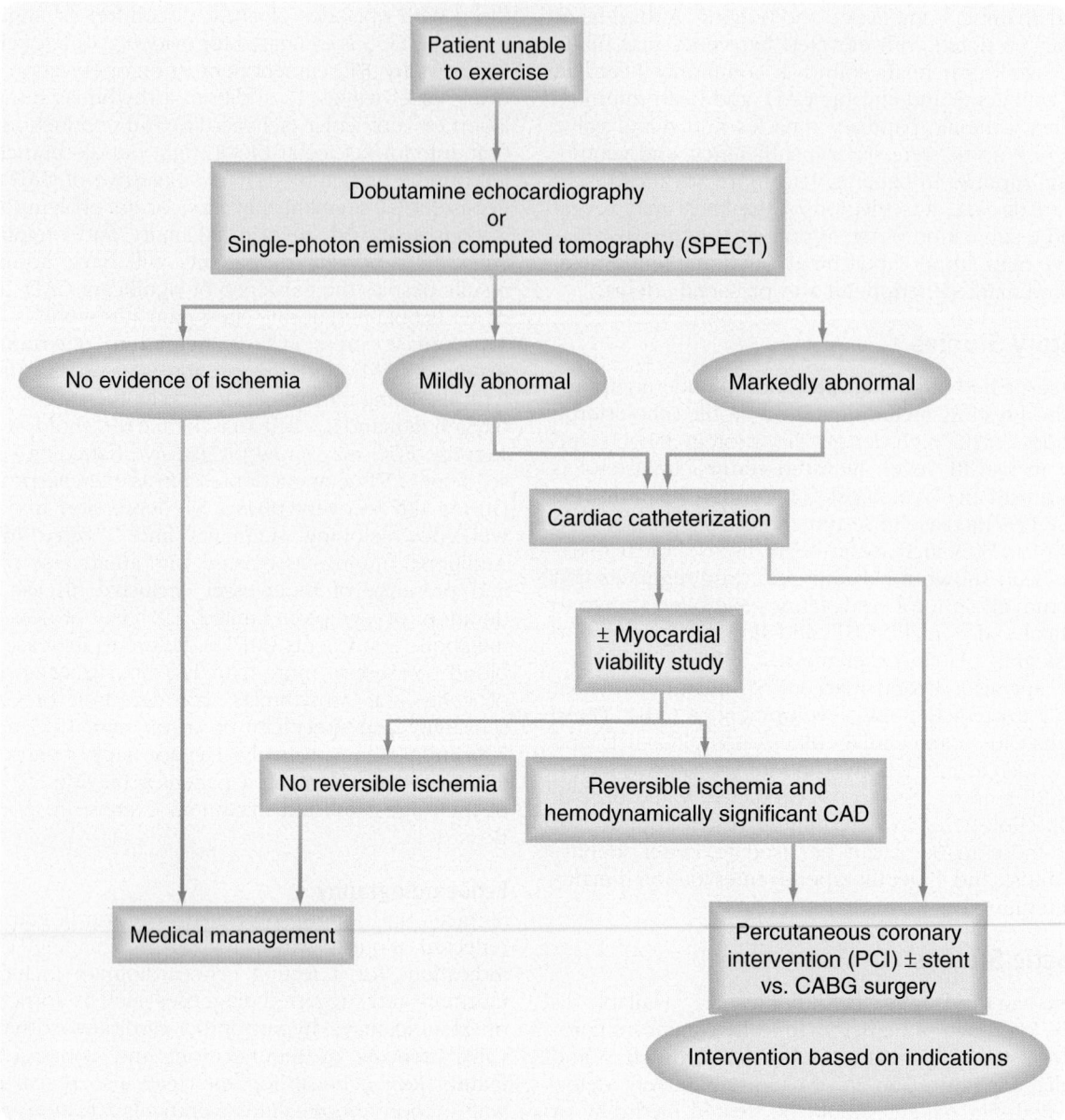

Figure 61-9 A strategy for evaluating patients with suspected coronary artery disease (CAD) and unable to exercise. **CABG,** coronary artery bypass grafting. (Courtesy of the Division of Cardiothoracic Surgery, University of Kentucky, 2003.)

left ventricular EF, and myocardial perfusion. For the patient who cannot exercise, administration of vasodilators (adenosine, dipyridamole) or inotropes (dobutamine) allows similar data acquisition with comparable sensitivity and specificity (see Box 61-1).

Positron Emission Tomography

PET scanning is a useful technique for assessing myocardial viability, metabolism, and the evaluation of myocardial blood flow. Because myocardial extraction of glucose is elevated in ischemic myocytes, the glucose-analogue radiotracer ^{18}F-2-fluoro-2-deoxyglucose (FDG) can be used to image the heart; PET is reported to be superior to thallium SPECT, ^{99m}Tc perfusion, and stress-dobuta-

mine echocardiography in the evaluation of myocardial viability. The positive predictive value (PPV) and negative predictive value (NPV) approach 95%. Perfusion of nonmetabolic tracers through the myocardium can identify two basic patterns: normal or uniform perfusion and underperfused myocardium. The combination of abnormal perfusion with a positive PET study indicates viable myocardium in an area of coronary artery stenosis. In addition, FDG PET is a highly accurate predictor of improvement in regional wall motion and global left ventricular EF after myocardial revascularization. For patients with abnormal perfusion and more than 75% of normal PET uptake, the PPV value of left ventricular recovery is 65% to 90%. Uptake less than 75% generally

Box 61-1 Strengths and Limitations of Diagnostic Techniques

Detecting Coronary Artery Disease and Assessing Prognosis

Exercise ECG

Strengths: Low cost; short duration; functional status evaluated; high sensitivity in three-vessel or left main coronary artery disease; prognostic (e.g., ischemia at low workload)

Limitations: Suboptimal sensitivity; low detection rate of one-vessel disease; nondiagnostic with abnormal baseline ECG; poor specificity in premenopausal women; must achieve ≥85% of maximum heart rate for accuracy

Exercise/Pharmacologic SPECT Perfusion Imaging

Strengths: Simultaneous evaluation of perfusion and function (gated SPECT); higher sensitivity and specificity than exercise ECG; high specificity with ^{99m}Tc; can be performed in most patients; added prognostic value; comparable accuracy with pharmacologic stress; viability and ischemia simultaneously assessed; quantitative image analysis

Limitations: Suboptimal specificity with ^{201}Tl; long procedure time with 99^{m}Tc; higher cost than exercise ECG; radiation exposure; poor-quality images in obese patients

Exercise/Pharmacologic Stress Echocardiography

Strengths: Higher sensitivity and specificity than exercise ECG; added prognostic value; comparable value with dobutamine stress; short examination time; identification of structural cardiac abnormalities; simultaneous evaluation of perfusion with contrast agents; relatively lower cost; no radiation

Limitations: Decreased sensitivity for detection of one-vessel disease or mild stenosis with postexercise imaging; inability to image all of the left ventricle in some patients; highly operator dependent; no quantitative image analysis; poor acoustic window in some patients (e.g., chronic obstructive lung disease); infarct zone ischemia less well detected

Assessment of Myocardial Viability

SPECT Imaging

Strengths: High sensitivity for predicting improved function after revascularization; quantitative objective criteria (e.g., >60% segmental uptake); LVEF quantitated on ^{99m}Tc-sestamibi or ^{99m}Tc-tetrofosmin imaging; predictive of clinical outcomes

Limitations: Reduced resolution and sensitivity compared to PET; less quantitative than PET; areas of attenuation (e.g., inferior wall on ^{99m}Tc-sestamibi scans) misconstrued as nonviability; cannot

differentiate endocardial from epicardial viability; no absolute measurement of blood flow; lower specificity than dobutamine echocardiography for predicting improved function after revascularization

PET Imaging

Strengths: Simultaneous assessment of perfusion and metabolism; more sensitive than other techniques; good specificity; no attenuation problems; absolute blood flow can be measured; predictive of outcomes

Limitations: Lower specificity than dobutamine echocardiography or MRI; cannot separate endocardial from epicardial viability; high cost and highly sophisticated technology; limited availability

Dobutamine Echocardiography

Strengths: Higher specificity than nuclear techniques; viability assessed at low doses and ischemia at higher doses; evaluation of mitral regurgitation on baseline echocardiography; predictive of outcomes; widely available; lower cost than dobutamine MRI

Limitations: Poor windows in 30% of patients; lower sensitivity than nuclear techniques; myocardium with poor flow may not show increase during stimulation; reliance on visual assessment of wall thickening

Contrast Echocardiography

Strengths: Microcirculatory integrity evaluated as well as systolic thickening; better estimation of extent of viability than functional assessment alone; precise delineation of area of necrosis; resolution of endocardial versus epicardial perfusion; viability assessed in presence of total coronary occlusion

Limitations: Difficult windows in 30% of patients; attenuation problems; scant clinical data available

Dobutamine MRI

■ *Strengths:* Evaluate inotropic reserve in endocardium with tagging; measurement of wall thickness more accurate than with TTE; better image quality than echocardiography for contractile reserve; simultaneous assessment of perfusion using contrast enhancement; good sensitivity and specificity for viability

■ *Limitations:* Higher cost than echocardiography; limited availability; less sensitive than nuclear techniques but may be more specific; imaging information not available in real time; patients with pacemakers or implantable cardioverter defibrillators cannot be imaged

---

ECG, electrocardiogram; LVEF, left ventricular ejection fraction; MRI, magnetic resonance imaging; PET, positron-emission tomography; SPECT, single-photon emission computed tomography; TTE, transthoracic esophageal echocardiography.

Adapted from Braunwald E, Zipes DP, Libby P (eds): Heart Disease: A Textbook of Cardiovascular Medicine, 6th ed. Philadelphia, WB Saunders, 2001, pp 435, 437.

---

indicates unlikely recovery of left ventricular function (NPV, 75%-95%) after revascularization. Limitations to PET include cost, availability of cardiac PET, and inability to interpret the study in diabetic patients who have significant insulin resistance (see Box 61-1).

Magnetic Resonance Imaging and Gadolinium Magnetic Resonance Imaging

Because of the radiation exposure of SPECT scanning and the limited availability of cardiac PET imaging, myo-

cardial first-pass perfusion magnetic resonance imaging (MRI) is a good alternative and may become the preferred technique for evaluating myocardial viability. One prospective study of 31 patients with confirmed CAD and reduced left ventricular function (EF<0.35) showed that MRI had a sensitivity and specificity of 86% and 94%, respectively, when PET was used as the standard for identifying segments of myocardium with matched flow or metabolism defects.[6] Quantitative assessment of infarct mass also correlated well with PET. In another study, 48 patients with CAD were prospectively evaluated with gadolinium-enhanced multislice hybrid echo-planar pulse sequence MRI versus PET and compared with 18 normal patients.[7] Receiver-operator characteristic analysis of CAD (as defined by PET) had a sensitivity and specificity of 91% and 94%, respectively. Compared with quantitative coronary angiography, MRI detected lesions greater than 50%, with a specificity and sensitivity of 87% and 85%, respectively. These findings suggest that cardiac MRI is an excellent alternative diagnostic method that can be used to determine the presence and extent of CAD and myocardial viability (see Box 61-1).

Electrocardiogram-Gated Multidetector Spiral Computed Tomography and Electron-Beam Computed Tomography

Computed tomography (CT) is a potential tool for functional and ischemic cardiac imaging. It can identify regional myocardial wall thinning and the presence of mural thrombus. Contrast-enhanced electron-beam CT is used to detect hemodynamically significant lesions, although 30% to 40% of patients cannot be imaged because of unacceptable cardiac motion artifact. There is variation in efficacy for specific coronary arteries, with an overall sensitivity and specificity of 90% and 80%, respectively. Electron-beam CT quantification of coronary artery calcium correlates with existing asymptomatic myocardial ischemia in clinically high-risk patients. This suggests that electron-beam CT may be a screening test for asymptomatic CAD in patients with intermediate risk.

Multidetector CT allows imaging of the coronary arteries and especially of coronary artery bypass grafts.[8] Studies indicate that sensitivity and specificity of multidetector CT approaches or exceeds that of other noninvasive methods of visualizing coronary artery anatomy.[8] Multidetector CT is especially useful for imaging proximal coronary artery disease and for imaging coronary artery bypass grafts. Newer technology improves on conventional multidetector CT by adding more arrays to the imaging process, such that 128-slice multidetector CT arrays are currently available. Newer machines with increased arrays provide increased sensitivity and specificity.[8] It remains to be seen whether multidetector CT or gadolinium MRI will supplant coronary angiography (discussed later) for routine diagnosis of CAD in symptomatic patients.

Cardiac Catheterization

Anatomy of the coronary arteries, ascending aorta, aortic and mitral valves, and left ventricle can be readily evaluated at the time of left heart catheterization. High-quality coronary angiography is essential for the identification of CAD and the assessment of its extent and severity. Cardiac catheterization that includes ventriculogram also permits assessment of systolic and diastolic function, diagnosis of intracardiac shunts, differentiation of myocardial restriction from pericardial constriction, and assessment of valve dysfunction. Right heart catheterization is used to measure central venous, right atrial, right ventricular, pulmonary artery, and pulmonary wedge pressures as well as cardiac output. It can also be used to evaluate the presence of intracardiac shunts, to assess arrhythmias, and to initiate temporary cardiac pacing.

INDICATIONS FOR CORONARY ARTERY BYPASS GRAFTING

The aim of medical treatment for patients with symptomatic CAD is to reduce the heart's demand for oxygen by slowing the heart rate, decreasing myocardial contractility, and reducing systemic vascular resistance.[9,10] The objective of interventional therapy is to increase the supply of oxygen and nutrients by dilating or bypassing the coronary artery obstructions. Although medical therapy can be effective, in many cases the optimal treatment is angioplasty with or without stents, CABG, or both. Because interventional therapy is not without risk, it is important to understand the relative survival benefits and risks associated with them. The survival benefit of CABG patients was initially studied in patients with chronic stable angina.

Chronic Stable Angina

CABG Versus Medical Management

In the 1970s and 1980s, several prospective randomized clinical trials evaluated the survival benefit of CABG in patients with chronic stable angina. These studies showed significant benefit and resulted in the widespread application of CABG for the treatment of patients with CAD. They also helped to identify specific categories of patients with angina who were most likely to benefit from CABG (Table 61-2), namely patients with left main coronary artery disease; one-, two-, or three-vessel disease with proximal LAD involvement; and three-vessel disease with impaired left ventricular function. These observations were confirmed in a meta-analysis of these studies (Fig. 61-10). It is important to note that these trials were conducted in an era in which fewer than 50% of patients were treated with β-blockers, less than 40% were administered aspirin (ASA), and less than 10% received an internal thoracic artery (ITA) graft. Also, calcium channel blockers, angiotensin-converting enzyme inhibitors, and lipid-lowering agents were not available. Women were excluded in all but one of the trials, and only patients younger than 65 years were studied. Nevertheless, as a direct result of these clinical studies, CABG is now accepted as an appropriate therapeutic modality for the treatment of specific subsets of patients with chronic stable angina (see Table 61-2).

PTCA Versus Medical Management

In the 1980s, PTCA was introduced as an alternative to CABG. The first successful PTCA was performed by Gruntzig and colleagues.[11] Initially, the procedure was performed in patients with single-vessel disease and isolated lesions. With improvements in catheter technology,

Table 61-2 Indications for CABG Surgery Alone in Patients With Stable Angina, Unstable Angina, and Acute Myocardial Infarction

CONDITION	CLASS*			
	I	IIa	IIb	III
Asymptomatic or mild angina	1. LMCA stenosis ≥60% 2. LMCA equivalent: proximal LAD and LCA stenoses >70% 3. 3VD (survival benefit >with abnormal LF function: EF ≤0.50)	Proximal LAD stenosis with 1VD or 2VD‡	1VD or 2VD not involving the proximal LAD‡	None
Chronic stable angina	1. LMCA stenosis ≥60% 2. LMCA equivalent: proximal LAD and LCA stenoses >70% 3. 3VD (survival benefit >with abnormal LV function: EF <0.50) 4. 2VD with significant proximal LAD stenosis: either EF <0.50 or ischemia on noninvasive testing 5. 1VD or 2VD without significant proximal LAD stenosis, but with a large area of viable myocardium and high-risk criteria on noninvasive testing 6. Disabling angina despite maximal medical therapy (acceptable-risk patient)	1. Proximal LAD stenosis with 1VD‡ 2. 1VD or 2VD without significant proximal LAD stenosis, moderate area of viable myocardium and demonstrable ischemia on noninvasive testing	None	1. 1VD or 2VD without significant proximal LAD stenosis, in patients who have mild symptoms that are unlikely due to myocardial ischemia or have not received an adequate trial of medical therapy and (1) have only a small area of viable myocardium or (2) no demonstrable ischemia on noninvasive testing 2. Borderline stenoses (50%-60%) other than in the LCMA, no demonstrable ischemia on noninvasive testing 3. <50% coronary stenosis
UA/NSTEMI	1. LMCA stenosis ≥60% 2. LMCA equivalent: proximal LAD and LCA stenoses >70% 3. Ongoing ischemia unresponsive to maximal nonsurgical therapy	1. Proximal LAD stenosis with 1VD or 2VD‡	1VD or 2VD not involving the proximal LAD‡	None
STEMI/AMI	Emergency or urgent CABG in patients with STEMI should be undertaken in the following circumstances: failed angioplasty with persistent pain or hemodynamic instability; persistent or recurrent ischemia refractory to medical therapy; at the time of surgical repair of postinfarction ventricular septal rupture or mitral valve insufficiency; cardiogenic shock in patients <75 years with ST-segment elevation or left bundle branch block or posterior MI who develop shock within 36 hours of MI; life-threatening ventricular arrhythmias in the presence of ≥50% left main stenosis and/or triple-vessel disease	CABG may be performed as primary reperfusion in patients who failed fibrinolysis/PCI and who are in the early hours (6-12 hours) of evolving STEMI. (CABG mortality is elevated for the first 3-7 days after infarction, and the benefit of revascularization must be balanced against this increased risk.)		Emergency CABG should not be performed in patients with persistent angina and a small area of myocardium at risk who are hemodynamically stable. Emergency CABG should not be performed in patients with successful epicardial reperfusion but unsuccessful microvascular reperfusion.

*Class I: Conditions for which there is evidence and/or general agreement that a given procedure/treatment is useful and effective.

Class IIa: Weight of evidence/opinion is in favor of usefulness/efficacy.

Class IIb: Usefulness/efficacy is less well established by evidence/opinion.

Class III: Conditions for which there is evidence and/or general agreement that the procedure/treatment is not useful/effective and in some cases may be harmful.

†Becomes class I if extensive ischemia documented by noninvasive study and/or a left ventricular ejection fraction <0.50.

‡If there is a large area of viable myocardium and high-risk criteria on noninvasive testing, becomes class I.

1VD, one-vessel disease; 2VD, two-vessel disease; CABG, coronary artery bypass grafting; LAD, left anterior descending coronary artery; LCA, left coronary artery; LMCA, left main coronary artery; MI, myocardial infarction; PCI, percutaneous coronary intervention; STEMI, ST-elevation myocardial infarction UA/NSTEMI, unstable angina/STEMI.

Data from Babapulle MN, Joseph L, Belisle P, et al: A hierarchical Bayesian meta-analysis of randomised clinical trials of drug-eluting stents. Lancet 364(9434):583-591, 2004; and Williams DO, Braunwald E, Thompson B, et al: Results of percutaneous transluminal coronary angioplasty in unstable angina and non-Q-wave myocardial infarction: Observations from the TIMI IIIB Trial. Circulation 94:2749-2755, 1996.

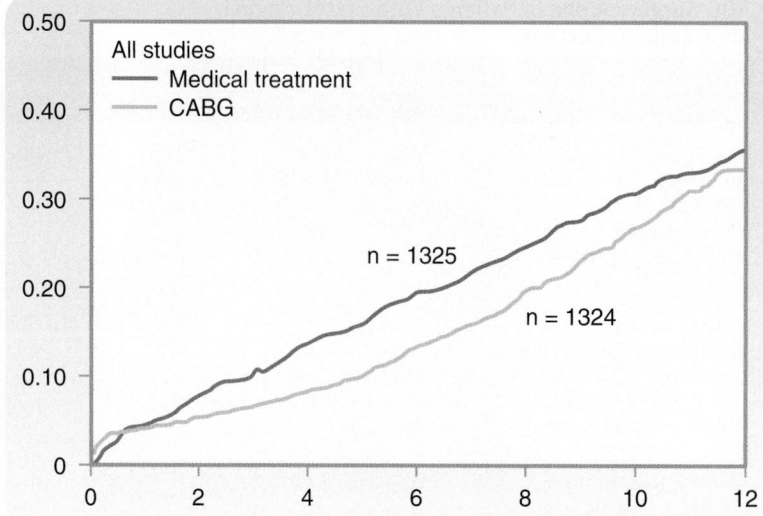

Figure 61-10 Cumulative total mortality for 12 years after coronary artery bypass grafting (CABG) surgery versus noninterventional management for patients with chronic stable angina. (Adapted from Yusuf S, Zucker D, Peduzzi P, et al: Effect of coronary artery bypass graft surgery on survival: Overview of 10-year results from randomised trials by the Coronary Artery Bypass Graft Surgery Trialists Collaboration. Lancet 344:563-570, 1994.)

increasing experience, and the advent of stent-based interventions, angioplasty is now performed in patients with multivessel disease. Although the short-term symptomatic success rate for PTCA approaches 85% to 90%, the role of PTCA in the management of patients with angina whose symptoms are adequately controlled with medical therapy remains controversial.[12,13] The efficacy of PTCA was compared with best medical management in 212 patients with proven ischemia, single-vessel disease, and stenoses greater than 70%.[14] In this study, patients undergoing PTCA demonstrated better relief from angina, reduced need for antianginal medications, better quality of life, and improved exercise tolerance; there was no difference in mortality. Some PTCA patients (19%), however, required additional catheter-based interventions, and 7% underwent CABG. In the medically managed group of patients, 11% progressed to PTCA, and none underwent CABG. At 4 years, the patients who were initially randomized to PTCA had a better quality of life and significantly fewer episodes of unstable angina. Thus, in this trial, the increased number of reinterventions in the first year and greater costs for the PTCA-treated group appeared to be justified by the lower incidence of late procedures and lower costs in the extended follow-up period. In the RITA-2 trial (Coronary Angioplasty versus Medical Therapy for Angina: The Second Randomised Intervention Treatment of Angina),[13] PTCA provided better early symptomatic relief from angina compared with medical treatment. This, however, was not sustained over time, and after 2.9 years, the PTCA group had a 3% greater risk for death or MI (Table 61-3).

A major limitation of these studies was the absence of preprocedural cardiac stress and myocardial viability testing. Without this information, it is difficult to know whether the PTCA and medical therapy groups were equally matched. It is also difficult to extrapolate the

findings to current practice because the studies were performed before the use of coronary stents. Nevertheless, it appears that patients with angina may be treated relatively safely with either medical management or PTCA intervention. The risk for early complications associated with PTCA, however, need to be taken into consideration before proceeding with the interventional approach in this group of patients.

CABG Versus PTCA

One of the first large-scale, prospective, randomized studies comparing PTCA and CABG was the Bypass Angioplasty Revascularization Investigation (BARI) trial reported in 1996.[15] Patients with multivessel disease were randomly assigned to either CABG (n = 914) or PTCA (n = 915) and followed for a mean of 5.4 years. In the short term, the incidence of Q-wave MI was higher in the CABG group (4.6% versus 2.1%); the stroke rates were similar (0.8% versus 0.2%). At the end of 5 years, the survival rate was 89.3% for the CABG cohort and 86.3% for the PTCA cohort (P = .19). Among the PTCA patients, however, 54% required additional revascularization procedures. Thirty-one percent underwent CABG, 34% underwent additional PTCA, and 11% underwent both interventions. In contrast, only 8% of the CABG patients required repeat revascularization. Thus, it appears that, although PTCA did not compromise the 5-year survival rate in patients with multivessel disease, subsequent revascularization including CABG was required more often. Among the diabetic patients, the 5-year survival rate for the CABG patients was markedly greater, 80.6% versus 65.5% (see Table 61-3). In the Emory Angioplasty versus Surgery Trial (EAST), the primary end points were death, MI, or the presence of a large myocardial ischemic defect after 3 years. Secondary end points included all-cause mortality and the requirement for repeat revascu-

Table 61-3   Pertinent Studies Comparing PTCA and CABG Surgery

STUDY, NO. OF PATIENTS (*N*), AND FOLLOW-UP (F/U)	REFERENCE	PURPOSE	FINDINGS
Arterial Revascularization Therapies Study (ARTS) *N*=205 F/U=400 days	J Am Coll Cardiol 39:559-564, 2002	Evaluated effectiveness of revascularization on event-free survival	Complete revascularization more frequently accomplished by CABG surgery. Patients randomized to stenting with incomplete revascularization had greater need for subsequent bypass surgery.
	N Engl J Med 344:1117-1124, 2001	Compared CABG surgery and stenting for multivessel disease	Coronary stenting was less expensive than bypass surgery ($3000/patient) and conferred same degree of protection against death, stroke, and myocardial infarction. Stenting was associated with greater need for repeat revascularization.
Bypass Angioplasty Revascularization Investigation (BARI) *N*=1829 F/U=5.4 yr	N Engl J Med 335:217-225, 1996	Compared CABG surgery with angioplasty inpatients with multivessel disease	Initial strategy of PTCA did not compromise 5-year survival of overall population but was associated with more frequent subsequent revascularizations. Five-year survival for treated diabetics was better after CABG surgery (PTCA, 65.5%; CABG, 80.6%).
	JAMA 277:715-721, 1997	Analyzed clinical and functional outcomes in patients with multivessel disease	Angina-free episodes were greater in CABG patients. Use of anti-ischemic medications was higher in PTCA group. Need for revascularization was greater in PTCA patients (52%) than CABG surgery (6%).
	Circulation 96:1761-1769, 1997	Assessed influence of diabetes in CABG and PTCA patients with multivessel disease	Patients with treated diabetes mellitus assigned to initial strategy of CABG had a marked improvement in survival (CABG, 94.2%; PTCA, 79.4%). Survival benefit of CABG surgery was confined to patients receiving at least one ITA graft.
	N Eng J Med 336:92-99, 1997	Analyzed cost and quality of life	CABG surgery was associated with better quality of life. PTCA had a lower 5-year cost than CABG surgery only in patients with two-vessel disease.
	Circulation 98:1279-1285, 1998	Analyzed outcome for women	The 5-year unadjusted mortality rates for women and men undergoing CABG and PTCA were similar. Because of higher risk profiles, female gender was an independent predictor of improved 5-year survival after adjusting for risk factors.
F/U=7.8 yr	J Am Coll Cardiol 35:1122-1129, 2000	Assessed long-term outcomes in diabetic patients	Survival benefit of CABG surgery over PTCA was more pronounced at 7 years (CABG, 76.4%; PTCA, 55.7%).
Emory Angioplasty versus Surgery Trial (EAST) *N*=392 F/U=8 years	J Am Coll Cardiol 35:1116-11121, 2000	Evaluated long-term outcome	Patients with proximal left anterior descending coronary artery stenosis and those with diabetes tended to have better late survival with CABG surgery (did not reach statistical significance).
Randomized Intervention Treatment of Angina (RITA)-1 *N*=1011 F/U=2.5 years	Lancet 341:573-580, 1993	Examined long-term effects of PTCA vs. CABG in patients with one-, two-, and three-vessel disease	Prevalence of angina was three times higher in the PTCA group at 6 months and 1.5 times higher at 2 years. Antianginal drugs were more frequent in the PTCA group. CABG surgery was associated with a lower risk for angina and fewer additional diagnostic and therapeutic interventions.
F/U=2 years	Lancet 344:927-930, 1994	Analyzed cost of intervention	Cost of PTCA was 80% of CABG surgery at 2 years.
F/U=6.5 years	Lancet 352:1419-1425, 1998	Analyzed clinical outcomes and cost	No difference in mortality. In the PTCA group, the prevalence of angina was higher, and 26% underwent CABG. PTCA and CABG surgery costs were similar after 5 years.
RITA-2 Coronary Angioplasty Versus Medical Therapy for Angina *N*=1018 F/U=2.7 years	Lancet 350:461-468, 1997	Compared long-term effects of PTCA and conservative care	Early intervention with PTCA was associated with greater symptomatic improvement but also with small but real excess hazard due to procedure-related complications.

CABG, coronary artery bypass grafting; LAD, left anterior descending coronary artery; ITA, internal thoracic artery; PTCA, percutaneous transluminal coronary angioplasty.

larization procedures after extended follow-up. After the 3-year anniversary visit, patients were contacted and medical records examined until death or the 8-year anniversary. The results showed that after 3 years, the number of repeat interventions was similar. At 8 years, the survival rate for both groups was also similar: angioplasty, 79.3%, and CABG, 82.7%. There was a tendency for patients with proximal LAD stenosis and those with diabetes to have better late survival with CABG (see Table 61-3). Because of the relatively small number of patients enrolled, however, the study was underpowered to detect significant survival differences.

A strength of the BARI trial was that the MI classification methodology was based on symptoms and ECG results obtained at predetermined time intervals, and a core laboratory was used to measure myocardial enzyme levels. The entry criteria, however, resulted in the selection of patients preferentially suited for PTCA. Thus, the findings may not be fully applicable to patients with complex multivessel disease. Also, in both the BARI and EAST studies, few CABG patients underwent extensive arterial grafting, and the studies were performed when stents and new pharmacologic agents, such as clopidogrel and other IIb/IIIa inhibitors, were not available. Despite these limitations, it appears that CABG clearly confers a survival benefit to diabetic patients that is superior to angioplasty. With respect to quality of life and economic issues, although the data collected in 934 of the 1829 patients enrolled in the BARI trial showed that PTCA patients returned to work sooner, CABG patients had better functional status scores (Duke Activity Status Index). Also, although the cost of angioplasty was 95% of that of CABG ($P = .047$), the actual difference between the two interventions was less than $3000, and this was observed only in patients with two-vessel disease. PTCA appeared to be more expensive in patients with three-vessel disease.

Since the BARI trial, at least nine randomized trials have been conducted to compare the short-term and long-term outcomes of CABG versus PTCA as primary treatment for multivessel disease. A meta-analysis of these nine randomized controlled trials revealed that survival was equivalent in these trials after 1 and 3 years of follow-up, but when CABG was the first intervention, there was a significant survival advantage at 5 and 8 years after intervention compared with percutaneous coronary intervention.[16] The 8-year mortality rate was 13.7% with CABG versus 17.1% with PTCA ($P < .03$). The relative mortality rate when PTCA was the initial intervention was 25% higher than when CABG was the initial intervention.

Randomized controlled trials (RCTs) of PTCA versus CABG are limited by highly selected enrollment, and any extrapolation of RCT results to entire populations of patients with multivessel disease is likely to be inappropriate.[17] Prospectively gathered data on the outcome of PTCA and CABG from an entire captive population provide useful information about how successfully practitioners applied the evidence from RCTs, meta-analyses, and uncontrolled trials to the real-world treatment of patients. A comparison of PTCA versus CABG in an entire captive population was reported from the New York State

Cardiac Procedure Registries.[18] Analysis of this large database of more than 50,000 patients found that during the 3-year follow-up, repeat revascularization was 11 times higher in the PTCA group (37% PTCA versus 3.3% CABG). Further, 3-year mortality was significantly higher in the PTCA group. For example, in patients with three-vessel disease, the 3-year adjusted mortality rate was 43% higher with primary PTCA than with CABG.

In the 1990s, coronary stents were introduced to address the problematic occurrence of restenosis after PTCA. Three major RCTs compared CABG to PTCA with stents:

1. Arterial Revascularization Therapies Study (ARTS) trial presented 5-year follow-up in 1205 randomized patients with multivessel disease.[18]
2. ERACI II reported 5-year follow-up of 450 patients randomized to PTCA with stenting versus CABG in seven Argentine centers.[19]
3. SoS trial reported results of CABG versus PTCA with stenting in 988 patients from 53 centers in Europe and Canada.[20]

Although there were methodologic variations in all the studies, a clear picture emerges that CABG confers a long-term reduction in major adverse events in patients randomized to CABG as the initial treatment.

Any benefit of CABG compared with stents for patients with multivessel disease was minimized by the interventional cardiology community with the advent of the drug-eluting stent (DES). DESs were introduced to reduce the rate of restenosis even further. The interventional cardiology community embraced DESs, claiming that improved technology made the results of RCTs favoring CABG obsolete. However, equivalent survival compared with CABG in patients with multivessel disease can be accomplished by DES only if the reduction in restenosis rate translates into reduced mortality. No mortality benefit of DES compared with bare metal stent has been demonstrated. A meta-analysis examined 11 RCTs of DES versus bare metal stent, and none of these trials found a mortality benefit for DES.[21] It is likely that use of DESs does not confer a mortality benefit because subsequent coronary events are often related to progression of disease in arteries other than the stented artery. Even if the restenosis rate in stented arteries were zero, most subsequent revascularizations would be in nonstented arteries. Hence, because restenosis in stented arteries is minimally related to intermediate-term and long-term mortality, and DESs have not shown a survival benefit, CABG remains the best option in patients with multivessel disease and in certain subgroups with one-vessel and two-vessel disease.

In summary, CABG confers a superior long-term survival benefit in patients with specific anatomic lesions (e.g., multivessel disease, left main CAD, one-vessel and two-vessel disease with proximal LAD obstruction) and is associated with an increased freedom from angina, a significant reduction in antianginal medications, and fewer subsequent interventions. CABG is the treatment of choice in diabetic patients. The economic impact appears to be comparable when the frequency of repeat

PCI is taken into consideration. Whether this will remain the case with DESs is unknown.

Acute Coronary Syndrome

Patients with acute coronary syndrome (ACS) represent a cohort of patients who have signs and symptoms that require expedited evaluation and treatment. ACS characterizes a constellation of clinical conditions that reflect acute myocardial ischemia and includes the categories of unstable angina (UA), non–ST-elevation myocardial infarction (NSTEMI), and ST-elevation myocardial infarction (STEMI). Unstable angina with an enzyme leak is considered an NSTEMI. More than 1.5 million patients with UA or NSTEMI are admitted to the hospital annually, and 800,000 are admitted with STEMI. Of those suffering an AMI, 213,000 will die, and half of these patients do so within an hour after onset of symptoms. Arrhythmias, usually ventricular fibrillation, are the cause of early death. The categories of AMI are NSTEMI, STEMI, non–Q-wave MI (NQWMI), and Q-wave MI (QWMI). Most patients with ST elevation go on to develop Q-wave AMI. Depending on presentation and diagnosis, the interventional management and outcomes may differ greatly among patients with UA/NSTEMI and STEMI/AMI.

UA/NSTEMI

PCI Versus Medical Management

The Thrombolysis in Myocardial Ischemia (TIMI) IIIB trial[22] studied the effectiveness of thrombolytic therapy with tissue plasminogen activator (t-PA) and early PTCA in the treatment of patients with unstable angina. The results showed that thrombolysis conferred no treatment benefit; in fact, there was some evidence that IV t-PA administration before PTCA increased the risk for periprocedural MI. PTCA, however, did achieve a high rate of angiographic success, and at 1-year follow-up, the cumulative mortality rate was only 2.0%. The recurrent ischemia rate, however, was frequent; rehospitalization was required in more than one third of the patients, and repeat revascularization was performed in 28%. Ten percent of the patients underwent CABG within 12 months. Thus, it appears that although PTCA may be an acceptable therapeutic option in patients with unstable angina, it is associated with the need for repeat revascularization procedures. It is also important to note that most patients in this study had single-vessel disease, and left ventricular function was only mildly compromised.

Adjunctive Therapy to PCI

To minimize the complications of acute coronary occlusion and restenosis after PTCA (35%-45% at 6 months), contemporary catheter-based revascularization now includes coronary stenting and the adjuvant use of platelet GP IIb/IIIa receptor inhibitors. The platelet GP IIb/IIIa receptor is a site for fibrinogen binding and promotes platelet aggregation. Binding of greater than 80% of these receptors results in potent antithrombosis. The ready availability of these inhibitors (abciximab, tirofiban, eptifi-

batide) has led to several multicenter clinical trials to address their efficacy. In the Evaluation of Platelet IIb/IIIa Inhibitor for Stenting (EPISTENT) trial, patients who underwent PTCA for UA/NSTEMI were randomized to stent use and abciximab therapy versus placebo.[23] The stent patients also received ASA and the thienopyridine ticlopidine. Adjunctive use of abciximab was associated with a reduction in death, MI, and urgent revascularization at 30 days. It was also associated, however, with a higher incidence of severe bleeding. After 1 year, the mortality rate for the stented patients with abciximab was also less in the diabetic patients. In contrast, in a meta-analysis of six randomized, placebo-controlled trials of patients with UA/NSTEMI receiving GP IIb/IIIa antagonists, there was only a slight reduction in death or MI in patients undergoing stenting. Major bleeding complications, however, remained a problem.

Thienopyridines, adenosine diphosphate (ADP) inhibitors like ticlopidine and clopidogrel, are also used to prevent the activation of platelets and thrombosis and have been studied in patients treated conservatively and with PCI. The Clopidogrel in Unstable Angina to Prevent Recurrent Ischemic Events (CURE) trial evaluated the effectiveness of clopidogrel in the noninterventional management of patients with UA.[24] Treatment was associated with a lower rate of death, MI, and stroke, but with a higher rate of major bleeding. In the PCI CURE trial, patients were randomized to clopidogrel and ASA, or placebo and ASA, preprocedurally and for 1 month after the procedure. PCI with adjuvant clopidogrel and ASA demonstrated a reduction in cardiac death and MI.[25] Although promising, it is premature to conclude that all patients with UA/NSTEMI with or without PCI should be treated with IIb/IIIa receptor or adenosine diphosphate inhibitors. This is due, in part, to the differences in clinical trial design that pertain to entry criteria and definable end points and the lack of sufficient long-term follow-up. It does appear, however, that coronary stenting and antiplatelet therapy improve the efficacy and durability of PCI in managing patients with UA/NSTEMI. A major advantage to using thienopyridines as adjunct therapy is the lower bleeding complication rates compared with the GP IIb/IIIa inhibitors.

CABG Versus Medical Management

One of the first studies to evaluate the role of CABG in the treatment of patients with UA/NSTEMI was reported by Parisi and colleagues.[12] Patients were stratified by clinical presentation and invasive evaluation of left ventricular function. Clinical presentations included progressive or new-onset angina and prolonged episodes of angina unrelieved by medication. *Abnormal left ventricular function* was defined as an EF of less than 0.50. Five-year follow-up revealed important survival differences in patients with three-vessel disease. The survival rate for the CABG patients was 89%, whereas it was only 75% for medically treated patients. CABG was also associated with fewer subsequent hospitalizations. At 8-years of follow-up, Sharma and colleagues reported that the cumulative survival rates for patients with severe rest angina associated with ST-T changes on the ECG and abnormal left ventricular function were higher in surgical patients than in medically treated patients (87% versus 54%).[26] In another analysis of the data, medical therapy was determined to be the preferred therapy with UA patients with only one- or two-vessel disease and normal EF, whereas surgery enhanced survival in patients with three-vessel disease or low EF.[27] These and other studies demonstrate that CABG is an effective treatment for the management of unstable angina and is associated with sustained symptom relief and excellent long-term survival (see Table 61-3).

CABG Versus PCI

With increasing evidence that PCI can be performed safely with good long-term survival rates in patients with chronic stable angina, PCI has now been expanded to treat patients with unstable angina. This has led to clinical trials designed to compare the survival rates between CABG and PCI for patients with UA/NSTEMI. The Angina with Extremely Serious Operative Mortality Evaluation (AWESOME) trial[28] randomized patients with medically refractory myocardial ischemia and risk factors for adverse outcomes with CABG into two groups: CABG or PCI. The 30-day survival rates for CABG and PCI were 95% and 97%, respectively. At 3 years, the survival rates were 79% and 80%. Thus, PCI appeared to be an acceptable alternative to CABG in patients with medically refractory myocardial ischemia. In a subanalysis of the ARTS trial, patients with multivessel disease and unstable angina were compared with patients with stable angina randomized to either PCI with stent implantation or CABG using arterial grafts.[29] Similar to the AWESOME trial, there was no difference in the rate of major adverse events at 1 year. The need, however, for repeat revascularization was higher in the stented PCI patients. As described earlier, the long-term mortality benefit seen with CABG favors the use of CABG over PCI as the first intervention for patients with unstable angina who have coronary anatomy amenable to bypass grafting.

STEMI/AMI

PCI Versus Medical Management for AMI

The role of primary angioplasty in the treatment of patients with STEMI/AMI is controversial. In a meta-analysis that included PTCA as an adjunct to primary thrombolysis, there was no improvement in survival with delayed PTCA after thrombolytics.[29] In this analysis, there was a trend toward an increase in the combined end points of death and MI for patients who underwent deliberate PTCA within a few days of infarction.

When PTCA as an initial therapy was compared with the use of thrombolytics; however, there was a significant reduction in both in-hospital and 6-week mortality and combined MI/mortality in the PTCA patients. These findings suggest that PTCA has a survival advantage over thrombolytics as an initial treatment for STEMI/AMI and that use of delayed PTCA as an adjunct to therapy, including thrombolytics, does not affect survival. In the Global Use of Strategies to Open Occluded Coronary Arteries in Acute Coronary Syndromes (GUSTO) IIb trial,[30] the com-

posite end point of death, nonfatal MI, and nonfatal disabling stroke at 30 days was 9.6% for PTCA and 13.7% for thrombolytics. At 6 months, however, the outcomes were similar. This study suggests that although PTCA may confer a short-term benefit over medical management and thrombolytics, the benefit does not persist over time. In contrast, a retrospective review of the National Registry of Myocardial Infarction (NRMI-2)[31] comparing PTCA and thrombolytic therapy for STEMI/AMI, showed no difference in in-house mortality (5.2% versus 5.4%) or reinfarction rates (2.5% versus 2.9%). However, in the cohort of patients who presented in cardiogenic shock, there was a survival advantage of 68% for PTCA versus 48% for thrombolytics. In general, however, there appears to be no major advantage to PTCA in patients with STEMI/AMI.

Role of CABG

In patients with AMI, CABG is usually performed in conjunction with an operation to treat a specific complication. Examples include refractory postinfarction angina, papillary muscle rupture with mitral regurgitation, and infarction ventricular septal defect. The rationale for urgent or emergent surgery is often based on high early mortality due to mechanical complications. Because there are an increasing number of patients who undergo catheterization early after AMI, it is not surprising that there has been an increase in the number of patients who are identified as candidates for surgery. The controversial aspect is the timing because the early operative mortality rate may be as low as 5% in patients with a subendocardial infarction or as high as 25% in patients with poor ventricular function.

In general, patients who were operated on early after AMI are sicker, are refractory to medical therapy, have a higher incidence of renal insufficiency, require IABP insertion, are older, or have sustained a previous MI. In one study, the mortality rates for patients undergoing urgent or emergent CABG less than 6 hours, 6 hours to 2 days, 2 to 14 days, 2 to 6 weeks, and more than 6 weeks after MI were 9.1%, 8.3%, 5.2%, 6.5%, and 2.9%, respectively.[32] There was also a twofold higher mortality rate in patients undergoing CABG in less than 48 hours versus more than 48 hours. The use of preoperative IABP was associated with an improvement in operative mortality. Thus, CABG after uncomplicated MI can be accomplished with acceptable mortality rates provided appropriate supportive interventions, including IABP, are used early to stabilize the patient before surgery. In STEMI/AMI patients who cannot be stabilized with aggressive medical therapy and nonsurgical interventional support, CABG should be entertained if the coronary anatomy is acceptable, and a specific mechanical defect can be corrected.

CABG and Special Patient Populations

Diabetes

Patients with diabetes mellitus are at increased risk for developing CAD. This is a significant problem because CAD accounts for 75% of deaths in diabetic patients.

Likewise, the mortality rate after CABG is higher in diabetic patients than it is for the general population. In the prospective, randomized BARI trial (see Table 61-3), CABG mortality rates in diabetic patients receiving saphenous vein grafts only or PTCA were high, 18.2% and 20.6%, respectively. The mortality rate was considerably lower, however, in surgery patients who received ITA grafts (2.9%). In the EAST trial (see Table 61-3), the findings were less conclusive, but there was a similar trend that favored surgery. Thus, CABG that includes ITA grafts appears to be the treatment of choice for diabetic patients. Currently, the Bypass Angioplasty Revascularization Investigation 2 Diabetes (BARI 2D) trial is underway to determine whether treatment targeted to attenuate insulin resistance can arrest or retard progression of CAD and whether early revascularization reduces the mortality and morbidity in patients with type II diabetes whose symptoms are mild and stable.[33]

Women

Although women in every age group have a lower incidence of CAD than men, CAD is still the leading cause of death in women in the United States. Historically, serious manifestations and associated complications of CAD in women were considered uncommon. This may explain, in part, why women have received less intensive management and invasive treatment. For these reasons, and the fact that the early studies evaluating the efficacy of CABG focused primarily on men, the objective of more recent studies has been to determine whether female gender is an independent risk factor for complications after interventional therapy. In the TIMI IIIB registry, the rates of MI and death at 6 weeks after thrombolytics and PCI for UA/NSTEMI were similar for women and men.[34] This was true even though the women were older and had significantly more comorbidities (hypertension, diabetes). Multivessel disease was, however, less common in women: women had fewer critical coronary lesions of 60% or more stenosis, and their mean EF was higher. This may explain why fewer women (19%) underwent CABG than men (27%). Among the CABG patients, the 6-week mortality rate, however, was higher for women (albeit the total number of deaths in the study was only 7). When age was factored into a multivariate analysis of the data, gender was not linked to outcome.

In contrast, examination of the Society of Thoracic Surgeons (STS) database in two separate studies revealed that the operative mortality rate was higher in women, namely 3.15% versus 2.61%.[35,36] The database consisted of 97,153 women and 247,760 men. In this analysis, the mean left ventricular function was better in women, and women received fewer ITA grafts, were older, and had more comorbidities (diabetes, hypertension, peripheral vascular disease) than men.

Similar findings were observed in a retrospective age-stratified analysis of 51,187 patients (number of women, 15,178 [29.7%]) in the National Cardiovascular Network database.[37] In this study, women experienced a nearly twofold increase in hospital mortality after CABG (5.3% versus 2.9%). Gender-based adjusted mortality, however, decreased inversely with age. Specifically, although women younger than 50 years had a twofold increase in mortality, this differential decreased with age and disappeared in patients older than 79 years. Women also experienced more postoperative complications, such as renal failure (5.0% versus 4.0%), neurologic complications (5.3% versus 3.8%), and postoperative MI (1.7% versus 1.3%). Although these findings suggest that women do experience more complications and are at a higher risk for death after CABG, it is unclear why the mortality rate was inversely related to age and the complication occurred most frequently in women younger than 50 years. It is also important to recognize that retrospective studies using a voluntary database have inherent limitations.

During the past decade, there has been a renewed interest in women's health, including important gender issues related to CABG. It is now well accepted that there are major differences in the risk profile of men compared with the profile of women undergoing CABG procedures.[35,37] Even when both genders share a common risk factor, the relative impact of a risk factor is often quite different in men than in women.[35] Furthermore, an intervention to medically address the same risk factor may evoke a very different response between the genders. Perhaps most importantly, a given postoperative complication appears to have a much more deleterious effect on women than on men who have the same complication. Because of possible gender-related differences in outcome from CABG, the STS Evidence Based Workforce undertook a study to summarize available evidence on gender differences in CABG-related outcomes. Table 61-4 summarizes key findings of this study.

Renal Disease

Renal insufficiency is also an independent risk factor for survival after CABG. A serum creatinine level greater than 2.0 mg/dL is associated with a twofold increase in mortality. It has been estimated that about 14% of patients undergoing CABG have some degree of *renal insufficiency* when it is defined as a serum creatinine level greater than 1.5 mg/dL. In one retrospective study[38] of 59,576 patients who underwent either CABG or PCI, a survival benefit with CABG in patients with a serum creatinine level of more than 2.5 mg/dL was demonstrated. The 1-, 2-, and 3-year survival rates were 84.1%, 77.4%, and 65.9%, respectively, for CABG compared with 70.8%, 51.9%, and 46.1% for PCI. This survival differential was not attributed to differences in left ventricular function, severity of CAD, and incidence of comorbidities. In another retrospective study[39] of 15,784 hemodialysis-dependent patients undergoing CABG, PTCA alone, and PTCA with stent, there was also a survival advantage for CABG. Although early mortality was higher for CABG (8.6%) versus PTCA (6.4%) or stenting (4.1%), mortality equalized at 6 to 9 months. At 2 years, survival was demonstrably better with CABG. Compared with PTCA, CABG provided a 20% reduction in death risk, whereas PTCA with stenting only provided a 6% survival advantage. This effect was more dramatic in diabetic patients, in which CABG was associated with a 27% lower risk for death. Thus, although CABG in patients with renal insuf-

Table 61-4 Gender-Specific Recommendations for Women Undergoing CABG

FINDING	RECOMMENDATION	CLASS	LEVEL OF EVIDENCE
The internal mammary artery is underutilized in women undergoing CABG procedures. The internal mammary artery confers a protective effect that is associated with a significant reduction in CABG mortality as compared with surgical revascularization with venous conduits alone.	Whenever it is technically possible, at least one internal mammary artery should be used in every CABG procedure.	I	B
Perioperative blood glucose >150 mg/dL is associated with increased operative morbidity and mortality.	Perioperative blood glucose levels should be maintained in the range of 100 to 150 mg/dL.	I	B
Intraoperative hematocrit levels below 22% are associated with an increased incidence of adverse outcomes.	Efforts should be made to ensure adequate intraoperative hematocrit levels.	IIa	B
There is no evidence to establish the superiority of OPCAB over conventional CABG using cardiopulmonary bypass.	The indications for OPCAB are the same for women as for men.	IIa	B
Low intraoperative levels of levothyroxine and free thyroxin are associated with a high CABG mortality rate in hypothyroid women.	Hypothyroid women undergoing CABG should be maintained in a euthyroid state during and after operation.	IIa	C
HRT is linked to several complications including serious thromboembolic events. Its use in CABG procedures is of questionable value.	HRT should not be used for postmenopausal women undergoing CABG.	III	B

CABG, coronary artery bypass grafting; OPCAB, off-pump coronary artery bypass; HRT, hormone replacement therapy.
From Mentzer RM Jr: Does size matter? What is your infarct rate after coronary artery bypass grafting? J Thorac Cardiovasc Surg 126(2):326-328, 2003.

ficiency and failure is associated with increased morbidity and mortality, CABG is associated with better survival when compared with PCI.

Obesity

Obesity is a known risk factor for CAD, diabetes, hypertension, and stroke and is associated with a 50% to 100% higher risk for all-cause mortality when compared with age-matched peers. Thus it is not surprising that obesity is generally assumed to be a risk factor for adverse events after CABG. It is important to note, however, that contrary to various assumptions, there is a lack of agreement as to whether obesity per se is an independent predictor of mortality. In one retrospective, multicenter study of 11,101 patients undergoing CABG,[40] the mortality was similar in *nonobese* (body mass index [BMI] <31), *moderately obese* (BMI 31-36), and *severely obese* (BMI >36) patients. Although sternal wound infections were more frequent in the moderately and severely obese patients, the incidence of bleeding complications and cerebral vascular accidents were the same.

In contrast, an adjusted multivariate analysis of data in the STS National Cardiac Database revealed that operative mortality was elevated in both the moderately and severely obese patient. In addition, the incidences of postoperative renal failure, prolonged ventilation, and sternal wound infection were also significantly higher. In this analysis, *obesity* was defined as follows: *normal/mild* (BMI <35), *moderate* (BMI 35-39.9), and *extreme* (BMI ≥40). Thus, although obesity may affect morbidity,

its impact on mortality is unclear. This may be due to the marked variability of the definition of obesity, a reliance on anecdotal experience, and the observational nature of the studies to date.

Reoperation for Coronary Artery Disease

Within 5 years, 15% of CABG patients experience a recurrence of symptoms, typically angina. This increases to about 40% within 10 years. Recurrent symptoms almost always indicate progression of disease in the native coronary circulation or graft disease. In most cases, the indications to proceed with coronary angiography, PCI with or without stenting, or repeat CABG are the same as for the first operation. Patients who are considered candidates for reoperative CABG are usually older, have more diffuse CAD, and have diminished ventricular function. Factors that increase the risk for reoperation include the absence of an ITA graft, younger age at the time of primary surgery, prior incomplete revascularization, congestive heart failure, and New York Heart Association class III or IV angina. Reoperative CABG differs from that of the primary procedure in that care is taken to avoid injury to the patent grafts. Manipulation of the old grafts is kept to a minimum to avoid distal coronary bed microembolization. The mortality rate of reoperative CABG may exceed that of primary CABG; in some series, it has been reported to be as high as 10%. Although reoperative CABG can be performed safely, overall patient survival and freedom from angina over time are diminished. Maximal survival and freedom from reoperation are best achieved in patients by aggressive management of risk factors such as diabetes mellitus, hypercholesterolemia, hypertension, and smoking.

Complications of Coronary Artery Disease Amenable to Surgery

A region of the ventricular wall that is akinetic or dyskinetic and results in a reduction in left ventricular EF is termed a *ventricular aneurysm*. Surgical treatment is designed to improve ventricular geometry and thus function, and often includes the use of prosthetic materials to restore normal ventricular geometry, chamber volume, and normalize ventricular wall tension. The incidence of ventricular aneurysm after AMI has been reported to be as high as 35%. This has been declining due, in part, to the early and aggressive application of interventional therapies. Ninety percent of left ventricular aneurysms are the result of a transmural MI secondary to an acute occlusion of the LAD. Patients may develop an aneurysm as early as 48 hours after infarction, but most patients do so within weeks. About two thirds of patients who develop ventricular aneurysms remain asymptomatic.

The 10-year survival rate of these patients may exceed 90%. In contrast, the 10-year survival rate for symptomatic patients is less than 50%. The most common causes of death are arrhythmias (>40%), congestive heart failure (>30%), and recurrent MI (>10%). Mortality is influenced by the patient's age, onset of heart failure, extent of CAD, presence of mitral regurgitation, incidence and types of ventricular arrhythmias, and reduced left ventricular function. The risk for thromboembolism is low, and long-term anticoagulation is not recommended, with the exception of those patients who have evidence of a mural thrombus. The diagnosis is usually made by echocardiography. Thallium imaging or PET is useful in detecting the extent of the aneurysm and viability of adjacent regions. In general, patients with symptoms of angina, congestive heart failure, or refractory arrhythmias should be considered candidates for CABG and resection of the aneurysm. Patients with a contained rupture or evidence of a false aneurysm should undergo surgery soon after the diagnosis is made because these have a tendency to rupture spontaneously. Patients experiencing thromboembolic events despite anticoagulation are also candidates for surgery. The most common cause of postoperative death is heart failure. The 5-year survival rate after surgery has been reported to range between 60% and 80%. In general, surgical repair or resection in conjunction with CABG results in angina relief and resolution of heart failure symptoms for most patients.

Another complication of AMI is a postinfarction ventricular septal defect (VSD). This occurs in about 5% of patients and is associated with an acute vessel occlusion. The defect is more common in men (3:2) and typically presents within 2 to 4 days of the infarction. The VSD is usually located in the anterior or apical aspect of the ventricular septum. About 25% of patients present with a defect in the posterior aspect of the ventricular septum. This is more commonly associated with an inferior wall MI and is secondary to an occlusion of the RCA system or a distal branch of the LCA. About one third of the patients have evidence of a transient AV conduction block before the onset of septal rupture. A new, loud systolic cardiac murmur after an MI suggests the diagnosis and is an indication for echocardiography. The echocardiogram is effective in determining the size and character of the VSD, as well as the degree of left-to-right shunting. Right heart catheterization typically shows a step up in oxygen saturation levels in the right ventricle and pulmonary artery. After the diagnosis is established, patients should undergo immediate left heart catheterization to characterize the degree of CAD, the magnitude of left ventricular dysfunction, and presence of mitral valve insufficiency. About 60% of patients with an infarction VSD have significant CAD in an unrelated vessel. The mortality rate in the untreated patient is high, with 25% of the patients dying within 24 hours from refractory heart failure. Patient survival rates at 1 week, 1 month, and more than 1 year are 50%, 20%, and less than 10%, respectively. Patients who are considered candidates for surgery should be managed early with closure of the defect and concomitant CABG. In the absence of refractory heart failure and hemodynamic instability, the survival rate may be as high as 75%.

Ischemic mitral regurgitation (IMR) may occur early or late and, depending on the severity of left ventricular dysfunction, may be life threatening. About 40% of patients who sustain an AMI develop IMR that is detectable by color-flow Doppler echocardiography. In 3% to 4% of cases, the degree of mitral regurgitation is moderate or severe. Acute IMR may occur as a result of papillary muscle necrosis and rupture due to occlusion of overlying epicardial arteries that give rise to penetrating vessels that supply the papillary muscles. The posterior papillary muscle is involved three to six times more often than the anterior muscle, and either the entire trunk of the muscle or one of the heads to which chordae attach may partially or totally rupture. Another cause of IMR is ischemic papillary muscle dysfunction. The pathogenesis of acute and chronic IMR in the absence of papillary muscle rupture is not completely understood but appears to be related to deformations of ventricular geometry. Patients usually present with chest pain and shortness of breath and evidence of pulmonary edema, hypotension, and a heart murmur that radiates into the left axilla. The chest x-ray shows signs of pulmonary congestion with interstitial pulmonary edema and cardiomegaly. Right heart catheterization demonstrates elevated pulmonary artery pressures with prominent v waves, low mixed venous oxygen saturation, and low cardiac output. Transthoracic or transesophageal echocardiography is often diagnostic, but left heart catheterization is helpful in defining coronary artery anatomy. In most cases, prompt surgical intervention provides the best chance for survival. Predictors of in-hospital death include congestive heart failure, renal insufficiency, and multivessel CAD. Emergent surgical treatment usually involves mitral valve replacement and concomitant CABG. The hospital mortality rate may be as high as 50%, although in selected patients, the mortality rate may be as low as 10% to 15%. The operation for chronic IMR is usually performed on an elective basis and more often consists of complete myocardial revascularization and mitral valve repair rather than replacement.

CORONARY ARTERY BYPASS OPERATIONS: TECHNICAL ASPECTS

Cardiopulmonary Bypass

The basic components of an extracorporeal heart pump circuit consist of one or more venous cannulas, a venous reservoir that collects blood by gravity, an oxygenator and heat exchanger, a perfusion pump, a blood filter in the arterial line, and an arterial cannula (Fig. 61-11). The cardiopulmonary bypass (CPB) machine is constructed from a variety of biocompatible materials that can include polycarbonate, polyvinylchloride, Teflon, polyethylene, stainless steel, titanium, silicone rubber, and polyurethane. The blood conduits are designed to minimize turbulence, cavitation, changes in blood flow velocity, and the volume of nonblood solutions necessary to prime the pump and tubing. The circuitry has multiple access ports or sites to obtain blood samples for laboratory studies and the infusion of blood, blood products, crystalloids, or drugs.

Supplemental components include a cardiotomy suction system to collect undiluted or "clean" blood from open cardiac chambers and the surgical field. This blood is filtered, de-aired, and returned to the bypass pump. Diluted field blood and blood that has been exposed to potentially harmful elements (e.g., inflammatory cytokines, fat) are collected through a separate system device that concentrates washed red cells before returning them directly to the patient. A cardioplegia infusion device consists of a separate pump, reservoir, and heat exchanger. It is used to deliver cold potassium-enriched blood or crystalloid solutions into the coronary circulation to protect the heart during ischemic arrest. About 2 liters of solution is required to prime the heart pump for adults. The priming solution consists of a balanced salt solution and often a starch solution. Homologous blood is not usually added unless the patient is anemic, that is, the hematocrit is less than 25. Use of CPB requires suppression of the clotting cascade with heparin because the components of the bypass pump and the surgical wound are powerful stimuli for thrombus formation. Systemic heparinization may, however, result in increased blood loss and the requirements for homologous blood and blood product transfusions. Heparin can also induce transient hypotension as a result of an allergic reaction.

The oxygen consumption of a patient on CPB at normal temperatures averages 80 to 125 mL/min/m², similar to the anesthetized adult not on bypass. Although a pump flow rate of 2.2 L/min/m² meets the metabolic needs of most patients and avoids acidosis, a flow rate of 2.5 L/min/m² ensures perfusion of the microcirculation and adds a margin of safety. If hypothermia is employed, the flow rate can be reduced to less than 2.2 L/min/m².

This is because the mean oxygen consumption of the body decreases by 50% for every 10°C decrease in body temperature. Below 28°C, a flow rate of 1.6 L/min/m² may be safe for as long as 2 hours. Significant disadvantages of using systemic hypothermia to accommodate lower flow rates include the extra time required to rewarm the patient and associated alterations that occur in the reactivity of blood elements, particularly platelets. The latter may result in a greater propensity for bleeding once the patient has been rewarmed. During CPB, the systemic blood pressure is maintained by adjusting the speed of the roller pump, manipulating the patient's intravascular volume, and adjusting the peripheral vascular resistance by infusing vasodilators such as nitroprusside or nitroglycerin or vasoconstrictors like ephedrine. In general, the mean normothermic blood pressure should be maintained between 50 and 70 mm Hg. The perfusion pressure may be maintained 10 to 15 mm Hg higher if a patient is known to have significant obstructive intracranial or carotid artery disease.

Myocardial Protection Techniques

With the advent of CABG, it was evident that some patients experienced varying degrees of myocardial injury and necrosis despite adequate myocardial revascularization. Many of these patients died from heart failure or experienced prolonged periods of low cardiac output. Ultimately, it was determined that this necrosis occurred as a result of ischemic damage sustained during the time of aortic cross-clamping and ischemic arrest. As a result, a number of methodologies and techniques have evolved during the past 50 years to prevent this complication (Table 61-5). The cornerstone, however, is the use of systemic hypothermia and the infusion of cold hyperkalemic crystalloid or blood solutions directly into the proximal ascending aorta after placement of the aortic cross-clamp. The latter results in diastolic arrest of the heart, a marked reduction in myocardial oxygen consumption, and a quiescent operative field.

Currently, there are a number of different ways to deliver cardioplegic solutions (Table 61-6). One technique involves a balanced approach, that is, the cardioplegic solution is administered first antegrade through the proximal ascending aorta, and then retrograde through a coronary sinus catheter inserted through a purse-string suture placed in the right atrium. The extensive collateralization among the coronary veins and arteries and the paucity of valves within the coronary vein system ensure a relatively homogeneous distribution of cardioplegia when the retrograde approach is used. Patients with high-grade proximal lesions, especially those with suboptimal collateral vessels, may benefit from the application of both techniques. After the initial administration of cardioplegia, additional doses are usually administered every 15 to 20 minutes. The temperature of the myocardium can be continuously monitored with an intracardiac probe. For patients with significant ventricular hypertrophy and those without obvious adequate collateral vessels, shorter intervals between infusions may be required.

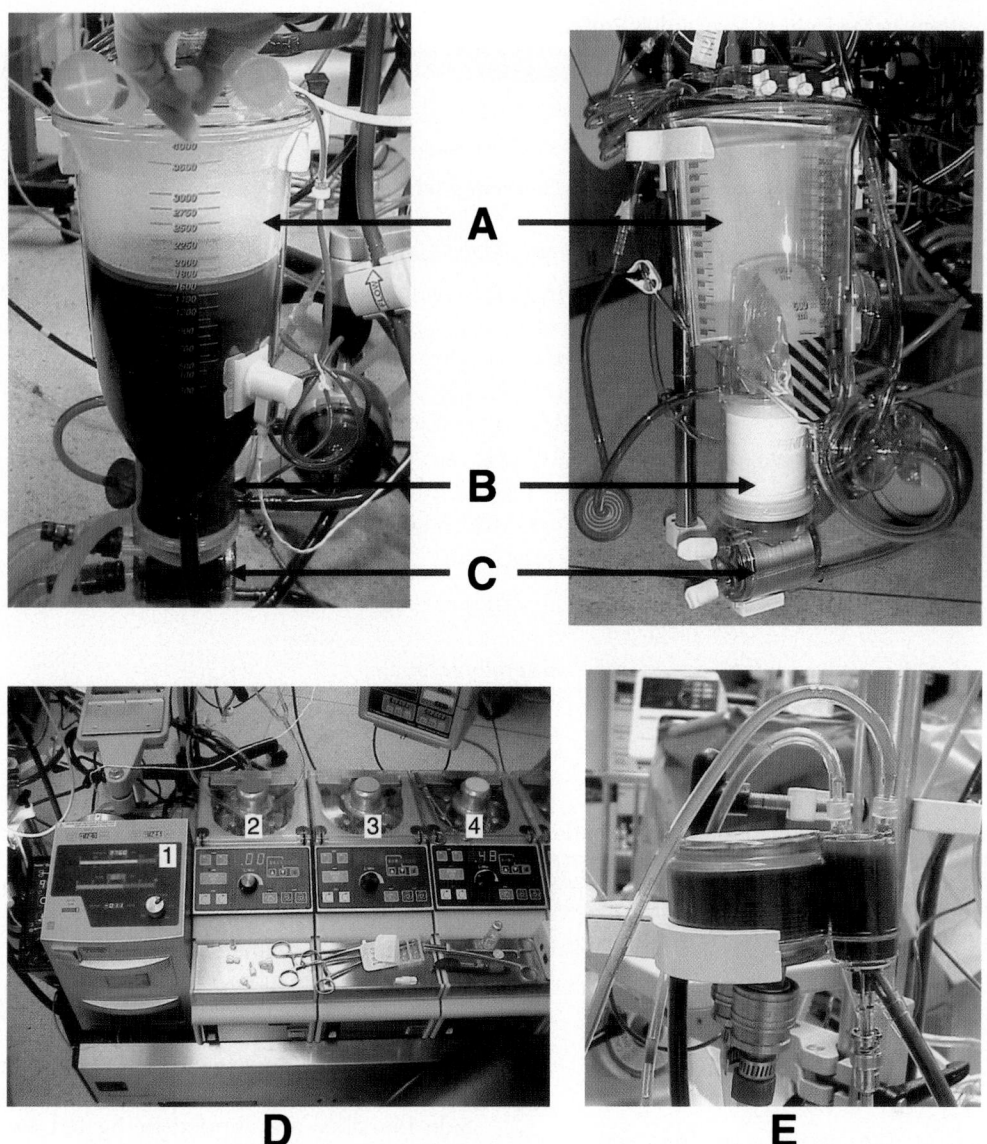

Figure 61-11 Components of cardiopulmonary bypass (CPB) system: *A* indicates the venous reservoir and blood filter; *B* indicates the membrane oxygenator; and *C* indicates the heat exchange coil. *D* shows the following components: (1) CPB control console, (2) roller pump for infusing oxygenated blood, (3) cardioplegia, and (4) controlling suction catheters. E is the cardioplegia reservoir and heat exchanger. (Courtesy of the Division of Cardiothoracic Surgery, University of Kentucky, 2003.)

Conduits for Coronary Artery Bypass Grafting

The internal thoracic arteries (ITAs, left and right) are the preferred conduits because their patency rates exceed 90% at 10 years.[41] The left ITA is generally used to graft the LAD, and reversed saphenous vein segments are used to graft the remaining vessels. The right ITA pedicle can be used to graft the RCA; if it is of sufficient length, it can be used to graft the PDA or branches of the LCA. The advantage of using these conduits must be weighed against the potential risks in specific subsets of patients. For example, diabetic patients may be at increased risk for infection. In these patients, bilateral ITA mobilization has been associated with a 14-fold increase in the risk for sternal wound infections. Because there is some evidence that there may be a survival benefit associated with using only arterial grafts, the radial artery is often used in conjunction with ITA grafts to revascularize the heart. Use of arterial grafts only has the added advantages of eliminating the need for lower extremity incisions and the risk for leg wound infections. Before making a forearm incision, an Allen test is performed, and the palmar arch is evaluated using ultrasound to confirm the presence of adequate collateral circulation in the hand. The radial artery is then procured using a no-touch technique. Before its removal, the adequacy of arterial flow to the respective hand can be assessed by direct compression of the proximal end of the vessel. Systemic

Table 61-5   Innovations in the Field of Myocardial Protection

INVESTIGATORS	YEAR	INNOVATION
Bigelow	1950	Studied the application of hypothermia to cardiac surgery in canines
Melrose & Bentall	1955	Introduced the concept of reversible chemical cardiac arrest in canines
Lillehei	1956	Detailed a method for delivering hypothermic crystalloid cardioplegia by cannulating coronary arteries
Gerbode & Melrose	1958	Used potassium citrate to induce cardiac arrest in humans
Bretschneider	1964	Developed a sodium-poor, calcium-free, procaine-containing solution to arrest the heart
Sondergaard	1964	Adopted Bretschneider's cardioplegic solution and was one of the first to routinely use it for myocardial protection in clinical practice
Gay & Ebert	1973	Credited with revival of potassium-induced cardioplegia; demonstrated that potassium solution could arrest a canine heart for 60 minutes without cellular damage
Hearse	1975	Emphasized preischemic infusions to negate ischemic injuries in rats; this formula became known as *St. Thomas solution No. 1*
Braimbridge	1975	One of the first to use St. Thomas solution No. 1 clinically
Buckberg	1979	Introduced the use of blood as the vehicle for infusing potassium into coronary arteries
Akins	1984	Utilized technique of hypothermic fibrillatory arrest for coronary revascularization without cardioplegia
Lichenstein & Salemo	1991	Introduced warm-blood cardioplegia

Table 61-6   Methods and Delivery of Cardioplegic Solutions

INFUSION TYPES	INFUSION TEMPERATURES	INFUSION INTERVALS
Antegrade	Tepid	Continuous
Retrograde	Warm	Intermittent
Combined retrograde and antegrade	Cold	

vasodilators, such as nitroglycerin, are frequently used during the dissection to minimize vasospasm. The free graft is then stored in a solution containing heparin and papaverine. Another pedicled arterial conduit that can be used is the gastroepiploic artery (GEA). This conduit is more appropriate for vessels in the inferior and lateral portions of the left ventricle. Limitations associated with the use of this graft include its predilection for vasospasm, twisting, kinking, and vulnerability to technical error at the anastomotic site due to its thin arterial wall. In general, use of the GEA is reserved for patients with limited conduit options.

The most commonly used conduit is the greater saphenous vein. Whether the right or left leg is chosen depends on a variety of factors such as evidence of previous saphenous vein stripping, venous stasis disease, arterial vascular insufficiency, presence of nonhealing wounds, varicose veins, or history of superficial thrombophlebitis. The adequacy of the vein can be assessed preoperatively using Doppler ultrasound. This technique can also be used to map the anatomic location of the vessel to minimize the extent of the lower extremity incision. Tech-

niques that are used to procure the saphenous vein include a single long incision over the vein, multiple small incisions with bridges of intact skin, and endoscopic dissection. In general, the ideal saphenous vein should have a diameter of 3.5 mm, with no varicosities or areas of stricture. The bridged or endoscopic technique minimizes the length of the skin incision and is associated with lower infection rates and less postoperative pain. Stretching or manipulation of the vessel is minimized to avoid endothelial injury and thrombosis. Side branches are clipped or ligated to avoid bleeding complications in the postoperative period. The leg incisions are closed in layers to eliminate dead space and avoid hematoma formation and decrease the risk for infection. The vein conduit is then stored in heparinized saline or blood until it is needed. Vein graft patency rates have been reported to be 88% early after grafting, 81% at 1 year, 75% at 5 years, and 50% at 15 years. Venous graft occlusion rate is about 2% per year.[42] If the saphenous vein is inadequate or unavailable, the lesser saphenous vein can be used.

Anesthesia for Myocardial Revascularization

Major advances in cardiac anesthesia during the past 5 years primarily reflect improvements in techniques and methodologies. For example, high-dose narcotic anesthesia, which was routinely used a decade ago, has evolved into a method of balanced anesthesia. This involves the judicious use of shorter-acting narcotics, such as remifentanil, supplemented by safer volatile agents, like sevoflurane, or short-acting IV agents, such as propofol. The use of short-acting agents has resulted in less ventilatory

Table 61-7   Foundation Studies of Patients With Stable Ischemic Heart Disease Used to Evaluate CABG Surgery Outcomes*

STUDY	REFERENCE	CONCLUSIONS
Veterans Administration Coronary Artery Bypass Surgery Cooperative Study Group: Eleven-year survival in the Veterans Administration randomized trial of coronary bypass surgery for stable angina	N Engl J Med 311:1333-1339, 1984	Survival advantage was associated with CABG surgery when CAD included LM and/or 3VD with impaired LV function.
Varnauskas E, European Coronary Surgery Study Group: Twelve-year European Coronary Surgery Study.	N Engl J Med 319:332-337, 1988	CABG surgery was associated with increased survival in patients with LM disease, 3VD, decreased LV function, and proximal LAD stenosis 12 years from randomization. Peak advantage was observed at 5 years.
Coronary Artery Surgery Study (CASS) principal investigators and associates: CASS: A randomized trial of coronary bypass surgery symptoms.	Circulation 68:939-950, 1983	CABG surgery and nonoperative management were associated with similar survival rates. Surgery could be safely deferred until onset of symptoms.
Norris RM, Agnew TM, Brandt PWT, et al: Coronary surgery after recurrent myocardial infarction: Progress of a trial comparing surgical with nonsurgical management for asymptomatic patients with advanced coronary disease.	Circulation 63:785-792, 1981	CABG surgery conferred survival advantage in patients with LM disease and/or 3VD with decreased LV function.
Mathur VS, Guinn GA: Prospective randomized study of the surgical therapy of stable angina.	Cardiovasc Clin 8:131-144, 1977	CABG surgery was associated with superior improvement in symptoms and quality of life.
Kloster FE, Kremkau EL, Ritzman LW, et al: Coronary bypass for stable angina.	N Engl J Med 300:149-157, 1979	CABG surgery resulted in greater functional improvement and less UA compared with medical therapy; there was no difference in death or myocardial infarction after 3 years.

*Used by Michels and Yusuf[29] in meta-analysis.

3VD, three-vessel disease; CABG, coronary artery bypass grafting; CAD, coronary artery disease; LAD, left anterior descending artery; LM, left main; LV, left ventricular; UA, unstable angina.

support time, shorter intensive care unit stay, and a decrease in hospital length of stay. There is also an increase in the use of supplemental techniques, such as regional, epidural, and paraspinal blocks to reduce the use of systemic agents, improve analgesic control, and improve postoperative pulmonary function. Maintaining control of the mean arterial blood pressure to preserve the cerebral perfusion pressure minimizes postoperative neuropsychometric and neurocognitive dysfunction. Also, real-time cerebral bispectral index monitoring, although somewhat controversial, can be used to predict anesthetic depth and avoid excess narcotic anesthesia. Adequate oxygen delivery is assured by maintaining a hematocrit of at least 25% during and after CPB. Finally, there is evidence that tight glycemic control in diabetic patients undergoing CABG may improve survival and decrease recurrent ischemic events. Perioperative serum glucose levels should be maintained between 100 and 150 mg/dL.

The use of intraoperative transesophageal echocardiography (TEE) represents another major advance in cardiac anesthesia. It is particularly useful in assessing myocardial function before and after CPB. Perioperative myocardial ischemia manifested by new regional wall motion abnormalities can often be detected before ischemic changes in the ECG and elevation in pulmonary artery pressures. TEE can also be used to determine the presence of intracavitary air and the ventricular response to increasing intravascular volume. This information can be helpful in deciding the optimum time to wean the patient from CPB.

With off-pump coronary artery bypass (OPCAB) surgery, there is, in general, a greater requirement for increased monitoring and circulatory support, particularly during cardiac manipulation and periods of isolated coronary occlusion. This includes a more dynamic administration of inotropic and chronotropic agents, intravascular volume loading and the administration of antiarrhythmic medications. This has enabled myocardial revascularization to be performed safely without CPB and is responsible, in part, for the wider application of OPCAB surgery (Table 61-7).

The Operation

Preparation for CABG includes the administration of preoperative antibiotics (e.g., cefuroxime 1.5 g IV or vancomycin 1.0 g IV for a patient with penicillin allergy) at least 30 minutes before making the skin incision. After

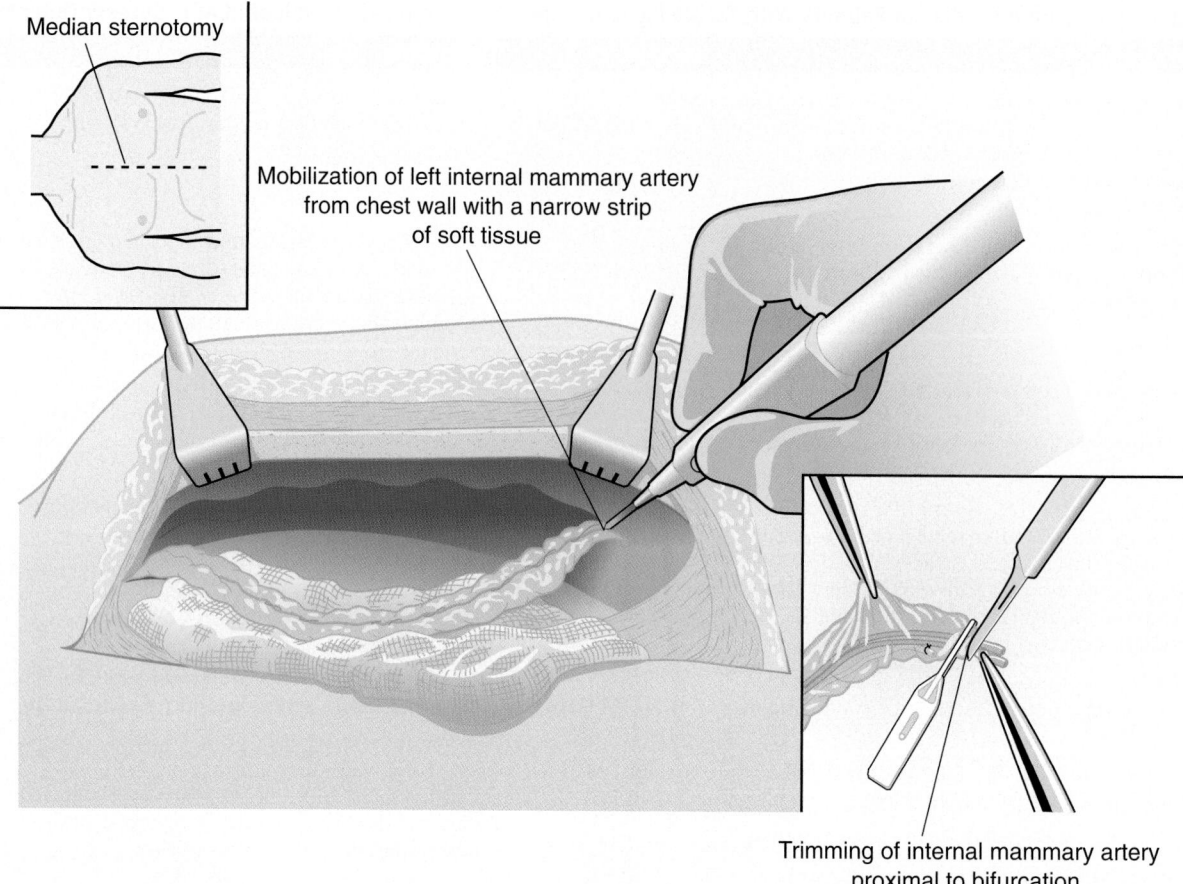

Median sternotomy

Mobilization of left internal mammary artery
from chest wall with a narrow strip
of soft tissue

Trimming of internal mammary artery
proximal to bifurcation

Figure 61-12 Coronary artery bypass procedures are performed through a median sternotomy (*left inset*). The divided sternum is lifted by controlled retraction that provides exposure but must not be so excessive as to fracture the sternum or ribs. Dissection proceeds proximally and distally until adequate length is obtained for the intended graft and usually terminates at the bifurcation of the internal mammary artery (*right inset*). Heparin is then administered systemically before the internal mammary artery is occluded. The internal mammary artery is prepared for grafting after transection. (From Jones RH: Coronary artery bypass grafts. In Sabiston DC Jr [ed]: Atlas of Cardiothoracic Surgery. Philadelphia, WB Saunders, 1995.)

the appropriate hemodynamic monitoring lines have been placed and a Foley catheter inserted, the patient is positioned in a frog-leg position and padded appropriately to minimize pressure points. The patient is prepared and draped, and a median sternotomy incision is performed (Fig. 61-12). Typically, the left half of the sternum is retracted and elevated to expose the ITA. Once identified and pulsatility verified, the endothoracic fascia is opened medial to the artery. Minimal traction and a no-touch technique are employed to protect the vessel.

The use of a headlight and magnification provided by surgical loupes allows precise dissection. A radiofrequency device or electrocautery can be used to mobilize the pedicle and identify the arterial and venous branches. The advantage of a radiofrequency device is the lack of transmitted thermal energy with its associated risk for heat-induced vascular injury. Side branches are clipped on the arterial side and the other side clipped or cauterized. The pedicle is mobilized from the subclavian artery and vein beneath the manubrium to the bifurcation of the superior epigastric and musculophrenic branches dis-

tally at the level of the diaphragm. After anticoagulation with heparin, the ITA is divided at the distal bifurcation and flow measured. A free flow rate greater than 60 mL/min is desirable. The vessel is then gently occluded distally with a clamp and the pedicle inoculated with a stream of papaverine solution to promote arterial dilation and prevent vascular spasm. The distal end of the vessel is prepared for grafting at this time or deferred to just before performing the anastomosis. If the diameter of the ITA appears adequate but the vessel lacks adequate inflow or pulsatility, the pedicle can be used as a free graft. In this case, the pedicle is divided at the level of the subclavian artery and stored in a papaverine solution until needed. Another surgical team can procure the greater saphenous vein or radial artery simultaneously.

Next, the patient is systemically heparinized (300 units/kg) with a target activated clotting time (ACT) greater than 400 seconds. The aorta is examined to detect areas of calcification and determine the site of cannulation and cross-clamping. Epiaortic echocardiography can be used to identify calcific plaques and help plan the site of cannulation to minimize disruption of atherosclerotic plaques and reduce the risk for embolization and stroke. The ascending aorta is then cannulated proximal to the innominate artery using double purse-string sutures placed anterolaterally. When the cannula is introduced into the aorta, it is important that the tip is directed distally. The aortic cannula is then secured in place by tightening the purse-string sutures with Rumel tourniquets; these are then secured to the side of the cannula. The open end of the cannula is back-flushed to de-air and remove any atherosclerotic debris in the cannula. It is then attached to the arterial perfusion line from the CPB machine. The proximal end of the aortic cannula is then secured to the wound edges. Venous cannulation is performed by introducing a cannula into the right atrium through a single purse-string suture in the right atrial appendage. If a dual-stage venous drainage cannula is used, the tip is directed into the inferior vena cava. The venous purse-string sutures are tightened using a Rumel tourniquet and then secured to the venous cannula. The open end is then interfaced with the venous tubing from the bypass pump. If retrograde cardioplegia is to be administered, a purse-string suture is placed near the AV groove, the atrium is incised, and a retrograde cardioplegia cannula is introduced into the coronary sinus.

After heparinization, the patient is placed on CPB and cooled to a core temperature of 30°C to 32°C. During cooling, a cardioplegic cannula can be inserted into the aorta through a separate purse-string suture. It is sufficiently distanced from the aortic cannula to allow room for the aorta to be cross-clamped. In addition to infusing cardioplegic solutions, the cannula can be used to decompress the left ventricle. After acceptable pump flows (2.2 L/min/m²) have been achieved, and the mean blood pressure stabilized (50-70 mm Hg), the aorta is cross-clamped, and cold cardioplegic solution is infused. The heart is also cooled topically using a saline slush solution. The phrenic nerve can be protected by covering it with an insulating pad. If both antegrade and retrograde cardioplegia are to be used, two thirds of the solution is administered antegrade, with the remainder given through the retrograde cannula. Antegrade or retrograde cold oxygenated blood cardioplegia is then administered intermittently, usually at 15- to 20-minute intervals, to ensure adequate myocardial protection during the period of ischemic arrest.

Distal Anastomoses

The target vessels can be identified and the sites of the distal anastomoses determined either before cross-clamping the aorta or afterward. The advantage of the former is that the coronary arteries are distended and appropriate graft length is easier to assess. The ideal anastomotic site is readily accessible, free of atherosclerotic disease, and has a diameter of at least 1.5 mm.

After the anastomotic site has been selected, a beaver blade is used to expose the anterior aspect of the coronary artery, and a small, sharp, pointed lance is used to puncture the vessel; the arteriotomy is then extended by using fine coronary scissors to create a 3- to 7-mm opening that is scaled to match the luminal diameter of

the conduit. Care must be taken not to injure the posterior wall. An endarterectomy of the coronary artery is avoided, if possible, because this is associated with a higher graft–to–native artery thrombosis rate.

When a reversed saphenous vein segment graft is used, the anastomosis is performed with either interrupted sutures or a continuous running 7-0 or 8-0 polypropylene suture. With the latter, care is taken to avoid purse-stringing the suture line and narrowing the anastomotic site. A 1.0- or 1.5-mm vessel probe is often used to evaluate the patency of the anastomosis. The graft is then pressurized with heparinized blood or cardioplegic solution to evaluate the anastomosis for hemostasis or evidence of stricture. If multiple vessels are to be grafted, a single conduit (e.g., saphenous vein) can be used by performing multiple side-to-side anastomoses (sequential grafting) in order to conserve graft length.

When using the ITA, the distal end of the vessel is beveled at a sharp angle and then the incision extended using fine iris scissors (Fig. 61-13). The arteriotomy of the native vessel is sized to match the opening of the ITA. The end-to-side anastomosis can be completed using a continuous running 8-0 polypropylene suture (Fig. 61-14). Upon completion of the anastomosis, both sides of the pedicle are sutured to the epicardium to minimize tension on the anastomosis or twisting of the graft when the patient is weaned from CPB and the lungs are ventilated.

Proximal Anastomoses

If the proximal anastomoses are completed after the distal anastomoses have been completed, this can be done either while the aortic cross-clamp is still in place or after it has been removed and replaced with a partial occlusion clamp. The latter allows the heart to be perfused and rewarmed. The advantage of the single cross-clamp technique is that it minimizes the number of times the aorta is manipulated, and theoretically reduces the risk for plaque disruption and embolization. With either approach, an aortic punch is used to excise buttons of aortic tissue and create the sites for the proximal graft anastomoses. The proximal opening of the conduits are then spatulated to create a hood, and each anastomosis is completed using a running 6-0 or 7-0 polypropylene suture. The same technique can be used if the proximal aortic anastomoses are performed before placing the patient on CPB using a partial aortic occlusion clamp. After completing the anastomoses, small bulldog clamps are placed on each graft, and the patient is placed in a head-down position. Pump flow is transiently reduced as the aortic cross-clamp is removed and the heart is reperfused. After the grafts have filled with blood, small punctures are made in the veins using a 25-gauge needle for de-airing. The bulldog clamps are then removed, and the heart is perfused through both the grafts and the native vessels. All anastomotic sites are re-examined and bleeding sites oversewn.

Termination of Cardiopulmonary Artery Bypass

Systemic rewarming is usually initiated after completion of the last distal anastomosis. Blood that has accumulated

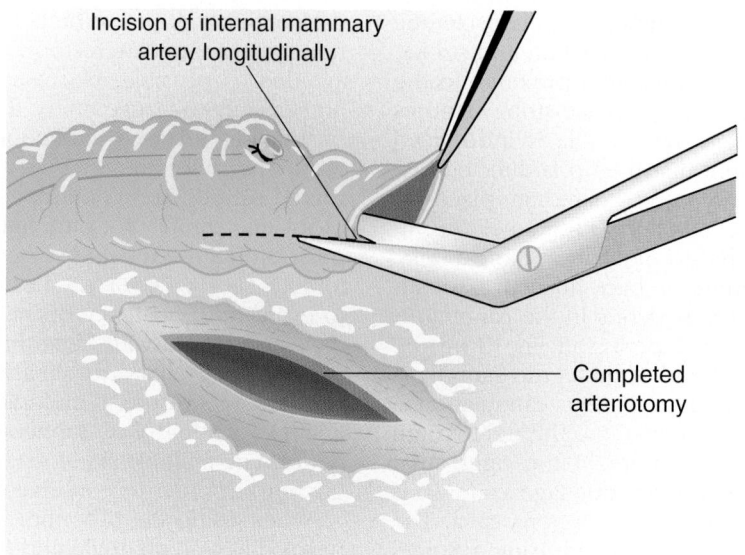

Incision of internal mammary
artery longitudinally

Completed
arteriotomy

Figure 61-13 The technique of anastomosis between the left internal mammary artery and the left anterior descending coronary artery illustrates the general principles used to construct all proximal and distal anastomoses. The graft is opened longitudinally to match or exceed the length of the coronary arteriotomy. This opening prevents kinking at the site of the anastomosis of the internal mammary artery and aorta to the saphenous vein. This opening is not necessary at the distal vein anastomotic site, but a slight bevel cut of the distal vein helps prevent kinking of the saphenous vein to the coronary artery anastomosis. (From Jones RH: Coronary artery bypass grafts. In Sabiston DC Jr [ed]: Atlas of Cardiothoracic Surgery. Philadelphia, WB Saunders, 1995.)

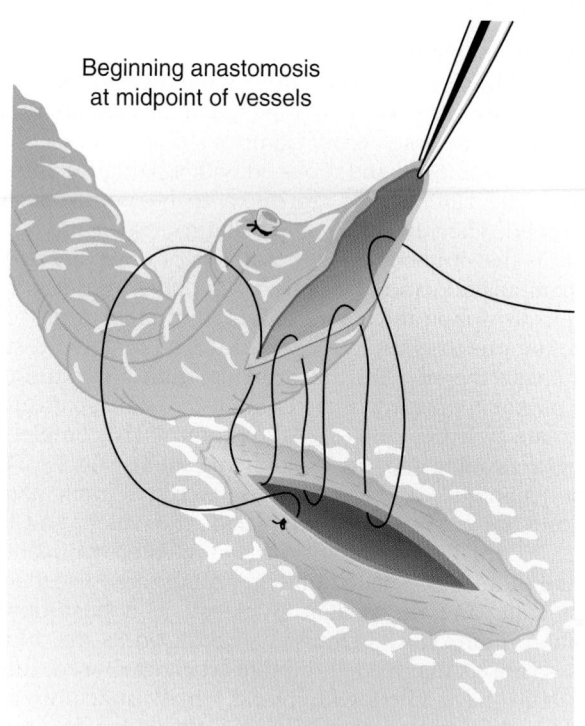

Beginning anastomosis
at midpoint of vessels

Figure 61-14 The anastomosis begins midway along the side of the graft so that the final knot will not be at the most distal or proximal portion of the anastomosis, thereby decreasing the chances of technical error that would impede graft flow. The polypropylene suture permits a portion of the anastomosis to be completed before the two vessels are joined. (From Jones RH: Coronary artery bypass grafts. In Sabiston DC Jr [ed]: Atlas of Cardiothoracic Surgery. Philadelphia, WB Saunders, 1995.)

in the pleural spaces is evacuated and reprocessed using a Cell Saver for later reinfusion. After removing the aortic cross-clamp, the heart usually starts to beat spontaneously within a short time. Although a normal sinus rhythm may develop, it frequently deteriorates into ventricular fibrillation and requires cardioversion using internal defibrillating paddles. If the heart rate is less than 70 beats/minute, temporary atrial and ventricular pacing wires can be attached to the surface of the heart, usually the right atrium or right ventricle, and pacing commenced at about 90 beats/minute.

When the patient has been adequately rewarmed (~36.5°C), normal sinus rhythm has been restored, and ventilation has been re-established, then the patient is weaned from CPB by gradually reducing the pump flow rates to zero while maintaining adequate intravascular volume through transfusion. It is often necessary to manipulate the contractile state of the heart and the peripheral vascular resistance (afterload) by infusing inotropic agents such as dobutamine and vasodilators or vasoconstrictors such as nitroglycerin and ephedrine, respectively. After the patient has been stabilized off CPB, protamine is administered to reverse the heparin-induced anticoagulation. The aortic and venous cannulas are removed and purse-string sutures tied. Pleural and mediastinal chest tubes are inserted (along with temporary epicardial atrial and ventricular pacing wires if not placed earlier) and after hemostasis has been achieved, the sternum is closed using large-caliber stainless steel wire in simple or figure-of-eight patterns. The presternal fascia and area around the xiphoid is then approximated with Vicryl sutures and the remaining tissue closed in layers.

The skin can be approximated with a running subcuticular monofilament suture, and Steri-Strips or staples. Dry sterile dressings are placed over all incisions, lines, wires, and drains, and the patient is transferred to the surgical intensive care unit.

Postoperative Care

Postoperative care begins with the transport of the patient to the cardiac surgery intensive care unit. A directed physical examination should be performed on arrival. This includes the assessment of level of consciousness, respiratory sounds, peripheral pulses, and body temperature. Mediastinal chest tube drainage should be recorded and assessed hourly. Initial ventilator settings should be set to match those in the operating room. Alternatively, the ventilator can be set at a tidal volume of 12 mL/kg, an intermittent mandatory ventilation rate of 8 to 10 breaths/minute, an FIO_2 of 60%, and a 5 cm H_2O of positive end-expiratory pressure to provide an adequate margin of safety. A portable chest radiograph is obtained to confirm the position of the endotracheal tube and identify a pneumothorax, atelectasis, pulmonary edema, or pleural effusions. Initial laboratory studies should include hemoglobin, hematocrit, electrolytes, blood urea nitrogen, creatinine, platelet count, prothrombin time, partial thromboplastin time, and arterial blood gases. With respect to continuous monitoring devices, the patient should have an ECG with the ability to assess ST-T-wave abnormalities, an arterial line to measure arterial blood pressure, and a line to measure central venous pressure, pulse oximetry, capnography, and a core temperature. In selected patients, pulmonary artery pressures and cardiac output are monitored continuously using a Swan-Ganz catheter.

The primary considerations during the first 12 hours after the operation should be the maintenance of adequate blood pressure, cardiac output, correction of coagulation defects, correction of ionized hypocalcemia, stabilization of intravascular volume, and normalization of the peripheral vascular resistance. This often involves the administration of crystalloid solutions, blood or blood products, inotropic agents, calcium, and vasodilators or vasoconstrictors.

In the immediate postoperative period, it is desirable to avoid marked elevations in blood pressure (mean arterial pressure >100 mm Hg). Significant hypertension results in increased myocardial oxygen consumption and tension on arterial suture lines. In patients with significant preexisting left ventricular dysfunction, this can also lead to a reduction in the cardiac index. The hypertension may be due to hypoxemia, hypercarbia, hypothermia with shivering, and inadequate sedation and analgesia. It can be treated by clearing the endotracheal tube of secretions, adjusting ventilator settings, warming the patient with forced hot-air blankets, administering analgesics, and infusing vasodilators. Because low cardiac output occurs frequently after CPB, a Swan-Ganz catheter can be used to assess the adequacy of systemic perfusion by measuring the cardiac index and monitoring mixed venous oxygenation. In general, the aim is to maintain a cardiac index of 2.2 L/min/m² and a mixed venous oxygenation of 60%. The most common causes of low cardiac output are myocardial ischemia, hypovolemia, abnormal heart rate and rhythm, myocardial dysfunction, and cardiac tamponade. Myocardial ischemia can range from asymptomatic ST-segment changes to infarction with profound hypotension. The former may be due to coronary artery spasm, ITA hypoperfusion, or early graft occlusion. Coronary artery spasm occurs in about 1% of patients and can be treated with IV nitroglycerin or calcium channel blockade. In the meantime, α-adrenergic agents may be required to support the blood pressure. If the ischemia is severe and the patient does not respond to pharmacologic support, the patient may require emergent coronary angiography or reoperation or regrafting. With hypovolemia, there is a variety of opinion as to which resuscitation fluid should be used postoperatively. Generally, lactated Ringer's solution is appropriate but can be supplemented with up to 1.5 liters of hydroxy ethyl starch (Hetastarch) or blood products. The latter depends on whether the patient is anemic or there is evidence of active bleeding.

In the immediate postoperative period, most patients are tachycardic. If they have been treated before surgery with β-blockers, they may be bradycardic (<60 beats/minute). In general, the desirable rhythm and heart rate is sinus and a rate between 70 and 100 beats/minute. A normal sinus rhythm ensures AV synchrony and maintenance of the atrial kick, which can contribute up to 25% of the cardiac output. If the patient is bradycardic or has evidence of heart block, atrial or AV pacing through temporary pacing wires should be initiated to increase the rate and restore synchrony. Arrhythmias are common and may result from abnormal electrolytes, acidosis, high circulating catecholamine levels, and myocardial ischemia. Supraventricular tachyarrhythmias associated with hemodynamic instability should be treated immediately with cardioversion. Hemodynamically stable patients with re-entrant supraventricular tachyarrhythmias should be treated with adenosine in incremental doses. Atrial flutter can be treated using overdrive pacing if the rapid atrial rate can be captured and controlled. Atrial fibrillation responds to IV digoxin, procainamide, diltiazem, β-blockers, amiodarone, and cardioversion. The hemodynamically unstable patient with ventricular arrhythmias needs immediate defibrillation and an IV bolus infusion of lidocaine followed by a continuous infusion. Other alternative agents include procainamide and bretylium.

Myocardial dysfunction is also common in patients after CPB and may be secondary to myocardial stunning (a transient reversible injury) or myocardial necrosis (infarction). If the heart rate, ventricular preload, rhythm, and afterload have been optimized and the patient still demonstrates a low cardiac output, the patient will most likely benefit from inotropic support. This support can be divided into catecholamine (epinephrine, norepinephrine, dobutamine, and dopamine) and noncatecholamine agents (milrinone). Epinephrine is an effective drug because of its α- and β-adrenergic properties. At low doses, epinephrine stimulates peripheral $β_2$ receptors and promotes mild vasodilation. At higher doses, α stimulation causes vasoconstriction and tachycardia. Norepinephrine has a more pronounced effect on the peripheral α receptors, with resultant vasoconstriction. These drugs are generally administered at doses between 0.01 and 0.10 µg/kg/min and adjusted according to the patient's response. Dobutamine and dopamine have comparable effects on cardiac output and are similar to epinephrine and norepinephrine but, in general, are less arrhythmogenic. Dobutamine is also a vasodilator and is used to reduce both left ventricular preload and afterload. Milrinone is a phosphodiesterase inhibitor and slows the degradation of cyclic adenosine monophosphate (cAMP). Its mechanism of action complements that of catecholamines, which stimulate cAMP. This drug is often used in combination with other inotropic agents to achieve a synergistic outcome.

Intra-aortic Balloon Pump

For patients who demonstrate profound myocardial dysfunction and are unresponsive to volume resuscitation, intense pharmacologic therapy treatment with an IABP may be indicated. Intra-aortic balloon pumping improves mean blood pressures and coronary artery perfusion and decreases cardiac work and oxygen demand. If the IABP was used to control chest pain preoperatively, it is often removed within 24 hours after the operation. However, if used preoperatively for hemodynamic instability, weaning from the IABP may be more difficult and require more time.

Tamponade

In the postoperative period, pericardial tamponade is due to formation of pericardial clot and compression of the heart. The condition should be suspected if the patient exhibits evidence of low cardiac output and hypotension, fails to respond to IV fluid infusions, and requires increasing levels of inotropic support. Often there has been a marked decline in mediastinal chest tube drainage before the onset of signs of tamponade. The diagnosis can be made on the basis of widening of the mediastinum on chest x-ray and evidence of a pericardial effusion by echocardiography. Surface echocardiography is helpful but may be compromised because of the presence of wound dressings and chest tubes. Transesophageal echocardiography is more reliable but may not be immediately available. If a Swan-Ganz catheter is in place and right and left heart pressures are monitored, the central venous pressure and pulmonary capillary wedge pressure are usually elevated and equal. After the diagnosis is made, the patient should be returned to the operating room for evacuation of the clot and relief of the compression. If the patient's condition is rapidly deteriorating, a simple subxyphoid approach can be performed at the bedside and result in a dramatic improvement in hemodynamics.

Postoperative Bleeding

The combination of heparinization, hypothermia, CPB, and protamine reversal is associated with increased risk for bleeding after CABG. Bleeding after CABG requiring transfusion or reoperation to stop the bleeding is associated with a significant increase in morbidity and mortality. A minority of patients having cardiac procedures (15%-20%) consume more than 80% of the blood products transfused at operation. Blood must be viewed as a scarce resource that carries significant risks and unproven benefits. There is a high-risk subset of patients who require multiple preventive measures to reduce the chance of postoperative bleeding. Six variables stand out as important indicators of risk:

1. Advanced age
2. Low preoperative red blood cell volume (preoperative anemia or small body size)
3. Preoperative antiplatelet or antithrombotic drugs
4. Reoperative or complex procedures
5. Emergency operations
6. Noncardiac patient comorbidities (e.g., renal failure, chronic obstructive pulmonary disease, diabetes, congestive heart failure)

Available evidence-based blood conservation techniques include the following:

1. Drugs that increase preoperative blood volume (e.g., erythropoietin) or decrease postoperative bleeding (e.g., aprotinin)
2. Devices that conserve blood (e.g., intraoperative blood salvage and blood sparing interventions)
3. Other interventions that protect the patient's own blood from the stress of operation (e.g., autologous predonation and normovolemic hemodilution)
4. Consensus, institution-specific blood transfusion algorithms supplemented with point-of-care testing
5. A multimodality approach to blood conservation combining all of the above, especially in high-risk patients (most important)

Despite efforts at blood conservation to limit perioperative bleeding and blood transfusion, 2% to 3% of patients will require re-exploration for bleeding, and as many as 20% will have excessive bleeding and blood transfusion after operation. Bleeding greater than 500 mL in the first hour or persistent bleeding greater than 200 mL/hour for 4 hours is an indication for mediastinal exploration. Exploration is also indicated if a large hemothorax is identified on chest x-ray or pericardial tamponade occurs. In as many as 20% of cases, a specific site of bleeding can be identified. The typical sources of surgical bleeding include the cannulation sites, the proximal and distal anastomoses, and branches of the ITAs and the vein grafts. Most of the time, however, a specific bleeding site is not identified, and it is related to inadequate heparin neutralization, qualitative or quantitative platelet dysfunction, fibrinolysis, and deficiencies in factors V, VIII, XIII, and fibrinogen and plasminogen. In the setting of suspected nonsurgical postoperative bleeding, one approach is to obtain an ACT and administer protamine to return the ACT to baseline. In general, red blood cells are administered if the patient is actively bleeding or anemic (Hgb = 7.0). Platelets are administered if there is evidence of clinical bleeding and abnormal clotting tests (preferably point-of-care tests such as PFA-100 platelet analyzer or thromboelastography). Cryoprecipitate can be used to treat low fibrinogen levels (<100 mg/dL). Drugs with blood-conserving properties such as aprotinin and lysine analogues (epsilon aminocaproic acid and tranexamic acid) are used frequently, especially in high-risk patients.

Extubation

It is desirable to initiate the process of ventilator weaning as soon as the patient awakens, is hemodynamically stable with minimal chest tube drainage, and can maintain a satisfactory spontaneous tidal volume and respiratory rate. In general, the cardiac index should be greater than or equal to 2.2 L/min/m², and the mean arterial pressure should exceed 70 mm Hg. The patient should be comfortable on continuous positive airway pressure support with minimal secretions and have a spontaneous respiratory rate of 20 breaths/min or less. The ability to maintain an arterial pH greater than 7.35 while the intermediate mandatory ventilation rate is reduced to zero is a reliable test. After extubation, the patient needs to be encouraged to breathe deeply and utilize incentive spirometry. Suboptimal postoperative pulmonary function may require additional therapy, including the use of bronchodilators, mucolytics, and chest physical therapy. After extubation, it is important to provide the patient with sufficient pain relief to minimize emotional distress, poor coughing, and the reluctance to begin ambulation. Unrelieved pain can also be a source of tachycardia, hypertension, and myocardial ischemia. Before leaving the ICU, unnecessary lines and catheters should be removed. Removal of temporary atrial and ventricular pacing wires is often deferred to the third postoperative day.

OUTCOME AND PROCESS ASSESSMENT FOR CORONARY ARTERY BYPASS GRAFTING

The operative techniques and technical components of CABG matured over the intervening years since the 1960s when the first operations were performed using cardiopulmonary bypass. Simultaneously, the results of operative intervention for CAD improved despite increased acuity of the patient population requiring operation. With increasing frequency of CABG came concern about outcomes and operative results, prompting surgeons, health care payers, and patients to focus on the quality of the services provided by surgeons who perform CABG. In an effort to address these concerns, many professional organizations sought to measure results of operation by using large databases to identify risk factors and sort patients according to their risk for an adverse outcome. It was immediately obvious that risk adjustment is essential for accurate comparison of providers (hospitals and surgeons). Table 61-8 is a partial listing of risk adjustment models used by various professional organizations for comparing mortality outcomes of providers. Because there are few absolute contraindications to CABG surgery, it is important to understand hospital mortality and morbidity in the context of preoperative risk. Examples of

risk adjusted, multi-institutional databases include the Department of Veterans Affairs (VA) Continuous Improvement in Cardiac Surgery Program (CICSP), the STS National Database, and the Northern New England (NNE) Database (see Table 61-8). Risk-stratified outcomes are provided to both participating institutions and surgeons. This information is then used as a screening tool to evaluate and improve quality of care and, increasingly, to compare providers.

In 2000, the Institute of Medicine issued a report that was highly critical of the U.S. health care system, suggesting that between 50,000 and 90,000 unnecessary deaths occur yearly because of errors in the health care system.[44] The Institute of Medicine reports created a heightened awareness of more global aspects of quality. For most of the history of cardiac surgery, quality was generally equated with operative mortality and, to a lesser extent, serious operative morbidity (i.e., outcome measures). A distinct change in the landscape of quality assessment occurred after the Institute of Medicine report appeared. The narrow focus on operative mortality gave way to a broader analysis that also included operative morbidity. The emphasis on these *outcomes measures* was further expanded to include the *process* of surgical care delivery. *Process measures* were developed to monitor the processes of care. These measures typically include the choice of medication, timing of administration, and other interventions considered appropriate for optimal care. *Structural measures* such as health information technology (HIT) and organizational design were also considered important elements in this more global model of medical quality. Donabedian[45] is credited with recognizing that outcome measures, process measures, and structural measures all contribute to quality of care. In keeping with the well-accepted Donabedian model, outcome measures, process measures, and structural measures are generally termed *performance measures*.

The following definitions are adapted from those proposed by the Joint Commission on Accreditation of Healthcare Organizations (JCAHO):

- *Performance Measure:* A quantitative entity that provides an indication of an organization's performance in relation to a specified process or outcome.
- *Outcome Measure:* A measure that indicates the results of process measures. Examples are operative mortality, the frequency of postoperative mediastinitis, renal failure, MI, and so forth.
- *Process Measure:* A measure that focuses on a process leading to a certain outcome. Intrinsic in this definition is a scientific basis for believing that the process will increase the probability of achieving a desired outcome. Examples include the rate of inferior mesenteric artery use in CABG patients or the fraction of CABG patients placed on β-blockers postoperatively.
- *Structural Measure:* A measure that assesses whether the appropriate number, type, and distribution of medical personnel, equipment, and facilities are in place to deliver optimal health care. Examples include enrollment in a national database or procedural volume.

Table 61-8 Recently Published Risk Models for Coronary Bypass Surgical Mortality

	NYS	TORONTO	USA	EMORY	VA	AUSTRALIA	CANADA	CLEVELAND	ISRAEL	STS	NNE	STROKE	PARSONNET	
No. of Patients	174,210	57,187	50,357	17,128	13,368	12,712	12,003	7491	4918	4835	3654	3055	2152	
No. of Risk Factors	*29*	*16*	*13*	*7*	*6*	*9*	*5*	*9*	*7*	*9*	*9*	*10*	*8*	*Sum*
Age	X	X	X	X	X	X	X	X	X	X	X	X		12
Gender	X	X	X	X	X		X	X		X		X		9
Surgical urgency	X		X		X	X		X		X	X	X		8
Ejection fraction	X	X			X		X	X		X	X	X		8
Renal dysfunction/Creatinine	X	X	X	X						X	X		X	7
Previous CABG	X		X	X				X			X	X		6
NYHA class	X	X	X	X		X				X				6
Left main disease	X	X						X		X	X	X		6
Diseased coronary vessels	X	X			X			X		X	X	X		6
Peripheral vascular disease	X		X			X		X	X					5
Diabetes mellitus	X	X			X					X			X	5
Cerebrovascular disease	X		X	X		X								4
Intraop/postop variables	X		X				X		X				X	4
Myocardial infarction	X	X	X	X										4
Body size	X	X	X											3
Preoperative IABP	X	X	X			X								3
Cardiogenic shock/unstable	X	X									X			3
COPD	X	X												2
PTCA	X		X											2
Angina		X					X							2
Intravenous nitrates	X					X								2
Arrhythmias	X	X							X					2
History of heart operation	X	X				X								

Risk factor						Grade
Charlson comorbidity score		X	X			2
Dialysis dependence	X					2
Pulmonary hypertension	X			X		2
Diuretics	X					2
Systemic hypertension			X			1
Serum albumin		X				1
Race	X					1
Previous CHF				X		1
Myocardial infarction timing	X					1
Cardiac index		X				1
LV end-diastolic pressure					X	1
CVA timing	X					1
Liver disease	X					1
Neoplasia/metastatic disease	X					1
Ventricular aneurysm	X					1
Steroids	X					1
Digitalis	X					1
Thrombolytic therapy					X	1
Arterial bicarbonate		X				1
Calcified ascending aorta					X	1

*Mortality risk models are sorted horizontally by the number of patients. The risk factors are sorted vertically by the sum of their appearances in these models.
CABG, coronary artery bypass grafting; CHF, congestive heart failure; COPD, chronic obstructive pulmonary disease; CVA, cerebrovascular accident; IABP, intraaortic balloon pump; LV, left ventricular; NYHA, New York Heart Association; PTCA, percutaneous transluminal coronary angioplasty.
From Grunkemeier GL, Zerr KJ, Jin R: Cardiac surgery report cards: Making the grade. Ann Thorac Surg 72:1845-1848, 2001.

Table 61-9 **Multivariate Factors Associated With Various Outcomes of Cardiac Surgery**

VARIABLE	RELATIVE RISK OF OUTCOME			
	Serious Morbidity (95%CI)	Mortality (95%CI)	Decreased Cost (95%CI)	Decreased LOS (95%CI)
Congestive heart failure	4.81 (2.16-5.98)	9.20 (6.02-14.0)	0.56 (0.51-0.63)	0.79 (0.73-0.85)
NYS predicted mortality risk		1.28 (1.16-1.41)	0.93 (0.89-0.97)	0.78 (0.76-0.80)
Type of operation		6.04 (3.48-10.5)	0.43 (0.40-0.47)	0.53 (0.48-0.59)
Creatinine >2.5 mg/100 mL			0.40 (0.33-0.49)	0.47 (0.38-0.58)
Priority		18.6 (7.42-46.6)	0.53 (0.50-0.56)	
Age/RBC volume (per 0.01 unit increase)	6.93 (3.21-11.5)		0.61 (0.55-0.67)	0.32 (0.30-0.36)
Reoperative procedure			0.68 (0.62-0.76)	
Preoperative IABP			0.65 (0.56-0.75)	
Hypertension	5.62 (2.11-15.2)		0.86 (0.81-0.92)	0.83 (0.78-0.89)
More than one prior MI			0.83 (0.75-0.91)	
Dialysis-dependent renal failure			0.61 (0.47-0.78)	
Peripheral vascular disease				0.85 (0.71-0.94)
Prior CNS disease	3.41 (2.99-4.91)			0.81 (0.72-0.92)
COPD				0.87 (0.79-0.94)

CNS, central nervous system; COPD, chronic obstructive pulmonary disease; IABP, intra-aortic balloon counterpulsation; LOS, length of stay; MI, myocardial infarction; RBC, red blood cell.

The STS took a leadership role in developing performance measures that incorporate structural, process, and outcome measures into a single gauge of quality. This quality measure will almost certainly be used by health care payers to judge cardiac surgery providers in coming years.

There are at least four clinical outcomes of interest to surgeons dealing with cardiac surgical patients: mortality, serious nonfatal morbidity, resource utilization, and patient satisfaction. Which patient characteristics constitute important risk factors may depend largely on the outcome of interest. For example, Table 61-9 lists the multivariate factors and odds ratios associated with mortality outcomes in patients having cardiac operations.[46] The clinical variables associated with increased resource use after operation are different from those associated with increased mortality risk. As a generalization, the risk factors associated with in-hospital death are likely to reflect concurrent, disease-specific variables, whereas factors associated with increased resource use reflect serious comorbid illness.[46] For example, mortality risk after CABG is associated with disease-specific factors such as ventricular ejection fraction, recent MI, and hemodynamic instability at the time of operation, whereas risk factors for increased resource use (as measured by length of stay and hospital cost) include comorbid illnesses such as peripheral vascular disease, renal dysfunction, hypertension, and chronic lung disease (see Table 61-9).

It is not surprising that comorbid conditions are important predictors of hospitalization charges because patients with multiple comorbidities often require prolonged hospitalization, not only for treatment of the primary surgical illness but also for treatment of complicating comorbid conditions.

Operative mortality is an easily defined, readily measured outcome, and its value to patients is undeniable. Most studies that have attempted to define effective care have focused on mortality as an outcome for the above reasons. Other outcomes such as resource utilization or quality-of-life indicators may be more relevant postoperative outcomes in many instances. Outcome measures other than operative mortality are particularly important when deciding how to spend health care dollars wisely.

Risk-adjusted databases are particularly helpful in identifying and prioritizing preoperative variables predictive of outcomes. A meta-analysis[47] of seven large databases of patients identified 7 core (unequivocally related to operative mortality) and 13 level 1 (likely relation to short-term CABG surgery mortality) risk factors. The core variables included acuity of operation, prior heart operation, age, EF, gender, severity of CAD, and presence of LMCA disease. These variables were acknowledged as predictive of mortality after CABG surgery in all seven databases. The presence of elevated serum creatinine levels, PTCA during index admission, recent MI less than 1 week, history of angina, ventricular arrhythmia, congestive heart failure, mitral regurgitation, diabetes, cerebro-vascular disease, peripheral vascular disease, chronic obstructive pulmonary disease, height, and weight were considered less predictive.

Mortality Indicators

By far, the bulk of available experience with risk stratification and outcome analysis in cardiothoracic surgery deals with risk factors associated with operative mortality, particularly in patients undergoing coronary revascularization. Most of the risk stratification analyses shown in Table 61-8 are used to evaluate life or death outcomes in surgical patients with ischemic heart disease, in part because mortality is such an easy end point to measure and track. Each of the risk stratification systems shown in Table 61-8 computes a risk score based on risk factors that are dependent on patient diagnosis. For the diagnosis of ischemic heart disease, Table 61-8 shows the significant risk factors found to be important for a spectrum of the risk stratification systems. The definition of operative mortality varies among the different systems (either 30-day mortality or in-hospital mortality), but the risk factors identified by each of the stratification schemes in Table 61-8 show many similarities. Some variables are risk factors in almost all stratification systems; some variables are never significant risk factors. Each of the risk models has been validated using separate data sets; hence, there is some justification in using any of the risk stratification methods both in preoperative assessment of patients undergoing CABG and in making comparisons among providers (either physicians or hospitals), but certain caveats exist about the validity and reliability of these models.

At present, it is not possible to recommend one risk stratification method over another. In general, the larger the sample size, the more risk factors can be found. An ideal model might include more variables than even the most robust model in Table 61-8. The regression diagnostics (e.g., receiver operating characteristic [ROC] curves and cross-validation studies) performed on the models included in Table 61-8 suggest that the models are good, but not perfect, at predicting outcomes. In statistical terms, this means that not all of the variability in operative mortality is explained by the set of risk factors included in the regression models. Hence, it is possible that inclusion of new putative risk factors in the regression equations may improve the validity and precision of the models.

New regression models and new risk factors are scrutinized and tested using cross-validation methods and other regression diagnostics before acceptance. It is uncertain whether inclusion of many more risk factors will significantly improve the quality and predictive ability of regression models. For example, the STS risk stratification model described in Table 61-8 includes many predictor variables, whereas the Canada risk adjustment scheme includes only five predictor variables. Yet the regression diagnostics for these two models are similar, suggesting that both models have equal precision and predictive

capabilities. This suggests that the models are effective at predicting population behavior but not necessarily suited for predicting individual outcomes.

Further work needs to be done, both to explain the differences in risk factors seen between the various risk stratification models and to determine which models are best suited for studies of quality improvement. Many critical features of any risk adjustment outcome program must be considered when determining quality of the risk stratification method or when comparing one to another (see later). Daley[48] provides a summary of the key features that are necessary to validate any risk adjustment model. She makes the point that no clear-cut evidence exists that differences in risk-adjusted mortalities across providers reflect differences in the process and structure of care.[49] This issue needs further study.

Many of the databases shown in Table 61-8 accumulate patient information on a voluntary basis. This implies that patient information is entered into the database voluntarily according to the wishes of each institution that participates in the database. Other databases enter patient data into the database because it is mandated by some overseeing organization (e.g. the Veteran's Administration or the New York state government). To determine differences between voluntary and mandatory databases, a 2001 10-year comparative analysis of CABG surgery risk factors and outcomes was performed using the voluntary STS National Database (*n*=1.1 million) and the mandatory VA Continuous Improvement in Cardiac Surgery Program (CICSP) (*n*=74,000).[41] Although there were differences in demographics, both data sets produced similar risk factors, with similar odds ratios for 30-day mortality after CABG surgery. The three strongest predictors of risk for mortality in the STS and VA databases were serum creatinine level higher than 3.0 mg/dL, need for preoperative IABP, and prior heart surgery. In the 1990s, CABG surgery mortality in both databases declined from 3.8% to 2.7% in the STS registry and from 4.3% to 2.7% in the CICSP registry. This occurred despite an increase in preoperative risk factors in both databases. This explains, in part, the significant decline over time in the observed-to-database predicted mortality ratios in both databases. These risk-adjusted databases provide an opportunity for hospitals and surgeons to identify system problems and address them with the intent to improve outcomes and enhance patient care. There are, however, subtle but important regional, institutional, and provider variances that cannot be entirely accounted for in a generalized model of risk stratification.

Risk Factors for Postoperative Morbidity and Resource Utilization

Patients with nonfatal outcomes after operations for ischemic heart disease make up more than 95% of the pool of patients undergoing operation. Of about 500,000 patients having CABG yearly, between 50% and 75% have what is characterized by both the patient and provider as an uncomplicated course after operation. The complications occurring in surviving patients range from serious organ system dysfunction to minor limitation or dissatisfaction with lifestyle, and account for a significant fraction of the cost of the procedures. One report estimates that as much as 40% of the yearly hospital costs for CABG are consumed by 10% to 15% of the patients who have serious complications after operation. This suggests that reducing morbidity in *high-risk* cardiac surgical patients has significant impact on cost reduction.

For many years, operative *mortality* was the sole criterion for a successful CABG procedure. This concept has given way to a broader focus on the entire hospitalization associated with CABG. There is universal agreement that nonfatal complications play a central role in the assessment of CABG quality, but many morbidity outcomes are relatively difficult to define and track. Risk adjustment is particularly difficult because of the fact that risk factors for most complications are not well established. The low frequency of some complications also creates statistical challenges.

Shroyer and coworkers[50] used part of the large national experience captured in the STS Database to examine five important postoperative CABG complications: stroke, renal failure, reoperation within 24 hours after CABG, prolonged (>24 hours) postoperative ventilation, and mediastinitis. For each of these complications, risk factors were identified using univariate screening followed by multivariate logistic regression analysis. Predictive models were developed for each of the five complications, thereby allowing one to use specific patient risk factors to adjust for severity of illness and determine profiles for providers. This, in turn, allows for meaningful comparisons of risk-matched populations between providers and a national benchmark.

For the purposes of morbidity estimates, more than 500,000 patients from the STS database were examined.[50] This allowed an accurate estimate of the frequency of each of these five postoperative complications. For example, the morbidity estimates in CABG patients from this large database are as follows:

1. Stroke—1.63%
2. Renal failure requiring dialysis—3.53%
3. Prolonged postoperative ventilation—5.96%
4. Mediastinitis—0.63%
5. Reoperation within 24 hours—7.17%

Predictor variables from the logistic regression for each complication demonstrated considerable overlap, but there were substantial differences in odds ratios associated with individual risk factors. The relative importance of specific risk factors differed depending on the outcome measure. For each of the complications, preoperative shock was invariably a major risk factor, as was any form of diabetes. Redo operations were associated with a high odds ratio for most postoperative morbidities, particularly for prolonged postoperative ventilation.

These models had good regression model diagnostics, indicating reasonable reliability of the models. The diagnostics are generally less than those seen with typical regression models of CABG operative mortality, suggesting that unmeasured factors may account for outcomes. Nevertheless, the ability to use validated models to risk-stratify patients in this context is invaluable. National quality organizations, such as the National Quality Forum (NQF), and large health care payers have clearly placed a high premium on the need for risk adjustment for most outcome measures, including both mortality and morbidity outcomes.

Risk Factors That Do Not Predict Outcomes

Occasionally, studies appear that suggest that a particular patient variable is *not* a risk factor for a particular patient outcome. Care must be exercised in interpreting negative results. Many putative risk factors labeled "no different from control" in studies using inadequate samples have not received a fair test. For example, Burns and associates[51] studied preoperative template bleeding times in 43 patients undergoing elective CABG. They found no increased postoperative blood loss in patients with prolonged skin bleeding times. Their study reports five patients whose bleeding times were prolonged greater than 8 minutes. In this small sample size, there was a trend toward more units of blood transfused, but differences between high and low bleeding time groups were reported as "not significant" by the authors at the $\alpha = 5\%$ level (i.e., $P = .05$). Using the author's data, it is possible to compute a β error for this negative observation of less than 0.5. This means that there is as much as a 50% chance that the negative finding is really a false-negative result. This high false-negative rate occurs because of the small sample size and the wide variation in the bleeding time values. We have found elevated bleeding time (>10 minutes) to be a significant multivariate risk factor for excessive blood transfusion after CABG in two different studies.[52,53] Although there is controversy about the value of bleeding time as a screening test, it is possible that discarding the bleeding time after an inconclusive negative trial, such as that of Burns and coworkers, may ignore a potentially important risk factor. Care must be taken in the interpretation of a negative finding, especially in a small study group. A similar cautionary note was sounded by Freiman and coauthors[54] after reviewing the medical literature over a 10-year period. These authors found that 50 of 71 "negative" randomized controlled trials could have missed a 50% therapeutic improvement from intervention because the sample size studied was too small.[54] Their conclusions were that many therapies discarded as ineffective after inconclusive negative trials may still have a clinically important effect. Negative findings in a literature report require scrutiny and an understanding of type II statistical errors.

ALTERNATIVE METHODS FOR MYOCARDIAL REVASCULARIZATION

Off-Pump Coronary Artery Bypass Grafting

The use of cardiopulmonary bypass is reportedly associated with a whole-body inflammatory response (WIR), a response mediated, in part, by activation of complement, macrophages, and cytokines. This phenomenon has been related to the contact of blood components with the surface of the bypass circuit. It has been hypothesized that the WIR contributes to postoperative bleeding, neurocognitive dysfunction, thromboembolism, fluid retention, and reversible organ dysfunction. In an attempt to minimize these complications, OPCAB is used with increasing frequency and is currently considered an acceptable alternative method for myocardial revascularization. A number of studies and clinical trials have been performed to evaluate the efficacy and safety of this operation and define the subsets of patient who are most likely to benefit from this approach (Table 61-10). The findings to date have been mixed.

In one retrospective multicenter analysis of 7867 registry patients published in 2001,[55] OPCAB patients had a lower incidence of IABP use (2.3% versus 3.41%), lower incidence of postoperative atrial fibrillation (21.2% versus 26.3%), and a shorter length of stay (5 versus 6 days) compared with CABG with CPB. The incidence of stroke, mediastinitis, and bleeding requiring reoperation were similar, however, and there was no difference in mortality, namely 2.5% for off-pump and 2.6% for on-pump. In another observational study involving 1570 patients, OPCAB surgery was associated with less blood loss, higher postoperative hemoglobin levels, and fewer blood transfusions, and the length of stay in the intensive care unit and hospital was shorter.[56] In this study, there was no difference in perioperative MI, use of inotropic agents, incidence of postoperative atrial fibrillation, neurologic complications, prolonged ventilation, renal failure, or death. Thus, it appears that the operation may be a safe alternative to conventional CABG with CPB.

To address CPB-mediated WIR more directly, Ascione and colleagues[56] conducted a prospective, randomized OPCAB surgery trial to examine the relationship between biomarkers of WIR and postoperative morbidity and mortality in OPCAB surgery and CABG patients (see Table 61-10). Serum neutrophil elastase, interleukin-8, and C3a and C5a levels were higher in the CABG with CPB group immediately after surgery. These elevated levels were also associated with a higher incidence of infection, longer intubation time, greater blood loss, greater transfusion requirements and longer intensive care unit and hospital lengths of stay. There was no difference, however, in the incidence of postoperative MI, acute renal failure, stroke, or death. The failure to demonstrate a reduction in the WIR and the incidence of death and MI could have been due, in part, to the relatively small number of patients studied. Alternatively, there may be no direct relationship between CPB-induced WIR, as assessed by certain biomarkers, and death and MI.

With respect to neurocognitive dysfunction, a prospective, randomized trial was performed to determine the possible relationship between the number of high intensive transient signals (HITS) using transcranial Doppler ultrasound (as a surrogate marker of cerebrovascular microemboli) in patients undergoing conventional CABG versus OPCAB.[57] The results suggested that the occurrence of microemboli and incidence of cognitive impairment were increased in the patients subjected to CPB. The median number of HITS in the OPCAB patients was

11, compared with 394 in the patients undergoing conventional CABG. This correlated with two of three neurologic tests, which indicated the incidence of neuropsychiatric and neurocognitive dysfunction was greater in the on-pump CABG patients. These findings support the hypothesis that OPCAB surgery is associated with a reduction in the occurrence of microemboli and adverse neurocognitive outcomes. Using a different approach, Patel and associates[58] studied 2327 consecutive patients and divided them into three groups: on-pump, off-pump with aortic manipulation (aorta used as source of graft inflow), and off-pump without aortic manipulation (pedicle-based inflow). In this study, CPB was a risk factor for focal neurologic deficit, but there were no differences in focal deficits between the OPCAB surgery patients with or without aortic manipulation. Although this study also supports the concept that CPB may be associated with more neurologic events, it does not appear to be related to *aortic manipulation* as defined by the investigators. Other investigators, however, have not demonstrated superior neurocognitive protection with OPCAB surgery (see Table 61-10). Whether OPCAB surgery results in greater cerebral protection will have to await the results of the VA Prospective Randomized Cooperative Study when it concludes in 2007.

Another rationale for performing OPCAB surgery is the potential for reducing the incidence of postoperative renal failure. In one prospective, randomized trial, patients were studied to determine whether OPCAB surgery patients were at lower risk for elevations in creatinine clearance and the urinary microalbumin-to-creatinine ratio in the immediate postoperative period.[59] In the OPCAB surgery patients, the values were lower, and N-acetyl-β-glucosaminidase (NAG) levels, a sensitive marker of renal injury, were less (see Table 61-10). This difference was observed despite the use of mannitol and the maintenance of normal mean arterial blood pressure in the patients undergoing conventional CABG. Neither group, however, demonstrated any clinical manifestations of renal failure. Thus, it is unclear whether OPCAB actually reduces the risk for significant clinical renal failure compared with CABG with CPB.

Robotics

Rapid advances in technology have led to the application of robotic CABG. Robotically assisted microsurgical systems have the theoretical advantage of enhancing surgical dexterity and minimizing the invasive nature of conventional coronary artery surgery.[60] One major system currently in use is the da Vinci system by Intuitive Surgical (Mountain View, CA). It consists of three major components: the surgeon-device interface module, the computer controller, and the specific patient interface instrumentation. They allow real-time surgical manipulation of tissue, advanced dexterity, and optical magnification of the operative field through minimal access ports. Although only a few preliminary studies have been initiated, the results to date suggest that CABG can be safely performed with satisfactory graft patency rates. Current limitations include its lack of applicability to all patients,

Table 61-10 Representative Prospective, Randomized Studies Comparing Results of OPCAB to CABG With CPB

STUDY, NO. OF PATIENTS (*N*), AND FOLLOW-UP (F/U)	REFERENCE	PURPOSE	FINDINGS
Low-Risk Patients			
Beating versus arrested heart revascularization: Evaluation of myocardial function in a prospective, randomized trial *N* = 80 F/U = 1 week	Eur J Cardiothorac Surg 15:685-690, 1999	Evaluated efficacy and safety	OPCAB is safe and effective and is associated with reduction in troponin I release.
On-pump versus off-pump revascularization: Evaluation of renal function *N* = 50 F/U = 1 week	Ann Thorac Surg 68:493-498, 1999	Analyzed postoperative renal function	Glomerular filtration, as assessed by creatinine clearance and microalbumin-to-creatinine ratio, was significantly reduced below preoperative levels in CABG patients and 48 hours after surgery. There were no instances of acute renal failure, death, or myocardial infarction in either group.
Economic outcome of off-pump coronary artery bypass surgery: A prospective, randomized study *N* = 200 F/U = 1 week	Ann Thorac Surg 66:2237-2242, 1999	Safety and cost analysis	OPCAB was safe and effective. On average, the cost was 30% lower with OPCAB. Total mean cost per patient for operating materials, bed occupancy, and transfusion requirements was $3731 for on-pump and $2615/patient for off-pump.
Inflammatory response after coronary revascularization with or without cardiopulmonary bypass *N* = 60 F/U = 1 week	Ann Thorac Surg 69:1198-1204, 2000	Effect of surgery on the inflammatory response	OPCAB was associated with reduced inflammatory response and postoperative infection (24 and 60 hr postoperatively).
Serum S-100 protein release and neuropsychologic outcomes during coronary revascularization on the beating heart: A prospective, randomized study *N* = 60 F/U = 12 weeks	J Thorac Cardiovasc Surg 119:148-154, 2000	Evaluated S-100 protein release up to 24 hours after operation and neuropsychological outcomes	Brain and/or blood-brain barrier may be more adversely affected during CABG surgery with CPB. This was not reflected in detectable neuropsychological deterioration at 12 weeks.
In-hospital outcomes of off-pump versus on-pump coronary artery bypass procedures: A multicenter experience	Ann Thorac Surg 72:1528-1534, 2001	Compared the preoperative risk profiles and in-hospital outcomes of patients done off-pump with those done by conventional coronary artery bypass with CPB	Patients undergoing OPCAB are not exposed to greater risk for short-term adverse outcomes. They have significantly lower need for intraoperative or postoperative IABP, lower rates of atrial fibrillation, and a shorter length of stay.
Cognitive outcome after off-pump and on-pump coronary artery bypass surgery *N* = 281 F/U = 3 and 12 months	JAMA 287:1405-1412, 2002	Analyze effect of procedures on cognitive outcome	OPCAB patients had improved cognitive outcomes 3 months after surgery, but effects were limited and became negligible at 12 months.
Complete revascularization in coronary artery bypass grafting with and without cardiopulmonary bypass *N* = 80 F/U = 2 weeks	Ann Thorac Surg 71:165-169, 2001	Evaluate the feasibility of CABG surgery without CPB to achieve complete revascularization	OPCAB was safe and effective, but the rate of incomplete revascularization was higher.
Early outcome after off-pump versus on-pump coronary bypass surgery *N* = 281 F/U = 1 month	Circulation 104:1761-1766, 2001	Evaluate cardiac outcome and quality of life	OPCAB is safe and results in a similar short-term cardiac mortality and quality-of-life outcome similar to CABG surgery with CPB. Note that creatine kinase-MB release was 41% less in the OPCAB group.

Table 61-10 Representative Prospective, Randomized Studies Comparing Results of OPCAB to CABG With CPB—cont'd

STUDY, NO. OF PATIENTS (*N*), AND FOLLOW-UP (F/U)	REFERENCE	PURPOSE	FINDINGS
On-pump versus off-pump coronary artery bypass surgery in a matched sample of women	Circulation 110(Suppl II): II1-6, 2004	Comparison of outcomes in a matched sample of women	Off-pump surgery led to decreased mortality and morbidity including bleeding complications.
Off-pump versus on-pump myocardial revascularization in low-risk patients with one- or two-vessel disease: Perioperative results in a multicenter randomized controlled trial *N* = 160 F/U = 2 weeks	Ann Thorac Surg 77:569-573, 2004	Evaluate hospital mortality and morbidity after myocardial revascularization, comparing CABG to OPCAB in a subset of patients with lesions in the left descending artery	No statistical difference in hospital mortality and morbidity using on-pump or off-pump techniques for low-risk patients.
Pulmonary outcome of off-pump versus on-pump coronary artery bypass surgery in a randomized trial (SMART Trial) *N* = 200 F/U = 30 days	Chest 127:892-901, 2005	Comparison of pulmonary outcomes after OPCAB versus CABG with CPB	OPCAB was associated with a greater reduction in postoperative respiratory compliance but no difference in chest radiographs, spirometry, or rates of death, pneumonia, pleural effusion, or pulmonary edema.
High-Risk Patients			
Different CABG methods in patients with chronic obstructive pulmonary disease *N* = 37 F/U = 2 months	Ann Thorac Surg 71:152-157, 2001	Determine effect of different CABG techniques on pulmonary function	OPCAB procedures were more advantageous than on-pump procedures for patients with chronic obstructive pulmonary disease.

CABG, coronary artery bypass grafting; CPB, cardiopulmonary bypass; OPCAB, off-pump coronary artery bypass.

prolonged operating room time, limited applicability to access all vessels, cost, and limited training opportunities.

Transmyocardial Laser Revascularization

Patients with chronic severe angina refractory to medical therapy who cannot be completely revascularized with either percutaneous catheter intervention or CABG surgery present clinical challenges. Transmyocardial laser revascularization (TMLR), either as sole therapy or as an adjunct to CABG surgery, may be appropriate for some of these patients.[61] TMLR uses a high-energy laser beam to create myocardial transmural channels that were originally thought to provide direct access to oxygenated blood in the left ventricular cavity. This is no longer considered the mechanism by which TMLR results in a reduction in symptoms of ischemic heart disease. Although some local neovascularization has been documented, the magnitude of changes do not account for any substantive increases in myocardial perfusion. Despite reports of anginal relief, ^{201}Tl SPECT imaging, PET imaging, and other perfusion studies have failed to show any significant improvement in regional blood flow. One mechanism that has been proposed relates to a local effect on cardiac neuronal signaling. It has been hypothesized that local tissue injury by TMLR damages ventricular sensory neurons and autonomic efferent axons, and this leads to

local cardiac denervation and anginal relief. Regardless of the mechanism, TMLR therapy is associated with a reproducible improvement in symptoms. Patients undergoing TMLR show a persistent improvement in angina class using the Canadian Cardiovascular System (CCS).[12] This improvement is achieved in 60% to 80% of patients within 6 months after the operation.

The procedure is usually performed on patients in conjunction with other revascularization procedures but can be done as a stand-alone procedure, especially with minimally invasive approaches. The STS Evidence-Based Workforce reviewed available evidence and recommends use of TMLR for patients with an EF greater than 0.30 and CCS class III or IV angina that is refractory to maximal medical therapy.[61] These patients should have reversible ischemia of the left ventricular free wall and CAD corresponding to the regions of myocardial ischemia. In all regions of the myocardium, the coronary disease must not be amenable to CABG or percutaneous coronary intervention as a result of one of the following:

1. Severe diffuse disease
2. Lack of suitable targets for complete revascularization
3. Lack of suitable conduits for complete revascularization

Randomized trials support this recommendation (level of evidence, A; class I recommendation). Patients with depressed ventricular function (EF<0.3), with unstable angina, or with lower levels of angina may also benefit from this procedure, but the supporting evidence is less well established.

Hybrid Procedures

Many interventional cardiologists are reluctant to recommend CABG in the era of DES, mostly because of the increased up-front mortality and significant morbidity. However, unbiased analysis of available evidence on mortality and morbidity associated with CABG suggests that operative mortality rates for isolated CABG are low (1%-2%) and approach those of PCI. Likewise, morbidity rates for primary CABG are decreasing. It is generally accepted that left internal mammary artery (LIMA) anastomosis to the left anterior descending artery (LAD) is a durable and effective treatment for CAD that confers long-term benefit in reduced mortality and freedom from reintervention. Furthermore, minimally invasive surgical approaches are highly successful in creating an LIMA-to-LAD anastomosis.

At the same time, catheter-based interventions are highly successful in opening blocked coronary arteries with a very low rate of restenosis. The confluence of these observations led several surgeons to suggest an integrated approach to coronary revascularization, termed the *hybrid procedure.* The hybrid procedure consists of a minimally invasive LIMA-to-LAD anastomosis in conjunction with DES to non–LAD-obstructed coronary arteries. This approach has met with initial success, but many potential pitfalls exist. The procedural costs may be greater than those of either CABG alone or DES implantation alone. The timing of which procedure to do first is uncertain. Long-term outcomes of the hybrid procedure are uncertain. These and other uncertainties make hybrid procedures a non–evidence-based intervention. Nevertheless, hybrid procedures have gained a place in the arena and may gain a greater acceptance as longer term results are published.

FUTURE DEVELOPMENTS

CABG has evolved into a mature treatment modality for the management of patients with ischemic heart disease. It is now the safest and most reliable method for completely revascularizing the ischemic heart and is associated with excellent medium and long-term outcomes. Preclinical and clinical studies are now underway to develop and evaluate new methodologies that will make the operation even safer and more effective. This includes use of less invasive techniques, testing of smaller extracorporeal circulation devices, and developing methods to improve myocardial protection and techniques to enhance graft patency. With respect to less invasive operative techniques, new enabling technologies are being developed to facilitate the performance of more precise surgical maneuvers within more confined spaces. There are already a variety of bypass graft coupling devices under investigation that are designed to facilitate proxi-

mal and distal coronary artery graft anastomoses. These include interrupted clips, magnetic docking ports, and specialized metallic intracoronary stents. Hopefully, a usable device will be available within the next few years. Also, clinical trials are underway to determine whether normalization of left ventricular geometry in patients with dilated ischemic heart disease will enhance the beneficial effects of complete myocardial revascularization. The development of smaller, more efficient ventricular assist devices, without a propensity for infection and thromboembolic complications, could lead to circulatory support systems that will obviate the need for orthotopic heart transplantation for ischemic left ventricular dysfunction. In regard to myocardial protection, there is increasing evidence that even mild necrosis during the CABG operation (as measured by CK and CK-MB) not only occurs more frequently than previously appreciated but is also associated with a decrease in medium and long-term survival. This has led to renewed interest in developing more effective methods for protecting the heart. One such strategy under intense investigation is to mimic the phenomenon of ischemic preconditioning pharmacologically.[62]

Finally, it is now known that vascular intimal hyperplasia (VIH) is an important component of vein graft occlusive disease. Gene-based therapies may make it possible to transfect human saphenous veins before grafting and to prevent VIH. It also may be possible to manipulate hs-CRP and slow the progression of the atherosclerotic heart disease process in native coronary arteries. Likewise, because statins have been shown to increase survival in patients with CAD, it may be possible to use these agents to promote endothelial protection and induce reversal of the inflammatory response cascade that leads to atherosclerotic plaque formation. If all these efforts are successful, it may be that the current survival benefit of CABG to patients with advanced CAD will be extended twofold within the near future.

References

1. Virmani R, Burke AP, Farb A, Kolodgie FD: Pathology of the unstable plaque. Prog Cardiovasc Dis 44:349-356, 2002.
2. Allen Maycock CA, Muhlestein JB, Horne BD, et al: Statin therapy is associated with reduced mortality across all age groups of individuals with significant coronary disease, including very elderly patients. J Am Coll Cardiol 40:1777-1785, 2002.
3. de Winter RJ, Heyde GS, Koch KT, et al: The prognostic value of pre-procedural plasma C-reactive protein in patients undergoing elective coronary angioplasty. Eur Heart J 23:960-966, 2002.
4. Solomon SD, Zelenkofske S, McMurray JJ, et al: Sudden death in patients with myocardial infarction and left ventricular dysfunction, heart failure, or both. N Engl J Med 352:2581-2588, 2005.
5. Boersma E, Mercado N, Poldermans D, et al: Acute myocardial infarction. Lancet 361(9360):847-858, 2003.
6. Klein C, Nekolla SG, Bengel FM, et al: Assessment of myocardial viability with contrast-enhanced magnetic resonance imaging: comparison with positron emission tomography. Circulation 105:162-167, 2002.

7. Schwitter J, Nanz D, Kneifel S, et al: Assessment of myo-cardial perfusion in coronary artery disease by magnetic resonance: A comparison with positron emission tomogra-phy and coronary angiography. Circulation 103:2230-2235, 2001.

8. Stein PD, Beemath A, Kayali F, et al: Multidetector com-puted tomography for the diagnosis of coronary artery disease: A systematic review. Am J Med 119:203-216, 2006.

9. Eagle KA, Guyton RA, Davidoff R, et al: ACC/AHA 2004 guideline update for coronary artery bypass graft surgery: A report of the American College of Cardiology/American Heart Association Task Force on Practice Guidelines (Com-mittee to Update the 1999 Guidelines for Coronary Artery Bypass Graft Surgery). Circulation 110:340-437, 2004.

10. Eagle KA, Guyton RA, Davidoff R, et al: ACC/AHA 2004 guideline update for coronary artery bypass graft surgery: summary article. A report of the American College of Car-diology/American Heart Association Task Force on Practice Guidelines (Committee to Update the 1999 Guidelines for Coronary Artery Bypass Graft Surgery). J Am Coll Cardiol 44:213-310, 2004.

11. Gruntzig AR, Senning A, Siegenthaler WE: Nonoperative dilatation of coronary-artery stenosis: Percutaneous translu-minal coronary angioplasty. N Engl J Med 301:61-68, 1979.

12. Parisi AF, Khuri S, Deupree RH, et al: Medical compared with surgical management of unstable angina: 5-year mor-tality and morbidity in the Veterans Administration Study. Circulation 80:1176-1189, 1989.

13. Coronary angioplasty versus medical therapy for angina: The second Randomised Intervention Treatment of Angina (RITA-2) trial. RITA-2 trial participants. Lancet 350(9076):461-468, 1997.

14. Hartigan PM, Giacomini JC, Folland ED, Parisi AF: Two- to three-year follow-up of patients with single-vessel coronary artery disease randomized to PTCA or medical therapy (results of a VA cooperative study). Veterans Affairs Coop-erative Studies Program ACME Investigators. Angioplasty Compared to Medicine. Am J Cardiol 82:1445-1450, 1998.

15. Influence of diabetes on 5-year mortality and morbidity in a randomized trial comparing CABG and PTCA in patients with multivessel disease: The Bypass Angioplasty Revascu-larization Investigation (BARI). Circulation 96:1761-1769, 1997.

16. Hoffman SN, TenBrook JA, Wolf MP, et al: A meta-analysis of randomized controlled trials comparing coronary artery bypass graft with percutaneous transluminal coronary angioplasty: One- to eight-year outcomes. J Am Coll Cardiol 41:1293-1304, 2003.

17. Hannan EL, Racz MJ, McCallister BD, et al: A comparison of three-year survival after coronary artery bypass graft surgery and percutaneous transluminal coronary angio-plasty. J Am Coll Cardiol 33:63-72, 1999.

18. Serruys PW, Ong AT, van Herwerden LA, et al: Five-year outcomes after coronary stenting versus bypass surgery for the treatment of multivessel disease: The final analysis of the Arterial Revascularization Therapies Study (ARTS) ran-domized trial. J Am Coll Cardiol 46:575-581, 2005.

19. Rodriguez AE, Baldi J, Fernandez Pereira C, et al: Five-year follow-up of the Argentine randomized trial of coronary angioplasty with stenting versus coronary bypass surgery in patients with multiple vessel disease (ERACI II). J Am Coll Cardiol 46:582-588, 2005.

20. SoS Investigators: Coronary artery bypass surgery versus percutaneous coronary intervention with stent implantation in patients with multivessel coronary artery disease (the

Stent or Surgery trial): A randomised controlled trial. Lancet 360(9338):965-970, 2002.

21. Babapulle MN, Joseph L, Belisle P, et al: A hierarchical Bayesian meta-analysis of randomised clinical trials of drug-eluting stents. Lancet 364(9434):583-591, 2004.

22. Williams DO, Braunwald E, Thompson B, et al: Results of percutaneous transluminal coronary angioplasty in unstable angina and non-Q-wave myocardial infarction: Observa-tions from the TIMI IIIB Trial. Circulation 94:2749-2755, 1996.

23. Topol EJ, Mark DB, Lincoff AM, et al: Outcomes at 1 year and economic implications of platelet glycoprotein IIb/IIIa blockade in patients undergoing coronary stenting: Results from a multicentre randomised trial. EPISTENT Investiga-tors. Evaluation of Platelet IIb/IIIa Inhibitor for Stenting. Lancet 354(9195):2019-2024, 1999.

24. Budaj A, Yusuf S, Mehta SR, et al: Benefit of clopidogrel in patients with acute coronary syndromes without ST-segment elevation in various risk groups. Circulation 106:1622-1626, 2002.

25. Mehta SR, Yusuf S, Peters RJ, et al: Effects of pretreatment with clopidogrel and aspirin followed by long-term therapy in patients undergoing percutaneous coronary intervention: The PCI-CURE study. Lancet 358(9281):527-533, 2001.

26. Sharma GV, Deupree RH, Khuri SF, et al: Coronary bypass surgery improves survival in high-risk unstable angina. Results of a Veterans Administration Cooperative study with an 8-year follow-up. Veterans Administration Unstable Angina Cooperative Study Group. Circulation 84(5 Suppl):III260-267, 1991.

27. Sharma GV, Deupree RH, Luchi RJ, Scott SM: Identification of unstable angina patients who have favorable outcome with medical or surgical therapy (eight-year follow-up of the Veterans Administration Cooperative Study). Am J Cardiol 74:454-458, 1994.

28. Morrison DA, Sethi G, Sacks J, et al: Percutaneous coronary intervention versus repeat bypass surgery for patients with medically refractory myocardial ischemia: AWESOME ran-domized trial and registry experience with post-CABG patients. J Am Coll Cardiol 40:1951-1954, 2002.

29. Michels KB, Yusuf S: Does PTCA in acute myocardial infarc-tion affect mortality and reinfarction rates? A quantitative overview (meta-analysis) of the randomized clinical trials. Circulation 91:476-485, 1995.

30. Berger PB, Ellis SG, Holmes DR Jr: Relationship between delay in performing direct coronary angioplasty and early clinical outcome in patients with acute myocardial infarc-tion: Results from the global use of strategies to open occluded arteries in Acute Coronary Syndromes (GUSTO-IIb) trial. Circulation 100:14-20, 1999.

31. Tiefenbrunn AJ, Chandra NC, French WJ, et al: Clinical experience with primary percutaneous transluminal coro-nary angioplasty compared with alteplase (recombinant tissue-type plasminogen activator) in patients with acute myocardial infarction: A report from the Second National Registry of Myocardial Infarction (NRMI-2). J Am Coll Cardiol 31:1240-1245, 1998.

32. Creswell LL, Moulton MJ, Cox JL, Rosenbloom M: Revascu-larization after acute myocardial infarction. Ann Thorac Surg 60:19-26, 1995.

33. Sobel BE, Frye R, Detre KM: Burgeoning dilemmas in the management of diabetes and cardiovascular disease: Ra-tionale for the Bypass Angioplasty Revascularization Inves-tigation 2 Diabetes (BARI 2D) Trial. Circulation 107:636-642, 2003.

34. Hochman JS, McCabe CH, Stone PH, et al: Outcome and profile of women and men presenting with acute coronary

syndromes: A report from TIMI IIIB. TIMI Investigators. Thrombolysis in Myocardial Infarction. J Am Coll Cardiol 30:141-148, 1997.

35. Edwards FH, Carey JS, Grover FL, et al: Impact of gender on coronary bypass operative mortality. Ann Thorac Surg 66:125-131, 1998.

36. Hartz RS, Rao AV, Plomondon ME, et al: Effects of race, with or without gender, on operative mortality after coronary artery bypass grafting: A study using The Society of Thoracic Surgeons National Database. Ann Thorac Surg 71:512-520, 2001.

37. Vaccarino V, Abramson JL, Veledar E, Weintraub WS: Sex differences in hospital mortality after coronary artery bypass surgery: Evidence for a higher mortality in younger women. Circulation 105:1176-1181, 2002.

38. Szczech LA, Reddan DN, Owen WF, et al: Differential survival after coronary revascularization procedures among patients with renal insufficiency. Kidney Int 60:292-299, 2001.

39. Herzog CA, Ma JZ, Collins AJ: Comparative survival of dialysis patients in the United States after coronary angioplasty, coronary artery stenting, and coronary artery bypass surgery and impact of diabetes. Circulation 106:2207-2211, 2002.

40. Birkmeyer NJ, Charlesworth DC, Hernandez F, et al: Obesity and risk of adverse outcomes associated with coronary artery bypass surgery. Northern New England Cardiovascular Disease Study Group. Circulation 97:1689-1694, 1998.

41. Grover FL, Shroyer AL, Hammermeister K, et al: A decade's experience with quality improvement in cardiac surgery using the Veterans Affairs and Society of Thoracic Surgeons national databases. Ann Surg 234:464-472; discussion 472-464, 2001.

42. Fitzgibbon GM, Kafka HP, Leach AJ, et al: Coronary bypass graft fate and patient outcome: Angiographic follow-up of 5,065 grafts related to survival and reoperation in 1,388 patients during 25 years. J Am Coll Cardiol 28:616-626, 1996.

43. Grunkemeier GL, Zerr KJ, Jin R: Cardiac surgery report cards: Making the grade. Ann Thorac Surg 72:1845-1848, 2001.

44. Kohn LT, Corrigan J, Donaldson MS, Institute of Medicine (U.S.): Committee on Quality of Health Care in America. To Err Is Human: Building a Safer Health System. Washington DC, National Academy Press, 2000.

45. Donabedian A: Explorations in Quality Assessment and Monitoring. Ann Arbor, MI, Health Administration Press, 1980.

46. Ferraris VA, Ferraris SP, Singh A: Operative outcome and hospital cost. J Thorac Cardiovasc Surg 115:593-602; discussion 602-603, 1998.

47. Jones RH, Hannan EL, Hammermeister KE, et al: Identification of preoperative variables needed for risk adjustment of short-term mortality after coronary artery bypass graft surgery. The Working Group Panel on the Cooperative CABG Database Project. J Am Coll Cardiol 28:1478-1487, 1996.

48. Daley J: Criteria by which to evaluate risk-adjusted outcomes programs in cardiac surgery. Ann Thorac Surg 58:1827-1835, 1994.

49. Daley J: Validity of risk-adjustment methods. In Iezzoni LI (ed): Risk Adjustment for Measuring Healthcare Outcomes, 2nd ed. Chicago, Health Administration Press, 1997, pp 331-363.

50. Shroyer ALW, Coombs LP, Peterson ED, et al: The Society of Thoracic Surgeons: 30-Day operative mortality and morbidity risk models. Ann Thorac Surg 75:1856-1864; discussion 1864-1865, 2003.

51. Burns ER, Billett HH, Frater RW, Sisto DA: The preoperative bleeding time as a predictor of postoperative hemorrhage after cardiopulmonary bypass. J Thorac Cardiovasc Surg 92:310-312, 1986.

52. Ferraris VA, Berry WR, Klingman RR: Comparison of blood reinfusion techniques used during coronary artery bypass grafting. Ann Thorac Surg 56:433-439; discussion 440, 1993.

53. Ferraris VA, Gildengorin V: Predictors of excessive blood use after coronary artery bypass grafting: A multivariate analysis. J Thorac Cardiovasc Surg 98:492-497, 1989.

54. Freiman JA, Chalmers TC, Smith HJ, Kuebler RR: The importance of beta, the type II error, and sample size in the design and interpretation of the randomized controlled trial. In Bailar JC, Mosteller F (eds): Medical Uses of Statistics, 2nd ed. Boston, NEJM Books, 1992, pp 357-373.

55. Hernandez F, Cohn WE, Baribeau YR, et al: In-hospital outcomes of off-pump versus on-pump coronary artery bypass procedures: a multicenter experience. Ann Thorac Surg 72:1528-1533; discussion 1533-1534, 2001.

56. Chamberlain MH, Ascione R, Reeves BC, Angelini GD: Evaluation of the effectiveness of off-pump coronary artery bypass grafting in high-risk patients: An observational study. Ann Thorac Surg 73:1866-1873, 2002.

57. Diegeler A, Hirsch R, Schneider F, et al: Neuromonitoring and neurocognitive outcome in off-pump versus conventional coronary bypass operation. Ann Thorac Surg 69:1162-1166, 2000.

58. Patel NC, Deodhar AP, Grayson AD, et al: Neurological outcomes in coronary surgery: Independent effect of avoiding cardiopulmonary bypass. Ann Thorac Surg 74:400-405; discussion 405-406, 2002.

59. Ascione R, Lloyd CT, Underwood MJ, et al: On-pump versus off-pump coronary revascularization: Evaluation of renal function. Ann Thorac Surg 68:493-498, 1999.

60. Shennib H, Bastawisy A, Mack MJ, Moll FH: Computer-assisted telemanipulation: An enabling technology for endoscopic coronary artery bypass. Ann Thorac Surg 66:1060-1063, 1998.

61. Bridges CR, Horvath KA, Nugent WC, et al: The Society of Thoracic Surgeons practice guideline series: Transmyocardial laser revascularization. Ann Thorac Surg 77:1494-1502, 2004.

62. Mentzer RM Jr: Does size matter? What is your infarct rate after coronary artery bypass grafting? J Thorac Cardiovasc Surg 126:326-328, 2003.

CHAPTER 62

Acquired Heart Disease: Valvular

David A. Fullerton, MD and Alden H. Harken, MD

Historical Perspective
Diagnostic Considerations
Mitral Valve
Aortic Valve
Operative Technique
Surgical Outcomes
Choice of Prosthetic Valves

Valvular heart diseases may be considered surgical diseases. Stenotic or regurgitant cardiac valves create hemodynamic demands on one or both ventricles of the heart. The compensatory mechanisms of the ventricles permit the heart to tolerate these lesions for varying periods of time, sometimes years, before surgical intervention is required. Significant valvular lesions, however, ultimately produce systolic or diastolic ventricular dysfunction, leading to heart failure. As a general rule, surgery for stenotic valve lesions may be deferred until the patient develops symptoms. Regurgitant valve lesions, however, may produce significant ventricular dysfunction before symptoms develop; surgery in patients who do not have symptoms may be indicated. Among the heart's valves, the aortic and mitral valves are by far the most likely to acquire disease; therefore, this chapter focuses on diseases of the aortic and mitral valves.

HISTORICAL PERSPECTIVE

Heart failure from mitral stenosis was well recognized by the late 19th century, and efforts at surgical correction began well before the heart-lung machine was available.[1] As early as 1897, Samways suggested (but never acted

on) the possibility of dilating the stenotic mitral valve. Based on his own postmortem studies of rheumatic heart disease in London, Brunton in 1902 proposed surgical intervention for mitral stenosis by passing a dilator through the wall of the left ventricle retrograde into the mitral valve orifice; his proposal was shunned by London physicians, and Brunton never tried this maneuver. The concept, however, was applied 20 years later in Boston when the first report of successful surgical correction of mitral stenosis appeared in 1923; Cutler and Levine reported successful relief of mitral stenosis by incision of the valve with a knife introduced through an apical left ventriculotomy. In 1925, Soutter performed the first successful closed mitral commissurotomy at the London Hospital by introducing his index finger through the left atrial appendage. Despite Soutter's success, he received no more patient referrals, and another 20 years elapsed before the procedure became widespread. In June 1948, Bailey in Philadelphia and Harken in Boston each performed a successful closed mitral commissurotomy. Thereafter, it became widely used for mitral stenosis.

By the mid-1970s, the closed technique was supplanted by open mitral commissurotomy. Although closed mitral commissurotomy did achieve good palliation of mitral stenosis for its era, open mitral commissurotomy offered several advantages. First, the valvuloplasty may be performed under direct vision. The primary reason for failure of closed mitral commissurotomy is residual stenosis, not restenosis. In up to 75% of patients, the subvalvular apparatus of the mitral valve contributes significantly to the stenosis. The open technique permits precise and maximal division of fused commissures as well as fused chordae. In addition, calcium may be sharply débrided from the valve, and any residual mitral insufficiency may be corrected at the time of operation. Finally, the closed technique has the disadvantage of potentially dislodging a left atrial thrombus, resulting in intraoperative embolization and stroke.

Surgical attempts to correct aortic stenosis also began in the early 20th century.[1] In 1912, Tuffier in Paris attempted transaortic digital dilation of a stenotic aortic valve. In 1947, Smithy (who died of aortic stenosis at 43 years of age) and Parker at the University of South Carolina described an experimental model of aortic valvotomy. Three years later in Philadelphia, Bailey reported successful aortic valvotomy by insertion of a mechanical dilator across the stenotic valve of patients to open fused commissures. In 1952, Hufnagel and Harvey at Georgetown University placed the first prosthetic ball valve into the descending aorta of a patient with aortic insufficiency. Surgery on the aortic valve under direct vision required the development of cardiopulmonary bypass by Gibbon in 1954. In 1955, Swann performed the first successful aortic valvotomy using hypothermia and inflow occlusion. Initially, open aortic valve operations were limited to aortic valve commissurotomy and débridement of calcified aortic valve leaflets. Harken in Boston in 1960 and Starr in Portland in 1963, however, reported replacement of the aortic valve with a ball-valve prosthesis. In 1962, Ross in London successfully performed orthotopic homograft valve replacement. In 1967, Ross performed the first pulmonary autograft procedure (Ross procedure) for correction of aortic stenosis. In the mid-1960s, stent-mounted porcine aortic valves were implanted, but these formaldehyde-fixed valves rapidly degenerated. In 1974, Carpentier in Paris reported superior longevity of the glutaraldehyde-preserved porcine valve.

DIAGNOSTIC CONSIDERATIONS

Valvular heart disease may be suggested by a patient's history or by a heart murmur detected on physical examination. Regardless of the valve lesion in question, echocardiography is employed to assess the severity of the stenosis, regurgitation, or both. Information available from the echocardiogram includes definition of valve anatomy, assessment of ventricular contractile function, determination of the magnitude of valve regurgitation using color-flow Doppler imaging, and determination of the severity of valve stenosis.

Transthoracic two-dimensional echocardiography is completely noninvasive and may provide the necessary information. If more information is needed, transesophageal echocardiography may provide better definition of aortic and mitral valve anatomy; it is also a more sensitive imaging modality for detection of mitral regurgitation.

Although most valve lesions may be accurately diagnosed by echocardiography, cardiac catheterization may be necessary to confirm the diagnosis or to provide additional information pertaining to ventricular function. Before surgery, it may be necessary to exclude the presence of coronary artery disease. Mitral or aortic valve areas may be determined at cardiac catheterization using the Gorlin formula,[2] which permits calculation of the valve area as follows:

Valve area = Flow across the valve ÷
$$(C \times \sqrt{\text{Mean transvalvular gradient}})$$

where C is an empiric constant: 44.5 for the aortic valve and 38 for the mitral valve

MITRAL VALVE

Surgical Anatomy of the Mitral Valve

The normal function of the mitral valve is dependent on coordinated interaction of the mitral valve apparatus, which includes the mitral valve annulus, the valve leaflets, the valve chordae tendineae, and the left ventricular papillary muscles. The normal mitral valve has two leaflets: the anterior (or aortic leaflet) and the posterior or (mural leaflet). Two papillary muscles arise from the left ventricular wall; the posterior (or posteromedial) and the anterior (or anterolateral). Each of the leaflets of the mitral valve is connected to each of the papillary muscles by tendons, the chordae tendineae.

The leaflets are suspended from the mitral annulus, a collagenous structure that encircles the orifice between the left atrium and ventricle. Although the two leaflets have about the same surface area, they have very different shapes (Fig. 62-1). The anterior leaflet is rectangular in shape. Its base is attached to the mitral annulus anteriorly, and the width of the base is about one third the circumference of the mitral annulus. This attachment of the anterior leaflet to the mitral annulus extends to the aortic annulus through fibrous tissue, providing "fibrous continuity" between the aortic and mitral valves; the anterior leaflet of the mitral valve is immediately visible as the surgeon looks down through the aortic valve. The posterior leaflet is rectangular in shape, and its attachment to the mitral annulus extends for about two thirds of the circumference of the mitral annulus. The two leaflets are separated by two distinct commissures.

There are three important surgical landmarks (see Fig. 62-1). First, the circumflex coronary artery runs along the epicardial surface of the heart overlying the posterior mitral annulus. Just millimeters of left atrial muscle separate the artery from the annulus, making it susceptible to injury during mitral valve surgery. Second, the aortic valve is in close approximation to the anterior leaflet of the mitral valve (aortomitral continuity). The noncoronary leaflet of the aortic valve is therefore susceptible to injury during mitral surgery. Third, the atrioventricular node is located deep to the posteromedial commissure of the mitral valve.

Mitral Stenosis

Etiology

Rheumatic fever is the principal cause of mitral stenosis, and about two thirds of patients with rheumatic mitral stenosis are female. Rheumatic fever usually occurs in childhood or adolescence (mean age, 8-12 years) and creates an inflammatory infiltration of the myocardium and valves. Perhaps because the disease afflicts young people and many years pass before symptoms are manifest, a prior history of rheumatic fever is often difficult to confirm. As the mitral valve heals after acute rheumatic fever, the mitral apparatus may slowly become deformed,

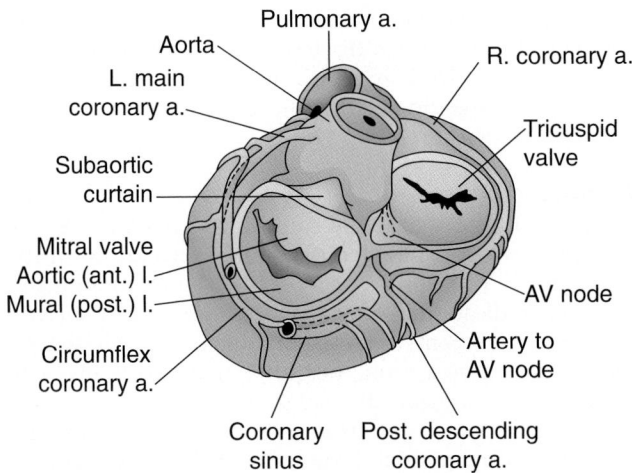

Aorta
Pulmonary a.
L. main coronary a.
R. coronary a.
Subaortic curtain
Tricuspid valve
Mitral valve Aortic (ant.) l.
Mural (post.) l.
AV node
Circumflex coronary a.
Artery to AV node
Coronary sinus
Post. descending coronary a.

Figure 62-1 Anatomy of the mitral valve as it relates to other cardiac structures. Important surgical landmarks include the relationship of the mitral valve to the aortic valve, the circumflex coronary artery, and the atrioventricular (AV) node. (From Buchanan SA, Tribble CG: Reoperative mitral replacement. In Kaiser LR, Kron IL, Spray TL [eds]: Mastery of Cardiothoracic Surgery. Philadelphia, Lippincott-Raven, 1998, p 351.

and the disease typically remains asymptomatic for at least 10 years; symptoms most commonly appear during the patient's third or fourth decade of life. Healing of the inflammation from rheumatic fever ultimately causes the cusps and commissures of the mitral valve to thicken and fuse, with concomitant fusion and shortening of the chordae tendineae. The structure of the valve apparatus then calcifies and narrows, becoming funnel shaped. Such thickening and fusion of the valve not only creates stenosis but also often prevents complete closure of the valve. In fact, of all patients with rheumatic mitral valve disease, about half have combined mitral stenosis and mitral regurgitation.

Other causes of mitral stenosis that are far less common than rheumatic fever include malignant carcinoid, systemic lupus erythematosus, and rheumatoid arthritis. Rarely, congenital malformation of the valve may cause mitral stenosis, and congenital mitral stenosis is almost never an isolated congenital cardiac lesion.

Pathophysiology

The cross-sectional area of the normal mitral valve is 4 to 6 cm². A mitral valve area of 2 cm² is considered "moderate" mitral stenosis, and an area of 1 cm² is considered "severe" mitral stenosis. Under normal conditions, there is no pressure gradient across the mitral valve, and the left atrial pressure is normally less than 15 mm Hg. As the mitral valve becomes more narrowed, an increasing pressure gradient is required to move the blood across the mitral valve from the left atrium into the left ventricle during diastole; a transvalvular gradient of 10 mm Hg indicates severe mitral stenosis. The significance of the transvalvular gradient is that left atrial pressure progressively increases, as the mitral valve becomes more stenotic. In turn, the increased left atrial pressure is

transmitted retrograde into the pulmonary veins, pulmonary capillaries, and ultimately pulmonary arteries. A left atrial pressure of about 25 mm Hg increases pulmonary capillary pressure enough to produce pulmonary edema.

The severity of obstruction across the valve is determined by the transvalvular gradient and the flow rate across the valve. The flow rate is a function of both the cardiac output and the heart rate; because flow across the mitral valve occurs during diastole and diastole is shortened as heart rate increases, a faster heart rate at any given cardiac output increases the transvalvular gradient and raises left atrial pressure. The contribution of the atrial contraction ("kick") to cardiac output is particularly important in mitral stenosis; it accomplishes as much as 30% of the transvalvular gradient. For these reasons, the onset of symptoms is generally associated with exertional activities or with the onset of atrial fibrillation.

To maintain adequate left ventricular filling across a 1-cm² valve, for example, a pressure gradient of 20 mm Hg is required. A normal left ventricular end-diastolic pressure of 5 mm Hg results in a left atrial pressure of 25 mm Hg. Left atrial pressure rises further if flow rate across the valve increases (increased cardiac output), transit time across the valve is shortened (decreased diastolic time), or atrial kick is lost (atrial fibrillation).

Pulmonary hypertension is an important component of the pathophysiology of mitral stenosis and, when severe, may dominate the clinical picture. At least three pathophysiologic mechanisms contribute to the pulmonary hypertension seen in long-standing mitral valvular disease:

1. Increased left atrial pressure transmitted retrograde into the arterial circulation
2. Vascular remodeling of the pulmonary vasculature in response to chronic obstruction to pulmonary venous drainage ("fixed component")
3. Pulmonary arterial vasoconstriction ("reactive component")

Diagnosis

Symptoms

Dyspnea is the principal symptom of mitral stenosis. Dyspnea is typically brought on with exertion or associated with the abrupt onset of atrial fibrillation. The increased cardiac output or heart rate with exertion or the loss of atrial kick and tachycardia with atrial fibrillation result in an increased transvalvular gradient. This in turn increases left atrial pressure, and the pulmonary veins and capillaries become engorged, producing the sensation of dyspnea and promoting pulmonary edema. If the left atrium enlargement is sufficient to compress surrounding structures, the patient may complain of dysphagia or hoarseness. Marked elevation in left atrial pressure may produce hemoptysis.

Physical Examination

The left ventricle is typically normal in size, and the apex is therefore not displaced. The murmur of mitral stenosis is best heard at the apex. It is a low-pitched, rumbling diastolic murmur that is decreased with inspiration and increased during expiration; it may be markedly decreased by Valsalva maneuver. An opening snap precedes the murmur, is heard at the apex, and represents the completed excursion of the mitral valve leaflets. If the mitral leaflets are stiff or calcified, an opening snap may not be heard. In patients with pulmonary hypertension, signs of elevated right ventricular and central venous pressure may dominate the clinical picture. Physical findings, such as distended neck veins, hepatomegaly, ascites, and peripheral edema, combined with a loud pulmonary valve component of the second heart sound (P_2) heard on cardiac auscultation, all suggest significant pulmonary hypertension.

Chest Radiograph

Several findings may be noted on the chest radiograph. The cardiac silhouette may be normal in size, but the left atrium is enlarged. The enlarged left atrium may be seen as a double density behind the right atrium on the posteroanterior projection, or it may be seen to displace the left main-stem bronchus superiorly. On the lateral projection, the enlarged left atrium may displace the esophagus posteriorly. Calcification of the mitral leaflets or the mitral annulus may be seen. Pulmonary venous hypertension is suspected when the pulmonary arteries are enlarged and there is cephalization of pulmonary blood flow.

Echocardiogram

The echocardiogram is the principal tool used to confirm the diagnosis. Using the echocardiogram, the mitral valve area may be determined by two mechanisms. First, the mitral valve area may be determined directly from the echocardiogram by planimetry. Second, measurement of the velocity of blood flow across the valve by Doppler echocardiography permits calculation of the transvalvular gradient. Because the transvalvular gradient persists longer with greater stenosis of the valve, the time required for the transvalvular gradient to decline may be measured and is referred to as the *pressure half-time.* The mitral valve area may then be calculated using the following formula:

$$\text{Mitral valve area} = 220 \div \text{Pressure half-time}$$

Cardiac Catheterization

Mitral stenosis may also be diagnosed by cardiac catheterization. In fact, before undergoing surgical correction of mitral stenosis, cardiac catheterization is performed in patients with a history of angina and in those who are older than 40 years to exclude coronary artery disease. At the time of cardiac catheterization, left atrial pressure may be determined directly (by transatrial puncture) or inferred from pulmonary capillary wedge pressure. Simultaneous measurement of the left ventricular diastolic pressure permits calculation of the transvalvular gradient; a transvalvular gradient of greater than 10 mm Hg is consistent with significant mitral stenosis. Using the Gorlin formula, the mitral valve area (MVA) may be calculated as follows:

$$\text{MVA} = F \div 38 \, (\sqrt{\Delta P})$$

where ΔP is the mean diastolic transvalvular gradient (mm Hg), F is the mean diastolic mitral flow in milliliters per second (derived from the measured cardiac output and a determination of diastolic duration), and 38 is a constant

Natural History

The natural history of mitral stenosis has been altered by successful surgical intervention. Data collected from the era before widespread surgery for mitral stenosis, however, indicate that after diagnosis, the mean survival time among patients with asymptomatic mitral stenosis was 15 to 20 years; on the other hand, patients with symptoms had a mean survival time of only 2 to 7 years.[3] Left atrial distention predisposes to atrial fibrillation and its associated intra-atrial thrombus formation. As many as 20% of patients with mitral stenosis and atrial fibrillation may sustain systemic embolization, especially strokes.

Treatment

The symptom-free patient in sinus rhythm requires only prophylaxis against bacterial endocarditis. When symptoms appear, medical treatment of mitral stenosis includes diuretics to lower left atrial pressure and efforts to maintain sinus rhythm with β-blocking agents or calcium channel blocking agents. Digoxin is helpful in controlling ventricular rate in patients who do go into atrial fibrillation. Patients in atrial fibrillation are anticoagulated with chronic warfarin sodium (Coumadin) therapy because the risk for systemic embolization is high.

Mechanical relief of mitral stenosis is considered when patients develop symptoms, when evidence of pulmonary hypertension appears, or when the mitral valve area is reduced to about 1 cm^2. Other conditions that prompt surgical consideration include systemic embolization, worsening pulmonary hypertension, and endocarditis. The options for mechanical relief of mitral stenosis include balloon mitral valvuloplasty, open surgical mitral valvuloplasty (commissurotomy), and mitral valve replacement.

Balloon Mitral Valvuloplasty

First performed in 1984, balloon mitral valvuloplasty has become the treatment of choice for selected patients with mitral stenosis.[4] Echocardiography may be used to determine patients considered to be good candidates, including those with pliable valve leaflets but without valvular calcification or deformation of the chordae tendineae. Contraindications to this procedure include the presence of moderate mitral regurgitation, thickening and calcification of the mitral leaflets, and scarring and calcification of the subvalvular apparatus.[5] Performed in the cardiac catheterization suite under fluoroscopic guidance, the technique entails advancement of one or two balloon catheters across the interatrial septum and inflation of the balloon within the stenotic mitral valve.

Balloon mitral valvuloplasty has provided good short-term and intermediate-term results in appropriately selected patients. Balloon inflation increases the mitral valve area to about 2 cm^2. This increase in mitral valve area is usually associated with a significant decline in left atrial pressure and transvalvular gradient and with at least a 20% increase in cardiac output. The mortality rate associated with balloon mitral valvuloplasty is 0.5% to 2%. Other risks associated with this procedure include systemic embolism, cardiac perforation, and creation of mitral regurgitation; the risk for each of these complications is about 1% to 2%. Increased pulmonary vascular resistance has been shown to normalize after successful balloon valvuloplasty. About 10% of patients are left with a residual interatrial septal defect. Three years after balloon valvuloplasty, at least 66% of patients are free of subsequent intervention. In appropriately selected patients, the results of balloon valvuloplasty compare favorably with surgical valvuloplasty.

Open Mitral Commissurotomy

Open surgical valvuloplasty (commissurotomy) permits careful examination of the mitral valve and the chordae tendineae under direct vision as well as removal of left atrial thrombus. Because thrombus typically originates in the left atrial appendage, its orifice may be surgically oversewn from within the left atrium, reducing the risk for subsequent embolization. The surgeon may then sharply divide fused commissures and leaflets, mobilize scarred chordae, and débride calcification. Further, reconstruction of the valve may eliminate preexistent mitral regurgitation. The presence of significant mitral regurgitation, however, prompts consideration of mitral valve replacement.

The mortality rate associated with open mitral valvuloplasty is less than 2%.[6] When performed in appropriately selected patients, the freedom from subsequent mitral valve intervention is about 75% at 5 years. Nonetheless, because of less procedure-related morbidity, balloon valvuloplasty is the procedure of choice.

Mitral Valve Replacement

The mitral valve is replaced when valvuloplasty is precluded by dense calcification of the leaflets or subvalvular apparatus or because of concomitant mitral regurgitation. Regardless of whether a tissue or mechanical prosthesis is implanted, efforts are made to preserve the continuity between the left ventricular apex and the mitral annulus provided by the chordae tendineae. This may be readily accomplished by preservation of the posterior leaflet of the native mitral valve.

The contribution of the mitral apparatus to overall left ventricular function is now well appreciated.[7] A mechanical advantage is afforded the left ventricle by the connection of its apex (by way of the papillary muscles) to the mitral annulus through the chordae tendineae; elimination of this connection by removal of the entire mitral apparatus leads to loss of left ventricular function. Convincing data from laboratory animals and humans demonstrate that preservation of at least some of the chordae tendineae at the time of mitral valve replacement results in much better long-term left ventricular function than mitral valve replacement with chordal separation. Therefore, if mitral valve replacement is required, efforts need to be made to preserve the posterior and, in some cases, the anterior leaflets of the native mitral valve.

The operative mortality rate associated with mitral valve replacement for mitral stenosis is 2% to 10%.[8] Operative mortality is increased with advanced age and the presence of coronary disease. Pulmonary hypertension typically resolves after valve replacement, but several weeks or months may be required. The 5-year survival rate after replacement is 70% to 90%.[6,9]

Mitral Regurgitation

Etiology

Competency of the mitral valve requires an intact mitral valve apparatus. Abnormalities of any component of the mitral valve apparatus may produce mitral regurgitation: the mitral leaflets, the chordae tendineae, the mitral valve annulus, or the papillary muscles. Worldwide, rheumatic fever remains the most common cause of mitral regurgitation; it results in deformity and retraction of the leaflets and shortening of the chordae. The leaflets may be perforated by trauma or infective endocarditis. Calcification of the mitral annulus may result in annular rigidity and may prevent valve closure, and mitral annular dilation resultant to left ventricular dilation may likewise preclude leaflet apposition during systole.

Chordal rupture may result from trauma, endocarditis, rheumatic fever, or diseases of collagen formation; chordae to the posterior leaflet rupture more frequently than those to the anterior leaflet. Mitral valve prolapse is found in about 2% of the U.S. population, and up to 5% of patients with mitral valve prolapse develop mitral regurgitation secondary to chordal elongation or rupture. Coronary arterial disease may produce infarction of the papillary muscle, resulting in mitral regurgitation. Infarction in the distribution of the anterior descending coronary artery may necrose the anterolateral papillary muscle, whereas the posteromedial muscle may infarct if blood flow through the posterior descending coronary artery is interrupted. Mitral regurgitation resultant to myocardial infarction typically presents as a new murmur several days after infarction.

Pathophysiology

The regurgitant mitral valve offers an alternative route by which blood may exit the left ventricle. During both isovolumetric contraction and systole, blood is preferentially ejected into the low-pressure left atrium. The volume of the regurgitant flow (regurgitant fraction) is dependent on the size of the regurgitant orifice and the pressure gradient between the left ventricle and left atrium.

Increased left ventricular afterload or decreased forward left ventricular stroke volume increases left ventricular pressure and thereby increases the pressure gradient between left ventricle and atrium. The mitral valve annulus is enlarged by dilation of the left ventricle. Therefore, the size of the regurgitant orifice is increased by diminished left ventricular contractility as well as increased left ventricular preload and increased afterload. Because the valve leaks during systole, the volume of regurgitant flow also increases as heart rate (number of systoles per minute) increases.

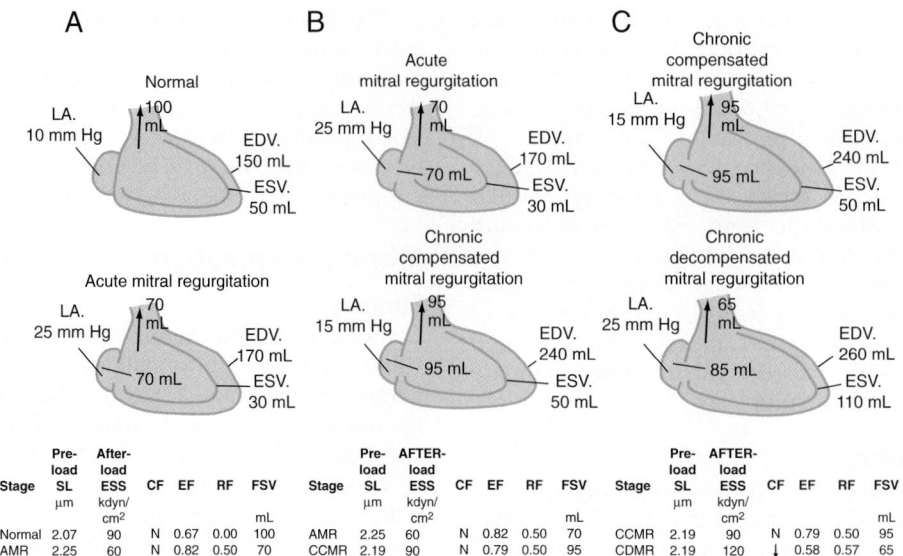

	A							B							C						
Stage	Pre-load SL μm	After-load ESS kdyn/cm²	CF	EF	RF	FSV mL	Stage	Pre-load SL μm	AFTER-load ESS kdyn/cm²	CF	EF	RF	FSV mL	Stage	Pre-load SL μm	AFTER-load ESS kdyn/cm²	CF	EF	RF	FSV mL
Normal	2.07	90	N	0.67	0.00	100	AMR	2.25	60	N	0.82	0.50	70	CCMR	2.19	90	N	0.79	0.50	95
AMR	2.25	60	N	0.82	0.50	70	CCMR	2.19	90	N	0.79	0.50	95	CDMR	2.19	120	↓	0.58	0.57	65

Figure 62-2 Pathophysiology and compensation for acute and chronic mitral regurgitation. **A,** With acute mitral regurgitation, end-diastolic volume (EDV) increases from 150 to 170 mL. Because the left ventricle ejects blood into both the aorta and the left atrium (LA), end-systolic volume (ESV) decreases from 50 to 30 mL. The ejection fraction (EF) therefore increases acutely, but because a significant percentage is ejected into the LA, the volume of blood flow into the aorta (forward stroke volume, FSV) decreases from 100 to 70 mL. The regurgitant volume into the LA increases LA pressure. **B,** Myocardial compensation for chronic mitral regurgitation includes eccentric left ventricular hypertrophy. Left ventricular EDV increases from 170 to 240 mL. The larger ventricle results in an increased total stroke volume as well as FSV. Enlargement of the LA increases its capacity, which accommodates the regurgitant volume at a lower pressure. The left ventricular EF is supernormal. **C,** Ultimately, the heart decompensates, and the contractile force (CF) of the left ventricle declines; the end-systolic volume increases from 50 to 110 mL. FSV declines. The left ventricle dilates, which further compromises the ability of the mitral valve apparatus to close; the regurgitant volume increases. The EF remains above normal until contractile function declines further. ESS, end-systolic stress; RF, regurgitant fraction; SL, sarcomere length. (From Carabello BA: Mitral regurgitation: Basic pathophysiologic principles. Mod Concepts Cardiovasc Dis 57:53,1988.)

The compensatory mechanism by which the left ventricle adapts to maintain an adequate systemic blood flow (forward cardiac output) is volume overload; it must pump the combined volume of systemic and regurgitant flows (Fig. 62-2). Volume overload leads to cardiac dilation as well as left ventricular hypertrophy. Because the left ventricle ejects into the reduced resistance of the left atrium, parameters of systolic function (ejection fraction [EF]) are *increased* in mitral regurgitation. As with aortic insufficiency, however, the left ventricle ultimately fails with chronic volume overload. In fact, *normal* parameters of systolic function indicate significant contractile dysfunction of the left ventricle. An EF of less than 40% in the setting of mitral regurgitation indicates significant left ventricular contractile dysfunction.

As in mitral stenosis, left atrial hypertension results from mitral regurgitation. This pressure is transmitted retrograde into the pulmonary circulation and, if high enough, produces pulmonary hypertension. The magnitude of the left atrial pressure is a function of the compliance of the left atrium. Normal or low compliance of the left atrium, such as may occur in acute mitral regurgitation, results in a relatively rapid rise in left atrial pressure. On the other hand, chronic, left atrial volume overload that develops slowly may create significant enlargement

of a compliant left atrium with relatively low left atrial pressure.

Diagnosis

Symptoms

The symptoms of mitral regurgitation are those of heart failure: shortness of breath, dyspnea on exertion, orthopnea, pulmonary edema, and diminished exercise tolerance. Symptoms are determined by the degree of mitral regurgitation, the rate of its progression, the degree of pulmonary hypertension, and the magnitude of left ventricular contractile dysfunction. For example, patients with mild mitral regurgitation may remain symptom-free for most of their lives. At the other extreme, patients with acute, severe mitral regurgitation, such as may occur with endocarditis or ruptured chordae tendineae, may have pulmonary edema and require urgent surgery. The onset of atrial fibrillation does impair the patient's functional status, but not to the same degree as with mitral stenosis. With chronic, moderate to severe mitral regurgitation, patients may be symptom-free for long periods of time. Lack of symptoms, however, may be very deceiving because the contractile function of the left ventricle may be slowly deteriorating from volume overload. When symptoms occur, left ventricular contractile dysfunction may be irreversible.

Physical Examination

On cardiac auscultation, a holosystolic murmur is heard best at the apex and radiates to the axilla and left scapular region. The pulmonary examination may be significant for rales and bronchospasm caused by increased pulmonary interstitial fluid. In fact, mitral valve pathology is considered in the differential diagnosis of patients with adult-onset asthma.

Electrocardiogram

The electrocardiogram is notable for left atrial enlargement and, frequently, atrial fibrillation.

Chest Radiograph

The chest radiograph is significant for cardiomegaly and left atrial enlargement. Pulmonary venous hypertension may manifest as cephalization of pulmonary blood flow and pulmonary edema.

Echocardiogram

The diagnosis is confirmed by echocardiography. Transesophageal echocardiography is particularly effective in providing an anatomic explanation for the regurgitation, such as perforated leaflets, poor leaflet coaptation, or ruptured chordae. Doppler echocardiography reveals a high-velocity jet of regurgitant blood flow into the left atrium during systole.

Unfortunately, the determination of the severity of mitral regurgitation is only semiquantitative. The severity of the regurgitation is gauged as a function of the distance from the mitral annulus that the jet can be visualized (e.g., into the pulmonary veins) and by the width of the regurgitant jet. The regurgitation is scored subjectively on a scale from 1 (mild) to 4 (severe). The chronicity of the regurgitation may be inferred from the size of the left atrium; an enlarged left atrium suggests chronic mitral regurgitation. Contrast ventriculography, performed at cardiac catheterization, likewise demonstrates mitral regurgitation during systole.

Natural History of Mitral Regurgitation

The natural history of the disease is variable, determined by the cause of mitral regurgitation, the regurgitant volume, and the magnitude of left ventricular systolic dysfunction. Patients with mild mitral regurgitation typically remain symptom-free for years and rarely go on to develop severe mitral regurgitation. As is the situation with most valve diseases, the natural history of mitral regurgitation is obscure because surgical intervention has effectively altered this history. In the presurgical era, however, about 80% of patients with severe mitral regurgitation survived 5 years, and 60% survived 10 years.[10,11] Patients with combined mitral stenosis and regurgitation had a worse prognosis, with a 5-year survival rate of only 67%.

Treatment

The cornerstone of medical management is diuresis and afterload reduction with angiotensin-converting enzyme inhibitors. The importance of afterload reduction cannot be overemphasized. Because blood leaving the left ventricle travels the path of least resistance, lowering systemic vascular resistance increases systemic cardiac output. In the setting of heart failure from acute mitral regurgitation, intravenous vasodilators (nitroprusside) may be needed. When a patient is stabilized, conversion to oral angiotensin-converting inhibitors may be achieved. Diuretics function not only to relieve pulmonary edema but also to reduce left ventricular diameter. The size of the mitral annulus is thereby diminished and the regurgitant fraction reduced.

The indications for surgical intervention include symptoms despite medical management; severe mitral regurgitation in the presence of an identified structural abnormality, such as a ruptured chorda tendinea; development of pulmonary hypertension; or evidence of deteriorating left ventricular contractile function as determined by echocardiography or contrast ventriculography.

It is difficult to judge left ventricular function in patients without symptoms, making close follow-up with serial echocardiograms essential. In fact, asymptomatic left ventricular dysfunction may develop insidiously. Two parameters of left ventricular function are useful in making the decision regarding timing of surgery: EF and end-systolic diameter (ESD). Because mitral regurgitation lowers the total impedance against left ventricular ejection, the EF should be supernormal in the presence of normal myocardial contractile function. An EF of less than 60% suggests myocardial dysfunction, and operative mortality increases.[12] The other useful parameter of left ventricular function is the left ventricular ESD.[12] ESD is less preload-dependent than is EF, and the information it implies is complementary. When left ventricular ESD exceeds 45 mm, the prognosis after surgery is worse.[13] Even in the absence of symptoms, therefore, patients are referred for surgery when the left ventricular EF is less than 60% or when the left ventricular ESD is more than 45 mm.[14]

In those cases, there are two surgical options: mitral valve repair or replacement. When possible, the valve needs to be repaired. The final decision about which of these options to employ is made intraoperatively after valve inspection. Mitral valve repair has several advantages over replacement. First, left ventricular function is better preserved after repair[15,16] (Fig. 62-3). Valve repair preserves the continuity between the mitral annulus and ventricular papillary muscle provided by the chordae tendineae; this provides the left ventricle a mechanical advantage and optimizes its function. When the chordae tendineae are sacrificed during a mitral valve replacement, the postoperative EF typically decreases (Fig. 62-4). Therefore, even when mitral valve replacement is necessary for mitral regurgitation, the chordae tendineae needs to be preserved if possible.[17]

Second, mitral valve replacement subjects the patient to the risks associated with the valve prosthesis, such as thromboembolism and the risk for prosthetic valve endocarditis. Bioprosthetic valves may ultimately experience structural deterioration, and mechanical prosthetic valves obligate the patient to lifelong anticoagulation with warfarin sodium. After mitral valve repair, patients in sinus

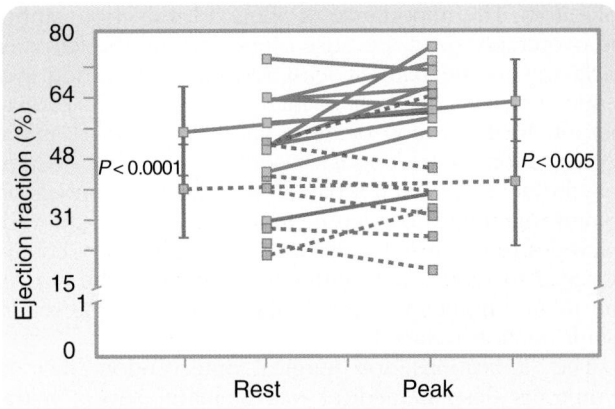

Figure 62-3 Left ventricular (LV) ejection fraction after mitral valve repair (*blue squares*) versus replacement (*pink squares*). Ejection fraction is greater at rest and with exercise after repair. (From Tishler MD, Cooper KA, Rowen M, LeWinter MM: Mitral valve replacement versus mitral repair: A Doppler and quantitative stress echocardiograph study. Circulation 89:132, 1994.)

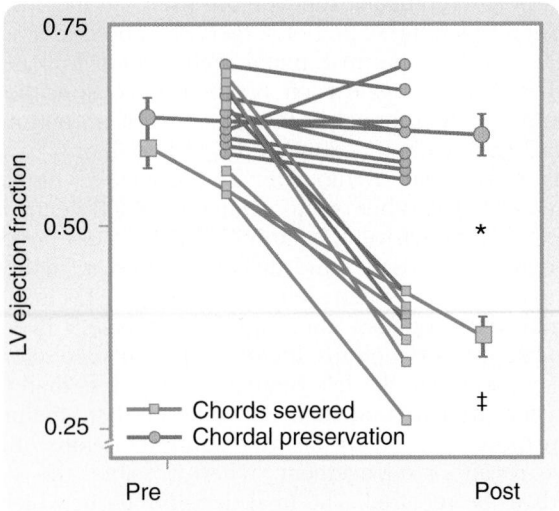

Figure 62-4 Postoperative ejection fraction after mitral valve replacement with (*circles*) and without (*squares*) preservation of the chordae tendineae. Ejection fraction decreases significantly with chords severed but is preserved with chordal preservation. (From Roseate JD, Carabello BA, Ushere BW, et al: Mitral valve replacement with and without chordal preservation in patients with chronic mitral regurgitation. Circulation 86:1718, 1992.)

rhythm do not require long-term warfarin sodium therapy.

Third, the operative mortality rate associated with mitral valve repair (0%-2%) is significantly less than that for replacement (4%-8%).[6] Long-term survival appears better with repair as well. These outcomes likely derive from the superior left ventricular function after mitral repair than after replacement.

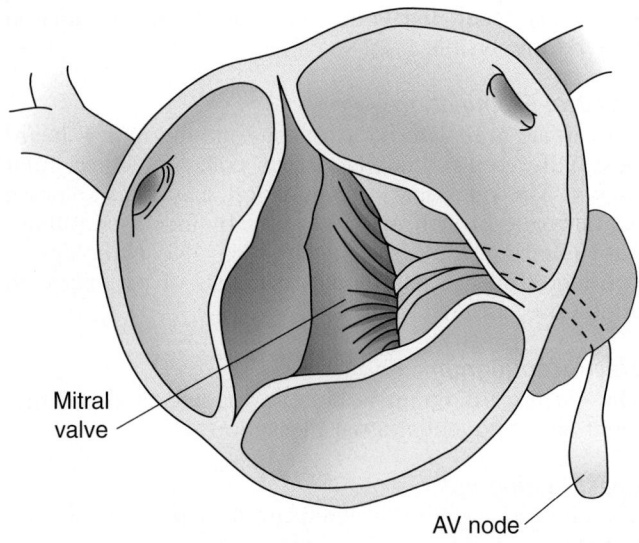

Mitral valve

AV node

Figure 62-5 Surgical anatomy of the aortic valve. The commissure between the noncoronary and the left coronary leaflets lies anterior to the left bundle of His. Injury to this conduction tissue during aortic valve surgery may result in heart block. AV, atrioventricular.

Significant left ventricular dysfunction has long been recognized as a significant risk factor for operative death after surgical correction for mitral regurgitation. Recently, however, several investigators have achieved excellent results with mitral valve repair even in patients with severe heart failure and left ventricular EFs below 20%.[18] Functional status of the patients has been significantly improved, and need for hospital admission for treatment of heart failure has been markedly decreased. Preservation of the mitral apparatus at the time of repair is essential to achieve those results.

AORTIC VALVE

Surgical Anatomy of the Aortic Valve

The normal aortic valve is composed of three thin, pliable leaflets, or cusps, attached to the heart at the junction of the aorta and the left ventricle. The leaflets are attached within the three sinuses of Valsalva of the proximal aorta and join together in three commissures, which create the shape of a coronet. Because the coronary arteries arise from two of the three sinuses of Valsalva, the aortic leaflets are named after their respective sinuses as the *left coronary leaflet,* the *right coronary leaflet,* and the *noncoronary leaflet*. There are two important surgical landmarks. First, the commissure between the left and noncoronary leaflets is positioned over the anterior leaflet of the mitral valve. Second, the commissure between the noncoronary and the right coronary leaflets is positioned over the left bundle of His. Injury to this conduction bundle during aortic valve surgery may create heart block (Fig. 62-5).

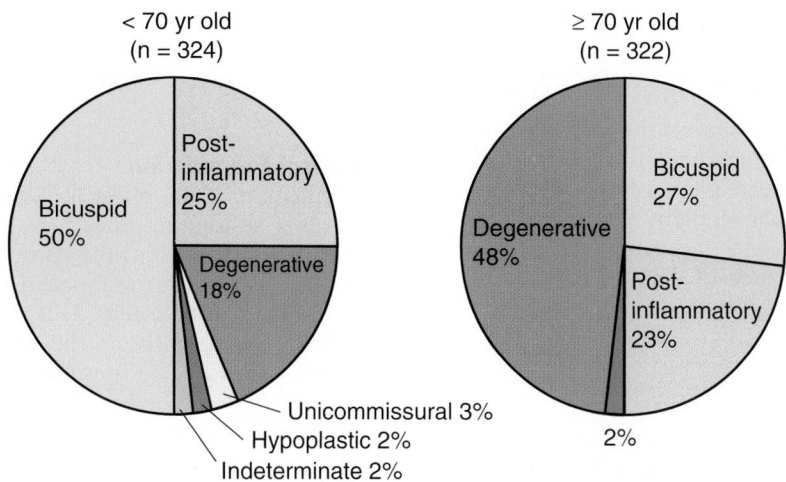

Figure 62-6 Causes of aortic stenosis as a function of age. (From Passik CS, Ackermann DM, Pluth JR, Edwards WD: Temporal changes in the causes of aortic stenosis: A surgical pathologic study of 646 cases. Mayo Clin Proc 62;119, 1987.)

Aortic Stenosis

Etiology

Acquired aortic stenosis usually results from calcification of the aortic valve associated with advanced age. Although the process is most often idiopathic,[19] rheumatic fever may affect the aortic valve in a process similar to that of the mitral valve. In rheumatic aortic stenosis, inflammation produces adhesions and fusion of the commissures and leaflets with thickening and calcification. Retraction of the leaflets often makes these valves both regurgitant and stenotic. The inflammatory process of rheumatic fever rarely involves the aortic valve alone, usually involving the mitral valve as well. In idiopathic degenerative or senile aortic stenosis, grossly normal leaflets become calcified as a result of normal leaflet stress at the flexion points causing leaflet immobility. This calcification may extend down onto the anterior mitral valve leaflet or upward along the aorta, occasionally causing coronary ostial stenosis.

Congenital valvular abnormalities may be clinically significant immediately after birth, as with unicuspid and dome-shaped valves. Patients born with a congenitally bicuspid aortic valve are uncommonly symptomatic in childhood but are prone to develop aortic stenosis early in adulthood. The bicuspid valve produces turbulent flow across the leaflets, leading to fibrosis, calcification, and stiffening. Patients with a bicuspid aortic valve are prone to develop aortic stenosis at an earlier age (fifth and sixth decades of life) than those with a tricuspid valve (seventh, eighth, and ninth decades) (Fig. 62-6).

Pathophysiology

In acquired aortic stenosis, there is a chronic, progressive narrowing of the aortic valve. As the valve narrows, the appropriate compensatory response of the left ventricle is hypertrophy. As the ventricle hypertrophies, it becomes stiffer as its compliance decreases; a higher left ventricular end-diastolic pressure is needed to maintain the same volume of cardiac output. To achieve a sufficiently high left ventricular end-diastolic pressure (diastolic loading), the heart becomes increasingly dependent on the atrial kick; loss of the atrial kick, as occurs with atrial fibrillation, may result in a significant decline in cardiac output and acute hemodynamic decompensation.

Although left ventricular hypertrophy is an appropriate biologic response to an increasing afterload, it has detrimental effects. The combined effects of any of the following will culminate in increased myocardial oxygen demand: greater left ventricular muscle mass; decreased left ventricular compliance, resulting in greater ventricular wall tension; higher systolic ventricular pressure; and longer systolic ejection time. At the same time, coronary artery blood flow is compromised by increased wall tension compressing the vessels and by higher left ventricular diastolic pressure, which lowers the coronary artery perfusion pressure. These factors contribute to inadequate coronary arterial perfusion of the subendocardium, leading to chronic ischemia. In turn, chronic ischemia leads to cell death and fibrosis.

Left ventricular hypertrophy may allow the heart to achieve a normal cardiac output under resting conditions.[20] To do so, however, a pressure gradient across the valve is required, and, as the aortic valve area (AVA) becomes smaller, the gradient across the valve from left ventricle to aorta increases. This relationship of flow across the valve, valve area, and transvalvular pressure gradient is expressed in the Gorlin formula,[2] as follows:

$$AVA = F \div 44.5 \, (\sqrt{\Delta P})$$

where ΔP is the mean pressure gradient across the valve; aortic valve flow (F) equals cardiac output in milliliters per minute, divided by systolic ejection period in seconds per minute; AVA is the aortic valve area in square centimeters; and C is an empiric orifice constant, 44.5.

For quick calculations, this simplifies to the following:

$$\text{AVA} = \text{Cardiac output} \div \sqrt{\text{Mean pressure gradient}}$$

The relationship of flow across the aortic valve and the transvalvular pressure gradient is shown in Figure 62-7. As the valve area decreases to 1 cm², there is little change in the transvalvular gradient needed to generate the same flow, and patients frequently experience no symptoms. With a valve area of 0.8 cm², patients invariably develop symptoms.

Diagnosis

Symptoms

The classic symptoms of aortic stenosis are angina, syncope, and heart failure. Patients may not develop symptoms until the aortic valve area is about 1 cm²; this usually requires years. When this degree of stenosis has been reached, however, it may quickly narrow further, with rapid onset of symptoms and occasionally sudden death.

Physical Examination

Auscultation of the chest in patients with aortic stenosis reveals a systolic murmur best heard at the base of the heart that radiates into the carotid arteries; it may be difficult to distinguish the murmur of aortic stenosis from a bruit in the carotid artery. This murmur is associated with a slow, prolonged rise in the arterial pulse, called *pulsus parvus et tardus*. The murmur of severe aortic stenosis is soft and high-pitched and is often described as a "sea gull" murmur.

Electrocardiogram

The electrocardiogram is notable for left ventricular hypertrophy in 85% of patients and evidence of left atrial enlargement in 80% of patients. T-wave inversion and ST-segment depression are common.

Chest Radiograph

The cardiac silhouette on the chest radiograph is usually normal but may reveal poststenotic dilation of the ascending aorta or calcification of the aortic valve. Patients with symptoms of heart failure may have visible evidence of pulmonary edema.

Echocardiogram

The severity of aortic stenosis may be accurately estimated by echocardiography. The peak transvalvular gradient may be calculated from velocity of blood traversing the valve by the following formula:

$$\text{Gradient} = 4V^2$$

where V is the maximal measured blood velocity (in meters per second) across the valve

Echocardiographic determination of the velocity across the valve may also be used to calculate the aortic valve area using the continuity equation[21] (Fig. 62-8).

Cardiac Catheterization

The most accurate measure of aortic stenosis is determined by cardiac catheterization. A catheter may be pulled back from the left ventricle to the aorta to determine the transvalvular pressure gradient. Simultaneous

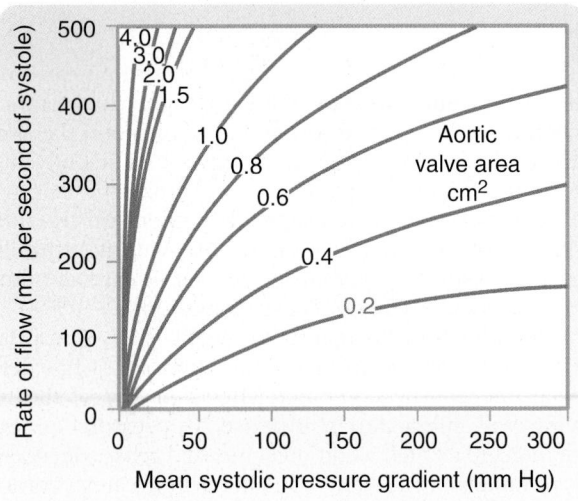

Figure 62-7 Chart illustrates the relationship between the mean systolic pressure gradient across the aortic valve and the rate of flow across the aortic valve per second of systole, as predicted by the Gorlin formula. As the valve area is reduced to about 0.7 cm², little increase in flow is achieved despite marked increases in mean gradient, thus defining "critical" aortic stenosis. (From Hurst JW, Logue RB, Schlant RC, Wenger NK [eds]: Hurst's The Heart: Arteries and Veins, 3rd ed. New York, McGraw-Hill, 1974, p 811.)

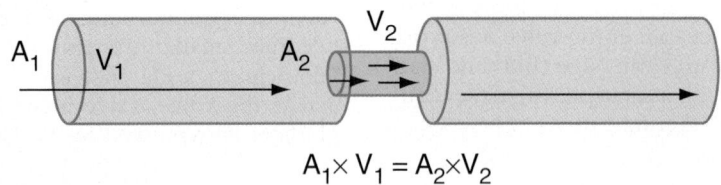

Figure 62-8 Determination of aortic valve area using the continuity equation. For blood flow ($A_1 \times V_1$) to remain constant when it reaches a stenosis (A_2), velocity must increase to V_2. Determination of the increased velocity V_2 by Doppler ultrasound permits calculation of both the aortic valve gradient and solution of the equation for A_2. A, area; V, velocity. (From Carabello BA: Aortic stenosis. In Crawford MH [ed]: Current Diagnosis and Treatment in Cardiology. Norwalk, CT, Appleton & Lange, 1995, p 87.)

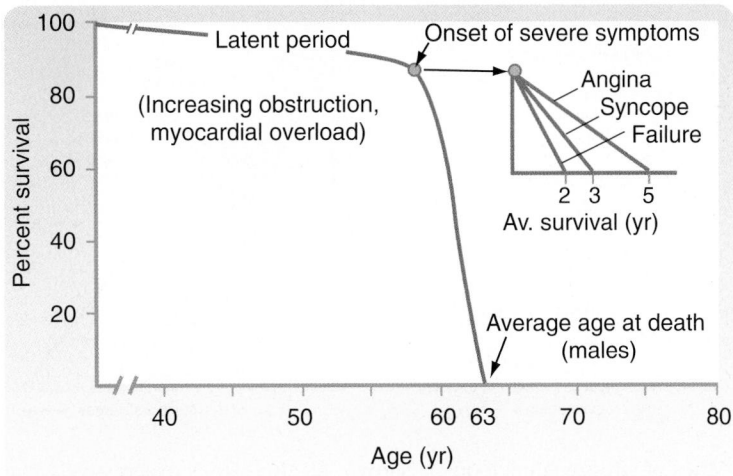

Figure 62-9 The natural history of medically treated aortic stenosis. (From Ross J Jr, Braunwald E: Aortic stenosis. Circulation 38:V61, 1968.)

aortic and ventricular pressure measurements are more precise, however, and they are in fact mandatory when the patient is in atrial fibrillation. Patients older than 40 years have coronary angiography before aortic valve surgery to exclude coronary artery disease.

Natural History

The natural history of aortic stenosis was reported by Ross and Braunwald.[22] Patient survival is not diminished until patients develop symptoms, which is associated with reduction in the aortic valve area from the normal 3 to 4 cm² to less than 1 cm². After symptoms develop, patient survival is limited. The three principal symptoms of aortic stenosis are angina, syncope, and congestive heart failure[22] (Fig. 62-9). Angina is usually the earliest symptom, and the mean survival of a patient with aortic stenosis and angina is 4.7 years. When a patient experiences syncope, survival is typically less than 3 years. Patients with dyspnea and congestive heart failure, in keeping with their associated left ventricular dysfunction, have a mean survival of 1 to 2 years. Congestive heart failure is the presenting symptom in nearly one third of patients.

Treatment

Aortic stenosis is a mechanical obstruction to flow from the left ventricle. The only effective therapy is aortic valve replacement. The existence of symptoms is an indication for valve replacement. Angina and syncope warrant elective surgical therapy, whereas congestive heart failure mandates urgent intervention. The issue of aortic valve replacement in patients with aortic stenosis who do not have symptoms is less clear. A small number of symptom-free patients do precipitously develop symptoms and then experience sudden death. Investigators agree, however, that in patients with aortic stenosis without symptoms, survival is excellent.[23-25] The risk for sudden death in symptom-free patients with a transvalvular gradient greater than or equal to 50 mm Hg or a valve area of less than 0.5 cm² is about 4% per year.[26]

In one study of 113 symptom-free patients with critical aortic stenosis, 38 developed symptoms within 2 years. There were no sudden cardiac deaths in 118 patient-years of follow up.[25] To identify better those symptom-free patients likely to develop symptoms, a group of 123 adults (mean age, 63 years) with asymptomatic aortic stenosis with an initial mean transvalvular gradient of 30 mm Hg were prospectively followed. During 2.5 years of follow-up, there were no sudden deaths. Among patients with an initial transvalvular velocity of more than 4 m/sec, however, only 21% were alive and free of valve replacement after 2 years of follow-up.[26] Therefore, aortic valve surgery is recommended to patients with symptomatic and asymptomatic disease who have evidence of left ventricular decompensation or a transvalvular gradient of more than 4 m/sec.

In patients with good ventricular function, aortic valve replacement is associated with an operative mortality rate of 2% to 8%.[28] Independent perioperative risk factors include age, left ventricular function, New York Heart Association class, and pulmonary function. After aortic valve replacement, the projected 10-year age-matched survival rate is 80% to 85%.[28] Symptoms are relieved in nearly all patients; however, improvement in EF and resolution of ventricular hypertrophy may require months to occur. Surgical mortality increases exponentially with decreasing left ventricular EF. Aortic valve replacement in patients with congestive heart failure carries a mortality rate of up to 24%.[28] In patients with aortic stenosis and coronary artery disease, valve replacement and myocardial revascularization are performed concurrently. Perioperative mortality is higher in patients who do not undergo simultaneous coronary artery bypass grafting.

For patients with severe aortic stenosis who are not candidates for aortic valve replacement, percutaneous aortic balloon valvuloplasty may provide some palliation of aortic stenosis. In this procedure, either one or two balloon catheters may be passed through the aortic orifice and then inflated in an effort to "crack" the calcium that is retarding leaflet motion. The immediate results show

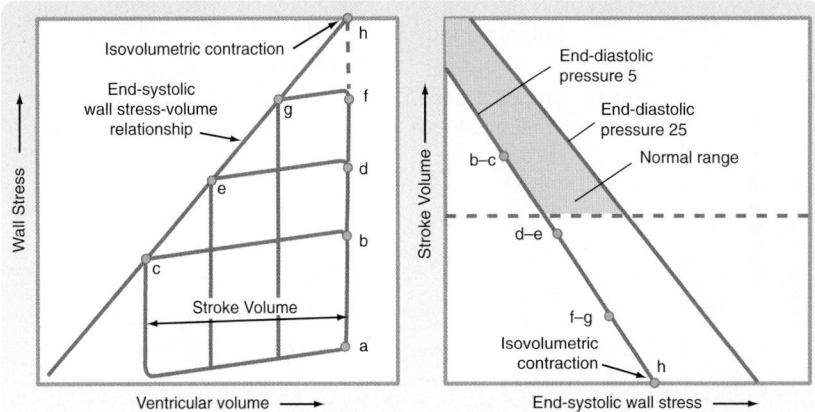

Figure 62-10 *Left,* A series of stress-volume loops is shown. As afterload is progressively increased, wall stress is increased such that ejection, which initially occurred at b, now occurs at d, and then f. Stroke volume diminishes from b-c to d-e, and then to f-g. At maximal wall stress h, there is no stroke volume but rather simply isovolumic contraction. *Right,* the inverse relationship between stroke volume and end-systolic wall stress is portrayed. The two negative slopes represent families of stroke volumes generated with a left ventricular end-diastolic pressure of 5 mm Hg. (From Weaver KT: The mechanics of ventricular function. Hosp Pract 18:113, 1983.)

an increase in the aortic valve area of only 50%, with a 3% to 10% mortality rate. The long-term results are even more disappointing: 30% to 35% of patients have recurrent symptoms within 6 months, and the mortality rate is 60% within 18 months after the procedure.[29] There is a recurrence of symptoms, death, aortic valve restenosis, or a combination of these in more than half of patients within 6 months. The only potential role of aortic balloon valvuloplasty may be in aged, frail, and possibly senile patients whose long-term survival is poor.

Aortic Insufficiency

Etiology

Aortic insufficiency may result from disease of the valve leaflets or of the aortic root. Rheumatic fever may affect the leaflets by shortening the distance from the leaflet-free edge to the aortic annulus rather than by leading to commissural fusion. This prevents coaptation of the leaflets during diastole and results in a central leak. Congenital bicuspid aortic valves typically lead to aortic stenosis but may become regurgitant if a leaflet prolapses. Endocarditis may destroy leaflets.

Dilation of the aortic root produces aortic regurgitation despite normal leaflet morphology by precluding leaflet coaptation. The most common of these conditions is annuloaortic ectasia, an idiopathic dilation of the aortic root and annulus; as the sinuses of Valsalva and the proximal aorta dilate, diastolic coaptation of the leaflets is precluded, resulting in valvular insufficiency. Similarly, myxoid degeneration of the aortic root may lead to dilation of the root, as seen in Marfan syndrome, Ehlers-Danlos syndrome, and cystic medial necrosis. Those conditions may lead to leaflet redundancy, progressive prolapse, and regurgitation. Trauma or dissection of the aortic wall may produce aortic regurgitation if it leads to loss of commissural suspension and leaflet prolapse.

Pathophysiology

The aortic valve leaks during diastole, which lowers diastolic pressure and widens the pulse pressure. Because coronary blood flow occurs primarily in diastole, the lower diastolic blood pressure lowers coronary perfusion pressure. Unlike aortic stenosis, in which the pathologic process is left ventricular pressure overload, the pathophysiology of aortic insufficiency derives from left ventricular volume overload. The increased left ventricular end-diastolic volume (preload) results from filling through the mitral valve as well as the incompetent aortic valve. Patients with chronic aortic insufficiency may have the greatest left ventricular end-diastolic volume of any form of heart disease. Because left ventricular compliance is often increased, however, left ventricular end-diastolic pressure may or may not be elevated. With left ventricular dilation, normal forward stroke volume and EF may be maintained by increased left ventricular end-diastolic and end-systolic volumes. According to the law of Laplace, this left ventricular dilation increases the left ventricular wall tension required to develop systolic pressure. Such increased wall stress not only increases myocardial oxygen demand but also initiates left ventricular hypertrophy and increases left ventricular wall mass. Ultimately, myocardial fibrosis occurs.

With well-compensated aortic insufficiency, exercise may be tolerated because peripheral vascular resistance declines, lowering left ventricular afterload and increasing effective forward flow. At the same time, heart rate increases, which shortens diastolic time, thereby decreasing the regurgitant flow. Because the ventricle ultimately decompensates, however, the left ventricular end-diastolic volume increases even without an increase in aortic regurgitant volume. The end-systolic volume increases as the forward stroke volume declines because ventricular emptying is impaired; the ventricle fails (Fig. 62-10).

In severe aortic regurgitation, increased myocardial oxygen demand exceeds myocardial oxygen supply, causing ischemia despite normal coronary arteries. Increased left ventricular mass and wall tension occur concurrently with low diastolic pressures (low coronary perfusion pressure). Consequently, and particularly with exercise when the diastolic period shortens, coronary blood flow may not meet demand.

Diagnosis

Symptoms
The compensatory mechanisms of aortic regurgitation may permit patients to remain symptom-free for long periods. When these compensatory mechanisms begin to fail, however, left ventricular dysfunction manifests, and patients experience symptoms of heart failure. Symptoms, generally the result of an elevation in left atrial pressure, include dyspnea on exertion, orthopnea, and paroxysmal nocturnal dyspnea. Nocturnal angina occurs occasionally as a result of a slow heart rate and an exceedingly low diastolic pressure with resultant poor coronary flow.

Physical Examination
The physical examination of patients with aortic regurgitation is distinctive because of the wide pulse pressure. The peripheral pulses rise and fall abruptly (Corrigan's or "water-hammer" pulse), the head may bob with each systole (de Musset's sign), and the capillaries visibly pulsate (Quincke's sign). Auscultation reveals a high-frequency decrescendo diastolic regurgitant murmur. A middle to late diastolic rumble may be heard (Austin-Flint murmur) and represents rapid antegrade flow across the mitral valve that closes prematurely as a result of rapid ventricular filling secondary to the aortic regurgitation.

Chest Radiograph
The chest radiograph typically reveals an enlarged cardiac silhouette with an enlarged left atrial shadow and chronic aortic regurgitation. With acute aortic regurgitation, however, the cardiac size may not be enlarged.

Electrocardiogram
The electrocardiogram is usually nonspecific but may reveal left ventricular hypertrophy and left atrial enlargement.

Echocardiography
Doppler echocardiography is the most accurate noninvasive technique to confirm the diagnosis of aortic regurgitation and to determine the severity of aortic insufficiency. As with mitral regurgitation, the severity is graded semiquantitatively as mild, moderate, or severe.

Cardiac Catheterization
The severity of the aortic regurgitation may be visualized angiographically at cardiac catheterization. As with echocardiography, the severity is graded subjectively from mild to severe.

Natural History
Because of the compensatory mechanisms discussed previously, patients with chronic aortic regurgitation may be symptom-free for long periods of time. In fact, patients with mild to moderate aortic regurgitation have an excellent long-term prognosis; 10-year survival rate after diagnosis is about 85% to 95%. Studies in which patients with severe aortic regurgitation have been included reveal a 70% 10-year survival rate and a 50% 20-year survival rate. After symptoms of congestive heart failure occur, survival is markedly decreased; almost 50% of patients with left ventricular failure die within 2 years.

Treatment
Medical therapy for aortic regurgitation is based on a combination of afterload reduction and diuretics. Afterload reduction with nifedipine has been demonstrated to delay the need for aortic valve replacement. Chronic use of angiotensin-converting enzyme inhibitors is more common for afterload reduction.

Patients with symptomatic aortic insufficiency require surgical therapy because their prognosis when treated medically is only a few years. Optimal timing of surgical intervention in patients with or without symptoms, however, may be a very difficult clinical decision.[30] Such patients may be successfully managed with diuretics and afterload reduction for long periods of time. Significant irreversible left ventricular systolic dysfunction may develop insidiously and before clinical evidence of congestive heart failure.

Therefore, symptom-free patients must be carefully followed noninvasively with serial echocardiography or radionuclide ventriculography for evidence of systolic dysfunction or decreasing EF. Aortic valve replacement is performed before the left ventricle has irreversibly dilated. An end-systolic dimension greater than 55 mm estimated by echocardiography has been associated with irreversible left ventricular dysfunction even after aortic valve replacement,[30] and aortic valve replacement needs to be performed before the ventricular dimension exceeds this. At cardiac catheterization, the end-systolic volume may help in determining management for these symptom-free patients. When end-systolic volume is less than 30 mL/m^2, prognosis after surgical therapy is excellent. Progressive systolic dysfunction with end-systolic volumes greater than 90 mL/m^2 have poor intermediate short-term and long-term results. When left ventricular dysfunction is noted in patients with diminished EF and good exercise tolerance, elective operation is recommended. Persistent medical management of these patients severely jeopardizes surgical outcome and ultimate prognosis.[14]

The mortality rate associated with aortic valve replacement for aortic insufficiency is about 4% to 6%.[14] Long-term survival is dependent on preoperative left ventricular function. Both early and late results are improved when surgical intervention precedes left ventricular decompensation.

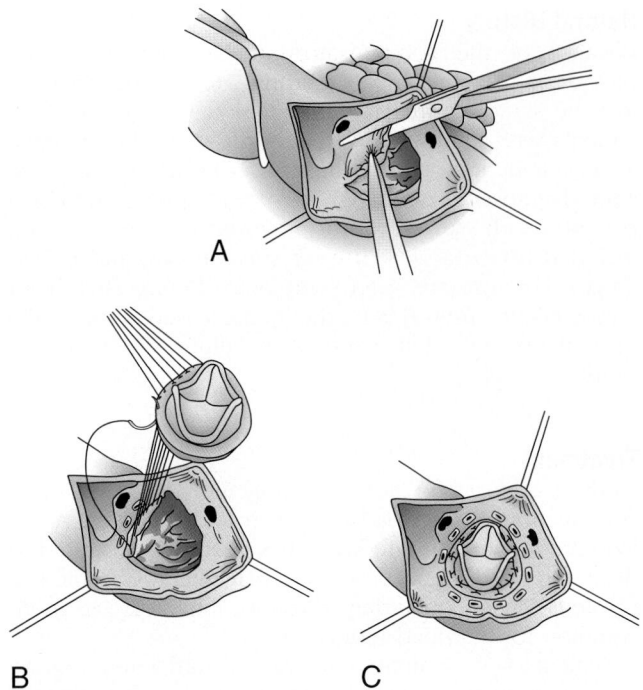

Figure 62-11 Aortic valve replacement. The diseased leaflets are excised (**A**), and the prosthetic valve is sewn in place with interrupted pledgeted mattress stitches (**B** and **C**). (From Albertucci M, Karp RB: Prosthetic valve replacement. In Al Zaibag M, Duran CMG [eds]: Valvular Heart Disease. New York, Marcel Dekker, 1994, p 615.)

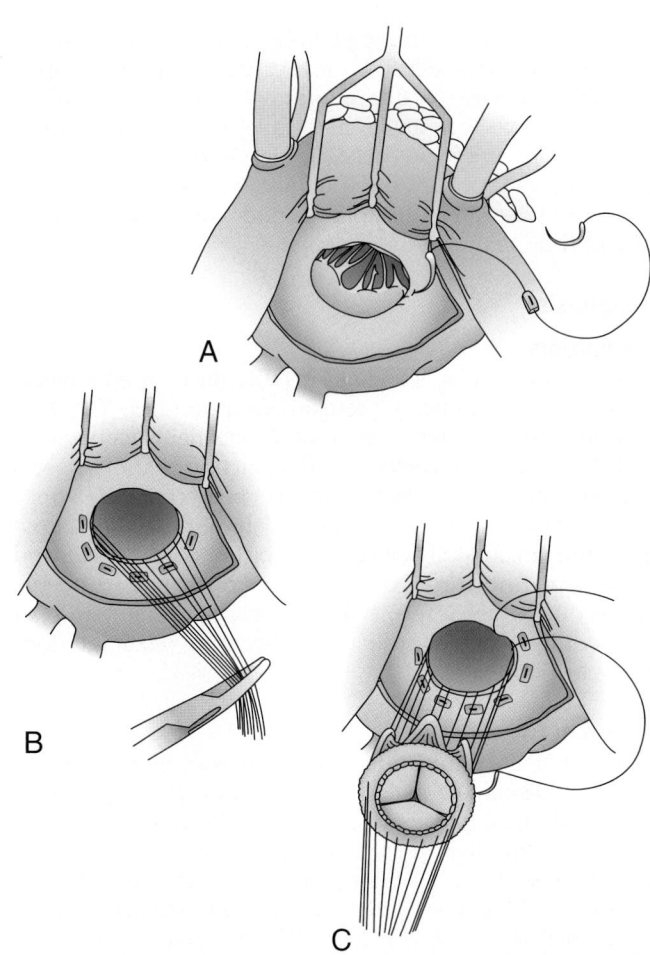

Figure 62-12 A to **C**, Mitral valve replacement with preservation of the posterior leaflet. This preserves the annular-apical connection by means of the chordae tendineae. (From Albertucci M, Karp RB: Prosthetic valve replacement. In Al Zaibag M, Duran CMG [eds]: Valvular Heart Disease. New York, Marcel Dekker, 1994, p 613.)

OPERATIVE TECHNIQUE

Aortic Valve Replacement

The standard incision for an aortic valve replacement is a median sternotomy. After the incision has been made, the patient is connected to the cardiopulmonary bypass circuit by cannulation of the distal ascending aorta and the right atrium. Myocardial protection is achieved by topical myocardial cooling and retrograde cardioplegia. Most surgeons employ moderate systemic hypothermia (28°C-32°C) during the operation.

After the heart fibrillates and the aortic cross-clamp has been applied, a transverse aortotomy is performed about 4 cm distal to the origin of the right coronary artery. The aortotomy is extended to the left and right, thus exposing the aortic valve (Fig. 62-11). The native aortic valve leaflets are excised, with great care to remove any particles of calcium. After the leaflets have been removed, an appropriately sized prosthetic valve is sewn in place (see Fig. 62-11). The aortotomy is closed, cardiac function is resumed, and the patient is weaned from cardiopulmonary bypass.

Mitral Valve Replacement and Repair

The standard incision for mitral valve replacement is a median sternotomy, although a right thoracotomy may sometimes be appropriate for reoperations. The patient is connected to the arterial limb of the cardiopulmonary bypass circuit by cannulation of the distal ascending aorta. Venous drainage for the cardiopulmonary bypass is established by cannulation of the superior and inferior vena cavae (bicaval cannulation). Myocardial protection is achieved by topical myocardial cooling and retrograde cardioplegia. Most surgeons employ moderate systemic hypothermia (28°C-32°C) during the operation.

Surgical exposure of the mitral valve may be particularly difficult and may be achieved by using several different incisions on the heart. The most common incision used to expose the valve is a transverse left atriotomy made in the right lateral wall of the left atrium, just anterior to the left pulmonary veins. An alternative surgical approach to the mitral valve is through an incision in the right atrium, then through the interatrial septum, which provides excellent exposure to the left atrium and the mitral valve.

After the mitral valve has been exposed, it must be carefully examined to determine whether it may be repaired or must be replaced. If the valve must be replaced, efforts need to be made to preserve the native

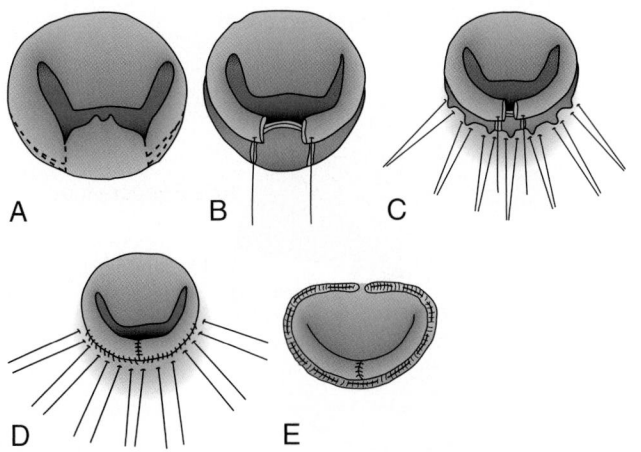

Figure 62-13 A to E, Example of mitral valve repair. In this example, the specific pathology is a flail posterior leaflet. It is repaired by resection of the flail segment, reapproximation of the leaflet, and reduction of the mitral annulus circumference using an annuloplasty ring. (From Perier P, Clausnizer B, Mistarz K: Carpentier "sliding leaflet" technique for repair of mitral valve: Early results. Ann Thorac Surg 57:383, 1994.)

Table 62-1 Operative Mortality Rates

	AVR	MVR	AVR/CAB	MVR/CAB
Society of Thoracic Surgeons	4.0	6.0	6.8	13.3
New York Cardiac Surgery Reporting System	3.3	6.2	7.1	12.8
Department of Veterans Affairs	3.9	5.9	7.3	11.8

AVR, aortic valve replacement; CAB, coronary artery bypass grafting; MVR, mitral valve replacement.

From Grover FL, Edwards FH: Similarity between STS and New York State databases for valvular heart disease. Ann Thorac Surg 70:1143, 2000.

Table 62-2 Independent Risk Factors for Operative Mortality (Odds Ratios) for Valve Replacements

RISK FACTOR	AVR	AVR+CAB	MVR	MVR+CAB
Salvage status	7.12	7.00	6.39	3.40
Dialysis-dependent renal failure	4.32	4.60	4.74	1.83
Emergency status	3.46	1.89	3.57	2.38
Non–dialysis-dependent renal failure	2.20	2.11	2.31	
First operation	1.70	2.40	1.45	1.31

AVR, aortic valve replacement; CAB, coronary artery bypass grafting; MVR, mitral valve replacement.

mitral valve apparatus if possible in order to preserve the mechanical continuity between the mitral valve annulus and the left ventricular apex. This may usually be accomplished by imbricating the leaflets of the mitral valve with sutures and placing an appropriately sized prosthetic valve within the annulus of the native valve (Fig. 62-12).

If the valve is repairable, a variety of surgical techniques may be applied to restore valve competency. In most cases, an incompetent portion of one or both of the mitral valve leaflets must be resected, and the leaflet then reapproximated (Fig. 62-13). At the time of mitral valve repair, the specific pathology responsible for the regurgitation is addressed. For example, a common cause of mitral regurgitation is a ruptured chordae tendinea. At the time of surgery, the prolapsed or flail leaflet subtended by the ruptured chorda tendineae is resected, the leaflet is primarily reapproximated, and the circumference of the mitral annulus is reduced by use of an annuloplasty ring. The adequacy of the repair is judged under direct vision by filling the left ventricle with saline under modest pressure. After the patient has been weaned from cardiopulmonary bypass, a final determination about the competency of the repair is made with use of intraoperative transesophageal echocardiography. The durability of a given mitral valve repair is largely dependent on the pathology responsible for the regurgitation. In most series, however, the failure rate of mitral valvuloplasty for mitral regurgitation is less than 1% per year. The mitral annulus is invariably dilated in surgical cases of mitral regurgitation, contributing to poor coaptation of the anterior and posterior mitral valve leaflets during systole. To return the enlarged mitral annular diameter to normal and to reinforce the leaflet repair, an annuloplasty ring is then sewn to the perimeter of the mitral annulus.

SURGICAL OUTCOMES

According to the Society of Thoracic Surgeons (STS) National Cardiac Surgery Database, about 70,000 valve operations are performed in the United States annually.[31] The operative mortality rate for valve replacement surgery is influenced by several variables, including which valve is replaced, whether coronary bypass surgery is performed at the same operation, and other patient-specific variables.

As shown in Table 62-1, the operative mortality rate in the STS Database for isolated aortic valve replacement is about 4%. On the other hand, the operative mortality rate for combined mitral valve replacement and coronary bypass grafting is much higher at 13%.[32,33] Other databases, including the New York State Department of Health Cardiac Surgery Reporting System and the Department of Veteran Affairs Cardiac Surgery Database, have found very similar mortality rates for cardiac valve operations.[34]

The inherent risks of all surgical procedures is influenced by patient-specific risk factors, and large databases such as those mentioned provide the statistical power to identify patient-specific factors contributing to the risks of valve surgery. Table 62-2 lists some of the major patient-specific risk factors for the most common valve operations from the STS Database.[31]

CHOICE OF PROSTHETIC VALVES

For replacement of either the aortic or mitral valves, there are two principal choices of cardiac valve prostheses: mechanical and bioprosthetic. Bioprosthetic valves are either porcine valves or bovine pericardial valves. The hemodynamic performances of the valves are similar. The operative risks associated with cardiac valve replacement are unassociated with the choice of prosthesis.

The choice of prosthetic valve must be patient specific. Mechanical valves have excellent durability and will perform indefinitely without structural deterioration. But because they are thrombogenic, mechanical valves obligate the patient to lifelong anticoagulation (warfarin sodium). Hence, the patient with a mechanical valve incurs the risks of chronic anticoagulation. Bioprosthetic valves do not require anticoagulation, but will undergo structural deterioration. The durability of a bioprosthetic valve is inversely related to the patient's age at the time the valve is implanted. Should a bioprosthetic valve structurally deteriorate, the patient will require reoperation and valve re-replacement. It is important to recognize that about 80% of all aortic and mitral valve replacements in the United States are performed in patients older than 60 years. The patient's age is considered because it may be dangerous to commit a geriatric patient to chronic anticoagulation.

The 10-year survival rate for patients after aortic valve replacement ranges from 40% to 70%, with an average in the literature of 50%.[35] The type of prosthesis does not affect survival, but other patient-specific factors, such as age at operation and presence or absence of coronary artery disease, do affect survival after valve replacement. Regardless of the type of prosthetic valve implanted, about one third of patients die of valve-related causes. An important consideration for the choice of valve for any patient is therefore how the individual patient may be affected by valve-related morbidity or mortality.

As shown in Figure 62-14, the principal causes of valve-related death following valve implantation include thromboembolism, reoperation, bleeding, and prosthetic valve endocarditis (PVE). The leading cause of valve-related death is thromboembolism. Largely because mechanical valves are thrombogenic, the risk for thromboembolism is greater with mechanical valves. Ten years after aortic valve replacement, the risk for thromboembolism is 20% for mechanical valves[36] and 9% for bioprosthetic valves.[37]

The risk for PVE is not different between mechanical or tissue valves. It is about 4% spread over the patient's lifetime. However, if PVE does occur, it is associated with a 50% mortality rate.[38]

The choice of prosthetic valve must consider the risks for anticoagulation (mechanical valve) and the likelihood and risks for reoperation for structural valve deterioration (bioprosthetic valve). The risk for bleeding complications from chronic anticoagulation is between 1% and 2% per

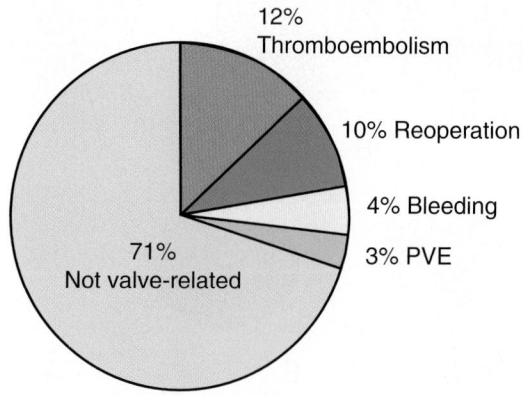

Causes of valve-related death

Figure 62-14 Causes of valve-related deaths following valve replacement surgery. Twenty-nine percent of all deaths following valve surgery are valve related; 71% are not valve related. Valve-related deaths are attributable to thromboembolism, reoperation, bleeding, and prosthetic valve endocarditis (PVE).

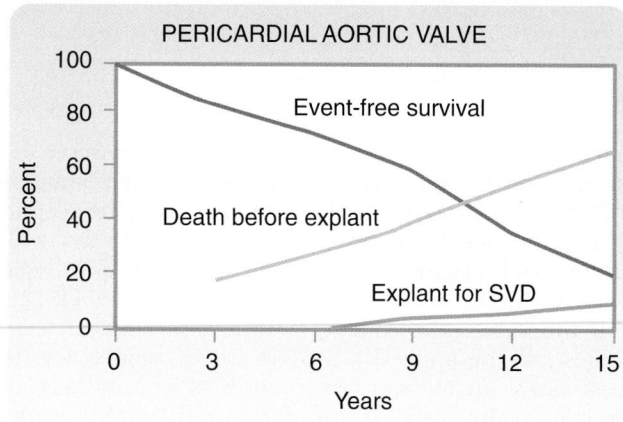

Figure 62-15 After aortic valve replacement with a bovine pericardial bioprosthesis, the risk for undergoing reoperation for structural valve deterioration (SVD) is less than 15% at 15 years. (From Banbury MK, Cosgrove DM 3rd, White JA, et al: Age and valve size effect on the long-term durability of the Carpentier-Edwards aortic pericardial bioprosthesis. Ann Thorac Surg 72:753, 2001.)

year. In fact, 4% of valve-related deaths result from bleeding (see Fig. 62-14). Bioprosthetic valves are indicated in patients with contraindications to anticoagulation because of occupation or because of coexistent medical conditions. Likewise, patients who are medically noncompliant or whose level of anticoagulation may not be closely monitored should not receive mechanical valves. Ten percent of valve-related deaths result from reoperation, and this fact steers some patients and physicians away from bioprosthetic valves. However, recent data demonstrate that if actual rather that actuarial statistical methodology is used to evaluate the likelihood of reoperation for structural valve deterioration of a bioprosthetic valve, the incidence of reoperation is less than 15% for patients older than 60 years[39] (Fig. 62-15). A joint task force from

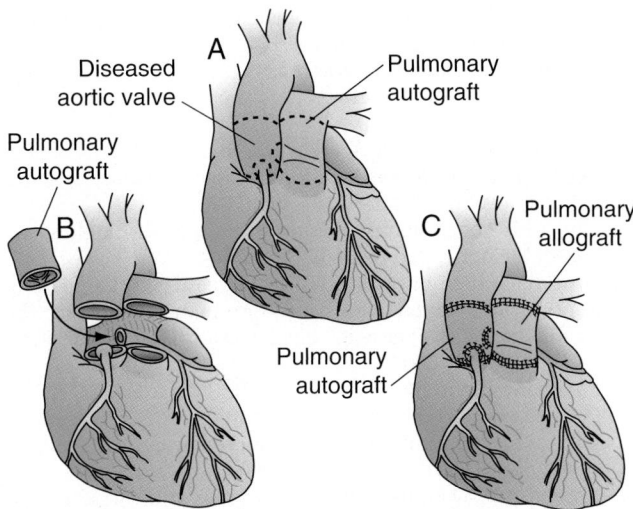

Figure 62-16 **A** to **C**, Pulmonary autograft (Ross) procedure. The diseased aortic valve and proximal aortic root are excised. The pulmonary valve and the main pulmonary artery (autograft) are excised, and the autograft is used to replace the aortic root. The coronary artery buttons are reimplanted into the pulmonary root. A pulmonary homograft is then used to reconstruct the right ventricular outflow tract. (From Kouchoukos NT, Davila-Roman VG, Spray TL, et al: Replacement of the aortic root with a pulmonary autograft in children and young adults with aortic-valve disease. N Engl J Med 330:1, 1994.)

the American Heart Association and the American College of Cardiology has provided some recommendations to help balance these risks. The task force recommended that tissue valves be placed in the aortic position in patients older than 65 years and in the mitral position in patients older than 70 years.[14]

An alternative treatment of aortic valve disease in young patients is the pulmonary autograft procedure (Ross procedure). Initially performed by Ross in 1967, the procedure has gained wider acceptance during the past 2 decades. The procedure entails use of the patient's own pulmonary root as an autograft to replace the diseased aortic valve and root. A cryopreserved pulmonary homograft is then used to replace the patient's pulmonary root (Fig. 62-16). Although it is a technically demanding procedure, the operative mortality rate associated with the Ross procedure is 5% or less and is not different from that associated with isolated aortic valve replacement when performed by experienced surgeons. Intermediate-term data suggest excellent function of the pulmonary autograft; need for autograft reoperation is rare within the first postoperative decade. The durability of the pulmonary homograft is excellent; 80% of patients are free of homograft dysfunction at 16 years. Chronic anticoagulation is not required, and the risk for valve-related complications is extremely low.[40]

Selected References

Bonow RO, Carabello B, De Leon AC, et al: ACC/AHA guidelines for the management of patients with valvular heart disease. J Am Coll Cardiol 32:1486, 1998.

This is an outstanding reference, which addresses virtually all aspects of valvular heart disease including indications for surgery.

Carabello BA: Modern management of mitral stenosis. Circulation 112:432-437, 2005.

The is a concise review and very easily understood.

Cardoso LF, Grinberg M, Rati MA, et al: Comparison between percutaneous balloon valvuloplasty and open commissurotomy for mitral stenosis. A prospective and randomized study. Cardiology 98:186-190, 2002.

This study confirmed balloon mitral valvuloplasty as the treatment of choice for mitral stenosis.

Banbury MK, Cosgrove DM 3rd, White JA, et al: Age and valve size effect on the long-term durability of the Carpentier-Edwards aortic pericardial bioprosthesis. Ann Thorac Surg 72:753, 2001.

This study illustrates the importance of using actual rather than actuarial statistical methodology in the assessment of valve-related events following prosthetic valve implantation. The paper highlights the fact that even though bioprosthetic valves may structurally deteriorate, the likelihood of reoperation is low because most patients may die before that event.

Grover FL, Edwards FH: Similarity between the STS and New York State databases for valvular heart disease. Ann Thorac Surg 70:1143-1144, 2000.

This paper confirms that surgical outcomes between large databases are comparable for valve surgery.

Classic References

Ross J Jr, Braunwald E: Aortic stenosis. Circulation 38:V61, 1968.

This classic study provides the natural history of aortic stenosis. It continues to guide therapy today.

Gorlin R, Gorlin SG: Hydraulic formula for calculation of area of stenotic mitral valve, other cardiac valves, and central circulatory shunts. Am Heart J 41:1, 1951.

This study provides the ability to determine valve orifice sizes.

Olesen KH: The natural history of 271 patients with mitral stenosis under medical treatment. Br Heart J 24:349, 1962.

This study provides the natural history of medically treated mitral stenosis.

References

1. Westaby S, Bosher C: Development of surgery for valvular heart disease. In Westaby S, Bosher C: Landmarks in Cardiac Surgery. Oxford, UK, Isis Medical Media, 1997, p 139.
2. Gorlin R, Gorlin SG: Hydraulic formula for calculation of area of stenotic mitral valve, other cardiac valves, and central circulatory shunts. Am Heart J 41:1, 1951.
3. Olesen KH: The natural history of 271 patients with mitral stenosis under medical treatment. Br Heart J 24:349, 1962.
4. Carabello BA: Modern management of mitral stenosis. Circulation 112:432-437, 2005.
5. Palacios IF, Sanchez PL, Harrell LC, et al: Which patients benefit from percutaneous mitral balloon valvuloplasty? Prevalvuloplasty and post valvuloplasty variables that

predict long-term outcome. Circulation 105:1465-1471, 2002.

6. Cardoso LF, Grinberg M, Rati MA, et al: Comparison between percutaneous balloon valvuloplasty and open commissurotomy for mitral stenosis: A prospective and randomized study. Cardiology 98:186-190, 2002.

7. Solomon NA, Pranav SK, Naik D, Sukumaran S: Importance of preservation of chordal apparatus in mitral valve replacement. Expert Rev Cardiovasc Ther 2:253-261, 2006.

8. Smerup M, Funder J, Nyboe C, et al: Strut chordal-sparing mitral valve replacement preserves long-term left ventricular shape and function in pigs. J Thorac Cardiovasc Surg 130:1675-1682, 2005.

9. Ruel M, Kulik A, Lma BK, et al: Long-term outcomes of valve replacement with modern prostheses in young adults. Eur J Cardiothorac Surg 27:425-433, 2005.

10. Rapaport E: Natural history of aortic and mitral valve disease. Am J Cardiol 35:221, 1975.

11. Buja P, Tatantini G, Del Bianco F, et al: Ischemic mitral regurgitation on the threshold of a solution: From paradoxes to unifying concepts. Circulation 112:745-758, 2005.

12. Heikkinen J, Biencari F, Satta J, et al: Quality of life after mitral valve repair. J Heart Valve Dis 14:722-726, 2005.

13. Bonow RO, Cheitlin MD, Crawford MH, Douglas PS: Task Force 3: Valvular heart disease. J Am Coll Cardiol 45:1334-1340, 2005.

14. Bonow RO, Carabello B, De Leon AC, et al: ACC/AHA guidelines for the management of patients with valvular heart disease. J Am Coll Cardiol 32:1486, 1998.

15. Adams DH, Anyanwu A: Pitfalls and limitations in measuring and interpreting the outcomes of mitral valve repair. J Thorac Cardiovasc Surg 13:523-529, 2006.

16. Borger MA, Adam A, Murphy PM, et al: Chronic ischemic mitral regurgitation: Repair, replace or rethink? Ann Thorac Surg 81:1153-1161, 2006.

17. Muthialu N, Varma SK, Ramanathan S, et al: Effect of chordal preservation on left ventricular function. Asian Cardiovasc Thorac Ann 13:233-237, 2005.

18. De Bonis M, Lapenna E, La Canna G, et al: Mitral valve repair for functional mitral regurgitation in end-stage dilated cardiomyopathy: Role of the "edge-to-edge" technique. Circulation 112(9 Suppl):I402-I408, 2005.

19. Rahimtoola SH: The year in valvular heart disease. J Am Coll Cardiol 47:427-439, 2006.

20. Anselmi A, Lotrionte M, Biondi-Zoccai GG, et al: Left ventricular hypertrophy, apoptosis, and progression to heart failure in severe aortic stenosis. Eur Heart J 26:2747, 2005.

21. Schroeder RA, Mark JB: Is the valve OK or not? Immediate evaluation of a replaced aortic valve. Anesth Analg 101:1288-1291, 2005.

22. Ross J Jr, Braunwald E: Aortic stenosis. Circulation 38:V61, 1968.

23. Carabello BA: Evaluation and management of patients with aortic stenosis. Circulation 105:1746-1750, 2002.

24. Rosenhek R, Binder T, Porenta, G: Predictors of outcome in severe, asymptomatic aortic stenosis. N Engl J Med 343:611-617, 2000.

25. Amato MCM, Moffa PJ, Werner KE, Ramires JAF: Treatment decision in asymptomatic aortic valve stenosis: Role of exercise testing. Heart 86:381-386, 2001.

26. Otto CM: Aortic stenosis: Listen to the patient, look at the valve. N Engl J Med 343:652-654, 2000.

27. Lung B, Gohlke-Barwolf C, Tornos P, et al: Working Group Report. Recommendations on the management of the asymptomatic patient with valvular heart disease. Eur Heart J 23:1253-1266, 2002.

28. Puvimanasinghe JP, Takkenberg JJ, Edwards MB, et al: Comparison of outcomes after aortic valve replacement with a mechanical valve or a bioprosthesis using microsimulation. Heart 90:1172-1178, 2004.

29. Andrus BW, O'Rourke DJ: Percutaneous and surgical treatment of aortic stenosis. Expert Rev Cardiovasc Ther 4:203-209, 2006.

30. Borer JS, Bonow RO: Contemporary approach to aortic and mitral regurgitation. Circulation 108:2432-2438, 2003.

31. Edwards FH, Peterson ED, Coombs LP, et al: Prediction of operative mortality after valve replacement surgery. J Am Coll Cardiol 37:885-892, 2001.

32. Grover FL, Edwards FH: Similarity between the STS and New York State databases for valvular heart disease. Ann Thorac Surg 70:1143-1144, 2000.

33. Edwards FH, Grover FL: Surgical risk assessment. Adv Card Surg 12:77-96, 2000.

34. Hannan EL, Racz MJ, Jones RH, et al: Predictors of mortality for patients undergoing cardiac valve replacements in New York State. Ann Thorac Surg 70:1212-1218, 2000.

35. Vesely I: Heart valve tissue engineering. Circ Res 97:743-755, 2005.

36. Takahashi T, Hasegawa Y, Ohshima K, et al: Long-term follow-up after aortic valve replacement with a small aortic prosthesis. Ann Thorac Cardiovasc Surg. 11:245-248, 2005.

37. Mistiaen W, Van Cauwelaert P, Muylaert P, et al: Thromboembolic events after aortic valve replacement in elderly patients with a Carpentier-Edwards Perimount pericardial bioprosthesis. J Thorac Cardiovasc Surg 127:1166-1170, 2004.

38. Mahesh B, Angelini G, Caputo M, et al: Prosthetic valve endocarditis. Ann Thorac Surg 80:1151-1158, 2005.

39. Banbury MK, Cosgrove DM 3rd, White JA, et al: Age and valve size effect on the long-term durability of the Carpentier-Edwards aortic pericardial bioprosthesis. Ann Thorac Surg 72:753-757, 2001.

40. Fullerton DA, Fredericksen JW, Sundaresan RS, Horvath KA: The Ross procedure in adults: Intermediate-term results. Ann Thorac Surg 76:471-476, 2003.

VASCULAR

Thoracic Vasculature With Emphasis on the Thoracic Aorta

Hazim J. Safi, MD   Anthony L. Estrera, MD   Charles C. Miller, III, PhD

Ali Azizzadeh, MD   and   Eyal E. Porat, MD

The thoracic vasculature includes the arterial, venous, and lymphatic structures contained within the thorax. The most significant structure with regard to surgical pathology, however, remains the thoracic aorta. For this reason, this chapter emphasizes the thoracic aorta: pathology, diagnosis, treatments, and outcomes of surgical management.

EMBRYONIC DEVELOPMENT

During embryonic development, the thoracic vasculature undergoes many stages of formation. Vascular connections may form then vanish, capillaries fuse and produce veins or arteries, and blood flow may reverse direction several times. None of the major vessels of the adult, other than the aorta, manifest as single trunks in the embryo. During this period, aortic anomalies may arise as a result of structures that fail to regress or to develop.[1]

The systemic arterial system originates from the heart and aortic sac as six pairs of ventrally situated arteries, or aortic arches, that pass laterally around the gut to form paired dorsal vessels, or dorsal aortae (Fig. 63-1). The two dorsal aortae are initially separated by the neural tube and notochord, which is in contact with the gut. With separation from the gut, cross connections develop between the two dorsal aortae until a plexus of vessels is formed. Progression of this plexus leads to coalescence and then fusion of the aorta dorsally.

The six paired embryonic aortic arches develop and regress during maturation to eventually become distinct structures of the thoracic aorta. The first and second arches are nearly gone by the time the third arch appears. The dorsal end of the second arch becomes the stem of the stapedial artery, whereas the remainder of this arch also disappears. The third pair of arches becomes the common carotid and proximal portion of the internal carotid arteries. The right fourth arch becomes the proximal portion of the right subclavian artery, whereas the left fourth arch constitutes a portion of the aortic arch between the left common carotid and left subclavian arteries. The fifth embryonic arch ultimately disappears on both sides. The right sixth arch becomes the proximal part of the right pulmonary artery, and the left sixth arch becomes the proximal part of the left pulmonary artery, whereas the distal portion persists as the ductus arteriosus.

Toward the end of the fourth week, the connection between the bulbus cordis, the foremost of the three parts of the primitive heart of the embryo, and the first pair of arches extends and becomes the truncus arteriosus. The truncus arteriosus becomes the aortic and pulmonary roots. The aortic sac becomes the ascending aorta, brachiocephalic artery, and aortic arch up to the origin of the left common carotid. The cranial portion of the right dorsal aorta becomes the right subclavian artery, and the left dorsal aorta becomes the distal arch. The

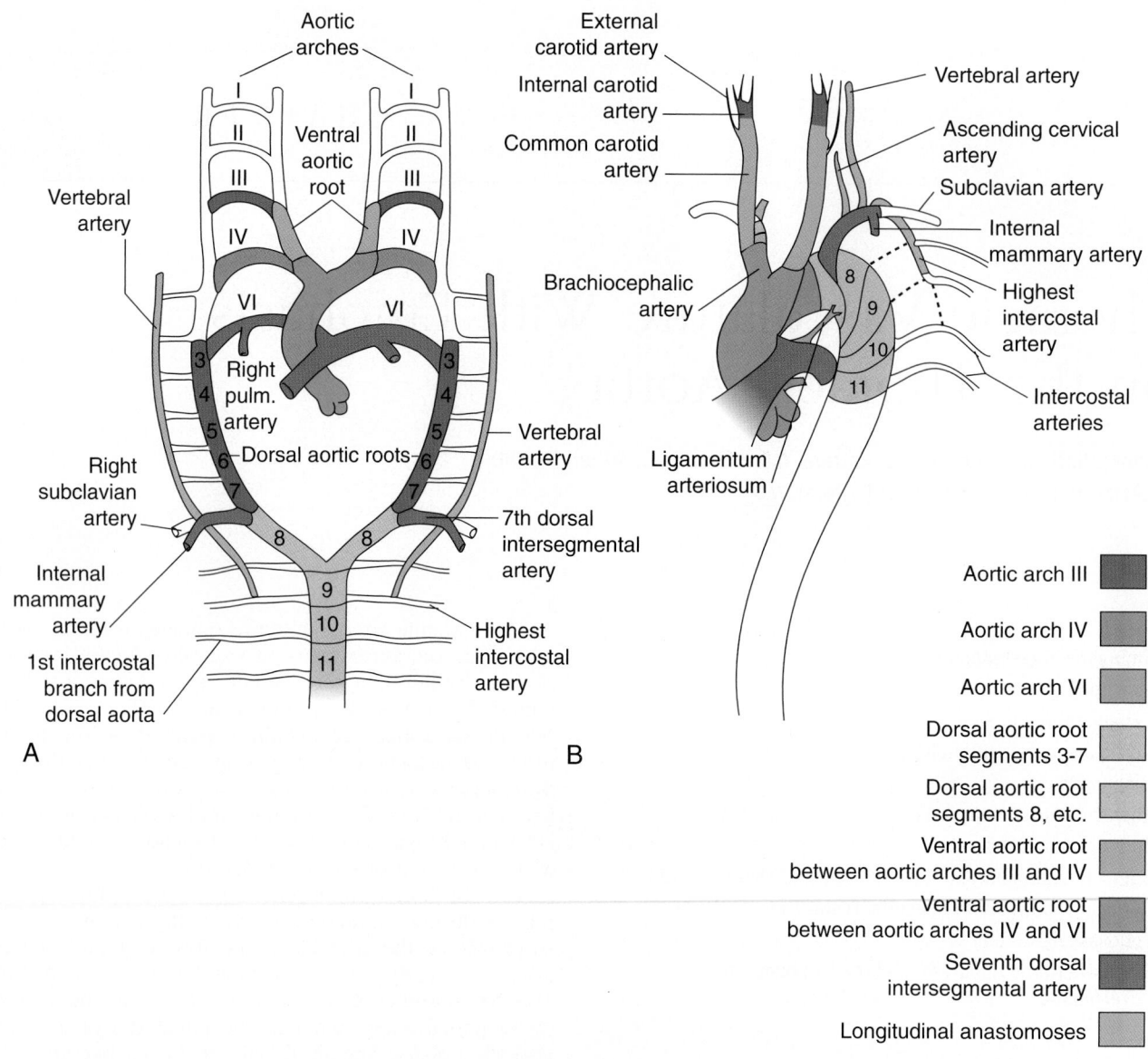

Figure 63-1 A diagram of the various components of the aortic arch in the human embryo (**A**). Portions that regress are noncolored; portions that develop into adult human aorta and branches (**B**) are depicted by coloring and are labeled.

remaining right and left dorsal aortae fuse to create the descending thoracic and abdominal aorta. The right and left seventh intersegmental arteries develop into the respective subclavian arteries.

Early embryonic veins can be segregated into three main groups: the vitelline, umbilical, and cardinal vein complexes. At about the same time as the arterial system develops, the venous system arises from a capillary network that eventually coalesces to form channels, then distinct vessels. The primitive cardinal system, from which the veins of the thorax arise, is formed by anastomoses with umbilical veins and vitelline veins at the posterior end of the developing heart. The early symmetrical disposition of the common cardinal vein, right and left pre-, post-, sub-, and supracardinal veins eventually enlarge,

combine, or retrogress to become the asymmetric arrangement of the inferior and superior venae cavae and the brachiocephalic, azygos, and homozygous veins.

FUNCTIONAL ANATOMY

The root of the aorta begins in the ventricular outflow tract of the heart and ends in the abdomen at the aortic bifurcation, which divides into the right and left common iliac arteries. The aortic root houses the aortic valve, sinuses of Valsalva, and right and left coronary arteries. The anterior tubular segment or ascending aorta emerges from the root. The ascending aorta curves posteriorly and to the left as the aortic arch, from which emerge the

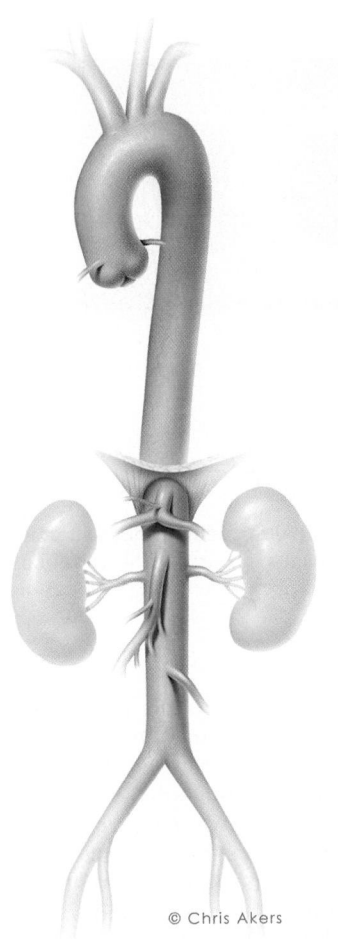

Figure 63-2 The normal aorta with major anatomic section colored for identification; in green is the aortic root and ascending aorta with coronary ostia, in pink is the aortic arch, in violet is the descending thoracic aorta, and in blue is the abdominal aorta. Together the sections colored violet and blue are known as the *thoracoabdominal aorta*. (© Chris Akers, 2006. Reprinted with permission.).

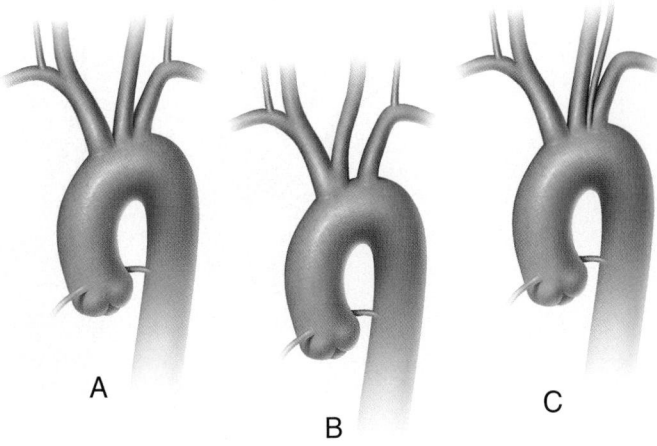

Figure 63-3 Branching patterns of the aortic arch. **A,** The most common pattern of brachiocephalic artery, left common carotid artery, and left subclavian artery. **B,** A less frequent pattern of the brachiocephalic and left common carotid arteries sharing a common origin from the arch proximal to the left subclavian artery (bovine arch). **C,** The least common pattern of separate starting points for the brachiocephalic, left common carotid, left vertebral, and left subclavian arteries. (© Chris Akers, 2006. Reprinted with permission.).

CONGENITAL ANOMALIES

Aortic anomalies are often multiple and frequently occur in siblings. The most common right-to-left branching pattern of the aortic arch is brachiocephalic artery, left common carotid artery, and left subclavian artery (75%). Less frequently (20%), the brachiocephalic and left common carotid arteries share a common origin from the arch proximal to the left subclavian artery (bovine arch). Least common (3%) are separate starting points for the brachiocephalic, left common carotid, left vertebral, and left subclavian arteries (Fig. 63-3). Fourteen other configurations have been described in cadavers with as many as four primary branches or as few as two primary branches.[2]

A vascular ring is a condition in which the anomalous configuration of the arch or associated vessels forms a partial or complete ring around the trachea or esophagus, causing compression. Anomalies of the aortic arch may be characterized as left, right, or double aortic arch. These arch configurations may be associated with a left or right ligamentum arteriosum, and left or right retroesophageal subclavian artery. Patients with a right aortic arch and left ligamentum frequently develop a diverticulum known as *Kommerell's diverticulum* associated with the left retroesophageal subclavian artery. An aberrant right subclavian artery (Fig. 63-4) forms as the result of a persistent right eighth segmental artery and regression of the right fourth aortic arch, which is the opposite of normal development. The aberrant right subclavian artery arises from the descending thoracic aorta, distal to the

brachiocephalic (or innominate), left common carotid, and left subclavian arteries. The descending thoracic aorta begins distal to the left subclavian artery and ends at the 12th intercostal space. Branches of the descending thoracic aorta are the intercostal, bronchial, and esophageal arteries. The artery of Adamkiewicz is the main source of blood to the lower part of the anterior spinal artery, which in turn supplies much of the blood to the spinal cord. There is significant variability in the origin of this critical artery, but it usually branches from an intercostal artery that connects to the aorta between the 9th and 12th intercostal spaces. As the aorta exits the thorax, it enters the abdomen through the aortic hiatus. The thoracoabdominal aorta refers to the entire descending thoracic and abdominal aorta. Figure 63-2 depicts a normal aorta with major anatomic sections colored for identification.

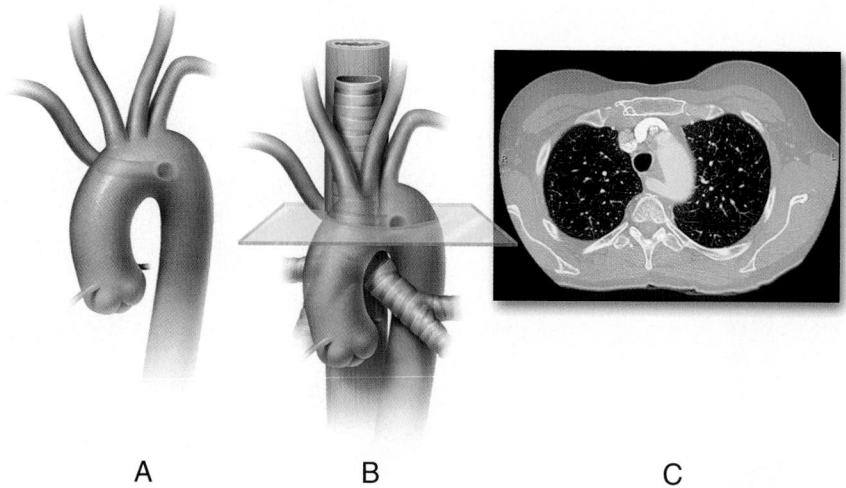

A   B   C

Figure 63-4 Illustrations of an aberrant right subclavian artery arising from the descending thoracic aorta, distal to the left subclavian artery (**A**), traversing posterior to the trachea and esophagus in front of the vertebral column (**B**), accompanied by a computed tomography image (**C**) of the same. (© Chris Akers, 2006. Reprinted with permission.).

left subclavian artery, traversing posterior to the trachea and esophagus in front of the vertebral column, and occurs with an incidence of 0.5% in the population.[3] As originally described by the English surgeon David Bayford in 1787, this anomaly may lead to compression of the esophagus by the right subclavian artery, promoting obstructed deglutition or dysphagia lusoria.[4]

Patent ductus arteriosus is the most common vascular anomaly, occurring with an incidence of 1 in 2000 live births and accounting for 5% to 10% of all types of congenital heart disease.[5] The ductus arteriosus, which carries fetal blood from the left pulmonary artery to the aorta, constricts at birth because of raised oxygen tension. At 1 month, the ductus arteriosus is usually obliterated, ultimately forming the fibrous ligamentum arteriosum. A patent ductus arteriosus can prompt shunting from the systemic to the pulmonary circulation, leading to pulmonary hypertension.

Coarctation refers to a narrowing of the aortic wall and lumen and accounts for 5% to 8% of congenital heart disease. The most common of these anomalies is the postductal type, which occurs distal to the ligamentum, compared with the preductal type, which occurs just proximal to a patent ductus arteriosus. The etiologic mechanism of coarctation is unknown, but constriction is thought to occur as the result of incorporation of oxygen-sensitive ductal tissue into the wall of the thoracic aorta. Chronic coarctation generates extensive formation of intercostal artery collaterals, proximal hypertension, and rib notching.

Venous Anomalies

Venous anomalies can occur in connections of either the systemic or pulmonary veins. The most common is persistent left superior vena cava, which drains into the right atrium through an enlarged orifice of the coronary sinus. The persistent left superior vena cava forms when the left anterior cardinal vein fails to regress, but communicates with the right atrium through the left horn of the sinus venosus, which becomes the coronary sinus. The absence of a left brachiocephalic vein (innominate vein) and a small right superior vena cava can signal the presence of persistent left superior vena cava. These vascular anomalies do not cause any inherent problems with circulation because the desaturated blood is eventually taken to the lungs. However, patent left superior vena cava can have implications during surgical procedures, such as complicating wire placement during transvenous endocardial pacemaker. Such situations require an astute surgeon who can recognize this anomaly intraoperatively because many patients with patent left superior vena cava undergo surgery for other intracardiac malformations with no knowledge of the presence of this anomaly.[6]

The most common anomaly of the inferior vena cava is an interruption of its abdominal course with drainage to the heart through the azygos or hemiazygos venous system. Anomalies of the pulmonary veins connect to sites individually or in combination. A totally anomalous connection is usually a confluence of veins behind the left atrium that join either to the superior vena cava, the coronary sinus, or the portal venous system crossing the diaphragm.

AORTIC DISEASES AND ETIOLOGY

Aortic Aneurysm and Dissection

The most common diseases of the aorta are aneurysm and dissection, which are classified by anatomic location (Figs. 63-5 to 63-7). An aortic aneurysm is defined as a localized or diffuse aortic dilation that exceeds 50% of the normal aortic diameter. Factors associated with aneurysm formation include advanced age, hypertension,

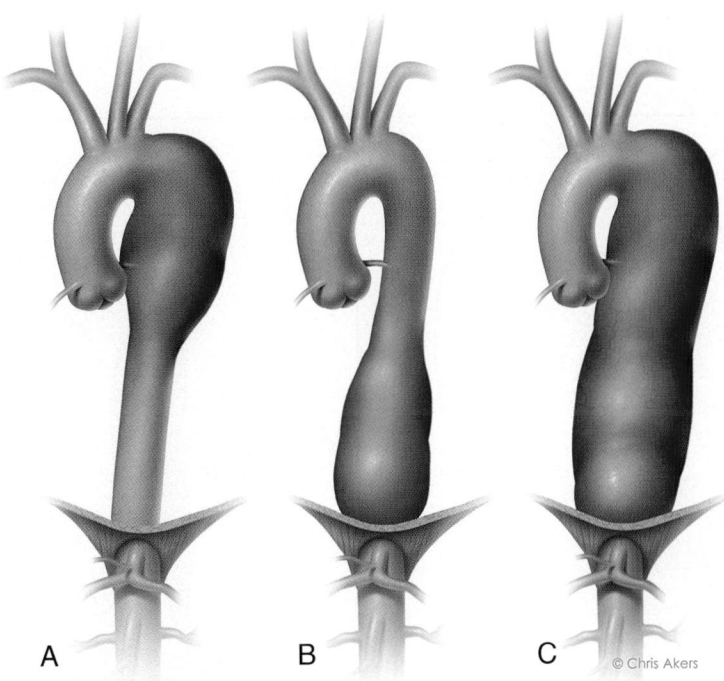

Figure 63-5 Classification, descending thoracic aortic aneurysm: type A, distal to the left subclavian artery to the sixth intercostal space (**A**); type B, sixth intercostal space to above the diaphragm (12th intercostal space) (**B**); type C, entire descending thoracic aorta, distal to the left subclavian artery to above the diaphragm (12th intercostal space) (**C**). (© Chris Akers, 2006. Reprinted with permission.).

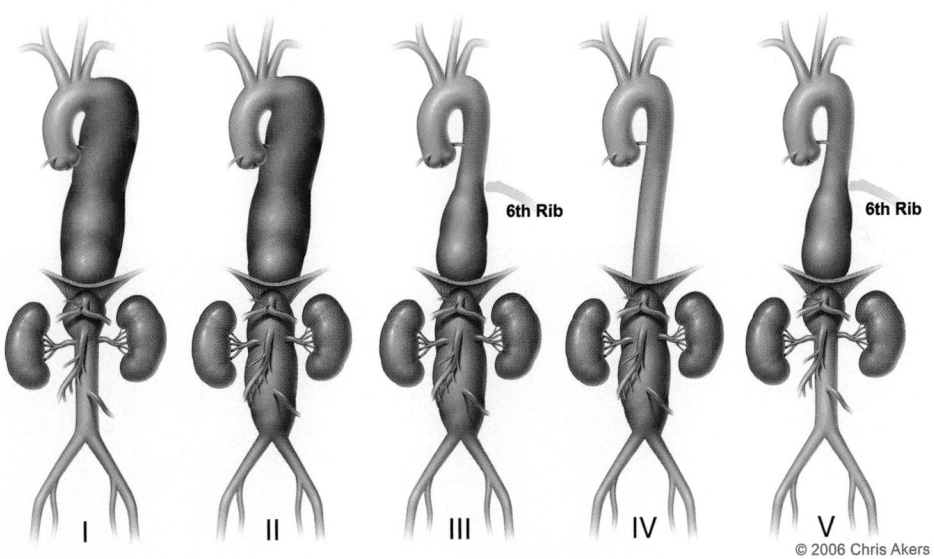

Figure 63-6 Normal thoracoabdominal aorta aneurysm classification. Extent I, distal to the left subclavian artery to above the renal arteries. Extent II, distal to the left subclavian artery to below the renal arteries. Extent III, from the 6th intercostal space to below the renal arteries. Extent IV, from the 12th intercostal space to the iliac bifurcation (total abdominal aortic aneurysm). Extent V, below the 6th intercostal space to just above the renal arteries. (© Chris Akers, 2006. Reprinted with permission.).

smoking, arteriosclerosis, and aortic dissection. Acute aortic dissection is thought to be most common catastrophic event of the aorta; however, a recent study suggests that acute aortic dissection and degenerative aortic aneurysm rupture may occur with similar frequency.[7] A tear in the intima allows blood to escape from the true lumen of the aorta, dissects the aortic layers, and reroutes some of the blood through a newly formed false channel. The weakened aortic wall is highly susceptible to acute rupture and chronically prone to progressive dilation.

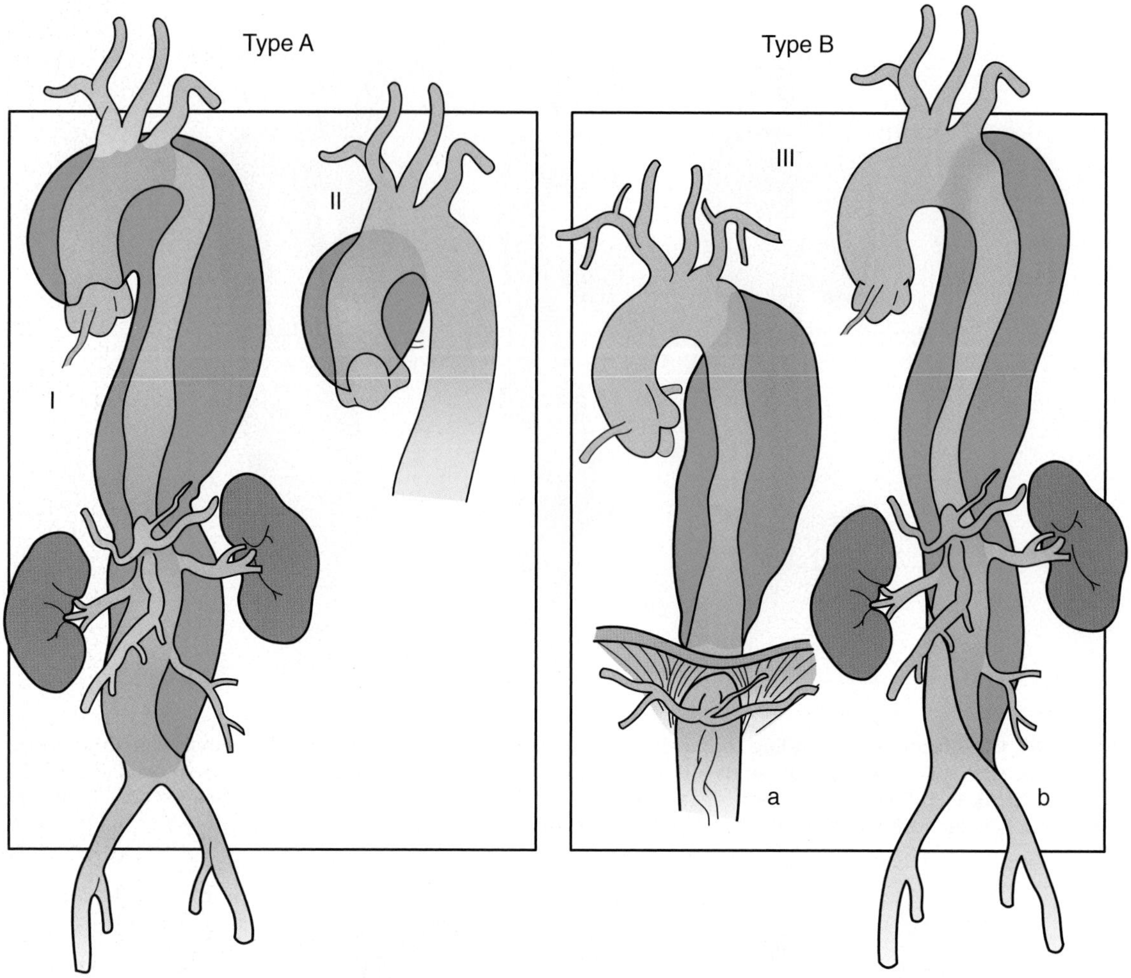

Type A

II

I

Type B

III

a

b

Figure 63-7 Aortic dissection classification based on the site of the intimal tear. *Left,* Stanford type A, DeBakey types I and II. *Right,* Stanford type B, DeBakey type III.

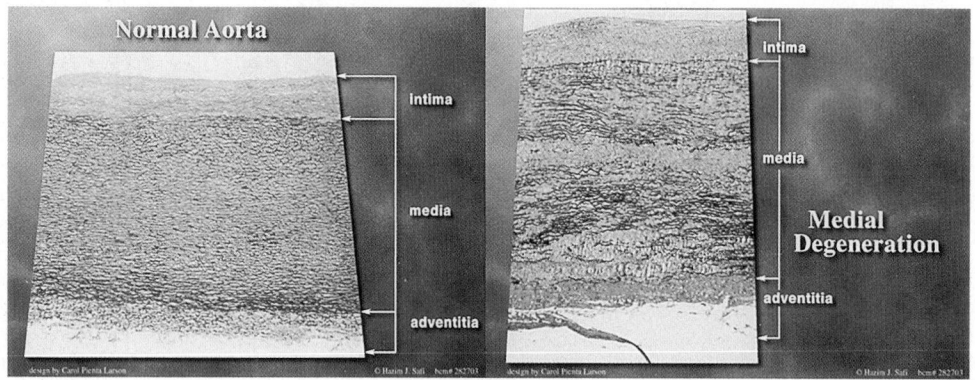

Figure 63-8 Normal (*left*) versus abnormal (*right*) aortic wall. (© Hazim J. Safi, 2006. Reprinted with permission.)

Arterial hypertension and connective tissue disorders (particularly Marfan syndrome) may predispose patients to dissection. The cause of the initial tear remains unknown, but the histology of the aortic wall typically exhibits medial degeneration (Fig. 63-8).

Aortic dissection is acute when clinical diagnosis is made within 14 days after the onset of symptoms, and chronic after 14 days. When a dissection involves the ascending aorta, it is commonly referred to as a Stanford type A. Dissection without involvement of the ascending aorta—most often with the intimal tear in the descending thoracic aorta—is referred to as a Stanford type B or DeBakey type III. DeBakey classification further distinguishes ascending aortic dissection *with* involvement of the descending thoracic aorta (DeBakey type I), from ascending aortic dissection *without* involvement of the descending thoracic aorta (DeBakey type II) (see Fig. 63-7).

About 20% of aortic aneurysms and dissections are related to hereditary connective tissue disorders.[8] Marfan syndrome is the most common of these disorders, occurring in the worldwide population at a frequency of 1 in 5000.[9] Skeletal, ocular, and cardiovascular complications characterize Marfan syndrome, with cardiovascular complications such as aneurysm and dissection the major cause of morbidity and mortality.

Aortic dilation observed in Marfan patients is the result of genetic defects in a specific component of elastic fibers known as fibrillin-1 (*FBN1*). Although inherited in an autosomal dominant manner, one fourth of patients do not have a family history and have the syndrome as the result of a new mutation. One hundred thirty-seven mutations have been entered in the international Marfan database (http://www.umd.necker.fr). Some patients who do not fulfill the usual diagnostic criteria may still have *FBN1* mutations and thoracic aortic aneurysm and dissection.[10]

A number of other known genetic syndromes predispose individuals to thoracic aortic aneurysm and dissection, such as Turner's syndrome, Ehlers-Danlos syndrome, and polycystic kidney disease. Mutations in fibrillin-2, or *FBN2*, cause congenital contractural arachnodactyly, a syndrome closely related to Marfan syndrome. Familial aggregation studies have indicated that up to 20% of thoracic aortic aneurysm and dissection patients without one of the genetic syndromes described earlier have other affected family members. These studies support the hypothesis that genetic factors predispose individuals who do not have a known genetic syndrome to thoracic aortic aneurysm and dissection.

Families in which multiple members have thoracic aortic aneurysm and dissection, or familial thoracic aortic aneurysm and dissection (TAAD), have been reported in the literature. Aortic imaging of family members of patients with TAAD has provided us with the best overview of the inheritance and features of this syndrome.[11] In most of these families, the phenotype for TAAD is inherited in an autosomal dominant manner, with marked variability in age at the onset of aortic disease and decreased penetrance. Most often, the condition is not due to mutations in *FBN1*. Mapping of TAAD on the locus to 3P24-25[12] has identified mutations in the transforming growth factor-β receptor type II associated with TAAD.[13]

Aortic Tumors

Primary tumors of the aorta are extremely rare, with fewer than 100 cases reported in the English literature.[14] Although tumors may be composed of varying histologic types, most are sarcomas, with malignant fibrous histio-cytoma predominating. Most primary sarcomas of the aorta and pulmonary artery (the elastic arteries) arise from the intima, growing along the lumen, forming polypoidal masses. Intimal tumors may present with symptoms related to vascular obstruction or distal embolization. Tumors that arise from the medial and adventitial layers occur less frequently. Symptoms are often nonspecific and include chest pain and dyspnea. Because tumors may mimic aneurysm or aortic occlusive disease, diagnoses are often made postmortem or intraoperatively.[15] Primary aortic tumors most commonly present between the sixth and seventh decades of life and involve the thoracic and abdominal aorta equally. Malignant tumors (i.e., sarcomas) are generally associated with a poor prognosis and respond poorly to chemotherapy or radiation. However, surgical resection of any sarcoma of the vasculature, when feasible, may result in cure or palliation of symptoms.

DIAGNOSTIC IMAGING

Before computed tomography (CT) scanning and, later, magnetic resonance imaging (MRI) became widely available, aortography was performed routinely in aortic aneurysm and aortic dissection patients. Images are produced by contrast media injected through a catheter positioned in the aorta hit by a rapid succession of radiographic images. In acute traumatic aortic injury, aortography typically can identify irregularity of the aorta, focal outpouching, and accumulation of contrast at the region of irregularity. The aortogram can detect aortic root dilation and define the condition of the smaller vessels. Aortography was the gold standard imaging modality for confirming the diagnosis of aortic dissection because it could identify the aorta's true and false lumen and determine tear sites and the extent of dissection. However, false-negative aortograms may occur when the false lumen is not opacified, when there is simultaneous opacification of the true and false lumen, and when the intimal flap is not seen. CT scan has replaced aortography for the evaluation of the thoracic aorta and its branches. Aortography is currently reserved for patients with suspected aortic branch occlusive disease and is often performed in conjunction with cardiac catheterization.

During the past decade, technical advances in CT and MRI have vastly improved thoracic vasculature imaging. CT, a digitally based radiographic technique, can quickly produce images of multiple slices of the body's soft tissue organs and is our preferred technique for imaging the thoracic aorta. It is less invasive, faster, safer, and less costly than aortography. CT evaluates systemic vasculature, defining aortic anomalies, dissection, aneurysm, clots, and calcification; and pulmonary vasculature, depicting lung disease and thoracic venous anomalies such as pulmonary arteriovenous malformation. Multidetector helical (spiral) CT has virtually supplanted conventional CT and provides three-dimensional reconstruction of the acquired CT images (Fig. 63-9). CT scan determines aneurysm extent by recording the aortic diameter serially, from the ascending aorta to the arch and

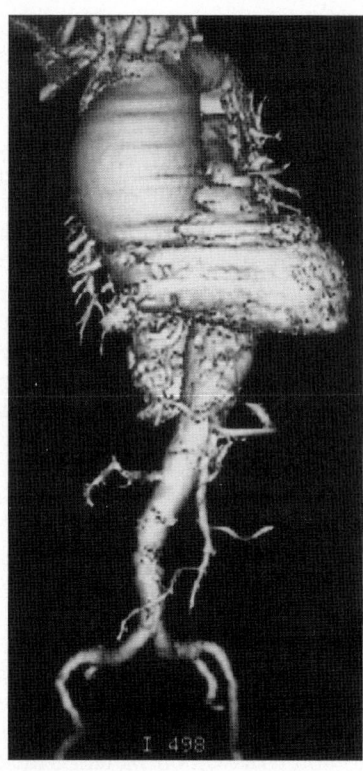

Figure 63-9 Reformatted three-dimensional computed tomographic angiogram of the aorta and its major branches in a patient with large ascending aortic aneurysm.

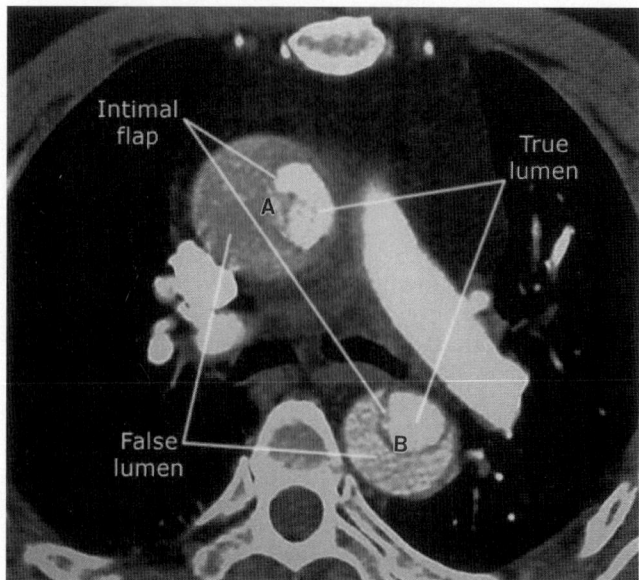

Figure 63-10 Computed tomography scan, type A aortic dissection with intimal flap in the ascending (A) and descending (B) segments of the aorta.

thoracoabdominal aorta. CT angiography (CTA) acquires axial images during the arterial phase following a bolus of intravenous (IV) contrast. CTA can distinguish the difference between the false and true lumen in aortic dissection and can accurately detect the proximal location of the intimal tear (Fig. 63-10). It can also reveal associated thrombus or inflammatory changes in the aortic wall. CT scans are indispensable for patient follow-up and tracking aortic aneurysm growth rate. Some patients may require additional preparation before undergoing CT scan, such as adequate hydration and premedication for renal insufficiency and contrast allergy. Figure 63-11 demonstrates a coronal CT image of a patient with chronic type B dissection.

MRI does not require iodinated contrast and can be performed safely in patients with impaired renal function. An image is detected by radiofrequency signals when the body's hydrogen atoms react to the MRI's strong magnetic field. MRI, particularly three-dimensional gadolinium-enhanced magnetic resonance angiography (MRA), can clearly identify the morphology of the aortic and pulmonary vasculature. MRI can reliably assess the site and extent of nonvalvular obstructive lesions of the aorta (i.e., coarctation, interruption of the aortic arch, and supravalvular stenosis). MRI is the imaging modality of choice for aortic tumors because of its diverse capabilities, which include multiplanar imaging for excellent anatomic definition of the heart, pericardium, mediastinum, and lungs, and improved morphologic differentia-

tion between tumor tissue and surrounding cardiovascular, mediastinal, or pulmonary tissues. Patients with internal metallic hardware (e.g., pacemakers, orthopedic rods) cannot undergo MRI. Higher cost and longer examination times (a particular concern for patients with claustrophobia) are limitations of MRI. Figure 63-12 demonstrates an MRI of a patient with chronic dissection.

Other imaging modalities for thoracic vasculature include transesophageal echocardiography, (TEE), intravascular ultrasound (IVUS), and intraoperative epiaortic ultrasound (IEUS). IVUS can provide an image of the anatomy within the aortic walls. A miniature catheter tip inserted percutaneously, incorporated with an ultrasound device, can identify intimal defects, atheromatous plaques, calcification, and laminated thrombi. TEE uses a miniature high-frequency ultrasound transducer placed on a probe and inserted into the lower esophagus. Because the lower esophagus is located close to the posterior of the heart, there is no image interruption by lung tissue. TEE has the advantage of portability and quick execution. TEE is highly sensitive in aortic pathology diagnosis (Fig. 63-13) and is an excellent intraoperative tool, able to report cardiac structure and function. It can assess ventricular function and reliably survey aortic valve disease, aortic dilation, ascending aortic aneurysm, dissection, thrombi, atherosclerotic disease, and mitral valve disease. Of particular value during cardiac operations that employ cardiopulmonary bypass, TEE and IEUS can detect atheromas of the thoracic aorta. Aortic aneurysms of the transverse aortic arch cannot be identified by TEE because of the interposition of the air-filled trachea and bronchi. Although TEE can be done at the bedside or intraoperatively, the technique requires a skilled cardiologist or anesthesiologist to interpret study data. Contraindications are esophageal obstruction, diverticulum, or varices,

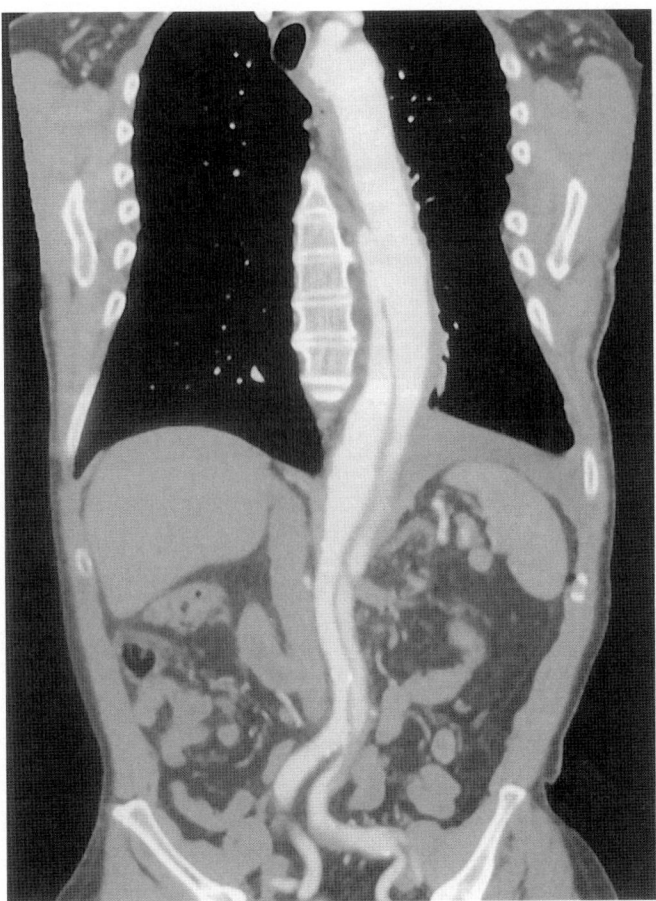

Figure 63-11 Coronal computed tomography image of a patient with chronic type B dissection.

active upper gastrointestinal bleed, or cervical spine disease.

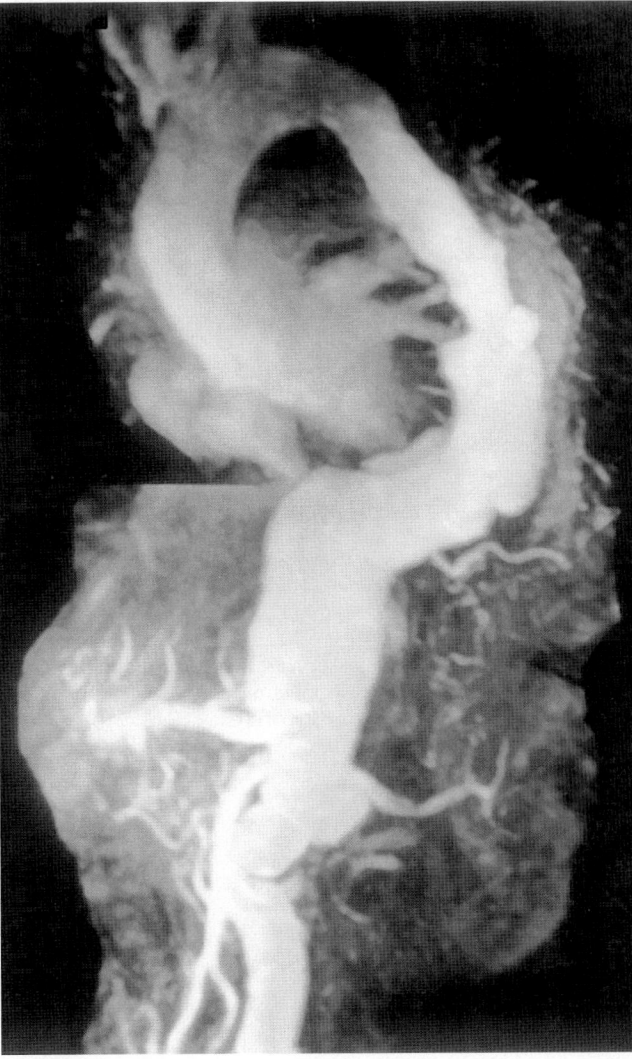

Figure 63-12 Magnetic resonance image demonstrating a thoracic aortic aneurysm with chronic dissection.

THORACIC AORTIC ANEURYSMS

Natural History and Incidence

Population screening for thoracic aneurysm is not a practical endeavor; consequently, we have no prospective or randomized analyses of the natural history of aortic aneurysms or dissection. However, population rates can be estimated by monitoring a defined population for health system utilization, which was the approach taken by Bickerstaff and colleagues[16] in the well-described population of Rochester, MN. The study was conducted on a population-based historical cohort from records collected between 1951 and 1980. Only 11% underwent surgical treatment. The time of diagnosis was abstracted from medical records, and patients were "followed" historically until death. This study reported a population incidence of detected thoracic aortic aneurysms estimated to be 5.9 new aneurysms per 100,000 person-years in 1982. In a follow-up to Bickerstaff's report, Clouse and associates studied the same Rochester, MN, cohort starting in 1980, when the previous study had left off, through 1994.[18]

These authors estimated the incidence to be 10.4 per 100,000 person-years, or three times higher than the 1951 to 1980 rates after age adjustment. The significant difference from the 1982 study was almost certainly due to improved case ascertainment brought about by the increased use of thoracic CT scanning after 1980.

Untreated, 75% to 80% of thoracic aortic aneurysms eventually rupture (Fig. 63-14). Five-year untreated survival rates range between 10% and 20%, with a median time to rupture in nondissecting aneurysms of 2 to 3 years. Although women develop thoracic aortic aneurysms 10 to 15 years later than men, rupture occurs more frequently in women. Significant alterations in the structure of the aortic wall occur with aging that are distinct from the formation of aneurysms. Age in thoracic aortic aneurysm patients, however, has been associated with increased risk for rupture. Aneurysm size significantly influences the rate of rupture. When an ascending aortic aneurysm reaches a diameter of 6 cm, the risk for rupture

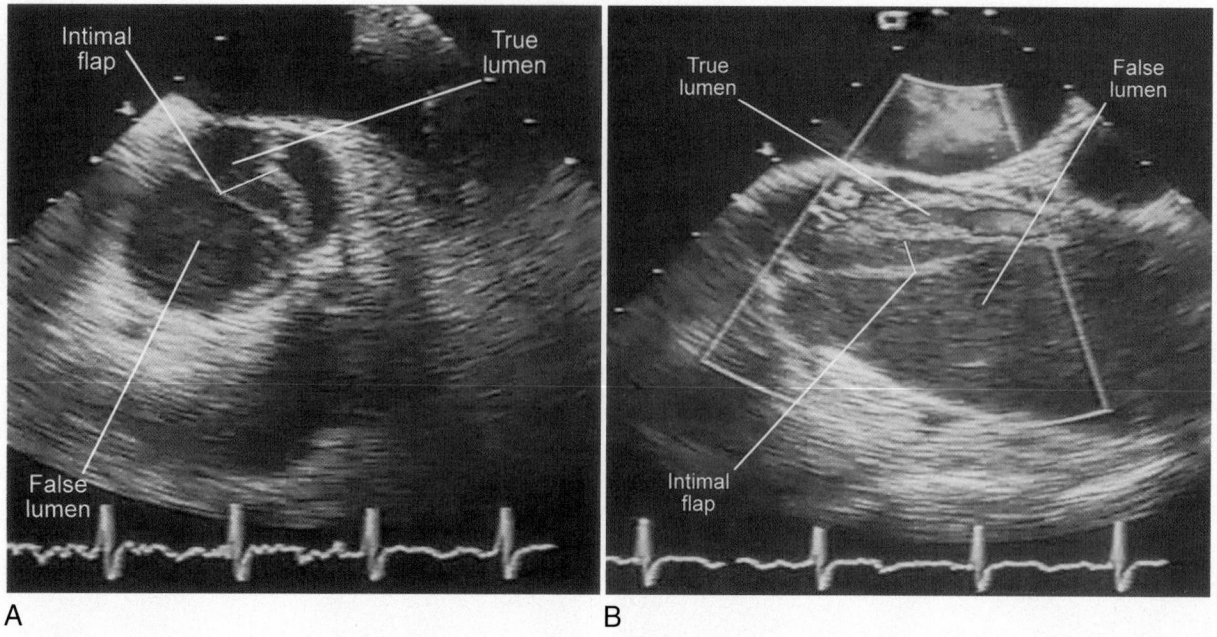

Figure 63-13 Transesophageal echocardiography of dissection of the ascending aortic aorta in cross section (**A**), and sagittal color-Doppler mode view demonstrates no flow in the large false lumen (**B**). (Courtesy of Mihai Croitaru, MD, University of Texas-Houston).

is 31%. For the descending thoracic aorta, the critical size is about 7 cm, with a 43% risk for rupture.[19]

Clinical Presentation

The clinical manifestations of thoracic aortic aneurysms vary widely. In most patients, an aortic aneurysm is discovered incidentally without specific symptoms because the slow growth of aneurysms is typically silent. Chronic back pain is a frequent complaint in patients, but pain related to musculoskeletal causes is usually difficult to differentiate from pain related to aneurysm. Large aortic aneurysms can put pressure on adjacent structures and can create symptoms such as hoarseness due to vocal cord paralysis related to compression of the left recurrent laryngeal or vagus nerves, dyspnea from mild to severe upper airway compromise from compression of the tracheobronchial tree, pulmonary hypertension due to pressure on the pulmonary artery, and dysphagia caused by compression of the esophagus. Direct erosion of the aneurysm into the adjacent tracheobronchial tree, esophagus, or both results in fistulization and bleeding (hemoptysis or hematemesis). A thoracoabdominal aortic aneurysm may press against the stomach and cause weight loss related to early satiety. Associated atherosclerotic occlusive disease of the visceral or renal arteries may cause intestinal angina or arterial hypertension, respectively. A widened pulse pressure with a diastolic murmur may alert the physician to an ascending aortic aneurysm with aortic valve insufficiency. A physician may also discover a thoracic aneurysm by incidental inspection of a chest x-ray (Fig. 63-15).

Indications for Operation

Patients who are diagnosed with aneurysms greater than or equal to 5 cm or with rapid aneurysm enlargement are considered for surgical repair. A sudden change in the characteristics or the severity of the pain is significant and alerts clinicians to the possibility of rapid aneurysm expansion, leakage, or rupture. When considering aneurysm growth rate and the risk for rupture, the Marfan patient or other patients with inherited collagen vascular disorders or familial patterns of aortic dissection must be given special attention. More than 90% of deaths in Marfan patients are related to complications of aneurysms or dissections of the thoracic aorta. Marfan patients and patients who are predisposed to dissection and rupture (familial TAAD), such as those with certain mutations in transforming growth factor-β receptor type II,[13] are often considered for surgery at an earlier stage of aneurysm development owing to faster rates of aneurysm growth and rupture at smaller diameters.[19]

THORACIC AORTIC DISSECTION

Clinical Presentation

Abrupt excruciating pain epitomizes the onset of acute aortic dissection.[20] Chest pain is present in about two thirds of patients, and back pain invariably accompanies dissections that begin distal to the aortic arch. Pain may migrate as the dissection progresses distally. Patients with ascending aortic dissections may have associated aortic valve insufficiency with dyspnea and a diagnostic loud

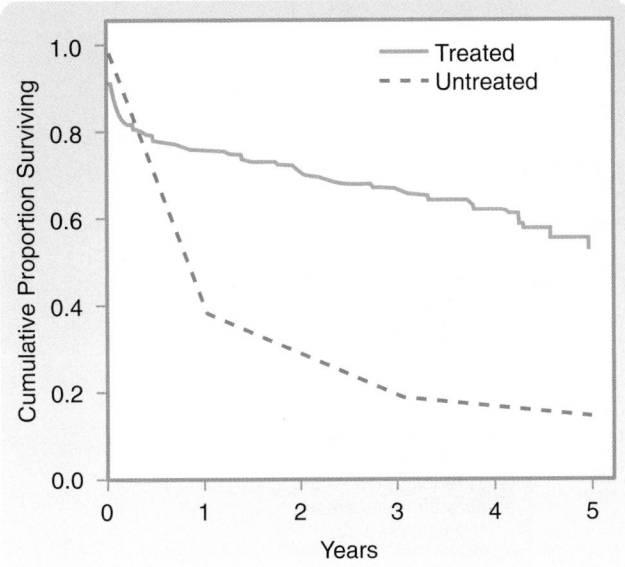

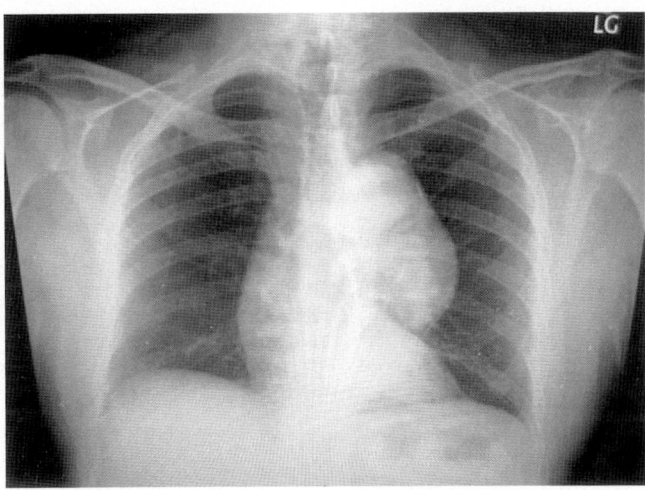

Figure 63-15 Chest x-ray of a patient with a thoracic aortic aneurysm.

Figure 63-14 Thoracoabdominal aortic aneurysm: comparison of survival rates in untreated (Bickerstaff and colleagues[16]) versus surgically treated patients (Safi and associates[17]).

pansystolic murmur. Other acute symptoms and signs related to aortic branch occlusion include cerebral infarction, myocardial infarction, abdominal vessel malperfusion, limb ischemia, and paraplegia. The distinctions between acute and chronic aortic dissections, types A and B, have important clinical implications (Fig. 63-16). The 14-day period after onset of dissection has been empirically designated the acute phase because mortality and morbidity rates are highest, and surviving patients usually stabilize at the end of this period. Serious life-threatening complications typically occur during the acute phase, and surgery on the acutely dissected aorta is high risk, associated with considerable bleeding because of the friability of the aortic wall.

Acute Phase

The natural history of acute type A aortic dissection is associated with a significant mortality rate, which has been reported as 1% per hour in the first 48 hours or about 50% at 2 days, 75% at 2 weeks, and 90% at 1 year.[21] Early death may occur as a result of malperfusion syndromes (cerebrovascular, visceral, renal, or peripheral ischemia), cardiac complications (acute aortic insufficiency, coronary ischemia, cardiac tamponade), or free rupture[22] (see Surgical Treatment and Results: Proximal Thoracic Aorta, later). The patient who is unstable with suspected type A acute aortic dissection is immediately transferred to the operating room and evaluated by TEE. If dissection is confirmed, repair is undertaken at once (Fig. 63-17). Surgery in the case of the hemodynamically stable patient is less urgent, and the patient is first transferred to an acute care setting until confirmation of the diagnosis is made.

For acute type B aortic dissection, the treatment of choice is generally medical therapy aimed at pain control and the correction of hypertension (see Medical Treatment, next). Patients are admitted to an intensive care unit and observed closely. Surgical repair is most often reserved for dissection complicated by aortic rupture, abdominal malperfusion, limb ischemia, intractable pain, or uncontrollable hypertension. About 16% of patients with acute type B aortic dissection require surgical therapy[23] (see Surgical Treatment And Results: Distal Thoracic Aorta, later).

Medical Treatment

We initiate antihypertensive or so-called anti-impulse therapy for all patients with acute dissection, whether type A or type B. An arterial line is placed for close monitoring of the systemic arterial blood pressure. We use esmolol for IV β-blockade (range, 50-300 µg/kg/min) titrated to heart rate (60-80 beats/min), systolic blood pressure (<120 mm Hg), and mean arterial blood pressure (80 mm Hg). We prefer esmolol, a β₁-selective agent, because of its ease of titration due to its short-acting nature. β-Blockade can also be achieved with propranolol, a nonselective β₁- and β₂-blocker (2-5 mg given IV every 4-6 hours) or labetalol, a nonselective β₁- and β₂-blocker as well as an α₁-blocker (20 mg IV slow injection followed by 40 mg IV every 10 minutes).

Patients whose hypertension is refractory to β-blockade may require combination therapy with other agents. Our choice with combination therapy includes a calcium channel blocking agent, nicardipine (5-15 mg/hr IV infusion), nitroglycerin (5 µg/min IV infusion), and sodium nitroprusside (0.5-5 µg/kg/min IV infusion). Because potent unloading agents such as sodium nitroprusside may actually cause an increase in the dP/dt when used alone, it is important to use them in combination with a β-blocking agent. In addition, sodium nitroprusside must be used with caution because it may be associated with cyanide toxicity and paraplegia.[24]

Chronic Phase

All patients who survive the acute phase of aortic dissection, whether type A or type B, must be followed closely.

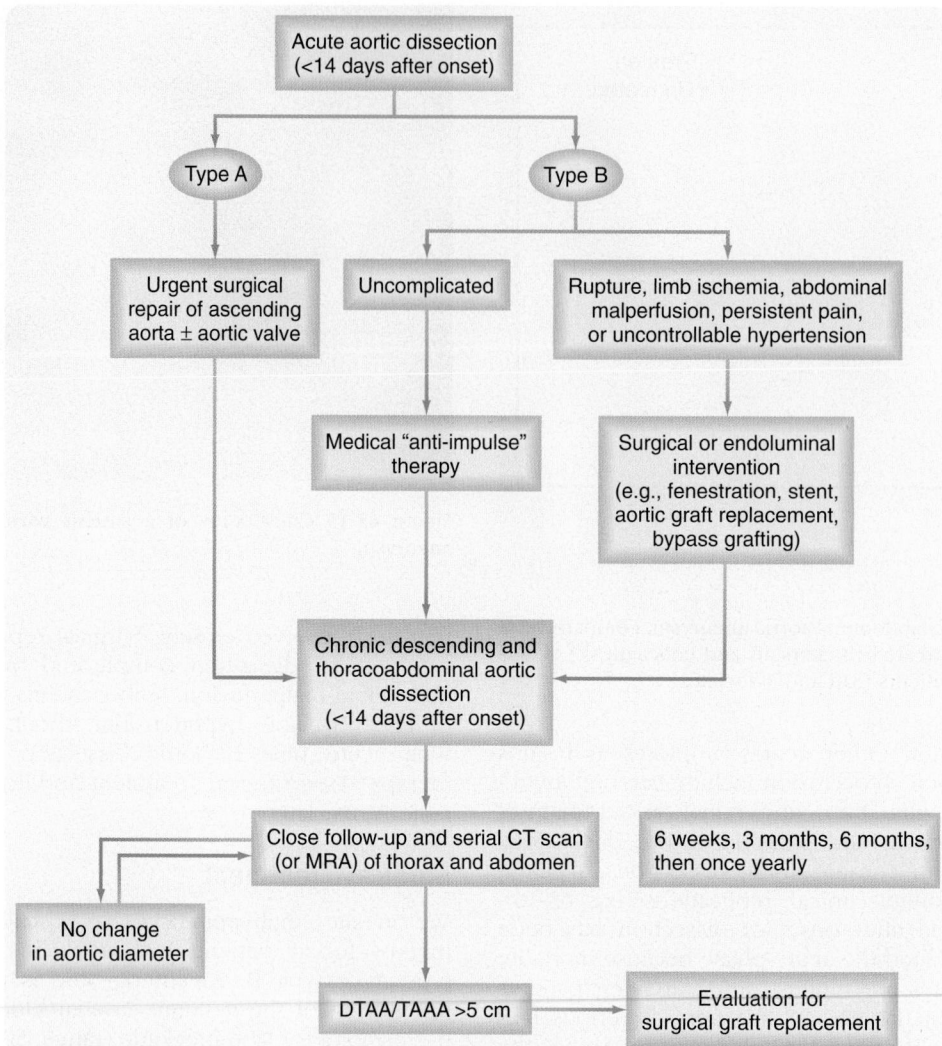

Figure 63-16 Algorithm for treatment of aortic dissection. CT, computed tomography; DTAA, descending thoracic aortic aneurysm; MRA, magnetic resonance angiography; TAAA, thoracoabdominal aortic aneurysm.

Serial imaging of the dissected aorta needs to be obtained before discharge from the acute care hospital and then at 6 weeks, 3 months, 6 months, 12 months, and yearly thereafter. Compliance with chronic antihypertensive therapy decreases the incidence of subsequent hospitalization and may reduce the progression of aortic dilation. In most patients, acute pain resolves, and symptoms subside. Recurrent chest and back pain may indicate sudden aortic expansion or impending rupture. All symptomatic patients are evaluated for surgical repair. About 20% to 40% of patients who survive the acute phase of aortic dissection develop significant aneurysmal dilation of the aorta within 2 to 5 years, requiring surgical graft replacement when the maximal aortic diameter reaches 5 to 6 cm to prevent rupture. The extent of surgical graft replacement will depend on the extent of the aortic aneurysm. In general, we replace all aneurysmal aortic segments, leaving the normal aorta (with or without dissection) in situ.

SURGICAL TREATMENT AND RESULTS: PROXIMAL THORACIC AORTA

Aortic Root

The technical innovations of the early 1950s permitted the first successful operations of the aortic root. Cardiopulmonary bypass, which replaces the pumping action of the heart and the gas exchange function of the lungs, was essential. The patient is placed on cardiopulmonary bypass after the chest is opened with a median sternotomy and either the ascending aorta or the axillary or femoral artery is cannulated. Retrograde cardioplegic perfusion through the coronary sinus provides myocardial protection throughout the procedure, keeping the myocardial temperature below 15°C. Venting through the left superior pulmonary vein prevents ventricular distention and allows optimal decompression of the left ventricle. Profound hypothermia and circulatory arrest are required

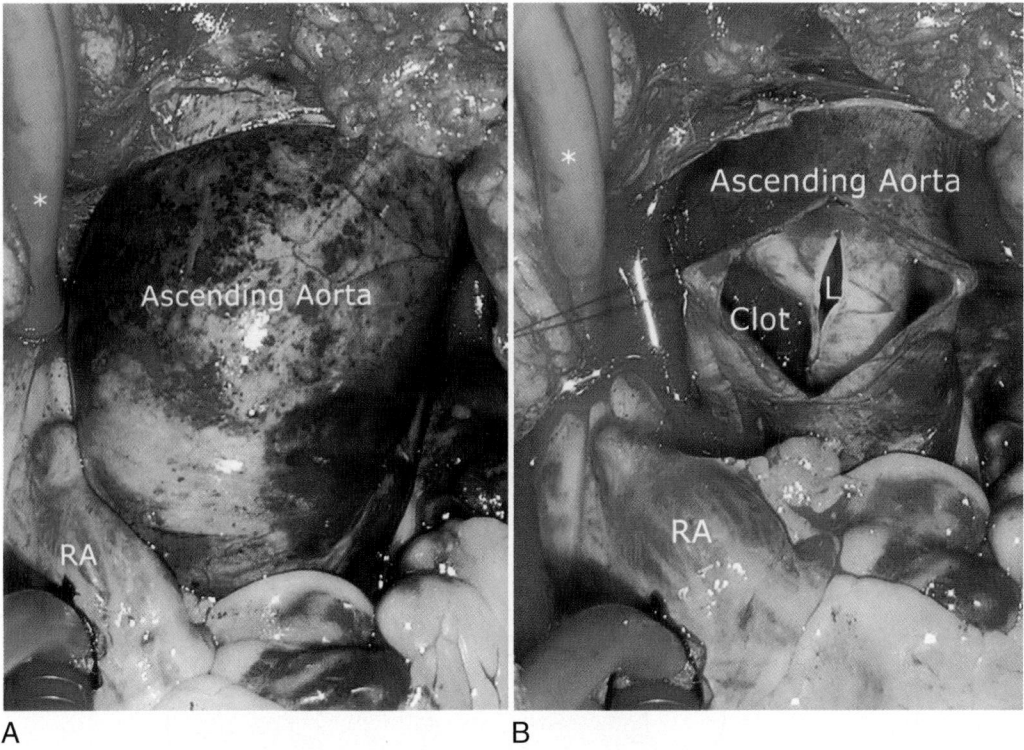

Figure 63-17 A, Operative photograph of acute type A aortic dissection with hematoma in the aortic wall. **B,** After opening the aorta, a large clot was cleared from the false lumen; true lumen (L) is seen after division of the intimal flap. RA, right atrium.

in cases of acute aortic dissection or aneurysms that extend into the aortic arch; otherwise, the ascending aorta can be safely clamped without profound hypothermia.

The extent of prosthetic valve or graft replacement or both depends on patient presentation and is determined at the time of surgery. Patients who have intrinsic abnormalities in the valve leaflets, bicuspid aortic valve, or Marfan syndrome may require aortic valve replacement. Valve replacement will depend on the degree of stenosis or insufficiency detected on preoperative echocardiography. Valve-sparing aortic root replacement may be performed when aortic valve function remains preserved. Separate valve and graft replacement, rather than a composite valved graft, may be applicable in patients with minor sinus dilation. Allograft (homograft) aortic root replacement may be suitable for physically active patients who do not wish to take anticoagulants or patients with native or prosthetic valve endocarditis. Aortic repair (by resuspension of the aortic valve commissures), rather than replacement, may be adequate in cases of acute aortic dissection and a normal aortic valve.

Bentall and de Bono in 1968 and Edwards and Kerr in 1970 created the composite valve graft. In the Bentall technique, a composite valve graft is placed in the aortic annulus after the walls of the aorta have been opened longitudinally and the aortic valve leaflets excised. The distal end of the graft is cut and sewn end-to-end to the distal ascending aorta. Openings are cut in the graft opposite the right and left coronary arteries. The coronary ostia are tightly sutured to their corresponding openings in the composite graft. However, the side-to-side attachment of the coronary arteries to the valve prosthesis can bring the anastomosis under tension, which can lead to pseudoaneurysm. Although a few groups continue to use the Bentall technique, the report of pseudoaneurysm in 7% to 25% of patients prompted many surgeons to adopt new techniques for coronary artery reattachment.[25] Christian Cabrol in 1981 devised a method for replacing the aortic root without having to mobilize the coronary arteries. A small Dacron tube graft is sutured to the left coronary ostium, passed behind the larger ascending aortic graft, and anastomosed to the right coronary ostium. The small Dacron graft is then anastomosed side-to-side to the composite graft. Bleeding is minimized because suture line tension is significantly reduced, but kinking can occur at the side-to-side anastomosis or right ostium. Modification of the Cabrol technique consists of an end-to-side anastomosis of the left main coronary Dacron graft, with a button attachment of the right coronary artery directly to the composite graft or replaced by separate vein or Dacron graft. Graft kinks or graft occlusion at the angle of the right coronary artery ostium are avoided because the smaller graft is not restrained by a side-to-side anastomosis. We most often use the button technique or Carrel patch for right and left coronary artery reattachment. It is more time consuming than the

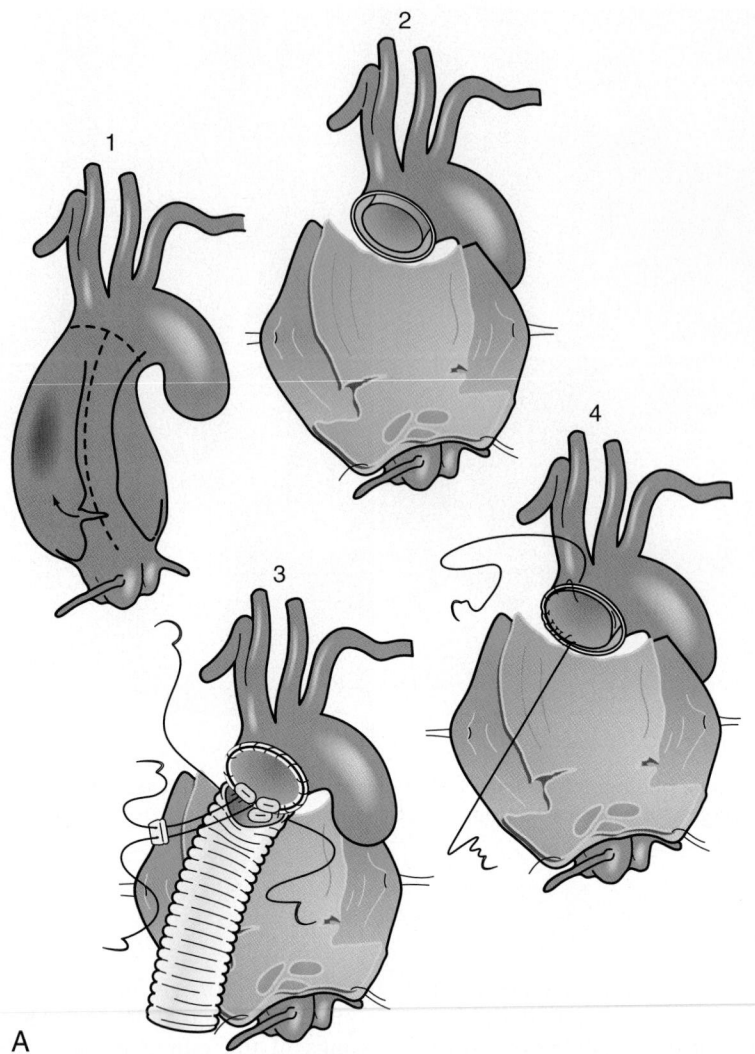

Figure 63-18 A, Ascending aortic dissection repair. Under circulatory arrest, the ascending aorta and transverse arch are opened, exposing the dissection (1, 2). The false lumen is obliterated (3). The graft is sutured to the transverse arch in an open distal anastomosis (4).

Cabrol technique, but complications are fewer. The right and left coronary artery ostia are dissected from the aorta, preserving a circle of tissue or button, and anastomosed directly to the composite graft.

Results: Aortic Root

A lack of reporting standards in the literature makes interpretation of aortic root surgical results difficult to summarize. In general, both etiology (dilation, Marfan syndrome, aortic dissection) and reconstructive technique (Cabrol, Wheat, Bentall, and button) appear to influence outcome. Repair of a diseased aortic root can be accomplished safely, depending on risk factors, with an overall operative mortality rate in the range of 2% to 15%. Major operative complications of the surgery are bleeding at the anastomotic site (requiring reoperation) and thromboembolism. Long-term complications include endocarditis, thromboembolic events, and pseudoaneurysm.

Ascending Aorta and Arch

If aneurysmal disease is limited to the tubular portion of the ascending aorta, profound hypothermia is not required, and we use the closed technique (i.e., with aorta clamped). If, however, the aneurysm extends beyond the ascending aorta into the arch, or there is acute dissection, we use the open distal anastomosis technique—with profound hypothermic circulatory arrest. The dry surgical field of the open technique permits the surgeon to clearly view all diseased portions of the ascending aorta to within a few millimeters of the great vessels. Cardiopulmonary bypass, circulatory arrest, and retrograde cerebral perfusion are also used. Retrograde

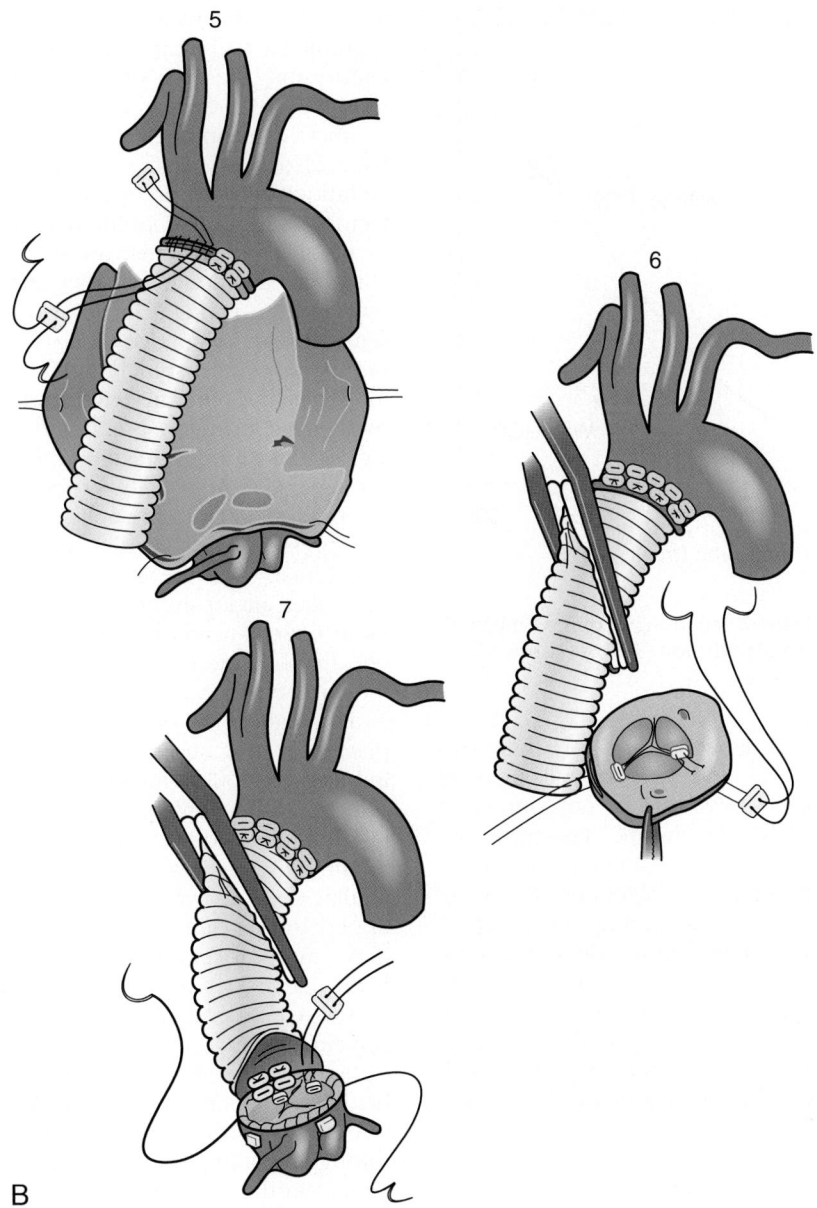

B

Figure 63-18, cont'd B, The distal anastomosis is reinforced (5). The aortic valve is resuspended (6). The proximal anastomosis is constructed (7).

cerebral perfusion is begun after the patient has been cooled to between 20°C and 15°C (nasopharyngeal temperature) and the electroencephalogram is reading isoelectric. Oxygenated blood is perfused in a retrograde direction through the superior vena cava to the brain. Another technique that has been used for cerebral protection during the circulatory arrest period is antegrade cerebral perfusion. This technique employs catheters inserted directly into the ostia of the innominate and left common carotid arteries or use of a cannula in the axillary artery with proximal clamping of the innominate artery during the period of arrest. Both approaches

have potential benefits, and efficacy continues to be debated.

The brachiocephalic, left common carotid, and left subclavian arteries are preserved as a patch while the ascending aorta and transverse arch are excised. After a graft is sutured to the descending thoracic aorta just distal to the left subclavian artery, the brachiocephalic arteries are anastomosed to a side hole cut in the superior arch portion of the graft. The aortic valve and aortic sinuses are inspected and repaired if necessary (see Aortic Root, earlier). The graft is then sutured to the supracoronary ascending aorta.

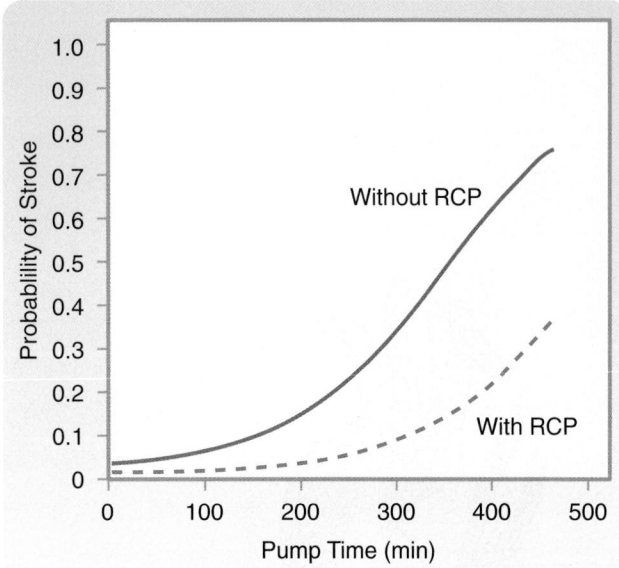

Figure 63-19 Probability of stroke according to pump time, with and without retrograde cerebral perfusion (RCP). (© Chris Akers, 2006. Reprinted with permission.)

Surgery for acute type A dissection and for aneurysms of the root, ascending aorta, and arch is similar except for the additional suturing necessitated by false lumen in aortic dissection (Fig. 63-18). In chronic dissection, the partition between the true and false lumen is opened. In the acute setting, the false lumen is obliterated by sewing together the dissected walls using running 4-0 polypropylene suture. The graft is sutured to the proximal aortic arch. The aortic arch is replaced if a hematoma, fragmentation of the aortic intima, or free rupture is identified. Intimal tears are either excised or repaired. The aortic root is reconstructed by placing 4-0 polypropylene pledgeted sutures along the sinotubular junction to prevent retrograde dissection.

Results: Ascending Aorta and Arch

Before profound hypothermic circulatory arrest became a regular part of aortic surgery, arch replacement carried an extremely high mortality rate of up to 75%. The introduction of profound hypothermia and circulatory arrest reduced operative mortality to between 10% and 15%. The development of additional circulatory adjuncts has reduced operative mortality to around 5%.[26] The major risk factors associated with stroke and encephalopathy following ascending/arch repair are circulatory arrest time and involvement of the transverse arch and the degree of atheromatous disease in the aorta (Fig. 63-19).

SURGICAL TREATMENT AND RESULTS: DISTAL THORACIC AORTA

In the past 15 years, remarkable strides have been made in the strategies to protect the spinal cord during repair of the descending thoracic and thoracoabdominal aorta

in an effort to lower the incidence of neurologic deficit (paraplegia or paraparesis). In even the most extensive aneurysms, the rate of neurologic deficit is about 4%. This has been achieved through the implementation of adjunctive techniques to protect the spinal cord. There have also been dramatic improvements in the surgical techniques and in preoperative evaluation of patient risk factors (e.g., cardiac, pulmonary, renal). Marked improvements in cardiovascular anesthesia, decreasing the mortality rate and length of stay in both the intensive care unit and the hospital, have also played a role. We have settled on an adjunctive therapy consisting of distal aortic perfusion, cerebrospinal fluid (CSF) drainage, and passive moderate hypothermia with intraoperative maneuvers to protect the kidneys, spinal cord, and viscera. Our rationale for this strategy relates to the state of the aorta after proximal clamping of the descending thoracic aorta. After the proximal clamp is applied, aortic pressure drops and CSF pressure rises, so that perfusion to the spinal cord is minimal. With the implementation of our strategy, we have seen major improvements in morbidity and mortality in patients undergoing repair. The use of our adjunct negates the side effects of the aortic clamping, allowing the surgeon to carry out the repair with greater care.

The patient is brought to the operating room and placed in the supine position. General anesthesia is induced. A double-lumen endotracheal tube is used for selective lung ventilation. This allows us to deflate the left lung in order to avoid damaging it during aortic repair. IV catheters are inserted into the left and right jugular veins, as well as in both radial arteries. A balloon-tipped thermodilution catheter is placed in the pulmonary artery for monitoring the hemodynamics of the heart. Electrodes are placed on the head for monitoring of the electroencephalogram and along the spine for somatosensory and motor evoked potentials. A Foley catheter is inserted; and, in most cases, we monitor bladder temperature. We may also monitor core temperature through the rectum and that of the spinal cord through nasopharyngeal temperature. We position the patient in the right lateral decubitus position with shoulder blades at a right angle to the surface of the operating table. The left groin and hip are tilted between 45 and 60 degrees to allow access to both common femoral arteries. The anesthesia team inserts a catheter at lumbar space 3 or 4, advancing it 5 cm. CSF pressure is maintained at less then 10 mm Hg for the duration of the surgery and for 3 days after surgery (Fig. 63-20). The patient is secured in position using bean bags and then prepared and draped in the usual sterile fashion.

We adapt the incision based on extent of the aneurysm (Fig. 63-21). For a thoracoabdominal aneurysm extending from the left subclavian to below the renal arteries, from the mid-descending aorta to below the renals, or for a total abdominal aortic aneurysm (i.e., extents II, III, and VI), we use a full thoracoabdominal incision; this begins parallel to the vertebral border of the scapula and curves along the sixth rib toward the umbilicus and then to the midline below the umbilicus. In patients with a descending thoracic aortic aneurysm or with extent I or V with involvement only to the celiac axis and not the superior

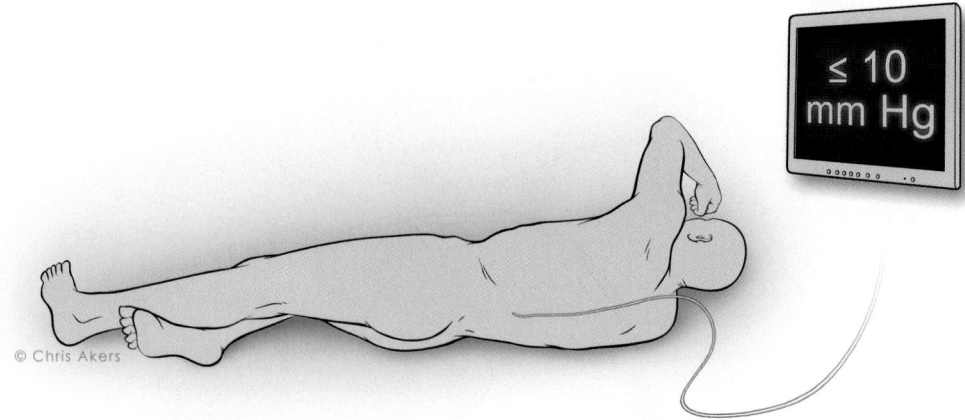

Figure 63-20 Cerebrospinal fluid (CSF) drainage is initiated intraoperatively and maintained for 3 days after surgery to keep CSF pressure below 10 mm Hg. (© Chris Akers, 2006. Reprinted with permission.)

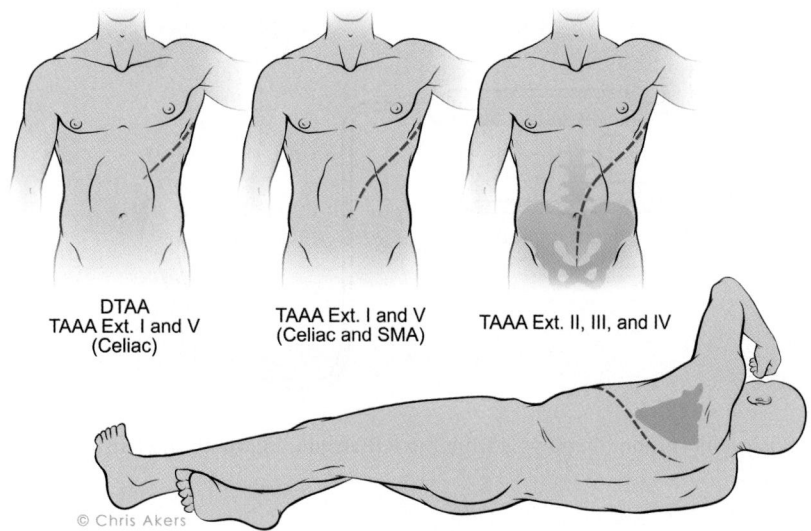

Figure 63-21 Incision is tailored to the extent of the thoracoabdominal aortic aneurysm. DTAA, descending thoracic aortic aneurysm; SMA, superior mesenteric artery; TAAA, thoracoabdominal aortic aneurysm.

mesenteric artery, we use the modified left thoracoabdominal incision. The sixth rib is removed. On rare occasions, we keep the rib and, instead, resect it.

In patients with extent I or V with superior mesenteric involvement, the abdominal incision is extended into the umbilicus. We dissect the abdominal aorta extraperitoneally to mobilize the viscera and the left kidney medially and extraperitoneally. The muscular portion of the diaphragm is cut, taking care not to injure the left phrenic nerve. We dissect the crus of the diaphragm around the aorta in order to expand the aortic hiatus. Self-retaining retractors are used to keep the chest and abdomen open. The patient is anticoagulated with 1 mg heparin per kilogram of body weight. We incise the pericardium parallel to the left phrenic nerve exposing the lower pulmonary vein. We use 3-0 pledgeted polypropylene sutures in a purse-string fashion. The left common femoral artery is exposed and cannulated. An aortic cannula is placed in

the left lower pulmonary vein, secured, and connected to the centrifugal BioMedicus pump and inline heat exchanger, which in turn is connected to the femoral line (Fig. 63-22). The proximal descending thoracic aorta is dissected. We begin at the hilum of the lung. Care must be taken not to injure the left vagus nerve. We therefore dissect between the vagus nerve and the descending thoracic aorta. This will continue cephalad until we come to the ligamentum arteriosum, a landmark for the left recurrent laryngeal nerve. We must take care to protect this nerve while transecting the ligamentum arteriosum. We dissect the proximal descending thoracic aorta circumferentially either proximal or distal to the left subclavian.

A site is chosen for placement of the proximal clamp. We use sequential clamping during our repair to minimize ischemic time (Fig. 63-23). We begin left heart bypass. A clamp is placed either proximal or distal to the

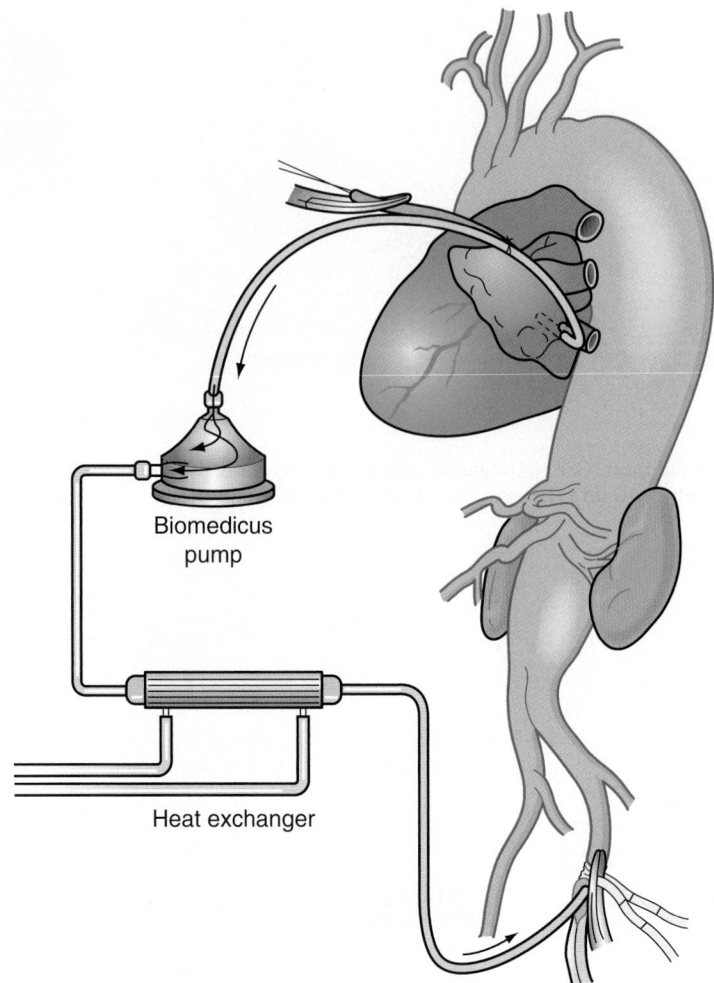

Figure 63-22 Distal aortic perfusion. Outflow is from the left atrium, inflow to the left femoral artery.

left subclavian and at the mid-descending thoracic aorta. The thoracic aorta is opened longitudinally between the two clamp sites. The walls of the aorta are retracted using No. 2 self-retracting sutures. Because of the danger of esophageal-graft fistula, we no longer use the inclusion technique of wrapping the graft within the aneurysmal aortic wall in the proximal anastomosis. Instead, we completely transect the proximal thoracic aorta to separate it from the underlying esophagus. We choose an appropriately sized, woven Dacron tube graft impregnated with collagen or gelatin. The graft is sutured to the descending thoracic aorta proximally using 3-0 polypropylene sutures. We reinforce the suture line with 3-0 polypropylene pledgeted sutures if needed. The distal clamp is moved to the abdominal aorta above the celiac axis, and the remainder of the thoracic aorta is opened longitudinally. We use No. 2 silk retracting sutures to retract the walls of the aorta. The upper intercostal arteries are ligated using 2-0 silk. We identify the lower intercostal arteries (T8-T12) to determine patency. We reattach these arteries if they are patent because we have previously found that their ligation increases risk for neurologic deficit.[27] If they are occluded, then we reattach the upper intercostal arteries rather than ligating. The intercostal arteries are reattached by an elliptical incision made in the Dacron graft. We reattach the graft to the thoracic aortic wall containing the orifices of the appropriate intercostal arteries using 3-0 polypropylene sutures. The proximal clamp is moved to the graft, distal to site of the intercostal artery reattachment. Any bleeding points are secured. In certain cases, such as those with acute type B (DeBakey type II) aortic dissection or severely calcified aorta with atheromatous plaque, intercostal artery reattachment is not advisable owing to the danger of bleeding and occlusion.

The graft is then passed through the aortic hiatus into the abdominal field. The infrarenal abdominal aorta is clamped, and the remainder of the abdominal aorta is opened. The walls are retracted using No. 2 silk retraction sutures. We inspect the celiac axis, superior mesenteric artery, and both renal arteries. In our experience, 5% of patients have atheromatous plaque or occlusive disease. In such cases, we perform an endarterectomy on those arteries. Otherwise, we perfuse the celiac axis, superior

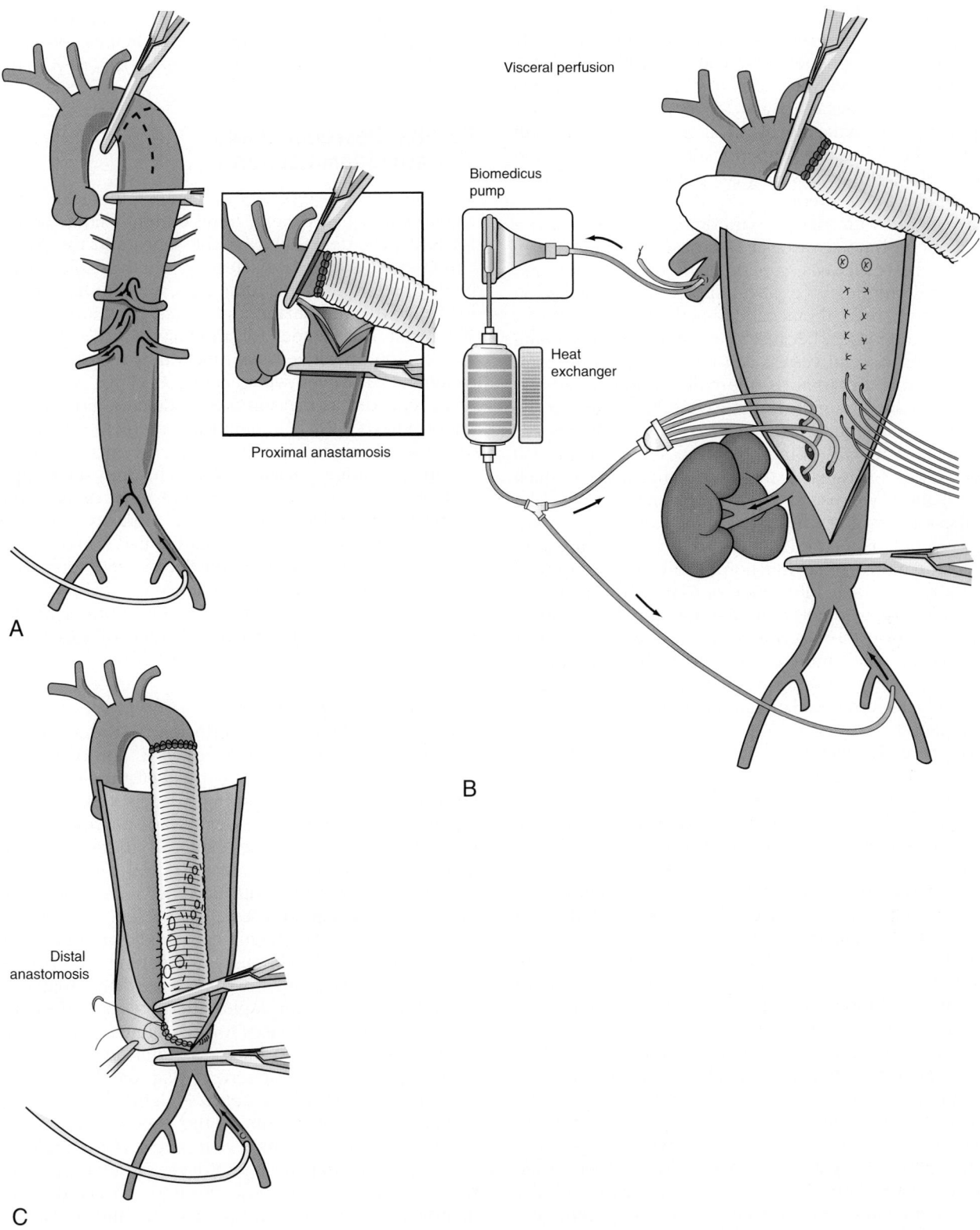

Figure 63-23 Sequential clamping, thoracoabdominal aortic aneurysm repair. **A,** The upper descending thoracic is clamped and the proximal aneurysm opened while the lower aorta and peripheral arteries continue to be perfused. **B,** The distal clamp is moved down the aorta. Bleeding from intercostal arteries can be controlled using 3-French balloon catheters, while the patent lower intercostals arteries are reattached. Visceral and renal perfusion is maintained using 9-French Pruitt catheters during reimplantation of the visceral and renal arteries. **C,** Distal anastomosis is completed, and the lower extremities remain perfused with the distal clamp on the aortic bifurcation.

mesenteric, and both renal arteries using either cold or tepid blood. The perfusion is carried out with a specially designed balloon-tip perfusing catheter with the ability to monitor the pressure distal to the perfusion. Renal artery pressure distal to the balloon is kept above 60 mm Hg. We make an elliptical incision in the graft opposite the celiac axis, superior mesenteric artery, and both renal arteries, and we use 3-0 polypropylene sutures to reimplant these arteries.

In patients with Marfan syndrome, we like to use a specially constructed vascular Dacron graft with sidearm grafts to the celiac axis, superior mesenteric artery, and both renal arteries. We also employ this strategy in patients with redo thoracoabdominal aortic aneurysms with enlarged viscera because using an elliptical opening opposite the visceral vessels is not feasible. Before completion of this anastomosis, the balloon-tipped catheter is removed and the graft flushed with the patient in the head-down position. We then restore flow to the viscera and renal arteries. Bleeding points are secured using 3-0 polypropylene sutures. If the wall of the aorta is thick and calcified, we use 2-0 polypropylene sutures. The anesthesiologist gives indigo carmine, and urinary dye clearance time is recorded and used to estimate immediate postoperative renal function. The clamp is applied either above the iliac bifurcation or to the left iliac artery. The graft is anastomosed to the infrarenal abdominal aorta just above the iliac bifurcation using either 3-0 or 2-0 polypropylene sutures. Before removal of the proximal clamp, the graft is again flushed, both distally and proximally, to remove all air and debris. The anastomosis is completed.

We proceed somewhat differently if the patient has a thoracic aortic aneurysm due to chronic dissection (type A or type B) and the distal abdominal aorta is not dilated. We repair only that portion of the descending thoracic aorta that is aneurysmal. We prefer to resect a wedge of the partition between the true and false lumen to allow perfusion to both channels. If the patient is suffering from acute dissection in the descending thoracic aorta, the intima of the proximal descending thoracic aorta will be sutured using fine 4-0 or 5-0 polypropylene sutures with liberal use of pledgeted sutures. Distally, we like to rechannel the blood flow into the true lumen after suturing the intima and the adventitia.

Upon completion of the final anastomosis, we first remove the distal clamp, and bleeding points are checked. Then the proximal clamp is removed. At the same time, the patient is rewarmed with the in-line heat exchanger. When the nasopharyngeal, bladder, or rectal temperature reaches 36°C, the patient is weaned from distal aortic perfusion. We then decannulate the patient, and the lower pulmonary vein is secured. We repair the left common femoral artery using 5-0 polypropylene suture, sewn in a running fashion. Protamine sulfate is administered (1 mg protamine per milligram of heparin given). The abdomen is closed in layers with polypropylene. We usually insert three 6-French chest tubes for drainage. We approximate the intercostal space and the muscular fascia using absorbable sutures. The skin is approximated using staples. The patient is placed in the supine position, and

the anesthesiologist exchanges the double-lumen tube for a single-lumen tube. In special circumstances, such as when the vocal cords are swollen, this step may be delayed.

Results: Descending and Thoracoabdominal Aorta

Mortality rates for repair of descending thoracic and thoracoabdominal aortic aneurysms currently range between 5% and 21%, depending on the series and the patient's condition at the time of surgery. Multivariable analyses by different groups, including ours, have found age, renal failure, and symptomatic and extent II aneurysms to be significant risk factors for mortality.[28-30] We previously assessed preoperative renal function by measuring serum creatinine. However, we recently found that preoperative renal function, as measured by estimated glomerular filtration rate (GFR), is a significant predictor of mortality in these patients, superior to assessments using gross serum creatinine measurements. In the subgroup of patients with no clinically apparent renal disease, those in the highest GFR quartile had a mortality rate of 5%, whereas those in the lowest quartile had a mortality rate of 27%.[31] Patients who undergo elective graft replacement at high-volume centers of excellence fare best, with mortality rates between 5% and 15%. Our current mortality rate for elective repair is between 5% and 12%, as opposed to rates of 20% to 25% in the early 1990s.

Spinal Cord Complications

The adjunct (distal aortic perfusion, CSF drainage, and moderate hypothermia) has reduced our overall incidence of immediate neurologic deficit to 2.4%[32] and, in particular, 0.8% for descending thoracic aortic aneurysm repair.[33] With the adjunct, our rate of neurologic deficit for the most troublesome extent II thoracoabdominal aortic aneurysms has also declined and is now between 7% and 12% compared with rates between 30% and 40% in the era of clamp-and-sew.[34] In the era of clamp-and-sew, clamp time was a significant predictor of neurologic deficit (Fig. 63-24). Although clamp time has increased steadily every year since we have used the adjunct (34 seconds per year), neurologic deficit rates have decreased. Although other risk factors for neurologic deficit remain, cross-clamp time is no longer a significant predictor of neurologic deficit in our series[32] (Fig. 63-25).

Immediate neurologic deficit is defined as paraplegia or paraparesis that occurs as the patient awakens from anesthesia. *Delayed-onset neurologic deficit* refers to paraplegia or paraparesis that develops after a period of normal neurologic function. We have observed delayed neurologic deficit as early as 2 hours and as late as 2 weeks after surgery (median, 2 days) in 2.4% of patients.[35] No single risk factor explains the onset of either deficit, but researchers have become more and more interested in how a patient can emerge from surgery neurologically intact but later develop paraplegia. Using multivariable analysis, we found that acute dissection, extent II thoracoabdominal aortic aneurysm, and renal insufficiency were independent preoperative predictors.[35]

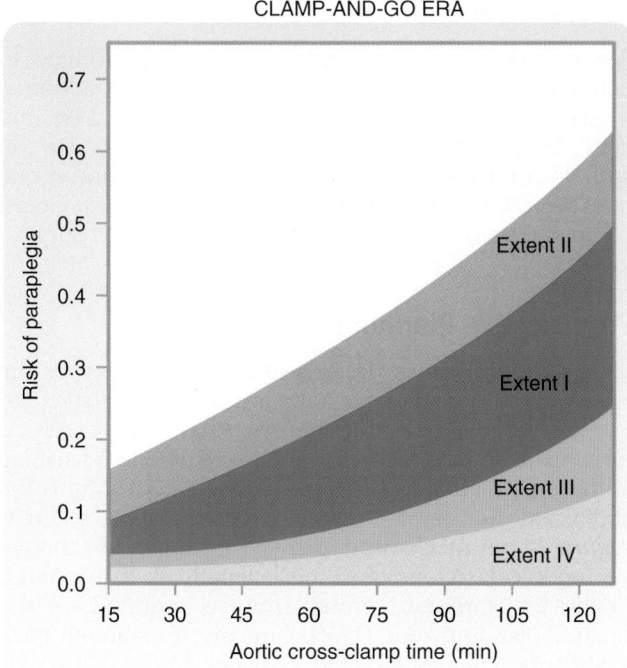

Figure 63-24 Multiple logistic regression analysis according to risk for neurologic deficit and aortic cross-clamp time without adjunct use.

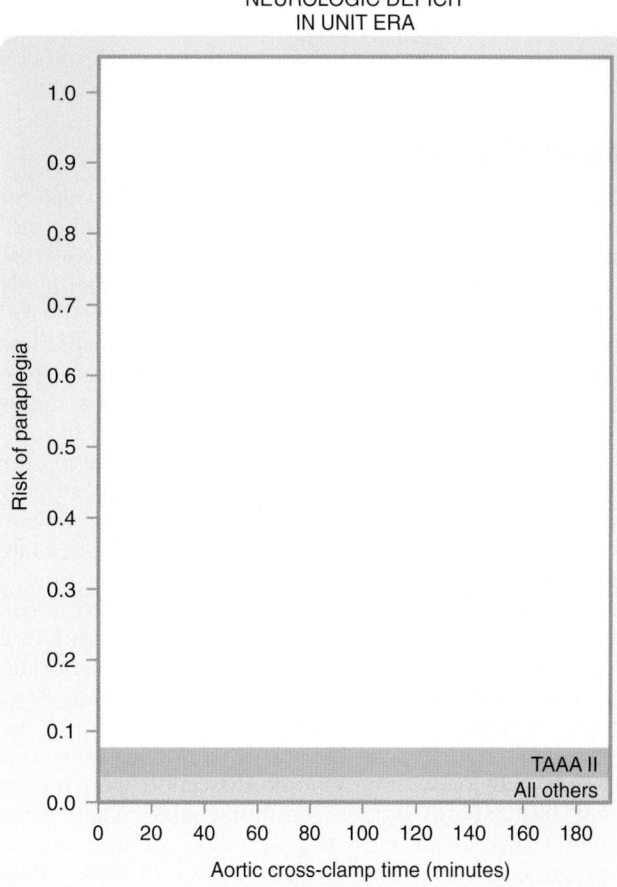

Figure 63-25 Multiple logistic regression analysis according to risk for neurologic deficit and aortic cross-clamp time with adjunct use. The incidence of neurologic deficit has decreased such that we now classify patient risk for neurologic deficit as extent II versus nonextent II. TAAA, thoracoabdominal aortic aneurysm.

In another study examining postoperative factors independent of preoperative risk factors, we found low postoperative mean arterial pressure (<60 mm Hg) and CSF drain complications to be significant predictors.[36] We speculate that delayed neurologic deficit after thoracoabdominal aortic repair may result from a "second hit" phenomenon. Although adjuncts may protect the spinal cord intraoperatively and reduce the incidence of immediate neurologic deficit, the spinal cord remains vulnerable during the early postoperative period. Additional ischemic insult caused by hemodynamic instability and CSF drainage catheter malfunction may constitute a second hit, causing delayed neurologic deficit. Because postoperative factors associated with delayed neurologic deficit are likely related to arterial blood pressure and oxygen delivery, we keep mean arterial pressure above 90 to 100 mm Hg, hemoglobin above 10 mg/dL, and cardiac index greater than 2.0 L/min. If delayed neurologic deficit occurs while the CSF drain is in place, the patient is placed in the supine position, and CSF is drained freely until the CSF pressure drops below 10 mm Hg. If the drain has been removed and delayed neurologic deficit occurs, the CSF drainage catheter is reinserted and drained for 72 hours. With this protocol, we have observed partial recovery from neurologic deficit in more than 50% of patients and complete recovery in 40%.[35]

Renal Failure

The incidence of renal failure after thoracoabdominal aortic repair ranges between 4% and 29%. Renal failure increases morbidity, length of stay, and mortality. We

have shown that the presence of preoperative renal insufficiency and the development of postoperative renal failure are associated with increased 30-day mortality and neurologic deficit.[31,37] Our current incidence of renal failure varies between 7% and 15%, depending on the extent of the aneurysm and the patient's preoperative renal function. About 15% of patients with postoperative renal failure require hemodialysis. Risk factors associated with renal failure are diminished GFR (<90 mL/min), direct left renal artery reattachment, and use of the simple cross-clamp technique. Good strategies to protect renal function during thoracoabdominal aortic repair remain elusive. Of great concern, though, is our finding of a higher incidence of subclinical renal disease (GFR 65-80 mL/min) than previously detected, which was significant for patient mortality.[31] The goals of perioperative renal protection are to maintain adequate renal oxygen delivery, reduce renal oxygen use, and reduce direct renal tubular injury. Thus far, these goals have been addressed most effectively by active renal cooling, directly maintaining renal perfusion, suppressing renal vasoconstriction, preventing micro-occlusion by particulate emboli, and preventing postischemic reperfusion injury. However, future efforts must focus on identifying the mechanism of renal impairment in these patients.

Impact of Dissection

Acute aortic dissection substantially raises the risk for paraplegia after graft replacement of the descending thoracic or thoracoabdominal aorta. Because dissection patients are critically ill and undergo surgery emergently with little time for preparation, the method of spinal cord protection during surgery for acute dissection is often less than optimal. Reported in-hospital death rates vary from 30% to 50%, compared with 10% to 20% of patients treated medically. Survival outcome for "uncomplicated" patients treated with early surgical repair resembles the outcome of patients treated medically. However, surgery during the acute phase is associated with more significant bleeding from the dissected aorta and with a higher rate of paraplegia (14%-32%).

Chronic dissection was previously considered a risk factor for paraplegia or paraparesis in patients undergoing repair of the descending thoracic and thoracoabdominal aorta, particularly during the era of clamp-and-sew. However, when we analyzed recent data, we found no appreciable difference in the rate of neurologic deficit for patients with or without chronic dissection who underwent descending thoracic or thoracoabdominal aortic repair, (3.6% versus 4.7%, respectively).[38] Chronic dissection undoubtedly makes surgical repair of descending thoracic and thoracoabdominal aortic aneurysms more difficult, but survival and neurologic outcome do not differ from those of aneurysm surgery without dissection. Several factors are likely responsible for the good neurologic outcome of our patients with chronic dissection, including better surgical techniques and anesthetic care and reimplantation of intercostal arteries. However, the key element in improved spinal cord protection is the use of the adjunct of distal aortic perfusion, CSF drainage, and moderate hypothermia.

ENDOVASCULAR REPAIR

Dake and colleagues reported the first endovascular treatment of a descending thoracic aortic aneurysm (DTAA) in 1994.[39] However, a relatively lower prevalence of DTAAs compared with abdominal aortic aneurysms, as well as technical and anatomic challenges, delayed the widespread use of this procedure. Technical considerations for thoracic endovascular aortic repair (TEVAR) include proximity of aneurysms to arch and visceral vessels, strong hemodynamic forces, large-profile devices, and highly tortuous anatomy. The first commercial device to obtain U.S. Food and Drug Administration (FDA) approval for TEVAR was the Gore Thoracic Aortic Graft (TAG) endoprosthesis (W. L. Gore, Flagstaff, AZ) (Fig. 63-26). Other devices currently undergoing trial are the Talent device (Medtronic AVE, Santa Rosa, CA) and the TX2 device (Cook, Bloomington, IN).

Pivotal Trial

A prospective, nonrandomized trial was performed to determine the safety and efficacy of the TAG endoprosthesis compared with open surgery.[40] Between 1999 and 2001, 139 patients were enrolled in the endovascular arm with 94 control subjects. Mortality, paraplegia, and stroke rates were 2.1%, 3%, and 4% in the endovascular patients, compared with 11.7%, 14%, and 4%, in the open surgical group.[25]

Preoperative Planning

Patients with fusiform DTAAs that are at least twice the size of the normal thoracic aorta are candidates for repair. For successful repair, the aneurysm has to be excluded proximally and distally. This requires fixation and sealing at the proximal and distal landing zones. *Fixation* is the ability of the device to resist displacement, whereas *sealing* is the mechanical barrier to prevent attachment site endoleak. A minimum neck length of 20 mm distal to the left common carotid artery is required for the proximal landing zone (PLZ). Similarly, a minimum neck length of 20 mm is required proximal to the celiac axis for the distal landing zone (DLZ).[41]

In some instances, the landing zone has been extended by coverage of arch or visceral vessels. Most centers revascularize the carotid, innominate, and visceral arteries before they are covered. Figure 63-27 demonstrates an MRA of a patient who underwent a carotid-carotid bypass before a TEVAR procedure. The left common carotid artery was excluded during this procedure. These procedures are often performed in a staged fashion. Left subclavian revascularization is now reserved for patients who develop left upper extremity ischemic symptoms, have a dominant left vertebral artery, or underwent a previous bypass requiring left subclavian flow. For example, patients who underwent previous coronary artery bypass procedures using the left internal mammary artery require adjunctive left subclavian transposition or bypass before endovascular repair.[42]

Other anatomic factors that require preoperative evaluation include the degree of atheroma in the aneurysm sac, the length of the aneurysm involving intercostal arteries, and the presence of thrombus or calcification in the proximal or distal neck. Finally, the size of the access vessels is critically important. Many patients with aneurysmal disease have underlying aortoiliac atherosclerotic disease. Delivery of a device for the TEVAR procedure requires placement of a large-profile 20- to 24-French (7.6-9.2 mm) sheath. In patients with borderline anatomy, early consideration is given to creation of an iliac conduit.

Imaging and Sizing

CTA is widely used for evaluation of DTAA. Three-dimensional reconstructions of these images are a valuable tool for sizing of endografts. Unusual anatomic characteristics of some DTAAs may make their measurements on axial images alone difficult. Center-line measurements on reconstruction images facilitate the measurement of aneu-

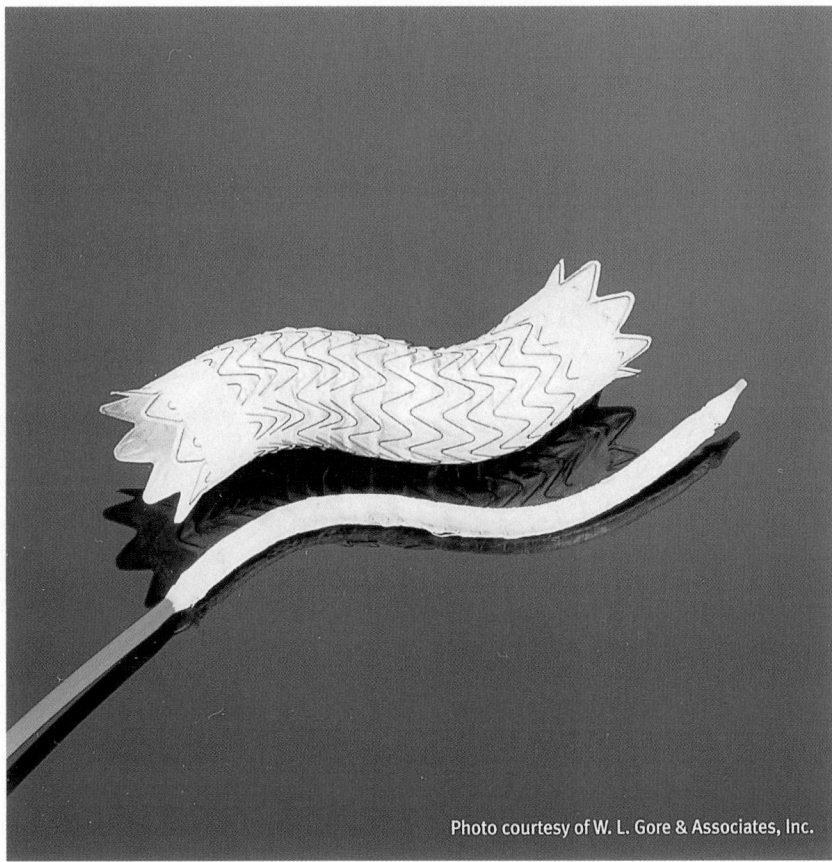

Photo courtesy of W. L. Gore & Associates, Inc.

Figure 63-26 The TAG Device. (Photo courtesy of W. L. Gore & Associates, Inc.)

rysm length, whereas vessel diameters are best measured from transverse images in a plane that is perpendicular to the central axis. Angiograms are only performed intraoperatively before device deployment except in unusual and complex aneurysms. In these rare circumstances, angiograms may provide valuable information for planning the procedure. IVUS is being increasingly used as an adjunctive tool, particularly in cases that involve aortic dissection.[43]

Accurate measurement and sizing is crucial in performing a successful TEVAR procedure. For the TAG device (W. L. Gore, Flagstaff, AZ), neck diameter measurements (inner wall to inner wall) ranging from 23 to 37 mm can be repaired using devices ranging from 26 to 40 mm. This allows for an oversizing of 6% to 19% compared with the vascular lumen. Stent grafts are available in lengths of 10, 15, and 20 cm.[41] In many instances, a combination of different length and diameter devices is necessary for complex repairs. In the TAG pivotal trial, 55% of patients required more than one device.[40] In general, the smaller-diameter or distal devices are deployed first. Adequate overlap (3-5 cm) is required in most circumstances. Overestimation or underestimation of the lumen may lead to improper sizing and a plethora of complications, including but not limited to endoleak, migration, aortic rupture, fistula, device kinking, and lumen occlusion.

Procedure

Appropriate patient selection and comprehensive preoperative planning are crucial to the efficiency and success of a TEVAR procedure. Hybrid operating rooms with fixed imaging equipment provide an ideal facility with combined open and endovascular capabilities. Regional and general anesthesia supportive equipment is often necessary. Perioperative CSF drainage can be performed at the discretion of the surgeon.[44] An accessible stockpile of guidewires, sheaths, catheters, and balloons to address various clinical circumstances is desirable. A groin cutdown procedure is often required for delivery of large sheaths; however, percutaneous techniques are performed by some investigators. Intraoperative diagnostic angiography is performed before placement of the device under live fluoroscopy. A completion angiogram is required to evaluate for aneurysm exclusion, arch and mesenteric vessel patency, and presence of endoleak. Figure 63-28 demonstrates reformatted three-dimensional CT reconstructions of the aorta before and after repair of a descending thoracic aortic aneurysm using an endovascular technique.

Complications

The most common complications in the TAG pivotal trial were vascular injury (14%), pulmonary disorder (10%),

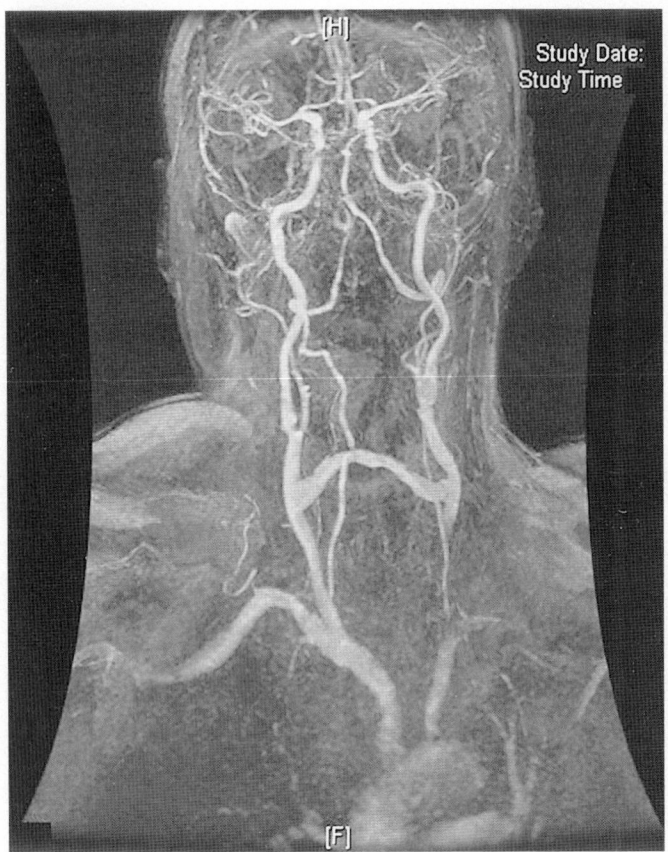

Figure 63-27 Magnetic resonance angiogram of a patient who underwent a carotid-carotid bypass before a thoracic endovascular aortic repair (TEVAR) procedure. The left common carotid artery was excluded during this procedure.

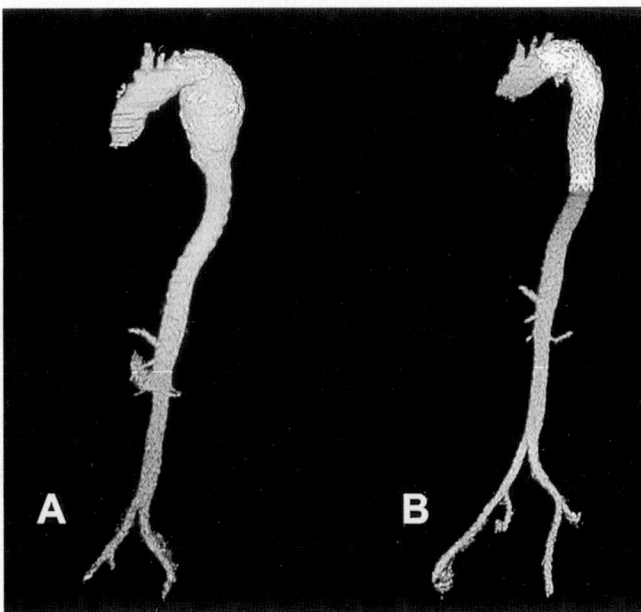

Figure 63-28 Reformatted three-dimensional computed tomography scans of an aorta before (**A**) and after (**B**) repair of a descending thoracic aortic aneurysm using an endovascular technique.

bleeding (9%), endoleak (4%), stroke (4%), cardiac (3%), paraplegia (3%), and death (2.1%).[40] Vascular injuries are often due to the introduction of relatively large introducer systems through the iliac system. Early consideration is given to creation of iliac conduits in patients with small vessels or severe iliac stenosis. The incidence of stroke was higher in patients with more proximal aneurysms, which required coverage of the left subclavian artery. All patients had undergone preoperative carotid-subclavian bypass. This makes atheroembolism secondary to manipulation of an atherosclerotic aortic arch a likely cause. The risk for paraplegia appears to increase with the extent of coverage of the descending thoracic aorta. Patients with compromised collateral circulation (previous abdominal aortic aneurysm repair, hypogastric artery occlusion, or planned left subclavian artery coverage) or perioperative hemodynamic compromise (hypotension, vascular injury) appear to be at increased risk.[44-46] Perioperative spinal cord drainage, performed either prophylactically or expectantly, has been used to prevent and treat paraplegia. The perioperative mortality in the TAG trial was related to cardiopulmonary and cerebrovascular complications. This is likely a reflection of the multiple medical comorbidities that are present in the aneurysm population.

Surveillance

All patients undergoing TEVAR require lifelong surveillance imaging. Our institutional protocol involves CTA performed at 1, 6, and 12 months, and yearly thereafter. Patients are evaluated for aneurysm size, endoleak, migration, and device fracture. Endoleaks are classified based on location: type I (proximal or distal landing zone), type II (retrograde flow from a branch such as an intercostal artery into the aneurysm sac), type III (component separation or structural failure in body of a graft), type IV (graft porosity), type V (endotension, or aneurysm expansion without an identifiable endoleak).[47] Type I and III endoleaks subject the aneurysm sac to systemic pressure and are repaired on diagnosis. Type II endoleaks may be observed closely if the aneurysm is stable or shrinking. Type IV endoleaks are often seen intraoperatively secondary to systemic anticoagulation and often resolve after reversal of heparin. Type V endoleaks may represent a failure of endovascular treatment and may require conversion to open repair.

Conclusion

Endovascular repair of DTAA is a less-invasive alternative to traditional open surgery in properly selected patients. Early results have been promising, with improved morbidity and mortality, but long-term data are lacking. The

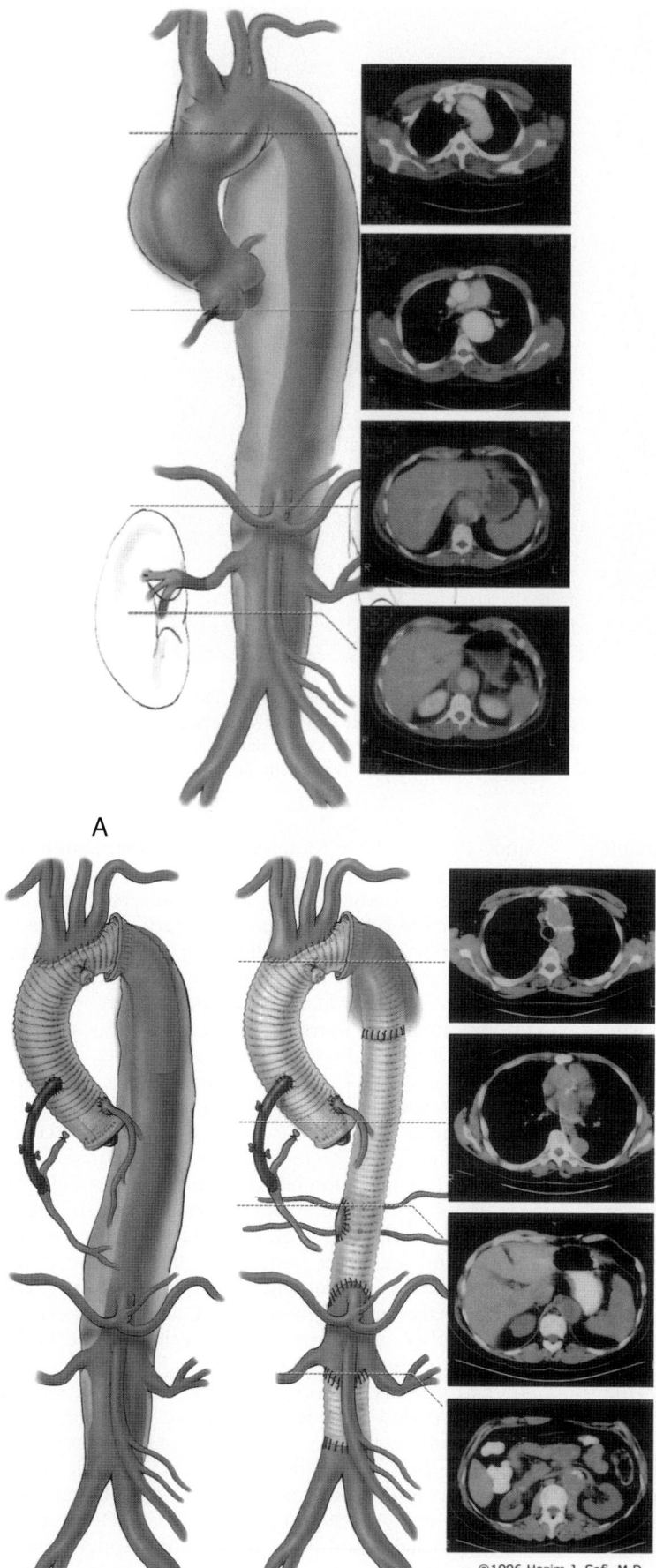

A

B

©1996 Hazim J. Safi, M.D.

Figure 63-29 Repair of extensive aortic aneurysm and chronic dissection. **A,** Artist's diagram (*left*), and corresponding computed tomography (CT) axial images (*right*) of preoperative aneurysm. **B,** Stage 1 "elephant trunk" repair with graft replacement of ascending/arch, reimplantation of great vessels, bypass of right coronary artery and Carrel patch of left coronary artery; the "trunk" is inside the descending thoracic aorta (*left*); stage 2 completion of "elephant trunk" repair with extent II thoracoabdominal aortic graft replacement, reattachment of lower intercostal arteries, reimplantation of visceral and renal arteries (*center*), and corresponding CT axial images (*right*). (Copyright © 1996 Hazim J. Safi, MD.)

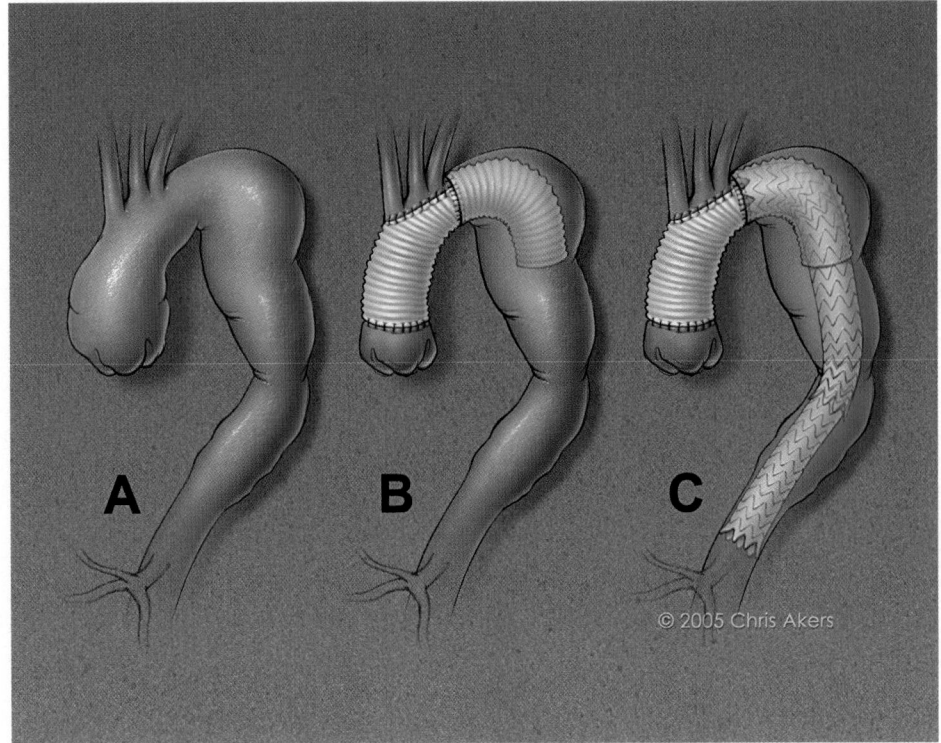

Figure 63-30 The hybrid elephant trunk technique for repair of extensive aortic aneurysms. **A,** The aneurysmal aorta. **B,** The ascending component is repaired using the traditional first-stage repair leaving the elephant trunk in the proximal descending aorta. **C,** The descending component is repaired using an endovascular technique, either at the time of first-stage repair or in a delayed fashion. (© Chris Akers, 2006. Reprinted with permission.).

wide application of this technology is currently limited by patient anatomy. The evolution of branched and fenestrated grafts may make endovascular repairs applicable to a wider range of patients in the future.

EXTENSIVE AORTIC ANEURYSM AND THE ELEPHANT TRUNK TECHNIQUE

Aneurysmal disease occurs in more than one part of the aorta in about 20% of cases. Extensive aortic aneurysm (also known as *mega aorta*) refers to aneurysmal involvement of the entire ascending, transverse aortic arch, and thoracoabdominal aorta. Although associated factors include Marfan syndrome and chronic aortic dissection, the cause of extensive aortic aneurysm remains unknown. Single-stage repair of extensive aneurysms can greatly increase risks. The patient is submitted to a lengthy procedure that requires multiple incisions, a daunting array of protective surgical adjuncts, protracted clamp times, and considerable blood loss. Staged repair would seem to be a logical solution. But before the introduction of the elephant trunk technique by Borst in 1983,[48] staged repair was fraught with complications, particularly excessive bleeding in the second stage. Because the elephant trunk technique permits the surgeon to avoid cross-clamping the proximal native descending thoracic aorta in the second stage, this problem was resolved.

Since 1991, we have routinely used the elephant trunk technique for extensive aortic aneurysm repair[49] (Fig. 63-29). The ascending aorta and transverse arch are usually operated first and, after a recovery period of 4 to 6 weeks, repair of the descending thoracic or thoracoabdominal aortic aneurysm is performed. The first stage is performed in a similar fashion to standard surgery of the ascending aorta and transverse arch (see Surgical Treatment and Results: Proximal Thoracic Aorta, earlier), except for graft replacement of the aortic arch. The replacement graft is partially inverted on itself, and the doubled graft is positioned 7 to 10 cm into the descending aorta. The folded edge of the graft is sutured to the descending thoracic aorta just distal to the left subclavian artery. When this anastomosis is completed, the inner portion of the tube graft is pulled out toward the ascending aorta, and the outer portion is left to dangle in the descending aorta (resembling an elephant's trunk). The brachiocephalic, left common carotid, and left subclavian arteries are then reimplanted to a side hole made in the superior arch portion of the graft.

After a recovery period of 4 to 6 weeks, the patient undergoes second-stage repair. The second stage of the elephant trunk technique is much like standard repair of descending thoracic or thoracoabdominal aortic aneurysms (see Surgical Treatment and Results: Distal Thoracic Aorta, earlier). CSF drainage is used. Distal aortic perfusion is established from the left atrial appendage or pulmonary vein to the left common femoral artery.

The proximal descending thoracic aorta is opened, and the elephant trunk portion of the graft (inserted in the descending thoracic aorta during stage 1), is promptly grasped and clamped. A new graft is sutured to the "elephant trunk." The elephant trunk technique obviates the need to clamp the proximal descending thoracic aorta and reduces the risk for excessive bleeding.

Results: Elephant Trunk Technique

As of December 2005, we have performed the elephant trunk procedure in 254 patients. Our 30-day mortality rate for the first-stage repair was 6.3%, and 30-day mortality was significantly associated with GFR ($P < .03$). Second-stage 30-day mortality was 8.7%; and although mortality in the second stage was not associated with GFR, we have previously shown that GFR is a predictor of mortality for repair of the descending thoracic and thoracoabdominal aorta.[31] During the interval between surgeries, or about 31 days to 6 weeks after stage 1, mortality was 2.9%. When we performed a 5-year follow-up of patients who failed to return for second-stage repair, we found that 32% had died. Although we were able to obtain the cause of death in only a small percentage of patients, most of these were due to aneurysm rupture.

Major complications for both stages have been relatively low, with stroke rates of about 2% in the first stage and no neurologic deficits in the second. Determining the optimum length of recovery time between stages has been difficult. Because these patients are vulnerable to rupture, we currently recommend a 4-week period of recovery before performing the second-stage procedure. Recently, a hybrid technique has been performed in which the descending component of the extensive aortic aneurysm was repaired using an endovascular technique[50,51] (Fig. 63-30). This endovascular portion may be repaired during the traditional first stage of the elephant trunk technique or in a delayed fashion, if necessary. This hybrid technique has the potential to reduce the morbidity associated with repair of the descending thoracic aorta by eliminating the traditional second-stage open repair. However, the durability of these stent grafts is unknown at this time.

ACKNOWLEDGMENTS

We are grateful to Dr. Dianna M. Milewicz for her contribution to the genetic section of this chapter, and thank our editor, Kirk Soodhalter, and our illustrator, Chris Akers.

Selected References

Clouse WD, Hallett JW Jr, Schaff HV, et al: Improved prognosis of thoracic aortic aneurysms: A population-based study. JAMA 280:1926-1929, 1998.

In this update of Bickerstaff's classic study on the natural history of thoracic aortic aneurysms, Clouse and colleagues examine the possible causes for the poor prognosis of this disease when untreated. From their population-based cohort study of 133 patients, they find an increased incidence of thoracic aortic aneurysm compared to Bickerstaff's study, but they also observe improved survival. They discuss the causes for these phenomena and provide a good look at a difficult and under-explored subject.

Hagan PG, Nienaber CA, Isselbacher EM, et al: The International Registry of Acute Aortic Dissection (IRAD): New insights into an old disease. JAMA 283:897-903, 2000.

Acute aortic dissection is a life-threatening medical emergency associated with high rates of morbidity and mortality. The International Registry of Acute Aortic Dissection culled the data of 464 patients from 12 international referral centers to increase our knowledge of the effect of recent technical advances on patient care and outcome. Physical findings previously regarded as typical are noted in only one third of patients, and clinicians are alerted to the wide range of manifestations in acute aortic dissection. A detailed analysis of data for type A and type B acute and chronic aortic dissection treated surgically or medically affords an excellent overview of the outcome of modern dissection patients.

Hasham SN, Willing MC, Guo DC, et al: Mapping a locus for familial thoracic aortic aneurysms and dissections (TAAD2) to 3p24-25. Circulation 107(25):3184-3190, 2003.

Milewicz and associates have extensively studied the molecular genetics of cardiovascular disease, particularly in the Marfan syndrome. This article explores the identity of genes that predispose patients without known syndromes to aortic aneurysms and dissections. The article provides a look at the future and how characterization of these genes will enhance our ability to determine persons at risk for aortic aneurysms and dissections.

Safi HJ, Estrera AL, Miller CC 3rd, et al: Evolution of risk for neurologic deficit after descending and thoracoabdominal aortic repair. Ann Thorac Surg 80(6):2173-2179; discussion 2179, 2005.

This article covers our 15-year experience with descending thoracic and thoracoabdominal aortic repair. With the adoption of the adjunct (distal aortic perfusion, CSF drainage, and moderate hypothermia), we have seen rates of neurologic deficit drop dramatically. Clamp time is no longer a significant risk factor for neurologic deficit in our series. The use of this adjunct has become the standard of care in our practice.

Safi HJ, Miller CC 3rd, Estrera AL, et al: Staged repair of extensive aortic aneurysms: Long-term experience with the elephant trunk technique. Ann Surg 240(4):677-684; discussion 684-685, 2004.

Borst introduced the elephant trunk technique in the 1980s, the two-stage repair of extensive aortic aneurysms that involve the ascending aorta, aortic arch, and descending or thoracoabdominal aorta. This article describes one of the largest series of elephant trunk patients from the group that continues to study the peculiar characteristics and surgical requirements of the patients with extensive aortic aneurysm or mega aorta. The article investigates patient outcome and provides a sound argument in favor of two-stage versus single-stage repair of the entire aorta.

Svensson LG, Crawford ES, Hess KR, et al: Experience with 1509 patients undergoing thoracoabdominal aortic operations. J Vasc Surg 17:357-368; discussion 368-370, 1993.

Svensson's study of E. Stanley Crawford's extensive patient series closely examines a wide range of risk factors associated with early death and postoperative complications in patients undergoing thoracoabdominal aortic operations. The size of the series permits solid comparisons of Crawford's four types of thoracoabdominal aortic aneurysm, and analysis of the effect of aneurysm extent on complications such as paraplegia and renal failure. The study is a classic and continues to be cited by thoracoabdominal aortic aneurysm researchers.

References

1. Gray H, William PL, Bannister LH: Embryology and development. In Gabella G (ed): Gray's anatomy: The anatomical basis of medicine and surgery, 38th ed. New York, Churchill Livingstone, pp 1609-1611.

2. McDonald JJ, Anson BJ: Variations in the origin of arteries derived from the aortic arch in American whites and negroes. Am J Phys Anthrop 27:97-107, 1940.

3. Skandalakis JE, Gray SW, Panagiotis S: The thoracic and abdominal aorta. In Skandalakis JE, Gray SW (eds): Embryology for Surgeons: The Embryological Basis for the Treatment of Congenital Anomalies, 2nd ed. Baltimore, Williams & Wilkins, 1994, pp 976-1030.

4. Bayford D: An account of a singular case of deglutition. Mem Med Soc Lond 2:275, 1794.

5. Mitchell SC, Korones SB, Berendes HW: Congenital heart disease in 56,109 births: Incidence and natural history. Circulation 43:323-332, 1971.

6. Skandalakis JE, Gray SW, Panagiotis S: Superior and inferior venae cavae. In Skandalakis JE, Gray SW (eds): Embryology for Surgeons: The Embryological Basis for the Treatment of Congenital Anomalies, 2nd ed. Baltimore, Williams & Wilkins, 1994, pp 1032-1051.

7. Clouse WD, Hallett JW Jr, Schaff HV, et al: Acute aortic dissection: Population-based incidence compared with degenerative aortic aneurysm rupture. Mayo Clin Proc 79:176-180, 2004.

8. Vaughan CJ, Casey M, He J, et al: Identification of a chromosome 11q23.2-q24 locus for familial aortic aneurysm disease, a genetically heterogeneous disorder. Circulation 103:2469-2475, 2001.

9. Dietz HC, Pyeritz RE: Mutations in the human gene for fibrillin-1 (FBN1) in the Marfan syndrome and related disorders. Hum Mol Genet 4(Spec No):1799-1809, 1995.

10. Milewicz DM, Michael K, Fisher N, et al: Fibrillin-1 (FBN1) mutations in patients with thoracic aortic aneurysms. Circulation 94:2708-2711, 1996.

11. Milewicz DM, Chen H, Park ES, et al: Reduced penetrance and variable expressivity of familial thoracic aortic aneurysms/dissections. Am J Cardiol 82:474-479, 1998.

12. Hasham SN, Willing MC, Guo DC, et al: Mapping a locus for familial thoracic aortic aneurysms and dissections (TAAD2) to 3p24-25. Circulation 107:3184-3190, 2003.

13. Pannu H, Fadulu VT, Chang J, et al: Mutations in transforming growth factor-beta receptor type II cause familial thoracic aortic aneurysms and dissections. Circulation 112:513-520, 2005.

14. Burke AP, Virmani R: Tumors of the heart and great vessels. In: Atlas of Tumor Pathology. Washington DC: Armed Forces Institute of Pathology, 1996, pp 1-11.

15. Estrera AL, Porat EE, Aboul-Nasr R, et al: Primary lymphoma of the aorta presenting as a descending thoracic aortic aneurysm. Ann Thorac Surg 80:1502-1504, 2005.

16. Bickerstaff LK, Pairolero PC, Hollier LH, et al: Thoracic aortic aneurysms: A population-based study. Surgery 92:1103-1108, 1982.

17. Miller CC 3rd, Porat EE, Esterera AL, et al: Number needed to treat: Analyzing the effectiveness of thoracoabdominal aortic repair. Eur J Vasc Endovasc Surg 28:154-157, 2004.

18. Clouse WD, Hallett JW Jr, Schaff HV, et al: Improved prognosis of thoracic aortic aneurysms: A population-based study. JAMA 280:1926-1929, 1998.

19. Davies RR, Goldstein LJ, Coady MA, et al: Yearly rupture or dissection rates for thoracic aortic aneurysms: Simple prediction based on size. Ann Thorac Surg 73:17-27; discussion 28, 2002.

20. Hagan PG, Nienaber CA, Isselbacher EM, et al: The International Registry of Acute Aortic Dissection (IRAD): New insights into an old disease. JAMA 283:897-903, 2000.

21. Hirst AE Jr, Johns VJ Jr, Kime SW Jr: Dissecting aneurysm of the aorta: A review of 505 cases. Medicine 37:217-219, 1958.

22. Estrera AL, Huynh TT, Porat EE, et al: Is acute type A aortic dissection a true surgical emergency? Semin Vasc Surg 15:75-82, 2002.

23. Estrera AL, Miller CC 3rd, Safi HJ, et al: Outcomes of medical management of acute type B aortic dissection. Circulation 114(1 Suppl):I384-389, 2006.

24. Shenaq SA, Chelly JE, Karlberg H, et al: Use of nitroprusside during surgery for thoracoabdominal aortic aneurysm. Circulation 70(3 Pt 2):17-10, 1984.

25. Kouchoukos NT, Marshall WG Jr, Wedige-Stecher TA: Eleven-year experience with composite graft replacement of the ascending aorta and aortic valve. J Thorac Cardiovasc Surg 92:691-705, 1986.

26. Estrera AL, Miller CC 3rd, Huynh TT, et al: Replacement of the ascending and transverse aortic arch: Determinants of long-term survival. Ann Thorac Surg 74:1058-1064; discussion 1064-1065, 2002.

27. Safi H, Miller CI, Carr C, et al: The importance of intercostal artery reattachment during thoracoabdominal aortic aneurysm repair. J Vasc Surg 27:58-68, 1998.

28. Cambria RP, Davison JK, Carter C, et al: Epidural cooling for spinal cord protection during thoracoabdominal aneurysm repair: A five-year experience. J Vasc Surg 31:1093-1102, 2000.

29. Estrera AL, Miller CC 3rd, Huynh TT, et al: Neurologic outcome after thoracic and thoracoabdominal aortic aneurysm repair. Ann Thorac Surg 72:1225-1230; discussion 1230-1231, 2001.

30. Svensson LG, Crawford ES, Hess KR, et al: Experience with 1509 patients undergoing thoracoabdominal aortic operations. J Vasc Surg 17:357-368; discussion 368-370, 1993.

31. Huynh TT, van Eps RG, Miller CC 3rd, et al: Glomerular filtration rate is superior to serum creatinine for prediction of mortality after thoracoabdominal aortic surgery. J Vasc Surg 42:206-212, 2005.

32. Safi HJ, Estrera AL, Miller CC, et al: Evolution of risk for neurologic deficit after descending and thoracoabdominal aortic repair. Ann Thorac Surg 80:2173-2179; discussion 2179, 2005.

33. Estrera AL, Miller CC 3rd, Chen EP, et al: Descending thoracic aortic aneurysm repair: 12-Year experience using distal aortic perfusion and cerebrospinal fluid drainage. Ann Thorac Surg 80:1290-1296; discussion 1296, 2005.

34. Safi HJ, Miller CC 3rd, Huynh TT, et al: Distal aortic perfusion and cerebrospinal fluid drainage for thoracoabdominal and descending thoracic aortic repair: Ten years of organ protection. Ann Surg 238:372-380; discussion 380-381, 2003.

35. Estrera AL, Miller CC 3rd, Huynh TT, et al: Preoperative and operative predictors of delayed neurologic deficit following repair of thoracoabdominal aortic aneurysm. J Thorac Cardiovasc Surg 126:1288-1294, 2003.

36. Azizzadeh A, Huynh TT, Miller CC 3rd, et al: Postoperative risk factors for delayed neurologic deficit after thoracic and thoracoabdominal aortic aneurysm repair: A case-control study. J Vasc Surg 37:750-754, 2003.

37. Safi HJ, Harlin SA, Miller CC, et al: Predictive factors for acute renal failure in thoracic and thoracoabdominal aortic

aneurysm surgery [published erratum appears in J Vasc Surg 25:93, 1997]. J Vasc Surg 24:338-344; discussion 344-345, 1996.

38. Safi HJ, Miller CC 3rd, Estrera AL, et al: Chronic aortic dissection not a risk factor for neurologic deficit in thoracoabdominal aortic aneurysm repair. Eur J Vasc Endovasc Surg 23:244-250, 2002.

39. Dake MD, Miller DC, Semba CP, et al: Transluminal placement of endovascular stent-grafts for the treatment of descending thoracic aortic aneurysms. N Engl J Med 331:1729-1734, 1994.

40. Makaroun MS, Dillavou ED, Kee ST, et al: Endovascular treatment of thoracic aortic aneurysms: Results of the phase II multicenter trial of the GORE TAG thoracic endoprosthesis. J Vasc Surg 41:1-9, 2005.

41. GORE TAG Thoracic Endoprosthesis Instructions for Use. (2006). Retrieved April 27, 2006, from http://www.goremedical.com/English/Products/TAG/Ifu.htm.

42. Matsumura JS: Worldwide survey of thoracic endografts: Practical clinical application. J Vasc Surg 43(Suppl A):20A-1A, 2006.

43. White RA, Donayre CE, Walot I, et al: Intraprocedural imaging: Thoracic aortography techniques, intravascular ultrasound, and special equipment. J Vasc Surg 43(Suppl A):53A-61A, 2006.

44. Cheung AT, Pochettino A, McGarvey ML, et al: Strategies to manage paraplegia risk after endovascular stent repair of descending thoracic aortic aneurysms. Ann Thorac Surg 80:1280-1288; discussion 1288-1289, 2005.

45. Mitchell RS: Endovascular stent graft repair of thoracic aortic aneurysms. Semin Thorac Cardiovasc Surg 9:257-268, 1997.

46. Sullivan TM, Sundt TM 3rd: Complications of thoracic aortic endografts: Spinal cord ischemia and stroke. J Vasc Surg 43(Suppl A):85A-88A, 2006.

47. Veith FJ, Baum RA, Ohki T, et al: Nature and significance of endoleaks and endotension: Summary of opinions expressed at an international conference. J Vasc Surg 35:1029-1035, 2002.

48. Borst HG, Walterbusch G, Schaps D: Extensive aortic replacement using "elephant trunk" prosthesis. Thorac Cardiovasc Surg 31:37-40, 1983.

49. Safi HJ, Miller CC 3rd, Estrera AL, et al: Staged repair of extensive aortic aneurysms: Long-term experience with the elephant trunk technique. Ann Surg 240:677-684; discussion 684-685, 2004.

50. Azizzadeh A, Estrera AL, Porat E, et al: The hybrid elephant trunk procedure: A single-stage repair of an ascending, arch, and descending thoracic aortic aneurysm. J Vasc Surg 44:404-407, 2006.

51. Karck M, Chavan A, Khaladj N, et al: The frozen elephant trunk technique for the treatment of extensive thoracic aortic aneurysms: Operative results and follow-up. Eur J Cardiothorac Surg 28:286-290; discussion 290, 2005.

Cerebrovascular Disease

Thomas Stuart Riles, MD and Caron B. Rockman, MD

The primary indication for performing cerebrovascular surgery is the prevention of stroke. As such, it is critically important to understand the prevalence of stroke as well as the relationship of stroke to existing cerebrovascular disease. Stroke is the third leading cause of death in the United States, exceeded only by heart disease and cancer. Each year, about 700,000 people experience a new or recurrent stroke in this country. About 83% of all strokes are ischemic, and 7.6% of these ischemic strokes result in the patient's death within 30 days. Additionally, it is estimated that 2% of the U.S. population, or more than 4.5 million individuals, are stroke survivors. As such, stroke is also a leading cause of serious, long-term disability. The estimated direct and indirect cost of caring for patients after stroke in the United States in 2002 was $49.4 billion. Certainly, no one would deny that stroke is a devastating illness, both from the patient's perspective and from a national health care cost perspective.[1]

More than 75% of patients who suffer a stroke survive their first stroke by at least 1 year. Of the 4.5 million stroke survivors in the United States, more than 1.1 million adults have resulting functional limitations and difficulty performing activities of daily living. To put this in perspective, of those older than 65 years who were observed 6 months after an ischemic stroke, 30% were unable to walk without some assistance, 19% had aphasia, 26% were institutionalized in a nursing home, and 35% had depressive symptoms. Each year, there are more than 900,000 stroke-related hospital admissions.

Unfortunately, treatment of stroke, once it has occurred, is generally unsuccessful.[1] About 30% of patients who have a stroke require long-term institutionalization, and an additional 30% require significant assistance with activities of daily living. Although early thrombolytic treatment of ischemic stroke has been reported,[2] this intervention is practically limited to the relatively small number of patients who can be treated at a major medical center within several hours of their initial symptoms.

Despite these staggering statistics and extensive research in this area, there is no consensus on how to best prevent ischemic stroke.[1] It is estimated that 20% to 75% of strokes in the United States are caused by cervical carotid artery disease, with the remainder caused by atrial fibrillation and hypertension[3] (Fig. 64-1). These three immediate causes of stroke often do not produce initial premonitory symptoms; in addition, appropriate early management of these conditions, when recognized, can prevent future strokes. It is clear that the optimal treatment for stroke is primary prevention.[1] From the point of view of cerebrovascular surgery, to prevent stroke, it is critical to understand the underlying causes of stroke, which patients are predisposed to having strokes, and what preventive therapies are effective and available.

EPIDEMIOLOGY OF STROKE AND CAROTID ARTERY ATHEROSCLEROSIS

The epidemiology of carotid atherosclerosis has been extensively studied. Individual risk factors for stroke include hypertension, atrial fibrillation, heart disease, diabetes, and smoking. Any combination of these factors

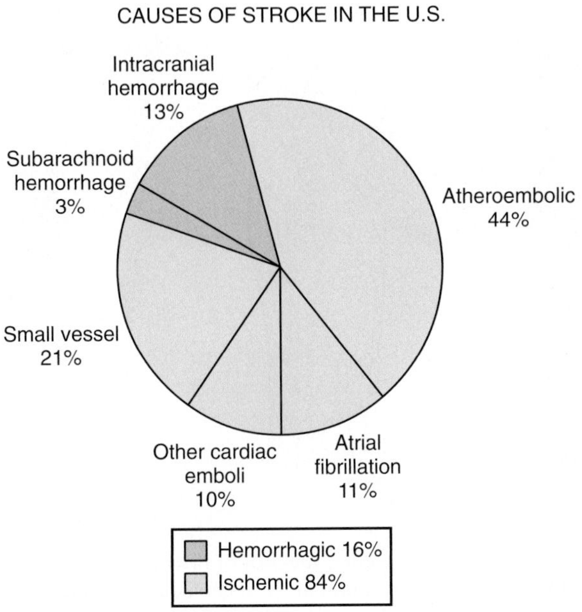

CAUSES OF STROKE IN THE U.S.

Intracranial
hemorrhage
13%

Subarachnoid
hemorrhage
3%

Atheroembolic
44%

Small vessel
21%

Other cardiac
emboli
10%

Atrial
fibrillation
11%

Hemorrhagic 16%
Ischemic 84%

Figure 64-1 Incidence of the various causes of stroke in the United States.

greatly increases the likelihood of stroke. Individuals who exercise vigorously have a decreased incidence of stroke.

In a subset of the Framingham Study involving 1116 patients, multivariate logistic regression revealed that age, cigarette smoking, systolic blood pressure, and cholesterol levels were independently related to carotid atherosclerosis.[4] However, the prevalence of significant carotid artery disease in the general population was low, about 8%. In the Tromso Study,[5] an analysis of 6727 patients who were screened for carotid artery disease reached similar conclusions, but additionally found that male gender was an independent predictor. In a further study of risk factors associated with internal carotid artery (ICA) occlusion, Bogousslavsky and colleagues found that smoking, a family history of stroke, and obesity were more prevalent than in age-matched and sex-matched patients without cerebrovascular disease.[6] Finally, the SMART study found that the prevalence of carotid artery disease increased as much as 50% in patients with peripheral arterial disease.[7] The incidence of stroke is higher for men than for women aged 65 to 75 years, but this gender difference is nonexistent at older ages. The overall mortality from stroke is actually higher among women because women generally have a longer life expectancy than men. African-American women have almost twice the risk for first-ever stroke as white women.

It is apparent from these studies that traditional atherosclerotic risk factors are associated with the development of carotid atherosclerotic disease. Although the incidence of stroke varies considerably among countries throughout the world, there is also a striking difference in the types of stroke that occur among various populations. In Japan and Korea, for example, nearly half of all strokes are hemorrhagic, compared with about 16% in the United States.

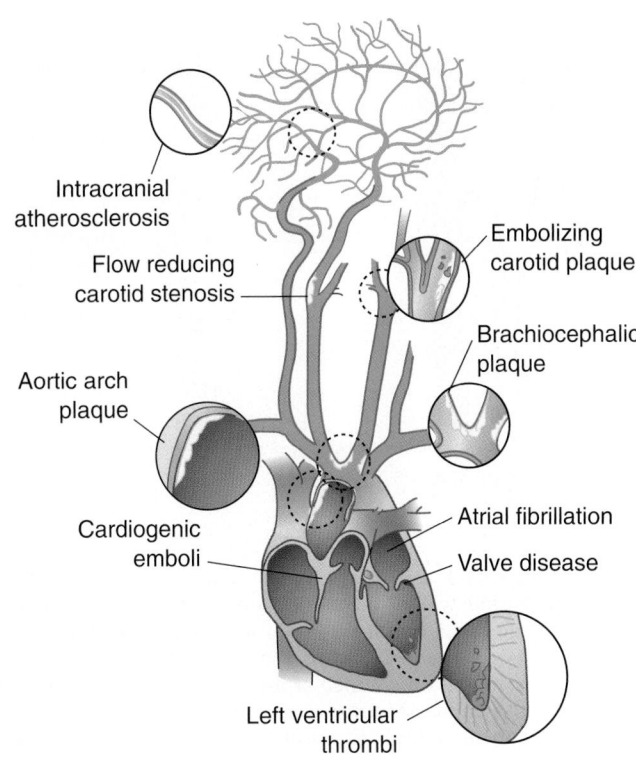

Figure 64-2 Cardiogenic and arterial atherosclerotic sources for stroke.

ETIOLOGY OF STROKE

Stroke is a broad term relating to any acute brain injury that results in a neurologic deficit of 24 hours or more. Although stroke may result from infections, trauma, tumors, or intrinsic neurologic disease, nearly 75% of cases are ischemic in nature, related to one of three underlying conditions: hypertension, atrial fibrillation, or cerebrovascular disease. Strokes are frequently classified as hemorrhagic or ischemic in nature. In the United States, 13% of strokes are due to intraparenchymal cerebral hemorrhage, and 3% are due to subarachnoid hemorrhage. Of the ischemic strokes that make up the remaining 84%, more than half are caused by atherosclerotic disease of the extracranial cerebrovascular vessels, including the aortic arch, the carotid artery, and the vertebral arteries (Fig. 64-2). About 10% of all strokes are due to embolization of mural thrombus in individuals with atrial fibrillation. An equal number are due to emboli from the left ventricle or valvular heart disease. Strokes related to chronic hypertension are generally caused by diffuse intracerebral small vessel disease.

CAROTID BIFURCATION DISEASE PATHOPHYSIOLOGY

Atherosclerotic disease at the bifurcation of the common carotid artery and extending into the internal and external carotid arteries is the most common cause of ischemic

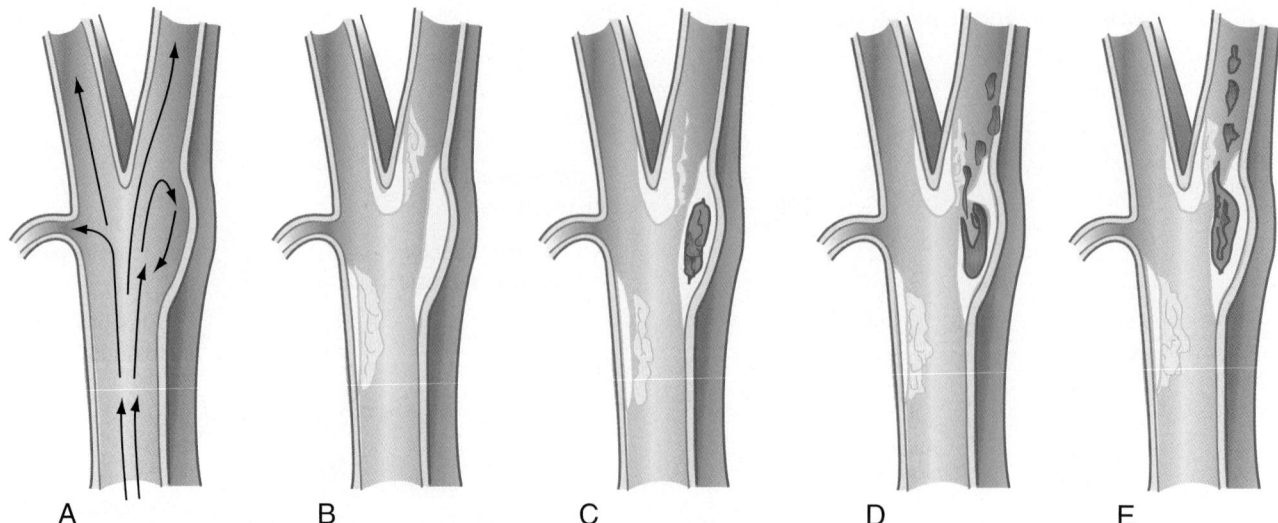

Figure 64-3 A, Simplified flow patterns at the carotid bifurcation demonstrate complex reversal of flow along the posterior wall of the carotid sinus. This region is most vulnerable to plaque development. **B,** Established plaque at the carotid bifurcation. **C,** Soft, central necrotic core with an overlying thin fibrous cap. This area is prone to plaque rupture. **D,** Disruption of the fibrous cap allows necrotic cellular debris and lipid material from the central core to enter the lumen of the internal carotid artery, thus becoming atherogenic emboli. The patient may experience symptoms (transient ischemia, stroke, or amaurosis fugax) or remain asymptomatic depending on the site of lodgment and the extent of tissue compromise. **E,** The empty necrotic core becomes a deep ulcer in the plaque. The walls of the ulcer are highly thrombogenic and reactive with platelets. This leads to thromboembolism in the internal carotid artery circulation.

stroke in the United States. The extraordinary prevalence of atherosclerotic plaque at this site has been the focus of much study. Some authors have correlated the shear forces on the arterial wall at the carotid bulb of flow with plaque formation[8] (Fig. 64-3). In addition to its shape, the carotid bifurcation has other unique features. Its innervation by the baroreceptors and embedded chemoreceptors may also have an association with the virulent plaque formation characteristic of the carotid bifurcation.

The early precursor to the carotid bifurcation plaque is a fibrous thickening of the intima of the artery due to a proliferation of smooth muscle cells (see Fig. 64-3). This may occur as early as the third or fourth decade of life. Later, lipid-laden macrophages may be found in the plaque giving rise to the characteristic atheroma. In time, the plaque may become calcified. Screening programs have shown that as many as 7% to 12% of individuals older than 65 years have plaque buildup at the carotid bifurcation.[1] Most of these cases are not clinically significant because they do not obstruct the blood flow, do not embolize plaque or thrombus to the brain, and therefore are not likely to cause a stroke.

As the plaque increases in thickness, a number of changes may occur that can lead to a stroke. The plaque can fragment or ulcerate, leading to embolization of plaque material to the intracranial arteries. Thrombus can form on the surface of the plaque. This too can embolize to the brain. Progression of the plaque or thrombus formation can reduce the blood flow to the brain by narrowing the lumen or completely occluding the ICA. Because of the rich collateral blood flow through the

circle of Willis, carotid occlusive disease rarely causes stroke by causing global cerebral hypoperfusion, resulting from flow restriction at the carotid bifurcation. Embolization of plaque material is the much more common cause of both transient ischemic attack and stroke related to extracranial carotid artery atherosclerosis.

CLINICAL MANIFESTATIONS OF CAROTID ARTERY DISEASE

Neurologic symptoms associated with carotid bifurcation disease are classified as strokes and transient ischemic attacks (TIAs). By convention, a stroke refers to symptoms that last more than 24 hours, whereas symptoms that resolve within 24 hours are classified as TIAs. In clinical practice, most TIAs last only seconds to minutes. It must be emphasized that these classifications are clinical and may not correlate with radiographic signs of a stroke. For example, an individual may experience a TIA or in fact be totally without symptoms, yet have evidence of a cerebral infarction on a computed tomography (CT) scan or magnetic resonance imaging (MRI) of the brain.

Most patients who are symptomatic describe classic focal symptoms related to ischemia of the ipsilateral cerebral hemisphere or retina. Most often, neurologic symptoms are the result of emboli from the carotid bifurcation plaque to more distal vessels. Less often an occlusion or severe stenosis can cause low flow and global ischemia to end-organ tissues. Right carotid territory symptoms, for example, may include left hemiplegia or monoparesis and right eye visual loss (Fig. 64-4). The

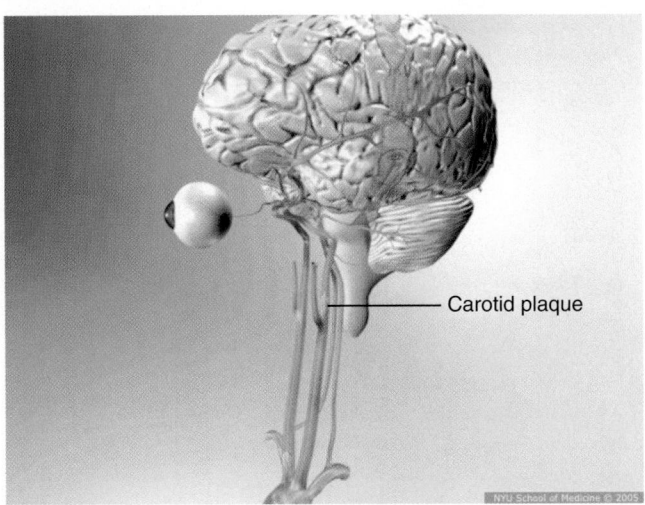

Figure 64-4 Representation of the distribution of the blood flow of the left internal carotid artery. Emboli from the bifurcation plaque may result in loss of motor strength or sensation in the contralateral side of the body, loss of speech if the speech center is on the left, and loss of vision in the ipsilateral eye. (Courtesy of New York University School of Medicine, © 2005. Reprinted with permission.)

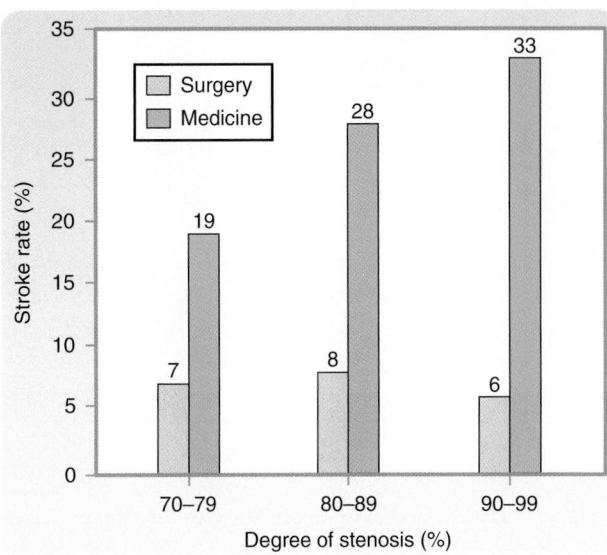

Figure 64-5 Data from the North American Symptomatic Carotid Artery Trial (NASCET) showing the risk for stroke in symptomatic patients with varying degrees of stenosis at the carotid bifurcation if treated with medical therapy alone. At 18 months, the incidences of stroke were 19%, 28%, and 33% for lumen diameter reductions of 70%-80%, 80%-90%, and 90%-99%, respectively.

weakness or paralysis of the contralateral face and limbs is due to ischemia of the motor strip of the cortex of the parietal lobe of the brain. Left-sided symptoms are the mirror image of the right-sided symptoms with the addition of aphasia—the loss of ability to speak or confusion of words—because the speech center is most commonly located in the left cerebral hemisphere. In a small percentage of the population, particularly in left-handed individuals, speech may be centered in the right hemisphere.

Visual symptoms related to carotid bifurcation disease are due to ischemia of the retina. These symptoms are typically caused by microemboli passing through the ipsilateral ophthalmic artery. If the monocular visual loss is transient, it is called *amaurosis fugax.* A patient who has experienced amaurosis fugax often describes the experience as a "window shade" coming down over one eye or a wedge defect in the visual field. Sometimes the symptoms are described as flashing lights or sparks in the visual field. If one examines the eye in a patient who has recently experienced amaurosis fugax, a small embolus may be seen lodged in a retinal artery. Retinal artery emboli, known as *Hollenhurst plaques,* also may be seen in patients without prior clinical symptoms. The finding of a Hollenhurst plaque is an indication for further evaluation of the carotid arteries because there is a high correlation with plaque at the carotid bifurcation.

Although the symptoms described are most typical, patients who complain of any new-onset neurologic symptoms, including light-headedness, disorientation, transient memory loss, slurring of speech, and unexplained loss of consciousness, must be thoroughly evaluated for carotid bifurcation disease as well as other causes of stroke.

RISK FOR STROKE FROM CAROTID BIFURCATION DISEASE

It is essential to understand the natural history of individuals with carotid bifurcation disease to determine which individuals will benefit from surgery or other therapy. The comparison of stroke rates for patients receiving best medical therapy versus surgical therapy has been the subject of a number of large, multi-institutional, randomized clinical trials. The medical arms of these trials provide us with some of the best information regarding the risk for carotid disease with medical therapy alone.

The North American Symptomatic Carotid Endarterectomy Trial (NASCET)[9] randomized individuals with prior neurologic symptoms consisting of TIA or stroke and carotid bifurcation disease into medical and surgical treatment groups. For those treated medically, the study showed that the risk for stroke correlated directly with the thickness of the plaque or, more precisely, the reduction in the size of the residual arterial lumen by the plaque. At 18 months, the incidences of stroke were 19%, 28%, and 33% for lumen diameter reductions of 70% to 80%, 80% to 90%, and 90% to 99%, respectively[10] (Fig. 64-5). The higher risk for stroke with the more significant plaque size appears to be due to the fact that advanced plaques are more likely to show elements of degeneration (ulceration, mural thrombus formation) that lead to embolization rather than the reduction in blood flow. Lending support to this concept is the observation that

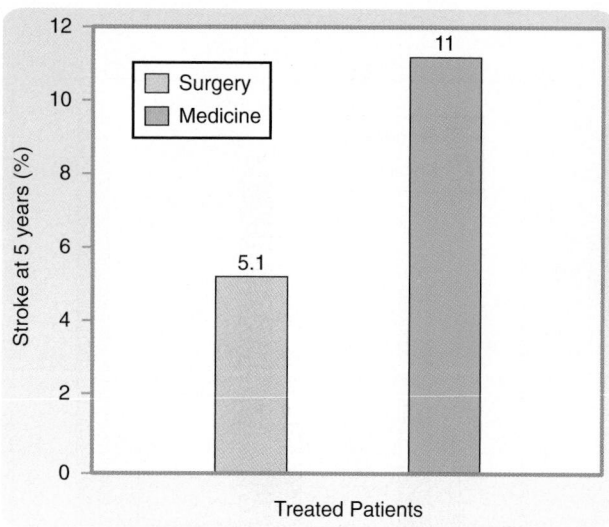

Figure 64-6 Data from the Asymptomatic Carotid Atherosclerosis Study (ACAS) show that, after 5 years, patients who were treated surgically had fewer strokes than those treated medically (5.1% versus 11%).

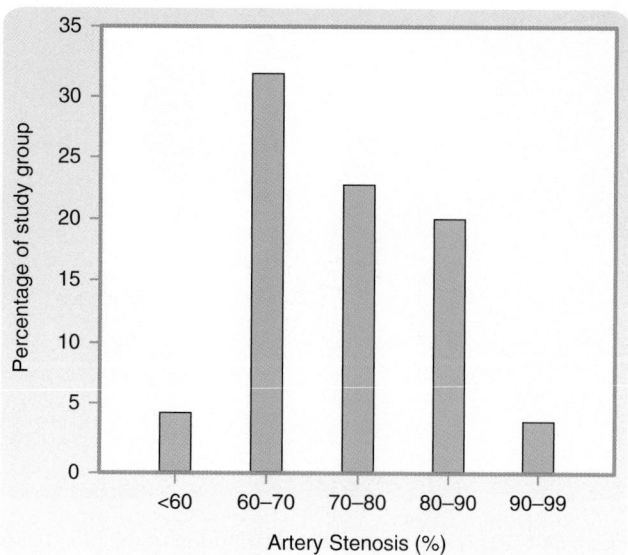

Figure 64-7 Data from the Asymptomatic Carotid Atherosclerosis Study (ACAS) show that most patients entered into the trial had moderate carotid artery stenosis (60%-80% diameter reduction). Relatively few individuals had more than 90% narrowing of the artery.

in individuals with high-grade stenosis and repetitive TIAs, the symptoms often stop if the artery goes on to complete occlusion.

The Asymptomatic Carotid Atherosclerosis Study (ACAS) was designed to give similar information regarding individuals with asymptomatic stenosis.[3] The overall risk for stroke in medically treated individuals with 60% to 99% diameter reduction of a carotid artery was found to be 11% at 5 years[3] (Fig. 64-6). In comparison, patients treated with carotid endarterectomy (CEA) had a risk for stroke of only 5.1% at 5 years. Although this clearly represents an overall risk reduction of greater than 50% for surgically treated patients, it must be emphasized that the risk for stroke among medically treated patients was only slightly more than 2% per year. However, most patients entered into the trial had a relatively moderate degree of carotid artery stenosis (60%-80%), with relatively few individuals having a stenosis of more than 90% (Fig. 64-7). The overall risk reduction for surgically treated patients was more meaningful for male patients than female patients, largely because of an increased risk for perioperative stroke among female patients in the study. Interestingly, the ACAS study also found a meaningful risk for stroke related to preoperative cerebral angiography alone of about 1%.

Before the NASCET[9] and ACAS[3] studies, a number of clinicians observed individuals with asymptomatic carotid disease in an effort to understand its natural history. Data from these early nonrandomized studies provide an additional picture regarding the risk for stroke in individuals with asymptomatic high-grade stenosis. From a collection of seven studies observing a total of 536 individuals with more than 75% narrowing for a mean period of 33 months, the risk for stroke was 5.4% per year.[11] From these observations, it appears that asymptomatic carotid plaques carry a far less risk for stroke than those associated with previous ipsilateral neurologic symptoms. For

both categories of patients, however, the risk is directly related to the severity of the diameter reduction of the lumen of the artery due to the plaque. As discussed in a later section, a clear understanding of the natural history of various conditions is essential to weighing the risks and benefits of a particular therapy. Several other observations are worthy of mention. From the NASCET study, it became clear that in patients with symptoms and appropriate carotid stenosis, the risk for stroke increases significantly if the contralateral carotid artery is occluded.[12] It has also been shown that the angiographic demonstration of ulceration in plaques increases the risk for stroke.[13]

INDICATIONS FOR WORKUP OF CAROTID OCCLUSIVE DISEASE

Any individual who has experienced a hemispheric stroke or TIA needs to be evaluated for possible carotid disease unless there is another clear cause such as an intracerebral bleed or tumor. The data supporting surgical treatment for stroke prevention in previously symptomatic patients is well established, provided the treatment offered, open surgical repair or angioplasty and stent placement, carries less than a 6% risk for stroke.[10] In a minority of symptomatic patients, a severe neurologic deficit or significant comorbidities such as advanced cancer may preclude intervention and therefore be a contraindication to further workup.

Indications for the evaluation of asymptomatic patients have not been well defined. The presence of a cervical bruit is probably the most common cause for an ultrasound diagnostic test for carotid artery disease. However, the presence of an audible bruit over the carotid bifurcation does not correlate well with the finding of significant stenosis. The presence of other vascular disease (e.g., coronary artery disease, intermittent claudication) or a family history of stroke or vascular disease is sufficient for some clinicians to asses the carotid arteries. At the present time, there is a growing movement for routine screening for carotid disease among individuals at risk. The limitations up to this point have been as follows:

1. Lack of definition of appropriate risk groups
2. High cost of diagnostic tests
3. Uncertainty in the minds of many clinicians as to the indications for interventions for asymptomatic individuals with carotid bifurcation plaques

Given the large numbers of strokes in the United States due to carotid disease and the fear of stroke among our aging population, it is likely that stroke screening will gain wider acceptance in the near future.

Although the cost-effectiveness of widespread screening for carotid artery disease remains an unavoidable issue, occult significant carotid stenosis was found to be the most common treatable cause of stroke discovered in a recent selected screening endeavor for the three most common treatable causes of stroke.[1] This, then, is presumed to be the most crucial area in which there is potential for aggressive intervention to prevent future stroke. Hypertension and atrial fibrillation, the other treatable causes of ischemic stroke, are more likely to be noted in a routine visit to a primary care practitioner, whereas carotid stenosis cannot be definitively diagnosed at physical examination alone. Certainly the diagnosis of occult carotid stenosis, even if it does not warrant CEA, prompts more vigorous risk factor modification, and perhaps the use of antiplatelet or anticholesterol medications.[1]

DIAGNOSTIC TESTS USED IN THE EVALUATION OF CAROTID ARTERY DISEASE

Evaluation of the neck with a stethoscope is the most simple and least costly means of evaluating an individual for carotid artery disease. The detection of a bruit in the neck is suggestive that an individual may have carotid stenosis and deserves further evaluation. Unfortunately, the finding of a bruit is neither very sensitive nor specific for carotid bifurcation disease. Of those with significant carotid stenosis, less than 70% will have a bruit. Of those with bruits, up to 30% will have no significant carotid stenosis.

Measurement of the Degree of Carotid Artery Stenosis

By convention, most investigators and clinicians have adopted *diameter reduction* as the measure to express a narrowing of an artery due to a plaque or some other disease process. For the carotid artery, this is a comparison of the diameter of the lumen at the most narrowed portion with the lumen of the artery several centimeters

DEGREE OF STENOSIS

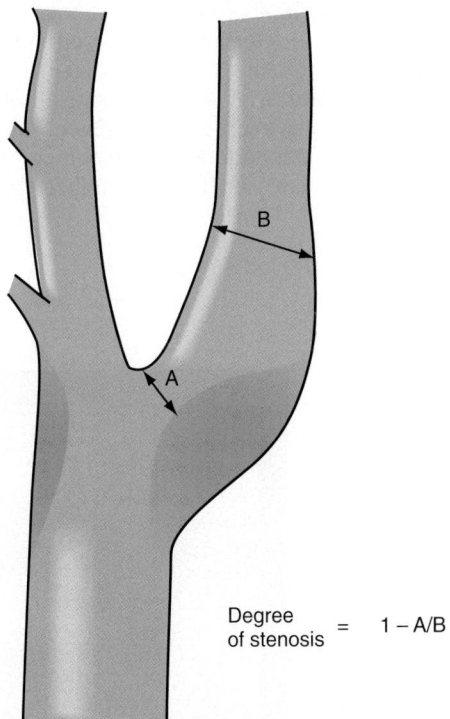

$$\text{Degree of stenosis} = 1 - A/B$$

Figure 64-8 The convention for describing carotid stenosis is to compare the lumen diameter at the most narrow point to the diameter of the internal carotid artery in a normal segment several centimeters distal to the stenosis.

above the carotid bifurcation where the artery is generally free of disease. It is understood that the carotid bulb is generally wider than the distal carotid artery, and therefore, the diameter reduction at that point may be considerably more than determined if one only considers the residual lumen. Also, clinicians are aware that the actual reduction in the area of the artery lumen is always greater than the diameter reduction. For clinical purposes, these inaccuracies are irrelevant because the reports that have been used to determine the risk for stroke with medical therapies have used the same diameter reduction criteria for classifying individuals within the study. Unless otherwise specified, a percentage stenosis of a carotid artery is the converse of the diameter of the residual lumen at the most narrowed point compared with a diameter of the ICA at a more distal point that is free of disease (Fig. 64-8).

Duplex Ultrasound

The duplex ultrasound is the most widely used test to assess the carotid arteries. The duplex, as the name suggests, uses both B-mode and Doppler ultrasound techniques to evaluate the cervical carotid arteries. The B-mode is used to visualize the artery and to center the focused Doppler beam in the center of the lumen. The Doppler mode assesses the velocity of flow at that point (Fig. 64-9). The more narrow the lumen of the artery, the higher the velocities during the systolic and diastolic phases of the cardiac cycle. Although criteria vary by Duplex machines and laboratories, commonly accepted criteria for determining different degrees of diameter reduction are shown in Table 64-1.[14]

Although the duplex scan is noninvasive and therefore safe, and it is readily available, it has several limitations. First, it is technician dependent. The accuracy of the test relies on the technician's ability to visualize the carotid arteries and to accurately measure the velocity of blood flow through the plaque. Calcification may make these assessments especially difficult. Second, the study is limited to the cervical portion of the carotid arteries. Assessment of the origin of the carotids and the intracranial portions is not possible. This aside, an experienced sonographer is generally able to determine the degree of stenosis of a carotid artery with an accuracy of more than 97%.

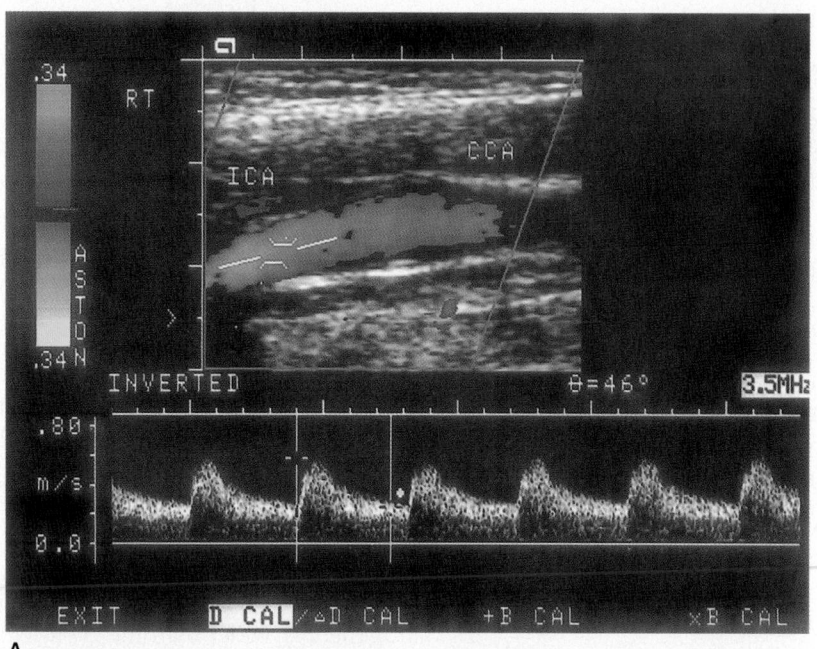

A

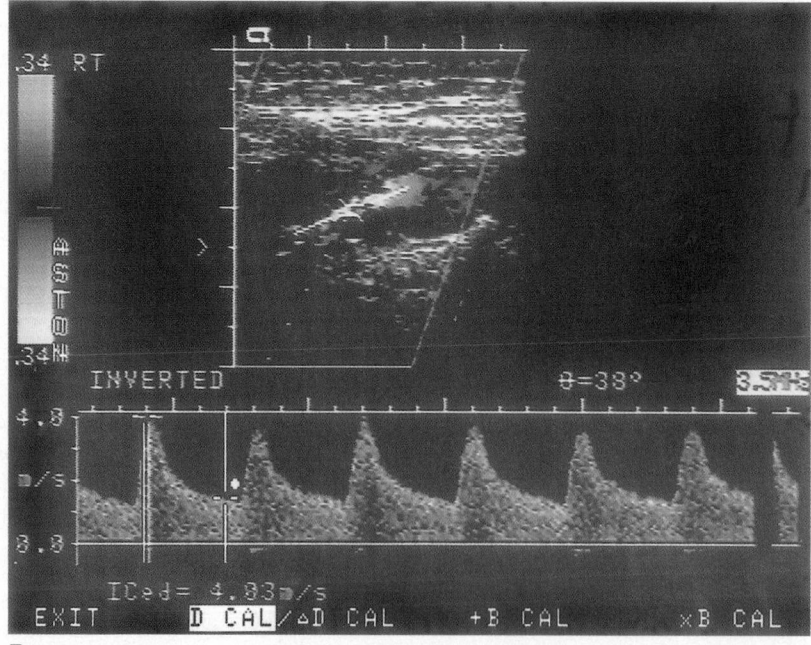

B

Transcranial Doppler

Transcranial Doppler is performed by insonating the middle cerebral artery through the temporal bone. The test can determine the quality of blood flow in the middle cerebral artery. Although it is most accurate in diagnosing an embolus to this artery, decreased flow can suggest carotid bifurcation disease. Given the limited information, it is seldom used as a first-line test for assessing individuals suspected of having carotid disease.

Table 64-1 Duplex Scan Criteria for Determining Different Degrees of Diameter Reduction

STENOSIS (%)	PEAK SYSTOLIC VELOCITY (cm/sec)	PEAK DIASTOLIC VELOCITY (cm/sec)	SPECTRAL BROADENING
0-15	<120	NA	None
16-49	<120	NA	Present
50-79	>120	<125	Marked
80-99	>120	>125	Marked
100	No flow noted	No flow noted	No flow noted

NA, not applicable.

Conventional Angiography

Although once the only means of imaging the extracranial vessels, and therefore serving as the gold standard for assessing newer imaging modalities, today catheter-directed cerebral angiography is seldom used solely for diagnosis of carotid disease. The risk for stroke from a femoral cerebral angiogram is as high as 1% in individuals with cerebrovascular disease. This risk is mostly due to the dislodgment of emboli during the manipulation of the catheter in the aortic arch and carotid vessels. There is also a risk for renal failure from the injection of iodinated dyes in patients with renal insufficiency. These risks and the introduction of simpler, safer, and less costly imaging modalities have led to fewer conventional angiograms being performed for diagnosing carotid artery disease. Angiography still can be of great value when other tests cannot be performed or fail to provide enough information to make an accurate diagnosis. Also, cerebral angiography is essential in the endovascular treatment of carotid disease. Catheter-directed images are a routine part of percutaneous balloon angioplasty, stent placement, and in some cases, thrombolytic therapy for thromboemboli of the intracranial vessels.

Magnetic Resonance Angiography

Magnetic resonance angiography (MRA) has become a reliable low-risk means of imaging the carotid arteries.

Figure 64-9 A duplex scan combines two diagnostic modalities. Anatomic information from the B-mode scan and the physiologic information of flow velocities from the Doppler scan define morphologic and hemodynamic abnormalities at the carotid bifurcation. Pulsed Doppler technology allows sampling of flow velocities within a particular area of the vessel lumen. Color-flow imaging allows determination of blood flow direction and velocity within the vessel lumen and is projected as colors displayed within the vessel image formed from the B-mode scan. Thus, vessels with blood flowing in the arterial direction are displayed as one color, generally *red,* and blood flow in the opposite direction (venous flow) is displayed as *blue.* Variations of color shading indicate changes in velocity, with lighter shades of color indicating higher velocities. This technology is useful in allowing the examiner to choose the areas of greatest disease and flow disturbance in the real-time B-mode image to measure velocities and perform spectral analysis at the point of maximal stenosis. Further information is derived from spectral waveform analysis. The returning Doppler signal consists of multiple frequencies that are representative of the velocities of the cellular elements of the blood within the sample volume. If the cells are moving at similar velocities and in similar directions, the resulting frequencies when displayed graphically as velocities on the Y axis produce a narrow waveform. This type of waveform is seen with unidirectional, laminar flow. Luminal irregularities, such as plaque, not only increase the peak velocities within the sample volume but also increase the range of frequencies within it, as the resulting flow disturbances cause variations in the velocity and direction of the cellular components of the blood. This results in broadening of the spectral waveform and is characteristic of significant stenosis of the lumen.
A, Arterial flow (*red*) is displayed in the internal (ICA) and common (CCA) carotid arteries. Sampling for flow velocities and spectral waveform analysis is carried out in the center stream of the ICA, as displayed on the diagram, and the waveform is shown below. Peak systolic and end-diastolic velocities are measured on a representative wave; in the example, these are 0.58 m/sec (58 cm/sec) and 0.25 m/sec (25 cm/sec), respectively. These are well within normal limits. **B,** The same general area is being interrogated in a diseased ICA. The lumen appears to narrow, and the *red* color becomes variegated and lighter. Arterial flow is sampled in the area of maximal disturbance and narrowing, and the resultant waveform is displayed below. The peak systolic velocities approach 4 m/sec (400 cm/sec), and the end-diastolic velocity is 1.41 m/sec (141 cm/sec). These values are elevated, indicating abnormally increased flow velocities in the area of stenosis. In addition, spectral analysis shows broadening from nonlaminar flow. These findings are characteristic of significant stenosis. By applying validated criteria, the severity of the stenosis can be estimated accurately.

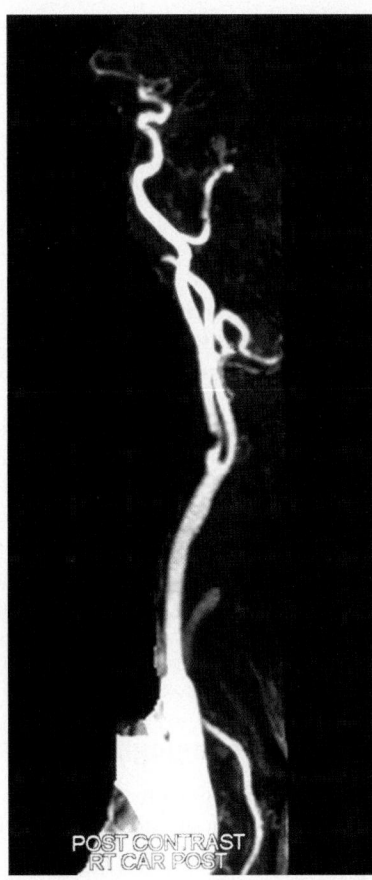

Figure 64-10 A representative image of the carotid artery with a stenosis at the origin of the internal carotid artery obtained with MRA using intravenous gadolinium.

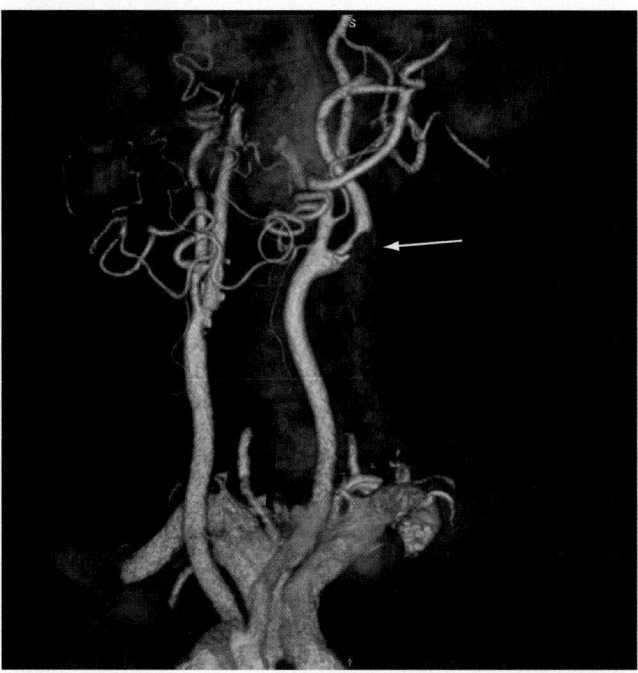

Figure 64-11 A representative image of the extracranial circulation obtained with CT angiography and three-dimensional reconstruction. The *arrow* points to the stenosis in the left internal carotid artery.

The advantages of MRA include the absence of risk and the ability to see the full extent of the carotid artery, including its origin from the aorta and the intracranial vessels. It is also a procedure that can be performed in convenient outpatient settings. Among the disadvantages are the inability to perform the test on individuals with pacemakers and other metallic implants and the fact that the machine is claustrophobic.

Fairly good images can be obtained in the cooperative patient with no contrast (Fig. 64-10). The inherent limitation to MRA is that turbulence of blood flow can make the lumen of the vessel appear narrower than it actually may be. For this reason, the MRA is not reliable to accurately measure the residual lumen of an artery. The addition of gadolinium, a noniodinated contrast material, to the bloodstream improves the sharpness of the images and, to some degree, the accuracy of the MRA for measuring lumen diameters.

Computed Tomography Angiography

CT angiograms have added yet another simple and relatively safe means of imaging the carotid arteries. Excellent three-dimensional images are rapidly becoming almost as accurate as conventional angiograms. Like MRA, CT angiography can be performed in an outpatient setting. It is not as claustrophobic as MRA and can be used in patients with metallic implants. Because the test requires iodinated contrast, it carries some risk for renal failure in individuals with compromised renal function (Fig. 64-11).

CAROTID ENDARTERECTOMY

Carotid endarterectomy, first performed in 1954 by Drs. Eastcott and Rob, is now the most frequently performed vascular operation in the United States. The role of carotid surgery has increased dramatically during the past 2 decades since the reporting of the several large, multicentered, randomized studies affirming the efficacy of surgery in reducing the risk for stroke in individuals with significant carotid artery disease. The increase in the numbers of procedures is also related to the ease of detecting carotid disease with newer diagnostic tests and the rapidly expanding elderly population. At present, more than 160,000 carotid operations are performed each year in the United States (Fig. 64-12).

Indications for Surgery

The indications for any intervention to the carotid artery are determined by the relative risk of the procedure and the natural history of the disease. At present, the absence or presence of focal neurologic symptoms and the degree of narrowing of the carotid lumen are the best indications of the risk for future stroke in a given individual. The randomized trials of NASCET,[9] ACAS,[3] and others, along

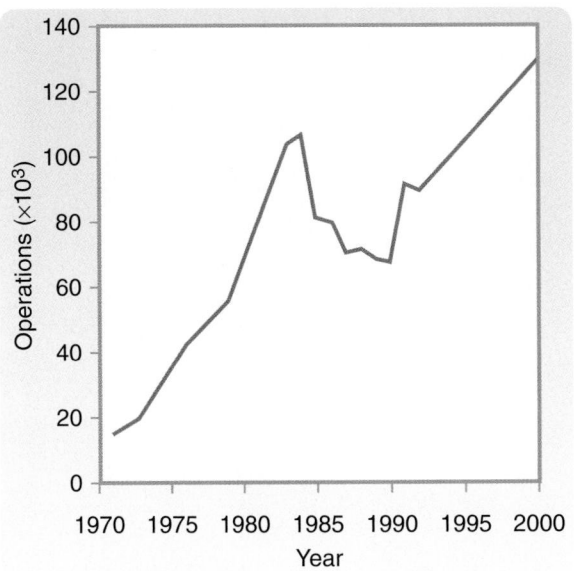

Figure 64-12 Number of carotid endarterectomies performed annually in the United States.

with other studies, have provided clinicians with a good understanding of the natural history of patients with a variety of clinical conditions and plaque characteristics. Generally accepted criteria based on these studies are (1) for symptomatic carotid arteries, more than 50% diameter reduction; and (2) for asymptomatic carotid arteries, more than 80% diameter reduction. Although ACAS recommended surgery for patients with more than 60% stenosis, many clinicians believe the benefit of surgery or angioplasty is not achieved for asymptomatic stenoses less than 80% because of the lower risk for stroke with lesser degrees of carotid stenosis and the relative risk of these interventions.

Other markers, including the ultrasonographic characteristic of the plaque (echo lucent or echo opaque), the absence or presence of ulceration or surface irregularity of the plaque, the presence of mobile thrombus, and the ability to cross-fill from one cerebral hemisphere to another through the circle of Willis have been used by some clinicians to determine which patients should have surgery or angioplasty of the carotid artery.

The NASCET and ACAS studies clearly showed that for individuals with similar degrees of stenosis at the carotid bifurcation, the risk for a future stroke is significantly increased in those who had already experienced an ipsilateral stroke or TIA compared with those who are asymptomatic. Although not substantiated by reliable data, most clinicians believe the higher the frequency and number of transient neurologic events in the territory of the carotid circulation, the greater the risk for imminent stroke and therefore the greater the indication for intervention.

Surgery is generally not indicated when a carotid artery is known to be completely occluded because the surgical risk for performing a thrombectomy of a chroni-

cally occluded ICA is high. Additionally, most patients do not experience recurrent symptoms after the artery has become completely occluded because embolization is unlikely to occur once the stream of blood flow over the plaque has ceased. In fact, many patients who are found to have a chronically completely occluded ICA have never manifested symptoms of a clinical stroke.

The comorbidities and general health of the individual also enter into the clinical decision. Factors such as severe heart or pulmonary diseases that may increase the risk of the procedure must be taken into account. Similarly, in as much as the risk for stroke in many individuals is calculated over years rather than months, the age and life expectancy based on the comorbidities may significantly affect the benefit of a prophylactic operation.

Finally, indications for surgery or angioplasty are based on the assumption that the risk for stroke and death from a procedure is less than 3% for asymptomatic patients and less than 6% for symptomatic patients. If the surgical team treating the patient cannot achieve these results, the benefit of the intervention cannot be justified based on available data.

Operative Management

Preoperative Evaluation

Once a decision has been made to perform surgery on a patient with carotid bifurcation disease, the preoperative assessment is essentially a history and physical examination, electrocardiogram, chest x-ray, and routine laboratory tests. Some clinicians operate on the basis of a duplex ultrasound scan alone, whereas others prefer to corroborate the ultrasound information with either MRA or CT angiography. Stress tests or other extensive cardiac testing is not necessary except for those individuals with severe angina, congestive heart failure, or other serious cardiac condition. Aspirin therapy (80-325 mg/day) is generally started as soon as the diagnosis is made and is continued up to the day of surgery and through the postoperative phase. This is based on data that have documented a reduction in thromboembolic events after carotid surgery for patients on antiplatelet therapy. Those who cannot take aspirin are given clopidogrel (Plavix), 75 mg/day, as an alternative.[15]

Anesthetic Considerations and Intraoperative Neurologic Monitoring Techniques

The choice of anesthetic for use during CEA has remained a matter of debate for more than 3 decades.[16] The initial rationale for using regional anesthesia was to observe the neurologic status of the awake patient during carotid artery clamping. A small but significant group of patients was found to be intolerant to clamping and required the insertion of a temporary shunt to reroute blood to the brain for cerebral protection during the surgery. For operations performed under general anesthesia, one of two methods could be used: a shunt could be used routinely, or some monitoring technique could be used to differentiate patients at risk for cerebral ischemia so that a shunt could be used selectively. Regional anesthetic was an essential tool to aid in the evaluation of various cerebral monitoring techniques and protective measures.[16]

Although excellent results have been achieved with general anesthesia and a variety of monitoring approaches, historically no single technique has correlated well with the neurologic status of the conscious patient. All the direct methods (electroencephalography, evoked potential responses) and indirect methods (carotid stump pressure measurement, transcranial Doppler ultrasound, jugular venous oxygen tension) of detecting cerebral ischemia during carotid clamping have been found at one time or another to lack either sensitivity or specificity when compared with the neurologic status of the awake patient.[16] Electroencephalogram (EEG), for example, may lead to as high as a 20% to 25% incidence of temporary shunting; the rate of selective shunting in a similar population of conscious patients is reported as low as 7%. Conversely, perioperative strokes have clearly occurred in the absence of any EEG changes.[16] Some surgeons use the mean pressure in the ICA distal to the clamp as a guide to selective shunting. Opinions differ as to the threshold for shunting, but in general, more than 50 mm Hg is considered safe for clamping without a shunt.

Advocates of regional anesthesia have proposed that neurologic complications should be less frequent because with regional anesthesia the need for shunting can be most accurately assessed. In addition, patients who have coronary and pulmonary disease presumably fare better without endotracheal intubation and general anesthesia. Although a number of reports have demonstrated improved results with regional as opposed to general anesthesia, several excellent large series reported in the literature demonstrate equally low neurologic and cardiopulmonary complication rates with general anesthesia using various forms of intracerebral monitoring.[16]

At our institution, regional anesthesia with selective shunting is the preferred method of carotid surgery and is used in about 85% of CEA procedures.[16] Claustrophobia, neurologic disorders including stroke, and language barriers have been relative contraindications if these factors make cooperation and communication difficult. Unexpected conversion to general anesthesia during the course of the surgery is rare, about 2% of cases. Data from our institution have revealed trends toward increased rates of perioperative mortality (2.0% versus 1.4%) and stroke (3.2% versus 2.0%) with general anesthesia as opposed to regional anesthesia. It is possible that patient selection also played a role in these results. Nevertheless, we believe that regional anesthesia can be used safely for CEA in most patients with excellent clinical results.[16]

From a practical point of view, there are advantages and disadvantages of each type of anesthesia for carotid surgery. General anesthesia is arguably more comfortable for the patient and the surgeon. It assures adequate access to the airway and avoids movement by the patient that could distract the surgeon. In patients with comorbidities such as pulmonary or cardiac disease, regional anesthesia may be safer. Also, some surgeons find that patients prefer to not have to undergo a general anesthetic to have their carotid artery repaired.

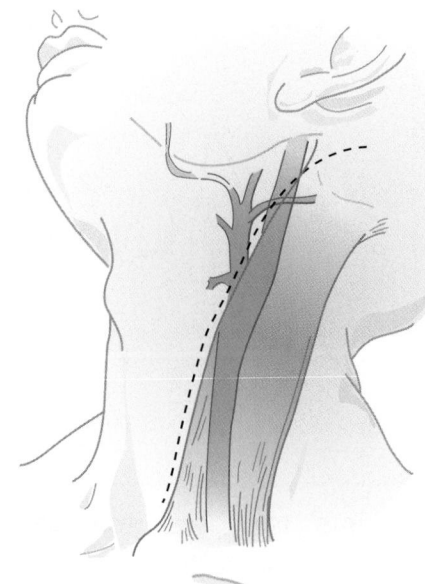

Figure 64-13 Position of incision for optimal exposure of the extracranial carotid artery.

Cerebral Monitoring and Protection

If the patient is awake, tolerance to the interruption of blood flow in the ICA can be easily discerned by asking the patient to move the contralateral hand and to count aloud. If the patient is intolerant of clamping, it usually is evident within several minutes if not seconds. Monitoring is continued throughout the procedure because changes in blood pressure, heart rate, and oxygen saturation may lead to cortical ischemia and cerebral dysfunction. From observations made on awake patients, if the contralateral carotid artery is patent, 92% of patients tolerate clamping of the operated artery without developing symptoms of cerebral ischemia.[16] Even when the contralateral carotid artery is completely occluded, more than half of patients tolerate clamping of the remaining carotid artery, presumably because of the excellent collateral flow from the posterior cerebral circulation.[17] For those patients who show signs of cerebral ischemia with clamping of the ICA, a temporary shunt from the common carotid artery to the ICA will provide sufficient blood flow to the brain while the repair is being done. For those who require a shunt, the interval between clamping of the artery and restoration of blood flow through the shunt should not be more than 4 minutes so as to prevent cerebral infarction from inadequate blood flow.

Operative Procedure

The patient is placed supine on the operating table with the head turned away from the operative side (Figs. 64-13 to 64-16). Slight extension of the neck is helpful if it can be tolerated. The incision of 5 to 10 cm is made along the anterior border of the sternocleidomastoid muscle. If additional cephalad extension is needed, the incision is directed posterior to the parotid gland and the ear. After dividing the platysma muscle, the sternocleidomastoid muscle is mobilized by dissecting the medial border until

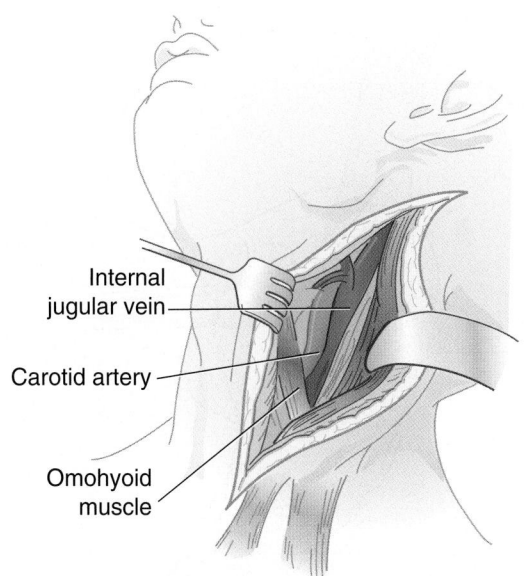

Figure 64-14 The sternocleidomastoid muscle is retracted posteriorly to expose the carotid sheath.

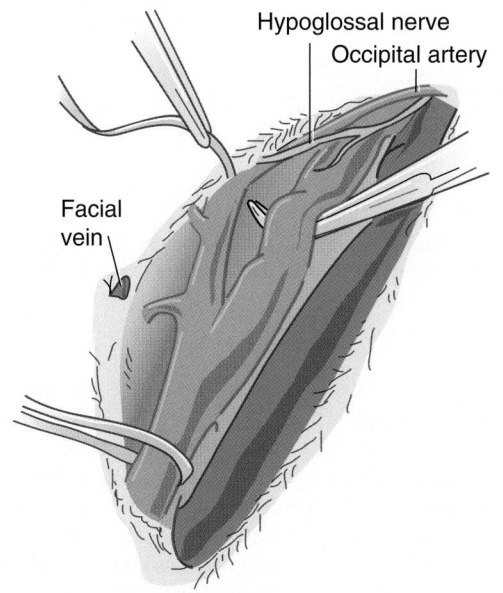

Figure 64-15 The common facial vein branch of the internal jugular vein marks the site of the carotid bifurcation. After dividing the facial vein, the internal jugular vein is retracted posteriorly to expose the carotid bifurcation.

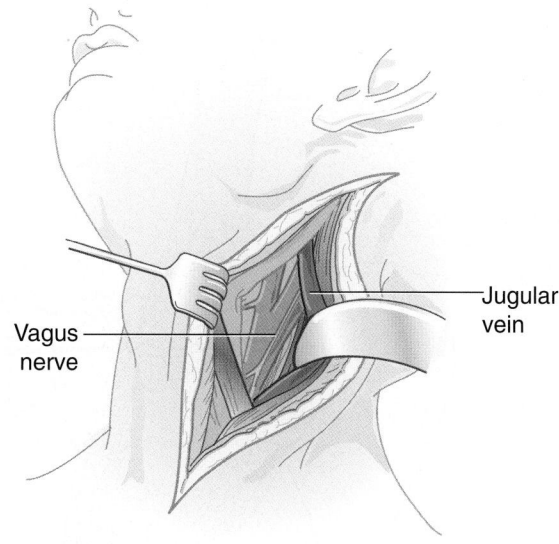

Figure 64-16 The common carotid, internal carotid, and external carotid arteries are exposed and mobilized with minimal dissection and manipulation of the disease-bearing segment of the distal, common, and proximal internal carotid arteries (carotid bulb).

venous structures are identified. Any crossing veins—the cervical, facial, or middle thyroid—can be traced to the jugular vein. These branches are divided between ties at their origin from the jugular.

With mobilization of the jugular vein laterally, the common carotid artery is exposed. The vagus nerve is usually found posterior to the carotid artery but occasionally is superficial to the carotid. Identification of the nerve is important to avoid injury during the dissection or clamping of the carotid artery.

At the superior portion of the dissection, the digastric tendon can be identified by dissecting below the parotid gland and above the cervical lymph nodes. The nodes are mobilized and reflected laterally, exposing the neurovascular structures below. The hypoglossal nerve is deep to the facial vein. The ansa cervicalis nerve branches from the hypoglossal nerve, where the hypoglossal changes course heading medially toward the pharynx. The ansa cervicalis can be helpful locating the hypoglossal if the dissection is difficult. Division of the facial vein, the sternocleidomastoid branch of the external carotid artery, and any other small crossing vessels exposes the hypoglossal and permits dissection of the ICA above the plaque. The ICA is in close proximity to the ascending portion of the hypoglossal nerve, the vagus nerve, and the jugular vein. Above and below the plaque, the carotid arteries are dissected and encircled with vessel loops. To avoid embolization of plaque material, dissection of the carotid bulb needs to be minimal until the intravenous heparin is given and the distal ICA is clamped.

The most common operation is a longitudinal arteriotomy from the common carotid to the ICA. For the eversion technique, the arteriotomy is made obliquely across the bulb onto the ICA. The plaque is removed by bluntly separating between the adventitia and the media. It is not necessary to remove the media, but if the media is not removed, care must be made to not leave loose fibers in the lumen that could embolize or serve as a nidus for thrombus formation.

The most common cause of postoperative stroke is a technical defect created at the time of the reconstruction of the artery. Defects, be they residual plaque, raised flaps of intima, narrowing of the lumen, clamp injuries, or kinks can lead to platelet aggregation, thrombus

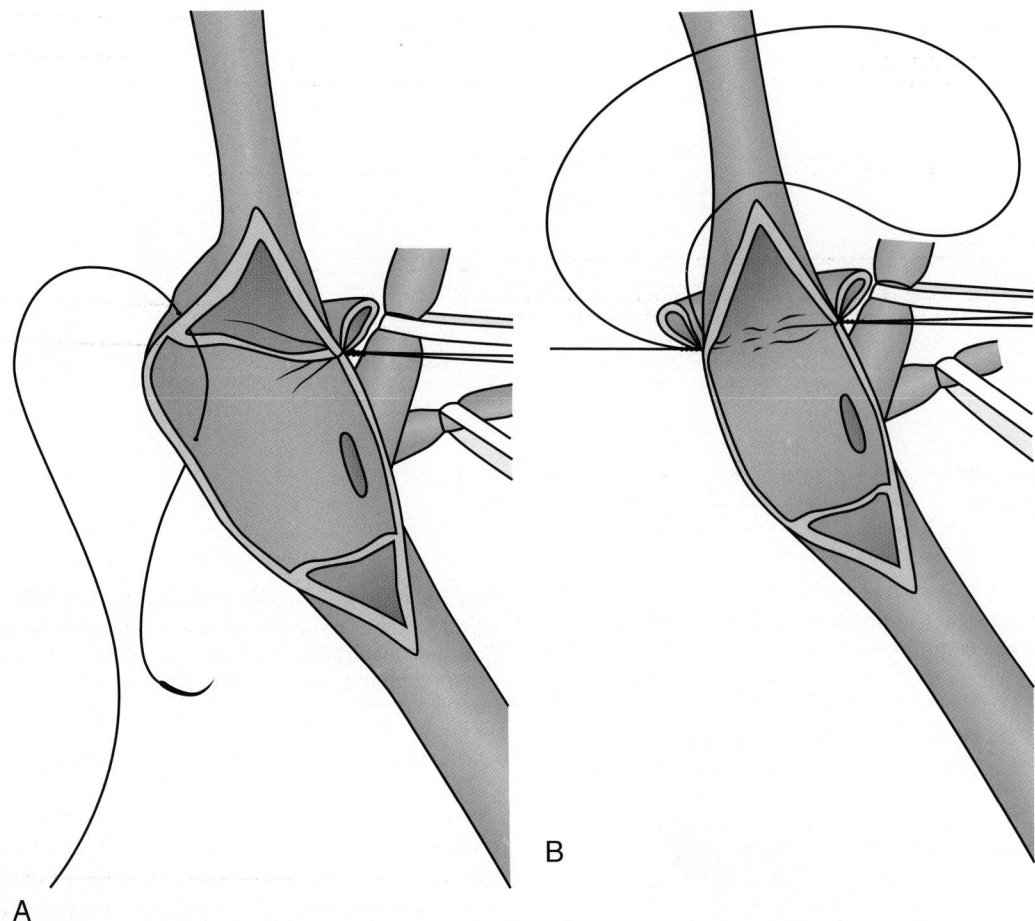

A

B

Figure 64-17 An illustration showing the operative technique for plicating the internal carotid artery to correct the redundancy resulting from the removal of a plaque from a tortuous vessel. **A** and **B,** The pleat is made with a suture on both sides of the ICA.

formation, embolization, and stroke. The technique for reconstruction must ensure that there is adequate lumen of the artery and that the lumen is smooth and free of defects that could lead to turbulence of blood flow.

Toward this end, it is important to make a sufficiently long arteriotomy to be sure there is no residual plaque or a raised flap of intima at the distal end of the endarterectomy. Either can be addressed by making a higher arteriotomy until a smooth transition point can be found, or by using tacking sutures of 6-0 Prolene and a patch to widen the lumen across the residual plaque.

Redundancy of the ICA can be a problem. If not addressed, what was previously a curve or coil in the artery can become a kink once the artery has been dissected and the rigid plaque has been removed. After the flow has been restored, a kink can cause turbulence and thrombosis. One technique for eliminating redundancy is to resect a portion of the ICA and reanastomose it with an arterial suture; another technique is to plicate the ICA making the redundant ICA extraluminal (Fig. 64-17). In either case, a patch is placed over the suture line rather than trying to close it primarily. Using the eversion technique, the ICA is simply transected from the carotid bulb with oblique incisions anteriorly and posteriorly

(Fig. 64-18). The arteriotomy in the ICA is continued past the point of the endarterectomy. The ICA is then pulled down to the bulb and reanastomosed with a running Prolene suture, effectively eliminating the redundancy.

Although the arteriotomy can be closed primarily with a running monofilament suture, most surgeons use an elliptical patch of some sort. Considerable evidence is available to show that patch closures are associated with a lower risk for preoperative stroke and a lower incidence of recurrent carotid stenosis. There appears to be little difference among patch materials—synthetic, autologous veins, bovine pericardium—with regard to early and late complications.

Arterial Closure Techniques During Carotid Endarterectomy

Arterial endarterectomy and reconstruction during CEA can be performed in a variety of ways, including standard endarterectomy with primary closure, standard endarterectomy with patch angioplasty, and eversion endarterectomy with reimplantation of the ICA. Furthermore, patch angioplasty can be performed with a diverse choice of both autologous and synthetic materials. Although excellent results have been independently reported with many

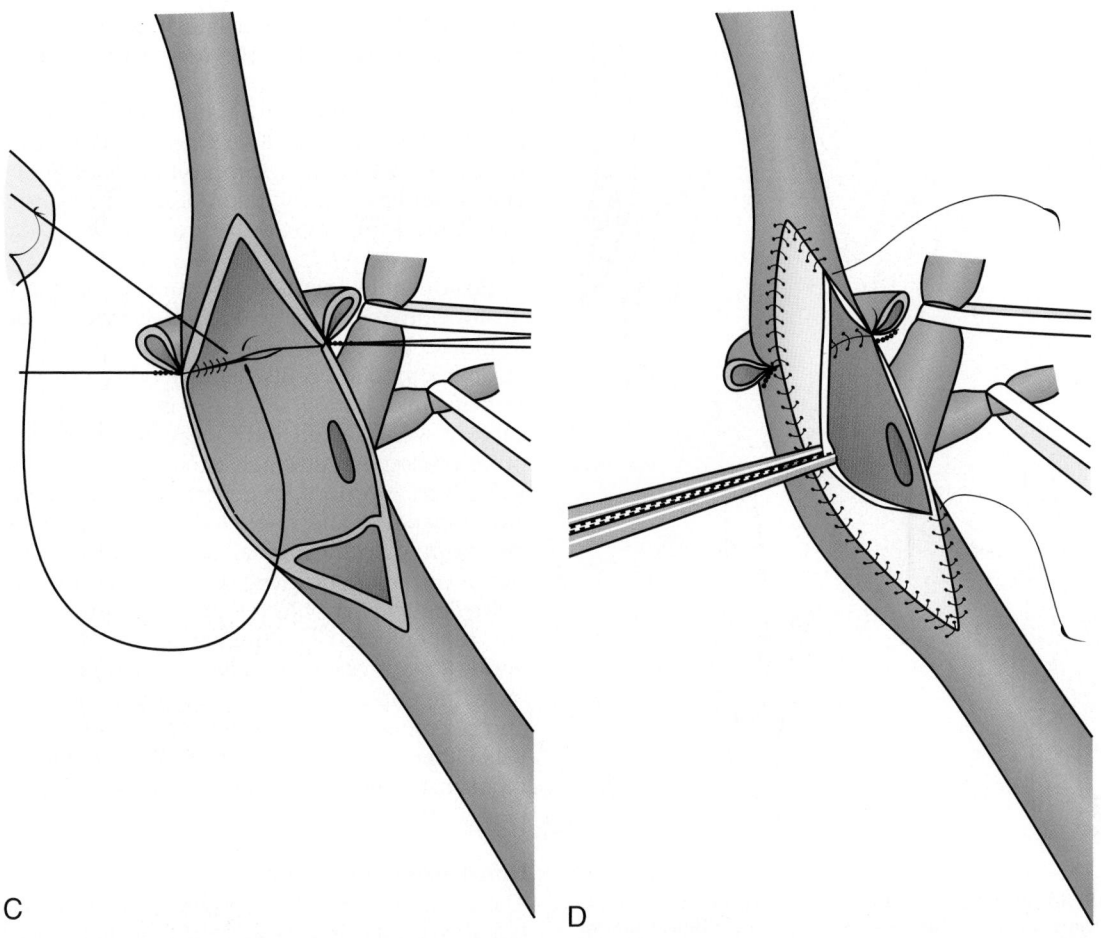

C   D

Figure 64-17, cont'd C, A monofilament suture is run from one side to the other to close the space. **D,** A patch is sewn to the arteriotomy to complete the reconstruction.

of these techniques, the optimal method of arterial reconstruction remains a matter of controversy. However, there is a large amount of data in the literature suggesting that either the patch angioplasty or eversion endarterectomy technique is superior to primary closure alone. Recently, a multivariate analysis of more than 10,000 carotid endarterectomies found that the use of patch angioplasty was associated with significantly lower perioperative risk than primary closure.[18] Similarly, several randomized controlled trials of patch angioplasty compared with primary closure during CEA have suggested that patch angioplasty decreases the risk for perioperative stroke or death.

From a physiologic viewpoint, in comparison with primary closure, patch angioplasty with vein has been shown to provide a partially endothelialized flow surface, a significantly greater cross-sectional area, and a relatively mild degree of wall shear stress. It has been hypothesized that all three of these factors may protect against both early postoperative thrombosis and significant late restenosis.[19] Patch angioplasty with prosthetic material is now also widely performed, with a number of studies showing equivalent outcomes to patch angioplasty with saphenous vein. In comparison to patch angioplasty, proponents of the eversion endarterectomy

mention possible improvement in the incidence of subsequent recurrent carotid stenosis, and a potential advantage in that there is no need for a longitudinal arteriotomy and placement of a patch on the artery.

Complications of Carotid Endarterectomy

Although the benefits of CEA over the medical treatment of patients with both symptomatic and asymptomatic carotid stenosis have been confirmed by randomized, prospective clinical trials, the advantage of surgical therapy is only achieved if the complications of carotid surgery are maintained at an extremely low level. Particularly in asymptomatic patients, in whom the margin of benefit in stroke prevention is less remarkable, reducing the incidence of post-CEA complications is critical. The most commonly discussed and analyzed complication of CEA is, of course, stroke. However, a variety of other complications can occur and can cause considerable morbidity to the patient in both the short and long term.

Stroke

Although many studies report the incidence of perioperative stroke following CEA, few reports have focused on the cause of the perioperative strokes. In a detailed report

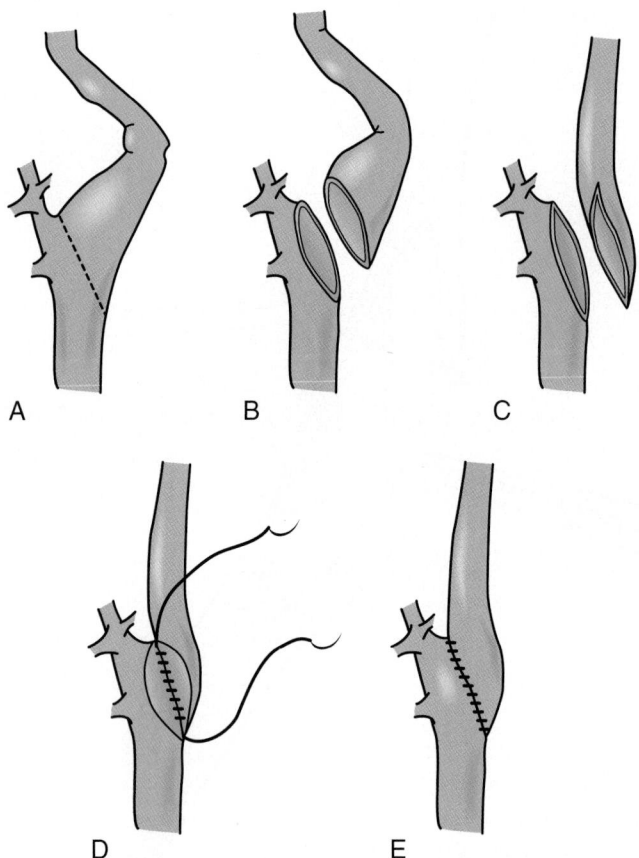

Figure 64-18 An illustration to show the technique for eversion endarterectomy and reconstruction of the carotid bulb to eliminate redundancy of the internal carotid artery (ICA). **A,** The arteriotomy is made obliquely over the carotid bulb. **B,** When the plaque is removed, the ICA is completely severed. **C,** The ICA is cut cephalad and the common carotid caudad the appropriate amount to remove the redundancy. **D** and **E,** The ICA is then reanastomosed to the common carotid artery effectively straightening the ICA by placing it in a new position.

from the NASCET study, it was found that thromboembolism stemming from technical error or imperfection at the site of the endarterectomy was the major cause of postoperative stroke following CEA.[20] At our institution, most CEA procedures have been performed in the awake patient. This technique has provided the opportunity to correlate the onset of perioperative strokes with the specific timing and events of the procedure. An extensive evaluation on the cause of the 66 (2.2%) perioperative strokes following 3062 carotid endarterectomies was undertaken.[21] Risk factors for the development of a perioperative stroke included hypertension, a history of a preoperative stroke, the use of a general anesthetic, and the use of an intra-arterial shunt during the surgery. The mechanisms of perioperative strokes could be grouped into several broad categories:

1. Ischemia during carotid artery clamping
2. Postoperative thrombosis or embolization
3. Intracerebral hemorrhage
4. Strokes from other mechanisms
5. Strokes unrelated to the reconstructed artery[21]

The most common cause of perioperative stroke was found to be postoperative thrombosis and thromboembolization, which was responsible for 38% of all perioperative strokes. Thromboembolization was usually related to technical imperfection or error at the endarterectomy site.[21]

Postoperative neurologic events occurring in the early postoperative period within 24 hours of surgery were found to be significantly more likely to be caused by thromboembolic events than by other causes of stroke.[22] Deficits manifesting after the first 24 hours following surgery were significantly more likely to be caused by other etiologies. Although each patient requires an individualized approach, in general we advocate for immediate reoperation and re-exploration in those patients who are neurologically normal at the end of the operation, but develop a neurologic deficit within the first 24 hours following surgery.[22] In patients who underwent immediate reoperation, intraluminal thrombus was noted in about 80% of cases, usually accompanied by some technical imperfection. After re-exploration, thrombectomy, and the repair of any noted technical imperfections, there was either complete resolution of or significant improvement in the neurologic deficit that had been present in nearly 70% of cases.[22]

Nonstroke Complications

The complications of CEA other than stroke can be additionally divided into neurologic and nonneurologic complications. Neurologic complications other than stroke include cranial nerve injury and cerebral hyperperfusion syndrome.

Cranial Nerve Injury

Although not a frank cerebral infarction, the rare permanent severe cranial nerve injury following CEA can have equally devastating consequences to a patient's quality of life. Fortunately, cranial nerve injury following CEA is usually a transient neurapraxia: the mechanism of injury is thought to be most often related to stretch, retraction, or clamping of the involved nerve rather than outright transection of the structure. Given the familiarity of most carotid surgeons with the anatomy of the neck, severe cranial nerve injuries most often occur in unusual circumstances such as reoperative carotid surgery or unusually high lesions. The reported incidence of cranial nerve dysfunction following CEA varies widely from 3% to 23% in representative series; the discrepancy in the reported incidence most likely depends on the exact methodology by which cranial nerve dysfunction is defined and diagnosed.[23] The true incidence of clinically significant cranial nerve injuries is more difficult to ascertain and is likely much lower.

The cranial and cervical nerves at risk curing CEA include the hypoglossal, vagus, recurrent laryngeal, marginal mandibular, superior laryngeal, glossopharyngeal, spinal accessory, transverse cervical, and greater auricular nerves.[23] Severe injury to the hypoglossal nerve can result in tongue clumsiness and biting, dysarthria, and impaired mastication and deglutition. Vagal or recurrent laryngeal nerve injury can result in vocal cord paralysis, hoarseness, or airway obstruction when bilateral. Glossopharyngeal injury most often results from unusually high dissection during CEA, especially if the posterior belly of the digastric muscle is divided. Symptoms of glossopharyngeal injury can range from dysphagia to recurrent aspiration, respiratory failure, and malnutrition. Tracheostomy and feeding jejunostomy rarely may be required. Injury to the superior laryngeal branch of the vagus can result in subtle voice changes that may be troublesome to singers or public speakers. Injury to the marginal mandibular branch of the facial nerve is usually transient and of mainly cosmetic concern.[23]

In summary, some degree of cranial nerve dysfunction following CEA is relatively common, but most injuries are transient and do not have great clinical significance. Treatment is expectant and supportive when required. In the case of planned bilateral procedures, care must be taken to document vocal cord recovery before proceeding with contralateral surgery. Severe cranial nerve injuries can best be avoided by excellent knowledge of the variations in cranial and cervical nerve anatomy, attention to detail in dissection and retractor placement, and meticulous placement of vascular clamps.[23]

Cerebral Hyperperfusion Syndrome

The cerebral hyperperfusion syndrome with potential resulting intracerebral hemorrhage (ICH) is one of the most feared complications by surgeons who perform CEA. Although relatively infrequent, this complication can have tremendous and often fatal sequelae and remains a significant cause of neurologic morbidity after CEA.[23] The proposed mechanism of hyperperfusion results from a lack of vascular autoregulation, and the common denominator in the pathophysiology of the syndrome appears to be reactive hyperemia.[23] In its less severe forms, hyperperfusion results in mild cerebral edema, headache, and seizures. When an abnormal, hyperperfused vessel ruptures, ICH results.

The true incidence of the hyperperfusion syndrome following CEA is unknown. The reported incidence from several large series ranges from 0.4% to 2%.[23] In our institution, an evaluation of 1500 CEAs performed identified 11 patients with ICH, for an incidence of 0.7%.[24] The mortality rate among these patients was 36%. ICH appears to account for as much as 13% to 15% of perioperative strokes after CEA.[24] Considering the severe morbidity of this particular complication, it is critically important to understand which patients are at increased risk.

The most commonly identified factors that predispose a patient to the development of cerebral hyperperfusion include a history of stroke, especially when recent; relief of a severely stenotic lesion (>90%); severe intraoperative or postoperative hypertension; anticoagulant use; severe chronic cerebral ischemia; and perhaps contralateral carotid occlusion.[24,25] Of course, one or more of these recognized factors are often present in many patients undergoing CEA, and clinically evident hyperperfusion does not occur in most patients in whom one or more

of these risk factors exists. However, awareness of the early symptoms of the syndrome is important in these cases.

In contrast to postoperative neurologic deficits related to thromboembolization, ICH following CEA tends to occur on postoperative day 3 or later. Patients present with headaches, seizures, progressive obtundation, or hemiparesis. The diagnosis of the syndrome is often clinical and rests heavily on the surgeon's suspicion in a patient with appropriate risk factors. CT scanning to evaluate for hemorrhage or edema is the test of choice in any patient who presents with severe frontoparietal or orbital pain or seizure activity. EEG may reveal lateralizing epileptiform discharges or frank seizure activity. Prophylaxis is difficult because it requires predicting which patients will sustain such an event. However, certain measures are reasonable in patients thought to be at risk: strict blood pressure control, judicious use of anticoagulants and antiplatelet agents, and close monitoring of the neurologic status. In patients with headaches only, simple analgesia may suffice. In patients with more severe symptoms, antihypertensives and anticonvulsant medications may be warranted. If cerebral edema is significant, diuretics and anti-inflammatory medications may be used. When petechial or small cerebral hemorrhages occur, the above measures often suffice. However, when massive hemorrhage occurs, neurosurgical intervention may be necessary, and the prognosis is exceedingly poor.

Vein Patch Rupture

Patch angioplasty reconstruction of the carotid artery after CEA is an accepted technique and may reduce the incidence of postoperative thrombosis, embolization, and recurrent carotid stenosis.[23] The greater saphenous vein has the advantages of being autologous, readily available, and easy to use. A rare but potentially life-threatening complication of its use is rupture of the vein patch. Its reported incidence ranges from 0% to 4.0%.[26] Manifestations of vein patch rupture in the early postoperative period include massive hemorrhage into the neck with airway compromise, respiratory arrest, and death. Possible predisposing factors include the use of ankle vein or the use of a small vein (<3.5 mm in diameter) when distended. The incidence of vein patch rupture can probably be reduced or nearly eliminated by using greater saphenous vein harvested from the thigh.[23,26]

Postoperative Hematoma

Wound hematoma after CEA can be life-threatening because of the risk for airway compromise with hemorrhage in the neck. The incidence reported in the literature varies form 1% to 4.5%. Risk factors reported include perioperative hypertension, lack of reversal of intraoperative heparinization with protamine sulfate, and postoperative resumption of anticoagulation with heparin or warfarin for treatment or prophylaxis of arterial or venous thromboembolization. At least one study found a significantly increased incidence of wound hematoma after CEA when protamine was not reversed.[27] The successful management of wound hematoma after CEA centers on immediate recognition of the complication and return to the operating room for hematoma evacuation. Even a hematoma that initially appears benign can rapidly progress to stridor and respiratory compromise. Although these hematomas are most often related to seemingly minor venous bleeding or diffuse bleeding from residual heparin effect, their consequences can be severe if not treated expeditiously.

Infectious Complications

Reports of vein patch rupture after CEA, as well as late aneurysmal degeneration of the vein patch, have led to investigations for alternative acceptable patch materials. Harvest site morbidity and the need for venous conduits for subsequent coronary or lower extremity revascularizations have also been cited as reasons to consider prosthetic patch options. Prosthetic patches, such as polytetrafluoroethylene (PTFE) and polyester, are attractive alternatives in that they are readily available and technically easy to use. Although several studies have shown that knitted polyester has been comparable to vein in rates of restenosis, potential drawbacks to prosthetic materials include possible increases in recurrent stenosis, increased thrombogenicity, and infection.

Although potential infectious complications remain a significant concern with prosthetic patches, there have been very few reported series of these after CEA, and their true incidence is unknown. From our institution, a series of 10 cases that required reoperation and management of postoperative Dacron patch infections after CEA was reported.[28] Half of the patients presented early with cellulitis and abscess formation within several weeks after the original surgery. However, the remaining half presented 1 to 2 years after surgery with draining sinus tracts. All patients had their carotid artery reconstructed with autologous material, with no significant morbidity occurring from the second operation. In our report as well as several others, all patients have remained free of infection after appropriate surgical and antibiotic management and removal of the prosthetic patch.[28]

Perioperative Blood Pressure Instability

Blood pressure instability after CEA may contribute to morbidity, increases length of hospital stay and costs, and occasionally results in mortality.[29] Carotid baroreceptor dysfunction and impaired cerebral autoregulation after manipulation of the carotid bulb and carotid sinus nerve have been implicated in the etiology of postoperative hypertension and hypotension. Potential reported risk factors of postoperative hypertension include having undergone an eversion endarterectomy and having undergone surgery under general as opposed to regional anesthesia. Postoperative hypertension in particular has been shown to be associated with increased postoperative stroke and death and with postoperative cardiac complications. Postoperative hypotension and bradycardia do not appear to correlate with perioperative outcome. Management of post-CEA patients must include aggressive treatment of hemodynamic instability so as to prevent secondary complications. In addition to potential cardiac complications, severe hypotension may theoretically predispose toward thrombosis of the arterial reconstruction,

and severe hypertension can increase the chance of cerebral hyperperfusion and intracranial hemorrhage.[23]

Myocardial Infarction

In addition to having systemic atherosclerosis, patients undergoing vascular surgery are typically elderly patients with past or current tobacco use, and often have medical comorbidities.[30] It is not surprising that cardiopulmonary complications are the most frequent perioperative problem facing this patient population. The pathophysiology of perioperative acute myocardial infarction (MI) is complex. Both surgery and anesthesia initiate processes that placed added stress on the myocardium, including catecholamine release, fluid shifts, blood pressure fluctuations, transient hypercoagulability, and tachycardia.[30] Interestingly, the incidence of postoperative MI following carotid artery surgery appears to be lower than the incidences following aortic surgery or infrainguinal arterial reconstruction. The reported incidences in the literature of acute MI after CEA range from 0.3% to 1.6%.[30]

It remains unclear whether this finding is secondary to the inherent lower degree of invasiveness and fluid shifts related to carotid surgery or to the more extensive nature of other major vascular procedures, or whether the patient population is truly different. However, the most critical factor for the surgeon is to perform a careful preoperative evaluation centered on the detection of unrecognized severe coronary artery disease that may become manifest in the perioperative period. The exact components of the appropriate preoperative cardiac workup remain controversial, with some investigators suggesting routine pharmacologic stress testing for nearly all patients who will undergo CEA, and others suggesting that this degree of widespread testing only rarely changes the course of the anticipated operation.

Special Situations

Contralateral Carotid Occlusion

Total occlusion of the contralateral ICA has often been considered to be a predictor of poor outcome after CEA for ipsilateral carotid stenosis.[17] Recently, advocates of carotid angioplasty and stenting (CAS) have suggested that this technique may be preferable in patients with contralateral occlusion (CO) because of the perceived poor outcome with surgery. At our institution, a study was undertaken to review a large series of CEAs in patients with CO to see whether results differed in patients with a patent contralateral artery.[17] Patients with CO were significantly more likely to be male, to have a history of cigarette smoking, and to have sustained a preoperative stroke than patients without CO. However, the incidence of perioperative stroke was 3.0% in patients with CO, compared with 2.1% in those without CO (*P* value not significant). When further examination of only asymptomatic patients was performed, the incidences of perioperative stroke in patients with and without CO were essentially equivalent at 1.8%.

Symptomatic patients with CO were found to be the subgroup with the highest perioperative stroke rate

(3.7%); however, this subgroup appears to have the worst prognosis when medical management is pursued as well. In conclusion, the presence of CO does not appear to significantly increase the perioperative risk for CEA. CEA can be performed safely in these patients and is not considered a high-risk condition for surgery in favor of CAS. However, the criteria for performing CEA for either symptomatic or asymptomatic patients with CO has remained the same, and the threshold for operating on an ipsilateral lesion in a patient with CO has not decreased.[17]

Redo Carotid Surgery

Estimates of the incidence of recurrent stenosis after prior CEA vary widely in the literature, ranging from 1.2% to 36% in a number of published series.[31] Investigators have focused on elucidating contributory risk factors, such as cigarette smoking, hypercholesterolemia, female gender, and the use of primary closure of the artery during the index CEA. The clinical significance of recurrent carotid stenosis remains an area of controversy. Recurrent stenosis generally occurs in two separate time periods after CEA: Early recurrent disease, occurring within 2 to 3 years after initial CEA, tends to be secondary to neointimal hyperplasia at the site of the prior endarterectomy. Later restenosis, occurring about 3 years after the index CEA, is usually caused by recurrent atherosclerotic disease at the carotid bifurcation. Some authors believe that the clinical course of recurrent stenosis is benign, especially when related to early neointimal hyperplasia. The arguments for the nonoperative management of recurrent carotid stenosis are on the basis of the presumed increased risk for a perioperative complication that exists with redo cases. Potential technical causes for increased risk in carotid reoperations include the formation of dense scar tissue, which could lead to difficulty in dissection, and inadvertent venous or cranial nerve injuries, inadvertent arterial injuries, technical difficulties in achieving an appropriate endarterectomy plane, technical difficulties in achieving distal control of the internal carotid in a reoperative field, and technical difficulties in shunt insertion, when required. Often during carotid reoperations, a formal second endarterectomy is not possible, and interposition grafting may be required.[31]

Despite these potential difficulties, there are many excellent reports of operative series for recurrent carotid stenosis. At our institution, the overall perioperative complication rate was low, with a combined permanent stroke and death rate of 3.7% after 82 carotid reoperations.[31] The rate of permanent cranial nerve injury was 1.2%. Unfortunately, the long-term durability of these 82 reoperations was not optimal, with late failures consisting of four significant cases of secondary restenosis requiring tertiary treatment, and five late cases of total occlusion. There was a trend toward improved long-term results with interposition grafting at the first reoperation as opposed to an attempt at redo endarterectomy and patch angioplasty. Interestingly, cases in which reconstruction was performed with vein had a significantly higher rate of late failures than those in which reconstruction was performed with prosthetic material.

Timing of Carotid Endarterectomy After Preoperative Stroke

It is generally accepted that symptomatic patients with previous TIA or stroke have an increased risk for perioperative stroke when compared with asymptomatic patients undergoing CEA. This is reflected in the American Heart Association guidelines on carotid surgery standards, which propose an "acceptable" stroke/death rate of 6% for symptomatic patients and less than 3% for asymptomatic patients.[32] Although the safety and efficacy of CEA in patients with hemispheric neurologic symptoms have been demonstrated in randomized, prospective clinical trials, the optimal timing of CEA after ipsilateral hemispheric stroke is controversial.[33] The initial CEA literature described the devastating conversion of pre-existing ischemic infarcts into fatal intracerebral hemorrhage after early revascularization with CEA for acute infarcts.[34] However, upon closer examination, several of these early studies reported on surgical patients with pre-existing profound neurologic deficits, or known acute ICA occlusion, patients at greatly increased risk for perioperative complications. The presumed mechanism was related to cerebral perfusion or hyperperfusion to an area of ischemic or infarcted brain that had lost its vascular autoregulatory control mechanisms. Nonetheless, based on these reports, as well as the poor experience of others with these patients, a waiting period of 4 to 8 weeks after acute stroke was recommended before revascularization.

More recently, other individual investigators have suggested that earlier CEA after a completed, stable stroke not only is safe but also may reduce the risk for recurrent infarction or the conversion of a severe stenosis to a complete occlusion during an arbitrarily defined waiting period.[35] Presumably the development of more sophisticated CT scanning as well as MRI of the brain allows for improved patient selection for early intervention. Analysis of data from NASCET[35] and the European Carotid Surgery Trial (ECST)[36] has suggested that early CEA may be safe as well. Several investigators have stressed the importance of proper patient selection for early revascularization after stroke, mentioning factors such as the severity and stability of the neurologic deficit and the size of the infarction on preoperative CT scans of the brain. Both preoperative infarct size and the initial stroke severity have been shown to be significant predictors of postoperative worsening of the neurologic status of the patient.

At our institution, a review of 1158 CEAs performed in symptomatic patients was conducted, of which 62.7% had TIAs and 37.3% had completed strokes.[33] Patients with TIAs were significantly more likely to undergo operation in an early time period, within 4 weeks of the presenting symptom, than were patients with cerebrovascular accident. Stroke patients operated on early had a significantly higher rate of perioperative stroke and perioperative death than stroke patients operated on in a delayed fashion (stroke, 9.4% versus 2.4%, $P = .003$; death, 2.2% versus 0%, $P < .04$). Of the 17 perioperative strokes that occurred in patients with prior strokes undergoing early CEA, 5 were due to intracerebral hemorrhage (29.4%), and 2 were secondary to extension of the pre-existing stroke presumably secondary to hyperperfusion (11.8%). This study concluded with a word of caution regarding early CEA in stroke patients.[33] However, it must be noted that most of the existing literature would suggest otherwise. Individualized decision making is recommended for the individual stroke patient, taking into account the severity of the stroke, stability of the neurologic condition, size of the infarct on preoperative imaging, and nature and severity of the carotid lesion. Delaying surgery for a period of about 4 weeks may be prudent if any of the above factors represents concern on the part of the clinician in an individual patient.[33]

Combined Carotid–Coronary Procedures

Atherosclerosis is a systemic disease, and many patients have significant disease in more than one vascular territory. The appropriate management of synchronous coronary artery disease and carotid artery disease remains an area of controversy. MI is a serious potential complication of and major cause of mortality after CEA, and stroke is a major potential complication of coronary artery bypass grafting (CABG). The true incidence of significant carotid artery disease in patients undergoing CABG is unknown; one large report of nearly 1800 screening carotid duplex scans performed in patients undergoing CABG found a 6.3% incidence of more than 75% carotid artery stenosis.[37] However, the etiology of stroke after CABG is multifactorial and may include atherosclerotic and cardioarterial embolization as well as carotid bifurcation disease. Furthermore, the approach to combined disease may be staged or simultaneous, and the literature varies widely as to recommendations for treatment strategies in different groups of patients. Most studies have demonstrated an increased incidence of stroke and death with combined CEA and CABG procedures; it is somewhat unclear whether this actually reflects the simple additive risks of two synchronous operative procedures, or the innately increased risk in patients with more extensive atherosclerotic disease.[37] Recent literature suggests that the latter is the case.[38]

Possible management strategies include staged procedures, with the symptomatic vascular territory taking preference, or simultaneous procedures. When the carotid lesion is symptomatic in the presence of stable, asymptomatic coronary artery disease, most practitioners elect to perform CEA first, with appropriate precautions applied in patients with known coronary artery disease. Some practitioners believe that CEA under locoregional anesthesia, or perhaps CAS, may be appropriate in this situation. Similarly, in the presence of active or unstable coronary disease and an asymptomatic carotid lesion, most practitioners elect to treat the coronary lesions primarily. The concern arises in those patients in whom CABG must be performed and in whom a preocclusive or symptomatic carotid lesion exists as well. There is concern that with the relative hypoperfusion that occurs with CABG on cardiopulmonary bypass, a preocclusive carotid lesion may go on to occlude or global cerebral hypoperfusion may result. This is especially concerning in patients with bilateral severe carotid stenosis and in those with unilateral carotid occlusion and contralateral severe stenosis. It is in these cases that a combined procedure may be most suitable.

In many combined CEA and CABG procedures, the sternotomy is performed first and cannulas may be placed, so that the option of beginning expedient cardiopulmonary bypass is available if the patient clinically deteriorates from a cardiac standpoint. Then, the CEA is performed in the usual fashion. Given the extreme degree of heparinization and the immediate availability of the harvested saphenous vein, many surgeons choose to perform vein patch angioplasty rather than using prosthetic material in these cases; prosthetic material with excessive heparinization can produce troublesome needle-hole bleeding, and the patient will require heparinization during the ensuing several hours while the cardiac procedure is being performed. The neck is usually left open during the CABG procedure, and is reinspected and closed after protamine is administered at the end of the CABG procedure.

Carotid Angioplasty and Stenting

Percutaneous transluminal balloon angioplasty and stenting of the coronary arteries has become a mainstay of treatment for coronary artery disease. Similarly, these percutaneous endovascular techniques have become widely used in the treatment of lower extremity arterial occlusive disease. Clear advantages of these techniques, as opposed to traditional CABG or lower extremity bypass surgery, include their less invasive nature, greatly improved ease of recovery, elimination of large incisions, decreased incidence of wound complications, and greater patient acceptance. It would seem natural to presume that percutaneous angioplasty and stenting of the carotid artery would offer similar advantages as compared with traditional CEA. However, before the initial development and use of CAS, there were several concerns. First, and most important, practitioners were greatly concerned about the risk for causing a stroke during the procedure as a result of atheroembolization related to the passage of endovascular wires and catheters across the atherosclerotic plaque. Additionally, many recognized that CEA, as an open operation, is a much less invasive surgery with a much easier recovery when compared with other open surgeries such as CABG. CEA can often be performed without general anesthesia, many patients undergoing CEA are discharged the morning after the procedure, and there is often little requirement for narcotic pain medications and few restrictions from normal activities. Finally, CEA in experienced hands carries generally excellent results, with an extremely low risk for severe morbidity or mortality. These results have been demonstrated consistently over nearly 50 years in both multi-institutional trials and single-center reports. As such, some practitioners were concerned that even percutaneous treatment of carotid artery disease might not offer such a dramatic advantage over CEA.

Nevertheless, CAS has gained some acceptance by many practitioners within the past decade. Although emerging as an alternative therapy, CEA remains the standard of care. The technique itself is similar in concept to balloon angioplasty and stenting in other areas of the vascular tree. A wire is passed endoluminally across the stenotic lesion, and a self-expanding metal stent is then passed over the wire, localized to the area of the lesion, and deployed. Balloon inflation and angioplasty usually complete the procedure. The development of "cerebral protection devices," consisting of a variety of filters and balloon catheters that can be gently positioned in the distal ICA before the actual angioplasty and stent deployment at the site of the lesion, has led to a decreased concern regarding intraprocedural atheroembolization and appears to have improved the overall results of the procedure.[39] The filter-based devices function to catch particles dislodged from the atherosclerotic plaque during the placement of the stent; these particles are then extracted when the filter device is removed. The balloon type of protection device serves to stop flow in the distal ICA during the stent deployment procedure, similar to the placement of a distal surgical clamp on the artery during open CEA. The patient must be similarly monitored for the development of cerebral ischemia during the period when the carotid artery flow is stopped. The static column of blood is then suctioned from the patient and examined for any atheromatous debris before deflation of the balloon and restoration of ICA blood flow. An additional newer type of protection device involves a system to reverse flow in the ICA during the stenting procedure, preventing any atheromatous debris from traveling to the brain.[40] Although these devices have generally become a routine part of CAS procedures, they do not completely eliminate the risk for embolic stroke during the procedure.

CAS remains in its development, and there are several large randomized controlled trials comparing the outcome of the newer procedure to traditional CEA currently in progress. Two areas of controversy and unanswered questions remain: First, which patients will benefit from the endovascular procedure as opposed to open surgery? And second, is the outcome of the endovascular procedure equally as good as the traditional treatment?

Carotid stenting was initially considered most applicable to patients considered at increased risk after CEA. Two categories of patients have been considered: patients at increased risk after surgery based on a high degree of medical comorbidities, and patients at increased risk after surgery because of anatomic complexity. For example, patients with severe coronary artery disease or congestive heart failure might be considered to have an increased risk for cardiac complications after CEA. On the other hand, patients with previous neck irradiation and those in need of reoperative carotid surgery might be considered at high risk for technical complications because of the degree of scar tissue present in the neck. Unfortunately, this concept of the patient at high-risk after CEA, who would presumably benefit from an endovascular procedure, has been somewhat difficult to establish precisely. One study reviewed CEAs performed in 228 patients who would not have met the inclusion criteria for the NASCET study based on their increased risk.[41] This study was also unable to demonstrate that these so-called high-risk patients actually had inferior outcomes

after CEA. An additional study of more than 13,000 endarterectomy procedures found that cardiopulmonary comorbid features did not increase the risk for perioperative stroke, death, or cardiac events.[42] Finally, many investigators have deemed patients older than 80 years, who were ineligible for the NASCET and ACAS trials, possibly at increased risk after open surgery. However, the interim results from the lead-in phase of the Carotid Revascularization Endarterectomy versus Stent Trial (CREST), an in-progress multicenter trial, surprisingly found that the risk for periprocedural stroke and death in patients undergoing carotid stenting was greatly increased among those older than 80 years. In fact, the risk for stroke or death among 99 patients aged 80 years or older after CAS was 12.1%.[43] It is counterintuitive that those patients deemed at high risk after open surgery might be at even higher risk for complications after the less-invasive endovascular procedure, and several explanations are possible. However, the point is well taken that it is not necessarily straightforward to define which patients might benefit from CAS secondary to an innate increased risk after open surgery.

At present, it remains unclear whether the results of carotid stenting are in fact equivalent to those of CEA. A number of trials comparing the outcome of CEA to carotid stenting have been completed. The Stenting and Angioplasty with Protection in Patients at High Risk for Endarterectomy (SAPPHIRE) trial randomly compared carotid artery stenting to endarterectomy in 334 patients with coexisting conditions that potentially increased the risk after endarterectomy.[44] Analysis of 30-day and 1-year outcomes, including death, stroke, or MI, found that carotid stenting was not inferior to CEA. However, the overall results in both arms of this trial were noted to be disturbingly high, with a risk of 12.2% among stenting patients and 20.1% among endarterectomy patients.[44] The Carotid Revascularization Using Endarterectomy or Stenting Systems (CaRESS) trial was a multicenter prospective but nonrandomized study comparing the two techniques.[45] This study of 397 patients also found that the 30-day and 1-year risks for death, stroke, or MI were equivalent between patients undergoing the two procedures. The Carotid and Vertebral Artery Transluminal Angioplasty Study (CAVATAS) trial randomly assigned 504 patients to the two treatments.[46] The incidences of major stroke or death in the 30 days following the procedure did not differ significantly: 6.4% for endovascular treatment and 5.9% for surgery. At 1 year, severe carotid restenosis was noted more frequently in the endovascular group (14% versus 4%, $P < .001$). Finally, the recently reported results of the SPACE (Stent-Protected Angioplasty Versus Carotid Endarterectomy) trial, which randomly assigned 1200 patients with symptomatic carotid artery stenosis to the two treatments, found a 30-day stroke or death rate of 6.9% after stenting as compared with 6.3% after endarterectomy.[47] This study concluded that the results failed to prove the noninferiority of carotid artery stenting compared with endarterectomy, and that the results did not justify the widespread use in the short-term for the treatment of carotid artery stenosis. An additional Cochrane systematic review of this topic, which included a meta-analysis of five trials involving 1269 patients, found that no significant differences in the major risks of the treatments were found, but that the wide confidence intervals made it impossible to exclude a difference in favor of one treatment.[48] This study also concluded that there is currently insufficient evidence to support a widespread change in clinical practice away from recommending CEA as the treatment of choice for appropriate carotid artery stenosis.

In summary, although the endovascular treatment of carotid artery disease with percutaneous angioplasty and stenting has emerged as a viable alternative to CEA, its precise role remains undefined at the time of this report. CEA is a procedure with excellent results whose superiority over medical treatment alone in stroke prevention has been repeatedly demonstrated in randomized prospective trials. However, as an evolving technology, the results of CAS may be likely to improve with time. Currently, there is no absolute consensus as to precisely which patients will benefit most from either technique, or as to whether their results are absolutely equivalent. Hopefully, the continued results from randomized prospective clinical trials will help to answer these questions definitively.

Vertebrobasilar Disease

Vertebrobasilar ischemia (VBI) is far less common than carotid territory ischemia. This is primarily for the following reasons:

1. The basilar artery can be adequately supplied by either vertebral artery.
2. The posterior communicating arteries in most individuals provide excellent collaterals to the basilar artery.
3. Disease of the vertebral and basilar arteries is less prevalent.

Nonetheless, under specific circumstances, VBI can lead to incapacitating symptoms, stroke, and sudden death. Patients with VBI may describe characteristic symptoms of diplopia, ataxia, dysarthria, and drop attacks. More difficult are those with nonspecific symptoms such as dizziness or ill-described visual symptoms. The clinician needs to consider VBI in those with such symptoms if no other obvious explanation exists. If transient symptoms are brought on by head rotation or neck extension, one needs to be suspicious of vertebrobasilar insufficiency. Strokes in the distribution of the cerebellum may result in severe visual deficits and speech disorders. Brainstem strokes may be fatal and are likely underdiagnosed as a cause of sudden death.

Although emboli from the heart or aortic arch or proximal subclavian artery disease may cause symptoms, it is generally thought that most cases of VBI are due to diminished blood flow through the vessels supplying the posterior brain. To have flow-related symptoms related to the vertebrobasilar system, generally there must be both an anatomic and a physiologic component.

Anatomic Considerations

In addition to stenosis or occlusions of the basilar artery and posterior communicating arteries, VBI may result from disease of the innominate artery, the subclavian arteries, and the vertebral arteries. With respect to the latter, in general, it is necessary to have occlusive disease of both vertebral systems. To put this differently, if one has unobstructed flow from the aorta to the basilar artery on at least one side, it is unlikely that the individual will have symptoms unless the remaining vertebral artery is temporarily occluded by kinking or compression of the artery with movement of the cervical vertebra.

Insufficient blood flow to the posterior cerebral circulation may result from a number of conditions, including anatomic anomalies, atherosclerotic disease, dissections, and bony compression of the vertebral arteries as they pass through the transverse processes of C2 through C7. Anomalies of the vertebral arteries are common. In up to 10% of the population, one vertebral artery may be smaller in size, fail to communicate with the basilar artery, or be absent entirely. Arch vessel anomalies, including the origin of the left vertebral from the aortic arch, are sufficiently frequent that one needs to consider them in evaluating the posterior cerebral circulation.

Atherosclerotic disease of the vertebrobasilar system may occur at any point but is most common at the origin of the vertebral arteries. Among individuals with arterial occlusive disease, the left subclavian artery is not uncommonly affected. Disease of the subclavian arteries more commonly produces arm symptoms but occasionally may lead to VBI.

Subclavian Steal Syndrome

Occlusion of the origin of either the subclavian or innominate artery may lead to reversal of flow in the ipsilateral vertebral artery, the vertebrobasilar system essentially serving as collateral flow to the affected arm. *Subclavian steal syndrome* refers to the reversal of vertebral artery flow due to a subclavian or innominate artery occlusion, resulting in VBI. Classically, symptoms occur when arm exercise increases the "steal" of blood flow from the brainstem. The exercise reduces peripheral resistance in the affected arm, lowering the blood pressure distal to the occlusion. This in turn results in increased retrograde flow from the vertebral artery. If the contralateral vertebral artery cannot keep up with the demand, the arm may "steal" blood from the basilar artery, lowering the pressure in the posterior cerebral circulation. The result may be transient VBI. Symptoms may also result from actions that occlude the contralateral vertebral artery or any condition that might result in reduced blood pressure or cardiac output.

Physiologic Factors

Assuming that an individual has marginal blood flow to the basilar artery due to some arterial occlusive process, transient neurologic symptoms may result from some physiologic change that effectively reduces the remaining blood flow through the system. This may be the result of a cardiac event such as an arrhythmia, a fall in blood pressure, or reduced cardiac output. It may also be the result of a change in the balance of blood flow through the patent vessels. Already described is the classic subclavian steal syndrome in which the physiologic change is initiated by the arm exercise. Kinking of the unobstructed vertebral artery with head turning is another common cause of vertebrobasilar TIA. If a patient describes symptoms with turning of the head to one side or with looking up, one needs to be alert to the possibility that these actions may be causing VBI.

Diagnosis

The first step in making the diagnosis of VBI is a careful history and a physical examination. The description of dizziness, speech symptoms, double vision, ataxia, and drop attacks should lead to further investigation for disease of the posterior cerebral circulation. The finding of a bruit over the clavicle may be a sign of subclavian or vertebral artery stenosis. Decreased blood pressure in one arm is diagnostic of subclavian or innominate artery occlusive disease. The finding of a "pulse lag" or delayed peak systolic pulse in the radial artery on the same side as the reduced blood pressure is a classic finding of a proximal subclavian artery stenosis with flow reversal in the ipsilateral vertebral artery. The pulse lag is due to the increased transit time as the pulse wave passes up the contralateral vertebral and down the ipsilateral vertebral to reach the affected arm.

An MRA with gadolinium or a CT angiogram can provide useful information regarding the vessels from the aortic arch to the basilar artery. More accurate imaging of the vertebral and basilar arteries usually requires a catheter-directed cerebral angiogram. Particularly difficult is visualization of the origins of the vertebral arteries. This often requires oblique views because these vessels usually arise from the posterior aspect of the subclavian arteries and may not be clearly seen with the classic anteroposterior view. If symptoms occur only with a particular position of the head, it is likely that the portion of the vertebral artery that passes through the transverse processes is being intermittently kinked or compressed. The diagnosis may be missed unless views are obtained with the head in the position associated with the symptoms.

If the patient has anatomic findings that support the diagnosis of VBI, the next step is to examine the potential physiologic factors that may produce the symptoms. A Holter monitor and a stress test may be needed to exclude arrhythmias and myocardial insufficiency. Although an individual may have vertebrobasilar disease, if the episodes are associated only with periods of bradycardia, a pacemaker may be all that is needed to control the symptoms. Overzealous treatment with antihypertensive medications may also precipitate VBI. Finally, one must exclude other causes of nonspecific symptoms such as hypoglycemia, hypercalcemia, hypothyroidism, and other intrinsic neurologic disorders.

Indications for Surgery

Unlike carotid artery disease, there is little evidence to link asymptomatic occlusive disease of the posterior cerebral circulation with a higher risk for stroke or death. In part, this may reflect the difficulty in recognizing a death due to brainstem infarction. On the other hand, clinical observation has shown that many individuals with occlu-

sive disease of the posterior cerebral circulation remain free of symptoms and die of unrelated causes. Because 90% of the blood flow to the brain is supplied by the anterior circulation, and usually there is excellent collateral flow through the circle of Willis, occlusive disease of the subclavian and vertebral arteries appears to be well tolerated by most. At present, there is no clear indication for surgical intervention in the asymptomatic patient with basivertebral occlusive disease. The possible exception is the rare asymptomatic patient with severe and unreconstructable occlusive disease of the carotids and diseased vessels supplying the posterior cerebral circulation. Under these circumstances, surgery to improve circulation to the vertebral arteries may be justified as a means of maintaining adequate blood flow to the brain.

If an individual has symptoms suggestive of VBI and has occlusive disease of both the carotid and vertebral circulation, attention is first focused on the correction of any flow-restrictive lesions of the carotid arteries. Because most individuals have excellent collateral circulation to the basilar artery and its branches through the posterior communicating arteries of the circle of Willis, carotid blood flow is usually sufficient to supply the entire brain. Correcting a severe carotid artery stenosis is all that is needed to arrest VBI symptoms in most cases. In general, surgical or endovascular intervention is reserved for patients who meet the following criteria:

- VBI symptoms or carotid territory symptoms ipsilateral to an occluded ICA
- Demonstrable occlusive disease that effectively restricts blood flow of both vertebral systems
- Carotid arteries either free of flow-restrictive lesions or totally occluded and inoperable
- Cardiac and metabolic causes of the symptoms excluded

For patients with these criteria, the likelihood of relief of symptoms with a procedure designed to improve the posterior cerebral circulation is excellent.

Surgical Procedures for Vertebrobasilar Disease

A wide range of surgical and endovascular procedures are available for the treatment of VBI. For each patient, consideration must be given to the following:

1. The particular combination of vascular diseases causing the symptoms
2. The morbidity associated with a specific procedure to address the problem
3. The durability of the procedure

VBI due to a subclavian steal syndrome offers an excellent example of the choices that must be made by the surgeon in planning a procedure.

Subclavian Artery Stenosis or Occlusion

Innominate or right subclavian artery occlusion can be managed by a limited sternotomy and direct repair with either endarterectomy or a synthetic interposition graft. This is seldom necessary because most patients can be managed with a variety of extra-anatomic reconstructions or angioplasty, both with excellent results and lower morbidity. The proximal left subclavian artery is one of the most difficult arteries to access because of its posterior position off of the aortic arch. Direct repair of this vessel is not recommended except under extraordinary circumstances.

For individuals with primarily innominate or subclavian artery occlusive disease, percutaneous transluminal angioplasty (PTA) and stent placement have been successful in recent years. De Vries and colleagues reported 110 patients treated with PTA, with clinical success in 102 (93%).[49] There were eight significant recurrent obstructions that required further intervention to relieve recurrent symptoms. Other series have shown similar results. Durability of the reconstruction needs to be considered when choosing PTA as a treatment for arch vessel disease.

Extra-anatomic procedures have long been used for treatment of VBI due to subclavian and innominate artery disease. In general, any patent arch vessel can be used as a donor artery for this purpose. Ipsilateral carotid-subclavian bypass and transposition of the subclavian artery into the side of the adjacent carotid have both been shown to be safe and durable procedures for proximal subclavian artery occlusions. Bypasses from vessels from the opposite side of the neck can be performed if the adjacent carotid is not suitable. Contralateral carotid-subclavian bypass or contralateral subclavian-subclavian bypass grafts can be tunneled retropharyngeally to avoid passing the graft anterior to the trachea. Axilloaxillary bypass, placing the graft in the subcutaneous tissue over the sternum, may also be used to manage this problem, but has the disadvantage of being in the way should a sternotomy be necessary at a future date. Synthetic grafts are most often used for these extra-anatomic bypasses because vein grafts tend to have a higher rate of restenosis over time.

Vertebral Artery Surgery

Although the vertebral artery can be diseased at any point along its course, the most common site of an atherosclerotic lesion is at its origin from the subclavian artery. This artery is accessible from a supraclavicular incision. The scalene fat pad and lymph nodes are mobilized inferiorly from the clavicle and medially from the jugular vein. Care must be taken to avoid or ligate the thoracic duct on the left to avoid a lymph leak. Below the fat pad, the phrenic nerve is identified crossing the anterior scalene muscle. The nerve must be mobilized in order to divide the muscle. After the muscle is divided, the subclavian artery is easily identified and dissected medially. In turn, the thyrocervical trunk, the mammary artery, and the vertebral artery are dissected.

The vertebral artery stenosis can be repaired directly by patch angioplasty. An L-shaped incision is made from the subclavian artery into the vertebral artery across the area of stenosis. A piece of saphenous vein can be sewn to the arteriotomy to enlarge the opening of the vertebral artery. Endarterectomy of the vertebral artery is not advised because the plaque usually extends into the subclavian artery, making it difficult to limit the extent of the endarterectomy.

Other operations that have been successful for managing proximal vertebral artery stenosis include transection and transposition of the vertebral artery to the side of the adjacent carotid artery or to a more distal point on the subclavian, and a bypass from one of these two vessels to the vertebral using a segment of saphenous vein.

If the vertebral artery is diseased in the V2 segment or the portion of the vertebral artery that passes through the transverse processes of C6 to C2, it is best to reconstruct the vertebral artery with a bypass from the carotid or subclavian artery to the segment of the vertebral artery between C1 and C2. Dr. Ramon Berguer, who first described this procedure, reports excellent results in selected patients.[50]

Although balloon angioplasty and stenting of the vertebral arteries has been described, the numbers of procedures performed is low, and the results have been mixed. At the time of writing this chapter, there are insufficient data to say whether angioplasty will be an important adjunct to the treatment of patients with VBI due to vertebral and basilar artery lesions.

Selected References

Coward LJ, Featherstone RL, Brown MM: Safety and efficacy of endovascular treatment of carotid artery stenosis compared with carotid endarterectomy: A Cochrane systematic review of the randomized evidence. Stroke 36:905-911, 2005.

> A recent meta-analysis of the existing trials comparing carotid angioplasty and stenting to carotid endarterectomy reported at the time of the writing of this chapter. Although the study did not find evidence for significant differences in the outcomes of the two procedures, it concluded that there is insufficient evidence to support a widespread change in clinical practice away from recommending carotid endarterectomy as the treatment of choice for appropriate carotid artery stenosis.

Executive Committee for the Asymptomatic Carotid Atherosclerosis Study: Endarterectomy for asymptomatic carotid artery stenosis. JAMA 273:1421-1428, 1995.

> The landmark multicenter randomized prospective trial comparing carotid endarterectomy to best medical therapy with regard to stroke prevention in patients with high-grade carotid artery stenosis who had never experienced TIAs or prior stroke. The study demonstrated the superiority of surgical treatment consisting of carotid endarterectomy to optimal medical management.

North American Symptomatic Carotid Endarterectomy Trial Collaborators: Beneficial effects of carotid endarterectomy in symptomatic patients with high-grade stenosis. N Engl J Med 325:445-453, 1991.

> The landmark multicenter randomized prospective trial comparing carotid endarterectomy to best medical therapy with regard to stroke prevention in patients with high-grade carotid artery stenosis who had already experienced prior TIA or stroke. The study demonstrated the superiority of surgery over best medical management in these patients, and confirmed the high risk for recurrent cerebrovascular events in patients with carotid stenosis who have already experienced an initial TIA or stroke.

Riles TS, Imparato AM, Jacobowitz GR, et al: The cause of perioperative stroke after carotid endarterectomy. J Vasc Surg 19:206-216, 1994.

An in-depth analysis of the causes of perioperative strokes after carotid endarterectomy from review of nearly 2500 consecutive cases. This study was notable for proving that most perioperative strokes following carotid surgery are related to technical imperfections at the site of the endarterectomy, establishing the need for absolute technical perfection in the performance of the surgery to ensure optimal results, and obtaining the best risk-to-benefit ratio with the performance of the surgery.

Zarins CK, Giddens DP, Bharadvaj BK, et al: Carotid bifurcation atherosclerosis: Quantitative correlation of plaque localization with flow velocity profiles and wall shear stress. Circ Res 53:502-514, 1983.

An in-depth analysis of 12 adult carotid artery bifurcations obtained from autopsy specimens. This study concludes that in the human carotid bifurcation, regions of moderate to high shear stress, where flow remains unidirectional and axially aligned, are relatively spared of intimal thickening. Intimal thickening and atherosclerosis develop largely in regions of relatively low wall shear stress, flow separation, and departure from axially aligned, unidirectional flow.

References

1. Rockman CB, Jacobowitz GR, Gagne PJ, et al: Focused screening for occult carotid artery disease: Patients with known heart disease are at high risk. J Vasc Surg 39:44-51, 2004.
2. Clark WM, Wissman S, Albers GW, et al: Recombinant tissue-type plasminogen activator (Alteplase) for ischemic stroke 3 to 5 hours after symptom onset. The ATLANTIS Study: A randomized controlled trial. Alteplase for acute noninterventional therapy in ischemic stroke. JAMA 282:2019-2026, 1999.
3. Executive Committee for the Asymptomatic Carotid Atherosclerosis Study: Endarterectomy for asymptomatic carotid artery stenosis. JAMA 273:1421-1428, 1995.
4. Fine-Edelstein JS, Wolf PA, O'Leary DH, et al: Precursors of extracranial carotid atherosclerosis in the Framingham Study. Neurology 44:1046-1050, 1994.
5. Mathiesen EB, Joakimsen O, Boaa KH, et al: Prevalence of and risk factors associated with carotid artery stenosis: The Tromso Study. Cerebrovasc Dis 12:44-51, 2001.
6. Bogousslavsky J, Regli F, Van Melle G: Risk factors and concomitants of internal carotid artery occlusion of stenosis: A controlled study of 159 cases. Arch Neurol 42:864-867, 1985.
7. Simos PCG, Algra A, Eikelboom BC, et al, for the SMART Study Group: Carotid artery stenosis in patients with peripheral arterial disease: The SMART study. J Vasc Surg 30:519-525, 1999.
8. Zarins CK, Giddens DP, Bharadvaj BK, et al: Carotid bifurcation atherosclerosis: Quantitative correlation of plaque localization with flow velocity profiles and wall shear stress. Circ Res 53:502-514, 1983.
9. North American Symptomatic Carotid Endarterectomy Trial Collaborators: Beneficial effects of carotid endarterectomy in symptomatic patients with high-grade stenosis. N Engl J Med 325:445-453, 1991.
10. Barnett HJM, Taylor DW, Eliasziw M, et al: Benefit of carotid endarterectomy in patients with symptomatic moderate or severe stenosis. North American Symptomatic Carotid Endarterectomy Trial Collaborators. N Engl J Med 339:1415-1425, 1998.
11. Riles TS, Fisher FS, Lamparello PJ, et al: Immediate and long-term results of carotid endarterectomy for asymptomatic high-grade stenosis. Ann Vasc Surg 8:144-149, 1994.
12. Gasecki AP, Eliasziw M, Ferguson GG, et al: Long-term prognosis and effect of endarterectomy in patients with symptomatic severe carotid stenosis and contralateral carotid stenosis or occlusion: Results from North American Symptomatic Carotid Endarterectomy Trial (NASCET) Group. J Neurosurg 83:778-782, 1995.
13. Eliasziw M, Streifler JY, Fox AJ, et al: Significance of plaque ulceration in symptomatic patients with high-grade carotid stenosis. North American Symptomatic Carotid Endarterectomy Trial. Stroke 25:304-308, 1994.
14. Taylor DC, Strandness DE Jr: Carotid artery duplex scanning. J Clin Ultrasound 15:635-644, 1987.
15. Taylor DW, Barnett HJM, Haynes RB, et al: Low-dose and high-dose acetylsalicylic acid for patients undergoing carotid endarterectomy: A randomized controlled Trial. ASA and Carotid Endarterectomy (ACE) Trial Collaborators. Lancet 353:2179-2184, 1999.
16. Rockman CB, Riles TS, Gold M, et al: A comparison of regional and general anesthesia in patients undergoing carotid endarterectomy. J Vasc Surg 24:946-956, 1996.
17. Rockman CB, Su W, Lamparello PJ, et al: A reassessment of carotid endarterectomy in the face of contralateral carotid occlusion: Surgical results in symptomatic and asymptomatic patients. J Vasc Surg 36:668-673, 2002.
18. Halm EA, Hannan EL, Rojas M, et al: Clinical and operative predictors of outcomes of carotid endarterectomy. J Vasc Surg 42:420-428, 2005.
19. Archie JP Jr: The geometry and mechanics of saphenous vein patch angioplasty after carotid endarterectomy. Tex Heart Inst J 14:396-400, 1987.
20. Ferguson GG, Eliasziw M, Barr HW, et al: The North American Symptomatic Carotid Endarterectomy Trial: Surgical results in 1415 patients. Stroke 30:1751-1758, 1999.
21. Riles TS, Imparato AM, Jacobowitz GR, et al: The cause of perioperative stroke after carotid endarterectomy. J Vasc Surg 19:206-216, 1994.
22. Rockman CB, Jacobowitz GR, Riles TS, et al: Immediate re-exploration for the perioperative neurologic event following carotid endarterectomy: Is it worthwhile? J Vasc Surg 32:1062-1070, 2000.
23. Rockman C, Riles TS: Nonstroke complications of carotid endarterectomy. In Towne JB, Hollier LH (eds): Complications in Vascular Surgery, 2nd ed. New York, Marcel Dekker, 2004, pp 475-482.
24. Pomposelli FB, Lamparello PJ, Riles TS, et al: Intracranial hemorrhage after CEA. J Vasc Surg 7:248-255, 1988.
25. Ouriel K, Shortell CK, Illig KA, et al: Intracerebral hemorrhage after carotid endarterectomy: Incidence, contribution to neurologic morbidity, and predictive factors. J Vasc Surg 29:82-89, 1999.
26. Archie JP: Carotid endarterectomy saphenous vein patch rupture revisited: Selective use on the basis of vein diameter. J Vasc Surg 24:346-352, 1996.
27. Treiman RL, Cossman DV, Foran RF, et al: The influence of neutralizing heparin after carotid endarterectomy on postoperative stroke and wound hematoma. J Vasc Surg 12:440-446, 1990.
28. Rockman CB, Wu WT, Domenig C, et al: Postoperative infection associated with polyester patch angioplasty following carotid endarterectomy. J Vasc Surg 38:251-256, 2003.
29. Nowak LR, Corson JD: Blood pressure instability after carotid endarterectomy. In Ernst CB, Stanley JD (eds):

Current Therapy in Vascular Surgery, 4th ed. St. Louis, Mosby, 2001, pp 71-73.

30. Clouse WD, Brewster DC: Cardiopulmonary complications related to vascular surgery. In Towne JB, Hollier LH (eds): Complications in Vascular Surgery, 2nd ed. New York, Marcel Dekker, 2004, pp 15-48.

31. Rockman CB, Riles TS, Landis, et al: Redo carotid surgery: An analysis of materials and configurations used in carotid reoperations and their influence on perioperative stroke and subsequent recurrent stenosis. J Vasc Surg 29:72-81, 1999.

32. Biller J, Feinberg WM, Castaldo JE, et al: Guidelines for carotid endarterectomy: A statement for healthcare professionals from a special writing group of the Stroke Council, American Heart Association. Stroke 29:554-562, 1998.

33. Rockman CB, Maldonado TS, Jacobowitz GR, et al: Early carotid endarterectomy in symptomatic patients is associated with poorer perioperative outcomes. J Vasc Surg 44:480-487, 2006.

34. Wylie EJ, Hein MF, Adams JE: Intracranial hemorrhage following surgical revascularization for treatment of acute strokes. J Neurosurg 21:212-216, 1964.

35. Gasecki AP, Ferguson GG, Eliasziw M, et al: Early endarterectomy for severe stenosis after a nondisabling stroke: Results from the North American Symptomatic Carotid Endarterectomy Trial. J Vasc Surg 20:288-295, 1994.

36. European Carotid Surgery Trialists' Collaborative Group. MRC European Carotid Surgery Trial. Interim results for symptomatic patients with severe (70-99%) or with mild (0-29%) carotid stenosis. Lancet 337:1235-1243, 1991.

37. Ricotta JJ, Faggioli GL, Castilone A, et al: Risk factors for stroke after cardiac surgery: Buffalo Cardiac-Cerebral Study Group. J Vasc Surg 21:359-364, 1995.

38. Ricotta JJ, Wall LP, Blackstone E: The influence of concurrent carotid endarterectomy on coronary bypass: A case-controlled study. J Vasc Surg 41:397-401, 2005.

39. Ohki T, Veith FJ, Grenell S, et al: Initial experience with cerebral protection devices to prevent embolization during carotid artery stenting. J Vasc Surg 36:1175-1185, 2002.

40. Parodi JC, Ferreira LM, Sicard G, et al: Cerebral protection during carotid stenting using flow reversal. J Vasc Surg 41:416-422, 2005.

41. Gasparis AP, Ricotta L, Cuadra SA, et al: High-risk carotid endarterectomy: Fact or fiction. J Vasc Surg 37:40-46, 2003.

42. Stoner MC, Abbott WM, Wong DR, et al: Defining the high-risk patient for carotid endarterectomy: An analysis of the prospective national Surgical Quality Improvement Program database. J Vasc Surg 43:285-296, 2006.

43. Hobson RW II, Howard VJ, Roubin GS, et al: Carotid artery stenting is associated with increased complications in octogenarians: 30-Day stroke and death rates in the CREST lead-in phase. J Vasc Surg 40:1106-1111, 2004.

44. Yadav JS, Wholey MH, Kuntz RE, et al, for the Stenting and Angioplasty with Protection in Patients at High Risk for Endarterectomy (SAPPHIRE) Investigators: Protected carotid-artery stenting versus endarterectomy in high-risk patients. N Engl J Med 351:1493-1501, 2004.

45. Carotid Revascularization Using Endarterectomy or Stenting Systems (CaRESS) Steering Committee: Carotid Revascularization Using Endarterectomy of Stenting Systems (CaRESS) phase I clinical trial: 1-Year results. J Vasc Surg 42:213-219, 2005.

46. Anonymous: Endovascular versus surgical treatment in patients with carotid stenosis in the Carotid and Vertebral Artery Transluminal Angioplasty Study (CAVATAS): A randomized trial. Lancet 357:1729-1737, 2001.

47. The SPACE Collaborative Group: 30-Day results from the SPACE trial of stent-protected angioplasty versus carotid endarterectomy in symptomatic patients: A randomized non-inferiority trial. Lancet 368:1239-1247, 2006.

48. Coward LJ, Featherstone RL, Brown MM: Safety and efficacy of endovascular treatment of carotid artery stenosis compared with carotid endarterectomy: A Cochrane systematic review of the randomized evidence. Stroke 36:905-911, 2005.

49. DeVries JP, Jager LC, Van Den Berg JC, et al: Durability of percutaneous transluminal angioplasty for obstructive lesions of the proximal subclavian artery: Long-term results. J Vasc Surg 41:19-23, 2005.

50. Berguer R: Distal vertebral artery bypass: Technique, the "occipital connection," and potential uses. J Vasc Surg 2(4):621-626, 1985.

CHAPTER 65

Aneurysmal Vascular Disease

Peter Gloviczki, MD   and   Joseph J. Ricotta, II, MD

The term *aneurysm* is derived from the Greek word *aneurysma* which means "widening" and can be defined as a permanent and irreversible localized dilation of a blood vessel, having at least a 50% increase in diameter compared with the expected normal diameter.[1] *Ectasia* is defined as a dilation less than 50% of the normal diameter. Normal diameter of the aorta and the arteries depends on age, gender, body size, and other factors. In men, the infrarenal aorta is normally between 14 and 24 mm, and in women, it is between 12 and 21 mm. Therefore, an abdominal aortic aneurysm (AAA) is diagnosed if the diameter is 3 cm or larger in a man or 2.6 cm or larger in a woman.

Aneurysms can develop at any location in the arterial tree but are most commonly located in the aorta, followed by the iliac, popliteal, and femoral arteries in decreasing order of frequency. Aneurysms can also develop in the innominate, subclavian, and carotid arteries; in arteries of the upper extremities; and in visceral and renal arteries. Intracranial aneurysms and those

affecting veins are not considered in this chapter, whereas thoracic and thoracoabdominal aortic aneurysms are discussed in a separate chapter in this volume.

HISTORICAL BACKGROUND

Arterial aneurysms have been recognized since ancient times. The Ebers Papyrus, a text from 2000 BC, contains a description of traumatic aneurysms of the peripheral arteries. Antyllus performed the first elective operation for treatment of an aneurysm in the 2nd century AD. He described ligation of the artery above and below the aneurysm, then incising the aneurysm sac and evacuating its contents. This description of aneurysm repair remained the basis of direct arterial operations for the next 1500 years. Hunter performed perhaps the most famous operation for an arterial aneurysm. In 1785, he treated a coachman with a pulsatile mass in the popliteal fossa, likely secondary to repetitive trauma against the coach seat. The patient also had claudication from arterial occlusion distal to the aneurysm, and Hunter concluded that collateral arteries had developed around the occlusion. Standard treatment at that time included amputation, but Hunter incised the medial thigh above the knee at a location now referred to as "Hunter's canal" and ligated the artery with four sutures. The patient survived, and Hunter went on to perform four similar operations. Hunter's most acclaimed disciple was Sir Astley Cooper, who was the first to repair a ruptured iliac artery aneurysm in 1817. His patient unfortunately died 2 days after an aortic ligation. Cooper also reported the first primary aortoenteric fistula and called attention to multiple aneurysms. In the late 1800s, Halsted first repaired successfully a subclavian aneurysm by proximal ligation in the chest. Matas, a legendary New Orleans surgeon, introduced the technique of endoaneurysmorrhaphy in 1906, which involved clamping above and below the aneurysm, opening it, ligating branches from within, and buttressing the wall with imbricating sutures. Matas performed the first successful proximal ligation of an aortic aneurysm in 1923, 106 years after Cooper's historic operation.

Modern vascular surgery was established by experiments of Carrell and Guthrie who developed techniques of successful vascular anastomoses in animals, a work for which Alexis Carrell won the Nobel Prize in 1912. It was not until 1951, however, that Charles Dubost performed the first successful replacement of an AAA using the retroperitoneal approach with a freeze-dried thoracic aortic homograft. In 1953, DeBakey and Cooley reported survival of five of six patients operated on for replacement of AAAs. In the same year, Bahnson from Johns Hopkins reported the first repair of a ruptured aortic aneurysm. Also in 1953, Vorhees introduced a prosthetic cloth graft for aortic replacement, whereas DeBakey used knitted Dacron in 1957. The first successful repair of a thoracoabdominal aortic aneurysm was described by Etheredge in 1955, followed by four cases in 1956 by DeBakey and colleagues. Throughout the 1960s, 1970s, and 1980s, Crawford perfected the treatment of thoracoabdominal aneurysms, and his contributions greatly reduced the risks associated with complex aortic surgery. In 1980, Williams and Ricotta described the extended retroperitoneal approach to the visceral aorta to treat aortic aneurysms. In 1988, Hollier reported excellent results using cerebrospinal fluid drainage to decrease paraplegia for thoracoabdominal aortic aneurysms.

Endovascular aortic aneurysm repair (EVAR) dates back to 1991 when Juan Parodi introduced this revolutionary treatment of AAA.[2] The technique involved transfemoral endovascular placement of a stented prosthesis into the aorta to exclude the aneurysm from circulation. EVAR offers the advantage of reduced morbidity by avoiding direct transabdominal or, in patients with thoracic aneurysm, transthoracic surgical exposure. The technique of EVAR has been continuously perfected during the past 2 decades, and currently in the United States, there are four devices approved by the U.S. Food and Drug Administration for AAA repair and one device approved for thoracic aneurysm repair.

CLASSIFICATION

Aneurysms are classified into two main groups: *true* and *false* aneurysms. In true aneurysms, all three layers of the vessel wall are involved, whereas false aneurysms or pseudoaneurysms do not have all three layers of a vessel wall. Aneurysms are also distinguished by both morphology and etiology. The most common aneurysms are spindle-shaped *fusiform* aneurysms, with symmetrical enlargement involving the whole circumference of the artery. Aneurysms that affect only part of the arterial circumference are termed *saccular*. These eccentric aneurysms are believed to have a higher risk for rupture than fusiform aneurysms.

Based on etiology, aneurysms most commonly distinguished are *degenerative* aneurysms, caused by athero-sclerotic changes in the vessel wall. The pathogenesis of aneurysms, as discussed later, is a multifactorial process involving genetic predisposition, aging, atherosclerosis, inflammation, and localized proteolytic enzyme activation. *Congenital* aneurysms and those associated with arteritides and connective tissue disorder are rare. Infected (mycotic) aneurysms are somewhat more common, and they frequently present as false aneurysms. Aneurysms may also occur with wall weakness caused by aortic or arterial dissection. Dissections lead to separation of the layers of the arterial wall due to a tear in the intima and varying thickness of the media. The term *dissecting aneurysm* is applied to dissections with aneurysmal dilation of the false lumen.

Aneurysmal enlargement can also result from post-stenotic dilation of an artery such as in the subclavian artery in patients with thoracic outlet syndrome or in aortic coarctation. Additional types of aneurysms include those associated with pregnancy and childhood. Etiologies of pseudoaneurysms include blunt or penetrating trauma, iatrogenic injury during arterial catheterization, and arterial graft anastomotic disruption.

The most frequent site of extracranial arterial aneurysms is the infrarenal aorta. In one large autopsy series of patients with aortoiliac aneurysms, the most frequent location was the abdominal aorta alone (65%), followed by the thoracic aorta alone (19%), the abdominal aorta and iliac arteries (13%), the thoracoabdominal aorta (2%) and iliac arteries alone (1%).[3] Peripheral arterial aneurysms are much less common. Popliteal aneurysms account for about 70% of all peripheral aneurysms, femoral aneurysms are less frequent, and carotids constitute less than 4%. Visceral (splanchnic) and renal artery aneurysms have been considered rare, although their reported incidence due to frequent abdominal imaging has increased recently.

Aneurysm size is described by their width (anteroposterior or lateral diameter) and by their length. It is the width of the aneurysm and not the length that is the most important predicting factor of rupture. *Arteriomegaly,* originally described by Leriche in 1943, refers to diffuse arterial enlargement without discrete aneurysm formation, involving several segments of the arterial tree including the aorta and the iliac, femoral, and popliteal arteries. Arteries that are normally not prone to develop aneurysm, such as the external iliac and profunda femoris artery, are frequently dilated as well. In nearly 6000 patients who underwent aortofemoral arteriography at the Mayo Clinic, arteriomegaly was found in 5%.[4] Three patterns were identified: type I, with aneurysms of the aorta to common femoral artery with more distal arteriomegaly; type II, with aneurysms of the femoropopliteal segment and more proximal arteriomegaly; and type III, with aneurysms of the aorta to popliteal artery with arteriomegaly of the intervening nonaneurysmal segments. Only males were affected, and they were about 5 years younger than the average-age patient with solitary aneurysms. This condition was distinct from multiple aneurysms that are separated by normal-diameter, nonectatic arterial segments, a condition often termed *aneurysmosis.* Gloviczki and associates reported on 102 patients with

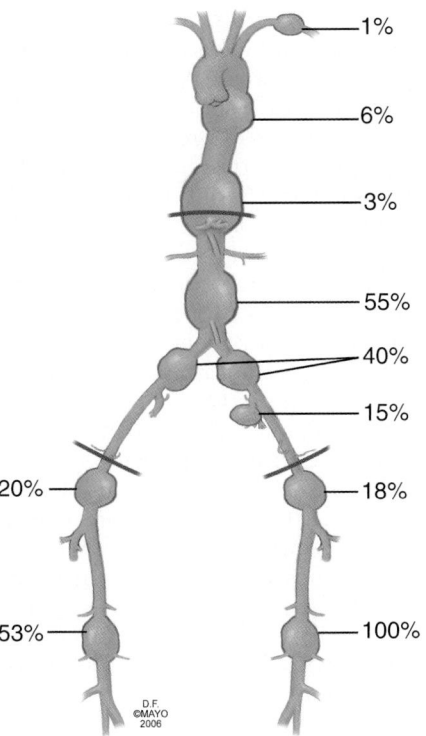

Figure 65-1 Prevalence of aneurysms in 368 patients with popliteal artery aneurysms. (From Huang Y, Gloviczki P, Noel AA, et al: Early complications and long-term outcome after open surgical treatment of popliteal artery aneurysms: Is exclusion with saphenous vein by-pass still the gold standard? J Vasc Surg 45:706-715, 2007. By permission of Mayo Foundation for Medical Education and Research. All rights reserved.)

multiple aortic aneurysms who underwent 201 aortic reconstructions.[5] Aneurysmosis was present in 3.4% of patients with aortic aneurysms, of whom 75% were men. Smoking history and abnormal electrocardiogram changes were present in 84%, hypertension in 75%, and obstructive lung disease in 61%. Eighteen percent with descending thoracic aortic aneurysms required surgical treatment of a second aortic aneurysm. In a population-based study by Bickerstaff and associates, 25% of patients with thoracic aneurysms had AAA.[6] Patients with AAAs have a proclivity for lower extremity aneurysms. In a review of nearly 1500 patients with aortoiliac aneurysms, 3.5%, all men, had aneurysms in the femoral, popliteal, or visceral arteries. The likelihood of detecting an AAA in a man with a femoral artery aneurysm was 92%, and it was 64% for men with a popliteal artery aneurysm.[7] In a recent Mayo Clinic review that included 141 (47%) unilateral and 158 (53%) bilateral popliteal artery aneurysms, AAA was present in 55% of patients, more frequently in those with bilateral than with unilateral popliteal artery aneurysms[8] (65% versus 43%; Fig. 65-1).

PATHOGENESIS

The pathogenesis of aneurysm formation is complex. Several theories have been proposed, but no single theory has been universally accepted. More than 90% of aneurysms are associated with atherosclerosis, which has traditionally been considered the primary cause. However, most patients (75%) with aneurysmal disease do not have occlusive vascular disease involving the aortoiliofemoral segments. In addition, induction of aneurysms in animals fed an atherogenic diet has not been predictable, yet regression of experimental atheromas has actually led to aneurysm formation in monkeys. These findings, as well as others, have led investigators to conclude that atherosclerosis is either a coincidental finding or a facilitating process rather than a primary cause of aneurysm formation. Rather than being termed *atherosclerotic*, AAAs are more accurately referred to as *degenerative*. Interaction of multiple factors rather than a single process is responsible for the destruction of the media of the aortic wall that leads to aneurysm formation.

The development of AAAs is associated with alterations in the connective tissue of the aortic wall. The normal aortic wall is made up of lamellar units that consist of elastin, collagen (mainly types I and III), and vascular smooth muscle cells. Elastin and collagen are the major structural components and act in a complementary fashion. Elastin fibers are most abundant in the media and are thought to be the main load-bearing component under most physiologic conditions and to provide elastic recoil. Collagen provides tensile strength; it helps maintain the structural integrity of the wall and acts as a "safety net," acquiring load-bearing functions at higher pressures or when elastin fails. Histologically, the aneurysm wall is thinned, with a marked decrease in the amount of medial elastin. Biochemical studies have shown decreased quantities of both elastin and collagen in the aneurysm wall, but an increased ratio of collagen to elastin.[9] Elastin fragmentation is the initial structural event, and elastin depletion is completed early in aneurysm formation. Aneurysms elongate as they enlarge, causing them to become bowed and tortuous. It is believed that the weakening and fragmentation of elastin is responsible for this elongation and tortuosity. Although elastin fragmentation is the most important characteristic of the wall of an aneurysm, the adventitial tissue, in which collagen is predominant, is responsible for the resistance of the aorta in the absence of medial elastin. Experimental studies demonstrated that enzymatic treatment with elastase leads to arterial dilation and stiffening at physiologic pressures, whereas treatment with collagenase leads to arterial rupture without dilation.[9] This suggests that elastin degradation is a key step in the development of aneurysms, but that collagen degradation is ultimately required for aneurysm rupture. Interestingly, there are fewer lamellar units in the abdominal aorta than the thoracic aorta, and there is even a further abrupt decrease in the number of lamellar units below the renal arteries. This relative paucity of elastin and collagen is thought to play a role, among other factors, in the predilection for aneurysm development in the infrarenal aorta. In addition, elastin is not synthesized in the adult aorta and has a half-life of 40 to 70 years, accounting for its reduction with age and the occurrence of AAAs in elderly patients.

Proteolytic enzymes have also been shown to play a role in aneurysm formation. There is increased expression and activity of matrix metalloproteinases (MMPs) in the wall of aortic aneurysms. Studies suggest that MMPs and other proteinases derived from macrophages and aortic smooth muscle cells are secreted into the extracellular matrix and are integral to aneurysm formation.[10] In AAAs, MMP activation favors elastin and collagen degradation. Interstitial collagen degradation accompanies increased expression of collagenases MMP-1 and MMP-13 in AAAs in humans. Elastases MMP-2, MMP-9, and MMP-12 also have an increased expression in aneurysmal aortic tissue.[11] MMP-12 is highly expressed along the proximal leading edge of AAAs in humans and may be important in aneurysm formation. MMP-2 is found in high concentrations in small aneurysmal aortas, suggesting a role during early aneurysm formation. MMP-9 is found in abundance in medial smooth muscle cells, and increased levels have been found in the aortic wall and serum in up to half of patients with aortic aneurysms, but not in those with aortic occlusive disease.[11] Interestingly, these increased serum levels return to normal after aneurysm repair. MMP-9 has also been found to have a threefold higher activity in aneurysms 5 to 7 cm in diameter compared with aneurysms smaller than 5 cm, consistent with the increased expansion rates observed for larger AAAs. The important role that MMP-9 plays in aneurysm formation is reinforced by the observation that MMP-9 knockout mice do not form experimental aneurysms. Wild-type bone marrow transplantation, however, restores the aneurysm phenotype. In addition, the expression of tissue inhibitors of MMPs (TIMPs) has been found to be decreased in the wall of aneurysms, thereby promoting overexpression of MMPs and consequently elastin and collagen degradation. Another protease inhibitor, α_1-antitrypsin, has been shown to be deficient in aortic aneurysms. This may explain the association of AAA ruptures with chronic obstructive pulmonary disease (emphysema patients with reduced α_1-antitrypsin levels). Based on this information, it can be concluded that during aortic aneurysm formation, the balance of vessel wall remodeling between MMPs, TIMPS, and other protease inhibitors favors elastin and collagen degradation.

Another prominent histologic feature of aortic aneurysms is the presence of an inflammatory infiltrate with a preponderance of plasma cells in the media and T cells in the adventitia. It is hypothesized that these cells subsequently release a cascade of cytokines that result in the activation of many different proteases. Exposed elastin degradation products may serve as a chemotactic agent for infiltrating macrophages. The concept that aneurysm formation is autoimmune is supported by the extensive lymphocytic and monocytic infiltrate in the media and adventitia, and deposition of immunoglobulin G (IgG) in the aortic wall. Macrophage- and lymphocyte-generated cytokines are increased in the wall of an aortic aneurysm. These inflammatory cytokines induce the expression and activation of MMPs and TIMPs. An infectious cause of aneurysm formation has also been suggested. As many as 55% of aortic aneurysms demonstrate *Chlamydia pneumoniae* by immunohistochemistry. *Chlamydia* has been shown to induce AAA in rabbits. Reactive oxygen species such as superoxide (O_2^-) also have been shown to be increased in human AAAs. Elastase infusion in animal models has been shown to increase nitric oxide synthase expression and decrease the expression of the antioxidant, superoxide dismutase. O_2^- levels in human aneurysmal tissue are 2.5-fold higher than adjacent nonaneurysmal aortic tissue and 10-fold higher than control aorta.

There is also considerable evidence that genetics play a role in aortic aneurysm formation. Familial clustering occurs in 15% to 25% of patients undergoing AAA repair. Inheritance patterns of autosomal dominant, autosomal recessive, and X chromosome linked have all been shown. Female siblings are at particularly high risk. Familial aneurysms do not appear to be anatomically or clinically distinguishable from those with no familial pattern, except that they develop earlier in life, have a decreased male-to-female ratio of 2:1 (more female prevalence), and appear to have a higher risk for aneurysm rupture. Specific genetic abnormalities that have been reported include decreased type III collagen in the aortic media of familial aneurysms, polymorphisms on the gene for pro–α chain of type III collagen and the Hp-2-1 haptoglobin allele, and deficiencies in α_1-antitrypsin. In addition, a deficiency in the copper-containing enzyme lysyl oxidase has been proved to cause aortic aneurysms in mice. Lysyl oxidase is important in collagen and elastin cross-linking and is sex chromosome linked. Genetic defects have also been linked to aneurysm formation in patients with Marfan syndrome (fibrillin gene on chromosome 15) and in patients with Ehlers-Danlos type 4 (COL3A1-procollagen type III gene).[12] The clinical implications of these genetic studies strongly support the screening of first-degree relatives of patients with aortic aneurysms. Genetic screening of patients at high risk for AAA will likely be available in the future.

Once an aneurysm develops, regardless of the cause, its enlargement is governed by physical principles, in particular the law of Laplace. Laplace's law, T = PR, describes the relationship between tangential stress (T) tending to disrupt the wall of a sphere, the radius (R), and the transmural pressure (P). Thus, for a given transmural pressure, the wall tension is proportionate to the radius. This explains why once dilation of the aorta has occurred, aortic enlargement is enhanced, and therefore large aneurysms are more prone to rupture than small ones. In addition, it explains why hypertension is an important risk factor for aneurysm rupture. Laplace's law, however, does not take into account wall thickness. Incorporating wall thickness (δ) into the equation now yields T = PR/δ. The tension within the arterial wall becomes greater when the pressure within the aneurysm increases, the radius of the aneurysm increases, or the thickness of the aortic wall decreases.

The pathogenesis of degenerative aortic aneurysms is multifactorial involving disordered remodeling of the extracellular matrix, activation of proteolytic enzymes, chronic inflammation, genetic predisposition, and biomechanical wall stress. Degenerative aneurysms account for more than 90% of AAAs. Less frequent causes include

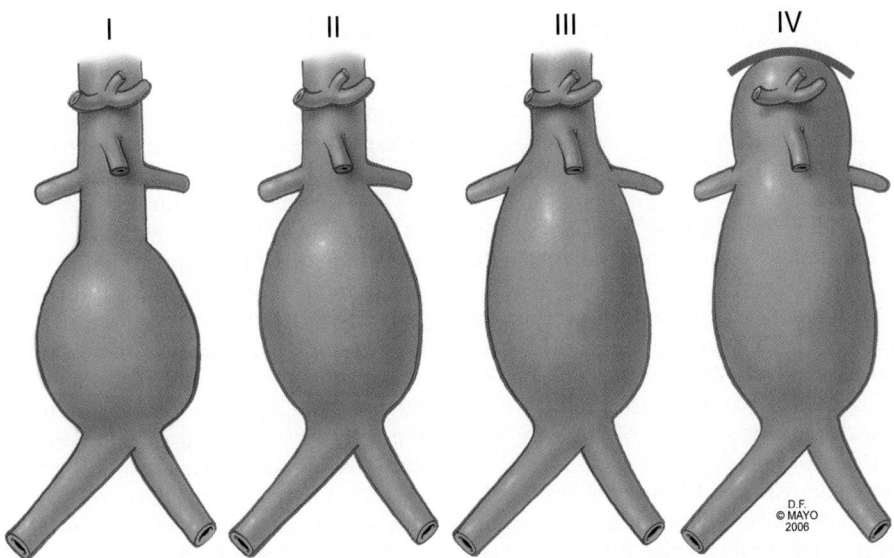

Figure 65-2 Classification of abdominal aortic aneurysms: infrarenal (I), juxtarenal (II), pararenal (III), and suprarenal (IV). (By permission of Mayo Foundation for Medical Education and Research. All rights reserved.)

infection, arteritis, cystic medial necrosis, trauma, inherited connective tissue disorders, and pseudoaneurysm from anastomotic disruption. Aortic aneurysms are rare in children and young adults and are of diverse etiologies, the most common of which is tuberous sclerosis, Behçet disease, Marfan syndrome, Ehlers-Danlos syndrome, and infection from umbilical artery catheters.

ABDOMINAL AORTIC ANEURYSMS

Epidemiology

Aortic aneurysms are most commonly located in the infrarenal aorta, and the segment immediately below the renal arteries is usually spared (Fig. 65-2). Aneurysms involving the immediate infrarenal segment are known as juxtarenal AAAs, whereas those involving the origin of the renal arteries are called *pararenal AAAs.* Suprarenal aneurysms extend above the renal arteries and correspond with the type IV thoracoabdominal aneurysm in Crawford's classification because these patients usually require thoracoabdominal approach for repair. The iliac arteries are involved in 40% of patients with AAAs. In 90% of these, the common iliac arteries are affected, whereas 10% involve the internal iliac arteries.

Aneurysms of the abdominal aorta are common. It is estimated that 1.7 million people have AAAs, 190,000 new cases are diagnosed each year, and more than 50,000 repairs are performed annually in the United States. The reported incidence has tripled since 1970, in part because of the aging of the population and the more frequent use of diagnostic screening modalities, but also because of an increase in the number of new cases. Large autopsy studies have demonstrated the prevalence of AAAs to be between 1.8% and 6.6%. It is estimated now that in the United States, between 3.5 and 6.6 per 1000 people have AAAs.[13,14]

Risk Factors

Although the exact cause is not known, multiple risk factors have been identified to contribute to the development of AAAs. The most important risk factors are age, gender, race, tobacco use, and a family history of aneurysmal disease.

The prevalence of AAAs increases with age. The frequency of aneurysms increases steadily in men older than 55 years, reaching a peak of 6% at 80 to 85 years. In women, there is a continuous increase after 70 years of age, reaching a peak at 4.5% at older than 90 years. The male:female ratio is 4:1 to 5:1 in the 60 to 70 year age group, but beyond age 80 it approaches 1:1.[15]

Male gender is an independent risk factor for AAA formation. In one large autopsy study from Sweden, the prevalence of AAAs was 4.3% in men and 2.1% in women. In a Veteran's Administration (VA) screening study of patients 50 to 79 years of age, a total of 122,272 men and 3450 women were screened for AAAs. The prevalence of AAAs 3 cm or larger was 4.3% in men and 1.0% in women.[16] More recently, Lederle and coworkers reported that AAAs are found in 4% to 8% of elderly men and 0.5% to 1.5% of elderly women.[15] In the Aneurysm Detection and Management (ADAM) study, women were six to eight times less likely to develop an AAA (odds ratio, 0.12-0.18).[14]

AAA is primarily a disease of elderly white men. White males are two to three times more likely to develop AAA than black males. The black race, much like the female gender, is considered a negative risk factor for AAA development (odds ratio, 0.53).[15]

Smoking is associated with 78% of AAAs, and there is an 8:1 preponderance of aneurysms in smokers compared with nonsmokers.[14] In the ADAM study, smoking was the risk factor most strongly associated with AAA formation and was associated with 75% of all AAAs 4.0 cm or larger. The prevalence of aneurysm formation is increased with tobacco smoking and is further increased with duration of smoking.[14,16] After the cessation of smoking, there is a slow decline in the risk for developing an AAA. The relative risk for death from AAA rupture is increased 4.6-fold for cigarette smokers and 2.4-fold for pipe and cigar smokers compared with nonsmokers.

A family history of aneurysmal disease is an important risk factor, and in first-degree relatives of patients with AAAs, there is an 11-fold increase in relative risk to develop AAA, with an incidence of 10% to 20%. Familial aneurysms affect patients at a younger age and affect women relatively more frequently than men. Aging brothers of patients with known AAAs have the highest risk for developing an AAA. The prevalence of AAA in siblings older than 60 years of age is 18%.

Patients with atherosclerosis are 1.6 times more likely to develop an AAA than those without atherosclerotic disease. Patients with peripheral arterial disease (PAD) have increased incidence of aortic aneurysm. The risk for aortic aneurysm formation is greater in patients with carotid stenosis. However, only patients without diabetes account for this increased prevalence. The prevalence of aneurysms is 10% to 12% in men with hypertension. Elevated diastolic pressure and elevated pulse pressure have been considered risks for AAA.

There is an inverse relationship between diabetes mellitus and development of an AAA. It is considered a negative risk factor. Patients with diabetes were two times less likely to develop an AAA than those without diabetes (odds ratio, 0.52).[15]

The prevalence of AAA in men with a history of an inguinal hernia is higher than in men without such history. This remains true when one adjusts for smoking history. Men with a history of an inguinal hernia are at increased risk for AAAs, most notably if they are cigarette smokers. As mentioned earlier, expansion of aortic aneurysms has been correlated with evidence of chronic *Chlamydia pneumoniae* infection. As many as 55% of aortic aneurysms demonstrate *C. pneumoniae* by immunohistochemistry. In several screening studies, a high prevalence of AAAs has been found among patients with COPD.

Natural History

The natural history of AAAs is continuous expansion. Rupture is the most frequent and lethal complication of AAAs. In the United States, aneurysm rupture is the cause of death in 1.2% of men and 0.6% of women. About 15,000 deaths each year are caused by ruptured AAAs, making AAA the 13th leading cause of death in the United States. It is the 10th leading cause of death in men. In a study of 231 ruptured aneurysms, 71% of patients did not know before rupture that they had an aneurysm.[17] Most ruptures occur into the retroperitoneal space, but free rupture of the anterior wall can result in herald bleeding into the abdominal cavity; rupture into the inferior vena cava or iliac vein causes aortocaval or aortoiliac arteriovenous fistula,[18] whereas rupture into the duodenum results in massive gastrointestinal bleeding due to a primary aortoduodenal fistula.

After rupture of an AAA, only half of patients arrive at the hospital alive. In one study, 50% reached the hospital alive, 7% died before surgery, 17% died during the operation, and 37% died within 30 days of surgery for an overall mortality rate for open surgical repair of 45%.[19] Although initial results of EVAR for ruptured AAA have been encouraging, about 25% to 30% of patients with a ruptured AAA will eventually survive. Occasionally, AAAs can lead to life- and limb-threatening conditions because of acute thromboembolism.

The growth rates of AAAs vary with aneurysm size, with a more rapid growth seen in aneurysms 5 cm or larger. Aneurysms smaller than 5 cm in diameter grow an average of 0.32 cm/year, whereas expansion for aneurysms greater than 5 cm was reported to be 0.4 to 0.5 cm per year. Cronenwett and colleagues found that the expansion rate was more accurately expressed as a function of aneurysm diameter rather than a fixed rate.[20] AAAs 3 to 6 cm in size expanded on average by 10% of their diameter per year. Eighty percent of AAAs grow, and of these, 20% grow at a rate greater than 0.5 cm per year.

The larger the aneurysm diameter, the greater the risk for rupture (Table 65-1). The annual risk for rupture of an AAA between 4 and 5.4 cm in size is about 0.5% to

Table 65-1 Risk Factors for Rupture of Abdominal Aortic Aneurysm

RISK FACTOR	LOW RISK	AVERAGE RISK	HIGH RISK
Diameter	<5 cm	5-6 cm	>6 cm
Expansion	<0.3 cm/yr	0.3-0.6 cm/yr	>0.6 cm/yr
Smoking, COPD	None, mild	Moderate	Severe/steroids
Family history	No relatives	One relative	Numerous relatives
Hypertension	Normal blood pressure	Controlled	Poorly controlled
Shape	Fusiform	Saccular	Very eccentric
Gender		Male	Female

1%. For AAAs between 5.5 and 6 cm, the annual rupture risk is estimated between 5% and 10%. AAAs between 6 and 7 cm have an estimated yearly rate of rupture of 10% to 20%.[13,21,22]

Factors other than size and growth rate also increase the risk for rupture. Cronenwett and colleagues demonstrated that chronic obstructive pulmonary disease (COPD) and systolic hypertension were predictors of rupture of small AAAs.[20] Increased pulse pressure was also associated with an increased rate of aneurysm growth and rupture. The ADAM and UK trials enrolled mostly good-risk surgical patients, but in both trials, cohorts were excluded because they were deemed unfit for surgical repair.[13-15,22] In both studies, the rupture rate was higher among the ineligible high-risk patients than those randomized (good-risk patients). There appears to be a seasonal variation in incidence of deaths from AAA rupture, with peak deaths in the cold winter months. The underlying cause is unknown, but hypertension and tobacco use are suspected because exposure to tobacco smoke is greater indoors in cold weather, and there is a winter peak of blood pressure in hypertensive patients.

Clinical Presentation

Most asymptomatic aneurysms are discovered on routine physical exam with the palpation of a pulsatile abdominal mass or during a radiographic study performed for aneurysm screening or for diagnosis of another abdominal, retroperitoneal, or pelvic pathology. Occasionally, an aneurysm is first discovered during an unrelated abdominal or pelvic operation.

Symptoms may be caused by contained or free rupture of the aneurysm, by thrombosis, or by distal embolism. Infected aneurysms have local or systemic signs of bacterial or fungal infection. Compression by a large aneurysm of the adjacent bowel can cause early satiety, or nausea and vomiting. Chronic vague abdominal or back pain is the most common symptom, present in up to 30% of patients. Severe back pain in the absence of rupture has been described as a result of erosion of a large aneurysm into the spine or in patients with inflammatory aneurysms. Acutely expanding aneurysms produce severe, deep back pain or abdominal pain radiating to the back. This may be associated with tenderness to palpation of the aneurysm. This presentation usually signifies impending rupture, and urgent evaluation and treatment is required.

The classic presentation of a ruptured AAA is the triad of sudden-onset midabdominal or flank pain, shock, and the presence of a pulsatile abdominal mass. However, only one third of patients with ruptured AAA present with this triad.[19] The pain may radiate into the groin or thigh and is usually severe, constant, and unaffected by position. It is more commonly located on the left side. Shock and abdominal distention are common, making it difficult to palpate a pulsatile abdominal mass. The severity of shock varies from mild to severe, and the duration of symptoms can vary from a few minutes to more than 24 hours. Delayed and contained ruptures may result in

misdiagnoses in the form of angina pectoris, perforated peptic ulcer, acute pancreatitis, acute cholecystitis, acute diverticulitis, mesenteric vascular occlusion, ureteral colic, symptomatic inguinal hernia, prolapsed lumbar intervertebral disk, and even sciatica. Most, if not all, contained ruptures progress to free rupture and must be urgently repaired.

Rarely, an AAA ruptures into the inferior vena cava or one of the iliac veins producing an aortocaval or aortoiliac fistula.[18] Patients may present with unilateral or bilateral lower extremity edema, high-output congestive heart failure, and a continuous abdominal bruit or palpable thrill. Gross hematuria from intravesicular venous hypertension is another characteristic sign of aortocaval fistula. An AAA may also rupture into the gastrointestinal tract, most frequently the fourth portion of the duodenum, producing a primary aortoenteric fistula, shock, and massive gastrointestinal bleeding.

Diagnosis

Physical examination will detect most large aneurysms in thin or normal-sized patients. An AAA can be detected as a firm, pulsatile abdominal mass where the gap between both hands placed on either side of the aneurysm widens with each systole. The aorta bifurcates at the level of the umbilicus and therefore can be palpated to the left and slightly above the umbilicus. Furthermore, if the superior bore of the aneurysm can be felt (at the level of the costal margin), the aneurysm is probably confined to the infrarenal aorta.

Physical examination in obese patients, especially in those with small aneurysms, is unreliable. Studies have shown that abdominal palpation for detecting an AAA has an overall sensitivity of 52%. Sensitivity increased with diameter from 29% for AAAs 3.0 to 3.9 cm, to 50% for AAAs 4.0 to 4.9 cm, to 76% for AAAs 5.0 cm or larger. Extension of the aortic aneurysm into the iliac arteries cannot be appreciated on physical exam. Large aneurysms of the hypogastric arteries can frequently be detected by rectal examination.

In about 70% of cases, AAAs can be diagnosed on plain abdominal or lumbar spine radiograph by the characteristic "eggshell" pattern of calcification. However, accurate determination of size is difficult, and a negative abdominal radiograph does not exclude the diagnosis. This is not a reliable method for diagnosis or exclusion.

Abdominal ultrasound is the most widely used noninvasive test for AAAs (Fig. 65-3). It provides structural detail of the vessel wall and atherosclerotic plaques and can accurately measure the size of the aneurysm in longitudinal as well as cross-sectional directions. Studies comparing ultrasound of the infrarenal aorta with intraoperative measurement demonstrated accuracy to within 3 mm. The thoracic and suprarenal aorta cannot be well visualized with ultrasound because of the overlying air-containing lung tissue. The quality of the examination may be influenced by patient factors such as obesity and bowel gas and by the expertise of the examiner.

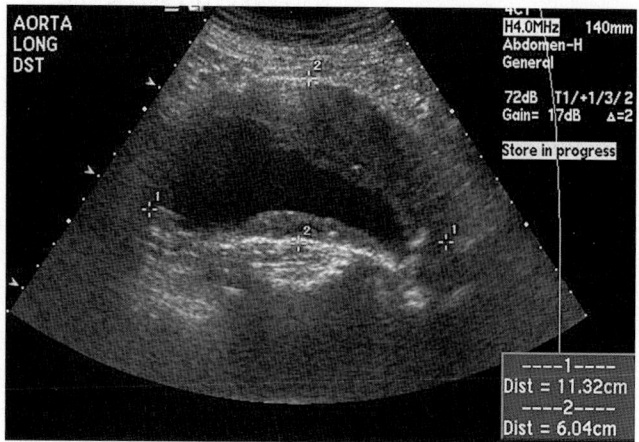

Figure 65-3 Ultrasound image of a 6-cm abdominal aortic aneurysm in the longitudinal plane. Note the large amount of thrombus in the aneurysm.

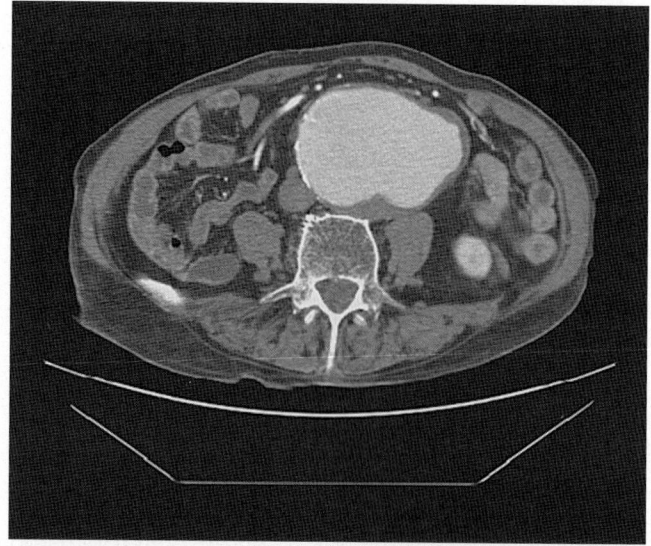

A

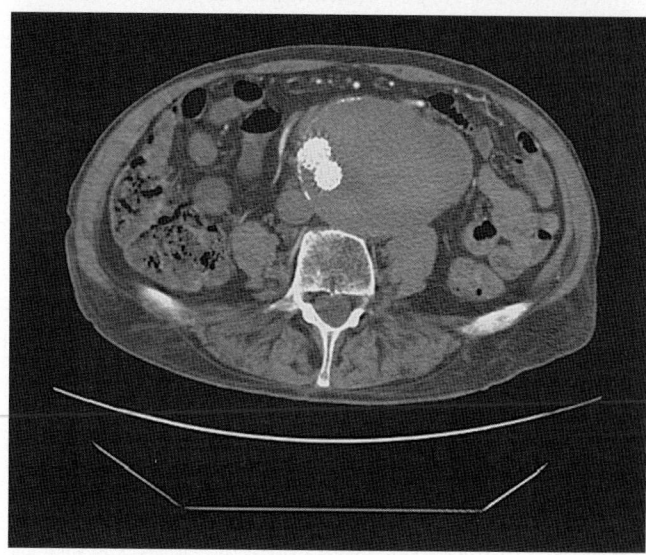

B

Figure 65-4 A, Cross sectional CT image of an 11-cm abdominal aortic aneurysm. **B,** CT image 3 months after endovascular repair. Note the thrombosed aneurysm and patent limbs of the AneuRx stent-graft.

Advantages of ultrasound are its noninvasiveness, low cost, wide availability, and lack of ionizing radiation. Thus, it is particularly suited for initial evaluation of patients with a suspected AAA, for screening, and for surveillance to determine increase in size. It is inconsistent in its ability to determine the dimensions of the neck of the aneurysm with respect to the renal arteries and is not reliable in visualizing the iliac arteries, accessory renal arteries or other anomalies. Therefore, it is less useful as a preoperative planning tool.

Computed tomography (CT) scan is the most precise test for imaging AAAs (Fig. 65-4). It can identify the proximal and distal extent of the aneurysm, including the thoracic portion; identify occlusive or aneurysmal disease in the renal, visceral, and iliac arteries; and identify the presence of multiple and accessory renal arteries. The size of the aortic lumen, amount and location of mural thrombus, and presence of calcific disease are all easily visualized. Adjacent retroperitoneal and intraperitoneal structures are easily identified, as are major venous structures and their anomalies.

If a dissection is present, it may assist in discerning the true from false lumen. It is also useful in identifying the retroperitoneal fibrosis that accompanies inflammatory aneurysms, as well as extravasation of contrast material, which is diagnostic of an aneurysm rupture.

Spiral CT scanners with multiplanar views and three-dimensional CT angiography (CTA) (Fig. 65-5) have largely replaced conventional angiography for evaluation of aortic aneurysmal disease. CT, especially with the availability of 64-view scanners, has become the optimal imaging modality for planning an AAA repair.

Magnetic resonance imaging (MRI) is a useful noninvasive imaging technique for evaluating aortic aneurysmal disease (Fig. 65-6). It obtains images in cross-sectional, longitudinal, and coronal planes without ionizing radiation or the need for contrast agents. Non-nephrotoxic contrast agents such as gadolinium have made it possible to produce high-quality images of the aorta and its vasculature that rival the CT scan. It is an imaging modality of choice for patients with AAA who have renal insufficiency.

Three-dimensional magnetic resonance angiography (MRA) accurately demonstrates aortoiliac aneurysmal disease and is useful for planning aneurysm repair and for follow-up of endovascular repair. However, it is less sensitive than CT in identifying accessory renal arteries and characterizing renal artery stenosis. In addition, the presence of monitoring equipment, cardiac pacemakers, or metallic surgical clips makes MRI impossible to perform. MRI is less widely available and more costly than either CT or ultrasound. MRI and MRA are reserved for use when planning aneurysm repair in patients with renal insufficiency.

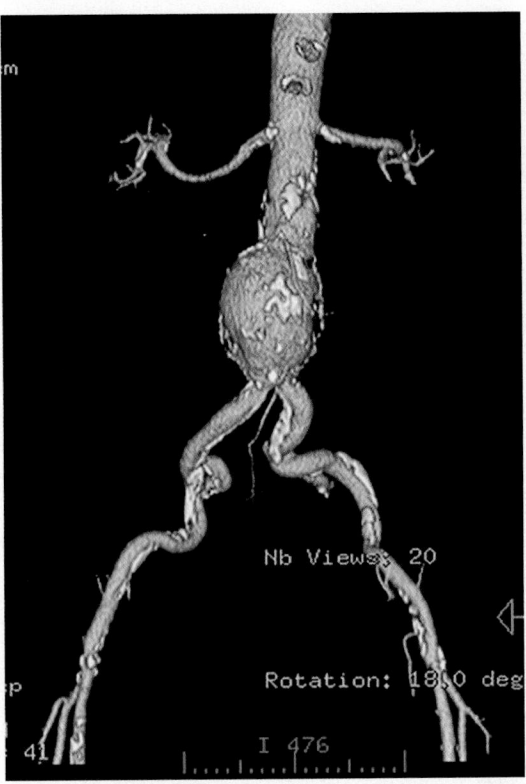

Figure 65-5 Three-dimensional colored CT angiography of a patient with abdominal aortic aneurysm.

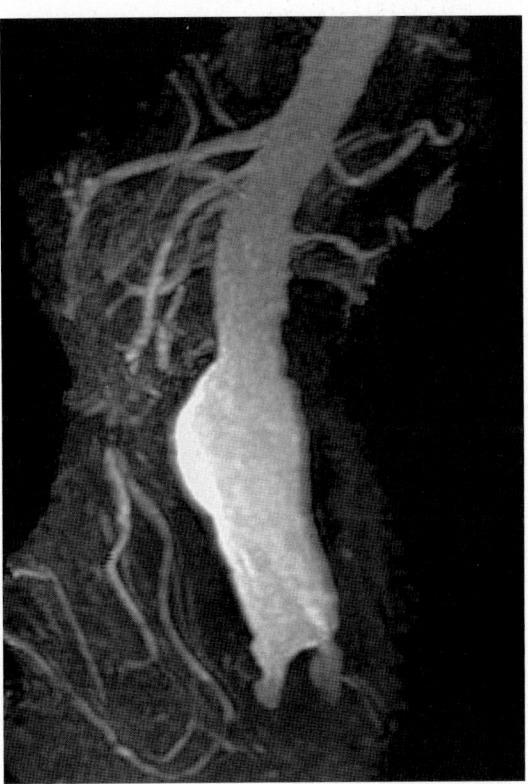

Figure 65-6 MRA demonstrates infrarenal aortic aneurysm.

Contrast arteriography (Fig. 65-7) provides reliable information on aortic lumen caliber and branch vessel disease. However, because most aneurysms contain a variable amount of mural thrombus, the aortic lumen is reduced to near normal in most patients, and assessment of the size of the aneurysm is unreliable. Despite this, arteriography can be helpful in the preoperative evaluation by providing the surgeon with accurate information about associated arterial disease involving the renal arteries, visceral branch vessels, and iliac and femoral arteries. Risks associated with arteriography include the nephrotoxic effects of contrast material, distal embolization from catheter manipulation, and hemorrhage or pseudoaneurysm formation at the puncture site. With the availability of high-quality three-dimensional CTA and MRA, contrast arteriography is being used less frequently for preoperative planning. The advantage of direct percutaneous arteriography over CTA and MRA is its ability to measure pressure gradients across occlusive lesions if present, and potentially to direct treatment.

Screening for Abdominal Aortic Aneurysms

AAAs remain asymptomatic for several years, and if left untreated, about one third will cause death from rupture. These aneurysms are readily detected by abdominal imaging, and elective repair can prevent rupture. Ultrasound is the preferred method of screening.

Four randomized trials of AAA screening using ultrasound including more than 125,000 men have been reported, and each trial observed a reduction in AAA-related mortality ranging from 21% to 68% as well as a 45% to 49% reduction in the incidence of ruptured AAA.

In the Multicentre Aneurysm Screening Study (MASS) from the United Kingdom,[23] 70,495 men aged 65 to 74 years were screened, and those with an AAA 5.5 cm or larger were referred for surgical repair. At 4 years, a 42% reduction in deaths from AAA was found in the screened versus the unscreened group.

In 2003, a consensus statement was issued by the Society for Vascular Surgery regarding screening for AAAs.[24] It recommended baseline ultrasound screening for AAA in men aged 60 to 85 years, women 60 to 85 years with cardiovascular risk factors, and men and women older than 50 years with a family history of AAA. Subsequent ultrasound is recommended annually for AAAs 4.0 to 4.5 cm and every 6 months for AAAs larger than 4.5 cm. The United States recently approved the Screening Abdominal Aortic Aneurysms Very Efficiently (SAAAVE) Act to provide AAA screening at age 65, for male ever-smokers and men and women with a family history of AAA, as recommended by the U.S. Preventive Services Task Force.[16]

Preoperative Evaluation

Patients with AAA often have associated cardiac, pulmonary, peripheral vascular, or renal disease. Assessment of these comorbidities is essential to determine the risk for

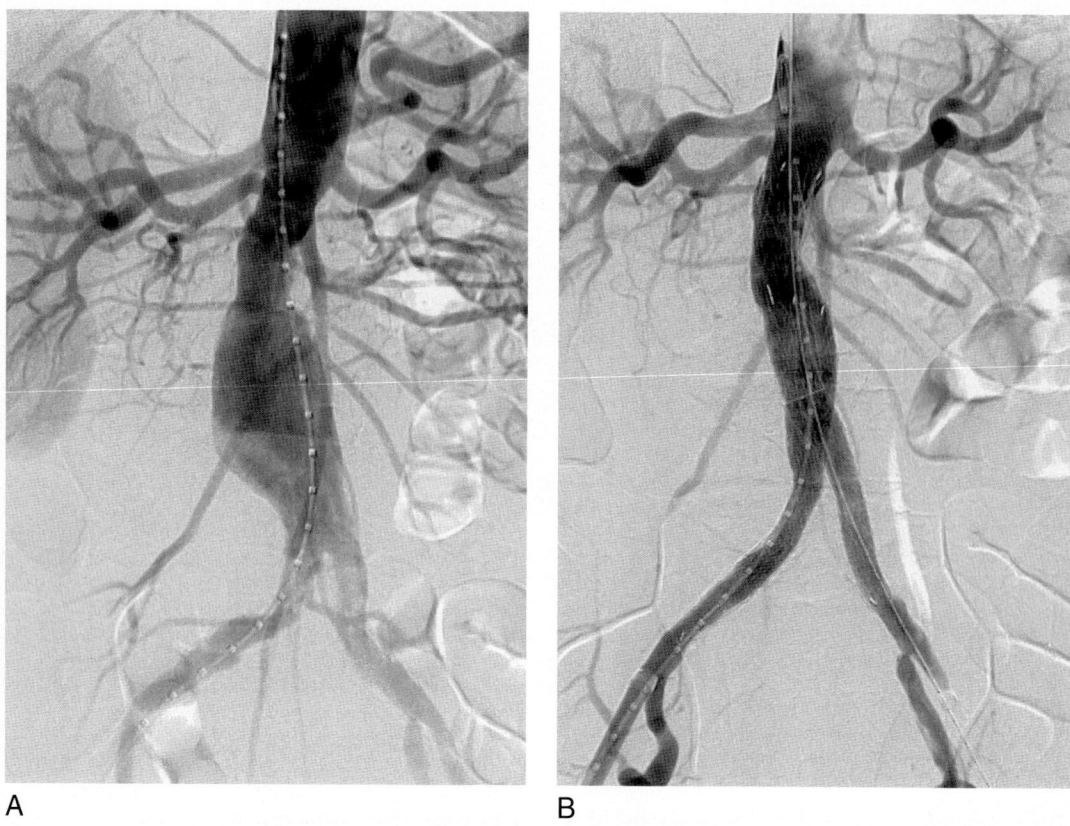

A   B

Figure 65-7 A, Conventional contrast aortography performed before endovascular aneurysm repair. **B,** Completion aortography after successful repair with endograft.

surgical repair and to plan preoperative interventions to reduce surgical risk (Table 65-2). A thorough history and physical exam are performed, including pulse examination and auscultation for carotid and abdominal bruits.

The pulse exam is important to establish associated peripheral occlusive or aneurysmal disease. There needs to be a low threshold of suspicion for other manifestations of atherosclerotic disease, such as coronary artery and cerebrovascular disease. Given the strong association between smoking and AAA, pulmonary disease is also a common comorbidity. Blood tests include measurements of serum electrolytes, creatinine level, complete blood count, coagulation parameters, urinalysis, electrocardiogram, and a two-view chest x-ray.

The most important step in reducing risks of operative repair is preoperative cardiac optimization given that cardiac complications are the most common cause of perioperative morbidity and mortality. The American College of Cardiology (ACC) has issued a consensus statement that categorizes the clinical risk into three levels: minor, intermediate, and major clinical predictors of cardiac risk. The decision to pursue further cardiac evaluation is based on these predictors and the patient's functional capacity. Patients with intermediate clinical predictors and those with minor clinical predictors but a poor functional capacity undergo preoperative cardiac stress testing in the form of exercise stress testing, dipyridamole-thallium scanning, or dobutamine stress echocardiography. Those patients with major clinical predictors of cardiac risk are considered for preoperative coronary angiography.

If the patient has a carotid bruit or prior history of transient ischemic attack or stroke, carotid duplex is performed. Patients with high-grade (70%-99%) internal carotid artery stenosis are considered for carotid endarterectomy before AAA repair.

In patients who are smokers and have a history of pulmonary insufficiency, preoperative evaluation includes pulmonary function testing, including response to β-adrenergic agonists and a room-air arterial blood gas measurement. All patients are encouraged and supported to stop smoking and educated on the health risks that tobacco smoking carries. Patients with severe pulmonary disease must be optimized with steroid or bronchodilator therapy before undergoing elective aneurysm repair.

Preoperative bowel preparation is performed using a mild cathartic to reduce colon caliber and luminal flora. Patients are treated with perioperative β-adrenergic antagonists (β-blockers), and automatic implantable cardiac defibrillators (AICDs) are deactivated. Perioperatively, a central venous catheter is placed for access and pressure measurements with or without the addition of a pulmonary artery catheter. An arterial line is placed as well as a urinary catheter, nasogastric tube, upper-body warming blanket, and administration of antibiotics (to be completed before incision).

Table 65-2   Risks of Open Surgical Repair of Abdominal Aortic Aneurysm

RISK FACTOR	LOW RISK	INTERMEDIATE RISK	HIGH RISK
Age	<70 yr	70-80 yr	>80 yr
Functional status	Active regular physical exercise	Sedentary, but otherwise independent	Minimally able to accomplish daily activities
Cardiac	No clinically overt cardiac disease	Stable coronary disease; remote MI; EF >35%	Significant coronary disease; recent MI; frequent angina; CHF; EF <25%
Pulmonary	No clinical disease	Mild COPD, $FEV_1 > 1$ L/sec	O_2 dependent; dyspnea at rest; FEV_1 <1 L/sec
Renal	Normal renal function	Creatinine 2.0-3.0	Creatinine >3.0
Other	Noninflammatory infrarenal AAA	Juxtarenal; suprarenal or inflammatory AAA	Child's class B or C liver failure; albumin <2
Anticipated operative mortality	1%-3%	3%-7%	At least 5%-10%. Each comorbid condition adding 3%-5% to overall risk

AAA, abdominal aortic aneurysm; CHF, congestive heart failure; COPD, chronic obstructive pulmonary disease; EF, ejection fraction; FEV_1, forced expiratory volume in 1 second; MI, myocardial infarction.

For patients with ruptured aneurysms, particularly those with hypotension, prompt operative intervention is indicated and usually the only opportunity for survival. These patients are taken directly to the operating room for emergent repair. The only essential test is a blood specimen for cross-matching. All patients have at least two large-bore intravenous (IV) lines and a urinary catheter in place. If possible, sedation is avoided until the patient is in the operating room with the abdomen prepared and draped with the surgeon ready to make incision. The anesthetic induction and skin incision do not begin until all resuscitative measures have been initiated.

Medical Management

For patients with low-risk AAAs (small diameter without other risk factors for rupture) being followed with serial size measurements, attempts are made to reduce expansion rate and rupture risk. This can be accomplished with risk factor modifications, including smoking cessation, blood pressure control, and reduction of cholesterol, triglycerides, and lipoproteins.

Despite initial promising results, recent randomized trials failed to confirm the beneficial effect of β-blockers in slowing growth of aortic aneurysms. Experimental studies have demonstrated that treatment with nonsteroidal anti-inflammatory drugs (NSAIDs, indomethacin) inhibits elastase-induced AAAs in rats through inhibition of cyclooxygenase-2 and reduction of prostaglandin E_2, interleukin-6, and matrix metalloproteinase-9 (MMP-9). Retrospective case-control studies in humans have found a significantly lower rate of aneurysm formation in those treated with NSAIDs. These findings demonstrate that NSAIDs may have the potential to reduce aneurysm growth.

MMP inhibitors have been proposed as another therapeutic approach to slow aneurysm expansion. Tetracycline derivatives, namely doxycycline, have been shown to be effective inhibitors of MMPs. In one study, patients undergoing open AAA repair who were treated preoperatively with oral doxycycline for 1 week exhibited a five-fold reduction in the amount of MMP-9 expressed within aneurysm wall tissue compared with controls. Another prospective, randomized placebo-controlled study examining the effects of doxycycline in patients with small asymptomatic AAAs demonstrated a significant difference in aneurysm expansion between the doxycycline group (7% of patients with AAA expansion >5 mm) as compared with the placebo group (41% of patients with AAA expansion >5 mm). Thus, these encouraging results strongly support further evaluation of doxycycline as a viable option in the medical management of AAA.[25]

Indications for Repair

The goal of elective AAA repair is to prevent rupture and prolong life. Careful assessment of factors that influence rupture risk, operative mortality, and life expectancy is essential, and patient preference receives increasing importance.

Level I evidence for the treatment of small AAAs has been provided by two randomized prospective clinical trials: the U.K. Small Aneurysm Trial[13] and the ADAM trial[22] conducted at Veterans Administration medical centers across the United States. Each trial examined more than 1000 patients with an AAA between 4.0 and 5.4 cm, randomly assigned to early elective open surgical repair versus ultrasonographic or CT surveillance every 3 to 6 months. The annual rupture rate for aneurysms in both trials was between 0.5% and 1%. Neither study demonstrated a difference in survival between patients who underwent early open surgical repair and those randomized to surveillance. The 6-year survival rate for both patient cohorts was 64% in the U.K. trial and about 70% in the ADAM trial. The U.K. trial demonstrated that death was attributable to aneurysm rupture in 5% of men but in 14% of women. The risk for rupture was four times higher among women. Investigators concluded that the AAA diameter threshold of 5.5 cm may be too large for women.

In 2003, the Joint Council of the Vascular Societies published guidelines for the treatment of AAAs.[21] They noted that treatment of AAAs is individualized and recommended operative repair for AAAs with a diameter of 5.5 cm or greater in men. Those aneurysms that expand at a rate of more than 1 cm/year or that are symptomatic must be repaired. However, subsets of younger, low-risk patients, with long projected life expectancy, may prefer earlier repair. If the surgeon's operative mortality rate is low, repair may be indicated at smaller sizes (4.5-5.4 cm) if that is the patient's preference. For women and patients with a greater than average rupture risk, an AAA diameter of 4.5 to 5.0 cm is an appropriate threshold for elective repair. Atypical aneurysms (dissecting, pseudoaneurysms, mycotic, saccular, and penetrating ulcers) may be an indication for surgical treatment regardless of size. For high-risk patients, delay in repair until larger diameter is warranted, especially if EVAR is not possible.

The guidelines recommended EVAR as the most appropriate option for patients at increased risk with conventional open repair. EVAR is preferred for older, high-risk patients; those with "hostile" abdomens; and patients with other clinical circumstance likely to increase the risk of open repair, if their anatomy is appropriate. It was emphasized that patient preference is of great importance. It is essential that the patients be well informed to make such choices.

Technique of Open Repair

For open repair, several exposures can be used, each with its own merits and disadvantages. Options include a transperitoneal approach, through a long midline incision or through a mini-laparotomy, or the retroperitoneal approach through a left flank incision.

Transperitoneal Approach

This approach affords the most flexibility for exposure of the AAA, renal arteries, and both iliac arteries (Fig. 65-8). A midline abdominal incision is made extending from the xiphoid to the pubis. Depending on the extent of the aneurysm, the length of the incision can be shortened. Upon entering the peritoneal cavity, a thorough abdominal exploration is performed. Proper placement of the nasogastric tube and bladder catheter is confirmed. The omentum and transverse colon are then retracted superiorly, and the small intestine is retracted to the patient's right. An effort is made to keep the small bowel within the abdominal cavity because this is thought to reduce the incidence of postoperative ileus. The posterior peritoneum between the inferior mesenteric vein and the fourth portion of the duodenum is then incised from the ligament of Treitz to the aortic bifurcation, exposing the infrarenal abdominal aorta. Care is taken to avoid injury to the inferior mesenteric artery (IMA) at its origin. The IMA usually arises off the left anterolateral aspect of the aorta halfway between the renal arteries and the aortic bifurcation. In inflammatory aneurysms, with redo aortic surgery, and in the face of pelvic infections or associated tumors placement of ureteral stents will help to avoid ureteral injury.

An abdominal, self-retaining retractor is placed to facilitate exposure. The dissection is carried superiorly

on the aorta until the left renal vein is identified. Mobilization of the left renal vein with ligation of its tributaries (left adrenal vein, left gonadal vein, and lumbar vein) is usually necessary for exposure of the suprarenal aorta. The renal arteries are identified, and the proximal infrarenal aneurysm neck is dissected free laterally and mobilized sufficiently to allow for infrarenal clamp placement. For an aneurysm that necessitates suprarenal clamping, both renal arteries must be dissected free. In patients who need suprarenal clamping, occlusion of the renal arteries with soft bulldog clamps or fine vessel loops is recommended to avoid atheroembolization.

Inferiorly, the dissection is carried down to the level of the aortic bifurcation, exposing both common iliac arteries. If the common iliac arteries are aneurysmal, both external and internal iliac arteries are dissected in a short segment to permit placement of vascular clamps. Excessive dissection of the aortic bifurcation and the proximal common iliac arteries, especially on the left side, is limited to avoid injury to the parasympathetic nerve plexus, which is critical in males to maintain normal ejaculatory function. The ureters are located near the iliac bifurcations, coursing along the anterior surface of the iliac arteries, and care is taken to avoid injury during dissection and clamping. Circumferential dissection of the iliac arteries is avoided to minimize the risk for injury to the iliac veins.

IV heparin is administered (60-70 U/kg), and mannitol (12.5 mg) is given to force diuresis before cross-clamping. The aortic clamp is placed in a location where the chance of loose thrombus causing renal embolization is minimal. A careful study of the CT scan is mandatory, and if the infrarenal aorta appears "shaggy," suprarenal or supraceliac clamping is needed. If suprarenal aortic clamping is done, and renal perfusion is interrupted for more than 30 minutes, perfusion of the kidney with iced heparinized saline is recommended.

Although some surgeons advocate placement of the iliac clamps first, this technique does not completely prevent retrograde embolization of thrombus material into the renal arteries. After proximal and distal clamping, the aneurysm sac is opened longitudinally, and thrombus is removed. Bleeding lumbar arteries are oversewn with polypropylene sutures, and bleeding from the IMA is controlled with a vessel loop or clamp. If the iliac arteries are not aneurysmal, a straight collagen or gelatin-coated zero porosity polyester (Dacron) graft is used for repair, usually 16 or 18 mm in diameter. Both proximal and distal anastomoses are performed with 3-0 polypropylene running sutures. When the common iliac arteries are involved, a 16- or 18-mm bifurcated graft is used and sutured to the distal common iliac arteries in an end-to-end fashion, using 4-0 polypropylene running sutures (Fig. 65-9). In patients with associated internal iliac aneurysms, at least one internal iliac artery is reconstructed with an 8-mm interposition graft from the iliac limb to the distal internal iliac artery. Associated external iliac artery occlusive disease is rare and is usually treated with aortofemoral bypass. Before declamping, the proximal and distal anastomoses are flushed of any thrombus, and the suture lines are completed. The aortic clamp is removed with caution to minimize hypotension and

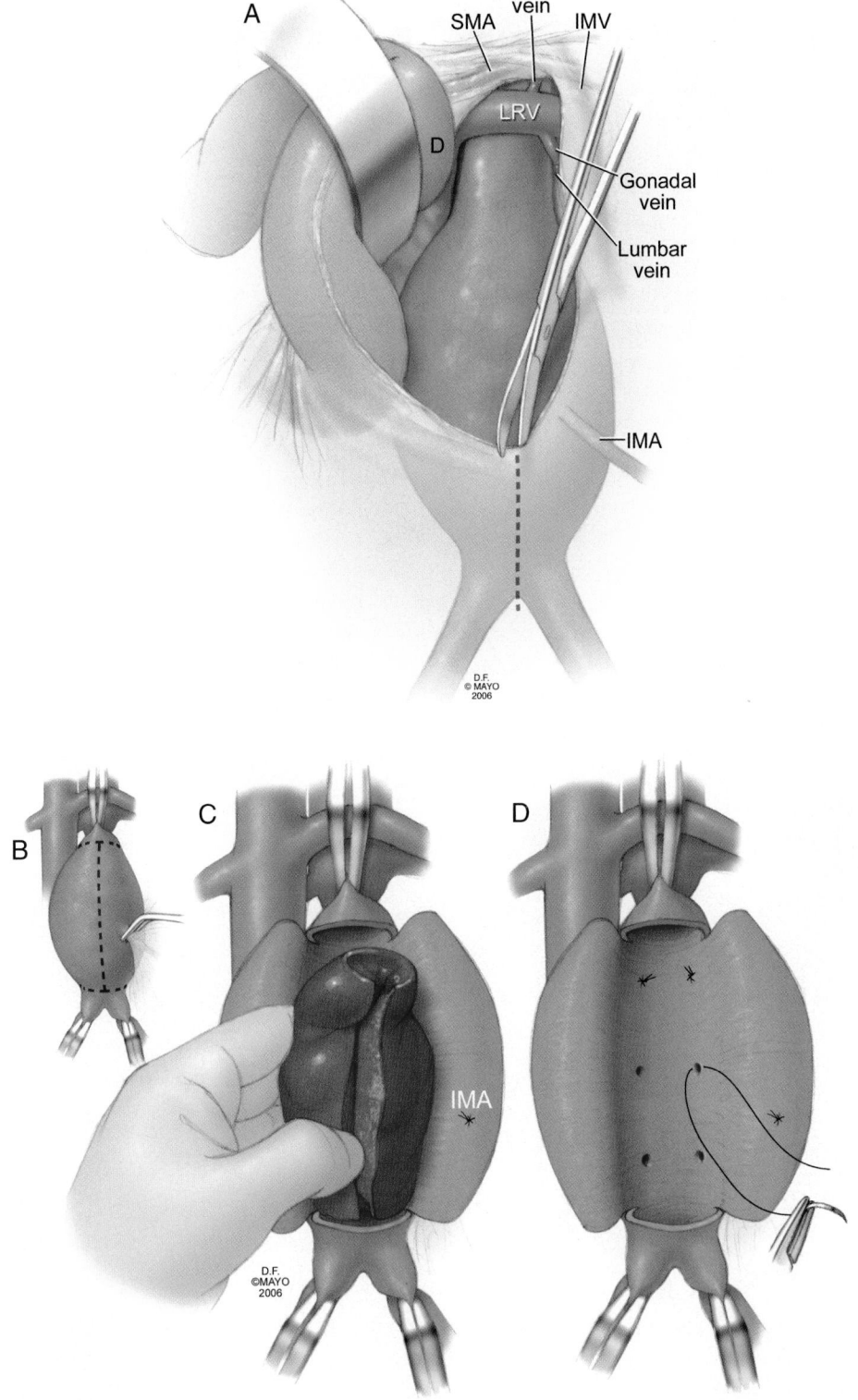

Figure 65-8 A to **J,** Operative technique of transperitoneal abdominal aortic aneurysm repair with a straight or a bifurcated prosthetic graft (see text for details). D, duodenum; IMA, inferior mesenteric artery; IMV, inferior mesenteric vein; LRV, left renal vein; SMA, superior mesenteric artery. (By permission of Mayo Foundation for Medical Education and Research. All rights reserved.)

Continued

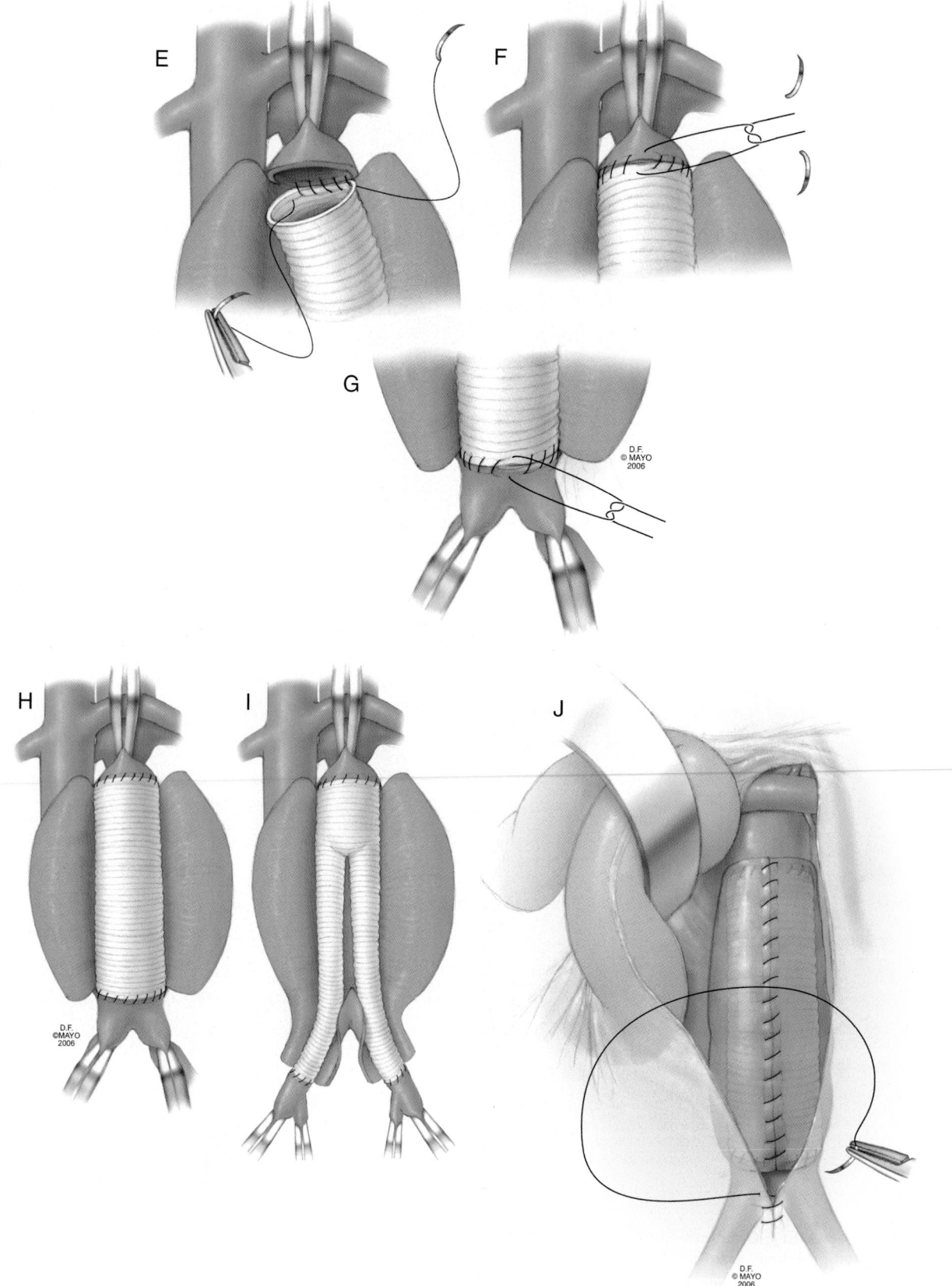

Figure 65-8, cont'd

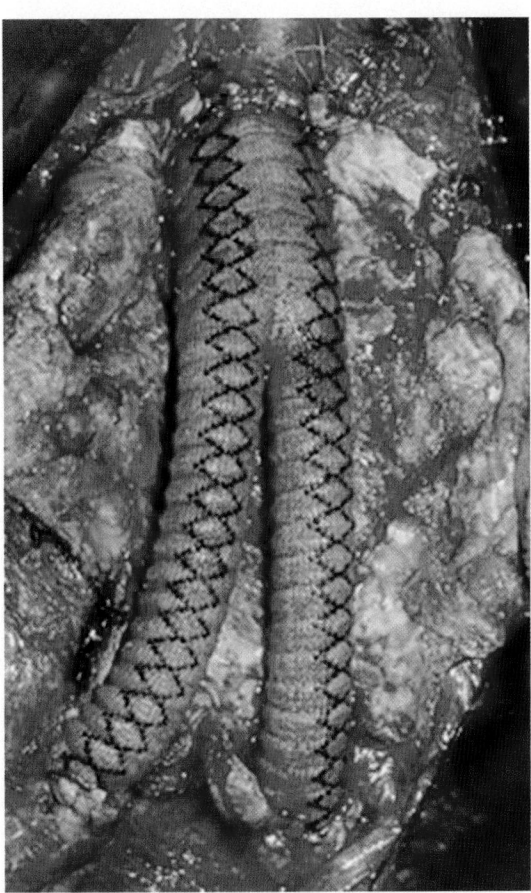

Figure 65-9 Bifurcated aortoiliac polyester graft used for abdominal aortic aneurysm repair.

allow anesthesia for adequate volume replacement. Any larger accessory renal artery is either incorporated into the proximal anastomosis or reimplanted into the graft separately. At this point, the IMA is assessed for backbleeding. If there is strong backbleeding (stump pressure >40 mm Hg), the IMA is ligated close to the aorta or oversewn from within the sac. Poor backbleeding from the IMA is a sign of insufficient collateral circulation to the sigmoid colon, and reimplantation of the IMA with a patch of the aorta into the aortic limb is warranted. A side-biting Satinsky clamp is used for the aortic graft, and the anastomosis is performed with running 4-0 polypropylene suture. If perfusion of the bowel is in question at the end of the procedure, we inject 2 ampules of fluorescein dye IV and assess the perfusion pattern with a Woods lamp.[26] If the pattern is patchy, perivascular, or absent, further revascularization or bowel resection has to be considered. When hemostasis is achieved, the aneurysm sac is closed over the graft with a running 3-0 polypropylene suture to separate the prosthesis from the duodenum and to help hemostasis. The retroperitoneum is then closed over the aneurysm sac, and the abdominal wall is closed in standard fashion.

Retroperitoneal Approach

The midline approach can be difficult in patients with a "hostile" abdomen with multiple prior operations or radiation treatment, suprarenal aneurysm extension, horseshoe kidney, peritoneal dialysis, inflammatory aneurysm, or ascites. In these situations, the retroperitoneal approach is preferred. It offers the advantage of avoiding the intraperitoneal contents entirely. It also has been reported to reduce gastrointestinal and pulmonary complications as well as length of intensive care unit and hospital stay. The disadvantage is that it provides poor accessibility to the distal right iliac arteries and the right renal artery.

For a retroperitoneal incision, the patient is positioned in a right lateral decubitus position, over a vacuum-operated beanbag (Fig. 65-10). The break of the operating table is halfway between the top of the iliac crest and the costal margin. The left arm is padded and protected on an arm support over the right side of the table. There is a 60-degree tilt at the shoulders and a 30-degree tilt at the hips to allow good exposure to the iliacs or even a right femoral artery, if needed. The operating table can be gently flexed in the middle to maximize the space between the iliac crest and the costal margin.

The incision originates at the 10th costal interspace beginning at the posterior axillary line and is extended medially to the lateral border of the rectus sheath toward a point midway between the umbilicus and pubic symphysis. The 12- to 15-cm incision can be prolonged both upward and downward if needed. The external oblique muscle is split bluntly along its fibers, and the internal oblique and transversus abdominis muscles are transected in the same plane with electrocautery. The dissection is kept lateral in the left lower quadrant, and the retroperitoneum is entered as lateral as possible to minimize the risk for entering the peritoneal cavity. The rectus sheath can be divided if needed. Care is taken to preserve the inferior epigastric vessels if possible, or to ligate them carefully if extension of the incision is needed. Blunt digital dissection is used to free the peritoneum laterally and posteriorly from the overlying muscle fascia. The peritoneum is retracted medially and superiorly, and the psoas muscle is identified. After this is accomplished, the iliac vessels and left ureter are identified. Two different techniques can be followed from this point. The dissection is continued over the left ureter, and the left kidney is preserved in its normal position. Care is taken to maintain the blood supply to the ureter and avoid excessive dissection of this structure. Injury to the descending colon is also avoided during dissection of the plane over Gerota's fascia. After the left renal vein is identified, it leads the surgeon to the neck of the aortic aneurysm, which is easily cross-clamped distal to the renal arteries. In patients with horseshoe kidney or inflammatory aneurysm and in those who likely need a suprarenal or supraceliac clamp, the ureter and the left kidney are retracted medially with the peritoneal cavity. The gonadal vein is divided to facilitate exposure of the aortic neck. The aortic neck and the iliac arteries are then clamped, and the repair and sac closure are carried out the same way as described for the transperitoneal approach. The abdominal wall muscles are closed in layers, followed by closure of the subcutaneous layer and the skin.

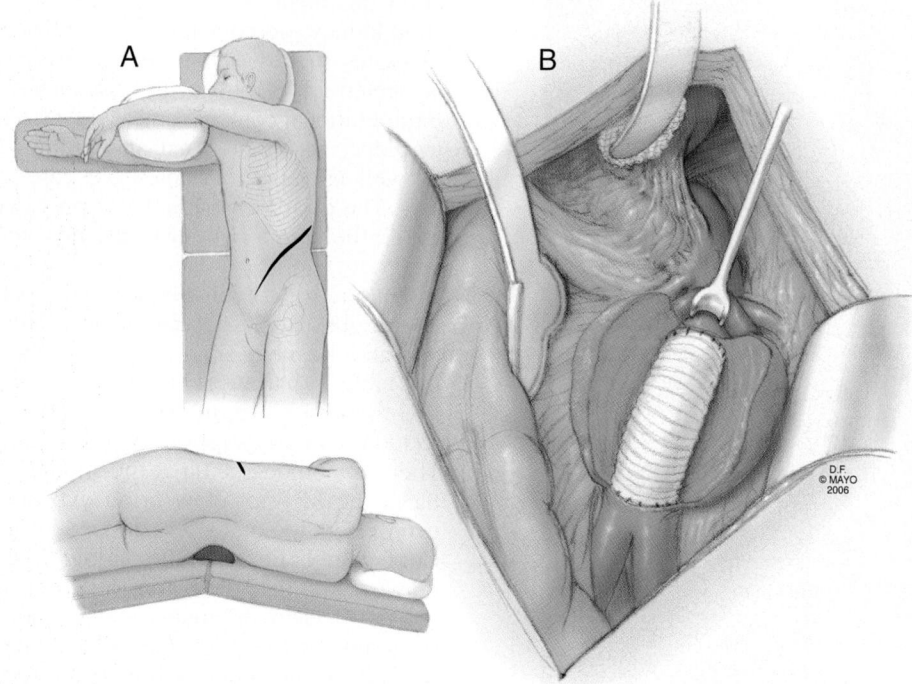

Figure 65-10 A and B, Operative technique of retroperitoneal abdominal aortic aneurysm repair with a straight infrarenal aortic prosthetic graft (see text for details). (By permission of Mayo Foundation for Medical Education and Research. All rights reserved.)

Minimal Incision Aortic Surgery

Patient selection is important because obese patients and those requiring bifurcated graft placement are not good candidates for this procedure. The length of the midline periumbilical incision is less than 12 to 15 cm, placing at least 9 cm of the incision proximal to the umbilicus (Fig. 65-11). The incision can be extended proximally or distally if needed. Abdominal exploration is limited, and retraction of the small bowel has to be done intra-abdominally with self-retaining retractors and large abdominal sponges. The aneurysm repair is performed much the same way as in a traditional transperitoneal repair, although retractors have to be readjusted after completion of the proximal anastomosis to gain adequate exposure for the distal anastomosis. The use of special, short aortic and iliac clamps (Cosgrove clamps) aids in keeping the visual field as large as possible.

Minimal incision aortic surgery (MIAS) has been shown to result in fewer cases of postoperative ileus, a reduction in postoperative pain requirement, and less incidence of incisional hernia as compared with the standard midline transperitoneal open repair. In a prospective nonrandomized study, Turnipseed and colleagues also reported shorter hospital stay and significant cost benefit of MIAS compared with standard open repair.[27]

Postoperative Management

Most patients are followed immediately after open surgical repair in the surgical intensive care unit. Close monitoring is necessary for proper response to hemodynamic changes and fluid shifts, assessment of respiratory and oxygenation status, and timely management of pain control. Some patients require a period of mechanical ventilation while coagulation is corrected and they are rewarmed. Laboratory analysis of blood includes arterial blood gas, complete blood count, basic metabolic profile, calcium, prothrombin and partial thromboplastin times, and lactate analysis. If supraceliac aortic clamping was performed, the blood is also sent to the laboratory for liver function tests and amylase and lipase levels. A chest x-ray is done to verify endotracheal tube position and central line placement. An electrocardiogram is done to compare with preoperative baseline, and this is repeated daily to observe for any changes. Routine serial troponin I measurements are done every 8 hours for the first 24 hours to evaluate for postoperative myocardial infarction. Close observation of the urine output, heart rate, blood pressure, and central venous pressure is important for evaluation of the patient's fluid status. β-Blockade is continued in the postoperative period to maintain a heart rate lower than 80 beats/minute. Urinary catheters are kept in place for assessment of fluid status. All patients need to have a mechanism for thromboembolic prevention, usually in the form of a lower extremity compression device and subcutaneous heparin. Nasogastric decompression is continued until the patient shows signs of restored gastrointestinal function. Gastric ulcer prophylaxis is administered with either histamine-2 receptor antagonists or proton pump inhibitors. Once extubated, the patient is encouraged to use an incentive spirometer and to cough as needed. Perioperative antibiotics are discontinued within 24 hours. Assessment of peripheral pulses is done at regular intervals.

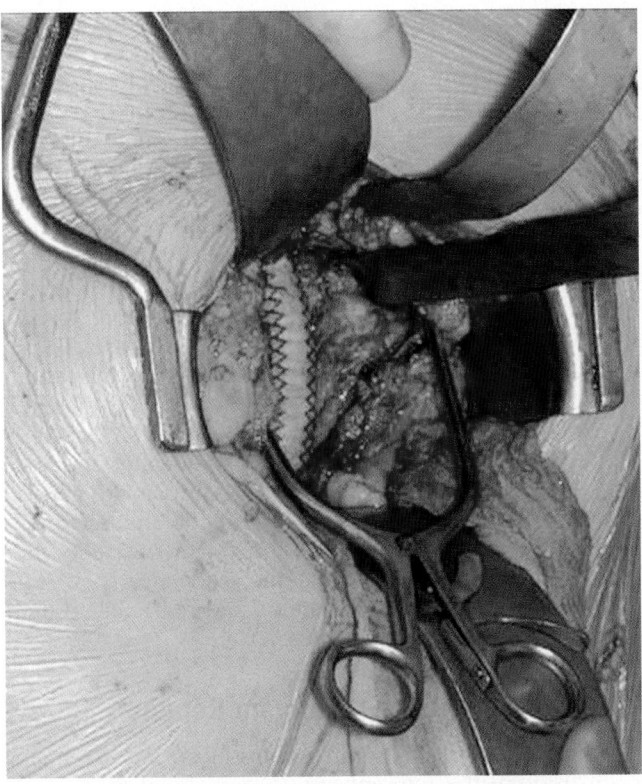

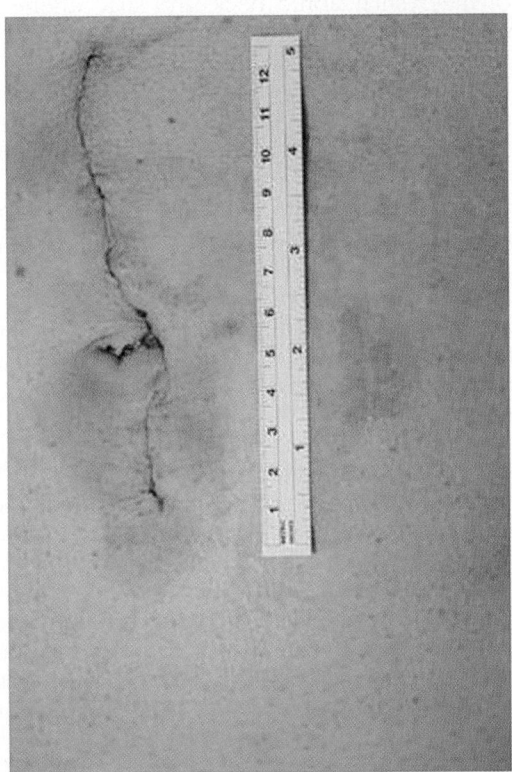

Figure 65-11 A, Straight aortic tube graft placed through mini-laparotomy. **B,** Closed skin incision of the 12-cm mini-laparotomy used for aneurysm repair.

Results of Open Repair

Early mortality for open elective AAA repair has greatly improved during the past 2 decades because of improvements in preoperative evaluation, intraoperative techniques, and perioperative care. Mortality rates of elective open infrarenal AAA repair in good-risk patients can be expected to be less than 5%; in high-volume centers, the mortality rate is between 1% and 3%.[28] The mortality rate in the ADAM trial was 1.8%. The most frequent cause of death is myocardial dysfunction, usually ischemic in origin.

Complications following elective open aortic aneurysm repair occur in 10% to 30% of cases. The most frequent complication is nonfatal myocardial infarction, which occurs in 3.1% to 16% (average 6.9%), usually within the first 48 hours after surgery.[29] Other cardiac complications include arrhythmias and congestive heart failure. Renal failure is the second most frequent complication, occurring in about 6% of cases and accounting for up to 12% of deaths.[30] It is more frequent in patients with preexisting renal disease and may occur as a result of hypoperfusion, suprarenal aortic clamping, atheroembolism, and contrast administration. Severe renal failure necessitating dialysis is rare. Renal failure after repair of a ruptured AAA occurs in 15% to 21% of patients and carries a high mortality rate. The postoperative pneumonia rate is about 5%. Early extubation and mobilization with aggressive pulmonary toilet can help prevent the onset of nosocomial pneumonia and pulmonary dysfunction.

Postoperative bleeding may occur from the anastomotic suture lines, from unrecognized venous injuries, and as a result of coagulopathy due to intraoperative hypothermia or blood loss. Evidence of ongoing bleeding prompts early re-exploration. Gastrointestinal complications of a functional nature occur regularly, but seldom last beyond 2 to 3 days. Occasionally, duodenal or small bowel obstruction persists longer. Postoperative pancreatitis may result from injury caused by retractors.

The most serious gastrointestinal complication is ischemia of the left colon and rectum. The incidence of transmural colonic ischemia after aortic reconstruction is between 0.6% and 2%, more frequent after operation for aneurysmal than for occlusive disease.[26] In patients with rupture, this complication rate can be as high as 30%. Intestinal ischemia develops when critical hypogastric arteries are not revascularized or when a patent IMA is ligated in the setting of superior mesenteric artery or bilateral hypogastric artery occlusion. Improper ligation of the IMA too far from the aneurysm wall can interfere with the collateral blood supply to the rectosigmoid and lead to ischemia. Postoperative hypotension and hemodynamic instability are contributory factors. It is important to maintain antegrade perfusion in at least one of the hypogastric arteries. The first indication of bowel ischemia may be a substantial IV fluid requirement in the first 8 to 12 hours after the operation. Diarrhea, usually bloody, typically follows within 48 hours. Abdominal distention, fever, or elevation of white blood cell count raises the suspicion for colonic ischemia and prompt immediate sigmoidoscopy. This typically reveals mucosal changes appearing abruptly between 10 and 20 cm above the anal verge. If necrosis is limited to the mucosa, treatment can be conservative with bowel rest, antibiotics, and fluid resuscitation. However, if the muscular layers are involved, segmental strictures may develop that eventually require resection. Full-thickness necrosis on sigmoidoscopy or signs of peritoneal irritation necessitate urgent reoperation with resection of all ischemic bowel and creation of an appropriate stoma. Only if the aortic graft is grossly contaminated is it removed and replaced with an extra-anatomic bypass (axillofemoral bypass). The mortality rate approximates 50%, and it is even higher when full-thickness bowel necrosis and peritonitis occur.

Lower extremity ischemia may result from embolization of mural thrombus or atherosclerotic plaque from the aneurysm, or thrombosis distal to the vascular clamp. It requires reoperation and thrombectomy. Occasionally, microembolization can occur, resulting in small patchy areas of ischemia, usually on the plantar aspect of the foot, referred to as "trash foot." This is manifested clinically with pain and muscle tenderness, frequently without loss of pedal pulses. In some patients with massive embolization, extensive buttock and lower extremity ischemia may develop and is associated with a high mortality rate.

Ischemic injury to the spinal cord or lumbosacral plexus is rare after infrarenal aortic reconstructions, with an incidence of 0.3%. It is much more frequent after ruptured AAA repairs (1.4%) than after elective open AAA repair (0.1%).[31] Preservation of the pelvic blood supply, avoiding prolonged suprarenal clamping, and carefully removing aortic thrombus from the aneurysm to prevent lumbar or internal iliac artery embolization are important to further decrease this devastating complication. The mortality rate associated with this complication can be as high as 50%.

Postoperative sexual dysfunction in males is more frequent and is due to injury to the autonomic nerves during para-aortic dissection and dissection of the iliac arteries. In addition, this could also result from reduction in pelvic blood flow secondary to hypogastric artery occlusion or embolization. Symptoms may include impotence and retrograde ejaculation. This complication has been reported to occur in as many as 25% of patients undergoing open AAA repair. Careful preservation of nerves, particularly as they course along the left side of the infrarenal aorta, around the IMA, and over the proximal left common iliac artery, has been shown to reduce this complication.

Deep venous thrombosis (DVT) can occur in as many as 18% of patients, although the number of clinically significant DVTs is lower. Perioperative prophylaxis with graduated compression stockings, intermittent pneumatic compression devices, and subcutaneous heparin will decrease the risk for both DVT and pulmonary embolism. Placement of prophylactic filters in those at high risk for pulmonary embolism needs to be considered.

Late complications after successful AAA repair are rare. In a population-based study by Hallett and associates,

only 7% experienced such complications within 5 years after aneurysm repair.[32] At a mean follow-up of 5.8 years, the most common complication was anastomotic pseudoaneurysm (3%), followed by graft thrombosis (2%), graft-enteric erosion or fistula (1.6%), graft infection (1.3%), anastomotic hemorrhage (1.3%), colonic ischemia (0.7%), and atheroembolism (0.3%). Late vascular complications after repair of ruptured aneurysm are more frequent, occurring in 17% of patients.[33]

Long-term survival after successful aortic aneurysm repair is less than that in the general population, primarily because of associated coronary artery disease. The 5-year survival rate after successful AAA repair is about 70%, compared with 80% for age- and gender-matched controls. The 10-year survival rate after AAA repair is about 40%, and the mean survival time after repair is 7.4 years. Causes of deaths after AAA repair are cardiac disease (44%), cancer (15%), rupture of another aneurysm (11%), and stroke (9%). Functional outcome after open repair is concerning; in one study nearly 3 years after surgery, one third of patients had not reached their preoperative functional status.

Endovascular Aortic Aneurysm Repair

During EVAR, the stent-graft is introduced into the aneurysm through the femoral arteries and fixed in place to the nonaneurysmal aortic neck and iliac arteries with self-expanding or balloon-expandable stents. Some of the stent-grafts have barbs, pins, or hooks to secure the stent, whereas some others have suprarenal fixation with self-expanding stents. A major abdominal incision is thus avoided, and procedure-related morbidity is reduced. An endovascular stent-graft excludes the aneurysm from blood flow and extends from the infrarenal aorta to both common iliac arteries, preserving flow to the internal iliac arteries.

The first EVAR was performed by Parodi and associates in 1991 using a Dacron graft sutured onto balloon-expandable Palmaz stents.[2] Since then, a number of commercially manufactured stent-graft devices have been developed and tested.[34-40] Presently, there are four U.S. Food and Drug Administration–approved endovascular devices for infrarenal AAA repair in the United States (Medtronic: AneuRx, Gore: Excluder, Cook: Zenith, Endologix: Powerlink) (Fig. 65-12). With the exception of the Powerlink stent-graft, which is a unibody device, the other three stent-grafts are multiple-component modular devices composed of self-expanding metallic stents attached to a thin polyester or polytetrafluoroethylene (PTFE) graft material. All three produce a seal at the proximal and distal attachment sites by the radial force produced by a deliberate oversizing of the device by 10% to 20%. The Zenith device has a proximal bare metal stent portion with small hooks for additional suprarenal fixation. The Powerlink device, which is a one-piece design incorporating PTFE graft material with a cobalt-chromium stent, is the only other graft that also offers this suprarenal fixation feature. The modular grafts require the successful deployment of multiple overlapping components, a bifurcated body, and one or two iliac

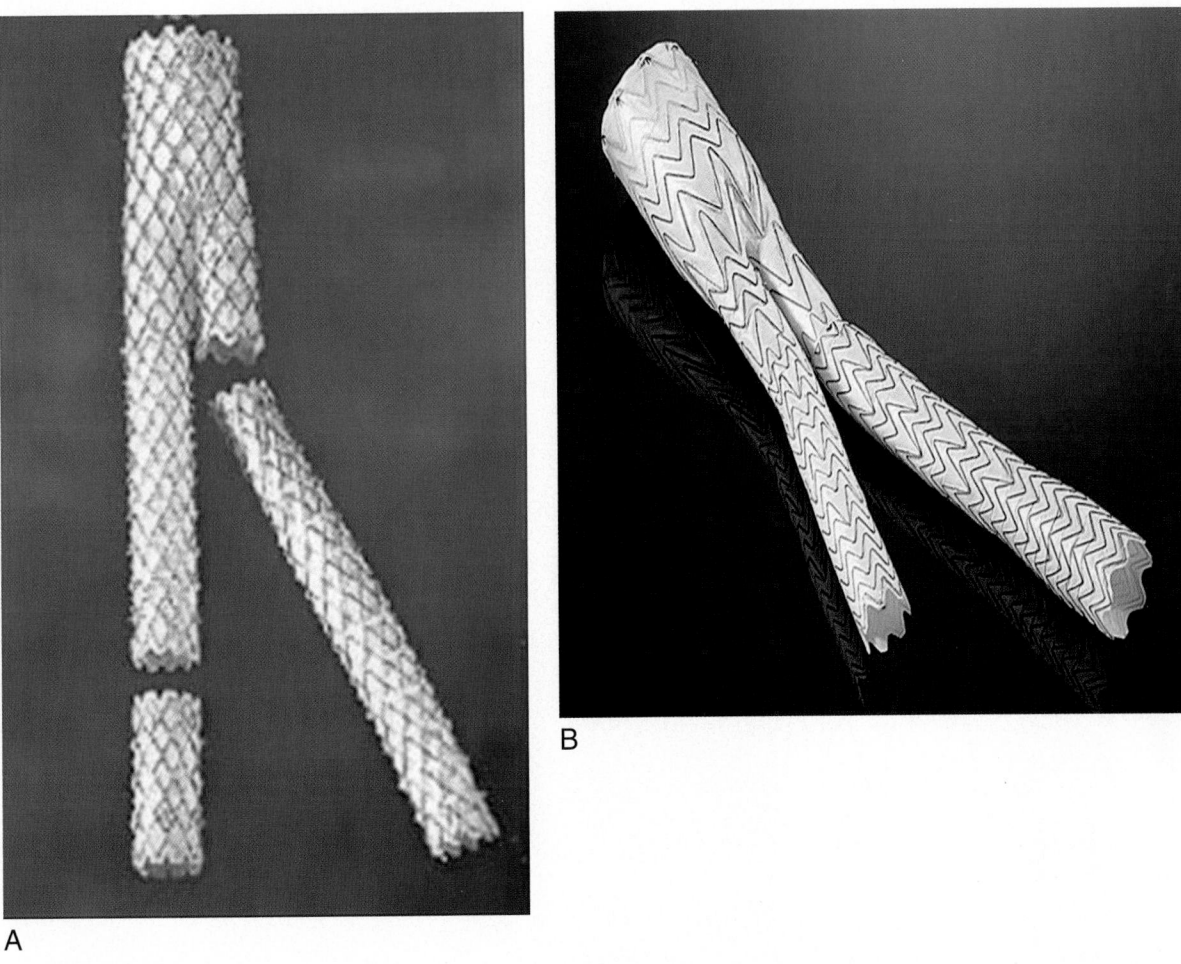

Figure 65-12 Endografts approved in the United States for abdominal aortic aneurysm repair. **A,** AneuRx (Medtronic). **B,** Excluder (W. L. Gore, Inc.).

Continued

components. Additional proximal or distal extension grafts can be added as necessary.

Patient Selection

In addition to risk and benefit considerations, patient selection for EVAR depends on accurate anatomic measurements of proximal and distal stent-graft attachment sites and of the "access" vessels (iliac and femoral arteries). The most important area of interest is the proximal aortic neck. A cylindrical neck distal to the renal arteries with a minimum length of 15 mm and a diameter of 28 mm or less is preferred. The neck needs to be relatively free of thrombus, allowing adequate room for proximal fixation. A conical, "reverse-tapered" neck flaring more than 4 mm from its proximal to distal end is less suitable for device placement. Neck angulation (the angle between the proximal neck and suprarenal aorta) of 60 degrees (45 degrees with the AneuRx device) or less is acceptable. Angles greater than 60 degrees carry an increased risk for inadequate sealing of the stent-graft. The second area of interest is the distal landing zone within the common iliac arteries. Distal attachment of the endograft requires common iliac artery landing zones of

less than 18 mm and about 2 cm in length. Large amounts of calcification or thrombus of the iliac arteries and angulation greater than 90 degrees may result in inadequate sealing. If the common iliac artery is short or the external iliac artery must be used as a landing zone, the hypogastric artery may be covered and will require embolization either before or during the procedure. One hypogastric artery can be sacrificed without causing pelvic or spinal ischemia provided that the contralateral hypogastric artery is patent. The third issue is the quality of the access vessels. The femoral and external iliac artery lumen diameters must allow access of the endograft deployment catheter. For the commercially available grafts, diameters of 7 mm or more are acceptable. Diameters smaller than 7 mm may prompt the need for a surgically constructed conduit onto the iliac artery through a flank incision. Heavy calcification and extreme tortuosity of the femoral and external iliac arteries can pose technical difficulties in even adequately sized lumens because of the stiffness of the deployment catheters.

Multiple methods of imaging are used to obtain these important anatomic data. The standard study is thin-slice (<3 mm) spiral CT scan with three-dimensional reconstructions. Diameters are measured from the individual

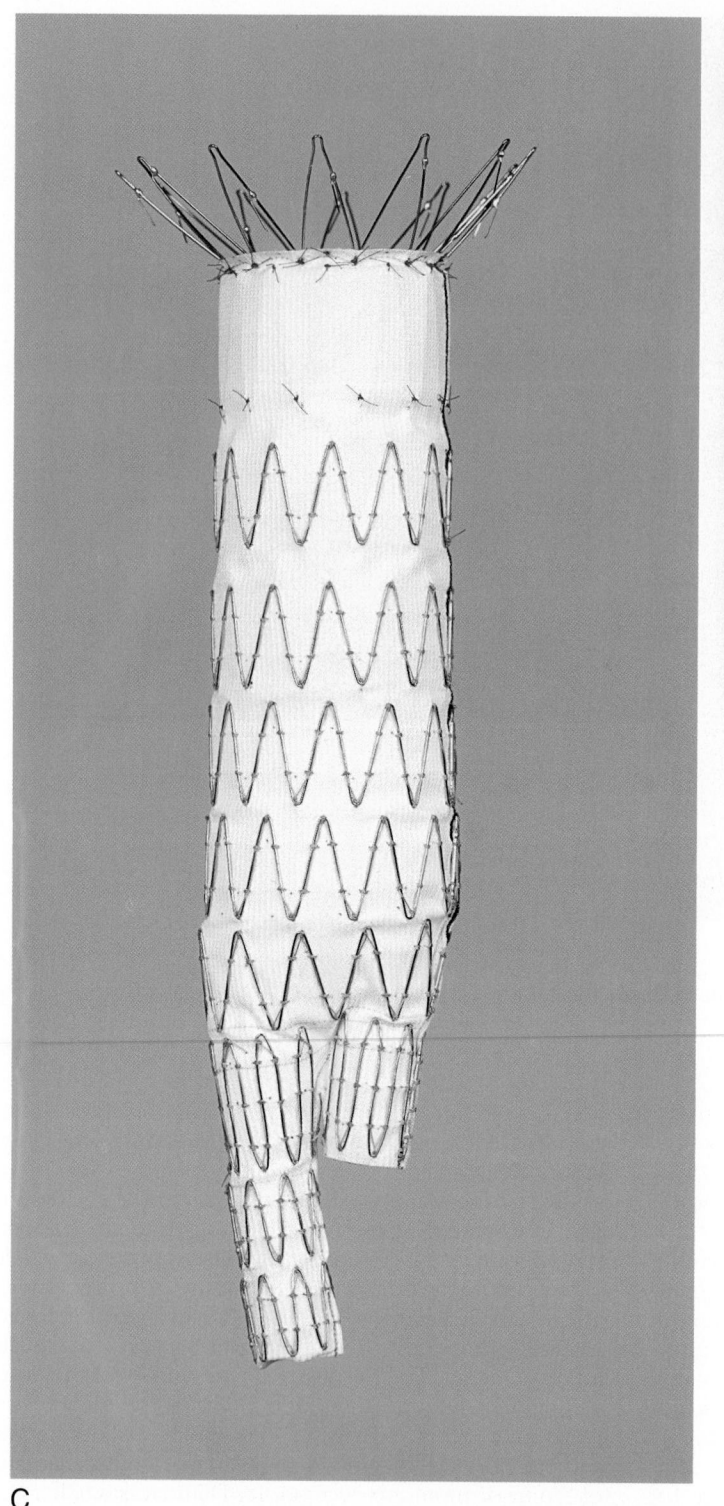

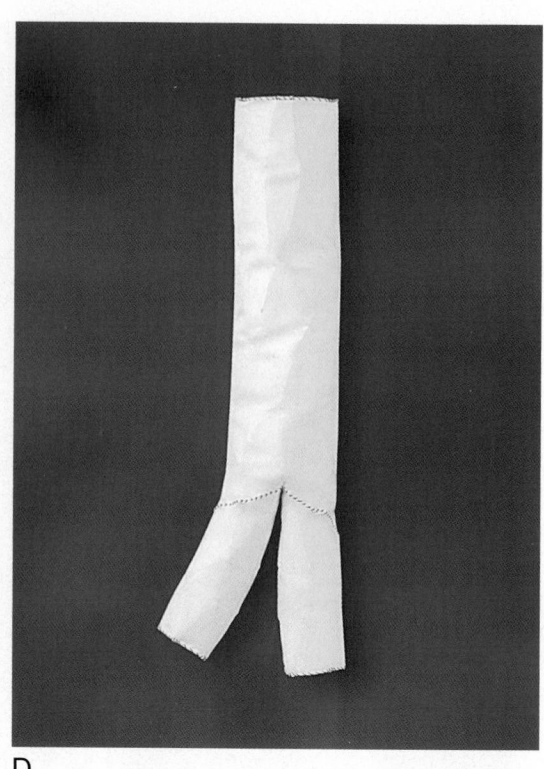

C

D

Figure 65-12, cont'd **C,** Zenith (Cook). **D,** Powerlink (Endologix).

transverse images, and lengths and angulations are calculated from the three-dimensional reconstructions. Intraoperative pre-reconstruction aortography with calibrated marking catheters can be used to measure length and evaluate neck angulation and iliac tortuosity. Intravascular ultrasound can be useful and may be the most

accurate means of aortic neck and iliac artery diameter measurement.

Technique of Endovascular Aortic Aneurysm Repair
The technical details of endovascular repair differ with each device, but the general principles are similar

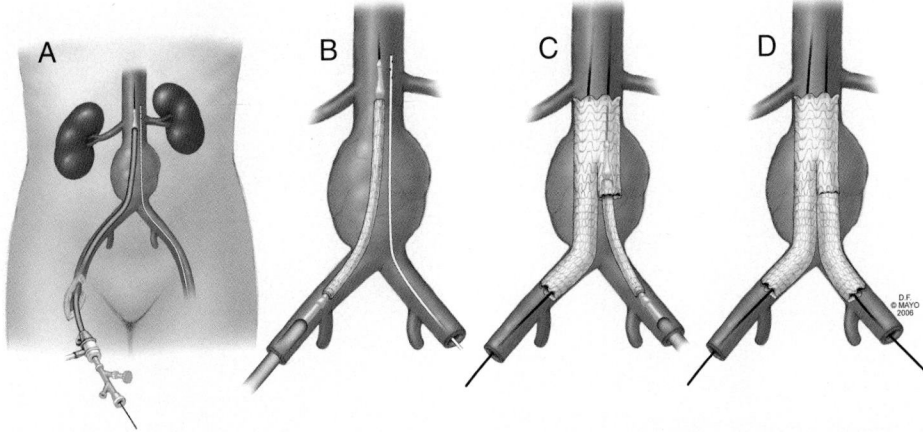

Figure 65-13 Technique of endovascular abdominal aortic aneurysm repair. **A** and **B,** Both common femoral arteries are cannulated. On the right, the device is advanced to the level of the renal arteries. Aortography through a multi-sidehole catheter, placed from the contralateral side, identifies the renal arteries before device deployment. **C,** The main body device is deployed in the aorta and right iliac artery. The left iliac limb is advanced into the main body device. **D,** The left iliac endograft limb is deployed. (By permission of Mayo Foundation for Medical Education and Research. All rights reserved.)

(Fig. 65-13). This procedure can be performed in a surgery-capable catheterization laboratory or a surgical suite equipped with a fixed or mobile angiography C-arm. This can be performed under general, regional, spinal, or local anesthesia. Both common femoral arteries are cannulated either percutaneously or more commonly with femoral artery cutdowns. Vascular sheaths are placed over guidewires under fluoroscopic guidance into both external iliac arteries. The patient is systemically heparinized, and a diagnostic aortogram is performed through a marker pigtail catheter placed just above the renal arteries. Appropriate measurements are taken. Super-stiff guidewires are then inserted into the thoracic aorta through both femoral sheaths. The endograft device is advanced into the aorta, usually through its own deployment sheath. A multi-sidehole catheter is advanced from the contralateral side to mark the level of the renal arteries, and the main body device is deployed just below the lowest renal artery. Distally, it is deployed to just above the iliac bifurcation, taking care not to cover the hypogastric artery unless preoperatively planned. The contralateral limb gate is then cannulated, and an appropriately chosen contralateral iliac limb endograft device is deployed from within the main device to just above the iliac bifurcation. Balloon dilation is performed of all attachment sites, and completion angiogram is done with attention paid to position and sealing of the graft attachment sites (Fig. 65-14).

Complications

Several complications can occur in the immediate post-operative period. These most commonly are groin and wound complications related to vascular access and include bleeding, hematoma, pseudoaneurysm formation, and wound infection. Distal embolization to the lower extremities can also result from manipulation of the endovascular devices within the aneurysm sac or the access vessels.

One of the principle reasons for endograft failure is the presence of endoleak. Endoleak is defined as persistence of blood flow outside of the graft and within the aneurysm sac. There are four types of endoleak (Table 65-3). Type I (attachment site leak) and III (disconnected device parts) endoleaks, if identified intraoperatively, are treated before leaving the procedure room. These are often treated with a second endoluminal procedure such as balloon dilation or placement of additional stents or aortic cuffs. Short and heavily calcified aneurysmal necks and large aneurysms are at increased risk for type I endoleak.[41] Type II endoleaks (patent lumbar or inferior mesenteric artery) can initially be managed with observation because most close spontaneously. A persistent type II endoleak, especially if it is associated with aneurysm sac enlargement, is treated with reintervention. This can be accomplished with coil embolization or *N*-butyl cyanoacrylate glue injection of the offending vessels. Alternatively, retroperitoneal endoscopic ligation of the lumbar arteries or IMA or open conversion in rare instances can be performed.

Endotension is a state of elevated pressure within the aneurysm sac. It is generally believed that for endotension to exist, an endoleak must also exist or must have recently sealed or clotted. Presently, CT scan is the only method of detecting endotension by noting sac enlargement. This is a crude method; however, work is being done to design micromachine pressure sensors to monitor aneurysm sac pressures.

Device migration is another complication of EVAR. It is defined as a more than 5-mm increase in the distance between the lowest renal artery and the cranial end of the device. Migration accounts for most type I endoleaks and is a significant factor for late rupture. It can occur

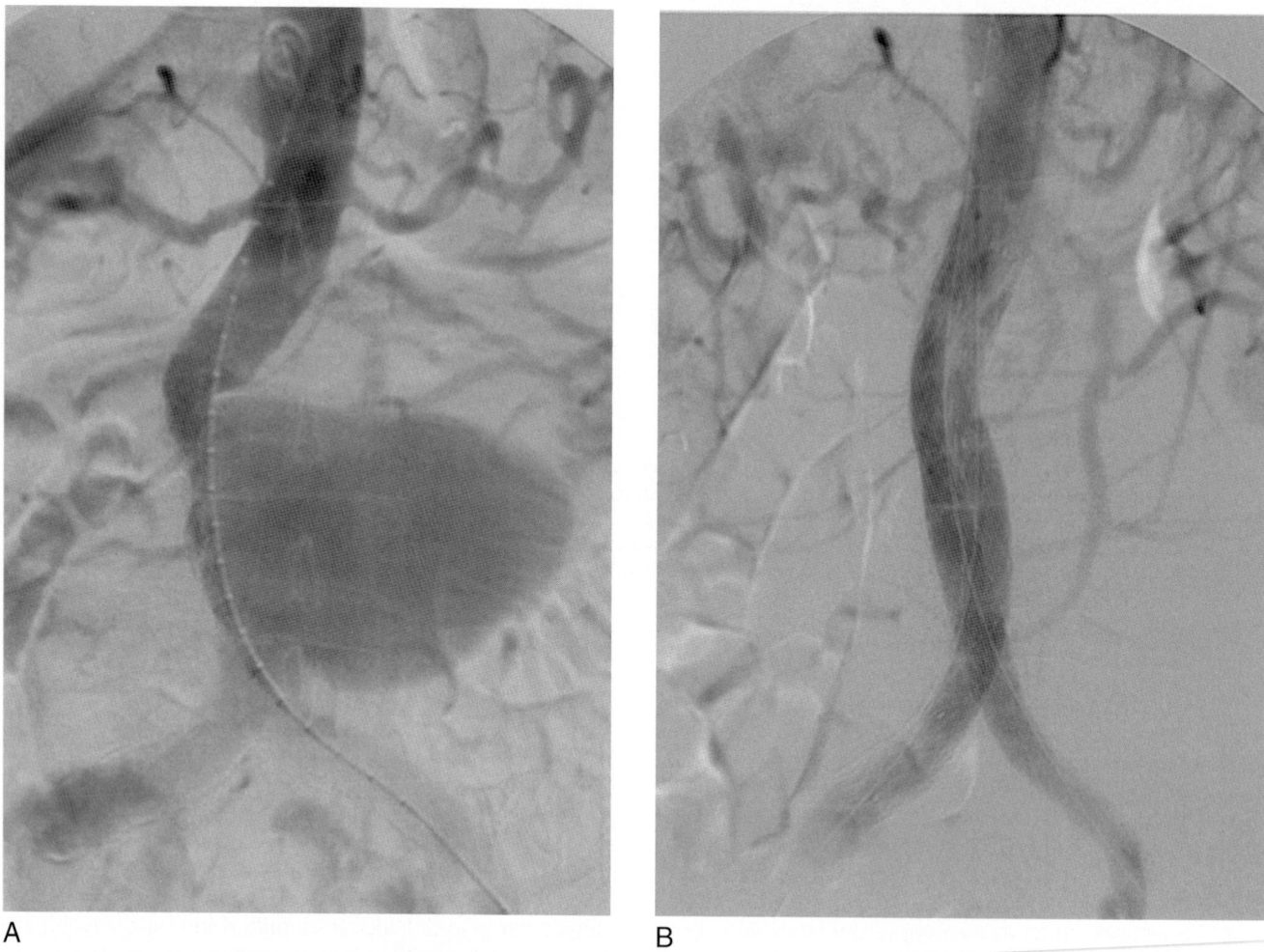

A   B

Figure 65-14 A, Aortography demonstrates a long aortic neck above a large abdominal aortic aneurysm. **B,** Aortography confirms a successful deployment of an endograft.

Table 65-3   Types and Treatments of Endoleak After Endovascular Aortic Aneurysm Repair

TYPE OF ENDOLEAK	CAUSES OF LEAK	TREATMENT OPTIONS
Type I	Inadequate seal of proximal or distal end of endograft	Balloon dilation Placement of additional stents or cuffs Open conversion
Type II	Flow from backbleeding arteries Patent lumbar, middle sacral, inferior mesenteric, hypogastric, accessory renal arteries	Observation Coil embolization or glue Laparoscopic ligation Open conversion
Type III	Fabric disruption or tear Module disconnection	Placement of additional stents or cuffs Secondary endograft Open conversion
Type IV	Flow from fabric porosity	Observation

when there is a fracture of hooks on the endograft or if there is initial failure of the attachment system to engage or penetrate the aortic wall. In addition, aortic neck remodeling and dilation after EVAR that alters the seal zone of the device has been suggested as another poten-

tial cause for graft migration. Device migration is associated with a threefold increased risk for type I endoleak and is associated with the degree of overlap between the device and infrarenal aorta (less overlap has a higher risk for migration). Device migration also depends on the

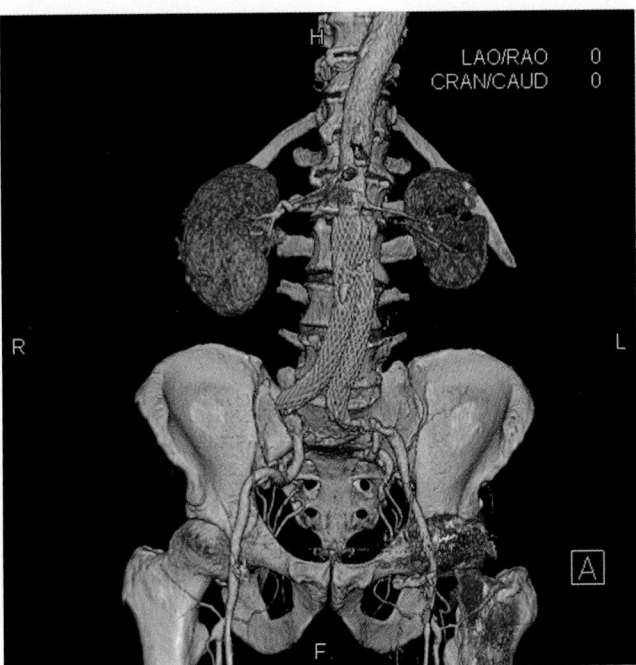

Figure 65-15 Three-dimensional CT angiography 6 months after endograft repair of abdominal aortic aneurysm.

length of aortic neck and the extent of proximal neck dilation.

Postoperative Surveillance

Surveillance is a key component of EVAR, and patient compliance needs to be considered. Surveillance allows for the identification of endoleaks, aneurysm sac growth, migration and position of endograft, kinks, and structural graft failure. A baseline CT scan is obtained 3 months after graft implantation. If there is no perigraft flow or endoleak identified on the initial postoperative CT scan, then CT scans can be obtained after 6, 12, and 18 months and then annually thereafter (Fig. 65-15). If there is perigraft flow other than a type I or II endoleak, suspicion of an endoleak, or failure of aneurysm sac shrinkage, CT scanning is done more frequently. In patients with type I or III endoleaks or aneurysm sac enlargement greater than 5 mm, angiographic evaluation and reintervention are considered.

Results

There are three large randomized controlled trials evaluating the efficacy of EVAR. The Endovascular Aneurysm Repair Trial 1 (EVAR-1) randomized 1082 patients with AAAs larger than 5.5 cm in diameter.[42] Early results showed a short-term survival benefit with endovascular repair, with a 30-day mortality rate of 1.7% in the EVAR group and 4.7% in the open repair group. However, 4 years after randomization, there was no difference between the two groups in all-cause mortality (~28%), although aneurysm-related death was 3% less after EVAR than after open surgery (4% versus 7%). Postoperative complications within 4 years were greater in the EVAR

group (41%) than the open repair group (9%). There was no difference in the quality of life, and hospital costs after up to 4 years were higher in the EVAR group.

The Dutch Randomized Endovascular Management (DREAM) trial randomized 351 patients with aneurysms of 5 cm or larger to EVAR and open surgical repair.[43] Thirty-day mortality favored the EVAR (1.2%) as opposed to open repair (4.6%). In addition, the combined rate of operative mortality and postoperative complications was 4.7% in the EVAR group and 9.8% in the open repair group. However, no overall survival difference was found at 2 years. Still, aneurysm-related death was higher after open repair (5.7%) than after EVAR (2.1%).

EVAR was presumed to be particularly effective in treatment of high-risk patients. This was studied in the EVAR-2 trial, which randomized 338 patients, unfit for open surgery, to EVAR versus observation.[44] Greenhalgh and colleagues did not find any benefit of EVAR over observation of aneurysms in high-risk patients unfit for open surgical repair. The 30-day mortality rate after EVAR was 9%, and the mortality rate after 4 years in the entire group was 64%. There was no difference in late overall mortality, nor was there a difference in aneurysm-related mortality between the two groups. Hospital costs were significantly higher in the EVAR group, and there was no health-related quality-of-life benefit. Several single-institution studies and the U.S. Lifeline Registry contradict these conclusions.[30,32,39]

A recent retrospective analysis of 355 patients from the Mayo Clinic who underwent treatment for AAA in the form of open repair or EVAR demonstrated that the 30-day mortality rate in the open repair group was 1.1%, as compared with 0% for EVAR.[32] Cardiac and pulmonary complications were less frequent after EVAR (11% and 3%) than after open surgical repair (22% and 16%), despite the higher number of high-risk patients who underwent EVAR. The trade-off of EVAR is a higher rate of graft-related complications, with more secondary interventions, late device-related problems, need for lifelong surveillance, and the high cost of the device.

Special Considerations for Abdominal Aortic Aneurysm Repair

A number of anatomic and pathologic conditions can complicate the management of AAAs and adversely affect the outcome. Occasionally, AAA repair is complicated by a concurrent disease process. Successful treatment requires careful evaluation and a correct decision about whether to treat the two entities sequentially or concurrently.

Pararenal Aortic Aneurysms

As many as 20% of AAAs are classified as pararenal, characterized by the absence of normal aorta between the upper extent of the aneurysm and the renal arteries (see Fig. 65-2). Although attempts to repair these using endovascular techniques or combined (hybrid) open and endovascular procedures have been encouraging, most pararenal aneurysms are repaired with open technique. West and coworkers reported on technique and results

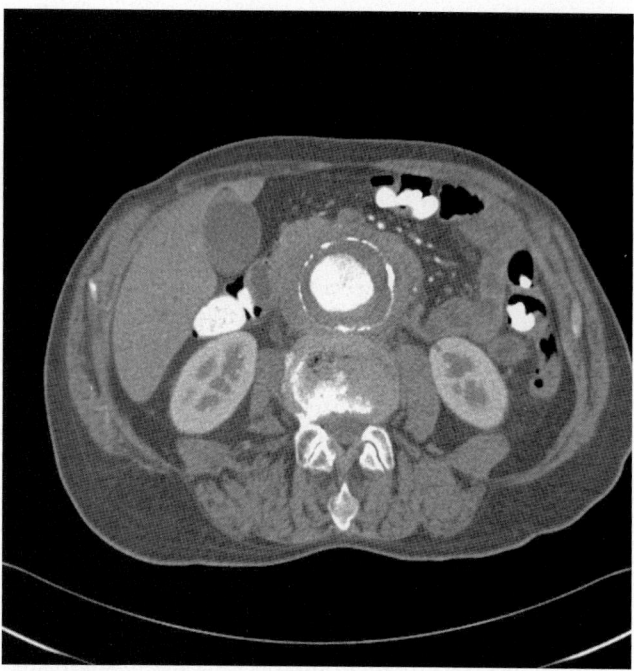

Figure 65-16 Cross-sectional image of a CT scan confirms inflammatory abdominal aortic aneurysm. Note the thick layer of vascularized inflammatory tissue around the aneurysm.

of 247 pararenal aortic aneurysm repairs.[45] The 30-day surgical and in-hospital mortality rates were 2.5% and 2.8%, respectively. The most common complication was renal insufficiency (22%); new dialysis was required in 3.7% of patients, and abnormal preoperative serum creatinine (>1.5 mg/dL) was predictive of the need for postoperative dialysis. Advanced age, increased mesenteric ischemic time, the need to perform renal artery bypass, and left renal vein ligation were significant predictors of cardiopulmonary and renal complications as well as prolonged hospital stay.

Inflammatory Aneurysm

Inflammatory aneurysms (Fig. 65-16) represent about 5% of all infrarenal AAAs. They typically have a dense fibrous, inflammatory rind that is usually adherent to the fourth portion of the duodenum and often involves the inferior vena cava and left renal vein. The ureters may also be involved. The etiology of inflammatory aneurysms is not fully understood. One theory is that lymphatic obstruction occurs during aneurysm expansion, producing stasis, edema, and secondary fibrosis. Other possibilities are infection, autoimmune disorder, and reaction from chronic, contained rupture. Inflammatory AAAs have a strong familial connection, and smoking plays an important role in the inflammatory response.[46]

Patients usually present with abdominal or flank pain and often have associated weight loss. The erythrocyte sedimentation rate is significantly elevated in 75% of cases. Aneurysm rupture is uncommon, likely because these aneurysms are often symptomatic and treated before rupture. Diagnosis is best made by CT scan (see

Fig. 65-16) and CTA, with four separate layers typically identified: aortic lumen, mural thrombus, thickened aortic wall, periaortic inflammatory tissue. Repair of these aneurysms can be technically challenging because of the involvement of adjacent structures. A retroperitoneal approach has been traditionally advocated because the risk for injury to the adherent duodenum or left renal vein using a transperitoneal approach is higher. The ureters need to be stented in most patients to minimize injury. Following these principles, results are generally good in elective repair.

Venous Anomalies

The most common anomalies are a left-sided vena cava and a retroaortic left renal vein. Anatomic variants of the left renal vein are estimated to be present in 10% of patients, with a retroaortic vein present 4% of the time. A circumaortic venous collar (two renal veins encircling the aorta) is found in up to 6% of cases. A double inferior vena cava, lying on each side of the aorta, is estimated to occur in 3% of patients, whereas a left-sided vena cava is only present in 0.5%. If abnormal anatomic variants of the left renal vein and vena cava are not recognized during aortic dissection and clamping, significant venous injury and subsequent exsanguinating hemorrhage may occur.

Aortocaval Fistula

Spontaneous perforation of an aortic aneurysm into the inferior vena cava has been reported in 0.2% to 1.3% of patients with AAA (Fig. 65-17). Its incidence is twice as high in patients presenting with a ruptured aneurysm. Signs of high-output cardiac failure are present in about half of patients. There is a continuous abdominal bruit in a patient with usually a large AAA. Manifestations of venous hypertension are present and include lower extremity edema, priapism, rectal bleeding, and hematuria. "Steal" by the fistula may result in decreased distal pulses or frank ischemia to the lower extremities. Treatment is surgical. Fistula closure is performed from within the aneurysm sac, paying careful attention to avoid pulmonary embolization. Venous bleeding is controlled with sponge sticks, finger pressure, or large balloon catheters. Repair is done with either direct suture or patch followed by AAA repair with a Dacron graft.[40] Inferior vena cava interruption is seldom warranted, although the use of removable filters makes this an attractive technique for perioperative embolus prevention. The mortality rate in elective cases is 6%.[18]

Horseshoe Kidney

Less than 0.3% of the population has horseshoe kidney. Its association with AAA is rare, but it complicates graft replacement because the kidney mass is usually fused anterior to the aorta. The collecting system and ureters are displaced inferiorly, and there are often multiple or anomalous renal arteries arising from the aorta.[47] The anomalous mass is apparent on preoperative CT, MRI, or ultrasound, but preoperative angiography is essential for the proper evaluation of the renal arteries. The isthmus of the kidney rarely needs to be divided and is avoided

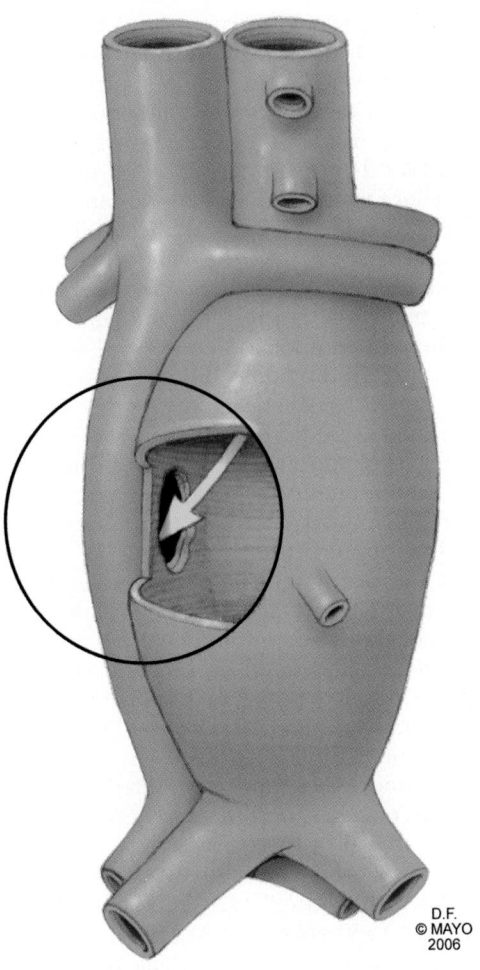

Figure 65-17 Aortocaval fistula. (By permission of Mayo Foundation for Medical Education and Research. All rights reserved.)

if possible because the aortic graft can be tunneled behind it. If the renal arteries arise from the aneurysm, they can be reimplanted into the graft as a patch. A left retroperitoneal approach is advocated because it allows easier management of the multiple accessory renal arteries (Fig. 65-18). Endovascular repair is difficult or not possible because of multiple renal arteries.

Associated Intra-abdominal Pathology

If an abdominal malignancy or other intra-abdominal pathology coexists with a symptomatic or ruptured AAA, treatment of the aneurysm must take precedence to ensure the immediate survival of the patient. Malignant tumors, most of them colonic, are found unexpectedly in 4% to 5% of patients undergoing operation for AAA. When a neoplasm coexists with an AAA, the most life-threatening problem is treated first. An obstructing, bleeding, or perforated colon cancer is resected before elective repair of a stable 5.5-cm AAA. Likewise, a symptomatic or ruptured aneurysm is repaired before an elective colon resection is carried out. When both entities are asymptomatic, treatment is based on the size of the aneurysm. If the AAA is 5 cm or larger, the aneurysm is repaired first, and the colonic resection can be performed 2 to 4 weeks later. If the aneurysm is small (<5 cm), the colonic lesion is repaired initially. If a symptomatic or ruptured AAA and an obstructing colonic cancer are encountered simultaneously, one strategy would be to repair the aneurysm and externalize a colonic loop proximal to the tumor for decompression at the same operation along with nasogastric tube decompression of the stomach. Maturation of the colostomy can be performed the following day to avoid contamination of the aortic graft.

The presence of asymptomatic gallstones is found unexpectedly in 5% to 20% of patients undergoing aortic

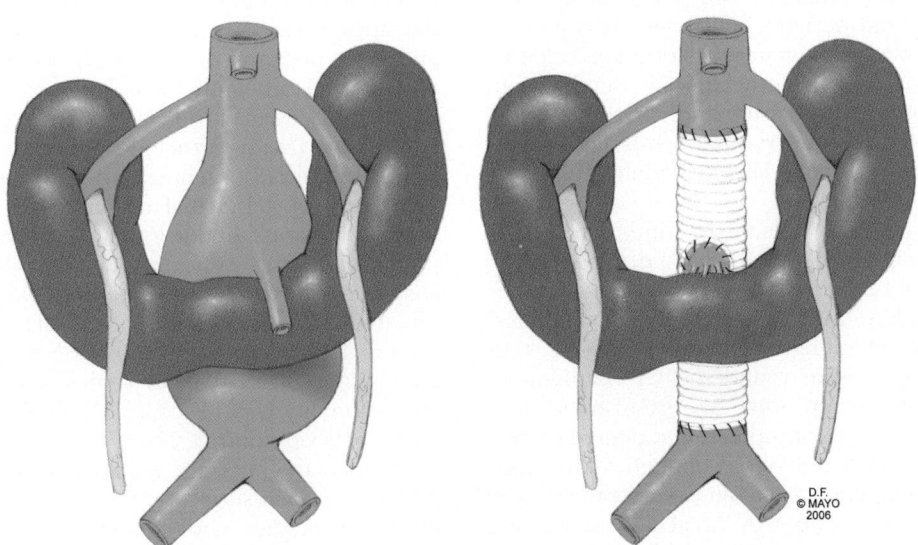

Figure 65-18 Abdominal aortic aneurysm repair in the setting of a horseshoe kidney. (By permission of Mayo Foundation for Medical Education and Research. All rights reserved.).

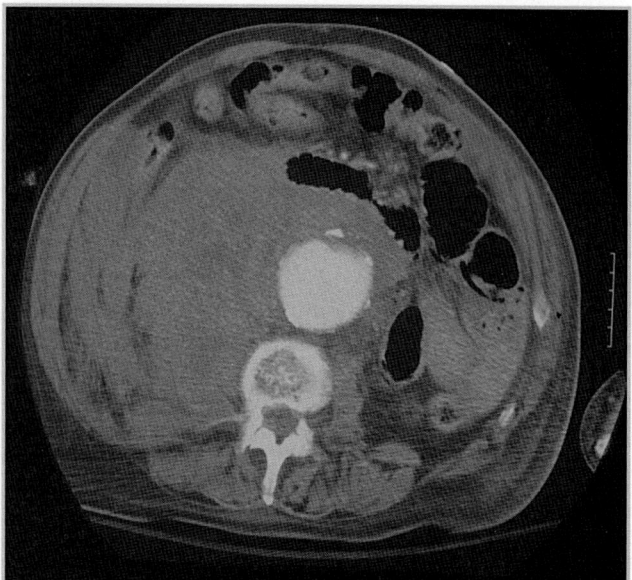

Figure 65-19 CT scan confirms a ruptured abdominal aortic aneurysm.

surgery. The incidence of positive bile cultures in patients with cholelithiasis is as high as 33%. As with colonic lesions, performance of elective cholecystectomy, which could lead to contamination of a newly implanted aortic graft, must not be performed in conjunction with AAA repair.

Ruptured Abdominal Aortic Aneurysm

The most dreaded complication of AAAs is aneurysm rupture (Fig. 65-19). Aneurysms can rupture freely into the peritoneal cavity or retroperitoneum. Free intraperitoneal rupture usually occurs anteriorly and is associated with immediate hemodynamic collapse and a very high mortality rate. Retroperitoneal ruptures are usually posterior and may be contained by the psoas muscle and adjacent periaortic and perivertebral tissue. This type of rupture can occur without significant blood loss initially, and the patient may be hemodynamically stable. Both types of rupture present with back and abdominal pain, pallor, diaphoresis, syncope, or other symptoms related to bleeding and hypovolemic shock. If untreated, AAA rupture is fatal in all cases.

Ruptured AAAs require immediate surgical repair. If the patient is unstable and an AAA has been previously diagnosed or a pulsatile mass is present, no further evaluation is needed, and the patient is transferred immediately to the operating room. Stable patients with a questionable diagnosis may undergo CT scanning to confirm the presence of an aortic aneurysm as well as demonstrate its extent, site of rupture, and degree of iliac involvement. In patients not stable enough to undergo CT scanning, an emergency room ultrasound can be used to confirm the presence of an AAA. An acutely expanding or symptomatic aneurysm is prone to rupture and also must be repaired expeditiously.

Open surgical repair of ruptured AAA is most commonly performed through the transperitoneal approach. The first priority is to control the hemorrhage by gaining proximal control of the aorta. Resuscitation is best done in the operating room rather than the emergency department, and blood pressure needs to be restored only to levels sufficient to maintain end-organ and cerebral perfusion before induction of anesthesia. The patient is prepped and draped with the surgical team poised to make incision before the induction of anesthesia because anesthesia induction can result in sudden, severe hypotension when the tamponade effects and reflex vasoconstriction are reversed by relaxation of the abdominal wall and administered anesthetic agents. In cases of contained rupture, proximal aortic control is best achieved at the supraceliac level through the lesser omentum (Fig. 65-20). After the aneurysm neck is dissected, the aortic clamp can be moved down to the infrarenal level. In cases of free rupture, the aorta can be quickly compressed at the diaphragmatic hiatus either manually or with a commercially available compression device. An infrarenal clamp or an intraluminal occluding balloon catheter can be substituted as soon as possible. When bleeding is controlled, adequate blood and volume resuscitation generally resume. The operation is then carried out in a manner similar to elective aneurysm repair. Heparin is unnecessary and is avoided. The aggressive use of blood, platelets, and fresh frozen plasma is essential for the survival of these patients.

In a study of 413 consecutive patients treated for a ruptured AAA, the overall early mortality rate was 45%. Advanced age (>80 years), APACHE II score, low initial hematocrit,[19] and preoperative cardiac arrest were associated with increased mortality. The cumulative survival rates after successful repair at 5 and 10 years are 64% and 33%, respectively. Two thirds of patients discharged from the hospital after ruptured AAA repair were alive after 5 years. Ruptured AAA is thought to be less suitable for EVAR because of the need for preoperative measurements of the aneurysm and arterial anatomy to determine the appropriate size and type of endograft to be used and also because of the delay in obtaining proximal aortic occlusion. Veith and colleagues reported the results of 29 endovascular repairs of ruptured AAAs.[48] Patients were treated with restricted fluid resuscitation (hypotensive hemostasis), urgent transport to the operating room, placement of a brachial or femoral guidewire into the supraceliac aorta under local anesthesia, and arteriography. EVAR was performed if aortoiliac anatomy was suitable; otherwise, patients underwent open surgical repair. A supraceliac balloon was placed and inflated for proximal aortic occlusion using the previously positioned guidewire only if circulatory collapse occurred. The operative mortality was 13%. Only 10 patients required supraceliac balloon control. There is increasing evidence that endovascular grafts are a better way to treat ruptured AAAs than open surgical repair. However, the number of published studies and patients remains small, and the final role of EVAR for the treatment of ruptured AAA is still to be determined.

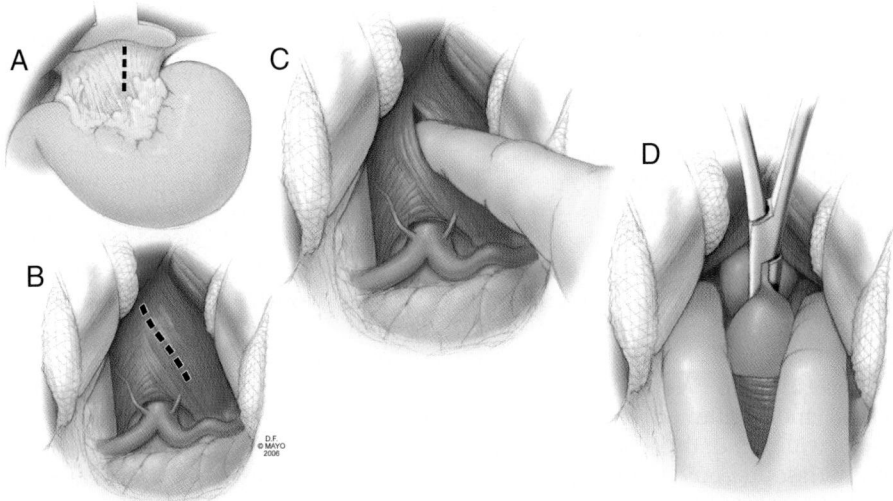

Figure 65-20 A to **D,** Supraceliac control of the aorta can be accomplished by dividing the gastrohepatic ligament and left crus of the diaphragm. Blunt finger dissection through the left diaphragmatic crus and laterally around the aorta allows proper clamp placement. (By permission of Mayo Foundation for Medical Education and Research. All rights reserved.)

ILIAC ARTERY ANEURYSMS

Iliac artery aneurysms occur in conjunction with aortic aneurysms in 40% of patients. Isolated iliac aneurysms are rare, accounting for less than 2% of all aortoiliac aneurysms. Much like aortic aneurysms, iliac aneurysms occur in association with atherosclerosis. However, they can also occur in pregnancy in the absence of atherosclerosis, as well as in patients with Marfan and Ehlers-Danlos syndromes, Kawasaki disease, Takayasu's disease, cystic medial necrosis, and arterial dissection. Most isolated iliac aneurysms involve the common iliac artery (70%) and the hypogastric (internal iliac) artery (20%). Isolated external iliac artery aneurysms are uncommon. Multiple iliac aneurysms occur in most patients and are bilateral in 33%. Because most occur in association with atherosclerosis, the average age at diagnosis is 69 years. Males are more commonly affected than females, with a ratio of 7:1, and left and right sides are involved equally.

The clinical presentation of iliac aneurysms is variable. Because of their location in the pelvis, they are not easily palpable on physical examination unless they are large. Many patients have symptoms in the absence of rupture. Symptoms are caused by compression of adjacent pelvic structures such as the bladder and ureter, colon and rectum, lumbosacral nerves, and pelvic veins. Consequently, patients often experience lower abdominal, flank, and groin pain. Diagnosis is usually made by CT or ultrasound performed because of symptoms or an unrelated condition. Large common iliac aneurysms can be palpated on abdominal exam, whereas hypogastric artery aneurysms are more readily palpable on rectal examination. Because these aneurysms often present with nonspecific symptoms, diagnosis is delayed in many cases. Therefore, iliac aneurysms tend to be large at

diagnosis. One study reported the average size of iliac aneurysms at diagnosis to be 5.6 cm with a rupture rate of 30%. The operative mortality rate in patients with ruptured iliac aneurysms is 40%.

Several studies suggest that isolated iliac aneurysms less than 3 cm in diameter can be treated conservatively by close observation with semiannual ultrasound or CT scan. Iliac aneurysms larger than 3.5 cm are repaired if possible. Common iliac artery aneurysms associated with aortic aneurysms, if larger than 2 cm, are repaired using a bifurcated graft at the time of aortic aneurysm repair.

Open repair of iliac artery aneurysms is by graft placement through open surgical incision. Because the external iliac artery is rarely aneurysmal, this operation can usually be confined to the abdomen. Bilateral common iliac aneurysms require reconstruction with a bifurcated aortoiliac graft. Hypogastric artery aneurysms can be treated with endoaneurysmorrhaphy. They are not treated with simple ligation of the neck because they will remain pressurized through collaterals, causing further aneurysmal enlargement. The advent of endovascular techniques has expanded the treatment options for iliac aneurysms. Common iliac aneurysms are treated percutaneously with a covered stent or stent-graft, thereby excluding the aneurysm, as in the endovascular repair of AAAs. Internal iliac artery aneurysms can be treated with catheter-based techniques by injecting embolization coils and other thrombogenic materials into the aneurysm sac and its branches.

FEMORAL ARTERY ANEURYSMS

Femoral artery aneurysms (FAAs) are the second most frequent peripheral artery aneurysms after popliteal aneurysms. They are bilateral in more than 50% of patients, and 92% of patients have a concomitant aortoiliac aneurysm. True aneurysms of the femoral arteries are almost always degenerative atherosclerotic aneurysms, whereas false FAAs may develop as a result of disruption of the graft-artery anastomosis following surgical revascularization with aortofemoral or femoropopliteal bypass. Femoral pseudoaneurysms (pulsatile hematoma) can also develop after percutaneous catheterization, whereas mycotic aneurysms can develop in patients who have infected graft sutured to the femoral artery or in IV drug users. The most common organisms causing mycotic aneurysms include *Staphylococcus aureus, Escherichia coli,* and *Salmonella* species.

The diagnosis of atherosclerotic FAA is usually made by physical examination and confirmed by ultrasound. In patients who present with femoral pseudoaneurysms after catheterization, ultrasound-guided compression, with or without thrombin injection, can also be used to treat the disease. In chronic true aneurysms, CTA or contrast aortography helps surgical planning, whereas in patients with mycotic aneurysms, more extensive preoperative evaluation, including blood cultures, local wound culture, and indium-labeled white blood cell scan, may be needed.

All true FAAs larger than 2 cm need to be considered for repair because of either risk for thromboembolic complications or an increased risk for rupture. Large femoral aneurysms, especially the false aneurysms and those involving the profunda femoris artery, have a high chance of rupture; in one study, 50% of the profunda femoris aneurysms ruptured.

Surgical treatment usually includes resection and replacement with a prosthetic interposition graft. An attempt is always made to revascularize the profunda femoris artery as well. In an infected field, reconstruction with femoral or saphenous vein graft or rifampin-soaked prosthetic graft is an option. Revascularization of the limb with an obturator bypass or an extra-anatomic axillofemoral or axillopopliteal bypass can also be considered. In these cases, the graft needs to be tunneled deep or lateral to the infected field, and the sterile part of the operation needs to be performed first, with the skin closed before removal of the infected artery or graft from the groin. Asymptomatic patients do very well after femoral aneurysm repair, but symptomatic patients have an amputation rate as high as 10% even in experienced hands, and many patients have residual symptoms due to decreased limb perfusion. The highest amputation rates have been reported in drug addicts who required treatment of infected femoral aneurysms. Reddy suggested autologous repair with a vein graft and immediate coverage with a sartorius muscle flap to decrease the rate of reinfection and recurrent bleeding.[49]

POPLITEAL ARTERY ANEURYSMS

Popliteal artery aneurysms (PAAs) are rare, occurring in less than 0.01% of hospitalized patients. They are the most common peripheral aneurysms and account for 70% of the peripheral artery aneurysms. Recognition of PAAs is important because of the risk for limb loss as a result of complications of the disease. Despite progress in therapy, amputation rates in patients with acute thromboembolism due to PAAs have ranged from 0% to 30%.[8]

Almost all patients (97%) with PAAs are male, and the disease is bilateral in 53%. In a study from the Mayo Clinic that included 368 PAAs treated in 299 patients, 40% were asymptomatic, 38% had chronic limb ischemia, and 22% presented with an acute thromboembolism that included popliteal artery thrombosis, tibial artery embolization, and blue toe syndrome.[8] Only 1 PAA ruptured.

Most PAAs can be diagnosed by careful physical examination. Duplex scanning confirms the diagnosis, and CTA, MRA, or contrast arteriography defines runoff and helps in the planning of open surgery or a more recently introduced endovascular management.

Acute and chronic symptoms are usually indications for intervention. In asymptomatic patients who are reasonable surgical risks and have an aneurysm of 2 cm or larger, have thrombus in the aneurysm, and have angiographic evidence of distal embolization, intervention is suggested.

Open surgical reconstruction with a saphenous vein bypass is the current gold standard for repair, whereas exclusion of the aneurysm is suggested using endoaneurysmorrhaphy to avoid late increase of the excluded aneurysm by feeding genicular arteries. In one study, 68% of the PAAs were repaired with saphenous vein and 26% with PTFE grafts. The medial approach is preferred by most surgeons, although the posterior approach is attractive if the proximal popliteal artery is of normal size (Fig. 65-21). Beseth and Moore used short PTFE grafts through this approach, with good runoff and excellent results.[50]

The early mortality rate of PAAs was 1% (3 of 368) in the Mayo Clinic study, all in patients with acute presentation.[8] The 30-day graft thrombosis rate was 4% (acute: 7/80, 10%; chronic: 5/142, 4%; asymptomatic: 1/146, 1%), and there were 5 early amputations following failed bypass (PTFE: 4; vein: 1), all with acute presentation. The 5-year graft patency rate was 86%, higher with saphenous vein graft (94%) than with PTFE graft (63%, $P \le .05$). The 5-year limb loss rate was 4% (16 of 368), and 14 of 16 amputations occurred with acute presentation (18%, 14/80). There was no limb loss in asymptomatic patients or those with chronic symptoms when saphenous vein graft was used for bypass.

In patients with acute limb ischemia, catheter-directed thrombolysis is considered. The tip of the catheter is placed into the distal popliteal artery, and no attempt is made to dissolve all thrombi in the aneurysm. Thrombolysis improves runoff for revascularization and decreases limb loss.

Recent publications show promise for endovascular treatment of PAAs with stent-grafts, especially for high-risk patients with good runoff. One study of 23 limbs reported a 74% patency of stent-grafts at 1 year, whereas a prospective randomized study of 30 patients reported a 2-year primary patency rate of 100% for open surgery, compared with 80% for endovascular treatment, without a statistically significant difference between the two

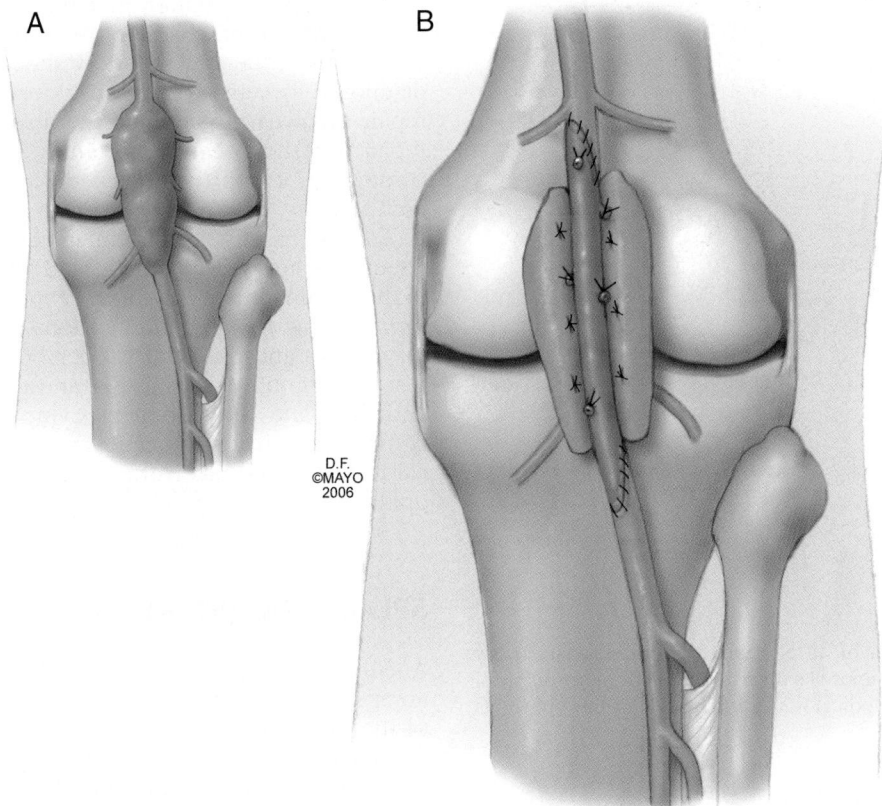

D.F.
©MAYO
2006

Figure 65-21 A, Popliteal artery aneurysm. **B,** Repair through a posterior approach using a saphenous vein interposition graft. The genicular arteries are interrupted from within the sac of the aneurysm. (By permission of Mayo Foundation for Medical Education and Research. All rights reserved.)

groups.[51] Further experience with larger number of patients and longer follow-up is needed with endovascular repair. Currently, repair of PAAs with saphenous bypass and endoaneurysmorrhaphy continues to be the gold standard.

UPPER EXTREMITY ANEURYSMS

Aneurysms of the upper extremity are rare, accounting for 1% of all peripheral aneurysms. However, they have the potential to lead to serious complications such as digit and limb loss, stroke from proximal embolization into the vertebral or carotid arteries, and exsanguinating hemorrhage. Therefore, prompt diagnosis and treatment are imperative.

Subclavian artery aneurysms are the most common of upper extremity aneurysms.[52] They are usually caused by atherosclerosis, trauma, compression at the thoracic outlet, and infection. Aneurysms of the proximal subclavian artery are most commonly associated with atherosclerosis, and as many as 50% have aneurysms elsewhere. Aneurysms of the distal subclavian artery are typically associated with a cervical rib or other causes of thoracic outlet syndrome. Patients may experience neck, chest, or shoulder pain from aneurysm expansion or rupture. The

primary complication with subclavian aneurysms is distal embolization to the upper extremity. Exertional fatigue of the arm, forearm, or hand may occur, as well as pain, paralysis, gangrene, or tissue loss as a result of chronic or acute ischemia. In addition, embolization may occur proximally into the vertebral and carotid arteries, and patients may experience transient ischemic attacks or stroke. Compression of the recurrent laryngeal nerve by aneurysm expansion can lead to hoarseness or respiratory insufficiency. Likewise, tracheal compression or compression of the brachial plexus may occur, causing respiratory distress or a brachial plexus palsy, respectively. Horner's syndrome may also result from compression of the stellate ganglion, and the aneurysm can erode into the lung, causing hemoptysis. A pulsatile mass may be palpated on physical exam, and a bruit may be present in the supraclavicular fossa or in the axilla. The diagnosis can be established by duplex ultrasound or CT scan. Aortic arch and upper extremity angiography is necessary to define the extent of the aneurysm; its position relative to the vertebral artery, common carotid artery (for right-sided aneurysms), and thoracic outlet structures; and the extent and nature of thromboembolic disease if present.

Subclavian aneurysms are considered potentially life- and limb-threatening and when detected should be

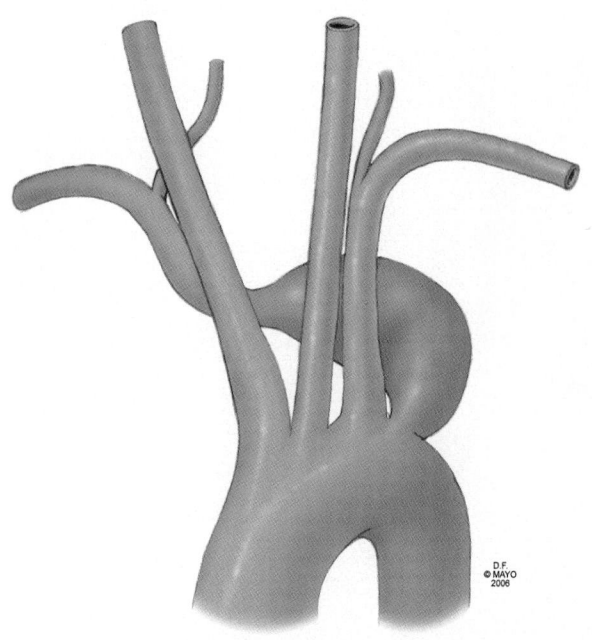

Figure 65-22 Aneurysm of an aberrant right subclavian artery with an associated Kommerell's diverticulum. (By permission of Mayo Foundation for Medical Education and Research. All rights reserved.)

repaired. Surgical repair involves resection of the aneurysm and reestablishment of arterial continuity, usually with an interposition graft. The vertebral artery should be preserved whenever possible. Aneurysms of the distal subclavian artery can be repaired through a supraclavicular or infraclavicular approach or a combination of the two. When the aneurysm is proximal enough so that proximal control cannot be safely obtained through these approaches, a median sternotomy (right-sided lesions) or left thoracotomy (left-sided lesions) is required. Midsubclavian lesions can often be managed through a supraclavicular or infraclavicular approach with or without medial resection of the clavicle. Extremity thromboembolism should be treated with balloon thrombectomy to restore distal perfusion. Endovascular repair can also be accomplished with a covered stent-graft and is particularly useful in high-risk patients. However, long-term results with this technique are unknown.

An aberrant right subclavian artery originating from the proximal descending thoracic aorta can be associated with aneurysmal change at the origin of the artery and is referred to as *Kommerell's diverticulum* (Fig. 65-22). Complications associated with this abnormality include dysphagia from esophageal compression (*dysphagia lusoria*), dyspnea from tracheal compression, pain from expansion and rupture, and ischemic symptoms of the upper extremity from thromboembolism. Repair of aberrant right subclavian arteries with Kommerell's diverticulum is recommended regardless of aneurysm size because of the risk for rupture and other distal embolization.

Axillary artery aneurysms are typically associated with blunt or penetrating trauma. Symptoms are related to nerve compression and ischemia from thrombosis or thromboembolism. Similar to subclavian aneurysms, aneurysms of the axillary artery should be repaired once diagnosed because of the risk for limb loss. Surgical repair involves resection of the aneurysm with primary repair if a short segment of artery is involved, or more commonly, reconstruction with an interposition vein graft.

Aneurysms can also form in the ulnar artery. Such aneurysms are typically associated with repetitive trauma to the dominant hand, a clinical entity termed *hypothenar hammer syndrome*. Complications include ulnar artery thrombosis and distal thromboembolism with associated rest pain, numbness, cyanosis, and gangrene of the hand and third and fourth fingers. Symptoms of ulnar nerve compression may also occur. Treatment consists of surgical resection and reconstruction with a vein interposition graft.

SPLANCHNIC ARTERY ANEURYSMS

Aneurysms of the visceral branches of the abdominal aorta are discovered with increasing frequency because of the more frequent use of abdominal imaging studies, particularly CT scans. They are three times as common as renal artery aneurysms, and their clinical significance is the high mortality of ruptured aneurysms. Up to 22% of cases present with "herald bleeding" or the so-called abdominal apoplexy, with a mortality rate that has ranged from 21% to 100% in published reports. Women of childbearing age are at the highest risk for rupture of a splanchnic artery aneurysm. Of 306 splanchnic artery aneurysms reported at the Mayo Clinic, Abbas and colleagues found that splenic artery aneurysms were the most common (71%).[53] At least one third of the splanchnic artery aneurysms are multiple.

Splenic Artery Aneurysms

Females are four times more likely to have splenic artery aneurysms than males; of 217 patients, Abbas and colleagues found that 71% were women and 29% men.[53] Splenic artery aneurysms are the most common splanchnic aneurysms, many are saccular in nature, and most are caused by degenerative atherosclerosis. High splenic artery flow is an important etiology, frequently a result of portal hypertension. Medial fibrodysplasia associated with renovascular hypertension and polyarteritis nodosa is another cause, whereas pancreatitis and septic emboli are the most frequent causes of mycotic false aneurysms. The incidence of splenic artery aneurysms is the highest in multiparous women: 40% or more of affected women had six or more pregnancies. They are also frequent in patients with splenomegaly and after orthotopic liver transplantation. The overall risk for rupture is 5% (10 of 217 patients studied). There is evidence in the literature that pregnant patients are at high risk for rupture of a splenic artery aneurysm.

Rupture is the most frequent complication and can present with hypotension, hemorrhagic shock, and left upper quadrant pain. Rupture in pregnancy can result in high (75%) maternal and even higher (95%) fetal mortality. The mortality rate after ruptured splenic aneurysm in transplant recipients is 50%. The mortality rate of patients with ruptured splenic artery aneurysms in the Mayo Clinic series was 20%.[53]

Plain radiographs may show curvilinear calcification of the aneurysm, but calcification does not protect from rupture. CT and contrast angiography reveal the aneurysm and help in the planning or initiation of treatment.

Percutaneous embolization of the splenic artery is the most frequently applied therapy. Open surgical splenectomy is rarely needed, but proximal and distal surgical ligation with open surgery or laparoscopy are good treatment options. Open ligation or transcatheter embolization should be considered for symptomatic aneurysms, for aneurysms 2 cm in diameter, or for any splenic artery aneurysm in a woman of childbearing age. Splenic infarct and recanalization of the artery treated with embolization are concerns, and these patients require follow-up with regular imaging. Most recently, stent-grafts and covered stents have been used with success to treat splenic artery aneurysms. Mycotic aneurysms may need open surgical treatment with splenectomy and pancreatectomy, and they frequently have a poor prognosis.

Hepatic Artery Aneurysms

Most extrahepatic aneurysms are true aneurysms, whereas most intrahepatic aneurysms are false, owing to the more frequently used transhepatic interventional procedures. Degenerative atherosclerosis and medial fibroplasia are the most frequent causes of extrahepatic aneurysms, followed by periarteritis nodosa, mycotic aneurysms (usually caused by pancreatitis), neurofibromatosis, liver transplantation, and Wegener's granulomatosis. Most symptomatic patients present with right upper quadrant pain or hypovolemic shock. Occasionally, gastrointestinal hemorrhage is caused by aneurysm rupture into the gastrointestinal tract. Rupture into the biliary tree results in the classic triad of biliary colic, hemobilia, and obstructive jaundice.

Most hepatic aneurysms require intervention because rupture is frequent and lethal.[53] Transcatheter embolization or proximal and distal ligation is suitable treatment if the gastroduodenal artery provides collateral circulation to the liver. Otherwise, a saphenous vein graft is advised because runoff is frequently poor owing to previous embolization from the aneurysm.

Stent-graft or covered stent placement is becoming an option in therapy. Occlusion of the proper hepatic artery may result in hepatic necrosis and usually should be avoided.

Superior Mesenteric Artery Aneurysms

Degenerative arteriosclerosis is the most common cause of superior mesenteric artery aneurysm, but septic emboli,

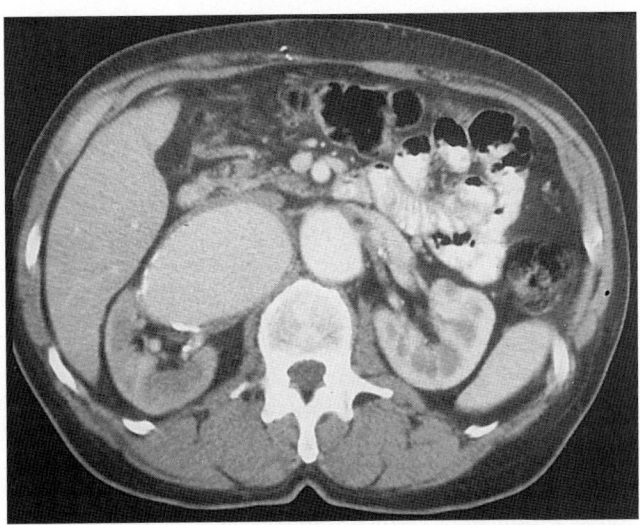

Figure 65-23 CT scan demonstrating a 6-cm degenerative right renal artery aneurysm. Note the associated small abdominal aortic aneurysm.

infected by nonhemolytic streptococcus, staphylococci, or gram-negative bacteria, are the cause in one third of patients. Polyarteritis nodosa, pancreatitis, neurofibromatosis, and traumatic and spontaneous dissections are additional causes. Herald bleeding and abdominal pain are the most typical presentations. Acute mesenteric ischemia due to thromboembolism is associated with rupture in 50% of patients. An aneurysm of any size should be considered for repair. Transcatheter embolization is a good option if collateral circulation is adequate; otherwise, proximal and distal ligation and surgical reconstruction with a bypass are indicated. There are successful case reports of stent-grafts or covered stents used for these aneurysms as well.

Pancreaticoduodenal and Gastroduodenal Aneurysms

Abdominal pain and bleeding from the pancreatic duct (hemosuccus pancreaticus) are typical presentations. They are frequently associated with pancreatic pseudocysts, and sudden enlargement or onset of pulsatility of the cyst warrants immediate therapy. Transcatheter embolization is typically used for acute treatment, although secondary infection of the embolic material is not uncommon. Proximal and distal ligation, usually without vascular reconstruction, is the definitive therapy in many patients.

RENAL ARTERY ANEURYSMS

Renal artery aneurysms are uncommon, and their rupture is rare. Most are saccular, and 75% occur at the bifurcation of the primary or secondary branches. Medial fibroplasia is the most frequent cause of true renal aneurysms, followed by degenerative atherosclerosis (Fig. 65-23) and polyarteritis nodosa. Spontaneous or traumatic dissection is the most frequent cause of false renal aneurysms. Patients are usually asymptomatic or have associated renal artery occlusive disease and renovascular hypertension or ischemic nephropathy. Rupture occurs in less than 3% of cases, but when the aneurysm ruptures in a pregnant woman, the fetal mortality rate is 75%, and the maternal mortality rate is 50%. Surgical indications are debated, but any aneurysm larger than 2 cm in a woman of childbearing age should be repaired.[54] The goals of surgical repair with a patch or bypass, occasionally using ex vivo reconstruction, are to prevent aneurysm rupture, preserve the kidney parenchyma, and treat any underlying renovascular hypertension. Ex vivo reconstruction may be needed for aneurysms involving the primary or secondary branches.[54] Transcatheter embolization can be attempted in patients not suitable for open repair and in those with a saccular aneurysm, in whom embolization may result in aneurysm occlusion without infarction of a significant portion of the kidney parenchyma. Patients who are followed for renal artery aneurysms at regular intervals should have thorough medical control of their blood pressure.

Selected References

Brewster DC, Cronenwett JL, Hallett JW Jr, for the Joint Council of the American Association for Vascular Surgery and Society for Vascular Surgery: Guidelines for the treatment of abdominal aortic aneurysms. Report of a subcommittee of the Joint Council of the American Association for Vascular Surgery and Society for Vascular Surgery. J Vasc Surg 37:1106-1117, 2003.

This important paper contains guidelines of the Society for Vascular Surgery on open surgical and endovascular treatment of abdominal aortic aneurysms.

EVAR Trial Participants: Endovascular aneurysm repair versus open repair in patients with abdominal aortic aneurysm (EVAR Trial 1): Randomised controlled trial. Lancet 365:2179-2186, 2005.

Report on 1082 patients who had abdominal aortic aneurysm of at least 5.5 cm in diameter and were randomized to open surgery or endovascular repair. Compared with open repair, endovascular repair did not offer advantage in this study with respect to all-cause mortality and quality of life, and it resulted in a greater number of complications and reinterventions. However, it resulted in a 3% better aneurysm-related survival. The author recommended ongoing surveillance and longer follow-up of patients to assess efficacy and durability of endovascular repair.

Lederle FA, Wilson SE, Johnson GR, et al, for the Aneurysm Detection and Management Veterans Affairs Cooperative Study Group: Immediate repair compared with surveillance of small abdominal aortic aneurysms. N Engl J Med 346:1437-1444, 2002.

This is a prospective multicenter study that randomized patients with abdominal aortic aneurysm of 4.0 to 5.4 cm in diameter to undergo immediate open surgical repair or surveillance every 6 months. The rate of aneurysm-related death was not different in the surgical group (3%) than in the surveillance group (2.6%). The study concluded that survival was not improved by immediate repair of small abdominal aortic aneurysms.

Noel AA, Gloviczki P, Cherry KJ Jr, et al: Ruptured abdominal aortic aneurysms: The excessive mortality rate of conventional repair. J Vasc Surg 34:41-46, 2001.

This retrospective study analyzed factors affecting survival in 413 consecutive patients treated at the Mayo Clinic for ruptured abdominal aortic aneurysm (AAA). The authors concluded that surgical mortality remains excessive, although improvement in the past decade was evident. Patients older than 80 years with shock or cardiac arrest have the highest mortality. Because the diagnosis of AAA was unknown in more than 70% of patients before rupture, the authors recommend screening of the high-risk population and early elective repair.

Zarins CK: Lifeline registry of endovascular aneurysm repair: Long-term primary outcome measure. J Vasc Surg 42:1-10, 2005.

This manuscript reviewed primary outcome measures of 2664 patients who underwent endovascular abdominal aortic aneurysm repair and compared data with those of 334 patients with open repair. Both techniques were effective in preventing aneurysm rupture at 1 year, and there was no difference in survival between the two groups at 4 years. The author concluded that endovascular aneurysm repair using FDA-approved devices is a safe, effective, and durable treatment for anatomically suited patients with infrarenal abdominal aortic aneurysms.

References

1. Johnston KW, Rutherford RB, Tilson MD, et al: Suggested standards for reporting on arterial aneurysms. Subcommittee on Reporting Standards for Arterial Aneurysms, Ad Hoc Committee on Reporting Standards, Society for Vascular Surgery and North American Chapter, International Society for Cardiovascular Surgery. J Vasc Surg 13:452-458, 1991.
2. Parodi JC, Palmaz JC, Barone HD: Transfemoral intraluminal graft implantation for abdominal aortic aneurysms. Ann Vasc Surg 5:491-499, 1991.
3. Bengtsson H, Sonesson B, Bergqvist D: Incidence and prevalence of abdominal aortic aneurysms, estimated by necropsy studies and population screening by ultrasound. Ann N Y Acad Sci 800:1-24, 1996.
4. Hollier LH, Stanson AW, Gloviczki P, et al: Arteriomegaly: Classification and morbid implications of diffuse aneurysmal disease. Surgery 93:700-708, 1983.
5. Gloviczki P, Pairolero P, Welch T, et al: Multiple aortic aneurysms: The results of surgical management. J Vasc Surg 11:19-27; discussion 27-28, 1990.
6. Bickerstaff LK, Pairolero PC, Hollier LH, et al: Thoracic aortic aneurysms: A population-based study. Surgery 92:1103-1108, 1982.
7. Dent TL, Lindenauer SM, Ernst CB, et al: Multiple arteriosclerotic arterial aneurysms. Arch Surg 105:338-344, 1972.
8. Huang Y, Gloviczki P, Noel AA, et al: Early complications and long-term outcome after open surgical treatment of popliteal artery aneurysms: Is exclusion with saphenous vein by-pass still the gold standard? J Vasc Surg 45:706-715, 2007.
9. Cohen JR, Mandell C, Chang JB, et al: Elastin metabolism of the infrarenal aorta. J Vasc Surg 7:210-214, 1988.
10. Ailawadi G, Eliason JL, Upchurch GR Jr: Current concepts in the pathogenesis of abdominal aortic aneurysm. J Vasc Surg 38:584-588, 2003.
11. McMillan WD, Pearce WH: Increased plasma levels of metalloproteinase-9 are associated with abdominal aortic aneurysms. J Vasc Surg 29:122-127; discussion 127-129, 1999.
12. Oderich GS, Panneton JM, Bower TC, et al: The spectrum, management and clinical outcome of Ehlers-Danlos syndrome type IV: A 30-year experience. J Vasc Surg 42:98-106, 2005.
13. The UK Small Aneurysm Trial Participants: Mortality results for randomised controlled trial of early elective surgery or

ultrasonographic surveillance for small abdominal aortic aneurysms. Lancet 352:1649-1655, 1998.

14. Lederle FA, Johnson GR, Wilson SE, et al: Prevalence and associations of abdominal aortic aneurysm detected through screening. Aneurysm Detection and Management (ADAM) Veterans Affairs Cooperative Study Group. Ann Intern Med 126:441-449, 1997.

15. Lederle FA, Johnson GR, Wilson SE, et al: The aneurysm detection and management study screening program: Validation cohort and final results. Aneurysm Detection and Management Veterans Affairs Cooperative Study Investigators. Arch Intern Med 160:1425-1430, 2000.

16. Fleming C, Whitlock EP, Beil TL, et al: Screening for abdominal aortic aneurysm: A best-evidence systematic review for the U.S. Preventive Services Task Force. Ann Intern Med 142:203-211, 2005.

17. Gloviczki P, Pairolero PC, Mucha P Jr, et al: Ruptured abdominal aortic aneurysms: Repair should not be denied. J Vasc Surg 15:851-857; discussion 857-859, 1992.

18. Davis PM, Gloviczki P, Cherry KJ Jr, et al: Aorto-caval and ilio-iliac arteriovenous fistulae. Am J Surg 176:115-118, 1998.

19. Noel AA, Gloviczki P, Cherry KJ Jr, et al: Ruptured abdominal aortic aneurysms: The excessive mortality rate of conventional repair. J Vasc Surg 34:41-46, 2001.

20. Cronenwett JL, Sargent SK, Wall MH, et al: Variables that affect the expansion rate and outcome of small abdominal aortic aneurysms. J Vasc Surg 11:260-268; discussion 268-269, 1990.

21. Brewster DC, Cronenwett JL, Hallett JW Jr, et al: Guidelines for the treatment of abdominal aortic aneurysms. Report of a subcommittee of the Joint Council of the American Association for Vascular Surgery and Society for Vascular Surgery. J Vasc Surg 37:1106-1117, 2003.

22. Lederle FA, Wilson SE, Johnson GR, et al: Immediate repair compared with surveillance of small abdominal aortic aneurysms. N Engl J Med 346:1437-1444, 2002.

23. Ashton HA, Buxton MJ, Day NE, et al: The Multicentre Aneurysm Screening Study (MASS) into the effect of abdominal aortic aneurysm screening on mortality in men: A randomised controlled trial. Lancet 360:1531-1539, 2002.

24. Kent KC, Zwolak RM, Jaff MR, et al: Screening for abdominal aortic aneurysm: A consensus statement. J Vasc Surg 39:267-269, 2004.

25. Steinmetz EF, Buckley C, Thompson RW: Prospects for the medical management of abdominal aortic aneurysms. Vasc Endovascular Surg 37:151-163, 2003.

26. Bergman RT, Gloviczki P, Welch TJ, et al: The role of intravenous fluorescein in the detection of colon ischemia during aortic reconstruction. Ann Vasc Surg 6:74-79, 1992.

27. Turnipseed WD, Carr SC, Hoch JR, et al: Minimal incision aortic surgery (MIAS). Ann Vasc Surg 17:180-184, 2003.

28. Rutherford RB, Krupski WC: Current status of open versus endovascular stent-graft repair of abdominal aortic aneurysm. J Vasc Surg 39:1129-1139, 2004.

29. Hertzer NR, Mascha EJ: A personal experience with factors influencing survival after elective open repair of infrarenal aortic aneurysms. J Vasc Surg 42:898-905, 2005.

30. Elkouri S, Gloviczki P, McKusick MA, et al: Perioperative complications and early outcome after endovascular and open surgical repair of abdominal aortic aneurysms. J Vasc Surg 39:497-505, 2004.

31. Gloviczki P, Cross SA, Stanson AW, et al: Ischemic injury to the spinal cord or lumbosacral plexus after aorto-iliac reconstruction. Am J Surg 162:131-136, 1991.

32. Hallett JW Jr, Marshall DM, Petterson TM, et al: Graft-related complications after abdominal aortic aneurysm repair: Reassurance from a 36-year population-based experience. J Vasc Surg 25:277-284; discussion 285-276, 1997.

33. Cho JS, Gloviczki P, Martelli E, et al: Long-term survival and late complications after repair of ruptured abdominal aortic aneurysms. J Vasc Surg 27:813-819; discussion 819-820, 1998.

34. Greenberg RK, Chuter TA, Sternbergh WC 3rd, et al: Zenith AAA endovascular graft: Intermediate-term results of the US multicenter trial. J Vasc Surg 39:1209-1218, 2004.

35. Matsumura JS, Brewster DC, Makaroun MS, et al: A multicenter controlled clinical trial of open versus endovascular treatment of abdominal aortic aneurysm. J Vasc Surg 37:262-271, 2003.

36. Moore WS, Matsumura JS, Makaroun MS, et al: Five-year interim comparison of the Guidant bifurcated endograft with open repair of abdominal aortic aneurysm. J Vasc Surg 38:46-55, 2003.

37. Carpenter JP: Multicenter trial of the PowerLink bifurcated system for endovascular aortic aneurysm repair. J Vasc Surg 36:1129-1137, 2002.

38. Zarins CK, White RA, Moll FL, et al: The AneuRx stent graft: Four-year results and worldwide experience 2000. J Vasc Surg 33:S135-145, 2001.

39. Lifeline registry of endovascular aneurysm repair: Long-term primary outcome measures. J Vasc Surg 42:1-10, 2005.

40. Greenberg RK, Lawrence-Brown M, Bhandari G, et al: An update of the Zenith endovascular graft for abdominal aortic aneurysms: Initial implantation and mid-term follow-up data. J Vasc Surg 33:S157-164, 2001.

41. Sampaio SM, Panneton JM, Mozes GI, et al: Proximal type I endoleak after endovascular abdominal aortic aneurysm repair: Predictive factors. Ann Vasc Surg 18:621-628, 2004.

42. Endovascular aneurysm repair versus open repair in patients with abdominal aortic aneurysm (EVAR trial 1): Randomised controlled trial. Lancet 365:2179-2186, 2005.

43. Blankensteijn JD, de Jong SE, Prinssen M, et al: Two-year outcomes after conventional or endovascular repair of abdominal aortic aneurysms. N Engl J Med 352:2398-2405, 2005.

44. Endovascular aneurysm repair and outcome in patients unfit for open repair of abdominal aortic aneurysm (EVAR trial 2): Randomised controlled trial. Lancet 365:2187-2192, 2005.

45. West CA, Noel AA, Bower TC, et al: Factors affecting outcomes of open surgical repair of pararenal aortic aneurysms: A 10-year experience. J Vasc Surg 43:921-927; discussion 927-928, 2006.

46. Nitecki SS, Hallett JW Jr, Stanson AW, et al: Inflammatory abdominal aortic aneurysms: A case-control study. J Vasc Surg 23:860-868; discussion 868-869, 1996.

47. de Virgilio C, Gloviczki P: Aortic reconstruction in patients with horseshoe or ectopic kidneys. Semin Vasc Surg 9:245-252, 1996.

48. Veith FJ, Ohki T, Lipsitz EC, et al: Treatment of ruptured abdominal aneurysms with stent grafts: A new gold standard? Semin Vasc Surg 16:171-175, 2003.

49. Reddy DJ: Treatment of drug-related infected false aneurysm of the femoral artery: Is routine revascularization justified? J Vasc Surg 8:344-345, 1988.

50. Beseth BD, Moore WS: The posterior approach for repair of popliteal artery aneurysms. J Vasc Surg 43:940-944; discussion 944-945, 2006.

51. Antonello M, Frigatti P, Battocchio P, et al: Open repair versus endovascular treatment for asymptomatic popliteal artery aneurysm: Results of a prospective randomized study. J Vasc Surg 42:185-193, 2005.

52. Bower TC, Pairolero PC, Hallett JW Jr, et al: Brachiocephalic aneurysm: The case for early recognition and repair. Ann Vasc Surg 5:125-132, 1991.

53. Abbas MA, Stone WM, Fowl RJ, et al: Splenic artery aneurysms: Two decades experience at Mayo Clinic. Ann Vasc Surg 16:442-449, 2002.

54. Dzsinich C, Gloviczki P, McKusick MA, et al: Surgical management of renal artery aneurysm. Cardiovasc Surg 1:243-247, 1993.

CHAPTER 66

Peripheral Arterial Occlusive Disease

Michael Belkin, MD   Christopher D. Owens, MD   Anthony D. Whittemore, MD

Magruder C. Donaldson, MD   Michael S. Conte, MD   and   Edwin Gravereaux, MD

BASIC CONSIDERATIONS

Arterial occlusive diseases are highly prevalent in Western societies, where they constitute the leading overall cause of death. Adverse events are due to the effects of impaired circulation on critical end organs (e.g., brain, heart, abdominal viscera) or extremities. In addition to death, which is most commonly caused by myocardial infarction or stroke, significant disability and loss of function are incurred at a substantial cost to society. Atherosclerosis accounts for the overwhelming majority of causative lesions and, with the increasing longevity and changing demographics of the U.S. population, assumes top priority as a national health issue.

Atherosclerosis

General Observations and Risk Factors

Atherosclerosis is a complex, chronic inflammatory process that affects the elastic and muscular arteries. The disease is both systemic and segmental, with clear predilections for certain locations within the arterial tree and relative sparing of others. The earliest lesions (i.e., fatty streaks) may be detected in childhood in susceptible individuals. Lesions progress through a series of well-characterized pathologic stages before clinical manifestations develop. Population-based studies have demonstrated a number of important risk factors that have become targets for preventive therapy as well as potential clues

into the pathogenesis of the disease (Table 66-1). The most important independent risk factors for atherosclerosis are hypercholesterolemia, hypertension, cigarette smoking, and diabetes mellitus.

Hypercholesterolemia (e.g., total serum cholesterol >200 mg/dL) is clearly associated with increased risk. Of great prognostic significance is the relative apportioning between the subclasses of cholesterol-carrying lipoproteins: the low-density fraction (LDL), which is atherogenic, and the high-density lipoprotein fraction (HDL), which exerts an atheroprotective effect by so-called reverse transport of cholesterol. Studies have demonstrated a strong positive correlation between atherosclerotic cardiovascular disease and elevated total and LDL cholesterol and an equally strong negative correlation with HDL levels. Despite these known relationships between serum lipid profiles and cardiovascular risk, the association with dietary intake remains complex in that individual metabolism is highly variable. Genetic variability in cholesterol metabolism provides one important mechanism for the well-known familial clustering of premature atherosclerotic disease. An important role for diet is strongly suggested by the variation in prevalence noted among different nations and ethnic groups, with a clear increase associated with consumption of the so-called Western diet (i.e., high fat, low fiber). The potential effects of numerous dietary components, both protective and atherogenic, have been intensely investigated with only limited consensus. Of these, a causative role of dietary lipid, particularly cholesterol and saturated fats, has been most well defined.

Cigarette smoking is strongly associated with the incidence of atherosclerosis, as well as with increased morbidity and mortality rates from its coronary, cerebral, and peripheral manifestations. The mechanism for the effects of smoking is likely to involve direct toxicity of tobacco metabolites on the vascular endothelium, probably by creating oxidant stress. Diabetic patients are also at

Table 66-1   Risk Factors for Atherosclerosis

Firmly Established
Hypercholesterolemia
Cigarette smoking
Hypertension
Diabetes mellitus

Relative
Advanced age
Male gender
Hypertriglyceridemia
Hyperhomocysteinemia
Sedentary lifestyle
Family history

Table 66-2   Guidelines for Risk Factor Modification

Lipid Management
Goal: Primary—serum LDL <100 mg/dL; secondary—HDL >35 mg/dL, TG <200 mg/dL
Approach: Diet: <30% fat, <7% saturated fat, <200 mg/day cholesterol; specific drug therapy targeted to lipid profile

Weight Reduction
Goal: <120% of ideal body weight
Approach: Physical activity, diet as outlined

Smoking
Goal: Complete cessation
Approach: Behavior modification, counseling, nicotine analogues

Blood Pressure
Goal: <140/90 mm Hg
Approach: Weight control, physical activity, sodium restriction, antihypertensive drugs

Physical Activity
Goal: At least 30 minutes of moderate exercise 3 to 4 times per week
Approach: Walking, cycling, jogging, lifestyle and work activities

HDL, high-density lipoprotein; LDL, low-density lipoprotein; TG, triglycerides.
Data from the American Heart Association Council Newsletter, Fall 1995.

markedly increased risk for atherosclerosis, often manifesting a particularly virulent form of the disease, leading to higher rates of myocardial events, stroke, and amputation. Hypertension is another important independent risk factor for coronary atherosclerosis, with a continuous increase in relative risk associated with each increment of pressure.

Age and gender also demonstrate an important influence. The implications of age as a risk factor are clear: prevalence will continue to increase with the advancing age of the U.S. population. In addition, initial end-organ manifestations tend to cluster at different ages, with coronary events often presaging peripheral disease by a decade or more. The increased risk associated with male gender and postmenopausal states in women has led to tremendous interest in the potential "atheroprotective" effects of estrogen. Hypertriglyceridemia, elevated serum fibrinogen, and hyperhomocysteinemia have also been associated with cardiovascular risk. Moderate amounts of daily physical activity appear to induce a protective effect, whereas a sedentary lifestyle has been associated with higher incidence of clinical disease. Guidelines for risk factor modification have been published and regularly updated by the American Heart Association (Table 66-2).

Pathology and Theories of Atherogenesis

The pathologic hallmark of atherosclerosis is the atherosclerotic plaque. There are several major components of plaque: smooth muscle cells, connective tissue (matrix), lipid, and inflammatory cells (predominantly macrophages). The presence of lipid within these lesions is a prominent distinguishing feature in comparison to other arteriopathies. Atherosclerotic lesions have been categorized by the varying extent of each of these components in addition to complicating features such as calcification and ulceration, which can occur in advanced plaques. An important concept linking plaque morphology with clinical events is the relationship between the fibrous cap—a layer of smooth muscle cells and connective tissue of variable thickness—and the underlying necrotic lipid core, composed of amorphous extracellular lipid, plasma proteins, and hemostatic factors.[1] The contents of this central region are markedly thrombogenic when

exposed to circulating blood, such as occurs when a thin fibrous cap ruptures or ulcerates. This phenomenon is thought to be an important mechanism whereby lesions of relatively mild hemodynamic significance may be responsible for acute thrombosis and downstream tissue infarction. In fact, this sequence may be more typical for some clinical end points (e.g., myocardial infarction) than slow progression of lesion size, producing hemodynamic failure downstream. Longitudinal study of plaque morphology has not been possible until recently, and with further refinements in ultrasound and magnetic resonance imaging, these types of data will assume an important role in clinical decision making. For the present, it is sufficiently clear that both the mechanical characteristics of the plaque and the degree of luminal encroachment (stenosis) it produces are of clinical importance.

The anatomic distribution of atherosclerosis is remarkably constant and is thought to reflect an important role for hemodynamic stresses.[2] An underlying influence of embryologic development (e.g., topographically distinct lineages of arterial smooth muscle cells in the developing circulatory system) may also be involved in this regional vulnerability. Plaques tend to be concentrated at bifurcations or bends, where local alterations in shear stress, flow separation, turbulence, and stasis are known to occur. The infrarenal abdominal aorta, proximal coronary arteries, iliofemoral arteries (especially the superficial femoral artery), carotid bifurcation, and popliteal arteries are commonly involved. Upper extremity vessels, as well

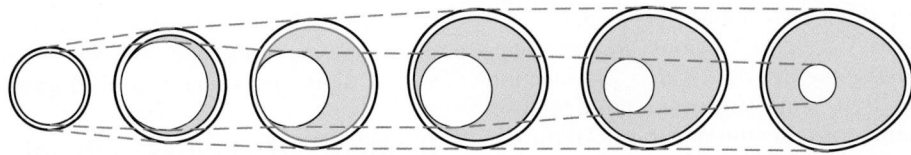

~40%
Stenosis

Figure 66-1 Adaptive arterial enlargement in atherosclerosis preserves luminal caliber until a critical plaque mass is reached. (Adapted from Glagov S, Weisenberg E, Zarins CK, et al: Compensatory enlargement of human atherosclerotic coronary arteries. N Engl J Med 316:1371-1375, 1987.)

as the common carotid, renal, and mesenteric arteries (beyond their origins), are usually spared.

Atherosclerotic plaques are dynamic lesions that may undergo progression or regression over time. Similarly, the underlying arterial wall also undergoes adaptive remodeling. Arterial enlargement is a well-established feature of atherosclerosis and often results in relative preservation of luminal area until plaque volume reaches a threshold size (~40% stenosis) beyond which compensation fails and lumen narrowing becomes progressive[3] (Fig. 66-1). Medial atrophy may also occur, in which case mechanical stability of the wall may be impaired. This has been suggested as one possible mechanism for the known association with aneurysmal disease.

The "response to injury" hypothesis and its more recent modifications, which include the concept of endothelial cell dysfunction, is the leading theory of pathogenesis.[4] This hypothesis incorporates important roles for lipid, inflammation, and thrombosis in addition to proliferation and dysfunction of the residing cells in the arterial wall. In the earlier versions of this theory, the triggering event was thought to be a focal denuding injury to the endothelium. More recently, a widened definition of endothelial injury has been espoused to include a mechanically intact but phenotypically altered endothelial monolayer as a substrate. The source of the initial mechanical or toxic injury may be variable, with a partial list including hemodynamic stress, toxic metabolites (e.g., cigarette smoke, homocysteine), hypoxia, or infectious agents (cytomegalovirus, *Chlamydia,* herpesvirus). The final common pathway is a loss of the numerous atheroprotective effects of normal endothelium, which include its barrier function, potent antiadhesive properties, and antiproliferative influence on the underlying smooth muscle cells.

The vascular smooth muscle cell (SMC) plays a central role in the developing lesion. Migration and proliferation of medial SMCs result in a cellular neointima. The intimal SMC undergoes a phenotypic change from a contractile to a secretory state, producing the extracellular matrix constituents of the plaque. Lipid entry and accumulation in the vessel wall is an important early event. Oxidation of lipid, particularly LDL particles, produces metabolites that potentiate the "activated" endothelial phenotype characterized by the expression of proinflammatory (e.g., leukocyte adhesion molecules) and procoagulant (e.g., tissue factor) molecules as well as producing a

decrease in protective substances (e.g., nitric oxide). Circulating monocytes are recruited by adhesion to activated endothelium or to exposed matrix, enter the wall to become macrophages, and scavenge lipid. T lymphocytes are also recruited, and together these inflammatory cells elaborate an array of cytokines (especially interleukin-1, tumor necrosis factor-α, and transforming growth factor-β), which potentiate the inflammation. In addition, macrophages are important sources of matrix degrading enzymes, which may be involved in wall remodeling and plaque stability.

Platelets may adhere to dysfunctional endothelium, exposed matrix, and monocytes-macrophages. An important role for platelets and their growth-promoting and vasoactive products has long been espoused. The prototypic growth factor known as platelet-derived growth factor (PDGF) is a potent stimulator of both migration and proliferation of SMCs, and it has been identified in abundance in atherosclerotic plaques. Platelets are not the only source of PDGF: different isoforms of PDGF may also be produced by endothelial cells and by SMCs themselves. Other locally produced growth factors, in particular basic fibroblast growth factor (bFGF), are likely to play a role in the SMC hyperplasia that occurs. Amplification occurs by means of numerous potential positive feedback loops between cytokines and growth factors (both autocrine and paracrine) in which persistent inflammatory activation is the central feature.

An alternative explanation is offered by the "monoclonal hypothesis," which hinges on the intriguing observation that many atherosclerotic plaques appear to contain a clonally expanded population of SMCs.[5] The developing plaque is viewed as a benign SMC neoplasm with an associated alteration in SMC phenotype to the secretory state. Even though the observation of plaque monoclonality remains intriguing, this theory falls short in explaining all of the epidemiologic and pathologic features of atherosclerosis and is currently less favored.

Other Arteriopathies

Other causes of arterial occlusive disease, although far less common than atherosclerosis in Western societies, must also be considered, especially in patients who do not fit the risk factor profile outlined. These include thromboangiitis obliterans (Buerger's disease), Takayasu's arteritis, giant cell or temporal arteritis, and other less common vasculitides. Each of these disorders has unique clinical, radiographic, and anatomic features.[6]

Buerger's disease is exclusively associated with cigarette smoking. The disease is more prevalent in the Middle East and Asia. Occlusive lesions are predominantly seen in the muscular arteries, with a predilection for the tibial vessels. Rest pain, gangrene, and ulceration are the typical presentations. Recurrent superficial thrombophlebitis (so-called phlebitis migrans) is a characteristic feature. The diagnosis is suspected in younger patients who are heavy smokers and do not have other atherosclerotic risk factors. Angiography often reveals diffuse occlusion of the distal extremity vessels. The arterial involvement appears to progress in a distal to proximal fashion. Revascularization options are therefore usually limited. The disease virtually always shows clinical remission if smoking cessation can be achieved. Sympathectomy has a limited role in patients with ulcerations.

Takayasu's arteritis (so-called pulseless disease) commonly afflicts younger female patients and has a higher prevalence in those of Eastern European or Asian descent. There is often a prodrome marked by systemic inflammatory signs and symptoms. The arterial pathology is focused on the aorta and its major branches; several patterns of involvement are described. The brachiocephalic vessels of the arch are often diffusely involved, leading to symptoms of global cerebral hypoperfusion or upper extremity claudication. Initial management focuses on the active inflammation and is predominantly medical. Surgical treatment is often indicated for ischemic manifestations and is only undertaken when active inflammation is under control (i.e., normalized erythrocyte sedimentation rate).

Temporal arteritis (sometimes referred to as *giant cell arteritis*) predominantly afflicts patients older than 50 years of age, with a slight (2:1) female preponderance. The incidence increases for each decade over age 50 years. The superficial temporal, vertebral, and major aortic arch branches may be involved. As in Takayasu's disease, there are often signs of systemic inflammation. Ischemic symptoms are common, including claudication of facial or extremity muscles and retinal ischemia. Headache is a common symptom. Blindness, usually irreversible, is a dreaded complication. When the clinical diagnosis is suspected, treatment must be prompt and consists of high-dose corticosteroid therapy. Surgery is rarely indicated except in cases of major aortic branch involvement with ischemic symptoms.

Raynaud's phenomenon is characterized by recurrent, episodic vasospasm of the digits brought on by cold exposure or emotional stress.[7] Exposure to cold initially produces pallor of the digits, followed by cyanosis, and is accompanied by pain and paresthesias. Rewarming leads to marked rubor caused by a hyperemic response. The clinical spectrum of severity is broad and may include ulceration or loss of digits in patients with protracted periods of ischemia. Progression to tissue loss implies persistent vascular occlusions beyond the vasospastic component. Primary (Raynaud's disease) and secondary causes are recognized. Secondary Raynaud's phenomenon has been associated with a variety of rheumatologic, hematologic, and traumatic disorders, as well as a number of drugs and toxins. Treatment is centered around minimizing exposure to the triggering stimulus and pharmacologic (calcium channel blockers, sympatholytics) therapy. Sympathectomy may play a role in patients with severe digital ischemia and ulceration.

Diagnostic Modalities in Peripheral Arterial Occlusive Disease

Noninvasive Hemodynamic Assessment

Atherosclerotic plaques produce local and downstream alterations in pressure and flow that may be quantitated by a variety of noninvasive methods. A key principle in the treatment of peripheral atherosclerosis is the hemodynamic assessment of circulatory impairment, which assumes paramount importance in comparison to the anatomic presence or distribution of lesions. In current practice, the noninvasive vascular laboratory is able to provide a combination of physiologic measurements and lesion mapping, which is critical for longitudinal surveillance, patient selection for interventions, and postprocedural follow-up.

In the lower extremities, measurement of pressure plays a central role in the assessment of disease severity. Segmental pressure measurements in the limb can be used to localize and grade hemodynamically significant lesions, as well as the overall degree of circulatory impairment. The single most useful index is the ankle pressure, which can be obtained simply at the bedside with a handheld Doppler probe and pressure cuff. The cuff is placed around the lower calf just above the malleolus, and the Doppler probe is positioned over the dorsalis pedis or posterior tibial arteries to obtain a flow signal. The cuff is inflated and then slowly deflated, and the examiner records the pressure at which the audible signal returns.

Because the ankle pressure varies with central aortic pressure, it is commonly indexed to the brachial artery pressure as a ratio (ankle-brachial index [ABI]). The ABI is quite reproducible in a given patient and is therefore extremely useful for longitudinal surveillance of obstructive disease. In normal resting subjects, the ABI is slightly greater than unity (1.0-1.2). There is a correlation between the severity of signs and symptoms of arterial insufficiency and the ABI (Fig. 66-2), such that claudicants usually fall in the 0.5 to 0.7 range, whereas critical ischemia (rest pain or tissue necrosis) most commonly is associated with an ABI less than 0.4. In addition to preoperative assessment, the ABI can be used to follow patients after arterial reconstruction as a measure of technical success or subsequent graft failure. The most common source of error in the ABI is false elevation resulting from extensive vascular calcification, as is common in diabetic patients or those with chronic renal failure. In these instances, other measures of distal perfusion (e.g., toe pressures, transmetatarsal pulse volume recording, transcutaneous oximetry) may be more reliable indicators of physiologic impairment.

A more complete assessment of infrainguinal arterial disease may be obtained by the segmental pressure tech-

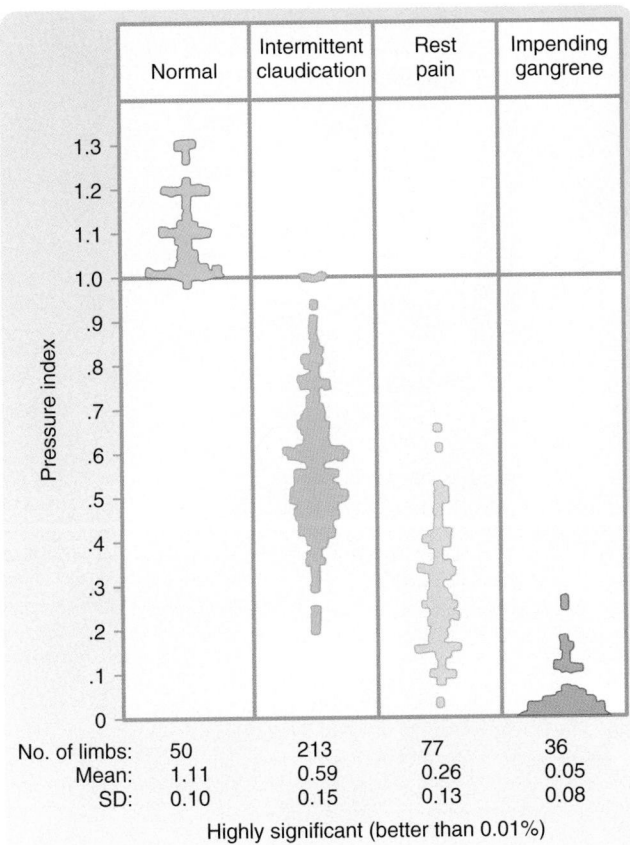

	Normal	Intermittent claudication	Rest pain	Impending gangrene
No. of limbs:	50	213	77	36
Mean:	1.11	0.59	0.26	0.05
SD:	0.10	0.15	0.13	0.08

Highly significant (better than 0.01%)

Figure 66-2 Correlation between signs and symptoms of lower extremity arterial insufficiency and the ankle-brachial index (ABI). (Adapted from Yao JST: Hemodynamic studies in peripheral arterial disease. Br J Surg 57:761, 1970.)

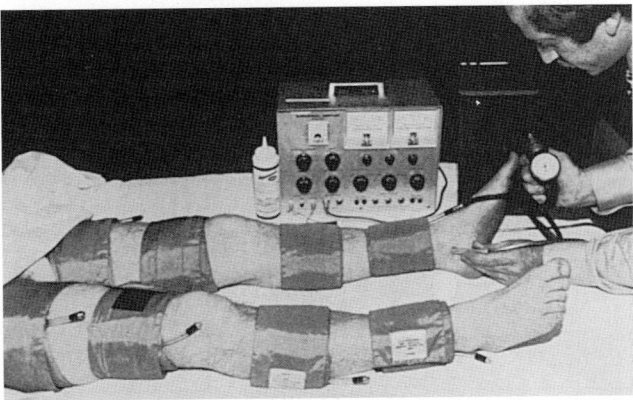

Figure 66-3 Technique of recording segmental limb pressures in the lower extremity. (From Summer DS, Thiele BL: The vascular laboratory. In Rutherford RB [ed]: Vascular Surgery, 4th ed. Philadelphia, WB Saunders, 1995, p 54.)

nique. Pneumatic cuffs are placed at several levels in the lower extremity, typically the upper thigh, lower thigh, calf, and ankle. The technique is facilitated by automated systems, which sequentially inflate and deflate the cuffs, while a Doppler probe is used to record distal flow as in the ABI technique (Fig. 66-3). Upper thigh pressures in normal patients exceed brachial pressure, and a high-thigh index of less than 1.0 is highly suggestive of aortoiliac disease. Pressure gradients between adjacent levels of 30 mm Hg or greater are usually indicative of occlusion of the intervening segment. Again, false-positive results may be obtained in patients with extensive calcification. Digital (finger or toe) pressures may be obtained with appropriately sized cuffs and the use of a photoplethysmography probe on the pulp of the distal digit. Digital pressures are useful in patients with disease confined to the distal vessels (e.g., advanced Raynaud's disease with fixed obstructive lesions) or, more commonly, to help predict the likelihood of healing of forefoot procedures, ulcerations, or toe amputations. A toe pressure of greater than 30 mm Hg is predictive of successful healing in about 90% of cases, whereas values less than 10 mm Hg are highly predictive of poor outcome. Values in the midrange of 10 to 30 mm Hg are not highly predictive and must be interpreted in the context of careful physical examination and clinical assessment.

Exercise (treadmill) testing may be used in patients with claudication. It is particularly useful in the evaluation of patients with atypical symptoms, normal resting pulse examinations, or clinical suspicion of lumbar spine disease, in which case both neurogenic and arterial causes may be present to varying extents. Patients with calf claudication resulting from superficial femoral arterial disease uniformly demonstrate a marked decrease in ankle pressure at the time of symptom occurrence as a result of the increased gradient produced by a fixed resistance in the setting of increased blood flow. A normal exercise test rules out arterial insufficiency explicitly. In addition, exercise testing has been used to quantify the degree of impairment in arterial claudication; self-reporting of walking distance is notoriously unreliable.

Limb plethysmography, which measures the fluctuation in limb volume during the cardiac cycle, is a useful adjunct to segmental pressure measurements. The most common technique involves segmental air plethysmograph cuffs, commonly referred to as a pulse volume recording (PVR). Waveform analysis (contour and amplitude) is highly predictive of upstream arterial stenosis or occlusion (Fig. 66-4). Transmetatarsal PVRs, obtained with a cuff across the forefoot, are particularly useful in diabetic patients with falsely elevated segmental limb pressures. In clinical practice, segmental pressures and PVRs are often obtained simultaneously and the information integrated by comparing adjacent segments as well as corresponding levels in the contralateral limb. Combined with a careful history and physical examination, these basic noninvasive studies usually provide adequate data for most clinical decision making regarding the selection of patients for lower extremity revascularization.

Doppler and Duplex Ultrasonography
Ultrasound technology has revolutionized vascular imaging. The availability of high-resolution portable scanners, with scan heads accommodating a range of tissue depths, allows for noninvasive longitudinal assessment of virtually the entire circulatory tree outside of the

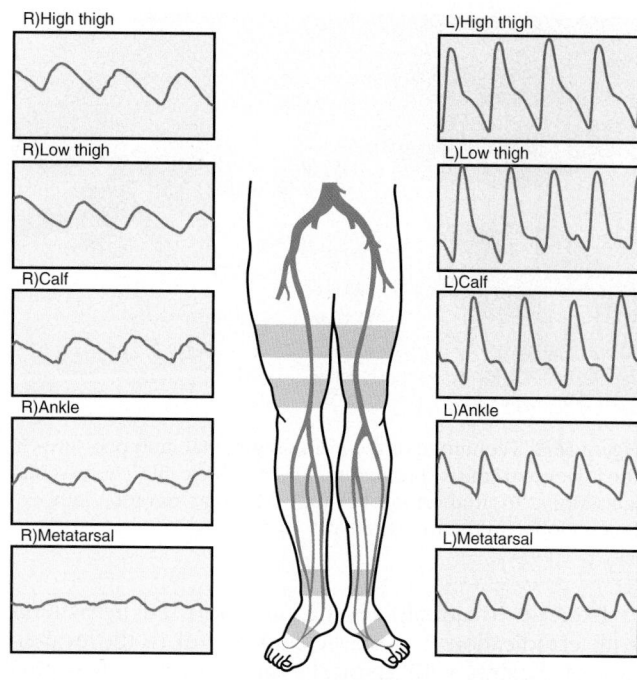

Figure 66-4 Example of PVR recordings from a normal lower extremity (*left*) and a patient with rest pain (*right*). The tracings on the right are consistent with combined aortoiliac and femoropopliteal disease with minimal distal collateralization.

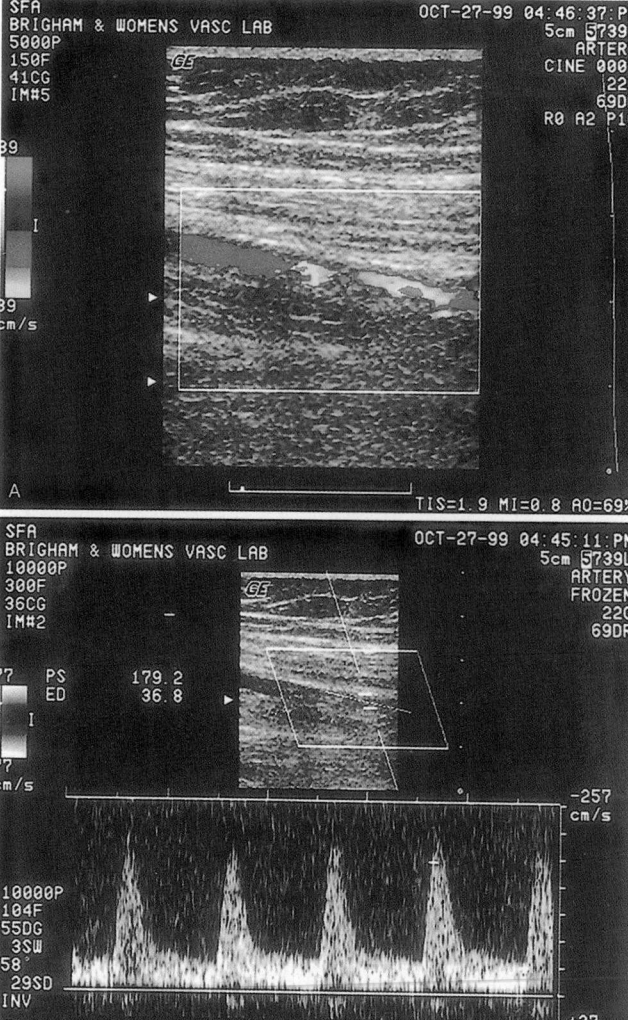

Figure 66-5 Color Duplex ultrasound images with Doppler velocity profiles. **A,** High-grade lesion in the superficial femoral artery as demonstrated by turbulent flow and high peak systolic velocities (PSV). **B,** A focal vein graft stenosis is identified by elevated PSV compared with adjacent segment.

thoracic aorta. Duplex ultrasound combines the traditional B-mode two-dimensional image with Doppler measurement of blood flow parameters. Doppler relies on a measured frequency shift, which correlates with the velocity of flow. The B-mode image is used to guide placement of the Doppler sampling volume at different locations, and the resulting frequency or velocity profile can be used to grade the severity of obstructive lesions. A color scale can also be used to visually assess locations of low velocity, high velocity, or turbulence (Fig. 66-5).

Duplex ultrasound plays a central role in several areas of vascular practice. The most common application is for carotid bifurcation disease, which is discussed in Chapter 64. In abdominal and extremity vascular disease, its use is continually expanding. Compared with the other noninvasive techniques discussed earlier, duplex scanning allows for precise anatomic localization of lesions, quantitates their severity, and, with the development of higher-resolution systems, can assess plaque morphology. Color-flow imaging facilitates the examination by allowing the technician to rapidly identify deeper vessels and by demonstrating areas of turbulence where high-grade lesions are likely to reside. Although the instrumentation has undergone tremendous technologic refinement, operator skill and training remains an important variable in accuracy. The abdominal aorta, renal and mesenteric vessels, iliac arteries, and infrainguinal vessels can all be visualized. Overlying bowel gas is a common technical limitation for the abdominal vessels. Lower extremity duplex arterial mapping has been touted as an imaging strategy to determine patient suitability for angioplasty or

bypass; however, the examination of an entire extremity is time-consuming and has significant operator-dependent variables. It does not provide the same global measure of limb perfusion as segmental pressures or PVRs, and it remains inferior to angiographic techniques for preoperative planning. In summary, duplex imaging is most useful to assess the anatomy and severity of native arterial lesions in defined locations within the vascular tree, particularly the carotid bifurcation and the renal and femoral arteries.

A critical application of duplex scanning is in the postoperative assessment of lower extremity vein bypass grafts. Numerous studies have demonstrated improved long-term graft patency and limb salvage when failing (i.e., stenotic) grafts are detected and revised before occlusion. Identification of patent but failing vein grafts by clinical examination alone, including serial ABI measurement, is relatively insensitive. Color-flow imaging of the entire graft, including proximal and distal arteries and anastomotic regions, provides a complete map of any flow disturbances or developing stenoses. Velocity criteria have been developed for high-grade lesions that may warrant either more intensive surveillance, arteriography, or intervention to prevent failure. Focal areas of high velocity (peak systolic velocity >300 cm/second or velocity ratio [lesion/upstream] >3.5) or overall low velocity (<40 cm/second) throughout the graft are usually indicative of a critical hemodynamic lesion.[8] By generating detailed velocity maps of a given graft, individual lesions can be followed over time for progression. In most high-volume vascular surgery practices, this technique has proved valuable in identifying and treating focal hyperplastic lesions with a variety of surgical (patch angioplasty, jump or interposition grafting) or radiologic (angioplasty) techniques, thereby improving long-term patency and reducing the need for difficult redo bypass surgery.

Transcutaneous Oximetry

Transcutaneous measurement of oxygen tension (tcPO$_2$) is another technique for assessing tissue perfusion. Small polarographic electrodes are applied to the skin in a number of locations, usually including the torso (control), thigh, calf, and dorsum of the foot. The electrodes measure oxygen diffused to the skin, which is a reflection of underlying tissue perfusion but is also affected by numerous other variables, including skin temperature, sympathetic tone, skin conditions such as cellulitis or hyperkeratosis, and edema. These variables limit the reproducibility of the examination. Nonetheless, tcPO$_2$ measurement has a role in the assessment of critical ischemia, particularly in diabetic patients with extensive vascular calcification. Normal tcPO$_2$ levels in the foot are in the 50 to 60 mm Hg range. Values greater than 40 mm Hg are predictive for healing of foot lesions or primary forefoot amputations; values less than 10 mm Hg are almost universally associated with failure to heal. As in the case of toe pressures, values in the middle range are not particularly useful as isolated measurements and must be placed in clinical context.

Arteriography

The modern era of arterial reconstruction was made possible by the development of contrast arteriography (Moniz, 1927; dos Santos, 1929), which allowed for anatomic localization of aneurysmal and occlusive lesions and their relationship to symptoms. Technologic advances in catheters, contrast agents, radiographic equipment, and image processing have led to greatly improved safety and high-resolution imaging of virtually the entire circulatory tree.

Aortic and lower extremity arteriograms are generally performed by needle puncture of the femoral or brachial arteries, followed by guidewire placement and catheter insertion using the Seldinger technique. Most diagnostic studies are performed using catheters passed through 5-French (1.7-mm outer diameter) sheaths. After fluoroscopic catheter positioning, radiopaque contrast medium

Table 66-3 **Complications of Contrast Arteriography**

Puncture Site or Catheter Related
Hemorrhage, hematoma
Pseudoaneurysm
Arteriovenous fistula
Atheroembolization
Local thrombosis
Contrast Agent Related
Major (anaphylactoid) sensitivity reaction
Minor sensitivity reactions
Vasodilation, hypotension
Nephrotoxicity
Hypervolemia (osmotic load)

is injected by a timed mechanical injector, and images are obtained rapidly by digital acquisition. Full examination of the abdominal aorta and lower extremities usually requires multiple injections because there is a need for different catheter positions, projections, and patient stations to obtain optimal images. A large variety of highly specialized guidewires and catheters have been developed to assist surgeons in selective cannulation of remote vessels (e.g., renal, mesenteric, cerebral, and pulmonary vasculature). Postprocessing of digital images allows for subtraction of overlying bone and other enhancements to facilitate visualization of the vessels and lesions in question.

Complications of arteriography can be divided into those related to the catheterization and those related to the injected contrast agent (Table 66-3). The major complications of catheter placement are atheroembolization and puncture site problems (bleeding, pseudoaneurysm, or arteriovenous fistula). Distal embolization may occur by dislodgment of plaque by the catheter as it is passed or manipulated within the arterial system. Atheroemboli from the proximal (thoracic or upper abdominal) aorta can produce devastating effects if they shower into the renal or mesenteric circulations where bowel infarction or renal failure may ensue. Debris traveling into the lower extremities usually lodges in the most distal vessels of the toes, resulting in the classic appearance of so-called blue toe syndrome. The skin lesions produced are usually exquisitely painful, and the extent of tissue loss, which is often overestimated by the initial appearance, may ultimately require toe or even forefoot amputation. This complication occurs in only a small fraction of cases.

Puncture site complications are relatively infrequent after diagnostic studies, being more commonly associated with the larger-caliber sheaths required for catheter-based interventions (i.e., angioplasty, stents). The key is prevention, which begins with appropriate selection of the arterial site for cannulation; a minimally traumatic needle, guidewire, or catheter insertion; and adequate management of hemostasis after catheter removal. Significant bleeding or pseudoaneurysm formation can almost always be attributed to either a technical difficulty or to the need for persistent systemic anticoagulant or antiplatelet drugs.

An arteriovenous fistula can result from inadvertent passage of the needle and guidewire through an adjacent vein en route to the artery. Diagnosis is suggested by the physical findings of a pulsatile mass or continuous bruit and is easily confirmed by duplex imaging. The management of these various puncture site complications is individualized and depends on the stability of the patient, the requirement for continuous anticoagulation, and other factors. Patients with hemodynamically significant bleeding, expanding hematomas, large pseudoaneurysms, or local complications caused by pressure on adjacent nerves or skin or patients requiring intensive continuous anticoagulation are best managed with early surgery. The vessel is exposed and the puncture site repaired by direct suture. Rarely, a prosthetic patch repair may be required, usually in the setting of severe injury to a badly calcified atherosclerotic vessel in which primary repair is either impossible or would produce narrowing. For stable pseudoaneurysms in patients without coagulopathy, ultrasound-guided compression has been highly successful as sole therapy. Most recently, ultrasound-directed thrombin injection into the sac has been reported as a rapid and highly successful technique for pseudoaneurysms.

Contrast agents may produce both minor and major adverse reactions. Conventional iodinated agents have direct toxic effects on endothelium because of their high osmolarity (five to eight times normal plasma osmolarity). Newer low-osmolarity (nonionic) agents have about one third the osmolarity of the older media. Intravascular injection of contrast agent causes vasodilation (sensation of heat) with a concomitant decrease in blood pressure. Many patients experience discomfort during injection, which is thought to be attributable to the osmolarity. Idiosyncratic reactions to the contrast medium occur in about 4% of patients. They are not dose related and may be either serious (anaphylaxis) or minor (nausea, urticaria, pruritus). Major reactions are rare; they must be recognized and treated promptly with airway control, corticosteroids, and cardiopulmonary support. The incidence of minor reactions appears to be reduced with low-osmolarity agents. Patients with a prior history of allergy to contrast agents or iodine (e.g., shellfish) or those with asthma are at higher risk.

Renal toxicity is an important adverse consequence of contrast arteriography. The mechanism is unknown and may involve renal ischemia resulting from the osmotic diuresis produced or direct toxic effects on tubular epithelium. Assessment of risk and preangiography preparation are critical. Factors associated with elevated risk include chronic renal insufficiency (baseline creatinine >1.5), diabetic nephropathy, multiple myeloma–associated nephropathy, dehydration, age older than 60 years, recent surgery, and larger doses of contrast medium. The risk factors appear additive. Iodinated contrast agents given to patients receiving metformin (dimethylbiguanide) can rarely result in lactic acidosis. Accordingly, this agent is held for 2 days before and then re-started 2 days after administration of the contrast agent if the renal function is stable. Maintenance of adequate hydration before, during, and after contrast injection is absolutely critical and is best accomplished by continu-

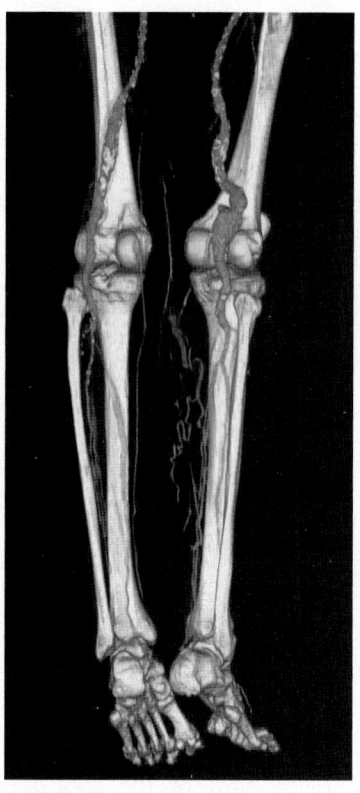

Figure 66-6 CT angiogram of lower extremity arteries with three-dimensional reconstruction reveals bilateral popliteal artery aneurysms. (Courtesy of Joseph Schoepf, MD, and Edgar K. Yucel, MD, Brigham and Women's Hospital.)

ous intravenous (IV) administration of isotonic sodium chloride or sodium bicarbonate.[9] Although controversial, the selective administration of *N*-acetylcysteine, a thiol-containing antioxidant, at a dose of 600 mg for 2 days before and after the procedure in individuals with evidence of renal impairment may offer the potential of renal preservation.[10] Nonionic agents appear to have less renal toxicity and are selected in high-risk patients. The major limitation of these agents is their markedly increased cost compared with conventional media.

Computed tomography (CT) with IV contrast medium administration can also delineate vascular anatomy. Specific protocols for timed injection and rapid image acquisition (i.e., spiral CT angiography) have improved the resolution. Three-dimensional reconstructions are possible that may be particularly helpful in highly tortuous vessels and aneurysms. The technique has been most useful for the thoracoabdominal aorta and carotid bifurcations (Fig. 66-6). Dissection and aneurysmal diseases of the aorta are particularly well suited, in that the pathologic process spans a longer segment and is less likely to be missed between adjacent slices. It has had limited use in aortoiliac or infrainguinal occlusive disease.

Magnetic resonance angiography (MRA) is an important technique that is gaining application by virtue of rapidly improving technology. It offers the distinct advantages of being noninvasive and avoiding contrast expo-

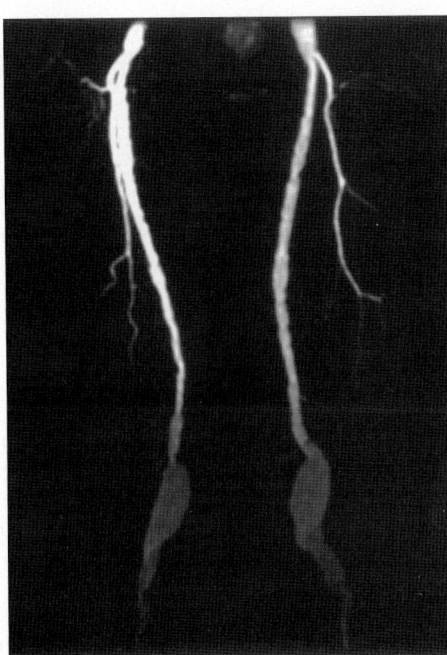

Figure 66-7 MRA with gadolinium enhancement of femoropopliteal vessels in a patient with bilateral popliteal artery aneurysm. (Courtesy of Servet Tatli, MD, and Edgar K. Yucel, MD, Brigham and Women's Hospital.)

sure. The most common technique used for obtaining vascular enhancement is time-of-flight (TOF), in which brightness is directly related to the velocity of blood entering the slice. As a result, lesion severity is often overestimated, which is an important limitation. The technique has had its greatest application thus far in evaluating the carotid and intracranial circulation, thoracoabdominal aorta, renal arteries, and lower extremity vessels (Fig. 66-7). It is the test of choice for studying arteriovenous malformations or the major abdominal veins (e.g., for planning portal decompression procedures). Lower extremity studies are primarily limited by the prolonged acquisition times required if the equivalent of an aortogram with leg runoff is needed. When the examination can be more limited, as in the preoperative assessment of distal runoff in a patient with a normal femoral pulse, its utility is increased. MRA is particularly useful in patients who are at high risk for contrast-induced nephropathy, particularly elderly diabetic patients.

Therapeutic Interventions in Arterial Occlusive Disease

The modern therapeutic armamentarium for treating arterial occlusive diseases is barely half a century old. Its development is marked by several key advances: the discovery of heparin, arteriography (Moniz, 1927), arterial homografts (DeBakey, 1950s), prosthetic grafts (Voorhees, 1952), balloon angioplasty (Gruntzig, 1974), and stents (Dotter, 1969), combined with a continuous improvement in instruments and suture materials to facilitate vascular anastomoses.

Medical Management

The medical management of atherosclerosis is targeted to reduce progression, induce regression, and prevent morbid end points of lesion formation. Risk factor management is the primary approach. Lipid-lowering therapy uses both dietary treatment and an increasing pharmacopeia with specific effects on different lipid subclasses. These drugs include niacin, bile acid–binding resins, HMG-CoA reductase inhibitors (the statins), clofibrate, and gemfibrozil. Newer agents inhibit cholesterol uptake at the small bowel brush border (ezetimibe) or increase the proficiency of "reverse-transport" by blocking the cholesterol ester transfer protein (torcetrapib). The specific dietary and drug regimen is tailored to the lipid profile abnormality of the individual patient. A recent practice guidelines statement published by the American College of Cardiology and the American Heart Association recommended that all patients with pulmonary artery disease reduce their LDL cholesterol levels to below 100 mg/dL and to below 70 mg/dL in individuals considered to be at very high risk for ischemic events, especially patients with diabetes mellitus, metabolic syndrome, or active coronary disease.[11] Smoking cessation is clearly of paramount importance. Newer nicotine analogues, available in a variety of sustained-release delivery forms, may be helpful, but long-term success hinges on behavior modification.

Antiplatelet therapy constitutes the other major medical treatment option. The goal is to prevent thrombosis, embolization, and perhaps even the progression of atherosclerotic disease given the possible role of platelets as an etiologic factor. Aspirin remains the cornerstone of antiplatelet therapy, with a well-established track record of compliance, low risk, and minimal cost. Large meta-analyses have demonstrated beneficial effects of aspirin in patients with prior myocardial infarctions, carotid atheroembolism, and peripheral arterial surgery.[12] Newer antiplatelet agents have been developed with ever-increasing potency and more specific antiaggregative effects. These include ticlopidine and clopidogrel, both of which have shown efficacy in reducing some cardiovascular end points. Oral antagonists of the platelet glycoprotein IIb/IIIa receptor for fibrinogen, the critical interaction required for aggregation, are being extensively studied primarily in patients with coronary interventions. The long-term roles for these newer agents remain to be defined, especially given their increased cost and lower safety profile as compared with aspirin. For the present, low-dose aspirin (325 mg/day) is the most widely accepted antiplatelet prophylaxis for patients with cardiovascular disease.

Basic Techniques of Arterial Surgery

Technical success in arterial reconstructive surgery hinges on the meticulous application of basic techniques of handling and suturing blood vessels. Arterial incisions are preferentially placed in soft areas of the vessel wall spared of disease. The choice of orientation (i.e., longitudinal or transverse) of the arteriotomy depends on the vessel size, the local extent of disease, and the reconstructive technique being used. Primary closure of

Table 66-4 Comparison of Arterial Reconstructive Techniques by Most Favorable Anatomic Features of Treated Lesions

	BYPASS	ENDARTERECTOMY	PTA, STENTING
Stenosis vs. occlusion	Either	Stenosis > occlusion	Stenosis > occlusion
Length of segment	Not a factor	Preferably short	Preferably short
Vessel caliber	>2 mm	Preferably >5-6 mm	Preferably >4 mm
Anatomic sites most suitable	Aortic arch through distal extremity	Carotid bifurcation, common femoral, aortic branch lesions	Distal abdominal aorta and iliac arteries, aortic branch lesions (?? femoral, popliteal, carotid)

PTA, percutaneous transluminal angioplasty; ??, controversial application of PTA.

longitudinal incisions may result in narrowing; hence these are often closed with a vein or prosthetic patch. In the case of thromboembolectomy of otherwise normal arteries, transverse incisions are often used in the larger (e.g., iliofemoral) vessels; longitudinal incisions with patch angioplasty are more forgiving in smaller vessels. In general, the longitudinal incision offers more flexibility for extension to deal with local disease or to accommodate a bypass graft anastomosis.

Suture materials for vascular surgery are nonabsorbable (e.g., polypropylene). A practice of minimal handling of the arterial wall, using specially designed vascular forceps (e.g., DeBakey), minimizes separation or fragmentation of plaque that can complicate the exercise. Suture bites must incorporate all layers of the vessel wall, with care taken to ensure the intima is included. The needle should pass through the wall at a right angle and then be gently rotated along its curvature to draw the suture through. Shallow angled bites, levering of the needle, or rough handling of the suture can produce a localized linear tear in an atherosclerotic vessel. In performing a primary closure of an arteriotomy, the bites are closely spaced and of appropriate depth to produce hemostasis without narrowing. Slight, gentle eversion of the edges is important and is facilitated by the assistant who maintains traction on the suture. In the case of a vein or prosthetic patch, the edges must be carefully everted onto the arterial wall to avoid leaks between sutures. The choice of suturing technique (i.e., continuous or interrupted) is dependent on vessel size and surgical preference. Interrupted sutures may be preferred in small-caliber vessels because they avoid the pursestring effect of a continuous stitch, which may produce a degree of narrowing. For larger arteries and in most cases of patch angioplasty or bypass grafting, a carefully done continuous suture works well and is more efficient. In either case, sutures are usually first placed at either corner of the arteriotomy, then progressively continued to the middle. Flushing and backbleeding by release of clamps is an important maneuver to be done before completing the anastomosis, to remove any small amounts of thrombus, air, or debris.

Surgical Bypass Grafting

Surgical bypass grafting has evolved as the most widely applicable technique for the treatment of arterial occlusive lesions. It has found broad application in the coro-

nary, abdominal, and peripheral vascular beds. In comparison to other techniques such as angioplasty, stenting, or endarterectomy, bypass is far less restrictive in terms of the anatomic nature of lesions amenable to treatment (Table 66-4). Although each of these other modalities is limited in treating longer occlusions and smaller-caliber vessels, these areas are precisely those where surgical bypass excels. The specific choice of percutaneous or surgical approach must be tailored to the individual patient, lesion, and the skill and experience of the operator. In current practice, a combination of these methods is frequently required to achieve the best therapeutic result; thus, familiarity with all the techniques is fundamental to the discipline of vascular surgery. A brief discussion of general techniques and graft materials follows; for more detailed technical descriptions, the reader is referred to one of the standard vascular surgical texts or atlases.[13]

Anatomic exposure of the selected inflow and outflow arteries is obtained through standard incisions in the abdomen or extremities. Complete circumferential dissection is not always required and, in some situations (e.g., aorta, iliac arteries, reoperative exposures), carries unnecessary additional risk because of the presence of immediately adjacent major venous structures. Despite arteriographic appearances, the presence of significant plaque or calcification may require modifying the original operative strategy. Whenever possible, segments bearing minimal disease are selected for anastomotic sites because this greatly facilitates both vascular occlusion as well as suturing. The outflow site is selected to be downstream from all hemodynamically significant disease, in the most readily accessible vessel that can provide downstream perfusion. Shorter grafts are preferable, particularly when autogenous vein conduit is in limited supply. Numerous techniques are available for occlusion and depend to great extent on the size of the vessel, the arterial pressure, and the presence or severity of plaque (especially calcification). These methods include the application of atraumatic vascular clamps, elastic vessel loops, intraluminal occluders, or an extremity tourniquet.

Systemic anticoagulation, by IV administration of heparin sodium, is achieved before vascular occlusion. Standard heparin doses are in the range of 70 to 100 units/kg as a bolus. Repeated doses may be necessary depending on the length of the operation and the requirement for additional periods of flow occlusion. The half-

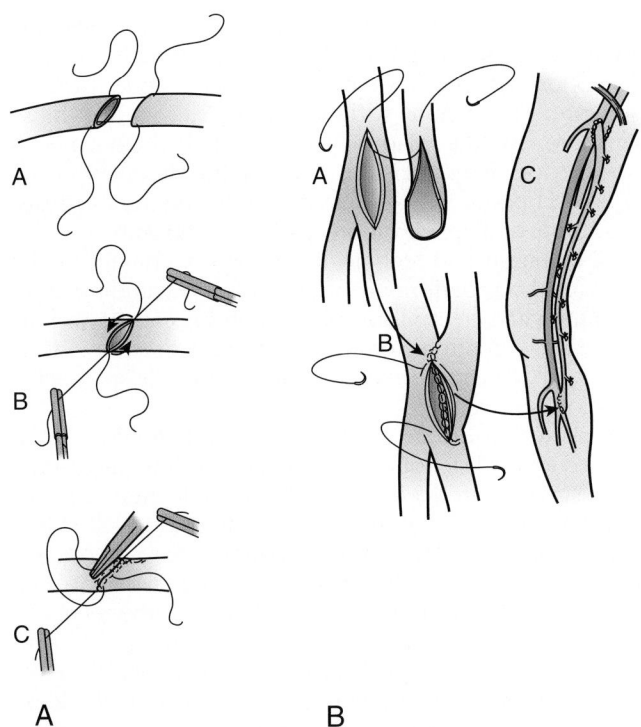

Figure 66-8 Techniques of constructing artery-to-graft anastomoses. **A,** End-to-end technique employing spatulation and corner sutures. **B,** End-to-side anastomosis employing a two-suture, continuous technique.

life of heparin ranges from 60 to 90 minutes in most patients, which is a suitable interval for redosing with smaller boluses (one third to one half the initial dose is typical). Measurement of the activated clotting time (ACT) is readily accomplished using standard equipment available in most cardiovascular operating suites and facilitates appropriate heparin dosing during longer procedures. For peripheral vascular operations, an ACT in the 250- to 350-second range is adequate. At the conclusion of the procedure, when hemostasis is desired, it may be necessary to reverse the effects of heparin by administration of protamine sulfate (dose: 1 mg/100 units of circulating heparin).

The arteriotomy is preferably made in a disease-free area; poorly chosen sites or ill-advised extension into areas of heavy plaque may greatly complicate the operation. Anastomoses are most commonly performed either in an end-to-side or end-to-end configuration (Fig. 66-8). The end-to-side approach has broader application and is somewhat more forgiving technically. End-to-end anastomoses are facilitated by slightly beveling the two ends (45 degrees) to enlarge the opening and by the use of interrupted sutures to avoid a pursestring effect of continuous suture. End-to-side configurations are usually made at an entry angle of less than 45 degrees to minimize turbulence. The graft is appropriately beveled, and the heel sutures are placed first. One or two sutures may be used to complete the anastomosis; in the two-suture technique, a separate stitch is placed at the toe, which

is the most critical point at which one must avoid narrowing.

Intraoperative assessment of the bypass is critical to both short- and long-term outcome. For lower extremity bypass, completion arteriography is the gold standard. Duplex scanning is finding an ever-increasing role in the operating suite and provides greater resolution of intraluminal defects as well as flow velocity mapping. In either case, the anastomotic sites, conduit, and distal runoff are examined for intraluminal defects (thrombus, valves, plaque, emboli), extrinsic compression or kinks (tunneling errors), and technical adequacy.

The optimal choice of graft material depends on the anatomic location, size, and hemodynamic environment of the bypass. The ideal vascular graft would be characterized by both its mechanical attributes and postimplantation healing responses. Mechanical strength is a paramount issue in that grafts placed in the arterial circulation must be capable of withstanding long-term hemodynamic stress without material failure, which might be catastrophic. Availability, suturability, and simplicity of handling are desirable for minimizing operating time, risk, and expense. The graft needs to be resistant to both thrombosis and infection and, optimally, would be completely incorporated by the body to yield a neovessel resembling a native artery in structure and function. Given the economic considerations, low cost and long-term durability are issues of great importance as well.

For large-caliber arterial reconstructions, currently available synthetic grafts made of either Dacron or expanded polytetrafluoroethylene (PTFE) offer a reasonable approximation of these ideals and proven clinical efficacy. Long-term results of synthetic grafts for replacement of the thoracic and abdominal aorta, arch vessels, and iliac and common femoral arteries for either aneurysmal or occlusive disease are generally excellent using any of a number of materials and manufacturing processes. Whereas graft infection, occlusion, and dilation are important clinical problems, most patients can expect durable patency and a low frequency of repeat procedures. However, prosthetic grafts have generally proved unfavorable as small-caliber (<6 mm) arterial substitutes. In these demanding, low-flow environments, the primary factor influencing long-term patency is the conduit itself, and the thromboresistance of endothelialized autogenous materials becomes paramount.

Autogenous vein, particularly the greater saphenous, has proved to be a durable and versatile arterial substitute. In the lower extremity, long-term results with saphenous vein bypass (used in either the in situ, reversed, or nonreversed configurations) to below-knee popliteal, tibial, and even pedal arteries have been excellent and serve as the standard of reference for other conduits. Ectopic (i.e., lesser saphenous, arm veins) or composite vein grafts for infrapopliteal bypass are generally inferior to a single segment saphenous vein, although they are still superior to the performance of synthetic grafts in the hands of most surgeons. Randomized trials of prosthetic grafts in the femoropopliteal position have demonstrated reasonable patency rates, particularly in the above-knee position, where they provide a viable alternative. Tibial bypass with prosthetics has generally achieved markedly inferior results and is only considered in extreme circumstances.

The most important complications of surgical bypass are graft occlusion and infection. Graft occlusion is covered in detail later in this chapter. Infection of vascular grafts may be catastrophic and poses immediate threat to both life and limb. Death may occur by sudden and massive hemorrhage internally or externally. Limb loss may result from secondary thrombosis or failure of attempted redo procedures after graft removal. Prosthetic grafts may become infected by break in sterile technique at implantation, hematogenous seeding from other sources, or wound complications resulting secondarily in exposure of the graft. By and large, these often require complete excision of the infected prosthetic and alternative revascularization approaches that avoid the contaminated field. Vein grafts are far less commonly afflicted by infection, which occurs almost exclusively in the context of a local wound complication resulting in exposed graft. These are best treated aggressively by operative wound débridement, segmental graft replacement if necessary, and adequate soft tissue coverage.

Surgical Endarterectomy

Endarterectomy is a direct disobliterative technique that takes advantage of the pathologic localization of atherosclerosis to the intima and inner media. This allows a cleavage plane to be easily developed between the plaque and the underlying deeper media (Fig. 66-9).

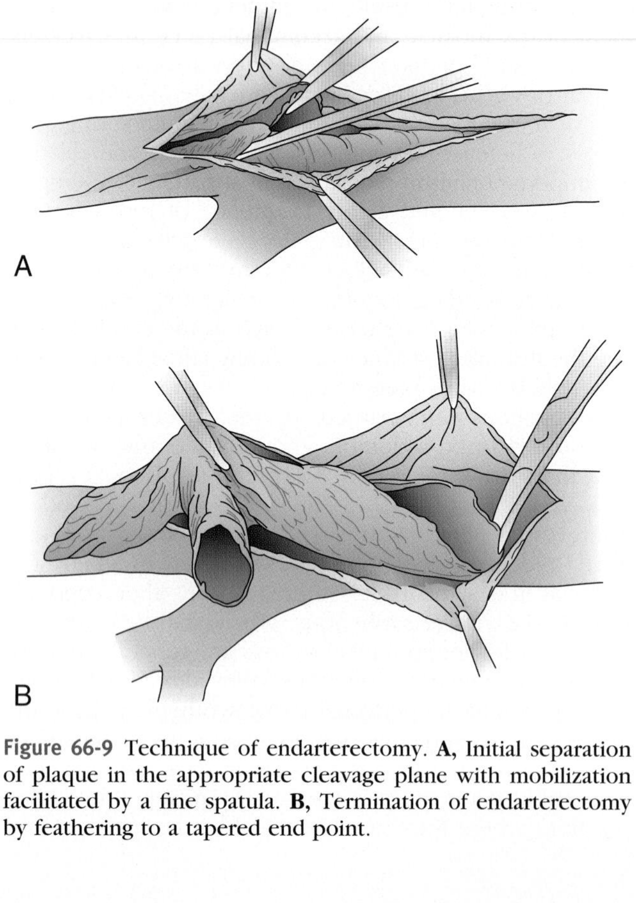

Figure 66-9 Technique of endarterectomy. **A,** Initial separation of plaque in the appropriate cleavage plane with mobilization facilitated by a fine spatula. **B,** Termination of endarterectomy by feathering to a tapered end point.

Surprisingly, the residual deep media and adventitia normally retain sufficient mechanical strength to resist disruption or progressive enlargement under arterial pressure. The various techniques used all involve blunt separation of the plaque, termination by spontaneous tapering or sharp division, and careful attention to the distal end point, which must be firmly adherent to resist dissection or flap elevation leading to thrombosis. The most common and technically simplest technique is the open method, performed by way of a longitudinal arteriotomy with direct vision of both end points as well as the entire endarterectomized surface. Extraction, eversion, and semiclosed methods are applicable in specific situations as well.

Endarterectomy is most feasible and durable when applied to focal stenotic lesions in large-caliber, high-flow vessels. The carotid bifurcation, visceral artery origins, and common femoral artery are particularly well suited to this approach. The use of endarterectomy for longer-segment disease in the aortoiliac and femoropopliteal systems has fallen into disfavor because of the technical difficulty, higher failure rates, and clear advantages demonstrated for bypass grafting in these locations. It offers the advantage of an autogenous reconstruction, avoiding the risk for infection associated with prosthetics. Early failures are due to technical problems with the imperfect end points or to in situ thrombosis on the exposed non-endothelialized surface. Platelet aggregation to the collagenous matrix is a particular problem, and antiplatelet therapy is usually used. Late failures are due to exuberant intimal hyperplasia, which is a more frequent occurrence in longer segments of muscular arteries (e.g., superficial femoral) (Fig. 66-10).

Percutaneous Angioplasty, Stenting, and Other Endovascular Techniques

Percutaneous techniques for treating arterial occlusions, including balloon dilation, stenting, and atherectomy, have undergone tremendous development in the past quarter century and are assuming an increasingly important role. Whereas the initial concepts of angioplasty and stenting can be first attributed to Dotter in the 1960s, it was the development of the double-lumen balloon catheter by Gruntzig in 1974 that initiated widespread clinical application. The use of balloon angioplasty in the treatment of coronary, renal, iliac, and lower extremity disease has come to be accepted as a standard alternative to open surgical therapy.

The mechanism of dilation in balloon angioplasty is thought to involve fracture and displacement of plaque and overstretch of the media and perhaps the adventitia as well. Specific guidewires, catheters, and balloons have been designed for different anatomic sites. The initial technical feat is to accomplish crossing of the lesion with a guidewire, followed by appropriate positioning of the balloon catheter. The balloon must be of adequate length to encompass the lesion and its diameter matched to that of the normal vessel to avoid overdistention (leading to rupture) or inadequate dilation. Low-profile balloon systems have allowed for smaller introducer sheaths, reducing puncture site complications.

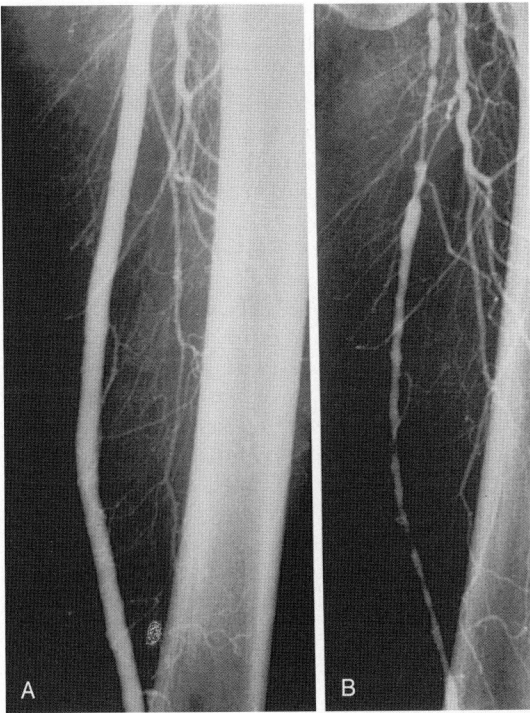

Figure 66-10 Restenosis after long-segment endarterectomy of the superficial femoral artery (SFA). **A,** Completion operative angiogram after semiclosed endarterectomy of SFA using a loop stripper. **B,** Follow-up arteriogram 8 months later, when symptoms of claudication had recurred. A vigorous intimal hyperplastic response is evident.

Similar to endarterectomy, percutaneous transluminal angioplasty (PTA) has found its greatest success in the treatment of focal stenoses in large-caliber, high-flow arteries. The 5-year patency rate for PTA (without stenting) of common iliac lesions, for example, is in the 70% to 80% range. Excellent results have also been reported for suitable aortic, arch vessel, renal, and mesenteric lesions. Results in the femoropopliteal system are inferior to bypass overall, but carefully selected lesions, primarily in patients presenting with claudication, may be durably treated. In all anatomic locations, both early and late success is increased for shorter lesions and stenoses as compared with occlusions.

Restenosis after angioplasty may be due to elastic recoil, constrictive remodeling (shrinkage), and intimal hyperplasia. In the coronary circulation, clinically significant restenosis may develop in as many as 40% of patients within the first year, necessitating repeat revascularization. Promising methods for limiting restenosis include the more liberal use of stents to minimize elastic recoil and constrictive remodeling and approaches targeting the cellular response by local delivery of antiproliferative agents (e.g., drug-eluting stents) or ionizing radiation (brachytherapy).

Intravascular stents have secured an important niche in the vascular armamentarium. The mechanical concept is to maintain luminal patency by exerting persistent radial force on the vessel. Metallic stents come in a variety of design configurations and sizes. For purposes of placement, they may be grouped into those that require balloon inflation (balloon-expandable) and those that do not (self-expanding,). Better and more accurate delivery systems, lower profile platforms, and overall ease of use are increasing their application as a primary modality. Newer nickel-titanium alloys (NITINOL—NIckel TItanium Naval Ordinance Laboratories) provide flexibility in multidimensions while preserving radial force that can serve not only as a mechanical scaffolding but also as a platform for pharmaceutical delivery. Localized, flow-limiting dissections, elastic recoil, or residual stenoses after PTA are situations in which stent placement can often improve the technical result. The superiority of stents over PTA alone remains to be proved but appears likely for longer-segment iliac lesions as well as ostial lesions of the aortic branch vessels, which tend to be heavily calcified and prone to elastic recoil. Recent interest has developed in the use of stents to treat carotid bifurcation disease, and in at least one randomized trial, they were not inferior to carotid endarterectomy.[14] The anatomic sites most suitable for stenting are similar to those mentioned for endarterectomy with the exception that stents placed over joints are susceptible to crimping or fracture due to excessive motion forces. At this time, it does not appear that stent placement extends longer-term patency in the femoropopliteal segments.[15] However, it does appear that prudent use of stents in the treatment of severe post-PTA dissection and residual stenosis of more than 30% may improve initial short-term results and avoid immediate occlusion. Clearly, more formal trials must be conducted with longer follow-up periods to ascertain their safety and indication profiles. As newer developments and technologies emerge, such as atherectomy, thermal devices, cutting balloons, and lasers, the vascular specialist must carefully weigh the risk-to-benefit ratio using available existing literature to make an informed and evidence-based decision when using these devices.

Thrombolytic Therapy

Fibrinolytic drugs enhance conversion of plasminogen to plasmin, which is then capable of degrading fibrin clot. These agents have been used in both systemic and local fashion to achieve lysis of both arterial and venous thrombi. Except for acute embolic events, thrombolytic therapy for arterial occlusive disease is not a sole modality. Rather, it is used as an important adjunct to PTA or surgical interventions that directly address the underlying atherosclerotic lesions, restoring perfusion to the downstream bed. The two major drugs in current use are urokinase and tissue plasminogen activator (tPA).

For arterial occlusions, regional therapy by means of an angiographically guided catheter is most effective. Compared with systemic administration, directed intraclot infusion has been shown to reduce the dose and duration of therapy required to achieve complete lysis. The catheter may be positioned just proximal to or directly into the thrombus. Different dosing regimens and catheters have been espoused for the available agents. Generally, an initial high-dose infusion (lacing dose) is followed by a lower-dose regimen, with frequent follow-up

Table 66-5 Contraindications to Thrombolytic Therapy

Absolute
Recent major bleeding
Recent stroke
Recent major surgery or trauma
Irreversible ischemia of end organ
Intracranial pathology
Recent ophthalmologic procedure

Relative
History of gastrointestinal bleeding or active peptic ulcer
  disease
Underlying coagulation abnormalities
Uncontrolled hypertension
Pregnancy
Hemorrhagic retinopathy

angiograms to document progressive lysis to a satisfactory end point. Systemic anticoagulation with continuous heparin administration must be maintained throughout, so that new thrombus is not formed on, around, or distal to the catheter as lysis is taking place. Because of the significant risk for bleeding as well as the need for careful monitoring of the infusion catheters, patients requiring extended therapy (in some cases up to 48 hours) are best managed in an intensive care setting. In some cases, lysis can be used in conjunction with a mechanical thrombectomy device, which uses the Bernoulli effect to create a vacuum to extract the clot. This can significantly shorten the duration of treatment and thus the patient's exposure to chemical thrombolysis.

Appropriate selection of patients is critical for reducing the incidence of serious complications and improving the likelihood of successful lysis. Even with regional delivery, a state of systemic fibrinolysis is induced; therefore, patients at high risk for serious bleeding are not candidates (Table 66-5). These include patients with recent surgery, trauma, gastrointestinal or other internal bleeding, intracranial tumors, pregnancy, or recent stroke. Relative contraindications include remote gastrointestinal bleeding, hemostatic disorders, severe hypertension, or intracardiac thrombus. The risk for serious bleeding (5%-15%) is increased with longer durations of therapy and a decrease in fibrinogen levels to less than 100 mg/dL or to less than 50% of baseline, which is associated with the development of a systemic lytic state. Fresh thrombi are the most easily lysed. Although no clear upper limit of chronicity has been established, most clinicians believe that thrombotic occlusions more than 2 weeks old are unlikely to respond well to lytic therapy.

An important consideration in evaluating patients for thrombolytic therapy is the severity of ischemia and the time interval for restoring perfusion before irreversible tissue injury has occurred. Patients with signs of irreversibility such as major neurologic impairment do not undergo attempted thrombolysis. In addition, patients with acute, rapid deterioration to advanced ischemia are often poorly collateralized and may not tolerate the time required to achieve reperfusion with this approach.

Recent large-scale trials have supported a potential useful role for thrombolytic therapy in the treatment of arterial occlusions, although many controversies remain concerning specific indications.[16] In appropriately selected patients and with a lesion-specific strategy of percutaneous or surgical intervention, thrombolytic therapy has an important role in the management of arterial occlusive disease.

ACUTE THROMBOEMBOLIC DISEASE

The management of acute extremity ischemia remains a major surgical challenge. Even with optimal surgical management, acute lower extremity ischemia resulting from thromboembolic disease continues to cause significant morbidity and mortality. Limb loss rates of 8% to 22% and perioperative mortality rates of 10% to 17% continue to be reported.[17-19] Maximization of limb salvage, although simultaneously minimizing associated morbidity and mortality, requires expeditious diagnosis and restoration of perfusion.

Pathophysiology

Compared with other organs and tissues, the extremities are relatively resistant to the effects of ischemia. Unlike the brain, which suffers infarction after only 4 to 8 minutes of ischemia, or the myocardium, which infarcts after 17 to 20 minutes, the lower extremity may be salvaged after up to 5 to 6 hours of profound ischemia.

Evaluation of the effect of ischemia on the extremity is complicated by the fact that the various tissues that comprise the extremity have different susceptibilities to ischemic injury, and they manifest this injury in different fashions. Skin and bone are relatively resistant to the effects of ischemia and may survive injuries that, by their effect on other tissues, have rendered the limb painful and useless. Nervous tissue is generally the most sensitive component of the extremity to the effects of ischemia. Significant morbidity may therefore result from isolated ischemic nerve injury in an otherwise intact limb.

Skeletal muscle is the major structural component of the extremity and, for a variety of reasons, plays a key role in the pathophysiology of extremity ischemia. Skeletal muscle constitutes more than 40% of the body mass and about 75% of the lower extremity weight. Although skeletal muscle has a relatively slow resting metabolic rate compared with other tissues, it accounts for 90% of the metabolic activity of the lower extremity. Skeletal muscle receives 71% of the resting lower extremity blood flow and a larger proportion during reperfusion hyperemia. Skeletal muscle plays a pivotal role in the numerous local and systemic manifestations of extremity ischemia-reperfusion injury.

Reperfusion Syndrome

The profound effects of revascularization of the ischemic lower extremity were described as early as the 1950s by Haimovici. As ischemic skeletal muscles reperfuse, a variety of intracellular ions, structural proteins, enzymes, and other components are released through the damaged sarcolemma into the circulation. The resulting myonephropathic syndrome, with its associated hemodynamic instability, lactic acidosis, and hyperkalemia, is well recognized by surgeons. Myoglobin released from injured muscle cells into the circulation is cleared through the kidneys, resulting in dark urine (without red blood cells). Myoglobinuria may persist for 2 to 4 days after reperfusion. Acute renal failure may ensue from myoglobin casts developing in the renal tubules as well as direct toxic effects of the myoglobin on the tubules. Serum creatine phosphokinase levels may increase dramatically (to >10,000 units) after reperfusion of ischemic muscle. Myocardial contractility may become depressed; increased cardiac irritability in the setting of electrolyte disturbances (typically hyperkalemia) may lead to life-threatening dysrhythmias.

When a lower extremity is subjected to severe ischemia, cellular membrane dysfunction results. In this setting, the reperfusion phase is marked by the development of both intracellular and interstitial edema. Intracellular edema results from membrane damage and failure of the membrane-bound adenosine triphosphatase (ATPase). Interstitial edema results from increased microvascular membrane permeability to ions, water, and proteins. This edema may appear within minutes, progressing significantly over the next 24 hours. The amount of edema is dependent on the period of ischemia, the underlying occlusive disease, and the adequacy of revascularization. When muscle edema occurs within the confines of an osseofascial compartment, interstitial pressure continues to increase. Acute compartment syndrome results as pressure increases beyond capillary perfusion pressure (30 mm Hg) and tissue perfusion is impaired. Unless recognized and decompressed by fasciotomy, compartment syndromes will lead to prolonged tissue ischemia despite apparent successful revascularization.

Occasionally, prolongation of the ischemic injury may also occur as a result of microvascular obstruction to blood flow. Endothelial cell edema may predispose to white blood cell and platelet sludging, leading to the so-called no-reflow phenomenon. Similarly, prolonged vascular occlusion can lead to small vessel thrombosis in the muscle and skin, which prevents tissue reperfusion when blood flow is restored to the larger vessels.

Although current understanding of the systemic effects of limb revascularization and compartment syndrome is well developed, understanding of ischemia-reperfusion injury at the tissue level is only beginning to evolve. The pathophysiology of the ischemic injury is complex and involves a variety of factors, including decreased cellular energy charge, inadequate oxygen and substrate delivery, altered ion compartmentalization, and membrane permeability changes. More recently, attention has focused on reperfusion injury (i.e., cellular injury that occurs or is manifested at the time perfusion is restored to ischemic tissue). Most of this injury is believed to be induced by oxygen-derived free radicals, which are formed as oxygen is reintroduced into ischemic tissue. These oxygen-derived free radicals are generated by neutrophils through an NADPH oxidase enzyme on the plasma membrane.

Table 66-6 Sources of Peripheral Emboli

SOURCE	PERCENTAGE
Cardiogenic	80
Atrial fibrillation	50
Myocardial infarction	25
Other	5
Noncardiac	10
Aneurysmal disease	6
Proximal artery	3
Paradoxical emboli	1
Other or Idiopathic	10

These radicals are highly reactive compounds that result from the univalent reduction of molecular oxygen. The most important free radical species include the superoxide radical, hydrogen peroxide, and the extremely reactive hydroxyl radical. These unstable compounds attack the unsaturated bonds of fatty acids within the phospholipid membranes, causing both mechanical and functional derangements within the reperfused tissue.

Etiology

Embolism

Embolic occlusion of a previously unobstructed vessel generally results in the most severe forms of acute ischemia. The most common sources of arterial emboli are reviewed in Table 66-6. About 80% of arterial emboli are cardiac in origin. In the past, most of these emboli were due to complications of rheumatic heart disease, including emboli from diseased valves as well as atrial fibrillation. More recently, atherosclerotic cardiovascular disease has become the major contributor. About 70% of patients with cardiogenic emboli have atrial fibrillation, with the emboli arising in atrial mural thrombus. Atrial fibrillation is currently the most common source of cardiogenic emboli. Acute myocardial infarction is the second most common cause of cardiogenic emboli, preceding about one third of peripheral embolic events. Ventricular mural thrombus, which occurs after acute myocardial injury, is often the source of emboli. Mural thrombus can form within hours of a myocardial infarction but may develop weeks after myocardial infarction and ultimately occurs in more than one third of cases. Peripheral embolization may often be the first sign of a previously "silent" myocardial infarction. Although readily available, standard echocardiographic techniques are often insensitive to the detection of thrombus within the atrium. Transesophageal echocardiography is more sensitive in the detection of both atrial and ventricular mural thrombus.

Although rheumatic valvular heart disease has declined in importance as a source of emboli, emboli from prosthetic heart valves have become an increasingly important source of embolization. Patients with prosthetic heart valves who have sudden onset of lower extremity ischemia are suspected of having valvular embolization, particularly in the setting of inadequate anticoagulation.

Bacterial or fungal endocarditis can result in peripheral embolization. Such emboli tend to be more peripheral and result in septic complications rather than large vessel occlusion and ischemia. IV drug abuse remains a major risk factor for endocarditis and subsequent embolic complications. These smaller emboli often result in digital lesions and peripheral infected pseudoaneurysms. More rare forms of cardiogenic emboli include embolization from intracardiac tumors, most commonly, atrial myxomas. Pathologic examination of unusual appearing emboli is essential for making the diagnosis in this situation. An unusual form of peripheral embolization, termed *paradoxical embolization,* may occur in the setting of patients with intracardiac defects (e.g., patent foramen ovale) and elevated right-sided cardiac pressures. In such patients, venous emboli to the heart may gain access to the arterial circulation through the patent foramen ovale and thereby embolize to the distal arterial circulation. Although rare, such emboli need to be considered in patients with concurrent deep venous thrombosis, pulmonary emboli, or appropriate cardiac defects.

Arterial-to-arterial embolization is another cause of extremity ischemia. Most of these cases arise from atherosclerotic plaque of the aorta. In most situations, such atheroembolization results in diffuse microembolization, resulting in the picture of painful, bluish discoloration of the toes with cutaneous gangrene, livedo reticularis, and often transient muscular pain. This so-called blue toe syndrome generally appears in the setting of palpable peripheral pulses right down to the pedal level. Although this syndrome most frequently occurs after intraluminal catheterization, it may occur spontaneously. Such microembolization may also affect the renal and mesenteric circulations, resulting in progressive renal failure and intestinal infarction. More rarely, artery-to-artery emboli may be sufficiently large to result in macroembolization with distal ischemia. This may result from mural thrombus or plaque from an atherosclerotic aorta or from the mural thrombus lining an aneurysmal artery.

In 10% to 15% of cases, the source of embolization ultimately cannot be determined. Such emboli are not designated as idiopathic until a detailed history and physical examination, as well as complete cardiac and peripheral imaging, fail to identify an embolic source.

The most common sites of embolization are reviewed in Table 66-7. Cardiogenic emboli most commonly travel to the distal aorta and lower extremities (70%-90% of all emboli). Within vessels, the emboli tend to lodge at branch points where vessel diameter decreases. About 10% to 15% of large cardiogenic emboli lodge at the aortic bifurcation (Fig. 66-11). Such "saddle emboli" may result in profound bilateral lower extremity ischemia as well as neurologic ischemic injury. Another 15% embolize to the iliac bifurcation. The most common site of lower extremity embolization is the femoral bifurcation (Fig. 66-12), constituting more than 40% of cases. Smaller emboli lodge at the distal popliteal artery level at the level of the tibioperoneal artery trunk (Fig. 66-13) in 10% to 15% of cases. The upper extremities are affected in about 10% of cases, in which the embolus most typically settles in the brachial artery.

Cardiogenic emboli are less likely to occur to the cerebral or visceral circulation. Embolization to the cerebral circulation occurs in about 13% of cases with potentially devastating results. Embolization to the mesenteric and renal vessels occurs in about 5% of peripheral emboli. Although often clinically silent, such emboli can result in acute catastrophes, such as mesenteric ischemia secondary to a superior mesenteric artery embolus.

Thrombosis

Acute thrombosis generally occurs in vessels affected by preexistent atherosclerosis. As such, there is generally some degree of collateral vessel development, and the resultant ischemia is often less severe than with acute embolic disease. The most common extremity vessel affected is the superficial femoral artery, which is often affected by long segments of atherosclerosis. Popliteal artery aneurysms are also prone to thrombosis and may result in severe ischemia, particularly when associated with embolization to the tibial vessels.

Table 66-7 Site of Peripheral Embolization

SITE	PERCENTAGE
Aortic bifurcation	10-15
Iliac bifurcation	15
Femoral bifurcation	40
Popliteal	10
Upper extremities	10
Cerebral	10-15
Mesenteric, visceral	5

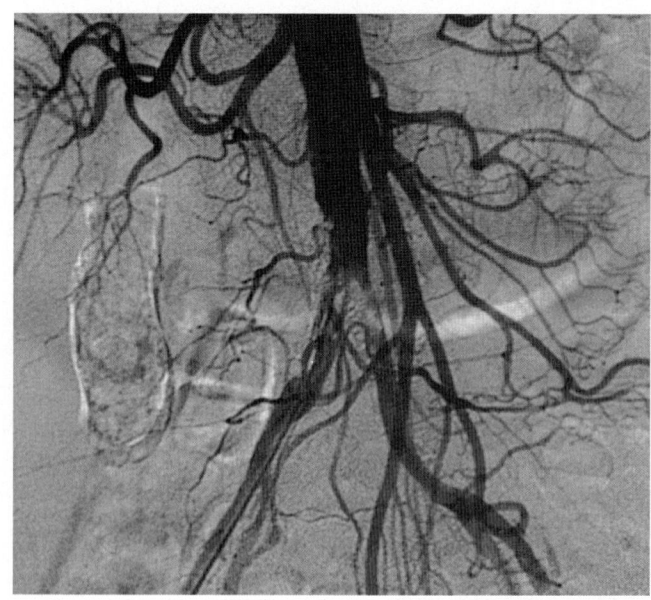

Figure 66-11 Large cardiogenic embolus lodged at the aortic bifurcation known as a "saddle embolus."

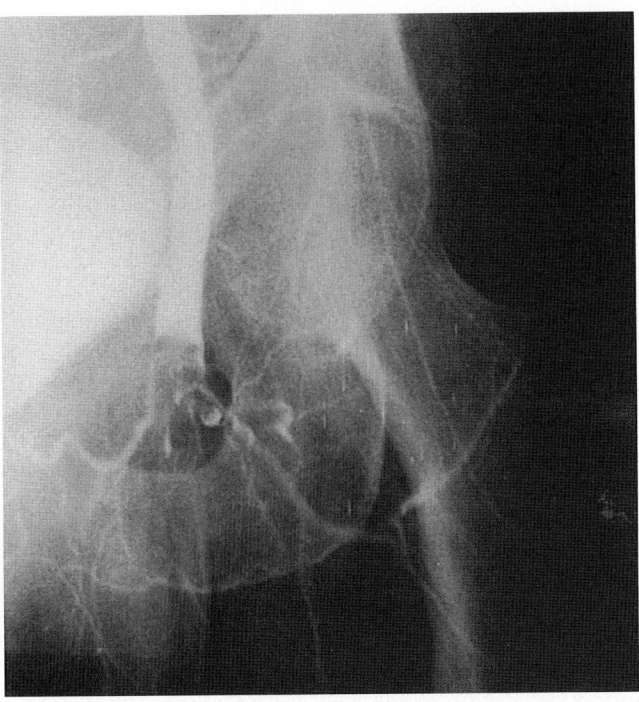

Figure 66-12 This arteriogram demonstrates an occlusive left femoral embolus with a typical rounded "meniscus" along its upper border.

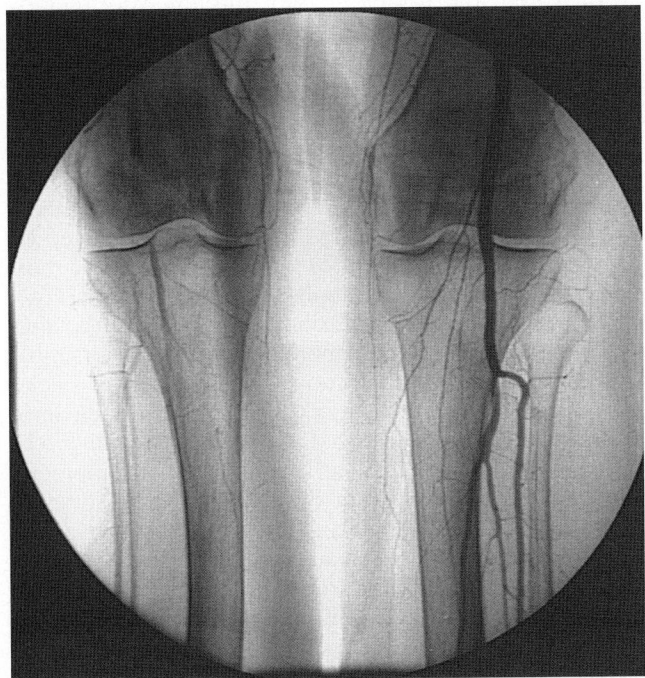

Figure 66-13 Distal embolus occluding the right popliteal artery.

A particularly severe form of ischemia results from distal vascular thrombosis of the extremities, which may occur in the setting of sepsis or with hypercoagulable states.[20] The most common hypercoagulable states associated with acute arterial thrombosis are hyperhomocyste-inemia, antithrombin III deficiency, lupus anticoagulant (antiphospholipid antibody), and protein C deficiency. Although usually associated with venous thrombosis, activated protein C resistance caused by the spontaneous mutations of factor V Leiden may also cause arterial thrombosis. Exposure to heparin may lead to heparin-induced thrombosis in patients with heparin-induced antibodies. These antibodies cross-react with the heparin–platelet factor 4 complex on the platelet surface, leading to granular, white, platelet-laden thrombi and thrombocytopenia.

Acute thrombosis of a previous arterial bypass graft may also lead to recurrent ischemia. The degree of ischemia depends on the location of the graft and the original indication for surgery. Early graft occlusions (within 2 months of surgery) are usually caused by technical or judgmental errors. Intermediate graft occlusions (within 2 years) are generally attributable to the formation of intimal hyperplasia at the anastomoses or within the graft (for vein grafts).

Presentation and Evaluation

The classic presentation of patients with acute ischemia of the extremities may be recalled by the "five Ps": *pain, pallor, pulselessness, paresthesias,* and *paralysis.*

Pain is the most common complaint in alert patients. The degree of pain depends on the severity of ischemia, which is generally determined by the location of the occlusion and the degree of collateral flow. Ischemic pain can be severe and difficult to relieve with even large doses of narcotics. The sudden onset of severe ischemic pain in a previously asymptomatic patient is most suggestive of an embolic occlusion. Patients with spontaneous thrombosis often have had chronic symptoms of claudication or various degrees of pain before the acute event. Obtunded patients may have severe ischemia without complaints of pain. This is most commonly encountered in intubated, postoperative patients with spontaneous or iatrogenic arterial thrombosis.

Pallor is a common but relative finding that depends on the degree of ischemia and the underlying skin color. A sudden and complete embolic occlusion may result in a cool, waxy-appearing white extremity with no signs of cutaneous blood flow. Conversely, a partial occlusion may result in only delayed capillary refill with pallor on elevation of the extremity and rubor on dependency.

The absence of arterial pulses on examination will alert the surgeon to both the location of the arterial occlusion and the degree of ischemia. Patients with acute arterial embolism generally have normal palpable pulses above the occlusion with a complete absence below. The pulse immediately above the occlusion (e.g., the common femoral pulse in a patient with a femoral bifurcation embolus) may be particularly prominent with a "water-hammer" quality that results from limited arterial outflow. The presence of normal arterial pulses in the contralateral extremity is most suggestive of an acute embolus because patients with acute thrombosis generally have some degree of symmetrical pulse deficit, owing to long-standing atherosclerosis. A handheld continuous-wave Doppler examination plays an important role in the initial evaluation of patients with acute vessel occlusion. The presence of even monophasic Doppler signals over the pedal vessels affirms distal vascular patency and at least short-term viability of the distal tissues. Conversely, a complete absence of arterial flow is most suggestive of profound ischemia and calls for immediate revascularization.

As mentioned previously, within the extremities, the peripheral nerve is the tissue that is most sensitive to ischemia. As such, the degree of neurologic dysfunction is a sensitive barometer of the degree of ischemia. With mild ischemia, the findings may be subjective and subtle. Early paresthesias may be characterized as a numbness of the toes or a slight decrease of sensation of the foot compared with the contralateral extremity to light touch or pinprick. With severe ischemia, however, profound sensory loss may lead to complete anesthesia of the foot, indicative of impending tissue loss without early revascularization. Paradoxically, these patients with the most severe ischemia and complete anesthesia complain of less pain than those with more mild ischemia and intact sensation.

Weakness of the extremity is another important sign of neurologic ischemia of the extremity. Mild ischemia results in a weakness or subjective stiffness of the toes and foot, which may be easily appreciated on physical examination. As ischemia becomes more progressively severe, the weakness may progress to frank paralysis of the effected extremity. It is not unusual for the patient with a sudden complete embolic occlusion to suffer the immediate onset of paralysis of the affected extremity. Patients with an aortic saddle embolus may have bilateral paralysis and anesthesia from the waist down. In patients with severe ischemia characterized by anesthesia and paralysis, it is important to distinguish reversible from irreversible ischemic changes. Patients with prolonged ischemia have palpable firmness to the extremity muscle and stiffness to the extremity indicative of muscle rigor. Reperfusion of such an extremity does not restore function and can result in severe systemic injury. Primary amputation is the safest form of management in such cases.

The acute embolic occlusion of an extremity artery can be accurately diagnosed by a careful history and physical examination in most cases; emboli to the cerebral and visceral bed may be more difficult to identify and treat. The diagnosis in these cases is based on a high index of suspicion based on the patient's complaints and history. For example, a patient with the sudden onset of severe aching abdominal pain coupled with risk factors for cardiogenic emboli and a relative lack of physical findings is presumed to have suffered a superior mesenteric artery embolus until proved otherwise.

Because evaluation of patients with acute arterial occlusion generally differs for patients who have suffered embolic versus thrombotic occlusion, it is important to make the appropriate clinical distinction. As outlined previously, patients with emboli tend to have risk factors (e.g., atrial fibrillation, recent myocardial infarction, prosthetic heart valve), a more sudden onset of symptoms (no prior claudication), and unilateral findings (normal

contralateral extremity). Despite these guidelines, the distinction can be difficult to make at times. Certainly, patients with recent myocardial infarctions or atrial fibrillation may have concurrent peripheral vascular occlusive disease and patients with peripheral vascular occlusive disease may suffer cardiogenic emboli. Thus, the evaluation of each patient must be individualized to supply enough information to effectively treat the patient without jeopardizing limb salvage or function by delaying revascularization.

When the history and physical examination implicates an embolus as the source of occlusion, the subsequent evaluation is simple and direct. Routine preoperative blood work and a chest radiograph are obtained, and a 12-lead electrocardiogram is performed to document atrial fibrillation, cardiac ischemia, or a previous (and perhaps unsuspected) myocardial infarction. Because arterial emboli are removed by direct arterial cutdown and removal of the embolus (as described later), there is generally no need for preoperative arteriography. When the diagnosis of embolus is questionable or the site for simple arterial cutdown and arteriotomy unclear, a preoperative arteriogram may be useful to define the anatomy and guide the revascularization procedure. The management of distal extremity emboli (below the brachial or popliteal artery) may be assisted by detailed preoperative angiograms in selected cases. For example, very distal emboli within the distal tibial or pedal vessels may be best treated by catheter-based thrombolytic therapy (described later) rather than surgical extraction. Arteriograms of intra-arterial emboli often demonstrate an abrupt cutoff of the artery with a rounded meniscus at the site of the embolus (see Fig. 66-12). Conversely, the embolus may appear as an intraluminal defect with partial flow around it (see Fig. 66-11). Postoperatively, when the embolus has been removed and the limb revascularized, and the patient is stable, the evaluation is completed by documentation of the source of the embolus. In most cases, this involves transesophageal echocardiography.

The surgical management of patients with acute arterial thrombosis is generally more complex than the simple arteriotomy and clot extraction used for embolic occlusion. Patients suffering thrombotic occlusion often have diffuse atherosclerotic disease at multiple arterial levels, various degrees of collateral blood vessel development, and unpredictable levels of distal arterial reconstitution. These patients are best evaluated with complete arteriography to define the optimal approach to revascularization. Rarely, arterial thrombosis results in such profound ischemia that the patient is taken immediately to the operating room and intraoperative arteriography is performed after arterial exposure.

Management

Embolic Occlusion

Patients with acute arterial occlusion are anticoagulated with an IV heparin bolus (5000-10,000 units) and begun on a continuous infusion at 1000 units/hour. The primary goal of anticoagulation is to prevent thrombosis resulting from stagnant flow beyond the primary embolic or thrombotic occlusion. Furthermore, short- and long-term anticoagulation is indicated in patients with cardiogenic emboli to prevent additional embolic events. Recurrent embolization occurs in about 7% of patients who are chronically anticoagulated versus 21% of those who are not.

The most important initial decision focuses on the viability and potential salvage in the ischemic limb. Rarely, patients have such long-standing and severe ischemia that irreversible ischemic injury to the extremity (manifesting as rigor of the muscles or frank gangrenous changes to the foot) has occurred. Such cases are best treated with primary extremity amputation.

In most cases, however, early revascularization for restoration of limb function is indicated. As mentioned earlier, immediate progression to the operating room after minimal and expeditious evaluation is indicated for patients who have suffered occlusive emboli to the extremities. For patients with emboli to the lower extremity, the entire extremity is prepped and draped into the field. This allows immediate evaluation of success of the revascularization as well as ready access for more distal arterial exposure if necessary to complete the procedure. Emboli to the iliac and femoral vessels are approached through a femoral cutdown. Femoral artery cutdowns can be performed under local anesthesia with IV sedation. Often, however, regional or general anesthesia is preferable, particularly when popliteal artery exposure is necessary.

A standard longitudinal or oblique skin incision is made, with the common femoral artery as well as profunda femoris and superficial femoral arteries all independently controlled. Normal arteries, free of significant atherosclerosis, are best incised transversely just above the femoral bifurcation. In patients with significant atherosclerosis, however, longitudinal arteriotomies afford the best exposure and most reliable closure (often with an arterial patch). Patients with iliac-level emboli often have an absence of a femoral pulse. Inflow is restored by retrograde passage of a No. 4 or 5 balloon thrombectomy catheter. The catheter is passed in 10-cm increments. Gentle inflation of the catheter as it is withdrawn engages and extracts the thrombus without causing arterial wall injury. Each passage extends an additional 10 cm until pulsatile arterial inflow is restored. Passages are continued until no additional thrombus is recovered. Attention is then turned to the outflow vessels. Antegrade passage of a No. 3 Fogarty catheter, 3 to 5 cm down the profunda, generally extracts any impacted thrombus and restores good backflow. The catheter is then passed down the superficial femoral artery in increments until no further thrombus is extracted. This may necessitate passage to the popliteal level or beyond. Blind passage of the Fogarty catheter from the groin to below the popliteal artery almost always results in cannulation of the peroneal artery. Specific cannulation of the anterior tibial and posterior tibial arteries requires more distal, below-knee popliteal artery exposure. Alternatively, selective passage of balloon catheters over guidewires using fluoroscopic control has facilitated selective cannulation of distal vessels. When good inflow and backbleeding have

been restored, the transverse arteriotomy is closed with 5-0 polypropylene sutures, and flow is restored.

For patients with a palpable popliteal pulse and distal emboli, exposure is best obtained at the level of the below-knee popliteal artery through a standard medial incision. The soleus muscle is carefully taken down off the tibia, exposing the tibioperoneal trunk. The anterior tibial veins may be divided to facilitate individual control of the anterior tibial, posterior tibial, and peroneal arteries. A distal popliteal arteriotomy may then be performed and retrograde passage of a No. 3 catheter used to restore normal inflow to the popliteal level. Selective cannulation of the anterior and posterior tibial vessels, as well as the peroneal artery, may be performed with a No. 2 or 3 thrombectomy catheter, restoring good backflow. At the conclusion of the embolectomy and closure of the arteriotomy, reperfusion of the extremity is assessed. In most cases, restoration of palpable pedal pulses and pink, well-perfused toes reassures the surgeon of a successful and complete embolectomy. In some cases, however, spasm of the distal vessels secondary to passage of the Fogarty catheter may delay the return of normal perfusion. Even in these cases, however, restoration of strong Doppler signals is present at the pedal level. After several minutes, palpable pulses and well-perfused skin are reestablished. In any case in which there is a doubt as to the success of the embolectomy, completion arteriography is performed to assess the distal vasculature for spasm and retained thrombus. For those rare patients who have restoration of patent vessels down to the mid-tibial level, with occlusions of the distal tibial and pedal vessels, direct intraoperative arterial infusion of urokinase (50,000-250,000 units) may help lyse distal thrombus and restore perfusion to the foot. Occasionally, direct cutdown and thrombectomy of the distal tibial and pedal levels is necessary to remove distally impacted thrombus.

Patients with a saddle embolus to the aortic bifurcation with bilateral lower extremity ischemia are approached through simultaneous bilateral femoral artery cutdowns. The femoral arteries are simultaneously clamped and opened, and retrograde thrombectomies are performed to both limbs simultaneously to prevent fragmentation of the thrombus and distal embolization to the extremity contralateral to the thrombectomy. After normal inflow is obtained, the remainder of the procedure is similar to that for an iliac-level embolectomy.

Patients with upper extremity emboli are approached in a similar fashion. The entire extremity is prepped and draped into the field. Usually the entire embolectomy can be performed under local anesthesia through a longitudinal incision performed just above the elbow. The brachial artery is carefully dissected from its companion structures, and a transverse arteriotomy is performed. Most emboli impact just above the elbow and are easily extracted by passage of a No. 3 Fogarty catheter both proximally and distally. Emboli that have lodged at the subclavian level are generally easy to remove by retrograde passage of the No. 3 Fogarty catheter from the elbow proximally to the subclavian level. Arterial closure and assessment are similar to that performed for the lower extremity.

Recently, several authors have reported on the adjunctive use of fluoroscopy for accurate passage of the thrombectomy catheter. Similarly, others have found angioscopy to be useful in the evaluation of completeness of the thrombectomy (particularly during thrombectomies of occluded prosthetic grafts).

Thrombotic Occlusion

As mentioned previously, patients with thrombotic arterial occlusion undergo an initial arteriogram to delineate the arterial anatomy and define the best mode of revascularization. In most cases, the site of thrombotic occlusion is well delineated. In patients with a satisfactory inflow and outflow vessel with a long segment of occluded vessel, the best option is generally to proceed to surgery and perform a surgical bypass procedure. Inflow to the femoral artery can be restored with either a direct aorto-femoral revascularization or various forms of extra-anatomic bypass (femorofemoral bypass, axillofemoral bypass, or iliofemoral bypass), depending on the patient's anatomy. Infrainguinal arterial occlusions are best treated with femoral-distal bypass operations with autogenous vein. When short-segment thrombotic occlusions are identified, a catheter-directed infusion of thrombolytic therapy may recanalize the vessel, revealing an appropriate underlying lesion for balloon angioplasty. Recent studies have suggested that aggressive thrombolytic therapy is most beneficial when the ischemic interval is short and that initial thrombolysis may reduce the magnitude of subsequent surgical procedures.[16,21] When the arteriogram reveals no distal arterial reconstitution appropriate for bypass, catheter-based thrombolysis may restore sufficient perfusion to establish or reveal a distal vessel suitable for bypass.

Compartment Syndrome

As described previously, extremities subjected to prolonged periods of ischemia followed by reperfusion suffer reperfusion injury manifesting as both intracellular and interstitial edema. This reperfusion injury occurs regardless of the cause of arterial occlusion (embolus or thrombosis) or mode of revascularization (balloon embolectomy, surgical bypass, or catheter-based thrombolytic recanalization). When muscular swelling occurs within the confines of an unyielding osseofascial bound space, increased compartmental pressures occur. These increased pressures can occur in either the arm or leg. In the lower extremity, the calf is the most frequently affected area. The anterior compartment of the calf and then the lateral, deep posterior, and superficial posterior compartments are involved with decreasing frequency. Within the thigh, the anterior quadriceps compartment is the most frequently involved area. In the upper extremity, the anterior or volar forearm compartment is most frequently involved, but the dorsal forearm, as well as hand and upper arm, may also be involved by reperfusion edema.

When the intracompartmental pressures increase to more than the level of capillary perfusion pressure, both venous outflow and capillary perfusion may become impaired. This may result in recurrent and prolonged ischemia unless the affected compartment is decompressed. As with the initial ischemic injury, the nerve tissue is most susceptible to the effects of compartment syndrome. The diagnosis of compartment syndrome is based on a high degree of suspicion and careful evaluation for signs and symptoms. Extremities that are revascularized after 4 to 6 hours of severe ischemia are most at risk for development of compartment syndrome. The early signs and symptoms must be carefully watched for, particularly in patients with decreased sensorium. The typical clinical findings of early compartment syndrome are severe pain that is disproportionate to the relative paucity of physical findings. Patients usually have marked tenderness on compression of the edematous calf and severe discomfort on passive extension of the calf with dorsiflexion or plantar flexion of the foot. Because the anterior compartment is the most commonly affected space within the calf, the first neurologic findings are often numbness in the area of the great toe web space, attributable to pressure on the deep peroneal nerve. Palpable pulses and strong Doppler signals may be well preserved despite progressive compartment syndrome and must not lead to a false sense of security. When the diagnosis of compartment syndrome is in question, direct measures of the pressure within the compartment may be performed. A needle cannula placed directly into the compartment and attached to a pressure transducer gives an accurate measure of the intracompartmental pressure. There are also portable, handheld devices designed for measurement of intracompartmental pressures. Although somewhat controversial, it is generally agreed that, as compartmental pressure reaches 30 mm Hg, capillary perfusion is impaired, and neurologic and muscular injury occurs.

Although significant calf swelling and increased compartment pressures can often be managed with extreme elevation of the extremity, marked elevation of compartment pressures with neurologic changes necessitates early and effective decompression to prevent a permanent and disabling injury. Most vascular surgeons prefer a two-incision, four-compartment fasciotomy. The medial-based longitudinal incision is made just posterior to the tibia and is carried down through the fascia into the superficial posterior space. The soleus muscle is then incised longitudinally, near its tibial insertion, and the deep fascia is incised longitudinally to decompress the deep posterior compartment. A second anterolateral calf incision is made longitudinally and carried down through the fascia into the anterior compartment. A second longitudinal fascial incision is made over the lateral compartment, decompressing the peroneus muscles. Severe compartment syndrome manifests by an immediate pouting of the muscles as they swell beyond the fascial incision. The skin incision needs to be long enough to prevent any restriction on the underlying muscle.

When patients undergo revascularization after a prolonged interval (≥6 hours) of severe ischemia, consideration for a prophylactic fasciotomy in anticipation of impending compartment syndrome needs to be entertained. Such prophylactic fasciotomies may be performed through more limited skin incisions with blind extension

Table 66-8 **Natural History of Intermittent Claudication**

STUDY	PATIENTS (n)	SURVIVAL (%)	FOLLOW-UP (yr)	STABLE OR IMPROVED (%)	AMPUTATION (%)
Boyd	1476	73	5	80	7.2
		38	10	60	12
Imparato	104	—	2.5	79	5.8
McAllister	100	89	6	78	7.0

Adapted from Braunwald E: Atlas of heart diseases. In Craeger MA (ed): Vascular Disease, vol VII. Philadelphia, Current Medicine, 1996, p 3.5.

of the fascial incisions by sliding a slightly opened Metzenbaum scissors along the cut edge of the fascia. The skin incisions can be extended later if full-blown compartment syndrome develops.

An alternative surgical approach to four-compartment fasciotomy, favored by many orthopedic surgeons, involves resection of a portion of the fibula or parafibular dissection of all soft tissues away from a section of the fibula. Because the fascia of all four compartments inserts on the fibula, disruption of these fibular attachments may adequately decompress the various calf compartments.

CHRONIC OCCLUSIVE DISEASE OF THE LOWER EXTREMITIES

Presentation and Natural History

Patients with arterial claudication suffer from reproducible ischemic muscle pain resulting from inadequate oxygen delivery during exercise. Studies suggest that patients with claudication, while having an increased risk for cardiovascular mortality, have a low risk for limb loss[22,23] (Table 66-8). Recent reports using noninvasive studies and multivariate analysis have more accurately defined the natural history of arterial claudication. The annual risk for mortality and limb loss in patients with claudication is about 5% and 1%, respectively. More than half of these patients either remain stable or have improvement in their symptoms with conservative management, consisting of increased exercise, weight loss, and risk factor modification. About 20% to 30% of patients with claudication come to operation within 5 years because of disease progression.

As opposed to the patient with claudication, who has cramping in the thigh, buttock, or calf with exercise, the patient with more advanced critical ischemia complains of pain at rest. Rest pain occurs when blood flow is inadequate to meet metabolic requirements. In the lower extremity, ischemic rest pain is localized to the forefoot and generally is easily distinguished from benign nocturnal muscle cramps in the calf, which are also common in older patients. The patient with rest pain is often awakened by severe discomfort in the forefoot and hangs the affected extremity off the bed for temporary relief of symptoms. Patients often have trophic changes, such as muscle wasting, thinning of skin, thickening of nails, and hair loss in the distal affected limb. Rest pain is an ominous symptom and usually requires revascularization because this form of advanced ischemia generally progresses to tissue loss.

The patient with critical ischemia is at risk for tissue infection or gangrene resulting from arterial insufficiency. Patients with diabetes or renal failure are more susceptible to the development of ischemic pedal ulcers. Minor trauma to the forefoot leads to ulcer formation and skin breakdown that, with diminished tissue perfusion, are unable to heal. The simple friction between adjacent ischemic toes may result in breakdown termed *kissing ulcers*. Bacterial superinfection of pedal and leg ulcers, as well as osteomyelitis of the underlying bone, frequently complicates the management of these patients. The depth and pattern of ulcer penetration, the degree of bone involvement, the location of the ulcer, the presence of infection, the presence of neuropathy, and the degree of arterial insufficiency all may affect management of the complex patient with lower extremity arterial insufficiency.

Evaluation

Vascular Laboratory

Noninvasive testing may aid in predicting the location and severity of atherosclerotic occlusive disease. Noninvasive evaluation is also helpful to establish a preoperative baseline assessment for subsequent comparison postoperatively. Routine segmental Doppler pressure ABI determinations are the standard studies, but results may be spuriously elevated in diabetic patients and those with renal failure. In this select group of patients with heavily calcified vessels, metatarsal and digital PVRs may be more helpful in evaluating peripheral vascular disease.

Patients with known risk factors and symptoms consistent with occlusive disease pose little diagnostic challenge. However, many patients with occlusive disease may have normal perfusion at rest and may require provocative testing to reproduce their symptoms and demonstrate abnormal laboratory findings. Treadmill testing may be used to enhance symptoms of claudication, at which point re-examination of the patient with measurement of PVRs and Doppler signals help delineate vascular insufficiency.

Angiography

The standard angiographic approach for patients with lower extremity occlusive disease is transfemoral catheterization. The aorta, iliac arteries, femoral arteries, and distal runoff arteries from both lower extremities need to be evaluated. The aorta must be imaged in two planes, and views of the celiac and superior mesenteric arteries are also obtained. If the hemodynamic significance of a lesion is called into question, pressure gradients across the lesion before and after infusion with a vasodilator (e.g., tolazoline [Priscoline] or nitroglycerin) need to be obtained. If the patient is an appropriate candidate for balloon angioplasty, interventional therapy may be performed at that time.

As discussed earlier, both MRA and duplex ultrasonography are assuming an increased role in the delineation of central and peripheral vascular anatomy. These noninvasive modalities may be of particular value in minimizing the use or dosage of contrast media in patients at risk for dye-induced nephropathy. An important limitation as compared with contrast arteriography is the inability to simultaneously treat lesions by catheter-based techniques (e.g., PTA). The use of duplex scanning or MRA as a screening test to predict the likelihood of a lesion amenable to PTA or stenting is another potential algorithm aimed at reducing the morbidity of conventional arteriography.

Cardiac Risk Assessment

Risk factors for occlusive disease are similar to those for atherosclerosis in general and include cigarette smoking, hypertension, hypercholesterolemia, diabetes, and male sex. Many of these patients have overt cardiac disease, and workup of these patients has been well described in the literature. Because myocardial ischemia remains the leading cause of death after vascular surgery, patients undergo preoperative risk factor assessment and selective stress testing before undergoing major vascular surgery. The initiation and optimization of medical therapy (particularly β-adrenergic blockade) before elective vascular surgery has been of paramount importance in minimizing perioperative morbidity and death in this group of patients. Indeed, in patients with stable coronary disease, preoperative cardiac revascularization does not offer any improvement in postoperative mortality benefit.[24]

Management

Aortoiliac Occlusive Disease

Many patients with aortoiliac occlusive disease (AOD) can be managed conservatively with risk factor modification and an aggressive walking regimen. Only patients who suffer disabling claudication or limb-threatening ischemia are considered for arteriography and intervention.

Percutaneous Transluminal Angioplasty

During the 1990s, the indications for PTA have become more liberal as the effectiveness of PTA of the iliac arteries has been increasingly well documented. PTA is performed under local anesthesia with minimal sedation, as a day surgery admission, with significantly less morbidity and productivity reduction. Although initially performed only in the common iliac artery for stenosis, PTA is routinely used to treat short-segment occlusions as well as external iliac lesions. Iliac artery PTA may be particularly useful to help improve inflow before a more distal surgical reconstruction.

The use of iliac artery stents has also begun to play an increasing role in the management of patients with AOD. Iliac artery stents are most useful after initial suboptimal results from PTA. Occasionally, however, they are used primarily in the treatment of complex lesions. For example, bilateral proximal common iliac lesions are problematic for standard PTA and are best managed with simultaneous bilateral common iliac stenting ("kissing" PTA and stenting technique). Overall, reports from numerous series suggest that the results of percutaneous therapies for aortoiliac disease are more favorable for common (versus external) iliac lesions and less favorable for long occlusions as opposed to short stenoses; stents appear to improve the results of isolated PTA in some situations, but the data are less clear. Application of advances in stent design and materials, as well as reduction in delivery profile, improved early patency results. Five-year patency rates for common iliac PTA alone are typically in the range of 80% and are notably inferior (50%-60%) for external iliac disease. Importantly, complication rates are low, and failure rarely changes the available surgical options.

When PTA is not an option, a number of surgical alternatives are available. The technique of combined open surgical common femoral artery exposure with endovascular recanalization and balloon angioplasty of severely diseased iliac artery segments has been described, primarily in patients with comorbidities prohibiting major surgery or general anesthesia. This treatment strategy includes femoral endarterectomy and subsequent endoluminal deployment of a stent-graft to reline the balloon-dilated artery, with the ability to postdilate the vessel to a larger caliber and to surgically fashion the distal anastomosis to the femoral outflow vessels. Depending on the condition of the patient and the patient's pathologic anatomy, the options include aortobifemoral (ABF) bypass, aortoiliac thromboendarterectomy, axillofemoral bypass, iliofemoral bypass, and femorofemoral bypass.

Aortofemoral Bypass

Aortofemoral bypass is performed under general endotracheal anesthesia. An epidural catheter is placed preoperatively to improve pain control and facilitate early postoperative extubation. The patient is prepped and draped from the chest to the mid thighs with the groins exposed. The femoral vessels are exposed first through bilateral longitudinal, oblique incisions. Preliminary exposure of the femoral vessels minimizes the time that the abdomen is open and improves the efficiency of the operation. In patients with significant occlusive disease of the femoral arteries, a broad exposure of the profunda femoris for potential profundaplasty is performed before entry into the abdomen. After the femoral vessels have been dissected, retroperitoneal tunnels are gently developed underneath the inguinal ligament on the anterior surface of the external iliac artery. The groins are packed with antibiotic-soaked sponges, and attention is turned to the abdomen. Either a direct transperitoneal or lateral (flank) retroperitoneal aortic exposure may be used; generally, the anterior approach is preferred because graft tunneling to the right groin is far easier. The abdomen is entered through a longitudinal midline incision, and the patient is explored for any intra-abdominal abnormalities. The transverse colon is pulled cephalad, and the entire small bowel is retracted to the right of the patient. The ligament of Treitz is incised, and the duodenum is mobilized to the right for standard infrarenal aortic exposure. The dissection is carried up to the level of renal vein to allow for optimal cross-clamping and improved conditions for a proximal anastomosis. The dissection is completed down to the level of the inferior mesenteric artery. Anticoagulation with heparin (5000-7000 units) is performed after creating retroperitoneal tunnels anterior to both iliac arteries and posterior to the ureters. Great care is taken to avoid trauma to the autonomic nervous plexus (particularly over the proximal left common iliac artery). Atraumatic vascular clamps are placed above the inferior mesenteric artery and below the renal arteries.

The proximal anastomosis may be completed with either an end-to-end or end-to-side configuration. The end-to-end technique is preferred in most cases and has the advantage of not requiring flow to be reestablished in the more distal aorta, thereby avoiding potential intraoperative emboli to the lower extremities. The end-to-end technique may also decrease the incidence of aortoenteric fistula postoperatively because retroperitonealization of the graft is facilitated. To perform an end-to-end proximal anastomosis, the aorta is divided in a beveled fashion just above the distal clamp. The distal aorta is closed with either a running nonabsorbable monofilament suture or a surgical stapler. If there is associated aneurysmal disease of the aorta, the aorta may be incised longitudinally and the bifurcation oversewn to achieve complete exclusion of the dilated segment. The end-to-side technique for the proximal anastomosis of the aortofemoral bypass graft is generally reserved for patients with occlusion of the external iliac arteries who would lack retrograde perfusion of important collaterals in the pelvis. The proximal anastomosis is completed using a running 3-0 polypropylene suture.

On completion, the proximal clamps are released and a vascular clamp is placed proximally across the graft limbs. The limbs of the graft are then passed through the previously created retroperitoneal tunnels to the femoral arteries. The femoral vessels are controlled in the groins with atraumatic vascular clamps. For those patients with normal femoral vessels and a widely patent profunda, the anastomosis is performed to the common femoral artery. Many patients with AOD have associated occlusive disease of the femoral arteries, and it is essential that blood flow to the profunda femoris artery be optimized. In this instance, the toe of anastomosis is placed onto the profunda femoris artery. If necessary, a complete profunda endarterectomy and profundaplasty may be performed. Before tying down the anastomosis, the inflow and outflow vessels are flushed in an attempt to remove any atherosclerotic debris or clot that may have collected in the graft or native vessels. On completion of

both anastomoses in the groin, the abdomen and proximal anastomosis are reinspected for evidence of bleeding. After hemostasis is attained, the proximal anastomosis and graft are covered with autogenous material. If an end-to-end anastomosis has been performed, the retroperitoneum is closed over the graft. If an end-to-side anastomosis was performed, the omentum may be used to wrap around the anastomosis and to partially cover the graft. The abdomen and groins are closed in a standard fashion.

ABF bypass grafting has generally resulted in patency rates among the highest reported for any major arterial reconstruction. Primary patency rates of ABF grafts at 5 years are reported to be 70% to 88% with 10-year rates of 66% to 78%. Patients operated on for claudication with good infrainguinal outflow have superior patency rates compared with those operated on for limb-threatening ischemia with associated infrainguinal occlusive disease. Studies have demonstrated that younger patients (<50 years) and those with smaller aortas have inferior patency rates to older patients and those with larger aortas.[25] In patients with significant profunda femoris disease, simultaneous profundaplasty improves graft patency. In addition to excellent patency rates after ABF bypass grafting, most patients have significant relief of their symptoms. Perioperative mortality rates average about 4% with a 5-year cumulative survival rate for patients undergoing ABF bypass grafting of 70% to 75%, which is significantly poorer than an age-matched control population but typical of claudicant patients in general.

Rarely, patients have isolated terminal aorta and proximal common iliac artery occlusive disease. These patients are primarily female smokers in their fourth or fifth decade of life. In these patients, when the AOD is localized at the aortic bifurcation, an aortoiliac endarterectomy may be performed. This procedure offers the advantage of not requiring prosthetic material; however, it is fraught with more numerous potential technical pitfalls and has largely been replaced by percutaneous options for such localized lesions. Aortoiliac endarterectomy is contraindicated in AOD patients with arterial ectasia or aneurysmal disease.

Extra-anatomic Bypass

Blaisdell[26] and others, using polyester (Dacron) grafts, pioneered the performance of extra-anatomic axillary to ipsilateral femoral artery bypass for occlusive disease. Originally, extra-anatomic bypasses were used for patients with complications after aortoiliac reconstruction. Currently, extra-anatomic bypasses are important alternatives in the selective management of AOD. Extra-anatomic bypass is most useful when femoral inflow is required and a direct transabdominal reconstructive approach is contraindicated because of patient comorbidities or intra-abdominal pathology, or because the aorta is thought to be an unsatisfactory inflow source. Extra-anatomic bypass grafting may also be preferable in patients with uncontrolled malignancy or in patients in whom other diseases might limit their life expectancy.

Axillofemoral (or bifemoral) bypass is performed with the patient under general anesthesia. The patient is placed in the supine position with the arm tucked or abducted no more than 90 degrees. The axillary artery on the side with the least evidence of upper extremity atherosclerosis (higher blood pressure, strongest pulse) is selected as the donor site. If the disease burden is equal in both upper extremities, the right axillary artery is used as the preferred donor vessel because it has a lower risk for developing subclavian occlusive disease than the left. Axillary exposure is gained through a transverse incision over the deltopectoral groove. The axillary artery, which is deep to the axillary vein and inferior to the brachial plexus, is identified and dissected free. Occasionally, division of the pectoralis minor tendon aids in axillary artery exposure. The femoral arteries are dissected in the standard fashion. A subcutaneous tunnel is made between the axillary and femoral artery with a tunneling device. The tunnel courses laterally from the axillary artery deep to the pectoralis major, inferiorly along the midaxillary line (superficial to the external oblique fascia), and then medial to the anterior superior iliac spine because this prevents kinking of the graft when the patient sits up. An extrafascial, suprapubic tunnel is then made between the two femoral incisions. After completion of the tunnels, the patient is anticoagulated with heparin. A 6- or 8-mm externally supported PTFE graft is the preferred conduit. The anastomoses are performed in a sequential fashion with the axillary anastomosis first, followed by the ipsilateral femoral artery and subsequently those of the femorofemoral bypass. If an axillobifemoral graft is to be performed, the inflow for the femorofemoral bypass originates off the hood of the femoral anastomosis of the axillofemoral graft. Flow is reestablished, hemostasis is attained, and the wounds are irrigated with antibiotic solution and closed with an absorbable suture. Because patients undergoing axillofemoral grafting often have increased comorbidities, the mortality rate after axillofemoral bypass grafting ranges up to 13%. Five-year primary patency rates vary widely in the literature and range from 19% to 79%, with secondary patency rates as high as 85%.

Femorofemoral Bypass

In the patient with unilateral iliac occlusive disease, the contralateral femoral artery may serve as a source of inflow. Even though a femorofemoral bypass is best performed under general or regional anesthesia, it may be completed under local anesthesia in selected circumstances. Bilateral groin incisions are made parallel to the femoral arteries, and the vessels are isolated. Before heparin is administered, a subcutaneous tunnel superficial to the external oblique fascia between the two incisions is created. Polyester (Dacron) or PTFE graft material may be used with similar results. If significant femoral occlusive disease is present, it is important to establish unrestricted flow to the profunda femoris. The graft is anastomosed to the femoral arteries in the standard fashion with a running monofilament suture. Cumulative patency rates range from 60% to 80% at 5 years after femorofemoral bypass.

Iliofemoral Bypass

In addition to femorofemoral bypass, iliofemoral bypass may be used to treat unilateral iliac artery disease. An iliofemoral bypass is best suited for patients with occluded or stenosed external iliac arteries and a relatively disease-free proximal common iliac artery. This procedure may be performed under general or regional anesthesia with the patient in the supine position. The common iliac artery is exposed through an oblique lower abdominal incision. The retroperitoneal plane is entered, the abdominal contents are retracted medially, and the proximal common iliac artery is isolated. A femoral incision is made as described previously. A tunnel under the inguinal ligament is created before heparin administration. The iliac artery anastomosis is performed first in an end-to-side fashion. PTFE or polyester (Dacron) grafts are equally suitable for use. The graft is passed under the inguinal ligament and anastomosed to the femoral artery as described earlier. The abdominal and femoral artery incisions are closed in a standard fashion after hemostasis is attained. Three-year patency rates for iliofemoral bypass are 90% or greater in several reports.

Infrainguinal Occlusive Disease

Infrainguinal arterial occlusive disease represents the most common manifestation of chronic arterial occlusive disease confronted by the vascular surgeon. Isolated superficial femoral artery occlusive disease generally presents as claudication of the calf muscles. Patients with multilevel occlusions of the superficial femoral, popliteal, and tibial arteries generally have rest pain or ischemic tissue loss. These ischemic ulcerations initially present as small, dry ulcers of the toes or heel area but may progress to frank gangrenous changes of the forefoot or heel. Most smokers initially have isolated superficial femoral artery occlusive disease and claudication. On the other hand, diabetic patients more often harbor distal occlusions of the popliteal and tibial arteries; these patients may initially have frank tissue necrosis with no prior history of claudication if the superficial femoral artery is spared.

Patients with symptoms of claudication are generally managed conservatively with risk factor modification and an aggressive walking regimen. Medical treatment has had a limited role, although newer agents (e.g., the phosphodiesterase III inhibitor cilostazol) currently being marketed may find a potential niche. Patients with truly disabling claudication, such as those who are unable to perform their occupation because of claudication symptoms, are considered for arteriography and interventional therapy. When the ischemic symptoms have progressed to the point of rest pain or tissue ulceration, surgical therapy is generally indicated for the purposes of pain relief and limb salvage. In the patient considered a candidate for interventional therapy, an arteriogram is performed to delineate the anatomy. Occasionally, patients have isolated lesions of the superficial femoral artery that may be appropriate for PTA (described later). In most cases, however, long-segment occlusions require femoral to distal artery bypass surgery to improve the distal circulation. Any such infrainguinal bypass operation requires normal inflow to the level of the groin. Patients with associated iliac occlusive disease have these lesions corrected with either PTA or surgical bypass before the infrainguinal reconstructive operation. In many cases, correction of the occlusions within the inflow vessels will relieve the patient's symptoms and obviate the need for infrainguinal reconstruction.

In general, infrainguinal bypass surgery is best performed with autogenous vein conduit, preferably the ipsilateral greater saphenous. The superiority of autogenous vein reconstructions is most evident for bypass grafts performed to the below-knee popliteal, tibial, or pedal vessels. When bypass grafts are performed to the above-knee popliteal artery for claudication, prosthetic grafts (i.e., Dacron or PTFE) may be used with the expectation of results approaching those achieved with greater saphenous vein.

Reversed Vein Graft

The original technique for infrainguinal bypass surgery, an approach still preferred by many surgeons, uses the greater saphenous vein in a reversed configuration. The operation may be performed under general or regional anesthesia. The patient's entire extremity from the umbilicus to the foot is prepped and draped into the wound. A longitudinal incision is made in the groin and deepened down through the fascia. The femoral vessels are carefully dissected from their companion veins and individually controlled.

Lymphatic tissue overlying the femoral vessels is best ligated and divided to prevent lymph fistulas or lymphoceles postoperatively. The greater saphenous vein is then dissected from the saphenofemoral junction and exposed through either a single, continuous, longitudinal incision along the thigh or through separate, shorter incisions leaving skin bridges between each incision. More recently, endoscopic saphenous vein harvest has allowed vein preparation through minimal incisions. Sufficient greater saphenous vein is exposed to reach the distal outflow vessel. The above-knee popliteal artery is exposed through a medial thigh incision and carried anterior to the sartorius muscle and posterior to the vastus medialis muscle entering the above-knee popliteal space. The popliteal artery is carefully dissected from its companion vein and nerves. Similarly, the below-knee popliteal artery is dissected through a medial upper calf incision just posterior to the tibia and is carried down through the fascia into the below-knee popliteal space. There, the below-knee popliteal artery is easily dissected from the companion structures. The tibioperoneal trunk may be exposed by dissecting distally and dividing the soleus insertion from the tibia. The posterior tibial and peroneal arteries are dissected through a similar, more distal medial incision, which is deepened down through the investing fascia of the calf. The soleus is then taken off the tibia, exposing the posterior tibial artery within the deep space of the calf. The peroneal artery is located more laterally and is exposed by reflecting the flexor hallucis longus muscle posteriorly. The anterior tibial artery is exposed through a separate, anterolateral calf incision, which is carried down through the fascia and just lateral to the

anterior tibialis muscle, thereby exposing the anterior tibial vessels lying directly over the interosseous membrane. After the proximal and distal vessels are exposed, the greater saphenous vein is gently removed from its bed by ligating its side branches with silk ties and gently dilating the vein with crystalloid solution containing heparin and papaverine. The patient is anticoagulated with 5000 to 10,000 units of heparin, and the femoral vessels are clamped and opened longitudinally. Because of the orientation of the greater saphenous vein valves, the vein is reversed such that the distal end of the vein is sewn to the proximal inflow artery and the proximal end of the vein is sewn to the outflow distal artery. The vein graft is spatulated appropriately, and the anastomosis is completed with 5-0 polypropylene suture, using standard anastomotic techniques. Before completion of the anastomosis, all vessels are flushed, and the anastomosis is tied down; flow is restored to the native vessels, and flow through the graft is assessed. The reversed vein graft may be placed directly in the subcutaneous plane as it travels from the proximal to distal anastomosis. Conversely, a more anatomic, subsartorial plane may be preferable, particularly in patients in whom wound healing may be a problem. When bypass grafts are performed at the below-knee popliteal artery, it is often preferable to tunnel the graft directly through the popliteal fossa to facilitate a favorable distal anastomotic configuration. Bypass grafts to the anterior tibial artery may be tunneled through the interosseous membrane or, if preferred, subcutaneously over the anterolateral thigh, lateral to the knee, and directly to the anterior tibial artery exposure site on the anterolateral calf. The distal vessels are clamped with atraumatic bulldog clamps and opened longitudinally. The vein graft is trimmed to an appropriate length and bevel, and the anastomosis is completed with 6-0 or 7-0 polypropylene suture. It is often preferable to "parachute" the heel of the distal anastomosis, particularly when the artery is deep within the calf. Before completion of the anastomosis, all vessels are flushed, and patency at each end of the anastomosis is verified with a fine coronary artery dilator. The anastomosis is tied down, and flow is restored. Recent reported results with reversed saphenous vein grafting using modern surgical techniques have been excellent, with 5-year primary and secondary patency rates of 75% and 80%, respectively, and limb salvage rates of 90%.[27]

In Situ Greater Saphenous Vein Bypass

The in situ greater saphenous vein bypass technique differs in that the saphenous vein is left in its own bed (i.e., in situ) rather than removing it and reversing its orientation. This approach requires disruption of the competent saphenous vein valves to allow flow down the vein. Although the in situ greater saphenous vein bypass was originally introduced in the 1960s, the tedious nature of the procedure and mixed results prevented its widespread adoption. In the early 1970s, however, Leather and colleagues[28] developed a new technique for lysing the valves, leading to new interest and eventual widespread adoption of this technique. Although there are a number of theoretical advantages to the in situ technique,

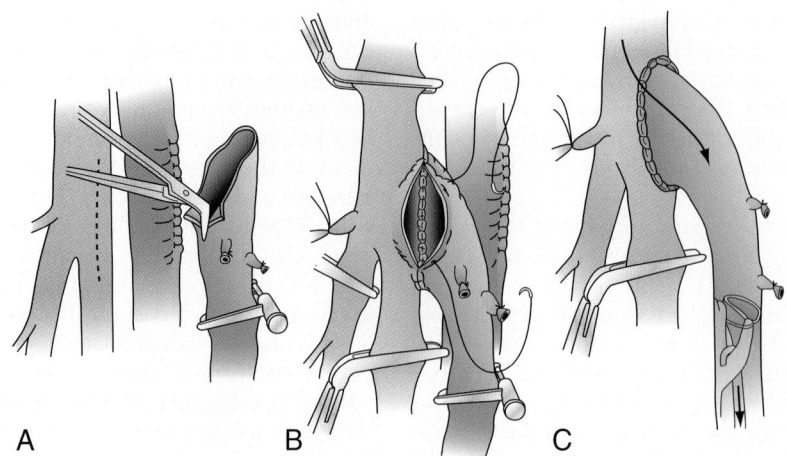

A   B   C

Figure 66-14 A, In the in situ method of infrainguinal reconstruction, the saphenofemoral junction is transected in the groin, the venotomy in the femoral vein is oversewn, and the proximal end of the saphenous vein is prepared for anastomosis. **B,** After the first venous valve is excised under direct vision, the graft is anastomosed end-to-side to the femoral artery. **C,** Flow is then restored through the vein graft, and the valvotome is inserted through side branches at appropriate intervals to lyse residual valve cusps.

including maintenance of the vasa vasorum and the endothelial layer of the vein graft, these have never been proved to offer a clear advantage in terms of patency or vein graft function. There are several practical advantages to the in situ technique, however, that offer technical benefits to the surgeon. Maintaining the vein graft in the in situ configuration allows the surgeon to sew the large end of the greater saphenous vein to the larger femoral vessels and to sew the smaller distal saphenous vein to the smaller tibial vessels. This size match at the proximal and distal ends facilitates the completion of precise technical anastomoses. Preservation of the saphenous vein hood offers particular advantages when sewing to a thick-walled, diseased femoral artery. Given these technical advantages, it is possible to successfully use smaller greater saphenous veins, which may not be serviceable for the reversed vein technique.

The preparation and arterial exposure for in situ bypass is similar to that for reversed vein bypass grafting. Most surgeons prefer to expose the entire greater saphenous vein through a continuous thigh and calf incision. After anticoagulation with heparin and performance of the arteriotomy, the saphenous vein hood is divided flush with the common femoral vein, using a Satinsky clamp. The common femoral vein is then oversewn with a 5-0 Prolene suture (Fig. 66-14). The proximal valve of the greater saphenous vein can be excised under direct vision with a fine forceps and Potts scissors. The proximal anastomosis of the saphenous vein hood to the femoral artery (see Fig. 66-14B) is performed with standard surgical techniques. Again, all vessels are flushed, and flow is restored to the femoral vessels after tying down the anastomosis.

Pulsatile flow is restored to the vein graft, and the first site of a competent valve is obvious as the vein graft distends to that point and remains decompressed below. A valvulotome is then used to lyse the valves and there-fore allow antegrade flow through the graft (see Fig. 66-14C). A number of valvulotomes are currently available. Most surgeons prefer the modified Mills valvulotome, which is a short, hockey-stick–shaped cutter that is serially introduced through side branches of the greater saphenous vein and pulled inferiorly, thereby lysing each pair of valves as they are encountered. The consistent orientation of the vein valves parallel to the skin facilitates precise, atraumatic valve lysis. The most distal valves are lysed by introducing the valvulotome through the open distal end of the vein graft and pulling inferiorly. A number of modifications of the in situ technique have been introduced to improve the simplicity and precision of the operation while decreasing morbidity. For example, long, self-centering valvulotomes, which may be introduced through the distal open end of the vein, may be used to lyse the valves in a single pass. When all of the valves have been lysed and excellent pulsatile flow through the graft is ensured, the various side branches of the greater saphenous vein must be occluded with surgical clips or ties to prevent the formation of arteriovenous fistulas. Most recently, intra-arterial angioscopy has been combined with specially designed valvulotomes and coil embolization of the side branches to allow the in situ technique to be performed through limited proximal and distal incisions without exposing the entire length of vein. Recent series using the in situ greater saphenous vein have reported 5-year cumulative graft patency rates in the 80% range, with limb salvage rates of 84% to 90%.[29]

On completion of the bypass with either a reversed or in situ saphenous vein, flow through the graft and the outflow arteries is assessed with a continuous-wave Doppler study. A completion arteriogram is performed by direct cannulation of the proximal graft to demonstrate the bypass conduit, distal anastomosis, and outflow bed. Unsuspected technical defects, such as intraluminal thrombus, kinking or twisting of the graft, or unlysed valves, are immediately repaired. More recently, intraoperative duplex ultrasonography has proved to be a sensitive completion study for detecting hemodynamically significant abnormalities at either anastomosis or within the graft conduit.

Prosthetic Bypass

As mentioned previously, both polyester (Dacron) and PTFE graft material may be selectively used for infrainguinal arterial reconstructive surgery, particularly when the distal anastomosis is to the above-knee popliteal artery. Better results can be anticipated when the operations are performed to large-caliber vessels with good outflow (two to three open tibial vessels). The conduct of the operation is similar to that of reversed vein greater saphenous vein bypass grafting except that the longitudinal incision for saphenous vein harvest is unnecessary. The ability to perform a prosthetic bypass graft through two small proximal and distal arterial exposure incisions is a distinct advantage of the technique. The arteriotomy and proximal anastomosis is performed using standard techniques, and the graft is tunneled through a subsartorial plane down to the above-knee popliteal artery. The distal anastomosis is then performed.

Aggressive flushing of the graft and native vessels is imperative when using prosthetic bypass materials. Depending on the size of the native vessels, a 6- or 8-mm graft may be desirable. Although prosthetic grafts are occasionally used for bypasses to the below-knee popliteal or tibial vessels, the results achieved in this setting are clearly inferior to those obtained with greater saphenous vein. A variety of surgical adjuncts, including the creation of a distal arteriovenous fistula, the patching of the distal prosthetic graft to native artery bypass with a vein patch, and the creation of a cuff of autogenous vein interposed between the native artery and prosthetic graft at the distal anastomotic site, have all been proposed as useful techniques for improving the results of prosthetic bypass grafts performed to the below-knee level.

Reoperative Bypass Surgery

Increasingly, patients are having failure of previous arterial reconstructions and recurrence of their limb-threatening ischemia symptoms. Reoperative infrainguinal arterial reconstruction offers a number of challenges. In most cases, the ipsilateral greater saphenous vein has previously been used and is no longer available for the secondary bypass procedure. Extensive scarring around the inflow and outflow vessels resulting from the previous surgical dissection complicates the surgical exposure. A number of strategies are useful in dealing with these complex cases. Whenever possible, alternative arterial inflow sites above or below the previous scarred arteries are used to avoid dissection in areas of previous scarring.

The contralateral greater saphenous vein, if available, constitutes the optimal conduit for secondary bypass surgery. Recent studies have also demonstrated minimal short- or long-term impact on the contralateral leg in

these situations.[30] Depending on the length of the bypass and the size of the greater saphenous vein, the graft may be used in either the reversed or nonreversed configuration with lysed valves. Frequently, however, because of contralateral bypass surgery or previous coronary artery bypass surgery, no greater saphenous vein is available for this secondary procedure. In these situations, a preliminary survey of the arm veins and lesser saphenous veins, using duplex ultrasound, reveals the best autogenous vein available for reconstruction. Although arm veins may be scarred or small below the elbows, the deeper upper arm veins, including cephalic and basilic veins, are often of excellent caliber and quality. Although these veins are thin walled and tedious to work with, they are strong and are generally of excellent caliber and quality. Because these various ectopic veins are usually relatively short, it is often necessary to perform a venovenostomy to create composite vein grafts of sufficient length to complete the arterial reconstruction.[31]

Ample spatulation of each vein and the use of fine monofilament sutures facilitate the completion of widely patent anastomoses within these composite vein grafts. Depending on the size and taper of these ectopic veins, they may be placed in either the reversed configuration or nonreversed configuration with lysed valves. When autogenous vein is in short supply, it is often advantageous to originate the bypass graft from a more distal vessel such as the distal superficial femoral or popliteal artery. Such distal origin grafts work particularly well in diabetic patients, who often have relative preservation of flow to the knee level.[32]

Despite improvements in operative techniques, the results of redo infrainguinal bypass surgery remain inferior to those obtained with primary operation. When autogenous vein is available for secondary bypass, 5-year patency rates of 60% and limb salvage rates of 72% have been achieved.[33]

After completion of any autogenous vein bypass graft, potential graft failure remains a major problem. Early failure of vein grafts (within 30 days) generally represents a judgmental or technical error within the conduct of surgery. These include simple technical errors, such as a kink or twist within the graft, or failure to completely lyse the valves. Judgmental errors include the use of a small or poor-quality vein conduit or the construction of an anastomosis to an inadequate outflow artery. Intermediate failures (30 days-2 years) are generally caused by intimal hyperplastic lesions that form at anastomotic sites or valve sites within the graft. Late graft failures (beyond 2 years) are most often caused by progression of atherosclerotic occlusive disease within the inflow or outflow vessels. Because of the importance of vein graft patency in maintaining both limb function and salvage, and because of the inability to restore durable patency to vein grafts after they have thrombosed, it is important to maintain a surveillance program to ensure that vein grafts are functioning well and not harboring stenotic lesions that threaten graft patency. Serial postoperative examinations with a duplex scan have proved extremely accurate in identifying significant vein graft lesions that threaten the graft patency. Recognition and repair of such lesions before graft thrombosis ensures continued durable graft patency in most cases.

Percutaneous Transluminal Angioplasty

The role of PTA in the management of infrainguinal occlusive disease is considerably more limited than in the management of AOD. The smaller vessel size, more diffuse nature of the disease, and more limited outflow significantly impair the long-term results of infrainguinal angioplasty compared with those achieved in the larger iliac vessels. Nevertheless, infrainguinal and even infra-popliteal PTA and stenting have recently been met with considerable enthusiasm by both vascular surgeons and other interventional specialists. This shift in practice patterns is largely fueled by single-center registries with relatively few patients and short follow-up periods. Despite lack of well-conducted randomized control trials,[34] there does seem to be a role for this therapy in very select patient populations. These include patients presenting with claudication and with short, isolated, stenotic lesions, or even short-segment occlusions within the superficial femoral artery. Patients with critical limb ischemia (rest pain or ulceration) often have complex, multisegmental disease extending below the popliteal artery that does not lend itself well to percutaneous approaches. Unlike the management of iliac lesions in which stents have proved to be useful after technically complicated angioplasties, stents have not significantly improved the patency of femoral or popliteal angioplasties. Newer and more flexible self-expanding stent design, smaller-caliber delivery systems, and medicated or drug-eluting stent technology may improve patency.[35] In patients with limited autogenous vein, a short-segment angioplasty of a superficial femoral artery lesion may allow the bypass graft to originate more distally from the superficial femoral artery or popliteal artery.

CHRONIC VISCERAL ISCHEMIA

Renovascular Occlusive Disease

Chronic occlusive disease of the main renal artery results in reduced blood flow to the kidney. When the level of occlusion exceeds 60% of the diameter of the main renal artery, changes in pressure and flow distally result in increased secretion of renin and subsequent shifts in peripheral vasoconstriction and extracellular fluid volume, which result in hypertension. It has been estimated that less than 5% of hypertensive people have renovascular hypertension. Patients with clinically apparent atherosclerosis have a somewhat higher prevalence of renal artery disease. For example, among patients with coronary disease who underwent abdominal arteriography, 11% had significant unilateral renal artery disease with stenosis greater than 50% and 4% had significant bilateral disease.[36] Among patients with diastolic blood pressure greater than 115 mm Hg, the prevalence of renovascular hypertension is 15% to 20%; and among children younger than 5 years of age, the prevalence approximates 75%.

Table 66-9 Causes of Renovascular Occlusive Disease

Atherosclerosis
Fibromuscular dysplasia
Takayasu's arteritis
Radiation vasculitis
Neurofibromatosis
Thromboembolism

When there is significant bilateral renal artery involvement, total glomerular filtration rate is reduced sufficiently to decrease creatinine clearance. Renal insufficiency from reduced renal perfusion is a late manifestation of advanced arterial occlusive disease involving both kidneys. It has been estimated that up to 30% of patients on dialysis for end-stage renal disease have significant renovascular occlusive disease as a contributing factor. Nephrosclerosis, diabetic nephropathy, atheroembolism, glomerulonephritis, and other conditions may coexist with renovascular disease in many patients with chronic renal insufficiency.

Recognition and correction of large artery renal occlusive disease can result in impressive improvement in blood pressure control and preservation of renal function.

Pathology

Atherosclerosis accounts for nearly 90% of cases of renovascular hypertension (Table 66-9). This cause is twice as common in men as in women, although as age increases, the sex distribution becomes more equal. Most commonly, the atherosclerotic process begins in the adjacent aorta with "spillover" plaque that encroaches into the proximal renal artery, resulting in "orificial" renal artery stenosis (Fig. 66-15). Plaque extends into the proximal third of the artery, but the more distal vessel remains relatively free of disease. Atherosclerosis involves the renal artery origins bilaterally in more than half of patients. Plaque is subject to fracture and subintimal hemorrhage with associated increase in stenosis or abrupt occlusion as well as atheroembolism, which produces small branch occlusion in the renal parenchyma. Studies using serial angiography and renal ultrasound have elucidated the natural history of atherosclerotic renal occlusive disease. Arteries detected to have more than 60% stenosis progress over the next several years to increased stenosis and ultimate occlusion.[37] The exact percentage that eventually go on to occlusion is unknown, but estimates of up to 18% over a 5-year period have been reported.[38]

Fibromuscular dysplasia is the second most common type of renal artery disease. Three subtypes are distinguished on the basis of the layer of the arterial wall most involved. Medial fibroplasia is by far the most common, accounting for 85% of dysplastic lesions. It nearly always affects women, most commonly appearing between the ages of 25 and 45 years. The etiology is unknown. The condition involves the main renal artery with either a

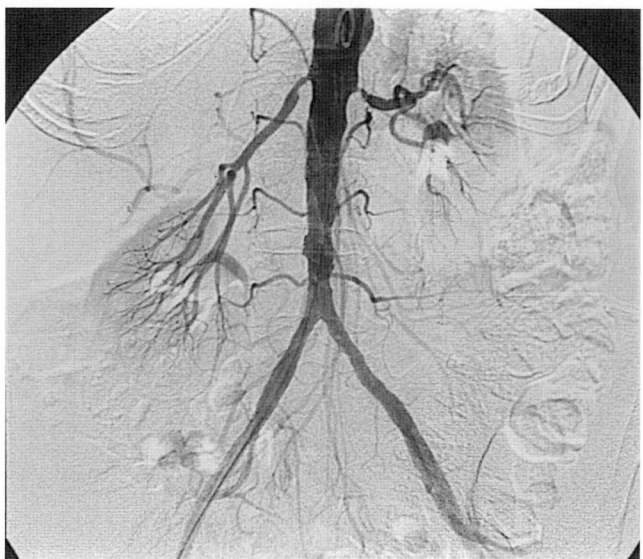

Figure 66-15 Arteriogram demonstrating proximal atherosclerotic involvement of both renal arteries. Most typically, aortic plaque encroaches on the renal ostium, as is seen in this example of bilateral orificial renal artery occlusive disease.

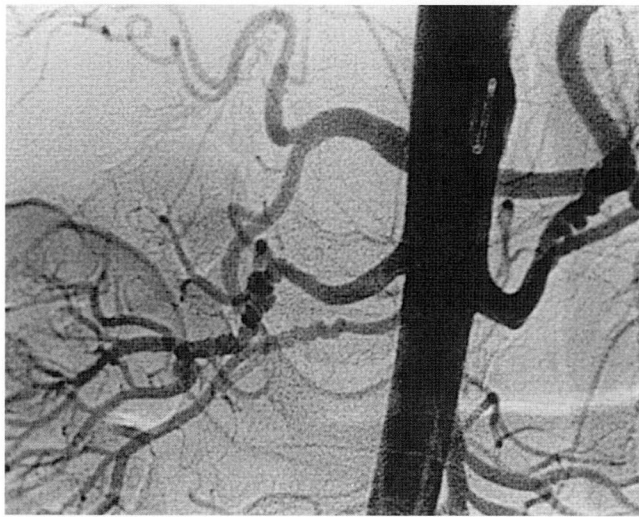

Figure 66-16 Arteriogram demonstrating bilateral fibromuscular dysplasia with involvement of the left renal artery and anomalous upper and lower pole arteries on the right. Note typical "string of beads" appearance in all three vessels.

solitary stenosis or multiple stenoses with intervening dilations that may appear as a string of beads (Fig. 66-16). True aneurysms may occur in about 10% of patients with this condition, most often at branch points of the peripheral arterial arcade. Lesions are bilateral in 70%, and medial fibroplasia can also affect other arteries, most commonly the internal carotid and external iliac arteries. Perimedial dysplasia accounts for about 10% of dysplastic lesions, also nearly exclusively in women between 30 and 50 years of age. Intimal fibroplasia accounts for the remaining 5% of dysplastic lesions. This subtype is more

common in children and young adults of either sex. Fibromuscular dysplasia is generally self-limited and does not progress after it reaches a clinically recognizable threshold.

A small number of patients in the pediatric age group have developmental anomalies that result in impaired renal artery flow. These lesions usually involve the origin of the renal artery with fibrous stricture, sometimes in association with abdominal aortic coarctation.

Pathophysiology

An association between hypertension and renal disease was noted in 1836. A pressor substance was discovered in the rabbit in 1897 and called *renin*. In 1934, Goldblatt showed that unilateral renal artery constriction produced hypertension in the dog. Cure of hypertension by nephrectomy was reported in 1937 and by restoration of flow to the kidney using thromboendarterectomy in 1954.

Hypertension occurs after reduction in mean renal artery perfusion pressure by greater than 60% diameter or 75% cross-sectional area of the proximal renal artery. Renal baroreceptors in the afferent arterioles sense the reduction in mean arterial pressure, leading to release of renin by the juxtaglomerular apparatus. Renin appears in the renal vein and hydrolyzes angiotensinogen, produced in the liver, to form angiotensin I. This decapeptide is inactive but is converted to the octapeptide angiotensin II in the lungs by angiotensin-converting enzyme (ACE). Angiotensin II is a strong vasoconstrictor with a half-life of 4 minutes and acts directly on vascular smooth muscle. ACE inhibitors such as captopril are particularly effective in treating hypertension related to high renin and subsequent high angiotensin II levels (Fig. 66-17).

Angiotensin II also facilitates formation of aldosterone by the adrenal cortex. Aldosterone causes conservation of salt and water by the kidney, resulting in increased extracellular fluid volume contributing to hypertension. Diuretics are beneficial in controlling hypertension because they help correct hypervolemia.

When one renal artery is involved with occlusive disease, increased renin secretion from the affected kidney results in hypertension, which suppresses renin secretion from the contralateral kidney. Increased glomerular filtration occurs in the normal kidney, resulting in relatively normal or low extracellular volume. When both kidneys are involved, or in circumstances of an affected solitary kidney, overall renal hypoperfusion results in hypervolemic hypertension. With increasing severity, decreased creatinine clearance occurs, and azotemia supervenes.

Renovascular hypertension has a significant impact on the heart and vascular tree. Nephrosclerosis develops in renal tissue "unprotected" by proximal renal artery disease and thus exposed to hypertension, as in a relatively normal kidney opposite a kidney with significant occlusive disease. Hypertension also contributes significantly to progression of atherosclerosis in the peripheral, coronary, and carotid arteries as well as to hypertensive retinopathy. The heart itself is affected with left ventricular hypertrophy and reduced ventricular compliance. In the

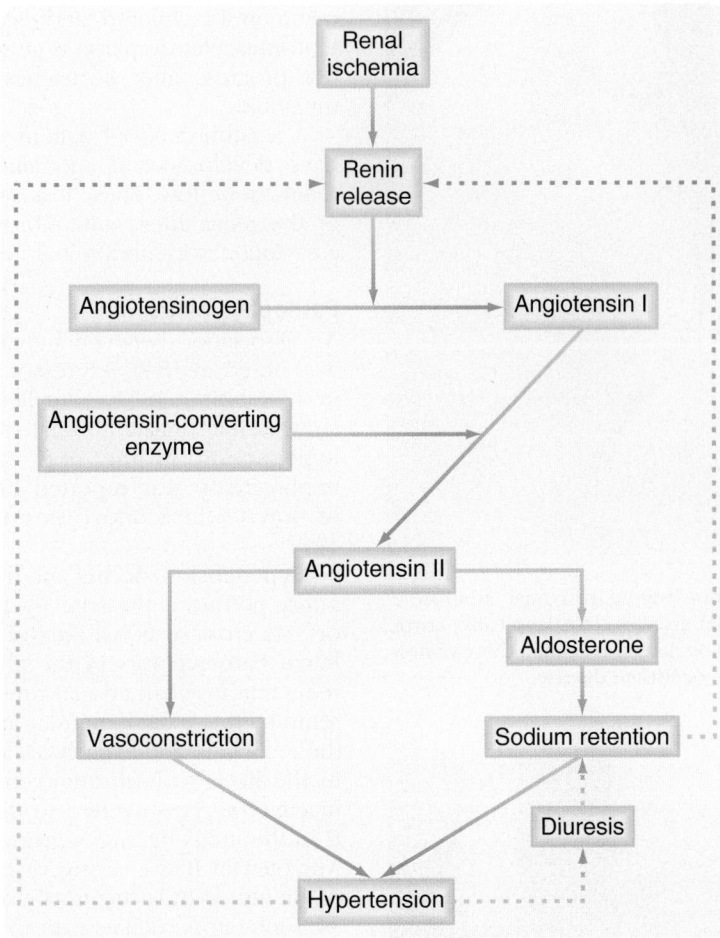

Figure 66-17 Consequences of renin hypersecretion as result of renal ischemia. *Dotted arrows* represent inhibitory influence. (Adapted from Pickering TG: Renal vascular disease. In Braunwald S, Creager MA [eds]: Atlas of Heart Diseases, vol 7. St Louis, CV Mosby, 1996, p 4.3.)

presence of bilateral renal artery occlusive disease and resulting hypervolemia superimposed on hypertension, a sudden hypertensive crisis may occur with acute left ventricular failure precipitating so-called flash pulmonary edema.

Diagnosis

Clinical Presentation

The clinical presentation is an important clue to the presence of renovascular occlusive disease (Table 66-10). Hypertensive patients in the pediatric age group, among whom renovascular causes are more prevalent, are investigated for correctable causes. Women between the ages of 25 and 50 years must be similarly considered. Patients in the older age group with recent significant change in blood pressure control or renal function and in whom there are coexistent risk factors for atherosclerosis also undergo screening. Patients who respond dramatically to ACE inhibitors are more likely to have high renin hypertension related to renovascular disease. If azotemia becomes worse on antihypertensive therapy, bilateral

renal artery disease is suspected. Patients with a hypertensive crisis and flash pulmonary edema and left ventricular failure are highly suspect, particularly if blood pressure control results in increased renal insufficiency.

Physiologic Tests

Much work has been done in an effort to perfect the use of the renin assay to make the diagnosis of renovascular hypertension. Selective sampling of blood from each renal vein and comparing each to samples from the infrarenal and suprarenal vena cava can indeed demonstrate unilateral hypersecretion of renin from the kidney affected by the diseased renal artery. The best accuracy requires cessation of β-blockers and stimulation of renin secretion by limiting sodium intake and administering a diuretic for a few days before the assay, as well as tilting the patient into an upright position during sampling. These logistical problems have made selective renin assay impractical in most centers. Peripheral venous renin assay has also been used, but values are most helpful only when similarly stimulated and indexed against serum

Table 66-10 Clinical Correlates of Increased Prevalence of Renovascular Disease

Severe hypertension—diastolic >115 mm Hg
Refractory hypertension
New onset of sustained hypertension at age <20 yr, female age <50 yr, either gender >50 yr
Hypertension and epigastric or flank bruit
Moderate progressive or severe hypertension in patients with manifestations of systemic atherosclerosis and unexplained stable or progressive renal insufficiency
Malignant hypertension or hypertensive crisis
Dramatic normalization of blood pressure by angiotensin-converting enzyme inhibitor
Increase in serum creatinine with blood pressure improvement

sodium balance. Because many antihypertensive drugs have an impact on renin and sodium and because such drugs must be stopped for as long as 3 weeks to obtain a precise measurement, this approach has also been generally impractical.

Demonstration of asymmetric renal function is another physiologic approach to diagnosis. Split renal function studies use selective ureteral catheterization to sample urine from each kidney. If decreased amounts of urine with higher concentrations of sodium, creatinine, or administered p-aminohippuric acid are detected on one side, the involved kidney is likely ischemic. This method is somewhat cumbersome and rarely used. Hypertensive IV pyelography can demonstrate delayed appearance of IV contrast dye in the involved kidney, a difference in renal size, and delayed hyperconcentration of contrast agent in the collecting system as well as occasional "nicking" of the ureter caused by large periureteral arterial collaterals.

More currently, radionuclide tracer is used to assess renal blood flow and excretory function. The ACE inhibitor captopril has enhanced the accuracy of radionuclide scanning. Angiotensin II in the involved kidney leads to selective vasoconstriction of the efferent arterioles, resulting in maintenance of relatively normal glomerular filtration despite proximal renal artery disease. When captopril is used to block angiotensin II, glomerular filtration decreases significantly. When renal scan is performed before and after captopril with findings of deterioration in filtration after the drug, the findings are highly suggestive of significant renovascular disease, with accuracy in the 90% to 95% range compared with arteriography.[39] Physiologic tests that rely on laterality are not applicable in the presence of bilateral disease, nor in cases in which the serum creatinine level is elevated above 3 mg/dL.

Anatomic Tests
Renal ultrasound is an important method of determining differential kidney size. In an adult, a kidney less than 10 cm in length is abnormally small, with proximal renal artery disease being one possible cause. Renal ultrasound is an important means of detecting other contributing causes of azotemia, such as renal cysts or hydronephrosis. Increasingly, duplex ultrasound has been used successfully to assess flow into the kidney. The renal artery can be imaged using B-mode ultrasound and Doppler imaging to characterize flow velocities, comparing the flow characteristics of the proximal renal artery with flow characteristics of the adjacent aorta and more distal renal artery. The so-called tardus-parvus phenomenon is typically observed in arteries with greater than 60% stenosis, causing delay and diminution in the flow waveform in the distal renal artery. Diastolic flow characteristics reflect vascular resistance in the renal parenchyma. In some noninvasive laboratories, duplex ultrasound is more than 90% accurate in detecting significant large vessel renal artery disease.[39] As with all ultrasound-dependent imaging technology, this is highly technician dependent for its accuracy and reproducibility.

MRI is becoming the anatomic imaging modality of choice in many centers where gadolinium-enhanced scanning has provided an expeditious, objective, and safe means of identifying renal artery disease.[40] Although tortuosity and obliquity of the renal artery origins may result in artifacts that may make images difficult to interpret, scans are generally sufficiently accurate to allow MRI an important role in the initial phases of patient evaluation. CT is also available, using spiral technique for high-resolution imaging of the renal arteries. This method is very accurate but requires use of IV contrast material with a small risk for renal toxicity.

Arteriography is the most precise diagnostic tool. IV digital subtraction arteriography, although less invasive, requires a relatively large dose of iodinated contrast and often yields comparatively poor images. Selective intra-arterial study using computer enhancement allows precise anatomic definition, usually with minimal dye exposure. An even safer variant involves use of carbon dioxide as a radiographic contrast medium in patients with advanced renal insufficiency.

Routine screening using a single laboratory study such as peripheral renin or a single anatomic study such as MRI on the broad population of hypertensive patients is inappropriate. Evaluation requires consideration of the clinical presentation and setting, followed by a logical sequence of confirmatory studies designed to uncover the diagnosis with minimal cost and risk. Because they are logistically cumbersome, physiologic studies have increasingly yielded to anatomic diagnosis, relying on ultrasound and MRI for initial detection of disease and then arteriography for confirmation and possible catheter-based intervention if appropriate (Table 66-11). In the proper clinical setting, the presence of a small kidney with arterial stenosis greater than 60%, poststenotic dilation, and evidence of delayed parenchymal function is highly predictive of therapeutic success after revascularization. Increasingly, percutaneous methods of revascularization are available with minimal risk to the patient, making absolute precision in diagnosis less compelling than it would be if the only therapeutic solution involved more risky and arduous surgery.

Table 66-11 Screening Studies for Renovascular Occlusive Disease

Renal ultrasound to assess kidney size, alternative diagnoses (cysts, hydronephrosis)
Renal artery duplex ultrasound
Renal scintigraphy with captopril
Magnetic resonance imaging
Arteriography

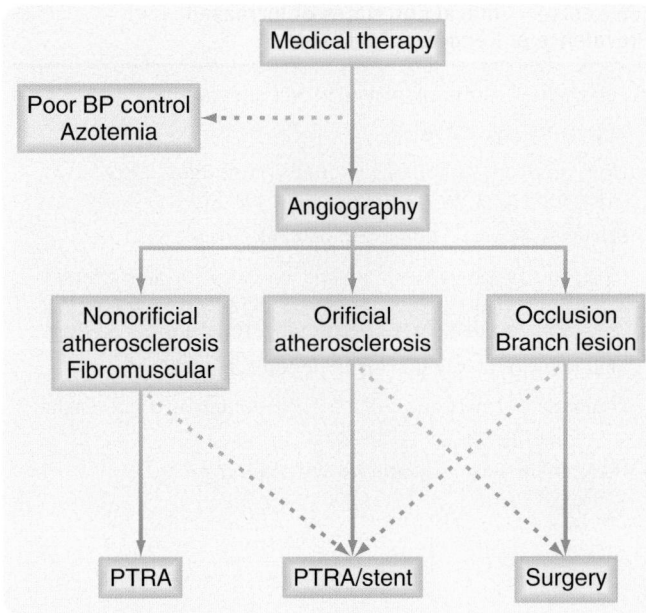

Figure 66-18 Therapeutic scheme for patients with proven renal artery occlusive disease. *Dotted arrows* represent secondary therapeutic options. BP, blood pressure; PTRA, percutaneous transluminal renal angioplasty.

Treatment

Initial therapy of renovascular hypertension is medical. β-Adrenergic blockers, diuretics, vasodilators, and ACE inhibitors are commonly used with success. A more aggressive therapeutic approach is justifiable if blood pressure control requires increasing doses of two or three medications or if renal function deteriorates while on antihypertensive medications, particularly ACE inhibitors (Fig. 66-18). Under these circumstances, noninvasive imaging with ultrasound or MRI is performed, followed by arteriography as appropriate, with plans to proceed at the same sitting with percutaneous endovascular renal artery therapy if favorable lesions are confirmed.

Percutaneous transluminal renal angioplasty is an important therapeutic tool. Access to the renal arteries can be approached from either the femoral or the brachial artery. Often a brachial approach is favorable given the natural downward-sloping direction of some renal arteries. Balloon dilation is the procedure of choice for patients with fibromuscular dysplasia involving the main renal artery, reserving surgical revascularization for more complicated lesions involving branches of the renal artery. Percutaneous transluminal renal angioplasty is also successfully applicable to patients with focal nonorificial atherosclerotic renal artery disease. Nonorificial atherosclerosis or dysplasia can be treated with a greater than 90% technical success rate and long-term benefit in 70% to 90% of cases.[13] Orificial atherosclerotic lesions are much less likely to respond to balloon dilation alone because they are essentially composed of aortic plaque, which cannot be effectively cracked and remodeled in a durable manner by a balloon alone. Technical success for orificial atherosclerosis is no greater than 50%, and the long-term success rate is 40% among those initially successfully treated by angioplasty.[41] The immediate and long-term success of balloon angioplasty can be improved by using arterial stenting[38,42] (Fig. 66-19). Although not necessary for most nonorificial lesions, stents have extended the usefulness of percutaneous therapy to orificial atherosclerosis.[43] Most practitioners use a pre-mounted, low-profile stent device to primarily stent renal artery stenotic lesions, with a technical success rate that approaches 100%. The morbidity rate after percutaneous therapy is below 10%, with severe morbidity including arterial rupture or occlusion occurring in 1% to 2%. At this time, long-term therapy with aspirin is standard of care after percutaneous renal artery stenting, although

trials are needed to determine the role of additional antiplatelet agents such as clopidogrel. The restenosis rate following renal artery stenting is about 15% to 17%, with a reported 5-year patency rate of 84.5%.[44]

A direct approach to the renal artery is possible using a variety of surgical techniques. Isolated renal endarterectomy may be performed in unusual circumstances to correct unilateral or bilateral renal artery disease. Transaortic endarterectomy is an effective and expeditious method to correct renal orificial disease at the time of surgery for aneurysmal or occlusive disease of the adjacent aorta. Occlusive lesions may be bypassed with proximal anastomosis on the aorta, iliac artery, or aortic prosthesis. Prosthetic material or autogenous vein is equally satisfactory for anastomosis to the proximal renal artery. Autogenous vein is preferred for more distal anastomoses or when small kidneys are involved. Because saphenous vein tends to dilate with time in the pediatric age group, it is preferable to use autogenous artery such as the internal iliac artery for renal bypass in children. To reduce operative morbidity in elderly patients who might not tolerate temporary clamping of the aorta during surgery, extra-anatomic alternatives including the hepatic and splenic arteries may be used as sites for the proximal anastomosis of a bypass graft to the right and left kidneys, respectively. In unusual circumstances, complicated vascular occlusive disease may require removal of the kidney for ex vivo reconstruction, with reimplantation in situ or in the pelvis using the iliac artery and vein as in a renal transplantation procedure. Major morbidity occurs in 5% to 10% of patients after contemporary surgery. Perioperative death is unusual in pediatric and dysplastic patients, and the mortality rate ranges between 0.9% and 5.8% in the older atherosclerotic group. Although it was initially

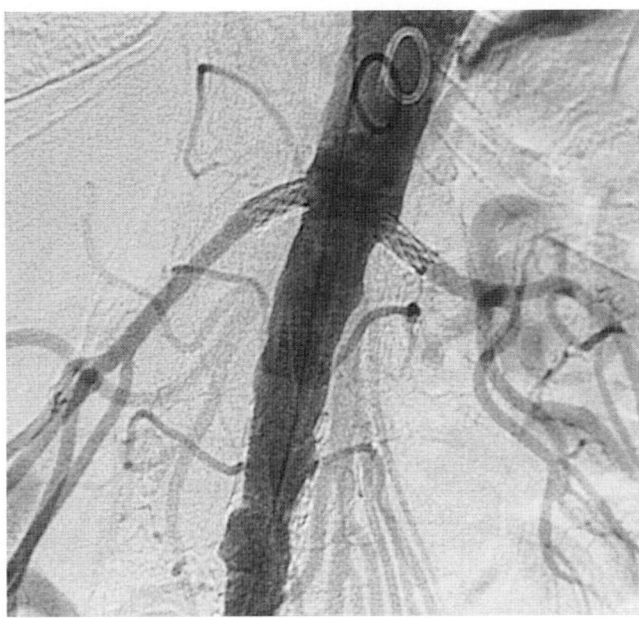

Figure 66-19 Completion arteriogram after percutaneous transluminal angioplasty and stenting for orificial left renal artery disease in patient illustrated in Figure 66-15.

thought that combining renal artery surgery with aortic surgery increased morbidity and mortality rates, recent experience indicates that renal artery endarterectomy can be performed in conjunction with aortic aneurysm resection or aortic bypass without increasing the mortality risk.

The presence of an occluded artery is not necessarily a contraindication to revascularization. Percutaneous therapy may be attempted, and, if a wire can be passed through the occlusion, balloon angioplasty and stent may succeed. More typically, surgery is necessary, at which time a short segmental occlusion is usually found, with reconstitution of a virtually normal artery within 1 to 2 cm. If the kidney is more than 7 to 8 cm in length, there is a significant chance of recovery of function and reduction in renin secretion after revascularization. Kidneys that are smaller than 6 cm are generally not salvageable, and nephrectomy may be considered. Nephrectomy is much less frequent than in past years because of the success of revascularization and the efficacy of ACE inhibitors for high-renin hypertension.

Results of Revascularization

Long-term results after percutaneous transluminal renal angioplasty are excellent for patients with fibromuscular dysplasia. Lesions involving branch arteries or bifurcation areas are less likely to be successfully treated and more likely to be associated with complications after attempted angioplasty. Among patients with atherosclerotic renal artery disease, appropriate selective use of balloon angioplasty and stents results in generally excellent success after several years, with cure of hypertension in 20% to 25% of cases, improvement or stabilization in 50% to 60%, and failure in 15% to 20%.[42,45,46]

Surgical revascularization for fibromuscular dysplasia results in cure or improvement of hypertension at rates similar to percutaneous therapy. Among children, surgical therapy is highly successful, resulting in cure of hypertension in 70% to 85% of cases and improvement in another 10% to 25%, with failure in less than 10%. Among patients with atherosclerosis, hypertension is cured in roughly one third and improved in 50%, with failure in 10% to 20%. Endarterectomy of the renal artery orifice is a very durable procedure. Serial study of bypass patency indicates that as many as 88% of grafts remain patent for as long as 20 years after surgery. Vein graft dilation occurs in 3% to 5%, particularly among the pediatric age group.

Renal function has been reported to improve in 40% of patients who had revascularization for azotemia. Such patients almost always underwent revascularization bilaterally or had a solitary kidney, with the therapeutic goal of increasing blood flow to as much renal parenchyma as possible. Follow-up evaluation of natural history indicates that, even among patients with no significant immediate improvement in renal insufficiency, the rate at which renal function deteriorates appears to be reduced by revascularization. On rare occasions, patients who have been placed on dialysis have been taken off support after intervention.

Renal artery occlusive disease is responsible for hypertension and renal failure in a significant number of patients. Clinical suspicion and appropriate diagnostic study may direct patients toward therapy designed to improve flow to the kidneys, increasingly using relatively safe percutaneous methods. Results of such therapy offer substantial benefit to carefully selected and managed patients.

Mesenteric Ischemia

Vascular occlusive disease of the mesenteric vessels is a relatively rare but often catastrophic problem. When acute occlusion of a major artery occurs, profound illness usually results, and survival is fortunate. Nonocclusive mesenteric insufficiency and mesenteric venous occlusion occur in the presence of severe concurrent illness of variable causes. Chronic intestinal ischemia often presents a diagnostic challenge, but results are gratifying with timely therapy.

Pathophysiology

Mesenteric arterial anatomy is notable for rich collateral flow (Fig. 66-20). As a result, gradual occlusion of one or even two of the main mesenteric trunks is usually tolerated, as long as there is time for a collateral vessel from uninvolved branches to enlarge. On the other hand, sudden occlusion of a main branch or more peripherally beyond the largest collateral vessels may be poorly tolerated, with profound consequences. Acute vascular occlusion results in tissue injury with release of intracellular contents and by-products of anaerobic metabolism to the general circulation. Compromised bowel mucosa allows unrestricted influx of toxic materials from the bowel lumen with systemic consequences. If serosal surfaces

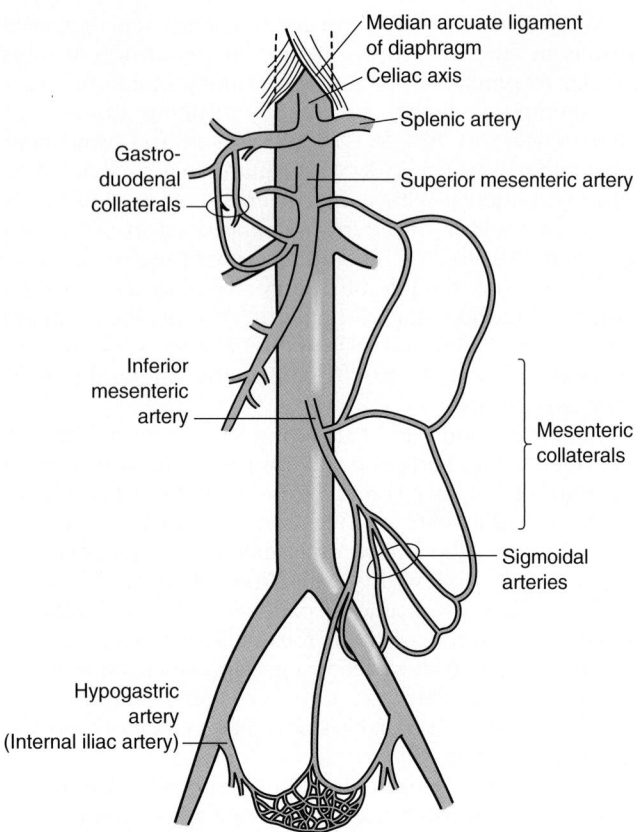

Figure 66-20 Mesenteric arterial anatomy demonstrating extensive collateral channels between major branches. (Adapted from Stoney RJ, Wylie EJ: Surgery of celiac and mesenteric arteries. In Haimovici HH [ed]: Vascular Surgery: Principles and Techniques. New York, McGraw-Hill, 1976, pp 668-679.)

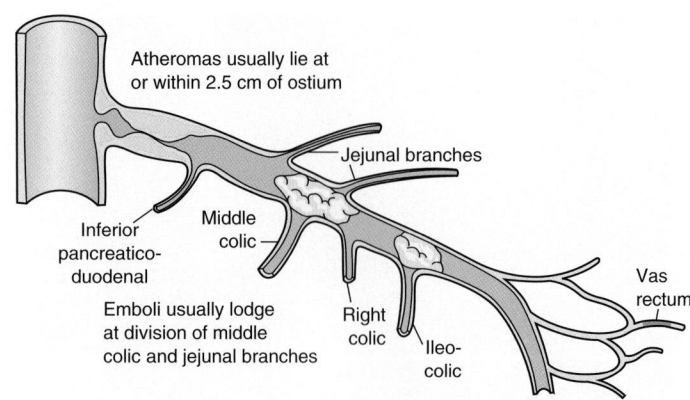

Figure 66-21 Typical location of superior mesenteric artery obstruction in patients with embolic and thrombotic occlusion. (From Donaldson MC: Mesenteric vascular disease. In Braunwald S, Creager MA [eds]: Atlas of Heart Diseases. St Louis, Mosby, 1996, p 56.)

Table 66-12 Extent of Obstruction in Chronic Mesenteric Arterial Insufficiency

SITE	PERCENTAGE
Celiac, SMA, IMA	41-75
Celiac, SMA	29-82
Celiac, IMA	2
SMA, IMA	5
Celiac	0-14
SMA	1.4-9

IMA, inferior mesenteric artery; SMA, superior mesenteric artery.

are affected by full-thickness necrosis, bowel perforation and peritonitis ensue. Associated heart disease or systemic atherosclerosis often compounds the complexity of acute arterial occlusion. Nonocclusive ischemia and mesenteric venous occlusion are usually complicated by significant or life-threatening concurrent abdominal or systemic illness.

Acute mesenteric artery occlusion most frequently results from a cardiogenic embolus and usually involves the superior mesenteric artery. Embolic occlusion most often occurs distal to the origin of the superior mesenteric artery because the embolus is pushed into the artery to a point at which arborization reduces the lumen to a diameter less than that of the embolus (Fig. 66-21). Less commonly, thrombotic occlusion at the site of chronic atherosclerotic plaque occurs at the origin of the vessel adjacent to ostial disease. In both instances, secondary stasis thrombosis may occur in adjacent proximal and distal vessels to the point at which flow from collaterals is maintained. Acute embolic occlusion is generally a more profound and damaging insult than thrombosis at the site of chronic disease because of the following:

1. Lack of protection by chronically enlarged collaterals from the other mesenteric arteries

2. Occlusion at levels beyond the point of inflow of larger collaterals
3. Occlusion of multiple branches to adjacent segments at the point of arterial arborization

Acute nonocclusive mesenteric insufficiency accompanies profound illness with sepsis and cardiovascular collapse, with consequent vasoconstriction of the mesenteric vascular bed. Use of vasopressors for hemodynamic support exacerbates the problem. If prolonged, such illness may result in hemodynamic compromise of nutrient flow to the bowel and mesenteric viscera. Mesenteric venous occlusion results in vascular compromise on the basis of reduced venous drainage of the bowel.

Chronic mesenteric insufficiency is almost exclusively a problem in the older age group with diffuse atherosclerosis that involves the aorta and the proximal mesenteric arteries. Because collaterals are usually abundant among the three main mesenteric vessels, at least two, most often the celiac and superior mesenteric artery, are severely compromised before symptoms arise (Table 66-12). Relative ischemia occurs after meals when there is increased demand for flow into the mesenteric bed. Vasodilation after eating reduces peripheral resistance, but flow cannot increase in the presence of proximal

Table 66-13   Presentation of Acute Mesenteric Ischemia

Concurrent cardiac or debilitating disease
Pain out of proportion to tenderness
Abdominal distention, gastrointestinal dysfunction
Evidence of third spacing—oliguria, hemoconcentration
Blood in stool
Elevated white cell count—often >20,000
Metabolic acidosis
Elevated serum enzymes
Bowel distention, wall thickening on kidney-ureter-bladder imaging and computed tomography
Endoscopic findings in colon
Specific findings on arteriogram

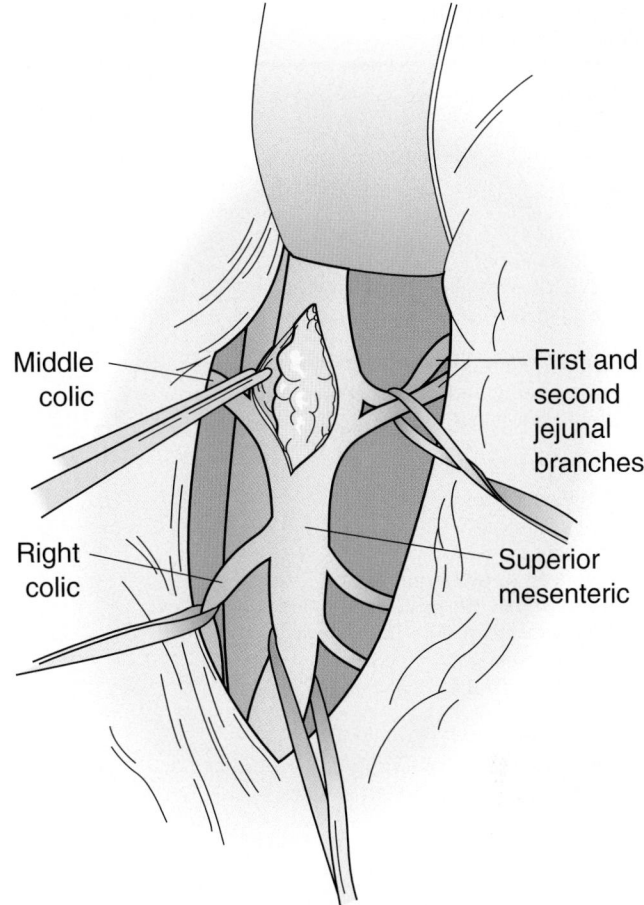

Figure 66-22 Longitudinal arteriotomy of the superior mesenteric artery for thromboembolectomy. Arteriotomy is closed either by patch angioplasty or by anastomosis to a bypass graft from a suitable source of inflow. (Adapted from Yao JST, Bergan JJ, Pearce WH, Flinn WR: Operative procedures in visceral ischemia. In Bergan JJ, Yao JST [eds]: Techniques in Arterial Surgery. Philadelphia, WB Saunders, 1990, pp 284-293.)

fixed occlusive lesions, creating transient ischemic pain that has been appropriately termed *intestinal angina.* Chronic abdominal pain occurs among an unusual group of generally younger and otherwise healthy patients who have compression of the celiac artery by the median arcuate ligament of the diaphragm.

Presentation and Management

Acute Mesenteric Arterial Occlusion

The most common cause of acute mesenteric arterial occlusion is embolus to the superior mesenteric artery and rarely the celiac artery. Severe pain is always present and prominent, centered in the periumbilical region (Table 66-13). Abdominal examination typically reveals relatively little tenderness during the early stages, only to become more impressive as ischemic bowel produces visceral peritonitis and finally parietal peritonitis. The white blood cell count is generally elevated, and metabolic acidosis may be present. A plain radiograph of the abdomen may demonstrate fluid-filled bowel loops with evidence of edema in the bowel wall. Underlying cardiac disease is responsible for the embolus in 90% of cases, and manifestations of arrhythmia, recent myocardial infarction, or valvular disease may be present.

Early management relies critically on prompt diagnosis, which requires a high index of suspicion. Alternative diagnoses such as acute pancreatitis, perforated viscus, ruptured aneurysm, or kidney stone must be rapidly excluded while fluid resuscitation and antibiotics are instituted. Arteriography can identify the site of occlusion but is not crucial if the patient has compelling clinical evidence and if surgical therapy will be inordinately delayed as a result.

Surgery offers the best chance of successful treatment.[47] Exploratory laparotomy allows rapid confirmation of the diagnosis and exclusion of other conditions. If the entire bowel is frankly necrotic, the likelihood of survival is virtually nil, and no further therapy is pursued in most cases. If there is patchy or segmental necrosis or generalized ischemia that appears reversible, the proximal superior mesenteric artery is exposed at the base of the transverse mesocolon. Pulsation and flow are assessed in the main artery and its arcades using intraoperative Doppler ultrasound.

In general, an embolus creates an accessible occlusion distal to the origin of the superior mesenteric artery, lodging in the first bifurcation point of the artery. Most often, the proximal superior mesenteric artery is opened longitudinally and thromboembolectomy performed using a patch angioplasty to close the artery (Fig. 66-22). If the artery is soft and free of atherosclerotic changes, a transverse arteriotomy may be used and closed primarily without a patch. In patients with significant associated chronic arterial disease in whom thrombosis has occurred, a simple thromboembolectomy may fail to restore normal inflow. In such cases, the superior mesenteric artery arteriotomy is used as the site for distal anastomosis of a bypass. Most often, autogenous vein is preferred to avoid the risk for infection of a prosthetic graft. The bypass may originate from the aorta or an iliac artery,

Table 66-14   Conditions Associated With Mesenteric Venous Thrombosis

Portal Hypertension
Cirrhosis
Congestive splenomegaly

Inflammation
Peritonitis
Inflammatory bowel disease
Pelvic or intra-abdominal abscess
Diverticular disease

Postoperative State and Trauma
Splenectomy and other postoperative states
Blunt abdominal trauma

Hypercoagulable States
Neoplasms (colon, pancreas)
Oral contraceptives
Pregnancy
Migratory thrombophlebitis
Antithrombin III, protein C, S deficiency
Peripheral deep vein thrombosis
Polycythemia vera
Thrombocytosis

Other Conditions
Renal disease (nephrotic syndrome)
Cardiac disease (congestive failure)

Table 66-15   Presentation of Mesenteric Venous Thrombosis

PRESENTATION	PERCENTAGE
Pain (insidious)	81
Gastrointestinal bleed	19
Guaiac-positive stool	63
Anorexia	44
Previous deep vein thrombosis	44
Pancreatic cancer	13
Hepatitis	25
Thrombocytosis	25
Increased fibrinogen	13
Decreased proteins C, S	50

depending on which is least involved with disease. After flow is established, frankly necrotic regions of bowel are resected. Regions where there is potential for recovery may be observed for 24 to 36 hours and reassessed at a "second look" operation. The mortality rate reported for patients undergoing surgery for acute intestinal ischemia is as high as 85%, although with aggressive diagnosis and intervention, mortality rates may be reduced to the range of 25%.[47]

Nonocclusive Mesenteric Insufficiency

Patients suffering from nonocclusive mesenteric insufficiency are frequently seriously ill and often have been in an intensive support setting before development of mesenteric insufficiency. If the patient is obtunded, intubated, or heavily narcotized, the presentation may be subtle and the diagnosis thus delayed. Diffuse abdominal pain is prominent and out of proportion to tenderness. Acidosis may be profound. Abdominal flat plate, ultrasound, and CT help to exclude other diagnoses such as perforated ulcer or acute cholecystitis. Arteriography is a valuable confirmatory diagnostic step. Classic arteriographic findings include absence of large vessel occlusion and a pattern of sequential focal vasospasm with "beading" of the major mesenteric branches and a pruned tree appearance to the distal vasculature.

In addition to making the diagnosis, arteriography facilitates valuable early therapy with continuous selective infusion of vasodilators such as papaverine into the superior mesenteric artery. Fluid resuscitation, withdrawal of vasoconstrictors, antibiotics to combat portal transmigration of bacteria, and angiographic monitoring of vasospasm are important components of patient management. Surgery is reserved for patients who experience clinical deterioration or evidence of peritonitis suggesting bowel infarction. Success is possible only with control of the underlying illness that precipitated the mesenteric insufficiency. Because of the complexity of the illness, patients with nonocclusive mesenteric insufficiency have a grim prognosis.

Mesenteric Venous Occlusion

Mesenteric venous occlusion occurs in patients with a number of concurrent illnesses, including liver disease and portal hypertension, pancreatitis, intraperitoneal inflammatory conditions, hypercoagulable states, and systemic low-flow states (Table 66-14). Venous thrombosis is less dramatic than arterial occlusion, and early diagnosis is typically difficult because the presentation is subtle[48] (Table 66-15). Abdominal pain is usually vague, and tenderness is mild or equivocal. CT may demonstrate thickened bowel wall with delayed passage of IV contrast agent into the portal system and lack of opacification of the portal vein. Arteriography may demonstrate venous congestion and lack of prompt filling of the portal system.

Therapy consists of hemodynamic support, anticoagulation, and serial examination. If peritonitis develops, exploratory laparotomy is appropriate to assess bowel viability with segmental bowel resection as necessary. Surgical thrombectomy is not likely to be successful. Fibrinolytic therapy is hazardous because the congested bowel wall is susceptible to hemorrhage. In general, prognosis is good because collateral venous outflow develops, and partial or even complete recanalization of the mesenteric veins may occur in many instances.

Chronic Mesenteric Insufficiency

Patients with advanced chronic mesenteric artery disease most commonly have a stereotypical pattern of postprandial pain in a periumbilical location that occurs within 30 minutes of a meal (Table 66-16). It gradually resolves

Table 66-16 Signs and Symptoms of Chronic Mesenteric Arterial Insufficiency

SIGN OR SYMPTOM	PERCENTAGE
Pain	100
Weight loss	80-98
Abdominal bruit	68-75
Nausea, vomiting	54-84
Diarrhea	35
Constipation	13-26
Hemoccult-positive stool	8

thereafter, only to recur with subsequent meals. Because eating causes pain, patients reduce the size of meals and develop a pattern of "food fear" abstinence that results in weight loss. Malabsorption is rarely, if ever, a component of this disease.

Diagnosis requires a careful history and exclusion of other illnesses such as malignancy, chronic pancreatitis, and gastric ulcer. Often, a series of diagnostic studies is performed to exclude these entities, and the diagnosis of chronic mesenteric ischemia is made late by exclusion. Duplex ultrasound has been used with increasing success to document occlusive disease in the proximal superior mesenteric artery and celiac arteries. The definitive diagnostic study is arteriography, which invariably reveals occlusion of at least two of the three major mesenteric arteries. Patterns of collateral vessels are often prominent, including a large meandering artery in the mesentery of the colon (Fig. 66-23).

In selected circumstances, revascularization by balloon angioplasty or stent placement may be successful, a strategy particularly applicable among elderly patients who may be poor candidates for surgery. However, restenosis and reintervention rates may be as high as 30% to 50% and 50%, respectively.[49] More commonly,[50] definitive therapy requires surgery using either a direct approach to proximal arterial occlusions through transaortic endarterectomy or bypass grafting. Bypass may be performed using a prosthetic graft originating in the supraceliac aorta and connecting to both the celiac and superior mesenteric arteries. Alternatively, retrograde bypass from the infrarenal aorta or iliac artery may be used. Surgical exploration and therapy are usually facilitated because the patient has lost a significant amount of weight preoperatively. Results of surgery are generally highly gratifying in properly selected patients, with rapid resolution of symptoms and return of weight. Long-term patency of the grafts is excellent, exceeding 90%.

A small subset of patients without atherosclerosis and generally of younger age experience postprandial pain on the basis of celiac artery compression from the median arcuate ligament of the diaphragm. In general, such patients have a long history of chronic complaints. They often have been evaluated by numerous physicians and may have developed dependency on pain medications. Evaluation using MRI or arteriography reveals extrinsic compression of the proximal celiac artery with postste-

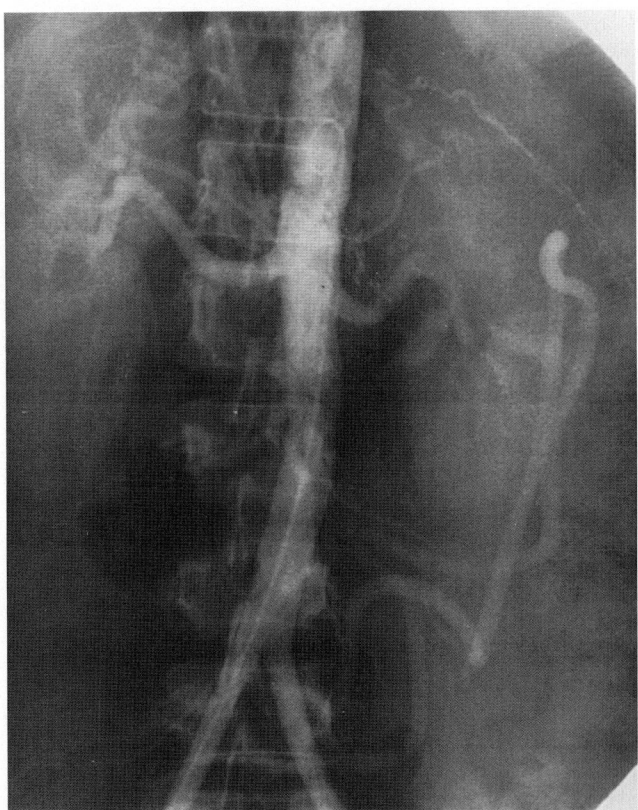

Figure 66-23 Arteriogram of patient with chronic intestinal ischemia demonstrating large meandering artery forming collateral within the mesentery of the colon.

notic dilation. Images during inspiration and expiration demonstrate a dynamic constriction of the artery. Therapy is directed at highly selected patients. Percutaneous methods are not successful in relieving extrinsic compression. Surgery involves release of the median arcuate ligament. A minority of patients may have secondary fibrous thickening of the proximal celiac artery, which is treated with a short bypass or patch angioplasty. A hemodynamic cause for pain is not always clear, and some therapeutic benefit may result from ablation of the celiac nerve plexus during surgery. Results of surgery are generally favorable in carefully selected patients.

Selected References

Antiplatelet Trialists' Collaboration: Collaborative overview of randomised trials of antiplatelet therapy. II. Maintenance of vascular graft or arterial patency by antiplatelet therapy. BMJ 308:159-168, 1994.

Second of a series of meta-analyses of published trials of antiplatelet therapy, focused on the issues of peripheral vascular disease and bypass grafts.

Boley SJ, Brandt LJ, Veith FJ: Ischemic disorders of the intestines. Curr Prob Surg 15:1-85, 1978.

This excellent overview emphasizes the important role of angiographic diagnosis and therapy, particularly for nonocclusive mesenteric disease.

Glagov S, Zarins C, Giddens DP, Ku DN: Hemodynamics and atherosclerosis: Insights and perspectives gained from studies of human arteries. Arch Pathol Lab Med 112:1018-1031, 1988.

> Authored by a pioneer in this field, this is an excellent introduction to the conceptual and experimental framework linking hemodynamic forces and atherosclerosis.

Goldblatt H: Studies on experimental hypertension. J Exp Med 59:347, 1934.

> This classic paper first describes the mechanism behind renovascular hypertension.

Haimovici H: Muscular, renal and metabolic complications of acute arterial occlusions: Myonephropathic-metabolic syndrome. Surgery 85:461-473, 1979.

> A classic description of the systemic effects of revascularization of the severely ischemic extremity.

Pohl MA: The ischemic kidney and hypertension. Am J Kidney Dis 21(Suppl 2):22-28, 1993.

> This paper is an excellent review of renovascular disease from the kidney's point of view.

Ross R: Atherosclerosis: An inflammatory disease. N Engl J Med 340:115-126, 1999.

> A concise, updated overview of current hypotheses of atherogenesis with an excellent reference list.

Sos T, Pickering T, Sniderman K, et al: Percutaneous transluminal renal angioplasty in renovascular hypertension due to atheroma or fibromuscular dysplasia. N Engl J Med 309:274, 1983.

> This paper was the first to carefully describe techniques and results of percutaneous therapy for renovascular disease, differentiating between ostial and nonostial disease.

STILE Investigators: Results of a prospective randomized trial evaluating surgery versus thrombolysis for ischemia of the lower extremity. The STILE Trial. Ann Surg 220:251-268, 1994.

> A large randomized evaluation of the role of thrombolysis in the management of acute lower extremity ischemia.

Stoney RJ, Cunningham CG: Acute mesenteric ischemia. Surgery 114:489-490, 1993.

> An authoritative review of a challenging subgroup of patients with mesenteric disease.

References

1. Fuster V: Syndromes of Atherosclerosis: Correlations of Clinical Imaging and Pathology. New York, Futura, 1996.
2. Glagov S, Zarins C, Giddens DP, Ku DN: Hemodynamics and atherosclerosis: Insights and perspectives gained from studies of human arteries. Arch Pathol Lab Med 112:1018-1031, 1988.
3. Glagov S, Weisenberg E, Zarins CK, et al: Compensatory enlargement of human atherosclerotic coronary arteries. N Engl J Med 316:1371-1375, 1987.
4. Ross R: Atherosclerosis: An inflammatory disease. N Engl J Med 340:115-126, 1999.
5. Benditt EP: Implications of the monoclonal character of human atherosclerotic plaques. Am J Pathol 86:693-702, 1977.
6. Porter JM, Taylor LM, Harris EJ: Nonatherosclerotic vascular disease. In Moore WS (ed): Vascular Surgery: A Comprehensive Review. Philadelphia, WB Saunders, 1991.
7. Creager MA, Halpern JL, Coffman JD: Raynaud's phenomenon and other vascular disorders related to temperature. In Loscalzo J, Creager MA, Dzau VJ (eds): Vascular Medicine. Boston, Little, Brown, 1996.
8. Bandyk DF, Schmitt DD, Seabrook GR, et al: Monitoring functional patency of in situ saphenous vein bypasses: The impact of a surveillance protocol and elective revision. J Vasc Surg 9:286-296, 1989.
9. Merten GJ, Burgess WP, Gray LV, et al: Prevention of contrast-induced nephropathy with sodium bicarbonate: A randomized controlled trial. JAMA 291:2328-2334, 2004.
10. Tepel M, van der Giet M, Schwarzfeld C, et al: Prevention of radiographic-contrast-agent-induced reductions in renal function by acetylcysteine. N Engl J Med 343:180-184, 2000.
11. ACC/AHA 2005 practice guidelines for the management of patients with peripheral arterial disease (lower extremity, renal, mesenteric, and abdominal aortic). Circulation 113:1474-1547, 2006.
12. Collaborative overview of randomised trials of antiplatelet therapy. II. Maintenance of vascular graft or arterial patency by antiplatelet therapy. Antiplatelet Trialists' Collaboration. BMJ 308:159-168, 1994.
13. Rutherford RB: Atlas of Vascular Surgery: Basic Techniques and Exposures. Philadelphia, WB Saunders, 1993.
14. Yadav JS, Wholey MH, Kuntz RE, et al: Protected carotid-artery stenting versus endarterectomy in high-risk patients. N Engl J Med 351:1493-1501, 2004.
15. Muradin GS, Bosch JL, Stijnen T, Hunink MG: Balloon dilation and stent implantation for treatment of femoropopliteal arterial disease: Meta-analysis. Radiology 221:137-145, 2001.
16. Results of a prospective randomized trial evaluating surgery versus thrombolysis for ischemia of the lower extremity. The STILE trial. Ann Surg 220:251-266; discussion 266-258, 1994.
17. Jivegard LE, Arfvidsson B, Holm J, Schersten T: Selective conservative and routine early operative treatment in acute limb ischaemia. Br J Surg 74:798-801, 1987.
18. Elliott JP Jr, Hageman JH, Szilagyi E, et al: Arterial embolization: Problems of source, multiplicity, recurrence, and delayed treatment. Surgery 88:833-845, 1980.
19. Baxter-Smith D, Ashton F, Slaney G: Peripheral arterial embolism: A 20 year review. J Cardiovasc Surg (Torino) 29:453-457, 1988.
20. Donaldson MC, Weinberg DS, Belkin M, et al: Screening for hypercoagulable states in vascular surgical practice: A preliminary study. J Vasc Surg 11:825-831, 1990.
21. Ouriel K, Veith FJ, Sasahara AA: A comparison of recombinant urokinase with vascular surgery as initial treatment for acute arterial occlusion of the legs. Thrombolysis or Peripheral Arterial Surgery (TOPAS) Investigators. N Engl J Med 338:1105-1111, 1998.
22. McAllister FF: The fate of patients with intermittent claudication managed nonoperatively. Am J Surg 132:593-595, 1976.
23. Boyd AM: The natural course of arteriosclerosis of the lower extremities. Proc R Soc Med 55:591-593, 1962.
24. McFalls EO, Ward HB, Moritz TE, et al: Coronary-artery revascularization before elective major vascular surgery. N Engl J Med 351:2795-2804, 2004.
25. Reed AB, Conte MS, Donaldson MC, et al: The impact of patient age and aortic size on the results of aortobifemoral bypass grafting. J Vasc Surg 37:1219-1225, 2003.

26. Blaisdell FW: Extraanatomical bypass procedures. World J Surg 12:798-804, 1988.
27. Taylor LM Jr, Edwards JM, Porter JM: Present status of reversed vein bypass grafting: Five-year results of a modern series. J Vasc Surg 11:193-205; discussion 205-206, 1990.
28. Leather RP, Shah DM, Chang BB, Kaufman JL: Resurrection of the in situ saphenous vein bypass: 1000 cases later. Ann Surg 208:435-442, 1988.
29. Donaldson MC, Mannick JA, Whittemore AD: Femoral-distal bypass with in situ greater saphenous vein: Long-term results using the Mills valvulotome. Ann Surg 213:457-464; discussion 464-465, 1991.
30. Chew DK, Owens CD, Belkin M, et al: Bypass in the absence of ipsilateral greater saphenous vein: Safety and superiority of the contralateral greater saphenous vein. J Vasc Surg 35:1085-1092, 2002.
31. Chew DK, Conte MS, Donaldson MC, et al: Autogenous composite vein bypass graft for infrainguinal arterial reconstruction. J Vasc Surg 33:259-264; discussion 264-265, 2001.
32. Reed AB, Conte MS, Belkin M, et al: Usefulness of autogenous bypass grafts originating distal to the groin. J Vasc Surg 35:48-54; discussion, 54-55, 2002.
33. Belkin M, Conte MS, Donaldson MC, et al: Preferred strategies for secondary infrainguinal bypass: Lessons learned from 300 consecutive reoperations. J Vasc Surg 21:282-293; discussion 293-295, 1995.
34. Adam DJ, Beard JD, Cleveland T, et al: Bypass versus angioplasty in severe ischaemia of the leg (BASIL): Multicentre, randomised controlled trial. Lancet 366:1925-1934, 2005.
35. Duda SH, Poerner TC, Wiesinger B, et al: Drug-eluting stents: Potential applications for peripheral arterial occlusive disease. J Vasc Interv Radiol 14:291-301, 2003.
36. Harding MB, Smith LR, Himmelstein SI, et al: Renal artery stenosis: Prevalence and associated risk factors in patients undergoing routine cardiac catheterization. J Am Soc Nephrol 2:1608-1616, 1992.
37. Zierler RE, Bergelin RO, Isaacson JA, Strandness DE Jr. Natural history of atherosclerotic renal artery stenosis: A prospective study with duplex ultrasonography. J Vasc Surg 19:250-257; discussion 257-258, 1994.
38. Zeller T: Renal artery stenosis: Epidemiology, clinical manifestation, and percutaneous endovascular therapy. J Interv Cardiol 18:497-506, 2005.
39. Davidson RA, Wilcox CS: Newer tests for the diagnosis of renovascular disease. JAMA 268:3353-3358, 1992.
40. Cambria RP, Kaufman JL, Brewster DC, et al: Surgical renal artery reconstruction without contrast arteriography: The role of clinical profiling and magnetic resonance angiography. J Vasc Surg 29:1012-1021, 1999.
41. Sos TA: Angioplasty for the treatment of azotemia and renovascular hypertension in atherosclerotic renal artery disease. Circulation 83:I162-166, 1991.
42. Rodriguez-Lopez JA, Werner A, Ray LI, et al: Renal artery stenosis treated with stent deployment: Indications, technique, and outcome for 108 patients. J Vasc Surg 29:617-624, 1999.
43. van de Ven PJ, Kaatee R, Beutler JJ, et al: Arterial stenting and balloon angioplasty in ostial atherosclerotic renovascular disease: A randomised trial. Lancet 353:282-286, 1999.
44. Blum U, Krumme B, Flugel P, et al: Treatment of ostial renal-artery stenoses with vascular endoprostheses after unsuccessful balloon angioplasty. N Engl J Med 336:459-465, 1997.
45. Lim ST, Rosenfield K: Renal artery stent placement: Indications and results. Curr Interv Cardiol Rep 2:130-139, 2000.
46. Tullis MJ, Zierler RE, Glickerman DJ, et al: Results of percutaneous transluminal angioplasty for atherosclerotic renal artery stenosis: A follow-up study with duplex ultrasonography. J Vasc Surg 25:46-54, 1997.
47. Park WM, Gloviczki P, Cherry KJ Jr, et al: Contemporary management of acute mesenteric ischemia: Factors associated with survival. J Vasc Surg 35:445-452, 2002.
48. Harward TR, Green D, Bergan JJ, et al: Mesenteric venous thrombosis. J Vasc Surg 9:328-333, 1989.
49. Brown DJ, Schermerhorn ML, Powell RJ, et al: Mesenteric stenting for chronic mesenteric ischemia. J Vasc Surg 42:268-274, 2005.
50. Kasirajan K, O'Hara PJ, Gray BH, et al: Chronic mesenteric ischemia: Open surgery versus percutaneous angioplasty and stenting. J Vasc Surg 33:63-71, 2001.

Vascular Trauma

Asher Hirshberg, MD   and   Kenneth L. Mattox, MD

CHALLENGE OF VASCULAR TRAUMA

Injuries to blood vessels are some of the most dramatic challenges facing trauma surgeons because the repair is often urgent, the surgeon has to decide between several management options (open or endovascular), and gaining control of and reconstructing a major arterial injury can be technically demanding. Furthermore, in an era of increasing subspecialization and markedly reduced exposure to vascular surgery in the general surgery training curriculum, increasing numbers of surgeons taking trauma call are now less comfortable dealing with these injuries. Yet major vascular trauma remains a crucial element of trauma surgery, and every general surgeon must be prepared to deal with them either definitively or using so-called bail-out vascular damage control tactics. A phone call to bring in a vascular surgeon from home is not a valid solution for the exsanguinating patient with an iliac vein injury.

The effective management of vascular injuries hinges on successfully merging the principles of modern trauma care with the current approach to vascular therapy as outlined in the previous chapters of this section. The fundamental difference between elective vascular surgery and vascular trauma is the physiology of the wounded patient. A lacerated major vessel is typically only one component of the multitrauma complex that includes injuries to other organs and systems. These patients are often critically ill and rapidly approaching a point of physiologic irreversibility.[1] In these dramatic clinical circumstances, the key to a favorable outcome is maintaining correct priorities.

The surgeon must keep in mind that although major hemorrhage (typical of truncal vascular injuries) is an immediate threat to the patient's life, ischemia (commonly from peripheral arterial injury) is a threat to limb viability, a much lower priority. Furthermore, although control of hemorrhage is usually mandatory and life-saving, the reconstruction of an injured vessel may be neither. As the injured patient is approaching the boundaries of his or her physiologic envelope, a simpler, sometimes temporary technical solution is often a safer option than a complex and time-consuming reconstruction.[2] In the severely traumatized patient, the best technically feasible definitive solution is not always in the patient's best interest.

The first part of this chapter focuses on fundamental principles in the diagnosis and management of vascular trauma. The second part deals with injuries to named vessels in specific anatomic locations. Both parts emphasize the modern convergence of innovative surgical strategies with cutting-edge imaging and endovascular technology, a convergence that offers the trauma surgeon an expanded and improved array of options for the management of injuries to major vessels.

GENERAL APPROACH TO VASCULAR TRAUMA

Injury Patterns

Vascular trauma occurs in a limited number of patterns, which are determined primarily by the mechanism of injury.[3] Penetrating trauma typically results in varying degrees of laceration or transection of the vessel. The severed ends of a completely transected artery often retract and undergo spasm with subsequent thrombosis. Therefore, a lacerated or incompletely transected vessel typically bleeds more profusely than a completely transected one.

Blunt trauma results in disruption of the arterial wall, ranging in severity from small intimal flaps to extensive transmural damage with either extravasation or thrombosis. Deceleration injury causes deformation of the arterial wall. In a small vessel (e.g., the renal artery), this leads to intimal disruption and subsequent thrombosis, whereas in a larger vessel, the result will be full-thickness injury with only a thin layer of adventitia temporarily bridging the gap, as typically occurs in the descending thoracic aorta.

Bleeding from a lacerated vessel can be free or contained, the latter leading to pseudoaneurysm formation. An arteriovenous fistula is the result of a traumatic communication between an injured artery and vein.

Limb loss is more likely to result from blunt trauma and high-velocity gunshot injuries, mainly because of the greater damage to bone and soft tissue of the injured extremity. Low-velocity gunshot injuries and stab wounds rarely lead to limb loss.

The rapidly increasing use of invasive diagnostic, monitoring, and therapeutic modalities in many fields of medicine has brought with it a corresponding dramatic increase in iatrogenic vascular trauma. Every cardiac catheterization or arterial line insertion is, in fact, a form of vascular injury, where the physician relies on the patient's hemostatic mechanism to plug the hole and repair the damage. Iatrogenic injury may occur either at the target site of the intervention (e.g., a coronary artery) or at the access site (e.g., the common femoral artery). The latter is more common and may require surgical repair.

Concept of Minimal Vascular Injury

Not all arterial injuries require operative management. During the past 2 decades, a series of studies have convincingly demonstrated that nonocclusive intimal flaps, segmental arterial narrowing, small false aneurysms, and small arteriovenous fistulas have a benign natural history and are very likely to either heal or improve without intervention. These asymptomatic angiographic findings that are neither occluding nor extravasating have been named minimal arterial injuries. Contrary to previous belief, only about 10% of minimal injuries progress to require a surgical or endovascular repair.[4] Nonoperative management with careful follow-up is therefore a safe and cost-effective course of action for these patients. However, currently there are no objective criteria to precisely define what constitutes a minimal lesion. The size of the angiographic defect, the patient's overall trauma burden, and most importantly, the patient's availability for follow-up are factors to consider in making a decision to treat a minimal lesion conservatively. In rare instances, when a nonocclusive minimal injury increases in size and

eventually requires operative or endovascular repair, morbidity is not increased by the delay.

Endovascular Management

With the rapid progress in endovascular therapy of arterial disease, it is not surprising that endovascular management options are gaining in popularity as alternatives to open repair in selected arterial injuries. In the hemodynamically stable patient with a nonbleeding traumatic arterial lesion, percutaneous placement of an endovascular stent-graft across a defect in the arterial wall is a low-morbidity solution to a problem that may otherwise require a technically challenging surgical procedure in a patient with a severely compromised physiology. In fact, endovascular therapy has revolutionized the management of delayed complications of trauma such as arteriovenous fistulas and pseudoaneurysms, especially in inaccessible sites.[5]

For some arterial injuries, the endovascular option is proving to be the preferred approach. The technical difficulties of gaining access to the vertebral artery inside the bony canal or obtaining distal control of a distal injury to the internal carotid artery make angiographic occlusion of the injured artery a very attractive alternative. In nonocclusive blunt injuries to the renal artery, endovascular stenting offers great expediency as compared with an open repair, albeit at the risk of yet unknown long-term patency. Similarly, blunt subclavian artery injury is often part of an injury complex involving multiple organ systems, and an endovascular stent-graft may well be the quickest and least hazardous solution for the patient.

The endovascular approach to blunt injuries to the descending thoracic aorta is rapidly gaining in popularity.[6-10] The clinical experience with endovascular stent-grafting of the aorta is showing promise, mainly because it is associated with low morbidity, and paraplegia, the dreaded complication of an open repair, has not been reported in endovascular repairs. The procedure is especially applicable in patients with multiple associated injuries who are poor candidates for a major aortic reconstruction. The major barriers to the adoption of endovascular repair as the procedure of choice for blunt aortic injury are technical problems with currently available devices[6,7] and the lack of prospective randomized studies.

OPERATIVE PRINCIPLES

Access, Exposure, and Control

Initial control of hemorrhage is achieved by direct pressure over the bleeding site using digital or manual compression. Blind clamping of a bleeding vessel is usually ineffective and may damage adjacent structures in the neurovascular bundle. The surgeon then chooses a definitive hemostatic technique from a wide array of available hemostatic options. These include, among others, hemostatic suture, ligation, reconstruction, and temporary shunt insertion.[11-13] Balloon catheter tamponade using a

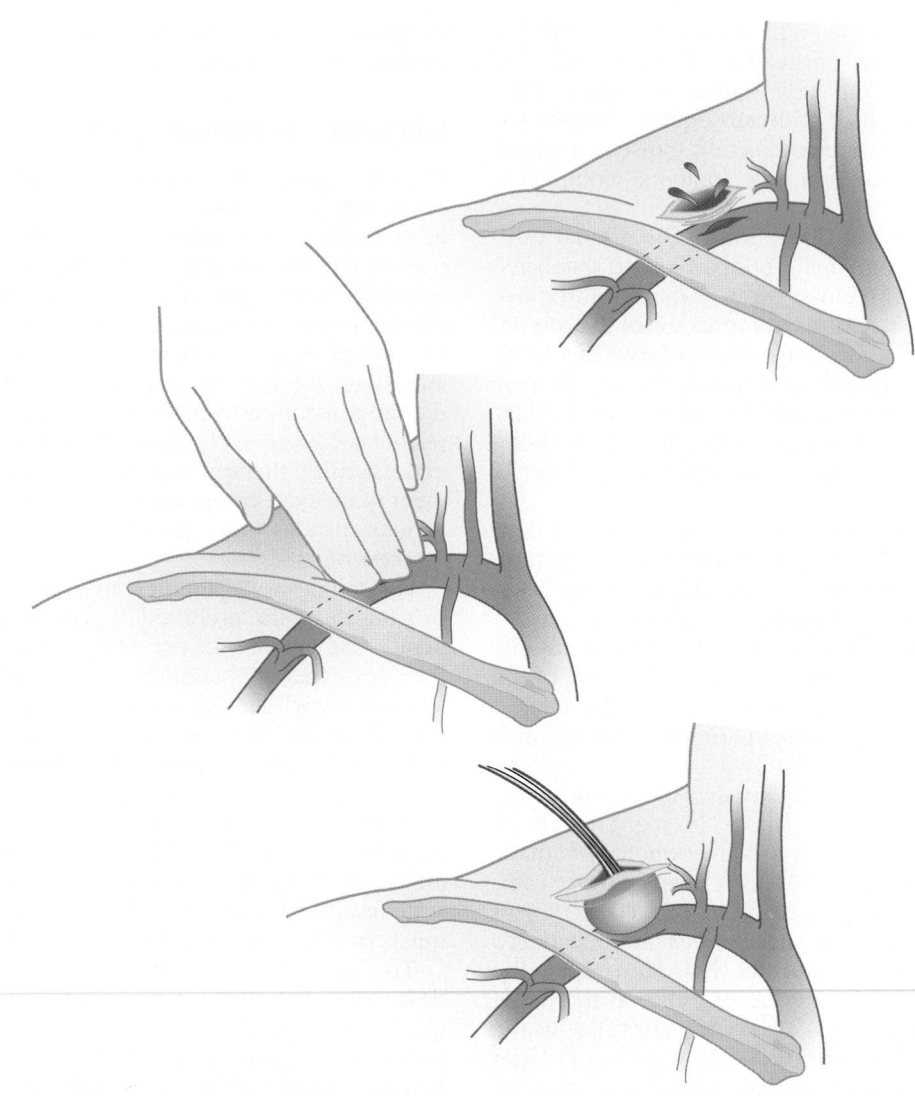

Figure 67-1 Use of a balloon tamponade for temporary hemostasis of subclavian artery injury. (Illustration by Jan Redden. © Kenneth L. Mattox, MD.)

Foley catheter inserted into the missile tract is a useful technique for obtaining rapid temporary control of torrential bleeding from a penetrating injury to an inaccessible vessel, such as high in the neck or deep in the pelvis (Fig. 67-1).

A cardinal operative principle in managing major vascular trauma is to first obtain proximal (and, if possible, also distal) control of the injured vessel before entering the hematoma. In the extremities and in the neck, control is achieved using standard extensile vascular exposure techniques.[13,14] In the chest, control of a vascular injury hinges on correct selection of a thoracotomy incision because each incision provides access to a different thoracic visceral compartment. In the abdomen, the major vessels are located in the retroperitoneum, and therefore exposure is based on operative maneuvers that rotate the intraperitoneal viscera off the underlying retroperitoneal structures.[15]

Assessing the Injury and the Patient

The anatomic extent of injury is revealed only when the traumatized vessel is carefully explored and opened. External inspection often does not reflect the full extent of intimal damage, especially in blunt trauma. The entire length of the injured segment must be precisely delineated at operation because leaving proximal or distal intimal damage will result in early failure of the reconstruction.

An important principle in the operative management of vascular trauma is that selection of the repair technique is heavily influenced not only by the anatomic situation but also by the patient's physiologic condition, associated injuries, and overall clinical trajectory. The massively bleeding patient incurs a rapidly increasing burden of physiologic insults. The marker of an irreversible (and lethal) physiology is a self-propagating triad of hypothermia, coagulopathy, and acidosis. From the vascular perspective, coagulopathy means that a suture line will continue to bleed after completion, and diffuse oozing will persist all over the operative field regardless of the technical success of the reconstruction. The hypothermia-coagulopathy-acidosis syndrome effectively marks the boundaries of the patient's physiologic envelope beyond which there is irreversible shock. The operative management of a vascular injury must therefore focus not only on restoration of anatomic integrity but also, more importantly, on the patient's physiologic envelope. The complexity and duration of the planned repair must be inversely proportional to the physiologic insult that the patient has already sustained.

Vascular Damage Control

These considerations have led to the introduction of so-called damage control surgery in trauma. The damage control approach replaces definitive and complex operation with a staged repair. The introduction of damage control was the most important innovation in trauma surgery in the last quarter of the 20th century. The damage control sequence begins with a rapid procedure in which simple temporary bail-out tactics are used to arrest hemorrhage, maintain distal perfusion, and control spillage. The patient is transferred to the surgical intensive care unit for resuscitation, rewarming, and reconstitution of the physiologic envelope. Definitive repair of the injuries is undertaken 24 to 48 hours later, during a planned reoperation.

The damage control approach has been applied to vascular injuries as well. Hemorrhage is controlled by ligation or balloon tamponade. Distal perfusion in an injured artery is maintained by means of a temporary intra-arterial shunt instead of a formal reconstruction.

Ligation of an injured vessel in a critically injured patient is a marker of good surgical judgment rather than an admission of defeat. All peripheral veins and most truncal veins can be ligated with impunity. The external carotid, celiac axis, and internal iliac arteries are examples of arteries that can be ligated with no adverse effects. The risk for amputation after ligation of the femoral vessels was 81% for the common femoral and 55% for the superficial femoral artery during World War II (before the advent of fasciotomy). The upper extremity is even more tolerant to ligation of the subclavian artery.

A temporary intraluminal shunt maintains distal perfusion through an injured artery.[16] Blood flow through the shunt is about half of the normal flow, enough to maintain limb viability. There are reports of temporary shunts remaining patent for more than 24 hours after insertion. A commercially available carotid shunt, endotracheal suction catheter, or sterile intravenous (IV) tubing trimmed to the appropriate length is inserted into both ends of a disrupted vessel and held in place with vessel loops or ligatures (Fig. 67-2). An intraluminal shunt can be used in three clinical situations:

1. As a damage control technique in a critically injured patient who is unlikely to survive a complex repair because physiologic reserves have been exhausted

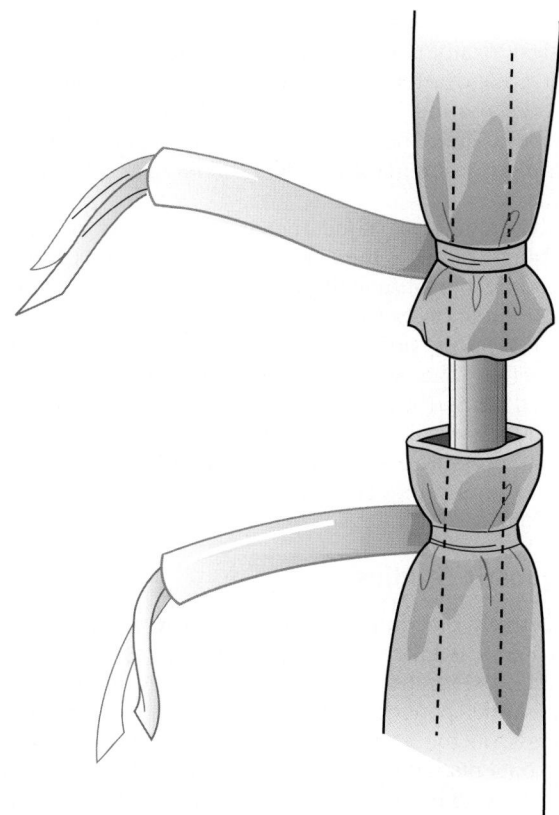

Figure 67-2 **Temporary intravascular shunt.** (Illustration by Jan Redden. © Kenneth L. Mattox, MD.)

2. Transfer of a patient with peripheral arterial injury from the field (or from a remote facility) for vascular reconstruction at a trauma center
3. Repair of combined vascular and orthopedic extremity injuries, when skeletal alignment is accomplished before vascular repair in an ischemic limb

NECK INJURIES

The anatomy of the neck consists of two large neurovascular bundles within the carotid sheaths, which are closely adherent to midline aerodigestive structures in a very compact arrangement. It is therefore not surprising that injuries to major cervical vessels are frequently associated with trauma to adjacent structures. An expanding cervical hematoma presents an immediate threat to the patient's airway. Major vascular injury occurs in one of every four patients with penetrating cervical trauma.[13] The most commonly injured vascular structure is the internal jugular vein, which is amenable to simple lateral repair or ligation.

Clinical Presentation and Immediate Concerns

Major cervical vascular injury may present as vigorous external bleeding, an expanding or stable cervical hematoma, or a hemispheric neurologic deficit. However, a major arterial injury may also remain asymptomatic, so physical examination alone cannot reliably exclude it. Blunt carotid artery injury is an uncommon but potentially devastating injury.[17-20] The only initial clinical clue may be a gross hemispheric neurologic deficit without computed tomographic (CT) evidence of cerebral trauma.

Two immediate concerns are the focus of clinical attention during the initial evaluation. The first is a rapidly expanding hematoma that requires immediate endotracheal intubation before the upper airway is shifted and compressed, making an orotracheal intubation difficult or impossible. The second immediate concern is severe external hemorrhage, which may lead to exsanguination. Vigorous external bleeding requires temporary control by manual pressure or balloon tamponade using a Foley catheter until proximal control is obtained in the operating room.

Diagnostic Studies

The actively bleeding unstable patient with a penetrating neck injury is taken immediately to the operating room for neck exploration. Management of the hemodynamically stable patient with a suspected vascular injury depends on the zone of cervical penetration. Asymptomatic patients with penetrating injuries to the base of the neck (zone 1) require four-vessel arch angiography either to exclude major arterial injury or to plan the operative approach if an injury is present. The same applies to penetrating injuries above the angle of the mandible (zone 3), where both exploration and distal control are technically difficult; therefore, an endovascular solution, if feasible, may be the safest option.

Patients with asymptomatic midcervical injuries (zone 2) may undergo either neck exploration (a straightforward procedure associated with very low morbidity) or a combination of four-vessel angiography, esophagoscopy, and barium swallow to rule out significant arterial and esophageal injury. Both pathways are acceptable alternatives, and thus choice between operative exploration and a sequence of diagnostic procedures reflects individual preferences or institutional policies.

Duplex ultrasonography is an excellent imaging modality for major cervical arterial trauma. However, lack of immediate availability around the clock in the trauma resuscitation area prevents it from becoming a practical substitute for angiography in most emergency centers.

Operative Management

Safe exploration of an anatomically hostile neck distorted by an expanding hematoma hinges on systematic progress from one key structure to the next using a so-called trail of safety. The standard cervical incision is along the anterior border of the sternocleidomastoid muscle. After division of the platysma, dissection proceeds to identify the first key structure: the anterior border of the sternocleidomastoid muscle. Dissection then progresses to identify the next key structure: the internal jugular vein. Dissection along the anterior border of this large vein identifies the facial vein, the gatekeeper structure of the

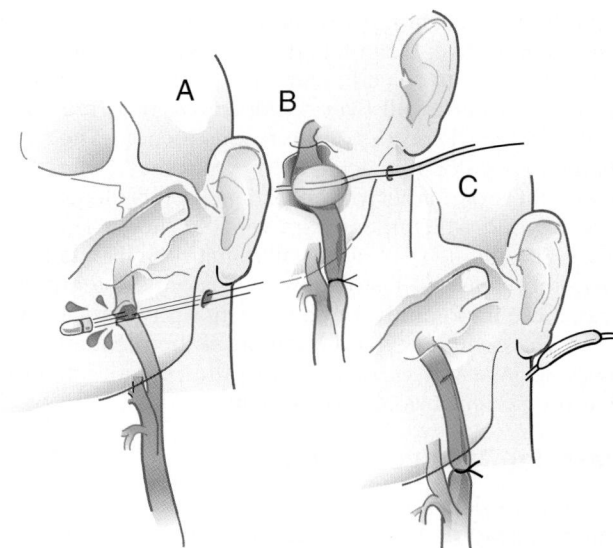

Figure 67-3 A to C, Balloon tamponade of inaccessible internal carotid artery injury. (© Baylor College of Medicine, 1980.)

carotid bifurcation. The facial vein is divided between ligatures to gain access to the carotid bifurcation.

The traumatized carotid arteries are reconstructed using standard vascular techniques. There are no good data to support preference for vein or synthetic interposition grafts in reconstructing the common or internal carotid artery, nor is there strong evidence to support routine shunting. A synthetic graft has the advantage of immediate availability, and a shunt can be threaded through the graft and then inserted into the internal and common carotids to facilitate construction of the anastomotic suture lines with the shunt in place. Control of the distal stump of an injured internal carotid artery at the base of the neck may be impossible even with adjunctive measures such as dividing the posterior belly of the digastric muscle, and an interventional angiographic solution is by far the best. Balloon catheter tamponade through the missile tract followed by ligation and division of the internal carotid artery at the carotid bifurcation, with removal of the balloon 3 days later, affords a simple solution to a difficult technical problem (Fig. 67-3). Another option is to insert an intraluminal Fogarty balloon catheter into the distal stump of the internal carotid, then clip and trim the catheter and leave the balloon inside the artery.

The need to reconstruct the carotid artery of a patient with a clear preoperative hemispheric neurologic deficit has long been a subject of controversy. Current evidence supports revascularization regardless of the patient's neurologic status, accepting that prognosis is poor in the presence of a profound neurologic deficit (i.e., coma) with or without revascularization.

Most vertebral artery injuries are diagnosed angiographically and are best managed by angiographic means. Rarely, it is encountered in the operative field as vigorous bleeding emanating from a hole between the transverse processes of the cervical vertebrae, posterolateral to the carotid sheath.[21-23] Although several elaborate techniques have been described for operative exposure of the extra-cranial vertebral artery, none is a practical option in the acute situation of severe hemorrhage. The artery is best controlled by simple means, such as tightly filling the bleeding hole in the transverse process with bone wax. If extravasation from the vertebral artery is encountered during arteriography, angiographic control of this inaccessible vessel is clearly the preferred course of action.

Blunt Cerebrovascular Trauma

The estimated incidence of clinically important blunt injury to the carotid and vertebral arteries is 1 to 3 patients per 1000 admitted to major trauma centers.[17-19,24] However, with increased awareness and a targeted screening protocol for asymptomatic patients, it is possible to identify these injuries in up to 1% of blunt trauma admissions. The typical mechanism is either hyperextension with contralateral rotation of the neck or a direct blow to the neck, but in some patients, no such mechanism can be elicited. The key pathophysiologic event is an intimal tear that can remain asymptomatic or progress to local thrombosis, embolization, distal dissection, and pseudoaneurysm formation.

The clinical hallmark of blunt carotid artery injury is a hemispheric neurologic deficit that is incompatible with CT findings. A salient clinical feature of this injury is that in about half of the patients, there is a latent period of hours or days before the neurologic deficit appears. Maintaining a high index of suspicion in patients with severe maxillofacial trauma, a mechanism of cervical hyperextension, and evidence of direct trauma to the neck or fractures of the skull base or cervical spine in proximity to the relevant vessels generally enables early diagnosis of these lesions. The standard diagnostic modality is angiography because duplex scanning is not sensitive enough. The sensitivity of CT angiography as a screening test for blunt cerebrovascular trauma is under investigation.

The treatment of blunt carotid and vertebral artery injury remains controversial and primarily nonoperative. Most patients are treated with systemic anticoagulation (if not prohibited by associated injuries), although the benefits of IV heparin are less clear in low-grade nonobstructing luminal irregularities. Hemodynamically significant dissection or inaccessible pseudoaneurysms are amenable to endovascular therapy, but there are several recent disturbing reports of high complication rates with endovascular therapy of blunt carotid artery injuries, so the role of endovascular therapy in these injuries is not well defined.

THORACIC VASCULAR INJURIES

Penetrating Thoracic Vascular Trauma

The patient with a major penetrating thoracic vascular injury typically presents in shock, with either a massive hemothorax or an expanding hematoma at the thoracic inlet. The need for urgent operation is usually obvious. Less commonly, the patient may be hemodynamically stable and a nonbleeding injury (e.g., a pseudoaneurysm, an arteriovenous fistula, or an occluded artery) is suspected on clinical grounds and then delineated angiographically.

Choice of Incision

The choice of thoracotomy incision is a central consideration in the management of thoracic vascular trauma because an incorrectly placed incision will often convert a straightforward procedure into a difficult one. In stable patients, the choice of incision is dictated by the angiographic findings. In the actively bleeding, hemodynamically unstable patient, the surgeon must base the incision on the presumed location of the vascular injury. As a general rule, an anterolateral thoracotomy on the injured side is the incision of choice for patients with ongoing bleeding into the pleural cavity. This incision, performed immediately below the nipple in men or below the manually retracted breast in women, does not require special patient positioning, nor does it limit access to the contralateral hemithorax or to the abdomen. The only exception is a penetrating injury to the right lower chest (below the nipple) where bleeding will most commonly emanate from an injured liver, so the operative approach begins with a midline laparotomy. An anterolateral thoracotomy can be rapidly extended across the sternum to provide access to the mediastinal great vessels and the contralateral hemithorax, albeit at the cost of additional morbidity associated with transecting the sternum.

Penetrating injuries to the base of the neck (thoracic outlet) present special access problems. Right-sided injuries to the base of the neck are approached through a median sternotomy, which provides access to the innominate artery and the proximal right carotid and subclavian arteries. The proximal part of the left subclavian artery is intrapleural and posterior, so the most expeditious way to obtain proximal control is through a separate left anterolateral thoracotomy incision through the third intercostal space (above the nipple).

A supraclavicular incision is used to gain access to the more distal parts of the subclavian artery. The incision entails careful division of two muscle layers: the sternocleidomastoid and the anterior scalene muscle behind it. The phrenic nerve, which crosses the latter muscle, is the key to the dissection and must be identified and preserved. In the actively bleeding patient with a grossly swollen upper chest, exposure of the subclavian vessels can be expedited by subperiosteal resection of the medial half of the clavicle.

Management of Specific Injuries

Penetrating injuries to the innominate vessels and proximal carotid arteries present intraoperatively as a mediastinal hematoma. Much like any other types of hematoma resulting from a major vascular injury, plunging into it without proximal control is a recipe for disaster. Proximal control can be obtained from within the pericardium where the anatomy is not obscured by the hematoma. Exposure is enhanced by division of the innominate vein.

The bypass exclusion technique for innominate artery injuries is described later.

In patients who are massively bleeding from pulmonary hilar injuries, the mortality rate is in excess of 70%. In practice, these injuries usually involve more than one element of the pulmonary hilum. Instead of attempting vascular repair of the pulmonary artery or vein in these exsanguinating patients, a rapid pneumonectomy using a linear stapler may prove lifesaving.

For injuries of the subclavian arteries, the exposure required is almost always more extensive than initially anticipated, and the incision can be extended laterally to expose the proximal axillary artery. Special care must be taken to avoid injury to the phrenic nerve and brachial plexus. Most subclavian artery injuries are repaired using a synthetic interposition graft. Subclavian vein injuries are repaired with lateral venorrhaphy or ligation of the vein. Penetrating injuries to the intrapericardial great vessels and to the vena cava are very rare, and repair requires cardiopulmonary bypass. In practice, these injuries are almost invariably fatal.

Blunt Thoracic Vascular Trauma

Aorta

Aortic injury is the great nemesis of blunt trauma, having caused or contributed to 10% to 15% of motor vehicle crash–related deaths for nearly 30 years.[25] It is a potentially lethal injury that provides the surgeon with a window of opportunity for effective intervention. This window may be missed because the injury remains asymptomatic until catastrophic bleeding suddenly occurs. Despite recent advances in diagnosis and management, mortality rates as high as 11% to 40% persist.[3-5,26] Paraplegia, the most dreaded complication of this injury, has been reported in roughly 13% of open repairs, but results vary considerably between institutions and individual surgeons.

In autopsy studies, injury location was reported at the proximal descending thoracic aorta in only 36% to 54% of cases; however, in surgical cases, this location is reportedly injured in 84% to 100%. Only 3% to 10% are reported to occur in the ascending aorta, arch, or distal descending thoracic aorta. Associated trauma to other cavities and organ systems is very common. In a multicenter report, 51% of patients with aortic injury had concomitant head injury, 46% had rib fractures, and 38% sustained lung contusions. Twenty to 35% of the patients had orthopedic injury, and abdominal injury was common. These multiple associated injuries often complicate or prohibit an urgent aortic repair, and the use of systemic heparin carries the potential for increased neurologic and hemorrhagic complications.

The dominant pathophysiologic event in blunt aortic injury is sudden deceleration with creation of a shear force between a relatively mobile part of the thoracic aorta and an adjacent fixed segment. The classic mechanism of blunt aortic injury is sudden deceleration during a frontal impact motor vehicle collision or a fall from height. However, recent data show a considerable number of cases secondary to other mechanisms, such as side-impact collisions, vehicular-pedestrian accidents, and crush and blast injuries. Certainly, the possibility of blunt aortic injury needs to be considered in all victims of motor vehicle collision, regardless of the point of impact.

It is important to keep in mind that a contained blunt aortic injury does not explain hemodynamic instability in the injured patient. If the patient with a suspected or proven blunt aortic injury is hemodynamically unstable, the explanation almost always lies in other associated injuries, typically in the abdomen. This source of active bleeding is an immediate threat to the patient's life and needs to be addressed before the aortic injury. Very rarely, the aortic disruption itself may present as an ongoing non-exsanguinating hemorrhage causing hemodynamic instability. The window of opportunity to salvage these patients is extremely narrow, and the surgeon is often forced to operate without an angiographic definition of the injury. The mortality rate in these patients is 90%.

Physical examination of the patient with blunt aortic injury is rarely helpful because the classically described signs such as upper extremity hypertension, diminished femoral pulses (called *pseudo-coarctation*), and an intrascapular murmur are distinctly uncommon. The most important aspect of the physical examination is to identify associated injuries that may have either priority over the aortic injury or a major impact on the operative risk.

Several radiographic findings on a supine chest radiograph suggest the diagnosis of blunt aortic injury. The most significant findings are a widened mediastinum (>8 cm), an obscured or indistinct aortic knob, deviation of the left main-stem bronchus, an off-midline position of a nasogastric tube, and obliteration of the aortopulmonary window. The diagnosis of blunt aortic injury remains notoriously elusive. In 5% of patients, the mechanism of injury is, in fact, the only clue to the diagnosis. In others, radiographic signs may be so subtle that even an experienced interpreter will not discern them.

The role of CT in the diagnosis of blunt aortic injury continues to be the focus of debate. Spiral or helical scan of the chest has a high negative predictive value and is a useful screening modality for aortic injury.[24,27-30] However, demonstration of a mediastinal hematoma does not obviate the need for subsequent aortography to clearly define the site and extent of injury. At least 10 aortic arch anomalies exist that are not demonstrated by CT, and the surgeon is best advised to know of these anomalies.

Helical CT angiography is rapidly becoming an imaging modality that rivals aortography as being more expedient and noninvasive. Three-dimensional reconstructions of the aorta provide accurate anatomic detail that obviates the need for a subsequent aortography. However, these reconstructions are time consuming and use massive computing resources. As this technology matures, it may replace aortography as the imaging modality of choice.

The correct and timely identification of blunt aortic injury hinges on a low threshold for aortography when the mechanism of injury, relevant physical findings, or an abnormal chest radiograph suggests the diagnosis. Aortography remains the gold standard imaging modality to which all other modalities are compared. It provides valuable information, not only about precise location and extent of the injury, but also about other details that may affect the operative plan. Two classic pitfalls in interpretation of aortograms are ductus diverticulum and vascular ring remnant.

The traditional management of blunt aortic injury is prompt repair of the injured aortic segment. However, in some patients, a purposeful delay or even nonoperative management may be indicated.[25,31,32] Patients with severe head injury or complex multisystem injury and those about to breach their physiologic envelope are bad candidates for an aortic reconstruction. The estimated risk for free rupture of 1% per hour pales into insignificance when compared with the risk of aortic surgery under these circumstances. Patients with severe comorbid factors are also poor candidates for aortic reconstruction. Evidence is now accumulating that in stable patients, purposeful delay of surgery combined with pharmacologic control of the blood pressure and afterload reduction (aiming for blood pressure values below preinjury levels) and careful monitoring of the mediastinal hematoma may be an acceptable course of action. This purposeful delay allows the surgeon to assess the total injury burden of the patient, select the optimal timing for intervention, and construct a tailor-made endograft when necessary. The concept that early blood pressure control and afterload reduction (typically using an IV β-blocker) converts these cases from urgent to delayed cases that can be repaired the next morning or even several days later is a paradigm shift that simplifies the management of these injuries and allows transfer of the patient to a center of excellence. In addition, minimal blunt aortic injuries, such as a small intimal flap or a small pseudoaneurysm, are probably amenable to nonoperative management. However, the long-term behavior of these minimal lesions is still not well defined, so careful follow-up by serial imaging is mandatory whenever nonoperative management is selected.

The use of endovascular stent-grafts to treat blunt aortic injury is rapidly gaining in popularity despite the conspicuous absence of data from randomized trials, long-term follow-up, and some serious technical problems with the endograft devices. Initially, such endografts were used in chronic transections. During the past 10 years, however, small series reporting use in acute aortic injury have been published.[6-9,25-28] At least 24 different custom and manufactured endografts and off-label use of components of abdominal aortic endografts have been used in the thoracic aorta.[6] Some radiologists and surgeons currently consider thoracic endografting to be as much a standard of care as open aortic reconstruction following trauma, despite the lack of controlled trials and long-term follow-up. This enthusiasm stems from the fact that although the reported mean mortality rate for post-traumatic open thoracic aortic repair is 13% (range, 0%-55%), and the paraplegia rates average 10% (range, 0%-20%), the mortality and paraplegia rates for selected blunt aortic injuries treated endovascularly is 3.8%, and only 1 out of 239 reported cases developed paraplegia. The endovascular option is particularly attractive for

patients with multiple associated injuries who cannot tolerate the single-lung ventilation required for an open repair or in whom systemic heparin is contraindicated because of associated injuries.

Several technical obstacles are still preventing endovascular repair from becoming the standard approach to blunt aortic injuries. One of the major obstacles is the issue of graft and aorta size discrepancy. The average diameter of a young patient's descending thoracic aorta is 19.3 mm. Commercially available endografts, originally designed for elderly patients with chronic aortic disease, are significantly larger. The smallest thoracic endograft approved in the United States is 26 mm in diameter. Inserting a larger endograft into a smaller aorta may lead to enfolding of the graft. This problem has led to the use of custom devices or off-label use of iliac endograft limbs, cuff extenders, and abdominal aortic endografts.

Other technical problems with currently available endografts are angulation at the junction of the aortic arch and the descending thoracic aorta (i.e., around the proximal fixation point of the endograft), which predisposes the endograft to endoleaks, and lack of a sufficient proximal neck to safely anchor the endograft proximal to the aortic tear. In addition, iatrogenic trauma at the insertion site and to the femoral and iliac arteries that must be traversed to insert the endograft adds to the morbidity of the procedure. Technologic advances and technical refinements will address most of these issues in the near future, enhancing the attractiveness of the endovascular repair over open reconstruction.

Open repair of the descending thoracic aorta is performed through a left posterolateral thoracotomy in the fourth intercostal space. The standard operative repair of aortic injuries uses clamp and direct reconstruction and can be achieved by using one of three adjuncts: pharmacologic control of central hypertension, a temporary passive shunt, or a pump-assisted atriofemoral bypass. The latter can be achieved either by a traditional pump bypass (which requires full heparinization) or by using a centrifugal pump without heparin.[26]

The use of temporary shunts or pump bypass is more complex than direct reconstruction with pharmacologic control. However, it has gained in popularity in recent years because of the perception among surgeons (unsupported by controlled clinical trials) that using a shunt or partial bypass may improve outcome and reduce the incidence of paraplegia.

Proximal control of the injury is obtained by encircling the subclavian artery and the aortic arch (between the carotid and left subclavian arteries). The latter is the most difficult part of the dissection. The pleura between the vagus and phrenic nerves is incised, and using a combination of blunt and sharp dissection, a plane is developed between the pulmonary artery and the inferior aspect of the aortic arch. A large curved vascular clamp can then be carefully brought around the aorta, making just enough space for an aortic clamp. The distal descending aorta is encircled after opening the mediastinal pleura, taking care not to injure an intercostal vessel. Clamps are placed on the isolated vessels, and extreme blood pressure fluctuations are avoided by careful pharmacologic control.

After clamping, the hematoma is entered, and the extent and configuration of the tear are assessed through a longitudinal aortotomy. Direct primary repair is possible in only 15% of patients, whereas the rest require an interposition graft.

The reported operative mortality following an open repair is 5%% to 25% and is related not only to the procedure itself but also to the presence of associated injuries and their late sequelae. The most dreaded complication is paraplegia or paraparesis, which occurs in about 8% of patients. The incidence of spinal cord damage is affected neither by choice of operative technique nor by the method chosen to deal with central hypertension and distal ischemia. There is also no direct proven correlation between aortic cross-clamp time and the incidence of spinal cord damage. As noted earlier, one of the most remarkable aspects of the endovascular repair option is that this dreaded complication does not occur.

Innominate Artery

The second most common blunt thoracic vascular injury is a tear at the origin of the innominate artery. The artery is either sheared off the aortic arch, as with blunt aortic injury, or pinched between the sternum and the spine during frontal impact. Blunt innominate artery injury is akin to a side hole in the thoracic aorta because operative repair requires obtaining control at the aortic arch.

The clinical presentation is similar to that of blunt aortic injury in that most patients are hemodynamically stable and asymptomatic. Radiologic evidence of mediastinal widening at the aortic outlet and leftward deviation of the trachea suggest the diagnosis, but angiography is the definitive diagnostic modality.

The operative repair of blunt innominate artery injury is based on the bypass and exclusion principle, eliminating the need for cardiopulmonary bypass, shunts, or the use of heparin.[20,25] After median sternotomy, the ascending aorta is exposed inside the pericardium while deliberately avoiding the traumatized segment. Using a partially occluding clamp on a segment of normal aorta, a graft is sewn to it in an end-to-side configuration, away from the injury. The distal innominate artery is then exposed and clamped, and the distal anastomosis is constructed (Fig. 67-4). Only then is the injured segment of the aortic arch addressed and repaired.

ABDOMINAL VASCULAR INJURIES

Most abdominal vascular injuries result from penetrating trauma and are associated with other abdominal injuries.[3] Vascular injuries are much more common after abdominal gunshot wounds (25% of patients) as compared with stab wounds (10%). Major abdominal vascular trauma presents clinically either as free intraperitoneal hemorrhage or as a contained retroperitoneal hematoma.[33,34] Most patients with major abdominal vascular trauma present with a contained or at least partially contained retroperitoneal hematoma because free bleeding from a major intra-abdominal artery usually results in death at the scene.

Occasionally there are clinical hints to the presence of an abdominal vascular injury. Examples are a bullet trajectory across the abdominal midline in a hypotensive patient or an absent femoral pulse. In most patients, the indication for urgent celiotomy is obvious and the diagnosis is made at operation. Time must not be wasted on unnecessary diagnostic tests or on futile attempts to stabilize the patient because volume loading before achieving surgical control of the bleeding vessel may augment bleeding and adversely affect the outcome.

Immediate Concerns

The typical situation encountered at celiotomy is vigorous bleeding or an expanding hematoma at a relatively inaccessible site, combined with other abdominal visceral injuries. Rapid temporary control of hemorrhage is the obvious first priority and is achieved by direct manual or digital pressure, whereas formal proximal and distal control is obtained later. After bleeding has been temporarily controlled, the surgeon needs to stop and organize the operative attack on the injury. The natural urge to immediately proceed with definitive repair is the worst possible mistake at this point. Instead, the time interval needs to be used to transfuse and resuscitate the patient, to obtain additional instruments and an autotransfusion device, to optimize exposure, and to organize the operating room team. Only then does the definitive repair begin.

Once the total injury burden of the patient is determined, the surgeon has to choose between the traditional operative profile of definitive repair and a damage control profile. The latter consists of a rapid initial operation wherein only temporary bail-out measures to control hemorrhage and spillage are employed. The patient is then transferred to the surgical intensive care unit for rewarming and stabilization, with definitive repair performed at a planned reoperation after 24 to 48 hours. This operative strategy is particularly suitable for the patient with major abdominal vascular injury in conjunction with hollow or solid abdominal visceral trauma, in whom formal repair of all injuries will not be tolerated by the patient's fragile physiology. In these circumstances, the surgeon may decide to address the vascular injury using only bail-out techniques such as ligation or temporary shunt placement. Another option is to perform a definitive repair of the vascular injury and use bail-out techniques for hollow visceral damage.

Aortic Clamping

Aortic cross-clamping is both an adjunct to resuscitation and a means of obtaining global proximal control to reduce torrential hemorrhage in the abdomen. The supraceliac aorta is most expediently clamped at the diaphragmatic hiatus. Rapid blunt creation of an opening in the lesser omentum allows the surgeon to approach the left diaphragmatic crus and open it longitudinally in the direction of its fibers. This is done by finger dissection, and the purpose is to create just enough space on both sides of the aorta to accommodate an aortic clamp. The

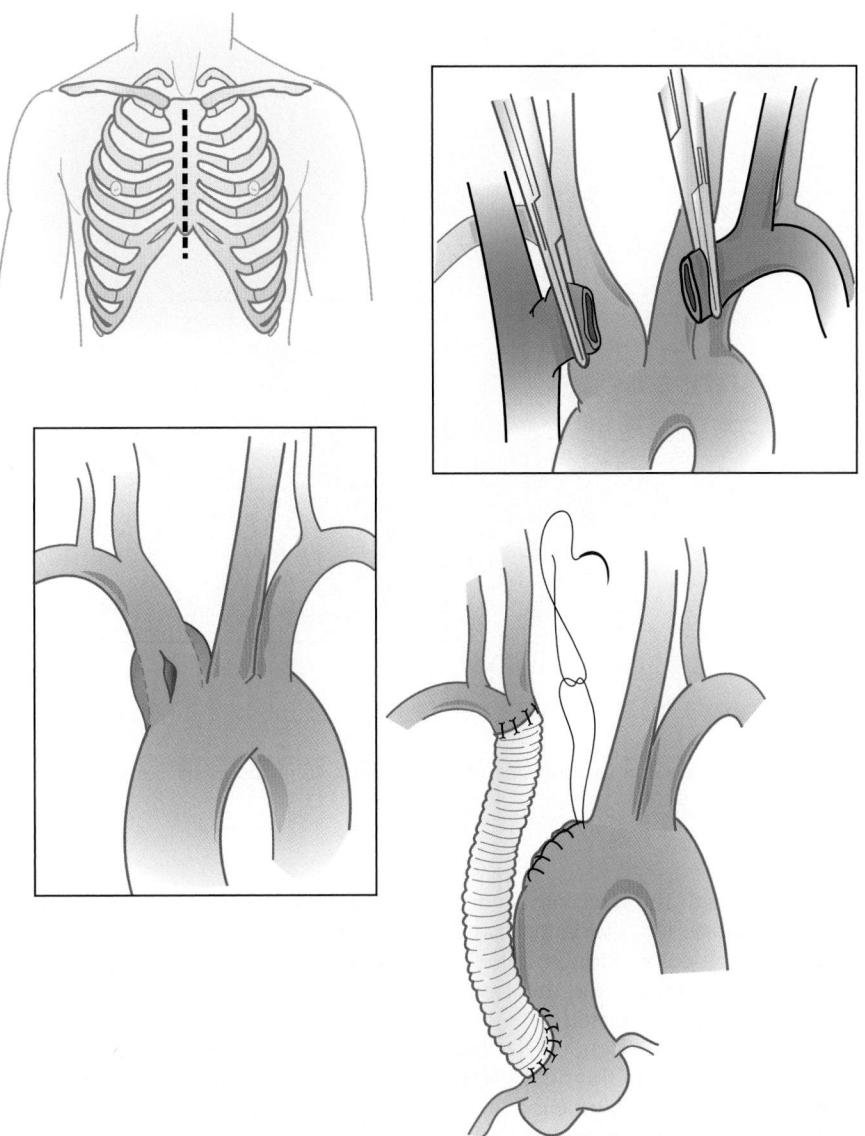

Figure 67-4 The "bypass and exclusion" technique for repair of innominate artery injuries. (Illustration by Jan Redden. © Kenneth L. Mattox, MD.)

transcrural route avoids the dense periaortic tissue of the suprarenal abdominal aorta. Clamping the aorta through the lesser sac is typically performed blindly in a pool of blood, and the dissection required is often far from simple, especially for the inexperienced. It is therefore much safer to compress the aorta manually at the hiatus than to risk iatrogenic damage to the celiac axis, esophagus, or even the aorta itself by a blindly and incorrectly placed clamp.

Aortic clamping has profound physiologic consequences. Although the maneuver elevates the patient's blood pressure, it also causes sudden afterload augmentation and visceral and peripheral ischemia, all of which are detrimental to the patient's borderline physiology. Thus, aortic clamping, although at times a lifesaving maneuver in a crashing patient, must be used judiciously and performed carefully.

Maneuvers for Retroperitoneal Exposure

The major abdominal vessels are retroperitoneal structures that lie posterior to the content of the peritoneal sac and close to the midline. Rapid exposure of these relatively inaccessible structures hinges on two mobilization maneuvers that rotate the abdominal visceral content off the midline retroperitoneal structures.

Left-sided medial visceral rotation (Mattox maneuver) exposes the entire length of the abdominal aorta and its branches (except the right renal artery).[15] The correct plane is entered by incising the lateral peritoneal attachment of the sigmoid and left colon. The hand is then swept upward lateral to the left colon, kidney, and spleen (Fig. 67-5). The presence of a retroperitoneal hematoma greatly facilitates the dissection. The plane of dissection is developed bluntly in front of the left common iliac

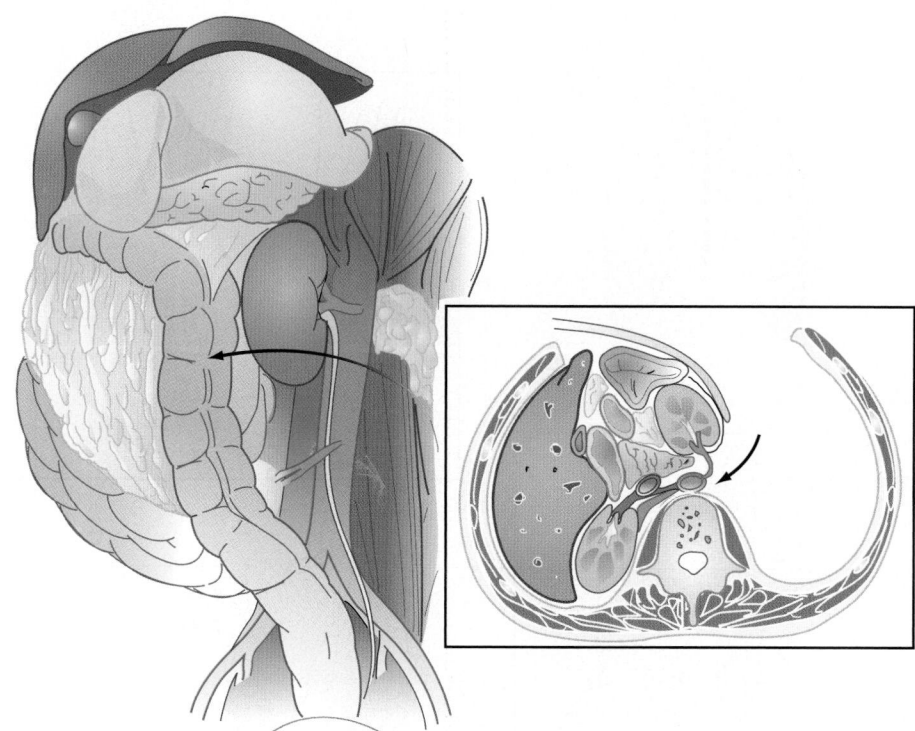

Figure 67-5 Left-sided medial visceral rotation (Mattox maneuver). (Illustration by Jan Redden after Jim Schmidt. © Kenneth L. Mattox, MD.)

vessels and behind the kidney, with the back of the dissecting hand sliding on the posterior abdominal wall muscles. The left-sided viscera (left colon, kidney, spleen, and pancreas) are brought to the midline, and the entire length of the abdominal aorta is thus exposed.

Right-sided medial visceral rotation (extended Kocher maneuver) consists of medial reflection of the right colon and duodenum by incising their lateral peritoneal attachments (Fig. 67-6). This exposure can be extended medially by detaching the posterior attachments of the small bowel mesentery toward the duodenojejunal ligament (Cattell-Braasch maneuver) (Fig. 67-7). The small bowel and the colon are reflected onto the lower chest, thus providing the widest possible exposure of the retroperitoneum, including the aorta, inferior vena cava, and iliac and renal vessels.

Approach to Retroperitoneal Hematoma

The location of a retroperitoneal hematoma and mechanism of injury guide the decision to explore the hematoma. The retroperitoneum is divided into three anatomic zones: the midline retroperitoneum (zone 1) (Fig. 67-8), the perinephric space (zone 2), and the pelvic retroperitoneum (zone 3).

Any hematoma in zone 1 mandates exploration for both penetrating and blunt injury because of the high likelihood and unforgiving nature of major vascular injury in this area. The transverse mesocolon is the dividing line between the supramesocolic and inframesocolic compartments. A central supramesocolic hematoma presents behind the lesser omentum, pushing the stomach forward, whereas an inframesocolic hematoma develops behind the root of the small bowel mesentery, pushing it forward in a configuration similar to that of a ruptured abdominal aortic aneurysm.[2,35]

This distinction between supramesocolic and inframesocolic hematoma has critical implications for proximal control and exposure. A supramesocolic hematoma is the result of injury to the suprarenal aorta, celiac axis, proximal superior mesenteric artery, or proximal part of a renal artery. Proximal control is obtained by clamping (or compressing) the aorta at the diaphragmatic hiatus, and the injured vessel is exposed by left-sided medial visceral rotation. A central inframesocolic hematoma is the result of injury to the infrarenal aorta or inferior vena cava. Proximal control is achieved at the supraceliac aorta, and exposure is provided by opening the posterior peritoneum in the midline, in much the same way as for an infrarenal aortic aneurysm.

A hematoma in zone 2 is the result of injury to the renal vessels or parenchyma and mandates exploration for penetrating trauma to assess the damage and repair the injuries. A nonexpanding stable hematoma resulting from a blunt trauma mechanism is better left unexplored because opening Gerota's fascia is very likely to result in further damage to the traumatized renal parenchyma and subsequent loss of the kidney. In the severely injured patient with a stable hematoma from a penetrating injury, it is advisable not to explore the injured kidney because the patient may not have the physiologic reserves to tolerate an elaborate and time-consuming repair.

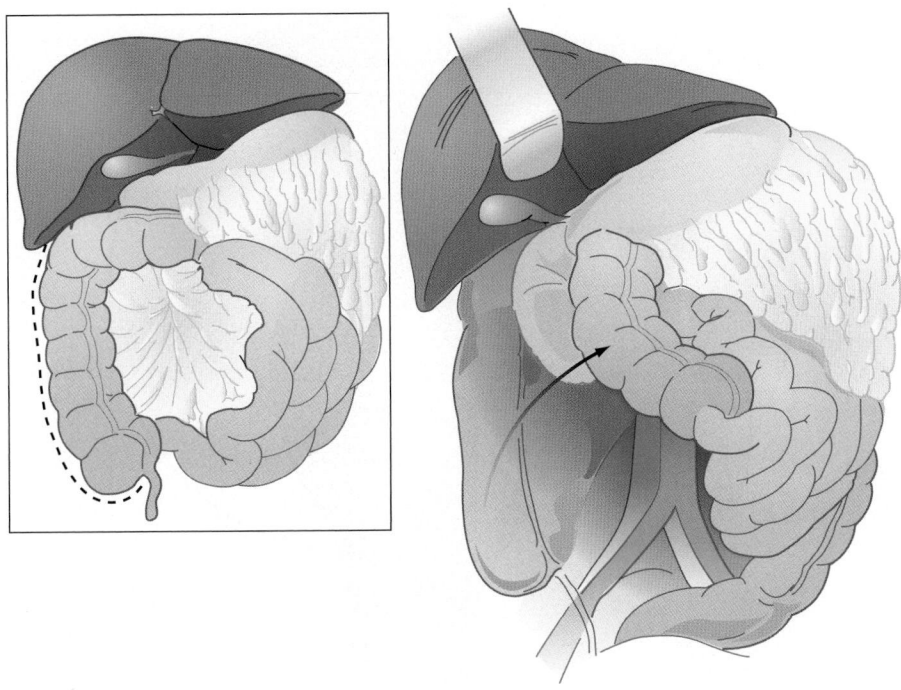

Figure 67-6 Right-sided medial visceral rotation (extended Kocher maneuver). (Illustration by Jan Redden. © Kenneth L. Mattox, MD.)

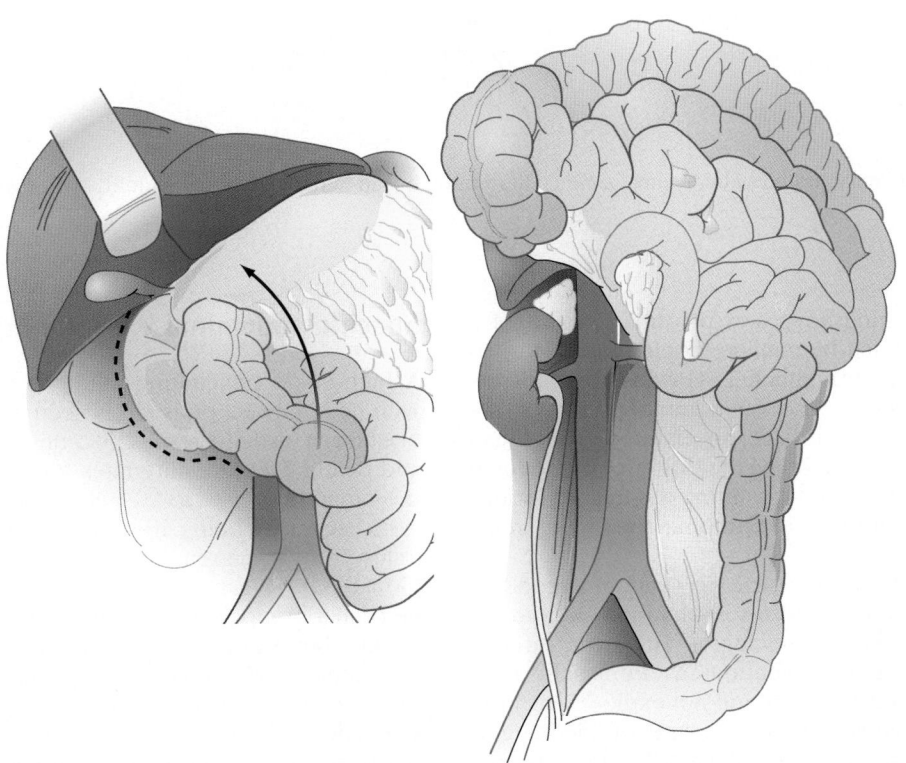

Figure 67-7 Extensive retroperitoneal exposure by the Cattell-Braasch maneuver. (Illustration by Jan Redden. © Kenneth L. Mattox, MD.)

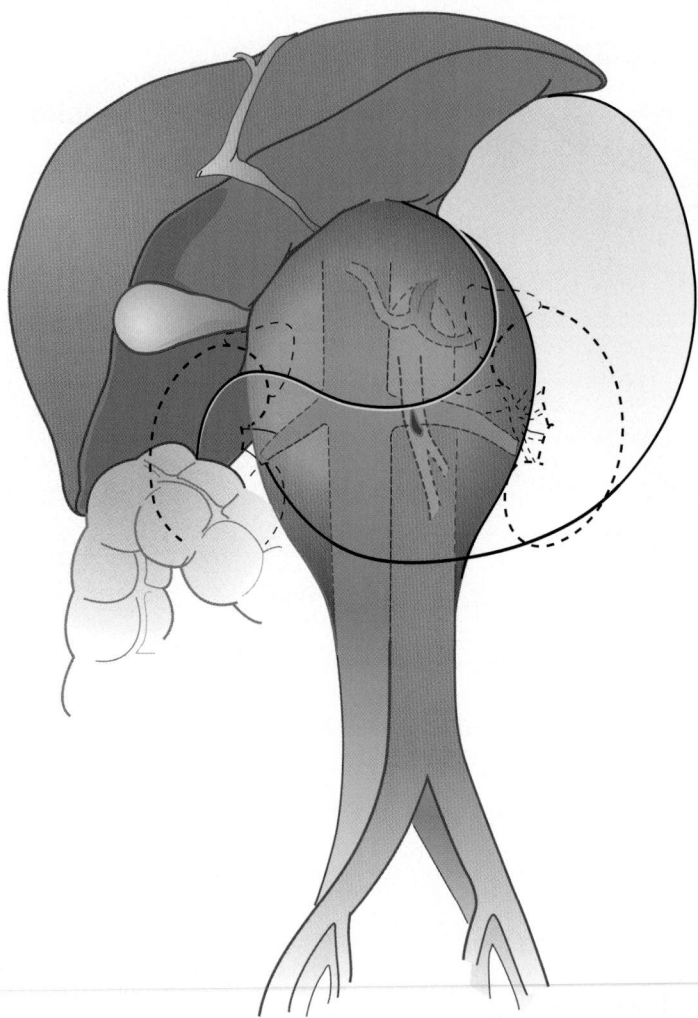

Figure 67-8 Retroperitoneal hematoma, zone 1. (Illustration by Jan Redden after Jim Schmidt. © Kenneth L. Mattox, MD.)

Traditional teaching advocates proximal control of a perinephric hematoma by midline looping of the ipsilateral artery and vein at the midline. However, this dissection is time-consuming and often unnecessary. In the presence of active hemorrhage, the injured kidney can be rapidly mobilized by incising the posterior peritoneum and Gerota's fascia lateral to it, lifting the injured kidney up and medially, and then clamping the entire renal hilum.

A pelvic retroperitoneal hematoma (zone 3) secondary to penetrating trauma mandates exploration because of the likelihood of iliac vessel injury. However, zone 3 hematomas resulting from blunt trauma are usually associated with pelvic fractures and are not explored because the effective management of this type of bleeding is based not on operative control (which rarely proves effective) but on external fixation or angiographic embolization of the bleeding vessels. The only exception is a rapidly expanding hematoma in which the surgeon suspects a major iliac vascular injury that requires operative repair.

Specific Abdominal Vascular Injuries

A high-grade penetrating injury to the abdominal aorta with near transection is rarely seen in the operating room because it usually results in immediate exsanguination and death. The mortality rates for abdominal aortic injuries range from 50% to 90%, with injuries to the perirenal aortic segment being the most lethal (>80% mortality), followed by suprarenal (50%-70%) and infrarenal injuries (50%-60%).[25] Clean lacerations of the aorta can sometimes be primarily repaired by transverse approximation of the lumen, but more often destruction of the aortic wall mandates prosthetic graft interposition. Despite theoretical concerns that spillage of intestinal content may cause synthetic graft infection, a synthetic graft is the only practical option, and graft infections after placement for penetrating trauma to the aorta have not been reported.

Blunt trauma to the abdominal aorta is very rare, usually the result of motor vehicle collision with impingement of the steering wheel or a seat belt. The most common location is the origin of the inferior mesenteric artery, and the clinical presentation is that of acute aortic thrombosis secondary to intimal disruption. The diagnosis is made at angiography, and operative repair usually requires a synthetic interposition graft.

Penetrating injuries to the iliac vessels carry high mortality rates (25%-40%) because exposure and control can be difficult, and associated injuries to adjacent abdominal organs are the rule rather than the exception.[36-38] Proximal control is initially obtained away from the injury, on the inframesocolic aorta and vena cava, and distal control is achieved on the external iliac vessels at the inguinal ligament by "towing in" with a large retractor to compress the iliac vessels against the edge of the bony pelvis. Reflection of the colon from its lateral peritoneal attachment on the relevant side unroofs the pelvic hematoma. Vascular control is then optimized by gradually advancing the clamps closer and closer to the injury as the dissection proceeds.

The iliac vessels are amenable to bail-out tactics such as temporary shunt insertion, balloon tamponade of a venous injury, or even arterial ligation with a delayed extra-anatomic reconstruction. Occasionally, the only way to gain access to an injured iliac vein is to divide the overlying common iliac artery and then reconstruct it after the venous repair has been completed.

The use of a synthetic graft for iliac artery reconstruction in the presence of peritoneal contamination is a cause for concern.[39] In the presence of limited spillage of small bowel content, use of a synthetic graft (after the bowel injury has been repaired and the field irrigated) is an acceptable option. However, with gross fecal contamination, ligation of the injured iliac artery and a subsequent femorofemoral bypass is the safe course of action.

A low threshold for fasciotomy is maintained after iliac vessel injuries because leg edema is common (particularly after iliac vein ligation) and repair of an iliac artery injury may be time-consuming and associated with prolonged ischemia. The hypotensive critically injured patient is particularly susceptible to the devastating effects of elevated compartment pressures.

Injuries to the superior mesenteric vessels present either as exsanguinating hemorrhage from the root of the mesentery, a supramesocolic central retroperitoneal hematoma, or ischemic bowel. The proximal segment of the superior mesenteric artery is exposed by left-sided medial visceral rotation, whereas the infrapancreatic segment is accessed by pulling the small bowel down and to the left and incising the peritoneum of the root of the mesentery. Another good option for exposure of the infrapancreatic segment is the Cattell-Braasch maneuver. The close proximity of the mesenteric vessels to the pancreatoduodenal complex, inferior vena cava, and the right renal pedicle means that severe associated injuries are the rule, opportunities for reconstruction are rare, and mortality is very high. The successful use of a temporary shunt in the superior mesenteric artery as a damage control technique has been reported. If graft interposition is required to reconstruct the superior mesenteric artery, a takeoff from the distal aorta above the bifurcation keeps

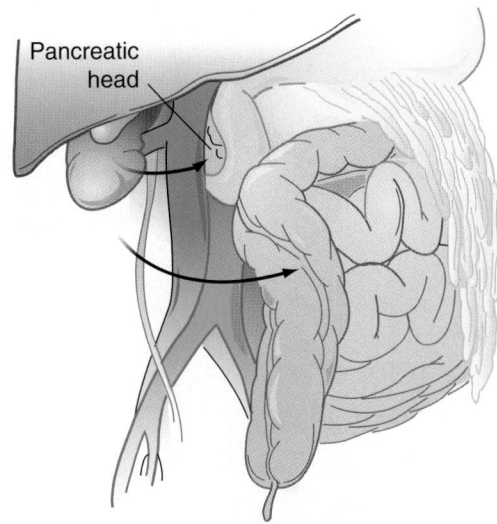

Figure 67-9 Right-sided medial rotation of the viscera to expose the inferior vena cava. (© Baylor College of Medicine, 1981.)

the suture line away from an injured pancreas. A second-look exploratory laparotomy is mandatory to assess the viability of the bowel. The injured superior mesenteric vein is repaired by lateral venorrhaphy when possible. Often the only technical option is ligation, which requires aggressive postoperative fluid resuscitation to compensate for ensuing massive splanchnic sequestration and may lead to venous gangrene of the bowel. A second-look laparotomy is mandatory.

Penetrating injuries to the renal arteries typically result in nephrectomy because associated injuries make complex vascular reconstruction of the renal artery an unattractive option. Blunt renovascular deceleration trauma is usually asymptomatic and is discovered when a kidney fails to opacify on CT. Arteriography is required for diagnosis and may document a spectrum of injuries ranging from intimal tear to complete renal artery thrombosis. Because blunt renovascular trauma is often associated with more life-threatening injuries, a significant diagnostic delay is common, and attempted renal salvage by major vascular reconstruction is usually not a practical option. For possible suitable operative candidates, the time limit that precludes a successful revascularization remains controversial. If 4 to 6 hours have elapsed since the injury and the renal artery is occluded, repair is not undertaken.

Injuries to the inferior vena cava (IVC) remain highly lethal, with mortality rates consistently in excess of 50%, particularly for the least accessible segments of the vein (iliac bifurcation, suprarenal and retrohepatic IVC).[2,40-44] The IVC is exposed by a right-sided medial visceral rotation (Fig. 67-9), and initial control is achieved by direct pressure above and below the injury (Fig. 67-10). The technical options for the infrarenal IVC are lateral repair or ligation.

Retrohepatic IVC injuries are especially unforgiving and difficult to access and control.[45] The typical operative findings are massive venous bleeding either through a deep hepatic wound or from the posterior aspect of a

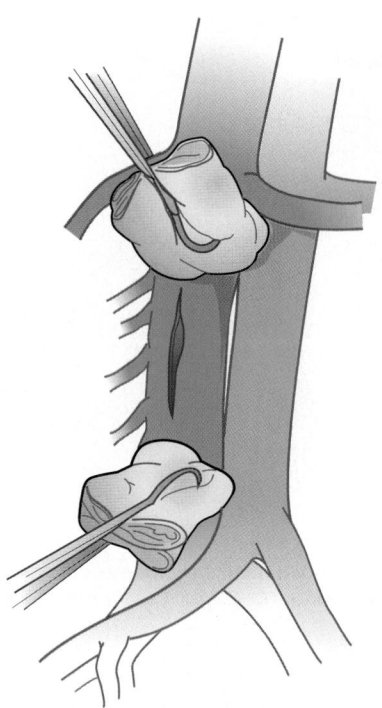

Figure 67-10 Compressing the inferior vena cava above and below the injury.

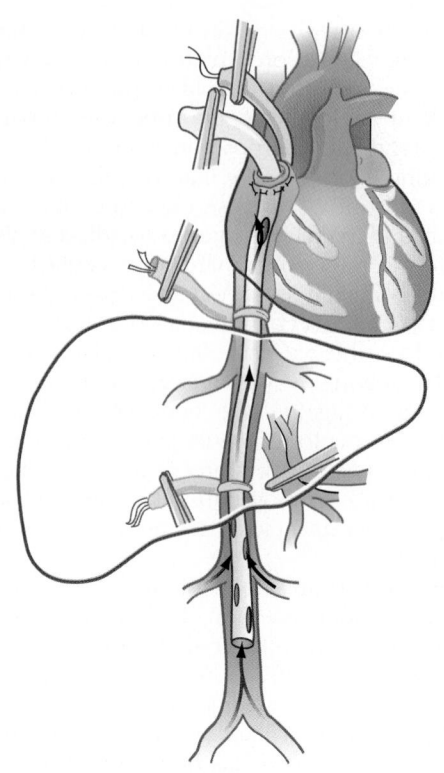

Figure 67-11 The atriocaval shunt. (© Baylor College of Medicine, 1984.)

severely injured liver. The bleeding is unaffected by a Pringle maneuver. Usually by the time the injury is recognized, the patient has already sustained massive blood loss and is in profound shock. Direct repair options for the retrohepatic IVC are complex and have dismal results. The most widely known technique is the atriocaval shunt first described by Schrock in 1968.[40,44,45] The atriocaval shunt uses either a chest tube or an endotracheal tube inserted through the right atrium to exclude the injured segment without compromising cardiac preload (Fig. 67-11). This technically demanding procedure requires familiarity with cardiac cannulation and is usually performed by two teams working simultaneously in the chest and abdomen. It is therefore not surprising that this elaborate technical maneuver, usually employed in dire circumstances, carries a reported mortality rate in excess of 80%. There is no optimal solution for the technical challenge of retrohepatic IVC trauma. Several authors have reported successful packing of these injuries, and this simple solution, if performed early and effectively, may prove the most practical solution for these inaccessible venous injuries.

PERIPHERAL VASCULAR TRAUMA

General Principles

Initial Assessment

Initial assessment and care of the patient with peripheral vascular trauma focuses on control of external hemorrhage and diagnosis of limb ischemia. In an ischemic extremity, assessing the severity of ischemia and identifying the arterial segment involved are the key considerations. It is extremely important to document the neurologic status of the injured extremity and to assess it for compartment syndrome. In the hemodynamically unstable trauma patient, a diminished arterial pulse or a cold and pale extremity is difficult to assess, so the diagnosis of ischemia often depends on comparison to the contralateral extremity.[24]

Although it is stated that restoration of arterial perfusion in less than 6 hours improves limb salvage rates, the window of opportunity for salvage is never a fixed interval but rather a flexible time frame that is heavily influenced by the site and nature of injury, the presence of efficient collaterals, and the patient's age and hemodynamic status. Of all the symptoms and signs of acute limb ischemia, a neurologic deficit conveys the greatest urgency because it signifies the imminent threat of an irreversible ischemic insult.

Noninvasive Vascular Diagnosis

The hand-held Doppler flow detector provides limited but useful qualitative information, especially in the hemodynamically unstable, cold, and vasoconstricted patient in whom diagnosis of limb ischemia is often difficult. The hand-held Doppler is a reliable screening tool for significant arterial obstruction after both blunt and penetrating trauma, and arteriography is indicated for any significant difference (>10 mm Hg) in ankle pressures between extremities. The hand-held Doppler is also useful in assessing severity of ischemia by determining the presence of an arterial and venous Doppler signal. Absence of the latter signifies grave ischemia.

Duplex scanning has an overall accuracy rate of about 98% in detecting clinically significant injuries. It can also detect minimal arterial injuries such as intimal flaps and small pseudoaneurysms. However, the routine use of Duplex ultrasonography in the acute admission area of many trauma centers is limited by logistical constraints. It remains a valuable tool for follow-up in patients with suspected or minimal vascular injuries, postoperative patients, and those with late complications of vascular trauma such as pseudoaneurysm and arteriovenous fistula.

Role of Arteriography

Arteriography is the definitive modality for diagnosing extremity arterial injuries in hemodynamically stable patients. It is indicated when the information gained can alter or facilitate the operative approach. In patients with multiple penetrations in an ischemic extremity and in those with blunt trauma (especially if several fractures are present), preoperative arteriography eliminates the need for extensive exposure and tedious exploration of the neurovascular bundle by precisely pinpointing the site of injury. In the actively bleeding patient, immediate surgical exploration without angiography is the correct course of action.

The use of arteriography to exclude arterial trauma in asymptomatic patients with penetrating wounds in proximity to the neurovascular bundle has changed in the past decade. Although previously considered a standard practice, it has been conclusively shown that physical examination accurately detects arterial injuries that require operative repair. If exclusion arteriography is routinely performed for proximity injuries, about 10% of patients will have an angiographic abnormality, but these lesions are minimal injuries that do not require operative repair and have a benign natural history. Based on these considerations, there is now conclusive evidence supporting a selective policy that avoids routine arteriography in asymptomatic patients with proximity injuries.

The Mangled Extremity

The decision to immediately amputate a severely wounded extremity (rather than attempt salvage) is difficult and emotionally charged, especially because vascular reconstruction is usually technically feasible, being one of the less problematic aspects of the injury. The *mangled extremity* is defined as injury that involves at least three of the four major tissue systems of a limb, consisting of bone, soft tissue, vessels, and nerves. Several scoring systems have been proposed to predict the ultimate fate of the limb based on the severity of injury and the patient's associated injuries and comorbid factors. However, in practice, the decision to proceed with amputation hinges on surgical judgment and the patient's specific circumstances. It is a team decision and is made only after careful examination and consideration. The decision is usually made in the operating room, where the mangled extremity can be meticulously examined

under optimal conditions. This is the only reliable way to assess the full extent of the damage, especially to nerve continuity, a critical factor in the decision process. Although the vascular injury itself is usually a less critical component than the neural damage or the ability to cover the vascular reconstruction with viable soft tissue, the total ischemia time is a major consideration in the decision to amputate. As a general rule, a totally interrupted distal innervation, extensive soft tissue destruction, and bone loss exceeding 6 cm in length all portend a grave prognosis for the limb.

Operative Technique

Although control of active hemorrhage is always a top priority, reconstruction of injured vessels must be carefully orchestrated with the management of bone and soft tissue injuries. It is preferable to achieve bone alignment before vascular reconstruction because orthopedic manipulation and reconstruction takes time and may disrupt the vascular repair. Thus, if the limb is not grossly ischemic, reduction and fixation of fractures is performed first. If the limb is ischemic, a temporary intraluminal shunt is inserted to maintain distal perfusion during the orthopedic procedure.

As in any type of vascular trauma, a key technical principle is to achieve proximal and distal control outside the hematoma and away from the area of active bleeding, using extensile exposure that can be carried proximally and distally as necessary.

The next step is to define the full extent of the injury and plan the necessary repair. In a contused vessel that remains in continuity, the key factor is integrity of the intima. An overlooked segment of injured intima can easily frustrate an otherwise meticulous arterial repair. The injury is carefully débrided and a reconstruction technique chosen depending on the specific circumstances in the operative field.

Because of the relatively small diameter of limb arteries, lateral repair is feasible only in a minority of patients: those with iatrogenic lacerations or a simple stab wound. Most injuries require end-to-end anastomosis or an interposition graft. The completely transected artery of a young patient typically retracts a surprising distance, making interposition graft the only practical option.

Before beginning the repair, a Fogarty thrombectomy is performed on both ends of the injured vessel to remove intraluminal clot and ascertain the presence of good inflow and backflow. The vessel ends are then irrigated with heparinized saline. Full systemic anticoagulation is often contraindicated in the patient with multiple injuries. If there is any uncertainty about the integrity or adequacy of the outflow tract, an intraoperative angiogram is performed before the reconstruction.

The small diameter of arteries in the arm and below the knee prohibits the use of synthetic material, making a segment of greater saphenous vein the ideal conduit in these locations. A synthetic graft is the preferred conduit in the thoracic outlet and above the groin. There is some controversy surrounding graft interposition of the femoral artery.[39] The traditional view that autogenous vein grafts have a better outcome in contaminated traumatic wounds is supported neither by clinical nor experimental data. Considerable evidence has accumulated to support the use of polytetrafluoroethylene (PTFE) grafts in a contaminated operative field because the material is resistant to dissolution by bacterial collagenase and fares better than a vein graft if soft tissue cover is lost. Use of a synthetic graft also expedites the operative procedure, an important consideration in severely injured patients.

Graft protection by adequate soft tissue cover is a fundamental principle in vascular surgery that is especially relevant in trauma. The graft must be routed through a noncontaminated field and must also be adequately covered with viable soft tissue. An exposed graft, even if patent, represents a serious threat, not only to the viability of the limb but also to the patient's life. Therefore, consideration of graft protection may dictate the use of a longer extra-anatomic route rather than a shorter but contaminated route and may also affect the operative sequence.

Vein Injuries

The need to repair injured peripheral veins and the long-term consequences of vein ligation in trauma patients remain the focus of active debate. The available evidence supports the repair of venous injuries encountered during exploration for an associated arterial trauma, but only if the patient is hemodynamically stable and the repair will not jeopardize or delay management of other significant injuries. Long-term patency rates of complex venous repairs (including interposition grafts using either saphenous vein or synthetic material) are poor. The best results are achieved by simple lateral repair that does not narrow the lumen or by end-to-end anastomosis. Contrary to previously held views, peripheral veins (including the popliteal vein) can be ligated without compromising adjacent arterial repairs or affecting limb salvage rates. The risk for long-term leg edema or chronic venous insufficiency is also very low.

Fasciotomy

Multiple factors contribute to the rapid dynamics of elevated compartment pressures in the patient with peripheral vascular injury: direct muscular trauma, hypotension, reperfusion of the ischemic extremity, and ligation of injured veins.[46,47] Compartment syndrome is common in these patients but is also notoriously difficult to diagnose early. Generalized edema, swelling of the injured extremity, and lack of communication with the patient all combine to deprive the surgeon of vital early clues. Arbitrary definitions of ischemic times are poor guidelines to the need for fasciotomy. Pressure measurement using a hand-held transducer is problematic in the hemodynamically labile patient, where the compartment pressure that compromises capillary perfusion may be significantly lower than in the stable patient. Therefore, the safest course of action is to maintain a low threshold for fasciotomy. Combined arterial and venous trauma, long delay between injury and revascularization, and extensive bone and soft tissue destruction are examples of clinical circumstances in which early fasciotomy is in the patient's best interest.

In lower extremity fasciotomy, the four compartments of the leg are all decompressed. This is most commonly achieved through two longitudinal incisions (Fig. 67-12). A longitudinal incision is made about 2 fingerbreadths lateral to the tibial crest, beginning immediately below the tibial tuberosity and extending to the ankle. Dividing the fascia along the line of incision decompresses the muscles of the anterior compartment, with special care

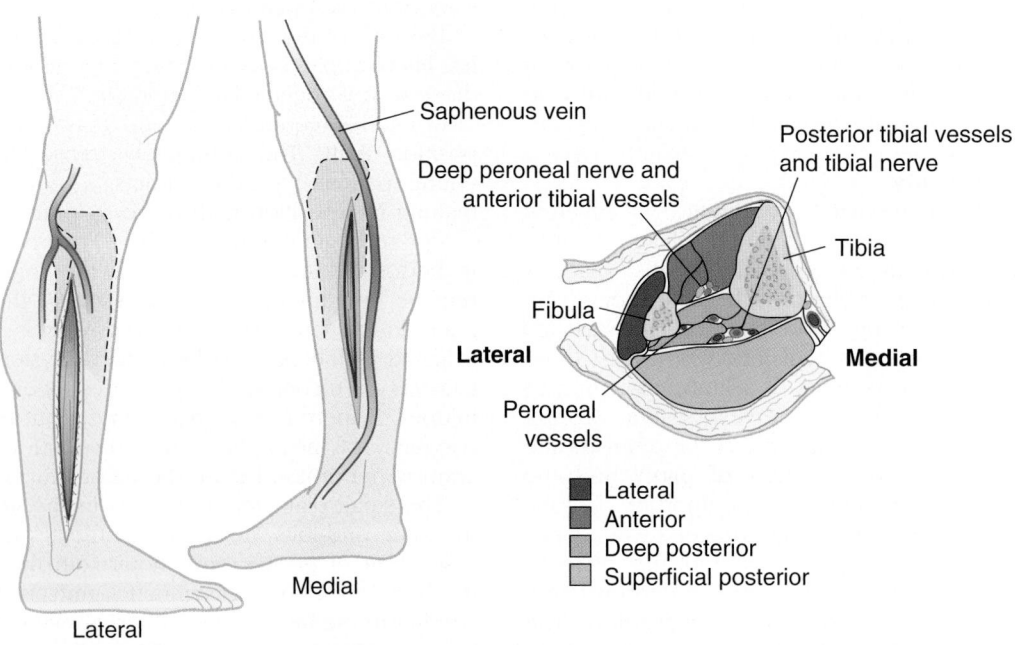

Figure 67-12 Fasciotomy.

being taken to divide the superior extensor retinaculum above the ankle. The surgeon then identifies the crural fascia between the anterior and lateral compartments and divides it along the entire length of the incision, taking care to avoid injury to the lateral peroneal nerve in the superior aspect of the incision, the most common iatrogenic injury during an anterior fasciotomy. The posterior compartments are decompressed through a separate medial incision placed immediately posterior to the posterior edge of the tibia, carefully avoiding injury to the long saphenous vein. The superficial posterior compartment is decompressed by incising the deep fascia. Detaching the soleus muscle from the posterior aspect of the tibia using the electrocautery opens the deep posterior compartment and completes the procedure.

Iatrogenic Trauma

Iatrogenic trauma to the femoral vessels in the groin can serve as a model of similar iatrogenic injuries in other anatomic locations. Bleeding from a groin puncture wound is often the result of inadequate groin compression after catheter removal. Ongoing hemorrhage into the subcutaneous tissue presents as an expanding hematoma, where the major concern is not massive blood loss but rather pressure necrosis of the overlying skin and compression of the cutaneous branches of the femoral nerve with a resulting painful neuralgia. The management is by operative decompression of the hematoma and repair of the injured femoral artery through a longitudinal groin incision. Proximal control can usually be obtained at or immediately above the inguinal ligament, and a simple hemostatic suture is all that is required.

An inadvertently high cannulation of the external iliac artery is difficult to compress effectively and may result in a large retroperitoneal hematoma. The patient typically presents with flank or groin pain and clinical signs of ongoing blood loss without a groin hematoma. Abdominal CT scan demonstrates the hematoma, and bleeding is usually self-limited. Rarely, hemodynamic deterioration leads to urgent operative repair of the injured external iliac artery.

Despite effective compression, a pseudoaneurysm may still develop at the puncture site. The typical presentation is groin pain and hematoma that may appear hours and even days after the arterial cannulation. With a large pseudoaneurysm, a pulsatile hematoma may be noted. Diagnosis of a pseudoaneurysm is made by color-flow Doppler ultrasound, and the initial treatment is by ultrasound-guided manual compression with the aim of inducing thrombosis of the pseudoaneurysm. The reported success rate of ultrasound-guided compression is 80% to 90% for small acute pseudoaneurysms but significantly lower for large ones and in anticoagulated patients. Thus, 20% to 30% of patients with iatrogenic femoral pseudoaneurysms still require operative repair.

Iatrogenic arteriovenous fistula is typically the result of a low groin puncture that perforates the superficial or deep femoral artery together with an adjacent vein. The resulting arteriovenous fistula is often asymptomatic and is incidentally discovered during color Doppler evaluation of a groin hematoma. A larger fistula may be associated with a continuous murmur and a palpable thrill. Small incidentally discovered fistulas usually have a benign natural history. They either close spontaneously or remain asymptomatic and do not require treatment. A large or symptomatic fistula may require surgical repair.

Arterial thrombosis is another frequently encountered type of iatrogenic injury. It is more common with large-bore cannulations in patients with atherosclerosis of the common femoral artery. The underlying mechanism is an intimal flap or fracture of a small segment of the arterial wall that leads to thrombosis. Understanding this mechanism of injury is the key to an effective repair because simple thrombectomy will not suffice. The underlying intimal injury must be identified and repaired, sometimes by means of a patch angioplasty.

Management of Specific Injuries

Most injuries to the common or superficial femoral arteries are penetrating. Proximal control for a high thigh or groin wound is usually obtained through a longitudinal groin incision using the inguinal ligament as a guide to dissection. The inguinal ligament limits the upward extension of a groin hematoma. Therefore, by carrying the dissection through the inguinal ligament and into the preperitoneal fat behind and above it, the surgeon can rapidly identify and control the distal external iliac artery before addressing the hematoma itself. Alternatively, the external iliac artery can be exposed through a separate oblique incision above and parallel to the inguinal ligament, using a retroperitoneal approach. Dissection can then proceed inside the femoral triangle to expose the injured vessels. The deep femoral artery needs to be identified and preserved during reconstruction of an injured common femoral artery.

The superficial femoral artery in Hunter's canal is exposed through a medial longitudinal thigh incision. The sartorius muscle is mobilized and retracted, exposing the roof of Hunter's canal. Special care must be taken to preserve the saphenous nerve lying on the anterior aspect of the artery.

Popliteal artery injuries result in limb loss more often than any other peripheral vascular injury. Amputation rates as high as 20% have been reported, especially from blunt trauma. The collateral arterial system around the knee is not well developed and is very susceptible to interruption by significant trauma, making delays in diagnosis and treatment particularly unforgiving. Posterior dislocation of the knee is associated with popliteal artery injury in one of every 3 to 5 patients, but other types of blunt trauma around the knee, such as a bumper injury to the proximal tibia or any injury that causes an unstable knee joint, are also likely to damage the artery. Most patients present with a clearly ischemic extremity, where the indication for an urgent surgical exploration is obvious. In the absence of associated injuries, some surgeons administer IV heparin preoperatively to prevent thrombosis of the distal capillary bed, a major concern with popliteal injuries. A full fasciotomy is performed before the vascular exploration in a grossly ischemic leg. In about 30% of patients, the clinical presentation is less clear because the limb is not grossly ischemic. The key to avoiding undue delays is a high index of suspicion and a low threshold for angiography whenever significant blunt trauma has affected the area around the knee.

The proximal popliteal artery is exposed through an incision along the anterior border of the sartorius muscle above the knee. The deep fascia is incised, and the sartorius is retracted, providing access to the popliteal space between the semimembranosus muscle and the adductor magnus tendon. The distal artery is approached through a medial incision immediately behind the posterior border of the tibia. The crural fascia is incised, and the popliteal space is entered between the medial head of the gastrocnemius and the soleus muscles. Wide exposure of the entire length of the popliteal artery can be achieved by joining the incisions and dividing the tendons of the semitendinosus, semimembranosus, gracilis, and sartorius and then dividing the medial head of the gastrocnemius. In most patients, the artery is repaired using a saphenous vein interposition graft from the contralateral extremity. On completion of the reconstruction, an intraoperative angiogram is obtained. An associated vein injury is repaired if the clinical circumstances allow, but venous reconstruction does not affect the eventual outcome of the arterial repair. In the absence of active bleeding from the injured popliteal artery, a more expedient approach is a bypass and exclusion technique. The proximal and distal popliteal artery is exposed and isolated through separate incisions, a saphenous vein graft is then tunneled between the exposed segments to bypass the injury and anastomosed proximally and distally using an end-to-end technique, thus excluding the injured segment without exposing it.

Penetrating injuries to the lower leg arteries below the popliteal trifurcation usually present with bleeding and progressive swelling of the calf. If one of the three shank arteries is involved, hemostasis can be achieved either by angiographic embolization or operative ligation. Patients with severe blunt trauma to the lower leg usually present with a combination of extensive bone and soft tissue damage as well as diminished or absent pedal pulses. Physical examination is unreliable under these circumstances, and angiography is used to diagnose or exclude an arterial injury. The traditional teaching to maintain patency of at least two shank arteries after blunt trauma is unproved. Exploration and repair of the lower leg arteries is technically difficult in the hostile circumstances created by adjacent bone and soft tissue injuries and can safely be avoided in the presence of a single patent artery. There is, however, evidence to suggest that if the only remaining intact vessel is the peroneal artery, this may not suffice to prevent foot ischemia.

Exposure of the lower leg arteries is best begun proximally, away from the area of injury (Fig. 67-13). The distal popliteal artery is exposed below the knee through a medial approach, and dissection is continued distally by detaching the soleus muscle from the posterior border of the tibia, thus providing access to the posterior tibial and peroneal arteries. The anterior tibial artery is approached through a separate anterolateral incision between the tibialis anterior and the extensor hallucis longus muscles.

Most axillary artery injuries are penetrating, resulting in hemorrhage or distal ischemia. In most published series, injuries to the subclavian and axillary vessels are treated as a single clinical entity. Extending a subclavian incision into the medial aspect of the abducted upper arm exposes the axillary artery. The incision is carried through the pectoral fascia, and the pectoralis major muscle can be either split or divided depending on the exposure required. The pectoralis minor muscle is then retracted or divided, and the clavipectoral fascia is opened, exposing the neurovascular bundle in the axillary sheath.

Injuries to the brachial artery account for 20% to 30% of peripheral arterial injuries, making this vessel the most frequently injured artery in the body. The artery is exposed through a medial arm incision in the groove between the biceps and triceps muscles. The first structure encountered in the neurovascular bundle is the median nerve, which must be isolated and preserved. If the brachial artery is exposed in the proximal arm, the deep brachial artery is identified and controlled at the lateral border of the teres major muscle.

Most isolated ulnar or radial artery injuries can be ligated with impunity. An ischemic hand (due to an incomplete palmar arch or injury to both arteries) requires an arterial reconstruction. In the presence of associated bone and soft tissue injury, it is often safest to begin the exposure of a radial artery proximally at the brachial bifurcation and then proceed distally to the injured segment. A lower medial arm incision is carried into the antecubital fossa in an S-shaped configuration to avoid a longitudinal incision across the antecubital skin crease. The bicipital aponeurosis is divided to expose the brachial bifurcation, and the radial artery is identified and isolated. Exposure of the ulnar artery in the proximal forearm is more difficult because of the deeper location of the artery at this level. It is found deep to the antebrachial fascia, between the flexor carpi ulnaris and flexor digitorum superficialis muscles.

CONCLUSION

There are several important differences between vascular trauma and other types of vascular disease. One salient feature of vascular trauma is the constant need to consider the injury and the various therapeutic options within the context of the patient's overall trauma burden. Purposeful delay in the operative repair of blunt aortic injury and the decision to employ damage control tactics during laparotomy for combined vascular and hollow visceral injury are but two examples of this key principle.

In the severely injured patient, management priorities change constantly, and the surgeon must not only tailor the technical solution to the specific clinical circumstances but also be prepared to modify it or improvise a new solution as the circumstances change. The sequencing of the orthopedic and vascular repairs in the severely wounded extremity illustrates this need for flexibility.

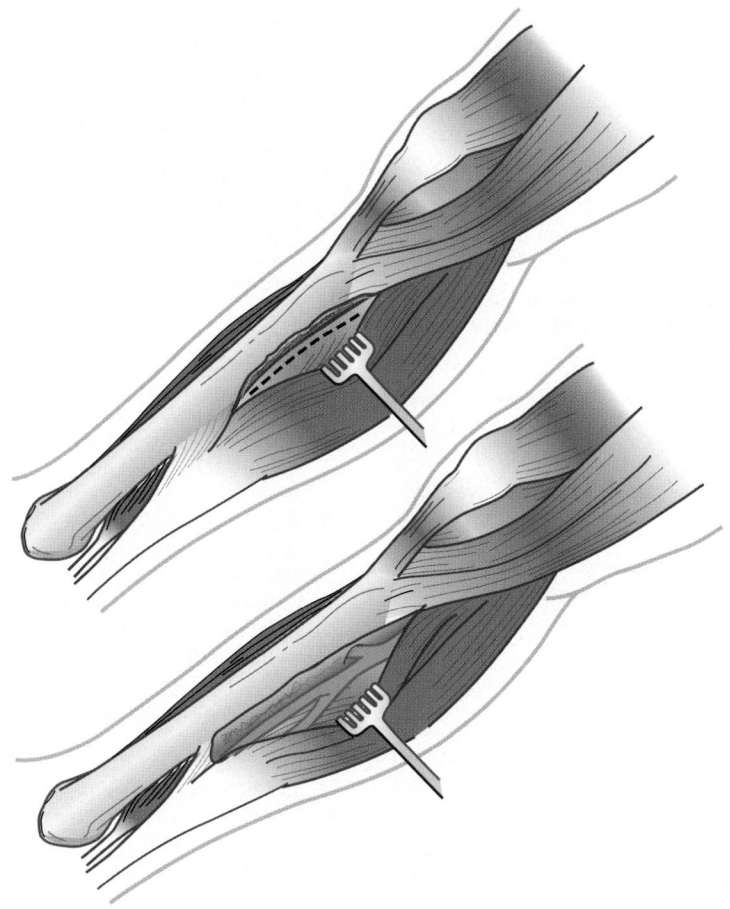

Figure 67-13 Exposure of tibial vessels. (Illustration by Jan Redden. © Kenneth L. Mattox, MD.)

The successful management of major vascular trauma hinges on the adaptation of standard vascular surgical techniques to nonstandard situations. The use of temporary intraluminal shunts and balloon catheter tamponade demonstrates how standard technical adjuncts have been adapted to provide new solutions in difficult situations.

Endovascular therapy offers a new array of management options for vascular trauma, and its minimally invasive nature is particularly suited to the critically injured patient with strained physiologic reserves. Endovascular solutions are playing an increasing role in the management of truncal vascular injuries in nonbleeding patients.

Current advances in understanding the pathophysiology of trauma and innovative technology for vascular diagnosis and therapy are rapidly converging to provide the trauma surgeon of the future with an exciting selection of new tools. These tools will be used to further push the therapeutic envelope and continuously improve outcome in the management of the patient with major vascular injury.

Selected References

Hirshberg A, Mattox KL: Top knife: The art and craft of trauma surgery. Shrewsbury, UK Publishing Ltd, 2004

A short and user-friendly manual of operative trauma surgery that includes detailed descriptions of the operative approach to major vascular injuries, with a special emphasis on vascular "damage control" techniques.

Rich NM, Mattox KL, Hirshberg A (eds): Vascular Trauma, 2nd ed. Philadelphia, Elsevier-Saunders, 2004.

The second edition of this classic textbook contains detailed discussions of every aspect of the modern management of major vascular injuries, operative and endovascular management options, techniques, and complications.

Bickell WH, Wall MJ Jr, Pepe PE, et al: Immediate versus delayed fluid resuscitation for hypotensive patients with penetrating torso injuries. N Engl J Med 331:1105-1109, 1994.

The only prospective randomized study in the literature that examined delayed fluid resuscitation in penetrating torso trauma and showed that delayed fluid resuscitation favorably affects outcome.

Buckner BA, DiBardino DJ, Cumbie TC, et al: Critical evaluation of chest computed tomography scans for blunt descending thoracic aortic injury. Ann Thorac Surg 81:1339-1346, 2006.

A critical evaluation of the utility of CT scanning as a screening versus a diagnostic test in patient with proximal descending aortic blunt injury

Burch JM, Richardson RJ, Martin RR, et al: Penetrating iliac vascular injuries: Recent experience with 233 consecutive patients. J Trauma 30:1450-1459, 1990.

The largest series in the literature, with a detailed discussion of the various technical options for control and repair of these devastating injuries.

Fabian TC, Richardson JD, Croce MA, et al: Prospective study of blunt aortic injury: Multicenter Trial of the American Association for the Surgery of Trauma. J Trauma 42:374-383, 1997.

This study showed that aortic clamp times under 30 minutes and bypass techniques that provide for distal aortic perfusion are associated with a lower risk for paraplegia.

Mattox KL, Feliciano DV, Burch J, et al: Five thousand seven hundred sixty cardiovascular injuries in 4459 patients: Epidemiologic evolution 1958 to 1987. Ann Surg 209:698-707, 1989.

The largest epidemiologic study in the literature on civilian vascular injuries.

Parker MS, Matheson TL, Rao AV, et al: Making the transition: The role of helical CT in the evaluation of potentially acute thoracic aortic injuries. AJR Am J Roentgenol 176:1267-1272, 2001.

Helical CT has a sensitivity and negative predictive value comparable to aortography.

Pratesi C, Dorigo W, Troisi N, et al: Acute traumatic rupture of the descending thoracic aorta: Endovascular treatment. Am J Surg 192:291-295, 2006.

A contemporary review of the utility and some of the difficulties encountered with using endografting as a standard treatment in thoracic aortic injury.

Valentine RJ, Wind GG: Anatomic Exposures in Vascular Surgery. Philadelphia, Lippincott Williams & Wilkins, 2003.

A modern text on exposure and access techniques in vascular surgery.

References

1. Bickell WH, Wall MJ Jr, Pepe PE, et al: Immediate versus delayed fluid resuscitation for hypotensive patients with penetrating torso injuries. N Engl J Med 331:1105-1109, 1994.
2. Asensio JA, Chahwan S, Hanpeter D, et al: Operative management and outcome of 302 abdominal vascular injuries. Am J Surg 180:528-534, 2000.
3. Mattox KL, Feliciano DV, Burch J, et al: Five thousand seven hundred sixty cardiovascular injuries in 4459 patients: Epidemiologic evolution 1958 to 1987. Ann Surg 209:698-707, 1989.
4. Hirshberg A, Wall MJ Jr, Allen MK, et al: Causes and patterns of missed injuries in trauma. Am J Surg 168:299-303, 1994.
5. Villas PA, Cohen G, Putnam SG III, et al: Wallstent placement in a renal artery after blunt abdominal trauma. J Trauma 46:1137-1139, 1999.
6. Mattox KL, Whigham C, Fisher RG, Wall MJ Jr: Blunt trauma to the thoracic aorta: Current challenges. In Lumsden AB, Lin PH, Chen C, and Parodi J (eds): Advanced Endovascular Therapy of Aortic Disease. London, Blackwell Publishing, 2007.
7. Lin P, Lumsden A: Traumatic thoracic aortic injury. Endovascular Today 5:58-66, 2006.
8. Pratesi C, Dorigo W, Troisi N, et al: Acute traumatic rupture of the descending thoracic aorta: Endovascular treatment. Am J Surg 192:291-295, 2006.
9. Tehrani HY, Peterson BG, Katariya K, et al: Endovascular repair of thoracic aortic tears. Ann Thorac Surg 82:873-878, 2006.
10. Orford VP, Atkinson NR, Thomson K, et al: Blunt traumatic aortic transection: The endovascular experience. Ann Thorac Surg 75:106-112, 2003.
11. Aucar JA, Hirshberg A: Damage control for vascular injuries. Surg Clin North Am 77:853-862, 1997.
12. Feliciano DV, Burch JM, Mattox KL, et al: Balloon catheter tamponade in cardiovascular wounds. Am J Surg 160:583-587, 1990.
13. Hirshberg A, Wall MJ, Johnston RH Jr, et al: Transcervical gunshot injuries. Am J Surg 167:309-312, 1994.
14. Valentine RJ, Wind GG: Anatomic Exposures in Vascular Surgery. Philadelphia, Lippincott Williams & Wilkins, 2003.
15. Mattox KL, McCollum WB, Jordan GL Jr, et al: Management of upper abdominal vascular trauma. Am J Surg 128:823-828, 1974.
16. Dawson DL, Putnam AT, Light JT, et al: Temporary arterial shunts to maintain limb perfusion after arterial injury: An animal study. J Trauma 47:64-71, 1999.
17. Biffl WL, Moore EE, Elliott JP, et al: The devastating potential of blunt vertebral arterial injuries. Ann Surg 231:672-681, 2000.
18. Biffl WL, Moore EE, Mestek M: Patients with blunt carotid and vertebral artery injuries. J Trauma 47:438-439, 1999.
19. Biffl WL, Moore EE, Ryu RK, et al: The unrecognized epidemic of blunt carotid arterial injuries: Early diagnosis improves neurologic outcome. Ann Surg 228:462-470, 1998.
20. Miller PR, Fabian TC, Bee TK, et al: Blunt cerebrovascular injuries: Diagnosis and treatment. J Trauma 51:279-286, 2001.
21. Giacobetti FB, Vaccaro AR, Bos-Giacobetti MA, et al: Vertebral artery occlusion associated with cervical spine trauma: A prospective analysis. Spine 22:188-192, 1997.
22. Weller SJ, Rossitch E Jr, Malek AM: Detection of vertebral artery injury after cervical spine trauma using magnetic resonance angiography. J Trauma 46:660-666, 1999.
23. Willis BK, Greiner F, Orrison WW, et al: The incidence of vertebral artery injury after midcervical spine fracture or subluxation. Neurosurgery 34:435-442, 1994.
24. Britt LD, Weireter LJ, Cole FJ: Newer diagnostic modalities for vascular injuries: The way we were, the way we are. Surg Clin North Am 81:1263-1279, xii, 2001.
25. Mattox KL: Red River anthology. J Trauma 42:353-368, 1997.
26. Weiman DS, Gurbuz AT, Gursky A, et al: Comparison of spinal cord protection using left atrial-femoral with femoral-femoral bypass in patients with traumatic rupture of the aortic isthmus. World J Surg 30:1638-1641, 2006.
27. Buckner BA, DiBardino DJ, Cumbie TC, et al: Critical evaluation of chest computed tomography scans for blunt descending thoracic aortic injury. Ann Thorac Surg 81:1339-1346, 2006.
28. Berland LL, Smith JK: Multidetector-array CT: Once again, technology creates new opportunities. Radiology 209:327-329, 1998.
29. Horrocks JA, Speller RD: Short communication. Helical computed tomography: Where is the cut? Br J Radiol 67:107-111, 1994.
30. Parker MS, Matheson TL, Rao AV, et al: Making the transition: The role of helical CT in the evaluation of potentially

acute thoracic aortic injuries. AJR Am J Roentgenol 176:1267-1272, 2001.

31. Fabian TC, Richardson JD, Croce MA, et al: Prospective study of blunt aortic injury: Multicenter Trial of the American Association for the Surgery of Trauma. J Trauma 42:374-383, 1997.

32. Pate JW, Fabian TC, Walker WA: Acute traumatic rupture of the aortic isthmus: Repair with cardiopulmonary bypass. Ann Thorac Surg 59:90-99, 1995.

33. Carrillo EH, Bergamini TM, Miller FB, et al: Abdominal vascular injuries. J Trauma 43:164-171, 1997.

34. Coimbra R, Hoyt D, Winchell R, et al: The ongoing challenge of retroperitoneal vascular injuries. Am J Surg 172:541-545, 1996.

35. Jurkovich GJ, Hoyt DB, Moore FA, et al: Portal triad injuries. J Trauma 39:426-434, 1995.

36. Burch JM, Richardson RJ, Martin RR, et al: Penetrating iliac vascular injuries: Recent experience with 233 consecutive patients. J Trauma 30:1450-1459, 1990.

37. Carrillo EH, Spain DA, Wilson MA, et al: Alternatives in the management of penetrating injuries to the iliac vessels. J Trauma 44:1024-1030, 1998.

38. Cushman JG, Feliciano DV, Renz BM, et al: Iliac vessel injury: Operative physiology related to outcome. J Trauma 42:1033-1040, 1997.

39. Feliciano DV, Mattox KL, Graham JM, et al: Five-year experience with PTFE grafts in vascular wounds. J Trauma 25:71-82, 1985.

40. Burch JM, Feliciano DV, Mattox KL: The atriocaval shunt: Facts and fiction. Ann Surg 207:555-568, 1988.

41. Burch JM, Feliciano DV, Mattox KL, et al: Injuries of the inferior vena cava. Am J Surg 156:548-552, 1988.

42. Kuehne J, Frankhouse J, Modrall G, et al: Determinants of survival after inferior vena cava trauma. Am Surg 65:976-981, 1999.

43. Porter JM, Ivatury RR, Islam SZ, et al: Inferior vena cava injuries: Noninvasive follow-up of venorrhaphy. J Trauma 42:913-918, 1997.

44. Schrock T, Blaisdell FW, Mathewson C Jr: Management of blunt trauma to the liver and hepatic veins. Arch Surg 96:698-704, 1968.

45. Cue JI, Cryer HG, Miller FB, et al: Packing and planned reexploration for hepatic and retroperitoneal hemorrhage: Critical refinements of a useful technique. J Trauma 30:1007-1113, 1990.

46. Feliciano DV, Cruse PA, Spjut-Patrinely V, et al: Fasciotomy after trauma to the extremities. Am J Surg 156:533-536, 1988.

47. Fainzilber G, Roy-Shapira A, Wall MJ Jr, et al: Predictors of amputation for popliteal artery injuries. Am J Surg 170:568-571, 1995.

Venous Disease

Julie A. Freischlag, MD   and   Jennifer A. Heller, MD

Anatomy
Primary Venous Insufficiency
Deep Venous Thrombosis of the Lower Extremity
Deep Venous Thrombosis of the Upper Extremity
Conclusion

An understanding of venous physiology provides the surgeon with valuable information with which to formulate a diagnosis and treatment plan. Recent technologic advances have broadened the therapeutic armamentarium. This chapter will provide the reader with a thorough overview of the physiology and pathophysiology of veins, followed by an evaluation of available diagnostic modalities and therapeutic interventions, and finally a discussion of specific venous disorders.

ANATOMY

To determine whether pathophysiology is present, precise knowledge of venous anatomy is essential. After the location and type of venous incompetence are determined, a therapeutic plan can then be constructed. Venous drainage of the legs is the function of two parallel and connected systems: the deep and the superficial systems. The nomenclature of the venous system of the lower limb has undergone a revision, and the most relevant changes are addressed here.[1] The revised nomenclature is delineated in Tables 68-1 and 68-2.

Superficial Venous System

The superficial veins of the lower extremity form a network that connects the superficial dorsal veins of the foot and the deep plantar veins. The dorsal venous arch, into which empty the dorsal metatarsal veins, is continuous with the greater saphenous vein medially and the lesser saphenous vein laterally (Fig. 68-1).

The greater saphenous vein, in close proximity to the saphenous nerve, ascends anterior to the medial malleolus, crosses, and then ascends medial to the knee (Fig. 68-2). It ascends in the superficial compartment and empties into the common femoral vein after entering the fossa ovalis. Before its entry into the common femoral vein, it receives medial and lateral accessory saphenous veins, as well as small tributaries from the inguinal region, pudendal region, and anterior abdominal wall. The posterior arch vein drains the area around the medial malleolus, and as it ascends up the posterior medial aspect of the calf, it receives medial perforating veins, termed *Cockett's perforators,* before joining the greater saphenous vein at or below the knee.

The lesser saphenous vein arises from the dorsal venous arch at the lateral aspect of the foot and ascends posterior to the lateral malleolus, and it empties into the popliteal vein after penetrating the fascia. The exact entry of the lesser saphenous vein into the popliteal vein is variable. The sural nerve closely accompanies the lesser saphenous vein.

Deep Venous System

The plantar digital veins in the foot empty into a network of metatarsal veins that compose the deep plantar venous arch. This continues into the medial and lateral plantar veins that then drain into the posterior tibial veins. The

Table 68-1 **Superficial Veins**

TERMINOLOGICA ANATOMICA	PROPOSED TERMINOLOGY
Greater or long saphenous vein	Great saphenous vein Superficial inguinal veins
External pudendal vein	External pudendal vein
Superficial circumflex vein	Superficial circumflex iliac vein
Superficial epigastric vein	Superficial epigastric vein
Superficial dorsal vein of clitoris or penis	Superficial dorsal vein of clitoris or penis
Anterior labial veins	Anterior labial veins
Anterior scrotal veins	Anterior scrotal veins
Accessory saphenous vein	Anterior accessory great saphenous vein Posterior accessory great saphenous vein Superficial accessory great saphenous vein
Smaller or short saphenous vein	Small saphenous vein Cranial extension of small saphenous vein Superficial accessory small saphenous vein Anterior thigh circumflex vein Posterior thigh circumflex vein Intersaphenous veins Lateral venous system
Dorsal venous network of the foot	Dorsal venous network of the foot
Dorsal venous arch of the foot	Dorsal venous arch of the foot
Dorsal metatarsal veins	Superficial metatarsal veins (dorsal and plantar)
Plantar venous network Plantar venous arch	Plantar venous subcutaneous network
Plantar metatarsal veins	Superficial digital veins (dorsal and plantar)
Lateral marginal vein	Lateral marginal vein
Medial marginal vein	Medial marginal vein

Table 68-2 **Deep Veins**

TERMINOLOGICA ANATOMICA	PROPOSED TERMINOLOGY
Femoral vein	Common femoral vein Femoral vein
Profunda femoris vein or deep vein of thigh	Profunda femoris vein or deep femoral vein
Medial circumflex femoral vein	Medial circumflex femoral vein
Lateral circumflex femoral vein	Lateral circumflex femoral vein
Perforating veins	Deep femoral communicating veins (accompanying veins of perforating arteries) Sciatic vein
Popliteal vein	Popliteal vein Sural veins Soleal veins Gastrocnemius veins Medial gastrocnemius veins Lateral gastrocnemius veins Intergemellar vein
Genicular veins	Genicular venous plexus
Anterior tibial veins	Anterior tibial veins
Posterior tibial veins	Posterior tibial veins
Fibular or peroneal veins	Fibular or peroneal veins Medial plantar veins Lateral plantar veins Deep plantar venous arch Deep metatarsal veins (plantar and dorsal) Deep digital veins (plantar and dorsal) Pedal vein

dorsalis pedis veins on the dorsum of the foot form the paired anterior tibial veins at the ankle.

The paired posterior tibial veins, adjacent to and flanking the posterior tibial artery, run under the fascia of the deep posterior compartment. These veins enter the soleus and join the popliteal vein, after joining with the paired peroneal and anterior tibial veins. There are large venous sinuses within the soleus muscle—the soleal sinuses—that empty into the posterior tibial and peroneal veins. There are bilateral gastrocnemius veins that empty into the popliteal vein distal to the point of entry of the lesser saphenous vein into the popliteal vein.

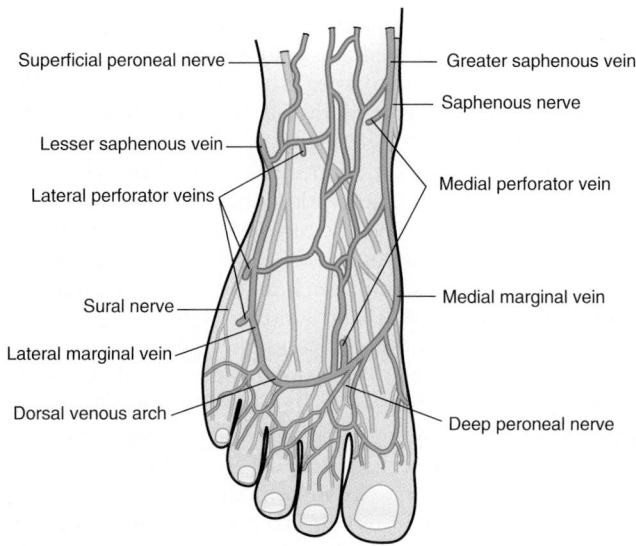

Figure 68-1 Venous drainage of the foot.

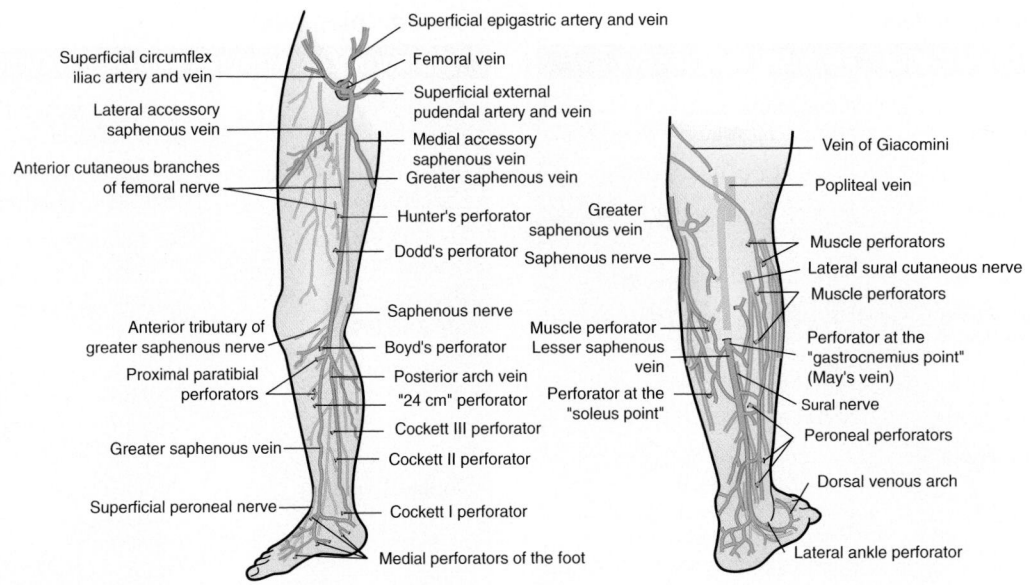

Figure 68-2 Venous drainage of the lower limb.

The popliteal vein enters a window in the adductor magnus, at which point it is termed the *femoral vein,* previously termed the *superficial femoral vein.* The femoral vein ascends and receives venous drainage from the profunda femoris vein, or the deep femoral vein, and after this confluence, it is the *common femoral vein.* As the common femoral vein crosses the inguinal ligament, it becomes the *external iliac vein.*

Perforating veins connect the superficial venous system to the deep venous system at various points in the leg: the foot, the medial and lateral calf, and the mid and distal thigh (Fig. 68-3). These perforating branches are extremely variable. The perforating veins in the foot are either valveless or have valves directing blood from the deep to the superficial venous system.

Normal Venous Histology and Function

The venous wall is composed of three layers: the intima, the media, and the adventitia. Vein walls have less smooth muscle and elastin than their arterial counterparts. The venous intima has an endothelial cell layer resting on a basement membrane. The media is composed of smooth muscle cells and elastin connective tissue. The adventitia of the venous wall contains adrenergic fibers, particularly in the cutaneous veins. Central sympathetic discharge and brainstem thermoregulatory centers can alter venous tone, as can other stimuli, such as temperature changes, pain, emotional stimuli, and volume changes.

The histologic features of veins vary depending on the caliber of the veins. The venules, the smallest veins ranging from 0.1 to 1 mm, contain mostly smooth muscle cells, whereas the larger extremity veins contain relatively few smooth muscle cells. These larger-caliber veins have limited contractile capacity in comparison to the thicker-walled greater saphenous vein. The venous valves prevent retrograde flow, and it is their failure or valvular incompetence that leads to reflux and its associated symptoms.

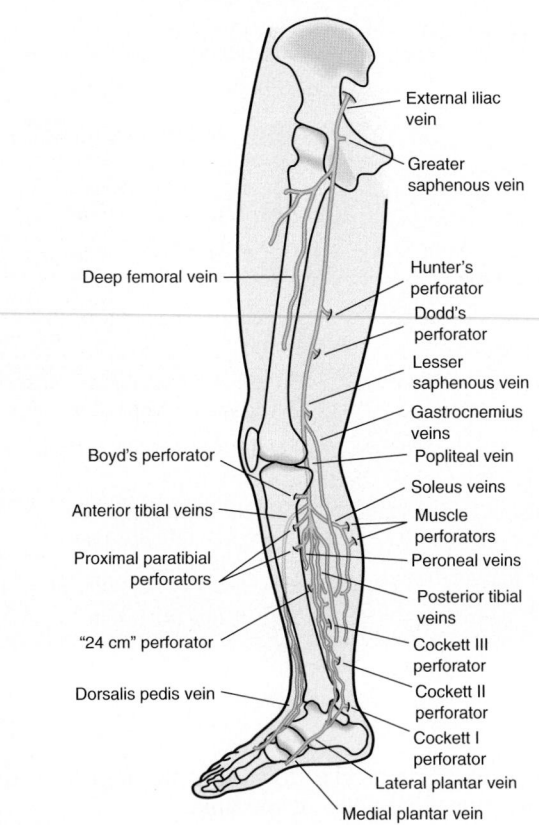

Figure 68-3 Perforating veins of the lower limb.

Venous valves are most prevalent in the distal lower extremity, whereas as one proceeds proximally, the number of valves decreases to the point that, in the superior vena cava and inferior vena cava (IVC), no valves are present.

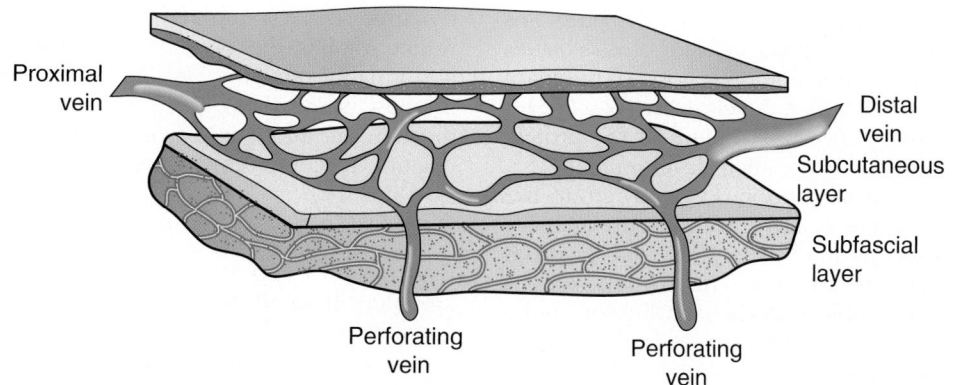

Figure 68-4 Dilation of superficial venous tributaries due to increased transmission of pressure by the perforating veins.

Most of the capacitance of the vascular tree is in the venous system. Because veins do not have significant amounts of elastin, veins can withstand large volume shifts with comparatively small changes in pressure. A vein has a normal elliptical configuration until the limit of its capacitance is reached, at which point the vein assumes a round configuration.

The calf muscles augment venous return by functioning as a pump. In the supine state, the resting venous pressure in the foot is the sum of the residual kinetic energy minus the resistance in the arterioles and precapillary sphincters. There is thus generated a pressure gradient to the right atrium of about 10 to 12 mm Hg. In the upright position, the resting venous pressure of the foot is a reflection of the hydrostatic pressure from the upright column of blood extending from the right atrium to the foot.

The return of the blood to the heart from the lower extremity is facilitated by the muscle pump function of the calf—a mechanism whereby the calf muscle, functioning as a bellows during exercise, compresses the gastrocnemius and soleal sinuses and propels the blood toward the heart. The normally functioning valves in the venous system prevent retrograde flow; it is when one or more of these valves become incompetent that symptoms of venous insufficiency can develop. During calf muscle contraction, the venous pressure of the foot and ankle drops dramatically. The pressures developing in the muscle compartments during exercise range from 150 to 200 mm Hg, and when there is failure of perforating veins, these high pressures are transmitted to the superficial system.

PRIMARY VENOUS INSUFFICIENCY

There are three main categories of primary venous insufficiency: telangiectasias, reticular veins, and varicose veins. Telangiectasias, reticular varicosities, and varicose veins all are physiologically similar despite the variations in caliber. The unifying end result is dilated, tortuous, elongated veins with dysfunctional or nonfunctional valves. Telangiectasias are very small intradermal varicosities. Reticular veins are subcutaneous dilated veins that enter the tributaries of the main axial or trunk veins. Varicose veins, such as the greater or lesser saphenous veins or their main tributaries, represent the largest-caliber veins of the superficial venous system.

Pathogenesis

Fundamental defects in the strength and characteristics of the venous wall enter into the pathogenesis of varicose veins. These defects may be generalized or localized and consist of deficiencies in elastin and collagen. Gandhi and colleagues[2] compared the collagen and elastin content of varicose veins with that of normal greater saphenous veins and discovered a significant increase in the collagen content and a significant reduction in the elastin content of varicose veins. No difference in proteolytic activity was demonstrated, thereby diminishing the likelihood that enzymatic degradation is an essential component of varicose vein formation. Cutaneous venectasia develops under these same influences and may become symptomatic. Textbooks of venous disease in the past and recent present have referred to venectasia as cosmetic and not symptomatic, yet ample documentation exists to the contrary. Effective treatment of venectasia can relieve symptoms of venostasis.

Anatomic differences in the location of the superficial veins of the lower extremities may contribute to the pathogenesis. For example, the main saphenous trunk is not always involved in varicose disease. Perhaps this is because it contains a well-developed medial fibromuscular layer and is supported by fibrous connective tissue that binds it to the deep fascia. In contrast, tributaries to the long saphenous vein are less supported in the subcutaneous fat and are superficial to the membranous layer of superficial fascia (Fig. 68-4). These tributaries also contain less muscle mass in their walls. Thus, these, and not the main trunk, may become selectively varicose.[3]

When these fundamental anatomic peculiarities are recognized, the intrinsic competence or incompetence of the valve system becomes important. For example, failure of a valve protecting a tributary vein from the pressures of the long saphenous vein allows a cluster of varicosities to develop. This is not an uncommon history for pregnant women, who describe a sudden development of a cluster of varicosities of unknown cause. Failure of the protective valve is the mechanism for such development.

The Middlesex Hospital (London, England) group has carried those observations into the clinical situation, where the micronized purified flavonoids were given as treatment for 60 days to patients with chronic venous disease.[4] Monitoring soluble endothelial adhesion molecules revealed that there was a reduction in the level of intercellular adhesion molecule-1, vascular cell adhesion molecules, and plasma lactoferrin.

Furthermore, communicating veins connecting the deep with the superficial compartment may have valve failure. Pressure studies show that two sources of venous hypertension exist. The first is gravitational and is a result of venous blood coursing in a distal direction down linear axial venous segments. This is referred to as *hydrostatic pressure* and is the weight of the blood column from the right atrium. The highest pressure generated by this mechanism is evident at the ankle and foot, where measurements are expressed in centimeters of water or millimeters of mercury. The second source of venous hypertension is dynamic. It is the force of muscular contraction, usually contained within the compartments of the leg. If a perforating vein fails, high pressures (range, 150-200 mm Hg) developed within the muscular compartments during exercise are transmitted directly to the superficial venous system. Here, the sudden pressure transmitted causes dilation and lengthening of the superficial veins. Progressive distal valvular incompetence may occur. If proximal valves such as the saphenofemoral valve become incompetent, systolic muscular contraction pressure is supplemented by the weight of the static column of blood from the heart. Furthermore, this static column becomes a barrier. Blood flowing proximally through the femoral vein spills into the saphenous vein and flows distally. As it refluxes distally through progressively incompetent valves, it is returned through perforating veins to the deep veins. Here, it is conveyed once again to the femoral veins, only to be recycled distally. Changes also occur at the cellular level. In the distal liposclerotic area, capillary proliferation is seen and extensive capillary permeability occurs as a result of the widening of interendothelial cell pores. Transcapillary leakage of osmotically active particles, the principal one being fibrinogen, occurs. In chronic venous insufficiency (CVI), venous fibrinolytic capacity is diminished, and the extravascular fibrin remains to prevent the normal exchange of oxygen and nutrients in the surrounding cells.[5,6] However, little proof exists for an actual abnormality in the delivery of oxygen to the tissues.[7] Instead, research suggests that many pathologic processes are involved, and at present, difficulty exists in identifying which are active and which are bystanders. Fundamental investigations into this problem in the future should improve the care of patients with severe venous stasis disease. An understanding of the source of venous hypertension and its differentiation into hydrostatic and hydrodynamic reflux is important. The presence of hydrostatic reflux implies the need for surgical correction of this abnormality, and the presence of hydrodynamic reflux implies the need for ablation of the perforating venous mechanism, allowing exposure of the subcutaneous circulation to compartment pressures.

Risk Factors

Risk factors for development of varicose veins include age older than 50 years, female sex hormones, heredity, gravitational hydrostatic force, and hydrodynamic force due to muscular contraction. Venous function is undoubtedly influenced by hormonal changes. In particular, progesterone liberated by the corpus luteum stabilizes the uterus by causing relaxation of smooth muscle fibers.[8,9] This effect directly influences venous function. The result is passive venous dilation, which, in many instances, causes valvular dysfunction. Although progesterone is implicated in the first appearance of varicosities in pregnancy, estrogen also has profound effects. It produces the relaxation of smooth muscle and a softening of collagen fibers. Further, the estrogen-to-progesterone ratio influences venous distensibility. This ratio may explain the predominance of venous insufficiency symptoms on the first day of a menstrual period when a profound shift occurs from the progesterone phase of the menstrual cycle to the estrogen phase. Although heredity is widely acknowledged as a risk factor for varicose vein development, the precise genetic mechanism has yet to be elucidated.

Symptoms

The patient with symptomatic varicose veins commonly reports heaviness, discomfort, and extremity fatigue. The pain is characteristically dull, does not occur during recumbency or early in the morning, and is exacerbated in the afternoon, especially after periods of prolonged standing. The discomforts of aching, heaviness, fatigue, or burning pain are relieved by leg elevation or elastic support. Cutaneous itching is also a sign of venous insufficiency. It is a manifestation of local congestion due to pooling of venous blood and may precede the onset of dermatitis. Females complain of symptom exacerbation during the early days of the menstrual cycle.

Physical Examination

The most important of all noninvasive tests available to study the venous system are the physical examination and a careful history that elucidates the symptoms previously described. Clinical examination of the patient in good light provides nearly all the information necessary. It determines the nature of the venous stasis disease and ascertains the presence of intracutaneous venous blemishes and subcutaneous protuberant varicosities, the location of principal points of control or perforating veins that feed clusters of varicosities, the presence and location of ankle pigmentation and its extent, and the presence and severity of subcutaneous induration. Visual examination can be supplemented by noting a downward-going impulse on coughing. Tapping the venous column of blood also demonstrates pressure transmission through the static column to incompetent distal veins.

After these facts have been obtained, the physician may turn to noninvasive techniques to corroborate the clinical impression.

Diagnostic Evaluation of Venous Dysfunction

The Perthes test for deep venous occlusion and the Brodie-Trendelenburg test of axial reflux have been replaced by in-office use of the continuous-wave, handheld Doppler instrument supplemented by duplex evaluation.[10] The handheld Doppler instrument can confirm an impression of saphenous reflux, and this, in turn, dictates the operative procedure to be performed in a given patient. A common misconception is belief that the Doppler instrument is used to locate perforating veins. Instead, it is used in specific locations to determine incompetent valves (e.g., the handheld, continuous-wave, 8-MHz flow detector placed over the greater and lesser saphenous veins near their terminations). With distal augmentation of flow and release, with normal deep breathing, and with performance of a Valsalva maneuver, accurate identification of valve reflux is ascertained. Formerly, the Doppler examination was supplemented by other objective studies. These included the photoplethysmograph, the mercury strain-gauge plethysmograph, and the photorheograph. These are no longer in common use.

Another instrument reintroduced to assess physiologic function of the muscle pump and the venous valves is the air-displacement plethysmograph.[11] This instrument was discarded after its use in the 1960s because of its cumbersome nature. Computer technology has allowed its reintroduction as championed by Christopoulos and coworkers.[12] It consists of an air chamber that surrounds the leg from knee to ankle. During calibration, leg veins are emptied by leg elevation, and the patient is then asked to stand so that leg venous volume can be quantitated and the time for filling recorded. The filling rate is then expressed in milliliters per second, thus giving readings similar to those obtained with the mercury strain-gauge technique.

Duplex technology more precisely defines which veins are refluxing by imaging the superficial and deep veins. The duplex examination is commonly done with the patient supine, but this gives an erroneous evaluation of reflux. In the supine position, even when no flow is present, the valves remain open. Valve closure requires a reversal of flow with a pressure gradient that is higher proximally than distally.[13] Thus, the duplex examination needs to be done with the patient standing or in the markedly trunk-elevated position.[14,15]

Imaging is obtained with a 10- or 7.5-MHz probe, and the pulsed Doppler consists of a 3.0-MHZ probe. The patient stands with the probe placed longitudinally on the groin. After imaging, sample volumes can be obtained from the femoral or saphenous vein. This flow can be observed during quiet respiration or by distal augmentation. Sudden release of augmentation allows assessment of valvular competence. The short saphenous vein and popliteal veins are similarly examined. Imaging improves the accuracy of the Doppler examination. For example, short saphenous venous incompetence can be differentiated from gastrocnemius venous valvular incompetence by the imaging and flow detection of the duplex or triplex scans.

Widespread use of duplex scanning has allowed a comparison of findings between standard clinical examinations with duplex Doppler studies.[16] In a study in which each patient was examined by three surgeons using different techniques (one using clinical examination, a second using the handheld Doppler instrument, and a third using a color duplex scanner), it was found that clinical examination failed in assessing main axial reflux at the saphenofemoral junction and saphenopopliteal junction. Whenever a Doppler instrument was added to the examination, the evaluation became more accurate. Based on preoperative assessments using clinical examination alone, inappropriate surgery would have been performed in 20% of the limbs. Clinical examination plus Doppler study would have produced a 13% incidence of inappropriate surgery.

Phlebography

In general, phlebography is unnecessary in the diagnosis and treatment of primary venous stasis disease and varicose veins. In cases of severe CVI, phlebography has specific utility. Ascending phlebography defines obstruction. Descending phlebography identifies specific valvular incompetence suspected on B-mode scanning and clinical examination.

Classification of Clinical Severity

The C-E-A-P classification is a recent scoring system that stratifies venous disease based on *c*linical presentation, *e*tiology, *a*natomy, and *p*athophysiology. This classification scheme, described in Table 68-3, is useful in helping the physician coherently and thoughtfully assess a limb afflicted with venous insufficiency and then arrive at an appropriate treatment plan.

Indications for Treatment of Primary Venous Insufficiency

Indications for treatment are pain, easy fatigability, heaviness, recurrent superficial thrombophlebitis, external bleeding, and appearance. After clinical and objective criteria have established the presence of symptomatic varicose veins, the next step is to plan a course of therapy.

Nonoperative Management

As previously described, symptoms of venous insufficiency are manifestations of valvular incompetence. Therefore, the objective of conservative management is to improve valve dysfunction. The first measure is external compression using elastic hose, 20 to 30 mm Hg, to be worn during the daytime hours. Although the exact mechanism by which compression is of benefit is not entirely known, a number of physiologic alterations have

Table 68-3   **Classification of Chronic Lower Extremity Venous Disease**

C	Clinical signs (grade$_{0-6}$), supplemented by "A" for asymptomatic and "S" for symptomatic presentation
E	Etiologic classification (congenital, primary, secondary)
A	Anatomic distribution (superficial, deep, or perforator, alone or in combination)
P	Pathophysiologic dysfunction (reflux or obstruction, alone or in combination)

Clinical Classification (C$_{0-6}$)

Any limb with possible chronic venous disease is first placed into one of seven clinical classes (C$_{0-6}$) according to the objective signs of disease.

Clinical Classification of Chronic Lower Extremity Venous Disease

Class 0   No visible or palpable signs of venous disease
Class 1   Telangiectasia, reticular veins, malleolar flare
Class 2   Varicose veins
Class 3   Edema without skin changes
Class 4   Skin changes ascribed to venous disease (e.g., pigmentation, venous eczema, lipodermatosclerosis)
Class 5   Skin changes as defined above with healed ulceration
Class 6   Skin changes as defined above with active ulceration

Limbs in higher categories have more severe signs of chronic venous disease and may have some or all of the findings defining a less severe clinical category. Each limb is further characterized as asymptomatic (A), for example, C$_{0-6,A}$, or symptomatic (S), for example, C$_{0-6,S}$. Symptoms that may be associated with telangiectatic, reticular, or varicose veins include lower extremity aching, pain, and skin irritation. Therapy may alter the clinical category of chronic venous disease. Limbs should therefore be reclassified after any form of medical or surgical treatment.

Etiologic Classification (E$_C$, E$_P$, or E$_S$)

Venous dysfunction may be congenital, primary, or secondary. These categories are mutually exclusive. Congenital venous disorders are present at birth but may not be recognized until later. The method of diagnosis of congenital abnormalities must be described. Primary venous dysfunction is defined as venous dysfunction of unknown cause but not of congenital origin. Secondary venous dysfunction denotes an acquired condition resulting in chronic venous disease, for example, deep venous thrombosis.

Etiologic Classification of Chronic Lower Extremity Venous Disease

Congenital (E$_C$)   Cause of the chronic venous disease present since birth
Primary (E$_P$)   Chronic venous disease of undetermined cause
Secondary (E$_S$)   Chronic venous disease with an associated known cause (post-thrombotic, post-traumatic, other)

Anatomic Classification (A$_S$, A$_D$, or A$_P$)

The anatomic site(s) of the venous disease should be described as superficial (A$_S$), deep (A$_D$), or perforating (A$_P$) vein(s). One, two, or three systems may be involved in any combination. For reports requiring greater detail, the involvement of the superficial, deep, and perforating veins may be localized by use of the anatomic segments.

Segmental Localization of Chronic Lower Extremity Venous Disease

SEGMENT NO.	VEIN(S)
SUPERFICIAL VEINS (A$_{S1-5}$)	
1	Telangiectasia/reticular veins
	Greater (long) saphenous vein
2	*Above knee*
3	*Below knee*
4	Lesser (short) saphenous vein
5	Nonsaphenous
DEEP VEINS (A$_{D6-16}$)	
6	Inferior vena cava
	ILIAC
7	*Common*
8	*Internal*
9	*External*
10	Pelvic: gonadal, broad ligament
	FEMORAL
11	*Common*
12	*Deep*
13	*Superficial*
14	Popliteal
15	Tibial (anterior, posterior, or peroneal)
16	Muscular (gastrointestinal, soleal, other)

Table 68-3   Classification of Chronic Lower Extremity Venous Disease—cont'd

Segment No.	Vein(s)
Perforating Veins (A$_{P17,18}$)	
17	Thigh
18	Calf

Pathophysiologic Classification (P$_{R,O}$)

Clinical signs or symptoms of chronic venous disease result from reflux (P$_R$), obstruction (P$_O$), or both (P$_{R,O}$).

Pathophysiologic Classification of Chronic Lower Extremity Venous Disease
Reflux (P$_R$)
Obstruction (P$_O$)
Reflux and obstruction (P$_{R,O}$)

been observed with compression. These include reduction in ambulatory venous pressure, improvement in skin microcirculation, and increase in subcutaneous pressure, which counters transcapillary fluid leakage. Patients are instructed to wear the hose during the day only, but to put on the stockings as soon as the day begins; swelling with standing will make stocking placement difficult. Care must be taken with patients who have concomitant arterial insufficiency because the compression stockings may exacerbate arterial outflow to the foot. Therefore, these patients require less compression, in some cases no compression whatsoever, depending on the severity of the arterial disease.

The second aspect of conservative therapy is to practice lower extremity elevation for two brief periods during the day, instructing the patient that the feet must be above the level of the heart, or "toes above the nose." With good compliance, these measures may ameliorate symptoms so that patients may not require further intervention.

Patients who exhibit venous stasis ulceration will require local wound care. A triple-layer compression dressing, with a zinc oxide paste gauze wrap in contact with the skin, is used most commonly from the base of the toes to the anterior tibial tubercle with snug, graded compression. This is an iteration of what is known most commonly as an *Unna boot*. A recent 15-year review of 998 patients with one or more venous ulcers treated with a similar compression bandage demonstrated that 73% of the ulcers healed in patients who returned for care. The median time to healing for individual ulcers was 9 weeks. In general, snug, graded-pressure, triple-layer compression dressings effect more rapid healing than compression stockings alone.

For most patients, well-applied, sustained compression therapy offers the most cost-effective and efficacious therapy in the healing of venous ulcers. After healing, most cases of CVI are controlled with elastic compression stockings to be worn during waking hours. Occasionally, patients who are elderly and those with arthritic conditions cannot apply the compression stocking required, and control must be maintained by triple-layer zinc oxide compression dressings, which can usually be left in place and changed once a week.

Venous Ablation: Sclerotherapy

Cutaneous venectasia with vessels smaller than 1 mm in diameter does not lend itself to surgical treatment. If the cause is saphenous or tributary venous incompetence, this condition can be treated surgically. The venectasia can be ablated successfully using modern sclerotherapy technique. Dilute solutions of sclerosant (e.g., 0.2% sodium tetradecyl) can be injected directly into the vessels of the blemish. Care must be taken to ensure that no single injection dose exceeds 0.1 mL but that multiple injections completely fill all vessels contributing to the blemish. When all of the ramifications of the blemish have been filled with sclerosant, and before the subsequent inflammatory reaction has progressed, a pressure dressing can be applied to keep vessels free of return blood for 24 to 72 hours. Fourteen to 21 days after injection, incision and drainage of entrapped blood are performed, and a second pressure dressing is applied for 12 to 18 hours. This liberation of entrapped blood is as important to success as the primary injection. Such therapy is remarkably successful in achieving an excellent cosmetic result and relief of stasis symptoms.

In allergic patients, a solution of hypertonic saline can be used for sclerotherapy. On the other hand, the use of newer technologies, such as the laser, in treatment of telangiectasia has proved disappointing. Venules larger than 1 mm and smaller than 3 mm in size can also be injected with sclerosant of slightly greater concentration (e.g., 0.5% sodium tetradecyl), but the amount injected needs to be limited to less than 0.5 mL. Pressure dressings for these venules must be in place for 72 hours or longer. Evacuation of entrapped blood is of paramount importance to prevent recanalization of these vessels after treatment.

Surgical Management

Varicose Veins and Superficial Venous Incompetence

Surgical treatment may be used to remove clusters with varicosities greater than 4 mm in diameter. Ambulatory phlebectomy may be performed using the stab avulsion technique with preservation of the greater and lesser saphenous veins, if they are unaffected by valvular

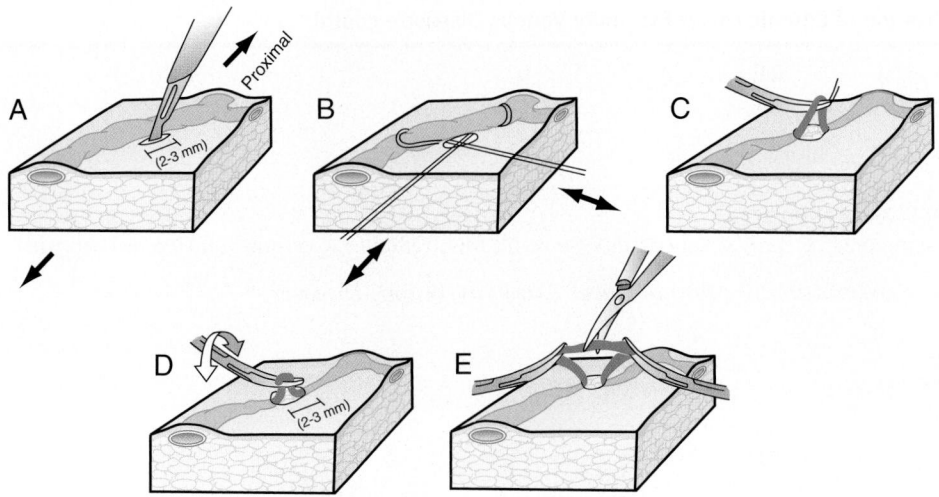

Figure 68-5 **A** to **E,** Technique of ambulatory phlebectomy, otherwise known as *stab avulsions of varicosities*.

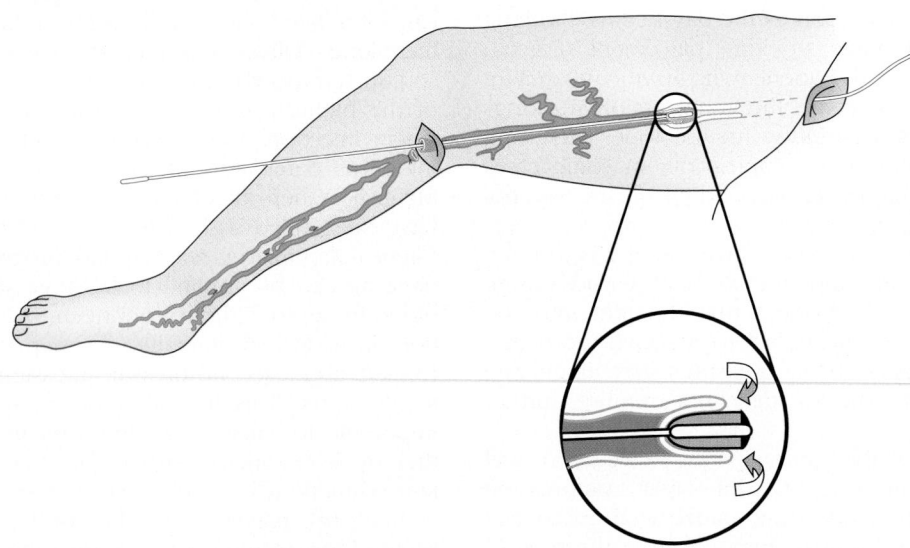

Figure 68-6 Inversion stripping of the saphenous vein for superficial venous reflux due to an incompetent saphenofemoral junction.

incompetence[17] (Fig. 68-5). When greater or lesser saphenous incompetence is present, the removal of clusters is preceded by limited removal of the saphenous vein (stripping). Stripping techniques are best done from above downward to avoid lymphatic and cutaneous nerve damage (Fig. 68-6). A number of techniques have been described that adapt new instruments to minimally invasive removal of the saphenous vein.[18,19]

At the present time, when the greater saphenous vein is used for coronary artery bypass and peripheral arterial reconstruction, there has been an interest in preserving the saphenous vein while relieving the symptoms of venous insufficiency, with little evidence to justify such an approach. However, a number of studies have shown

the advantage of stripping in prevention of varicose vein recurrence.

The question of preservation or stripping of the saphenous vein is an important one; therefore, a 5-year clinical and duplex scan follow-up examination of a group of patients has been performed.[20] Patients were randomized to stripping of the long saphenous vein during varicose vein surgery versus saphenofemoral ligation with stab avulsion of varices. It was found that reoperation, either done or awaited, was necessary for only 3 of 52 legs that underwent stripping, as compared with 12 of 58 limbs in which proximal ligation had been done. Neovascularization at the saphenofemoral junction was responsible for 10 of 12 recurrent varicose veins that underwent reoperation, and it was the cause of recurrence of saphenofemoral incompetence in 12 of the 52 limbs that were stripped versus 30 of the 58 limbs in which ligation was done. Clearly, the problem of neovascularization and recurrent varicose veins was not solved by the stripping operation, but stripping reduced the risk for reoperation by two thirds after 5 years of observation. It was the conclusion of the authors of the study that stripping "should be routine for primary long saphenous varicose veins."[20]

Modern treatment of varicose veins is fundamentally centered on the principle of ablation of the reflux source, sometimes termed the *escape point*. In most cases, this escape point is the incompetent valve at the saphenofemoral junction. It is clear to those who study this disease that unless the anatomic problem of reflux and the source of the reflux are dealt with, secondary procedures such as injection sclerotherapy are plagued with a high rate of recurrence. For this reason, the fundamental precept in the treatment of superficial venous insufficiency is to treat the escape point and then treat the secondary varicosities.

Recent advances in ablation of the incompetent greater saphenous vein have included radiofrequency closure and endovenous laser ablation. Both methods employ a duplex-guided percutaneous access to the greater saphenous vein, usually at the level of the knee. "Closure" of the vein is accomplished with either radiofrequency heat or laser. Confirmation of closure is obtained with postprocedure duplex at the conclusion of the intervention. Advantages of these procedures are that they are percutaneous and are performed on an outpatient basis. No anesthesia is necessary. Patients can return to baseline activities within a day or so. Risks of the procedures include development of a deep venous thrombosis (DVT) or pulmonary embolism, skin burn, thrombophlebitis, paresthesias, and recurrence. A 2-year follow-up study compared endovenous radiofrequency closure with ligation and vein stripping. The findings of this study revealed similar closure rates of the greater saphenous vein. Interestingly, the authors did not find that ligation of the vein at the saphenofemoral junction improved long-term outcome. However, patients' quality-of-life index was superior in the endovenous radiofrequency group. Although initial findings are promising in both the radiofrequency and endovenous laser therapies, to date, there is no prospective randomized trial to compare these three modalities[21,22] (Box 68-1).

Surgery for Severe Chronic Venous Insufficiency

While conservative therapy is being pursued or ulcer healing achieved, appropriate diagnostic studies generally

---

> **Box 68-1   Indications for Varicose Vein Intervention**
>
> Cosmesis
> Symptoms refractory to conservative therapy
> Bleeding from a varix
> Superficial thrombophlebitis
> Lipodermatosclerosis
> Venous stasis ulcer

---

reveal patterns of venous reflux or segments of venous occlusion so that specific therapy can be prescribed for the individual limb being evaluated. Imaging by duplex suffices for detection of reflux if the examination is carried out in the standing individual. Such noninvasive imaging may prove the only testing necessary beyond the handheld, continuous-wave Doppler instrument if superficial venous ablation is contemplated. If direct venous reconstruction by bypass or valvuloplasty techniques is planned, ascending and descending phlebography is required.[23]

Surprisingly, superficial reflux may be the only abnormality present in advanced chronic venous stasis. Correction goes a long way toward permanent relief of the chronic venous dysfunction and its cutaneous effects. Using duplex technology, Hanrahan and colleagues found that in 95 extremities with current venous ulceration, 16.8% had only superficial incompetence, and another 19% showed superficial incompetence combined with perforator incompetence.[24] Similarly, the Middlesex group, in a study of 118 limbs, found that "in just over half of the patients with venous ulceration, the disease was confined to the superficial venous system."[25]

A significant proportion of patients with venous ulceration have normal function in the deep veins, and surgical treatment is a useful option that can definitively address the hemodynamic derangements. Maintaining that all venous ulcers are surgically incurable is not reasonable when data suggest that superficial vein surgery holds the potential for ameliorating the venous hypertension. A randomized trial comparing compression therapy and surgery for superficial reflux versus conservative management alone revealed significant improvement in those patients who had undergone the surgical component.[25] Early success in patients with CVI and superficial valvular incompetence and venous ulceration has been obtained with both the endovenous radiofrequency and endovenous laser therapies.

In the early 1940s, Linton[27] emphasized the importance of perforating veins, and direct surgical interruption of these was advocated. This has fallen into disfavor because of a high incidence of postoperative wound healing complications. However, video techniques that allow direct visualization through small-diameter scopes have made endoscopic subfascial exploration and perforator vein interruption the desirable alternative to the Linton technique, minimizing morbidity and wound complications. The connective tissue between the fascia cruris and the underlying flexor muscles is so loose that this potential space can be opened up easily and dissected with the endoscope. This operation, done with a vertical proximal incision, accomplishes the objective of perforator vein interruption on an outpatient basis.

The availability of subfascial endoscopic perforator vein surgery had an impact on the care of venous ulcers in Western countries, albeit not as dramatic as its proponents had hoped. As patient limbs with severe CVI were studied accurately, the phrase *post-thrombotic syndrome* had to give way to the term *chronic venous insufficiency*, and a link to platelet and monocyte aggregates in the circulation reflected the leukocytic infiltrate of the ankle skin with its lipodermatosclerosis and healed and open ulcerations.[28]

Data regarding leukocytes in CVI accumulated and were consistent, showing that the activation of leukocytes sequestered in the cutaneous microcirculation during venous stasis was important to the development of the skin changes of CVI. This is reflected in the finding of adhesion markers between leukocytes and endothelial cells and an increased production of leukocyte degranulation enzymes and oxygen free radicals. Nevertheless, experimental evidence was still required for decisive proof of the leukocyte hypothesis.

In the United States, several groups have performed perforating vein division using laparoscopic instrumentation. Initial data suggested that perforator interruption produced rapid ulcer healing and a low rate of recurrence. The North American Registry, which voluntarily recorded the results of perforating venous surgery, confirmed a low 2-year recurrence rate of ulcers and a more rapid ulcer healing.[29]

A comparison of the three methods of perforator vein interruption, including the classic Linton procedure, the laparoscopic instrumentation procedure, and the single open-scope procedure, revealed that the endoscopic techniques produced results comparable with those of the open Linton operation, with much less scarring and much greater tendency toward a fast recovery. More perforating veins were identified with the open technique. However, the mean hospital stay and the period of convalescence were more favorable with the scope procedures.[30]

In general, the registry reports and individual institution clinical experience showed that patients with true post-thrombotic limbs were disadvantaged by the procedure, enough so that at Leicester (England), the students of the procedure said, "We conclude that perforating vein surgery is not indicated for the treatment of venous ulceration in limbs with primary deep venous incompetence."[30] Nevertheless, studies were reported in which previous superficial reflux was corrected with failures of such treatment. Rescue of such limbs with perforating vein division produced satisfactory results and verified that perforating veins are important in the genesis of venous ulceration and that their division accelerates healing and may reduce recurrence of ulceration.

Part of the difficulty in understanding the need for perforating vein division is the disparity between venous hemodynamics and the severity of cutaneous changes. This is not surprising because the cutaneous changes of CVI are dependent on leukocyte-endothelial interactions, and these may not be directly related to venous hemodynamics. Yet, endoscopic perforator vein division has improved venous hemodynamics in some limbs, as would be expected, by removing superficial reflux and perforating vein outflow. In an effort to eliminate incompetent perforator veins without the associated morbidity described in the aforementioned procedures, ultrasound-guided sclerotherapy has been developed as an alternative technique. Early study results are promising and reveal improved wound healing rates compared with the

SEPS. More data will be required before definitive recommendations can be made.[31]

Direct Venous Reconstruction

Historically, the first successful procedures done to reconstruct major veins were the femorofemoral crossover graft of Eduardo Palma and the saphenopopliteal bypass described by him and used also by Richard Warren of Boston.[33] These operations were elegant in their simplicity, use of autogenous tissue, and reconstruction by a single venovenous anastomosis.

With regard to femorofemoral crossover grafts, the only group to provide long-term physiologic data on a large number of patients is Halliday and colleagues from Sydney, Australia.[33] Although phlebography was used in selecting patients for surgery, no other details of preoperative indications are given. These investigators were able to document that 34 of 50 grafts remained patent in the long term as assessed by postoperative phlebography. They believed the best clinical results were achieved in relief of postexercise calf pain, but they had the impression that a patent graft also slowed the progression of distal liposclerosis and controlled recurrent ulceration. No proof of this was given in their report. The history of application of bypass procedures for venous obstruction is a fascinating one. Nevertheless, the advent of endovascular techniques has made those operations nearly obsolete.[34]

Perforator interruption, combined with superficial venous ablation, has been effective in controlling venous ulceration in 75% to 85% of patients. However, emphasis on failures of this technique led to Kistner's significant breakthrough in direct venous reconstruction with valvuloplasty in 1968 and the general recognition of this procedure after 1975.[35] Late evaluation of direct valve reconstruction indicates good to excellent long-term results in more than 80% of the patients.[36]

One cannot overestimate the contributions of Kistner. The technique of directing the incompetent venous stream through a competent proximal valve by venous segment transfer was his next achievement. After Kistner's contributions, surgeons were provided with an armamentarium that included Palma's venous bypass, direct valvuloplasty (of Kistner), and venous segment transfer (of Kistner). Moreover, external valvular reconstruction as performed by various techniques, including monitoring by endoscopy, holds the promise of a renewed interest in this form of treatment of venous insufficiency.

Axillary-to-popliteal autotransplantation of valve-containing venous segments has been considered since the early observations of Taheri and colleagues.[37] Verification in the long term of some preliminary excellent results has not been accomplished.

The advent of perforator vein surgery and the fine results achieved with it have displaced direct valvuloplasty into a position of less importance and even less interest than the procedure had called for during the 1980s.

DEEP VENOUS THROMBOSIS OF THE LOWER EXTREMITY

Acute DVT is a major cause of morbidity and mortality in the hospitalized patient, particularly in the surgical patient. The triad of venous stasis, endothelial injury, and hypercoagulable state first posited by Virchow in 1856 has held true a century and a half later.

Acute DVT poses several risks and has significant morbid consequences. The thrombotic process initiating in a venous segment can, in the absence of anticoagulation or in the presence of inadequate anticoagulation, propagate to involve more proximal segments of the deep venous system, thus resulting in edema, pain, and immobility. The most dreaded sequel to acute DVT is that of pulmonary embolism, a condition of potentially lethal consequence. The late consequence of DVT, particularly of the iliofemoral veins, can be CVI and ultimately post-thrombotic syndrome, as a result of valvular dysfunction in the presence of luminal obstruction.

For these reasons, understanding the pathophysiology, standardizing protocols to prevent or reduce DVT, and instituting optimal treatment promptly all are critical to reducing the incidence and morbidity of this unfortunately common condition.

Etiology

The triad of stasis, hypercoagulable state, and vessel injury all exist in most surgical patients. It is also clear that increasing age places a patient at a greater risk, with those older than 65 years representing a higher-risk population.

Stasis

Labeled fibrinogen studies in patients, as well as autopsy studies, have demonstrated quite convincingly that the soleal sinuses are the most common sites of initiation of venous thrombosis. The stasis may contribute to the endothelial cellular layer contacting activated platelets and procoagulant factors, thereby leading to DVT. Stasis, in and of itself, has never been shown to be a causative factor for DVT.

The Hypercoagulable State

Our knowledge of hypercoagulable conditions continues to improve, but it is still undoubtedly embryonic. The standard array of conditions screened for when searching for a "hypercoagulable state" is listed in Box 68-2. Should

---

Box 68-2 Hypercoagulable States

Factor V Leiden mutation
Prothrombin gene mutation
Protein C deficiency
Protein S deficiency
Antithrombin III deficiency
Homocysteine
Antiphospholipid syndrome

---

any of these conditions be identified, a treatment regimen of anticoagulation is instituted for life, unless specific contraindications exist. It is generally appreciated that the postoperative patient, following major operative procedures, is predisposed to formation of DVT. After major operations, large amounts of tissue factor may be released into the bloodstream from damaged tissues. Tissue factor is a potent procoagulant expressed on the leukocyte cell surface as well as in a soluble form in the bloodstream. Increases in platelet count, adhesiveness, changes in coagulation cascade, and endogenous fibrinolytic activity all result from physiologic stress, such as major operation or trauma, and have been associated with an increased risk for thrombosis.

Venous Injury

It has been clearly established that venous thrombosis occurs in veins that are distant from the site of operation; for instance, it is well known that patients undergoing total hip replacement frequently develop contralateral lower extremity DVT.

In a set of elegant experiments,[38,39] animal models of abdominal and total hip operations were used to study the possibility of venous endothelial damage distant from the operative site. In these experiments, jugular veins were excised after the animals were perfusion fixed. These experiments demonstrated that endothelial damage occurred after abdominal operations and were much more severe after hip operations. There were multiple microtears noted within the valve cusps that resulted in the exposure of the subendothelial matrix. The exact mechanism by which this injury at a distant site occurs and what mediators, whether cellular or humoral, are responsible are not clearly understood, but that the injury occurs and occurs reliably is evident from these and other studies.

Diagnosis

Incidence

Venous thromboembolism occurs for the first time in about 100 persons per 100,000 each year in the United States. This incidence increases with increasing age, with an incidence of 0.5% per 100,000 at 80 years of age. More than two thirds of these patients have DVT alone, and the rest have evidence of pulmonary embolism. The recurrence rate with anticoagulation has been noted to be 6% to 7% in the ensuing 6 months.

In the United States, pulmonary embolism causes 50,000 to 200,000 deaths per year. A 28-day case fatality rate of 9.4% after first-time DVT and of 15.1% after first-time pulmonary thromboembolism has been observed. Aside from pulmonary embolism, secondary CVI (that resulting from DVT) is significant in terms of cost, morbidity, and lifestyle limitation.

If the consequence of DVT, in terms of pulmonary embolism and CVI, is to be prevented, the prevention, diagnosis, and treatment of DVT must be optimized.

Clinical Diagnosis

The diagnosis of DVT requires, to use an overused phrase, a high index of suspicion. Most are familiar with Homans' sign, which refers to pain in the calf on dorsiflexion of the foot. It is certainly true that although the absence of this sign is not a reliable indicator of the absence of venous thrombus, the finding of a positive Homans' sign prompts one to attempt to confirm the diagnosis. Certainly, the extent of venous thrombosis in the lower extremity is an important factor in the manifestation of symptoms. For instance, most calf thrombi may be asymptomatic unless there is proximal propagation. This is one of the reasons that radiolabeled fibrinogen testing demonstrates a higher incidence of DVT than incidence studies using imaging modalities. Only 40% of patients with venous thrombosis have any clinical manifestations of the condition.

Major venous thrombosis involving the iliofemoral venous system results in a massively swollen leg with pitting edema, pain, and blanching, a condition known as *phlegmasia alba dolens*. With further progression of disease, there may be such massive edema that arterial inflow can be compromised. This condition results in a painful blue leg, the condition called *phlegmasia cerulea dolens*. With this evolution of the condition, unless flow is restored, venous gangrene can develop.

Venography

Injection of contrast material into the venous system is obviously and understandably the most accurate method of confirming DVT and the location. The superficial venous system has to be occluded with a tourniquet, and the veins in the foot are injected for visualization of the deep venous system. Although this is a good test for finding occlusive and nonocclusive thrombus, it is also invasive, subject to risks of contrast, and requires interpretation with 5% to 10% error rate.

Impedance Plethysmography

Impedance plethysmography measures the change in venous capacitance and rate of emptying of the venous volume on temporary occlusion and release of the occlusion of the venous system. A cuff is inflated around the upper thigh until the electrical signal has plateaued. When the cuff is deflated, there is usually rapid outflow and reduction of volume. With a venous thrombosis, one notes a prolongation of the outflow wave. It is not very useful clinically for the detection of calf venous thrombosis and in patients with prior venous thrombosis.

Fibrin, Fibrinogen Assays

The basis of fibrin or fibrinogen can be assayed by measuring the degradation of intravascular fibrin. The D-dimer test measures cross-linked degradation products, which is a surrogate of plasmin's activity on fibrin. It is shown that in combination with clinical evaluation and assessment, the sensitivity exceeds 90% to 95%. The negative predictive value is 99.3% for proximal evaluation and 98.6% for distal evaluation. In the postoperative patient, D-dimer is causally elevated due to surgery, and,

as such, a positive D-dimer assay for evaluating for DVT is of no use. However, a negative D-dimer test in patients with suspected DVT has a high negative predictive value, ranging from 97% to 99%.[40]

Duplex Ultrasound

The modern diagnostic test of choice for the diagnosis of DVT is the duplex ultrasound, a modality that combines Doppler ultrasound and color-flow imaging. The advantage of this test is that it is noninvasive, comprehensive, and without any risk of contrast angiography. This test is also highly operator dependent, and this is one of the potential drawbacks.

The Doppler ultrasound is based on the principle of the impairment of an accelerated flow signal due to an intraluminal thrombus. A detailed interrogation begins at the calf with imaging of the tibial veins and then proximally over the popliteal and femoral veins. A properly done examination evaluates flow with distal compression that results in augmentation of flow and with proximal compression that should interrupt flow. If any segment of the venous system being examined fails to demonstrate augmentation on compression, venous thrombosis is suspected.

Real-time B-mode ultrasonography with color-flow imaging has improved the sensitivity and specificity of ultrasound scanning. With color-flow duplex imaging, blood flow can be imaged in the presence of a partially occluding thrombus. The probe is also used to compress the vein. A normal vein is easily compressed, whereas in the presence of a thrombus, there is resistance to compression. In addition, the chronicity of the thrombus can be evaluated based on its imaging characteristics, namely, increased echogenicity and heterogeneity. Duplex imaging is significantly more sensitive than indirect physiologic testing.

Magnetic Resonance Venography

With major advances in technology of imaging, magnetic resonance venography has come to the forefront of imaging for proximal venous disease. The cost and the issue of patient tolerance due to claustrophobia limit the widespread application, but this is changing. It is a useful test for imaging the iliac veins and the IVC, an area where duplex ultrasound is limited in its usefulness.

Prophylaxis

The patient who has undergone either major abdominal surgery or major orthopedic surgery, has sustained major trauma, or has prolonged immobility (>3 days) represents an elevated risk for the development of venous thromboembolism. The specific risk factor analysis and epidemiologic studies dissecting the etiology of venous thromboembolism are beyond the scope of this chapter. The reader is referred to more extensive analysis of this problem.[41]

The methods of prophylaxis can be mechanical or pharmacologic. The simplest method is for the patient to walk. Activation of the calf pump mechanism is an effective means of prophylaxis, as evidenced by the fact that few active people without underlying risk factors develop venous thrombosis. A patient who is expected to be up and walking within 24 to 48 hours is at low risk for developing venous thrombosis. The practice of having a patient "out of bed into a chair" is one of the most thrombogenic positions that one could order a patient into. Sitting in a chair with the legs in a dependent position causes venous pooling, which in the postoperative milieu could easily be a predisposing factor in the development of thromboembolism.

The most common method of prophylaxis in the surgical universe has traditionally revolved around sequential compression devices, which periodically compress the calves and essentially replicate the calf bellows mechanism. This has clearly reduced the incidence of venous thromboembolism in the surgical patient. The most likely mechanism for the efficacy of this device is prevention of venous stasis. There is some literature that suggests that fibrinolytic activity systemically is enhanced by a sequential compression device. However, this is by no means established because there are a considerable number of studies demonstrating no enhancement of fibrinolytic activity.[42]

Another traditional method of thromboprophylaxis is the use of low-dose unfractionated heparin. The dose traditionally used was 5000 units of unfractionated heparin every 12 hours. However, analysis of trials comparing placebo versus fixed-dose heparin shows that the stated dose of 5000 units subcutaneously every 12 hours is no more effective than placebo. When subcutaneous heparin is used on an every-8-hour dosing, rather than every 12 hours, there is a reduction in the development of venous thromboembolism.

More recently, a wealth of literature has revealed the efficacy of fractionated low-molecular-weight heparin (LMWH) for prophylaxis and treatment of venous thromboembolism. LMWH inhibits factor Xa and IIA activity, with the ratio of anti–factor Xa to anti–factor IIA activity ranging from 1:1 to 4:1. LMWH has a longer plasma half-life and has significantly higher bioavailability. There is much more predictable anticoagulant response than in fractionated heparin. No laboratory monitoring is necessary because the partial thromboplastin time (PTT) is unaffected. A variety of analyses, including a major meta-analysis, have clearly shown that LMWH results in equivalent, if not better, efficacy with significantly less bleeding complications.

Comparison of LMWH with mechanical prophylaxis demonstrates superiority of LMWH in reduction of the development of venous thromboembolic disease.[43-45] Prospective trials evaluating LMWH in head-injured and trauma patients have also proved the safety of LMWH, with no increase in intracranial bleeding or major bleeding at other sites.[46] In addition, LMWH shows significant reduction in the development of venous thromboembolism compared to other methods.

In short, LMWH is considered the optimal method of prophylaxis in moderate- and high-risk patients. Even the traditional reluctance to use heparin in high-risk groups such as the multiply injured trauma patient and the head-injured patient must be re-examined, given the efficacy and safety profile of LMWH in multiple prospective trials.

Treatment

After a diagnosis of venous thrombosis has been established, a treatment plan must be instituted. Complications of calf DVT include proximal propagation of thrombus in up to one third of hospitalized patients and post-thrombotic syndrome. In addition, untreated lower extremity DVT carries a 30% recurrence rate.

Any venous thrombosis involving the femoropopliteal system is treated with full anticoagulation. Traditionally, the treatment of DVT centers around heparin treatment to maintain the PTT at 60 to 80 seconds, followed by warfarin therapy to obtain an International Normalized Ratio (INR) of 2.5 to 3.0. If unfractionated heparin is used, it is important to use a nomogram-based dosing therapy. The incidence of recurrent venous thromboembolism increases if the time to therapeutic anticoagulation is prolonged. For this reason, it is important to reach therapeutic levels within 24 hours. A widely used regimen is 80 U/kg bolus of heparin, followed by a 15 U/kg infusion. The PTT needs to be checked 6 hours after any change in heparin dosing. Warfarin is started the same day. If warfarin is initiated without heparin, the risk for a transient hypercoagulable state exists because protein C and S levels fall before the other vitamin K–dependent factors are depleted. With the advent of LMWH, it is no longer necessary to admit the patient for intravenous heparin therapy. It is now accepted practice to administer LMWH to the patient as an outpatient, as a bridge to warfarin therapy, which also is monitored on an outpatient basis.

The recommended duration of anticoagulant therapy continues to undergo evolution. A minimum treatment time of 3 months is advocated in most cases. The recurrence rate is the same with 3 versus 6 months of warfarin therapy. If, however, the patient has a known hypercoagulable state or has experienced episodes of venous thrombosis, then lifetime anticoagulation is required, in the absence of contraindications. The accepted INR range is 2.0 to 3.0; a recent randomized, double-blind study confirmed that a goal INR of 2.0 to 3.0 was more effective in preventing recurrent venous thromboembolism than a low-intensity regimen with a goal INR of 1.0 to 1.9.[47] Additionally, the low-intensity regimen did not reduce the risk for clinically important bleeding.

Oral anticoagulants are teratogenic and thus cannot be used during pregnancy. In the case of the pregnant patient with venous thrombosis, LMWH is the treatment of choice, and this is continued through delivery and can be continued postpartum as indicated.

Thrombolysis

The advent of thrombolysis has resulted in increased interest in thrombolysis for DVT. The purported benefit is preservation of valve function with subsequently lesser chance of developing CVI. However, to date, few definitive, convincing data exist to support the use of thrombolytic therapy for DVT.

One exception is the patient with phlegmasia in whom thrombolysis is advocated for relief of significant venous obstruction. In this condition, thrombolytic therapy probably results in better relief of symptoms and less long-term sequelae than heparin anticoagulation alone. The alternative for this condition is surgical venous thrombectomy. No matter which treatment is chosen, long-term anticoagulation is indicated. The incidence of major bleeding is higher with lytic therapy.[48]

DEEP VENOUS THROMBOSIS OF THE UPPER EXTREMITY

Upper extremity DVT is much less common than its lower extremity counterpart, constituting only about 5% of all documented DVTs. Although not as common, it is a serious problem; pulmonary embolism occurs in up to one third of all patients with an upper extremity DVT. Upper extremity DVT usually refers to thrombosis of the axillary or subclavian veins. The syndrome can be divided into two categories: primary/idiopathic and secondary.

Primary etiologies include Paget-Schroetter syndrome and idiopathic upper extremity DVT. Patients with Paget-Schroetter syndrome develop effort thrombosis of the extremity due to compression of the subclavian vein, the venous component of thoracic outlet syndrome. A classic presentation involves a young athlete who uses the upper extremity in a repetitive motion, such as swimming, which causes repetitive extrinsic compression of the subclavian vein. In these patients, anatomic anomalies such as a cervical rib or myofascial bands cause the venous compression. Plain films are one of the first diagnostic tests used to confirm thoracic outlet syndrome. Treatment with initial thrombolysis followed by first rib resection is standard of care. Idiopathic upper extremity DVT is sometimes eventually attributed to an occult malignancy, and therefore a diagnosis of idiopathic upper extremity DVT warrants evaluation for an undetected malignancy.

Secondary etiologies of upper extremity DVT are more common and include indwelling central venous catheter, pacemaker, thrombophilia, or malignancy.

Classic findings on physical examination include unilateral swelling, pain, extremity discomfort, erythema, and a palpable cord. Diagnosis is confirmed by duplex ultrasonography. Because the clavicle obscures the midportion of the subclavian vein, venography or magnetic resonance venography may be required, and these constitute second-line imaging modalities. Treatment of upper extremity DVT involves anticoagulation therapy. Therapeutic dosing parameters are the same as for lower extremity DVT. Long-term complications of upper extremity DVT include recurrence and post-thrombotic syndrome. Post-thrombotic syndrome is treated with extremity elevation and graduated elastic compression.[49,50]

Vena Caval Filter

The most worrisome and potentially lethal complication of DVT is pulmonary embolism. The symptoms of pulmonary embolism, ranging from dyspnea, chest pain, and

---

Box 68-3	Indications for a Vena Cava Filter

Recurrent thromboembolism despite adequate anticoagulation
Deep venous thrombosis in a patient with contraindications to anticoagulation
Chronic pulmonary embolism and resultant pulmonary hypertension
Complications of anticoagulation
Propagating iliofemoral venous thrombus in anticoagulation

---

hypoxia to acute cor pulmonale, are nonspecific and require a high index of suspicion. The gold standard remains the pulmonary angiogram, but increasingly, this is being displaced by the computed tomographic angiogram.

Adequate anticoagulation is usually effective in stabilizing venous thrombosis, but if a patient should develop a pulmonary embolism in the presence of adequate anticoagulation, a vena cava filter is indicated. The general indications for a caval filter are listed in Box 68-3. The modern filters are placed percutaneously over a guidewire. The Greenfield filter, with the most extensive use and data, has a 95% patency rate and a 4% recurrent embolism rate. This high patency rate allows for safe suprarenal placement if there is involvement of the IVC up to the renal veins or if it is placed in a woman of childbearing potential.

The device-related complications are wound hematoma, migration of the device into the pulmonary artery, and caval occlusion due to trapping of a large embolus. In the latter situation, the dramatic hypotension that accompanies acute caval occlusion can be mistaken for a massive pulmonary embolism. The distinction between the hypovolemia of caval occlusion and the right heart failure from pulmonary embolism can be made by measuring filling pressures of the right side of the heart. The treatment of caval occlusion is volume resuscitation.

Retrievable Vena Caval Filters

Although generally safe, IVC filters are not without risk and significant morbidity. Therefore, permanent placement of a caval filter, particularly in a young patient who may only require short-term caval protection, is not generally accepted. Retrievable filters entered the field as a potential solution for the patient with temporary indications for pulmonary embolus prophylaxis. There are three retrievable IVC filters that have U.S. Food and Drug Administration approval: the Recovery filter, the OptEase filter, and the Gunther-Tulip filter. These filters vary slightly with respect to shape and length. All can be deployed from the internal jugular vein or femoral vein and retrieved from the right jugular vein (Gunther-Tulip and Recovery) or the right femoral vein (OptEase). Before retrieval, a venogram is performed to ensure there is no nidus of IVC thrombus in the filter. These filters can be placed either in an angiography suite or at the bedside using intravascular ultrasound. A major advantage to retrievable filters is that they may be removed when the patient either no longer requires pulmonary embolism protection or is able to undergo anticoagulation. Patient groups that may benefit from retrievable filters include multiple-trauma patients and high-risk surgical patients. Insertion complications reported include vena cava perforation, filter migration, and venous thrombosis at the insertion site. Retrieval complications include failure to retrieve the filter, thrombus embolization from the filter, vein retrieval site thrombus, and groin hematoma. However, the role of retrievable filters continues to be a work in progress. Further investigation is required before definitive practice guidelines are established[51,52] (Box 68-4).

Superficial Thrombophlebitis

Superficial thrombophlebitis is a common disorder, diagnosed both in the hospital and in the outpatient setting. In hospitalized patients, superficial thrombophlebitis is usually due to an indwelling catheter. In the clinic, patients with thrombophlebitis report common predisposing risk factors such as recent surgery, recent childbirth, venous stasis, varicose veins, or intravenous drug use. Patients who deny any of the aforementioned factors may be classified with idiopathic thrombophlebitis. In these cases, care must be taken to ensure that the patient does not harbor an occult hypercoagulable state or an occult malignancy. Indeed, in 1876, Trousseau identified the phenomenon of migratory thrombophlebitis and malignancy, particularly involving the tail of the pancreas. Mondor's disease involves superficial thrombophlebitis of the superficial veins of the breast. Diagnosis of superficial thrombophlebitis can be easily made by physical examination of an erythematous palpable cord coursing along a superficial vein, more commonly located along the lower extremities. Duplex ultrasonography is used if there is suspicion of proximal propagation into the deep venous system. With this diagnosis of DVT, anticoagulation is indicated. If, however, thrombus abuts the saphenofemoral junction, treatment of this more elusive condition is controversial. Some authors recommend serial ultrasound, others anticoagulation; another alternative is operative ligation at the junction.

Treatment of localized, noncomplicated thrombophlebitis involves conservative therapy, which consists of anti-inflammatory medication and compression stockings. When the thrombophlebitis involves clusters of varicosities, particularly in the lower extremities, excision is indicated. Selective removal of the entire vein along its course is only indicated in the rare instance of sup-

purative septic thrombophlebitis after all other sources of sepsis have been excluded.

CONCLUSION

The spectrum of venous disease is widespread and diverse, providing surgeons who fully understand the unique physiology of veins a rewarding and rich arena for future investigation.

Selected References

American Venous Forum: Classification and grading of chronic venous disease in the lower limb: A consensus statement. Vasc Surg 30:5, 1996.

> Interpretation based on external evidence alone, with regard to chronic venous disease, can be highly error prone, and this consensus statement by an international group of experts in chronic venous disease is an attempt to clearly identify the etiologic, anatomic, pathophysiologic, and clinical features of the limb with chronic venous disease.

Caggiati A, Bergan JJ, Gloviczki P, et al: Nomenclature of the veins of the lower limbs: An international interdisciplinary consensus statement. J Vasc Surg 36:416-422, 2002.

> A revision in the nomenclature of the venous system that seeks to eliminate some confusion about the superficial and the deep venous system, as commonly understood. It is unclear whether this advances the cause, but it is an attempt to standardize the nomenclature.

Christopoulus D, Nicolaides AN, Cook A, et al: Pathogenesis of venous ulceration in relation to the calf muscle pump function. Surgery 106:829, 1989.

> Ulceration due to venous insufficiency is accompanied by increasing reflux and decreasing calf ejection fraction. The authors elegantly demonstrate that the combination of venous reflux and ejection fraction with exercise, expressed as the residual volume fraction, correlated well with the incidence of ulceration and the measurement of ambulatory venous pressure.

Lippman HI, Fishman LM, Farrar RH, et al: Edema control in the management of disabling chronic venous insufficiency. Arch Phys Med Rehabil 75:436, 1994.

> A 15-year experience demonstrating the efficacy of compression therapy, in particular Unna's boot, in healing ulceration of the limb, with 90% success in healing in compliant patients.

Rutgers PH, Kitslaar PJ: Randomized trial of stripping versus high ligation combined with sclerotherapy in the treatment of the incompetent saphenous vein. Am J Surg 168:311, 1994.

> This study demonstrated convincingly that the saphenous vein ligation and stripping in combination with stab avulsions were superior to high ligation without stripping and sclerotherapy with regard to cosmetic, functional, and duplex outcome criteria.

References

1. Caggiati A, Bergan JJ, Gloviczki P, et al: Nomenclature of the veins of the lower limbs: An international interdisciplinary consensus statement. J Vasc Surg 36:416-422, 2002.
2. Gandhi RH, Irizarry E, Nackman GB, et al: Analysis of the connective tissue matrix and proteolytic activity of primary varicose veins. J Vasc Surg 18:814-820, 1993.

3. Mashiah A, Rose SS, Hod I: The scanning electron microscope in the pathology of varicose veins. Isr J Med Sci 27:202-206, 1991.

4. Shoab SS, Porter J, Scurr JH, et al: Endothelial activation response to oral micronised flavonoid therapy in patients with chronic venous disease: A prospective study. Eur J Vasc Endovasc Surg 17:313-318, 1999.

5. Burnand KG, O'Donnell TF Jr, Thomas ML, et al: The relative importance of incompetent communicating veins in the production of varicose veins and venous ulcers. Surgery 82:9-14, 1977.

6. Burnand KG, Whimster I, Clemenson G, et al: The relationship between the number of capillaries in the skin of the venous ulcer-bearing area of the lower leg and the fall in foot vein pressure during exercise. Br J Surg 68:297-300, 1981.

7. Scurr JH, Coleridge-Smith PD: Pathogenesis of venous ulceration. Phlebologie 1(Suppl):3-16, 1992.

8. Wahl LM: Hormonal regulation of macrophage collagenase activity. Biochem Biophys Res Commun 74:838-845, 1977.

9. Woolley DE: On the sequential changes in levels of oestradiol and progesterone during pregnancy and parturition and collagenolytic activity. In Pez KA, Eddi AH (eds): Extracellular Matrix Biochemistry. New York, Elsevier, 1984.

10. Hoare MC, Royle JP: Doppler ultrasound detection of saphenofemoral and saphenopopliteal incompetence and operative venography to ensure precise saphenopopliteal ligation. Aust N Z J Surg 54:49-52, 1984.

11. Christopoulos D, Nicolaides AN: Noninvasive diagnosis and quantitation of popliteal reflux in the swollen and ulcerated leg. J Cardiovasc Surg (Torino) 29:535-539, 1988.

12. Christopoulos D, Nicolaides AN, Szendro G: Venous reflux: Quantification and correlation with the clinical severity of chronic venous disease. Br J Surg 75:352-356, 1988.

13. van Bemmelen PS, Beach K, Bedford G, et al: The mechanism of venous valve closure: Its relationship to the velocity of reverse flow. Arch Surg 125:617-619, 1990.

14. van Bemmelen PS, Bedford G, Beach K, et al: Quantitative segmental evaluation of venous valvular reflux with duplex ultrasound scanning. J Vasc Surg 10:425-431, 1989.

15. Vasdekis SN, Clarke GH, Nicolaides AN: Quantification of venous reflux by means of duplex scanning. J Vasc Surg 10:670-677, 1989.

16. Singh S, Lees TA, Donlon M, et al: Improving the preoperative assessment of varicose veins. Br J Surg 84:801-802, 1997.

17. Bishop CCR, Jarrett PEM: Outpatient varicose vein surgery under local anaesthesia. Br J Surg 73:821-822, 1986.

18. Conrad P: Groin-to-knee downward stripping of the long saphenous vein. Phlebology 7:20-22, 1992.

19. Neglen P, Einarsson E, Eklof B: The functional long-term value of different types of treatment for saphenous vein incompetence. J Cardiovasc Surg (Torino) 34:295-301, 1993.

20. Dwerryhouse S, Davies B, Harradine K, et al: Stripping the long saphenous vein reduces the rate of reoperation for recurrent varicose veins: Five-year results of a randomized trial. J Vasc Surg 29:589-592, 1999.

21. Sybrandy JE, Wittens CH: Initial experiences in endovenous treatment of saphenous vein reflux. J Vasc Surg 36:1207-1212, 2002.

22. Marston WA, Owens LV, Davies S, et al: Endovenous saphenous ablation corrects the hemodynamic abnormality in patients with CEAP clinical class 3-6 chronic venous insufficiency due to superficial reflux. Vasc Endovasc Surg 40:25-30, 2006.

23. Bergan JJ: New developments in the surgical treatment of venous disease. Cardiovasc Surg 1:624-631, 1993.

24. Hanrahan LM, Araki CT, Rodriguez AA, et al: Distribution of valvular incompetence in patients with venous stasis ulceration. J Vasc Surg 13:805-812, 1991.

25. Gohel MS, Barwell JR, Earnshaw JJ, et al: Randomized clinical trial of compression and surgery versus compression alone in chronic venous ulceration (ESCHAR study) haemodynamic and anatomical changes. Br J Surg 92:291-297, 2005.

26. Walsh JC, Bergan JJ, Beeman S, et al: Femoral venous reflux abolished by greater saphenous vein stripping. Ann Vasc Surg 8:566-570, 1994.

27. Linton RR: The communicating veins of the lower legs and the operative technique for their ligation. Ann Surg 107:582, 1938.

28. Powell CC, Rohrer MJ, Barnard MR, et al: Chronic venous insufficiency is associated with increased platelet and monocyte activation and aggregation. J Vasc Surg 30:844-851, 1999.

29. Gloviczki P, Bergan JJ, Rhodes JM, et al: Mid-term results of endoscopic perforator vein interruption for chronic venous insufficiency: Lessons learned from the North American Subfascial Endoscopic Perforator Surgery Registry. The North American Study Group. J Vasc Surg 29:489-502, 1999.

30. Murray JD, Bergan JJ, Riffenburgh RH: Development of open-scope subfascial perforating vein surgery: Lessons learned from the first 67 cases. Ann Vasc Surg 13:372-377, 1999.

31. Masuda EM, Kessler DM, Lurie F, et al: The effect of ultrasound-guided sclerotherapy of incompetent perforator veins on clinical severity and disability scores. J Vasc Surg 43:551-556, 2006.

32. Rhodes JM, Gloviczki P, Canton L, et al: Endoscopic perforator vein division with ablation of superficial reflux improves venous hemodynamics. J Vasc Surg 28:839-847, 1998.

33. Palma EC, Esperon R: Vein transplants and grafts in the surgical treatment of the postphlebitic syndrome. J Cardiovasc Surg (Torino) 1:94-107, 1960.

34. Sillesen H, Just S, Jorgensen M, et al: Catheter-directed thrombolysis for treatment of iliofemoral deep venous thrombosis is durable, preserves valve function, and may prevent chronic venous insufficiency. Eur J Vasc Endovasc Surg 30:556-562, 2005.

35. Kistner RL: Surgical repair of the incompetent femoral vein valve. Arch Surg 110:1336-1342, 1975.

36. Kistner RL: Late results of venous valve repair. In Yao JST, Pearce WL (eds): Long-Term Results of Vascular Surgery. Philadelphia, WB Saunders, 1993, p 451.

37. Taheri SA, Lazar L, Elias S, et al: Surgical treatment of postphlebitic syndrome with vein valve transplant. Am J Surg 144:221-224, 1982.

38. Schaub RG, Lynch PR, Stewart GJ: The response of canine veins to three types of abdominal surgery: A scanning and transmission electron microscopic study. Surgery 83:411, 1978.

39. Stewart GJ, Alburger PD, Stone EA, Soszka TW: Total hip replacement induces injury to remote veins in a canine model. J Bone Joint Surg Am 65:97, 1983.

40. Kovacs MJ, MacKinnon KM, Anderson D, et al: A comparison of three rapid D-dimer methods for the diagnosis of venous thromboembolism. Br J Haematol 115:140-144, 2001.

41. Anderson FA Jr, Spencer FA: Risk factors for venous thromboembolism. Circulation 107:I9-I16, 2003.

42. Killewich LA, Cahan MA, Hanna DJ, et al: The effect of external pneumatic compression on regional fibrinolysis in a prospective randomized trial. J Vasc Surg 36:953-958, 2002.

43. Bernardi E, Prandoni P: Safety of low-molecular-weight heparins in the treatment of venous thromboembolism. Expert Opin Drug Saf 2:87-94, 2003.

44. Couturaud F, Julian JA, Kearon C: Low-molecular-weight heparin administered once versus twice daily in patients with venous thromboembolism: A meta-analysis. Thromb Haemost 86:980-984, 2001.

45. Mismetti P, Laporte S, Darmon JY, et al: Meta-analysis of low-molecular-weight heparin in the prevention of venous thromboembolism in general surgery. Br J Surg 88:913-930, 2001.

46. Norwood SH, McAuley CE, Berne JD, et al: Prospective evaluation of the safety of enoxaparin prophylaxis for venous thromboembolism in patients with intracranial hemorrhagic injuries. Arch Surg 137:696-702, 2002.

47. Kearon C, Ginsberg JS, Kovacs MJ, et al: Comparison of low-intensity warfarin therapy with conventional-intensity warfarin therapy for long-term prevention of recurrent venous thromboembolism. N Engl J Med 349:631-639, 2003.

48. Sillesen H, Just S, Jorgensen M: Catheter-directed thrombolysis for treatment of iliofemoral deep venous thrombosis is durable, preserves valve function, and may prevent chronic venous insufficiency. Eur J Vasc Endovasc Surg 30: 556-562, 2005.

49. Joffe HV, Goldhaber SZ: Upper-extremity deep vein thrombosis. Circulation 106:1874-1880, 2002.

50. Martinelli T, Battaglioni P, Bucciarelli SM, et al: Risk factors and recurrence rate of primary deep vein thrombosis of the upper extremities. Circulation 110:566-570, 2004.

51. Offner PJ, Hawkes A, Madayag R, et al: The role of temporary IVC filters in critically ill surgical patients. Arch Surg 138:591-595, 2003.

52. Rosenthal D, Wellons ED, Lai KM, et al: Retrievable inferior vena cava filters: Initial clinical results. Ann Vasc Surg 20: 157-165, 2006.

The Lymphatics

Iraklis I. Pipinos, MD   and   B. Timothy Baxter, MD

EMBRYOLOGY AND ANATOMY

The primordial lymphatic system is first seen during the sixth week of development in the form of lymph sacs located next to the jugular veins. During the eighth week, the cisterna chyli forms just dorsal to the aorta, and at the same time, two additional lymphatic sacs corresponding to the iliofemoral vascular pedicles begin forming. Communicating channels connecting the lymph sacs, which will become the thoracic duct, develop during the ninth week.

From this primordial lymphatic system sprout endothelial buds that grow with the venous system to form the peripheral lymphatic plexus (Fig. 69-1). Failure of one of the initial jugular lymphatic sacs to develop proper connections and drainage with the lymphatic and, subsequently, venous system may produce focal lymph cysts (cavernous lymphangiomas) also known as *cystic hygromas*.[1] Similarly, failure of embryologic remnants of lymphatic tissues to connect to efferent channels leads to the development of cystic lymphatic formations (simple cap-illary lymphangiomas) that, depending on their location, are classified as truncal, mesenteric, intestinal, or retroperitoneal lymphangiomas. Hypoplasia or failure of development of drainage channels connecting the lymphatic systems of extremities to the main primordial lymphatic system of the torso may result in primary lymphedema of the extremities.

Lymphangiogenesis appears to be regulated by the vascular endothelial factors C and D (VEGF-C, VEGF-D) their receptor VEGFR-3, and their binding protein neurophilin-2 (Nrp2). Consistent with these findings, Nrp2-deficient mice have lymphatic hypoplasia and heterozygous inactivating mutation of VEGFR-3 is found in Chy mice, an animal model of primary lymphedema, and appears to be the underlying problem in patients with Milroy's disease (congenital familial lymphedema).[2]

FUNCTION AND STRUCTURE

The lymphatic system is composed of three elements:

1. Initial or terminal lymphatic capillaries, which absorb lymph
2. Collecting vessels, which serve primarily as conduits for lymph transport
3. Lymph nodes, which are interposed in the pathway of the conducting vessels, filtering the lymph and serving a primary immunologic role

The terminal lymphatics have special structural characteristics that allow entry not only of large macromolecules but also of cells and microbes. Their most important structural feature is a high porosity resulting from a very small number of tight junctions between endothelial cells, a limited and incomplete basement membrane, and anchoring filaments (4-10 nm) tethering the interstitial matrix to the endothelial cells. These filaments, once the

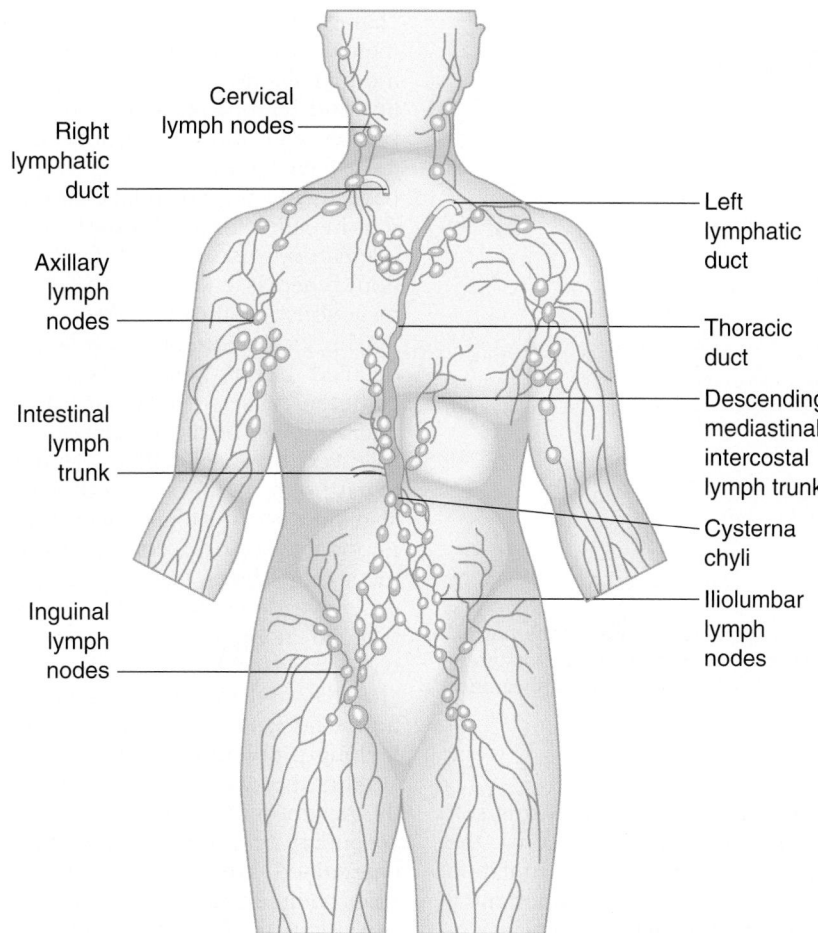

Right
lymphatic
duct

Cervical
lymph nodes

Axillary
lymph
nodes

Intestinal
lymph
trunk

Inguinal
lymph
nodes

Left
lymphatic
duct

Thoracic
duct

Descending
mediastinal-
intercostal
lymph trunk

Cysterna
chyli

Iliolumbar
lymph
nodes

Figure 69-1 Major anatomic pathways and lymph node groups of the lymphatic system

turgor of the tissue increases, are able to pull on the endothelial cells and essentially introduce large gaps between them that allow for low-resistance influx of interstitial fluid and macromolecules into the lymphatic channels. The collecting vessels ascend alongside the primary blood vessels of the organ or limb, pass through the regional lymph nodes, and drain into the main lymph channels of the torso. These channels eventually empty into the venous system through the thoracic duct. There are additional communications between the lymphatic and venous systems. These smaller lymphovenous shunts mostly occur at the level of lymph nodes and around major venous structures, such as the jugular, subclavian, and iliac veins. Several structures in the body contain no lymphatics. Specifically, lymphatics have not been found in the epidermis, the cornea, the central nervous system, the cartilage, tendon, and muscle.

The lymphatic system has three main functions. First, tissue fluid and macromolecules ultrafiltrated at the level of the arterial capillaries are reabsorbed and returned to the circulation through the lymphatic system. Every day, 50% to 100% of the intravascular proteins are filtered this way in the interstitial space. Normally, they then enter the terminal lymphatics and are transported through the collecting lymphatics back into the venous circulation. Second, microbes arriving in the interstitial space enter

the lymphatic system and are presented to the lymph nodes, which represent the first line of the immune system. Last, at the level of the gastrointestinal tract, lymph vessels are responsible for the uptake and transport of most of the fat absorbed from the bowel.

In contrast to what happens with venous forward flow, lymph's centripetal transport occurs mainly through intrinsic contractility of the individual lymphatic vessels, which in concert with competent valvular mechanisms, is effective in establishing constant forward flow of lymph. In addition to the intrinsic contractility, other factors, such as surrounding muscular activity, negative pressure secondary to breathing, and transmitted arterial pulsations, have a lesser role in the forward lymph flow. These secondary factors appear to become more important under conditions of lymph stasis and congestion of the lymphatic vessels.

PATHOPHYSIOLOGY AND STAGING

Lymphedema is the result of an inability of the existing lymphatic system to accommodate the protein and fluid entering the interstitial compartment at the tissue level.[3] In the first stage of lymphedema, impaired lymphatic drainage results in protein-rich fluid accumulation in the

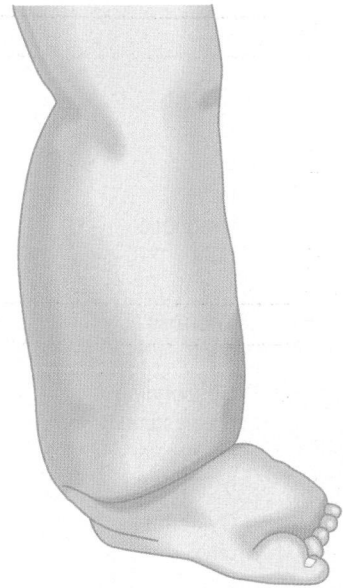

Figure 69-2 Lymphedema with characteristic loss of the normal perimalleolar shape resulting in a tree trunk pattern. Dorsum of the foot is characteristically swollen, resulting in the appearance of the buffalo hump.

interstitial compartment. Clinically, this manifests as soft pitting edema. In the second stage of lymphedema, the clinical condition is further exacerbated by accumulation of fibroblasts, adipocytes, and perhaps most importantly, macrophages in the affected tissues, which culminate in a local inflammatory response. This results in important structural changes from the deposition of connective tissue and adipose elements at the skin and subcutaneous level. In the second stage of lymphedema, tissue edema is more pronounced, is nonpitting, and has a spongy consistency. In the third and most advanced stage of lymphedema, the affected tissues sustain further injury as a result of both the local inflammatory response and recurrent infectious episodes that typically result from minimal subclinical skin breaks in the skin. Such repeated episodes injure the incompetent, remaining lymphatic channels, progressively worsening the underlying insufficiency of the lymphatic system. This eventually results in excessive subcutaneous fibrosis and scarring with associated severe skin changes characteristic of lymphostatic elephantiasis.

DIFFERENTIAL DIAGNOSIS

In most patients with second- or third-stage lymphedema, the characteristic findings on physical exam can usually establish the diagnosis. The edematous limb has a firm and hardened consistency. There is loss of the normal perimalleolar shape resulting in a so-called tree trunk pattern. The dorsum of the foot is characteristically swollen, resulting in the appearance of the so-called buffalo hump, and the toes become thick and squared (Fig. 69-2). In advanced lymphedema, the skin undergoes

characteristic changes such as lichenification, development of peau d'orange, and hyperkeratosis.[3] Additionally, the patients give a history of recurrent episodes of cellulitis and lymphangitis after trivial trauma and frequently present with fungal infections affecting the forefoot and toes. Patients with isolated lymphedema usually do not have the hyperpigmentation or ulceration one typically sees in patients with chronic venous insufficiency. Lymphedema does not respond significantly to overnight elevation, whereas edema secondary to central organ failure or venous insufficiency does.

The evaluation of a swollen extremity starts with a detailed history and physical examination. The most common causes of bilateral extremity edema are of systemic origin. The most common etiology is cardiac failure, followed by renal failure.[4] Hypoproteinemia secondary to cirrhosis, nephrotic syndrome, and malnutrition can also produce bilateral lower extremity edema. Another important cause to consider with bilateral leg enlargement is lipedema. Lipedema is not true edema but rather excessive subcutaneous fat found in obese women. It is bilateral, nonpitting, and greatest at the ankle and legs, with characteristic sparing of the feet. There are no skin changes, and the enlargement is not affected by elevation. The history usually indicates that this has been a lifelong problem that "runs in the family."

After the systemic etiologies of edema are excluded in the patient with unilateral extremity involvement, edema secondary to venous and lymphatic pathology must be entertained. Venous pathology is overwhelmingly the most common cause of unilateral leg edema. Leg edema secondary to venous disease is usually pitting and is greatest at the legs and ankles, with a sparing of the feet. The edema responds promptly to overnight leg elevation. In the later stages, the skin is atrophic with brawny pigmentation. Ulceration associated with venous insufficiency occurs above or posterior to and beneath the malleoli.

CLASSIFICATION

Lymphedema is generally classified as primary when there is no known etiology and secondary when its cause is a known disease or disorder.[5] Primary lymphedema has generally been classified on the basis of the age of onset and presence of familial clustering. Primary lymphedema with onset before the first year of life is called *congenital*. The familial version of congenital lymphedema is known as *Milroy's disease* and is inherited as a dominant trait. Primary lymphedema with onset between the ages of 1 and 35 years is called *lymphedema praecox*. The familial version of lymphedema praecox is known as *Meige's disease*. Finally, primary lymphedema with onset after the age of 35 years is called *lymphedema tarda*. The primary lymphedemas are relatively uncommon, occurring in 1 of every 10,000 individuals. The most common form of primary lymphedema is praecox, which accounts for about 80% of the patients. Congenital and tarda lymphedemas each account for the remaining 10%. Worldwide, the most common cause of secondary lymphedema is infestation of the lymph nodes by the parasite *Wuchereria bancrofti* in the disease state called *filariasis*. In developed countries, the most common causes of secondary lymphedema involve resection or ablation of regional lymph nodes by surgery, radiation therapy, tumor invasion, direct trauma, or less commonly, an infectious process.

DIAGNOSTIC TESTS

The diagnosis of lymphedema is relatively easy in the patient who presents in the second and third stages of the disease. It can, however, be a difficult diagnosis to make in the first stage, particularly when the edema is mild, pitting, and relieved with simple maneuvers such as elevation.[6,7] For patients with suspected secondary forms of lymphedema, computed tomography (CT) and magnetic resonance imaging (MRI) are valuable and indeed essential for exclusion of underlying oncologic disease states.[8,9] In patients with known lymph node excision and radiation treatment as the underlying problem of their lymphedema, additional diagnostic studies are rarely needed except as these studies relate to follow-up of an underlying malignancy. For patients with edema of unknown etiology and a suspicion for lymphedema, lymphoscintigraphy is the diagnostic test of choice. When lymphoscintigraphy confirms that lymphatic drainage is delayed, the diagnosis of primary lymphedema is never made until neoplasia involving the regional and central lymphatic drainage of the limb has been excluded through CT or MRI. If a more detailed diagnostic interpretation of lymphatic channels is needed for operative planning, contrast lymphangiography may be considered.

Lymphoscintigraphy has emerged as the test of choice in patients with suspected lymphedema.[10-12] It cannot differentiate between primary and secondary lymphedemas; however, it has a sensitivity of 70% to 90% and a specificity of nearly 100% in differentiating lymphedema from other causes of limb swelling. The test assesses lymphatic function by quantitating the rate of clearance of a radiolabeled macromolecular tracer (Fig. 69-3). The advantages of the technique are that it is simple, safe, and reproducible with low exposure to radioactivity (~5 mCi). It involves the injection of a small amount of radioiodinated human albumin or ^{99m}Tc-labeled sulfide colloid into the first interdigital space of the foot or hand. Migration of the radiotracer within the skin and subcutaneous lymphatics is easily monitored with a whole body gamma camera, thus producing clear images of the major lymphatic channels in the leg as well as measuring the amount of radioactivity at the inguinal nodes 30 and 60 minutes after injection of the radiolabeled substance in the feet. An uptake value that is less than 0.3% of the total injected dose at 30 minutes is diagnostic of lymphedema. The normal range of uptake is between 0.6% and 1.6%. In patients with edema secondary to venous disease, isotope clearance is usually abnormally rapid, resulting in more than 2% ilioinguinal uptake. Importantly, variation in the degree of edema involving the lower extremity

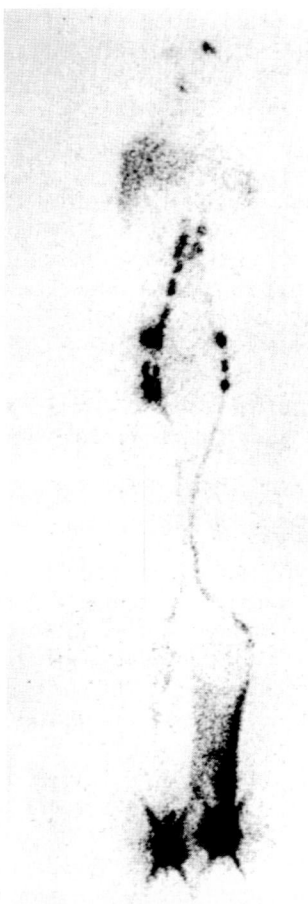

Figure 69-3 Lymphoscintigraphic pattern in primary lymphedema. Note area of dermal backflow on the left and diminished number of lymph nodes in the groin. (From Cambria RA, Gloviczki P, Naessens JM, Wahner HW: Noninvasive evaluation of the lymphatic system with lymphoscintigraphy: A prospective, semiquantitative analysis in 386 extremities. J Vasc Surg 18:773-782, 1993.)

does not appear to significantly change the rate of the isotope clearance.

Direct-contrast lymphangiography provides the finest details of the lymphatic anatomy.[13] However, it is an invasive study that involves exposure and cannulation of lymphatics at the dorsum of the forefoot, followed by slow injection of contrast medium (ethiodized oil). The procedure is tedious, the cannulation often necessitates aid of magnification optics (frequently an operating microscope is needed), and the dissection requires some form of anesthetic. After cannulation of a superficial lymph vessel, contrast material is slowly injected into the lymphatic system. A total of 7 to 10 mL of contrast is ideal for lower extremity evaluation, and 4 to 5 mL for upper extremity evaluation. Potential complications include damage of the visualized lymphatics, allergic reactions, and pulmonary embolism if the oil-based contrast enters the venous system through lymphovenous anastomoses. Lymphangiography in the present practice of vascular surgery is used infrequently and reserved for the preoperative evaluation of selected patients who are candidates for direct operations on their lymphatic vessels.

THERAPY

Most lymphedema patients can be treated with a combination of limb elevation, a high-quality compression garment, complex decongestive physical therapy, and compression pump therapy. A new class of medications known as *benzopyrones* is still under investigation in the United States but may find a place in the care of lymphedema in the near future. Operative treatment may be considered for patients with advanced, complicated lymphedema who fail management with nonoperative means.

General Therapeutic Measures

All patients with lymphedema need to be educated in meticulous skin care and avoidance of injuries.[14] Patients must always be instructed to see their physicians early for signs of infection because these may progress rapidly to serious systemic infections.[15] Infections must be aggressively and promptly treated with appropriate antibiotics directed at gram-positive cocci.[16] Eczema at the level of the forefoot and toes requires treatment, and hydrocortisone-based creams may be considered. Additionally, basic range-of-motion exercises for the extremities have been shown to be of value in the management of lymphedema in the long term. Finally, the patients must make every effort to maintain ideal body weight.

Elevation and Compression Garments

For lymphedema patients in all stages of disease, management with high-quality elastic garments is necessary at all times except when the legs are elevated above the heart.[17,18] The ideal compression garment is custom-fitted and delivers pressures in the range of 30 to 60 mm Hg. Such garments may have the additional benefit of protecting the extremity from injuries such as burns, lacerations, and insect bites. Patients need to avoid standing for prolonged periods and must elevate their legs at night by supporting the foot of the bed on 15-cm blocks.

Complex Decongestive Physical Therapy

Complex decongestive physical therapy (CDP) is a specialized massage technique for patients with lymphedema designed to stimulate the still-functioning lymph vessels, evacuate stagnant protein-rich fluid by breaking up subcutaneous deposits of fibrous tissue, and redirect lymph fluid to areas of the body where lymph flow is normal.[19] The technique is initiated on the normal contralateral side of the body, evacuating excessive fluid and preparing first the lymphatic zones of the nonaffected extremity, followed by the zones in the trunk quadrant adjacent to the affected limb, before attention is turned to the swollen extremity. The affected extremity is massaged in a segmental fashion with the proximal zones being massaged first, proceeding to the distal limb. The technique is time-consuming but effective in reducing the volume of the lymphedematous limbs.[20] After the massage session is complete, the extremity is wrapped with a low-stretch wrap, and the limb is placed in the custom-fitted garment to maintain the decreased girth obtained with the massage therapy. This kind of therapy is appropriate for patients with all stages of lymphedema.[21]

When the patient is first referred for CDP treatment, the patient undergoes daily to weekly massage sessions for up to 8 to 12 weeks. Limb elevation and elastic stockings are a necessary adjunct in this phase. After maximal volume reduction is achieved, the patient returns for maintenance massage treatments every 2 to 3 months.

Compression Pump Therapy

Pneumatic compression pump therapy is another effective method of reducing the volume of the lymphedematous limb using a similar principle to massage therapy. The device consists of a sleeve containing several compartments. The lymphedematous limb is positioned inside the sleeve, and the compartments are serially inflated so as to "milk" the stagnant fluid out of the extremity.[22]

When a patient with advanced lymphedema is first referred for therapy, an initial approach with hospitalization for 3 to 4 days involving strict limb elevation, daily CDP, and compression pump treatments may be necessary to achieve optimal control of the lymphedema. Patients with cardiac or renal dysfunction are monitored for fluid overload. After this initial period of intensive therapy, patients are fitted with a high-quality compression garment to maintain the limb volume. Maintenance sessions are then prescribed on an as-needed basis.

Drug Therapy

Benzopyrones have attracted interest as potentially effective agents in the treatment of lymphedema. This class of medications, which includes coumarin (1,2-benzopyrone), is thought to reduce lymphedema through stimulation of proteolysis by tissue macrophages and stimulation of the peristalsis and pumping action of the collecting lymphatics. Benzopyrones have no anticoagulant activity. The first randomized, crossover trial of coumarin in patients with lymphedema of the arms and legs was reported in 1993.[23] The study concluded that coumarin was more effective than placebo in reducing volume; other important parameters, including skin temperature, attacks of secondary acute inflammation and discomfort of the lymphedematous extremities, and skin turgor and suppleness, were also improved with coumarin. A second randomized, crossover trial was reported in 1999.[24] This study focused on effects of coumarin in women with secondary lymphedema after treatment for breast cancer. The trial investigators found that coumarin was not effective therapy for the specific group of women. Because of the disagreement between these two major trials, the enthusiasm for use of benzopyrones in the United States has been tempered. Additional trials need to be undertaken to clarify the potential effects of the medications on primary and secondary lymphedemas in different extremities and stages.

Diuretics may temporarily improve the appearance of the lymphedematous extremity with stage I disease, leading patients to request continuous therapy. However, other than producing temporary intravascular volume depletion, there is no long-term benefit. Thus, diuretics have no role in the treatment of lymphedema at any stage.

Operative Treatment

Ninety-five percent of patients with lymphedema can be managed nonoperatively. Surgical intervention may be considered for patients with stage II and III lymphedema who have severe functional impairment, recurrent episodes of lymphangitis, and severe pain despite optimal medical therapy. Two main categories of operations are available for the care of patients with lymphedema: reconstructive and excisional.

Reconstructive operations[25-27] are considered for those patients with proximal (either primary or secondary) obstruction of the extremity lymphatic circulation with preserved, dilated lymphatics distal to the obstruction. In these patients, the residual dilated lymphatics can be anastomosed to nearby veins or to transposed healthy lymphatic channels (usually mobilized or harvested from the contralateral extremity) in an attempt to restore effective drainage of the lymphedematous extremity. Treatment of selected lymphedema patients with lymphovenous anastomoses has resulted in objective improvement in 30% to 60% of the patients, with an average initial reduction in the excess limb volume of 40% to 50%.[28,29]

For those patients with primary lymphedema who have hypoplastic and fibrotic distal lymphatic vessels, such reconstructions are not an option. For such patients, surgical strategy involving transfer of lymphatic-bearing tissue (portion of the greater omentum) into the affected limb has been attempted. This is intended to connect the residual hypoplastic lymphatic channels of the leg to competent lymphatics in the transferred tissue. Omental flap operations have been found to have poor results.[30] Alternatively, a segment of the ileum can be disconnected from the rest of the bowel, stripped of its mucosa, and mobilized to be sewn onto the cut surface of residual ilioinguinal nodes in an attempt to bridge lower extremity with mesenteric lymphatics. When this enteromesenteric bridge procedure was applied to a group of eight carefully selected patients, the outcomes were promising, with six patients showing sustained clinical improvement in long follow-up.[31]

Excisional operations are essentially the only viable option for patients without residual lymphatics of adequate size for reconstructive procedures. For patients with recalcitrant stage II and early stage III lymphedema in whom the edema is moderate and the skin is relatively healthy, an excisional procedure that removes a large segment of the lymphedematous subcutaneous tissues and overlying skin is the procedure of choice. This palliative procedure was introduced by Kontoleon in 1918 and was later popularized by Homan as "staged subcutaneous excision underneath flaps" (Fig. 69-4). The operative approach starts with a medial incision extending from the level of the medial malleolus through the calf into the midthigh.[32-34] Flaps about 1 to 2 cm thick are elevated anteriorly and posteriorly, and all subcutaneous tissue beneath the flaps, along with the underlying medial calf deep fascia, is removed with the redundant skin. The sural nerve is preserved. After the first-stage procedure is completed, and if additional lymphedematous tissue removal is necessary, then a second operation is performed, usually 3 to 6 months later. The second-stage operation is performed using similar techniques through an incision on the lateral aspect of the limb.

In a recent long-term follow-up study, 80% of patients undergoing staged subcutaneous excision underneath flaps had significant and long-lasting reduction in extremity size associated with improved function and extremity contour. Wound complications were encountered in 10% of the patients.[32]

When the lymphedema is extremely pronounced and the skin is unhealthy and infected, the simple reducing operation of Kontoleon is not adequate. In this case, the classic excisional operation originally described by Charles in 1912 is performed (Fig. 69-5). The procedure involves complete and circumferential excision of the skin, subcutaneous tissue, and deep fascia of the involved leg and dorsum of the foot.[35] The excision is usually performed in one stage, and coverage is provided preferably by full-thickness grafting from the excised skin. In a follow-up report, patients subjected to Charles' operation had immediate volume and circumference reduction. Skin graft take was 88%, and complications of operation consisted primarily of wound infections, hematomas, and necrosis of skin flaps. The hospital stay was 21 to 36 days.[36] Although this is a successful and radically reducing operation, the behavior in the healing skin graft is unpredictable. Between 10% and 15% of the grafted segments do not take and can be difficult to manage because of frequent localized sloughing, excessive scarring, focal recurrent infections, and hyperkeratosis or dermatitis. These complications appear to be worse in patients in whom leg resurfacing is performed using split-thickness grafts from the opposite extremity. In advanced cases, the exophytic changes within the grafted skin, chronic cellulitis, and skin breakdown may eventually lead to leg amputation.[37]

CHYLOTHORAX

Chylous pleural effusion is usually secondary to thoracic duct trauma (usually iatrogenic after chest surgery) and rarely a manifestation of advanced malignant disease with lymphatic metastasis.[38] Presence of chylomicrons on lipoprotein analysis and a triglyceride level of more than 110 mg/dL in the pleural fluid are diagnostic. Initially, patients can be treated nonoperatively with tube thoracostomy and medium-chain triglyceride diet or total parenteral nutrition. For patients with thoracic duct injury and an effusion that persists after 1 week of drainage, video-assisted thoracoscopy or thoracotomy is employed to identify and ligate the thoracic duct above and below the leak. The site of the leak can be identified if cream

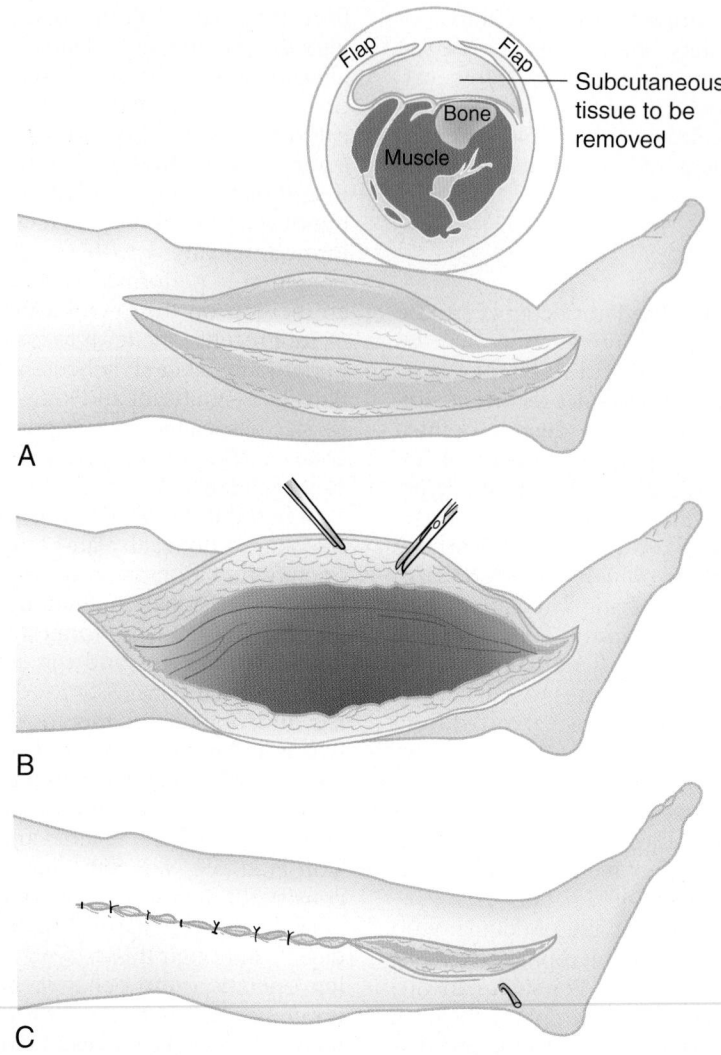

Figure 69-4 A to **C,** Schematic representation of Kontoleon's or Homans' procedure. Relatively thick skin flaps are raised anteriorly and posteriorly, and all subcutaneous tissue beneath the flaps and the underlying medial calf deep fascia is removed along with the necessary redundant skin.

is given to the patient a few hours before operation. For patients with cancer-related chylothorax and persistent drainage despite optimal chemotherapy and radiation therapy, pleurodesis is highly successful in preventing recurrences.[39]

CHYLOPERITONEUM

In contrast to chylothorax, the most common cause of chylous ascites is congenital lymphatic abnormalities in children and malignancy involving the abdominal lymph nodes in adults. Operative injury to abdominal lymphatics resulting in chylous ascites is rare.[40] Presence of chylomicrons on lipoprotein analysis and a triglyceride level of more than 110 mg/dL are diagnostic. Initial treatment includes paracentesis followed by medium-chain triglyceride diet or total parenteral nutrition. In patients with postoperative chyloperitoneum, if ascites does not respond after 1 to 2 weeks of nonoperative management,

exploration is employed to identify and ligate the leaking lymphatic duct. Congenital and malignant causes are given longer periods (up to 4-6 weeks) of nonoperative management. If ascites persists in patients with congenital ascites, lymphoscintigraphy or lymphangiography is performed before making an attempt to control the leak with celiotomy. At the time of exploration, control of the leak can be achieved by ligation of leaking lymphatic vessels or resection of the bowel associated with the leak. Patients with malignancies receive aggressive management of their underlying disease, which generally is effective at controlling the chyloperitoneum.

TUMORS OF THE LYMPHATICS

Lymphangiomas are the lymphatic analogue of the hemangiomas of blood vessels. They are generally divided into two types: (1) simple or capillary lymphangioma and (2) cavernous lymphangioma or cystic hygroma.[41] They

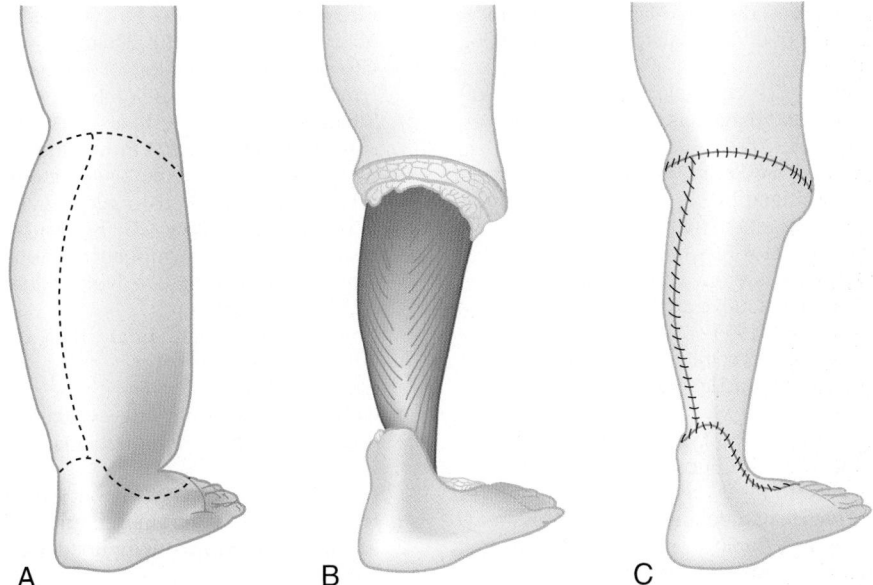

Figure 69-5 A to C, Schematic representation of Charles' procedure. It involves complete and circumferential excision of the skin, subcutaneous tissue, and deep fascia of the involved leg and dorsum of the foot. Coverage is provided preferably by full-thickness grafting from the excised skin.

are thought to represent isolated and sequestered segments of the lymphatic system that retain the ability to produce lymph. As the volume of lymph inside the cystic tumor increases, they grow larger within the surrounding tissues. Most of these benign tumors are present at birth, and 90% of them can be identified by the end of the first year of life. The cavernous lymphangiomas almost invariably occur in the neck or the axilla and rarely in the retroperitoneum. The simple capillary lymphangiomas also tend to occur subcutaneously in the head and neck region as well as the axilla. Rarely, however, they can be found in the trunk within the internal organs or the connective tissue in and around the abdominal or thoracic cavities. The treatment of lymphangiomas is surgical excision, taking care to preserve all normal surrounding infiltrated structures.

Lymphangiosarcoma is a rare tumor that develops as a complication of long-standing (usually more than 10 years) lymphedema.[42] Clinically, patients present with acute worsening of the edema and appearance of subcutaneous nodules that have a propensity toward hemorrhage and ulceration. The tumor can be treated, as other sarcomas, with preoperative chemotherapy and radiation followed by surgical excision, which usually takes the form of radical amputation. Overall, the tumor has a poor prognosis.[43]

Selected References

Gloviczki P: Principles of surgical treatment of chronic lymphoedema. Int Angiol 18(1):42-46, 1999.
Nagase T, Gonda K, Inoue K, et al: Treatment of lymphedema with lymphaticovenular anastomoses. Int J Clin Oncol 10:304-310, 2005.

These comprehensive reviews summarize the important elements in the management of patients with lymphedema.

Tiwari A, Cheng KS, Button M, et al: Differential diagnosis, investigation, and current treatment of lower limb lymphedema. Arch Surg 138:152-161, 2003.
Rockson SG: Lymphedema. Curr Treat Options Cardiovasc Med 8:129-136, 2006.

These two reviews illustrate the current knowledge and controversies in the pathophysiology, classification, natural history, differential diagnosis, and treatment of lymphedema.

Wyatt LE, Miller TA: Lymphedema and tumors of the lymphatics. In Moore WS (ed): Vascular Surgery: A Comprehensive Review. Philadelphia: WB Saunders, 1998, pp 829-843.

This authoritative treatise provides a succinct summary of the diagnosis and treatment of lymphatic disorders.

References

1. Levine C: Primary disorders of the lymphatic vessels: A unified concept. J Pediatr Surg 24:233-240, 1989.
2. Alitalo K, Tammela T, Petrova TV: Lymphangiogenesis in development and human disease. Nature 438(7070):946-953, 2005.
3. Browse NL, Stewart G: Lymphoedema: Pathophysiology and classification. J Cardiovasc Surg (Torino) 26:91-106 1985.
4. Cho S, Atwood JE: Peripheral edema. Am J Med 113(7):580-586, 2002.
5. Szuba A, Rockson SG: Lymphedema: Classification, diagnosis and therapy. Vasc Med 3:145-156, 1998.
6. Tiwari A, Cheng KS, Button M, et al: Differential diagnosis, investigation, and current treatment of lower limb lymphedema. Arch Surg 138:152-161, 2003.
7. Rockson SG: Lymphedema. Curr Treat Options Cardiovasc Med 8:129-136, 2006.
8. Marotel M, Cluzan R, Ghabboun S, et al: Transaxial computer tomography of lower extremity lymphedema. Lymphology 31:180-185, 1998.

9. Werner GT, Scheck R, Kaiserling E: Magnetic resonance imaging of peripheral lymphedema. Lymphology 31:34-36, 1998.

10. Burnand KG, McGuinness CL, Lagattolla NR, et al: Value of isotope lymphography in the diagnosis of lymphoedema of the leg. Br J Surg 89:74-78, 2002.

11. Szuba A, Shin WS, Strauss HW, et al: The third circulation: Radionuclide lymphoscintigraphy in the evaluation of lymphedema. J Nucl Med 44:43-57, 2003.

12. Cambria RA, Gloviczki P, Naessens JM, et al: Noninvasive evaluation of the lymphatic system with lymphoscintigraphy: A prospective, semiquantitative analysis in 386 extremities. J Vasc Surg 18:773-782, 1993.

13. Weissleder H, Weissleder R: Interstitial lymphangiography: Initial clinical experience with a dimeric nonionic contrast agent. Radiology 170:371-374, 1989.

14. Cohen SR, Payne DK, Tunkel RS: Lymphedema: Strategies for management. Cancer 15:92(4 Suppl):980-987, 2001.

15. Harris SR, Hugi MR, Olivotto IA, et al, for the Steering Committee for Clinical Practice Guidelines for the Care and Treatment of Breast Cancer: Clinical practice guidelines for the care and treatment of breast cancer. 11. Lymphedema. CMAJ 164:191-199, 2001.

16. Bernas MJ, Witte CL, Witte MH: The diagnosis and treatment of peripheral lymphedema: Draft revision of the 1995 Consensus Document of the International Society of Lymphology Executive Committee for discussion at the September 3-7, 2001, XVIII International Congress of Lymphology in Genoa, Italy. Lymphology 34(2):84-91, 2001.

17. Yasuhara H, Shigematsu H, Muto T: A study of the advantages of elastic stockings for leg lymphedema. Int Angiol 15:272-277, 1996.

18. Badger CM, Peacock JL, Mortimer PS: A randomized, controlled, parallel-group clinical trial comparing multilayer bandaging followed by hosiery versus hosiery alone in the treatment of patients with lymphedema of the limb. Cancer 88:2832-2837, 2000.

19. Lerner R: What's new in lymphedema therapy in America? Int J Angiol 7:191-196, 1998.

20. Franzeck UK, Spiegel I, Fischer M, et al: Combined physical therapy for lymphedema evaluated by fluorescence micro lymphography and lymph capillary pressure measurements. J Vasc Res 34:306-311, 1997.

21. Ko DS, Lerner R, Klose G, et al: Effective treatment of lymphedema of the extremities. Arch Surg 133:452-458, 1998.

22. Richmand DM, O'Donnell TF Jr, Zelikovski A: Sequential pneumatic compression for lymphedema: A controlled trial. Arch Surg 120:1116-1119, 1985.

23. Casley-Smith JR, Morgan RG, Piller NB: Treatment of lymphedema of the arms and legs with 5,6-benzo-[alpha] pyrone. N Engl J Med 329:1158-1163, 1993.

24. Loprinzi CL, Kugler JW, Sloan JA, et al: Lack of effect of coumarin in women with lymphedema after treatment for breast cancer. N Engl J Med 340:346-350, 1999.

25. Campisi C, Boccardo F: Lymphedema and microsurgery. Microsurgery 22:74-80, 2002.

26. Gloviczki P: Principles of surgical treatment of chronic lymphoedema. Int Angiol 18(1):42-46, 1999.

27. Tanaka Y, Tajima S, Imai K, et al: Experience of a new surgical procedure for the treatment of unilateral obstructive lymphedema of the lower extremity: Adipo-lymphatico-venous transfer. Microsurgery 17:209-216, 1996.

28. O'Brien BM, Mellow CG, Khazanchi RK, et al: Long-term results after microlymphaticovenous anastomoses for the treatment of obstructive lymphedema. Plast Reconstr Surg 85:562-572, 1990.

29. Nagase T, Gonda K, Inoue K, et al: Treatment of lymphedema with lymphaticovenular anastomoses. Int J Clin Oncol 10:304-310, 2005.

30. Goldsmith HS: Long term evaluation of omental transposition for chronic lymphedema. Ann Surg 180:847-849, 1974.

31. Hurst PA, Stewart G, Kinmonth JB, Browse NL: Long-term results of the enteromesenteric bridge operation in the treatment of primary lymphoedema. Br J Surg 72:272-274, 1985.

32. Miller TA, Wyatt LE, Rudkin GH: Staged skin and subcutaneous excision for lymphedema: A favorable report of long-term results. Plast Reconstr Surg 102:1486-1498, 1998.

33. Wyatt LE, Miller TA: Lymphedema and tumors of the lymphatics. In Moore WS (ed): Vascular Surgery: A Comprehensive Review. Philadelphia: WB Saunders, 1998, pp 829-843.

34. Miller TA: Surgical management of lymphedema of the extremity. Plast Reconstr Surg 56:633-641, 1975.

35. Dellon AL, Hoopes JE: The Charles procedure for primary lymphedema: Long-term clinical results. Plast Reconstr Surg 60:589-595, 1977.

36. Dandapat MC, Mohapatro SK, Mohanty SS: Filarial lymphoedema and elephantiasis of lower limb: A review of 44 cases. Br J Surg 73:451-453, 1986.

37. Miller TA: Charles procedure for lymphedema: A warning. Am J Surg 139:290-292, 1980.

38. Johnstone DW: Postoperative chylothorax. Chest Surg Clin N Am 12:597-603, 2002.

39. Romero S: Nontraumatic chylothorax. Curr Opin Pulm Med 6:287-291, 2000.

40. Aalami OO, Allen DB, Organ CH Jr: Chylous ascites: A collective review. Surgery 128:761-778, 2000.

41. Fonkalsrud EW: Congenital malformations of the lymphatic system. Semin Pediatr Surg 3:62-69, 1994.

42. Nakazono T, Kudo S, Matsuo Y, et al: Angiosarcoma associated with chronic lymphedema (Stewart-Treves syndrome) of the leg: MR imaging. Skeletal Radiol 29:413-416, 2000.

43. Sordillo PP, Chapman R, Hajdu SI, et al: Lymphangiosarcoma. Cancer 48:1674-1679, 1981.

CHAPTER 70

Access and Ports

Frank M. Parker, DO   Michael C. Stoner, MD   and   Carl E. Haisch, MD

Vascular Access
Peritoneal Dialysis

VASCULAR ACCESS

History

Access to the vascular system is necessitated by the therapy required for the complex medical conditions that occur in many patients. Frequent access to the bloodstream is required for patients undergoing parenteral nutrition, chemotherapy for malignant disease, plasmapheresis, and short-term and long-term dialysis.

Without adequate vascular access, hemodialysis would not have developed as we know it today. The first significant research to investigate dialysis was begun in the 19th century by Thomas Graham. George Haas, in 1924, continued Graham's work when he attempted dialysis in the first human patient. The patient tolerated the procedure well, but the amount of dialysis was inadequate for the patient to gain a therapeutic effect, and the patient died. In the early 1940s, Willem Johan Kolff designed a dialysis machine using cellulose tubing, and when heparin became available, he dialyzed his first patient. The patient eventually died after 26 days of treatment when vascular access became unavailable after repeated surgical cutdowns.

The breakthrough in long-term access for dialysis occurred when Quinton and colleagues used a Teflon conduit to construct arteriovenous connections in 1960. This advance allowed the first long-term dialysis of patients and was not improved on until 1966, when Brescia and associates[1] constructed a natural arteriovenous fistula between the radial artery and the cephalic vein. The Brescia-Cimino fistula is still considered the gold standard for dialysis. For patients without an adequate cephalic vein, saphenous vein was used but found to be unsatisfactory. Artificial materials were eventually developed, and the current standard material is polytetrafluoroethylene (PTFE).

The need to infuse irritating solutions into a patient required a high-flow system. Aubaniac used the subclavian vein for vascular access in 1952, and Dudrick and Wilmore used it later for nutritional support. This vein was selected for its high flow and easy accessibility. The Broviac catheter and, later, the Hickman catheter were used for nutritional support and for chemotherapy and blood drawing, respectively. Currently, double-lumen and triple-lumen catheters are available for access in monitoring, dialysis, and numerous other applications. Catheters such as the Port-A-Cath and Infus-A-Port are designed so that the entire catheter and access port are totally covered by skin. To use these catheters, access is gained through a septum in an access port with a special needle.

Indications

Hemoaccess through a fistula, jump graft, or external angioaccess is appropriate when frequent access to the vascular system is required, when a high-flow system is needed, when the ability to withstand multiple needle punctures is required, or when highly sclerotic solutions are administered intravenously (IV). The most common uses are for acute and chronic renal failure, administration of chemotherapeutic agents and other drugs, hyperalimentation, and administration of blood and blood products. Angioaccess is also frequently required in patients with AIDS who need medications for treatment of cytomegalovirus infection or who need access for blood drawing.

Vascular access is an extremely important part of medicine. In the end-stage renal disease budget, maintaining and placing vascular access devices and fistulas cost more than $1 to 2 billion per year in the United States. This amount constitutes up to 17% of the budget for patients with end-stage renal failure. An estimated 300,000 patients require dialysis, and the number continues to increase, as does the age of these patients. Currently, 40% of all patients who undergo dialysis are 65 years old or older, and the percentage of patients older than 65 years continues to increase.

External Angioaccess

Dialysis

The first successful shunt for repeated hemodialysis was the Scribner shunt, which used a Teflon tip inserted into both the artery and the vein. Silastic tubing, attached to the Teflon tip, was placed through the skin by means of a skin incision, both ends were connected, and continuous blood flow was established. These shunts are used infrequently now, primarily for plasmapheresis or for acute, continuous renal replacement therapy.

Dialysis Through Major Vessels

Short-term angioaccess for hemodialysis may be obtained by insertion of a nontunneled catheter into the subclavian, external jugular, internal jugular, or femoral vein. These percutaneously placed catheters may make construction of an autogenous or internal arteriovenous fistula more difficult or impossible secondary to central venous stenosis. After placement of a subclavian catheter for even as short a period as 2 weeks, up to 50% of subclavian veins have a significant stenosis that causes either clotting of the fistula or a swollen arm after fistula placement. The incidence of stenosis is much lower, less than 10%, with use of the internal jugular vein, but this complication must be considered nonetheless. Stenoses may not be clinically evident because of collateral circulation, but a fistula will make the stenosis evident because of the high flow rate. While the patient is undergoing dialysis, the fistula or graft may have a high venous pressure. If the patient has had a subclavian or internal jugular catheter, peripherally inserted central catheter line, pacemaker, or total parenteral nutrition line in place, a Doppler study of the central veins is done before an internal access is placed. The gold standard is still a venogram, which allows the subclavian vein to be seen behind the clavicular head. Femoral catheters may be placed at the patient's bedside; ideally, they are removed after dialysis, to prevent infection or venous thrombosis. Repeated use of these catheters may result in iliofemoral thrombosis, local bleeding, or arterial puncture and injury.

The most commonly used catheters today are dual-lumen, silicone rubber, and polyurethane catheters. These catheters are soft and therefore are usually placed percutaneously in the external jugular or internal jugular vein, with the help of a peel-away sheath. A cutdown will be necessary infrequently. These catheters can be placed in the veins listed earlier, but they also have been

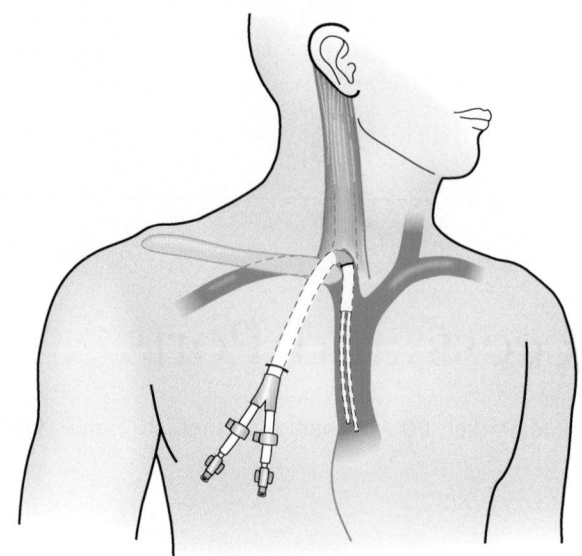

Figure 70-1 Position of a soft Silastic internal jugular catheter for dialysis. (From Uldall R, DeBruyne M, Besley M, et al: A new vascular access catheter for hemodialysis. Am J Kidney Dis 21:270, 1993.)

placed in the inferior vena cava using a translumbar or transhepatic approach. The dual-lumen design imparts a low incidence of recirculation (2%-5%), except when short catheters are placed in the femoral vein, where recirculation is unacceptably high (18% to almost 40% at higher blood flows of 400 mL/min) (Fig. 70-1). Because these catheters are soft and pliable, endothelial damage is less than with stiff catheters and the incidence of thrombosis is lower.

Patients who will require long-term access have a tunneled catheter placed while awaiting internal access or, better, have internal access planned before the acute need for dialysis. Dialysis Outcomes Quality Initiative (DOQI) guidelines state that internal access needs to be attempted first. The Dacron cuff allows tissue ingrowth, which helps reduce the risk for infection when compared with noncuffed catheters. Many different types of catheters can be used in patients who are undergoing dialysis. Most catheters have both lumens in a single unit; however, the Tesio catheter is really two separate catheters that are placed through two separate needle sticks. These catheters allow blood flows of up to 400 mL/min and thus allow high-flux dialysis. The catheter tip is in the right atrium to prevent recirculation and decrease the incidence of clot forming on the catheter tip. Stiff catheters are placed at the junction of the right atrium and the superior vena cava to prevent arrhythmias or venous puncture. The incidence of central stenosis is about the same with these soft catheters as it is with the stiffer catheters described earlier. Some patients are not candidates for placement of a fistula or a PTFE graft. In these patients, a silicone rubber catheter may be adequate. McLaughlin and colleagues[2] showed that about 50% of catheters placed in the right subclavian position survive for 1 year. This finding is consistent with the data of

Mosquera and associates,[3] who showed that the cumulative PermCath survival rate was 74% at 1 year and 43% at 2 years. One of the major problems with these catheters is that they become dysfunctional because of clot or fibrin sheath formation. The use of tissue plasminogen activator for opening the catheters has been discussed. This agent is safe and nonallergenic and, although expensive, may prolong catheter life. Newer thrombolytic therapy is being developed to replace urokinase.

Nutrition, Blood Access, and Chemotherapy

Access to the venous system for chemotherapy, parenteral nutrition, antibiotics, and blood products is most frequently obtained through the central vessels such as the subclavian, internal jugular, external jugular, or basilic vein. When no other site can be found, a catheter can be placed in the inferior vena cava by using a translumbar or transhepatic approach. If a patient has had multiple previous catheters, ultrasound-guided access to collateral veins with fluoroscopically monitored central advancement can assist in catheter placement as well as recanalization of occluded central veins. Venography done before attempted catheter placement is unnecessary because this can be done concomitantly. The catheters used are either totally implantable, such as Port-A-Cath or Infus-A-Port, or external, such as Broviac, Hickman, and Groshung catheters. Groshung catheters have a valve on the end to prevent blood flow into the catheter. These catheters can be placed in the operating room or can be safely placed in the angiography suite with no increased infectious risk.

The peripherally inserted central catheter line is placed through an arm vein at the bedside. This catheter may have an open tip and may require heparin, or it may have a Groshung tip. These catheters are constructed with a port, similar to that of a Port-A-Cath, which is placed under the skin. These peripherally inserted catheters have no fewer infectious complications than do central lines.

Complications

Complications can be divided into those that occur secondary to catheter placement and those that occur later. The early complications of subclavian or internal jugular placement include pneumothorax, hemothorax, arterial injury, thoracic duct injury, air embolus, inability to pass the catheter, bleeding, nerve injury, and great vessel injury. These complications all decrease in incidence as the physician gains more experience in placing these catheters. A chest radiograph must be taken after catheter placement to rule out pneumothorax and injury to the great vessels and to check for position of the catheter. The incidence of pneumothorax is 1% to 4%, and the incidence of injury to the great vessels is less than 1%.[4] A widened mediastinum is an indication of injury to the great vessels. Injury most commonly occurs when the catheter is placed from the right side. In patients who have had catheters placed previously or in whom finding the vein is difficult, ultrasonography is recommended. This allows determination of the anatomic location of the vein and pathologic processes that may be present from previous invasive procedures, such as occlusion, thrombosis, or stenosis. The use of ultrasound in one study resulted in successful venous cannulation in 100% of patients.[5]

Other complications are mechanical, thrombotic, and infectious. Mechanical complications include catheter malposition, inability to pass fluid or withdraw blood, and catheter shearing between the clavicle and the first rib. If one has a question regarding the catheter lumen or the inability to flush the catheter secondary to potential shearing between the clavicle and first rib, the catheter must be removed to prevent division of the catheter and the need to retrieve it from the heart.

Thrombotic complications occur in 4% to 10% of patients. Thrombosis may occur secondary to venous wall irritation caused by the catheter, as a result of a hypercoagulable state, or from irritation to the venous wall by the chemotherapeutic agents. The initial sign of thrombosis is the inability to draw blood from the catheter. However, the catheter may draw up against the vessel wall and thereby may also cause an inability to withdraw blood. Tissue plasminogen activator (tPA) can be used in an attempt to lyse clot in the catheter. If this is unsuccessful, a contrast radiograph is indicated to determine catheter position and integrity. When fresh thrombus surrounds the catheter but patient care requirements preclude its removal, mechanical or pharmacologic thrombectomy are considered to lyse venous clot. If the catheter can be removed and placed elsewhere, the patient will still need to be treated for the deep venous thrombosis.

The second most common catheter problem is infection. It may occur soon after placement (3-5 days) or late in the life of the catheter and may be at the exit site or be the cause of catheter-related sepsis. Despite the use of antibiotics, infection can be a catastrophic complication and result in epidural abscess, osteomyelitis, bacterial endocarditis, or septic arthritis. The diagnosis of infection is difficult. The best techniques to determine whether a catheter is infected require that the catheter be removed. Maki and associates (as reported by Whitman[4]) described a semiquantitative culture that is considered positive with 15 colony-forming units. Another technique calls for a Gram stain and culture of the catheter tip.[4] A third technique quantifies colony counts of bacteria in blood cultures taken from the central venous catheter and from a peripheral IV catheter. If the ratio is 10:1 catheter to blood colonies, the catheter is considered infected.

The exact incidence of catheter-related infection is difficult to ascertain, but reports indicate a rate of between 0.5 and 3.9 episodes per 1000 catheter-days. Many patients who have catheters in place are immunocompromised secondary to chemotherapy, nutritional status, or underlying disease. Multilumen catheters and catheter thrombosis both increase the incidence of catheter sepsis.[4]

When the catheter is placed, strict sterile technique must be used. A report by Darouiche and colleagues[6] indicated that catheters with minocycline and rifampin on the external and luminal surfaces had a lower infection rate than those with chlorhexidine and silver sulfadiazine on the external surface only. This finding indicates that the antibiotic combination may be important but also that the intraluminal route remains important in central catheter–related bloodstream infections.

Infections are most often caused by skin flora. Early infection (3-5 days) most often results from infection of the subcutaneous tract. Later infections may have the same cause or may occur by hematogenous spread. The most common bacteria are *Staphylococcus epidermidis* and *Staphylococcus aureus*. *Candida* species can also be involved but less frequently. The exit site is covered with dry gauze impregnated with iodophor ointment. This method is effective against both bacteria and fungi, and the dressing can be changed three times a week.

The most common therapy for suspected catheter infection is removal of the catheter. However, because catheter sites may be few, consideration has been given to catheter exchange over a guidewire. Beathard[7] outlined an approach to catheter exchange. The exit site was examined; if clean, the catheter was simply changed over a guidewire. If the exit site was thought to have an infection, a guidewire was used for the catheter, but a new exit site was chosen. When the infection was severe, the catheter was removed, the patient was allowed to improve, and a new catheter was placed.

Internal Angioaccess

Natural Fistulas
Prosthetic material, regardless of type, has a greater tendency toward thrombosis than autogenous tissue and therefore costs 30% to 50% more per year to maintain than does an autogenous fistula. Thus, the development of arteriovenous fistulas by direct anastomosis without the use of intervening prosthetic material represented one of the major advances in the management of patients undergoing hemodialysis. The fistula most frequently used, the standard by which all other fistulas are measured, is the Brescia-Cimino fistula. An Allen test is performed before operation to ensure adequate collateral flow from the ulnar artery to minimize hand ischemia. The artery and vein are isolated through a longitudinal incision, with care taken to avoid the superficial branch of the radial nerve. The artery and vein can be anastomosed in a number of ways, including from side artery to side vein, from end artery to side vein, from side artery to end vein, or from end artery to end vein (Fig. 70-2). A side-to-side anastomosis can cause venous hypertension in the hand, which can be corrected by ligation of the vein distal to the anastomosis. The end-to-end anastomosis appears to be accompanied by a higher initial thrombosis rate because fewer collateral channels are present. Dilation of the artery and vein at the time of creation of the fistula by insertion of a coronary dilator appears to diminish the initial thrombosis rate of these anastomoses.

Types of Natural Fistulas
Arteriovenous fistulas have several different anastomotic possibilities, the names of which have been standardized.[8] In addition to the autogenous radial-cephalic direct wrist access (Brescia-Cimino fistula), other possibilities

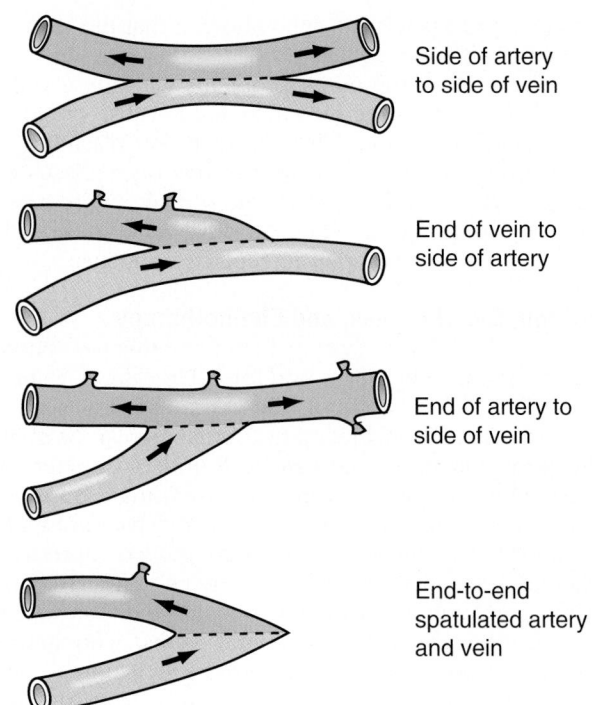

Figure 70-2 Four different anastomoses commonly constructed between the radial artery and cephalic vein. (From Ozeran RS: Construction and care of external arteriovenous shunts. In Wilson SE, Owens ML [eds]: Vascular Access Surgery. Chicago, Year Book Medical, 1980.)

Side of artery to side of vein

End of vein to side of artery

End of artery to side of vein

End-to-end spatulated artery and vein

include the autogenous posterior radial branch–cephalic direct access (snuffbox fistula), autogenous ulnar-cephalic forearm transposition, autogenous forearm radial-basilic transposition fistula (Feinberg), autogenous brachial-cephalic upper arm direct access (antecubital vein to the brachial artery), and autogenous brachial-basilic upper arm transposition (basilic vein transposition). The last fistula calls for dissection of the basilic vein and transfer to a superficial position on the medial portion of the upper extremity (Fig. 70-3). New reports of brachial artery to brachial vein fistula at primary procedure with secondary superficialization have been noted in the literature.[9]

There are also reports of transposing saphenous vein to upper arm as a conduit or transposing a loop in the thigh to create natural fistula access.[10] Superficial femoral vein transfer has also been reported but carries a high rate of initial as well as late complications and is reserved for limited cases.[11] The use of Nitinol U clips has shown higher maturation rates in forearm fistulas but no improvement in maturation rates of upper arm fistulas when compared with conventional continuous sutured anastomosis. If at all possible, all autologous options must be exhausted before nonautogenous material is used for dialysis access.

Because of the high propensity for infection among patients with acquired immunodeficiency syndrome (AIDS), natural vein is the preferred conduit for construction of vascular access for hemodialysis. Frequently, these

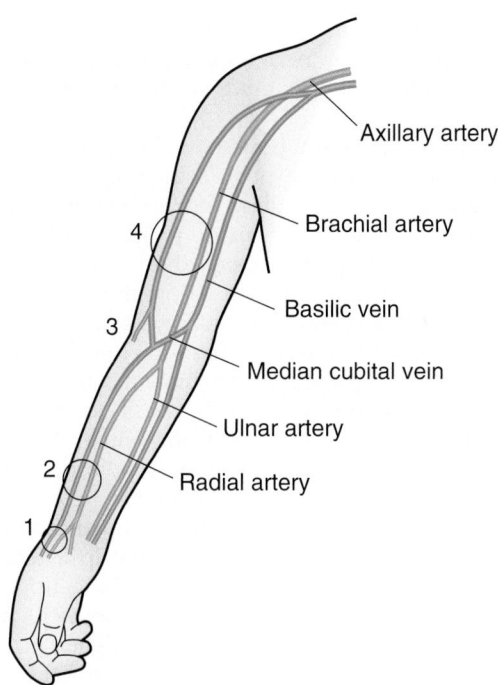

Figure 70-3 Four possible anastomotic sites for arteriovenous fistulas in the upper extremity. (Redrawn from Tilney NL, Lazarus JM [eds]: Surgical Care of the Patient with Renal Failure. Philadelphia, WB Saunders, 1982; as shown in Haisch CE: Chronic vascular and peritoneal access. In Davis JH, Sheldon GF [eds]: Clinical Surgery. St Louis, CV Mosby, 1995.)

patients have no usable veins in their arms. Gorski and colleagues[12] described their experience using the saphenous vein in the lower leg in these patients. The vein was dissected free of its bed and was anastomosed to the superficial femoral artery just below the profunda femoris to form a loop of saphenous vein to be used for dialysis.[12]

At present, the number of natural fistulas is thought to be too low. Therefore, the National Kidney Foundation's Dialysis Outcome Quality Initiative Guidelines have called for a much higher use of natural fistulas.[13] The Fistula First Initiative has set a goal 50% of new accesses being fistulas and 40% of patients on dialysis using a fistula long term. Doppler mapping of vessels has been done to determine what vessels can be used for the construction of a natural fistula. Silva and colleagues[14] showed that an artery had to be 2 mm or more in diameter and a vein had to be 2.5 mm or more in diameter to be useful for a fistula. Using these size criteria based on Doppler studies, the authors were able to improve patency rates of natural fistulas. Allon and Robbin[15] have described an approach to venous mapping and planning access. These authors have also shown that venous mapping has improved maturation rates in diabetic patients and women but have also shown that certain patients have inadequate veins for fistula construction. Investigators also believe that this type of information will make possible a greater number of natural fistulas.

The patency of these fistulas depends on the anatomic type. The autogenous radial-cephalic direct wrist access (Brescia-Cimino arteriovenous wrist fistula) has a patency at 2 years of 55% to 89%. One analysis combined a collective series of more than 1400 autogenous radial-cephalic direct wrist accesses and found an overall patency rate of 65% at 1 year.[16] Studies 20 to 25 years ago showed a failure rate of 10% after construction of a fistula, compared with more recent studies, which have shown failure rates of up to 50%.[15] This failure rate is attributed to poor vessels in an aging population, poor venous outflow, excessive dehydration, or hypotension. The patency rate for autogenous brachial-cephalic upper arm direct accesses (brachiocephalic fistulas) is about 80%. The use of the autogenous brachial-basilic upper arm transposition (basilic vein transposition) is also impressive, with a 24-month patency rate of 73%. All patients who are potential candidates for dialysis should have an arm vein preserved for future placement of dialysis access.

Complications

Several complications occur with arteriovenous fistulas. The most common is failure to mature (i.e., enlarge to a size that can be used for dialysis). After the fistula has been in place, the most common complication is stenosis at the proximal venous limb (48%). Aneurysms (7%) and thrombosis (9%) are the next most common complications.[16] Aneurysms from repeated needle punctures are more likely to occur when venous access is obtained repeatedly in the same location, a maneuver that weakens the vessel wall. Heart failure can occur in those patients with a marginal cardiac reserve and a fistula flow rate of more than 500 mL/min. The cardiac failure may be reversed by placing a Teflon band around the outflow tract of the fistula until the blood flow is decreased to less than 500 mL/min. Occasionally, the fistula requires ligation. The arterial steal syndrome and its ensuing ischemia occur in about 1.6% of patients with arteriovenous fistulas. This problem is unusual in patients with wrist fistulas (0.25%), but it is relatively common in patients with the more proximal fistulas (~30%).[17] The steal syndrome is caused by blood flow from the anastomosed artery to the low-resistance vein, with additional blood flowing in retrograde fashion from the hand and forearm to create ischemia.

The complication of venous hypertension distal to the fistula results from high-pressure arterial blood flow into the low-pressure venous system; this situation causes venous hypertension with distal tissue swelling, hyperpigmentation, skin induration, and eventual skin ulceration similar to that seen in the legs of patients with venous stasis.[17] With normal unobstructed venous outflow, this is a rare condition. When there is a proximal venous stenosis in a side-to-side anastomosis, this condition can occur. Both the steal syndrome and distal venous hypertension occur more frequently in patients with side-to-side anastomosis. Ligation of the distal limb of a side-to-side shunt corrects the problem, but this maneuver often causes shunt occlusion because the proximal vein is usually at least partially occluded. This proximal partial occlusion can be detected clinically by ballottement of the vein to feel a transmitted pulse wave in the proximal vein or by using duplex scanning to map the veins of the arm.[18] These complications can be avoided by performing an end-venous to side-arterial anastomosis in all cases. Infection of an autogenous radial-cephalic direct wrist access (Brescia-Cimino arteriovenous fistula) is rare (<3%). Rarely, a patient develops clinical steal syndrome characterized by pain, weakness, paresthesia, muscle atrophy, and, if left untreated, gangrene. These conditions can be reversed by closure of the fistula.

Prosthetic Grafts

The construction of vascular access using subcutaneously placed prosthetic material to join an artery to a vein is becoming increasingly necessary in patients with poor peripheral veins or previously failed arteriovenous fistulas. The material ideally is easy to handle and to suture, allows graft-host biocompatibility, is minimally thrombogenic, and resists infection. It also should be inexpensive, seal after repeated needle punctures, and allow tissue ingrowth.

Several different prosthetic materials were used for jump grafts in the past, including Dacron, bovine graft, and PTFE. PTFE is the most popular material. It permits ingrowth of tissue through the interstices of the graft and thus incorporates the graft into viable tissue. A neointima formed in the graft presumably lessens the likelihood of thrombosis and infection. PTFE grafts have a lower incidence of aneurysm formation than do bovine grafts, and PTFE grafts do not always have to be removed when they become infected. Heparin-bonded PTFE has recently been introduced, and the patency rates are yet to be determined. In addition, the use of a vein cuff or a pre-cuffed prosthetic graft may improve patency by allowing a more favorable geometry and reducing compliance mismatch.[19]

Technique of Prosthetic Jump Grafts

Successful creation of vascular access using prosthetic material requires good arterial inflow and venous outflow. Duplex scanning can help outline the arterial and venous vasculature. In patients who have had multiple venous punctures and subsequent venous stenosis, the site of the venous anastomosis must be chosen carefully so that it is proximal to these areas of obstruction. Rotation or pinching of the graft in the tunnel must be avoided. The graft must be large enough to permit needle puncture readily. The usual sizes used are a 6-mm graft and a rapid-taper 4- to 7-mm graft. The latter gives about 20% of the maximum flow of the straight 6-mm graft at the same pressure and length. A number of studies comparing graft sizes have been reported. A recent randomized trial comparing 4- to 7-mm taper with 6-mm straight showed no difference in patency or flow rates.[20] Another trial comparing 6-mm straight and 6- to 8-mm taper showed better patency and flow rates in the larger grafts in selected patient populations.[21] Dialysis can usually be performed relatively promptly after the graft has been placed; however, hematoma formation from bleeding at the puncture site is a serious complication because of the propensity for infection and pressure occlusion of the graft. Allowing the graft to mature for 1 to 2 weeks minimizes this problem by permitting tissue ingrowth, which facilitates sealing of the graft at the needle puncture site.

Several graft configurations have been developed for dialysis, and names have been standardized.[8] Just as in natural arteriovenous fistulas, the nondominant arm is used first, and an attempt is made to start as distal in the arm as possible. A graft between the radial artery at the wrist and the cephalic vein just below the elbow accomplishes this end. This graft has the lowest primary patency rate of any configuration because of the low flow through the radial artery. A prosthetic brachial-antecubital forearm loop access (forearm loop graft) is easily constructed to join the brachial artery to the cephalic vein or the brachial vein at the elbow. In the upper arm, an approach from the brachial artery to the axillary vein may be used (prosthetic brachial-axillary access [new nomenclature]). A loop between the axillary artery and the ipsilateral axillary vein is also possible (Fig. 70-4). These upper arm grafts have a high flow rate and a low incidence of thrombosis. However, they do have a higher incidence of ischemia in the hand compared with other grafts because of preferential flow of arterial blood through the graft rather than to the peripheral circulation (Fig. 70-5). After graft placement, swelling is frequently seen secondary to surgical trauma and changes in venous outflow. Both these problems usually resolve with arm elevation and time.

Interposition grafts in the lower extremity are used for patients who have no usable vessels available in the upper arms. A loop graft in the thigh (superficial femoral artery to saphenous vein; prosthetic femoral-saphenous looped inguinal access [new nomenclature]) and a jump graft between the popliteal artery and the femoral vein are the two most common configurations. They are especially poor choices in patients with diabetes and in elderly patients, who frequently have peripheral arterial insufficiency. When a leg graft is considered in a patient with no other sites for construction of a jump graft, one must realize that 18 months after graft placement, one third of these patients will have died of the systemic complications of renal failure.[22]

In patients who have exhausted all previously described sites, other sites can be used for the creation of an arteriovenous jump graft. These possibilities include grafting from the axillary artery to the axillary vein across the chest, creating a loop on the anterior chest, grafting from the axillary artery to the iliac vein, or grafting from artery to artery (Fig. 70-6). The last type of graft requires narrowing the artery between the graft anastomoses with the prosthesis to allow adequate flow through the graft itself and thus to prevent graft thrombosis, which would potentially result in acute limb-threatening ischemia.

Complications

Early hemorrhage can occur at the anastomotic site, whereas late hemorrhage is usually secondary to needle puncture of the graft and bleeding into the perigraft space. Early thrombosis usually occurs for technical reasons, such as narrowing of inflow or outflow. Later

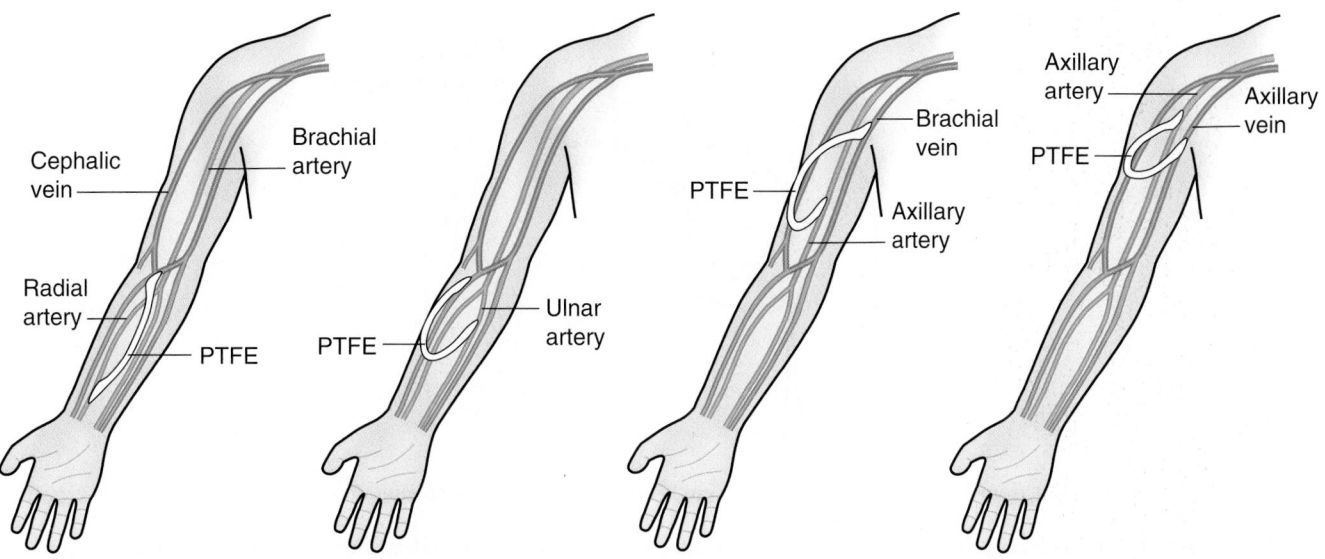

Figure 70-4 Four most common sites for placement of a jump graft in the upper extremity. PTFE, polytetrafluoroethylene. (From Haisch CE: Chronic vascular and peritoneal access. In Davis JH, Sheldon GF [eds]: Clinical Surgery. St Louis, CV Mosby, 1995.)

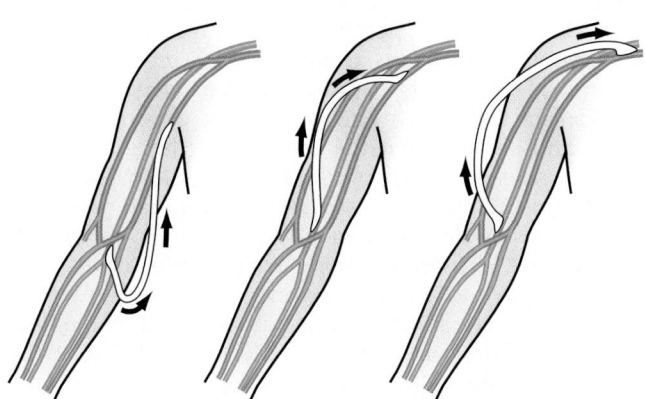

Figure 70-5 Three possible graft configurations for jump grafts in which standard sites have been used. (Redrawn from Tilney NL, Lazarus JM [eds]: Surgical Care of the Patient with Renal Failure. Philadelphia, WB Saunders, 1982; as shown in Haisch CE: Chronic vascular and peritoneal access. In Davis JH, Sheldon GF [eds]: Clinical Surgery. St Louis, CV Mosby, 1995.)

thrombosis is secondary to venous intimal hyperplasia at or distal to the anastomosis. Outflow stenosis or occlusion may be repaired by a patch graft, balloon dilation of the strictured area, or graft bypass of the obstruction.

Low blood pressure or excessive external pressure applied to graft puncture sites can contribute to the incidence of thrombosis. Thrombosis unaccompanied by narrowing of either inflow or outflow is often corrected by simple thrombectomy of the graft or by simple thrombolytic injection into the graft. Occasionally, no anatomic or blood pressure–related reason exists for a patient to have recurrent episodes of thrombosis. The cause is frequently thought to be hypercoagulability. Pharmacologic intervention for prevention of thrombosis has been largely

unsuccessful. Some early studies indicated that dipyridamole was of use in new grafts but was of no use in preventing subsequent clotting. The Dialysis Outcomes and Practice Patterns Study showed that aspirin increased secondary graft patency by 30%; however, use of both aspirin and clopidogrel after graft placement resulted in unacceptable bleeding complications, thought to be caused by uremic platelets.[23] One approach to a patient whose graft seems to clot for no anatomic reason has been to perform a coagulation evaluation and then to treat with an appropriate medication. These studies include evaluations of protein S, protein C, antithrombin III, plasminogen, factor V Leiden, and antiphospholipid antibodies. No pharmacologic interventions have satisfactorily prevented intimal hyperplasia; however, both cilostazol (Pletal) and clopidogrel (Plavix) have been shown to reduce the incidence of intimal hyperplasia in animal models. Local application of numerous agents bound to stents as well as brachytherapy are being investigated, and results are promising.

Infection is a major problem in patients with prosthetic jump grafts. Local drainage and wound care may resolve the problem in a number of grafts, if the suture line is not involved. In some cases, the infected area may be bypassed with a short graft or may be covered with a skin flap. The major reasons for removal of the entire graft for infection are involvement of the suture line, tunnel infection, clotting of the graft, or lack of success with local wound therapy. If the suture line is involved with the infection, the entire graft must be removed and the artery reconstructed. The salvage rate of infected grafts is low (25%-50%). Old clotted prosthetic grafts can be a source of future infection, especially in patients who have a low serum albumin concentration. Nassar and Ayus speculate that leaving old clotted PTFE grafts in place may predispose a number of hemodialysis patients to the risk for developing a serious infection that

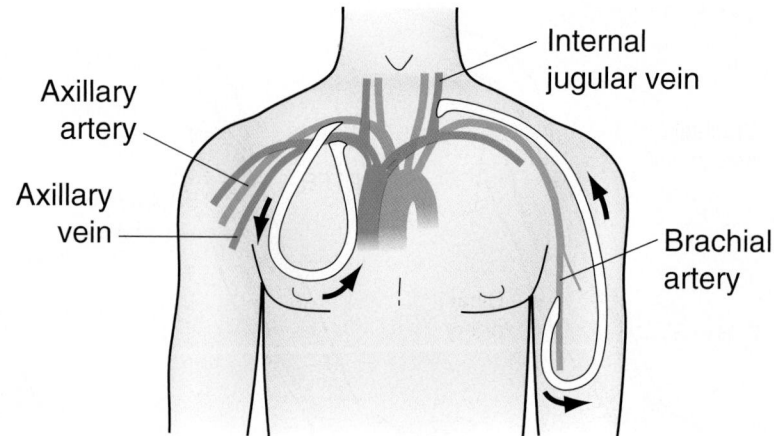

Figure 70-6 **A graft from axillary artery to axillary vein with a loop on the chest.** (Redrawn from Haimov M: Vascular access for hemodialysis: New modifications for the difficult patient. Surgery 92:109, 1982; as shown in Haisch CE: Chronic vascular and peritoneal access. In Davis JH, Sheldon GF [eds]: Clinical Surgery. St Louis, CV Mosby, 1995.)

originates from the PTFE graft.[24] In patients infected with human immunodeficiency virus (HIV), the leading complication is infection; 32% of grafts in these patients become infected within 30 days. The organisms are *S. aureus* or coagulase-negative staphylococcal species. Patients with a history of IV drug use and those with AIDS have an infection rate with PTFE grafts in place of about 40%.[25]

PTFE and other prosthetic materials are also associated with false aneurysms, usually secondary to laceration of the graft material with the dialysis needle; these can be bypassed or treated with endovascular technique using covered stents. The hemodynamic complications of venous hypertension, congestive heart failure, vascular steal, and vascular access neuropathy may occur with jump grafts as they do with natural fistulas. These complications can be decreased by use of a rapid-taper 4- to 7-mm graft. This method decreases the flow rate in the graft and has been used in elderly patients and in those with diabetes. The steal syndrome is more likely to occur in upper arm fistulas than in forearm fistulas. Tordoir and colleagues[26] have reviewed the use of the distal revascularization and interval ligation procedure in seven studies. A saphenous vein graft was placed proximal to the arterial anastomosis of the graft. The distal end of the saphenous vein was placed distal to the arterial takeoff of the graft. The artery was then ligated between the arterial takeoff of the graft and the distal end of the saphenous vein graft. This technique resolved the steal syndrome in more than 85% of patients in the studies. Most of the studies showed patency of the access to be more than 80%.[26]

Patency

The patency rate of jump grafts is less than that of autogenous arteriovenous fistulas. Marx and colleagues,[16] in an evaluation of numerous articles, showed that the 1-year secondary patency rate for PTFE grafts is 80% and the 2-year rate is 69%. This is about the same rate as for natural fistulas; however, most of the losses, as with natural fistulas, are early, and the rate of loss decreases after the first 3 to 6 months. Therefore, a natural fistula is always attempted if vessels are available. Raju[18] reported a 93% patency of PTFE at 1 year and a 77% patency at 2 years. Munda and associates[27] analyzed their experience with PTFE and showed that the location of the graft affects patency rates. In an upper arm location, the patency rate was 60% at 12 months; a straight forearm graft produced a 35% patency rate at 12 months, compared with a 78% patency for a forearm loop. Thigh grafts have been shown to have a 12-month patency rate of 80%. Overall, the patency rate appears to be related to the magnitude of arterial inflow and the size and distensibility of the venous outflow.

Radiographic Intervention and Screening for Stenosis

Schwab and associates[28] showed that early intervention for graft stenosis with percutaneous transluminal angioplasty reduced the incidence of graft thrombosis. These investigators measured venous pressure with an inline three-way stopcock attached to a 16-gauge venous return needle. The measurements were performed with a flow rate in the dialysis machine of 200 to 250 mL/min. A pressure greater than 150 mm on three separate occasions correlates with a venous stenosis of 50% or greater. Monitoring of grafts and fistulas has included Doppler examination, checking venous pressure, checking for recirculation, and feeling for a thrill. If the thrill is felt throughout the length of the graft, then the blood flow is greater than 450 mL/min. A change in the thrill means that the blood flow has decreased. Hemodynamically significant stenoses of greater than 50% need to be dilated; however, no data suggest that stenoses greater than 50% without hemodynamic abnormalities need to be dilated or repaired. There is no clear consensus whether radiographic intervention before thrombosis

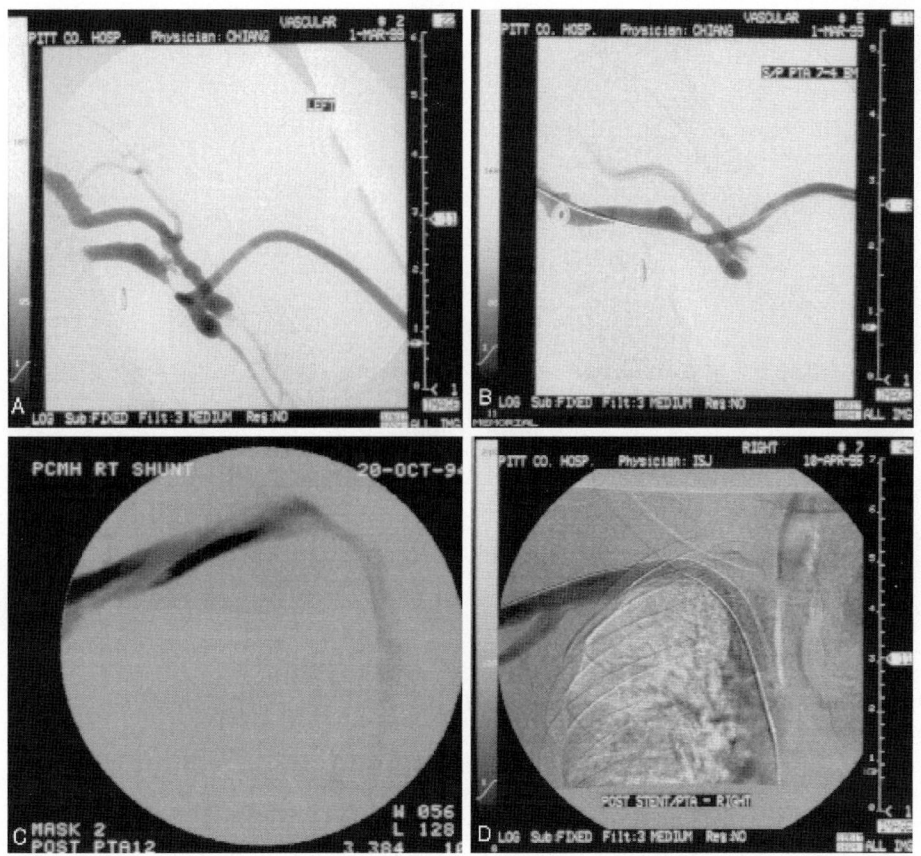

Figure 70-7 A, A fistulogram showing a short-segment stenosis of a dialysis access graft that has caused thrombosis of the graft. **B,** Balloon dilation that shows stenotic "waist." **C,** Successful postdilation view with resolution of stenosis. **D,** Subclavian vein stenosis caused by a central catheter. This stenosis is so significant that collateral vessels have been formed.

Continued

leads to increased graft survival. Because of its lower cost and noninvasive nature, color Doppler ultrasonography is suggested in grafts with suspected stenosis and can be used to direct and refine interventional technique on these grafts.

The superiority of surgical intervention over percutaneous angioplasty of peripheral lesions is yet to be determined. Dilation is performed using a balloon inflated for up to 10 to 15 minutes at a pressure up to 30 atm. A residual stenosis of 30% or less is considered an adequate result. Peripheral dilation by angioplasty has a good success rate with both long and short stenotic lesions. The diameter of the balloon used may also be important for long-term results (a 6-mm graft distal stenosis may need dilation to 7 or 8 mm). The restenosis-free time interval varies, but at 90 days, patency was 90%, and at 1 year, it was 40%. Most series have published a 6-month patency of 40% to 50% without additional intervention. In contrast to the findings of other investigators, Beathard[29] was able to show that subsequent dilations gave the same patency rate as did initial dilations (Fig. 70-7). In addition, there is a clear subset of patients with venous stenosis recalcitrant to traditional balloon angioplasty. Cutting balloons, covered stents, and drug-eluting stents have all been proposed as useful adjuncts in these cases; however, random-

ized data are lacking.[30] Balloon cryotherapy, which has been shown to reduce intimal hyperplasia, has also been used to treat outflow stenosis.[31]

When a graft is clotted, the clot can be dissolved with a thrombolytic therapy, broken up mechanically, removed with a rheolytic catheter, or removed with a Fogarty catheter through an open method. The technical success rate of mechanical and pharmacologic therapies approaches 95%. Some of these treatments may result in pulmonary emboli, which can be significant in patients with compromised pulmonary reserve. A series of pharmacomechanical endovascular devices, such as the Trellis Peripheral Infusion System, are now available, which propose to decrease the dose of thrombolytic agent and the rate of pulmonary emboli. Some studies have shown no significant difference in success or long-term patency between those grafts opened surgically and those treated percutaneously. A recent meta-analysis examining surgical versus endovascular treatment of clotted access grafts found seven acceptable studies with a total of 479 patients and showed a clear superiority of surgical therapy at 30, 60, and 90 days and 1 year.[32]

Few studies have compared surgery and radiology in a randomized prospective manner. Marston and colleagues[33] showed that in patients with both venous

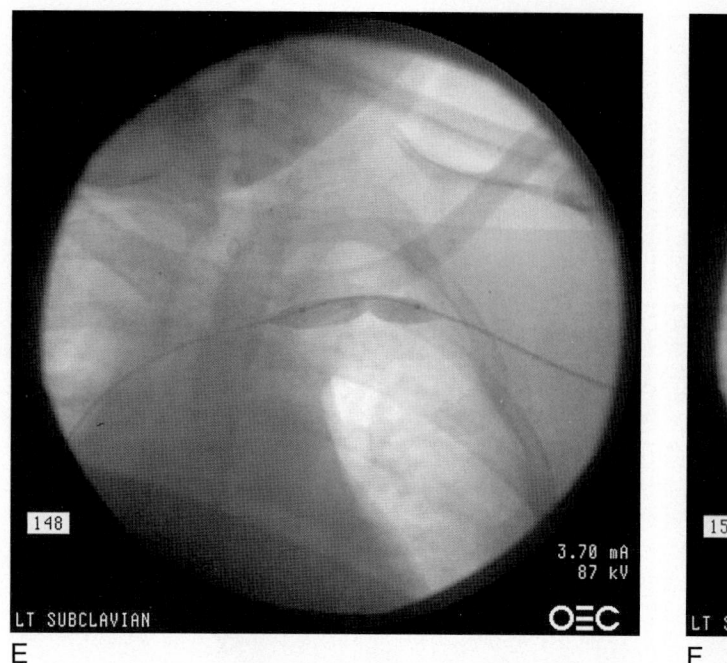

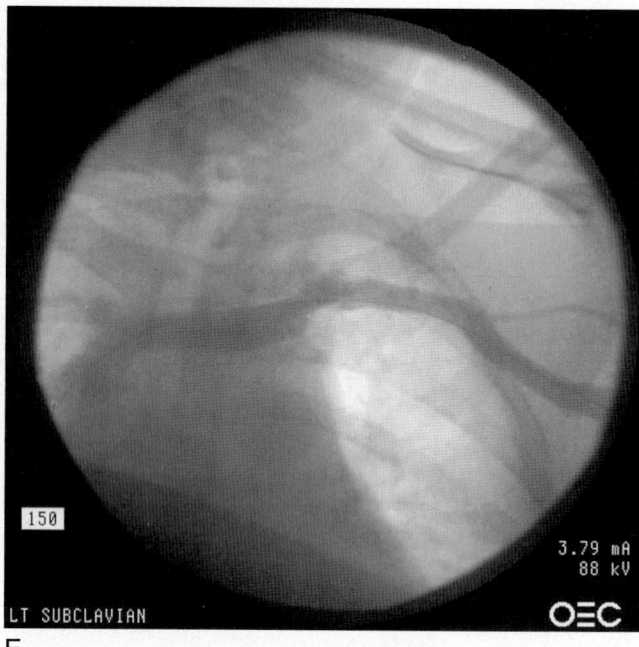

Figure 70-7, cont'd **E**, Large-diameter balloon with "waist." **F**, Successful dilation of the stenosis. Collaterals are no longer seen, indicating no residual gradient.

stenosis and long-segment venous outflow stenosis, surgical therapy resulted in a longer functional life of the graft when compared with the endovascular group (36% versus 11% at 6 months). The arguments against surgical therapy are that additional vein is used and that surgery requires central catheters before the access is reused. This article indicates a possible place for both types of therapy, and selection of the best type of therapy for both long stenotic lesions and short lesions at the anastomosis is yet to be determined.[33] Despite shorter patency of endovascular therapy in the present studies, surgical jump graft revision may still be employed after failure of endovascular therapy. Hence, using the two techniques as complementary may potentially extend the life span of an access site.

Percutaneous intervention plays an important role in central as well as peripheral stenoses. Because these patients frequently have many comorbidities, high-risk surgical intervention is undertaken only when no percutaneous alternatives exist. Lumsden and associates[34] showed that balloon dilation was successful in 17 of 22 patients with central stenosis, with a 42% patency at 6 months. The authors used a stent in 5 patients and had good initial success.[34] The most common cause of stent failure is intimal hyperplasia in or around the stent. These stents appear to be most effective in patients with a large vein without a venous confluence, such as occurs in the central venous system (see Fig. 70-7). Venous stenosis in the periphery has been treated by a number of modalities, including cutting balloon, stent, covered stent, and brachytherapy. In small, nonrandomized studies, some of these modalities demonstrate superiority; however, further research is needed.[35,36]

Physiology

The physiologic consequences of arteriovenous fistulas depend on the size of the proximal and distal arteries and veins, the collateral flow around the fistula, and the diameter of the fistula. The length of the fistula has little influence on the flow when this length is less than 20% or greater than 75% of the arterial diameter. Between these two values, however, small changes in the size of the fistula can change flow dramatically. Most fistulas for clinical use are constructed so that the fistula is larger than the arterial diameter to allow some margin for subsequent stenosis. Blood flow through a side-to-side or an end vein–to–side artery wrist fistula is contributed by both the proximal arteries and the distal arteries, with as much as one third of the flow coming from the distal artery.

A large, functioning arteriovenous fistula may cause a fall in both systolic and diastolic blood pressure, an increase in cardiac output, an increase in venous blood pressure both proximal and distal to the fistula, an increase in pulse rate, and a slight increase in the size of the heart. Increases also occur in blood volume in patients with chronic arteriovenous fistulas. These changes are all reversible with fistula closure.

Platelets and fibrin may accumulate in a chronic fistula, with eventual closure of the lumen. Patients with a larger fistula usually have progressive lengthening and dilation of both the proximal artery and the vein. The proximal artery elongates and dilates, and smooth muscle hypertrophy occurs. Eventually, smooth muscle atrophy develops, and additional elongation and dilation occur. This situation produces an aneurysmal dilation and a tortuous vessel. The outflow vein has increases in smooth muscle, fibrous tissue, and collagen and also enlarges significantly. Blood flow around the fistula is increased to maintain flow distal to the fistula. A corresponding increase in temperature also occurs. However, blood flow distal to the fistula may be decreased, with resultant cool temperatures, particularly in the hand.

Pathophysiology of Venous Hyperplasia

The turbulent flow at the anastomosis of an arteriovenous fistula or PTFE graft has an influence on venous hyperplasia. The Reynolds number changes when the flow of fluid is not straight. When a fistula or an H graft between an artery and vein is in place, the Reynolds number will increase. An increased Reynolds number correlates with increased turbulence and consequent hyperplasia. Haruguchi and Teraoka[37] reviewed wall-shear stress data and showed that with decreased wall-shear stress, the amount of intimal hyperplasia is decreased.

The changes that occur at the molecular level at the anastomosis of the arteriovenous fistula and the venous end of a PTFE graft have been examined. Stracke and colleagues[38] have compared levels of transforming growth factor-β (TGF-β) and insulin growth factor-1 (IGF-1) in stenotic veins of arteriovenous fistulas and nonstenosed control veins from patients who were uremic but not on dialysis. Another control was from normal saphenous veins of patients who had undergone coronary artery bypass grafting. The stenosed veins showed markedly increased levels of TGF-β and IGF-1 in the neointimal and medial layers compared with control veins. Both of these growth factors have been shown to correlate with neointimal formation and are known to be involved with local inflammation.

Changes in the venous intima have also been examined in the PTFE-vein anastomosis from patients with intimal hyperplasia with a PTFE graft in place. Several descriptive studies found an increase in the amount of platelet-derived growth factor (PDGF), basic fibroblast growth factor (bFGF), and vascular endothelial growth factor (VEGF) compared with the unaffected vein. These factors were expressed in the smooth muscle cells in the neointima of the vein and in the macrophages lining the PTFE graft.[39] This understanding in molecular biology has led to a proposed clinical trial using gene therapy to prevent intimal hyperplasia at the graft-vein anastomotic site.[40]

Novel approaches to preventing and treating intimal hyperplasia are being considered. Brachytherapy has shown improved patency at 6 months in patients who had a venous stenosis dilated.[41] Local gene therapy has been considered, as has the use of drug-eluting stents. The experimental use of a perivascular delivery of paclitaxel again has shown promise but has not been used clinically.[42]

Summary

The development of convenient vascular access made long-term hemodialysis possible. Clearly, the three major improvements in the development of adequate vascular

access were the development of the external shunt with prosthetic material penetrating the skin, the development of the arteriovenous wrist fistula, and the use of a subcutaneous prosthetic material to connect the artery and the vein. These techniques have been associated with an increasing success rate and decreasing morbidity. However, for some patients, hemodialysis is not clinically appropriate. For patients with these and other indications, peritoneal dialysis is now widely used.

PERITONEAL DIALYSIS

Physiology

The exact surface and mechanism responsible for hemofiltration in peritoneal dialysis remain unknown. Investigators widely believe that the capillary vessels in the peritoneum are critical, with diffusion across the capillary membrane being the primary transport barrier. The peritoneal surface approximates the total body surface area. The effective surface area depends on the number of transcellular pores available for transport corresponding to the number of perfused capillaries. Much of our understanding of peritoneal membrane diffusion comes from comparison with hemodialysis, in which the exact membrane pore size and surface area are known. Clearance of various molecules is different between the two techniques. For example, clearance of urea exceeds 100 L/wk in hemodialysis, whereas continuous ambulatory peritoneal dialysis (CAPD) yields 70 L/wk of urea clearance (604 L/wk for normal kidneys).[43] The current targets for weekly dialysis is a Kt/V of greater than 2 and a creatinine clearance of more than 60 L/1.73m². The differences are well documented and can be summarized by stating that CAPD appears more effective at removal of large solutes (>500 daltons) and less effective at removal of small solutes than does hemodialysis.[43] The peritoneal lymphatics and mesothelial cells play a lesser role in ultrafiltration. Measurement of lymphatic absorption can be accomplished using intraperitoneally administered macromolecular tracer. Regardless of the exact contributions, overall ultrafiltration in CAPD depends on Starling forces and lymphatic drainage.

Indications

The only absolute indication for peritoneal dialysis as renal replacement therapy is the inability to undergo hemodialysis. Poor vascular access, an unstable cardiovascular system, and bleeding diatheses are the most frequent reasons to avoid hemodialysis. CAPD therapy has many relative advantages, including increased patient mobility and independence, fewer dietary restrictions, increased patient satisfaction, and no requirement for systemic anticoagulation.

The absolute contraindications for CAPD are few and include obliteration of the peritoneal space from previous surgery, inadequate peritoneal clearance, and lack of diaphragmatic integrity. Relative contraindications include respiratory insufficiency secondary to dialysate infusion, large abdominal hernias, or malignant peritoneal disease.

Technical Procedures

Several types of catheters are available for use in peritoneal dialysis. Three frequently used types are the Tenckhoff catheter, the Toronto Western catheter, and the curl-tip catheter. Variations on catheter design include straight versus coiled intra-abdominal configurations, single and double cuffs, and preformed intercuff bends (swan neck). Prospective studies have not demonstrated significant differences in catheter survival or catheter complications between coiled and straight catheters.

Peritoneal dialysis catheters can be placed using open surgical technique, percutaneously, or laparoscopically. In experienced hands, percutaneous placement is safe and can be accomplished at the bedside. The catheter is inserted aseptically below the umbilicus and using local anesthesia is directed toward the pelvis. The catheter is brought out through a subcutaneous tunnel on the side of the insertion site, with the Dacron cuff placed in the tunnel at least 1 inch from the skin surface. The percutaneous approach is being used more frequently by interventionalists in the interventional suite but still requires a 2-cm long incision for the deep cuff placement.[44] Surgeons typically can perform an open placement through an incision of the same size.

In the surgical approach, the Tenckhoff or curl-tip catheter is placed by making a paramedian incision below the umbilicus longitudinally through the anterior rectus sheath and muscle. The posterior fascia and the peritoneum are exposed, and a purse-string suture is placed. The catheter is directed toward the pelvis with a metal guide. Care is taken to avoid bowel or bladder injury. The deep Dacron cuff is left in the muscle just above the posterior fascia and is sutured into place with the purse-string suture. The anterior fascia is closed, and the second cuff is placed in the subcutaneous tunnel with the catheter exiting distally. This approach results in a decreased number of pericatheter leaks and hernias. If necessary, placement and fixation of the catheter in the pelvis under direct vision may decrease the incidence of nonfunctioning straight catheters. Omentectomy may also be necessary in some instances (Fig. 70-8).

The role of laparoscopy in peritoneal dialysis catheter placement is being developed. Single-port and double-port laparoscopic techniques have been successfully described for catheter placement.[45] Patency and complication rates are comparable to those seen with the open approach. However, the cost-effectiveness of the laparoscopic approach has not been evaluated. Peritoneoscopy has a definite role in evaluation and salvage of malfunctioning catheters. The incidence of catheter malfunction ranges from 12% to 73% of patients, and obstruction is a common cause of catheter loss. Multiple studies have demonstrated successful laparoscopic manipulation of obstructed catheters, with salvage rates between 50% and 80%.

Dialysis Fluids

Dialysis fluids are glucose based and vary in concentration. As stated earlier, peritoneal dialysis depends on

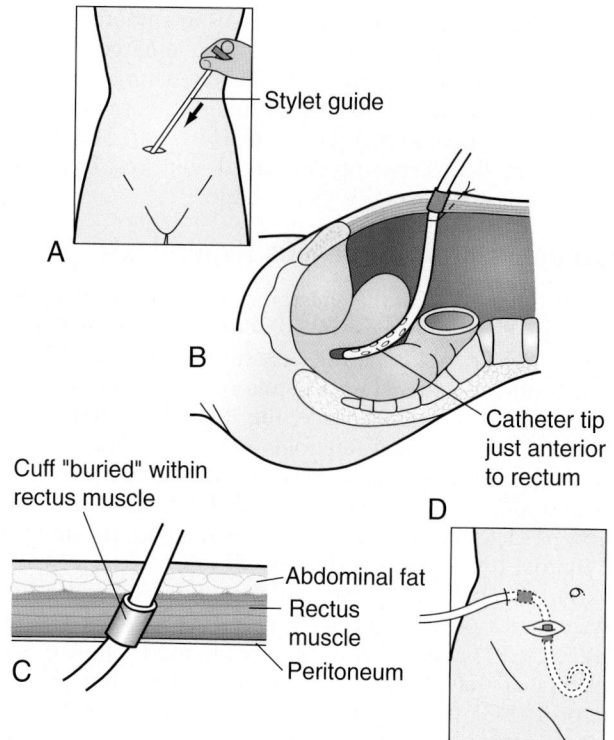

Figure 70-8 Location of the chronic ambulatory peritoneal dialysis catheter. **A,** Location of the surgical incision. **B,** Location of the catheter in the pelvis. **C,** Dacron cuff at the level of the posterior rectus sheath. **D,** Exit site shown with final placement. (Redrawn from Simmons RL, Finch ME, Ascher NL, Najarian JS [eds]: Manual of Vascular Access, Organ Donation and Transplantation. New York, Springer-Verlag, 1984; as shown in Haisch CE: Chronic vascular and peritoneal access. In Davis JH [ed]: Clinical Surgery. St Louis, CV Mosby, 1987.)

Starling forces. The largest contribution in peritoneal dialysis comes from osmotic forces. Therefore, dialysis fluid with low osmolarity (1.5%) causes little fluid removal (200 mL per 2-L exchange), whereas the greatest concentration (4.5%) treats or prevents fluid overload (800 mL per 2-L exchange). High-concentration dialysis fluid is more irritating to the peritoneal surface. Glycosylation of the peritoneal vascular walls occurs over time and reduces the intrinsic filtering ability of the peritoneum. These changes are likely similar to the microangiopathy that occurs in patients with diabetes. Lower-concentration dialysis fluid is used routinely when possible. Glucose polymers have been in clinical trials since the early 1990s, with emphasis on reducing the glucose concentration.[46] Electrolyte components are adjusted based on the patient's needs. A typical exchange is 2 L four times per day.

Research is ongoing to produce more biocompatible dialysis fluids. Insulin is often added to the dialysis fluid of patients with diabetes to allow for steady absorption. Intraperitoneal amino acids are being studied in an attempt to reduce malnutrition in patients undergoing peritoneal dialysis.[46] Administration of glycosaminoglycans has improved ultrafiltration in animal models, but results in humans are inconclusive.

Complications

Complications can be divided into those related to surgical placement of the catheter and those occurring after catheter placement. Technical problems related to placement include leakage of dialysate, intraperitoneal bleeding, bowel or bladder perforation, subcutaneous bleeding with hematoma formation from tunnel construction, and ileus. All these complications, except ileus, are preventable with close attention to surgical technique.

Complications occurring after catheter placement include exit-site infection, mechanical failure, and peritonitis. Peritonitis is a potentially life-threatening complication with an average incidence of 1.3 to 1.4 episodes per patient-year.[47] Peritonitis rates have decreased in some series to 0.9 episode per patient-year with the introduction of Y-set dialysis systems that allow flushing of the catheter before use.[48] At least half the peritonitis episodes are experienced by only 25% of patients undergoing peritoneal dialysis.[48] Five routes of infection are recognized: through the dialysis tubing and peritoneal catheter; from tissue around the catheter; from fecal contamination, such as in diverticulitis; blood-borne infections; and ascending infection from the fallopian tubes in women. The use of a closed system with a Y-set or twin-bag system has been shown in multiple studies to decrease the incidence of peritonitis. Peritonitis is usually caused by a single pathogen. In 60% to 70% of cases, gram-positive cocci are the culprit, with coagulase-negative staphylococcus the most common pathogen.[47] Gram-negative bacilli account for 20% to 30% of the cases of peritonitis. *Pseudomonas aeruginosa* is not uncommon, occurring in 5% to 10% of the cases. Uncommon causes are tuberculosis and fungal infection. However, fungal peritonitis is increasing in relative frequency. Risk factors for fungal peritonitis include recent hospitalization, immunologic compromise, and bacterial peritonitis. Combination therapy using both peritoneal and parenteral antibiotics treats peritonitis. Therapy is directed by Gram stain and culture of peritoneal fluid. Synergistic double coverage is indicated for *P. aeruginosa* peritonitis. A biofilm containing microorganisms is thought to be the reason that some catheter infections are refractory to therapy. In these cases, catheter removal is required. Catheter removal is also required for fungal infections.[47]

Exit-site infections occur at a rate of 0.80 per patient-year. Most are caused by gram-positive organisms (80%), with *S. aureus* accounting for 90% of these cases. Catheter infection precedes peritonitis in about 20% of cases.

Catheter malfunction may be caused by a number of factors and is manifested by poor inflow or total obstruction. Poor inflow is caused by displacement, omental wrapping, or partial blockage of the catheter holes. Total obstruction is caused by kinking of the catheter, blockage of all catheter holes, or omental wrapping of the entire intra-abdominal portion of the catheter. If the catheter flips out of the pelvis, it can be repositioned under fluoroscopic guidance or with peritoneoscopy. Other complications such as hernia formation, fluid loculation, or dialysate leaks can be detected using CT.[49]

Catheter Longevity

CAPD catheters function for 1 year in 85% of patients with an expectation of a 3-year catheter survival rate of 80%. However, catheter survival is significantly shorter in patients with diabetes than in other patients. Infection is the leading reason for discontinuation of CAPD. Abdominal surgical events and social reasons have surpassed infection as a cause of treatment failure in some centers.

Summary

Peritoneal dialysis allows the patient to be at home and to work with minimal disruption of activities. This approach to the management of chronic renal failure is gaining popularity because of the decreasing incidence of catheter infections, the decrease in cardiac complications, the lower incidence of anemia, and the greater convenience than hemodialysis. Some studies indicate a slight decrease in mortality relative to hemodialysis.[50] Infection and mechanical failure are the major factors that cause patients to switch to hemodialysis. Because these techniques may produce uncertain results, renal transplantation is still the therapy of choice for suitable patients with end-stage renal failure. Superb patient compliance is a basic requirement of paramount importance.

Selected References

Brescia MJ, Cimino JE, Appel D, Harwich BJ: Chronic hemodialysis using venipuncture and a surgically created arteriovenous fistula. N Engl J Med 275:1089, 1966.

> This article is the original description of the wrist fistula, which revolutionized dialysis and allowed patients long-term vascular access with fewer complications than occurred with external shunts. The article describes the fistula against which all other methods of vascular access for dialysis are measured.

Davidson IJA: Access for Dialysis: Surgical and Radiologic Procedures, 2nd ed. Georgetown, TX, Landes Biosciences, 2002.

> This book has information on management of hemodialysis access procedures and radiologic approaches to access for dialysis. There are a large number of case reports as learning exercises. There is also a section on coding for access procedures.

Eerola R, Kaukinen L, Kaukinen S: Analysis of 13,800 subclavian vein catheterizations. Acta Anaesthesiol Scand 29:193, 1985.

> The results of a large study are presented on the practice of subclavian catheterization. Complications are discussed.

Gray RJ, Sands JJ (eds): Dialysis Access: A Multidisciplinary Approach. Philadelphia, Lippincott, Williams & Wilkins, 2002.

> A comprehensive volume covering surgery, radiology, and peritoneal dialysis.

Haimov M, Baez A, Neff M, Slifkin R: Complications of arteriovenous fistulas for hemodialysis. Arch Surg 110:708, 1975.

> This article reports on a group of more than 400 patients with more than 500 arteriovenous fistulas. The vascular complications are examined. Complications including ischemia, steals, gangrene, aneurysms, and venous hypertension are outlined, and their incidence is noted. The therapy and outcome are discussed for these complications.

Henry ML: Vascular Access for Hemodialysis IX. Los Angeles, WL Gore and Associates Bonus Books, 2005.

> The publication is from a meeting on dialysis access held in 2004. The symposium reviewed physiology, pathology, and results of clinical care of dialysis patients. This good review covers a wide variety of topics.

National Kidney Foundation: Dialysis outcomes quality initiatives (DOQI) guidelines. Am J Kidney Dis 37(Suppl):137-179, 2001.

> These are group guidelines that recommend care to be given to patients in renal failure. These include peritoneal dialysis guidelines and care to be given to patients who need vascular access through a fistula or a graft.

Nolph KD: Peritoneal anatomy and transport physiology. Mion CM: Practical use of peritoneal dialysis. In Drukker W, Parson FM, Maher JF (eds): Replacement of Renal Function by Dialysis. Boston, Martinus Nijhoff, 1983.

> These two chapters give an excellent overview of peritoneal physiology and anatomy and the practical uses and limitations of peritoneal dialysis. The chapter on physiology compares peritoneal dialysis with hemodialysis and gives its limitations. The chapter on the use of peritoneal dialysis includes sections on solutions and catheter insertion, complications, and catheter longevity.

References

1. Brescia MJ, Cimino JE, Appel K, et al: Chronic hemodialysis using venipuncture and a surgically created arteriovenous fistula. N Engl J Med 275:1089-1092, 1966.
2. McLaughlin K, Jones B, Mactier R, et al: Long-term vascular access for hemodialysis using silicon dual-lumen catheters with guidewire replacement of catheters for technique salvage. Am J Kidney Dis 29:553-559, 1997.
3. Mosquera DA, Gibson SP, Goldman MD: Vascular access surgery: A 2-year study and comparison with the Permcath. Nephrol Dial Transplant 7:1111-1115, 1992.
4. Whitman ED: Complications associated with the use of central venous access devices. Curr Probl Surg 33:309-378, 1996.
5. Denys BG, Uretsky BF, Reddy PS: Ultrasound-assisted cannulation of the internal jugular vein: A prospective comparison to the external landmark-guided technique. Circulation 87:1557-1562, 1993.
6. Darouiche RO, Raad II, Heard SO, et al: A comparison of two antimicrobial-impregnated central venous catheters. Catheter Study Group. N Engl J Med 340:1-8, 1999.
7. Beathard GA: Management of bacteremia associated with tunneled-cuffed hemodialysis catheters. J Am Soc Nephrol 10:1045-1049, 1999.
8. Sidawy AN, Gray R, Besarab A, et al: Recommended standards for reports dealing with arteriovenous hemodialysis accesses. J Vasc Surg 35:603-610, 2002.
9. Angle N, Chandra A: The two stage brachial artery-brachial vein autogenous fistula for hemodialysis: An alternative autogenous option for hemodialysis access. J Vasc Surg 42:806-810, 2005.
10. Pierre-Paul D, Williams S, Lee T, Gahtan V: Saphenous vein loop to femoral artery arteriovenous fistula: A practical alternative. Ann Vasc Surg 18:223-227, 2004.
11. Huber TS, Hirneise CM, Lee WA, et al: Outcome after autogenous brachial-axillary translocated superficial femoropopliteal vein hemodialysis access. J Vasc Surg 40:311-318, 2004.
12. Gorski TF, Nguyen HQ, Gorski YC, et al: Lower-extremity saphenous vein transposition arteriovenous fistula: An alternative for hemodialysis access in AIDS patients. Am Surg 64:338-340, 1998.
13. National Kidney Foundation: Dialysis outcomes quality initiative (DOQI) guidelines. Am J Kidney Dis 37:S139-S179, 2001.
14. Silva MB Jr, Hobson RW II, Pappas PJ, et al: A strategy for increasing use of autogenous hemodialysis access procedures: Impact of preoperative noninvasive evaluation. J Vasc Surg 27:302-308, 1998.
15. Allon M, Robbin ML: Increasing arteriovenous fistulas in hemodialysis patients: Problems and solutions. Kidney Int 62:1109-1124, 2002.
16. Marx AB, Landmann J, Harder FH: Surgery for vascular access. Curr Probl Surg 27:1-48, 1990.
17. Haimov M, Baez A, Neff M, et al: Complications of arteriovenous fistulas for hemodialysis. Arch Surg 110:708-712, 1975.
18. Raju S: PTFE grafts for hemodialysis access: Techniques for insertion and management of complications. Ann Surg 206:666-673, 1987.
19. Lin PH, Bush RL, Nguyen L, et al: Anastomotic strategies to improve hemodialysis access patency: A review. Vasc Endovascular Surg 39:135-142, 2005.
20. Dammers R, Planken RN, Pouls KP, et al: Evaluation of 4-mm to 7-mm versus 6-mm prosthetic brachial antecubital forearm loop access for hemodialysis: Results of a randomized multicenter clinical trial. J Vasc Surg 37:143-148, 2003.
21. Polo JR, Ligero JM, Diaz-Cartelle J, et al: Randomized comparison of 6 mm straight grafts versus 6- to 8- mm tapered grafts for brachial-axillary dialysis access. J Vasc Surg 40:319-324, 2004.
22. Taylor SM, Eaves GL, Weatherford DA, et al: Results and complications of arteriovenous access dialysis grafts in the lower extremity: A five-year review. Am Surg 62:188-191, 1996.
23. Kaufman JS, O'Connor TZ, Zhang JH, et al: Randomized controlled trial of clopidogrel plus aspirin to prevent hemodialysis access graft thrombosis. J Am Soc Nephrol 14:2313-2321, 2003.
24. Nassar GM, Ayus JC: Infectious complications of the hemodialysis access. Kidney Int 60:1-13, 2001.
25. Brock JS, Sussman M, Wamsley M, et al: The influence of human immunodeficiency virus infection and intravenous drug abuse on complications of hemodialysis access surgery. J Vasc Surg 16:904-912, 1992.
26. Tordoir JHM, Dammers R, van der Sandi FM: Upper extremity ischemia and hemodialysis vascular access. Eur J Vasc Endovasc Surg 27:1-5, 2004.
27. Munda R, First MR, Alexander JW, et al: Polytetrafluoroethylene graft survival in hemodialysis. JAMA 249:219-222, 1983.
28. Schwab SJ, Raymond JR, Saeed M, et al: Prevention of hemodialysis fistula thrombosis: Early detection of venous stenoses. Kidney Int 36:707-711, 1989.
29. Beathard GA: Percutaneous transvenous angioplasty in the treatment of vascular access stenosis. Kidney Int 42:1390-1397, 1992.
30. Clark TW, Rajan DK: Treating intractable venous stenosis: Present and future therapy. Semin Dial 17:4-8, 2004.
31. Rifkin BS, Brewster UC, Aruny JE, Perazella MA: Percutaneous balloon cryoplasty: A new therapy for rapidly recurrent anastomotic venous stenoses of hemodialysis grafts? Am J Kidney Dis 45:e27-32, 2005.
32. Green LD, Lee DS, Kucey DS: A meta-analysis comparing surgical thrombectomy, mechanical thrombectomy, and pharmacomechanical thrombolysis for thrombosed dialysis grafts. J Vasc Surg 36:939-945, 2002.

33. Marston WA, Criado E, Jaques PF, et al: Prospective randomized comparison of surgical versus endovascular management of thrombosed dialysis access grafts. J Vasc Surg 26:373-381, 1997.

34. Lumsden AB, MacDonald MJ, Isiklar H, et al: Central venous stenosis in the hemodialysis patient: Incidence and efficacy of endovascular treatment. Cardiovasc Surg 5:504-509, 1997.

35. Singer-Jordan J, Papura S: Cutting balloon angioplasty for primary treatment of hemodialysis fistula venous stenoses: Preliminary results. J Vasc Interv Radiol 16:5-7, 2005.

36. Vogel PM, Parise C: Comparison of SMART stent placement for arteriovenous graft salvage versus successful graft PTA. J Vasc Interv Radiol 16:1619-1626, 2005.

37. Haruguchi H, Teraoka S: Intimal hyperplasia and hemodynamic factors in arterial bypass and arteriovenous grafts: A review. J Artif Organs 6:227-235, 2003.

38. Stracke S, Konner K, Kostlin I, et al: Increased expression of TGF-beta1 and IGF-I in inflammatory stenotic lesions of hemodialysis fistulas. Kidney Int 61:1011-1019, 2002.

39. Roy-Chaudhury P, Kelly BS, Miller MA, et al: Venous neointimal hyperplasia in polytetrafluoroethylene dialysis grafts. Kidney Int 59:2325-2334, 2001.

40. Fuster V, Charlton P, Boyd A: Clinical protocol. A phase IIb randomized, multicenter, double-blind study of the efficacy and safety of Trinam (EG004) in stenosis prevention at the graft-vein anastomosis site in dialysis patients. Hum Gene Ther 12:2025-2027, 2001.

41. Roy-Chaudhury P, Zuckerman D, Duncan H, et al: Endovascular radiation therapy reduces venous stenosis in PTFE dialysis access grafts. J Am Soc Nephrol 15:61A, 2004.

42. Masaki T, Rathi R, Zentner G, et al: Inhibition of neointimal hyperplasia in vascular grafts by sustained perivascular delivery of paclitaxel. Kidney Int 66:2061-2069, 2004.

43. Nolph KD: Comparison of continuous ambulatory peritoneal dialysis and hemodialysis. Kidney Int Suppl 24:S123-131, 1988.

44. Georgiades CS, Geschwind JF: Percutaneous peritoneal dialysis catheter placement for the management of end-stage renal disease: Technique and comparison with the surgical approach. Tech Vasc Interv Radiol 5:103-107, 2002.

45. Nijhuis PH, Smulders JF, Jakimowicz JJ: Laparoscopic introduction of a continuous ambulatory peritoneal dialysis (CAPD) catheter by a two-puncture technique. Surg Endosc 10:676-679, 1996.

46. Medcalf JF, Walls J: New frontiers in continuous ambulatory peritoneal dialysis. Kidney Int Suppl 62:S108-110, 1997.

47. Johnson CC, Baldessarre J, Levison ME: Peritonitis: Update on pathophysiology, clinical manifestations, and management. Clin Infect Dis 24:1035-1045; quiz 1046-1037, 1997.

48. Stippoli GFM, Tong A, Johnson D, et al: Catheter-related interventions to prevent peritonitis in peritoneal dialysis: A systematic review of randomized, controlled trials. J Am Soc Nephrol 15:2735-2746, 2004.

49. Hollett MD, Marn CS, Ellis JH, et al: Complications of continuous ambulatory peritoneal dialysis: Evaluation with CT peritoneography. AJR Am J Roentgenol 159:983-989, 1992.

50. Fenton SS, Schaubel DE, Desmeules M, et al: Hemodialysis versus peritoneal dialysis: A comparison of adjusted mortality rates. Am J Kidney Dis 30:334-342, 1997.

SPECIALTIES IN GENERAL SURGERY

Pediatric Surgery

Brad W. Warner, MD

Pediatric surgery is a subspecialty that is both exciting and rewarding for multiple reasons. First, the range of problems encountered may be quite dramatic and is not limited to specific anatomic boundaries. Further, the pathogenesis of many significant pediatric surgical conditions remains unknown. As such, the challenge for intense, active investigation is ever-present. Finally, the approach to the child, interactions with concerned parents, and lifelong consequences of operative interventions demand a unique sensitivity and attention to detail, the impact of which is often profound.

This chapter seeks to emphasize the most important components of the more common pediatric surgical conditions. A discussion of several common pediatric conditions (e.g., appendicitis, inflammatory bowel disease) is intentionally omitted to avoid redundancy with other chapters.

NEWBORN PHYSIOLOGY

General

The newborn infant is both physically and physiologically distinct from the adult patient in several respects. The smaller size, immature organ systems, and differing volume capacities present unique challenges toward perioperative management. In utero, the cardiovascular system essentially pumps blood from the placenta and bypasses the lungs through the patent foramen ovale and the ductus arteriosus. With clamping of the umbilical cord at the time of delivery, the foramen ovale closes, and there is an abrupt fall in pulmonary arterial pressure. The ductus arteriosus begins to close soon thereafter. These factors serve to promote pulmonary blood flow. Persistent pulmonary hypertension, which is associated with hypoxemia, acidosis, or sepsis, may contribute to ductal patency, and right-to-left shunting may occur. In addition, prematurity is a risk factor for failure of the ductus arteriosus to close. As such, attempts to close the ductus pharmacologically using indomethacin or by direct surgical ligation may be necessary. Before the ductus is closed, there may be a higher partial pressure and saturation of oxygen in the blood when sampled from the right arm (preductal), as compared with the other extremities (postductal), owing to the flow of unoxygenated blood from the pulmonary artery through the ductus into the aorta.

Cardiovascular

Cardiac perfusion is best monitored clinically by capillary refill, which ideally is less than 1 second. A capillary refill longer than 1 to 2 seconds is associated with significant shunting of blood from the skin to the central organs as may occur with cardiogenic shock or significantly reduced intravascular volume from dehydration or bleeding. In neonates, the size of the liver is a reasonable gauge of intravascular volume. Finally, cardiac output in the newborn period is rate dependent, and the heart has a limited capacity to increase stroke volume to compensate for bradycardia.

Pulmonary

The lungs are not completely developed at birth and continue to form new terminal bronchioles and alveoli until about 8 years of age. In premature infants, lung immaturity is one of the greatest contributors to morbidity and mortality. In addition to reduced alveoli, immature lungs have reduced production of surfactant, which is critical for maintaining surface tension within the alveoli and gas exchange. A major contribution in the management of premature infants has therefore been the ability to provide exogenous surfactant. This has resulted in improved survival and less *bronchopulmonary dysplasia* (defined as the need for supplemental oxygen beyond the first 28 days of life). In addition to pulmonary parenchymal issues, the airway of the newborn is quite small (tracheal diameter, 2.5-4 mm) and easily plugged with secretions. The respiratory rate for a normal newborn may range from 40 to 60 breaths/min. Respiratory distress is heralded by nasal flaring, grunting, intercostal and substernal retractions, and cyanosis. Finally, infants preferentially breathe through their nose and not their mouth.

Cold Stress

Newborn infants must be maintained in a neutral thermal environment because they are at great risk for cold stress. The major risk factors for the development of hypothermia in infants include their relatively large body surface area, lack of hair and subcutaneous tissue, and increased insensible losses. Neonates who are cold stressed respond by nonshivering thermogenesis. Metabolic rate and oxygen consumption are augmented by brown fat mobilization. Continued cold exposure leads to decreased perfusion and acidosis. Radiant heat warmers are usually necessary in very small premature infants, and this may contribute to further insensible water losses.

Infection

The neonate is relatively immunodeficient, with reduced levels of immunoglobulins and the C3b component of complement. As such, premature infants are at significantly increased risk for severe infection. Sepsis may result from multiple interventions that are necessary to care for these premature infants, including prolonged endotracheal intubation and central vein or bladder catheterization. Empiric antibiotic therapy to prevent overwhelming sepsis may be lifesaving and may be based on simple clinical judgment of subtle alterations in factors such as reduced tolerance of enteral feeding, temperature instability, reduced capillary refill, tachypnea, or irritability.

FLUIDS, ELECTROLYTES, AND NUTRITION

Several basic principles must be understood before assuming the responsibility for the metabolic needs for an infant or child. First, the margin for error is narrower when compared with adults. The consequences of too much or too little intravenous (IV) glucose in a neonate may be devastating and even life threatening. As such, the fluid, electrolyte, and parenteral nutrition orders are considered as important as writing for any medication that has the potential for serious side effects. Second, on a body weight basis, protein and energy requirements are much greater in younger children, and decrease with age. Not only are calories utilized for higher baseline metabolic rates, but also a significant proportion of energy in the diet must be allocated for growth. Third, in contrast with adults, daily weight gain in neonates is an important indicator of providing sufficient calories. Infants who are losing weight, or even failing to gain weight, mandate a careful reassessment of metabolic needs and amount of nutrition provided.

Fluid Requirements

Because of increased insensible water losses through thinner, less mature skin, the fluid requirements for premature infants are substantial. Insensible water losses are directly related to gestational age and range from 45 to 60 mL/kg/day for premature infants weighing less than 1500 g to 30 to 35 mL/kg/day for term infants. In contrast, insensible water losses in an adult are roughly 15 mL/kg/day. Other factors such as radiant heat warmers, phototherapy for hyperbilirubinemia, and respiratory distress further increase losses.

At 12 weeks' gestation, 94% of the fetal body weight is composed of water. This amount declines to roughly 78% by term (40 weeks' gestation) and reaches adult levels (60%) by $1\frac{1}{2}$ years of age. In the first 3 to 5 days of life, there is a physiologic water loss of up to 10% of the body weight of the infant. This is the singular exception to the general principle that infants are expected to gain weight each day. As such, fluid replacement volumes are less over the first several days of life. Recommended fluid volume replacements are shown in Table 71-1. These fluid volumes are regarded as estimates and may change given differing environmental or patient factors.

Table 71-1 Daily Fluid Requirements for Neonates and Infants

WEIGHT	VOLUME
Premature <2.0 kg	140-150 mL/kg/day
Neonates and infants 2-10 kg	100 mL/kg/day for first 10 kg
Children 10-20 kg	1000 mL + 50 mL/kg/day for weight 10-20 kg
Children >20 kg	1500 mL + 20 mL/kg/day for weight >20 kg

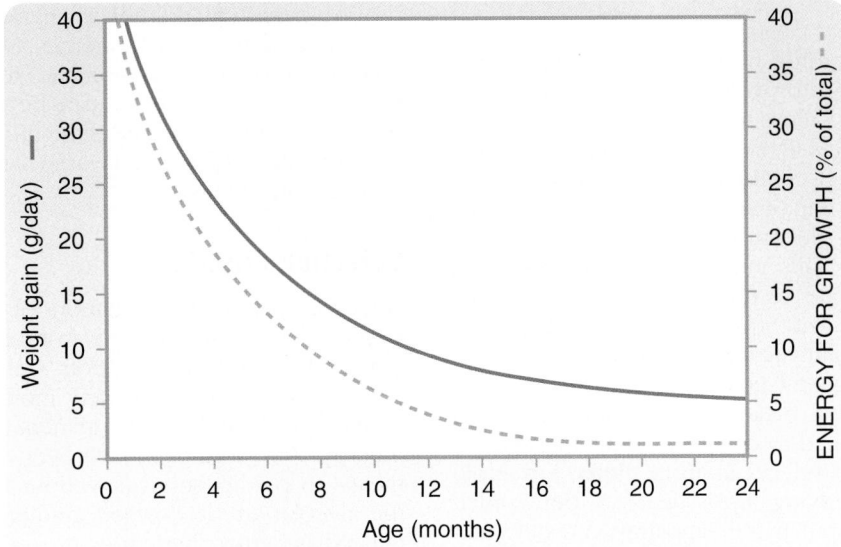

Figure 71-1 Daily gain in body weight and percentage of energy intake utilized for growth at 2 weeks to 2 years of age. Solid line, weight gain (g/day); dashed line, % of energy utilized for growth. (From Anderson TA: Birth through 24 months. In Rudolph AM [ed]: Pediatrics, 18th ed. Norwalk, CT, Appleton & Lange, 1987, p 158.)

The best two indicators of sufficient fluid intake are urine output and osmolarity. The minimum urine output in a newborn and young child is 1 to 2 mL/kg/day. Although adults can concentrate urine in the 1200 mOsm/kg range, an infant responding to water deprivation is only able to concentrate urine to a maximum of 700 mOsm/kg. Clinically, this means that greater fluid intake and urine output are necessary to excrete the solute load presented to the kidney during normal metabolism.

Electrolyte Requirements

In general, the daily requirements for sodium are 2 to 4 mEq/kg and for potassium are 1 to 2 mEq/kg. These requirements are usually met with a solution of 5% dextrose in 0.2% normal saline with 20 mEq KCl added per liter at the calculated maintenance rate, as noted previously.

Caloric Requirements

Energy requirements from birth through childhood are partitioned into maintenance of existing body tissues, growth, and physical activity. As depicted in Figure 71-1, the amount of energy from the diet required for growth alone may be as high as 40% in neonates. The parameter that is most indicative of sufficient provision of calories in neonates is daily weight gain. As such, infants gain roughly 30 g/day. The expected daily weight gain decreases with age. Total daily caloric requirements also decrease with age, and guidelines are listed in Table 71-2.

Protein

The average intake of protein makes up about 15% of the total daily calories and ranges from 2 to 3.5 g/kg/day

Table 71-2 Average Energy Requirement by Age

AGE (mo)	AVERAGE ENERGY REQUIREMENT* (kcal/kg/d)
0-1	124
1-2	116
2-3	109
3-4	103
4-5	99
5-6	96.5
6-7	95
7-8	94.5
8-9	95
9-10	99
10-11	100
11-12	104.5

*Based on measured intakes.
From Beaton GH: Nutritional needs during the first year of life: Some concepts and perspectives. Pediatr Clin North Am 32:275, 1985.

in infants. This protein requirement is reduced in half by age 12 years and approaches adult requirement levels (1 g/kg/day) by 18 years of age. The provision of greater amounts of protein, relative to nonprotein, calories will result in rising blood urea nitrogen levels. The nonprotein calorie (carbohydrate plus fat calories) to protein calorie ratio (when expressed in grams of nitrogen) therefore is not less than 150:1. For infants receiving parenteral nutrition, the amount of protein provided is usually begun at 0.5 g/kg/day and advanced in daily increments of 0.5 g/kg/day to the target goal.

Carbohydrate

When oral nutrition cannot be provided to infants, it is critical that IV fluids are provided to supply water, electrolytes, and glucose. Failure to provide glucose for prolonged periods will result in the rapid (within hours) development of hypoglycemia. In turn, this may lead to seizures, neurologic impairment, or even death. The absolute minimum IV glucose infusion rate for neonates is 4 to 6 mg/kg/min. This rate needs to be calculated daily for every neonate receiving parenteral nutrition. During total parenteral nutrition, the amount of glucose provided is increased daily to a maximum of 10 to 12 mg/kg/min. These are general guidelines and must be tailored to each individual patient. The amount of weight gain will dictate the need to continue advancing glucose calories. Further, hyperglycemia from either too rapid advancement or underlying sepsis needs to be avoided because it leads to rapid hyperosmolarity and dehydration. In contrast with adults, the addition of insulin to the parenteral nutrition solution in children is very high risk and is generally not indicated in routine practice.

Fat

In adults, parenteral fat is provided as a daily infusion as a source of calories or is given intermittently to prevent the development of essential fatty acid deficiency. In the pediatric population, fat is always provided as a daily infusion for both purposes. The lipid requirements for growth are significant, and fat is a robust caloric source. Similar to protein, fat infusions are started at 0.5 g/kg/day and advanced up to 2.5 to 3 g/kg/day. In infants with unconjugated hyperbilirubinemia, fat administration is done with caution because fatty acids may displace bilirubin from albumin. The free unconjugated bilirubin may then cross the blood-brain barrier and lead to kernicterus and resultant mental retardation.

EXTRACORPOREAL LIFE SUPPORT

Extracorporeal life support (ECLS), formerly referred to as extracorporeal membrane oxygenation (ECMO), is a type of heart-lung bypass that provides short-term (days to weeks) support for the critically ill patient with acute life-threatening respiratory or cardiac failure. ECLS is a purely supportive, nontherapeutic intervention that maintains adequate gas exchange and circulatory support while resting the injured lungs or heart. Although the use of ECLS has been described in both pediatric and adult populations, the greatest experience has been reported in neonatal respiratory failure.[1] Since the mid-1970s when the first neonatal survival was reported, ECLS has become the standard of care for neonatal respiratory failure unresponsive to maximum conventional medical management. It is practiced in more than 90 centers worldwide, with an overall survival rate of 80%.

Indications

The major indications for initiation of neonatal ECLS include meconium aspiration, respiratory distress syndrome, persistent pulmonary hypertension, sepsis, and congenital diaphragmatic hernia. Occasionally, neonates with congenital cardiac anomalies may be supported with ECLS until surgical repair can be accomplished. Meconium aspiration syndrome is the most common indication for neonatal ECLS and is associated with the highest survival rate (>90%).

Selection Criteria

Selection criteria for initiation of neonatal ECLS vary slightly from institution to institution and are usually derived from historical controls. Generally, an infant must have at least 80% predicted mortality with continued conventional medical management to justify this high-risk therapy. Two formulas have been historically used as a means to predict survival without ECLS. One formula is the alveolar-arterial oxygen gradient ($AaDO_2$) and is calculated as (atmospheric pressure $- 47) - (PaO_2 + PaCO_2)$. An $AaDO_2$ that is greater than 620 for 12 hours or an $AaDO_2$ greater than 620 for 6 hours associated with extensive barotrauma and severe hypotension requiring inotropic support are considered to be criteria for ECLS. The other formula is the oxygen index (OI) and is calculated as the fraction of inspired oxygen (usually 1.0) multiplied by the mean airway pressure times $100 \div PaO_2$. If the OI is more than 40, 80% mortality may be assumed. Additional inclusion criteria include gestational age greater than 34 weeks, birth weight more than 2 kg, and a reversible pulmonary process. Exclusion criteria include the presence of cyanotic congenital heart disease or other major congenital anomalies that preclude survival, intractable coagulopathy or hemorrhage, sonographic evidence of a significant intracranial hemorrhage (>grade I intraventricular hemorrhage), and more than 10 to 14 days of high-pressure mechanical ventilation. Before initiation of ECLS, all infants must undergo a cardiac echocardiogram to rule out congenital heart disease and a cranial ultrasound to exclude the presence of significant intracranial hemorrhage.

Extracorporeal Life Support Circuit

The basic concept of ECLS is to drain venous blood, remove carbon dioxide, and add oxygen through the artificial membrane lung, and then return warmed blood to the arterial (venoarterial) or venous (venovenous) circulation. Venoarterial bypass provides both cardiac and respiratory support, whereas venovenous bypass provides only respiratory support. Venoarterial bypass is used most commonly, and the right internal jugular vein and common carotid artery are typically chosen for cannulation because of their large size, accessibility, and adequate collateral circulation. The ECLS circuit (Fig. 71-2) is composed of a silicone rubber collapsible bladder (which collapses if venous return is diminished), a roller pump, a membrane oxygenator, a heat exchanger, tubing, and connectors. Venous blood from the right atrium drains through the venous cannula to the bladder and is pumped to the membrane oxygenator, where carbon dioxide is removed and oxygen is added. The

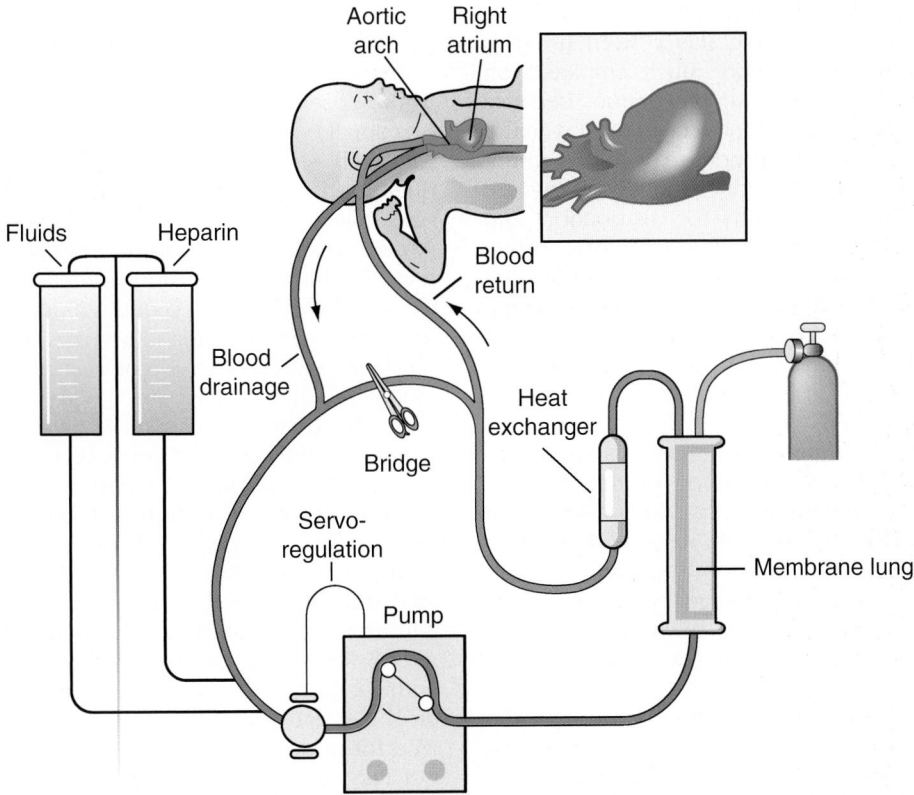

Figure 71-2 Diagrammatic representation of venoarterial extracorporeal life support circuit. (From Shanley CJ, Bartlett RH: Extracorporeal life support: Techniques, indications, and results. In Cameron JL [ed]: Current Surgical Therapy [4th ed]. St Louis, Mosby–Year Book, 1992, pp 1062-1066.)

oxygenated blood then passes through the heat exchanger and is returned to the patient through the arterial cannula.

To prevent clotting of the ECLS circuit, systemic anticoagulation is maintained. The fully heparinized patient is at risk for serious bleeding complications. As such, hematocrit levels are followed closely. Similarly, platelet counts and fibrinogen level must be monitored and normal levels maintained. Daily cranial ultrasound evaluations are obtained to monitor for hemorrhage.

Weaning From Extracorporeal Life Support

Extracorporeal flow is gradually weaned as native cardiac or pulmonary function improves. Indicators of lung recovery include an increasing PaO_2, improved lung compliance, and clearing of the chest x-ray. Once the extracorporeal flow rates are at minimal levels, the venous and arterial cannulas may be clamped to give the patient a trial off bypass. If the patient remains hemodynamically stable with adequate oxygenation and ventilation while the cannulas are clamped, the cannulas are surgically removed, and conventional ventilatory support is continued. The mean duration of ECLS in neonates is roughly 5 to 6 days. Patients with congenital diaphragmatic hernia and sepsis tend to have the longest required duration of bypass.

Complications

In addition to bleeding, ECLS is associated with significant morbidity and mortality. Multiple factors contribute to the risk of this technology and include ligation and cannulation of the right common carotid artery and right internal jugular vein, systemic heparinization, exposure to multiple blood products, and potential for mechanical failure of the circuit. Bleeding is the most common complication and may be either medical (e.g., too few platelets, too much heparin, intracranial) or surgical (e.g., neck cannulation site, intrathoracic, gastrointestinal). Birth weight and gestational age are the most significant correlates of intracranial hemorrhage on ECLS, and infants weighing less than 2.2 kg and younger than 35 weeks' gestational age are at highest risk. Other significant complications associated with ECLS include seizures, neurologic impairment, renal failure requiring hemofiltration or hemodialysis, hypertension, infection, and mechanical malfunction (e.g., failure of the membrane oxygenator, pump, heat exchanger).

TRAUMA

In children between 1 and 15 years of age, trauma is the leading cause of death. Although motor vehicle crashes account for most traumatic deaths, falls, bicycle accidents, and child abuse constitute a substantial component as well. Violence-related penetrating injury from firearms is becoming increasingly common. Much emphasis on trauma research is directed toward prevention. Because a large percentage of motor vehicle crash–related injury occurs because of absent or improper use of child restraint devices, community outreach education programs are vital. Along these lines, programs for distribution and education on the use of safety helmets for bike riding and skateboarding and on the safest location within the car for children[2] are extremely important in reducing injury severity. Finally, active participation by pediatric surgeons in legislative efforts toward factors such as firearm safety locks and use of all-terrain vehicles by young children are critical.

The management of trauma in children is similar to that of adults and beyond the scope of the chapter. However, several caveats are important to consider. Just as in adults, the priorities during the resuscitation phase are airway, breathing, and circulation. In general, a child who is crying on arrival to the emergency department is reassuring because the airway and breathing are more than likely to be intact. If endotracheal intubation is required, an uncuffed endotracheal tube is used in children younger than 8 to 10 years of age because of the small size of the trachea. The appropriate endotracheal tube size can be estimated visually as being equivalent to the diameter of the child's little finger. Alternatively the appropriate endotracheal tube inner diameter can be calculated by the following formula: $4 + ($patient's age in years$) \div 4$. Because of the soft and easily injured trachea of young children, surgical cricothyroidotomy must never be attempted in a child who is younger than 12 years of age.

With regard to fluid resuscitation, crystalloid is given as a rapid IV bolus in increments of 20 mL/kg. The ability to secure reliable IV access in young children may be quite challenging. In children younger than 6 years of age in whom an IV line cannot be secured within a reasonable period, intraosseous access is considered. This is accomplished with a specially designed needle placed under sterile conditions through the flat, anteromedial surface of the tibia, 1 to 2 cm below the anterior tibial tuberosity. Virtually any IV drug or fluid that may be required during resuscitation can be safely administered by the intraosseous route. Blood transfusion is warranted in pediatric trauma patients who demonstrate persistent evidence of hypovolemic shock after two boluses (total of 40 mL/kg) of crystalloid fluid. An estimate of a child's entire blood volume is roughly 80 mL/kg. As a general rule, if the need for blood transfusion within the first 24 hours after blunt abdominal trauma exceeds half the estimated blood volume, active hemorrhage is presumed and is usually an indication for laparotomy.

Imaging of the pediatric blunt trauma patient is predominately by computed tomography (CT) of the abdomen and pelvis. The indications for CT include the presence of a distracting injury such as an associated arm or leg fracture, significant closed head injury, if the examination is unclear or cannot be obtained because of an uncooperative or very young child, or if the serum glutamic-oxaloacetic transaminase or serum glutamic-pyruvic transaminase levels are higher than 200 or 100 IU/L, respectively. A significant amount of peritoneal fluid in the absence of solid organ injury raises the suspicion of a small bowel injury and prompts further investigation. Although significant spleen and liver injuries are frequently identified, the need for operative intervention is rare. The major indications for laparotomy in these circumstances include obvious hemodynamic instability, the need for blood transfusion in amounts greater than half the child's calculated blood volume (40 mL/kg) within the first 24 hours after injury, or obvious extravascular blush of IV administered contrast material. Specific treatment guidelines based on CT grade of liver or spleen injury have been prospectively validated by the Liver/Spleen Trauma Study Group of the American Pediatric Surgical Association and are more focused to the pediatric population.[3] According to these guidelines, a patient with an isolated grade I liver or spleen injury may be managed without the need for admission to an intensive care unit (ICU), require no more than 2 days of hospitalization, and resume full activities and contact sports after 3 weeks. At the other end of the spectrum, patients with isolated grade IV injuries are carefully monitored in an ICU for at least the first 24 hours and remain hospitalized for no less than 5 days. Return to full activities does not take place until 6 weeks after injury. Regardless of the injury grade and in the absence of specific indications, follow-up imaging either at the time of discharge or before resumption of normal activities is not indicated.

LESIONS OF THE NECK

Cystic Hygroma

A cystic hygroma is a lymphatic malformation that occurs as a result of a maldeveloped localized lymphatic network, which fails to connect or drain into the venous system. Most (75%) involve the lymphatic jugular sacs and present in the posterior neck region (Fig. 71-3). Another 20%

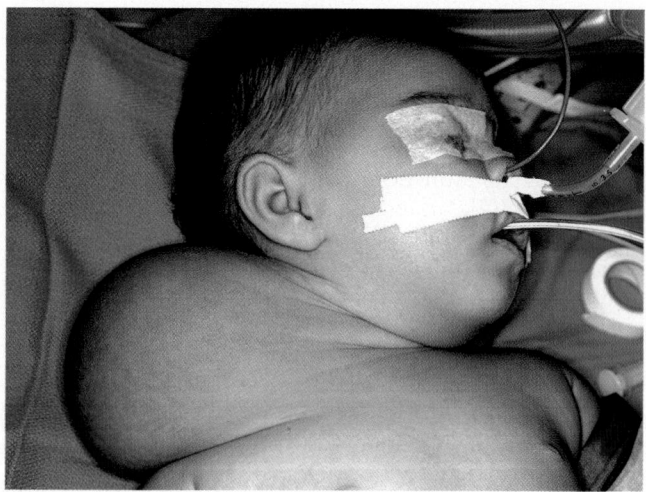

Figure 71-3 Cystic hygroma.

occur in the axilla, and the remainder are found throughout the body, including the retroperitoneum, mediastinum, pelvis, and inguinal area. Roughly 50% to 65% of hygromas present at birth, and most become apparent by the second year of life.

Because hygromas are multiloculated cystic spaces lined by endothelial cells, they usually present as soft, cystic masses that distort the surrounding anatomy. The indications for therapy are obviously cosmetic. In addition, the hygroma may expand to compress the airway, resulting in acute airway obstruction. Prenatal recognition of a large cystic mass of the neck is associated with significant risk to the airway, greater association with chromosomal abnormalities, and higher mortality rates.[4] Improved fetal imaging modalities may allow for intervention at the time of delivery based on principles of pharmacologic maintenance of placental circulation until endotracheal intubation is achieved. This technique is referred to as the *ex utero intrapartum therapy* (EXIT) procedure[5] and is discussed later in this chapter. In addition to accumulating lymph fluid, hygromas are prone to infection and hemorrhage within the mass. Thus, rapid changes in the size of the hygroma may necessitate more urgent intervention.

Complete surgical excision is the preferred treatment; however, this may be impossible because of the hygroma infiltrating within and around important neurovascular structures. Careful preoperative magnetic resonance imaging (MRI) to define the extent of the hygroma is crucial. Operations are routinely performed with the aid of loupe magnification and a nerve stimulator. Because hygromas are not neoplastic tumors, radical resection with removal of major blood vessels and nerves is not indicated. Postoperative morbidity includes recurrence, lymphatic leak, infection, and neurovascular injury.

Injection of sclerosing agents such as bleomycin or the derivative of *Streptococcus pyogenes* OK-432 have also been reported to be effective in the management of cystic hygromas. Intracystic injection of sclerosants appears to be most effective for macrocystic hygromas, as opposed to the microcystic variety.

Branchial Cleft Remnants

The mature structures of the head and neck are embryologically derived from six pairs of branchial arches, their intervening clefts externally, and pouches internally. Congenital cysts, sinuses, or fistulas result from failure of these structures to regress, persisting in an aberrant location. The location of these remnants generally dictates their embryologic origin and guides the subsequent operative approach. Failure to understand the embryology may result in incomplete resection or injury to adjacent structures.

By definition, all branchial remnants are present at the time of birth, although they may not become clinically evident until later in life. In children, fistulas are more common than external sinuses, which are more common than cysts. In adults, cysts predominate. The clinical presentation may range from a continuous mucoid drainage from a fistula or sinus to the development of a cystic

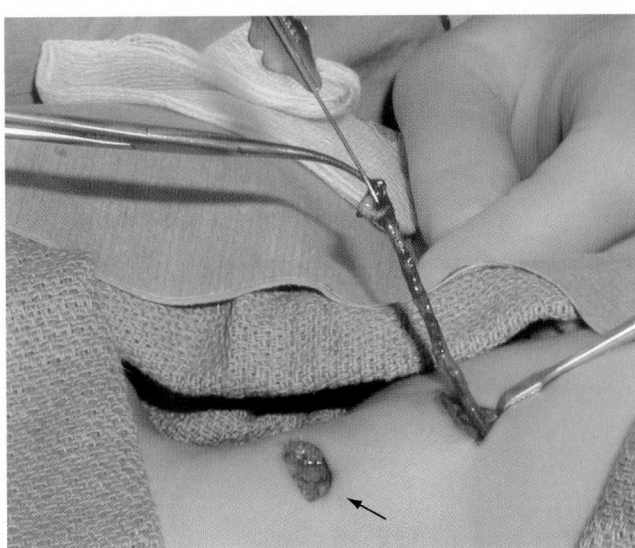

Figure 71-4 Branchial cleft fistula. The original site of the fistula in the lower neck (*arrow*) has been elliptically excised, and a stepladder counterincision has been made higher in the neck to remove the entire tract. A lacrimal probe has been inserted into the tract to define its course.

mass that may become infected. Branchial remnants may also be palpable as cartilaginous lumps or cords corresponding with a fistulous tract. Dermal pits or skin tags may also be evident.

First branchial remnants are typically located in the front or back of the ear, or in the upper neck in the region of the mandible. Fistulas typically course through the parotid gland, deep, or through branches of the facial nerve, and end in the external auditory canal.

Remnants from the second branchial cleft are the most common. The external ostium of these remnants is located along the anterior border of the sternocleidomastoid muscle, usually in the vicinity of the upper half to lower third of the muscle. The course of the fistula must be anticipated preoperatively because stepladder counterincisions are often necessary to excise the fistula completely (Fig. 71-4). Typically, the fistula penetrates the platysma, ascends along the carotid sheath to the level of the hyoid bone, and then turns medially to extend between the carotid artery bifurcation. The fistula then courses behind the posterior belly of the digastric and stylohyoid muscles to end in the tonsillar fossa.

Third branchial cleft remnants usually do not have associated sinuses or fistulas and are located in the suprasternal notch or clavicular region. These most often contain cartilage and present clinically as a firm mass or as a subcutaneous abscess.

Thyroglossal Duct Cyst

One of the most common lesions in the midline of the neck is the thyroglossal duct cyst, which most commonly presents in preschool-aged children. Thyroglossal remnants are involved with the embryogenesis of the thyroid gland, tongue, and hyoid bone and produce midline

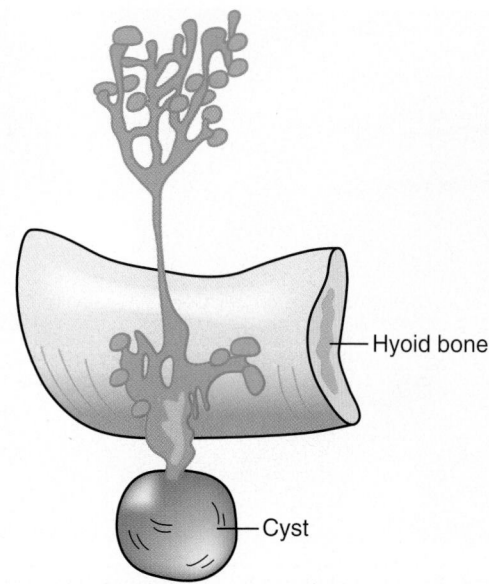

Figure 71-5 Thyroglossal duct cyst. There are usually branches from the cyst that are intimate with the hyoid bone and extend cephalad for variable distances. The Sistrunk procedure, which involves en bloc removal of the cyst, central portion of the hyoid bone, and tissue above to the base of the tongue is required to minimize recurrence. (From Horisawa M, Niinomi N, Ito T: What is the optimal depth for core-out toward the foramen cecum in a thyroglossal duct cyst operation? J Pediatr Surg 27:710-713, 1992).

masses extending from the base of the tongue (foramen cecum) to the pyramidal lobe of the thyroid gland. Complete failure of thyroid migration results in a lingual thyroid. Ultrasound or radionuclide imaging may therefore be useful to identify the presence of a normal thyroid gland within the neck. This information would be useful to prevent performing an inadvertent complete thyroidectomy during treatment of a presumed thyroglossal remnant.

Thyroglossal duct cysts may be located in the midline of the neck anywhere from the base of the tongue to the thyroid gland. Most, however, are found at or just below the hyoid bone. The indications for surgery include increasing size, the risk for cyst infection, or the presence (1%-2%) of carcinoma. The classic treatment has remained unchanged since it was described by Sistrunk in 1928 and involves complete excision of the cyst in continuity with its tract, the central portion of the hyoid bone, and the tissue above the hyoid bone extending to the base of the tongue. Failure to remove these tissues will result in a high risk for recurrence because multiple sinuses have been histologically identified in these locations (Fig. 71-5).

Torticollis

Torticollis simply refers to a twisted neck, which may be either congenital or acquired. In infants with congenital torticollis, the head is typically tilted toward the side of the affected muscle and rotated in the opposite direction. In many cases, a mass can be palpated within the affected muscle. Although the true etiology is unknown, birth trauma is most frequently considered. The typical onset of congenital torticollis is 4 to 6 weeks of age in an otherwise healthy infant. The diagnosis is purely clinical.

Treatment of congenital torticollis is initially conservative. Range-of-motion exercises consist of passive stretching of the affected muscle and are curative in most infants. The average duration of required treatment is 4.7 months. Surgical resection or division of the involved muscle is rarely necessary, but is indicated if symptoms persist beyond 1 year.

Congenital torticollis must be distinguished from acquired torticollis. In the former, the onset is fairly soon (within weeks) after birth, and associated problems are rare. Acquired torticollis occurs later and is associated with a range of conditions, including acute myositis, brainstem tumors, atlantoaxial subluxation, or infectious causes such as retropharyngeal abscess, cervical adenitis, or tonsillitis.

Cervical Lymphadenopathy

Enlarged cervical lymph nodes occur frequently in the pediatric population, and referral to a surgeon for biopsy is common. The etiology is overwhelmingly infectious; however, it is important to be aware of several other causative factors. Decisions regarding diagnostic testing and therapy are based largely on clinical judgment and must be derived from a thoughtful history and physical examination.[6]

The distribution of enlarged lymph nodes is important because most healthy children have small, mobile, rubbery, palpable lymph nodes in the anterior cervical triangle. On the other hand, nontender, fixed nodes in the supraclavicular region are worrisome for malignancy. Further, concern is raised regarding nodes that are larger than 2 cm, hard, nontender, and fixed to surrounding structures. Additional concerns for an underlying neoplasm are raised by a history of weight loss, night sweats, and progressive nodal enlargement.

If a diagnostic lymph node biopsy is indicated, a preoperative chest radiograph is performed to exclude associated mediastinal adenopathy. If enlarged anterior mediastinal nodes are seen, CT of the chest is done to determine whether there is airway compression. Failure to recognize this preoperatively may result in life-threatening airway obstruction during the induction of general anesthesia. If significant airway compression is seen, every attempt is made to perform the biopsy under local anesthesia. Because this may not be feasible in some children, preoperative discussion of the CT findings with the anesthesiologist is critical. Anesthetic caveats for this patient population include preservation of spontaneous ventilation during intubation, induction in the sitting position, securing IV access in a lower extremity, and changing the patient's position whenever cardiorespiratory compromise is apparent. Access to fiberoptic and rigid bronchoscopy, a skilled bronchoscopist, and longer endotracheal tubes must be immediately available.

Patients with acute, bilateral cervical lymphadenitis are usually managed conservatively because infection with

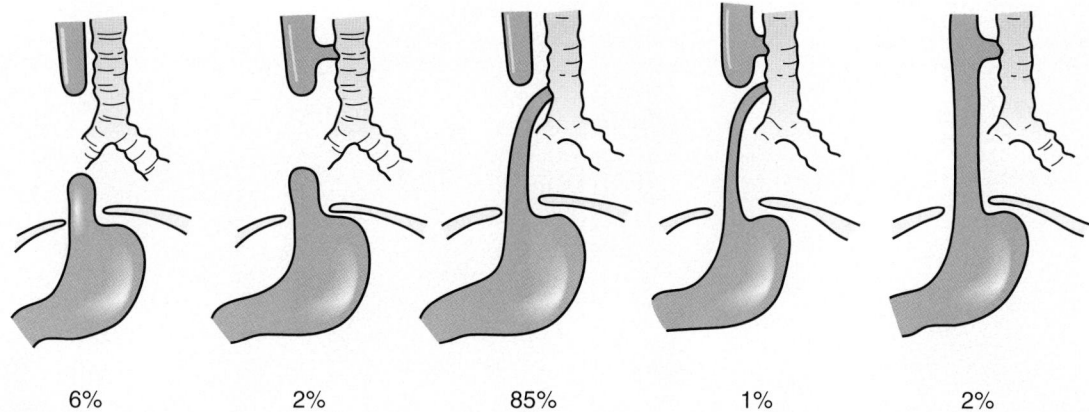

6%   2%   85%   1%   2%

Figure 71-6 The main anatomic variants and incidence of esophageal atresia and tracheoesophageal fistula.

respiratory viruses is so common. These viruses include adenovirus, influenza virus, and respiratory syncytial virus and are often associated with symptoms of cough, rhinorrhea, and sinus congestion. Acute unilateral pyogenic lymphadenitis is caused by *Staphylococcus aureus* and group A *Streptococcus* species in more than 80% of cases. In early cases, an oral antibiotic directed primarily toward gram-positive organisms is indicated. After the nodes become fluctuant, needle aspiration or incision and drainage will be necessary.

Cat-scratch disease is thought to account for as much as 3% of acute cervical lymphadenopathy and is caused by the organism *Bartonella henselae*. A history of exposure to cats is helpful, but not always present. The diagnosis may be made by polymerase chain reaction from nodal tissue. Antibiotic therapy is not recommended because the disease is self-limited in most cases.

A less common infectious cause for cervical lymphadenitis is nontuberculous *Mycobacteria* infection. Typically, the nodes are fluctuant, and the overlying skin has a violaceous appearance, but is not particularly tender. Occasionally, the nodes will drain spontaneously with the formation of mature sinus tracts. The diagnosis is made by positive cultures for nontuberculous acid-fast bacilli together with a positive tuberculin skin test. Because most of the nontuberculous *Mycobacteria* are resistant to conventional chemotherapy, surgical excision is the treatment of choice.[7] Incision and drainage alone are associated with a high rate of recurrence and poor healing of the wound. In contrast with patients with active tuberculous infections, there is no indication for isolation of patients with nontuberculous lymphadenitis.

ALIMENTARY TRACT

Esophageal Atresia and Tracheoesophageal Fistula

Esophageal atresia (EA) is a congenital interruption or discontinuity of the esophagus resulting in esophageal obstruction. Tracheoesophageal fistula (TEF) is an abnor-

mal communication (fistula) between the esophagus and trachea. Esophageal atresia may be present with or without a TEF. Alternatively, a TEF can occur without EA. The incidence and range of anatomic variants is depicted in Figure 71-6. The prevalence of EA or TEF is 2.6 to 3 per 10,000 births, with a slight male predominance.

Associated Anomalies

The etiology of the disturbed embryogenesis is presently unknown. Roughly one third of infants with EA or TEF have low birth weight, and two thirds of infants have associated anomalies. There is a nonrandom, nonhereditary association of anomalies in patients with EA or TEF that must be considered under the acronym VATER (*v*ertebral, *a*norectal, *t*racheal, *e*sophageal, *r*enal or *r*adial limb). Another acronym that is commonly used is VACTERL (*v*ertebral, *a*norectal, *c*ardiac, *t*racheal, *e*sophageal, *r*enal, and *l*imb).

Clinical Presentation

The diagnosis of EA is entertained in an infant with excessive salivation along with coughing or choking during the first oral feeding. A maternal history of polyhydramnios is often present. In a baby with EA and TEF, acute gastric distention may occur as a result of air entering the distal esophagus and stomach with each inspired breath. Reflux of gastric contents into the distal esophagus will traverse the TEF and spill into the trachea, resulting in cough, tachypnea, apnea, or cyanosis. The presentation of isolated TEF without EA may be more subtle and often beyond the newborn period. In general, these infants have choking and coughing associated with oral feeding.

Diagnosis

The inability to pass a nasogastric tube into the stomach of the neonate is a cardinal feature for the diagnosis of EA. If gas is present in the gastrointestinal tract below the diaphragm, an associated TEF is confirmed (Fig. 71-7A). On the other hand, inability to pass a nasogastric tube in an infant with absent radiographic evidence for gastrointestinal gas is virtually diagnostic of an isolated EA without TEF (see Fig. 71-7B). These simple rules provide the correct

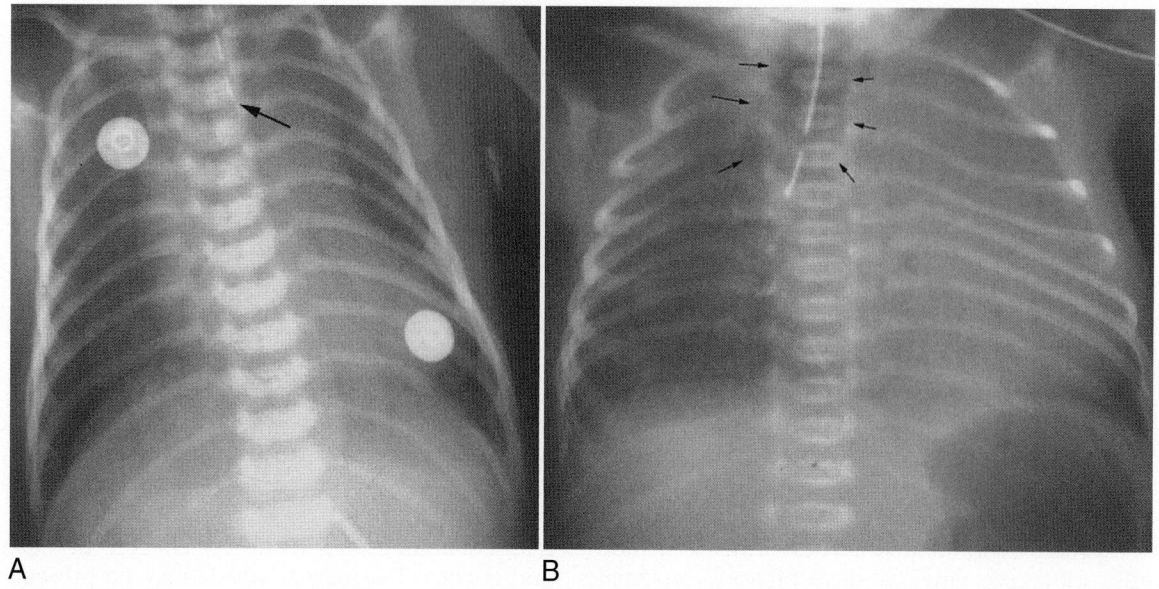

A   B

Figure 71-7 A, Plain chest radiograph of infant with pure esophageal atresia. Note the inability to pass the nasogastric tube (*arrow*) into the stomach and absence of gas within the abdomen. **B,** Plain chest radiograph of infant
with esophageal atresia and tracheoesophageal fistula (TEF). The esophageal atresia is suggested by the inability
to pass the nasogastric tube into the stomach and the surrounding gas-filled proximal esophagus (*arrows*). The
TEF is verified by the presence of gas within the abdomen.

diagnosis in most cases. Occasionally, a small amount of
isotonic contrast may be given by mouth to demonstrate
the level of the proximal EA pouch or the presence of a
TEF, but this is rarely necessary. In fact, the risk for aspiration with studies of this type is generally high.

Preoperative Evaluation and Management

The immediate care of an infant with EA or TEF includes
decompression of the proximal EA pouch with a sump
type of tube placed to continuous suction. This will
prevent spillover of oral secretions into the trachea. The
presence of the TEF may be life threatening; positive-
pressure ventilation may be inadequate to inflate the
lungs because air is directed into the TEF through the
path of least resistance. Ventilation may further be compounded by the resultant gastric distention. In these circumstances, manipulation of the endotracheal tube distal
to the TEF (e.g., right main-stem intubation) may minimize the leak and permit adequate ventilation. Further,
placement of an occlusive balloon (Fogarty) catheter into
the fistula through a bronchoscope may be useful. Finally,
urgent thoracotomy with direct ligation of the fistula, but
without repair of the EA, may be required. In these cases,
performance of a gastrostomy to decompress the distended stomach is avoided because it may result in the
abrupt inability to ventilate the patient.

In the preoperative period, it is necessary to perform
a thorough physical examination with particular attention
to the aforementioned VACTERL anomalies. A preoperative echocardiogram is essential to evaluate the presence
or absence of congenital heart disease as well as to define
the side of the aortic arch. A right thoracotomy is typically
done for the repair of EA or TEF in patients with a normal
left-sided aortic arch. However, for infants with a right-

sided arch, a left thoracotomy would be preferred, and
a higher incidence of aortic arch anomalies (vascular
rings) and postoperative complications must be anticipated.[8] Additional preoperative imaging studies include
ultrasonography of the spine and kidneys.

Surgical Management

The traditional surgical treatment of the most common
EA or TEF involves an extrapleural thoracotomy through
the fourth intercostal space. More recently, thoracoscopic
repair has been described by several pediatric centers
with advanced minimally invasive expertise.[9] A bronchoscopy is performed to identify the relative site of the
fistula, exclude the presence of a second fistula, and
delineate the bronchial anatomy. On the right side, the
azygos vein is divided to reveal the underlying TEF. The
TEF is dissected circumferentially and then ligated using
interrupted, nonabsorbable sutures. The proximal esophageal pouch is then mobilized as high as possible to
afford a tension-free esophageal anastomosis. The blood
supply to the upper esophageal pouch is generally robust
and based on arteries derived from the thyrocervical
trunk. On the other hand, the blood supply to the lower
esophagus is more tenuous and segmental, originating
from intercostal vessels. As such, significant mobilization
of the lower esophagus is not done, so as to avoid ischemia at the site of the esophageal anastomosis. The
anastomosis is performed using either a single- or double-
layer technique. The rates of anastomotic leak are slightly
higher with the single-layer anastomosis, whereas the
rates of esophageal stricture are higher with the double-
layer technique.

If the two ends of the esophagus cannot be joined
without significant tension, there are several options. The

first is to suture the divided end of the distal esophagus to the prevertebral fascia, mark its location with a metal clip, and close the thoracotomy. Over time (2-3 months), the proximal esophageal pouch may grow such that a subsequent thoracotomy may permit a primary esophageal anastomosis. A circular or spiral esophagomyotomy[10] of the upper pouch may also be done to gain esophageal length and facilitate a primary anastomosis. Another technique involves placement of traction sutures through the proximal and distal ends of the esophagus, brought out through the chest. These sutures are progressively tightened, and a primary esophageal anastomosis is performed after several days.[11] Alternatively, a cervical esophagostomy may be constructed and a formal esophageal replacement performed at a later date.

In patients with pure EA, the gap between the two esophageal ends is frequently wide, thus preventing a primary anastomosis in the newborn period. In these patients, the traditional approach is to perform a cervical esophagostomy for drainage of oral secretions and insertion of a gastrostomy for enteral feeding. An esophageal replacement using the stomach, small intestine, or colon is then performed at about 1 year of age. More recently, it has become apparent that the two ends of the esophagus may spontaneously grow such that a primary anastomosis may be accomplished by 4 months of age.[12] Thus, insertion of a gastrostomy in the neonatal period for feeding may be the only necessary intervention. The swallowing of saliva may actually promote elongation of the upper pouch, and an esophagostomy is therefore avoided.

In patients with pure TEF without EA, the site of the TEF is usually in the region of the thoracic inlet. As such, the surgical approach is through a cervical incision. After the induction of anesthesia, but before making the incision, it is often helpful to cannulate the TEF with a guidewire to facilitate identification of the TEF.

Outcome

The mortality rate of EA or TEF is directly related to the associated anomalies—particularly cardiac defects and chromosomal abnormalities. In the absence of these factors, survival of more than 95% of patients is expected.[13] Postoperative complications unique to EA or TEF include esophageal motility disorders, gastroesophageal reflux (25%-50%), anastomotic stricture (15%-30%), anastomotic leak (10%-20%), and tracheomalacia (8%-15%).

Gastroesophageal Reflux

Vomiting during infancy is a common occurrence and can be difficult to distinguish from chronic gastroesophageal reflux (GER) that ultimately requires surgical correction. Although the diagnosis and surgical management of GER are similar between adults and children, there are several major differences that must be understood.

Clinical Presentation

Although the symptoms of GER can often be obtained easily in adults, the recognition of symptoms in young children may be more subtle. Rather than complain of heartburn, children tend to associate pain with eating. As such, they may be irritable during or after feeding, or limit their formula intake altogether. This may be identified by failure to thrive (FTT). Another cause of FTT in infants with GER is the nutritional consequences of reduced caloric intake due to protracted emesis. Other unique symptoms include life-threatening episodes of apnea, termed *near-miss sudden infant death syndrome* (SIDS). In a child with documented GER, an episode of near-miss SIDS is an absolute indication for antireflux surgery. Respiratory symptoms of GER in children may manifest as chronic cough, hoarseness, recurrent pneumonias, or asthma. Persistent asthma may be due to GER in up to 75% of children, a significant proportion of whom have no other apparent symptoms of GER. Acid suppression alone has not been shown to alleviate the asthma symptoms, and operative therapy in these patients may be considered sooner.[14]

Many children referred for antireflux surgery are neurologically impaired, usually secondary to such factors as metabolic conditions, head trauma, or birth asphyxia. As such, most of these patients require permanent feeding access in the form of a gastrostomy tube. Thus, antireflux surgery is often entertained at the time of the gastrostomy tube insertion, especially in patients who are unable to reliably protect their airway, or who already have significant vomiting associated with intragastric tube feeding.

Preoperative Evaluation

The evaluation of the child with GER involves several studies, each designed to provide different information. The initial study includes an upper gastrointestinal (UGI) radiographic series. The UGI does not correlate well with the presence or absence of GER but is important to exclude other causes of vomiting in children. These would include malrotation, antral web, foregut duplication cysts, and pyloric or duodenal stenosis. The gold standard test for delineating pathologic from physiologic GER is continuous (18-24 hour) esophageal pH monitoring.[15] Risk assessment for the development of esophagitis can be derived from a reflux index, which takes into account the percentage of time the lower esophageal pH is less than 4. A reflux index of greater than 11% in infants up to 1 year of age, or greater than 6% in older children, is considered pathologic. The limitation of this study is that it nicely delineates risk for acid injury to the esophagus but may fail to detect pathologic GER in patients who have symptoms related to pulmonary aspiration. In these circumstances, the episode of reflux may be of sufficient magnitude to cause pneumonia or bronchospasm, but cleared efficiently from the esophagus so as to be interpreted as normal. Multichannel intraluminal impedance studies have been demonstrated to be equivalent to pH probe testing and may add benefit for the detection of reflux of gastric contents that are nonacidic.[16] Nuclear scintigraphy involves labeling food or formula with a radioisotope and then measuring the number of postprandial episodes of GER and aspiration events. The advantages of this technique include the ability to identify nonacid GER events and to quantitate gastric emptying. A drawback is that it is extremely sensitive and therefore is unable to distinguish between pathologic and non-pathologic GER. Further, normative data for the pediatric population are lacking. Finally, endoscopic visualization of the esophagus, larynx, and trachea are all complementary studies to confirm the presence of acid injury.

Conservative Management

Nonoperative measures to reduce GER include thickening of formula with cereal, reducing the volume of feeding, and postural maneuvers. In addition, pharmacologic acid suppression may be useful. Indications for surgical intervention include severe GER that is unresponsive to aggressive medical management. In addition, surgery is generally warranted in patients with life-threatening near-miss SIDS episodes, FTT, or esophageal stricture. Other relative indications include those requiring complex surgical airway reconstruction,[17] neurologic impairment requiring permanent feeding access, or a history of recurrent pneumonias or persistent asthma.

Operative Management

As in adults, multiple operations have been designed for children with GER. The gold standard procedure remains Nissen's fundoplication. In the pediatric population, this can be done open or laparoscopically with similar results. In severely neurologically impaired patients, a complete esophagogastric disconnection with Roux-en-Y esophagojejunostomy has been proposed but is associated with significant morbidity.[18]

Outcome

The overall results for antireflux surgery in children are excellent. The risk for recurrent GER is elevated in the neurologically impaired population, in the presence of severe underlying lung disease, or with a history of prematurity.[19]

Hypertrophic Pyloric Stenosis

Hypertrophic pyloric stenosis (HPS) is one of the most common gastrointestinal disorders during early infancy, with an incidence of 1 in 3000 to 4000 live births. This condition is most common between the ages of 2 and 8 weeks. In HPS, hypertrophy of the circular muscle of the pylorus results in constriction and obstruction of the gastric outlet. Gastric outlet obstruction leads to nonbilious, projectile emesis; loss of hydrochloric acid with the development of hypochloremic, metabolic alkalosis; and ultimately dehydration. Treatment of this condition is by surgical mechanical distraction of the pyloric ring. There is currently no place for medical management of HPS.

Etiology

The cause for pyloric stenosis is unknown, and multiple factors have been implicated. Ethnic origin is important because the highest incidence is found among whites of Scandinavian decent and lowest risk among African Americans and Chinese. Males outnumber females in every series by a ratio of 4:1 or 5:1. There is a higher risk for developing HPS in offspring of parents with this

condition, and in many series, first-born males are frequently encountered.

Clinical Presentation

Infants with HPS typically present with projectile emesis or frequent episodes of nonbilious emesis. Occasionally, the vomitus may be brown or blood streaked, but it is always nonbilious. Visible gastric peristalsis may be seen as a wave of contraction from the left upper quadrant to the epigastrium. The infants usually feed vigorously between episodes of vomiting.

Diagnosis

Palpation of the pyloric tumor (also called the *olive*) in the epigastrium or right upper quadrant by a skilled examiner is pathognomonic for the diagnosis of HPS. If the olive is palpated, no additional diagnostic testing is necessary. When the olive cannot be palpated, the diagnosis of HPS can be made with an ultrasound exam or fluoroscopic UGI series. These imaging tests are similar in terms of sensitivity and specificity for the diagnosis of HPS. The UGI is useful for the evaluation of other causes of vomiting, whereas the absence of radiation exposure and cost make the ultrasound the usual preferred study. A persistent pyloric muscle thickness of more than 3 to 4 mm or pyloric length of more than 15 to 18 mm in the presence of functional gastric outlet obstruction is generally considered diagnostic.[20] Recently, it was demonstrated that preoperative palpation of an olive did not affect the frequency of ultrasound imaging.[21]

Treatment

Treatment of HPS is by a pyloromyotomy. This consists of cutting across the abnormal pyloric musculature while preserving the underlying mucosa (Fig. 71-8). This can be done through a traditional right upper quadrant incision, through a periumbilical incision, or laparoscopically

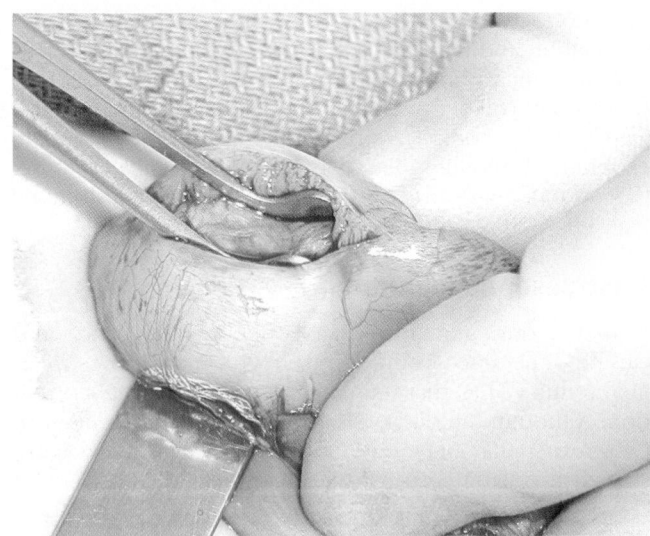

Figure 71-8 Pyloromyotomy for hypertrophic pyloric stenosis. The thickened pyloric musculature has been cut and then spread apart to reveal the underlying mucosa.

with similar outcomes.[22] Before surgery, it is important that the infant is hydrated with IV fluids to establish a normal urine output. It is important that the underlying metabolic alkalosis is slowly corrected with normal saline. Potassium is not given until the intravascular volume has been restored and normal urine output has resumed. Because the infant with underlying metabolic alkalosis will compensate with respiratory acidosis, postoperative apnea may occur. Thus, the serum HCO_3^- needs to be normalized before surgery.

Postoperatively, infants are usually allowed to resume enteral feedings. Vomiting after surgery occurs frequently but is usually self-limited. Complications specific to the pyloromyotomy include incomplete myotomy, mucosal perforation (usually at the duodenal end), and wound infection.

Intestinal Atresia

Duodenal Atresia

In contrast with more distal intestinal atresias, duodenal atresia (DA) is thought to occur as a result of failure of vacuolization of the duodenum from its solid cord stage. The range of anatomic variants includes duodenal stenosis, mucosal web with intact muscular wall (so-called windsock deformity), two ends separated by a fibrous cord, or complete separation with a gap within the duodenum.

Associated Anomalies

DA is associated with several conditions, including prematurity, Down syndrome, maternal polyhydramnios, malrotation, annular pancreas, and biliary atresia. Other anomalies, such as cardiac, renal, esophageal, and anorectal anomalies, are also common. In most cases, the duodenal obstruction is distal to the ampulla of Vater, and infants present with bilious emesis in the neonatal period. In patients with a mucosal web, the symptoms of postprandial emesis may occur later in life.

Diagnosis

The classic plain abdominal radiograph of DA is termed the *double-bubble sign* (air-filled stomach and duodenal bulb; Fig. 71-9). In cases in which there is no distal air, the diagnosis is secured, and no further studies are necessary. On the other hand, if distal air is present, an upper gastrointestinal contrast study is performed fairly rapidly. This study is important not only to confirm the diagnosis of duodenal stenosis or atresia but also to exclude midgut volvulus, which would constitute a surgical emergency.

Treatment

The management of DA is by surgical bypass of the duodenal obstruction as either a side-to-side or proximal transverse–to–distal longitudinal (diamond-shaped) duodenoduodenostomy. When the proximal duodenum is markedly dilated, a tapering duodenoplasty may be performed to reduce the duodenal caliber and may improve postoperative gastric emptying. In patients with a duodenal mucosal web, the web is excised transduodenally. The ampulla is often associated with the web itself and

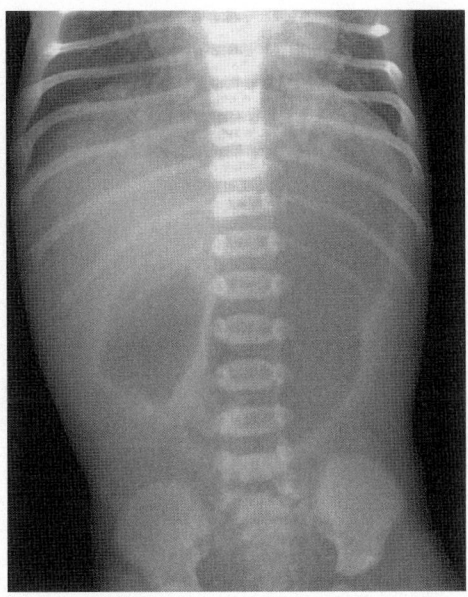

Figure 71-9 Plain abdominal radiograph demonstrating the typical double-bubble appearance of duodenal atresia. The large gas-filled stomach is visualized along with the dilated proximal duodenum. There is no gas beyond the duodenum.

must therefore be identified and preserved during the web excision.

Jejunoileal Atresia

Although several mechanisms have been proposed to explain the findings of jejunoileal atresia (JIA), the prevailing theory is that of an intrauterine focal mesenteric vascular accident. The spectrum of gross pathologic findings includes simple stenosis, complete interruption of the intestinal lumen with or without a fibrous cord attached to the distal bowel, a missing segment of bowel and mesentery, or multiple atresias. One final type is referred to as the *apple-peel* or *Christmas tree deformity* (Fig. 71-10). This atresia is unique from the standpoint that the obstruction is usually in the proximal jejunum, which is supplied by the entire superior mesenteric artery (SMA). There is then a gap in the mesentery, and the remainder of the small intestine is coiled around the ileocolic branch of the SMA, which is perfused retrograde from the middle colic artery. This tenuous blood supply has obvious implications for reanastomosis and the potential for ischemic necrosis due to an antenatal volvulus. As such, many of these infants with this type of atresia are born with reduced intestinal length.

Clinical Presentation

The clinical presentation is typically dependent on the level of obstruction. In proximal atresia, abdominal distention is less frequent, and bilious emesis is usually present. Plain abdominal radiographs typically reveal air-fluid levels with absent distal gas. If the atresia is distal, abdominal distention may be present. A preoperative barium enema may be useful to exclude multiple atresias, which may be present in 10% to 15% of cases. In contrast

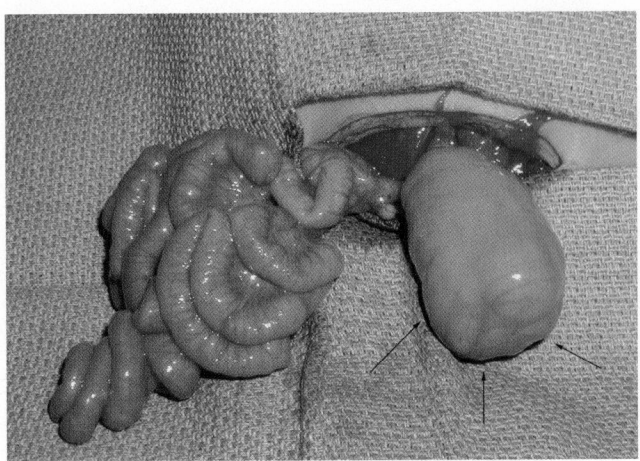

Figure 71-10 Proximal jejunal atresia of the apple-peel or Christmas tree variant. The dilated proximal jejunum (*arrows*) is supplied by the superior mesenteric artery (SMA). There is a gap in the mesentery, and the remainder of the small intestine is coiled around the ileocolic branch of the SMA, which is perfused retrograde from the middle colic artery.

with DA, JIA is usually not associated with other anomalies. One exception is cystic fibrosis, which may be present in roughly 10% of cases.

Management

The treatment of JIA is to reestablish intestinal continuity. In the presence of multiple atresias, it is imperative to preserve as much intestinal length as possible. This may require multiple anastomoses over an endoluminal stent. If the proximal intestine is significantly dilated, peristalsis will be perturbed. As such, on the one hand a tapering enteroplasty of the dilated bowel is performed if the remnant intestinal length is short. On the other hand, the dilated bowel needs to be resected if the remnant small bowel length is normal. The overall survival for infants with JIA atresia is more than 90%[23] and unrelated to the type of atresia encountered. The most significant associated morbidity is the short gut syndrome.

Anomalies of Intestinal Rotation and Fixation

Most intestinal rotation and fixation abnormalities become clinically evident during infancy and childhood. The true incidence of rotational anomalies of the midgut is difficult to determine and has been reported to occur with a frequency of 1 in 6000 live births. An understanding of the embryology of the intestine is essential in the recognition and appropriate surgical management of these conditions.

Normal Intestinal Rotation

The midgut normally herniates out of the abdominal cavity through the umbilical ring at about the fourth week of development in all human fetuses. By the 10th week of gestation, the intestine returns to the abdominal cavity and rotates around the axis of the SMA for 270 degrees in a counterclockwise direction. The final position of the ligament of Treitz is in the left upper quadrant and the cecum in the right lower quadrant of the abdomen. Interruption or reversal of any of these coordinated movements permits an embryologic explanation for the range of anomalies seen.

Abnormal Intestinal Rotation

Complete nonrotation of the midgut is the most frequently encountered anomaly and occurs when neither the duodenojejunal limb nor the cecocolic limb undergoes rotation. As a result, there is no duodenal C-loop, and the ligament of Treitz is located on the right side of the abdomen. Likewise, the cecum has failed to rotate and is present in the left side of the abdomen. In nonrotation, the proximal jejunum and ascending colon are fused together as one pedicle, through which the blood supply to the entire midgut (SMA) is located. It is this pedicle on which a midgut volvulus occurs, leading to ischemic necrosis of the entire midgut.

Nonrotation of the duodenojejunal limb followed by normal rotation and fixation of the cecocolic limb will result in duodenal obstruction due to mesenteric (Ladd's) bands originating from the colon and extending over the duodenum to end in the retroperitoneum. In this situation, a midgut volvulus is less likely because the base of the mesentery is relatively wide and fixed to the posterior abdomen. Duodenal obstruction from Ladd's bands is usually heralded by bilious emesis. Several other abnormalities are possible with any combination of incomplete, absent, or reverse rotation of the duodenojejunal limb followed by varied rotation patterns of the cecocolic limb.

Clinical Presentation

Rotational anomalies may manifest clinically in several different ways; however, the main symptom complexes may be grouped together as those related to volvulus, duodenal obstruction, or intermittent or chronic abdominal pain, or as an incidental finding in an otherwise asymptomatic patient. Most patients develop symptoms during the first month of life.

Midgut volvulus is a true surgical emergency because delay in operative correction is associated with a high risk for intestinal necrosis and subsequent death. The sudden appearance of bilious emesis in a newborn is the classic presentation. Although bilious emesis is most often due to other causes, it is critical to exclude midgut volvulus. When clinical signs of intestinal compromise begin to appear, the ability to salvage the patient or any significant length of small bowel may be gone.

Midgut volvulus may also be incomplete or intermittent. Patients may have chronic abdominal pain, intermittent episodes of emesis (which may be nonbilious), early satiety, weight loss, failure to thrive, or malabsorption and diarrhea. With partial volvulus, the resultant mesenteric venous and lymphatic obstruction may impair nutrient absorption and produce protein loss into the gut lumen as well as mucosal ischemia and melena as a result of arterial insufficiency.

Diagnosis

The preoperative evaluation of a child with a suspected rotational anomaly of the intestine includes plain abdominal radiographs and a UGI contrast series. Occasionally, plain abdominal radiographs may reveal evidence of intestinal obstruction; however, the most common findings are nonspecific. The UGI contrast series remains the gold standard for the diagnosis. A key element in the diagnosis of rotational abnormalities of the intestine is the position of the ligament of Treitz. This is normally located to the left of midline and at the level of the gastric antrum. In the presence of a volvulus, the site of obstruction is usually the third portion of the duodenum and has the appearance of a bird's beak.

In the acutely ill child with midgut volvulus and obstruction, urgent operative correction is indicated, and little time is available for IV fluid resuscitation, placement of a nasogastric tube and Foley catheter, type and crossmatch for blood, and administration of broad-spectrum antibiotics. Time is critical in terms of intestinal salvage.

Operative Management: Ladd's Procedure

Surgical management of most rotational anomalies of the intestine is Ladd's procedure. On entering the peritoneal cavity, the entire bowel is immediately exposed. If a volvulus is encountered, it needs to be remembered that in most cases, the volvulus twists in a clockwise direction and thus needs to be untwisted in a counterclockwise manner. After detorsion, the intestine may be congested and edematous, and some areas may appear necrotic. Placement of warm sponges and observation for a period of time may improve the appearance of the intestine when the vascular integrity has been compromised. If areas of the bowel are obviously necrotic, resection with creation of a stoma is performed. Because it is imperative to preserve as much intestine as possible, marginal or questionable segments of bowel are left in place and a second-look procedure performed within 24 to 36 hours. Next, Ladd's bands are divided as they extend from the ascending colon across the duodenum and attach to the posterior aspect of the right upper quadrant. To prevent extramural compression of the duodenum and recurrent obstruction, the bands must be lysed completely on both lateral and medial aspects of the duodenum. In dividing the medial bands, the distance between the duodenum and ascending colon is increased. Broadening this mesenteric base will reduce the incidence of volvulus. There has been no demonstrated benefit to pexing the cecum or duodenum to the abdominal wall. In neonates, a balloon catheter may be passed through the mouth and advanced beyond the pylorus into the distal duodenum to exclude an intraluminal obstruction. An incidental appendectomy is then performed because the cecum will ultimately lie on the left side of the abdomen after this procedure. The intestine is replaced into the abdominal cavity with the small bowel lying entirely on the right side while the colon is positioned on the left.

Outcome

Recurrent volvulus is relatively infrequent but must be of prime concern in patients presenting with obstructive symptoms at any time postoperatively. More commonly, the cause for postoperative obstruction is adhesive bands. Gastrointestinal motility disturbances are also frequent. Midgut volvulus accounts for roughly 18% of cases of short gut syndrome in the pediatric population. Urgent recognition and management is the most important factor in preventing this complication.

Necrotizing Enterocolitis

Necrotizing enterocolitis (NEC) is the most common gastrointestinal emergency in the neonatal period. Prematurity is the single most important risk factor, although other factors such as ischemia, bacteria, cytokines, and enteral feeding are all likely significant. The advent of exogenous surfactant and improved methods of mechanical ventilation are contributing to greater numbers of premature infants at risk for developing NEC. Despite the tremendous impact of NEC on neonatal morbidity and mortality, progress in understanding this condition is hampered by the fact that a reliable animal model for NEC does not exist.

Clinical Presentation

The development of NEC is unusual in the first few days of life. About 80% of cases, however, occur within the first month of life. The clinical presentation of NEC is often nonspecific and unpredictable. Clinical signs include irritability, temperature instability, poor feeding, or episodes of apnea or bradycardia. More specific signs include abdominal distention, vomiting, feeding intolerance, or passage of a bloody stool. As NEC progresses, systemic sepsis develops with cardiorespiratory deterioration, coagulopathy, and death. The radiographic hallmark of NEC is pneumatosis intestinalis (Fig. 71-11). Pneumatosis is composed of hydrogen gas generated by bacterial fermentation of luminal substrates. Other radiographic findings may include portal venous gas, ascites, fixed loops of small bowel, or free air. The distal ileum and ascending colon are the usual sites affected, although the entire gastrointestinal tract (NEC totalis) may also be involved.

Conservative Management

After the diagnosis of NEC has been established, initial management consists of bowel rest with nasogastric tube decompression, fluid resuscitation, blood and platelet transfusion, and administration of broad-spectrum antibiotics. Medical management continues for 7 to 10 days and is successful in roughly half of cases. The absolute indication for operative management of NEC is the presence of intestinal perforation as revealed by the identification of free air on plain abdominal radiographs. Other relative indications for surgery include overall clinical deterioration, abdominal wall cellulitis, worsening acidosis, falling white blood cell or platelet count, palpable abdominal mass, or a persistent fixed loop on repeated abdominal radiographs. The decision to proceed with

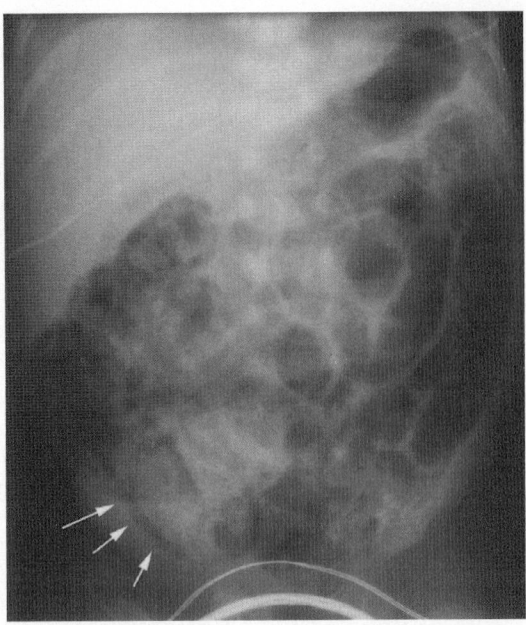

Figure 71-11 Plain abdominal radiograph of an infant with necrotizing enterocolitis demonstrating diffuse pneumatosis intestinalis. In addition to the typical ground-glass appearance, linear gas corresponding with the submucosal plane of the bowel wall is easily visualized (*arrows*).

surgery can be difficult and must be weighed against the risks of laparotomy in an already compromised premature infant.

Surgical Management

The general principles of surgical management of NEC include resection of all nonviable segments of intestine with creation of a stoma. All efforts need to be made to preserve as much intestinal length as possible. As such, it may be necessary to resect multiple sites of necrotic bowel, preserve intervening segments of viable intestine, and create multiple stomas. In cases in which the bowel is ischemic, but not frankly necrotic, a second-look operation may be performed after 24 hours. Bowel resection with primary reanastomosis may be considered in the rare infant with focal involvement of NEC and minimal peritoneal contamination who is very stable in the operating room. The risks for anastomotic leak and stricture formation have tempered widespread enthusiasm for this approach.

Another, more recent operative approach to the management of the infant with NEC whose intestine has perforated is bedside placement of peritoneal drains under local anesthesia. Drainage of the contaminated peritoneal fluid may improve ventilation and halt the progression of sepsis in select very ill, preterm infants. Surprisingly, drainage of the peritoneum may be the only necessary intervention in a few patients. The data to support peritoneal drainage as an accepted mode of treatment for NEC were recently established in a multicenter, randomized prospective clinical trial.[24] In this study, survival, need for parenteral nutrition, and length

of hospital stay were similar for NEC infants weighing less than 1500 g treated by either peritoneal drainage or laparotomy.

Outcome

The overall mortality rate for surgically managed NEC ranges from 10% to 50%. NEC is currently the single most common cause of short gut syndrome in children.[25] Intestinal strictures may develop after either medical or surgical management of NEC in roughly 10% of infants. The most common site of involvement is the splenic flexure of the colon. Because of the risk for stricture, a radiographic contrast study of the distal intestine needs to be done before elective stoma closure. Neurodevelopmental delay is also a frequent long-term problem in these infants.

Meconium Syndromes

The meconium syndromes of infancy represent a complex group of gastrointestinal conditions associated with cystic fibrosis (CF), with considerable overlap in clinical presentation and management. Cystic fibrosis results from a mutation within the cystic fibrosis transmembrane regulator (*CFTR*) gene and is autosomal recessive. Therefore, both parents must be carriers. It is estimated that 3.3% of the white population in the United States are asymptomatic carriers of the mutated CF gene. The abnormal chloride transport in patients with CF results in tenacious, viscous secretions affecting a wide variety of organs, including the intestine, pancreas, lungs, salivary glands, reproductive organs, and biliary tract. The clinical presentation of the meconium syndromes ranges from a meconium plug to simple and complicated meconium ileus.

Meconium Plug

Meconium plug syndrome is a frequent cause of neonatal intestinal obstruction and associated with multiple conditions, including Hirschsprung's disease, maternal diabetes, hypothyroidism, and CF. Although most children with meconium plug syndrome are normal, further studies to exclude Hirschsprung's disease and CF are warranted. Typically, affected infants are often preterm and present with signs and symptoms of distal intestinal obstruction. Abdominal distention is a prominent feature. Plain abdominal radiographs reveal multiple dilated loops of intestine. The diagnostic and therapeutic procedure of choice is a water-soluble contrast enema. This often results in the passage of a plug of meconium and relief of the obstruction (Fig. 71-12).

Simple Meconium Ileus

Meconium ileus in the newborn represents the earliest clinical manifestation of CF and affects roughly 15% of patients with this inherited disease. In North America, virtually all white neonates with meconium ileus have CF. In simple meconium ileus, the terminal ileum is dilated and filled with thick, tarlike, inspissated meconium. Smaller pellets of meconium are found in the more distal ileum, leading into a relatively small colon. In

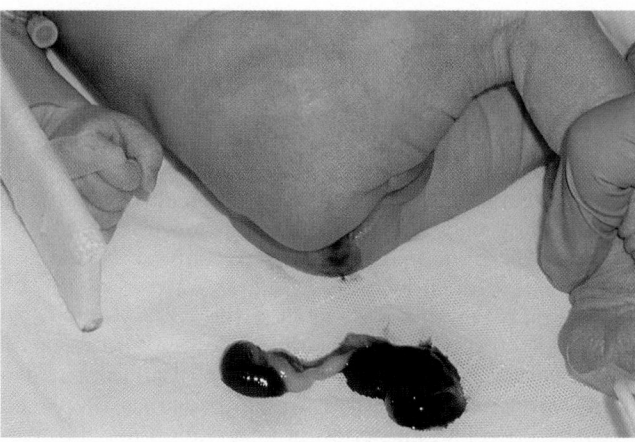

Figure 71-12 Meconium plug. This plug of meconium was passed following a contrast enema performed in an infant with abdominal distention and obstipation for 48 hours. After passage of the plug, the infant began to pass stool normally.

patients with simple meconium ileus, important plain abdominal radiographic findings include dilated, gas-filled loops of small bowel, absence of air-fluid levels, and a mass of meconium within the right side of the abdomen mixed with gas to give a ground-glass or soap bubble appearance.

The initial diagnostic study of choice is a contrast enema using water-soluble, ionic contrast solution. The exact type of contrast material is inconsistent among pediatric radiologists; however, Gastrografin is probably the most frequently used. Because the contrast agents are typically hypertonic relative to serum, it is important that the infants are well hydrated and electrolytes and vital signs carefully monitored following the procedure. It is important that the contrast reach the ileum into the area of inspissated meconium. This is successful in relieving the obstruction in up to 75% of cases, with a bowel perforation rate of less than 3%.

Operative Management

The operative management of simple meconium ileus is required when the obstruction cannot be relieved with contrast enema. Historically, the dilated terminal ileum was resected, and various types of stomas were created. This allowed for a very sick neonate to recover who would have otherwise died. More recently, simple evacuation of the luminal meconium without the need to create a stoma is all that is necessary in most cases. This is accomplished by open laparotomy, and a small enterotomy is made in the dilated terminal ileum. A red rubber catheter is used to irrigate the proximal and distal bowel with either warmed saline solution or 4% *N*-acetylcysteine. The latter solution serves to break the disulfide bonds within the meconium and facilitate separation from the bowel mucosa. The meconium is either manipulated into the distal colon or removed through the enterotomy, with care taken to avoid peritoneal contamination. After the obstruction is relieved, the procedure is concluded by closure of the enterotomy in two layers. In cases in which

the meconium evacuation is incomplete, a T tube may be left in place within the ileum to facilitate continued postoperative irrigation.

Complicated Meconium Ileus

Meconium ileus is considered complicated when perforation of the intestine has taken place. This may occur in utero or the early neonatal period. Meconium within the peritoneal cavity results in severe peritonitis with a dense inflammatory response and calcification. The presentation of complicated meconium ileus is variable and includes formation of a meconium pseudocyst, adhesive peritonitis with or without secondary bacterial infection, or ascites.

The diagnosis of CF is usually confirmed in the postoperative period. The pilocarpine iontophoresis sweat test revealing a chloride concentration greater than 60 mEq/L is the most reliable and definitive method to confirm the diagnosis of CF. This test may not be reliable in infants and is usually performed later. A more immediate test includes detection of the mutated *CFTR* gene. This test, coupled with a careful family history and clinical presentation, permits confirmation of the diagnosis in most infants.

Outcome

The long-term outcome of patients with CF with or without meconium ileus is probably not different, although gastrointestinal complications continue throughout life. A meconium ileus equivalent (distal ileal obstructive syndrome) may develop as a consequence of noncompliance with oral enzyme replacement therapy or bouts of dehydration. This is managed nonoperatively in most patients with enemas or oral polyethylene glycol purging solutions. Other diagnoses must also be considered, including simple adhesive intestinal obstruction. Further, with the introduction of enteric-coated, high-strength pancreatic enzyme replacement therapy, a fibrosing cholangiopathy has been described. Resection of the inflammatory colon stricture may be necessary.

Intussusception

Intussusception is the telescoping of one portion of the intestine into the other and is the most common cause of intestinal obstruction in early childhood. In most pediatric intussusceptions, the cause is unknown, the location is at the ileocecal junction, and there is no identifiable pathologic lead point. Invariably, there is marked swelling of the lymphoid tissue within the region of the ileocecal valve. It is unknown whether this represents the cause or the effect of the intussusception. Evidence to implicate a role for lymphoid swelling in the pathogenesis of intussusception is suggested by the association of this condition with a history of recent episodes of viral gastroenteritis, upper respiratory infections, and recently, administration of rotavirus vaccine.

Etiology

The incidence of a pathologic lead point is up to 12% in most pediatric series and increases directly with age. The most common lead point for intussusception is Meckel's diverticulum; however, other causes must be considered, including polyps, the appendix, intestinal neoplasm, submucosal hemorrhage associated with Henoch-Schönlein purpura, foreign body, ectopic pancreatic or gastric tissue, and intestinal duplication. Intussusception may also occur within the small bowel in the absence of a lead point in children who undergo abdominal surgery for a variety of reasons. This diagnosis is entertained in a child with crampy abdominal pain and emesis in the early postoperative period.

Clinical Presentation

Intussusception classically produces severe, cramping abdominal pain in an otherwise healthy child. The child often draws the legs up during the pain episodes and is usually quiet during the intervening periods. After some time, the child becomes lethargic. Vomiting is almost universal. Although frequent bowel movements may occur with the onset of pain, the progression of the obstruction results in bowel ischemia with passage of dark blood clots mixed with mucus commonly referred to as *currant jelly stool*. An abdominal mass may be palpated.

Diagnosis

In about half of cases, the diagnosis of intussusception can be suspected on plain abdominal radiographs. Suggestive radiographic abnormalities include the presence of a mass, sparse gas within the colon, or complete distal small bowel obstruction. In cases in which there is a low index of suspicion for intussusception based on clinical findings, an abdominal ultrasound may be the initial diagnostic test. The characteristic sonographic findings of intussusception include the target sign of the intussuscepted layers of bowel on transverse view or the pseudokidney sign when seen longitudinally.

Nonoperative Management

When the clinical index of suspicion for intussusception is high, hydrostatic reduction by enema using contrast or air is the diagnostic and therapeutic procedure of choice. Contraindications to this study include the presence of peritonitis or hemodynamic instability. Further, an intussusception that is located entirely within the small intestine is unlikely to be reached by enema and more likely to have an associated lead point. Hydrostatic reduction using barium has been the mainstay of therapy; however, more recently, the use of air enema has become more widespread. Successful reduction is accomplished in more than 80% of cases and confirmed by resolution of the mass, along with reflux of air into the proximal ileum. To avoid radiation exposure altogether, intussusception reduction by saline enema under ultrasound surveillance may be employed. Recurrence rates after hydrostatic reduction are roughly 11% and usually occur within the first 24 hours. Recurrence is usually managed by another attempt at hydrostatic reduction. A third recurrence is usually an indication for operative management.

Operative Management

The indications for operation in patients with intussusception include the presence of peritonitis or a clinical exam consistent with necrotic bowel. The presence of complete small bowel obstruction, small bowel location, failure of hydrostatic complete reduction, or history of several recurrences also directs surgical intervention. Laparoscopy may be useful as a first step to confirm the presence of an incompletely reduced intussusception and to facilitate reduction, thus avoiding a larger incision.[26] The intussusceptum is delivered through a transverse incision in the right side of the abdomen and reduced by squeezing the mass retrograde from distal to proximal until completely reduced. Warm lap pads may be placed over the bowel and a period of observation may be warranted in cases of questionable bowel viability. Adhesive bands around the ileocecal junction are divided, and an appendectomy is then performed. Invariably, the lymphoid tissue within the ileocecal valve region is thickened and edematous and may be mistaken for a tumor within the small bowel. Experience with this condition may prevent an unnecessary bowel resection. The recurrence rates are very low after surgical reduction. Bowel resection is required in cases in which the intussusception cannot be reduced, the viability of the bowel is uncertain, or a lead point is identified. An ileocolectomy with primary reanastomosis is the usual procedure performed.

Hirschsprung's Disease

Hirschsprung's disease occurs in 1 out of every 5000 live births and is characterized pathologically by absent ganglion cells in the myenteric (Auerbach's) and submucosal (Meissner's) plexus. This neurogenic abnormality is associated with muscular spasm of the distal colon and internal anal sphincter resulting in a functional obstruction. Hence, the abnormal bowel is the contracted, distal segment, whereas the normal bowel is the proximal, dilated portion. The area between the dilated and contracted segments is referred to as the *transition zone*. In this area, ganglion cells begin to appear, but in reduced numbers. The aganglionosis always involves the distal rectum and extends proximally for variable distances. The rectosigmoid is affected in roughly 75% of cases, splenic flexure or transverse colon in 17%, and the entire colon with variable extension into the small bowel in 8%. The risk for Hirschsprung's disease is greater if there is a positive family history and in patients with Down syndrome.

Clinical Presentation

Most infants with Hirschsprung's disease have symptoms within the first 24 hours of life with progressive abdominal distention and bilious emesis. Failure to pass meconium in the first 24 hours is a highly significant and cardinal feature of this condition. In some infants, diarrhea may develop as a result of enterocolitis. The diagnosis of Hirschsprung's disease may also be overlooked for prolonged periods. In these cases, older children may present with a history of poor feeding, chronic abdominal

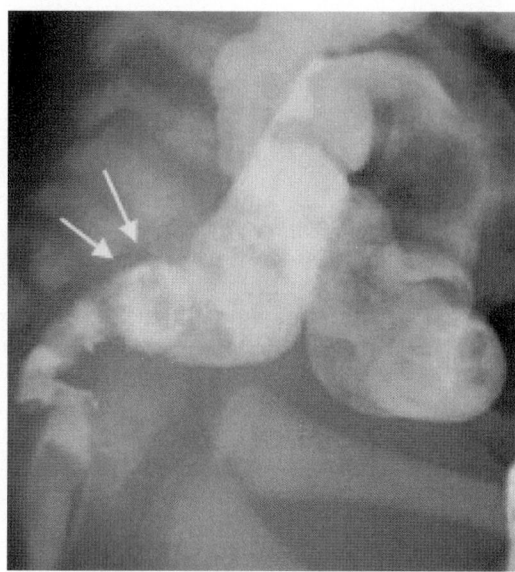

Figure 71-13 Hirschsprung's disease. A barium enema demonstrating the zone of transition (*arrows*) from the dilated proximal normal colon to the reduced caliber of the distal aganglionic colon.

distention, and a history of significant constipation. Because constipation is a common problem among normal children, referral for surgical biopsy to exclude Hirschsprung's disease occurs relatively frequently. Enterocolitis is the most common cause of death in patients with uncorrected Hirschsprung's disease and may manifest as diarrhea alternating with periods of obstipation, abdominal distention, fever, hematochezia, and peritonitis.

Diagnosis

The initial diagnostic step in a newborn with radiographic evidence of a distal bowel obstruction is a barium enema. Before this study, rectal examination and enemas are avoided so that they do not interfere with the identification of a transition zone. In a normal barium enema study, the rectum is wider than the sigmoid colon. In patients with Hirschsprung's disease, spasm of the distal rectum usually results in a smaller caliber when compared with the more proximal sigmoid colon. Identification of a transition zone may be quite helpful (Fig. 71-13); however, determination of the location of the transition zone is considered to be relatively inaccurate. Failure to completely evacuate the instilled contrast material after 24 hours would also be consistent with Hirschsprung's disease and may provide additional diagnostic yield. An important goal of this study is to exclude other causes of constipation in the newborn, such as meconium plug, small left colon syndrome, and atresia.

Anorectal manometry may also suggest the diagnosis of Hirschsprung's disease. The classic finding is failure of the internal sphincter to relax when the rectum is distended with a balloon. The advantage of this method is that it can be done in an outpatient setting, without the need for general anesthesia. This is more often useful in an older patient and is seldom used in neonates.

A rectal biopsy is the gold standard for the diagnosis of Hirschsprung's disease. In the newborn period, this is done at the bedside with minimal morbidity using a special suction rectal biopsy instrument. It is important to obtain the sample at least 2 cm above the dentate line to avoid sampling the normal transition from ganglionated bowel to the paucity or absence of ganglia in the region of the internal sphincter. In older children, because the rectal mucosa is thicker, a full-thickness biopsy is obtained under general anesthesia. Absent ganglia, hypertrophied nerve trunks, and robust immunostaining for acetylcholinesterase are the pathologic criteria to make the diagnosis.

Surgical Management

Multiple surgical options exist for the management of Hirschsprung's disease. Traditionally, a leveling procedure is done, followed by proximal diversion. This consists of a formal laparotomy, which is usually performed through a small incision in the left lower quadrant of the abdomen. The location of the transition zone is then identified and confirmed by multiple seromuscular biopsies. A diverting colostomy is then performed in the region of normal ganglionated bowel. A definitive procedure is then performed later.

The definitive management of Hirschsprung's disease involves variations among three main procedures. In the Swenson procedure, the aganglionic bowel is removed down to the level of the internal sphincters and a coloanal anastomosis is performed on the perineum. In the Duhamel procedure, the aganglionic rectal stump is left in place, and the ganglionated, normal colon is pulled behind this stump. A GIA stapler is then inserted through the anus with one arm within the normal, ganglionated bowel posteriorly and the other in the aganglionic rectum anteriorly. Firing of the stapler therefore results in formation of a neorectum that empties normally because of the posterior patch of ganglionated bowel. Finally, the Soave technique involves an endorectal mucosal dissection within the aganglionic distal rectum. The normally ganglionated colon is then pulled through the remnant muscular cuff and a coloanal anastomosis performed. More recently, these procedures have been performed in the newborn period as a primary procedure and without an initial ostomy. Further, the same procedure has been described in infants completely through a transanal approach with or without laparoscopic guidance.[27] The overall survival of patients with Hirschsprung's disease is excellent; however, long-term stooling problems are not infrequent. Constipation is the most frequent postoperative problem followed by soiling, incontinence, and enterocolitis.

Imperforate Anus

The spectrum of anorectal malformations ranges from simple anal stenosis to the persistence of a cloaca; incidence ranges from 1 in 4000 to 5000 live births and is slightly more common in boys. The most common defect

Table 71-3 Classification of Congenital Anomalies of the Anorectum

Female	
High	Anorectal agenesis with or without rectovaginal fistula
	Rectal atresia
Intermediate	Anorectal agenesis with or without rectovaginal fistula
	Anal agenesis
Low	Anovestibular or anocutaneous fistula (anteriorly displaced anus)
	Anal stenosis
Cloaca	
Male	
High	Anorectal agenesis with or without rectoprostatic urethral fistula
	Rectal atresia
Intermediate	Anorectal agenesis with or without rectobulbar urethral fistula
	Anal agenesis
Low	Anocutaneous fistula (anteriorly displaced anus)
	Anal stenosis

is an imperforate anus with a fistula between the distal colon and the urethra in boys or the vestibule of the vagina in girls.

Anorectal Embryology

By 6 weeks of gestation, the urorectal septum moves caudally to divide the cloaca into the anterior urogenital sinus and posterior anorectal canal. Failure of this septum to form results in a fistula between the bowel and urinary tract (in boys) or the vagina (in girls). Complete or partial failure of the anal membrane to resorb results in an anal membrane or stenosis. The perineum also contributes to development of the external anal opening and genitalia by formation of cloacal folds, which extend from the anterior genital tubercle to the anus. The perineal body is formed by fusion of the cloacal folds between the anal and urogenital membranes. Breakdown of the cloacal membrane anywhere along its course results in the external anal opening being anterior to the external sphincter (i.e., anteriorly displaced anus).

Classification of Anorectal Anomalies

An anatomic classification of anorectal anomalies is based on the level at which the blind-ending rectal pouch ends in relationship to the levator ani musculature (Table 71-3). Historically, the level of the end of the rectal pouch was determined by obtaining a lateral pelvic radiograph (i.e., invertogram) after the infant is held upside-down for several minutes to allow air to pass into the rectal pouch. This examination is very subjective and no longer used. Inspection of the perineum alone determines the pouch level in 80% of boys and 90% of girls. Clinically, if an anocutaneus fistula is seen anywhere on

the perineal skin of a boy or external to the hymen of a girl, a low lesion can be assumed, which allows a primary perineal repair procedure to be performed, without the need for a stoma. Most other lesions are high or intermediate, and they require proximal diversion by a sigmoid colostomy. This is followed by a definitive repair procedure at a later date. If required, the level of the rectal pouch can be detailed more definitively by ultrasonography or MRI.

Rectal atresia refers to an unusual lesion in which the lumen of the rectum is either completely or partially interrupted, with the upper rectum being dilated and the lower rectum consisting of a small anal canal. A *persistent cloaca* is defined as a defect in which the rectum, vagina, and urethra all meet and fuse to form a single, common channel. In girls, the type of defect may be determined by the number of orifices at the perineum. A single orifice would be consistent with a cloaca. If two orifices are seen (i.e., urethra and vagina), the defect represents either a high imperforate anus or, less commonly, a persistent urogenital sinus comprising one orifice and a normal anus as the other orifice.

Associated Anomalies

Congenital anorectal anomalies often coexist with other lesions, and the VATER or VACTERL association must be considered. Bony abnormalities of the sacrum and spine occur in about one third of patients and consist of absent, accessory, or hemivertebrae or an asymmetric or short sacrum. Absence of two or more vertebrae is associated with a poor prognosis for bowel and bladder continence. Occult dysraphism of the spinal cord also may be present and consists of tethered cord, lipomeningocele, or fat within the filum terminale.

Preoperative Evaluation

Clinical evaluation includes plain radiographs of the spine as well as an ultrasound of the spinal cord. Genitourinary abnormalities other than the rectourinary fistula occur in 26% to 59% of patients. Vesicoureteral reflux and hydronephrosis are the most common, but other findings such as horseshoe, dysplastic, or absent kidney, as well as hypospadias or cryptorchidism, also must be considered. In general, the higher the anorectal malformation, the greater the frequency of associated urologic abnormalities. In patients with a persistent cloaca or rectovesical fistula, the likelihood of a genitourinary abnormality is about 90%. In contrast, the frequency is only 10% in children with low defects (i.e., perineal fistula). Radiographic evaluation of the urinary tract includes renal ultrasonography and voiding cystourethrography; a rectourinary fistula (if present) likely will be demonstrated by the latter procedure.

In addition to the other tests described previously, a plain chest radiograph and careful clinical evaluation of the heart are conducted. If a cardiac defect is suspected, echocardiography is performed before any surgical procedure. Before feeding, a nasogastric tube is placed and its presence within the stomach confirmed to exclude esophageal atresia.

Low Lesions

The newborn infant with a low lesion can have a primary, single-stage repair procedure without need for a colostomy. Three basic approaches may be used. For anal stenosis in which the anal opening is in a normal location, serial dilation alone is usually curative. Dilations are performed daily by the caretaker, and the size of the dilator is increased progressively (beginning with 8-9 French and increased slowly to 14 to 16 French). If the anal opening is anterior to the external sphincter (i.e., anteriorly displaced anus) with a small distance between the opening and the center of the external sphincter, and the perineal body is intact, a *cutback* anoplasty is performed. This consists of an incision extending from the ectopic anal orifice to the central part of the anal sphincter, thus enlarging the anal opening. Alternatively, if there is a large distance between the anal opening and the central portion of the external anal sphincter, a *transposition* anoplasty is performed in which the aberrant anal opening is transposed to the normal position within the center of the sphincter muscles, and the perineal body is reconstructed.

High or Intermediate Lesions

Infants with intermediate or high lesions traditionally require a colostomy as the first part of a three-stage reconstruction. The colon is completely divided in the sigmoid region, with the proximal bowel as the colostomy and the distal bowel as a mucous fistula. Complete division of the bowel minimizes fecal contamination into the area of a rectourinary fistula, and it may lessen the risk for urosepsis. Furthermore, the distal bowel can be evaluated radiographically to determine the location of the rectourinary fistula. The second-stage procedure usually is performed 3 to 6 months later and consists of surgically dividing the rectourinary or rectovaginal fistula with pull-through of the terminal rectal pouch into the normal anal position. A posterior sagittal approach as championed by Peña is the procedure most frequently performed.[28] This consists of determination of the location of the central position of the anal sphincter by electrical stimulation of the perineum. An incision is then made in the midline extending from the coccyx to the anterior perineum and through the sphincter and levator musculature until the rectum is identified. The fistula from the rectum to the vagina or urinary tract is divided. The rectum is then mobilized and the perineal musculature reconstructed. The third and final stage is closure of the colostomy, which is performed a few months later. Anal dilations are begun 2 weeks after the pull-through procedure and continue for several months after the colostomy closure.

More recently, a single-stage procedure using a transabdominal laparoscopic approach has been described for treatment of intermediate and high imperforate anus anomalies.[29] This technique offers the theoretic advantages of placement of the neorectum within the central position of the sphincter and levator muscle complex under direct vision and avoids the need to cut across these structures. The long-term outcome of this new approach when compared with the standard posterior sagittal method is presently unknown.

Most of the morbidity in patients with anorectal malformations is related to the presence of associated anomalies. Fecal continence is the major goal regarding correction of the defect. Prognostic factors for continence include the level of the pouch and whether the sacrum is normal. Globally, 75% of patients have voluntary bowel movements. Half of this group still soil their underwear occasionally while the other half are considered totally continent.[30] Constipation is the most common sequela. A bowel management program consisting of daily enemas is an important postoperative plan to reduce the frequency of soilage and improve the quality of life for these patients.

ABDOMINAL WALL

Abdominal Wall Defects

Defects of the anterior abdominal wall are a relatively frequent anomaly managed by pediatric surgeons. During normal development of the human embryo, the midgut herniates outward through the umbilical ring and continues to grow. By the 11th week of gestation, the midgut returns back into the abdominal cavity and undergoes normal rotation and fixation, along with closure of the umbilical ring. If the intestine fails to return, the infant is born with abdominal contents protruding directly through the umbilical ring, termed an *omphalocele* (Fig. 71-14A). Most commonly, a sac is still covering the bowel, thus protecting it from the surrounding amniotic fluid. Occasionally, the sac may be torn at some point in utero, creating confusion with the other major type of abdominal wall defect termed *gastroschisis* (see Fig. 71-14B). In contrast with omphalocele, the defect seen with gastroschisis is always on the right side of the umbilical ring with an intact umbilical cord, and there is never a sac covering the abdominal contents. Major morbidity and mortality with either anomaly are not as high with surgical repair of the abdominal defect as with the associated abnormalities. In the absence of other major anomalies, long-term survival is excellent.[31]

Omphalocele

The abdominal contents with an omphalocele are covered with a membrane composed of the peritoneum on the inside and amnion on the outside. The size of the defect is variable, ranging from a small opening through which a small portion of the intestine is herniated to a large one in which the entire bowel and liver are included. In contrast with gastroschisis, karyotype abnormalities are present in roughly 30% of infants, including trisomies 13, 18, and 21. More than half of infants with omphalocele have other major or minor malformations, with cardiac being the most common, followed by musculoskeletal, gastrointestinal, and genitourinary. There is also a close

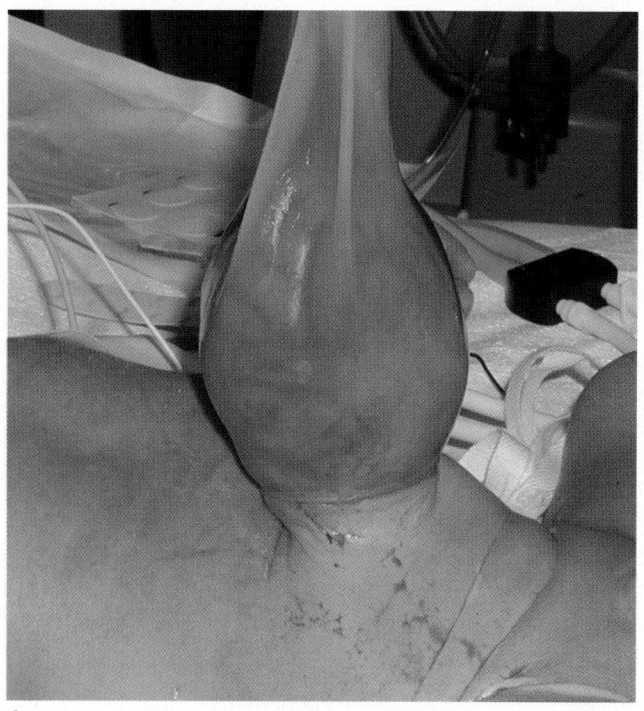

A

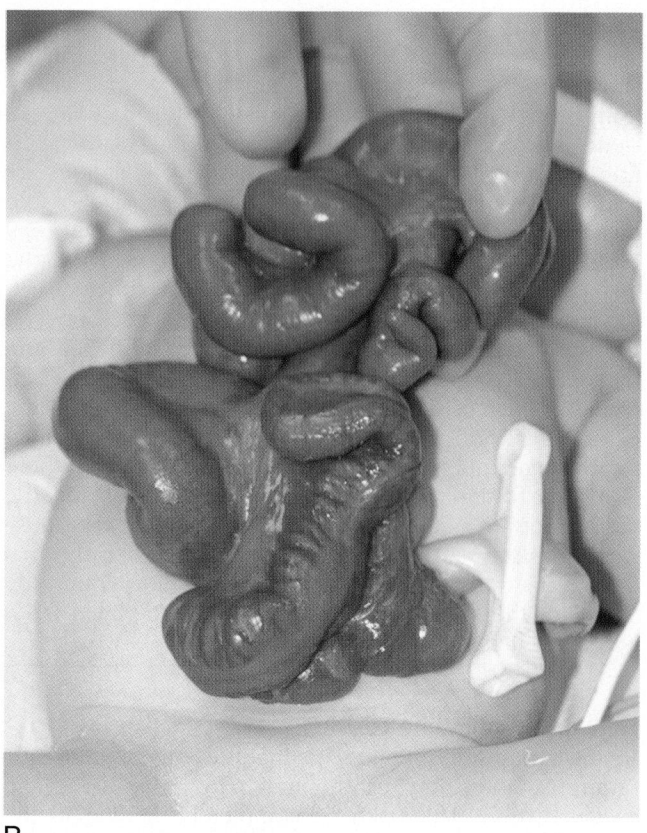

B

Figure 71-14 The two major abdominal wall defects. An omphalocele (**A**) originates in the center of the umbilical ring and contains a sac covering the bowel. There is a high incidence of other associated anomalies in the infant. In contrast, a gastroschisis (**B**) defect originates on the right side of the umbilical ring, there is no sac covering the viscera, and associated anomalies are relatively infrequent.

association with Beckwith-Wiedemann syndrome (omphalocele, hyperinsulinemia, and macroglossia).

Preoperative Evaluation and Management

The immediate treatment of an omphalocele consists of nasogastric or orogastric tube decompression for prevention of visceral distention due to swallowed air. An IV line is secured for administration of fluids and broad-spectrum antibiotics. The sac is covered with a sterile, moist dressing and the infant transported to a tertiary care pediatric surgery facility. Before operative repair, the infant is evaluated for potential chromosomal and developmental anomalies by a careful physical examination, plain chest radiograph, echocardiography if the physical examination suggests underlying congenital heart disease, and renal ultrasonography. Because the viscera are covered by a sac, operative repair of the defect may be delayed to allow thorough evaluation of the infant.

Surgical Management

Several options exist for the surgical management of an omphalocele and are largely dictated by the size of the defect. In most cases, the contents within the sac are reduced back into the abdomen, the sac is excised with

care to individually ligate the umbilical vessels, and the fascia and skin are closed. Fascial closure may be facilitated by stretching the anterior abdominal wall as well as milking out the contents of the bowel proximally and distally.

In giant omphaloceles, the degree of visceroabdominal disproportion prevents primary closure, and the operative management becomes more challenging. Construction of a Silastic silo allows for gradual reduction of the viscera into the abdominal cavity over a several-day period. Monitoring of intra-abdominal pressure during reduction may prevent the development of an abdominal compartment syndrome. After the abdominal contents are returned to the abdomen, the infant is taken back to the operating room for formal fascia and skin closure. Occasionally, closure of the fascia may be impossible. In these cases, the skin is closed, and a large hernia is accepted. This is repaired after 1 or 2 years. When the skin cannot be closed over the defect, several options exist, including the topical application of an antimicrobial solution to the outside of the sac, such as silver nitrate or silver sulfadiazine. Over time, this will result in granulation tissue and subsequent epithelialization of the sac. A repair of the large hernia is then performed a few years after this.

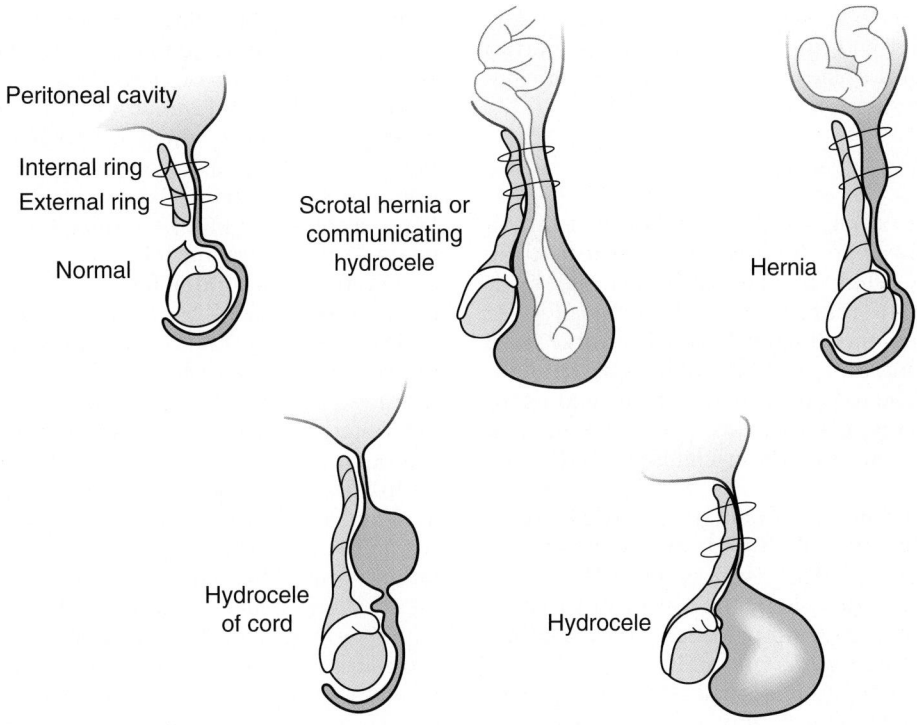

Figure 71-15 Anatomic variants of inguinal hernia and hydrocele. (From Cox JA: Inguinal hernia of childhood. Surg Clin North Am 65:1331-1342, 1985).

Gastroschisis

In contrast to patients with an omphalocele, the risk for associated anomalies with gastroschisis is low. One major exception to this general rule is the association of gastroschisis with intestinal atresia, which may be present in up to 15%. Atresias may involve the small and large intestine. The cause of gastroschisis is presently unknown, but a prevailing theory is that it results from an abdominal wall defect associated with normal involution of the second umbilical vein. In addition, babies with gastroschisis are more often small for gestational age and born to mothers with a history of cigarette, alcohol, and recreational drug use and intake of aspirin, ibuprofen, and pseudoephedrine during the first trimester; there is also an 11-fold increase in risk in mothers younger than 20 years.

The surgical management of gastroschisis is similar to omphalocele. Considerations for third-space fluid losses from the exposed intestine and risk for infection dictate more expedient coverage. The presence of atresia in a patient with gastroschisis may be managed in a number of ways. The bowel can simply be placed into the abdomen with a planned reoperation after several weeks. Another approach would be to perform a proximal diverting stoma. Finally, a primary anastomosis may be attempted. This is rarely advised because of the possibility of other atresias as well as the overall condition of the bowel.

In patients with gastroschisis, the intestine is often thickened, edematous, matted together, and foreshortened. It is unclear whether this represents damage from the amniotic fluid or ischemia from the small, constricting abdominal wall defect. The short gut syndrome may be a consequence of the attenuated intestinal length. Even with adequate length, the remnant bowel may be damaged to the point that motility, digestion, and absorption are markedly impaired. This prenatal intestinal injury accounts for most of the postoperative morbidity and mortality. Virtually all infants have a prolonged postoperative ileus. Parenteral nutrition is lifesaving but is also associated with the development of cholestasis, cirrhosis, portal hypertension, and ultimate liver failure.

Inguinal Hernia

Repair of an inguinal hernia (IH) represents one of the most common surgical procedures performed in the pediatric age group. Virtually all IHs in children are indirect and congenital in origin. The variable persistence of the embryonic processus vaginalis offers a spectrum of abnormalities, including a scrotal hernia, communicating hydrocele, hydrocele of the cord, or simple hydrocele (Fig. 71-15).

Incidence

The incidence of IH has been reported to range between 0.8% and 4.4%, which roughly translates into 10 to 20 per 1000 live births. In preterm infants, the incidence may be as high as 30%. About one third of children with IH are younger than 6 months, and males are affected about six times more often than females. The right side is involved in 60% and the left in 30% of patients; bilateral hernias are seen in 10%. The higher incidence on the right side compared with the left is probably related to the later descent and obliteration of the processus vaginalis of the right testis.

Diagnosis

Most IHs present as a bulge in the region of the external ring extending downward for varying distances to the scrotum or labia. Often, the hernia is detected by a pediatrician during a routine physical examination or observed by the parents. Inguinal pain may also be a presenting complaint. Incarceration and possible strangulation are the most feared consequences of IH and occur more frequently in premature infants. Because of the risk for these complications, all IHs in children need to be repaired.

Hydroceles represent fluid around the testicle or cord. A hydrocele that fills with fluid from the peritoneum is termed *communicating*. This is distinguished from a *noncommunicating* hydrocele by the history of variation in size throughout the day and palpation of a thickened cord above the testicle on the affected side. A communicating hydrocele is basically a small IH in which fluid, but not peritoneal structures, traverses the processus vaginalis. As such, all communicating hydroceles are repaired in the same manner as an indirect IH. In contrast, noncommunicating hydroceles are common in infants and can be observed for several months. The indications for repair of a noncommunicating hydrocele include failure to resolve and increase in size to one that is large and tense. The acute development of a hydrocele might be associated with the onset of epididymitis, testicular tumor, trauma, and torsion of a testicular appendage. An ultrasound of the scrotum may provide important diagnostic information in cases of an acute hydrocele in which examination of the testicle is difficult.

The timing of IH repair in premature infants is controversial. Early repair may be associated with a higher risk for injury to the cord structures, greater recurrence rate, and anesthetic-related apnea. These factors must be weighed against the higher risk for incarceration and strangulation, the potential for losing the patient during follow-up, and the development of a larger IH with loss of domain in the abdominal cavity. Taking these factors into account, most pediatric surgeons perform herniorrhaphy before the neonate is discharged home from the nursery.[32] If the infant has already been discharged home, most pediatric surgeons wait until the infant is older than 50 weeks postconception (gestational age+postnatal age). After this age, the risk for postoperative apnea is diminished.

The timing of repair of incarcerated IH is another important point and depends on the sex of the patient and contents within the hernia sac. In girls, the most common structure present in an IH that cannot be reduced is an ovary. The ovary within the sac is at significant risk for torsion and strangulation. Although this is not a true surgical emergency, IH repair needs to be done relatively soon (within a few days).

In patients with incarcerated IH containing bowel, attempts must be made to reduce the hernia, unless there is clinical evidence of peritonitis. This may require IV sedation and careful monitoring. If the reduction is successful, the child is admitted and observed for 24 to 48 hours. The IH repair is done after the period of observation to allow for tissue edema to subside. On the other hand, if the IH cannot be reduced, the child is promptly taken to the operating room for inguinal exploration. If an intestinal resection is required, it can usually be done through the opened hernia sac before IH repair.

There is much controversy over the management of the opposite groin of the child with a unilateral IH. The major advantage of contralateral exploration is that it determines the presence of a patent processus vaginalis. Although a patent processus is not the same as an IH, an indirect IH cannot occur without it. Because there is a higher incidence of a contralateral patent processus within the first year of life, many surgeons restrict exploration of the other side to children younger than 1 year. In addition, many surgeons believe that contralateral exploration must be performed in all girls presenting with a clinically obvious unilateral IH because the likelihood of injury to reproductive structures is rare. Laparoscopic evaluation of the contralateral groin through the opened sac at the time of repair may be a safe and accurate method of identifying the presence of a patent processus vaginalis.[33]

The technical details of IH repair in infants have been well described and consist of high ligation of the hernia sac at the level of the internal ring. A repair of the floor of the inguinal canal is usually not necessary. In most cases, this is an outpatient procedure with minimal morbidity. Recurrence, injury to the vas deferens, wound infection, and postoperative hydrocele are recognized complications associated with IH repair but occur with a frequency of less than 1%.

Umbilical Hernia

An umbilical hernia (UH) occurs as a result of persistence of the umbilical ring. Complete closure of this ring can be anticipated by the age of 4 to 6 years in up to 80% of cases. In contrast with IH, a UH is rarely associated with significant complications. As such, most pediatric surgeons defer UH repair until the child is old enough to begin kindergarten. Exceptions to this general rule are a large UH defect (>2 cm) because the likelihood for spontaneous resolution is lower. History of incarceration, a large skin proboscis, and a ventriculoperitoneal shunt are other relative indications for repair. The technique for UH repair generally involves an infraumbilical semicircular incision, separation of the hernia sac from the overlying umbilical skin, repair of the fascial defect, pexing the base of the umbilical skin to the fascia, and skin closure.

Epigastric Hernia

Epigastric hernias (EH) represent the third most common hernia in children. These are found anywhere along the midline of the abdomen between the umbilicus and xiphoid process. Not to be confused with a broad defect of a diastasis rectus, the fascial defect of an EH is quite small but allows herniation of properitoneal fat through the defect. Although this does not pose significant risk to the patient, strangulation of the fat often results in pain, redness, and swelling. This scenario often directs urgent operative exploration to exclude incarceration of other, more important structures. Because of this and the likelihood for continued enlargement, most pediatric surgeons recommend elective repair. This is accomplished through a small transverse incision overlying the palpable mass. The herniated fat is excised and the fascia repaired.

Umbilical Abnormalities

The most significant abnormalities of the umbilicus are generally associated with an abnormal communication with the gastrointestinal tract or urinary bladder. In the newborn period, failure of separation of the umbilical cord, prolapsed mucosa or granulation tissue at the base of the umbilicus, or drainage of urine or stool from the umbilicus suggest these abnormalities.

Communication of the gastrointestinal tract to the umbilicus occurs through a patent omphalomesenteric duct. When the remnant of this duct is not connected to the abdominal wall, it is referred to as Meckel's diverticulum. Stool may be identified in the base of the umbilicus when the communication is open. The connection between the ileum and umbilicus may also be nonpatent, in which the remnant band may serve as a nidus for an intestinal volvulus or obstruction. If the connection is patent and stool is noted, umbilical exploration is warranted, and no further imaging is needed. The omphalomesenteric duct remnant is excised down to the antimesenteric side of the ileum, where it is divided.

Communication of the urinary bladder to the umbilicus occurs through a patent urachus. A urachal connection extends from the dome of the bladder in a retroperitoneal plane along the midline of anterior abdominal wall, where it connects to the base of the umbilicus. As such, the diagnosis may be easily made by ultrasonography of the infraumbilical abdominal wall. This test is warranted if there is clear umbilical drainage to suggest urine or prolapsed mucosa or granulation tissue after the umbilical stalk has separated. Treatment involves an umbilical exploration with dissection of the urachus down to the top of the bladder, where it is divided and removed. Occasionally, there is only a sinus, which extends for variable distances from the umbilicus to the bladder, but without a frank communication. Because of the propensity for infection, abnormal urothelium contained in the sinus, and mucoid drainage from the umbilicus, it needs to be excised in the same manner as for a patent urachus. Finally, a cyst may be contained within a urachal remnant that does not communicate with either the umbilicus or the bladder. These cysts most commonly present as urachal abscess. After percutaneous or open drainage of the abscess for initial treatment, the entire urachal remnant is excised.

GENITOURINARY

Cryptorchidism

Cryptorchidism (undescended testes [UDT]) is the most common disorder of sexual differentiation and occurs in about 2% of human male births. The consequences of cryptorchidism include degeneration of the testes with impaired fertility and an increased risk for germ cell testicular tumors. Despite the significance of this problem, the cause of UDT has not been clarified in most patients. It is presently unclear whether the peculiar pathologic change in the cryptorchid testes occurs as a result of a primary defect in testicular development or that a normal testis fails to descend with the high temperature inducing a secondary change.

A true UDT must be distinguished from a retractile testis. Retractile testes can usually be manipulated from the inguinal canal to a scrotal position. These testes can be expected to spontaneously descend into a normal scrotal position over time. Thus, no specific therapy is needed beyond careful long-term follow-up.

When a unilateral gonad is palpated in the inguinal canal, but cannot be manipulated into a scrotal position, an orchidopexy is performed. In most pediatric centers, this is done when patients have reached about 6 months of age. This early intervention may permit postnatal germ cell development to proceed normally. The orchidopexy is done through an inguinal incision. In about 90% of cases of UDT, there is an associated inguinal hernia, which is repaired at the same time. The testicle and its blood supply are mobilized into the scrotal position. A pouch is created within the dartos fascia through a separate scrotal incision, and the testicle is sutured to this fascia.

If the testicle is unable to be brought into a scrotal position after mobilization alone, a Fowler-Stephens technique may be applied. In this procedure, the tethering spermatic blood vessels are divided. At a second stage, the testicle may be placed into the scrotum after collateral blood supply to the testicle has developed. Alternatively, the testicular artery and vein can be divided and reanastomosed using microvascular techniques to permit placement of the gonad into the scrotum.

In the event that the gonad cannot be palpated on one side, ultrasonography or MRI may be used to locate the testicle. This localization is typically followed by laparoscopy to either facilitate the orchidopexy or to remove the atrophic gonad. When congenital UDT presents beyond puberty, removal of the gonad is usually indicated to prevent the development of malignancy.

Intersex Abnormalities

In all mammalian embryos, both male and female primordial reproductive ducts coexist for a short period of time. In the absence of testes, the uterus, fallopian tubes, and upper third of the vagina form autonomously. Similarly, the external genitalia develop autonomously into a clitoris, labia majora, and labia minora. The development of male external genitalia requires the reduction of testosterone by the enzyme 5α-reductase into dihydrotestosterone. Although autonomous female development can occur without ovaries, the development of a male phenotype requires a functional Y chromosome and androgenic steroids.

A baby born with ambiguous genitalia mandates an expeditious and thoughtful evaluation to establish an optimal gender assignment. This dictates a multidisciplinary approach with input from experienced physicians in endocrinology, neonatology, genetics, and pediatric surgery. Inaccurate and hasty gender assignment can be psychologically devastating to the parents and child with lifetime consequences. Significant advances in genitourinary reconstruction have provided multiple acceptable options to harmonize the appearance and function of the external genitalia with the sex of rearing. Three major categories of developmental abnormalities account for ambiguous genitalia in newborns and are discussed next.

Female Pseudohermaphroditism
In the first category, genetic females become masculinized because of an overproduction of androgenic steroids. The most common cause of this is an enzyme defect involved in the conversion of progesterones to glucocorticoids and mineralocorticoids. Mutations in the *CYP21* gene (previously referred to as the *gene encoding 21-hydroxylase*) are noted in 90% of cases. This genetic defect results in the syndrome known as *congenital adrenal hyperplasia,* also known as *adrenogenital syndrome,* also referred to a *female pseudohermaphroditism.* Although this syndrome may be seen in both males and females, ambiguous genitalia are only observed in female infants. Because of timing of internal organ formation relative to adrenal function in the developing embryo, the external genitalia of female infants are most significantly masculinized, whereas the internal structures (uterus, fallopian tubes, and ovaries) are normal.

Male Pseudohermaphroditism
The second group of developmental abnormalities results from deficient production, response to, or conversion of androgen in genetic males. Defective synthesis of at least five different enzymes needed for the successful conversion of cholesterol to testosterone has been characterized as leading to the development of ambiguous genitalia in males. Androgen insensitivity results from point mutations in both coding and noncoding regions of the androgen receptor gene leading to a variable phenotype. The complete form of androgen insensitivity is known as *testicular feminization syndrome.* This condition most commonly presents at the time of inguinal hernia repair in a presumed female patient. The presence of bilateral inguinal hernia sacs containing palpable, reducible gonads suggests this diagnosis. Intraoperatively, testicles are discovered, and vaginoscopy reveals a shortened, blind-ending vagina and no cervix. In these cases of complete androgen insensitivity, the child continues to be raised as a female and will ultimately require testicular

removal to avoid the potential for malignancy. Although these children do not have a uterus, exogenous estrogen is typically required at the age of puberty to facilitate secondary sexual development. Finally, defective production of the 5α-reductase type 2 gene prevents the conversion of testosterone to dihydrotestosterone in genital tissues and permits feminization of the developing genetic male.

Defective Gonadal Differentiation
The third and final set of abnormalities involves gene mutations causing absent, incomplete, or asymmetric gonad differentiation. In these conditions, gonadal dysgenesis may involve both gonads (pure) or one gonad on one side combined with a streak remnant on the other (mixed). A true hermaphrodite is represented typically with a normal testis on one side and a gonad containing both testicular and ovarian tissue (ovotestes) on the other side. Various other gonadal combinations have been described.

CONGENITAL DIAPHRAGMATIC HERNIA

Congenital diaphragmatic hernia (CDH) represents one of the most enigmatic diseases encountered in pediatric surgery. The reported incidence of CDH is in the range of 1 in 2000 to 5000 live births. Most CDH defects are on the left side (80%); however, up to 20% may occur on the right side. A CDH may also be bilateral, but this is distinctly rare. Despite multiple innovative treatment strategies, including in utero diaphragm repair, fetal tracheal occlusion, high-frequency oscillation or partial liquid ventilation, ECLS, exogenous surfactant, and inhaled nitric oxide, survival rates for this condition have not been significantly impacted. The exact survival rate for CDH is difficult to determine but in the range of 70% to 90%.[34] Calculation of true survival is complicated by the fact that many infants with CDH are stillborn, and many reports tend to exclude infants with complex associated anomalies from survival calculations.[35]

Pathogenesis
The cause for CDH is unknown, but it is thought to result from failure of normal closure of the pleuroperitoneal canal in the developing embryo. As a result, abdominal contents herniate through the resultant defect in the posterolateral diaphragm and compress the ipsilateral developing lung. The posterolateral location of this hernia is known as *Bochdalek's hernia* and is distinguished from the congenital hernia of the anteromedial, retrosternal diaphragm, which is known as *Morgagni's hernia.* Compression of the lung results in pulmonary hypoplasia involving both lungs, with the ipsilateral lung being the most affected. In addition to the abnormal airway development, the pulmonary vasculature is distinctly abnormal in that the medial muscular thickness of the arterioles is excessive and extremely sensitive to the multiple local and systemic factors known to trigger vasospasm. Thus, the two main factors that affect morbidity and

mortality are pulmonary hypoplasia and pulmonary hypertension.

Clinical Presentation

The most frequent clinical presentation of CDH is respiratory distress due to severe hypoxemia. The infant appears dyspneic, tachypneic, and cyanotic, with severe retractions. The anteroposterior diameter of the chest may be large, and the abdomen may be scaphoid. There are three general presentations of infants with CDH. In the first scenario, signs of severe respiratory distress are present immediately at the time of birth. As such, if the diagnosis is known prenatally, delivery within an institution capable of providing ECLS, high-frequency ventilation, and sophisticated neonatal care is crucial. In these infants, pulmonary hypoplasia may be severe enough to be incompatible with life. The infant may also have a reversible cause for immediate hypoxia such as hypovolemia or severe pulmonary vasospasm. Unfortunately, there are no known criteria for distinguishing infants with severe lung hypoplasia from those with reversible conditions. As such, many infants with irreversible lung hypoplasia are placed on ECLS for prolonged periods before it becomes apparent that their underlying lung condition is incurable.

In the second and most common presentation, the infant does well for several hours after delivery (the so-called honeymoon period) and then begins to deteriorate from a respiratory standpoint. Patients in this category may benefit from therapy to reduce pulmonary hypertension and hypoxemia. Theoretically, these patients are ideal candidates for ECLS because their lung development has progressed enough to sustain life. Unfortunately, this is not always the case because many infants in this group do not survive, even with ECLS support.

The third and final clinical presentation of CDH is beyond the first 24 hours of life, which occurs in about 10% to 20% of cases. Many of these children present with feeding difficulties, chronic respiratory disease, pneumonia, or intestinal obstruction. This group of patients enjoys the best prognosis.

Diagnosis

The diagnosis of CDH is frequently made at the time of a prenatal ultrasound during an otherwise unremarkable pregnancy. The postnatal diagnosis is relatively straightforward; a plain chest radiograph demonstrates the gastric air bubble or loops of bowel within the chest (Fig. 71-16). There may also be a mediastinal shift away from the side of the hernia or polyhydramnios from the obstructed stomach. Rarely is an upper gastrointestinal contrast study necessary.

Preoperative Management

The management of CDH that has been detected in utero has directed open fetal surgery as a strategy to remove the compression of the abdominal viscera and allow for improved lung development. Unfortunately, this intervention is high risk to both the mother and fetus and has

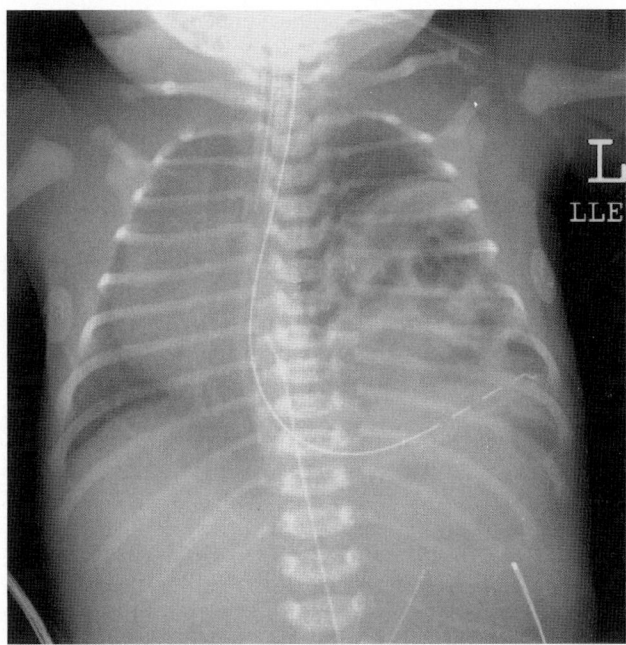

Figure 71-16 Congenital diaphragmatic hernia. The tip of the nasogastric tube and obvious loops of gas-filled bowel are located in the left hemithorax.

failed to demonstrate any survival advantage.[36] Subsequent to this was the realization that occlusion of the fetal trachea might result in accumulation of lung fluid with stimulation of lung growth. Although several techniques for occlusion of the trachea have been described, including the use of balloons, sponges, or external clip application, the overall result is larger, but persistently abnormal lungs and survival are not significantly improved.[37] Currently, there appears to be no rationale for fetal intervention in the diagnosis of CDH.

The postnatal management of CDH is complex, but all efforts need to be directed toward stabilization of the cardiorespiratory system, while minimizing iatrogenic injury from therapeutic interventions. Endotracheal intubation is critical to optimize ventilation. Placement of a nasogastric tube is also important to prevent gastric distention, which may worsen the lung compression, mediastinal shift, and ability to ventilate. Acute deterioration of an infant with CDH may be due to a number of factors, including inadvertent extubation. However, it is important to remember that a pneumothorax may develop during aggressive attempts at ventilation. As such, it is important to remember that the pneumothorax in patients with CDH always occurs on the side *contralateral* to the side of the CDH. Needle decompression of the contralateral chest during an acute deterioration event may be lifesaving and necessary before a chest radiograph can be obtained.

Although used traditionally, pharmacologic pulmonary vasodilators (tolazoline), surfactant, high-frequency ventilation, and inhaled nitric oxide have all demonstrated inconsistent success. One of the more important recent contributions to the management of infants with CDH has been the concept of gentle ventilation with permissive hypercapnia and stable hypoxemia (tolerance of preductal oxygen saturations above 80%.). Using this strategy, Stolar and colleagues reported a survival rate of 75.8%.[38]

Surgical Management

Historically, the surgical repair of a CDH was considered to be a surgical emergency because it was thought that the abdominal viscera within the chest prevented the ability to ventilate. More recently, it has become evident that the physiologic stress associated with early repair probably adds more insult and that survival is not improved when compared with delayed repair. Thus, most pediatric surgeons wait for a variable period of time (24-72 hours) to allow for stabilization of the infant before embarking on surgical repair.

Most pediatric surgeons repair a posterolateral CDH through an abdominal subcostal incision, although a thoracotomy will also provide adequate exposure. The viscera are reduced into the abdominal cavity, and the posterolateral defect in the diaphragm is closed using interrupted, nonabsorbable sutures. In most cases (roughly 80%-90%), a hernia sac is not present. If identified, however, it is excised at the time of repair. Occasionally, the defect is too large to permit primary closure, and a number of reconstructive techniques are available, including various abdominal or thoracic muscle flaps. The use of prosthetic material such as Gore-Tex has become more widespread. The advantage of a prosthetic patch is that a tension-free repair can be frequently obtained. The major problems with prosthetic patches are the risk for infection and recurrence of the hernia. Occasionally, the abdominal compartment may be too small to accommodate the viscera, which have developed within the thoracic cavity. In these circumstances, an abdominal silo may need to be constructed, as in the management of congenital abdominal wall defects.

Beyond the early postoperative period, many infants with CDH have continued morbidity, which demands careful long-term follow-up.[39] Many children who survive aggressive management of severe respiratory failure manifest neurologic problems, such as abnormalities in both motor and cognitive skills, developmental delay, seizures, and hearing loss. Other problems include a high incidence of foregut gastroesophageal reflux and foregut dysmotility. Other morbidity associated with CDH survivors includes chronic lung disease, scoliosis, growth retardation, and pectus excavatum deformities.

CONGENITAL CHEST WALL DEFORMITIES

Although several categories of congenital chest wall deformities exist, the two major types are *pectus excavatum* and *pectus carinatum* (Fig. 71-17). Pectus excavatum is also referred to as a funnel or sunken chest and is the most common deformity encountered (roughly five times more common than carinatum deformities). It is three

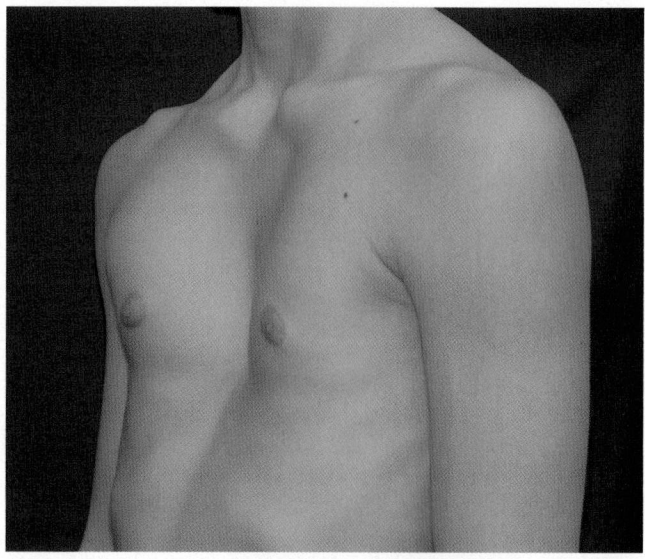

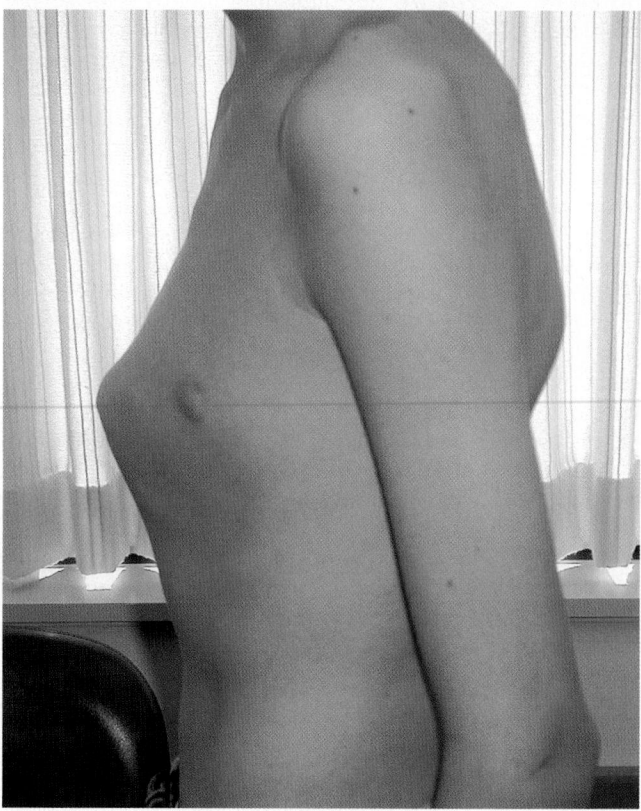

Figure 71-17 Pectus excavatum (**A**) and pectus carinatum (**B**).

times more frequent in males and is identified in the first year of life in roughly 90% of cases.

Etiology

Although the etiology is unknown, abnormalities of costal cartilage development have been most frequently implicated. Several conditions are known to be associated with pectus excavatum and must be considered in the preoperative evaluation. Roughly 15% of patients have scoliosis. In addition, the possibility of Marfan syndrome must be considered, and ophthalmologic evaluation, along with an echocardiogram, obtained. Mitral valve prolapse may be seen in about half of patients and structural congenital heart disease in roughly 2%. Asthma is also common, but it is unknown whether asthma contributes to the development of the defect or occurs as a result of it.

Indications for Surgery

The most common indication for surgery in patients with pectus deformities is cosmetic. This is not a minor issue, particularly for adolescents with significant concerns regarding body image and development of self-esteem. Theoretically, correction of a severe excavatum deformity will significantly improve cardiopulmonary function. However, notwithstanding many decades of experience with this condition, no appreciable consensus has been reached regarding the degree of cardiopulmonary impairment, if any, that this common chest wall deformity produces. Despite this, it is important to screen for underlying cardiopulmonary conditions before embarking on operative correction.

Preoperative Evaluation

A standard anteroposterior and lateral chest radiograph is essential to serve as a baseline of the degree of deformity as well as to detect the presence of thoracic scoliosis. Pulmonary function studies are important to document either restrictive or obstructive abnormalities. The latter is particularly important if this component is reversible with bronchodilators. If a heart murmur is detected on physical examination, an echocardiogram is indicated. Finally, a CT scan permits the calculation of a Haller index by dividing the measured transverse diameter of the chest by the anteroposterior diameter to more objectively document the severity of the defect. This measurement is affected by both age and gender.[40]

Surgical Treatment

The surgical correction of a pectus excavatum is not done before the age of 5 years because a severe, postoperative restrictive chest wall deformity may result. Presently, there are two main methods for operative correction. The first technique was originally described in 1949 by Ravitch and remains the standard to which all other procedures are compared. This procedure is applied to patients with either excavatum or carinatum deformities and consists of a transverse skin incision overlying the deformity, bilateral subchondral resection of abnormal costal cartilages, sternal osteotomy, and anterior fixation of the sternum with a retrosternal stainless steel strut. The strut is removed as a secondary procedure in 6 months to a year. The results with this operation are excellent.

More recently, a minimally invasive technique has been described for excavatum defects in which a C-shaped bar is passed in a retrosternal plane from one hemithorax into the other through two lateral intercostal

incisions. The bar is then "flipped" such that the convexity is outward, and the chest wall defect is immediately corrected. As described by Nuss,[41] this technique avoids the creation of pectoral flaps, cartilage resection, and sternal osteotomy. The bar must be left in place for 2 years after which it is removed. Although this new technique has gained considerable popularity among the lay public, the advantages of this technique over the standard Ravitch procedure has yet to be conclusively demonstrated. A multicenter, prospective trial to address this issue is currently ongoing. Treatment of pectus carinatum is done by open costal cartilage resection and sternal fixation in the same way as for pectus excavatum. More recently, success has been described with external brace application to correct carinatum deformities.[42]

BRONCHOPULMONARY MALFORMATIONS

Dramatic improvements in prenatal ultrasonography have led to a more frequent recognition of developmental abnormalities of the lungs and major bronchi. Some lesions may be associated with in utero death unless fetal intervention is performed, some infants may have respiratory compromise at birth, and some patients may present later in life with a persistent infection or neoplasm.

Bronchogenic Cyst

These cysts are usually solitary and lined by cuboidal or columnar ciliated epithelium and mucus glands. Roughly two thirds of cysts are within the lung parenchyma, and the remainder are found within the mediastinum. Cysts within the pulmonary parenchyma typically communicate with a bronchus, whereas those in the mediastinum usually do not. Although up to one third of patients are asymptomatic and the diagnosis is made on a routine chest radiograph, many patients present with respiratory complaints, including recurrent pneumonia, cough, hemoptysis, or dyspnea. Because of these symptoms, as well as the reports of neoplasm occurring within these cysts, treatment for all bronchogenic cysts is resection. Frequently, mediastinal cysts may be amenable to resection using minimally invasive techniques.

Pulmonary Sequestration

Sequestrations represent malformations of the lung in which there is usually no bronchial communication and there is frequently an aberrant systemic blood supply. Sequestrations are discriminated on the basis of being either intralobar, in which they reside within the lung parenchyma, or extralobar, in which they are surrounded by a separate pleural covering. Intralobar sequestrations are infrequently associated with other anomalies and are found within the medial or posterior segments of the lower lobes, with about two thirds occurring on the left side. In about 85% of cases, the intralobar sequestration is supplied by an anomalous systemic vessel arising from the infradiaphragmatic aorta and located within the inferior pulmonary ligament. Anticipation of this structure is therefore critical during attempted resection of this malformation. The venous drainage is usually through the inferior pulmonary vein, but may also occur by way of systemic veins. Because of the risk for infection and bleeding, intralobar sequestrations are usually removed, either by segmentectomy or lobectomy. Historically, angiography was considered an important preoperative study before embarking on resection of a sequestration. More recently, CT and MRI have replaced the need for angiography and provide excellent mapping of the blood supply.

In contrast with those that are intralobar, extralobar sequestrations occur predominantly in males (3:1 male-to-female ratio) and are found three times more frequently on the left side. In roughly 40% of cases, multiple other anomalies are encountered, including posterolateral diaphragmatic hernia, eventration of the diaphragm, pectus excavatum and carinatum, enteric duplication cysts, and congenital heart disease. Extralobar sequestrations are usually asymptomatic, and because there is usually no bronchial communication, the risk for infection is low. As such, many of these malformations may be observed. Frequently, their discovery during other procedures or inability to make the correct diagnosis by noninvasive imaging dictates their removal.

Congenital Lobar Emphysema

Congenital lobar emphysema (CLE) results from overdistention of one or more lobes within a histologically normal lung due to abnormal cartilaginous support of the feeding bronchus. This focal area of bronchial collapse results in a check-valve with air trapping and a progressive increase in lobar distention. Most often, the cartilage within the bronchus is abnormal; however, extrinsic compression of the bronchus from an aberrant vessel may also cause the same findings. The left upper lobe is involved in roughly half of cases, with the remainder evenly distributed between the right middle and lower lobes.

The symptoms of CLE range from none to severe respiratory distress within the neonatal period. Asymptomatic patients are often identified during a routine chest radiograph as an area of hyperlucency. In these cases, observation without pulmonary resection may be prudent. Occasionally, CLE is identified in a patient with recurrent of persistent pneumonia or with progressive dyspnea. Resection of the involved lung is therapeutic and well tolerated. The presentation of CLE in a neonate may include severe respiratory distress. In these cases, the clinical and radiographic picture may mimic a tension pneumothorax with severe mediastinal shift. Inadvertent placement of a chest tube into the distended lung would be catastrophic. Immediate thoracotomy with resection of the involved lobe may be lifesaving.

Congenital Cystic Adenomatoid Malformation

A congenital cystic adenomatoid malformation (CCAM) typically involves a single lobe and represents a multicys-

tic mass of pulmonary tissue in which there is proliferation of bronchial structures at the expense of alveoli. Unlike sequestrations, a CCAM typically has a bronchial communication, and the arterial and venous drainage is classically from the normal pulmonary circulation. There are three general types segregated on the basis of cyst size. A type I CCAM is considered the macrocystic variety and includes single or multiple cysts greater than 2 cm. Type I lesions account for roughly 50% of all cases and usually have no associated anomalies. A type II CCAM contains respiratory epithelium–lined cysts, but less than 1 cm in size. Type II lesions are associated with other anomalies such as renal agenesis, cardiac malformations, CDH, or skeletal abnormalities. The outcome of patients with type II CCAM depends on the associated conditions. A type III CCAM is considered microcystic and on gross inspection may appear solid, but microscopic analysis shows multiple cysts. Type III CCAMs are often associated with mediastinal shift, the development of nonimmune hydrops, and a generally poor prognosis. In utero surgery has been applied with some success in the management of large CCAMs. The development of nonimmune hydrops is one of the main predictors of survival and in utero intervention (thoracoamniotic shunting, fetal thoracotomy) may be indicated.[43] The postnatal management of the symptomatic patient is relatively straightforward by pulmonary resection in the newborn period. In asymptomatic patients with small lesions detected by fetal ultrasound, the rationale for resection becomes less clear. Because there have been reports of malignancy developing within these lesions, as well as the potential for infection and enlargement, they probably all need to be resected.

HEPATOBILIARY

Neonatal Jaundice

Many children with chronic or life-threatening liver disease present in the neonatal period. As such, early recognition is important for apt diagnosis, treatment, and improved outcome. Jaundice is the most common symptom associated with neonatal liver disease. Physiologic (unconjugated) jaundice of the newborn is the most common cause of jaundice and seen in up to 15% of term infants by 2 weeks of age. Cholestasis is defined as a pathologic state of reduced bile formation or flow. Because of the relative immaturity of enzymes involved with bile formation and transport, the neonate is particularly prone to develop cholestasis in response to a wide variety of insults that would not normally be associated with cholestasis in adults. As such, the differential diagnosis of cholestasis is broader in neonates when compared with adults.

Definition of Pathologic Hyperbilirubinemia

The possibility of liver disease is considered in any infant who is jaundiced beyond 2 weeks of age. Hyperbilirubinemia is considered pathologic if the direct (conjugated fraction) serum bilirubin is greater than 1.0 mg/dL or

Table 71-4 Most Common Causes of Cholestasis in Infants Younger Than 2 Months

OBSTRUCTIVE CHOLESTASIS	HEPATOCELLULAR CHOLESTASIS	GENETIC AND METABOLIC DISORDERS	TOXIC OR SECONDARY
Biliary atresia	Idiopathic neonatal hepatitis	α_1-Antitrypsin deficiency	Parenteral nutrition–associated cholestasis
Choledochal cysts	Viral infection	Tyrosinemia	
Gallstones or biliary sludge	Cytomegalovirus	Galactosemia	
Alagille syndrome	HIV	Hypothyroidism	
Inspissated bile	Bacterial infection	Progressive familial intrahepatic cholestasis (PFIC)	
Cystic fibrosis	Urinary tract infection	Cystic fibrosis	
Neonatal sclerosing cholangitis	Sepsis	Panhypopituitarism	
Congenital hepatic fibrosis (Caroli's disease)	Syphilis		

From Moyer V, Freese DK, Whitington PF, et al: Guideline for the evaluation of cholestatic jaundice: Recommendations of the North American Society of Pediatric Gastroenterology, Hepatology and Nutrition. J Pediatr Gastroenterol Nutr 39:115-128, 2004.

represents more than 20% of the total bilirubin when the total bilirubin level is great than 5 mg/dL. Any infant beyond 2 weeks of life with this level of direct hyperbilirubinemia needs to undergo a thorough investigation.

Differential Diagnosis

Although the list of conditions associated with neonatal cholestasis is long, fewer than 15 disorders account for greater than 95% of neonatal cholestasis. Idiopathic neonatal hepatitis accounts for roughly 30% to 40% of cases and is characterized histologically by identification of giant cell transformation in the absence of evidence of other causes of neonatal cholestasis. Treatment is supportive. Biliary atresia is the second most common cause of neonatal cholestasis. Treatment for this condition is urgent and requires surgical intervention to reestablish bile flow (discussed later). The third most common cause of neonatal cholestasis is α_1-antitrypsin deficiency. This autosomal recessive disorder results in a misfolded protein that cannot traverse the secretory pathway. Additional causes of cholestasis in infants younger than 2 months are shown in Table 71-4.

Evaluation

In the assessment of neonatal liver disease, it is important to distinguish between hepatocellular, physiologic, medical treatment and obstructive, anatomic, surgical treatment of cholestasis. In an ill-appearing infant, the primary cause (e.g., sepsis, hypothyroidism, metabolic disorder) needs to be investigated and corrected. In the absence of underlying liver disease, treatment of the causal condition results in resolution of the cholestasis. Further testing includes urine for reducing substances, serum for α_1-antitrypsin and albumin, and a complete blood count with coagulation studies.

A hepatobiliary ultrasound is performed simultaneously with the previously mentioned diagnostic tests. An absent gallbladder would be suggestive of biliary atresia, whereas a cystic hilar mass would suggest the diagnosis

of a choledochal cyst. Other less common conditions in which an ultrasound would be useful include gallstones or biliary sludge or the presence of an obstructing hilar tumor. The final diagnostic procedure in the evaluation of the cholestatic infant is a percutaneous liver biopsy. This modality provides the greatest accuracy for diagnosing neonatal liver disease. Hepatobiliary scintigraphy scans, although historically useful, add little to the combination of ultrasonography and percutaneous liver biopsy and are no longer routinely employed.

Biliary Atresia

Biliary atresia (BA) is characterized by progressive (not static) obliteration of the extrahepatic and intrahepatic bile ducts. The cause is presently unknown, and the incidence is about 1 in 15,000 live births. Presently, there is no medical therapy to reverse the obliterative process, and patients who are not offered surgical treatment uniformly develop biliary cirrhosis, portal hypertension, and death by 2 years of age.

Pathology

Pathologically, the biliary tracts contain inflammatory and fibrous cells surrounding miniscule ducts that are probably remnants of the original ductal system. Bile duct proliferation, severe cholestasis with plugging, and inflammatory cell infiltrate are the pathologic hallmarks of this disease. Over time, these changes progress to fibrosis with end-stage cirrhosis. This histology is usually distinct from the giant cell transformation and hepatocellular necrosis that are characteristic of neonatal hepatitis, the other major cause of direct hyperbilirubinemia in the newborn. There are variants of BA ranging from fibrosis of the distal bile ducts with proximal patency (5%, considered *correctable* form), fibrosis of the proximal bile ducts with distal patency (15%), or fibrosis of both proximal and distal bile ducts (80%).

Diagnosis

A serum direct bilirubin level of more than 2.0 mg/dL or greater than 15% of the total bilirubin level defines cholestasis, is distinctly abnormal, and further evaluation is mandatory. Delay in diagnosis of BA is associated with a worse prognosis. Success with surgical correction is much improved if undertaken before 60 days of life and related to the degree of hepatic fibrosis.[44] Thus, the initial opportunity for success in the management of this disease relies on the *early* recognition of abnormal direct hyperbilirubinemia.

The list of potential causes for cholestasis in infants is relatively long; however, an organized, systematic approach usually permits the establishment of an accurate diagnosis within a few days. In addition to a careful history and physical examination, blood and urine are obtained for bacterial and viral cultures, reducing substances in the urine to rule out galactosemia, serum immunoglobulin M (IgM) titers for syphilis, cytomegalovirus, herpes, and hepatitis B, serum α_1-antitrypsin level and phenotype, serum thyroxine level, and a sweat chloride test done to exclude cystic fibrosis.

Ultrasonography of the liver and gallbladder is important in the evaluation of the infant with cholestasis. In BA, the gallbladder is typically shrunken or absent, and the extrahepatic bile ducts cannot be visualized. The next diagnostic step is to perform a percutaneous liver biopsy if the hepatic synthetic function is normal. This is well tolerated under local anesthesia, and the diagnostic accuracy is in the range of 90%.[45] In cases in which the ultrasound and biopsy findings are inconclusive, hepatobiliary scintigraphy, using iminodiacetic acid analogues, may demonstrate normal hepatic uptake, but absent excretion into the intestine. Pretreatment of the infant with phenobarbital may improve the sensitivity of this test.

Surgical Management

If the needle biopsy or abdominal ultrasound is consistent with BA, exploratory laparotomy is then performed expeditiously. The initial goal at surgery is to confirm the diagnosis. This requires the demonstration of the fibrotic biliary remnant and definition of absent proximal and distal bile duct patency by cholecystocholangiography. The classic technique for correction of BA is the Kasai hepatoportoenterostomy. In this procedure, the distal bile duct is transected and dissected proximally up to the level of the liver capsule, whereby it is excised, along with the gallbladder remnant (Fig. 71-18). A Roux-en-Y hepaticojejunostomy is then constructed by anastomosis of the jejunal Roux limb to the fibrous plate above the portal vein. Some surgeons prefer to monitor postoperative bile flow by constructing a distal double-barrel stoma. Although it has been considered that this may lessen the risk for cholangitis, this has yet to be definitively established.

Postoperative Management

Postoperatively, the use of oral choleretic bile salts such as ursodeoxycholic acid may facilitate bile flow.[46] In

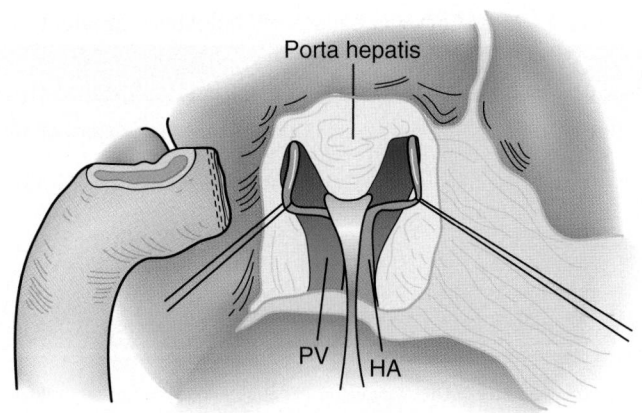

Figure 71-18 Kasai's hepatoportoenterostomy procedure for biliary atresia. The extrahepatic bile ducts and gallbladder have been removed. The fibrous plate of the hepatic duct is transected above the bifurcation of the portal vein (PV) and hepatic artery (HA), and a Roux limb of jejunum is sewn to this plate to achieve drainage of bile. (From Grosfeld JL, Fitzgerald JF, Predaina R, et al: The efficacy of hepatoportoenterostomy in biliary atresia. Surgery 106:692-700, 1989).

addition, methylprednisolone is employed as an anti-inflammatory agent, and trimethoprim sulfamethoxazole is administered for long-term antimicrobial prophylaxis. Cholangitis is a serious but common problem after hepatoportoenterostomy and may be associated with cessation of bile flow. Episodes of cholangitis are managed by hospitalization, rehydration, broad-spectrum IV antibiotics, steroids, and occasionally surgical exploration of the portoenterostomy.

Outcome

About 30% of infants undergoing hepatoportoenterostomy before 60 days of age will have a long-term successful outcome and not require liver transplantation. Older children and those with preoperative evidence for bridging fibrosis seen on liver biopsy will predictably do less well. As such, some surgeons may forgo performing a portoenterostomy procedure and simply place the patient on a waiting list for liver transplantation. The remaining patients undergoing portoenterostomy will develop progressive hepatic fibrosis with resultant portal hypertension and progressive cholestasis. In this group, liver transplantation is lifesaving and associated with a 79% survival rate.[47] Biliary atresia currently represents the most common indication for pediatric liver transplantation.

Choledochal Cyst

A cystic enlargement of the common bile duct is referred to as a *choledochal cyst*. The initial anatomic organization was proposed by Alonso-Lej in 1959 and has been updated to the current classification as depicted in Figure 71-19. Type I cysts represent 80% to 90% of cases and are simply cystic dilations of the common bile duct. Type II cysts are represented as a diverticulum arising from the common bile duct. Type III cysts are also referred to as

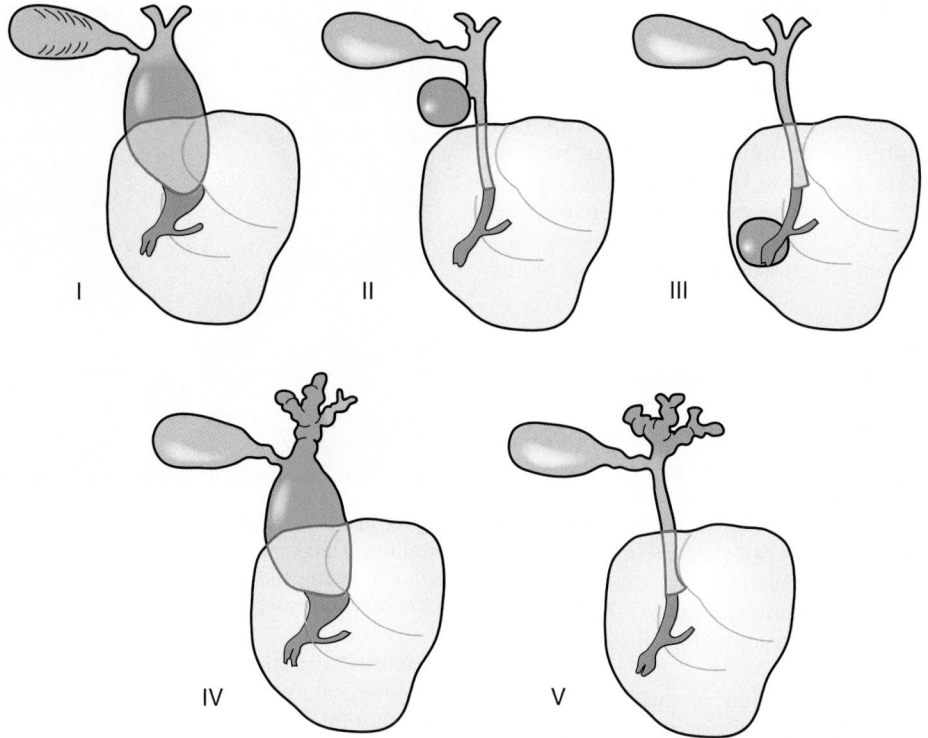

Figure 71-19 The anatomic classification of choledochal cyst. (From Sigalet DL: Biliary tract disorders and portal hypertension. In Ashcraft KW, Sharp RJ, Sigalet DL, Snyder CL [eds]: Pediatric Surgery, 3rd ed. Philadelphia, WB Saunders, 2000, p 588.)

choledochoceles and are isolated to the intrapancreatic portion of the common bile duct and frequently involve the ampulla. Type IV cysts are second in frequency and represent dilation of both intrahepatic and extrahepatic bile ducts. In Type V cysts, only the intrahepatic ducts are dilated.

The pathophysiology of choledochal cysts remains poorly understood. In one theory, reflux of pancreatic digestive enzymes into the bile duct through an anomalous pancreaticobiliary ductal junction results in damage to the duct. In another theory, persistent or transient obstruction of the distal bile duct may be present.

Clinical Presentation

Although choledochal cysts can produce symptoms in any age group, most become clinically evident within the first decade of life. The triad of a right upper quadrant mass, abdominal pain, and jaundice is highly suggestive of the diagnosis. In some patients, pancreatitis may be present. In older children and adults, the presentation may be more insidious and include choledocholithiasis, cholangitis, and cirrhosis with progression to portal hypertension. Malignant degeneration is also found in up to 16% of adults with choledochal cysts.

Preoperative Evaluation

In addition to routine measurement of serum bilirubin, alkaline phosphatase, and amylase levels, the most useful diagnostic test for choledochal cysts is ultrasonography.

Once dilation of the extrahepatic biliary ducts is demonstrated, no further testing is usually necessary in children. Although seldom necessary, preoperative endoscopic retrograde cholangiopancreatography (ERCP) may provide addition information regarding the pancreaticobiliary ductal anatomy to guide intraoperative decision making.

Operative Management

Total cyst excision with Roux-en-Y hepaticojejunostomy is the definitive procedure for management of type I and II choledochal cysts. In cases in which there is significant inflammation, it may be impossible to safely dissect the entire cyst away from the anterior surface of the portal vein. In these circumstances, the internal lining of the cyst can be excised, leaving the external portion of the cyst wall intact. Type III cysts are typically approached by opening the duodenum, resecting the cyst wall with care to reconstruct and marsupialize the remnant pancreaticobiliary ducts to the duodenal mucosa. In type IV cysts, the bile duct excision is coupled with a lateral hilar dissection to perform a jejunal anastomosis to the lowermost intrahepatic cysts. If the intrahepatic cysts are confined to a single lobe or segment, hepatic resection may be indicated. The treatment of type V cysts involving both lobes is usually palliative with transhepatic or U-tubes until liver transplantation can be performed. The postoperative outcomes following excision of choledochal cysts are excellent.[48]

CHILDHOOD SOLID TUMORS

Neuroblastoma

Neuroblastoma (NBL) is the most common abdominal malignancy in children, accounting for 6% to 10% of all childhood cancers and 15% of all pediatric cancer deaths in the United States. The overall incidence in an unscreened population is 1 case per 10,000 persons with roughly 525 new cases diagnosed in the United States each year.

Sites of Involvement

These tumors are of neural crest origin and as a result may arise anywhere along the sympathetic ganglia or within the adrenal medulla. Although these tumors may occur at any site from the brain to the pelvis, 75% originate within the abdomen or pelvis, and half of these occur within the adrenal medulla. Twenty percent of NBLs originate within the posterior mediastinum, and 5% are within the neck. The median age at diagnosis is 2 years. Nearly 35% occur in children younger than 1 year, and less than 5% of cases present after the age of 10 years.

NBL is an enigmatic tumor that is capable of rapid progression in some children and spontaneous regression in others, particularly those younger than 1 year. About 25% of patients present with a solitary mass that may be cured by surgical therapy, whereas most present with extensive locoregional or metastatic disease. In this latter group of patients, the prognosis is generally poor, with an overall survival rate of less than 30%.

Clinical Presentation

The presenting symptoms of NBL are dependent on several factors, including the site of the primary tumor, the presence of metastatic disease, the age of the patient, and the metabolic activity of the tumor. The most common presentation is a fixed, lobular mass extending from the flank toward the midline of the abdomen. Although the abdominal mass may be noted in an otherwise asymptomatic child, patients may complain of abdominal pain, distention, weight loss, or anorexia. Bowel or bladder dysfunction may arise from direct compression of these structures by the tumor. Cervical tumors may be discovered as a palpable or visible mass or be associated with stridor or dysphagia. Posterior mediastinal masses are usually detected by plain chest radiographs in a child with Horner's syndrome, dyspnea, or pneumonia. Further, the tumor may extend into the neural foramina and cause symptoms of spinal cord compression. Neuroblastoma tends to metastasize to cortical bones, bone marrow, and liver. As such, patients may present with localized swelling and tenderness, lump, or refusal to walk. Periorbital metastasis accounts for proptosis and ecchymosis (so-called panda or raccoon eyes). Marrow replacement by tumor may result in anemia and weakness. In infants, liver metastasis may rapidly expand, causing massive hepatomegaly and respiratory distress requiring mechanical ventilation and surgical decompression. Metastatic lesions to the skin produce a characteristic blueberry muffin appearance.

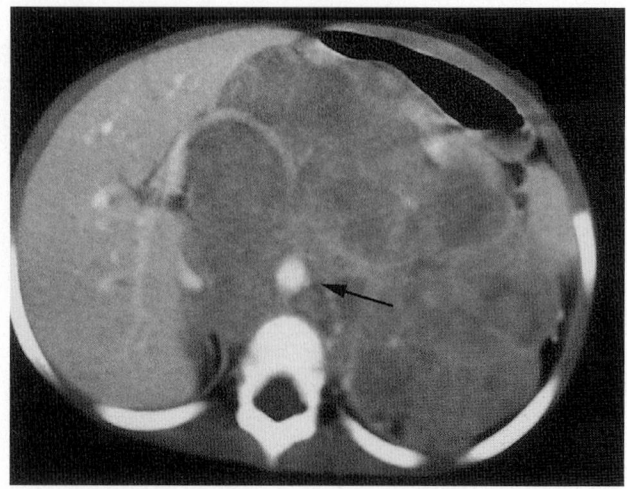

Figure 71-20 Neuroblastoma. A CT scan of the abdomen demonstrating a large neuroblastoma surrounding the aorta (*arrow*) and displacing the liver to the right. Punctate areas of calcium can be seen dispersed throughout the tumor.

Numerous paraneoplastic syndromes can occur in conjunction with NBL. Cerebellar ataxia, involuntary movements, and nystagmus are the hallmark of the "dancing eyes and feet" syndrome. Excess secretion of vasoactive intestinal polypeptide may stimulate an intractable watery diarrhea. Hypertension may be significant, owing to excessive catecholamine production by the tumor.

Preoperative Evaluation

Although histologic evaluation of tissue is necessary for establishing the definitive diagnosis, a high level of suspicion may arise from the history and physical examination. Initial laboratory evaluation includes a complete blood count, serum electrolytes, blood urea nitrogen, creatinine, and liver function studies. A spot urine test is done for the catecholamine metabolites homovanillic and vanillylmandelic acid. In addition, several other biochemical markers harbor prognostic significance. A serum lactic dehydrogenase level greater than 1500 IU/mL, serum ferritin level above 142 ng/mL, and neuron-specific enolase levels greater than 100 ng/mL correlate with advanced disease and reduced survival.

CT and MRI are the preferred modalities for characterizing the location and extent of the neuroblastoma. This tumor frequently infiltrates vascular structures (Fig. 71-20). As such, many tumors that cross the midline are generally not resectable. A CT scan of the chest is done to exclude pulmonary metastasis and a bone scan to identify potential bone metastasis. In addition, radiolabeled metaiodobenzylguanidine (MIBG) is one of the single best studies to document the presence of metastatic disease. Finally, a bone marrow aspirate and biopsy complete the staging evaluation. The international NBL staging system is depicted in Table 71-5.

Although imaging at the time of presentation of most tumors reveals unresectability, the definitive diagnosis requires tissue. This can be obtained by an incisional or needle biopsy of the tumor. Neuroblastoma identified

Table 71-5 International Neuroblastoma Staging System

STAGE	DEFINITION
1	Localized tumor with complete gross excision, with or without microscopic residual disease; representative ipsilateral lymph nodes negative for tumor microscopically (nodes attached to and removed with the primary tumor may be positive)
2A	Localized tumor with incomplete gross excision; representative ipsilateral nonadherent lymph nodes negative for tumor microscopically
2B	Localized tumor with or without complete gross excision, with ipsilateral nonadherent lymph nodes positive for tumor; enlarged contralateral lymph nodes must be negative microscopically
3	Unresectable unilateral tumor with contralateral regional lymph node involvement; or midline tumor with bilateral extension by infiltration (unresectable) or by lymph node involvement
4	Any primary tumor with dissemination to distant lymph nodes, bone, bone marrow, liver, skin, and/or other organs (except as defined for stage 4S)
4S	Localized primary tumor (as defined for stage 1, 2A, or 2B), with dissemination limited to skin, liver, and/or bone marrow (limited to infant <1 yr of age)

Table 71-6 Schema of Clinical Factors Combined for Patient Risk Group Assignment in Future Neuroblastoma Studies*

RISK GROUP		FACTORS
Low	Stage 1	
	Stage 2	<1 yr
		>1 yr, low N-*myc*
		>1 yr, amplified N-*myc*; favorable histology
	Stage 4S	favorable biology
Intermediate	Stage 3	<1 yr, low N-*myc*
		>1 yr, favorable biology
	Stage 4	<1 yr, low N-*myc*
	Stage 4S	Low N-*myc*
High	Stage 2	>1 yr, all unfavorable biology
	Stage 3	<1 yr, amplified N-*myc*
		>1 yr, any unfavorable biology
	Stage 4	<1 yr, amplified N-*myc*
		>1 yr
	Stage 4S	Amplified N-*myc*

*Favorable biology denotes low N-*myc*, favorable histology, and hyperdiploidy (infants).

within bone marrow aspirate or biopsy may also be sufficient.

Prognostic Factors

Cytogenetic studies provide significant prognostic information that may affect treatment. Amplification of the N-*myc* oncogene is one of the classic factors associated with rapid tumor progression and poor prognosis. In addition, gain of genetic material from chromosome arm 17q is associated with deletion of chromosome 1p and N-*myc* amplification and is highly predictive of poor outcome.[49] Diploid tumors have an unfavorable prognosis, whereas hyperdiploid tumors have a better prognosis. Further, expression of the *TRK* proto-oncogene is inversely associated with N-*myc* amplification and has a more favorable prognosis. Finally, expression of the multidrug resistance–associated protein (MRP) is associated with a poor outcome. In addition to the cytogenetic studies, prognosis may be derived from the pathologic classification as proposed by Shimada and colleagues,[50] taking into account the degree of differentiation, the mitotic-karyorrhexis index, and the presence or absence of stroma.

Treatment

Current therapy for NBL is multimodal, incorporating surgery, chemotherapy, radiation, and occasionally immunotherapy. Surgical resection of the primary tumor and adjacent lymph nodes is the goal and may be curative for localized stage 1 and 2 disease. In most situations in which the tumor is unresectable, exploration with inci-

sional biopsy is the initial procedure, with re-evaluation for resection following a course of adjuvant therapy. After cytoreductive therapy, attempts at resection may be the only option for long-term survival. Meticulous dissection of major blood vessels, which often course through the tumor, is required. These procedures are frequently prolonged and associated with significant blood loss.

Survival

Children of any age with localized neuroblastoma and infants younger than 1 year with advanced disease and favorable disease characteristics have a high likelihood of long-term, disease-free survival. Older children with advanced-stage disease, however, have a significantly decreased chance for cure despite intensive therapy. Prognosis resides in stratification of patients into low-, intermediate-, and high-risk categories (Table 71-6). These are associated with survival rates of greater than 90%, greater than 80%, and 10% to 20%, respectively.[51]

Wilms' Tumor

Wilms' tumor (WT) is an embryonal tumor of renal origin and is the most common primary malignant kidney tumor of childhood. Roughly 500 new cases of WT are diagnosed in the United States each year. This tumor is most frequently seen in children between the ages of 1 and 5 years (~80%), with a peak incidence between 3 and 4 years. Bilateral WT is present in up to 13% of cases and, when present, is synchronous in 60%.

Etiology

Despite the number of genes implicated in the genesis of this neoplasm, hereditary WT is uncommon. Specific germline mutations in one of these genes (Wilms' tumor gene-1, *WT1*) located on the short arm of chromosome 11, are not only associated with WT but also cause a variety of genitourinary abnormalities such as cryptorchidism and hypospadias. A gene that causes aniridia is located near the *WT1* gene on chromosome 11p13, and deletions encompassing the *WT1* and aniridia genes may explain the association between these two conditions. There appears to be a second WT gene at or near the Beckwith-Wiedemann gene locus, also on chromosome 11. Children with Beckwith-Wiedemann syndrome (omphalocele, visceromegaly, macroglossia, and hypoglycemia) are at increased risk for WT. About one fifth of patients with Beckwith-Wiedemann syndrome who develop WT present with bilateral disease at the time of diagnosis.

Clinical Presentation

Most patients (60%) with WT present clinically with a palpable abdominal mass (Fig. 71-21). Often, the patient has no symptoms, and the parents discover the mass during bathing, or the pediatrician discovers it during a routine physical examination. Hypertension is present in about 25% of patients and hematuria in 15%. Because WT is associated with several syndromes, including the Denys-Drash syndrome (WT, intersex disorder, and progressive nephropathy), WAGR syndrome (WT, aniridia, genitourinary anomalies, mental retardation), and Beckwith-Wiedemann syndrome, patients with these phenotypes need to be screened closely into adulthood for the potential development of WT.

Preoperative Evaluation

The initial evaluation of the child with an abdominal mass and suspected WT is by ultrasonography. This is useful in confirming not only that the mass originates from the kidney, but also whether the mass is cystic or solid, and in the detection of potential tumor thrombus within the renal vein and inferior vena cava (IVC). Frequently, it is difficult to distinguish WT from NBL. Both CT and MRI are frequently useful in this regard (Fig. 71-22) because WT originates in the kidney and NBL develops in the adrenal or sympathetic ganglia. In cases in which the origin of the mass is difficult to determine, urinary catecholamine measurements can distinguish WT from NBL; they are elevated in most cases of NBL, but not in WT. CT and MRI are also indicated preoperatively to identify bilateral WT, characterize potential invasion into surrounding structures, document liver or lung metastasis, and detect tumor thrombus within the IVC. A preoperative plain chest radiograph is also necessary for staging purposes.

Surgical Management

After the preoperative evaluation is completed as outlined earlier, exploratory laparotomy is crucial for both staging and treatment of WT. Preoperative chemotherapy may be indicated in cases in which WT is present in a solitary or horseshoe kidney or in both kidneys, with the presence of respiratory distress from extensive metastatic tumor, or when IVC tumor thrombus has extended above the level of the hepatic veins. In these situations, chemotherapy-induced tumor shrinkage may allow for a more complete resection with less morbidity and with the potential to salvage maximal functional renal parenchyma.

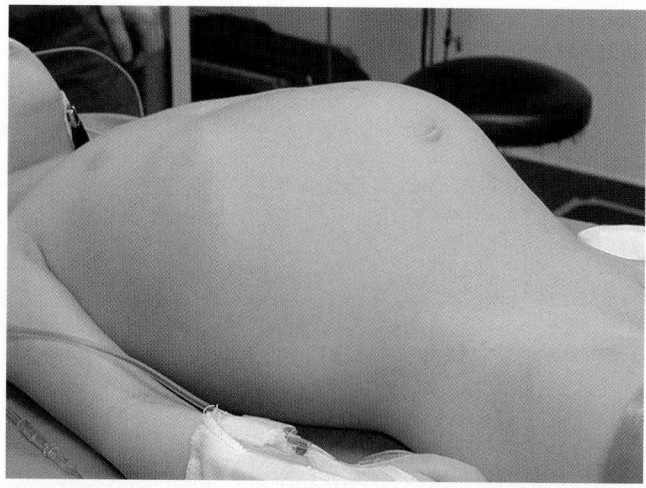

A

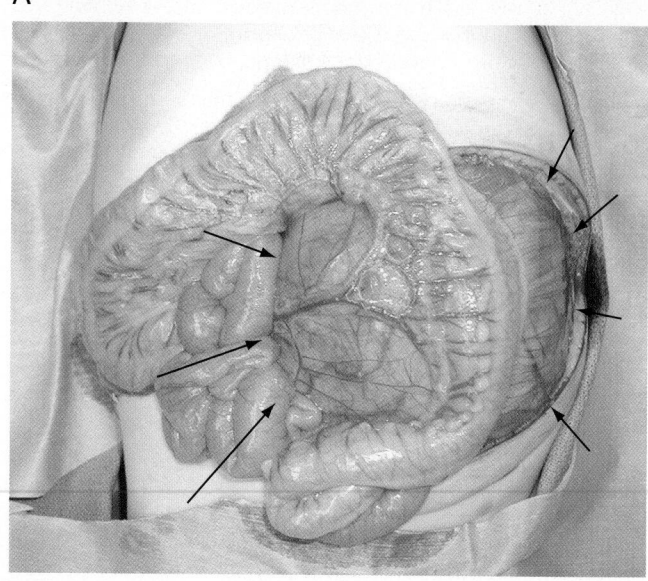

B

Figure 71-21 Wilms' tumor. The large left-sided flank mass is obvious on visual inspection (**A**). Upon entering the peritoneal cavity (**B**), the large Wilms' tumor within the left kidney (outlined by *arrows*) can be seen behind the descending colon, displacing it anterior and medially.

The goals of operative therapy for WT are to confirm the diagnosis, assess the opposite kidney and other abdominal organs for metastatic spread, and completely resect the primary tumor, ureter, and adjacent lymph nodes. These are achieved through a generous transverse or midline transperitoneal incision. At some point during the exploration, Gerota's fascia of the opposite kidney must be opened to more definitively exclude bilateral tumor. The anterior and posterior surfaces of the opposite kidney must be carefully inspected and palpated. Despite the large size of the tumor, complete resection by radical nephroureterectomy can be safely performed. Care must be taken to avoid tumor rupture because this increases the stage of the tumor and mandates additional postoperative adjuvant therapy. Frequently, the ipsilateral adrenal gland is removed en bloc with the kidney. Inva-

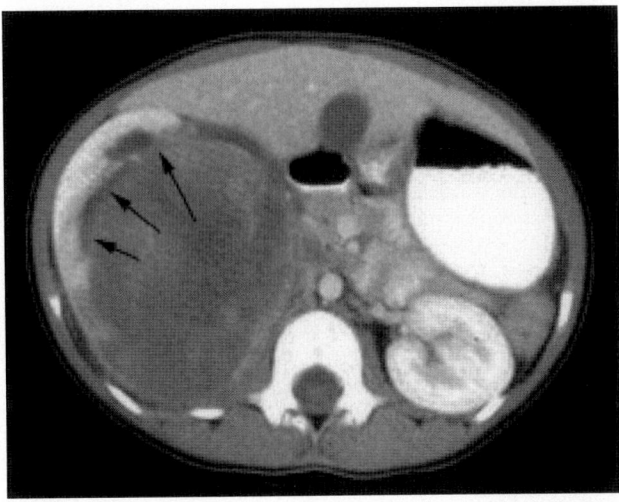

Figure 71-22 CT scan of a Wilms' tumor involving the right kidney. Remnants of the remaining functional kidney (*arrows*) are noted at the periphery of the tumor.

sion into surrounding organs such as the pancreas, spleen, or liver may direct their removal as well.

Surgical exploration, coupled with the preoperative imaging studies and histology, permits accurate staging of WT, which correlates with prognosis and guides postoperative adjuvant therapy. The pathologic evaluation of WT involves inspection of the three elements of normal renal development (blastemal, epithelial, and stromal) and identification of the absence or presence of anaplasia, which distinguishes the classification of either favorable (FH) or unfavorable (UH) histology, respectively. The current staging scheme as proposed by the National Wilms' Tumor Study (NWTS) group is depicted in Table 71-7.

Survival

Treatment of WT represents one of the greatest triumphs in the field of pediatric oncology. In contrast with what used to be a lethal malignancy, the current overall survival rate exceeds 85%. The successful treatment of this tumor is a direct result of collaboration between multiple disciplines to form two major associations (NWTS and the International Society of Pediatric Oncology) in which there has been a systematic organization of multicenter trials designed to address focused, highly relevant questions. The recommended treatment of WT based on stage is shown in Table 71-8. The survival rates of patients with stage I or II FH or stage I UH are both about 95%. For all stages, the overall survival rate of patients with FH is 90%. For patients with UH, stages II, III, and IV are associated with 70%, 56%, and 17% 4-year survival rates, respectively.[52]

Rhabdomyosarcoma

Rhabdomyosarcoma (RMS) is a soft tissue malignant tumor of skeletal muscle origin and accounts for about 3.5% of the cases of cancer among children younger than 14 years. It is a curable disease in most children, with more than 60% surviving 5 years after diagnosis. The most common primary sites for RMS are the head and

Table 71-7 Staging System Used by the National Wilms' Tumor Study Group

STAGE	DEFINITION
I	Tumor limited to the kidney and completely excised without rupture or biopsy. Surface of the renal capsule is intact.
II	Tumor extends through the renal capsule but is completely removed with no microscopic involvement of the margins. Vessels outside the kidney contain tumor. Also placed in stage II are cases in which the kidney has undergone biopsy before removal or where there is "local" spillage of tumor (during resection) limited to the tumor bed.
III	Residual tumor is confined to the abdomen and of nonhematogenous spread. Also included in stage III are cases with tumor involvement of the abdominal lymph nodes, "diffuse" peritoneal contamination by rupture of the tumor extending beyond the tumor bed, peritoneal implants, and microscopic or grossly positive resection margins.
IV	Hematogenous metastases at any site.
V	Bilateral renal involvement.

Table 71-8 NWTS-5 Treatment Recommendations for Wilms' Tumor*

Stage I (FH): Surgery, no radiotherapy, dactinomycin+vincristine for 18 wk

Stage I focal anaplasia: Surgery, no radiotherapy, dactinomycin+vincristine for 18 wk

Stage II (FH): Surgery, no radiotherapy, dactinomycin+vincristine for 18 wk

Stage II focal anaplasia: Surgery, 1080 cGy to tumor bed, dactinomycin+vincristine+doxorubicin for 24 wk

Stage III (FH): Surgery, 1080 cGy to tumor bed, dactinomycin+vincristine+doxorubicin for 24 wk

Stage III focal anaplasia: Surgery, 1080 cGy to tumor bed, dactinomycin+vincristine+doxorubicin for 24 wk

Stage IV (FH) focal anaplasia: Surgery, 1080 cGy to tumor bed according to local tumor stage, 1200 cGy to lung and/or other metastatic sites, dactinomycin+vincristine+doxorubicin for 24 wk

Stage II-IV diffuse anaplasia: Surgery, radiotherapy (whole lung; abdominal 1080 cGy), cyclophosphamide+ etoposide+vincristine+doxorubicin+mesna for 24 wk

Stage I-IV (clear cell sarcoma): Surgery, radiotherapy (abdominal 1080 cGy; whole lung, stage IV only), cyclophosphamide+etoposide+vincristine+ doxorubicin+mesna for 24 wk

Stage I-IV (rhabdoid tumor): Surgery, radiotherapy, carboplatin+etoposide+cyclophosphamide+mesna for 24 wk

*Infants <11 mo are given half the recommended dose of all drugs. Full doses lead to prohibitive hematologic toxicity in this age group. Full doses of chemotherapeutic agents should be administered to those >12 mo.

NWTS, National Wilms' Tumor Study.

neck (parameningeal, orbit, pharyngeal), the genitourinary tract, and the extremities. Other, less common primary sites include the trunk, gastrointestinal (including liver and biliary) tract, and intrathoracic or perineal region. Most cases of RMS occur sporadically with no recognized predisposing factors, although a small proportion are associated with other genetic conditions. These include the Li-Fraumeni cancer susceptibility syndrome (with germline *p53* mutations), neurofibromatosis type I, and Beckwith-Wiedemann syndrome.

The prognosis for a child or adolescent with RMS is related to patient age, site of origin, extent of tumor at time of diagnosis or after surgical resection, and tumor histology.[53] Age less than 10 years is considered a more favorable prognosis. With regard to tumor site, a more favorable prognosis is afforded when tumors are located in the orbit and nonparameningeal head and neck, genitourinary system (excluding bladder and prostate), and biliary tract.

Patients with smaller tumors (<5 cm) have improved survival when compared with that of children with larger tumors, whereas children with metastatic disease at diagnosis have the worst prognosis. The prognostic significance of metastatic disease is further modulated by tumor histology, patient age, and primary site. Patients younger than 10 years with metastatic disease and with embryonal histology have 5-year survival rates greater than 50%, whereas those older than 10 years or with alveolar histology have a much poorer outcome. The presence of regional lymph node involvement is also associated with a worse prognosis. The ability to resect the tumor completely is associated with a better outcome when compared with gross residual disease after initial surgery.

From a histologic standpoint, the botryoid and spindle cell subtypes are associated with a more favorable outcome. Embryonal and pleomorphic subtypes are intermediate, and alveolar or undifferentiated subtypes are generally associated with a worse prognosis. Favorable prognostic groups have been identified by previous Intergroup Rhabdomyosarcoma Studies, and treatment plans have been designed based on assignment of patients to different groups according to prognosis (Table 71-9).

The diagnostic workup generally involves CT or MRI. Because there are no useful markers at present, an accurate diagnosis depends on incisional biopsy of the tumor. In the extremity, the direction of the incision must allow it to be incorporated into the wound created by a subsequent wide local excision.

All children with RMS require multimodality therapy. This entails surgical resection, if possible, followed by chemotherapy, followed by second-look surgery for some patients with initially unresectable tumors, and depending on original histologic type, extent of disease, and extent of resection, radiation therapy.

The basic surgical principles for the treatment of RMS are complete resection of the primary tumor with a surrounding margin of normal tissue, coupled with sampling of the adjacent lymph nodes. This may not be feasible in patients with obvious metastatic disease but is done if possible. Because RMS can arise from so many primary muscle sites, surgical care must be tailored to the unique

Table 71-9 Staging for Rhabdomyosarcoma

Group I: Localized disease that is completely resected with no regional node involvement (13%)

Group II: (~20%)
  IIA: Localized, grossly resected tumor with microscopic residual disease but no regional nodal involvement.
  IIB: Locoregional disease with tumor-involved lymph nodes with complete resection and no residual disease.
  IIC: Locoregional disease with involved nodes, grossly resected, but with evidence of microscopic residual tumor at the primary site and/or histologic involvement of the most distal regional node (from the primary site).

Group III: Localized, gross residual disease including incomplete resection, or biopsy only of the primary site (~48%).

Group IV: Distant metastatic disease present at the time of diagnosis (~18%).

aspects of each site. Surgical management of the more common primary sites is described next.

Head and Neck

For those tumors that are superficial and nonorbital, wide excision of the primary tumor with ipsilateral neck lymph node sampling of clinically involved nodes is appropriate. Because of cosmetic and functional concerns, margins smaller than 1 mm are acceptable. For patients with tumors that are considered unresectable, chemotherapy and radiation therapy become the primary management. Rhabdomyosarcomas of the orbit require a biopsy to establish diagnosis and then chemotherapy and radiation therapy. Orbital exenteration is reserved for the small number of patients with local, persistent, or recurrent disease.

Extremity

The definitive surgical procedure involves wide local excision with en bloc of normal tissue. If it is anatomically feasible, a re-excision procedure is associated with better outcome in patients whose initial surgical procedure left microscopic residual disease on pathologic examination. Amputation is reserved for selected patients with lesions involving major neurovascular structures in addition to the muscle of origin. Because of the significant incidence of nodal spread for extremity primary tumors (often without clinical evidence of involvement), and because of the prognostic and therapeutic implications of nodal involvement, surgical assessment for regional nodal involvement is important.[54] For clinically negative nodes, axillary or femoral node sampling is done for upper or lower extremity tumors, respectively. If clinically positive nodes are present, biopsy of more proximal nodes is recommended before sampling of the involved nodal region.

Trunk

As with RMS in other locations, wide local excision and an attempt to achieve negative microscopic margins is the goal. Reconstruction may require use of prosthetic materials. Extremely large masses undergo biopsy initially, followed by a course of chemotherapy with or without radiation. This may shrink the tumor enough to permit a subsequent margin-negative resection with successful reconstruction.

Genitourinary

The initial surgical procedure in most patients consists of a biopsy, which often can be performed using a cystoscope, transanally, or under direct vision. Bladder salvage is an important goal of therapy for patients with tumors arising in the prostate and bladder. Occasionally, when the tumor is confined to the dome of the bladder, it can be completely resected. Otherwise, pre-resection chemotherapy and radiation therapy allow preservation of a functional bladder in most patients. For patients with a biopsy-proven residual malignant tumor after chemotherapy and radiation therapy, appropriate surgical management may include partial cystectomy, prostatectomy, or anterior exenteration.

Testis or spermatic cord RMS are removed by radical orchiectomy and resection of the entire spermatic cord. Resection of hemiscrotal skin may be necessary when there is tumor fixation or invasion, or if a previous transscrotal biopsy has been performed. Because paratesticular tumors are associated with a relatively high incidence of lymphatic spread, all patients with paratesticular primary tumors have thin-cut abdominal and pelvic CT scans with contrast to evaluate nodal involvement. Retroperitoneal lymph node sampling is needed for patients with suggestive or positive CT scans who are younger than 10 years. In contrast, an ipsilateral retroperitoneal lymph node dissection is required for all children older than 10 years with paratesticular RMS for staging.

Liver Tumors

Liver cancer is rare in childhood and essentially is either hepatoblastoma (HBL) or hepatocellular carcinoma (HCC). Several important differences exist between these two subtypes. HBLs usually occur before 3 years of age, whereas HCC may be found in children and adults of all ages. Hepatoblastoma is most often unifocal, whereas HCC is often extensively invasive or multicentric at the time of diagnosis. Complete resection is therefore more often possible in patients with HBL. Childhood HBL frequently involves associated mutations in the β-catenin gene, the function of which is closely related to the development of familial adenomatous polyposis. In addition, HBL is associated with hemihypertrophy, very low birthweight, and Beckwith-Wiedemann syndrome. In contrast, HCC is associated with a history of perinatally acquired hepatitis B and C infection, mutations in the hepatocyte growth factor receptor gene (c-*met*), and tyrosinemia, biliary cirrhosis, and α$_1$-antitrypsin deficiency. The serum tumor marker α-fetoprotein levels parallel disease activity for both HBL and HCC. The overall survival rate for children with HBL is 70%, as compared with 25% for HCC. A general staging scheme for hepatic tumors in children is depicted in Table 71-10. Children

Table 71-10 Liver Tumor Staging

STAGE	DEFINITION
I	No metastases, tumor completely resected.
II	No metastases, tumor grossly resected with microscopic residual disease (i.e., positive margins); or tumor rupture, or tumor spill at the time of surgery.
III	No distant metastases, tumor unresectable or resected with gross residual tumor, or positive lymph nodes.
IV	Distant metastases regardless of the extent of liver involvement.

diagnosed with stage I and II HBL have a cure rate of greater than 90%, whereas stage III is associated with a 60% survival rate. Children with stage IV disease have a survival rate of roughly 20%. Children diagnosed with stage I HCC generally have a good outcome. Stage II is too rarely seen to predict outcome, and stages III and IV are usually fatal.

Complete resection of the primary tumor with negative surgical margins is one of the most critical factors in prognosis. Preoperative chemotherapy can convert an unresectable tumor into one that is resectable and may lessen the incidence of postoperative morbidity.[55] Preoperative chemotherapy is more effective in the treatment of HBL than HCC. Surgical resection of distant disease has also contributed to the cure of children with hepatoblastoma. Resection of pulmonary metastases is recommended when the number of metastases is limited. Liver transplantation may be useful therapy in patients with unresectable hepatic tumors.[56] Five-year survival rates approximating 83% for children with HBL and 63% for children with HCC have been reported. Because of the worse prognosis in patients with HCC, liver transplantation is considered early in the course for disorders such as tyrosinemia and familial intrahepatic cholestasis before the development of liver failure and malignancy. The fibrolamellar variant of HCC may have a better prognosis with liver transplantation than other types.

Teratoma

Teratomas are tumors that contain elements derived from more than one of the three embryonic germ layers. In addition, teratomas must contain tissue that is foreign to the anatomic site in which they occur. Teratomas can occur anywhere in the body and present as cystic, solid, or mixed lesions. When they occur during infancy and early childhood, they are most commonly extragonadal. In contrast, in older children, teratomas most frequently involve the gonads.

Teratomas occur most frequently in the neonatal period, and the sacrococcygeal region is the most common site. Sacrococcygeal teratoma (SCT) is four times more common in females and is most often an obvious external

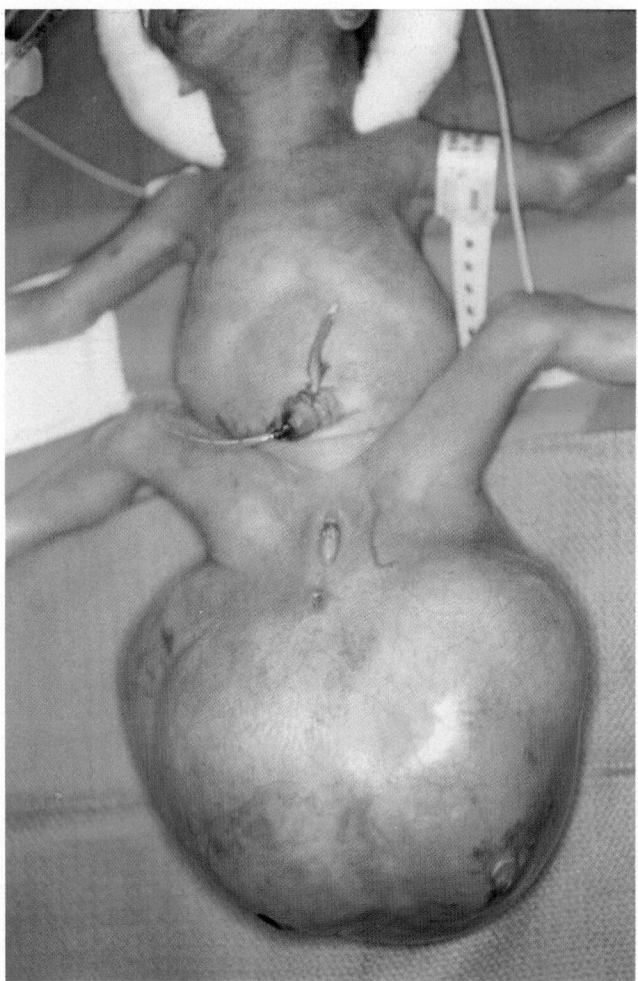

Figure 71-23 Sacrococcygeal teratoma. Despite its large size, this tumor is benign in most cases.

presacral mass (Fig. 71-23). Although most of the tumor is usually external, with a minimal intrapelvic presacral component, there is a spectrum of tumor distribution, to the extent of being entirely presacral, with no visible external component. As such, a digital rectal examination of a neonate with care to feel the normal presacral space may be an important screening technique. Occasionally, SCTs are identified during routine prenatal ultrasonography. It is important that these lesions be carefully followed with serial sonography until delivery because the blood supply to the tumor may grow to the point of stealing a significant proportion of placental blood flow to the fetus. The development of hydrops or placentomegaly is associated with a poor prognosis. In these situations, in utero resection of the tumor may be lifesaving.[57]

Most neonatal SCTs are benign. The incidence of malignancy is related to age at time of diagnosis and is most frequently represented as endodermal sinus tumors (yolk sac tumors) or embryonal carcinomas. The presence of trophoblasts is associated with choriocarcinoma. The likelihood of malignancy is slightly increased in males.

Treatment of SCT is complete surgical excision through a chevron-shaped buttock incision. Most tumors can be completely removed using a sacral approach. If preoperative imaging demonstrates significant intra-abdominal extension of the tumor, a combined abdominal-sacral approach may be needed. Resection of the coccyx is critical because failure to remove this structure results in significantly higher local recurrence rates. Care must be taken to individually ligate the vessels supplying the tumor, including the middle sacral artery and branches of the hypogastric arteries. After the tumor is excised, the levator muscle complex is secured to the presacral fascia, and the remaining wound is closed in layers. Careful follow-up is necessary because recurrence may be significant, even for benign tumors.

FETAL SURGERY

The motivation for fetal surgical intervention has been the realization that with certain congenital anomalies, irreversible changes have already occurred by the time of birth. In utero intervention therefore could theoretically prevent continued progression of the anomaly, reverse the pathophysiology, and prevent fetal demise. At present, there are a few indications for open fetal surgery, which needs to be performed only at centers with multidisciplinary expertise in this area. As with open surgery in general, the indications for minimally invasive fetal surgical intervention are expanding.

Fetal Imaging

Ultrasonography remains the mainstay of imaging modalities for the fetus. It is rapid, noninvasive, and applied in most pregnancies. Although three-dimensional ultrasound has added little to what can be seen by conventional ultrasound, four-dimensional ultrasound may provide tomographic assessment of the fetus in three dimensions, which may significantly enhance diagnostic capabilities. Ultrafast MRI is complementary to ultrasound imaging. In particular, MRI has proved superior in the assessment of central nervous system lesions.

Open Fetal Surgery

One of the major conditions that have been systematically evaluated with regard to open fetal surgery has been congenital diaphragmatic hernia. Initial attempts at in utero repair demonstrated some success, but outcomes were no different for low-risk patients when compared with contemporary postnatal management. In high-risk patients (liver up in the chest, a right lung-to-head circumference ratio [LHR]<1.4), open fetal surgery was associated with poor survival, primarily because of kinking of the hepatic veins and IVC when the liver was moved into the abdomen. At present, open fetal surgery for congenital diaphragmatic hernia has been abandoned. Occlusion of the fetal trachea by either external clips or intraluminal balloons has been shown to induce lung growth; however, outcomes have not been significantly improved.[39]

Although congenital cystic adenomatoid malformation often presents as a benign pulmonary mass in infants and children, a few fetuses have extremely large lesions associated with the development of hydrops fetalis. Without intervention, these infants die in utero. Careful ultrasound surveillance of large lesions is therefore necessary to detect the first signs of hydrops. Fetal pulmonary resection has been successful in preventing this complication. For lesions consisting of a single large cyst, thoracoamniotic shunting may be useful.

Another condition in which open fetal surgical intervention has been valuable is sacrococcygeal teratoma. In large teratomas, increased blood flow to the tumor is associated with high-output heart failure in the fetus (hydrops) as well as placentomegaly. The development of these two findings is associated with dismal survival. Open fetal resection of the teratoma has been reported in a few cases to reverse the hydrops and to salvage the fetus.

Although it has been initially assumed that the spinal cord in infants with myelomeningocele is intrinsically abnormal, recent work has suggested that much of the neurologic damage may be due to in utero exposure and trauma to the spinal cord. At present, a randomized prospective multicenter trial is underway to determine the potential benefit of in utero repair on need for postnatal ventricular decompressive shunting and neurocognitive development.

Fetal Endoscopic Surgery

With the explosion of minimally invasive technology, the applications to fetal surgical intervention are also expanding. Fetal urethral obstruction is most commonly due to posterior urethral valves in males and ureteral atresia in females. Urethral obstruction results in oligohydramnios, pulmonary hypoplasia, and renal dysplasia. In fetuses with a good prognosis (fetal urine $Na^+ < 100$ mEq/L, $Cl^- < 90$ mEq/L, and osmolarity <210 mOsm/L), percutaneous vesicoamniotic shunt or fetocystoscopic ablation of urethral valves may restore amniotic fluid volume and prevent death from pulmonary hypoplasia. Whether these approaches can preserve renal function is less clear.

Fetoscopic intervention appears to have had the greatest impact on complications associated with monochorionic (single placenta) twins. In cases in which there is spontaneous or imminent demise of one twin with lethal anomalies, death of the normal twin may rapidly follow. In this scenario, fetoscopic ligation of the cord to the anomalous twin prevents deterioration of the normal twin. Twin reversed arterial perfusion (TRAP) sequence is a rare situation in which one twin is acardiac and acephalic. Without intrinsic cardiac function, blood flow thorough this fetus is entirely drained from the normal heart of the so-called pump twin, resulting in cardiac failure and death. Diathermic occlusion or radiofrequency ablation of the umbilical cord going to the acardiac and acephalic twin will therefore halt the progression of cardiac failure in the opposite twin. Finally, the single most commonly performed fetal surgical procedure is fetoscopic photocoagulation of communicating placental blood vessels in twin-twin transfusion syndrome. This intervention will arrest the development of a steal phenomenon of blood flow from one twin to the other. A comparison of this method with the standard treatment of serial amnioreduction for polyhydramnios in hope of prolonging the pregnancy has just been completed.

Ex Utero Intrapartum Treatment

Lesions that compromise the fetal airway constitute an immediate threat at the time of delivery for hypoxia, ischemic brain injury, and death. These include large cervical teratomas, vascular malformations, and laryngeal atresia. As such, a strategy known as the EXIT procedure has converted these potentially catastrophic events into a more controlled and safe procedure for establishment of an airway. The basic premise of the EXIT procedure is controlled uterine hypotonia to facilitate uteroplacental circulation. Thus, appropriate time can be taken to secure a safe airway just before clamping the umbilical cord and delivery of the fetus. In contrast with a typical cesarean birth in which uterine tone is maximized to prevent postpartum hemorrhage and minimal inhalation agents are used for fear of neonatal depression, the EXIT procedure employs deep inhalation anesthesia and tocolytic agents to maximize uterine relaxation, uterine volume is preserved to prevent placental abruption, and a surgical level of anesthesia is achieved in the fetus. During this time, endotracheal intubation can be achieved. For large lesions, division of the strap muscles of the neck, subtotal tumor resection, or tracheotomy may be needed before cord clamping. The congenital high airway obstruction syndrome (CHAOS) is associated with hydrops in which nearly complete or complete intrinsic obstruction of the fetal airway prevents egress of lung fluid from the tracheobronchial tree. These children may benefit from an EXIT strategy. Further, the EXIT procedure may be applied during the transition to ECLS in cases of known severe cardiac anomalies as a bridge to postnatal intervention.

Selected References

Ashcraft KW, Holcomb GW III, Murphy JP (eds): Pediatric Surgery (4th ed). Philadelphia, Elsevier/Saunders, 2005.

> This is an excellent reference source for most pediatric surgical conditions. Although most topics are not covered as in-depth as in the Grosfeld text mentioned next, this book is easy to read and serves as an outstanding practical resource.

Grosfeld JL, O'Neill JA, Fonkalsrud EW, Coran AG (eds): Pediatric Surgery (6th ed). Philadelphia, Mosby Elsevier, 2006.

> This two-volume monograph provides a very comprehensive review of the field of pediatric surgery. This book is considered to be the most authoritative and traditional textbook for pediatric surgeons.

Mattei P (ed): Surgical Directives: Pediatric Surgery. Philadelphia, Lippincott Williams & Wilkins, 2003.

> This is an outstanding reference text for senior surgery residents, fellows, and general surgeons. The chapters are short, to the point, and written to provide a reasonable approach to most of the common pediatric surgery conditions.

Oldham KT, Colombani PM, Foglia RP, Skinner MA (eds): Principles and Practice of Pediatric Surgery. Philadelphia, Lippincott Williams & Wilkins, 2005.

This is a superb reference book that tends to integrate more pathophysiology and basic science discussions of pediatric surgical conditions.

Ziegler MM, Azizkhan RG, Weber TR (eds): Operative Pediatric Surgery. New York, McGraw-Hill, 2003.

This is a beautifully illustrated text that emphasizes various pediatric surgical techniques. This is especially valuable for review of the more commonly done pediatric surgery procedures.

References

1. Dalton HJ, Rycus PT, Conrad SA: Update on extracorporeal life support 2004. Semin Perinatol 29:24-33, 2005.
2. Brown JK, Jing Y, Wang S, et al: Patterns of severe injury in pediatric car crash victims: Crash Injury Research Engineering Network database. J Pediatr Surg 41:362-367, 2006.
3. Stylianos S, Egorova N, Guice KS, et al: Variation in treatment of pediatric spleen injury at trauma centers versus nontrauma centers: A call for dissemination of American Pediatric Surgical Association benchmarks and guidelines. J Am Coll Surg 202:247-251, 2006.
4. Gallagher PG, Mahoney MJ, Gosche JR: Cystic hygroma in the fetus and newborn. Semin Perinatol 23:341-356, 1999.
5. Hedrick HL: Ex utero intrapartum therapy. Semin Pediatr Surg 12:190-195, 2003.
6. Leung AK, Robson WL: Childhood cervical lymphadenopathy. J Pediatr Health Care 18:3-7, 2004.
7. Flint D, Mahadevan M, Barber C, et al: Cervical lymphadenitis due to non-tuberculous mycobacteria: Surgical treatment and review. Int J Pediatr Otorhinolaryngol 53:187-194, 2000.
8. Allen SR, Ignacio R, Falcone RA III, et al: The effect of a right-sided aortic arch on outcome in children with esophageal atresia and tracheoesophageal fistula. J Pediatr Surg 41:479-483, 2006.
9. Holcomb GW III, Rothenberg SS, Bax KM, et al: Thoracoscopic repair of esophageal atresia and tracheoesophageal fistula: A multi-institutional analysis. Ann Surg 242:422-428, 2005.
10. Livaditis A: Esophageal atresia: A method of overbridging large segmental gaps. Z Kinderchir 13:298-306, 1973.
11. Foker JE, Kendall TC, Catton K, et al: A flexible approach to achieve a true primary repair for all infants with esophageal atresia. Semin Pediatr Surg 14:8-15, 2005.
12. Seguier-Lipszyc E, Bonnard A, Aizenfisz S, et al: The management of long gap esophageal atresia. J Pediatr Surg 40:1542-1546, 2005.
13. Lopez PJ, Keys C, Pierro A, et al: Oesophageal atresia: Improved outcome in high-risk groups? J Pediatr Surg 41:331-334, 2006.
14. Stordal K, Johannesdottir GB, Bentsen BS, et al: Acid suppression does not change respiratory symptoms in children with asthma and gastro-oesophageal reflux disease. Arch Dis Child 90:956-960, 2005.
15. Lee P, Rudolph C: Gastroesophageal reflux in infants and children. Adv Pediatr 48:301-329, 2001.
16. Rosen R, Lord C, Nurko S: The sensitivity of multichannel intraluminal impedance and the pH probe in the evaluation of gastroesophageal reflux in children. Clin Gastroenterol Hepatol 4:167-172, 2006.
17. Dedivitis RA, Camargo DL, Peixoto GL, et al: Thyroglossal duct: A review of 55 cases. J Am Coll Surg 194:274-277, 2002.
18. Buratti S, Kamenwa R, Dohil R, et al: Esophagogastric disconnection following failed fundoplication for the treatment of gastroesophageal reflux disease (GERD) in children with severe neurological impairment. Pediatr Surg Int 20:786-790, 2004.
19. Diaz DM, Gibbons TE, Heiss K, et al: Antireflux surgery outcomes in pediatric gastroesophageal reflux disease. Am J Gastroenterol 100:1844-1852, 2005.
20. Rohrschneider WK, Mittnacht H, Darge K, Troger K: Pyloric muscle in asymptomatic infants: Sonographic evaluation and discrimination from idiopathic hypertrophic pyloric stenosis. Pediatr Radiol 28:429-434, 1998.
21. Helton KJ, Strife JL, Warner BW, et al: The impact of a clinical guideline on imaging children with hypertrophic pyloric stenosis. Pediatr Radiol 34:733-736, 2004.
22. Kim SS, Lau ST, Lee SL, et al: Pyloromyotomy: A comparison of laparoscopic, circumumbilical, and right upper quadrant operative techniques. J Am Coll Surg 201:66-70, 2005.
23. Kumaran N, Shankar KR, Lloyd DA, et al: Trends in the management and outcome of jejuno-ileal atresia. Eur J Pediatr Surg 12:163-167, 2002.
24. Moss RL, Dimmitt RA, Barnhart DC, et al: Laparotomy versus peritoneal drainage for necrotizing enterocolitis and perforation. N Engl J Med 354:2225-2234, 2006.
25. Spencer AU, Neaga A, West B, et al: Pediatric short bowel syndrome: Redefining predictors of success. Ann Surg 242:403-409, 2005.
26. Kia KF, Mony VK, Drongowski RA, et al: Laparoscopic vs open surgical approach for intussusception requiring operative intervention. J Pediatr Surg 40:281-284, 2005.
27. Dasgupta R, Langer JC: Transanal pull-through for Hirschsprung disease. Semin Pediatr Surg 14:64-71, 2005.
28. Pena A, Hong A: Advances in the management of anorectal malformations. Am J Surg 180:370-376, 2000.
29. Lima M, Tursini S, Ruggeri G, et al: Laparoscopically assisted anorectal pull-through for high imperforate anus: Three years' experience. J Laparoendosc Adv Surg Tech A 16:63-66, 2006.
30. Levitt MA, Pena A: Outcomes from the correction of anorectal malformations. Curr Opin Pediatr 17:394-401, 2005.
31. Salihu HM, Emusu D, Aliyu ZY, et al: Mode of delivery and neonatal survival of infants with isolated gastroschisis. Obstet Gynecol 104:678-683, 2004.
32. Wiener ES, Touloukian RJ, Rodgers BM, et al: Hernia survey of the Section on Surgery of the American Academy of Pediatrics. J Pediatr Surg 31:1166-1169, 1996.
33. Sozubir S, Ekingen G, Senel U, et al: A continuous debate on contralateral processus vaginalis: Evaluation technique and approach to patency. Hernia 10:74-78, 2006.
34. Javid PJ, Jaksic T, Skarsgard ED, et al: Survival rate in congenital diaphragmatic hernia: The experience of the Canadian Neonatal Network. J Pediatr Surg 39:657-660, 2004.
35. Colvin J, Bower C, Dickinson JE, et al: Outcomes of congenital diaphragmatic hernia: A population-based study in Western Australia. Pediatrics 116:e356-e363, 2005.
36. Cass DL: Fetal surgery for congenital diaphragmatic hernia: The North American experience. Semin Perinatol 29:104-111, 2005.
37. Harrison MR, Keller RL, Hawgood SB, et al: A randomized trial of fetal endoscopic tracheal occlusion for severe fetal congenital diaphragmatic hernia. N Engl J Med 349:1916-1924, 2003.
38. Boloker J, Bateman DA, Wung JT, et al: Congenital diaphragmatic hernia in 120 infants treated consecutively with

permissive hypercapnea/spontaneous respiration/elective repair. J Pediatr Surg 37:357-366, 2002.

39. Cortes RA, Keller RL, Townsend T, et al: Survival of severe congenital diaphragmatic hernia has morbid consequences. J Pediatr Surg 40:36-45, 2005.

40. Daunt SW, Cohen JH, Miller SF: Age-related normal ranges for the Haller index in children. Pediatr Radiol 34:326-330, 2004.

41. Croitoru DP, Kelly RE Jr, Goretsky MJ, et al: The minimally invasive Nuss technique for recurrent or failed pectus excavatum repair in 50 patients. J Pediatr Surg 40:181-186, 2005.

42. Frey AS, Garcia VF, Brown RL, et al: Nonoperative management of pectus carinatum. J Pediatr Surg 41:40-45, 2006.

43. Wilson RD, Hedrick HL, Liechty KW, et al: Cystic adenomatoid malformation of the lung: Review of genetics, prenatal diagnosis, and in utero treatment. Am J Med Genet A 140:151-155, 2006.

44. Shteyer E, Ramm GA, Xu C, et al: Outcome after portoenterostomy in biliary atresia: Pivotal role of degree of liver fibrosis and intensity of stellate cell activation. J Pediatr Gastroenterol Nutr 42:93-99, 2006.

45. Sokol RJ, Mack C, Narkewicz MR, et al: Pathogenesis and outcome of biliary atresia: Current concepts. J Pediatr Gastroenterol Nutr 37:4-21, 2003.

46. Meyers RL, Book LS, O'Gorman MA, et al: High-dose steroids, ursodeoxycholic acid, and chronic intravenous antibiotics improve bile flow after Kasai procedure in infants with biliary atresia. J Pediatr Surg 38:406-411, 2003.

47. Hung PY, Chen CC, Chen WJ, et al: Long-term prognosis of patients with biliary atresia: A 25 year summary. J Pediatr Gastroenterol Nutr 42:190-195, 2006.

48. Yamataka A, Oshiro K, Okada Y, et al: Complications after cyst excision with hepaticoenterostomy for choledochal cysts and their surgical management in children versus adults. J Pediatr Surg 32:1097-1102, 1997.

49. Tajiri T, Tanaka S, Higashi M, et al: Biological diagnosis for neuroblastoma using the combination of highly sensitive analysis of prognostic factors. J Pediatr Surg 41:560-566, 2006.

50. Shimada H, Ambros IM, Dehner LP, et al: The International Neuroblastoma Pathology Classification (the Shimada system). Cancer 86:364-372, 1999.

51. Haase GM, Perez C, Atkinson JB: Current aspects of biology, risk assessment, and treatment of neuroblastoma. Semin Surg Oncol 16:91-104, 1999.

52. Shamberger RC: Pediatric renal tumors. Semin Surg Oncol 16:105-120, 1999.

53. Raney RB, Anderson JR, Barr FG, et al: Rhabdomyosarcoma and undifferentiated sarcoma in the first two decades of life: A selective review of intergroup rhabdomyosarcoma study group experience and rationale for Intergroup Rhabdomyosarcoma Study V. J Pediatr Hematol Oncol 23:215-220, 2001.

54. Neville HL, Andrassy RJ, Lobe TE, et al: Preoperative staging, prognostic factors, and outcome for extremity rhabdomyosarcoma: A preliminary report from the Intergroup Rhabdomyosarcoma Study IV (1991-1997). J Pediatr Surg 35:317-321, 2000.

55. Schnater JM, Aronson DC, Plaschkes J, et al: Surgical view of the treatment of patients with hepatoblastoma: Results from the first prospective trial of the International Society of Pediatric Oncology Liver Tumor Study Group. Cancer 94:1111-1120, 2002.

56. Tiao GM, Bobey N, Allen S, et al: The current management of hepatoblastoma: A combination of chemotherapy, conventional resection, and liver transplantation. J Pediatr 146:204-211, 2005.

57. Kitano Y, Flake AW, Crombleholme TM, et al: Open fetal surgery for life-threatening fetal malformations. Semin Perinatol 23:448-461, 1999.

Neurosurgery

Joel T. Patterson, MD   Fadi Hanbali, MD   Robbi L. Franklin, MD
and   Haring J. W. Nauta, MD, PhD

Intracranial Dynamics
Cerebrovascular Disorders
Central Nervous System Tumors
Traumatic Brain Injury
Degenerative Disorders of the Spine
Functional and Stereotactic Neurosurgery
Hydrocephalus
Pediatric Neurosurgery
Central Nervous System Infections

Neurosurgery is defined as surgery of the brain, spinal cord, peripheral nerves, and pituitary gland and of their supporting structures, including the blood supply, and protective elements, the spinal fluid spaces, bony cranium, and spine. Although it may be intuitive to think of neurosurgery as mostly concerned with the neural tissue itself, it is common that the pathophysiology and opportunity for therapy involve its infrastructure. Thus, it is easy to understand that neurosurgeons are often focused on intracranial pressure (ICP), cerebrospinal fluid (CSF) dynamics, cerebral blood flow, and compression syndromes of the spinal cord, nerve roots, and peripheral nerves. Whatever may be happening to the neural tissue, whose complexity often defies direct intervention, its environment must be optimized for improvement or recovery to occur. The rigid closed space around the brain and spinal cord is often said to set neurosurgery apart from other branches of surgery. A prime example is the contrast between intra-abdominal and intracranial hemorrhage. Whereas bleeding in the abdomen may focus concern on blood loss and hypotension, bleeding within the closed space of the cranium causes problems with raised ICP with attendant decreased cerebral blood flow, infarction, edema, and obstruction of spinal fluid absorption. These intracranial mechanisms can be lethal at volumes of intracranial bleeding that have no effect on systemic blood pressure through the mechanism of hypovolemia.

The chapter is intended for non-neurosurgeons who want to initiate a framework on which to add further knowledge and experience. It hopefully will also help someone at a community hospital emergency room, or a medical student on the ward for the first time, communicate patient problems efficiently to neurosurgeons. The chapter is laid out to first provide a brief overview of the underlying principles of neurosurgery with focus on intracranial dynamics. The remaining space is divided in subsections: cerebrovascular disorders, which include subarachnoid hemorrhage, intracerebral hemorrhage, aneurysm, and arteriovenous malformation (AVM); central nervous system (CNS) tumors, which include neoplasms of the brain, cranial nerves, spinal cord, and their coverings, and lesions of the skull base; traumatic head injury; degenerative diseases of the spine; functional neurosurgery, which includes stereotaxis, epilepsy surgery, surgery for the management of pain and movement disorder, and stereotactic radiosurgery; hydrocephalus and pediatric neurosurgery; and neurosurgical management of CNS infections. The field of neurosurgery is simply too broad to make a detailed encyclopedic overview realistic, but some introduction to these subdivisions will hopefully be useful to the reader.

INTRACRANIAL DYNAMICS

A few basic principles concerning intracranial dynamics, CSF, cerebral blood flow, and ICP are essential to grasp at the outset and are summarized here for quick review. Some of these principles are obvious; others are frankly counterintuitive.

The *first principle* is obvious: the cranial cavity has a fixed volume that is filled by various things:

1. Brain tissue
2. CSF

Table 72-1 Intracranial Excess Volume Syndromes and Therapy

	EXCESS VOLUME SYNDROME	SPECIFIC THERAPY
Brain tissue	Edema: cytotoxic, vasogenic, perineoplastic, inflammatory	Diuretics: mannitol, furosemide, hypertonic saline; steroids for perineoplastic and inflammatory edema
Vascular	Elevated P_{CO_2}; hyperperfusion state with loss of autoregulation as in severe hypertension, after trauma, after arteriovenous malformation removal; relative venous obstruction	Increased ventilation, diuretics (but in hyperperfusion state, avoid mannitol), barbiturates; clear venous obstruction, elevate head of bed (to reduce venous volume)
Cerebrospinal fluid (CSF)	Impaired absorption with congenital, posthemorrhagic, or postinfectious hydrocephalus, communicating or obstructive; loculations; arachnoid or periventricular cysts; rare increased production of CSF with choroid plexus papilloma	Ventricular external drainage (or lumbar drainage only if no threat of herniation) or shunt; with flocculation, or with some kinds of obstructive hydrocephalus, endoscopic fenestration or third ventriculostomy may be possible; acetazolamide and steroids may temporarily decrease CSF production.
Mass lesion	Tumor, cyst, abscess, hematoma, radiation necrosis, or cerebral infarction necrosis	Remove, fenestrate, aspirate lesion (often with stereotactic guidance); less commonly, it may be warranted to enlarge intracranial volume by decompression

3. Blood vessels and intravascular blood volume
4. Volume associated with any pathologic process, which can include tumor, cyst, abscess, hemorrhage, edema, necrosis

Because the volume of the cranial cavity is rigidly fixed, an increase in one component must be accompanied by some decrease in other components or the ICP will rise precipitously.[1,2] The clinical implications are also straightforward. For each intracranial component, there is a family of pathologic conditions of excess volume, and a means to improve that excess, as summarized in Table 72-1.

A consequence of this principle is that if there is an elevation in the volume of any one compartment, there is a stage of compensation in which the volume of one or more other compartments can be reduced to avoid elevations in ICP.

The *second principle* is not obvious and may seem counterintuitive: The spinal fluid is produced at a constant rate (~15-20 mL/hr) largely by the choroid plexus of the ventricles by an energy-dependent, physicochemical process. It is essential to understand that the production is affected hardly at all by any intracranial "back pressure," so that the CSF production continues unabated even to lethal elevations of intracranial pressure. Since production is nearly always constant, it follows that derangement of CSF dynamics almost always involves some aspect of impeding CSF absorption, either through obstruction along the CSF pathways inside the brain, the subarachnoid spaces at the basal cisterns or cerebral convexity, or arachnoid granulations from which most absorption occurs. In the sections on tumors, infection, intracranial hemorrhage, and trauma that follow, many examples will become apparent whereby impaired CSF absorption contributes to the pathologic condition. The only exceptions to the nearly constant CSF production are the excess production associated with the very rare choroid plexus papilloma tumor, and the occasional

decreased CSF production seen with some gram-negative bacterial meningitides with ventriculitis, usually in neonates.

The *third basic principle* is that the cerebral blood flow (CBF) normally varies over a wide range (30-100 mL per 100 g brain tissue per minute), depending on metabolic demand from neuronal activity within a particular area of the brain. The CBF may be considered in aggregate or of specific small regions, pathologic or normal.

For any brain region

$$CBF = \frac{\text{cerebral perfusion pressure}}{\text{cerebral vascular resistance}}$$

The blood flow to any brain area is commonly luxuriant, exceeding demand by a wide margin, so that O_2 extraction ratios are often low. The brain vasculature matches the blood flow to tissue metabolic demand, and the CBF generally maintains what is needed despite wide variations in systemic blood pressure by a phenomenon known as *autoregulation* (Fig. 72-1). Chronic hypertension and elevated arterial P_{CO_2} shift the curve as indicated. If tissue demand exceeds autoregulation, or if CBF declines for pathologic reasons, the first defense is that the O_2 extraction goes up. The tissue begins to dysfunction at levels below 25 mL per 100 g brain tissue per minute, and infarction with attendant swelling can gradually occur at levels below 20. The lower the CBF falls below 20, the quicker the infarction (Fig. 72-2). Complete loss of blood flow to any brain area results in infarction (irreversible damage) within a few minutes. Swelling of the infarcted tissue takes days to peak and weeks to resolve.

An important implication is that if brain dysfunction is occurring clinically because compensatory mechanisms (autoregulation changing the vascular resistance, or the capacity to elevate mean systemic arterial pressure, or the ability to increase O_2 extraction) have been exceeded, the tolerance for further decline in blood flow is low, and tissue damage is seriously threatened. Therapy to

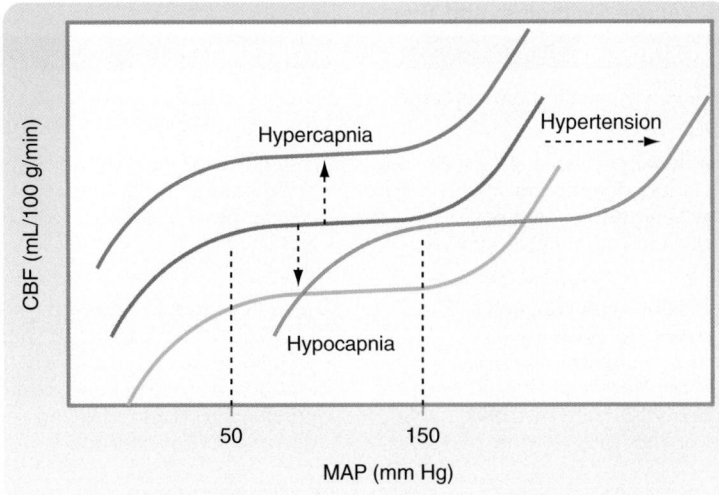

Figure 72-1 Cerebral blood flow (CBF) as a function of mean arterial pressure (MAP). Note the upward and downward shifts with hypercapnia and hypocapnia, respectively. The curve is shifted to the right with chronic hypertension.

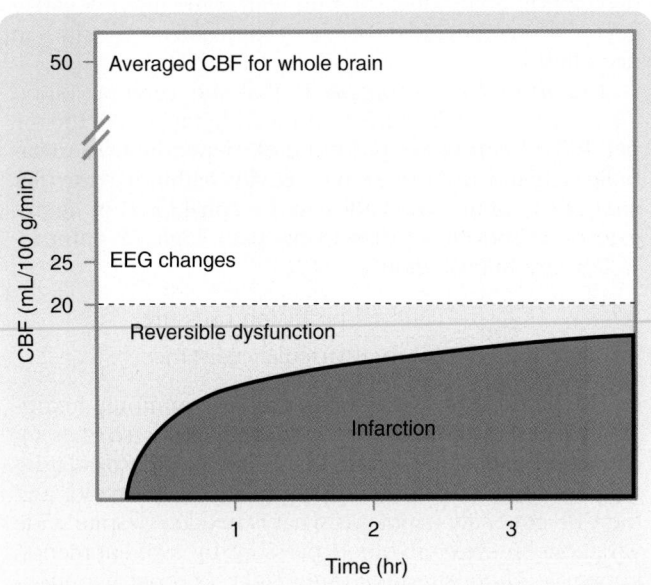

Figure 72-2 Electroencephalogram (EEG) changes, reversible injury, and infarction seen with cerebral blood flow (CBF) changes as a function of time.

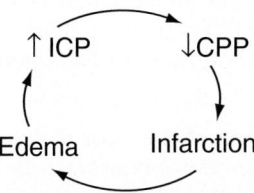

Figure 72-3 The vicious cycle. CPP, cerebral perfusion pressure; ICP, intracranial pressure.

increase blood pressure or decrease ICP may be urgently needed. When time permits because the dysfunction fluctuates chronically, it may sometimes be appropriate to measure O_2 extraction ratios as one index of the overall adequacy of the CBF. At low CBFs, O_2 extraction is increased with lower venous PO_2. It is interesting to note that the variations in CBF and extraction ratios related to neuronal activity are said to underlie the ability to image function by functional magnetic resonance imaging (MRI), a technique that is finding wider usage in the clinical neurosciences.

A *fourth principle* derives from the other three and the fact that injured tissue swells, making obvious the poten-

tial for a cascading injury by a vicious cycle (Fig. 72-3). If the stage of compensation mentioned earlier, even with therapy, is exceeded and ICP is elevated high enough by whatever mechanism so that cerebral perfusion pressure (CPP) declines, CBF can decline to levels where tissue injury occurs.

Cerebral perfusion pressure (CPP)=
    mean systemic arterial pressure (MAP)−ICP

Brain edema swelling within the closed cranium will lead to further increases in ICP with even further decreases in CPP in a stage of decompensation. When the capacity for autoregulation is exceeded or damaged so that it can no longer play a role, the CBF is linked directly to the CPP.

In the management of intracranial pathology, ICP and CPP are easy to measure continuously and thus serve as highly practical surrogates for the more fundamental, but much more difficult to measure, CBF. Clearly, however, these are not equivalent, and the limitations these parameters have in guiding therapy need to be kept in mind. Regardless of causation, when concern arises about the possibility of cascading injury, every effort is made to keep the CPP in the 60 to 80 mm Hg range and the ICP below 20 to 25 mm Hg if possible.

A *fifth principle* concerns focal mass effect and its progression within the complex anatomy of the cranial cavity. The cranial cavity is not just a hollow spherical space but contains several almost knifelike projections of folded dura, the falx and tentorium, which divide the cavity into a right and left supratentorial compartment and an infratentorial compartment, the posterior fossa. The sphenoid wing is a prominent, mostly bony ridge that separates the anterior fossa containing the frontal lobe from the middle fossa containing the temporal lobe. A narrow opening, the incisura, edged by the tentorium, surrounds the midbrain and is the only passage between the supratentorial and infratentorial compartments. Apart from the small openings for the cranial nerves and arteries, the foramen magnum is the only sizable opening from the cranial cavity as a whole.

The condition that classically illustrates the expanding mass lesion is the acute epidural hematoma, seen after trauma with skull fracture. Regardless of the source, however, the progression can be similar and has been dubbed *rostrocaudal decay* to reflect the early and late stages as listed in order below:

Focal distortion only
Effacement of gyri and sulci
Compression of the lateral (or other) ventricle
Midline shift
Subfalcial herniation
Temporal lobe tentorial herniation
　Third nerve compression (unilateral dilated pupil)
　Obliteration of basal cisterns
　Midbrain compression
　Midbrain infarction, Duret's hemorrhages (both pupils dilate with irreversible damage to midbrain)
Further brainstem compression
　Loss of brainstem reflexes
　　Progression from flexor posturing to extensor posturing
　　Vestibulo-ocular and oculocephalic reflexes
　　Corneal reflexes
　Medullary compression syndrome
　　Respiratory reflexes
　　Vasomotor reflexes, Cushing's reflex with elevation of the systolic blood pressure, widening of the pulse pressure, and bradycardia.
Foramen magnum herniation

At stages beyond tentorial herniation, it is unusual for focal mass effects not to be accompanied by an overall increase in ICP. The point at which focal mass effect evolves to include a rise in overall ICP depends largely on the compliance within the cranial cavity. Young patients with so-called tight brains can develop raised ICP even with relatively small volumes of mass that produce only effacement of the cortical gyri. On the other hand, patients with advanced cerebral atrophy can, for example, tolerate large frontal intracerebral hematomas or chronic subdural hematomas with compression of the lateral ventricle and midline shift while maintaining tolerable ICP and a surprising degree of intact neurologic function.

The Glasgow Coma Score (see Traumatic Brain Injury, later) provides a clinical functional measure of the degree of mass effect and advanced raised ICP. Although it is a good, standardized functional measure of the more advanced stages of mass effect or raised ICP, it was never really intended to be focused on the more subtle functional changes that might be seen at the earliest stages.

A *sixth principle* concerns the separateness of the phenomenology of the following:

1. Focal mass effect (as described earlier)
2. Diffuse raised ICP
3. Ventriculomegaly (enlargement of the cerebral ventricles)

Although these three processes often occur in combination, the notion that they are separable comes from the observation that there is a pure form of each. The ability to recognize these separate phenomena clinically is not an esoteric exercise but is often useful in deciding priorities in diagnosis and treatment. This requires some explanation. The pure form of raised ICP (without focal mass lesion, and without enlargement of the ventricular system) is a condition known as *pseudotumor cerebri,* whereas the pure form of ventriculomegaly is a condition known as *normal-pressure hydrocephalus* (NPH). The pure form of the focal mass lesion without either increased ICP or ventriculomegaly is quite common and occurs with tumors too small to raise ICP on their own and not situated to cause interference with CSF pathways. Instead, such focal mass lesions are typically discovered incidentally or because of symptoms from focal neurologic deficit or seizure disorder.

Normal ICP varies over a wide range, with generally accepted values between 0 and 20 mm Hg. *Diffuse raised ICP,* in the fully evolved pure form, results in a clinical picture that may include *symptoms* of headache, nausea and vomiting, double vision, and obscurations of vision. The accompanying clinical *signs* may include papilledema and sixth cranial nerve palsy with lateral rectus weakness and side-by-side diplopia, initially worse on far vision or gaze directed toward the side of the palsy. The papilledema is a mostly chronic phenomenon and is not seen acutely. The sixth nerve palsy of raised ICP can occur regardless of the cause of the increased ICP and does not imply direct involvement by a mass lesion, large or small, on the sixth nerve. In this situation, the sixth nerve palsy is a false localizing sign. With raised ICP, there may also be obscurations of vision, in which patients report the vision temporarily fades or becomes gray in combination with headache. Again, these obscurations are due to the effect of diffusely increased ICP on the sensitive optic nerves. They do not imply the presence of a focal mass lesion directly affecting the optic nerves or pathways. Intuitively, it seems that if there is a slow increase in a process raising ICP, the pressure would also rise slowly and evenly in pace with the evolving process. However, as first shown by Lundberg in 1960, the intermediate stages of decompensation are characterized by transient pronounced elevations in ICP (to 60 mm Hg) that characteristically plateau for up to 45 minutes and then cycle down again transiently to a more normal range.[3]

The archetype of this condition of chronic diffuse raised ICP is known by the old term *pseudotumor cerebri*

Table 72-2 **Intracranial Hypertension Syndromes**

RAISED INTRACRANIAL PRESSURE	SMALL MASS LESION	LARGE MASS LESION	VENTRICULOMEGALY	ARCHETYPE
+ + + +	0	0	0	Pseudotumor cerebri
0	0	0	+ + + +	Normal pressure hydrocephalus
+ + +	0	0	+ + + +	Typical hydrocephalus, communicating or noncommunicating, requiring shunt or ventriculostomy
+ + + +	+	0	+ + + +	Small tumor such as colloid cyst obstructing the foramen of Monroe
+ + +	+	0	0	Subdural empyema in which widespread inflammatory cerebral swelling dominates over the small mass of empyema itself
+ + +	0	+ + +	0	Frontal brain tumor reaching large size because the local effects are on "functionally silent" brain
0	+	0	0	Typical small tumor with only focal mass effect and focal dysfunction or seizure disorder

or the more descriptive *idiopathic intracranial hypertension.* Because it is often not benign (causing disabling chronic headache and visual loss sometimes even to permanent blindness), the term *benign intracranial hypertension* is falling out of favor. The basis for the condition is not entirely understood. It occurs most commonly in obese young women. Treatment is with acetazolamide diuretics, steroids, and intermittent lumbar puncture. Severe cases with threatened permanent visual loss may require CSF shunt, lumboperitoneal or ventriculoperitoneal, or optic nerve fenestration in which the meninges around the optic nerves are opened to vent CSF in the orbit.

Pure *ventriculomegaly,* specifically enlargement of the lateral ventricles, is characterized by gait disturbance and incontinence early in the clinical picture. As the process worsens, cognitive disturbances may be added on. The early appearance of gait disturbance and urinary incontinence is attributed to dysfunction of the medial cerebral hemispheres where the leg area of the primary motor cortex and the bladder control area reside. Nerve fiber pathways inside the brain must pass around the lateral ventricles to reach these areas on the medial hemisphere and therefore are especially vulnerable to pressure or distortion by the enlarged ventricle. This syndrome is called *NPH.* The usual diagnostic difficulty is in differentiating the condition from cerebral atrophy. Ventricular enlargement more prominent than enlargement of the CSF subarachnoid spaces over the cerebral convexity is typical in NPH. The clinical impression that gait disturbance and incontinence occur early and predominate over dementia is considered an important feature of NPH. Treatment is with CSF shunt (either lumboperitoneal or ventriculoperitoneal). The differentiation between NPH and cerebral atrophy is important because of the increased risk for subdural hematoma with shunting in cerebral atrophy.

Table 72-2 summarizes the relationships among ICP, mass lesions, and ventriculomegaly.

Table 72-3 **Cerebral Vascular Disease**

Congenital
Arteriovenous malformation and fistula
Cavernous malformation
Telangiectasis
Venous anomaly (angioma)

Acquired
Traumatic
Some arteriovenous fistulas (type I carotid cavernous fistula)
Traumatic aneurysm
Some arterial dissections

Degenerative
Atherosclerotic, occlusive disease
Most cerebral ("berry") aneurysms
Some arterial dissections
Spontaneous intracerebral hemorrhage

Infectious
Mycotic aneurysms

Idiopathic
Moyamoya
Some arteriovenous fistulas: the dural arteriovenous malformation–like, or type 2 carotid cavernous fistula

CEREBROVASCULAR DISORDERS

Cerebrovascular disorders encompass a host of disorders, both congenital and acquired, as outlined in Table 72-3.

Arteriovenous Malformation and Fistula

In the early embryo, the circulatory system does not yet have capillaries between the arterial and venous sides. Instead, there are vascular channels on the order of 200 μm in diameter that must undergo further development and maturation to form the capillary bed. There is reason to believe that when this does not occur perfectly, a focal failure of maturation can lead to a nidus of persistent embryonic, low-resistance vessels connecting the arteries and veins. Over time, the high blood flow in these circuits leads to secondary changes enlarging the nidus as well as the afferent arteries and efferent veins, often to impressive proportions. The high flow in the nidus, afferent, and efferent vessels predisposes to degenerative events, sometimes with aneurysm formation, causing hemorrhage, either intracerebral, subarachnoid, or both. Brain tissue at the edge or intermixed with the abnormal vessels may develop dysfunction to become an epileptic focus, or less commonly, progressive ischemic deficits occur as the low-resistance AVM draws blood flow away from adjacent areas with normal vascular resistance.

It follows that AVMs can have a wide variety of configurations and sizes, depending on which part or parts of the vascular bed fail to mature, and which consequences of the increased flow occur over time. If the venous outflow is restricted, the venous side of the complex may enlarge disproportionately and form a venous varix, of which the so-called vein of Galen "aneurysm" is the prime example. Here the vein of Galen, restricted by the downstream outflow limitations of the stiff dura-contained straight sinus, dilates, sometimes to massive proportions, and can cause obstructive hydrocephalus in the newborn, often together with high-output heart failure. More commonly, the venous outflow channels enlarge to a moderate degree and become thickened in the vessel wall, or arterialized. They do not, as a rule, cause symptoms by mass effect.

Clinical presentation is most commonly that of a hemorrhagic stroke picture, typically either intracerebral or subarachnoid hemorrhage, or some combination thereof. The patient complains of sudden-onset severe headache with or without focal neurologic deficit, and with or without meningismus. These symptoms can occur in all degrees of severity, but are less commonly fatal than after aneurysmal subarachnoid hemorrhage into the basal cisterns. Investigation usually begins in the emergency department with a computed tomography (CT) scan showing the hemorrhage. MRI or magnetic resonance angiography (MRA) studies typically follow, often showing enlarged afferent and efferent vessels. The role of CT angiography is evolving. Regardless of the mode of presentation, diagnosis is ultimately made by conventional catheter cerebral angiography (Fig. 72-4) and is based on demonstration of arteries and veins on the same conventional angiographic image, proving the high-flow shunting of blood through the nidus network or fistulous vessels. In an arteriovenous fistula, the shunting occurs through short, sparse, larger-diameter channels such that a cloud-like nidus of smaller vessels is not evident. Instead, the enlarged afferent arteries appear to connect directly with the enlarged efferent veins. In the typical AVM, there is a cloudlike nidus, or network of smaller vessels, well seen on angiography and not necessarily fully appreciated on MRI or MRA. The AVM can occur in all locations and with all degrees of size, complexity, and compactness.

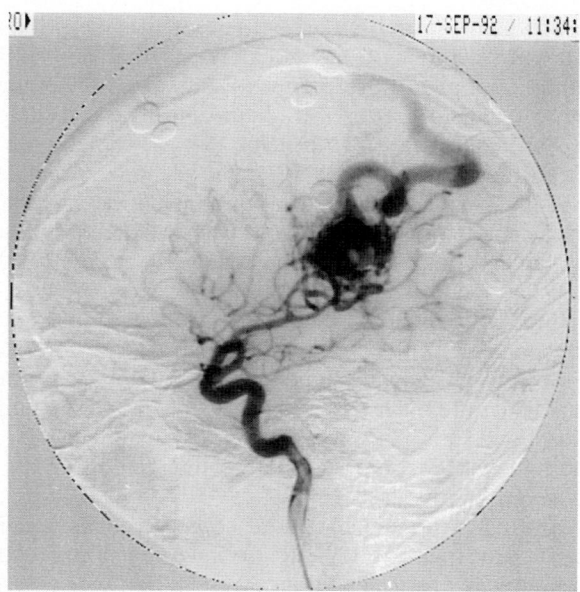

Figure 72-4 Subtracted carotid angiogram shows an arteriovenous malformation fed by the middle cerebral artery and drained by a superficial vein into the superior sagittal sinus.

When the patient presents with new-onset seizure, the next most common presentation, the investigation typically begins with brain MRI showing enlarged afferent and efferent vessels. The MRI, however, may not suggest the diagnosis if the afferent and efferent vessels are not grossly enlarged; however, this is rare in lesions presenting with seizure. Again, definitive diagnosis is with conventional catheter angiography, but this may sometimes be omitted if the diagnosis is sufficiently suggestive on MRI alone and there is reluctance to consider surgery with only anticonvulsant treatment planned.

It is important to pay attention to the nidus or fistula as the prime mover of the process and realize that the secondary changes in the afferent and efferent vessels, however impressive they may seem, will generally revert to normal once the nidus or fistula is resected or occluded. The assessment of AVM size refers to the size of the nidus and not the conglomeration of large feeding or draining vessels.

Therapy can fall into one or a combination of three categories: surgical excision; endovascular embolization of the nidus; or stereotactic radiosurgery. The decision to embark on any treatment depends on the assessment of the patient's treatment risk in comparison with the natural risk. Thanks to the work of Ondra and colleagues,[4] the natural risk is fairly well characterized. Hemorrhage occurs with a frequency of about 4% per year, and because only about 25% of these are severe with permanently severe disability or death, the catastrophe risk is only about 1% per year. The treatment risk, therefore, must be favorably low to justify action in most situations, and delays in treatment to allow for patient acceptance and to optimize the circumstances for therapy are understandable and reasonable. The main reason to recommend treatment is that the treatment may offer a lower risk over the long term. Younger patients have the most to gain by such an assessment. It may be possible to define features of individual AVMs that adjust the natural risk upward or downward, but so far these have been difficult to prove, and for the purposes of clinical decision making, the hemorrhage risk is generally taken "across the board" for all AVMs as a starting point. An across-the-board assessment of treatment risk, however, is clearly not warranted because each AVM is as unique as a finger print. Size, location relative to access by the treatment method considered, and location relative to proximity to deficit-prone brain structures are all important variables to consider. Another feature is the compactness of the AVM, with some forming a tightly clustered nidus with little brain tissue in between, and others being diffuse and rambling with scattered small clusters of nidus vessels encompassing large intervening areas of functional brain.

Obviously, the smaller, more compact AVMs located superficially in areas of "silent" brain function are the most attractive for open surgical resection. Diffuse, large AVMs encompassing deficit-prone areas of brain are least attractive to open surgery and other methods. Spetzler and Martin[5] devised a grading system for assessing risk with open operation. However, any decision is ultimately based on how an individual neurosurgeon assesses the risk for that unique AVM in that unique patient with his or her limits of risk tolerance. Surgical excision is carried out by craniotomy and almost always with microsurgical technique. The lesions are evident at operation as a bright-red blood–containing network of vessels. Feeding arteries are thicker walled than the generally larger, thinner-walled draining veins. Nidus vessels are thin, bright red, and very thin walled, such that they resist coagulation. This feature makes it important to remain just at the edge of the lesion if at all possible. Entry into the AVM nidus results in vigorous bleeding, which is time-consuming to control. Recent innovations in surgical therapy include the more common use of "frameless stereotaxy" or "neuronavigation," which allows more accurate localization and definition of the margins and important feeders and draining veins. Also, newer bipolar cautery instruments with advanced nonstick features have been helpful. A risk of open surgery is the unintended occlusion of vessels passing through the lesion to supply important functional areas of brain. Also, there is the potential to inadvertently leave part of the nidus behind, leaving the hemorrhage risk unpredictable. A postprocedure angiogram is essential to perform, either at the end of the procedure or as soon as possible thereafter. Residual AVM is addressed as soon as practical. Another category of concern is with hemorrhage resulting from a sudden increased blood flow at the periphery of the resected lesion, exceeding the limited autoregulatory capacity there. For the larger, more complex AVM, intentionally staged surgery is sometimes an option and is probably reasonably safe as long as with each stage, the remaining venous drainage of the AVM stays in balance with its residual afferent blood supply.

Stereotactic radiosurgery (SRS) is most attractive for small (<2.5 cm diameter), deep lesions that are difficult to access by open surgery. The method has the obvious attraction that hospitalization and craniotomy can be avoided, and patient acceptance is often high. Size of the nidus is the major limitation, however, such that the smaller the nidus, the higher the dose of radiation that can be given safely, and the more effective the treatment is likely to be. Negative considerations are that the radiation is not immediately effective, and the risk for hemorrhage during the latent interval must be factored in. About 60% of treated AVMs will obliterate in 1 year, and about 80% are expected to do so by 2 years. The obliteration rate is probably higher in younger patients and in those with nidus vessels of smaller diameter. The larger normal vessels generally escape obliteration by SRS even when passing through the treatment volume to supply distant areas of brain. However, this may also mean that the more fistulous type of AVM with sparse large-diameter nidus channels is less likely to be treated successfully. When an AVM reacts to SRS, there may be a period of edema in the surrounding or intervening brain. Most often, the edema evident by MRI is not symptomatic. However, the edema can be quite extensive and sometimes is temporarily disabling for up to several months. Steroids may be helpful in this setting. Seizures may also be more likely during a reactive interval and require upward adjustments of anticonvulsant medication, but the eventual seizure risk is not increased. Overall risk for permanent neurologic deficit with SRS is low, on the order of a few percent, when pooling large numbers of patients. But, as with other modalities of treatment, the risk for permanent deficit is dependent on proximity to deficit-prone structures. The optic nerves and chiasm and the brainstem are particular concerns with radiation. It is safest not to target lesions within 5 mm of the optic pathways, and this limits its application in treating parasellar or pituitary lesions.

Endovascular therapy is a rapidly evolving field, making it difficult to assess in terms of predicting actual patient outcomes with currently available methods. Whatever criticisms apply currently may be overcome with newer methods, but that remains to be proved. It is increasingly being carried out by neurosurgeons, although the familiarity with catheter angiography has made it largely the domain of the interventional neuroradiologists. Endovascular therapy has the allure of avoiding open surgery, but the likelihood of obliterating an entire AVM by this method alone is currently limited. To be effective in any permanent way, the embolic material must reach the nidus vessels but not pass readily through to the venous side. This can be more difficult than would seem intuitive because the diameter of the nidus vessels may not be uniform. Initially, the high blood flow to the nidus draws the embolic material to it, but as the nidus progressively occludes, the embolic material is progressively more likely to reflux into normal vessels, and the risk for stroke increases. The method is safest in situations in which there is a long segment of feeding vessel dedicated to the AVM because then reflux to the normal circulation is less likely. As with any endovascular technique, some areas of the circulation are easier to access than others. The method can be effective alone in treating the smaller, more fistulous lesions with single feeding and draining vessels. Such lesions are rare, however, and the method is more often used to reduce the size or complexity of an AVM just before open surgical resection. Afferent vessel occlusion alone without penetration of the nidus is not effective in any other context, however. Over time, an occluded feeding vessel recruits a network of replacement channels that may make it even more difficult to treat definitively. When used in conjunction with radiosurgery, the embolic material must reach the nidus, reducing the nidus volume permanently in a dimension, making radiosurgery of the remainder more effective. Risks for permanent deficit with embolization have been described as high as 5% per embolization session, but these numbers are based on older techniques. The problem with clinical decision making is that we do not know accurately the risks with evolving current techniques.

Cavernous Angioma (Cavernous Malformation)

The cavernous angioma is a highly characteristic, usually nearly spherical, discrete lesion, composed of a cluster of vascular sinusoids fed by small vessels in the arteriolar size range or smaller. Unlike the AVM, large feeding arteries and draining veins are not seen, and diagnosis by catheter angiography is not possible. The sinusoids are tightly compacted, and there is no intervening brain tissue (a diagnostic feature). At surgery, they often appear as a discrete mulberry-like collection of thin-walled vascular sinusoids with a greenish hemosiderin rim in the surrounding brain edge. When incised, bleeding from the lesion is minimal and easy to control, unlike the AVM, which bleeds vigorously if entered. The sinusoids often seem admixed with small chronic hematomas containing blood in various stages of decomposition. Many are older and contain birefringent yellow cholesterol crystals. Early autopsy studies[6] pointed out that they should be more common than recognized clinically. However, the lesions were not usually evident on CT or conventional catheter angiography available at that time. The clinical entity was not fully appreciated until the more widespread availability of MRI in the 1980s. The lesions are easily seen on MRI, where their appearance is diagnostic. They show a center containing some small, high-intensity signal foci surrounded by a null signal corona, dark on both T1- and T2-weighted images, that corresponds to hemosiderin deposition in the adjacent brain.

Like the true AVM, cavernous angiomas can present with symptomatic hemorrhage or new-onset seizures. Unlike AVM, they can also present as a slowly growing mass lesion. At least part of this growth appears to result from the accumulation of multiple small hemorrhagic foci in various stages of healing. The lesion can be particularly problematic in this manner when located in the brainstem. The hemorrhage frequency is not understood completely, in part because probably most hemorrhages are small and asymptomatic and not recorded as events. When located in the cerebral cortex or medial temporal lobe structures, they can be a focus of seizures. They can be solitary or multiple, incidental or symptomatic. The multiple form is more common in women and in persons of Latin American descent and has been linked to a specific gene on a specific chromosome. Cavernous angioma can appear de novo in patients with earlier completely negative MRI scans. Because of these features, cavernous angiomas occupy a position somewhere between congenital vascular malformation and vascular tumor. The term *angioma* probably reflects this tumor-like nature better than the term *malformation* and is preferred here for that reason.

Many lesions are followed conservatively with interval MRI scans for years without signs of activity. At the other extreme, they can sometimes bleed to produce a large, symptomatic or life-threatening intracerebral or brainstem hematoma, but that is relatively uncommon. The threat of such hemorrhage is generally not held out as a reason to operate, as it is for the true AVM. Surgical excision is usually reserved for lesions that are problematic, either because of hemorrhage, demonstrated growth, or seizures difficult to control with medication alone. Surgical excision is practical in most locations because of the distinct margins and minor bleeding encountered at operation. Lesions in the brainstem can pose major challenges, but even there, surgical resection is not ruled out as long as access can be achieved without needing to traverse crucial structures anticipated to produce major new deficit. Intraoperative ultrasound and either frame-based or frameless stereotaxy can be helpful in locating the lesions if small and situated in deep locations. Radiosurgery can be performed for these lesions but is not of demonstrated benefit. The hazards of radiosurgery in critical brainstem locations remain a concern.

Capillary Telangiectasia

The telangiectasis is composed of vascular channels with extremely thin walls reminiscent of dilated capillaries. These are usually grouped in small clusters with prominent intervening brain tissue as the rule. They are often clinically silent and generally do not appear on imaging studies. They are not evident on conventional catheter angiography unless large, and then only in the capillary venous phase. They clearly differ from an AVM in that flow through the lesion is not fast enough to demonstrate arteries and veins in the same conventional angiographic image. These lesions are not treated surgically.

Developmental Venous Anomaly ("Venous Angioma")

These lesions are composed of an abnormally configured venous drainage system converging on a single enlarged venous outflow channel. The typical appearance is that of a hydra with radially converging veins. A characteristic feature of this lesion appears to be that the abnormal venous bed is poorly collateralized. The abnormal venous drainage may or may not be fully adequate to the needs of the brain tissue supplied. Slowly evolving degenerative changes in the brain tissue supplied can occur as a result, but unfortunately, this is not helped by any known intervention. However inadequate, the venous anomaly represents the only venous drainage available to that area of brain, and it is for this reason that removal of the venous anomaly is not recommended. Doing so could lead to a venous infarction with swelling and hemorrhage, the consequences of which are particularly dangerous in the posterior fossa.

Traumatic Arteriovenous Fistula

Both the internal carotid artery and the vertebral artery enter the cranial cavity immediately after passing through a venous network. The internal carotid artery passes through the cavernous sinus, which communicates with the superior ophthalmic vein; the petrosal sinus; and the sphenoparietal sinus. The vertebral artery passes through a venous plexus at the occipital-C1 epidural space, which communicates with the jugular vein; the epidural venous plexus; and a paraspinal venous plexus. Trauma leading to a tear in either the carotid or vertebral artery at its tether point passing through the skull base can lead to fistula with the surrounding venous plexus. The consequences may vary in severity and suddenness but typically include periorbital swelling, with proptosis and scleral edema in the case of the carotid-cavernous fistula (CCF), and prominent pulsatile bruit in the case of the vertebral-jugular fistula. Intraocular pressure measurement by tonometry can guide the urgency in treating CCF. These lesions are usually treated by endovascular techniques. A catheter is advanced through the tear in the artery into the venous side of the fistula. The high flow and large fistulous channel facilitate this process. Embolic material, coil, or detachable balloon is then used to occlude the venous side of the fistula. Occasionally, neurosurgical assistance is required to provide access to the fistula for endovascular therapy.

Atherosclerotic Occlusive Disease

Patients with ischemic strokes are usually managed primarily by the medical service, often with consultation by the neurology service. In centers with an active "brain attack" approach, extraordinary efforts are made to diagnose the condition as promptly as possible and begin treatment with fibrinolytics when indicated. The faster the indications can be established and treatment started, the better the results are likely to be. Unfortunately the optimal therapeutic window between ischemic stroke onset and treatment is on the order of a few hours, and during that time, the patient must be transported to the emergency department, triaged, examined and assessed clinically, and investigated with at least a CT scan to rule out hemorrhagic stroke. Most stroke patients coming to the emergency department fall outside this window or have some contraindication to therapy. The challenges are even greater for patients who would be candidates for some early endovascular treatment.

The role of the neurosurgeon in the management of ischemic stroke is also evolving. The literature now clearly supports the use of large decompressive craniectomy for large ischemic strokes if performed early, well before swelling becomes symptomatic with raised ICP. Numerous reports point out that both survival and func-

tional outcome can be improved. Patient and family acceptance, however, is not high for a procedure of this magnitude under these circumstances, and often delays in both referral and family and patient decision making frustrate that potential for benefit. Resection of the infarcted cerebral tissue for decompression is generally not recommended in the supratentorial compartment.

A special consideration is the cerebellar hemisphere infarction. Here the swelling of the infarcted cerebellar hemisphere can be fatal from direct brainstem compression, whereas functional recovery is generally very good with decompression and resection of infarcted cerebellar tissue. Ventricular drainage is often begun before craniotomy but with some caution to the possibility of upward transtentorial herniation.

Because many strokes occur as artery-to-artery emboli, a search for a source is part of the evaluation. Carotid artery stenosis and vertebral artery stenosis are potentially amenable to endarterectomy or bypass. The indications are discussed in another chapter.

Cerebral Saccular ("Berry") Aneurysms

The saccular or "berry" cerebral aneurysms form as a degenerative change in the wall of the larger intracranial arteries in and around the circle of Willis. They are very rare in children, and occur with increased frequency in older age groups, sooner in patients with connective tissue defects, such as polycystic kidney disease, Marfan syndrome, and Ehlers-Danlos syndrome. The likelihood of having multiple intracranial aneurysms is estimated to be around 20%. The aneurysms form in relation to defects in the smooth muscle–containing media layer. Such defects are common at branch points in the arteries and can also occur in relation to shear forces at the edge of stiffened parts of the vessel wall containing atheroma. The defect in the media then allows the intima to stretch outward, fragmenting the internal elastic lamina in the process and carrying the connective tissue of the external adventitial layer outward with it. The connective tissue in the dilating intima and adventitia is capable of proliferation such that the aneurysm can reach a size considerably larger than stretching alone would allow. The Laplace equation predicts that at any given pressure, the stretching force on the wall of the aneurysm increases as the diameter increases. The process is therefore inherently not self-limited but progressive. With robust connective tissue proliferation in the wall, a minority of aneurysms enlarge to surprising dimensions, and hence the blood flow within slows to allow thrombus formation, usually in concentric layers to form a partly solid mass of much greater outer diameter than the lumen would suggest on angiography alone. Distal embolization of clot material is a rare occurrence. Calcification can occur in the wall in advanced cases, and the adjacent brain can become gliotic from chronic pressure, making seizures also a possible presentation. An enlarging aneurysm can also compress an adjacent cranial nerve, the optic and third nerves being most commonly affected by this mechanism. Overall, however, it is much more common for an aneurysm to present with subarachnoid hemorrhage. The proliferative ability of the connective tissue in the dome of the forming aneurysm can be exceeded by the stretching force leading to rupture. The onset is unpredictable and overall appears to occur at a surprisingly low rate. Incidentally discovered unruptured aneurysms bleed at a rate depending on size. Those smaller than 1 cm bleed at a rate of 0.05% to 0.5% per year, whereas those larger than 1 cm bleed at a rate of 1% to 2%. Treatment recommendations for unruptured aneurysms smaller than 5 mm in diameter vary widely based on patient preference, aneurysm accessibility to treatment, and the surgeon's assessment of risk. Once hemorrhage from an aneurysm occurs, the situation changes dramatically. Bleeding of highly oxygenated arterial blood occurs suddenly into the surrounding CSF-containing subarachnoid space, which initially offers little back pressure. Aneurysmal subarachnoid hemorrhage can occur in all gradations of severity. In most patients, accumulated blood in the basal spinal fluid cisterns leads to a coagulum that spontaneously stops the bleeding. In 10% to 15% of patients, the bleeding is so severe at the outset that death occurs before even reaching a hospital. About 40% die following the initial hemorrhage but at a later stage. Rebleeding occurs with a peak incidence in the first 24 hours after the initial event. If the aneurysm is left unsecured, the rebleed rate is 20% in the first 2 weeks, 50% in the first 6 months, and thereafter 3% to 4% per year. Rebleeding is the principal cause of death, usually by raised ICP.

Subarachnoid hemorrhage with or without increased ICP sets in motion a series of problems that can cause complications and poor outcomes regardless of the technical success of treating the aneurysm itself. First, the blood can interfere with the spinal fluid circulation such that acute hydrocephalus contributes to raised ICP and reduced cerebral perfusion. The hydrocephalus is evident as ventricular enlargement on CT and can usually be readily treated with ventricular drainage. Second, the highly oxygenated blood coagulum surrounds the vessels traversing the subarachnoid space. Whereas usually these vessels enjoy an environment of clear, colorless CSF, they now are marinated in a broth of decomposing blood, triggering activation of lysosomal and proteolytic enzymes and generating chemically active free radicals. The smooth muscle coating of the otherwise intact vessels can become irritated to trigger vasospasm, at first reversible but in severe cases evolving to a damaged and swollen arterial wall with persistent luminal narrowing. The vessels eventually remodel over 3 to 6 weeks and return to a normal configuration, but all too often, ischemic deficits in the supplied brain occur in the interim. Unfortunately, such ischemic neurologic deficits are not rare and are the single major cause of serious morbidity after successful aneurysm treatment after subarachnoid hemorrhage. The blood coagulum eventually clears from the subarachnoid space but sometimes sets in motion a progressive slow fibrosis that results in delayed hydrocephalus, distinct from the early hydrocephalus caused by the coagulum itself. Treatment of the vasospasm includes elevating the blood pressure, blood volume, and cardiac output in an attempt to bring more blood flow past the narrowing in the vessels (Box 72-1). The calcium channel blocker

---

Box 72-1 Management of Vasospasm

Prevention of arterial narrowing
   Subarachnoid blood removal
   Prevention of dehydration and hypotension
   Calcium-channel blockers (nimodipine)
Reversal of arterial narrowing
   Intra-arterial papaverine
   Transluminal balloon angioplasty
Prevention and reversal of ischemic neurologic deficit
   Hypertension, hypervolemia, and hemodilution

---

nimodipine appears to reduce the incidence of ischemic deficits, probably through opening collaterals to the ischemic brain. Its direct effect on the vasospasm is still in question.

Investigation of patients with suspected aneurysmal subarachnoid hemorrhage begins with an assessment of the history. Because the hemorrhage occurs into the subarachnoid space and not in the brain tissue, there is usually not a focal neurologic deficit. Symptoms of sudden-onset headache with meningismus are classic and reflect a sudden rise in ICP and irritation of the basal meninges by the blood. In severe cases, the patient may be comatose or uncooperative. Report of a strokelike picture of sudden onset of neurologic signs and symptoms prompts a CT scan showing blood filling the subarachnoid cisterns (Fig. 72-5A). Because the hemorrhage can occur in all gradations of severity, the difficulty comes in recognizing the patient with the small "sentinel hemorrhage" who arrives in good condition with only the report of alarmingly severe sudden onset of headache. Headache from increased ICP may be only transient until compensatory mechanisms occur. Residual headache and neck stiffness from meningismus, although usually present, may not be impressive. A high index of suspicion is required in such patients. It is important to focus on the suddenness of the symptom onset rather than the severity because the reports of severity are more subjective or may be tainted by a strong psychological overlay of denial or exaggeration, or the headache caused by a very small hemorrhage may be dissipating to some extent naturally by the time the patient is finally assessed. If the headache onset is truly instantaneous or nearly so, lumbar puncture is usually advised in cases in which the CT scan is negative. Blood in the CSF with xanthochromia in the supernatant is diagnostic.

If the CT scan or lumbar puncture is positive for subarachnoid blood, the next step is usually conventional catheter cerebral angiography (see Fig. 72-5B). CT angiography with bolus intravenous (IV) contrast is becoming increasingly convenient and accurate, and thus its role is increasing. Newer scanners are capable of large numbers of simultaneous slices so that three-dimensional reconstruction with good registration and surprising detail is possible. With selections in density windowing, the relation of the aneurysm to any blood clot can also be visualized.

Treatment of a cerebral aneurysm can be performed in a variety of ways:

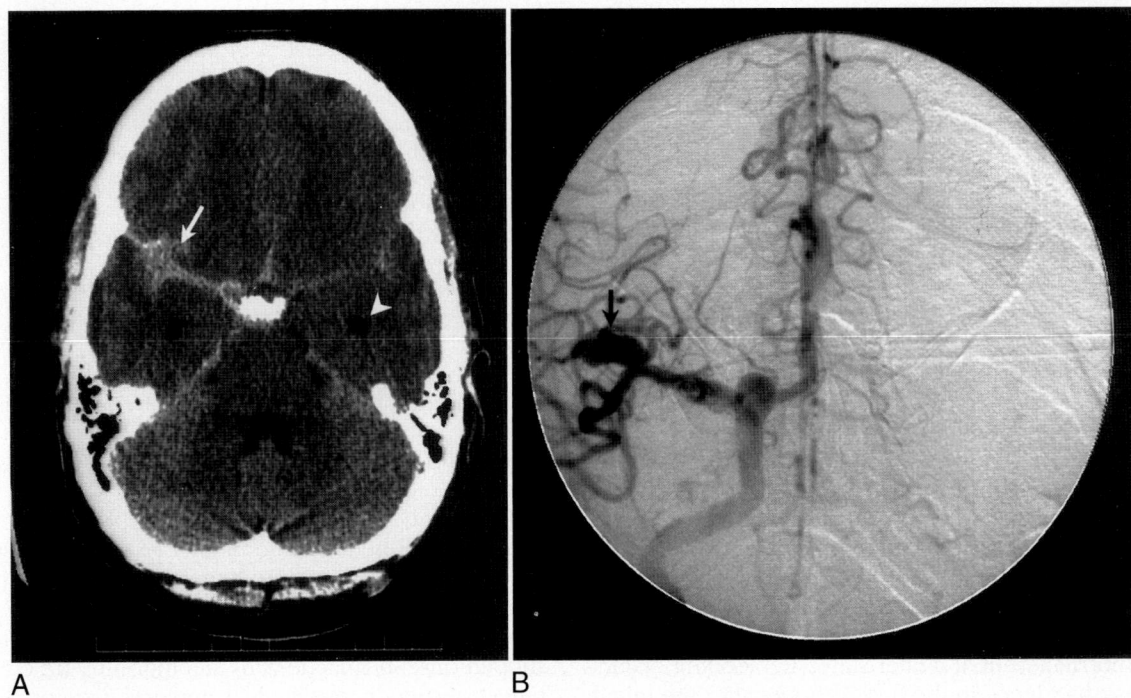

A   B

Figure 72-5 A, CT scan of brain showing subarachnoid blood in the basal cisterns. A focal deposition of blood in the distal sylvian fissure (*arrow*) suggests a middle cerebral artery aneurysm. Dilated temporal horns (*arrowhead*) indicate the presence of hydrocephalus. **B,** Cerebral angiogram shows a right middle cerebral artery aneurysm (*arrow*).

1. Open craniotomy with microdissection and clipping of the neck (Fig. 72-6)
2. Endovascular occlusion with detachable coil placement in the fundus (Fig. 72-7)
3. Elimination from the circulation by segmental occlusion of the parent artery proximal and distal to the aneurysm neck, with or without bypass

The segmental occlusion and bypass are usually reserved for those most awkward to treat by any other method. The choice of endovascular coil occlusion versus open surgical clipping has, on the other hand, become a complex issue.

In terms of the aneurysm configuration, a narrow neck is a favorable attribute for treatment by either open surgical clipping or endovascular embolization methods. Wide-necked or sessile aneurysms with a high neck-to-fundus ratio make it difficult to contain coils in the fundus without protrusion into the parent artery. A stent placed in the parent artery may provide a way around this problem, but the technology is evolving, and stenting is currently practical only in more proximal locations. Generally, wide-necked aneurysms gravitate toward open surgical treatment.

In terms of aneurysm location, it is probably fair to say that the more proximal the aneurysm, the easier it is to reach by endovascular means, whereas the more distal it is, the more difficult it is to reach and treat effectively by that method. Aneurysms in the cavernous sinus are considered difficult to reach by any open surgical method and are generally only treated by endovascular means, or parent artery occlusion with bypass. Aneurysms of the

internal carotid artery (ICA) at the level of the ophthalmic artery origin can be treated by open surgery or endovascular methods, as can most aneurysms of the ICA, proximal middle cerebral artery (MCA), and anterior cerebral artery (ACA) as far as the anterior communicating artery. The more distal MCA aneurysms, at the trifurcation in the sylvian fissure and beyond, and ACA aneurysms distal to the anterior communicating artery are more difficult to treat by endovascular methods and generally come to open surgical clipping. The basilar artery termination and midbasilar area can usually be reached easily by endovascular methods, whereas open surgery is possible but not attractive in these locations. The vertebral artery aneurysms can be reached easily by either method.

In situations in which the aneurysm location or configuration presents a clear advantage of one method over the other, the decision making is fairly easy, even at centers where all current methods are available.

The problems in decision making focus on aneurysms that are favorably situated and configured such that they would be attractive to treat by either open surgical clipping or endovascular coil occlusion. In the past, open surgical clipping was considered first, and the patient was referred for endovascular coil occlusion only if there were reasons to avoid open surgery. However, since the European prospective randomized trial of surgery versus open clipping, this paradigm is now open to question, and it is becoming increasingly common to consider endovascular treatment ahead of open surgical clipping in aneurysms attractive to treat by either method.[7] Increasingly, the patient is treated by a team approach in which all treatment methods are available and considered in

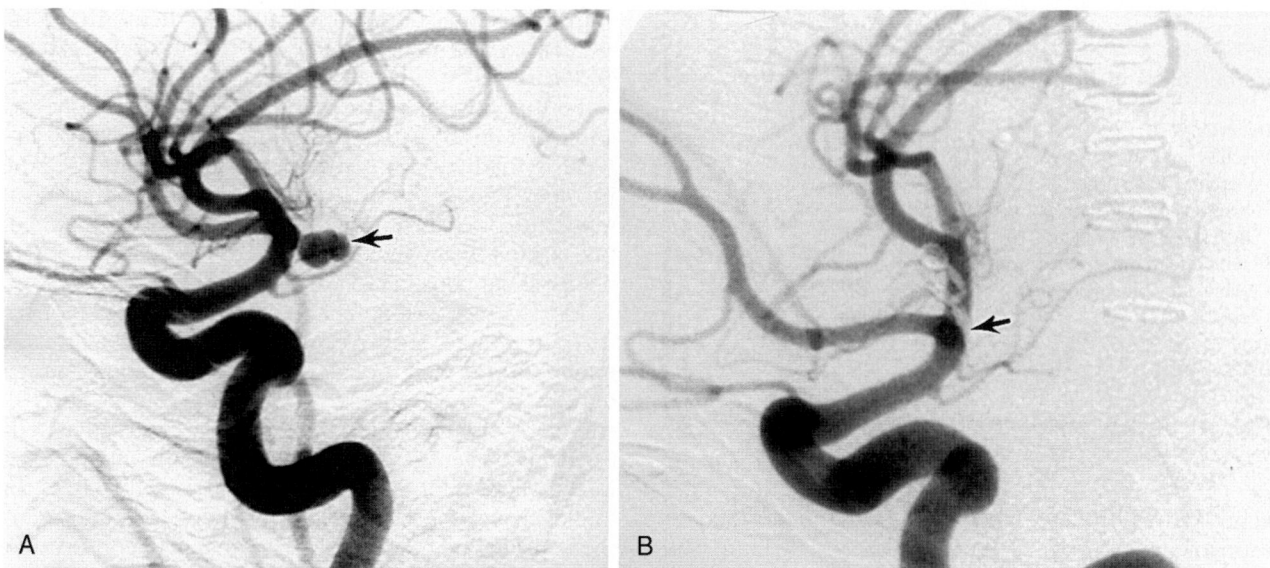

Figure 72-6 A, Subtraction carotid angiogram shows a 4-×6-mm berry aneurysm (*arrow*) originating from the distal internal carotid artery. **B,** Postoperative carotid angiogram shows clip placement (*arrow*) with total obliteration of the aneurysm.

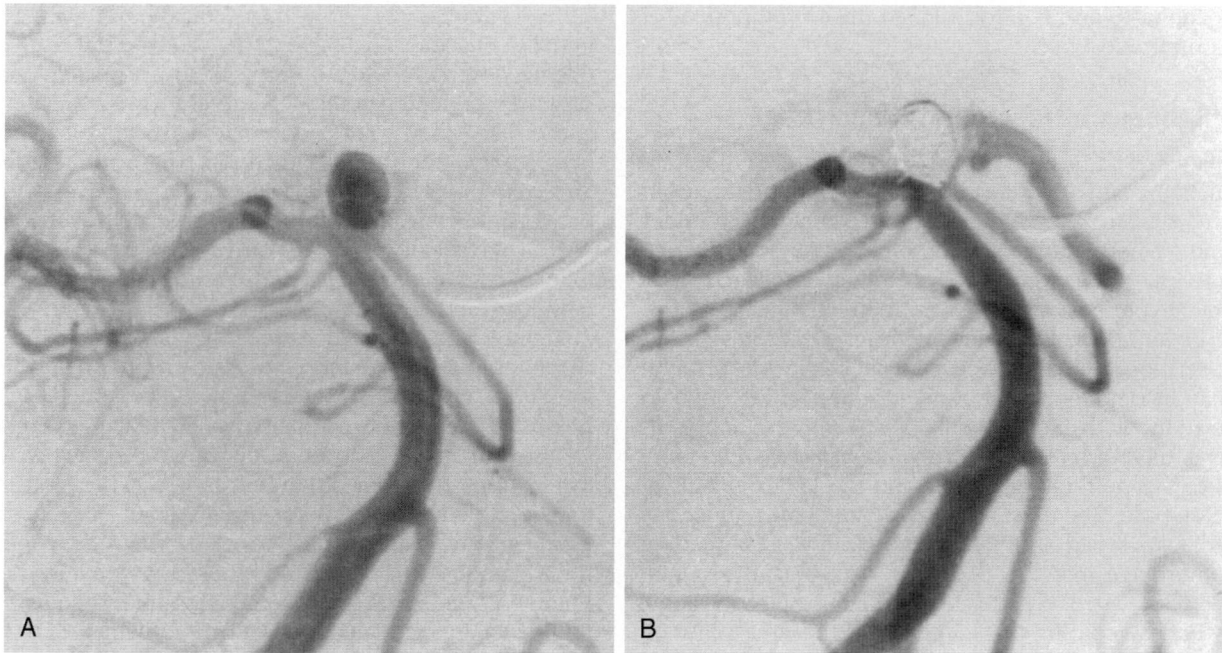

Figure 72-7 A, Subtraction vertebral angiogram shows a basilar tip aneurysm. **B,** Subtracted vertebral angiogram after the placement of coils demonstrates excellent obliteration of the aneurysm and preservation of adjacent vessels.

light of the patient's aneurysm location, configuration, general medical condition, and expressed personal or family preferences. Endovascular treatment avoids craniotomy, but an uncomfortable aspect remains with an aneurysm recurrence rate of 15% or higher. The recurrence rate after open surgical clipping appears to be much lower.

As for results, treatment of unruptured aneurysms is generally good, by whatever method, but these are usually a carefully selected group in whom conditions

for treatment are favorable, and most importantly, there is no aftermath of subarachnoid hemorrhage to overcome. These good results in patients with unruptured aneurysms, without subarachnoid hemorrhage, contrast markedly with the overall disappointing outcomes in patients with aneurysmal subarachnoid hemorrhage. Treated by whatever means, the opportunity for disabling ischemic complications from cerebral vasospasm and hydrocephalus are much higher in patients with subarachnoid hemorrhage. Patients with aneurysmal subarachnoid hemorrhage who present at the hospital in reasonable condition, at least awake and talking, still have only a 60% chance of returning home without functional deficit. The treatment contributes about 5% to the complications. Vasospasm and its comorbidities associated with prolonged treatment account for most of the rest. Infection from ventriculostomy needed to treat hydrocephalus and control ICP is a minor component of the complication rate.

Spontaneous Intracerebral Hemorrhage

Spontaneous intracerebral hemorrhages are into the brain parenchyma and are quite common, accounting for about 10% of all strokes. They are most common in older patients, where they usually come from degenerative changes in the cerebral vessels often associated with chronic hypertension (Box 72-2). In younger patients, they are more likely related to drug abuse or vascular malformation. They can occur anywhere in the cerebral circulation or brainstem but are classically described in association with very small degenerative aneurysms (known as *Charcot-Bouchard aneurysms*) at the junctions of the perforating vessels and the larger vessels at the skull base. The most typical are on the MCA junctions with the small perforating lenticulostriate vessels, leading to hemorrhage into the putamen. The clinical presentation is with a stroke pattern of sudden-onset neurologic signs and symptoms that depend on the area of brain affected. Symptoms are more likely to include headache than with ischemic stroke. The diagnosis is with CT scan, usually done in an emergency department setting. The size and location of the acute hematoma are well seen with CT as well as any associated brain shift or hydrocephalus (Figs. 72-8A and 72-9). In older patients with a well-known history of hypertension and a classic CT appearance of a hematoma in the putamen, thalamus, cerebellum, or pons, further diagnostic studies are usually not indicated. Rehemorrhage is unlikely in that setting. However, further investigation is probably warranted in cases of atypical hematoma location or appearance, especially if there is any component of subarachnoid blood. Also, investigation is usually recommended in younger patients without known hypertension and in patients

with a potential underlying cause for hemorrhage such as a history of neoplasm, blood dyscrasias, or bacterial endocarditis.

Further investigation is most commonly done with contrast MRI or MRA. Any suggestion of aneurysm or AVM is followed by conventional catheter angiography. In older patients with a history of early dementia and multiple episodes of more peripherally located intracerebral hematomas, the diagnosis of amyloid angiopathy needs to be considered.

Most cases of spontaneous intracerebral hemorrhage do not require surgery. Many hemorrhages are small enough to be well tolerated and do not require surgery. Others are devastatingly large at the outset such that surgery is of little benefit. Relief of any obstructive hydrocephalus by ventricular drainage is usually offered except in the most impossible cases. Patients who obey commands and can be monitored by changes in their neurologic exam are generally fit to manage conservatively with observation in hospital for at least 5 to 7 days. Peak swelling and decompensation are probably most likely to occur within that time frame. Surgery for evacuation of the hematoma may be appropriate in a small group of patients with intermediate-sized hemorrhages in accessible locations who appear to tolerate the hematoma initially but then deteriorate in delayed fashion with edema despite medical therapy. Steroids not have demonstrated benefit. Attempts to predict which patients will deteriorate based solely on hematoma volume have been frustrated by the broad spectrum of intracranial compliance exhibited by different patients. Generally, younger patients with smaller ventricles and small subarachnoid spaces have a lower compliance with lower tolerance than older patients with cerebral atrophy and generous ventricles and subarachnoid spaces.

If indicated, surgical evacuation is usually done by craniotomy over the most accessible part of the hematoma (see Fig. 72-8B). Intraoperative ultrasound is often helpful in finding hematomas that do not quite come to the cortical surface and in monitoring the progress of the evacuation. The goal of surgery is decompression more than complete removal but is usually done as far as safely practical. The wall of the hematoma cavity is inspected for any underlying cause, and biopsy is taken if indicated. Putamen hemorrhage can sometimes be evacuated with minimal surgical damage to the overlying brain by a trans-sylvian fissure, transinsular approach. Stereotactic aspiration and methods with fibrinolytic agents are under development and are especially a consideration for patients with hematomas in deep locations otherwise difficult to access.

A special situation to consider is the patient with cerebellar hemorrhage (see Fig. 72-9). Surgery is offered more readily in such cases because the danger of sudden deterioration from brainstem compression is more of a concern and because even extensive damage to the cerebellum itself is generally survivable with good functional outcome. Patients with fourth ventricular obstruction and hydrocephalus from cerebellar hemorrhage can sometimes be treated with ventricular drainage alone but more often are offered surgical evacuation of the hematoma

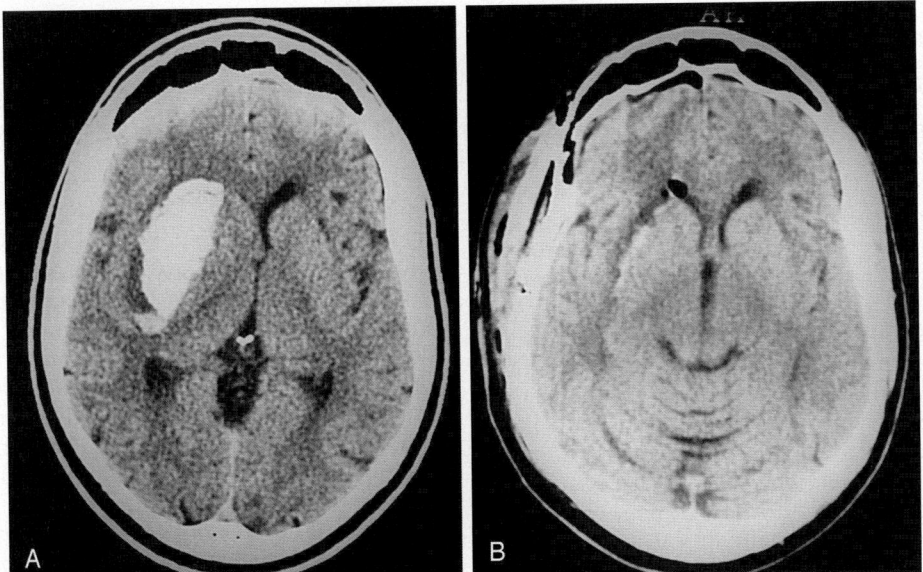

Figure 72-8 Nonenhanced CT scan of the head. **A,** Spontaneous hypertensive intracerebral hematoma in the non-dominant hemisphere. **B,** Immediate postoperative CT scan shows near-total removal of intracerebral hematoma.

by suboccipital craniotomy because of the risks for brainstem compression.

Mycotic Aneurysms

These aneurysms are associated with a systemic infection capable of showering small particles of bacterial infected material into the cerebral vascular bed. Subacute bacterial endocarditis and some pulmonary infections can do this. A distinguishing feature of these aneurysms is that they are generally found more distal in the cerebral vascular bed, as opposed to the berry aneurysms, which are usually found on larger vessels near the circle of Willis. They too can be multiple in nature. When the bacterial emboli lodge in distal cerebral arterial branches, they can erode through the wall of these smaller vessels, often creating a hemorrhage contained by the perivascular tissue. Of course, maximal antibiotic treatment is essential to begin with. The presence of an intracerebral hematoma may force immediate craniotomy for evacuation. Operation on the aneurysm at this early stage often reveals both a component of subarachnoid hemorrhage and an early inflammatory reaction in the subarachnoid space with only a blood collection covering the erosion defect in the wall of the small artery. Attempts to dissect and define a neck are frustrated by a lack of developed fibrous tissues and intraoperative hemorrhage is then common. Typically the diseased arterial segment must be occluded and resected when operated in this early stage. The need for arterial bypass to maintain blood flow to critical cerebral areas should be anticipated, but this is not always possible.

If the mycotic aneurysm or aneurysms are discovered or treated at some later stage, a fibrous wall to the aneurysm may have had time to develop, and clipping can then be a possibility, although the surgeon needs to be forewarned that it may be difficult to find the aneurysm

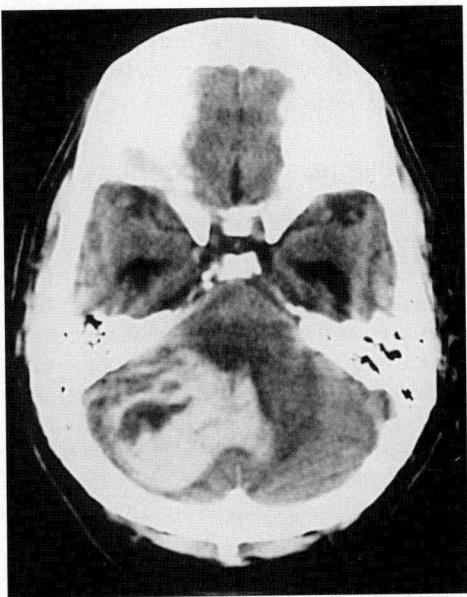

Figure 72-9 Nonenhanced CT scan of brain shows a large hypertensive intracerebellar hematoma with obstruction of the fourth ventricle and enlargement of the temporal horns indicating obstructive hydrocephalus.

in a distal location, often buried deep in a cerebral sulcus thickened with reactive fibrous scar tissue.

Moyamoya Disease

Moyamoya disease is a cerebrovascular disorder characterized by an idiopathic, nonatherosclerotic narrowing or occlusion of major intracranial blood vessels with the development of a conspicuous compensatory collateral rete vessel network allowing continued cerebral perfusion around the occluded or severely narrowed segment. The disorder is usually bilateral, although not necessarily exactly symmetrical. Although generally rare, the disease is more common in persons of Asian ancestry and was first recognized from cases studied with angiography in Japan before the advent of CT and MRI. The term *moyamoya* comes from the Japanese word for "puff of smoke" or mist. The true disease is sometimes confused with the less conspicuous collateral vascular networks seen around severe narrowing of common atherosclerotic origin in persons of Western origin. In the juvenile form, moyamoya typically presents as cognitive decline with deteriorating school performance with a multi-infarct picture. Angiography reveals the ICA, proximal MCA, or proximal ACA with severe narrowing or occlusion and usually multiple clusters of fine collateral vessels. In the adult form of moyamoya disease, the rete vessels cause subarachnoid or basal ganglia hemorrhage, the most common presentations. The hemorrhage can usually be treated conservatively. Some form of extracranial-to-intracranial bypass is usually offered in an attempt to take the load off the collateral vascular network. In the juvenile group, the results are good, with an onlay interposition of the superficial temporal artery sewed into the dura after a strip craniotomy. A feature of the disorder is the vigor with which collaterals form from the onlay transposed vessel. In the adult form, a microvascular anastomosis with the superficial temporal artery or grafted vessel may be preferred.

Dural Arteriovenous Malformations

Dural AVMs, of which the type 2 CCF is a subtype, are not seen with any frequency in juvenile patients. The lesions seem to occur only in adults and probably are acquired lesions that follow a dural sinus thrombosis usually of the cavernous sinus or the sigmoid-transverse sinus junction area. With subsequent healing, the thrombosed segment triggers a neovascular response that evolves to an AVM configuration with fistulous channels that can gradually enlarge. Usually there is associated stenosis of the affected dural segment, suggesting the earlier thrombosis. The lesions are generally not dangerous unless they produce retrograde venous drainage into the cerebral circulation. The risk for intracranial hemorrhage is then fairly high, and it is important to at least separate the dural AVM drainage from the cerebral circulation when that is appreciated to occur. In the case of transverse-sigmoid sinus dural AVM, the patient usually complains of a bruit, and embolization or resection is optional depending on symptom tolerance. In the case of type 2 CCF, the problem is usually intraocular and intraorbital venous hypertension, with proptosis, chemosis, and sometimes threatened vision. Ocular tonometry offers some measure of the threat to vision. Treatment of type 2 CCF involves endovascular embolization of prominent feeders followed by occlusion of the affected venous dural sinus. As long as the dural AVM drainage is separated from the cerebral circulation, occlusion of the affected venous drainage is safe and curative. The affected stenotic transverse-sigmoid sinus segment can be reached by endovascular techniques through the jugular vein. The cavernous sinus can be reached by the petrosal sinus or, with neurosurgical assistance, through the superior orbital vein.

CENTRAL NERVOUS SYSTEM TUMORS

Intracranial Tumors

Intracranial tumors can be classified in different ways: primary versus secondary, pediatric versus adult, by cell of origin, or by location in the nervous system. Primary tumors arise from tissues within the nervous system, whereas secondary tumors originate from tissues outside the nervous system and metastasize secondarily to the brain. They may represent local extension of regional tumors like chordoma or scalp cancer but, more commonly, may reach the nervous system through the hematogenous route.

In general, the incidence of primary brain tumors is higher in whites than in blacks, and mortality is higher in males than in females. According to the Central Brain Tumor Registry of the United States (CBTUS), the overall incidence of primary brain tumors was 14.8 per 100,000 person-years between 1998 and 2002 (CBTUS statistical report, 2005-2006). On the other hand, secondary tumors outnumber primary brain tumors by 10 to 1 and occur in 20% to 40% of cancer patients.[8] Because no national cancer registry documents brain metastases, the exact incidence is unknown, but it has been estimated that 98,000 to 170,000 new cases are diagnosed in the United States each year.[9]

Clinical Presentation

The clinical manifestations of various brain tumors can best be divided into those due to focal compression and irritation by the tumor itself and those attributed to the secondary consequences, namely increased ICP, peritumoral edema, and hydrocephalus. Most commonly, symptoms are caused by a combination of these factors.

The clinical presentation does not differ much by tumor histology but rather by rate of growth and location of the tumor. A meningioma peripherally located in a relatively silent area of the brain, with a slow rate of growth, may enlarge to a significant size in a neurologically intact patient because the brain can accommodate to a slowly growing lesion. On the other hand, a small metastatic lesion at the foramen of Monro or in the sensorimotor strip can cause acute hydrocephalus or seizures, respectively.

Headache occurs in 50% to 60% of primary brain tumors and in 35% to 50% of metastatic tumors. It is classically described as being worse in the morning, probably due to hypoventilation during sleep with consequent elevation of PCO_2 and cerebrovascular dilation. The headache is associated with nausea and vomiting in 40% of patients and may be temporarily relieved by vomiting, as a result of hyperventilation. Seizures may be the first symptom of a brain tumor. Patients older than 20 years presenting with a new-onset seizure are aggressively investigated for a brain tumor.

Infratentorial lesions may present with headache, nausea and vomiting, gait disturbance and ataxia, vertigo, cranial nerve deficits leading to diplopia (abducens nerve), facial numbness and pain (trigeminal nerve), unilateral hearing deficit and tinnitus (vestibulocochlear nerve), facial weakness (facial nerve), dysphagia (glossopharyngeal and vagus nerves), and CSF obstruction causing hydrocephalus and papilledema. Supratentorial lesions may present with different symptoms depending on the location. Frontal lobe lesions manifest as personality changes, dementia, hemiparesis, or dysphasia. Temporal lobe lesions may present with memory changes, auditory or olfactory hallucinations, or contralateral quadrantanopsia. Patients with parietal lobe lesions may develop contralateral motor or sensory impairment, apraxias, and homonymous hemianopsias, whereas those with occipital lobe lesions may show contralateral visual field deficits and alexia.

Radiology

The initial workup usually involves a relatively inexpensive diagnostic tool, namely a CT scan of the brain. CT scan provides a rapid means of evaluating changes in brain density like calcifications, hyperacute hemorrhages (<24 hours old), and skull lesions. MRI of the brain, however, is the gold standard modality for diagnosis, presurgical planning, and post-therapeutic monitoring of brain tumors. Gadolinium contrast enhancement with MRI is much more sensitive in demonstrating defects in the blood-brain barrier and localizing small metastases (up to 5 mm). It can be used in patients allergic to iodine and in those with renal failure. Recent advances in MRI technique have evolved from a strictly morphology-based imaging to one that encompasses function, physiology, and anatomy. Diffusion-weighted imaging can help in the distinction between gliomas and abscesses, and perfusion-weighted imaging can predict response to radiotherapy in low-grade gliomas. Functional MRI can be used in the planning of surgery for tumors in eloquent areas of the brain to enable radical resection with less morbidity. Diffusion tensor imaging can demonstrate the effect of a tumor on white-matter tracts. MRA is more routinely used as a noninvasive modality to evaluate the vascularity of a tumor or the anatomic relationship of a tumor to normal cerebral vasculature.[10]

Surgery

Dexamethasone is recommended in the management of brain tumors because of its propensity to reduce peritumoral edema by stabilizing the cell membrane. An antiepileptic drug is also recommended for tumors close to the sensorimotor strip.

A number of technical advances have made tumor surgery safer and more effective. The intraoperative microscope provides superior illumination and magnification, thereby allowing the surgeon to resect tumors from critical areas through small cranial openings. The cavitational ultrasonic surgical aspirator (CUSA) simultaneously breaks up and sucks away firm tumors while protecting vital neural and vascular structures. Intraopera-

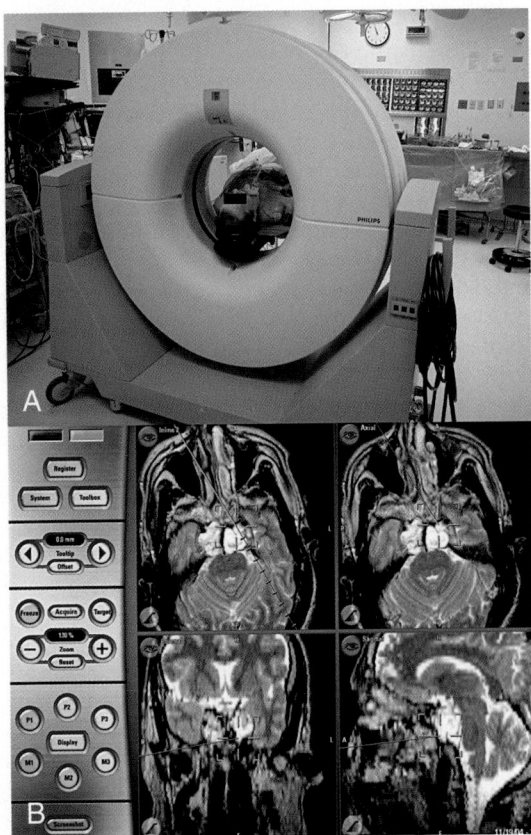

Figure 72-10 Technologic advances in the operating room. **A,** An intraoperative CT scan. **B,** Computer-guided surgical navigation showing real-time location of a surgical probe tip on the preoperative MRI study during resection of clival chordoma.

tive ultrasonography provides real-time images of tumors and cysts in subcortical and deep areas of the brain. Intraoperative CT or MRI is now standard practice in some centers, enabling on-table imaging of the extent of resection (Fig. 72-10A). CT and MRI also allow real-time visualization of a biopsy needle within a target. Image-guided (CT or MRI) frameless surgical navigation allows instant and accurate localization of the tip a probe during a craniotomy by displaying that point on a preoperative CT or MRI (see Fig. 72-10B).

The primary goals of surgery include histologic diagnosis and reduction of ICP by removing as much tumor as is safely possible to preserve neurologic function. The decision between a needle biopsy and a more radical surgical resection depends on the location and the size of the tumor, its sensitivity to radiation or chemotherapy, the preoperative Karnofsky performance score of the patient, and the systemic status of the primary cancer in case of metastatic brain lesions.

Primary Brain Tumors

Primary tumors of the brain are divided into intra-axial (those arising from within the brain parenchyma) or extra-axial (those arising from outside the brain parenchyma).

Intra-axial Brain Tumors

Intra-axial brain tumors develop from the glia, or supportive structures, of the neurons and are collectively called *gliomas*. Total surgical resection of gliomas is extremely rare because of their ability to infiltrate widely along the white-matter tracts and to cross the corpus callosum into the contralateral hemisphere. Radiation therapy and chemotherapy options vary according to the histology of the brain tumor. Therapy involving surgically implanted carmustine-impregnated polymer combined with postoperative radiation therapy has a role in the treatment of de novo and recurrent high-grade gliomas. Novel biologic therapies under clinical evaluation for patients with brain tumors include dendritic cell vaccination, tyrosine kinase receptor inhibitors, farnesyl transferase inhibitors, viral-based gene therapy, and oncolytic viruses. An ideal therapy will target rapidly growing malignant glioma cells along with infiltrating tumor cells, with minimal toxicity to normal cells. This will require the therapeutic vehicle of choice to have access to all cells in the brain and to be able to distinguish invasive or quiescent tumor cells from normal cells.[11]

The World Health Organization (WHO) classifies intra-axial brain tumors by cell type and grades them on a scale of I to IV based on light microscopy characteristics that include degree of cellularity, pleomorphism, mitotic figures, endothelial proliferation, and necrosis. The higher the grade, the more aggressive and malignant the tumor.

Astrocytoma

Astrocytomas arise from astrocytes and account for 50% of all primary brain tumors. Grade I astrocytomas, also called *pilocytic astrocytomas,* are a special group of tumors that are discrete appearing, contrast enhancing, and often cystic with a mural nodule. The mean age of occurrence is lower than for typical astrocytomas, usually in the first two decades of life. Patients have a median survival time of 8 to 10 years. Astrocytomas represent the most common glioma in children, representing 10% of cerebral and 85% of cerebellar astrocytomas. They tend to occur in the cerebellum, optic tract, and hypothalamus. These lesions are usually curable by radical resection. Radiation therapy and chemotherapy have no role in their treatment.[12]

Low-grade, or grade II, astrocytomas tend to occur in children and young adults. Most present with seizures. They typically demonstrate one histologic criterion, usually nuclear atypia; have a low degree of cellularity; and manifest preservation of normal brain elements. They appear hypointense on T1-weighted MRI sequence and hyperintense on T2, and fail to show contrast enhancement. The ultimate behavior of these tumors is usually not benign. Treatment is controversial and can include observant management and follow-up, radiation with or without chemotherapy, and surgery. Surgery is not curative because most of these tumors are infiltrative with no clear margins. The median survival time is 7 to 8 years.

Grade III (anaplastic) and grade IV (glioblastoma multiforme, GBM) astrocytomas are considered high-grade tumors. The presence of endothelial proliferation or necrosis on histology makes the tumor grade IV. A number of papers have suggested correlations between the presence of *p53* mutations on chromosome 17p and a number of findings, including increased likelihood of anaplastic progression, longer survival time, correlation with the presence of aneuploidy, young age at diagnosis, and correlation with subsets of GBM.[13] These tumors are seen in older patients (>50 years). Malignant astrocytomas may develop from low-grade astrocytomas by dedifferentiation. GBM is the most common primary brain tumor. Anaplastic astrocytomas tend to have irregular enhancement on MRI (Fig. 72-11), whereas GBMs will have ring enhancement with central necrosis (Fig. 72-12).

The optimal treatment includes a cytoreductive surgery followed by external-beam radiation therapy (EBRT) to a dose of 60 Gy. The extent of tumor resection has a significant effect on time to tumor progression and median survival. All chemotherapeutic agents in use have no more than a 30% to 40% response rate, and most have a 10% to 20% response rate.[14] Carmustine (BCNU) and cisplatin have been the primary agents used against malignant gliomas. More recently, temozolomide, an oral alkylating agent, has shown some promise in the management of newly diagnosed and recurrent GBM, with an overall survival time of 13.6 months.[15] Median survival time for anaplastic astrocytoma is 2 to 3 years, and for GBM, it is less than 1 year.

Oligodendroglioma

This tumor frequently presents with seizures, has a predilection for the cortex and white matter of the cerebral hemispheres (frontal lobe in 50%-65%), and has a classic histologic feature of "fried egg" cytoplasm, "chicken wire" vasculature, and microscopic calcifications. The most frequent genetic alterations include loss of heterozygosity (LOH) on chromosome 19q followed by LOH on chromosome 1p. These alterations are usually associated with a better prognosis.[12] Brain CT may show tumoral calcifications, and MRI findings are similar to those with the astrocytomas. This tumor is classified into low and high grade. Chemotherapy is the primary modality of treatment after an appropriate surgical resection. Median survival times ranging from 3 to 5 years have been reported for patient with oligodendroglial tumors of all histologic grades. Benefits of radiation therapy are controversial.

Ependymoma

These neoplasms arise from the ependymal lining of the cerebral hemispheres and from the remnants of the central canal of the spinal cord. They manifest predominantly in children (within the fourth ventricle) and young adults. MRI findings include a well-circumscribed lesion with varying degrees of enhancement. Ventricular or brainstem displacement and hydrocephalus are frequent features. Optimal treatment includes maximal possible resection without causing neurological deficits followed by EBRT (45-56 Gy). Ependymomas have the potential to spread through the neuraxis by seeding of the CSF; craniospinal radiation is recommended in this case.

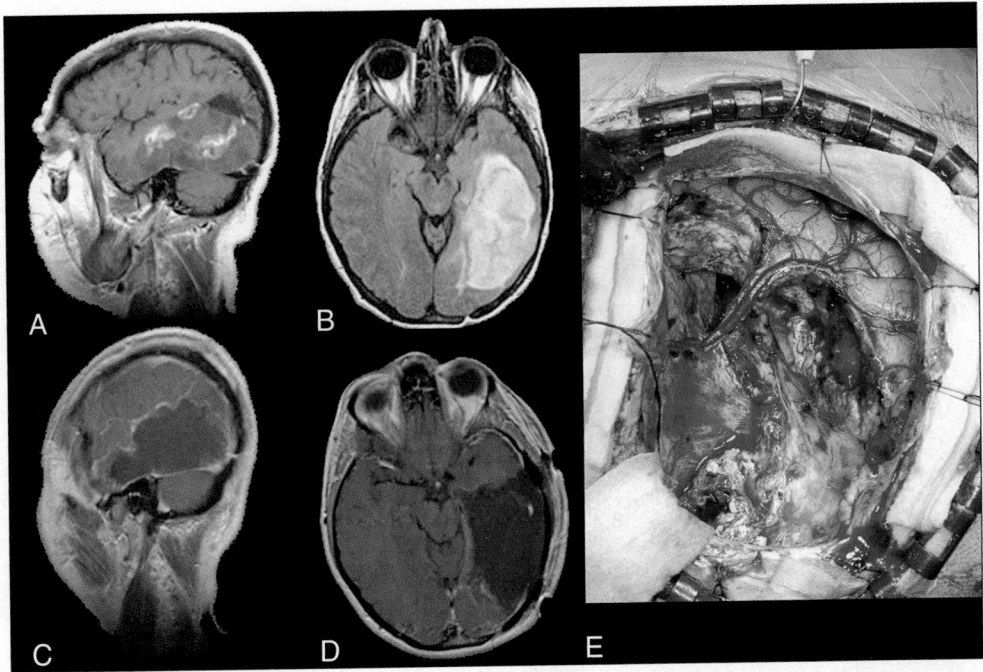

Figure 72-11 Radiographic and intraoperative pictures of a patient with a left temporal anaplastic astrocytoma. **A,** A partially enhancing tumor is noted in the left temporal lobe on this gadolinium-enhanced sagittal MRI study. **B,** FLAIR-sequence axial MRI shows the extent of the tumor. Postoperative gadolinium-enhanced sagittal (**C**) and axial (**D**) MRI showing near-total resection of the tumor. **E,** An intraoperative picture showing the surgical field after resection of the tumor.

Primitive Neuroectodermal Tumors

Primitive neuroectodermal tumors (PNETs) originate from primitive neuroectodermal cells (actual cell of origin is unknown) and encompass medulloblastoma (the most common PNET), retinoblastoma, pineoblastoma, neuroblastoma, esthesioneuroblastoma, and ependymoblastoma. These tumors also have a tendency to seed through the CSF. Medulloblastoma is the most common pediatric brain malignancy, usually arises in the roof of the 4th ventricle (often producing hydrocephalus), and may invade the brainstem. The treatment of choice includes maximal surgical debulking followed by craniospinal irradiation. BCNU and vincristine are primarily used for recurrences, in poor-risk patients, and in children younger than 3 years to avoid radiation therapy. Patients without a residual tumor on postoperative MRI and with negative CSF seeding have more than a 75% 5-year survival rate.

Hemangioblastoma

Hemangioblastoma represents the most common primary intra-axial tumor in the adult posterior fossa, is histologically benign, and may be associated with erythrocytosis. Hemangioblastomas may be solid or cystic with a mural nodule. They may occur sporadically, and 20% of cases may be associated with von Hippel-Lindau disease (hemangioblastomas, retinal angiomas, renal cell carcinoma, pheochromocytoma, renal and pancreatic cysts). These lesions may also occur in the brainstem and the spinal cord. The optimal surgical treatment involves

resection of the mural nodule in case of a cystic lesion (cyst wall need not be removed). Solid lesions tend to be more difficult to remove.

Primary Central Nervous System Lymphoma

The incidence of CNS lymphoma is rising relative to other brain lesions. This is in part due to the high frequency of CNS lymphoma in AIDS patients and transplant recipients. The median age at diagnosis is 52 years (younger in the immunocompromised population). It has a predilection for periventricular areas, deep nuclei, and the frontal lobes. It may also occur in the cerebellum. Primary CNS lymphoma is also known as *ghost-cell tumor* because of its tendency for partial to complete resolution on CT after the administration of steroids. A stereotactic needle biopsy is indicated when the index of suspicion for CNS lymphoma is high because these lesions are highly sensitive to radiation. In non-AIDS cases, chemotherapy combined with EBRT prolongs survival compared with EBRT alone. Without therapy, median survival time is 1.8 to 3.3 months. With radiation, median survival time is 10 months. In AIDS-related cases, the median survival time is only 3 to 5 months.

Extra-axial Brain Tumors

Meningiomas

Meningiomas can occur anywhere where arachnoid cap cells are found (surface of brain and cord, ventricles). They are slow growing, usually benign tumors, most

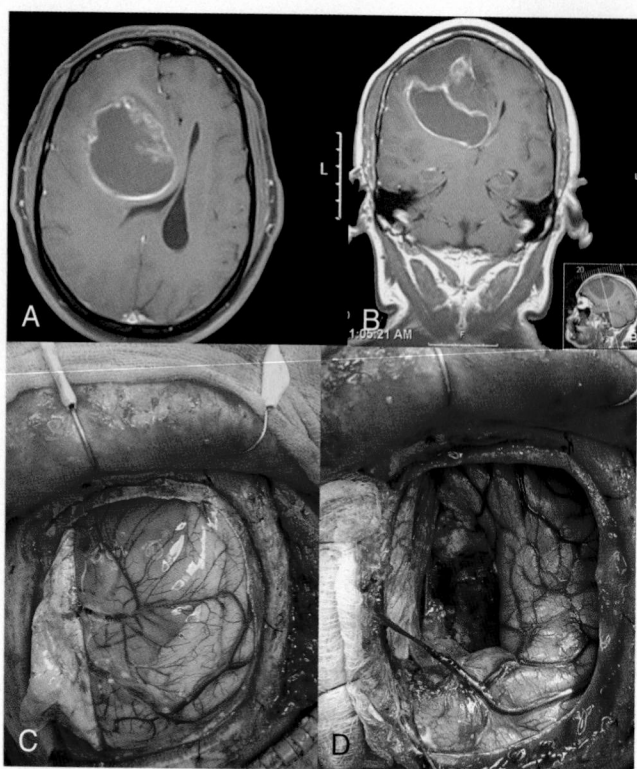

Figure 72-12 MRI and intraoperative pictures of a patient with a glioblastoma multiforme. Gadolinium-enhanced axial (**A**) and coronal (**B**) MRIs show a large tumor with ring enhancement causing a 1-cm subfalcine shift of midline structures. Intraoperative pictures show the yellowish tumor surrounded by normal brain gyri (**C**) and the surgical field after a resection of the tumor (**D**).

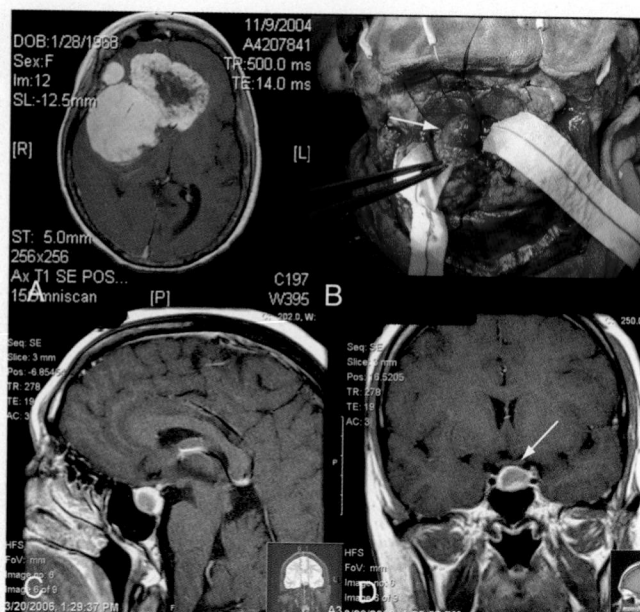

Figure 72-13 A, A large homogeneously enhancing meningioma can be seen in this gadolinium-enhanced axial MRI study. **B,** An intraoperative picture showing the dissection of the meningioma (*arrow*) from the surrounding gyri. Gadolinium-enhanced sagittal (**C**) and coronal (**D**) MRIs of a patient with a pituitary macroadenoma showing impingement on the optic chiasm (*arrow*).

commonly located along the falx, convexity, or sphenoid bone, and can cause hyperostosis of adjacent bone. They tend to occur more in women, with a peak incidence at age 45 years. In one series, 32% of primary brain tumors seen on imaging were meningiomas, and 39% of these were asymptomatic.[16] They are characterized histologically by the presence of psammoma bodies. Meningiomas appear isointense on T1- and T2-weighted sequences on MRI but enhance strongly and homogeneously (Fig. 72-13A). A dural tail is a common finding on MRI (Fig. 72-14A and B). Surgery is the treatment of choice for symptomatic meningiomas, with the extent of resection being the most important factor in the prevention of recurrence. Recurrence after gross total resection occurs in 11% to 15% of cases. Radiation therapy (either conventional fractionated or more commonly radiosurgery using gamma knife or linear accelerator) may be of benefit in subtotally resected tumors located in critical areas (petroclival region, cavernous sinus), in patients whose age or medical condition would prohibit surgery, and in those with tumor recurrence after previous surgery.[17]

Schwannomas

Schwannomas are benign tumors that arise from Schwann cells of the myelin sheath around cranial and spinal

nerves after they emerge from the brainstem and the spinal cord. Vestibular schwannomas, the most common type, arise from the superior division of the vestibulocochlear nerve and manifest as unilateral sensorineural hearing loss, tinnitus, and disequilibrium. Characteristic findings on MRI include a round or oval enhancing tumor centered on the internal auditory canal (see Fig. 72-14C and D). Treatment options include expectant management with MRI and hearing audiometrics to detect tumor growth, surgical resection, and radiation therapy either in the form of EBRT or radiosurgery (alone or in conjunction with surgery). A complete surgical resection may result in a cure; however, the primary risks of surgery include cranial nerve deficits, namely the facial nerve. In one series of 157 patients with tumors smaller than 3 cm treated with radiosurgery with a median follow-up of 9.1 years, 73% of patients had a decrease in the tumor size, 95% maintained normal facial function, and hearing remained at serviceable levels in 50%.[18,19] Vestibular schwannomas are at least 95% unilateral. Bilateral occurrence is associated with a neurocutaneous disorder, neurofibromatosis type 2, an autosomal dominant disorder (gene, 22q12.2). Other commonly affected cranial nerves include the facial nerve, the trigeminal nerve, and the glossopharyngeal and vagus nerves.

Pituitary Adenomas

Pituitary adenomas arise primarily from the anterior pituitary gland and are classified as either functional (secreting) or nonfunctional (nonsecreting) tumors, with the

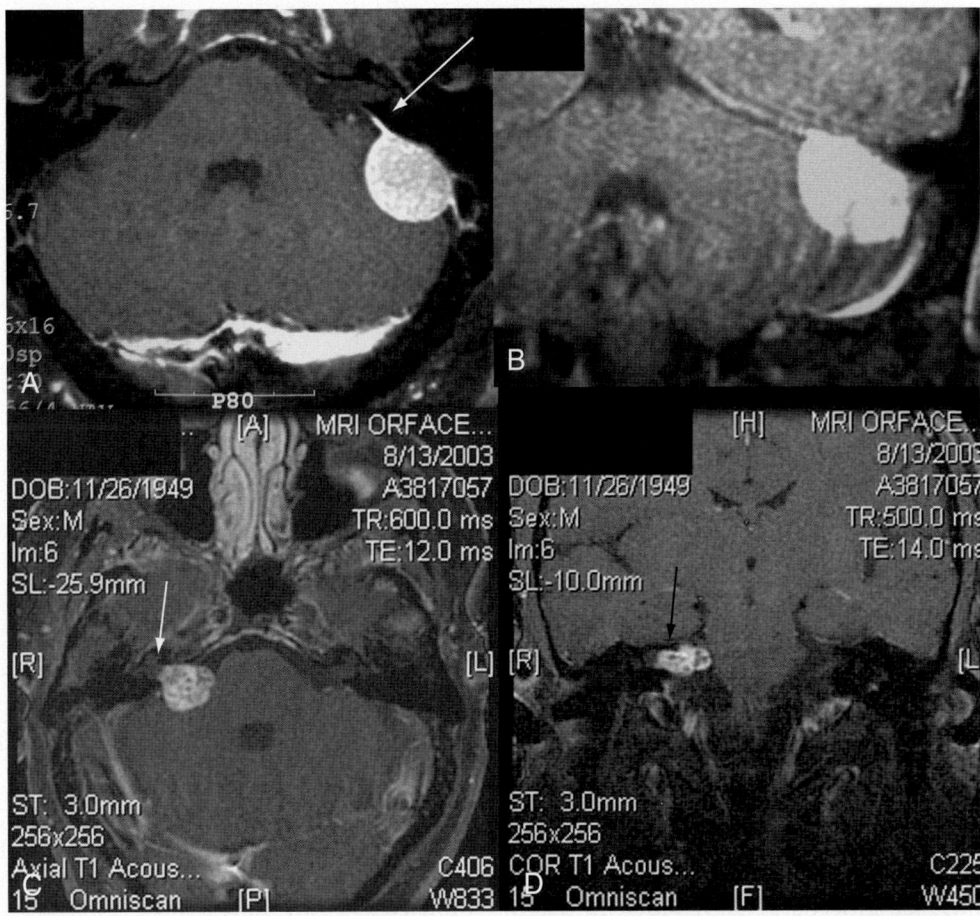

Figure 72-14 MRI studies of two patients presenting with cerebellopontine angle tumors. Gadolinium-enhanced axial (**A**) and coronal (**B**) MRI studies show a well-circumscribed, homogeneously enhancing tumor with a dural tail (*arrow*) arising from the tentorium. Gadolinium-enhanced axial (**C**) and coronal (**D**) MRIs show a vestibular schwannoma extending into the internal auditory meatus (*arrow*).

former presenting earlier with symptoms caused by physiologic effects and the latter presenting when of sufficient size to cause neurologic deficits by mass effect on the chiasm with consequent bitemporal hemianopsia. Tumors smaller than 1 cm in diameter are called *microadenomas,* and the rest are considered *macroadenomas;* 50% of pituitary tumors are smaller than 5 mm at the time of diagnosis. Their incidence is increased in multiple endocrine neoplasia. They occur commonly in the third and fourth decades of life and affect both sexes equally. The most common functional tumor is the prolactinoma, which causes amenorrhea and galactorrhea in women. Oversecretion of adrenocorticotropic hormone by the adenoma may lead to Cushing's disease, characterized by centripetal obesity, moon facies, hypertension, buffalo hump, hyperpigmentation, hyperglycemia, and psychiatric disturbances. Overproduction of growth hormone by the tumor manifests as acromegaly with resultant skeletal overgrowth, deformities of the hands and feet, hypertension, cardiomyopathy, hyperglycemia, soft tissue swelling, and peripheral nerve entrapment syndromes. The latter two may be reversible with normalization of growth hormone (GH) levels. Thyrotropin- and gonadotropin-secreting adenomas are rare.

MRI is the imaging test for pituitary tumors, providing information about location and invasion or compression of nearby structures like the optic chiasm and the cavernous sinus (see Fig. 72-13C and D). Typically, the pituitary gland enhances rapidly owing to lack of blood-brain barrier. As a result, the microadenoma may appear as a nonenhancing area within the gland. Diagnostic workup includes a full endocrinologic profile and a formal visual fields test. Oral administration of a dopamine agonist, bromocriptine, can shrink prolactinomas in 75% of patients with macroadenomas in 6 to 8 weeks, but only as long as therapy is maintained. Bromocriptine may also work on GH-secreting tumors with tumor shrinkage in less than 20%. Octreotide, a somatostatin analogue, can reduce GH levels in 71% of patients, with a significant reduction in tumor volume in 30% of cases.

Surgical treatment is indicated as an initial treatment for most GH-secreting tumors, for primary Cushing's disease, for nonprolactin-secreting macroadenomas causing symptoms by mass effect, and in any adenoma causing acute visual deterioration. Surgery is indicated in prolactinomas only if the prolactin level is less than 500 ng/mL in tumors that are not extensively invasive, or if the prolactin level is more than 500 ng/mL in tumors

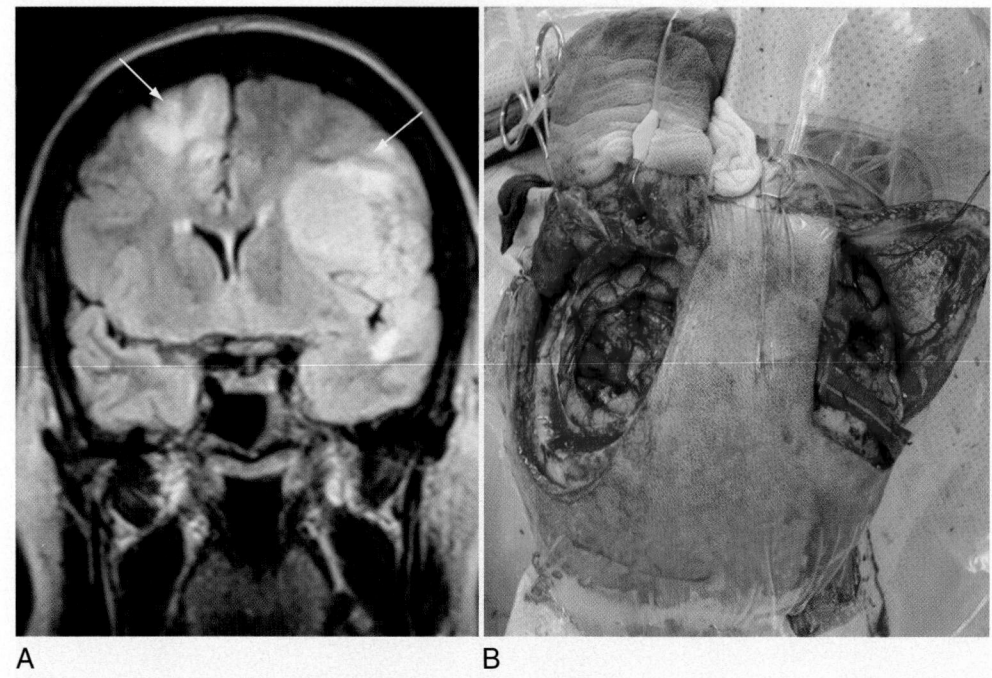

A   B

Figure 72-15 A, A FLAIR-sequence coronal MRI of a patient with two simultaneous metastatic tumors along the right and left frontal lobes (*arrows*). **B,** Simultaneous right and left frontal craniotomies for resection of both metastatic lesions.

not controlled medically. The surgical approach of choice is a sublabial or intranasal trans-sphenoidal approach, which is an extracranial procedure that requires no brain retraction. This procedure can be done either using the microscope or through an endoscopic technique. It is a minimally invasive procedure that allows access to the sella through the sphenoid sinus. Care is taken to avoid injury to the carotid arteries located within the cavernous sinus, which constitutes the lateral margins of the sella turcica. A transcranial approach is sometimes chosen to operate on a primarily suprasellar tumor or residual suprasellar component after a subtotal trans-sphenoidal resection.

The incidence of recurrence is about 12%, with most recurring 4 to 8 years after surgery. Consequently, patients are followed up with yearly MRIs. Radiosurgery can also be used either as primary therapy, as an adjuvant therapy after subtotal resection, or for recurrent disease. The main dose-limiting structure is proximity to the optic chiasm and optic nerves (within 3-5 mm). In this case, fractionated EBRT may be indicated as an adjuvant therapy.

Secondary Brain Tumors

Metastatic Brain Tumors

Metastatic brain tumors are the most common tumors of the brain. They outnumber primary brain tumors by 10 to 1. In patients with no cancer history, a brain metastasis was the presenting symptom in 15%. The distribution of metastases in the brain is directly related to the amount of blood flow to each part of the brain. Eighty percent of brain metastases occur in the cerebral hemispheres,

mainly the frontal lobes; 15% occur in the cerebellum; and 5% occur in the brainstem. The most common primary sites are lung (50%), breast cancer (15%-20%), unknown primary cancer (10%-15%), melanoma (10%), and colon cancer (5%). Metastases to the brain are multiple in more than 70% of cases, but solitary metastases do occur. Dural metastases may constitute as much as 9% of total CNS metastases.[20]

MRI with gadolinium enhancement is the diagnostic study of choice for metastases (Fig. 72-15). It shows a lesion at the gray-matter and white-matter junction, well circumscribed, surrounded by edema. Planning of therapy depends on the number of lesions, their location in deep or eloquent areas of the brain, their size, the radiosensitivity of the primary cancer, the systemic status of the primary cancer, and the Karnofsky performance score of the patient. Surgery is recommended for accessible lesions (up to three) causing mass effect followed by whole-brain radiation therapy (WBRT) to eradicate micrometastases. Stereotactic radiosurgery followed by WBRT has also been shown to be as effective as surgery in the management of metastatic brain tumors (<3 cm). The median survival time with optimal treatment remains 7 to 12 months. Chemotherapy is not useful in most brain metastases except small cell lung cancer and seminomas.

Regional Tumors

Brain involvement can occur with cancers of the nasopharyngeal region by direct extension along the cranial nerves or through the foramina at the base of the skull. Skull base tumors may cause symptoms of headache, diplopia, or other cranial nerve deficits. Clival chordoma, a remnant of the primitive notochord, is a skull base tumor that is locally invasive. Treatment consists of surgery followed by proton-beam radiotherapy.

Intraspinal Tumors

Intraspinal tumors are commonly divided into three groups: extradural, intradural extramedullary, and intramedullary.

Extradural Tumors

These tumors originate in the vertebral body, or less commonly the epidural space. Most tend to be malignant and represent metastatic tumors, particularly from the lung, breast, and prostate. Spinal epidural metastases occur in up to 10% of cancer patients. Other common extradural tumors include lymphomas and multiple myelomas. Pain is usually the first symptom and may be exacerbated by recumbency, especially at night; by movements; and by coughing or sneezing. Pathologic fractures are common. The pain may be mechanical or axial owing to an inherent instability in the diseased spine, or may be radicular or referred owing to epidural extension and compression of radicular nerves. As the tumor enlarges and compresses the spinal cord, myelopathic signs may be evident in the form of paraparesis or paraplegia, hyperreflexia, and spasticity. A sensory level appropriate to the spinal level in question may also be found.

Diagnostic workup includes CT scan to visualize the extent of bony destruction and MRI with gadolinium to visualize the neural elements and soft tissue invasion. A CT-guided needle biopsy is also recommended to establish the diagnosis in case of an absent primary cancer. A metastatic workup includes a chest x-ray; CT of the chest, abdomen, and pelvis; bone scan; serum prostate-specific antigen; and a mammogram in women. Treatment consists of surgery with or without EBRT, depending on the radiosensitivity of the tumor. Surgery is indicated in patients with the following:

1. Progressive neurologic deficit
2. Excruciating axial pain resistant to pain medications
3. Progressive kyphotic deformity
4. Radioresistant tumor (melanoma, renal cell carcinoma)

The surgical approach is directed toward the tumor area whether it involves a simple laminectomy posteriorly or a posterolateral thoracotomy or thoracoabdominal approach for a vertebrectomy. Stabilization in the form of instrumentation is always recommended in radical spinal oncology surgery (Fig. 72-16).

Intradural Extramedullary Tumors

These tumors are located within the dura, but outside the substance of the spinal cord. Most are benign and arise from the meninges (meningioma) or nerve roots (schwannomas and neurofibromas). Metastatic tumors may also seed this area through subarachnoid spreading (lymphoma, ependymoma, medulloblastoma). Lymphomatous spread into the subarachnoid space may lead to meningeal carcinomatosis, typically diagnosed with CSF cytology through a lumbar puncture.

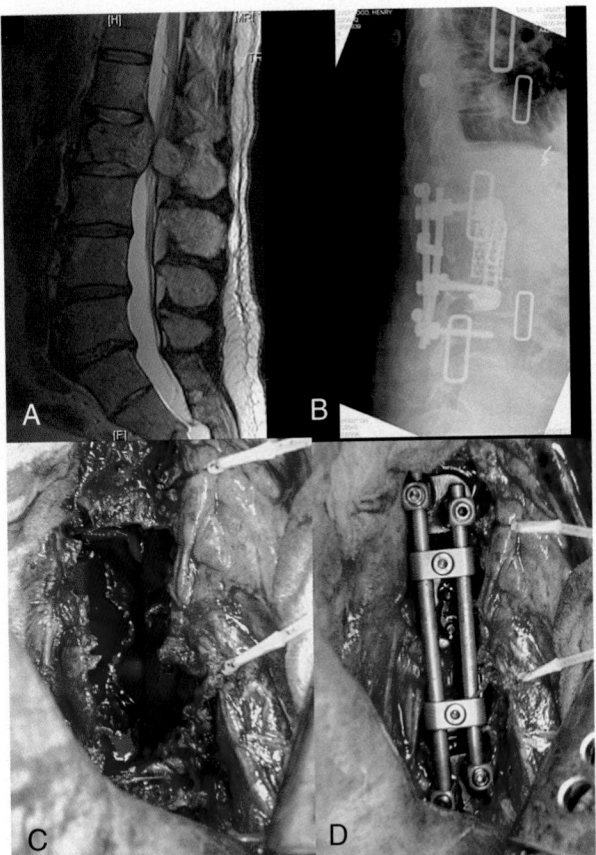

Figure 72-16 Radiographic and intraoperative pictures of a patient presenting with metastatic renal cell carcinoma to L2. **A,** An expansile bony lesion with an epidural component at L2 causing obliteration of the spinal canal can be seen on this T2-weighted sagittal MRI study. **B,** A postoperative lateral radiograph shows the spinal instrumentation with posterior L1, L3, and L4 pedicle screws-rod system, and anterior L1 to L3 titanium cage with a lateral L1 to L3 vertebral body screws-rod system. Intraoperative pictures show the surgical field after L2 vertebrectomy (**C**) and the implanted cage at the vertebrectomy site covered by the lateral L1 to L3 screws-rod system (**D**).

Spinal meningiomas (Fig. 72-17C and D) are more common in females and involve mainly the thoracic region (82%). They tend to occur lateral (68%), posterior (18%), and anterior (15%) to the spinal cord. Schwannomas and neurofibromas can originate anywhere there is a nerve root. Schwannomas usually develop from the sensory portion of the nerve root (dorsal), thereby sparing the motor portion (anterior). They may extend through the nerve root foramen into the extraspinal space, giving the shape of a dumbbell appearance on MRI. These lesions are best evaluated by an MRI with gadolinium, which shows the relationship of the tumor to the spinal cord and roots. These lesions are frequently amenable to surgical resection with minimal morbidity. Sacrifice of the dorsal root during resection of a nerve sheath tumor is sometimes warranted without any significant complications.

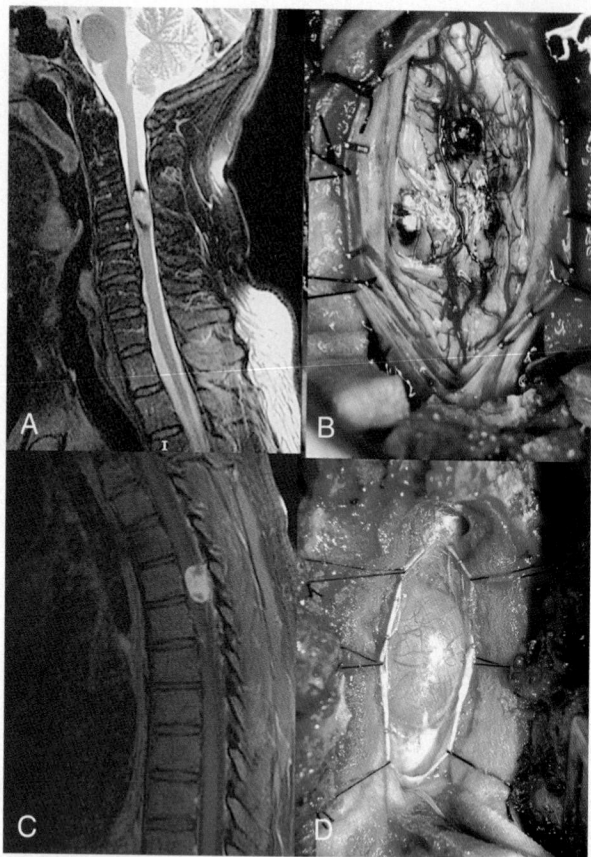

Figure 72-17 Radiographic and intraoperative pictures of patients with spinal intradural tumors. **A,** A T2-weighted sagittal MRI study shows an intramedullary cervical cord ependymoma at the C3-C4 level with a small rostral and caudal syrinx. **B,** An intraoperative picture shows the dura splayed open with the ependymoma showing in the cord. **C,** A gadolinium-enhanced sagittal MRI shows a T4 meningioma. **D,** An intraoperative picture shows the spinal cord and the overlying meningioma.

Intramedullary Tumors

These tumors originate from the substance of the spinal cord. Patients usually experience myelopathy and sensory disturbances below the level of involvement. The two most common tumors are astrocytoma and ependymoma. MRI with gadolinium is the preferred imaging study. The treatment of intramedullary tumors is laminectomy followed by maximal tumor resection without causing significant neurologic deficits. The CUSA and the operating microscope are indispensable tools in this type of surgery. Ependymomas are the most common glioma of the lower cord, conus, and filum (50%). The next most common location is the cervical cord (see Fig. 72-17A and B). They are usually slow growing and benign. They are typically encapsulated with a cleavage plane between the tumor and normal cord, which makes gross total resection feasible.[21] Astrocytomas, on the other hand, tend to be more infiltrative and less amenable to a total resection without significant neurologic deficits. EBRT is offered for residual ependymomas, if total resection was not possible, and most astrocytomas. Other, less common intramedul-

lary tumors include dermoid and epidermoid neoplasms, lipomas, and hemangioblastomas.

TRAUMATIC BRAIN INJURY

This section considers traumatic brain injury. The goal of this section is not to present a comprehensive review of the epidemiology, basic science research, and outcome studies on brain injury, but rather to present a practical, common sense approach to the management of injuries of the brain. There is bound to be overlap between this section of the chapter and other parts of this text. Guidelines for the management of severe head injury were first published by the Brain Trauma Foundation in 1995.[22] These evidence-based guidelines have been a tremendous aid to the practitioner caring for brain-injured patients. The following discussion on the management of severe traumatic brain injury is based largely on these guidelines. As with all practice guidelines, they can and need to be modified, as dictated by the experience of the treating physician and in accordance with the needs of the patient. This publication and the protocols laid out in the Advanced Trauma Life Support guidelines, published by the American College of Surgeons Committee on Trauma, are also invaluable resources for the student and practitioner.

We first consider severe traumatic brain injury. We discuss the epidemiology, pathophysiology, prehospital and emergency management, and definitive treatment of severe traumatic brain injury. Concussion and mild to moderate brain injury are then discussed.

Epidemiology

Depending on the source of information, it is estimated that there are anywhere from 500,000 to well over 1 million cases of head injury every year. Most of these are classified as mild injuries, with about 20% classified as moderate to severe. About half of the 150,000 trauma deaths every year are caused by head injury. It is estimated that 5.3 million people are living with brain injury–related disabilities, and the estimated cost to society exceeds $4 billion per year. The social, medical, and economic implications are profound. Fortunately, prevention programs appear to be decreasing the incidence of severe traumatic brain injury.

Pathophysiology

Traumatic brain injury can be classified into primary and secondary injuries. Primary injury occurs at impact and is considered first. It includes bone fracture, intracranial hemorrhage, and diffuse axonal injury (DAI). Fractures of the cranial vault and skull base are indicative of the forces applied to the skull at the time of impact. Fractures of the skull base may be associated with cranial nerve deficit, arterial dissection, and CSF fistula formation. Fractures of the cranial vault are classified as follows:

Table 72-4 Scoring with the Glasgow Coma Scale

EYE-OPENING RESPONSE		VERBAL RESPONSE		MOTOR RESPONSE	
Score	Response	Score	Response	Score	Response
4	Spontaneous	5	Oriented	6	Obeys commands
3	To speech	4	Confused	5	Localizes to painful stimulus
2	To pain	3	Inappropriate responses	4	Withdraws to painful stimulus
1	No response	2	Incomprehensible responses	3	Flexion to painful stimulus
		1	No response	2	Extension to painful stimulus
				1	No response

1. Open or closed
2. Depressed or nondepressed
3. Linear or comminuted

Any fracture of the cranial vault can cause disruption of the underlying meningeal arteries or dural venous sinuses, which can lead to intracranial bleeding. Intracranial hemorrhage can be classified as epidural, subdural, subarachnoid, and intraparenchymal or intracerebral. Epidural hemorrhage occurs between the dura and the skull and is usually the result of a skull fracture causing the laceration of a meningeal artery.

Rarely, a fracture crossing a dural venous sinus can cause a venous epidural hematoma, especially in children. Subdural hemorrhage occurs in the potential space between the dura and the arachnoid. This usually is the result of shearing of the bridging veins between brain and the dural venous sinuses. Sometimes, it comes from injury to cortical vessels, which then bleed into the subdural space. Subarachnoid hemorrhage from trauma consists of bleeding into the spinal fluid spaces surrounding the blood vessels feeding the cerebral cortex. Trauma is the most common cause of subarachnoid hemorrhage. Rupture of an intracranial aneurysm is the second most common cause of subarachnoid hemorrhage and is usually distinguished from traumatic SAH by history and sometimes by the distribution of blood on CT. Intraparenchymal or intracerebral hemorrhage is bleeding into the brain itself. This can run the spectrum from small contusions (bruises of the brain) to large intracerebral clots that require emergent surgical evacuation. These usually are the result of coup and contrecoup injuries. Although often small and nonsurgical at first, these can "blossom" and become life-threatening over a period of hours to days. DAI is a rotational acceleration-deceleration injury to the white-matter pathways of the brain. This results in a functional or anatomic disruption of these pathways and is cited as the cause of loss of consciousness in patients without mass lesions. DAI can occur with or without other primary injuries such as an epidural or subdural hematoma. In addition to being one of the many primary injuries seen in severe traumatic brain injury, DAI can also be seen as one of the secondary injuries, which are to be considered next.

Secondary injury to the brain occurs as a result of decreased oxygen delivery to the brain, which in turn sets off a cascade of events that causes even more damage than the initial injury. In the face of severe traumatic brain injury, there can be an alteration in cerebral vessel autoregulation. Systemic hypotension in the face of this altered autoregulation results in decreased cerebral blood flow and decreased oxygen delivery. This ischemia is exacerbated even further by systemic hypoxemia. Add intracranial hypertension, which even further decreases cerebral blood flow, and a cascade of events involving mediators of inflammation, excitotoxicity, calcium influx, and Na^+,K^+-ATPase dysfunction leads to neuronal cell dysfunction and death. The prevention of secondary injury is therefore thought to lead to increased cell survival and improved outcome. This is achieved by preventing hypotension and hypoxia, while taking measures to control ICP and maintain cerebral perfusion pressure.

Prehospital and Emergency Department Management

The prehospital and emergency department management of the traumatized patient is reviewed in other chapters and other texts. We will deal more specifically with those issues critical to the patient with severe brain injury in this chapter. The ABCs must always be addressed first, regardless of the severity of the patient's injury. Attention is first paid to securing a patent airway, establishing adequate ventilation and oxygenation, and maintaining adequate circulation. By doing this, one may avoid hypotension and hypoxia, and in so doing, avoid or minimize secondary brain injury. In patients with severe traumatic brain injury, a systolic blood pressure of less than 90 mm Hg or a PaO_2 of less than 60 mm Hg is a predictor of poor outcome. Appropriate spine precautions are observed in the initial resuscitation of the patient with a severe traumatic brain injury.

Once airway, breathing, and circulation have been addressed, neurologic evaluation may proceed. The Glasgow Coma Scale (GCS) is a time honored, simple, reproducible method of neurologic assessment. It is also used to grade traumatic brain injury as mild, moderate, or severe. The GCS consists of three components: intensity of stimulus required to cause eye opening, verbal response, and motor response (Table 72-4). Pupillary size and reactivity are also essential components of the initial neurologic examination. Hypoxia, hypotension, alcohol, and drugs may all contribute to an abnormal neurologic examination. In the absence of hypotension and hypoxia, an abnormal exam is considered to be a primary brain injury until proved otherwise. Once all life-threatening injuries have been addressed and stabilized, the patient with a suspected traumatic brain injury is taken to CT. The CT scan is used to evaluate the presence or absence of fracture, epidural and subdural hematomas, intracerebral hematomas and contusions, shift of the midline structures, and the appearance of the basal and perimesencephalic cisterns. In many centers with multislice scanners, routine scanning of the cervical spine is also performed to rule out acute fractures or traumatic dislocations. If life-threatening injuries elsewhere necessitate transport of the patient immediately to the operating room, and the patient has a suspected intracranial hematoma (e.g., unilateral fixed and dilated pupil on one side with a contralateral hemiparesis), exploratory burr holes may be performed in the operating room simultaneous to the laparotomy or thoracotomy.

Not infrequently, trauma patients with brain injury will require transfer to a hospital equipped to provide those patients with a higher level of care. In preparing these patients for transfer, the practitioner needs to follow the Advanced Trauma Life Support guidelines and secure the airway, ensure adequate ventilation, and maintain circulation. Anemia is treated with transfusion as necessary. Hypoxia and hypotension need to be avoided. Adequate immobilization with a back board and cervical collar are mandatory. In those patients with obvious intracranial hypertension or mass lesions, treatment with mannitol may be considered after neurosurgical consultation. Vigilance and attention to detail, as well as communication between the transferring and accepting physicians, is the key to the successful transfer and treatment of these patients.

Treatment

When the workup of a patient reveals an intracranial mass lesion and deficits thought to be related to that lesion, operative intervention is indicated. In general, any clot or contusion greater than 30 cc is thought to be operable. Epidural and subdural hematomas (Fig. 72-18) are addressed with similar approaches, with the craniotomy centered on the clot. Intracerebral hematomas are addressed through appropriately located craniotomies. ICP monitors are often placed at operation. These can be intraventricular drains, intraparenchymal monitors, or devices placed in the epidural or subdural spaces. The decision about when to place an ICP monitor depends on the patient's preoperative exam, the appearance of the brain at operation, and the potential risk for deterioration. In general, all patients with a GCS of 8 or less have ICP monitors placed. Some patients with moderate traumatic brain injury may also benefit from ICP monitoring. Postoperatively, the patient is managed similarly to those with nonoperable traumatic brain injury, as described later.

The following is a simplified algorithm for the management of intracranial hypertension in the intensive care setting. The head of the bed is elevated to 30 degrees with the head placed in a neutral position. Care is taken to ensure that any cervical spine immobilization device is not obstructing jugular venous flow because this can increase ICP. The goal of treatment is to try to keep the ICP less than 20 to 25 mm Hg and to maintain cerebral perfusion pressure at or above 70 mm Hg. Remember that cerebral perfusion pressure is MAP minus ICP. If the ICP is persistently elevated above 20 to 25 mm Hg, it is treated. CSF drainage is now the first line of therapy in decreasing ICP. This is accomplished by an external ventricular drain, or ventriculostomy. This is a drain placed in the operating room or at the bedside in the intensive care unit in an appropriately monitored patient. If ICP remains persistently elevated despite CSF drainage, the patient can be sedated and even pharmacologically paralyzed to keep the ICP down. The practitioner is dependent on the pupillary exam and ICP reading in this situation. If the ICP changes rapidly, or the pupillary exam changes (i.e., blown pupil), emergent CT of the head is indicated. Sedation and paralysis can be discontinued to allow for an adequate neurologic evaluation from time to time in this situation.

If the ICP remains persistently elevated despite the above interventions, mannitol and other diuretic agents may be used. Mannitol is administered as an IV bolus of 0.25 to 1 g/kg every 4 to 6 hours. Serum osmolality is followed closely when giving mannitol, and the drug is withheld if the serum osmolality exceeds 320. It is also important to maintain euvolemia in these patients. If ICP is still elevated, judicious use of hyperventilation to a $PaCO_2$ of 30 to 35 mm Hg may be used. At this point, second-tier therapeutic interventions (hypertonic saline, high-dose barbiturate therapy, decompressive craniectomy) may be considered.[23,24] Serial CT scans are critical throughout this treatment algorithm, and their use is tailored to the individual patient.

Several comments regarding nutrition, steroids, anticonvulsants and $PaCO_2$ are in order. Energy requirements after traumatic brain injury are increased. The nonparalyzed patient requires replacement of 140% of their resting metabolism expenditure, and the paralyzed patient requires 100%. Fifteen percent of this is protein. Feeding begins within 7 days of injury. Steroids have no proven benefit in the management of traumatic brain injury and are not used. Prophylactic use of anticonvulsant drugs (phenytoin, carbamazepine, phenobarbital) is not indicated for the prevention of late post-traumatic seizures. Anticonvulsants may, however, be used to prevent early post-traumatic seizures, primarily in patients at high risk for early seizures who may suffer adverse effects if they were to seize early in their hospital course. They can usually be tapered after 1 week of therapy. Hyperventilation causes a decrease in ICP by lowering $PaCO_2$, which causes vasoconstriction and decreases intracranial blood volume. Unfortunately, it also causes decreased cerebral blood flow. If hyperventilation to a $PaCO_2$ of less than 30 mm Hg is required for the maintenance of an acceptable ICP and CPP, then monitoring of cerebral blood flow is strongly recommended by some. Jugular venous O_2 saturation and cerebral oxygen extraction may also be of use in this clinical scenario.

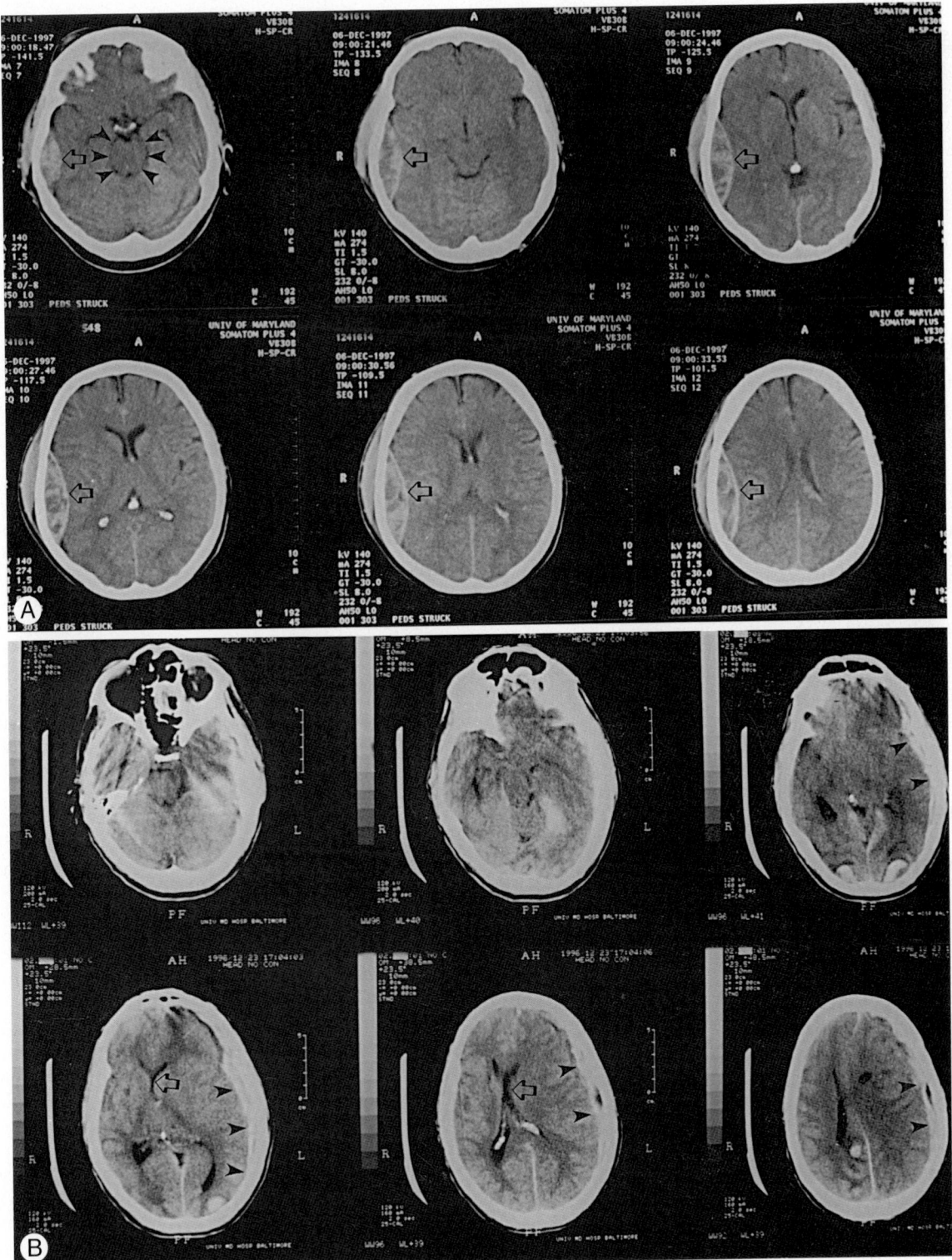

Figure 72-18 CT scans of two patients with closed head injury. **A,** This patient has a right temporal epidural hematoma (*arrows*). The mesencephalic cisterns are patent in the *top left,* indicating a lack of brainstem compression despite mass (*arrowheads*). **B,** This patient has suffered an acute left subdural hematoma (*arrowheads*) with midline shift (*arrows*).

Table 72-5   Clinical Findings in Common Lumbar Disk Herniations

DISK	INCIDENCE (%)	ROOT	PAIN DISTRIBUTION	MUSCLE INVOLVED	SENSORY DEFICITS	REFLEX LOSS
L3-L4	3-10	L4	Anterior thigh	Quadriceps femoris	Medial malleolus and medial foot	Knee jerk
L4-L5	40-45	L5	Posterolateral thigh and leg	Tibialis anterior Extensor hallucis longus	Large toe web and dorsum of foot	None
L5-S1	45-50	S1	Posterolateral thigh and leg down to ankle	Gastrocnemius	Lateral malleolus Lateral foot	Ankle jerk

Mild Brain Injury

Data suggest that most of brain-injured patients have mild brain injuries (GCS > 13). Many of these are young people involved in athletic competition. Many never seek medical attention. There are at least three published grading scales for concussion or mild head injury.[25-27] All use loss of consciousness, confusion, and post-traumatic amnesia in different combinations to classify concussions into mild, moderate, and severe. Although no system has been conclusively shown to be better than the other, there is agreement on one thing: individuals who are symptomatic from their concussion must not return immediately to full activity, or play, in the case of athletes. There is mounting neuropsychometric evidence that repeated mild brain injury may have significant long-term neurologic ramifications.[28,29]

DEGENERATIVE DISORDERS OF THE SPINE

Degenerative Disease of the Lumbar Spine

According to the National Institute of Neurological Disorders and Stroke, 25.9 million Americans complain of low back pain per year, with a cumulative expense of about $50 billion per year. Low back pain is the most common cause of job-related disability and a leading contributor to missed days at work. Back pain is the second most common neurologic ailment in the United States—only headache is more common.

A good understanding of the normal anatomy of the spine is of utmost importance for the appreciation of spinal disorders. The lumbar spine consists of five lumbar vertebrae with five intervening intervertebral disks (IVDs). Each vertebra is made up of an anterior vertebral body and a posterior neural arch. Each neural arch is, in turn, composed of pedicles, facet joints, transverse processes, laminae, and a spinous process. The IVD consists of three components:

1. Cartilaginous end plates for the purpose of nutrition and anchoring
2. Anulus fibrosis made of concentric sheets of collagen for the purpose of containing the pressurized nucleus
3. Nucleus pulposus made of a soft, semigelatinous collagen that can absorb axial compressive loads

The spinal cord ends at the L1 level, beyond which lumbar and sacral nerve roots, collectively called the *cauda equina,* continue distally and exit at their corresponding neural foramen. At each segmental level, a nerve root containing both motor and sensory components exits the thecal sac, crosses the IVD space, travels a short distance within the lateral recess of the spinal canal, and passes underneath the pedicle on its way to exit the spine through the intervertebral foramen.

Biomechanically, as we age, the nucleus loses its ability to bear compressive loads. The load transfer, then, shifts to the anulus, a structure that is poorly suited to withstand compression, thereby causing fatigue failure, fissuring, and possibly rupture. A herniation of a fragment of the nucleus pulposus may follow. As the mechanical integrity of the nucleus further deteriorates, the load transfer is concentrated at the periphery of the vertebral end plates, leading to osteophyte formation, a process called *spondylosis.* Subsequently, as the degenerating disk becomes less able to resist rotations and shear, additional stresses are transferred to the posterior elements with resultant facet arthrosis and hypertrophy, and thickening and buckling of the ligamentum flavum.

Lumbar Radiculopathy

Disk herniations can occur in any direction but most commonly follow a posterolateral direction at the site where the posterior longitudinal ligament is thinnest. Disk material extruded in this location can compress a nerve root, leading to low back pain and radicular symptoms in a specific dermatomal distribution (Table 72-5). The back pain is usually a minor component. Large, more central disk herniations may compress the cauda equina with resultant cauda equina syndrome, consisting of saddle anesthesia, urinary retention with possible overflow incontinence, and significant motor weakness. In this case, it is advisable to decompress the thecal sac within 24 hours of onset of symptoms.

An initial period of nonsurgical management for at least 4 to 8 weeks is indicated unless the patient presents with cauda equina syndrome, progressive neurologic deficit, recurrent episodes of incapacitating pain, or profound motor weakness. Conservative therapy includes rest, activity modification, physical therapy, weight loss, analgesics, muscle relaxants, oral steroids, and epidural steroid injections. If conservative measures fail to control the pain, imaging of the spine is indicated. MRI is the

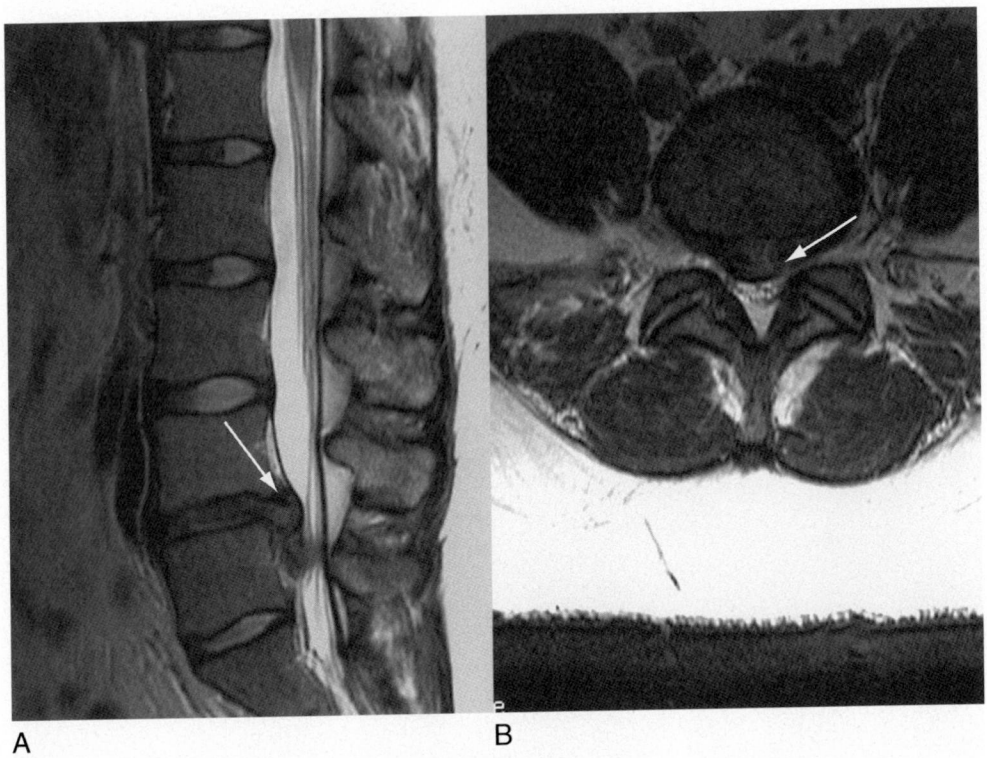

A   B

Figure 72-19 A, A T2-weighted sagittal MRI study showing a herniated lumbar disk fragment (*arrow*) at the L4-L5 level. **B,** T2-weighted axial MRI showing the same fragment (*arrow*) compressing the thecal sac.

diagnostic test of choice (Fig. 72-19); a postmyelography CT may be indicated in patients who have pacemakers.

The standard treatment of these herniations involves a midline approach centered over the affected interspace followed by a hemilaminectomy to expose the thecal sac and nerve root. The herniated fragment is usually located medial to the root along its shoulder. Removal of the herniated or extruded fragment is sufficient to relieve the symptoms. A minimally invasive procedure through a 1-cm paramedian incision with a muscle-splitting technique can also be used under either microscopic or endoscopic visualization with less postoperative morbidity. Most patients experience good results immediately after surgery. A recurrent herniated disk at the same level may occur in 3% to 19% of patients, with the higher rates usually in series with long-term follow-up.

Lumbar Spinal Stenosis

Advanced degeneration of the lumbar spine may result in spondylosis with arthrosis and hypertrophy of the facet joint as well as thickening and buckling of the ligamentum flavum. These changes lead to narrowing of the spinal canal with resultant constriction of the thecal sac and development of neurologic deficits. Patients classically present with neurogenic claudication: unilateral or bilateral dermatomal discomfort precipitated by standing or walking or prolonged maintenance of the same posture, and characteristically relieved by a change in posture like sitting, squatting, or recumbency. This discomfort may be in the form of pain, weakness, or paresthesias. Neurogenic claudication is thought to arise

from ischemic changes of roots as a result of increased metabolic demands from exercise in the presence of a vascular compromise of the root from the surrounding constriction. The clinical history is important if spinal stenosis is suspected because most of these patients have nonspecific neurologic findings like absent or reduced reflexes. Again, MRI is the diagnostic test of choice for lumbar stenosis and typically shows an hourglass appearance on T2-weighted sagittal sequence. Nonsteroidal anti-inflammatory drugs, analgesics, and physical therapy are the mainstays of nonsurgical management. Surgical decompression is warranted in patients with recurrent and disabling pain that limits their daily activity. Laminotomies or laminectomies of the involved levels with undercutting of the superior articular facet are required to decompress the nerves in the foramina. Wide aggressive decompression of the spinal canal may result in lumbar instability.

Lumbar Instrumentation and Fusion

The instrumentation is an adjunct to the fusion. It provides immediate rigid fixation while the spine completes the process of bony fusion that ensures long-term stabilization. Spondylolisthesis (vertebral body subluxation) is the most common indication for fusion and instrumentation. Lumbar fusion can be a potential adjunct to disk excision in cases of a herniated disk or a recurrent herniated disk in patients with evidence of preoperative lumbar spinal deformity or instability or in patients with chronic mechanical and diskogenic back pain.[30] Lumbar fusion is also recommended for carefully selected patients with

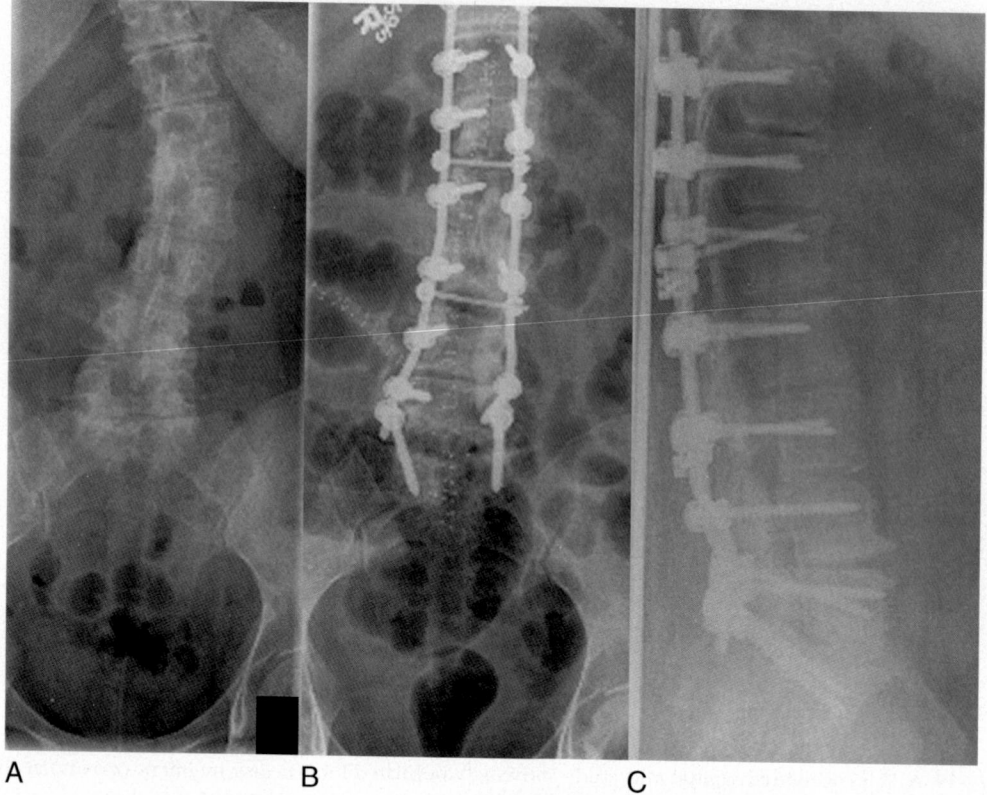

A   B   C

Figure 72-20 A, A posteroanterior (PA) x-ray of a patient with degenerative scoliotic deformity of the thoracolumbar spine. Postoperative PA (**B**) and lateral (**C**) x-rays show correction of the deformity using a long pedicle screws-rod construct from T11 to S1.

disabling low back pain due to one- or two-level degenerative disease without stenosis or spondylolisthesis.

Lumbar fusion and instrumentation can be performed through a number of approaches:

1. Posterolateral fusion (PLF), whereby the transverse processes of the involved segments are decorticated and covered with a mixture of bone autograft or allograft
2. Pedicle screw fixation (PSF), whereby screws are inserted into the pedicles of the involved segments and then attached to each other under compression with a rod (Fig. 72-20), either alone or in conjunction with PLF
3. Posterior lumbar interbody fusion (PLIF), whereby an intervertebral body spacer, either a bone allograft or a cage packed with bone, is inserted in the disk space through a laminotomy on each side of the midline, together with PSF, either alone or in conjunction with PLF
4. Transforaminal interbody fusion (TLIF), whereby the facet joint and the isthmus on one side are removed and a single bone graft or cage is introduced into the disk space in an oblique fashion, together with unilateral or bilateral PSF, either alone or in conjunction with PLF
5. Anterior lumbar interbody fusion (ALIF), whereby the interbody space is fused using either a bone graft or a cage augmented by a metallic interbody plate through an anterior retroperitoneal approach

Bony fusion can also be augmented with bony extenders or substitutes like demineralized bone matrix or recombinant human bone morphogenetic protein (rhBMP-2) in an attempt to avoid harvesting autologous bone grafts.

Degenerative Diseases of the Cervical Spine

The pathophysiology of the degenerative changes of the cervical spine is essentially similar to that of the lumbar spine. An important distinction is that the spinal canal in the cervical spine contains the spinal cord rather than the cauda equina, and consequently, minor reduction in the canal space may lead to compression of the spinal cord with devastating neurologic results. There are seven cervical vertebrae, but eight pairs of cervical nerves.

Cervical Radiculopathy

The most common scenario for patients with herniated cervical disk is that the symptoms were present upon awakening in the morning without identifiable trauma or stress. The pain usually radiates from the proximal arm distally, together with numbness and paresthesia, in a dermatomal distribution. The pain may be intensified by neck movements. In severe cases, a motor weakness along the same nerve may be noticed. On examination, pain with downward pressure on the vertex while tilting

Table 72-6 Clinical Findings in Common Cervical Disk Herniations

DISK	INCIDENCE (%)	ROOT	PAIN DISTRIBUTION	MUSCLE INVOLVED	REFLEX LOSS
C4-C5	2	C5	Shoulder	Deltoid	Deltoid
C5-C6	19	C6	Upper arm, thumb, radial forearm	Biceps, extensor carpi radialis	Biceps, brachioradialis
C6-C7	69	C7	Fingers 2 and 3, all fingertips	Triceps	Triceps
C7-T1	10	C8	Fingers 4 and 5	Hand intrinsics	Finger jerk

the head toward the symptomatic side (Spurling's sign) is a mechanical sign of disk herniation. Nerve root compression in the upper cervical spine is unusual. Compression of C2 root causes occipital neuralgia, whereas compression of C3 and C4 may lead to nonspecific neck and shoulder pain. Compression of the other cervical roots leads to the manifestations noted in Table 72-6.

Cervical Myelopathy

Compression of the cervical cord, either acutely by a large herniated disk fragment or chronically by osteophytic bony spurs as a result of advanced spondylosis or stenosis, causes cervical myelopathy. Myelopathy is manifested by spasticity, hyperreflexia, increased deep tendon reflexes, clonus, and the Babinski and Hoffman signs. Patients also complain of clumsiness in their hands as a result of poor muscle coordination. If left untreated, patients may become quadriparetic and wheelchair bound.

Diagnosis and Treatment

MRI is the study of choice for the initial evaluation of a herniated cervical disk. A CT myelogram is indicated for patients who cannot undergo MRI or when anatomic bony details are required. MRI is less accurate than CT myelogram for identifying foraminal fragments but is less invasive. A cervical spine x-ray is always recommended to evaluate the degree of spondylosis in the cervical spine before surgery. Electromyography and nerve conduction studies can be useful when other causes need to be excluded, such as plexopathies or peripheral nerve entrapment.

More than 90% of patients with acute cervical radiculopathy as a result of disk herniation can improve without surgery. Conservative therapy includes a combination of oral steroids, nonsteroidal anti-inflammatory drugs, analgesics, muscle relaxants, intermittent cervical traction, and physical therapy. Surgery is indicated for those who fail to improve and those with progressive neurologic deficit while undergoing the conservative therapy. The aim of the surgery is to decompress the nerve root. This can be accomplished through an anterior or a posterior approach. Both procedures carry an excellent outcome in the range 90% to 96% improvement in preoperative symptoms.

With anterior pathology (paracentral herniation or large uncovertebral osteophyte), an anterior cervical diskectomy, nerve root decompression, and fusion are indicated (Fig. 72-21). The approach is fairly simple through the avascular plane between the carotid sheath and the tracheoesophageal complex. The operative microscope is used to remove the IVD, decompress the thecal sac, and free the nerve roots. A bone graft, more commonly an allograft, is applied in the disk space. Next, a metallic plate can be applied between the two vertebral bodies, thereby accomplishing a rigid fixation and minimizing the need for a postoperative cervical collar.

A posterior approach, also called *keyhole foraminotomy,* is indicated in patients with unilateral radiculopathy with soft disk herniation or small lateral osteophyte, in professional speakers or singers who want to avoid the small risk for permanent injury to the recurrent laryngeal nerve (5%), and in patients with a short thick neck. With the aid of an operating microscope, a small foraminotomy is performed with a high-speed drill to unroof the nerve root. The disk fragment can be removed, if accessible.

Patients with cervical spondylosis and myelopathy present a difficult problem. The approach is tailored to the patient's specific pathology. Patients who suffer from multiple disks or osteophytes with myelopathy and those with significant cervical stenosis in addition to a superimposed disk herniation can benefit from posterior cervical laminectomy; this, in turn, may need to be reinforced by lateral mass instrumentation and fusion, depending on the degree of spinal instability (Fig. 72-22). Patients with chronic spondylosis who manifest anterior as well as posterior compression may require complex surgery. In this case, the patients may undergo a staged surgical approach with an initial anterior exposure for multiple cervical diskectomies or even cervical corpectomies with reconstruction with bone grafts or cages followed by an anterior cervical plate. Next, the patient would undergo posterior cervical laminectomies reinforced with lateral mass plating. Unfortunately, the outcome from surgery for cervical spondylosis with myelopathy is often disappointing. The aim of the surgery is to arrest the progression of the myelopathy. In one series, 66% of patients had relief from radicular pain, whereas only 33% had improvement in sensory or motor complaints.[31]

FUNCTIONAL AND STEREOTACTIC NEUROSURGERY

Functional neurosurgery is concerned with the anatomic or physiologic alteration of the nervous system to achieve a desired effect. This can be done with focal electrical stimulation procedures, ablative procedures, or the

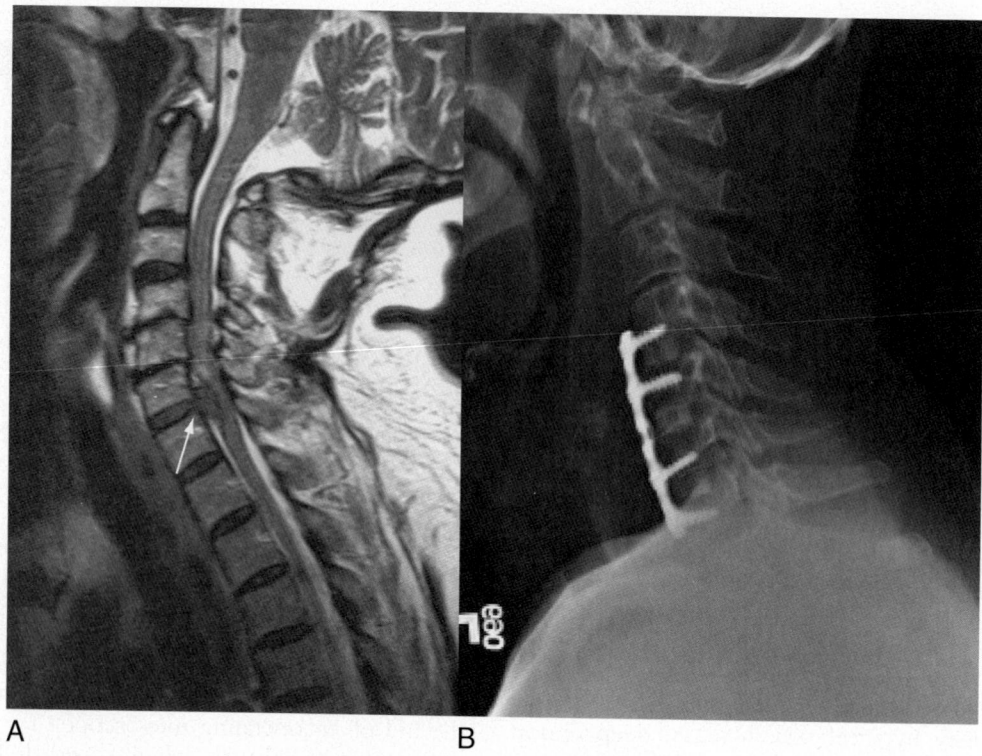

Figure 72-21 A, T2-weighted sagittal MRI study of a patient with advanced cervical spondylosis and stenosis from C3-C4 down to C6-C7 with an acute herniated disk fragment at C6-C7 (*arrow*) after cervical spine manipulation. **B,** Postoperative lateral x-ray showing C4-C5, C5-C6, and C6-C7 anterior cervical diskectomy and fusion using bone allograft and a titanium plate and screws.

implantation of pumps to deliver drugs, usually to the CSF but potentially the parenchyma as well. The field of functional neurosurgery deals primarily with the treatment of pain, movement disorders, epilepsy, and some psychiatric disorders when refractory to conventional treatments. These disorders all have in common an overfunction or deranged function of some part or parts of CNS. Sometimes the overfunction results from a loss of function in some other part of the brain. An example of this is the overfunction in the output pathways of the globus pallidus that occurs when the dopamine system in the brain degenerates, as occurs with Parkinson's disease. The transmitter of the overactive globus pallidus output system is inhibitory, and it turns out that the overall effect on the motor system is also inhibitory. The physiology of each functional disorder is usually quite complex and only partly understood. It is not the focus of this discussion to describe in detail what is known about the mechanism underlying each of these disorders. Instead, the focus is on the surgery, especially the stereotactic techniques and the possible interventions at the target site. This section also discusses stereotactic radiosurgery in general terms.

In considering brain stimulation, if the reader could image the consequences of placing two electrodes on the central processing unit of a computer and running a pulsatile "stimulating current" across it, not many would expect that the functioning of the computer would be enhanced by that. Rather, we would expect part of the

computer to not work at all as a result. Although we talk about "neuroaugmentation" as if it were always adding something to the function of the nervous system, in fact, most of the interventions are actually effective because they stop certain unwanted activity in the brain. It comes as a surprise to many, but in most situations, brain stimulation results in a temporary "lesion" of the stimulated structure. In almost all situations in which a focal lesion was found effective in the older neurosurgical literature, modern stimulation of that same structure is also effective. The difference is that a lesion is permanent and static in size and location. The advantage of stimulation is that it can be turned on or off, increased or decreased, and, in the case of an implanted electrode array, changed in location somewhat depending on which of the several contacts are activated. Thus, stimulation provides a reversible, scalable, and somewhat moveable, functional lesion. There are exceptions to the idea that stimulation is equivalent to a functional lesion. The frequency of stimulation can determine its overall effect, and the neurotransmitters at the site of stimulation can also have an effect. The cerebral cortex, with its high concentrations of excitatory neurotransmitters, may actually "turn on" with stimulation. Thus, certain crude visual prostheses may be effective on that basis.

Stereotaxis as applied to neurosurgery is concerned with the localization of a target in three-dimensional space. The target deep in the brain is not seen directly at surgery. This can be a tumor, a white-matter pathway,

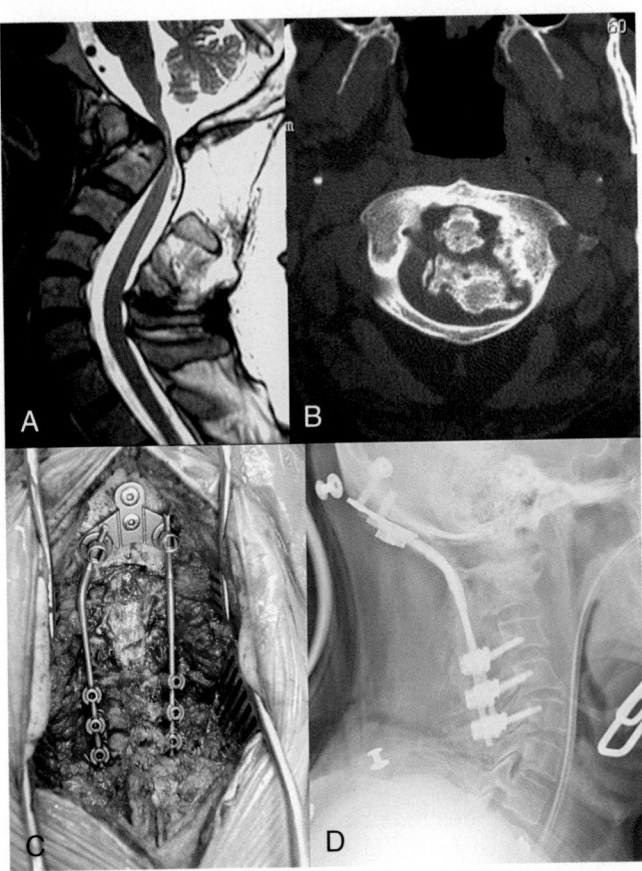

Figure 72-22 Radiographic and intraoperative pictures of a patient presenting with C2 odontoid fracture. A T2-weighted sagittal MRI study (**A**) and an axial CT image at the level of C1 (**B**) showing an odontoid fracture with anterior displacement of the odontoid fragment and settling of C2 body into the C1 ring, resulting in significant compromise of the spinal canal and cord. Intraoperative picture (**C**) and lateral radiograph of the cervical spine (**D**) show an occipitocervical fusion after an anterior transoral approach for a C2 vertebrectomy.

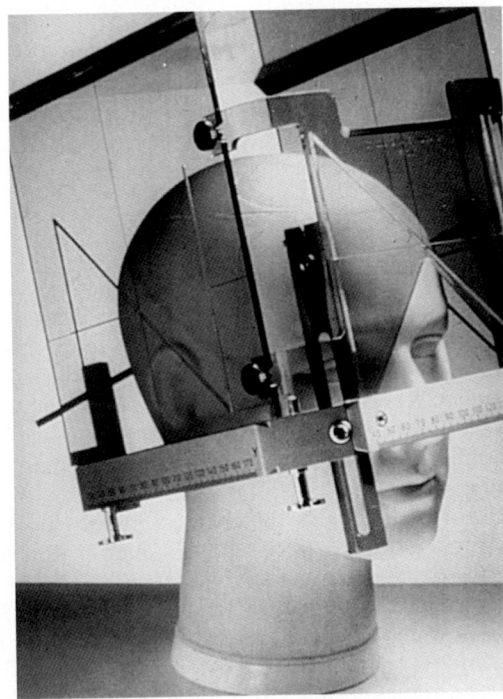

Figure 72-23 The Leskell stereotactic coordinate frame is rigidly attached to the head by four threaded pins. The fiducial box is mounted on the frame during the imaging (MRI or CT) study. *X, Y,* and *Z* coordinates are determined directly from the imaging study. The center of the frame is arbitrarily given the coordinates 100, 100, 100.

a cranial nerve, a vascular malformation, or a nucleus deep within the brain. The field has evolved using both frame-based systems and frameless systems, but in each case, a calculated inference is used to reach the target accurately.

Frame-based systems use a rigid frame attached to the skull by pins that penetrate the outer table of the skull (Fig. 72-23). This can easily be done under local anesthesia, with the patient wide awake. The patient is then taken to CT or MRI with a localizer on the frame. Using cartesian coordinates, the x, y, and z coordinates of the target can then be determined. In other words, the position of the target in relation to the frame is known. Using an arc system, which is mounted on the frame, the target can be accessed by different trajectories. When the target is a vascular lesion, an arteriogram can be performed with a localizing frame and the position of the vascular lesion in three-dimensional space determined. Frame-based systems are used for brain biopsies, deep brain stimulation, ablative procedures, and stereotactic radiosurgery.

Stereotactic radiosurgery involves the delivery of a concentrated dose of radiation to a defined volume in the brain. The dose of radiation delivered would be toxic if given in a broad field to the entire brain. When delivered in multiple collimated beams from numerous different angles, or in arcs at different angles, the effect on the surrounding brain is minimized. Two methods of frame-based stereotactic radiosurgery are currently widely used. The gamma knife uses cobalt-201 radiation sources focused on one point. Once the target is localized in three dimensions, it is placed at this point, and different collimators are used to focus the radiation. Modified linear accelerators deliver the radiation dose in multiple arcs, thereby minimizing the effect on surrounding brain tissue. Both systems use multiple isocenters in the treatment of irregularly shaped lesions. Stereotactic radiosurgery has been used in the treatment of just about every intracranial lesion but is commonly used in the treatment of metastatic tumors, benign lesions of the cranial nerves, arteriovenous malformations, and, recently, trigeminal neuralgia.[18,32,33] The primary risks of stereotactic radiosurgery are radiation necrosis and radiation injury to surrounding structures.

Frameless stereotactic techniques use advanced imaging techniques and fiducials and reference markers in place of a fixed frame. Robotic arms, infrared reflectors, and light-emitting diodes provide the surgeon with real-time information about the anatomy at hand. This technology can also be fused with a display from the operating microscope, aiding in the operative dissection. It is useful for the planning of incisions and craniotomies and, when combined with intraoperative ultrasound, may be of use in determining the extent of tumor resection. Frameless stereotactic radiosurgical devices are commercially available.[34,35]

Brain Stimulation

Electrical stimulation of the nervous system is used in the treatment of movement disorders, pain, and epilepsy. Stimulation involves placement of an electrode, which is then connected to a subcutaneously placed generator. Here we briefly discuss neurostimulation as it applies to the treatment of movement disorders, chronic pain states, and epilepsy.

Parkinson's disease is the most common movement disorder for which patients have surgery. Stereotactic techniques developed in the 1950s were used to create lesions in the pallidum and thalamus. These ablative procedures fell by the wayside for a time with the introduction and widespread use of L-dopa. In the early 1990s, there was a renewed interest in the use of surgical techniques for Parkinson's patients who had become unresponsive to pharmacologic agents or intolerant of their side effects. Lesions of the internal segment of the globus pallidus (GPi) saw a tremendous resurgence. With improvements in imaging and intraoperative microelectrode recording, deep brain stimulation soon replaced ablative procedures in the surgical treatment of these patients. Stimulation induces a reversible inhibition of neuronal activity, which can be adjusted as the clinical situation demands. The subthalamic nucleus has replaced the GPi as the target of choice. Subthalamic nucleus stimulation is most effective for the treatment of rigidity and akinesia. Tremor is best addressed with stimulation of the ventralis intermedius nucleus of the thalamus.

Spinal cord stimulation is used in the treatment of chronic pain as well as dystonia and bladder dysfunction. Patients typically undergo a trial of stimulation in which wire electrodes are placed percutaneously and attached to an external generator. If symptoms improve, permanent wire electrodes or paddle electrodes are placed and connected to a programmable generator placed subcutaneously. The precise mechanism of action is unknown. The most common indication is that of the so-called postlaminectomy syndrome, especially when leg pain is worse than back pain. There is also some benefit in those patients with chronic regional pain syndrome. It has not been found to be routinely effective in the treatment of cancer pain.

Vagal nerve stimulation is approved by the U.S. Food and Drug Administration for the treatment of intractable seizures and severe depression. The mechanism of action is not clear but is thought to be due to afferent stimulation of higher cortical centers in the hypothalamus, amygdala, insular cortex, and cerebral cortex through the nucleus of the solitary tract. Stimulation of the left vagus nerve decreases seizure frequency by about 50%. It rarely makes patients seizure-free.[36]

Implantable Pumps

Implantable pumps are used in the treatment of chronic pain and spasticity. An intrathecal catheter is inserted into the lumber spinal canal and a trial infusion used to gauge response. Many patients with cancer pain will respond favorably to intrathecal administration of narcotics through a programmable pump. Baclofen is the agent of choice for the treatment of spasticity with this modality.

Destructive Lesions

Ablative lesioning of the CNS in the treatment of pain, movement disorders, epilepsy, and psychiatric diseases has a long history. Before the advent of antipsychotic drugs, institutionalization and "psychosurgery" were thought by some to be the most efficient way of curing and controlling some patients with severe psychiatric disease. Before the development of some of the technologies elucidated earlier, lesioning of different pathways in the brain and spinal cord was the only way we had to treat patients with chronic pain and movement disorders. Even though neuroaugmentative procedures and drug infusion technology have replaced many of the neuroablative procedures formerly in widespread use, there still remain a few ablative procedures that retain their clinical utility.

Dorsal root entry zone lesions are particularly useful in patients with deafferentation pain related to brachial plexus injury and, to a lesser extent, patients with spinal cord injury who have "end zone" pain. In these conditions, deafferentation of the spinothalamic tract neurons results in spontaneous firing and the sensation of pain. The procedure creates lesions of the dorsal horn of the affected levels using a thermocoupled probe. Extension of this concept has been applied to the caudal nucleus of the trigeminal nerve for the treatment of facial pain syndromes.

Myelotomy has traditionally been used in the treatment of bilateral cancer pain and involves sectioning of the anterior commissure at and above the involved levels. This interrupts pain fibers on their way to the contralateral spinothalamic tract. Recently, a modified technique that only interrupts the median raphe of the dorsal columns has been described.[37] This presumably interrupts the recently described second-order visceral pain pathway demonstrated to travel up the mammalian dorsal funiculus.[38]

Cordotomy involves lesioning the anterolateral quadrant of the spinal cord at cervical levels, thereby eliminating input from the spinothalamic tract on the contralateral side of the body. Historically, it was most useful in the treatment of unilateral cancer pain. Bilateral lesioning increases the risk for neurologically mediated sleep apnea (Ondine's curse). It can be performed either percutaneously or as an open procedure.

Sympathectomy involves surgical interruption of the sympathetic chain at either the high thoracic or lumbar levels. A variety of endoscopic, thoracoscopic, radiofrequency, and open techniques are used. It is primarily used in patients with hyperhidrosis, sympathetically mediated pain, causalgia, chronic regional pain syndrome, and Raynaud's disease. There are disagreement and debate about the clinical utility of this procedure. Its use is tailored to the individual patient.

Nerve block or neurectomy. Local anesthetic, sometimes with corticosteroids can be injected into the tissues surrounding a peripheral nerve, blocking conductivity and relieving pain. This can result in a long-lasting effect but typically is short lived. Neurolytic agents (phenol or absolute alcohol) can also be used. Nerves can also be surgically divided or interrupted using radiofrequency techniques. There is a significant risk for recurrence with ablative neurectomy. Local nerve blocks are typically used in diagnostic procedures but can be repeated as necessary for the relief of pain. Ablative neurectomy is usually reserved for short-term relief in patients with a poor prognosis and short life expectancy.

Epilepsy

Epilepsy is not a distinct clinical entity with an identifiable cause, but rather a complex collection of disorders of the brain that all share seizures as part of the complex. Seizures are classified as partial, generalized, or unclassified. Partial seizures are either simple (consciousness not impaired) or complex (consciousness impaired). Generalized seizures are either convulsive or nonconvulsive. Incidence rates in developed countries (40-70 per 100,000) are lower than those in developing countries (100-190 per 100,000). About 20% to 40% of patients with seizures do not respond to anticonvulsant therapy. Failure to respond to three anticonvulsant medications prompts referral to a center specializing in epilepsy evaluation and treatment. About 1.33% to 4.50% of those patients are candidates for surgical intervention.[39]

The goal of the workup of the patient who is a potential candidate for the surgical treatment of epilepsy is to identify the cortical area responsible for the onset of the seizure. When the radiographic workup (MRI, CT, or both) reveals an obvious lesion causing the seizure (tumor, vascular malformation), the treatment is relatively straightforward and involves removal of the lesion. In other cases, the offending lesion is not as obvious on imaging, and intensive and often invasive monitoring is necessary to determine the epileptogenic focus. It is also important to determine language dominance and areas of the brain that are functionally abnormal during the interictal period. Noninvasive techniques that are becoming more available and better characterized include magnetoencephalography, positron emission tomography, single-photon emission CT, and functional MRI. Invasive modalities used in the evaluation of patients for seizure surgery include Wada's test for language dominance, stereotactically implanted depth electrode, implanted strip electrodes, and implanted grid electrodes. Any or all of these techniques may be useful in brain mapping. It has long been possible to map critical speech and limb movement areas in awake, local anesthetized craniotomy patients at the time of seizure focus resection.

Based on the information obtained in a noninvasive workup, the patient may be taken to surgery. Dominant hemisphere lesions are often operated on with the patient

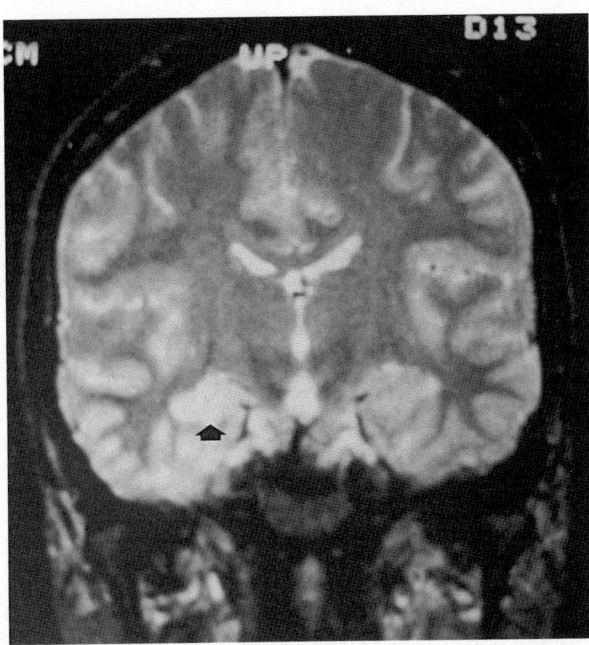

Figure 72-24 T2-weighted coronal MRI study shows gliosis of mesial temporal structure (*arrow*).

awake to allow for intraoperative confirmatory brain mapping. This is accomplished by stimulating the cortex and observing and monitoring the patient's response, looking for speech arrest, anomia, or limb weakness or numbness. The most common surgical procedures performed for epilepsy are anterior temporal lobectomy, focal cortical resection, multiple subpial transection, hemispherectomy, and corpus callosotomy.

Anterior temporal lobectomy is the most operation for seizures. An entirely unilateral interictal focus is the ideal indication (Fig. 72-24). The anterior temporal lobe, anterior hippocampus, and amygdala are excised. If the epileptogenic focus is not completely excised, the patient may continue to experience intractable seizures. If too much temporal lobe is resected, it can result in a contralateral superior quadrantanopsia or, in dominant hemisphere lesions, speech and language dysfunction.

Focal cortical resection is usually performed in the frontal cortex. The results are more variable than those with temporal lobectomy.

Multiple subpial transection is used in more eloquent areas of the brain and involves making cortical incisions perpendicular to the surface of the gyrus in question. This presumably preserves descending fibers and function, while interrupting spread of any epileptogenic activity within the cortical mantel itself.

Corpus callosotomy is used to prevent the rapid spread of seizures, rather than eliminate the focus. It is primarily useful in seizures that suddenly generalize, resulting in atonic "drop attacks," as in Lennox-Gastaut syndrome.

Hemispherectomy is usually reserved for young children with seizures restricted to one hemisphere but threatening the good hemisphere by secondary effects of repeated seizures, as in Rasmussen's syndrome. There is usually some abnormality of cellular migration. In the past, the entire cortex was removed, leaving the basal

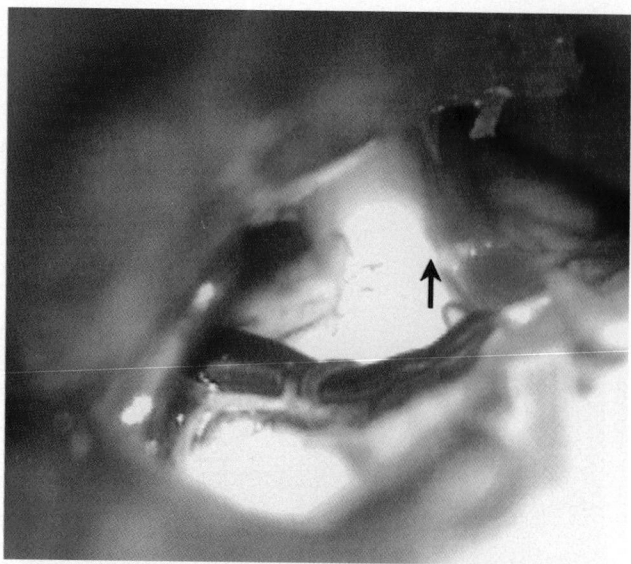

Figure 72-25 An intraoperative photograph through the operative microscope in a patient with typical trigeminal neuralgia. The left trigeminal nerve is compressed superiorly by an arterial branch of the superior cerebellar artery (*arrow*).

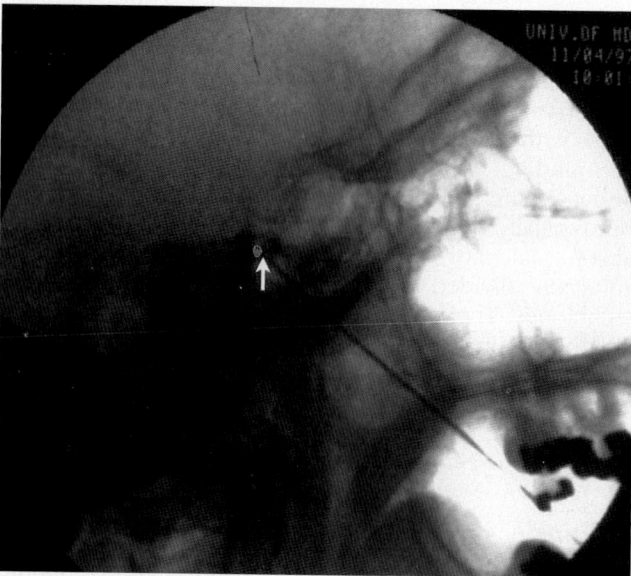

Figure 72-26 A lateral skull film in a patient undergoing glycerol rhizotomy for typical trigeminal neuralgia. A 20-gauge spinal needle is directed to the foramen ovale, and nonionic contrast agent is injected to outline the trigeminal ganglion (*arrow*).

ganglia intact. Even though there was a significant decrease in seizure activity, the procedure led to a high complication rate, with ex vacuo brain shifts. A newer technique now involves preservation of portions of the cortex and its blood supply while disconnecting them from the rest of the brain by extensive undercutting of the adjacent white matter.[40]

Trigeminal Neuralgia

Trigeminal neuralgia affects about 4 in 100,000 people and is characterized by brief episodes of severe, lancinating pain in one or more of the three divisions of the trigeminal nerve, usually V2 and V3. Patients often describe that it is precipitated by touch or extremes of temperature. In extreme cases, a patient may refuse to eat or shave to avoid triggering the severe jolts of pain. Sensation usually remains intact, and significant numbness or jaw weakness leads to suspicion of a compressive mass lesion such as tumor. Often, the patients are referred with an already established diagnosis. It is reassuring if the patient did respond at some point to carbamazepine or appropriate medication. Patients have an MRI to rule out posterior fossa tumors and multiple sclerosis, which can present with related symptoms. Most patients respond to the oral administration of carbamazepine. Baclofen and gabapentin also have some clinical utility in the medical management. The most common mechanism is presumed to be related to vascular compression of the fifth cranial nerve as it enters the brainstem (Fig. 72-25). With aging, the arteries elongate and can then begin to loop against the cranial nerves. At its entry to the pons, the fifth nerve has lost its peripheral nerve supportive architecture, the reticulin and mesenchymal elements that toughen the nerve more peripherally. Focal, pulsatile pressure of the artery against this vulnerable part of nerve results in

ephaptic transmission from large myelinated fibers to small myelinated (A delta) and unmyelinated fibers.

Surgical therapy is usually reserved for patients who fail medical management. Microvascular decompression involves a small suboccipital craniotomy for microsurgical exploration of the dorsal root entry zone of the trigeminal nerve on the affected side. The offending vessel (usually the superior cerebellar artery) is then dissected off the nerve and a barrier (Teflon or PVA sponge) is placed between the vessel and the nerve to prevent continued pulsatile focal compression. In especially favorable situations, the offending artery can be dissected free to loop away from the nerve without need for padding. A small sling of arterial patch graft material can also be sewn to hold the artery loop away from the nerve.

Percutaneous trigeminal rhizotomy techniques generally involve either radiofrequency heat lesioning of the trigeminal ganglion, glycerol injection (Fig. 72-26) into the spinal fluid of Meckel's cave (which causes an osmotic damage preferentially to the smaller pain-carrying nerve fibers), or mechanical trauma to the nerve or ganglion by transient inflation of a No. 4 Fogarty catheter balloon. Each method has its own proponents along with advantages and disadvantages.

Stereotactic radiosurgery has recently been described in the treatment of trigeminal neuralgia.[18] Although initial results are encouraging, long-term efficacy has yet to be determined.

HYDROCEPHALUS

Hydrocephalus, defined as enlargement of the cerebral ventricles, occurs when production of CSF outpaces the body's ability to absorb that fluid. This can be related to obstruction of flow of the CSF through the ventricular system (obstructive hydrocephalus) or the inability of the body to reabsorb CSF at the level of the arachnoid granulations (so-called communicating hydrocephalus). The distinction between communicating and obstructive hydrocephalus is determined by the nature of CSF flow disruption. If there is free flow of spinal fluid through the ventricular system to the level of the arachnoid granulations, then hydrocephalus is referred to as communicating. If there is obstruction to flow anywhere in the ventricular system, the hydrocephalus is referred to as obstructive. Rarely, a tumor of the choroid plexus, the structure responsible for CSF production, will cause overproduction of the spinal fluid, outpacing the body's ability to absorb it. Obstructive hydrocephalus is typically congenital but can be related to intraventricular or periventricular masses (neoplastic and non-neoplastic). It typically presents with imaging demonstrating enlargement of some ventricles, but not others, indicating an obstruction in the flow of spinal fluid from one part of the ventricular system to another. Communicating hydrocephalus is typically acquired, is usually secondary to infection or hemorrhage, and demonstrates more uniform enlargement of all four ventricles.

Hydrocephalus is usually discussed in conjunction with pediatric neurosurgery because this is one of the more common conditions treated by neurosurgeons specializing in the treatment of infants and children. In fact, hydrocephalus is quite common in the adult population, and it behooves the adroit practitioner to be familiar with its pathophysiology and treatment. In this section, we concentrate on the types of hydrocephalus affecting the adult population. Pediatric hydrocephalus is discussed later.

Posthemorrhagic hydrocephalus is caused by obstruction of the arachnoid granulations with blood cells. This results in hydrocephalus of the communicating variety. *Postinfectious hydrocephalus* is also communicating and results from meningeal infection and altered CSF absorption.

Normal-pressure hydrocephalus is a condition characterized by the clinical triad of gait ataxia, incontinence, and dementia. Imaging reveals ventriculomegaly out of proportion to brain atrophy. This condition is most commonly seen in the elderly population and does respond to CSF diversion. Many techniques have been used to predict whether patients will respond to CSF diversion. Many believe that the clinical presentation of ataxia, incontinence, and dementia, in that order, is the best predictor of response to shunting.

Hydrocephalus and pregnancy is seen when women with ventriculoperitoneal or lumboperitoneal shunts become pregnant. In general, treatment and management must be tailored to the individual patient. Headache, nausea, vomiting, seizures, and lethargy may be the presenting signs of shunt failure. In gravid patients, this may be due to an increased incidence of distal malfunction. These signs and symptoms are also seen in pre-eclampsia, which must be ruled out. Patients undergoing cesarean birth receive prophylactic antibiotics. Shunt externalization may be necessary for grossly contaminated cases.

Abdominal surgery in patients with ventriculoperitoneal shunts must be individualized. In grossly contaminated cases, shunt externalization is recommended.[41] Prophylactic antibiotics are recommended for percutaneous gastrostomy tube placement in patients with shunts because there is an increased incidence of shunt infection in these patients.[42,43]

PEDIATRIC NEUROSURGERY

Pediatric neurosurgery is that aspect of the discipline that deals with infants and children. As mentioned earlier, a large portion of the pediatric neurosurgeon's time is spent dealing with hydrocephalus. In addition, pediatric neurosurgery is concerned with the treatment of other congenital anomalies, neurotrauma, functional problems such as spasticity and epilepsy, cerebrovascular disorders in children, brain tumors, and congenital defects of the spine and spinal cord. In this section, we briefly discuss some of these disease processes and their treatment.

Hydrocephalus in newborns manifests by an increased head circumference, full and tense fontanelles, and widened cranial sutures. The child may demonstrate lethargy and poor feeding and have abnormalities of the extraocular apparatus resulting in poor upgaze. Diagnosis is made with ultrasound, MRI, or CT.

The etiology of hydrocephalus in infants and newborns is either congenital or acquired. Congenital hydrocephalus is typically obstructive, whereas acquired hydrocephalus is usually communicating. Acquired hydrocephalus in newborns is usually postinfectious (meningitis, intrauterine toxoplasmosis infection, cytomegalovirus infection) or related to prematurity (intraventricular hemorrhage). Congenital conditions that can cause hydrocephalus include aqueductal stenosis, Chiari II malformation (discussed later), Dandy-Walker malformation, vein of Galen aneurysms, tumors, and arachnoid cysts. Aqueductal stenosis causes obstructive hydrocephalus by impeding flow of spinal fluid from the third ventricle to the fourth ventricle. Chiari II malformation causes fourth ventricular outflow obstruction. Dandy-Walker malformation is associated with absence of the cerebellar vermis, cystic expansion of the fourth ventricle, and hydrocephalus. Vein of Galen aneurysms, tumors, and arachnoid cysts cause hydrocephalus through an obstructive mechanism (Fig. 72-27).

The treatment of hydrocephalus is primarily concerned with the prevention of neurologic injury, which may occur if the condition is left untreated. In some cases, neurologic deficit can be reversed. Treatment typically involves treatment of the offending lesion (resection of the tumor or treatment of the infection) and CSF diversion. The distal terminus for most shunts is the peritoneal cavity. Other sites include the pleural cavity or superior vena cava. CSF diversion procedures are not without complications, and 5% to 15% of all shunts become infected. Treatment of shunt infections usually involves externalization or removal of the device, sterilization of the spinal fluid, and eventual replacement of the shunt.

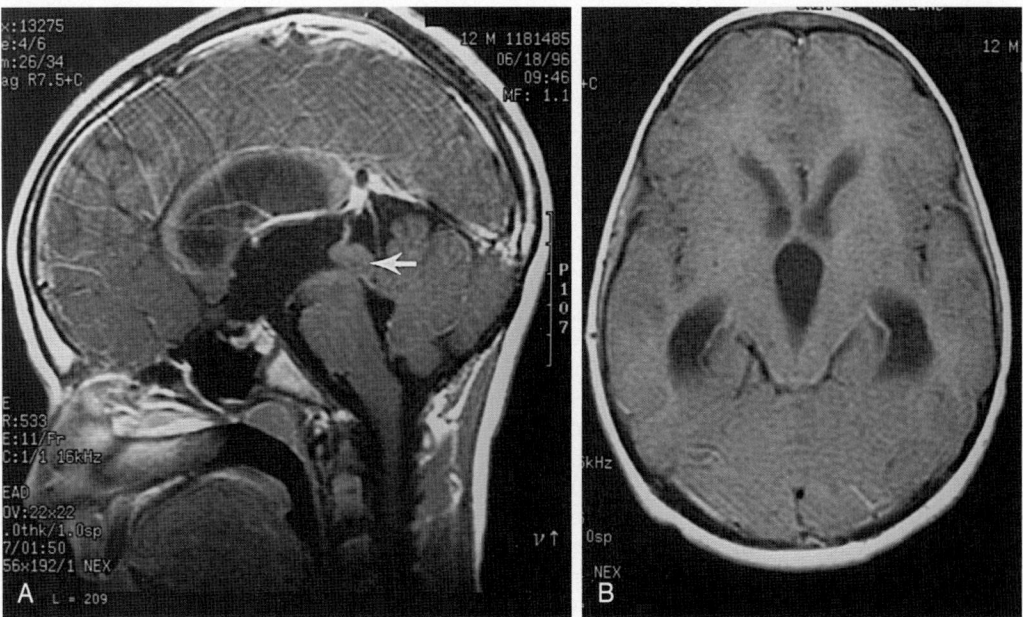

Figure 72-27 MRI studies in a 12-year-old boy with hydrocephalus. **A,** Sagittal T1-weighted MRI study demonstrates a small tectal glioma (*arrow*) causing aqueductal stenosis and the typical pattern of triventricular hydrocephalus. **B,** Axial MRI study demonstrating a dilated third ventricle and enlarged temporal horns.

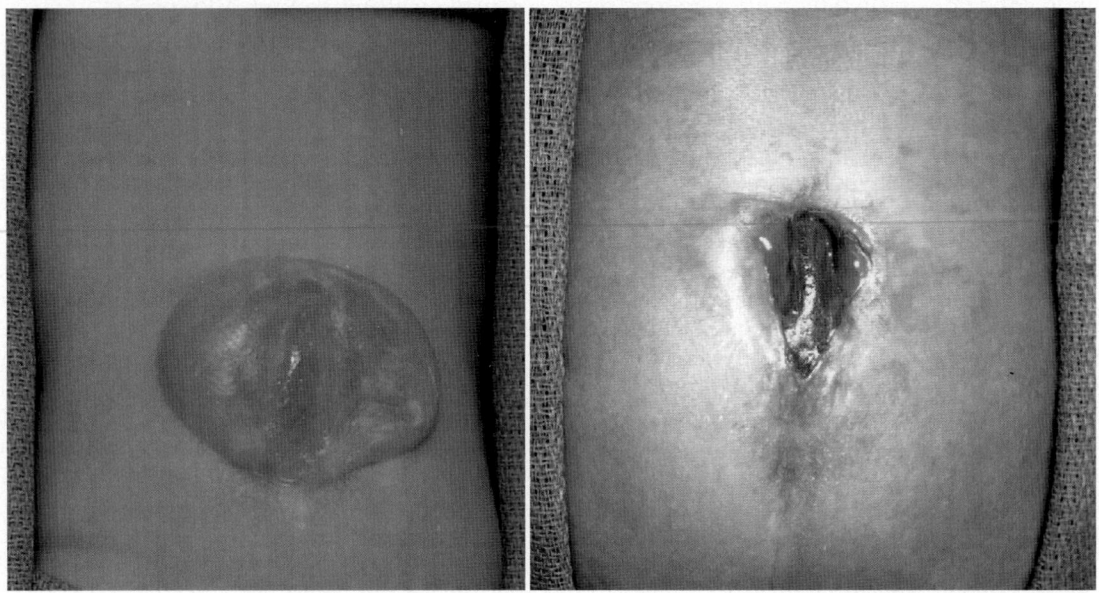

Figure 72-28 Two examples of myelomeningoceles. The neural placode, a flat plate of dysraphic neural elements, is exposed.

Other neurosurgical conditions affecting infants and children include a variety of congenital anomalies affecting the nervous system. Myelomeningocele (Fig. 72-28) is an anomaly related to failure of the neural tube to close, with deficient meningeal, skeletal, and muscular development. The resultant neural placode is present without skin covering and is usually associated with a sac or enlarged subarachnoid space. Treatment consists of closure and reconstruction of the different layers. Neurologic deficit distal to the defect is common, as

are hydrocephalus and Chiari malformation (discussed later).

Encephaloceles (Fig. 72-29) are the result of disordered closure of the cranial neuropore. Occipital encephaloceles are more commonly seen in Western populations, whereas frontal lesions are more common in southeastern Asia. The lesion may or may not have neural tissue within it. The brain that is involved is usually dysplastic. There is frequently an associated intracranial abnormality. Occult spinal dysraphism often manifests cutaneously in

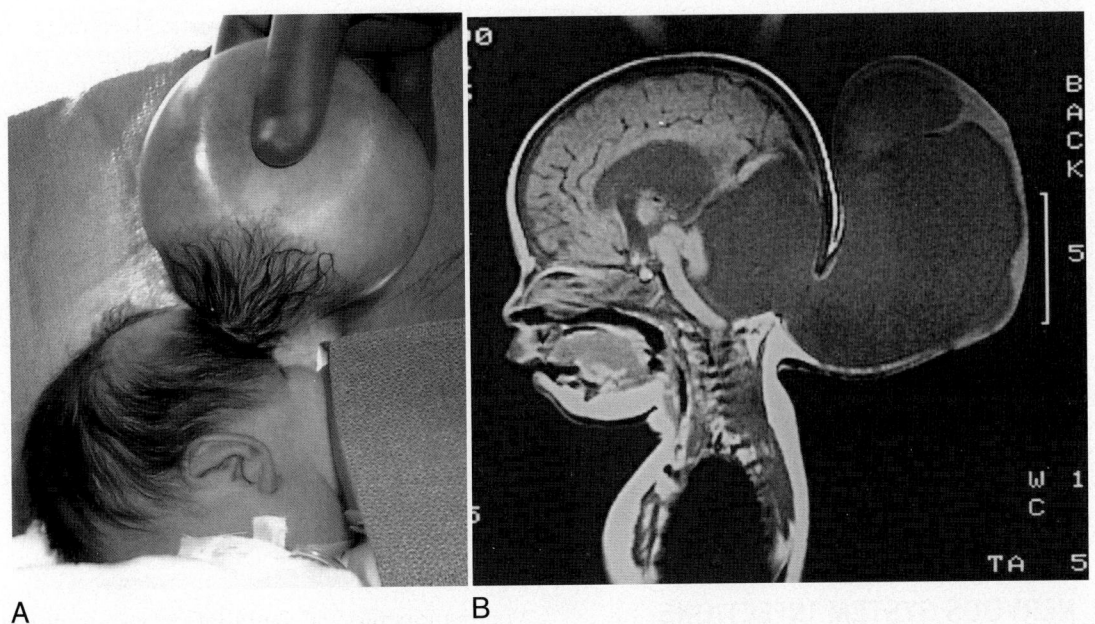

Figure 72-29 An infant with a large occipital encephalocele. **A,** The large skin-covered encephalocele is visible. **B,** A sagittal MRI study in a newborn with a large occipital encephalocele. At surgery, the sac contained herniated dysplastic cerebellar tissue as well as cerebrospinal fluid.

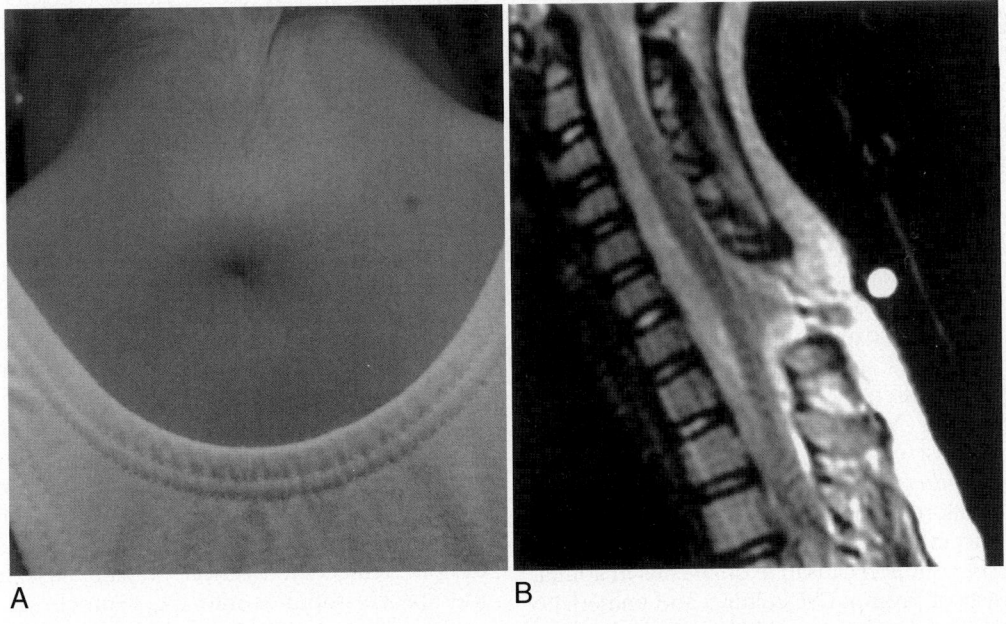

Figure 72-30 A, Dermal sinus tract in a 10-year-old girl who presented with purulent drainage. **B,** Sagittal T2-weighted MRI study shows a connection of the sinus tract with the thecal sac.

the lumbosacral area. Hemangiomas, hair tufts, dermal sinus tracts, and lipomatous masses are frequently seen. This condition is frequently associated with tethered cord syndrome. This syndrome clinically manifests as back and leg pain, gait difficulty, weakness, orthopedic deformity of the feet, voiding dysfunction, and sexual dysfunction. Diastematomyelia is a dysraphic state in which there is duplication of the spinal cord at one or more continuous levels. Dermal sinus tracts are squamous-lined fistulas, often associated with small cutaneous pits in the

midline. They are often associated with intradural dermoid or epidermoid tumors (Fig. 72-30). Treatment is usually surgical with excision of the fistula and removal of the dermoid or epidermoid component.

Chiari malformations (also known as *Arnold-Chiari malformations*) consist of four different hindbrain abnormalities that are probably unrelated. Types I and II are considered here. Chiari I malformation is usually diagnosed in adults and involves downward displacement of the cerebellar tonsils into the foramen magnum. It may also be associated with syringomyelia of the cervical spinal cord. Downward displacement of the medulla is typically absent. Patients present with occipital headache exacerbated by Valsalva maneuver and may also have signs of foramen magnum compression, central cord syndrome, or cerebellar syndrome. Some patients also present with signs of intracranial hypertension. Diagnosis is made with MRI and CT. Sagittal MRI gives an accurate assessment of the extent of tonsillar descent. Treatment consists of bony decompression of the occiput with removal of the posterior arch of C1 and sometimes C2. The dura is then opened and a dural patch graft sewn into place, thus creating more room for the neural elements. Chiari II malformation is usually associated with myelomeningocele. The medulla, cervicomedullary junction, and fourth ventricle are caudally displaced. These children can present with stridor, dysphagia, and apnea. Operative intervention is indicated in these cases.

CENTRAL NERVOUS SYSTEM INFECTIONS

This section addresses infections of the CNS and its surrounding structures. Timely diagnosis and treatment of CNS infections are critical because failure to diagnose and appropriately treat can have long-lasting and devastating consequences.

Meningitis

Acute bacterial meningitis is an infection of the subarachnoid spaces and meninges. Symptoms and signs include fever, malaise, altered mental status, neck stiffness, and headache. Symptoms result from leptomeningeal irritation and increased ICP. The causative organism varies with the patient's age. Neonatal meningitis is caused by group B streptococcus, *Escherichia coli,* or *Listeria* species infection. "Late" neonatal meningitis can be caused by any of these, as well as staphylococci or *Pseudomonas aeruginosa*. In children, *Streptococcus pneumoniae* (pneumococcus) and *Neisseria meningitidis* (meningococcus) are the most common causative organisms. In the past, *Haemophilus influenzae* was a common cause of meningitis in children, but its prevalence has decreased secondary to vaccination. Pneumococci and meningococci are the most common causative organisms in adults. Treatment consists of prompt CSF cultures and immediate IV administration of antibiotics. Altered mental status secondary to communicating hydrocephalus may necessitate placement of an external ventricular drain and eventual placement of a ventriculoperitoneal shunt once the CSF is sterilized. Recurrent episodes of bacterial meningitis prompt investigation into abnormal communication between the CNS and the outside world (dermal sinus or CSF fistula).

Postoperative Infections

Infections of the CNS occurring after neurosurgical procedures are typically caused by staphylococcal species. Enteric organisms and pseudomonal and streptococcal species can also be problematic. Treatment, as with any infection, involves the identification of the causative organism and appropriate antibiotic administration. Postoperative abscesses are addressed with drainage, surgery, or both, as dictated by the clinical situation.

Post-traumatic Meningitis

Meningeal infection after head injury is typically related to CSF fistula. Most post-traumatic fistulas stop spontaneously within days of injury. The incidence of meningitis increases if a leak persists for longer than 7 days. Clinically obvious leaks manifest as CSF rhinorrhea or otorrhea. The prophylactic antibiotic treatment of CSF fistula is controversial and needs to be tailored to the clinical situation.[44,45] A persistent post-traumatic CSF fistula is addressed surgically to prevent the risk associated with recurrent bouts of meningitis.

Shunt Infections

Ventriculoperitoneal shunt infections are typically due to colonization of the shunt tubing by staphylococci (*S. aureus* and *S. epidermidis*). The clinical presentation can be somewhat nonspecific and involve fever, malaise nausea, vomiting, irritability, and signs of shunt malfunction. Infection with more virulent species of bacteria can be associated with ventriculitis and meningitis. The reported rate of shunt infection varies from 3% to 20%. If shunt infection is suspected, treatment consists of CSF culture and administration of antibiotics. Most authors advocate externalization or removal of the infected hardware with replacement when the CSF is sterilized,[46] although there are reports of sterilization without removal or externalization.

Brain Abscess

Cerebral abscesses present with signs and symptoms related to an expanding mass lesion. Patients can present with altered mental status, focal neurologic deficit, headache, nausea and vomiting, or seizures. Fever, elevated white blood cell count, and signs of meningeal irritation are often absent. Contrast-enhanced CT and MRI reveal a ring-enhancing lesion usually at the gray-white interface with surrounding edema. This can be confused with tumor. Acute deterioration of patients can occur when the abscess ruptures into the ventricle or subarachnoid space with resultant ventriculitis or meningitis. Brain abscesses develop by either contiguous spread from adjacent structures (paranasal sinuses and petrous bone) or hematogenous spread from a distant site. They can be either solitary or multiple. Causative organisms are extremely varied and include both aerobic and anaerobic organisms, fungi, and parasites. Principles of treatment revolve around the accurate identification of the causative organism, relief of mass effect, administration of appropriate antibiotic therapy, and treatment of the underlying cause (e.g., paranasal sinus infection, dental caries, ear infection, bronchiectasis). Controversy exists as to whether surgical excision or aspiration of the abscess yields better results.

Subdural Empyema

Subdural empyema is a collection of pus in the subdural space. It is typically related to contiguous spread from the paranasal sinuses or ear infection. Patients can present with fever, meningeal signs, headache, seizures, focal neurologic deficits, and altered mental status. It is often heralded by a rapid clinical deterioration. Diagnosis is made based on index of suspicion and the presence of a subdural fluid collection, sometimes adjacent to a known focus of sinus infection. Often, the collection is interhemispheric. Prompt institution of surgical (drainage and irrigation) and medical (antibiotics) therapy is critical in the treatment of this disease.

Spinal Infections

Spinal infections can be divided into those affecting the bone (vertebral osteomyelitis), the disk space (diskitis), and the epidural space (spinal epidural abscess). Occasionally, infectious processes can involve more than one, or even all three.

Osteomyelitis of the bone is most commonly seen in IV drug users, diabetic patients, hemodialysis patients, and older adults. The causative organism is usually *S. aureus,* and spread is hematogenous, although postoperative infections are also seen. These infections can and do affect the integrity of the bone, resulting in collapse. This in turn can result in pain and neurologic compromise. Treatment consists of organism identification, appropriate long-term antibiotics, and maintenance of anatomic spinal alignment, with or without surgical intervention.

Diskitis often occurs concomitantly with osteomyelitis and is seen in the same patient population. Fever, back pain, and an elevated sedimentation rate or C-reactive protein are often seen. The white blood cell count may or may not be elevated. This may occur spontaneously or postoperatively. Treatment may or may not be surgical. Long-term antibiotic therapy is usually indicated.

Spinal epidural abscess usually occurs in the setting of an infectious process elsewhere in the body. Spread occurs either hematogenously or by direct extension. Patients present initially with localized back pain and possible radiculopathy. Spinal cord compromise can follow rapidly with paraplegia or quadriplegia. Predisposing factors are the same as those for osteomyelitis and diskitis. Diagnosis is made with contrast-enhanced MRI. When spinal cord compression is evident, surgery is usually performed for decompression and diagnosis. Spinal epidural abscess can sometimes be managed medically, with close neurologic observation and imaging studies. This is usually reserved for cases in which the causative organism is known, the abscess is small, and there is no neurologic compromise. As in all fields of medicine, treatment must be tailored to the individual patient.

Acquired Immunodeficiency Syndrome

The most common CNS opportunistic infection in patients with AIDS is toxoplasmosis caused by *Toxoplasma gondii.* These lesions usually present with ring enhancement on contrast-enhanced imaging studies and are usually in the basal ganglia. They may be solitary or multiple. Primary CNS lymphoma occurs in about 10% of AIDS patients and presents as an irregularly enhancing mass (target lesion). Progressive multifocal leukoencephalopathy presents with hypodense nonenhancing white-matter lesions. Fungal abscess and viral encephalopathy are not uncommon in this patient population. Even though the incidence of CNS opportunistic infections has decreased with the widespread use of highly active antiretroviral therapy (HAART), the treatment of these problems remains a challenge.

Selected References

Albright AL, Pollack IF, Adelson PD: Principles and Practice of Pediatric Neurosurgery. New York, Thieme, 1999.

This multiauthored reference extensively covers the subject of pediatric neurosurgery. The editors emphasize "clinical pearls" following each chapter, and extensive bibliographies are provided for more detailed reference.

Apuzzo MLJ (ed): Malignant Cerebral Glioma. Park Ridge, IL, American Association of Neurological Surgeons, 1990.

This single volume provides an excellent review of malignant gliomas, including pathology, surgical results, radiation therapy, and chemotherapy.

Benzel EC: Spine Surgery: Techniques, Complication Avoidance, and Management. Philadelphia, Churchill Livingstone, 1999.

This multiauthored text emphasizes the fundamentals of spine surgery and practical considerations in the management of spinal disorders. A large number of expert authors provide an excellent discussion of the subjects as well as extensive references for further study.

Bullock R, Chestnut RM, Clifton G, et al: Guidelines for the management of severe head injury. Brain Trauma Foundation, 2000 (Updates 2003).

Evidence-based guidelines for use in the management of brain injury.

Engel J Jr, Pedley TA (eds): Epilepsy: A Comprehensive Textbook, Vols. 1-3. Philadelphia, Lippincott-Raven, 1998.

A three-volume comprehensive epilepsy text.

Germano IM (ed): Neurosurgical Treatment of Movement Disorders. Park Ridge, IL, American Association of Neurological Surgeons, 1998.

An excellent review of all aspects of movement disorder surgery. Detailed chapters describe a variety of surgical approaches, including implantation of neurostimulators.

References

1. Kellie G: The kind of appearances observed in the dissection of two or three individuals . . . with some reference to the pathology of the brain. Trans Med Chi Edin 84-169, 1824.
2. Monro A: Observation on the Structure and Function of the Nervous System. Edinburgh, Creech and Johnson, 1783.
3. Lundberg N: Continuous recording and control of ventricular fluid pressure in neurosurgical practice. Acta Psychiatr Scand Suppl 36:1-193, 1960.

4. Ondra SL, Troupp H, George ED, et al: The natural history of symptomatic arteriovenous malformations of the brain: A 24-year follow-up assessment. J Neurosurg 73:387-391, 1990.
5. Spetzler RF, Martin NA: A proposed grading system for arteriovenous malformations. J Neurosurg 65:476-483, 1986.
6. McCormick WF, Hardman JM, Boulter TR: Vascular malformations ("angiomas") of the brain, with special reference to those occurring in the posterior fossa. J Neurosurg 28:241-251, 1968.
7. Molyneux A, Kerr R, Stratton I, et al: International Subarachnoid Aneurysm Trial (ISAT) of neurosurgical clipping versus endovascular coiling in 2143 patients with ruptured intracranial aneurysms: A randomised trial. Lancet 360:1267-1274, 2002.
8. Patchell RA: The management of brain metastases. Cancer Treat Rev 29:533-540, 2003.
9. Levin VA, Leibel SA, Gutin PH: Neoplasms of the central nervous system. In DeVita VT Jr, Hellman S, Rosenberg SA (eds): Cancer: Principles and Practice of Oncology, 6th ed. Philadelphia, Lippincott Williams & Wilkins, 2001, pp 2100-2160.
10. Rees J: Advances in magnetic resonance imaging of brain tumours. Curr Opin Neurol 16:643-650, 2003.
11. Kew Y, Levin VA: Advances in gene therapy and immunotherapy for brain tumors. Curr Opin Neurol 16:665-670, 2003.
12. Kleihues P, Cavenee WK: Pathology and Genetics of Tumours of the Nervous System. Lyon, International Agency for Research on Cancer, 2000.
13. Henson JW: Early genetic events in the formation of astrocytomas. Curr Opin Neurol 13:613-617, 2000.
14. Kornblith PL: The role of cytotoxic chemotherapy in the treatment of malignant brain tumors. Surg Neurol 44:551-552, 1995.
15. Galanis E, Buckner JC: Chemotherapy of brain tumors. Curr Opin Neurol 13:619-625, 2000.
16. Kuratsu J, Kochi M, Ushio Y: Incidence and clinical features of asymptomatic meningiomas. J Neurosurg 92:766-770, 2000.
17. Suh JH, Vogelbaum MA, Barnett GH: Update of stereotactic radiosurgery for brain tumors. Curr Opin Neurol 17:681-686, 2004.
18. Kondziolka D, Lunsford LD, Flickinger JC, et al: Emerging indications in stereotactic radiosurgery. Clin Neurosurg 52:229-233, 2005.
19. Kondziolka D, Nathoo N, Flickinger JC, et al: Long-term results after radiosurgery for benign intracranial tumors. Neurosurgery 53:815-821; discussion 821-812, 2003.
20. Suki D: The epidemiology of brain metastases. In Sawaya R (ed): Intracranial Metastases: Current Management Strategies. Malden, MA, Blackwell, 2004, pp 20-35.
21. Hanbali F, Fourney DR, Marmor E, et al: Spinal cord ependymoma: Radical surgical resection and outcome. Neurosurgery 51:1162-1172; discussion 1172-1174, 2002.
22. Narayan RK: Development of guidelines for the management of severe head injury. J Neurotrauma 12:907-912, 1995.
23. Ogden AT, Mayer SA, Connolly ES Jr: Hyperosmolar agents in neurosurgical practice: The evolving role of hypertonic saline. Neurosurgery 57:207-215; discussion 207-215, 2005.
24. Rutigliano D, Egnor MR, Priebe CJ, et al: Decompressive craniectomy in pediatric patients with traumatic brain injury with intractable elevated intracranial pressure. J Pediatr Surg 41:83-87; discussion 83-87, 2006.
25. Quality Standards Subcommittee: Practice parameter: The management of concussion in sports (summary statement). Neurology 48:581-585, 1997.
26. Cantu RC: Return to play guidelines after a head injury. Clin Sports Med 17:45-60, 1998.
27. Kelly JP, Nichols JS, Filley CM, et al: Concussion in sports: Guidelines for the prevention of catastrophic outcome. JAMA 266:2867-2869, 1991.
28. Gosselin N, Theriault M, Leclerc S, et al: Neurophysiological anomalies in symptomatic and asymptomatic concussed athletes. Neurosurgery 58:1151-1161; discussion 1151-1161, 2006.
29. McClincy MP, Lovell MR, Pardini J, et al: Recovery from sports concussion in high school and collegiate athletes. Brain Inj 20:33-39, 2006.
30. Resnick DK, Choudhri TF, Dailey AT, et al: Guidelines for the performance of fusion procedures for degenerative disease of the lumbar spine. Part 8: Lumbar fusion for disc herniation and radiculopathy. J Neurosurg Spine 2:673-678, 2005.
31. Lunsford LD, Bissonette DJ, Zorub DS: Anterior surgery for cervical disc disease. Part 2: Treatment of cervical spondylotic myelopathy in 32 cases. J Neurosurg 53:12-19, 1980.
32. Chang SD, Adler JR Jr: Current treatment of patients with multiple brain metastases. Neurosurg Focus 9:e5, 2000.
33. Flickinger JC, Barker FG 2nd: Clinical results: Radiosurgery and radiotherapy of cranial nerve schwannomas. Neurosurg Clin N Am 17:121-128, vi, 2006.
34. Kuo JS, Yu C, Petrovich Z, et al: The CyberKnife stereotactic radiosurgery system: Description, installation, and an initial evaluation of use and functionality. Neurosurgery 53:1235-1239; discussion 1239, 2003.
35. Romanelli P, Schaal DW, Adler JR: Image-guided radiosurgical ablation of intra- and extra-cranial lesions. Technol Cancer Res Treat 5:421-428, 2006.
36. Groves DA, Brown VJ: Vagal nerve stimulation: A review of its applications and potential mechanisms that mediate its clinical effects. Neurosci Biobehav Rev 29:493-500, 2005.
37. Nauta HJ, Soukup VM, Fabian RH, et al: Punctate midline myelotomy for the relief of visceral cancer pain. J Neurosurg 92:125-130, 2000.
38. Willis WD Jr, Westlund KN: The role of the dorsal column pathway in visceral nociception. Curr Pain Headache Rep 5:20-26, 2001.
39. Zimmerman RS, Sirven JI: An overview of surgery for chronic seizures. Mayo Clin Proc 78:109-117, 2003.
40. Devlin AM, Cross JH, Harkness W, et al: Clinical outcomes of hemispherectomy for epilepsy in childhood and adolescence. Brain 126:556-566, 2003.
41. Gassas A, Kennedy J, Green G, et al: Risk of ventriculoperitoneal shunt infections due to gastrostomy feeding tube insertion in pediatric patients with brain tumors. Pediatr Neurosurg 42:95-99, 2006.
42. Ein SH, Miller S, Rutka JT: Appendicitis in the child with a ventriculo-peritoneal shunt: A 30-year review. J Pediatr Surg 41:1255-1258, 2006.
43. Sane SS, Towbin A, Bergey EA, et al: Percutaneous gastrostomy tube placement in patients with ventriculoperitoneal shunts. Pediatr Radiol 28:521-523, 1998.
44. Eftekhar B, Ghodsi M, Nejat F, et al: Prophylactic administration of ceftriaxone for the prevention of meningitis after traumatic pneumocephalus: Results of a clinical trial. J Neurosurg 101:757-761, 2004.
45. Friedman JA, Ebersold MJ, Quast LM: Post-traumatic cerebrospinal fluid leakage. World J Surg 25:1062-1066, 2001.
46. Kestle JR, Garton HJ, Whitehead WE, et al: Management of shunt infections: A multicenter pilot study. J Neurosurg 105:177-181, 2006.

CHAPTER 73

Plastic Surgery

John L. Burns, MD   and   Steven J. Blackwell, MD

General Plastic Surgical Principles and Techniques
Head and Neck: Congenital and Craniomaxillofacial
Head and Neck
Trunk and External Genitalia
Lower Extremity
Breast and Aesthetic Surgery
Conclusion

Plastic surgery takes its name from the Greek term *plas-tikos,* which means to mold and reshape. Plastic surgery is an extremely diverse surgical specialty whose chief purpose is to restore form and function. The American Board of Plastic Surgery stated, "the specialty of plastic surgery deals with the repair, replacement, and reconstruction of physical defects of form or function involving the skin, musculoskeletal system, craniomaxillofacial structures, hand, extremities, breast and trunk, and external genitalia. It uses aesthetic surgical principles not only to improve undesirable qualities of normal structures, but in all reconstructive procedures as well."

The diverse nature of this discipline lends itself to many areas of further specialization. These include, but are not limited to, hand and microvascular surgery, craniomaxillofacial surgery, acute and reconstructive burn surgery, and aesthetic surgery. Several of these areas, including hand surgery, burns, wound care, and cutaneous malignancies, are covered in separate chapters. Herein we offer medical students, residents, and general surgeons only an overview of plastic surgery with an emphasis on reconstruction.

GENERAL PLASTIC SURGICAL PRINCIPLES AND TECHNIQUES

Skin Incisions and Excisions

As plastic surgery is a specialty dealing with difficult wounds and wound problems, meticulous attention is focused on wound closure and avoidance of unsightly scars. Skin incisions are carefully planned to avoid an obvious scar. Skin creases and hair-bearing areas are useful places to camouflage incisions. For example, facial incisions can be hidden in the pretragal crease, subciliary crease, or nasolabial fold. Breast incisions can be hidden in the periareolar skin, the inframammary crease, or the axilla.

Tension is avoided across skin incisions because it will result in wide and unsightly scars. In 1861, Carl Langer noted that tension is unevenly distributed in skin and that human skin is less distensible in the direction of tension lines than across them. *Langer's lines* can be used to design skin incisions and diminish tension across the incision. When possible, incisions are placed perpendicular to the long axis of the underlying muscle. Relaxed skin tension lines (RSTLs) are lines of minimal tension, which often appear as wrinkle lines, or natural skin lines.[1] RSTLs lie perpendicular to the underlying muscle and are accentuated by contraction of the muscle (Fig. 73-1). An example of this principle is transverse wrinkling of the forehead, which is perpendicular to the underlying vertically oriented frontalis muscle. Anatomic areas where tension is excessive are avoided if possible. The shoulders, back, and anterior chest are high tension and mobile areas where wide scarring is difficult to avoid. Patients are also questioned as to propensity for development of hypertrophic scars or keloid formation. Ears, anterior chest, and shoulders are areas prone to these problematic scars.[2,3]

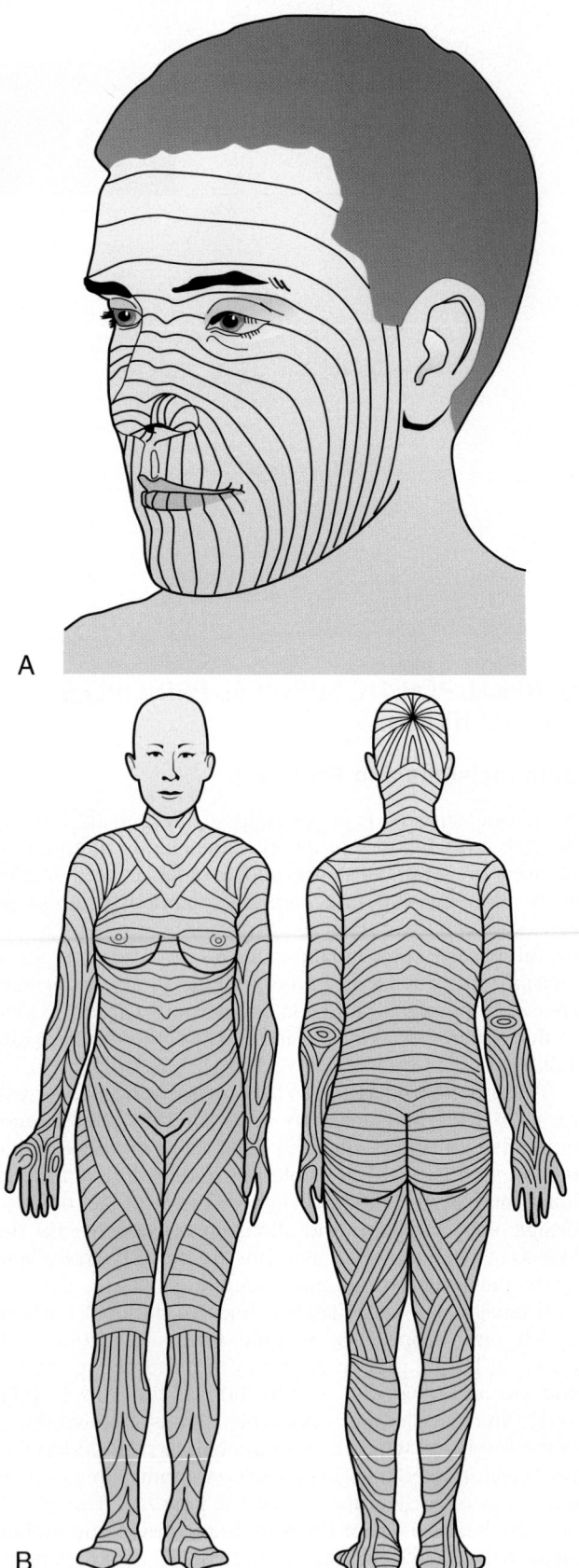

When possible, incisions are not placed over weight-bearing or high-use surfaces. Incisions placed on the palm of the hand, sole of the foot, or fingertips occasionally result in painful and functionally impairing scars. Linear scars will contract up to 20% in the longitudinal direction. For this reason, cutaneous scars that cross the flexor surface of joints can restrict the ability of the joint to extend. This problem is obviated by designing elective incisions across flexor creases in a zigzag pattern.

The most favorable excision design is the double lenticular or elliptical design with a 4:1 length-to-width ratio. This will result in an ability to close the wound without a mound of skin at the extremes of the incision (dog-ear deformity). A circular excision will deform spontaneously to an ovoid defect according to Langer's principle, allowing an elliptical pattern to be easily implemented for a more aesthetic closure. In certain instances in which the length of the scar is a concern, circular defects can be closed in a purse-string fashion, and the resultant unfavorable scar can be revised in several months. The purse-string design is particularly useful on the face where the skin is loose and circular defects are common.

Open Wounds

Wound closure by primary healing or first intention involves closure of the wound by direct skin approximation, flap, or skin graft. The result is transformation of an open to a closed wound in a single operative session. Spontaneous healing, or secondary intention, involves wound healing without surgical manipulation. Tertiary healing, healing by third intention, or delayed primary closure combines tenets of both primary healing and spontaneous healing. In this case, a contaminated wound is left open for a period of several days to allow the normal host defenses to débride the wound. The wound is then closed primarily, and tensile strength develops normally.

An open wound undergoing spontaneous healing can be induced to heal if etiologic factors are recognized and treatments optimized. Wound healing is negatively affected by systemic, regional, or local factors (Fig. 73-2). Systemic factors include active history of tobacco use, diabetes, malnutrition, anemia, hypoxemia, congestive heart failure or coronary artery disease, immunosuppression, cancer, and genetic factors. Regional factors include peripheral atherosclerosis, venous hypertension, and peripheral neuropathy. Local causes include trauma, burns, pressure, infection, radiation, and infiltration. These issues must be recognized when evaluating an open wound, and treatment must address both the open wound and any factors that threaten to impair healing.

Two common problems encountered in chronic open wounds are malnutrition and bacterial inoculation. Larger chronic open wounds can serve as a source of protein loss. A serum albumin of less than 2.5 g/dL reflects inadequate nutritional reserve and impaired ability to heal a wound. Careful attention to diet and protein replacement is critical for normal wound healing to occur.

Figure 73-1 A, Facial relaxed skin tension lines (RSTLs). **B,** RSTLs of the entire body. (From Trott A: Wounds and Lacerations: Emergency Care and Closure, 2nd ed. St Louis, Mosby, 1997, p 51.)

ETIOLOGIES   DIAGNOSIS   TREATMENTS

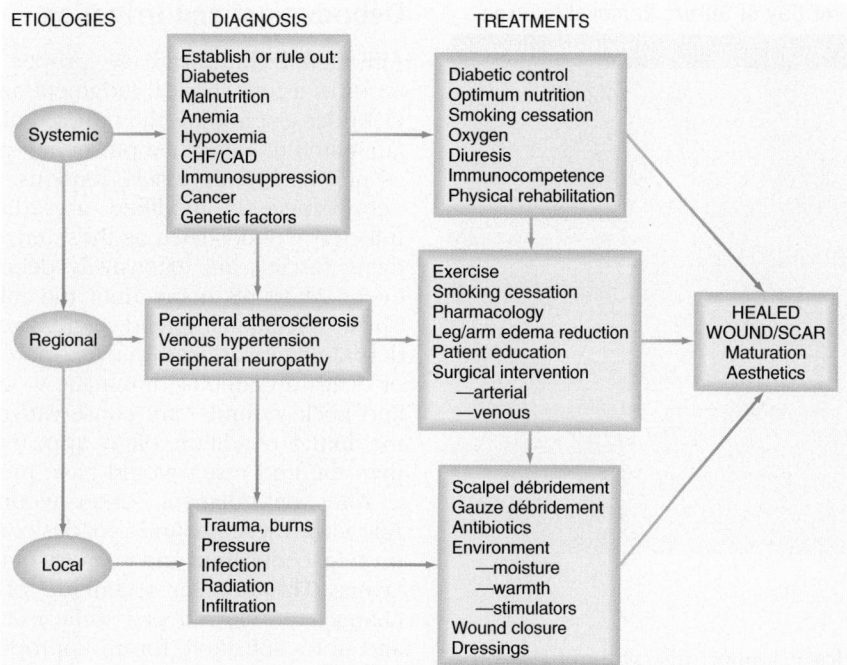

Figure 73-2 Impediments to wound healing. CHF, congestive heart failure; CAD, coronary artery disease. (From Russel R [ed]: Plastic Surgery Educational Foundation: Instructional Courses, Vol. 4. St Louis, Mosby, 1991, p 252.)

Because of the fear of bacterial invasion, primary wound closure beyond 6 to 8 hours after injury was historically proscribed. However, several scientific studies have since shown that when blood supply to a wound is adequate and bacterial invasion is absent, wounds can be safely closed at any time after proper débridement and irrigation.[4] Routine swab cultures of wound surfaces offer both inadequate and inaccurate reflections of the risk for wound infection. Quantitative bacteriology is a highly effective test whereby a biopsy of viable wound tissue can accurately assess the risk for unfavorable outcome for contemplated wound closure (>10^3 bacteria/g of tissue for β-hemolytic streptococcus and >10^5 bacteria/g of tissue for all other bacterial species). Wounds with counts below those stated can be expected to heal.

Wound Closure

In general, expeditious closure of wounds is one of the goals of plastic surgery and follows a reconstructive ladder beginning with the simple and advancing to the complex as the wound dictates (Table 73-1). An optimal linear closure is seen when the skin edges are coapted under minimal tension without redundant skin mounds (dog-ears) at the incisional poles. Undermining adjacent skin, either just deep to the dermis or just superficial to the fascia, is commonly used to alleviate tension. Layered closure of wounds describes the technique whereby the separate anatomic planes of the wound are reapproximated, like with like. Dermal approximation is of paramount importance because it bears most of the tension

Table 73-1 Reconstructive Ladder

Linear closure
Skin grafts
Skin flaps
Myocutaneous flaps
Free flaps

dispersed across the skin interface. Dermal sutures are placed with the knot buried. Dermal sutures can be placed vertically, obliquely, or horizontally to approximate the dermis. Upon completion of a correct dermal closure, the skin edges are perfectly aligned, even slightly everted, along the length of the wound.

Epidermal skin sutures function for fine alignment of skin edges. Interrupted sutures are less constrictive than running sutures. The needle enters and exits the skin at 90 degrees in order to evert the skin edges. These skin sutures are removed as soon as adequate intrinsic bonding strength is sufficient. Skin sutures left in place too long result in an unsightly track pattern. On the other hand, sutures removed prematurely risk wound dehiscence. Nonabsorbable sutures on the face are typically removed after 5 days. Sutures in the hand, foot, or across areas that are acted on by motion are left for 14 days or longer (Table 73-2). Alternatively, by employing the running intradermal suturing technique, the time constraints of suture removal may be disregarded, and these sutures

Table 73-2 Guidelines for Day of Suture Removal by Area

BODY REGION	REMOVAL (DAYS)
Scalp	6-8
Ear	10-14
Eyelid	3-4
Eyebrow	3-5
Nose	3-5
Lip	3-4
Face (other)	3-4
Chest, abdomen	8-10
Back	12-14
Extremities	12-14
Hand	10-14
Foot, sole	12-14

may be left in place for a longer time without risking a track pattern scar. Finally, epidermal approximation can be achieved without suture using a medical-grade cyanoacrylate adhesive such as Dermabond. Such adhesives are applied across the coapted skin edges only and contribute no tensile strength. Tape closure strips such as Steri-Strips can be applied at the completion of wound closure to help splint the coapted skin edges.

Subsequent follow-up visits are necessary to survey for infection, monitor adequacy of healing, remove sutures, and assess scar maturation. Infection is detected and treated early. Erythema at the suture line is considered bacterial cellulitis, not suture reaction, and is treated with appropriate antibiotic therapy and topical antimicrobials. Undiagnosed infection can lead to dehiscence of the wound and problematic scars. Patients are instructed to avoid ultraviolet radiation exposure to immature scars because it risks local hyperpigmentation changes. Although barrier protection is best, sunscreens can also be used. For patients with firm and tender scars, scar massage using moisturizing lotion can soften the scar and lessen the discomfort.

Certain patients may demonstrate a propensity for hypertrophic or keloid scar formation. Preoperative discussion must review the increased risk for untoward scar consequences in these susceptible patients. When wounds demonstrate these tendencies, several treatment options are available. Antipruritic medication is often necessary to manage complaints of itching of the scar. Scar massage with lotion can be used to soften and soothe these scars. Although the mechanism is still in question, topical application of silicone gel strips or sheets has shown value for improving such problematic scars. Intralesional injection of steroids into a keloid scar can inactivate and shrink the scar; such therapy is not indicated for hypertrophic scars. Interval follow-ups are necessary to gauge therapeutic response. In extreme cases, radiation therapy can be used to treat severe keloid scars such as those that cause functional impairment.

Débridement and Irrigation

Although technically easy, proper wound débridement requires astute surgical judgment and careful inspection. Débridement implies the removal of devitalized and contaminated tissues while preserving critical structures such as nerves, blood vessels, tendons, and bone. Extent of débridement is modified according to wound type. Infected wounds such as those encountered with necrotizing fasciitis are extensively débrided and redébrided every 24 to 48 hours until the infection is controlled. These infections spread aggressively, and conservative débridement can lead to even more extensive tissue loss or death. In contrast, traumatic wounds (especially head and neck wounds) are conservatively débrided because the initial condition often appears much more severe than the end result would have predicted.

After débridement, open wounds are kept moist. Allowing these wounds to desiccate results in loss of proteinaceous fluid and necrosis of the superficial wound layers. The popular technique of wet-to-dry dressing changes are viewed as a surface débridement technique and not a substitute for an appropriate wound dressing. The wet-to-dry dressing technique when used on a clean and viable wound bed may cause injury to granulation tissue and delay wound healing.

In addition to débridement, wound irrigation, with or without antibiotics, is a mainstay of infection control. Wounds suspected of harboring bacteria are evaluated using quantitative bacteriology, as discussed earlier. Numerous jet lavage systems are available (Fig. 73-3) that forcefully apply irrigant to the wound surface and act to decrease the bacterial load. As a general rule, jet lavage irrigation decreases the bacterial load on the wound surface by 10^2. The amount of irrigant used averages 1.5 liters, with larger wounds requiring a greater volume of irrigant.

Grafts and Flaps

As a rule, the surgeon applies the concept of a reconstructive ladder when assessing possibilities for wound closure (see Table 73-1). The reconstructive ladder is followed so that simple options are used before complex solutions are considered. A secondary plan needs to be available in case the primary plan fails. This ensures that the surgeon does not compromise a future option while performing an initial closure.

Ascending the reconstructive ladder, skin grafts follow only linear closure in complexity. Skin grafts can be divided based on thickness: full-thickness and split-thickness grafts (Fig. 73-4). Full-thickness grafts include epidermis with the entirety of the dermis; the donor site must be closed separately. Split-thickness grafts vary in the amount of dermis included in the graft. The modern power-driven dermatome allows precise selection of graft thickness. Typically, a split-thickness graft is harvested at 10/1000 of an inch. For split-thickness grafts, the donor site is most often closed with an occlusive or medication impregnated meshed gauze. The donor site re-epithelializes spontaneously. Because of this healing ability of the

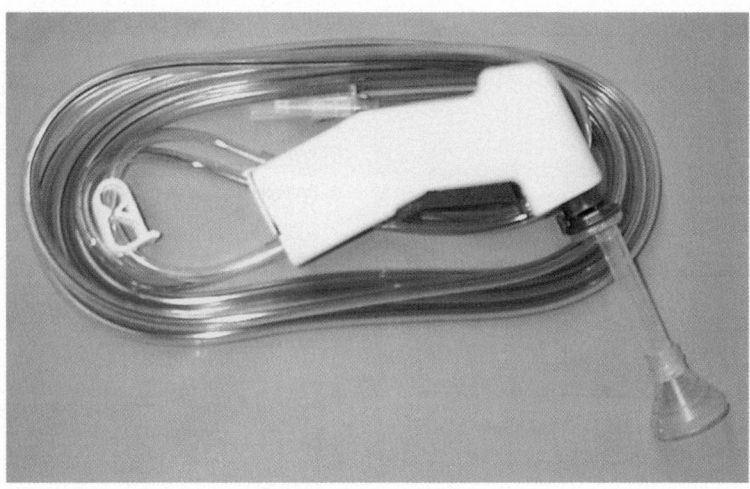

Figure 73-3 Example of jet lavage system used for wound irrigation.

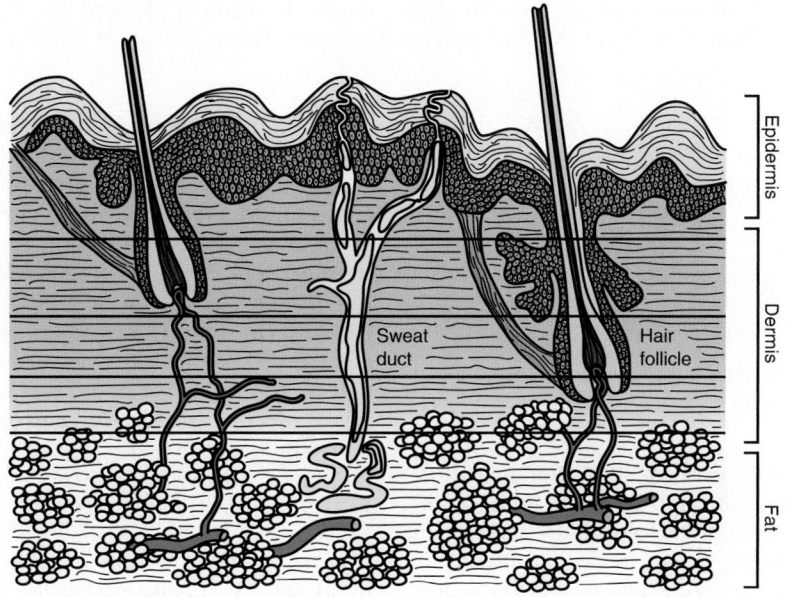

Figure 73-4 Cross section of skin depicting levels contained in split-thickness and full-thickness skin grafts.

donor site, split-thickness grafts are especially valuable to close larger wounds. Because split-thickness donor sites can be reharvested after re-epithelialization, this method of wound closure is the workhorse for burn injuries. Thin split-thickness grafts contract to a greater extent than thick split-thickness or full-thickness grafts. Full-thickness grafts resist deformation more than thinner split-thickness grafts and are therefore more suitable for reconstruction when late contracture is expected to compromise the functional or aesthetic outcome.

The skin graft must be applied to a well-vascularized recipient wound bed. It will not adhere to exposed bone, cartilage, or tendon devoid of periosteum, perichondrium, or peritenon, respectively, or devoid of its vascularized perimembranous envelope. There are three steps in the "take" of a skin graft: imbibition, inosculation, and

revascularization. Imbibition occurs up to 48 hours after graft placement and involves the free absorption of nutrients into the graft. Inosculation designates the time period when donor and recipient capillaries become aligned. There remains a debate as to whether new channels are formed or if preexisting channels reconnect. Finally, after about 5 days, revascularization occurs, and the graft demonstrates both arterial inflow and venous outflow.

Reasons for skin graft failure are well understood. The most common causes of skin graft failure are hematoma (or seroma), infection, and movement (shear).[5] Hematoma is most often the consequence of inadequate intraoperative hemostasis and can be identified before irreversible damage has occurred. By examining the skin graft before the fourth postoperative day, a hematoma or seroma can be evacuated, and the mechanical

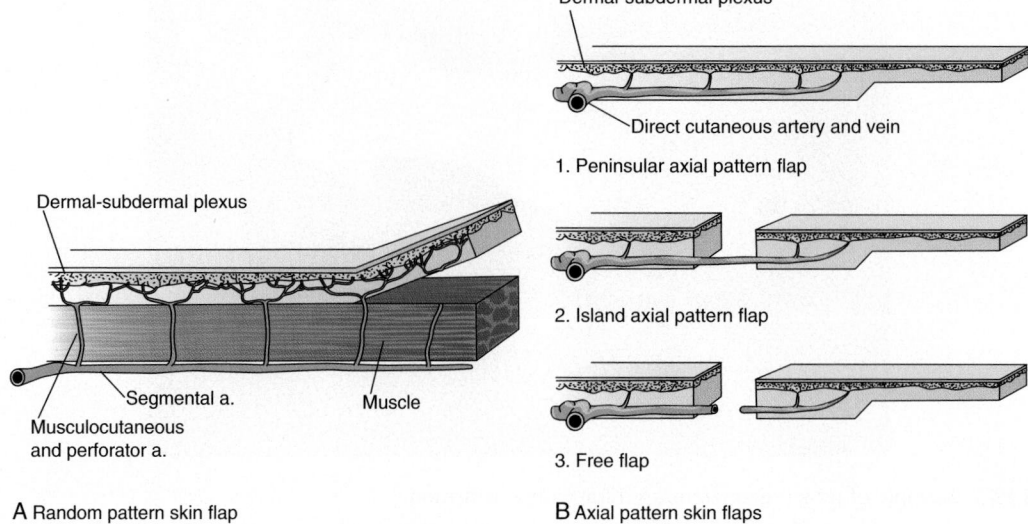

Figure 73-5 **Vascular patterns of random pattern (A) and axial pattern (B) skin flaps.** (From Place MJ, Herber SC, Hardesty RA: Basic techniques and principles in plastic surgery. In Aston SJ, Beasley RW, Thorne CHM [eds]: Grabb and Smith's Plastic Surgery, 5th ed. Philadelphia, Lippincott-Raven, 1997, p 21.)

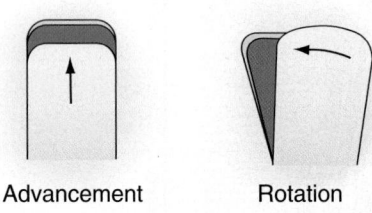

Figure 73-6 **Graphic representation of commonly used local flaps: advancement and rotation flaps.**

obstruction to revascularization of the graft is thus removed. Some surgeons make stab incisions in the graft preemptively to create small outlets for fluid to drain from beneath the graft, a technique know as *pie crusting.* Others might use a mesh expander device, which creates a chain-link fence pattern in the graft. Although these methods may provide egress portals for serous fluid or blood, an unsightly meshed pattern results, making this technique unsuitable for aesthetic reconstruction. Bacterial contamination of a wound will result in graft loss. Topical or systemic antimicrobials or both can be used to control bacterial proliferation. Finally, movement of the graft will result in shearing of delicate capillary alignments and graft loss. Graft immobilization is critical to graft take and can be accomplished with a variety of methods, including a bolster dressing, light compression wraps, or a vacuum-assisted closure device, just to name a few.

Special considerations in choosing a skin graft donor site include skin quality and color from the donor region that will best match the recipient site. For example, skin harvested from the blush zone above the clavicles is best suited for facial grafting. Skin grafts harvested from areas caudal to the waist will result in tallow discoloration and possible unwanted hair growth. Because split-thickness donor sites will permanently scar, it is wise to choose a donor site that can be concealed. When a large amount of graft is needed, the thighs and buttocks are areas that can be hidden with everyday clothes. The inner arm and groin crease are each fine sources for full-thickness grafts because both areas offer relatively glabrous skin sources, the donor sites of which can be easily hidden with clothes. One often overlooked split-thickness donor site is the scalp, taking extreme care to avoid taking the graft below the level of the hair follicle; this donor site heals quickly, painlessly, and with imperceptible scar consequences.

Flaps

Flap reconstruction represents the next order of complexity along the reconstructive ladder (Fig. 73-5). A *flap* is defined as a partially or completely isolated segment of tissue perfused with its own blood supply. Flaps are the reconstructive option of choice when a padded and durable cover is needed to reconstruct an integumentary defect over vital structures, tissues devoid of perivascular membrane, or implants. Flaps vary greatly in terms of complexity from simple skin flaps with a random blood supply to microvascular free flaps containing composite tissue. Numerous schemes exist to classify flaps. Flaps may be classified based on the type of tissue contained in the flap: fasciocutaneous, musculocutaneous, or osteocutaneous flaps.[6,7] Flaps are also described based on their design and method of transfer: advancement, rotation, transposition, interpolation, or pedicled flaps. Flaps may be further defined by the source of their blood supply: random, axial, or free. Random flaps rely on the low perfusion pressures found in the subdermal plexus to sustain the flap and not a named blood vessel.[8] Nevertheless, random flaps are used widely in reconstruction of cutaneous defects, including those resulting from Mohs

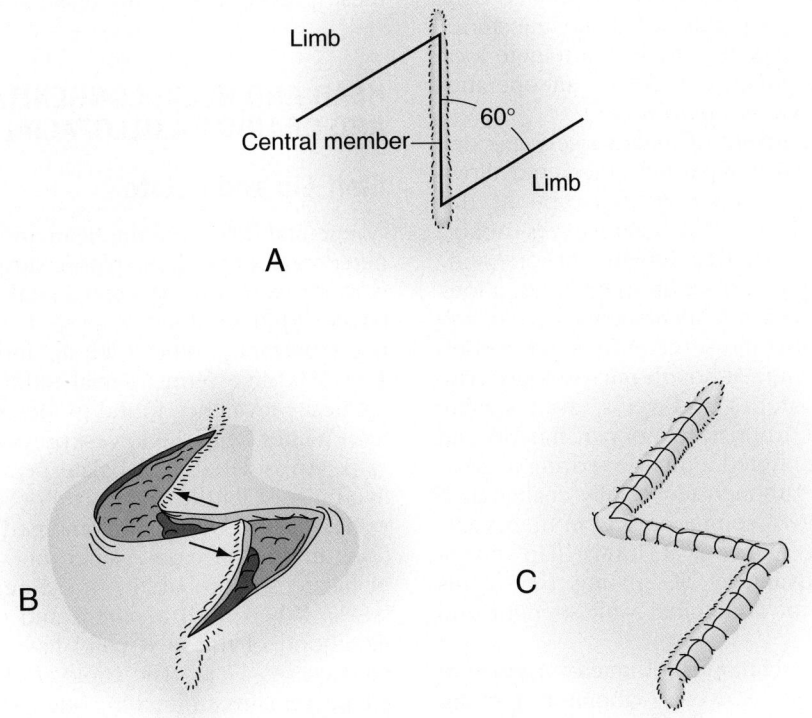

Figure 73-7 Graphic representation of the Z-plasty transposition flap commonly used for scar contracture release. (From Aston SJ, Beasley RW, Thorne CHM [eds]: Grabb and Smith's Plastic Surgery, 5th ed. Philadelphia, Lippincott-Raven, 1997, p 20.)

excision of cutaneous malignancies. These local flaps recruit adjacent tissue based on geometric design patterns.

Advancement and rotation flaps represent commonly used random-pattern skin flaps (Fig. 73-6). The Z-plasty, bilobed flap, rhomboid, and V-Y (or Y-V) advancement flaps are commonly used random flaps. Z-plasty involves transposing two adjacent triangular flaps to redirect and lengthen an existing scar (the central limb) (Fig. 73-7). The angles of the Z-plasty can be increased to provide greater length. Typically a 60-degree angle is used that lengthens the central limb by 75%.[9] The bilobed flap is commonly used for nasal reconstruction; here, a larger primary and smaller secondary flap are transposed into adjacent defects borrowing the loose adjacent tissue to close the defect (Fig. 73-8). The rhomboid flap described by Limberg uses a 60- and 120-degree parallelogram to transpose tissue into a diamond-shaped defect. It is an extremely versatile flap option and the workhorse for most plastic surgeons. Finally, the V-Y (or Y-V) advancement flaps are commonly used to lengthen scars around the nose and mouth. A backcut at the base of a flap may decrease tension at a flap's tip, creating a greater arc of rotation; overzealous back cut or tension at flap inset can each cause ischemia to the flap and threaten its survival.

An axial flap is based on a named blood vessel and can provide a reproducible and stable skin or skin-

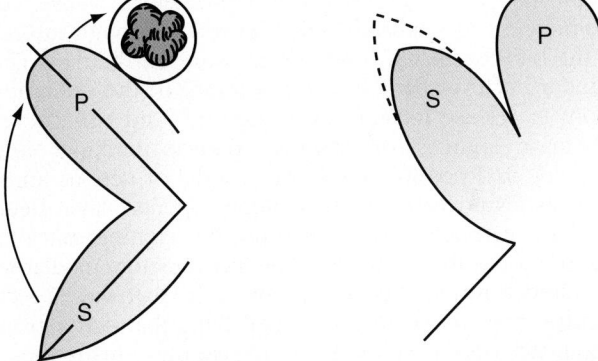

Figure 73-8 Graphic representation of the bilobed flap commonly used for nasal reconstruction. P, primary flap; S, secondary flap. (From Aston SJ, Beasley RW, Thorne CHM [eds]: Grabb and Smith's Plastic Surgery, 5th ed. Philadelphia, Lippincott-Raven, 1997, p 23.)

muscle (myocutaneous) flap. Flaps can also be raised with the underlying fascia (fasciocutaneous), which recruits the fascial blood supply, thereby increasing the predictable vascularity to the flap. Because of its reliable blood supply, the axial flap can be used to provide much needed length and bulk, which the random flap cannot. An axial flap that remains attached to its proximal blood supply and is transposed to a defect is known as a *pedicled flap*. Alternately, the vascular pedicle can be completely transected and the paddle of tissue transferred and reanastomosed to recipient vessels in a remote location. This technique requires the use of an operating microscope and is known as *microsurgery*.

The relatively recent advent of microsurgery has dramatically altered the practice of plastic surgery and allows the surgeon a plethora of reconstructive options that were not previously available.[10] The human eye is capable of visualizing objects as small as 100 μm. An operating microscope can magnify an object up to 40 times, allowing the surgeon precise control. Microsutures vary in size from 8-0 to 11-0 and allow the surgeon to suture vessels less than 1 mm in diameter. Although microsurgery typically involves named arteries and veins, even smaller vessels that pierce and arborize to nourish muscle and the overlying skin have offered a muscle-sparing alternative for tissue transfer. Although technically challenging, perforator flaps are now commonplace in transverse rectus abdominis myocutaneous (TRAM) flap breast reconstruction. The advantage of sparing the rectus muscle is preservation of abdominal wall strength and integrity.[11]

The principles and techniques of microsurgery are similar to vascular surgery. However, laboratory training with an operating microscope using small animals is essential before progressing into clinical surgery. In addition, experience in recognizing the causes and solutions of flap failure is mandatory. Despite numerous techniques, such as Doppler probing and temperature monitoring, clinical assessment remains the gold standard for free flap monitoring. The most common cause of flap failure is venous congestion. If a problem is suspected, the first response must include removal of enough sutures at the bedside that will relieve pressure on the flap. The standard of care dictates a rapid return to the operating room to release tension, evacuate any fluid collections, eliminate sources of vascular pedicle kinking, and examine and possibly revise the arterial or venous anastomosis. Numerous pharmacologic agents have been used to manipulate vascular tone, the clotting cascade, and to reduce the ill effects of the inflammatory mediators liberated through the arachidonic acid pathway. Leech therapy may on occasion salvage flaps that suffer from significant venous congestion. Despite these many therapies, nothing can replace meticulous operative technique and diligent postoperative clinical assessment.

Recent advances in microsurgical technique have been combined with advances in transplant immunology to make possible replacement of missing or nonfunctional anatomic subunits. Advancing the pioneering work of plastic surgeon and Nobel laureate Joseph Murray, who performed the first kidney transplant, decades of refinements in antirejection therapy have made reality of complete hand and partial face transplantation.[12-14] Although ethical debate over elective transplantation continues, there is no question that for devastating hand injuries and face disfigurement, transplantation offers hope for the best solution. However, the lifetime risk for rejection, cancer risk from chronic immunosuppression,

and social and identity issues (face transplantation) make these procedures controversial at this time.

HEAD AND NECK: CONGENITAL AND CRANIOMAXILLOFACIAL

Cleft Lip and Palate

Congenital defects of the head and neck make up a large percentage of pediatric plastic surgery. Here, no problem is more common than congenital clefting of the lip and palate. Epidemiologic analysis is important when advising expectant parents. Cleft lip and palate occur in about 1 in 1000 live births. Racial differences are noted, with greatest prevalence found in Mesoamericans and Asians, then whites, with the lowest prevalence in African Americans. An isolated cleft palate occurs in about 1 in 2000 live births. Cleft lip and palate occur as an isolated event in 86% of cases but are combined with other malformations in 14% of cases. When one sibling has a cleft lip or palate, the probability of the next child being affected is 4%. When both a parent and child are affected, the likelihood of the next child having a cleft lip or palate increases to 17%.[15] The etiology of clefting of the lip and palate remains unknown, but a multifactorial combination of heredity and environmental factors seems most plausible. Suspected environmental agents based purely on animal studies have implicated phenytoin, ethanol, and folate deficiency.

For those born with a cleft lip or palate, a multidisciplinary team approach provides the highest level of care. Cleft patients require a wide variety of specialists, including a plastic surgeon, otolaryngologist, pediatric dentist, orthodontist, oral surgeon, speech therapist, audiologist, nutritionist, pediatrician, psychologist, and social worker. Such organized teams generally employ more experienced surgeons who perform a large number of these procedures and are more familiar with variant cases. The timing of cleft repair is important, and a general recommendation is lip repair at 3 months, palate repair by 12 months, and alveolar bone grafting at about 9 years which coincides with partial eruption of the canine teeth.[9] The child will likely require other surgeries to address speech impediments not responsive to speech therapy, the residual bony deficit and oronasal fistula at the gum line, nasal airway obstruction, malocclusal relationships, and distortional stigmata. Because eustachian tube dysfunction is found in most children with cleft palate, placement of myringotomy tubes to prevent recurrent otitis media and preserve hearing is commonplace.

Principles of cleft lip repair include layered repair of the skin, muscle, and mucous membrane to restore symmetric length and function. Presurgical orthodontic nasoalveolar molding has been offered as a measure to assist in preoperative alignment of the unrepaired segments. However, this process requires specialized orthodontic skills and frequent follow-up visits for adjustments, making this modality impractical for many cleft centers with outlying patient populations. The Millard rotation-advancement unilateral cleft lip repair (Fig. 73-9) has become a widely applied and reproducible model.[16] An initial correction of the nasal deformity is frequently performed at the time of the lip repair. Even though the preoperative defects are more severe, repair of a bilateral cleft lip (Fig. 73-10) often results in better symmetry, a status more accepting to the casual eye.

The goal of cleft palate repair is to establish a competent valve that can isolate the oral and nasal cavities, thus recreating the muscular sling necessary for palatal elevation. Just before school age, both speech assessment and speech diagnostic studies determine whether there is residual hypernasal speech; additional surgery of pharyngeal flap or pharyngoplasty might be necessary to remedy the problem.

Other Congenital Anomalies

Embryologic development of the head and neck begins at the fourth week with the formation of the branchial apparatus. Branchial cleft cyst, sinus, or fistula represents remnants from epithelial-lined tracts in the lateral neck along the anterior border of the sternocleidomastoid muscle. Clinically, the sinus or fistula may connect with

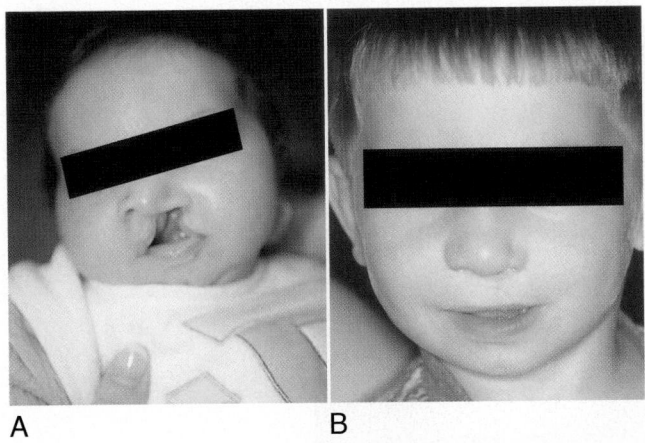

Figure 73-9 A, Three-month-old boy with a unilateral cleft lip and palate. **B,** Postoperative photograph, age 5 years, after Millard rotation-advancement cleft lip repair.

the skin or oropharynx, and later in life, if surgical excision is not carried out, malignant transformation or infection may occur.

The thyroid develops embryologically at the base of the tongue and descends along a midline tract to its final pretracheal position in the neck. Thyroglossal duct cysts arise from remnant tissue left during the embryonic descent of the thyroid tissue. Usually, the thyroglossal duct disappears with development. However, duct remnants may be present as sinuses or cysts along the migration pathway. These are most commonly present in the midline at the level of the hyoid bone and are treated with excision.

Ear deformities are commonly encountered in newborn infants and vary widely in severity. Anotia (complete absence) and microtia (vestigial remnants or absence of part of the ear) require extensive surgery and can be associated with other craniofacial deformities. Minor abnormalities in ear shape can sometimes be overcome with early splinting or taping of the newborn's ear; this is possible because the effect of maternal estrogen makes the ear cartilage extremely pliable and amenable to reshaping in the neonate. For anotia or microtia, surgical repair may be initiated by age 7 years. By this age, the contralateral ear has developed to near adult size, and the child will begin to experience the expectations of schoolmates. Although numerous synthetic implants exist for reconstruction of an absent ear, the gold standard remains autologous rib cartilage graft taken from the contralateral cartilaginous portion of the ribs[17] (Fig. 73-11). The graft is shaped and placed into a subcutaneous pocket over a suction drain. Autologous rib grafts have been shown to be superior to synthetic implants because of their resistance to extrusion and infection.

Prominent ears provide a frequent source of peer teasing in school-age children. When ears protrude excessively from the temporal scalp, otoplasty provides the surgical correction. Ear prominence must be carefully analyzed because it can result from conchal constriction or hypertrophy, a poorly defined or absent antihelical fold, or a conchoscaphal angle greater than 90 degrees. Knowledge of normal ear position is critical to attaining an acceptable

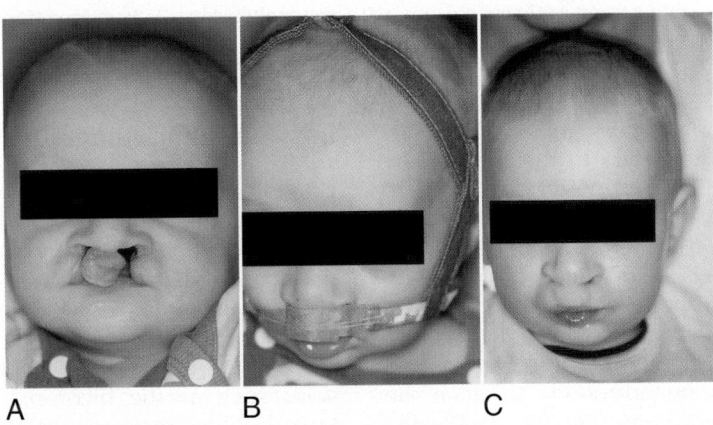

Figure 73-10 A, Preoperative photographs of a 3-month-old boy with a bilateral cleft lip and palate. **B,** Wearing orthodontic appliance to push back prominent premaxilla. **C,** Postoperative view 6 months after lip repair.

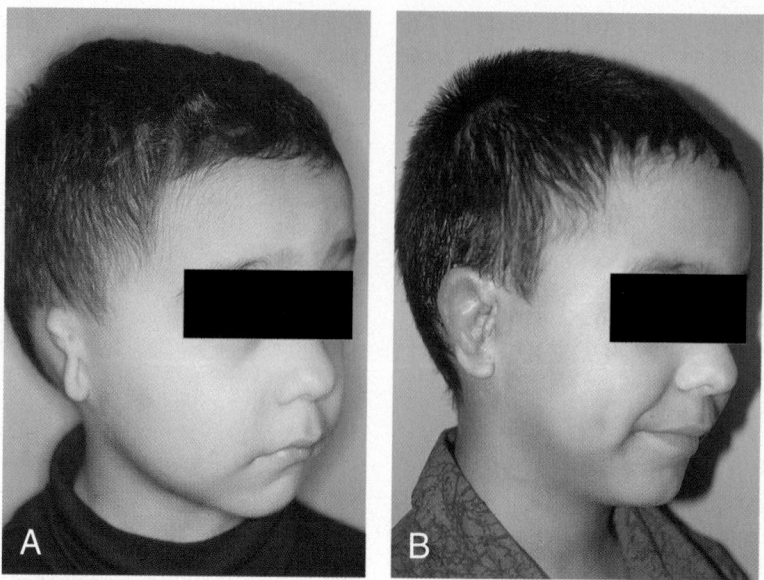

Figure 73-11 **A,** Preoperative photograph of 3-year-old boy with microtia. **B,** Postoperative photograph, age 7 years, 1 year after ear reconstruction with autologous rib graft and subsequent ear lobule rotation.

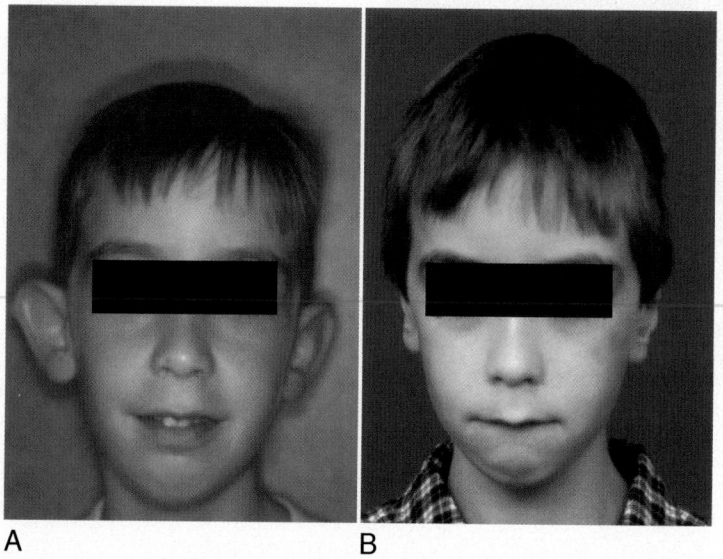

Figure 73-12 A, Preoperative view of 7-year-old boy with prominent ears. B, Postoperative view 3 months after otoplasty.

postoperative result. A normal ear's anatomic bounds extend from the eyebrow superiorly to the base of the nasal columella inferiorly; it inclines posteriorly about 20 degrees off vertical and protrudes at its midpoint 16 to 18 mm from the scalp. For conchal excess, an ellipse of conchal cartilage can be excised adjacent to the mastoid, and the reduced concha can be recessed additionally by suture fixation to the mastoid fascia.[18] The antihelical fold is recreated using both scoring anteriorly to weaken the cartilage and mattress suturing posteriorly to attain the desired natural-appearing convexity (Fig. 73-12). Ideally, it is better to overcorrect a bit because most patients are sensitive to even minor residual prominence.

Less Common Anomalies

Craniofacial surgery is a reconstructive discipline that addresses the skull, the facial skeleton, and soft tissues of the face. Using this approach, both neurosurgeon and plastic surgeon are able to address pathology due to congenital anomalies, post-traumatic deformities, and defects after tumor ablation. Access to the craniofacial skeleton is accomplished through inconspicuous incisions such as the bicoronal, lower eyelid, and upper buccal sulcus incisions. After craniotomy, the dura and brain are retracted to provide safe exposure that will allow selective osteotomies of the craniofacial skeleton that are repositioned and then rigidly fixed using plates and screws.

Congenital anomalies involving the skull and facial skeleton are rare but severely deforming. Premature fusion of the cranial sutures is known as *craniosynostosis* and occurs in 1 in 2000 live births.[19] Craniosynostosis can limit the skull's volume and increase intracranial pressure.[20] Skull deformities may also arise from extrinsic causes such as torticollis or as a result of intrauterine head molding during pregnancy. These skull deformities may be responsive to serial orthotic helmet compression therapy alone, without the need for surgery. When synostosis also affects the cranial base, the conditions are called *craniofacial syndromes*. Here, restricted skull and facial growth result in a constricted and deformed cranial vault, shallow orbits with exorbitism, and midface retrusion, which manifests as nasopharyngeal airway narrowing and severe dental malocclusion. Examples of such syndromes include Apert's (craniosynostosis, exorbitism, midface hypoplasia, and complex syndactyly) and Crouzon's (similar to Apert's but without syndactyly). When premature skull fusion is documented, surgical correction is performed in conjunction with a neurosurgeon. This involves removing the involved portion of the skull, reshaping the skull, and replacing the reshaped portion with resorbable plates and screws; best outcomes are obtained when this surgery is carried out before 1 year of age.[21] Other conditions that may require craniofacial surgery include facial clefts that extend beyond the lip and palate, hemifacial microsomia, and various rare craniofacial syndromes.

Distraction osteogenesis is a technique employed by some craniofacial surgeons that is based on original work by Ilizarov. In distraction osteogenesis, a controlled osteotomy is made in the designated facial bones, and an internal or external fixator device is applied. The device is activated by a jackscrew mechanism that allows 1 mm per day distraction of the divided bone ends until a desired length is achieved. New bone is formed at the osteotomy site, and the distractor is removed several weeks after completion of the distraction process. In the midface, this technique is often employed with Le Fort osteotomies to reposition the maxilla. Distraction has also been successfully applied to the surgical correction of unilateral or bilateral conditions of mandibular hypoplasia.

Maxillofacial surgery addresses dental occlusion with selective osteotomies of facial bones. Preoperative management usually involves cephalometric analysis of the facial skeleton as it relates to dentition. Dental relationships are commonly represented by Angle's classification. Class I is centric (normal) occlusion, class II is mandibular retrusion with significant overbite, and class III is prognathic mandible with significant underbite. Preoperative orthodontic alignment of the teeth with dental models is also necessary. When the maxilla is implicated, a maxillary osteotomy (Le Fort I osteotomy) can be performed to advance or impact the maxilla with its dentition. Likewise, the mandible can be osteotomized with its intact dentition to restore centric or normal occlusion. Similar procedures can be used to address facial asymmetry.

Trauma

Facial soft tissue injuries are frequently encountered in the emergency department. Common etiologies include abrasions, lacerations, blast injuries, and human or animal bites. For more severe injuries, a trauma evaluation is mandatory with establishment of a secure airway and cervical spine clearance before management of the facial injury.[22] Patients with extensive facial bony fractures deserve special attention because traumatic edema and intraoral bleeding can quickly compromise the airway, as seen with bilateral subcondylar mandible fractures. Radiologic evaluation is mandatory to rule out bony fractures. Physical exam includes careful attention to facial nerve (cranial nerve VII) function and parotid duct integrity. Foreign bodies are removed and the wound irrigated, but radical débridement of damaged tissue is never indicated because facial soft tissues have an exceptional blood supply. Meticulous reapproximation of the anatomy is undertaken as soon as the patient's general medical condition allows. This includes careful realignment of the eyebrows, eyelids, and vermillion border of the lips. When possible, facial wounds are irrigated and closed within 8 hours of the injury. Primary closure may be delayed up to 24 hours if the wounds are irrigated, sterile dressings are applied, and antibiotics are instituted. Tetanus prophylaxis is administered. Treatment of dog and cat bites usually includes a single antibiotic (e.g., amoxicillin or doxycycline), but for human bites, a second antibiotic aimed at anaerobic coverage is prescribed.

Common fractures of the facial skeleton include nasal fractures, mandible fractures, zygomatic complex, maxilla (Le Fort I, II, and III), naso-orbital-ethmoid complex (NOE), and frontal sinus fractures.[23] Nasal fractures are the most common facial fractures. The diagnosis is most frequently made clinically, and x-ray study offers little added value. On physical exam, it is mandatory to assess the nasal septum for a possible septal hematoma left undrained; septal hematoma may result in necrosis and erosion of the nasal septum. Most nasal fractures can be treated with closed reduction and splinting, including intranasal packing. Postoperatively, these patients are covered with appropriate antibiotics because toxic shock syndrome has been reported with intranasal packing. NOE fractures are the result of a high-energy impact. These patients classically present with a complex nasal fracture, including a saddle nose deformity, a wide nasal root with loss of anterior projection, and telecanthus (wide interpupillary distance resulting from a fracture of the medial orbital wall and ethmoids with displacement of the medial canthal tendons laterally). NOE fractures can involve damage to the nasolacrimal duct, which can be repaired over a stent. In addition, care must be taken to accurately reposition the medial canthal tendons and restore nasal projection.

Fractures of the frontal sinus are most frequently seen in association with NOE fractures. In such injuries, damage to the nasofrontal duct and posterior wall of the frontal sinus must be identified. When nasofrontal duct injury is missed, duct obstruction and future mucocele may occur. When recognized, obliteration of the sinus

Le Fort I level

Le Fort III level

Le Fort II level

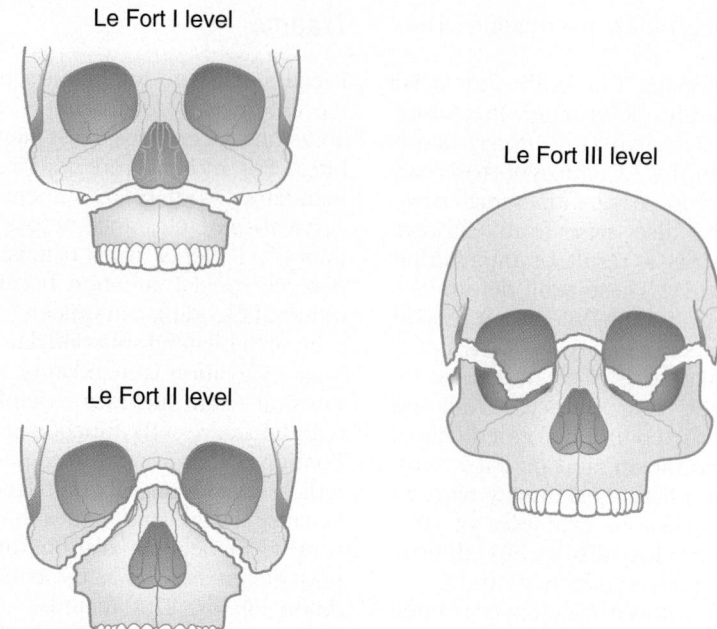

Figure 73-13 **Representation of facial fractures at the Le Fort I, II, and III levels.** (From Manson PN: Facial injuries. In McCarthy JG [ed]: Plastic Surgery, Vol. 2, The Face. Philadelphia, Saunders, 1990, pp 867-1141.)

remains the mainstay of treatment and includes stripping the sinus of all mucous lining and packing the sinus with autologous bone or fat.[24] Cerebrospinal fluid rhinorrhea indicates fracture involvement of the posterior wall of the frontal sinus. Here, neurosurgical comanagement is essential. Selection of a proper surgical plan takes into account the forehead deformity, potential for nasofrontal duct obstruction, and evidence of breached bony confines of the anterior cranial fossa.

Midface fractures involving the zygoma and maxilla often result in loss of facial height and symmetry. Facial height and projection depend on a complex bony buttressing system. These buttresses represent the thickest bony supports for the facial skeleton. In the vertical dimension, the nasomaxillary, zygomaticomaxillary, and pterygomaxillary buttresses maintain facial height. Anterior projection of the face is maintained by the horizontal buttresses: the mandible, palate, orbital rims, and frontal bar. The primary goals of repairing midface fractures are restoration of facial height, projection, and symmetry. Once the fractures are anatomically reduced, plates and screws placed across the buttresses allow for rigid union. In the pediatric population, resorbable plates and screws have demonstrated comparable strength to titanium, and because they ultimately dissolve, they will not restrict future facial growth.

Fractures of the zygoma, or malar bone, are known as *zygomatic complex fractures*. Because of the zygoma's anatomic contribution to the bony orbit, these patients present with eye findings such as periorbital ecchymosis, subconjunctival hemorrhage, paresthesia of the infraorbital nerve, tenderness at the infraorbital rim, and enophthalmos. Axial and coronal view CT imaging is the most valuable study for assessing the damage. Classically, these fractures involve the lateral orbital wall (zygomati-

cofrontal region), infraorbital rim, zygomaticomaxillary buttress, and zygomatic arch. Surgical reduction and plate fixation are challenging; the three-dimensional spacial relationships must be anatomically perfect because volumetric changes within the orbit can cause permanent double vision and enophthalmos. Isolated zygomatic arch fractures can be approached by incising below the deep temporal fascia and placing a lever below the fractured arch to lift the depressed segment: the Gilles approach. For fractures involving the orbital floor, indications for surgical exploration include diplopia, extraocular muscle entrapment, and enophthalmos. Orbital injury that affects the superior orbital fissure is a surgical emergency. The resulting set of nerve palsies is called *superior orbital fissure syndrome:* eyelid ptosis, globe proptosis, motionless globe (cranial nerve III, IV, and VI paralyses), and ophthalmic division (cranial nerve V_1) anesthesia. If blindness is seen in addition to these findings, the term *orbital apex syndrome* is used.

Midface fractures involving the maxilla can be classified by fracture patterns know as Le Fort I, II, and III (Fig. 73-13). These patterns also represent progressive gradation of severity and reflect increasing causal impact energies. Le Fort I fractures traverse the maxilla horizontally at the level of the piriform rim. Le Fort II fractures involve the nasofrontal junction, nasal process of the maxilla, medial portion of the inferior orbital rim, and across the anterior maxilla. Le Fort III fractures refer to complete disjunction of the facial skeleton from the skull base. Operative reduction of maxillary fractures begins with placement of arch bars to the maxillary and mandibular dentition. The dentition is then brought into normal occlusion before the fractures are plated. This procedure, known as *interdental* or *intermaxillary fixation* (IMF), is necessary to reestablish the proper dento-

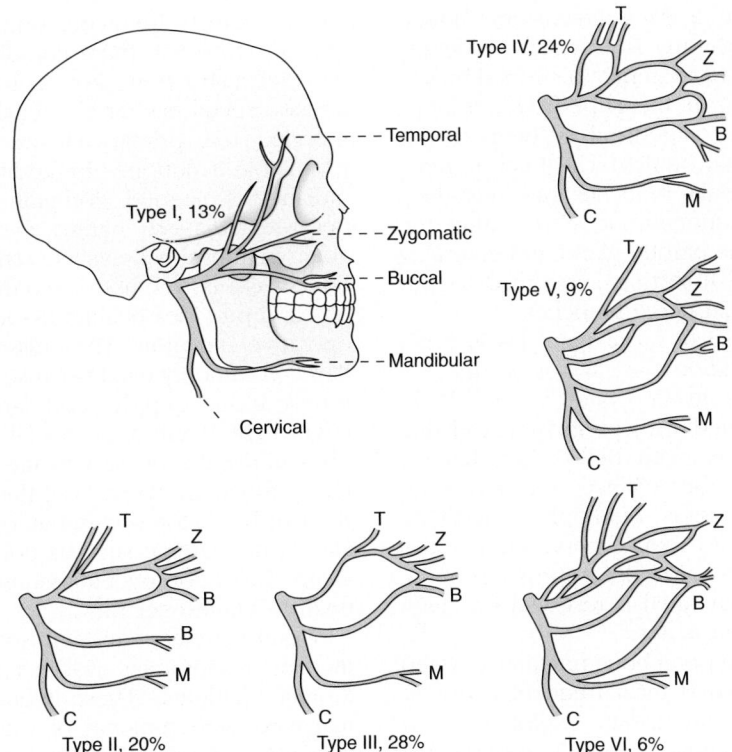

Figure 73-14 Facial nerve anatomy and common branching patterns. (From May M: The Facial Nerve. New York, Thieme, 1986, p 55.)

skeletal relationships, immobilize the fractured bones, and ensure normal postoperative occlusion. Facial buttresses are then plated to restore normal facial height and projection.[25]

Mandible fractures are second only to nasal fractures in frequency. Because the mandible is the largest and strongest of the facial bones, the force required to fracture the mandible can also damage the cervical spine. C-spine clearance is recommended because up to a 10% coincidence of C-spine trauma is reported in association with mandible fractures.[22] In addition, the airway can be compromised in patients with bilateral subcondylar mandible fractures because support for the posterior oropharynx is lost. Recommended radiographic evaluation of a mandible fracture includes a panoramic radiograph (Panorex) and Towne's view x-ray. As in midface fractures, restoration of dental occlusion forms the foundation for fracture management. Intermaxillary fixation before fracture exposure and plating is necessary. Most mandibular fractures can be plated using intraoral incisions. If necessary, a small stab incision can be made for a percutaneous approach to the fracture. This technique, which requires intraoral exposure and an externally placed trocar, eliminates the need for a larger external incision. If an external incision is necessary, care must be taken to avoid trauma to the marginal mandibular branch of the facial nerve. Many patients with mandibular fractures experience trauma to the inferior alveolar nerve (a branch of the trigeminal nerve), which runs through a canal within the body of the mandible and terminates in the lower lip as the mental nerve. These patients may experience permanent numbness of the lower lip and teeth on the affected side. Fractures of the coronoid process of the mandible can result in trismus (inability to open the mouth) because the coronoid process normally passes beneath the zygomatic arch with mouth opening. Condylar and subcondylar mandible fractures are most often treated by IMF alone. Surgical exposure of the temporomandibular joint places the facial nerve at risk and exposes the joint to possible injury and dysfunction. Medical management of mandibular fractures involves a purée-type diet, interdental fixation for several weeks, 1% chlorhexidine mouth rinses, and antibiotics.

HEAD AND NECK

Facial Nerve Palsy

The facial nerve, cranial nerve VII, is responsible for innervating muscles of facial expression (mimetic muscles). Facial expression is a unique trait of each individual, and loss of facial nerve function is psychologically and functionally problematic. Facial nerve anatomy is complex and oftentimes variable.[26] Detailed knowledge of facial nerve anatomy is paramount in facial surgery to avoid iatrogenic injury. There are five distinct branches of the facial nerve: frontal (temporal), zygomatic, buccal, marginal mandibular, and cervical. After the facial nerve exits the stylomastoid foramen, it can branch in a variety of patterns (Fig. 73-14). Despite differing arborization patterns, the branches are always found in precise anatomic planes. Therefore, a three-dimensional understanding of facial nerve anatomy is essential to identify or protect a nerve branch. For example, the frontal branch of the facial nerve travels in the superficial temporal fascia. Dissecting in planes superficial or deep to this layer will protect the frontal branch. The buccal, zygomatic, and marginal mandibular branches travel just deep to the superficial musculoaponeurotic system after traversing the substance of the parotid gland and emerging from its anterior border. Dissecting superficial to this layer will protect these facial nerve branches.

The most common cause of facial paralysis is Bell's palsy. In most cases, it is idiopathic, and it occurs in 1 in 5000 individuals per year in the United States.[27] Bell's palsy is commonly associated with pregnancy and diabetes mellitus. Most patients with Bell's palsy have a complete remission, but the chance for remission decreases with age. Bell's palsy is commonly treated with corticosteroids in an effort to reduce nerve edema and restore normal circulation. Surgical decompression of the nerve within the bony facial canal is reserved for cases refractory to conservative measures.[28]

Trauma in the form of temporal bone fractures or deep facial lacerations is the second most frequent cause of facial palsy. When possible, immediate exploration and primary repair of the facial nerve affords the best chance to regain nerve function. If primary repair is not possible because of a nerve gap, then nerve grafting is attempted. When this is not possible, cross-face nerve grafting may be indicated. To accomplish this, a minor branch of the nerve on the normal side is sectioned, and the proximal end of this branch is then anastomosed to the distal nerve end on the paralyzed side with the use of nerve grafts. The sural nerve is most commonly used as a nerve graft, resulting in paresthesia of the heel and lateral foot. Other alternatives include muscles transfers, such as the temporalis or masseter muscle, to provide motion to the corner of the mouth. Free innervated tissue transfer has been successful using the gracilis muscle. As a two-stage procedure, cross-face nerve grafting is performed at least 6 months before the gracilis free muscle transfer. Alternatively, a nerve branch to the masseter muscle can be used in a single-stage procedure. For elderly and very ill patients, static procedures can be implemented. These include gold implants in the upper eyelid with tightening of the lower lid to allow eyelid closure. Tensor fasciae latae and dermis grafts offer autogenous donor sources that can be used to statically suspend the corner of the mouth. Although techniques to reestablish facial balance in repose are largely successful, obtaining facial symmetry with animation has remained an elusive outcome.

TRUNK AND EXTERNAL GENITALIA

Chest Wall Reconstruction

Chest wall defects most frequently occur as a consequence of ablative tumor resection or from extensive trauma. The resulting defects range from soft tissue only to complex defects involving skin, muscle, and bone.

Simple defects involving only soft tissue can be skin grafted. However, more complex defects usually require flap reconstruction. For example, advanced cases of breast cancer mandate extensive resection of skin and muscle. Here primary closure or skin grafting may be unsuitable solutions. In addition, when postoperative radiation is planned, skin graft coverage is a poor choice because radiation changes and breakdown are predictable. In these patients, selecting a myocutaneous flap offers vascularized tissue into the defect to cover exposed ribs and provides healthy tissue, which can sustain postoperative radiation. The latissimus dorsi myocutaneous flap is commonly used because of its wide arc of rotation, robust blood supply, and large surface area. Defects larger than 10 cm with loss of more than three adjacent ribs can risk flail chest with attendant compromised respiratory function. To prevent this outcome, skeletal integrity can be restored using autogenous split rib grafts, or alloplastic material such as polypropylene mesh.[29] Once again, muscle or myocutaneous flaps are used to provide final coverage over this.

Wound infection and dehiscence occur in about 2% of median sternotomies and increase morbidity for cardiothoracic patients. These wounds can be successfully managed with removal of sternal wires, generous débridement of necrotic bone and cartilage, culture-based antimicrobial therapy, and flap closure. In addition to providing soft tissue coverage, a muscle flap will also recruit much needed blood supply to the area to assist in healing and controlling infection. Muscle flaps most frequently used for closure of sternal wounds include the pectoralis major or rectus abdominis. Release of sternal wire fixation has not been shown to result in chest wall instability and is generally well tolerated.

Breast Reconstruction

Breast cancer is the most common malignant neoplasm in women, affecting about 1 in 8 women in the United States. Although the loss of a breast can be a psychosocially devastating reality, the opportunity to reconstruct the breast is rewarding for both the plastic surgeon and the patient.[30] Because it has been conclusively shown that postmastectomy reconstruction does not adversely influence survival outcomes or recurrence rates, preoperative consultation is offered to all women desiring breast reconstruction, and the option of not reconstructing the breast is also discussed.[31]

With rare exception, the nipple-areolar complex is excised with the breast. After removal of the breast, there is usually only enough skin to close the defect over a flat chest wall. The reconstructive surgeon must account for this deficient skin envelope in an attempt to recreate the breast mound. With the advent of immediate breast reconstruction, a team approach between the ablative and reconstructive surgeon has produced an improved aesthetic outcome for many women. When possible, a skin-sparing mastectomy is performed so as to provide a sufficient skin envelope to support a reconstructed breast. Immediate breast reconstruction has been shown to be safe, and the psychological benefit of waking from

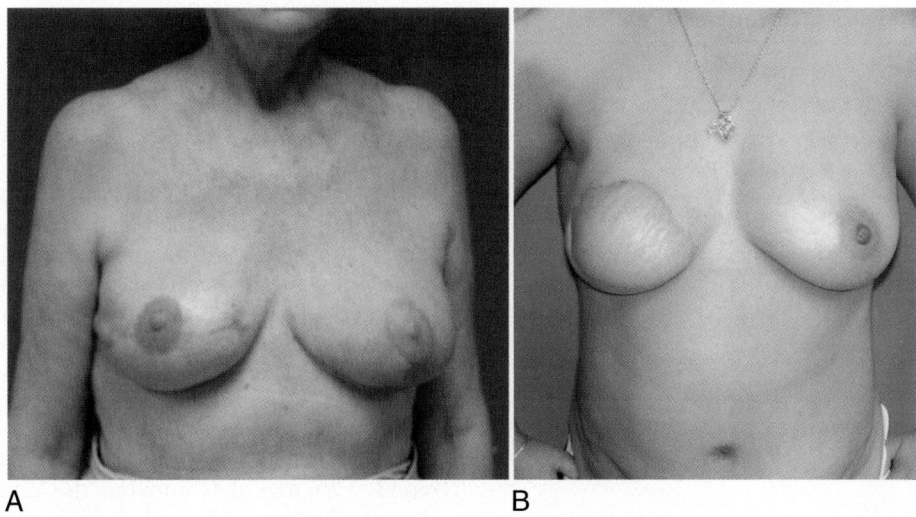

A   B

Figure 73-15 A, A 63-year-old woman after right mastectomy with tissue expander followed by implant reconstruction, right nipple reconstruction with tattooing of the nipple-areolar complex, and contralateral full-scar mastopexy. **B,** A 43-year-old woman after right mastectomy with autologous tissue reconstruction with a transverse rectus abdominis myocutaneous flap.

anesthesia with a reconstructed breast mound cannot be underestimated. When postmastectomy x-ray therapy is planned, the adverse consequences of ionizing radiation on the reconstruction site must be predicted. Adverse effects of radiation include flap distortion due to fat necrosis, skin envelope contracture and scarring, and implant capsular contracture.[32]

The simplest form of breast reconstruction is tissue expansion followed by placement of permanent breast implants (Fig. 73-15). A tissue expander is an inflatable silicone implant that contains an integrated or remote port for access during expansion using injectable saline. This implant is placed into a dissected cavity just overlying the ribs but covered with the pectoralis major muscle superiorly and medially and the serratus muscle inferiorly and laterally. These muscles are raised from the chest wall and sutured together over the uninflated tissue expander. The skin is closed and allowed to heal for 2 to 3 weeks. Inflation of the tissue expander is performed weekly until a volume slightly larger than desired is reached. The skin is allowed to remodel for several weeks. In a separate procedure, the expander is exchanged for a permanent breast implant. Tissue expansion has the benefit of a relatively short procedure, limiting other body scars, and no sacrifice of muscle to support a flap. Drawbacks include difficulty creating natural breast ptosis, capsular contracture, weekly office visits for expansion, and the need for a second procedure. This is the most popular mode of breast reconstruction.

The breast mound can be created using myocutaneous flaps such as the TRAM flap (see Fig. 73-15) or the latissimus dorsi myocutaneous flap. The TRAM flap uses the infraumbilical and suprapubic fat, which derives its blood supply from the underlying rectus abdominis muscle. This flap may be executed in a pedicled fashion based on the superior epigastric vessels. This technique can leave the patient with a bothersome epigastric bulge. In

addition, the entire rectus muscle must be sacrificed to support the flap. Using microvascular technique, the TRAM flap can be transferred as a free flap based on the deep inferior epigastric vessels or smaller perforator vessels, which are anastomosed to branches of the thoracodorsal in the axilla or the internal mammaries at the sternocostal junction.[33] The perforator-free TRAM flap has the advantage of sparing the underlying rectus muscle, thus preserving the abdominal wall integrity and strength.[11] However, blood flow is less robust compared with the deep inferior epigastric vessels, and long-term fat necrosis can be problematic in larger flaps. Alternatively, the lateral third of the rectus muscle can be spared using the deep inferior epigastric vessels (muscle-sparing technique), leaving some native rectus strength. Free TRAM flaps have been shown to have a more robust blood supply than pedicled TRAM flaps and can be used in patients who smoke. Advantages of the TRAM flap include ability to create a natural breast appearance that contains a generous volume of autogenous fat, virtually identical to the resected breast. In addition, many women like the flattened appearance of their abdomen, which is similar to that achieved with abdominoplasty. Drawbacks to the TRAM flap include a longer operative time, a visible scar on the lower abdomen, and a slight weakening of the abdominal wall.

The latissimus dorsi muscle can be used with a skin paddle to make up for the deficient skin envelope after mastectomy. Based on the thoracodorsal vessels, this method of reconstruction commonly requires placement of a small breast implant beneath the flap in order to achieve adequate size. Natural breast appearance and ptosis can be achieved in a single procedure using the latissimus dorsi flap. Implants covered by the latissimus dorsi muscle undergo less capsular contracture after postoperative radiation treatment as compared with primary expander and implant reconstructions as mentioned

Table 73-3 Classification System for Pressure Ulcers

Stage I: Nonblanchable erythema of intact skin; impending skin ulceration

Stage II: Partial-thickness skin loss involving epidermis and/or dermis; ulcer is superficial and presents clinically as an abrasion, blister, or shallow crater

Stage III: Full-thickness skin loss involving damage or necrosis of subcutaneous tissue that may extend down to, but not through, underlying fascia; ulcer presents clinically as a deep crater with or without undermining of adjacent tissue

Stage IV: Full-thickness skin loss with extensive destruction, tissue necrosis, or damage to muscle, bone, or supporting structures

earlier. Disadvantages include sacrifice of the latissimus dorsi muscle, a wide scar on the back, and difficult operative positioning. In addition to breast reconstruction, the latissimus dorsi is commonly relied on for other chest wall reconstructive needs.

The contralateral breast is always considered as part of the total reconstructive procedure. When needed, reduction mammaplasty or mastopexy are performed to match the reconstructed breast. At times, breast augmentation may be necessary if the reconstructed breast is larger. Nipple reconstruction using local flaps and tattooing of the nipple-areola complex (NAC) are performed after the breast mound reconstruction has been completed. Using these techniques, a natural-appearing breast mound can be created, and symmetry can be restored.

Abdominal Wall Reconstruction

The abdominal wall is a complex structure strengthened by a precise arrangement of abdominal wall musculature and fascia. Abdominal wall defects are frequently encountered and may or may not include a hernia component. Prosthetic fabrics such as PTFE and polypropylene are widely used to span preperitoneal defects. Exposure of such alloplastic material results in the harboring of bacteria in the interstices of the mesh fabric. In the case of infection, the mesh must be removed and the infection cleared before closure is attempted. Temporary (interim) closure is often achieved using autogenous skin graft placed directly on the well-vascularized bowel serosa. Final and permanent closure requires fascial, muscular, and skin reconstruction. Lower abdominal defects can be closed using a tensor fasciae latae or rectus femoris flap. Large abdominal hernias that have failed mesh repair, may be amenable to closure by component separation.[34] In this procedure, muscular layers of the abdominal wall are meticulously separated and allowed to slide, making mobilization possible to cover large defects. Postoperative issues of increased intra-abdominal pressure and respiratory insufficiency can be expected, and appropriate ventilator support may be required for a time. To foster uneventful healing and maintenance of the repair integrity, use of an abdominal binder or compression

garment and avoidance of strenuous activity are necessary.

Pressure Sores

One of the most costly problems in modern medicine is pressure sores, which are derived from prolonged immobility. Patients with spinal cord injuries and paralysis, elderly nursing home patients, and severely ill intensive care patients are most commonly at risk for pressure sores. Prevention of pressure sore formation requires a high level of patient compliance and support from ancillary staff. Given today's economic environment and nursing shortage, this level of care is frequently not available for these high-demand patients. Prevention of pressure sores requires pressure relief in the form of specialized mattresses and wheelchair cushions combined with manually moving the patient. Skin is kept clean and dry.

Pressure sores commonly occur over pressure-bearing surfaces such as the occipital scalp, elbows, heels, iliac crests, greater trochanters, ischial tuberosities, and sacrum. Pressure sores result from tissue ischemia occurring from prolonged pressure exceeding capillary arterial pressure of 32 mm Hg. In the supine position, pressures of 40 to 60 mm Hg occurs over the occiput, sacrum, and heel. In the sitting position, pressures of 100 mm Hg occur over the ischial tuberosities. Constant pressure applied for 2 hours can result in muscle necrosis.

Numerous grading schemes have been devised to classify pressure sores (Table 73-3). The simplest involves four grades: grade I (skin erythema), grade II (skin ulceration with necrosis into subcutaneous tissue), grade III (necrosis involving the underlying muscle), and grade IV (exposed bone or joint). On inspection, a pressure sore usually appears much smaller than it actually is. This occurs because deeper tissues adjacent to bone are exposed to higher pressure than the cutaneous tissue. The deep (muscle) layer is more susceptible to ischemic insult than the overlying fat or skin. Surgical débridement discloses the true extent of pressure-induced injury.

Treatment of these wounds requires a multidisciplinary approach with focus on prevention of reoccurrence. Initially, a pressure sore is débrided of nonviable tissue to include quantitative microbiologic testing. Antibiotic therapy is culture-based with the knowledge that wounds with more than 10^5 organisms/g of living tissue are infected and will not heal. Wound care is initiated with appropriate topical antimicrobials. The patient is given a pressure-relieving mattress and seat cushion and the caregiver instructed to turn the patient a minimum of every 2 hours. The nutritional status of the patient must be assessed, including nutrition consultation and serum protein and albumin levels. Nutritionally depleted patients cannot heal their wounds regardless of the quality of care.

Surgical closure of these wounds involves flap closure to pad bony prominences, and myocutaneous flaps may be chosen to recruit blood supply to the wound. Unfortunately, numerous studies have demonstrated that most surgically closed wounds eventually reoccur.[35] For ambulatory patients, surgical closure should never compromise the patient's ability to mobilize. Most ambulatory patients will heal with good local wound care, nutritional support, and avoidance of pressure.

The recent advent of vacuum-assisted closure (VAC) devices has dramatically improved the outcomes for many of these difficult wounds.[36] Using a specialized suction apparatus applied over a sponge and occlusive dressing, VAC therapy can shrink these wounds and stimulate the formation of granulation tissue and healing by secondary intention without the need for flap surgery closure. This form of therapy is notably proprietary and requires the use of a specialized device and additionally trained health care personnel. However, many third-party payers have come to accept VAC therapy as a cost-effective means of managing these wounds.

External Genitalia

Deformities of the external genitalia can be congenital or secondary to trauma, neoplastic defects, and infections. For those infants with ambiguous external genitalia, gender reassignment (usually female) is done by 18 months of age. Causes of ambiguous genitalia include hormonal imbalance (congenital adrenal hyperplasia), maternal drug use, and hermaphroditism. Of primary importance in gender reassignment is functional anatomic potential, with lesser consideration given to potential fertility and karyotype.

After cutaneous avulsion injury to the male genitalia, a temporizing measure of burying the penis and testes in adjacent soft tissues of the upper thigh allows salvage until permanent reconstruction is possible. Both the penile shaft and testes are amenable to split-thickness skin graft coverage. If the injury is sharp in nature, the penis can be replanted using microvascular technique. Total penile reconstruction is complex because of the need to reestablish both external and internal (urethral) function. Urethral reconstruction can be accomplished with free grafts of buccal mucosa or glabrous skin. The standard for penile shaft reconstruction is the free radial forearm flap microvascular transfer. Penile rigidity can be obtained using either an external device or an implanted prosthesis. Vaginal reconstruction performed by plastic surgeons is most often accomplished using pudendal groin flaps or skin grafts.

Infections in the groin region can be problematic. Hidradenitis suppurativa results from chronic infection of apocrine sweat glands. Incision and drainage or wide excision is often necessary in addition to culture-directed antibiotic therapy to reduce the bacterial load in these wounds. Skin graft success to cover these wounds can be compromised if infection is incompletely controlled and if the skin grafts are inadequately immobilized. Fournier's gangrene is a mixed aerobic and anaerobic infection that spreads rapidly along fascial planes. Diabetic patients are particularly susceptible. Radical surgical débridement and jet lavage irrigation are mandatory in addition to antibiotic therapy. Patients so affected frequently require serial operating room sessions for débridement before the wound bed is deemed ready for definitive wound coverage. When the infection is controlled, closure is achieved with skin grafts or local flaps.

Table 73-4   Gustilo Classification of Open Fractures of the Tibia

TYPE	DESCRIPTION
I	Open fracture with a wound <1 cm
II	Open fracture with a wound >1 cm without extensive soft tissue damage
III	Open fracture with extensive soft tissue damage
IIIA	III with adequate soft tissue coverage
IIIB	III with soft tissue loss with periosteal stripping and bone exposure
IIIC	III with arterial injury requiring repair

LOWER EXTREMITY

Trauma

Trauma to the lower extremity is frequently complex and can require a team of specialists to include orthopedic, plastic, and vascular surgery disciplines to deliver all the care needs. Reestablishment of normal or near-normal ambulation in a sensate extremity is the goal in lower extremity trauma. Patients presenting with traumatic injuries to the lower extremity frequently have other life-threatening injuries mandating strict adherence to Advanced Trauma Life Support protocol. Of foremost concern is assuring good vascular supply to the affected extremity. Fasciotomy is often required to prevent ischemic changes in muscle and nerve tissues following high-energy or crush injuries. When necessary, revascularization by primary repair or bypass grafting can salvage a compromised extremity.[37] Degloved tissue is conservatively débrided and its viability carefully assessed clinically or with the aid of intravenous fluorescein testing whereby cutaneous survival can be predicted. Copious jet lavage irrigation always accompanies initial débridement. Thigh injuries can generally be managed with delayed primary closure or skin grafting alone. Extensive soft tissue loss may require reconstruction using muscle or myocutaneous local flaps to cover exposed bone, blood vessels, or nerves.

Lower leg trauma is more complex because of the paucity of tissue surrounding the anterior tibia. Fractures of the lower leg are most often classified according to the Gustilo system[37] (Table 73-4). The proximal third of the lower leg, including the knee joint, is amenable to closure using the medial or lateral head of the gastrocnemius muscle. Defects involving the middle third of the lower leg can be closed using a pedicled soleus muscle flap with or without addition of the flexor digitorum longus muscle as well.[37] Distal-third defects, those defects above the ankle, are problematic and do not infrequently necessitate free tissue transfer to provide adequate soft tissue coverage with a reliable blood supply.[38] Foot wounds can often be closed with local flaps such as the sural artery island flap for heel defects.

Venous Stasis, Ischemic, and Diabetic Ulcers

Lower extremity ulcers may have a similar appearance but often have differing etiologies and treatment needs. Treatment success and healing depend on proper identification of the underlying problem, good wound hygiene, and surgical intervention that addresses all the pathologic issues.

Venous stasis ulcers result from venous hypertension, which is usually caused by valvular incompetence. These ulcers are characteristically present over the medial malleolus and are usually nontender but may be associated with pruritus. Other typical findings include increased lower extremity edema and hyperpigmentation in the adjacent skin resulting from increased hemosiderin deposition. Treatment regimens focus on increasing venous return and decreasing edema. Compression stockings or wraps, combined with frequent elevation of the extremity and avoidance of prolonged standing, are commonly prescribed. The wound is kept clean by washing, and judicious use of topical antimicrobials is instituted. Either surgical or enzymatic débridement of nonviable tissue acts to facilitate wound healing. Importantly, arterial inflow is checked using noninvasive Doppler studies that record the ankle-brachial index. Compression techniques need to be avoided for those patients with an ankle-brachial index of less than 0.8 because vascular compromise may ensue.

Ischemic lower extremity ulcers are due to arterial insufficiency from proximal arterial occlusion. These are typically painful, are punched out in appearance, demonstrate minimal edema, and have no change in surrounding pigmentation. They are typically located in a more distal location than venous ulcers, such as the lateral aspects of the great and fifth toes, as well as the dorsum of the foot. These ulcers indicate advanced peripheral vascular disease and are associated with very low ankle-brachial index readings between 0.1 and 0.3. Typically, these ulcers will not heal without surgical revascularization of the extremity. Once revascularized, these wounds can be expected to heal with either simple wound care or skin grafting.

Diabetic ulcers commonly result from decreased protective sensation. Diabetic peripheral neuropathy is common in the hands and feet (stocking-and-glove distribution). Diabetic ulcers are usually found on the plantar surface of the foot over the metatarsal heads or heel. Edema is usually mild with no change in surrounding pigmentation. Treatment is focused on preventing further damage to the area with devices such as custom-fitted orthopedic shoes to eliminate pressure over the metatarsal heads. Necrotic tissue must be judiciously débrided, and topical antimicrobials are needed to control local infection. In some cases, resection of the underlying bony prominence may improve wound healing. Diabetic patients must be educated to examine their feet routinely. This is paramount to prevent recurrence of these problematic wounds.

Lymphedema

Lymphedema is an accumulation of protein and fluid in the subcutaneous tissue. Functional disability and gross disfigurement can occur. Congenital lymphedema is seen in 10% of cases. When the condition presents first in early puberty, it is called *lymphedema praecox*. Lymphedema tarda is congenital lymphedema that becomes manifest only in middle age. The most common cause of secondary lymphedema in developed nations is resection of regional nodal basins for cancer. In subtropical and tropical underdeveloped nations, filariasis accounts for the primary etiology of secondary lymphedema. Treatment of lymphedema is difficult and often frustrating for both patient and surgeon alike. Nonoperative management includes compression garments, intermittent compression machines or manual lymphatic massage, elevation of the affected extremity, antiparasitic medications when appropriate, and systemic antibiotics to treat recurrent bouts of cellulitis. Surgical techniques offer only symptomatic relief, and there is no procedure that reliably produces a cure. The most common procedures include circumferential excision and skin grafting, serial excision of subcutaneous tissues, or serial liposuction reduction of the subcutaneous tissues. Microlymphatic bypass has been attempted but has met with only marginal success. The postsurgical leg deformities can be nearly as grotesque as the presenting swelling; however, functional improvement with both decreased weight of the affected extremity and reduced cutaneous infection incidence offer net gains in quality of life.

BREAST AND AESTHETIC SURGERY

Because plastic surgery is a specialty that deals with outwardly visible concerns, the psychological state of a patient must be considered. In this specialty, in which outward appearance remains a benchmark for success, it is necessary to maintain an objective but compassionate perspective. It is difficult to put an accurate value on a patient's self esteem. As humans, our psyche is intimately related to our perception of the way we appear to those around us. Although cosmetic or aesthetic surgery is medically unnecessary, its importance to the overall well-being of patients cannot be underestimated. Patient selection is paramount, and realistic postoperative outcomes must be carefully explained.

Elective breast surgery addresses both functional and aesthetic concerns. Breasts can be reduced, enlarged, or lifted to produce a more normal appearance. Macromastia (abnormally large breasts) is a functionally difficult and psychologically devastating problem for some women (Fig. 73-16). From a functional standpoint, macromastia can result in functional difficulty with exercise, neck and back pain, painful bra strap shoulder grooving, inframammary intertrigo, and difficulty finding appropriate clothing. Breast reduction surgery (reduction mammaplasty) involves resection of wedges of breast and fatty tissue as

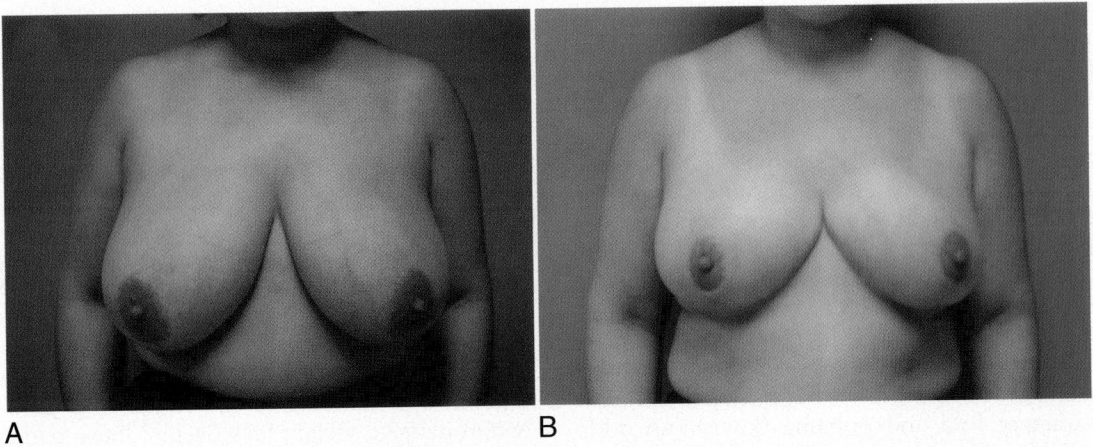

A   B

Figure 73-16 A 35-year-old woman with macromastia before (**A**) and after (**B**) reduction mammaplasty using an inferior pedicle with Wise (keyhole) pattern.

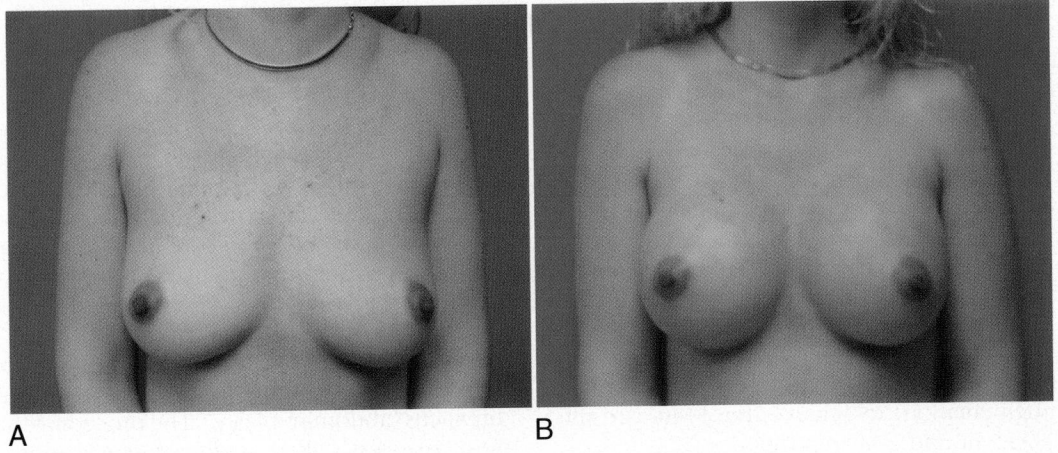

A   B

Figure 73-17 A, Preoperative view of a 28-year-old G0P0 woman. **B,** Postoperative view 6 months after a bilateral submuscular augmentation mammaplasty through an inframammary approach.

well as relocating the nipple and areola to a position on the chest wall opposite the inframammary fold, a position known as *Pitanguy's point.* The NAC may remain attached to the native underlying breast or in gigantomastia (extremely large breasts) may be transferred as a full-thickness graft. The keyhole pattern represents the most popular incisional design to achieve the desired recontouring. Alterations in nipple sensation and compromised ability to breast-feed infants may be experienced. Despite these potential risks, most patients are happily relieved from both the discomfort and psychological concerns associated with abnormally large breasts.[39]

For males, the problem of large breasts (gynecomastia) can be psychologically devastating. Most adolescents will experience some degree of breast tissue enlargement. However, if this does not resolve by the late teens or early 20s, surgery may be indicated. It is important to remember that breast cancer can occur in males and suspicious masses (hard, unilateral, or nodular) must undergo biopsy. Gynecomastia can be due to abnormal hormone levels, and assessment of the endocrine system is advisable. Most cases of gynecomastia are amenable to simple liposuction with minimal glandular resection through a periareolar incision as necessary. Redundant skin will usually redrape over the chest in a cosmetically acceptable manner, thereby limiting the need for skin resection to extreme cases only.

On the opposite extreme, many women suffer from concern surrounding abnormally small breasts, micromastia (Fig. 73-17). For appropriate candidates, breast augmentation can restore a feminine ideal of sexual attractiveness. Breast augmentation is usually accomplished through discrete incisions placed around the areola, at the inframammary fold, or in the axilla. Breast implant volume is determined by a woman's breast diameter. Most breast implants are constructed of a silicone envelope that is filled with sterile saline. Silicone-filled breast implants are today used only by select centers and physicians to reconstruct mastectomy defects and for exchange of previous silicone-filled implants. The past concerns about silicone-induced autoimmune disease have been disproved in the scientific literature, and U.S. Food and Drug Administration approval for use of silicone breast implants on a wide-scale basis is imminent.

Breast implants can be inserted above or below the pectoralis major muscle. The decision of which approach to use is influenced by the need to better camouflage the implant, associated breast ptosis, concern about potential capsular contracture, and doctor or patient preference.[40]

With age and child bearing, breasts will sag below the level of the inframammary crease, resulting in breast ptosis. Breast ptosis is graded based on the position of the NAC in relation to the inframammary crease. In addition, breasts may involute with childbearing and age resulting in worsening ptosis. Breast ptosis is classified as grade I (NAC position at the level of the inframammary fold), grade II ptosis (NAC position below the inframammary fold), and grade III ptosis (NAC position well below the inframammary fold and pointing down). An additional classification known as *pseudoptosis* indicates that a significant portion of the breast gland resides below the inframammary fold despite an anatomically correct nipple position. The goal of breast lifting or mastopexy is to restore a normal position of the NAC in relation to the inframammary fold. For grade I ptosis, simple breast augmentation may restore upper pole breast volume and also correct NAC position. For grades II and III ptosis, skin recontouring and NAC complex repositioning are necessary. Mastopexy incisions can involve a superior NAC incision (crescent mastopexy), circumareolar incision (donut mastopexy) with or without a vertical component, or a keyhole incision, which involves skin excision in the vertical and horizontal dimensions (anchor mastopexy) similar to the pattern used for breast reduction surgery. Some women may require a combination of both incisional recontouring (mastopexy) and implant placement (augmentation) to achieve the desired result: volume replacement and NAC reposition.

Lipodystrophy, excess fatty deposits in distinct anatomic areas, and redundant skin can be addressed through suction-assisted lipectomy (SAL) or excisional techniques, respectively. Body contouring involves creating a more ideal body shape given a patient's preoperative anatomy and goals. Many patients present complaining of an inability to lose fatty deposits in problem areas such as the infraumbilical region, hips, flanks, buttocks, thighs, and knees. Patients who are candidates for SAL have good skin turgor without abundant laxity or striae. Liposuction will not remedy cellulite. After infiltration of a tumescent solution containing a dilute mixture of local anesthetic with epinephrine, specialized hollow cannulas attached to tubing that connects to a vacuum aspirator device are used to extract the targeted areas of excess subcutaneous fat. Up to 30 mg/kg of lidocaine is typically injected first into the targeted areas to be liposuctioned. This is well tolerated because the solution contains epinephrine, which slows absorption and is injected directly into fat, which has a minimal blood supply. Ultrasound-assisted liposuction (UAL) involves passing an ultrasonic probe through the proposed tissues to be liposuctioned, which disrupts adipocyte membranes before extraction of the fat emulsion through a liposuction cannula. Proponents of this technique argue that it facilitates removal of large amounts of fat with reduced physical effort on the part of the surgeon. Reported complications include

end-hit burns of skin and cutaneous hyperesthesias. UAL can also be useful for areas containing fibrofatty tissue such as in gynecomastia and the upper back as in buffalo hump deformity. Although large-volume liposuction has been reported in the literature, the surgeon must be cautious because large intravascular fluid shifts may occur when volumes in excess of 5000 mL are aspirated.[41,42] Severe infections that spread along fascial planes can occur when sterile technique is compromised. The recent increase in bariatric surgery in the United States has created a unique and difficult new patient population. These patients who are morbidly obese can lose massive amounts of weight after bariatric procedures such as laparoscopic banding of the stomach or gastric bypass. When massive weight loss occurs, these patients experience profound deflation of the skin envelope without compensatory shrinkage. This typically manifests in sagging and redundant skin involving the face, arms, breasts, abdomen, thighs, and buttocks.

Excision techniques are necessary in cases in which redundant skin, abundant striae, or ptotic changes are present (e.g., in the large-volume weight loss patient).[43] When this procedure is performed to address the upper inner arm, it is called *brachioplasty,* whereas for the upper inner thigh, it is commonly referred to as a *thigh lift.* For the abdomen, when a patient presents with a hanging abdominal apron of skin and fat, simple amputation of this overhang (panniculectomy) will suffice. After weight loss or multiple pregnancies, there is often the problem of loose, hanging skin or lower abdominal stretch marks that require excision of skin redundancy, tightening of lax rectus fascia, and repositioning of the umbilicus (abdominoplasty). The procedure that addresses these issues is called *abdominoplasty*. Skin and fat are excised as a modified transverse ellipse from the lower abdomen, and an abdominal flap is raised to the costal margin laterally and the xiphoid centrally. The underlying fascia may be plicated to correct any diastasis between the paired rectus muscles. The umbilicus is left attached to its underlying vascular stalk and then relocated through a midline stab incision as the abdominal flap is closed devoid of the wrinkled infraumbilical and suprapubic skin and fat. In extreme cases, the incision will need to be extended across the back because the excess of tissue cannot be adequately removed through an anterior approach. This technique, known as *belt lipectomy,* requires both supine and prone positioning strategies in the operating room.

Body contouring, especially in excisional surgery, requires judicious monitoring of the patient and close communication with the anesthesiologist. Large volume shifts can occur because of the amount of tissue being removed.[42] Exposure of a large surgical field to room temperature for an extended time may pose a risk for hypothermia. In addition, these procedures may place the patient at an increased risk for deep venous thrombosis and potential pulmonary embolus. Thus, deep venous thrombosis prophylaxis measures are essential.

Facial rejuvenation is a complex area of plastic surgery requiring a detailed understanding of facial anatomy. Facial aging, although unavoidable, can be drastically hastened with sun exposure, smoking, and poor skin care. The effects of facial aging are the result of three mechanisms: actinic damage, dynamic muscle activity, and gravitational changes.

Actinic damage refers to environmental damage to the skin such as ultraviolet light and smoking. Dyschromia (mottled appearing skin), lentigenes (age spots), and telangiectasias (broken capillaries) are common manifestations of actinically damaged skin. Treatment focuses on good moisturizing skin care, strict sun avoidance using sun-blocking agents, and avoidance of environmental toxins such as cigarette smoke. Many authors advocate retinoic acid (Retin A) as an essential component of skin care regimens because of its proven ability to increase collagen turnover and thicken the dermis. Lasers (single wavelength) and other light sources (broadband intense pulsed light devices) can also be useful in improving actinic damage.

Dynamic muscle activity over time produces a characteristic and predictable aging pattern. Beginning in the third decade of life, vertical scowl lines at the glabella, transverse forehead rhytids, and fine-line crow's feet may be seen. These dynamic rhytids (wrinkles) can be treated using botulinum toxin (Botox), which temporarily paralyzes the underlying mimetic muscle in a process known as *chemodenervation*. In addition, Botox has shown success when injected into the frontalis to treat migraine headaches.[44] Botox injections are one of the most common aesthetic plastic surgical procedures in the United States today. Injections performed for cosmetic effacement of dynamic wrinkles must be repeated every 4 months or so for optimal effect. For static, established wrinkles or fine lines, or to de-emphasize folds such as the nasolabial fold, soft tissue fillers have enjoyed success. Examples include collagen, hyaluronic acid derivatives, polylactic acid, and autologous fat. They are usually injected below a fold or wrinkle in a deep dermal or subdermal plane. Most synthetic fillers offer correction that may last in excess of 6 months. Success with autologous fat injection appears to be operator and recipient site dependent.

Gravitational facial aging is associated with descent of facial fat, brow ptosis, deepening of the nasolabial fold, jowling, and loss of the cervicomental angle. Isolated excesses of skin and fat in the upper or lower eyelids can be addressed with a blepharoplasty, excision of skin and fat from the upper or lower eyelids. If the eyebrows have fallen below the superior orbital rim, a browlift is needed to bring the brow back to its normal position and rejuvenate the forehead region as well. The browlift can be performed in an open technique (transcoronal) or with limited incisions (endoscopic browlift). When facial or neck resuspension cannot be accomplished with nonsurgical means, a rhytidectomy or facelift needs to be considered. Using a combination of temporal, preauricular, and postauricular incisions, the facial skin with or without the underlying submuscular aponeurotic system fascia is undermined, advanced, and finally secured to rid facial rhytids and sagging neck and to resuspend facial fat. As with browlifts, endoscopic techniques can be employed for midface suspension. Sometimes, to maximize the refinement sought for recontouring the neck,

additional liposuction and tightening by plication of the platysma muscle is necessary. These procedures alone or in combination are successful toward achieving a well-rested and more youthful facial appearance.[45]

Although there is still no substitute for astute surgical technique in facial rejuvenation, many patients are unwilling to accept the risk and downtime associated with aesthetic surgery. The recent trend toward minimally invasive modalities needs to be carefully understood both in terms of their benefits and limitations. The so-called lunchtime face lift relies on several barbed polypropylene sutures introduced percutaneously and sinuously threaded through the loose soft tissues of the cheeks and forehead. Optimal vector lift is achieved during tension adjustment.

In the field of laser surgery, there are noninvasive, moderately invasive, and ablative techniques that can be used. The minimal and moderate alternatives refer to the fact that the epidermis remains intact. This reduces downtime and allows the procedure to be performed by a specially trained physician extender. For this reason, these alternatives are popular in outpatient skin care facilities. These modalities can significantly improve actinic damage but demonstrate only limited ability to improve wrinkles. No single moderate modality has been proved superior.

Ablative techniques include dermabrasion, deep chemical peels such as phenol and croton oil, and CO_2 and erbium lasers. Dermabrasion uses mechanical sheer to remove epidermis and superficial dermis. Phenol and croton oil peels also penetrate to the reticular dermis but require cardiac monitoring because of potential side effects. CO_2 and erbium lasers ablate tissue using water as the chromophore (target) for the laser light (specific wavelength). All ablative modalities require antiviral prophylaxis. Although these ablative modalities require extensive downtime for the skin to re-epithelialize (10-14 days), they are vastly superior to the nonablative alternatives in terms of improving both actinic damage and wrinkles.

Finally, nasal deformities can be corrected with rhinoplasty.[46] An open technique using a transcolumellar incision is preferred when moderate sculpting of the nasal alar cartilage is necessary and when septal surgery is needed at the same time. Alternatively, a closed approach using intranasal incisions can be used for more minor corrections. Careful preoperative assessment of the deformity and nasal airway is essential. Different techniques exist to shape the nose, including suture plication,[47,48] cartilage resection, cartilage grafting, controlled fracturing of the nasal bones, and rasping of cartilage or bone. Nasal obstruction can be corrected by removing the offending buckle of a deviated septum and internally splinting the dorsal septum with a septal cartilage graft. Postoperative nasal packing is instilled to prevent hematomas, and antibiotics are given to prevent staphylococcal infection. Postoperative nasal edema takes months to completely resolve, and revision surgery is not considered before a 12-month period has elapsed because the distortion from postsurgical induration and swelling will not have cleared before then.

CONCLUSION

Plastic surgery is an extremely diverse surgical specialty whose primary goal is to restore both form and function. Important areas of plastic surgery such as thermal injury, hand and upper extremity surgery, and wound care are covered in other chapters within this text. Herein, we have offered only a superficial overview of the realm of plastic surgery.

Selected References

Achauer B, Eriksson E, Guturon B, et al (eds): Plastic Surgery: Indications, Operations and Outcomes. St Louis, Mosby, 2000.

A five-volume comprehensive text of plastic and reconstructive surgery.

Aston SJ, Beasley RW, Thorne CH (eds): Grabb and Smith's Plastic Surgery, 5th ed. Philadelphia, Lippincott-Raven, 1997.

A concise single volume text of plastic and reconstructive surgery.

Borges A: Elective Incisions and Scar Revision. Boston, Little, Brown, 1973.

A concise review of designing elective incision and scar treatment with particular attention to local flaps such as the Z-plasty.

Bostwick J: Plastic and Reconstructive Breast Surgery. St Louis, Quality Medical, 2000.

An excellent single-author text dedicated to aesthetic and reconstructive breast surgery.

Gill PS, Hunt JP, Guerra AB, et al: A 10-year retrospective review of 758 DIEP flaps for breast reconstruction. Plast Reconstr Surg 113:1153, 2004.

A large case series detailing experience with microvascular breast reconstruction using perforator vessel technique.

Henriksen T, Holmich L, Friis S, et al: The Danish registry for plastic surgery of the breast: Establishment of a nationwide registry for prospective follow-up, quality assessment, and investigation of breast surgery. Plast Reconstr Surg 112:2182, 2003.

The Danish experience investigating outcomes and analysis of plastic surgery on the breast.

Jackson IT: Local Flaps in Head and Neck Reconstruction. St Louis, Mosby, 1985.

An excellent and concise overview of local flaps for head and neck reconstruction with clear visual explanations.

Kenkel JM, Brown SA, Love EJ, et al: Hemodynamics, electrolytes, and organ histology of larger volume liposuction in a porcine model. Plast Reconstr Surg. 113:139, 2004.

Excellent physiologic investigation of large volume liposuction in a porcine model.

Mathes S, Nahai F: Reconstructive Surgery: Principles, Anatomy, and Technique. New York, Churchill Livingstone, 1997.

A clear and clinically relevant text dedicated to flap-based reconstructive surgery.

Millard D: Cleft Craft: The Evolution of Its Surgery. Boston, Little, Brown, 1976.

A comprehensive review of the history and techniques of cleft lip and palate surgery.

Tessier P, Kawamoto H, Matthews D, et al: Autogenous bone grafts and bone substitutes: Tools and techniques. A 20,000-case experience in maxillofacial and craniofacial surgery. Plast Reconstr Surg 116(5):6S, 2003.

Large craniomaxillofacial experience with bone grafts and bone substitutes.

References

1. Borges AF: Relaxed skin tension lines (RSTL) versus other skin lines. Plast Reconstr Surg 73:144-150, 1984.
2. Atkinson JA, McKenna KT, Barnett AG, et al: A randomized, controlled trial to determine the efficacy of paper tape in preventing hypertrophic scar formation in surgical incisions that traverse Langer's skin tension lines. Plast Reconstr Surg 116:1648-1656; discussion 1657-1658, 2005.
3. Chan KY, Lau CL, Adeeb SM, et al: A randomized, placebo-controlled, double-blind, prospective clinical trial of silicone gel in prevention of hypertrophic scar development in median sternotomy wound. Plast Reconstr Surg 116:1013-1020; discussion 1021-1022, 2005.
4. Hamer ML, Robson MC, Krizek TJ, et al: Quantitative bacterial analysis of comparative wound irrigations. Ann Surg 181:819-822, 1975.
5. Teh BT: Why do skin grafts fail? Plast Reconstr Surg 63:323-332, 1979.
6. Cormach GC, Lamberty GGH: A classification of fasciocutaneous flaps according to their patterns of vascularization. Br J Plast Surg 37:80, 1984.
7. McCraw JB, Vasconez LO: Musculocutaneous flaps: Principles. Clin Plast Surg 7:9-13, 1980.
8. Yousif NJ, Ye Z, Grunert BK, et al: Analysis of the distribution of cutaneous perforators in cutaneous flaps. Plast Reconstr Surg 101:72-84, 1998.
9. Stal S, Klebuc M, Taylor TD, et al: Algorithms for the treatment of cleft lip and palate. Clin Plast Surg 25:493-507, vii, 1998.
10. Armstrong MB, Masri N, Venugopal R: Reconstructive microsurgery: Reviewing the past, anticipating the future. Clin Plast Surg 28:671-686, vi, 2001.
11. Gill PS, Hunt JP, Guerra AB, et al: A 10-year retrospective review of 758 DIEP flaps for breast reconstruction. Plast Reconstr Surg 113:1153-1160, 2004.
12. Huang JI, Zuk PA, Jones NF, et al: Chondrogenic potential of multipotential cells from human adipose tissue. Plast Reconstr Surg 113:585-594, 2004.
13. Ulusal BG, Ulusal AE, Ozmen S, et al: A new composite facial and scalp transplantation model in rats. Plast Reconstr Surg 112:1302-1311, 2003.
14. Dragoo JL, Lieberman JR, Lee RS, et al: Tissue-engineered bone from BMP-2-transduced stem cells derived from human fat. Plast Reconstr Surg 115:1665-1673, 2005.
15. Jones MC: Facial clefting: Etiology and developmental pathogenesis. Clin Plast Surg 20:599-606, 1993.
16. Millard DR: Extensions of the rotation-advancement principle for wide unilateral cleft lips. Plast Reconstr Surg 42:535-544, 1968.
17. Brent B: Technical advances in ear reconstruction with autogenous rib cartilage grafts: Personal experience with

1200 cases. Plast Reconstr Surg 104:319-334; discussion 335-338, 1999.

18. Mustarde JC: The treatment of prominent ears by buried mattress sutures: A ten-year survey. Plast Reconstr Surg 39:382-386, 1967.

19. Mulliken JB, Gripp KW, Stolle CA, et al: Molecular analysis of patients with synostotic frontal plagiocephaly (unilateral coronal synostosis). Plast Reconstr Surg 113:1899-1909, 2004.

20. Renier D, Sainte-Rose C, Marchac D, et al: Intracranial pressure in craniostenosis. J Neurosurg 57:370-377, 1982.

21. Fong KD, Warren SM, Loboa EG, et al: Mechanical strain affects dura mater biological processes: Implications for immature calvarial healing. Plast Reconstr Surg 112:1312-1327, 2003.

22. Manson P: Management of facial fractures. Perspect Plast Surg 2(2):1, 1988.

23. Yaremchuk MJ: Facial skeletal reconstruction using porous polyethylene implants. Plast Reconstr Surg 111:1818-1827, 2003.

24. Tessier P, Kawamoto H, Matthews D, et al: Autogenous bone grafts and bone substitutes—tools and techniques. I. A 20,000-case experience in maxillofacial and craniofacial surgery. Plast Reconstr Surg 116:6S-24S; discussion 92S-94S, 2005.

25. Markowitz BL, Manson PN: Panfacial fractures: Organization of treatment. Clin Plast Surg 16:105-114, 1989.

26. Freilinger G, Gruber H, Happak W, et al: Surgical anatomy of the mimic muscle system and the facial nerve: Importance for reconstructive and aesthetic surgery. Plast Reconstr Surg 80:686-690, 1987.

27. Merren MD: Nonepidemic incidence of Bell's palsy. Am J Otol 9:159, 1988.

28. Wells MD, Manktelow RT: Surgical management of facial palsy. Clin Plast Surg 17:645-653, 1990.

29. Arnold PG, Pairolero PC: Chest-wall reconstruction: An account of 500 consecutive patients. Plast Reconstr Surg 98:804-810, 1996.

30. Henriksen TF, Holmich LR, Friis S, et al: The Danish Registry for Plastic Surgery of the Breast: Establishment of a nation-wide registry for prospective follow-up, quality assessment, and investigation of breast surgery. Plast Reconstr Surg 111:2182-2189; discussion 2190-2191, 2003.

31. Shons AR, Cox CE: Breast cancer: Advances in surgical management. Plast Reconstr Surg 107:541-549; quiz 550, 2001.

32. Kronowitz SJ, Robb GL: Breast reconstruction with post-mastectomy radiation therapy: Current issues. Plast Reconstr Surg 114:950-960, 2004.

33. Schusterman MA, Kroll SS, Miller MJ, et al: The free transverse rectus abdominis musculocutaneous flap for breast reconstruction: One center's experience with 211 consecutive cases. Ann Plast Surg 32:234-241; discussion 241-242, 1994.

34. Shestak KC, Edington HJ, Johnson RR: The separation of anatomic components technique for the reconstruction of massive midline abdominal wall defects: Anatomy, surgical technique, applications, and limitations revisited. Plast Reconstr Surg 105:731-738; quiz 739, 2000.

35. Disa JJ, Carlton JM, Goldberg NH: Efficacy of operative cure in pressure sore patients. Plast Reconstr Surg 89:272-278, 1992.

36. Wanner MB, Schwarzl F, Strub B, et al: Vacuum-assisted wound closure for cheaper and more comfortable healing of pressure sores: A prospective study. Scand J Plast Reconstr Surg Hand Surg 37:28-33, 2003.

37. Byrd HS, Spicer TE, Cierney G 3rd: Management of open tibial fractures. Plast Reconstr Surg 76:719-730, 1985.

38. Khouri RK, Shaw WW: Reconstruction of the lower extremity with microvascular free flaps: A 10-year experience with 304 consecutive cases. J Trauma 29:1086-1094, 1989.

39. Collins ED, Kerrigan CL, Kim M, et al: The effectiveness of surgical and nonsurgical interventions in relieving the symptoms of macromastia. Plast Reconstr Surg 109:1556-1566, 2002.

40. Hidalgo DA: Breast augmentation: Choosing the optimal incision, implant, and pocket plane. Plast Reconstr Surg 105:2202-2216; discussion 2217-2218, 2000.

41. Hetter GP: Blood and fluid replacement for lipoplasty procedures. Clin Plast Surg 16:245-248, 1989.

42. Kenkel JM, Brown SA, Love EJ, et al: Hemodynamics, electrolytes, and organ histology of larger-volume liposuction in a porcine model. Plast Reconstr Surg 113:1391-1399, 2004.

43. Hurwitz DJ: Single-staged total body lift after massive weight loss. Ann Plast Surg 52:435-441; discussion 441, 2004.

44. Guyuron B, Tucker T, Davis J: Surgical treatment of migraine headaches. Plast Reconstr Surg 109:2183-2189, 2002.

45. Pitanguy I: Facial cosmetic surgery: A 30-year perspective. Plast Reconstr Surg 105:1517-1526; discussion 1527, 2000.

46. Sheen JH: Rhinoplasty: Personal evolution and milestones. Plast Reconstr Surg 105:1820-1852; discussion 1853, 2000.

47. Guyuron B, Behmand RA: Nasal tip sutures part II: The interplays. Plast Reconstr Surg 112:1130-1145; discussion 1146-1149, 2003.

48. Behmand RA, Ghavami A, Guyuron B: Nasal tip sutures part I: The evolution. Plast Reconstr Surg 112:1125-1129; discussion 1146-1149, 2003.

74 | CHAPTER

Hand Surgery

David Netscher, MD   and   Nicholas Fiore, MD

Although hand surgery fellowships traditionally receive trainees primarily with backgrounds in orthopedic surgery or plastic surgery, fellowship training in hand surgery may also be undertaken by those having completed a residency in general surgery. Basic tenets of hand surgery must be acquired by all general surgeons. Depending on the practice locale (rural or urban), type of hospital, and residency rotations (e.g., surgical intern covering the emergency department), or even for the purposes of board examinations, an ability to evaluate and manage hand injuries and problems is a necessary skill for the general surgeon. The purpose of this chapter is not to provide the general surgeon with an exhaustive study of hand surgery, as specialty texts are more appropriate, but to provide an overview of hand pathology encountered more commonly by the general surgeon, and especially to emphasize basics in anatomy, physical examination, and management of common hand and upper extremity emergencies.

BASIC ANATOMY

The arm and hand are divided into volar or palmar, and also dorsal, aspects. Distal to the elbow, structures are termed either *radial* or *ulnar* to the middle finger axis rather than lateral and medial, respectively, because with forearm *pronation* and *supination,* the latter terms become confusing. Nomenclature of digits has become standardized. The hand has five digits, namely the thumb and four fingers (the thumb is not called a finger). The four fingers are respectively termed the *index, long (middle), ring,* and *small (little) fingers.* The use of numbers to designate digits is no longer accepted (Fig. 74-1). Within the hand, those structures close to the fingertips are termed *distal,* whereas those further up toward the wrist are termed *proximal.* Motion in a palmar direction is flexion, whereas dorsal motion is termed *extension.* Finger motion away from the long finger axis is termed *abduction,* whereas motion toward the axis of the long finger is adduction. The description of motion of the thumb is sometimes confusing. Extension of the thumb is in the plane of the palm of the hand, whereas palmar abduction of the thumb is the motion that occurs at 90 degrees away from the plane of the palm. Finally, side-to-side motion of the wrist is termed *radial* and *ulnar deviation.*

Intrinsic muscles of the hand are those that have their origins and insertions in the hand, whereas the extrinsic muscles have their muscle bellies in the forearm and their tendon insertions in the hand. The intrinsic muscles that make up the thenar eminence are the abductor pollicis brevis (APB), flexor pollicis brevis (FPB), opponens pollicis (OP), and adductor pollicis (AP). There are four dorsal interossei that arise from adjacent sides of each metacarpal and provide abduction of the metacarpophalangeal (MP) joints of the index, middle, and ring fingers. There are three palmar interossei that adduct the index, ring, and little fingers toward the middle finger. Four lumbricals originate on the flexor digitorum profundus

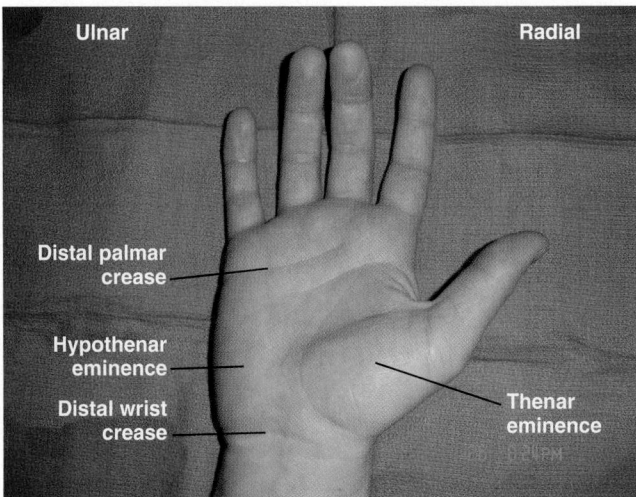

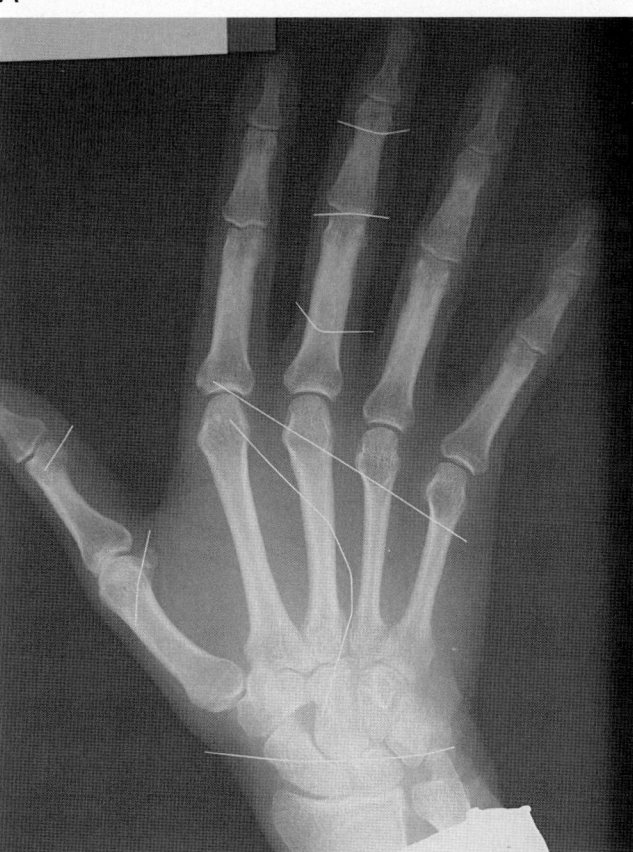

Figure 74-1 Surface anatomy of the hand. **A,** Hand surfaces and nomenclature. **B,** Skin creases of the hand superimposed on the skeletal structures.

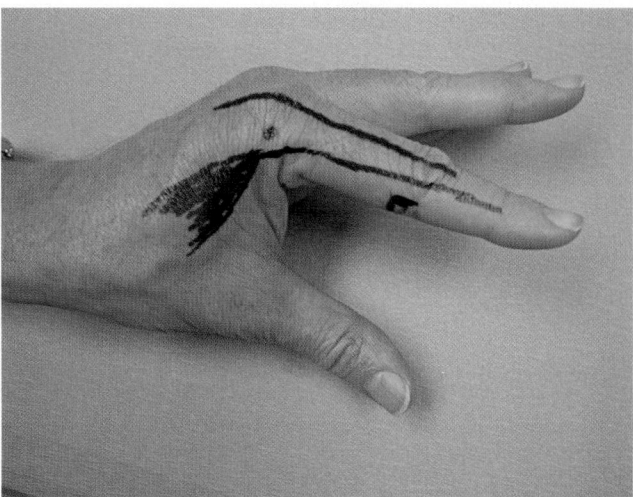

Figure 74-2 Outline of first dorsal interosseous muscle on the index finger shows how it passes volar to the fulcrum of flexion of metacarpophalangeal joint (MP) and dorsal to interphalangeal joints. Interossei flex MP joints and extend proximal and distal interphalangeal joints. Long extrinsic extensor tendon passes dorsal to all joints.

The hypothenar muscles consist of the flexor digiti minimi (FDM), which flexes the little finger at the MP joint, as well as the abductor digiti minimi (ADM) and the opponens digiti minimi (ODM). A small muscle called the *palmaris brevis* is located transversally in the subcutaneous tissue at the base of the hypothenar imminence. It is innervated by the ulnar nerve and puckers the skin and helps in cupping the skin of the palm during grip (Table 74-1).

The extrinsic muscles originate proximal to the wrist and comprise the long flexors and extensors of the wrist and digits. The extensors are located dorsally and are divided into three subgroups. The radial-most subgroup is termed the *mobile wad* and comprises the brachioradialis (BR), extensor carpi radialis longus (ECRL), and the extensor carpi radialis brevis (ECRB). The ECRL and ECRB extend the wrist and deviate it radially. The second group is located in a more superficial layer and comprises three muscles, namely the extensor carpi ulnaris (ECU), extensor digiti minimi/quinti (EDM/Q), and extensor digitorum communis (EDC). The ECU deviates the wrist in an ulnar direction and extends the wrist, whereas the EDM and EDC extend the MP joints of the fingers. The third and deeper subgroup comprises four muscles, three of which act on the thumb, and the remaining muscle influences the index finger. The abductor pollicis longus (APL), extensor pollicis longus (EPL), and extensor pollicis brevis (EPB) provide function to the thumb, and the extensor indicis proprius (EIP) extends the MP joint to the index finger. Last of the deep muscles is the supinator, which is located proximally in the forearm (Table 74-2).

The extensor tendons pass through six compartments deep to the extensor retinaculum at the dorsum of the wrist. From radial to ulnar side, these tendons and compartments are arranged as follows: The first compartment contains the APL and EPB, which also form the radial

(FDP) tendons in the palm and insert on the radial sides of the extensor mechanisms of the four fingers. They, together with the interossei, bring about both flexion of the MP joints and extension of the interphalangeal (IP) joints of the fingers (Fig. 74-2). The FPB flexes the thumb at the MP joint, in contrast with the extrinsic flexor pollicis longus (FPL), which flexes the thumb IP joint.

Table 74-1   Extrinsic Muscles of the Volar Forearm

MUSCLE	INNERVATION*	FUNCTION
Pronator teres (PT)	Median	Pronation
Flexor carpi radialis (FCR)	Median	Flexion and radial deviation of the wrist
Palmaris longus (PL)	Median	Flexion of the wrist
Flexor carpi ulnaris (FCU)	Ulnar	Flexion and ulnar deviation of the wrist
Flexor digitorum superficialis (FDS)	Median	Flexion of the proximal interphalangeal (PIP) joint
Flexor digitorum profundus (FDP)	Median and ulnar	Flexion of the distal interphalangeal (DIP) joint
Pronator quadratus	Median	Pronation
Flexor pollicis longus (FPL)	Median	Flexion of the thumb

*All muscles of the volar forearm are innervated by the median nerve and its branches *except* the two ulnar digits of the FDP and the FCU, which are innervated by the ulnar nerve.

Table 74-2   Extrinsic Muscles of the Dorsal Forearm

MUSCLE	INNERVATION*	FUNCTION
Extensor pollicis brevis (EPB)	Radial	Abducts the hand and extends the thumb at the proximal phalanx
Abductor pollicis longus (APL)	Radial	Abducts the hand and thumb
Extensor carpi radialis longus (ECRL)	Radial	Extends and radially deviates the hand
Extensor carpi radialis brevis (ECRB)	Radial	Extends and radially deviates the hand
Extensor pollicis longus (EPL)	Radial	Extends the distal phalanx of the thumb
Extensor digitorum communis (EDC)	Radial	Extends the fingers and the hand
Extensor indicis proprius (EIP)	Radial	Extends the index finger
Extensor digiti minimi/quinti (EDM/Q)	Radial	Extends the small finger
Extensor carpi ulnaris (ECU)	Radial	Extends and ulnarly deviates the wrist
Supinator	Radial	Supination
Brachioradialis	Radial	Flexes the forearm

*All muscles of the dorsal forearm are innervated by the radial nerve and its respective branches.

boundary of the so-called anatomic snuffbox. The second compartment consists of the ECRL and ECRB, and the third compartment (which also forms the ulnar boundary of the anatomic snuffbox) contains the EPL. The EIP and EDC pass through the fourth compartment and the EDM through the fifth compartment, where they overlie the distal radioulnar joint. The sixth compartment contains the ECU (Fig. 74-3).

At the level of the MP joints, the long extrinsic extensor tendons broaden out to form the extensor hood. The proximal part of the hood at this level is called the *sagittal band.* It loops around the MP joint and blends into the volar plate and thus forms a lasso around the base of the proximal phalanx, through which it extends the MP joint. The insertions of the interossei and lumbricals enter into the extensor hood as the lateral bands. These lateral bands insert distal and dorsal to the axis of the PIP joint, and it is through this distal insertion that the intrinsic muscles, namely the interossei and lumbricals, are flexors of the MP joints and yet extensors of the IP joints. The extensor hood inserts to the base of the middle phalanx, which is termed the *central slip,* and

finally proceeds on to the base of the distal phalanx, where it inserts through the terminal slip, thus extending the distal interphalangeal (DIP) joint (Fig. 74-4).

The extrinsic flexor muscles are located on the volar aspect of the forearm and are arranged in three layers. The superficial layer comprises four muscles, pronator teres (PT), flexor carpi radialis (FCR), flexor carpi ulnaris (FCU), and palmaris longus (PL). This latter muscle may be absent as frequently as in 10% to 12% of persons. These muscles originate from the medial humeral epicondyle in the proximal forearm and function to flex the wrist and pronate the forearm. The intermediate layer consists of the flexor digitorum superficialis (FDS), which allows independent flexion of the proximal interphalangeal (PIP) joints of the fingers. In the deep layer, there are three muscles: the FPL, which flexes the IP joint to the thumb; the FDP, which flexes the DIP joints of the fingers; and a distal quadrangular muscle that spans between the radius and ulna termed the *pronator quadratus,* which helps in pronation of the forearm (Table 74-3).

Nerve supply to the hand is by three nerves: the median, ulnar, and radial nerves. A knowledge of the

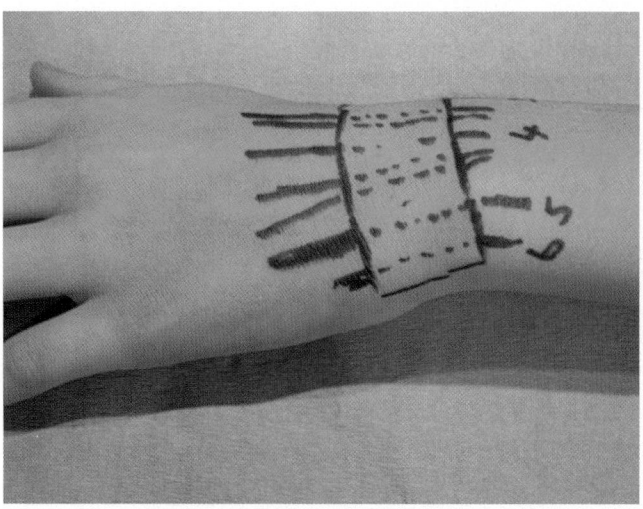 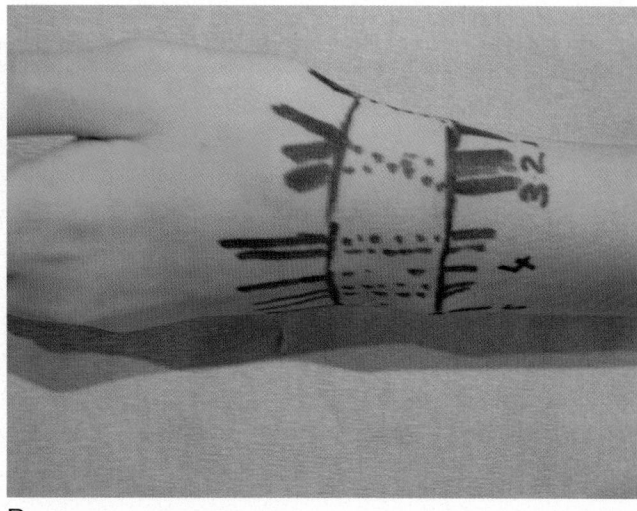

A B

Figure 74-3 **A** and **B,** Surface anatomy of the six dorsal extensor compartments at the wrist. Note that the first (abductor pollicis longus and extensor pollicis brevis) and third (extensor pollicis longus) compartments form the radial and ulnar boundaries, respectively, of the "anatomic snuffbox."

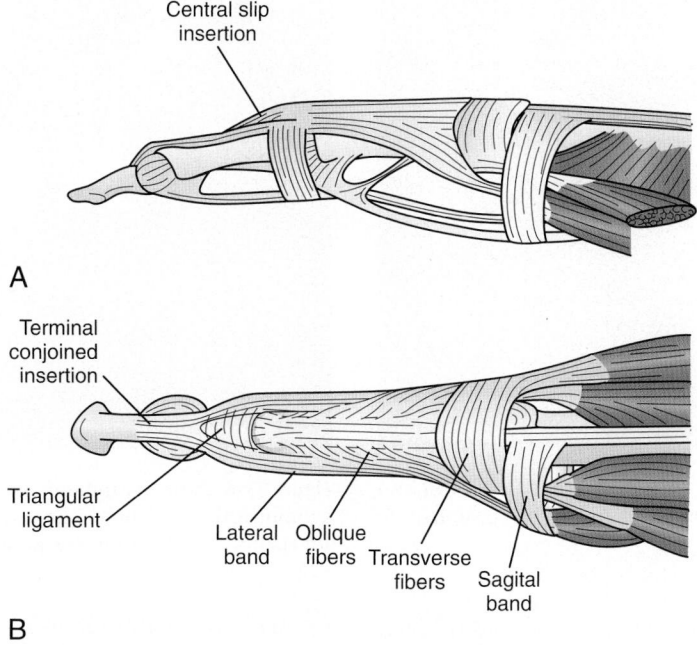

A

Central slip
insertion

Terminal
conjoined
insertion

Triangular
ligament

Lateral
band
Oblique
fibers
Transverse
fibers
Sagittal
band

B

Figure 74-4 Extensor mechanism of the fingers. **A,** Lateral view. **B,** Dorsal view.

surface anatomy of nerves helps to evaluate specific lacerating injuries (Fig. 74-5). The ulnar attachment to the flexor retinaculum is to the pisiform and hook of the hamate, and the radial attachment is to the scaphoid and ridge of the trapezium. The median nerve passes through the carpal tunnel between these landmarks. It gives sensation to the thumb, index finger, middle finger, and radial half of the ring finger. The palmar cutaneous branch of the median nerve originates from its radial side 5 to 6 cm proximal to the wrist, providing sensation to the palmar triangle. The ulnar nerve travels to the radial side of the

pisiform and passes to the ulnar side of the hook of the hamate in its passage through Guyon's canal. It gives sensation to the little finger and the ulnar half of the ring finger, and the dorsal branch of the ulnar nerve (arising proximal to the wrist and curving dorsally around the head of the ulna) supplies the same digits on their dorsal aspects. The superficial radial sensory nerve emerges from under the brachioradialis in the distal forearm, dividing into two or three branches proximal to the radial styloid, which then proceed in a subcutaneous course across the anatomic snuffbox, innervating the skin of the dorsum of

Table 74-3 **Intrinsic Muscles of the Hand**

MUSCLE	INNERVATION*	FUNCTION
Abductor pollicis brevis (APB)	Median	Abducts the thumb
Flexor pollicis brevis (FPB)	Median	Flexes the thumb
Opponens pollicis (OP)	Median	Opposes the thumb
Lumbricals	Median and ulnar	Flexes metacarpal phalangeal (MCP) joints and extends interphalangeal (IP) joints
Palmaris brevis	Ulnar	Wrinkles the skin on the medial (ulnar) side of the palm
Adductor pollicis (AdP)	Ulnar	Adducts the thumb
Abductor digiti minimi (ADM)	Ulnar	Abducts the small finger
Flexor digiti minimi (FDM)	Ulnar	Flexes the small digit
Opponens digiti minimi (ODM)	Ulnar	Opposes the small finger
Dorsal interossei	Ulnar	Abducts the fingers; flexes MCP joints and extends the IP joints
Palmar interossei	Ulnar	Adducts the fingers; flexes MCP joints and extends the IP joints

*All the thenar intrinsic muscles are supplied by the median nerve *except* the AdP; all the remaining intrinsic muscles are supplied by the ulnar nerve *except* the two radial lumbricals.

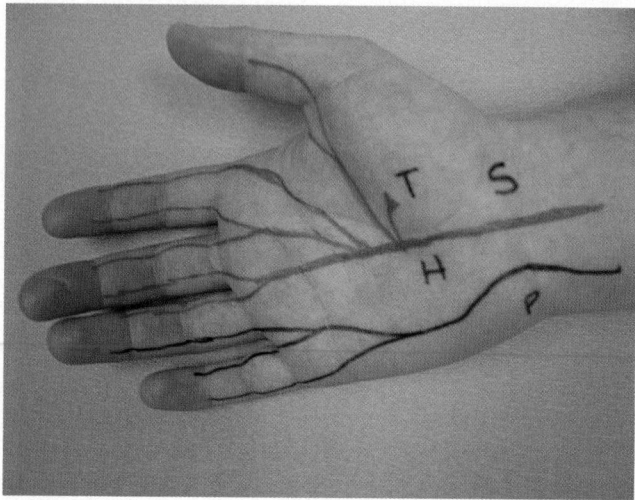

Figure 74-5 Surface anatomy of median (*red*) and ulnar (*black*) nerves. T, trapezium; H, hook of hamate; P, pisiform; S, scaphoid.

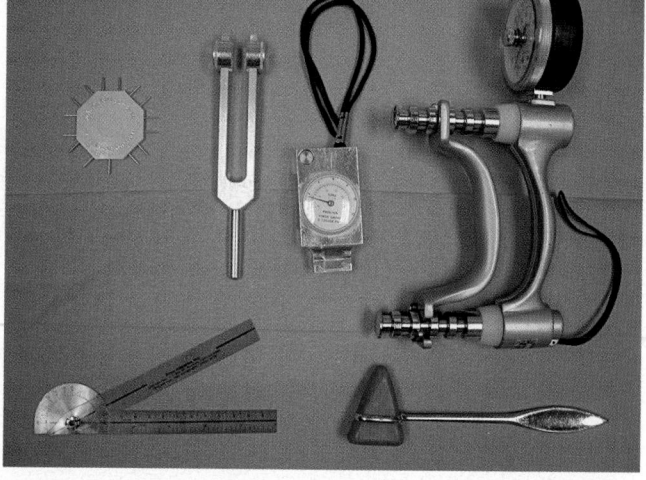

Figure 74-6 Basic instruments used in hand examination include a tuning fork, pinch meter, grip dynamometer, 2-point discriminator (paper clip also suffices), goniometer, and patella hammer.

the first webspace. The number of fingers served by each nerve is variable. However, as an absolute rule, the palmar surfaces of the index and little fingers are always served by the median and ulnar nerves, respectively.

With regard to the motor supply of these nerves, the ulnar nerve supplies the hypothenar muscles, interossei, ulnar two lumbricals, adductor pollicis, and deep head of the flexor pollicis brevis. The median nerve supplies the abductor pollicis brevis, opponens pollicis, radial two lumbricals, and superficial head of the flexor pollicis brevis. In summary, the median nerve thus supplies all of the extrinsic digit flexors and wrist flexors (except the FDP to the ring and little fingers and the FCU, which are supplied by the ulnar nerve) and all the thumb intrinsic muscles (except the AP innervated by the ulnar nerve). The ulnar nerve supplies all the interossei, all the lum-

bricals (except the radial two, supplied by the median nerve), and the adductor of the thumb. The radial nerve innervates all of the wrist, finger, and thumb extrinsic long extensors.

EXAMINATION AND DIAGNOSIS

Observation

Examination of the resting posture of the hand can provide valuable information (Fig. 74-6). If a finger flexor tendon is severed, that affected finger does not assume its normal resting position in line with the natural flexion cascade of the adjacent digits (Fig. 74-7). Extensor tendon

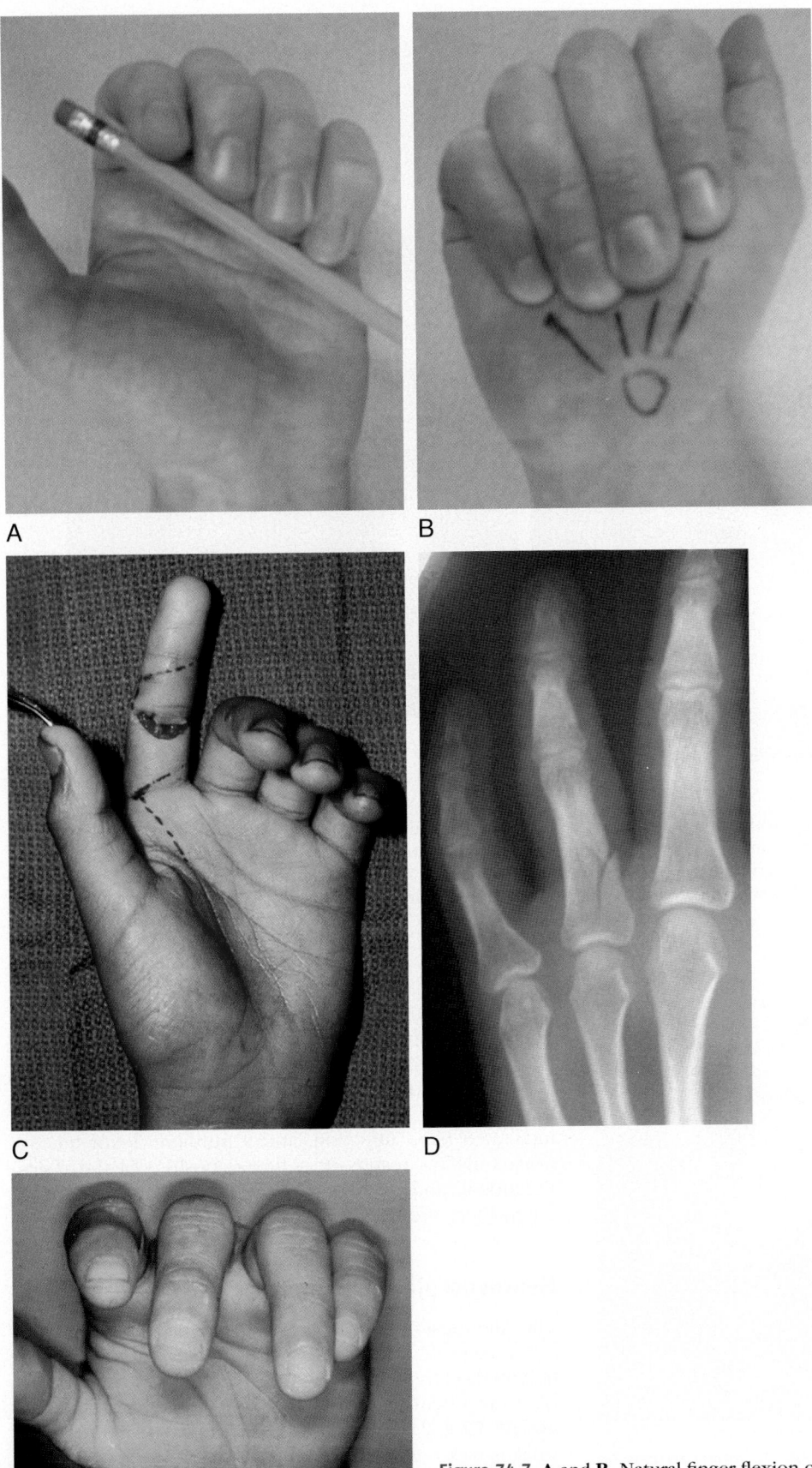

Figure 74-7 A and **B,** Natural finger flexion cascade of the hand in repose. Note the fingertips pointing to the distal pole of the scaphoid. **C,** With flexor tendon injury, the affected digit does not adopt this resting flexed posture. **D** and **E,** Spiral finger fractures produce a rotational deformity, which is also noted as an interruption in the finger flexion cascade.

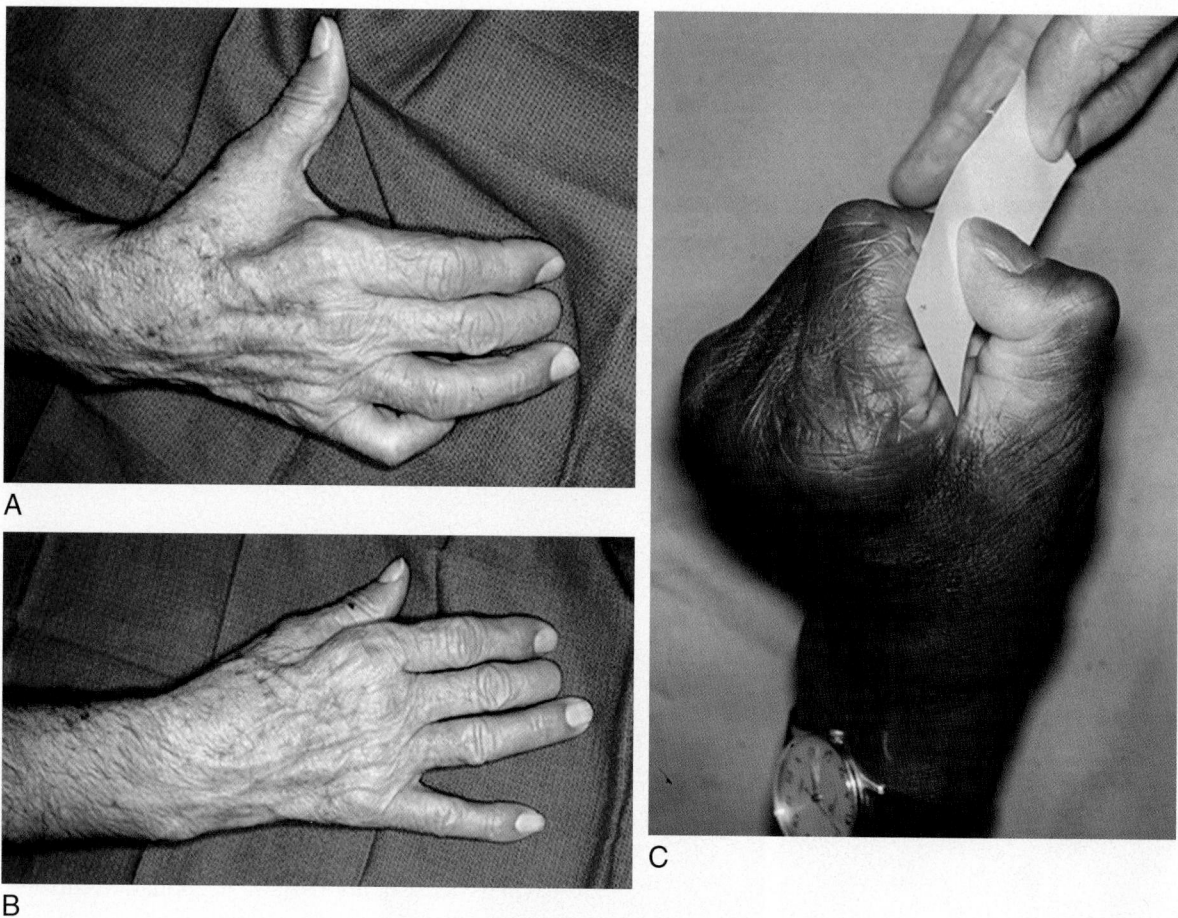

A

B

C

Figure 74-8 A, Marked atrophy in the first webspace dorsal interosseous muscle is noted with ulnar nerve palsy with clawing of the little and ring fingers. **B,** The little finger assumes an abducted position and cannot be adducted to the adjacent fingers (Wartenberg's sign). **C,** Because thumb adduction is weak, attempts to grasp a piece of paper between the adducted thumb and index finger produce compensatory thumb interphalangeal joint flexion (Froment's sign).

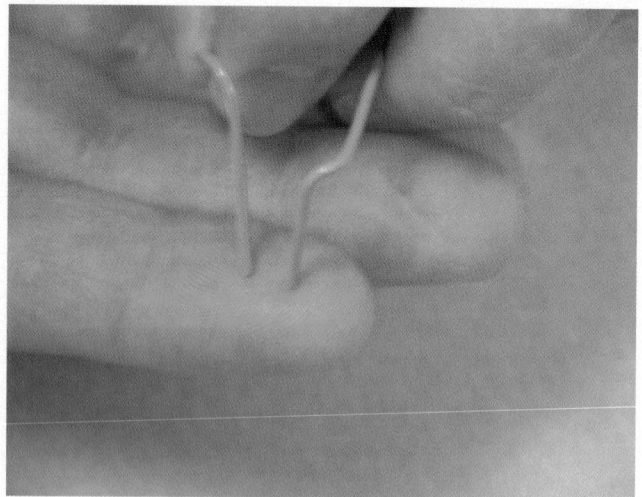

Figure 74-9 Two-point discrimination on the fingertip can be tested with a bent paper clip with the tips of the paper clip set specific distances apart.

injuries may be indicated by a droop at the affected joint. A clawed posture of the little and ring fingers may be characteristic of an ulnar nerve injury (Fig. 74-8). Absence of sweating at the fingertips may imply a nerve injury in that particular distribution. Swelling and erythema may indicate a hand infection, and a purulent flexor tenosynovitis always results in a flexed posture of the digits. Rotational and angular digital deformities may occur when there are underlying fractures.

Neurovascular Examination

The Allen test confirms patency of ulnar and radial arteries. Two-point sensory discrimination is the most sensitive method for testing for sensory loss and is easily done by using a bent paperclip (Fig. 74-9). The paper clip ends are set to a distance of about 5 mm apart for fingertip pulp sensory testing. The points are aligned along the axis of the finger. If this test is not reproducible because of an uncooperative patient, suspicion of a nerve injury

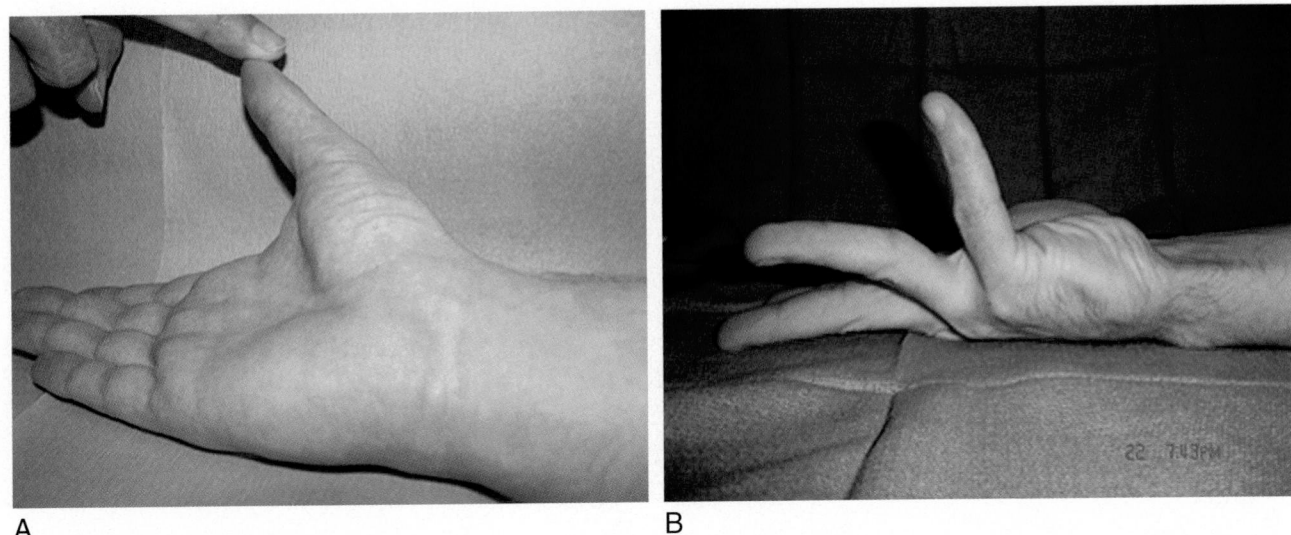

Figure 74-10 Motor innervation of muscles of the hand. **A,** Thumb abduction tests median motor nerve function. **B,** Little finger flexion at the metacarpophalangeal joint with simultaneous interphalangeal joint extension tests ulnar motor nerve function.

can be confirmed by the tactile adherence test in which a plastic pen is passed back and forward gently across the pulp on either side of each finger. Adhesion, because of the presence of sweat, is shown by slight but definite movement of the finger being examined (an anesthetic finger pulp will not sweat).

There are two muscle tests that may provide the examiner with an absolute diagnosis of median or ulnar nerve injury. The motor function of the abductor pollicis brevis tests the median nerve. With the hand flat and facing palm up, the patient is asked to touch with the thumb the examiner's finger held directly over the thenar eminence (Fig. 74-10). The FDM muscle function will test the motor supply of the ulnar nerve. In the same hand position, the patient raises the little finger vertically, flexing the MP joint to a 90-degree angle with the IP joint held straight. Tests for radial nerve function and its branches require wrist extension, thumb extension, and finger extension at the MP joint.

Musculoskeletal Examination

Integrity of tendons is individually tested (Fig. 74-11). Flexion at distal joints of the thumb and fingers confirms that FPL and FDP, respectively, are intact. Testing of FDS tendons is more complex. It is not possible to flex the DIP joints independently of one another because of a common origin of the FDP tendons. Thus, the other fingers are fixed in extension by the examiner, and the patient is asked to flex the remaining digits. Movement is produced by the FDS and occurs at the PIP joint. In about one third of patients, the FDS cannot produce little finger flexion. In half of these, in turn, there is a common origin with the ring finger, and so flexion will occur if the ring finger is permitted to flex simultaneously. More

uncommonly, there is no profundus tendon to the little finger, and the superficialis inserts into both the middle and distal phalanges. The long and short extensors (EPL and EPB) and long abductor of the thumb are tested by asking the patient to extend the thumb against resistance, whereas these tendons are individually palpated. Long extensors of the fingers are tested by asking the patient to extend against resistance applied to the dorsum of the proximal phalanx.

Special Investigations

Radiographs are necessary in almost every case. These help in diagnosis and evaluation of fractures and also in investigation of foreign bodies. Multiple radiographic views of the affected part are required to define the precise pathology or fracture pattern. Glass is often seen on plain radiographs, and if not seen but suspected, they may be visualized by computed tomography (CT) or magnetic resonance imaging (MRI). If plastic is painted, it may be seen on routine radiographs but is generally poorly visualized with CT scan and can be clearly seen with MRI. Wood foreign bodies may be seen by CT or MRI, but not by routine radiography.

Various stress radiographic views and cineradiography may be useful for demonstrating dynamic wrist instability patterns, especially scapholunate separation. Arthrography may detect ligamentous tears by extravasation of contrast material between the radiocarpal, distal radioulnar, and midcarpal joints. This is best combined with MRI scanning, especially for the detection of triangular fibrocartilage tears at the ulnocarpal joint. Radionuclide bone scanning may help in a diagnosis of osteomyelitis, but in the hand, a false-positive result may occur because of close proximity of soft tissue infections to the bones.

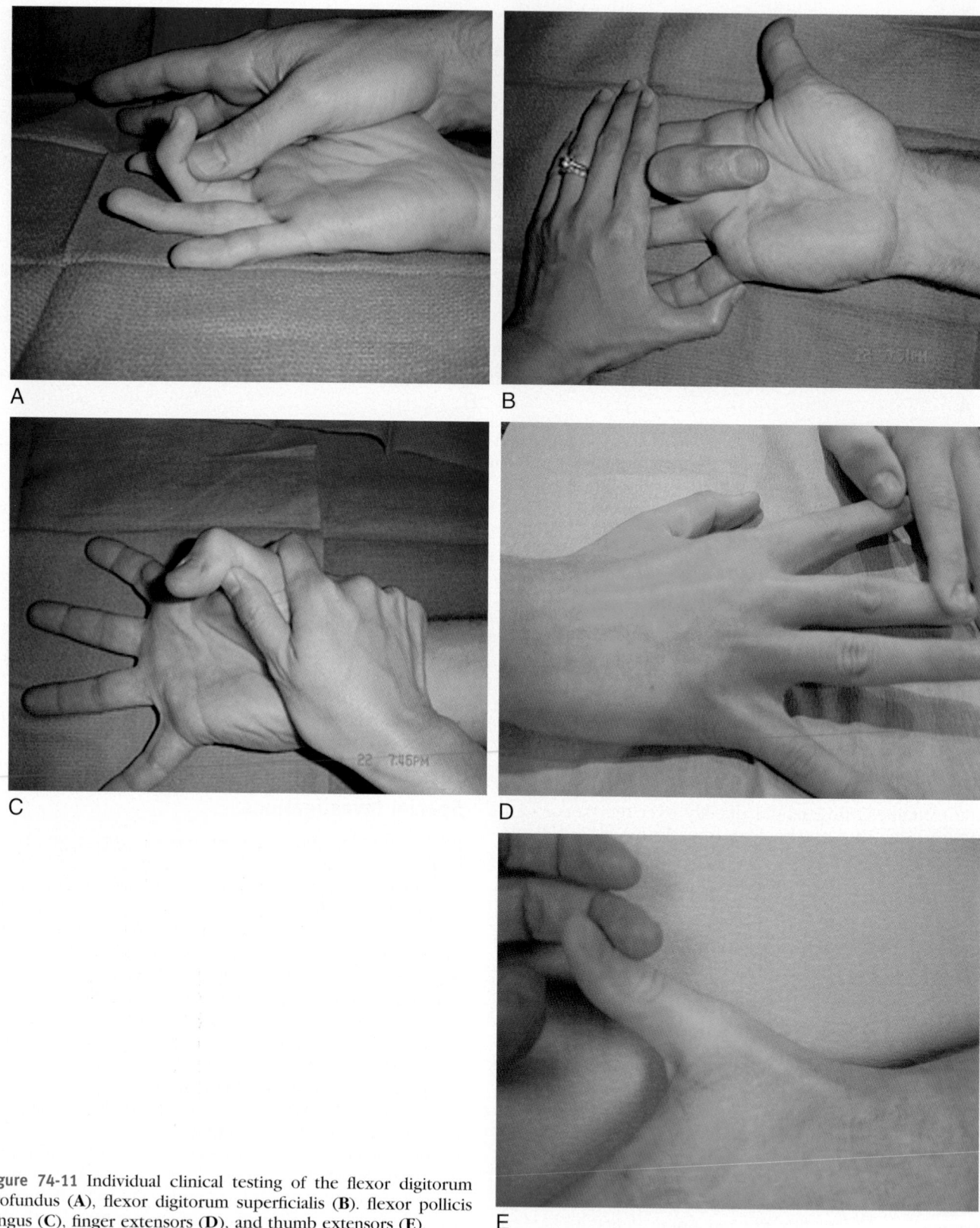

Figure 74-11 Individual clinical testing of the flexor digitorum profundus (**A**), flexor digitorum superficialis (**B**). flexor pollicis longus (**C**), finger extensors (**D**), and thumb extensors (**E**).

Occult wrist fractures may be localized by increased radionuclide uptake, but a false-positive test evaluating for a fracture may also occur with ligamentous injuries. CT scanning may be the best modality for diagnosing suspected carpal fractures, such as a scaphoid fracture that may not be seen on a routine radiograph.

Wrist arthroscopy has been recently introduced and is useful as a diagnostic and therapeutic modality for a number of wrist problems, especially for disorders of the triangular fibrocartilage. Minimally invasive surgery with arthroscopic guidance has added a new dimension to treatment of acute wrist disorders such as scaphoid and distal radius intra-articular fractures.

Patients with ischemic problems often require noninvasive vascular studies. Doppler pressure measurements help to localize the site of a vascular lesion. Angiography in the upper extremity is always done in the presence of a vasodilator (e.g., tolazoline [Priscoline] or nitroglycerin) or an axillary block in order to differentiate apparent vessel occlusion from vasospasm. Subtraction radiographs with magnification help to improve the detail and definition of the vascular study (especially in the distal forearm and hand).

PRINCIPLES OF TREATMENT

In the case of injuries, treatment is directed at the specific structures damaged: skeletal, tendon, nerve, vessel, and integument. In emergency situations, the goals of treatment are to maintain or restore distal circulation, obtain a healed wound, preserve motion, and retain distal sensation. Stable skeletal architecture is established in the primary phase of care because skeletal stability is essential for effective motion and function of the extremity. This also results in reestablishing skeletal length, straightening deformities, and correction of compression or kinking of nerves and vessels. Arteries are also repaired in the acute phase of treatment to maintain distal tissue viability. Additionally, extrinsic compression on arteries must be released emergently such as in compartment pressure problems. In clean-cut injuries, tendons can be repaired primarily. In situations in which there is a chance that tendon adhesions may form, such as when there are associated fractures, it is nonetheless better to repair tendons primarily with preservation of their length and if necessary at a later date to perform tenolysis. However, when there are open and contaminated wounds or a severe crushing injury, it is best to delay repair of both tendon and nerve injuries.

In clean-cut sharp wounds, primary nerve repair lessens the possibility of nerve end retraction and therefore the need for later nerve grafting. However, primary nerve repair must not be performed in situations in which there is contusion of the nerve (gunshot wounds, power saw injuries, blunt crushing trauma) because the extent of proximal axonal injury may not be immediately evident. If nerve repair is performed before this is apparent, it may result in abnormal nerve ends being reattached, negating the chance for functional return.

In severe soft tissue injuries, wound closure may not be immediately possible. Initial open treatment of the wound is directed to prevent an infection and protect critical deep structures by proper dressing and wound management (Fig. 74-12). Adequate débridement is essential, but appropriate soft tissue coverage must be achieved as soon as possible thereafter. The sooner the soft tissue coverage can be achieved, the less likely there will be a secondary deformity due to fibrosis and joint contractures. The more rapidly one can start hand therapy, the better the chances for maximizing functional return. The treatment regimen must consist of débridement, rigid skeletal fixation, and early soft tissue resurfacing (possibly even requiring microvascular soft tissue reconstruction), followed by protected range-of-motion exercises as soon as possible. It has been shown that early soft tissue reconstruction results in improved function, decreased morbidity, and shortened hospital stay.

Appropriate treatment of upper extremity problems requires a thorough knowledge of local and regional anesthesia, use of a tourniquet to provide a bloodless field, correct placement of incisions to minimize later scar contracture, and appropriate use of dressings and splints to reduce edema and maintain a functional position, and above all, a clear knowledge of the unique anatomy of the hand and upper extremity that not only aids accurate clinical diagnosis, but also enables safe performance of surgery.

Anesthesia

The choice of general, regional (e.g., intravenous Bier block, or brachial plexus block that might be either a supraclavicular or axillary block), or local anesthesia is governed by the extent and length of the operation. An upper arm or forearm tourniquet can be used in the unanesthetized extremity with only local anesthetic field infiltration or digital block for 30 to 45 minutes in a relaxed, cooperative patient provided that the arm is well exsanguinated. After this time, tourniquet pain will not permit more extensive local anesthetic procedures. If one has to operate in other areas, such as for harvesting of bone, nerve, tendon, or skin graft, or if more extensive surgical procedures are planned, general anesthesia will be required.

A digital block or median, ulnar, or radial wrist nerve block may be very useful, especially for more limited emergency room procedures (Fig. 74-13). Digital nerve blocks as a rule do not include epinephrine, which could lead to vasospasm, but recent evidence implies the safety of distal blocks using an epinephrine solution. A maximum safe dose of lidocaine is 4 mg/kg.

Tourniquet Application

The tourniquet is used to provide a bloodless field so that clear visualization of all structures in the operative field is obtained. Penrose drains, rolled rubber glove fingers, or commercially available tourniquets can be used on digits. Great care must be taken in using any constrictive device on digits because narrow bands cause

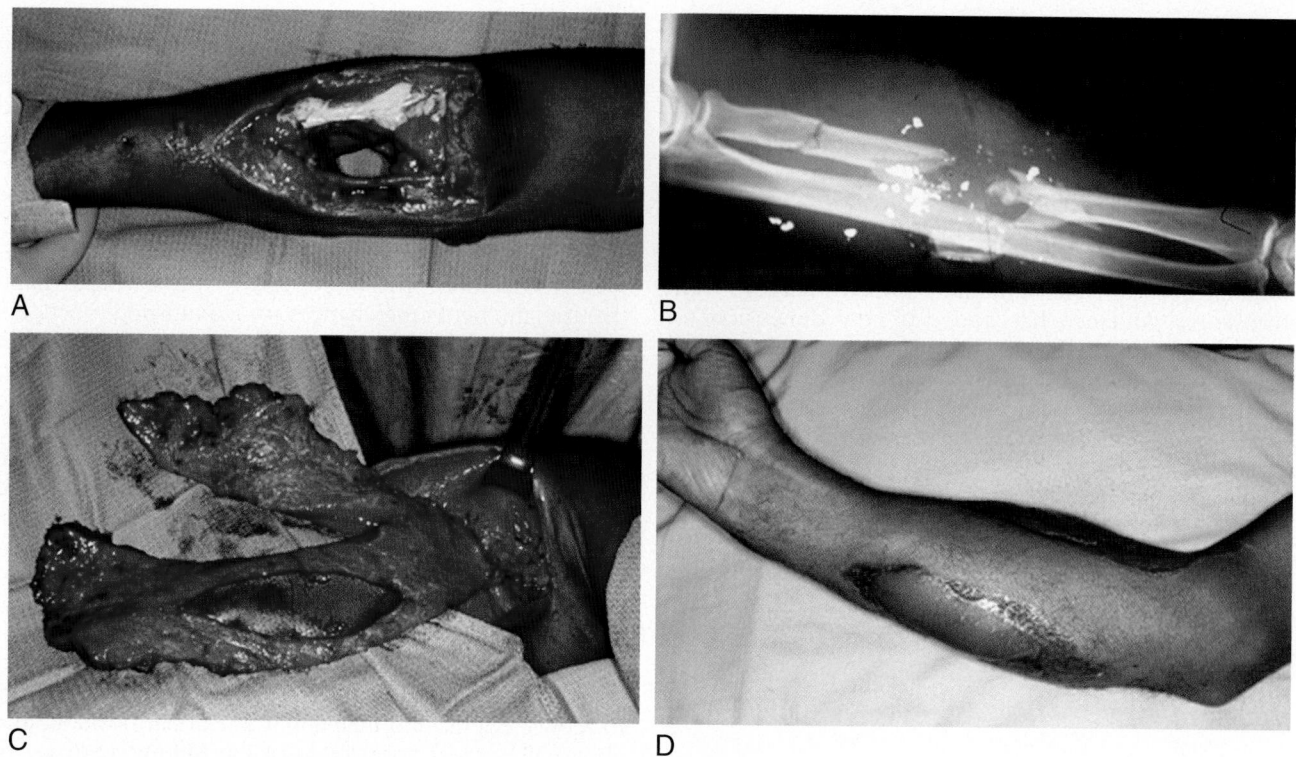

Figure 74-12 A, Gunshot wound of forearm showing extensive soft tissue injury. **B,** Initial radiograph. **C,** Microvascular reconstruction using a bilobed latissimus dorsi musculocutaneous flap was done in association with fracture fixation. **D,** Long-term follow-up of reconstructed forearm that also required sural nerve grafting to a segmental injury of the median nerve.

direct injury to underlying nerves and digital vessels. With the use of an arm tourniquet, the skin beneath the cuff must be protected with several wraps of cast padding. During skin preparation, this area must be kept dry to prevent blistering of the skin under an inflated cuff over moist padding. The cuff selected needs to be as wide as the diameter of the arm. Standard pressures used are 100 to 150 mm Hg greater than systolic blood pressure. The cuff is deflated every 2 hours for 15 to 20 minutes (5 minutes of reperfusion for every 30 minutes of tourniquet time) to revascularize distal tissues and to relieve pressure on nerves locally before reinflating the cuff for more extensive procedures.[1,2] Exsanguination of the extremities is performed by wrapping the extremity with a Martin's bandage in all cases, except those involving infection or tumors. In these latter cases, because of the possibility of embolization by mechanical pressure, exsanguination by bandage wrapping needs to be avoided. Simple elevation of the extremity for a few minutes before tourniquet inflation suffices.[3,4]

Incisions

Incisions are of the Bruner zigzag or midaxial type or combinations of these in order to avoid longitudinal motion-restricting scars that cross palmar flexion creases

(Fig. 74-14). The marginal edge of a skin graft with healthy skin is also a potential scar line, and so the margin of the skin graft is designed to be in these same lines to prevent contractures across flexion creases. Palmar incisions follow the pattern of skin creases. Dorsal incisions on the fingers and wrist and also incisions on the forearm may follow longitudinal straight lines.

Dressings and Splints

The purposes of dressings are to protect wounds, absorb drainage, and help splint repaired structures. The first layer consists of a nonadherent dressing and may contain an antibiotic. The next layer is soft and bulky and is usually followed by a firmer, more conforming external wrap. Conforming compression is useful, but constriction is harmful. Splints are made to protect only the part necessary to be immobilized and must not prevent motion in the remainder of the extremity. Often patients keep the injured, operated, or infected hand in a flexed wrist position, and this automatically causes the MP joints to extend thereby placing the collateral ligaments in their shortest lengths. Edema fluid collects dorsally, and the resulting dorsal hand swelling causes stiff joints. Thus, a splint that keeps the hand in the protected position extends the wrist 40 to 50 degrees, maintaining the MP

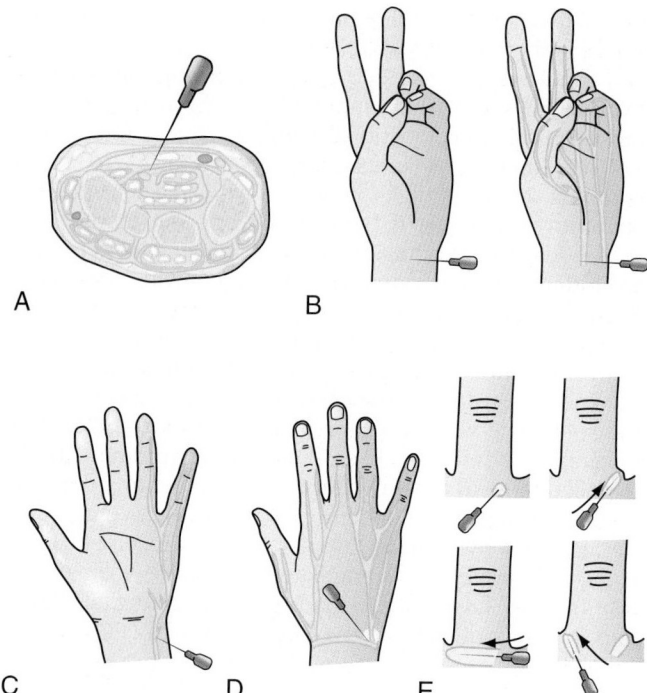

Figure 74-13 A, Median nerve block is done at the wrist where the median nerve is superficial to all the flexor tendons in the carpal tunnel. **B,** At the wrist, when a median nerve block is performed, the needle is directed between the palmaris longus and flexor carpi radialis tendons. **C,** Ulnar nerve block at the wrist is done by passing the injecting needle around the ulnar deep aspect of the flexor carpi ulnaris tendon just proximal to the pisiform. Intravascular injection into the immediately adjacent ulnar artery is avoided by first aspirating before injection. **D,** Dorsal branches of the ulnar nerve and superficial sensory radial nerve are anesthetized by raising a broad weal of local anesthetic across the dorsum of the wrist. **E,** A dorsal approach to the finger can be used for digital nerve block.

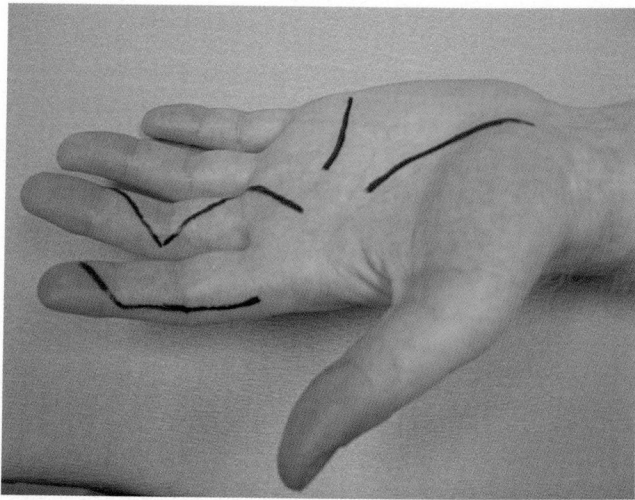

Figure 74-14 Incisions used on the palmar surface of the hand must respect the creases. These may be zigzag Bruner incisions or midaxial incisions of the digits.

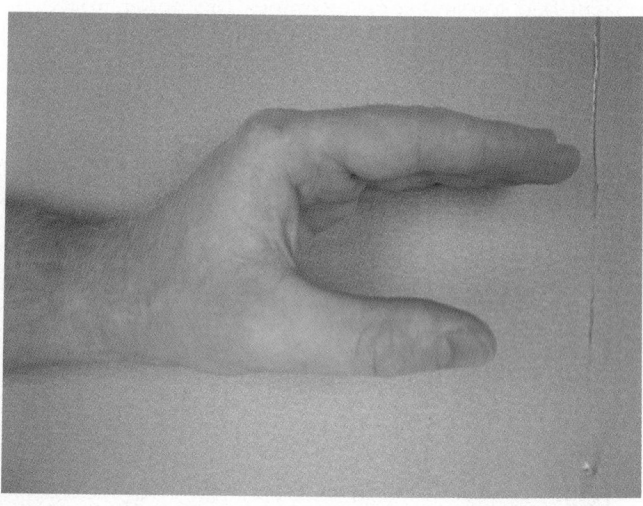

Figure 74-15 Application of a splint and dressings to demonstrate the "safe" or "protected" position of the wrist, hand, and digits. The thumb is palmar abducted.

joints at 70 degrees of flexion and the IP joints in a neutral position (Fig. 74-15). Postoperative hand elevation is essential to reduce edema.

TRAUMA

Lacerations and Fingertip and Complex Soft Tissue Injuries

Although it is tempting to look within a wound to determine whether any tendon or nerve injuries exist, the same information can be obtained by careful physical examination without further violating a potential operative field and causing the patient extreme discomfort. A combination of knowledge of anatomy, the presence of sensory or motor deficits, and the presence or absence of radial or ulnar pulses can narrow the differential diagnosis of injured structures to a minimum. Control of bleeding is attempted by direct pressure with dressings and not by blind clamping of vessels because vital structures may be inadvertently injured in the depths of the wound. However, a tourniquet may be used if the initial pressure fails. Tourniquets are generally not used initially because the entire limb will be ischemic during the patient transportation time. If the trauma has caused complete obliteration of anatomy, incisions can be extended into nonviolated areas where control of bleeding vessels and delineation of injured tendons and nerves may be easier, using the previously stated guidelines for extremity incisions.

All patients who present with extremity injuries have radiographs. Fractures of the distal phalanx are among the more commonly encountered hand fractures.[5] A distal phalangeal fracture is appropriately splinted, reduced to improve alignment, or occasionally fixated internally if the fracture is unstable. Internal fixation is most commonly provided by simply placing a longitudinal 0.028-inch Kirschner wire. Appropriate antibiotics are administered because technically these are open fractures.

The least severe injury of the dorsum of the fingertip is a nail bed hematoma. When seen early, the hematoma can be decompressed by perforating the nail plate after administration of a digital local anesthetic block. Both fingertip and nail bed injuries can be managed with a digital block anesthesia and use of a Penrose drain at the base of the finger as a tourniquet. After the nail plate has been stripped, simple gentle removal of the nail to examine the underlying nail bed is next done, and suture repair of the nail bed is performed using loupe magnification and a 6-0 catgut suture. Once the nail bed has been repaired, it is best to place the thoroughly cleansed nail back under the nailfold, where it both serves as a rigid splint for an underlying distal phalangeal fracture and also prevents adhesions from forming between the adjacent surfaces of the nailfold, which would potentially lead to an unsightly split nail deformity. If there is a piece of nail bed missing, one examines the undersurface of the avulsed nail plate. Frequently, the missing piece may still be adherent to the nail, and it can be gently removed and replaced as a nail bed graft. Some fingertip injuries may be so severe that amputation revision may be the most sensible and functional solution.

Volar fingertip injuries range from simple to more complex. Multiple digits may be involved such as with lawnmower injuries. If bone is not exposed and a soft tissue defect of the finger pulp is smaller than 1 cm, the wound is best left open and managed with dressings. Such an injury will heal with excellent functional and cosmetic results. Larger soft tissue defects of the fingertip pulp are more appropriately treated with a small full-thickness skin graft. However, if bone is exposed, and the soft tissue wound is larger, one considers either flap coverage or revision of amputation by trimming back exposed bone to obtain soft tissue coverage. In a dorsally angulated fingertip amputation, soft tissue coverage can be achieved by a neurovascular V-Y advancement flap. If the soft tissue loss is angulated in a more volar direction, a cross finger flap, an adjacent finger digital island flap, or homodigital flap may be performed (Figs. 74-16 to 74-18).

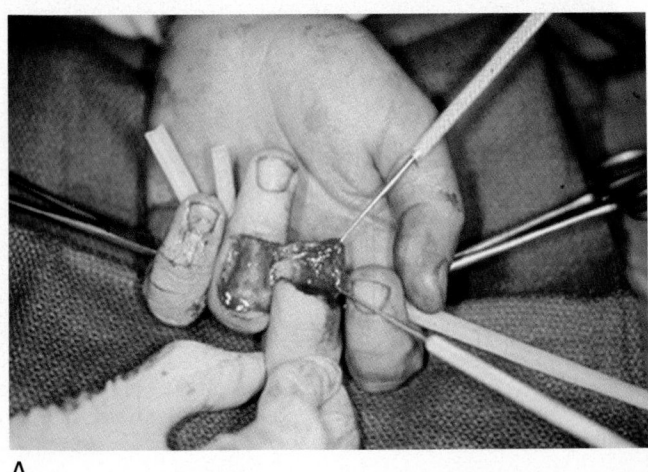

A

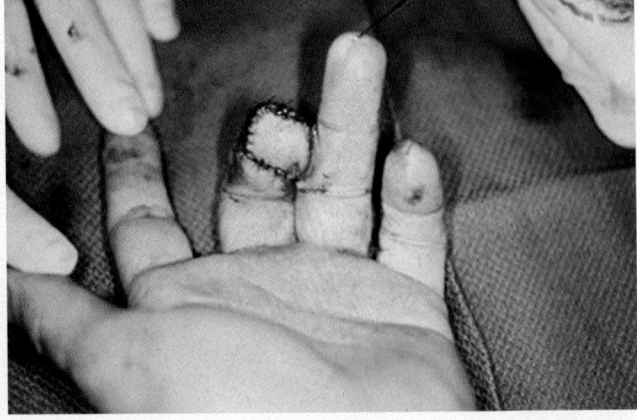

B

C

Figure 74-16 A and **B,** Volar angulated fingertip injury with loss of pulp pad and bone exposed was treated with a traditional cross-finger flap from the dorsum of the adjacent finger. **C,** Excellent healing is seen in the long term after flap division.

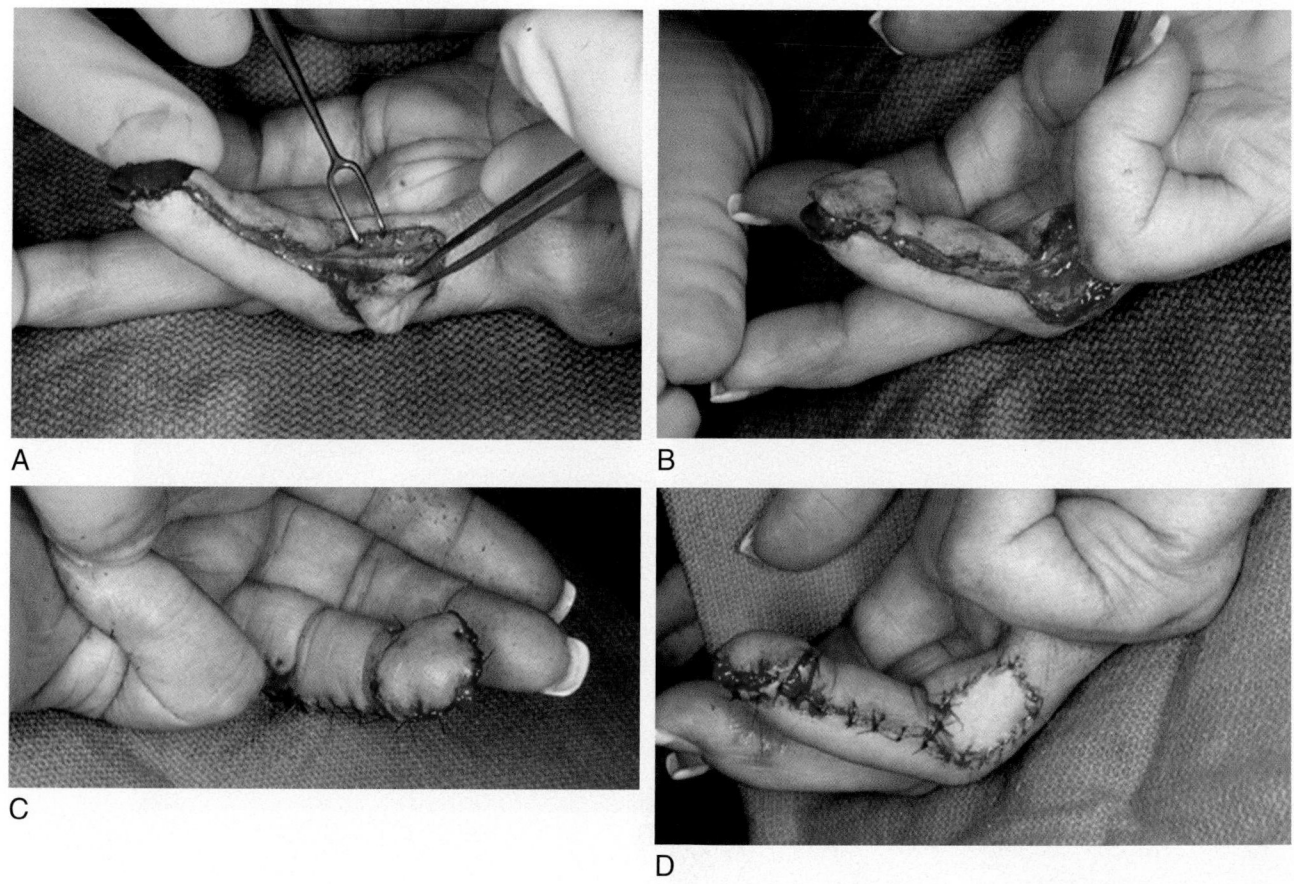

Figure 74-17 A to **D,** More recent understanding of the vascular skin territories of the finger and hand enable "intrinsic" flap coverage of fingertip injuries and avoid the cumbersome tethering of adjacent fingers, as is done with cross-finger flaps. In this patient, a distally based turnover vascular island flap reconstructs an avulsed fingertip. The reverse-flow perforating vessels at the proximal interphalangeal joint cross from the opposite side to nourish this flap.

Tendon Injuries

Flexor Tendons

Flexor tendon injuries most commonly result from lacerations or puncture wounds on the palmar surface of the hand though flexor tendons can be avulsed from their distal bony insertions by sudden violent contractions. They are best treated by a surgeon experienced in the management of these injuries. Flexor tendon injuries are divided into five zones (Fig. 74-19). In zones 1, 2, and 4, each tendon is surrounded by a synovial sheath and contained within a semirigid fibro-osseous canal, either within the flexor tendon sheath of the digit or within the carpal tunnel. In the other zones, the flexor tendons are surrounded by loose areolar (paratenon) tissue. Healing those parts devoid of a fibrous sheath is usually excellent because of the good blood supply from the paratenon. Tendons in the carpal tunnel (zone 4) have their rich blood supply provided by the mesotenon; however, zones 2 and 1 have a precarious blood supply through the vincula, and complementary nutritional support is provided by the synovial fluid in these latter two zones. In order for tendon gliding to occur, the mesotenon has

disappeared in the digital flexor sheath except at the sites of the vincula that carry the vessels from the periosteum to the tendons (Fig. 74-20). Tendon zones to the thumb are T1 through T3.

Primary tendon repair undertaken within a few hours of injury is generally reserved for cleanly cut tendons. Delayed primary repair is performed from several hours up to 10 days after injury and is indicated for tidy, but potentially contaminated, wounds to allow for prophylaxis against infection before the tendon repair. Relative contraindications to immediate tendon repair are listed:

1. Injuries more than 12 hours old
2. Crush wounds with poor skin coverage
3. Contaminated wounds, especially human bites
4. Tendon loss greater than 1 cm
5. Injury at multiple sites along the tendon
6. Destruction of the pulley system

After 4 weeks, a later secondary repair is generally not possible because of retraction of the musculotendinous unit so that reapproximation of tendon ends produces undesirable joint flexion. Under such a situation, tendon

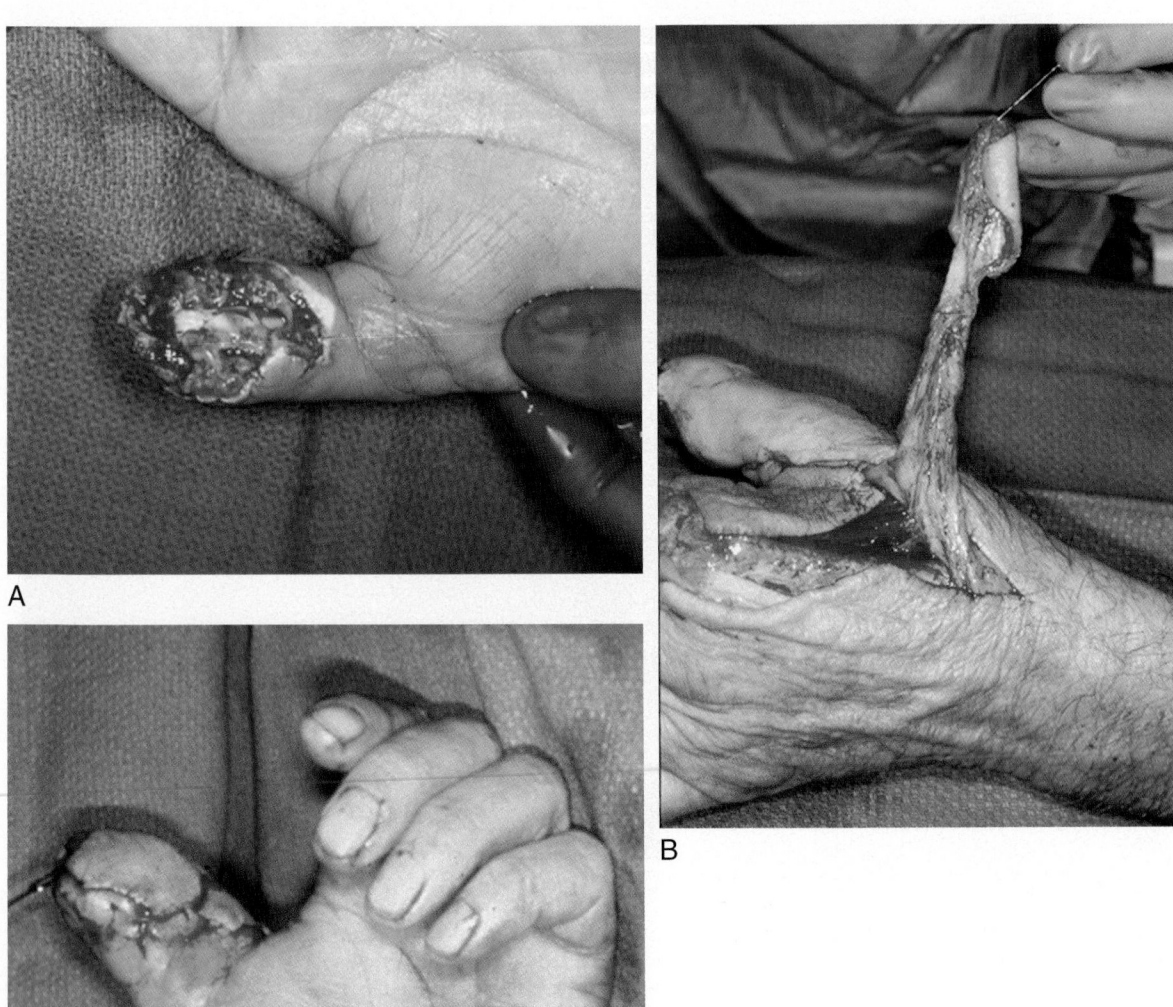

A

B

C

Figure 74-18 **A** to **C,** The first dorsal metacarpal artery flap is a vascularized island flap that is transposed from the dorsoradial aspect of the index finger to the distal pulp of the thumb following a crushing injury.

graft repair may be required. Surgeons' endeavors are directed at avoiding the four major complications that interfere with smooth gliding and the integrated action of tendons: adhesions, attenuation of the repair, repair rupture, and joint and soft tissue contractures. Prerequisites for tendon repair are aseptic conditions in an operating room with good lighting, good instruments, adequate anesthesia, and loupe magnification. A well-performed technical operation can be futile without proper postop-

erative hand therapy, splinting, and excellent patient compliance.[6]

Appropriate treatment of partial flexor tendon injuries is necessary to produce a smooth juncture at the injury site. Prevention of complications requires exploration of all wounds likely to cause partial flexor tendon lacerations. A partial tendon injury of 50% or less is treated by simple trimming of the lacerated portion. Those injuries greater than 50% are repaired. Failure to diagnose a

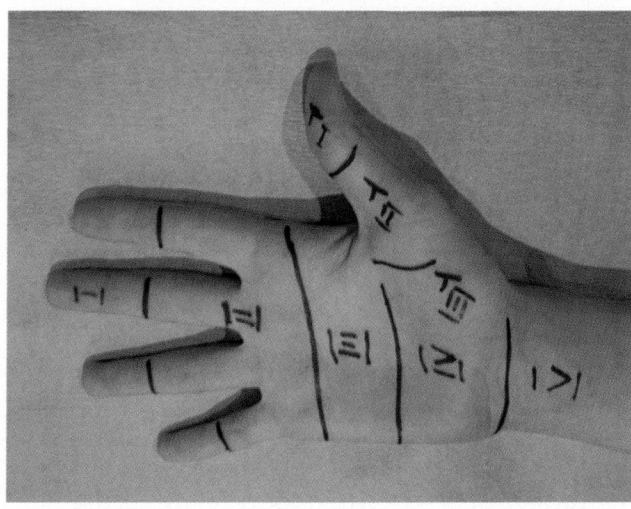

Figure 74-19 Zones of flexor tendon injuries on the fingers, thumb, and hand.

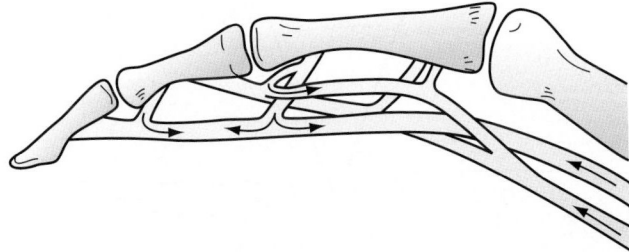

Figure 74-20 Complex arrangement of flexor digitorum superficialis and flexor digitorum profundus tendons in the flexor sheath of the fingers. Blood supply to the tendons travels through the vincula from the dorsal aspects of the tendons.

partial flexor tendon laceration at the time of primary repair may lead to delayed tendon rupture, entrapment between the tendon laceration and the laceration in the flexor sheath, or trigger finger.

Zone 2 flexor tendon injuries require special attention. This zone is also called *no-man's land* of Bunnell. There are three tendons (profundus and two slips of superficialis) that traverse zone 2, and they constantly interchange their mutual spatial relationships. Tendon injury in this region requires opening the existing laceration in the flexor tendon sheath by making a longitudinal trap door so that a flap of tendon sheath can be elevated. Care must be taken to avoid excising annular pulleys, especially A2 and A4, because bowstringing of the tendons can result in ineffective finger flexion. It is often difficult to repair both profundus and superficialis tendons if they are injured in zone 2. Nonetheless, both are repaired because resection of the superficialis reduces overall grip strength, predisposes to a recurvatum and swan neck deformity at the PIP joint, and damages the vincula supply to the profundus.

Usually skin wounds have to be extended proximally and distally in a zigzag fashion in order to display the retracted divided tendon ends. Tendon ends are handled with fine-tooth forceps and the tendon surface is never touched. The wrist is flexed, and a small Keith needle is passed transversely through the proximal tendon, about 2 cm from the end, transfixing it to the skin and tendon sheath. In this way, immobilization of the tendon end facilitates a tension-free repair. Ragged tendon ends may be squared off sharply, but no more than 1 cm is resected or permanent finger contracture will result. The tendon ends are brought together by a single tension-holding locking core suture. A variety of such locking core suture techniques have been described, but more commonly, a modified Kessler type suture is placed. A specifically placed locking loop increases by 10% to 50% the ultimate tensile strength of the tendon repair compared with a

simple mattress suture. If this is not done, tension on the suture line can open up the repair, increasing the propensity for tendon gapping at the repair site. The ideal suture material for tendon repairs has not been found. A 4-0 coated polyester or braided nylon is the best material for the core suture. Increasing the number of suture strands that cross the tendon repair site and obtaining suture bites of at least 0.7 cm will increase the overall tensile strength of the actual repair.[7] However, the more suture strands that are added, the greater will be the friction and edema within the flexor tendon sheath. Either a four-stranded core repair or six-stranded core repair appears to provide the optimum repair strength and yet not excessively increase stiffness and friction at the repair site. Some achieve a four-stranded core repair by means of simply using a double-stranded type of suture material, whereas others place a second core suture with a single-stranded material. Such a four-stranded core repair permits light protected composite grip during the entire postoperative healing. Additionally, a running circumferential epitenon suture repair is also placed (Fig. 74-21). This not only helps to smooth the repair but also adds to the ultimate tensile strength at the repair site and reduces gap formation. A peripheral 6-0 nylon suture serves this purpose.[8]

Zone 1 flexor tendon injury may be caused by a penetrating injury. However, closed-traction injury may also cause profundus tendon avulsion, which most frequently involves the ring or middle finger. In repair of zone 1 injury, a pullout suture is necessary if distal tendon length is insufficient to repair the tendon securely (Fig. 74-22), although suture bone anchors have now facilitated this mode of tendon repair into bone at the base of the distal phalanx.

Postoperatively, hand elevation is important to reduce edema. The wrist is placed in about 20 degrees of flexion and the MP joint at about 60 to 70 degrees of flexion. The splint is molded against the fingers with the IP joints fully extended. A system of rubber-band dynamic traction may be used as described by Kleinert following repair of flexor tendons in zone 2, with good results obtained in more than 80% of cases. Differential excursion between the two digital flexors is dramatically increased by a synergistic splint that allows for wrist extension and finger flexion. This position of wrist extension and MP

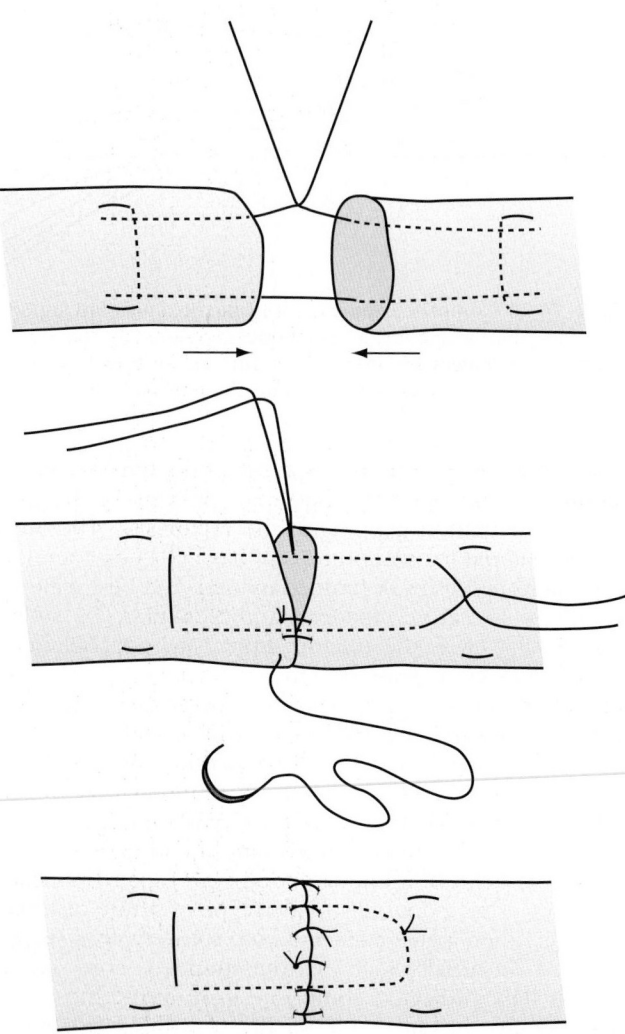

Figure 74-21 One technique of performing a four-strand flexor tendon core suture repair is demonstrated in association with a peripheral running suture.

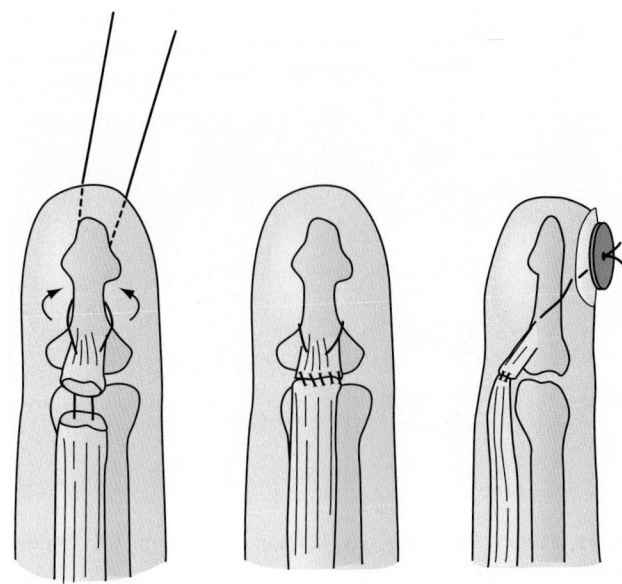

Figure 74-22 Zone 1 flexor tendon repair to reattach tendon to bone.

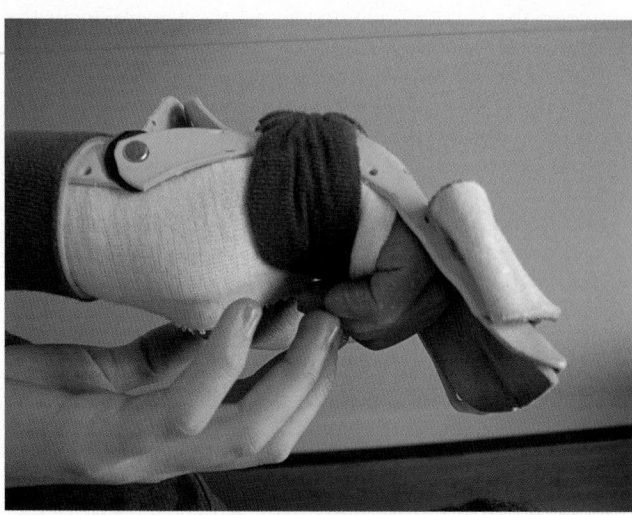

Figure 74-23 Flexor hinge brace with place-and-hold technique of finger mobilization is one of the preferred methods for postoperative rehabilitation after flexor tendon repair.

joint flexion produces the least tension on a repaired flexor tendon during active digital flexion; thus, we have come to use the flexor hinge brace technique advocated by Strickland and the so-called place-and-hold protocol (Fig. 74-23). A tenodesis brace with a wrist hinge is fabricated to allow for full wrist flexion, wrist extension of 30 degrees, and maintenance of MP joint flexion of at least 60 degrees. After composite passive digital flexion, the wrist is extended, and passive finger flexion is maintained. The patient actively maintains digital flexion and holds that position for about 5 seconds. The patient is instructed to use the lightest muscle power necessary to maintain digital flexion. Wrist flexion and finger extension follow. This type of protected motion postoperative protocol is continued for 6 weeks.

Extensor Tendons

Proper diagnosis of extensor tendon injuries requires full knowledge of the relatively complex anatomy of the extensor mechanism of the dorsum of the finger. The subcutaneous location of extensor tendons makes them susceptible to crush, laceration, and avulsion injuries. The presence of juncturae tendinum prevents proximal retraction of the EDC tendons. Extensor tendon injuries have been divided into nine zones that ascend numerically from the dorsum of the DIP joints to the forearm. The odd-numbered zones begin at the DIP joint and are located over the joints, whereas the even-numbered zones are located between the joints.

Extensor tendons are thinner than flexor tendons and over the dorsum of the digits are spread out to form the extensor hood. It may occasionally be possible to use conventional tendon repair techniques in the proximal

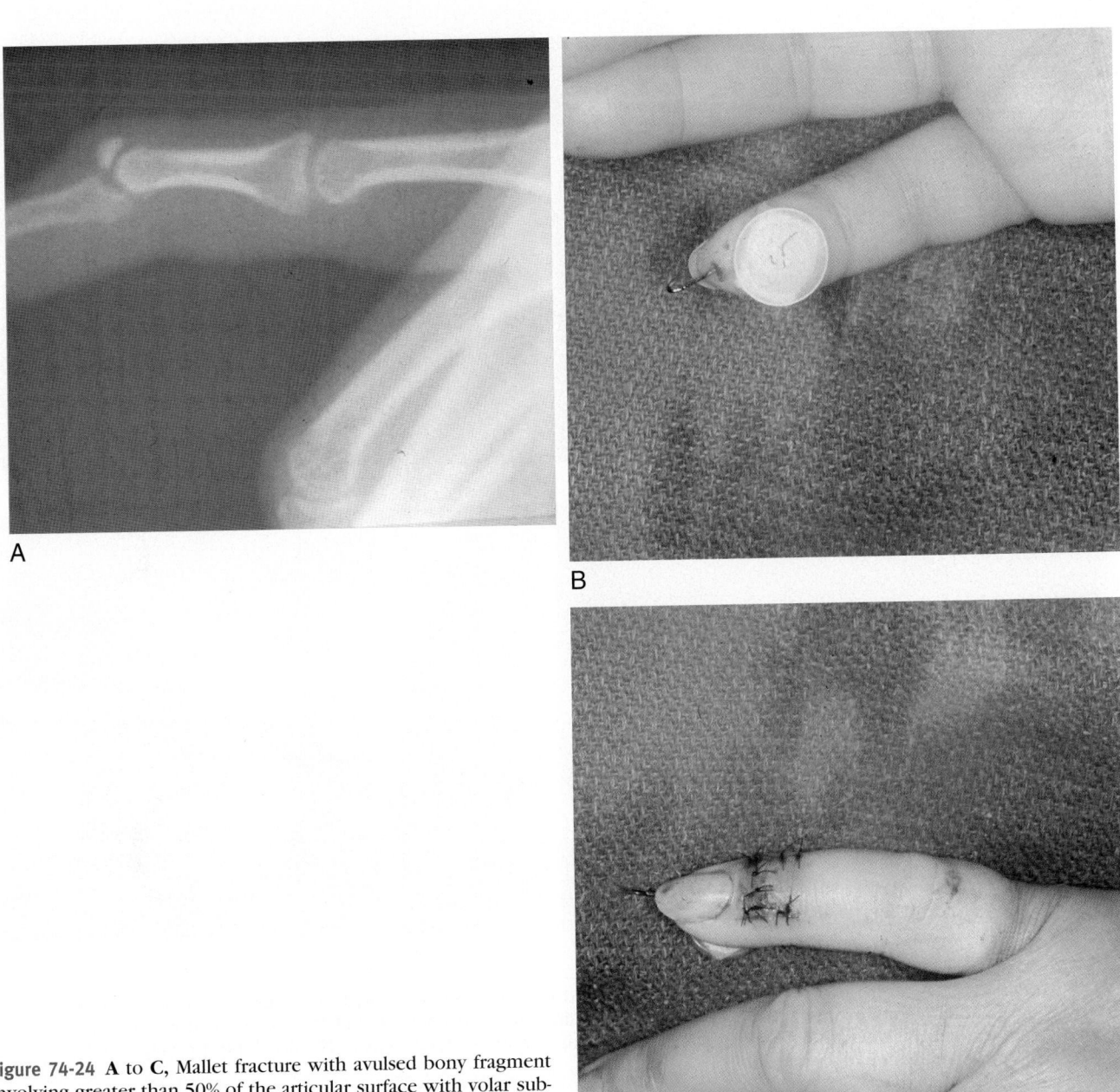

A

B

C

Figure 74-24 A to **C,** Mallet fracture with avulsed bony fragment involving greater than 50% of the articular surface with volar subluxation of the distal phalanx. The bony fragment is reapproximated with a tie-over volar suture and a longitudinal pin traversing the distal interphalangeal joint.

parts of the tendons, but this is usually not the case in the extensor hood region. Here, horizontal mattress sutures or figure-of-eight mattress sutures may be needed. All lacerations are repaired if 50% or more of the tendon is divided.

Extensor tendon avulsions are most likely to occur at the DIP joint from a jamming type of injury that results in a mallet finger deformity (Fig. 74-24). If a bone fragment representing 50% or more of the articular surface is involved, or if there is volar subluxation of the DIP joint, an open reduction with internal fixation is performed. If there is a tendon rupture only or a small piece of bone is avulsed with the tendon, good results can be obtained by 6 weeks of continuous splinting with the

DIP joint in extension (Fig. 74-25). After this period of splinting, the DIP joint is further protected during sleeping hours for 2 more weeks.

Closed tears through the triangular ligament may be caused by PIP joint subluxation or a jamming type of injury that results in a boutonniere deformity. The central slip attachment at the base of the middle phalanx is disrupted, so that extension of that joint is altered. The lateral bands lose their support dorsal to the PIP joint axis and slip volar and become flexors at the PIP joint and extensors of the DIP joint. The consequent deformity is one of flexion at the PIP joint and hyperextension at the DIP joint. Within 6 weeks of injury, these can be treated satisfactorily by extension splinting

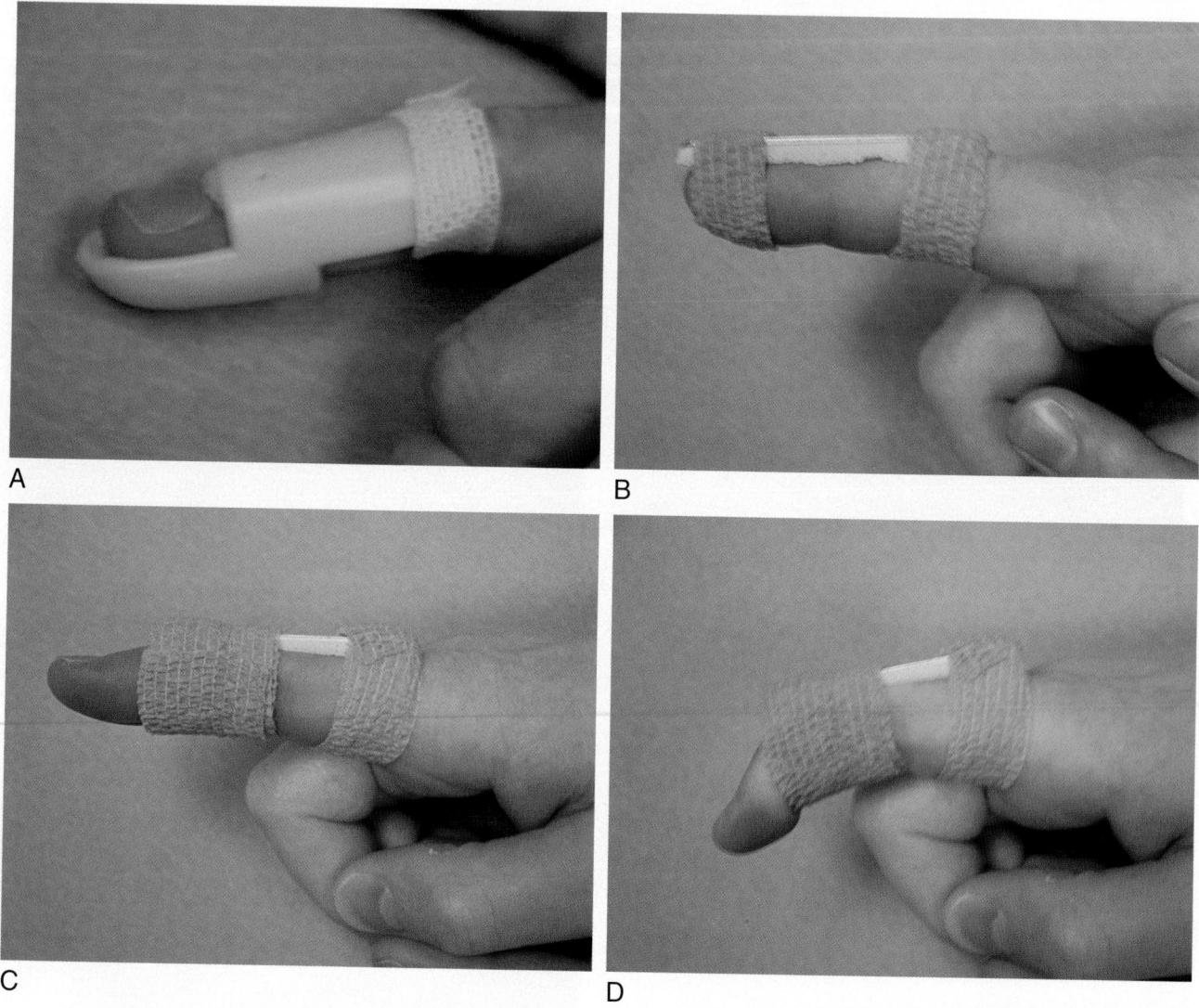

Figure 74-25 A, Prefabricated stack splint may be used for the closed treatment of a mallet finger. **B,** A simple dorsal aluminum splint may serve equally well for mallet finger treatment. **C** and **D,** Dorsal splinting across the proximal interphalangeal joint enables closed treatment of a boutonniere injury. The distal interphalangeal joint is left free for flexion and extension.

at the PIP joint, maintaining the DIP joint free for active flexion and extension (see Fig. 74-25). If there is an open laceration to the central slip mechanism and adjacent triangular ligament, direct suture repair or reinsertion into bone by means of bone anchor minisutures is performed, followed by the same postoperative protocol.

Extensor tendon injuries proximal to the PIP joint result in a drop finger (Fig. 74-26). These are repaired and splinted for 4 weeks. Common extensor tendon injuries over the dorsum of the hand and at the wrist must be repaired and then treated postoperatively by one of a number of different controlled motion protocols, one of which is a dynamic rubber-band extension outrigger brace or use of a relative motion splint in which the affected digit is kept at a more dorsal pitch to the adjacent

fingers, thus relaxing the repaired tendon. This latter splint causes minimal interference with day-to-day activities during rehabilitation[9] (Fig. 74-27).

Nerve Injuries

There are a variety of classifications of nerve injuries depending on the extent of injury. The Sunderland classification of injuries describes three types: neuropraxia, axonotmesis, and neurotmesis. *Neuropraxia* is a physiologic block of impulse conduction without anatomic destruction of nerve fibers. Neuropraxia can occur in association with a closed injury such as may be the case with the radial nerve in the spiral groove associated with a midshaft humerus fracture. Neuropraxia may also be seen after prolonged pressure on a nerve, as may occur

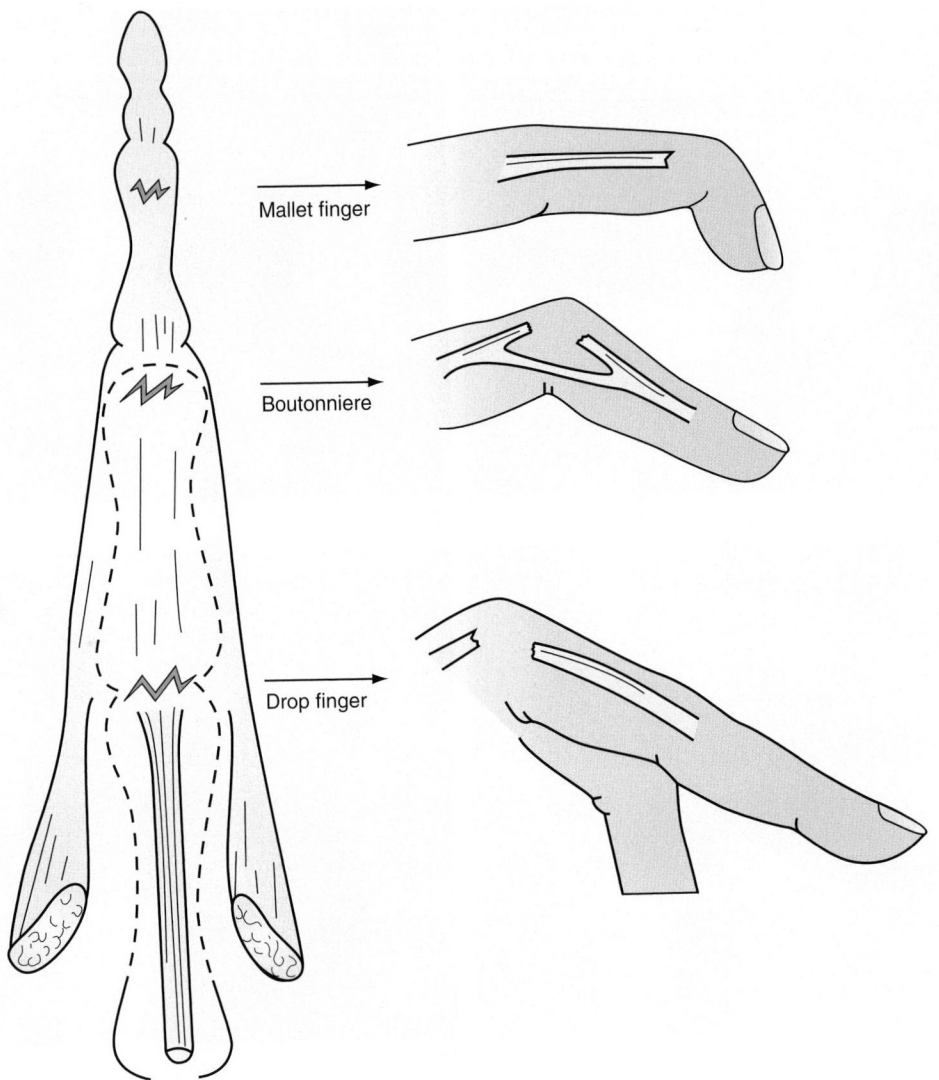

Figure 74-26 Extensor tendon injuries on the dorsum of the finger. Injury at the distal insertion causes a mallet finger and at the central slip over the proximal interphalangeal (PIP) joint causes a boutonniere deformity. Proximal to the PIP joint, over the proximal phalanx, injury results in a drop finger.

after prolonged use of a tourniquet or compression in confined places such as carpal tunnel syndrome. Once the offending cause has been removed, spontaneous recovery is generally the rule but can take as long as 3 months. *Axonotmesis* refers to injuries in which the axonal fibers are completely divided but the covering neural tubes are intact. Such injuries usually accompany traction on nerves that rupture the weaker axons, leaving the stronger nerve sheaths intact. *Neurotmesis* is the most severe degree of nerve injury and refers to a complete transection of the nerve. This may be the result of a direct sharp trauma or a very violent traction injury. Accurate approximation of the cut nerve ends and meticulous repair are required for the best possible recovery. Traction injuries may result in a mixture of all these. A distally progressing Tinel's sign following repair is indicative of a successful repair. Axonal regen-

eration following axonotmesis or following a successful nerve repair for neurotmesis occurs at a rate of 1 mm/day.

Severance of a peripheral nerve involves an acute loss of sensory, motor, and sympathetic functions. Knowledge of the motor and sensory distribution of the nerve allows for a clinical evaluation of the injury. However, associated injury such as fractures and muscle and tendon lacerations may complicate the evaluation. Loss of pseudomotor activity occurs within 30 minutes of the nerve injury. Loss of sweating can be demonstrated with a ninhydrin test. Nerve conduction studies, on the other hand, are not helpful immediately after injury. They become useful 3 weeks after injury. They demonstrate fibrillation and denervation potentials in muscles that are completely denervated, so that in a closed injury, they may differentiate between a neuropraxia and neurotmesis. Later, nerve

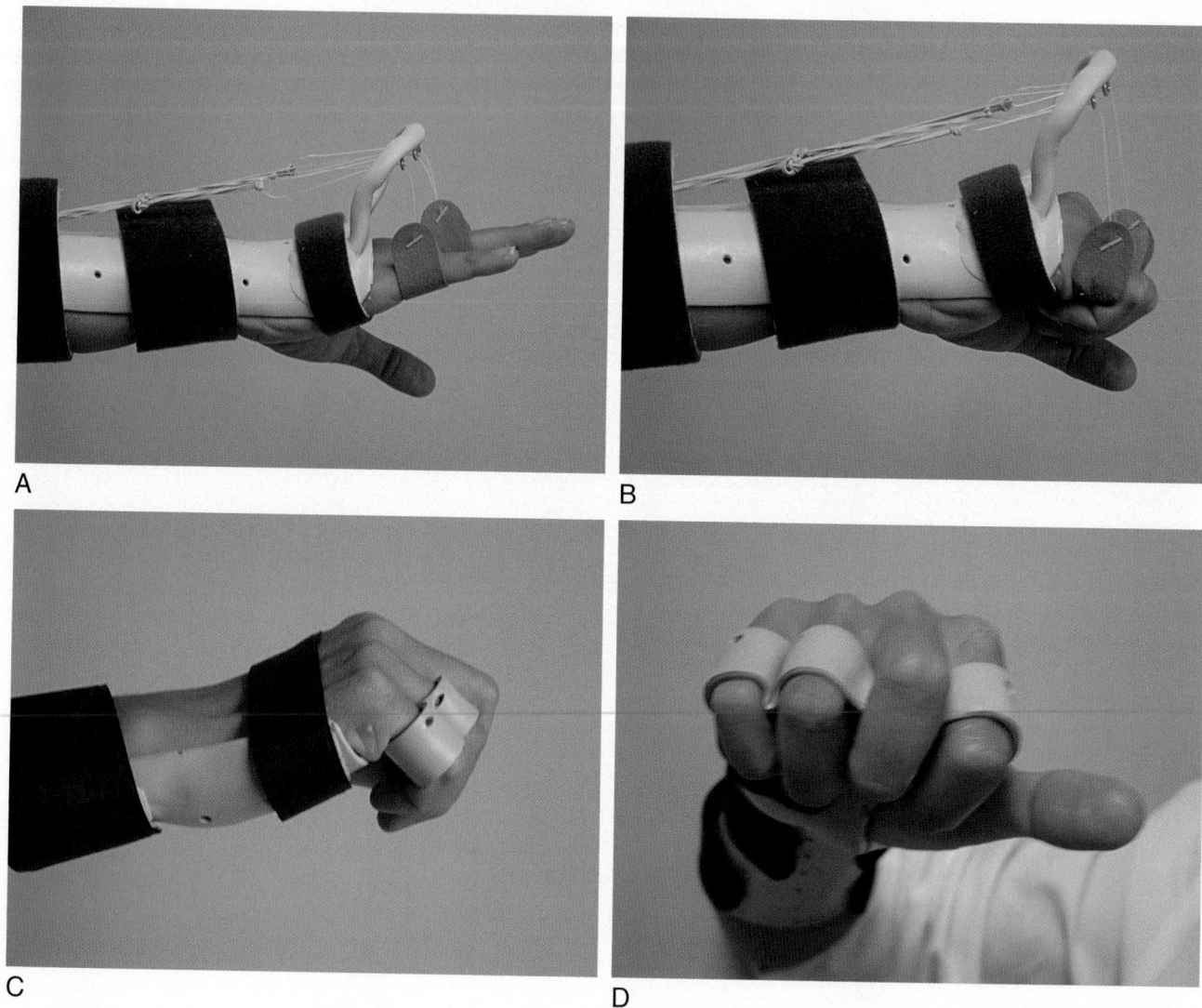

Figure 74-27 A and **B,** An extension outrigger dynamic splint commonly used for extensor tendon injuries postoperatively (extension and flexion views). **C** and **D,** Relative motion splint has the advantage of being low profile and causes minimal interference with daily activities and yet provides protection to the freshly repaired extensor tendon.

conduction studies may help monitor nerve regeneration following repair.

Primary nerve repair is done within 72 hours of injury, delayed primary repair from 72 hours to 14 days, and secondary nerve repairs 14 days or more after injury. Primary neurorrhaphy is recommended in the following situations:

1. The nerve is sharply incised.
2. There is minimal wound contamination.
3. There are no injuries that preclude obtaining skeletal stability or adequate skin cover.
4. The patient is medically stable to undergo an operation.
5. Appropriate facilities and instrumentation are available.

In a completely severed nerve, wallerian degeneration occurs in the entire segment distal to the injury and 1 to 2 cm proximal to it. In closed injuries, when the severity of the nerve injury is unknown, repeat clinical evaluation and electrical studies every 3 to 6 weeks help distinguish between neuropraxia and axonal injury. In most cases, surgical exploration with repair is indicated after 3 months if no clinical recovery is detected.

The nerve repair needs to be tension free. With sharp nerve lacerations, an epineurial repair provides as good a functional recovery as fascicular repair provided that anatomic landmarks such as vasa nervorum allow an accurate and precise matching of the cut nerve ends. Current investigation suggests that optimum nerve regeneration and proximal and distal axonal matching result from a combination of neurotropism and contact guidance. A critical distance must exist between proximal and distal nerve segments to obtain maximum benefits of neurotropism. With nerve grafting, the fascicular matching, when chosen by the surgeon, may not always be appropriate. With a small nerve gap, probably up to 2 cm in humans, experimental evidence suggests that it might be more appropriate to place a polyglycolic acid tube to bridge the gap rather than to perform nerve grafting.

If a nerve gap exists, it may be overcome by proximal and distal mobilization of the nerve ends, or in the case of the ulnar nerve, anterior nerve transposition in front of the elbow may be done. If there is judged to be too much tension on the nerve repair (cannot be held together with 8-0 nylon suture), nerve grafting (or in some incidences, placement of a nerve tube) must be done. Donor sources for nerve grafting most frequently are from the posterior interosseous nerve or the medial antebrachial cutaneous nerve for small digital nerves and the sural nerve for nerve gaps involving larger nerves.

After nerve repair, the affected part is splinted for 3 weeks to protect the repair site in the position of least tension. At the nerve repair, Tinel's sign is followed distally as an index of progressive recovery.

Vascular Injuries

Acute vascular injuries may follow closed or penetrating trauma or iatrogenic injury. Fractures or dislocations may be causes of vascular injury. Indirect vascular trauma may be caused by traction injuries, which can avulse vessels, or by intimal damage or repetitive microtrauma from vibratory tools, which can lead to thrombosis. The latter usually affects the ulnar artery in Guyon's canal at the wrist and is called the *hypothenar hammer syndrome.* Irrespective of their cause, vascular injuries may lead to a critical compromise of circulation in the extremity. With a closed injury, the onset of symptoms may be delayed, as the culmination of swelling, hypotension, and intimal injury all combine to result in late thrombosis and vascular insufficiency.

Following an acute arterial injury, symptoms result from a combination of the adequacy of collateral circulation, post-traumatic sympathetic tone, and vasomotor control mechanisms. Patients with an upper extremity arterial injury who have adequate collateral circulation and normal vasomotor control may have minimal symptoms, so that reconstruction is not necessarily mandatory and can be treated with simple arterial ligation. If there is a noncritical arterial injury such as to the radial artery alone, reconstruction may be advocated to restore parallel flow in case of future arterial injury, to enhance nerve recovery, to facilitate healing, and to prevent cold intolerance. However, reported patency rate, even with microvascular techniques for single vessel repairs, varies from 47% to 82%. The following injuries are optimally managed by vascular repair and reconstruction: axillary or brachial artery injury, combined radial and ulnar artery injury, and radial or ulnar artery injury associated with poor collateral circulation. Relative indications for repair of a noncritical vascular injury are extensive distal soft tissue injury, technical ability to achieve repair without compromising patient well-being, and a combined vascular and neural injury. The need for arterial reconstruction necessitates

assessment of adequacy of collateral circulation, and this is based primarily on initial clinical judgment. However, the final decision regarding arterial reconstruction is often made in the operating room after exploration. Once the injured structures have been isolated and potential bleeding sites controlled and hematoma evacuated, the distal extremity can be more adequately assessed. At this time, lacerated vessel ends are controlled by atraumatic vascular clamps, and a tourniquet can be released. Capillary refill and perfusion of the distal extremity can then be assessed, as can backflow from the distal lacerated vessel ends. Digital blood pressure can be quantified with a sterile Doppler probe and cuff, and a digital brachial index of 0.7 or greater suggests adequate perfusion. If there is poor collateral flow, then arterial reconstruction is performed. At this time, standard of care does not require arterial repair of isolated noncritical vessels. In combined radial and ulnar artery injuries, one or both vessels are reconstructed. If possible, both vessels are repaired.[10,11]

Muscles often swell after prolonged periods of ischemia. This can lead to an increase of pressure within the closed compartment of the forearm, resulting in a compartment syndrome. It is hence the practice of most surgeons to perform a routine fasciotomy to decompress the forearm compartment after a true revascularization procedure has been performed. During the period of ischemia to the muscles, there may be a buildup of lactic acid. Furthermore, myonecrosis might occur. Restoration of circulation to such a limb can cause a sudden flooding of the circulation with myoglobin, lactic acid, and other toxic substances. This is called *reperfusion syndrome* and can lead to multiorgan failure, especially affecting the renal and cardiac systems.

Replantation and Amputations

It can often be frustrating for the beginner general surgeon being told by a replant surgeon in the middle of the night that a consultation was obtained inappropriately or not soon enough. General indications do exist for replantation of amputated parts, but the overriding decision is still to save life before limb. Although patients and their respective family members may desire (and in some cases have even been promised by members of the primary team) replantation, it is not performed in patients with severe associated medical problems or injuries. Replantation is also generally not considered under the following circumstances:

1. Severe crush or multilevel injury of the amputated part
2. A psychotic patient who has willfully self-amputated the part
3. Amputation of a single digit proximal to the FDS distal insertion (zone 2), except for single-digit amputations in children or in those with demanding professions such as musicians
4. Amputation in patients with severely atherosclerotic arteries (sometimes only able to be determined when exploring the vessels in the operating room)[1,12,13]

Indications for replantation of amputated parts are as follows:

1. Whenever possible for a thumb amputation (it provides >40% of the overall hand function)[13]
2. Single digits that have been amputated distal to the FDS insertion (a manual worker may likely desire revision of amputation and desires to return to work quickly)
3. Multiple digits
4. Most amputations in children, including single digit amputations
5. Guillotine-sharp clean amputations at the hand, wrist, or distal forearm

Replantation is reattachment of the part that has been completely amputated. Revascularization requires reconstruction of vessels in a limb that has been severely injured or incompletely severed in such a way that vascular repair is necessary to prevent distal necrosis, but some soft tissue (skin, tendon, nerve) is still intact. Revascularization generally has a better success rate than replantation because venous and lymphatic drainage may be intact.

Minor replantation is a reattachment at the wrist, hand, or digital level, whereas major replantation is that performed proximal to the wrist. This clinical distinction exists because in the case of major replantations, ischemic time is crucial to viability of muscle and to functional outcome. Ischemic muscle may result in myonecrosis, myoglobinemia, and infection that may threaten the patient's life as well as limb. There are three types of amputations:

1. Guillotine amputation, whereby the tissue is cut with a sharp object and is minimally damaged
2. Crush amputation, in which a local crushing injury can be converted into a guillotine injury simply by débriding back the edges, although this may not be possible in a diffusely crushing amputation
3. Avulsion amputation, which is the most unfavorable type for replanting because structures are injured at different levels

Avulsion amputation may occur, for example, with a so-called ring avulsion injury. The extensor tendons are shredded, flexor tendons are often avulsed at the musculotendinous junctions, and nerves are stretched and may be ripped from end organs.

Ischemia time is also an important consideration when evaluating a patient for replantation. For amputated digits, more than 12 hours of warm ischemia is a relative contraindication. Promptly cooling the part to 4°C dramatically alters the ischemia factor, but even ischemia exceeding 24 hours does not necessarily preclude successful digital replantation. Ischemia time is more crucial for replantation above the proximal forearm, and reimplantation is not considered after more than 6 to 10 hours of warm ischemia time. Single digits in adults, other than the thumb in zone 2, are generally not reattached because of the consequent adverse overall functional result on the hand with a single stiff finger.[13]

Amputation is not an outmoded operation; rather, it is necessary where replantation might not be indicated. When primary amputation is performed, the stump is preserved with as much length as possible. Exception might be made if there is only a very short segment of proximal phalanx. A short proximal phalangeal remnant at the index finger position may serve as an impediment for thumb-to–middle finger prehension, and one might consider a formal ray amputation in such a case to improve overall hand function. The ends of the cut nerve are cut sharply and allowed to retract to minimize the occurrence of painful neuromas at the amputation tip. Tendons also are divided sharply and allowed to retract. The practice of suturing flexor and extensor tendons over the ends of the middle, ring, or small finger stump seriously impairs the motion of the uninjured fingers owing to the common origin of the flexors. There will be an active flexion deficit in the uninjured digits, which is called the *quadriga syndrome* and is corrected simply by release of the flexor tendon remnant at the injured amputated digit.

If it is anticipated that the amputated part will be considered for replantation, it is critical to transport both the patient and the part in an appropriate manner. The amputated part is placed in a clean, dry, plastic bag, which is sealed and placed on top of ice in a Styrofoam container. This keeps the part sufficiently cool at 4° to 10° C without freezing. The amputated part is wrapped in a lightly moistened saline gauze to prevent tissue drying.

With only a few minor variations, the sequence of replantation has been standardized. Preliminary exploration of the distal amputated part under a microscope by an initial surgical team not only determines whether a replantation is technically feasible but also can be started while the patient is being prepared for the operating room. Bone shortening allows skin to be débrided back to where it is free of contusion and where direct tension-free closure can be achieved. In the thumb, bone shortening is minimized to less than 10 mm. The order of repair is usually bone, tendons, muscle units, arteries, nerves, and finally veins. Establishment of arterial flow before venous flow clears lactic acid from the replanted part. The functional veins can now also be detected by spurting bleeding. However, blood loss must be closely monitored.

For major replantations, reestablishing arterial circulation as rapidly as possible is crucial to limiting ischemia time. A dialysis shunt or carotid shunt may be placed between arterial ends. Intermittent clamping of the shunt may be necessary to restrict blood loss. In the upper extremity, bone shortening can be aggressive to achieve primary skin closure and primary nerve repair. Judicious use of anticoagulants may enhance the success of replantation. Topical application of 2% lidocaine or papaverine may help relieve vasospasm. Postoperative dressings consist of nonadherent mesh gauze, loose flap gauze, and a plaster splint with postoperative elevation to minimize edema and venous congestion. The patient's room must be kept warm, and smoking is forbidden postop-

Table 74-4   Comparison of Methods of Skeletal Fixation

METHOD OF FIXATION	PROS	CONS
Kirschner wires	Come in varying diameters Can be applied percutaneously or open Second surgery not required for removal Require less soft tissue dissection than plates and screws	Pins can loosen Cannot provide rigid fixation Soft tissue may be transfixed (but can be avoided by careful placement) Infection can occur along pin tracks
Screws	Have high stability Allow for early finger mobilization	Frequently require open approach (although not always)
Plates	Can be used when fracture line is not oblique enough for screws Allow for early finger mobilization	Require open approach Require extensive soft tissue dissection Have relatively high profile and may be palpable through the skin and soft tissue on the dorsum of fingers and hand May promote extensor tendon adhesions by their relative bulk and dissection required for placement

eratively. Aside from antibiotics and analgesics, one aspirin tablet a day for its retarding effect on platelet aggregation is suggested. Postoperative monitoring is done hourly for color, pulp turgor, capillary refill, and digital temperature.

Fractures and Dislocations

Pain, swelling, limited motion, and deformities suggest the presence of a fracture or dislocation. Standard anteroposterior and lateral x-rays may miss some fractures and dislocations, and multiple views may be necessary to establish the exact diagnosis. Fractures may be rotated, angulated, telescoped, or displaced. Angulation is described by the direction in which the apex of the fracture is pointing, and displacement is described by the direction of the distal fragment. Fractures may be open or closed depending on whether or not a wound is involved. They may also be complete, incomplete, or comminuted (>2 pieces). Fractures are also described by their pattern and may be transverse, longitudinal, oblique, or spiral. Open fractures need to be thoroughly irrigated and débrided urgently. Displaced fractures or dislocations are repositioned as soon as possible. A dislocation is described according to the direction of the displacement of the distal bone in the involved joint. The separation of joints may be complete or incomplete (subluxed) depending on the severity of the capsular injury.[5,14-16]

Displaced fractures or dislocations are repositioned as soon as possible to decrease soft tissue injury, decompress nerves that might be stretched, and relieve kinking of blood vessels. Good bony contact and stability are necessary for fractures to heal. Some fractures are stable and require only external support in a splint or cast, others are unstable and require internal support, which can be provided by Kirschner wires, internal wire sutures through drill holes in the fracture fragments, screws, or plates, or even external fixation devices (Table 74-4). The more complicated the fixation, the more dissection is required to apply that fixation and therefore the greater the potential for scarring around adjacent tendons and consequential stiffness. Plates and screws, however, can nonetheless establish a degree of rigid fixation that allows early motion of the part and so potentially reduces the risk for cicatricial stiffness. Intra-articular fractures require accurate reduction to preserve motion and minimize the risk for later development of arthrosis. Persistent rotational deformity and significant lateral angular deformity generally do not remodel with time and can be avoided by observing the alignment of the injured fingers as compared with adjacent digits while passively gently flexing into a fist after reduction is attained. If they do not fit comfortably adjacent to each other and do not point toward the distal pole of the scaphoid, a fresh attempt at reduction must be performed. A thorough neurovascular examination is always performed both before and after fracture reduction has been completed.

Distal Phalangeal Fractures

Fractures of the distal phalanx are the most frequent hand fractures and represent half of all hand fractures. Most result from crush injuries with associated nail bed injuries. Precise reduction is generally not required, and treatment typically consists of splinting alone. However, unstable shaft fractures with overriding fragments are indications for reduction and longitudinal Kirschner wire fixation.

Most closed mallet fractures can be managed by splinting the DIP joint in extension provided the fracture involves less than 50% of the joint surface and is not associated with DIP joint subluxation. If fixation is required, the fracture fragment is held in place with a monofilament wire or a nonabsorbable suture passed through to the palmar aspect of the finger through the distal phalanx. Transarticular longitudinal Kirschner wire is used to keep the joint in neutral position. A so-called jersey finger is an avulsion fracture of the insertion of the FDP tendon into the distal phalanx. It occurs after a pull of the FDP against resistance, as can occur when a footballer catches onto the jersey of an opponent. Occasionally, the avulsed fragment may lie as far proximally as the palm. This fracture fragment generally requires open reduction and internal fixation.[5]

Middle Phalanx and Proximal Phalanx Fractures

Fractures may involve the head, neck, shaft, or base of the respective bone. Head and base fractures may be intra-articular. A middle phalangeal shaft fracture is displaced according to the forces exerted by the insertions of the FDS and the central slip mechanism. If the fracture lies distal to the FDS insertion, the proximal fragment is flexed by this muscle, resulting in a volar angulation. In contrast, if the fracture is proximal to the FDS insertion, the proximal fragment is extended by the central slip, whereas the distal part is flexed by the FDS. This results in a dorsal angulation. Most shaft fractures of the proximal phalanx tend to angulate volarward because the interossei reflect the proximal fragment and the central slip (through the PIP joint) extends the distal fragment. Displaced and unstable shaft fractures require open reduction followed by fixation with Kirschner wires or plates and screws.

Metacarpal Fractures

Stable metacarpal fractures may be treated with splinting alone. Fractures with dorsal or volar angulation can be stabilized by percutaneous insertion of intramedullary fixation pins. If they are displaced or unstable, such as oblique, spiral, or multiple metacarpal fractures, open reduction and internal fixation of these metacarpal fractures are performed. The internal fixation can be achieved with Kirschner wires, lag screws, or plate and screws, depending on the fracture pattern configuration. Dorsally angulated fractures at the neck of the little finger metacarpal, the so-called boxer's fracture, do not require reduction if the dorsal angulation is less than 30 degrees. The mobility of the carpometacarpal joint will compensate for this degree of angulation. The index and middle finger metacarpals are less mobile than the ring and little finger metacarpals. Therefore, a maximum of 15 degrees of angular deformity can be tolerated in the index and middle finger metacarpals.[17]

Oblique fractures at the base of the thumb metacarpal (Bennett's fracture) result in the small proximal fragment being held in position by the volar oblique ligament to the trapezium. The remaining portion of the thumb metacarpal is displaced dorsally and radially because of the pull of the abductor pollicis longus tendon (Fig. 74-28). These fracture fragments must be properly reduced and secured with internal fixation, either with Kirschner wires or with a screw. Comminuted fractures at the base of the thumb metacarpal (Rolando's fracture) are infrequently treated by closed reduction. If the fragments are large and badly displaced, an open reduction is indicated so

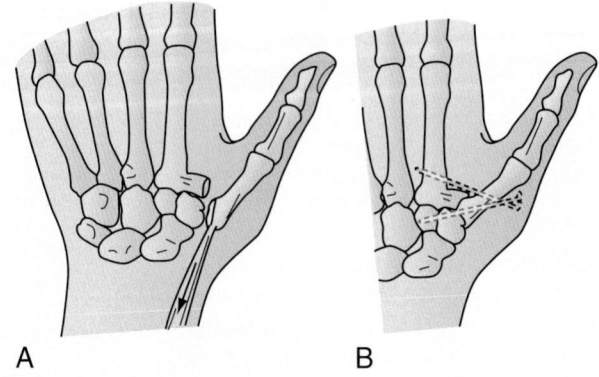

Figure 74-28 A, Fracture-dislocation at the base of the thumb metacarpal is called *Bennett's fracture.* The deforming force is produced by the pull of the abductor pollicis longus muscle. **B,** Open reduction and pinning of the fracture are frequently required.

that accurate restoration of the joint surface at the base of the thumb metacarpal is restored. Fractures of the shaft of the thumb metacarpal tend to become displaced by the opposing muscle forces of the abductor and the adductor on the proximal and distal fragments, respectively. Even undisplaced fractures may with time become progressively more displaced and angulated, necessitating an internal fixation. If initial splint immobilization is chosen for such an undisplaced thumb metacarpal fracture, then close scrutiny in follow-up is required to detect the earliest signs of displacement and instability. Fracture at the base of the little finger metacarpal is analogous to the Bennett's fracture of the thumb. It is sometimes called a *reverse Bennett's fracture.* This results in a fracture dislocation, with the deforming force being the insertion of the extensor carpi ulnaris tendon.[18,19]

Scaphoid Fractures

The scaphoid is by far the most common carpal bone fracture and accounts for about 60% of all carpal injuries. Clinical examination shows tenderness over the anatomic snuffbox and also over the scaphoid tubercle. If a scaphoid fracture is suspected, the initial radiographic examination includes not only the standard three views of the wrist but also a scaphoid view, which is a posteroanterior image with the wrist in full ulnar deviation. Frequently, immediate postinjury radiographs may not reveal a fracture. A CT or MRI scan may help in such situations, or one may elect to apply a splint and repeat the radiographs in 2 weeks.[20]

Treatment of a nondisplaced scaphoid fracture is with a long-arm cast that includes the thumb. The thumb spica cast is maintained for 6 weeks, followed by a short-arm cast until radiographic healing has occurred. More recently, there has been a trend toward percutaneous screw fixation of even, undisplaced scaphoid fractures.

Displaced scaphoid fractures require open reduction with internal fixation, most frequently using a compression screw. Complications with inadequately treated scaphoid fractures are notorious. The blood vessels enter

SALTER-HARRIS CLASSIFICATION

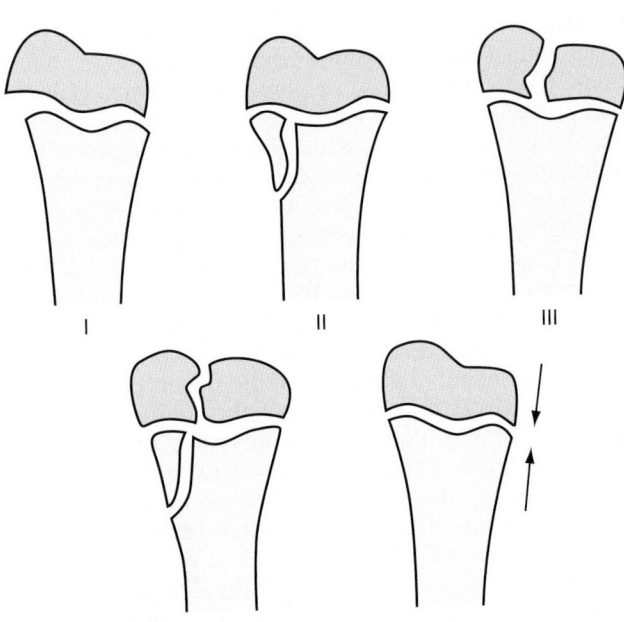

I   II   III

IV   V

Figure 74-29 Salter Harris fracture patterns involving the epiphysis in children.

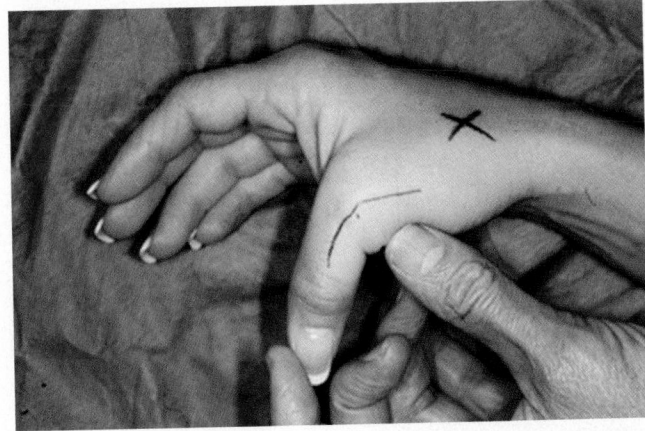

A

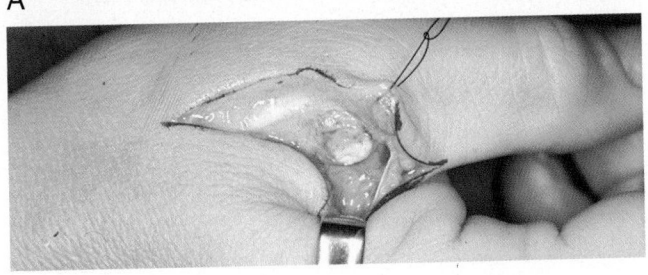

B

Figure 74-30 A, Instability of the ulnar collateral ligament of the metacarpophalangeal joint of the thumb. **B,** Stener's lesion shows that the distal insertion of the collateral ligament has avulsed proximal to the extensor hood and is thus blocked from spontaneous reattachment. Open operation is required to reanchor the collateral ligament insertion to the base of the proximal phalanx.

the scaphoid mainly through its distal half, and fractures through the waist of the scaphoid may deprive the proximal half of its blood supply, leading to avascular necrosis of the proximal pole of the scaphoid. Nonunion also occurs with relative frequency, and such cases need to be treated with cancellous bone grafting or even a pedicle vascularized bone graft. Early diagnosis of scaphoid fractures is essential so that appropriate treatment is instituted to reduce the risks for these complications. Modern cannulated compression screws, intraoperative fluoroscopy, and arthroscopy have allowed minimally invasive percutaneous fixation of some of these scaphoid fractures, resulting in the trend toward more aggressive surgical management of these fractures.

Fractures in Children

The Salter-Harris classification describes five types of epiphyseal injuries (Fig. 74-29). Pediatric bones are still growing and so permit a greater degree of remodeling. Hence, moderate angular and translational displacement of fractures tends to correct with age. However, rotational deformities never correct in the hand and are totally unacceptable even in children. Implants that cross the epiphysis must have minimal potential for damage. Hence, smooth Kirschner wires are generally used for fixation of pediatric skeletal injuries, and threaded screws are usually avoided.

Dislocations

Dislocations are more frequently seen at the PIP joint. A closed dislocation of the PIP joint can frequently be managed by closed reduction and splinting. If the joint

is unstable after reduction, it needs exploration for collateral ligament repair. The most common type of PIP joint dislocation is a dorsal dislocation. A PIP joint volar dislocation is often associated with a tear in the triangular ligament of the extensor mechanism through which the head of the proximal phalanx protrudes and becomes trapped. Attempts at closed reduction fail because they tighten the fibers of the lateral bands and central slip around each side of the protruding proximal phalangeal neck, and these injuries often require open reduction with repair of the extensor tear.

Palmar dislocations of the head of the index finger metacarpal often require open reduction. The head of the metacarpal becomes trapped between the superficial transverse metacarpal ligament, the flexor tendons, and lumbrical muscles, whereas the volar plate becomes trapped between the metacarpal head and the base of the proximal phalanx. Attempts at closed reduction are fruitless because of the entrapment resulting from this arrangement.

MP joint dislocation of the thumb often results from jamming it in a radial direction, thus tearing the ulnar collateral ligament. The ulnar collateral ligament may pull proximally and come to rest dorsal to the extensor hood (Stener's lesion) (Fig. 74-30). This cannot heal spontaneously because the ulnar collateral ligament is prevented

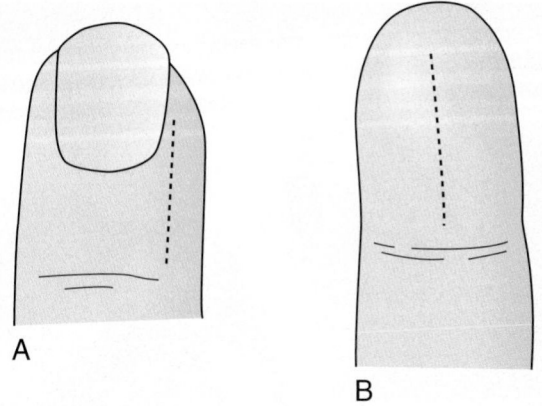

Figure 74-31 Incisions for paronychia (**A**) and felon (**B**).

from reattaching to bone. This so-called ski pole injury may then require operative repair. Stress radiograph (sometimes enabled only after anesthetizing the digit with a metacarpal block) may be required to facilitate diagnosis of a complete ulnar collateral ligament injury of the thumb metacarpal joint.

INFECTIONS

Hand infections commonly present to the surgical resident covering the emergency room. When diagnosed and treated properly initially, most patients do well. The extent of deep palmar infections may often be underestimated during the early phases because the volar aspect of the hand does not show edema as readily as the dorsal aspect of the hand. Hand infections can result in significant morbidity and severe functional compromise if not appropriately diagnosed and treated. Some of the more common types of infections are discussed next.

Superficial Paronychial Infections

Paronychia is the most common infection of the hand and usually results from trauma to the eponychial or paronychial region. The infection localizes around the nail base, advances around the nail fold, and burrows beneath the base of the nail. If pus is trapped beneath the nail, pressure on the nail evokes exquisite pain. The most common causative organism is *Staphylococcus aureus*. Treatment for early cases is with antibiotics, preferably penicillin in combination with a β-lactamase inhibitor such as sulbactam or clavulanic acid. After an abscess develops, surgical drainage is required. The surgical approach to an acute paronychia depends on the extent of the infection. Incisions may not be necessary. A Freer elevator is used to lift about one fourth of the nail adjacent to the infected perionychium, extending proximally to the edge of the nail. This portion of the nail is transected and gauze packing inserted beneath the nail fold. A single incision to drain the affected perionychium also allows elevation of the eponychial fold when both eponychium and paronychium are involved[21-23] (Fig. 74-31).

Infections of the Intermediate-Depth Spaces

Infections of the intermediate-depth spaces are pulp space infections (felons) and also deep webspace infections. The former may involve the terminal pulp or middle or proximal volar pulp spaces and may result from direct implantation with a penetrating injury or may represent spread from a more superficial subcutaneous infection. The volar pulp of the distal digital segment is a fascial space closed proximally by a septum joining the distal flexion crease to the periosteum, where the long flexor tendon is inserted. This space is also partitioned by fibrous septa. Tension in the distal digital segment can become so great that the arteries to the bone are compressed, resulting in gangrene of the fingertip and necrosis of the distal three fourths of the terminal phalanx. With infection of the digital pulp space, one must not wait for fluctuance before making the decision for surgery because of the danger of ischemic necrosis of the skin and bone. Clinical diagnosis is made by rapid onset of throbbing pain, swelling, and exquisite tenderness of the affected pulp space. Surgical drainage is required. Either a single volar longitudinal incision or a unilateral longitudinal incision may be used (see Fig. 74-31). Postoperative care includes packing of the wound and elevation of the extremity. Use of antibiotics is guided by the Gram stain. Similar to a paronychia, *S. aureus* is the most common etiologic agent. Spread from a pulp space infection may move into a joint space or the underlying bone, or burst through the septum proximally to involve the rest of the finger. More proximally, a pulp space infection at the base of the finger can travel through the lumbrical canal into the palm to create a deep palmar space infection.[24]

Webspace abscesses result from either direct implantation or spread from a pulp space. An inflamed and tender mass in the webspace separates the fingers. There is loss of the normal palmar concavity with a widened space between the fingers. Dorsal swelling is present and must not be mistaken for the infection site. A surgical incision is placed transversely across the webspace, and a counter longitudinal incision may be placed dorsally between the bases of the proximal phalanges; a generous communication is established between these two incisions (Fig. 74-32).

Deep Infections

Deep Palmar Space Infections

These infections are localized to the deep space of the hand between the metacarpals and the palmar aponeurosis. A transverse septum to the metacarpal of the middle finger divides the deep space into an ulnar midpalmar space and the radial thenar space. The transverse head of the adductor pollicis partitions the thenar space from the retroadductor space. There may be ballooning of the palm, thenar eminence, or posterior aspect of the first webspace depending on which of the affected spaces is involved with an abscess. The dorsal subaponeurotic space of the hand deep to the extensor tendons may also be affected by an isolated infection, generally as the result of direct implantation (Fig. 74-33A). For a thenar space infection, the preferred approach to surgical drainage is a dual volar and dorsal incision (see Fig. 74-33B). On the volar side, an incision is made adjacent and parallel to the thenar crease. Great care is taken to avoid injury to the palmar cutaneous branch of the median nerve in the proximal part of the incision and the motor branch of the median nerve in a deeper plane. A second, slightly curved, longitudinal incision is made on the dorsum of the first webspace. Dissection is continued more deeply into this area between the first dorsal interosseous muscle and the adductor pollicis. A drain is placed in the incision after thorough exploration of the respective spaces. With midpalmar space infections, dorsal swelling of the hand will be present (as is the case with all palmar infections) and must not be mistaken for the infection site. Motion of the middle and ring fingers is limited and painful. A longitudinal curvilinear incision is the preferred approach for drainage of this space (see Fig. 74-33B).

Infection of Parona's space occurs in the potential space deep to the flexor tendons in the distal forearm and superficial to the pronator quadratus muscle. It is usually the result of spread from the adjacent contiguous midpalmar space or from the radial or ulnar bursa. Swelling, tenderness, and fluctuation will be present in the distal volar forearm. A midpalmar infection may be associated. Active digital flexion is painful, as is passive finger extension. A surgical incision must be planned so as to leave the median nerve adequately covered with soft tissue.

Pyogenic Flexor Tenosynovitis

Kanavel's cardinal signs include the following characteristics: the finger is held flexed because this position allows the synovial sheath its maximum volume and eases pain; symmetrical fusiform swelling of the entire finger is present with edema of the back of the hand; the slightest attempt at passive extension of the affected digit produces exquisite pain; and the site of maximum tenderness is at the proximal cul-de-sac of the index, middle, and ring finger synovial sheaths in the distal palm or in the case of infection of the sheaths of the thumb and little finger more proximally in the palm (see Fig. 74-33). The radial and ulnar bursae communicate in about 80% of cases and may be simultaneously infected. Bursal infections may spread into the forearm space of Parona, deep to the flexor tendons in the distal part of the forearm, creating a horseshoe abscess.

Pyogenic flexor tenosynovitis may be aborted with parenteral antibiotics, extremity elevation, and hand immobilization if the patient is seen within the first 24 hours of onset of infection. If this course is unsuccessful, or if the patient is seen more than 48 hours after onset of infection, surgical drainage is undertaken. The preferred surgical approach is through two separate incisions, with the first being a midaxial incision made on the finger, usually on the ulnar side of the digit (on the radial side of the thumb or little finger); the digital artery and nerve remain in the volar flap with the dissection proceeding directly to the tendon sheath. Synovium between A3 and A4 pulleys is incised, and cloudy fluid

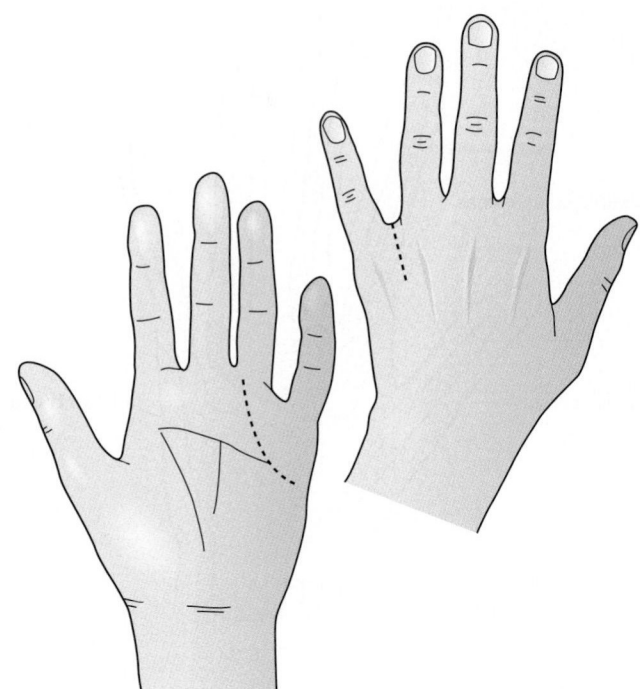

Figure 74-32 Incisions for webspace abscess between the little and ring fingers.

is encountered. A second incision is made in the palm over the tendon to drain the cul-de-sac. A 16-gauge polyethylene catheter is inserted beneath the A1 pulley into the sheath, and the sheath is flushed manually with sterile saline every 2 hours after surgery; a bulky hand dressing absorbs the drainage. Recent studies have found that postoperative catheter drainage may not always be necessary.[25,26]

Chronic and Atypical Infections

Chronic paronychia are generally the result of *Candida albicans* (>95%) infection and are not bacterial. When bacteria are involved, they are more commonly atypical mycobacteria or gram-negative organisms. These chronic paronychia generally respond to treatment with topical antifungal agents, although oral antifungal agents are sometimes used. Occasionally, surgical treatment by means of marsupialization of the eponychial fold is required. If the lesion is refractory to treatment, the possibility of a malignancy is entertained.

Chronic tenosynovitis can occur either in the flexor tendons or in the dorsum of wrist and extensor tendons. It is usually of a granulomatous type and is caused by mycobacteria or fungi. Treatment includes surgical excision of the involved synovium as well as prolonged treatment with the appropriate antimicrobial agents. Chronic infected tenosynovitis must be differentiated from other causes of chronic granulomatous synovitis, such as sarcoidosis, amyloidosis, gout, and rheumatoid arthritis.

Herpetic "Whitlow"

Herpetic Whitlow is caused by type I or II herpes simplex virus and may be confused with a paronychia. Infection

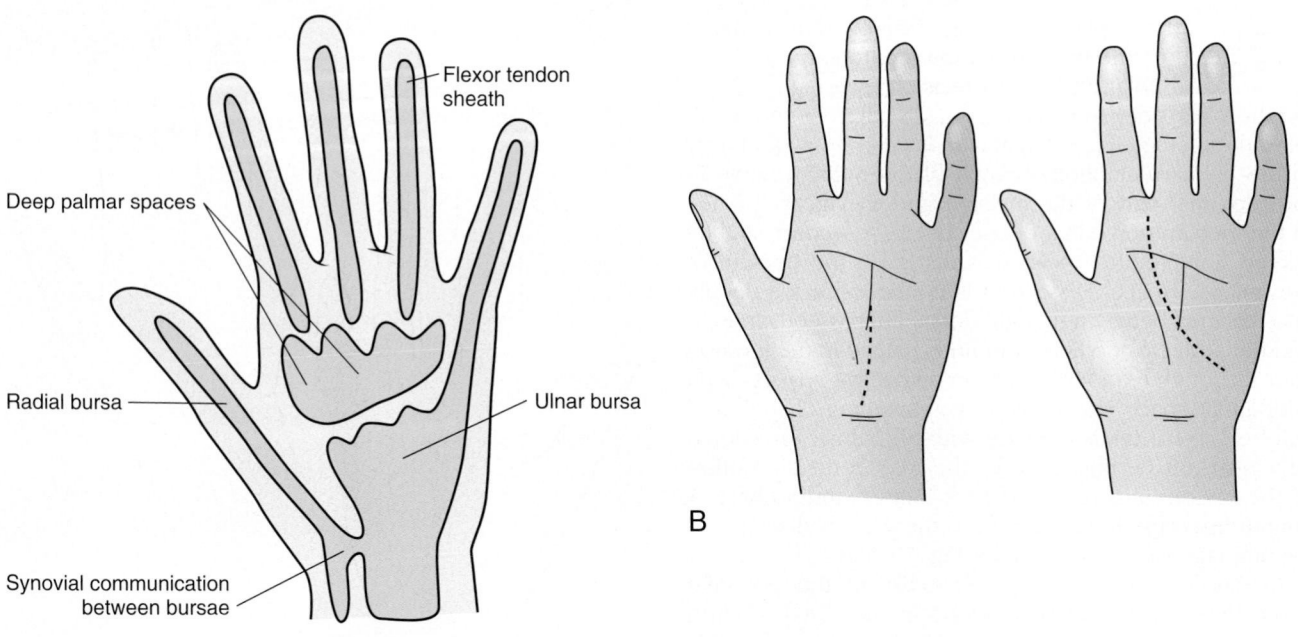

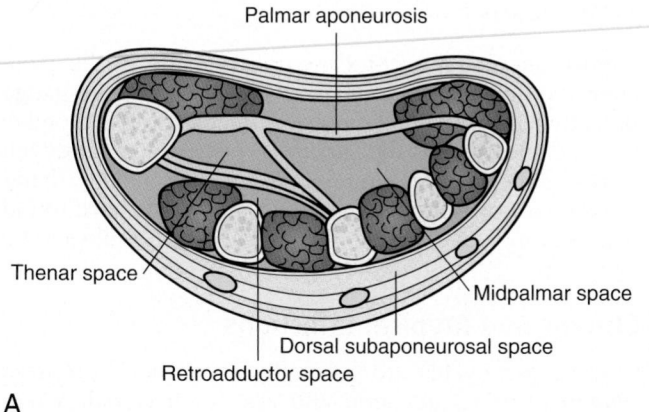

Figure 74-33 A, Deep spaces of the hand and synovial bursae. Infections may be bound by these spaces or may track along anatomic dissection planes between these spaces. **B,** Incision for thenar space infection. A dorsal first webspace incision is also often required. Incision for midpalmar space abscess.

begins with the appearance of small clear vesicles with localized swelling, erythema, and intense pain. The vesicles may subsequently appear turbid and coalesce over the next few days before ulcerating. Diagnosis is confirmed by culturing the virus from the vesicular fluid, assessing immunofluorescent serum antibody titers, or performing a Tzanck smear. However, these measures are rarely required because clinical diagnosis is usually sufficient. Infection can occur from either autoinoculation from an oral or genital lesion or exposure as a health care worker. Pain is often out of proportion to physical findings. Treatment is generally nonoperative because this infection is usually self-limited. Antivirals such as acyclovir or famciclovir may be of some benefit if started within the first 48 hours of symptom onset. Surgical incision and drainage can lead to systemic involvement and possible viral encephalitis.

Animal and Human Bites

The most striking difference in the microbial flora of human and animal bite wounds is the higher number of bacterial isolates per wound in human bites, the difference being mostly due to the presence of anaerobic bacteria. Human bites can occasionally transmit other infectious diseases such as hepatitis B, tuberculosis, syphilis, or actinomycosis. The incidence of *Eikenella corrodens* in human bite infections of the hand has been reported to vary between 7% and 29%. Most commonly isolated organisms from infected human bite wounds are, as in animal bites, α-hemolytic streptococcus and *S. aureus,* β-lactamase-producing strains of *S. aureus,* and *Bacteroides* species. Anaerobic bacteria are more prevalent in human bite infections than previously recognized, including *Bacteroides, Clostridium, Peptococcus,* and

Veillonella. Most studies of animal bite wounds are focused on the isolation of *Pasteurella multocida,* disregarding the role of anaerobes. Recent studies show that dog bite wounds point toward multiple organisms, with *P. multocida* being isolated from only 26% of dog bite wounds in adults. Most animal bites cause mixed infections of both aerobic and anaerobic bacteria.

Pyogenic joint infections usually result from trauma, such as a bite wound from a tooth when the assailant's hand impacts the jaw. A tooth impacting the clenched fist of an attacker penetrates the skin, tendon, joint capsule, and metacarpal head. Once the finger is extended, the four puncture wounds separate from each other to create a closed space within the joint. All such so-called fight bite wounds of the MP joint need to be explored surgically, débrided, and thoroughly lavaged. Human bite wounds are not closed primarily and are treated with appropriate antibiotics.

COMPARTMENT SYNDROME, HIGH-PRESSURE INJECTION INJURIES, AND EXTRAVASATION INJURIES

High-pressure injection injuries to the hands are relatively uncommon, but consequences of a misdiagnosis are serious. Urgent treatment is required. High-pressure injection guns are used for painting, lubricating, cleaning, and mass farm animal vaccinations. Materials that may be injected with these devices include paint, paint thinners, oil, grease, water, plastic, vaccines, and cement. These high-pressure injection guns may generate pressures ranging between 3000 and 12,000 PSI. Injection injuries can also be caused by other sources such as defective lines and valves and also from pneumatic hoses and hydraulic lines. The type of material injected is the most important prognostic factor. Oil-based paints and paint thinners can generate significant early inflammation leading to severe fibrosis. Because tendon sheaths at the index, middle, and ring fingers end at the level of the MP joints, material injected at either the DIP or PIP flexion creases will remain within these digits. However, tendon sheaths at the thumb and little finger extend all the way into the radial and ulnar bursae. Thus, material injected at the little finger or at the IP flexion crease of the thumb may potentially extend all the way into the forearm and even cause a compartment syndrome.

Initial presentation of a patient with a high-pressure injection may be benign and subtle. This may result in mismanagement by minimizing the patient's complaints. The break in the skin may be a very benign-looking pinhole-sized puncture site. However, within several hours, the digit becomes increasingly more painful, swollen, and pale. Prompt recognition and realization of the severity of injury are paramount. Radiographs may help determine the extent and dispersion of the injected material, either in the form of subcutaneous emphysema or with lead-based paints appearing as radiopaque soft tissue densities. The entire digit must be surgically decompressed and all foreign material and necrotic tissue

débrided. Wounds are closed loosely over Penrose drains or in a delayed manner. Appropriate antibiotics must be administered. Despite prompt recognition and treatment, many such injuries result ultimately in surgical amputation of the digits.

In the past, extravasation injuries of chemotherapeutic agents frequently affected the upper extremity. However, subcutaneously tunneled central lines have now reduced the incidence of these injuries. If extravasation is suspected, infusion must be stopped immediately. Cold packs are applied for 15 minutes four times a day and the extremity elevated over the next 48 hours. This treatment is generally effective for most extravasation injuries. However, if blistering, ulceration, and pain occur in the damaged tissue, progressive necrosis to the limits of the extravasation will then follow, and surgical excision of all damaged tissue is necessary. Most subsequent wounds can generally be treated with delayed split-thickness skin grafting, although the options for wound coverage after débridement depend on the extent of the débridement that was required.

Compartment syndrome results in symptoms and signs occurring from increased pressure within a limited space that compromises circulation and function of the tissues in that space. Volkmann's ischemic contracture is the sequel of untreated compartment syndrome and results in muscle that is fibrosed, contracted, and functionless, and nerves that are insensible. A variety of injuries are known to cause compartment syndrome:

1. Decreased compartment volume (externally applied tight dressings or casts; lying on a limb in a comatose state)
2. Increased compartment content (from bleeding or trauma with fractures or finger injuries; increased capillary permeability such as reperfusion after ischemic injury; and electrical burn injuries
3. Other injuries such as snake bites and high-pressure injection injuries[27]

The diagnosis of compartment syndrome is based primarily on clinical evaluation. Although it is possible to measure intracompartment pressure, the decision to perform fasciotomy is based on a high degree of clinical suspicion. Compartment ischemia may be severe and still not affect the color or temperature of the distal fingers, and the distal pulses are rarely obliterated by compartment swelling. However, circulation in the muscle and nerve may be greatly reduced. Muscle ischemia that lasts for more than 4 hours leads to muscle death and may also give rise to significant myoglobinuria. After 8 hours of total ischemia, irreversible nerve changes are complete. The hallmark of muscle and nerve ischemia is pain, which is progressive and persistent. The pain is accentuated by passive muscle stretching, and this is the most reliable clinical test for making a diagnosis of compartment syndrome. The next most important clinical finding is diminished sensation, which indicates nerve ischemia. The closed compartments of the forearm and hand are also palpated and are found to be tense and tender, confirming the diagnosis of compartment syndrome. A passive muscle stretch test elicits severe pain in the

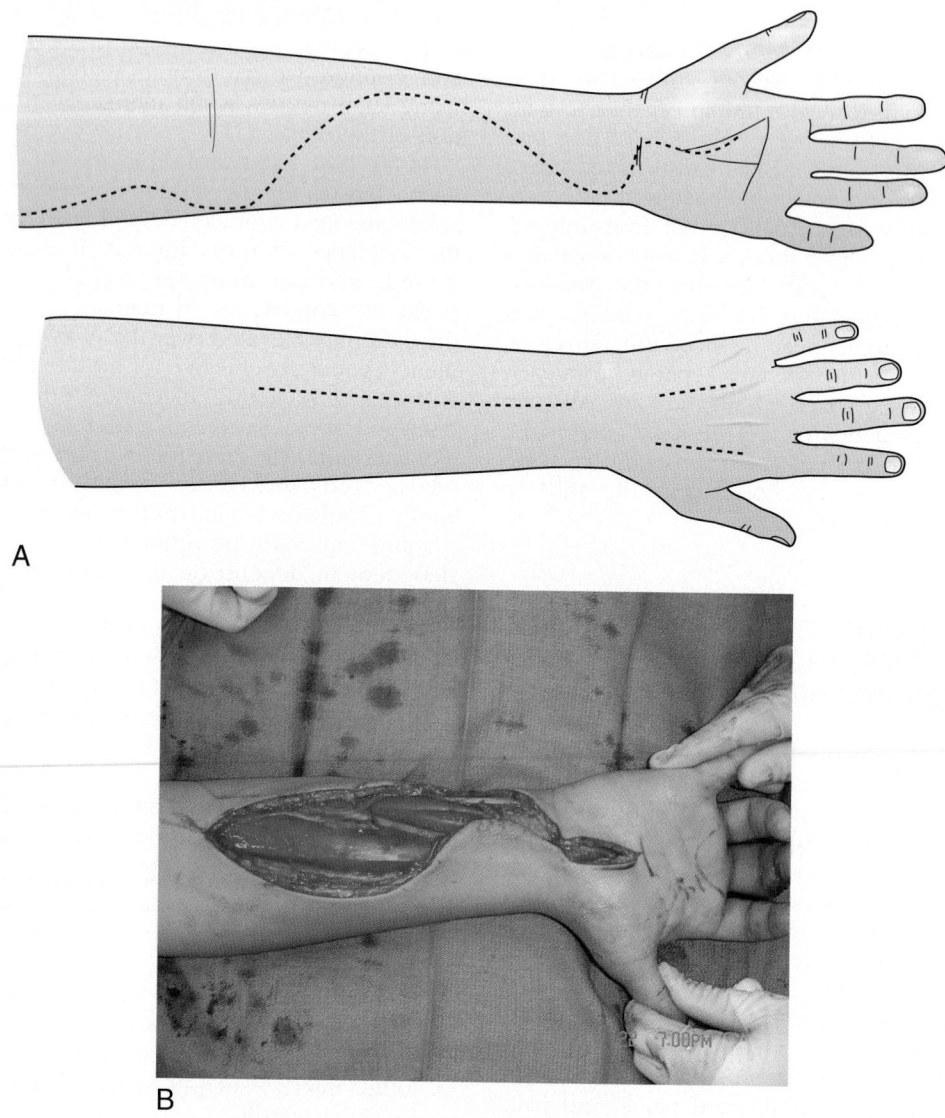

Figure 74-34 A, Incisions for forearm fasciotomy. **B,** Fasciotomy in a child for compartment syndrome following a snakebite.

presence of compartment syndrome. An arterial injury and nerve injury need to be distinguished in the differential diagnosis of compartment syndrome. All three of these injuries produce paresthesias and paresis; pain with passive stretch is present in compartment syndrome and arterial occlusion, but not in neuropraxia; and pulses are intact in compartment syndrome and neuropraxia, but not with arterial occlusion. In situations in which the clinical diagnosis is difficult because the patient cannot cooperate either through inebriation or unconsciousness, compartment pressure can be measured.

Release of forearm compartment syndrome always requires carpal tunnel release (Fig. 74-34). The palmar incision starts in the valley between the thenar and hypothenar muscles, and the incision then curves transversely across the flexion crease of the wrist at the ulnar border. This incision must avoid the palmar cutaneous branch of

the median nerve and must prevent flexion contracture across the wrist crease. It also provides an opportunity to release Guyon's canal. The incision then extends proximally up the forearm before curving back in a radial direction so as to have a large skin flap that will cover the median nerve and distal forearm tendons. At the elbow, the incision for the flap then curves again across the antecubital fossa providing cover for the brachial artery and the median nerve as well as preventing linear contracture across the antecubital fossa. The dorsal and so-called mobile wad compartments of the forearm are readily released through a straight incision as needed. Appropriate release of the various intrinsic compartments of the hand may also be required. Most wounds can be partially closed at 5 days. If the skin cannot be closed secondarily within 10 days, a split-thickness skin graft can be applied.

TENOSYNOVITIS

de Quervain's Disease

de Quervain's disease is a stenosing tenosynovitis of the first dorsal compartment of the wrist and is a common cause of pain and disability. Diagnosis is easily made from a history of pain localized to the radial side of the wrist and aggravated by movement of the thumb. There is frequently a history of chronic overuse of the wrist and hand. Other features are local tenderness and swelling over the first dorsal compartment of the wrist and a positive Finkelstein's test (the patient clasps the thumb, and brisk ulnar deviation to the hand elicits extreme pain). Crepitus may be palpable. This condition must be differentiated by radiographic and physical examination from arthritis of the thumb carpometacarpal joint.

Nonoperative treatment includes local steroid injection, thumb and wrist immobilization, local heat, and systemic anti-inflammatory medications. If these nonoperative measures fail, surgical decompression of the first dorsal compartment at the wrist is performed. Care must be taken to protect the radial sensory nerve branches during the course of the operation because these branches traverse just under the skin in this area, and trauma or transection may lead to painful disabling neuromas.

Intersection Syndrome

This condition is not well understood but is characterized by pain and crepitus at the point where the APL and EPB tendons cross over the tendons of the second dorsal compartment (ECRL and ECRB) (Fig. 74-35). Initial treatment is by splinting, local corticosteroid injection, and anti-inflammatory medications. Refractory cases require surgical release at the second dorsal compartment and excision of involved tenosynovial membranes.

Trigger Thumb and Fingers

Trigger finger is a constricting tenosynovitis of the flexor tendons generally at the level of the A1 pulley. The patient can flex the digit, but an apparent nodule catches at the proximal edge of the A1 pulley, locking the PIP joint (or the IP joint of the thumb) in this flexed position. Attempts at extending the digit cause it to suddenly snap back, much like the trigger of a gun. Often, the patient needs to use the opposite hand to unlock and extend the digit. In its most severe form, the constriction is so tight that the patient cannot flex the digit or it gets fixed in a flexed position and can no longer be fully extended. A congenital form of trigger thumb or finger presents in infants, but most cases resolve by the time the patient reaches 1 year of age; if not, an operation is indicated.

Nonoperative treatment in adults includes local injection of corticosteroids. If this regimen fails, the A1 pulley is longitudinally divided by surgery.[28]

Other Sites of Tenosynovitis

Other sites include the FCR and FCU tendons. They can frequently be treated by splinting and local corticosteroid injection, although surgery occasionally may be required. Inflammation of the ECU may also be an enigmatic cause of ulnar-sided wrist pain. Diagnosis is made by eliciting tenderness along the ECU tendon, as well as pain on active-resisted extension and ulnar deviation of the wrist.

NERVE COMPRESSION SYNDROMES

Along the length of the upper extremity, nerves pass through a number of anatomic bottlenecks. These are all possible sites of nerve entrapment and lead to characteristic distal sensory and motor deficits. The most common sites of nerve compression, from proximal to distal along the length of the extremity, are at the nerve root secondary to cervical disk disease or cervical degenerative arthritis, thoracic outlet compression at the level of the clavicle, ulnar nerve entrapment at the elbow (cubital tunnel syndrome), entrapment of the posterior interosseous nerve in the proximal forearm (radial tunnel syndrome and posterior interosseous syndrome), entrapment of the median nerve and its branches in the proximal forearm (the so-called pronator syndrome and also the anterior interosseous nerve syndrome), and, finally, entrapment of the median nerve at the wrist (carpal tunnel syndrome) and the ulnar nerve in Guyon's canal (ulnar tunnel syndrome).

In most cases of nerve entrapment, no specific aggravating etiologic factor is found. An increasing incidence of compression neuropathy is reported in work-related patients who undergo chronic repetitive stress (e.g., assemblers and chicken cutters). In some, there may be a clearly defined extrinsic compressive problem on the nerve or an aggravating factor. These include the following:

- Trauma that can produce bony compression, for example, carpal tunnel following carpal dislocations or a distal radius malunion (median) and supracondylar humerus fractures that increase the elbow carrying angle (ulnar nerve at the elbow)

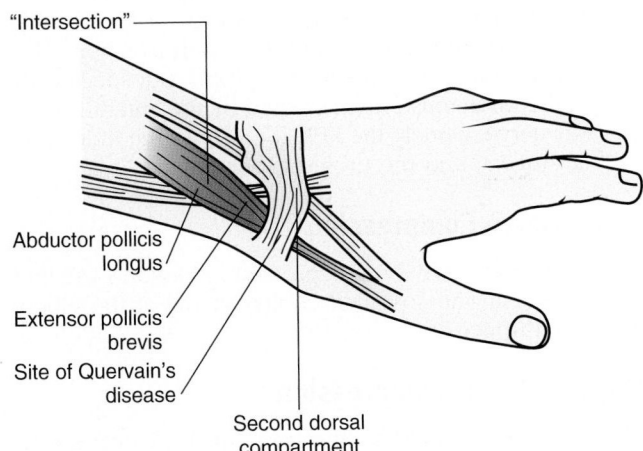

Figure 74-35 Anatomic locations for de Quervain's stenosing tenosynovitis and intersection syndrome.

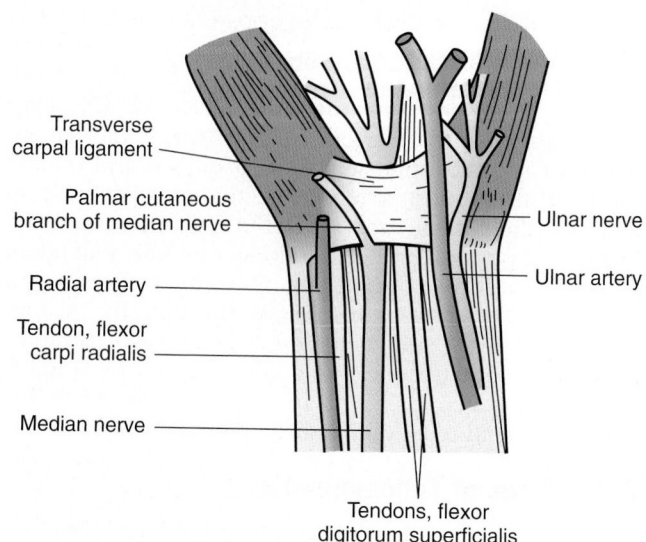

Transverse carpal ligament

Palmar cutaneous branch of median nerve

Radial artery

Tendon, flexor carpi radialis

Median nerve

Ulnar nerve

Ulnar artery

Tendons, flexor digitorum superficialis

Figure 74-36 Anatomy of the carpal tunnel. The transverse carpal ligament (flexor retinaculum) is divided longitudinally during a carpal tunnel release.

- Synovial thickening of the bursa in rheumatoid arthritis, either in the carpal tunnel (median) or at the elbow (posterior interosseous)
- Tumor such as giant cell tumor in Guyon's canal (ulnar) or a lipoma in the radial tunnel (posterior interosseous)
- Developmental with anomalous muscles present in the carpal tunnel (median), in Guyon's canal (ulnar), or in the forearm (median)
- Metabolic, in which disturbances of fluid balance cause increased pressure on the nerve, particularly at the carpal tunnel (e.g., in myxedema, pregnancy)

Carpal tunnel syndrome is the most common peripheral nerve entrapment syndrome, and it is next followed by ulnar nerve entrapment at the elbow.[29] The other entrapment syndromes are less common.

Carpal Tunnel Syndrome

The carpal tunnel is a packed fibro-osseous tunnel at the wrist that is traversed by the median nerve and nine long extrinsic digital flexor tendons (Fig. 74-36). Its floor is formed by the carpal bones and roofed by the flexor retinaculum (transverse carpal ligament). Normal pressures in this tunnel are 20 to 30 mm Hg. A rise in pressure above this causes a chronic compressive ischemic injury to the nerve segment, resulting first in demyelination and eventually in axonal death. There is progressive conduction block in the nerve with subsequent sensory and motor dysfunction. The earliest symptoms are pain and paresthesias, which are characteristically more obvious at night, after prolonged activity, and with positional postural changes at the wrist such as when driving, using a blower hairdryer, or reading a book. The patient may complain of clumsiness and a tendency to drop objects. The paresthesias characteristically follow the distribution of the median nerve, including the thumb and index and

middle finger. Physical examination consists of compressing the carpal canal, percussing the median nerve, and hyperflexing the wrist to produce paresthesias (Durkin's sign, Tinel's sign, and Phalen's test, respectively). Sensory evaluation reveals hypoesthesia in the distribution of the median nerve and may reveal a widened two-point sensory discrimination. Thenar weakness or muscle wasting is a late finding. Nerve conduction studies and electromyography are useful adjuncts to the clinical examination.

Initial treatment of carpal tunnel syndrome includes use of wrist splints (especially at night), occasionally local corticosteroid injections, and modification in work patterns. If symptoms persist, or if the initial presentation shows severe carpal tunnel syndrome, surgical decompression is required. This is performed by longitudinally dividing the flexor retinaculum by either open or endoscopic means. Both the Agee (single portal) and the Chow (two portal) have shown similar efficacy to the open approach.[30,31] Synovectomy and removal of any mass lesion may also be required if that is the cause for the problem.[32,33]

Pronator Syndrome

In the proximal forearm, the median nerve may be compressed at the fibrous arch between the two heads of the FDS, the two heads of the pronator teres, the lacertus fibrosis (bicipital aponeurosis at the elbow), and the ligament of Struthers. Compression at any or all of these sites is loosely grouped under the pronator syndrome. The symptoms produced are similar to those of carpal tunnel, although nocturnal symptoms are uncommon. The palm may also feel numb because the palmar cutaneous branch is involved, but is specifically spared in carpal tunnel syndrome because that nerve branch passes superficial to the flexor retinaculum and arises proximal to the retinaculum. Symptoms may be reproduced or worsened by attempting pronation against resistance and by resisted flexion of the middle finger. However, it may be difficult to precisely locate the compressive cause in the pronator syndrome, and surgical decompression often involves release of all four potential sites of compression.

The anterior interosseus nerve branch of the median nerve may occasionally be compressed in isolation. This does not produce any sensory symptoms, but specifically targets the three muscles innervated by the anterior interosseous nerve, namely the FPL, the FDP to the index and middle fingers, and the pronator quadratus.

Ulnar Nerve Compression

The ulnar nerve may be compressed in Guyon's canal at the wrist or in the so-called cubital tunnel at the elbow and distal upper arm.

Guyon's Canal Compression

This canal is bounded by the hook of the hamate, pisiform, pisohamate ligament, and palmar carpal ligament. Compression by mass lesions may occur at this site, including a ganglion, giant cell tumor, ulnar artery thrombosis, or ulnar artery aneurysm (as in the hypothenar hammer syndrome). Compression at this site may also be idiopathic. Distal ulnar deficits may be in either the motor or sensory distribution or both, depending on where in the canal the compression occurs relative to the takeoff of the deep motor branch of the ulnar nerve. There may be a positive Tinel's sign and worsening of symptoms by direct compression over Guyon's canal. Treatment is surgical and consists of dividing the palmaris brevis muscle and the palmar carpal ligament, as well as removing any offending mass in this region.

Cubital Tunnel Syndrome

The cubital tunnel is a long tunnel starting in the distal upper arm and extending into the proximal forearm. As the ulnar nerve passes into the forearm, it curves tightly around the grooved posterior and inferior surfaces of the medial epicondyle of the humerus. This groove is bridged by the aponeurosis between the two heads of the FCU, the leading edge of which may be thickened and fibrosed, called *Osborne's ligament.* More proximally, the ulnar nerve passes from the anterior compartment of the arm into the posterior compartment, and this may be bridged by a long tunnel called the *arcade of Struthers.* The medial intermuscular septum in the upper arm may also cause ulnar nerve compression. The most distal fibro-osseous tunnel is more accurately termed the *cubital tunnel.* However, compression on the ulnar nerve can occur at any of these sites proximal to distal starting in the upper arm and extending into the forearm. Motor and sensory symptoms develop in the distribution of the ulnar nerve and are worsened by adopting a flexed position at the elbow. Examination reveals a positive Tinel's sign over the tunnel. Paresthesias are described in the distribution of the ulnar nerve to the little and ring fingers and ulnar border of the hand. A differential diagnosis includes thoracic outlet syndrome, compression of the ulnar nerve in Guyon's canal, and nerve root compression in the neck.

Initial treatment consists of splinting the elbow in extension at night. Use of soft extension elbow pads prevents elbow flexion and direct pressure on the nerve. Failure of nonoperative measures, together with significant changes in electrodiagnostic studies, are indications for surgical decompression. Most frequently, all the fibrous restraints on the ulnar nerve around the elbow are released, and the nerve is transposed anteriorly to the medial epicondyle into either a subcutaneous or submuscular position.

Radial Nerve Compression

The radial nerve may be compressed proximally in the triangular space in the axilla (specifically involving the axillary branch), the spiral groove posterior to the humerus in the arm, and the lateral intermuscular septum proximal to the elbow. More distally in the forearm, the posterior interosseous nerve (the principle motor division of the radial nerve) can be compressed in the so-called radial tunnel starting at the leading fibrous edge of the supinator (ligament of Frohse). There may be a variable degree of interosseous nerve paresis, or there may be pain radiating down the dorsoradial aspect of the forearm (the latter is called *radial tunnel syndrome*). Initial treatment is nonoperative with splinting, but if this fails, surgical decompression may occasionally be required.

Thoracic Outlet Compression

The thoracic outlet is a narrow space at the base of the neck bounded by the first rib medially, the scalenus anterior muscle and clavicle anteriorly, and the scalenus medius muscle posteriorly. All elements of the brachial plexus, as well as the subclavian artery and vein, pass through this narrow space and can be potentially compressed at this site. A positive Tinel's sign can often be elicited at both the supraclavicular and infraclavicular regions. A Roos test is performed by asking the patient to hold both arms overhead in a surrender position while opening and closing the fists. This reproduces symptoms within 1 minute, and if continued, the arm collapses at the side. Adson's test involves palpating the radial pulse while the patient turns the chin toward the same side, inhales deeply, and holds the breath. The radial pulse either disappears or diminishes. The costoclavicular compression test involves sustained downward pressure on the clavicle, and the symptoms are reproduced. Radiographic evaluation may reveal a cervical rib. Nerve conduction studies are often normal.

Thoracic outlet compression may occur in association with other peripheral sites of nerve compression, a condition termed *double-crush syndrome.* Treatment is primarily nonoperative, involving posture-improving exercises and avoidance of aggravating activities. If symptoms persist, especially if associated with vascular compression, the thoracic outlet may be surgically decompressed. This is accomplished by a transcervical or transaxillary resection of the first rib, often with release of the scalene muscles.

SOFT TISSUE TUMORS

Ganglia and mucous cysts represent 60% to 70% of hand tumors, followed in frequency by inclusion cysts, warts (verrucae), giant cell tumors in tendon sheaths, foreign body granulomas, lipomas, hemangiomas, and pyogenic granulomas. Benign tumors account for 95% of hand neoplasms. Squamous cell carcinoma is the most frequent primary malignancy of the hand; basal cell carcinoma is quite rare; and melanoma is relatively uncommon in the upper extremity. Acral lentiginous melanoma (palms, soles, nail beds) has a tendency toward early metastasis. Primary bone tumors of the hand are generally benign, the most common being enchondromas and osteochondromas, except in the terminal phalanges, where the most common is the inclusion cyst. Giant cell tumors of bone are rare in the hand, occurring most commonly in the distal radius. They are locally aggressive and may occasionally metastasize. Of malignant bone tumors, only 1.2% affect the hand. Although bone metastases in other parts of the body are relatively common, bones of the

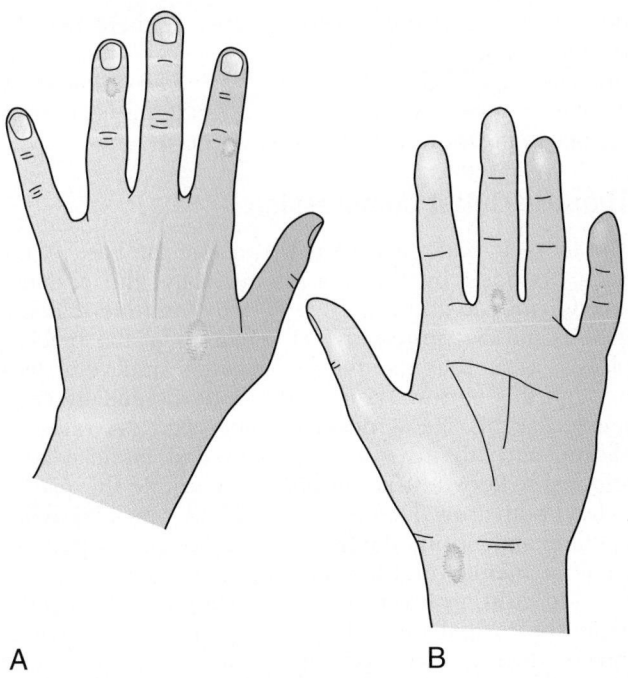

Figure 74-37 Dorsal (**A**) and ulnar (**B**) aspects of the hand and wrist showing common presenting sites for ganglion cysts.

hand are rarely affected by metastases from elsewhere.[34,35]

Soft tissue sarcomas are rare, representing 1% of all malignancies of the body, excluding skin tumors. Although uncommon, certain types predominate in the hand. Epithelioid, synovial, and clear cell sarcomas are relatively rare in other sites, but by comparison are more common in the hand.

Within the spectrum of benign and malignant tumors, there is a group with intermediate malignancy, the giant cell and desmoid tumors (of soft tissue), with a propensity for local recurrence after surgical excision. Their histologic patterns may belie their behavior. Juvenile aponeurotic fibroma and nodular fasciitis may appear histologically more aggressive than desmoid tumors, yet are self-limiting. The tiny glomus tumor is uncommon but has a propensity for the fingertips and subungual regions. It may be an enigmatic cause of severe and exquisite pain at the fingertips. It may be recognized by a pinpoint site of extreme local tenderness and a violaceous hue deep to the nail plate. An MRI may on occasion detect these tiny lesions at the fingertip.

If a lesion is thought to be benign, excision without further workup (except perhaps for routine radiographs) is appropriate. However, if a primary malignancy of bone or soft tissue is suspected, additional studies must be done before biopsy. A CT scan may help to delineate tumor boundaries. Desmoid tumors have radiographic density identical to that of muscle and are better demonstrated by MRI.

Ganglion Cysts

Ganglions are formed by an outpouching of the synovial membrane from a joint or tendon sheath and contain thick jelly-like mucinous material similar in composition to synovial fluid. Sixty percent of ganglions occur on the dorsal aspect of the wrist, arising in the region of the scapholunate ligament. Other sites for ganglions to occur in the hand are at the volar wrist arising from one of the scaphoid articulations, the flexor tendon sheath at the area of the A1 pulley, and at the dorsum of the DIP joint (called a *mucous cyst*), where they are often associated with osteoarthritis of that DIP joint (Fig. 74-37). In the latter location, the ganglion cyst can exert pressure on the general matrix of the nail bed, resulting in a deformed or grooved nail.

Ganglions are most common in women in the third decade of life. They are innocuous and can often be left alone. However, treatment may be required for cosmetic purposes or to relieve pressure effects on adjacent structures. The dorsal wrist ganglion can sometimes be quite painful as a result of pressure on the posterior interosseous nerve at that location. A very small impalpable dorsal wrist ganglion can become quite painful, the so-called occult ganglion, and on occasion may be best diagnosed by MRI. Treatment of dorsal wrist ganglions may be performed by aspiration of the mucinous substance with a large-bore needle. If this fails, the ganglion can then be surgically excised. Care must be taken to trace and resect the pedicle of the ganglion all the way down to the joint or tendon sheath from which it arises. A volar wrist ganglion may often be closely related to the radial artery. Aspiration of volar wrist ganglions is seldom advised because of potential risk for injury to the radial artery. At the level of the DIP joint, optimal treatment includes not only meticulous excision of the ganglion but also removal of associated osteophytes from the joint. Arthroscopic decompression of dorsal wrist ganglions has been described.[36]

Giant Cell Tumor

Giant cell tumor is also called *pigmented villonodular synovitis* (PVNS). It is the second most common hand tumor and also arises from synovial membrane of joints or tendon sheaths. It is yellow-brown in color and histologically contains multinucleated giant cells. Giant cell tumors can envelope digital neurovascular structures and extend along tendon sheaths. The tumor is benign and often asymptomatic. Its large size can produce notching of adjacent bones by pressure. Treatment is surgical excision. There is a reported local recurrence rate that may be as high as 10%. If necessary, the tumor is pursued into the joint from which it might seem to arise, and a synovectomy of that joint may be necessary.

Epidermal Inclusion Cysts

Epidermal inclusion cysts are also known as *implantation dermoids* and occur after trauma. Epidermal cells become lodged in the subcutaneous tissue and form a cystic mass containing a thick toothpaste-like material made of desquamated cells. They occur more commonly in men, especially in manual laborers, and most frequently involve the palm of the hand and the fingertips. They may also occur in previous surgical scars. Treatment is surgical excision, and recurrence is rare.

Lipoma

Lipomas occur most commonly on the thenar eminence. They are often painless but may become symptomatic by compression on adjacent nerves. They may reach a large size and insinuate into the deep palmar spaces. Treatment is by resection.

Pyogenic Granuloma

Pyogenic granuloma is a misnomer for an exuberant outburst of highly vascular granulation tissue at the site of previous relatively trivial trauma. These lesions are very friable, bleed easily, and may grow rapidly. They respond to either curettage or simple excision. They occur most commonly on the fingertips.

Verruca Vulgaris

Verrucae vulgaris are viral warts associated with human papillomavirus. They most commonly occur on the digits as hyperkeratotic lesions. They may also occur in the nail bed region. They may be treated by topical chemicals, oral cimetidine, cryotherapy, and duct tape but are most effectively treated by curettage. They may occur especially in immunocompromised patients such as after transplantations. In such patients, they may be at multiple digital sites. Recurrence is relatively common.[37]

Vascular Malformations and Hemangiomas

Hemangiomas are hamartomas. They have a rapid growth phase in the first year of life (although most are not present at birth) and histologically show endothelial mitotic activity and increased mast cell counts. Most hemangiomas involve by age 7 years, and therapeutic intervention is seldom required. By contrast, vascular malformations show normal endothelial growth characteristics and normal mast cell counts, grow commensurately with the child, are present at birth, and do not undergo spontaneous involution. Vascular malformations are subclassified according to flow dynamics. Capillary, venous, and lymphatic elements predominate in low-flow lesions. Arteries and arteriovenous fistulas predominate in high-flow lesions and may grow to large proportions, at which stage they are difficult to treat surgically because the hemodynamic characteristics may simply open up more proximal arteriovenous connections after excision.

Lymphaticovenous malformations may also be associated with generalized hypertrophy of an extremity. Compression garments can be tried but give unpredictable results, although may be helpful symptomatically. Vascular malformations may cause pain as a result of vascular engorgement, or thrombosis with phlebitis. Large size can hamper hand function. Embolization has been described with mixed reports.[38] Surgical debulking may on occasion be required.[39]

CONGENITAL ANOMALIES

The causes of congenital hand anomalies may be genetic, teratogenic, or idiopathic and may also have syndromic association with anomalies elsewhere in the body. Knowledge of these associations is important because frequently the more life-threatening associated problems need to be treated first before the hand and upper extremity reconstruction can be performed. Such an association is found in a constellation of problems that occur in the VACTERL association of congenital defects (*v*ertebral anomalies, *a*nal atresia, *c*ardiac abnormalities, *t*racheoesophageal fistula, *r*enal agenesis, and *l*imb anomalies). A number of factors must be considered in optimizing the timing of each surgical procedure to the upper extremity, including the psychosocial development of the child, the presence of other illnesses, the size of the structures to be operated on, and the normal growth and development of the hand. Modern technologic advances allow us to operate on smaller structures; the timing of the procedure can now be guided by our knowledge of the anatomy and development of the growing hand. Optimal function is the primary goal of surgery. Principles of management of congenital hand anomalies recognize that infant immunity to infection develops over time, that early surgery prevents the emotional scarring associated with a child's awareness of the deformity, and that some congenital problems may not be apparent in the neonate. The hand surgeon must work closely with the pediatrician to identify general conditions that may affect the child's health. Some congenital anomalies of the extremities, especially those with the radial ray, may be associated with bone marrow failure (Fanconi's syndrome) or heart defects that may not be immediately apparent in the neonate. Children with congenital anomalies will attempt to keep up with their peers and often develop successful hand substitution techniques. However, once a child experiences the cruel ridicule of playmates or the unintentional but sometimes overly solicitous supervision of a teacher, his or her deformity becomes very important. Generally plans for surgical reconstruction are designed to be completed by school age, so that the child may adapt to and fully use the reconstructed limb.[40]

The rationale for early surgery includes the avoidance of deformity and malfunction and the optimal use of infantile tissue plasticity. Because hand length nearly doubles during the first 2 years of life, a digit tethered to another digit that fails to grow can produce a major deformity during the early growth spurt. Thus, for example, with separation of syndactyly that involves the border digits of the hand, because of adjacent tethering to a digit of unequal length, surgical separation of the syndactyly is required at an early age, as early as 6 months, to avoid secondary angular deformity of the digits.

In rare circumstances, urgent treatment in the neonate is required. The distal lymphedema of a severe constriction band syndrome may be so marked as to inhibit function totally or even threaten distal viability. This may require urgent release. The unusual clinical entity of aplasia cutis may result in exposure of vital structures, requiring urgent soft tissue coverage, even in the neonatal period.

Early operation, though not urgent, may be required not only because of the rapid growth that occurs in the first 2 years of life but also because of functional consequences. Surgery at a young age is considered mandatory in children with malformations in which hand function may be altered by surgery or in children who are at risk for developing certain grasping habits that would have to be unlearned after corrective surgery. An older child, 12 to 14 years of age, has developed grasp patterns that would have to be altered by prolonged periods of physical therapy after corrective surgery.[41,42]

The ability to place the upper limbs in space (a cortical function) and development of a strong grasp are established by 1 year of age, as are grasp and pinch maneuvers between the thumb and fingers. Accuracy of prehension and refinement of coordination continue until 3 years of age. Surgery must be performed early to allow the affected parts to develop differently when the function of the parts of the hand is altered by transposition (e.g., pollicization of an index finger for thumb aplasia). Duplicated thumb correction is carried out before 1 year of age, well in advance of the development of integrated thumb grasp patterns.

Finally, the physical ability of infant bone and soft tissues to adapt to change produced by surgery is also a key factor in deciding when to operate. In the early pollicization of the index finger, the first dorsal interosseous muscle hypertrophies to form a thenar eminence, and the first metacarpal (formerly the proximal phalanx of the index finger) broadens. If centralization of the wrist for radial dysplasia (formerly radial club hand) has been undertaken early, the head of the ulna broadens to resemble the distal end of the radius.

Thus, multiple issues are taken into consideration when deciding on the optimum time for surgical reconstruction for congenital hand and upper extremity anomalies. Among the more common hand anomalies are syndactyly, polydactyly, constriction band syndrome, and absent or hypoplastic thumb.

Syndactyly results from failure of programmed cell death (apoptosis) between the individual finger rays. Consequently, there is a resulting fusion of adjacent digits. It can involve part or all of the length of the digits (incomplete or complete) and may be limited to skin and soft tissue only (simple syndactyly) or can also involve skeletal fusion (complex syndactyly). Apert's syndrome also involves craniofacial anomalies and is a severe form of bilaterally symmetric complex syndactyly. Surgical treatment involves digit separation using a local flap to reconstruct the depths of the commissure between the fingers and release of the finger borders with zigzag incisions and use of full-thickness skin grafts (Fig. 74-38A).

Polydactyly is the presence of extranumerary digits on the hand. Preaxial (radial) polydactyly involves the thumb. It is not as common as postaxial (ulnar) polydactyly, which is the most frequent congenital hand anomaly occurring amongst African Americans. Polydactyly can be as simple as the presence of a skin tag–like structure or may have a complex arrangement of shared vessels, nerves, and bones. Thumb polydactyly is not merely a duplication, but is a splitting of a single digit with vari-

able degrees of development in each of the separate parts. It is typically classified into seven subtypes using the Wassel classification. This classification is based on the specific duplication progressing from distal to proximal. Type IV is the most common type, with total duplication of proximal and distal phalanges and a shared metacarpophalangeal joint. Type VII refers to associated triphalangia with a duplication. Reconstructive goals include stabilization without sacrificing mobility, proper alignment of joints along the longitudinal axis of the thumb, balanced motor units, and a cosmetically acceptable nail plate (see Fig. 74-38B, C).

The Blauth classification categorizes thumb hypoplasia as type I, which represents minor hypoplasia, to type V, which is a total thumb absence. Surgical correction ranges from reconstruction of the existing hypoplastic thumb to pollicization (creating a thumb from the index finger) for a complete absence or the more severe types of hypoplasia (Fig. 74-39).

Clinodactyly is a curving of the digits in a radial or ulnar direction. It is common, particularly involving the little finger in many individuals, but a curvature of greater than 10 degrees is considered abnormal. The distal phalanx is most commonly affected, and a delta phalanx may be associated. A delta phalanx occurs when the epiphysis forms a C shape around the metaphyseal core in the middle phalanx. Most cases present little or no functional or cosmetic deformity, and operative intervention is seldom required. If there is a functionally impairing deviation of the finger, corrective osteotomy can be done.

Camptodactyly is a congenital flexion deformity of digits. It occurs most commonly in the little finger PIP joint. The exact cause is unclear, and the etiology has been attributed to a variety of different structures around the PIP joint, including a skin pterygium, collateral ligaments, volar plate, flexor tendon, abnormal insertions of lumbrical and interosseous muscles, and the size and shape of the head of the proximal phalanx. Treatment is most commonly nonoperative and may involve serial splinting. Should no improvement occur and if the flexion deformity is sufficient to cause a functional problem, surgical intervention may be required, which includes correction of the deformity with Z-plasty and possibly grafts. One author reported that all of his patients who had reconstructive surgery on one hand did not ask for corrective surgery on an opposite affected hand.

Constriction band syndrome is secondary to intrauterine amniotic bands (see Fig. 74-38D). These can act like tourniquets and threaten the viability of digits and even limbs, resulting in congenital amputation. Infants may suffer from a similar problem from the external ligature effect of cotton strands coming off protective booties and even from a human hair. This is termed the *hair-thread-tourniquet syndrome*.

OSTEOARTHRITIS AND RHEUMATOID ARTHRITIS

Osteoarthritis may be primary or post-traumatic (secondary). Primary osteoarthritis is a degenerative joint disease

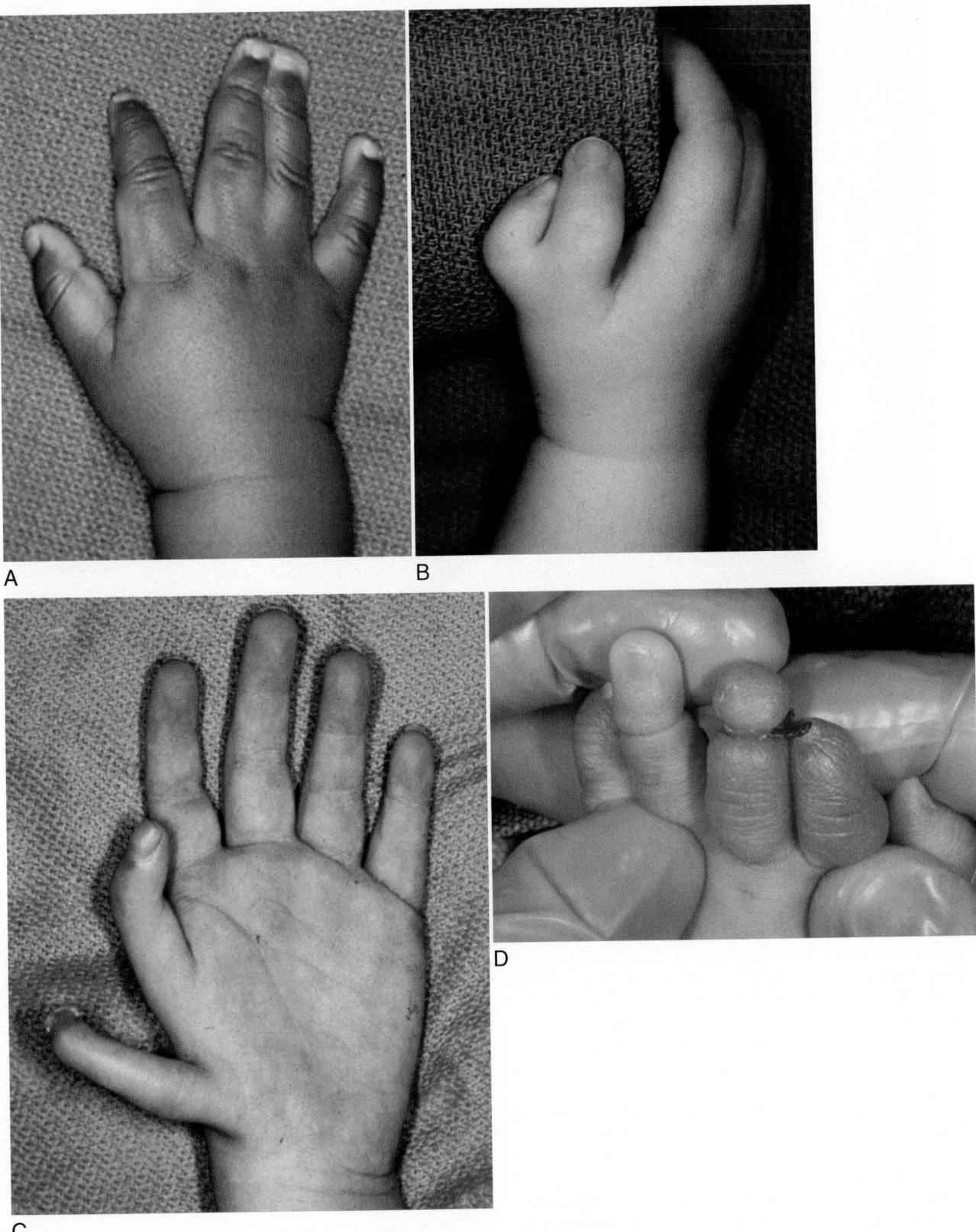

Figure 74-38 Some congenital hand anomalies include syndactyly (**A**), Wassel type IV thumb polydactyly (**B**), Wassel type VI polydactyly (**C**), and constriction band (**D**).

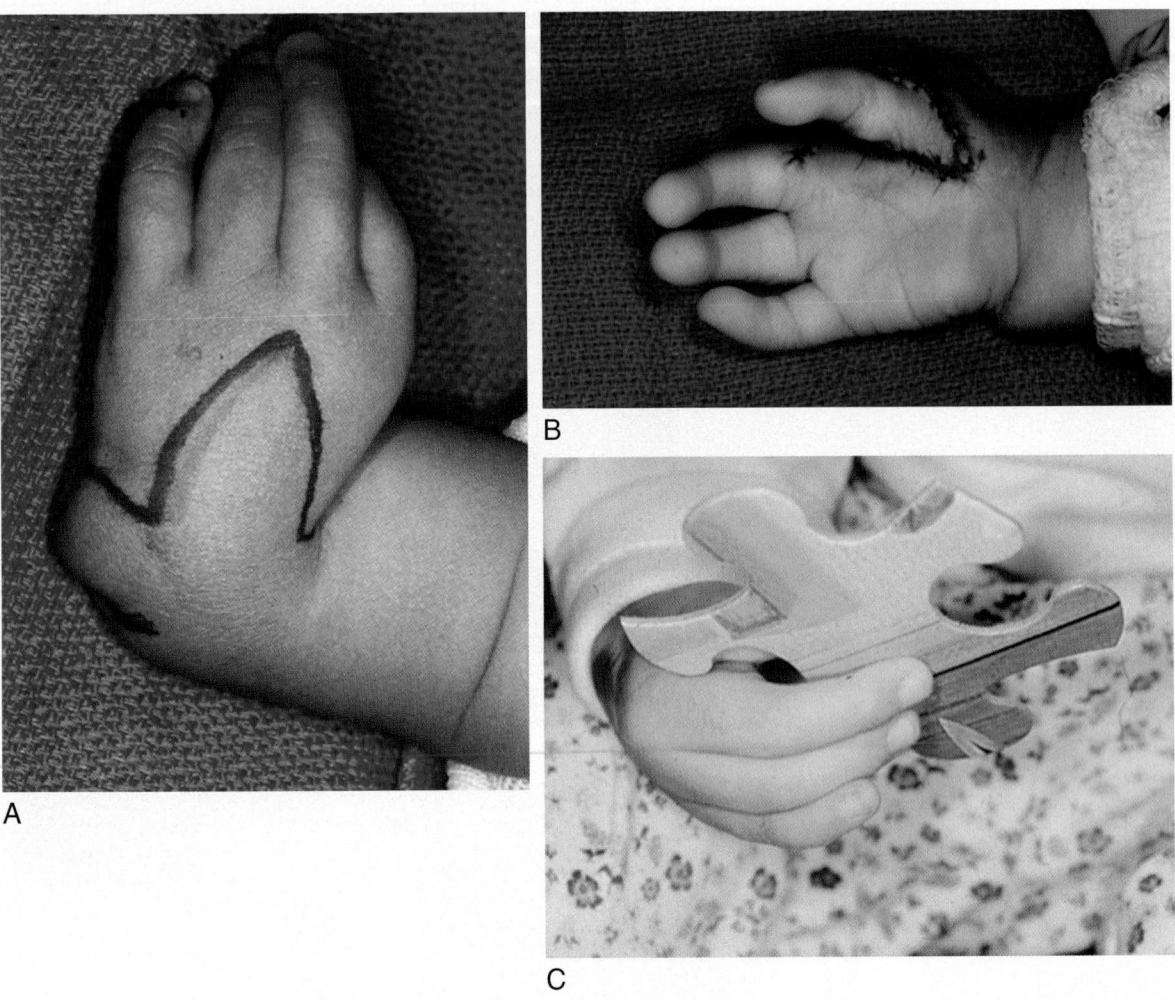

A

B

C

Figure 74-39 A, Patient with radial dysplasia and absent thumb. **B,** After centralization of the wrist on the distal ulna, pollicization of the index finger is performed. **C,** Natural prehension has been restored to this three-finger hand with a reconstructed wrist and thumb.

occurring in later life. An injury that leaves articular surfaces of a joint incongruous can precipitate secondary osteoarthritis. Osteoarthritis begins with biochemical alteration of the water content of articular cartilage. The cartilage weakens and develops cracks (called *fibrillation*). Progressive erosion and thinning of the cartilage results, and the subchondral bone becomes sclerotic (termed *eburnation*). New bone forms around the edges of the articular cartilage, and these outcroppings are call *osteophytes* (Fig. 74-40).

The joints most commonly affected in the hand are the DIP and PIP joints of the fingers and the carpometacarpal joint at the base of the thumb. Osteophytes at the DIP joint are called *Heberden's nodes,* and those at the PIP joint are *Bouchard's nodes.* The involved joints may be painful, stiff, deformed, or subluxated. Radiographs reveal narrowing of the joint space, sclerosis of subchondral bone, and presence of osteophytes.

Initial treatment may be symptomatic and include splinting and even local corticosteroid injections. Nonsteroidal anti-inflammatory medications may be helpful, and

chondroprotective medications such as glucosamine and chondroitin sulfate have demonstrated ability to reduce symptoms. In advanced cases, the DIP joints respond best to arthrodesis. The PIP joints may be surgically treated by replacement arthroplasty or by means of arthrodesis (Fig. 74-41). The thumb carpometacarpal joint may be treated by arthrodesis, which is favored particularly in the young patient who might have post-traumatic arthritis following, for example, an improperly treated Bennett's or Orlando's fracture. In an older patient with primary osteoarthritis at the thumb base, excision of the trapezium followed by tendon suspension (interposition) arthroplasty may be preferred. This uses local tendons for construction of a sling arthroplasty with interposition of tendon material.

Rheumatoid arthritis is an autoimmune process by which destruction of the musculoskeletal system may occur. Synovial inflammation results in pain, joint destruction, tendon ruptures, and characteristic deformities. Some of the more common deformities associated with rheumatoid arthritis include a swan neck deformity

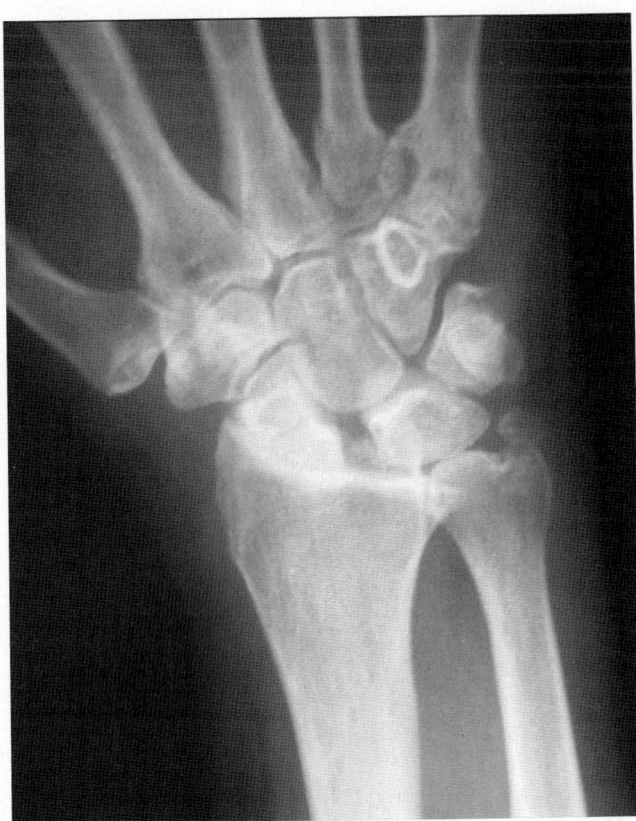

Figure 74-40 Radiograph of a patient with scapholunate advanced collapse wrist showing post-traumatic osteoarthritis at the radioscaphoid junction. This is many years after a wrist "sprain" in which the scapholunate ligament was torn; there is a wide scapholunate gap visible on radiograph.

(hyperextension of the PIP joint with concurrent flexion at the DIP joint), a boutonniere deformity (flexion at the PIP joint with concurrent hyperextension at the DIP joint), joint subluxation, radial deviation of the wrist, and ulnar deviation and flexion of the fingers (Fig. 74-42). Rheumatoid arthritis is primarily a medical illness for which multiple medications are currently available. For this reason, excellent lines of communication must exist with the rheumatologist and the surgeon. Nonsteroidal anti-inflammatory drugs are used, as well as the newer disease-modifying antirheumatoid drugs. Rheumatoid arthritis is a progressive disorder, and ongoing slow destruction may be anticipated despite surgery (Fig. 74-43). Some of the more common surgical procedures include joint synovectomy, tenosynovectomy, tendon transfers, joint replacements (especially at the MP and PIP joints), and arthrodesis (more commonly at the wrist and thumb MP joint).[43]

CONTRACTURES

Volkmann's ischemic contracture develops as a result of myofascial contractures in response to prolonged ischemia. This most common contracture results from unat-

tended compartment syndrome of the forearm and hand. The muscles necrose and become replaced by fibrous scar tissue. The FDP and FPL muscles are most commonly affected, being in the deepest forearm volar compartment, and digits are characteristically flexed with passive extension of the wrist worsening the flexion deformity of the digits. Intrinsic contractures can occur in the hand, and these are tested by Bunnell's test, in which passive extension of the MP joint makes passive flexion of the PIP joint more difficult.

In the milder forms of Volkmann's ischemic contracture, serial splinting and passive stretching exercises may resolve the problem. In more severe contractures, Z-type lengthening of tendons may be required, and a flexor pronator muscle slide, in which subperiosteal elevation of the common flexor origin from the medial epicondyle of the humerus and also from the ulna, allows the muscles to slide distally until the contracture is corrected. In the most severe form, all the muscles of the volar forearm may be affected, requiring tendon transfers, even microvascular functional muscle transfers to provide some functional return.

Post-traumatic contractures are by far the most common type of contracture. These can be prevented by appropriate treatment of the primary injury and especially with attention to detail in the manner in which the hand and upper extremity are splinted and immobilized. Once contractures have developed, if they are mild, they may be able to be stretched out by exercises and hand therapy. If these contractures are severe and functionally deforming, surgical release of joint contractures and release of tendon adhesions may be required.

Dupuytren's contracture is a disease process of contracting collagen affecting the palmar fascia, which can also affect the dorsum of the fingers (knuckle pads), soles of the feet, and penis (Peyronie's disease). It is thought to be a hereditary mendelian dominant disorder and is bilateral in 65% of cases. It is six times more frequent in males and predominantly involves the ring and little fingers (Fig. 74-44).

The process of Dupuytren's contracture occurs in the normal bands of collagen tissue that form the palmar fascia, natatory ligaments, and digital sheaths. Nodules containing myofibroblasts and immature collagen (type III) develop either in these tissues or in the dermis. The nodules progressively increase in size, leading to thickened contractures and shortened fascial bands that develop into cords extending up the digits. Treatment is surgical excision and is indicated in metacarpophalangeal contractures of 30 degrees or more (when the patient fails the so-called tabletop test and cannot place the palm of the hand flat on a surface) and whenever there is a PIP joint contracture. Careful surgical technique is necessary to avoid complications such as skin necrosis, hematoma, and digital nerve injuries. Collagenase injections using enzyme derived from *Clostridium histolyticum* have been attempted and show some promise in the treatment of Dupuytren's contracture. However, long-term follow-up in patients who had these injections is still required.[44-46]

Text continued on p 2196

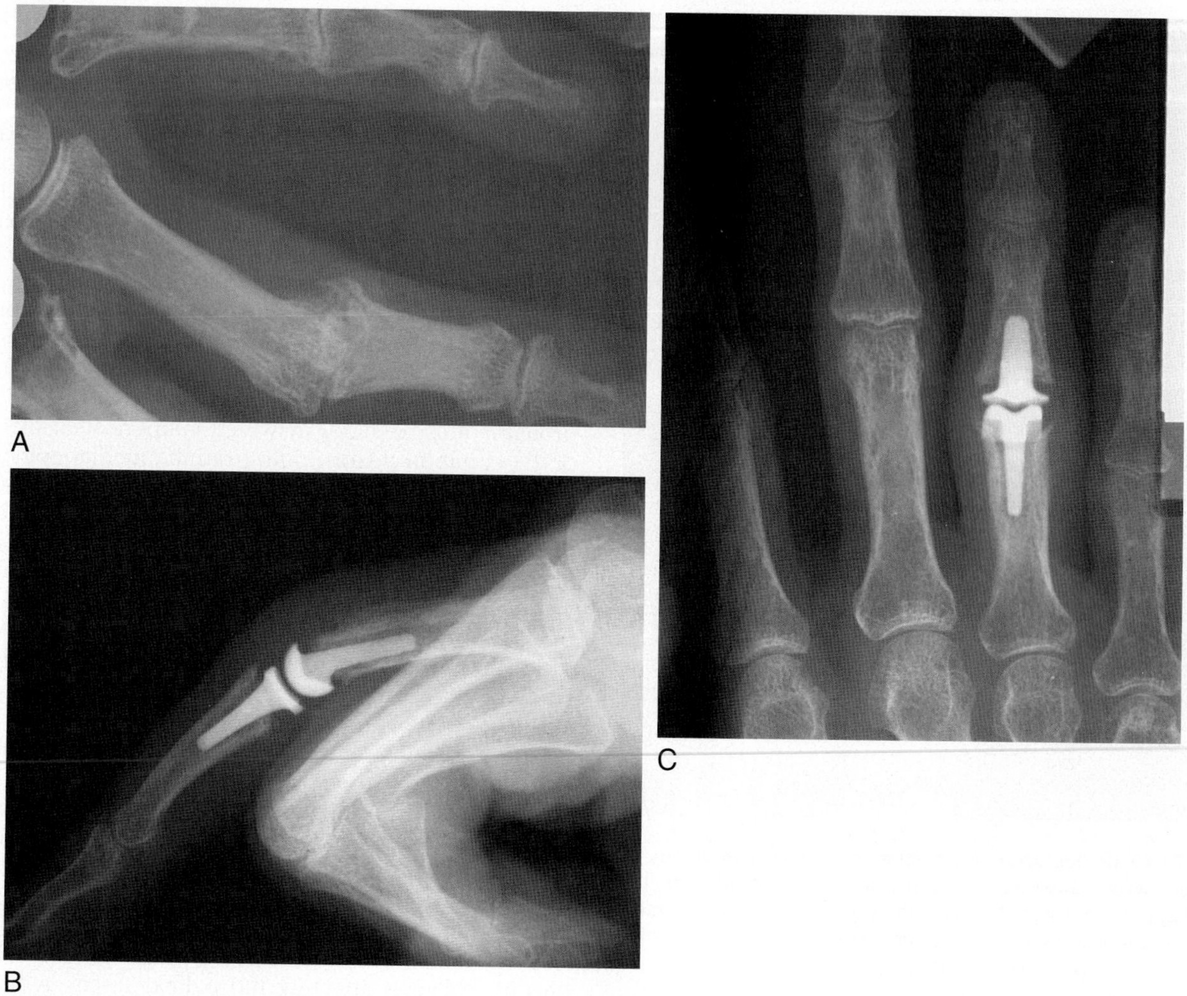

A

B

C

Figure 74-41 A, Patient with painful and unstable proximal interphalangeal joint from osteoarthritis. **B** and **C,** Reconstruction is performed by implant arthroplasty. An advantage over arthrodesis is that motion is retained, although there remains a potential for future recurrent joint instability and wear of the artificial joint.

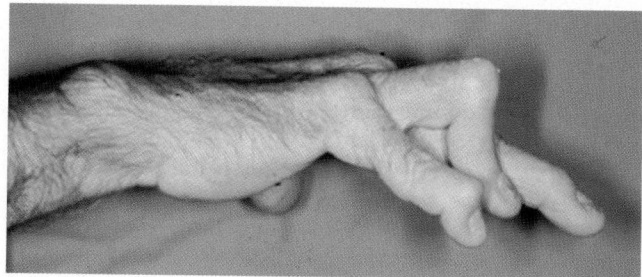

Figure 74-42 Patient with inflammatory arthritis has both boutonniere deformity and swan neck deformity on the same hand.

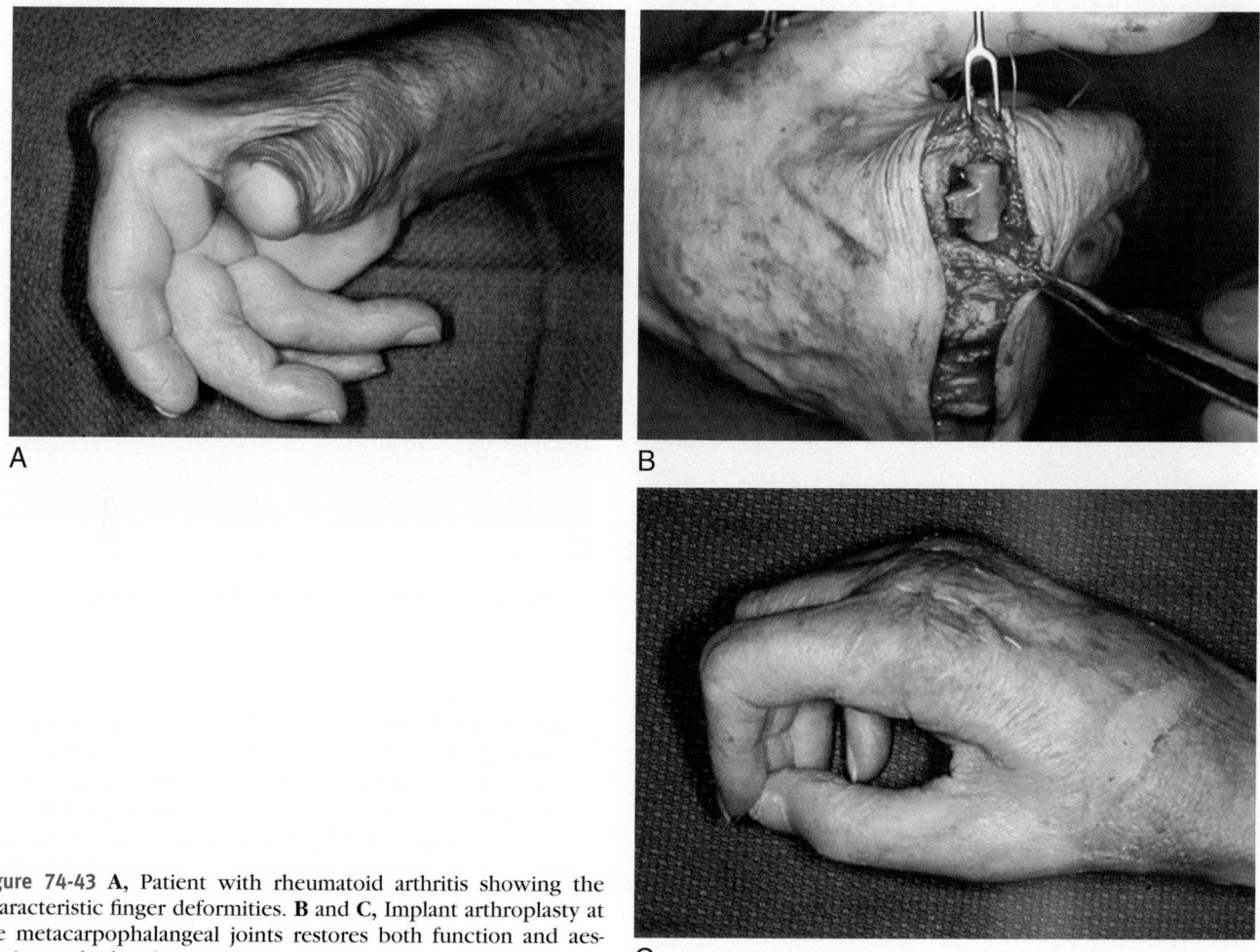

Figure 74-43 A, Patient with rheumatoid arthritis showing the characteristic finger deformities. **B** and **C,** Implant arthroplasty at the metacarpophalangeal joints restores both function and aesthetics to the hand.

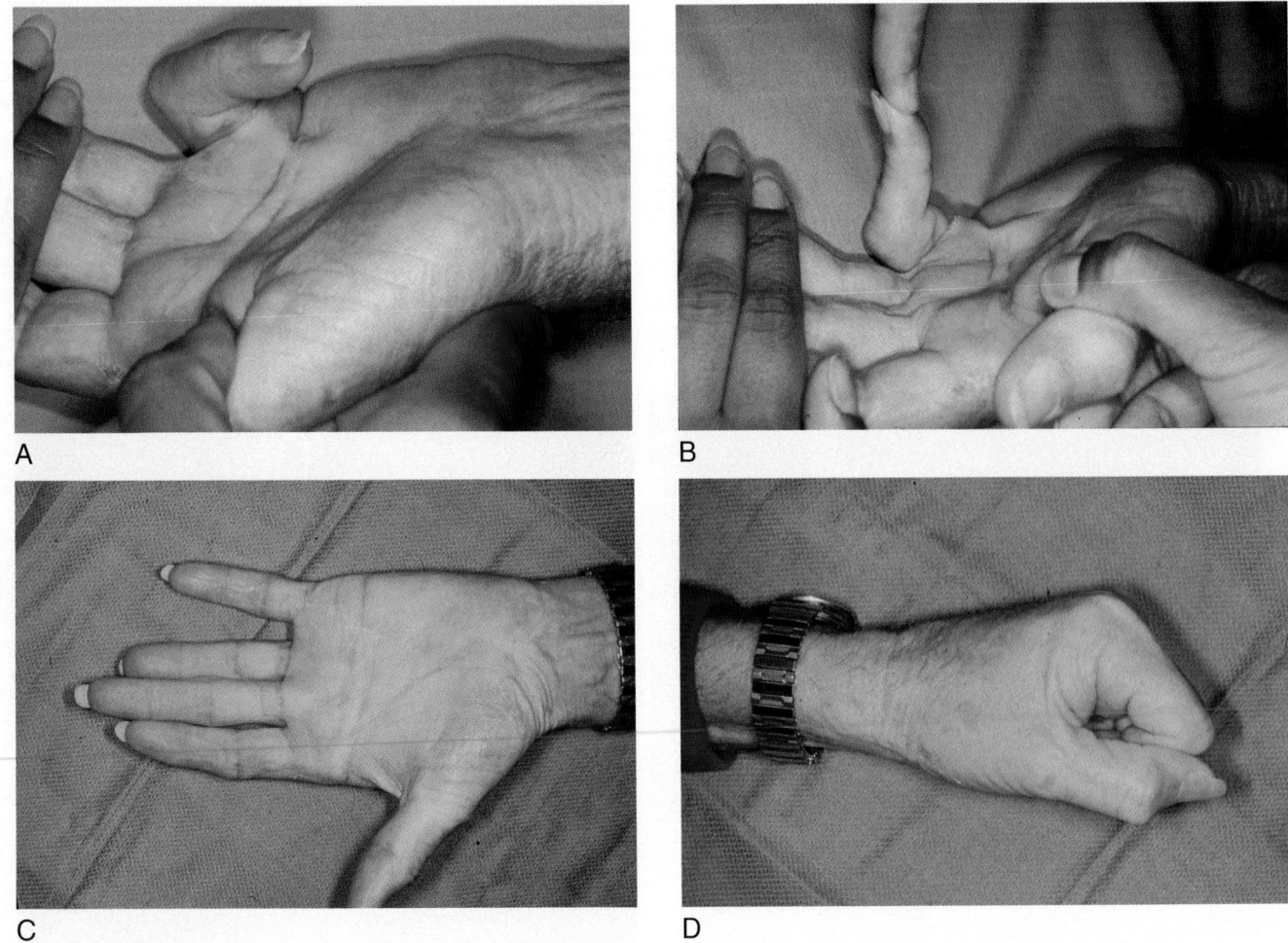

Figure 74-44 A to **D,** Patient with Dupuytren's contracture is treated by regional palmar and digital fasciectomy, and good hand function is restored.

CONCLUSION

The specialty of hand surgery is exhaustive, and multiple specialty textbooks on the subject are available. Although general surgeons may be responsible for the basic tenets of hand surgery, knowledge of minute details is often not necessary, and thus, most details have been omitted from this chapter because the purpose of the chapter is to see the big picture in regard to hand surgery. Those topics of hand surgery with which the general surgeon is most likely to be confronted have been emphasized, particularly with regard to knowledge of anatomy, physical examination, and emergency treatments. Taking this into consideration, Table 74-5 includes some high-yield facts relevant to hand surgery that have been compiled from various general surgery review books as well as topics discussed on the ABSITE. A list of these facts is added for the convenience of general surgeons preparing for ABSITE or board examinations (Table 74-5).

Table 74-5 Board Review Topics

TOPIC	ANSWER
Fracture of the distal radius	Injury to the median nerve
Innervation of the flexor digitorum profundus (FDP) to the ring and small fingers	Ulnar nerve
Injury to the ulnar nerve at the elbow	Weakness in abduction and adduction of the index through small digits
Midshaft humeral fracture	Associated with radial nerve injury
Distal phalanx fractures	>50% of all hand fractures
Joint involved in Bennett's fracture	Carpometacarpal (CMC) joint of the thumb
Common name for a metacarpal fracture of the small finger	Boxer's fracture
Most frequently fractured carpal bone	Scaphoid
Complications associated with displaced fractures of the scaphoid	Avascular necrosis and nonunion
Axonal nerve growth rate	1 mm/day
Common maximum intraoperative tourniquet time in hand surgery	2 hr
Single digits that are primarily replanted	Thumbs in adults and children, all digits whenever possible in children
Maximal period of anoxia compatible with replantation	Finger—8 hours (warm ischemia), but longer times have been anecdotally reported Upper/lower extremity—6 hr
Proper method for transportation of an amputated body part to maximize replantation success	Cleaned of debris, wrapped in a sterile towel or gauze, moistened with sterile lactated Ringer's solution, placed in a sterile plastic bag, and transported in an insulated cooler with ice water (ideal temperature, 4°C)
Complications if nerve repair is delayed >2 wk	Retraction of the nerve's ends resulting in the need for nerve grafting
Zone 2/"no man's land"	Area of flexor tendon injury between the metacarpal phalangeal (MCP) and flexor digitorum superficialis (FDS) insertion
Mallet finger	Injury to the extensor mechanism at the level of the distal interphalangeal (DIP) joint
Gamekeeper's thumb	Rupture of the ulnar collateral ligament of the thumb MCP joint with resultant instability of the joint to radial-directed force
Most common organism resulting in hand infections	*Staphylococcus aureus*
Classic symptoms of carpal tunnel syndrome	Paresthesias in the median nerve distribution often waking the patient at night
Most effective therapy for full-thickness burns of the hand	Early excision and grafting
Most common location of ganglion cysts	Scapholunate interosseous ligament at the dorsal wrist
Treatment of de Quervain's stenosing tenosynovitis after failed nonoperative management	Surgical release of the first extensor compartment
Etiology of trigger fingers	Stenosing tenosynovitis in the region of the MCP joint/A1 pulley
Late findings of rheumatoid arthritis	Subluxation of involved joints resulting in deformity
Swan neck deformity	Hyperextension of the proximal interphalangeal (PIP) joint with flexion of the DIP joint
Boutonniere deformity	Flexion of the PIP joint with hyperextension of the DIP
Nonoperative measures of Dupuytren's contracture	Exercise, local steroid injections, collagenase injections, and radiotherapy
Digits most commonly affected in Dupuytren's contracture	Ring and small fingers
Etiology of Dupuytren's contracture	Proliferation and fibrosis of the palmar fascia
Fractures likely to cause compartment syndrome/Volkmann's ischemic contracture	Supracondylar fracture of the humerus
Artery and nerve compromised in Volkmann's ischemic contracture	Median nerve and anterior interosseous artery
Complication of cast placement for supracondylar fractures of the humerus	Volkmann's ischemic contracture

Selected References

General

Omer, GE: Development of hand surgery: Education of hand surgeons. J Hand Surg [Am] 25:616-628, 2000.

This article traces the development of hand surgery from the publication of Kanavel's classic book on infections of the hand, published in 1916, through the recognition of the specialty of hand surgery, to the training of modern-day hand surgeons and their educational requirements. The article is peppered with historical vignettes and mentions many giants in hand surgery.

Soft Tissue

Foucher G, Khouri RK: Digital reconstruction with island flaps. Clin Plast Surg 24:1-32, 1997.

New knowledge of the "intrinsic flaps" of the hand enables ingenious soft tissue reconstructions using local tissues from the hand and fingers as pedicled, vascularized, island flaps. A thorough knowledge of the vasculature of the hand is required outside of that published in standard anatomy texts.

Godina M: Early microsurgical reconstruction of complex trauma of the extremities. Plast Reconstr Surg 78:285-292, 1986.

This paper emphasizes the concept of primary repair and reconstruction of all damaged tissues (including microvascular soft tissue coverage) acutely following major trauma.

Martin D, Bakhach J, Casoli V, et al: Reconstruction of the hand with forearm island flaps. Clin Plast Surg 24:33-48, 1997.

Knowledge of the vascular anatomy of the forearm enables an array of pedicled flaps to be performed for soft tissue reconstruction of the hand, thus avoiding the need to employ microvascular anastomoses.

Flexor Tendons

Hunter JM, Salisbury RE: Flexor tendon reconstruction in severely damaged hands: A two stage procedure using a silicone Dacron reinforced gliding prosthesis prior to tendon grafting. J Bone Joint Surg 53:829-858, 1971.

This paper introduces the concept of two-stage flexor tendon repair in cases in which the flexor tendon sheath is scarred in a late repair. A tendon spacer is placed as a preliminary procedure to later tendon grafting. This remains a time honored way of dealing with late flexor tendon reconstructions.

Kleinert H, Kutz JE, Atasoy E, Stormo A: Primary repair of flexor tendons. Orthop Clin North Am 4:865-876, 1973.

This article was the first substantive evidence that flexor tendons could be safely and effectively repaired in "no man's land," emphasizing the importance of postoperative controlled mobilization of the fingers.

Strickland JW: Development of flexor tendon surgery: Twenty-five years of progress. J Hand Surg 25:214-235, 2000.

This excellent review article describes the current state of the art for treatment of flexor tendon injuries.

Nerve Injuries

Millesi H, Meissel G, Berger A: The interfascicular nerve-grafting of the median and ulnar nerves. J Bone Joint Surg 54:727-750, 1972.

This landmark article emphasizes the importance of tension-free nerve repair, matching of proximal and distal fascicular groups, and the use of nerve grafts in cases of a large nerve gap injury.

Lundborg G: A 25 year perspective of peripheral nerve surgery: Evolving neuroscientific concepts and classical significance. J Hand Surg 25:391-414, 2000.

This excellent article establishes the experimental basis and neuroscience behind nerve repair and nerve regeneration. The rationale for nerve conduits is discussed. The future holds exciting prospects.

Weber RV, Mackinnon S: Nerve transfers in the upper extremity. J Am Soc Surg Hand 4:200-213, 2004.

The innovative use of nerve transfers is described to bypass and overcome long nerve gaps following nerve injury to hasten and improve functional recovery.

Replantation

Buncke HJ: Microvascular hand surgery—transplants and replants—over the past 25 years. J Hand Surg 25:415-428, 2000.

This article traces the history of microvascular surgery as it applies to the upper extremity and outlines many of the milestones achieved. Its value also lies in the potential myriad microvascular reconstructive options that are available for free tissue transfer and microvascular toe-to-hand transfers. It also evaluates potential anticipated survival and functional outcome for replantation surgery.

Fractures

Stern PJ: Management of fractures of the hand over the last 25 years. J Hand Surg 25:817-823, 2000.

Fluoroscopic imaging has greatly facilitated operative management of hand fractures. The evolution from Kirschner wires to plates and screws is discussed. New innovations include self-tapping screws, low-profile plates, and cannulated screws with the goal of achieving rigid bone fixation to enable restoration of early digital motion to minimize the risk for tendon adhesions and joint contractures.

Russe O: Fracture of the carpal navicular: Diagnosis, non-operative, and operative treatment. J Bone Joint Surg [Am] 42:759-768, 1960.

Although new innovations of cannulated compression screw and minimally invasive surgery have changed the management of scaphoid fractures, this manuscript has stood the test of time and laid the foundation for modern understanding and treatment of scaphoid fractures and their complications.

Infections

Kanavel AB: An anatomical, experimental, and clinical study of acute phlegmons of the hand. Surg Gynecol Obstet 1:221-259, 1905.

This is a classic paper that describes the anatomic spaces of the hand. It changed the course of infection treatment and also saw the origins of hand surgery. The clinical outcome was changed from amputation to surgical management that preserved function of structures, emphasizing that hand surgery is founded in a sound knowledge of anatomy. The basic principles of this article, written in the preantibiotic era, remain as true today as they were then.

Compartment Syndrome

Mubarak SJ, Hargens AR: Acute compartment syndromes. Surg Clin North Am 63:539-565, 1983.

This excellent article describes the pathogenesis of acute compartment syndrome, including the diagnosis and surgical management in the upper extremity.

Entrapment Neuropathy

Koo JT, Szabo RM: Compression neuropathies of the median nerve. J Am Soc Surg Hand 4:156-175, 2004.

This comprehensive article gives excellent anatomic descriptions of all the anatomic sites in the upper extremity where chronic compression of the median nerve can occur. Nonsurgical and surgical management guidelines are outlined for each.

Phalen GS: The carpal-tunnel syndrome: Seventeen years' experience in diagnosis and treatment of six hundred fifty-four hands. J Bone Joint Surg 48:211-228, 1966.

This is a classic paper written by a founder and past president of the American Society for Surgery of the Hand. This article gives an understanding of median nerve compression at the wrist that is surgically treated simply by decompression and release of the transverse carpal ligament. The most common procedure performed by hand surgeons today is median nerve decompression.

Vascular Tumors

Mulliken JB, Glowacki J: Hemangioma and vascular malformations in infants and children: A classification based on endothelial characteristics. Plast Reconstr Surg 69:412-422, 1982.

The authors attempt to unify the classification of hemangiomas and vascular malformations. Suggested classifications fall into six broad categories: embryology, histology, clinical features, dynamics of growth, hemodynamic patterns, and cell biology. A classification is useful only if it has diagnostic applicability and aids in planning therapy and in understanding of the pathogenesis.

Congenital

McCarroll HR: Congenital anomalies: A 25 year overview. J Hand Surg [Am] 25:1007-1037, 2000.

This excellent review identifies the more commonly treated congenital hand anomalies. It also identifies some of the newer developments in surgical treatment to include distraction lengthening, pollicization, microvascular surgery, and the potential for in utero interventions. Useful classifications for treatment management are provided.

Netscher DT, Scheker LR: Timing and decision making in the treatment of congenital upper extremity deformities. Clin Plast Surg 17:113-131, 1990.

This review describes commonly treated congenital hand anomalies and provides a rational basis for timing of surgical interventions to meet critical hand functional milestones.

Osteoarthritis

Burton RI, Pellegrini VD: Surgical management of basal joint arthritis of the thumb. Part II. Ligament reconstruction with tendon interposition arthroplasty. J Hand Surg [Am] 11:324-332, 1986.

An excellent description of the pathogenesis and surgical management of basilar joint osteoarthritis of the thumb. This is the most commonly performed surgical procedure for carpometacarpal joint osteoarthritis of the thumb.

Eaton RG, Littler JW: Ligament reconstruction for the painful thumb carpometacarpal joint. J Bone Joint Surg [Am] 55:1655-1666, 1973.

One of the most common joints affected by osteoarthritis is at the base of the thumb. This operation originally described by Eaton and Littler for surgical management forms the basis of surgical treatment today with few modifications in technique and has stood the test of time.

Rheumatoid Arthritis

Swanson AB: Flexible implant arthroplasty for arthritic finger joints: Rationale, technique, and results of treatment. J Bone Joint Surg [Am] 54:435-455, 1972.

A landmark article that changed the course of treatment for rheumatoid arthritis. In this paper, Swanson introduced small joint arthroplasty.

Contractures

Curtis RM: Capsulectomy of the interphalangeal joints of the fingers. J Bone Joint Surg [Am] 36:1219-1232, 1954.

This classic article changed the course of treatment of the stiff hand. Curtis kindled interest in the complex anatomy of the proximal interphalangeal joint. He was meticulous in his technique and insisted on rigid postoperative therapy.

McFarlane RM: Patterns of the diseased fascia in the fingers in Dupuytren's contracture: Displacement of the neurovascular bundle. Plast Reconstr Surg 54:31-44, 1974.

This article clearly outlines the pathology, anatomy, and proposed surgical treatment for Dupuytren's contracture. The author describes the patterns of diseased fascia in the palm and fingers and how displacement of the digital neurovascular bundle may occur.

References

1. Idler RS, Manktelow RT: The Hand: Primary Care of Common Problems, 2nd ed. Philadelphia, Churchill Livingstone, 1990.
2. Kleinert HE, Jejurikar SS, Miller JH: Hand surgery. In Townsend CM, Beauchamp RD, Evers BM, et al (eds): Sabiston Textbook of Surgery. Philadelphia, WB Saunders, 2001, pp 1570-1588.
3. Green DP: Basic principles. In Green DP, Pederson WC, Hotchkiss RN, et al (eds): Green's Operative Hand Surgery. Philadelphia, Elsevier/Churchill Livingstone, 2005, pp 3-24.
4. Klenerman LA: Tourniquet time: How long? Hand 12:231-232, 1980.
5. Netscher DT, Cohen V: Phalangeal fractures. In Evans GRD (ed): Operative Plastic Surgery. New York, McGraw-Hill, 2000, pp 979-991.
6. Hunter JM, Salisbury RE: Flexor-tendon reconstruction in severely damaged hands. A two-stage procedure using a silicone-Dacron reinforced gliding prosthesis prior to tendon grafting. J Bone Joint Surg Am 53:829-858, 1971.
7. Tang JB, Zhang Y, Cao Y, et al: Core suture purchase affects strength of tendon repairs. J Hand Surg [Am] 30:1262-1266, 2005.
8. Boyer MI: Flexor tendon injuries. In Green DP, Pederson WC, Hotchkiss RN, et al (eds): Green's Operative Hand Surgery. Philadelphia, Elsevier/Churchill Livingstone, 2005, pp 219-240.
9. Netscher DT: Extensor tendon injuries. In Goldwyn RM, Cohen MN (eds): The Unfavorable Result in Plastic Surgery. Philadelphia, Lippincott Williams & Wilkins, 2001, pp 751-770.
10. Koman LA, Ruch DS, Smith BP: Vascular disorders. In Green DP, Pederson WC, Hotchkiss RN, et al (eds): Green's Operative Hand Surgery. Philadelphia, Elsevier/Churchill Livingstone, 2005, pp 2265-2313.
11. Idler RS, Manktelow RT: The Hand: Examination and Diagnosis, 3rd ed. Philadelphia, Churchill Livingstone, 1990.

12. Goldner RD, Urbaniak JR: Replantation. In Green's Operative Hand Surgery, Philadelphia, Elsevier/Churchill Livingstone, 2005, pp 1569-1586.

13. Soucacos PN: Indications and selection for digital amputation and replantation. J Hand Surg [Br] 26:572-581, 2001.

14. Stern PJ: Fractures of the metacarpals and phalanges. In Green DP, Pederson WC, Hotchkiss RN, et al (eds): Green's Operative Hand Surgery. Philadelphia, Elsevier/Churchill Livingstone, 2005, pp 277-342.

15. Netscher DT, Cohen MN: Metacarpals and phalanges. In Evans GRD (ed): Operative Plastic Surgery. New York, McGraw-Hill, 2000, pp 959-978.

16. Trumble TE: Hand fractures. In Trumble TE (ed): Principles of Hand Surgery and Therapy. Philadelphia, WB Saunders, 2000, pp 41-89.

17. Dye TM: Metacarpal fractures. Retrieved April 4, 2006, from http://www.emedicine.com/orthoped/topic193.htm.

18. Priano SV, Baratz ME: Bennett fracture. Retrieved April 7, 2006, from http://www.emedicine.com/orthoped/topic19.htm.

19. Walsh JJ: Rolando fracture. Retrieved April 6, 2006, from http://www.emedicine.com/orthoped/topic288.htm.

20. Kumar S, O'Connor A, Despois M, et al: Use of early magnetic resonance imaging in the diagnosis of occult scaphoid fractures: The CAST Study (Canberra Area Scaphoid Trial). N Z Med J 118:U1296, 2005.

21. Clark DC: Common acute hand infections. Am Fam Physician 68:2167-2176, 2003.

22. Stevanovic MV, Sharpe F: Acute infections in the hand. In Green DP, Pederson WC, Hotchkiss RN, et al (eds): Green's Operative Hand Surgery. Philadelphia, Elsevier/Churchill Livingstone, 2005, pp 55-93.

23. Rockwell PG: Acute and chronic paronychia. Am Fam Physician 63:1113-1116, 2001.

24. Trumble TE, Hashisaki P: Hand infections. In Trumble TE (ed): Principles of Hand Surgery and Therapy. Philadelphia, WB Saunders, 2000, pp 214-221.

25. Lille S, Hayakawa T, Neumeister MW, et al: Continuous postoperative catheter irrigation is not necessary for the treatment of suppurative flexor tenosynovitis. J Hand Surg [Br] 25:304-307, 2000.

26. Mollitt DL: Infection control: Avoiding the inevitable. Surg Clin North Am 82:365-378, 2002.

27. Kare JA: Volkmann contracture. Retrieved April 4, 2006, from http://www.emedicine.com/orthoped/topic578.htm.

28. Patel MR, Bassini L: Trigger fingers and thumb: When to splint, inject, or operate. J Hand Surg [Am] 17:110-113, 1992.

29. Trumble TE: Compressive neuropathies. In Trumble TE (ed): Principles of Hand Surgery and Therapy. Philadelphia, WB Saunders, 2000, pp 324-342.

30. Trumble TE, Diao E, Abrams RA, et al: Single-portal endoscopic carpal tunnel release compared with open release: A prospective, randomized trial. J Bone Joint Surg [Am] 84:1107-1115, 2002.

31. Brown RA, Gelberman RH, Seiler JG 3rd, et al: Carpal tunnel release: A prospective, randomized assessment of open and endoscopic methods. J Bone Joint Surg [Am] 75:1265-1275, 1993.

32. Goodyear-Smith F, Arroll B: What can family physicians offer patients with carpal tunnel syndrome other than surgery? A systematic review of nonsurgical management. Ann Fam Med 2:267-273, 2004.

33. Mackinnon SE, Novak CB: Compression neuropathies. In Green DP, Pederson WC, Hotchkiss RN, et al (eds): Green's Operative Hand Surgery. Philadelphia, Elsevier/Churchill Livingstone, 2005, pp 999-1046.

34. Netscher DT, Hildreth DH, Kleinert HE: Tumors of the hand. In Georgiade GS, Riefkohl R, Levin LS (eds): Plastic, Maxillofacial, and Reconstructive Surgery. Baltimore, Williams & Wilkins, 1997, pp 1046-1070.

35. Athanasian EA: Bone and soft tissue tumors. In Green DP, Pederson WC, Hotchkiss RN, et al (eds): Green's Operative Hand Surgery. Philadelphia. Elsevier/Churchill Livingstone, 2005, pp 2211-2265.

36. Cohen V, Netscher DT: Excision of ganglion cysts. In Evans GRD (ed): Operative Plastic Surgery. New York, McGraw-Hill, 2000, pp 924-935.

37. Rinker MH, Shenefelt PD: Warts, nongenital. Retrieved April 3, 2006, from http://www.emedicine.com/derm/topic457.

38. Sofocleous CT, Rosen RJ, Raskin K, et al: Congenital vascular malformations in the hand and forearm. J Endovasc Ther 8:484-494, 2001.

39. Koman LA, Ruch DS, Paterson SB: Vascular disorders. In Green DP, Pederson WC, Hotchkiss RN, et al (eds): Green's Operative Hand Surgery. Philadelphia, Elsevier/Churchill Livingstone, 2005, pp 2265-2313.

40. Trumble TE: Congenital hand deformities. In Trumble TE (ed): Principles of Hand Surgery and Therapy. Philadelphia, WB Saunders, 2000, pp 579-602.

41. Netscher DT: Congenital hand problems: Terminology, etiology, and management. Clin Plast Surg 25:537-552, 1998.

42. McCarroll HR: Congenital anomalies: A 25-year overview. J Hand Surg [Am] 25:1007-1037, 2000.

43. Feldon P, Terrono AL, Nalebluff EA: Rheumatoid arthritis and other connective tissue diseases. In Green DP, Pederson WC, Hotchkiss RN, et al (eds): Green's Operative Hand Surgery. Philadelphia, Elsevier/Churchill Livingstone, 2005, pp 2049-2136.

44. Saar JD, Grothaus PC: Dupuytren's disease: An overview. Plast Reconstr Surg 106:135-136; quiz 135-126, 2000.

45. Reilly RM, Stern PJ, Goldfarb CA: A retrospective review of the management of Dupuytren's nodules [Abstract]. J Hand Surg [Am] 30:1014-1018, 2005.

46. Hurst LC, Badalamente MA: Nonoperative treatment of Dupuytren's disease. Hand Clin 15:97-107, vii, 1999.

47. Blecha M, Brown A: Orthopedic and hand surgery pearls. In Pearls of Wisdom: General Surgery Review. Lincoln, MA, Boston Medical Publishing, 2004, pp 217-224.

48. Deziel DJ, Witt TR, Bines SD: Hand surgery. In Rush Review of Surgery. Philadelphia, WB Saunders, 2000, pp 579-589.

CHAPTER 75

Gynecologic Surgery

Stephen S. Entman, MD   Cornelia R. Graves, MD   Barry K. Jarnagin, MD
and   Gautam G. Rao, MD

Pelvic Embryology and Anatomy
Reproductive Physiology
Clinical Evaluation
Management of Preinvasive and Invasive Disease of the
   Female Genital Tract
Alternatives to Surgical Intervention
Technical Aspects of Surgical Options
Surgery During Pregnancy

Gynecology, along with the co-specialty of obstetrics, represents the art and science of the female reproductive tract. The global knowledge base for the specialty demands an understanding of embryology and anatomy of female pelvic organs, the hypothalamic-pituitary-ovarian hormonal axis, ovulation, the endometrial response to the hormonal milieu, oocyte fertilization and implantation, embryogenesis, fetal health and development, maternal adaptation to pregnancy, and labor and delivery. Additionally, obstetric and gynecologic care requires knowledge of functional and pathologic variations and abnormalities in these processes, including dysfunctional hormonal and endometrial cycling, ovarian accidents, pelvic infection, benign and malignant neoplasms, abnormal pregnancy implantation, teratogenesis, fetal and maternal complications of pregnancy, and abnormal labor. The full range of this knowledge is beyond the scope of one chapter. Instead, the focus will be to provide the surgeon with sufficient understanding of the basic information for effective care of the female patient in need of surgical evaluation and care. The potential settings for this care are as follows:

- Evaluation of women with abdominopelvic complaints in the emergency setting
- Request for intraoperative assistance or consultation by a gynecologic surgeon
- Unanticipated pelvic pathology in the operative setting
- Emergency surgical care in the absence of an obstetrician-gynecologist
- Surgical care of the pregnant patient

To these ends, this chapter is structured to provide the following information:

- Anatomy, with attention to surgical anatomic relationships
- Reproductive physiology
- Clinical evaluation of the female patient, including important elements of the history, physical examination, and ancillary tests
- Surgical technique for common gynecologic procedures, vulnerabilities for surgical injury, and specific issues related to surgical judgment
- Special considerations related to gynecologic malignancies
- Physiologic changes in pregnancy and perioperative and intraoperative care of the pregnant patient
- Surgical technique for obstetric procedures
- Medical alternatives to surgical management of common gynecologic conditions

PELVIC EMBRYOLOGY AND ANATOMY

Embryology

The female external genitalia are derived embryologically from the genital tubercle, which, in the absence of testosterone, fails to undergo fusion and devolves to the

Table 75-1 Selected Anatomic Abnormalities as a Result of Disrupted Embryogenesis

ORGAN	ABNORMALITY
Ovary	Duplication of ovary; secondary ovarian rests; paraovarian cysts (wolffian remnants)
Tube	Congenital absence; paratubal cyst (hydatid of Morgagni)
Uterus	Agenesis; complete or partial duplication of the uterine fundus
Cervix	Agenesis; complete or partial duplication of the cervix
Vagina	Agenesis; transverse or longitudinal septum; paravaginal (Gartner's duct) cyst
Vulva	Fusion; hermaphroditism; cyst of the canal of Nuck (round ligament cyst)

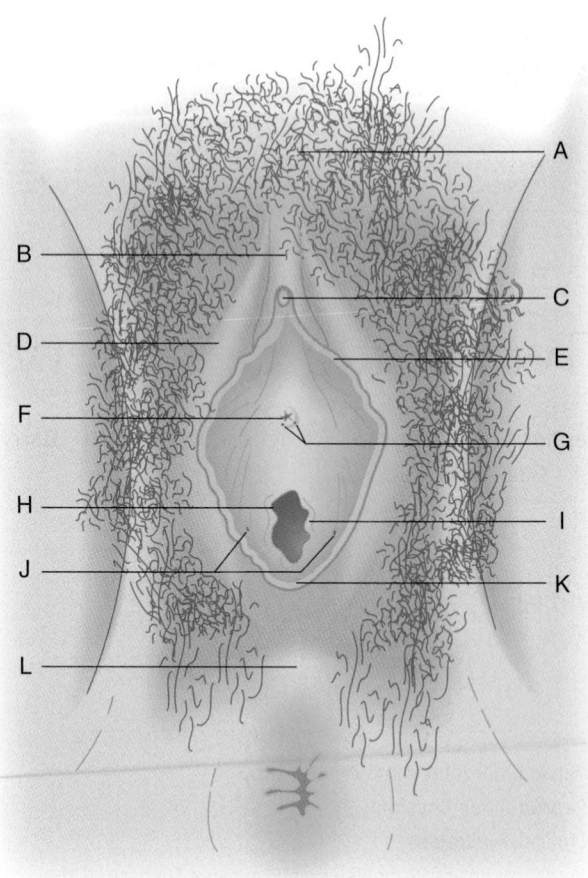

Figure 75-1 The external genitalia: A, mons pubis; B, prepuce; C, clitoris; D, labia majora; E, labia minora; F, urethral meatus; G, Skene's ducts; H, vagina; I, hymen; J, Bartholin's glands; K, posterior fourchette; L, perineal body.

vulvar structures. The labial structures are of ectodermal origin. The urethra, vaginal introitus, and vulvar vestibule are derived from uroepithelial entoderm. The lower third of the vagina develops from the invagination of the urogenital sinus.

The internal genitalia are derived from the genital ridge. The ovaries develop from the incorporation of primordial germ cells into coelomic epithelium of the mesonephric (wolffian) duct, and the tubes, uterus, cervix, and upper two thirds of the vagina develop from the paramesonephric (mullerian) duct. The embryologic ovaries migrate caudad to the true pelvis. Primordial ovarian follicles develop but remain dormant until stimulation in adolescence by gonadotropins. The paired mullerian ducts migrate caudad and medially to form the fallopian tubes and fuse in the midline to form the uterus, cervix, and upper vagina. The Wolffian ducts regress. Failure or partial failure of these processes can result in distortions of anatomy and potential diagnostic dilemmas (Table 75-1).

Anatomy

External Genitalia

The external genitalia consist of the mons veneris, labia majora, labia minora, clitoris, vulvar vestibule, urethral meatus, and ostia of the accessory glandular structures (Fig. 75-1). These structures overlie the fascial and muscle layers of the perineum. The perineum is the most caudal region of the trunk and includes the pelvic floor and those structures occupying the pelvic outlet. It is bounded superiorly by the funnel-shaped pelvic diaphragm and inferiorly by the skin covering the external genitalia, anus, and adjacent structures. Laterally, the perineum is bounded by the medial surface of the inferior pubic rami, the obturator internus muscle below the origin of the levator ani muscle, the coccygeus muscle, the medial surface of the sacrotuberous ligaments, and the overlapping margins of the gluteus maximus muscles (Fig. 75-2).

The pelvic outlet can be divided into two triangles separated by a line drawn between the ischial tuberosi-

ties. The anterior or urogenital triangle has its apex anteriorly at the symphysis pubis, and the posterior or anal triangle has its apex at the coccyx.

The urogenital triangle contains the urogenital diaphragm, a muscular shelf extending between the pubic rami and penetrated by the urethra and vagina, and the external genitalia, consisting of the mons pubis, the labia majora and minora, the clitoris, and the vestibule. The mons pubis is a suprapubic fat pad covered by dense skin appendages. The labia majora extend posteriorly from the mons, forming the lateral borders of the vulva. They have a keratinized stratified squamous epithelium with all of the normal skin appendages and extend posteriorly to the lateral perineum. Within the confines of the labium are fat and the insertion of the round ligament. Medial to the labia majora are interlabial grooves and the labia minora, of similar cutaneous origin, but devoid of hair follicles. The labia minora are richly vascularized, with an erectile venous plexus. The bilateral roots of the clitoris fuse in the midline to form the glans at the lower edge of the pubic symphysis. The labia minora fuse over the clitoris to form the hood and, to a variable degree, below to create the clitoral frenulum.

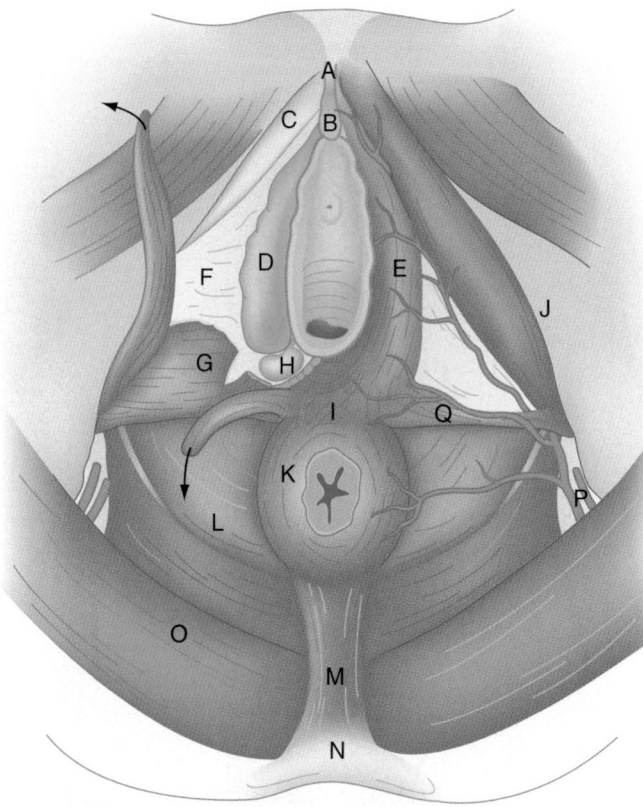

Figure 75-2 The muscles and fascia of the perineum: A, suspensory ligament of clitoris; B, clitoris; C, crus of clitoris; D, vestibular bulb; E, bulbocavernosus muscle; F, inferior fascia of urogenital diaphragm; G, deep transverse perineal muscle; H, Bartholin's gland; I, perineal body; J, ischiocavernosus muscle; K, external anal sphincter; L, levator ani muscle; M, anococcygeal body; N, coccyx; O, gluteus maximus muscle; P, pudendal artery and vein; Q, superficial transverse perineal muscle.

Contiguous to the medial aspect of the labia minora, demarcated by Hart's line, is the vulvar vestibule extending to the hymeneal sulcus. The vestibular surface is a stratified, squamous mucous membrane that shares embryology and has similar characteristics to the distal urethra and urethral meatus. The Bartholin's glands at 5 and 7 o'clock, the paraurethral Skene's glands, and minor vestibular glands positioned around the lateral vestibule are all under the vestibular bulb, subjacent to the bulbocavernosus muscle. The ostia of these glands pass through the vestibular mucosa, directly adjacent to the hymeneal ring.

The muscles of the external genitals consist of the deep and superficial transverse perineal muscles, the paired ischiocavernosus muscles that cover the crura of the clitoris, and the bulbocavernosus muscles lying on either side of the vagina covering the vestibular bulbs.

The anal triangle contains the anal canal with surrounding internal and external sphincters; the ischiorectal fossa, filled with fatty tissue; the median raphe; and the overlying skin.

Blood supply to the perineum is predominantly from a posterior direction from the internal pudendal artery, which, after arising from the internal iliac artery, passes

through Alcock's canal, a fascial tunnel along the obturator internus muscle below the origin of the levator ani muscle. Upon emerging from Alcock's canal, the internal pudendal artery sends branches to the urogenital triangle anteriorly and to the anal triangle posteriorly. Anteriorly, there is blood supply to the mons pubis from the inferior epigastric, a branch of the femoral artery. Laterally, the external pudendal artery arises from the femoral artery and supplies the lateral aspect of the vulva. Venous return from the perineum accompanies the arterial supply and, therefore, drains into the internal iliac and femoral veins.

It is important for the surgeon dissecting the external genitalia to be cognizant of the variability of direction from which the blood supply of the operative field is derived.

The major nerve supply to the perineum comes from the internal pudendal nerve, which originates from S2 to S4 anterior rami of the sacral plexus and travels through Alcock's canal in company with the internal pudendal artery and vein. Anterior branches supply the urogenital diaphragm and the external genitalia, whereas posterior branches, the inferior rectal nerve, supply the anus, the anal canal, the ischiorectal fossa, and the adjacent skin. Branches of the posterior femoral cutaneous nerve from the sacral plexus innervate the lateral aspects of the ischiorectal fossa and adjacent structures. The mons pubis and anterior labia are supplied by the ilioinguinal and genitofemoral nerves from the lumbar plexus; they travel through the inguinal canal and exit through the superficial inguinal ring. All of these paired nerves routinely cross the midline for partial innervation of the contralateral side. The visceral efferent nerves responsible for clitoral erection are derived from the pelvic splanchnic nerves and reach the external genitalia in company of the urethra and vagina as they pass through the urogenital diaphragm.

Surgical injury to the pelvic nerve plexus can result in neuropathic pain, and diminished sexual, voiding, and excretory function.

The lymphatic drainage of the perineum, including both the urogenital triangle and anogenital triangle, travels for the most part with the external pudendal vessels to the superficial inguinal nodes. The deep parts of the perineum, including the urethra, the vagina, and the anal canal, drain in part through the lymphatics that accompany the internal pudendal vessels and into the internal iliac lymph nodes.

The fascia and fascial spaces of the perineum are important regarding spread of extravasated fluids and both superficial and deep infections. Fascia covers each of the muscles bounding the perineum, including the deep surface of the levator ani, obturator internus, and coccygeus, as well as other perineal muscles such as the urogenital diaphragm. The fascia of the levator ani muscles fuses with the obturator internus fascia and the pubic rami, creating well-defined fascial spaces, the ischiorectal fosse. Beneath the skin of the external genitalia is a layer of fat, and deep to this is Colles' fascia, which is attached to the ischiopubic rami laterally and the posterior edge of the urogenital diaphragm.

Anteriorly, Colles' fascia of the vulva is continuous with Colles' fascia of the anterior abdominal wall.

Infections or collections of extravasated urine deep to the urogenital diaphragm are usually confined to the ischiorectal fossa, including the anterior recess, which is superior to the urogenital diaphragm. Collections of fluid or infections superficial to the urogenital diaphragm may pass to the abdominal wall deep to Colles' fascia. Because of various fascial fusions, infections spreading from the vulva to the anterior abdominal wall do not spread into the inguinal regions or the thigh.

Internal Genitalia

The internal genitalia consist of the ovaries, fallopian tubes, uterus, cervix, and vagina with associated blood supply and lymphatic drainage (Figs. 75-3 to 75-5).

Ovary

The oblong ovaries, glistening white in color, vary in size, which is dependent on age and status of the ovulatory cycle. In the prepubescent girl, the ovary will appear as a white sliver of tissue less than 1 cm in any dimension. The ovary of a woman during her reproductive years will vary in size and shape. The size of the nonovulating ovary will typically be in the range of 3×2×1 cm. When a follicular or corpus luteum cyst is present, the size may extend up to 5 to 6 cm. A follicular cyst is an asymmetrical, translucent, clear structure. A corpus luteum cyst will generally be characterized by areas of golden yellow, and occasionally with hematoma. The ovaries are suspended from the lateral side wall of the pelvis below the pelvic brim by the infundibulopelvic ligament and attach to the superolateral aspect of the uterine fundus with the utero-ovarian ligament.

The primary blood supply to the ovary is the ovarian artery. It arises directly from the aorta and courses with the vein through the infundibulopelvic ligament into the medulla on the lateral aspect of the ovary. The right ovarian vein generally drains to the inferior vena cava, and the left drains to the common iliac vein; however, variations commonly occur. There is a rich, anastomotic arterial complex arising from the uterine artery that spreads across the broad ligament and the mesosalpinx. The venous return accompanies that arterial supply. There is no somatic innervation to the ovary, but the autonomic fibers arise from the lumbar sympathetic and sacral parasympathetic plexuses. Lymphatic drainage parallels the iliac and aortic arteries.

There are three important relationships to be considered in surgical dissection. The infundibulopelvic ligament, with the ovarian blood supply, crosses over the ureter as it descends into the pelvis. As the surgeon divides and ligates the ovarian vessels, it is critical that this relationship be identified to avoid transecting, ligating, or kinking the ureter. The risk for ureteral injury is greater with a more proximal dissection of the ligament. Additionally, in its natural position, the suspended ovary drops along the pelvic sidewall along the course of the midureter. If there are adhesions between the ovary and the peritoneum of the pelvic sidewall, careful dissection is necessary to avoid tenting the peritoneum with the

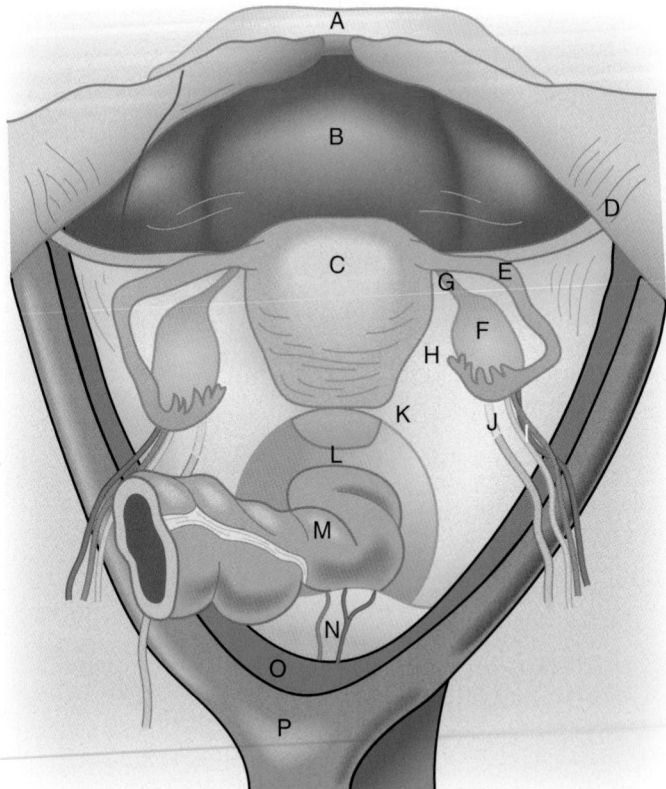

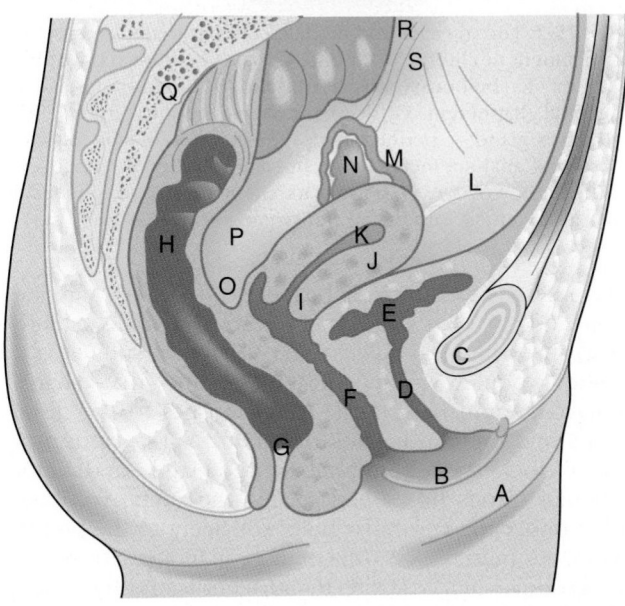

Figure 75-3 The internal genitalia. *Front view:* A, symphysis pubis; B, bladder; C, corpus uteri; D, round ligament; E, fallopian tube; F, ovary; G, utero-ovarian ligament; H, broad ligament; I, ovarian artery and vein; J, ureter; K, uterosacral ligament; L, cul-de-sac; M, rectum; N, middle sacral artery and vein; O, vena cava; P, aorta. *Side view:* A, labium majus; B, labium minus; C, symphysis pubis, D, urethra; E, bladder; F, vagina; G, anus; H, rectum; I, cervix uteri; J, corpus uteri; K, endometrial cavity; L, round ligament; M, fallopian tube; N, ovary; O, cul-de-sac; P, uterosacral ligament; Q, sacrum; R, ureter; S, ovarian artery and vein.

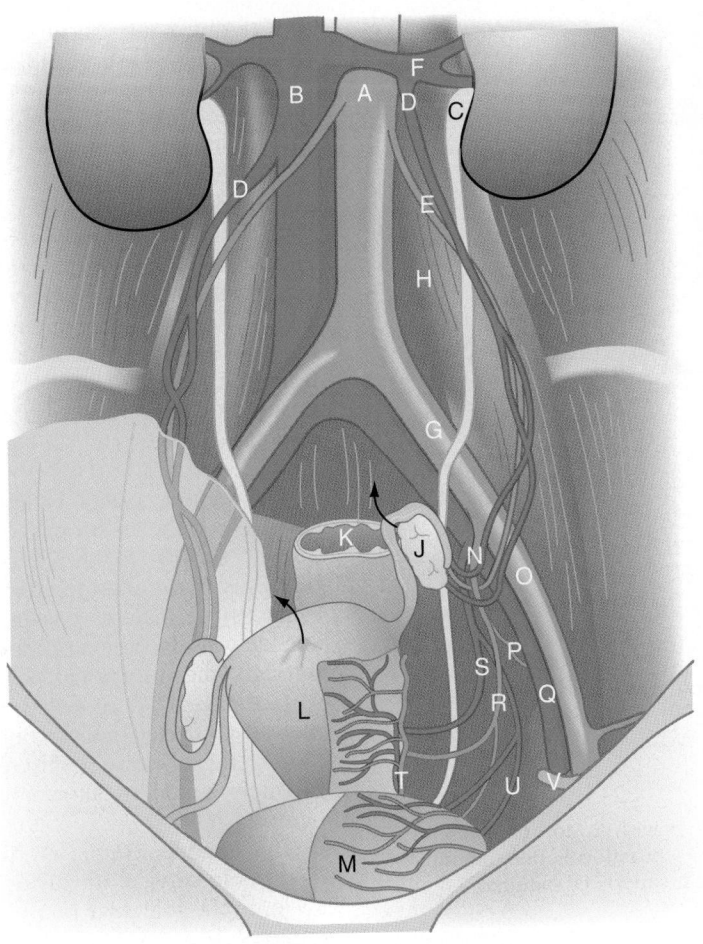

Figure 75-4 Blood supply of the pelvis: A, aorta; B, inferior vena cava; C, ureter; D, ovarian vein; E, ovarian artery; F, renal vein; G, common iliac artery; H, psoas muscle; J, ovary; K, rectum; L, corpus uteri; M, bladder; N, internal iliac (hypogastric) artery, anterior branch; O, external iliac artery; P, obturator artery; Q, external iliac vein; R, uterine artery; S, uterine vein; T, vaginal artery; U, superior vesicle artery; V, inferior epigastric artery.

attached ureter and creating injury. The third surgical relationship is the complex of external iliac vessels and the femoral nerve, which course along the iliopsoas muscle, directly below the course of the ovarian vessels; with anterior adhesions of an ovary, these structures may be subjacent to the malpositioned ovary.

Fallopian Tubes

The fallopian tubes are cylindrical structures about 8 cm in length. They originate at the uterine cavity in the uterine cornua, with an intramural segment of 1 to 2 cm and a narrow isthmic segment of 4 to 5 cm, flaring over 2 to 3 cm to the funnel of the infundibular segment, and terminating in the fimbriated end of the tube. The fimbria are fine, delicate mucosal projections that are positioned to allow for capture of the extruded oocyte to promote the potential for fertilization. The blood supply to the tube is derived primarily from branches of the uterine artery, with a delicate cascade of vessels in the mesosalpinx. There is a secondary supply from the anastomosis with the ovarian vessels.

The surgeon must be aware of the fragility of the fallopian tube and handle this structure delicately, especially in women wishing to preserve their fertility. The mucosa lining the tubal lumen, especially at the fimbriated end, is highly specialized to facilitate transport of the oocyte and the fertilized zygote. Traumatic manipulation of the tube can induce tubal infertility or predispose to later tubal pregnancy, either through damage to the mucosa or by distortion of tubal position by adhesions, thereby interfering with the access or transport mechanisms.

Uterus and Cervix

The uterus with the cervix is a midline, pear-shaped organ suspended in the midplane of the pelvis by the cardinal and uterosacral ligaments. The cardinal ligaments are dense fibrous condensations arising from the fascial covering of the levator ani muscles of the pelvic floor and inserting into the lateral portions of the uterocervical junction. The uterosacral ligaments arise posterolaterally from the uterocervical junction and course

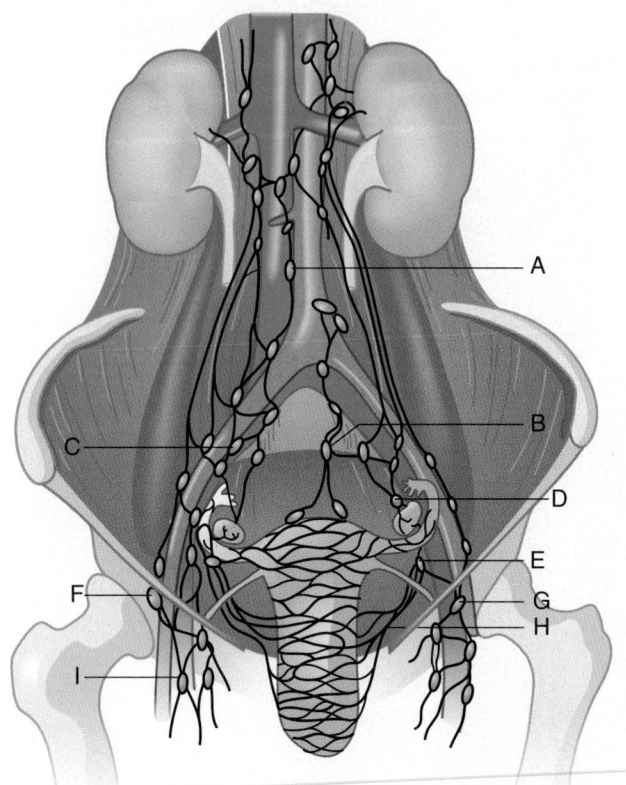

Figure 75-5 Lymphatics of the pelvis: A, aortic; B, sacral; C, common iliac; D, hypogastric; E, obturator; F, deep inguinal; G, Cloquet's node; H, parametrial; I, superficial inguinal.

obliquely in a posterolateral direction to insert into the parietal fascia of the pelvic floor at the sacroiliac joint. The round ligaments of the uterus arise from the anterolateral superior aspect of the uterine fundus, course anterolaterally to the internal inguinal ring, and insert into the labia majora. The round ligaments are highly stretchable and serve no function in pelvic organ support. The broad ligaments are composed of a visceral peritoneal surface containing loose adventitious tissue. These ligaments also provide no pelvic organ support, but do allow access to an avascular plane of the pelvis through which the retroperitoneal vasculature and ureter can be exposed.

The size of the uterus is influenced by age, hormonal status, prior pregnancy, and common benign neoplasms. The normal uterus during the reproductive years is about 8×6×4 cm and weighs about 100 g. The prepubertal and postmenopausal uterus is substantially smaller. The mass of the uterus is almost exclusively made up of myometrium, a complex of interlacing bundles of smooth muscle. The uterine cavity is 4 to 6 cm from the internal cervical os to the uterine fundus, shaped as an inverted triangle, 2 to 3 mm wide at the cervix, and 3 to 4 cm across the fundus, extending from cornua to cornua. It is only a few millimeters of depth between anterior and posterior walls, with no defined lateral walls in the nonpregnant state. The most common reason for variation in size is current pregnancy followed by uterine fibroids.

If during a surgical procedure, the surgeon encounters an enlarged uterus, undiagnosed pregnancy must be considered. The morphologic differences between a uterus enlarged by a pregnancy and one enlarged by fibroid include symmetrical enlargement in pregnancy with generally asymmetric enlargement with fibroids. If symmetrical, consider the origin of the round ligaments. With pregnancy, the round ligaments stretch as the uterus grows and continue to originate from the normal site; even with an apparently symmetrical fibroid uterus, the origin of the round ligaments is frequently displaced from the top of the uterine fundus or asymmetrical course through the pelvis. Finally, the pregnant uterus is usually dusky and soft, whereas fibroids are generally firm, and nodular masses can be palpated in the myometrial wall.

The uterine cavity is lined by the endometrium, a complex epithelial-stromal-vascular secretory tissue. The arterial supply to the endometrium is derived from branches of the uterine artery that perforate the myometrium to the inactive basalis layer. There they form the arcuate vessels, which produce radial branches extending through the functional layer toward the compacted surface layer. There will be further description of the menstrual cycle below; but during the postovulatory phase, these vessels differentiate into spiral arteries, uniquely suited to allow menstruation and subsequent hemostasis.

The uterine cervix is histologically dynamic, with changes in cervical mucus production during the ovarian cycle. In the follicular phase, under estrogen stimulation, copious clear mucus is produced that facilitates the transport of sperm through the cervical canal to ascend through the uterine cavity to the fallopian tubes. During progesterone-dominant states, either luteal phase or with exogenous hormones, the mucus becomes viscous and plugs the cervix. The secretory epithelium of the endocervical canal has a dynamic metaplastic interaction with the stratified squamous epithelium of the portio vaginalis of the ectocervix under hormonal stimulation.

Because the cervical canal is continuous with the vagina, surgical procedures involving the uterus and tubes are considered to be clean-contaminated cases.

The major sources of blood supply for the uterus and cervix are the uterine arteries, which are branches of the anterior division of the internal iliac (hypogastric) arteries. Although the origin of the uterine artery is usually a single, identifiable vessel, it divides into multiple ascending and descending branches as it courses medially to the lateral margins of the cervicouterine junction. The distance from the uterus at which this division occurs is highly variable. Venous return from the uterus flows into the companion internal iliac vein. Lymphatics from the cervix and upper vagina drain primarily through the internal iliac nodes, but from the uterine fundus, drainage occurs primarily along a presacral path directly to the para-aortic nodes.

The primary surgical consideration for managing the uterine vessels is the close proximity of the ureter, which courses about 1 cm below the artery and 1 cm lateral to the cervix. If the surgeon loses control of one of the branches of the vessel, it is important to use techniques that avoid clamping or kinking the ureter. Often, the most prudent way to secure the uterine artery is to expose its origin and place hemostatic clips on the vessel.

Innervation of the uterus and cervix is derived from the autonomic plexus. Autonomic pain fibers are activated with dysmenorrhea, in labor, and with instrumentation of the cervix and uterus.

In the retroperitoneal space lateral to the uterus is the obturator nerve, arising from the lumbosacral plexus and passing through the pelvic floor by way of the obturator canal to innervate the medial thigh. With relatively normal pelvic anatomy, it is unlikely to be subjected to injury; but under circumstances in which the surgeon must dissect the retroperitoneal or paravaginal spaces, this relatively subtle structure can be injured with significant neuropathic residual.

Vagina

The vagina originates at the cervix and terminates at the hymeneal ring. The anatomic axis of the upper vagina is posterior to anterior in a caudad direction. The anterior and posterior walls of the upper two thirds of the vagina are normally apposed to each other to create a transverse potential space, distensible through pliability of the lateral sulci. The lower third of the vagina has a relatively vertically oriented caudad lumen. The mucosa of the vagina is nonkeratinized, stratified, squamous epithelium that responds to estrogen stimulation.

The blood supply to the vagina is provided by descending branches of the uterine artery and vein and ascending branches of the internal pudendal artery and its companion vein. These vessels course along the lateral walls of the vagina. Innervation is derived from the autonomic plexus and the pudendal nerve, which track with the vessels.

Traumatic lacerations of the vagina are most commonly located along the lateral sidewalls, and the degree to which there is major injury to the vessels can be associated not only with significant evident hemorrhage but also with concealed hemorrhage. Spaces in which a hematoma can be concealed are the retroperitoneum of the broad ligaments, paravesical and pararectal spaces, and ischiorectal fossa. Because of the proximity of the pudendal nerve, attempts to ligate the vessels require maintaining orientation to the location of Alcock's canal to avoid creating neuropathic injury. In the absence of an accumulating hematoma, often the best approach to management is a bulk vaginal pack to achieve tamponade. To accomplish this requires significant sedation or anesthesia and an indwelling urinary catheter.

The uterus, cervix, and vagina with their fascial investments comprise the middle compartment of the pelvis. The structures of the anterior compartment, the bladder and urethra, and of the posterior compartment, the rectum, are each invested with a fascial layer. Avascular planes of loose areolar tissue separate the posterior fascia of the bladder and the anterior fascia of the vagina and also the anterior fascia of the rectum and the posterior fascia of the vagina. Anteriorly, the bladder is attached to the lower uterine segment by the continuous visceral

peritoneum. This vesicouterine fold can be incised transversely with minimal difficulty to expose the plane and allow dissection of the bladder from the cervix and vagina. Posteriorly, the proximity of the rectum to the posterior vagina is significant only below the peritoneum of the cul-de-sac of Douglas, unless the cul-de-sac anatomy is distorted by dense adhesions.

Operative technique for gynecologic procedures is optimized by careful identification of these planes to separate and protect the adjacent organs from operative injury. The surgeon can create an incidental cystotomy, which may or may not be recognized, or devitalize the bladder wall with a crush or stitch, with delayed development of a vesicovaginal fistula.

In the lower pelvis, the ureter courses anteromedially after it passes under the uterine vessels and progresses toward the trigone of the bladder through a fascial tunnel on the anterior vaginal wall. The fixation of the ureter by the tunnel precludes effective displacement from the operative site by retracting. Although the location of the fascial tunnel is generally 1 to 2 cm safely below the usual site for vaginotomy during hysterectomy, in cases with a large cervix, a distorting uterine myoma, a prior cesarean birth, or bleeding from the bladder base or vaginal wall, the ureter can be transected, crushed, or kinked with a stitch.

The rectovaginal septum is surgically relevant during repair of episiotomy or obstetric laceration, repair of rectovaginal fistula, or pelvic support procedures. Identification of the fascial layers investing the subjacent structures and using the tissue strength is critical to an optimal repair.

REPRODUCTIVE PHYSIOLOGY

The development of a differential diagnosis of gynecologic complaints is facilitated by an understanding of the reproductive cycle and eliciting a careful menstrual history. Many conditions are a direct consequence of aberrations in the hypothalamic-pituitary-ovarian cycle and the effects of the hormonal milieu on the endometrium. Others tend to be mere variation in the presentation of different phases of the cycle. A detailed description of the cycle is beyond the scope of this text, but the surgeon needs to have a basic understanding of the relationships in this complex process in order to elicit an adequate history, interpret the findings on physical examination, use ancillary tests appropriately, and formulate the differential diagnosis (Fig. 75-6).

Ovarian Cycle

Under the stimulus of hypothalamic secretion of gonadotropin-releasing hormone (GnRH) to the pituitary gland, follicle-stimulating hormone (FSH) is released into the systemic circulation. During this secretory phase of the ovarian cycle, the primordial follicles of the ovary are targeted and stimulated toward growth and maturity. Multiple follicles are recruited each cycle; but generally, only one follicle becomes dominant, destined to reach

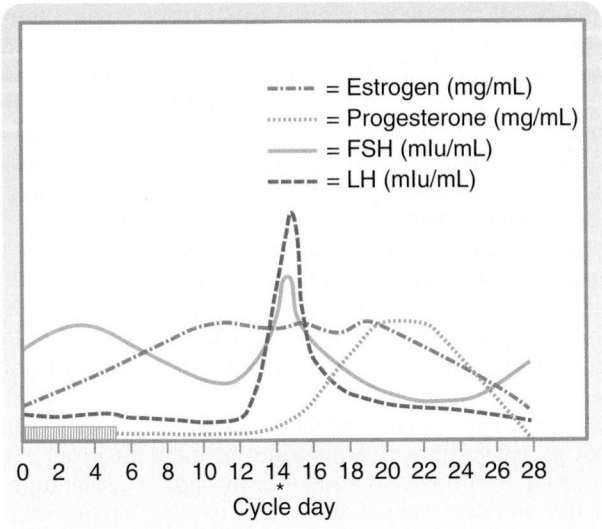

Figure 75-6 Hormonal changes during the menstrual cycle. Menses, days 0-5; ovulation, day 14. FSH, follicle-stimulating hormone; LH, luteinizing hormone.

maturity and extrusion at ovulation. The effects of the maturation process include not only the completion of the meiotic germ cell development but also the stimulation of the granulosa cells that surround the follicle to secrete estradiol and other estrogenic compounds and inhibin. As the estradiol level increases in the circulation, it has a positive regulatory effect on GnRH, which in turn stimulates the pituitary gland to release a surge of luteinizing hormone (LH). The LH surge stimulates the release of the oocyte from the follicle. After the release, the follicle site converts to the corpus luteum, and the dominant hormone secreted during this luteal phase is progesterone. This sequence of hormonal events prepares the cervix, uterus, and tubes for sperm transport into the upper genital tract, fertilization, implantation, and support of the early gestation. In the absence of conception, through mechanisms not yet known, the corpus luteum undergoes atresia, and the next ovarian cycle begins.

Endometrial Cycle

The hormonal sequence of the ovarian cycle controls the physiologic changes in the endometrium. By convention, each endometrial cycle begins on *day 1,* defined as the onset of menses. In an idealized cycle, the LH surge and ovulation occur on day 14. Atresia of the corpus luteum occurs on day 28, and menses begin the next day, day 1 of the new cycle.

During the follicular phase of the ovarian cycle, estrogen exerts a stimulatory effect on the endometrium, producing the proliferative phase of the endometrial cycle. The endometrial tissues that are affected include the surface and glandular epithelium, the stromal matrix, and the vascular bed. The stromal layer thickens, the

glandular elements elongate, and the terminal arterioles of the endometrial circulation extend from the basalis toward the endometrial surface. The mucous secretions of the glands of the endometrium (and the endocervix) become profuse and watery, facilitating ascent of spermatozoa for potential fertilization.

During the luteal phase of the ovarian cycle, corresponding to the secretory phase of the endometrial cycle, progesterone domination converts the endometrium toward receptivity for implantation of the fertilized oocyte. Several endometrial changes occur under progesterone stimulation. The growth of the endometrial stroma is terminated, the surface layer of the endometrium becomes compacted, the glandular secretions become more viscous, and the terminal arterioles become coiled, creating the spiral arterioles. Cervical mucus similarly becomes more viscous and tenacious, creating a relative barrier between the vagina and the uterine cavity.

In the absence of fertilization, and with the withdrawal of progesterone due to atresia of the corpus luteum, there is a complex sequence of arteriolar spasm, leading to ischemic necrosis of the endometrial surface and endometrial shedding, or menses. Normal menses, in the absence of structural pathology, is an orderly process because these arteriolar changes occur in the entire mucosa simultaneously and universally, with vasospasm and coagulation occluding the terminal vessels. Bleeding associated with normal menses is notable for the absence of clotting because of fibrinolysis within the uterine cavity before flow. With fertilization and implantation, menses are absent (amenorrhea). Alternatively, a disordered ovarian cycle leads to a disordered endometrial cycle and abnormal uterine bleeding patterns.

Early Pregnancy

A brief description of the events leading to pregnancy is useful for understanding the possible complications of early pregnancy. Coitus during the 48 hours before ovulation or within the periovulatory period establishes the conditions for fertilization. As noted earlier, sperm transport is facilitated by the estrogenic environment, and the spermatozoa ascend through the cervix and uterine cavity to the fallopian tube. When a mature oocyte and spermatozoa come into contact in the distal fallopian tube, fertilization can occur. This usually occurs 3 to 5 days after ovulation. During tubal transport, the zygote undergoes multiple divisions to reach the stage of the morula by the time it reaches the cavity. Implantation generally occurs about 5 to 7 days after fertilization.

There are two significant clinical implications to delay in the fertilization-transport sequence. If the zygote has not matured adequately before reaching the endometrial cavity, implantation will not occur, and a preclinical, unrecognized pregnancy will be lost. If there is delay in the fertilization-transport sequence, whether because of the randomness of coital timing or because of altered tubal structure or function, the zygote can reach the stage at which it is programmed to adhere to genital mucosa while still in the fallopian tube, resulting in an ectopic pregnancy.

Amenorrhea and Abnormal Menses

A disrupted sequence of the hypothalamic-pituitary-ovarian interaction has profound effect on the endometrium and menses. There are two broad classes of amenorrheic disorders: hypogonadotropic and anovulatory. Although the details of the pathology and evaluation are beyond the scope of this text, hypogonadotropic conditions result from central disruption of the hypothalamic-pituitary axis. Common etiologies for this condition include stress, hyperprolactinemia, and low body mass (anorexia nervosa; athletes such as distance runners, gymnasts, ballerinas). Because of the hypogonadotropic state, follicles are not stimulated, estrogen is not secreted, and endometrial proliferation does not occur. The result is an atrophic endometrium.

Atrophic endometrium can be identified with ultrasound, measuring the endometrial bilayer. Although local equipment and operator experience will vary, an endometrial bilayer of less than 5 mm in a young amenorrheic woman is highly supportive of the diagnosis. This must then be followed by a thorough investigation of the entire axis.

Anovulation results from a disrupted sequence of the axis from failure of the feedback loop to trigger the LH surge. The patient may have normal or elevated FSH levels, but FSH continues to stimulate continuous production of estrogen from the granulosa cells. The chronic unopposed estrogen promotes continuous proliferation of the endometrium, without the maturing sequence induced by progesterone. The proliferation of the endometrium results in excessive thickness. This becomes clinically manifest by prolonged amenorrhea, often followed by prolonged and profuse uterine bleeding (hypermenorrhea, menorrhagia). The most common etiology for this presentation is polycystic ovarian disease, but physiologic or social stress can produce a similar clinical scenario.

Ultrasound measurement of the endometrial bilayer can exceed 20 mm. Patients with chronic anovulation with chronic unopposed estrogen are at risk for endometrial hyperplasia and even endometrial cancer. The evaluation of the patient must address both the etiology for the chronic anovulation and the endometrial consequences. Histologic diagnosis requires an endometrial biopsy or curettage.

After prolonged amenorrhea with excessive proliferation of the endometrial lining, hypermenorrhea and menorrhagia may occur because of four parallel mechanisms. The growth of tissue from basalis to surface extends beyond the terminal branches of the arterioles, resulting in surface ischemia and necrosis. The volume of endometrial tissue is obviously increased. The normal hemostatic mechanisms of the spiral arterioles in the menstrual cycle are absent. Finally, the shedding of the endometrial surface is not a universal event, but rather is random and leads to multiple foci of bleeding that are dyssynchronous and occur over a prolonged time. Frequently, the rate of bleeding exceeds the capacity of the normal intracavitary fibrinolytic processes, and blood clots are common in the flow.

CLINICAL EVALUATION

In the urgent or acute setting, the gynecologic history focuses on the variation from normal ovarian and menstrual physiology as it relates to the reproductive life cycle. Patients will typically present with aberrant bleeding patterns, pelvic-abdominal pain or ill-defined discomfort, or a combination of these symptoms. With a focused history, the differential diagnosis can be constructed with further refinement from physical findings and ancillary tests. The key elements to be elicited are age, pregnancy history, recent and past menstrual history, sexual history, contraception, prior gynecologic disease and procedures, and the evolution of the current complaints.

History

Age
Patient age is primarily relevant because of the phases of the reproductive life cycle: menarche at adolescence, perimenopause in middle age, and menopause.

At time of menarche, the synchrony of the hypothalamic-pituitary-ovarian axis is immature, and the sequence of hypergonadotropic anovulatory amenorrhea-hypermenorrhea is common. Similarly, this is the age group in which emotional stress, anorexia nervosa, and excessive athleticism commonly occur, and the amenorrheic patient may have hypogonadotropic amenorrhea. Finally, however, the young patient may be fertile and sexually active, so pregnancy with complications must always be considered.

In the perimenopausal years, the ovary is less responsive to the gonadotropic stimulus, and anovulation with the amenorrhea-hypermenorrhea sequence is common. In this age group, however, anatomic abnormalities such as uterine leiomyomas or endometrial polyps may confound the presentation.

Menopause is defined as cessation of menses for 1 year or more. Any postmenopausal woman who presents with uterine bleeding must be presumed to have uterine pathology and needs to undergo an appropriate evaluation for possible hyperplastic or neoplastic endometrial pathology.

Pregnancy History
The commonly used notation for describing pregnancy history is G, T, P, A, L—for *g*ravidity (number of pregnancies), *t*erm births, *p*reterm births, abortions (spontaneous, induced, or ectopic), and *l*iving children. Additional comment is made if there have been recurring spontaneous abortions, ectopic pregnancies, or multiple gestation.

Although any pregnancy can develop complications, the patient with a history of poor outcomes in prior pregnancies will be at higher risk for another adverse outcome. In the acute setting, with pain or bleeding, pregnancy complications must be considered.

Menstrual History
The date of the last menstrual period (LMP) and the prior menstrual period (PMP) must be determined as accu-

rately as possible. It is often necessary to elicit menstrual events over several prior months to establish a pattern. Additionally, it is important to obtain a description of any variation from the patient's normal pattern of quantity and duration of menstrual flow. Within the context of this menstrual history, one can place the current complaints of bleeding and pain in perspective.

The amenorrhea-hypermenorrhea sequence has been described previously. The patient who describes "two periods this month" may merely be describing a normal 28-day cycle beginning early and then late in the same calendar month. Alternating episodes of light bleeding with normal flow may suggest breakthrough bleeding at time of ovulation or on oral contraceptives. Excessive flow (menorrhagia) associated with regular cycles at normal intervals suggests structural abnormalities of the endometrial cavity, most commonly submucous leiomyomas or endometrial polyps. Random or intermittent bleeding episodes during the cycle prompts consideration of a lesion of the cervix, endometrial hyperplasia, or occasionally, adenocarcinoma of the endometrium.

Dysmenorrhea (menstrual cramps) is generally considered to occur only with ovulatory cycles. The patient who typically has dysmenorrhea but who currently denies cramps, even with a current episode of heavy flow, may be having an anovulatory bleeding episode, regardless of the interval between periods. Patients with high-volume flow, with insufficient intracavitary fibrinolysis, may experience cramps as the uterus contracts to expel the clot. Bleeding associated with threatened pregnancy loss or from an extrauterine pregnancy must be considered, whether heavy or light flow, continuous or episodic, whether anteceded by reported normal cycles or occurring after amenorrhea. Bleeding after menopause demands consideration of endometrial pathology and appropriate workup to rule out hyperplasia or carcinoma. Postcoital bleeding suggests cervical lesions, including cervicitis, polyps or neoplasia.

Sexual History

As a sensitive and personal subject that is often difficult to elicit reliably in the acute setting, sexual activity may significantly influence the formulation of the differential diagnosis. Beyond the possibility of pregnancy, the patient who will acknowledge unprotected coitus with casual sexual partners is considered to be at high risk for sexually transmitted diseases (STDs). Reliable reports of the use of barrier contraception reduce, but do not eliminate, the possibility of an STD.

Pregnancy must be ruled out in any circumstance in which there is a clinical presentation that is not inconsistent with complications of pregnancy.

Contraception

Reliable use of contraception does not totally preclude the possibility of pregnancy but raises other possible diagnoses to a higher level in the differential.

Breakthrough bleeding on hormonal contraception is typically low volume and is rarely associated with cramps

or pain. In the presence of other symptoms, pregnancy complications and genital tract infections need to be considered. Patients with an intrauterine contraceptive device (IUD) may have spotting and cramping, but because the IUD increases the risk for endometrial infection, and because a disproportionate percentage of pregnancies that are conceived with an IUD are extrauterine, these patients need careful evaluation.

Patients with previous tubal sterilization have a 1% to 3% lifetime risk for pregnancy, with a disproportionate number of extrauterine pregnancies. Irregular bleeding associated with pain mandates careful evaluation.

Prior Gynecologic Diseases and Procedures

Past gynecologic history may give direction to recurring conditions suggesting lifestyle issues that create risk for recurrence or raise consideration of complications of previous interventions.

Tubal ligation, prior tubal injury from an ectopic pregnancy, endometriosis, and pelvic inflammatory disease (PID) all increase the risk for extrauterine pregnancy. Endometriosis with an intraperitoneal inflammatory response may cause significant pain. Patients with a history of functional ovarian cysts with or without intraparenchymal hemorrhage have a higher risk for recurrence. Previous pelvic surgery with periovarian adhesions can cause significant pain even with benign, self-limited ovarian cyst accidents, but also may predispose to ovarian torsion.

The ovarian remnant syndrome is an interesting and confusing entity. It can cause pelvic pain in ill-defined patterns. The etiology of the syndrome is a retained fragment of ovarian capsule after previous ovarian surgery. The fragment is adherent to the peritoneum and remains viable through a parasitic blood supply. Active follicles can be recruited through gonadotropin stimulation, and the dynamics of peritoneal inflammation can be severely symptomatic. These remnants are most commonly found after resection of a densely adherent ovary with endometriosis or purulent infection of the pelvis. They are frequently located along the course of the ureter and may present with flank pain from urinary obstruction.

History of Present Illness

The surgeon elicits the historical elements described above to construct the evolution of the presenting complaint and formulate a plan for further evaluation and treatment. This section will focus on the most common emergency presentations: bleeding and pain.

Bleeding

- When did bleeding begin?
- How does the current flow compare to normal? Are there clots in the menstrual flow normally? Currently?
- How did the timing of onset relate to previous menses? Was there any prolongation of the interval between the last period and the onset of the current bleeding event?
- Were recent menses normal? Expected timing, flow, duration?

- Are menstrual periods normally associated with menstrual cramps? Is the current episode associated with similar cramps? No cramps? More intense discomfort?

Pain

- When did the pain begin? Relationship to last menses? Ovulatory?
- What is the character of the pain? Cramping? Sharp? Pressure? Stabbing? Colicky?
- What is the pattern of the pain? Constant? Intermittent? Episodic?
- Where is the pain located? Generalized? Midline suprapubic? Lateralized?
- Does the pain radiate? Vagina? Rectum? Legs? Back? Upper abdomen? Shoulder?
- Were there changes in the character, pattern, or location of the pain over time? For example, did cramping midline pain become acute sharp lateralized pain, followed by relief, evolving to generalized abdominal pain radiating to the shoulder? Did lateralized constant intense pressure evolve to acute sharp pain or intermittent colicky pain?
- Is there exacerbation of the pain with movement? Intercourse? Coughing?
- Are there any urinary tract symptoms? Dysuria?
- Are there any intestinal symptoms? Constipation? Obstipation? Diarrhea?

Physical Examination

The approach to the physical examination of the gynecologic patient must account for the threat to dignity and modesty that genital examination poses. In the emergency setting, against a background of fear or pain, and especially among the young and the elderly patients, the patient must be afforded maximum comfort. This includes an adequate sense of physical privacy, the continuous presence of a chaperone, a comfortable examination table on which to assume the lithotomy position, and patience by the examiner.

Although the chief complaint might suggest that only a focused pelvic examination is necessary, the examiner will enhance comfort and trust by a more general examination before the pelvic exam. The examiner must remember that the patient cannot see and cannot anticipate what she will experience next; the examiner or the assistant informs the patient at every step in the process what the next sensation will be.

At the beginning of the pelvic exam, the examiner encourages relaxation and exposure by having the patient relax her medial thighs to allow the knees to drop out toward laterally placed hands. The knees must never be pushed apart by the examiner. Before contacting the genitalia, gentle touch of the gloved hand on the medial thigh, with gentle pressure and movement toward the vulva, will orient the patient to the progress of the exam. The external genitalia are inspected for lesions and evidence of trauma. This is followed by the insertion of a properly sized, lubricated vaginal speculum. The patient needs to be prepared for the speculum by placing a

finger on the perineum and exerting gentle pressure with encouragement to relax the introital muscles. The speculum is placed at the hymeneal ring at a 30-degree angle from the vertical in order to minimize lateral or urethral pressure. After the leading edge is through the introitus, the speculum is rotated to the horizontal plane as it is advanced toward the apex of the vagina. The blades are gently separated as the midvagina is approached so that the cervix can be visualized, and the blades are spread to surround the cervix. During the advancement and subsequent withdrawal, the walls of the vagina are visualized for lesions or trauma. The cervix is inspected for lesions, lacerations, dilation, products of conception, or purulent discharge. Support of the pelvic structures in the anterior, posterior, and superior compartments is evaluated. Vaginal swabs for microscopic wet mount examination of the vaginal environment, for gonorrhea and chlamydia, and for a Papanicolaou (Pap) test is obtained as indicated.

After the speculum examination, the index and middle fingers of the dominant hand are inserted into the vagina. Before placing the abdominal hand, the examining fingers gently palpate the vaginal walls to elicit tenderness or to detect fullness or mass. The cervix is palpated for size and consistency. The examining fingers are placed sequentially along the side in all four quadrants of the cervix, and gentle pressure is exerted to move the cervix in the opposite direction to elicit cervical motion tenderness.

Because the major supporting structures for the uterus are the cardinal and uterosacral ligaments that insert at the cervicouterine junction, the junction serves as the fulcrum for leverage. As the cervix is moved in one direction, it is likely that the uterine fundus is being displaced in the opposite direction. Tenderness with cervical motion may be related to traction on the ligamentous attachments, collision of the cervix against a structure in the direction to which the cervix is being displaced, or collision of the fundus against a structure on the opposite side.

The bimanual examination is performed with gentle pressure from the nondominant hand systematically mobilizing pelvic contents against the vaginal fingers. Except with large masses that are palpable on abdominal examination, the primary information gathered is detected by the vaginal fingers. Specifically note lateralized tenderness and masses. The rectovaginal examination provides additional perspective, especially for the cul-de-sac and adnexal structures.

Very young women and some elderly women will not tolerate insertion of two fingers, or occasionally even one. Under these circumstances, a rectal finger along with the abdominal placement of the other hand can simulate a bimanual examination.

Diagnostic Considerations

Although there are always atypical crossover presentations for any of the possible diagnoses, the most common considerations for the differential diagnosis of symptom complexes are as follow:

Bleeding Without Pain

- Anovulatory cycle
- Threatened or spontaneous abortion (miscarriage of intrauterine pregnancy)
- Vaginal laceration
- Vaginal or cervical neoplasm

Bleeding Associated With Midline Suprapubic Pain

- Dysmenorrhea
- Threatened or spontaneous abortion (miscarriage of intrauterine pregnancy)
- Endometritis associated with pelvic infection
- Uterine fibroids
- Early presentation of a complication of extrauterine pregnancy
- Vaginal laceration

Bleeding Associated With Lateralized Pelvic Pain

- Extrauterine pregnancy, prerupture
- Functional ovarian cyst
- Ruptured functional ovarian cyst
- Ruptured corpus luteum with or without an intrauterine pregnancy
- Vaginal trauma

Bleeding Associated With Generalized Pelvic Pain

- Ruptured extrauterine pregnancy
- Ruptured corpus luteum with or without an intrauterine pregnancy
- Septic spontaneous or induced abortion
- Vaginal trauma

Midline Pelvic Pain Without Bleeding

- Endometritis or PID
- Endometriosis
- Pelvic neoplasm
- Urinary tract infection
- Constipation

Lateralized Pelvic Pain Without Bleeding

- Extrauterine pregnancy
- Functional ovarian cyst, with or without intraparenchymal hemorrhage
- Functional ovarian cyst with rupture
- Functional or neoplastic ovarian cyst with intermittent torsion
- Pedunculated paratubal or paraovarian cyst with intermittent torsion
- Endometriosis
- Ovarian remnant syndrome
- Ureteritis
- Constipation

Generalized Abdominal Pain Without Bleeding

- Ruptured extrauterine pregnancy
- Ruptured ovarian cyst
- PID with pelvic peritonitis
- Endometriosis

Obstipation

- Cul-de-sac hematoma
- Cul-de-sac adnexal mass
- Posterior uterine fibroid
- Pelvic abscess
- Endometriosis

Flank Pain

- Pyelonephritis
- Ureteral obstruction
- Ovarian remnant syndrome with or without ureteral obstruction

Other Acute Clinical Presentations

Acute vulvovaginitis is a common presenting emergency complaint. Presenting symptoms are intense pruritus or cutaneous pain with discharge. The most frequent pathogens are mycotic or herpes simplex. Mycotic infections are generally characterized by a thick, white, cottage cheese–like discharge. Primary herpetic infections often present with profuse watery discharge, inguinal adenopathy, and signs of a viremia. In contrast, other common vaginal infections, such as bacterial vaginosis and trichomoniasis, may cause irritative symptoms and malodorous discharge, but rarely cause pain.

Common acute vulvar complaints include infection of skin appendages: folliculitis, furunculosis, and cellulitis. The ostium of the Bartholin's gland may become occluded, with or without infection. Sterile cysts are only minimally uncomfortable, but a Bartholin's cyst abscess is exquisitely painful.

Necrotizing fasciitis is a life-threatening infection that can occur in the vulva. It can begin as a cellulitis, from infected skin appendages, or following biopsy or episiotomy. Once established, it can quickly extend through the fascial planes. Women at risk are patients with obesity, diabetes, and steroid or other immunosuppressive drug use. Management is immediate surgical débridement. Patients may require several débridements to determine the extent of the fascial involvement. Skin grafts are often needed to repair large defects. It is very important that women with risk factors for necrotizing fasciitis who present with a vulvar cellulitis be admitted for intravenous (IV) antibiotics and possible surgical treatment.

Pelvic Masses

Masses identified in the pelvis can be functional, congenital, neoplastic, hemorrhagic, or inflammatory and can arise from the ovary or the uterus. Additionally, the anatomy of the cul-de-sac of Douglas in its dependent position in the pelvis facilitates restriction of pelvic infection as collections or abscesses to that location.

Common ovarian masses include functional cysts, hemorrhagic cysts, paraovarian or paratubal woolfian remnants, endometrioma, and benign or malignant tumors (epithelial, germ cell, stromal). The most common neoplastic mass in young women is the benign cystic teratoma. Because of the sebaceous content of these lesions, they frequently "float" to the anterior cul-de-sac between the uterus and the bladder. Diagnostic considerations for differentiating among ovarian masses of the various etiologies are discussed in detail in the later section on ovarian cancer.

Common uterine masses include leiomyoma, adenomyoma, and bicornuate uterus. Common inflammatory masses are tubo-ovarian abscess (TOA), pelvic collection, and appendiceal or diverticular abscesses.

Inflammatory masses in the anterior cul-de-sac most commonly originate from sigmoid diverticular disease.

Ancillary Tests

Imaging
The single most effective and efficient modality for assessing pelvic anatomy and pathology is real-time ultrasound, especially with a transvaginal transducer. This technique not only allows assessment of the size and relationship of the pelvic structures, but also, by clear delineation of echogenicity, can provide strong suspicion of the nature of pathology. With real-time Doppler flow assessment, blood flow to an organ or mass and fetal heart motion are readily apparent.

Axial tomography and magnetic resonance imaging (MRI) rarely provide additional information for benign pelvic pathology but are valuable techniques for assessing malignancies.

IV pyelography may be useful if ultrasound assessment of the urinary tract is inadequate to delineate obstruction or anatomic distortion.

Pregnancy Tests
There are two endocrine tests that are useful for determining the presence and health of a pregnancy: human chorionic gonadotropin (HCG) and progesterone.

Modern pregnancy tests measure the β subunit of HCG, and the sensitivity of the qualitative urine assay can be as low as 20 mIU/mL. This is sufficiently low as to virtually exclude all but the earliest of gestations. Unless a viable fetus can be detected clinically or by ultrasound, a positive urine test in the clinical setting that could suggest an ectopic pregnancy must be followed with a quantitative serum radioimmunoassay. A result less than 5 mIU/mL is a negative test. In most laboratories, and depending on the quality of the ultrasound equipment and the experience of the sonographer, a healthy intrauterine pregnancy that has produced 2000 mIU/mL of β-HCG is generally visualized. In the absence of that threshold, serial β-HCG tests are scheduled at 2-day intervals.[1]

In the so-called typical healthy intrauterine pregnancy, serum β-HCG levels double every 48 hours. However, this description is based on pooled, aggregated data; within the data sets, there are many patients with successful pregnancies who will have intervals with a lower slope of rise followed by an interval with steep rise. A decline in value over a 2-day period is always ominous and, therefore, demands a clinical decision about intrauterine versus extrauterine failed pregnancy. The greater challenge occurs when the rate of increase is less than 60% over 48 hours. This is ambiguous, and if the β-HCG

is below the discriminatory value of 2000 mIU, clinical presentation and clinical judgment are vital to determine whether continued observation or intervention is the appropriate course.[2]

Note that there are three commonly used reference standards for β-HCG, as well as significant interlaboratory variation in test results. It is critical to understand the standard used and to be certain that the sequential tests are performed in the same laboratory. If a change in laboratories is necessary, repeated parallel testing in the new lab using the residual serum from the original sample will resolve the question. Significantly elevated β-HCG levels raise suspicion of a hydatidiform mole or a germ cell tumor.

Serum progesterone can be a useful adjunct in assessing the viability of a pregnancy. The quantitative relationship with pregnancy status is not as discrete, and cutoff values must be established in each laboratory. Progesterone levels less than 5 ng/mL are rarely associated with successful pregnancies. A recent report demonstrated 100% sensitivity for ectopic pregnancy and 100% negative predictive value for a progesterone level cutoff of 22 ng/mL, but specificity and positive predictive value were poor. The role of progesterone assay results in the clinical management of the acute patient is not yet clear.[3]

Serum Hormone Assays
Other than the assessment of pregnancy, there is relatively little value to ordering reproductive hormone levels in the acute setting. These tests are relatively expensive, and the sequence of ordering them is determined by the clinical findings. The laboratory turn-around time is rarely less than a day.

Cervicovaginal Cultures, Gram Stain, and Wet Prep
Because the healthy vagina is a polymicrobial environment, there are only four organisms for which cervicovaginal cultures are clinically useful: gonococcus, *Chlamydia trachomatis*, herpes simplex, and, in pregnancy, group B β-hemolytic streptococcus. Current technology links the tests for gonococcus and chlamydia in a single swab-medium kit for molecular analysis of the organisms.

Gram stain of purulent cervical discharge is useful in the emergency setting for identification of the gram-negative intracellular diplococci, diagnostic of gonococcus. The test may also be useful in helping identify trichomonas vaginalis. Culture and Gram stain of purulent material from an abscess of Bartholin's gland may allow the physician to select a narrow spectrum antibiotic as an adjunct to drainage.

The vaginal wet mount is useful in diagnosis of the offending organism in acute vaginitis. A sample of discharge is taken, both from the vaginal pool and by rubbing the vaginal walls with a cotton swab. The swab is placed in 1 to 2 mm of saline in a tube to create a slurry. A drop of the slurry is placed on a slide with a cover slip and viewed examined under low- and high-power light microscopy for polymorphonuclear leukocytes, clue cells, trichomonads, hyphae, and budding yeast forms. If hyphae and budding yeast forms are not identified, a second slide is prepared by mixing a drop of the slurry with a drop of potassium hydroxide, which will lyse the epithelial cells and highlight the fungal organisms.

The clue cell is an epithelial cell with densely adherent bacteria, creating a stippled effect. To make this diagnosis, the density of bacteria must obscure cell margins in a substantial percentage of the cells. These, along with a strong amine odor, are diagnostic of bacterial vaginosis. There is rarely a significant white cell response to this condition because it is not an infection per se, but rather, a shift in the normal vaginal ecosystem.

Trichomonads are often obvious as flagellated, motile organisms similar in size to white blood cells. The organism is fragile, however, and motility can be inhibited by severe infection or cooling of the specimen during a delay before inspecting.

Lower Genital Cytology

The Pap cytology technique has had significant public health impact, reducing the incidence of invasive cervical cancer. Although the processing time for the smear limits usefulness in the acute setting, there are two important reasons to consider obtaining the sample. The first is to take the opportunity of the visit to test a previously noncompliant patient. The second is to satisfy any significant concern about a high-grade cervical lesion before surgical manipulation of the cervix (see "Special Considerations in Management of Cervical Cancer and Treatment Complications," later).

There are two fundamental approaches to obtaining and preparing the specimen. In the older technique, a cervical spatula is placed in the cervical os and rotated circumferentially against the cervical epithelium. This is followed by a cotton swab placed in the cervical canal and rotated on its long axis. As each step is completed, the instrument is wiped across a glass slide, and spray fixative is applied. In the more recent technique, the specimen from the instrument is swirled in a fluid-based preservative, which is processed to provide a more homogeneous slide for Pap staining. Although the cost of the fluid-based technique is greater, the improved accuracy and the reduction of both false-positive and false-negative results makes this more cost-effective.

MANAGEMENT OF PREINVASIVE AND INVASIVE DISEASE OF THE FEMALE GENITAL TRACT

Staging guidelines for various types of neoplasia may be found at the website for the Federation of International Gynecologic Oncology, www.figo.org; see also the Selected References at the end of this chapter.[4]

Preinvasive Vulvar Squamous Lesions

Dysplasia of the vulva usually presents with persistent symptoms of vulvar pruritus, occasionally because the patient has seen a visible lesion and rarely because of bleeding. Vulvar dysplasia and condylomata tend to be multifocal and can involve any area on the vulva (Fig.

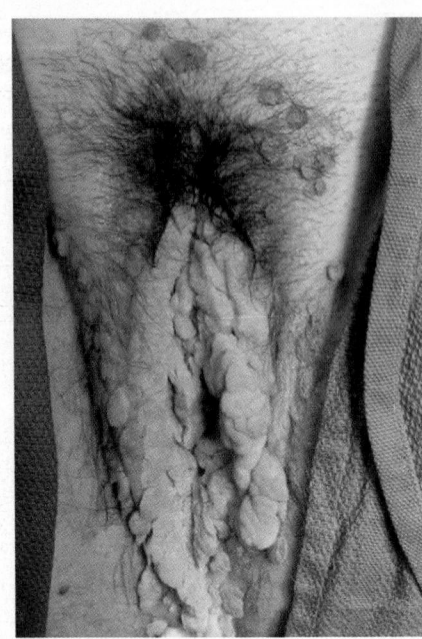

Figure 75-7 Condylomata. (Courtesy of Lynn Parker, MD, Vanderbilt University Medical Center.)

75-7). On physical exam, the dysplasia can appear as white thickened epithelium, pigmented, erythematous, exophytic, or a combination of the above. Because appearance can be variable, a 4- or 5-mm punch biopsy sample is taken to differentiate dysplasia from an invasive lesion. Vulvar dysplasia is related to exposure to the human papillomavirus (HPV); but unlike cervical cancer, there is not a direct relationship between preinvasive disease and cancer.

Evaluation of the patient with vulvar dysplasia includes colposcopy of the vulva, vagina, and cervix because 15% to 20% of patients have dysplasia in more than one of these sites. Colposcopy is the use of a microscope to better visualize the area of concern. A 4% acetic acid solution is applied to the skin to make more apparent any areas of preinvasive disease. Changes can appear as thickened white epithelium, vascular changes, or any of the possible appearances described previously. A biopsy sample is taken of any suspicious lesion and sent to pathology. Pathologic classification is based on the extent of epithelial involvement: involvement up to one third of the epithelium is called *vulvar intraepithelial neoplasia type I* (VIN I); up to two thirds, VIN II; and greater than two thirds, VIN III.

Treatment of dysplasia of the vulva includes wide local excision with a 5-mm margin around the lesion and little, if any, removal of the underlying subcutaneous tissue. This approach is best used in patients with a focal lesion. Patients who have multifocal disease will benefit from laser ablation with CO_2 laser. Depth of ablation depends on whether of not the area is hair bearing. Hair-bearing areas require ablation to a depth of 2 to 2.5 mm. Non-hair-bearing areas are ablated to a depth of 1 to 2 mm. Postoperative care of the treatment area includes silver sulfadiazine (Silvadene) cream applications three times a day.

Table 75-2 Treatment of Vulvar Cancer

DIAGNOSIS	TREATMENT
Invasion <1 mm	Wide local excision
Stage I or II lesion, lateral location	Wide radical excision + unilateral inguinofemoral lymphadenectomy
Stage I or II midline lesion	Wide radical + bilateral inguinofemoral lymphadenectomy
Lesion with extension into vagina, anus, or distal urethra	Wide radical excision with bilateral inguinofemoral lymphadenectomy or chemoradiation followed by excision of residual tumor
Any size lesion with groin nodes	Excision of groin followed by chemoradiation therapy
Distant metastases	Palliative chemotherapy

An alternative treatment is imiquimod (Aldara) cream. The mechanism of action is thought to be stimulation of the patient's immune system to reverse the effect of the HPV virus. The most common side effect of the cream is an area of irritation involving the treatment area.

Invasive Vulvar Squamous Lesions

The most common vulvar cancer is squamous cell carcinoma (90%). It tends to present in women older than 65 years. Other risk factors include immunocompromised state, cigarette smoking, obesity, and lichen sclerosis. Patients may present with a visible lesion, bleeding, pain, or dysuria. The lesion may be exophytic, ulcerative, or nodular. Any suspicious lesion on the vulva undergoes a 3- or 4-mm punch biopsy to rule out malignancy. Any lesion with greater than 1 mm depth of invasion requires treatment not only of the primary lesion but also evaluation of the inguinal lymph nodes.

Treatment of vulvar cancer is primarily surgical. For early-stage disease, primary therapy is wide radical excision, which is removal of a 1.5- to 2-cm margin around the primary tumor, and removal of the subcutaneous tissue down to the level of the endopelvic fascia. If the lesion is lateralized, the ipsilateral inguinal lymph nodes only need to be removed. If the lesion is midline, bilateral inguinal lymph nodes are removed. If more than two lymph nodes are positive, the patient receives postoperative radiation therapy. If one node is positive and only ipsilateral nodes were done, the other groin is dissected. For advanced-stage disease (stage III or IV), chemotherapy and radiation are treatments of choice. Although if there are large inguinal lymph nodes, surgical debulking may have value before chemoradiation (Table 75-2).

Vulvar cancer may recur locally or distally. With local recurrence, wide radical excision can be used with removal of ipsilateral nodes if they have not previously been removed. Distal sites can include nodal areas, liver, lung, and subcutaneous nodules in the skin. Unless there is an isolated lesion that can be excised, distal disease is best treated with chemotherapy.

Verrucous carcinoma is a specific variant of vulvar carcinoma that presents as a fungating mass. It has a papillary architecture with pushing borders. Microscopically, there is little or mild nuclear atypia, which distinguishes it from warty squamous cell carcinomas. In general, this type of vulvar cancer is best treated with surgery. As opposed to other vulvar malignancies, it may get larger if treated with radiation therapy.

Melanoma of the Vulva

Melanoma is the second most common type of malignancy involving the vulva, primarily occurring in older women. Clinical presentation and appearance are similar to melanoma at other sites, and lesions are staged by the same criteria. Standard treatment is wide local excision with a 2-cm margin around the lesion. Melanomas of the vulva follow lymphatic pathways just as they do in other locations in the body, but the role of lymphadenectomy in the treatment of vulvar melanoma is controversial. Lymphadenectomy in this disease appears to be prognostic instead of therapeutic, and helps identify patients who would benefit from adjuvant therapy.

Bartholin's Gland Carcinoma

Bartholin's gland carcinomas can be adenocarcinomas arising from the gland itself, squamous cell carcinomas that arise from the duct, or adenoid cystic carcinomas. Histologically, there must be a transition between normal gland or duct and cancer to make the diagnosis. Unlike squamous cells cancers, lymph node involvement is common and can be bilateral. Treatment is wide radical excision with bilateral lymph node dissection.

Basal Cell Carcinoma

Just like basal cell carcinomas in other locations, vulvar basal cell carcinoma is a local tumor with little risk for lymph node metastasis. Therefore, treatment includes wide local excision only.

Paget's Disease of the Vulva

Paget's disease of the vulva occurs in postmenopausal women. It presents as a red, velvety lesion with pruritus and, occasionally, bleeding. It can occur anywhere on the vulva. Microscopically, the disease extends far beyond the visible lesion. Paget's disease may be intraepithelial, invasive beyond the basement membrane, or Paget's with an underlying adenocarcinoma (Paget's cells involving the epithelium plus an adenocarcinoma in the subcutaneous tissue). Paget's disease of the vulva is also associated with coexisting malignancies such as breast, colon, or genitourinary locations. Workup of patients with this diagnosis includes screening for other malignancies. Treatment is wide local excision for patients with intraepithelial Paget's, but wide radical excision and lymph node dissections are considered in patients with invasive Paget's or intraepithelial Paget's with an underlying adenocarcinoma.

Vulvar Sarcomas

Vulvar sarcomas can occur with many histologic subtypes. In general, the treatment is wide radical excision followed by radiation therapy and in some cases postoperative chemotherapy.

Preinvasive Vaginal Lesions

Dysplasia of the vagina, with or without overt condylomata, typically presents with an abnormal Pap smear. On colposcopic exam, lesions appear as thickened white epithelium or areas of vascular change. In patients with a uterus intact, vaginal dysplasia is typically seen in conjunction with cervical dysplasia. Therefore, colposcopy of the cervix also includes evaluation of the vagina. Any abnormal area on colposcopy undergoes biopsy to confirm the diagnosis and rule out invasion.

Treatment of vaginal dysplasia includes laser ablation or wide excision of the vaginal mucosa. An alternative treatment for women who are poor surgical candidates is intravaginal 5-fluorouracil (5-FU).

Invasive Vaginal Lesions

Although far less common than squamous cell carcinomas of the cervix or vulva, this lesion is the most common type of cancer in the vagina. Tumors may be identified through an abnormal Pap smear or by a visible lesion. They can occur at any location in the vagina but are most likely to occur at the vaginal apex. These tumors can present as a second primary site in patients with previous cervical carcinoma. Diagnosis is made with biopsy or wide local excision. It is important to exclude a cervical cancer with vaginal involvement and recurrent cervical or endometrial carcinoma. If a vaginal primary is confirmed, staging is based on examination and evaluation of the paravaginal areas and sidewall. If the disease is apical, pelvic nodal disease is the most likely site of spread. If the disease is in the lower vagina, inguinal node involvement must be ruled out. Computed tomography (CT) scans of the abdomen and pelvis are done to rule out nodal involvement. A chest x-ray must be done to rule out pulmonary metastasis.

Treatment options for vaginal cancer include surgical resection or chemoradiation for stage I tumors and chemoradiation for more advanced disease. Recurrence can be local or remote. If recurrence is local after radiation, pelvic exenteration can be considered. For remote recurrence, chemotherapy is used.

Vaginal adenocarcinomas occur rarely. Most well known is the correlation of clear cell carcinoma of the vagina in patients who were exposed in utero to diethylstilbestrol (DES). Because DES has not been used for many years, this diagnosis has decreased in occurrence. Other epithelial types can include endometrioid or papillary serous carcinomas. Treatment of adenocarcinomas is the same as outlined for squamous malignancies. Neuroendocrine carcinomas can occur in the vagina. Evaluation for metastasis includes not only the chest, abdomen, and pelvis but also the head and bones. As opposed to squamous malignancies, chemotherapy and radiation therapy are most appropriate.

Melanomas can occur in the vagina, with the same variations of presentation as other body sites. Treatment options include anterior or posterior exenteration depending on the location of the lesion in the vagina. Pelvic irradiation can also be considered. Prognosis is poor for these patients even if surgical margins are negative.

Rhabdomyosarcoma can occur in the vagina and mainly occurs in young girls. Combined-modality therapy with surgery, chemotherapy, and radiation therapy has been the most effective in treating this tumor.

Preinvasive Disease of the Cervix

HPV is a DNA virus that has an affinity for cells in the junction of squamous and glandular cells in the cervix (transformation zone). High-risk HPV types, most notably types 16 and 18, enter the cell and use the cell's system to produce viral products like E6 and E7. These viral products interfere with the cell's natural apoptotic mechanism, which makes the cell immortal. This is the mechanism for the transition to malignancy for HPV-related cancers. Dysplasia or precancer can occur in the cervix and typically arises in the transformation zone.

Pap smears are a screening test for dysplasia and malignancy. Over the years, there have been several classifications of Pap smears, of which the most recent is the revised Bethesda Classification. In that classification, patients who require further evaluation with colposcopy include those with glandular lesions, atypical cells and inability to rule out a high-grade lesion, or low-grade or high-grade squamous intraepithelial lesions. Biopsy at the time of colposcopy can confirm the histologic diagnosis of mild, moderate, or severe dysplasia. At the time of colposcopy, comment is made as to whether the entire lesion and transformation zone can be seen. If the patient has an adequate colposcopic exam, a low-grade lesion (mild dysplasia), and is compliant, she can be expectantly managed because regression may occur in up to 70% of patients over 2 years. If the patient is noncompliant or has other concerning factors, treatment could include cryotherapy, large-loop excision of the transformation zone (LEEP), or laser ablation. For high-grade lesions such as moderate or severe dysplasia, LEEP or laser is a consideration.

Cone biopsy is recommended for patients who have glandular lesions, a Pap smear causing concern for invasion or microinvasion, a positive endocervical curetting, inadequate colposcopy, or a two-step discrepancy between Pap smear and biopsy results. The technique for cone biopsy is discussed later.

Invasive Disease of the Cervix

Ninety percent of invasive cancers of the cervix are squamous cell carcinomas. Other histologic types include adenocarcinoma, adenosquamous carcinoma, neuroendocrine carcinoma, basal cell carcinoma, and rarely signet ring cell carcinoma. Patients may present with postcoital bleeding, irregular bleeding, malodorous discharge, abnormal Pap smear, or visible lesion. Advanced lesions

Table 75-3   Treatment of Cervical Cancer

DIAGNOSIS	TREATMENT
Stage IA1	Simple hysterectomy
Stage IA2	Modified radical hysterectomy and pelvic lymphadenectomy
Stage IB1	Radical hysterectomy and pelvic lymphadenectomy; or pelvic radiation therapy followed by brachytherapy
Stage IB2	Chemoradiation therapy
Stage IIA-IVA	Chemoradiation therapy
Stage IVB	Palliative radiation with chemotherapy

may present with symptoms of sidewall involvement, which include back pain that radiates down the leg, unilateral edema of the leg, or flank pain. Whether there is a grossly visible lesion or abnormal cytology and abnormal colposcopy, diagnosis requires tissue biopsy. Cervical cancer is staged clinically. These lesions invade into the stroma of the cervix, then expand into the lymphatics accompanying the ligamentous supporting tissues of the cervix and upper vagina. As they extend, pelvic sidewall involvement may cause ureteral obstruction and hydronephrosis. The bladder or rectum may become involved. Although lymphatic spread is common, staging criteria do not include node involvement. That being said, however, metastasis to lymph nodes significantly affects prognosis.

When the diagnosis of cervical cancer is made from a LEEP or a cone biopsy, it is important to determine as accurately as possible the depth of invasion involved. The type of treatment recommended varies significantly based on depth of invasion.

Once the diagnosis is confirmed histologically, bimanual and rectovaginal exam is done to determine whether there is any vaginal, parametrial, or pelvic sidewall extension. This completes clinical staging. Other evaluation includes a chest radiograph, either a CT scan or IV pyelogram to rule out hydronephrosis, and either a CT scan or lymphangiogram to rule out lymph node involvement.

Treatment varies with stage of disease (Table 75-3). For example, a tumor with 1 to 3 mm of invasion is a microinvasive cancer of the cervix that can be treated with simple hysterectomy or, in selected cases, with a cone biopsy in patients who strongly desire fertility. However, a tumor with greater than 5 mm depth of invasion or 7 mm on horizontal extent is a stage IB1 tumor with 10% risk for pelvic lymph node metastasis and requires a radical hysterectomy for treatment. Therefore, if depth of invasion cannot be accurately determined, or if the invasive component involves the endocervical margin, a repeat cone biopsy is done.

Treatment of Stage IA1 Disease
Stage IA1 disease is typically a total abdominal hysterectomy. However, some European studies have described treating this disease with cold-knife cone biopsy in

patients who strongly desire fertility and will be compliant with follow-up.

Treatment of Stage IA2 Disease
Stage IA2 disease is treated with modified radical hysterectomy. Modified radical hysterectomy differs from radical hysterectomy in that the uterine artery is ligated at the level of the ureter instead of at the origin.

Treatment of Stage IB1 Disease
Patients with stage IB1 disease have equal cure rates with radiation therapy or radical hysterectomy with pelvic lymphadenectomy. Radiation therapy includes 45 to 50 Gy of whole pelvic radiation followed by brachytherapy. The goal dose is 85 to 90 Gy to point A, which is a point measured 2 cm above and 2 cm lateral to the cervix. Radical hysterectomy involves removal of the uterus, parametrial tissue, and 1 cm of the upper vagina. *It does not necessarily include oophorectomy.* Cure rates are between 85% and 90%. Risks and benefits of both treatment options are discussed with the patient and a treatment plan agreed on.

Pelvic lymphadenectomy involves removal of all visible lymph tissue from the level of the bifurcation of the iliac arteries down to the transverse circumflex iliac vein. Laterally, the tissue is separated from the genitofemoral nerve and the external iliac artery and vein. The bundle is then separated medially from the hypogastric and superior vesical artery. Inferiorly, the bundle is separated from the obturator nerve.

In patients who have more than one positive pelvic lymph node, deep invasion of the cervix, or a positive margin, pelvic radiation is recommended postoperatively.

Treatment of Stage IB2 Disease
Stage IB2 or bulky IB2 disease can be treated in a variety of ways. Some would favor radical hysterectomy with a high likelihood of postoperative radiation therapy. Others would favor chemoradiation as primary treatment. Finally, some patients respond to pelvic radiation and one brachytherapy followed by extrafascial hysterectomy.

Treatment of Stages IIA to IVA
Stage IIA disease can be treated with radical hysterectomy, but most gynecologic oncologists would currently treat these patients with chemoradiation. For stage IIB to IVA tumors, treatment is a combination of radiation therapy with cisplatin-based chemotherapy. In 1999, Morris and colleagues compared extended-field radiation therapy versus chemotherapy and radiation in stage IB2 to IVA tumors. There was a survival advantage seen for patients receiving chemoradiation. Current regimens include cisplatin, possibly in combination with 5-FU.

Treatment of Stage IVB Disease
Stage IVB disease involves distant metastasis. Most commonly seen is lung or liver. In this instance, radiation therapy is changed to palliative, and chemotherapy is the focus of treatment. First-line agents typically include cisplatin or 5-FU.

Treatment of Patients with Enlarged Lymph Nodes

When enlarged lymph nodes are seen on initial CT evaluation, patients may benefit from retroperitoneal lymph node dissection to remove the bulky disease. Radiation therapy alone cannot sterilize bulky adenopathy. Retroperitoneal node dissection allows the nodes to be debulked and to determine whether para-aortic lymph nodes are involved. Para-aortic lymph node involvement is a poor prognostic factor. Nodal dissection is undertaken with a retroperitoneal approach through a paramedian or midline incision. A retroperitoneal approach has a much lower risk for fistula formation or bowel obstruction than an intraperitoneal approach.

Treatment of Neuroendocrine Tumors

Neuroendocrine carcinomas of the cervix are among the most rare and aggressive types. Five-year survival rates have been reported in the 5% to 10% range. As with other neuroendocrine tumors, the disease can metastasize to bone, brain, lung, or liver. Assessment includes evaluation of these areas before treatment. As opposed to other cervical cancers, chemoradiation regimens can include other agents in addition to cisplatin such as etoposide.

Treatment of Recurrent Disease

If the patient has evidence of local recurrence on pelvic exam, distant disease must be ruled out by imaging studies. After this has been completed, sidewall involvement must be ruled out on exam. Patients with central recurrence of cervical cancer who have received previous radiation therapy can be cured with pelvic exenteration (Fig. 75-8). Survival rates are between 30% and 40%.

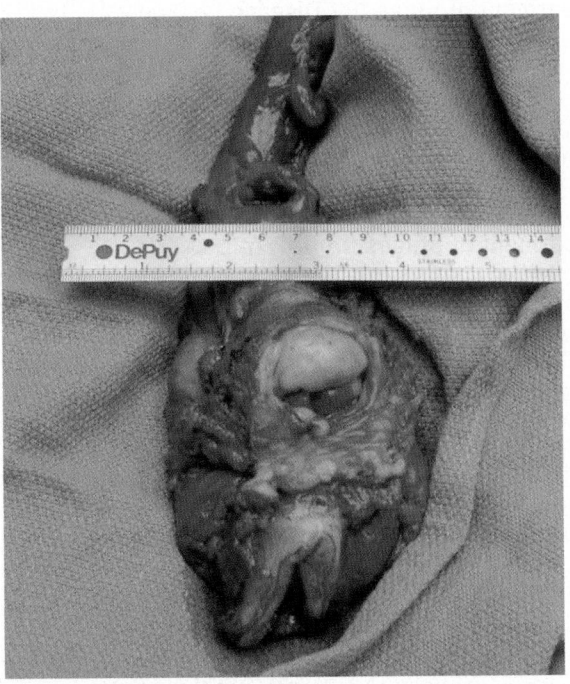

Figure 75-8 Pelvic exenteration. (Courtesy of Lynn Parker, MD, Vanderbilt University Medical Center.)

Postoperative morbidity and mortality rates for the procedure can be as high as 10%. Isolated distant metastasis, such as a single lung lesion or an incisional recurrence, may be treated with surgical resection followed by radiation therapy. In patients with multiple, distant metastases or sidewall involvement, chemotherapy is palliative, and an average life expectancy is 9 to 12 months.

Special Considerations in Management of Cervical Cancer and Treatment Complications

Inappropriate Surgical Management

One of the most frequent and deleterious errors in surgical management of cervical cancer is failure to recognize the importance of block dissection of the tumor. The so-called cut-through procedure, in which the surgeon transects active cancer extending beyond the cervix, results in a reduction of 5-year survival rates from the 50% to 85% range to the 20% to 30% range. This error may occur because of inadequate preoperative evaluation of the diagnosed cancer or be encountered at the time of hysterectomy for presumed (and perhaps, coexistent) benign disease.

Treatment of the Pregnant Patient

Cervical cancer diagnosed early in pregnancy is a difficult situation. By continuing the pregnancy, the mother may be risking her own life. Recommendations in the first trimester are to consider radical hysterectomy in stage IB1 lesions and chemoradiation in higher-stage lesions. If the radiation is given, spontaneous abortion will occur in 4 to 6 weeks. In the second trimester and later, the patient may be expectantly managed until maturity of the fetus, with plans for treatment after delivery. Typically, delivery is expedited at 34 weeks once lung maturity is confirmed.

Management of the Cervical Cancer Patient With Acute Hemorrhage

Some patients with cervical cancer present with acute hemorrhage. When this occurs, *do not attempt a surgical resection.* The vagina is packed with Monsel's solution applied to the gauze and a Foley catheter is placed. The patient is transfused, then transferred to a center that can begin evaluation and treatment.

Management of Radiation Complications

Typical complications after radiation therapy include hemorrhagic cystitis, hemorrhagic proctitis, small bowel obstruction, and fistula formation.

Hemorrhagic cystitis can be managed with placement of a large three-way Foley catheter with continuous bladder irrigation. Hydrocortisone can be added as well. Cystoscopy and focal cauterization can also stop focal bleeding sites. Transfusion is commonly required.

Hemorrhagic proctitis can be managed with cortisone enemas and transfusion. Colonoscopy with focal cautery can also be used. *However, biopsies are avoided owing to the risk for fistula formation.* In some cases, colostomy with resection of the affected bowel may be indicated.

Small bowel obstruction tends to occur in the ileum in patients who had previous surgery before radiation. When conservative management fails, laparotomy with small bowel resection and reanastomosis may be required. Sharp dissection is important to use to avoid injury to surrounding structures.

Fistula formation occurs in 3% to 5% of patients treated with radiation therapy. Patients at higher risk include diabetic patients and patients with peripheral vascular disease or collagen vascular disease. Rectovaginal fistula in a radiated field typically is not treatable with more conservative surgeries, and colostomy is required. In vesicovaginal fistulas, a urinary conduit is usually required.

Endometrium

The patient who presents with postmenopausal bleeding or abnormal bleeding after chronic anovulatory amenorrhea must be evaluated for endometrial hyperplasia or endometrial carcinoma. Although suspicion may be heightened by an abnormal endometrial ultrasound, diagnosis of these lesions requires tissue confirmation. Ultrasound measurement of the thickness of endometrial stripe can assist in avoiding unnecessary biopsies. The postmenopausal woman who has an endometrial bilayer stripe less than 5 mm without an irregularity in the cavity is very unlikely to have a carcinoma. If patient comfort or cervical stenosis precludes office endometrial biopsy, dilation and curettage (D&C) may be necessary to make the diagnosis.

Hyperplasia

Endometrial hyperplasia is an overgrowth of the lining of the uterus. There are several different histologic types, including simple hyperplasia, simple hyperplasia with atypia, complex hyperplasia, and complex hyperplasia with atypia. These are listed in an order of increasing risk of development into endometrial adenocarcinoma. Patients with complex hyperplasia with atypia have a 20% to 30% chance of developing or having a coexisting adenocarcinoma. Risk factors for hyperplasia include obesity, hypertension, diabetes, anovulation, and unopposed estrogen use. Simple hyperplasia can be managed with progestin therapy followed by a repeat endometrial biopsy after 3 months. In patients with complex atypical hyperplasia who have completed childbearing, hysterectomy is recommended.

Endometrial Adenocarcinoma

There are many histologic types of endometrial cancer. The most common type is endometrioid, but other types include papillary, papillary serous, squamous, clear cell, and neuroendocrine. Papillary serous, clear cell, and neuroendocrine tumors behave aggressively with high risk for recurrence of disease.

Because bleeding is an early symptom, most patients present with early-stage disease, and potential for survival is high. Staging of endometrial adenocarcinoma is surgical. The procedure involves obtaining pelvic washings upon entering the abdomen, total abdominal hyster-

Table 75-4 Treatment of Endometrial Cancer

DIAGNOSIS	TREATMENT
Grade 1 or 2, stage IA or IB, <30% myometrial invasion, no lymph or vascular invasion	No further therapy
Grade 1, 2 with one third to two thirds myometrial invasion; or grade 1 or 2 with cervical involvement; no lymph or vascular invasion	Vaginal brachytherapy
Grade 1, 2 with more than two thirds myometrial invasion; grade 3 with myometrial invasion and lymph or vascular invasion	Whole pelvic radiation therapy
Stage IIIC disease	Extended-field radiation therapy
Stage IV B disease	Postoperative chemotherapy

ectomy with bilateral salpingo-oophorectomy, and possible bilateral pelvic and para-aortic lymphadenectomy. Recently, gynecologic oncologists have begun treating and surgically staging endometrial cancer with laparoscopic surgery. Results from clinical trials have shown similar outcomes to laparotomy and improved quality of life.[5] Table 75-4 outlines the patients who require lymphadenectomy as well as those who require postoperative radiation therapy. However, management of patients with advanced stage disease is variable, with chemotherapy, radiotherapy, and even adjunctive surgical debulking of tumor.

Risk factors for recurrence include grade of tumor, depth of invasion, lymphovascular space invasion, cervical involvement, stage of disease, and histologic subtype. Table 75-4 outlines treatment recommendations for postoperative vaginal brachytherapy or pelvic radiation.

Papillary serous adenocarcinoma of the endometrium behaves more like an ovarian carcinoma than an endometrial cancer. Most patients experience recurrence with intra-abdominal disease and carcinomatosis. This is a rare histologic type, and the numbers reported in the literature are small. Postoperative chemotherapy is indicated.

Treatment options for local recurrence of endometrial cancer in the pelvis include radiation therapy in the unradiated patient or pelvic exenteration in the radiated patient. Remote disease must be ruled out before undertaking these therapies. Half of patients who did not receive postoperative radiation can be salvaged in this situation. Isolated metastases involving the abdominal wall, lung, or bone can be treated with surgical resection or focused radiotherapy. Multifocal remote or nodal disease is treated with hormonal therapy or chemotherapy.

Endometrial Cancer in Young Women

If a young woman still desires children, she may be treated with high-dose progestins and followed with hysteroscopy and D&C. These patients must have no evidence of myometrial invasion on MRI. They also must actively pursue pregnancy, at times with the help of a reproductive endocrinologist, once the cancer has been cleared because of their risk factors for recurrence.

Endometrial Sarcomas

Endometrial sarcomas can present with vaginal bleeding or a rapidly growing uterus. The sarcoma can be homologous (arising from tissue normally found in the uterus such as smooth muscle) or heterologous (arising from tissue normally not found in the uterus such as cartilage). Sarcomas are classified based on tissue type, necrosis, and degree of atypia. Leiomyosarcoma is the most common type. Diagnosis is made on hypercellularity, moderate nuclear atypia, high mitotic rate (10 mitotic figures per 10 high-power fields), and tumor necrosis. Two of the last three are required for diagnosis.

Endometrial stromal sarcomas tend to occur in younger women and are low grade, with typically less than 3 mitotic figures per high-power field. High-grade endometrial sarcomas are rare and tend to be aggressive.

Management of these patients is surgical, with staging performed as noted for endometrial adenocarcinomas. These tumors are vascular, and patients often require intraoperative transfusion. Unlike endometrial adenocarcinomas, these tumors spread hematogenously and can recur in the pelvis, lung, or liver. Postoperative radiation therapy decreases risk for pelvic recurrence, but does not improve overall survival.

Mixed Mullerian Tumors of the Uterus

Malignant mixed mullerian tumors of the uterus (MMMTs) are a combination of epithelial adenocarcinoma and sarcoma that coexist in the uterus. The most common epithelial component is papillary serous carcinoma. It is the epithelial component that metastasizes, typically to the abdomen with carcinomatosis, lung, or liver. Staging is performed as in other endometrial cancers with the addition of omental biopsy because abdominal metastases are common. In patients with stage I and II disease, Molpus and colleagues[6] reported an increased survival in patients who received postoperative radiation therapy. For comparison, the 5-year survival rate with endometrioid adenocarcinoma stage I is about 90%, but in patients with MMMT, the 5-year survival rate is 50%. In patients with advanced disease, multiagent chemotherapy is indicated.

Management of a Pelvic Mass

When a pelvic mass is discovered on examination, ultrasound can be helpful in determining characteristics that are worrisome for malignancy. In general, a simple cyst in a premenopausal patient will not be cancerous. However, a mass with complex features such as septations, papillations, and solid components is more worrisome. Several benign lesions such as endometriomas, hemorrhagic corpus lutea, and dermoid cysts can have these features and must be in the differential diagnosis (Table 75-5). TOA can also appear worrisome on ultra-

Table 75-5 Differential Diagnosis of Ovarian Masses

MASS	DIFFERENTIAL DIAGNOSIS
Benign disease	Hemorrhagic corpus luteum; endometrioma; tubo-ovarian abscess; ectopic pregnancy; serous or mucinous cystadenoma; cystadenofibroma; fibroma; Brenner's tumor; dermoid
Malignant: epithelial	Serous borderline tumor; mucinous borderline tumor; invasive cancer (papillary serous; endometrioid; transitional cell; clear cell; neuroendocrine or small cell; malignant mixed mullerian tumor)
Germ cell	Dysgerminoma; endodermal sinus tumor; choriocarcinoma; immature teratoma; embryonal carcinoma; polyembryoma
Stromal	Sertoli-Leydig cell tumor; granulosa cell tumor
Metastasis	Colon cancer; stomach cancer; breast cancer; lymphoma

sound, so the clinical scenario is important in determining the treatment plan.

In a premenopausal patient with a simple cyst, an ultrasound is repeated in 6 to 8 weeks to determine whether it is a hemorrhagic corpus lutea. However, in a postmenopausal patient with a complex adnexal mass, evaluation includes CT scan to rule out omental disease or other site of primary tumor, and barium enema to rule out colon involvement or primary.

CA-125 is a glycoprotein that is produced by certain tumors. It unfortunately is not specific for ovarian cancer and may be elevated in lung, appendiceal, and signet ring cell carcinomas, as well as other malignancies. In the premenopausal patient, benign findings such as leiomyomas, endometriosis, menstruation, pregnancy, and PID may elevate CA-125. Other diseases such as cirrhosis of the liver may also elevate the value. CA-125, therefore, is not checked in the premenopausal patient with a pelvic mass because the false-positive rate is too high. However, in the postmenopausal patient with a pelvic mass and an elevated CA-125, ovarian cancer is diagnosed in 80% of these patients. This is the population in which the test is helpful.

Definitive diagnosis of a pelvic mass requires visual inspection and histologic diagnosis. Laparoscopy or laparotomy can be done depending on the clinical suspicion of malignancy. In patients with potential for carcinomatosis, laparoscopy is not done because of port site metastasis that occurs quickly and can make debulking difficult. At the time of surgery, pelvic washings are done, and the mass is visually inspected to augment prior information from ultrasound. If all indications are that the lesion is benign, ovarian cystectomy or drainage (see "Technical Aspects of Surgical Options") are indicated, with evaluation of cyst cytology or gross or microscopic evaluation of the tissue to confirm a benign lesion. If there is a higher level of suspicion or the patient is menopausal, oophorectomy is performed, and frozen section histologic diagnosis provided.

Serous and mucinous cystadenomas are very common benign tumors of the ovary that can occur in any age group. Treatment can be cystectomy or oophorectomy, depending on the amount of ovary involved. Brenner's tumors are benign transitional cell tumors of the ovary that can also be managed in a similar fashion.

If the lesion is an invasive, epithelial ovarian cancer, treatment includes a hysterectomy, bilateral salpingo-oophorectomy, omentectomy, peritoneal biopsies of the diaphragm, bilateral paracolic gutters, bilateral pelvis, and cul-de-sac and lymph node sampling. If the cell type is mucinous, an appendectomy is also performed to rule out a metastasis from the appendix. Attention has turned toward minimally invasive (laparoscopic) and fertility-sparing surgical approaches. Interval laparoscopic staging of newly diagnosed ovarian tumors, with no suspicion of carcinomatosis, may be performed in selected patients.[7]

Extensive disease mandates tumor debulking to remove all possible tumor. Patients who undergo optimal tumor reductive surgery (<2 cm of visible disease) have a survival advantage over patients who cannot be or are not optimally debulked. Complete staging is very important because patients who have a grade 1 or 2 stage 1A ovarian cancer do not require chemotherapy. With other stages, surgery is followed by chemotherapy.

Borderline tumors do not behave like invasive ovarian cancers. Typically, they are treated with surgery alone and do not require chemotherapy. They tend to occur in younger women. If found at frozen section and the patient is finished with childbearing, pelvic washings, hysterectomy, bilateral salpingo-oophorectomy, omentectomy, peritoneal biopsies, and lymph node biopsies are performed. If the patient desires future fertility, a unilateral oophorectomy, omentectomy, peritoneal biopsies, and lymph node biopsies on the side of the tumor can be performed. The other ovary can then be monitored with ultrasound. Staging is done in the event an invasive ovarian cancer is found at the time of final pathology. Mucinous borderline tumors have also been associated with abnormalities in the appendix. Therefore, an appendectomy is performed in conjunction with other staging.

Other types of ovarian tumors include sex-cord stromal tumors such as granulosa cell tumors or Sertoli-Leydig cell tumors. These typically appear solid but occasionally have a cystic appearance. Hysterectomy, bilateral salpingo-oophorectomy, and staging are performed. For stage I tumors of adult type, no further therapy is needed. For patients with higher stages, postoperative chemotherapy or radiation therapy is added.

Among girls and young women, germ cell tumors must be considered. The most common cell type is a dysgerminoma. Ninety percent of dysgerminomas are diagnosed at stage I. Conservative surgery with unilateral oophorectomy and staging can be performed, leaving the uterus and other tube and ovary in place. No further therapy is needed.

Other germ cell tumors include endodermal sinus tumor, choriocarcinoma, immature teratoma, and embryonal carcinoma. A mixture of these cancers can be present. Tumor markers such as β-HCG, alpha-fetoprotein, and lactate dehydrogenase (LDH) may be detected in certain germ cell tumors. Patients who have a gonadoblastoma must be evaluated with chromosomes. If XY chromosomes are discovered, the gonads are removed to prevent development of dysgerminoma. This may occur in 20% of patients with gonadoblastoma.

Because these are potentially very aggressive tumors, postoperative chemotherapy is implemented with the diagnoses of teratoma (stage IA, grade 2 or 3 immature teratoma or any higher stage), dysgerminoma (stage II and above), any endodermal sinus tumor, or choriocarcinoma.

ALTERNATIVES TO SURGICAL INTERVENTION

There are valid indications for medical or observational management of many acute gynecologic conditions, even if there is also a surgical option available. Because acute pelvic pathology is often accompanied by severe pain or bleeding to a degree that the general surgeon would consider it a surgical emergency in the upper abdomen, we provide some guidance to the clinical judgment to allow the surgeon to avoid, or defer, surgery. We also provide an overview approach to the medical management and the points to observe during follow-up observation.

Dysfunctional Uterine Bleeding

As described earlier, dysfunctional uterine bleeding condition is a manifestation of dys-synchronous endometrial physiology. In the acute setting, medical management does not require a tissue or even ultrasound diagnosis. Emergency implementation of D&C is not necessary. The episode can be truncated by inducing acute proliferation and regeneration of the endometrium with high-dose estrogens, followed by induction of a secretory endometrium with a progestin.

An oral or IV bolus of estrogens (e.g., conjugated estrogens, 5 mg orally every 6 hours for 4-6 doses, or 25 mg IV in 2 doses 6 hours apart) with simultaneous administration of an active progestin (micronized progesterone, 100 mg orally twice daily or medroxyprogesterone, 10 mg four times a day) will stabilize the endometrium. The progestin must be continued for at least 7 days, and then withdrawn to simulate atresia of the corpus luteum. This will mimic the orderly menses of an ovulatory cycle, although perhaps with heavy bleeding. The patient receives oral contraceptives for several months to stabilize iron stores, allow for orderly evaluation of structural pathology, and initiate a plan to assess underlying hypothalamic-pituitary-ovarian cycle pathology.

Spontaneous Abortion

First-trimester pregnancies fail 10% to 15% of the time, often with minimal symptoms. For the patient who does present with pain or bleeding, confirm that this is an early gestation. On inspection of the cervix, observe whether there is placental tissue in the dilated cervical os; if so, it can often be removed with a sponge forceps and resolve the event. The need for acute surgical intervention with curettage is wholly dependent on the amount of blood loss and intensity of pain. The patient who is hemodynamically stable and has pain control may spontaneously complete her miscarriage without a procedure.

Ectopic Pregnancy

Ruptured ectopic pregnancy is a surgical emergency, but there are two other tubal pregnancy scenarios that are amenable to less aggressive management in the patient who is hemodynamically stable and has limited intraperitoneal blood loss: the tubal abortion and the unruptured ectopic pregnancy. The tubal abortion results when the pregnancy is extruded from the fimbriated end of the tube. Pain is often described as lateralized cramping, and the volume of blood identified in the cul-de-sac is only 100 mL or so. These events may be self-limited, and if pain and hemodynamic status are under control during observation, surgery may be avoided.

A patient may present with pain and vaginal bleeding, and an intact tubal pregnancy is identified by ultrasound. There are varying sets of criteria for medical management of the unruptured tubal pregnancy, based on gestational size (<3 cm or <5 cm) and the presence of fetal cardiac activity, but the physician must actively consider medical rather than surgical management.

Surgical procedures for managing an ectopic pregnancy include salpingectomy, salpingostomy, or segmental resection. For the patient desiring to maintain maximal future fertility, preservation of the tube is preferable.

Medical management of tubal pregnancy relies on the cytotoxic effect of methotrexate. Several protocols for dosage (e.g., 1 mg/kg) and follow-up are available. Consultation with an experienced gynecologist before initiation is advisable.

Pelvic Infection

The diagnosis of PID can be challenging. Most commonly, the differential diagnosis includes appendicitis, urinary tract infection, ruptured ovarian cyst, or ectopic pregnancy, all of which share some of the signs and symptoms of PID. The diagnosis of PID is made only when the patient has fever, leukocytosis, purulent discharge from the cervix, bilateral adnexal tenderness on gentle palpation, and peritoneal signs limited to the pelvis. Appendicitis is differentiated by anteceding gastrointestinal symptoms, the evolving pain pattern, absence of cervical discharge, and generalized peritonitis. Lower urinary tract infection is distinguished by dysuria and obvious pyuria. Rarely do ovarian cysts or ectopic pregnancy present with significant fever or leukocytosis. In a classic study, Wolner-Hanssen and associates[8] concluded that the sensitivity and specificity of clinical assessment for PID was so poor that laparoscopic inspection of the pelvis is necessary to make a firm diagnosis. Although

that may be unduly aggressive in many cases, this diagnosis must be applied cautiously because it is stigmatizing and labels the patient, disproportionately among women of color, from lower socioeconomic status, or with counterculture lifestyles.

Acute PID, as a polymicrobial infection, is a medical, not a surgical, disease. The major acute complication of this disease is a TOA. In contrast to abscesses related to the intestine, however, initial management of a TOA is with broad-spectrum IV antibiotics. Indications for surgical intervention are ruptured TOA with generalized peritonitis or failure to respond to medical therapy.

A pelvic inflammatory collection is a clinical variant of a TOA. Whereas an abscess is an infectious process bounded by inflammatory response across natural tissue planes, the collection, which may be indistinguishable on ultrasound or CT scan, is bounded by anatomic surfaces of the posterior cul-de-sac, rectum, uterus, and intestine. Pelvic collections are more common than true abscesses and are much more likely to respond to medical therapy than abscesses.

Functional Ovarian Cysts

Rupture of a follicle or corpus luteum cyst or intraparenchymal hemorrhage in the corpus luteum can result in extreme pain, with signs of localized peritoneal irritation. If ultrasound evaluation reveals a simple cyst and does not demonstrate significant intraperitoneal bleeding, and if Doppler flow rules out an ovarian torsion, this acute condition will resolve in 12 to 24 hours. Fluids and analgesic support are all that is necessary.

If the event is on the right ovary, the acuity clearly will force consideration of appendicitis, but prior gastrointestinal symptoms, fever, and leukocytosis are rarely present.

Ovarian torsion is a surgical emergency and sometimes mandates oophorectomy. However, unless the ovary is obviously necrotic at the time of laparoscopic inspection, the surgeon needs to untwist the ovarian pedicle and directly observe for return of blood flow before considering removal.

Uterine Leiomyomas

Uterine leiomyomas are benign myometrial tumors present in up to 40% of women, more prevalent among women of African descent. With clinical or ultrasound confirmation of the diagnosis, observation for stability over time is indicated. Surgical intervention is warranted if the patient has unresponsive menorrhagia, intolerable pressure symptoms, rapid growth, or change in consistency of palpable masses. Leiomyosarcoma is a sufficiently rare event that hysterectomy or myomectomy to rule out malignancy carries greater statistical risk than the lesion itself.

Observational management is especially valid in women who are approaching menopause because leiomyomas are estrogen dependent, and with the decline in estrogen production, typically the lesions will decrease in size. Continued observation is important after menopause because progressive growth in this time period may reflect malignant transformation.

Endometriosis and Endometriomas

Endometriosis is a complex disease created by the presence of ectopic endometrial tissue in the peritoneal cavity or adnexa. This endometrial tissue transforms and bleeds with the ovarian cycle. This process induces a sterile inflammatory response, resulting in pain, pelvic adhesions, and when located within the ovary, a complex hemorrhagic mass, known as an *endometrioma*. First-line therapy for this disease is medical induction of temporary menopause and suppression of ovarian estrogen. Surgical management for younger women is conservative, with local destruction of lesions and maximum conservation of reproductive organs. Women who have completed their reproductive plans will benefit from hysterectomy and oophorectomy.

TECHNICAL ASPECTS OF SURGICAL OPTIONS

Surgery for Menorrhagia or Abnormal Uterine Bleeding

D&C is the classic gynecologic procedure for the evaluation and possible therapeutic treatment of menorrhagia, menometrorrhagia, and abnormal uterine bleeding. It is now understood that its therapeutic success is 25% or less and usually temporary. Because it is a blind procedure, it is difficult to ensure that the entire endometrium is curetted uniformly, much like attempting to scoop cake batter out of a bowl with a spoon. Therefore, more commonly now, hysteroscopy is utilized in conjunction with D&C so that the cavity can be visualized and any pathology seen can be directly resected or removed. The combination of the two adds to both the evaluation and the therapeutic success.

In addition, ablative techniques now are being used for improved therapy for nonstructural bleeding abnormalities.[9,10] These ablative techniques (rollerball, thermal balloon, hydrotherapy, cryotherapy, microwave) are advanced techniques best reserved for a surgeon with extensive experience in hysteroscopy and the evaluation and manipulation of the endometrial cavity.

Technique: Fractional Dilation and Curettage

A weighted speculum and anterior retracting blade or a bivalve Graves speculum are used in the vagina to visualize the cervix. The cervix is grasped transversely on the anterior lip with a single-toothed tenaculum. A Kevorkian curette is used to curette the endocervix for a specimen. A sound is placed through the cervix and into the uterus and gently tapped on the fundus of the uterus to measure the depth of the cavity. This step is important to help prevent or recognize uterine perforation for the remainder of the procedure. The cervix is dilated with graduated dilators of increasing diameter. At this time, if hysteroscopy is going to be performed, the hysteroscope is introduced through the cervix and into the uterus for visualization of the endometrial cavity; glycine or saline

is commonly used as a distention medium. The curettage phase is performed. A sharp curette (the largest diameter that will easily fit through the cervix) is introduced gently into the cervix and endometrial cavity. This is done without excessive pressure or undue force. The fundus is found, and a firm withdrawal stroke is applied until the curette reaches the cervicouterine junction. This is repeated while moving circumferentially around the uterine cavity, attempting to curette as much of the endometrial cavity as possible. The procedure is terminated; the instruments are removed with careful attention to the cervix, which may bleed when the tenaculum is removed. The bleeding usually stops with pressure, silver nitrate, or Monsel's solution.

Potential Complications

As with any surgical procedure, infection from instrumenting the cavity or bleeding from the denuded endometrial lining can occur. In addition, perforation of the uterine cavity is possible and can occur in any of the phases of the procedure. However, it occurs most commonly during the sounding of the uterus, and bleeding from the perforated area can result. The perforation is usually midline and self-limited. Usually, observation for 24 hours is all that is required. If there is continued bleeding, as evidenced by decreasing hemoglobin or increased abdominal pain, or if other symptoms present, exploration by laparoscopy or laparotomy may be required. Injury to the bowel is possible, although rare, with perforation.

Treatment of Bartholin's Gland Cyst or Abscess

Large, symptomatic Bartholin's gland cysts or painful abscesses may not respond to conservative treatment. The surgical treatment options follow:

1. Incision and drainage with Word catheter placement
2. Marsupialization
3. Excision of the gland itself

Excision of the gland is rarely indicated. Typically, incision and drainage with appropriate follow-up, with or without marsupialization, is all that is needed to treat this condition.

Incision and drainage generally is done on the vestibular side at the hymeneal ring in a lower dependent portion of the cyst or abscess using a sharp knife. The cyst is stabilized, and an incision is made into the cyst itself. A small Word catheter is placed into the cyst for drainage and is re-evaluated on a weekly basis. Patients with abscesses are pretreated with antibiotics.

To perform a marsupialization, an elliptical incision is made in the vestibular mucosa down to the wall of the gland. The wall of the gland is incised the entire length of the ellipse. The contents are evacuated, and the wall of the cyst is sutured to the vestibular mucosa with 3-0 synthetic absorbable sutures, either in an interrupted fashion or using a baseball stitch (Fig. 75-9). The patient is placed on a regimen of hot sitz baths. If the lesion is an abscess, the patient is covered with antibiotics. Whether marsupialization or incision and drainage have been per-

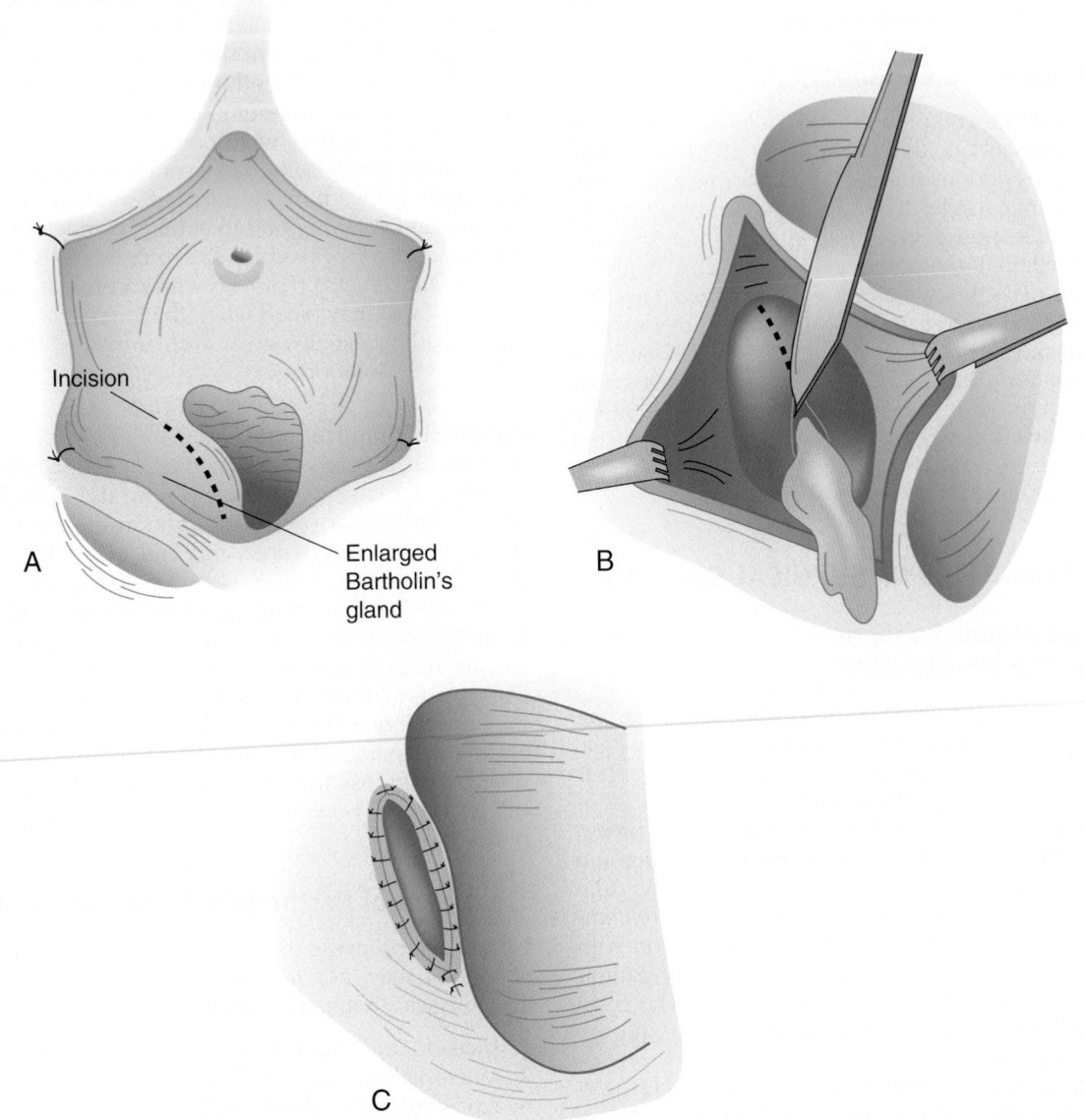

A

Incision

Enlarged
Bartholin's
gland

B

C

Figure 75-9 Bartholin's gland marsupialization. **A,** Retraction of the labia and incision over the mucosa of the vagina. **B,** Wall of the gland is excised. **C,** Completed marsupialization. (Modified from Mitchell CW, Wheeless CR: Atlas of Pelvic Surgery, 3rd ed. Philadelphia, Lippincott Williams & Wilkins, 1997.)

formed, sexual intercourse is avoided until the area has completely healed.

Cone Procedure

Conization can be performed with a cold knife or a LEEP. A LEEP conization entails removal of the transformation zone with an ectocervical loop followed by removal of an endocervical specimen with an endocervical loop. This is called a *top-hat procedure* and allows for sampling of the canal. If a cold-knife conization is done in the operating room, a single-tooth tenaculum is placed on the anterior lip of the cervix. Figure-of-eight retention sutures of 0-0 Vicryl are placed at 3 and 9 o'clock. A circumferential incision is made around the transformation zone and the lesion. The specimen is grasped with Allis

clamps to maintain orientation, and a deeper circumferential incision is made in the cervix. The specimen is removed with a scalpel or mayo scissors. A marking stitch is placed at 12 o'clock on the specimen, and an endocervical curetting is performed above the cone biopsy. Risk for recurrence of dysplasia is dependent on the status of the endocervical and ectocervical margins as well as on whether the endocervical curetting is positive for dysplasia.

Surgery for Ovarian Cysts

Ovarian cysts are common, especially functional cysts. Benign ovarian cysts have been discussed previously. When found, the decision is, "What management is most appropriate?" Treatment is individualized to each patient, depending on the clinical scenario. When an ovarian cyst is an incidental finding at the time of other surgery, it is important to know what, if any, the patient's symptoms are, and to have knowledge of where the patient is in her menstrual cycle, and what size of follicle is normal for that part of the cycle.

It is critical to remember that any time surgery is performed on the adnexal structures, there is a risk for adhesion formation that might inhibit fertility. If the patient has been asymptomatic with a small functional cyst, observation, especially in the younger patient, is most appropriate. If the functional ovarian cyst is large (>5-6 cm) or symptomatic, aspiration may be considered. If the cyst is larger or is not consistent with a functional lesion, oophorectomy may be considered if the patient is closer to menopause. As an alternative, ovarian cystectomy may be considered. This option removes the cyst but preserves the function of the ovary. It also reduces the risk for recurrence as compared with ovarian cyst drainage.

Technique

Ovarian Cyst Drainage
It is imperative, before considering drainage, that the ovarian cyst is benign and functional in nature. With this being noted, a hollow needle can be used, by laparoscopy or exploratory laparotomy, to pierce the cyst at a 90-degree angle to the cyst and to suction the fluid from the cyst through tubing and a syringe connected to the needle. Suction is performed until all the fluid is removed. The fluid is sent to pathology to ensure accurate diagnosis. The needle is removed, and the procedure is terminated.

Oophorectomy With or Without Salpingectomy
When oophorectomy is desired, the infundibulopelvic (IP) ligament is identified and isolated. The ipsilateral ureter must be identified and noted to be remote from the area of the IP ligament to be ligated. With the IP ligament isolated, the following strategies can be followed:

1. Clamp, cut, and suture ligate the IP ligament.
2. Ligate the IP ligament with one or two Endoloops, then surgically dissect it.
3. Cauterize the IP ligament with bipolar cautery and sharply dissect it.

If the ipsilateral tube is to be removed, the dissection across the mesosalpinx is performed, either with clamp, sharp dissection, and suture ligation or with bipolar coagulation and sharp dissection. If the uterus is present, attention is directed to the utero-ovarian ligament. This ligament is dissected in a similar fashion, as described previously, through bipolar cautery or the clamping technique. The ovary, completely dissected, possibly in conjunction with the fallopian tube, can be removed.

Ovarian Cystectomy
To begin an ovarian cystectomy, a surgical line into the ovarian capsule is developed sharply over the area of the cyst, on the antimesovarian side of the ovary. After the incision into the capsule, the cyst is dissected away from the capsule using sharp or blunt dissection. Scissors, knife, Kitner, hydrodissection, or a combination of these may be used for this dissection, taking care to avoid rupture of the cyst. After the cyst is removed in toto, the base of the ovarian capsule usually has some bleeding. Hemostasis can be obtained at the base, either with electrocautery or by suturing. After hemostasis is obtained, most surgeons do not suture the capsule, but rather approximate the edges loosely together to heal spontaneously on its own. It is believed that this reduces the risk for adhesion formation. Interceed or other adhesion barriers can be used at this time to reduce adhesion formation.

Potential Complications
Bleeding from the large vascular pedicles is the most dangerous potential risk. If hemostasis is not completely obtained, the large vessels can bleed profusely very quickly. The more chronic complication from adnexal surgery is adhesion formation with infertility or subfertility. Injury to the ureter is always a concern during this surgery if the ureteral course is not monitored appropriately.

Surgery for the Fallopian Tube or Ectopic Pregnancy

There are many options for treatment of ectopic pregnancy. Surgical options include salpingostomy, segmental resection, or salpingectomy, depending on desire for future fertility and if the tube is salvageable. As in prior discussions, these procedures can be performed by laparoscopy, laparotomy, or mini-laparotomy.

Technique

Salpingostomy
With a salpingostomy, a linear incision is made in the antisalpingetic line over the pregnancy. This is usually performed with a monopolar needle. The pregnancy is removed from the tube. "Milking" the pregnancy from the tube has been discussed in the past; however, it is no longer recommended because of an increased risk for retained tissue. After the pregnancy is completely removed, hemostasis is achieved with monopolar or bipolar cautery. The tube is not sutured, but rather left open to heal spontaneously. This has been shown to improve patency rates and fertility (Fig. 75-10).

Segmental Resection
In segmental resection, the portion of the tube encompassing the products of conception is resected, and the proximal and distal ends are left in situ. This gives the option of reanastomosis at a later date if the patient chooses. The mesosalpinx is perforated in an avascular space. Ligatures are placed on each side of the pregnancy. The segment is sharply resected within the ligatures, and the vessels of the mesosalpinx are inspected for injury, and secured if necessary.

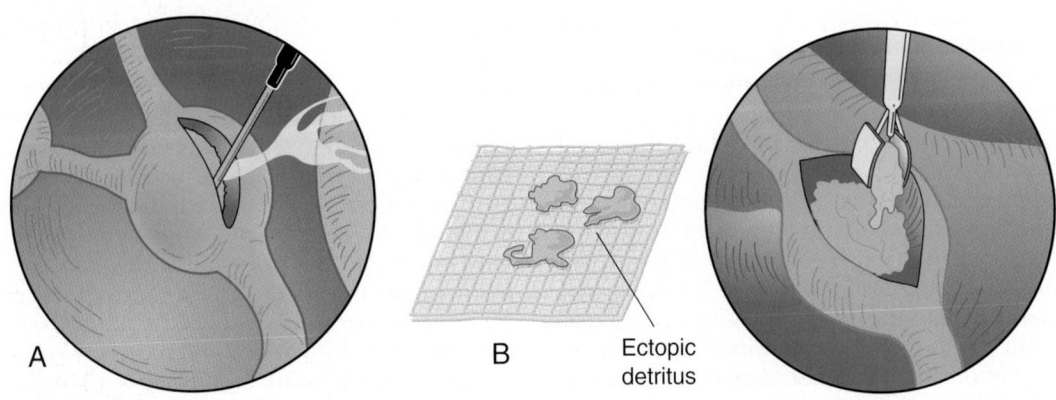

Figure 75-10 Salpingostomy. **A,** Fallopian tube is opened in a longitudinal manner. **B,** Trophoblastic tissue removed in pieces. (Modified from Mitchell CW, Wheeless CR: Atlas of Pelvic Surgery, 3rd ed. Philadelphia, Lippincott, Williams & Wilkins, 1997.)

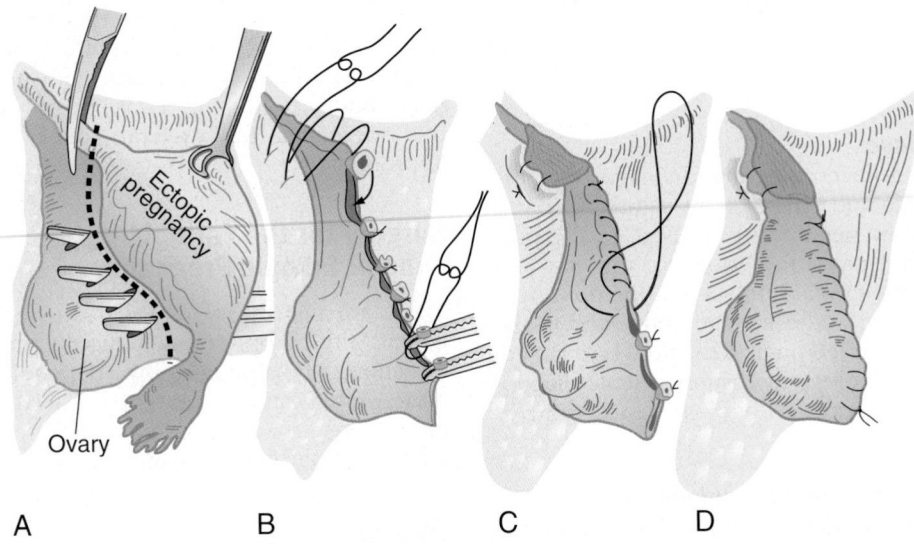

Figure 75-11 Salpingectomy. **A,** Tube is excised from the cornual portion across the mesosalpinx to the fimbria. **B,** Pedicles are tied, peritoneal lining is reestablished, and cornual portion of the tube is buried into the posterior segment of the uterine cornu. **C,** Mesosalpinx is reperitonealized. **D,** Mesosalpinx is closed and the procedure completed. (Modified from Mitchell CW, Wheeless CR: Atlas of Pelvic Surgery, 3rd ed. Philadelphia, Lippincott, Williams & Wilkins, 1997.)

Salpingectomy

In salpingectomy, the tube is grasped, and the mesosalpinx is secured using bipolar cautery, an Endoloop, or clamps with a suture ligation. The tube is sharply excised. The area is examined closely for hemostasis (Fig. 75-11).

In rare cases, the ectopic pregnancy is in the abdomen and not in the fallopian tube. In these cases, the fetus is removed with ligation of the umbilical cord near its insertion into the placenta. Because of the vascularity of the placenta, the placenta is left in situ, with subsequent medical therapy with methotrexate.

Potential Complications

The vascular supply of the tube in pregnancy is markedly increased; therefore, bleeding is a risk both during and after the surgery is completed. If the tube is preserved,

there is a risk for subsequent recurrent ectopic pregnancy. Also, there is a risk for retained placental tissue in the tube and persistent ectopic pregnancy. Adhesions of the affected adnexa are also a significant risk, whether the tube is preserved or removed.

Hysterectomy

Hysterectomy is one of the most common procedures performed. The route of hysterectomy depends on the indication for surgery, the size of the uterus, the descent of the cervix and uterus, the shape of the vagina, the size of the patient, and the skill and preference of the surgeon. Surgical routes for hysterectomy include total abdominal hysterectomy (TAH), total vaginal hysterectomy (TVH), laparoscopically assisted vaginal hysterectomy (LAVH), and two newer techniques: total laparoscopic hysterectomy (TLH) and laparoscopic supracervical hysterectomy (LSH).[11]

Because of the significant impact of the transvaginal approach on appreciating anatomic relationships, vaginal hysterectomy and laparoscopically assisted hysterectomy must only be performed by an experienced vaginal surgeon.

Technique

Any lower abdominal incision (vertical, Pfannenstiel, Maylard, Cherney) can be used. The bowel is packed from the pelvis and the patient placed in Trendelenburg position. The ureters are identified, and the following steps are performed bilaterally (Fig. 75-12).

The round ligament is identified, incised between clamps, and ligated with 0-0 absorbable suture. The leaves of the broad ligament are sharply opened anteriorly and posteriorly, with the anterior leaf open to the vesicouterine fold. If the ovary is to be preserved, the proximal tube and utero-ovarian ligament are clamped, incised, and ligated. If the tube and ovary are to be removed, the infundibulopelvic ligament is doubly clamped, incised, and doubly ligated with a 0-0 absorbable tie and a 0-0 synthetic absorbable suture, as described in detail previously.

After this has been performed bilaterally, the vesicoperitoneal fold is elevated and incised. The filmy attachments of the bladder to the pubovesical fascia are sharply dissected, mobilizing the bladder off the cervix. The filmy adventitious tissue surrounding the uterine vessels is skeletonized sharply, dissecting the tissue to expose the uterine vessels. The uterine vessels are clamped, incised, and ligated at the level of the lower uterine segment. This is accomplished by placing the tip of the clamp on the uterus at a right angle to the axis of the cervix and sliding or stepping off the uterus. The pedicle is incised, and a simple absorbable 0-0 suture ligature is placed. The cardinal and uterosacral ligaments are sequentially clamped, incised, and suture-ligated with a Haney double transfixion suture. Each clamp is placed medial to the previous pedicle to allow for the ureter to passively retract laterally. The anterior vagina can be entered by a stab incision and cut across with either a scalpel or scissors. Alternatively, right-angle clamps can be used to clamp the angle of the vagina, below the distal cervix. The tissue above this angle clamp is then incised and ligated with a Haney stitch. With the lumen of the vagina now exposed, sharp dissection is used to complete the vaginal transection. The vaginal wall, incorporating perivaginal fascia, muscularis, and mucosal edge, is closed with a series of figure-of-eight 0-0 absorbable sutures with the angle stitches incorporating the ipsilateral uterosacral ligament. Ligatures need to be snug, but they must not strangulate the vaginal edges. The pelvic peritoneum does not need to be closed. The pelvis is irrigated, hemostasis assured, and the abdominal incision closed routinely.

Potential Complications

Because of the proximity of the ureter to the cervix, uterine vessels, and infundibulopelvic ligament, the ureter can be injured during the hysterectomy, and with the

dissection necessary between the bladder and cervix, injury to the bladder is likewise a common complication. It is imperative that these injuries be recognized and repaired intraoperatively, if possible. Fistulas, such as vesicovaginal or ureterovaginal, likewise can form postoperatively secondary to ischemic injury caused by denudation of the bladder muscularis or partial entrapment with a vaginal closure stitch.

The vascular supply to the uterus and ovaries is rich. Intraoperative and postoperative bleeding is a concern. A previously secure pedicle can begin to bleed acutely in the postoperative period. A vaginal stump vessel, missed because of operative vasospasm, can cause a pelvic cuff hematoma. Thromboembolism originating from the pelvic vasculature is also a potential postoperative problem. Hysterectomy is considered a clean-contaminated procedure because of entering the vagina. Pelvic cuff infection is common, despite the routine use of prophylactic antibiotics.

There has been increased discussion recently regarding the effect of hysterectomy on the pelvic floor. Failure to reapproximate the endopelvic fascia or failure to heal results in a large, apical endopelvic fascial defect. This results in an apical enterocele that progresses in size over time. It is estimated that 60% of women by 60 years of age have significant pelvic support defects.

Radical Hysterectomy

Radical hysterectomy can be performed through a vertical, Cherney, or Maylard incision. After the pelvis is entered, the retroperitoneal space is opened, and the paravesical and pararectal spaces are developed. The boundaries of the paravesical space are the symphysis pubis anteriorly, cardinal ligament posteriorly, obliterated umbilical artery medially, and external iliac vein laterally. The boundaries of the pararectal space are the cardinal ligament anteriorly, sacrum posteriorly, ureter medially, and hypogastric artery laterally. The bladder flap is then developed to the level of the vagina. The uterine arteries are isolated back to the origin and are ligated. The ureter is then separated from the medial leaf of the broad ligament, and the parametrial tunnel is developed. The ureter is separated from the parametrial tissue and is rolled laterally. The rectovaginal space is then entered, and the uterosacral ligaments are transected two thirds of the way to the sacrum. The amount of postoperative urinary retention is related to how close to the sacrum the uterosacral ligament is ligated. The parametria are then taken at the sidewall. The specimen is removed when the vagina is entered 1 cm below the cervix. The angle sutures are secured with 0-0 Vicryl Heaney sutures, and the cuff is closed with 0-0 Vicryl figure-of-eight sutures. New surgical techniques for the management of cervical cancer include total laparoscopic radical hysterectomy with lymphadenectomy and fertility-sparing vaginal radical trachelectomy.[12,13]

SURGERY DURING PREGNANCY

About 0.1% to 2.2% of pregnant women require surgery during pregnancy. Changes in maternal-fetal physiology,

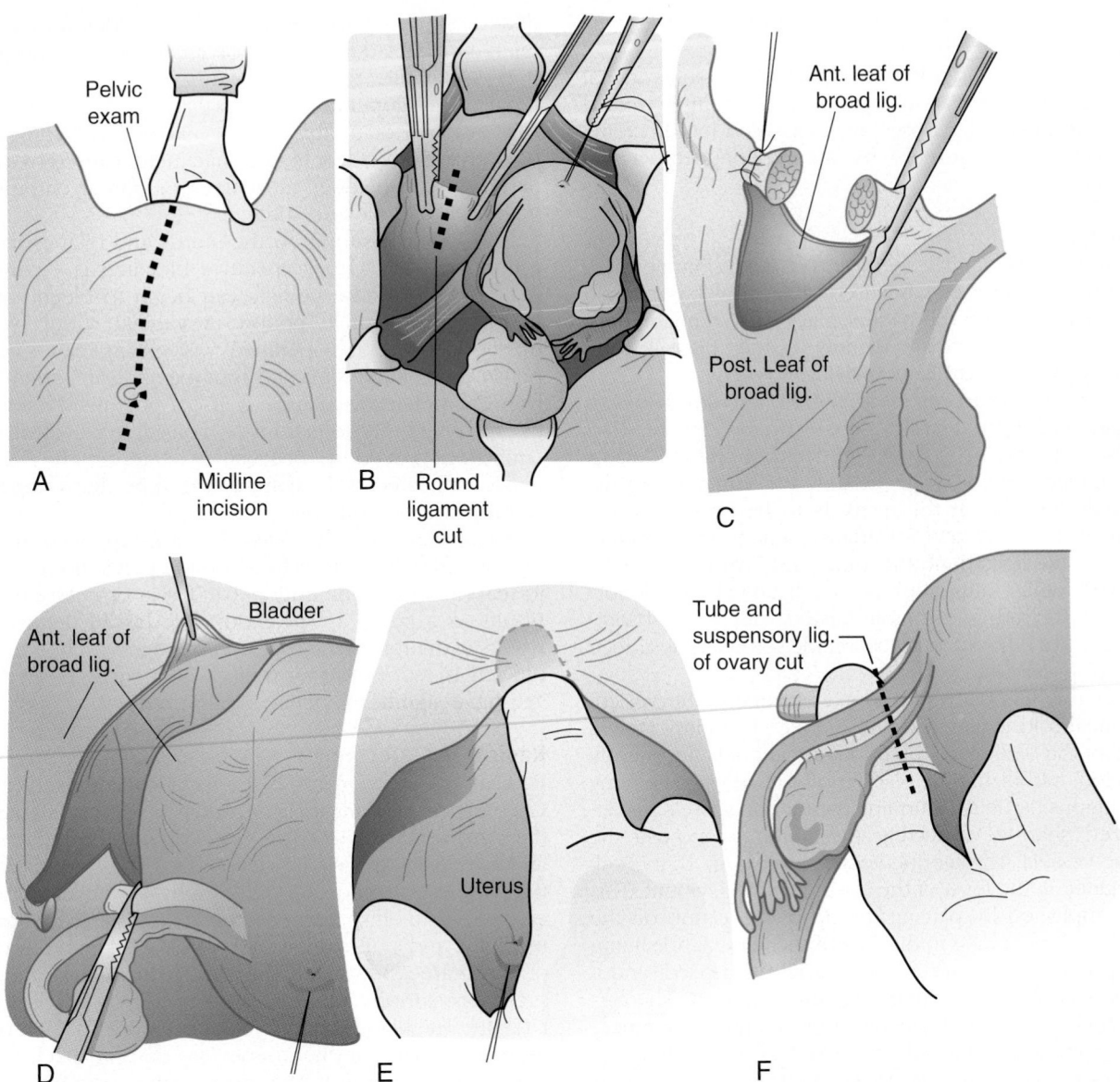

Figure 75-12 A to N, Hysterectomy. (Modified from Mitchell CW, Wheeless CR: Atlas of Pelvic Surgery, 3rd ed. Philadelphia, Lippincott, Williams & Wilkins, 1997.)

the enlarging gestation, and changes in maternal organ placement can make diagnosis and treatment challenging. In this section, we address important issues for the surgeon to consider before proceeding to the operating room.

Physiologic Changes

During pregnancy, multisystem adaptions result in altered physiology.

Cardiovascular System

Blood volume increases by 45% to 50% at term. Placental hormone production stimulates maternal erythropoiesis, which increases red cell mass by about 20%. This results in a functional hemodilution manifested by a physiologic anemia. Therefore, pregnancy needs to be considered a hypervolemic state.

Maternal heart rate increases as early as 7 weeks' gestation. In late pregnancy, maternal heart rate is increased by about 20% over antepartum values.

Systemic vascular resistance decreases by 20%, but gradually increases near term. This results in a decrease in systolic and diastolic blood pressure during pregnancy, with a gradual recovery to nonpregnant values by term. Because there is increased pressure in the venous system, there is decreased return from the lower extremities, resulting in dependent edema.

Respiratory System

In pregnancy, minute volume is increased, whereas functional residual volume is decreased (Table 75-6). Although it seems intuitive that lung volume would be decreased

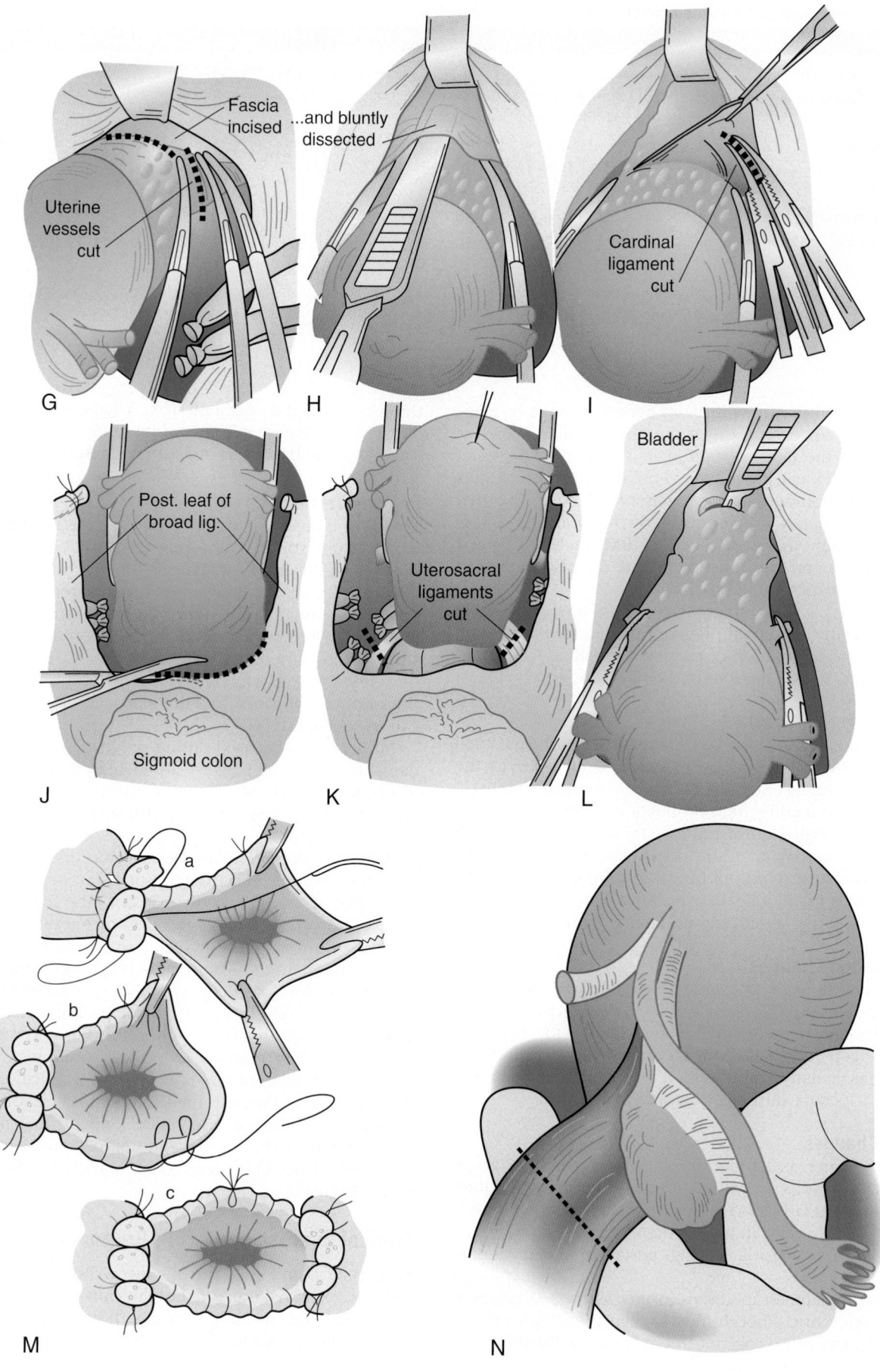

Figure 75-12, cont'd

Table 75-6 **Physiologic Changes of Pregnancy**

SYSTEMS	CHANGES	RESULT
Cardiovascular, hemodynamic	Blood volume increased by 50%; red cell mass increased by 20%; cardiac output increased by 50%; heart rate increased by 20%; systemic vascular resistance decreased by 20%	High-output cardiac state with a hemodilutional anemia
Respiratory	Minute volume increased by 20%; functional residual capacity decreased by 15%; tidal volume increased by 20%-30%; oxygen consumption increased by 20%	Compensated respiratory alkalosis
Gastrointestinal	Smooth muscle relaxation; delayed gastrointestinal emptying	Full stomach; constipation
Coagulation	Fibrinogen increased by 30%; protein S decreased by 30%-40%	Hypercoagulable state regardless of risk factors
Renal	Glomerular filtration rate increased by 50%; serum creatinine decreased 40%; physiologic hydronephrosis	Increased urination; increased risk for upper tract infection

during pregnancy, an increase in minute volume in association with an expansion of the anterior and posterior diameter of the chest results in increased tidal volume, thereby also increasing minute ventilation. These changes result in a compensated respiratory alkalosis. Normal PCO_2 in pregnancy ranges from 28 to 35 mm Hg. PO_2 is usually greater than or equal to 100 mm Hg. Oxygen consumption and basal metabolic rate are also increased during pregnancy by about 20%.

These physiologic changes result in less pulmonary reserve for the acutely ill pregnant patient, reducing time needed for deterioration of respiratory distress to respiratory failure. Early intervention is mandatory.

Gastrointestinal Tract

During pregnancy, there is a decrease in gastrointestinal motility. This is caused by mechanical changes in the abdomen with the enlarging uterus and the smooth muscle relaxation induced by high production of progesterone in pregnancy. Gastric emptying may be delayed for up to 8 hours. Pregnant women are considered to have a functionally full stomach at all times. In addition, a decrease in large intestine motility may result in constipation severe enough to cause significant abdominal pain.

Coagulation Changes

Pregnancy is a hypercoagulable state. Fibrinogen is increased about 30% over baseline values. The hypercoagulable state of pregnancy is associated with increased risk for deep venous thrombosis and pulmonary embolus. This is particularly compounded when bed rest or immobilization occurs during the gestational period.

Renal Changes

Pregnancy increases blood flow to the renal pelvis about 50%. This results in an increased glomerular filtration rate. Frequent urination is common. Serum creatinine is about 40% less than in a nonpregnant state. Therefore, a creatinine of 1 mg/dL during gestation is considered abnormal.

Ureteral diameter increases in pregnancy secondary to compression and smooth muscle relaxation. Peristalsis is delayed, and reflux occurs freely from the bladder into the lower ureteral segment. This results in an increased incidence of pyelonephritis during pregnancy. Therefore, asymptomatic bacteriuria must be aggressively treated.

Imaging Techniques

The most common imaging technique used during pregnancy is ultrasound. Ultrasound is considered the safest modality and is used for fetal assessment. In patients with abdominal pain, an ultrasound is considered the first-line diagnostic test. During ultrasound, the presence of an intrauterine pregnancy needs to be documented if possible. In addition, evaluation of the cul-de-sac for fluid, the ureter for dilation or stones, the gallbladder for the presence of gallstones, and the placenta for abnormalities can be obtained.

MRI also can be used during pregnancy. There are, to date, no data that suggest an increased risk from this modality; in fact, MRI is now used to diagnose fetal abnormalities, especially abnormalities of the central nervous system.

Although there are theoretical risks associated with ionizing radiation, most diagnostic x-ray procedures are associated with minimal or no risk to the fetus. Existing evidence suggests that there is no increased risk to the fetus with regard to congenital malformations, growth restriction, or abortion from x-ray procedures that expose the fetus to doses of 5 cGy or less. In 1995, the American College of Obstetrics and Gynecology published guidelines regarding diagnostic imaging during pregnancy. These published outlines reflect our opinions. Women need to be reassured that concern about radiation exposure must not prevent medically indicated diagnostic procedures. It cannot be stressed enough that maternal well-being is of the utmost importance, and appropriate diagnostic procedures need to be obtained to facilitate a rapid diagnosis.

Clinical Evaluation During Pregnancy

Abdominal pain during pregnancy can be confusing to the clinician. It is natural for the clinician to attribute most abdominal pain to the pregnancy; however, other organ systems during pregnancy are affected at the rate of the

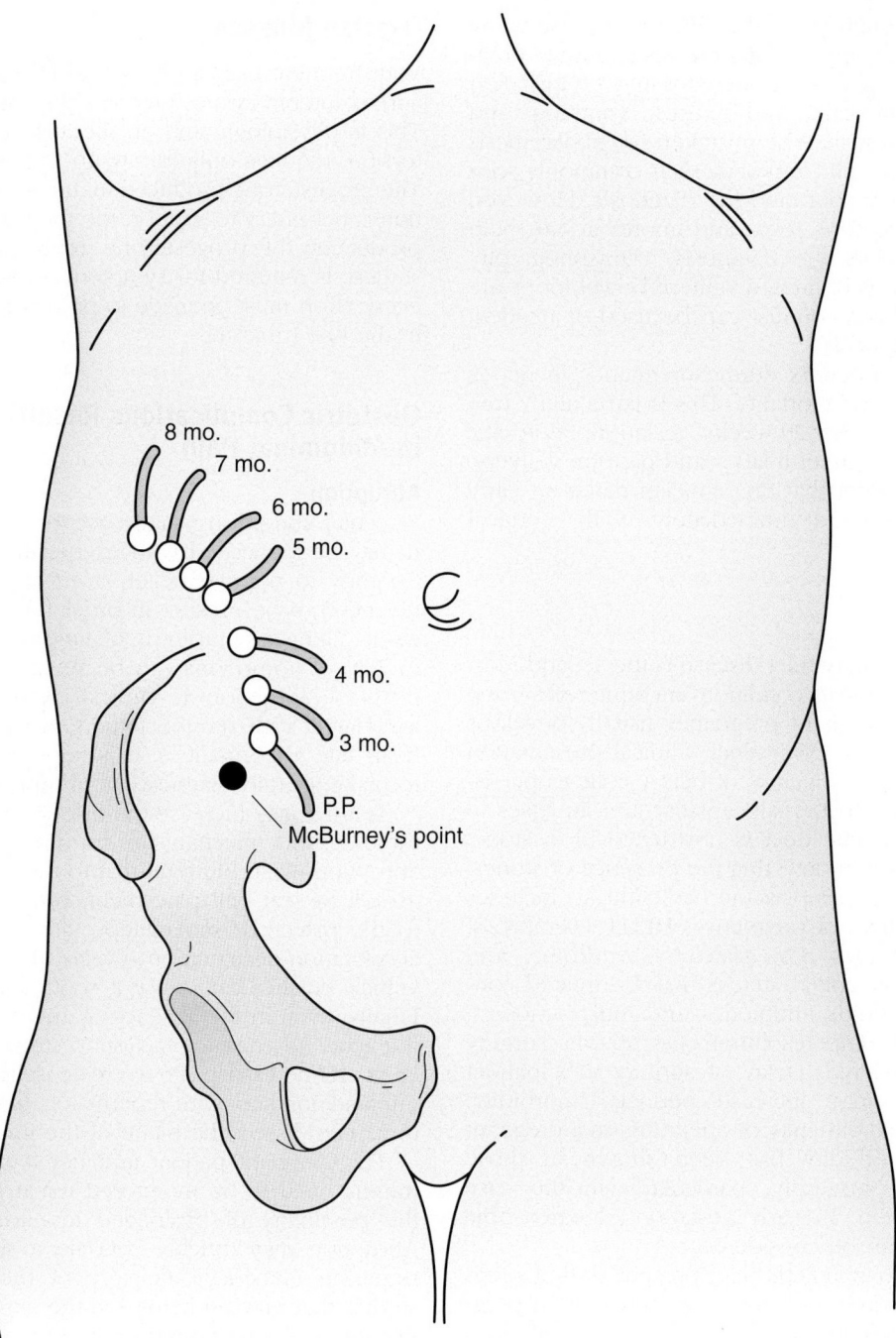

Figure 75-13 Location of the appendix in pregnancy. As modified from Bauer and colleagues (JAMA, 1932), the approximate location of the appendix during succeeding months of pregnancy is diagrammed. In planning an operation, it is better to make the abdominal incision over the point of maximum tenderness unless there is a great disparity between that point and the theoretical location of the appendix. (From Ludmir J, Stubblefield PG: Surgical procedures in pregnancy. In Gabbe S, Neibyl JR, Simpson JL [eds]: Obstetrics: Normal and Problem Pregnancies, 4th ed. Philadelphia, Churchill Livingstone, 2002, p 617.)

general population. In addition to these diagnoses, diagnosis specific to pregnancy also needs to be considered.

Appendicitis

Appendicitis is one of the most common surgical complications of pregnancy, with an incidence of about 2 per 1000 pregnant women. This incidence is not higher than that of the general population; however, appendiceal location during pregnancy changes with the upward displacement of the appendix with advancing gestation[14] (Fig. 75-13). Nevertheless, the most common presenting symptom is pain in the right lower quadrant. This presents regardless of gestational age. The diagnosis of appendicitis in pregnancy may be difficult because many of the symptoms of appendicitis are seen during pregnancy. Pain in the right lower quadrant may be mistaken for round ligament pain, and nausea, vomiting, and abdominal discomfort may be mistaken for hyperemesis gravidarum. Because mild leukocytosis is commonly seen in pregnancy, it may confound the diagnosis. However, other symptoms, such as fever and anorexia, can help the clinician establish the diagnosis. Ultrasonography may be used, but it is of limited value if bowel loops are distended. CT without contrast can be used, if needed, to assist in the diagnosis.

Rupture of the appendix during pregnancy increases perinatal morbidity and mortality. This is particularly true when rupture occurs after 20 weeks' gestation. Peritonitis increases the risk for preterm labor and preterm delivery. Therefore, it is prudent that the clinician make an early diagnosis and proceed immediately with surgical intervention.

Cholelithiasis

After appendicitis, biliary tract disease is the second most common general surgical condition encountered during pregnancy. Cholelithiasis of pregnancy usually develops from obstruction of the cystic duct. Clinical presentation ranges from intermittent attacks of biliary colic to persistent pain radiating into the subcapsular area in cases in which the common bile duct is obstructed by a stone. Ultrasound is helpful in detecting the presence of stones. The differential diagnosis of acute cholelithiasis includes acute pain in the liver of pregnancy, HELLP (*h*emolysis, *e*levated *l*iver enzymes, *l*ow *p*latelets) syndrome, and severe preeclampsia. Initial attacks may be treated conservatively with IV fluids, antibiotics, and antispasmodics; however, without prompt resolution of symptoms, surgery needs to be considered. Delay of surgery in a patient with cholecystitis may increase perinatal morbidity. Despite the potential difficulty of operating on a pregnant woman, lower morbidity has been shown in those patients managed surgically, particularly in the case involving obstruction. In early gestations, laparoscopic cholecystectomy can be considered.

Although rare, pancreatitis may present during pregnancy. The most common cause of pancreatitis in pregnant women is cholelithiasis. However, pancreatitis can be a complication of severe preeclampsia or HELLP syndrome. Pancreatitis caused by milk-alkali toxicity may be seen in patients with excessive intake of antacids.[15]

Intestinal Obstruction

The incidence of intestinal obstruction in pregnant women is similar to that of the general population. Patients present with classic symptoms of abdominal colicky pain associated with hyperactive peristalsis. Nausea and vomiting are present in about 80% of cases. Bowel distention is marked. Laparotomy needs to be performed before bowel necrosis and perforation occur. If perforation occurs during pregnancy, there is a significant increase in maternal and perinatal morbidity and mortality.

Ovarian Masses

With frequent use of ultrasound in early pregnancy, the corpus luteum cyst of pregnancy is frequently identified. This is physiologic and, in the absence of symptoms of torsion, requires only follow-up to ensure the diagnosis. The progesterone produced in the first 14 weeks of gestation is necessary to support the pregnancy until placental production of progesterone replaces it. Therefore, if surgery is required for symptoms of torsion or bleeding, every effort must be made to preserve the corpus luteum in the first trimester.

Obstetric Complications Resulting in Abdominal Pain

Abruption

Placental abruption usually occurs in the third trimester. It may be associated with excruciating abdominal pain. Contrary to popular belief, overt vaginal bleeding does not need to be present in order for the diagnosis to be made. Ultrasonography is of little use because only 5% to 10% of abruptions can be seen. Therefore, the diagnosis of abruption is clinical. Abruptions are usually associated with uterine hypertonicity, resulting in fetal heart rate abnormalities. It is important for the clinician to make a rapid diagnosis of abruption.

Trauma may increase the risk for abruption. There are three distinct mechanisms for post-traumatic placental abruption. First, blunt trauma to the uterus, for example, assault or seat belt placement, can cause a direct injury to the placental implantation site. Second, the sudden acceleration-deceleration cycle that occurs in motor vehicle crashes can cause a contrecoup shearing injury. Finally, even in the absence of any overt physical injury, the acute adrenergic reaction to stress can result in sufficient uterine vasospasm to create ischemic necrosis at the implantation site; with reperfusion, a subplacental hematoma can dissect the plane of the implantation site.

The pregnant patient and her fetus who experience trauma need to be monitored for at least 4 hours, with the possibility of prolonged monitoring for 24 hours. Abruption may quickly become a surgical emergency, requiring immediate delivery of the fetus. Laboratory studies that may be helpful in the diagnosis of abruption include a platelet count and fibrinogen. As the retroplacental hematoma expands, clotting factors, especially fibrinogen and platelets, are consumed. This may assist the clinician in the diagnosis in occult cases.

Pregnancy-related Hepatic Complications

HELLP syndrome and acute fatty liver of pregnancy can present as right upper quadrant pain and nausea and vomiting. HELLP is a form of severe preeclampsia. It is important that the clinician not mistake this for cholelithiasis or other gastrointestinal pathology. Progression of this disease can result in rupture of the hepatic capsule and maternal death if the diagnosis is missed.

Acute fatty liver of pregnancy, which also carries a serious risk for maternal and fetal morbidity and mortality, can present in similar fashion. Laboratory studies are useful in the diagnosis of these entities to include an LDH, serum glutamic-oxaloacetic transaminase (SGOT), platelet count, creatinine, uric acid, and hematocrit. SGOT and LDH will be elevated, platelets will be decreased, and the hematocrit may be increased, especially when seen in association with intravascular volume depletion. In patients with acute fatty liver, glucose may also be decreased. It is important that the clinician remember the physiologic changes in interpreting values that are discussed at the beginning of this chapter.

Trauma

Trauma from accidental injuries occurs in 6% to 7% of all pregnancies. In addition to the risk for placental abruption noted previously, blunt trauma may increase the risk for preterm labor and preterm rupture of the membranes. It is important that pregnant trauma patients be assessed for the same spectrum of injuries as nonpregnant patients. Multiple studies have established that fetal-maternal hemorrhage is increased in women who have suffered trauma. Women who are RhD negative need to have a quantitative assessment of the volume of fetal cells in maternal circulation and an appropriate dose of anti-D immune globulin administered. Peritoneal lavage is not contraindicated in pregnancy and can be performed safely in those patients in whom the possibility of a ruptured viscus is suspected.

Common Obstetric Surgical Procedures

The most common obstetric procedure that the surgeon will encounter is the cesarean birth. Most cesarean births are performed through a Pfannenstiel incision; however, a vertical subumbilical midline incision can be used, especially in obese patients and in patients in whom rapid entry into the abdominal cavity is indicated. After the placement of a bladder catheter, entry into the peritoneal cavity can be undertaken. In most cases, the peritoneum of the vesicouterine fold is transected transversely, and the bladder is gently dissected from the lower uterine segment. The lower uterine segment is palpated to check for malrotation to ensure that a transverse uterine incision centers on the midline. The underlying fetal part is palpated. If the presenting part is the fetal head, the incision is marked 1 to 2 cm above the original margin of the bladder. A small transverse incision is made with a scalpel across the midline of the lower uterine segment down to the fetal membranes. The incision may be extended in a transverse fashion using bandage scissors or in blunt fashion. The membranes are then ruptured. The nondominant hand is placed into the cavity below the fetal head to provide leverage that redirects the vertex through the incision. The vertex is delivered through the uterine and abdominal incisions. The remainder of the infant is delivered using gentle fundal pressure. The cord is clamped and cut, and the fetus is handed to the receiving team.

In cases in which the fetus presents in a transverse or breech presentation, a low vertical cesarean birth is per-

formed. A vertical incision is made into the lower uterine segment and extended downward toward the bladder and upward toward the fundus using the bandage scissors. It is generally preferred that the incision is not taken into the contractile portion of the uterus; but, should head entrapment occur, extension of the incision in a cephalad direction is appropriate.

Although not commonly performed, a classic cesarean birth with an incision over the anterior and superior uterine fundus can be used in those patients in which obstruction of the lower uterine segment occurs secondary to uterine fibroids or in very early gestations.

After the infant is delivered through the incision of choice, closure of the uterine incision may be aided by removing the uterine fundus through the abdominal incision. Delivery of the fundus also facilitates uterine massage. Oxytocin is administered via IV. It is recommended that 20 units be placed into a liter bag of IV fluid, with care taken not to run the fluids at a rate greater than 200 mL/hour in most cases. The uterine incision is closed using an interlocking suture of 1-0 Vicryl or chromic. A second imbricating layer may be used to achieve hemostasis. After the uterus incision is reapproximated and completed, care is taken to investigate for bleeding. The abdomen may be irrigated if there is spillage of meconium or vernix outside the operative field. There is no need to reapproximate the peritoneum or the rectus muscles. The abdominal wall is closed in the usual fashion with absorbable suture.

It is possible that the surgeon may be called to assist with a patient with postpartum hemorrhage. Therefore, it is important to recognize factors that may be unique to pregnancy. As mentioned at the beginning of the chapter, blood volume is increased during pregnancy. *Hemorrhage in pregnancy* is defined as blood loss in excess of 1000 mL. Because of the increase in blood volume by term, however, the patient may lose 1500 to 2000 mL of blood before symptoms. The most common cause of postpartum hemorrhage is uterine atony. Risk factors for uterine atony include prolonged labor, uterine infection, cesarean birth, and overdistention of the uterus. Hemorrhage can also be seen in abruption of the placenta and in patients with placenta previa, either before or after delivery. It is recommended that therapy be initiated after the loss of 600 mL.

The first step is to assess for vaginal, cervical, or uterine lacerations. If negative, and uterine atony is the mechanism, manual exploration of the uterus is initiated to ensure complete removal of the placenta and aggressive fundal massage begun. If this is unsuccessful, the administration of a solution of oxytocin, 20 units in 1 liter of physiologic saline solution at a rate of 200 mL/hour, may assist with uterine contractility. A rate of as high as 500 mL in 10 minutes can be administered without significant cardiovascular complications; however, maternal hypotension may occur with an IV bolus injection of as low as 5 units.

When oxytocin fails to provide adequate response, a synthetic 15-methyl-$F_{2\alpha}$ prostaglandin (carboprost) is administered intramuscularly or in the uterine wall. In addition, methylergonovine maleate (Methergine), 0.2 mg given intramuscularly, may be administered. Methergine is contraindicated in patients with hypertension. Prostaglandin $F_{2\alpha}$ is contraindicated in patients with asthma. Misoprostol (Cytotec) has also uterotonic properties and can be used at a dose of $1000\,\mu g$ per rectum.

When pharmacologic measures fail to control hemorrhage, then surgical measures are undertaken. If the hemorrhage is secondary to uterine atony, ligation of the uterine vessels may be successful. The first step in ligating the uterine arteries is at the anastomosis of the uterine and the ovarian artery high on the fundus just below the utero-ovarian ligament. A large suture on the atraumatic needle can be passed from the uterus around the vessel and tied. If bilateral utero-ovarian vessel ligation does not stop the bleeding, temporary atraumatic occlusion of the ovarian arteries in the infundibulopelvic ligaments may be attempted. By decreasing perfusion pressure, thrombosis in the vascular bed may produce hemostasis.

If conservative measures are unsuccessful, cesarean hysterectomy may need to be performed before sequelae of coagulopathy and hemorrhagic shock occur. In the case of postpartum hemorrhage, supracervical hysterectomy is often the procedure of choice. As in the gynecologic hysterectomy described previously, the superior attachments of the uterus are separated, but following the ligation of the uterine arteries, the fundus of the uterus is amputated from the cervix, which is closed with figure-of-eight sutures. This procedure also maintains the integrity of the uterosacral ligaments.

It is difficult to remove the cervix, especially after a vaginal delivery secondary to dilation of the lower uterine segment. Only surgeons who are skilled in this procedure can proceed without consultation.

Other Procedures

On rare occasions, the surgeon may be consulted to assist with repair of an episiotomy and extension. Episiotomy is an incision into the perineal body made to help facilitate delivery. Most episiotomies are cut in the midline from posterior fourchette toward the rectum. Although more comfortable for the patient, these incisions may extend through the anal sphincter (third degree) or through the rectal wall (fourth degree). An inappropriate repair may result in a rectovaginal fistula. These fistulas present with the same symptoms as seen in other rectal fistulas associated with Crohn's disease but are much easier to repair and have a lower rate of recurrence.

Repair of an episiotomy requires reapproximation of the vaginal tissue and the perineal body. Repair of the anal sphincter requires that the fascial capsule that usually retracts posteriorly be identified and reapproximated. If the rectal wall has been compromised, a multilayer closure, using 2-0 or 3-0 absorbable sutures, of mucosa, muscularis, rectovaginal fascia, anal sphincter, vaginal muscularis, and vaginal mucosa will provide the best opportunity to avoid a fistula. Due to the increased vascularity associated with pregnancy, with an adequate closure without stitch-induced tissue necrosis, healing is not usually a problem.

Selected References

Baggish MS, Karram M (eds): Atlas of Pelvic Anatomy and Gynecologic Surgery, 2nd ed. Philadelphia, WB Saunders, 2006.

> Detailed pelvic anatomy and comprehensive coverage of gynecologic procedures are presented.

Clarke S, Phelan JP, Cotton DB (eds): Critical Care Obstetrics, 3rd ed. Boston, Blackwell Science, 1997.

> This book provides a comprehensive pathophysiology of pregnancy.

Greene FL (ed): American Joint Committee on Cancer Staging Manual, 6th ed. New York, Springer, 2002.

> Comprehensive cancer staging is described.

Mitchell CW, Wheeless CR Jr (eds.): Atlas of Pelvic Surgery, 3rd ed. Baltimore, Williams & Wilkins, 1997.

> Detailed pelvic surgical procedures are presented.

Rock J, Jones HWJ III (eds): TeLinde's Operative Gynecology, 9th ed. Philadelphia, Lippincott Williams & Wilkins, 2003.

> Encyclopedic coverage addresses all areas of gynecologic surgery with an expanded oncology section.

Speroff L, Glass RH, Kase NG (eds): Clinical Gynecologic Endocrinology and Infertility, 7th ed. Philadelphia, Lippincott Williams & Wilkins, 2005.

> A comprehensive description of reproductive physiology is presented.

References

1. Kadar N, Friedman M, Zacher M: Further observations on the doubling time of human chorionic gonadotropin in early asymptomatic pregnancies. Fertil Steril 54:783-787, 1990.
2. Keith SC, London SN, Weitzmen GA, et al: Serial transvaginal ultrasound scans and β-human chorionic gonadotropin levels in early singleton and multiple pregnancies. Fertil Steril 59:1007-1010, 1993.
3. Buckley RG, King KJ, Disney JD, et al: Serum progesterone testing to predict ectopic pregnancy in symptomatic first-trimester patients. Ann Emerg Med 36:95-100, 2000.
4. Federation of International Gynecology and Obstetrics. FIGO Staging of Gynecologic Cancer. Available at: http://www.figo.org, 2006.
5. Zullo F, Palomba S, Russo T, et al: A prospective randomized comparison between laparoscopic and laparotomic approaches in women with early stage endometrial cancer: A focus on the quality of life. Am J Obstet Gynecol 193:1344-1352, 2005.
6. Molpus KL, Redlin-Frazier S, Reed G, et al: Postoperative pelvic irradiation in early stage mixed mullerian tumors. Eur J Gynaecol Oncol 19:541-546, 1998.
7. Spirtos NM, Eisenkop SM, Boike G, et al: Laparoscopic staging in patients with incompletely staged cancers of the uterus, ovary, fallopian tube, and primary peritoneum: A Gynecologic Oncology Group (GOG) study. Am J Obstet Gynecol 193:1645-1649, 2005.
8. Wolner-Hanssen P, Mardh P-A, Svensson L, et al: Laparoscopy in women with chlamydial infection and pelvic pain: A comparison of patients with and without salpingitis. Obstet Gynecol 61:299-303, 1983.

9. Loffer FD: Three-year comparison of thermal balloon and rollerball ablation in treatment of menorrhagia. J Am Assoc Gynecol Laparosc 8:48-54, 2001.

10. Loffer FD, Grainger D: Five-year follow-up of patients participating in a randomized trial of uterine balloon therapy versus rollerball ablation for treatment of menorrhagia. J Am Assoc Gynecol Laparosc 9:429-435, 2002.

11. Parker WH: Total laparoscopic hysterectomy and laparoscopic supracervical hysterectomy. Obstet Gynecol Clin N Am 31:523-527, 2004.

12. Ramirez PT, Slomovitz BM, Soliman PT, et al: Total laparoscopic radical hysterectomy and lymphadenectomy: The M. D. Anderson Cancer Center Experience. Gynecol Oncol (in press).

13. Plante M, Renaud M-C, Hoskins IA, et al: Vaginal radical trachelectomy: A valuable fertility-preserving option in the management of early-stage cervical cancer. A series of 50 pregnancies and review of the literature. Gynecol Oncol 98:3-10, 2005.

14. Ludmir J, Stubblefield PG: Surgical procedures in pregnancy. In Gabbe S, Neibyl JR, Simpson JL (eds): Obstetrics: Normal and Problem Pregnancies, 4th ed. Philadelphia: Churchill Livingstone, 2002, p 368.

15. Marcovici I, Marzano D: Pregnancy-induced hypertension complicated by postpartum renal failure and pancreatitis: A case report. Am J Perinatol 19:177-179, 2002.

Surgery in the Pregnant Patient

Dean J. Mikami, MD   Paul R. Beery, MD   and   E. Christopher Ellison, MD

The pregnant patient presents a unique clinical challenge. An estimated 1% to 2% of pregnant women require surgical procedures, with nonobstetric surgery necessary in up to 1% of pregnancies in the United States each year. A recent review by Cohen-Kerem and associates evaluated the effects of nonobstetric surgical procedures on maternal and fetal outcomes (see Selected References). In a review of 44 papers and 12,452 patients, a maternal death rate of .006% and a miscarriage rate of 5.8% were reported. Most indications for surgical intervention are common for the patient's age group and unrelated to pregnancy, such as acute appendicitis, symptomatic cholelithiasis, breast masses, or trauma. Changes in maternal anatomy and physiology and safety of the fetus are among the issues of which the surgeon must be cognizant. The presentation of surgical diseases in the pregnant patient may be atypical or may mimic signs and symptoms associated with a normal pregnancy, and a standard evaluation may be unreliable because of pregnancy-associated changes in diagnostic tests or laboratory values. Finally, many physicians may be more conservative in diagnostic evaluation and treatment. Any of these factors may result in a delay in diagnosis and treatment, adversely affecting maternal and fetal outcome. Although consultation with an obstetrician is ideal when caring for a pregnant patient, the surgeon needs to be aware of certain fundamental principles when such a resource is unavailable. This chapter discusses the key points in caring for the pregnant patient who presents with nonobstetric surgical disease.

PHYSIOLOGIC CHANGES OF PREGNANCY

Progesterone and estrogen, two of the principal hormones of pregnancy, mediate many of the maternal physiologic changes in pregnancy. Normal laboratory values differ in the gravid compared with the nonpregnant patient. The diaphragm can be elevated in pregnancy up to 4 cm, and the lower chest wall can widen up to 7 cm.[1] These changes may also mimic similar pathophysiology that occurs in nonpregnant individuals who have cardiac or liver disease. Elevated progesterone levels, as well as decreased serum motilin, result in smooth muscle relaxation, producing multiple effects in several organ systems. In the stomach, this decreased smooth muscle tone results in diminished gastric tone and motility. The lower esophageal sphincter tone is also decreased, and when combined with increased intra-abdominal pressure, this results in an increase in the incidence of gastroesophageal reflux. Small bowel motility is reduced, increasing small bowel transit time. Absorption of nutrients, however, remains unchanged, with the exception of iron absorption, which is increased because of increased iron requirements. In the colon, pregnancy-related changes usually manifest as constipation. This is due to a combination of increased colonic sodium and water absorption, decreased motility, and mechanical obstruction by the gravid uterus. An increase in portal venous pressure, and therefore an increase in the pressure in the collateral venous circulation, results in dilation of the veins at the gastroesophageal junction. This is of importance only if the patient had esophageal varices before becoming pregnant. The most common result of the increased portal venous pressure is the dilation of the hemorrhoidal veins leading to the well-known complaint of hemorrhoids by the patient.

In addition to alterations in smooth muscle tone and motility, other notable changes occur in the gastrointestinal tract. The function of the gallbladder is altered, as is the chemical composition of bile. During the second and third trimesters, the volume of the gallbladder may be twice that found in the nonpregnant state, and gallbladder emptying is markedly slower. Up to 4% of pregnant patients have gallstones on routine obstetric ultrasounds.[2] Still, only 1 out of every 1000 pregnant patients develops symptoms. It is unknown whether the increased biliary stasis, changes in bile composition, or a combination of the two factors results in an increased risk for gallstone formation, but the risk for developing gallstones increases with multiparity. However, the incidence of symptomatic cholelithiasis during pregnancy is similar to the incidence in age-related nonpregnant patients.

Some of the changes of pregnancy closely resemble liver disease. These include spider angiomas and palmar erythema from elevated serum estrogen levels. Hypoalbuminemia is also seen, along with elevated serum cholesterol, alkaline phosphatase, and fibrinogen levels. Serum bilirubin and hepatic transaminase levels remain unchanged during pregnancy.

In the cardiovascular system, peripheral vascular resistance is decreased as a consequence of diminished vascular smooth muscle tone. Cardiac output increases by as much as 50% during the first trimester of pregnancy. Initially, this is due to an increased stroke volume resulting from an increase in plasma volume and red blood cell mass, but a gradual increase in maternal heart rate also contributes. Cardiac output falls back to nearly normal late in pregnancy, usually during the 36th to 40th weeks of gestation. During the third trimester, cardiac output is dramatically decreased when the mother is lying supine. This is due to compromised venous return from the lower extremity from compression of the inferior vena cava by the gravid uterus. In the supine position, the inferior vena cava may be completely occluded; venous drainage of the lower extremities is through collateral channels. With this drop in preload, an increase in sympathetic tone usually maintains peripheral vascular resistance and blood pressure. However, up to 10% of patients may experience supine hypotensive syndrome, in which the sympathetic response is not adequate to maintain blood pressure. During anesthesia induction in the operating room, anesthetic agents may inhibit the compensatory sympathetic response, causing a more precipitous fall in blood pressure. From a surgeon's perspective, it may be necessary to place the patient in the left lateral decubitus position during procedures performed during the third trimester, relieving caval compression by the enlarged uterus.

Inguinal swelling secondary to varicosities of the round ligament is also a phenomenon that occurs during pregnancy. The increase in swelling is a result of hormonal and mechanical changes. It is often mistaken for an inguinal or femoral hernia. The appropriate management includes careful physical examination and ultrasound if needed. The varicosities generally resolve postpartum.

Oxygen consumption increases during pregnancy. Minute ventilation increases by 50%, owing to an increase in tidal volume, which appears to be a result of elevated serum progesterone level.[1] Progesterone not only increases the sensitivity of the respiratory centers to CO_2 but also acts as a direct stimulant to the respiratory centers. As a consequence of the increased minute ventilation, maternal PaO_2 levels during late pregnancy range from 104 to 108 mm Hg, and maternal $PaCO_2$ ranges from 27 to 32 mm Hg. Renal compensation maintains normal maternal pH. The decreased $PaCO_2$ increases the CO_2 gradient from the fetus to the mother, facilitating CO_2 transfer from the fetus to the mother. The oxygen-hemoglobin dissociation curve of maternal blood is shifted to the right; this, coupled with the increased affinity for oxygen of fetal hemoglobin, results in increased oxygen transfer to the fetus. Elevation of the diaphragm by as much as 4 cm results in a decrease in total lung volume by 5%. Diminished expiratory reserve volume and residual volume result in a functional residual capacity that is 20% lower than that in the nonpregnant woman. Vital capacity and inspiratory reserve volume remain stable.

In the kidney, there is an increase in the glomerular filtration rate by 50% that accompanies a 75% increase in renal plasma flow. Urinary glucose excretion increases as a direct consequence of the increased glomerular filtration rate. Blood urea nitrogen decreases by 25% during the first trimester and maintains at that level for the remainder of pregnancy. Serum creatinine also decreases by the end of the first trimester from a nonpregnant value of 0.8 mg/dL to 0.7 mg/dL and may be as low as 0.5 mg/dL by term. A 5- to 10-fold increase in serum renin occurs with a subsequent 4- to 5-fold increase in angiotensin. Although the pregnant patient is apparently less sensitive to the hypertensive effects of the increased angiotensin, elevated aldosterone levels result in an increase in sodium reabsorption, overcoming the natriuresis produced by elevated progesterone. Serum sodium levels are decreased, however, because the increase in sodium reabsorption is less than the increase in plasma volume. Serum osmolality is decreased to 270 to 280 mOsm/kg.[1]

The increase in plasma volume and red blood cell mass is accompanied by a progressive rise in the leukocyte count during pregnancy. During the first trimester, the white blood cell count ranges from 3000 to 15,000 cells/mm^3, increasing to a range of 6000 to 16,000 cells/mm^3 during the second and third trimesters.[1] Platelet count progressively declines throughout pregnancy, whereas the mean platelet volume tends to increase after

Table 76-1 Fetal Radiation Exposure With Radiographic Imaging

EXAMINATION TYPE	ESTIMATED FETAL RADIATION EXPOSURE (cGy)
Two-view chest radiograph	0.00007
Cervical spine radiograph	0.002
Pelvis radiograph	0.04
Head CT	<0.050
Abdomen CT	2.60
Upper GI series	0.056
Barium enema	3.986
Hepatobiliary (HIDA) scan	0.150

CT, computed tomography; GI, gastrointestinal.

28 weeks' gestation. As previously stated, fibrinogen levels are elevated to a range of 400 to 500 mg/dL. Plasma levels of factors VII, VIII, IX, and X also rise progressively, whereas levels of factors XI and XIII decline, and levels of factors II, V, and XII remain unchanged. Despite these alterations in the coagulation cascade and platelet count, bleeding time and clotting time are unchanged.

RADIOLOGY SAFETY CONCERNS IN PREGNANCY

Radiographic studies remain useful diagnostic tools in the pregnant patient. Of greatest concern with radiation exposure is the risk to the fetus from the exposure. The accepted maximum dose of ionizing radiation during the entire pregnancy is 5 cGy. The fetus is at the highest risk from radiation exposure from the preimplantation period to about 15 weeks' gestation. Primary organogenesis occurs during this time, and the teratogenic effects of radiation, particularly to the developing central nervous system, are at their highest. Perinatal radiation exposure has also been associated with childhood leukemia and certain childhood malignancies. The radiation dose that has been associated with congenital malformation is higher than 10 cGy.[3] As demonstrated in Table 76-1, radiation exposure to the fetus with the doses from the more common radiology procedures is well below that threshold. Nonetheless, prudence on the part of the clinician is required to avoid unnecessary fetal exposure to ionizing radiation, especially during the first trimester and early second trimester, when the risk from exposure is greatest.

Magnetic resonance imaging (MRI) avoids exposure to ionizing radiation but poses an unknown risk to the fetus. Animal studies have shown no teratogenic effect or increased incidence of fetal death or congenital malformations from the electromagnetic radiation, static magnetic field, radiofrequency magnetic fields, or intravenous (IV) contrast agents used during MRI. Theoretically, the gradient magnetic fields may produce electric currents within the patient, and the high-frequency currents induced by radiofrequency fields may cause local generation of heat. The long-term effect of exposure is not known.[4] Currently, the National Radiological Protection Board advises against the use of MRI during the first trimester of pregnancy.

Ultrasonography is routinely used by obstetricians during pregnancy. Although tissue heating and cavitation are theoretical effects of ultrasound exposure, such effects have never been reported. Ultrasound may be a helpful alternative diagnostic tool when trying to avoid exposure to ionizing radiation, but it does have some limitations. Deeper structures are difficult to visualize and may be obscured by superficial structures that are more echodense. Ultrasound imaging has a limited field of view and is highly operator dependent. Despite these limitations, certain disease processes, such as a palpable breast mass, may be evaluated effectively and safely.

ANESTHESIA SAFETY CONCERNS IN PREGNANCY

Anesthesia concerns during pregnancy include the safety of both the mother and the fetus. The fetus may be affected by exposure to teratogenic effects of anesthetic agents, risk for preterm labor, and the risk from changes in maternal physiology as a consequence of anesthesia. Changes in uterine blood flow and maternal acid-base status may result in hypoxemia or asphyxia for the fetus. These can be a result of maternal hypotension or hypoxia, maternal hyperventilation, or the placental passage of anesthetic agents that affect the fetal central nervous or cardiovascular systems.

The effects of anesthesia during pregnancy can be divided into direct, or active, and indirect, or passive, effects. The direct effects relate to the possible teratogenic or embryotoxic properties of the drugs used for anesthesia, some of which cross the placenta. The indirect effects are those mechanisms by which an anesthetic agent or surgical procedure may interfere with maternal or fetal physiology and in doing so harm the fetus. For the most part, the fetus experiences indirect effects as a consequence of anesthetic agents administered to the mother and hemodynamic changes of the mother from blood loss or anesthetic agents. The most profound effects on the fetus are related to decreased uterine blood flow or decreased oxygen content of uterine blood. Unlike circulation to other vital organs, most notably the brain, the uterine circulation is not autoregulated. During the third trimester, uterine circulation represents nearly 10% of cardiac output. When treating maternal hypotension, vasopressors such as dopamine and epinephrine, while increasing the maternal systemic pressure, have little or no effect on uterine circulation. Phenylephrine and metaraminol are α-agonists that are effective in maintaining maternal blood pressure and preventing fetal acidosis.[5] Other maneuvers, such as fluid bolus, Trendelenburg position, compression stockings, and leg elevation, have a larger impact on increasing uterine blood flow.

In addition to the risks related to maternal hypoxia or hypotension, the risk for spontaneous abortion and teratogenesis related to anesthetic agents is of major concern. Many nonhuman studies have demonstrated different teratogenic effects with similar agents but have not led to definitive conclusions regarding teratogenic potential in humans. For a congenital defect to result, exposure to the teratogen must occur during the vulnerable differentiation stage of the affected organ system. As previously noted, differentiation of the major organ systems occurs during the first trimester of human embryonic development. Therefore, delaying semielective surgical procedures until after the first trimester may reduce the risk for teratogenicity. However, large survey studies have demonstrated an increased risk for spontaneous abortions, intrauterine growth retardation, and low-birth-weight neonates in women who require surgery during pregnancy. These studies lacked information on the indications for the nonobstetric surgical procedures.

Elective surgical procedures are delayed until at least 6 weeks after delivery, when maternal physiology has returned to the nonpregnant state and when the impact on the fetus is no longer a concern. When emergent procedures are required, obviously, the life of the mother takes priority, although an experienced anesthesiologist will be able to modify the anesthesia used according to maternal physiology and fetal well-being. For semielective surgical procedures, attempts are made to delay surgery until after the first trimester whenever possible. This needs to be determined on an individual case basis because continued exposure to the underlying disease process may be more harmful than the operative risk to both the mother and the fetus. During the second trimester, after organ system differentiation has occurred, there is almost no risk for anesthetic-induced malformation or spontaneous abortion. Later in pregnancy, during the third trimester, the risk for preterm delivery is at its highest.

When the pregnant patient requires surgical intervention, consultation with the obstetrician and possibly a perinatologist is essential. The specialist is helpful in determining the optimum technique to monitor fetal status and is able to assist with perioperative management and diagnose and manage preterm labor. Typically, when emergent surgery occurs during the first trimester or early second trimester, fetal heart tones are obtained before and after anesthesia exposure. During the late second trimester and third trimester, when the fetus is of viable age, continuous intraoperative monitoring is performed when possible. Transvaginal ultrasound can be used when the surgical field involves the abdomen. Continuous monitoring is used if a significant blood loss is possible or anticipated to assess fetal well-being.

Fetal heart rate for fetal status and tocometer monitoring for uterine activity are obtained before and after the procedure, even if intraoperative monitoring is not believed necessary or is not available.

Postoperative pain control in the pregnant patient needs to be monitored closely. Nonsteroidal anti-inflammatory drugs are not used in pregnancy because of the risk for premature closure of the ductus arteriosis.[6] Morphine and fentanyl are both good IV choices postoperatively. Morphine does have a higher associated incidence of nausea and vomiting, but most surgeons have extensive experience with it. A patient-controlled analgesia pump after surgery may be the best choice because of the associated low incidence of maternal respiratory depression and drug transfer to the fetus.

Postoperative oral narcotic use is generally considered safe in pregnancy. Narcotic analgesics have not been found to cause birth defects in humans in normal dosages. Oxycodone, hydrocodone, and codeine are commonly used narcotics and can be safely used in moderation. Chronic use of narcotics during pregnancy may cause fetal dependency. It is recommended that the pregnant postsurgical patient be weaned off narcotic use as soon as possible.

PREVENTION OF PRETERM LABOR

The incidence of preterm labor associated with nonobstetric surgery is related to both gestational age and the indication for surgery. Studies have suggested that the rate of premature labor induced by nonobstetric surgical intervention is 3.5%. Gestational age at treatment and severity of the underlying disease are the most predictive indicators of patients at risk for preterm labor. The later in gestation the patient is, the higher the risk for preterm contractions or preterm labor. Intraperitoneal surgeries and disease processes with intraperitoneal inflammation are the most likely to have postoperative courses complicated by preterm contractions and preterm labor. In multiple studies, a significant difference was found in the number of patients with preterm contractions based on the average time from onset of symptoms to operative intervention. A delay in treatment appears to increase the chance of preterm labor, likely related to the primary disease process. Laparoscopic and open techniques have an equal associated incidence of preterm labor.

There is no general consensus on the use of prophylactic tocolytics after nonobstetric surgery during pregnancy. Tocolytic use varies widely between centers and among physicians. Most studies suggest that tocolytics only be used if contractions are noted during postoperative monitoring or are appreciated by the patient. Tocolytics used as needed are generally successful at preventing preterm labor and preterm delivery when postoperative contractions are detected. Terbutaline, magnesium, and indomethacin (Indocin) all have been used in different studies with equivalent results. Nearly 100% of patients with postoperative contractions were successfully tocolyzed and delivered at term. In general, for patients with postoperative contractions before 32 weeks, indomethacin would be a reasonable treatment, whereas terbutaline could be used first line for patients at more than 32 weeks' gestation. The use of prophylactic tocolysis is individualized, depending on the patient's gestational age and the underlying disease process.

ABDOMINAL PAIN AND THE ACUTE ABDOMEN IN PREGNANCY

When the pregnant patient presents with abdominal pain, it may be difficult to distinguish a pathophysiologic cause from normal pregnancy-associated symptoms. Changes in the position and orientation of abdominal viscera from the enlarging uterus, as well as alterations in physiology already described, may modify the perception or manifestation of an intra-abdominal process. If early in the pregnancy, the woman may not know that she is pregnant. Additionally, some intra-abdominal processes are exclusive to pregnancy, such as ectopic pregnancy, HELLP (*h*emolysis, *e*levated *l*iver enzymes, *l*ow *p*latelets) syndrome, or acute fatty liver of pregnancy. Third, both patient and physician may attribute the patient's complaints to normal pregnancy, resulting in a delay in evaluation and treatment. These delays in diagnosis and definitive intervention are the most serious adverse event affecting maternal and fetal outcome. It is usually not the treatment but the delay in diagnosis and severity of the primary disease process that poorly affect outcomes.[7] Table 76-2 lists the more common causes of abdominal pain in the pregnant patient, classified according to location.

MINIMALLY INVASIVE SURGERY IN PREGNANCY

When laparoscopic techniques were initially described, pregnancy was considered a contraindication to laparoscopy. Effects of CO_2 pneumoperitoneum on venous return and cardiac output, uterine perfusion, and fetal acid-base status were unknown. Laparoscopy was safely used in several series to evaluate pregnant patients for ectopic pregnancy. Those patients with an intrauterine pregnancy had no increase in fetal loss or observed negative effect on long-term outcome.[8,9] When comparing laparoscopic and open techniques in nonpregnant patients, those patients who underwent laparoscopic procedures had decreased pain, shorter hospital stays, and a quicker return to normal activity.

Major concerns of laparoscopy during pregnancy include injury to the uterus, decreased uterine blood flow, fetal acidosis, and preterm labor from increased intra-abdominal pressure. During the second trimester, the uterus is no longer contained within the pelvis. The open technique for abdominal access reduces the risk for injury. Utilizing a Veress needle for insufflation is discouraged after the first trimester because of the increased risk for puncturing the uterus. Decreased uterine blood flow from pneumoperitoneum remains theoretical because significant changes in intra-abdominal pressure occur normally during pregnancy with maternal Valsalva maneuvers. The risk for pneumoperitoneum may also be less than the risk for direct uterine manipulation that occurs with laparotomy. Fetal respiratory acidosis with subsequent fetal hypertension and tachycardia were observed in a pregnant ewe model but were reversed by maintaining maternal respiratory alkalosis.[10] Additionally, in the small series comparing laparoscopy and open techniques, no significant difference in preterm labor or delivery-related side effects was observed.[11] Table 76-3 illustrates the general comparison between laparoscopic and open technique.

The Society of American Gastrointestinal Endoscopic Surgeons recommends the following guidelines for laparoscopic surgery during pregnancy:

Table 76-2 Common Causes of Abdominal Pain in the Pregnant Patient

Right Upper Quadrant
Gastroesophageal reflux
Peptic ulcer disease
Acute cholecystitis
Biliary colic
Acute pancreatitis
Hepatitis
Acute fatty liver of pregnancy
HELLP syndrome
Preeclampsia
Pneumothorax
Pneumonia
Acute appendicitis
Hepatic adenoma
Hemangioma

Right Lower Quadrant
Acute appendicitis
Ectopic pregnancy
Renal or ureteral colic
Pelvic inflammatory disease
Tubo-ovarian abscess
Endometriosis
Adnexal torsion
Ruptured ovarian cyst
Ruptured corpus luteum

Lower Abdomen
Threatened, incomplete, or complete abortion
Abruptio placentae
Preterm labor
Pelvic inflammatory disease
Tubo-ovarian abscess
Inflammatory bowel disease
Irritable bowel syndrome
Pyelonephritis

Flank
Pyelonephritis
Hydronephrosis of pregnancy
Acute appendicitis (retrocecal appendix)

Diffuse Abdominal Pain
Early acute appendicitis
Small bowel obstruction
Acute intermittent porphyria
Sickle cell crisis

HELLP, hemolysis, elevated liver enzymes, low platelets.

Table 76-3 Advantages and Disadvantages of Use of Laparoscopy Instead of Laparotomy in Pregnancy

Advantages
Decreased fetal depression secondary to decreased narcotic requirement
Lower rates of wound infections and incisional hernias
Diminished postoperative maternal hypoventilation
Decreased manipulation of the uterus
Faster recovery with early return-to-normal function
Decreased risk for ileus
Disadvantages
Possible uterine injury during trocar placement
Decreased uterine blood flow
Preterm labor risk secondary to the increased intra-abdominal pressure
Increased risk of fetal acidosis and unknown effects of CO_2 pneumoperitoneum
Decreased visualization with gravid uterus

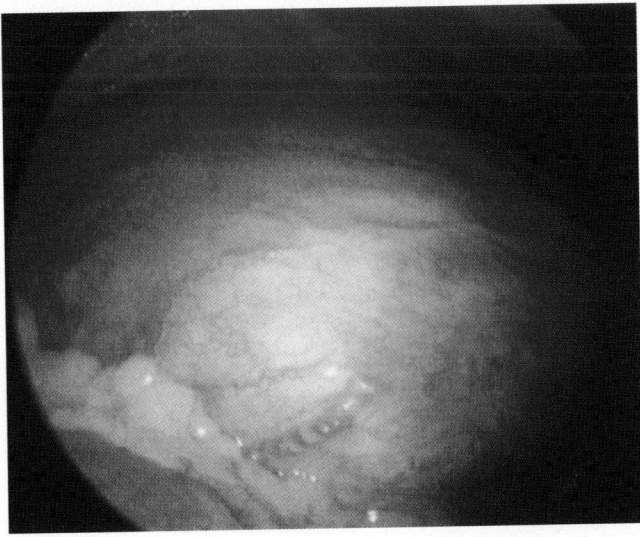

Figure 76-1 Intraoperative image of a 24-week gravid uterus taken with a 5-mm, 30-degree, high-definition camera.

1. Obstetric consultation is obtained preoperatively.
2. When possible, operative intervention is deferred until the second trimester, when fetal risk is lowest.
3. Pneumoperitoneum enhances lower extremity venous stasis already present in the gravid patient, and pregnancy induces a hypercoagulable state. Therefore, pneumatic compression devices are used whenever possible.
4. Fetal and uterine status, as well as maternal end-tidal CO_2 and arterial blood gases, needs to be monitored.
5. The uterus needs to be protected with a lead shield if intraoperative cholangiography is a possibility. Fluoroscopy is used selectively.
6. Given the enlarged gravid uterus, abdominal access is attained using an open technique.
7. Dependent positioning is used to shift the uterus off the inferior vena cava.
8. Pneumoperitoneum pressures are minimized to 8 to 12 mm Hg and not allowed to exceed 15 mm Hg.[12,13]

Trocar placement in the pregnant patient does not differ radically from placement in the nonpregnant patient early in pregnancy. Later in pregnancy, the camera port must be placed in a supraumbilical location, and the remaining ports are placed under direct camera visualization. The gravid uterus enlarges superiorly (Fig. 76-1); adjustments in trocar placement must be made to avoid uterine injury and to improve visualization. An angled scope may aid in viewing over or around the uterus. The uterus should be manipulated as little as possible.

BREAST MASSES IN PREGNANCY

Pregnancy-associated breast cancer is defined as breast cancer that is diagnosed during pregnancy or within 1 year after pregnancy. It has become increasingly more prominent as more women delay childbearing until they are in their 30s and 40s; the incidence of breast cancer is higher in women of those age groups. Overall, pregnancy-associated breast cancer has been reported to occur in 1 in 10,000 to 1 in 3000 pregnant women.[14,15]

It is the most common nongynecologic malignancy associated with pregnancy. It usually presents as a painless palpable mass with or without nipple discharge. Recent studies have demonstrated that pregnancy-associated breast cancer may be more common in women with a genetic predisposition to breast cancer. In a group of 292 women diagnosed with breast cancer before age 40 years, those with a known *BRCA1* or *BRCA2* gene mutation were more likely to develop cancer during pregnancy.[16] In a group of 383 women in Japan, a family history of breast cancer was three times more common in patients who were diagnosed with breast cancer while pregnant or lactating when compared with nonpregnant patients with breast cancer.[17] As is true in nonpregnant patients, ductal carcinoma is the most common pathologic type of tumor, accounting for 75% to 90% of breast cancers in pregnant patients.[18]

Delays in diagnosis and treatment are common, although this has recently improved. Previous studies demonstrated delays in diagnosis of nearly 6 months, but more recent data show a mean delay of 1 to 2 months. Given a tumor doubling size of 130 days, a delay in diagnosis and treatment of 1 month increases the risk for nodal metastasis by 0.9%, whereas a delay of 6 months increases the risk by 5.1%.[18] Although the initial reports of pregnancy-associated breast cancer more than 100 years ago proposed a dismal prognosis, more recent literature has suggested that this is due to a more advanced stage at the time of diagnosis.[15,19] When compared with age-matched nonpregnant controls, women with pregnancy-associated breast cancer present with a larger primary tumor and a higher risk for positive axillary lymph nodes.[19] However, women with pregnancy-associated breast cancer have a similar stage-related prognosis compared with nonpregnant controls. Overall, these women bear a worse prognosis because of the more advanced disease at presentation. Pregnancy is a hyperestrogenic state and may correlate with rapid tumor proliferation and axillary lymph node metastases,[20] although pregnant women and nonpregnant young women have a higher percentage of estrogen receptor–negative cancers than older women.[21] In a series comparing 75 patients with pregnancy-associated breast cancer and 182 nonpregnant patients with breast cancer, 42% of cancers were estrogen receptor negative in the pregnant group, and 21% were estrogen receptor negative in the nonpregnant control group.[22] This higher incidence of estrogen receptor–negative cancer is likely due to a down-regulation of estrogen receptors during pregnancy. Physiologic changes of breast engorgement, rapid cellular proliferation, and increased vascularity make a reliable physical examination difficult; masses of similar size that would be easily palpable in the nonpregnant state may be obscured, or palpable masses may be attributed to normal pregnancy-related changes. Benign breast lesions such as galactoceles, mastitis, abscesses, lipomas, fibroadenomas, lobular hyperplasia, and lactational adenomas account for 80% of breast masses that occur during pregnancy or during lactation. However, any palpable mass that persists for 4 weeks or longer needs to be evaluated.

Because of the changes in the breast tissue with pregnancy, imaging modalities may be difficult to interpret. If used with appropriate shielding, mammography carries a limited risk to the fetus. Mammography has a high false-negative rate due to the increased density of the fibroglandular breast tissue, however, so it has limited usefulness in the evaluation of the pregnant patient. Ultrasonography can safely be performed as an initial evaluation or in conjunction with mammography. Ultrasound is able to distinguish solid from cystic lesions in 97% of patients and is helpful in guiding fine-needle aspiration or biopsy. MRI of the breast is highly sensitive but only moderately specific and is being used more frequently in the nonpregnant patient. Its usefulness in the pregnant patient is yet to be determined. Although MRI does not use ionizing radiation, the two main risks to the fetus from the magnetic field and electromagnetic radiation are heating and cavitation. The gadolinium contrast is listed as a pregnancy category C drug, to be used only if the potential benefit outweighs the potential risk. Gadolinium crosses the placenta and has been associated with fetal abnormalities in rats. With other reliable imaging modalities available, MRI is not currently recommended for breast imaging in the pregnant patient.[2]

Tissue diagnosis is essential. Core-needle biopsy with or without ultrasound guidance is a safe and reliable method for obtaining tissue. The major risks are hematoma formation and milk fistula development. A pressure dressing is applied following the biopsy to minimize the risk for hematoma from the hypervascularity of the breasts. The risk for milk fistula may be reduced by stopping lactation for several days before biopsy and by emptying the breast of milk just before the procedure. If the biopsy is done postpartum, a 1-week course of bromocriptine may also be given before biopsy. Fine-needle aspiration may be a reliable alternative to core-needle or open biopsy. It can be performed safely with ultrasound guidance under local anesthesia without exposing the patient and fetus to the risks involved with general anesthesia, but its accuracy is dependent on the pathologist's experience in distinguishing the proliferative changes of pregnancy from cancer. In a series of 214 patients, none of the patients with negative fine-needle aspiration cytology developed cancer during the 18- to 24-month follow-up period.[21]

The mainstay of therapy for pregnancy-associated breast cancer is surgical resection. Modified radical mastectomy has long been considered the appropriate choice for local control. It eliminates the need for adjuvant radiation and its risk to the fetus. More recent data have suggested that the combination of local control and adjuvant therapy may be tailored to the patient according to the stage of pregnancy as well as the stage of the cancer.[18] In stages I and II cancer, mastectomy with axillary dissection is preferred. Axillary dissection is necessary because of the aggressive nature of pregnancy-associated breast cancer and the higher incidence of nodal metastasis. Sentinel node biopsy poses an unknown risk to the fetus and is avoided until the safety of the radioisotope is determined.

In patients diagnosed during the late second trimester or later, immediate breast-conserving lumpectomy and axillary dissection followed with radiation postpartum is a treatment option. If the diagnosis of breast cancer is made in the first or early second trimester of pregnancy, lumpectomy and axillary dissection can be followed by chemotherapy after the first trimester and radiation after delivery. Chemotherapy is indicated for node-positive cancers or node-negative tumors greater than 1 cm. Current chemotherapeutic regimens are relatively safe after the first trimester, when the teratogenic risk is greatest. The increased plasma volume, the hypoalbuminemia, and the fact that almost all chemotherapeutic agents cross the placenta change the pharmacokinetics of the drugs and make accurate dosing difficult. Antimetabolites such as methotrexate are avoided because of the high risk for spontaneous abortion even after the first trimester. Other agents have been associated with congenital malformations and complications such as preterm delivery, low birth weight, hyaline membrane disease, transient leukopenia, transient tachypnea of the newborn, and intrauterine growth retardation, but most of these effects occurred when the chemotherapeutic agent was administered during the first trimester. Twenty-four patients with pregnancy-associated breast cancer were given a chemotherapeutic regimen during the second and third trimester that included fluorouracil, cyclophosphamide, and doxorubicin. None of the infants had congenital malformations, and the median age at delivery was 38 weeks.[23] Long-term effects of the chemotherapeutic agents used for pregnancy-associated breast cancer on growth and development of children are not known. Cyclophosphamide and doxorubicin can enter breast milk; breast-feeding is contraindicated during chemotherapy.

Radiation is typically not offered during pregnancy because of its teratogenic risk and its risk for induction of childhood malignancies. The risk is directly related to

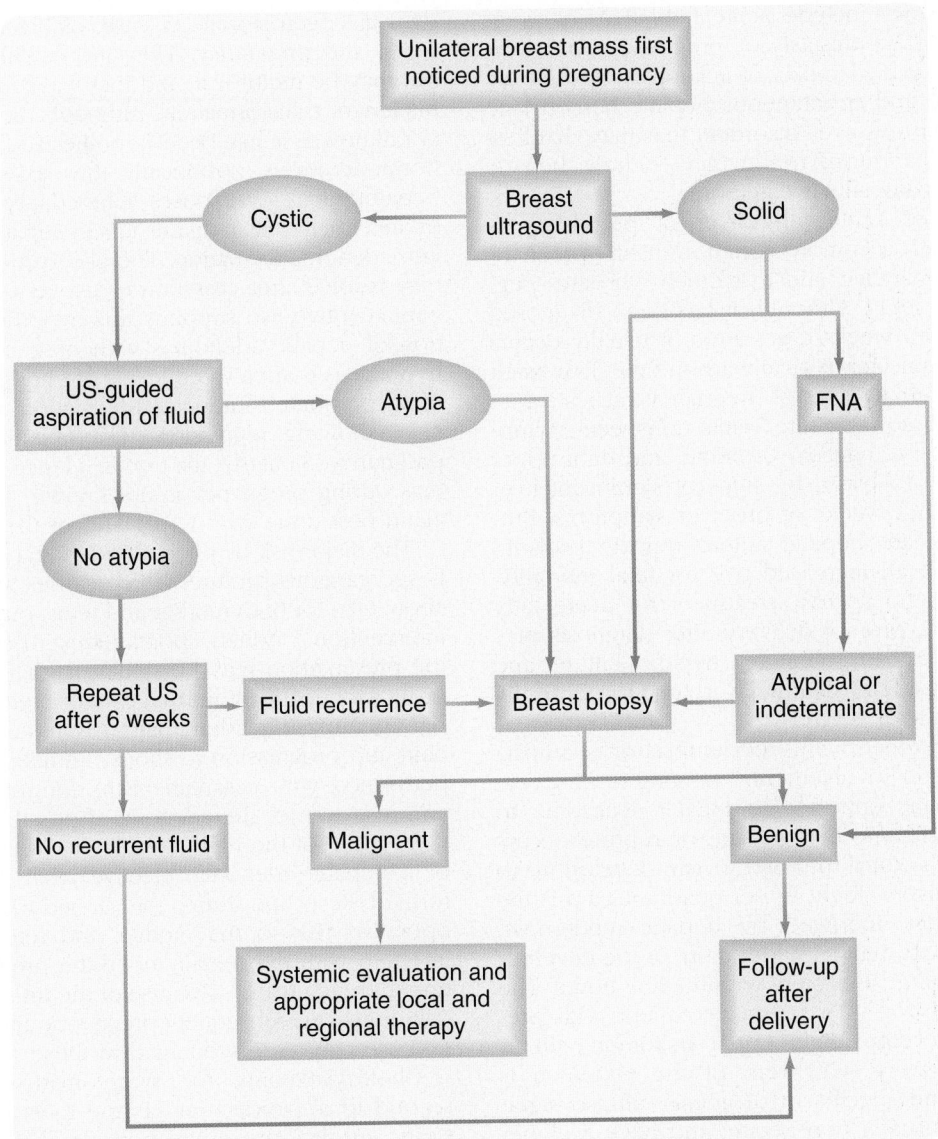

Figure 76-2 Algorithm for the management of a breast mass during pregnancy. US, ultrasound; FNA, fine-needle aspiration.

both dose and developmental stage. During the preimplantation stage and continuing to 15 weeks after conception, during organogenesis, the rapidly proliferating cells of the fetus are most sensitive to radiation, and exposure greater than 1 Gy during this period has a high likelihood of causing fetal death. The standard therapeutic course of 50 Gy results in a varying exposure to the fetus, depending on the gestational age and proximity of the gravid uterus to the radiation bed. Even with abdominal shielding, the greatest fetal exposure is due to scatter. Although there are several case reports of healthy infants born after maternal radiation exposure, radiation is not recommended during pregnancy because of the risks to the fetus.

Elective termination of the pregnancy to receive appropriate therapy without the risk for fetal malformation is no longer routinely recommended because no improvement in survival has been demonstrated.[18] With the treatment options available to the pregnant patient with breast cancer, a combined approach among the patient, surgeon, oncologist, and maternal-fetal medicine specialist ensures optimal treatment of the disease while minimizing risk to the patient and the fetus. A suggested algorithm for the management of breast masses in pregnancy is shown in Figure 76-2.

HEPATOBILIARY DISEASE IN PREGNANCY

Liver abnormalities during pregnancy can be classified as occurring exclusively during pregnancy as a direct result of conditions during pregnancy, occurring simultaneously but not exclusively during pregnancy, or developing before the pregnancy. Examples of liver disorders unique to pregnancy include acute fatty liver of pregnancy, intrahepatic cholestasis of pregnancy, and liver disease related to preeclampsia or eclampsia, specifically HELLP syndrome and spontaneous hepatic hemorrhage or rupture. Preexisting liver disorders that may manifest with complications during pregnancy include hepatic adenoma and hepatocellular carcinoma.

The etiology of acute fatty liver of pregnancy is unknown, although it is more common in first pregnancies, in twin pregnancies, and in women who are pregnant with a male fetus. Although it has been diagnosed as early as the 26th week of gestation, it usually occurs during the third trimester, typically around the 35th week of gestation. Acute fatty liver of pregnancy carries a 20% maternal and fetal mortality rate. Initial nonspecific symptoms such as malaise, nausea, vomiting, and right upper quadrant pain are followed by signs of significant liver dysfunction within 2 weeks of onset of symptoms. Progression to fulminant hepatic failure quickly leads to preterm labor and an increased risk for fetal mortality. Although there is no specific treatment for acute fatty liver of pregnancy, prompt delivery after diagnosis may prevent progression to fulminant hepatic failure and reduce the risk for fetal death. Liver function typically returns to normal after delivery.

About 10% of women with preeclampsia or eclampsia have associated liver involvement,[24] ranging from severe elevation of hepatic enzymes to HELLP syndrome to hepatic rupture. Hepatic hemorrhage or rupture occurs primarily during the third trimester or can develop up to 48 hours after delivery. Right upper quadrant pain is the initial manifestation, followed by hepatic tenderness, peritonitis, chest and right shoulder pain, or the development of hemodynamic instability within a few hours. The diagnosis is suspected in a pregnant patient with preeclampsia who develops right upper quadrant pain. A computed tomography (CT) scan of the abdomen is highly sensitive and specific in diagnosis; ultrasonography findings are usually nonspecific and have a higher incidence of false-negative studies. The diagnosis may also be made during cesarean section.[25] Management depends on suspicion of ongoing intraperitoneal hemorrhage or vascular instability. Hepatic hematomas without evidence of ongoing bleeding in hemodynamically stable patients may be managed nonoperatively with serial imaging and close monitoring, and these lesions typically heal without intervention. If there is evidence or suspicion of rupture, immediate intervention is required because maternal and fetal mortality rates from hepatic hemorrhage are 60% and 85%; respectively.[24] Immediate laparotomy with either abdominal packing or hepatic artery ligation reduces maternal and fetal mortality. Coagulopathy must be corrected aggressively. If the patient is relatively stable or abdominal packing has been unsuccessful in controlling hemorrhage, angiography with selective embolization may be performed. Angiography is most useful when the diagnosis is made postpartum.[25]

Hepatic adenomas are uncommon, benign lesions that are usually associated with oral contraceptive use in young women.[26] Hepatic adenomas are also associated with glycogen storage disease, diabetes, exogenous steroids, and pregnancy. They are usually solitary lesions but may be multifocal, and they have a low potential for malignant transformation. Although the specific etiology is unknown, it has been hypothesized that a change in hormone levels, specifically the sex steroids, leads to hepatotoxicity or exposes a hereditary defect in carbohydrate metabolism that results in hepatocyte hyperplasia and adenoma formation. The observation that adenomas may resolve after cessation of exogenous steroid or oral contraceptive use supports this hypothesis. The association of hepatic adenomas with pregnancy supports the hypothesis that elevated levels of endogenous hormones may contribute to adenoma formation, although no data exist showing regression of a hepatic adenoma after pregnancy. Similarly, the true incidence of hepatic adenomas during pregnancy is not known. Diagnosis is once again best done with CT or MRI of the liver.[27]

The major risk of a hepatic adenoma during pregnancy is spontaneous rupture, which carries a mortality rate of about 60% for both mother and fetus, even with operative intervention.[28] When spontaneous rupture does occur, the presentation may be similar to that described previously for hepatic hemorrhage associated with preeclampsia: right upper quadrant pain with referred right shoulder pain and progression to shock. Immediate laparotomy is performed with cesarean birth, control of hemorrhage, and resection of the adenoma if possible.

Because of the high mortality associated with rupture of a hepatic adenoma, elective resection may be performed. Resection during the second trimester minimizes operative risk to the mother and fetus and does not interfere with the remainder of the pregnancy or subsequent pregnancies.[26] Because of the unknown recurrence risk, however, subsequent pregnancy and oral contraceptive use may be discouraged in these patients.

Cholecystectomy for symptomatic cholelithiasis is second to appendectomy as the most common nonobstetric surgical procedure performed during pregnancy. As stated earlier, pregnancy is associated with an increased incidence of cholelithiasis. Most pregnant women are asymptomatic. Although an estimated 2% to 4% of pregnant women may be found to have gallstones by ultrasound, only 0.05% to 0.1% of those women will be symptomatic. The symptoms of biliary colic are the same in pregnant and nonpregnant patients. In patients with symptoms consistent with cholelithiasis, ultrasound is the diagnostic examination of choice. In pregnant patients, ultrasound is as accurate in identifying gallstones and signs of inflammation as it is in nonpregnant patients.

Historically, pregnant patients with a clear operative indication, such as obstructive jaundice, gallstone pancreatitis, and choledocholithiasis, underwent cholecystectomy regardless of gestational age. Patients with recurrent biliary colic or acute cholecystitis that responded to medical management were treated expectantly until after delivery, at which time they underwent cholecystectomy. As it has become understood that adverse maternal and fetal outcomes are related more to the disease process and not the surgical intervention, management patterns have changed.[29] Additionally, complications from nonoperative management of gallstone disease result in an increase in maternal and fetal mortality. With gallstone pancreatitis during pregnancy, a maternal mortality rate of 15% and a fetal mortality rate of 60% have been reported. In a study of 63 patients who were admitted with symptomatic cholelithiasis, surgical management reduced the need for labor induction, rate of preterm deliveries, and fetal mortality.[30] Therefore, surgical intervention is considered as primary management of gallstones in pregnancy.

The timing of cholecystectomy for biliary colic depends on the gestational age and the severity of symptoms. A spontaneous abortion rate of 12% with open cholecystectomy during the first trimester falls to 5.6% and 0% during the second and third trimesters, respectively. The risk for preterm labor is nearly 0% during the second trimester and 40% during the third trimester.[2] The optimum time for cholecystectomy is the second trimester, when the risks for spontaneous abortion and preterm labor are the lowest, unless the patient develops a complication of cholelithiasis.

Laparoscopic cholecystectomy is relatively safe during the second trimester. The gravid uterus is not usually large enough at this gestational age to interfere with visualization; the uterus also is less likely to be inadvertently instrumented at this size. The open technique using the Hasson trocar is recommended for obtaining access to the abdomen. If intraoperative cholangiography or endoscopic retrograde cholangiopancreatography is indicated for choledocholithiasis, the uterus needs to be protected with appropriate shielding. If the severity of symptoms prevents delaying surgical intervention until after delivery, laparoscopic cholecystectomy can be safely performed during the third trimester, although the risk for preterm labor is substantially increased. In several small series of patients, preterm labor was successfully managed with tocolytics, and the patients delivered healthy term infants.[31]

ENDOCRINE DISEASE IN PREGNANCY

Adrenal

Pheochromocytomas originate from chromaffin cells in the adrenal medulla or from extramedullary paraganglion cells. They are hormonally active tumors, secreting the catecholamines norepinephrine, epinephrine, and, less commonly, dopamine. Pheochromocytomas are usually described by the "rule of 10," which states that 10% of pheochromocytomas are extra-adrenal, 10% are bilateral, 10% are malignant, and 10% are familial. These tumors can occur sporadically or as part of a syndrome, such as multiple endocrine neoplasia (MEN) type 2A, MEN 2B, or von Hippel-Lindau disease.

Although pheochromocytomas are uncommon in pregnancy, they have devastating effects for both mother and fetus. Pheochromocytomas that remain undiagnosed during pregnancy have a postpartum maternal mortality as high as 55%, with fetal mortality also exceeding 50%. The greatest risk occurs from the onset of labor to 48

hours after delivery. The index of suspicion must be high in any patient with preeclampsia, paroxysmal hypertension, or unexplained fever after delivery. With diagnosis and appropriate treatment, the maternal mortality rate is reduced to nearly 0%, and the fetal mortality rate is decreased to 15%.[32] Diagnosis is made by elevated urine catecholamines; urinary catecholamines in the pregnant patient without a pheochromocytoma are the same as in the nonpregnant patient. Lack of proteinuria also helps eliminate preeclampsia as a cause of hypertension. Metaiodobenzylguanidine (MIBG) imaging is not recommended during pregnancy because the small molecule may cross the placenta; use of MIBG imaging has not been evaluated in pregnancy.

Surgical resection needs to be performed before 20 weeks' gestation, when spontaneous abortion is less likely and the size of the gravid uterus does not interfere with the procedure. If the diagnosis is made late in the second trimester or during the third trimester, medical management followed by combined cesarean birth and resection of the pheochromocytoma may be an option. It is unknown if the standard preoperative management with α-blockade or calcium-channel blockade followed by perioperative β-blockade in nonpregnant patients is safe during pregnancy. The long-term effects of the α-blocker phenoxybenzamine on the fetus have not been determined, although calcium channel blockers are safe to use during pregnancy. β-Blockers are frequently used during pregnancy with close monitoring for intrauterine growth retardation. Consultation with a maternal-fetal medicine specialist is essential to determine the preoperative management that will ensure the optimal postoperative result for the patient and fetus. In nonpregnant patients, the method of approach depends on suspected malignancy, unilateral versus bilateral tumors, extra-adrenal location, size of the tumor, and surgeon's preference and experience. In all series comparing the different approaches, including open versus laparoscopic technique, pregnant patients were not included. In a small series, two pregnant patients who underwent transperitoneal laparoscopic adrenalectomy delivered healthy infants at term.[33]

Thyroid

Thyroid diseases during pregnancy can be categorized into three groups: hypothyroidism, hyperthyroidism, and thyroid cancer. Hypothyroidism is found in 2.5% of pregnancies. Of these, only 20% to 30% of patients develop symptoms. The first step is to obtain a serum thyroid-stimulating hormone (TSH) concentration. This will help categorize primary hypothyroidism versus hypothyroidism resulting from pituitary or hypothalamic causes.

Current guidelines from Lebeau and Mandel for treatment of hypothyroidism during pregnancy are as follows (see Selected References):

1. Check serum TSH.
2. Initial levothyroxine dosage is based on severity of symptoms. Levothyroxine is started at 2 μg/kg/day. If TSH is less than 10 mU/L, dose is adjusted to 0.1 mg/day.

3. For previously diagnosed hypothyroidism, monitor TSH every 3 to 4 weeks.
4. Goal TSH level is less than 2.5 mU/L.
5. Monitor serum TSH and total every 3 to 4 weeks with each dose change.

Hyperthyroidism during pregnancy has an incidence of 0.1% to 0.4%.[34] Gestational thyrotoxicosis is a multifactorial phenomenon. High serum concentrations of human chorionic gonadotropin (HCG) during pregnancy activate the TSH receptors. Elevated serum-free T_4 and low-serum TSH levels are seen with this form of thyrotoxicosis. Gestational thyrotoxicosis is usually self-limited and spontaneously resolves by 20 weeks' gestation, when the HCG level declines. Repeat evaluation is warranted if thyrotoxicosis persists. Most cases of hyperthyroidism are a result of Graves' disease. After the diagnosis is made, medical treatment with thionamides (propylthiouracil and methimazole) is the mainstay of treatment. Iodides are avoided, except in patients preparing for thyroidectomy during pregnancy. Subtotal thyroidectomy for Graves' disease is reserved for patients who are taking high-dose propylthiouracil (>600 mg/day) or methimazole (>40 mg/day), are allergic to thionamides, are noncompliant, or have compressive symptoms because of goiter size. Surgery is performed during the second trimester before 24 weeks' gestation to minimize the risk for miscarriage. A 2-week course of a β-adrenergic agent, along with potassium iodide, is implemented before surgery to minimize perioperative complications. Radioactive iodine therapy is contraindicated during pregnancy.

Because of hormonal changes, thyroid nodules may have a higher prevalence during pregnancy, but thyroid cancers do not. Thyroid cancers are worked up in the traditional fashion during pregnancy. Fine-needle aspiration, along with ultrasonic evaluation, remains the cornerstone of diagnosis. If cytology shows thyroid cancer, surgery is recommended during the second trimester, before 24 weeks' gestation. If thyroid cancer is found after the second half of pregnancy, surgery can be performed after delivery. Postoperative radioactive iodine therapy also needs to be delayed until after delivery.

SMALL BOWEL DISEASE IN PREGNANCY

Intestinal obstruction is the third most common nonobstetric surgical issue in pregnancy, after acute appendicitis and acute cholecystitis. The incidence of small bowel obstruction during pregnancy has been reported to be between 1 in 1500 to 17,000 pregnancies.[35] Small bowel obstructions usually occur during the second and third trimesters. Adhesions resulting from prior abdominal and pelvic surgeries are the most frequent causes for intestinal obstruction in pregnancy, accounting for 53% to 59% of cases. Other causes of small bowel obstruction in the pregnant patient include volvulus, intussusception, malignancy, or hernia, although the displacement of the small bowel out of the pelvis by the enlarging uterus makes this a rare cause.

The symptoms of an obstruction are identical to those in the nonpregnant patient and consist of the triad of abdominal pain, vomiting, and obstipation. Pain, present in 85% to 98% of cases, is usually colicky in nature and located in the midabdomen, although the character and duration are highly variable. Nausea and vomiting are seen in 80% of pregnant patients with small bowel obstruction; however, nausea and vomiting are not uncommon during the first trimester of normal pregnancy. Nausea and vomiting that persist or begin later in pregnancy should arouse suspicion and be evaluated. Bowel distention may be marked but difficult to assess because of the gravid uterus. Diagnosis is made by serial examination and plain abdominal radiograph.

Treatment for small bowel obstruction in pregnancy is identical to that in the nonpregnant patient. Therapy consists of nasogastric decompression and IV fluids. However, a lower threshold for operative management is necessary. If, after 6 to 8 hours of nonoperative treatment, there is no satisfactory patient response, a laparotomy is performed before perforation or bowel necrosis occurs. Maternal mortality ranges from 6% to 20% due to sepsis and multisystem organ failure, and fetal loss is as high as 26% to 50%.[35] To avoid the risk to the mother and fetus, a more aggressive approach is used.

Midgut volvulus remains a dreaded diagnosis during the postpartum period. Midgut volvulus is usually more common in the pregnant patient if she has undergone previous abdominal surgery; however, spontaneous midgut volvulus may occur. A case report of maternal death caused by midgut volvulus after bariatric surgery has been reported.[36] The key is increased vigilance for all the parties involved in the patient's care. Early exploration is warranted if the diagnosis is unclear.

COLON AND RECTAL DISEASE IN PREGNANCY

Acute appendicitis is the most common nonobstetric surgical problem in the pregnant patient, occurring in 1 in 1500 pregnancies. The incidence of acute appendicitis is fairly evenly distributed among the trimesters of pregnancy, with a slight predominance during the second trimester. Timely and accurate diagnosis is challenging because the typical clinical findings of nausea, vomiting, abdominal pain, and mild leukocytosis may be findings in a normal pregnancy. Delay in diagnosis results in an increased perforation rate of 10%. This has significant consequences for the patient and fetus. Fetal mortality increases from 1.5% in acute appendicitis to 35% in perforated appendicitis.[37] Preterm labor and premature delivery rates are as high as 40% in perforated appendicitis,[37-39] compared with a 13% rate of preterm labor and 4% rate of premature delivery in acute appendicitis.[40]

In 1932, Baer studied 78 normal pregnant women with radiographic studies at regular intervals from the second month of pregnancy to 10 days postpartum. As the uterus enlarges, the appendix is driven upward with a counterclockwise rotation. Baer concluded that early in pregnancy, pain is low, and that as the gestation progresses, pain is located higher in the abdomen.[41] A review of 45 pregnant patients with acute appendicitis demonstrated that pain in the right lower quadrant is the most common symptom, regardless of gestational age (first trimester, 86%; second trimester, 83%; third trimester, 85%).[40] Despite the inconsistency, acute appendicitis needs to be included in the differential diagnosis of every pregnant woman who presents with right-sided abdominal pain. Treatment of suspected acute appendicitis in the pregnant patient is emergent appendectomy. Although helical CT scans have demonstrated higher than 90% sensitivity and specificity in the diagnosis of acute appendicitis, few data are available in pregnant patients. In nonpregnant patients, a 10% to 15% negative laparotomy rate is considered acceptable. Because of the increased risk to both mother and fetus with appendiceal perforation, a negative rate of 30% to 33% is acceptable. The debate is then for open or laparoscopic technique. The argument for open appendectomy is that the laparoscopic approach exposes the fetus to the risks for pneumoperitoneum and trocar placement without the benefit of a significantly smaller incision. The laparoscopic technique enables examination of a larger portion of the abdomen with less uterine manipulation and allows location of the appendix as it is pushed into the right upper quadrant by the enlarging uterus.

Colonic pseudo-obstruction, or Ogilvie's syndrome, is a functional obstruction, or adynamic ileus, without a mechanical etiology. Ten percent of all cases of Ogilvie's syndrome occur in postpartum patients. It is characterized by massive abdominal distention with cecal dilation. Although neostigmine is an effective first-line therapy in nonpregnant patients, its safety in pregnancy is unknown. It can be used safely in the postpartum period. Colonoscopic decompression has been described in postpartum patients, with laparotomy indicated only in suspected perforation.

VASCULAR DISEASE IN PREGNANCY

Of more than 400 cases of ruptured splenic artery aneurysms in the literature, about 100 cases of ruptured splenic artery aneurysm during pregnancy have been reported, with only 12 cases of maternal and fetal survival.[42] Rupture occurred during the third trimester in two thirds of the cases and was typically misdiagnosed as splenic rupture or uterine rupture. The maternal mortality rate was 75%, with a fetal mortality rate of 95%. Increased portal pressures, high splenic artery flow due to distal aortic compression, and progressive arterial wall weakening are contributing factors. Multiparity may increase the risk; 78% of patients with ruptured splenic artery aneurysms have been in their third pregnancy. Survival is most likely related to a "two-stage rupture," in which the lesser sac temporarily tamponades the bleeding aneurysm.

When treated electively in nonpregnant patients, the mortality rate is only 0.5% to 1.3%. When the diagnosis is made in a woman of childbearing age or in a pregnant patient, a splenic artery aneurysm of 2 cm or larger is treated electively because of the increased risk for rupture during pregnancy.[42]

Acute iliofemoral venous thrombosis is six times more frequent among pregnant than nonpregnant patients. Pregnancy may increase the risk for thrombosis through a number of factors, including mechanical obstruction of venous drainage by the enlarging uterus, decreased activity in late pregnancy and at time of delivery, intimal injury from vascular distention or surgical manipulation during cesarean section, and abnormal levels of coagulation factors already described.[43] Additionally, a wide spectrum of pathologic abnormalities such as the presence of lupus anticoagulant antibodies and deficiencies of proteins C and S may further increase the risk for thrombotic disease. Protein S serves as a cofactor for activated protein C, which has anticoagulant activity. Therefore, a deficiency of protein S leads to spontaneous, recurrent thromboembolic complications in nonpregnant adults. Even in normal individuals, protein S levels are substantially reduced during pregnancy.

The management of acute iliofemoral venous thrombosis during pregnancy is controversial because thrombolytic therapy poses hazards to the fetus. The risk for pulmonary thromboembolism with manipulation of the clot during thrombectomy would have catastrophic effects on both the patient and the fetus. Techniques that have been described include interruption of the inferior vena cava through a right retroperitoneal approach or interruption of the inferior vena cava passage of a Fogarty catheter through the unaffected contralateral femoral vein. The disadvantage of the retroperitoneal approach is that an extensive dissection is required. The disadvantages of the Fogarty catheter are that the catheter may still dislodge clots that have extended into the vena cava and that once the catheter is removed, an inferior vena cava filter must still be placed. However, the most effective technique is filter placement in the inferior vena cava through the internal jugular vein using ultrasound guidance, followed by thrombectomy.

TRAUMA IN PREGNANCY

Trauma is the leading nonobstetric cause of maternal mortality and occurs in about 5% of pregnancies.[44] The most common mechanisms of injury are from falls or from motor vehicle crashes.[45] When compared with age-matched pregnant controls, pregnant women who sustained trauma had a higher incidence of spontaneous abortion, preterm labor, fetomaternal hemorrhage, abruptio placentae, and uterine rupture.[46] Multiple studies have attempted to identify risk factors that predict morbidity and mortality in the pregnant trauma patient. The maternal Injury Severity Score, mechanism of injury, and physical findings are unable to adequately predict adverse outcomes such as abruptio placentae and fetal loss. Pregnant patients with severe head, abdominal, thoracic, or lower extremity injuries are at high risk for pregnancy loss.[47] Early involvement of an available obstetrician is important to evaluate both maternal and fetal well-being.

In the management of the pregnant trauma patient, the critical point is that resuscitation of the fetus is accomplished by resuscitation of the mother. Therefore, the initial evaluation and treatment of the pregnant injured patient is identical to that of the nonpregnant injured patient. Rapid assessment of the maternal airway, breathing, and circulation, as well as ensuring an adequate airway, avoids maternal and fetal hypoxia. In the later stages of pregnancy, as already described, uterine compression of the vena cava may result in hypotension from diminished venous return, thus the pregnant trauma patient needs to be placed in a left lateral decubitus position. If spinal cord injury is suspected, the patient may be secured to a backboard and then tilted to the left.

The increased blood volume associated with pregnancy has important implications in the trauma patient. Signs of blood loss such as tachycardia and hypotension may be delayed until the patient loses nearly 30% of her blood volume. As a result, the fetus may be experiencing hypoperfusion long before the mother manifests any signs. Early and rapid fluid resuscitation is administered even in the pregnant patient who is normotensive.

As with the primary survey, the secondary survey proceeds in a fashion similar to that in the nonpregnant patient. Special attention is given to the abdominal examination. The uterus remains protected by the pelvis until about 12 weeks' gestation and is relatively well sheltered from the abdominal injury until that time. As the uterus grows, it becomes more prominent and more vulnerable to injury. Measurement of fundal height provides a rapid approximation of gestational age. At 20 weeks' gestation, it is at the level of the umbilicus and is about 1 cm per week of gestation. Intrauterine hemorrhage or uterine rupture may result in a discrepancy in measurement. A pelvic examination is performed, by an obstetrician if possible, to evaluate for vaginal bleeding, ruptured membranes, or a bulging perineum. Vaginal bleeding may indicate abruptio placentae, placenta previa, or preterm labor. Rupture of the amniotic fluid may result in umbilical cord prolapse, which compresses the umbilical vessels and compromises fetal blood flow. This requires immediate cesarean birth. If cloudy white or greenish fluid is seen from the cervical os or perineum, the presence of amniotic fluid is confirmed by Nitrazine paper, which changes from green to blue.

The Kleihauer-Betke (K-B) test for the assessment of fetomaternal transfusion is useful after maternal trauma and is ordered with the initial laboratory studies that include a type and crossmatch. Because of the sensitivity of the K-B test, a small amount of fetomaternal transfusion may be undetected. Therefore, all Rh-negative pregnant trauma patients are considered for Rh immunoglobulin (RhoGAM) therapy.

The most common cause of fetal death after blunt injury is abruptio placentae. Deceleration of the fetal heart rate may be the earliest sign of abruption. The uterus needs to be evaluated for contractions, rupture, and abruptio placentae. Early initiation of cardiotocographic fetal monitoring adequately warns of deterioration in the condition of the fetus.

SUMMARY

Pregnant patients are susceptible to the same surgical diseases as nonpregnant patients of similar age. Maternal physiologic changes, as well as the enlarging uterus, may result in atypical presentation of surgical disease, or symptoms may be attributed to normal pregnancy. A delay in diagnosis and treatment of surgical illnesses in pregnancy poses a greater risk to maternal and fetal well-being than the risks of anesthesia or of surgical intervention. Early consultation with an obstetrician, maternal-fetal medicine specialist, and perinatologist can ensure optimal outcomes and avoid pitfalls. Laparoscopy is becoming increasingly accepted in the pregnant patient, and future advances should make it even safer for obstetric patients. Preterm labor prevention needs to be individualized given the patient's gestational age and underlying disease process.

Selected References

Babler EA: Perforative appendicitis complicating pregnancy. JAMA 51:1310, 1908.

Landmark article first describing appendicitis in pregnancy.

Baer JL: Appendicitis in pregnancy. JAMA 98:1359, 1932.

Landmark article illustrating the change in appendiceal location during pregnancy.

Brodsky JB, Cohen EN, Brown BW Jr, et al: Surgery during pregnancy and fetal outcome. Am J Obstet Gynecol 138:1165, 1980.

Large series that first looked at fetal outcomes in nonobstetric surgery.

Cohen-Kerem R, Railton C, Oren D, et al: Pregnancy outcome following non-obstetric surgical intervention. Am J Surg 190:3, 2005.

Large series that looked at nonobstetric surgical pregnancy outcomes in 12,452 patients reported in 44 papers. Maternal death rate was .006%. Miscarriage rate was 5.8%.

LeBeau SO, Mandel SJ: Thyroid disorders during pregnancy. Endocrinol Metab Clin N Am 35:117, 2006.

Comprehensive review of all the major thyroid abnormalities that occur during pregnancy.

Mourad J, Elliott JP, Erickson L, et al: Appendicitis in pregnancy: New information that contradicts longheld clinical beliefs. Am J Obstet Gynecol 182:1027, 2000.

This paper, which retrospectively reviewed more than 66,000 deliveries and found 45 pregnant patients with appendicitis, challenged the original landmark paper by Baer regarding the presentation of acute appendicitis in pregnant patients.

Society of American Gastrointestinal Endoscopic Surgeons: Guidelines for laparoscopic surgery during pregnancy. Surg Endosc 12:189, 1998.

Current guidelines for laparoscopy in pregnancy.

Tarraza HM, Moore RD: Gynecologic causes of the acute abdomen and the acute abdomen in pregnancy. Surg Clin North Am 77:1371, 1997.

Current review that accurately describes the increased risk to the mother and fetus due to the underlying pathology as opposed to the risk imposed by surgical intervention.

Woo JC, Yu T, Hurd TC: Breast cancer in pregnancy. Arch Surg 138:91, 2003.

The most current comprehensive review of breast cancer in pregnancy, including the ongoing trends in treatment.

References

1. Chesnutt AN: Physiology of normal pregnancy. Crit Care Clin 20:609-615, 2004.
2. Melnick DM, Wahl WL, Dalton VK: Management of general surgery problems in the pregnant patient. Am J Surg 187:170-180, 2004.
3. Kal HB, Struikmans H: Radiotherapy during pregnancy: Fact or fiction. Lancet Oncol 6:328-333, 2005.
4. Harrison BP, Crystal CS: Imaging modalities in obstetrics and gynecology. Emerg Med Clin N Am 21:711-735, 2003.
5. Ni Mhuireachtaigh R, O'Gorman DA: Anesthesia in pregnant patients for nonobstetric surgery. J Clin Anesth 18:60-66, 2006.
6. Schecter WP, Farmer D, Horn JK, Peitrocola DM: Special considerations in perioperative pain management: Audio-visual distraction, geriatrics, pediatrics, and pregnancy. J Am Coll Surg 201:612-618, 2005.
7. Cappell MS, Friedel D: Abdominal pain during pregnancy. Gastroenterol Clin North Am 32:1-58, 2003.
8. Shay DC, Bhavani-Shankar K, Datta S: Laparoscopic surgery during pregnancy. Anesth Clin North Am 19:1, 2003.
9. Stepp K, Falcone T: Laparoscopy in the second trimester of pregnancy. Obstet Gynecol Clin North Am 31:485-496, 2004.
10. Hunter JG, Swanstrom L, Thornburg K: Carbon dioxide pneumoperitoneum induces fetal acidosis in a pregnant ewe model. Surg Endosc 9:272, 1995.
11. Curet MJ: Special problems in laparoscopic surgery: Previous abdominal surgery, obesity, and pregnancy: Surg Clin North Am 80:1093, 2000.
12. Society of American Gastrointestinal Endoscopic Surgeons: Guidelines for laparoscopic surgery during pregnancy. Surg Endosc 12:189, 1998.
13. Uen Y, Liang A, Lee H: Randomized comparison of conventional carbon dioxide insufflation and abdominal wall lifting for laparoscopic cholecystectomy. J Laparoendosc Surg 12:7, 2002.
14. Keleher AJ, Theriault RL, Gwyn KM, et al: Multidisciplinary management of breast cancer concurrent with pregnancy. J Am Coll Surg 194:54-64, 2002.
15. Falkenberry SS: Breast cancer in pregnancy. Obstet Gynecol Clin North Am 29:225, 2002.
16. Johannsson O, Loman N, Borg A, Olsson H.: Pregnancy-associated breast cancer in BRCA1 and BRCA2 germ-line mutation carriers. Lancet 352:1359, 1998.
17. Ishida T, Yokoe T, Kasumi F, et al: Clinicopathological characteristics and prognosis of breast cancer patients associated with pregnancy and lactation: Analysis of case-control study in Japan. Jpn J Cancer Res 83:1143, 1992.
18. Woo JC, Yu T, Hurd TC: Breast cancer in pregnancy. Arch Surg 138:91, 2003.
19. Gemignani ML, Petrek JA, Borgen PI, et al: Breast cancer and pregnancy. Surg Clin North Am 79:1157, 1999.
20. Leslie KK, Lange CA: Breast cancer and pregnancy. Obstet Gynecol Clin North Am 32:547-558, 2005.
21. Gupta R, McHutchinson A, Dowle C, et al: Fine-needle aspiration cytodiagnosis of breast masses in pregnant and lactating women and its impact on management. Diagn Cytopathol 9:156, 1993.
22. Bonnier P, Romain S, Dilhuydy J, et al: Influence of pregnancy on the outcome of breast cancer: A case-control study. Int J Cancer 72:720, 1997.
23. Berry D, Theriault R, Holmes F, et al: Management of breast cancer during pregnancy using a standardized protocol. J Clin Oncol 17:855, 1999.
24. Doshi S, Zucker SD: Liver emergency during pregnancy. Gastroenterol Clin North Am 32:1213-1227, 2003.
25. Wicke C, Pereira PL, Neeser E, et al: Subcapsular liver hematoma in HELLP syndrome: Evaluation of diagnostic and therapeutic options—a unicenter study. Am J Obstet Gynecol 190:160-112, 2004.
26. Cobey FC, Salem RR: A review of liver masses in pregnancy and a proposed algorithm for their diagnosis and management. Am J Surg 187:181-191, 2004.
27. Guntupalli SR: Hepatic disease in pregnancy: An overview and of diagnosis and management. Crit Care Med 33:S332-339, 2005,
28. Rosel HD, Baier A, Mesewinkel F: Exsanguination caused by liver cell adenoma and rupture of the hepatic capsule as cause of maternal death. Zentralbl Gynakol 112:1363, 1990.
29. Kahaleh M, Hartwell G, Arseneau K, et al: Safety and efficacy of ERCP in pregnancy. Gastrointest Endosc 60:287-292, 2004.
30. Lu EJ, Curet MJ, El-Sayed YY, Kirkwood KS: Medical versus surgical management of biliary tract disease in pregnancy. Am J Surg 188:755-759, 2004.
31. Eichenberg BJ, Vanderlinden J, Miguel C, et al: Laparoscopic cholecystectomy in the third trimester of pregnancy. Am Surg 62:874, 1996.
32. Janetschek G, Finkenstedt G, Gasser R, et al: Laparoscopic surgery for pheochromocytoma: Adrenalectomy, partial resection, excision of paragangliomas. J Urol 160:330, 1998.
33. Janetschek G, Neumann HPH: Laparoscopic surgery for pheochromocytoma. Urol Clin North Am 28:1, 2001.
34. Mandel SJ: Thyroid disease and pregnancy. In: Copper DS (ed): Medical Management of Thyroid Disease. New York, Marcel Dekker, 2001, pp 38-418.
35. Malangoni MA: Gastrointestinal surgery and pregnancy. Gastroenterol Clin North Am 32:181-200, 2003.
36. Loar PV, Sanchez-Ramos L, Kaunitz AM: Maternal death caused by midgut volvulus after bariatric surgery. Am J Obstet Gynecol 191:1748-1749, 2005.
37. Rollins MD, Chan KJ, Price RR: Laparoscopy for appendicitis and cholelithiasis during pregnancy. Surg Endosc 18:237-241, 2004.
38. Challoner K, Incerpi M: Nontraumatic abdominal surgical emergencies in the pregnant patient. Emerg Med Clin North Am 21:4 971-985, 2003.
39. Wu JM: Laparoscopic appendectomy in pregnancy. J Laparoendosc Adv Surg Tech A 15:447-450, 2005.
40. Mourad J, Elliott JP, Erickson L, et al: Appendicitis in pregnancy: New information that contradicts long-held clinical beliefs. Am J Obstet Gynecol 182:1027, 2000.
41. Baer JL: Appendicitis in pregnancy. JAMA 98:1359, 1932.
42. Herbeck M, Horbach T, Putzenlechner C, et al: Ruptured splenic artery aneurysm during pregnancy: A rare case with both maternal and fetal survival. Am J Obstet Gynecol 181:763, 1999.
43. Neri E, Civeli L, Benvenuti A, et al: Protected iliofemoral venous thrombectomy in a pregnant woman with

pulmonary embolism and ischemic venous thrombosis. Tex Heart Inst J 29:130, 2002.

44. Mattox KL, Goetzl L: Trauma in pregnancy. Crit Care Med 20:3310, 2005.

45. Schiff MA, Holt VL, Daling JR: Maternal and infant outcomes after injury during pregnancy in Washington State from 1989 to 1997. J Trauma 53:939, 2002.

46. Pak LL, Reece EA, Chan L: Is adverse pregnancy outcome predictable after blunt abdominal trauma? Am J Obstet Gynecol 179:1140, 1998.

47. Ikossi DG, Lazar AA, Morabito D: Profile of mothers at risk: An analysis of injury and pregnancy loss in 2295 trauma patients. J Am Coll Surg 9:16, 2004.

Urologic Surgery

Aria F. Olumi, MD   and   Jerome P. Richie, MD

The field of urology has undergone unprecedented advances during the past decade. Advances in treatment of erectile dysfunction, laparoscopic and minimally invasive surgery, and reconstructive urology are some of the highlights. This chapter focuses on general urologic issues with special emphasis on issues pertinent to the general surgeon. It reviews anatomy of the genitourinary system, urologic trauma, emergent urologic conditions, nephrolithiasis, neurogenic bladder, benign prostatic hyperplasia, scrotal masses, and urologic malignancies.

ANATOMY

Retroperitoneum

The retroperitoneum is bounded anteriorly by the peritoneal sac and its contents (Fig. 77-1), is separated from the thorax superiorly by the muscular diaphragm, and is contiguous with the extraperitoneal portions of the pelvis inferiorly. The body wall creates the posterior and lateral limits of the retroperitoneum, and incisions through the posterolateral abdominal wall, or flank, provide the most direct routes to the structures of the retroperitoneum.

Adrenal Glands

The adrenal, or suprarenal, glands are paired, yellow-orange, solid endocrine organs that lie within the perirenal (Gerota's) fascia superomedial to either kidney, buried within the perinephric fat. Although closely applied to the upper poles of the kidneys, the adrenals are embryologically and functionally distinct and are physically separated from the kidneys by connective tissue septa in continuity with Gerota's fascia as well as by varying amounts of perinephric adipose tissue. Thus, in cases of renal ectopia, the adrenal is usually found in approximately its normal anatomic position and does not follow the kidney. Similarly, in cases of renal agenesis, the adrenal on the involved side is typically present (in >90% of such cases).

The normal adult adrenal gland weighs about 5 g and measures 3 to 5 cm in its greatest transverse dimension. In the neonate, the adrenals are relatively much larger in size compared with total body mass and may be one third the size of the kidney at birth (Fig. 77-2). Both adrenals are somewhat flattened in the anteroposterior axis, the left more so than the right. The right gland assumes a more pyramidal shape and rests more superior to the upper pole of the right kidney. The left gland has a more crescentic shape and rests more medial to the upper pole of the left kidney; in fact, it may lie directly atop the renal vessels at the left renal hilum. The right adrenal thus tends to lie more superiorly in the retroperitoneum than does the left adrenal. This is in contradistinction to the fact that the right kidney lies, in general, slightly more inferiorly than the left, and this fact must be taken into account in the planning of incisions for adrenal surgery.

Each adrenal is a composite of two separate and functionally distinct glandular elements: cortex and medulla. The medulla, which forms the central core of each adrenal, consists of chromaffin cells derived from the neural crest and is intimately related to the sympathetic nervous system. The cells of the medulla produce neuro-active catecholamines, primarily epinephrine and nor-epinephrine, which are released directly into the blood stream through an extensive venous drainage system. The adrenal cortex is mesodermally derived, completely surrounds and encases the medulla, and forms the bulk of the adrenal gland—80% to 90% by weight. Three cell layers can be identified in the cortex. The outermost layer is the zona glomerulosa, which produces aldosterone in response to stimulation by the renin-angiotensin system. Centripetally located are the zona fasciculata and zona reticularis, which produce glucocorticoids and sex steroids, respectively. Unlike the zona glomerulosa, these latter functions are regulated by pituitary release of adrenocorticotropic hormone (ACTH). The substance of the adrenal gland is inherently quite friable but is enclosed by a thick, collagenous capsule; yet it still can be readily torn with aggressive handling at time of operation.

The adrenals, concordant with their key role in the body's hormonal milieu, are highly vascularized. The arterial supply is relatively symmetrical bilaterally. Multiple small arteries supply each adrenal gland. These are branch vessels, which can be traced to three major arterial sources for each gland:

1. Superior branches from the inferior phrenic artery
2. Middle branches directly from the aorta
3. Inferior branches from the ipsilateral renal artery

In contrast to the multiple arteries, usually a single large adrenal vein exits each gland from its hilum anteromedially. On the right side, this vein is very short and enters directly into the inferior vena cava (IVC) on its posterolateral aspect. The adrenal vein on the left is more elongated and is typically joined by the left inferior phrenic vein before entering the superior aspect of the left renal vein. The adrenal lymphatics in general exit the glands along the course of the venous drainage and eventually empty into para-aortic lymph nodes.

The adrenal medulla receives greater autonomic innervation than any other organ in the body. Multiple preganglionic sympathetic fibers enter each adrenal along the course of the adrenal vein and synapse with chromaffin cells in the medulla. This rich sympathetic innervation of the medulla reaches the adrenal through the splanchnic nerves and celiac ganglion. In contrast, the adrenal cortex is believed to receive no innervation.

Kidneys and Ureters

The kidneys are paired solid organs that lie in the retroperitoneum along the borders of the psoas muscle (see Fig. 77-1). The kidneys and associated adrenal glands are surrounded by perirenal fat, which is enclosed in perinephric fascia, known as *Gerota's fascia.* The Gerota's fascia forms an important anatomic barrier around the kidney and tends to contain pathologic process originating from the kidney. Superiorly, Gerota's fascia fuses and tapers to disappear over the inferior diaphragmatic surface. Medially, Gerota's fascia extends across the midline and is contiguous with Gerota's fascia on the contralateral side, although the anterior and posterior leaves are generally fused and inseparable as they cross the great vessels. Inferiorly, Gerota's fascia remains an open potential space, containing the ureter and gonadal vessels on either side.

Each kidney is positioned obliquely, and awareness of the anatomic relationship of the kidneys to the surrounding organs is paramount. The posterior relations of the kidneys to the abdominal wall musculature are relatively symmetrical (Fig. 77-3). The 12th rib crosses the upper third of each kidney. Because the left kidney lies more cephalad than the right kidney, the 11th rib lies directly posterior to the upper aspect of the left kidney

Figure 77-1 A and **B,** The retroperitoneum dissected. The anterior perirenal fascia (Gerota's fascia) has been dissected. 1, diaphragm; 2, inferior vena cava; 3, right adrenal gland; 4, upper pointer at celiac artery, lower pointer at celiac autonomic nervous plexus; 5, right kidney; 6, right renal vein; 7, Gerota's fascia; 8, pararenal retroperitoneal fat; 9, perinephric fat; 10, upper pointer at right gonadal vein, lower pointer at right gonadal artery; 11, lumbar lymph node; 12, retroperitoneal fat; 13, right common iliac artery; 14, right ureter; 15, sigmoid colon (cut); 16, esophagus (cut); 17, right crus of diaphragm; 18, left inferior phrenic artery; 19, upper pointer at left adrenal gland, lower pointer at left adrenal vein; 20, upper pointer at superior mesenteric artery, lower pointer at left renal artery; 21, left kidney; 22, upper pointer at left renal vein, lower pointer at left gonadal vein; 23, aorta; 24, perinephric fat; 25, aortic autonomic nervous plexus; 26, upper pointer at Gerota's fascia, lower pointer at inferior mesenteric ganglion; 27, inferior mesenteric artery; 28, aortic bifurcation into common iliac arteries; 29, left gonadal artery and vein; 30, left ureter; 31, psoas major muscle covered by psoas sheath; 32, cut edge of peritoneum; 33, pelvic cavity. **C** and **D,** The retroperitoneum dissected. Kidneys and adrenal glands have been sectioned and the inferior vena cava has been excised over most of its intra-abdominal course. 1, inferior vena cava (cut); 2, diaphragm; 3, right inferior phrenic artery; 4, right adrenal gland; 5, upper pointer at celiac artery, lower pointer at superior mesenteric artery; 6, right kidney; 7, upper pointer at right renal artery, lower pointer at right renal vein (cut); 8, lumbar lymph node; 9, transversus abdominis muscle covered with transversalis fascia; 10, right ureter; 11, anterior spinous ligament; 12, inferior vena cava (cut); 13, right common iliac artery; 14, right ureter; 15, right external iliac artery; 16, esophagus (cut); 17, left adrenal gland; 18, celiac ganglion; 19, left kidney; 20, upper pointer at left renal artery, lower pointer at left renal vein (cut); 21, left renal pelvis; 22, aorta; 23, aortic autonomic nervous plexus; 24, inferior mesenteric ganglion; 25, left ureter; 26, inferior mesenteric artery; 27, psoas major muscle covered by psoas sheath. (From Kabalin J: Surgical anatomy of the retroperitoneum, kidneys, and ureters. In Walsh PC, Retik AB, Vaughan ED Jr, et al [eds]: Campbell's Urology, 8th ed. Philadelphia, Elsevier, 2002, pp 4-7.)

and not the right kidney (see Fig. 77-3). As a result of the contour of the psoas muscle, both kidneys lie obliquely with the upper pole more medially located than the lower pole. In addition, each kidney does not lie in a simple coronal plain, and the lower pole is pushed more anteriorly than the upper pole of each kidney.

In contrast to the similarities of posterior anatomic relations in each kidney, the anterior relation of each kidney is significantly different. The right kidney lies behind the liver, and it is separated from the liver by reflection of the peritoneum, except for a small area of its upper pole, which comes into direct contact with the liver's retroperitoneal bare spot. The extension of parietal peritoneum that bridges between the perirenal fascia covering the upper pole of the right kidney and the posterior aspect of the liver is called the *hepatorenal*

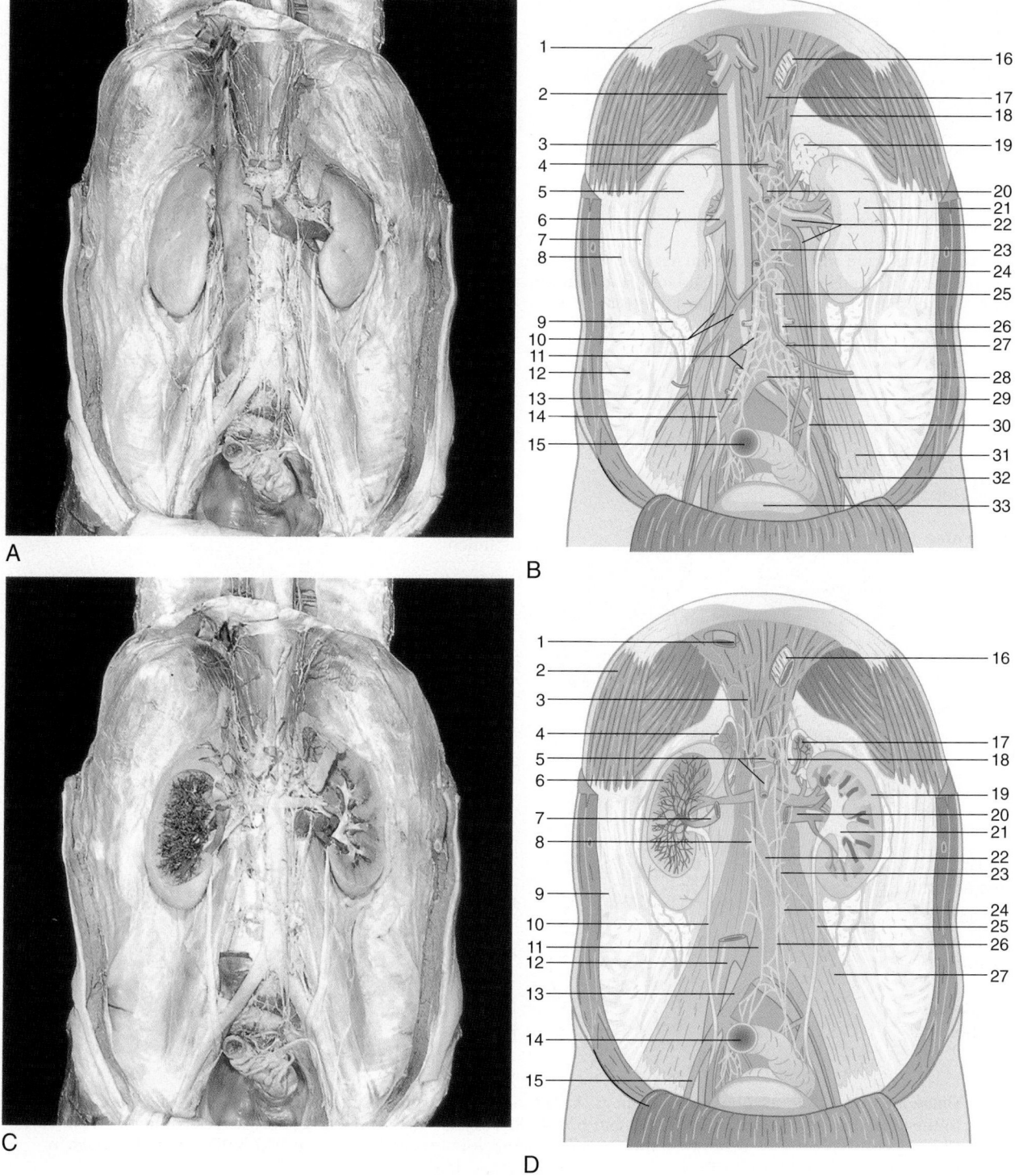

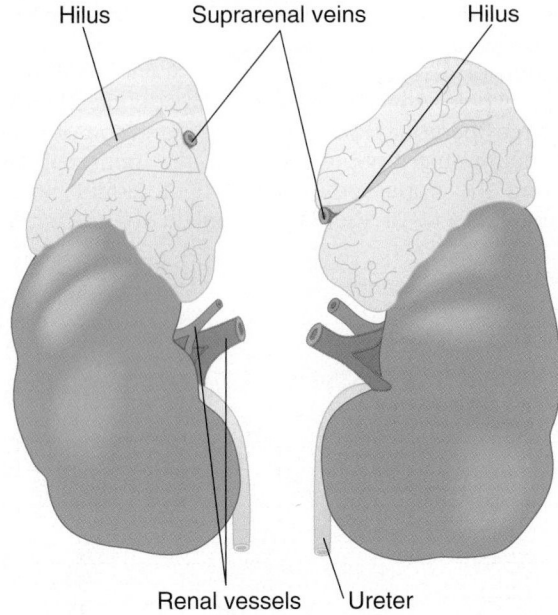

Figure 77-2 Kidneys and adrenal glands from neonate. Note large size of the adrenal glands relative to the kidneys, and note the fetal lobation of the kidneys. (From Kabalin J: Surgical anatomy of the retroperitoneum, kidneys, and ureters. In Walsh PC, Retik AB, Vaughan ED, et al [eds]: Campbell's Urology, 8th ed. Philadelphia, Elsevier, 2002, p 21.)

ligament. Excessive traction on this attachment or the hepatocolic ligament during right renal surgery may produce hepatic parenchymal tears. The duodenum is applied directly to the medial aspect and hilar structures of the right kidney (see Figs. 77-1 and 77-3). The hepatic flexure of the colon, which also is extraperitoneal, crosses the lower pole of the right kidney. The adrenal gland covers the superomedial aspect of the upper poles of both right and left kidneys, as already discussed.

On the left, the retroperitoneal tail of the pancreas and the related splenic vessels are applied directly to the upper to middle portion and hilum of the kidney. Superior to the pancreatic tail, the left kidney is covered by peritoneum of the lesser sac and here is related to the posterior gastric wall. Below the pancreatic tail, the medial aspect of the kidney is covered by peritoneum of the greater sac and is related to the jejunum. The lower pole of the left kidney is crossed by the splenic flexure of the colon, generally in an extraperitoneal position. The spleen is separated from the upper lateral portion of the left kidney by peritoneal reflection. However, there is typically a peritoneal extension between the perirenal fascia covering the upper pole of the left kidney and the inferior splenic capsule, called the *splenorenal,* or *lienorenal, ligament.* Just as with the adjacent and often contiguous splenocolic ligamentous attachment, care must be taken not to exert undue tension on the splenorenal ligament during operative procedures on the left

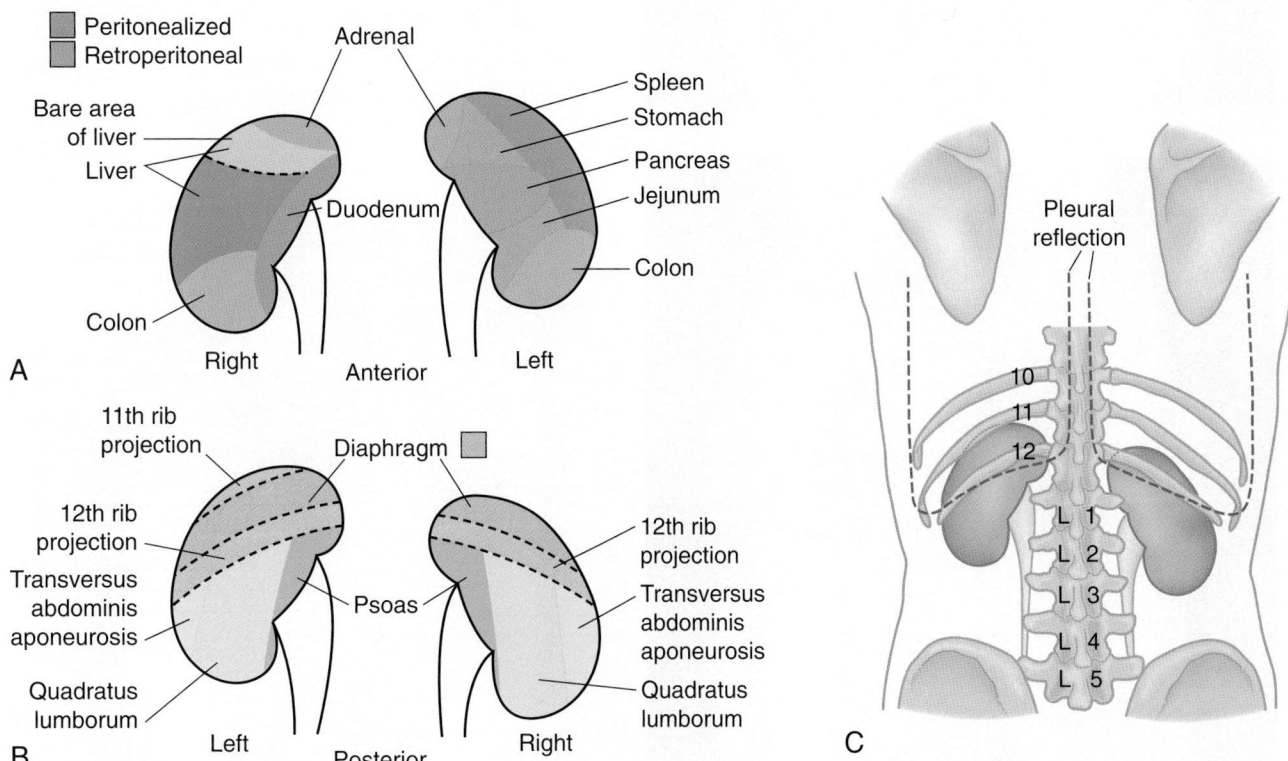

Figure 77-3 Anatomic relations of the kidneys. **A,** Anterior relations to the abdominal organs. **B,** Posterior relations to the muscles of the posterior body wall and ribs. **C,** Relations to the pleural reflections and skeleton posteriorly. (From Kabalin J: Surgical anatomy of the retroperitoneum, kidneys, and ureters. In Walsh PC, Retik AB, Vaughan ED Jr, et al [eds]: Campbell's Urology, 8th ed. Philadelphia, Elsevier, 2002, pp 49-87.)

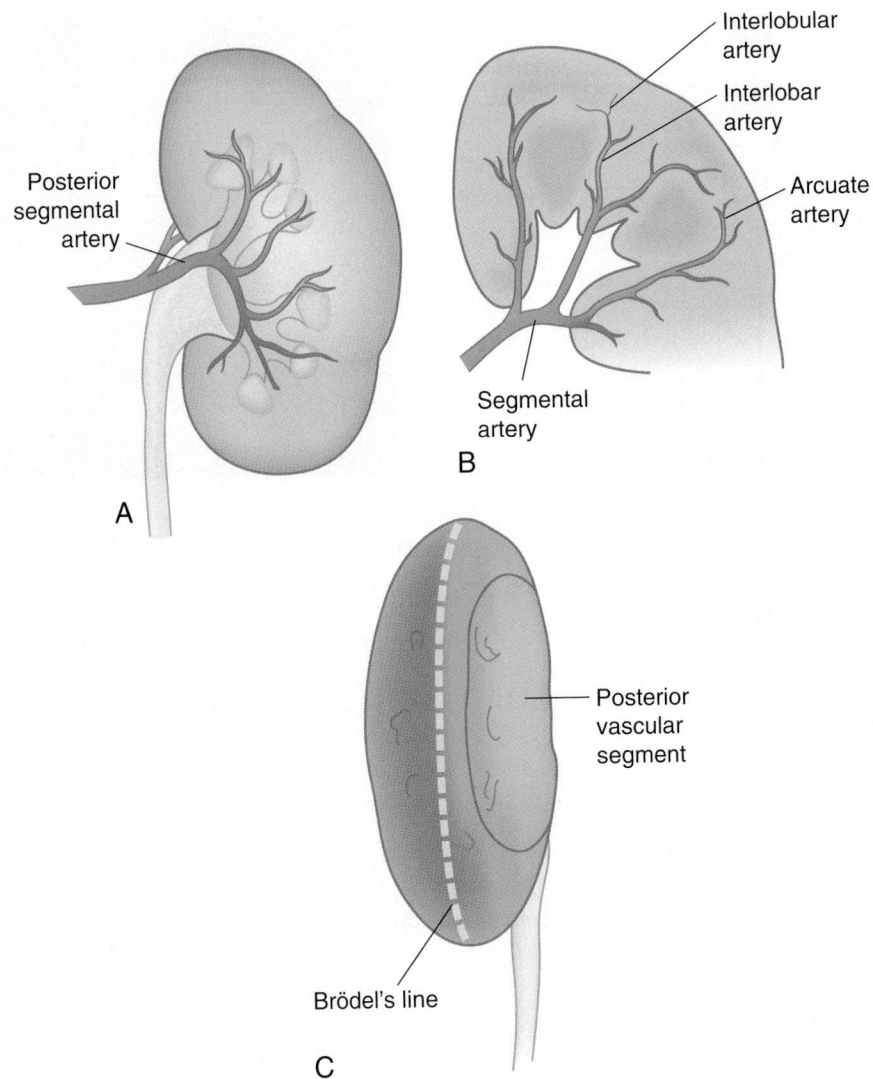

Figure 77-4 **A,** The posterior branch of the renal artery and its distribution to the central segment of the posterior surface of the kidney. **B,** Branches of the anterior division of the renal artery supplying the entire anterior surface of the kidney as well as the upper and lower poles at both surfaces. The segmental branches lead to interlobar, arcuate, and interlobular arteries. **C,** The lateral convex margin of the kidney. Brödel's line, which is 1 cm from the convex margin, is the bloodless plane demarcated by the distribution of the posterior branch of the renal artery. (A and C, From Tanagho E: Anatomy of the genitourinary tract. In Smith's General Urology, 14th ed. Norwalk, CT, Appleton & Lange, 1995, pp 1-16. With permission of the McGraw-Hill Company.)

kidney, in order to avoid inadvertent tearing of the spleen. Such tearing may necessitate splenectomy during left nephrectomy. Both splenocolic and splenorenal ligaments, and the contralateral hepatocolic and hepatorenal ligaments, are typically avascular and can safely be sharply divided.

The renal artery and vein typically branch from the aorta and IVC, respectively, to supply each kidney (see Fig. 77-1). The renal vein is more anterior than the renal artery, whereas the urinary collecting system (i.e., the renal pelvis) is the most posteriorly located structure of the renal hilum. The renal arteries and veins typically branch from the aorta and IVC at the level of the second lumbar vertebral body, below the level of the anterior takeoff of the superior mes-

enteric artery. The right renal artery passes behind the IVC in its course and is considerably longer than the left renal artery. The main renal artery typically divides into segmental vessels, with five branches most commonly described. The first and most constant segmental division is a posterior branch, which usually exits the main renal artery before it enters the renal hilum and proceeds posteriorly to the renal pelvis to supply a large posterior segment of the kidney. The remaining anterior division of the main renal artery typically branches as it enters the renal hilum (Fig. 77-4). The renal arteries are end branch vessels and do not communicate with each other. This is in contrast to the renal venous system that contains many intrarenal anastomoses.

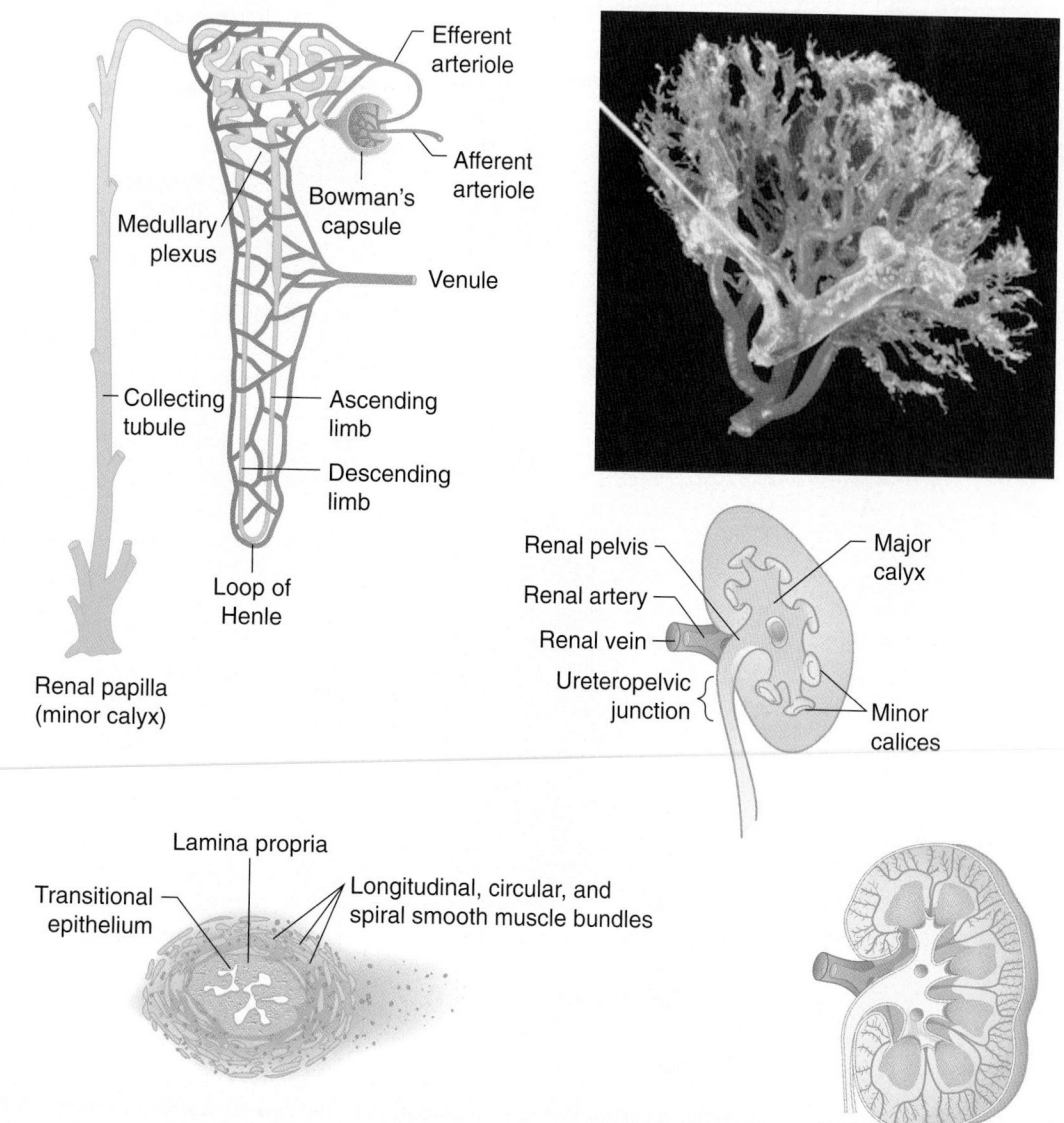

Figure 77-5 Anatomy and histology of the kidney and ureter. *Upper left,* Diagram of the nephron and its blood supply. *Upper right,* Cast of the pelvic calyceal system and the arterial supply of the kidney. *Middle,* Renal calyces, pelvis, and ureter (posterior aspect). *Lower left,* Histology of the ureter. The smooth muscle bundles are arranged in both a spiral and a longitudinal manner. *Lower right,* Longitudinal section of kidney showing calyces, pelvis, ureter, and renal blood supply (posterior aspect). (From Tanagho E, McAninch JW [eds]: Smith's General Urology, 15th ed. New York, McGraw-Hill, 2000. Reproduced with permission of the McGraw-Hill Company.)

The right renal vein is short (2-4 cm) and enters the right lateral aspect of the IVC directly, usually without receiving other venous branches. The left renal vein is generally three times the length of the right (6-10 cm) and must cross anterior to the aorta to reach the left lateral aspect of the IVC (see Fig. 77-1). Lateral to the aorta, the left renal vein typically receives the left adrenal vein superiorly, a lumbar vein posteriorly, and the left gonadal vein inferiorly.

The renal collecting system includes the calyces, the renal pelvis, and the ureter (Fig. 77-5). There are usually 8 to 12 minor calyces that unite to form two to three major calyces, which in turn join to form the renal pelvis. The renal pelvis tapers to form the ureter inferomedially.

The adult ureter is usually 25 to 30 cm in length. The ureter is arbitrarily divided into segments for the purposes of surgical or radiographic demonstration. The "abdominal" ureter extends from the renal pelvis to the iliac vessels, and the "pelvic" ureter extends from the iliac vessels to the bladder (Fig. 77-6). For radiographic purposes, the ureter is divided into three segments. The upper, middle, and lower ureter are commonly described from the renal pelvis to the upper border of sacrum, from the upper border to the lower border of sacrum, and from the lower border of sacrum to the bladder, respectively. There are three areas of relative narrowing in the ureter that are of clinical importance: the ureteropelvic junction, the point where the ureter crosses anterior to

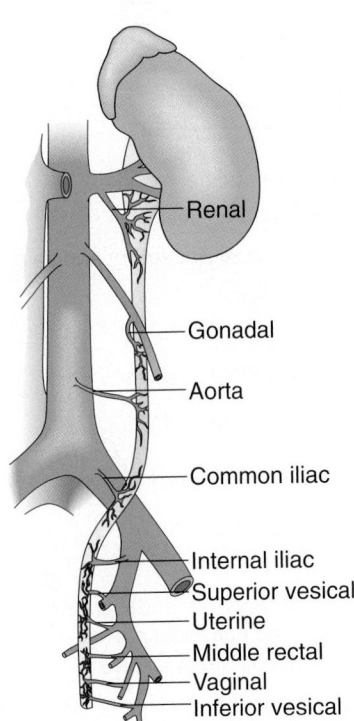

Figure 77-6 Sources of arterial blood supply to the ureter. (From Kabalin J: Surgical anatomy of the retroperitoneum, kidneys, and ureters. In Walsh PC, Retik AB, Vaughan ED Jr, et al [eds]: Campbell's Urology, 8th ed. Philadelphia, Elsevier, 2002, pp 49-87.)

the iliac vessels, and the ureterovesical junction. For example, spontaneous passage of ureteral stones can be hampered at these areas of relative narrowing.

The ureters lie on the psoas muscle, pass medially to the sacroiliac joints, and cross the iliac vessels anteriorly. An important anatomic landmark for easy identification of the ureters is at the site where the ureters cross anterior to the iliac vessels. After crossing the iliac vessels, the ureters swing laterally near the ischial spines before passing medially to penetrate the base of the bladder. In males, the vasa deferentia pass anterior to the ureters as they exit the internal inguinal ring. In females, the uterine arteries are closely related to the lower ureters.

The blood supply to the calyces, pelvis, and upper ureter is derived from the renal arteries (see Fig. 77-6). The lower ureter obtains its blood supply from the common and internal iliac, internal spermatic, and vesical arteries.

Bladder

The bladder is a hollow muscular organ that functions to store and evacuate urine. In adulthood, it has a capacity of about 500 mL. The cephalad portion of the bladder is attached to the anterior abdominal wall by the urachus, a fibrous remnant of the cloaca that attaches the bladder to the anterior abdominal wall. The obliterated umbilical artery in the medial umbilical fold serves as an important landmark for the surgeon (Fig. 77-7). It may be traced to

its origin from the internal iliac artery in order to locate the ureter, which lies on its medial side. The superior aspect of the bladder is covered by peritoneal reflection. Inferiorly, the bladder is attached to the pubic bone by dense condensations to the posterior aspect of the pubic bone, known as the *puboprostatic ligaments* in males and *pubovesical ligaments* in females.

The superior, middle, and inferior vesical arteries, which are branches of the hypogastric artery, are the major source of blood supply to the bladder. In females, additional branches from the vaginal and uterine arteries supply the bladder. The veins of the bladder coalesce into the vesicle plexus and drain into the internal iliac vein. Lymphatics from the lamina propria and muscularis drain to channels on the bladder surface, which run with the superficial vessels within the thin visceral fascia. Small paravesical lymph nodes can be found along the superficial channels. The bulk of the lymphatic drainage passes to the external iliac lymph nodes. Some anterior and lateral drainage may go through the obturator and internal iliac nodes, whereas portions of the bladder base and trigone may drain into the internal and common iliac groups.

A transitional epithelial layer lines the bladder mucosa. Lamina propria, a thin elastic connective tissue, lies between the transitional epithelial cell layer and the muscularis propria. The muscularis propria, also known as the *detrusor muscle,* is composed of interlacing smooth muscle bundles with no distinct layers.

Prostate and Seminal Vesicles

The prostate is a fibromuscular organ that lies just inferior to the bladder. The normal prostate weighs about 20 g and contains the prostatic urethra. The prostate is supported anteriorly by the puboprostatic ligament and inferiorly by the urogenital diaphragm (Fig. 77-8). The ejaculatory ducts exit in the posterior portion of the prostate across the verumontanum, a mound within the prostate gland (see Fig. 77-8). The prostate has a peripheral zone, a central zone, and a transitional zone; an anterior segment; and a preprostatic sphincteric zone (Fig. 77-9). Benign prostatic hyperplasia develops from the periurethral glands at the site of the median or lateral lobes, whereas the posterior lobe is prone to cancerous formation. Prostate is separated from the rectum by the two layers of Denonvilliers' fascia, serosal rudiments of the pouch of Douglas, which once extended to the urogenital diaphragm (Fig. 77-10).

The arterial supply to the prostate is derived from the inferior vesical, internal pudendal, and middle rectal (hemorrhoidal) arteries. The veins from the prostate drain into the periprostatic plexus, which has connections with the deep dorsal vein of the penis and the internal iliac (hypogastric) veins.

The neurovascular bundles responsible for erection are located near the posterolateral surface of the urethra and prostate gland (see Prostate Carcinoma, later, for a detailed anatomic picture; see also Fig. 77-29, later). Special care in preserving these nerves is crucial to maintaining potency after radical prostatectomy.[1]

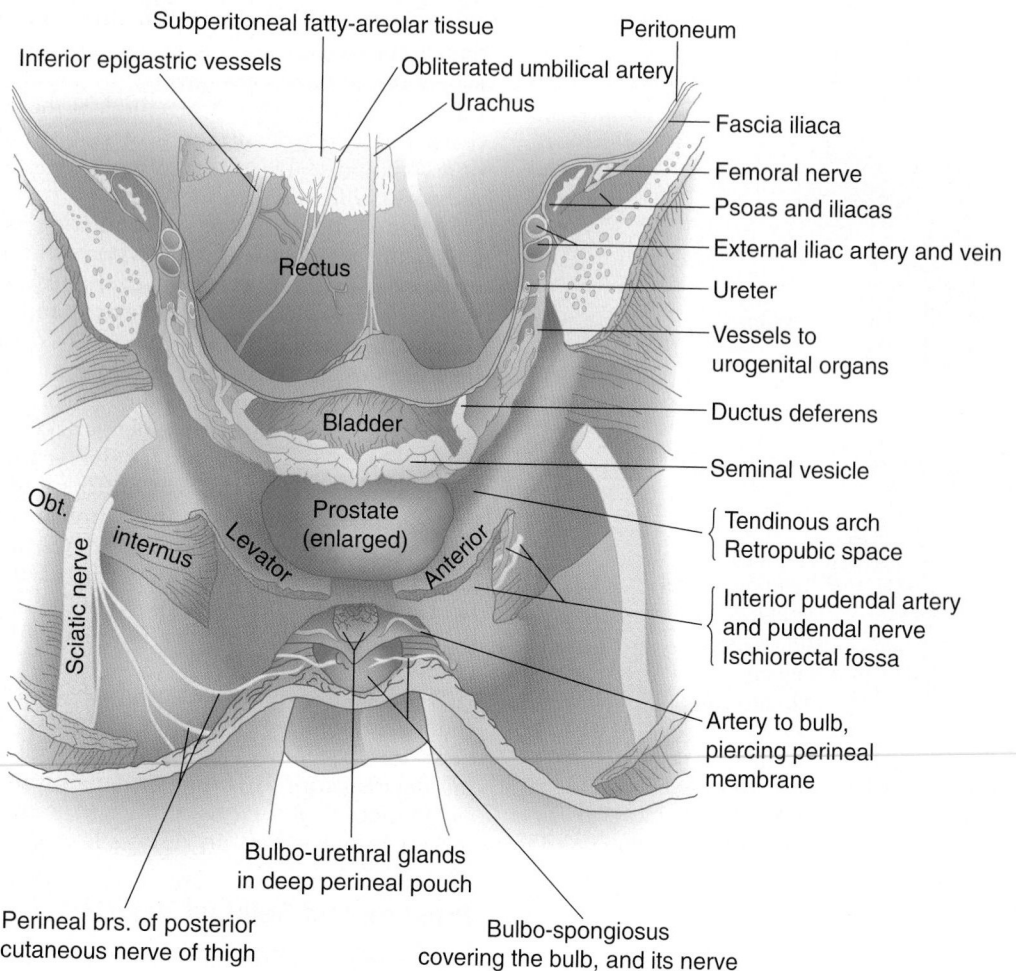

Figure 77-7 Male pelvis and anterior abdominal wall viewed from behind. The sacrum and ilia have been removed. (From Brooks JD: Anatomy of the lower urinary tract in male genitalia. In Walsh PC, Retik AB, Vaughan ED Jr, et al [eds]: Campbell's Urology, 8th ed. Philadelphia, Elsevier, 2002, pp 41-80.)

The seminal vesicles lie just cephalad to the prostate under the base of the bladder. They are about 6 cm long and quite soft. Each vesicle joins its corresponding vas deferens to form the ejaculatory duct. The ureters lie medial to each, and the rectum is contiguous with their posterior surfaces.

Penis and Urethra

The penis is composed of two corpora cavernosal bodies (responsible for erectile function of the penis) and one corpora cavernosum through which the urethra courses. Each corporal body is covered by tunica albuginea (Fig. 77-11), and collectively all corporal bodies are covered by a thick layer of Buck's fascia. All corporal bodies are capped by the glans of the penis (see Fig. 77-10).

The male urethra, about 20 cm in length, is divided into four different anatomic sections: prostatic, membranous, bulbous, and penile urethra. The voluntary external urinary sphincter lies within the urogenital diaphragm and is an important anatomic landmark to preserve the function of

the urinary sphincter after prostatic or urethral surgery. The female urethra is about 4 cm in length and lies below the pubic symphysis and anterior to the vagina.

Spermatic Cord, Epididymis, and Testes

The two spermatic cords extend from the internal rings through the internal canals to the testicles. Each cord contains the vas deferens, the internal and external spermatic arteries, artery of the vas, the spermatic vein, lymphatics, and nerves.

The epididymis is connected to the testis by efferent ducts from the testis. The epididymis consists of a markedly coiled duct. At its lower pole, the epididymis becomes continuous with the vas deferens (Fig. 77-12).

The average testis is $4 \times 3 \times 2.5$ cm in diameter. Tunica albuginea, which is a dense fascial covering, overlies the testis. The tunica albuginea forms a dense fibrous mediastinum that connects with the lobules within the testis (see Fig. 77-12). The testis is covered anteriorly and laterally by the visceral layer of the serous tunica vaginalis.

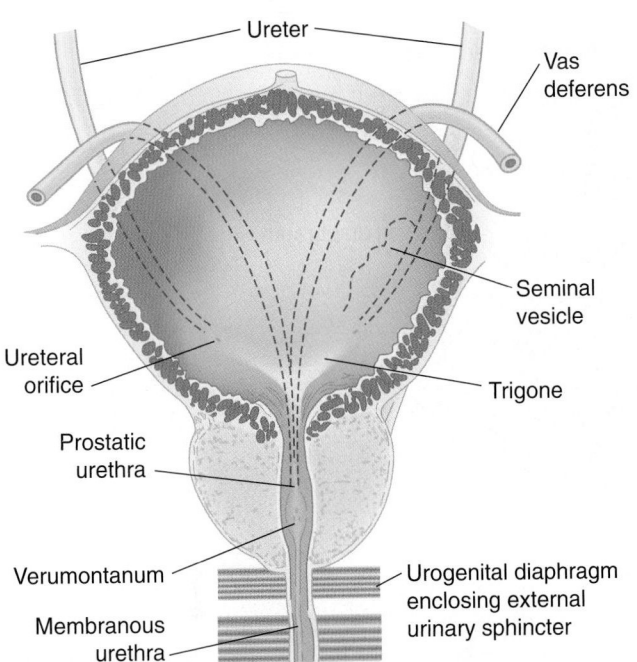

Figure 77-8 Anatomy and relations of the ureters, bladder, prostate, seminal vesicles, and vasa deferentia (anterior view). (From Tanagho EA, McAninch JW [eds]: Smith's General Urology, 15th ed. New York, McGraw-Hill, 2000)

UROLOGIC TRAUMA

About 10% of all injuries seen in the emergency room involve the genitourinary system to some extent. Many of the injuries are subtle and difficult to define and require great diagnostic expertise. Initial assessment in order of importance includes A, airway with cervical spine protection; B, breathing; C, circulation and control of external bleeding; D, disability or neurologic status; E, exposure (undress) and environment (temperature control).

Resuscitation may require intravenous (IV) lines and urethral catheterization in seriously injured patients. In males, before the Foley catheter is inserted, the urethra is carefully inspected for the presence of any blood.

A detailed history and description of the accident is obtained. In cases of gunshot wounds, the type and caliber of the weapon needs to be determined because high-velocity projectiles cause much more extensive damage than low-velocity ones.

Renal Trauma

The urologic examination focuses on the abdomen and genitalia. Fractures of the lower ribs are often associated with renal injuries to the retroperitoneum (see Fig. 77-3), whereas pelvic fractures can be accompanied by bladder and urethral injuries.

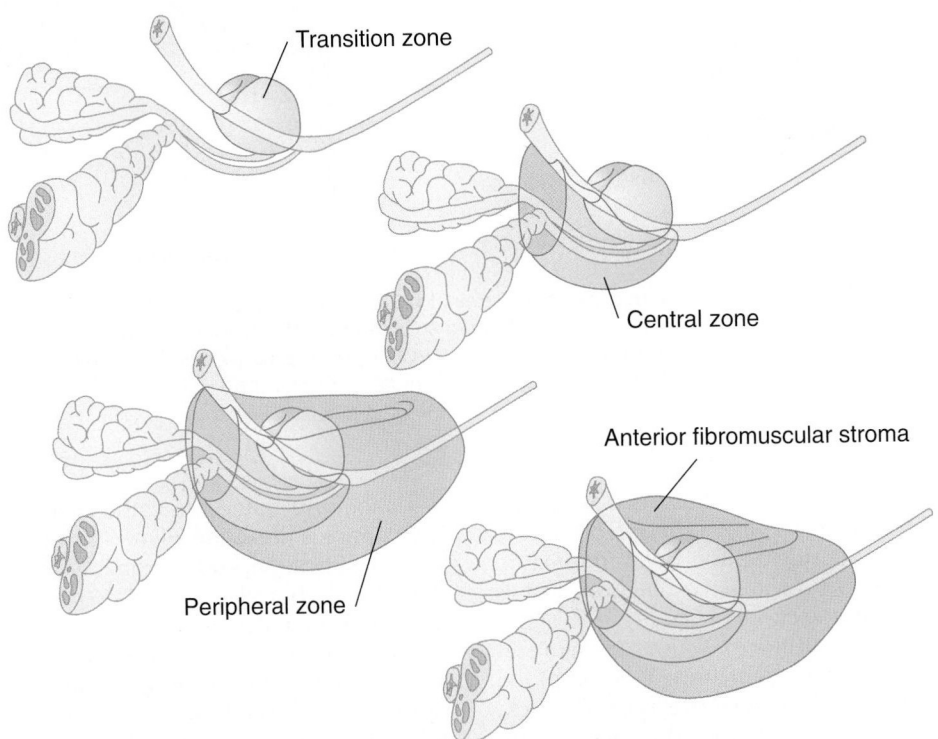

Figure 77-9 Zonal anatomy of the prostate as described by J. E. McNeal (Am J Surg Pathol 12:619-633, 1988). The transition zone surrounds the urethra proximal to the ejaculatory ducts. The central zone surrounds the ejaculatory ducts and projects under the bladder base. The peripheral zone constitutes the bulk of the apical, posterior, and lateral aspects of the prostate. The anterior fibromuscular stroma extends from the bladder neck to the striated urethral sphincter. (From Brooks J: Anatomy of the lower urinary tract and male genitalia. In Walsh PC, Retik AB, Vaughan ED Jr, et al [eds]: Campbell's Urology, 8th ed. Philadelphia, Elsevier, 2002, p 112.)

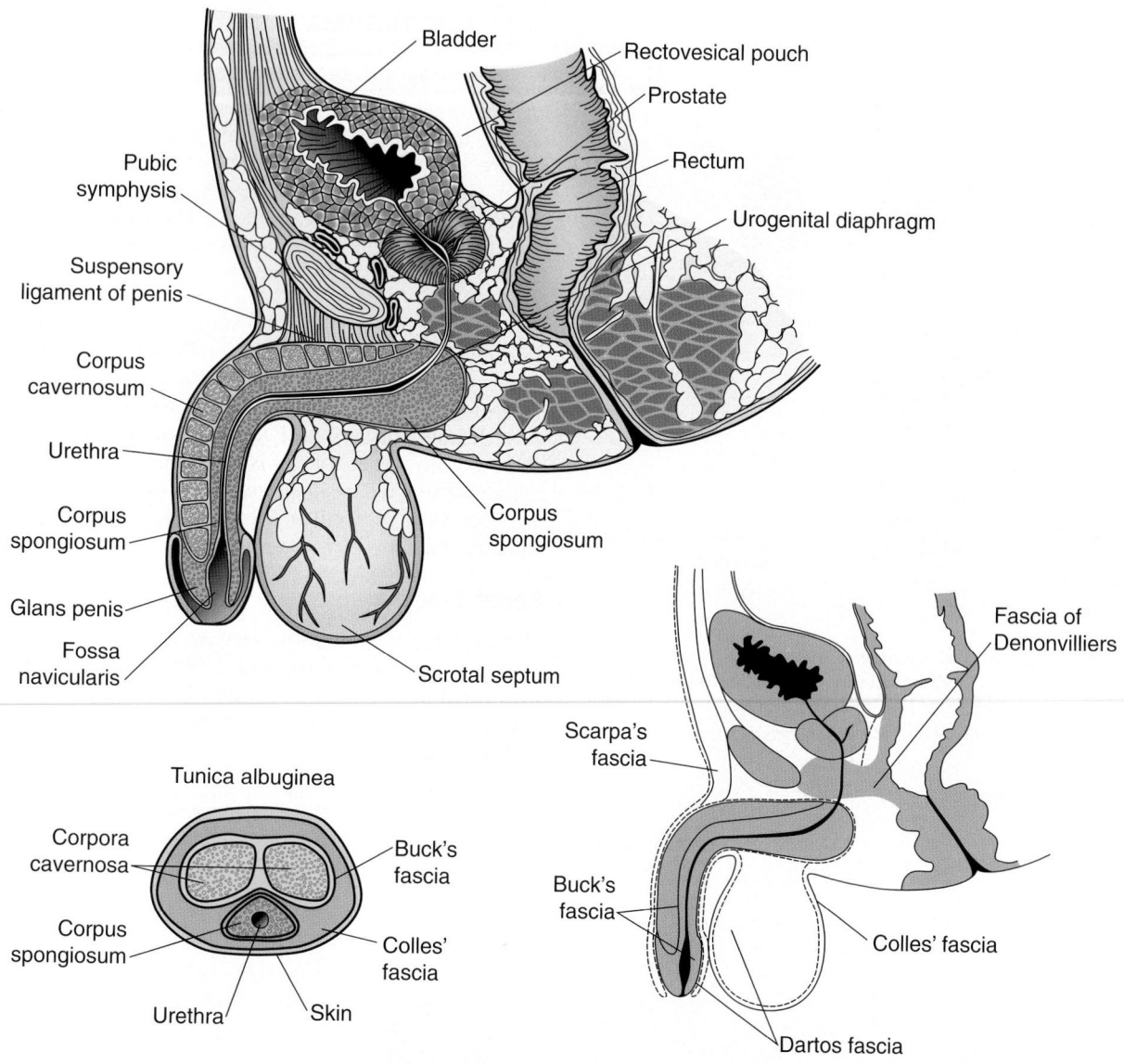

Figure 77-10 *Top,* Relations of the bladder, prostate, seminal vesicles, penis, urethra, and scrotal contents. *Lower left,* Transverse section through the penis. The paired upper structures are the corpora cavernosa. The single lower body surrounding the urethra is the corpus spongiosum. *Lower right,* Fascial planes of the lower genitourinary tract. (From Tanagho EA, McAninch JW [eds]: Smith's General Urology, 15th ed. New York, McGraw-Hill, 2000.)

The assessment of the extent of injury is done in an orderly fashion for proper staging. The algorithm in Figure 77-13 outlines the staging for blunt trauma in adults as it pertains to the urologic evaluation and is further discussed in a later section.

Hematuria is the best indicator of traumatic injury to the urinary system. Microscopic hematuria (>5 red blood cells per high-power field), heme-positive urine dipstick, and gross hematuria are the strongest indicators of genitourinary injury. However, the degree of hematuria does not necessarily correlate with degree of injury. The combination of systemic shock (systolic blood pressure <90 mm Hg) and microscopic hematuria is strongly associated with severe renal injuries. The best urine sample for assessment of hematuria in the trauma patient is the

first aliquot of voided or catheterized specimen because later samples are often diluted by diuresis.

A classification and grading system for renal injuries (Fig. 77-14; see also Fig. 77-13) has helped in proper identification and better communication of the extent of injury between different members of the trauma team. Use of appropriate imaging studies enables the trauma team to appropriately stage the extent of the renal injury. All blunt trauma patients with gross hematuria and those patients with microscopic hematuria and shock (systolic blood pressure <90 mm Hg any time during evaluation and resuscitation) undergo renal imaging, usually computed tomography (CT) with IV contrast. Adult patients with microscopic hematuria and without shock can be followed clinically without imaging studies because an

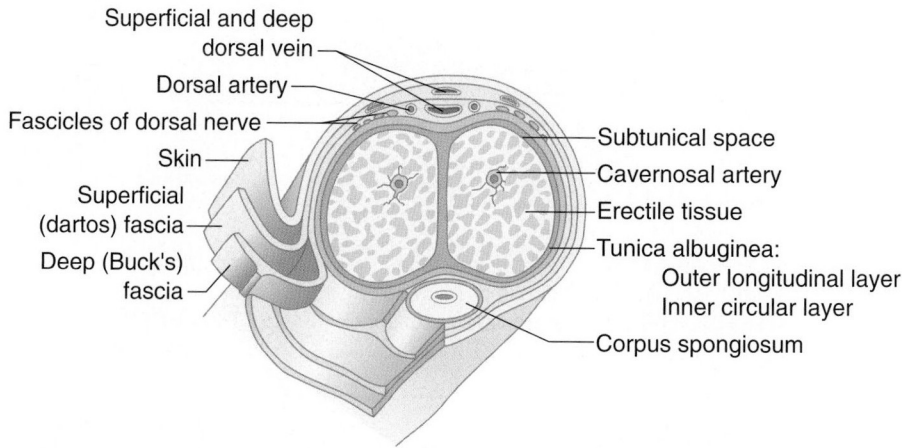

Figure 77-11 Cross section of the penis, demonstrating the relationship between the corporeal bodies, penile fascia, vessels, and nerves. (From Devine CJ, Angermeier KW: Anatomy of the penis and male perineum, part I. AUA Update Series 13(2):10, 1994.)

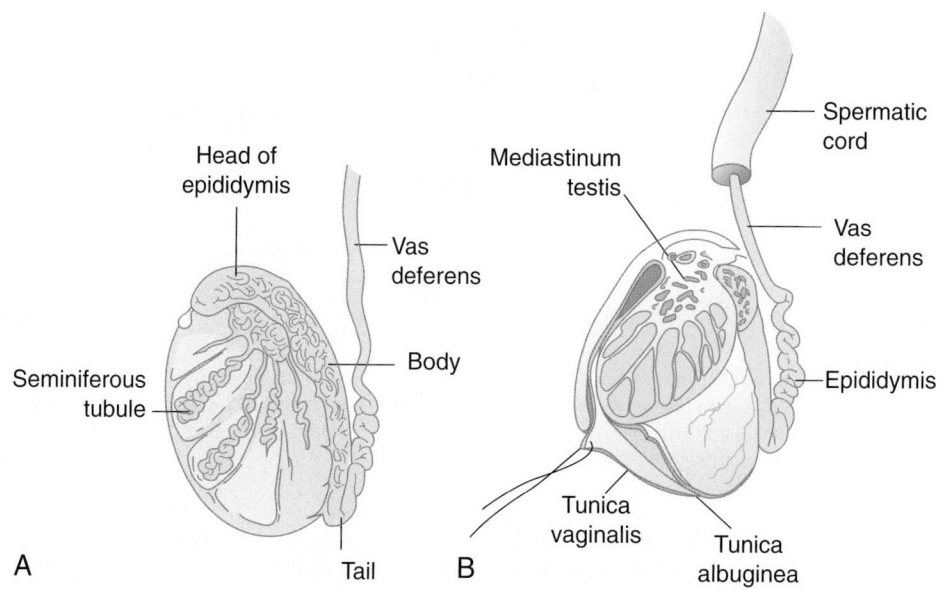

Figure 77-12 Testis and epididymis. **A,** One to three seminiferous tubules fill each compartment and drain into the rete testis in the mediastinum. Twelve to 20 efferent ductules become convoluted in the head of the epididymis and drain into a single coiled duct of the epididymis. The vas is convoluted in its first portion. **B,** Cross section of the tunica vaginalis, showing the mediastinum and septations continuous with the tunica albuginea. The parietal and visceral tunica vaginalis are confluent where the vessels and nerves enter the posterior aspect of the testis. (From Brooks J: Anatomy of the lower urinary tract and male genitalia. In Walsh PC, Retik AB, Vaughan ED Jr, et al [eds]: Campbell's Urology, 8th ed. Philadelphia, Elsevier, 2002, pp 89-128.)

extremely low percentage of these patients (<0.0016%) have significant renal injury.[2] In contrast, pediatric patients with blunt trauma and microscopic hematuria require an imaging modality (CT scan or ultrasound). Children have a high catecholamine output; therefore, shock is not a good predictor of the degree of renal injury.

Excretory urography used to be the imaging modality for assessment of renal trauma, but it has been replaced for the most part by contrast enhanced CT imaging in most emergency rooms. Occasionally, single-shot

excretory urography is used for immediate intraoperative assessment of renal trauma.[3]

Significant injuries (grades II through V) are found in only 5.4% of renal trauma cases[3] (see Fig. 77-14). More than 98% of all renal injuries can be managed nonoperatively. More often, high-grade renal injuries (grades IV and V) require surgical management; however, with proper staging of the renal injury and careful patient selection, even these injuries can be managed nonoperatively.

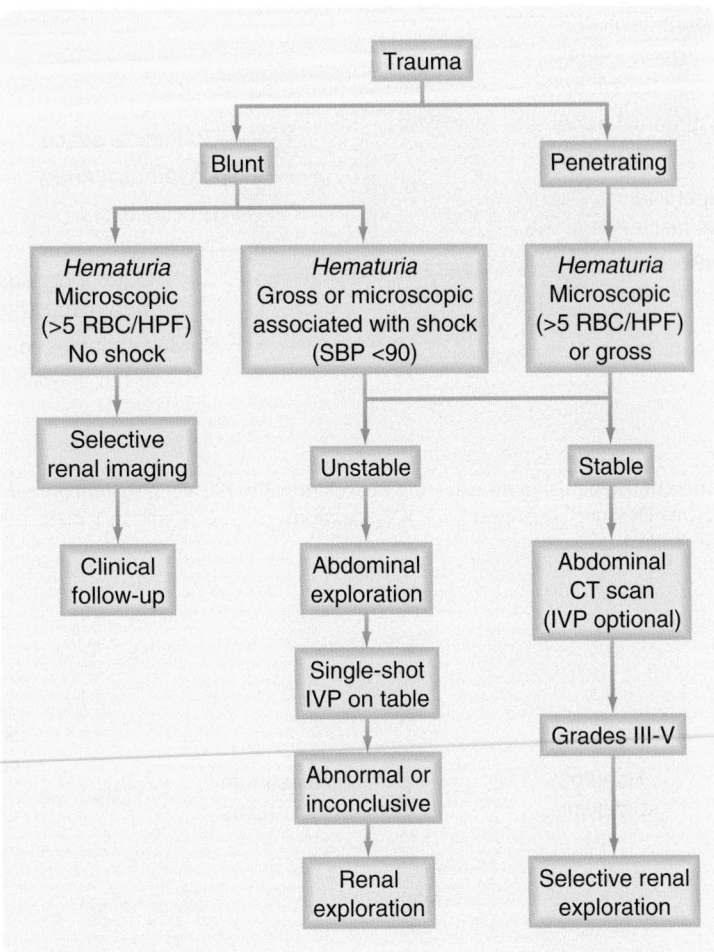

Figure 77-13 Flow chart for adult renal injuries to serve as a guide for decision making. CT, computed tomography; HPF, high-power field; IVP, intravenous pyelography; RBC, red blood cell; SBP, systolic blood pressure. (From McAninch JW, Santucci RA: Genitourinary trauma. In Walsh PC, Retik AB, Vaughan ED Jr, et al [eds]: Campbell's Urology, 8th ed. Philadelphia, Elsevier, 2002, p 3711.)

Indications for renal exploration after trauma can be separated into absolute and relative. Absolute indications include evidence of persistent renal bleeding, expanding perirenal hematoma, and pulsatile perirenal hematoma. Relative indications include urinary extravasation, nonviable tissue, delayed diagnosis of arterial injury, segmental arterial injury, and incomplete staging.

Segmental renal artery injury with an associated renal laceration results in a substantial amount of nonviable tissue (usually >20%), and such injuries usually resolve more quickly with surgical reconstruction and tissue removal. This approach often avoids the high complication rate noted when this group is followed without renal exploration.

When surgical exploration for renal trauma is indicated, it is recommended to use a transabdominal approach and early exploration of the renal hilum and vasculature before exploring the retroperitoneum (Fig. 77-15). Retroperitoneal incision over the aorta medial to the inferior mesenteric artery allows identification of the left and right renal hilum and enables the surgeon to obtain early vascular control before exploring the injured

kidney, which often has an associated large retroperitoneal hematoma. Renal bleeding is a major cause of nephrectomy in the renal trauma patient. Early vascular control has been shown to decrease the rate of nephrectomy from 56% to 18%.

Nephrectomy is indicated in the unstable patient who has a normal contralateral kidney. Packing the wound to control bleeding, correcting metabolic and coagulation abnormalities, and planning for corrective surgery in 24 hours when the patient is stabilized provides a good option for delayed renal reconstructive repair. Immediate nephrectomy is indicated when the patient's life is threatened as a result of severe uncontrolled bleeding and when reconstructive surgery may not be technically feasible.

Ureteral Injuries

Ureteral injuries occur in less than 4% and 1% of all penetrating and blunt traumas, respectively. Ureteropelvic junction (UPJ) disruption after blunt trauma is rare and can be missed because patients often do not exhibit hematuria. Diagnosis of UPJ disruption is made by a high

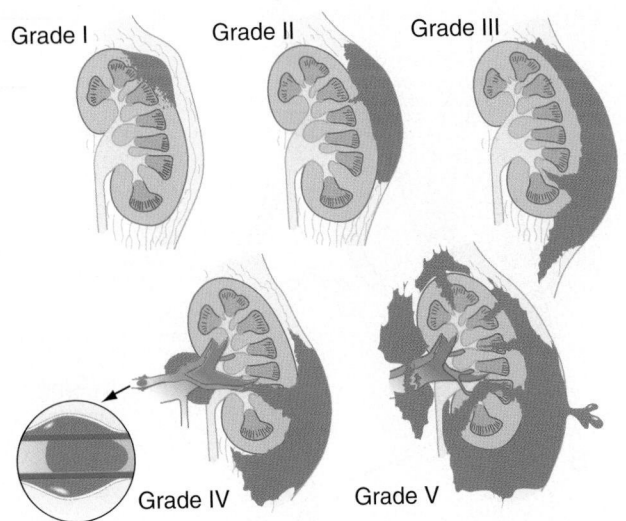

Figure 77-14 Classification of renal injuries by grade (based on the organ injury scale of the American Association for the Surgery of Trauma). (From McAninch JW, Santucci RA: Genitourinary trauma. In Walsh PC, Retik AB, Vaughan ED Jr, et al [eds]: Campbell's Urology, 8th ed. Philadelphia, Elsevier, 2002, p 3709.)

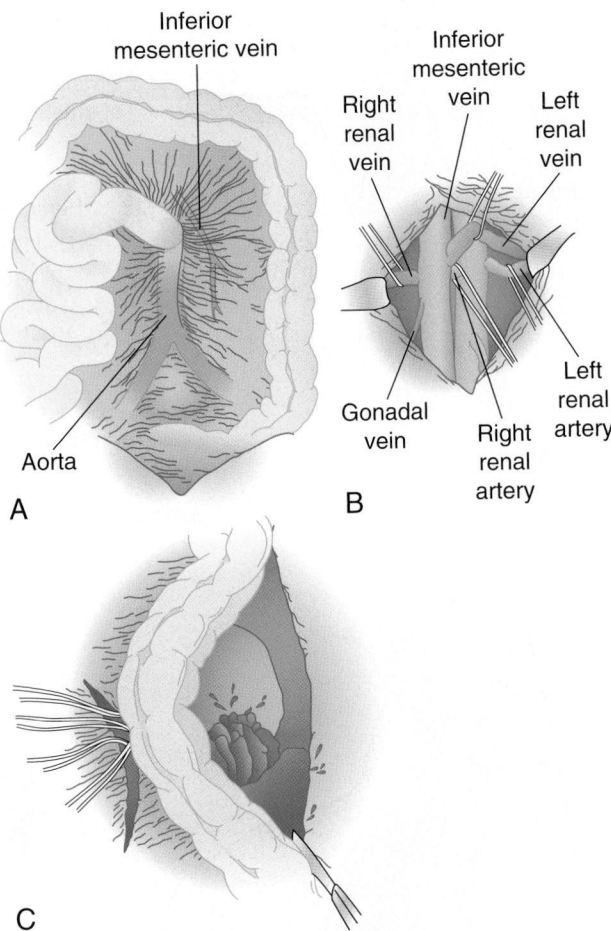

Figure 77-15 The surgical approach to the renal vessels and kidney. **A,** Retroperitoneal incision over the aorta medial to the inferior mesenteric vein. **B,** Anatomic relationships of the renal vessels. **C,** Retroperitoneal incision lateral to the colon, exposing the kidney. (From McAninch JW: Surgery for renal trauma. In Novick AC, Pontes ES, Streem SB [eds]: Stewart's Operative Urology, 2nd ed. Baltimore, Williams & Wilkins, 1989.)

index of suspicion in cases of high deceleration injury. Delayed CT contrast images that visualize the renal collecting system and proximal ureter with excreted contrast material are the best mode of assessing UPJ integrity. When delayed contrast images are not possible because of hemodynamic instability, an intraoperative one-shot (2 mg/kg IV contrast material given 10 minutes before flat plate abdominal x-ray) IV pyelogram (IVP) is recommended in patients with hypotension or a history of significant deceleration, despite absence of gross hematuria. Intraoperative palpation of the UPJ is usually not sensitive enough to assess any UPJ disruption.

Iatrogenic Ureteral Injury

Management of iatrogenic ureteral injuries is dependent on timing and location of the ureteral injury. Ureteral injuries are rare. Iatrogenic ureteral injuries are often associated with large pelvic masses (benign or malignant) that may displace the ureter from its normal anatomic position. Inflammatory pelvic disorders such as endometriosis may encase the ureter in a similar way and account for inadvertent ureteral injury during pelvic surgery. Extensive carcinoma of the colon may invade areas outside the colon wall and directly involve the ureter; thus, resection of the ureter may be required along with resection of the tumor mass. Devascularization may occur with extensive pelvic lymph node dissections or after radiation therapy to the pelvis for pelvic cancer. In these situations, ureteral fibrosis and subsequent stricture formation may develop along with ureteral fistulas.

Injuries to the lower third of the ureter allow several options in management. The procedure of choice is reimplantation into the bladder combined with a psoas hitch procedure to minimize tension on the ureteral anastomosis.[4] The bladder is dissected after catheter

instillation of saline. The urachus and contralateral obliterated umbilical artery are divided (Fig. 77-16A). Peritoneum is mobilized off the anterior and posterior aspect of the bladder. These maneuvers allow more extensive mobilization of the bladder. The bladder is incised in midline or obliquely to allow mobilization of the bladder to the ipsilateral psoas muscle (see Fig. 77-16B). The bladder is sutured to the psoas muscle, but care is taken to avoid the genitofemoral nerve on the surface of muscle or the femoral nerve deep in the psoas muscle (see Fig. 77-16C). An antireflux ureteral anastomosis is done when possible to minimize potential damage to the upper urinary tract from long-standing urinary reflux (see Fig. 77-16D).

Primary ureteroureterostomy can be used in lower-third injuries when the ureter has been ligated without transection. The ureter is usually long enough for this type of anastomosis. A bladder tube flap (Boari flap) can be used when the ureter is shorter.

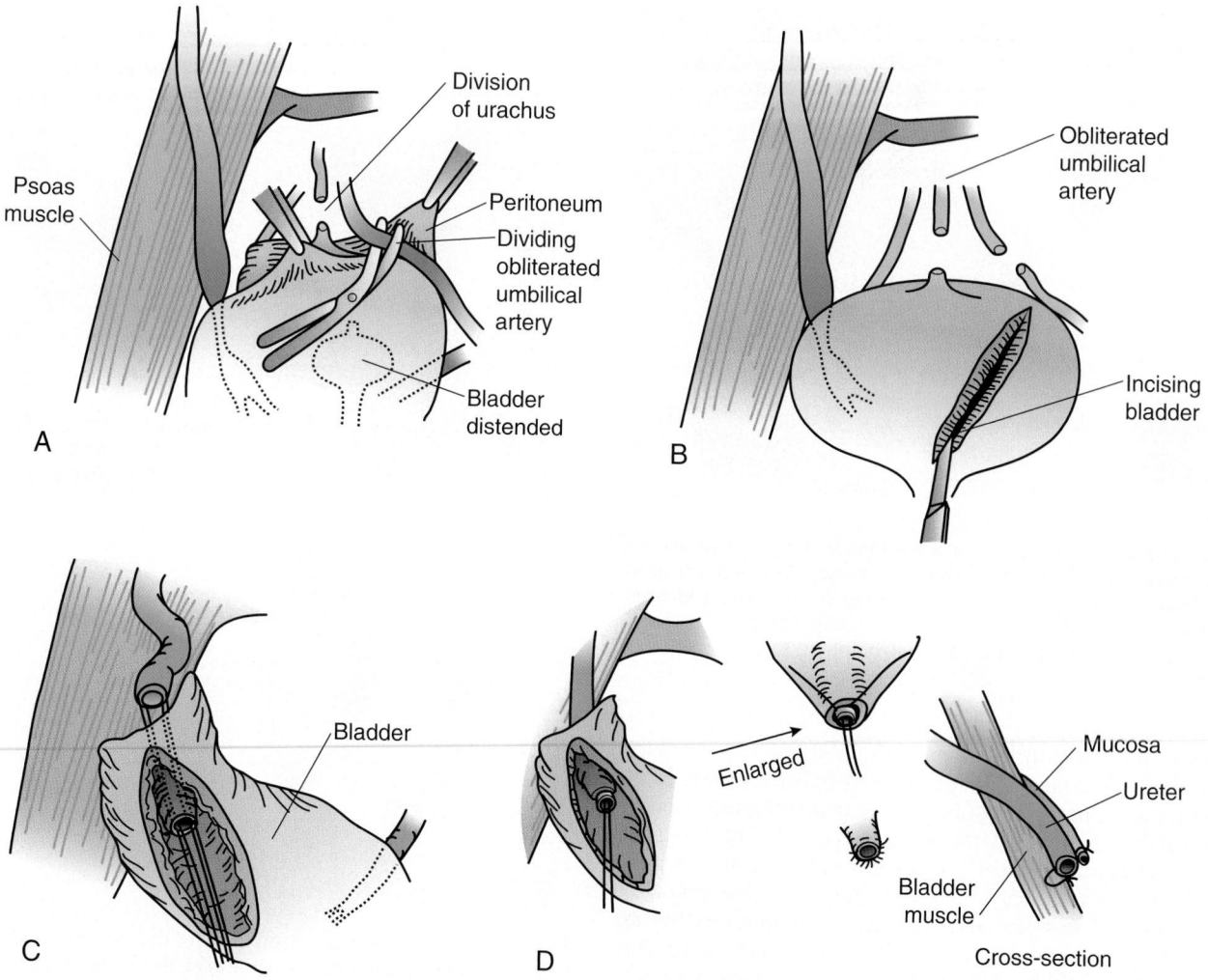

Figure 77-16 A, After the midline incision is made, a retroperitoneal approach delineates the bladder. The bladder is dissected after catheter instillation of saline. The urachus and contralateral obliterated umbilical artery are divided. The peritoneum is mobilized off the posterior aspect of the bladder. These maneuvers allow more extensive mobilization of bladder. **B,** The bladder is incised in midline or obliquely to allow mobilization of bladder to right psoas muscle. **C,** The bladder is sutured to psoas muscle, but care is taken to avoid genitofemoral nerve on surface of muscle. It is important not to place the sutures too deeply in psoas muscle because femoral nerve branches can be injured. **D,** Antireflux submucosal ureteral reimplantation is then constructed. The ureter is advanced in a submucosal tunnel. Anchoring absorbable sutures are placed in mucosa and muscle. (Modified from Mathews R, Marshall F: Versatility of the adult psoas hitch ureteral reimplantation. J Urol 158:2078-2082, 1997.)

Transureteroureterostomy may be used in lower-third injuries if extensive urinoma and pelvic infection have developed. This procedure allows anastomosis and reconstruction in an area away from the pathologic processes. Caution must be taken to prevent tension on the normal recipient ureter.

Midureteral injuries can be managed with primary ureteroureterostomy if there is not a significant loss of viable ureter between the proximal and distal sites of injury; otherwise, transureteroureterostomy is a good option.

Upper ureteral injuries are best managed by primary ureteroureterostomy. If there is extensive loss of the ureter, autotransplantation of the kidney and transposition of bowel to replace the ureter are potential surgical options.

Bladder Injuries

Bladder injury after blunt trauma is relatively rare owing to the protected intrapelvic position of the bladder. Bladder injuries are associated with 6% to 10% of all pelvic fractures. Conversely, in the presence of a bladder injury, most patients (83%-100%) suffer from other pelvic fractures. Bladder injuries can be classified into two types: extraperitoneal and intraperitoneal. Extraperitoneal ruptures are thought to result from direct laceration, usually by bone spicules from the fractured pelvis. Extraperitoneal bladder rupture can most commonly be managed conservatively with catheter drainage leading to spontaneous healing of the bladder injury. However, some authors have listed several contraindications to such conservative management: bone fragment

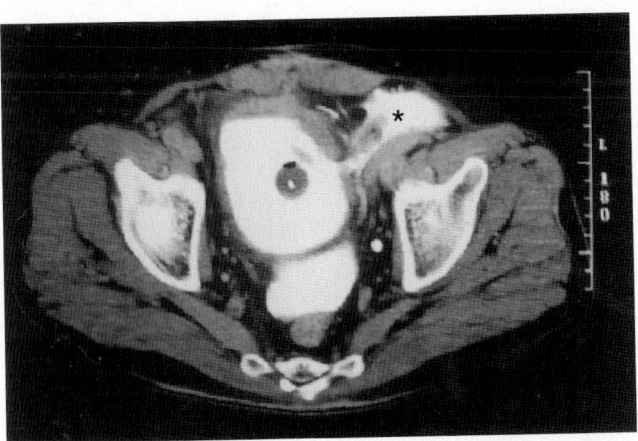

Figure 77-17 Extraperitoneal bladder injury. Contrast agent is extravasated to the space of Retzius (*asterisk*) after retrograde filling of the bladder through the indwelling Foley.

projecting into the bladder (which is unlikely to heal), open pelvic fracture, and rectal perforation. Another relative indication for surgical repair of extraperitoneal bladder injury is concomitant abdominal or pelvic injuries requiring surgical management. In this setting, surgical repair of the bladder injury can potentially decrease the risk for vesicocutaneous fistula.[5]

Intraperitoneal bladder rupture accounts for 25% of all bladder injuries. The postulated mechanism of intraperitoneal bladder injury is thought to be rapid rise of intra-abdominal pressure during a blunt trauma.[6] In contrast to extraperitoneal bladder injuries, intraperitoneal bladder rupture requires operative repair with two-layer closure of the bladder injury and placement of a perivesical drain.

Retrograde cystography is the traditional imaging modality to diagnose bladder rupture. It is critical to obtain filling and drainage cystography films because 13% of bladder injuries are diagnosed by these plain films. CT scan can also be used for diagnosis of bladder injury (Fig. 77-17). The preferred method of assessing bladder injury is by retrograde filling of the bladder with 300 to 400 mL of contrast material (or until patient experiences discomfort) through a Foley catheter, obtaining images during both the filled and drained phases of the study.

Urethral Injuries

Urethral injuries are associated with 4% to 14% of all pelvic fractures and are more common in cases of bilateral pelvic injuries.[7] Diagnosis of urethral injury is made by a high index of suspicion in the presence of blood at the urethral meatus, inability to urinate, or a palpable full bladder on abdominal examination. When blood is present at the meatus, retrograde urethrography aids in the diagnosis of urethral injury. In the presence of minor urethral injury, a catheter can be placed by an experienced urologist with or without the aid of a cystoscope.

Urethral injuries are classified as those confined to the posterior urethra (above the urogenital diaphragm) or the anterior urethra (below the urogenital diaphragm). Posterior urethral injuries are further subclassified as type I (urethral stretch), type II (urethral disruption proximal to the urogenital diaphragm), or type III (proximal and distal disruption of the urogenital diaphragm).

For treatment of posterior urethral injuries, early endoscopic realignment has become more accepted as an excellent initial option.[8] Realignment of the damaged urethra with a stented Foley catheter can lead to either complete healing of the urethral injury or need for future endoscopic treatment of developed urethral strictures. If realignment of the damaged urethra cannot be achieved, then suprapubic catheterization, followed by delayed combined antegrade and retrograde endoscopic repair or open surgical repair, is undertaken.

In contrast to posterior urethral injuries, which are often associated with many other pelvic injuries, anterior urethral injuries are often isolated and associated with straddle injuries. The bulbar urethra is typically the site of injury. The best initial treatment modality for anterior urethral injuries is not well defined; however, most would agree that primary realignment with a Foley catheter is the best initial treatment. In cases of severe anterior urethral injury, a suprapubic catheter may be required, followed by delayed open surgical repair.

External Genitalia Injuries

The most common cause of penile amputation is genital self-mutilation. If the amputated penis is available, reattachment of the penis is recommended by most; however, the clinician is often challenged by the overriding psychiatric issues that led to the act of penile amputation. Psychiatric consultation is always sought to assess the risk for further self-mutilation.

Penile "fracture" or rupture of the corpus cavernosum (see Figs. 77-10 and 77-11) from trauma to the erect penis most commonly occurs by striking the symphysis pubis or the perineum during sexual intercourse. Presentation of penile fracture includes trauma to the erect penis, followed by a "popping" sound, pain, and immediate detumescence. Penile fractures are associated with urethral injuries in 38% of cases.[9] Therefore, urethrography is performed in suspected cases when the patient has blood at the meatus, gross hematuria, or inability to void. Immediate repair of the penile injury is recommended because there is lower risk for penile deformity, faster recover, and less morbidity.[10]

The risk for testicular rupture after blunt trauma to the scrotum is greater than 50%. The most common causes are assaults, sports injuries, and motor vehicle crashes. Surgical exploration and repair of significant hematocele, intratesticular hematoma, or rupture of tunica albuginea is recommended.[11]

EMERGENT UROLOGIC CONDITIONS

Fournier's Gangrene

Fournier's gangrene is a necrotizing fasciitis of the male genitalia and perineum that primarily involves subcutaneous tissues. The disease can rapidly progress and, although mortality is dependent on severity of disease, it has exceeded 50% in some series.[12] The most common cause of Fournier's gangrene is infection of the colon, rectum, or lower genitourinary tract or cutaneous infection of the genitals, perineum, or anus. The most common risk factors are diabetes mellitus, alcohol use, and immunocompromised states. Infections can spread along the dartos, Collie's, and Scarpa's fascia because these fascial planes are continuous. The spread of infection rarely involves the deep fascial planes and musculature.

Both aerobic and anaerobic organisms can cause the infection. The most common isolated organism is *Escherichia coli;* other commonly cultured organisms include enterococci, staphylococci, streptococci, *Bacteroides fragilis,* and *Pseudomonas aeruginosa.*

The presenting sign is usually a painful swelling and induration of the penis, scrotum, or perineum. Cellulitis, eschar, necrosis, crepitus, foul odor, and fever may be accompanying signs.

Aggressive surgical débridement of all necrotic, ischemic, and infected tissue, along with copious irrigation, are critical. Infected tissue is cultured and initial broad-spectrum IV antibiotic coverage (e.g., ampicillin, gentamicin, and clindamycin) instituted. Suprapubic catheter placement can help divert the urine and decrease the risk for further bacterial seeding of the wound.

If a colonic source is the suspected cause, proctoscopy under general anesthesia can be performed, and if necessary, diverting colostomy may be indicated. Additional débridement in 24 hours after the initial débridement may be necessary. Careful attention to wound care, frequent dressing changes, strict control of diabetes and metabolites, and adequate nutritional support are critical to proper wound healing.

Testicular Torsion

Testicular torsion is a urologic emergency that requires rapid diagnosis and intervention in order to maintain viability to the testicle. There are two types of testicular torsion: extravaginal and intravaginal. Extravaginal torsion is diagnosed in newborns and is caused by nonadherence of tunica vaginalis to the dartos layer. As a result, the spermatic cord and tunica vaginalis are rotated as a unit. Intravaginal torsion is usually diagnosed in boys 12 to 18 years of age, but it can occur at any age. The etiology of intravaginal torsion is malrotation of the spermatic cord with the tunica vaginalis. Both extravaginal (newborn) and intravaginal (adolescent) types of testicular torsion lead to strangulation of blood supply to the testis.

Presentation of testicular torsion is acute onset of testicular pain or swelling. Some patients may have episodic symptoms of pain suggestive of intermittent torsion. Physical examination may reveal a tender firm testicle, high riding testicle, horizontal lie of testicle, absent cremasteric reflex, and no pain relief with elevation of the testicle. The spermatic cord may appear thickened. The posteriorly positioned epididymis may be positioned differently.

Table 77-1 Causes of Low- and High-Flow Priapism

Low-Flow
Sickle cell trait and disease
Leukemia (especially chronic myelogenous leukemia
Total parenteral nutrition (especially with 20% lipid infusion)
Medications (e.g., sildenafil, trazodone, chlorpromazine, topical and systemic cocaine)
Intracavernosal injections
Malignant penile infiltration
Hyperosmolar intravenous contrast
Spinal cord injury (usually self-limiting with no treatment required)
Spinal or general anesthesia (usually self-limiting with no treatment required)

High-Flow
Perineal or penile trauma

Diagnosis of testicular torsion is made mainly by clinical suspicion. When uncertain, color Doppler ultrasound or a nuclear testicular scan may help with the diagnosis. In the case of epididymo-orchitis, Doppler ultrasound would demonstrate increased blood flow, and radionuclide can would show increased radionuclide activity. In the case of testicular torsion, however, Doppler would show no blood flow, and radionuclide scan would show poor radionuclide tracer uptake.

Immediate surgical exploration is indicated if testicular torsion is suspected. If treated within the first 4 to 6 hours of onset of symptoms, the chance of testicular salvage is high. During surgical exploration, the testicle is rotated to its normal position to restore blood flow to the testicle. If viable, orchiopexy of the affected and the contralateral testicle is completed. If the affected testicle is nonviable, orchiectomy of the affected testicle and orchiopexy of the contralateral side are performed.

If an operating facility is not immediately available, manual detorsion by external rotation of the testicle toward the thigh for intravaginal (adolescent) torsion can be attempted.

Priapism

Priapism is a pathologic condition of a penile erection that persists beyond or is unrelated to sexual stimulation. Except in cases of the nonischemic type, priapism is often accompanied by pain and tenderness. It can occur in all age groups, including the newborn, but the peak incidence is seen from ages 5 to 10 and 20 to 50 years. In the younger group, priapism is most often associated with sickle cell disease or neoplasm; in the older group, priapism is often caused by pharmacologic agents. Low-flow (veno-occlusive, or type I) priapism accounts for most cases (Table 77-1). Because of decreased venous outflow and increased intracavernosal pressure, low-flow priapism is associated with a painful, fully erect penis, causing local hypoxia and acidosis. In addition, the penile glans is engorged.

Table 77-2 Intracavernous Vasoconstrictor Therapy for Low-Flow Priapism*

DRUG	RECOMMENDED DOSAGE
Epinephrine	10-20 µg
Phenylephrine	250-500 µg
Ephedrine	50-100 mg

*Intracavernous injection every 5 minutes until detumescence after aspiration of 10-20 mL of blood.

In contrast to low-flow priapism, high-flow (type II) priapism is associated with increased arterial inflow without increased venous outflow resistance, thus resulting in high inflow and high outflow (see Table 77-1). As a result, the penis is erect but nontender in high-flow priapism states. The penile glans is usually soft and nontender.

Low-flow priapism can be distinguished from high-flow priapism by obtaining a corporal blood gas. Measurements of PO_2 <30, PCO_2 >60, and pH <7.25 are consistent with low-flow priapism. If the patient has a history of sickle cell disease (or trait), IV hydration, alkalinization with bicarbonate in IV fluid, analgesia, and supplemental oxygen can help reduce the veno-occlusive state in the corporal bodies. If the low-flow priapism persists in the sickle cell patient, red blood cell transfusion to increase the hemoglobin above 10 and reduce the hemoglobin S below 30% of total hemoglobin can help reduce the severity of priapism.

Low-flow priapism may require corporal irrigation with normal saline. The mid shaft of the penis can be injected with a small-gauge butterfly needle and irrigated with 10 to 20 mL of normal saline. After irrigation with normal saline, α-adrenergic intracorporal injections every 5 minutes until detumescence can be used to correct low-flow priapism (Table 77-2). The patient's blood pressure and pulse are monitored during intracorporeal α-adrenergic treatments. In severe cases when intracorporal α-adrenergic treatment fails to treat low-flow priapism, surgical procedure with shunts (corporoglandular, corporospongiosal, or corporosaphenous) may be necessary to divert the occluded corporal blood.

High-flow priapism can be confirmed by a perineal Doppler ultrasound or arteriography performed to identify an arterial-lacunar fistula responsible for the priapism. High-flow priapism can be treated expectantly, and if not resolved, arterial embolization or open surgical arterial ligation may be required.

NEPHROLITHIASIS

The prevalence of renal calculi varies with the population studied, and rates of nephrolithiasis vary regionally. About 3% to 12% of the population will develop symptomatic nephrolithiasis during their lifetime. Eighty percent of patients with nephrolithiasis form calcium stones, most of which are composed primarily of calcium oxalate or, less often, calcium phosphate.[13] The other main types include uric acid, struvite (magnesium ammonium phosphate), and cystine stones. A combination of different stone types may exist within a single stone.

Stone formation occurs when normally soluble material (e.g., calcium) supersaturates the urine and begins the process of crystal formation. It is not clear how crystals formed in the tubules become a stone, rather than being washed away by the high rate of urine flow. It is presumed that crystal aggregates become large enough to be anchored (usually at the end of the collecting ducts), and then slowly increase in size over time. This anchoring is thought to occur at sites of epithelial cell injury, perhaps induced by the crystals themselves.

Major risk factors associated with idiopathic nephrolithiasis, which accounts for most symptomatic stones, include the following:

- Low urine volume
- Hypercalciuria
- Hyperoxaluria
- Hyperuricosuria
- Dietary factors
  - Low fluid intake
  - Types of fluid intake—sodas, apple juice, grapefruit juice
  - High sodium chloride intake
  - High protein intake
  - Low calcium intake
- History of prior nephrolithiasis
- Hyperoxaluria (enteric hyperoxaluria, short bowel syndrome)
- Type I renal tubular acidosis

Patients may occasionally be diagnosed with asymptomatic nephrolithiasis when a radiologic imaging study of the abdomen is performed for other purposes. Symptoms are usually produced when stones pass from the renal pelvis into the ureter. Pain is the most common symptom and varies from a mild and barely noticeable ache to severe pain requiring parenteral analgesics. Pain typically waxes and wanes in severity, and develops in waves or paroxysms that are related to movement of the stone in the ureter and associated ureteral spasm. The site of obstruction from the stone generally determines the location of pain. The referred pain associated with the renal colic usually originates from the flank and radiates to the front upper abdomen for kidney-related pain or radiates to the front toward the groin (Fig. 77-18). Often microscopic hematuria and less commonly gross hematuria are associated with the patient with acute nephrolithiasis; however, lack of hematuria does not rule out nephrolithiasis.

The diagnosis of nephrolithiasis is initially suspected by the clinical presentation. Confirmatory radiologic tests include abdominal plain film (kidney-ureter-bladder), IVP, ultrasonography, and non–contrast-enhanced CT scan. At our institution, non–contrast CT is the test of choice for accurate and rapid diagnosis of symptomatic nephrolithiasis (Fig. 77-19).

Many patients with acute renal colic can be managed conservatively with pain medication and hydration until the stone passes spontaneously. Based on axial

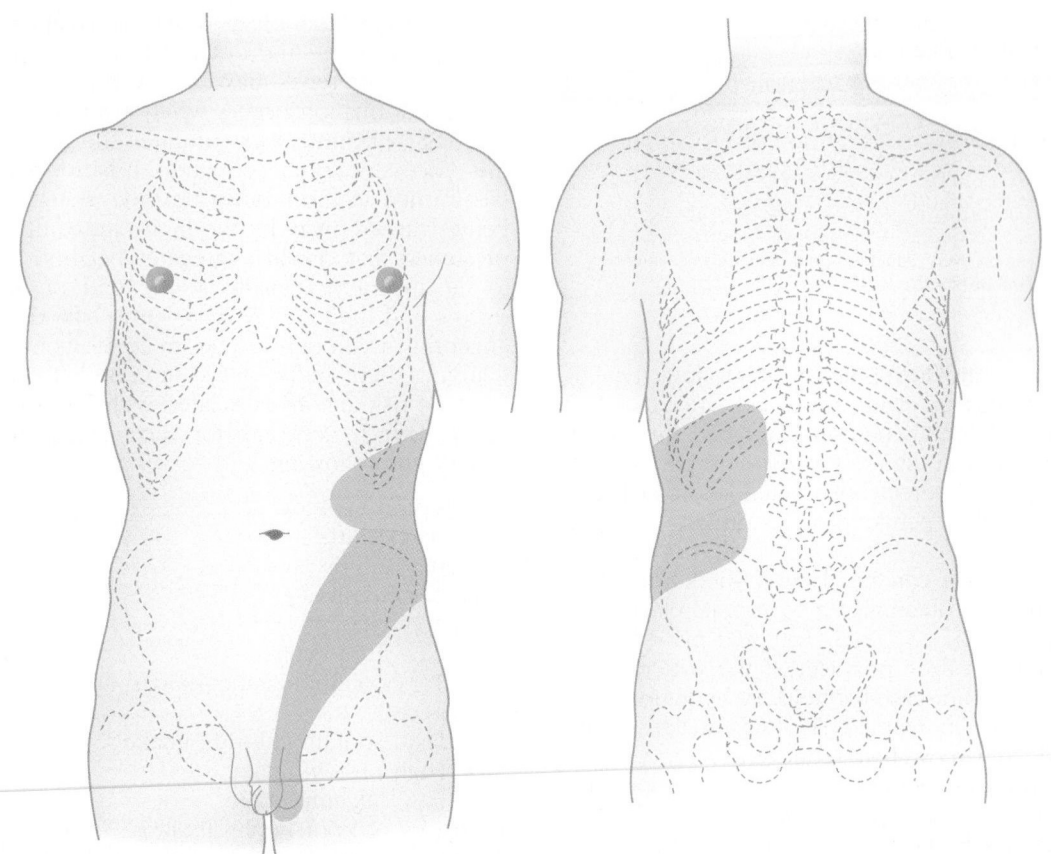

Figure 77-18 Referred pain from kidney (*dotted areas*) and ureter (*shaded areas*). (From Tanagho E, McAninch JW [eds]: Smith's General Urology, 15th ed. New York, McGraw-Hill, 2000.)

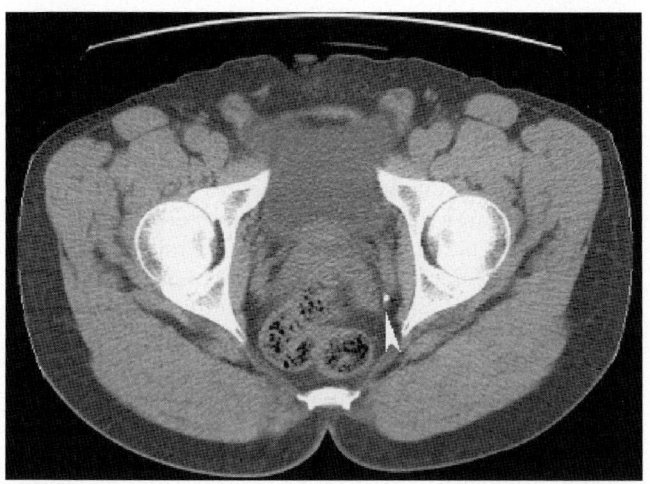

Figure 77-19 CT scan of the pelvis demonstrating ureterolithiasis in the distal left ureter (*arrowhead*).

Table 77-3 Spontaneous Rate of Stone Passage Based on Size and Location of Stone

STONE SIZE (mm)	STONES PASSED (%)
1	87
2-4	76
5-7	60
7-9	48
>9	25

STONE LOCATION	STONES PASSED (%)
Proximal ureter	48
Mid ureter	60
Distal ureter	75
Ureterovesical junction	79

From Coll DM, Varanelli MJ, Smith RC: Relationship of spontaneous passage of ureteral calculi to stone size and location as revealed by unenhanced helical CT. AJR Am J Roentgenol 178:101-103, 2002.

dimension of the stone determined by CT scan, the spontaneous rate of stone passage is dependent on the stone size and location of the stone[14] (Table 77-3). Recent evidence suggests that α-adrenergic blockers, which are usually used for treatment of bladder outlet obstruction in men, can potentiate the likelihood of ureteral stone expulsion during an acute ureteral colic episode in both men and women.[15-17]

Treatment of urinary lithiasis is dependent on the size and location of the stone in addition to the severity of symptoms associated with the stone. Patients who are suspected of having uric acid stones (those with urine pH <6.5, radiolucent calculi on plain films) can be treated with oral bicarbonate or potassium citrate supplementation to alkalinize the urine. If urine pH is alkalinized above 7.0, the chance of spontaneous dissolution of stone by 3 months is great. Open surgery for nephrolithiasis is seldom performed in the United States because of advances in minimally invasive techniques using extracorporeal shock-wave lithotripsy (mainly used for renal and proximal ureteral stones <2 cm), percutaneous litho­tripsy (mainly used for renal stones >2 cm), and ureteroscopy (used in treatment of renal and ureteral stones).

NEUROGENIC BLADDER

Micturition is a complex process involving the central nervous system, autonomic nervous system, and detrusor and sphincter muscle systems. The storage phase of micturition requires a bladder that can accommodate large urine volumes with low bladder pressure, which is accomplished by reflex inhibition of detrusor muscle. The relationship between change in bladder volume and bladder pressure is referred to as *compliance* of the bladder. Normal micturition begins with relaxation of external sphincter followed by relaxation and opening of the bladder neck and contraction of the detrusor. Complex interactions in the central nervous system are coordinated between cerebral motor cortex, basal ganglia, cerebellum, pontine nuclei, and sacral cord nuclei. Disruption in any of the central nervous system, autonomic nervous system, or the detrusor-sphincter mechanisms can lead to a neurogenic bladder.

To determine which particular pathway is responsible for a neurogenic bladder, a detailed history, physical examination, and evaluation of the voiding pattern using a voiding diary are essential. Detailed questioning about the sensation of filling and urgency assesses sensory function. Urodynamics evaluations, which include a cystometrogram, help to analyze the strength and timing of detrusor contraction and bladder compliance. Cystometrogram can assess the presence of any uninhibited or hyperreflexic bladder contractions. The urinary sphincter is assessed by urethral pressure profiles and electromyography. Postvoid residual volume can help determine the efficiency of voiding. Fluoroscopic voiding studies help to determine the anatomic position of the bladder and the urethra during the storage and the micturition phases. Renal ultrasound assesses for any potential hydronephrosis associated with high bladder pressures.

The primary therapeutic goal of treating patients with neurogenic bladder is preservation of renal function and restoring normal urinary patterns. Anticholinergic therapy can help in decreasing the frequency and severity of any uninhibited bladder contractions and improving bladder compliance. α-Adrenergic compounds can be used to increase sphincteric resistance when necessary. Clean intermittent catheterization is an efficient, relatively easy, and safe method of ensuring bladder emptying with a wide range of applications. Because of a lower rate of urinary tract infection, clean intermittent catheterization is the preferred method of ensuring efficient bladder emptying over chronic indwelling urethral catheterization. Many patients may require a combination of medicines and manipulations to minimize urinary incontinence, improve bladder emptying, prevent urinary infections, and preserve renal function.

Patients with severe bladder dysfunction who develop high-pressure, poorly compliant bladders secondary to a variety of causes such as bladder extrophy, myelomeningocele, or spinal cord injuries may require augmentation cystoplasty (usually performed by using gastrointestinal segments as donor tissue for cystoplasty) to maximize the bladder volume and minimize the bladder pressures.[18,19] Recent advances in tissue engineering may prove useful by using patients' autologous bladder cells in combination with collagen-based scaffolds to maximize bladder volume and reduce pressure in patients who would otherwise be treated by standard gastrointestinal cystoplasty techniques.[20]

BENIGN PROSTATIC HYPERPLASIA

Benign prostatic hyperplasia (BPH) is a common entity among elderly men and is responsible for significant disability; however, it is an infrequent cause of death. In men 20 to 30 years of age, the prostate weighs about 20 g; however, the mean prostatic weight increases after the age of 50. The prevalence of histologically diagnosed prostatic hyperplasia increases from 8% in men aged 31 to 40 years, to 40% to 50% in men aged 51 to 60 years, to more than 80% in men older than age 80 years. The Baltimore Longitudinal Study of Aging compared the age-specific prevalence of pathologically defined BPH at autopsy with the clinical prevalence based on history and the results of digital rectal examination. There was good agreement between the clinical prevalence and autopsy incidence in men of all ages.

The natural history of BPH as studied by a population-based study in Olmstead County, Minnesota demonstrated that lower urinary tract symptoms associated with BPH increase with age.[21] In most men, symptoms are progressive and eventually require medical or surgical treatment. Men with symptomatic BPH who are not treated have a 2.5% risk per year for developing urinary retention. Predictive risk factors associated with chance of developing urinary retention include age, symptoms, urinary flow rate, and prostate size.[21]

Race has some influence on the risk for BPH severe enough to require surgery. Although the age-adjusted relative risk for BPH necessitating surgery is similar in black and white men, black men younger than 65 years may need treatment more often than white men. In the American Male Health Professional Study, men of Asian ancestry were less likely (relative risk, 0.4; 95% confidence interval, 0.2-0.8) to undergo surgery for BPH as compared with white men, and black men had risk similar to white men.[22]

Androgens are necessary for both normal and abnormal development of the prostate. Testosterone is converted to a more potent androgen, dihydrotestosterone (DHT), by the enzyme 5-α reductase type 2. The type 1 form of the enzyme is present in liver and skin.

Men who congenitally lack 5-α reductase type 2 enzyme have normal serum testosterone levels but lack dihydrotestosterone.[23] Men with this disorder have a rudimentary prostate throughout life but rarely experience bladder outlet obstruction secondary to BPH. These findings suggest that the active androgen, DHT, is important in promoting growth of prostate that would eventually lead to symptomatic BPH.

Most of the prostatic nodules responsible for the bladder outlet obstructive symptoms associated with BPH arise in the periurethral tissue (see Fig. 77-9). The hyperplastic nodules comprise primarily stromal components and to a lesser degree epithelial cells; stereologic measurements have revealed a fourfold increase in stroma and a twofold increase in glandular components. It has been suggested that the stromal-epithelial component of prostatic tissue significantly increases in men with symptomatic BPH. Because BPH is primarily a disease of the stroma, the stroma might have intrinsic properties that enable it to proliferate and also to induce hyperplasia of the epithelium. In the presence of androgen, mesenchymal tissue derived from the urogenital sinus can induce differentiation of prostate epithelium.[24] In contrast, stroma lacking functional androgen receptors cannot induce differentiation of normal epithelium. These observations emphasize the importance of the stroma in development of the prostate.

The common symptoms of BPH are increased frequency of urination, nocturia, hesitancy, urgency, and weak urinary stream. These symptoms typically appear slowly and progress gradually over a period of years. However, they are not specific for BPH. Furthermore, the correlation between symptoms and the presence of prostatic enlargement on rectal examination is poor. This discrepancy probably results from changes in bladder function that occur with aging and from enlargement of the transitional zone of the prostate that is not always evident on rectal examination (see Fig. 77-9).

It is critical to exclude causes of lower urinary tract symptom other than BPH before institution of any medical or surgical treatment. The differential diagnosis of lower urinary tract symptoms in addition to BPH includes the following:

- Urethral stricture
- Bladder neck contracture
- Carcinoma of the prostate
- Carcinoma of the bladder
- Bladder calculi
- Urinary tract infection and prostatitis
- Neurogenic bladder

Physical examination includes a detailed examination of the abdomen; genitalia; and prostate size, consistency, nodularity, and symmetry. Urinalysis, serum prostate specific antigen (PSA), and serum creatinine are routine laboratory evaluations for men with lower urinary tract symptoms.

Clinical testing with uroflowmetry and assessment of postvoid residual can help the clinician determine the severity of bladder outlet obstruction. In some cases, detailed urodynamics evaluations that include pressure flow studies, cystometrogram, and cystourethroscopy may be helpful in the diagnosis of causes of lower urinary tract symptoms other than BPH. The American Urological Association (AUA) symptom score was developed to better assess the severity of patients' lower urinary tract symptoms secondary to BPH[25] (Table 77-4). The AUA symptom score can be a useful tool to compare a patient's urinary symptoms before and after initiating therapy.

Medical treatment for BPH has played a major role in improving the symptoms associated with bladder outlet obstruction. Although 1 decade ago, surgical treatment may have been at the forefront of therapy for BPH, medical treatment is now the first line therapy for BPH. Medical therapy focuses on two aspects of the pathophysiology of BPH:

- A dynamic (physiologic, reversible) component related to the tension of prostatic smooth muscle in the prostate, prostate capsule, and bladder neck
- A fixed (structural) component related to the bulk of the enlarged prostate impinging on the urethra

The two classes of drugs, α-adrenergic antagonists (release smooth muscle tension) and 5-α reductase inhibitors (reduce the enlarged prostate size), act on each of these components mentioned.

The three most common α-adrenergic antagonists used in the United States are terazosin, doxazosin, and tamsulosin. α_1-Adrenergic antagonists act against the dynamic component of bladder outlet obstruction. Prostatic tissue contains two types of α-adrenergic receptors: α_1 and α_2. α_1 Receptors are abundant in the prostate and base of the bladder and sparse in the body of the bladder.[26] The density of these receptors is increased in hyperplastic prostatic tissue. In one report, there was a direct relationship between the smooth muscle content of prostatic tissue and the increase in maximal urinary flow rate in men with BPH treated with terazosin.

The most common 5-α reductase inhibitor used in the United States is finasteride. It acts by blocking the conversion of testosterone to the more potent androgen, DHT. The decreased serum and per-prostatic levels of DHT lead to reduction in prostatic size over time.

α Adrenergic blockers have been shown to be more efficacious than 5-α reductase inhibitors by improving the lower urinary tract symptoms associated with BPH. In a Veterans Administration Cooperative trial, 1229 men with BPH were randomly assigned to receive placebo, terazosin (10 mg/day), finasteride (5 mg/day) or combination of terazosin and finasteride.[27] The study concluded the following:

- Terazosin lowered the symptom score by 6.1 points (from 16.2-10.1) versus 2.6 points with placebo.
- Terazosin increased the peak urinary flow rate by 2.7 mL/second versus 1.4 mL/second with placebo.
- Finasteride alone was no better than placebo.
- The combination of finasteride and terazosin was no better than terazosin alone.

Although the Veterans Administration Cooperative trial did not find a benefit to combination of finasteride and terazosin after only 1 year of therapy,[27] the Medical Therapy of Prostatic Symptoms (MTOPS) study

Table 77-4   American Urological Association Urinary Symptom Score

1. Incomplete emptying: Over the past month, how often have you had a sensation of not emptying your bladder completely after you finished urinating?

Not at all	Less than 1 time in 5	Less than half the time	About half the time	More than half the time	Almost always	Your Score
0	1	2	3	4	5	

2. Frequency: Over the past month, how often have you had to urinate again less than 2 hours after you finished urinating?

Not at all	Less than 1 time in 5	Less than half the time	About half the time	More than half the time	Almost always	Your Score
0	1	2	3	4	5	

3. Intermittency: Over the past month, how often have you found that you stopped and started again several times when you urinated?

Not at all	Less than 1 time in 5	Less than half the time	About half the time	More than half the time	Almost always	Your Score
0	1	2	3	4	5	

4. Urgency: Over the past month, how often have you found it difficult to postpone urination?

Not at all	Less than 1 time in 5	Less than half the time	About half the time	More than half the time	Almost always	Your Score
0	1	2	3	4	5	

5. Weak-stream: Over the past month, how often have you had a weak stream?

Not at all	Less than 1 time in 5	Less than half the time	About half the time	More than half the time	Almost always	Your Score
0	1	2	3	4	5	

6. Straining: Over the past month, how often have you had to push or strain to begin urination?

Not at all	Less than 1 time in 5	Less than half the time	About half the time	More than half the time	Almost always	Your Score
0	1	2	3	4	5	

7. Nocturia: Over the past month or so, how many times did you get up to urinate from the time you went to bed until the time you got up in the morning?

None	1 time	2 times	3 times	4 times	5 or more times	Your Score
0	1	2	3	4	5	

Add up your scores for total AUA score = _____

Quality of Life Due to Urinary Symptoms: If you were to spend the rest of your life with your urinary condition just the way it is now, how would you feel about that? (Bold, Highlight, or Underline)

Delighted	Pleased	Mostly satisfied	Mixed	Mostly dissatisfied	Unhappy	Terrible

was designed as a multicenter randomized, placebo-controlled, double-masked clinical trial with a 4-year follow-up to assess whether combination of finasteride and terazosin was beneficial in reducing the risk for progression of BPH.[28] The MTOPS trial demonstrated that finasteride and combination of finasteride and doxazosin (another α-blocker equivalent to terazosin) significantly reduced the risk for BPH progression to the point of requiring invasive therapy (Fig. 77-20).

Surgical Treatments for Benign Prostatic Hyperplasia

Transurethral Resection of Prostate

Transurethral resection of prostate (TURP) is a proven surgical technique that significantly improves lower urinary tract symptoms associated with BPH.[29] This intervention is most commonly recommended in the patient with symptoms of bladder outlet obstruction and irritability that are moderate to severe, bothersome, and interfere with the patient's quality of life. Although symptoms constitute the primary reason for recommending intervention, in patients with an obstructing prostate, there are some absolute indications. These are acute urinary retention, recurrent infection, recurrent hematuria, and azotemia.

Transurethral resection (TUR) syndrome is an immediate postoperative complication that happens in 2% of TURP patients. Glycine, which is a hypotonic solution, is used during TURP. Excessive systemic absorption of glycine can lead to dilutional hyponatremia. The symptoms associated with TUR syndrome include con-

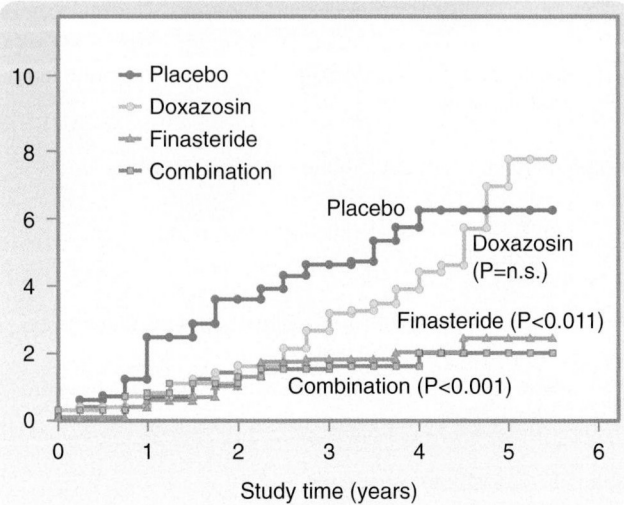

CUMULATIVE INCIDENCE OF BPH-RELATED INVASIVE THERAPY (%)

Figure 77-20 Medical Therapy of Prostatic Symptoms (MTOPS) trial demonstrating that finasteride when used alone or in combination with doxazosin (an α-adrenergic blocking agent) can reduce the cumulative incidence of invasive therapy related to benign prostatic hypertrophy. (Courtesy of Dr. Claus Roehrborn, University of Texas, Southwestern Medical Center.)

fusion, nausea, vomiting, hypertension, bradycardia, and visual disturbance. Usually, the patient does not become symptomatic until the serum sodium concentration reaches 125 mEq/dL. The risk is increased if the gland is larger than 45 g, the resection time is longer than 90 minutes, or the irrigant fluid is greater than 70 cm H_2O above the patient. All these factors lead to greater fluid absorption and increase the risk for the syndrome. Other potential causes of TUR syndrome include conversion of glycine to glycolic acid and ammonium. Glycolytic acid and ammonium, which are byproducts of glycine, may be responsible for some of the side effects of confusion and metabolic abnormalities observed in these patients.

Furosemide (Lasix) can be used to treat the hyponatremia associated with TUR syndrome. Combination of diuretic and decreasing fluid overload gradually treats the hyponatremia over 8 to 12 hours. In severe cases, slow infusion of 3% saline can be used to slowly correct the hyponatremia.

To avoid TUR syndrome associated with the standard TURP, newer technologies that use isotonic saline as opposed to hypotonic solutions have emerged.[30] Because these newer technologies use isotonic saline, systemic fluid absorption is not associated with hyponatremia as is the case with standard TURP. Therefore, larger prostate glands can be resected with less perioperative risk.

Open Prostatectomy

Indications for open prostatectomy are the same as for TURP. Open prostatectomy instead of TURP is the preferred technique for treatment of bladder outlet obstruction from BPH when the prostate is estimated to weight

more than 100 g. Open prostatectomy also needs to be considered when a man presents with ankylosis of the hip or other orthopedic conditions, preventing proper positioning in dorsal lithotomy for TURP.

Open prostatectomy can be performed by a retropubic or a suprapubic approach. With either technique, the prostatic adenoma (periurethral central zone) is removed while the prostatic capsule or the peripheral zone of the prostate remains behind (see Fig. 77-9). After open prostatectomy, patients remain at risk for developing prostate cancer in the peripheral zone of the prostate and need to continue to be monitored.

Minimally Invasive Therapy for Benign Prostatic Hyperplasia

During the past few years, minimally invasive therapies that use some form of thermotherapy have been developed, including transurethral needle ablation (TUNA)[31] and transurethral microwave therapy (TUMT),[32] for ablation of the enlarged prostate gland. The advantage of these procedures is that they have less morbidity than TURP and open prostatectomy. Most notably, prostate thermotherapy for treatment of BPH has fewer sexual side effects (e.g., retrograde ejaculation) than TURP and open prostatectomy. However, results of long-term efficacy, safety, and retreatment are lacking at this time. Minimally invasive therapies are particularly useful in patients taking anticoagulants, patients who are poor surgical candidates, and younger men who are sexually active and would like to avoid the risk for retrograde ejaculation commonly encountered with surgical therapies for BPH.

SCROTAL MASSES

In order for the clinician to differentiate between the emergent and urgent scrotal conditions such as testicular torsion and testis cancer, knowledge of the anatomy of the scrotum and potential scrotal masses is essential. Scrotal and paratesticular masses are mostly benign conditions.

Hydrocele

A hydrocele consists of a collection of fluid within the tunica or processus vaginalis. Although it may occur within the spermatic cord, it is most often seen surrounding the testis (Fig. 77-21). Surgical correction is only required if the patient has symptoms secondary to the size of or discomfort associated with the hydrocele. Communicating hydrocele of infancy and childhood is secondary to a patent processus vaginalis, which is continuous with the peritoneal cavity. It is also a form of indirect inguinal hernia. Most communicating hydroceles spontaneously close by 1 year of age. However, persistent communicating hydroceles and presence of bowel content within the hydrocele sac may require surgical correction.

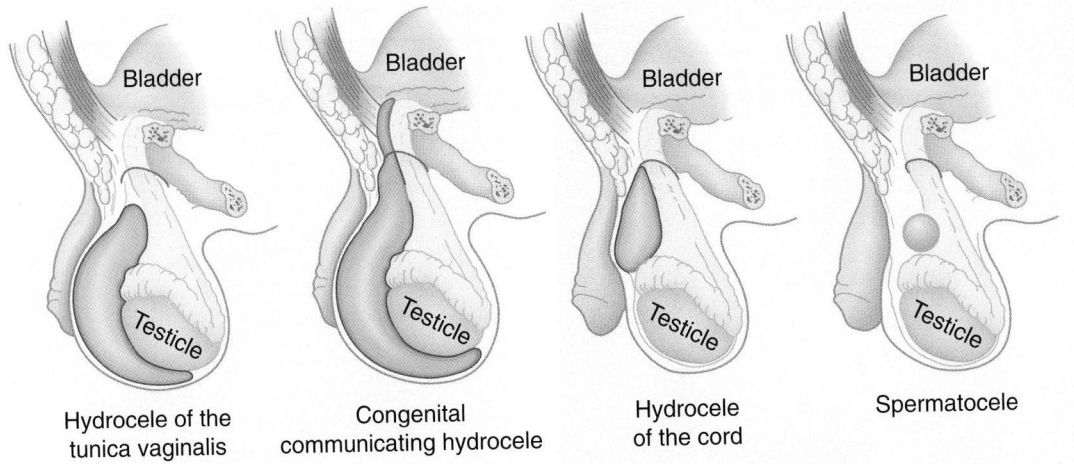

Figure 77-21 Hydrocele of the tunica vaginalis and cord; spermatocele. (From Tanagho E, McAninch JW [eds]: Smith's General Urology, 15th ed. New York, McGraw-Hill, 2000.)

Spermatocele

A spermatocele is a painless fluid-filled sac with sperm that is often located above and posterior to the testicle. Although most spermatoceles are smaller than 1 cm, some may become large and hard, mimicking a solid neoplasm. Spermatocele is differentiated from hydrocele of the tunica vaginalis in that the latter covers the entire anterior surface of the testicle. Spermatoceles do not require intervention unless the patient experiences discomfort associated with it.

Torsion of Testicular Appendix and Epididymis

At the upper pole of the testis and epididymis, there are small vestigial appendices that can spontaneously undergo torsion. A very reactive inflammatory reaction leading to testicular and scrotal swelling can follow ischemic necrosis of the appendix testis. It may be difficult to differentiate between torsion of the testicular appendix and torsion of the spermatic cord. If clinical diagnosis is uncertain, immediate surgical exploration is necessary because in the case of spermatic cord torsion, time is of the essence to restore blood supply to a viable testis.

Varicocele

Varicocele is a result of dilation of veins that drain into the internal spermatic veins. About 10% of young men have varicoceles, with the left side most commonly affected. Typically, varicoceles arise secondary to incompetent internal spermatic vein valves. However, the presence of unilateral right-sided varicocele raises the suspicion of poor drainage at the junction of the right testicular vein and right renal vein, which could be secondary to a large right-sided renal mass. In addition, the sudden onset of varicocele in an older man raises the suspicion of a retroperitoneal mass leading to inadequate drainage of the testicular veins.

Examination of a man with varicocele when he is upright reveals a mass of dilated, tortuous veins lying posterior to and above the testis. It may extend up to the external inguinal ring, and the Valsalva maneuver can increase the degree of dilation.

Sperm concentration and motility is significantly decreased in 65% to 75% of subjects. Infertility is observed in a higher percentage of individuals with varicoceles than the rest of the population. Surgical ligation for the dilated internal spermatic veins may restore fertility; however, in the absence of infertility, poor testicular growth in the adolescent, or patient discomfort, surgical intervention is not indicated.

UROLOGIC MALIGNANCIES

Renal Cell Carcinoma

Renal cell carcinomas, which originate within the renal cortex, are responsible for 80% to 85% of all primary renal neoplasms. Transitional cell carcinomas of the renal pelvis are the next most common (~8%). Other parenchymal epithelial tumors, such as oncocytomas, collecting duct tumors, and renal sarcomas, occur infrequently. Nephroblastoma or Wilms' tumor is common in children (5%-6% of all primary renal tumors).

Patients with renal cell carcinoma present with a range of symptoms, but many are asymptomatic until the disease is advanced. At presentation, about 25% of individuals have either distant metastases or significant local disease. Other patients, despite having only localized disease, present with a wide array of symptoms and laboratory abnormalities. Fever, cachexia, amyloidosis, anemia, hepatic dysfunction, and hormonal abnormalities are some of the features of the paraneoplastic syndrome complex associated with renal cell carcinoma. Renal cell carcinomas may produce a host of hormones, including erythropoietin, parathyroid hormone–related protein (PTHrP), gonadotropins, human chorionic somatomammotropin, an ACTH-like substance, renin, glucagon, and insulin. Because of this unusual paraneoplastic characteristic, renal cell carcinoma has been labeled the *internist's tumor*. The *classic triad of renal cell carcinoma,* which

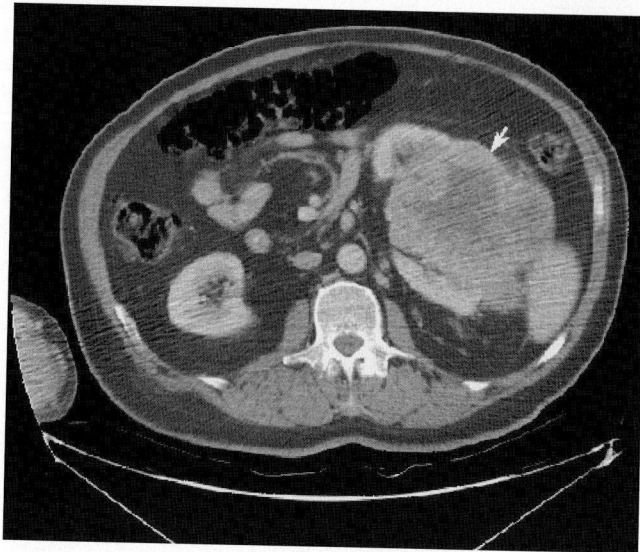

Figure 77-22 CT scan of abdomen demonstrates a large enhancing left renal mass consistent with renal cell carcinoma (*arrow*).

Table 77-5	TNM Classification for Renal Cell Carcinoma

Primary Tumor (T)	
TX	Primary tumor cannot be assessed
T0	No evidence of primary tumor
T1	Tumor 7 cm or less in greatest dimension, limited to the kidney
T1a	Tumor 4 cm or less in greatest dimension, limited to the kidney
T1b	Tumor more than 4 cm but not more than 7 cm in greatest dimension, limited to the kidney
T2	Tumor more than 7 cm in greatest dimension, limited to the kidney
T3	Tumor extends into major veins or invades adrenal gland or perinephric tissues but not beyond Gerota's fascia
T3a	Tumor directly invades adrenal gland or perirenal and/or renal sinus fat but not beyond Gerota's fasica
T3b	Tumor grossly extends into the renal vein or its segmental (muscle-containing) branches, or vena cava below the diaphragm
T3c	Tumor grossly extends into vena cava above diaphragm or invades the wall of the vena cava
T4	Tumor invades beyond Gerota's fascia

Regional Lymph Nodes (N)	
NX	Regional lymph nodes cannot be assessed
N0	No regional lymph node metastases
N1	Metastases in a single regional lymph node
N2	Metastases in more than one regional lymph node

Distant Metastasis (M)	
MX	Distant metastasis cannot be assessed
M0	No distant metastasis
M1	Distant metastasis

is defined as flank pain, hematuria, and a palpable abdominal renal mass, is uncommon (9% of patients); when present, it strongly suggests metastatic disease.

With increasing use of radiologic modalities, there has been a significant rise in the incidence of renal cancer in the United States. During the past decade, CT scan has replaced IVP and ultrasound as the radiologic modality of choice to evaluate renal masses. Characteristic features of renal cell carcinoma on CT scan include enhancement of the lesion after injection of IV contrast (Fig. 77-22), thickened irregular walls, thickened or enhanced septa within the mass, or multilocular mass. Magnetic resonance imaging (MRI) can be used for defining poorly characterized renal masses on CT scan, or when CT scan is contraindicated in cases of allergy to IV contrast or poor renal function. In addition, MRI is very helpful in defining tumor extension into the renal vein or IVC.

Clinical staging (Table 77-5) using the best available radiologic modality is crucial before therapy. Surgical therapy is principally offered to patients with early renal cell carcinoma in whom it may be curative. This includes patients in whom preoperative staging suggests that the tumor is either stage I or II, representing small (<7 cm) or large (>7 cm) growths limited to the kidney without evidence of lymph node or metastatic disease.

Slightly different surgical considerations involve patients in whom preoperative evaluation suggests that the renal cell carcinoma is stage III. Patients with this stage of disease include those with tumor invasion into the adrenal gland or perinephric tissues (but not extending beyond Gerota's fascia), those with enlarged abdominal lymph nodes, and those with invasion of the major veins (renal vein or IVC).

Among those with radiologic evidence of abdominal lymph node involvement, a standard radical nephrectomy is offered as a possible curative procedure because many nodes initially suspected of harboring tumor radiologically are enlarged only because of reactive inflammation.

Patients with stage IV disease have large tumors extending beyond Gerota's fascia, obvious evidence of extensive disease in regional lymph nodes, and frank metastases. Nephrectomy may be indicated for palliative reasons or as a component of clinical trials.

Renal cancer is not responsive to radiation and chemotherapy; therefore, radical nephrectomy remains the cornerstone of treatment for localized renal cancer. Radical nephrectomy consists of early ligation of the renal artery and vein and excision of the kidney and Gerota's fascia. Routine removal of the ipsilateral adrenal gland is uncommon, unless the tumor involves a large portion of the upper pole of the kidney or there is suggestion of adrenal gland involvement on preoperative radiologic exams.[33]

Immunotherapy[34] and new targeted kinase inhibitors[35] and antiangiogenic agents[36] have resulted in modest response in patients with advanced renal cancer, and their utility is under intense investigation. Cytoreductive nephrectomy followed by systemic therapy may be beneficial for patients with metastatic renal cell carcinoma.[37,38]

Urothelial Carcinoma

The epithelial lining comprising the renal pelvis, ureter, bladder, and proximal urethra is from transitional cell epithelium. Transitional cell carcinomas (TCCs) make up more than 90% of all urothelial cancers in the United States. Adenocarcinoma (2%), squamous cell carcinoma (5%-10%), undifferentiated carcinomas (2%), and mixed carcinomas (4%-6%) are other types of urothelial malignancies. TCCs commonly appear as papillary and exophytic lesions.

TCC of the renal pelvis or ureter accounts for less than 5% of all renal tumors and less than 1% of genitourinary neoplasms. The ratio of tumors of the bladder to those of the renal pelvis to those of the ureter is 51:3:1. However, in the Balkan countries (Bulgaria, Greece, Romania, Yugoslavia), an endemic familial nephropathy predisposes to renal pelvic neoplasms, which account for almost 50% of all renal tumors. The incidence of upper tract urothelial neoplasms has modestly increased during the past 20 years in the United States. The age-adjusted annual incidence in the National Cancer Institute Surveillance, Epidemiology and End Results (SEER) database increased from 0.69 to 0.73 per 100,000 person-years over the time period of 1973 to 1996.[39]

Cancer of the bladder is the 4th most common cancer in men and the 10th in women. More than 56,000 people (41,500 males and 15,000 females) develop bladder cancer each year in the United States, and 12,600 individuals (8600 males and 4000 females) are expected to die from the disease.

The surface epithelium (urothelium) that lines the mucosal surfaces of the entire urinary tract is exposed to potential carcinogens that may be excreted in the urine, or activated in the urine by hydrolyzing enzymes. Environmental exposures are thought to account for most cases of urothelial cancer. For example, a link between environmental factors and TCC of the urothelium was first suggested by the increased incidence of TCC in industrialized societies and urban dwellers. In addition, an increased incidence of renal pelvis and bladder carcinoma has been reported in aniline dye workers. Exposure to chemicals used in the aluminum, dye, paint, petroleum, rubber, and textile industries has been estimated to account for up to 20% of all bladder cancer cases.[40] Hairdressers and barbers have an excess risk for bladder cancer that is thought related to long-term exposure to permanent hair dyes. In most cases, the suspect carcinogens are arylamines or their derivatives, which take several years to accumulate, thus accounting for the long latency period before the development of bladder cancer.

Clinical manifestations of urothelial carcinoma include gross or microscopic hematuria, which is the most common symptom at the time of presentation, occurring in 70% to 95% of patients. For renal pelvis and ureteral malignancies, flank pain occurs in 8% to 40% of cases and may be precipitated by obstruction of the ureter or UPJ by the tumor mass. Bladder irritation and constitutional symptoms occur in less than 10% of patients with urothelial malignancies.

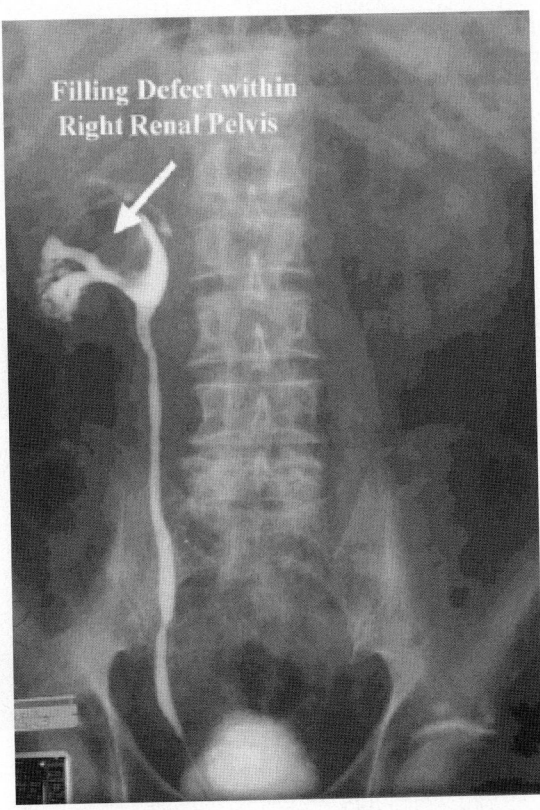

Figure 77-23 Retrograde pyelography demonstrating a filling defect in the right renal pelvis consistent with transitional cell carcinoma of renal pelvis.

In patients with a renal pelvis or ureteral tumor, diagnosis is commonly made by radiologic modalities that may include CT scan, IVP, or retrograde pyelography (Fig. 77-23). Ureteroscopy has been used for confirming upper urinary tract malignancies when radiologic modalities are not confirmatory. Cystoscopy is the main procedure used for diagnosing bladder carcinoma (Fig. 77-24).

Staging of urothelial malignancy is dependent on the depth of invasion of the tumor through the submucosal musculature or adjacent organs. Figure 77-25 demonstrates the staging system most commonly used for bladder carcinoma. More than 70% of all newly diagnosed bladder cancers are superficial, about 50% to 70% are Ta, 20% to 30% are T1, and 10% are carcinoma in situ.

The standard treatment of renal pelvis and upper ureteral urothelial carcinomas includes complete nephroureterectomy with excision of the distal ureteral cuff from the bladder. Distal ureteral tumors can be treated with segmental resection followed by reimplantation of the remainder of the ureter into the bladder. The initial treatment options for bladder carcinoma are dictated by the tumor stage, grade, size, and number of tumors detected. In general, low-grade, superficial tumors are treated by TUR of the bladder tumor with or without intravesical treatment, whereas muscle invasive tumors (stage T2 or higher) are treated with radical cystectomy with or without systemic chemotherapy (see Fig. 77-25 for staging of bladder carcinoma). Bacille Calmette-Guérin (BCG) is an attenuated strain of *Mycobacterium bovis* rendered completely avirulent by long-term cultivation on bile-glycero-potato medium, used in BCG vaccine for immunization against tuberculosis. BCG introduced intravesically has been shown to induce a major histocompatibility complex–mediated immunoresponse against bladder cancer. Intravesical treatment with BCG has been shown to decrease the rate of bladder cancer recurrence and risk for tumor progression. Table 77-6 summarizes the general guidelines for treatment of bladder carcinoma.

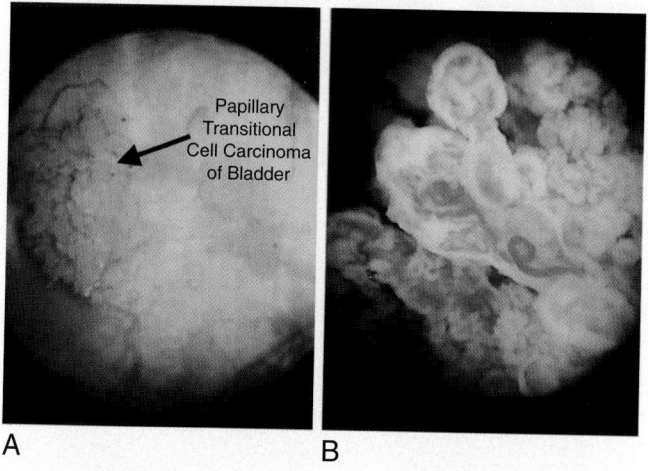

Figure 77-24 Cystoscopic views of papillary transitional cell carcinoma of the bladder with low (**A**) and high (**B**) magnifications.

Table 77-6 Guidelines for the Treatment of Transitional Cell Carcinoma of the Bladder

CANCER STAGE	INITIAL TREATMENT OPTION
Tis	TUR + intravesical immunotherapy (BCG)
Ta (single, small focus)	TUR
Ta (large, multifocal)	TUR + BCG or intravesical chemotherapy
T1 (low grade)	TUR + BCG or intravesical chemotherapy
T1 (high grade)	TUR + (BCG or intravesical chemotherapy) or radical cystectomy
T2-T4	Radical cystectomy Neoadjuvant chemotherapy + radical cystectomy Radical cystectomy + adjuvant chemotherapy Neoadjuvant chemotherapy + chemotherapy + irradiation
Any T, N+, M+	Systemic chemotherapy followed by selective surgery or irradiation

BCG, bacille Calmette-Guérin; TUR, transurethral resection.

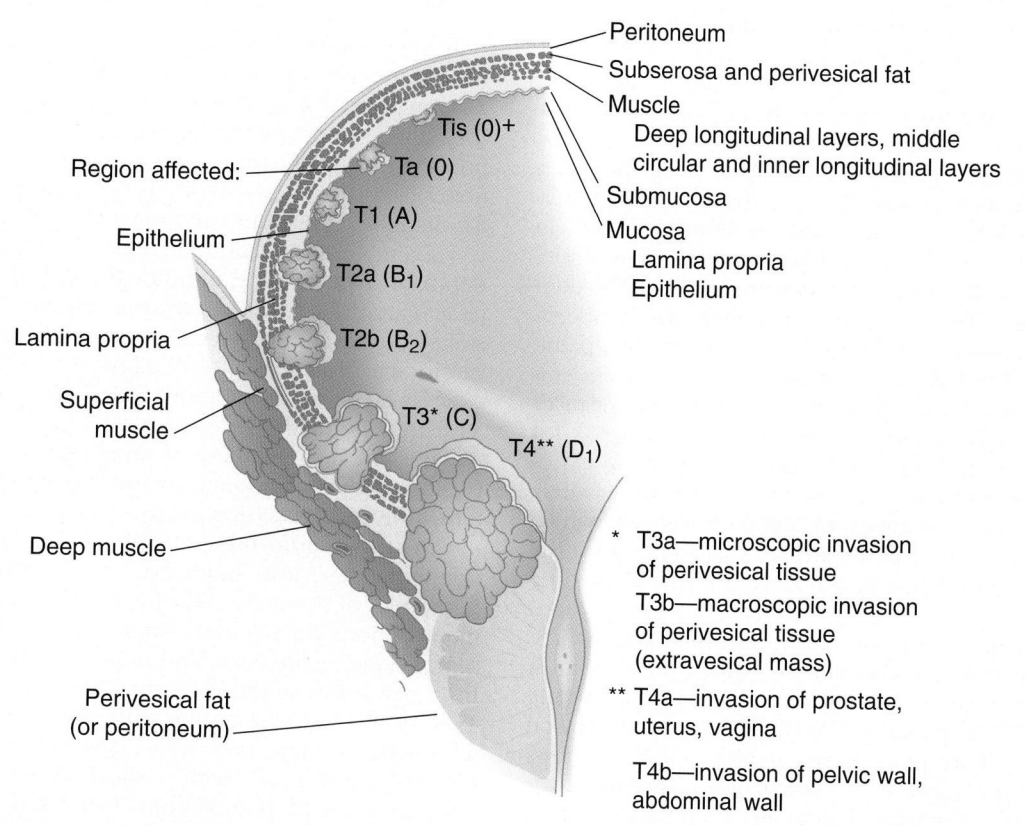

Figure 77-25 Staging of bladder cancer. (From Tanagho E, McAninch JW [eds]: Smith's General Urology, 15th ed. New York, McGraw-Hill, 2000.)

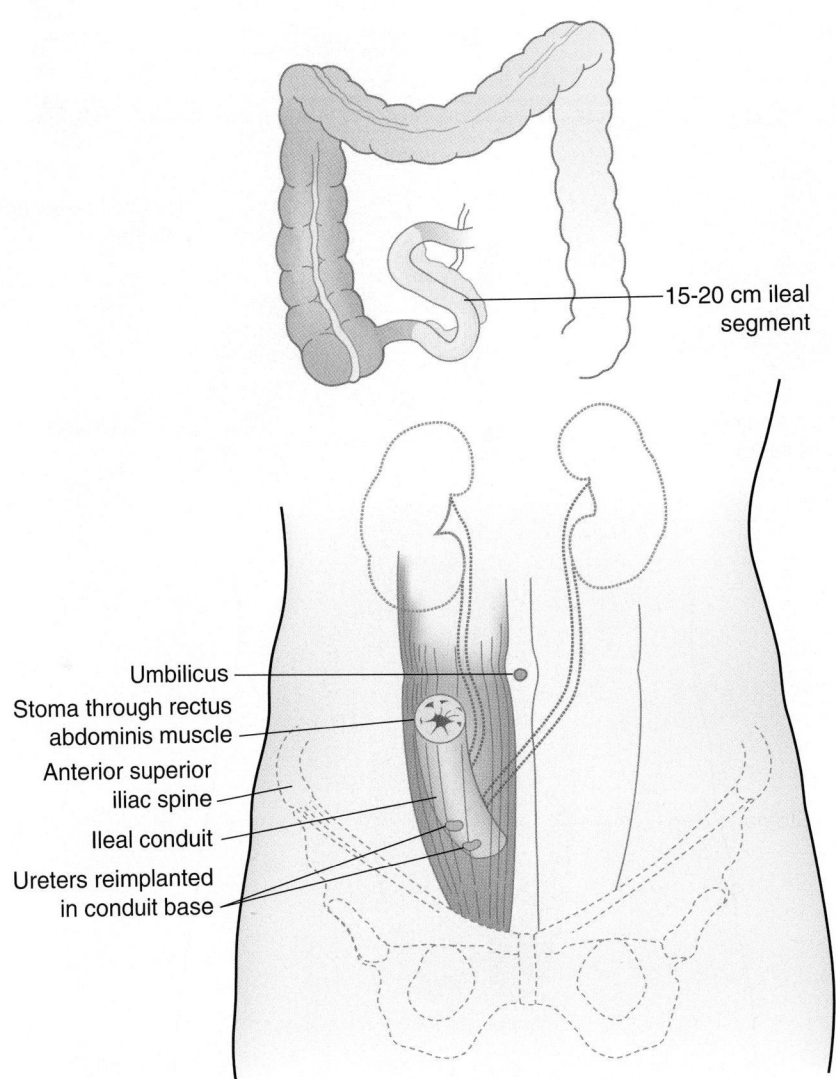

15-20 cm ileal segment

Umbilicus
Stoma through rectus abdominis muscle
Anterior superior iliac spine
Ileal conduit
Ureters reimplanted in conduit base

Figure 77-26 **Ileal conduit urinary reservoir.** (From Tanagho E, McAninch JW [eds]: Smith's General Urology, 15th ed. New York, McGraw-Hill, 2000.)

After radical cystectomy, a portion of small bowel, large bowel, or both is often used for diversion of the urine. Knowledge of the anatomy and potential metabolic complications associated with various urinary diversions is important for proper management of patients after urinary diversion. Ureteroileal urinary diversion is the most common method of urinary diversion in the United States. The conduit is constructed from a segment of the ileum about 15 to 20 cm proximal to the ileocecal valve (Fig. 77-26). In contrast to the ileal loop urinary diversion that requires constant drainage of urine into a drainage bag, continent urinary reservoirs (Fig. 77-27) are catheterized four to six times per day to drain the urine and do not require application of an abdominal urinary stoma. The biggest advance in urinary diversion during the past 2 decades has been the ability to perform continent orthotopic urinary diversion (Fig. 77-28) in both male and female patients.[41]

Early complications after urinary diversion include excessive bleeding, intestinal obstruction, urinary extrav-asation, and rupture and infection. Late complications include metabolic disorders, stomal stenosis, pyelonephritis, and formation of calculi. Metabolic abnormalities associated with colonic urinary diversions are dependent on the length and segment of bowel used in the urinary diversion. In general, when ileum or large bowel is used for urinary diversion, hyperchloremic metabolic acidosis may manifest. A potential complication of chronic long-term metabolic acidosis may be decreased bone calcium content and osteomalacia.

Prostate Carcinoma

Prostate cancer is the most common cancer in men in the United States except for nonmelanoma skin cancer. It is estimated that 234,460 men were diagnosed with prostate cancer in 2006 and that 27,350 deaths occurred. Prostate cancer has been detected with increasing frequency. The increase in detection is due in part to the widespread availability of tests for serum PSA and to

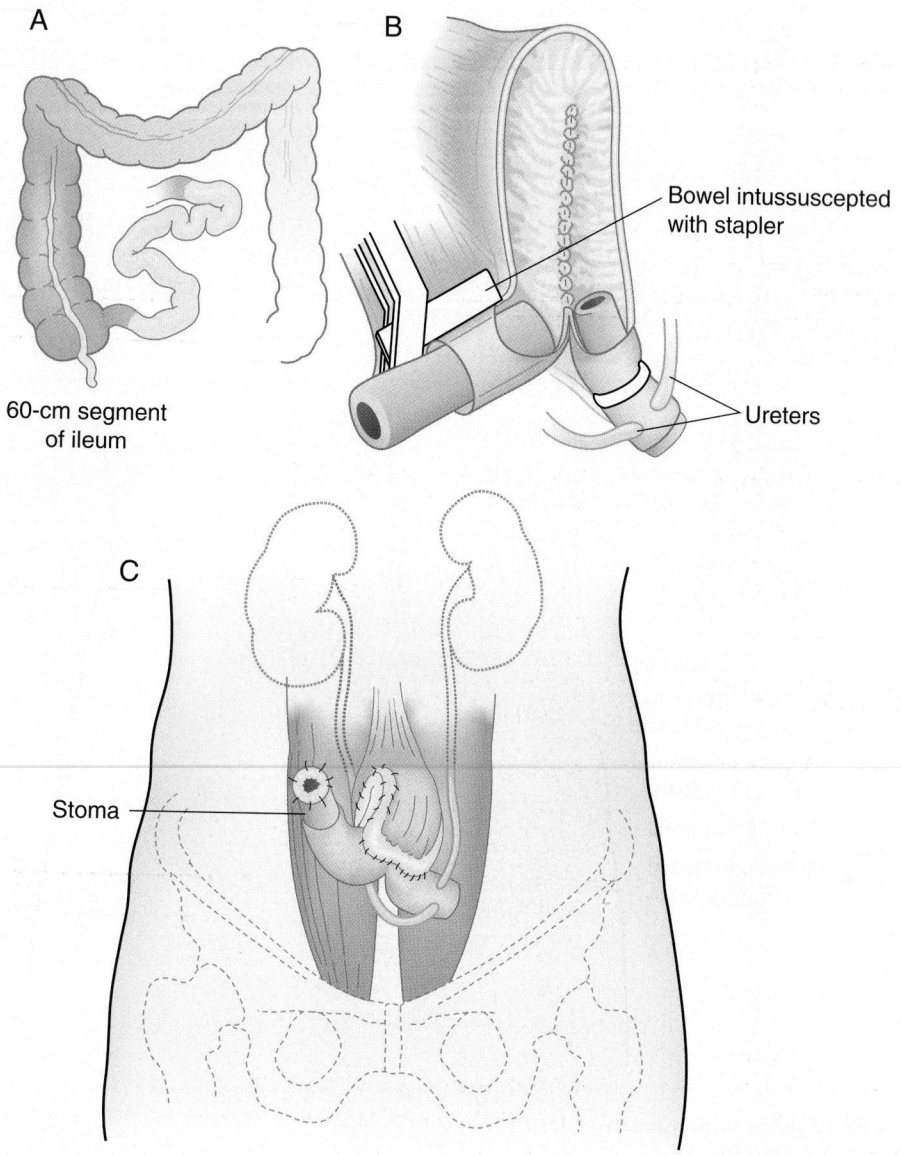

Figure 77-27 Continent catheterizable Kock pouch urinary reservoir. **A,** Sixty centimeters of small intestine selected. **B,** Afferent (nonrefluxing) limb for ureteral reimplantation and efferent limb for stoma fashioned using stapling devices. **C,** Completed reservoir. (From Tanagho E, McAninch JW [eds]: Smith's General Urology, 15th ed. New York, McGraw-Hill, 2000.)

increased public awareness and increased screening for the disease.

The clinical presentation of prostate cancer has significantly changed ever since the introduction and wide use of PSA. Fifteen years ago, before common use of PSA, prostate cancer was first detected by digital rectal examination or because the patient had urinary symptoms. Urinary symptoms could include urgency, nocturia, frequency, and hesitancy, clinical symptoms similar to those of BPH. Since the 1990s, prostate cancer is often diagnosed after a man has been found to have a high serum PSA concentration with a normal prostate exam. Only 20% of newly detected prostate cancers are associated with an abnormal digital rectal exam as the first clinical sign of prostate cancer.

Serum PSA elevation is often the first sign of prostatic pathology. Both BPH and prostate cancer can lead to an elevation of serum PSA; however, the rate of rise of PSA associated with prostate cancer is usually higher than that of BPH.[42] Other causes of elevated PSA include prostate inflammation and perineal trauma.

A total serum PSA concentration of more than 4.0 ng/mL is considered abnormal in most assays and is suspicious for prostate cancer. To improve the accuracy of PSA as a cancer screening tool, age-related and race-related PSA values have been recommended and are widely used by clinicians for early diagnosis of prostate cancer, as follows:

Normal Range for Age-Related PSA Levels[43]

- 40 to 49 years-old—0 to 2.5 ng/mL
- 50 to 59 years-old—0 to 3.5 ng/mL

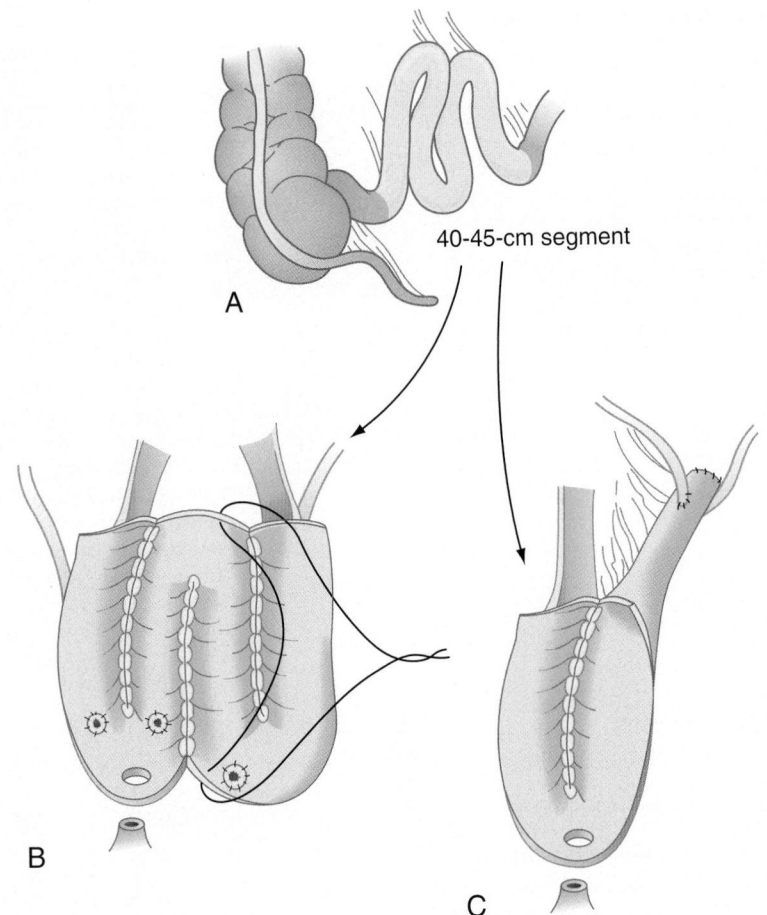

40-45-cm segment

A

B

C

Figure 77-28 Orthotopic neobladder. Bladder substitutes constructed entirely of small intestine. **A,** From 40 to 45 cm of small intestine is selected. **B,** Small intestine is opened and fashioned into a W. The ureters are reimplanted into the second and third limbs of the reservoir, and the reservoir is attached to the urethra. **C,** Small intestine is folded into a J, with the most proximal portion of the segment not opened. The ureters are reimplanted into the intact ileal segment of the reservoir, and the reservoir is attached to the urethra. (From Tanagho EA, McAninch JW [eds]: Smith's General Urology, 15th ed. New York, McGraw-Hill, 2000.)

- 60 to 69 years-old—0 to 4.5 ng/mL
- 70 to 79 years-old—0 to 6.5 ng/mL

Normal Range for Age- and Race-Related PSA Levels[44]

- 40 to 49 years-old—0 to 2.0 ng/mL (blacks); 0 to 2.5 (whites)
- 50 to 59 years-old—0 to 4.0 ng/mL (blacks); 0 to 3.5 (whites)
- 60 to 69 years-old—0 to 4.5 ng/mL (blacks); 0 to 3.5 (whites)
- 70 to 79 years-old—0 to 5.5 ng/mL (blacks); 0 to 3.5 (whites)

Prostate biopsy is the gold standard for prostate cancer diagnosis. Transrectal biopsy is a relatively simple office technique that can be performed without sedation or analgesia. If a prostate biopsy specimen is interpreted as containing carcinoma, additional evaluation or clinical staging may be required to determine the extent of spread. Clinical and pathologic staging of prostate cancer is listed in Table 77-7.

The most effective therapy for an individual man with early-stage prostate cancer is not clear. Management options include surgery, radiation therapy (external-beam or brachytherapy, with or without hormone therapy), or observation, also termed *watchful waiting*. Issues to be considered in making the choice between treatments include the following:

- The man's general medical condition, age, and comorbidity
- The histologic grade (Gleason score) of the tumor on prostate biopsy
- Pretreatment serum PSA
- Extent of tumor involving the prostate biopsy needle cores
- The clinical stage of the disease and the likelihood of the cancer being confined to the prostate gland, and, therefore, potentially amenable to cure
- An estimation of the outcome associated with the alternative treatments for prostate cancer
- The potential side effects associated with the different forms of treatment for early-stage disease

Table 77-7   TNM Classification for Prostate Carcinoma

Pathologic: Primary Tumor (T)		Clinical	Primary Tumor (T)	
pT2	Organ confined		TX	Primary tumor cannot be assessed
pT2a	Unilateral, one half of one lobe or less		T0	No evidence of primary tumor
pT2b	Unilateral, involving more than one half of lobe but not both lobes		T1	Clinically inapparent tumor neither palpable nor visible by imaging
pT2c	Bilateral disease		T1a	Tumor incidental histologic finding in 5% or less of tissue resected
pT3	Extraprostatic extension		T1b	Tumor incidental histologic finding in more than 5% of tissue resected
pT3a	Extraprostatic extension		T1c	Tumor identified by needle biopsy (e.g., because of elevated PSA)
pT3b	Seminal vesicle invasion		T2	Tumor confined within prostate
pT4	Invasion of bladder, rectum		T2a	Tumor involves one half of one lobe or less
			T2b	Tumor involves more than one half of one lobe but not both lobes
			T2c	Tumor involves both lobes
			T3	Tumor extends through the prostate capsule
			T3a	Extracapsular extension (unilateral or bilateral)
			T3b	Tumor invades seminal vesicle(s)
			T4	Tumor is fixed or invades adjacent structures other than seminal vesicles: bladder neck, external sphincter, rectum, levator muscles, and/or pelvic wall

Regional Lymph Nodes (N)		Regional Lymph Nodes (N)	
pNX	Regional nodes not sampled	NX	Regional lymph nodes were not assessed
pN0	No positive regional nodes	N0	No regional lymph node metastasis
pN1	Metastases in regional node(s)	N1	Metastasis in regional lymph node(s)

Clinical	Pathologic	Distant Metastasis (M)	
		MX	Distant metastasis cannot be assessed (not evaluated by any modality)
		M0	No distant metastasis
		M1	Distant metastasis
		M1a	Nonregional lymph node(s)
		M1b	Bone(s)
		M1c	Other site(s) with or without bone disease

For purposes of this chapter, only an overview of the surgical treatment (radical retropubic prostatectomy) will be explained. After gaining access to the retropubic space of Retzius, the endopelvic fascia is incised (Fig. 77-29A) and the puboprostatic ligament is divided. Incision of the dorsal venous complex is followed by obtaining hemostasis and incision of the urethra (see Fig. 77-29B). After incising the urethra and releasing the rectourethralis fascia, care is taken not to harm the neurovascular bundle that is responsible for maintaining potency (see Fig. 77-29C). Excision of the lateral pelvic fascia is followed by division of the bladder neck and excision of the seminal vesicles (see Fig. 77-29D). Reconstruction of the bladder neck and anastomosis to the remnant urethra (see Fig. 77-29E) complete the procedure.

Because prostate cancer has a high prevalence in elderly men, prostate cancer prevention is an attractive treatment strategy. In a recent large randomized trial that included 18,000 men, the effect of finasteride as a chemopreventive agent on development of prostate cancer was examined.[45] It has been long appreciated that prostate cancer is an androgen-dependent cancer, and removal of androgens reduces the progression of prostate cancer. Finasteride blocks the conversion of testosterone to the more potent androgen DHT by blocking the enzyme 5-α reductase type 2. The hypothesis of this study was to determine whether elimination of DHT would reduce the risk for developing prostate cancer. The study determined that finasteride may prevent or delay the appearance of prostate cancer; however, men using finasteride are at increased risk for developing more advanced high-grade prostate cancers. The study concluded that the potential benefits of finasteride are in reducing or delaying prostate cancer and improving lower urinary tract symptoms. However, the potential benefits need to be weighed against the sexual side effects and the increased risk for developing high-grade prostate cancer.[45]

Testis Carcinoma

Testicular cancer, although relatively rare, is the most common malignancy in men in the 15- to 35-year age group and evokes widespread interest for several reasons. Testicular cancer has become one of the most curable

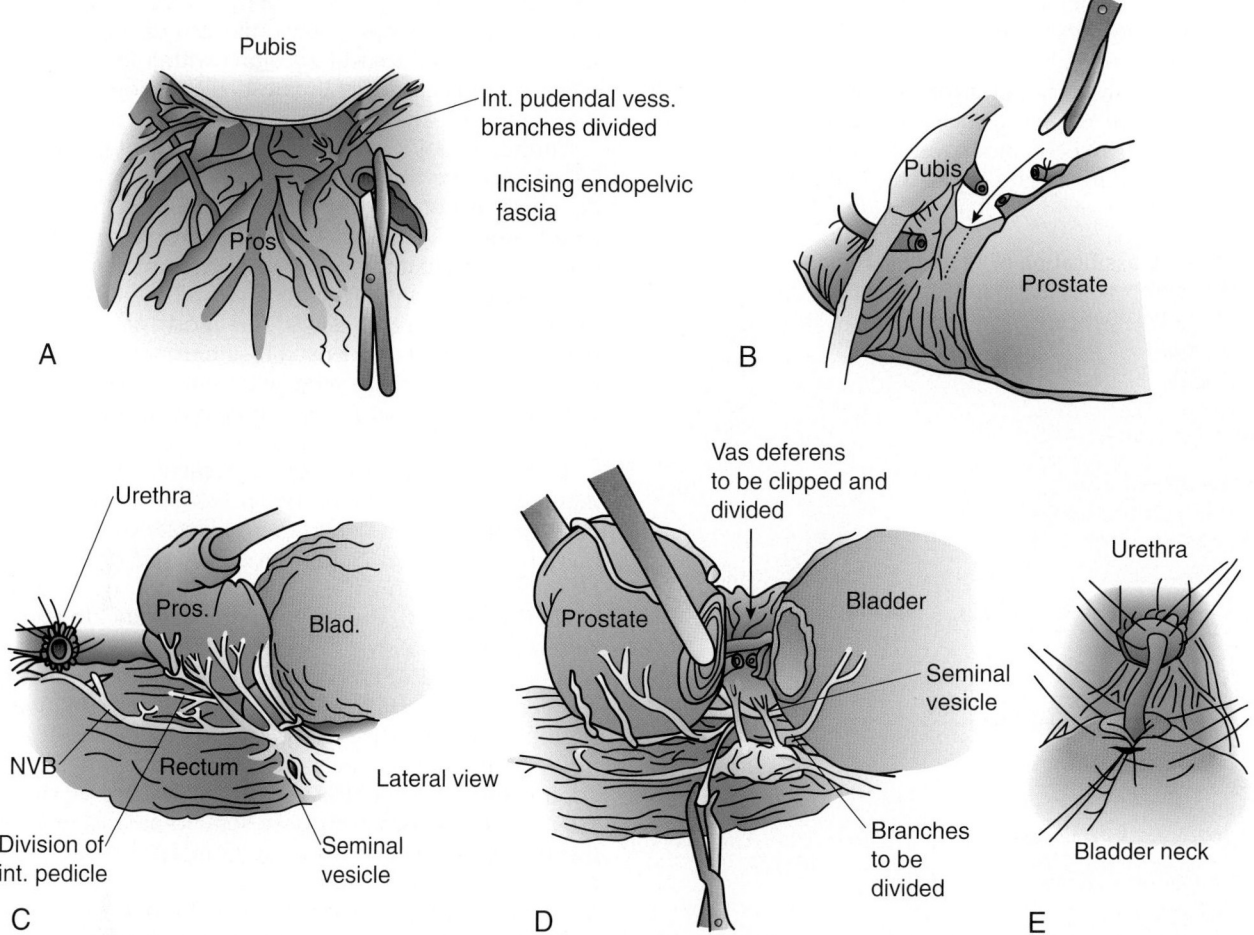

Figure 77-29 Anatomic radical retropubic prostatectomy. **A,** The incision in the endopelvic fascia is made at the junction with the pelvic sidewall well away from the prostate and bladder. Anteriorly, near the puboprostatic ligaments, small arterial and venous branches from the internal pudendal vessels are often encountered. These are clipped and divided. **B,** Transection of the puboprostatic ligaments and exposure of the anterior urethra. **C,** Posterior dissection of the prostate gland (*side view*) by reflecting the prostate off of the rectum. Special care is taken to preserve the neurovascular bundle (NVB). **D,** Transection of the prostate from the bladder neck and transection of the vas deferens. **E,** Anastomosis between the bladder neck and the urethra after removal of the prostate and seminal vesicles. (From Walsh PC, Retik AB, Vaughan ED Jr, et al [eds]: Campbell's Urology, 8th ed. Philadelphia, Elsevier, 2002, pp 3113-3126.)

solid neoplasms and serves as a paradigm for the multimodal treatment of malignancies. The dramatic improvement in survival resulting from the combination of effective diagnostic techniques, improved tumor markers, effective multidrug chemotherapeutic regimens, and modifications of surgical technique has led to a decrease in patient mortality from more than 50% before 1970 to less than 5% in 1997.[46] Germ cell tumors (GCTs) account for 95% of testicular cancers (Table 77-8). They may consist of one predominant histologic pattern, or represent a mix of multiple histologic types. For treatment purposes, two broad categories of testis tumors are recognized: pure seminoma (no nonseminomatous elements present), and all others, which together are termed *non-seminomatous germ cell tumors* (see Table 77-8).

Testicular cancer has become one of the most curable cancers in the United States because of advances in

medical and surgical therapy since the 1970s. Cisplatin-based chemotherapy regimens have improved the response rates for testis cancer.[47] In addition, detailed identification of the retroperitoneal lymph nodes and metastatic landing sites has been a major advance in surgical treatment of patients at high risk for advanced cancers.[48]

Testicular tumors usually present as a nodule or painless swelling of one testicle, which may be noted incidentally by the patient or by his sexual partner.[46] Occasionally, a man with a previously small atrophic testis will note enlargement. About 30% to 40% of patients complain of a dull ache or heavy sensation in the lower abdomen, perianal area, or scrotum, whereas acute pain is the presenting symptom in 10%. Gynecomastia, which occurs in about 5% of men with testicular GCTs, is a systemic endocrine manifestation of these neoplasms.

Examination includes a detailed evaluation of the neck, chest, and abdominal contents. Patients with testicular tumors often have a palpable parenchymal testis mass, which can be better appreciated if compared with the contralateral normal testicle. The examiner needs to differentiate between intraparenchymal testis masses, which are often malignant, and extraparenchymal testicu-lar masses, which are often benign (see earlier section, Scrotal Masses). Scrotal ultrasound can distinguish intrinsic from extrinsic testicular lesions with a high degree of accuracy and can detect intratesticular lesions as small as 1 to 2 mm in diameter (Fig. 77-30).

Further radiologic workup includes a high-resolution CT scan of the abdomen and pelvis and a chest x-ray. Regional metastases first appear in the retroperitoneal lymph nodes. Although CT is the imaging modality of choice to evaluate the retroperitoneum, false-negative rates as high as 44% have been described. Occult micro-metastases are responsible for most of these false-negative results, as evidenced by a retroperitoneal relapse rate of 20% to 25% in men with clinical stage I disease who do not undergo retroperitoneal lymph node dissection (RPLND).[49]

In men suspected of having testicular tumor, serum markers of α-fetoprotein, the sβ subunit of human chorionic gonadotropin (β-HCG), and lactate dehydrogenase (LDH) are obtained. Serum levels of AFP or β-HCG are elevated in 80% to 85% of men with nonseminomatous GCTs (Table 77-8), even when nonmetastatic. In contrast, serum β-HCG is elevated in fewer than 20% of testicular seminomas, and AFP is not elevated in pure seminomas. Neither serum β-HCG nor AFP alone or in combination is sufficiently sensitive or specific to establish the diagnosis of testicular cancer in the absence of histologic confirmation. Serum LDH concentrations are elevated in 30% to 80% of men with pure seminoma and in 60% of those with nonseminomatous tumors. LDH is a less sensitive and less specific tumor marker than β-HCG or AFP for men with nonseminomatous GCTs, but it may be the only marker that is elevated in seminomas. In addition, a significantly elevated serum LDH has independent prognostic value in men with advanced seminoma.

A radical inguinal orchiectomy with high ligation of the spermatic cord near the internal inguinal ring is performed to permit histologic evaluation of the primary tumor and to provide local tumor control. Scrotal violation through a scrotal incision or an attempt to biopsy the testicle must be avoided because of concern for

Table 77-8 Classification of Testicular Tumors

Germ Cell Tumors
Seminoma
Classic (typical)
Atypical
Spermatocytic

Nonseminomatous
Embryonal carcinoma
Teratoma
Mature
Immature
Mature or immature with malignant transformation
Choriocarcinoma
Yolk sac tumor (endodermal sinus tumor)

Sex Cord and Stromal Tumors
Sertoli's cell tumor
Leydig's cell tumor
Granular cell tumor
Mixed types (e.g. Sertoli-Leydig tumor)

Mixed Germ Cell and Stromal Elements
Gonadoblastoma

Adnexal and Paratesticular Tumors
Adenocarcinoma of rete testis
Mesothelioma

Miscellaneous Tumors
Carcinoid
Lymphoma
Testicular metastasis

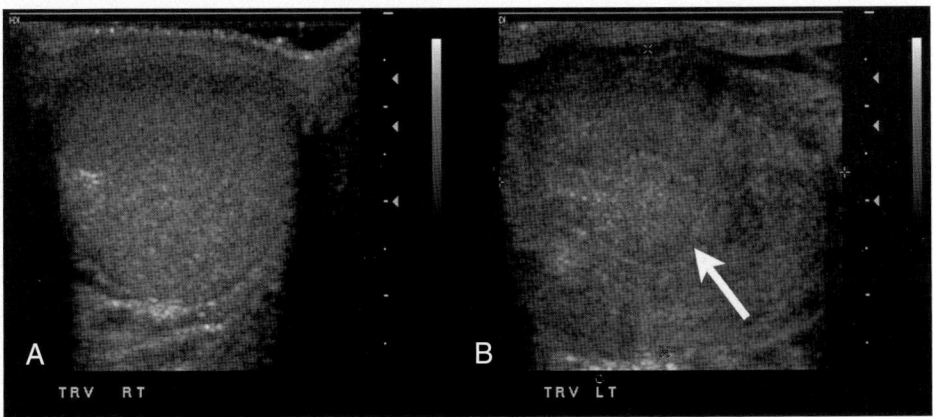

Normal right testis   Heterogeneous mass in left testis

Figure 77-30 A, Normal ultrasound image of testis. **B,** Heterogeneous mass in left testicle (*arrow*) that is very irregular. Pathology was consistent with embryonal cell carcinoma with extensive lymphovascular invasion.

Table 77-9   TNM Classification for Testis Cancer

Pathologic	**Primary Tumor (T)**	
	pTX	Primary tumor cannot be assessed (if no radical orchiectomy has been performed, TX is used)
	pT0	No evidence of primary tumor (e.g., histologic scar in testis)
	pTis	Intratubular germ cell neoplasia (carcinoma *in situ*)
	pT1	Tumor limited to the testis and epididymis without vascular/lymphatic invasion; tumor may invade into the tunica albuginea but not the tunica vaginalis
	pT2	Tumor limited to the testis and epididymis with vascular/lymphatic invasion, or tumor extending through the tunica albuginea with involvement of the tunica vaginalis
	pT3	Tumor invades the spermatic cord with or without vascular/lymphatic invasion
	pT4	Tumor invades the scrotum with or without vascular/lymphatic invasion

Clinical	**Primary Tumor (T)**	
	Tumor stage is generally determined after orchiectomy at which time a pathologic stage is assigned.	

Pathologic	**Regional Lymph Nodes (N)**		Clinical	**Regional Lymph Nodes (N)**
	pNX	Regional lymph nodes cannot be assessed	NX	Regional lymph nodes cannot be assessed
	pN0	No regional lymph node metastasis	N0	No regional lymph node metastasis
	pN1	Metastasis with a lymph node mass 2 cm or less in greatest dimension and less than or equal to 5 nodes positive, none more than 2 cm in greatest dimension	N1	Metastasis with a lymph node mass 2 cm or less in greatest dimension; or multiple lymph nodes, none more than 2 cm in greatest dimension
	pN2	Metastasis with a lymph node mass more than 2 cm but not more than 5 cm in greatest dimension; or more than 5 nodes positive, none more than 5 cn; or evidence of extranodal extension of tumor	N2	Metastasis with a lymph node mass more than 2 cm but not more than 5 cm in greatest dimension; or multiple lymph nodes, any one mass greater than 2 cm but not more than 5 cm in greatest dimension
	pN3	Metastasis with a lymph node mass more than 5 cm in greatest dimension	N3	Metastasis with a lymph node mass more than 5 cm in greatest dimension

Distant Metastasis (M)

MX	Distant metastasis cannot be assessed
M0	No distant metastasis
M1	Distant metastasis
M1a	Nonregional nodal or pulmonary metastasis
M1b	Distant metastasis other than to nonregional lymph nodes and lungs

Serum Tumor Markers (S) (*N indicates the upper limit of normal for the LDH assay*)

SX	Marker studies not available or not performed
S0	Marker study levels within normal limits
S1	LDH $< 1.5 \times N$ *and* hCG (mIu/mL) <5000 *and* AFP (ng/ml) <1000
S2	LDH $1.5\text{-}10 \times N$ *or* hCG (mIu/mL) $5000\text{-}50,000$ *or* AFP (ng/ml) $1000\text{-}10,000$
S3	LDH $> 10 \times N$ *or* hCG (mIu/mL) $>50,000$ *or* AFP (ng/mL) $>10,000$

changing the lymphatic channels available to the testis tumor and potential for a poorer outcome.

The serum half-lives of HCG and AFP are 18 to 36 hours and 5 to 7 days, respectively. If testicular cancer produces any of these serum markers, following their progressive change after radical orchiectomy is an important consideration in determining the adequacy of therapy. As an example, rapid normalization after orchiectomy for stage I disease suggests elimination of the tumor, whereas persistence of tumor markers after the period during which normalization is expected to occur may be the only evidence of persistent occult disease.

After determination of the histologic subtype of the testis cancer, several parameters may identify patients at high risk for metastasis to the retroperitoneum despite absence of lymphadenopathy on the staging CT scan. For nonseminomatous germ cell tumors, those factors include the following:

1. Vascular or lymphatic invasion
2. Primary tumor (T) stage T2-T3 (Table 77-9)
3. Embryonal carcinoma component greater than 40% of total tumor volume

Patients with these risk factors who have no bulky retroperitoneal lymphadenopathy and have normal tumor makers after radical orchiectomy may be candidates for RPLND.

The principles underlying the modern surgical treatment of testicular GCT are based on the stepwise predictable metastatic pattern of these tumors, with the notable exception of choriocarcinoma. RPLND is the only reliable method to identify nodal micrometastases and is the gold

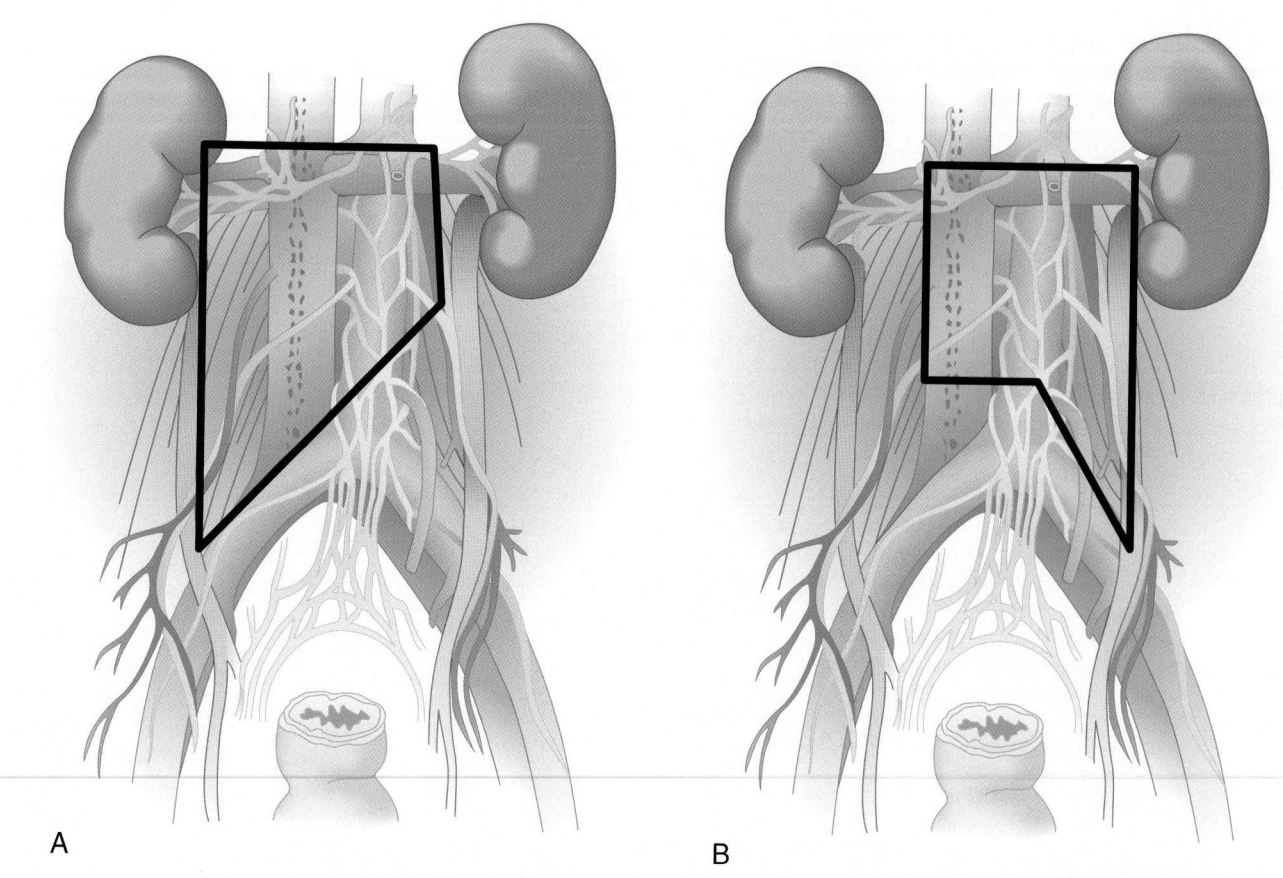

Figure 77-31 Surgical template for modified, left-sided (**A**) and right-sided (**B**) retroperitoneal lymph node dissection. (From Sheinfeld J, McKierman J, Bosl GJ: Surgery of testicular tumors. In Walsh PC, Retik AB, Vaughan ED Jr, et al [eds]: Campbell's Urology, 8th ed. Philadelphia, Elsevier, 2002, pp 2926-2927.)

standard for providing accurate pathologic staging of the retroperitoneum. Both the number and size of involved retroperitoneal lymph nodes have prognostic importance (see Table 77-9). As surgical therapy for metastatic testicular cancer has evolved, the full bilateral RPLND used in the past evolved first to a template-type (Fig. 77-31) dissection and then to a nerve-sparing modification with a unilateral template.[50] The evolution of the modified nerve-sparing RPLND has resulted in decreased morbidity, with ejaculatory dysfunctions commonly observed with bilateral RPLND. Adjuvant chemotherapy may be considered after RPLND in patients with resected stage II disease, or as an alternative to RPLND in men with low-stage testis cancer.

Selected References

Barry MJ, Fowler FJ Jr, O'Leary MP, et al: The American Urological Association symptom index for benign prostatic hyperplasia. The Measurement Committee of the American Urological Association. J Urol 148:1549-1557, 1992.

The American Urological Association (AUA) symptom index was developed to standardize and assess men's obstructive lower urinary tract symptoms due to benign prostatic hyperplasia in a quantitative manner. The AUA symptom index questionnaire includes seven questions covering frequency, nocturia, weak urinary stream, hesitancy, intermittency, incomplete emptying, and urgency. The questionnaire is used to assess a patient's urinary symptoms before any medical or surgical therapy. After initiation of the therapy, the AUA symptom score can be used again to assess the efficacy of the treatment.

Bretan PN Jr, McAninch JW, Federle MP, Jeffrey RB Jr: Computerized tomographic staging of renal trauma: 85 consecutive cases. J Urol 136:561-565, 1986.

Staging has greatly helped in proper management of renal trauma patients. Accurate staging of renal injuries by CT scan has significantly helped in proper management of renal trauma patients. This article is one of the first that described staging of renal injuries using CT scan.

Carter HB, Pearson JD, Metter EJ, et al: Longitudinal evaluation of prostate-specific antigen levels in men with and without prostate disease. JAMA 267:2215-2220, 1992.

This was a case-control prospective longitudinal study that assessed the rate of prostate specific antigen change in men with and without prostate diseases. This study was one of the first studies to demonstrate that the rate of PSA change can be an early determinant of differentiating between benign prostatic hyperplasia and prostate.

Coll DM, Varanelli MJ, Smith RC: Relationship of spontaneous passage of ureteral calculi to stone size and location as revealed by unenhanced helical CT. AJR Am J Roentgenol 178:101-103, 2002.

Noncontrast CT has become an important imaging modality in diagnosis and management of acute renal colic. This study nicely demonstrates the likelihood of spontaneous passage of renal/ureteral stones in relation to the size and location of the stone.

Einhorn LH, Donohue JP: Improved chemotherapy in disseminated testicular cancer. J Urol 117:65-69, 1977.

Testicular cancer has become one of the most curable cancers in the United States because of advances in medical and surgical therapy since the 1970s. Addition of cisplatin to chemotherapy regimens significantly improved the long-term survival and curability of metastatic testicular cancer. This reference is a classic landmark article demonstrating the efficacy of platinum based chemotherapy for testicular cancer patients.

Thompson IM, Goodman PJ, Tangen CM, et al: The Influence of finasteride on the development of prostate cancer. N Engl J Med 349:215-224, 2003.

This large randomized prospective clinical trial included 18,000 men and the investigators examined the effect of finasteride in development of prostate cancer. It has been long appreciated that prostate cancer is an androgen-dependent cancer, and removal of androgens reduces the progression of prostate cancer. Finasteride blocks the conversion of testosterone to the more potent androgen dihydrotestosterone by blocking the enzyme 5-α reductase type 2. The hypothesis of this study was to determine whether elimination of the more potent androgen, dihydrotestosterone, would reduce the risk for developing prostate cancer. The study determined that finasteride may prevent or delay the appearance of prostate cancer; however, men using finasteride are at increased risk for developing more advanced high-grade prostate cancers. The study concludes that the potential benefits of finasteride are reducing/delaying prostate cancer and improving the men's lower urinary tract symptoms. However, the potential benefits need to be weighed against the sexual side effects and the increased risk for developing high-grade prostate cancer.

References

1. Walsh PC, Lepor H, Eggleston, JC: Radical prostatectomy with preservation of sexual function: Anatomical and pathological considerations. Prostate 4:473-485, 1983.
2. Miller KS, McAninch JW: Radiographic assessment of renal trauma: Our 15-year experience. J Urol 154:352-355, 1995.
3. Morey AF, McAninch JW, Tiller BK, et al: Single shot intraoperative excretory urography for the immediate evaluation of renal trauma. J Urol 161:1088-1092, 1999.
4. Mathews R, Marshall FF: Versatility of the adult psoas hitch ureteral reimplantation. J Urol 158:2078-2082, 1997.
5. Kotkin L, Koch MO: Morbidity associated with nonoperative management of extraperitoneal bladder injuries. J Trauma 38:895-898, 1995.
6. Peters PC: Intraperitoneal rupture of the bladder. Urol Clin North Am 16:279-282, 1989.
7. Koraitim MM, Marzouk ME, Atta MA, et al: Risk factors and mechanism of urethral injury in pelvic fractures. Br J Urol 77:876-880, 1996.
8. Asci R, Sarikaya S, Buyukalpelli R, et al: Voiding and sexual dysfunctions after pelvic fracture urethral injuries treated with either initial cystostomy and delayed urethroplasty or immediate primary urethral realignment. Scand J Urol Nephrol 33:228-233, 1999.
9. Zargooshi J: Penile fracture in Kermanshah, Iran: Report of 172 cases. J Urol 164:364-366, 2000.
10. Mellinger BC, Douenias R: New surgical approach for operative management of penile fracture and penetrating trauma. Urology 39:429-432, 1992.
11. Altarac S: Management of 53 cases of testicular trauma. Eur Urol 25:119-123, 1994.
12. Morpurgo E, Galandiuk S: Fournier's gangrene. Surg Clin North Am 82:1213-1224, 2002.
13. Moe OW: Kidney stones: Pathophysiology and medical management. Lancet 367:333-344, 2006.
14. Coll DM, Varanelli MJ, Smith RC: Relationship of spontaneous passage of ureteral calculi to stone size and location as revealed by unenhanced helical CT. AJR Am J Roentgenol 178:101-103, 2002.
15. Dellabella M, Milanese G, Muzzonigro G: Efficacy of tamsulosin in the medical management of juxtavesical ureteral stones. J Urol 170:2202-2205, 2003.
16. Yilmaz E, Batislam E, Basar MM, et al: The comparison and efficacy of 3 different alpha1-adrenergic blockers for distal ureteral stones. J Urol 173:2010-2012, 2005.
17. Dellabella M, Milanese G, Muzzonigro G: Randomized trial of the efficacy of tamsulosin, nifedipine and phloroglucinol in medical expulsive therapy for distal ureteral calculi. J Urol 174:167-172, 2005.
18. Snodgrass WT, Adams R: Initial urologic management of myelomeningocele. Urol Clin North Am 31:427-434, viii, 2004.
19. Kiddoo DA, Carr MC, Dulczak S, et al: Initial management of complex urological disorders: Bladder exstrophy. Urol Clin North Am 31:417-426, vii-viii, 2004.
20. Atala A, Bauer SB, Soker S, et al: Tissue-engineered autologous bladders for patients needing cystoplasty. Lancet 367:1241-1246, 2006.
21. Girman CJ, Jacobsen SJ, Guess HA, et al: Natural history of prostatism: Relationship among symptoms, prostate volume and peak urinary flow rate. J Urol 153:1510-1515, 1995.
22. Platz EA, Kawachi I, Rimm EB, et al: Race, ethnicity and benign prostatic hyperplasia in the health professionals follow-up study. J Urol 163:490-495, 2000.
23. Imperato-McGinley J, Gautier T, Zirinsky K, et al: Prostate visualization studies in males homozygous and heterozygous for 5 alpha-reductase deficiency. J Clin Endocrinol Metab 75:1022-1026, 1992.
24. Cunha GR, Donjacour AA, Cooke PS, et al: The endocrinology and developmental biology of the prostate. Endocrine Rev 8:338-363, 1987.
25. Barry MJ, Fowler FJ Jr, O'Leary MP, et al: The American Urological Association symptom index for benign prostatic hyperplasia. The Measurement Committee of the American Urological Association. J Urol 148:1549-1557; discussion 1564, 1992.
26. Lepor H: Alpha blockade for the treatment of benign prostatic hyperplasia. Urol Clin North Am 22:375-86, 1995.
27. Gormley GJ, Stoner E, Bruskewitz RC, et al: The effect of finasteride in men with benign prostatic hyperplasia. The Finasteride Study Group. N Engl J Med 327:1185-1191, 1992.
28. Bautista OM, Kusek JW, Nyberg LM, et al: Study design of the Medical Therapy of Prostatic Symptoms (MTOPS) trial. Control Clin Trials 24:224-243, 2003.
29. Wasson JH, Reda D, Bruskewitz R, et al: A comparison of transurethral surgery with watchful waiting for moderate symptoms of benign prostatic hyperplasia. The Veterans Affairs Cooperative Study Group on Transurethral Resection of the Prostate. N Engl J Med 332:75-79, 1995.
30. Gupta N, Sivaramakrishna, Kumar R, et al: Comparison of standard transurethral resection, transurethral vapour resection and holmium laser enucleation of the prostate for managing benign prostatic hyperplasia of >40 g. BJU Int 97:85-89, 2006.
31. Cimentepe E, Unsal A, Saglam R: Randomized clinical trial comparing transurethral needle ablation with transurethral

resection of the prostate for the treatment of benign prostatic hyperplasia: Results at 18 months. J Endourol 17:103-107, 2003.

32. Osman Y, Wadie B, El-Diasty T, et al: High-energy transurethral microwave thermotherapy: Symptomatic vs urodynamic success. BJU Int 91:365-370, 2003.

33. Tsui KH, Shvarts O, Barbaric Z, et al: Is adrenalectomy a necessary component of radical nephrectomy? UCLA experience with 511 radical nephrectomies. J Urol 163:437-441, 2000.

34. Atkins MB: Interleukin-2: Clinical applications. Semin Oncol 29:12-17, 2002.

35. Schoffski P, Dumez H, Clement P, et al: Emerging role of tyrosine kinase inhibitors in the treatment of advanced renal cell cancer: A review. Ann Oncol 17:1185-1186, 2006.

36. Yang JC, Haworth L, Sherry RM, et al: A randomized trial of bevacizumab, an anti-vascular endothelial growth factor antibody, for metastatic renal cancer. N Engl J Med 349:427-434, 2003.

37. Flanigan RC, Salmon SE, Blumenstein BA, et al: Nephrectomy followed by interferon alfa-2b compared with interferon alfa-2b alone for metastatic renal-cell cancer. N Engl J Med 345:1655-1659, 2001.

38. Mickisch GH, Garin A, van Poppel H, et al: Radical nephrectomy plus interferon-alfa-based immunotherapy compared with interferon alfa alone in metastatic renal-cell carcinoma: A randomised trial. Lancet 358:966-970, 2001.

39. Munoz JJ, Ellison LM: Upper tract urothelial neoplasms: Incidence and survival during the last 2 decades. J Urol 164:1523-1525, 2000.

40. Jung I, Messing E: Molecular mechanisms and pathways in bladder cancer development and progression. Cancer Control 7:325-334, 2000.

41. Hautmann RE, Mille K, Steiner U, et al: The ileal neobladder: 6 years of experience with more than 200 patients. J Urol 150:40-45, 1993.

42. Carter HB, Pearson JD, Metter EJ, et al: Longitudinal evaluation of prostate-specific antigen levels in men with and without prostate disease. JAMA 267:2215-2220, 1992.

43. Oesterling JE, Jacobsen SJ, Chute CG, et al: Serum prostate-specific antigen in a community-based population of healthy men: Establishment of age-specific reference ranges [see comments]. JAMA 270:860-864, 1993.

44. Morgan TO, Jacobsen SJ, McCarthy WF, et al: Age-specific reference ranges for prostate-specific antigen in black men. N Engl J Med 335:304-310, 1996.

45. Thompson IM, Goodman PJ, Tangen CM, et al: The influence of finasteride on the development of prostate cancer. N Engl J Med 349:215-224, 2003.

46. Bosl GJ, Motzer RJ: Testicular germ-cell cancer. N Engl J Med 337:242-253, 1997.

47. Einhorn LH, Donohue JP: Improved chemotherapy in disseminated testicular cancer. J Urol 117:65-69, 1977.

48. Richie JP: Clinical stage 1 testicular cancer: The role of modified retroperitoneal lymphadenectomy. J Urol 144:1160-1163, 1990.

49. Gels ME, Hoekstra HJ, Sleijfer DT, et al: Detection of recurrence in patients with clinical stage I nonseminomatous testicular germ cell tumors and consequences for further follow-up: A single-center 10-year experience. J Clin Oncol 13:1188-1194, 1995.

50. Donohue JP, Foster RS, Rowland RG, et al: Nerve-sparing retroperitoneal lymphadenectomy with preservation of ejaculation. J Urol 144:287-291, discussion 291-292, 1990.

Note: Page numbers followed by b refer to boxes; page numbers followed by f refer to figures; and page numbers followed by t refer to tables.

M

Reproduction, 2207–2209. *See also* Pregnancy
  endometrial cycle in, 2208
  ovarian cycle in, 2207–2208, 2208f
Respiration. *See also* Respiratory failure;
    Respiratory system
  age-related changes in, 375–376
Respiratory distress, in congenital
    diaphragmatic hernia, 2073
Respiratory failure. *See also* Acute lung injury;
    Acute (adult) respiratory distress
    syndrome
  in burn injury, 578
  in critical care patient, 613–616, 614f
  in fail chest, 496
  in pulmonary contusion, 497
  parenteral nutrition in, 186
  postoperative, 256, 257t, 258t, 337
  treatment of, 340
Respiratory inversion point, 1060, 1061f
Respiratory system
  in pregnancy, 2228, 2230, 2230t
  postoperative infection of, 310–311
  preoperative evaluation of, 253t, 256, 257t,
    258t, 337
    in bariatric surgery patient, 403
    in elderly patients, 380
Restriction nucleases, 31, 31f
Resuscitation. *See also* Fluid therapy
  in burn injury, 567–569
  in gastrointestinal hemorrhage, 1201
  in hemorrhagic shock, 100–101, 130
  in septic shock, 103–106, 104t, 106b
  in shock, 94
  in variceal hemorrhage, 1530–1531
RET gene
  in multiple endocrine neoplasia 2, 1037–
    1038, 1038t, 1039–1040
  in thyroid cancer, 935–936, 935f, 936t, 943,
    1039–1040
Retained antrum syndrome, 1255
Retention cyst, appendiceal, 1345
Reticular veins, 2005
Retina, ischemia of, 1885, 1885f
Retinoblastoma, 751t, 752, 752f
Retinopathy, diabetic, pancreatic
    transplantation and, 723
Retroperitoneum
  abscess of, 1150–1151, 1150f, 1150t
  anatomy of, 1149, 2251, 2253f
  fibrosis of, 1151
  hematoma of, 1151, 1990, 1992, 1992f
  infection of, 309–310
  malignancy of, 1151–1153, 1152f
  operative approaches through, 1149
  sarcoma of, 794–795, 1152–1153, 1152f
  surgical exposure of, 1989–1990, 1990f,
    1991f
REV procedure, 1771
Rewarming therapy, in postoperative
    hypothermia, 335
Reynolds, pentad of, 1553
Rhabdomyosarcoma, 2083–2085, 2084t
  extremity, 2084
  genitourinary, 2085
  head and neck, 2084
  mediastinal, 1694
  trunk, 2084–2085
  vaginal, 2216
Rheumatic fever, valvular heart disease after,
    1834–1835, 1841. *See also* Aortic valve,
    stenosis of; Mitral valve, stenosis of
Rheumatoid arthritis
  adalimumab in, 55
  anakinra in, 55

Rheumatoid arthritis *(Continued)*
  aortic valve stenosis and, 1841
  etanercept in, 55
  infliximab in, 55
  of hand, 2192–2193, 2194f, 2196f
Rhinoplasty, 2151
Rhoads, Jonathan E., 17, 18f
Rhytids, 2151
Rib(s)
  absence of, 1658
  anatomy of, 1655, 1699, 1699f
  aneurysmal bone cyst of, 1660
  eosinophilic granuloma of, 1660
  fibrous dysplasia of, 1659
  first, 1699, 1699f
    resection of, 1664, 1746
  fracture of, 496, 496f, 1664
  osteochondroma of, 1659–1660
  osteoid osteoma of, 1660
Riboflavin
  hepatic metabolism of, 1483
  in severe illness, 164t
Ribonucleic acid (RNA)
  messenger (mRNA), 29–30
  synthesis of, 28–30, 29f, 30
  translation of, 29–30, 30t
Ribonucleic acid (RNA) splicing, 29, 29f
Ribonucleic acid (RNA) viruses, 758, 758b
Ribonucleic (RNA) interference, 33, 33f
Richmond Agitation and Sedation Scale, 605,
    605t
Richter, August, 10
Riedel's struma, 927
Right ventricle, single. *See* Hypoplastic left
    heart syndrome
Rings
  esophageal, 1076–1078, 1077f, 1078f
  vascular, 1708, 1783–1784, 1784f
Riolan, arc of, 1354, 1355f, 1357f
Ripstein repair, in rectal prolapse, 1419–1420
Rituximab, in transplantation, 679, 701
Robodoc, 468
Robot(s), 464–473
  active, 467–469
  camera holder, 467–468
  definition of, 465
  long-distance, 465–467, 466f, 469–473, 470f
  master-slave, 469–473, 470f, 471f
    for abdominal surgery, 471
    for cardiothoracic surgery, 471–473
  neurosurgery, 468–469
  orthopedic, 468
  passive, 467
  semiactive, 467
  synergistic, 467
  urology, 469
Rocuronium, 436–437, 437t, 606
Roentgen, Wilhelm, 8
Roos test, 1663
Ropivacaine, 451
Ross procedure, 1774–1775, 1774f, 1848,
    1849f
Round ligament, 1132
  in pregnancy, 2237
Roux-en-Y gastric bypass, 408–412, 409b,
    409f–413f
  anastomotic stenosis after, 424–425
  complications of, 422t, 423–425, 424t
  failure of, 426
  follow-up after, 418
  results of, 419t, 420–421, 420t
Roux-en-Y hepaticojejunostomy, 1578, 2079
Rovsing's sign, 1186, 1187t, 1334
RU-486, in cachexia, 186

Rubber band ligation, in hemorrhoids, 1441,
    1441f
Rubens flap, 910–911, 910f
Ruvalcaba-Myhre-Smith syndrome,
    1402t–1403t

S

S protein, 61
Sacrococcygeal teratoma, 2085–2086, 2086f
Sacrum
  fracture of, 541, 542f
  radiography of, 431
Safety, surgical, 237–246
  characteristics of, 239, 239b
  checklists for, 243–244, 243f, 244b
  economic factors and, 241–242, 241f
  fellowships in, 246
  for bedside procedures, 632, 633b, 634f
  historical perspective on, 237–238
  improvement of, 242–246
  information technology for, 244–245, 244b
  observational studies of, 245, 245t, 246t
  problem of, 238–239, 238b
  procedure-specific risks and, 237–238
  site-specific risks and, 237, 238
  system-related errors and, 239–242, 240b,
    240f, 241f
  systems engineers for, 245–246
  team development for, 242
  tight-coupling–related errors and, 241–242
  time-out procedure for, 244, 244b
  workload factors and, 241–242, 241f, 245,
    246t
Salivary glands, 834
  tumors of, 822, 834–836, 835b, 836f
Salmonella infection, 1307
Salmonella typhi infection, 1389
Salmonella typhosa infection, 1307
Salpingectomy, 2226, 2226f
Salpingostomy, 2225, 2226f
Santorini, duct of, 1590
Saphenous vein
  anatomy of, 2002, 2004f
  for cardiopulmonary bypass grafting, 1814,
    1817
  for coronary artery bypass grafting, 1830
  for infrainguinal arterial occlusive disease
    treatment, 1965–1967, 1966f
  for peripheral artery bypass, 1951–1952
  for popliteal artery grafting, 1934, 1935f
  laser ablation of, 2011
  radiofrequency closure of, 2011
  stripping of, 2010, 2010f
Sarcoidosis, 1736
Sarcoma
  abdominal wall, 1137
  aortic, 1859
  endometrial, 2220
  esophageal, 1105
  gastric, 1271–1272
  hepatic, 1507
  Kaposi's, 783
  osteogenic, 802t, 805, 806f, 1660
  pulmonary, 1727
  retroperitoneal, 1152–1153, 1152f
  skeletal, 800, 804–806, 805f, 806f
  soft tissue. *See* Soft tissue sarcoma
  vulvar, 2216
Satisfaction surveys, for outcomes research,
    233t, 234
Sauerbruch, Ernst, 17
Scaffolds, in wound healing, 241